Fourth Edition

Harwood-Nuss' Clinical Practice of Emergency Medicine

Fourth Edition

Harwood-Nuss' Clinical Practice of Emergency Medicine

Editor-in-Chief

Allan B. Wolfson, MD

Professor of Emergency Medicine
Program Director, Affiliated Residency in Emergency Medicine
University of Pittsburgh
Pittsburgh, Pennsylvania

Associate Editors

Gregory W. Hendey, MD

Associate Professor of Clinical Medicine
Emergency Medicine Research Director
University of California San Francisco,
Fresno Medical Education Program
Fresno, California

Phyllis L. Hendry, MD

Associate Professor of Pediatrics and
Emergency Medicine
University of Florida Health Science
Center/Jacksonville
Director, Pediatric Emergency Services
Shands Jacksonville
Jacksonville, Florida

Christopher H. Linden, MD

Professor
Department of Emergency Medicine
Division of Medical Toxicology
University of Massachusetts
Worcester, Massachusetts

Carlo L. Rosen, MD

Assistant Professor of Medicine
Harvard Medical School
Program Director
Beth Israel Deaconess Medical Center
Harvard Affiliated Emergency Medicine Residency
Boston, Massachusetts

Jeffrey Schaider, MD

Interim Chairman
Department of Emergency Medicine
Cook County Hospital
Associate Professor of Emergency Medicine
Rush Medical College
Chicago, Illinois

Assistant Editors

Ghazala Q. Sharieff, MD

Associate Clinical Professor
Children's Hospital and Health Center
University of California, San Diego
Director of Pediatric Emergency Medicine,
Palomar-Pomerado/California Emergency Physicians
San Diego, California

Jeffrey R. Suchard, MD

Associate Clinical Professor
Department of Emergency Medicine
University of California Irvine Medical Center
Orange, California

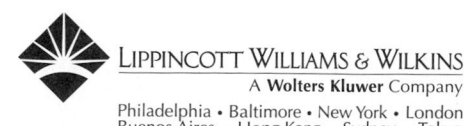

LIPPINCOTT WILLIAMS & WILKINS
A **Wolters Kluwer** Company
Philadelphia • Baltimore • New York • London
Buenos Aires • Hong Kong • Sydney • Tokyo

Acquisitions Editor: Anne M. Sydor
Developmental Editor: Michelle M. LaPlante
Project Manager: Alicia Jackson
Senior Manufacturing Manager: Benjamin Rivera
Marketing Manager: Angela Panetta
Cover Designer: Becky Baxendell
Production Service: TechBooks
Printer: Courier, Westford

© 2005 by LIPPINCOTT WILLIAMS & WILKINS
530 Walnut Street
Philadelphia, PA 19106 USA
LWW.com

3rd edition Lippincott Williams & Wilkins, 2001
2nd edition Lippincott-Raven, 1996
1st edition J.B. Lippincott, 1991

Printed in the USA

Library of Congress Cataloging-in-Publication Data

Harwood-Nuss' clinical practice of emergency medicine / editor-in-chief, Allan B.
    Wolfson ; associate editors, Gregory W. Hendey . . . [et al.].– 4th ed.
      p. ; cm.
    Rev. ed. of: The clinical practice of emergency medicine. 3rd ed. c2001.
    Includes bibliographical references and index.
    ISBN 0-7817-5125-X (hardbound)
    1. Emergency medicine.   I. Wolfson, Allan B.   II. Harwood-Nuss, Ann.   III. Title:
    Clinical practice of emergency medicine.
    [DNLM: 1. Emergencies.   2. Emergency Medicine.]
  RC86.7.C534   2005
  616.02′5—dc22
                                                        2005002918

Care has been taken to confirm the accuracy of the information presented and to describe generally accepted practices. However, the authors, editors, and publisher are not responsible for errors or omissions or for any consequences from application of the information in this book and make no warranty, expressed or implied, with respect to the currency, completeness, or accuracy of the contents of the publication. Application of this information in a particular situation remains the professional responsibility of the practitioner.

The authors, editors, and publisher have exerted every effort to ensure that drug selection and dosage set forth in this text are in accordance with current recommendations and practice at the time of publication. However, in view of ongoing research, changes in government regulations, and the constant flow of information relating to drug therapy and drug reactions, the reader is urged to check the package insert for each drug for any change in indications and dosage and for added warnings and precautions. This is particularly important when the recommended agent is a new or infrequently employed drug.

Some drugs and medical devices presented in this publication have Food and Drug Administration (FDA) clearance for limited use in restricted research settings. It is the responsibility of the health care provider to ascertain the FDA status of each drug or device planned for use in their clinical practice.

10 9 8 7 6 5 4 3 2 1

Dedications

To my family; to my friends; to my mentors; and to the many residents and students who have taught me so much.
Allan B. Wolfson, MD

To my wife, Lisa, and my boys, Eric and Adam, with whom all things are possible, and without whom little else matters; and to the residents and students I have had the honor of teaching and learning from over the years.
Gregory W. Hendey, MD

To my God, family, friends, neighbors, colleagues, fellows, residents, and patients who have taught me life's true lessons and always believed in me. To Dr. Robert Luten, my first mentor in Pediatric Emergency Medicine.
Phyllis L. Hendry, MD

To my family, friends, mentors, colleagues, and students, past, present, and future.
Christopher H. Linden, MD

To my wife Cathy, daughter Sofia, and my parents for their support; to Drs. Rich Wolfe, Peter Rosen, and Jonathan Edlow for their guidance and for the opportunities; and to the Emergency Medicine residents and faculty at Beth Israel Deaconess Medical Center with whom I am proud to work.
Carlo L. Rosen, MD

Special thanks to the Cook County Emergency Medicine residents and staff who keep the shifts fun and challenging! To my wife, Anna, and children, Jacob and Isaac, who have always supported and inspired me. Final thank you to Dr. Robert Simon who has served as a role model and mentor in emergency medicine to me throughout my career.
Jeffrey Schaider, MD

To my dear sweet husband Javaid, my beautiful daughters Mariyah and Aleena, my mom, Afroz, and all of my friends and family who have made it possible for me to pursue my dreams. Your sacrifices, never ending love and gentle encouragement mean more to me than you could ever know.
Ghazala Q. Sharieff, MD

To Emma, Madeline, and Julianna, for graciously allowing me access to the computer during this (and many other) projects.
Jeffrey R. Suchard, MD

Contents

SECTION XIV   PSYCHIATRIC EMERGENCIES
Jeffrey Schaider, MD

SECTION XV   DERMATOLOGIC EMERGENCIES
Jeffrey Schaider, MD

SECTION XVI   ALLERGIC AND IMMUNOLOGIC EMERGENCIES
Jeffrey Schaider, MD

SECTION XVII   INFECTIOUS DISEASE EMERGENCIES
Jeffrey Schaider, MD

SECTION XVIII   HEMATOLOGIC/ ONCOLOGIC EMERGENCIES
Jeffrey Schaider, MD

SECTION XIX   ENDOCRINE AND METABOLIC EMERGENCIES
Jeffrey Schaider, MD

SECTION XX   TRAUMA
Carlo L. Rosen, MD

PART I.   General Considerations

PART II.   Specific Injuries

PART III.   Orthopaedic Trauma

SECTION XXI   PEDIATRICS
Phyllis L. Hendry, MD *and Ghazala Q. Sharieff,* MD

PART V.   *Administrative and Clinical Issues*

SECTION XXII   TOXICOLOGY
Christopher H. Linden, MD and
Jeffrey R. Suchard, MD

PART I.   *General Considerations*

PART II.   *Alcohol-Related Agents and Conditions*

PART III.   *Analgesics and Related Conditions*

SECTION XXIII   ENVIRONMENTAL EMERGENCIES
Christopher H. Linden, MD and Jeffrey R. Suchard, MD

SECTION XXIV   ADMINISTRATIVE AND SPECIAL CLINICAL CONSIDERATIONS
Carlo L. Rosen, MD

SECTION XXV   APPENDICES
Christopher H. Linden, MD

Contributing Authors

Cynthia K. Aaron, MD, FACMT
New England Center for Toxicology at
    UMass
UMass Memorial Medical
    Center–University Campus
Department of Emergency Medicine
Worcester, Massachusetts

Lina Abujamra, MD
Clinical Instructor of Pediatrics
Feinberg School of Medicine
Attending Physician
Children's Memorial Hospital
Chicago, Illinois

Norberto Adame, Jr., MD
Interim Chairman
Department of Emergency Medicine
Maricopa Medical Center
Phoenix, Arizona

James G. Adams, MD
Professor and Chair
Department of Emergency Medicine
Feinberg School of Medicine
Northwestern University
Northwestern Memorial Hospital
Chicago, Illinois

Stephen L. Adams, MD
Professor of Medicine and Chief
Division of Sports Medicine
Chief Emeritus
Division of Emergency Medicine
Department of Medicine
Northwestern University Feinberg School
    of Medicine
Medical Director
Emergency Preparedness/Disaster
    Services
Northwestern Memorial Hospital
Team Physician
Chicago Cubs National League Baseball
    Club
Chicago, Illinois

David H. Adler, MD, MPH
Assistant Clinical Professor
Department of Medicine
University of California, San Francisco
Attending Physician
Department of Emergency Medicine
Highland Hospital–Alameda County
    Medical Center
Oakland, California

Steven E. Aks, MD
Department of Emergency Medicine
Cook County Hospital
Chicago, Illinois

Timothy E. Albertson, MD, MPH, PhD
California Poison Control System,
    Sacramento Division
University of California, San Francisco
    School of Pharmacy
Division of Pulmonary and Critical Care
    Medicine
Division of Emergency Medicine and
    Clinical Toxicology
University of California, Davis School of
    Medicine
Sacramento, California

Judith A. Alsop, PharmD
Director
California Poison Control System,
    Sacramento Division
University of California, San Francisco
    School of Pharmacy
Division of Pulmonary and Critical Care
    Medicine
University of California, Davis School of
    Medicine
Sacramento, California

Janet G. Alteveer, MD
Associate Professor of Emergency
    Medicine
UMDNJ–Robert Wood Johnson Medical
    School
Associate Medical Director/Attending
Department of Emergency Medicine
Cooper University Hospital
Camden, NJ

David Amponsah, MD
Assistant Professor of Emergency
    Medicine
Case Western Reserve University
Cleveland, Ohio
Senior Staff Attending
Department of Emergency Medicine
Henry Ford Health Systems
Detroit, Michigan

James T. Amsterdam, MD
Professor of Clinical Emergency
    Medicine
The Pennsylvania State University College
    of Medicine
Chair and Service Line Director
Department of Emergency Medicine
Hershey, Pennsylvania

Christine Anderegg, MD
Department of Emergency Medicine
Harbor–UCLA Medical Center
Torrance, California

Eric Anderson, MD, MBA
Assistant Clinical Professor of Emergency
    Medicine
The Ohio State University
Associate Director of Operations
Quality Review Officer
Department of Emergency Medicine
The Cleveland Clinic Foundation
Cleveland, Ohio

Ilene B. Anderson, PharmD
Associate Clinical Professor
University of California, San Francisco
    School of Pharmacy
Senior Toxicology Management Specialist
California Poison Control System, San
    Francisco Division
San Francisco, California

Paul S. Auerbach, MD
Clinical Professor of Surgery
Division of Emergency Medicine
Stanford University School of Medicine
Stanford, California

Mark J. Ault, MD
Professor of Clinical Medicine
University of California, Los Angeles
    School of Medicine
Cedars–Sinai Medical Center
Los Angeles, California

Jeffrey R. Avner, MD
Professor of Clinical Pediatrics
Albert Einstein College of Medicine
Director
Pediatric Emergency Service
Children's Hospital at Montefiore
Bronx, New York

John Bailitz, MD
Department of Emergency Medicine
Cook County Hospital
Assistant Professor of Emergency Medicine
Rush Medical College
Chicago, Illinois

Katherine Bakes, MD
Assistant Professor of Surgery
Division of Emergency Medicine
Department of Surgery
University of Colorado
Attending Emergency Medical Physician
Denver Health Medical Center
Denver, Colorado

Steven T. Baldwin, MD
Associate Professor
Department of Pediatrics and Emergency
    Medicine
University of Alabama School of Medicine
Birmingham, Alabama

Jill M. Baren, MD
Assistant Professor of Emergency Medicine
and Pediatrics
University of Pennsylvania School of
Medicine
Department of Emergency Medicine
Hospital of the University of Pennsylvania
Division of Emergency Medicine
Department of Pediatrics
The Children's Hospital of Philadelphia
Philadelphia, Pennsylvania

Robert A. Barish, MD
Senior Associate Dean for Clinical Affairs
Professor of Surgery and Medicine
University of Maryland School of Medicine
Baltimore, Maryland

Tobias D. Barker, MD
Instructor in Medicine/Emergency
Medicine
Harvard Medical School
Associate Physician
Department of Emergency Medicine
Brigham and Women's Hospital
Boston, Massachusetts

Roger M. Barkin, MD
Professor of Surgery
Division of Emergency Medicine
University of Colorado Health
Sciences Center
Denver, Colorado

Fermin Barrueto, Jr., MD
Assistant Professor
Division of Emergency Medicine
Department of Surgery
University of Maryland
Baltimore, Maryland

Christopher B. Beach, MD
Assistant Professor of Emergency Medicine
Northwestern University–The Feinberg
School of Medicine
Associate Director of Clinical Operations
Department of Emergency Medicine
Northwestern Memorial Hospital
Chicago, Illinois

Marc A. Bellazzini, MD
Clinical Assistant Professor of Medicine
University of Wisconsin Medical School
Attending Physician
Section of Emergency Medicine
University of Wisconsin Hospital and
Clinics
Madison, Wisconsin

Kip Benko MD, FACEP
Clinical Instructor
Affiliated Residency in Emergency
Medicine
University of Pittsburgh
Staff Clinical Physician
Mercy Hospital of Pittsburgh
Pittsburgh, Pennsylvania

Theodore I. Benzer, MD, PhD, FACEP
Instructor in Medicine
Harvard Medical School
Director of Clinical Operations
Massachusetts General Hospital
Boston, Massachusetts

Howard A. Bessen, MD
Department of Emergency Medicine
Harbor–UCLA Medical Center
Torrance, California

Phillip I. Bialecki, MD, MHE
Assistant Professor
Department of Emergency Medicine
Ohio University College of Medicine
Athens, Ohio

Daan Biesbroeck, MD
Attending Physician
Department of Emergency Medicine
Onze Lieve Vrouwe Gasthuis
1090 HM Amsterdam
The Netherlands

Louis S. Binder, MD
Professor of Emergency Medicine
Case Western Reserve University
Associate Residency Director and Director
of Education
Department of Emergency Medicine
MetroHealth Medical Center
Cleveland, Ohio

Dale S. Birenbaum, MD
Academic Director
Florida Emergency Physicians
Department of Emergency Medicine
Florida Hospital
Clinical Assistant Professor
Florida State University College of
Medicine
Orlando, Florida

Adrienne J. Birnbaum, MD
Associate Professor of Clinical Emergency
Medicine
Director
Residency Program
Albert Einstein/Jacobi and Montefiore
Medical Center
Bronx, New York

Diane M. Birnbaumer, MD
Professor of Medicine
University of California, Los Angeles
Associate Program Director
Department of Emergency Medicine
Harbor–UCLA Medical Center
Torrance, California

Herbert Bivins, MD
Clinical Professor of Medicine/Emergency
Medicine
Univerity of California, San Francisco,
Fresno Emergency Medicine Program
University Medical Center
Fresno, California

Paul Blackburn, DO, FACEP
Residency Director
Department of Emergency Medicine
Maricopa Medical Center
Phoenix, Arizona

Michael A. Bohrn, MD
Clinical Assistant Professor
The Pennsylvania State University College
of Medicine
Associate Program Director
York Hospital/The Pennsylvania State
University
Emergency Medicine Residency
York, Pennsylvania

Eric T. Boie, MD
Assistant Professor
Department of Emergency Medicine
Mayo Medical School
Staff Physician
Department of Emergency Medicine
Mayo Clinic–Saint Mary's Hospital
Rochester, Minnesota

Edward B. Bolgiano, MD
Assistant Professor
Departments of Surgery and Medicine
University of Maryland School of Medicine
Chairman
Emergency Medicine
Bon Secours Hospital
Baltimore, Maryland

G. Randall Bond, MD
Professor
Departments of Emergency Medicine and
Pediatrics
Medical Director
Drug and Poison Information Center
Cincinnati Children's Hospital Medical
Center and University of Cincinnati
Cincinnati, Ohio

Pierre Borczuk, MD
Instructor in Medicine
Harvard Medical School
Assistant in Emergency Medicine
Massachusetts General Hospital
Boston, Massachusetts

Keith Borg, MD
Assistant Professor
Department of Emergency Medicine
Emory University
Atlanta, Georgia

Rodney B. Boychuk, MD
Clinical Professor
Departments of Surgery and Pediatrics
Kapiolani Medical Center
Honolulu, Hawaii

William P. Bozeman, MD
Assistant Professor
Associate Director of Research
Department of Emergency Medicine
Wake Forest University Baptist Medical
Center
Winston-Salem, North Carolina

G. Richard Braen, MD
    Chair and Professor
    Department of Clinical Emergency
        Medicine
    School of Medicine and Biomedical
        Sciences
    University of Buffalo
    Buffalo, New York

Darren Braude, MD, MPH, FACEP
    Assistant Professor
    Department of Emergency Medicine
    University of New Mexico School of
        Medicine
    Albuquerque, New Mexico

John A. Brennan, MD, FAAP, FACEP
    Director of Pediatric Emergency Medicine
    Senior Vice President, Clinical and
        Emergency Services
    Saint Barnabas Health Care System
    West Orange, New Jersey

Jeffrey Brent, MD, PhD
    Clinical Professor of Medicine
    University of Colorado Health Science
        Center
    Toxicology Associates
    Denver, Colorado

Kerry B. Broderick, MD
    Associate Residency Director
    Denver Health Medical Center
    Denver, Colorado

Geoffrey Broocker, MD
    Walthour-DeLaPerriere Professor of
        Ophthalmology
    Emory University School of Medicine
    Chief of Service
    Grady Memorial Hospital
    Atlanta, Georgia

Daniel E. Brooks, MD
    Assistant Professor of Medical Toxicology
        and Emergency Medicine
    Director
    Medical Toxicology Service
    Co-Medical Director
    Pittsburgh Poison Center
    University of Pittsburgh Medical Center
    Pittsburgh, Pennsylvania

Tonia J. Brousseau, DO
    Department of Emergency Medicine
    University of Florida College of Medicine
    Jacksonville, Florida

David F. M. Brown, MD
    Assistant Professor of Medicine
    Division of Emergency Medicine
    Harvard Medical School
    Associate Chief
    Department of Emergency Medicine
    Massachusetts General Hospital
    Boston, Massachusetts

Lance Brown, MD, MPH
    Associate Professor
    Department of Emergency Medicine
    Loma Linda University Medical Center
    Chief
    Division of Pediatric Emergency Medicine
    Loma Linda University Children's
        Hospital
    Loma Linda, California

Kathleen Brown, MD
    Assistant Professor
    Children's National Medical Center
    Washington, DC

Richard Bruno, MD
    Department of Emergency Medicine
    Thomas Jefferson University Hospital
    Philadelphia, Pennsylvania

James H. Bryan, MD, PhD
    Assistant Professor
    Department of Emergency Medicine
    Oregon Health and Science University
    Assistant Chief
    Emergency Medicine Service
    Veterans Affairs Medical Center
    Portland, Oregon

Robert G. Buckley, MD, MPH, FACEP
    Captain, Medical Corps, US Navy
    Residency Program Director
    Department of Emergency Medicine
    Naval Medical Center San Diego
    San Diego, California

E. Bradshaw Bunney, MD, FACEP
    Associate Professor
    Department of Emergency Medicine
    University of Illinois at Chicago
    Chicago, Illinois

Michael D. Burg, MD
    Assistant Clinical Professor
    Department of Emergency Medicine
    University of California, San Francisco,
        Fresno University Medical Center
    Fresno, California

Keith K. Burkhart, MD
    Professor of Emergency Medicine and
        Pharmacology
    Department of Emergency Medicine
    The Milton S. Hershey Medical Center
    The Pennsylvania State University
    Hershey, Pennsylvania

Michael Joseph Burns, MD
    Assistant Professor of Medicine
    Harvard Medical School
    Co-Director
    Division of Toxicology
    Department of Emergency Medicine
    Beth Israel Deaconess Medical Center
    Boston, Massachusetts

Michael James Burns, MD
    Clinical Professor of Emergency Medicine
    Division of Infectious Diseases
    University of California, Irvine Medical
        Center
    University of California, Irvine College of
        Medicine
    Orange, California

Jonathan L. Burstein, MD
    Assistant Professor of Medicine
    Department of Emergency Medicine
    Harvard Medical School
    Assistant Professor of Population and
        International Health
    Harvard School of Public Health
    Boston, Massachusetts

Laurie J. Burton, MD
    Assistant Professor
    Department of Pediatrics
    Emory University
    Attending Physician
    Division of Pediatric Emergency Medicine
    Children's Healthcare of Atlanta
    Hughes Spalding Children's Hospital
    Atlanta, Georgia

Richard Byyny, MD
    Clinical Instructor
    Research Fellow
    UCLA School of Medicine
    Los Angeles, California

Clifton W. Callaway, MD, PhD
    Assistant Professor
    Department of Emergency Medicine
    University of Pittsburgh
    Pittsburgh, Pennsylvania

Michelle J. Canham, MD
    Attending Physician
    Department of Emergency Medicine
    John H. Stroger Jr. Hospital of Cook
        County
    Chicago, Illinois

Donna Caniano, MD
    Department of Pediatric Surgery
    Columbus Children's Hospital
    Columbus, Ohio

Richard M. Cantor, MD
    Associate Professor
    Department of Emergency Medicine
    SUNY Upstate Medical Center
    Syracuse, New York

Thomas R. Carraccio, MD, PharmD
    Associate Professor of Emergency Medicine
    State University of New York at Stony
        Brook;
    Director Long Island Regional Poison and
        Drug Information Center
    Winthrop University Hospital
    Mineola, New York

Leslie S. Carroll, MD, ABMT
  Assistant Professor
  Department of Emergency Medicine
  Temple University Hospital
  Philadelphia, Pennsylvania

Austen Chai, MD
  Department of Emergency Medicine
  Cook County Hospital
  Assistant Professor of Emergency Medicine
  Rush Medical College
  Chicago, Illinois

Andrew K. Chang, MD
  Assistant Professor
  Department of Emergency Medicine
  Montefiore Medical Center
  Bronx, New York

Michael E. Chansky, MD
  Chairman
  Department of Emergency Medicine
  Associate Professor of Emergency Medicine
    and Internal Medicine
  Robert Wood Johnson Medical School
  Cooper University Hospital
  Camden, New Jersey

Michelle Charfen, MD
  Department of Emergency Medicine
  Harbor–UCLA Medical Center
  Torrance, California

William K. Chiang, MD
  Associate Director, Emergency Department
  Bellevue Hospital Center
  Assistant Professor of Emergency Medicine
  New York University School of Medicine
  New York, New York

Brian Chinnock, MD
  Assistant Clinical Professor of Medicine
    Department of Emergency Medicine
  University of California, San Francisco,
    Fresno Medical Education Program
  University Medical Center
  Fresno, California

Theodore A. Christopher, MD
  Associate Professor and Chairman
  Department of Emergency Medicine
  Thomas Jefferson University Hospital and
    Jefferson Medical College
  Philadelphia, Pennsylvania

Carl R. Chudnofsky, MD
  Associate Professor and Chairman
  Department of Emergency Medicine
  Albert Einstein Medical Center
  Philadelphia, Pennsylvania

Joseph A. Church, MD
  Professor
  The Saban Research Institute
  Children's Hospital of Los Angeles
  Los Angeles, California

James E. Cisek, MD
  Associate Clinical Professor of Internal
    Medicine and Preventive Medicine
  Virginia Commonwealth University
  Richmond, Virginia

David M. Cline, MD
  Associate Professor
  Department of Emergency Medicine
  Wake Forest University School of Medicine
  Director of Research
  Department of Emergency Medicine
  Baptist Medical Center
  Winston-Salem, North Carolina

Joseph E. Clinton, MD
  Professor and Head
  Department of Emergency Medicine
  University of Minnesota Medical School
  Minneapolis, Minnesota

Wendy C. Coates, MD
  Director
  Medical Education
  Harbor–UCLA Medical Center
  Department of Emergency Medicine
  Associate Professor of Medicine
  Vice-Chair
  Acute Care College
  Geffen School of Medicine at UCLA

James Colletti, MD
  Senior Associate Consultant
  Department of Emergency Medicine with
  Joint Appointment in Department of
    Pediatric and Adolescent Medicine
  Assistant Residency Program Director
  Department of Emergency Medicine
  Instructor in Pediatrics
  Mayo Medical School
  Mayo Clinic
  Rochester, Minnesota

Stephen Colucciello, MD
  Clinical Professor of Emergency Medicine
  University of North Carolina Medical
    School–Chapel Hill
  Associate Chair, Department of Emergency
    Medicine
  Carolinas Medical Center
  Charlotte, North Carolina

Christopher B. Colwell, MD
  Assistant Professor
  Division of Emergency Medicine
  Department of Surgery
  University of Colorado Health Sciences
    Center
  Faculty
  Denver Health Medical Center Residency
    in Emergency Medicine
  Denver, Colorado

James A. Comes, MD
  Assistant Clinical Professor
  Department of Emergency Medicine
  University of California, San Francisco,
    Fresno Medical Education Program
  Fresno, California

William F. Coombs, MD
  Attending Physician
  Emergency Services
  Miami Children's Hospital
  Miami, Florida

Anna Kate Corbin, MD
  Department of Emergency Medicine
  The Ohio State University
  Columbus, Ohio

Karen S. Cosby, MD
  Assistant Professor
  Department of Emergency Medicine
  Rush Medical University
  Senior Attending Physician
  Department of Emergency Medicine
  John H. Stroger Jr. Hospital of Cook County
  Chicago, Illinois

Sandra A. Craig, MD
  Clinical Instructor
  University of North Carolina at Chapel Hill
    School of Medicine
  Chapel Hill, North Carolina
  Clinical Faculty
  Department of Emergency Medicine
  Carolinas Medical Center
  Charlotte, North Carolina

Barbara Insley Crouch, PharmD, MSPH
  Professor (Clinical)
  Department of Pharmacotherapy
  Director
  Utah Poison Control Center
  University of Utah
  Salt Lake City, Utah

Steven C. Curry, MD
  Associate Professor of Clinical Medicine
  University of Arizona College of Medicine
  Director
  Department of Medical Toxicology
  Banner Good Samaritan Medical Center
  Phoenix, Arizona

Catherine B. Custalow, MD, PhD
  Assistant Professor
  Department of Emergency Medicine
  University of Virginia Health System
  Charlottesville, Virginia

Rita K. Cydulka, MD, MS
  Associate Professor and Vice-Chair
    Department of Emergency Medicine
  Case Western Reserve University-Metro
    Health Medical Center
  Cleveland, Ohio

Richard C. Dart, MD, PhD
  Director, Rocky Mountain Poison and Drug
    Center;
  Professor of Surgery (Emergency Medicine)
  University of Colorado Health
  Sciences Center
  Rocky Mountain Poison and Drug Center
  Denver, Colorado

Benjamin Davies, MD
Instructor of Urology
Department of Urology
University of Pittsburgh Medical
Center
Pittsburgh, Pennsylvania

Peter M.C. DeBlieux, MD
Residency Program Director
Section of Emergency Medicine
Professor of Clinical Medicine
Charity Hospital
New Orleans, Louisiana

Wyatt W. Decker, MD
Chair
Department of Emergency Medicine
College of Medicine
Mayo Clinic
Rochester, Minnesota

Atima Chumpa Delaney, MD
Instructor in Pediatrics
Harvard Medical School
Assistant in Medicine
Children's Hospital
Boston, Massachusetts

Theodore R. Delbridge, MD, MPH
Associate Professor of Emergency Medicine
and Health Policy & Management
University of Pittsburgh
Senior Medical Advisor
STAT-MedEvac
Pittsburgh, Pennsylvania

David Della-Giustina, MD
Adjunct Assistant Professor of Military and
Emergency Medicine
Uniformed Services University of the
Health Sciences
Bethesda, Maryland
Assistant Professor of Medicine
University of Washington School of
Medicine
Seattle, Washington
LTC, United States Army
Chairman
Department of Medicine
Madigan Army Medical Center
Tacoma, Washington

William R. Dennis, MD
Staff Physician
Emergency Medicine Department
Naval Medical Center Portsmouth
Portsmouth, Virginia

Deborah Diercks, MD
Assistant Professor
Department of Emergency Medicine
University of California, Davis Medical
Center
Sacramento, California

Ann M. Dietrich, MD
Clinical Associate Professor
Department of Pediatrics
The Ohio State University College of
Medicine and Public Health
Attending Physician
Pediatric Emergency Medicine
Children's Hospital
Columbus, Ohio

Valerie Ann Dobiesz, MD
Associate Residency Director
Department of Emergency Medicine
Universiry of Illinois at Chicago
Chicago, Illinois

Michele L. Dorfsman, MD, FACEP
Assistant Professor
Department of Emergency Medicine
University of Pittsburgh
Attending Physician
Department of Emergency Medicine
University of Pittsburgh Medical Center,
Presbyterian Hospital
Pittsburgh, Pennsylvania

Robert P. Dowsett, BM, BS, FACEM
Medical Director
Department of Emergency Medicine
Westmead Hospital
Sydney
Australia

Jeffrey Dubin, MD
Medical Director
Department of Emergency Medicine
Washington Hospital Center
Assistant Professor of Clinical Emergency
Medicine
Georgetown University School of Medicine
Washington, DC

Ellen M. Dugan, MD, FACEP
Associate Professor
Department of Emergency Medicine
Georgetown University Medical Center
Washington, DC

Susan M. Dunmire, MD
Department of Emergency Medicine
University of Pittsburgh School of
Medicine
Pittsburgh, Pennsylvania

Jo Ellen Dyer, PharmD
Associate Clinical Professor
University of California, San Francisco
California Poison Control System, San
Francisco Division
San Francisco, California

Sophia Dyer, MD
Department of Research, Training and
Quality Improvement
Boston EMS
Boston, Massachusetts

Pamela L. Dyne, MD
Associate Clinical Professor
Department of Internal
Medicine/Emergency Medicine
David Geffen School of Medicine at UCLA
Los Angeles, California
Associate Clinical Professor
Department of Emergency Medicine
Olive View–UCLA Medical Center
Sylmar, California

Philip A. Edelman, MD
Office of the Director
Centers for Disease Control and Prevention
(OTPER)
Senior Medical Advisor to the Assistant
Secretary
Public Health Emergency Preparedness
Department of Health and
Human Services
Washington, District of Columbia

Jonathan A. Edlow, M.D. FACEP
Associate Professor of Medicine
Harvard Medical School
Vice Chairman
Department of Emergency Medicine
Beth Israel Deaconess Medical Center
Boston, Massachusetts

Erin E. Endom, MD
Assistant Professor
Section of Emergency Medicine
Department of Pediatrics
Baylor College of Medicine
Texas Children's Hospital
Houston, Texas

Brianna Enriquez, MD
Pediatric Emergency Medicine Fellow
Harbor UCLA
Torrance, California

Jeffrey A. Evans, MD
Instructor in Medicine
Department of Medicine
Division of Emergency Medicine
Harvard Medical School
Boston, Massachusetts
Attending Physician
Department of Emergency Medicine
Mount Auburn Hospital
Cambridge, Massachusetts

James A. Feldman, MD
Vice Chair of Research
Department of Emergency Medicine
Boston Medical Center
Associate Professor of Emergency
Medicine,
Boston University School of Medicine
Boston, Massachusetts

Susan S. Fish, PharmD, MPH
Associate Director
Office of Clinical Research
Boston University Medical Center
Boston, Massachusetts

Susan Mumm Fitzgerald, MD
Staff Physician
Department of Emergency Medicine
Highland Hospital–Alameda County
Medical Center
Oakland, California

Alan Forstater, MD
Clinical Assistant Professor of Emergency
Medicine
Vice Chair, Clinical Affairs
Department of Emergency Medicine
Thomas Jefferson University
Philadelphia, Pennsylvania

Marla J. Friedman, DO
Attending Physician
Department of Emergency Medicine
Miami Children's Hospital
Miami, Florida

R. Brent Furbee, MD, FACMT
Medical Director, Indiana Poison Center
Methodist Hospital of Indiana
Indiana University School of Medicine
Indianapolis, Indiana

Brendan R. Furlong, MD
Assistant Professor of Clinical Emergency
Medicine
Georgetown University School of Medicine
Clinical Chief of Emergency Medicine
Georgetown University Hospital
Washignton, DC

Ronald A. Furnival, MD
Associate Professor
Pediatric Emergency Medicine
Primary Children's Medical Center and
Department of Pediatrics
University of Utah School of Medicine
Salt Lake City, Utah

Gregory G. Gaar, MD
Clinical Professor of Pediatrics
University of South Florida College of
Medicine
Medical Director
Florida Poison Information Center
Tampa, Florida

E. John Gallagher, MD
Professor of Medicine
Albert Einstein College of Medicine
Chairman
Department of Emergency Medicine
Jacobi Medical Center
New York, New York

Gus M. Garmel, MD, FACEP, FAAEM
Co-Director
Stanford/Kaiser Emergency Medicine
Residency Program
Stanford University School of Medicine
Palo Alto, California
Senior Staff Emergency Physician
Department of Emergency Medicine
Kaiser Permanente Medical Center
Santa Clara, California

Pierre Gaudreault, MD, FRCPC
Clinical Associate Professor
Department of Pediatrics
University of Montreal Chief
Clinical Pharmacology/Toxicology Unit
CHU Sainte-Justine
Montréal, Québec Canada

Marianne Gausche-Hill, MD, FACEP,
FAAP
Professor of Clinical Medicine
David Geffen School of Medicine at UCLA
Director, Emergency Medical Services and
EMS Fellowship
Director, Pediatric Emergency Medicine
Fellowship
Department of Emergency Medicine
Harbor-UCLA Medical Center
Torrance, California

Michael Gayle, MD
Associate Professor
University of Florida College of Medicine
Director of Pediatric Transport
Wolfson Children's Hospital
Jacksonville, Florida

Joel M. Geiderman, MD
Clinical Professor of Medicine
David Geffen UCLA School of Medicine
Co-Chair
Department of Emergency Medicine
Ruth and Harry Roman Emergency
Department
Cedars–Sinai Medical Center
Los Angeles, California

Richard J. Geller, MD, MPH, FACMT
Associate Clinical Professor
Department of Emergency Medicine
University of California, San Francisco
Medical and Acting Managing Director
California Poison Control System,
Fresno/Madera
Children's Hospital Central California
Madera, California

Charles J. Gerardo, MD
Assistant Clinical Professor
Division of Emergency Medicine
Duke University
Director
Graduate Education
Division of Emergency Medicine
Duke University Medical Center
Durham, North Carolina

Richard D. Gerkin, Jr., MD, MS
Department of Medical Toxicology
Banner Good Samaritan Medical Center
Phoenix, Arizona

Michael A. Gibbs, MD
Chief
Department of Emergency Medicine
Maine Medical Center
Portland, Maine

Timothy G. Givens, MD
Associate Professor of Emergency Medicine
and Pediatrics
Associate Director
Pediatric Emergency Medicine
Vanderbilt University Medical Center
Nashville, Tennessee

Steven Andy Godwin, MD, FACEP
Assistant Professor
Director of Medical Education
Residency Program Director
Department of Emergency Medicine
University of Florida HSC
Jacksonville, Florida

William Goldberg, MD
Assistant Professor
New York University School of Medicine
Department of Emergency Medicine
Bellevue Hospital
New York, New York

Javier A. Gonzalez del Rey, MD
Associate Professor of Pediatrics
Associate Director
Division of Emergency Medicine
Director
Pediatric Residency Program
Cincinnati Children's Hospital Medical
Center
Cincinnati, Ohio

Collin S. Goto, MD
Assistant Clinical Professor
Children's Hospital and Health Center
University of California, San Diego
San Diego, California

John E. Gough, MD
Professor
Department of Emergency Medicine
East Carolina University
Greenville, North Carolina

Deepi G. Goyal, MD
Assistant Professor
Department of Emergency Medicine
Mayo Clinic College of Medicine
Staff Physician
Department of Emergency Medicine
Mayo Clinic–Saint Mary's Hospital
Assistant Program Director
Mayo Emergency Medicine Residency
Rochester, Minnesota

Louis Graff, MD, FACEP, FACP
Professor of Emergency Medicine
Clinical Professor of Medicine
University of Connecticut School of
Medicine
Assistant Professor, Section of Emergency
Medicine
Department of Surgery
Yale University School of Medicine
Medical Director of Quality
Associate Director Emergency Medicine
New Britain General Hospital
New Britain, Connecticut

Andis Graudins, MD
Conjoint Senior Lecturer
Faculty of Medicine
University of New South Wales.
Division of Clinical and Experimental
Toxicology
Staff Specialist
Department of Emergency Medicine
Prince of Wales Hospital, Randwick
Australia

Michael I. Greenberg, MD, MPH
Professor of Emergency Medicine
Professor of Public Health
Drexel University College of Medicine
Clinical Professor of Emergency
Medicine
Temple University School of Medicine
Philadelphia, Pennsylvania

Constance S. Greene, MD, MHPE, FACEP
Associate Professor of Emergency
Medicine
Rush Medical School
Chicago, Illinois

Howard A. Greller, MD
Fellow
Medical Toxicology
New York University School of
Medicine/Bellevue Hospital Center
New York City Poison Control Center
New York, New York

Lauren Grossman, MD
Division of Emergency Medicine
University of Colorado Health Sciences
Center
Denver, Colorado

Steven Guillen, MD
Department of Emergency Medicine
Temple University Hospital
Philadelphia, Pennsylvania

Gregory T. Guldner, MD, MS
Program Director
Emergency Medicine Residency Program
Loma Linda University Medical Center
Loma Linda, California

Alan H. Hall, MD
Clinical Assistant Professor of Preventive
Medicine and Biometric
University of Colorado Health Sciences
Center
Denver, Colorado

Christine Haller, MD
Assistant Adjunct Professor of Medicine
and Laboratory Medicine
University of California, San Francisco
Chief
Toxicology Service
San Francisco General Hospital Clinical
Laboratories
San Francisco, California

Luis H. Haro, MD
Instructor
Department of Emergency Medicine
Mayo Clinic College of Medicine
Staff Physician
Department of Emergency Medicine
Mayo Clinic–Saint Mary's Hospital
Rochester, Minnesota

Rachel Haroz, MD
Department of Emergency Medicine
Drexel University College of Medicine
Philadelphia, Pennsylvania

David Hartman, MD
Department of Emergency Medicine
Michigan State University Kalamazoo
Center for Medical Studies
Kalamazoo, Michigan

Richard S. Hartoch, MD
Assistant Professor
Department of Emergency Medicine
Oregon Health & Science University
Portland, Oregon

Steven C. Hartsell, MD
Associate Professor of Surgery
Division of Emergency Medicine
University of Utah School of Medicine
Salt Lake City, Utah

Stephen R. Hayden, MD
Associate Professor of Medicine
Program Director
Emergency Medicine Residency
UCSD Medical Center
San Diego, California

Kennon Heard, MD
Assistant Professor of Surgery
Division of Emergency Medicine
University of Colorado
Section Chief
Medical Toxicology
University of Colorado Health Sciences
Center
Attending Physician
Rocky Mountain Poison and Drug Center
Denver, Colorado

Alan C. Heffner, MD
Naval Medical Center Portsmouth
Portsmouth, Virginia

Michael Heller, MD
Clinical Professor of Medicine
Temple University School of Medicine
Philadelphia, Pennsylvania
Department of Emergency Medicine
St. Luke's Hospital
Bethlehem, Pennsylvania

Sean O. Henderson, MD
Associate Professor
Department of Emergency Medicine
Keck School of Medicine of the University
of Southern California
Los Angeles, California

Gregory W. Hendey, MD
Associate Professor of Clinical Medicine
University of California, San Francisco
Emergency Medicine Research Director
University of California, San Francisco,
Fresno Medical Education Program
Fresno, California

Phyllis L. Hendry, MD
Associate Professor of Pediatrics and
Emergency Medicine
University of Florida Health Science Center
Director
Pediatric Emergency Services
Shands Jacksonville
Jacksonville, Florida

Philip L. Henneman, MD
Professor and Chair
Department of Emergency Medicine
Baystate Health Systems
Tufts University School of Medicine
Boston, Massachusetts

Fred M. Henretig, MD
Poison Control Center
Children's Hospital of Philadelphia
Philadelphia, Pennsylvania

Mel Herbert, MD
Associate Professor of Clinical Emergency
Medicine
Keck School of Medicine
Department of Emergency Medicine
USC/LAC Medical Center
Los Angeles, California

H. Gene Hern, Jr., MD, MS
Associate Residency Director
Highland Hospital–Alameda County
Medical Center
Oakland, California

Robert D. Herr, MD
Medical Director, Utilization Management
Department of Emergency Medicine
Group Health Cooperative of Puget Sound
Seattle, Washington

Robert W. Hickey, MD
Associate Professor of Pediatrics
Department of Pediatrics
Division of Pediatric Emergency Medicine
University of Pittsburgh
Children's Hospital of Pittsburgh
Pittsburgh, Pennsylvania

Kendall Ho, MD, FRCPC
Associate Dean of Medicine
Assistant Professor
Division of Emergency Medicine
The University of British Columbia
Vancouver General Hospital
Vancouver, British Columbia
Canada

Robert S. Hockberger, MD
Professor of Medicine
David Geffen School of Medicine at UCLA
Chair
Department of Emergency Medicine
Harbor–UCLA Medical Center
Torrance, California

Dee Hodge III, MD
Associate Professor of Pediatrics
Washinton University School of Medicine
Associate Director
Clinical Affairs
St. Louis Children's Hospital
St. Louis, Missouri

Cynthia C. Hoecker, MD
Associate Clinical Professor of Pediatrics
(Voluntary)
University of California, San Diego School
of Medicine
Attending Physician
Children's Hospital, San Diego
San Diego, California

Gwendolyn L. Hoffman, MD
Associate Professor
Department of Emergency Medicine
Michigan State University College of
Human Medicine
East Lansing, Michigan
Chairman
Department of Emergency Medicine
Spectrum Hospital
Grand Rapids, Michigan

Jerome R. Hoffman, MD, MA
Professor
Department of Medicine/Emergency
Medicine
Univerity of California, Los Angeles School
of Medicine
Attending Physician
Emergency Medical Center
University of California, Los Angeles
Los Angeles, California

Robert S. Hoffman, MD
Associate Professor
Department of Emergency Medicine
New York University School of Medicine
Director
New York City Poison Control Center
New York, New York

Judd E. Hollander, MD
Professor
Clinical Research Director
Department of Emergency Medicine
Hospital of the University of Pennsylvania
Philadelphia, Pennsylvania

Mark A. Hostetler, MD, MPH
Chief, Section of Pediatric Emergency
Medicine
University of Chicago Children's Hospital
Chicago, Illinois

Debra Houry, MD, MPH
Assistant Professor and Attending
Physician
Department of Emergency Medicine
Emory University
Atlanta, Georgia

Hoori Hovanessian, MD
Assitant Clinical Professor
Departments of Medicine and Emergency
Medicine
University of San Francisco
University Medical Center
Fresno, California
Staff Emergency Physician
Presbyterian Intercommunity Hospital
Whittier, California

John M. Howell, MD
Clinical Professor
Department of Emergency Medicine
The George Washington University
Washinton, DC
Director of Academic Affairs
Department of Emergency Medicine
INOVA Fairfax Hospital /Best Pracices, Inc.
Falls Church, Virginia

David S. Howes, MD
Professor
Department of Medicine/Emergency
Medicine
Program Director
Section of Emergency Medicine
University of Chicago
Chicago, Illinois

Kathleen C. Hubbell, MD
Clinical Associate Professor
Department of Medicine/Emergency
Medicine
Director
Accident Room
Medical Center of Lousiana–Charity
Hospital
New Orleans, Louisiana

J. Stephen Huff, MD
Associate Professor
Emergency Medicine and Neurology
Department of Emergency Medicine
University of Virginia Health Systems
Charlottesville, Virginia

Matthew J. Hunt, MD
Department of Emergency Medicine
University of California Irvine Medical
Center
Orange, California

Sabiha Hussain, MD
University of Medicine & Dentistry of
New Jersey
Robert Wood Johnson University Medical
Group
Department of Medicine
New Brunswick, New Jersey

Daniel J. Isaacman, MD
Professor of Pediatrics
Eastern Virginia Medical School
Chief
Division of Pediatric Emergency Medicine
Children's Hospital of the King's
Daughters
Norfolk, Virginia

Alexander P. Isakov, MD, MPH
Assistant Professor of Emergency
Medicine
Co-Director
Section of Prehospital and Disaster
Medicine
Department of Emergency Medicine
Emory University
Atlanta, Georgia

Jennifer L. Isenhour, MD
Associate Program Director
Department of Emergency Medicine
Carolinas Medical Center
Charlotte, North Carolina

Kenneth V. Iserson, MD, MBA
Professor of Emergency Medicine
Director, Arizona Bioethics Program
University of Arizona
Emergency Physicians
University Medical Center
Tucson, Arizona

Kenneth C. Jackimczyk, MD
Attending Physician
Department of Emergency Medicine
Maricopa Medical Center
Phoenix, Arizona

Dag Jacobsen, MD, PhD
Director and Professor
Department of Acute Medicine
Ullevaal University Hospital
Oslo
Norway

Sheldon Jacobson, MD, FACP, FACEP
Chairman and Professor
Mount Sinai School of Medicine
New York, New York

Cynthia Jacobstein, MD, MSCE
Clinical Assistant Professor of Pediatrics
University of Pennsylvania School of
Medicine
Division of Emergency Medicine
The Children's Hospital of Philadelphia
Philadelphia, Pennsylvania

David M. Jaffe, MD
Division of Pediatric Emergency
Medicine
St. Louis Children's Place
St. Louis, Missouri

Andy Jagoda
  Professor
  Vice Chair of Academic Affairs
  Residency Director
  Department of Emergency Medicine
  Mount Sinai School of Medicine
  New York, New York

David Anthony Jerrard, MD
  Associate Professor of Surgery and
    Medicine
  University of Maryland
  Division of Emergency Medicine
  Baltimore, Maryland

Ian D. Jones, MD
  Assistant Professor of Emergency
    Medicine
  Director, Adult Emergency Department
  Vanderbilt University Medical Center
  Nashville, Tennessee

Madeline Matar Joseph, MD
  Clinical Associate Professor
  Department of Emergency Medicine
  University of Florida
  Jacksonville, Florida

Steven M. Joyce, MD
  Professor of Surgery
  Division of Emergency Medicine
  University of Utah School of Medicine
  Salt Lake City, Utah

Amy Kaji, MD
  Clinical Instructor of Medicine
  David Geffen School of Medicine at UCLA
  Research Fellow
  Department of Emergency Medicine
  Harbor–UCLA Medical Center
  Torrance, California

Richard M. Kaplan, MD, MS
  Clinical Associate Professor
  Department of Emergency Medicine
  University of Pittsburgh
  Staff Physician
  Department of Emergency Medicine
  Western Pennsylvania Hospital
  Pittsburgh, Pennsylvania

John S. Kashani, MD
  Department of Medical Toxicology
  Banner Good Samaritan Medical Center
  Phoenix, Arizona

Thomas E. Kearney, PharmD
  Professor
  Department of Clinical Pharmary
  University of California, San Francisco
    School of Pharmacy
  Managing Director
  California Poison Control System, San
    Francisco Division
  San Francisco, California

John J. Kelly, DO
  Associate Professor of Emergency Medicine
  Jefferson Medical College
  Adjunct Associate Professor of Emergency
    Medicine
  Drexel University School of Medicine
  Philadelphia College of Osteopathic
    Medicine
  Associate Chair
  Department of Emergency Medicine
  Albert Einstein Medical Center
  Philadelphia, Pennsylvania

John L. Kendall, MD, FACEP
  Assistant Professor
  Division of Emergency Medicine
  Department of Surgery
  University of Colorado Health Sciences
    Center
  Attending Physician
  Department of Emergency Medicine
  Denver Health Medical Center
  Denver, Colorado

Christopher S. Kennedy, MD
  Division of Pediatric Emergency Medicine
  Children's Mercy Hospital
  Kansas City, Missouri

B. Nazeema Khan, MD
  Pediatric Emergency Medicine Fellow
  University of Florida, Jacksonville
  Jacksonville, Florida

Naghma S. Khan, MD
  Assistant Professor
  Department of Pediatrics
  Emory University School of Medicine
  Atlanta, Georgia

George S. Kim, MD
  Department of Emergency Medicine
  MetroHealth Medical Center
  Cleveland, Ohio

Joseph D. Kim, MD*

Brent R. King, MD
  Professor of Emergency Medicine and
    Pediatrics
  Chairman
  Department of Emergency Medicine
  The University of Texas Health Science
    Center at Houston Medical School
  Service Chief
  Emergency Medicine
  Memorial Hermann Hospital Emergency
    Center
  Houston, Texas

Christopher King, MD
  Associate Professor of Emergency
    Medicine and Pediatrics
  University of Pittsburgh School of Medicine
  Pittsburgh, Pennsylvania

*Deceased

Donna Kinser, MD
  Clinical Professor
  Division of Emergency Medicine
  University of California, Davis School of
    Medicine
  Sacramento, California

J. Douglas Kirk, MD
  Associate Professor and Vice-Chair
  Department of Emergency Medicine
  University of Califirnia, Davis School of
    Medicine
  Director of Clinical Operations
  Department of Emergency Medicine
  University of Califiornia, Davis Medical
    Center
  Sacramento, California

Niranjan Kissoon, MD
  Professor and Chief
  Department of Pediatrics
  University of Florida
  Jacksonville, Florida

Christine A. Kletti, MD
  Assistant Professor
  Department of Emergency Medicine
  University of Minnesota
  Attending Physician
  Hennepin County Medical Center
  Minneapolis, Minnesota

Andrew L. Knaut, MD, PhD
  Associate Program Director
  Denver Health Medical Center Residency
    in Emergency Medicine
  Denver, Colorado

Kevin J. Knoop, MD
  Director for Medical Education
  Office of Alumni and Academic Affairs
  Naval Medical Center
  Portsmouth, Virginia

Christine E. Koerner, MD
  Associate Professor of Emergency Medicine
  The University of Texas Health Science
    Center at Houston
  Chief
  Division of Pediatric Emergency Medicine
  Memorial Hermann Hospital and LBJ
    General Hospital
  Houston, Texas

Paul Kolecki, MD
  Assistant Professor
  Department of Emergency Medicine
  Director of Medical Student Education
  Thomas Jefferson University
  Philadelphia, Pennsylvania

Michele E. Krajicek, M.D.
  Chief Resident
  Mayo Emergency Medicine Residency
  Mayo School of Graduate Medical
    Education
  Rochester, Minnesota

David A. Kramer, MD
Clinical Associate Professor
Department of Emergency Medicine
The Pennsylvania State University
Program Director
York Hospital
York, Pennsylvania

Richard S. Krause, MD
Residency Director and Assistant Professor
of Clinical Emergency Medicine
School of Medicine and Biomedical
Sciences
University of Buffalo
Buffalo, New York

Joel Kravitz, MD
Assistant Program Director
Department of Emergency Medicine
Albert Einstein Medical Center
Philadelphia, Pennsylvania

Robert D. Kregenow, MD
Washington University School of Medicine
St. Louis Children's Hospital
Department of Pediatrics
Division of Emergency Medicine
St. Louis, Missouri

Kenneth W. Kulig, MD
Associate Clinical Professor
Division of Emergency Medicine and
Trauma
Department of Surgery
University of Colorado
Denver, Colorado

Kenneth T. Kwon, MD
Associate Clinical Professor
Department of Emergency Medicine
University of California, Irvine School of
Medicine
Director of Pediatric Emergency
Medicine
Department of Emergency Medicine
UC Irvine Medical Center
Orange, California

Joseph Lang, MD
Assistant Director
Emergency Department
Maryview Medical Center
Portsmouth, Virginia

William G. Langston, II, MD
The Parkinson's Institute
Sunnyvale, California

James L. Larson, MD
Assistant Professor
Clinical Director
Assistant Residency Director
Department of Emergency Medicine
University of North Carolina at
Chapel Hill
Chapel Hill, North Carolina

Eric L. Legome, MD
Assistant Professor
Director, NYU/Bellevue EM Residency
Department of Emergency Medicine
New York University School of Medicine
Emergency Department
Bellevue Hospital
New York, New York

William J. Levin, MD, FACEP
Associate Professor of Clinical Emergency
Director of Faculty Development
Department of Emergency Medicine
New York Medical College/Metropolitan
Hospital
Valhalla, New York

William J. Lewander, MD
Director of the Division of Pediatric
Emergency Medicine
Associate Professor
Department of Pediatrics
Brown Medical School
Providence, Rhode Island

Christopher A. Lewandowski, MD
Assistant Professor
Department of Internal Medicine
Case Western Reserve University
Cleveland, Ohio
Program Director
Department of Emergency Medicine
Henry Ford Hospital
Detroit, Michigan

Matthew R. Lewin, MD, PhD
Assistant Professor of Medicine
Department of Emergency Medicine
University of California, San Francisco
San Francisco, California

Ivan E. Liang, MD
Division of Medical Toxicology
Department of Emergency Medicine
University of Massachusetts Medical
School
Worcester, Massachusetts

Christopher H. Linden, MD
Professor
Division of Medical Toxicology
Department of Emergency Medicine
University of Massachusetts Medical
School
UMass Memorial Medical Center
Worcester, Massachusetts

Jeffrey F. Linzer, MD
Assistant Professor of Pediatrics and
Emergency Medicine
Emory University School of Medicine
Associate Medical Director for Compliance
Emergency Pediatric Group
Attending Physician
Children's Healthcare of Atlanta at
Egleston and Hughes Spalding
Children's Hospital
Atlanta, Georgia

Grant S. Lipman, MD
Wilderness Medical Fellow
Clinical Instructor
Division of Emergency Medicine
Stanford University School of Medicine
Palo Alto, California

Shahram Lotfipour, MD
Assistant Clinical Professor of Emergency
Medicine
Director of Undergraduate Medical
Education
Department of Emergency Medicine
University of California, Irvine
Irvine, California

Heather Long, MD
Attending Physician
North Shore University Hospital
Manhasset, New York

Bernard L. Lopez, MD
Associate Professor of Emergency Medicine
Vice Chair, Academic Affairs
Jefferson Medical College
Philadelphia, Pennsylvania

John W. Love, MD
Lieutenant Commander, Medical Corps,
US Navy
Attending Faculty, Residency Program
Department of Emergency Medicine
Naval Medical Center San Diego
San Diego, California

Douglas W. Lowery, MD
Vice Chair for Clinical Operations
Associate Professor of
Emergency Medicine
Emory University School of Medicine
Atlanta, Georgia

Robert C. Luten, MD
Professor
Department of Pediatrics and Emergency
Medicine
University of Florida
Jacksonville, Florida

Binh T. Ly, MD
Assistant Clinical Professor of Medicine
UCSD Division of Medical Toxicology
Department of Emergency Medicine
UCSD Medical Center
California Poison Control System, San
Diego Division
San Diego, California

Sharon E. Mace, MD
Associate Professor
Department of Emergency Medicine
Ohio State University School of Medicine
Director
Observation Unit and
Director
Pediatric Education/QI-Cleveland Clinic
Foundation
Faculty
Metro Health Medical Center
Emergency Medicine Residency
Cleveland, Ohio

Jayne MacLaughlin, MD
   Chief Resident
   Department of Emergency Medicine
   Carolinas Medical Center
   Charlotte, North Carolina

Swaminatha V. Mahadevan, MD
   Assistant Professor
   Department of Surgery
   Stanford University School of
      Medicine
   Associate Chief and Medical
      Director
   Division of Emergency Medicine
   Stanford University Medical Center
   Palo Alto, California

Brian D. Mahoney, MD, FACEP
   Clinical Associate Professor
   Department of Emergency
      Medicine
   University of Minnesota
   Medical Director
   Emergency Medical Services
   Hennepin County Medical Center
   Minneapolis, Minnesota

Kelli A. Maiers, MD
   Fellow
   Division of Pediatric Emergency
      Medicine
   Children's Hospital of The King's
      Daughters
   Clinical Instructor of Pediatrics
   Eastern Virginia Medical School
   Norfolk, Virginia

Beth H. Manning, PharmD
   Assistant Clinical Professor of Pharmacy
   University of California, San Francisco
   Toxicology Management Specialist
   California Poison Control System, San
      Francisco Division
   San Francisco, California

Anthony S. Manoguerra, PharmD
   Professor of Clinical Pharmacy
   University of California, San Diego
   School of Pharmacy and Pharmaceutical
      Sciences
   Clinical Professor of Pediatrics and
      Pharmacology
   University of California, San Diego School
      of Medicine
   San Diego, California

Catherine A. Marco, MD
   Clinical Professor
   Department of Suregry
   Medical College of Ohio
   Attending Physician
   Depatrment of Emergency
      Medicine
   St. Vincent Mercy Medical Center
   Toledo, Ohio

Steven M. Marcus, MD
   Professor of Preventive Medicine and
      Community Health
   Associate Professor of Pediatrics
   New Jersey Medical School of the
      University of Medicine of New Jersey
   Executive Director
   New Jersey Poison Information and
      Education System
   Newark, New Jersey

Vincent J. Markovchick, MD
   Professor
   Department of Surgery
   Division of Emergency Medicine
   University of Colorado
   Director
   Emergency Medical Services
   Denver Health Medical Center
   Denver, Colorado

Kathy Marquardt, PharmD
   California Poison Control System,
      Sacramento Division
   University of California, San Francisco
      School of Pharmacy
   Division of Pulmonary and Critical Care
      Medicine
   University of California, Davis School of
      Medicine
   Sacramento, California

Michelle Marsala, MD
   Department of Emergency Medicine
   University of Missouri-Kansas City School
      of Medicine
   Truman Medical Center
   Kansas City, Missouri

Marcus L. Martin, MD
   Professor and Chairman
   Department of Emergency Medicine
   University of Virginia
   Charlottesville, Virginia

Thomas P. Martin, MD
   Clinical Assistant Professor
   Department of Emergency Medicine
   University of Pittsburgh School of Medicine
   Attending Physician
   Department of Emergency Medicine
   Western Pennsylvania Hospital
   Pittsburgh, Pennsylvania

Jorge A. Martinez, MD, JD
   Clinical Professor of Medicine, Pediatrics,
      and Public Health
   Louisiana State University Health Science
      Center
   Director
   Emergency Medical Services
   Medical Center of Louisiana
   Co-Director
   Louisiana State University Combined
      Internal Medicine/Emergency Medicine
      Residency Program
   Adjunct Professor of Law
   Louisiana State University School of Law
   Metairie, Louisiana

John A. Marx, MD
   Chair and Chief
   Department of Emergency Medicine
   Carolinas Medical Center
   Charlotte, North Carolina

Michael J. Matteucci, MD
   Research Coordinator
   Emergency Medicine Residency
   Naval Medical Center
   Portsmouth, Virginia

Thom A. Mayer, MD
   Professor of Emergency Medicine and
      Pediatrics
   Georgetown University and The George
      Washington University School of
      Medicine
   Washington, DC

Kathryn McCans, MD
   Assistant Professor of Emergency Medicine
      and Pediatrics
   Department of Pediatric Emergency
      Medicine
   UMD NJ–Robert Wood Johnson Medical
      School
   Attending
   Cooper University Hospital Cam Den, New
      Jersey

Ian McCaslin, MD
   Clinical Associate Professor
   Department of Pediatrics
   University of California San Diego School
      of Medicine
   Chief Pediatric Emergency Medicine
   Children's Hospital and Health Center
   San Diego, California

Maureen D. McCollough, MD, MPH
   Assistant Professor of Medicine
   University of California, Los Angeles
      School of Medicine;
   Director of Pediatric Emergency Medicine
   OliveView-University of California, Los
      Angeles Medical Center
   Los Angeles, California

Lynne McCullough, MD
   Assistant Professor of Medicine
   Division of Emergency Medicine
   University of California, Los Angeles
   David Geffen School of Medicine at UCLA
   Associate Program Director
   UCLA/Olive View–UCLA Medical Center
   Emergency Medicine Residency Program
   Los Angeles, California

Robin B. McFee, MD
   Department of Preventive Medicine
   SUNY-Stony Brook, University Medical
      Center
   Stony Brook, New York
   The Long Island Regional Poison Control
      Center at Winthrop
   University Hospital
   Mineola, New York

Douglas L. McGee, MD
Assistant Professor
Thomas Jefferson University
Program Director
Emergency Medicine Residency
Albert Einstein Medical Center
Philadelphia, Pennsylvania

Erin McNutt, MD
Clinical Instructor
Department of Medicine
University of California, San Francisco
School of Medicine
Emergency Services
San Francisco General Hospital
San Francisco, California

Moss H. Mendelson, MD, FACEP
Associate Professor
Emergency Medicine Department
Eastern Virginia Medical School
Norfolk, Virginia

Carrie D. Mendoza, MD
Resident
Denver Health Residency in
Emergency Medicine
Denver Health Medical Center
Denver, Colorado

Marc Mickiewicz, MD
Clinical Instructor
Department of Emergency Medicine
Vanderbilt University Medical
Center
Nashville, Tennessee

Leslie Mihalov, MD
Assistant Professor of Clinical
Pediatrics
Department of Pediatrics
The Ohio State University
Chief
Section of Emergency Medicine
Children's Hospital
Department of Pediatrics
Medical Director
Division of Emergency Medicine
Department of Emergency Medicine
The Ohio State University
Columbus, Ohio

Scott A. Miller, MD
Clinical Instructor
Emergency Medicine
Rush University Medical Center
Chicago, Illinois
Senior Director, Epidemiology
Wyeth Research
Collegeville, Pennsylvania

Stephan J. Miller, MD
Instructor
Department of Emergency Medicine
Mayo Clinic College of Medicine
Rochester, Minnesota

Steve Miller, MD
Instructor of Emergency Medicine
Mayo Clinic College of Medicine
Mayo Clinic–Saint Mary's Hospital
Rochester, Minnesota

Daniel Mines, MD
Adjunct Assistant Professor of Medicine
University of Pennsylvania School of
Medicine
Philadelphia, Pennsylvania

Howard C. Mofenson, MD
Professor of Emergency Medicine and
Pediatrics Director
Departments of Pediatrics and Emergency
Medicine
Long Island Regional Poison Control
Center Winthrop University Hospital
Long Island, New York

Mary E. Moffatt, MD
Olathe Health System, Inc.
Kansas City, Missouri

Kathy W. Monroe, MD
Associate Professor
Department of Pediatrics
University of Alabama
Birmingham, Alabama

Gregory J. Moran, MD
Professor of Clinical Medicine
UCLA School of Medicine
Department of Emergency Medicine and
Division of Infectious Diseases
Olive View–UCLA Medical Center,
Sylmar, California

Lawrence Mottley, MD, MHSA
Assistant Professor
Harvard Medical School
Vice Chairman
Department of Emergency Medicine
Beth Israel Deaconess Medical Center
Boston, Massachusetts

William R. Mower, MD, PhD
Associate Professor
Department of Medicine/Emergency
Medicine
University of California, Los Angeles
Associate Professor and Attending
Physician
Department of Medicine/Emergency
Medicine
UCLA Center for the Health Sciences
Los Angeles, California

Walter H. Mullen, PharmD, CSPI
Assistant Clinical Professor
University of California, San Francisco
School of Pharmacy
Toxicology Management Specialist
California Poison Control System, San
Francisco Division
San Francisco General Hospital
San Francisco, California

Michael F. Murphy, MD, FRCPC
Clinical Assistant Professor of Emergency
Medicine
University of North Carolina at Chapel Hill
Denver, North Carolina
Clinical Chief Anesthesiology
Lincoln Medical Center
Lincolnton, North Carolina
Staff Emergency Physician
Carolinas Medical Center
Charlotte, North Carolina

Patricia M. Murphy, MD, CCFP, EM
Fellow in Clinical Toxicology
Indiana University School of Medicine
Indianapolis, Indiana

Lewis S. Nelson, MD
Assistant Professor
Department of Emergency Medicine
Fellowship and Associate Director
New York City Poison Control Center
New York University School of
Medicine/Bellevue Hospital Center
New York, New York

Kenneth Neuburger, MD
Clinical Assistant Professor of Emergency
Medicine
Director of Travel Medicine
Department of Emergency Medicine
Thomas Jefferson University
Philadelphia, Pennsylvania

Ann P. Nguyen, MD
Assistant Professor
Department of Emergency Medicine New
York University School of Medicine
Attending Physician
Department of Emergency Medicine
Bellevue Hospital Center and New York
University Medical Center
New York, New York

Constance G. Nichols, MD
Assistant Professor of Emergency
Medicine
Department of Emergency Medicine
University of Massachusetts Medical
School
Worcester, Massachusetts

James T. Niemann, MD
Professor of Medicine,
David Geffen School of Medicine at UCLA
Torrance, California

Flavia Nobay, MD
Assistant Clinical Professor of Medicine
Division of Emergency Medicine
University of California, San Francisco
San Francisco, California
Attending Physician
Department of Emergency Medicine
Highland Hospital–Alameda County
Medical Center
Oakland, Californa

Valerie C. Norton, MD
  Assistant Clinical Professor of Medicine
  Division of Emergency Medicine
  University of California, San Diego
  Director of Quality Improvement
  Department of Emergency Medical Services
  Scripps Mercy Hospital
  San Diego, California

Joanne L. Oakes, MD
  Assistant Professor of Emergency Medicine
  Assistant Residency Program Director
  Department of Emergency Medicine
  University of Texas Health Science Center
    at Houston
  Houston, Texas

Yasuharu Okuda, MD
  Clinical Instructor and Assistant Residency
    Site Director
  Department of Emergency Medicine
  Mount Sinai Medical Center
  New York, New York

Jonathan S. Olshaker, MD, FAAEM,
FACEP
  Chief, Emergency Department
  Boston Medical Center
  Professor and Chairman
  Department of Emergency Medicine
  Boston University School of Medicine
  Boston, Massachusetts

Kent R. Olson, MD
  Medical Director
  San Francisco Division
  California Poison Control System
  San Francisco, California

Jennifer A. Oman, MD
  Assistant Clinical Professor of Emergency
    Medicine
  Program Director
  University of California, Irvine
  Irvine, California

Joseph P. Ornato, MD
  Professor and Chairman
  Department of Emergency Medicine
  Virginia Commonwealth University
    Medical Center
  Richmond, Virginia

David T. Overton, MD
  Emergency Medicine Program Director
  Michigan State University Kalamazoo
    Center for Medical Studies
  Professor and Chairman of Emergency
    Medicine
  Michigan State University College of
    Human Medicine
  Kalamazoo, Michigan

S. Margaret Paik, MD
  Section of Pediatric Emergency Medicine
  The University of Chicago
  Chicago, Illinois

Lisa R. Palivos, MD
  Assistant Professor
  Department of Emergency Medicine
  Rush Medical College
  John H. Stroger Jr. Hospital of Cook County
  Chicago, Illinois

Robert Palmer, MD
  Woodland Heights Medical Center
  Memorial Hospital
  Lufkin, Texas

Edward A. Panacek, MD, MPH
  Professor of Medicine in Emergency
    Medicine
  University of California, Davis School of
    Medicine
  Sacramento, California

Sharad Pandit, MD, FACEP, UD (Hon.)
  Diplomate American Board of Emergency
    Medicine, FACEM
  Consultant, Emergency Medicine
  Royal Adelaide Hospital
  Adelaide, Australia

Paul M. Paris, MD, FACEP, UD (Hon.)
  Professor and Chair
  Department of Emergency Medicine
  University of Pittsburgh, School of
    Medicine
  Pittsburgh, Pennsylvania

Steven J. Parrillo, DO
  Assistant Professor of Emergency Medicine
  Philadephia College of Osteopathic
    Medicine
  Assistant Professor of Emergency Medicine
  Thomas Jefferson University
  Attending Physician and Residing Faculty
  Albert Einstein Medical Center
  Philadelphia, Pennsylvania

Andrew D. Perron, MD, FACEP
  Residency Program Director
  Department of Emergency Medicine
  Maine Medical Center
  Portland, Maine

Jeanmarie Perrone, MD, FACMT
  Associate Professor
  Department of Emergency Medicine
  University of Pennsylvania
  Attending Physician
  Department of Emergency Medicine
  Hospital of the University of Pennsylvania
  Philadelphia, Pennsylvania

Shawna J. Perry, MD
  Assistant Professor and Assistant Chair
  Director of Clinical Operations Emergency
    Medicine Department
  University of Florida Health Science
    Center/Shands Jacksonville
  Case Western Reserve University School of
    Medicine
  Jacksonville, Florida

Anne L Peters, MD
  Director of the Clinical Diabetes Programs
  Professor of Medicine
  University of Southern California, Keck
    School of Medicine
  Los Angeles, California

Howard A. Peth, Jr., MD, JD
  Assistant Clinical Professor
  Department of Emergency Medicine
  University of Missouri School of Medicine
  Columbia, Missouri

Erin Doherty Phrampus, MD
  Fellow
  Pediatric Emergency Medicine
  University of Pittsburgh School of Medicine
  Pittsburgh, Pennsylvania

Paul E. Phrampus, MD, FACEP
  Assistant Professor of Emergency Medicine
  Assistant Director of Emergency Medical
    Programs
  Peter M. Winter Institute for Simulation,
    Education and Research
  University of Pittsburgh
  Pittsburgh, Pennsylvania

Paul A. Pitel, MD
  Department Chair
  Department of Pediatrics
  Division of Hematology/Oncology
  Nemours Children's Clinic-Jacksonville
  Jacksonville, Florida

Rick C. Place, MD
  Department of Emergency Medicine
  Inova Fairfax Hospital
  Falls Church, Virginia

Stephen J. Playe, MD, FACEP
  Assistant Professor, Emergency Medicine
  Tufts University School of Medicine
  Residency Program Director
  Department of Emergency Medicine
  Baystate Medical Center
  Springfield, Massachusetts

Peter T. Pons, MD
  Department of Emergency Medicine
  Denver Health Medical Center
  Professor of Emergency Medicine
  Division of Emergency Medicine
    Department of Surgery
  University of Colorado Health Science
    Center
  Denver, Colorado

Robert S. Porter, MD, FACEP
  Clinical Assistant Professor
  Department of Emergency Medicine
  Thomas Jefferson University
  Philadelphia, Pennsylvania

Louis G. Poulos, MD*

*Deceased

Susan B. Promes, MD
Associate Clinical Professor
Residency Program Director
Division of Emergency Medicine
Duke University
Durham, North Carolina

Kimberly S. Quayle, MD
Division of Pediatric Emergency Medicine
St. Louis Children's Place
St. Louis, Missouri

Bruce Quinn, MD
Clinical Assistant Professor
Department of Medicine
University of Miami School of Medicine
Attending Physician
Pediatric Emergency Department
Jackson Memorial Hospital
Miami, Florida

Cyrus Rangan, MD
Director, Toxics Epidemiology Unit
Los Angeles Department of Health Services
Assistant Medical Director and Director of
    Los Angeles Medical Toxicology
    Education, California Poison Control
    System
Attending Staff, Children's Hospital Los
    Angeles
Toxics Epidemiology Unit
Health Assessment and Epidemiology
Los Angeles, California

Mobeen H. Rathore, MD
Professor and Assistant Chairman
Department of Pediatrics
Chief
Pediatric Infectious Diseases and
    Immunology
University of Florida Health Science
    Center
Jacksonville, Florida

Eileen M. Raynor, MD
Assistant Professor of Otolaryngology
Shands Jacksonville
Jacksonville, Florida

Eric F. Reichman, MD, PhD
Assistant Professor of Emergency
    Medicine
Residency Program Director
Department of Emergency Medicine
University of Texas at Houston
Houston, Texas

Marc C. Restuccia, MD
Assistant Professor of Emergency Medicine
Medical Director
LifeFlight and Emergency Medical
    Services
UMass Memorial Department of
    Emergency Medicine
Worcester, Massachusetts

David Richardson, MD
Clinical Assistant Professor
Department of Medicine
The Pennsylvania State University College
    of Medicine
Hershey, Pennsylvania
Emergency Department Director
Lehigh Valley Hospital–Muhlenberg
Lehigh Valley Hospital and Health
    Network
Allentown, Pennsylvania

Renee L. Riggs, DO
Emergency Medicine
Robert Wood Johnson Medical School
    Cooper University Hospital
Camden, New Jersey

Emanuel P. Rivers, MD
Director of Research
Department of Emergency Medicine
Henry Ford Health Systems
Detroit, Michigan
Associate Professor of Emergency Medicine
    and Surgery
Case Western Reserve University
Cleveland, Ohio

James R. Roberts, MD, FAAEM, FACEP,
FACMT
Vice Chair, Department of Emergency
    Medicine
Director, Division of Toxicology
Drexel University College of Medicine
Chair, Department of Emergency Medicine
Director, Division of Toxicology
Mercy Catholic Medical Center
Philadelphia, Pennsylvania

Rebecca R. Roberts, MD
Director of Research Division
Department of Emergency Medicine
Cook County Hospital
Chicago, Illinois

Luis E. Rodriguez, MD
Assistant Clinical Professor
East Carolina University
Greenville, North Carolina
Director of Emergency Medicine
Roanoke Chowan Hospital
Ahoskie, North Carolina

Robert M. Rodriguez, MD
Clinical Associate Professor of
    Medicine–UCSF
Department of Emergency Medicine
Alameda County Medical Center
Oakland, California

S. Rutherfoord Rose, PharmD
Clinical Toxicologist and Director
Virginia Poison Center;
Associate Professor of Medicine and
    Pharmacy
Department of Clinical Toxicology
School of Virginia Commonwealth
    University Pharmacy
Richmond, Virginia

Carlo L. Rosen, MD
Assistant Professor of Medicine
Harvard Medical School
Program Director
Beth Israel Deaconess Medical Center
Harvard Affiliated Emergency Medicine
    Residency
Boston, Massachusetts

Peter Rosen, MD
Senior Lecturer in Medicine
Division of Emergency Medicine
Harvard Medical School
Attending Physician
Beth Israel Deaconess Medical Center
Teaching Attending
Massachusetts General Hospital
Attending Physician
St. John's Hospital Jackson Hole Wyoming
Visiting Professor
Emergency Medicine
University of Arizona School of Medicine
Beth Israel Deaconess Medical Center
Director of Education, Emergency Medicine
Boston, Massachusetts

Tina Rosenbaum, MD
Department of Emergency Medicine
George Washington Unversity
Washington, DC

Steven Rosenzweig, MD
Director, Jefferson Center for Integrative
    Medicine
Thomas Jefferson University and Hospital
Philadelphia, Pennsylvania

Christopher Ross, MD
Assistant Professor
Department of Emergency Medicine
Rush University
Assistant Program Director
Department of Emergency Medicine
John H. Stroger Jr. Hospital of Cook County
Chicago, Illinois

Todd C. Rothenhaus, MD, FACEP
Assistant Professor of Emergency Medicine
Assistant Residency Program Director
Director of Medical Informatics
Boston University Medical Center
Boston, Massachusetts

Richard Rothman, MD
Assistant Professor
Director, Research Fellowship
Director, Residency Research
Department of Emergency Medicine
John Hopkins Medical Center
Baltimore, Maryland

Scott E. Rudkin, MD, MBA
Assistant Clinical Professor of Emergency
    Medicine
Director of Medical Informations
Assistant Program Director
University of California, Irvine
Irvine, California

Douglas A. Rund, MD
  Professor and Chair
  Department of Emergency Medicine
  Associate Dean College of Medicine and
    Public Health
  The Ohio State University
  Columbus, Ohio

Richard J. Ryan, MD
  Assistant Professor
  Department of Emergency Medicine
  University of Cincinnati
  Medical Director
  Department of Emergency Medicine
  The Jewish Hospital
  Vice President, Clinical Operations
    Vanguard Medical, Inc.

Alfred Sacchetti, MD
  Chief Emergency Services
  Our Lady of Lourdes Medical Center
  Camden, New Jersey
  Assistant Clinical Professor of Emergency
    Medicine
  Thomas Jefferson University
  Philadelphia, Pennsylvania

Annie T. Sadosty, MD
  Assistant Professor
  Department of Emergency Medicine
  Mayo Clinic College of Medicine
  Program Director
  Mayo Emergency Medicine Residency
  Rochester, Minnesota

Philip N. Salen, MD
  Clinical Assistant Professor
  Department of Emergency Medicine
  Temple University School of Medicine
  Attending, Emergency Residency
  St. Luke's Hospital

Leon D. Sanchez, MD, MPH
  Department of Emergency Medicine
  Beth Israel Deaconess Medical Center
  Boston, Massachusetts

Robert E. Sapien, MD
  Department of Emergency Medicine
  University of New Mexico
  Albuquerque, New Mexico

Radu V. Saveanu, MD
  Professor and Chairman
  Department of Psychiatry
  Columbus, Ohio

Eric A. Savitsky, MD
  Associate Professor
  Department of Emergency Medicine
  UCLA Emergency Medicine Residency
    Program
  UCLA Medical Center
  Los Angeles, California

David Schaeffer, MD
  Division Chief
  Nemours Children's Clinic–Jacksonville
  Division of Pulmonology/Allergy and
    Immunology
  Department of Pediatrics
  Jacksonville, Florida

Jeffrey Schaider, MD
  Associate Chairman
  Department of Emergency Medicine
  Cook County Hospital
  Associate Professor
  Rush Medical College
  Chicago, Illinois

Neil Schamban, MD
  Director, Department of Emergency
    Medicine
  Newark Beth Israel Medical Center
  Newark, New Jersey

Jay L. Schauben, PharmD, DABAT, FAACT
  Clinical Professor
  Department of Emergency Medicine
  University of Florida Health Science Center
  Director
  Florida Poison Information Center
  Shands Jacksonville
  Jacksonville, Florida

Frederick M. Schiavone, MD, FACEP
  Associate Professor
  Department of Emergency Medicine
  University Medical Center School of
    Medicine
  Stony Brook, New York

Joshua G. Schier, MD
  Assistant Professor of Emergency Medicine
  Emory University School of Medicine
  Consultant
  Georgia Poison Center
  Atlanta, Georgia

Eric W. Schmidt, MD
  Assistant Professor of Emergency Medicine
  Department of Emergency Medicine
  University of Massachusetts Medical
    School
  Worcester, Massachusetts

Joseph Schmidt, MD
  Associate Residency Director
  Baystate Medical Center Emergency
    Medicine Residency
  Assistant Professor of Emergency Medicine
  Tufts University School of Medicine
  Boston, Massachusetts

Robert E. Schneider, MD
  Clinical Associate Professor
  Department of Emergency Medicine
  University of North Carolina at Chapel Hill
  Chapel Hill, North Carolina
  Faculty
  Department of Urology
  Carolinas Medical Center
  Charlotte, North Carolina

Robert A. Schwab, MD
  Professor and Chair
  Department of Emergency Medicine
  UMKC School of Medicine
  Kansas City, Missouri

Theresa M. Schwab, MD
  Attending
  Advocate Christ Medical Center
  Oak Lawn, Illinois

Phillip A. Scott, MD
  Assistant Professor
  Department of Emergency Medicine
  University of Michigan
  Ann Arbor, Michigan

David C. Seaberg, MD
  Department of Emergency Medicine
  University of Florida
  Gainesville, Florida

Charles M. Seamens, MD
  Assistant Professor
  Department of Emergency Medicine
  Vanderbilt University Medical Center
  Nashville, Tennessee

Timothy Seay, MS, MD
  Regional Medical Director
  Department of Emergency Medicine
  Greater Houston Emergency Medicine
  Houston, Texas

Steven M. Selbst, MD
  Professor of Pediatrics
  Vice-Chair for Education
  Pediatric Residency Program Director
  Jefferson Medical College
  Thomas Jefferson University
  Philadelphia, Pennsylvania
  Attending Physician
  Division of Emergency Medicine
  Alfred I. duPont Hospital for Children
  Wilmington, Delware

Clare T. Sercombe, MD, FACEP
  Staff Emergency Physician
  North Memorial Medical Center
  Robbinsdale, Minnesota

Harry W. Severance, MD, FACEP
  Asssistant Research Director
  Division of Emergency Medicine
  University of South Florida
  Attending Physician
  Department of Emergency Medicine
  Tampa General Hospital
  Tampa, Florida

Kaushal Shah, MD
  Physician Attending
  St. Luke's–Roosevelt Hospital
  Department of Emergency Medicine
  New York, New York

Nathan I. Shapiro, MD, MPH
Research Director
Department of Emergency Medicine
Beth Israel Deaconess Medical Center
Instructor of Medicine
Harvard Medical School
Boston, Massachusetts

Ghazala Q. Sharieff, MD, FACEP, FAAEM, FAAP
Associate Clinical Professor
Children's Hospital and Health Center
University of San Diego, California
Director of Pediatric Emergency Medicine
Palomar-Pomerado Hospitals
California Emergency Physicians
San Diego, California

Adhi N. Sharma, MD
Assistant Professor
Department of Emergency Medicine
Mount Sinai School of Medicine
New York, New York
Director
Division of Toxicology
Department of Emergency Medicine
Elmhurst Hospital Center
Elmhurst, New York

Kathy Shaw, MD
Professor of Pediatrics
University of Pennsylvania School of Medicine
Chief
Division of Emergency Medicine
The Children's Hospital of Philadelphia
Philadelphia, Pennsylvania

Philip Shayne, MD
Associate Professor
Residency Program Director
Department of Emergency Medicine
Emory University School of Medicine
Atlanta, Georgia

Peter Shearer, MD
Assistant Professor
Emergency Medicine
Mount Sinai School of Medicine
Mount Sinai Hospital
New York, New York
Elmhurst Hospital Center
Elmhurst, New York

Suzanne Moore Shepherd, MD
Department of Emergency Medicine
University of Pennsylvania Health System
Philadelphia, Pennsylvania

Scott C. Sherman, MD
Assistant Professor of Emergency Medicine
Rush Medical College
Assistant Program Director
Cook County Emergency Medicine
Residency
Chicago, Illinois

Robert Shesser, MD, MPH
Professor and Chair
Department of Emergency Medicine
The George Washington University
Chair
Department of Emergency Medicine
The George Washington University
Hospital
Washington, DC

Richard D. Shih, MD
Program Director
Department of Emergency Medicine
Morristown Memorial Hospital
Morristown, New Jersey
Associate Professor of Surgery
UMONJ–New Jersey Medical School
Newark, New Jersey

Lee W. Shockley, MD
Associate Professor
The University of Colorado Health Sciences
Center
Residency Program Director
Denver Health Medical Center Residency
in Emergency Medicine
Denver, Colorado

Jan Marie Shoenberger, MD
Assistant Professor of Clinical Emergency
Medicine
Keck School of Medicine of the University
of Southern California
Assistant Director of Residency
Los Angeles County and University of
Southern California
Los Angeles, California

John A. Siefert, MD, Captain
Medical Corps, USN
Fellow, American College of Emergency
Physicians
Department of Emergency Medicine
Naval Medical Center of San Diego
San Diego, California

Robert Sigillito, MD
Assistant Professor of Clinical Medicine
Section of Emergency Medicine
Charity Hospital
New Orleans, Louisiana

Harold K. Simon, MD
Assistant Professor
Department of Pediatrics
Emory University School of Medicine
Atlanta, Georgia

Robert R. Simon, MD, FAAEM
Professor and Chairman
Department of Emergency Medicine
Cook County Hospital
Rush Medical College
Chicago, Illinois

Adam J Singer, MD
Professor and Vice Chairman for Research
Department of Emergency Medicine
Stony Brook University Hospital
Stony Brook, New York

Jonathan I. Singer, MD
Professor of Emergency Medicine and
Pediatrics
Vice-Chair and Associate Program
Director
Department of Emergency Medicine
Wright State University School of
Medicine
Dayton, Ohio

Marco L.A. Sivilotti, MD, MSc, FRCPC, FACEP, FACMT
Assistant Professor
Departments of Emergency Medicine and
of Pharmacology and Toxicology
Queens University
Kingston, Ontario
Consultant
Ontario Regional Poison Control
Information Centre
The Hospital for Sick Children
Toronto, Ontario
Canada

Corey M. Slovis, MD, FACP, FACEP
Professor of Emergency Medicine and
Medicine
Chairman, Department of Emergency
Medicine
Vanderbilt University Medical Center
Nashville, Tennessee

Mark Smith, MD
Chair
Department of Emergency Medicine
Washington Hospital Center
Chair and Professor of Emergency
Medicine
Georgetown University School of
Medicine
Washington, DC

Matthew P. Smith, MD
Clinical Instructor of Medicine
University of California, San Francisco
School of Medicine
Attending Physician
Department of Emergency Medicine
San Francisco General Hospital
San Franscico, California

Eric Snoey, MD
Program Director
Department of Emergency Medicine
Highland Hospital–Alameda County
Medical Center
Associate Clinical Professor
University of California, San Francisco
Medical Center
Oakland, California

Brian K. Snyder, MD
Assistant Clinical Professor of Medicine
Department of Emergency Medicine
Hyperbaric Medicine Center
University of California, San Diego
San Diego, California

Peter E. Sokolove, MD, FACEP
Associate Professor
Department of Emergency Medicine
University of California–Davis School of
Medicine
Davis, California
Vice Chair of Education
Residency Program Director
Department of Emergency Medicine
University of California–Davis Medical
Center
Sacramento, California

Annalise Sorrentino, MD
Assistant Professor
Department of Pediatrics
Division of Emergency Medicine
University of Alabama
Birmingham, Alabama

Mark Spektor, D.O.
Director, Emergency Services
VA—NYHHCS
Assistant Professor
Department of Emergency Medicine
SUNY–Downstate
Brooklyn, New York

Mark T. Steele, MD
Professor
Associate Dean
Chief Medical Officer
Truman Medical Center
University of Missouri-Kansas City, School
of Medicine
Kansas City, Missouri

Mardi Steere, MBBS
Pediatric Emergency Medicine Fellow
Department of Emergency Medicine
University of Florida Health Science Center
Jacksonville, Florida

C. Keith Stone, MD
Professor and Chairman
Department of Emergency Medicine
Texas A&M University System Health
Science Center
Scott & White Memorial Hospital
Temple, Texas

Mark Su, MD
Assistant Professor and
Director of Medical Toxicology
Department of Emergency Medicine
SUNY–Downstate Medical Center/Kings
County Hospital Center
Brooklyn, New York

Jeffrey R. Suchard, MD
Associate Clinical Professor of Emergency
Medicine
Director of Medical Toxicology
Department of Emergency Medicine
University of California Irvine Medical
Center
Orange, California

John B. Sullivan, Jr., MD
Associate Dean for Clinical Affairs
Associate Professor of Emergency Medicine
University of Arizona Health Sciences
Center
Tucson, Arizona

Matthew D. Sztajnkrycer, MD, PhD
Assistant Professor
Department of Emergency Medicine
Mayo Clinic College of Medicine
Rochester, Minnesota

Jeffrey A. Tabas, MD
Assistant Professor
San Francisco General Hospital
Emergency Services
University of California, San Francisco
School of Medicine
San Francisco, California

David A. Talan, MD, FACEP, FIDSA
Professor of Medicine
UCLA School of Medicine
Chairman, Department of Emergency
Medicine
Faculty, Division of Infectious Diseases
Olive View–UCLA Medical Center
Sylmar, California

David A. Tanen, MD
Assistant Program Director
Research Director
Emergency Medicine Residency
Naval Medical Center
San Diego, California

Milton Tenenbein, MD
Professor of Pediatrics, Pharmacology,
Medicine and Community Health
Sciences;
Director, Emergency Services
Children's Hospital, Winnipeg
Director, Manitoba Poison Control Center
Children's Hospital
Winnipeg, Manitoba
Canada

Harold A. Thomas, Jr. MD
Professor
Department of Emergency Medicine
Oregon Health Sciences University
Portland, Oregon

Stephen H. Thomas, MD, MPH
Associate in Emergency Services
Massachusetts General Hospital
Assistant Professor of Surgery
Harvard Medical School
Boston, Massachusetts

Carrie D. Tibbles, MD
Associate Program Director
Beth Israel Deaconess Medical Center
Harvard Affiliated Emergency Medicine
Residency
Boston, Massachusetts

Michael K. Tibbles, MD
Department of Emergency Medicine
Boston Medical Center
Boston, Massachusetts

Tri C. Tong, MD
Assistant Clinical Professor of Medicine
UCSD Division of Medical Toxicology
Department of Emergency Medicine
UCSD Medical Center
California Poison Control System, San
Diego Division
San Diego, California

Susan P. Torrey, MD
Assistant Professor of Emergency Medicine
Tufts University School of Medicine
Boston, Massachusetts

Alexander T. Trott, MD
Professor
Director, Alliance Clinical Effectiveness
University Hospital Associate Chief of Staff
University Hospital Attending
Department of Emergency Medicine
Cincinnati, Ohio

Stephen Trzeciak, MD
Assistant Professor
Department of Emergency Medicine
and the Section of Critical Care Medicine
UMDNJ-Robert Wood Johnson Medical
School
Cooper University Hospital
Camden, New Jersey

Michael A. Turturro, MD, MPH
Clinical Associate Professor of Emergency
Medicine
University of Pittsburgh School of Medicine
Vice Chair and Director of Academic
Affairs
Department of Emergency Medicine
The Mercy Hospital of Pittsburgh
Pittsburgh, Pennsylvania

Edward Ullman, MD
Attending Physician
Beth Israel Deaconess Medical Center
Department of Emergency Medicine
Boston, Massachusetts

Federico E. Vaca, MD, MPH
Associate Professor of Clinical Emergency
Medicine
Director, Center for Trauma and Injury
Prevention Research
Department of Emergency Medicine
University of California, Irvine
Irvine, California

Phyllis A. Vallee, MD
Associate Program Director
Department of Emergency Medicine
Henry Ford Hospital
Detroit, Michigan
Assistant Professor
Department of Internal Medicine
Case Western Reserve University
Cleveland, Ohio

Paul B. Vanderbeek, MD
Department of Emergency Medicine
Albert Einstein Medical Center
Philadelphia, Pennsylvania

Larissa I. Velez, MD
The University of Texas Southwestern
Department of Surgery
Division of Emergency Medicine
Dallas, Texas

Gary M. Vilke, MD, FACEP, FAAEM
Associate Professor of Clinical Medicine
Department of Emergency Medicine
University of California, San Diego Medical
Center
Medical Director, San Diego County EMS
San Diego, California

John Vinen, MD
Director Emergency Support Services
RNSH
Sydney, Australia

Robert J. Vissers, MD
Residency Director
Assistant Professor
Department of Emergency Medicine
University of North Carolina at
Chapel Hill
Chapel Hill, North Carolina

Gregory A. Volturo, MD
Associate Professor and Vice Chairman
Department of Emergency Medicine
University of Massachusetts Medical
School
Worcester, Massachusetts

Scott R. Votey, MD
Professor of Medicine/Emergency
Medicine
Assistant Dean for Graduate Education
David Geffen School of Medicine at UCLA
UCLA Medical Center
Los Angeles, California

Richard Y. Wang, DO
Department of Emergency Medicine
Emory University School of Medicine
Atlanta, Georgia

Kevin R. Ward, MD
Associate Professor and Director of
Research
Department of Emergency Medicine
VCU Reanimation Engineering Shock
Center
Virginia Commonwealth University
Richmond, Virginia

Craig R. Warden, MD, MPH
Associate Professor
Emergency Medicine and Pediatrics
Chief
Pediatric Emergency Services
Oregon Health Science University
Doernbecher Children's Hospital
Portland, Oregon

Gary S. Wasserman, DO
Professor of Pediatrics
Department of Medicine
University of Missouri–Kansas City School
of Medicine
Chief
Section of Medical Toxicology
Children's Mercy Hospitals and Clinic
Kansas City, Missouri

William A. Watson, PharmD
Associate Director
Toxicosurveillance
American Association of Poison Control
Centers
Washington, DC

Paul M. Wax, MD
Department of Medical Toxicology
Phoenix, Arizona

Robert L. Wears, MD, MS
Professor
Department of Emergency Medicine
University of Florida
Staff Physician
Department of Emergency Medicine
Shands Jacksonville
Jacksonville, Florida

Joseph M. Weber, MD
Clinical Instructor
Department of Emergency Medicine
Rush Medical College
Cook County
Chicago Illinois

Lori Weichenthal, MD
Assistant Clinical Professor
University of California, San Francisco,
Fresno
Fresno, California

Larry D. Weiss, JD, MD
Albert J. Lauro Professor of Medicine
Clinical Professor of Law
Assistant Chief for Academic Affairs
Section of Emergency Medicine
Louisville State University
New Orleans, Louisiana

Howard A. Werman, MD
Professor of Clinical Emergency
Medicine
The Ohio State University
College of Medicine and Public Health
Medical Director
MedFlight of Ohio
Columbus, Ohio

J. M. Whitworth, MD
Professor
University of Florida School of Medicine
State Consultant to Child Protection
Teams
Jacksonville, Florida

Robert A. Wiebe, MD, FACEP, FAAP
The Sarah and Charles E. Seay
Distinguished Chair
Professor
Director Division of Pediatric Emergency
Medicine
University of Texas
Southwestern Medical Center
Director
Emergency Services
Children's Medical Center of Dallas
Dallas, Texas

Sage W. Wiener, MD
Senior Fellow
Medical Toxicology
New York City Poison Control Center
New York, New York

James A. Wilde, MD, FAAP
Associate Professor of Emergency Medicine
and Pediatrics
Section Chief, Pediatric Emergency
Medicine
Research Director, Department of
Emergency Medicine
Medical College of Georgia
Augusta, Georgia

Brandon Wills, DO, MS
Fellow of Clinical Toxicology and
Clinical Instructor
Department of Emergency Medicine
University of Illinois at Chicago
Chicago, Illinois

Lance D. Wilson, MD
Assistant Professor
Department of Emergency Medicine
Case Western Reserve
University–MetroHealth Medical Center
Cleveland, Ohio

Michael D. Witting, MD, MS
Assistant Professor
University of Maryland
Staff Physician
Merry Medical Center
Baltimore, Maryland

Stephen J. Wolf, MD
Assistant Professor
Department of Surgery
Division of Emergency Medicine
University of Colorado School of
Medicine
Staff Physician
Department of Emergency Medicine
Denver Health Medical Center
Denver, Colorado

Richard E. Wolfe, MD
  Associate Professor of Medicine
  Harvard Medical School
  Chief of Emergency Medicine
  Beth Israel Deaconess Medical Center
  Boston, Massachusetts

Allan B. Wolfson, MD
  Professor of Emergency Medicine
  Program Director, Affiliated Residency in
    Emergency Medicine
  University of Pittsburgh
  Pittsburgh, Pennsylvania

Deborah R. Wong, MD
  Physician, Emergency Department
  Mount Auburn Hospital
  Cambridge, Massachusetts

Alan D. Woolf, MD, MPH
  Associate Professor
  Harvard Medical School
  Director
  Program in Environmental Medicine
  Children's Hospital
  Boston, Massachusetts

Martha S. Wright, MD
  Associate Professor
  Department of Pediatrics
  Case Western Reserve University
  Division of Emergency Medicine
  Rainbow Babies and Children's Hospital
  Cleveland, Ohio

Daniel T. Wu, MD
  Assistant Professor
  Department of Emergency Medicine
  Emory University School of Medicine
  Atlanta, Georgia

Todd Wylie, MD
  Department of Emergency Medicine
  University of Florida
  Jacksonville, Florida

Loren G. Yamamoto, MD, MPH, MBA
  Professor of Pediatrics
  University of Hawaii
  John A. Burns School of Medicine
  Pediatric Emergency Medicine Director
  Kaprolani Medical Center for Women and
    Children
  Honolulu, Hawaii

Samuel Yang, MD
  Assistant Professor
  Department of Emergency Medicine
  Johns Hopkins University
  Baltimore, Maryland

Donald M. Yealy, MD
  Professor and Vice-Chair of Emergency
    Medicine
  University of Pittsburgh
  Pittsburgh, Pennsylvania

Robert D. Yniguez, MD
  Olathe Health System, Inc.
  Kansas City, Missouri

Robert Zalenski, MD
  Professor of Emergency Medicine and
    Internal Medicine
  Wayne State University School of Medicine
  Detroit Receiving Hospital
  John D. Dingell Veterans Hospital
  Detroit, Michigan

Elisa Alter Zenni, MD
  Associate Professor and Associate
    Residency Director
  Department of Pediatrics
  University of Florida Health Science Center
  Jacksonville, Florida

Noel S. Zuckerbraun, MD
  Fellow, Pediatric Emergency Medicine
  Division of Pediatric Emergency Medicine
  Children's Hospital of Pittsburgh
  Pittsburgh, Pennsylvania

David N. Zull, MD
  Associate Professor of Medicine
  Northwestern University Medical School
  Co-Director
  Emergency Medicine Department
    Observation Unit
  Northwestern Memorial Hospital
  Chicago, Illinois

CD-ROM CONTRIBUTORS

Daniel E. Brooks, MD
  Assistant Professor of Medical Toxicology
    and Emergency Medicine
  Director
  Medical Toxicology Service
  Co-Medical Director
  Pittsburgh Poison Center
  University of Pittsburgh Medical Center
  Pittsburgh, Pennsylvania

Michael D. Burg, MD
  Assistant Clinical Professor
  Department of Emergency Medicine
  University of California, San Francisco,
    Fresno University Medical Center
  Fresno, California

Hoori Hovanessian, MD
  Assistant Clinical Professor
  Departments of Medicine and Emergency
    Medicine
  University of San Francisco
  University Medical Center
  Fresno, California
  Staff Emergency Physician
  Presbyterian Intercommunity
    Hospital
  Whittier, California

Christopher Ross, MD
  Assistant Professor
  Department of Emergency Medicine
  Rush University
  Assistant Program Director
  Department of Emergency Medicine
  John H. Stroger Jr. Hospital of
    Cook County
  Chicago, Illinois

Scott C. Sherman, MD
  Assistant Professor of Emergency
    Medicine
  Rush Medical College
  Assistant Program Director
  Cook County Emergency Medicine
    Residency
  Chicago, Illinois

Carrie D. Tibbles, MD
  Associate Program Director
  Beth Israel Deaconess Medical Center
  Harvard Affiliated Emergency Medicine
    Residency
  Boston, Massachusetts

Stephen J. Traub, MD
  Instructor in Medicine
  Harvard Medical School
  Co-Director
  Division of Toxicology
  Department of Emergency Medicine
  Beth Israel Deaconess Medical
    Center
  Boston, Massachusetts

Vincent Wang, MD
  Assistant Professor of Clinical
    Pediatrics
  Keck School of Medicine of the University
    of Southern California
  Fellowship Director
  Division of Emergency Medicine
  Children's Hospital Los Angeles
  Los Angeles, California

Preface

Harwood-Nuss' Clinical Practice of Emergency Medicine is designed to be used both as a source of readily accessible information and as a concise yet comprehensive summary of current knowledge and practice in emergency medicine. The editors hope that it will assist clinicians in their daily practice and also serve as an educational resource for physicians in training and for those preparing for board examination.

One of the most useful features of the book is its uniform format, which in each chapter directs the reader to clear discussions of basic disease processes, clinical presentations, differential diagnosis, and the details of emergency evaluation, management, and disposition decisions. The Pitfalls section draws attention to common errors in the care of the emergency patient.

A new feature in this edition, Critical Interventions, further highlights the most important elements of care. The table of contents also has been reorganized into a more user-friendly format so that medical and surgical emergencies can be found within sections for each organ system.

The editors have made every effort to ensure that this fourth edition is clinically focused and evidenced-based, conveying both what is currently accepted and what is controversial or has yet to be investigated. With few exceptions, contributing authors are practicing emergency physicians who bring years of practical experience and academic expertise to their subjects. Their extraordinary efforts and commitment to excellence are deeply appreciated.

Finally, this book exists because of the prodigious efforts of Dr. Ann Harwood-Nuss, Editor-in-Chief of the first three editions. Her dedication and masterful stewardship continue to inspire us.

ALLAN B. WOLFSON, MD

Fourth Edition

Harwood-Nuss' Clinical Practice of Emergency Medicine

INTRODUCTION

The Approach to the Emergency Department Patient

Robert L. Wears

... in the physician or surgeon, no quality takes rank with imperturbability.... Imperturbability means coolness and presence of mind under all circumstances, calmness amid storm, clearness of judgment in moments of grave peril, immobility, impassiveness, or, to use an old and expressive word, *phlegm.* It is the quality which is most appreciated by the laity though often misunderstood by them; and the physician who has the misfortune to be without it, who betrays indecision and worry, and who shows that he is flustered and hurried in ordinary emergencies, loses rapidly the confidence of his patients.

—Sir William Osler, *Æquanimitas*

INTRODUCTION

It is one thing to practice medicine in an emergency department (ED); it is quite another to practice emergency medicine. The effective practice of emergency medicine requires an approach, a way of thinking that differs from other medical specialties.

Its physical limitation to the ED is perhaps the least important of emergency medicine's characteristics. Five factors have led emergency physicians to develop a unique approach to the patient: the pressure of time and volume, the variety of conditions faced, the paucity of information, the limitation of therapeutic options, and the constraint of disposition.

Time and Volume Pressure

More than any other specialty, emergency physicians experience clinical work as turbulent flow in a constricted channel. In a true emergency, seconds to minutes may make the difference between life and death or serious disability. In these situations, emergency physicians, contrary to much of their previous training, must be prepared to "treat first and ask questions later."

Also, the time available for an emergency physician to evaluate and think about any given patient is severely limited by the demands of other patients being managed concurrently. In most practices, during the busiest part of the day, an emergency physician has on average only 10 to 15 minutes per patient for evaluation, testing, treatment, disposition, and documentation. Whether this is adequate or not is immaterial; the reality is that no more time is available.

The combination of time and volume pressures forces emergency physicians to be much more aware of priorities among patients. Although trauma surgeons occasionally face triage conditions, emergency physicians are the only practitioners who routinely make (at least mental) triage decisions every day.

Variety of Conditions

As a specialty in breadth rather than depth, emergency physicians must manage a wider variety of conditions than any other specialists, save perhaps family practitioners. In addition, unlike other specialists, emergency physicians must shift domains rapidly. Practicing emergency medicine is like carefully lining up a putt, then dropping the putter, picking up a tennis racket to return a volley or two, quickly side-stepping an onrushing tackler, and then returning to sink the putt.

Paucity of Information

Emergency physicians frequently deal with episodes of real or perceived crises in patients of whose past course they are unaware. Old records are often unavailable and patients' memories are limited in scope and reliability. The information-gathering options available in the ED are similarly limited. Only a small subset of the vast diagnostic armamentarium is available to the emergency physician within a reasonable time.

Limited Therapeutic Options

Options for treatment are limited as well. Often, emergency physicians can provide only temporizing or symptomatic treatment, while definitive management must be deferred to another specialist. In addition, in emergency situations, the tolerance for therapeutic failures or misadventures is more limited than in nonemergencies.

Although one may not realize it when viewing the chaotic, turbulent activity of a busy ED, emergency medicine possesses a certain elegance enforced by these constraints. There is an attractive intellectual simplicity in meeting the challenge of providing timely, accurate care using primarily one's own hands and brain, supplemented by a few, limited laboratory and imaging tests.

Constraint of Disposition

Every patient interaction an emergency physician has must soon be ended. This forces emergency physicians to focus on the "bottom line." No matter how uncertain the diagnosis or how much extended observation or testing might help, every patient encounter in the ED ultimately reduces to three binary decisions: Is the patient sick or not sick? If sick, should I treat or not treat? Should I admit or discharge? These questions must be answered despite the lack of definitive information, the lack of time to collect or consider additional information, or the lack of availability of advice from colleagues and consultants.

A FRAMEWORK FOR APPROACHING THE EMERGENCY DEPARTMENT PATIENT

Because there are many sources outlining the mechanics of history taking and physical examination, this section does not discuss those areas in detail; instead, it concentrates on how they are different in emergency medicine.

The first question to be asked on initial approach to a patient in the ED is, "Do I need to resuscitate this patient?" Corollaries to this question are, "How great is the threat?" and "How soon must I act?" The first question is usually answered in the first few seconds at the bedside and is as often based on an overall *gestalt* of the chief complaint and patient's general appearance as on specific complaints or vital sign abnormalities.

In true emergencies, the usual sequence of history, physical examination, laboratory testing, and treatment is altered by the need to take rapid action. In the most extreme cases, the sequence becomes treatment, physical examination, laboratory testing, and history.

When action is urgently required, the emergency physician must commit to it unhesitatingly. This requires mental preparedness; there is no time to ponder the benefits and risks of the various options for managing acute upper airway obstruction. The thinking required must be invested ahead of time, and a plan of action internalized by the physician before the situation requiring it arises.

If action is to be effective, it often must be initiated before all the information bearing on the decision is available. This requires a "bias toward action" in the emergency physician's mind. While this is occasionally a source of criticism from other specialists who fail to understand emergency medicine, in the proper circumstances it can save lives. A simplistic example of bias toward action is putting a patient with chest pain on a cardiac monitor on arrival to the ED; clearly the diagnosis of heart disease has not yet been made, so it is not certain that the monitor is truly "needed," but we anticipate a potential need and act without waiting for confirmation. A more dramatic example is sudden upper airway obstruction, where the decision to perform a cricothyroidotomy must be made promptly; to wait until the need is clear may be to wait too long.

Part of the art of emergency medicine is the ability to reliably discriminate between cases requiring urgent action and those allowing a more measured approach. Maintaining a bias toward action should not be used as an excuse for an indiscriminate, "shoot-from-the-hip" approach to the patient; it is a tool that the emergency physician must learn to use effectively.

Bedside Evaluation

If resuscitation or other urgent interventions are not required, then the usual framework for patient evaluation (history, physical, laboratory, treatment, disposition) can be used. In the ED, certain factors require more or less emphasis or alteration, however (Table I.1).

Patients and physicians in EDs are generally complete strangers, and thus patients have legitimate questions about the emergency physicians they have just met: Are they capable? Can they be trusted? Consequently, the first task faced by the emergency physician, even before information gathering begins, is to build a working relationship with the patient right away (7).

The initial contact the physician makes should be social—an introduction. This should include everyone in the room, and should be accompanied by physical contact—a handshake or touch. This establishes a tone of personal respect for the patient and helps enlist the family, if present, in an alliance with the physician. As early as possible the physician should show empathy with the patient by acknowledging recognition of an ap-

TABLE I.1   Rules to Guide the Bedside Evaluation of the
Emergency Department Patient

Introduce yourself to everyone
Shake hands
Sit down
Relieve pain early
Don't interrupt
Provide information
Explain what will happen
Provide updates
Be helpful

parent need. This can be done by an offer to relieve apparent pain, if appropriate.

The body language of the physician–patient encounter is important. Often in the ED, the standing physician presides over the supine, frequently disrobed patient, presenting an authoritarian image that can be threatening to patients. As often as possible, therefore, the physician should sit while conducting the initial interview, ideally bringing his or her head to the same level as the patient's. This is especially important in dealing with children, but should not be neglected in adult patients.

The information-gathering phase of the encounter should begin with a general, open-ended question, such as, "How can I help you?" It is important to remember that both parties, not just the physician, are interested in gathering information at this time. Patients' desires for information, explanation, and reassurance are great, but are seldom met by physicians (1,8). One way emergency physicians can meet this almost insatiable need for information early in the encounter is by commenting about findings during the physical examination: "Your heart sounds normal," or "Your throat looks red" (7).

Given the time pressures of emergency medicine, physicians typically fear losing control of the interview and attempt to keep the patient focused and on target. Observations of physician–patient interactions show that patients are interrupted by the physician on average about 18 seconds after they begin to relate their history, but that if uninterrupted, 80% can get their story out within 1 minute (2). Physicians' time concerns are real, but if the physician dominates the interview, the patient will become passive and volunteer little (4); the physician will then have to spend additional time extracting information later. In addition, the chief complaint may not always be mentioned first; failure to wait for the true chief complaint to emerge can lead to false trails and lost time (7). Considering the gain in rapport with the patient and the potential for mischief with early interruption, it seems wise for emergency physicians to discipline themselves to be quiet for the first 60 seconds of the interview.

Disposition

Once the initial assessment is complete, the physician should outline the plan to the patient, and should give an honest estimate of about how long it will take. It is also useful to provide some anticipatory guidance about the probable outcome, particularly in complex, chronic problems that are unlikely to be resolved in an ED evaluation. During the wait for laboratory results, consultations, or observation, the patient and family should be updated periodically on progress and asked if there is anything they need.

Finally, once a disposition is reached, the plan should be carefully and clearly communicated to the patient and family. Particularly if the patient is to be discharged, specific instructions about followup and reasons to return to the ED should be covered. Because patients are likely to have difficulty remembering a series of detailed explanations or instructions, it is most helpful if patients are given instructions in writing. Having a printed instruction sheet does not relieve the physician of the obligation to instruct the patient, but it does help to reinforce those instructions once the patient has left the ED.

A FRAMEWORK FOR DECISION MAKING IN EMERGENCY MEDICINE

Medicine is essentially about making decisions; in emergency medicine, this general property of medicine is intensified. Because a great deal of medical decision making occurs at a subconscious level, it is surprising to many to learn that there is a formalism for making and assessing the quality of medical decisions. Although it seems unrealistic to expect clinicians to adopt a formal decision-making model in their practices, some useful insights into the nature of decision making in the ED can be gained by such models.

Management, Not Diagnosis

Traditionally, medicine has focused on diagnosis as the central important task of the clinician. Emergency medicine makes it clear that this is erroneous: In medicine in general, and especially in emergency medicine, the central task is not diagnosis, but management. Often a diagnosis cannot be made under the constraints of an ED evaluation; the great insight that emergency physicians have contributed to their colleagues in other specialties is the notion that there need not always be a diagnosis. If one can be made, it is extremely helpful, but if not, decisions must still be made and actions must still be taken.

In addition, patients want more than simply a diagnosis. They want explanation and reassurance. For example, parents will not be satisfied to know that their child's abdominal pain is caused by gastroenteritis; they want to know that it is not appendicitis. Simply providing the diagnosis, however correct, dismisses the parents' concerns and leaves them unsatisfied. By empathizing with their fears, the physician can strengthen rapport with the family and take a position as their friend and ally, rather than as a remote authority. Thus the intellectual task is to devise a reasonable plan of management, which may include, but not be limited to, making a diagnosis.

Decision Thresholds

The concept of "decision threshold" (6) clarifies many decisions emergency physicians make and adds specificity to the often used but vaguer concept of "index of suspicion." Consider the following hypothetical scenario of the simplest possible situation in emergency medicine: there is only one disease under consideration and there are only two possible actions—to treat or not treat—based on the emergency physician's assessment of the patient. In this scenario, there are four possible outcomes: The patient either has the disease and may be treated or not treated, or does not have the disease and is treated or not treated. The optimal management decision depends on the values of these outcomes and on the probability that a particular patient (or group of patients) actually has the disease in question.

If the patient is almost certainly nondiseased (i.e., the probability of disease is near zero), then the correct decision is to not treat, because treatment entails costs and risks of its own. Conversely, if the patient surely has the disease (probability near 1), then the correct decision is to treat, because the costs and risks of treatment are outweighed by the negative consequences of failing to treat. Therefore, there must be some *threshold* probability between 0 and 1 at which the decision is a toss-up; that is, either choice will produce about the same outcome. This treatment threshold need not (and often does not) coincide with the diagnostic thresholds that clinicians traditionally have been taught. Consequently, the clinician's task is not necessarily to make a diagnosis, but to discover whether the probability of disease is clearly over or clearly under the treatment threshold, and to act accordingly.

The threshold approach can be extended to more complex problems. For example, a more realistic scenario allows use of a diagnostic test to improve the physician's initial assessment. Now there are two decision thresholds. At very low probabilities of disease, it is better not to test and not to treat, because the outcome of large numbers of false positives erroneously treated outweigh that of the occasional diseased patient detected. Similarly, at very high probabilities, it is better not to test, but to treat everyone, because the consequences of large numbers of false negatives erroneously denied treatment outweigh the occasional nondiseased patient spared unnecessary treatment. At intermediate probabilities, testing and treating only those patients with a positive test will produce the best overall outcome. Thus, the clinician's task is to decide whether a given patient's probability of disease lies either below the no treat–test threshold, or above the test–treat threshold. Testing is useful only in changing the management decision in the area between the two thresholds. While there may be other benefits to testing besides producing a change in management (e.g., reducing uncertainty or clarifying prognosis), the threshold approach provides a rationale for understanding physicians' differing choices when faced with seemingly similar clinical scenarios.

In framing decision making in this way, it is important to note that a very broad idea of "test" is used. Anything that helps physicians revise their probability assessments is considered a test in this sense, so therapeutic trials, periods of observation, clinical scoring systems, or practice guidelines could all be considered "tests" because they help physicians sort out the probabilities of diseases. McNutt and associates (5) have provided interesting evidence that physicians' diagnostic and management performance improves when they receive the nonverbal cues that accompany face-to-face communication, even though this "test" occurs largely at a subconscious level.

The way in which emergency physicians determine whether they have crossed an action threshold seems to be by the use of naturalistic or "event-driven" decision making (4). This contrasts strongly with the algorithmic or analytical decision-making process taught in medical school. Naturalistic decision making is effective in settings characterized by ill-defined problems; dynamic, uncertain environments; shifting, unclear, or competing goals; tight but nonlinear or hidden coupling between actions and their effects; time pressure; high stakes; and scant opportunity for learning by trial and error.

The decision-making process can be divided into several phases. First, the physician classifies the current situation as typical or atypical, based on matching critical cues to stored patterns or schemata. If the situation is typical, the stored patterns will evoke a customary set of responses. If it is not typical, variations of customary responses are considered first, and then novel, "one-of-a-kind" responses are considered. Clearly, experience is critical in developing a sufficiently rich set of stored schemata such that the vast majority of clinical problems can be recognized and dealt with by a preplanned response.

Next, the physician engages in serial evaluation of the available courses of action, beginning with the most typical response, and evaluating each by mentally simulating the expected outcomes. Once a sufficiently satisfying action is discovered, it is implemented. In other words, there is generally not a search for the best of all possible responses, but for a sufficiently good response. The payoff for accepting a good, but not necessarily best, response is that decisions can be quick and almost effortless. In fact, a great deal of physicians' expertise seems to lie in their ability to constructively perceive the problem, which seems to lead automatically to a solution without much conscious effort. This contrasts sharply with the slow and laborious analytic approach of exhaustively considering all the possibilities and eliminating them one by one until the best option is identified.

Learning this method of decision making is not easy. It can be gained with experience, and is generally communicated by narratives of meaningful cases (3). It does not appear to be attainable through application of formal analytical methods. Such methods have their place, but they have not proven useful in helping medical students or residents to become physicians.

COMMON PITFALLS

There are three common pitfalls in the approach to the patient in the ED.

✔ The first is tunnel vision. Here the physician, in single-minded pursuit of the disposition, fastens onto a single complaint (typically the first offered) without waiting to be sure that the patient's *chief* complaint has been elicited. A related error is the premature closure of hypothesis generation (e.g., assuming that chest pain is caused by myocardial ischemia without first mentally ruling out the possibilities of aortic dissection, esophageal rupture, or pericarditis)

✔ The second pitfall is just the opposite: an inability to see the forest for the trees. Here the physician fails to rank findings in any order of importance, is reluctant to close off hypothesis generation, or is unable to integrate the findings into a small number of possible explanations. This is frequently manifested by procrastination in decision making, perhaps hidden behind a cascade of laboratory testing. The ability to simultaneously entertain a modest number of possible expla-nations for the patient's problem without prematurely settling on one, or letting the number in contention grow too large, is the "golden mean" between these two problems

✔ The final pitfall is failure to attend to the patient. Time "gained" by failing to attend to the social interaction with patient and family is likely to be lost later, as missing information may not be extracted except by persistent questioning, leaving the physician at risk of pursuing many false leads before happening across the true trail

References

1. Adamson TE, Tschann JM, Gullin DS, et al. Physician communication skills and malpractice claims: a complex relationship. *West J Med* 1989;150:356–360.
2. Beckman HB, Frankel RM. Effect of physician behavior on the collection of data. *Ann Intern Med* 1984;101:692–696.
3. Klein GA. *Sources of power: how people make decisions.* Cambridge, MA: MIT Press, 1998.
4. Klein GA, Orasanu J, Calderwood R, et al., eds. *Decision making in action: models and methods.* Norwood, NJ: Ablex Publishing, 1993.
5. McNutt RA, Evans AT, Wallsten TS, et al. The effect of visual information on physicians' estimates of acute ischemic heart disease and their decisions to admit. *Med Decis Making* 1993;13:393(abst).
6. Pauker SG, Kassirer JP. The threshold approach to clinical decision making. *N Engl J Med* 1980;302:1109–1117.
7. Rosenzweig S. Emergency rapport. *J Emerg Med* 1993;11:775–778.
8. Waitzkin H. Doctor-patient communication: clinical implications of social science research. *JAMA* 1984;252:2441–2446.

SECTION I

Section Editor: Jeffrey Schaider

Resuscitation

CHAPTER 1
Airway Management

Michael F. Murphy

Airway evaluation and management continues to be the first priority of resuscitation and takes precedence over other interventions. Concurrent evaluation and management activities should occur while the airway management is undertaken. It is widely recognized that a conceptual framework focused on rapid airway evaluation, critical action analysis and performance, and facility with an array of airway management techniques minimizes the risk of failure and improves outcome (2).

Both the identification of an inadequate airway and the decision that active airway intervention is required are usually reached quickly by emergency physicians. The failure to maintain a patent airway and the failure to affect adequate gas exchange are the cornerstones of this decision. Subsequent decisions with respect to *how and when* the airway will be managed depend on the integration of numerous factors including the skills and knowledge of the physician, the equipment available, the condition of the patient, and the anatomy of the airway.

By the early 1970s endotracheal intubation had become a skill necessary to those practicing in the fledgling field of emergency medicine. It was generally accomplished either nasally or orally with varying degrees of brute force. By the mid to late 1990s most emergency practitioners employed neuromuscular blockade in some form most of the time to facilitate oral endotracheal intubation. It had become evident that neuromuscular blockade not only made the technical task of intubation easier and faster, but that the complication rates were lower and the success rates higher. However, for many practitioners, the need to evaluate the airway for difficulty and the development of a systematic method for doing so lagged behind the clinical introduction of rapid sequence intubation (RSI). There was also the need to expand the rescue options beyond cricothyrotomy. Bag and mask ventilation, the cornerstone of airway management, is discussed in Chapter 2 and is a critically important skill in emergency medicine (18).

The current challenges facing emergency airway managers include:

- Which patients should not receive paralytics?
- How is the airway best rescued in the event intubation and/or ventilation is impossible or has failed?

THE DECISION TO INTUBATE

The following are the five generally accepted indications to secure an airway by endotracheal intubation in emergency medicine practice:

1. Failure of the patient to maintain a patent airway.
2. Failure of the patient to adequately protect the airway from aspiration.
3. Failure of the patient to maintain adequate gas exchange (oxygen and carbon dioxide).
4. The employment of paralytic agents or therapeutic hyperventilation is indicated.
5. Inability of the patient to adequately clear secretions.

A sixth indication that is frequently invoked is *intubation prior to transport*, where it is reasonably anticipated that while an indication to intubate does not exist now, one may develop during the transport. This risk-to-benefit analysis recognizes the practicalities of intubating in a transport vehicle.

The decision to intubate is ordinarily easily made. The timing of the intubation may be more problematic, particularly in patients who are barely holding their own, because it is important to intervene before the respiratory failure precipitates an adverse cardiac event. There are probably few other situations in emergency practice where judgment and knowledge of the *anticipated clinical course* of a disorder are as crucial to the emergency physician.

EVALUATION OF THE PATIENT

Human beings protect their airway at virtually all costs. Endotracheal intubation stimulates an extreme autonomic response. As such, potent medications are generally employed to attenuate the adverse responses to intubation such as hypertension, tachycardia, increased intracranial pressure (ICP), and bronchospasm, among others. The emergency physician must attempt to balance the anticipated aggression of the response to intubation by selecting appropriate classes and dosages of medication to mitigate them. Underdosing may fail to mitigate an aggressive response; overdosing may produce hypotension or premature apnea.

The evaluation of the patient to be intubated is focused on the three crucial organ systems: the central nervous system (CNS), the cardiovascular system, and the respiratory system. The response to laryngoscopy and intubation dictates which medications and what dose are required to maintain stability through the procedure.

APPROACH TO THE AIRWAY: HOW TO PROCEED

Once one has decided that intubation is indicated, the thinking progresses rapidly to identify exactly what kind of airway is present, and how one will proceed:

- Is this a *crash airway* where the patient is unconscious, unresponsive, and near death?
- Is this a *difficult airway* where one anticipates difficulty with bag-mask ventilation, laryngoscopy, and intubation or cricothyrotomy?
- If neither of these exists, *RSI* is reasonable.
- Has a *failed airway* supervened?

This systematic approach to airway management in the emergency department encompasses all possible presentations. Identifying the type of airway to be intubated permits the practitioner to select an appropriate course of action. Algorithms are presented below for each of these clinical presentations. Figure 1.1 depicts this conceptual framework (21).

Crash Airway Algorithm

The patient who presents in an unresponsive state, or is deemed unlikely to respond in any way to direct laryngoscopy, is said to have a *crash airway*, and the crash airway algorithm (Fig. 1.2) is employed (21). Noteworthy points in the crash airway algorithm include:

- Bag-mask ventilation is occurring as preparations are made to intubate.
- The initial action is to attempt oral intubation immediately by direct laryngoscopy without pharmacologic assistance.

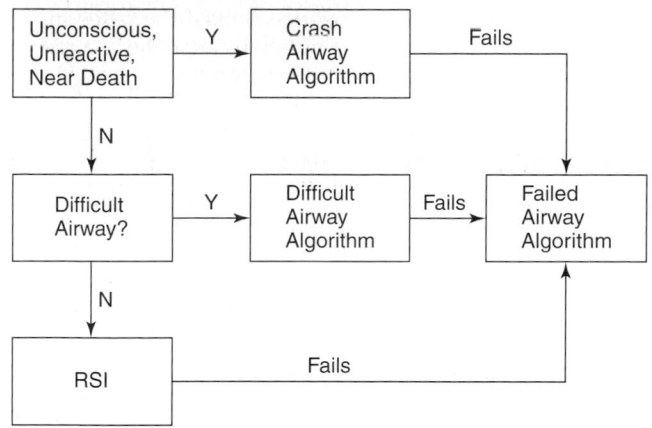

Figure 1.1. Airway management algorithm. RSI, rapid sequence intubation.

- If this first attempt is unsuccessful, it is assumed that the patient is not optimally relaxed and succinylcholine is administered in an increased dose.
- If bag-mask ventilation is unsuccessful at any time, and if intubation has failed, a failed airway is present, and one proceeds to the failed airway algorithm (Fig. 1.3).
- Once three attempts have failed, one proceeds to the failed airway algorithm (Fig. 1.3).

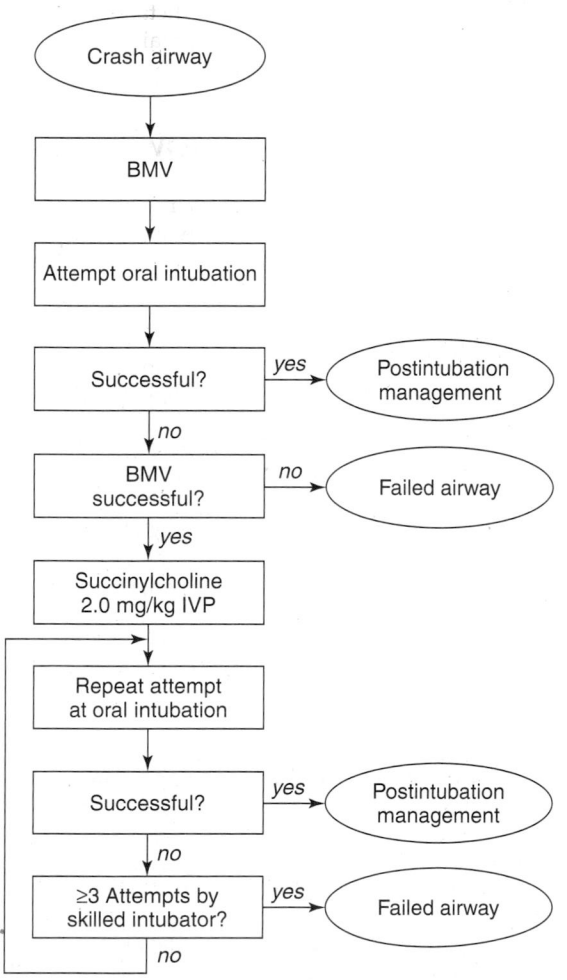

Figure 1.2. The crash airway algorithm. BMV, bag-mask ventilation; IVP, intravenous push.

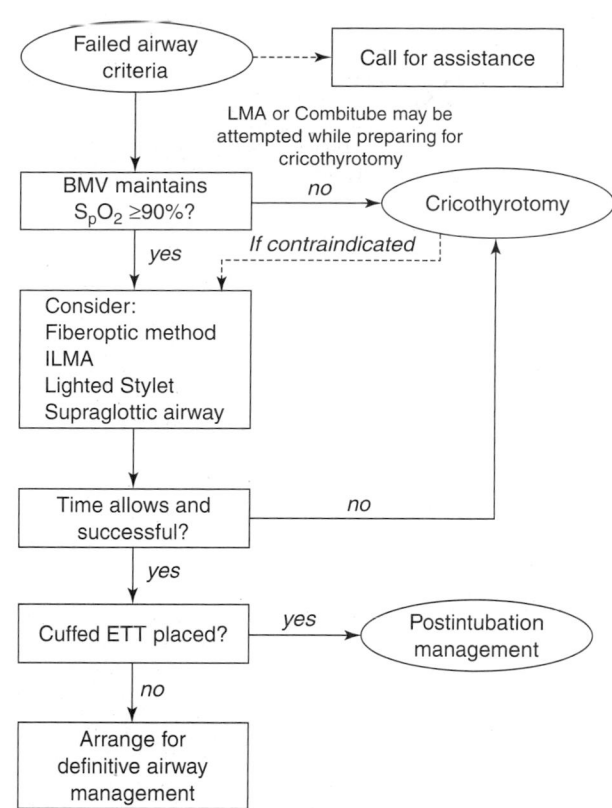

Figure 1.3. The failed airway algorithm. BMV, bag-mask ventilation; ETT, endotracheal tube; ILMA, intubating laryngeal mask airway; LMA, laryngeal mask airway.

Difficult Airway Algorithm

Should the situation not be a crash airway, one must determine whether it is a *difficult airway*. Although all emergency intubations are difficult to some degree, the evaluation of the airway for those features that reliably predict difficult bag-mask ventilation, difficult laryngoscopy, or difficult cricothyrotomy is extremely important. In the event that the airway is judged to be difficult, the difficult airway algorithm (Fig. 1.4) is used (21). The evaluation for difficulty is presented in the next section.

Noteworthy points in the difficult airway algorithm include:

- How much time is available: If ventilation and oxygenation are adequate then a careful assessment and a planned approach can be undertaken. If not, does bag-mask ventilation provide adequate ventilation? If not, the situation is equivalent to a "can't intubate; *can't* oxygenate" failed airway, and one proceeds to the failed airway algorithm (see Fig. 1.3) (21).
- If the patient can be adequately oxygenated, the next step is to consider RSI. If bag-mask ventilation is deemed unlikely to succeed or if success at laryngoscopy and intubation is felt to be questionable, RSI is not recommended.
- *Awake* laryngoscopy is the cornerstone of difficult airway management. An "awake look" is intended to either intubate the nonparalyzed patient orally, or identify whether the patient can be safely paralyzed and intubated using an RSI technique. An awake look in an emergency airway situation relies *virtually entirely* on the intravenous titration of systemically active sedation (15).
- If at any time oxygenation and ventilation become inadequate, the situation has become a failed airway. If oxygenation remains adequate, several options remain, all of which place a cuffed (in adults) endotracheal tube in the trachea.

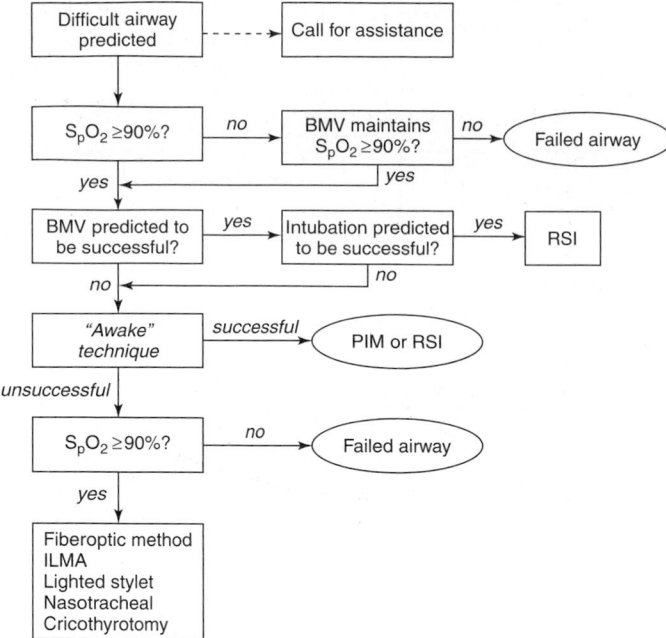

Figure 1.4. The difficult airway algorithm. BMV, bag-mask ventilation; ILMA, intubating laryngeal mask airway; PIM, post intubation management; RSI, rapid sequence intubation; SpO₂, arterial oxyhemoglobin saturation.

In the absence of an identified crash or difficult airway, RSI is the method of choice for airway management in the emergency department.

Failed Airway Algorithm (21)

The failed airway is easily defined:

1. Three failed attempts at orotracheal intubation by a skilled intubator or
2. Failure to maintain acceptable oxygen saturations

The problem in day-to-day practice is recognizing failure when it occurs and changing gears rapidly to deal with it appropriately. Clinically, the failed airway presents itself in two ways:

1. Time available: "can't intubate; *can* oxygenate"
2. Immediate action required: "can't intubate; *can't* oxygenate"

Noteworthy points in the failed airway algorithm (see Fig. 1.3) (21) include:

- Unlike the difficult airway, where the placement of a cuffed tube in the trachea is the goal, the failed airway calls for immediate action to provide emergency oxygenation by whatever appropriate maneuvers are available, regardless of whether this results in a secure, protected airway. Thus the devices considered for the failed airway are somewhat different from, but inclusive of, the devices used for the difficult airway.
- When a failed airway has been determined to be present, the response is dictated by whether bag-mask ventilation is possible and adequate.
- A "can't intubate; *can't* oxygenate" situation mandates immediate cricothyrotomy. The airway manager may elect to attempt to rapidly place an alternative device, such as the Combitube or intubating laryngeal mask airway (ILMA), *simultaneously* with the preparation for a cricothyrotomy, to convert the "can't intubate; *can't* oxygenate" situation into a "can't intubate; *can* oxygenate" situation (21).

- If at any time during the management of the failed airway adequate oxygenation and ventilation cannot be assured, immediate performance of a cricothyrotomy is mandated.

EVALUATION OF THE AIRWAY

Airways that are difficult to manage are fairly common in emergency practice with some estimates being as high as 20% of all emergency intubations. However, the incidence of intubation failure is quite uncommon, being in the 0.5% to 2.5% range. Moreover, the disastrous situation of being able to neither intubate nor ventilate rarely occurs (0.1% to 0.5%) (15).

The most important way to avoid airway management failure is to predict those airways that might be difficult to intubate, bag-mask ventilate, or perform a cricothyrotomy on, particularly if one is relying on the latter two techniques to rescue the airway in the event that oral intubation proves impossible.

Unlike the failed airway, the difficult airway is not so easily defined, although many have tried. Rather than a *definition*, the concept of the difficult airway has the following four "dimensions" (15):

1. Difficult bag-mask ventilation (BMV)
2. Difficult laryngoscopy
3. Difficult intubation
4. Difficult cricothyrotomy

These four dimensions can be reduced to the following three technical operations (15):

1. Difficult BMV
2. Difficult laryngoscopy and intubation
3. Difficult cricothyrotomy

The evaluation of the airway for difficulty in an emergency must be done quickly, with care taken not to omit anything important. Like well-constructed algorithms, mnemonics are efficient memory aid strategies, so one for each technical operation has been crafted to permit a rapid and complete evaluation.

Difficult Bag-Mask Ventilation

If the airway manager is uncertain that neuromuscular blockade facilitated orotracheal intubation (RSI) will be successful, the airway manager must be confident that BMV is possible, or at the very least that a cricothyrotomy can be rapidly performed. The five indicators of difficult BMV (9) can be easily recalled for rapid use in the emergency setting by using the mnemonic MOANS (15) (Table 1.1).

- **M** *Mask seal:* Bushy beards, crusted blood on the face or a disruption of lower facial continuity are the most common examples of conditions that may make an adequate mask seal difficult.
- **O** *Obese or Obstructed:* Patients that are obese (body mass index [BMI] >26 kg/m²) are often difficult to ventilate adequately by bag and mask. Parturients at term, patients with angioedema, Ludwig's angina, upper airway abscesses (e.g., peritonsillar), epiglottitis, and others ought to be considered at this juncture.
- **A** *Advanced age:* Patient age older than 55 years is associated with a higher risk of difficult bag-mask ventilation, perhaps because of a loss of muscle and tissue tone in the upper airway with increased age.
- **N** *No teeth:* An adequate mask seal may be difficult in the edentulous patient because the face tends to cave in.

TABLE 1.1. Airway Mnemonics

Difficult Bag-Mask Ventilation: MOANS
• Mask seal
• Obese or Obstructed
• Advanced age
• No teeth
• Stiff

Difficult Laryngoscopy and Intubation: LEMON
• Look externally
• Evaluate 3-3-2
• Mallampati score
• Obstruction
• Neck mobility

Difficult Cricothyrotomy: SHORT
• Surgery/disrupted airway
• Hematoma or infection
• Obese/access problem
• Radiation
• Tumor

• **S** *Stiff:* Patients with high airway resistance or diminished pulmonary compliance are exceedingly difficult to adequately manage with a bag and mask.

Difficult Laryngoscopy and Intubation

Difficult laryngoscopy and intubation ordinarily implies that the operator had a poor view of the target, that is, the glottis. Cormack and Lehane provided some clarity to the way we think of the "difficult airway" by parsing the act of intubation into its two subcomponents: laryngoscopy and intubation. They also introduced the most widely used system of categorizing the degree of visualization of the larynx during laryngoscopy (4) (Fig. 1.5).

Cormack-Lehane view grades 3 (epiglottis only visible) and 4 (no glottic structures at all visible) are often used as surrogates to represent difficult laryngoscopy and to predict difficult intubation. View grades 1 (visualization of the entire laryngeal aperture) and 2 (visualization of the posterior cords and arytenoids) are not typically associated with difficult intubation, although some grade 2s may be very anterior and difficult or impossible to intubate.

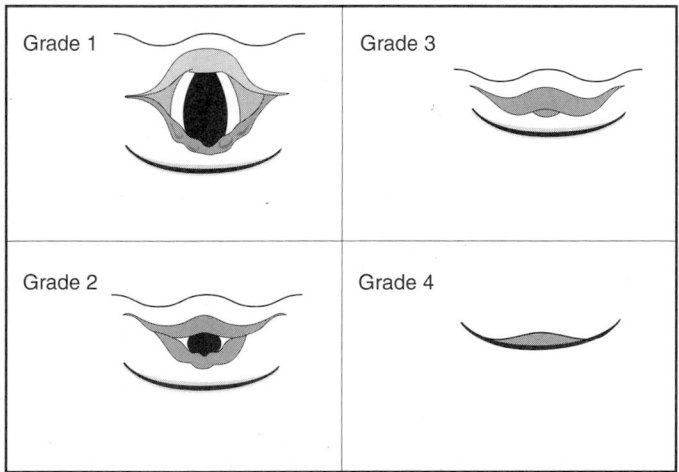

Figure 1.5. Cormack and Lehane system of categorizing the degree of visualization of the larynx during laryngoscopy.

The mnemonic LEMON (15) (see Table 1.1) is a useful guide to identifying as many of the risks as possible as quickly as possible to meet the demands of an emergency situation.

• **L** *Look externally*: meaning that if the airway looks difficult, it probably is! A litany of physical features is associated with difficult laryngoscopy and intubation, making the glottic aperture difficult to visualize. A small mandible may indicate that the tongue is "retrofitted" over the larynx; a large tongue elongates the pharyngeal axis, serving to extend the distance to the larynx beyond the visible horizon. Buck teeth block access to the oral cavity and also elongate the length of the oral axis. A high, arched palate is often associated with a long narrow oral cavity, making access a problem. A short neck may mean the larynx is positioned higher in the neck relative to the base of the tongue, making it more difficult to bring the glottis into view. Lower facial disruption is inconsistent with adequate mask seal and may make the glottis impossible to find.

• **E** *Evaluate 3-3-2:* This step recognizes the importance of the geometric relationships of various parts of the airway to successful intubation (3,17). One ought to be able to open his mouth enough to accomodate three of their own fingers; be able to accommodate three of their own fingers between the tip of the mentum and the hyoid bone; and fit two fingers between the hyoid bone and the thyroid notch. The first "3" assesses the adequacy of oral access. The second "3" addresses the capacity of the *mandibular space* to accommodate the tongue on laryngoscopy. More than, or less than, three fingers are both associated with greater degrees of difficulty in visualizing the larynx at laryngoscopy. The former because the length of the oral axis is elongated; the latter because the mandibular space may be too small to accommodate the tongue, leaving it to obscure the view of the glottis. The final "2" identifies the location of the larynx in relation to the base of the tongue. If more than two fingers are accommodated, the larynx is further below the base of the tongue beyond the visible horizon. Fewer than two fingers may mean that the larynx is tucked up under the base of the tongue and may be difficult to expose. This condition is often called *anterior larynx*.

• **M** *Mallampati score:* Mallampati determined that the degree to which the posterior oropharyngeal structures are visible is loosely associated with intubation success (13,14). He had patients sit on the side of the bed, open their mouth as widely as possible, and protrude their tongue as far as possible, without phonating. Figure 1.6 depicts how the scale is constructed. Although classes I and II patients are associated with low intubation failure rates, the importance with respect to the wisdom of using neuromuscular blockade rests with those in classes III and IV, particularly those in class IV where intubation failure rates may exceed 10%. By itself the scale is neither sensitive nor specific; however, it is easily performed in an emergency and may reveal important information about access to the oral cavity and the potential for difficult glottic visualization.

• **O** *Obstruction:* Upper airway obstruction is always a difficult airway. The three cardinal signs of upper airway obstruction are muffled voice ("hot potato voice"), difficulty swallowing secretions (either because of pain or obstruction), and stridor. The first two signs do not ordinarily herald imminent total upper airway obstruction; stridor does. The presence of stridor is generally considered to indicate that the airway has been reduced to roughly 10% of its normal caliber. Upper airway obstruction should always be managed with extreme care. The administration of small doses of opioids and benzodiazepines to manage anxiety may induce total obstruction as the tone of the upper airway musculature stenting the airway open relaxes.

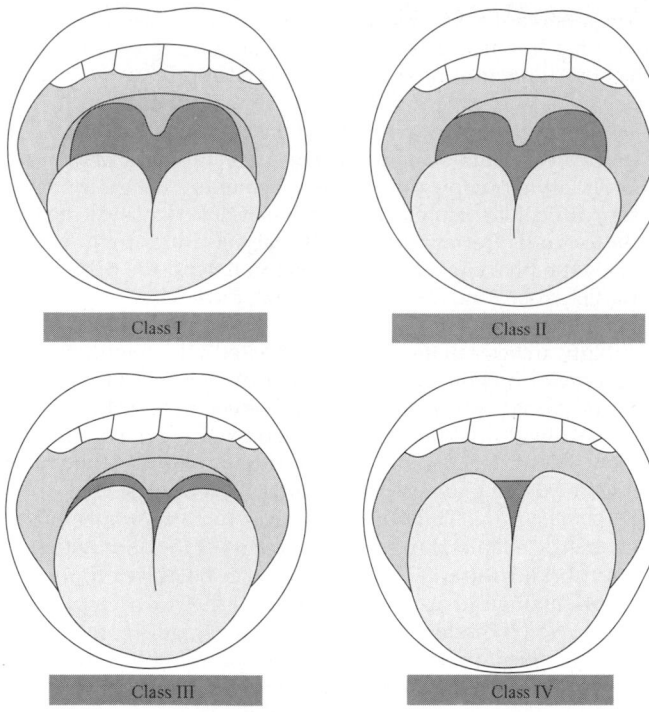

Figure 1.6.   Mallampati score.

- **N** *Neck mobility:* The ability to position the head and neck is one of the factors employed to achieve an optimal view of the larynx. Although cervical spine immobilization, of and by itself, may not automatically lead one to drop RSI from consideration, it ought to turn on an amber light, and be considered in light of additional features indicating difficulty.

Difficult Cricothyrotomy

There really are no absolute contraindications to performing an emergency cricothyrotomy. However, some conditions may make it difficult or impossible to perform the procedure, making it imperative to identify those conditions up front, particularly in the event one is relying on a rapidly performed cricothyrotomy as a rescue technique. The mnemonic SHORT (15) (see Table 1.1) is used to quickly assess the patient for features that may indicate that a cricothyrotomy might be difficult.

- **S** *Surgery/disrupted airway:* The anatomy may be distorted making the airway difficult to find, or access to it difficult.
- **H** *Hematoma or infection:* An infective process in the direct path of the cricothyrotomy may make the procedure technically difficult, but should never be considered a contraindication in a life-threatening situation.
- **O** *Obese/access problem:* Obesity should be considered a surrogate for any problem that makes percutaneous access to the anterior neck problematic. A fixed flexion deformity of the cervical spine, halo traction, and other situations come to mind.
- **R** *Radiation:* Past radiation therapy may distort tissues, making the procedure difficult.
- **T** *Tumor:* Tumor in or around the airway may present difficulty from an access perspective, as well as bleeding.

No single indicator, combination of indicators or even weighted scoring system of indicators can be relied on to assure success or predict failure when it comes to oral intubation.

Thus emergency physicians must evaluate the airway for difficulty, identify those factors known to increase the degree of difficulty, match them to the skill, experience, and judgment of the individual performing the intubation, and make a decision: Does this airway meets the threshold of being sufficiently difficult to warrant using the difficult airway algorithm, or is it safe to proceed directly to RSI?

RAPID SEQUENCE INTUBATION

RSI is defined as the virtually simultaneous administration of an induction agent and a neuromuscular blocking agent to facilitate endotracheal intubation (23). Attenuating the adverse responses to intubation, maintaining adequate oxygen saturations, and protecting the airway from aspiration are integral to the procedure.

The adage in anesthesia with respect to neuromuscular blockade to facilitate the orotracheal intubation of a patient that has some effective spontaneous ventilation has always been: "Don't take anything away from the patient that you cannot replace." Although such a rigid principle is not always consistent with the realities of emergency airway management (some patients need to be paralyzed even in the face of anticipated difficulty), it is a useful one to remember.

The use of neuromuscular blocking agents assumes that the operator is entirely versed in

Bag and mask ventilation.
Airway evaluation for difficulty.
The use of rescue devices and the performance of a surgical airway.

Walls has referred to the steps of RSI as the "Seven Ps of RSI" (23). It is a useful framework for discussing the procedure:

- *Preparation*
- *Preoxygenation:* This is a crucial step, permitting oxygen saturations to remain acceptable during the period of apnea as the neuromuscular blocking agent becomes fully effective. The goal is to replace the nitrogen in the patient's functional residual capacity (FRC; normally 30 mL/kg) with oxygen. The ability to do so varies with the time available, the ability of the oxygen delivery apparatus to deliver high concentrations oxygen used, and the patient's condition.
- *Pretreatment:* The goal of pretreatment is to attenuate the adverse responses to intubation, particularly the surges in heart rate, blood pressure, ICP, and airway resistance. Ideally, the pretreatment medications ought to precede the induction agent by 3 minutes to be optimally effective. Not all patients are equally at risk from these responses. Based on the best available evidence and expert recommendations at least the following patients should be pretreated:
  - Those suspected of having elevated ICP and imperfect autoregulation: lidocaine 1.5 mg/kg and fentanyl 3 to 13 µg/kg (ordinarily 3 to 5 µg/kg) (7).
  - Those with significant ischemic heart disease, or major vessel dissection or rupture: fentanyl 3 to 13 µg/kg (ordinarily 3 to 5 µg/kg). Caution ought to be exercised in administering fentanyl to patients with compensated or uncompensated shock.
  - Adults with significant existing reactive airways disease: lidocaine 1.5 mg/kg (22).
  - Children up to the age of 10 years, or any patient with potentially hemodynamically significant bradycardia where succinylcholine is to be used: atropine 0.01 to 0.02 mg/kg (minimum 0.1 mg; maximum 0.5 mg).

TABLE 1.2.   Induction Agents and Dosage Selection

	Stable Patient	Unstable Patient	Unstable Patient*
Etomidate (mg/kg)	0.3	0.15–0.2	0.1
Propofol (mg/kg)	1.0	0.5	0
Midazolam (mg/kg)	0.3	0.1	0.01–0.02
Pentothal (mg/kg)	3.0	1.5	0
Ketamine (mg/kg)	1.5	1.0	0.5

*The recommended doses are empiric and intended to produce amnesia in patients that are severely ill. Some practitioners may elect to administer none of these agents in this situation.

- *Paralysis with induction:* Both of these agents are rapidly administered intravenously. Induction agents have profound effects on all three vital organ systems: the CNS, cardiovascular system, and ventilation. These effects depend on the particular drug, the patient's underlying physiologic condition, and the dose and speed of injection of the drug. Because RSI requires rapid administration of the sedative–induction agent, the choice of drug and the dose *must be tailored* to capitalize on desired effects, while minimizing those that might adversely affect the patient (Table 1.2). In some cases, an amnestic dose may be selected, rather than an induction dose. While the sedative–induction dose might be tailored, the dose of the neuromuscular blocking agent is not (e.g., succinylcholine 1 to 2 mg/kg;, rocuronium 1 to 1.5 mg/kg).
- *Protection and Positioning:* Cricoid pressure to prevent regurgitation and aspiration is maintained until proper placement of the endotracheal tube is confirmed. Premature release of cricoid pressure is a common error, and places the patient at risk of aspiration, particularly if an inadvertent esophageal intubation has occurred. Cricoid pressure must be released immediately should active vomiting occur, otherwise there is danger of esophageal rupture. Most experts on airway management agree that positioning the head and neck is an important step in gaining the best view of the larynx with conventional laryngoscopy. It has long been taught that the "sniffing the morning air" or "sipping English tea" positioning of the head and neck, when possible, is best. Although there is some dissension as to whether this positioning does indeed deliver the best view of the larynx, most agree that it is a reasonable place to start (1,10).
- *Pass the tube*
- *Postintubation management*

RESCUE DEVICES

Airway rescue devices can be divided into the following two groups depending on the situation:

1. *"Can't Intubate; Can't Oxygenate":* Cricothyrotomy is the standard method of airway management in this situation. However, devices that can be inserted rapidly and are associated with high success rates include the Combitube and the ILMA (Fastrack). It is likely that the King LT Airway will be useful in this situation as well. The advantage of the Fastrack over the Combitube and the King LT Airway is the ability to intubate through the Fastrack.
2. *"Can't Intubate; Can Oxygenate":* Flexible and rigid fiberoptic devices, lightwands (e.g., Trachlight), and nasotracheal intubation require time to perform and are inappropriate in an emergency situation where ventilation and oxygenation cannot be guaranteed.

CONFIRMATION TECHNIQUES

Fiberoptic bronchoscopy remains the gold standard of verifying correct endotracheal tube placement by permitting direct visualization of tracheal rings (5). Visualization of the endotracheal tube entering the larynx also provides a highly reliable method of verifying intratracheal placement.

Detection of expired carbon dioxide provides reliable evidence of tracheal rather than esophageal intubation, and is the standard of care in emergency medicine. In nonarrested patients, carbon dioxide detection is highly reliable, indicating correct placement 99% to 100% of the time (11,16,20). Soft drinks in the stomach that contain carbon dioxide may mimic the exhaled carbon dioxide from the lungs for a couple of breaths, the so-called Cola-complication, although this confounding result ought not to persist beyond six breaths (25).

The migration of an endotracheal tube from the trachea to the esophagus during the tosses and turns of transport is an ever-present hazard. It has been demonstrated that the continuous monitoring of exhaled carbon dioxide during the prehospital phase of care minimizes the risk of such displacement going unrecognized (19).

As might be expected, carbon dioxide detection techniques tend to be less accurate in identifying correct placement of the endotracheal tube (ETT) in patients with circulatory arrest, with reported false-negative rates (carbon dioxide not detected, tube in the trachea) as high as 30% to 35% (12). In this circumstance, the endotracheal placement of the tube can be evaluated by an esophageal detector device (EDD) that consists of a self-inflating suction bulb or syringe armed with an adapter to fit a standard endotracheal tube connector. The collapsed bulb or syringe rapidly fills with air if the ETT is in the trachea; it does not inflate if the tube is in the esophagus, with a specificity of approximately 99% (24). Use of this device *instead of* carbon dioxide detection is not recommended because of its failure to detect esophageal intubation in as many as 20% of cases (6).

Physical examination techniques used to confirm intratracheal placement of an endotracheal tube, although neither sensitive nor specific, remain important adjuncts to more elaborate techniques, particularly in the cardiopulmonary arrested patient. Auscultation of the chest for breath sounds and of the epigastrium for absence of air entry into the stomach, observation of chest motion during ventilation, and condensation inside the ETT during extubation are common, but notoriously unreliable, methods of ascertaining proper endotracheal tube placement (8).

In summary, although carbon dioxide detection remains the most reliable method of verifying tracheal placement of the endotracheal tube in prehospital care, the incorporation of multiple methods of confirmation is superior to any single method.

CONCLUSIONS

RSI by emergency practitioners is associated with high success rates and low complication rates. The challenge now has become how to recognize those patients that ought not to be paralyzed, and to develop alternative skills to successfully manage those airways.

There is no "recipe" of RSI pretreatment and induction medications that can be sanguinely applied in every case. A careful assessment of risk and benefit in each individual patient is required to select the appropriate medication and its dose to minimize adverse outcomes.

Emergency airway managers must possess an array of airway management skills to be able to appropriately manage difficult airways and rescue failed airways.

CRITICAL INTERVENTIONS

- Evaluate the airway prior to airway management
- Pre-oxygenate patients prior to rapid sequence intubation
- Perform cricothyrotomy or insert intubating LMA in patients who cannot be ventilated or intubated
- Know which drugs and what doses ought to be employed
- Know when *not* to paralyze a patient
- Expertise at bag/mask ventilation is crucial
- Recognize airway management failure immediately

References

1. Adnet F, Baillard C, Borron SW, et al. Randomized study comparing the "sniffing position" with simple head extension for laryngoscopic view in elective surgery patients. *Anesthesiology* 2001;95:836–841.
2. Benumof JL. *The ASA difficult airway algorithm: new thoughts and considerations.* 51st annual refresher course lectures and clinical update program, #235 of the American Society of Anesthesiologists, 2000.
3. Cass NM, James NR, Lines V. Difficult direct laryngoscopy complicating intubation in anaesthesia. *Br Med J* 1956;1:488–490.
4. Cormack RS, Lehane J. Difficult tracheal intubation in obstetrics. *Anaesthesia* 1984;39:1105–1111.
5. Grmec S. Comparison of three different methods to confirm tracheal tube placement in emergency intubation. *Intensive Care Med* 2002;28:701–704.
6. Hendey GW, Shubert GS, Shalit M, et al. The esophageal detector bulb in the aeromedical setting. *J Emerg Med* 2002;23:51–55.
7. Jagoda A, Bruns J. Increased intracranial pressure. In: Walls RM, Murphy MF, Luten RC, eds. *Manual of emergency airway management.* 2nd ed. Philadelphia: Lippincott Williams and Wilkins, 2004:262–269.
8. Katz SH, Falk JL. Misplaced endotracheal tubes by paramedics in an urban emergency medical services system. *Ann Emerg Med* 2001;37:32–37.
9. Langeron O, Masso E, Huraux C. Prediction of difficult mask ventilation. *Anesthesiology* 2000;92:1229–1236.
10. Levitan RM, Ochroch AE, Hollander J, et al. Assessment of airway visualization: validation of the percent of glottic opening (POGO) scale. *Acad Emerg Med* 1998;5:919–923.
11. Li J. Capnography alone is imperfect for endotracheal tube placement confirmation during emergency intubation. *J Emerg Med* 2001;20:223–229.
12. MacLeod BA, Heller MB, Gerard J, et al. Verification of endotracheal tube placement with colorimetric end-tidal CO$_2$ detection. *Ann Emerg Med* 1991;20:267–270.
13. Mallampati SR. Clinical sign to predict difficult tracheal intubation (hypothesis). *Can Anaesth Soc J* 1983;30:316–317.
14. Mallampati SR, Gatt SP, Gugino LD, Murphy MF, Luten RC. A clinical sign to predict difficult intubation: a prospective study. *Can Anaesth Soc J* 1985;32:429–434.
15. Murphy MF, Walls RM. Identification of the difficient and failed airway. In: Walls RM, Murphy MF, Luten RC, eds. *Manual of emergency airway management.* 2nd ed., Philadelphia: Lippincott Williams and Wilkins, 2004:70–81.
16. Ornato JP, Shipley JB, Racht EM, et al. Multicenter study of a portable, hand-size, colorimetric end-tidal carbon dioxide detection device. *Ann Emerg Med* 1992;21:518–523.
17. Savva D. Prediction of difficult tracheal intubation. *Br J Anaesth* 1994;73:149–153.
18. Schneider RM, Murphy MF. Bag/mask ventilation and endotracheal intubation. In: Walls RM, Murphy MF, Luten RC, eds. *Manual of emergency airway management.* 2nd ed. Philadelphia: Lippincott Williams and Wilkins, 2004:43–69.
19. Silvestri S, Ralls G, Rothrock S, et al. Improvement in misplaced endotracheal tube recognition within a regional EMS system. *Soc Acad Emerg Med* 2003 (abst submitted).
20. Takeda T, Tanigawa K, Tanaka H, et al. The assessment of three methods to verify tracheal tube placement in the emergency setting. *Resuscitation* 2003;56:153–157.
21. Walls RM. The emergency airway algorithms. In: Walls RM, Murphy MF, Luten RC, eds. *Manual of emergency airway management.* 2nd ed. Philadelphia: Lippincott Williams and Wilkins, 2004:8–21.
22. Walls RM. Lidocaine and rapid sequence intubation. *Ann Emerg Med* 1996;27:528–529.
23. Walls RM. Rapid sequence intubation. In: Walls RM, Murphy MF, Luten RC, eds. *Manual of emergency airway management.* 2nd ed. Philadelphia: Lippincott Williams and Wilkins, 2004:22–32.
24. Wee MY. The oesophageal detector device. Assessment of a new method to distinguish oesophageal from tracheal intubation. *Anaesthesia* 1988;43:27–29.
25. Zbinden S, Schüpfer G. Detection of oesophageal intubation: the cola complication. *Anaesthesia* 1989;44:81.

CHAPTER 2
Airway Procedures

Eric F. Reichman

Airway management is one of the most basic, crucial, and important aspects of emergency medicine (15). Without oxygen, the brain begins to die within minutes. The mission for airway management is to ensure airway patency, to protect the airway from contamination (blood, fluids, and/or food), to provide supplemental oxygen, and to institute positive pressure ventilation when spontaneous respirations are inadequate or absent. Airway management can be as simple as lifting a snoring patient's chin, or as involved as awake fiberoptic-guided endotracheal intubation.

A thorough understanding of anatomy is essential for the performance of any medical procedure. Untoward events related to a procedure are often the result of inexperience and/or an inadequate understanding of the regional anatomy, and the airway procedures are no exception. From the evaluation of external anatomic landmarks to the performance of nerve blocks for fiberoptic intubation, understanding the anatomy of the airway will result in fewer attempts at intubation and improved success with fewer iatrogenic misadventures.

CLINICAL PRESENTATION

Airway intervention is required if there is uncertainty about whether the patient's airway patency, respiratory drive, or oxygenation can be maintained without intervention. Inadequate ventilation may occur for a variety of reasons. Spontaneously breathing patients may develop an airway obstruction caused by food, blood, or secretions, or from tissue obstruction as a result of the loss of the normal pharyngeal tone. Unconscious patients should have their airway secured, as well as receive mechanical ventilation. Despite spontaneous respiration, the unconscious patient is at risk for aspiration of gastric contents. The conscious patient with airway obstruction is in obvious distress and is more likely to have an obstruction caused by a foreign body, tissue swelling from an infection, laryngeal edema, cancer, or laryngospasm.

Endotracheal intubation can be performed to administer resuscitation medications, ensure a patent airway, deliver oxygen, isolate the airway, reduce the risk of aspiration of gastric or oral contents, suction the trachea, ventilate the patient, or to apply positive pressure ventilation. Other indications include altered mental status, head injury requiring hyperventilation, hypoxemia, hypoventilation, apnea, lack of a gag reflex, and unconsciousness.

EMERGENCY DEPARTMENT EVALUATION

Evaluation of the airway includes an internal and external examination. The internal examination should evaluate the patient's dentition, palate, and tongue. Note any protuberant incisors, loose teeth, broken teeth, dental work, and dental devices. Determine if the palate is normal, high and arched, or cleft. Determine if the tongue is elevated, larger, or wider than normal in comparison to the oral cavity. A common classification used by anesthesiologists to grade the difficulty of laryngoscopy and intubation involves the identification of the size the tongue in relation to the faucial pillars, the soft palate, and the uvula (7). External evaluation of the airway is a critical step to a successful intubation. External inspection should include mouth opening, atlanto-occipital extension, and thyromental distance. External inspection should also identify obvious problems (e.g., cervical collars, face and/or neck trauma, severe micrognathia, massive obesity, etc.). Please refer to Chapter 1, "Airway Management," for a more detailed discussion of this topic.

There are numerous differences between the adult's and the child's airway (14). The head-to-body ratio is larger in the child, which results in neck flexion when the child is supine. Placing a rolled towel under the child's shoulders will correct the flexion. Children have a small mouth with a relatively large tongue when compared to an adult, making orotracheal intubation difficult. The presence of adenoidal tissue in the child makes nasotracheal intubation difficult and orotracheal intubation the preferred method. The most important difference is that the narrowest portion of the infant and child's airway is below the vocal cords at the cricoid cartilage. In an adult, the narrowest point is the vocal cords. An endotracheal tube may pass through the vocal cords of a young child but might not advance past the cricoid cartilage because of normal anatomy. Forcing an endotracheal tube past the vocal cords might result in trauma to the airway and subsequent tracheal stenosis. The child's laryngeal inlet is narrow and more susceptible to obstruction. The U-shaped epiglottis and a more acute angle between the epiglottis and glottis causes the aryepiglottic folds to be more midline. Children have a relatively shorter trachea, making both right main bronchial intubation and accidental extubation much easier. The narrower diameter of the trachea with smaller spaces between the cartilaginous rings makes a tracheostomy more difficult to perform. To avoid injury and subsequent subglottic stenosis, uncuffed endotracheal tubes should be used in children who are younger than 8 years of age.

EMERGENCY DEPARTMENT MANAGEMENT

Basic Airway Management

Basic airway management is a fundamental skill that must be mastered by all caregivers. With an oxygen source, a means to deliver positive pressure ventilation, attention to detail in positioning, and the use of airway adjuncts, it is usually possible to prevent hypoxia and hypercarbia in the apneic patient.

Patient Positioning

The first goal of airway management is the establishment of a patent airway. The importance of proper positioning cannot be overemphasized. The success of airway management is predicated on this very basic, but often overlooked, issue. Placing the patient in the "sniffing" position may correct many upper airway obstructions because of soft-tissue impingement. The "sniffing" position is achieved by flexing the cervical spine approximately 15 degrees and extending the atlanto-occipital joint maximally. This position can also be achieved with the chin-lift or jaw-thrust maneuvers. If the patient is obese or has large breasts, the normal sniffing position is often insufficient for relieving an airway obstruction. A ramp or shoulder roll placed under the upper back will result in the "sniffing" position.

Jaw-Thrust Maneuver

The jaw thrust is one of the most basic maneuvers and an initial method of establishing a patent airway. The jaw-thrust maneuver

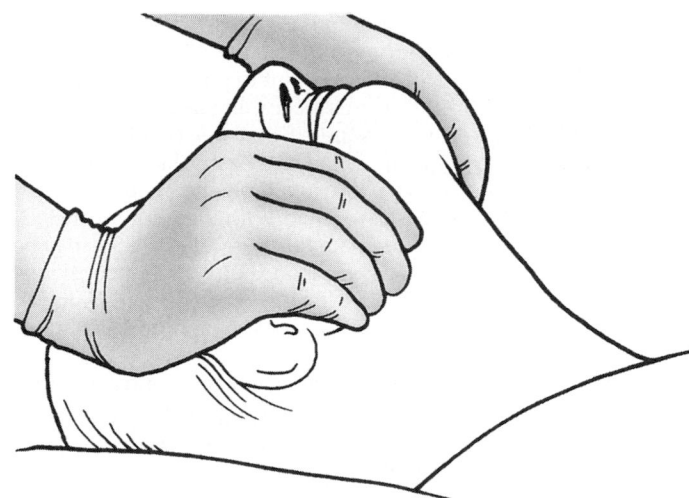

Figure 2.1.   The jaw-thrust maneuver. (From Reichman EF, Simon RR. *Emergency medicine procedures.* New York: McGraw-Hill, 2004 with permission.)

is a two-handed technique. The operator is positioned at the head of the patient and places his or her fingers on the angles of the mandible bilaterally, displacing it anteriorly (Fig. 2.1). A face mask may be simultaneously held in place with the operator's thumbs and index fingers.

Chin-Lift Maneuver

The chin lift is also one of the most basic maneuvers to establish a patent airway. This is performed by placing the fingers under the tip of the mandible and lifting the chin in an anterior and cephalic direction (Fig. 2.2). Do not place the fingers on the soft tissue of the submandibular space, because this will elevate the tongue and cause further obstruction. The patient's head may be tilted slightly posterior to aid in opening the airway.

Nasopharyngeal Airways

In addition to proper positioning, one can use various aids to overcome pharyngeal obstruction and facilitate effective

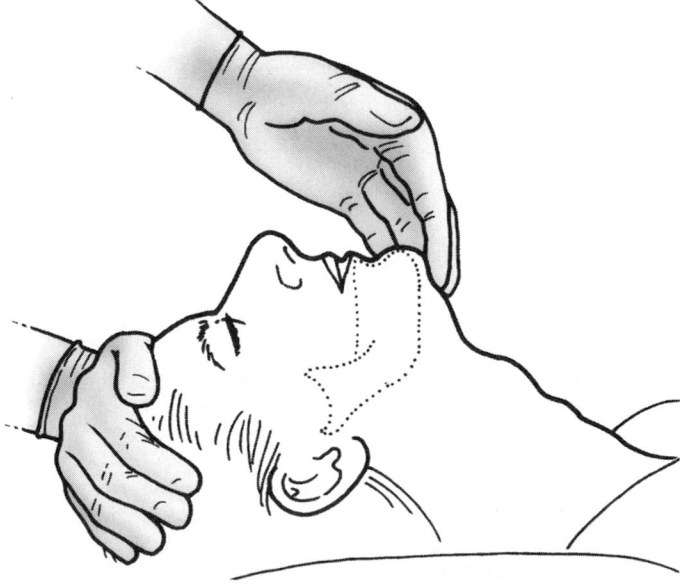

Figure 2.2.   The chin-lift maneuver. (From Reichman EF, Simon RR. *Emergency medicine procedures.* New York: McGraw-Hill, 2004 with permission.)

ventilation (1). The most commonly used devices are oropharyngeal (oral) and nasopharyngeal (nasal) airways. Regardless of which device is chosen, it is important to place a large enough airway to bridge the area of soft-tissue impingement on the pharynx. Nasopharyngeal airways are soft-rubber or plastic tubes that are inserted through the nostril and into the oropharynx, just above the epiglottis. They are available in numerous sizes; the larger inner diameter is associated with the longer tubes. A size 30- to 32-French is appropriate for most adults. They can be safely placed in the conscious, semiconscious, and unconscious patient. They can also be used when an oropharyngeal airway cannot be placed (e.g., in cases of oral trauma, braces, seizures, trismus, etc.).

Insertion of a nasopharyngeal airway is a quick and rapid procedure. Choose the proper size nasopharyngeal airway. The correct size is estimated by placing the airway next to the patient's face. Place the flared end of the airway near the tip of the patient's nose. Its tip should be at the external auditory canal. Liberally apply water-soluble lubricant or anesthetic jelly to the nasopharyngeal airway. If not contraindicated, apply a vasoconstrictor to the patient's nasal mucosa. Gently insert the nasopharyngeal airway with the beveled tip against the nasal septum to prevent it from getting caught on the turbinates. Insert it completely until the flared tip is against the nostril and rotate it 90 degrees so that it is concave upward. Slight rotation often facilitates the passage of the airway if resistance is encountered during insertion. Supplementary oxygen or positive pressure ventilation with a bag-valve-mask device can be started after the insertion of the airway.

Insertion of a nasopharyngeal airway is associated with complications. If too long, it may cause laryngospasm and vomiting. It may also be placed with its tip in the esophagus, resulting in gastric distention and subsequent aspiration. Nasal mucosal injury upon insertion can cause epistaxis and aspiration of blood.

Oropharyngeal Airways

The oropharyngeal airway is a semicircular plastic device that holds the tongue up and away from the posterior pharyngeal wall. It is less traumatic and more easily placed than a nasopharyngeal airway. An oropharyngeal airway must only be used in an unconscious patient or it may cause laryngospasm and vomiting. An 8-, 9-, or 10-cm oral airway is appropriate for most adults.

Insertion of the oropharyngeal airway is a quick and simple procedure. Choose the proper size oropharyngeal airway. The correct size is estimated by placing the airway next to the patient's mouth. The distal tip should lie just above the angle of the mandible. Clear the mouth and oropharynx of any blood, secretions, or vomit. Open the patient's jaw and separate the teeth. Insert the oropharyngeal airway curved side down. The tip will slide along the palate. After insertion, rotate it 180 degrees so that the curve of the oropharyngeal airway follows the curvature of the tongue. An alternative method is to use a tongue blade to depress the tongue and then insert the oropharyngeal airway as above. If the tongue blade is used, the oropharyngeal airway may also be inserted with the curve side upward. Supplementary oxygen or positive pressure ventilation with a bag-valve-mask device can be started after the insertion of the airway.

Insertion of an oropharyngeal airway is not a benign procedure. It can push the tongue posteriorly and further obstruct the oropharynx if not inserted properly. Significant lacerations can occur if the lips or tongue are caught between the teeth and the oral airway. It can force the epiglottis closed against the vocal cords if it is too long, resulting in complete airway obstruction. Too small an airway will force the tongue against the pharynx, producing an obstruction.

Mask Ventilation

Once mastered, expertise with bag-mask ventilation (BMV) allays the urgency to intubate and permits one to rescue a failed intubation. It is a prerequisite to the use of neuromuscular blocking agents to facilitate intubation. Provided one takes steps to minimize the risks of gastric aspiration, BMV for prolonged periods is not unreasonable if intubation is not possible.

Face masks are made of clear plastic, have a soft seal, and have an anatomic shape that conforms to the contours of the patient's face. Typical adult sizes are 3, 4, or 5. The size must be large enough to completely cover the nose and mouth but not be so large as to allow a leak. The key to effective mask ventilation is ensuring a continually patent airway. This is initially achieved by placing the patient in the "sniffing" position coupled with a combination of chin lift, jaw thrust, oral airway, or nasal airway. Neglecting this key maneuver results in using excessive positive pressure ventilation in an attempt to compensate for an obstructed upper airway. A bag-mask device can deliver 50 to 100 cm of water pressure to the upper airway with an adequate mask seal, more than sufficient pressure to insufflate the stomach if the airway is not optimally opened.

There are two ways to properly hold a face mask (1). The one-handed technique is performed with the nondominant hand (Fig. 2.3). Place the little, ring, and middle fingers under the side of the patient's mandible. Place the index finger and thumb on the bottom and top portion of the mask. This technique allows the operator to simultaneously lift the mandible and extend the atlanto-occipital joint while applying enough downward pressure to create an airtight seal. The dominant hand is used to ventilate the patient with the bag-valve device. The bag-valve device is used to provide positive pressure ventilation. It consists of a self-inflating bag connected to oxygen on one end and a one-way (nonrebreathing) valve on the other. The valve is connected to the mask, or other airway device, to allow one-way flow of oxygen.

A two-handed, two-person technique may be necessary in patients with facial hair, and in those who are obese, elderly, or edentulous. Both of the operator's hands are applied to the face mask to aid in the creation of a tight seal and proper airway

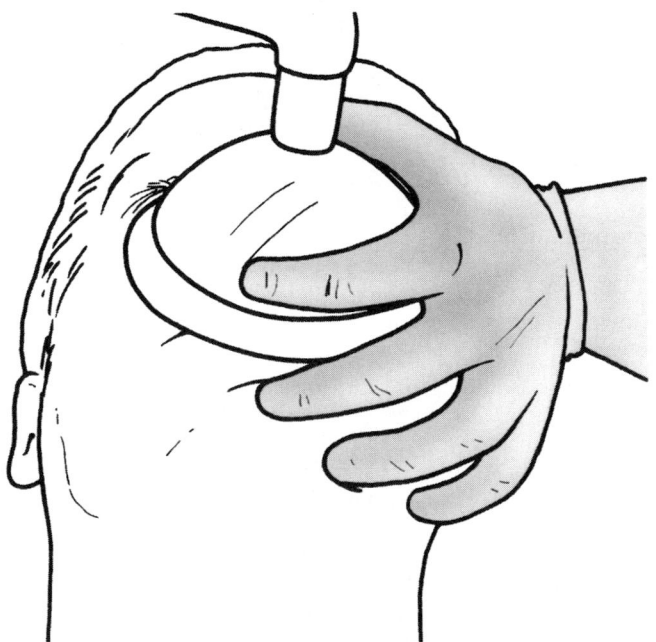

Figure 2.3. The one-handed, one-person, mask-ventilation technique. (From Reichman EF, Simon RR. *Emergency medicine procedures*. New York: McGraw-Hill, 2004 with permission.)

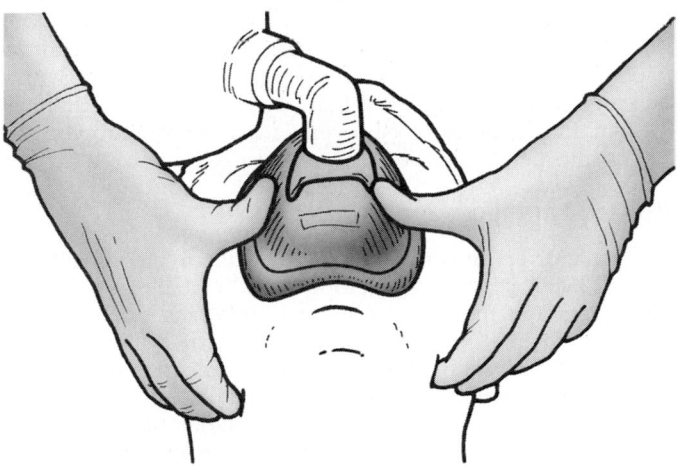

Figure 2.4. The two-handed, two-person, mask-ventilation technique. (From Reichman EF, Simon RR. *Emergency medicine procedures*. New York: McGraw-Hill, 2004 with permission.)

alignment (Fig. 2.4). Place the index, middle, ring, and small fingers of the left hand on the body of the left half of the mandible. Position the right hand similarly on the right half of the mandible. Place the face mask on the patient's face. Apply both thumbs to the mask and apply pressure to create a seal. Anteriorly elevate the mandible to perform the jaw-thrust maneuver. The second person applies positive pressure through the bag-valve device.

A standard adult resuscitation bag is 1,500 mL. The goal is to deliver 500 to 600 mL of tidal at a rate of 24 breaths per minute. Provided the airway is patent, significant insufflation of the stomach is unlikely. The cadence should be similar to the "squeeze ... release ... release" cadence recommended by advanced cardiac life support (ACLS) but at a slightly faster pace.

The specific type of bag employed in bag-mask ventilation is also important (1). Recent studies demonstrate that bags that minimize dead space, incorporate unidirectional air flow valves (e.g., "duck bill" inspiratory valves), and use one-way expiratory valves to prevent the entrainment of room air during inspiration will deliver 90% to 97% oxygen to spontaneously breathing or ventilated patients. This is in sharp distinction to improperly configured bags that will provide high oxygen concentration during active bagging, but deliver only 30% oxygen during spontaneous patient breathing as a result of the entrainment of room air.

Complications of Basic Airway Management

The most serious complication of basic airway management is aspiration of gastric contents, resulting in an acute chemical pneumonitis. It is a significant risk when airway management is needed emergently or routinely in the pregnant, trauma, diabetic, or obese patient. Less-serious complications include soft-tissue trauma to the lips, tongue, oral cavity, and eyelids. Tooth fractures or avulsion are uncommon but possible. Facial nerve dysfunction caused by pressure effects of the mask are transient. Corneal abrasions, conjunctival chemosis, and increased intraocular pressure are common with masks that are too large.

Orotracheal Intubation

Orotracheal intubation is both common and life saving. It is the primary and preferred method of airway management that every emergency physician must master (10). With proper preparation, definitive control of the airway can be obtained. This assures that the patient can be oxygenated and ventilated when the patient cannot do this on his or her own.

Orotracheal intubation is relatively contraindicated in patients who do not need it, are likely to be injured by the procedure, whose injuries make success unlikely, or where less-invasive techniques may suffice. It may be difficult in patients with likely cervical spine injuries, severe arthritis, severe orofacial injuries, deep airway obstruction, gross deformities of the head and neck, or a quickly changing obstruction (edema or an expanding hematoma). Choose a surgical airway if the manipulation or time required for oral endotracheal intubation puts the patient at risk for spinal injury or hypoxia.

The evaluation, preparation, and technique for orotracheal intubation are complex and essential. Firmly grasp the laryngoscope in the left hand. Insert the tip of the laryngoscope blade into the right side of the patient's mouth. Smoothly advance the blade inward while keeping pressure against the tongue. Move the blade toward the midline to trap and push the tongue to the left, "clearing a path" for your gaze.

Lift the patient's airway up and forward exactly along the long axis of the laryngoscope handle (Fig. 2.5). Do not "cock" or "crank back" on the laryngoscope handle with the wrist or the back of the laryngoscope blade may break the maxillary incisors. If intubating with the curved Macintosh blade, advance the tip into the vallecula, lift the laryngoscope handle to raise the tongue-jaw-epiglottis unit (Fig. 2.5), visualize the vocal cords, and insert the endotracheal tube. If intubating with the straight Miller blade, insert the blade completely, lift the laryngoscope handle to raise the tongue-jaw-epiglottis unit, visualize the vocal cords and airway, and insert the endotracheal tube. Advance the endotracheal tube until the cuff passes through the vocal cords and 2 to 3 cm into the trachea. Inflate the cuff, assess for proper placement, and secure it in place.

Numerous complications are associated with orotracheal intubation (10). Hypoxia often results from prolonged intubation attempts and misplaced endotracheal tubes. Bradycardia can be produced by pharyngeal manipulation. It may be especially

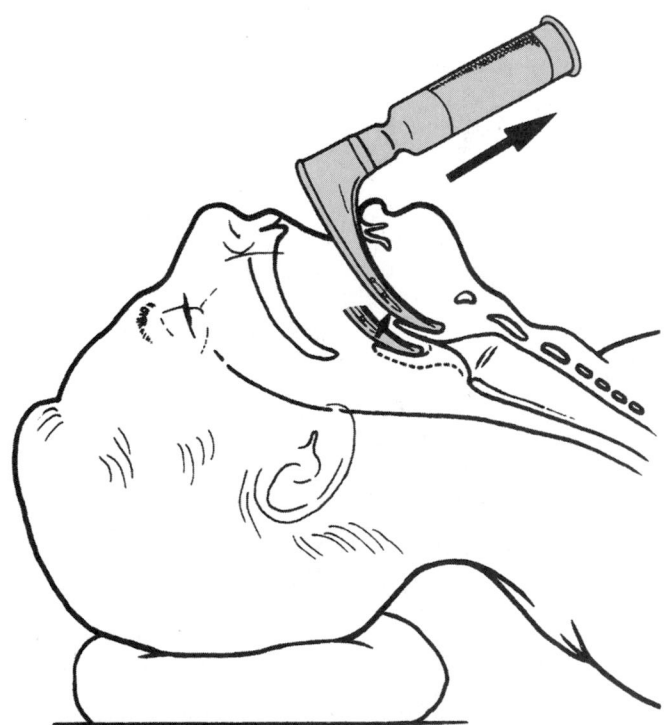

Figure 2.5. Intubation with the Macintosh blade. It is inserted into the vallecula to elevate the mandible, tongue, and epiglottis as a unit. (From Reichman EF, Simon RR. *Emergency medicine procedures*. New York: McGraw-Hill, 2004 with permission.)

pronounced in children because of their higher vagal tone. Pretreatment with atropine (0.02 mg/kg with minimum dose of 0.15 mg) in children younger than 6 years of age can avoid this. Increased intracranial pressure that is transient can occur as a result of the direct laryngoscopy. Direct mechanical complications from the laryngoscope include lacerations of the lips, trauma to the pharyngeal wall, broken teeth, or dentures that may be aspirated. Vomiting and aspiration can cause subsequent chemical and bacterial pneumonitis. Prolonged stimulation of the pharynx may cause apnea, bronchospasm, or laryngospasm.

Digital (Tactile) Orotracheal Intubation

Digital (tactile) intubation is a viable alternative airway management technique with which every practitioner of emergency medicine should be familiar (6). It is a rapid and safe method to intubate a patient. It is an ideal method for intubating a comatose or paralyzed patient if the patient's upper airway cannot be visualized because of secretions or blood. Digital intubation also should be considered when intubating the patient with a known or suspected cervical spine fracture because this technique requires minimal head and neck movement. It is also a variable method for out-of-hospital intubation. The main danger of this procedure is to the health care worker performing the intubation who is at risk for having his or her fingers bitten. This technique should only be performed on patients who are paralyzed or unconscious.

The intubator should stand to the patient's right side and be facing the patient. Insert the right index and middle fingers into the right side of the patient's mouth. Elevate the epiglottis with the index finger (Fig. 2.6). Insert the endotracheal tube into the patient's mouth between the two fingers and advance the tip into the trachea. Advance the endotracheal tube an additional 3 to 4 cm. Inflate the cuff, begin ventilation, confirm proper tube placement, and secure the tube.

Bullard Laryngoscope Intubation

The Bullard laryngoscope is a rigid structure composed of a handle, blade, stylet, and fiberoptic bundle. It allows for direct visualization of the vocal cords and endotracheal tube placement despite no direct line of sight (16). It may be used for routine and difficult intubations. This includes patients with congenital malformations, cervical spine immobilization, actual or potential cervical spine injuries, oromaxillofacial trauma, and trismus. It allows endotracheal tube placement with little manipulation of the cervical spine and minimal mouth opening. Its similarity in structure and use to traditional laryngoscopes make it easier to master and faster to use than flexible fiberoptic intubating bronchoscopes. Any proximal obstruction that would prevent passage of an endotracheal tube would preclude using the Bullard laryngoscope. The optical port may become obstructed by particulate matter, thick secretions, or vomitus, making visualization difficult. In these cases, a standard laryngoscope and a Yankauer tip attached to wall suction may be more appropriate.

Assemble the Bullard laryngoscope and apply an endotracheal tube. The intubator should stand at the head of the bed. The

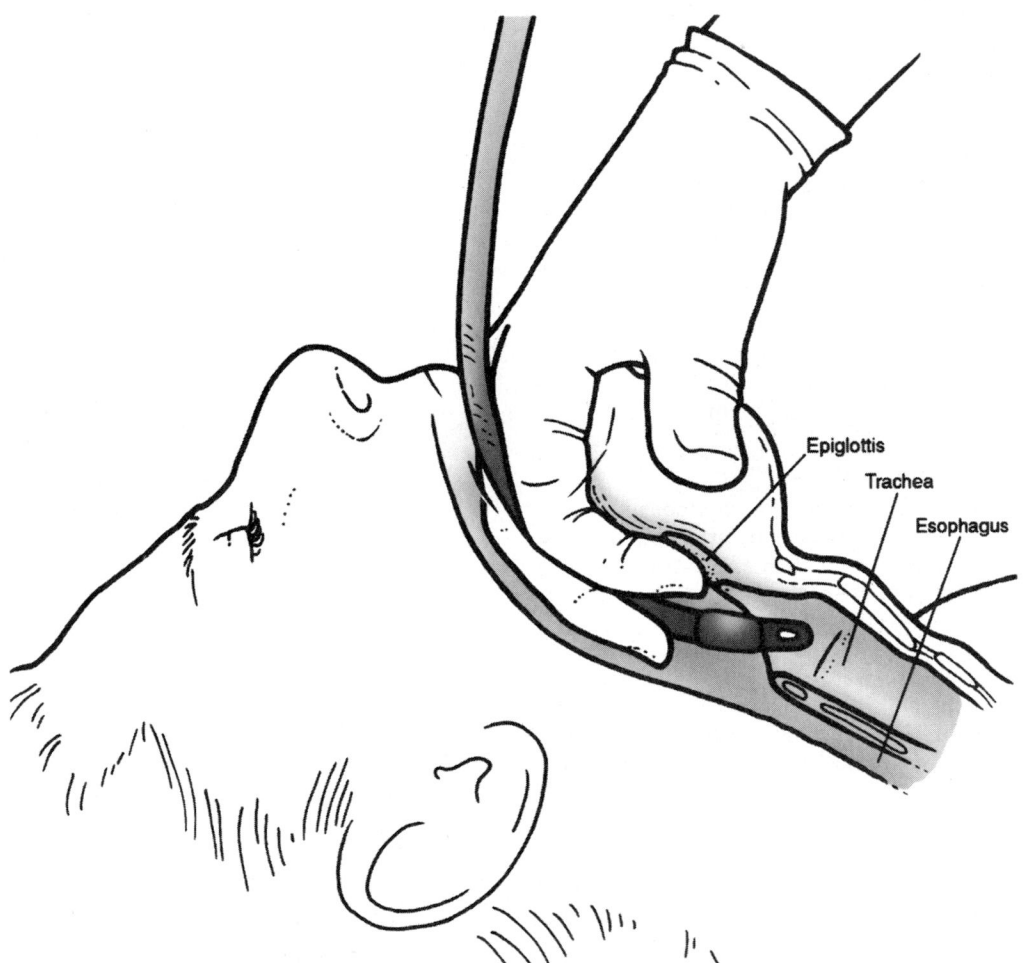

Figure 2.6.   Digital orotracheal intubation. (From Reichman EF, Simon RR. *Emergency medicine procedures.* New York: McGraw-Hill, 2004 with permission.)

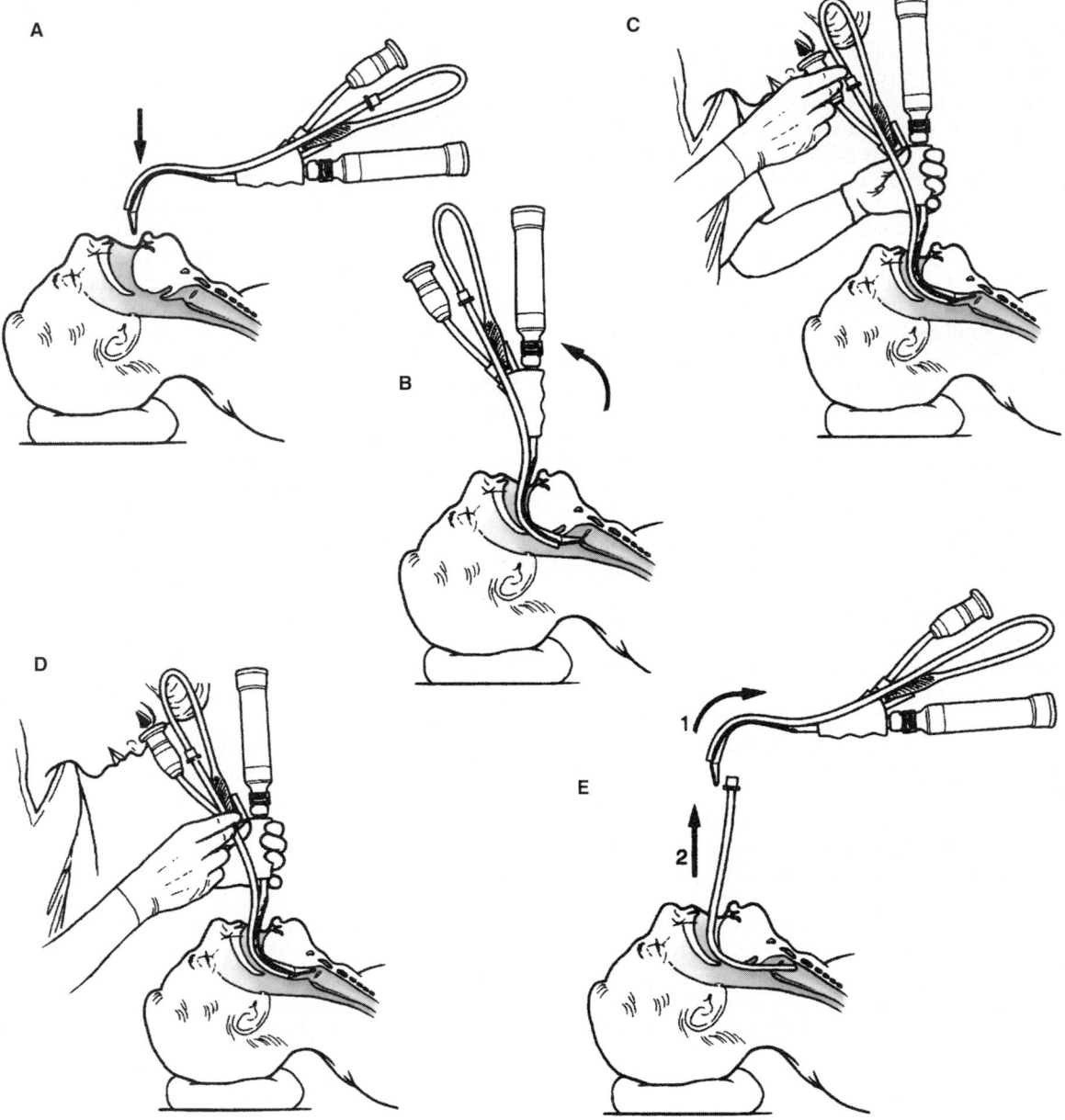

Figure 2.7.   Intubation with the Bullard laryngoscope. (From Reichman EF, Simon RR. *Emergency medicine procedures.* New York: McGraw-Hill, 2004 with permission.)

blade is introduced similar to that of an oral airway, rather than a traditional Macintosh blade. Hold the handle of the Bullard laryngoscope parallel to the patient and toward the patient's feet (Fig. 2.7A). Insert the blade directly into the center of the patient's mouth. Lift the laryngoscope handle upward (Fig. 2.7B). Slightly elevate the Bullard laryngoscope to lift up the tongue (Fig. 2.7C). Visualize the airway through the fiberoptic port. Advance the endotracheal tube under direct visualization (Fig. 2.7D). Securely hold the endotracheal tube at the patient's teeth. Remove the Bullard laryngoscope by reversing the technique of insertion (Fig. 2.7E).

The majority of complications mirror those of endotracheal intubation. Potential problems may arise that are specific to the Bullard laryngoscope (16). The vocal cords may not be visible if the view is obscured by blood, fluid, or vomitus. The loaded endotracheal tube may slip underneath the blade. The stylet may cause abrasions, bleeding, and lacerations to the walls of the oral cavity, oropharynx, and laryngopharynx. These can be prevented with proper assembly of the Bullard laryngoscope.

Lighted Stylet Intubation

The lighted stylet is an innovative alternative that provides a safe, rapid, relatively easy, and indirect approach for airways that cannot be easily visualized by direct laryngoscopy (3). The concept first appeared in the late 1950s. There are two models of lighted stylets available today. The Tube-Stat (Medtronic Xomed, Jacksonville, FL) is the simplest. It incorporates a stylet, power source, and light bulb in a single piece. The unit is inserted into the endotracheal tube in place of the stylet. The second available model is the Trachlight (Laerdal Medical Corporation, Wappingers Falls, NY). It is comprised of a battery-powered handle, the lightwand, and a separate stylet that inserts into the lightwand.

Light-guided intubation is primarily used in difficult airways when direct laryngoscopy is likely to fail. It is a blind and indirect technique that is particularly useful when anatomic variations prevent easy visualization of the vocal cords; the cervical spine is immobilized or its movement restricted; there is limited mobility of the jaw; there is significant maxillofacial trauma; in the presence of extensive dental work or loose teeth; or excess secretions impair direct visualization. Patients with laryngeal trauma should have direct laryngeal visualization for intubation rather than a blind technique that may cause additional trauma. As a blind technique, it should not be used if there is any active infection or known tumor of the posterior pharynx or upper airway. The presence of epiglottitis, retropharyngeal abscess, tracheal stenosis, laryngeal polyp or tumor, or airway foreign body precludes the use of this technology.

The trachea lies anterior to most structures of the neck and is covered anteriorly only by skin, subcutaneous tissue, and pretracheal fascia. A light source positioned within the trachea will transilluminate a bright and discrete glow that can be easily seen on the surface of the neck. In contrast, the esophagus lies posteriorly and is surrounded by numerous soft tissue structures. A light source directed within the pharynx and esophagus will be diffused by the surrounding tissue and appear dull. At the bedside, the examiner can easily discriminate between the dull, diffuse transillumination of an esophageal light source and the more discrete, intense signal transmitted from within the trachea. A submental, superior to the hyoid bone, glowing light indicates that the tip is positioned in the vallecula. A lateral glowing light indicates placement in the pyriform sinus.

The exact technique used depends on the type of lighted stylet or lightwand used. This text describes the general guidelines for the lighted stylets. Assemble the lighted stylet and check the light source. Load the endotracheal tube over the lighted stylet. Measure the mandibular–hyoid distance in the patient. Bend the tip of the endotracheal tube and stylet sharply (90 to 120 degrees) at a site that approximates the mandibular–hyoid distance between the bend and the junction of the lighted tip. The lighted stylet can be held in either hand. Lift upward and inferiorly to open the patient's jaw, elevate the tongue, and elevate the epiglottis. Grasp the lighted stylet with the dominant hand and turn it on.

Introduce the endotracheal tube from the side of the patient's mouth and bring it to the midline (Fig. 2.8A). Advance the tip by moving the handle in a vertical arc toward the patient's head (Fig. 2.8B). A bright light will be seen in the midline of the neck just below the hyoid bone. If the glowing light is malpositioned,

simply withdraw the endotracheal tube, reposition it in the midline, and advance it again. Advance the endotracheal tube while observing the transilluminating light march down the neck to the suprasternal notch (Fig. 2.8C). The light will disappear as the tube passes behind the suprasternal notch. Remove the lighted stylet, ventilate the patient, confirm proper tube positioning, and secure the tube.

Lighted intubating stylets are relatively free of complications. The literature cites a handful of complications over the last 30 years (3). This includes two reports of accidental bulb dislodgment, two arytenoid dislocations, one case of stylet fracture, a lacerated frenulum, and varied reports of mild soft-tissue trauma, sore throat, and hoarseness that are not statistically different than intubations done by direct laryngoscopy. Success rates with lighted stylet intubation are comparable with other techniques. The American Society of Anesthesiologists includes use of lighted stylets in its recommendations for management of difficult airways.

Esophageal–Tracheal Combitube Intubation

The Esophageal–Tracheal Combitube (ETC; Kendall Sheridan, Mansfield, MA) is a double-lumen, double-tubed, and double-cuffed airway device that can be blindly inserted into the unconscious and unresponsive patient (13). It is most often used in the prehospital setting by emergency medical technicians not trained in standard orotracheal intubation and by paramedic-level rescuers as an alternative when standard orotracheal intubation fails.

The ETC is inserted blindly into a patient's airway. If the distal tip enters the trachea, the patient is ventilated through the shorter tube and the distal cuff prevents aspiration of gastric contents into the trachea. If the distal tip enters the esophagus, the patient is ventilated through the longer tube whose proximal ports lie in the hypopharynx while the distal cuff will occlude the esophagus.

Certain contraindications exist and should be addressed. The ETC should not be used on patients with an intact gag reflex. The size limits of the standard ETC prevent its use in patients shorter than 5 feet in height. The smaller SA model can be used in shorter adults and adolescent patients from 4 to 5.5 feet in

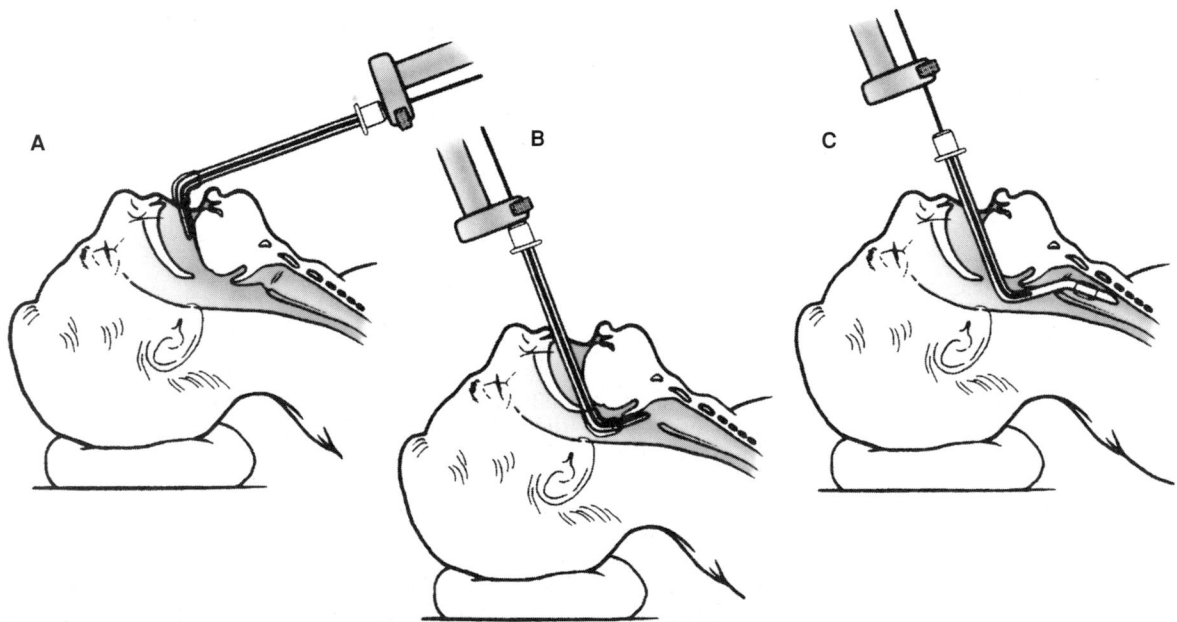

Figure 2.8. Intubation with the lighted stylet. (From Reichman EF, Simon RR. *Emergency medicine procedures.* New York: McGraw-Hill, 2004 with permission.)

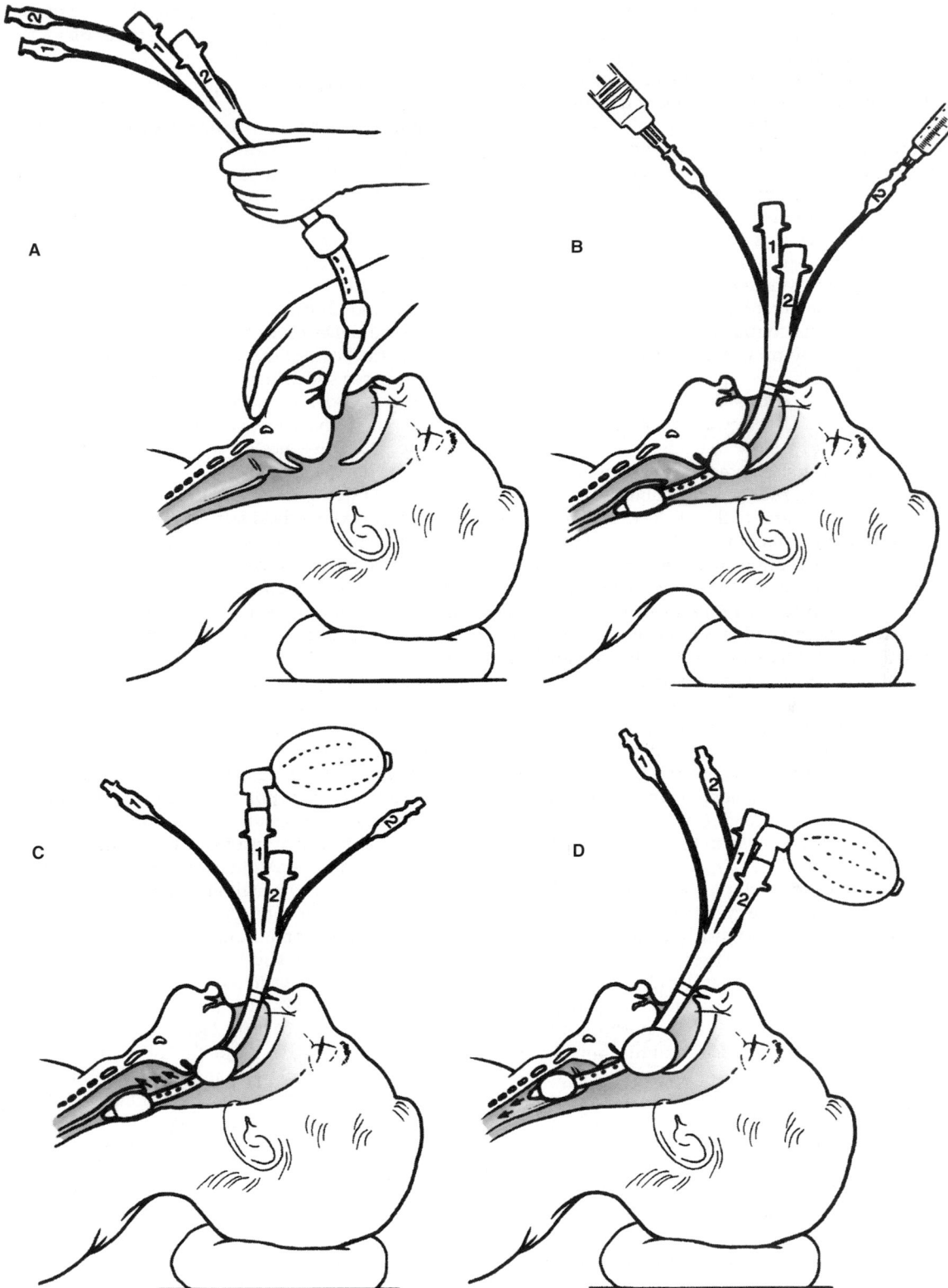

Figure 2.9. Intubation with the Esophageal–Tracheal Combitube. (From Reichman EF, Simon RR. *Emergency medicine procedures.* New York: McGraw-Hill, 2004 with permission.)

height. Neither model can be used in people shorter than 4 feet in height. The ETC is contraindicated if the patient has known esophageal disease or airway obstruction.

Insert the ETC into the midline of the patient's open mouth (Fig. 2.9A). Advance the ETC in a downward curved motion until the patient's teeth or alveolar ridge lie between the two printed bands (Fig. 2.9B). Inflate the pharyngeal cuff with air. The ECT

will slightly withdraw from the patient's mouth. Inflate the distal cuff with air.

Because most intubations are esophageal, begin ventilation through the longer blue tube labeled No. 1 (Fig. 2.9C). Auscultation of breath sounds, symmetric use of the chest, fogging in the tube for more than six breaths, and lack of gastric insufflation confirm placement within the esophagus and ventilation through the proximal ports (Fig. 2.9C). If no breath sounds are auscultated and gastric insufflation occurs, the trachea is intubated (Fig. 2.9D). Begin ventilation through the shorter clear tube and verify by auscultation the presence of breath sounds. Secure the ETC using the standard method of taping or a commercially available endotracheal tube holder.

Despite the potential utility of the ETC in acute situations, several disadvantages must be kept in mind (13), including its high cost and bulky packaging. A rigid cervical collar might cause great difficulties in the proper placement of this device. There is a risk of esophageal injury. There is no way to suction the trachea with the open distal port in the esophagus. It is important to note that resuscitation drugs that can be routinely given through an endotracheal tube cannot be given through the ETC positioned with the tip in the esophagus. Significant soft-tissue injury can occur as a consequence of the tip of the device or the balloons containing too much air.

Fiberoptic Endoscopic Intubation

The flexible fiberoptic bronchoscope has become a popular and useful instrument for placing endotracheal tubes in awake and nonparalyzed patients. It is unique in that its flexible cord allows it to conform to the patient's anatomy, making intubation possible in a variety of clinical situations when direct laryngoscopy is likely to be difficult or impossible. When performed properly, awake fiberoptic tracheal intubation is more accepted by patients and is associated with fewer hemodynamic changes than awake laryngoscopy. It may be used to orally or nasally intubate a patient (8). It provides excellent visualization of the airway.

A fiberoptic intubation is indicated when it is anticipated that a direct laryngoscopy might be difficult to perform as, for example, in morbidly obese patients; in patients with a limited mandibular opening, an unstable or immobile cervical spine, macroglossia, or micrognathia; in patients who appear to have pathologic airway anatomy (tracheal deviation, stenosis, tumors, trauma); and in patients who appear to be at increased risk for dental damage (4).

Proficiency in the skills required for fiberoptic intubation requires both instruction and practice. In most instances, it is a lack of expertise with the fiberoptic bronchoscope that results in technical problems and inadequate patient preparation, and prevents the successful completion of fiberoptic intubation. Successful intubation is also prevented by blood or secretions obstructing the fiberoptic port. Patients who are hypoxic or require assisted ventilation by mask are poor candidates. Contraindications specific to nasal fiberoptic intubation include coagulopathy, significant midface trauma, severe intranasal pathology, cribriform plate fracture, and cerebrospinal fluid leak.

Prepare the fiberoptic bronchoscope. Apply antifog solution to the insertion cord tip or place the tip in warm water. Apply a thin film of silicone spray or water-soluble lubricant over the insertion cord. Insert the flexible insertion cord completely through the endotracheal tube.

Insert and navigate the insertion cord tip through the nose or mouth until the glottic opening comes into view. Advance the fiberoptic bronchoscope tip toward and past the vocal cords. Advance the insertion cord tip further to bring the bifurcation of the trachea at the carina into view. Advance the endotracheal tube over the fiberoptic bronchoscope and into the trachea. Securely hold the endotracheal tube and remove the bronchoscope. Inflate the endotracheal tube cuff, begin ventilation, confirm proper tube placement, and secure the tube.

While the fiberscope is passed through the glottis and into the trachea under direct vision, the tracheal tube is passed blindly over the fiberoptic bronchoscope tip. It is possible to cause injury to the arytenoids. The endotracheal tube may also be blocked in the nasal cavity or larynx, resulting in epistaxis, nasal turbinate fracture, and tearing of the tracheal tube cuff.

Nasotracheal Intubation

Nasotracheal intubation is an alternative to orotracheal intubation to secure an airway in the spontaneously breathing patient (12). It allows awake intubations while the patient maintains protective airway reflexes and avoids the risks of paralytic agents. It is a fairly simple procedure that should be considered in patients with spontaneous respirations in whom an oral airway is considered difficult and in those with an anticipated short intubation period. Nasotracheal intubation is well tolerated by most patients and produces less reflex salivation than orotracheal intubation, thus leading to fewer attempts of self-extubating.

Nasotracheal intubation is contraindicated in patients with apnea, severe facial, or maxillofacial fractures, basilar skull fractures, head injury with an elevated intracranial pressure, nasal or nasopharyngeal obstruction, patients receiving thrombolytics, the presence of a coagulopathy, or those receiving parenteral anticoagulants. It is also contraindicated in patients with neck injuries as the procedure may increase morbidity and mortality. Nasotracheal intubation should not be performed in neonates, infants, and young children.

Prepare for the procedure. Apply a topical vasoconstrictor to shrink the nasal mucosa. Apply a topical anesthetic to the nasal mucosa. Dilate the nasal passage with your little finger or a series of increasingly larger size nasopharyngeal airways. Choose an endotracheal tube. The proper size tube should be at least 0.5 to 1.0 mm smaller than the size chosen for orotracheal intubation of the same patient.

Insert the endotracheal tube into the nostril with the bevel facing the septum (Fig. 2.10A). Advance the endotracheal tube with gentle pressure along the nasal floor to pass it through the nasal cavity (Fig. 2.10B). Continue advancing the tube as resistance is met while the tube makes a 90-degree change of direction into the oropharynx. Advance the endotracheal tube through the oropharynx and into the laryngopharynx (Fig. 2.10C). Listen for breath sounds through the proximal end of the endotracheal tube while advancing it. As soon as an exhalation is heard, the patient will take a breath and advance the endotracheal tube during inhalation. The vocal cords are opened their widest during inspiration, which facilitates passage of the endotracheal tube. Inflate the cuff (Fig. 2.10D), begin ventilation, confirm proper positioning, and secure the endotracheal tube.

The immediate complications of nasotracheal intubation include epistaxis, laryngeal and tracheal trauma, mucosal avulsion, retropharyngeal laceration, turbinate avulsion, intracranial placement, bacteremia, esophageal intubation, and prolonged attempts to place the tube. Many of these can be prevented by choosing the appropriate-size endotracheal tube, nasal mucosal vasoconstriction, and the liberal application of lubricant to the endotracheal tube. Long-term complications include maxillary sinusitis, retropharyngeal abscess, mediastinitis, nasal mucosal necrosis, and cellulitis.

Retrograde Guidewire Intubation

Retrograde guidewire intubation is an alternative airway management technique that should be familiar to those involved with emergency airway management (5). It should be considered in any patient in whom endotracheal intubation may be difficult, contraindicated, or has failed. It is useful when bleeding obstructs visualization of the glottis. The major contraindication to retrograde intubation is the ability to control the airway with less-invasive techniques. Other contraindications include an anterior neck mass, infectious or cancerous process overlying the

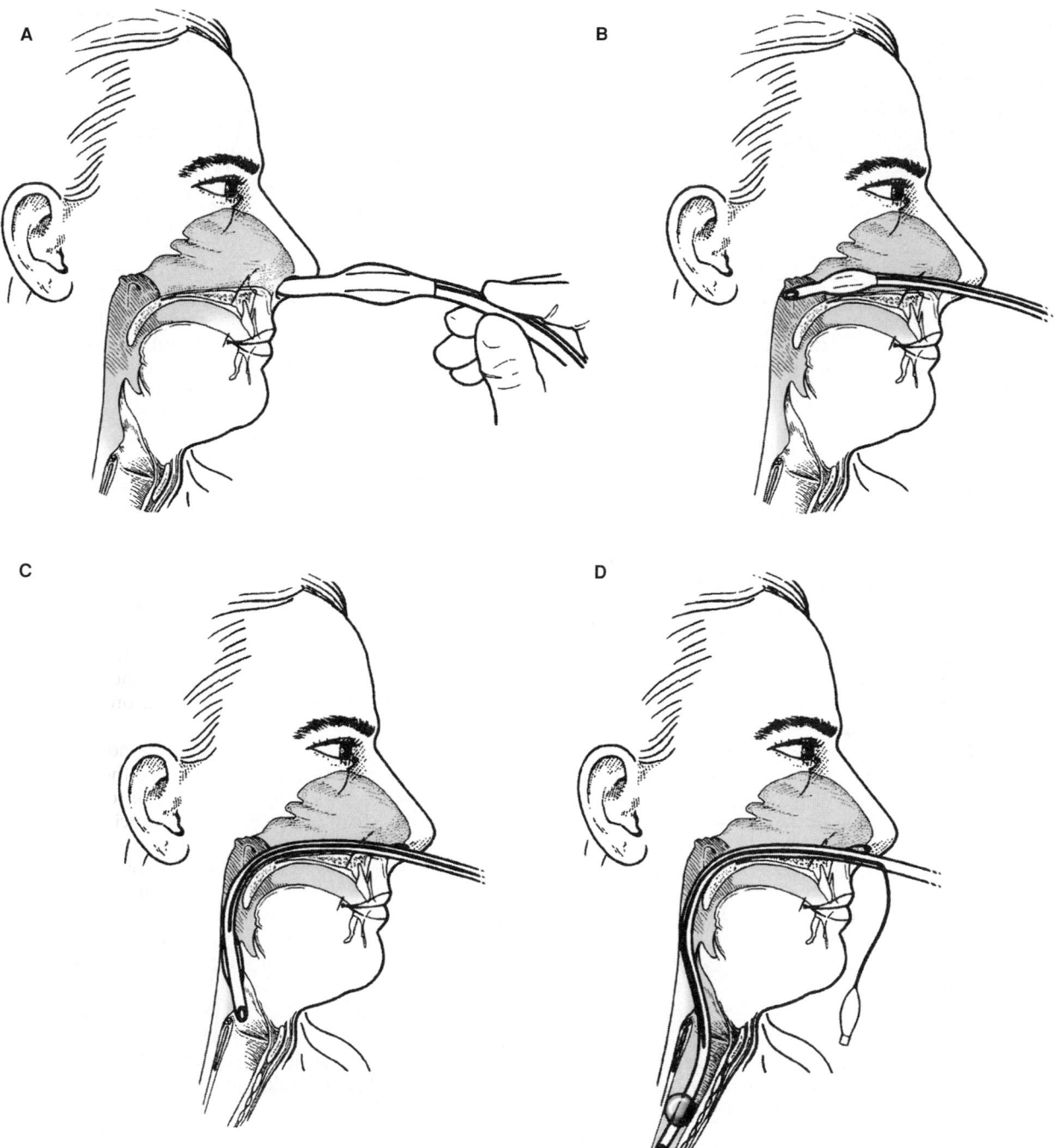

Figure 2.10.   Nasotracheal intubation. (From Reichman EF, Simon RR. *Emergency medicine procedures.* New York: McGraw-Hill, 2004 with permission.)

cricothyroid membrane, or trismus. Apneic patients who cannot be ventilated with a bag-valve-mask device should receive a cricothyrotomy.

The procedure is relatively simple in theory but difficult to perform "in the heat of battle" (5). Stabilize the patient's larynx and identify the cricothyroid membrane. Insert a 16- to 18-gauge catheter-over-the-needle at a 20- to 30-degree angle upward and through the cricothyroid membrane (Fig. 2.11A). Advance the guidewire through the catheter, into the oropharynx, and out of the mouth (Fig. 2.11B). Carefully remove the catheter while firmly holding the guidewire in place. Pass the introducer catheter over the guidewire guide, exiting the mouth until the tip is inside the cricothyroid membrane (Fig. 2.11C). Advance the well-lubricated endotracheal tube over the intro-

ducer and guidewire (Fig. 2.11D). Securely hold the endotracheal tube and simultaneously withdraw the guidewire and introducer catheter while advancing the endotracheal tube into the trachea (Fig. 2.11E). Inflate the endotracheal tube cuff, begin ventilation, confirm proper placement, and secure the tube. The patient should receive standard wound care and dressing of the neck skin entrance site.

Complications of retrograde guidewire intubation include those of standard endotracheal intubation. Complications can occur from the needle traversing the cricothyroid membrane. Hypoxia caused by prolonged intubation time or incorrect endotracheal tube placement remains an important complication. Retrograde intubation carries additional complications as a consequence of use of the guidewire.

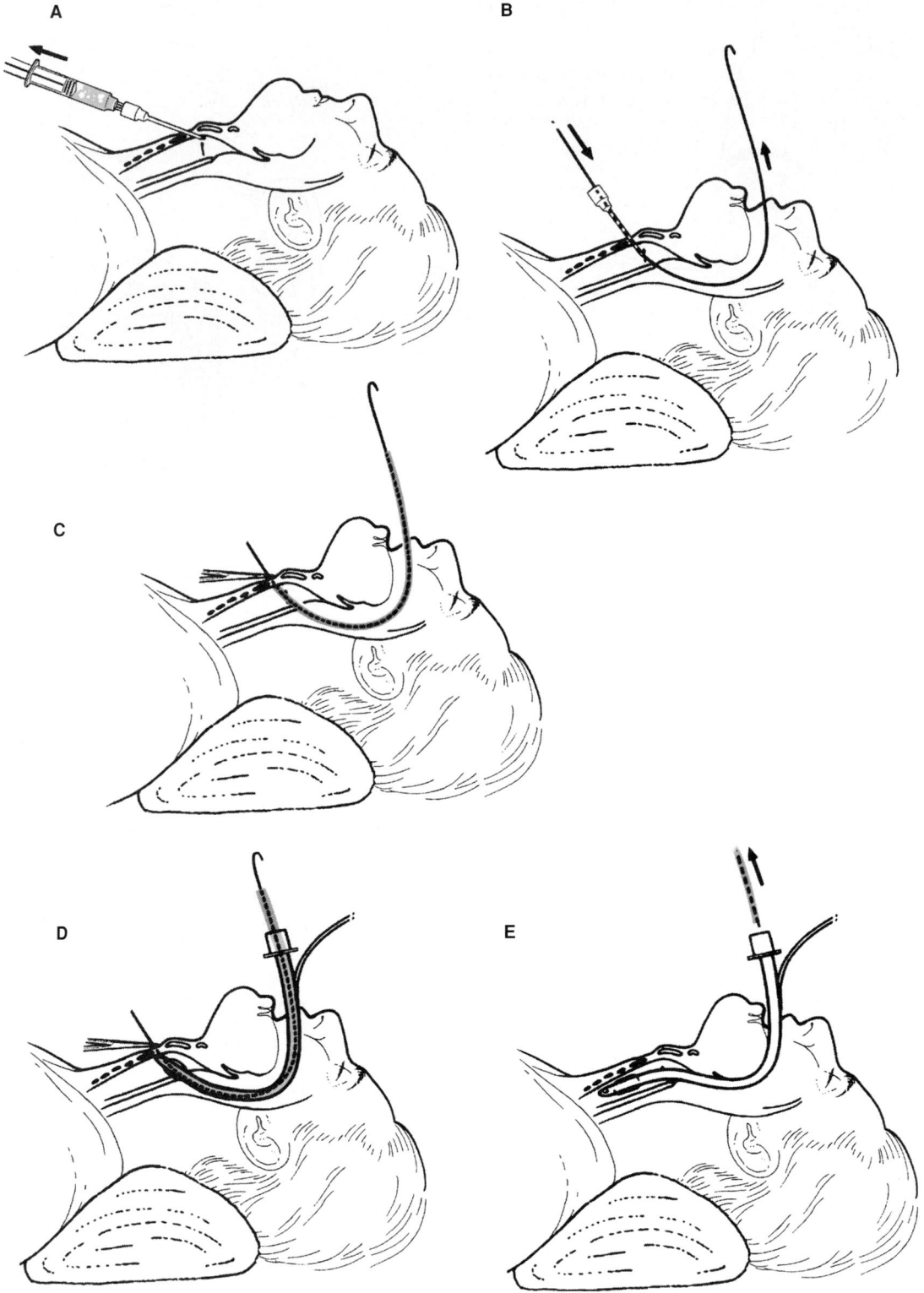

Figure 2.11.   Retrograde guidewire intubation. (From Reichman EF, Simon RR. *Emergency medicine procedures.* New York: McGraw-Hill, 2004 with permission.)

Laryngeal Mask Airway and Intubating Laryngeal Mask Airway

The laryngeal mask airway (LMA) is a novel device, which fills the gap in airway management between that of endotracheal intubation and the use of a face mask (9). The LMA was designed primarily as a means of providing ventilatory support while avoiding the fundamental disadvantage of the need to visualize and penetrate the vocal cords with an endotracheal tube. The LMA is blindly introduced into the hypopharynx to form a low-pressure seal around the laryngeal inlet and to permit positive pressure ventilation.

Many disadvantages of the standard LMA became apparent with widespread use of the device. The intubating laryngeal mask airway (ILMA) was developed through the aid of analysis of magnetic resonance images of the human pharynx and laboratory testing of endotracheal tubes (4).

The indications for the use of the LMA and the ILMA parallel the general indications for active airway management. Either the LMA or the ILMA may be used in the event of failed endotracheal intubation. They have a role in securing the airway preemptively in patients with an "anteriorly" situated larynx. However, there is a conspicuous absence of airway protection from aspiration.

There are no absolute contraindications to the use of either the LMA or the ILMA. However, there are several relative contraindications, including patients at an increased risk of regurgitation or aspiration; with airway obstruction at or below the larynx; with low pulmonary compliance or high airway resistance (morbidly obese, bronchospasm, pulmonary edema, pulmonary fibrosis or thoracic trauma); and who cannot open their mouth at least 1.5 cm. It is relatively contraindicated in cases of pharyngeal pathology. This includes, but is not limited to, abscesses, hematomas, or tissue disruptions.

The LMA is a disposable unit that conforms to the contours of the hypopharynx with its lumen facing the glottic opening (Fig. 2.12). It consists of an airway tube, inflation line, and mask. The technique for inserting the LMA is rather simple (9). Position the patient's head as for endotracheal intubation in the "sniffing" position. Insert and advance the LMA into the oral cavity in one smooth movement following the curvature of the pharynx until it enters the hypopharynx until resistance is felt. Inflate the cuff with the recommended volume of air. When correctly positioned, the tip of the LMA cuff lies at the base of the hypopharynx against the upper esophageal sphincter, the sides lie in the pyriform fossae, and the upper border of the mask lies at the base of the tongue, pushing it forward (Fig. 2.12). Secure the LMA in fashion similar to that used to secure an endotracheal tube.

The form of the ILMA was derived from head and neck sagittal magnetic resonance imaging studies. It consists of an anatomically curved steel tube connected to the standard LMA cuff. The ILMA has several significant modifications that make it different from the LMA. This includes a stainless steel airway tube covered with silicone rubber, a handle fused to the airway tube, a larger inner diameter (13 mm vs. 9 mm) than the LMA. The mask of the ILMA is similar to that of the LMA with two major modifications. A ramp inside the distal airway tube directs an endotracheal tube into the center of the aperture and into the

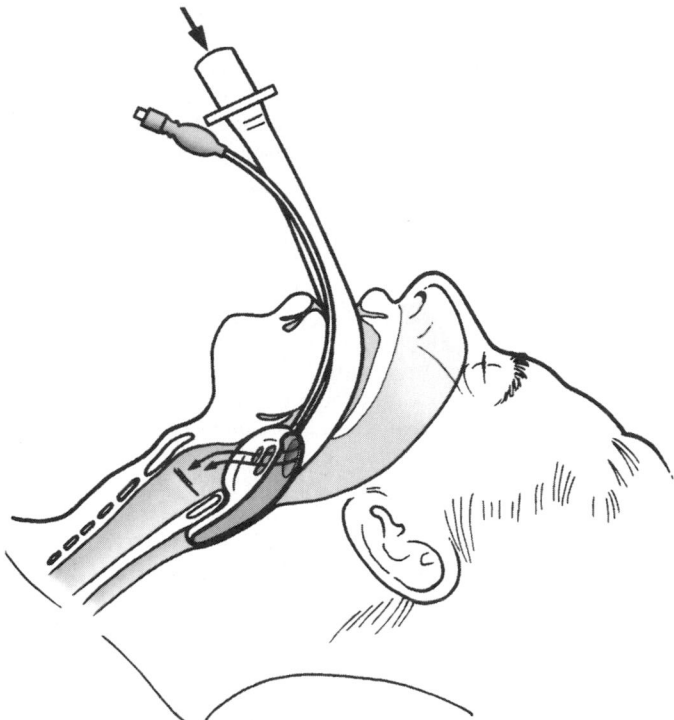

Figure 2.12.   Sagittal view of the airway demonstrating correct placement of the laryngeal mask airway. (From Reichman EF, Simon RR. *Emergency medicine procedures*. New York: McGraw-Hill, 2004 with permission.)

patient's airway. It has a large, single, and stiff epiglottic elevating bar designed to lift the epiglottis away from the path of the advancing endotracheal tube.

The insertion of the ILMA is not too dissimilar from the standard LMA (9). Confirm proper placement of the ILMA with a bag-valve device attached to the proximal end of the airway tube and ventilate the patient. The ILMA may be left like this (Fig. 2.13A). Alternatively, an endotracheal tube can be inserted through the ILMA and into the trachea (Fig. 2.13B).

There are numerous documented complications associated with the use of the LMA and ILMA. An obvious complication, and potentially the most devastating, is the failure to successfully

A   **B**

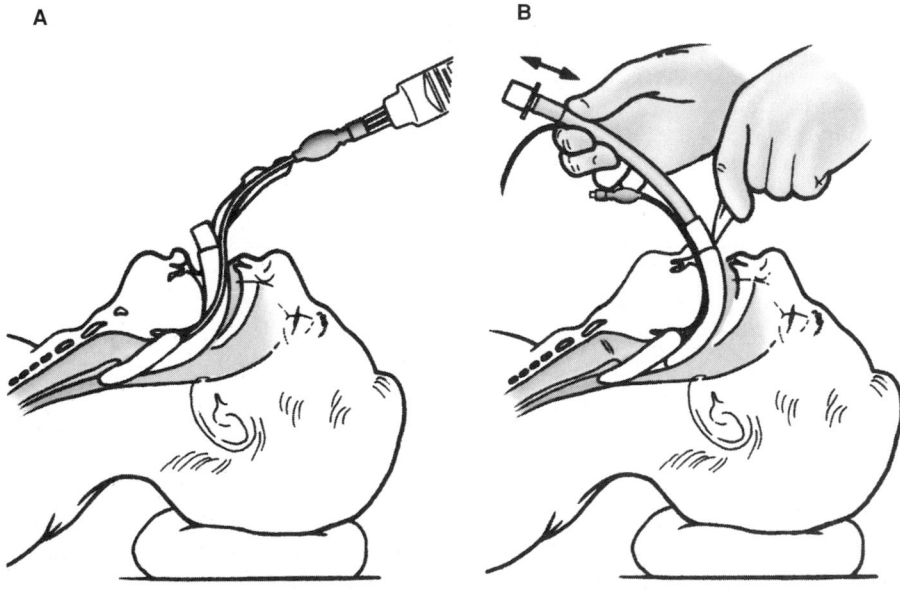

Figure 2.13.   Insertion of the intubating laryngeal mask airway. (From Reichman EF, Simon RR. *Emergency medicine procedures*. New York: McGraw-Hill, 2004 with permission.)

place the device or to attain a satisfactory laryngeal seal. The incidence of failure to attain satisfactory ventilation is quite low. Other complications include aspiration, cuff herniation, contusions, lingual nerve injury, tongue numbness, parotid gland swelling, hypoglossal nerve palsy, unilateral vocal cord paralysis, dental trauma, laryngospasm, bronchospasm, and cardiac arrhythmias.

Percutaneous Transtracheal Jet Ventilation

Percutaneous transtracheal jet ventilation (PTTJV) provides emergency ventilatory support in patients who cannot be adequately ventilated with a bag-valve-mask device (with oral or nasal airways) or endotracheally intubated (2). This includes patients with upper airway foreign bodies or neoplasms, maxillofacial trauma, laryngeal edema, or infection. Placement of a catheter through the cricothyroid membrane and attached to a high-pressure oxygen source will provide adequate oxygenation and ventilation until a more definite airway can be established. This is a rapidly performed airway management technique that should be considered as a backup rescue technique.

PTTJV serves as a simple, relatively safe, and effective alternative to cricothyrotomy (2). This is especially true in pediatric patients who are younger than 5 years of age in whom a cricothyrotomy is contraindicated. PTTJV has a large number of advantages when compared with an emergent cricothyrotomy. It is easier and faster to perform. The technique is simpler to learn. The need for a large number of instruments, surgical preparation and technique, and an assistant is eliminated. The complications of bleeding, glottic stenosis, subglottic stenosis, and tracheal erosion are significantly lessened. If the patient survives, PTTJV causes less cosmetic disfigurement. Finally, PTTJV can direct secretions and foreign bodies out of the proximal trachea.

PTTJV is contraindicated in patients that can be orally or nasally intubated. Anterior neck trauma is a relative contraindication to PTTJV. Lower tracheal or proximal bronchial tree disruption can result in an increased risk of pneumothorax and pneumomediastinum with high-pressure ventilation. Complete airway obstruction is an absolute contraindication to PTTJV.

Stand at the side of the bed and adjacent to the patient's head and neck. Identify the cricothyroid membrane. Attach a 12- to 16-gauge catheter-over-the-needle to a 10 mL syringe containing 5 mL of sterile saline. Insert the catheter-over-the-needle through the cricothyroid membrane, directed inferiorly and at a 30- to 45-degree angle (Fig. 2.14A). Apply negative pressure within the syringe and advance it until air bubbles are visible in the syringe and a loss of resistance is felt (Fig. 2.14B). Hold the needle and syringe stationary while advancing the catheter until the hub is against the skin and then remove the needle and syringe (Fig. 2.14C). Attach high-pressure-oxygen tubing to the catheter (Fig. 2.14D) and begin ventilation until a definitive airway is established.

Complications are fewer than with a cricothyrotomy, but they do occur and must be anticipated. Subcutaneous emphysema occurs most commonly when the transtracheal catheter is misplaced, becomes dislodged into the soft tissues of the neck during ventilation, or is against the mucosa of the posterior tracheal wall. Barotrauma may present as a pneumothorax, pneumomediastinum, or pneumopericardium. Catheter obstruction or misplacement and pulmonary aspiration are other potential complications.

Cricothyrotomy

Cricothyrotomy is a technique that has been in use since the early 1900s. It has evolved into the surgical airway of choice for emergent situations in which other less-invasive intubation methods

have failed or are contraindicated (11). There are numerous advantages to performing a cricothyrotomy over a tracheostomy. A cricothyrotomy is easier, faster, and safer to perform. It can be performed in less than 2 minutes. It can be performed by those with little to no surgical training. It does not require the support of an operating room and a large amount of equipment. The anatomic landmarks are superficial, easily seen, and palpated. It does not require a deep dissection. The cricothyroid membrane is not covered by any structures that would interfere with the procedure. A cricothyrotomy can be performed with the neck in a neutral position. The procedure has fewer associated complications than a tracheostomy.

There are a few absolute contraindications to performing a cricothyrotomy. The most important is if the patient can be endotracheally intubated by less-invasive methods. Partial or complete transection of the airway is a contraindication to a cricothyrotomy. In these cases, a tracheostomy is the preferred method to secure the airway. Finally, it should not be performed in cases of significant injury or fracture of the cricoid cartilage, larynx, and/or thyroid cartilage. Relative contraindications to performing a cricothyrotomy are the presence of a coagulopathy, massive neck swelling, or a hematoma in the neck, which all increase the risk of bleeding and distortion of the anatomy.

Stabilize the large thyroid cartilage. The immobilization of the larynx cannot be overemphasized. If the larynx is not secure and thus the landmarks are lost, the procedure will fail. Identify the anatomic landmarks necessary to perform this procedure. This is critical to the performance of a cricothyrotomy.

There are numerous techniques to perform a cricothyrotomy (11). The surgical techniques require a skin incision carried down through the cricothyroid membrane (Fig. 2.15A). This is followed by grasping the thyroid cartilage with a tracheal hook to control the airway (Fig. 2.15B). The tract is dilated (Fig. 2.15C) and a tracheostomy tube or endotracheal tube is inserted into the trachea (Fig. 2.15D). A percutaneous kit is available and uses a modified Seldinger technique to perform a cricothyrotomy. A needle cricothyrotomy is performed in children, instead of the surgical approach. The technique is similar to percutaneous transtracheal jet ventilation.

Complications following a cricothyrotomy can be classified as early or late based on when they occur. Early complications will be recognized either immediately after insertion of the tracheostomy tube or within a few hours. These include malposition, laryngeal injury, bleeding, and infection. Late complications may not be apparent for weeks to months following the procedure. These include progressive airway obstruction and chronic voice changes.

Cricothyrotomy is a potentially life-saving technique. It is an important procedure for the emergency physician to be skilled in because it may represent the only access to the patient's airway. It can be used to provide oxygenation and ventilation to a patient when other less-invasive airway control methods have failed or are contraindicated. It is a relatively safe, simple, and reliable procedure that can be performed within a few minutes. Knowledge of the anatomy of the anterior neck is essential to minimize early complications.

Tracheostomy

The tracheostomy is an ancient and time-honored technique for securing and maintaining an artificial airway. Modern emergency physicians have many options for airway management (15). They are skilled in a variety of invasive, noninvasive, and surgical procedures to optimize the management of a patient's airway. The role of tracheostomy for emergent airway access has diminished as newer, safer, and equally effective techniques have evolved. Familiarity with the methods for tracheostomy,

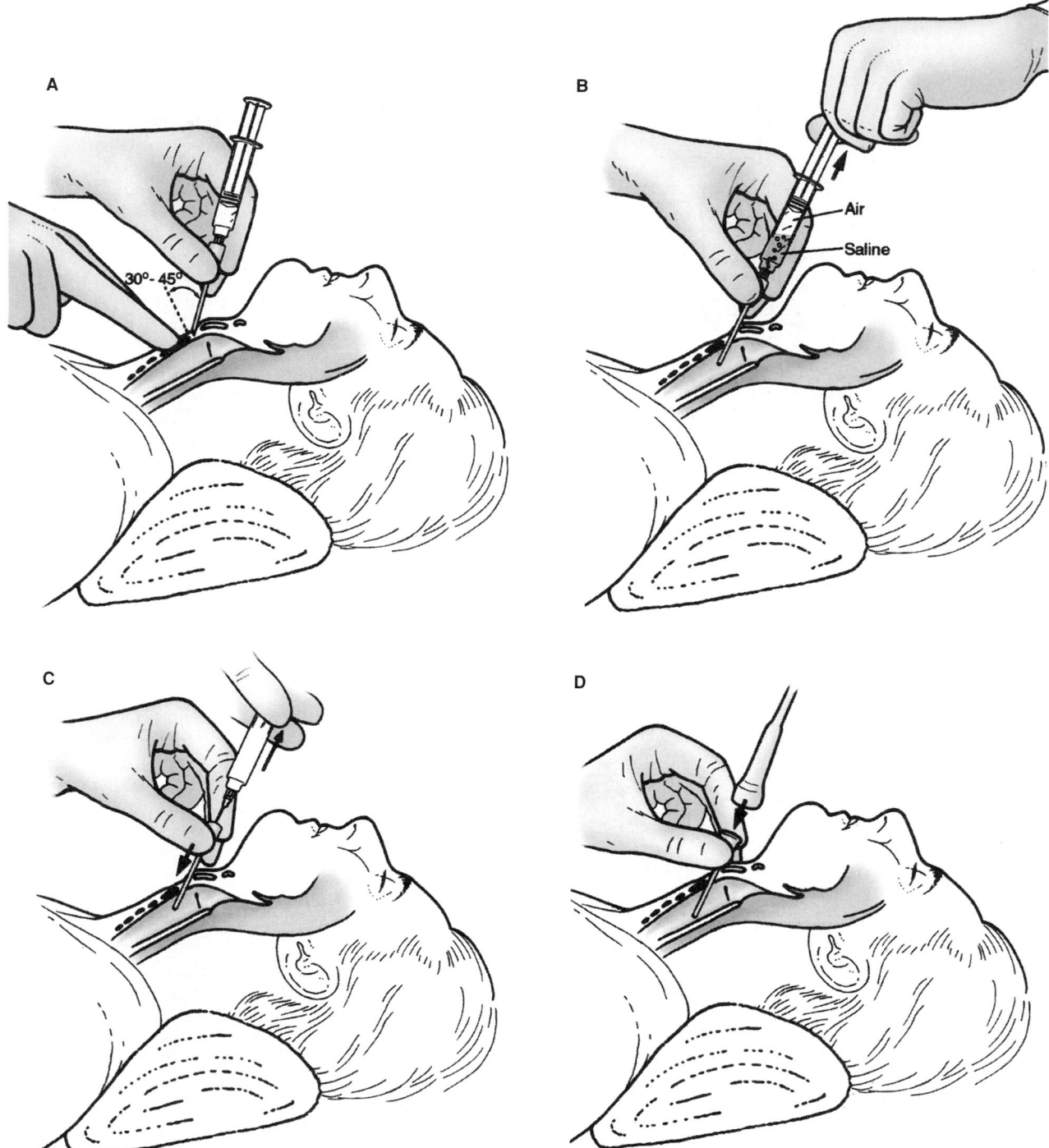

Figure 2.14. Percutaneous transtracheal jet ventilation. (From Reichman EF, Simon RR. *Emergency medicine procedures.* New York: McGraw-Hill, 2004 with permission.)

however, is still valuable (4). Knowledge of proper techniques, possible indications, limitations, and likely complications will guide one's judgment in critical moments when it most counts. Understanding the procedure for a tracheostomy allows emergency physicians to properly care for a problem or complication when a patient with a tracheostomy tube presents to the emergency department.

When performed under emergency circumstances, it is fraught with danger. There are only three clinical settings in which emergency tracheostomy should be considered (4). The first is laryngotracheal injuries with airway disruption. The second is the need for a surgical airway in an infant or small child where a cricothyrotomy is contraindicated. The third is the need for an airway when all other methods have failed.

Cricothyrotomy is the procedure of choice when an invasive approach to the trachea is needed. Compared with tracheostomy, the cricothyrotomy is faster, more direct, relies predominantly on external landmarks, requires only a single operator, can be done with ambient lighting, and requires a limited amount of equipment. In contrast, tracheostomy is a procedure requiring multiple steps. It involves direct visualization to dissect through vascular structures and requires better light than is commonly present at the bedside. It is easier, and thus faster, if one has an assistant, proper suctioning equipment, and electrocautery.

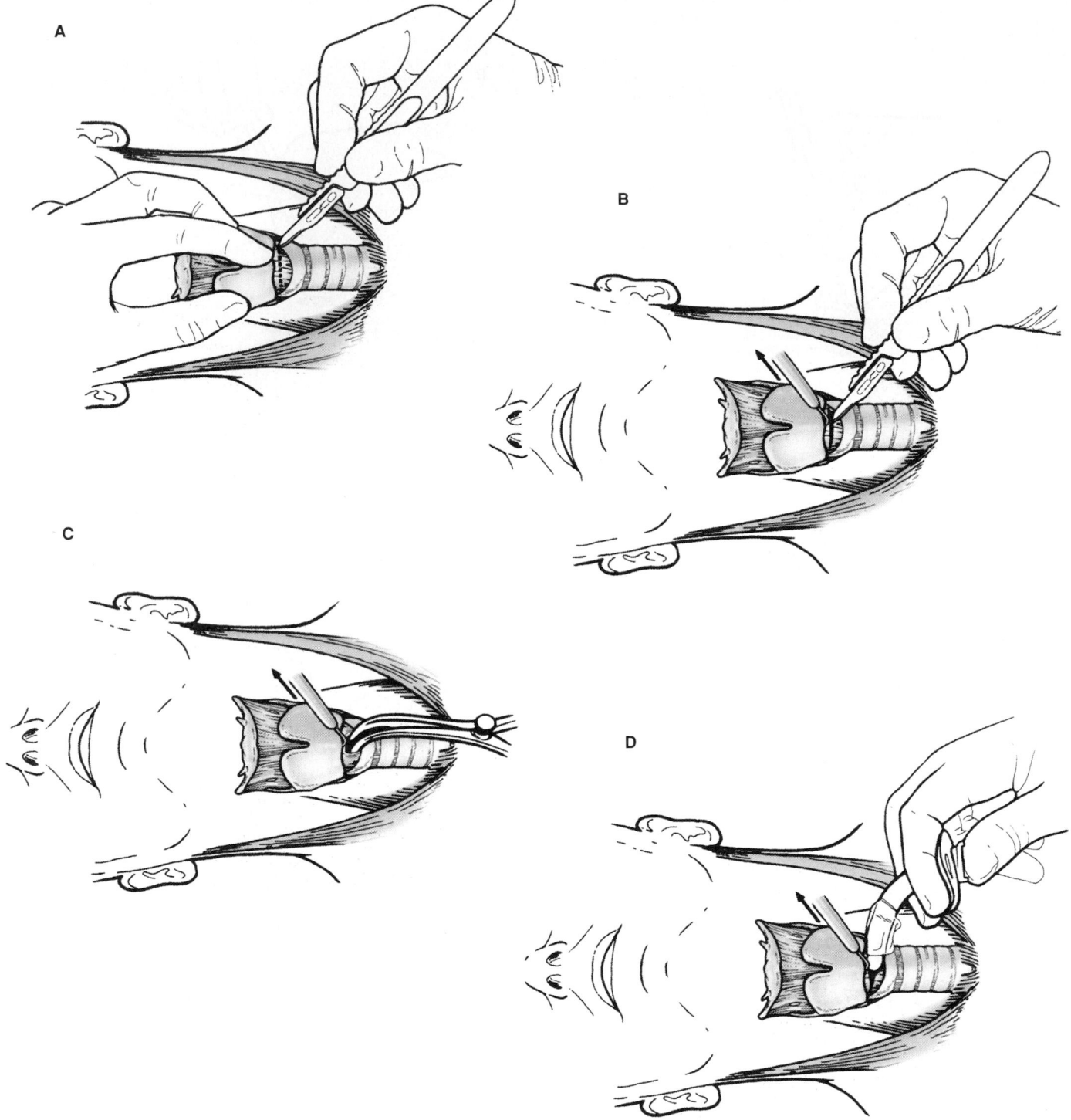

Figure 2.15.   Cricothyrotomy. (From Reichman EF, Simon RR. *Emergency medicine procedures.* New York: McGraw-Hill, 2004 with permission.)

Without these advantages, the technique is difficult and likely to be complicated. The average time to establish an airway by tracheostomy is too long for the true emergency in a patient who lacks an airway.

DISPOSITION

Almost all patients who require the airway management techniques as described in this chapter will be admitted to an intensive care unit setting. The patient who is intoxicated, has taken too much medication, or used illicit substances may be the exception to admission.

COMMON PITFALLS

✔ Proper patient positioning is very basic but often overlooked
✔ Simple maneuvers using the jaw thrust, chin lift, nasopharyngeal airways, or oral airways can prevent hypoxia and hypercarbia in the apneic patient
✔ Orotracheal intubation is the airway of choice

✔ The emergency physician must know several alternative techniques for airway management when orotracheal intubation fails or is contraindicated

✔ The cricothyrotomy is the preferred surgical airway in an emergency

References

1. Bird DJ, Markey JR. Basic airway management. In: Reichman EF, Simon RR, eds. *Emergency medicine procedures.* New York: McGraw-Hill, 2004:10–18.
2. Cabel JR. Percutaneous transtracheal jet ventilation. In: Reichman EF, Simon RR, eds. *Emergency medicine procedures.* New York: McGraw-Hill, 2004:94–100.
3. Cosby KS. Lighted stylet intubation. In: Reichman EF, Simon RR, eds. *Emergency medicine procedures.* New York: McGraw-Hill, 2004:58–64.
4. Cosby KS. Tracheostomy. In: Reichman EF, Simon RR, eds. *Emergency medicine procedures.* New York: McGraw-Hill, 2004:118–132.
5. Gimbel R, Petri R. Retrograde guidewire intubation. In: Reichman EF, Simon RR, eds. *Emergency medicine procedures.* New York: McGraw-Hill, 2004:87–93.
6. Ma OJ, Hoffmann ME. Digital (tactile) orotracheal intubation. In: Reichman EF, Simon RR, eds. *Emergency medicine procedures.* New York: McGraw-Hill, 2004:49–51.
7. Mallampati SR, Gugino LD, Desai SP, et al. A clinical sign to predict difficult tracheal intubation: a prospective study. *Can Anaesth Soc J* 1985;32(4):429–434.
8. Markey JR, Bird DJ. Fiberoptic endoscopic intubation. In: Reichman EF, Simon RR, eds. *Emergency medicine procedures.* New York: McGraw-Hill, 2004:71–79.
9. Meeks SL, Candido KD. Laryngeal mask airways. In: Reichman EF, Simon RR, eds. *Emergency medicine procedures.* New York: McGraw-Hill, 2004:141–153.
10. Morocco M, Reichman EF. Orotracheal intubation. In: Reichman EF, Simon RR, eds. *Emergency medicine procedures.* New York: McGraw-Hill, 2004:37–48.
11. Nagy K. Cricothyrotomy. In: Reichman EF, Simon RR, eds. *Emergency medicine procedures.* New York: McGraw-Hill, 2004:101–117.
12. Nasr IF, Nasr NF. Nasotracheal intubation. In: Reichman EF, Simon RR, eds. *Emergency medicine procedures.* New York: McGraw-Hill, 2004:80–86.
13. Pearlman K, Cromwell HH. Esophageal—Tracheal Combitube intubation. In: Reichman EF, Simon RR, eds. *Emergency medicine procedures.* New York: McGraw-Hill, 2004:65–70.
14. Pedicini EL, Candido KD, Nasr NF. Essential anatomy of the airway. In: Reichman EF, Simon RR, eds. *Emergency medicine procedures.* New York: McGraw-Hill, 2004:3–9.
15. Reichman EF, Simon RR, eds. *Emergency medicine procedures.* New York: McGraw-Hill, 2004.
16. Schubel PT, Reichman EF. Bullard laryngoscope intubation. In: Reichman EF, Simon RR, eds. *Emergency medicine procedures.* New York: McGraw-Hill, 2004: 52–57.

CHAPTER 3
Cardiopulmonary Arrest

Christopher Ross and Theresa M. Schwab

The triad of unconsciousness, apnea and pulselessness defines cardiopulmonary arrest. The majority of patients who die suddenly of natural causes succumb primarily to cardiac disorders. It is estimated that more than 500,000 of the 2 million nontraumatic deaths per year that occur in the United States are caused by sudden cardiac death (SCD) (27,36). SCD is defined as an unexpected natural death from a cardiac cause that occurs instantaneously or within 1 hour from the onset of an abrupt change in clinical status in a person without a prior condition that would appear to be fatal (14,42).

Resuscitation was described more than 100 years ago. It was only in the late 1950s that closed-chest cardiac massage, mouth-to-mouth ventilation, and electrical defibrillation were incorporated into practice guidelines in an attempt to improve survival (36,43,59). Although advances in emergency medical services and in the field of resuscitation have occurred, the rate of survival of cardiac arrest victims that are neurologically intact remains a dismal 3% to 8% (37). The concept of extending treatment into the community is a fairly new phenomenon. In the 1970s was it demonstrated that advanced cardiac life support (ACLS) by trained paramedics could significantly improve resuscitation and survival in patients suffering cardiac arrest (15). Training laypersons in the community to deliver cardiopulmonary resuscitation (CPR) has been shown to increase survival of SCD. The availability of automatic external defibrillators to trained persons such as police and flight attendants, and its use by these people prior to emergency medical services (EMS) intervention, also increases survival (50).

The epidemiology of SCD parallels that of ischemic heart disease. The incidence increases with age and cardiac risk factors such as smoking, diabetes, left ventricular hypertrophy, and hypercholesterolemia. The biggest risk factor for SCD is previous coronary artery disease (CAD), especially if there is associated left ventricular dysfunction. The more cardiac risk factors and electrocardiogram (ECG) abnormalities present, the higher the risk of SCD (22).

Blacks are more likely than whites to experience SCD in excess of their risk of CAD and are less likely to survive SCD (6). Men are three to four times more likely than women to experience SCD. This difference can be explained by the difference in the incidence of CAD and the hormonal protection women have before menopause (42). Recent major life changes, women who are not married or who have no children or few children, high life stress, and type A personality are all factors that increase the risk for SCD, although the validity of some of these claims remains controversial (17). There may be both seasonal and circadian patterns for risk assessment in SCD because SCD is more likely to occur in the winter months. SCD, like acute myocardial infarction, is most likely to occur in the first few hours after awakening from sleep as a consequence of increased sympathetic stimulation (12).

The ECG can identify patients at an increased risk for SCD. ECG findings consistent with previous ischemic disease such as old myocardial infarction (MI), left ventricular hypertrophy, interventricular conduction delay, or repolarization abnormality are significant predictors of SCD. Some studies report that a powerful predictor of SCD is three or more premature ventricular contractions (PVCs) (10). Other studies state that high-risk forms of PVCs such as multifocal, bigeminy, short coupling with R-on-T phenomenon, and three or more consecutive ectopic beats are more predictive (35). There are also specific ECG findings such as interventricular conduction delays, QT prolongation, delta waves, and an increase in resting heart rate of more than 90 beats per minute (bpm) that place patients at a higher risk (58).

Multiple factors trigger SCD in a susceptible myocardium but the final mechanisms for triggering the fatal ventricular dysrhythmias is unclear. Significant coronary stenosis is the most common abnormality found in SCD patients, although more than half of SCD patients have no previous history of CAD (23). Less than half of all SCDs occur during an acute myocardial infarction (AMI). In fact, cardiac arrest during AMI is associated with an improved outcome when compared to cases not occurring in this setting (9). Other factors involved include other structural abnormalities and transient electrophysiologic disturbances (Table 3.1). In the majority of cases, the terminal rhythm of ventricular fibrillation has occurred from the initiating event of a ventricular tachydysrhythmia (5).

TABLE 3.1.   Risks Associated with Sudden Cardiac Death

Structural Abnormalities
- Coronary Artery Disease and Acute Myocardial Infarction
- Hypertrophic Cardiomyopathy
- Valvular Heart Disease
- Dilated Cardiomyopathy
- Inflammatory and Infiltrative disorders

Primary Electrophysiologic Abnormalities
- Congenital Long QT Syndrome
  - Jervell, Lange-Nielsen
  - Roman Ward
- Acquired Long QT Syndrome
  - Antidysrhythmics (class IA, class III)
  - Antihistamines (terfenadine, astemizole)
  - Antimicrobials (erythromycin, clarithromycin, azithromycin, ketoconazole, chloroquine)
  - Antipsychotics (phenothiazine, haloperidol, risperidone)
  - Antidepressants (tricyclic antidepressants, ketanserin, zindeline)
  - Antimotility (cisapride)
  - Electrolytes (hypokalemia, hyponatremia, hypocalcemia, hypomagnesemia)
  - Organophosphates
  - Intracranial Hemorrhage and Trauma
  - Bradydysrhythmias
  - Dietary (anorexia nervosa, liquid protein diets)
- Wolf-Parkinson-White Syndrome
- Brugada's syndrome
- Idiopathic Ventricular Tachycardia
- Specialized Conduction System Abnormalities
  - Lenegre's disease
  - Lev's disease

Prolongation of the QT interval on the ECG increases the risk of SCD as a consequence of the increased risk of polymorphic ventricular tachycardia. This prolongation predisposes myocardium to reentry phenomenon. Reentry is the major mechanism by which a dysrhythmia is created and maintained, although triggered activity and increased automaticity are also important. A minority of cases of SCD begin with a bradydysrhythmia or an organized rhythm without a pulse (pulseless electrical activity [PEA]). Ventricular fibrillation (VF) usually begins with a run of sustained or nonsustained ventricular tachycardia (VT), which then degenerates to VF.

The net result of the dysrhythmia is global cessation of blood flow and corresponding ischemic injury to various organs. Resultant hypoxia and hypotension cause cessation of aerobic metabolism within seconds. Anaerobic metabolism occurs that cannot meet the metabolic demands of the tissues and subsequent cell death ensues if spontaneous circulation is not resumed. The time before irreversible cell death is dependent on the metabolic rate of the organ system. Both the heart and brain have high metabolic rate and are very sensitive to ischemic insults. Thus the probability of achieving successful resuscitation from cardiac arrest is related to the interval from onset to institution of resuscitative efforts, the setting in which the event occurs, the mechanism (VF, VT, PEA, or asystole) and the clinical status of the patient prior to the cardiac arrest.

CLINICAL PRESENTATION

Patients suffering from SCD do not have any more specific complaints than those suffering any major cardiac or pulmonary event. Symptoms such as increasing angina, dyspnea, palpitations, easy fatigability, and other nonspecific complaints are experienced by these patients in the preceding days to months of the event. However, the onset of the terminal event of SCD, if

instantaneous or abrupt, is cardiac in origin in more than 95% of patients. Dysrhythmic events are characterized by a high likelihood of patients being awake and active immediately prior to the event, are dominated by VF as the electrical mechanism, and have a short duration of terminal illness. Patients who have circulatory failure deaths tend to have more systemic medical problems and present with a higher incidence of asystole and PEA. A cardiac arrest may be characterized by symptoms such as prolonged angina or the pain of an MI, acute shortness of breath, palpitations, and lightheadedness (34). The complete loss of consciousness is the sine qua non in cardiac arrest. The natural history of cardiac arrest is to progress to death within minutes unless expedient interventions are undertaken.

EMERGENCY DEPARTMENT EVALUATION AND MANAGEMENT

Return of spontaneous circulations (ROSC) is dependent on restoration of adequate cardiac function. Restoration of normal brain function is the defining factor of a successful resuscitation. The attainment of both of these goals decreases with each passing minute of the cardiac arrest. Health care providers need to orchestrate simultaneous assessment and management of a cardiac arrest victim.

Patients require airway and ventilatory support, control of cardiac dysrhythmias, and cardiac output stabilized in order to restore organ perfusion. Endotracheal intubation, defibrillation–cardioversion, pacing, pressor agents, and insertion of an intravenous line incorporated with CPR carries out these goals in resuscitation. The final goal is to restore ROSC before irreversible neurologic damage occurs. If the patient is resuscitated, rapid diagnosis and proper management of the pathologic condition that precipitated and resulted from the arrest are essential for optimal outcome.

Basic Cardiopulmonary Resuscitation

Americans spend more than $500 million dollars a year on some form of CPR training or retraining. Yet the utility of this training is limited in the field because of the poor outcome of community cardiac arrests. CPR alone is of little value for restoring effective circulation and preventing brain death. The survival from SCD is dependent on a series of actions represented by the American Heart Association's (AHA) Chain of Survival: early access to 911, early CPR, early defibrillation, and early advanced care (28).

An allorhythmic process approach to the unresponsive victim is used (Fig. 3.1). The function of basic CPR is to provide some blood flow to vital organs until more definitive treatment, such as defibrillation, can be initiated. The activation of the EMS system to allow patients rapid access to ACLS protocols is the first step in the graduated response to care for the cardiac arrest victim.

Most studies show a benefit of layperson CPR in the resuscitation of victims of cardiac arrest, especially when initiated early. The earlier the CPR is applied, the better the outcome (1). Cardiac output generated by standard chest compressions is less than 10% to 30% of baseline and decreases precipitously with both time to initiation and duration of chest compressions (13). Endogenous mechanisms direct blood flow preferentially to the heart and brain during the early minutes of resuscitation. This distribution of blood flow is ideal during CPR because the goal is to generate myocardial perfusion adequate to restore organized electrical activity and effective mechanical function of the heart while minimizing ischemic brain injury. This response becomes ineffective within minutes of circulatory arrest so early intervention is key.

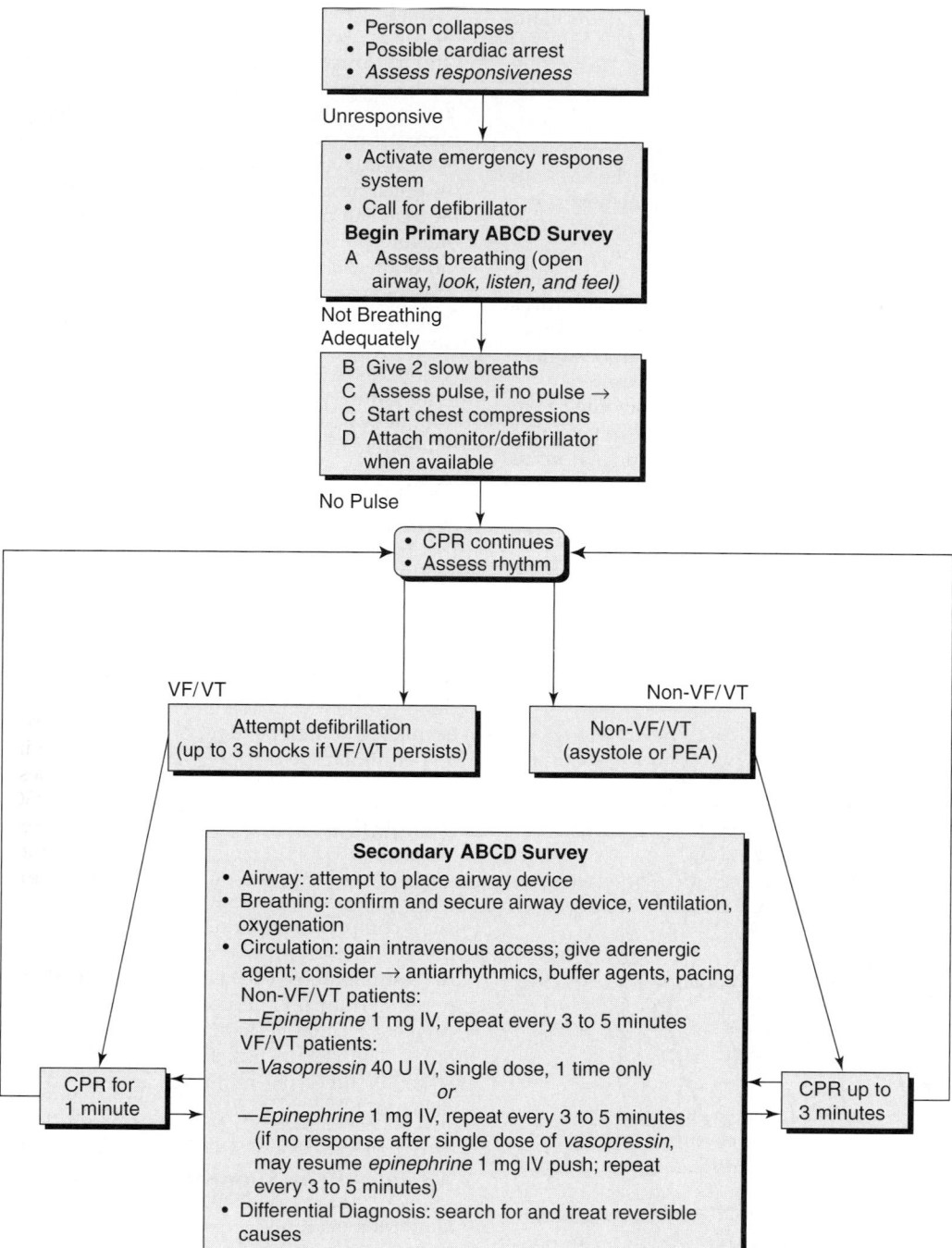

Figure 3.1. Initial emergency cardiac therapy. (From the American Heart and Stroke Association.)

The mechanism of blood flow during closed-chest compressions has been continuously debated. The major theories include (a) direct cardiac compression model in which CPR squeezes the heart between the sternum and the thoracic spine, creating a pressure gradient between the ventricles and the great arteries, and (b) the thoracic pump mechanism in which the thorax acts as a pump when the chest is compressed, generating pressure gradients between intrathoracic and extrathoracic structures. In either method, the valve system in the heart allows forward rather than retrograde blood flow (20).

Which mechanism to use to stimulate blood flow back to the heart is controversial. It was recently recognized that a small vacuum occurs in the thorax after each chest compression (31). New devices have been developed to increase this vacuum effect, such as the vest approach, active compression–decompression,

and an impedance threshold valve. Using these adjuncts for resuscitation in this manner has been tried, but clinical results have proven disappointing for many reasons, including an inability to implement the mechanism and an inability to overcome the standard CPR mind-set. Thus, CPR has changed very little in the last 20 years (46).

The *precordial thump* was originally advocated for use in a witnessed cardiac arrest scenario. A forceful precordial thump can convert patients from VF/pulseless VT into a perfusing rhythm. Patients can also be converted from coordinated cardiac activity to VF/pulseless VT or asystole. There is little recent literature in the form of peer-reviewed studies, but there are numerous case reports of both benefit and risk. The latest recommendation for the precordial thump is that it is an acceptable intervention for health care providers, not laypersons, to use for a witnessed cardiac arrest when the victim has no pulse and no defibrillator is available (4).

Airway

After assessing a cardiac arrest victim's unresponsiveness and activating the response system (in the community, the EMS system is activated and the code team in a hospital), the next step is airway management if there is no immediate access to a defibrillator. In a cardiac arrest victim, the most common reason for airway obstruction is from the tongue falling back in the oropharynx. The airway can be opened by performing either a jaw-thrust or head-tilt–chin-lift maneuver (see Chapter 2, "Airway Procedures"). The jaw thrust is the better maneuver if any trauma is suspected, or if cervical spine immobilization is required.

If the airway is still obstructed after these maneuvers, one must be concerned about an obstructed airway from another cause. The *Heimlich maneuver,* or subdiaphragmatic abdominal thrust, is the recommended procedure for clearing the obstructed airway of a foreign body. The rescuer's hand is positioned between the patient's xiphoid and naval, and several quick thrusts are administered in an attempt to relieve the foreign-body obstruction. If the victim is unconscious, like a victim of SCD, the Heimlich maneuver may be accompanied by attempts to visualize the foreign body in the pharynx and by finger sweeps to remove the foreign body (Fig. 3.2).

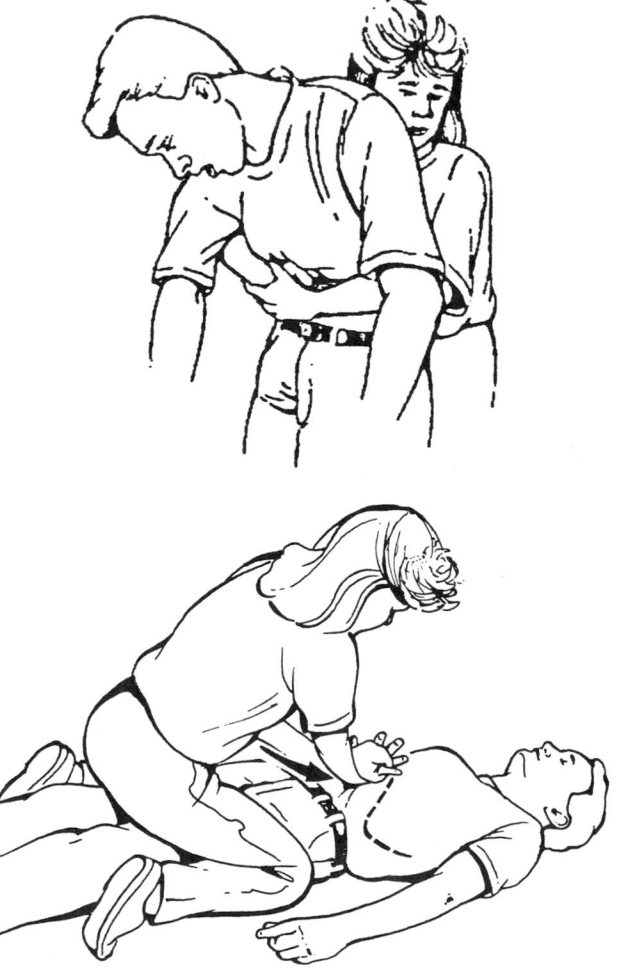

Figure 3.2. Administration of the Heimlich maneuver to conscious (*top*) and unconscious victims (*below*). (From Emergency Cardiac Care Committee and Subcommittee, AHA. Guidelines for cardiopulmonary resuscitation, I. *JAMA* 1992;268:2172, with permission.)

Breathing

Once the airway is open, the rescuer looks, listens and feels for an exchange of air. Rescuers in the field use airway adjuncts such as oropharyngeal and nasopharyngeal airways to avoid unnecessary exposure. Without specialized equipment available, however, layperson mouth-to-mouth respiration is performed by pinching the victim's nostrils and blowing slowly into the mouth. The patient should receive 2 slow and steady breaths delivered over 2 seconds. The rescuer watches for the rise and fall of the chest during ventilation. The AHA recommends that 1 rescuer use a ratio of 15 compressions to 2 ventilations and that 2 rescuers use a ratio of 5 compressions to 1 ventilation in the cardiac arrest victim with ongoing CPR.

Bag-mask ventilation is the first choice for basic life support ventilation but should give way to alternative airway ventilation methods once ACLS providers are available. Tracheal intubation remains the procedure of choice for the unconscious, apneic patient. This skill is not without significant challenges and ACLS guidelines recommend intubation be performed by those experienced in the procedure (24). Correct tube placement in the trachea can be confirmed by physical examination, an end-tidal carbon dioxide detector, or an esophageal detection device.

Other airway maneuvers recommended over bag-valve masking are the laryngeal mask airway or the esophageal-tracheal Combitube (see Chapter 2, "Airway Procedures"). Once definitive airway management has occurred, the ventilations are administered independent of the chest compressions at a rate of 12 per minute.

Circulation

The carotid pulse should be checked because it is the most reliable pulse to check in low-flow states. If no pulse is detected, chest compressions should be instituted. The victim needs to be placed on a firm surface or backboard to assist mechanically with the compressions. The heel of the hand is placed on the lower half of the sternum and depressed 1.5 to 2.0 inches in the adult. Children have a compression depth of 1.0 to 1.5 inches and neonates are at 0.5 to 1.0 inches. The recommended compression rate is 80 to 100 times per minute in adults and 100 for children and neonates (2).

Advanced Life Support

Defibrillation

The passage of current through the heart causes defibrillation with the goal of restoring a perfusing cardiac rhythm. If energy and current are too low, the delivered shock will not terminate the dysrhythmia; if energy and current are too high, myocardial damage may result. Because of ischemia, acidosis, and electrophysiologic deterioration, a longer duration of ventricular fibrillation correlates with a higher defibrillation threshold (45).

Modern-day defibrillators deliver electrical shocks in one of two ways. Monophasic waveforms deliver current in one direction through the heart. Biphasic waveforms are used to deliver current through the heart, reverse polarity, and return through the myocardium. As a result, the energy needed for successful conversion of tachydysrhythmias with biphasic technology is often significantly less than that required with monophasic waveforms. The latest defibrillators and automated external defibrillators use biphasic waveform technology (40).

Current is directly related to the energy set on the defibrillator and inversely related to the transthoracic impedance. The transthoracic impedance can be minimized by attention to several factors, including position of the defibrillation paddles, amount of energy selected on the defibrillator, firm pressure on the paddles, the use of conductive material between the skin and paddles, employing sets of shocks, and coordinating the shock with the end-expiratory phase of ventilation (1).

Defibrillation–cardioversion should be used quickly because delay will reduce the effectiveness of the resuscitation. If ventricular fibrillation is corrected within 1 minute, there is a survival rate of greater than 90%; however, the survival rate falls by 10% per minute following the initiating event (33). In this fashion, public access defibrillation (PAD) has the potential to be one of the greatest advances in the treatment of SCD since the development of CPR. The mechanism for PAD is in the form of an automated external defibrillator (AED). AEDs are computerized devices that are simple and reliable to operate; they allow lay rescuers with minimal training to administer this life-saving intervention. Self-adhesive electrode pads are provided with application diagrams; voice and text prompts guide the rescuer through a few simple steps. A dysrhythmia analysis algorithm automatically interprets the rhythm and either recommends countershock, to be given by the push of a button, or no countershock. After the shock, the device immediately reevaluates the rhythm and determines whether to recommend an additional shock. Flight attendants, security personnel, sports trainers, police officers, firefighters, lifeguards, family members, and many other trained laypersons have used AEDs successfully in the field (48). One study trained security guards in 36 Las Vegas casinos to use AEDs. The witnessed VF survival for that study was 53% (51).

The hospital setting, with its highly trained health care personnel, uses defibrillators with manual settings for more precise control. If a defibrillator is immediately available and VF or pulseless VT is evident, a 200-joule (J) shock should be delivered *preceding* airway management and intravenous line placement. If VF and pulseless VT are sustained after the initial 200-J shock, higher energies of 300 and 360 J are tried.

Pharmacologic Therapy

Pressor Agents

Historically, catecholamine-induced adrenergic receptor stimulation is the therapy most commonly used in cardiac arrest, with epinephrine being the drug used most often. *Epinephrine* stimulates α_1 and α_2 receptors almost equally, and β_1 and β_2 receptors in a ratio of 1 to 4. We now realize that trials validating the use of epinephrine in cardiac arrest are not well defined because there are no prospective clinical trials. "High-dose" epinephrine was recently endorsed in cardiac arrest if regular-dose epinephrine was unsuccessful in resuscitation, only to have the endorsement rescinded by the AHA when larger numbers revealed no benefit and potential harm with such administration (2). Some studies found that patients may have a higher incidence of ROSC with high-dose epinephrine, but no improvement in neurologic outcome. Patients with irreparable central nervous system (CNS) injury may result in significant burden on families and health care resources. At present, meta-analyses have not determined if high-dose epinephrine is better, worse, or the same as standard dose (39). The current recommended dose is epinephrine 1 mg initially, with repeated doses every 3 to 5 minutes, but the optimal dose has not been established.

Vasopressin, also termed *antidiuretic hormone*, has entered the treatment armamentarium for the cardiac arrest victim that has VF or pulseless VT. Circulating endogenous vasopressin concentrations were high in patients undergoing CPR, and levels in successfully resuscitated patients are significantly higher than in patients who died (30). A study showed improved survival at 24 hours after the event but no difference at hospital discharge, with vasopressin as compared to epinephrine (29). Vasopressin produces the same positive effects as epinephrine in terms of vasoconstriction and increasing the blood flow to the brain and heart during CPR. Vasopressin does not have the adverse effects on the heart that epinephrine does such as increased ischemia and irritability and, paradoxically, the propensity for VF. The AHA has given vasopressin a class IIb recommendation for VF/pulseless VT arrests (Table 3.2). Vasopressin is given as a single one-time dose (40 U intravenously), because of the much longer half-life of 10 to 20 minutes.

Vasopressin and epinephrine are equivalent in ROSC in cardiac arrest victims in in-hospital patients (49). There is limited experience with vasopressin in PEA or asystole, so epinephrine remains the pressor of choice empirically (54). The future of pressor agents may be in combination of current drugs. Promising results have been shown in combination of epinephrine and vasopressin in cardiac arrest patients (39).

Antidysrhythmic Agents

The role of antidysrhythmic drugs is to suppress premature ectopic complexes and improve symptoms related to palpitations. The literature supporting use of antidysrhythmic drugs in cardiac arrest is sparse and no studies show that using them increases survival with good neurologic outcome. Most of the antidysrhythmic agents raise the fibrillation threshold and are thus useful for preventing recurrent ventricular fibrillation in patients who were successfully defibrillated. *Amiodarone* is categorized as a class III antidysrhythmic but contains characteristics of all four Vaughn Williams classes. The AHA has included amiodarone in the VF/pulseless VT algorithm since the updated guidelines were published in 2000. Amiodarone increases the percentage of cardiac arrest patients admitted to the hospital. One study demonstrated no difference between the amiodarone and placebo groups in hospital discharge of patients with good neurologic functioning, although the study was underpowered for these observations (26). Amiodarone was compared to lidocaine in out-of-hospital cardiac arrests and found to be superior in survival to hospital discharge, substantiating the AHA guidelines. The dosage of amiodarone in VF/pulseless VT arrests is 300 mg intravenous (i.v.) push.

Lidocaine has been used to treat VF/pulseless VT but with little evidence to support its use. The only evidence for its use is from a large historical trial in which receipt of the drug was associated with improved resuscitation and admission alive to hospital. This study had nursing staff present only for the lidocaine cohort, which could explain the difference in survival alone (21). Lidocaine has thus taken an indeterminate role in ACLS. The initial recommended dosage of lidocaine is 1.0 to 1.5 mg/kg i.v. push. This dose can be followed with 0.5 to 0.75 m/kg every 5 to 10 minutes for refractory VF to a maximum of 3 mg/kg.

Procainamide is an effective agent for suppressing ectopic ventricular complexes and ventricular tachycardia, as well as other ventricular dysrhythmias. Procainamide has a limited use in cardiac arrest because of the slow loading to therapeutic doses. Its use is primarily in treating VT with a pulse and other ventricular dysrhythmias (25). Procainamide is administered in an infusion of up to 50 mg/min to a total maximum of 17 mg/kg.

Magnesium has an unclear mechanism of action in treatment of dysrhythmias. Its primary use is in the management of torsades de pointes, although this indication has not had formalized trials. There have been studies that show a correlation between normal magnesium levels and successful resuscitation, but the administration of supplemental magnesium to patients in arrest has not been studied (11). Most studies performed showed no benefit associated with its routine administration unless a documented hypomagnesemic state existed (25). The dosage of magnesium is 1 to 2 g i.v. push in this specific subset of patients.

Bretylium was removed from the ACLS guidelines because it is not superior to any other antidysrhythmic agent. Bretylium has a higher incidence of hypotension and hemodynamic deterioration than other agents and has limited availability to hospital personnel.

Guidelines for Cardiac Arrest

The AHA developed guidelines for treatment of patients in cardiac arrest. Every few years the protocols are updated to include the latest in cardiovascular literature, so clinicians should be aware of the most recent version. In 2000, the guidelines were revised using evidence-based medicine and international experts for the first time. Although the ACLS treatment for patients in cardiac arrest is based on the ECG monitor rhythm, the clinician must always consider the etiology of the arrest in developing a treatment plan. Cardiac arrest is an end point of a physiologic process that results in the loss of circulation and ventilation. Etiologies such as respiratory failure, asthma, medication toxicity, hypovolemia, pulmonary embolism, sepsis, trauma, acute myocardial infarction, anaphylaxis, metabolic abnormalities, and others may be treated specifically while going through the ACLS algorithms. The treatment modalities were classified by a consensus of experts based on the scientific evidence of the efficacy and safety of the modalities (Table 3.2).

Ventricular Fibrillation and Pulseless Ventricular Tachycardia

The key to the treatment of patient with VF or pulseless VT (Fig. 3.3) is to remember that successful resuscitation depends on electrical defibrillation. All other treatments, including CPR, intubation, and drugs, are merely attempts to prepare the patient for successful defibrillation. Defibrillation should be attempted with up to three shocks as soon as the diagnosis is made. Shocking the patient several times successively decreases the transthoracic impedance and increases the chance for successful defibrillation.

If defibrillation is unsuccessful, CPR is initiated, the trachea is intubated and an intravenous line is placed as soon as possible. Epinephrine or the more recently endorsed vasopressin is the first recommended pharmacologic agent. After administration of the drug, attempts at defibrillation should occur. Antidysrhythmic drugs may be useful in preventing refibrillation once the patient has been electrically defibrillated. Amiodarone in recommended as the first antiarrhythmic agent. Subsequent treatment with magnesium, procainamide or lidocaine may be used if first line medications are ineffective. Treatment with sodium bicarbonate should be initiated if there is clinical suspicion of hyperkalemia, tricyclic antidepressants or preexisting acidosis. Shock-resistant VF develops in only 10% to 25% of all cardiac arrests, yet 87% to 98% of these patients die (45).

Asystole

Asystole (Fig. 3.4) is a cardiac arrest rhythm associated with no discernible electrical activity on the ECG. The asystolic patient has a poor prognosis for resuscitation. The single most impor-

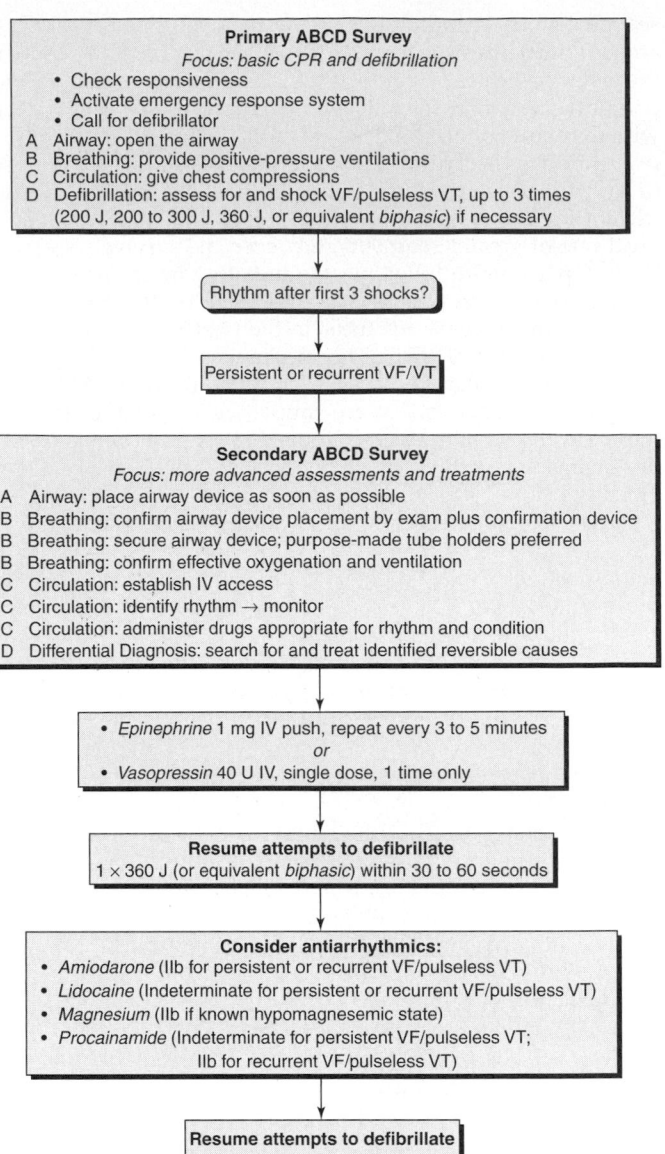

Figure 3.3.   Ventricular fibrillation/pulseless ventricular tachycardia algorithm. (From the American Heart and Stroke Association.)

tant therapy for asystole is to search for, identify, and reverse any treatable cause. The asystolic patient may actually be in fine ventricular fibrillation when using confirmation in another lead on the monitor. The diagnosis of asystole should thus be confirmed by checking a straight-line rhythm on three leads. If there is any suspicion of fine ventricular fibrillation masking as asystole, clinician should proceed to immediate defibrillation. As in VF, the clinician must consider the underlying process that precipitated asystole and focus treatment in this specific area while following ACLS protocols (Table 3.3). These conditions cause only the clinical deterioration of these conditions; they do not cause the rhythm.

An important minority of SCD events begin with a bradydysrhythmia that degenerates to asystole (38). Bradyasystole occurs when there is an intrinsic failure of the heart's electrical system. This failure can be in the form of failure to generate or propagate an adequate number of ventricular depolarizations per minute to sustain consciousness and other vital functions. It is unclear why bradyasystole, which uses very little myocardial oxygen and should have enough high-energy phosphate stores to initiate a return of spontaneous circulation, has such a dismal outcome in the majority of cases. Certainly, the underlying myocardial and valvular dysfunction in conjunction with systemic

---

TABLE 3.2.   Levels of Evidence for Interventions

Class I	Definitely helpful
Class IIA	Acceptable, probably helpful
Class IIB	Acceptable, possibly helpful
Class III	Not indicated, may be harmful
Class Indeterminate	No recommendation until further evidence available

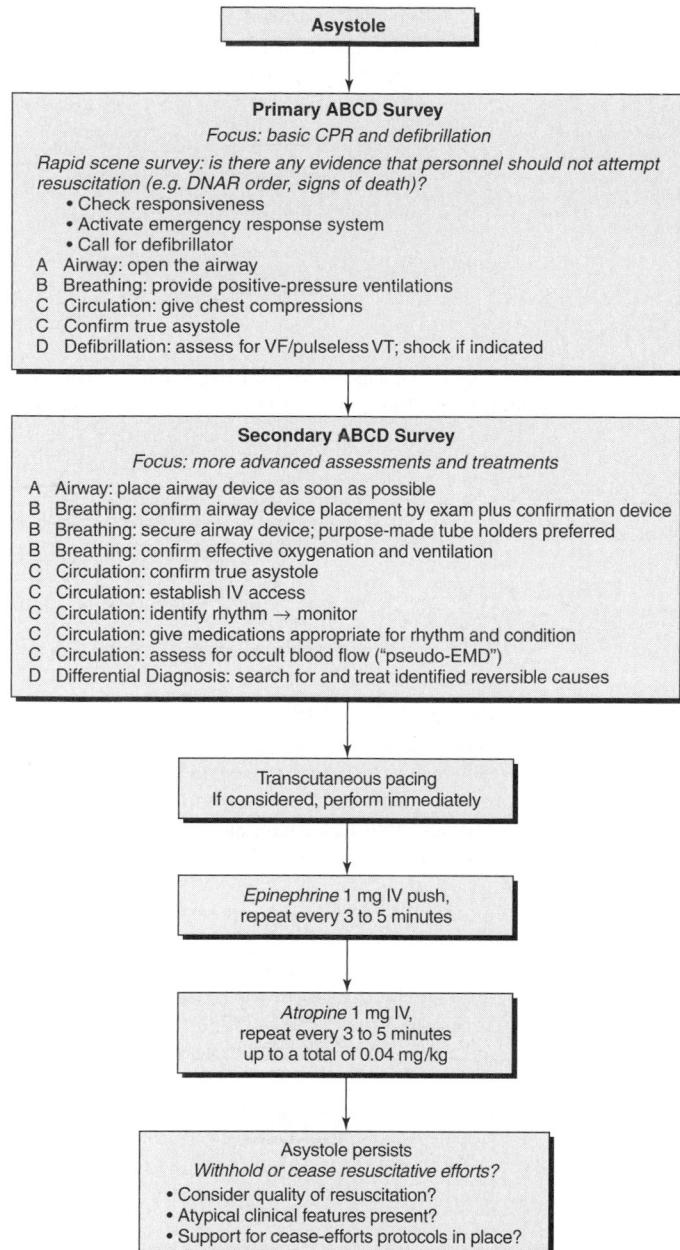

Figure 3.4. Asystole algorithm. (From the American Heart and Stroke Association.)

insults are entwined in this process. Several studies that used cardiac pacing in this setting showed poor outcomes. To be effective, pacing must be initiated in the first few minutes after arrest. Pharmacologic treatment of asystole involves the use of epinephrine to improve myocardial and cerebral blood flow during CPR, and atropine to antagonize parasympathetic stimulation (36).

Pulseless Electric Activity

PEA (Fig. 3.5) is coordinated electrical activity of the heart (other than VT or VF) without a palpable pulse. In this scenario, either the heart cannot pump at all (true electrical–mechanical dissociation [EMD]) or myocardial contractions do occur but without a palpable pulse (pseudo-EMD). PEA is the term used to describe both true and pseudo EMD. Primary PEA, like asystole, has a very poor prognosis. The differential of causes of PEA are the same as for asystole (Table 3.3).

PEA is the result of a primary disorder of electromechanical coupling in myocardial cells. It is most often associated with global myocardial energy depletion and acidosis resulting from

TABLE 3.3. Most Frequent Causes of Asystole and Pulseless Electrical Activity

Hypovolemia	Tension pneumothorax
Hypoxia	Cardiac Tamponade
Acidosis	Myocardial Infarction
Hyperkalemia/	Pulmonary Embolism
Hypokalemia	Drug Ingestion (beta-blockers, Ca++
Hypothermia	channel blockers, digoxin)

ischemia or hypoxia. Pseudo-EMD is a transient state in the progression to EMD and has the same etiology. In these cases of severely decreased flow, patients must be evaluated for cardiac and extracardiac causes of severe shock.

Intubation and ventilation with 100% oxygen plus an intravenous fluid bolus can begin the resuscitation. Careful consideration of the common causes of PEA should dictate subsequent interventions. Bedside ultrasonography might allow the treating physician to determine whether or not the heart is beating and whether or not pericardial fluid is present. Alternatively, the placement of an arterial line can be used to differentiate severe shock states from true EMD. In cases where these modalities are unavailable, the clinician must consider the differential and decide whether or not needle thoracostomy and

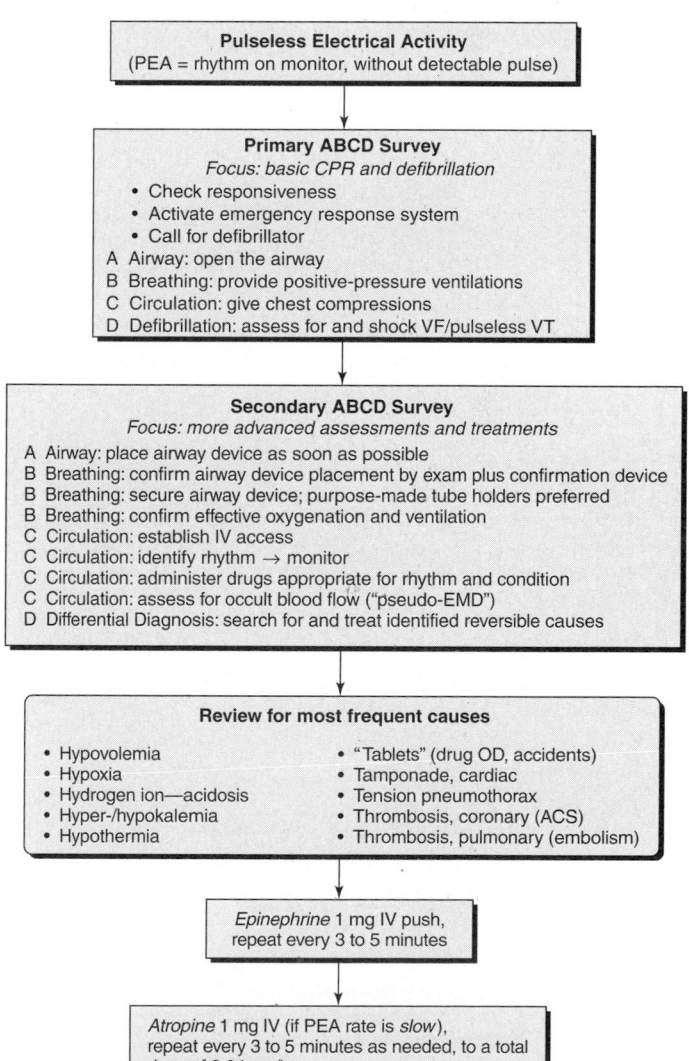

Figure 3.5. Pulseless electrical activity algorithm. (From the American Heart and Stroke Association.)

pericardiocentesis are indicated. Once extracardiac causes of EMD are excluded, treatment recommendations include epinephrine to improve myocardial and cerebral blood flow during cardiac arrest, and atropine if the ECG shows bradycardia.

Initiating and Discontinuing Resuscitation Efforts

It was classically taught that CPR should be instituted for all patients in cardiac arrest, except in two circumstances: (a) the patient made it clear, while competent and informed, that he or she did not want resuscitation efforts to be instituted; and (b) successful resuscitation would be futile because the patient has clear signs of irreversible death, such as rigor mortis, dependent lividity, or decapitation.

In the last 15 years, several studies challenged the usefulness of initiating ACLS protocols in all patients. In most geographic areas, all cardiac arrest patients are transported to the nearest emergency department for definitive care despite the futility of the resuscitation efforts and the attendant hazards to motorists, pedestrians, and EMS personnel. Transportation of all patients to the nearest emergency department can limit the availability of EMS personnel to care for other patients, increase patient waiting time, decrease emergency department (ED) and hospital bed and equipment availability, and increase the costs (18).

Termination of resuscitation (TOR) guidelines can identify nonsalvageable patients. There is ample evidence that patients that fail out-of-hospital ACLS interventions do not survive to hospital discharge, and that ED interventions in this patient population changes survival with good neurologic outcome in less than 1% of patients (53). No survivors of asystolic patients have been documented in normothermic patients with a call to arrival time by EMS personnel greater than 8 minutes (41). Once undertaken, resuscitation efforts are generally continued until it is clear that the patient is not responding to them. The longer the patient remains in cardiac arrest without response, the worse is the prognosis for survival. After 30 minutes of resuscitation attempts, the prognosis is very poor. Consequently, the clinician must exercise his or her judgment as regards termination of resuscitation.

Hypothermia (see Chapter 349, "Hypothermia") patients should have ongoing resuscitative efforts while the rewarming process continues. Cardiopulmonary bypass should be considered for these patients. Only when the patient is warmed and ACLS interventions are ineffective should termination of resuscitation be considered.

Emergency physicians and paramedics are obligated to respect patients' wishes regarding resuscitation. In most cases, these wishes may be known through documentation on advance directives. The patient and patient's health care provider should update these forms and have them ready for paramedics or ED personnel so that they can be used in an emergency situation. Many communities have developed a standardized "do not resuscitate" form that patients and their physicians can fill out. These forms document the patients' wishes and provide guidance for both EMS and hospital personnel.

There are three cardiac arrest characteristics that are associated with survival to hospital discharge: ROSC prior to transport, a shock given prior to transport, and cardiac arrest witnessed by EMS personnel (53). In any case of cardiac arrest, the decision to either not initiate or terminate advanced care is determined by the clinician using his or her best clinical judgment and knowledge of futility situations.

Invasive Cardiopulmonary Resuscitation

Studies in animal models show that techniques of invasive CPR, such as open chest CPR and cardiopulmonary bypass, and the use of direct mechanical-assist devices improve hemodynamics, resuscitation, and the chances of surviving cardiac arrest. It has also been demonstrated that when invasive CPR is applied late in the treatment protocol (after more than 15 minutes of total arrest time), there is no improvement in resuscitation. The resources required to provide many of the interventions, principally invasive perfusion technologies, cannot be justified unless there is clear benefit. The allocation of such resources to provide intensive resuscitation and postresuscitation support needs to be addressed from both medical and societal viewpoints (32).

Quality of Resuscitation Efforts

How well CPR is performed and ACLS delivered does make a difference in the outcome for patients in cardiac arrest. Unfortunately, the performance of CPR is frequently not optimal (52). There are many ways to measure the quality of resuscitation efforts but practicality inhibits some of these measures. The use of capnometry to monitor end-tidal CO_2 levels during CPR provides a noninvasive assessment of the cardiac output generated by CPR (44). Other measures, such as invasive hemodynamic parameters, although useful, aren't realistic in an acute resuscitation setting. The quality of resuscitation efforts should also be assessed retrospectively by systemically tracking key variables and the outcome of resuscitation efforts in both the in-hospital and out-of-hospital setting (12).

Postresuscitation

The resuscitation of a cardiac arrest victim does not end with a ROSC. The underlying medical conditions leading to the arrest as well as the complications of prolonged global ischemia must be carefully managed to result in an optimal outcome. Although the neurologically intact victim of a cardiac arrest is rare, there is no reliable way to determine the prognosis of an individual patient immediately after resuscitation.

Because the majority of patients have a cardiac etiology for their arrest, immediate focus in the early postresuscitation period should involve looking for an acute coronary syndrome. An ECG should be performed to look for evidence of myocardial infarction. Administration of all cardiac therapies can be initiated if ischemic heart disease is the presumptive diagnosis. Heparin, aspirin, thrombolytics, and angioplasty can all be considered. Antidysrhythmic therapy for all patients that presented with VF/pulseless VT should also be initiated. Patients with high-risk conduction abnormalities, such as right bundle-branch blocks associated with a hemiblock, second-degree type II blocks, third-degree heart blocks, or new left bundle-branch block, should have transthoracic pacing pads placed and used if necessary (19).

Controversy is renewed about controlling hypothermia in the postcardiac arrest victim for improved neurologic outcome. The original studies from the 1950s had small patient numbers but the authors concluded that the clinical use of hypothermia after cardiac arrest seemed justified (7,55). More recent studies used larger controlled trials in an attempt to ascertain if there is a neurologic benefit to induced resuscitative hypothermia. Patients in the postarrest resuscitative phase were sedated and paralyzed to prevent shivering and subsequently cooled to between 32°C (89.6°F) and 34°C (93.2°F) over the course of the subsequent several hours. The absolute number of survivors and their neurologic outcome were compared to normothermic resuscitations. Each of these studies did show some improved survival and favorable neurologic outcome (3,8,56,57).

Mild hypothermia seems to be a sufficient compromise between the beneficial effects of mitigation of ischemic membrane damage and reperfusion injury and the adverse risks of dysrhythmic, inflammatory, hemodynamic, and coagulation disorders. Therefore mild hypothermia holds the potential of being the first direct therapy for the brain after cardiac arrest apart from hemodynamic stabilization. There is limited definitive evidence of a beneficial effect of resuscitative hypothermia because of a lack of prospective, randomized controlled trials and only small patient numbers (16).

DISPOSITION

Patients who survive should be admitted to the intensive care unit where invasive monitoring can be continued or in some cases, initiated. Postresuscitation patients who have evidence of an acute coronary syndrome may be moved to the catheterization lab.

COMMON PITFALLS

✔ *Failure to stay calm and approach the patient in an organized fashion.* It is important to remember that resuscitation efforts require a well-disciplined team in which each member plays a role. Optimal patient care depends on management in a well-controlled, calm environment that is focused on each individual task. The emergency physician should take control of the situation and lead all players in the resuscitation

✔ *Erroneously administering amiodarone, bicarbonate, magnesium, and procainamide endotracheally.* The only medications that can be administered via the endotracheal tube are epinephrine, atropine, lidocaine and naxolone

✔ *Erroneously giving intracardiac medications.* There are no current indications to give intracardiac medications

✔ *Failure to suspect hyperkalemia in renal failure patients for patients in cardiac arrest.* Resuscitation of these patients should include calcium gluconate, bicarbonate, and insulin with glucose. Be sure to look for monitor and ECG manifestations of hyperkalemia such as a hyperacute T waves, prolongation of the QRS complex, or a sine wave pattern

✔ *Failure to defibrillate in the appropriate manner.* The majority of patients in VF can be defibrillated. If unsuccessful, review your technique. One paddle should be placed to the right of the sternum below the right clavicle, and the other in the midaxillary line at the level of the nipple. If the paddles are too close together, the skin, rather than the heart, may be getting the current. Alternatively, the anteroposterior position may be used over the left precordium. Firm pressure of approximately 25 lb should be applied to each paddle, and the appropriate contact gel must be used. The shocks should be given in pairs or triplets to decrease the transthoracic impedance and improve the chances of successful defibrillation

✔ *Mistaking torsade de pointes for ventricular tachycardia or fibrillation.* Although antidysrhythmic drugs are commonly ineffective in terminating torsades, electrical cardioversion is usually successful. Further treatment with magnesium sulfate, isoproterenol, or overdrive pacing decreases the QT interval and prevents recurrence

Acknowledgments

Thanks to previous edition chapter author Arthur B. Sanders.

References

1. Standards and guidelines for cardiopulmonary resuscitation and emergency cardiac care. *JAMA* 1992;281:1175–1181.
2. Cummins RO. Case 3: VF/pulseless VT: persistent/refractory/recurrent/shock resistant. In: *ACLS Provider Manual.* American Heart Association, 2002:75–96.
3. Mild therapeutic hypothermia to improve the neurologic outcome after cardiac arrest. *N Engl J Med* 2002;346(8):549–556.
4. Part 1: introduction to the International Guidelines 2000 for CPR and ECC: a consensus on science. *Circulation* 2000;102[8 Suppl]:I1–I11.
5. Bayes de Luna A, Coumel P, Leclercq JF. Ambulatory sudden cardiac death: mechanisms of production of fatal arrhythmia on the basis of data from 157 cases. *Am Heart J* 1989;117(1):151–9.
6. Becker LB, Han BH, Meyer PM, et al. Racial differences in the incidence of cardiac arrest and subsequent survival. The CPR Chicago project. *N Engl J Med* 1993;329(9):600–606.
7. Benson DW, Williams GR Jr, Spencer FC, et al. The use of hypothermia after cardiac arrest. *Anesth Analg* 1959;38:423–428.
8. Bernard SA, Jones BM, Horne MK. Clinical trial of induced hypothermia in comatose survivors of out-of-hospital cardiac arrest. *Ann Emerg Med* 1997;30(2):146–153.
9. Beuret P, Feihl F, Vogt P, et al. Cardiac arrest: prognostic factors and outcome at one year. *Resuscitation* 1993;25(2):171–179.
10. Bigger JT Jr, Fleiss JL, Kleiger R, et al. The relationships among ventricular arrhythmias, left ventricular dysfunction, and mortality in the 2 years after myocardial infarction. *Circulation* 1984;69(2):250–258.
11. Cannon LA, Heiselman DE, Dougherty JM, et al. Magnesium levels in cardiac arrest victims: relationship between magnesium levels and successful resuscitation. *Ann Emerg Med* 1987;16(11):1195–1199.
12. Cummins RO, Chamberlain D, Hazinski MF, et al. Recommended guidelines for reviewing, reporting, and conducting research on in-hospital resuscitation: the in-hospital "Utstein style." American Heart Association. *Circulation* 1997;95(8):2213–2239.
13. Del Guercia LRM, et al. Comparison of blood flow during external and internal cardiac massage in man. *Circulation* 1965;31/32[Suppl I]:171.
14. Dunbar SB, Ellenbogen K, Eptstin AE.In: *Sudden cardiac death: past, present, and future.* Futura, 1997.
15. Eisenberg MS, Bergner L, Hallstrom A. Cardiac resuscitation in the community. Importance of rapid provision and implications for program planning. *JAMA* 1979;241(18):1905–1907.
16. Eisenburger P, Sterz F, Holzer M, et al. Therapeutic hypothermia after cardiac arrest. *Curr Opin Crit Care* 2001;7(3):184–188.
17. Gillum RF. Sudden coronary death in the United States: 1980–1985. *Circulation* 1989;79(4):756–765.
18. Gray WA, Capone RJ, Most AS. Unsuccessful emergency medical resuscitation—are continued efforts in the emergency department justified? *N Engl J Med* 1991;325(20):1393–1398.
19. Gunnar RM, Passamani ER, Bourdillon PD, et al . Guidelines for the early management of patients with acute myocardial infarction. A report of the American College of Cardiology/American Heart Association task force on assessment of diagnostic and therapeutic cardiovascular procedures (subcommittee to develop guidelines for the early management of patients with acute myocardial infarction). *J Am Coll Cardiol* 1990;16(2):249–292.
20. Halperin HG. Mechanisms of forward flow during CPR. Cardiac arrest: the science and practice of resuscitation medicine. 1996.
21. Herlitz J, Ekstrom L, Wennerblom B, et al. Lidocaine in out-of-hospital ventricular fibrillation. Does it improve survival? *Resuscitation* 1997;33(3):199–205.
22. Kannel WB, Cupples LA, D'Agostino RB. Sudden death risk in overt coronary heart disease: the Framingham study. *Am Heart J* 1987;113(3):799–804.
23. Kannel WB, Schatzkin A. Sudden death: lessons from subsets in population studies. *J Am Coll Cardiol* 1985;5[6 Suppl]:141B–149B.
24. Kern KB, Halperin HR, Field J. New guidelines for cardiopulmonary resuscitation and emergency cardiac care: changes in the management of cardiac arrest. *JAMA* 2001;285(10):1267–1269.
25. Kudenchuk PJ. Advanced cardiac life support antiarrhythmic drugs. *Cardiol Clin* 2002;20(1):79–87.
26. Kudenchuk PJ, Cobb LA, Copass MK, et al. Amiodarone for resuscitation after out-of-hospital cardiac arrest due to ventricular fibrillation. *N Engl J Med* 1999;341(12):871–878.
27. Kuller L, Lilienfeld A, Fisher R. An epidemiological study of sudden and unexpected deaths in adults. *Medicine (Baltimore)* 1967;46(4):341–361.
28. Larsen MP, Eisenberg MS, Cummins RO, et al. Predicting survival from out-of-hospital cardiac arrest: a graphic model. *Ann Emerg Med* 1993;22(11):1652–1658.
29. Lindner KH, Dirks B, Strohmenger HU, et al. Randomised comparison of epinephrine and vasopressin in patients with out-of-hospital ventricular fibrillation. *Lancet* 1997;349(9051):535–537.
30. Lindner KH, Strohmenger HU, Ensinger H, et al. Stress hormone response during and after cardiopulmonary resuscitation. *Anesthesiology* 1992;77(4):662–668.
31. Lurie K, Voelckel W, Plaisance P, et al. Use of an inspiratory impedance threshold valve during cardiopulmonary resuscitation: a progress report. *Resuscitation* 2000;44(3):219–230.
32. Manning JE, Katz LM. Cardiopulmonary and cerebral resuscitation. *Crit Care Clin* 2000;16(4):659–679.
33. Marenco JP, Wang PJ, Link MS, et al. Improving survival from sudden cardiac arrest: the role of the automated external defibrillator. *JAMA* 2001;285(9):1193–1200.
34. Myerburg RJ, Castellanos A. Cardiovascular collapse, cardiac arrest, and sudden cardiac death. In: Braunwald E, et al., eds. *Harrison's principles of internal medicine,* 15th ed. New York: McGraw-Hill, 2001:228–233.
35. Myerburg RJ, Kessler KM, Luceri RM, et al. Classification of ventricular arrhythmias based on parallel hierarchies of frequency and form. *Am J Cardiol* 1984;54(10):1355–1358.
36. Neumar R, Ward K.Adult resuscitation. In: Marx J, Hockberger R, Walls R, eds. *Rosen's emergency medicine: concepts and clinical practice,* 5th ed. St. Louis: Mosby, 2003:64–82.
37. Ornato J. Sudden cardiac death. In: Tintinalli J, ed. *Emergency medicine: a comprehensive study guide,* 5th ed. New York: McGraw-Hill, 2003:39–44.
38. Ornato JP, Peberdy MA. The mystery of bradyasystole during cardiac arrest. *Ann Emerg Med* 1996;27(5):576–587.

39. Paradis NA, Wenzel V, Southall J. Pressor drugs in the treatment of cardiac arrest. *Cardiol Clin* 2002;20(1):61–78, viii.
40. Peberdy MA. Defibrillation. *Cardiol Clin* 2002;20(1):13–21, vii.
41. Petrie DA. Termination-of-resuscitation guidelines in a basic life support-defibrillation system. *Acad Emerg Med* 2002;9(12):1460–1461.
42. Rasekh A, Munir Z, Massumi A.Sudden cardiac death. In: Willerson J, Cohn J, eds. *Cardiovascular medicine*, 2nd ed. Churchill-Livingstone, 2000:1710–1738.
43. Safar P, Escarraga LA, Elam JO. A comparison of the mouth-to-mouth and mouth-to-airway methods of artificial respiration with the chest-pressure arm-lift methods. *N Engl J Med* 1958;258(14):671–677.
44. Sanders AB, Kern KB, Otto CW, et al. End-tidal carbon dioxide monitoring during cardiopulmonary resuscitation. A prognostic indicator for survival. *JAMA* 1989;262(10):1347–1351.
45. Sarkozy A, Dorian P. Strategies for reversing shock-resistant ventricular fibrillation. *Curr Opin Crit Care* 2003;9(3):189–193.
46. Schwab TM, Callaham ML, Madsen CD, et al. A randomized clinical trial of active compression—decompression CPR vs. standard CPR in out-of-hospital cardiac arrest in two cities. *JAMA* 1995;273(16):1261–1268.
47. Sirbaugh PE, Pepe PE, Shook JE, et al. A prospective, population-based study of the demographics, epidemiology, management, and outcome of out-of-hospital pediatric cardiopulmonary arrest. *Ann Emerg Med* 1999;33(2):174–184.
48. Sommers AL, Slaby JR, Aufderheide TP. Public access defibrillation. *Emerg Med Clin North Am* 2002;20(4):809–824.
49. Stiell IG, Hebert PC, Wells GA, et al. Vasopressin versus epinephrine for inhospital cardiac arrest: a randomised controlled trial. *Lancet* 2001;358(9276):105–109.
50. Stiell IG, Wells GA, Field BJ, et al. Improved out-of-hospital cardiac arrest survival through the inexpensive optimization of an existing defibrillation program: OPALS study phase II. Ontario prehospital advanced life support. *JAMA* 1999;281(13):1175–1181.
51. Valenzuela TD, Roe DJ, Nichol G, et al. Outcomes of rapid defibrillation by security officers after cardiac arrest in casinos. *N Engl J Med* 2000;343(17):1206–1209.
52. van Hoeyweghen RJ, Bossaert LL, Mullie A, et al. Quality and efficiency of bystander CPR. Belgian Cerebral Resuscitation Study Group. *Resuscitation* 1993;26(1):47–52.
53. Verbeek PR, Vermeulen MJ, Ali FH, et al. Derivation of a termination-of-resuscitation guideline for emergency medical technicians using automated external defibrillators. *Acad Emerg Med* 2002;9(7):671–678.
54. Wenzel V, Ewy GA, Lindner KH. Vasopressin and endothelin during cardiopulmonary resuscitation. *Crit Care Med* 2000;28[11 Suppl]:N233–N235.
55. Williams GR Jr, Spencer FC. The clinical use of hypothermia following cardiac arrest. *Ann Surg* 1958;148(3):462–468.
56. Yanagawa Y, Ishihara S, Norio H, et al. Preliminary clinical outcome study of mild resuscitative hypothermia after out-of-hospital cardiopulmonary arrest. *Resuscitation* 1998;39(1–2):61–66.
57. Zeiner A, Holzer M, Sterz F, et al. Mild resuscitative hypothermia to improve neurological outcome after cardiac arrest. A clinical feasibility trial. Hypothermia After Cardiac Arrest (HACA) Study Group. *Stroke* 2000;31(1):86–94.
58. Zipes DP, Wellens HJ. Sudden cardiac death. *Circulation* 1998;98(21):2334–2351.
59. Zoll PM, Linenthal AJ, Gibson NW, et al. Termination of ventricular fibrillation in man by externally applied electric countershock. *N Engl J Med* 1956;254(16):727–732.

for the care of patients in the United States with septic shock is approximately $17 billion. Mortality from shock remains high, despite better understanding of the underlying pathophysiology and aggressive treatment. Approximately 30% to 45% of patients in septic shock, and 60% to 90% for those with cardiogenic shock, die within 1 month of presentation. The presentation may be as subtle as the patient with compensated heart failure (3), or as obvious as the ultimate shock state of cardiac arrest. It is estimated that 15% of patients with undetected severe sepsis and septic shock are admitted to general medical floors, which frequently leads to lethal consequences after hospital admission (4,5). Irrespective of the type of ED presentation, timely diagnosis and aggressive intervention significantly improves survival (5).

The principles of oxygen delivery and utilization are paramount to the understanding of shock. A maximum of four molecules of oxygen is loaded onto each molecule of hemoglobin as it passes through the lungs. If all available oxygen sites are occupied (four per molecule of hemoglobin), then the arterial oxygen saturation (SaO_2) is 100% (Fig. 4.1). Arterial oxygen concentration (CaO_2) is the amount of oxygen bound to hemoglobin plus the amount dissolved in plasma. Oxygen delivery (DO_2) is the product of the CaO_2 and cardiac output (CO). Oxygen consumption (VO_2) reflects a sensitive balance between supply and demand. Normally, the tissues consume about 25% of the oxygen carried on hemoglobin, and venous blood returning to the right heart is about 75% saturated venous oxygen saturation (S_{vo2}). When oxygen supply is insufficient to meet demand, the first compensatory mechanism is an increase in CO. If the increase in CO is inadequate, the amount of oxygen extracted from hemoglobin by the tissues increases, reflected in a decrease in S_{vo2}.

When compensatory mechanisms fail to correct the imbalance between tissue supply and demand, anaerobic metabolism occurs, resulting in the formation of lactic acid (normally between 0.5 and 1.5 mM/L). An elevated lactate level is associated with an S_{vo2} <50%. Most cases of lactic acidosis are caused by inadequate oxygen delivery, but lactic acidosis occasionally can develop from an excessively high oxygen demand, as, for example, in status epilepticus. In other cases, lactic acidosis occurs because of impairment in tissue oxygen utilization, as in septic shock and immediately after resuscitation from cardiac arrest. A normal S_{vo2} and adequate oxygen delivery with an elevated lactate indicates such an impairment. Elevated lactate is a marker of impaired oxygen delivery or utilization and correlates with short-term prognosis of critically ill patients in the ED (6). S_{vo2} can also be used as a measure of the balance between tissue oxygen supply and demand. S_{vo2} is measured through a pulmonary artery catheter, but similar information can be obtained from the

CHAPTER 4

Shock

Emanuel P. Rivers and David Amponsah

More than 1 million cases of shock are estimated to present to U.S. emergency departments (EDs) each year. The number of patients with shock continues to rise yearly, particularly in patients older than 65 years. The incidence of septic shock, for example, increased markedly over a 22-year period (1979 to 2000), with an annualized increase of 8.7% (1). The annual economic burden

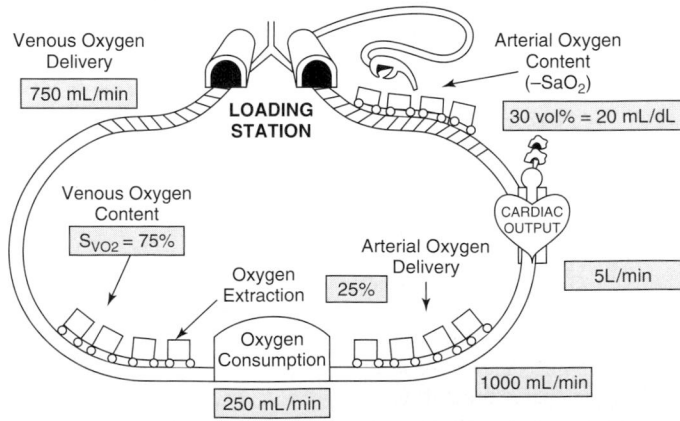

Figure 4.1. Oxygen saturation, content, and delivery.

central venous blood saturation Sc_{vo2}, which correlates well with S_{vo2} and is more easily obtained in the ED setting (7).

Shock is circulatory insufficiency caused by tissue oxygen delivery that is insufficient to meet oxygen demands. The result of shock is global hypoperfusion or tissue hypoxia and is manifested by a decreased venous oxygen content and metabolic acidosis (lactic acidosis). Global tissue hypoxia alone can independently activate the inflammatory response and serve as a comorbid variable in the pathogenesis of all forms of shock (9). The failure to diagnose and treat global tissue hypoxia in a timely manner leads to an accumulation of an oxygen debt, the magnitude of which correlates with increased mortality.

CLINICAL PRESENTATION

History

The clinical presentation of shock can range from dramatic to subtle. It can be instantly apparent, as with acute myocardial infarction, anaphylaxis, or hemorrhage, whereas some patients may have few symptoms other than generalized weakness, lethargy, or altered mental status. Symptoms that suggest volume depletion include bleeding, vomiting, diarrhea, excessive urination, insensible losses as a result of fever, or orthostatic lightheadedness. A history of cardiovascular disease is important, particularly episodes of chest pain or symptoms of congestive heart failure. Prior neurologic diseases can render patients more susceptible to complications from hypovolemia. Use of medications, both prescribed and nonprescribed, is important. Some medications cause volume depletion (e.g., diuretics), whereas others depress myocardial contractility (e.g., β-blockers and calcium channel blockers) and others are vasodilators (e.g., niacin or antiimpotence drugs). The possibility of an anaphylactic reaction to a new medication should also be considered.

Physical Examination

The clinical presentation of shock varies depending on the underlying cause. Although not specific, physical findings taken as a composite may be useful in the assessment of patients in shock (Table 4.1) No single vital sign or physical finding is diagnostic of shock, as vital signs are insensitive in detecting and assessing the severity of tissue hypoperfusion. Measurement of blood pressure can be particularly difficult because of peripheral vascular disease, tachycardia with a small pulse pressure, and arrhythmias such as atrial fibrillation. Shock is usually, but not always, associated with systemic arterial hypotension; that is, systolic blood pressure less than 90 mm Hg. Because blood pressure is the product of flow and resistance (mean arterial pressure [MAP] = CO × systemic vascular resistance [SVR]), the blood pressure may not fall in the presence of decreased cardiac output if there is increase in peripheral vascular resistance (Fig. 4.2). The insensitivity of blood pressure in detecting inadequate flow to tissues and global tissue hypoxia has been repeatedly confirmed. Thus, shock may occur with a normal blood pressure, and hypotension may occur without shock.

The onset of shock provokes a myriad of autonomic responses, many of which serve to maintain perfusion pressure to vital organs. Stimulation of the carotid baroreceptor stretch reflex activates the sympathetic nervous system leading to (a) arteriolar vasoconstriction, resulting in redistribution of blood volume from the skin, skeletal muscle, kidneys, and splanchnic viscera; (b) an increase in heart rate and contractility that increases cardiac output; (c) constriction of venous capacitance vessels, which augments venous return; (d) release of the vasoactive hormones epinephrine, norepinephrine, dopamine, and

TABLE 4.1.   Clinical Findings in Shock

Temperature
- Hyperthermia, hypothermia, or afebrile, especially in the elderly

Skin
- Pale, dusky, clammy, cyanosis
- Sweaty
- Altered temperature
- Decreased capillary refill

Central nervous system
- Acute delirium or brain failure
- Restlessness, disorientation, confusion, psychosis
- Coma

Neck
- Neck vein distention or flattening

Respiratory
- Tachypnea
- Increased minute ventilation
- Increased dead space
- Bronchospasm
- Hypocapnia, respiratory failure, adult respiratory distress syndrome
- Respiratory alkalosis

Cardiovascular
- Tachycardia; S3 may result from high output states
- Dysrhythmias
- Hypotension
- Increased then decreased pulse pressure
- Pulsus paradoxus
- Elevated shock index (heart rate: systolic blood pressure >1.0)
- β-Blockers may blunt response

Gastrointestinal
- Ileus
- Gastrointestinal bleeding
- Pancreatitis
- Acalculous cholecystitis
- Mesenteric ischemia from low flow states

Renal
- Oliguria, anuria, and unexplained metabolic acidosis; Paradoxical polyuria

Heme
- Hemoconcentration
- Decreased platelets
- Decreased fibrinogen
- Increased fibrin-split products
- Increased D-dimers

cortisol to maintain arteriolar and venous tone; and (e) release of antidiuretic hormone and activation of the renin–angiotensin axis to enhance water and sodium conservation to maintain intravascular volume. These compensatory mechanisms attempt to maintain Do_2 to the most critical organs: the coronary and cerebral circulation. During this process, blood flow to other organs, such as to the kidneys and gastrointestinal tract, may be compromised.

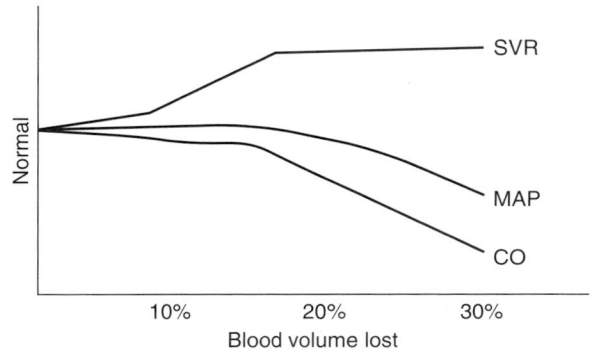

Figure 4.2. Relationship between SVR (systemic vascular resistance), MAP (mean arterial pressure), and CO (cardiac output) with volume loss.

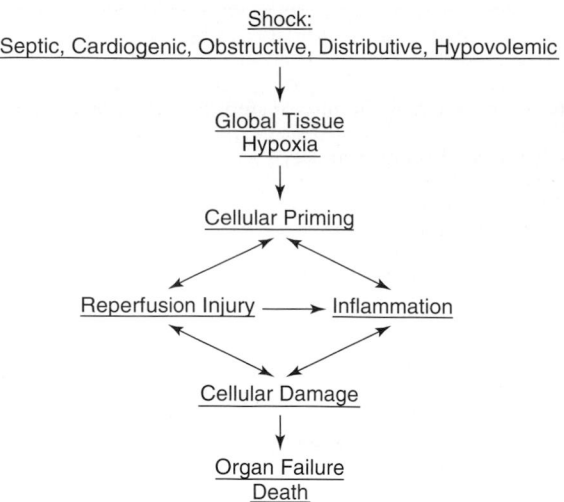

Shock:
Septic, Cardiogenic, Obstructive, Distributive, Hypovolemic

↓

Global Tissue
Hypoxia

↓

Cellular Priming

↗   ↖

Reperfusion Injury ⟶ Inflammation

↘   ↙

Cellular Damage

↓

Organ Failure
Death

Figure 4.3.   Mechanism of cell death.

The cellular response to decreased Do_2 is adenosine triphosphate (ATP) depletion, leading to ion pump dysfunction, influx of sodium, efflux of potassium, and reduction in membrane resting potential. Cellular edema occurs secondary to increased intracellular sodium while cellular membrane receptors become poorly responsive to the stress hormones insulin, glucagon, cortisol, and catecholamines. As shock progresses, lysosomal enzymes are released into the cells with subsequent hydrolysis of membranes, deoxyribonucleic acid, ribonucleic acid, and phosphate esters. As the cascade of shock continues, the loss of cellular integrity and the breakdown in cellular homeostasis result in cellular death (Fig. 4.3).

These pathologic events give rise to the metabolic features of hemoconcentration, hyperkalemia, hyponatremia, prerenal azotemia, metabolic acidosis, hyper- or hypoglycemia, and lactic acidosis.

The clinical presentation of early shock is often characterized as a syndrome called the systemic inflammatory response syndrome (SIRS). It is defined as the presence of two or more of the following features: (a) temperature greater than 38°C (100.4°F) or less than 36°C (96.8°F); (b) heart rate faster than 90 beats per minute; (c) respiratory rate faster than 20 breaths per minute; and (d) white blood cell count greater than $12.0 \times 10^9/L$, less than $4.0 \times 10^9/L$, or with greater than 10% immature forms or bands. SIRS may occur in any shock state. The stimulus for SIRS is a complex elaboration of humoral and cellular pro- and antiinflammatory products, which induces a pan-endothelial cell disruption or generalized inflammation within the vast capillary network in each organ. The hemodynamic consequence of SIRS is the generation of global tissue hypoxia from hypovolemia, vasodilation, and myocardial suppression. There is an increase in oxygen demands secondary to fever or an increased work of breathing. Cytopathic tissue hypoxia develops when there is a defect in the peripheral utilization of oxygen in the tissues (8).

As SIRS progresses, organ dysfunction and the multiorgan dysfunction syndrome (MODS) ensue. This is characterized by adult respiratory distress syndrome, disseminated intravascular coagulation, hepatic failure, and adrenal and renal failure, among others. Early detection and interruption of these hemodynamic perturbations are key for improving survival. Table 4.2 compares shock states.

DIFFERENTIAL DIAGNOSIS

The four classifications of shock are based on etiology:

- Hypovolemic (caused by inadequate circulating volume), as in hemorrhagic shock
- Cardiogenic (caused by inadequate cardiac pump function), as in anterior wall acute myocardial infarction
- Distributive (caused by peripheral vasodilatation and maldistribution of blood flow), as in sepsis, anaphylaxis, or spinal cord injury
- Obstructive (caused by extracardiac obstruction to blood flow), as in a pulmonary embolus.

Although there may be an initial predominant cause of shock, as the shock state persists or progresses to irreversible end-organ damage, other pathophysiologic mechanisms become operative and can create a mixed picture.

EMERGENCY DEPARTMENT EVALUATION

Ancillary Studies

The clinical presentation and the presumptive etiology of shock dictate the use of ancillary studies. A battery of standard arterial blood gas, hematologic, coagulation, and biochemical tests usually provides an assessment of each organ function and may detect an abnormality that requires specific treatment. A wide range of laboratory abnormalities may be encountered in shock, but most abnormal values merely point to the particular organ system that is either contributing to or being affected by the shock state. No single laboratory value is sensitive or specific for shock. Additional studies, including an ECG, a chest radiograph (CXR), and source-specific plain radiographs or computerized tomography (CT), should be done.

TABLE 4.2.   Comparison of Shock States

	MAP	CVP	Sc_{vo2}	Lactate	CI	SVR	Comment
Cardiogenic	↓	↑	↓	↑	↓	↑	Myocardial infarction or decompensated heart failure
Obstructive	↓	↑	↓	↑	↓	↑	Pulmonary embolus or pericardial tamponade
Hypovolemic	↓	↓	↓	↑	↓	↑	Hemorrhagic or hypovolemic
Septic							
Stage 1	↓ or Normal	↓	↓	↑	↓	↑	Early sepsis, hypovolemia
Stage 2	↓	Normal	↑	↑	↑	↓	Compensated
Stage 3	Normal	↑	↓	↑	Normal	Normal	Myocardial suppression
Stage 4	↓	Normal	↑	↑	↓	↑	Impaired tissue oxygen utilization or cytopathic tissue hypoxia
Distributive	↓	↓	↓	↑	↓	↓	Anaphylaxis, spinal shock

CI, cardiac index; CVP, central venous pressure; MAP, mean arterial pressure; SVR, systemic vascular resistance.

TABLE 4.3.   Adjuncts that Guide Therapeutic Interventions

Base deficit	Base deficit is an indicator of metabolic acidosis and is an index of hemodynamic and tissue perfusion changes in shock. Predicts illness severity in intraabdominal hemorrhage and blunt trauma.
Invasive blood pressure monitoring	Intense vasoconstriction caused by sympathetic activity or vasopressors given will cause the cuff pressure to underestimate true blood pressure. A Doppler used in conjunction with a sphygmomanometer may provide a more accurate measure of systolic blood pressure once Korotkoff sounds are no longer audible. Intraarterial pressure measurement is preferable because vasoactive drugs can cause rapid swings in blood pressure and multiple blood samplings typically are required.
Central venous pressure (CVP)	Aid in assessing volume status. Preferred for the long-term administration of vasopressor therapy and provides rapid access to the heart if pacemaker placement is required. May not reliably reflect the left ventricular filling pressure in clinical states such as pulmonary embolus, obstructive airway disease, right ventricular infarction, and pericardial effusion. Common iliac venous pressure can approximate CVP.
Central venous oximetry (Sc_{vo2})	Sc_{vo2} closely approximates mixed venous O_2 saturation (Sm_{vo2}) and can be monitored continuously using infrared oximetry. This technology enables the clinician to detect clinically unrecognized global tissue hypoperfusion in the treatment of myocardial infarction, general medical shock, trauma, hemorrhage, septic, hypovolemic, end-stage heart failure, cardiogenic shock during and after cardiopulmonary arrest.
Arterial-central venous P_{co2} difference	Increased arterial-mixed venous carbon dioxide gradients, or $(a-v)P_{co2}$, are seen in acute circulatory failure, and inversely correlate with the cardiac index (CI). Central venous and mixed venous carbon dioxide values can be interchanged to determine cardiac index.
Pulmonary artery catheterization	The standard of care for assessing cardiac status. Valuable in determining left-sided heart filling and pulmonary artery pressure, and for assessing the cause of pulmonary edema. Can obtain cardiac output and mixed venous oxygen saturation. Will be able to calculate hemodynamic (i.e., systemic vascular resistance) and oxygen transport variables (Vo_2 and Do_2). The effectiveness of this monitoring technique on improving outcome is questionable.
Noninvasive cardiac output	Cardiac output can be measured by transesophageal Doppler, cutaneous bioimpedance, and lithium dilution.
Gastric tonometry and sublingual capnography	Serial measurements of gastric and sublingual mucosal blood flow are base on hydrogen ion diffusion and carbon dioxide elimination. Inadequate visceral perfusion, as evidenced by persistently low intramucosal pH or increased sublingual carbon dioxide concentration after resuscitation, is associated with subsequent organ dysfunction and death.
Retinal venous O_2 saturation	Retinal venous O_2 saturation ($SraO_2$) correlates with blood volume, central venous O_2 saturation, and arterial O_2 saturation.
Metabolic cart	Directly measured VO_2 without a pulmonary artery catheter. A reduction in VO_2 after acute myocardial infarction predicts cardiogenic shock and mortality after human cardiac arrest.

Hemodynamic monitoring is important in the assessment of patients in shock and evaluation of response to treatment. Monitoring capabilities vary from institution to institution, but should include pulse oximetry; electrocardiographic monitoring; continuous, noninvasive, but preferably intraarterial, blood pressure monitoring; end-tidal CO_2 monitoring; central venous pressure (CVP) monitoring; and continuous central venous oximetry. Because hemodynamic measurements are physiologic values, they should be used to answer specific physiologic questions rather than to serve as therapeutic end points. Table 4.3 outlines adjuncts to aid in the evaluation patients in shock.

EMERGENCY DEPARTMENT MANAGEMENT

The *ABCDE* tenets of shock resuscitation are fundamental to deliver enough oxygen to the tissues to meet the metabolic demands of the tissues (Fig. 4.4). This includes establishing an *Airway*, providing and controlling the work of *Breathing*, optimizing the *Circulation*, assuring adequate oxygen *Delivery*, and achieving *End* points of resuscitation.

Establishing Airway

Airway control is best obtained through endotracheal intubation for airway protection, positive pressure ventilation (oxygenation), patency, and pulmonary toilet. Sedatives, which are frequently used to facilitate intubation, can exacerbate hypotension through arterial vasodilatation, venodilation, and myocardial suppression. Furthermore, positive pressure ventilation reduces preload and cardiac output. The combination of these

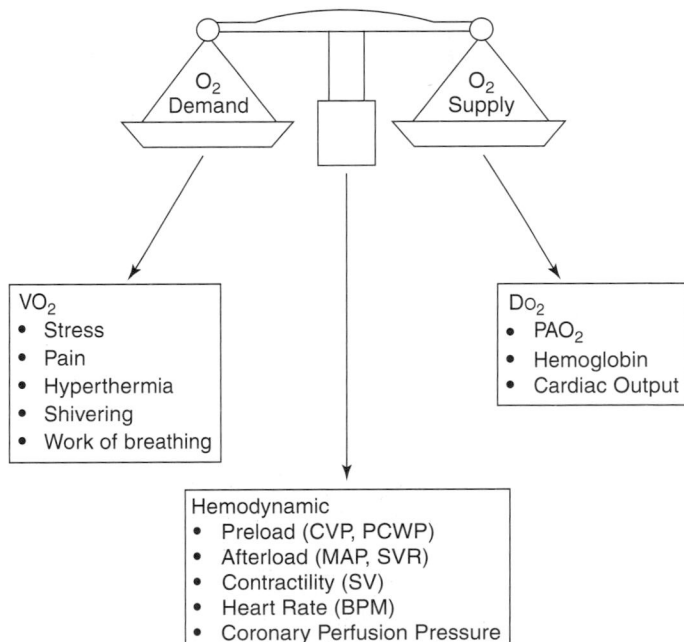

Figure 4.4.   Balance between oxygen supply and demand. BPM, beats per minute; CVP, central venous pressure; MAP, mean arterial pressure; PCWP, pulmonary capillary wedge pressure; SV, stroke volume; SVR, systemic vascular resistance.

interventions can lead to hemodynamic collapse. Volume resuscitation or application of vasoactive agents may be required prior to intubation and positive pressure ventilation.

Controlling the Work of Breathing

Control of breathing is required when tachypnea accompanies shock. Respiratory muscles are significant consumers of oxygen during shock and contribute to lactate production. Mechanical ventilation and sedation decrease the work of breathing and have been shown to improve survival. SaO_2 should be restored to greater than 93% and ventilation controlled to maintain an arterial carbon dioxide pressure ($PaCO_2$) of 35 to 40 mm Hg. Attempts to normalize pH above 7.3 by hyperventilation are not beneficial. Mechanical ventilation not only provides oxygenation and corrects hypercapnia, but it assists, controls, and synchronizes ventilation, which ultimately decreases the work of breathing. Neuromuscular blocking agents are used as adjuncts to further decrease respiratory muscle fatigue, oxygen consumption and preserve Do_2 to vital organs.

Optimizing the Circulation

In restoring the balance between systemic oxygen delivery and demands, optimization of circulatory dysfunction begins with a thoughtful manipulation of preload, afterload, contractility, and coronary perfusion pressure, while maintaining an optimal heart rate.

Circulatory or hemodynamic stabilization begins with intravascular access through large-bore peripheral venous lines. Trendelenburg positioning, historically considered necessary for maintaining perfusion in the hypotensive patient does not improve cardiopulmonary performance in comparison with the supine position. It may worsen pulmonary gas exchange and predispose to aspiration. If a volume challenge is urgently required, an alternative to the Trendelenburg position is to raise the patient's legs above the level of the heart with the patient supine. Central venous access aids in assessing volume status (preload) and monitoring Sc_{vo2}. It is the preferred route for the long-term administration of vasopressor therapy, and provides rapid access to the heart if pacemaker placement is required.

Fluid resuscitation begins with isotonic crystalloid; the amount and rate are determined by an estimate of the hemodynamic abnormality. Except for the patient in cardiogenic shock with pulmonary edema, most patients in shock have either an absolute or relative volume deficit. Fluid is given rapidly in set quantities (e.g., 500 or 1,000 mL), with reassessment of the patient after each amount. Patients with a modest degree of hypovolemia usually require an initial 20 mL/kg of isotonic crystalloid. More fluids may be necessary with profound volume deficits.

The colloid-versus-crystalloid resuscitation controversy remains despite evidence that there is a slight increase in mortality when colloids are used for volume replacement in critically ill patients. Some studies have found a lower incidence of pulmonary edema and possibly greater benefit in elderly patients with colloid resuscitation, although survival is not statistically improved. In the acute situation with severe shock, colloids may be considered to achieve rapid plasma expansion using less volume than crystalloids. Without invasive hemodynamic monitoring, noncardiogenic pulmonary edema may be difficult to differentiate from cardiogenic pulmonary edema in the ED. Even though the former may respond to fluids, fluids should be minimized in a patient with clinical or radiographic evidence of pulmonary edema until appropriate monitoring is established.

Vasopressor agents (Table 4.4) are used when there has been an inadequate response to volume resuscitation or when a patient has contraindications to volume infusion. They are most effective when the vascular space is "full" and least effective when the vascular space is depleted. However, vasopressors may be necessary early in the treatment of shock, before volume resuscitation is complete, in order to prevent potentially lethal consequences of prolonged systemic arterial hypotension. This is especially important in elderly patients with significant coronary and cerebrovascular disease. Rapidly restoring the MAP to 60 mm Hg or systolic pressure to 90 mm Hg might avoid the coronary and cerebral complications of decreased blood flow. Vasopressor agents have variable effects on the α- and β-adrenergic receptors (10).

Using vasopressors has potential pitfalls. While improving perfusion pressure in the large vessels, they may decrease capillary blood flow in certain tissue beds, especially the bowel. Vasopressors also may alter the relationship between volume and pressure measurements through their effect on the pulmonary and peripheral vascular beds. In other words, vasopressors will falsely elevate intracardiac filling pressures (i.e., CVP). They should be used judiciously, generally only after volume resuscitation. Volume assessment should be a dynamic process. When multiple vasopressors are used, they should be simplified as soon as the most therapeutic agent is identified.

Assuring Adequate Oxygen Delivery

Once blood pressure is stabilized through optimization of preload and afterload, Do_2 can be assessed and further manipulated. Arterial saturation should be returned to physiologic levels (93% to 95%) and hemoglobin maintained above 10 g/dL. If cardiac output can be assessed, it should be increased using volume infusion and inotropic agents in incremental amounts until venous oxygen saturation (S_{vo2} or Sc_{vo2}) and lactate are normalized.

The control of VO_2 is important in restoring the balance of oxygen supply and demand to tissues. A hyperadrenergic state results from the compensatory response to shock, physiologic stress, pain, and anxiety. Shivering frequently results when a patient is unclothed for examination and then left inadequately covered in a cold resuscitation room. The combination of these variables increases systemic oxygen consumption. Pain further suppresses myocardial function, thus impairing Do_2 and VO_2. Providing analgesia, muscle relaxation, warm covering, anxiolytics, and even paralytic agents, when appropriate, decreases this inappropriate VO_2.

Tissue oxygen extraction assesses adequacy of the resuscitation in meeting the oxygen needs of the tissues. Sequential examination of lactate and S_{vo2} or Sc_{vo2} is a method to assess adequacy of tissue oxygen extraction. Continuous measurement of S_{vo2} or Sc_{vo2} through fiberoptic technology can be used in the ED (7). Other technologies also have the potential to assess tissue perfusion during resuscitation.

Achieving End Points of Resuscitation

Normalization of blood pressure, heart rate, and urine output are traditional end points. Global tissue hypoxia can still persist in patients resuscitated from shock even with normalization of vital signs (11) and urine output (12). Because these underestimate the degree of remaining hypoperfusion and oxygen debt, more physiologic end points have been investigated (13). No therapeutic end point is universally effective, and only a few have been tested in prospective trials, with mixed results. The goals of resuscitation are to maximize survival and to minimize morbidity by using objective hemodynamic and physiologic values to guide therapy. A goal-directed approach at achieving

TABLE 4.4. Commonly Used Vasoactive Agents

Drug	Dose/Mixture	Action	Effects				Side Effects/Comments
			Cardiac Stimulation	Vasoconstriction	Vasodilation	Cardiac Output	
Dopamine	0.5–25 μg/kg/min 200–400/250 mL	α, β, and dopaminergic	++ at 2–10 μg/kg/min	++ at 7 μg/kg/min	+ at 0.5–5.0 μg/kg/min	Usually increases	Tachydysrhythmias; increases myocardial O_2 consumption; a cerebral, mesenteric, coronary, and renal vasodilator
Norepinephrine	0.01–0.5 μg/kg/min 4 mg/250 mL	primarily α_1, some β_1	++	++++	0	Slight decrease	Dose-related, reflex bradycardia; useful when loss of venous tone predominates; spares the coronary circulation
Phenylephrine	0.15–0.75 μg/kg/min 10 mg/250 mL	pure α	0	++++	0	Decrease	Reflex bradycardia, headache, restlessness, excitability, rarely dysrhythmias; ideal for patients in shock with tachycardia or supraventricular dysrhythmias
Ephedrine	5–25 mg	α and β	+++	++	+	Increase	Causes palpitations, hypertension, cardiac arrhythmias; an indirect-acting central nervous system stimulant; limited long-term value as therapy for shock
Vasopressin	0.01 to 0.04 U/min	α		++++			Primarily α; outcome data of its use is lacking. Infusions of >0.04 U/min may lead to adverse, likely vasoconstriction-mediated events; reserved for refractory hypotension
Epinephrine	0.01–0.75 μg/kg/min 1 mg/250 mL	α and β	++++ at 0.03–0.15 μg/kg/min	++++ at 0.15–0.30 μg/kg/min	++	Increase	Causes tachydysrhythmia and leukocytosis; increases myocardial oxygen consumption
Dobutamine	2.0–20 μg/kg/min 250 mg/250 mL	β_1, some β_2, and α_1 in large dosages	+++	+	++	Increase	Causes tachydysrhythmia, occasional gastrointestinal distress, an increase in myocardial oxygen consumption, and hypotension in volume-depleted patient; has less peripheral vasoconstriction than dopamine; can cause fewer arrhythmias than isoproterenol
Isoproterenol	0.01–0.02 μg/kg/min 1 mg/250 mL	β_1 and some β_2	++++	0	+++	Increase	Causes tachydysrhythmia, facial flushing, and hypotension in hypovolemic patients; increases myocardial oxygen consumption; never use alone in patient in shock

urine output ≥ 0.5 mL/kg/h, CVP 8 to 12 mm Hg, MAP 65 to 90 mm Hg, and $Sc_{vo2} \geq 70\%$ during ED resuscitation of septic shock significantly decreases mortality (5).

Bicarbonate Use in Shock

The primary treatment for acidosis in shock is to reverse the underlying cause. Because this goal is not rapidly attainable, intravenous bicarbonate is often administered. The rationale for giving bicarbonate is that it diminishes myocardial depression and counteracts the insensitivity to endogenous catecholamines attributed to acidosis. However, experimental data indicate that exogenous bicarbonate can actually worsen intracellular acidosis and prospective studies do not show any benefit from its use. Bicarbonate also shifts the oxygen–hemoglobin dissociation curve to the left and impairs tissue unloading of hemoglobin-bound oxygen. However, many clinicians are reluctant to withhold bicarbonate. A compromise is to partially correct the metabolic acidosis over time. The bicarbonate deficit is determined, which is equal to

$$(\text{normal } HCO_3^- - \text{the patient's } HCO_3^-) \times 0.4 \times \text{body weight in kilograms}$$

Half of this amount is infused slowly with the remainder infused over 6 to 8 hours to achieve a pH of no greater than 7.25.

Resuscitative Adjuncts

Adjuncts that can guide therapeutic interventions are evolving. A variety of invasive and noninvasive adjuncts (see Table 4.3) are available to monitor the response to shock resuscitation.

DISPOSITION AND PROGNOSIS

Pathogenic mechanisms such as cytopathic tissue hypoxia (a form of irreversible shock) can occur within the first few hours of an ED stay, rendering therapy in the intensive care unit less effective (8). Current national increases in ED patient acuity and overcrowding have resulted in extending the golden hour into hours and even days, consequently requiring the provision of critical care in the ED. The benefit of timely ED intervention in nontraumatic critical illness is significant; standard ED care can significantly decrease morbidity and predicted mortality in as little as 6 hours of treatment (16). In addition, application of an algorithmic approach to optimize hemodynamic end points with early goal-directed therapy in the ED reduces mortality by an absolute 16% in patients with severe sepsis or septic shock (5).

Documentation and communication are important. Resuscitation in the ED is commonly performed in "ordered chaos." Even though resuscitation is systematic and thoughtful, miscommunication with the critical care specialist accepting the patient can undo the benefits of initial treatment. A system-oriented problem list with an assessment and plan, including all procedures and complications, should be verbally communicated and written or dictated prior to transfer. For prolonged ED stays, notations regarding patient status, diagnostic and therapeutic intervention, and sentinel events should be provided frequently.

Outcome prediction at ED disposition has not been fully studied; however, some clinical variables, for example, severity of shock, temporal duration, underlying cause, preexisting vital organ dysfunction, and reversibility, are associated with poor outcome. Persistently elevated lactate level, base deficits, sublingual capnography, and decreased Sc_{vo2} are prognostic for morbidity and mortality in trauma, septic shock, and after cardiac arrest (18). Outcome predictions using physiologic scoring systems in the ED are also being studied.

COMMON PITFALLS

- ✔ Failure to appropriately monitor patients: Be aware of arterial blood pressure monitoring malfunctions that occur, such as dampening of the arterial line or disconnection from the transducer
- ✔ Failure to adequately volume resuscitate patients: Studies show that persistent global tissue hypoxia may still persist even after resuscitation to normal vitals signs (14) and urine output (15). The hospital mortality in this subset of patients can be >50% (5). The early use of vasopressors may "falsely" elevate CVP and disguise hypovolemia
- ✔ Problems with vasopressor administration: Is the intravenous tubing into which the vasopressors are running properly connected? Are the vasopressor infusion pumps working? Are the vasopressors mixed adequately?
- ✔ Failure to recognize a pneumothorax after placement of central venous access
- ✔ Not recognizing an occult penetrating injury (a bullet hole or stab wound) or occult bleeding (from a ruptured spleen or ectopic pregnancy)
- ✔ Failure to recognize anaphylactic shock caused by just-administered medication (e.g., penicillin) or by medication taken before arrival
- ✔ Failure to diagnose cardiac tamponade in the chronic renal failure patient on dialysis or in the cancer patient
- ✔ Failure to recognize adrenal insufficiency. The incidence of adrenal dysfunction can be as high as 20% in this subset of patients (2)

References

1. Martin GS, Mannino DM, Eaton S, et al. The epidemiology of sepsis in the United States from 1979 through 2000. *N Engl J Med* 2003;348:1546–1554.
2. Rivers EP, Blake HC, Dereczyk B, et al. Adrenal dysfunction in hemodynamically unstable patients in the emergency department. *Acad Emerg Med* 1999;6:626–630.
3. Ander DS, Jaggi M, Rivers E, et al. Undetected cardiogenic shock in patients with congestive heart failure presenting to the emergency department. *Am J Cardiol* 1998;82:888–891.
4. Angus DC, Linde-Zwirble WT, Lidicker J, et al. Epidemiology of severe sepsis in the United States: analysis of incidence, outcome, and associated costs of care. *Crit Care Med* 2001;29:1303–1310.
5. Rivers E, Nguyen B, Havstad S, et al. Early goal-directed therapy in the treatment of severe sepsis and septic shock. *N Engl J Med* 2001;345:1368–1377.
6. Aduen J, Bernstein WK, Khastgir T, et al. The use and clinical importance of a substrate-specific electrode for rapid determination of blood lactate concentrations. *JAMA* 1994;272:1678–1685.
7. Rivers EP, Ander DS, Powell D. Central venous oxygen saturation monitoring in the critically ill patient. *Curr Opin Crit Care* 2001;7:204–211.
8. Fink MP. Cytopathic hypoxia. Is oxygen use impaired in sepsis as a result of an acquired intrinsic derangement in cellular respiration? *Crit Care Clin* 2002;18:165–175.
9. Karimova A, Pinsky DJ. The endothelial response to oxygen deprivation: biology and clinical implications. *Intensive Care Med* 2001;27:19–31.
10. Kellum JA, Pinsky MR. Use of vasopressor agents in critically ill patients. *Curr Opin Crit Care* 2002;8:236–241.
11. Rady MY, Rivers EP, Nowak RM. Resuscitation of the critically ill in the ED: responses of blood pressure, heart rate, shock index, central venous oxygen saturation, and lactate. *Am J Emerg Med* 1996;14:218–225.
12. Cortez A, Zito J, Lucas CE, Gerrick SJ. Mechanism of inappropriate polyuria in septic patients. *Arch Surg* 1977;112:471–476.
13. Pinsky MR. Targets for resuscitation from shock. *Minerva Anestesiol* 2003;69:237–244.
14. Rady MY, Smithline HA, Blake H, et al. A comparison of the shock index and conventional vital signs to identify acute, critical illness in the emergency department. *Ann Emerg Med* 1994;24:685–690.
15. Lucas CE, Harrigan C, Denis R, et al. Impaired renal concentrating ability during resuscitation from shock. *Arch Surg* 1983;118:642–645.

16. Nguyen HB, Rivers EP, Havstad S, et al. Critical care in the emergency department: a physiologic assessment and outcome evaluation. *Acad Emerg Med* 2000;7:1354–1361.
17. Rady MY, Edwards JD, Rivers EP, et al. Measurement of oxygen consumption after uncomplicated acute myocardial infarction. *Chest* 1993;104:930–934.
18. Weil MH, Nakagawa Y, Tang W, et al. Sublingual capnometry: a new noninvasive measurement for diagnosis and quantitation of severity of circulatory shock. *Crit Care Med* 1999;27:1225–1229.

CHAPTER 5
Vascular Access

Eric F. Reichman and Joanne L. Oakes

The practice of Emergency Medicine frequently requires access to the venous, and sometimes the arterial circulation of a patient (10). Vascular access allows for blood sampling, medication administration, blood product administration, hydration, patient monitoring (arterial lines and pulmonary artery catheters), and insertion of cardiac pacing wires. Peripheral venous puncture is the most common invasive procedure performed in the Emergency Department. Peripheral vein cannulation is performed on a daily basis and is the cornerstone of circulatory resuscitation.

EMERGENCY DEPARTMENT EVALUATION

There are numerous techniques to access a patient's venous or arterial circulation. Venous puncture (venipuncture) or arterial puncture with a needle is only indicated for the sampling of blood. Medications may be administered as a one-time dose via this technique but the risk of extravasation is high. Venous cannulation (i.v. placement) is indicated for repeated sampling of venous blood. It is also performed for the administration of medications, fluid solutions, blood products, and nutritional support.

Arteries and veins should not be accessed through infected skin. Do not withdraw venous blood from a vein proximal to a running intravenous infusion. The blood sample will be tainted or diluted by the infused solution. A hole in the vein may allow blood, infused solutions, and medications to extravasate into the surrounding tissues.

Venipuncture and venous cannulation of veins in an extremity with an arteriovenous fistula should be avoided. Veins in the upper extremity that may be needed for arteriovenous fistula construction for hemodialysis in the future should not be punctured unless absolutely necessary.

Complications specific to each technique and site are discussed more fully in this chapter. Venous and arterial catheters should be assessed immediately after their placement and be reassessed frequently. The assessment must include the skin puncture site, catheter function, the neurovascular status of the distal extremity, and the patient's overall condition.

EMERGENCY DEPARTMENT MANAGEMENT

General Principles for Intravenous Access

While veins can dilate and constrict somewhat on their own, they do so mostly in response to the pressure within them. The use of venous tourniquets, dependent positioning, "pumping" via muscle contraction, and the local application of heat or nitroglycerin ointment all contribute to venous engorgement. These maneuvers can be used to aid in the performance of a venipuncture or peripheral venous access.

The vascular anatomy can affect access (3). Deficient perivascular connective tissue permits the vein to "roll" from side to side and evade the needle. Tough connective tissue can impede the entry of a flexible catheter while serving to stabilize the vein and prevent its collapse. Venous valves allow unidirectional flow and prevent blood from pooling in the dependent portions of the extremities. Valves can block the passage of a catheter through and into a vein. Valves are more numerous at the points where tributaries join larger veins and in the lower extremities. Valves are almost absent within the large central veins, the veins of the head, and the veins of the neck.

Peripheral veins are easiest to access at the apex of the "Y," formed when two tributaries merge into a larger vein or where the vein is straight and free of branches and valves for 2 cm or so proximal to the site of puncture. These sites tend to be anchored and "roll" less than other sites.

The angle of insertion of the needle varies depending on the depth of the vein being punctured. A shallow angle (30°–45°) should be used for small and superficial veins. A more obtuse angle (60°) should be used to access deeper veins. Very small and superficial veins should be entered at a very acute (15°–30°) angle.

Fluid Flow Considerations

Both the diameter and the length of the infusion device affect the flow rate through the catheter. Viscous fluids (e.g., blood products and albumin) infuse more slowly than less viscous fluids (e.g., saline). These relationships can be seen in the solution of Poiseuille equation for ideal fluid flow through a cylindrical tube. The pressure gradient and resistance to flow is inversely proportional to the length of the catheter tubing. Flow rates decrease as catheter length increases. Using the shortest possible catheter permits the highest fluid infusion rates. Catheter diameter changes will have the most effect on flow rates. The flow rate increases to the fourth power as the catheter internal radius increases. Maximal flow rates result from using the largest internal diameter (smallest gauge) catheter that will fit inside the vein. Large-bore venous catheters are preferred for high volume infusions.

Venous Cannulation

There are four main techniques of venous cannulation (3). The first is the needle-only using a butterfly-type needle. This is seldom used today. The catheter-over-the-needle is the most commonly used technique for peripheral venous cannulation. The catheter-through-the-needle technique is occasionally used but not very popular. The Seldinger wire-guided technique is most commonly used for central venous access.

Identify the vein to be cannulated and the site of the skin puncture. Clean the area of any dirt and debris. Cleanse the skin with isopropyl alcohol or povidone iodine. Apply a tourniquet to the extremity, proximal to the venous cannulation site, to engorge the vein. Additional engorgement of the vein can be accomplished by placing the extremity in a dependent position, "pumping" via muscle contractions of the extremity, and the application of heat or nitroglycerin ointment over the vein. A small subcutaneous wheal of local anesthetic solution may be placed at the skin puncture site to provide comfort to the patient.

The needle-only technique is used occasionally for short-term venous access in young children and elderly patients with fragile veins. This system is prone to malposition and infiltration. The tip of the needle can easily lacerate the vein if the needle is not secure and allowed to move. This technique is therefore not recommended.

The catheter-over-the-needle systems are the most commonly used for venous access (Fig. 5.1). The infusion catheter fits closely over a hypodermic needle. Placement of these catheters is usually quick and simple. Several considerations should always be kept in mind when using a catheter-over-the-needle. Intravascular placement is indicated by a flash of blood in the hub of the needle. If the patient's venous pressure is very low or if the needle is long and narrow, both sides of the vessel may be traversed (through-and-through) before the practitioner realizes that the needle was within the vein. If the tip of the needle is withdrawn from the

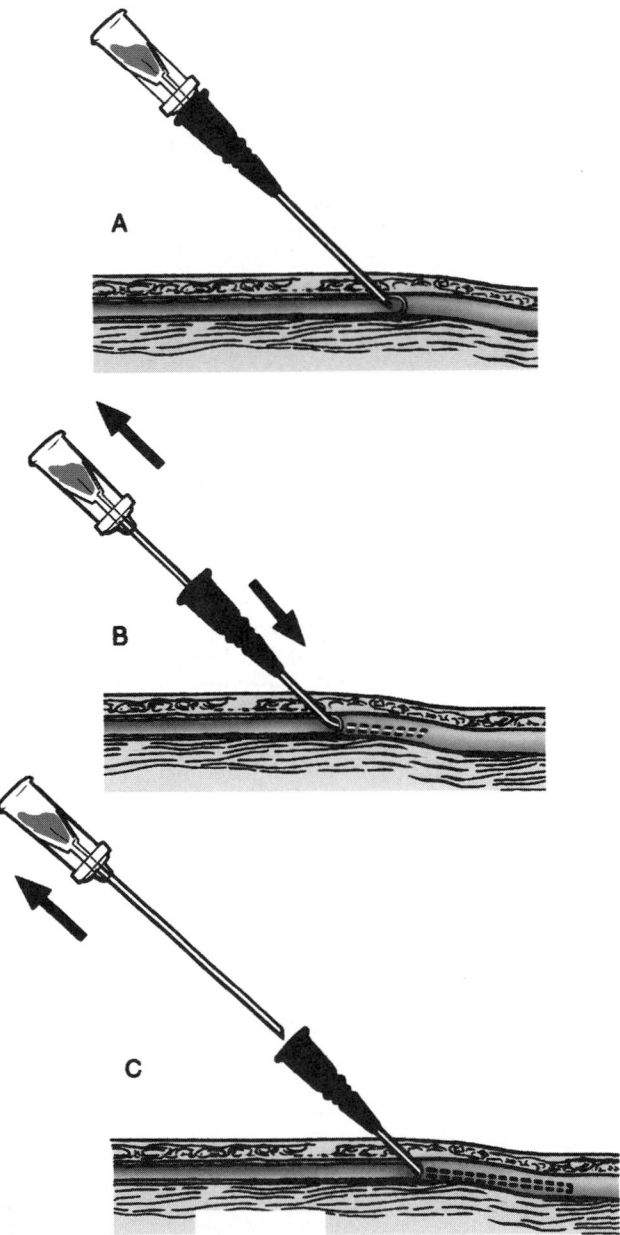

Figure 5.1.   The catheter-over-the-needle technique. (Reprinted with permission from Reichman EF, Simon RR. *Emergency medicine procedures.* New York: McGraw-Hill, 2004.)

vein, the catheter will not advance. If the catheter is advanced when the tip of the needle but not the catheter is within the vein, the catheter will not advance. The catheter will push the vein off the needle. Depress the skin just distal to the puncture site and pull it distally to prevent the vein from "rolling."

As opposed to the over-the-needle approach, the catheter-through-the-needle technique eliminates the need for a needle that is as long as the catheter and eliminates the possibility of pushing the vein off the end of the needle when the catheter is advanced (3). The main disadvantage of this technique is the possibility of the needle tip shearing off the catheter resulting in a catheter embolism. This is prevented by using proper technique. Another disadvantage is an increased risk of hematoma formation since the needle used for venipuncture must be larger in diameter than the catheter.

The Seldinger technique allows for the placement of a catheter over a wire rather than directly over a needle. The wire used must be longer than the catheter. The needle used to insert the wire can be short and of a smaller gauge than the catheter. The Seldinger technique is most commonly used for central venous catheter insertion.

Venipuncture and Peripheral Intravenous Access

The upper extremity is preferred to the lower extremity for vein cannulation (4). Distal placement should be attempted before moving more proximal (4). Avoid veins overlying a joint. These simple principles allow the patient maximum mobility and increase the chance of successfully cannulating a vein. It is easiest to insert a venous cannula where two tributaries merge and form a "Y." Choose a straight portion of vein without branches to minimize the chance of hitting valves within the vein and make threading the catheter easier.

Peripheral Venipuncture

Stabilize the vein with the nondominant hand. Insert the needle attached to a syringe or vacuum tube adapter, with the bevel upward, into the vein at a 45° to 60° angle. Lower angles, at times nearly parallel to the skin, are often required to enter very narrow or superficial veins. Apply negative pressure to the syringe. A flashback of blood in the hub of the needle indicates that the tip of the needle is within the vein. Pulsatile blood indicates an arterial puncture. Unless venous blood is specifically needed for a test, collect the necessary samples before removing the needle. No additional harm will be done by withdrawing a blood sample from an artery that has already been punctured.

If no blood is obtained, slowly advance the needle until it is deeper than the judged depth of the vein. The tip of the needle can collapse the vein and prevent the flashback of blood (Fig. 5.2A). Slowly withdraw the needle to just beneath the skin. The vein will often have been punctured through-and-through (Fig. 5.2B). If this is the case, blood will flash back into the catheter as the needle is withdrawn (Fig. 5.2C). If no blood is obtained by the time the needle is withdrawn to just beneath the skin, re-direct the needle and make another attempt at puncturing the vein. Never sweep the point of the needle around without withdrawing it as the sharp bevel can lacerate nearby structures.

Peripheral Intravenous Cannulation

Vein cannulation begins with a successful venipuncture (3). Insert the catheter-over-the-needle through the skin and into the vein (Fig. 5.1A). A flash of blood in the hub of the needle confirms that the tip of the needle is within the vein. Advance the catheter-over-the-needle an additional 2–3 mm to ensure that the catheter is within the vein. Securely hold the hub of the needle. Advance the catheter until its hub is against the skin (Fig. 5.1B).

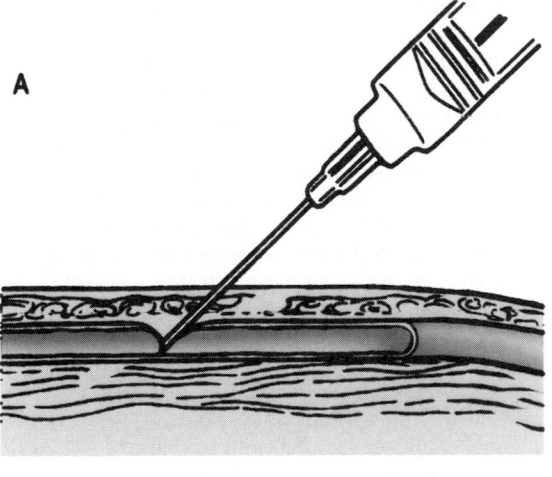

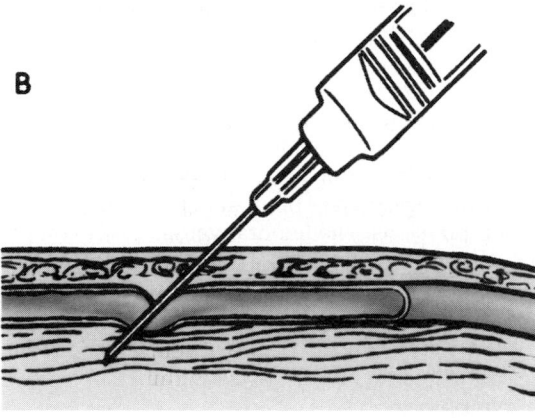

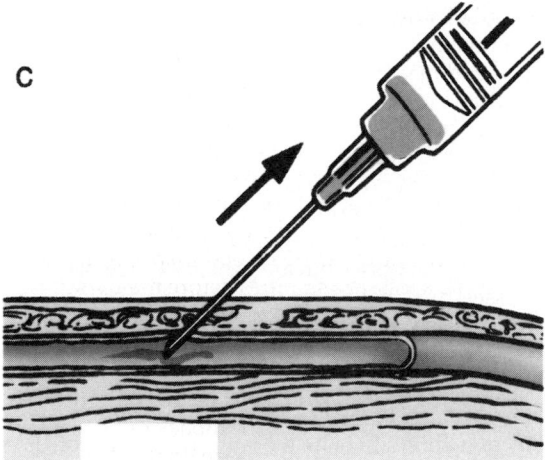

Figure 5.2. Through-and-through puncture of a vein. (Reprinted with permission from Reichman EF, Simon RR. *Emergency medicine procedures.* New York: McGraw-Hill, 2004.)

Withdraw the needle leaving the catheter in place (Fig. 5.1C). Apply pressure, with the nondominant index finger, over the catheter to prevent blood from exiting the catheter. Attach intravenous tubing to the catheter hub and begin the infusion. Secure the catheter with tape.

A modified Seldinger technique (described later in this chapter) with a radial artery catheterization kit is very useful for deep brachial and external jugular venous catheterization (4). The depth of the deep brachial vein combined with overlying skin (which is often scarred from previous venous punctures) makes catheterization with the usual 1 1/4" catheter difficult.

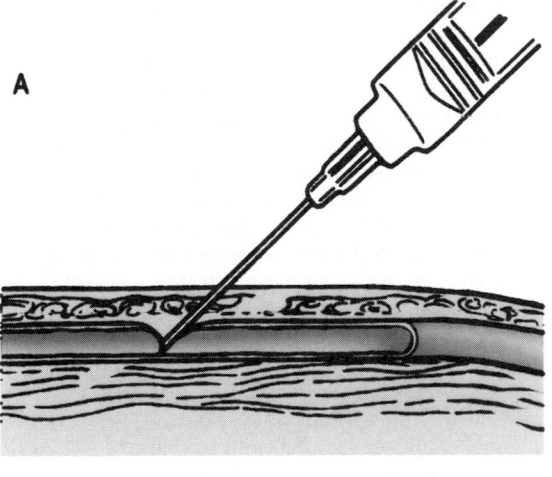

The external jugular vein is quite mobile and the overlying tissues are fairly tough. This can make threading an over-the-needle catheter into the vein, without pushing the vein off the end of the needle, quite difficult.

External Jugular Vein Cannulation

Place the patient in the Trendelenburg position to distend the external jugular vein. Turn the patient's head toward the opposite side. Clean and prep the skin of the neck. Place the nondominant thumb or index finger above the midportion of the clavicle to obstruct outflow and distend the external jugular vein. Align the catheter-over-the-needle parallel to the vein with the bevel of the needle upward. Enter the vein midway between the angle of the mandible and the mid-clavicle. Insert the catheter-over-the-needle during inspiration, when the valves of the external jugular vein are open. Be sure to cover the hub of the needle or catheter with a finger at all times to prevent an air embolism. The remainder of the technique is similar to that described previously.

Deep Brachial Vein Cannulation

Extend the patient's arm. Identify by palpation the brachial artery pulse in the antecubital fossa. Clean and prep the skin of the antecubital fossa. Place a tourniquet on the upper arm. Re-identify the brachial artery pulse. Place a catheter-over-the-needle onto a 5-mL syringe. Insert the catheter-over-the-needle just medial or lateral to the brachial artery pulse and at a 30° to 45° angle to the skin with the tip of the needle pointing cephalad. Advance the catheter-over-the-needle while applying negative pressure to the syringe. A flash of blood in the syringe indicates that the vein has been entered. The remainder of the technique is similar to that described previously.

Pediatric Considerations

Venipuncture and peripheral venous access can be quite a challenge in the infant and small child (4). Proper restraint of the extremity will greatly aid the process. Aside from the techniques discussed above, there are a few techniques that can aid pediatric vascular access. The scalp veins can be used for venous access in newborns (Fig. 5.3). They are most easily cannulated with a small (23–25 gauge) butterfly needle or catheter. A rubber band can be placed about the baby's head as a tourniquet. Other veins commonly used include those of the antecubital fossa, dorsal hand, dorsal foot, external jugular vein, and saphenous vein at the knee or groin. For small and superficial veins, place a small bend at the hub of the catheter-over-the-needle assembly. This provides a less acute angle and easier entry into the vein. The best guide to the gauge (diameter) of catheter to use is to compare the catheter to the vein. The catheter should be, at least, slightly smaller than the vein. In practice, the smallest readily available catheters are 24 gauge. Keeping a peripheral intravenous line from being pulled out by an active toddler is quite a challenge. Each institution has its own "recipe" for securing pediatric IV's including taping securely, covering the catheter with a cut plastic medicine cup, and covering the whole assembly with a gauze roll or stockinette.

Assessment

The line should flush easily. Any infusions should flow by gravity alone. Progressive swelling at the catheterization site indicates a hematoma formation or extravasation of infused fluids. Peripheral infusions of vasopressors, intravenous contrast, and caustic solutions require the skin puncture site to be assessed frequently and carefully as extravasation may lead to extensive local soft tissue necrosis. Pain at the intravenous access site must be taken seriously and should prompt a search for the cause.

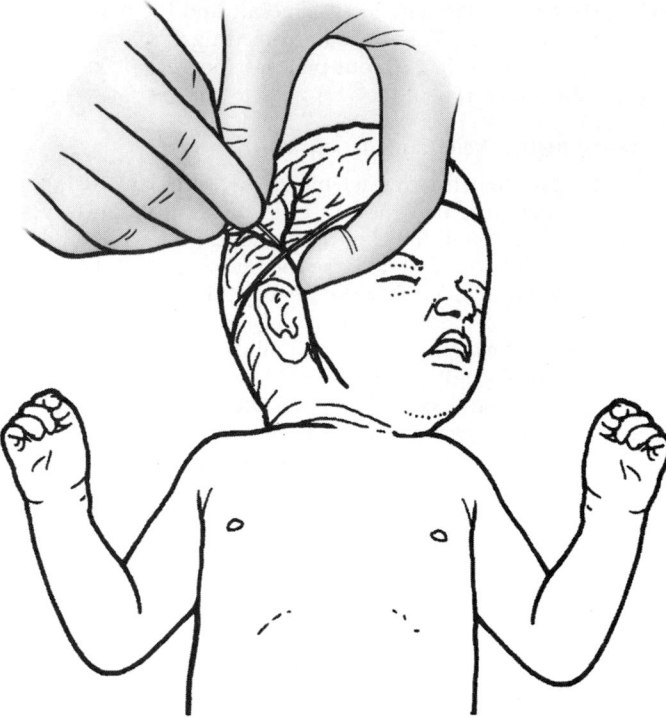

Figure 5.3.   Scalp vein cannulation in the neonate. (Reprinted with permission from Reichman EF, Simon RR. *Emergency medicine procedures.* New York: McGraw-Hill, 2004.)

Complications

The main complications of venipuncture are pain and hematoma formation. Other complications include nerve injury and usually reversible paresthesias. Infection is uncommon from simple venous sampling. In addition to these complications, venous catheters have additional risks. Intravenous catheters increase the risk of superficial venous thrombosis and thrombophlebitis. It is possible to injure a number of structures in the neck or cause a pneumothorax during external jugular vein cannulation with inadvertent deep penetration. Extravasation of some intravenous solutions can cause local skin necrosis. Extravasation of large volumes into a muscle compartment can lead to compartment syndrome, although this is rare with superficial peripheral venous lines. Infections can often be prevented by using aseptic technique, sterile dressings, and changing peripheral catheters every 48 to 72 hours. The rare complications of peripheral nerve palsies, pressure necrosis, and compromised peripheral circulation do occasionally occur. They can be prevented with frequent neurovascular checks to any restrained extremity, padding all pressure points, and avoiding the placement of circumferential tape on an extremity.

Central Venous Access

Percutaneous cannulation of the central veins is an essential technique for both long-term and emergent medical care (2). Access to the major veins of the torso allows rapid high-volume fluid resuscitation, administration of concentrated ionic and nutritional solutions, and hemodynamic measurements. The right internal jugular vein is generally preferred to the left internal jugular vein as the site of central venous cannulation. The right internal jugular vein provides a nearly direct route to the superior vena cava. The dome of the right lung is somewhat lower than that of the left lung and thus decreases the chance of a pneumothorax during catheter placement. The thoracic duct is relatively large and lies high in the left chest. These anatomic considerations favor the right internal jugular approach to central venous cannulation to minimize complications.

The internal jugular route is acceptable for central venous access in most cases. It allows ready access to the superior vena cava for long-term central venous access, caustic or concentrated infusions, and central venous pressure monitoring. Pulmonary artery catheters and transvenous pacing wires can be introduced through the right internal jugular vein. The internal jugular vein is accessible without terminating CPR efforts, although chest compressions and the lack of carotid pulsations make accessing it difficult. The risk of a pneumothorax is probably less with the internal jugular vein cannulation as opposed to the subclavian vein route, although patient mobility is less and discomfort is greater. In a coagulopathic patient, the internal jugular vein puncture site is compressible but hematoma formation may lead to compromise of the airway.

The subclavian vein is the preferred route for longer-term central venous access. This site allows for ambulation (unlike a femoral line) and neck movement without discomfort (unlike a jugular line). The catheter is concealable under clothing making outpatient use more acceptable.

The femoral vein is often the preferred route for emergency central venous cannulation in many patients. The femoral vein is not a suitable route for ambulatory patients beyond the initial resuscitation and stabilization period. Femoral venous access is relatively easy during CPR and often does not require the cessation of chest compressions. The femoral vein is easily compressible. This makes it preferable to the subclavian vein in coagulopathic patients or those undergoing thrombolysis, although peripheral access would be preferred in these cases.

Internal Jugular Vein

Central Approach

Place the patient in the Trendelenburg position with their head down 15° to 30°. Rotate the patient's head away from the side that will be cannulated. Excessive rotation will distort the anatomic landmarks and may bring the internal jugular vein closer to the carotid artery.

Insert the needle at a 30° to 60° angle at the apex of the triangle formed by the sternal and clavicular heads of the sternocleidomastoid muscle and the clavicle (Fig. 5.4). Direct the needle toward the ipsilateral nipple. Shallower angles cause a greater amount of subcutaneous tissues and structures to be traversed before entering the vessel, but are generally necessary in children whose vessels are smaller. Steeper angles make insertion of the catheter over the guidewire difficult as the guidewire tends to kink.

Anterior Approach

The skin puncture site is at the anterior border of the sternal head of the sternocleidomastoid muscle, just lateral to the carotid artery (Fig. 5.5). Enter the skin at a 45° to 60° angle. Direct the needle toward the ipsilateral nipple. The internal jugular vein should be encountered within 3 to 5 cm in an adult. If the vein is not encountered by 5 cm, withdraw the tip of the needle to the subcutaneous space and redirect it slightly medially.

Posterior Approach

Enter the skin at the posterior edge of the sternocleidomastoid muscle, one-third of the way from the clavicle to the mastoid process (Fig. 5.6). Alternatively, the point where the external jugular vein crosses the lateral border of the sternocleidomastoid muscle can be used. Direct the needle under the muscle at a 30° to 45° angle to the skin and toward the sternal notch. Place the index finger of the nondominant hand in the sternal notch to provide a landmark with the patient draped. The internal

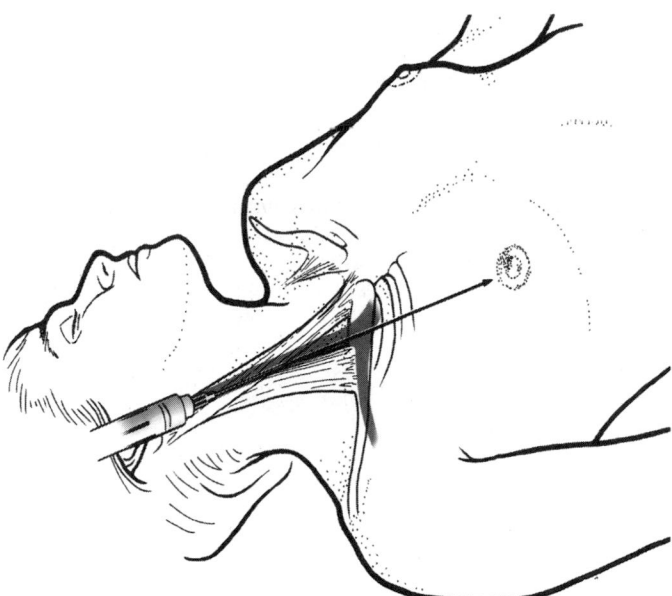

Figure 5.4. Central approach to the right internal jugular vein. (Reprinted with permission from Reichman EF, Simon RR. *Emergency medicine procedures*. New York: McGraw-Hill, 2004.)

jugular vein should be encountered within 5 cm in an adult. This approach is not recommended in children.

Subclavian Vein

Infraclavicular Approach

The infraclavicular approach to the subclavian vein is the most commonly used. It is easier to perform and less likely to result

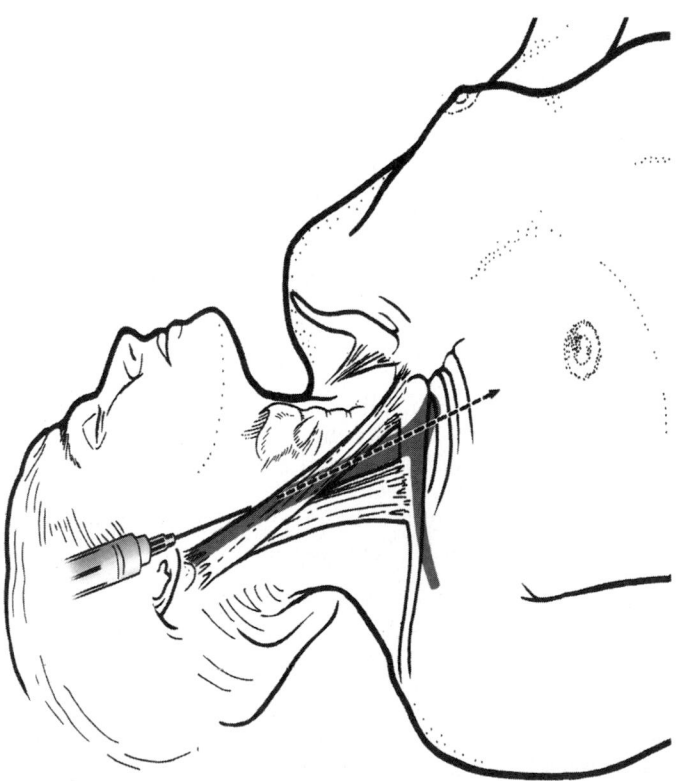

Figure 5.5. Anterior approach to the right internal jugular vein. (Reprinted with permission from Reichman EF, Simon RR. *Emergency medicine procedures*. New York: McGraw-Hill, 2004.)

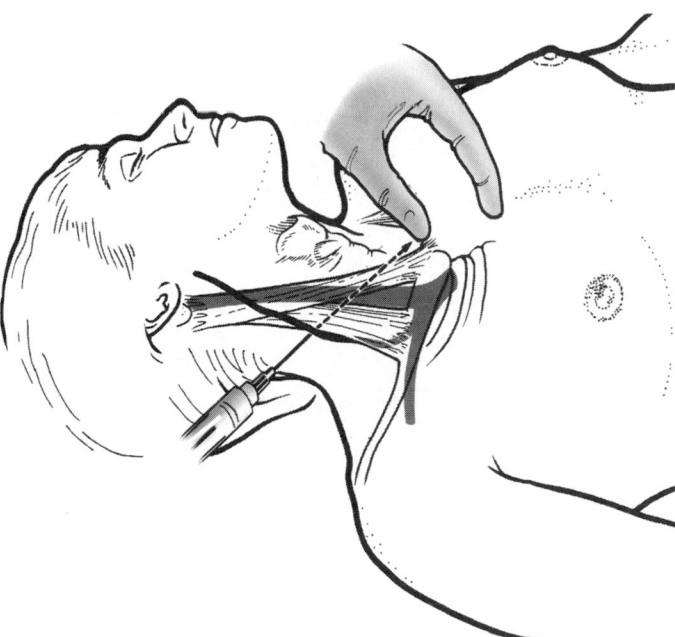

Figure 5.6. Posterior approach to the right internal jugular vein. (Reprinted with permission from Reichman EF, Simon RR. *Emergency medicine procedures*. New York: McGraw-Hill, 2004.)

in a pneumothorax than the supraclavicular approach. Several different skin entry sites have been described (2). Some feel that the preferred entry site is 1 cm caudal to the junction of the medial third and middle third of the clavicle. The subclavian vein lies just posterior to the clavicle at this site. Direct the needle just superior and posterior to the suprasternal notch while staying as close to the frontal (coronal) plane as possible. The needle and syringe should be parallel to the bed (Fig. 5.7). Placing the nondominant index finger in the sternal notch will help to guide placement (Fig. 5.7).

Some practitioners prefer to enter the skin inferior to the clavicle at the deltopectoral groove, or the point just lateral to the mid-clavicular line along the inferior surface of the clavicle. This is the point where the skin may be maximally depressed. Direct the needle parallel to the bed and towards the sternal notch. This entry site may make it easier to keep the needle in the coronal plane. The distance before entering the subclavian vein is longer than in the preceding approach and the protection offered by the first rib is lost.

An additional alternative landmark exists. Palpate the bony tubercle, or protrusion, on the inferior surface of the clavicle and approximately one-third to one-half the length of the clavicle from the sternoclavicular joint. The advantage of this site is that it is a definitive landmark and avoids approximating distances as described for the other sites previously. The needle is inserted parallel to the bed and aimed just posterior to the sternal notch.

Supraclavicular Approach

While most practitioners are more comfortable with the infraclavicular approach to the subclavian vein, the supraclavicular approach offers some advantages (2). These include: the subclavian vein being closer to the skin, the route from a right-sided skin puncture site to the superior vena cava is more direct, it avoids the hazards of a left-sided puncture (i.e., the thoracic duct), and the skin entry site is more accessible during CPR. The complication rate for the supraclavicular approach is probably lower than that for the infraclavicular approach with experience.

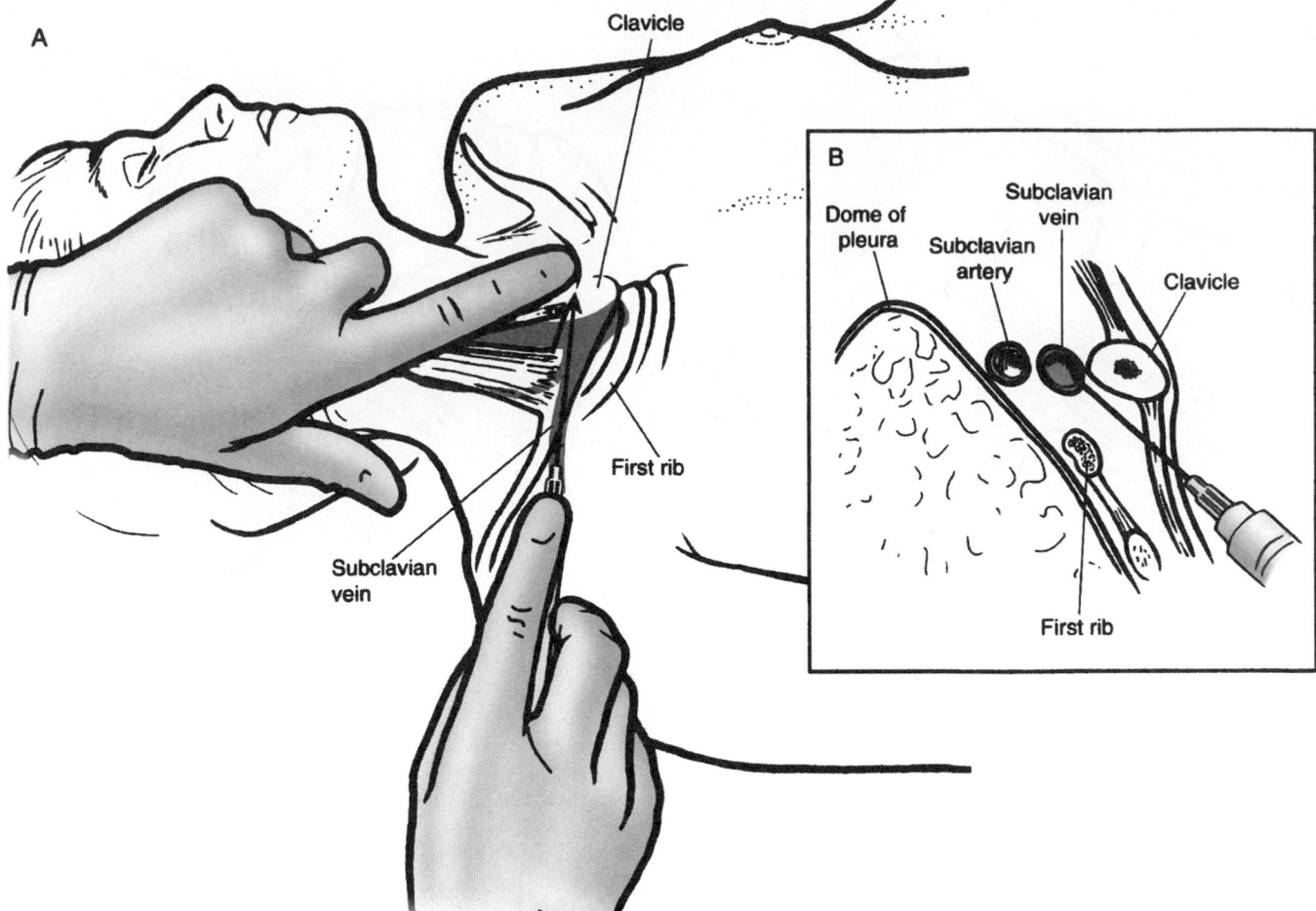

Figure 5.7.   Infraclavicular approach to subclavian vein cannulation. (Reprinted with permission from Reichman EF, Simon RR. *Emergency medicine procedures.* New York: McGraw-Hill, 2004.)

The skin is entered at a point 1 cm lateral to the lateral border of the clavicular head of the sternocleidomastoid muscle and 1 cm superior to the clavicle (Fig. 5.8). The needle should bisect the angle formed by the clavicle and the lateral border of the sternocleidomastoid muscle (Fig. 5.8A). Direct the needle toward the contralateral nipple or a point just superior and posterior to the sternal notch. Orient the needle bevel medially. The subclavian vein should be entered within 2 to 3 cm in an adult. The length of catheter inserted will be a few centimeters less than that for the infraclavicular approach.

Alternative skin entry sites and approaches have been described. Enter the skin 1 cm medially and 1 cm superiorly to the midpoint of the clavicle with the needle directed toward the ipsilateral sternoclavicular joint. The skin can be entered just posterior to the clavicle, at the junction of the medial third and middle third of the clavicle, with the needle directed toward the ipsilateral sternoclavicular joint and parallel to the coronal plane. This last approach is probably the simplest although the study cited was performed on cadavers rather than live patients.

Femoral Vein Catheterization

Premeasuring from the insertion site to the xiphoid process will give the maximum catheter insertion depth. The needle should enter the skin 2 to 4 cm inferior to the midpoint of the inguinal ligament and 1 cm medial to the femoral artery pulse (Fig. 5.9). The needle should enter the skin 1 to 2 cm inferior to the inguinal ligament and 0.5 cm medial to the femoral artery pulse in an infant or young child.

Two site-specific considerations deserve mention. The use of a "finder" needle is unnecessary since there are no vital structures in the area other than the femoral artery that is compressible if it is punctured. The introducer needle is directed at a 45° to 60° angle to the skin and parallel to the long axis of the thigh. Shallower angles may be necessary in very small and thin patients. Use caution to avoid puncturing the posterior wall of the vein above the inguinal ligament since this can result in a retroperitoneal hemorrhage.

Seldinger Technique

There are numerous anatomic approaches to obtain central venous access (2). This includes three approaches to the internal jugular vein, two approaches to the subclavian vein, and one approach to the femoral vein. A more detailed discussion of the anatomy and approaches can be found elsewhere (2,10). Regardless of the approach, the Seldinger technique is the preferred method.

Clean, prep, and drape the area. Position the patient based on which central vein is to be accessed. Several cardinal rules for the insertion of the catheter should be observed. Always occlude the open hub of a needle or catheter in a central vein to prevent an air embolism. Never let go of the guidewire to prevent its embolization into the central venous circulation. Never apply excessive force to the guidewire on insertion or removal if resistance is met. Doing so may injure the vessel, break the guidewire, or embolize the guidewire.

Attach the thin-walled needle to a 5-mL syringe containing 1 ml of sterile saline. Insert the needle while applying negative

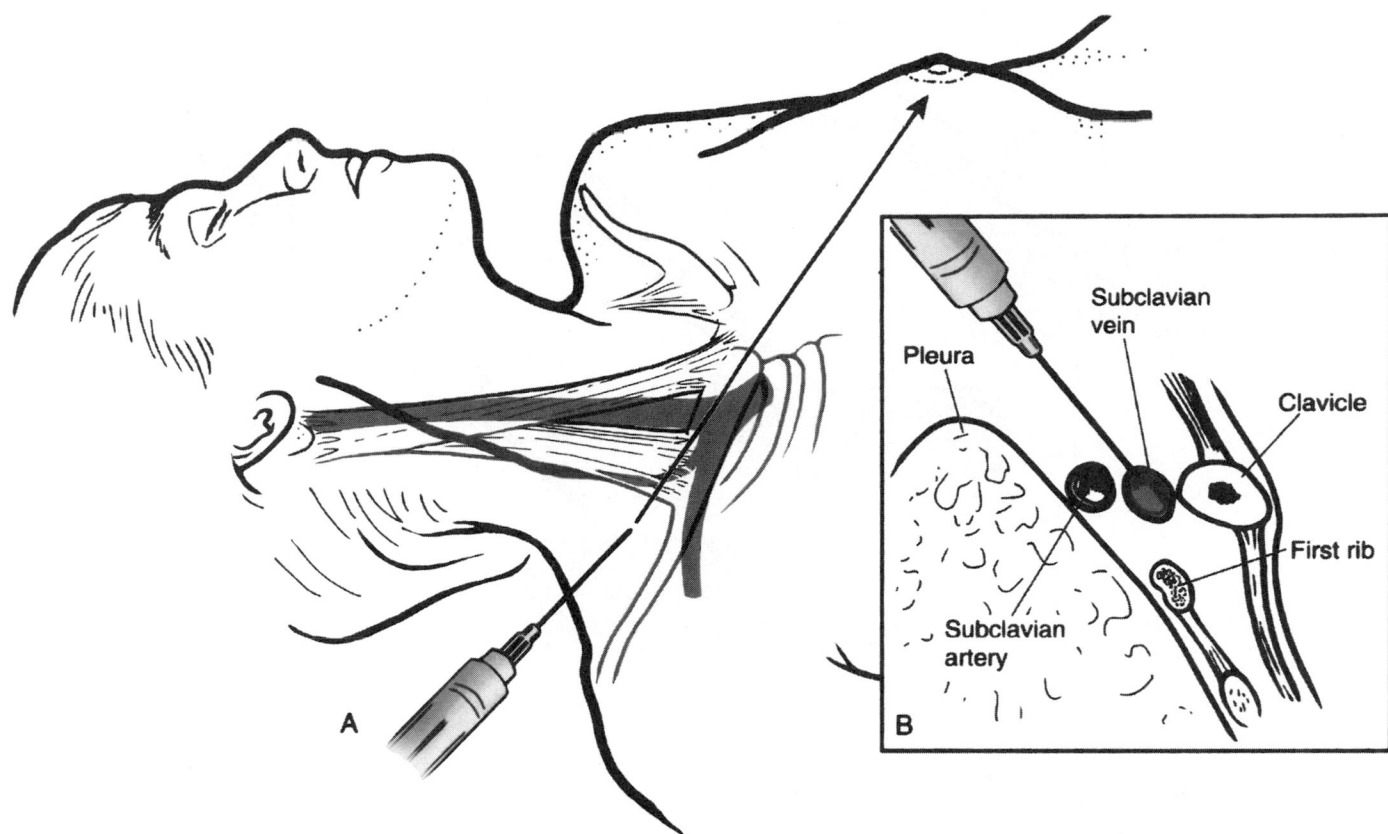

Figure 5.8. Supraclavicular approach to subclavian vein cannulation. (Reprinted with permission from Reichman EF, Simon RR. *Emergency medicine procedures.* New York: McGraw-Hill, 2004.)

pressure to the syringe by withdrawing the plunger. Advance the needle into the vein (Fig. 5.10A). If the vein is not located within 3 to 5 cm, stop advancing the needle. Withdraw the needle slowly while continuing to aspirate. Often, the vessel will have been completely traversed upon insertion and blood will flash back into the syringe as the needle is withdrawn. Stabilize and

hold the needle perfectly still with the nondominant hand once blood returns in the syringe. Remove the syringe. Occlude the open hub of the needle with the thumb of the nondominant hand while keeping the small finger of the hand in contact with the patient's skin.

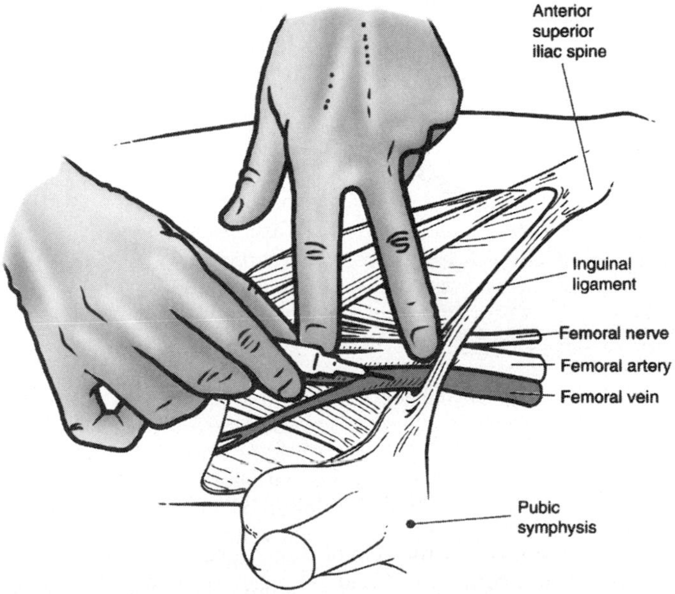

Grasp the guidewire and its sleeve with the dominant hand. Slide the sleeve forward to straighten out the "J" of the guidewire. Insert the wire sleeve into the hub of the needle (Fig. 5.10B). Advance the guidewire through the needle and into the vein (Fig. 5.10B). The guidewire should advance easily into the vein. Withdraw the needle and guidewire sleeve over the guidewire while securely holding the guidewire (Fig. 5.10C). Grasp the guidewire with the nondominant hand as soon as the guidewire is visible between the tip of the needle and the skin.

Make a small incision in the skin adjacent to the guidewire using a #11 scalpel blade (Fig. 5.10D). Place the dilator over the guidewire and advance it into the vein (Fig. 5.10E). Continue to advance the dilator until its hub is against the skin. Do not release hold of the guidewire at any time. Remove the dilator over the guidewire. Place the catheter tip over the guidewire. Advance the catheter over the guidewire and into the vein to the desired depth (Fig. 5.10F). The depth is typically 10 to 15 cm for the internal jugular or subclavian approaches, or completely to the hub for femoral central venous lines. Securely hold the catheter in place and remove the guidewire (Fig. 5.10G). Occlude the open catheter lumen with a sterile-gloved finger to prevent air embolization and excessive blood loss.

Attach a syringe to the catheter hub and aspirate blood to confirm that the catheter is within the vein. Withdraw any necessary blood samples. Attach infusion tubing or a heparin lock to the port and flush the catheter to prevent a blood clot from obstructing the lumen. Securely attach the catheter to the skin with nylon or silk sutures. Cover the skin puncture site with a sterile dressing. Obtain a chest radiograph to evaluate for

Figure 5.9. Femoral vein cannulation. (Reprinted with permission from Reichman EF, Simon RR. *Emergency medicine procedures.* New York: McGraw-Hill, 2004.)

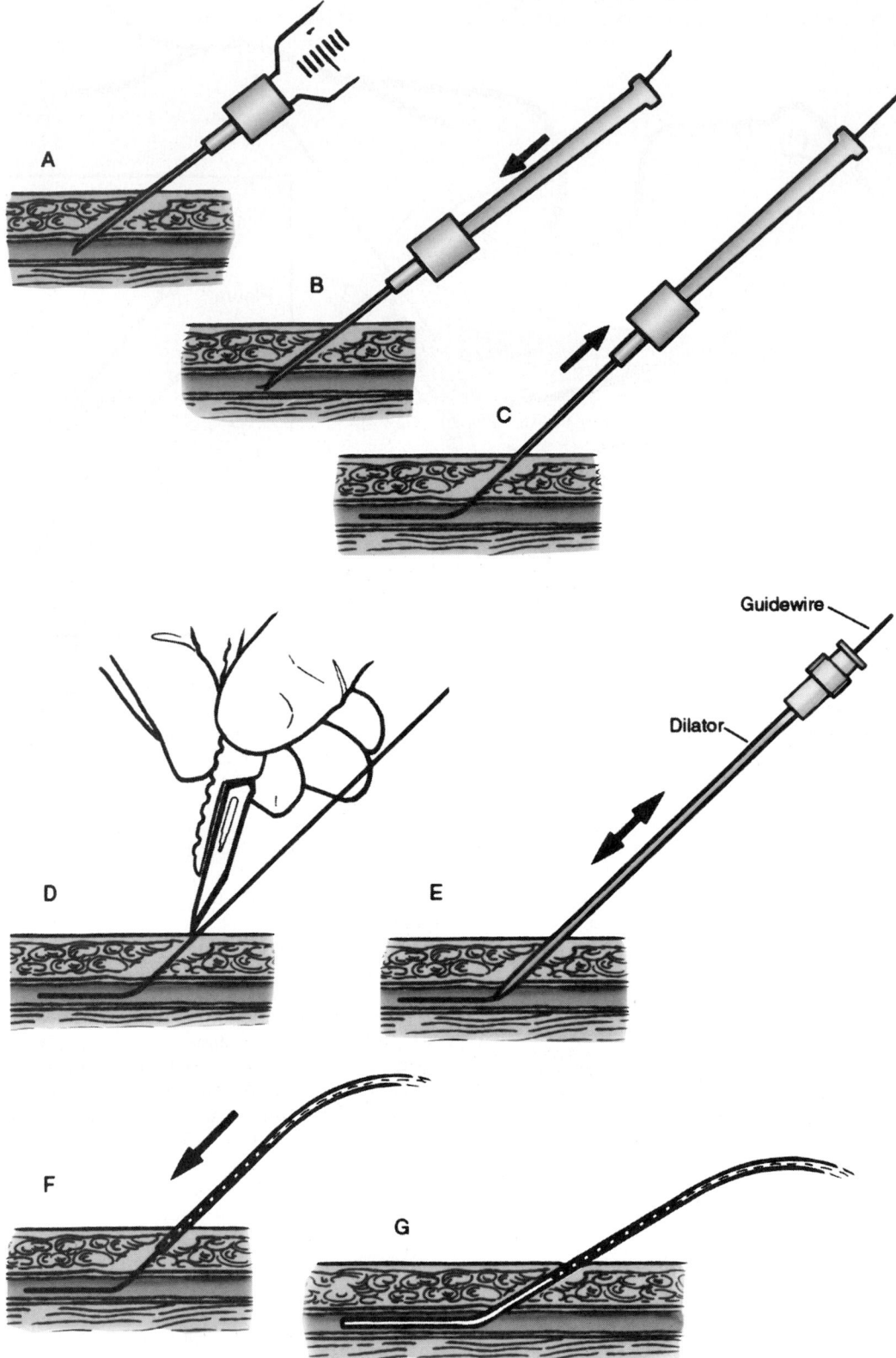

Figure 5.10.   The Seldinger technique for central venous access. (Reprinted with permission from Reichman EF, Simon RR. *Emergency medicine procedures.* New York: McGraw-Hill, 2004.)

central line placement complications such as a pneumothorax, hemothorax, hematoma, and/or line malpositioning.

Pediatric Considerations

The anterior or central approach to the internal jugular vein is preferred for children. Appropriate catheter sizes and lengths are shown elsewhere (2). The child must be sedated and immo-

bilized prior to attempts at cannulation of the internal jugular or subclavian vein.

The femoral vein is the vein of choice if central venous access is needed in a combative child who cannot be completely restrained. The patient need not be in Trendelenburg position, the consequences of a misdirected needle are less severe, and the procedure is less threatening as the face is not draped. A shallower angle of skin entry is necessary to access the femoral vein compared to an adult. Enter the skin 1 to 2 cm inferior to the inguinal ligament and 0.5 mm medial to the femoral artery.

Assessment

Examine the patient after central line placement. Examine the lung fields carefully to exclude a significant pneumothorax. Vital signs should be re-checked. Obtain a portable anteroposterior chest radiograph to verify line tip placement in the superior vena cava and to rule out a procedural-related pneumothorax. Check the catheter site for hematoma formation or hemorrhage along the dilated catheter track. Control any hemorrhage with direct pressure. Check the function of the catheter by aspiration and infusion through all ports.

Most femoral vein catheters can be fully inserted. Premeasurement is recommended to make sure that the catheter tip will not reach the right atrium. If there is any doubt about the catheter position, postinsertion abdominal and chest radiographs should be obtained. The tip of the catheter must be at or below the xiphoid process of the sternum. Reassess the lower extremity distal to the catheter in order to determine any change in the neurovascular status after line placement.

Removal of the Central Venous Catheter

Place the patient in the Trendelenburg position when removing a central venous catheter from the internal jugular or subclavian vein. Place the patient supine to remove a femoral vein catheter. Remove the dressing overlying the skin puncture site. Cut the suture securing the catheter to the skin. Ask the patient to exhale and hold his breath. Briskly remove the catheter and cover the puncture site with a gauze dressing. Apply an occlusive dressing to the site for the first 1 to 2 days after the catheter has been removed and if the catheter had a large diameter or had been in place for more than 2 to 3 days. The skin puncture site should be observed for signs of infection twice a day for 48 hours.

Complications

Complications associated with central venous access are numerous. The internal jugular and subclavian access has a myriad of potential complications (2,10). These include infection, vessel laceration, catheter malposition, pneumothorax, hemothorax, chylothorax, carotid artery puncture, stroke, airway compromise, air embolism, cardiac dysrhythmias, cardiac puncture, pericardial tamponade, and death. The guidewire can become entrapped, necessitating surgical or interventional radiology removal. Thrombosis of the catheter or vein may lead to pulmonary embolism. Infection may result in septic emboli or endocarditis. Complications during catheterization occur in proportion to the operator's inexperience (12). If the patient is unlikely to survive a mistake, the most experienced person available should perform the procedure!

Deep venous thrombosis of the femoral and more distal veins is a recognized complication of femoral venous lines (8). Inadvertent cannulation of the femoral artery may occur. This is particularly true during an episode of severe hypotension or cardiac arrest during central venous line placement. If intraarterial placement is unrecognized, infusion of vasopressors into the artery may result in ischemic injury to the distal limb.

Accessing Indwelling Central Venous Lines

A variety of indwelling central venous access devices have been developed to avoid repeated venipunctures and permit direct access to the central circulation (1). These devices may be partially or completely implanted under the patient's skin and include tunneled catheters, Permacaths, Hickman catheters, Groshong catheters, and Mahukar catheters. The Emergency Physician must be able to access these devices to administer medications and withdraw blood samples without damaging the device or causing it to thrombose. The most important elements after accessing indwelling lines are to prevent the central venous line from clotting off and to avoid contaminating the line.

There are several contraindications to accessing indwelling central venous lines. Fully implanted devices should not be accessed through infected skin. Phenytoin and diazepam cannot be given via silicone indwelling central venous lines as they can crystallize and permanently obstruct the catheter lumen. Devices used for hemodialysis should only be accessed in a true emergency and if no other method of venous access can be readily obtained. This guideline is intended to prevent loss of the patient's dialysis access.

Accessing a partially implanted central venous catheter is simple and similar to accessing a heparin-locked peripheral intravenous catheter. The Luer cap can be removed entirely and the catheter lumen accessed directly with a syringe if an infusion is to be subsequently started.

A noncoring Huber-type needle must be used to access subcutaneous injection ports. A small-gauge standard hypodermic needle can be used in a dire emergency if a noncoring needle is not available. The diaphragm covering the injection reservoir can be damaged by a standard hypodermic needle, leading to subcutaneous hemorrhage and requiring surgical replacement of the implanted device.

It is extremely important to prevent the indwelling central venous catheter from becoming thrombosed after it is used. Flush the Hickman and Broviac catheters with 3 to 5 mL of heparinized saline (100 units/mL). Flush the Groshong catheter with 5 mL of normal saline. Flush dialysis catheters with the volume printed on the catheter (usually ≤ 2 mL) with heparinized saline (1000 units/mL). Flush fully implanted catheters with 3 to 5 mL of heparinized saline (100–200 units/mL). Heparin, however, may be contraindicated in some patients due to bleeding or thrombocytopenia. Sterile saline is an alternative but may result in catheter thrombosis.

Peripheral Venous Cutdown

Venous access in the critically ill patient is of the utmost importance. Peripheral venous access can be extremely difficult due to vascular collapse from shock, previous injury to the vessel, obesity, or scars. Direct visualization of the vein to be cannulated will often times be quicker and more successful than indirect visualization with central venous lines (9). To perform peripheral venous cutdowns, one must understand the anatomy and details of venous cannulation (9). Practicing the cutdown technique before its critical need will help with placement in the emergent setting. Emergency Physicians should be knowledgeable of the anatomy of the saphenous vein at the ankle, the saphenous vein at the groin, and the basilic vein at the elbow.

The primary indication for a peripheral venous cutdown is the need for venous access in a patient with no peripheral access and in whom central access is not obtainable or contraindicated (9). This is the ideal procedure for the intravenous drug user with no peripheral veins, burn patients, the patient in cardiorespiratory arrest, or the hypovolemic trauma patient. This is also an excellent technique for emergent pediatric vascular access after other access attempts (interosseous access, central venous access, peripheral venous access—including scalp veins) have failed.

Greater Saphenous Vein Isolation at the Ankle

The saphenous vein is easily found and isolated at the ankle (Fig. 5.11). Extend and externally rotate the lower extremity. Identify the medial malleolus of the tibia. Find the spot 2.5 cm anterior and 2.5 cm superior to the medial malleolus. The greater saphenous vein will be found at this site. Alternatively, the vein will

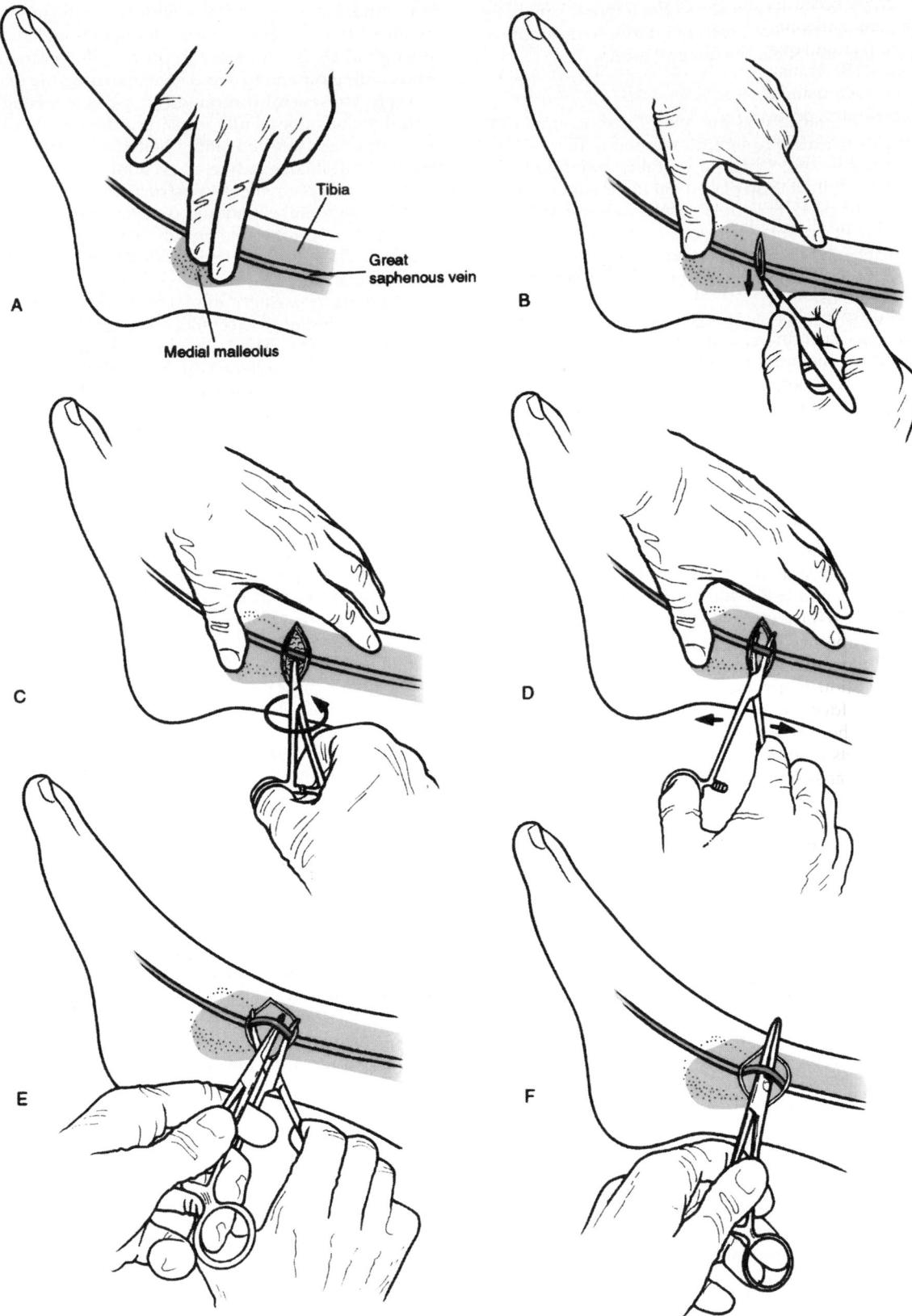

Figure 5.11. Isolation of the greater saphenous vein at the ankle. (Reprinted with permission from Reichman EF, Simon RR. *Emergency medicine procedures.* New York: McGraw-Hill, 2004.)

be found two finger breadths above and two finger breadths in front of the medial malleolus (Fig. 5.11A).

Stretch the skin taught over the distal tibia with the nondominant hand (Fig. 5.11B). Transversely incise the skin overlying the great saphenous vein using a #10 scalpel blade, from the anterior tibial border to the posterior tibial border (Fig. 5.11B). This incision should be superficial to expose only the subcutaneous tissue. An incision into the subcutaneous tissue may transect the vein causing significant bleeding, difficulty visualizing the surgical field, and difficulty finding the ends of the vein which may retract proximally and distally.

Isolate the greater saphenous vein. Insert a curved hemostat along the posterior border of the tibia and scrape the tip along the tibia. Advance the hemostat along the tibia while scraping the periosteum until the tip reaches the anterior border of the tibia (Fig. 5.11C). Widely open the arms of the hemostat (Fig. 5.11D). This will open the jaws of the hemostat and separate the saphenous vein from the saphenous nerve and fibrous strands of connective tissue. Insert a straight hemostat (Kelly clamp) between the jaws of the curved hemostat and below the greater saphenous vein (Fig. 5.11E). Remove the curved hemostat to leave the straight hemostat elevating the greater saphenous vein (Fig. 5.11F).

Greater Saphenous Vein Isolation at the Groin

The groin vasculature offers the potential for massive infusion of blood or fluids in a matter of minutes. These vessels are closer to the central circulation and large enough to easily accommodate intravenous tubing, cut off at a 45° angle, as a catheter. The greater saphenous vein is superficial at the groin and lies in a meshwork of subcutaneous tissue, superficial to the femoral artery and vein.

Identify the location where the scrotal or labial fold meets the thigh (Fig. 5.12). Identify the lateral edge of the mons pubis. Identify the point where a vertical line from the lateral edge of the mons pubis meets a horizontal line from the scrotal/labial fold. Make a 6-cm transverse, medial to lateral incision with a #10 scalpel blade on the patient's thigh starting where the scrotal or labial fold meets the thigh. Extend the incision laterally until it meets the vertical line from the lateral edge of the mons pubis. Dissect the subcutaneous tissue to locate the greater saphenous vein.

Basilic Vein Isolation at the Elbow

The basilic vein may be used for a peripheral venous cutdown. This is often performed when the greater saphenous vein can-

not be accessed due to lower extremity amputation, deformity, injury, or trauma. This site is not ideal as it may interfere with resuscitative efforts. The vein is deep, small, and often hard to find.

Techniques for Cannulation of the Vein

There are a number of techniques to cannulate a vein after it has been isolated (9). Either of the following techniques can be used to cannulate the greater saphenous vein or basilic vein. The techniques include a surgical technique using intravenous tubing, a Seldinger technique, a modified Seldinger technique, and an intravenous catheter technique. It is important to realize that this may be a lifesaving procedure in an emergent setting and the rapid and definitive cannulation of the vessel is the primary goal and not the technique chosen.

The complications of a peripheral venous cutdown include arterial injury, nerve injury, phlebitis, thromboembolism, wound dehiscence, and wound infection. The incidence of complications ranges from 2% to 15% (9). The difficulty in reporting complications is that there is a high mortality rate in patients undergoing this procedure due to the underlying problem requiring emergent vascular access (i.e., hypovolemia, sepsis, shock, trauma, etc.).

Intraosseous Infusion

Obtaining peripheral vascular access in the critically ill pediatric patient may be difficult and time consuming. An alternative route to intravenous infusion for blood, drug, and fluid administration is to insert an intraosseous line (5). Intraosseous infusion is quick, safe, and effective in compromised neonates and adults when other vascular access techniques fail or are contraindicated (5). The procedure is technically straightforward.

The intraosseous needle is inserted through the cortex and into the bone marrow (medullary) cavity of a long bone. Numerous anatomic sites can be used to access the medullary cavity. The most traditional site, which is favored in pediatric patients, is the flat anteromedial surface of the proximal tibia. The distal tibia just above the medial malleolus is the preferred site in adults. It is easier to penetrate the cortex of the medial malleolus in the adult than the thicker cortex of the proximal tibia. A third site for intraosseous access is the flat anterior surface of the distal femur. The sternum can be used, but this route is difficult and associated with numerous complications. A new system has recently been developed to perform intraosseous infusion through the sternum (Pyng Medical, Richmond, BC, Canada). This system cannot be recommended at this time until further information and trials of its effectiveness and safety are available.

Intraosseous line placement is contraindicated in diseased or osteoporotic bone. Avoid placement of an intraosseous line through areas of cellulitis, abscess, or burns. Fractures in the ipsilateral bone increase the risk of extravasation-induced compartment syndrome and nonunion of the fractures. Failed placement of an intraosseous line in the same bone is a relative contraindication.

Use only specifically designed intraosseous needles for this procedure. Spinal needles bend, do not penetrate the cortex, and have increased resistance to fluid flow. Standard hypodermic needles often bend and do not penetrate the cortex of the bone. Both these types of needles may break while being inserted and may injure the healthcare provider.

Identify the landmarks and stabilize the extremity with the nondominant hand (Fig. 5.13A). Firmly grasp the intraosseous needle with the dominant hand. Insert the needle perpendicularly or slightly angulated (10°–15° angle) to the long axis of the bone. Advance the needle through the skin and subcutaneous

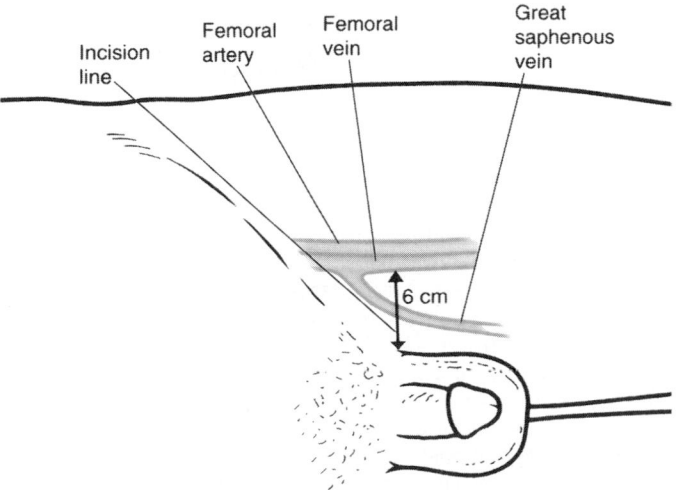

Figure 5.12. Isolation of the greater saphenous vein at the groin. (Reprinted with permission from Reichman EF, Simon RR. *Emergency medicine procedures.* New York: McGraw-Hill, 2004.)

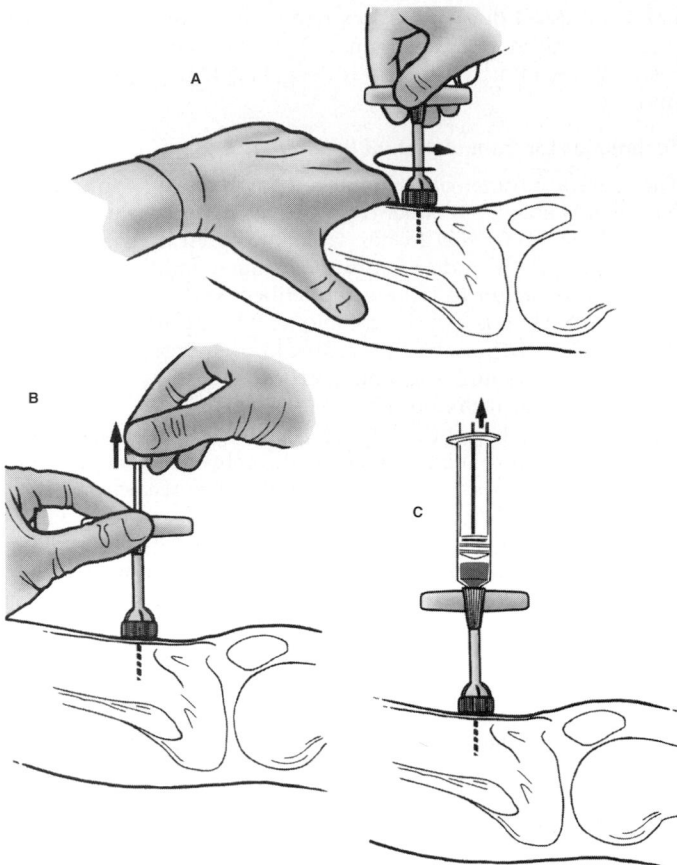

Figure 5.13. Intraosseous line placement. (Reprinted with permission from Reichman EF, Simon RR. *Emergency medicine procedures.* New York: McGraw-Hill, 2004.)

tissue until the bone is contacted. Advance the intraosseous needle through the bone with a twisting or rotary motion to cut through the cortex of the bone (Fig. 5.13A). A significant reduction in the resistance to forward motion will be encountered when the cortex is penetrated and the needle enters the medullary canal. Remove the stylet when the medullary canal is entered (Fig. 5.13B).

Attach a 5- to 10-mL syringe to the hub of the intraosseous needle (Fig. 5.13C). Aspirate blood from the medullary canal to confirm proper placement of the needle. Any samples obtained may be sent to the laboratory for subsequent analysis. A second sign of correct placement is to assess whether the intraosseous needle will stand erect without support. Finally, flush the intraosseous line. The ability of the fluid to flow without inducing soft tissue swelling can also be used to confirm proper placement. Check the firmness of the calf compartment often during the infusion to avoid a compartment syndrome.

Attach intravenous tubing to the hub of the intraosseous needle and begin the infusion of fluids. Medications can be administered through the injection port of the intravenous tubing. Apply a sterile dressing around the skin puncture site and secure the device. The intraosseous line should be removed once the resuscitation is complete and another form of secure vascular access has been obtained.

The most common complication of intraosseous infusion is extravasation of fluid. Localized infections may occur after intraosseous needle placement. Injury to the growth plate and bone marrow embolism are possible. The flow rate of fluid through an intraosseous line is slower than that through a peripheral intravenous line.

Umbilical Vessel Catheterization

Umbilical vessel catheterization can be used as a reliable method for vascular access, fluid resuscitation, blood transfusion, medication administration, frequent blood sampling, and cardiovascular monitoring. Either the umbilical artery or vein may be used for vascular access (6). The artery can usually be accessed within the first 24 hours of life. It is occasionally possible to use the umbilical artery up to 7 days after birth. The umbilical vein can be accessed for up to 2 weeks of age.

Umbilical artery catheterization is more desirable than umbilical vein catheterization because it allows frequent arterial blood gas sampling and continuous blood pressure monitoring in addition to fluid, blood, and medication administration. Unfortunately, umbilical artery catheterization is more difficult and time consuming to perform, especially in unskilled hands. Therefore, umbilical vein catheterization is the preferred procedure for the infant in shock in need of rapid resuscitation. Arterial access can be obtained later in a more controlled environment, such as in the neonatal intensive care unit.

The umbilical vein and arteries can easily be differentiated by examination of a cross section of the umbilical cord. The umbilical vein is a single vessel with thin walls and a large lumen. It is usually flattened in one direction. There are two thick-walled umbilical arteries that are significantly smaller in diameter than the umbilical vein. Occasionally, only a single umbilical artery is present.

Umbilical vessel catheterization in the Emergency Department should only be performed on severely ill neonates in whom peripheral vascular access attempts have failed. Never insert an umbilical catheter if there are any signs of infection on or around the remnant of the umbilical cord. It is contraindicated if a neonate is older than the above stated ages or an abdominal abnormality exists.

Arterial Puncture and Cannulation

Arterial blood gas sampling is an essential component of the care of many Emergency Department patients (11). It provides key information regarding a patient's oxygenation and acid-base status. Arterial cannulation allows for continuous and accurate blood pressure monitoring and frequent blood gas sampling in the care of the critically ill patient. A modified Allen test should be performed to assess the adequacy of the collateral circulation to the hand prior to radial artery puncture or cannulation. An alternative method of evaluating the collateral circulation involves the use of a pulse oximeter with a visual pulse waveform display.

The preferred site for the initial attempt at arterial puncture or cannulation is the radial artery. Other acceptable second attempt sites of access include the femoral, dorsalis pedis, brachial, posterior tibial, and superficial temporal arteries. Arterial puncture may be performed to obtain a single blood sample.

Arterial cannulation can be accomplished by numerous techniques (10,11). The catheter-over-the-needle technique is the most basic method, yet possibly the one associated with the lowest rate of successful cannulation. It is the direct introduction of the catheter-over-the-needle in a manner similar to that of inserting an intravenous catheter. The second technique for arterial cannulation is a Seldinger-type technique (catheter-over-the-wire) utilizing one of a number of prepackaged commercially available kits. A double arterial wall puncture technique may offer an advantage in passing the guidewire and catheter into the true arterial lumen. This technique for cannulation theoretically may be associated with greater vascular damage. Finally, a cutdown technique may be performed to cannulate an artery. This technique is primarily used for the brachial or radial arteries but may be used to access other peripheral arteries.

Arterial puncture and catheterization are generally safe procedures with an incidence of clinically significant complications under 5% (7). The primary complications of arterial catheterization are infection, bleeding, arterial injury, and intraarterial thrombosis. Infection is usually limited to the site of catheterization. Nerve injury can occur from direct puncture or neuropathy as a result of a hematoma formation and subsequent nerve compression. Small hematomas are common after arterial puncture. Major bleeding is unusual. Rare complications include the formation of a pseudoaneurysm or arteriovenous fistula.

COMMON PITFALLS

✔ Know the anatomy and common variations of the major veins used for vascular access
✔ Be familiar with the equipment and techniques for venous access prior to performing the procedure
✔ Have a back-up plan for an alternative vascular access site if the attempts at the primary site are unsuccessful
✔ Anticipate difficult central venous line placement or complications due to a particular patient's anatomic variation from the "norm"

References

1. Feldman R. Accessing indwelling central venous lines. In: Reichman EF, Simon RR, eds. *Emergency medicine procedures*. New York: McGraw-Hill, 2004;342–348.
2. Feldman R. Central venous access. In: Reichman EF, Simon RR, eds. *Emergency medicine procedures*. New York: McGraw-Hill, 2004;314–337.
3. Feldman R. General principles of intravenous access. In: Reichman EF, Simon RR, eds. *Emergency medicine procedures*. New York: McGraw-Hill, 2004;285–296.
4. Feldman R. Venipuncture and peripheral intravenous access. In: Reichman EF, Simon RR, eds. *Emergency medicine procedures*. New York: McGraw-Hill, 2004;297–313.
5. Hoffmann ME, Ma OJ. Intraosseous infusion. In: Reichman EF, Simon RR, eds. *Emergency medicine procedures*. New York: McGraw-Hill, 2004;383–389.
6. Kang I, Reichman EF. Umbilical vessel catheterization. In: Reichman EF, Simon RR, eds. *Emergency medicine procedures*. New York: McGraw-Hill, 2004;390–397.
7. Lodato RF. Arterial pressure monitoring. In: Tobin MJ, ed. *Principles and practice of intensive care monitoring*. New York: McGraw-Hill, 1998;733–747.
8. Meridith JW, Young JS, O'Neil EA, Snow DC, Hansen KJ. Femoral catheters and deep venous thrombosis: a prospective evaluation with venous duplex sonography. *J Trauma* 1993;35(2):187–191.
9. Nobay F. Peripheral venous cutdown. In: Reichman EF, Simon RR, eds. *Emergency medicine procedures*. New York: McGraw-Hill, 2004;367–382.
10. Reichman EF, Simon RR, eds. *Emergency medicine procedures*. New York: McGraw-Hill, 2004.
11. Stroud S, Rodriguez R. Arterial puncture and catheterization. In: Reichman EF, Simon RR, eds. *Emergency medicine procedures*. New York: McGraw-Hill, 2004;398–410.
12. Sznajder JI, Zveibil FR, Bitterman H, Weiner P, Bursztein S. Central vein catheterization: failure and complication rates by three percutaneous approaches. *Arch Int Med* 1986;146:259–261.

SECTION

II

Section Editor: Carlo L. Rosen

High-Risk Chief Complaints

CHAPTER 6
Chest Pain

Robert J. Zalenski and Rebecca R. Roberts

The challenge in accurately diagnosing chest pain arises from several important neuroanatomic facts. First, neither the quality nor the intensity of pain produced by the nerves coming from the thoracic viscera is specific for any single organ system. Spasm of the esophagus, ischemia of the heart, or distention of the great vessels can produce feelings of pressure, aching, or burning. Pain can be severe, minimal, or even absent during the course of life-threatening conditions such as an acute myocardial infarction.

Second, the location and radiation of the pain do not reliably identify the specific organ system involved. Thoracic organ pathology can produce pain that is referred outside the thorax to the epigastrium, neck, or jaw. Conversely, cervical pathology from a ruptured cervical disk can produce pain in the shoulder and around the clavicle. Abdominal pathology, such as a ruptured ectopic pregnancy, can produce chest and scapular pain due to diaphragmatic irritation.

The anatomic explanation for referred pain is simple. Somatic afferent nerves from the skin and muscle of the arms enter the same dorsal root nerve pools as the visceral afferent nerves from the heart, esophagus, and other thoracic organs. Activation of this nerve pool by visceral afferents can stimulate the somatic afferent nerves. The brain interprets the pain as coming from the arm, muscle, or joint innervated by the pooled somatic afferents. Pain from the heart can be perceived as pain in the upper inner arm, forearm, or axilla, because both areas synapse in the dorsal roots T1–T5 (10). Also, because dorsal nerve segments overlap three segments above and below a particular level, thoracic pain can be referred to the neck or abdomen. Therefore, to identify the organ system and the disease process, the physician must rely on the duration and frequency of the pain, the setting in which it occurs, the aggravating and relieving factors, and associated symptoms.

The five major thoracic organ systems are listed in Table 6.1. The most common etiologies that affect these organs can be categorized as structural disruption, infarction or ischemia, infection, and inflammation.

CLINICAL PRESENTATION

The historical features of chest pain are useful in establishing the "pretest" probability for each disease in the differential diagnosis. Such probabilities guide the choice and interpretation of further diagnostic tests.

Acute myocardial infarction (AMI) produces a nonlocalized pressure, ache, or burning, the intensity of which ranges from minimal discomfort to severe pain. The pain is usually substernal and in the left chest, but can occur between the umbilicus and the neck. It frequently radiates to the shoulder or left arm and lasts several hours.

Stuttering presentations may last 12 to 24 hours. Determining the onset of constant pain is essential in deciding whether the patient is eligible for acute reperfusion therapy. Dyspnea, diaphoresis, nausea, and weakness are frequently associated symptoms. Occasionally, pain is felt only in a referred area, such as the arm, or via the vagus nerve, in the ear. Patients with AMI, particularly the elderly and diabetic patients, often present without pain (1), and this diagnosis must be suspected with the presentation of syncope or confusion.

Pain features not suggestive of AMI include stabbing, knife-like sensations or radiation to areas outside of cervicothoracic nerve segments, such as the legs or flanks (6). Very brief pain (lasting less than 5 seconds) or pain that is clearly pleuritic or exactly reproduced by bending or palpation is very unlikely to be of coronary origin (12).

The pain of angina is similar to that of AMI but is of shorter duration. A clear exertional pattern is helpful to the diagnosis; pain can also be provoked by effort, emotion, or exposure to cold. Prompt relief within 5 minutes from sublingual nitroglycerin is suggestive of angina but can also occur with esophageal spasm or placebo. Pain that is relieved with exertion and brought on by rest is not anginal. Angina is unstable when it increases in severity (duration, intensity, frequency), occurs with reduced activity or at rest, or has been present for less than 4 weeks. This diagnosis requires hospital admission or risk stratification prior to discharge from the ED.

Aortic dissection classically produces a severe tearing pain in the anterior chest radiating to the back, flank, or arm. The patient sometimes feels pain traveling down the back or flank as the dissection extends distally. The pain is frequently described as being migratory. Its onset is sudden, but it may be intermittent or wax and wane. Uncommonly, it presents as a myocardial infarction or as a chronic pain that has become worse. The pain has no relieving factors, and writhing, diaphoresis, dyspnea, nausea, and vomiting are commonly associated. A common error is to dismiss the diagnosis of aortic dissection because the pain gets better with nitroglycerin. This may be due to a decrease in the intraluminal pressure of the aorta after nitroglycerin. Associated symptoms, such as weakness, paralysis, syncope, and numbness or pain in an extremity, are also common and more specific for dissection.

Pericarditis produces a sharp or aching pain in the precordium that may radiate to the scapula, neck, or shoulder. Unlike AMI, it has a long duration (days), and can be continuous and severe or pleuritic. It is usually made worse by lying down or breathing; thus, the associated "shortness of breath." Patients may insist on leaning forward to make themselves more comfortable.

Myocarditis can present with associated pericarditis. It also uncommonly masquerades as a myocardial infarction (13). Antecedent viral illness and younger age are diagnostic clues, but an in-hospital evaluation is necessary for definitive diagnosis of this uncommon cause of chest pain.

The most common presentation of *pulmonary embolism* (PE) is dyspnea, pleuritic pain, or hemoptysis (20). About 85% of cases of PE present with one or more of these nonspecific symptoms. Tachypnea is common, but tachycardia is found in only a minority of proven cases of PE. Large pulmonary emboli can produce circulatory collapse with syncope due to acute pulmonary hypertension and right heart failure. PE is mistaken for AMI about 7% of the time (20). Chest pain that is strictly reproducible is not consistent with PE, but rarely is present in these patients.

Pneumothorax may produce a severe, sudden stabbing pain in the affected side, or it may be asymptomatic. It has no characteristic pain radiation. It is made worse by breathing, is relieved by splinting, and is associated with shortness of breath and nonproductive cough. *Pleurisy*, an inflammation of the parietal pleura, is similar but does not have the associated symptoms or radiographic findings. *Pneumonia* can also cause pleuritic pain, but its association with productive cough, shortness of breath (at rest or exertion), and fever is often a helpful differentiating feature.

Pain may be due to an esophageal source. Pain from *esophageal spasm* is often indistinguishable from angina in quality, intensity, location, and radiation. Spasm has been described as a perfect mimic of acute myocardial ischemia. Esophageal reflux is a

TABLE 6.1.   Common Causes of Chest Pain

Organ System/Etiology	Chest Pain	Associated Symptoms
CARDIOVASCULAR		
Acute myocardial infarction	Pressure, aching, burning	Dyspnea, palpitations, nausea, diaphoresis, radiation
Aortic dissection	Sudden, severe, tearing	Back pain, neurovascular deficits
Unstable angina	Same as AMI except episodic	Same as AMI
Pericarditis	Sharp, pleuritic, positional	Fever, dyspnea
Myocarditis	Same as AMI or pericarditis	Dyspnea, palpitations, CHF
RESPIRATORY		
Pulmonary embolus	Sharp pleuritic or central ache	Dyspnea, cough, hemoptysis, leg swelling, risk factors
Pneumothorax	Sudden, sharp, pleuritic	Dyspnea, cough
Pneumomediastinum	Variable	Risks: cocaine, COPD, iatrogenic procedures
Pneumonia	Sharp, pleuritic	Cough, fever, dyspnea
Pleuritis	Sharp, pleuritic	Cough, fever
Mediastinitis	Variable	Fever, dyspnea, sepsis
Tumor	Chronic, variable	Weight loss
ESOPHAGEAL		
Rupture: Boerhaave	Sudden, severe	Vomiting, hematemesis
Esophageal spasm	Similar to AMI	Reflux, nausea
Reflux esophagitis	Burning, worse supine	Reflux, nausea, sore throat
ABDOMINAL DISORDERS		
Gastrointestinal	Constant, related to food	Vomiting, abdominal pain, GI bleeding
Cholecystitis	Constant or colicky	Vomiting, abdominal pain, jaundice, fever
Ruptured ectopic pregnancy	Sharp, pleuritic	Abdominal pain, vaginal bleeding, shoulder pain
MUSCULOSKELETAL		
Ruptured cervical disc	Pain on neck movement	Neurologic signs, pain referred in root distribution
Costochondritis	Sharp, pleuritic	Localized tenderness and inflammation
Herpes zoster	Burning, lancinating	Dermatomal distribution of pain, rash, paresthesias
Postherpetic neuralgia	Burning, lancinating	History of zoster

AMI, acute myocardial infarction; CHF, congestive heart failure; GI, gastrointestinal.

midline epigastric discomfort usually described as indigestion or burning. It lasts minutes to hours, and is worse after eating and lying down. It is associated with belching but not shortness of breath, and tends to be chronic; it may be associated with an acid taste.

Relief with antacids does not reliably rule out pain from cardiac ischemia. Esophageal rupture produces pain in the anterior chest, back, or epigastrium. Rupture occurs in the setting of increased barotrauma from retching or prolonged vomiting or coughing. Vomiting that occurs before the pain suggests esophageal rupture, not AMI (14). Dysphagia and occasionally hemoptysis are the initial symptoms. Life-threatening mediastinitis and sepsis develop if esophageal rupture goes untreated.

DIFFERENTIAL DIAGNOSIS

The following immediately or potentially life-threatening diseases of the thoracic organ systems must be considered in every patient who presents to the emergency department with chest pain.

Acute Myocardial Infarction and Ischemia

Occlusion of a coronary vessel resulting in death of heart muscle can present as a catastrophic condition, with malignant dysrhythmias, pump failure, or myocardial rupture, or as a completely compensated minimally painful state. It is by far the most

common chest pain emergency, accounting for 40 of 1,000 hospital admissions (2). Although the Framingham study risk factors of smoking, hypertension, diabetes, family history, and elevated cholesterol further increase the likelihood of developing AMI or angina over a period of years, they are not helpful in excluding or confirming the diagnosis in the acute care setting. Nevertheless, the physician should document, for medicolegal purposes, the presence of risk factors in all patients with chest pain. The symptoms of coronary vasospasm may be very similar to those of AMI or angina due to occlusive disease.

Emergency physicians frequently evaluate patients with pain associated with recent cocaine use (9,24). Such patients commonly have vasospasm, and indeed have a lower confirmed rate of myocardial infarction than non–cocaine-related admissions (4). Vasospastic ischemic pain is more common than AMI. In patients with cocaine-associated chest pain, even in those without ischemia, ST segment elevation is present much of the time due to repolarization abnormalities (9). Unless the presentation of AMI is classic, these abnormal baseline findings make it helpful to have an old electrocardiogram (ECG) without ST elevation, or serial ECGs showing evolving ST elevation in the emergency department, before giving thrombolytic therapy. Cardiac catheterization is the optimal diagnostic and potentially therapeutic maneuver.

In AMI, thrombolytic therapy, percutaneous coronary interventions, adjunctive treatment with antithrombotic and antiplatelet agents, and treatment in the coronary care unit have significantly lowered case fatality and reinfarction rates, making it imperative to diagnose an acute coronary syndrome in the emergency department. Unstable angina is just as important to recognize, because 10% to 20% of confirmed cases proceed to infarction. Heparin, glycoprotein IIB/IIIA and ACE inhibitors, and vasodilators, or more invasive procedures such as coronary revascularization, may be required to treat recurrent pain or associated heart failure or shock (see Chapter 41, Acute Coronary Syndromes).

Dissection of the Thoracic Aorta

This disruption in the intimal layer of the aorta allows blood to track within the media. Aortic rupture is an ever-present threat. Untreated dissection has a mortality rate of 90%; fortunately, it is responsible for less than 1 in 1,000 hospital admissions (2). Progression of the dissection can cause severe organ damage to the spine (sometimes misclassified as stroke), brain, kidneys, bowel, and heart, including AMI and cardiac tamponade. The patient must be carefully examined for evidence of these complications. Hypertension is the most common risk factor, although younger patients with Marfan or Ehlers-Danlos syndromes may have dissection due to cystic medial necrosis (see Chapter 55, Thoracic Aortic Dissections and Aneurysms).

Pulmonary Embolism

Pulmonary embolism is an obstruction of the pulmonary arterial system due to clot, which usually embolizes from deep femoral or pelvic veins. In addition to dyspnea, pleuritic pain, and hemoptysis, it can produce acute respiratory failure or right-sided heart failure, as evidenced by cyanosis, hypotension, increased jugular venous pressure, and a loud S2 or right heart gallop. The hospitalization rate is 2 in 1,000 (2). Mortality from PE itself is uncommon and is usually due to recurrent emboli. Recognition of such predisposing conditions as immobilization, recent surgery, hypercoagulability, and low-flow circulatory states is critical to raising the clinician's diagnostic suspicion. A high degree of suspicion is especially important, because PE often presents with subtle, nonspecific findings (see Chapter 38, Pulmonary Embolism).

Tension Pneumothorax

Tension pneumothorax occurs when air escapes from the lung into the thoracic cavity, shifting the mediastinum to one side and compromising right-sided heart filling. Dyspnea, diaphoresis, tachycardia, tachypnea, and hypotension commonly result. Jugular vein distention, tracheal deviation, decreased breath sounds, and percussion tympany are noted on physical examination. Pneumothorax may be spontaneous or secondary to trauma, infection (such as tuberculosis and AIDS), or the rupture of emphysematous blebs. Patients with tension pneumothorax require immediate needle thoracostomy and subsequent placement of a chest tube (see Chapter 37, Spontaneous Pneumothorax and Pneumomediastinum and Chapter 183, Penetrating Chest Trauma).

Esophageal Rupture

Esophageal rupture can occur in the cervical esophagus, but it usually occurs in the distal esophagus. Conditions associated with retching, vomiting, and coughing, such as ethanol abuse, hyperemesis gravidarum, and status asthmaticus, predispose patients to this rare but important disease (21)(see Chapter 58, Esophageal Disease).

DIAGNOSTIC APPROACH

After verifying or establishing initial patient stability, the diagnostic approach proceeds from a consideration of age, sex, specific clinical presentation, and preexisting conditions or risk factors for the specific emergency diagnoses. The history and physical examination are essential for differentiating these conditions and detecting their complications.

The chest x-ray is key to the detection of pneumothorax, heart failure, pneumonia, and a widened mediastinum, as seen in aortic dissection. Mediastinal or subcutaneous air can be a clue to devastating conditions such as mediastinitis or esophageal rupture. Diagnosis of certain entities may require more advanced imaging modalities, such as CT scanning, MRI, angiography, or echocardiography. Transesophageal echocardiography is sensitive, specific, and practical for the emergency department diagnosis of aortic dissection (11).

Diagnosing PE continues to be clinically challenging, as ECG, arterial blood gas, and chest radiography are all nondiagnostic tests. Arterial blood gas studies are useful to assess the severity of hypoxemia, but a normal PO_2 is present about 10% of the time in the patient with PE. The fundamental approach is to risk stratify patients into high, medium, and low probabilities of disease (3,25). Clinical probability then guides test selection. An assay for d-dimers is a sensitive test, and thus can serve to exclude the diagnosis in patients with low clinical probability of disease (3). For those with high or moderate probability, imaging with thin-slice spiral CT is overtaking V/Q scanning as the confirmatory test of choice (22). However, a negative V/Q scan virtually excludes pulmonary emboli whereas a negative spiral CT does not exclude the presence of smaller, subsegmental clots. Optimal evaluations are guided by risk stratification and local availability of specific tests (3,8,25).

Bedside risk stratification is also the fundamental approach to the diagnosis of acute coronary syndromes. The history, physical exam, and 12-lead ECG are the basis for dividing patients into high and low probability of disease (6,18). In the patient with chest pain or other suggestive symptoms of cardiac ischemia, ST-segment deviation (elevation or depression, or left bundle branch block) or positive troponin testing indicates a high-risk patient.

The ECG is particularly instructive. Regional ST elevation of 1 mm (0.1 mV) in two leads is the indication for coronary reperfusion therapy, and assessment of ST-segment depression in leads opposite (i.e., reciprocal) to the ST-segment elevation is helpful in confirming subtle ST elevation. Serial ECGs are useful with recurrent pain in higher risk patients to detect AMI evolution or reperfusion (5). The ECG pattern can also provide information favoring other elements of the differential diagnosis. Diffuse ST-segment elevation with associated PR depression (most frequent in lead II) suggests pericarditis; low-voltage or electrical alternans suggests an effusion. Anterior T-wave inversions can be present in myocardial ischemia or pulmonary embolism (17). The ECG may reveal ischemia or an infarction pattern in the inferior leads in patients with aortic dissection, as the right coronary artery may be involved in the dissection. The most common ECG finding in pulmonary embolism is sinus tachycardia, followed by right precordial T-wave inversion, a strain pattern (17). The $S_1Q_3T_3$ pattern has greater specificity, but is uncommon in pulmonary embolism.

The emergency department ECG is also a simple prognostic indicator for in-hospital complications. In stable, pain-free patients who are being admitted to rule out AMI, an ECG without ST-segment changes, Q waves, T-wave inversion, or left bundle-branch block is associated with a very low (less than 1%) incidence of life-threatening complications. When an ST-segment elevation of 0.1 mV is present in the right ventricular lead V4R in the setting of inferior AMI, suggesting coincident right ventricular infarction, complication rates are higher than when it is absent (26).

In addition to bedside risk stratification, formal diagnostic decision tools, such as the algorithm for risk assessment in AMI (6) or a computer-generated numerical probability for acute ischemia (18), have been developed and validated. They are not yet in widespread clinical use. For prognosis, a formal algorithm developed by Goldman and associates can predict short-term complication rates using ECG findings, presence of heart failure, low blood pressure, and worsening angina (7).

The tools and technologies are now well established for the relatively rapid diagnostic assessment of acute cardiac ischemia (15,16,23,24,27). For low probability patients, in the setting of an in-hospital or short stay ED observation bed, serial ECGs (5) followed by serial cardiac markers can confirm or exclude myocardial necrosis (15). Further assessment with provocative testing, such as stress echocardiography or stress nuclear imaging complete the work-up to exclude an acute coronary syndrome (23). Such testing also provides valuable prognostic information (4,7,15,23,25,26). Newer cardiac biomarkers not based on cardiac muscle death, such as an albumin-based assay for coronary ischemia, aim to be the "holy grail" of an early marker of ischemia rather than just necrosis; however, such an assay has not been validated (19). It is now widely accepted by emergency physicians and their in-hospital colleagues that a large portion of chest pain patients can only be evaluated by serial rather than cross-sectional testing. This realization has likely contributed to decreased rates of "missed" ischemia and improved patient care.

CRITICAL INTERVENTIONS

All patients with acute chest pain should have a rapid ($\leq$ 10 minutes) ECG and then continuous cardiac ECG monitoring, chest radiography, intravenous access, and oxygen. Aspirin, nitroglycerin, and beta-blockers are indicated for suspected ischemic pain. Most patients with unstable angina should also receive low-molecular weight or unfractionated heparin. Patients with MI and high risk ECGs (ST-segment elevation, left or right bundle-branch block, ST-depression with ongoing ischemic pain) should have an immediate cardiology consultation. Patients with suspected pulmonary embolism receive a similar diagnostic approach, but oxygen and low-molecular weight or unfractionated heparin are the initial treatments. Patients with aortic dissection must have immediate blood pressure control with both a beta-blocking agent and a vasodilator, and no anticoagulation. Tension pneumothorax with cardiovascular compromise (absent breath sounds, distended neck veins, tracheal deviation) is a clinical diagnosis and requires immediate decompression with a 16-gauge angio-catheter followed by chest tube insertion and hospitalization.

DISPOSITION

All of the life-threatening elements in the differential diagnosis of chest pain must be excluded prior to discharge from the ED. Chest pain with features typical for active acute ischemia requires the initiation of antithrombotic and antiischemia therapies in the ED with continuation in the hospital. Cardiac consultation and coronary care unit admission is indicated for all such patients. Transfer to percutaneous transluminal coronary angioplasty (PTCA) capable institutions should be considered for patients in need of reperfusion (ST-segment elevation or left bundle-branch block) but ineligible for thrombolytic therapy,

and for those with active ischemic pain. Patients with lower probabilities of ischemia and complications can be safely and effectively ruled out in an emergency department or in-hospital observation unit. This can be done over a 6- to 9-hour period with serial biomarkers, followed by a cardiovascular stress test prior to discharge or within 2 to 3 days of discharge. Patients with pulmonary embolism may need ICU admission if they are hemodynamically unstable or have refractory hypoxemia; for smaller emboli, admission to a telemetry bed or the medical floor is appropriate. Patients with pericarditis should undergo echocardiography if pericardial effusion or tamponade are suspected, and may require a period of observation in the hospital. However, stable patients with pericarditis can be discharged from the ED.

COMMON PITFALLS

✔ Ordering a single cardiac biomarker or enzyme to exclude myocardial infarction

✔ Failure to order serial ECGs in patients with a negative ECG and a history suggestive of an acute coronary syndrome

✔ Believing that right bundle-branch block prevents detection of ST-segment elevation

✔ Believing that therapeutic maneuvers of sublingual NTG or antacids have diagnostic value

✔ Failure to consider the diagnosis of esophageal rupture and palpate the soft tissue of the neck for subcutaneous emphysema

✔ Failure to consider the diagnosis of aortic dissection in patients with anterior or posterior chest pain

✔ Believing that pain relief with sublingual nitroglycerin excludes aortic dissection

✔ Failure to examine the chest x-ray for the absence of pulmonary vascular markings extending to the parietal pleura

References

1. Canto JG, Shlipak MG, Rogers WJ, et al. Prevalence, clinical characteristics, and mortality among patients with myocardial infarction presenting without chest pain. *JAMA* 2000;283:3223–3229.
2. Ehxhauser A, Andrews RM, Fox SF. Clinical classifications for health policy research: discharge statistics by principal diagnosis and procedure. *Agency Health Care Policy Res* 1993;93:43.
3. Fedullo PR, Tapson VF. The evaluation of suspected pulmonary embolism. *N Engl J Med* 2003;349:1247–1256.
4. Feldman JA, Fish SS, Beshansky JR, Griffith JL, Woolard RH, Selker HP. Acute cardiac ischemia in patients with cocaine-associated complaints: results of a multicenter trial. *Ann Emerg Med* 2000;36:469–476.
5. Fesmire FM. Which chest pain patients potentially benefit from continuous 12-lead ST-segment monitoring with automated serial ECG? *Am J Emerg Med* 2000;18:773–778.
6. Goldman L, Cook EF, Brand DA, et al. A computer protocol to predict myocardial infarction in emergency department patients with chest pain. *N Engl J Med* 1988;318:797.
7. Goldman L, Cook EF, Johnson PA, et al. Prediction of the need for intensive care in patients who come to emergency departments with acute chest pain. *N Engl J Med* 1996;334:1498–1504.
8. Holbert JM, Costello P, Federle MP. Role of spiral computed tomography in the diagnosis of pulmonary embolism in the emergency department. *Ann Emerg Med* 1999;33:520–528.
9. Hollander JE. The management of cocaine-associated myocardial ischemia. *N Engl J Med* 1995;333:1267–1272.
10. Horwitz L, Groves B. *Signs and symptoms in cardiology.* Philadelphia: JB Lippincott Co, 1985:5.
11. Hwang JJ, Shyu KG, Chen JJ, et al. Usefulness of transesophageal echocardiography in the treatment of critically ill patients. *Chest* 1993;104:861.
12. Lee TH, Cook EF, Weisberg M, et al. Acute chest pain in the emergency room. *Arch Intern Med* 1985;65:60.
13. Narula-Jagat AU, Khaw-Ban AN, William DEC Jr, et al. Recognition of acute myocarditis masquerading as acute myocardial infarction. *N Engl J Med* 1993;328:100.
14. Nehra D, Beynon J, Pye JK. Spontaneous rupture of the oesophagus (Boerhaave's syndrome). *Postgrad Med J* 1993;69:214.
15. Newby LK, Storrow AB, Gibler WB, et al. Bedside multimarker testing for risk stratification in chest pain units: the chest pain evaluation by

creatine kinase-MB, myoglobin, and troponin I (CHECKMATE) study. *Circulation* 2001;103:1832–7.

16. Roberts RR, Zalenski RJ, Mensah EK, et al. Costs of an emergency department-based accelerated diagnostic protocol vs hospitalization in patients with chest pain. *JAMA* 1997;278:1670–1676.

17. Sashara AA, Hyers TM, Cole CM, et al. The urokinase pulmonary embolism trial: a national cooperative study. *Circulation* 1990;47:11–86.

18. Selker HP, Beshansky JR, Griffith JL, et al. Use of the acute cardiac ischemia time-insensitive predictive instrument to assist with triage of patients with chest pain or other symptoms suggestive of acute cardiac ischemia. A multicenter, controlled trial. *Ann Intern Med* 1998;129:845–855.

19. Sinha MK, Roy D, Gaze DC, Collinson PO, Kaski JC. Role of "Ischemia Modified Albumin," a new biochemical marker of myocardial ischaemia, in the early diagnosis of acute coronary syndromes. *Emerg Med J* 2004;21:29–34.

20. Stein PD, Terrin ML, Hales CA, et al. Clinical, laboratory, roentgenographic, and electrocardiographic findings in patients with acute pulmonary embolism and no pre-existing cardiac or pulmonary disease. *Chest* 1991;199:598.

21. Taylor MB. *Gastrointestinal emergencies*. Baltimore: Williams & Wilkins, 1992.

22. Trowbridge RL, Araoz PA, Gotway MB, Bailey RA, Auerback AD. The effect of helical computed tomography on diagnostic and treatment strategies in patients with suspected pulmonary embolism. *Am J Med* 2004;116:84–90.

23. Udelson JE, Beshansky JR, Ballin DS, et al. Myocardial perfusion imaging for evaluation and triage of patients with suspected acute cardiac ischemia: a randomized controlled trial. *JAMA* 2002;288:2693–2700.

24. Weber JE, Shofer FS, Larkin GL, Kalaria AS, Hollander JE. Validation of a brief observation period for patients with cocaine-associated chest pain. *N Engl J Med*. 2003;348:510–517.

25. Wells PS, Anderson DR, Rodger M, et al. Excluding pulmonary embolism at the bedside without diagnostic imaging: management of patients with suspected pulmonary embolism presenting to the emergency department by using a simple clinical model and d-dimer. *Ann Intern Med* 2001;135:98–107.

26. Zalenski RJ, Rydman RJ, Sloan EP, et al. ST segment elevation and the prediction of hospital life-threatening complications: the role of right ventricular and posterior leads. *J Electrocardiol*. 1998;31(S):164–171.

27. Zalenski RJ, McCarren M, Roberts F, et al. An evaluation of a chest pain diagnostic protocol to exclude acute cardiac ischemia in the emergency department. *Arch Intern Med* 1997;157:1085–1091.

CHAPTER 7
Abdominal Pain

Michelle Charfen, Diane M. Birnbaumer, and Sheldon Jacobsen

Abdominal pain is one of the most frequent chief complaints in emergency medicine, and one of the most challenging. Abdominal pain accounts for 5% of the greater than 105 million annual emergency department visits (18). Abdominal pain can be caused by benign processes that present with severe pain or by fatal processes that present with subtle findings. Patients with abdominal pain continue to be diagnostically challenging despite improving imaging modalities. Even in patients who have undergone an appropriate work up, approximately 30% of patients will be discharged with the diagnosis of undifferentiated abdominal pain (18).

CLINICAL PRESENTATION

The importance of a thorough history and physical examination cannot be overemphasized, as it helps narrow the vast differen-

tial diagnosis and focus on the diagnostic testing. A review of malpractice cases relating to abdominal conditions shows that failure to actually gather and chart patient data (history and physical exam) is a more frequent cause of misdiagnosis than is misinterpretation of the data gathered (21).

When obtaining the history and performing a physical examination it is important to understand that there are three major types of abdominal pain: *visceral, somatic* and *referred* pain. They differ based on the anatomic pathway relaying the pain signal.

Visceral pain is relayed by afferent visceral fibers that are located in the walls of hollow organs and capsules of solid organs. These fibers are stimulated by stretching, distension and excessive contraction. The visceral pain fibers are unmyelinated, originate from both sides of the spinal column, and enter the spinal column at multiple levels. This results in the perception of a poorly localized, midline pain that is described as dull or aching.

The specific abdominal location of visceral pain is determined by the embryologic origin of the abdominal organs. During embryologic development the gastrointestinal (GI) tract is divided into the foregut, midgut, and hindgut. Each of these divisions has its own innervation and blood supply. The *foregut* derives its blood supply from the superior mesenteric artery and includes the stomach, proximal duodenum, liver, and pancreas. Diseases of these organs cause *upper abdominal or epigastric pain*. The *midgut* derives its blood supply from the celiac artery and includes the distal duodenum, jejunum, ileum, appendix, ascending colon, and proximal two-thirds of the transverse colon. Diseases of the midgut cause *periumbilical pain*. The *hindgut* derives its blood supply from the inferior mesenteric artery and consists of the distal third of the colon, rectum, and urogenital system. Diseases of the hindgut cause *lower abdominal pain*.

Somatic pain results from irritation of the parietal peritoneum. Pain is relayed by myelinated, unilateral afferent fibers that travel to a specific level in the spinal cord making this pain more localized. It is usually described as sharp, intense and well localized. Somatic pain is responsible for the physical findings of tenderness to palpation, guarding and rebound.

Abdominal pain often begins as visceral pain and then progresses to somatic pain as the inflammation spreads to involve the parietal peritoneum. As an example, the early epigastric pain of gallbladder distension is characteristic of visceral pain while the right upper quadrant pain caused by local peritoneal inflammation with cholecystitis is deep somatic pain.

Referred pain is discomfort perceived at a site distant from the diseased organ. The diseased organ and the body area to which the pain is referred have overlapping transmission pathways at the level of the spinal cord. A common example of referred pain is shoulder pain caused by irritation of the diaphragm from free air or blood. In the same manner extraabdominal organs may cause referred pain to the abdomen, such as myocardial ischemia or pneumonia causing epigastric pain.

History

When evaluating the patient with abdominal pain, a thorough history of the abdominal pain is crucial. Specifically, the physician should determine the onset, time course, character, location, aggravating and alleviating factors, associated symptoms and if there are previous episodes of abdominal pain. The general medical and social history should also be obtained, including past medical and surgical history, medications, allergies, tobacco, alcohol and illicit drug exposure, recent travel and toxic exposures.

Onset. Sudden onset of severe pain is very concerning and is assumed to be due to a surgical condition, until proven otherwise. Vascular emergencies such as mesenteric ischemia or a ruptured abdominal aortic aneurysm, and intestinal perforation or torsion of a viscous may all present this way. Sudden onset of severe pain with an unimpressive physical exam is typical for a vascular catastrophe or torsed organ. Nonsurgical causes of abrupt onset of abdominal pain include renal colic and myocardial infarction. The physician should determine what the patient was doing when the pain began. Pain related to eating may be secondary to peptic ulcer disease, gallbladder disease or mesenteric ischemia (intestinal angina). Pain that began during physical activity may be caused by rectus abdominal muscle tear and hematoma, or myocardial ischemia.

Progression of pain. The physician should question the patient about whether the pain is constant or intermittent, and, if constant, whether it has been increasing or decreasing in severity. Pain that begins slowly and gradually progresses is typical of an inflammatory or infectious process such as appendicitis or salpingitis. Pain that is improving over time is less likely to be surgical in nature.

Location. In addition to onset, location may be one of the most useful pieces of information in determining the etiology of pain. Figure 7.1 shows the different etiologies of abdominal pain by location. Visceral pain is perceived either as epigastric, periumbilical or infraumbilical depending on the embryologic origin of the involved organ. Visceral pain tends to be poorly localized and midline while parietal pain tends to be well localized and

unilateral. It is important to determine if the location has changed over time or radiates to a distant site.

Character. The severity and character of the pain are important historical factors. Dull aching pain is more likely to be visceral, and sharp pain is more likely to be somatic. Crampy intermittent pain is typically due to bowel obstruction. Severe tearing back pain is classic for aortic dissection.

Aggravating and alleviating factors. The patient should be asked about how the pain changes with food, movement, position or medications. Pain that is intensified by the car ride to the hospital or other movement is indicative of peritoneal irritation. The pain of pancreatitis is often exacerbated by lying in the supine position. The pain of myocardial ischemia may be relieved with rest.

Associated symptoms. The physician should determine the presence or absence of fever, nausea, vomiting, diarrhea, constipation, hematemesis, hematochezia, melena, dysuria, or hematuria. It is important to ask women about abnormal or increased vaginal discharge or vaginal bleeding, and to ask men about testicular or penile complaints (swelling or pain). When patients complain of vomiting and abdominal pain, it is useful to determine which came first. Typically, in surgical diseases the abdominal pain almost always precedes the vomiting while the converse is true in 75% of cases of gastroenteritis and nonspecific causes. Since both cardiac and pulmonary processes can present with

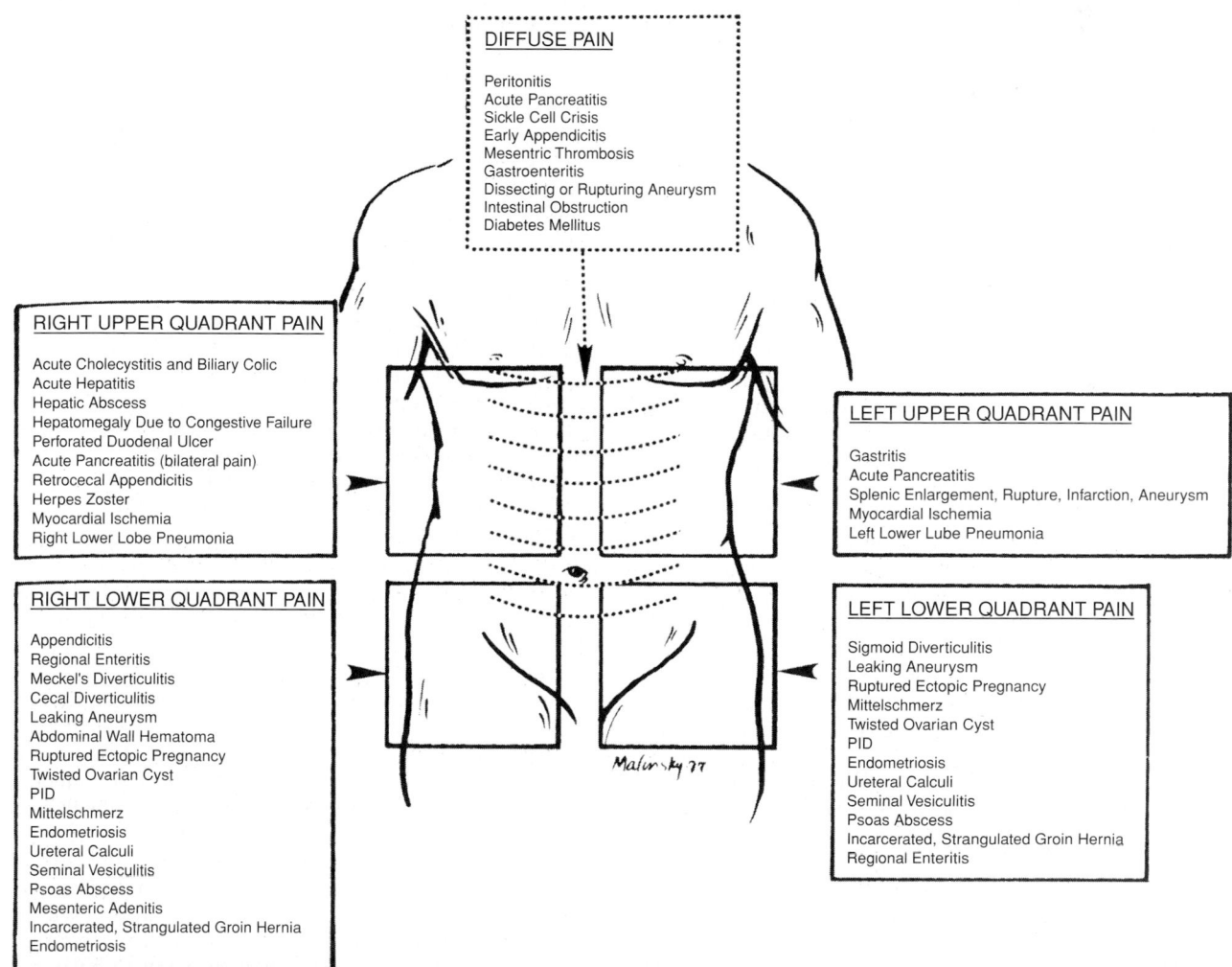

Figure 7.1. Differential diagnosis of acute abdominal pain by location. (From Wagner DK: Approaches to the patient with acute abdominal pain. Current Topics (a program of the Medical College of Pennsylvania) 1L3, 1978. Used by permission.)

abdominal pain, an appropriate history should include questions about the presence of chest pain, shortness of breath or cough. Also, the patient should be asked about the presence of flank or back pain. Patients with abdominal aortic aneurysm or renal colic may have pain that radiates to these areas.

Previous episodes. Previous episodes of the pain should be investigated. Chronic recurrent abdominal pain involves a wide differential diagnosis; when obtaining the history the physician should try to identify triggers of the abdominal pain. If the patient has undergone diagnostic studies in the past there may be no point in repeating the work up. If pain is recurrent, it may be related to the menstrual cycle. Pain that begins 2 weeks after the start of the menstrual cycle is suggestive of mittelschmerz.

Past medical history. Cardiovascular diseases including hypertension, atrial fibrillation and valvular disease place patients at higher risk for vascular diseases such as mesenteric ischemia, abdominal aortic aneurysm and myocardial infarction. A gynecologic history should be obtained including menstrual history, history of sexually transmitted diseases and previous ectopic pregnancy.

Past surgical history. Previous abdominal surgeries place patients at greater risk for conditions such as bowel obstruction resulting from adhesions.

Medications. A medication history should be obtained including herbal supplements, and recent antibiotic (may lead to *Clostridium difficile* infection) or steroid use. Certain drugs place patients at higher risk for hepatitis and pancreatitis.

Social history. Alcohol abuse increases the risk of GI bleeds, pancreatitis, hepatitis and cirrhosis. Heroin withdrawal may present with abdominal pain, nausea, and vomiting.

Other. Recent traumatic events such as motor vehicle collisions or blows to the abdominal wall or back can result in rectus sheath hematoma, intraperitoneal bleeding, duodenal hematoma, or traumatic pancreatitis. A history of recent food intake, sick contacts and travel is important for patients with suspected gastroenteritis. Finally, a history of any toxic exposures (e.g., lead) may also reveal the cause of the abdominal pain.

Physical Examination

The physical examination should begin with an evaluation of the vital signs. When interpreting the vital signs, the emergency physician should take into account any medications that may affect heart rate or blood pressure (i.e., beta-blockers). Tachycardia and hypotension should alert the physician to possible sepsis, dehydration from volume loss or third spacing, or hemorrhage from an abdominal aortic aneurysm or ruptured ectopic pregnancy. Fever makes an infectious etiology more likely, although absence of a fever should not be used to rule out an infectious cause of the pain. This is especially true in the elderly who may present with infectious etiologies, but no fever. Since an oral temperature may be falsely low (14), the more reliable rectal temperature should be obtained if infection is suspected. Tachypnea may be secondary to pain, hypoxia, sepsis, anemia or metabolic acidosis. Pulse oximetry should be obtained to assess for hypoxia.

The general appearance of the patient may reveal clues to the diagnosis. A patient with peritonitis will lie still while a patient with renal colic may present writhing in the bed. The patient's level of alertness, mental status and orientation are also important. Lethargy and confusion are concerning for toxic ingestions, sepsis or other causes of hypoperfusion.

The patient's skin should be carefully examined. Pale, diaphoretic skin suggests shock or a low volume state (dehydration or bleeding). Jaundice may be present in patients with biliary or hepatic disease. The skin should be examined for rashes. Skin findings such as petechiae and spider hemangiomas are suggestive of liver disease. Whether the mucous membranes are moist or dry should be noted; dry membranes suggest dehydration. Oral thrush or hairy leukoplakia may indicate undiagnosed immunocompromise.

When examining the heart and lungs, the physician should listen for rales, rhonchi, wheezing or other abnormal breath sounds that indicate a pulmonary etiology of abdominal pain. Atrial fibrillation and valvular disease put patients at risk for mesenteric ischemia caused by emboli.

The abdominal exam should start with inspection. The physician should look for distention, hernias and the presence of surgical scars and auscultate for bowel sounds noting their frequency, quality, and pitch. Obstruction and processes that cause inflammation within the GI tract result in increased bowel sounds while processes that cause inflammation outside of the GI tract such as peritonitis result in diminished bowel sounds. With obstruction, high-pitched tinkling bowel sounds are present; in patients with an ileus, bowel sounds may be absent. Percussion may aid in the diagnosis of ascites, obstruction, or perforation, and tenderness to percussion may indicate peritonitis.

When palpating the abdomen the physician should assess for location of tenderness, the presence of voluntary and involuntary guarding and peritoneal signs. It is recommended to begin with gentle palpation starting farthest away from the suspected location of tenderness. If the patient is able to tolerate gentle palpation, then deeper palpation should be used to localize the area of tenderness. Palpation at one location may cause pain at a separate location. An example of this is seen in patients with appendicitis and is referred to as *Rovsing's sign* (pain experienced at *McBurney's point* during deep palpation of the left lower quadrant). The physician should examine for masses or organomegaly. In assessing for right upper quadrant (RUQ) pathology, the physician should note the presence of a *Murphy's sign*. During deep palpation of the RUQ the patient is asked to take a deep breath. If inspiration is arrested in mid-cycle this is suggestive of cholecystitis (positive *Murphy's sign*). In elderly patients the physician should assess for an abdominal aortic aneurysm by listening for bruits and assessing for the presence of an infra-epigastric pulsating mass.

Voluntary guarding may be due to anxiety, fear, or discomfort. Maneuvers that aid in relieving voluntary guarding include warming of the hands, examination with the patient's thighs flexed, deep inspiration and reassurance from the physician. Involuntary guarding or rigidity will not resolve with these maneuvers and is more indicative of surgical disease. *Peritoneal signs* are markers of surgical disease. Classically, peritonitis was assessed by examining for the presence of *rebound tenderness*, increased tenderness when the examiner let go after deep palpation of the abdomen. Studies have shown that rebound tenderness is often present even in the absence of peritonitis and given that it is painful for the patient, some advocate using other methods to look for peritonitis (15). Other methods include the *cough test* (the abdominal pain will worsen abruptly when the patient coughs), jostling the gurney, or striking the patient's heels. Rigidity and peritoneal signs may be absent in the elderly even in the presence of peritoneal irritation. This may be attributed to the relatively thin musculature of the abdominal wall in older patients.

Carnett's test can be used to help determine whether abdominal pain arises from the abdominal wall. While in the supine position the patient is asked to lift the head off the table and the abdomen is palpated. If the source of the pain is intraabdominal the contracted musculature of the abdominal wall will provide shielding and diminish tenderness. If the source of pain is the abdominal wall the tenderness will be the same or even increased (8).

It is important to examine for umbilical, inguinal, femoral and surgical incision hernias, especially in the elderly. In this age group, approximately 10% of cases of obstruction are due to hernias, and they are often undiagnosed (25).

Examination of the back is necessary to check for costovertebral angle tenderness that may indicate either pyelonephritis or ureteral obstruction.

Women of childbearing age with lower quadrant pain should undergo a pelvic examination to aid in differentiating salpingitis or ovarian pathology from appendicitis or diverticulitis. The results of the pelvic exam should be interpreted carefully as women with appendicitis may also have cervical motion tenderness and adnexal tenderness. Mucopurulent discharge from the cervical os suggests pelvic inflammatory disease. In women with right upper quadrant pain, particularly if laboratory evaluation for gall bladder disease is negative, the pelvic exam may also be helpful. *Fitz-Hugh Curtis* syndrome, a perihepatitis caused by pelvic inflammatory disease, may present with complaints of upper abdominal pain and the patient may have no pelvic complaints. The diagnosis can be missed if the pelvic examination is not performed.

The digital rectal examination is helpful in assessing for guaiac positive stool, melena or hematochezia, and it may also aid in the diagnosis of prostate disease, perirectal disease and rectal foreign bodies. A testicular exam should be performed to assess for torsion, epididymitis, or masses.

Patients with abdominal pain may remain in the emergency department for hours during their evaluation and work up. Repeat abdominal examination is very useful in these patients as changes over time may clarify the cause of their illness.

DIFFERENTIAL DIAGNOSIS

The differential diagnosis of abdominal pain is extensive and includes both intraabdominal and extraabdominal sources of pain (Tables 7.1 and 7.2). A thorough history and physical exam are crucial in determining the etiology of the pain and narrowing down this vast list of possible causes. The location of the pain is very useful in narrowing the differential diagnosis. Figure 7.1 lists the differential diagnosis by location.

It is of utmost importance to rule out the immediately life-threatening causes of abdominal pain. These include ruptured or leaking abdominal aortic aneurysm, splenic rupture, perforated viscous, intestinal obstruction, mesenteric ischemia, pancreatitis, ruptured ectopic pregnancy and myocardial infarction. Once the life threat is ruled out, focus should be placed on diagnosing emergent surgical entities such as testicular and ovarian torsion, incarcerated hernia, ascending cholangitis, appendicitis, cholecystitis, and diverticulitis.

TABLE 7.1. Surgical Causes of Abdominal Pain

Abdominal aortic aneurysm**
Mesenteric ischemia**
Ectopic pregnancy**
Perforated viscus**
Aortic dissection**
Appenditicis†
Diverticulitis†
Ovarian torsion†
Cholecystitis
Cholelithiasis
Ascending cholangitis
Ovarian cysts

**Immediate life threat
†Surgical urgency

TABLE 7.2. Nonsurgical Causes of Abdominal Pain

Myocardial infarction
Diabetic ketoacidosis
Pneumonia
Inflammatory bowel disease
Irritable bowel syndrome
Esophagitis
Prostatitis
Intraabdominal malignancy
Mesenteric lymphadenitis
Gastroenteritis
Peptic ulcer disease
Gastritis
Hepatitis
Pelvic inflammatory disease
Tubo-ovarian abscess
Mittelschmerz
Endometriosis
Herpes zoster
Abdominal wall contusion
Acute glaucoma
Acute intermittent porphyria
Heavy-metal poisoning
Abdominal tabes (Dietl crisis)
Abdominal epilepsy
Abdominal migraine
Black widow spider bite
Vasculitis
Abdominal angina
Intestinal pseudoobstruction
Sickle cell crisis
Right-sided colonic diverticulitis
Meckel's diverticulitis
Familial Mediterranean fever
Massive intravascular hemolysis
Narcotic withdrawal
Factitious or drug-seeking behavior
Psychogenic abdominal pain
Addisonian crisis
Spastic colon

Although many causes of abdominal pain originate from the abdominal organs, extraabdominal causes of abdominal pain also occur. Upper abdominal pain may have a pulmonary etiology such as pneumonia, pneumothorax or pulmonary embolism or a cardiac etiology such as myocardial infarction. Lower abdominal pain may be of genitourinary or pelvic origin.

Certain groups of patients presenting with abdominal pain deserve special attention because of their higher rates of misdiagnosis and increased morbidity and mortality. These groups include the elderly, patients with human immunodeficiency virus (HIV) infection, women of childbearing age and the very young. The pediatric patient with abdominal pain is discussed in Chapter 214, Abdominal Pain.

Abdominal Pain in the Elderly

The conditions causing abdominal pain in elderly patients are usually more serious and urgent, but despite this they may present with a relatively benign history and physical examination. The elderly often have comorbid illnesses confusing the clinical situation and may have hearing loss or underlying dementia making obtaining an adequate history more difficult. Elderly patients may be unable to physiologically mount the typical response to pain and infection. They may lack fevers despite surgical disease and laboratory values may be normal. As the risk of mortality in patients presenting with abdominal pain increases with each decade of life, the clinician's suspicion for serious disease must be higher in elderly patients. The spectrum of disease is also different in elderly patients, with acute cholecystitis being the most common disease and nonspecific abdominal pain accounting for only 15% of patients over the age of 50. This compares with an incidence of nonspecific abdominal pain of greater than 33% for patients under the age of 50. Elderly patients are also at increased risk for abdominal catastrophes such as mesenteric ischemia, ruptured abdominal aortic aneurysm and intestinal volvulus.

Abdominal Pain in Patients With HIV

HIV-positive patients with abdominal pain are at risk for unusual conditions related to their immunocompromised state and associated disease processes and side effects caused by the antiretroviral medications. In the HIV-positive patient with abdominal pain, the pain is attributable to the immunocompromised state or medications in 65% of cases (17); the three most common disorders are GI non-Hodgkin's lymphoma, pancreatitis, and cytomegalovirus (CMV) enterocolitis (17). CMV enterocolitis may be life-threatening as it can cause a toxic megacolon and colonic perforation. Drug-induced pancreatitis may be fulminant and has a mortality rate of approximately 10% (17). This complication is most often associated with didanosine but is also reported with the use of lamivudine (especially in children), zalcitabine, or stavudine (27) (see Chapter 147, Human Immunodeficiency Virus Infection and Related Disorders).

Women of Childbearing Age

Women of childbearing age presenting with abdominal pain are often among the most challenging patients. During early evaluation of these patients a pregnancy test is of utmost importance, as a positive result raises the possibility of ruptured ectopic pregnancy. The differential diagnosis of abdominal pain in this group is complicated by other possible genito-urinary and pelvic pathology (ovarian torsion, ovarian cysts, ruptured ovarian cyst, mittelschmerz, pelvic inflammatory disease, ectopic pregnancy), complicating the diagnostic work up and potentially leading to misdiagnosis. The difficulty in accurately diagnosing these patients is underscored by the fact that up to 33% of nonpregnant women of childbearing age with appendicitis are initially misdiagnosed (20).

In pregnant women, the gravid uterus becomes an intraabdominal organ later in pregnancy and may shift the anatomic location of other organs resulting in confusing presentations. By the second half of pregnancy the appendix has moved out of the right lower quadrant and into the right upper quadrant, so appendicitis may present with tenderness under the ribs or over the right flank. For more information on abdominal pain and pelvic pain in women of childbearing age see Chapter 88, Pelvic Pain.

Several other causes of abdominal pain deserve special mention.

Familial Mediterranean Fever

Familial Mediterranean fever (FMF) is a disease that is most common in non-Ashkenazi Jews, Turks, Armenians, and Middle Eastern Arabs, but generally not in other Mediterranean populations (13,22). It is characterized by bouts of abdominal pain with signs of peritonitis. Fever and pleuritis are very common, and arthritis and migratory skin lesions can also occur. It can mimic an acute abdomen and be accompanied by an elevated white cell count with a left shift and a high erythrocyte sedimentation rate. Episodes of the disease generally last 24 to 72 hours. The

diagnosis is usually made by the second decade of life, and very rarely after the age of 40. A family history cannot always be obtained, as the transmission is autosomal recessive. Diagnosis is clinical, although work on genetic markers may someday make a laboratory diagnosis possible (13). A diagnosis of FMF should never be definitively made in the ED. Patients with suspected FMF should be admitted and observed, given the possibility of misdiagnosis.

Porphyria

The porphyrias affect the biosynthesis of heme and result in the accumulation of excessive porphyrins and their precursors. They are inherited enzyme disorders, almost always autosomal dominant with poor penetrance. They are characterized by abdominal pain with or without manifestations of autonomic dysfunction or neuropsychiatric symptoms. Other presenting conditions in patients with porphyria include demyelinating syndromes, SIADH, hypertensive crisis, and acute psychosis. There are many variants depending on the particular enzyme deficiency and the heme precursor accumulated. The most common porphyria that causes abdominal pain is acute intermittent porphyria (7,24). Many drugs can precipitate attacks; potentially harmful drugs are listed in Table 7.3 (18).

The diagnosis is difficult, given the low prevalence. The pain of porphyria is usually out of proportion to physical signs, and fever is usually absent. A family history is helpful but not always present. Although not totally sensitive or specific, a Watson-Schwartz urine test should be ordered to look for porphobilinogen (7,24). The urine dipstick for urobilinogen yields a strong false-positive result. The diagnosis is made by a finding of elevated 24-hour levels of urine and stool porphyrins.

Abdominal Vasculitis

Abdominal vasculitis occurs in several disease processes, but polyarteritis nodosa, systemic lupus erythematosus, and Henoch-Schönlein purpura are probably the most common. The spectrum of presentation varies from acute severe ischemia to mild pain, malabsorption, and abdominal angina.

Patients with abdominal vasculitis may have peripheral manifestations of vasculitis as well. The abdominal pain may be epigastric or periumbilical, reflecting ischemia of the foregut or midgut, respectively. Fever is prominent in some cases. The key issue in these conditions is considering the diagnosis and then obtaining appropriate tests, such as angiography. Abdominal vasculitis should always be considered in patients with abdominal pain who also have a history of rheumatologic disease.

TABLE 7.3. Drugs That May Precipitate Attacks of Acute Porphyria

Barbiturates	Succinimides
Sulfonamide antibiotics	Carbamazepine
Meprobamate	Valproic acid
Glutethimide	Pyrazolones
Methyprylon	Griseofulvin
Ethchlorvynol	Ergots
Phenytoin	Danazol
Mephenytoin	Alcohol
Chlorpropamide	Estrogens and progestins

From *Cecil Textbook of Medicine*, 19th ed. Chap. 191, Philadelphia: WB Saunders, 1992.

Angioedema

Hereditary angioneurotic edema is transmitted as an autosomal dominant trait. Symptomatic patients have low levels of C1' esterase inhibitor (type 1), or they have a dysfunctional inhibitor (type 2); either condition allows activation of the complement system (3). Initial symptoms usually arise in adolescence but can have their onset in later life.

Classically, patients with angioedema do not have urticaria. Angioneurotic edema of the skin involves the deeper portions of the dermis and the subcutaneous layers, as well, and does not cause pruritus, whereas urticaria results from edema in the superficial layers of the skin and is pruritic.

Attacks of hereditary angioneurotic edema may begin with abdominal pain due to angioedema of the bowel wall. The pain is often colicky and is associated with nausea and vomiting, but there are scant physical findings in the abdomen. Fever is usually absent, and white blood cell counts are normal. During an attack, serum levels of C2 and C4 are low. Between attacks, the diagnosis can be established by assaying for the presence of the C1' esterase inhibitor. Attacks of angioedema are self-limited but generally last 24 to 72 hours.

Use of angiotensin-converting enzyme inhibitors (ACE inhibitors) has also been associated with angioedema of the small bowel. Strong consideration should be given to withholding ACE inhibitors in patients with persistent, unexplained abdominal pain. See Chapter 132, Angioedema.

Intestinal Pseudoobstruction

Intestinal pseudoobstructions are a group of diseases that present as bouts of recurrent abdominal distention, obstipation, and, on occasion, colicky abdominal pain. The presentation can be identical to that of small bowel mechanical obstruction. Pseudoobstruction can be caused by a primary disorder of the myenteric plexus or the smooth muscle itself, or may be secondary to a host of systemic diseases. The diagnosis is made by ruling out other causes of abdominal pain and motility disorders, including adult Hirschsprung disease and mechanical obstruction. The differential diagnosis also includes toxic megacolon, typhlitis, and idiopathic colonic dilation of the elderly (Ogilvie syndrome). Definitive diagnosis requires manometric and electrophysiologic testing, as well as biopsy.

Sickle Cell Disease

Patients with sickle cell disease and vasoocclusive painful crisis can present with pain almost anywhere in the body, including the abdomen. What is not commonly appreciated is that a few patients with homozygous sickle cell disease have their first painful crisis in their late teens or early 20s, frequently presenting with cryptogenic abdominal pain. Patients with established sickle cell disease can also pose a diagnostic challenge because their abdominal pain can be caused by a vasoocclusive event involving any of the abdominal viscera or the abdominal wall.

In addition, almost all patients with sickle cell disease have gallstones; acute cholecystitis, common duct obstruction, and ascending cholangitis are ever-present dangers in these immunocompromised patients. Abdominal pain also can develop for reasons unrelated to sickle cell disease, but the primary process may be misdiagnosed as crisis pain.

The laboratory evaluation of sickle cell patients with abdominal pain is often misleading. Many vasoocclusive crises are not associated with fever, and the white blood cell count is typically chronically elevated in these patients, commonly with a left shift. In addition, many sickle cell disease patients are icteric because of chronic hemolysis. Many have intrinsic liver disease as well, but liver function test abnormalities are not helpful unless there is a significant deviation from baseline values. For patients presenting with right upper quadrant pain, diagnosis can be assisted by the use of abdominal ultrasonography, nuclear scans of the biliary system, or abdominal CT scanning. See Chapter 154, Sickle Cell Disease.

Chronic Lead Intoxication

Chronic lead intoxication can present as a painful abdominal crisis (lead colic). Abdominal pain can be slowly progressive or subacute in onset. There is abdominal tenderness with voluntary guarding, but true peritoneal findings are rare. Patients commonly complain of fatigue, weakness, musculoskeletal pains, irritability, and constipation. Hemolytic anemia is usually evident, and the red blood cells show basophilic stippling. An occasional patient may have the triad of lead nephropathy, "saturnine" gout, and hypertension. The diagnosis is made by determining blood lead and erythrocyte protoporphyrin levels. See Chapter 314, Lead Poisoning.

Addison's Disease

Addison's disease can present as a dramatic acute syndrome with vasomotor collapse, altered mental status, and characteristic electrolyte abnormalities. A subacute-to-chronic form of the disease, however, can present with recurrent abdominal pain, often associated with nausea and vomiting and usually with a negative abdominal examination.

The most common cause of primary adrenal insufficiency is idiopathic or autoimmune destruction of the gland. Patients with AIDS have a high incidence of adrenal gland involvement from a number of mechanisms. Other presenting complaints include salt craving, anorexia, weight loss, and generalized weakness. Characteristic physical findings include orthostatic hypotension, freckling and hyperpigmentation of the skin, and surgical scars. Classic laboratory findings include hyperkalemia, hyponatremia, mild azotemia, mild metabolic acidosis, and hypoglycemia. See Chapter 164, Adrenal and Pituitary Disorders.

Narcotic Withdrawal

Narcotic withdrawal frequently produces crampy abdominal pain, often associated with nausea, vomiting, and diarrhea. Diagnosis of this syndrome is frequently difficult unless the patient admits to narcotic addiction. Other signs and symptoms of narcotic withdrawal (e.g., mydriasis, rhinorrhea, piloerection) may be present, but these features are rarely prominent.

Psychogenic Abdominal Pain

Psychogenic abdominal pain involves a diverse group of psychiatric disturbances, including somatoform disorders, eating disorders, conversion reactions, depression, and hypochondriacal neurosis. Abdominal pain can also occur as a somatic delusion or as a hallucinatory phenomenon, but it generally is found in association with bizarre symptoms and evidence of underlying thought disorder. Women represent a disproportionately large percentage of patients with psychogenic abdominal pain in several studies. Early psychiatric consultation is important, but it must be kept in mind that psychogenic abdominal pain must always remain, to some degree, a diagnosis of exclusion.

DIAGNOSTIC APPROACH

Appropriate labs and imaging tests should be ordered in the context of the history and physical examination.

Laboratory Testing

Women of childbearing age should have a pregnancy test; sensitive and rapid bedside urine pregnancy tests can be used. A positive pregnancy test in a patient with abdominal pain should raise the concern for an ectopic pregnancy.

A complete blood count, although frequently ordered, should be interpreted with caution. A normal white blood cell count should not be used to rule out appendicitis. Studies have shown that the white blood cell count is often normal early in the course of the disease; even checking serial white blood cell counts may not aid in making the diagnosis (16). Although low hemoglobin suggests occult blood loss, it may be normal initially in rapid, acute blood loss.

The urinalysis should also be interpreted with caution. Any process adjacent to the ureters that is inflammatory (such as appendicitis) can cause a positive urinalysis in the absence of a urinary tract infection. Twenty to thirty percent of patients with appendicitis present with blood, leukocytes, or bacteria in the urine (2,23). Hematuria may be due to a urinary tract infection, nephrolithiasis, trauma, tumor or ruptured abdominal aortic aneurysm. Hematuria in patients with an abdominal aortic aneurysm may be misleading and can delay the diagnosis while a urinary work up is performed (1). Therefore, a patient with risk factors for abdominal aortic aneurysm who presents with flank or abdominal pain and hematuria should undergo a work up for the aneurysm as well as a work up of the urinary tract. If there is concern that the patient may become hemodynamically unstable, a rapid bedside ultrasound should be performed to assess for the aneurysm. If there is little concern that the patient may become unstable, then abdominal computed tomography can assess for both conditions.

The measurement of serum electrolytes (sodium, potassium, chloride, bicarbonate, blood urea nitrogen and creatinine) is helpful in determining hydration status, in guiding volume replacement, and in diagnosing metabolic disturbances. The creatinine is necessary to determine renal function and whether a patient can receive intravenous contrast for imaging. Assessing the blood glucose may help diagnose new onset or poorly controlled diabetes. Diabetic ketoacidosis can present with abdominal pain and nausea and vomiting.

A lipase should be ordered when pancreatitis is suspected. Lipase is a more sensitive and specific indicator of pancreatitis than amylase, and an elevation of three times the normal value of the lipase is suggestive of pancreatic inflammation. Less sensitive and specific than lipase, amylase levels may be elevated in many disease processes including peptic ulcer disease, small bowel obstruction or ischemia, common duct stone, ectopic pregnancy, renal failure, alcohol intoxication, or facial trauma (salivary amylase).

Serum transaminases, bilirubin, alkaline phosphatase, and coagulation studies are useful in certain patients with a tender right upper quadrant or symptoms suggestive of biliary or liver disease. However, these studies may not be abnormal in patients with biliary colic or cholecystitis. Thus, if biliary colic or cholecystitis is suspected, an ultrasound should be performed to make the diagnosis.

Other studies may be useful when specific diagnoses are considered. For instance, the serum lactate is elevated in patients with mesenteric ischemia.

Radiographic Studies

Plain films are primarily useful when certain disease processes are suspected: obstruction, perforation and foreign body. The acute abdominal series includes supine and upright views of the abdomen and a single upright chest view. Of these three views, the upright chest x-ray is the single most useful view to assess for free air, although free air may be absent on plain films in one-third to one-half of patients with visceral perforation (4). Diagnostic accuracy may be improved by inserting 500 cc of air down a nasogastric tube prior to obtaining radiographs. The chest x-ray can also help to diagnose pneumonia, pleural effusion or other pulmonary causes of abdominal pain. If the patient is unable to stand upright, a left lateral decubitus film can be obtained to look for air fluid levels and free air. The kidney, ureter, and bladder film (KUB) in combination with ultrasound may be helpful in evaluating urinary stone disease. The finding of hydronephrosis or calcification over the ureters is almost as sensitive and specific as intravenous pyelogram (IVP) (9). This approach is still inferior to the sensitivity of helical computed tomography (CT).

Ultrasound images intraabdominal organs such as the liver, spleen, pancreas, gallbladder, kidneys, uterus and ovaries. It is the imaging modality of choice in the patient with right upper quadrant pain or presumed pelvic pathology. Other conditions that ultrasound can detect include aortic aneurysm, pancreatic pseudocyst, and ureteral obstruction. Transvaginal ultrasound can help determine intrauterine versus ectopic pregnancy. Appendicitis can be diagnosed with good accuracy in the hands of an experienced ultrasonographer, although CT is the modality of choice in making this diagnosis unless radiation is a concern (e.g., in a pregnant woman). In many hospitals emergency physicians perform goal-oriented ultrasonography in an attempt to reduce time to diagnosis and improve patient care for patients with abdominal pain. Emergency physicians can accurately diagnose cholelithiasis (11), as well as ruptured ectopic pregnancy, abdominal aortic aneurysm, and hydronephrosis as an indicator of ureteral colic (6).

Computed tomography is useful in the diagnosis of many diseases presenting with abdominal pain. Helical CT can identify kidney stones, abdominal aortic aneurysm, appendicitis, diverticulitis, splenic or liver lacerations or infarctions, intraabdominal abscesses and free air. Most patients require intravenous and oral contrast for detecting appendicitis, diverticulitis, mesenteric ischemia, and intraabdominal abscess. Some institutions use rectal contrast as a rapid method of detecting appendicitis and diverticulitis. In patients with suspected abdominal aortic aneurysm, CT without oral or intravenous contrast should be performed, as it is a fast, accurate method of identifying the pathology. Such patients can be transported to the radiology suite without waiting for the creatinine to return or oral contrast to be administered. In addition, CT to diagnose ureteral stone does not require contrast administration. CT is now considered the imaging procedure of choice for patients with suspected mesenteric ischemia (12). Although angiography remains the gold standard for diagnosing thromboembolism, it is an invasive, time-consuming, potentially nephrotoxic and costly procedure and should be performed only when acute mesenteric ischemia cannot be established by noninvasive modalities (12).

Patients presenting with epigastric pain and a nontender abdomen who are over the age of 50 or have cardiac risk factors should have an electrocardiogram. In addition, unstable patients and the elderly should have an electrocardiogram as part of their work up for abdominal pain. Relief of pain after "GI cocktail" does not preclude myocardial ischemia and should not be used to rule out cardiac disease.

CRITICAL INTERVENTIONS

In patients presenting with acute abdominal pain the major goals are to stabilize the patient, replenish volume loss, transfuse if necessary, treat the pain, control emesis and administer antibiotics when indicated. In patients with a condition requiring urgent surgical evaluation (appendicitis, ruptured viscous, bowel obstruction, diverticulitis, mesenteric ischemia, abdominal aortic aneurysm, gallbladder disease) appropriate surgical consultation should be obtained early. If ruptured ectopic pregnancy is suspected, an emergent gynecology consultation should be obtained.

In the hemodynamically unstable patient, life-threatening conditions should be rapidly ruled out; these include ruptured abdominal aortic aneurysm, myocardial infarction, ruptured ectopic pregnancy, adrenal insufficiency, perforated viscous, and sepsis. Immediate resuscitation should start with the airway, breathing and circulation first. This includes supplemental oxygen, intravenous access with two large bore IVs and continuous cardiac monitoring. Volume resuscitation should begin with crystalloid infusion and then packed red blood cell transfusion when bleeding is suspected. If the patient remains hypotensive, vasopressors may be necessary. In the hypotensive patient who does not respond to volume replacement, acute adrenal crisis may be the cause. If adrenal insufficiency is suspected a stress dose of intravenous steroids (hydrocortisone 100 mg or dexamethasone 10 mg) should be administered; dexamethasone may be preferable as using it will not interfere with diagnostic testing for adrenal insufficiency.

Medications are indicated to treat pain and nausea and vomiting. Traditionally, pain medication was withheld from patients with undifferentiated abdominal pain for fear of masking physical exam findings and hindering diagnosis. Although some controversy remains surrounding this issue, multiple studies have shown that treating undifferentiated abdominal pain with judicious amounts of narcotic analgesia does not affect diagnostic accuracy (26). Morphine in 2- to 5-mg increments or fentanyl in 50- to 100-μg increments can be titrated to the desired effect. When infections are a consideration, appropriate antibiotics should be initiated in a timely fashion. If sepsis from an undifferentiated abdominal source is a concern then broad-spectrum antibiotics should be started, covering gram-positive, gram-negative, and anaerobic bacteria.

Patients with familial Mediterranean fever can be treated with oral colchicine 0.6 mg q1h for three doses, and then 0.6 mg q2h for an additional dose. Intravenous colchicine is not recommended unless the patient is unable to tolerate oral medications. Long-term prophylactic treatment with colchicine reduces the rate of recurrence and also helps prevent amyloidosis, the long-term complication of FMF. Opiates can be used to treat the pain. Patients should be admitted for observation, and surgical consultation obtained.

Management of porphyria is largely supportive. Intravenous glucose infusion may abort attacks. Intravenous hematin also may be helpful, although studies have not been large enough to prove its efficacy (10).

In patients with angioedema, because the upper airway can be involved acutely, a major clinical concern is sudden upper airway obstruction requiring epinephrine administration, intubation, or cricothyrotomy. Management is otherwise supportive.

DISPOSITION

Patients with surgical or gynecologic disease should be evaluated by a surgeon or gynecologist and may require admission for treatment and operative intervention. The more challenging dispositions arise in patients with abdominal pain of unclear etiology. If possible it is prudent to observe these patients for 6 to 12 hours before discharge, particularly if they are elderly. Observation may be helpful in differentiating surgical from nonsurgical disease. Patients with abdominal pain of uncertain cause

that improves while in the emergency department can be discharged to home with close follow up. In these patients the most accurate and appropriate discharge diagnosis is abdominal pain of unclear etiology; it is important to resist labeling these patients with a more specific and sometimes speculative diagnosis.

COMMON PITFALLS

✔ Failure to obtain a thorough and accurate history and physical examination
✔ Failure to diagnose an abdominal aortic aneurysm in patients who present with flank pain and hematuria
✔ Failure to order a pregnancy test in all women of childbearing age to rule out the possibility of ectopic pregnancy
✔ Relying on a normal white blood cell count to rule out the diagnosis of appendicitis or other infectious causes of abdominal pain, particularly in the elderly
✔ Failure to recognize that the urinalysis may be abnormal in patients with processes that inflame the ureters, such as appendicitis or salpingitis

Acknowledgments

Thanks to the authors from the previous edition's Chapters 34 and 161.

References

1. Acheson AG, Graham AN, Weir C, et al. Prospective study on factors delaying surgery in ruptured abdominal aortic aneurysms. *J Royal Coll Surg Edinburgh* 1998;43:183–184.
2. Arnbjornsson E. Bacteriuria in appendicitis. *Am J Surg* 1988;155:356–358.
3. Borum ML, Howard DE. Hereditary angioedema. Complex symptoms can make diagnosis difficult. *Postgrad Med* 1998;104:251, 255–256.
4. Campbell JP, Gunn AA. Plain abdominal radiographs and acute abdominal pain. *Br J Surg* 1988;75:554–556.
5. Colucciello SA, Lukens TW, Morgan DL. Assessing abdominal pain in adults: a rational, cost-effective, and evidence-based strategy. *Emerg Med Pract* 1999;1(1):1–20.
6. Durham B. Emergency medicine physicians saving time with ultrasound. *Am J Em Med* 1996;14:309–313.
7. Elder GH, Hill RJ, Meissner PN. The acute porphyries. *Lancet* 1997;349:1613–1617.
8. Gallegos NC, Hobsley M. Abdominal wall pain, an alternative diagnosis. *Br J Surg* 1990;77:1167–1170.
9. Gorelick U, Ulish Y, Yagil Y. The use of standard imaging techniques and their diagnostic value in the workup of renal colic in the setting of intractable flank pain. *Urology* 1996;47:637–642.
10. Herrick AL, McColl KEL, Moore MR, et al. Controlled trial of haem arginate in acute hepatic porphyria. *Lancet* 1989;i:1295–1297.
11. Kendall JL, Shimp RJ. Performance and interpretation of focused right upper quadrant ultrasound by emergency physicians. *J Em Med;* 21(1):7–13.
12. Kim AY, Ha HK. Evaluation of suspected mesenteric ischemia: efficacy of radiologic studies. *Radiol Clin North Am* 2003;41:327–342.
13. Koopman WJ. Arthritis and allied conditions, 13th ed. Baltimore: Williams & Wilkins, 1997:1280–1287.
14. Kresovich-Wendler K, Levitt MA, Do, Yearly L. An evaluation of clinical predictors to determine the need for rectal temperature measurement in the emergency department. *Am J Emerg Med* 1989;7:391–394.
15. Liddington MI, Thompson WH. Rebound Tenderness Test. *Br J Surg* 1991; 78(7):795–796.
16. Lyons D, Waldron R, Ryan T, et al. An evaluation of the clinical value of the leucocyte count and sequential counts in suspected acute appendicitis. *Br J Clin Pract* 1987;41:794–796.
17. Parente F, Cernushi M, Antinoti S, et al. Severe abdominal pain in patients with AIDS: frequency, clinical aspects, causes and outcome. *Scand J Gastroenterol* 1994;29:511–515.
18. Powers RD, Guertler AT. Abdominal pain in the ED: stability and change over 20 years. *Am J Em Med* 1995;13:301–303.
19. Reynolds SL, Jaffee DM. Diagnosing abdominal pain in a pediatric emergency department. *Pediatr Emerg Care* 1992;8(3):126.
20. Rothrock SG, Green SM, Dobson M, et al. Misdiagnosis of appendicitis in nonpregnant women of childbearing age. *J Em Med* 1995;13:1–8.
21. Rusnack RA, Borer JM, Fastow JS. Misdiagnosis of acute appendicitis: common features discovered in cases after litigation. *Am J Emerg Med* 1994;12:397–402.

22. Samuels J, Aksentijevich I, et al. Familial Mediterranean Fever in the millennium. Clinical spectrum, ancient mutations, and a survey of 100 American referrals to the national Institutes of Health. *Medicine* 1998;77:268–297.

23. Scott JH 3rd, Amin M, Harty JI. Abnormal urinalysis in appendicitis. *J Urol* 1983;129:1015.

24. Tefferi A, Colgan JP, Solberg LA. Acute porphyries: diagnosis and management. *May Clin Proc* 1994;69:991–995.

25. Telfer S, Fenyo G, Holt PR, de Dombal FT. Acute abdominal pain in patients over 50 years of age. *Scand J Gastroenterol* 1988;23(suppl 144):47–50.

26. Thomas SH, Silen W, Cheema F, et al. Effect of morphine analgesia on diagnostic accuracy in emergency department patients with abdominal pain: a prospective randomized trial. *J Am Coll Surg* 2003;196:18–31.

27. Yarchoan R, Broder S. Treatment of HIV infection and AIDS. In: Goldman L, Bennet JC. *Cecil Textbook of Medicine*. Philadelphia: W.B. Saunders Company, 2000;1936.

CHAPTER 8
Shortness of Breath

C. Keith Stone

Shortness of breath refers to difficult, labored, or uncomfortable breathing. It is a symptom of many disorders that involve alterations or abnormalities in gas exchange, pulmonary circulation, respiratory mechanics, O_2-carrying capacity of the blood, or cardiovascular function. Shortness of breath results when ventilatory demand exceeds respiratory function. A mismatch between supply and demand of oxygen and failure of CO_2 elimination is the mechanism that produces the sensation of shortness of breath.

An individual with normal breathing capacity may require a large increase in ventilatory demand before shortness of breath is produced. Conversely, in a person with a preexisting diminished respiratory capacity, a small increase in ventilatory demand may produce significant shortness of breath. Because the perception of shortness of breath is also mediated by psychological and cultural factors (6), it may be helpful to assess breathing difficulty in terms of diminished ability to perform specific daily functions such as housework or climbing stairs.

The pathophysiology of shortness of breath is complex. However, an understanding of the basic principles behind respiration is necessary to understand the cause and treatment of shortness of breath in any given disorder. Chemoreceptors in the blood and brain, as well as mechanoreceptors in the airways, lungs, and chest wall, are involved in the automatic regulation of the depth and pattern of breathing (6). The carotid and aortic bodies and central chemoreceptors in the medulla sense changes in the partial pressure of oxygen (PO_2), partial pressure of carbon dioxide (PCO_2), and pH of the blood and transmit signals back to brainstem respiratory centers that adjust breathing to maintain blood–gas and acid–base homeostasis (6). In most individuals, the most profound stimulus to the central nervous system respiratory control center is normally the arterial carbon dioxide tension (PCO_2). An increase in PCO_2 of 1.5 mm Hg from the normal level of 40 mm Hg may produce a doubling of ventilation. Arterial oxygen tension and pH are other factors that significantly influence ventilation. In the patient with chronic obstructive pulmonary disease (COPD) and hypercarbia, the arterial oxygen tension may be the most influential factor affecting respiratory drive.

Afferent impulses from vagal receptors in the airways and lungs also exert important influences on the depth and pattern of breathing. Feedback of afferent information from lung and chest wall mechanoreceptors provides respiratory motor and premotor neurons with important information regarding the mechanical status of the ventilatory pump, as well as changes in length and force of contraction of the respiratory muscles (6). Elastic resistance of the lung to stretch, airway flow resistance, and tissue friction must be overcome for breathing to proceed. Elastic resistance is the most significant of these factors at normal respiratory rates. At rates faster than 15 breaths per minute, airway resistance becomes more important.

Shortness of breath may result from respiratory, cardiovascular, hematologic, neuromuscular, metabolic, or psychogenic disorders. Table 8.1 details the most frequently encountered causes and the most common etiologies of acute shortness of breath seen in the emergency department (ED). Most commonly, cardiovascular and respiratory disorders are the cause, with the degree of derangement proportional to the resultant shortness of breath.

TABLE 8.1.   Causes of Acute Shortness of Breath

UPPER AIRWAY OBSTRUCTION

Angioedema
Epiglottitis
Foreign body
Vocal cord paralysis/spasm

CARDIOVASCULAR

Congestive heart failure
Pulmonary edema
Cardiac tamponade
Acute coronary ischemia
Cardiac dysrhythmias
Pulmonary embolus

PULMONARY

Aspiration
Asthma
COPD exacerbation
Pneumonia
Pneumothorax
Pleural effusion
Adult respiratory distress syndrome
Toxic inhalation

NEUROMUSCULAR

Guillain-Barré syndrome
Myasthenia gravis

METABOLIC/SYSTEMIC

Anaphylaxis
Anemia
Hyperthyroidism
Sepsis
Acidosis
Salicylate intoxication
Obesity

PSYCHOGENIC

Hyperventilation syndrome

CLINICAL PRESENTATION

Patients commonly present to the ED complaining of shortness of breath. Depending on their preexisting respiratory problems, they may appear comfortable or may exhibit varying degrees of respiratory distress. Once the initial assessment assures that the airway is patent and oxygenation is adequate, a thorough history should be obtained.

Pertinent questions in the history can provide valuable information and diagnostic clues to the cause of the shortness of breath. The duration and onset of the sensation of shortness of breath; associated chest pain or palpitations; precipitating factors such as exertion, exercise, or anxiety; associated paresthesias of the mouth and fingers; the number of pillows the patient uses to sleep; concomitant coughing or sputum production; exercise tolerance; tobacco use; recreational drug use; and occupational history are several important factors that can help narrow the differential diagnosis (24). Past medical history of asthma, COPD, congestive heart failure, coronary artery disease and valvular heart problems should be sought. Trepopnea, the presence of shortness of breath in one lateral position but not the other, may be the result of unilateral lung disease, unilateral pleural effusion, or, occasionally, COPD. Paroxysmal nocturnal dyspnea (PND), breathlessness that occurs while sleeping, is usually associated with left ventricular failure. Orthopnea, the presence of shortness of breath in the recumbent position, is also associated with left ventricular failure, but can be associated with COPD.

Although, in most patients, the degree of shortness of breath may be readily apparent to the examiner, certain populations are not able to relay a history. The very young, the elderly, and those with diminished mental capacity may present only with tachypnea or an altered level of consciousness. In these patients, it is important to keep respiratory difficulty in the differential diagnosis. On physical examination, the patient's vital signs, mental status, body position, use of accessory muscles, conjunctival and mucous membrane color, skin and nailbed color, upper airway examination, neurologic examination, cardiovascular and pulmonary examinations may give valuable clues to the etiology. Problems with oxygenation may be easily revealed by pulse oximetry, and difficulty with CO_2 elimination may be revealed by arterial blood gas determination in the patient who is unable to relay an adequate history.

DIFFERENTIAL DIAGNOSIS

Upper Airway Obstruction

Obstruction of the upper airway may be the consequence of a diverse group of entities, including foreign-body aspiration, epiglottitis, croup, angioedema, peritonsillar or retropharyngeal abscess, or neuromuscular dysfunction. The nature of the presenting picture depends on the site and degree of the obstruction, as well as the underlying cause. Cough, stridor, shortness of breath, aphonia, or hoarseness may be present. Although many of these conditions do not usually cause complete airway obstruction, rapid deterioration is possible in these patients, and the emergency physician must be ready to provide immediate airway intervention. Alternative techniques to conventional direct laryngoscopy may be necessary to include blind nasotracheal intubation, lighted or optical stylets, flexible or rigid fiberoptic scopes, retrograde intubation and surgical airways (26).

Epiglottitis is an important life-threatening cause of respiratory distress due to upper airway obstruction. However, it is seen significantly less frequently with the use of the HiB vaccine; the incidence in children less than 5 years old has decreased from 41 cases per 10,000 children in 1987 to 1.3 cases per 10,000 in 1997 (28). The onset is characteristically abrupt, with a mild upper respiratory infection progressing within hours to high fever, lethargy, and difficulty in swallowing oral secretions or drooling. Respiratory distress and stridor are the most consistent signs. Restlessness, anxiety, and tachycardia are also often present.

In adults, the presentation of epiglottitis is typically less dramatic, and the shortness of breath may be minimal or absent. Fever and sore throat are the most common complaints. Consequently, the diagnosis is often delayed in adults.

Pneumothorax

Pneumothorax, or air in the pleural cavity, can occur spontaneously or as the result of trauma. Normally, the visceral and parietal pleura are in close apposition, but when the potential space between the two is occupied by gas, the lung can no longer fully expand. Depending on the amount of air within the pleural space, respiratory compromise can result. Spontaneous pneumothorax typically occurs in tall, thin, young males and smoking increases the likelihood (13). The cause of the pneumothorax is the rupture of a subpleural bleb, which is usually apical in location. Spontaneous pneumothorax also may be seen in patients with asthma, COPD, and tuberculosis and in AIDS patients with *Pneumocystis carinii* pneumonia (PCP). Traumatic pneumothorax results from blunt or penetrating trauma to the chest. Hemothorax, pulmonary contusion, and bronchial rupture are injuries that may accompany the pneumothorax (33).

Patients may present to the ED in obvious respiratory distress or may complain of shortness of breath and pleuritic chest pain. Auscultation may reveal unilateral diminution of the breath sounds associated with increased tympany on percussion. Subcutaneous emphysema also may be present. Signs of imminent cardiovascular collapse such as hypotension, mediastinal shift and the aforementioned findings may herald a tension pneumothorax, prompting swift needle chest decompression prior to any further examination or diagnostic studies. One of the earliest signs of tension pneumothorax is hypoxia. Chest radiography may reveal an obvious pneumothorax or may only show subtle findings. In the supine patient, the only sign of a pneumothorax may be an abnormally prominent costophrenic angle on the AP or PA view. A spontaneous pneumomediastinum also may present as shortness of breath or chest pain. It is a benign entity that responds to conservative treatment of bed rest, oxygen, and analgesics (15).

Congestive Heart Failure

Congestive heart failure (CHF) is a clinical condition that develops when cardiac output becomes insufficient to meet systemic metabolic tissue demands at normal ventricular-filling pressures (2). Acute failure of the left ventricle to eject a normal quantity of blood may cause fluid to accumulate in the pulmonary interstitium, alveoli, and bronchioles, thereby producing pulmonary edema. In addition to interfering with gas exchange, transudation of fluid into the perialveolar spaces reduces pulmonary compliance. In response, the body attempts to use compensatory mechanisms to maintain adequate perfusion of tissues. These include release of neurohumoral factors (endothelin-1, tumor necrosis factor α, interleukin-6 and natriuretic peptides) (23), stimulation of the sympathetic nervous system, activation of the renin-angiotensin-aldosterone system and local vasoregulation (2). These compensatory mechanisms are initially beneficial but eventually have a detrimental effect on left ventricular remodeling and an increase in myocardial oxygen demand which ultimately results in further worsening of cardiac function (2). Acute precipitating factors of CHF include increased sodium intake, noncompliance with medications, acute myocardial infarction (MI), dysrhythmia or anemia. The most common causes of CHF are coronary artery disease and hypertension, valvular heart disease and cardiomyopathy.

Pertinent information obtained on history includes the presence of orthopnea or PND relieved by standing or walking, peripheral edema, and fatigue. The physical examination may reveal jugular venous distention (JVD), rales, cardiac S3 gallop, and peripheral edema (30). Pulmonary edema may also lead to bronchospasm and wheezing, often termed "cardiac asthma." Chest radiography may reveal cardiomegaly, pulmonary vascular redistribution, Kerley B lines, pleural effusion, and peribronchial cuffing. The measurement of b-type natriuretic peptide (BNP) has become a useful tool in the diagnosis of CHF. BNP is synthesized as preproBNP in the cardiac ventricles and is released as a result of left ventricular wall stress (23).

Other cardiac causes of shortness of breath include valve rupture and papillary muscle ischemia. An uncommon but quickly fatal cardiac cause of shortness of breath is ventricular septal rupture post-MI. This generally occurs within the first week after infarction (9). Although rare, prompt diagnosis is crucial if potential life-saving measures, such as surgery, are to be employed (34).

Chronic Obstructive Pulmonary Disease

The American Thoracic Society defines COPD as a disease state characterized by the presence of airflow obstruction due to chronic bronchitis or emphysema (5). The airflow obstruction is often continuous and progressive and, in contrast to asthma, the shortness of breath is usually always present. Chronic bronchitis is defined as the presence of a chronic, productive cough for 3 months in each of 2 successive years in which other causes of chronic cough have been eliminated (5). Emphysema is defined as abnormal permanent enlargement of the air spaces distal to the terminal bronchioles, accompanied by destruction of bronchiolar walls but without obvious fibrosis (5). Although COPD is a chronic disorder, acute exacerbations of diminished respiratory function often bring patients to the ED.

COPD exacerbations are usually caused by a worsening of airflow obstruction due to increased bronchospasm, increased sputum production from superimposed respiratory infection, environmental irritants (such as tobacco smoke), or cardiovascular deterioration. The patient may present with progressive shortness of breath, increased sputum production, and audible wheezing. Hypoxemia, tachypnea, cyanosis, and agitation may be seen. Signs of hypercarbia such as confusion, stupor, inadequate respiratory effort or apnea, may be seen and indicate severe compromise with impaired gas exchange (5). These patients attempt to improve ventilation by sitting forward, using pursed-lip exhalation and accessory muscles of respiration in order to overcome the increase in airflow resistance that accompanies bronchoconstriction and dynamic airway collapse (22). Auscultation may reveal a combination of diminished breath sounds, a prolonged expiratory phase, wheezes or rales. The chest radiograph may reveal an increased anterior–posterior diameter, flattened diaphragms, hyperinflated lungs, attenuation of the peripheral lung markings, and, in cases of superimposed infection, an infiltrate.

Asthma

Asthma is a chronic inflammatory disease, clinically characterized by recurrent episodes of wheezing, chest tightness and discomfort, shortness of breath, and cough. Exacerbation is characterized by an early phase, which chiefly consists of bronchospasm, edema, and obstruction; and a late phase, which is caused primarily by the inflammatory response. Triggers cause mast cell degranulation and release of inflammatory mediators leading to mucosal edema, bronchial smooth muscle contraction, mucous production and impaired mucociliary transport (1). Duration of symptoms for greater than 24 hours suggests a greater component of inflammation in the absence of any evidence of infection.

Patients with an asthma exacerbation present to the ED with the complaints of shortness of breath, wheezing, and cough (1). The physical examination may reveal an increased AP diameter of the chest due to air trapping, tachypnea, wheezing and mild-to-severe respiratory distress. Auscultation may be misleading in the case of severe obstruction; wheezing may be absent, as bronchial airflow is diminished to such an extent that no sound is audible. Chest radiographs may be normal, reveal signs of airway obstruction (such as in COPD), demonstrate a pneumothorax, pneumomediastinum or, in the case of a precipitating infection, reveal an infiltrate.

Pulmonary Embolism

Pulmonary embolism (PE) is an obstruction of the pulmonary artery or one of its branches by an embolus, usually a blood clot derived from the deep venous system of the leg or pelvic veins. The diagnosis of PE is often subtle and may be difficult to make. Estimates are that the diagnosis is missed more than 400,000 times each year (29).

The most common symptoms in a patient with PE are shortness of breath and chest pain, although dizziness, syncope, and cough are also frequent complaints (32). Frequent clinical signs of PE include tachypnea and tachycardia. Although embolism may present as pulmonary infarction, with the acute onset of pleuritic pain, hemoptysis, and an audible pleural friction rub, such a presentation is uncommon. PE may also mimic other entities. Associated fever and cough may suggest pneumonia, while associated rib tenderness or pleuritic chest pain may suggest a musculoskeletal etiology.

Clinical suspicion plays a key role in the decision to pursue an evaluation for acute PE. Patients at high risk include those who have had a previous PE or DVT, recent surgery or immobilization; those with a malignancy or cardiopulmonary disease; those with lower extremity or pelvic trauma; and women during pregnancy or in the postpartum period (29). PE rule out protocols stratify patients into a low risk category based on low pretest probability assessment along with a negative d-dimer assay. Protocols based on a negative d-dimer assay plus a normal alveolar dead space have also been proposed to preclude the use of ventilation-perfusion scans or spiral CT on all patients (19). Laboratory analysis may include an arterial blood gas, which may reflect hypoxemia or hypocarbia. The arterial–alveolar (A-a) oxygen gradient is generally increased but has been shown to be an inadequate screening test due to the low sensitivity and specificity (18). A ventilation–perfusion scan, spiral computed tomography scan, and pulmonary angiogram, used in conjunction with the clinical pretest probability, d-dimer assay and duplex Doppler evaluation of the lower extremities, will help the physician determine the likelihood of the presence of PE and the necessity of anticoagulation and admission.

Pneumonia

Pneumonia classically presents as an acute febrile illness with cough and purulent sputum production. Shortness of breath results from alveolar obstruction secondary to sputum production, bronchiole obstruction due to mucous plugging, increased work of breathing, and hypoxia.

Pneumonia should be suspected in patients with newly acquired lower respiratory symptoms (cough, sputum production, or shortness of breath), especially if these symptoms are accompanied by fever, altered breath sounds, and rales (7). *Streptococcus pneumoniae* remains the most common etiology of community-acquired pneumonia, even in the immunocompromised host (7). Patients with atypical pneumonia caused by *Mycoplasma pneumoniae, Legionella pneumophila, Chlamydia psittaci* and *Bordetella pertussis* may present with an insidious or subacute onset, moderate fever, and less purulent sputum. Headache, nonproductive cough, myalgias, arthralgias, and malaise may predominate (7). Immunosuppressed patients may present with staphylococcal pneumonia or pneumonia caused by opportunists such as *Pneumocystis carinii*, mycobacteria, or fungal organisms.

The physical examination in pneumonia may reveal rales, egophony, vocal resonance, increased vocal fremitus or bronchial breath sounds. A chest radiograph may demonstrate lobar consolidation, as in bacterial pneumonia; patchy infiltrates, suggesting staphylococcal pneumonia, *Haemophilus influenzae,* or gram-negative pneumonia; interstitial infiltrates, suggesting *Mycoplasma, Legionella,* or *Pneumocystis;* or cavitary lesions, as in tuberculosis (12) or, as seen in up to 30% of *Pneumocystis carinii* pneumonia (PCP), it may be entirely normal (7). In community-acquired pneumonia, the utility of sputum gram stain and culture and blood cultures are low and should only be obtained in the ED if the patient is going to be hospitalized (3). Early recognition is important, so that appropriate empiric antibiotic treatment may be selected and administered promptly.

Anaphylaxis

Anaphylaxis is a severe allergic reaction involving one or more body systems that produces symptoms such as hives, flushing, pruritis, angioedema, stridor, shortness of breath, bronchospasm, tachycardia, and hypotension. Death from anaphylaxis usually results from respiratory obstruction or cardiovascular collapse. Symptoms typically occur within minutes of exposure to the triggering antigen but occasionally may occur as late as one hour (14) (see Chapter 131, Anaphylaxis).

Psychogenic Causes

Shortness of breath can also occur as a somatic manifestation of psychiatric disorders, such as anxiety disorder, with resultant hyperventilation (24). Patients with hyperventilation syndrome are often seen in the ED. Tachypnea and anxiety are the predominant findings. The patient may complain of paresthesias around the mouth and the fingers. Carpopedal spasm also may be present. The patient may give a history of obtaining relief of shortness of breath with exertion, which is not a typical feature of organic disorders producing difficulty breathing. The presence of respiratory alkalosis without hypoxemia on arterial blood–gas analysis is characteristic, as is a normal arterial–alveolar oxygen gradient. Given that a number of important processes produce respiratory alkalosis (e.g., salicylate intoxication, PE, and anemia), psychogenic hyperventilation should be a diagnosis of exclusion.

Vocal cord dysfunction (VCD) is a paradoxic closure of the cords during inspiration or expiration when the cords should remain open. This entity is often misdiagnosed as asthma and has a very large psychologic component. VCD is most commonly seen in adolescent females who present with acute onset of shortness of breath or a choking sensation and inspiratory stridor. Attacks can be managed with oxygen, Heliox or sedation (20).

DIAGNOSTIC APPROACH

The most important initial step in the evaluation and treatment of shortness of breath is to secure the airway and assure oxygenation and circulation. In cases of obvious severe distress, this may mean noninvasive positive pressure ventilation or endotracheal intubation and mechanical ventilation; whereas mild-to-moderate distress may warrant only the use of oxygen initially. Once the ABCs have been addressed, the physician should perform a rapid, complete history and physical examination, to elucidate the cause of the shortness of breath (pulmonary, cardiac or other etiology) and formulate a diagnostic plan if the etiology is not readily identified (30).

It is important to remember that many of the common diseases that produce shortness of breath share many physical findings. Intermittent adventitial sounds (crackles or rales) are heard in a variety of illnesses, such as COPD, CHF, and pulmonary fibrosis, and are not specific for any one disease entity. Continuous adventitial sounds (wheezes) are also produced by a variety of illnesses (Table 8.2) and are almost always a sign of airflow obstruction. Stridor (a loud and harsh-sounding wheeze with a crowing or musical sound of fixed pitch) can be heard, predominantly during inspiration, when the trachea, bronchus, or larynx is obstructed. The presence of other signs and symptoms, such as fever and purulent sputum production in pneumonia, or JVD and gallop rhythm in CHF, significantly supplement the auscultatory findings in establishing the diagnosis in the patient with shortness of breath.

Pulse oximetry is an easy, noninvasive monitoring technique that allows low cost, continuous, reliable measurements of oxygen saturation (30). Every person that presents to the ED complaining of shortness of breath should have his or her oxygen saturation recorded. Use of the pulse oximeter does have limitations, however. First, because of the shape of the oxyhemoglobin dissociation curve, measurement of oxygen saturation is relatively insensitive in detecting changes in PaO_2 at high levels of oxygenation. In patients receiving supplemental oxygen, for example, a substantial drop in PaO_2 may be unaccompanied by any change in saturation. In addition, the curve has a steep

---

TABLE 8.2.   Causes of Wheezing

UPPER RESPIRATORY TRACT

Angioedema
Foreign body
Tumor
Infection

LOWER RESPIRATORY TRACT

Anaphylaxis
Asthma
Aspiration
Bronchiolitis
COPD
Foreign body

VASCULAR

Adult respiratory distress syndrome
Congestive heart failure
Pulmonary embolus

EXTRATHORACIC

Carcinoid
Factitious

downward slope normally commencing at a saturation of 91% corresponding to a PaO_2 of 60 mm Hg. Even relatively modest desaturation below this level represents a significant decline in PaO_2 (31). The curve may also shift due to changes in body temperature and pH. Pulse oximetry may be inaccurate in reflecting oxygen saturation in the presence of high carboxyhemoglobin levels, methemoglobinemia, and low-perfusion states (30). Finally, pulse oximetry does not relay any information regarding PCO_2.

Arterial blood gas measurement may be necessary in evaluating patients who present with shortness of breath. Blood gases demonstrate the severity of gas exchange impairment and are useful as diagnostic tools, as well as for establishing a baseline for monitoring therapy. In disease states such as COPD and asthma, measurement of the carbon dioxide level and degree of acidosis can provide valuable information about the severity of the exacerbation and may be more helpful than oxygen saturation in guiding treatment. The physician should use discretion, however, when obtaining blood gases. In cases of mild shortness of breath due to asthma or COPD exacerbation, a normal oxygen saturation on room air pulse oximetry, and other noninvasive diagnostic studies, such as spirometry forced expiratory volume (FEV1) or forced vital capacity (FVC), are often adequate.

If a blood gas is obtained, the A-a oxygen gradient may be calculated. The most common formula used for calculation is as follows:

$$A\text{-}a = [150 - (1.2 \times PCO_2)] - \text{arterial } PO_2.$$

This formula is accurate at sea level, where the alveolar partial pressure of oxygen is 150 mm Hg. The normal gradient should be approximately 10 in a young person and may increase to no more than 20 as a person ages. A quick way to calculate a patient's normal A-a gradient is to add one-tenth of the patient's age plus 10. Patients, in whom hypoxemia is caused by alveolar hypoventilation alone, such as those with drug overdose or neuromuscular disease, have a normal A-a gradient. The calculated A-a gradient is increased in patients with hypoxemia produced by ventilation–perfusion mismatch, right-to-left shunting and diffusion barrier, which typically occurs in COPD, parenchymal lung disease, PE, and pneumonia.

The chest radiograph is a valuable diagnostic tool in elucidating the cause of shortness of breath and should be obtained in most cases. Diagnostic radiographic findings can be expected in certain entities, such as pneumonia, PE, and pneumothorax. However, the chest radiograph may be entirely normal, even when significant illness is manifested by shortness of breath.

Chest radiographic findings may also be minimal in certain conditions, such as aspiration or toxic inhalation, when the study is obtained as part of the initial evaluation. Also, the presence of radiographic abnormalities does not necessarily imply that a given illness is producing the current episode of shortness of breath. For example, the radiograph of the patient with COPD manifests various abnormalities, but a given episode of shortness of breath may be unrelated to the chronic findings displayed on the radiograph. In addition, the presence of chronic radiographic changes in such instances may render the appearance of acute disease processes, such as CHF or pneumonia, less apparent. Patients with a PE may have a normal chest radiograph.

Special views of the chest may be helpful in certain circumstances. An expiratory view may accentuate the presence of a small pneumothorax, because the constant volume of the intrapleural air is accentuated by the reduced size of the hemithorax on expiration (33). The lateral decubitus view may confirm the presence of a pleural effusion. Inspiratory–expiratory or positional films may indicate a bronchial foreign body. Other radio-

graphic studies, such as a lateral view of the neck in suspected epiglottitis, also may be appropriate.

The measurement of BNP can play an important role in the diagnosis of undifferentiated dyspnea. Twenty percent of cardiomegaly diagnosed on echocardiography is missed on chest x-ray and pulmonary vascular congestion can be minimal or absent in patients with significantly increased pulmonary wedge pressures (10). A BNP of 100 pg/dL or greater is consistent with the diagnosis of CHF with a sensitivity of 90%, specificity of 76%, and an accuracy of 83% for differentiating CHF from other causes of dyspnea (21). A recent study demonstrated that the measurement of BNP in the ED used in conjunction with other clinical data resulted in a reduced time to initiation of treatment in the ED, decreased need for hospitalization, decreased ICU admission rate and hospital length of stay, and lower total cost of treatment (25). In addition, following BNP levels in response to therapy has been shown to be beneficial (10), suggesting routine testing for BNP in the emergency department for patients with CHF may be appropriate.

Peak-flow meters are inexpensive instruments that provide a rapid bedside measure of airway function, and may provide additional useful information during the management of asthmatic patients (1). With proper instruction on use and good patient cooperation, the physician can make a rapid and objective assessment of the patient's condition and can also use sequential peak-flow measurements as an additional measure of the effectiveness of therapy.

Other diagnostic studies may be helpful when evaluating a patient with shortness of breath. An ECG can show abnormalities of heart rate and rhythm, or evidence of ischemia, injury, or infarction (24). An ECG also may be helpful in evaluating patients with a suspected pulmonary embolus, although suggestive changes are present in only a minority of patients. Anemia is an important cause of shortness of breath (17), and a check of the patient's hemoglobin or hematocrit may be useful as part of the work up. Rarely, bedside laryngoscopy or bronchoscopy may provide a definitive diagnosis, especially in the case of upper airway obstruction or suspected foreign body.

CRITICAL INTERVENTIONS

Management of the patient with shortness of breath in the ED depends on the patient's baseline respiratory status, the cause of the current respiratory decline, and the degree of respiratory distress. The goal of the treatment is to correct the underlying disorder causing the symptoms. Unfortunately, in many patients, treatment of the underlying cause is ineffective or only partly effective, and the shortness of breath will persist (22).

Every patient who complains of shortness of breath should have pulse oximetry performed and, at least initially, be provided with supplemental oxygen. If the clinical condition warrants consideration of mechanical ventilation, the physician should determine whether or not the patient is a candidate for noninvasive positive pressure ventilation (30). The selection criteria include at least two of the following: moderate to severe dyspnea, accessory respiratory muscle use, paradoxical abdominal movements, respiratory rate > 25 and respiratory acidosis with the pH < 7.35 and a pCO_2 > 45 (4). Absolute contraindications include respiratory arrest; severe cardiorespiratory instability; uncooperative patients; recent craniofacial trauma or burns; anatomic abnormalities of the nasopharynx; recent facial, esophageal or gastric surgery; the inability to protect the airway; and the inability to manage secretions (4). If noninvasive positive pressure ventilation is not appropriate, endotracheal intubation should be performed.

Once a preliminary diagnosis is made, treatment should be appropriately tailored to alleviate the patient's shortness of breath. A patient in CHF may require therapy with diuretics, nitroglycerin, inotropes or nesiritide (a recombinant form of BNP) (2). Nesiritide has been shown to improve hemodynamic function and clinical status in patients with acute decompensated heart failure (11). However, the only published study comparing nesiritide versus nitroglycerin when added to standard treatment found slightly improved hemodynamic measurements at 3 hours but no significant difference in patient assessment of dyspnea (27). The cost of nesiritide and the paucity of data to show that it is clinically superior to standard treatment has made its routine use controversial.

Patients with COPD or asthma exacerbation may benefit from inhaled beta-adrenergic agents, anticholinergic agents and intravenous or oral steroids (16). Patients with severe asthma may require subcutaneous epinephrine injection. Patients with pneumonia should receive appropriate prompt antibiotic therapy based on the probable etiology. Pneumothorax usually requires either aspiration or chest tube placement. Patients with pulmonary embolism require anticoagulation. Specific therapies can be found in the chapters devoted to each of the differential diagnoses.

In patients with anaphylaxis, a patent airway must be established and maintained. Immediate treatment with parental epinephrine (1:1000 dilution in a dose of 0.3-0.5 ml intramuscularly [IM] or subcutaneously [SC]) is the cornerstone of therapy. The intramuscular route has been shown to be superior to the subcutaneous administration (14). Intravenous epinephrine (1:10,000 dilution) is reserved for patients in shock. The dose may be repeated every 5 to 15 minutes until there is resolution of the symptoms or the patient exhibits signs of hyperadrenalism (14). Additional treatment includes antihistamines to block both H1 and H2 receptors and steroids. Observation after treatment is needed due to the second phase of reactivity that may occur. A period of 24 hours of observation in a monitored setting is prudent.

DISPOSITION

The disposition of the dyspneic patient depends on the cause of the respiratory difficulty, the severity of the respiratory compromise, and the success of the ED treatment. Any patient with continuing shortness of breath, despite treatment, should be admitted for further evaluation and treatment. Depending on the clinical condition and diagnosis, the patient may need observation on the general ward, on telemetry, or in the intensive care unit. The patient may be safely discharged home if he or she has improvement in or resolution of shortness of breath and an appropriate diagnosis, such as an asthma exacerbation, has been made. When considering discharge in dyspneic patients, it is important to assure that they are back to their baseline respiratory status, will be able to obtain the medications prescribed, are capable of caring for themselves at home, and will have adequate, prompt followup care.

COMMON PITFALLS

✔ Relying on pulse oximetry alone to gauge a patient's respiratory status; it gives no information about pCO_2
✔ Waiting for radiographic confirmation before decompressing the pleural space, in patients with clinical signs of a tension pneumothorax
✔ Withholding oxygen for fear of blunting the hypoxic respiratory drive in a patient with COPD; correct the hypoxia first
✔ Relying on a normal chest radiograph to rule out the diagnosis of PE
✔ Failure to realize that absence of wheezing in a patient with asthma or COPD in respiratory distress indicates severely obstructed airways

References

1. Adams BK, Cydulka RK. Asthma evaluation and management. *Emerg Med Clin North Am* 2003;21:315–330.
2. Almeda FQ, Hollenberg SM. Update on therapy for acute and chronic heart failure. *Postgrad Med* 2003;113:36–38, 41–44, 47–48.
3. American College of Emergency Physicians. Clinical policy for the management and risk stratification of community-acquired pneumonia in adults in the emergency department. *Ann Emerg Med* 2001;38:107–113.
4. American Respiratory Care Foundation. Consensus conference: noninvasive positive pressure ventilation. *Resp Care* 1997;42:364–369.
5. American Thoracic Society. Standards for the diagnosis and care of patients with chronic obstructive pulmonary disease. *Am J Respir Crit Care Med* 1995;152:S78–S106.
6. American Thoracic Society. Dyspnea. Mechanisms, assessment, and management: a consensus statement. *Am J Respir Crit Care Med* 1999;159:321.
7. Bartlett JG, Breiman RF, Mandell LA, File TM. Community-acquired pneumonia in adults: guidelines for management. *Clin Infect Dis* 1998;26:811–838.
8. Barton ED. Tension pneumothorax. *Curr Opin Pulm Med* 1999;5:269–274.
9. Birnbaum Y, Fishbein MC, Blanche C, Siegel RJ. Current Concepts: ventricular rupture after acute myocardial infarction. *N Engl J Med* 2992;347:1426–1432.
10. Collins SP, Ronan-Bentle S, Storrow AB. Diagnostic and prognostic usefulness of natriuretic peptides in emergency department patients with dyspnea. *Ann Emerg Med* 2003;41:532–545.
11. Colucci WS, Uui E, Horton DP, et al. Intravenous Nesiritide, a natriuretic peptide, in the treatment of decompensated congestive heart failure. *N Eng J Med* 2000;343:246–253.
12. Cunha BA. TB pneumonia. *Emerg Med* 1998;30:102–111.
13. Cunnington J. Spontaneous pnuemothorax. *Clin Evid* 2003;7:1384–1390.
14. Ellis AK, Day JH. Diagnosis and management of anaphylaxis. *CMAJ* 2003;169:307–311.
15. Gerazounis M, Athanassiadi K, Kalantzi N, Moustardas M. Spontaneous pneumomediastinum: a rare benign entity. *J Thorac Cardiovasc Surg* 2003;126:774–776.
16. Gibbs MA, Camargo CA, Rowe BH, Silverman RA. State of the art: therapeutic controversies in severe acute asthma. *Acad Emerg Med* July 2000;7:800–815.
17. Hetzel TM, Losek JD. Unrecognized severe anemia in children presenting with respiratory distress. *Am J Emerg Med* 1998;16:386–389.
18. Kline JA, Johns KL, Colucciello SA, Israel EG. New diagnostic tests for pulmonary embolism. *Ann Emerg Med* 2000;35:168–180.
19. Kline JA, Wells PS. Methodology for a rapid protocol to rule out pulmonary embolism in the emergency department. *Ann Emerg Med* 2003;35:266–276.
20. Leggit J. Vocal cord dysfunction. *Am Fam Physician* 2004;69:1045–1046.
21. Maisel AS, Krishnaswamy P, Nowak RM, et al. Rapid Measurement of b-type natriuretic peptide in the emergency diagnosis of heart failure. *N Engl J Med* 2002;347:161–167.
22. Manning HL, Schwartzstein RM. Pathophysiology of dyspnea. *N Engl J Med* 1995;333:1547–1553.
23. McCullough PA, Omland T, Maisel AS. B-type natriuretic peptides: a diagnostic breakthrough for clinicians. *Rev Cardiovasc Med* 2003;4:72–80.
24. Morgan WC, Hodge HL. Diagnostic evaluation of dyspnea. *Am Fam Physician* 1998;57:711–716.
25. Mueller C, Scholer A, Laule-KilianK, et al. Use of b-type natriuretic peptide in the evaluation and management of acute dyspnea. *N Engl J Med* 2004;350:647–654.
26. Orebaugh SL. Difficult airway management in the emergency department. *J Emerg Med* 2002;22:31–48.
27. Publication Committee for the VMAC Investigators. Intravenous neiritide vs nitroglycerin for the treatment of decompensated congestive heart failure: a randomized trial. *JAMA* 2002;287:1531–1540.
28. Rotta AT, Wiryawan. AT, Respiratory emergencies in children. *Resir Care* 2003;48:248–258.
29. Sadosty AT, Boie ET, Stead LG. Pulmonary embolism. *Emerg Med Clin North Am* 2003;21:363–384.
30. Sigillito RJ, DeBlieux PM. Evaluation and initial management of the patient in respiratory distress. *Emerg Med Clin North Am* 2003;21:239–258.
31. Schnapp LM, Cohen NH. Pulse oximetry uses and abuses. *Chest* 1990;98:1244–1249.
32. Susec O, Boudrow D, Kline JA. The clinical features of acute pulmonary embolism in ambulatory patients. *Acad Emerg Med* 1997;4:891–897.
33. Ullman EA, Donley LP, Brady WJ. Pulmonary trauma emergency department evaluation and management. *Emerg Med Clin North Am* 2003;21:291–313.
34. Yahia S, Brodyn NE, Rokosz GJ, Doskow J. Emergency use of echocardiography in a post-myocardial infarction patient with acute shortness of breath. *Am J Emerg Med* 1996;14:33–36.

CHAPTER 9
Syncope

Thomas P. Martin

Syncope is the sudden transient loss of consciousness associated with an inability to maintain postural tone that resolves without intervention (13). Syncope is not an illness but rather is a manifestation of numerous entities spanning a spectrum from life-threatening disease processes to adverse medication reactions and psychiatric illness. The diagnostic effort, therefore, has two primary components. First, when possible, the goal is to establish a cause of the syncopal episode and direct the therapy and disposition dictated by that diagnosis. Second, in patients in whom a diagnosis is not possible, the goal is to identify the subset of patients who are likely to benefit from further inpatient evaluation and therapy, through risk assessment. As is common in the practice of emergency medicine, this group of high-risk patients represents only a small fraction of the entire population who present with syncope. The challenge of accurately identifying this small group is formidable.

The incidence of syncope depends on the population studied. The Framingham study evaluated 7,814 men and women aged 20 to 96 years for an average of 17 years. A total of 822 participants reported an episode of syncope. The overall incidence rate of a first report of syncope was 6.2 per 1,000 patient years. Incidence rates, however, varied widely with age. Young men aged 20 to 29 had an incidence of 2.6 episodes per 1,000 patient years, while men and women aged 80 and above had incidence rates of 16.9 and 19.5 episodes per 1,000 patient years, respectively (26).

While prior epidemiologic studies frequently labeled significant proportions of patients as having "unexplained syncope" or "syncope of unknown origin," broader use of event monitoring, tilt-table testing, and psychiatric evaluation, as well as recognition that syncope is often multifactorial in the elderly, have substantially reduced the number of patients without a diagnosis.

CLINICAL PRESENTATION

History and physical examination are the most important elements of the evaluation of patients presenting with syncope. The history should focus on the events and symptoms before, during, and after the syncopal episode, as well as on the past medical and medication histories. Patients, witnesses and prehospital care providers are vital sources of information. Patients are often able to provide key information that assists the physician in determining the cause of syncope and identifying the patients at high risk for adverse, short-term outcome. Syncope associated with exertion may prompt the physician to look for evidence of cardiac outflow obstruction. Patients can describe what actions or events immediately preceded the loss of consciousness, including standing (orthostatic hypotension); coughing, urinating or defecating (situational syncope); or painful or emotionally charged situations (vasovagal or psychiatric causes of syncope). Diaphoresis and nausea (vasovagal syncope), headache (subarachnoid hemorrhage), abdominal pain (ectopic pregnancy, abdominal aortic aneurysm), chest pain (thoracic aortic dissection)

or shortness of breath (pulmonary embolism) may be reported either immediately preceding or following the loss of consciousness. Patients and bystanders can also provide information that will assist the physician in differentiating syncope from other causes of a loss of consciousness. Tongue-biting, the presence of a postictal period or urinary incontinence may suggest seizure rather than syncope caused the patient's symptoms.

The value of symptoms in identifying patients at risk for cardiac dysrhythmia and death has been examined. Traditionally, an absence of prodromal symptoms has been associated with dysrhythmia as the cause of syncope. In a population of both inpatients and outpatients with syncope, in whom a diagnosis could not be made by history and physical exam, only an absence of nausea and vomiting was a reliable symptom in predicting syncope caused by dysrhythmia (odds ratio 7:1). Symptoms surrounding the event could not be used to predict mortality or reccurrence (25). Family history should be explored for cases of unexplained sudden death.

Physical examination should focus on the vital signs and a careful cardiovascular (murmurs, pulses, signs of congestive heart failure) and neurologic evaluation. The examination may also reveal asymmetric upper extremity blood pressures and lead to consideration of aortic dissection or subclavian steal.

Although orthostatic vital signs are a part of the physical examination for a patient with syncope, there is little agreement on the definition of orthostatic hypotension. An increase in the heart rate of 30 beats or more on standing correlates with an acute blood loss of 1,000 mL, but smaller degrees of volume loss do not reliably correlate with orthostatic changes (3,15). Even symptoms of dizziness on standing correlate poorly with orthostatic changes or volume depletion. Thus, the diagnosis of postural syncope is best made by a history of syncope on standing. If hypovolemia is profound, then orthostatic vital signs will be reliably abnormal.

Physical exam may also identify cardiac murmurs or a diminished carotid upstroke, suggesting significant valvular heart disease. Pulmonary examination may reveal a pleural rub associated with pulmonary embolism. Examination of the abdomen may disclose a pulsatile mass alerting the physician to the possibility of an abdominal aortic aneurysm. Rectal or vaginal bleeding may identify gastrointestinal hemorrhage or ectopic pregnancy as the cause of the syncopal episode.

DIFFERENTIAL DIAGNOSIS

The pathophysiology common to most causes of syncope is a sudden, transient reduction in cerebral blood flow (Table 9.1). Impaired function results either in the area of the brainstem thought to be responsible for the conscious state (reticular activating system) or in both cerebral hemispheres simultaneously. In the few causes of syncope in which cerebral blood flow is not markedly reduced, glucose is not utilized because of a sudden, dramatic reduction in cerebral metabolism secondary to acute brain injury or subarachnoid hemorrhage. The sudden increase in intracranial pressure associated with these conditions may limit cerebral blood flow as well, and may also deform the neural structures involved in the maintenance of consciousness.

Transient tachyarrhythmias (ventricular or supraventricular) may produce syncope by decreasing ventricular filling and stroke volume, resulting in systemic hypotension and decreased cerebral blood flow. Loss of consciousness may also occur as a result of transient bradyarrhythmias. Although bradyarrhythmias are often an incidental finding and asymptomatic, some episodes of syncope are related to sinus node dysfunction, particularly in the elderly (18). Medications can also produce an inappropriate bradycardia as well as vasodilatation and

TABLE 9.1.   Differential Diagnosis of Syncope

CARDIAC CAUSES

Arrhythmias
  Bradyarrhythmias: second- and third-degree heart block, sinus
    node dysfunction, pacemaker malfunction
  Tachyarrhythmias: ventricular tachycardia, ventricular fibrillation,
    SVT, torsade de pointes
Pump failure
  Myocardial infarction, cardiac ischemia
Obstruction to flow
  Aortic stenosis, hypertrophic cardiomyopathy, pulmonary
    hypertension, pulmonary embolism, prosthetic valve
    dysfunction
Impairment of venous return
  Pericardial tamponade
Other cardiovascular causes
  Aortic dissection, Brugada Syndrome

REFLEX-MEDIATED

Vasovagal/vasodepressor syncope
Situational syncope
  Micturition, defecation
Other
Carotid sinus hypersensitivity

ORTHOSTATIC HYPOTENSION

Hypovolemia, acute blood loss, dehydration, medications

NEUROLOGIC

Subarachnoid hemorrhage, posterior circulation TIA, subclavian
  steal, peripheral and autonomic neuropathies, seizure

MEDICATIONS

Vasodilators, calcium channel blockers, beta-blockers, nitrates,
  diuretics, antiarrhythmics, ACEIs

PSYCHIATRIC DISEASE

Major depression, somatization disorder, panic disorder, substance
  abuse

OTHER CAUSES

Hypoglycemia

  SVT, supraventricular tachycardia; TIAs, transient ischemic attacks;
ACEI, angiotensin converting enzyme inhibitors.

depressed left ventricular output. In pacemaker-dependent patients, pacemaker malfunction has been reported to produce syncope as a result of bradyarrhythmias or pacemaker-induced tachycardia. Of note, studies in patients with chronic bifascicular block and syncope have shown that in fewer than 20% are the two related. In fact, ventricular tachycardia rather than bradyarrhythmia is responsible for more episodes of syncope in these patients (20).

Syncope may also be a manifestation of cardiovascular disease producing an obstruction to blood flow. Exertional syncope may be the first clue to a diagnosis of aortic stenosis or hypertrophic cardiomyopathy. In these disorders, the conventional explanation of decreased cardiac output as a result of left ventricular outflow obstruction has been supplemented by findings that tachyarrhythmias occur frequently in these patients and may be particularly compromising to those who depend on adequate ventricular filling to overcome the obstruction. In addition, paradoxical vasodilation has been shown to occur in

patients with aortic stenosis and may contribute to the syncopal episodes common to this disease.

Mitral valve disease may also cause syncope. Severe mitral valve stenosis may be associated with syncope, most commonly during periods of atrial fibrillation. Various tachyarrhythmias and neuropsychiatric complaints occur in patients with mitral valve prolapse, which may be associated with syncope. Left atrial myxoma is a rare tumor that causes an abrupt decrease in cardiac output, often when a change in position causes the tumor to occlude the mitral orifice.

Acute pulmonary hypertension causes functional acute obstruction to pulmonary flow, and thus abruptly decreases left ventricular preload and cardiac output. This event may occur with massive pulmonary embolism. In patients with chronic pulmonary hypertension, activities that acutely raise intrathoracic pressure, such as coughing or the Valsalva maneuver during defecation, produce the same phenomenon. Air embolism may produce syncope by obstructing flow through the heart, lungs, or carotids, causing myocardial infarction by occluding coronary flow or by inducing ventricular dysrhythmias.

Other causes of cardiac-related syncope include sudden left ventricular dysfunction or ventricular dysrhythmias associated with myocardial ischemia or infarction (4). Patients with pericardial tamponade, constrictive pericarditis, and constrictive myocardial disease may develop impairment of venous return, leading to decreased left ventricular output. This may also result in syncope.

Reflex-mediated syncope is a common cause of syncope in all populations. Vasovagal syncope (precipitated by painful or emotional situations), carotid sinus hypersensitivity, and situational syncope (with micturition or defecation) may share components of a common pathophysiologic mechanism (23). Until recently, the explanation for the findings of hypotension or bradycardia was anchored in a cardiac mechanoreceptor mechanism. The orthostatic stress of upright posture, causing an underfilled left ventricle, or the emotional stress of phlebotomy, for example, leads to vigorous left ventricular contraction and stimulation of arterial and cardiopulmonary mechanoreceptors. Stimulation of these receptors leads to the transmission of vagal afferent signals to the ventral lateral medulla. The result is a withdrawal of sympathetic efferents (producing peripheral vasodilation and hypotension) and increased vagal efferents to the heart (producing bradycardia) in susceptible individuals (10,23).

The finding that vasovagal syncope occurs in individuals following cardiac transplantation, as well as information from animal studies, has led to recognition that a purely cardiac mechanoreceptor mechanism is inadequate to explain the physiologic changes of reflex-mediated syncope. Increasingly, the importance of neurohumoral factors, including the renin-aldosterone–angiotensin system, vasopressin, serotonin, pancreatic polypeptides, endogenous opioids, and nitric oxide, is being recognized. The exact contributions of each of these factors and the nature of their interaction remain to be elucidated (10,23).

Syncope may be a manifestation of psychiatric illness. Studies have documented a high prevalence of psychiatric illness among patients with syncope, particularly patients with syncope of unknown origin. Psychiatric disorders included somatoform disorders, mood disorders (including major depressive disorder), anxiety disorders (including panic attacks), and substance abuse (24). Psychiatric disease may be associated with syncope by several mechanisms, including exacerbation of coexisting medical illness, by leading to hyperventilation, by triggering a vasovagal response, or as a presenting complaint in a somatic disorder. Syncope may also be the result of volume depletion or cardiac ischemia produced by alcohol or cocaine abuse, respectively (24).

True seizures also cause a transient loss of consciousness. Distinguishing a seizure disorder from syncope is usually straightforward by history. Postictal disorientation is the most reliable discriminator, occurring in most patients with seizures and very rarely in patients with syncope. Brief (usually less than 10 seconds) tonic–clonic seizure activity can accompany syncope of any etiology, especially vasodepressor syncope. This activity is not accompanied by postictal disorientation, and it does not represent true seizure activity.

Transient ischemic attacks and stroke rarely cause syncope (16). For cerebrovascular disease to cause a loss of consciousness, either both cerebral hemispheres or the brainstem must be deprived of blood flow. In a patient with a prior hemispheric infarction, marked ischemia or infarction on the contralateral side may cause a loss of consciousness, but it is unlikely that this alteration in consciousness would be transient and resolve spontaneously. Similarly, vertebrobasilar ischemia may cause syncope, but not in isolation. Other manifestations of brainstem dysfunction (diplopia, vertigo, or nausea) are required to make this rare diagnosis. Most investigators agree that syncope is rarely a manifestation of neurologic disease (16).

Subarachnoid hemorrhage can produce syncope, presumably as a result of a sudden increase in intracranial pressure and a sudden transient decrease in cerebral metabolism. Another possible mechanism is suggested by the association of torsade de pointes and prolonged Q-T syndrome in patients with subarachnoid hemorrhage (5). The complaint of headache or the appearance of focal neurologic findings in a patient with syncope raises this possibility.

Medications can produce syncope by several mechanisms. Certain medications result in volume depletion, orthostasis, gastrointestinal hemorrhage, or depressed left ventricular function. Other medications have a proarrhythmic effect that may result in syncope. Medications and the interaction of multiple medications, particularly in the elderly, are important considerations in the evaluation of syncope (18).

Other causes of syncope include orthostasis secondary to acute blood loss, dehydration, and third-spacing of fluid, as well as disorders of autonomic function, including peripheral neuropathies and central nervous system disease. Finally, a simple cause of syncope is hypoglycemia.

DIAGNOSTIC APPROACH

The emergency physician should have several goals when evaluating patients presenting with syncope. First, the clinician must identify the subgroup of syncope patients presenting with life-threatening or other causes of syncope requiring emergent or urgent diagnosis and treatment (e.g., subarachnoid hemorrhage, abdominal aortic aneurysm, myocardial infarction). Second, the clinician must be able to identify other recognizable causes of syncope that will benefit from specific treatment or other intervention (e.g., volume depletion, adverse effects of medications). Third, in the patients who remain without a diagnosis despite a thorough emergency department evaluation, the emergency physician must identify those who require further evaluation. Finally, the physician must determine whether the most appropriate setting for that evaluation is as an inpatient or outpatient.

History, physical examination, and the initial electrocardiogram (ECG) are the crucial elements in determining a cause of syncope and in stratifying the risk of those patients in whom it is not possible to make a diagnosis during the emergency department visit. These three components established the diagnosis in 88% of patients who eventually received a diagnosis according to two large studies (7,14). In addition, specific abnormalities revealed in this evaluation led to the performance of other tests, which established the diagnosis in another 5% of patients. This resulted in a net diagnostic yield of 93% from a directed emergency department evaluation. A history of exercise-induced syncope, for example, suggests hypertrophic cardiomyopathy or aortic stenosis and justifies echocardiography, while a history of sudden-onset headache with syncope suggests an intracranial hemorrhage and justifies computed tomography of the brain and lumbar puncture.

Dysrhythmias on ECG direct the evaluation down the path of a cardiac etiology. The ECG is analyzed for dysrhythmias, conduction abnormalities, signs of ischemia or infarction, QT prolongation and evidence of accessory pathways. Brugada syndrome, a recently recognized, new clinical entity characterized by ST segment elevation in the right precordial leads and associated with episodes of sudden death, may also be identified by ECG (2).

Screening laboratory studies have been shown to add little in establishing a cause of syncope. In most cases, hypoglycemia was clinically suspected, abnormal electrolytes never accounted for a loss of consciousness, and anemia from bleeding was clinically evident (7). Thus, there is no "standard" emergency department workup for syncopal patients beyond history, physical examination, and ECG. Further studies are indicated only for selected patients as determined by the initial evaluation.

Although there are reports of syncope as the initial complaint in elderly patients with acute myocardial infarction, there are no convincing reports of acute myocardial infarction presenting solely with syncope (4). Often patients whose painless infarction was "ushered in by a syncopal attack," all had other symptoms or signs (acute severe dyspnea or cardiovascular collapse) or ECG changes that were diagnostic of myocardial infarction at the time of their first evaluation (4). More recent reports of syncope as the initial symptom of myocardial infarction in the elderly have also stressed that these patients are often pain-free on presentation. Diagnoses were made nevertheless on the basis of other symptoms, signs, and ECG findings available to the initial examining physician. Therefore, admission to the hospital to "rule out myocardial infarction" for the patient whose syncope is unexplained is not warranted (unless indicated for other reasons).

Similarly, syncope is described as the initial symptom in patients with aortic dissection, ruptured aortic aneurysm, pulmonary embolism, subarachnoid hemorrhage, and ruptured ectopic pregnancy. However, careful evaluation directed by findings on initial history, examination, and ECG is usually sufficient to make the diagnosis in all cases.

Attributing syncope to transient dysrhythmias, unless they are identified on the initial ECG or monitor strip, can be problematic. Long-term, continuous ECG (Holter) monitoring has inadequate specificity to provide useful results; the vast majority of abnormalities detected cause no symptoms and are of no particular significance (9,14). Invasive electrophysiologic studies may be indicated for a small group of patients who are at high risk for sudden death (those with a history of ventricular tachycardia or fibrillation, myocardial infarction, congestive heart failure, or valvular or hypertrophic heart disease) (8). Consultation with a cardiologist is desirable when deciding on disposition in this setting.

Upright tilt-table testing has become a useful adjunct in the further evaluation of patients with suspected vasovagal or neurocardiogenic syncope. Tilt-table testing reveals abnormalities in 20% to 70% of patients whose ED evaluation leaves them without a diagnosis. A positive test in patients with a recurrent syncope may guide therapy with a beta-blocker, anticholinergic agent, fludrocortisone or dual-chamber pacing. Treatment has been shown to be effective in preventing recurrence of syncope in the majority of patients with positive tests (10).

CRITICAL INTERVENTIONS

As with the emergency department evaluation, the management of patients with syncope also requires a tiered approach. For patients presenting with symptoms, physical examination findings or ECG findings that allow identification of a cause of the syncopal episode, management is directed toward that entity. Bedside determination of the patient's blood sugar should be performed at presentation. Adequacy of oxygenation must be assessed by pulse oximetry and electrocardiographic monitoring should be instituted in all ill-appearing patients and in patients in whom a cardiac etiology of syncope is being considered. Patients with hypotension, evidence of hypovolemia or significant blood loss should have appropriate intravenous access established and undergo immediate resuscitation with crystalloid solutions and packed red blood cells, as clinically indicated. Institution of thrombolysis should be considered in patients with massive pulmonary embolism. Immediate consultation with surgeons, obstetrician-gynecologists, cardiologists and other key specialists must be obtained when the clinical picture is consistent with life-threatening emergencies such as ruptured abdominal aortic aneurysm, ruptured ectopic pregnancy or pericardial tamponade.

DISPOSITION

Once conditions posing an immediate threat to patient well-being have been excluded, the emergency physician must identify those patients requiring admission for treatment and those who require an admission to facilitate a timely evaluation. Admission for treatment is recommended for patients with acute severe volume loss or chronic, severe orthostatic hypotension, and for discontinuation or adjustment of medications producing adverse reactions. Elderly patients with coexisting medical problems often require admission (9).

For patients who remain without a diagnosis at the end of the emergency department visit, the need for expedited evaluation is predicated on an assessment of risk. The job of the emergency physician, however, is complicated by deficiencies in the available medical literature. First, no information is available concerning the risk of adverse outcome (significant dysrhythmia or cardiovascular mortality) in the time typically covered by hospitalization surrounding an acute syncopal episode. Second, no literature supports the conclusion that hospital admission results in a benefit to patients or a change in outcome. Despite these shortcomings, some guidance is available concerning the question of disposition in patients with syncope. Left ventricular function is a clear determinant of outcome. Studies have documented left ventricular function as a significant predictor of dysrhythmia, cardiovascular mortality, and sudden death (19,21,22). In populations matched for age and comorbid illnesses, syncope was not a risk factor for overall and cardiac mortality or for cardiovascular events. Rather, age, male sex, and congestive heart failure were the factors predictive of these end points (12).

Two emergency department studies have reported prediction rules for identifying patients at risk for adverse outcome at 1 year. One study (19) found that the risk of dysrhythmia and 1-year mortality could be stratified by the presence of the following: (1) age greater than 45 years, (2) a history of congestive heart failure, (3) a history of ventricular ectopic activity, and (4) an abnormal ECG, defined as any finding other than sinus tachycardia, sinus bradycardia, or nonspecific ST and T-wave changes. Dysrhythmias and death within 1 year occurred in 4% to 7% of patients without any risk factors and in 57% to 80% of patients with three or four risk factors (19). The European Society of Cardiology has reported similar findings, in a multicenter trial, identifying: (1) age >65 years, (2) cardiovascular disease in the clinical history,

(3) syncope without prodrome, and (4) an abnormal ECG as predictors of 12-month mortality. Risk could be stratified based on the number of factors present. All-cause mortality varied from 0% in patients with no risk factors to 52.9% to 57.1% in patients with all four risk factors. No deaths were reported in the 6 months following enrollment in the groups with 0 to 1 risk factors (6).

Given the high stakes involved in evaluating the emergency department patient with syncope and our imperfect ability to predict outcome, the decision to hospitalize a patient in whom the history, physical examination, and initial ECG are unrevealing must often be individualized. This decision must be predicated on a careful assessment of the risk of adverse outcome and the potential benefit to the patient of inpatient evaluation. Patients should be admitted for expedited evaluation if they have any of the following: (1) a history of congestive heart failure, left ventricular dysfunction; valvular heart disease or congenital heart disease; (2) a history of ventricular dysrhythmias; (3) historical factors or physical examination findings suggestive of structural heart disease, left ventricular dysfunction, dysrhythmia, ischemia or conduction system disease; (4) ECG findings of ischemia, conduction system disease, dysrhythmia, prolonged QT interval, accessory pathways, ST elevation in the right precordial leads or pacemaker malfunction; (5) syncope related to exertion; or (6) if they are taking medications that may predispose to dysrhythmia (1,6,9,17,19). A patient's age and a family history of sudden death are additional factors that should be considered in the admission decision (1).

Patients with no suspicion of structural heart disease and a single episode of syncope may often be closely followed without other testing, while those with recurrent episodes should be referred for tilt-table testing, event monitoring, or psychiatric evaluation (16).

In patients for whom emergency department discharge is considered, the ability of the patient to provide for basic needs, the safety of ambulation, and the availability of necessary supports following discharge should be assured.

COMMON PITFALLS

- ✔ Attributing syncope to a vasovagal or unknown cause because of a failure to take a detailed history of the syncopal event
- ✔ Attributing syncope to an incidentally found, asymptomatic dysrhythmia
- ✔ Attributing syncope to a transient ischemic attack
- ✔ Attributing syncope to any finding when the causal relation is tenuous
- ✔ Failure to take seriously the finding of an aortic outflow murmur in a patient with syncope
- ✔ Admission of patients with isolated syncope of unknown cause to "rule out myocardial infarction" when no other historical, physical examination, or electrocardiographic finding supports this management strategy
- ✔ Failure to recognize the following catastrophic scenarios: syncope with headache (subarachnoid hemorrhage), syncope with chest pain (myocardial infarction, aortic dissection, pulmonary embolism, pulmonary hypertension), syncope with exertion (aortic stenosis, hypertrophic cardiomyopathy), and syncope with abdominal pain (abdominal aortic aneurysm, ruptured ectopic pregnancy)

Acknowledgments

Previous edition's author Jay M. Goldman.

References

1. American College of Emergency Physicians. Clinical policy: critical issues in the evaluation and management of patients presenting with syncope. *Ann Emerg Med* 2001;37:771.

2. Antzelevitch C, Brugada P, Brugada J, Brugada R, Towbin JA, Nademanee K. Brugada syndrome: 1992–2002. A historical perspective. *J Am Coll Cardiol* 2003;41:1665.

3. Atkins D, Hanusa B, Sefcik T, et al. Syncope and orthostatic hypotension. *Am J Med* 1991;91:179.

4. Bayer AJ, Chadha JS, Farag RR, et al. Changing presentation of myocardial infarction with increasing age. *J Am Geriatr Soc* 1986;34:263.

5. Carruth JE, Silverman ME. Torsade de pointe atypical ventricular tachycardia complicating subarachnoid hemorrhage. *Chest* 1980;78:886.

6. Colivicchi F, Ammirati F, Melina D, Guido V, Imperoli G, Santini M. Development and prospective validation of a risk stratification system for patients with syncope in the emergency department: the OESIL risk score. *European Heart J* 2003;24:811.

7. Day SC, Cook EF, Funkenstein H, et al. Evaluation and outcome of emergency room patients with transient loss of consciousness. *Am J Med* 1982;73:15.

8. Dennis AR, Rodd DL, Richards DA, et al. Electrophysiologic studies in patients with unexplained syncope. *Int J Cardiol* 1992;35:211.

9. Kapoor WN. Syncope. *N Engl J Med* 2000;343:1856.

10. Kapoor WN. Using a tilt table to evaluate syncope. *Am J Med Sci* 1999;317:110.

11. Kapoor WN, Cha R, Peterson JR, et al. Prolonged electrocardiographic monitoring in patients with syncope. *Am J Med* 1987;82:20.

12. Kapoor WN, Hanusa BH. Is syncope a risk factor for poor outcome? Comparison of patients with and without syncope. *Am J Med* 1996;100:646.

13. Kapoor WN, Karpf M, Maher Y, et al. Syncope of unknown origin. *JAMA* 1982;247:2687.

14. Kapoor WN, Karpf M, Wieand S, et al. A prospective evaluation and follow-up of patients with syncope. *N Engl J Med* 1983;309:197.

15. Koziol-McLain J, Lowenstein S, Fuller B. Orthostatic vital signs in emergency department patients. *Ann Emerg Med* 1991;20:606.

16. Linzer M. Syncope. *South Med J* 1987;80:545.

17. Linzer M, Yang EH, Estes M, et al. Diagnosing syncope. Part 2: unexplained syncope. *Ann Intern Med* 1997;127:76.

18. Lipsitz LA, Wei JY, Rowe JW. Syncope in an elderly, institutionalized population: prevalence, incidence and associated risk. *Q J Med* 1985;55:45.

19. Martin TP, Hanusa BH, Kapoor WN. Risk stratification of patients with syncope. *Ann Emerg Med* 1997;29:459.

20. McAnulty JH, Rahimtoola SH, Murphy E, et al. Natural history of "high-risk" bundle branch block: final report of a prospective study. *N Engl J Med* 1982;307:137.

21. Middlekauff HR, Stevenson WG, Saxon LA. Prognosis after syncope: impact of left ventricular function. *Am J Heart* 1993;125:121.

22. Middlekauff HR, Stevenson WG, Stevenson LW, et al. Syncope in advanced heart failure: high risk of sudden death regardless of the origin of syncope. *J Am Coll Cardiol* 1993;21:110.

23. Morillo CA, Ellenbogen KA, Pava LF. Pathophysiologic basis for vasodepressor syncope. *Cardiol Clin* 1997;15:233.

24. Oh JH, Kapoor WN. Psychiatric illness and syncope. *Cardiol Clin* 1997;15:269.

25. Oh JH, Hanusa BH, Kapoor WN. Do symptoms predict cardiac arrythmias and mortality in patients with syncope? *Arch Intern Med* 1999;159:375.

26. Soteriades, ES, Evans, JC, Larson, et al. Incidence and prognosis of syncope. *N Engl J Med* 2002;347:878.

CHAPTER 10
Fever

James H. Bryan and Harold A. Thomas Jr.

"Humanity has but three great enemies: fever, famine, and war; of these, by far the greatest, by far the most terrible, is fever."

—Sir William Osler

Fever is one of the oldest and most widely recognized signs of disease and accounts for numerous adult visits and an estimated 25% of pediatric visits to the emergency department (27). While the exact temperature that constitutes a fever is debatable, most consider a rectal temperature of 38°C in children and a temper-

ature of 38.3°C in adults to represent a fever. Although fever has been recognized as a pathologic sign for at least 2,500 years, and despite Sir William Osler's acclamation, it is still unclear whether fever represents the physician's ally or foe.

Regulation of body temperature is under the control of the preoptic area of the anterior hypothalamus. This area acts like a thermostat, continuously balancing heat production and heat loss. Heat production is controlled by altering the basal metabolic rate by varying the level of circulating thyroxine, which increases cellular metabolism. In addition, the fastest and most sensitive way in which the body increases heat production is by increasing muscle activity (shivering when cold or the shaking chill of a fever).

The principal method of body heat loss is to vary the volume of blood flowing to the skin's surface. The exocrine sweat glands can also contribute to heat loss. Sweating cools the body by vaporization.

The hypothalamic thermostat has an inherent set-point of about 37°C. The normal circadian rhythm exhibits daily variations of up to 2°C. Temperatures are lowest around 4 a.m. and then gradually increase until they peak between 6 and 10 p.m. Most fevers follow this pattern; the fever is higher in the evening and lower in the morning.

Elevation of the hypothalamic set-point appears to be mediated by cytokines. Exogenous pyrogens such as microorganisms, as well as toxins and metabolic byproducts of these organisms, act to stimulate the release of cytokines from lymphocytes, monocytes, and macrophages. Cytokines are believed to travel via the bloodstream to the hypothalamus, where they act to increase prostaglandin synthesis, primarily prostaglandin E2 (PGE2). The resulting increase in prostaglandins causes an elevated cyclic adenosine monophosphate (cAMP) level, resulting in an elevated hypothalamic set-point. This elevated set-point increases body temperature by affecting peripheral vasoconstriction and internal heat production. Fever is maintained until pyrogen levels fall or until prostaglandin production is inhibited. Aspirin, ibuprofen, and acetaminophen exert their antipyretic effects by blocking central hypothalamic prostaglandin synthesis, without any effect on circulating endogenous pyrogen. Corticosteroids can block the release of endogenous pyrogen as well as inhibit prostaglandins, but are nevertheless relatively weak antipyretics.

Cytokines produced in response to pyrogens include interleukins (ILs), tumor necrosis factor (TNF), and interferons (IFNs). It is generally believed that bacteria and their products of metabolism typically provoke release of IL-1. In contrast, viral proteins appear to stimulate IFN. IL-1 induces the liver to produce acute phase reactants, including C-reactive protein (CRP), which are responsible for the elevated erythrocyte sedimentation rate (ESR) associated with some fevers. IFN, although a potent pyrogen, does not enhance production of acute-phase reactants. Although not supported by data, this is the rationale behind the expectation of an elevated ESR and CRP level with a bacterial fever but not with one of viral etiology.

Not all elevations of body temperature necessarily constitute a fever. A true fever is an elevation of body temperature caused by a change in the hypothalamic set-point. This new elevated set-point causes the body to engage its normal heat-generating mechanisms to elevate the temperature until the new set-point is reached. In contrast, in hyperthermia a true fever does not exist; rather, the body attempts to maintain a normal temperature, but its homeostatic mechanisms are overwhelmed. Some causes of hyperthermia include heat exhaustion or heat stroke, vigorous exercise (marathon runners may have temperatures as high as 41°C), hyperthyroidism, hypothalamic stroke or tumor, burns, malignant hyperthermia, and the use of amphetamines, phenothiazines, or anticholinergic drugs. Temperatures greater than 41°C (106°F) almost always represent hyperthermia and not a true fever (21,26). Additionally, in middle-aged to elderly patients who present with what appears to be a septic syndrome, chronic salicylate intoxication should be considered. Fever above 38°C, an elevated white blood cell count with an associated bandemia, decreased systemic vascular resistance, and evidence of multisystem organ failure all have been documented in cases of chronic salicylate intoxication. A careful inquiry into a history of a chronic inflammatory condition or chronic use of one of the myriad salicylate-based antiinflammatory agents (e.g., aspirin, Pepto-Bismol, salsalate, oil of wintergreen) is important in avoiding the significant morbidity and mortality associated with this condition.

The phenomenon of night sweats represents a nocturnal fluctuation in the hypothalamic set-point, causing a slight rise in body temperature that leads to reactive perspiration. Night sweats are most commonly related to tuberculosis or lymphoma, but are also seen in elderly patients with disorders of catecholamine excess and in solid malignancies. Evaluation of temperature fluctuations in patients with Hodgkin's disease who complained of night sweats found that their body temperature rose 0.5°C to 1.5°C within 30 minutes before sweating began (14).

Many metabolic abnormalities are associated with the febrile state. Fever increases both the oxygen tension (PO_2) and the carbon dioxide tension (PCO_2), and shifts the oxyhemoglobin dissociation curve to the right, resulting in lower oxygen saturation. Fever also seems to lower the seizure threshold, causing febrile seizures in children without a predisposition to epilepsy. Fever also can cause reactivation of latent herpes simplex infections (fever blisters).

The value of fever to the host remains a subject of debate, but evidence suggests that fever may have a significant protective effect (21). Neutrophils, macrophages and lymphocytes are most active at elevated temperatures. In addition, higher temperatures decrease the level of serum iron, a substrate that many bacteria need in order to replicate. When iron levels are experimentally kept in the normal range, increased mortality is noted for a given inoculum of bacteria. Fever also seems to inhibit certain viruses, such as coxsackievirus and poliovirus. There is, however, some evidence that argues against a protective effect of fever. Mice infected with tetanus spores or *Streptococci* had decreased survival with an elevation of temperature. Mice and possibly humans are more susceptible to pneumococcal infections when febrile.

CLINICAL PRESENTATION

Most febrile patients present to the emergency department with a chief complaint of fever. However, some patients may present with more generalized complaints. Elderly patients may complain of general malaise or not feeling well; parents may bring in infants who are eating poorly or appear lethargic. In these patients, fever may be an incidental finding.

In children, fevers documented at home should be treated as real, even in the absence of a documented fever in the emergency department. Additionally, in children with subjective fevers, one study showed that mothers have an overall accuracy of 79% for detecting fever by palpation, with positive and negative predictive values of 68% and 88%, respectively (15). Further, bundling of infants has been shown to have no effect on the rectal temperature of healthy infants, so elevated rectal temperatures should not be attributed to bundling (16). In the elderly, basal body temperature may be lower than the established mean of 37°C. One study found that lowering the definition of fever to 37.8°C (100°F) increases the sensitivity of predicting an infection to 70% (versus 40% if 38.3°C is used), while the specificity remained at 90% (8).

A patient with a low-grade fever may suffer from an acute, life-threatening condition, and elderly patients may have bacterial infections and mount no febrile response. Other patients with much higher temperatures may have a benign viral infection. The source of the fever may be readily apparent, or it may remain undiagnosed after weeks of sophisticated evaluation. While pediatric patients often require a more extensive evaluation, history and physical examination alone can identify the etiology of a fever in the majority of adults. In many cases, a patient's appearance and history may be as important as the measurement of a fever.

History

Important points in the history include:

1. Associated symptoms (e.g., vomiting, dysuria, cough, shortness of breath, joint pain, rashes)
2. Duration and magnitude of fever
3. Close contacts with similar illness
4. Occupational, travel, or recreational exposure
5. History of diseases associated with immunocompromise (e.g., HIV), diabetes, chronic renal failure, blood dyscrasia, alcohol or drug abuse, chronic lung disease, or cardiac valve disease
6. Presence of medical hardware (e.g., prosthetic valves)
7. History of recent hospitalizations, which might suggest nosocomial infections
8. Current medications, particularly antibiotics and antipyretics, and duration of use
9. Allergies

Physical Examination

The most important observation on the physical examination is the general overall appearance and mental status of the patient. Specifically, does the patient look well or toxic? Does the patient have an altered mental status, which might indicate infection or sepsis, especially in the elderly? Vital signs should be obtained, including pulse oximetry in selected patients with respiratory signs or symptoms. In the presence of a fever, the pulse can be expected to increase by 18 beats per minute for each 1°C increase in temperature (11). Some diseases are associated with a relative bradycardia for the degree of fever (pulse–temperature dissociation). This dissociation is classically seen with typhoid fever, although one study found it does not occur in children with enteric fever (11). A pulse-temperature dissociation may also be seen in legionnaires' disease, mycoplasmal infections, drug fever, factitious fever, and some viral syndromes. In addition, patients taking beta-blockers may have no change in their pulse in response to a fever. The earliest sign of septic shock is an inappropriately elevated pulse. Tachypnea and dyspnea are suggestive of pulmonary disease, while tachypnea without dyspnea may indicate sepsis or metabolic acidosis of any cause. In a study of nursing home patients, tachypnea greater than 25 was the highest predictor of disease, with a sensitivity of 90% and a specificity of 95% for pneumonia (2).

The history will frequently direct the physician to the most likely source of the infection. In the absence of localizing symptoms, a thorough examination should be undertaken. The entire body should be examined for rashes, skin breakdown or decubiti, cellulitis, "track marks," or lymphadenopathy. Rashes may suggest a viral exanthem, vasculitis, meningococcemia, Rocky Mountain spotted fever, Lyme disease, or toxic shock syndrome (staphylococcal or streptococcal). Lymphadenopathy associated with fever may suggest malignancy, autoimmune disorders, or infection. Tender, localized adenopathy is usually associated with an infection in the region drained by the involved nodes.

The most common cause of acute generalized adenopathy is infectious mononucleosis. Nodes secondary to malignancy are usually painless, rubbery, and firm.

The head and neck should be examined for scleral icterus, which might indicate hepatitis, cholecystitis, or ascending cholangitis. Examination in and around the ears may reveal otitis externa or media, or suggest mastoiditis. The oropharynx may show evidence of pharyngitis, peritonsillar or retropharyngeal abscess, or periodontal infection. Sore throat, drooling, and fever may suggest epiglottitis in children or adults. While children should be examined in the operating room, in adults epiglottis may be visualized by direct or indirect laryngoscopy in the ED. Although epiglottitis is rare since the introduction of the *Haemophilus influenzae* type b (Hib) vaccine, clinicians should still retain a high level of suspicion, especially in children from foreign countries. While most of North America, Central America, South America, Australia and Western Europe have national vaccination programs, Eastern Europe and Asia (including Japan, China, and the Soviet Union) do not routinely vaccinate for Hib.

The chest should be examined for indications of a pulmonary or cardiac cause of fever. Localized rales or rhonchi suggest pneumonia. As x-ray findings frequently lag behind physical findings, an early pneumonia may not be visible on x-ray. A pericardial rub is indicative of pericarditis, and a new heart murmur should suggest endocarditis, especially in intravenous (IV) drug users. However, functional murmurs may increase due to fever-induced tachycardia.

The abdomen should be examined for signs of peritoneal irritation or ascites. Localized pain may suggest cholecystitis, appendicitis, pancreatitis, or diverticulitis. Suprapubic pain suggests a urinary tract infection. A rectal examination may demonstrate evidence of a perirectal abscess or prostatitis. In patients with a urethral discharge, a detailed sexual history should be obtained. A swollen or painful testicle suggests epididymoorchitis or torsion. In women, a pelvic examination should be performed to evaluate for sexually transmitted diseases and cervical motion tenderness suggestive of pelvic inflammatory disease or tuboovarian abscesses.

Examination of the musculoskeletal system is often overlooked in febrile patients, but examination of the spine may reveal tenderness suggestive of osteomyelitis, discitis, or epidural abscess (especially in IV drug users). A detailed examination of the extremities may demonstrate a septic or inflamed joint, or it may suggest osteomyelitis, myositis, or deep venous thrombosis. In IV drug users, skin-popping and track-mark sites should be examined for evidence of cutaneous abscesses, crepitation suggestive of soft-tissue infection, and infected pseudoaneurysms.

DIFFERENTIAL DIAGNOSIS

Infection

Infection is the most common cause of fever. Infection may originate in any portion of the body and lead to a febrile response. Much of the emergency physician's time is spent ascertaining the source of the fever and attempting to differentiate a viral from a bacterial etiology.

Drug-Induced Hyperthermia

Drug-induced hyperthermic syndromes include neuroleptic malignant syndrome (NMS), malignant hyperthermia (MH), and serotonin syndrome (SS). Because all three syndromes share similar presentations, with severe muscle contraction and hyperpyrexia, they share common complications of rhabdomyolysis, myoglobinemia, and intravascular hemolysis. Temperatures above 42°C cause central nervous system (CNS) damage, initially

---

TABLE 10.1.   Diagnostic Criteria for Neuroleptic Malignant Syndrome

PATIENT TAKING NEUROLEPTIC WITH

Fever, muscle rigidity, and elevated CPK

OR TWO OF THE ABOVE, PLUS FOUR OF THE FOLLOWING:

Tachycardia
Abnormal blood pressure
Tachypnea
Altered mental status
Diaphoresis
Leukocytosis

CPK, creatine phosphokinase.

---

to the more sensitive cerebellum and eventually to the cerebral cortex, brainstem, and spinal cord. Patients may also develop pulmonary embolism, cardiovascular collapse, myocardial infarction, and acute respiratory failure.

NMS is a rare idiosyncratic reaction to neuroleptic medications. It has also been reported in patients taking lithium. NMS is thought to result from dopamine depletion in the brain, possibly in combination with increased anticholinergic activity. Diagnostic criteria for NMS are presented in Table 10.1. In general, NMS presents with altered mental status, autonomic instability, hyperpyrexia, and muscular rigidity, which develop rapidly over 1 to 3 days. Temperature in excess of 41°C has been reported. Muscular rigidity of the thorax may impair breathing. Autonomic dysfunction may cause severe variations of both blood pressure and pulse, and some patients may develop seizures.

Malignant hyperthermia is a rare, genetically determined reaction to inhaled anesthetic gases, depolarizing muscle relaxants (e.g., succinylcholine) and other agents. Succinylcholine is more likely to cause MH than are inhaled anesthetic gases. In affected patients, the offending agent triggers the release of calcium by the sarcoplasmic reticulum, resulting in increased muscle contraction and oxygen consumption. Masseter muscle spasm is generally noted initially, and then generalized muscle rigidity leads rapidly to hyperpyrexia. Some patients develop recurrent symptoms 48 hours after the initial episode.

Serotonin syndrome (SS) is a reaction to serotonin-active agents and most commonly occurs after an increase in dosage of a drug or with the addition of a new drug to another serotonin-active agent. Common drugs that may cause serotonin syndrome are listed in Table 10.2. SS involves an alteration in mental status, autonomic dysfunction, and increased neuromuscular activity, the latter causing a rise in temperature. Diagnostic criteria for SS are presented in Table 10.3. Mental status changes may be manifested as agitation, confusion, drowsiness, coma, or seizures. Autonomic dysfunction may produce nausea, salivation, tachycardia, diaphoresis, diarrhea, hyperthermia, hypertension, and mydriasis. Reported neuromuscular findings include ankle clonus, hyperreflexia, rigidity, tremor, ataxia and myoclonus. Symptoms can be seen within 15 minutes of ingestion and can last for up to 6 hours. The duration of symptoms in other cases is dependent on drug half-life, but, in severe cases, symptoms can persist for up to 6 weeks.

Pulmonary Embolus

Research using patient data from the Prospective Investigation of Pulmonary Embolism Diagnosis (PIOPED) study found, after eliminating other sources of fever, 24% of patients with a pulmonary embolus were febrile. While the fever in the majority of these patients was low grade, 6% had a temperature ≥ 38.3°C and 2% had a temperature ≥ 38.9°C (31).

TABLE 10.2. Drugs That Cause Serotonin Syndrome

SELECTIVE INHIBITORS OF SEROTONIN UPTAKE

Fluoxetine (Prozac), Paroxetine (Paxil)
Sertraline (Zoloft), Trazodone
Meperidine, Dextromethorphan
Fluvoxamine (Luvox)

SPECIFIC SEROTONIN AGONISTS

Buspirone
LSD, Mescaline

NONSPECIFIC SEROTONIN AGONISTS

Bromocriptine, Bupropion
Phenytoin, Tryptophan
Levodopa, Lithium

OTHER DRUGS

Chlorpheniramine, Brompheniramine
Ginseng, St. John's wort
Tramadol

NONSPECIFIC INHIBITORS OF SEROTONIN REUPTAKE

Clomipramine (Anafranil)
Venlafaxine (Effexor)
Nefazodone (Serzone)

AGENTS THAT INCREASE SEROTONIN RELEASE

Amphetamine, MDMA (Ecstasy)
Cocaine, Codeine
Reserpine

MONOAMINE OXIDASE INHIBITORS

Pargyline (Eutonyl)
Phenelzine (Nardil)
Selegiline (Eldepryl)
Isocarboxazid (Marplan)
Procarbazine (Matulane)
Tranylcypromine (Parnate)
Isoniazid
Moclobemide

Drug Ingestion

Drugs associated with elevated temperature include cocaine, amphetamines, belladonna alkaloids, tricyclic antidepressants, and monoamine-oxidase inhibitors. As discussed previously, elderly patients with chronic salicylate poisoning are also prone to fever.

TABLE 10.3. Diagnostic Criteria for Serotonin Syndrome

THE ADDITION OR INCREASE IN DOSAGE OF A SEROTONERGIC AGENT, PLUS THREE OF THE FOLLOWING:

Agitation
Mental status changes
Diaphoresis
Diarrhea
Myoclonus
Fever
Tremor
Hyperreflexia
Incoordination
No neuroleptic has been involved

Central Nervous System Lesions

Structural lesions, head trauma, and strokes can cause elevated temperature either by direct destruction of the hypothalamic thermoregulatory center (hypothermia is more likely) or, more commonly, by blood irritating the central receptors in the preoptic area. Acute subdural hematomas may elevate body temperature; nonaccidental trauma should be considered in an irritable infant with unexplained fever, especially if circumstances raise suspicion of possible abuse.

Rheumatologic and Connective Tissue Disorders

Fever may be the only initial manifestation of many connective tissue and rheumatologic disorders. In systemic lupus erythematosus (SLE), fever is the initial symptom in 5% of cases. In older patients, temporal arteritis may present as recurrent fevers with no identifiable source.

Drug Fever

While any drug can cause a febrile reaction, penicillin and penicillin analogues are the most frequent causative agents. The fever typically begins 7 to 10 days after the patient starts taking the drug, and there is an associated rash in 18% of cases and eosinophilia in 22% of cases. Drugs that are commonly associated with a drug fever are listed in Table 10.4. Drug fever should always be a diagnosis of exclusion.

TABLE 10.4. Drugs Commonly Associated with Drug Fevers

ANTIBIOTICS

Cephalosporins
Isoniazid
Nitrofurantoin
Penicillins
Rifampin
Sulfonamides

ANTICANCER DRUGS

Bleomycin
Streptozocin

ANTICONVULSANTS

Carbamazepine
Phenytoin
Barbiturates

CARDIAC DRUGS

Hydralazine
Methyldopa
Nifedipine
Procainamide
Quinidine

NSAIDs

Ibuprofen
Salicylates

OTHERS

Cimetidine
Iodides

Neoplastic Diseases

While many different malignancies and tumors may produce fever, leukemia, Hodgkin's disease and non-Hodgkin's lymphoma, hepatoma, and atrial myxoma are the most common. However, because the underlying disease or its treatment often leaves the patient immunosuppressed, it is important to eliminate occult infection as the etiology of the fever.

Factitious Fever

Factitious or self-induced fever should be suspected if the history is suspicious, if other vital signs do not correlate with the degree of fever, or if the patient does not appear ill. Patients may have an underlying psychiatric disorder, such as a personality disorder or psychosis, or there may be an issue of secondary gain (e.g., work avoidance). Factitious fever is most common in females, and many are health care professionals or have a medical background. The easiest way to detect a factitious fever is to simultaneously measure temperatures at two or more body sites (e.g., oral and rectal), or measure the temperature of a freshly voided urine sample, which should reflect the true core temperature.

DIAGNOSTIC APPROACH

At presentation, it is important to obtain an accurate temperature measurement. Unfortunately, this measurement is commonly circumvented for the sake of convenience. Recorded temperatures may vary widely depending on the method used to obtain them. Rectal temperatures have long been the gold standard, but because of the invasiveness and relative difficulty of obtaining them, easier methods, such as oral, axillary, tympanic, pacifier and temporal artery thermometers are often employed. Multiple studies have shown that none of these alternative methods consistently provides a temperature comparable to the rectal temperature. In addition, there appears to be no standard correction factor that may be used to improve their accuracy.

The rectal temperature, which most accurately reflects the core temperature, tends to be, on average, 0.7°C higher than a simultaneously obtained oral temperature. Oral temperatures can, in fact, vary more than 1.6°C, depending on where the probe is positioned in the mouth. In addition, an increase in respiratory rate results in decreased oral temperatures.

While axillary temperatures are generally felt to be approximately 1°C lower than rectal temperatures, they have repeatedly been shown to be unreliable and miss many patients with significant fevers. In addition, studies have shown there is no reliable correction factor that would allow conversion of axillary to rectal temperatures.

The tympanic thermometer is frequently employed because it is noninvasive and rapid; however, numerous studies in both adults and children have shown that temperatures obtained tympanically are a poor reflection of the rectal temperature. A recent meta-analysis of 31 studies involving over four thousand children found the difference between rectal and tympanic techniques too great to rely on tympanic measurements (10). Like oral and axillary temperatures, no single correction factor will allow conversion of tympanic to rectal temperatures, and discrepancies exist in spite of using the rectal equivalency setting on the tympanic thermometer.

Newer innovations for obtaining temperatures are the pacifier and temporal artery thermometers. Pacifier thermometers measure supralingual temperatures and are relatively sensitive for detecting fevers (after adding a 0.5°F correction factor). However, they are impractical in the clinical setting because they take

approximately 4 minutes to produce a reading (28). Temporal artery thermometers measure infrared emissions through the skin over the temporal artery and are better for detecting higher fevers than low grade fevers. Studies are currently lacking to recommend their routine use (28).

Laboratory Evaluation

While no test exists that easily identifies patients with serious infections, a thorough understanding of certain basic laboratory tests can greatly enhance patient evaluation. The white blood cell (WBC) count is the oldest and best-known screening test used to differentiate serious bacterial infections from other disorders. In adults as well as children, however, its discriminatory value is not as great as most expect. In a study of adults with unexplained fever after careful physical examination, only 15% had a WBC count $\geq$ 15,000/μL, and only 56% of those patients were subsequently shown to have a bacterial source (23). In addition, an elevated WBC count is nonspecific. Neutrophilia may occur secondary to emotional or physical stress, acute or chronic inflammation, benign or malignant tumors, myeloproliferative disorders, asthma, seizures, or medications such as steroids, lithium, or epinephrine. Neutrophil counts over 30,000/μL have been reported secondary to strenuous exercise, seizures, and lithium use (35). In addition, patients with low WBC counts (less than 1,000/μL) are at significant risk for occult bacterial infections.

A "left shift" is only slightly more useful. A total neutrophil band count greater than 1,500/μL was found in approximately one-third of adult patients with unexplained fever, of which only half proved to have bacterial infections (23). Several noninfectious processes including burns, fractures, steroids, diabetic ketoacidosis and Addison's disease can increase the WBC count. From these data, it is apparent that the WBC count is neither sensitive nor specific for bacterial infection.

In febrile infants 1 to 3 months old, the WBC count has often been used as a discriminator of those needing a full septic work up versus less complete evaluations. Two recent studies from Children's Hospital, Boston reveal, however, that the peripheral WBC count is an inaccurate screen for meningitis and bacteremia in young infants (4,5). There was no statistical difference in the WBC count of those with or without bacteremia; and, using a cutoff of 15,000/μL, the sensitivity for detecting bacteremia or meningitis was 45% and 27%, respectively. One drawback of these studies was the inclusion of infants less than 1 month old, a patient population that would usually receive a full septic work up regardless of their WBC count.

Certain changes in neutrophil morphology are associated with bacterial infections. Toxic granulations are small, dark cytoplasmic inclusions found in 75% of bacteremic patients. They can also be seen in patients with vasculitis and in those who are on chemotherapy. Döhle bodies are round or oval cytoplasmic inclusions seen in 29% of bacteremic patients, as well as in patients with burns, trauma, neoplasms, or during pregnancy. In one study, 91% of patients with more than 10% cytoplasmic vacuolization had bacteremia. Cytoplasmic vacuolization has not been proven to be useful in pediatric patients.

The occurrence of thrombocytopenia in septic patients has been recognized for many years. Studies have shown longer stays in the intensive care unit and a higher mortality rate in patients with thrombocytopenia. The role of platelets in sepsis is complex and is believed to be related to their ability to modulate their own function as well as that of cells around them (33).

Measurement of acute-phase reactants, erythrocyte sedimentation rate (ESR) and C-reactive protein (CRP), is often used to help recognize patients with serious occult infections. The results can be misleading, as these tests are neither sensitive nor specific. The ESR is often used as a screening test for temporal arteritis, bacterial endocarditis, tuberculosis, osteomyelitis, septic joints, and occult bacteremia in children (18). A major disadvantage of the ESR is the 1-hour time to complete the test; ESR is the distance, in millimeters, that red blood cells in citrated blood fall in 1 hour.

CRP is more sensitive and specific and rises faster than the ESR, but it is also not particularly useful in the emergency department. While many small studies have indicated that an elevated CRP may be useful in detecting acute intraabdominal infections, a metaanalysis of 22 studies using CRP to aid in the diagnosis of appendicitis found a combined sensitivity and specificity of only 62% and 66%, respectively (17). The individual studies showed a wide range of sensitivities (40% to 99%) and specificities (27% to 90%), believed to be due in part to the wide variation of cut-off values used. With the few exceptions noted previously, both the ESR and CRP are probably best used for following the resolution of a known disease.

While there is no consensus on the value of screening for streptococcal pharyngitis in febrile patients with a sore throat, many guidelines recommend some variation on the Centor criteria [history of fever, anterior cervical lymphadenopathy, tonsillar exudate, absence of cough] (9). Most commonly, it is recommended that patients with 0-1 criterion receive no testing and no antibiotics and those with 2-3 criteria undergo rapid streptococcal antigen testing and treatment instituted only for those with positive tests. Patients meeting all 4 criteria are generally felt to qualify for empiric antibiotics without antigen testing, but this results in a substantial number of patients receiving antibiotics that do not have the disease (3). In addition, using this system of treatment only applies to streptococcal disease and will miss other causes of pharyngitis, such as *Gonococcus, Chlamydia,* or *Mycoplasma.*

An appropriately performed urinalysis demonstrating pyuria and bacteriuria in patients with suprapubic pain, dysuria, frequency, or hesitancy supports a diagnosis of urinary tract infection (UTI). In young adult women, urine cultures are probably not necessary at the time of initial diagnosis. In older women, men, children, and patients with comorbid diseases, and in cases resistant to therapy, urine cultures are recommended. In a recent study of fever in infants less than 3 months of age, 19% of uncircumcised males and 13% of females had UTIs (25). Another study of infants less than 60 days old found an 85% sensitivity for a dipstick urinalysis positive for either nitrite or leukocyte esterase, an 80% sensitivity for a Gram stain showing an organism, and a 65% sensitivity for microscopy showing 5 or more WBC/hpf (12). In addition, in adults in whom there is a high clinical suspicion but a negative urinalysis, urine cultures should be obtained and initial treatment based on the degree of suspicion. The formation of significant levels of nitrites or leukocytes in the urine occurs over time (up to 6 hours), and therefore, patients with urinary frequency may have a falsely negative urinalysis. Conversely, 10% to 50% of nursing home patients have chronic asymptomatic bacteriuria (essentially 100% in those with indwelling catheters), so the diagnosis of UTI as a cause of fever or mental status changes should be made with some caution (2).

Because acute diarrhea is usually self-limited or viral in nature, stool evaluation is rarely helpful or necessary unless the patient is febrile, systemically ill, dehydrated, or has blood or pus in their stool. In ill patients, stool culture for *Salmonella, Shigella, Campylobacter,* and *E. coli O157:H7* is indicated. In developed countries, testing for fecal leukocytes is 73% sensitive and 84% specific for inflammatory diarrhea (32). Stool should be tested for *Clostridium difficile* toxin if there is a history of recent hospitalization or antibiotic use. The presence of ova or parasites is indicative of a parasitic etiology for diarrhea. An enzyme immunoassay is also available for Giardia and has a sensitivity of 95% (32). In travelers from malarious areas, malaria should also

be considered, as it may present with fever, gastrointestinal (GI) symptoms, and anemia, but without cells in the stool.

Like many laboratory tests, there is no consensus on the value of routine blood cultures in febrile patients. The incidence of bacteremia in the emergency department has been reported to vary from 2.6% to as high as 10.7% of febrile patients. The higher figures generally come from tertiary referral centers, the lower figures from community hospitals. Most community hospitals report approximately equal numbers of gram-positive and gram-negative bacteremia, whereas university centers report a much higher incidence of gram-negative bacteremia. Mortality from bacteremia ranges from 20% to 40%; there are no data, however, on mortality for clinically unsuspected bacteremia.

Several studies have shown that blood culture results rarely alter the treatment of patients with either community-acquired pneumonia (CAP) or nosocomial pneumonias. In one study of adult patients admitted for CAP, cultures were positive in only 5.7% of patients, and of those, the culture results altered therapy to a less resistant antibiotic in only 0.4% of the total patients (7).

Sklar and Rusnak (30) examined the value of outpatient blood cultures in febrile adults discharged from the emergency department. In this study, 5 of 86 patients subsequently proved to have positive blood cultures. All were contacted, and four were subsequently admitted. No long-term morbidity was noted. Of these patients, three were diagnosed with endocarditis and one with pyelonephritis. The fifth patient, who refused to return for admission, had presumed pneumococcal endocarditis. Each of the patients with endocarditis had identifiable risk factors (two with murmur and a history of rheumatic fever, one on dialysis and with a murmur, and one IV drug abuser). Other studies have shown that patients with underlying illnesses, most commonly diabetes, are at greater risk for bacteremia, and this study seems to support those findings. Therefore, it is prudent to limit outpatient blood cultures to febrile patients who have underlying diseases or risk factors (e.g., murmurs, IV drug use, immunosuppression, diabetes).

For inpatients, the current recommendations are to obtain cultures in patients with fever and signs of sepsis (hypotension, tachycardia, chills), in those with altered mental status, in ill-appearing patients with unexplained leukocytosis, and in immunocompromised patients. In addition, some recommend blood cultures to identify the causative organism in pneumonia, osteomyelitis, meningitis, or septic arthritis, but in general, it is preferable to obtain cultures directly from the infected site. Blood cultures are rarely helpful adjuncts in the management of immunocompetent patients with simple infections such as cellulitis, orchitis, dental infections, and most CAPs.

The management of neutropenic cancer patients (absolute neutrophil count < 500 cells/mm^3 or a count $< 1,000$ cells/mm^3 with a predicted decrease to < 500 cells/mm^3) presenting with a fever is evolving. Whereas previous guidelines recommended admission and IV antibiotics for all of these patients, recent strategies focus on early oral therapy, outpatient management, and discontinuation of antibiotics in low risk patients (19). Recommended evaluation of febrile neutropenic patients includes a thorough history and physical exam to localize a source of fever, CBC with differential, liver and renal function tests (necessary for antibiotic choices), and blood cultures for bacteria and fungi (one set from any central venous access device and one peripheral set). Urinalysis should be performed, as well as urine culture, if urinalysis is abnormal, there are signs or symptoms of a urinary tract infection, there is an indwelling catheter, or for pediatric patients. Chest radiograph should be obtained only if indicated by respiratory signs or symptoms or if there is consideration of outpatient therapy. Site-directed studies based on history and physical (e.g, lumbar puncture, aspiration and culture of abscesses) are also recommended.

TABLE 10.5. Factors Favoring Low Risk of Infection in Adults with Febrile Neutropenia (19)

Age <60 years
Absolute neutrophil and monocyte counts ≥ 100 cells/mm^3
Normal chest radiograph
Normal or near normal hepatic and renal function tests
Outpatient status at time of fever onset
Duration of neutropenia <7 days or expected resolution in <10 days
No IV catheter site infection
Early evidence of bone marrow recovery
Malignancy in remission
Peak temperature < 39°C
No prior history of fungal infection or treatment for fungal infections
Asymptomatic or non-ill appearing
Absence of neurologic or mental status changes
Absence of abdominal pain
No comorbid conditions or complications (e.g., diabetes, lung disease, hypotension)

Because patients with bacterial infections cannot reliably be distinguished from noninfected patients at presentation, empiric IV antibiotics should be administered promptly. After evaluation, patients that look well, have no focus of bacterial infection (including vomiting or diarrhea) and are felt to be at low risk for severe infection may be considered for outpatient antibiotic therapy if they can be carefully observed at home and have prompt access to health care 24 hours a day. Factors favoring a low risk of infection in adults are listed in Table 10.5. Children may be considered for outpatient therapy if they meet these same criteria, but are disqualified for outpatient treatment if they are < 5 years of age, ≤ 12 months post stem-cell transplant, appear irritable or if they have a previous history of sepsis or bacteremia from neutropenia, a diagnosis of leukemia or leukemia in relapse, rigors with flushing of a central venous line, or mucositis (24).

Lumbar puncture to obtain cerebrospinal fluid (CSF) for analysis is recommended in patients with fever, headache, photophobia, and signs of meningeal irritation such as nuchal rigidity, Kernig's sign (with the thigh flexed at the hip, there is pain or resistance with knee extension) or Brudzinski's sign (passive flexion of the head onto the chest induces flexion of the lower limbs). However, since signs of meningeal irritation are frequently absent, especially in the very young or old, one must have a low threshold to perform a lumbar puncture in these patients. The CSF should be routinely analyzed for protein, glucose, Gram stain, and cell count with differential. In selected cases, a VDRL/RPR for syphilis, viral cultures, or tests for bacterial antigens should be added.

Various antigenic tests are available; they have the advantage of identifying a specific organism when positive. Latex agglutination is rapid, economical, and noninvasive. Better results are obtained with urine than with serum or CSF, presumably because the antigens are more concentrated in urine. Unfortunately, these tests historically have had a high specificity (greater than 99%) but a low sensitivity. The sensitivity is best for *Haemophilus influenzae* type b (Hib) and *Group B streptococci* (61% and 67%, respectively) and much worse for *Streptococcus pneumoniae* (7%) (1). The importance of detecting Hib has diminished with the decline in documented cases as a result of the introduction of the Hib vaccine. While there may be a theoretical advantage in identifying the causative organism, one study has shown that, in clinical practice, treatment and disposition decisions are made without utilizing the latex agglutination results (1). Latex agglutination is less useful in adults because they are at risk for many more pathogens. Commercial reagents are available only for *Streptococcus pneumoniae*, *Neisseria meningitidis*, *H. influenzae*, and *Group B streptococci*.

Enzyme-linked immunosorbent assay (ELISA), an immunologic test, is much more sensitive in detecting pneumococci than is latex agglutination. An ELISA assay is also used to detect West Nile virus IgM, but this test may be falsely negative if tested too early as IgM takes time to develop. Quicker means of identifying organisms grown in blood cultures are also available. DNA probes have been developed that, when mixed with the growth from positive blood culture bottles, directly and rapidly identify *Staphylococcus aureus*, *Streptococcus pneumoniae*, *Escherichia coli*, *H. influenzae*, *Enterococcus* sp., and *Streptococcus agalactiae*. This method uses a chemiluminescent probe that detects the rRNA of the target organism.

Polymerase chain reaction (PCR) is useful in diagnosing viral meningitis and has a high sensitivity and specificity for *Herpes* simplex type I, Epstein-Barr virus, *Enterovirus*, and *Cytomegalovirus* (considered the gold standard for CMV). PCR can also detect tuberculosis and acute neurosyphilis.

Radiologic Studies

Routine chest radiographs are commonly obtained in patients who present with fever without an obvious source. This practice is probably based on studies that show a lack of auscultatory findings in patients with infiltrates on chest radiographs. In one study, physical exams performed by an experienced internist, pulmonologist, and infectious disease subspecialist were only 47% to 69% sensitive in detecting radiographically proven pneumonia. However, all of these patients had symptoms suggestive of pneumonia and did not represent patients with a fever and no source (34). In infants and children, chest radiographs are currently recommended in patients with fever and signs or symptoms of a lower respiratory tract infection (e.g., rales, rhonchi, wheezing, retractions, tachypnea, stridor, and cough). In one study of 197 febrile infants less than 3 months old, 40 had no respiratory signs or symptoms (6). Radiographs in these 40 were normal in all but four, and the only abnormality present in these four was hyperinflation.

Signs or symptoms should guide the need for other radiologic studies. Plain films may reveal osteomyelitis in patients with fever and bone pain, but bone scans and magnetic resonance imaging (MRI) are more sensitive. Abdominal radiographs may identify free air (bowel perforation), appendicoliths or focal ileus (appendicitis), thumbprinting or gas in the bowel wall (mesenteric ischemia), or pneumobilia or gallstones (cholecystitis). Patients with fever and abdominal pain may benefit from an ultrasound to evaluate for the presence of cholecystitis or a tuboovarian abscess. Computed tomography scans should be used in selected patients to evaluate for appendicitis, abdominal abscess, or diverticulitis. Magnetic resonance imaging should be considered in IV drug abusers with back pain and fever to rule out epidural abscess.

CRITICAL INTERVENTIONS

The choice of antibiotics should, when possible, be based on the type and site of infection. Patients with suspected meningitis should receive antibiotics immediately unless the lumbar puncture can be performed without delaying treatment. Most commonly, treatment is initiated with ceftriaxone 50 mg/kg IV in pediatric patients and 2 grams IV in adult patients. Neonates are treated with cefotaxime 50 mg/kg IV with the addition of ampicillin 50 mg/kg IV to treat *Listeria*. Immunocompromised adults (e.g., alcoholics) should also receive ampicillin 2 grams IV in addition to ceftriaxone to cover *Listeria*. Vancomycin 15 mg/kg (maximum 1 gram) IV should be added to these treatments if drug-resistant *Streptococcus pneumoniae* is suspected.

Septic patients should be started on broad-spectrum antibiotics after appropriate specimens for culture are obtained. It is probably best not to initiate antibiotics in febrile patients with an unknown source who appear nontoxic and are not thought to be septic. Suggested antibiotic regimens for the initial treatment of sepsis in immunocompetent and neutropenic cancer patients are listed in Table 10.6. Although trials testing outpatient oral antibiotics in low risk children with febrile neutropenia are ongoing, this strategy is currently recommended only for low risk adult patients. Low risk children may be treated as outpatients using a broad-spectrum parenteral antibiotic, usually once daily ceftriaxone.

In addition to antibiotic therapy, a recent study by Rivers, et al., showed that septic patients treated in the emergency department for at least 6 hours with goal-directed therapy had a significantly lower mortality than patients treated with standard therapy (30.5% vs. 46.5%, respectively) (29). Goal-directed therapy consisted of adjusting cardiac preload, afterload and contractility in an effort to balance oxygen delivery with demand. Patients randomized to goal-directed therapy received a central venous catheter capable of measuring central venous oxygen saturation and were treated with boluses of IV crystalloid, vasopressors or vasodilators, red cell transfusions, dobutamine, and intubation as needed in order to optimize oxygen delivery and consumption.

Antipyretics are frequently used in febrile patients who are significantly uncomfortable or tachycardic. Many patients and parents, as well as practitioners, believe that fever is harmful or likely to cause harm. A survey of pediatricians in Massachusetts showed that 58% felt fever greater than 104°F could cause seizures and 10% felt brain damage could occur (22). Similarly, a survey of emergency department nurses found 57% felt seizures were the primary concern in a child with fever and 29% felt permanent brain damage or death could occur (27). In spite of these beliefs, no studies have shown true fevers to be harmful, and the use of antipyretics has not been shown to decrease the recurrence rate of febrile seizures in children (13). Finally, the response to antipyretics does not allow the differentiation between serious (e.g., bacterial) and nonserious (e.g., viral) infections (26). In addition, some practitioners believe there is an unwarranted phobia of fever in children, resulting in knee-jerk administration of antipyretics without first judging the overall appearance of the child (i.e., when febrile, does the child look toxic, or is he or she active and playful?). Most parents report that their practice of giving antipyretics at the first sign of fever was influenced by the practice of health care providers. Parental anxiety is greatly reduced if they are educated on the risks and benefits of fever and the need for proper management. It should be noted, however, that the rise in core body temperature associated with fever must be differentiated from temperature elevations secondary to hyperthermia. Interestingly, while hyperthermia may cause severe metabolic and neurologic compromise or death, pyogenic cytokines are not directly involved and standard antipyretic therapy is usually ineffective (26).

If the decision is made to use antipyretics to treat discomfort (rigors, chills, headache, malaise) and there are no contraindications, adults should receive oral doses of acetaminophen 650 to 1000 mg or ibuprofen 800 mg. Children should receive 15 to 20 mg/kg acetaminophen orally or rectally. Some providers give an initial, single rectal loading dose of 30 to 40 mg/kg, although studies vary as to the efficacy and toxicity of this higher dose. Ibuprofen dosed at 10 mg/kg orally may be used in children over 6 months of age. Because of the potential for dehydration in febrile infants less than 6 months old, ibuprofen is not recommended because it may increase the risk of kidney damage.

Once the symptoms of malignant hyperthermia are identified, treatment should be instituted as outlined in Table 10.7. Dantro-lene, the mainstay of treatment, is a muscle relaxant that decreases the release of calcium by the sarcoplasmic reticulum. The dosage is 2.5 mg/kg IV q6h, up to a maximum of 10 mg/kg/d. Agents safe for use in patients with MH include vecuronium, pancuronium, etomidate, propofol, opiates, barbiturates, and benzodiazepines.

In addition, all patients with hyperthermia > 41°C, whether from malignant hyperthermia, neuroleptic malignant syndrome, or serotonin syndrome, should be cooled rapidly with cool IV fluids, fans, cool-water spray, or cooling blankets. Patients should be monitored for rhabdomyolysis or treated prophylactically with sodium bicarbonate.

Specific treatment for neuroleptic malignant syndrome is not well established. Neuroleptic agents should be discontinued. Dantrolene appears to be most useful in patients with prominent muscle contraction (see above). Bromocriptine mesylate, a dopamine agonist, is widely used alone or in combination with dantrolene; the dosage is 2.5 to 7.5 mg orally q8h. Bromocriptine is most useful when hyperthermia is not accompanied by dramatic muscle rigidity. Levodopa and carbidopa–levodopa are useful in many patients, particularly those in whom NMS is associated with the recent withdrawal of these medications.

Treatment of SS consists of discontinuing the offending medication and providing supportive care. Benzodiazepines have been useful in decreasing hyperactivity.

DISPOSITION

When considering the disposition of the febrile patient, the single most important consideration is age and general health. Infants less than 90 days old require an extensive evaluation, and selected patients 30 to 90 days old may be discharged with close follow up within 24 hours. Most of these patients are routinely treated with ceftriaxone 50 to 100 mg/kg IM prior to discharge. For a discussion of the management of infants and children with a fever, see Chapter 224, Fever of Acute Onset.

Children and young adults who appear nontoxic and have no medical problems have a very slight chance of developing a serious infection (with the exception of IV drug abusers). As the age and presence of underlying medical problems increase, the chance of serious occult infection increases and makes admission advisable. Keating and associates (20) found that 95% of patients who were older than 60 years and had a temperature above 101°F (38.3°C) on admission to the emergency department had a serious infection, and 92.5% required admission.

Any patient with unexplained fever and neutropenia or malignancy should be admitted for a full "septic" work up. Patients with diabetes are at special risk, as are patients who are taking corticosteroids. Alcoholics are also considered to be immunosuppressed and at increased risk. They have many alterations in their host defenses and may require admission for infections that are often treated on an outpatient basis among other populations.

The postsplenectomy patient is at special risk for developing clinically inapparent bacteremia, usually from *S. pneumoniae*. Such patients often have fever and a flu-like syndrome as their only complaints. Even when these patients are promptly diagnosed and started on antibiotics, there is a 50% to 75% mortality; these patients should all be encouraged to be immunized against *S. pneumoniae*.

If good follow up can be arranged, specimens for cultures can be obtained in the emergency department, and the nontoxic, low-risk patient can be discharged and rechecked in 24 hours when initial culture results become available. Continued follow up or contact is necessary until cultures are confirmed to be negative.

TABLE 10.6.   Suggested Antibiotic Regimens for the Initial Treatment of Septic Patients

Patient	Antibiotic
Neonate (1 wk–2 mo)	Cefotaxime 50 mg/kg IV *plus* ampicillin 50 mg/kg IV
Infant/child	Cefotaxime 50 mg/kg IV *or* ceftriaxone 50–100 mg/kg IV
Adult	Ticarcillin/clavulanic acid 3.1 g IV plus gentamicin 2 mg/kg IV *or* Piperacillin/tazobactam 3.375 g IV plus gentamicin 2 mg/kg IV *or* Imipenem 500–1,000 mg IV or meropenem 1 g IV
PCN allergic patients (Adults and children)	Vancomycin 15 mg/kg IV (max. 1 g) plus gentamicin 2 mg/kg IV or Aztrednam 30 mg/kg IV (max. 1–9)
Neutropenic patients (Adults and children)	Gentamicin 2 mg/kg IV or tobramycin 2 mg/kg IV Plus Ticarcillin/clavulanic acid 50 mg/kg IV (max. 3.1 g) or piperacillin/tazobactam 80 mg/kg IV (max. 3.375 g) or ceftazidime 50 mg/kg IV (max. 2 g) or cefepime 50 mg/kg IV (max. 2 g) or imipenem (> 3 months old) 25 mg/kg IV (max. 1 g) or meropenem 40 mg/kg IV (max. 1 g) Plus (if indicated*) Vancomycin 15 mg/kg IV (max. 1 g)
Outpatient oral therapy (low-risk adults only)	Amoxicillin-clavulanate 875 mg po bid plus ciprofloxacin 750 mg po bid

*Vancomycin is indicated if central IV access is infected, suspected drug resistant *Streptococcus pneumoniae* (DRSP) or methicillin resistant *Staphylococcus aureus* (MRSA), hypotension or blood culture positive for gram-positive cocci.

TABLE 10.7.   Treatment of Malignant Hyperthermia

Discontinue precipitating agent
Administer dantrolene 2.5 mg/kg IV, up to 10 mg/kg/d
Infuse saline with sodium bicarbonate to maintain urinary output
　　Monitor systemic pH to prevent alkalosis
Cool patient with cooling blanket, ice packs, or evaporation
Monitor for electrolyte imbalance and cardiac dysrhythmias
　　Avoid the use of calcium antagonists or digoxin

COMMON PITFALLS

✔ Failure to obtain a rectal temperature when a fever is important to the evaluation and management of a pediatric patient
✔ Ignoring parental reports of fever in infants who are afebrile on arrival to the emergency department
✔ Attributing fever in infants to overbundling
✔ Relying on the WBC count to determine the presence or seriousness of an infection
✔ Relying on the response to antipyretics to help differentiate serious from nonserious infections
✔ Failure to immediately cool patients with severe hyperthermia (greater than 41°C), regardless of the underlying etiology
✔ Failure to monitor and treat hyperthermic patients for rhabdomyolysis, renal failure, and other end-organ damage
✔ Administering serotonin-active drugs, including such commonly prescribed medications as meperidine and dextromethorphan, to patients receiving serotonin agonists

Acknowledgments

Thanks to the previous edition's chapter author of "Drug-Induced Hyperthermic Syndromes," *Sandra M. Schneider.*

References

1. Adcock PM, Paul RI, Marshall GS. Effect of urine latex agglutination tests on the treatment of children at risk for invasive bacterial infection. *Pediatrics* 1995;96:951–954.
2. Bentley DW, Bradley S, High K, Schoenbaum S, Taler G, Yoshikawa TT. Practice guideline for evaluation of fever and infection in long-term care facilities. *J Am Geriatr Soc* 2001;49:210–222.
3. Bisno AL, Peter GS, Kaplan EL. Diagnosis of strep throat in adults: are clinical criteria really good enough? *Clin Infect Dis* 2002;35:126–129.
4. Bonsu BK, Harper MB. Utility of the peripheral blood white blood cell count for identifying sick young infants who need lumbar puncture. *Ann Emerg Med* 2003;41:206–214.
5. Bonsu BK, Harper MB. Identifying febrile young infants with bacteremia: is the peripheral white blood cell count an accurate screen? *Ann Emerg Med* 2003;42:216–225.
6. Bramson RT, Meyer TL, Silbiger ML, Blickman JG, Halpern E. The futility of the chest radiograph in the febrile infant without respiratory symptoms. *Pediatrics* 1993;92:524–526.
7. Campbell SG, Marrie TJ, Anstey R, Dickinson G, Ackroyd-Stolarz S. The contribution of blood cultures to the clinical management of adult patients admitted to the hospital with community-acquired pneumonia: a prospective observational study. *Chest* 2003;123:1142–1150.
8. Castle SC, Yeh M, Toledo S, Yoshikawa TT, Norman DC. Lowering the temperature criterion improves detection of infections in nursing home residents. *Aging Immunol Infect Dis* 1993;4:67–76.
9. Centor RM, Witherspoon JM, Dalton HP, Brody CE, Link K. The diagnosis of strep throat in adults in the emergency room. *Med Decis Making* 1981;1:239–246.
10. Craig JV, Lancaster GA, Taylor S, Williamson PR, Smyth RL. Infrared ear thermometry compared with rectal thermometry in children: a systematic review. *Lancet* 2002;360:603–609.
11. Davis TME, Makepeace AE, Dallimore EA, Choo KE. Relative bradycardia is not a feature of enteric fever in children. *Clin Infect Dis* 1999;28:582–586.
12. Dayan PS, Bennett J, Best R, et al. Test characteristics of the urine Gram stain in infants ≤ 60 days of age with fever. *Pediatr Emerg Care* 2002;18:12–14.
13. El-Radhi AS, Barry W. Do antipyretics prevent febrile convulsions? *Arch Dis Child* 2003;88:641–642.
14. Gobbi PG, Pieresca C, Ricciardi L, et al. Night sweats in Hodgkin's disease. *Cancer* 1990;65:2074–2077.
15. Graneto JW, Soglin DF. Maternal screening of childhood fever by palpation. *Pediatr Emerg Care* 1996;12:183–184.
16. Grover G, Berkowitz CD, Lewis RJ, Thompson M, Berry L, Seidel J. The effects of bundling on infant temperature. *Pediatrics* 1994;94:669–673.

17. Hallan S, Åsberg A. The accuracy of C-reactive protein in diagnosing acute appendicitis-a meta-analysis. *Scand J Clin Lab Invest* 1997;57:373–380.
18. Harrow C, Singer AJ, Thode HC. Facilitating the use of the erythrocyte sedimentation rate in the emergency department. *Acad Emerg Med* 1999;6:658–660.
19. Hughes WT, Armstrong D, Bodey GP, et al. 2002 guidelines for the use of antimicrobial agents in neutropenic patients with cancer. *Clin Infect Dis* 2002;34:730–751.
20. Keating HJ, Klimek JJ, Levine DS, Kiernan FJ. Effect of aging on the clinical significance of fever in ambulatory adult patients. *J Am Geriatr Soc* 1984;32:282–287.
21. Knoebel EE, Narang AS, Ey JL. Fever: to treat or not to treat. *Clin Pediatr* 2002;41:9–16.
22. May A, Bauchner H. Fever phobia: The pediatrician's contribution. *Pediatrics* 1992;90:851–854.
23. Mellors JW, Horwitz RI, Harvey MR, Horwitz SM. A simple index to identify occult bacterial infection in adults with acute unexplained fever. *Arch Intern Med* 1987;147:666–671.
24. Orudjev E, Lange BJ. Evolving concepts of management of febrile neutropenia in children with cancer. *Med Pediatr Oncol* 2002;39:77–85.
25. Pantell RH, Newman TB, Bernzweig J, et al. Management and outcomes of care of fever in early infancy. *JAMA* 2004;291:1203–1212.
26. Plaisance KI, Mackowiak PA. Antipyretic therapy: physiologic rationale, diagnostic implications, and clinical consequences. *Arch Intern Med* 2000;160:449–456.
27. Poirier MP, Davis PH, Gonzalez-del Rey JA, Monroe KW. Pediatric emergency department nurses' perspectives on fever in children. *Pediatr Emerg Care* 2000;16:9–12.
28. Rideout ME, First LR. Fever: Measuring and managing a sizzling symptom. *Contemp Pediatr* 2001;18:42–50.
29. Rivers E, Nguyen B, Havstad S, et al. Early goal-directed therapy in the treatment of severe sepsis and septic shock. *N Engl J Med* 2001;345:1368–1377.
30. Sklar DP, Rusnak R. The value of outpatient blood cultures in the emergency department. *Am J Emerg Med* 1987;5:95–100.
31. Stein PD, Afzal A, Henry JW, Villareal CG. Fever in acute pulmonary embolism. *Chest* 2000;117:39–42.
32. Thielman NM, Guerrant RL. Acute infectious diarrhea. *N Engl J Med* 2004;350:38–47.
33. Vincent JL, Yagushi A, Pradier O. Platelet function in sepsis. *Crit Care Med* 2002;30[suppl.]:S313–S317.
34. Wipf JE, Lipsky BA, Hirschmann JV, et al. Diagnosing pneumonia by physical exam: relevant or relic? *Arch Intern Med* 1999;159:1082–1087.
35. Young GP. CBC or not CBC? That is the question. *Ann Emerg Med* 1986;15:367–371.

CHAPTER 11
Altered Mental Status and Coma

Marcus L. Martin and J. Stephen Huff

Consciousness is the sum of the activities and interactions between the reticular activating system and the cerebral cortex. A useful model is to think of the general state of alertness and wakefulness occurring in the reticular activating system, a group of neurons in the brainstem. Cognitive functions and a higher awareness of the environment are cerebro-cortical functions. For a human to be fully conscious, both of these systems must be intact anatomically and functionally.

CLINICAL PRESENTATION

An altered level of consciousness may be clinically characterized along a spectrum. Drowsiness or lethargy is a minor change; there is slightly decreased wakefulness and decreased interaction with the environment and the patient may be aroused by verbal stimuli or light touch. Coma is the state in which the patient cannot be awakened by any environmental stimuli. The comatose patient has complete failure of the arousal system, no spontaneous eye opening, and is unable to be awakened by vigorous sensory stimulation. Obtundation and stupor are intermediate stages in which the patient may be awakened only briefly by energetic stimulation. Delirium is a state of disturbed consciousness with restlessness and disorientation. A description of the stimulus and the patient's response to the stimulus is preferred to the use of inexactly employed clinical terms.

Some other persistent disorders of consciousness include the persistent vegetative state characterized by complete absence of self or environmental awareness but preserved capacity for spontaneous or stimulus-induced arousal. Sleep-wake cycles are present in the persistent vegetative state. The locked-in syndrome is a mimic of altered consciousness in which damage to efferent motor tracts causes the patient to appear unresponsive. Though quadriplegic and unable to speak, cognition and emotion are preserved. Sometimes vertical eye-movements are the only remnant of voluntary motor activity. Recently the "minimally conscious state" has been described in patients with inconsistent but discernible evidence of partial consciousness; these patients may demonstrate sustained visual fixation and limited motor function, including localizing stimuli and automatic movements such as scratching. Often clinicians underestimate the degree of an injured or disabled patient's awareness when that patient's responses to environmental stimulation are impaired.

Central nervous system (CNS) dysfunction from the cellular level to gross anatomic pathologic changes may cause altered mental status. If impaired at an anatomic structural level, there may be focal injury or dysfunction of CNS structures. This may result from increased intracranial pressure with mechanical compression of CNS structures or reduction in cerebral perfusion pressure, or from direct destruction due to tumors, trauma, stroke or hemorrhage. Dysfunction in almost any of the organ systems may impair CNS function at a cellular level. This dysfunction may occur with hypothyroidism or adrenal insufficiency; with disturbances of electrolyte regulation, which produce hypo- or hypernatremia or hypercalcemia; or with other metabolic disturbances, such as hypoglycemia or hyperosmolar states. Illnesses resulting in renal or hepatic damage may cause uremic and hepatic encephalopathy. Impairment of neurotransmitters may be the mechanism of some of these encephalopathies. Hypoxia from a pulmonary or cardiac etiology may also affect CNS function. Hypotension with decreased intracerebral perfusion may result from a primary cardiac etiology, sepsis, or volume loss from gastrointestinal (GI) bleeding or trauma. External environmental or toxic insults may also cause CNS depression at the cellular level through a direct toxic effect or secondarily through damage to specific organ systems.

In general, when the CNS function is impaired at a cellular level, diffuse CNS depression ensues and focal findings such as hemiparesis or abnormal extraocular movements are not present on clinical examination. Among the exceptions are hypoglycemia, hyperglycemia, and hepatic failure in which focal findings may be seen on occasion. Pupillary light reflexes generally remain intact with toxic and metabolic causes of altered mental status, except when the CNS depression is caused by certain toxins that affect pupillary size, such as anticholinergics or opiates.

There may be focal findings on examination when a destructive process causes structural damage to a specific area of the CNS. However, a localized problem may also cause a secondary diffuse process. This may be seen with the postictal state following a seizure, in cerebral edema secondary to a tumor, or in a subarachnoid hemorrhage secondary to a ruptured aneurysm.

DIFFERENTIAL DIAGNOSIS

The differential diagnosis of altered mental status and coma is extensive. In the emergency department, history and physical examination will help narrow the possibilities. History will usually suggest a likely cause and all historical sources—family, witnesses, EMS providers, and medical records—should be consulted if possible. The list of etiologies may be divided into several groups (Table 11.1). The high-risk conditions that result in altered mental status and coma are discussed below.

Hypoxia and Hypoglycemia

In the evaluation of any patient with mental status changes or coma, failure of substrate supply necessary for neuronal function must always be considered and ruled out. After evaluating for hypoxia and initiating oxygen supplementation, another common cause of altered mental status that is readily reversible and detectable should be considered—hypoglycemia. Hypoglycemia is most common in patients on insulin therapy. It may be due to dosage errors, missed meals, a change in exercise pattern, or erratic absorption from injection sites. Interaction with other drugs, such as alcohol, beta-blockers, or salicylates, may also lead to hypoglycemia. The oral hypoglycemic agents, including the first- and second-generation sulfonylureas and newer agents such as troglitazone, may also produce hypoglycemia. The half-life of these agents is long, so the patient should be admitted for appropriate glucose supplementation and careful monitoring if long-acting oral agents are thought to be the cause of the hypoglycemia. Hypoglycemia may also occur with alcohol intoxication and some other toxins.

The following drugs may potentiate the action of the oral hypoglycemics: clonidine, ethanol, beta-blockers, monoamineoxidase inhibitors, sulfonamides, coumarin anticoagulants, and salicylates. Salicylates may by themselves induce hypoglycemia. The predominant cause of hypoglycemia until age 2 is salicylate ingestion; alcohol predominates in the succeeding 8 years. Insulin and the oral hypoglycemics, alone or with alcohol, predominate until age 50. Over age 60, the oral hypoglycemics are the usual cause.

Renal or hepatic disease with impairment of function also increases the risk that a patient will develop hypoglycemia. Betablockers may inhibit some of the warning signs and symptoms for hypoglycemia, although sweating is minimally affected. Hypoglycemia may also be seen in other medical conditions, such as sepsis.

When blood glucose levels begin to fall (50–70 mg/dL), symptoms of CNS excitation appear; these may include anxiety, tremor, sweating, and occasionally hallucinations. With a fall to the range of 20 to 50 mg/dL, further symptoms may appear, including convulsions, loss of consciousness, hyperreflexia, pupillary dilation, and tachycardia. As the glucose level continues to fall, progressive CNS depression and coma may occur. Brain stem reflexes are preserved until late. Primitive movements such as sucking and pouting movements of the lips, forced grasping, or extensor plantar responses may be seen as cortical control is removed. Loss of consciousness is usually preceded by a period of confusion but it can occur suddenly. Hypoglycemia may also cause focal neurologic signs including hemiplegia and should be considered early in the differential diagnosis of stroke.

Hyperglycemia

At the other end of the glycemic spectrum is diabetic ketoacidosis (DKA). This may be seen in the emergency department as the initial presentation of new-onset juvenile diabetes, in a known diabetic with poor compliance, or in a diabetic with a precipitating stressful event, such as infection. Acute myocardial infarction or treatment with steroids may also be a factor. A history of polyuria, polydipsia, nausea, vomiting, or abdominal pain may be obtained. Weight loss may be a complaint in new-onset diabetes. The patient is dehydrated. Acetone breath or Kussmaul respirations may be present. Mental status changes, including coma, may be seen.

TABLE 11.1. Differential Diagnosis of Altered Mental Status and Coma

METABOLIC CAUSES

Electrolyte Disorders
  Hypernatremia
  Hyponatremia
  Hypercalcemia
  Hypoglycemia
  Hypermagnesemia (coma due to respiratory depression, hypoxia, hypotension)
Diabetic ketoacidosis
Hyperosmolar states
Hypothyroidism
Thyrotoxicosis
Adrenal insufficiency
Hepatic encephalopathy
Uremia
Thiamine deficiency (Wernicke's encephalopathy)

VASCULAR CAUSES

Hypertension
Hypotension
Vasculitis
Stroke (thrombotic or hemorrhagic)
Subarachnoid hemorrhage (aneurysm or AVM)

NEUROLOGIC ETIOLOGIES

Tumor
Hydrocephalus
Status epilepticus

TRAUMA

Subdural hematoma
Epidural hematoma
Cerebral contusion
Diffuse cerebral edema

INFECTIOUS ETIOLOGIES

Meningitis
Encephalitis
Intracranial abscess
Sepsis

TOXICOLOGIC ETIOLOGIES

Carbon monoxide
Ethanol, methanol, isopropyl alcohol, ethylene glycol
Drug abuse and overdose

ENVIRONMENTAL ETIOLOGIES

Heatstroke
Hypothermia
High-altitude cerebral edema (HACE)
Near-drowning
Dysbarism

AVM, arteriovenous malformation.

Hyperosmolar hyperglycemic nonketotic coma is typically seen in an older patient with undiagnosed or mild type II diabetes who experiences another illness. Gram-negative pneumonia, uremia with vomiting and acute viral illnesses are the most commonly reported predisposing conditions. The patient often has a longer history of symptoms before admission than in DKA and may present in coma. Mortality figures vary from 40% to 70%, in contrast to 1% to 10% for DKA.

Hypertension

In a patient with severe hypertension who presents with mental status changes, common causes include intracerebral hemorrhage or hypertensive encephalopathy. Hypertensive encephalopathy is a diagnosis of exclusion and requires evidence of retinal hemorrhages as well as high blood pressure and confusion or transient neurologic complaints. A subarachnoid hemorrhage due to a ruptured aneurysm or an arteriovenous malformation usually presents with diffuse findings on examination. The spectrum of presentation includes mild mental status changes to coma. The classic history is the sudden onset of a severe headache associated with nausea and vomiting. A patient may give a history of prodromal headaches in the preceding weeks. Sudden transient loss of consciousness is seen in 45% of patients. In a small percentage of patients with subarachnoid hemorrhage, the CT scan is normal. If a subarachnoid hemorrhage is suspected and the computed tomography (CT) scan is negative, a lumbar puncture must be performed.

Toxic Causes

Overdose of a wide variety of medications or illicit substances may produce a variety of mental status changes. Appropriate diagnosis requires an adequate history and familiarity with the constellation of signs and symptoms that may appear in specific toxicologic emergencies.

High doses of benzodiazepines may produce sedative–hypnotic effects. Cardiac depression is usually minor, as is respiratory depression. However, respiratory depression may become a problem if benzodiazepines are combined with other CNS depressants, in the elderly, or in patients with underlying respiratory disease. Opiates and barbiturates produce more severe respiratory depression. Hypotension may be seen with barbiturate overdoses and may also be seen with opiates. Miosis is usually present with opiates (an exception is meperidine, in which mydriasis may be seen). Glutethimide, formerly used as a sedative–hypnotic, has properties similar to those of the barbiturates; patients generally present with dilated pupils, and the drug tends to produce a fluctuating level of consciousness. The coma may be prolonged, lasting up to several days. Pulmonary edema is most commonly seen with intravenous heroin overdose, but may be present in other opiate or barbiturate intoxications. Cutaneous bullae and hypothermia may occur with barbiturate overdoses with prolonged unresponsiveness.

Alcohol intoxication may produce a somnolent, difficult-to-arouse patient with varying degrees of respiratory depression. Ingestion of substitute substances such as methanol, ethylene glycol, or isopropyl alcohol may also occur. Ingestion of isopropyl alcohol can present as stupor in a known alcoholic or as an encephalopathy of unknown cause in persons with hidden addictions. Along with CNS depression, GI effects (abdominal pain, gastritis, nausea, or vomiting) and cardiac toxicity can occur. The major metabolite of isopropyl alcohol is acetone; as such, the severe anion-gap metabolic acidosis seen in methanol and ethylene glycol poisoning is not seen with isopropyl poisoning. In methanol intoxication, the patient may present with visual changes ranging from blurred vision to blindness. Calcium ox-

alate crystals may be present in the urine of patients who have ingested ethylene glycol. The osmolal gap should be calculated and any discrepancy that cannot be attributed to ethanol ingestion must be considered.

Ingestion of tricyclic antidepressants may produce rapid mental status changes, seizures, and cardiovascular effects. Sinus tachycardia is most commonly noted. The QRS complex may become widened and atrial or ventricular dysrhythmias may occur. Anticholinergic effects such as delayed gastric emptying, decreased bowel sounds, and mydriasis may be present.

A history of prior tinnitus and vomiting may lead the clinician to suspect salicylate intoxication. Chronic salicylism in the elderly is often subtle. Respiratory alkalosis in adults or metabolic acidosis in children may be seen. Acetaminophen and salicylate levels should always be obtained in the patient comatose from an ingestion of any unknown substance or known ingestion of acetaminophen or salicylates. Carbon monoxide or cyanide inhalation should be suspected if the patient has been involved in a fire. Carbon monoxide poisoning should also be suspected in colder weather, particularly if the patient or others in the household have experienced flu-like symptoms. Arterial blood gas levels may show a normal PO_2, but the measured hemoglobin saturation may be low. Co-oximetry should be performed to quantitate carboxyhemoglobin and to look for other abnormal hemoglobin complexes. Cyanide interferes with the cellular use of oxygen; therefore, mixed venous PO_2 will be high, as cells cannot use the available oxygen. Cyanide also causes a severe metabolic lactic acidosis.

Seizures

Convulsive seizures usually offer little difficulty in recognition though the clinician must always remember that the seizures may be a symptom of another disease process, injury, ingestion, or withdrawal, and that epilepsy is largely a diagnosis of exclusion. Patients are often described as "postictal" yet there is no definition or test for this condition or any consensus as to the duration of the condition. Patients who are postictal following generalized convulsions often have altered mental status. However, it may be an underlying disease state causing the alteration in consciousness and the clinician must always consider possible etiologies or complications of the seizures particularly if the patient is not becoming more alert 20 to 30 minutes following cessation of the convulsions. Should the patient not be awakening following cessations of generalized convulsions, the possibility of "subtle" status epilepticus exists in which the abnormal electrical seizure activity is continuing in the absence of motor movements. Nonconvulsive status epilepticus may also present in the patient with altered mental status. These uncommon seizures with clouded consciousness or confusion require a high level of suspicion for recognition; typically there is a history of generalized seizures. Neurology consultation and electroencephalographic evaluation may be required for recognition.

Adrenal and Thyroid Emergencies

Adrenal and thyroid emergencies are not commonly seen in the emergency department, but are important in the differential diagnosis of coma since treatment may be life-saving. In a patient with suspected myxedema coma, history may reveal symptoms or prior treatment of hypothyroidism. Prior treatment of hyperthyroidism with radioactive iodine is associated with a relatively high incidence of eventual hypothyroidism. A surgical scar on the neck might alert the physician to the possibility of thyroid or parathyroid dysfunction. A history of noncompliance with thyroid medications may be obtained from the family.

Clinically, hypothermia to 36°C or lower may be seen, hypotension is common though blood pressure may be normal, and bradycardia is generally present. Periorbital and pretibial nonpitting edema may be present. The patient's hair may be dry with loss of the lateral eyebrows. The cardiac examination may be consistent with a pericardial effusion. On neurologic examination, the muscle relaxation phase of the deep tendon reflexes is classically delayed. Laboratory studies may reveal hyponatremia, hypoosmolarity, and an elevated creatine phosphokinase as well as abnormalities in the thyroid panel.

Thyroid storm rarely presents as coma. Confusion, agitation, or occasionally hallucinations are more common presentations. Hyperthermia above 38°C and tachycardia, with or without cardiac failure, may be present. Often a precipitating event such as trauma or infection is present.

Acute adrenal crisis may occur due to an acute exacerbation of chronic adrenal insufficiency, rapid cessation of chronic steroids, or adrenal hemorrhage. Physiologic stressors such as infection, trauma, or surgery may precipitate an adrenal crisis. Nausea, vomiting, abdominal pain, and fever may be noted. Hypovolemic shock may develop and the mental status may deteriorate into lethargy or coma. A patient with adrenal insufficiency or Addison's disease maintained on chronic glucocorticoid replacement may not develop dehydration and hypotension until late in the course of adrenal crisis, as mineralocorticoid secretion is usually preserved.

DIAGNOSTIC APPROACH

The initial assessment of a patient presenting with coma or transient loss of consciousness should be performed in a relatively short time and should be combined with stabilization procedures. The state of consciousness is determined by functioning of both the cerebral cortex and the ascending reticular activating system. Key observations will often help determine whether the disease is of the brainstem or cerebral hemispheres.

Before the patient arrives in the emergency department, field personnel should assist with airway support and administer oxygen. The spine is immobilized and stabilized if there is any possibility of trauma. Intravenous access is obtained, and cardiac monitoring is initiated. Bedside evaluation of blood sugar is performed when possible, and the patient should receive glucose if hypoglycemic. Any of the support mechanisms not performed by field personnel are initiated in the emergency department.

The history, physical examination, and serial neurologic examinations are all of importance. However, life-threatening and reversible processes causing coma or altered level of consciousness should be considered and addressed before a detailed history and physical are performed; these include hypoxia, hypoglycemia, poisoning, infections, and increased intracranial pressure secondary to trauma or other mechanisms. Evaluation of the cardiorespiratory status and blood glucose takes precedence over investigation of other potential etiologies. A large glucose load given to a patient with stroke or other brain injury may theoretically worsen the injury process and should be avoided when possible.

Obtaining historical information proceeds while stabilizing the patient. Information should include the abruptness of change in mental status, preceding events, medical history, current medications, and use of toxic agents. The clothing should be checked for suicide notes and drug bottles, and any medical alert tags should be noted. After the ABCs have been addressed, the patient is evaluated for signs of head trauma, including pupillary asymmetry and reactivity, hemotympanum, and Battle sign. The level of consciousness is documented, and the Glasgow Coma Scale used to quantify the patient's condition. Vital signs, including a core body temperature, are assessed.

Examination of the patient's eyes may be the single most important assessment in the evaluation of coma. An unresponsive patient who has open eyes may actually be in a persistent vegetative state or have the locked-in syndrome. The "locked-in syndrome" refers to patients who are paralyzed but in fact awake. This syndrome is often due to pontine infarction, but high cervical spinal cord injuries and severe drug-related dystonias may simulate the syndrome. The fundi are examined for lack of venous pulsation or evidence of papilledema, which might suggest increased intracranial pressure.

The shape and size of pupils and their reactions are recorded. Reactive asymmetric pupils differing in size by 1 to 2 mm (physiologic anisocoria) may be seen in 10% of normal people. Pupils are more likely to remain equal and reactive in cases of metabolic and drug etiology; a fixed, unilaterally dilated pupil in an unresponsive patient suggests transtentorial herniation. Local trauma or topical mydriatics can also cause unilateral dilation. The patient with a possible head or neck injury presents a problem with the performance of the doll's-eye maneuvers (oculocephalic reflex).

Ice water caloric testing (oculovestibular reflex) may be performed to detect the presence of nystagmus. The slow phase of reflex extraocular movements is driven by the brainstem and the fast jerk-like phase (the visible nystagmus) is driven by the cortex. The presence of nystagmus in an unresponsive patient indicates cortical functioning and suggests pseudocoma. Caloric testing performed correctly in a comatose patient may also help differentiate a brain stem lesion from a hemispheric lesion. If the brainstem is normal, the eyes will deviate conjugately toward the side where ice water is flushed into the ear. This is the slow phase of the eye movement. If the hemispheres are intact and functioning, the slow phase of eye movement will be followed by a fast jerking phase, in which the eyes move away from the side of the water infusion. The cold caloric response involves the vestibular system, the afferent functions of cranial nerve VIII, brainstem interneurons, and efferent functions of cranial nerve III (adduction of eyes) and cranial nerve VI (abduction). Stimulation of the cornea is another method to evaluate brainstem function and will cause an eye blink if the fifth and seventh cranial nerves are intact and the coma is light.

Respirations should be observed. Apneustic breathing, characterized by deep inspiration followed by a long apneic phase and occurring only a few breaths per minute, suggests brainstem failure. Irregular ataxic breathing is an ominous sign of brainstem failure. Normal or Cheyne-Stokes respiration indicates good brainstem function. However, Cheyne-Stokes respiration may be due to bilateral dysfunction of structures deep in the cerebral hemispheres, bilateral cerebral infarctions, congestive heart failure, hypertensive encephalopathy, or other systemic causes.

The neck should be flexed to check for nuchal rigidity, if there is no possible injury or contraindication to this maneuver. Rigidity of the neck or resistance to flexion suggests meningeal inflammation due to meningitis or subarachnoid hemorrhage. Empiric antibiotic coverage should be promptly initiated in cases highly suspicious of meningitis. Antibiotic coverage should not be delayed by the diagnostic workup (i.e., inability to perform lumbar puncture due to delay in obtaining a head CT). It is important to note that the absence of nuchal rigidity cannot reliably exclude meningitis or other processes of meningeal irritation.

The patient's posture is observed and the response to stimulation is noted. Decorticate and decerebrate posturings are abnormal postures that may be present in the deeply comatose patient. Decorticate or flexor posturing is characterized by flexion of the upper extremities with extension in the lower extremities and may suggest injury to the brain above the level of the midbrain.

Decerebrate or extensor posturing is characterized by arms that are extended, adducted, and hyperpronated, and legs that are extended with feet plantar flexed. Decerebrate posturing occurs in patients with infarcts of the brainstem rostral to the midpons and also in patients with large cerebral hemorrhages that destroy or compress the lower thalamus and midbrain. This motor pattern typically emerges in the wake of lesions of the internal capsule or cerebral hemisphere that interrupt the corticospinal pathways. Clinical disease patterns often cloud the demarcation between flexor and extensor posturing, and motor responses may shift back and forth depending on the location of the lesion and pressure effects on the upper brain stem.

Elderly patients with altered mental status are a challenge for the emergency physician. Aside from the usual suspects previously mentioned, seemingly mild infections (UTIs, urosepsis, pneumonias) may cause mental status changes in this age group. Thus, a systematic approach should be taken that includes a fever work up (chest x-ray, urinalysis, and blood cultures). In addition, an ECG should be obtained to evaluate for myocardial infarction or ischemia as a cause of mental status change in the elderly.

CRITICAL INTERVENTIONS

Suggested steps in the management of the comatose patient are as follows:

1. Establish and maintain the airway and protect the patient from aspiration.
2. Administer oxygen.
3. Provide adequate ventilation.
4. Support circulation.
5. Establish intravenous access and draw blood for rapid glucose determination; other laboratory evaluation may include electrolytes, calcium, and renal and liver function; drug screen; arterial blood gas determination; complete blood count; thyroid function studies; or platelet count depending upon the clinical situation.

If indicated by the rapid glucose determination, administer glucose as 25 to 50 mL of 50% dextrose solution to adults and 2 mL per kilogram of 25% dextrose solution to children. To avoid precipitating acute Wernicke's disease in a thiamine-depleted patient, 100 mg thiamine IV is given in conjunction with the glucose. An electrocardiogram is obtained, pulse oximetry applied, and a Foley catheter placed.

If a narcotic toxidrome is present or if a narcotic overdose is suspected, 2 to 4 mg of naloxone is given intravenously in adults, and 0.01 to 0.1 mg per kilogram in children. In cases of suspected elevated intracranial pressure, measures to transiently decrease intracranial pressure include hyperventilation to reduce PCO_2 to about 35 mm Hg and administration of intravenous mannitol (0.5 to 1.0 g per kilogram). Fluid restriction may be necessary; cerebrospinal fluid may need to be drained by intraventricular catheter. Seizures are treated and seizure precautions observed; if generalized seizures are present a benzodiazepine (lorazepam or diazepam) is considered the initial drug of choice (see Chapter 113, Seizures for further information). If extreme hypothermia or hyperthermia is present, the cause of this should be sought and appropriate environmental issues initiated to bring the temperature towards normal. After the initial treatment of reversible causes and stabilization, definitive work up and therapy are instituted to prevent further CNS damage. In addition to diagnostic laboratory studies, plain radiographs (cervical spine series, chest x-ray), and head CT scan may prove helpful. Lumbar puncture should be performed in suspected cases of meningitis, encephalitis, or subarachnoid hemorrhage; this typically follows a cranial

TABLE 11.2. Mnemonic for Coma and Transient Loss of Consciousness

A —alcohol
E —epilepsy, electrolytes, encephalopathy
I —insulin
O —opium
U —urea (metabolic)
T —trauma
I —infection
P —psychiatric
P —poison
S —shock

T for tumor, and **E** for environmental causes such as heatstroke, hypothermia, and high-altitude injuries should also be considered.

CT in patients with suspected subarachnoid hemorrhage or if focal neurologic findings are present. Magnetic resonance imaging may be useful in some cases but is typically not available on an urgent basis.

There are three primary pathologic processes that produce coma: expanding mass lesions that affect the reticular activating system, brainstem lesions that directly damage the reticular activating system, and metabolic disorders that disrupt global CNS function.

The approach to coma and alterations in consciousness must be systematic. Orderly evaluation, with simultaneous stabilization, is of the utmost importance. Early recognition and correction of reversible causes and prevention of further brain damage by definitive intervention are the basic principles of treatment in patients with altered consciousness. The mnemonic AEIOU-TIPPS (Table 11.2) helps organize the approach for specific treatment and antidote administration. CT scanning will aid in identifying operable lesions that need neurosurgical treatment. In carbon monoxide poisoning, patients immediately receive high-flow oxygen. Hyperbaric treatment may also be indicated in patients with CO toxicity. Patients suspected of meningitis receive intravenous antibiotics promptly when the diagnosis is considered. Patients intoxicated with ethanol receive supportive care and careful observation, and determination that methanol, ethylene glycol, or isopropyl alcohol is not responsible for their presentation. All metabolic causes, such as hypothyroidism, adrenal insufficiency, and electrolyte abnormalities, receive specific treatment. See Chapter 163, Thyroid Emergencies, Chapter 164, Adrenal and Pituitary Disorders, and Chapters 165–167 for a discussion of the management of electrolyte abnormalities.

DISPOSITION

All patients with significantly altered mental status require admission after definitive diagnosis for continued evaluation and treatment. Consultation is immediately required on any potentially operable focal lesions, and immediate contact with a neurosurgeon or transfer to an appropriate facility is essential if the brain is to be saved. Rapid transfer to a center with neurologic and neurosurgical diagnostic and treatment capabilities is essential in patients with potentially surgically treatable disease. When transferring comatose patients, it is important to provide advanced life support. Such patients generally require definitive airway control before transfer. In patients in whom there is no surgically treatable disease, consultation with either a neurologist or internist for intensive care unit admission is indicated if a rapidly reversible cause of the coma is not identified.

COMMON PITFALLS

✔ Delay in obtaining neurosurgical or neurologic consultation in patients with a focal abnormality requiring immediate intervention

✔ Delay in establishment of an airway, cardiovascular support, and provision of adequate oxygen and glucose to the patient with severely altered mental status

✔ Failure to reexamine the patient at intervals and detect changes in patient condition

✔ Failure to consider other causes of mental status change in a patient who appears to be exhibiting postictal behavior

Acknowledgments

The authors would like to thank Dr. Rebecca A. Seip and Dr. Gregory L. Henry for their contributions in prior editions of this book.

References

1. Bernat JL. Questions remaining about the minimally conscious state (editorial). *Neurology* 2002;58:337–338.
2. Bruno A, Levine SR, Frankel MR, et al. Admission glucose level and clinical outcomes in the NINDS rt-PA stroke trial. *Neurology* 2002;59:669–674.
3. Giacino JT, Ashwal S, Childs N, et al. The minimally conscious state: definition and diagnostic criteria. *Neurology* 2002;58:349–353.
4. Glauser JM. Coma: a systematic approach to patient evaluation and management. *Emergency Medicine Reports* 2003;24:147–162.
5. Henry GL, Jagoda A, Little NE, Pelligrino TR. Altered states of consciousness and coma. In: *Neurologic emergencies: A symptom-oriented approach,* 2nd ed. New York: McGraw-Hill, 2003:49–79.
6. Plum F, Posner JB. The pathologic physiology of signs and symptoms of coma. In: Plum F, Posner JB, eds. *The diagnosis of stupor and coma,* 3rd ed. Philadelphia: FA Davis Co., 1980:1–86.
7. Young GB. Major symptoms of impaired consciousness. In: Young GB, Ropper AH, Bolton CF, eds. *Coma and impaired consciousness: A Clinical Perspective.* New York: McGraw-Hill, 1998:39–78.

CHAPTER 12
Headache

Jonathan A. Edlow

CLINICAL PRESENTATION

Headache is the reason for approximately 2% to 4% of all emergency department (ED) visits (7,8,24). This large number of patients can be divided into two groups–those with benign causes (about 95%), and those with treatable illnesses that are life, limb, vision, or brain threatening (about 5%). These two groups are not always easily distinguished, and delay in the diagnosis of meningitis and subarachnoid hemorrhage (SAH) remains an important reason for malpractice payments in emergency medicine (16).

The brain parenchyma is insensate (11,12). Head pain results from tension, traction, distention, dilation or inflammation of the pain-sensitive structures external to the skull, portions of the dura, and the blood vessels (11). However, each of these mecha-nisms is likely mediated by a final common biochemical pathway that results in pain. Because of this, a favorable response to analgesics or even the more specific "antimigraine" agents should not be used to judge the cause of an individual headache (7,8,12,28).

These basic facts highlight two points; headache is common, and the potential for serious diagnostic error exists. Given that emergency physicians work under both time and resource utilization pressures, physicians must develop a logical, practical and accurate approach to distinguish between the two groups of patients.

Physicians have three tools to make this critical distinction– the history, the physical examination and other diagnostic tests.

DIFFERENTIAL DIAGNOSIS

The differential diagnosis of headache can be organized in several ways. The International Headache Society method (Table 12.1) (1), although comprehensive, is cumbersome for use in the emergency department. Another method of sorting the differential diagnosis is by temporal pattern. For example, is the current headache a chronic recurring one, or is it a new-onset unusual event? Still a third method, and one that is consistent with the way emergency physicians work, is the division of headaches into the two groups above. The problems that are life, limb, brain or vision threatening are referred to as "cannot miss items" (8). These disorders result in serious morbidity or mortality if untreated (Table 12.2).

Overall, primary headache disorders such as migraine, cluster and tension headache are by far the most common causes of headache (31). Detailed discussions of the primary headache syndromes and the other individual disease entities are discussed in other chapters (Chapter 110, Headache and Chapter 111, Subarachnoid Hemorrhage). This chapter will focus on strategies to avoid missing these "cannot miss" diagnoses.

DIAGNOSTIC APPROACH

The physician has two parallel and related goals–correct diagnosis and effective treatment, with the first goal facilitating the second. Not only is it perfectly acceptable to begin treating the pain before the diagnosis is made, but it may be preferable. The patient may be more relaxed when a subsequent lumbar puncture is performed. Faster pain control results in greater patient satisfaction and more rapid disposition.

Because most patients have benign causes of their headaches, and because of the limiting issues of both time and cost, many patients do not require further evaluation beyond history and physical examination. Physicians must decide who requires further evaluation and who can be safely treated and discharged with appropriate follow up.

All patients with acute headache and new neurologic deficits must be evaluated sufficiently to explain the cause of those deficits. The same is true for those with abnormal HEENT examinations and significant abnormalities in vital signs. However, the more common and more difficult situation is the patient whose physical examination is normal. In this group of patients, physicians must use the history, past medical and family history and other epidemiologic factors (see below) to decide upon further evaluation. As with any painful symptom, the standard attributes of the pain–location, severity, quality, onset, timing and duration, associated symptoms, alleviating and exacerbating factors, are used to try to make the distinction between benign and "cannot miss" diagnoses. Each of these factors must be factored into the equation. There is no single response to any single question that automatically triggers a work up.

TABLE 12.1. International Headache Society Classification

Diagnostic Group—Headache Associated with:	Comments
Migraine	Requires five or more attacks of a specific nature. For migraines with neurologic deficits (e.g., ophthalmoplegic), other etiologies should be excluded
Tension-type	Requires 10 or more attacks of specific nature. Absence of nausea, vomiting, and photophobia
Cluster and chronic paroxysmal hemicrania	Always unilateral. Periorbital location lasting minutes to hours. Associated with eye, nose, or face symptoms (e.g., rhinorrhea)
Miscellaneous headaches unassociated with structural lesions	This group includes a variety of brief (idiopathic stabbing headache), situational (cough, exertional, coital) headache syndromes
Head trauma	This group includes the minor postinjury headaches
Vascular disorders	A very important group for emergency physicians which includes brain ischemia and infarction, and all forms of intracranial hemorrhage, venous sinus thromboses, giant cell arteritis, arterial dissections, and hypertensive encephalopathy
Nonvascular intracranial disorders	Includes idiopathic intracranial hypertension, post-LP headache and headaches from meningitis, encephalitis, and brain abscess and tumor
Substances or their withdrawal	Includes drugs and food additives (e.g., monosodium glutamate headache, or Chinese restaurant syndrome); also includes headache from carbon monoxide poisoning
Noncephalic infection	Includes pain due to febrile illnesses (e.g., pyelonephritis, pneumonia and acute viral syndromes)
Metabolic disorder	Includes headaches from hypercarbia or high altitude illness
Disorders of HEENT—associated (includes dental)	Includes narrow angle closure glaucoma. Note that for sinus headache to be confidently diagnosed, specific criteria must be followed. Chronic sinusitis should not cause headache
Cranial neuralgias, nerve trunk and deafferentation pain	Most of these are cranial neuropathies and herpes zoster
Not-classifiable	Others

HEENT, head, eyes, ears, nose and throat.

The *location* of pain is less helpful in making this distinction than it is with other types of pain; there is significant overlap between benign and serious causes (7,8). Some recommend working up patients whose headaches are always on the same side (10). *Severity* of pain also has limitations. While the "worst of life" headache suggests a more serious problem, most severe headaches in the ED have benign causes (18,21). This is partly because of the variability of patients' pain thresholds and partly because overall, most headaches have benign causes. That said, increasing severity should lower one's threshold for further diagnostic testing, and most patients with a "worst of life" headache should be evaluated for SAH (7,8). Defining the *quality* of pain is crucial (7,8). It is important to ask in detail about the patient's prior headaches. A new headache that is qualitatively unique and unusual for the patient may be more significant than the "worst ever" headache in another patient with frequent similar quality headaches. *Onset* is another important feature that drives decision-making. Abrupt or "thunderclap" onset suggests intracranial hemorrhage or cerebral venous sinus thrombosis, although once again, most abrupt onset headaches are benign. For abrupt onset headaches, the activity at onset sometimes suggests the etiology, for example, in coital headache or benign exertional headache (14,23). However while these activities are sensitive for the corresponding diagnoses, they are not specific; SAH must be ruled out in both cases. The converse is also true; many SAH patients develop their headache during quiet activity or even sleep (27).

Defining the *timing* and *duration* of the pain is useful. Worrisome features include new acute headache, or a subacute headache that is increasing in severity. Long-standing duration (years) headache or a similarly long history of intermittent headaches is less likely to be due to a "cannot miss" cause, assuming that sufficient history is taken to ensure that there is nothing new or different to the prior headache pattern. Very fleeting headaches, termed "jabs and jolts" that last seconds are benign (22).

Similarly, *associated symptoms* can be important. Nausea and vomiting occur with migraine, but also suggest intracranial mass, blood or infection. Again, comparison with prior headaches is important. The significance in a patient with migraines who always vomits with them is different from the migraineur who is now vomiting for the first time. The same is true of photophobia. Visual abnormalities suggest migraine, idiopathic intracranial hypertension, temporal arteritis, and pituitary apoplexy. Diplopia from a pupil-involving third nerve palsy suggests a cerebral aneurysm, or other mass. Diplopia from a sixth nerve palsy is seen with elevated intracranial pressure of any cause, presumably due to stretching of the sixth cranial nerve. Syncope, seizure, or any focal neurologic symptoms associated with a new headache should prompt an evaluation.

Exacerbating and *alleviating* factors are less helpful with headache. For example, the classic history that a headache from brain tumor increases on awakening is neither specific nor sensitive (6). It is also seen in patients with chronic lung disease

TABLE 12.2.   "Cannot Miss" Causes of Headache (see text for definition)

Diagnosis	Suggestive History & Physical Findings	Diagnostic Testing
Meningitis and encephalitis	Fever, stiff neck, jolt accentuation, altered mental status, seizure	LP (If preceded by a CT because of concern for raised intracranial pressure, give antibiotics before CT)
Subarachnoid hemorrhage	Abrupt onset of severe headache, stiff neck, 3rd nerve palsy	CT scan LP if CT is nondiagnostic
Stroke (ischemic or hemorrhagic)	Abrupt onset and focal neurologic deficit conforming to an arterial territory	CT scan; MRI if available will give more information (should not delay thrombolytic therapy)
Dissection of craniocervical arteries	Neck pain, abrupt onset, variable presence of neurologic deficit Possible Horner syndrome	MRA, CT angiography, or conventional angiography
Hypertensive encephalopathy	Severe (usually chronic) hypertension Often papilledema and other signs of end-organ damage	Careful, titratable lowering of BP to ~ 25% off the peak BP will decrease the headache
Idiopathic intracranial hypertension	Obese, female patient Papilledema, often 6th nerve palsy	LP (following an imaging study, that by definition will be normal)
Giant cell arteritis	Nearly always age > 50 years Symptoms of polymyalgia rheumatica Abnormal scalp vessels on exam	ESR Temporal artery biopsy
Acute angle closure glaucoma	Painful red eye with mid-position pupil and corneal edema	Tonometry
Intracranial mass (tumor, abscess, hematoma)	Any neurologic finding, focal or generalized	CT scan; if available, MR will give more information
Cerebral venous sinus thrombosis	Hypercoagulable state of any type	MRI and MRA with venous phase
Carbon monoxide poisoning	Cluster of cases, winter season	COHb level
Pituitary apoplexy	Visual acuity or field abnormalities. Known pituitary tumor	MRI

BP, blood pressure; CT, computed tomography; ESR, erythrocyte sedimentation rate; LP, lumbar puncture; MRA, magenetic resonance angiography; MRI, magnetic resonance imaging.

and hypercarbia (which worsens during sleep). Headache from intracranial hypotension (postlumbar puncture headache) tends to worsen on standing upright, and headache due to sinusitis often worsens on bending forward with the head dependent. In terms of alleviating factors, diagnostic significance should not be ascribed to pain relief, even with over-the-counter medications. New medications or the discontinuation of a medication may also be diagnostically relevant in some patients (20).

Patients frequently use the word "migraine" inaccurately to refer to any "bad" headache, or "sinusitis" to refer to any frontal headache. Unless these diagnoses have been substantiated by a prior medical evaluation, it is preferable to simply use the less specific, but more accurate word "headache" (7). Sinusitis is a relatively uncommon cause of headache (5). Tension headache and migraine are very common. The lifetime incidence of migraine is about 11% (12); therefore, even patients with true histories of tension headache or migraine may develop new headaches of another cause. This fact underscores the importance of carefully exploring the difference between a patient's prior headache and the one that led to the current ED visit.

The epidemiologic context is important. A family or past history of cerebral aneurysm increases the likelihood of an aneurysmal cause. Poorly treated hypertension may lead to hypertensive encephalopathy. Vascular risk factors can result in stroke. Hypercoagulability or a past or family history of thromboembolic events should raise the possibility of cerebral venous sinus thrombosis. Obesity increases the possibility of idiopathic intracranial hypertension (pseudotumor cerebri), especially in women. New-onset headache at older ages also suggests a secondary cause (24). Most migraine headaches begin before age 20 and very few begin after age 50. Therefore, physicians must have a lower threshold to work up older patients with new headaches. Specifically giant cell arteritis, tumors, subdural hematoma and medication-related headache should be considered in this group.

Patients who are HIV positive or have a history of cancer represent other groups in whom a lower threshold to pursue evaluation seems justified. Winter season and common source clusters are associated with carbon monoxide poisoning.

The International Headache Society definition of tension and migraine headaches requires multiple episodes to definitively diagnose migraine or tension headache (1). Migraine is defined by 5 or more episodes of a particular kind of throbbing headache and tension headache is defined as 10 or greater episodes. Although all of these patients must have their first headache at some point in time, most do not present to the ED. Therefore, diagnosing a patient with a new, different headache with a primary headache disorder opens the door to misdiagnosis.

The physical examination starts with the general appearance and vital signs. General appearance can be deceiving and is, at least in part, a function of a given patient's pain threshold. Nevertheless, the patient who is shielding his eyes from the light, while consistent with migraine, also suggests meningeal irritation. Fever is not a symptom of migraine and suggests infection, or a several-day old subarachnoid hemorrhage (SAH). Hypertension is an uncommon cause of headache. Conversely, many secondary causes of headache result in a high blood pressure reading, either from pain and stress, or due to the presence of intracranial pathology. In some causes of headache, such as stroke, over-zealous blood pressure reduction can be detrimental (32). In the case of hypertensive encephalopathy, reduction of the blood pressure by about 25% of its peak value is usually followed by rapid improvement of the patient's symptoms. The emergency physician should have a low threshold for brain imaging (and possibly lumbar puncture) in patients with hypertension and headache.

The emergency physician should look for signs of meningeal irritation. Meningismus, stiffness on passive flexion of the neck, is seen from infections (meningitis) or irritation (SAH). However

TABLE 12.3.   Common HEENT Findings That Suggest Particular Diagnoses

Finding	Diagnosis	Comments
Vesicles on scalp	Herpes zoster of upper two cervical roots or V-1 root of trigeminal nerve	Usually unilateral pain Must examine scalp carefully
Vesicles on tip of nose	Herpes zoster of V-1 root of trigeminal nerve	Carefully examine the cornea with slit-lamp
Vesicles in external ear canal	Ramsay-Hunt syndrome	Carefully examine the 7th and 8th cranial nerves
Temporal artery nodules, tenderness or thickening	Giant cell arteritis	Ask patients about visual symptoms; order ESR; and consider empiric steroid use and arranging temporal artery biopsy
Red eye and corneal edema	Acute narrow angle glaucoma	Pupil is usually mid-position Consult ophthalmology
Proptosis of eye Chemosis of conjunctiva	Cavernous sinus thrombosis	Neurosurgical consultation and MRA with venous phase

ESR, erythrocyte sedimentation rate.

this finding is not reliably present in either condition and its absence does not exclude these diagnoses. The same is true of Kernig and Brudzinski signs (see Chapter 138, Meningitis and Encephalitis). One physical finding that is found more reliably in meningitis is "jolt accentuation." This sign is positive if, when the patient is asked to turn their head horizontally two to three rotations per second, the baseline headache increases (2).

The head, eyes, ears, nose and throat (HEENT) examination may reveal the headache's cause (Table 12.3). Vesicles on the scalp, tip of the nose, or external ear canal suggest herpes zoster. Scalp lesions suggest a first or second cervical root involvement; tip of the nose lesions suggest that the first division of the trigeminal nerve is involved and should prompt a careful slit-lamp exam for corneal involvement. Vesicles in the ear canal are associated with the Ramsay-Hunt syndrome (herpes zoster infection causing 7th nerve palsy). Temporal artery tenderness, nodularity or thickening is seen with giant cell arteritis. A red eye with an edematous cornea and mid-position pupil suggests narrow angle closure glaucoma. A proptotic eye or chemosis suggests a cavernous sinus thrombosis.

The physician should perform a complete neurologic examination on patients with headache. New neurologic abnormalities should trigger a work up beyond history and physical examination, although some migraine patients, specifically those with aura, will have neurologic deficits. An abnormal mental status with a new headache always must be explained, and suggests increased intracranial pressure or a diffuse process such as meningitis, encephalitis or severe carbon monoxide poisoning. Several cranial nerve findings suggest particular causes of a headache (Table 12.4).

The remainder of the neurologic examination, power, sensation, cerebellar function, gait, and reflexes should be performed. Abnormalities in these areas suggest a mass lesion or focal brain ischemia or infarction; the specific findings are a function of the location of the pathology. The ocular fundi should be inspected for signs of raised intracranial pressure, but the appearance of papilledema can be delayed and is not always present. Physicians should also look for venous pulsations in the retina. Their presence is strongly indicative of normal intracranial pressure, while the converse is not true. Two aspects of the neurological exam that are frequently omitted are visual fields and gait testing. Both are important in that they cover a large amount of neuro-anatomic territory. Field cuts are seen in pituitary apoplexy (3). Horner syndrome, meiosis, ptosis but usually without anhydrosis at this level is associated with carotid artery dissection. A new

headache, especially occipital, associated with ataxia suggests a cerebellar stroke. Gait abnormalities may also have an impact on safe disposition from the ED.

Based on the history and physical examination, patients will fall into one of three categories. The first is patients who have abnormal physical examinations in whom the need for further diagnostic testing is unambiguous. The second is patients whose exams are normal and whose histories do not suggest the presence of a "cannot miss" diagnosis. The last category is patients with normal physical examinations and worrisome histories that trigger further diagnostic testing. Separating out these last two categories is largely a matter of experience, judgment, and meticulous attention to detail in the history (Table 12.5).

Once the decision has been made to pursue other diagnoses, there are a limited number of tests to be performed. The choice of which tests, and what sequence, is partly a function of the specific differential diagnosis, and the intrinsic limitations of the tests. This latter point cannot be over-emphasized. All tests have some limitations that the physician must factor into the decision-making. Once again, the response to analgesics of any class must not be assigned any diagnostic significance.

Brain imaging has revolutionized the diagnosis of patients with headache. Computed tomography scanning (CT) and magnetic resonance imaging (MRI) allow diagnosis of conditions much earlier and with far greater precision. CT scanning is widely available, extremely rapid, and there is a great deal of experience with its interpretation amongst radiologists and emergency physicians. A noncontrast CT scan is extremely sensitive for acute intraparenchymal blood and very sensitive for subarachnoid blood, but small or older subarachnoid bleeds may not be visible. Physicians may miss subtle findings (9). Some tumors and abscesses will not show on a scan performed without intravenous contrast, although most masses large enough to cause a significant headache will be associated with some abnormality on a noncontrast head CT.

In general, MRI is superior to CT, especially in evaluating vascular and neoplastic lesions, infections and pathology at the cervico-medullary junction and in the posterior fossa (10). When MRI is not available and if it is indicated, the emergency physician should consider transferring the patient or performing CT with intravenous contrast.

MRI permits even greater detail of the brain anatomy, and physiology. Blood vessels, both arterial and venous, can now be evaluated by MR angiography (MRA). Brain tumor, abscess and pituitary apoplexy are easily visible. Carotid and vertebral

TABLE 12.4.   Common Cranial Nerve Findings of Diagnostic Significance in Patients with Headache

Finding	Diagnosis	Comments
Decreased visual acuity	Giant cell arteritis Acute narrow angle closure glaucoma	Carefully examine the eye and the temporal arteries Send ESR in patients > 50 years old
Visual field cut	Mass lesion Pituitary apoplexy Stroke	Location depends on the specific field cut (this may be a parenchymal problem rather than a cranial neuropathy)
3rd nerve palsy	SAH Cavernous sinus thrombosis	Check the pupil (usually involved in SAH; usually spared in "diabetic" 3rd nerve palsy)
6th nerve palsy	Any condition associated with increased or decreased ICP Basilar meningitis (e.g., Lyme, tuberculous, cyptococcal, etc.) Cavernous sinus thrombosis	Look for papilledema. Consider pseudotumor or cerebral venous sinus thrombosis Consider LP if brain imaging is negative
Direction changing nystagmus	Cerebellar or brainstem stroke	This can occur with any central lesion causing vertigo
Lower motor neuron 7th nerve palsy	Bell palsy Ramsay-Hunt syndrome	This may present with severe ear or retroauricular pain
8th nerve palsy (diminished hearing or vertigo)	Ramsay-Hunt syndrome	See above; also look for vesicles in the external auditory canal
Partial Horner syndrome	Carotid dissection	Meiosis and ptosis are present but anhydrosis is generally absent in lesions of the carotid

ESR, erythrocyte sedimentation rate; ICP, intracranial pressure; LP, lumbar puncture; SAH, subarachnoid hemorrhage.

artery dissections, cerebral aneurysms, and cerebral venous sinus thromboses are diagnosed with MRA. However, like any other test, it is not perfect. One article documented two cases in which a cerebral aneurysm was missed by MRA. This occurred despite the fact that both patients presented with a 3rd nerve palsy, and the clinician expressed his concern for a posterior communicating artery aneurysm to an experienced neuroradiologist, who carefully reviewed the films (15). This underscores the fact that even in the face of negative imaging studies, it is important to pursue hard physical findings.

Despite the development of these sophisticated neurodiagnostic tests, there is still a role for the lumbar puncture (LP). For cases of subarachnoid hemorrhage in which the CT scan is nondiagnostic, and for suspected meningitis, an LP will establish those diagnoses with nearly 100% sensitivity. However, like all tests in medicine, even the LP has limitations. Rare cases of meningitis can be associated with no white blood cells (26), and late-presenting cases of SAH may have no red blood cells (7,8). After two weeks, even xanthochromia may disappear. Measuring the opening pressure may help to distinguish traumatic LP from true subarachnoid hemorrhage, as well as help with the diagnosis of idiopathic intracranial hypertension and cerebral venous sinus thrombosis (8).

On specific occasions, other tests are diagnostic. Measurement of the erythrocyte sedimentation rate (ESR) is useful in diagnosing giant cell arteritis. Tonometry can rule in acute narrow angle

TABLE 12.5.   Factors Suggesting Further Evaluation Should Be Pursued Beyond History and Physical Examination

Headache-Related or Patient-Related Factors	Diseases to Be Considered	Evaluation
First or worst HA	All diseases in Table 12.2	Varies (see Table 12.2)
Increasing frequency or severity	Mass lesion	Consider brain imaging
Associated with altered mental status	Elevated ICP SAH Encephalitis and meningitis Carbon monoxide poisoning	Brain imaging, LP if negative results of imaging
Associated with new neurological deficits	Any of the intracerebral diagnoses	Varies, but includes brain imaging
Visual symptoms	Idiopathic intracranial hypertension, pituitary apoplexy, migraine with aura	Brain imaging LP for idiopathic intracranial hypertension (Note: if visual symptoms classic of migraine aura, other testing may not be necessary)
With fever & meningismus	Meningitis, SAH	LP, (CT first in many cases—see text)
New onset over 50 years of age	Tumor, SDH, giant cell arteritis	Brain imaging ESR
New onset in HIV + patients	Meningitis, lymphoma, opportunistic infections	Varies, but usually includes both brain imaging and LP
New onset in patients with cancer	Tumor or cerebral venous sinus thrombosis	Brain imaging, ideally MRI but CT may suffice

CT, computed tomography; HA, headache; ICP, intracranial pressure; LP, lumbar puncture; SAH, subarachnoid hemorrhage; SDH, subdural hematoma.

closure glaucoma, and carboxyhemoglobin levels are useful when carbon monoxide poisoning is suspected. Standard pulse oximetry may be falsely normal in patients with carbon monoxide poisoning.

Given the limitations of individual tests, it should be clear that sometimes a series of tests is necessary. For example, if a CT scan is negative in a possible subarachnoid hemorrhage patient, an LP should be performed. If an ESR is normal in an elderly patient with a new headache, the physician should consider performing a brain imaging test since giant cell arteritis is much less likely. If a CT scan is negative in a patient with a clear-cut focal neurologic finding, an MRI should be considered.

One other "test" to be considered is a neurologic consultation. Although the emergency physician should be able to diagnose the vast majority of patients with headache who seek care in the ED, there may be times when a neurologist can supply a useful perspective, either in real time or in follow up. The timing of consultation is a function of the specific differential diagnosis, the pace of the patient's illness, and the availability of that service. In patients with a new, definite neurologic finding on physical examination and normal results of brain imaging, the physician should consider urgent or emergent consultation to sort out the possibilities.

Once the decision has been made to evaluate for SAH, an LP should follow any CT scan that is negative, equivocal or technically inadequate. Many physicians are reluctant to perform LPs; and many patients are reluctant to have the procedure. The LP will sometimes diagnose conditions such as idiopathic intracranial hypertension, meningitis, or a small SAH, which cannot be diagnosed in any other way. Occasional patients thought to have viral meningitis will have SAH. Despite the fact that approximately 15% of LPs are traumatic (30), there are a number of techniques for distinguishing traumatic LP from true SAH. The most useful is the presence or absence of xanthochromia (29).

Giant cell arteritis may lead to blindness and brain infarction. While the decision to start steroids should ideally be made in consultation with the patient's primary care physician, the emergency physician should remember that this intervention can be vision saving. Several days of prednisone, 1 mg/kg per day, will not negate a temporal artery biopsy's diagnostic utility (10).

CRITICAL INTERVENTIONS

It is unusual for headache patients to require airway intervention. When the need does occur, however, it is usually in patients with impending herniation from a mass lesion or massive intracranial bleeding. The standard rapid sequence intubation can be used in these patients. Agents such as lidocaine and fentanyl should be administered to try to blunt the transient rise in intracranial pressure (ICP) that accompanies tracheal intubation, although this practice is not clearly proven by data. Emergency brain imaging is important to determine if there is an urgent surgical problem such as a cerebellar hemorrhage or mass. Occasionally, in a comatose patient who has had a severe headache, ocular or retinal hemorrhages are a clue that the patient has had a SAH (8).

In other patients, if bacterial meningitis is a serious consideration, the physician must decide whether to proceed to LP directly or perform a CT first. In patients who have new focal neurological findings, papilledema, abnormal mental status, or are HIV positive, the CT should be performed first. However, this intermediate step should never delay administering appropriate antibiotics prior to CT. In the absence of these findings, performing the LP directly is usually safe, especially in patients with normal venous pulsations on fundoscopy.

The impulse to lower the blood pressure pharmacologically in headache patients who are hypertensive should be resisted. Frequently, the high blood pressure is either a nonspecific response to pain, or the brain's autoregulation to preserve cerebral blood flow. The emergency physician should think of the high blood pressure as a clue that a serious problem exists, not a number to be treated or a diagnosis to be made. Interfering with the body's autoregulatory function often leads to worse outcomes; this is certainly true in stroke (32). There are, however, three situations in which rapid pharmacologic blood pressure management in headache patients is indicated—hypertensive encephalopathy, aneurysmal SAH before the aneurysm is definitively treated, and parenchymal intracranial hemorrhage. Hypertensive encephalopathy, relatively uncommon nowadays, is associated with evidence of end-organ damage to the brain, eyes, heart and kidney. Reduction of the mean arterial pressure by 25% from its peak, using parenteral titratable agents such as nitroprusside, should rapidly improve the headache. In the setting of a ruptured cerebral aneurysm, prior to surgery, most neurosurgeons prefer to have the systolic blood pressure lower than 120 mm Hg, using either labetalol or nitroprusside. The AHA has published a different set of guidelines for patients with parenchymal intracerebral hemorrhage (4).

DISPOSITION

Most patients with headache will be discharged after successful treatment of their acute pain. This includes patients with the diagnoses of primary headache disorders and those who have had a negative evaluation. For patients with suspected subarachnoid hemorrhage, for example, five studies looking at outcomes after negative CT scans and normal spinal fluid examination have all found that these patients do not develop subarachnoid hemorrhage after this work up (13,17–19,33). However, because occasional patients are outliers (25), and because abnormal tests are occasionally incorrectly interpreted as normal, follow up is important.

Because time can sometimes be an effective diagnostic tool, arranging follow up for patients with headache is important. This may be with their primary care physician or a neurologist. However in patients with abnormal physical examinations, this evaluation should take place urgently if not emergently, and in consultation with the physician who will be doing the follow up.

COMMON PITFALLS

✔ Failure to inquire about prior headache details, and how they compare to the current one
✔ Failure to understand that some patients with serious pathology will not appear very ill
✔ Relying on a past history of migraine or sinusitis, in the absence of a substantiated diagnosis. Patients may use words like "migraine" and "sinusitis" without knowing what they mean
✔ Failure to perform complete neurologic and HEENT examination
✔ Failure to realize that there is no diagnostic significance to successful treatment of the pain with any kind of analgesic or antimigraine drug
✔ Failure to perform a lumbar puncture after a nondiagnostic head CT in the evaluation of SAH
✔ Failure to know that hypertension rarely is the cause of a new headache
✔ Failure to explain new neurological findings. If the first test (e.g., a CT scan) is negative, consider a second test (e.g., MRI

or neurological consultation), since the physical finding is still present and requires explanation

References

1. Anonymous. Classification and diagnostic criteria for headache disorders, cranial neuralgias and facial pain. *Cephalgia* 1988;8 (supp 7):1–73.
2. Attia J, Hatala R, Cook DJ, et al. The rational clinical examination. Does this adult patient have acute meningitis? *JAMA* 1999;282:175–181.
3. Bills DC, Meyer FB, Laws ER, Jr, et al. A retrospective analysis of pituitary apoplexy. *Neurosurger* 1993;33:602–609.
4. Broderick JP, Adams HP, Jr, Barsan W, et al. Guidelines for the management of spontaneous intracerebral hemorrhage: a statement for healthcare professionals from a special writing group of the Stroke Council, American Heart Association. *Stroke* 1999;30:905–915.
5. Cady RK, Schreiber CP. Sinus headache or migraine? Considerations in making a differential diagnosis. *Neurology* 2002;58:S10–S14.
6. Dodick D. Headache as a symptom of ominous disease. What are the warning signals? *Postgrad Med* 1997;101:46–50, 55–56, 62–64.
7. Edlow JA. Diagnosis of subarachnoid hemorrhage in the emergency department. *Emerg Med Clin North Am* 2003;21:73–87.
8. Edlow JA, Caplan LR. Avoiding pitfalls in the diagnosis of subarachnoid hemorrhage. *N Engl J Med* 2000;342:29–36.
9. Edlow JA, Wyer PC. How good is a negative cranial computed tomographic scan result in excluding subarachnoid hemorrhage? *Ann Emerg Med* 2000;36:507–516.
10. Evans R. Diagnostic testing for the evaluation of headaches. *Neurol Clin* 1996;14:1–26.
11. Gelb D, Ashok H, Fales W. Headache. In: Shah S, Kelly K (eds): *Emergency Neurology: principles and practice.* New York: Cambridge University Press, 1999:105–121.
12. Goadsby PJ, Lipton RB, Ferrari MD. Migraine—current understanding and treatment. *N Engl J Med* 2002;346:257–270.
13. Harling DW, Peatfield RC, van Hille PT, et al. Thunderclap headache: is it migraine? *Cephalgia* 1989;9:87–90.
14. Imperato J, Burstein J, Edlow JA. Benign exertional headache. *Ann Emerg Med* 2003;41:98–103.
15. Johnson MR, Good CD, Penny WD, et al. Lesson of the week: playing the odds in clinical decision making: lessons from berry aneurysms undetected by magnetic resonance angiography. *BMJ* 2001;322:1347–1349.
16. Karcz A, Holbrook J, Burke M, et al. Massachusetts emergency medicine closed malpractice claims: 1988–1990. *Ann Emerg Med* 1993;22:553–559.
17. Landtblom AM, Fridriksson S, Boivie J, et al. Sudden onset headache: a prospective study of features, incidence and causes. *Cephalalgia* 2002;22:354–360.
18. Linn FH, Wijdicks EF, van der Graaf Y, et al. Prospective study of sentinel headache in aneurysmal subarachnoid haemorrhage. *Lancet* 1994;344:590–593.
19. Markus HS. A prospective follow-up of thunderclap headache mimicking subarachnoid hemorrhage. *J Neurol Neurosurg Psychiatry* 1991;54:1117–1125.
20. Mathew NT. Drug-induced headache. *Neurol Clin* 1990;8:903–912.
21. Morgenstern LB, Luna-Gonzales H, Huber JC, Jr, et al. Worst headache and subarachnoid hemorrhage: prospective, modern computed tomography and spinal fluid analysis. *Ann Emerg Med* 1998;32:297–304.
22. Pareja JA, Ruiz J, de Isla C, et al. Idiopathic stabbing headache (jabs and jolts syndrome). *Cephalalgia* 1996;16:93–96.
23. Pascual J, Iglesias F, Oterino A, et al. Cough, exertional, and sexual headaches: an analysis of 72 benign and symptomatic cases. *Neurology* 1996;46:1520–1524.
24. Ramirez-Lassepas M, Espinosa CE, Cicero JJ, et al. Predictors of intracranial pathologic findings in patients who seek emergency care because of headache. *Arch Neurol* 1997;54:1506–1509.
25. Raps EC, Rogers JD, Galetta SL, et al. The clinical spectrum of unruptured intracranial aneurysm. *Arch Neurol* 1993;50:265–268.
26. Ris J, Mancebo J, Domingo P, et al. Bacterial meningitis despite normal CSF findings. *JAMA* 1985;254:2893–2894.
27. Schievink WI, Karemaker JM, Hageman LM, et al. Circumstances surrounding aneurismal subarachnoid hemorrhage. *Surg Neurol* 1989;32:266–272.
28. Seymour JJ, Moscati RM, Jehle D. Response of headache to nonnarcotic analgesics resulting in missed intracranial hemorrhage. *A J Emerg Med* 1995;13:43–45.
29. Shah KH, Edlow JA. Distinguishing traumatic lumbar puncture from true subarachnoid hemorrhage. *J Emerg Med* 2002;23:67–74.
30. Shah KH, Richard KM, Nicholas S, et al. Incidence of traumatic lumbar puncture. *Acad Emerg Med* 2003;10:151–154.
31. Stewart WF, Lipton RB, Celentano DD, et al. Prevalence of migraine headache in the United States. Relation to age, income, race, and other sociodemographic factors. *JAMA* 1992;267:64–69.
32. Vlcek M, Schillinger M, Lang W, et al. Association between course of blood pressure within the first 24 hours and functional recovery after acute ischemic stroke. *Ann Emerg Med* 2003;42:619–626.
33. Wijdicks EFM, Kerkhoff H, vanGijn J. Long-term follow-up of 71 patients with thunderclap headache mimicking subarachnoid hemorrhage. *Lancet* 1988;ii:68–69.

CHAPTER 13
Weakness

Andy Jagoda and Yasuharu Okuda

Patients presenting to the emergency department with a complaint of weakness pose a great diagnostic challenge for the emergency physician. This nonspecific complaint has a myriad of causes, and a systematic evaluation is critical. Specific attention to potentially life-threatening etiologies is the principal focus, and diligence in data gathering is essential to the establishment of a diagnosis. A detailed history and physical examination guide the selection of diagnostic studies in these challenging cases. Though rarely encountered, when approaching the patient with a complaint of weakness, consideration is given to disorders such as botulism, myasthenia gravis, and Guillain-Barré syndrome because of their associated high morbidity and mortality. The emergency physician should consider these and all other disorders that can precipitously compromise the respiratory and functional status of the patient when approaching a patient with the chief complaint of weakness.

The complaint of "dizziness" may accompany that of "weakness," and, at times, patients use these terms interchangeably. There is considerable overlap in their etiologies. In the ambulatory care setting, dizziness is the most common presenting complaint in patients over the age of 75 (1). *Weakness* is defined as a decrease in muscle strength or power. It may be a focal symptom, involving a single muscle group, or it may be generalized. Dizziness is imprecisely interpreted by patients and may be used to describe lightheadedness, disequilibrium, disorientation, confusion, or vertigo (see Chapter 14, Dizziness and Chapter 31, Vertigo and Labrynthine Disorders). The emergency physician must appreciate the distinction between these symptoms and attempt to understand the patient's intended meaning. This chapter specifically addresses those patients who present with a complaint of "weakness."

CLINICAL PRESENTATION

The historical features that are important when assessing the patient with weakness are the acuity of onset and duration of symptoms, exacerbating and mitigating factors, and presence of associated symptoms (8). Sudden onset of weakness may suggest botulism, while a slower progression of symptoms from days to weeks may suggest Guillain-Barré syndrome or myasthenia gravis, although these illnesses may also have accelerated courses (14). The weakness of myasthenia gravis may fluctuate, and a careful history is needed to elicit a progression of symptoms throughout the day or an association with exercise or repeated activity, such as chewing or combing one's hair. Recent illness, other medical problems, recent vaccination, occupational history, travel history, history of tick bites, use of medications, and use of recreational drugs are important factors in assessing the patient complaining of weakness. A thorough review of systems should include inquiry about recent weight loss, fever or sweats, visual changes (including diplopia), difficulty swallowing, joint or muscle pain, palpitations, change in bowel habits, and skin rashes. Eliciting a history of severe vomiting, diarrhea, rhinorrhea, and urinary incontinence in a farmer presenting with weakness and respiratory failure will enable the clinician to decontaminate and treat the acute organophosphate poisoned patient. Symmetric ascending weakness in a patient with a recent respiratory illness or influenza vaccine will aid in the diagnosis of Guillain-Barré syndrome.

The patient's age is an important consideration in developing the differential diagnosis in a patient with weakness. The elderly have a higher incidence of comorbid medical conditions than do their younger counterparts and are at higher risk of acute central nervous system and cardiovascular events. They are more likely to present with occult infections and metabolic disorders that are symptomatically manifested as weakness (8). In the pediatric age group, infantile botulism and intussusception are two rare but important considerations. Infantile botulism may be seen in children days old to over 1 year of age. This variant of botulism is much more common than food-borne or wound botulism; it presents with weakness, poor tone, poor suck, or constipation.

On the physical examination, orthostatic monitoring and oxygen saturation should be included in the vital signs. Supplemental oxygen is indicated if hypoxemia is present; the airway must be secured if there is a potential for imminent compromise. Tachycardia, with or without hypotension, suggests volume depletion or toxic drug ingestion. Rectal temperature measurement is particularly important, because infection frequently presents with nonspecific complaints, such as weakness. A blood glucose level should be obtained early during the evaluation, as hypoglycemia may present with an array of symptoms, including weakness. The ears, sinuses, thyroid, and cardiac status should be assessed, and there should be a careful evaluation for signs of trauma, which may suggest physical abuse. A rectal examination, including a guaiac test for occult blood, is recommended.

The neurologic examination begins early in the course of the patient's evaluation with an assessment of the mental status. Altered mental status, including confusion, slowness, or agitation, may represent underlying disease or toxic exposure such as in carbon monoxide poisoning and organophosphate exposure; suspicion of cognitive defects should prompt a formal mental status evaluation. Abnormal neuropsychiatric testing in a patient with carbon monoxide poisoning may increase the need for hyperbaric oxygen therapy. Cranial nerve testing in the patient with a complaint of weakness focuses on the motor examination. Ptosis, usually symmetric but sometimes unilateral, can be an early sign of myasthenia gravis. When myasthenia is a consideration, having the patient hold an upward gaze for several minutes is helpful in assessing for fatigue. Difficulty with accommodation can be the earliest sign of weakness due to botulism and does not occur with myasthenia. Diplopia due to weak oculomotor muscles should be assessed, with an emphasis on the evaluation of the sixth cranial nerve. The abducens is the longest cranial nerve and the most sensitive to toxins such as botulism or to increased pressure from intracranial mass lesions.

The remainder of the neurologic examination in the patient complaining of weakness concentrates on motor strength, deep tendon reflexes, and assessment for muscle atrophy and fasciculations. Table 13.1 lists the motor strength grading system (from 0 to 5), which permits standardization of documentation of the motor exam between examiners. Deep tendon reflexes are graded on a scale from 0 indicating areflexia to 4 signifying hyperreflexia with 2 being normal. *Upper motor neuron* diseases, such as multiple sclerosis, will typically present with hyperactive reflexes in comparison to the diminished or absent reflexes seen in diseases of the *lower motor neuron*, as in Guillain-Barré syndrome. Acute spinal cord lesions, such as in cauda equina, can often initially present with areflexia early in its course. Cauda equina syndrome is due to impingement of the lumbar and sacral nerve roots, commonly from a ruptured vertebral disk. These patients

TABLE 13.1. Motor Strength Grading System (MRC Scale)

Grade	Definition
5	Normal strength
4	Active movement against gravity and resistance
3	Active movement against gravity (no resistance from physician)
2	Active movement with gravity eliminated (no resistance from physician)
1	Flicker or trace contraction
0	No visible or palpable contraction

MRC, medical research council.

will present with distal motor weakness, areflexia, urinary retention, and anesthesia in the saddle distribution.

Both upper and lower motor neuron diseases can initially present with the complaint of weakness. The important distinguishing characteristics are listed in Table 13.2. *Upper motor neurons* arise in the cerebral cortex and their axons extend through the subcortical white matter, internal capsule, brainstem, and spinal cord, where they synapse directly with lower motor neurons or interneurons, fine-tuning motor activity. *Lower motor neuron* cell bodies lie in the brainstem motor nuclei and anterior horn of the spinal cord. Their axons extend to the skeletal muscles they innervate.

The weakness of *upper motor neuron* disease is generally unilateral, the Babinski sign is present, muscle tone is increased, deep tendon reflexes are increased, and no fasciculations are visible or palpable. In general, distal muscle groups are more severely affected than are proximal groups. Lower motor neuron disease affects single muscle groups. Flexors and extensors are equally compromised in an extremity. Deep tendon reflexes and muscle tone are decreased with lower motor neuron disease. Muscle atrophy and fasciculation are long-term results of lower motor neuron lesions. Amyotrophic lateral sclerosis (ALS) is a combined upper and lower motor neuron disease that can clinically present as a mixed picture. The etiology of ALS is unclear but it is a disease involving the destruction of the anterior horn cells in the spinal column and the Betz cells in the motor cortex of the CNS. The clinical presentation is of asymmetric weakness in the distal motor groups with sensory sparing. Patients often have muscle fasciculations of lower motor neuron disease but associated positive Babinski signs and hyperreflexia as seen in upper motor neuron disorders.

Lower motor neuron diseases can arise from a muscle-based disorder, a neuropathic-based disorder, or a myoneural junction source. Table 13.3 illustrates several symptoms, physical signs, and laboratory findings that distinguish the etiologies

TABLE 13.2. Upper Versus Lower Motor Neuron Weakness

Clinical	Upper Motor Neuron	Lower Motor Neuron
Weakness	Weakness greater in the arm extensors and leg flexors; weakness often unilateral	Weakness often in one muscle group; extensor same as flexor
Deep tendon reflexes	Increased	Decreased
Muscle tone	Increased	Decreased
Fasciculation	None	Present
Muscle atrophy	None	Severe
Babinski sign	Present	Absent

TABLE 13.3. Myopathy Versus Neuropathy Versus Myoneural Junction Disease

Clinical	Myopathy	Neuropathy	Myoneural Junction
Distribution	Proximal > distal	Distal > proximal	Diffuse, especially bulbar and respiratory muscles
Reflexes	Decreased	Decreased	Normal
Sensory involvement	−	+	−
Atrophy	±	±	−
Fatigue	±	±	+
Serum CPK	Normal to elevated	Normal	Normal
Example	polymyositis	Guillain-Barré syndrome	myasthenia gravis

CPK, creatine phosphokinase.

of lower motor neuron weakness. Weakness due to a myopathy tends to involve proximal muscle groups, while neuropathic disease (Guillain-Barré syndrome) affects distal muscle groups. Myoneural junction diseases have a more distal distribution and are particularly inclined to affect respiratory and bulbar muscle groups (myasthenia gravis and botulism).

Spinal cord disorders from compressive or traumatic injury can also present with weakness involving motor function distal to the defect, as well as sensory and autonomic nerve dysfunction. In comparison to atraumatic cord disorders, such as in multiple sclerosis, traumatic cord lesions generally present acutely with distinct sensory and motor findings, as seen with the saddle anesthesia in patients with cauda equina syndrome. Autonomic dysfunction is also seen more commonly in spinal cord injuries manifesting with hypotension or priapism. Detailed history including anticoagulation, recent fall or trauma, immune status, fever, intravenous drug abuse, spinal procedure or surgery is often necessary to make the diagnosis. An uncommon and occasionally overlooked diagnosis of spinal epidural abscess can be made in the setting of a patient with a history of intravenous drug abuse presenting with severe back pain, fever, and progressive lower extremity weakness.

When psychogenic weakness is considered in the differential diagnosis, several maneuvers may be helpful. Weak muscles give way to pressure in a smooth fashion, but psychogenic weakness usually results in a jerking or sudden release. In a patient with upper extremity weakness from organic disease, making a fist should not result in wrist extension (unless there is an isolated lesion of the flexor tendons); in functional states, the wrist extends as the patient tries to make a fist. In patients with psychogenic bilateral lower extremity weakness, attempts to lift one leg against resistance result in the other leg firmly thrusting downward, while in patients with organic disease, the downward thrust is diminished or absent.

DIFFERENTIAL DIAGNOSIS

The differential diagnosis of the weak patient is extensive. Division of the etiologies into broad categories, such as metabolic, toxic, infectious, structural, endocrinologic, cardiac, and rheumatologic, permits a more organized approach to this extensive list. In this section, the diagnoses are also presented in order from high risk to low risk. Detailed history taking and careful examination should direct the physician to one of these categories. Diagnostic testing may then be used to narrow the

differential diagnosis and determine the management plan for the patient's condition.

Metabolic

Metabolic derangements that can present with weakness include hypoxia, hyperthermia, and alterations in serum glucose, potassium, sodium, and calcium (12). Hypokalemia may be induced by medications such as diuretics, gastrointestinal losses; it also rarely occurs in association with genetic disorders such as familial periodic paralysis. This disorder presents with generalized weakness and paralysis and is due to a dysfunction of potassium regulation (5,7). During summer months, elderly patients with heat exhaustion will frequently present to the emergency department with weakness due to dehydration and inability to autoregulate their temperature.

Cardiac and Vascular

Weakness may be the only complaint in the elderly patient with acute myocardial infarction and must be in the differential diagnosis for all geriatric patients presenting with nonspecific complaints. In one study of symptoms of myocardial infarction in the elderly with autopsy-proven MI, 20% of the patients initially presented with weakness (8,18). As the population ages, more patients will present with atypical complaints of myocardial infarction such as weakness or shortness of breath (17). Other cardiovascular causes of weakness associated with lightheadedness or presyncope can be caused by transient decreased cerebral perfusion. These disorders include postural hypotension, carotid and vertebral artery insufficiency, cardiac dysrhythmias, vasovagal events, and states of decreased cardiac output.

Structural Lesions

Structural lesions often cause focal weakness. Lesions in the spinal canal as seen in cases with epidural hematoma and abscess as well as metastatic cancer can result in weakness that is symmetric and distal to the site of compromise. Transverse myelitis is an infrequent yet debilitating demyelinating disease of the spinal cord presenting with an acute onset of back pain, lower extremity weakness or paralysis, and sensory deficit below the level of involvement. The etiology is unknown but thought to be related to a recent viral infection or autoimmune disorder. The clinician should suspect this disease in a patient with a recent viral illness presenting with both weakness and sensory deficit below a cord level. This disease should not be confused with Guillain-Barré syndrome. Though also preceded by a viral syndrome, the physical examination findings of Guillain-Barré syndrome will typically demonstrate sparing of the anal sphincter and hyporeflexia with progressive weakness in an ascending pattern over days to a week. Clinical findings of transverse myelitis generally progress over 24 hours and include diminished or absence of strength and sensation below the level of involvement, sphincter dysfunction, hyperreflexia, and urinary incontinence or retention. Lesions in the frontal lobes, basal ganglia, and cerebellum can cause disequilibrium. Brainstem infarcts can present with difficulty swallowing, talking, or breathing, in addition to weakness.

Specific Neuromuscular Diseases

The patient with myasthenia gravis will present with weakness of a specific muscle group associated with blurred vision, diplopia, and ptosis. Patients with Guillain-Barré present with generalized ascending paralysis with variable sensory deficits

(10,14). Amyotrophic lateral sclerosis is a disease that affects both upper and lower motor neurons and can present with a mixed picture. Myopathies caused by metabolic derangements, medications, and inflammatory states may present with symmetric proximal muscle weakness with preservation of sensory function.

Infections

All infections can potentially cause weakness, either through nonspecific mechanisms, such as those seen with mononucleosis or hepatitis, or from specific toxins affecting neuromuscular function, such as those in poliomyelitis, botulism, Guillain-Barré, or tick paralysis. Sinus and ear infections can affect the labyrinthine system and produce lightheadedness or vertigo. The human immunodeficiency virus can directly or indirectly cause the full spectrum of weakness, from nonspecific fatigue to neuropathies and myelopathies. Chronic fatigue syndrome, thought to be viral in origin, requires an extensive work up to exclude all other processes before the diagnosis can be established. This diagnosis should not be made in the emergency department (15).

Medications and Toxins

Prescription mediations can produce generalized weakness (Table 13.4). There are usually no focal findings on examination. In one study of 106 patients with a chief complaint of weakness and dizziness, 9% of all patients and 20% of those over age 60 had symptoms attributed to prescription medications (16). Drugs associated with vasodilatation, bradycardia, or diuresis can produce orthostatic blood pressure changes often giving the patient the feeling of weakness.

Toxins can present with the sudden onset of weakness leading to acute respiratory compromise. Other toxins present with a slowly progressive course and subtle complaints. Organophosphates and carbamates act at the neuromuscular junction by inhibiting acetylcholinesterase. Patients present with a constellation of symptoms including lacrimation, defecation, salivation, and weakness, which can progress rapidly to paralysis and respiratory failure. The ability to recognize this toxidrome is critical to early medical treatment and public health intervention (4,6). In contrast, poisonings from heavy metals can be subtle and present with a slowly progressive course. In these cases a thorough history is necessary to elucidate the cause of the patient's symptoms. Carbon monoxide exposure still remains the leading cause of death from poisoning in the United States (3,11). The patient may present with only the complaint of weakness and headache. The emergency physician should consider this diagnosis in patients presenting with weakness especially during the winter months.

Endocrine

Hypothyroidism is the most common endocrine cause of weakness and is often initially misdiagnosed (see Chapter 163, Thyroid Emergencies). Thyrotoxic periodic paralysis can present with weakness as a primary complaint, probably mediated through hypokalemia (2,13). Adrenal insufficiency, perhaps the most life-threatening endocrine etiology of weakness, may present with hypotension, hyperkalemia, and hyponatremia (see Chapter 164, Adrenal and Pituitary Disorders). It is a diagnosis that must be considered in weak patients on chronic steroid therapy. The diabetic patient with hyperglycemia can present with generalized weakness from diabetic ketoacidosis or nonspecific neurological deficits secondary to hypoglycemia (Chapters 159–162).

Rheumatologic

Weakness is a prominent complaint of most rheumatologic diseases and occasionally is the primary presenting symptom. Systemic lupus erythematosus, polymyositis, dermatomyositis, polymyalgia rheumatica, and particularly myasthenia gravis must all be considered in patients presenting with symmetric weakness.

Psychogenic Weakness

This diagnosis should be made after an exhaustive search for the cause of weakness has excluded both metabolic and systemic diseases. Patients with conversion disorder may present with paralysis of a specific muscle group that is not anatomically consistent. The symptoms of these patients are subconscious which is in contrast to the malingering patient whose actions are purposeful and often have secondary gain. Although the evaluation of this group of patients can often be difficult and resource consuming, the diagnosis of psychogenic weakness should be one of exclusion after other diagnoses have been considered (9).

DIAGNOSTIC APPROACH

An exhaustive history and physical examination should be performed to uncover the subtle details essential in establishing the cause of a patient's complaint of weakness. The patient's definition of *weakness* must first be clarified. Whether the weakness is focal muscle weakness or generalized fatigue must be determined early in the evaluation. If the patient complains of muscular weakness, then the clinician must determine whether it is focal or generalized, proximal or distal. The information gathered from the history and physical examination guides further testing. In general, a complete blood count, serum chemistry, and urinalysis should be obtained. A sedimentation

---

TABLE 13.4.   Commonly Used Drugs and Other Substances Associated with Weakness

MYOPATHIES

Steroids
Alcohol
Heroin
Clofibrate
Epsilon-aminocaproic acid
Diuretics
Laxatives
Amphotericin
D-penicillamine
Cimetidine
Procainamide

NEUROPATHIES

Carbon monoxide
Heavy metals
Polychlorinated biphenyls
Isoniazid
Nitrofurantoin
Gold

NEUROMUSCULAR JUNCTION DISEASE

Organophosphates
Carbamates

rate is helpful if rheumatologic disease is suspected. A Monospot test, liver function tests, and thyroid function tests are sometimes indicated. Heavy metal screening and red blood cell acetylcholinesterase level are required in selected cases, but these are rarely available to the emergency physician while the patient is in the department. Carboxyhemoglobin is indicated in suspected cases of carbon monoxide poisoning. A serum creatine phosphokinase and aldolase are helpful in cases of suspected myopathy.

Pulse oximetry and arterial blood gas analysis are indicated in cases of suspected pulmonary dysfunction. Pulmonary function testing, including vital capacity and maximum inspiratory force, is recommended when respiratory muscle compromise is suspected as in patients with myasthenia gravis and Guillain-Barré syndrome. An electrocardiogram and cardiac monitoring have a low diagnostic yield in patients with generalized weakness, though they may be helpful when dysrhythmias or electrolyte abnormalities are suspected. In the elderly patient without other sources of weakness, an electrocardiogram should be obtained to rule out a cardiac source. Rarely, more specialized laboratory testing is indicated in the evaluation of the weak patient in the emergency department. Lumbar puncture and CSF analysis for gram stain and culture can be a useful diagnostic tool when suspecting infection as a cause of weakness. In the setting of a fever and headache without a source or an immunocompromised patient with unknown fever and weakness, lumbar puncture is imperative. If there is a suspicion of increased intracranial pressure in a patient with fever and headache, a CT scan, prior to LP, should be performed to exclude an intracranial mass. The lumbar puncture can also aid in the diagnosis or exclusion of specific neurologic disorders. Multiple sclerosis will typically have a pleocytosis on CSF examination and electrophoresis may demonstrate oligoclonal bands of IgG that is highly suggestive of the disease. Guillain-Barré syndrome characteristically exhibits fewer than 50 lymphocytes per milliliter, a normal sugar, and an elevated protein. A tensilon test should be considered in patients with suspected myasthenia gravis.

Computed axial tomography or magnetic resonance imaging with intravenous contrast best evaluates structural lesions in the brain or spinal canal. The CT is a useful tool to diagnose intracerebral lesions and edema as a cause of weakness, such as in tumors, toxoplasmosis, cerebral bleeds, and infarcts. Patients may present with global cognitive deficits as in the case of massive bleeds or subtle upper motor neuron findings as seen with minor cerebral infarcts or infections. In patients requiring an LP, a pre-procedure noncontrast CT may be indicated if there is a high suspicion of increased intracranial pressure. Clinical history and physical examination can be used to guide the clinician on this decision. An HIV-positive patient with fever and headache or a patient with global mental status change and fever have an increased risk for elevated cerebral pressures. If there are no focal neurologic findings in a patient with normal mental status and a careful fundoscopic examination reveals no signs of papilledema with adequate venous pulsations, an LP can be performed safely without a CT. Imaging using CT is also useful in patients with physical examination findings suggestive of upper motor neuron disease associated with symptoms such as headache, nausea, and vomiting. Unfortunately the CT is not as sensitive in the evaluation of spinal cord lesions such as in spinal epidural hematomas and abscesses. If a patient presents with distinct weakness and sensory deficit below a cord level with associated back pain and the diagnosis of a spinal cord lesion is considered, the MRI is the test of choice. The MRI is also a useful imaging modality in the diagnosis of cauda equina syndrome as a cause of the lower extremity weakness in the setting of urinary dysfunction, saddle anesthesia, and impotence. Because most hospitals have limited MRI availability, if it cannot be obtained, the patient should be stabilized and transferred to the appropriate facility.

CRITICAL INTERVENTIONS

The focus of the emergency physician's approach to the patient complaining of weakness is to rule out the life-threatening diagnoses, specifically those diagnoses that can progress to cardiopulmonary or respiratory compromise (Table 13.5). After airway patency is established, patients should be assessed for adequacy of respiration. Certain patients, based on the history and physical examination, must be assessed for hypoxemia, hypercapnia, or carboxyhemoglobinemia. Assessment of pulmonary function with measurements of tidal volume and vital capacity may be valuable, especially in patients with suspected myasthenia gravis or Guillain-Barré syndrome; patients with a vital capacity less than 1.5 L are possible candidates for intubation.

The patient will need intubation and mechanical ventilation when respiratory failure is imminent. Signs of respiratory compromise are seen with declining oxygen saturations, increasing hypercapnea if capnometry is available, changes in mental status such as confusion or lethargy, and the increased use of accessory muscles for the work of breathing. Upon preparation for rapid sequence intubation, careful thought should be given to the medications used. If intracerebral mass lesion is suspected, premedication with lidocaine and fentanyl with a defasciculating dose of a nondepolarizing agent should be considered. In a patient suspected of organophosphate poisoning, paralysis using a nondepolarizing agent such as rocuronium is preferred. Organophosphates decrease the amount of plasma pseudocholinesterase and prolong activation of succinylcholine at the neuromuscular junction. Using a depolarizing agent in the paralysis of a suspected myasthenic patient should be attempted with caution because of increased sensitivity and possible exaggerated response to succinylcholine. Hyperkalemia can also result from using succinylcholine in association with patients with multiple sclerosis and amyotrophic lateral sclerosis and should be avoided.

Potentially unstable patients require intravenous access, pulse oximetry, and cardiac monitoring. Regular reassessment throughout the emergency department stay is necessary to avoid missing deterioration in the patient's status. Specific interventions depend on the diagnosis. Both plasmapheresis and intravenous IgG have been shown to improve outcome and shorten the course of disease in patients presenting with Guillain-Barré syndrome (14) Sedating drugs should be avoided in anxious patients who are hypoxemic. Drugs that interfere with myoneural junction function, such as the aminoglycosides, should be avoided in patients with suspected myasthenia gravis. Hypoglycemia is treated with dextrose, and hypokalemia with potassium. Hydrocortisone, 100 mg intravenously, should be given to patients with suspected adrenal insufficiency. Patients with periodic paralysis do not have a total body deficit of potassium, but instead have an alteration in intra- and extracellular potassium levels. Therefore, potassium should be carefully corrected to avoid inducing hyperkalemia. Patients who are weak due to toxins require specific antidotes when available. Significant carbon monoxide poisoning is an indication for hyperbaric oxygen treatment. Organophosphate poisoning requires the use of atropine and pralidoxime. Heavy metal poisoning is treated with chelation therapy.

DISPOSITION

Patients with progressive symptoms or those with suspected or confirmed disease that have a progressive course or risk of respiratory compromise, such as myasthenia gravis, Guillain-Barré, or botulism, should be admitted to an intensive care setting regardless of their initial appearance. Early consultation

TABLE 13.5.   Acute Life-Threatening Causes of Weakness

Cause	History	Physical	Laboratory	Treatment
Myasthenia gravis	Chronic weakness, improves with rest	Double vision, muscle fatigue, improves with rest	Positive Tensilon test	Thymectomy, AChE inhibitors
Guillain-Barré	Recent infection, progressive weakness distal to proximal	Distal motor and +/− sensory loss, absent reflexes, no visual deficits	CSF with elevated protein, < 50 WBCs	Supportive care, plasma exchange, gamma globulin
Botulism	Acute onset; canned, pickled, smoked food	Blurred or double vision	None	Supportive care, equine antitoxin
Adrenal insufficiency	Acute weakness associated with stress	Hypotension, hyperpigmentation	Hyperkalemia, hyponatremia	Hydrocortisone
Organophosphate poisoning	Occupational exposure, progressive weakening	Miosis, fasciculations, muscarinic dysfunction	Decreased RBC AChE	Atropine, pralidoxime
Carbon monoxide poisoning	Occupational or social exposure	Nausea, vomiting, coma, headache, dizziness	Elevated carboxyhemoglobin	100% oxygen, hyperbaric oxygen
Hypokalemia	Familial, GI, or renal loss	Diffuse weakness	Low serum potassium	Potassium

AChE, acetylcholinesterase; CSF, cerebrospinal fluid; WBCs, white blood cells; RBC, red blood cell; GI, gastrointestinal.

with a neurologist or neurosurgeon is recommended, and a comprehensive management plan should be determined. Laboratory tests should not be ordered unless the results will be available before emergency department discharge or careful follow up has been arranged.

COMMON PITFALLS

✔ Failure to perform a detailed history and physical examination

✔ Failure to obtain a drug and toxin exposure history and failure to detect an occupational exposure, drug-induced myopathy, or drug-induced adrenal insufficiency

✔ Diagnosing a psychogenic etiology or the chronic fatigue syndrome in the emergency department

✔ Failure to recognize absent reflexes as an early manifestation of the Guillain-Barré syndrome

✔ Failure to distinguish periodic paralysis from hypokalemia induced by drugs, gastrointestinal loss, or other etiologies

References

1. Baloh R. Dizziness in older people. *J Am Geriatr Soc* 1992;40:713.
2. Bergeron L, Sternbach G. Thyrotoxic periodic paralysis. *Ann Emerg Med* 1988;17:843.
3. Braun R. Environmental emergencies. *Emerg Med Clin North Am* 1997;15:451.
4. Brennan R. Chemical warfare agents: emergency medical and emergency public health issues. *Ann Emerg Med* 1999;34:191–204.
5. Cannon L, Bradford J, Jones J. Hypokalemic periodic paralysis. *J Emerg Med* 1986;4:287.
6. CDC. Nosocomial poisoning associated with emergency department treatment of organophosphate toxicity-Georgia. *JAMA* 2001;285:527–528.
7. Chau T, Lin S, Chiu J, Hsu C. A simple and rapid approach to hypokalemic paralysis. *Am J Em Med* 2003;21:487–491.
8. Chew W, Birnbaumer D. Evaluation of the elderly patient with weakness: an evidence based approach. *Emerg Med Clin North Am* 1999;17:265.
9. Gaufberg S, Glick T, Workman T. Suspected conversion disorder: Foreseeable risks and avoidable errors. *Acad Emerg Med* 2000;11:1272–1277.
10. Jagoda A, Feuer H. Myasthenia gravis presenting as a unilateral abducens nerve palsy. *Am J Em Med* 2001;19:410–412.
11. Jerrard D, Kuo D. Environmental insults: smoke inhalation, submersion, diving, and high altitude. *Emerg Med Clin N Am* 2003;21:475–497
12. Knochel J. Neuromuscular manifestations of electrolyte disorders. *Am J Med* 1982;72:521.
13. Lin S, Lin Y, Wu C, Pei D, Chu S. Diagnosing thyrotoxic periodic paralysis in the ED. *Am J Em Med* 2003;21:339–342.
14. LoVecchio F, Jacobson S. Approach to generalized weakness and peripheral neuromuscular disease. *Emerg Med Clin North Am* 1997;15:605.
15. Schluederberg A, Straus S, Peterson P, et al. Chronic fatigue syndrome research: definition and medical outcome assessment. *Ann Intern Med* 1992;117:325.
16. Skiendzielewski J, Martyak G. The weak and dizzy patient. *Ann Emerg Med* 1980;9:353.
17. Tresch D. Management of the older patient with acute myocardial infarction. *J Am Geriatr Soc* 1998;46:1157.
18. Wroblewski M. Symptoms of myocardial infarction in old age. *Age Ageing* 1986;15:99.

CHAPTER 14
Dizziness

Michele E. Krajicek and Wyatt W. Decker

The prevalence of dizziness in the general population ranges from 1.8% in young adults to over 30% in those over 65 years old (13). It is also one of the most challenging chief complaints facing the emergency physician. The complaint itself is vague and can imply many different symptom profiles. The word "dizzy" has different meanings for different people. Some patients will use this word to describe feelings of abnormal motion, such as spinning or unsteadiness. Others intend the word to mean light-headedness, weakness, or generalized malaise. A good history of the present illness will often allow the physician to categorize the dizziness, and thus direct further work-up.

The symptom of dizziness has an extensive differential diagnosis including emergent causes that require immediate intervention. The focus of the emergency department work-up of the dizzy patient is to identify emergent causes and provide appropriate intervention. Less acute causes of dizziness can result in significant morbidity if left undiagnosed and untreated. An attempt should be made to identify potentially treatable conditions, or to provide appropriate disposition and referral when these causes are suspected. A standardized, symptom-based approach to the dizzy patient is the key to sorting through the large differential diagnosis.

CLINICAL PRESENTATION

A thorough history is pivotal in attempting to categorize a patient's dizziness. The initial step is to obtain a full, unprompted description of the symptoms experienced by the patient. This description should include the dizziness symptoms and any associated symptoms, such as auditory, neurologic, and autonomic complaints. Onset, duration, exacerbating and relieving factors, and frequency of occurrence should be established. It is important to note if symptoms occurred in relationship to head or neck trauma.

Dizziness is commonly categorized into four broad subtypes. These include *vertigo, presyncope, disequilibrium,* and *"other"* for miscellaneous causes. *Vertigo* describes the sensation of movement of a patient or of his or her surroundings when no actual movement exists. It can occur in episodes or be continuous. The feeling of spinning and the feeling of falling are often associated with vertigo. Symptoms brought on by movement, such as head turning, are typical. Autonomic symptoms, including nausea and vomiting, are also common with vertigo.

Once dizziness has been classified as vertigo, it can be further divided into *peripheral* or *central* vertigo based on the history and physical examination (Table 14.1). This is an important distinction because some causes of central vertigo are life threatening and require immediate intervention. Typically, symptoms of peripheral vertigo are more intense and more sudden in onset. Central vertigo tends to have an insidious onset, often includes gait instability, and eventually includes central nervous system symptoms.

Presyncope, which has also been called *near-syncope* or *near-fainting,* refers to a light-headed, faint feeling with the sense of impending loss of consciousness. Symptoms of presyncope are typically episodic. Patients often describe diminished or tunnel vision. Presyncope may be associated with changes in vertical position, such as moving from sitting to standing. It may also be associated with cardiac symptoms such as palpitations, shortness of breath or chest discomfort.

Disequilibrium is a sense of unsteadiness or imbalance, typically experienced when walking. The course of this symptom tends to be continuous, but it may wax and wane. The lower extremities are typically described as being unsteady. It generally presents with complaints of difficulty with gait, and is relieved by sitting down.

Some dizzy patients will defy categorization, and may describe a generalized feeling of floating, "wooziness" or other nonspecific symptoms. These patients require a more generalized approach and have a broad differential diagnosis. Important subgroups within the *"other"* category include psychophys-

iologic, metabolic, and drug-induced or toxic causes. Feelings of anxiety or panic are common with psychophysiologic dizziness.

The past medical history is helpful in assessing a patient's risk for certain causes of dizziness. The physician should determine if the patient has had any type of dizziness before and if the current symptoms are similar or different. Careful review of past neurologic and cardiovascular problems is necessary in order to determine the likelihood that diseases involving these systems are the cause of the dizziness symptoms. For example, of patients with acute myocardial infarction, 4% present to the emergency department with only symptoms of dizziness, weakness or syncope (6). In these patients, a history of cardiovascular disease is critical information.

A review of patient medications is helpful in determining the cause of dizziness. An extensive list of medications can cause dizziness (Table 14.2). However, it is important not to stop the work up if one of these medications is found. The work up should focus on serious causes of dizziness; only when these are ruled out should medications be considered as the causative factor.

Physical examination in the dizzy patient is directed by the initial history obtained by the physician. The physical examination should begin with assessment of vital signs. This may include blood pressure and pulse measurements in both upper extremities; these may be unequal in patients with aortic dissection or subclavian steal syndrome. Orthostatic blood pressure measurements may be helpful in patients with presyncope. The most useful orthostatic measurements in confirming suspected blood loss are severe postural dizziness preventing upright measurements and pulse increase of 30 beats/minute or more in the standing position (9). General examination of the heart, lungs, abdomen and extremities should be performed in all patients. The neck should be auscultated for bruits in the carotid and vertebral artery distributions in older patients.

In patients with vertigo, the examination should focus on the auditory, neurologic and vestibular systems. Examination of the ears may reveal foreign body, infection, or perilymphatic fistula. Hearing should be screened, followed by Weber and Rinne testing when abnormalities are found. The cranial nerves should be tested. Examination of the eyes, especially for nystagmus, is important in diagnosing vertigo. The characteristics of the nystagmus are helpful in differentiating central from peripheral vertigo (Table 14.1).

Evaluation of cerebellar function is an essential part of the examination, especially in patients complaining of disequilibrium. Gait should be observed for abnormalities. Patients with

---

TABLE 14.1.   Central Versus Peripheral Vertigo

Type of Vertigo	Central	Peripheral
Autonomic symptoms	Infrequent	Frequent, severe
Onset	Gradual	Sudden
Duration	Continuous	Intermittent
Intensity	Mild-Moderate	Severe
CNS symptoms	Common	None
Nystagmus: Direction	Multidirectional, horizontorotary or vertical	Unidirectional, horizontal or rotary (not vertical)
Fatigable	No	Yes
Suppressed with visual fixation	No	Yes

TABLE 14.2.   Medications That Can Cause or Contribute to Dizziness

Subtype of Dizziness	Probable Mechanism of Dizziness	Class of Medication
Vertigo, Disequilibrium	Vestibulotoxicity	Alcohols, aminoglycosides, anticonvulsants, aspirin, cisplatin, erythromycin, loop diuretics, minocycline, quinine, quinidine, quinolones
Dysequilibrium	CNS depression	Alcohol, anticonvulsants, narcotics
Presyncope	Orthostatic hypotension	Antihypertensives, diuretics, antidepressants, antiparkinsonians
	Arrhythmias	Class 1a antiarrhythmics
Other	Hypoglycemia	Oral sulfonylureas

peripheral causes tend to have imbalance, but are able to walk. Patients with central lesions often cannot stand or walk without falling. The patient should be tested for dysdiadochokinesia with rapid alternating movements and for dysmetria with finger-to-nose pointing; either finding indicates that the cerebellum is the likely cause.

DIFFERENTIAL DIAGNOSIS

A categorical approach to the differential diagnosis is appropriate if a subtype of dizziness has been determined by the history and physical exam. Within each category, it is imperative to first consider acute life-threatening causes of dizziness (Table 14.3). Once these diagnoses have been either identified and treated or ruled out, the work up can be expanded to include less serious causes of dizziness.

Age is an important consideration in forming a differential diagnosis. The elderly are more susceptible to dizziness due to a reduction in sensory receptors in the inner ear, proprioceptive end organs, and retina. Some authors have suggested that the multiple etiologies and increased susceptibility to dizziness in older patients may constitute a syndrome of "geriatric dizziness" (14). However, it is important to remember that this does not imply that there is not a single specific cause for dizziness in elderly patients. These patients are also more likely to have cardiovascular disease as a cause of the dizziness symptoms.

In children, determining a subtype of dizziness is more difficult due to their inability to characterize their symptoms. In children who are unable to communicate the details of their dizziness, the physical examination is critical. The examination may include findings specific for children. For example, prolonged skinfold, sunken eyes, and dry oral mucosa correlate with dehydration, which suggests a presyncope subtype of dizziness (3). The distribution of causes of dizziness in children is different from adults. As in adults, the life-threatening etiologies should be considered first. The emergent causes of dizziness in children include infection, such as meningoencephalitis and labyrinthitis; central lesions, such as tumor or hematoma; cardiac dysrhythmias, such as long QT syndrome, hypovolemia; and head trauma (15). The most common cause of dizziness in children is migraine headache, followed by benign paroxysmal vertigo, vestibular neuronitis, and anxiety (12).

Vertigo is caused by imbalance in tonic vestibular signals. The differential diagnosis includes lesions in the auditory and vestibular systems. The acute, life-threatening causes of vertigo are typically central in origin. These include infection, vascular insufficiency, infarction, hemorrhage, and neoplasm (Table 14.3). Head and neck trauma can lead to vertigo. These injuries include mild closed-head injury (concussion) and can present acutely or up to 7 days after the initial trauma. Vertigo is a presenting symptom in about 5% of patients with multiple sclerosis (11). Migraine headache is the cause of dizziness in up to 7% of patients presenting to ambulatory clinics (10). Another cause of centrally mediated vertigo is temporal lobe epilepsy. Peripheral vertigo is typically associated with more benign causes. These include benign paroxysmal peripheral vertigo (BPPV), Meniere's disease, perilymphatic fistula, vestibular neuronitis, labyrinthitis, and more serious causes such as ototoxicity and acoustic neuroma.

Presyncope occurs because of decreased blood flow to the entire brain. This is the same mechanism as true syncope, and therefore the causes of presyncope and syncope are the same. Decreases in mean arterial pressure challenge the cerebral autoregulatory mechanisms, resulting in fainting or near-fainting (16). Acute, life-threatening causes of presyncope include acute cardiac ischemia, hypovolemia, obstruction of blood flow and cardiac dysrhythmias. In patients with a history of syncope and presyncope studied by loop recorder, dysrhythmia was recorded in 18% of those with presyncope alone (8). Common causes of presyncope include vasodepressor (vasovagal) response, autonomic failure, and orthostatic hypotension.

TABLE 14.3. Emergent Causes of Dizziness

Dizziness Subtype	Condition	Findings
Vertigo	Infection (encephalitis, meningitis, abscess)	Febrile, toxic patient, Head CT scan findings
	Vertebrobasilar insufficiency	Neurologic deficits often present, but initial exam may be normal, MRA may show lesion
	Cerebellar hemorrhage or infarction	Gait and balance disturbance; CT shows hemorrhage; MRI is better for evaluating posterior fossa and shows infarct
	Brain stem infarction:	Asymmetric cerebellar dysfunction
	Lateral Medullary (posterior inferior cerebellar artery) (Wallenberg syndrome)	Nausea, ipsilateral facial numbness, contralateral loss of pain and temp. sense, Horner syndrome
	Lateral pontomedullary (anterior inferior cerebellar artery)	Nausea, unilateral hearing loss, tinnitus, facial paralysis
	Intracranial mass lesion (neoplasm or hematoma)	Headache, deafness, ataxia, ipsilateral facial weakness, loss of corneal reflex, cerebellar signs
Presyncope	Acute ischemic heart disease	Chest pain, dyspnea, nausea, diaphoresis, ECG findings
	Cardiac dysrhythmias	Palpitations, dyspnea, ECG findings
	Obstruction of blood flow:	
	Aortic stenosis, hypertrophic cardiomyopathy, PE	Dyspnea, murmur, ECG findings
		Dyspnea, chest pain, CT, VQ, U/S or angio findings
	Aortic dissection	Chest pain radiating to back, CT/angio/TEE findings
	Tamponade	Distended neck veins, hypotension, muffled heart sounds, echocardiographic findings
	Hypovolemia	Hypotension, signs of active bleeding or dehydration
Disequilibrium	Motor (frontal lobe) lesions	Weakness, rigidity, tremor
	Cerebellar lesions	Wide-based gait, Ataxia
Other	Toxin exposure	Toxidrome symptoms, presence of toxin in urine or blood screen

CT, computed tomography; ECG, electrocardiogram; MRA, magnetic resonance angiography; MRI, magnetic resonance imaging; PE, pulmonary embolism; TEE, transesophageal echocardiography; US, ultrasound; VQ, ventilation-perfusion.

Disequilibrium is caused by loss of sensori-motor control. The differential diagnosis includes lesions in the peripheral nerves, spinal cord, visual or central nervous system. Acute, life-threatening causes include lesions of the motor cortex and cerebellar lesions. Other causes include proprioception and somatosensory loss, which is common in patients with diabetes, renal failure, cervical spine disease, and peripheral neuropathy. Disequilibrium is a typical symptom in patients with Parkinson's disease.

The causes of dizziness in the "*other*" category typically are not associated with life-threatening causes. The exception to this is toxic exposures. Toxic causes of dizziness include carbon monoxide and alcohol. *Psychophysiologic dizziness* is caused by impaired central integration of sensory signals. These include hyperventilation syndrome, panic disorder, and psychiatric dizziness. In patients with chronic dizziness, the frequency of psychophysiologic dizziness ranges from 20% to 50% (4). Dizziness is the second most common symptom during a panic attack, occurring in 50% to 90% of patients with panic disorder (5). Metabolic causes of dizziness include hypoglycemia and hypo- or hyperthyroidism.

For patients in whom a specific subtype of dizziness cannot be identified, a broad work up investigating the serious causes of dizziness from each category must be pursued. If a definite cause is not discovered, and acute causes are ruled out, the patient may have a dizziness syndrome, such as geriatric dizziness or psychiatric dizziness. These are diagnoses of exclusion, and can be further delineated in the outpatient setting.

DIAGNOSTIC APPROACH

The diagnostic approach to the dizzy patient is directed by the findings from the history and physical examination (Fig. 14.1).

This approach is focused on identifying the emergent causes of dizziness. In some cases the history and physical examination provide enough information to diagnose and treat a patient. In others, ancillary testing is necessary. Patients with central vertigo need imaging to look for infarction, hemorrhage, or neoplasm. CT is helpful for excluding hemorrhage but is notoriously poor at visualizing the posterior fossa. When tumors or infarction are suspected, MRI is the modality of choice for imaging the dizzy patient (2). Patients with unknown causes of disequilibrium may also require neurologic imaging if a central lesion is suspected. Patients with suspected infection will need laboratory work up including blood and cerebrospinal fluid counts and cultures. BPPV may be identified in the emergency department by use of diagnostic maneuvers such as the *Dix-Hallpike maneuver*. In this maneuver, the patient's head is held on both sides and turned 45 degrees to the side, and then the patient is quickly lowered from sitting to supine so that the head is hanging at 45 degrees off the head of the examination table. A positive test induces nystagmus and reproduction of the symptoms (7).

Patients with presyncope symptoms or any patient with cardiac symptoms associated with the dizziness should have an ECG and monitoring while in the ED to search for indications of cardiac ischemia or dysrhythmia. These patients may require chest x-ray to look for pulmonary or cardiac disease; echocardiography to look for effusion, functional abnormalities, valve disease or thrombus; chest CT to look for pulmonary embolism or thoracic aortic dissection; and laboratory tests including cardiac biomarkers to look for evidence of cardiac ischemia. Patients with orthostatic hypotension should have a complete blood count to look for anemia, which may then lead to further tests to discover the cause of anemia. Electrolytes, glucose, renal function and thyroid tests can be helpful in evaluating other causes of dizziness. The use of these

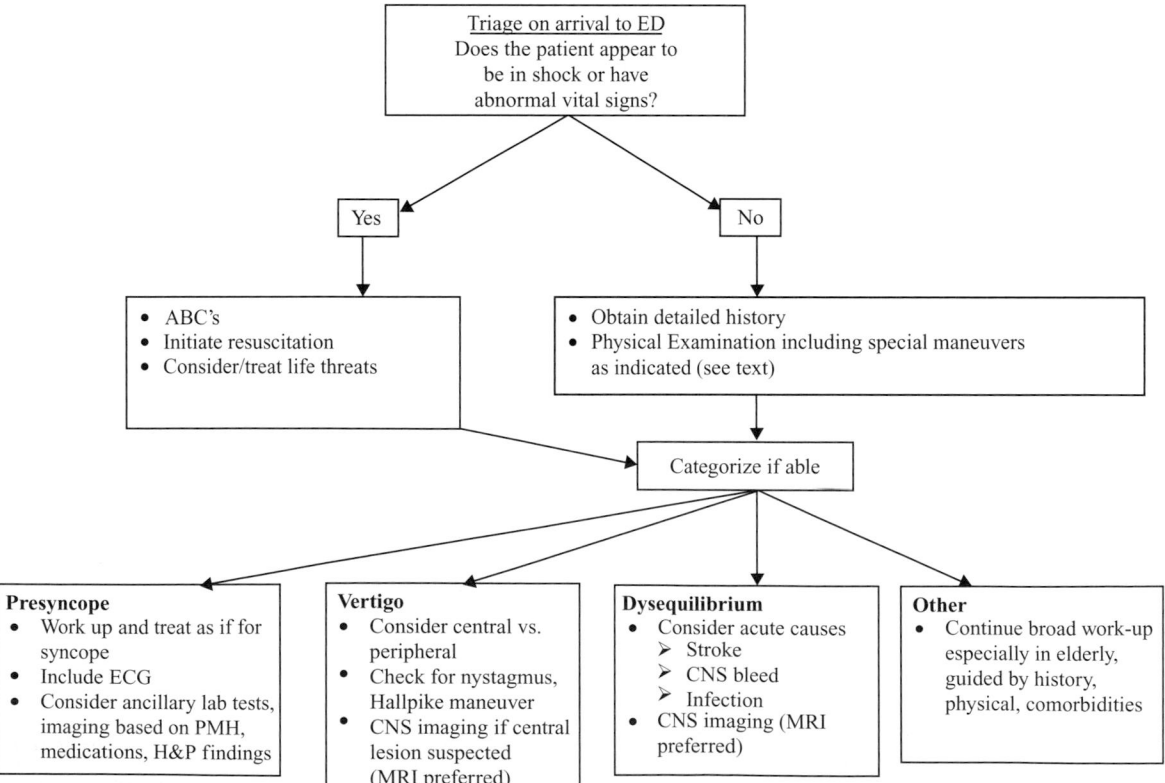

Figure 14.1. Diagnostic approach to patients with dizziness.

tests should be guided by specific causes, as they are often not indicated.

CRITICAL INTERVENTIONS

The initial management of all patients presenting with dizziness begins with assessment and stabilization of the airway, breathing and circulation. Emergent causes of dizziness are identified, stabilized and appropriate consulting services notified. Some patients with less acute causes of dizziness may benefit from treatment of their symptoms. Vestibular suppressant drugs are antihistamines, including dimenhydrinate, cyclizine, meclizine, and promethazine; benzodiazepines, including diazepam and lorazepam; butyrophenones, including droperidol; phenothiazines, including prochlorperazine; and benzamides, including metoclopramide. Most of these medications are useful to treat both vertigo and the associated nausea. However, other antiemetics can also be added. The method of determining which medication or combination of medications to use is determined by the effects of each drug and the time course and severity of the patient's symptoms (1). Patients with BPPV may benefit from canalith-repositioning maneuvers. The more complicated Epley maneuver is based on a series of head movements designed to reposition the offending canalith within the semicircular canals and utricle (7). For a discussion on the work up and management of vertigo see Chapter 31, Vertigo and Labyrinthine Disorders.

DISPOSITION

Patients without emergent causes of dizziness may be referred for outpatient work up. Once serious causes have been ruled out, it is important to determine that the patient has appropriate follow up scheduled. Follow up should start with the primary care provider and may involve neurology and otolaryngology. In addition, it is necessary to determine whether or not the patient can function in the outpatient setting. Some patients have such severe dizziness symptoms that they are unable to function at home, and these patients need to be admitted to the hospital.

COMMON PITFALLS

✔ Assuming dizziness has a benign cause before ruling out emergent causes
✔ Failure to take a good history and get an accurate description of what the patient means by the word "dizzy"
✔ Labeling a patient with a dizziness syndrome such as "geriatric" or "psychiatric" dizziness in the acute setting
✔ Discharging a patient with severe symptoms who is unable to safely function at home

Acknowledgments

Thanks to the previous edition's chapter authors Phillip G. Fairweather and Andy Jagoda upon whose chapter some of this material was based.

References

1. Asmundson GJ, Larsen DK, Stein MB. Panic disorder and vestibular disturbance: an overview of empirical findings and clinical impressions. *J Psychosomatic Res* 1998;44(1):107–120.
2. Baloh R. Dizziness: neurologic emergencies. *Neurol Clin* 1998;16:305–321.
3. Becker K, Craig BJ, Monsein LH. Vertebrobasilar thrombosis: diagnosis, management, and the use of intra-arterial thrombolytics. *Neurol Crit Care* 1996;24:1729–1742.
4. Duggan C, et al. How valid are clinical signs of dehydration in infants. *J Ped Gastroenterology and Nutrition* 1996;2256–61.
5. Furman J, Jacob R. Psychiatric dizziness. *Neuro* 1997;48:1161–1166.
6. Gupta M, et al. Presenting complaint among patients with myocardial infarction who present to an urban, public hospital emergency department. *Ann Emerg Med* Aug 2002;40:180–186.
7. Koelliker Paul, et al. Benign paroxysmal positional vertigo: Diagnosis and treatment in the emergency department—a review of the literature and discussion of canalith-repositioning maneuvers. *Ann Emerg Med* 2001;37:392–398.
8. Krahn A, Klein GJ, Yee R., Skanes AC. Predictive value of presyncope in patients monitored for assessment of syncope. *Am Heart J* 141:817–821.
9. McGee S, et al. Is this patient hypovolemic. *JAMA* 1999;281:1022–1029.
10. Neuhauser H, et al. The interrelations of migraine, vertigo, and migrainous vertigo. *Neurology* 2001;56:436–441.
11. Rae-Grant A, et al. Sensory symptoms of multiple sclerosis: a hidden reservoir of morbidity. *Multiple Sclerosis* 1999;5:179–183.
12. Ravid S, et al. A simplified diagnostic approach to dizziness in children. *Ped Neuro* 29:317–320.
13. Sloane P, et al. Dizziness: state of the science. *Ann Int Med* 2001;134:823–832.
14. Tinetti M, et al. Dizziness among older adults: a possible geriatric syndrome. *Ann Int Med* 2000;132:337–344.
15. Tusa RJ, et al. Dizziness in childhood. *J Child Neurol* 1994;9:261–724.
16. Van Lieshout J, et al. Syncope, cerebral perfusion, and oxygenation. *J Applied Physiol* 2003;94:833–848.

Section Editor: Gregory W. Hendey

Eye Emergencies

CHAPTER 15
The Ophthalmic Examination

Geoffrey Broocker

Ocular emergencies can cause a great deal of anxiety for both the patient and the physician, but a systematic approach to the history and physical exam should help lead one to the correct diagnosis (Fig. 15.1).

EMERGENCY DEPARTMENT EVALUATION

History

The history often provides enough information to establish a reasonable differential diagnosis, allowing the physician to focus on the appropriate segment of the visual system. Key historical points include age, trauma, family history, systemic illnesses, occupation, allergies, and ocular history. It is essential to know whether the patient had any previous visual problems or wears glasses or contact lenses.

Pain and Discomfort

It is often difficult to identify the source of pain because of the sensory overflow from various segments of the fifth cranial nerve. Discomfort may be localized according to specific symptoms. Discomfort related to the anterior ocular surface or lids usually involves burning, itching, tearing, and foreign-body sensation. Orbital or periorbital discomfort may involve eye muscle fatigue, sinus congestion, and vascular headaches, all of which are nonocular causes. These, along with ocular and intracranial pathology, are best described as dull aches or pressure. Ocular inflammatory disorders (including uveitis, episcleritis, scleritis, and acute glaucoma) are more commonly associated with these kinds of pains than intracranial pathology (arteritis, aneurysm, pituitary apoplexy, and tumors).

Photophobia

Photophobia is a common type of discomfort particular to ophthalmic disease. It is the hallmark of uveal inflammation (e.g., iritis or uveitis of any cause). It may also occur in corneal, retrobulbar, and meningeal inflammatory conditions. This dull, achy pain (which may be quite severe) must be differentiated from light sensitivity (mild discomfort from bright lights, e.g., car headlights).

Discharge and Tearing

Discharge is due primarily to anterior surface disorders, such as infections (Chapter 20, Diplopia). Tearing, most often reflex in origin, indicates abnormal surface irritation from dysfunctional lubrication (chemical and infectious sources) and injured epithelium (corneal foreign body or abrasion, Chapter 18).

Redness and Swelling

Redness and swelling are signs of congestion; they may be due to the release of inflammatory mediators. Allergens and infectious agents contribute to anterior surface signs. The orbital outflow disorders (congestive) are of concern; they include trauma, thyroid ophthalmopathy, orbital cellulitis, orbital inflammatory syndromes, cavernous sinus thrombosis, and fistulas. Intraocular inflammation tends to cause circumlimbal redness (ciliary flush) or generalized redness, but usually does not cause swelling. Exceptions to this are endophthalmitis and some cases of scleritis.

Changes in Appearance

A sense of urgency arises most often when there is an acute change in appearance. A common example is the subconjunctival hemorrhage. Although usually benign, it may be more ominous in the setting of possible penetrating trauma. Swelling and mass effect are noted with chalazia and dacryocystitis (over the lacrimal crest region). Proptosis may be due to a retrobulbar mass effect (thyroid ophthalmopathy, mucocele, tumor, and fistula).

Visual Disturbances

Visual disturbances are a frequent complaint and are often related to a nonocular cause, as discussed in Chapter 19. Blurred vision may originate from refractive errors all the way through the visual system to occipital cortex disorders. A good clinician should use the history as a starting point in the evaluation. *Glare* or *halos* are common disturbances. They are usually the result of light-scatter phenomena from unclear ocular media (mucinous tear film, corneal edema of any cause, corneal epithelial abnormalities, cataract, or vitreous haze). *Spots* or *floaters* are commonly degenerative opacities within the vitreous; they may, however, indicate red or white blood cells or pigment granules in the aqueous or vitreous. The sudden appearance of floaters may be clinically important.

Transient visual loss is a potentially serious problem. If monocular, consider the anterior circulation and pathways. If binocular, consider generalized hypoperfusion, posterior circulation, or pathways from the chiasm back to the occipital cortex.

Diplopia

Diplopia may be due to serious underlying disease (Chapter 20, Diplopia). A major point is whether it is monocular or binocular (Does it disappear when one eye is covered?). Monocular diplopia is generally due to pathology within the cornea or lens, while binocular diplopia is caused by ocular motility disturbances (cranial nerve palsies or muscle disorders). Whether the diplopia is horizontal or vertical may be key information. Horizontal diplopia is significant and may imply possible intracranial pathology (3rd- or 6th-nerve palsies caused by increased intracranial pressure, tumor, or aneurysm). Vertical diplopia after blunt orbital trauma may indicate orbital floor fracture with entrapment of the inferior rectus. Painful ophthalmoplegias are important and suggest intracranial disease. Pupil-sparing third-nerve palsies are usually vascular in origin (diabetes).

THE OCULAR EXAMINATION

Visual acuity is the key vital sign in ophthalmology. A Snellen chart (or equivalent), near card, or description of visual ability from any source (e.g., finger counting or newsprint) is necessary before proceeding with further examination. It is critical to evaluate each eye separately. Most physicians tend to focus only on the symptomatic eye. The physician must be certain that the non-examined eye is completely covered while checking the vision in the other eye. Patients often look around hands and through fingers in an attempt to perform well. Carefully document the visual acuity, and note whether it was checked with or without glasses. If the vision is subnormal, consider rechecking the

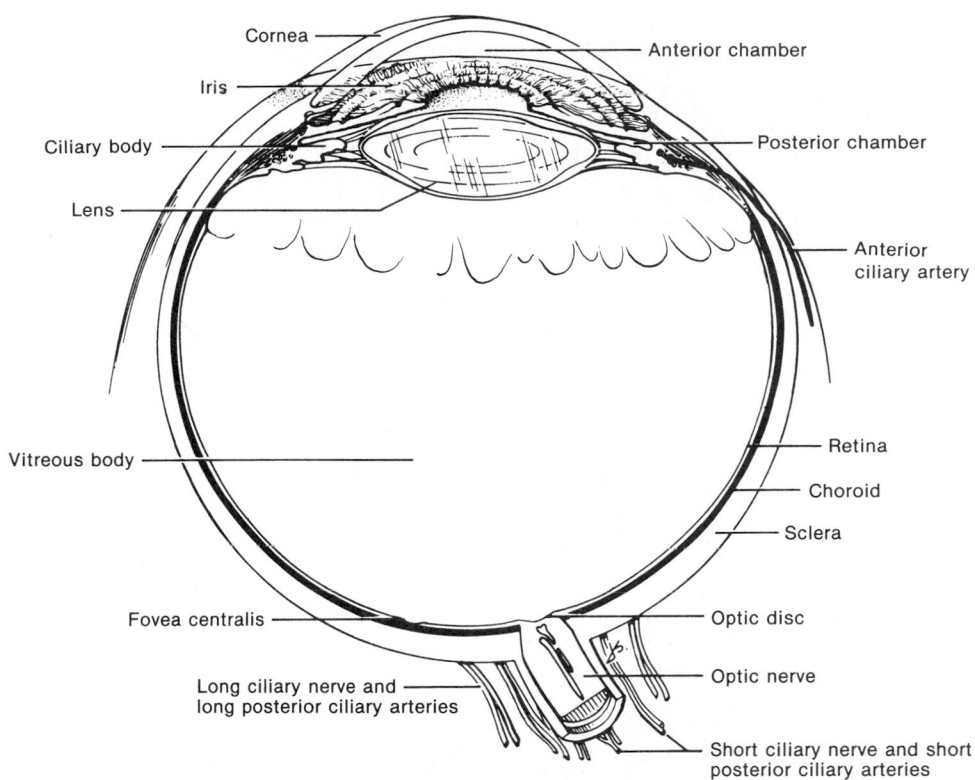

Figure 15.1.   Cross-section of the eye.

vision through pinholes, which optically correct most refractive errors. If the vision improves significantly, one must consider a refractive abnormality.

A "step back and look" approach to the inspection of the eye and adnexa is critical. By going right to the slit lamp or direct ophthalmoscope, one may not detect key findings such as small puncture wounds in the eyelid. Evert the upper lids to look for retained foreign bodies. An applicator stick can be used to provide a fulcrum for the lid. The lid margins are often a source for anterior surface disorders of the eye and should be carefully inspected for erythema, crusting, lash loss, and irregularity. A marginal laceration, especially near the nasal canthus, should be referred for proper repair.

The pupillary examination, often labeled PERRLA (pupils equal, round, reactive to light, and accommodation), is one of the most important tests of the integrity of the anterior visual pathway. Iris color and pupil size and shape are important. Drugs and trauma (blunt or sharp) affect these circumstances. Iritis tends to cause miosis as well as adhesions to the lens (posterior synechiae). Systemic and topical medications may dilate or constrict the pupil, depending on parasympathetic or sympathetic effects. Narcotics, barbiturates, psychotropics, and psychedelic drugs affect the pupil size, depending on their toxicity and whether the patient is in withdrawal. Essential anisocoria (inequality in diameter of pupils) occurs in a significant percentage of the normal population. *Horner syndrome* and tonic pupil (*Adie's pupil*) cause anisocoria. The anisocoria of Horner syndrome may be accentuated in dim illumination and diagnosed pharmacologically. Adie's pupil has light-near dissociation (minimal light reaction, greater for accommodation) and is generally larger than the *Argyll Robertson pupil*. Dorsal midbrain syndromes also create this finding but are associated with paresis of upward gaze and retraction nystagmus. Trauma may cause pupillary dilation through sphincter injury or miosis from traumatic iritis. Ruptures can be seen on slit-lamp examination. Corneoscleral lacerations are often plugged with a segment of iris, creating a peaked pupil toward the laceration.

The deafferented, or *Marcus Gunn*, pupil has ocular and neurologic significance. Using a bright light, the physician should check the pupils individually for size, shape, and direct reaction. The physician can view the consensual response in the other eye. By swinging the light directly from one eye to the other and back again, the midbrain can sample the intensity of input from each eye. For example, in retrobulbar neuritis, if the light swings from the normal eye to the eye with the problem, the midbrain quickly interprets a relative reduction in input and the efferent response is subsequently less. The examiner will see the pupil dilate instead of constrict. One must be careful not to confuse this with hippus (rhythmic wavering pupil). A bright light and a notable initial constriction differentiate these two. If both optic nerves are equally damaged, the examiner cannot demonstrate the Marcus Gunn pupil because there is no *relative* difference.

Ocular position and motility are part of the "step back and look" approach. Exophthalmos and enophthalmos are usually obvious. Enophthalmos is commonly seen in severe orbital floor fractures. A tethered inferior rectus causing marked upgaze restriction may also be seen. The extraocular movements involve a complex coordination of fronto-mesencephalic and cerebello-mesencephalic interactions through the third, fourth, and sixth cranial nerves. Any disturbance in intracranial processing or in midbrain or cranial nerve function, or an intraorbital or cranial nerve or muscle abnormality may result in an imbalance in ocular position response. This includes abnormalities in primary gaze (straight ahead) or congruity of gaze in the six cardinal positions (left, right, up and right, up and left, down and right, down and left). Esotropia (cross-eye) can be seen by observing the light reflex off the cornea to be temporal to the central cornea; exotropia (walleye) can be seen by observing the light reflex nasal to the central cornea. This can be documented by the cover–uncover test. Ask the patient to fixate on a distant object or target; cover and then uncover each eye. The deviated eye straightens when the normal eye is covered (opposite to the direction of the original deviation). An esotropic eye moves temporally when the normal eye is covered. Vertical deviations can be noted by the

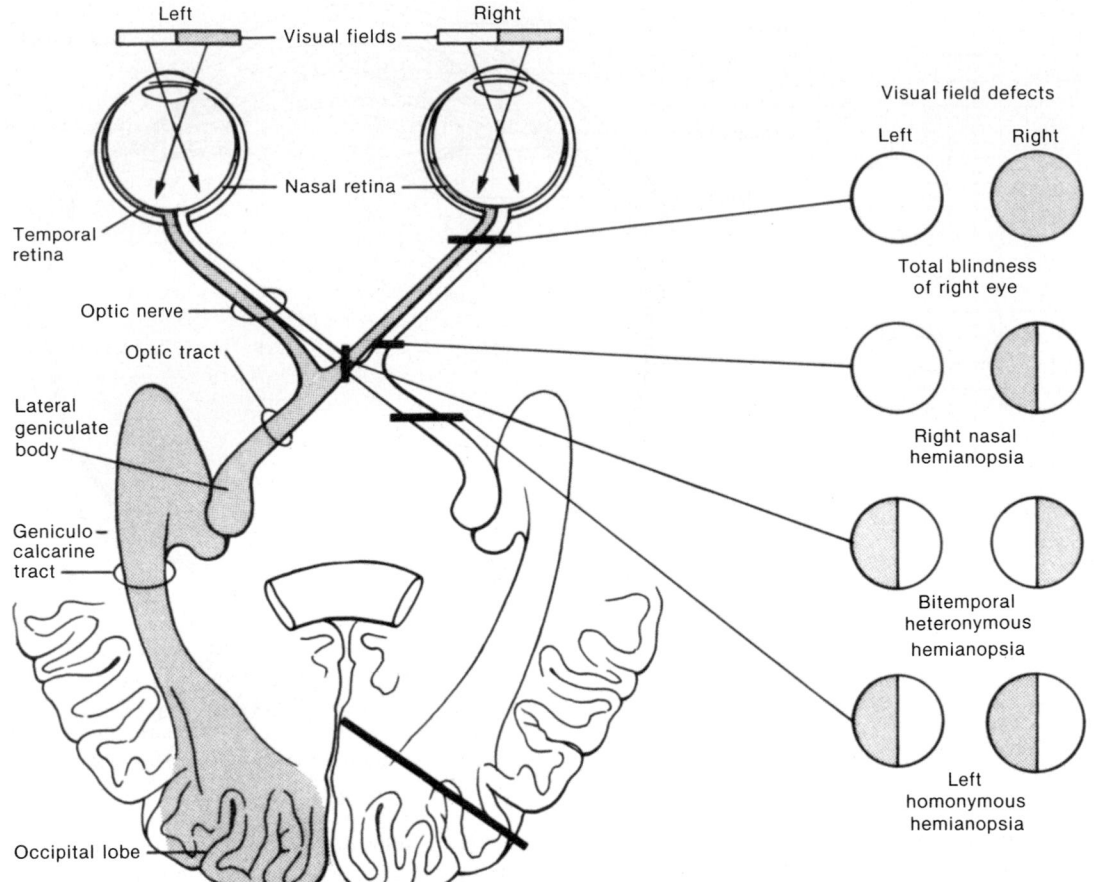

Figure 15.2.   Lesions in the optic pathways.

higher eye, which is labeled a hypertropia. The light reflex is lower on the cornea in the hypertropic eye than in the other eye. During cover testing, that eye moves downward when the normal eye is covered. It is a challenge to determine whether the origin of the motility disturbance is inherited, acquired, neural, muscular, or some combination.

The eyes are just the anterior-most extension of the visual system. The most important test of the "total" system is the visual field. Defects in the visual field may indicate injury anywhere from the retina to the occipital cortex (Fig. 15.2). Abnormalities in visual field testing may occur before the patient has actual visual complaints. Performing formal visual field assessment by perimetry is difficult in the emergency setting, but simple confrontation fields (Fig. 15.3) may produce the information required for localization. The examiner is the "control" and faces the patient. Targets (e.g., fingers) in 45-degree intervals are used to test the peripheral field, one eye at a time. Gross hemianopic defects (homonymous or bitemporal), as well as isolated defects, can be easily described. The Amsler grid (Fig. 15.4) is an ancillary test that assesses the visual field of the central 10 degrees of vision. Because this is the macular projection of the retina, it provides useful information on central retinal disorders (hemorrhage, edema, and degeneration). The Amsler grid is essentially a "tile floor" pattern with a central dot. Using one eye at a time, the patient fixates on this dot and is asked to describe wavy lines or missing areas. Principal findings are metamorphopsia (wavy distortion) and scotomas (blind spots) of macular lesions or optic nerve disorders (e.g., toxic amblyopia and optic neuritis).

Because the central retina and optic nerve are essentially a color projection system, even simple analysis of color perception may help isolate the problem. Color vision testing can be performed using many techniques, but in the emergency setting, the testing of the central red saturation is a good way to localize the problem to the central retina or optic nerve. Using the red bottle top of a dilating or cycloplegic agent (e.g., tropicamide [Mydriacyl] or phenylephrine hydrochloride [Mydfrin]), the examiner can ask the patient to quantitate the "degree" of red seen in each eye ("If this is a dollar's worth of red in the good eye, how much is it worth in the other?"). If the response reveals desaturation, macular or optic nerve disease may be present.

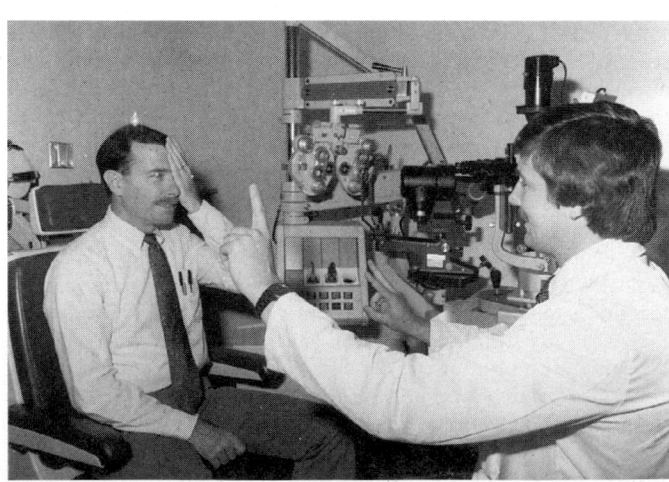

Figure 15.3.   Performing confrontation fields.

AMSLER RECORDING CHART

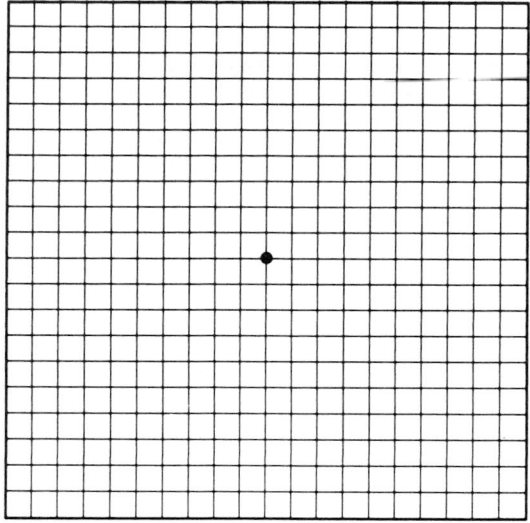

Figure 15.4. Amsler grid.

Finally, *intraocular pressure* should be evaluated. The intraocular pressure is to the eye what the blood pressure is to the cardiovascular system. Normal values range from 10 to 21 mm Hg, and are measured in various ways:

Indentation tonometry. The Schiøtz tonometer is cumbersome, can spread infection, and may create its own trauma, but it is relatively easy to use.

Applanation tonometry. The applanation tonometer is accurate, easy to use, and mounted on most slit lamps. Figure 15.5 shows the hand-held model.

Tonometer pens are electronic devices that are easy to use and relatively accurate, but very expensive (see Fig. 15.5).

Noncontact tonometers are for screening only; they may be inaccurate.

Pneumotonometers are effective and relatively easy to use, but somewhat expensive to maintain; they must be calibrated.

Manual assessment of the intraocular pressure may be crude and inaccurate but may provide a quick, rough estimate in certain situations (e.g., suspected angle closure glaucoma). The eyeball is palpated through closed lids in a gentle balloting motion. Comparison may be made with the unaffected eye, or with the examiner's eye. This method should be avoided in recently operated on globes or if lacerations are suspected.

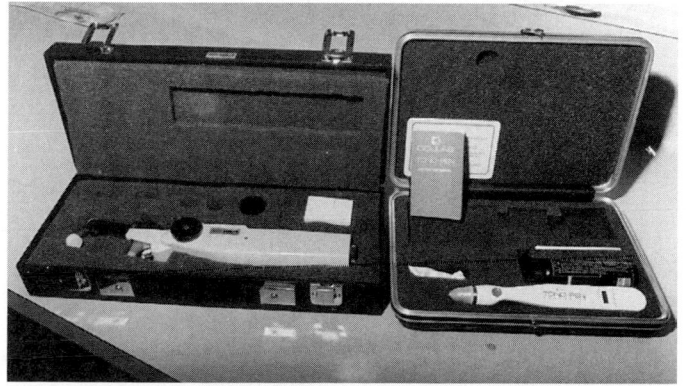

Figure 15.5. Hand-held applanation tonometer (**left**) and tonometer pen (**right**).

A bright penlight is helpful for pupil evaluation and is also useful in assessing the lids and anterior surface of the eye. The light should be moved across the eye to perceive the glassy reflective surface of the cornea. Epithelial abrasions and edema can be identified from the discontinuity in the reflections. It is useful to compare the findings with those of the other eye. The patient should be asked to look up while the lower lid is pulled down to evaluate the lower cornea and globe. *Foreign bodies* commonly are located under the upper lid. The examiner should look for discharge and areas of inflammation.

Fluorescein dye is picked up by damaged or absent epithelial cells (corneal abrasion). It changes color in the presence of pH changes. A dark flow in a green-yellow background is seen if aqueous humor is present from a corneal laceration (aqueous has a different pH than the tear film). Some penlights are equipped with a cobalt blue filter that can be used with fluorescein application.

Slit-Lamp Examination

The anterior segment of the eye is best examined with the slit-lamp biomicroscope. The view of the anterior segment anatomy is astounding under high magnification. In the presence of injury or infection, the slit-lamp examination is mandatory. The patient's head is positioned in the chin rest, with the forehead against the bar. The black line on the right vertical pole next to the patient's face is aligned with the level of the eyes. The examiner sets the oculars (usually to 0) and then adjusts the interpupillary distance, as with binoculars. The light source is moved to 45 degrees from the examiner–patient axis, and the chassis is adjusted forward or backward to bring the eye into focus. The examination is started on low magnification (10×). Once the eye is in focus, the magnification may be increased. Fine adjustments are made with the joystick. On some models, the up–down control is on the joystick. The beam is adjusted to a slit rather than a full circle. The three-dimensional box seen on the cornea shows the 0.5-mm thickness. With the slit lamp, the extent and level of corneal injuries can be assessed. The lids, conjunctiva, cornea, anterior chamber, and irises of both eyes should be examined systematically.

The *lid margins* may demonstrate information related to "the red eye." Lacerations may be appreciated, especially in the nasal canthal region, where the identification of a canalicular laceration is critical.

The *conjunctiva* has epibulbar and tarsal components. The examiner should look for discharge, follicles (cobblestone-like lymphoid aggregates characteristic of certain viral, toxic, or allergic conditions), chemosis (subconjunctival fluid swelling), and hyperemia. Small foreign bodies can be swept from under the upper lid during the slit-lamp examination.

The examination of the *cornea* involves the following:

1. Epithelium: to detect abrasions, edema, ulcers, and foreign bodies
2. Stroma: to detect primarily edema, but also deep ulcers, deep scars and vascularization, and penetration
3. Endothelium: to detect keratitic precipitates (white cells on the endothelium). These precipitates are a hallmark of iritis. Penetration through this layer is called a *laceration*.

The size and shape of the findings should be noted, and it is helpful to draw the findings in the medical record.

The *anterior chamber* is bounded by the cornea and iris and is filled with aqueous. Its depth can be assessed by adjusting the slit beam. By narrowing the beam into a small column of light, the examiner may see iritis with a cellular reaction as well as flare (light scatter caused by inflammatory proteins in the aqueous).

Red or white blood cells may be present in the anterior chamber. Red blood cells usually result from trauma; the layering of these cells in the anterior chamber is called a *hyphema*. Sometimes, pigment dispersion (granules of pigment) is difficult to differentiate from mild diffuse red blood cells. White blood cells are present in iritis; the visible layering of these cells in the anterior chamber is called a *hypopyon*.

The *iris–lens* examination involves noting pupil dysfunction, which may include traumatic tears in the sphincter or adhesions to the anterior lens capsule (posterior synechiae). The iris may plug corneoscleral lacerations (thereby peaking the pupil) or be torn at its root (iridodialysis). Note the presence of blood vessels growing on the iris surface (rubeosis iridis), which is usually due to proliferative retinopathies (e.g., diabetic). Opacities of the lens are defined as cataract opacities and may be due to many causes. Injury to the anterior capsule of the lens in penetrating trauma has diagnostic and surgical significance, because these lenses generally become rapidly opaque and incite tremendous inflammation.

The Ocular Fundus Evaluation

The ophthalmoscope can be used to magnify the anterior surface of the eye, using the higher, black (or green)-numbered lenses. Impaired view may be due to cloudy media (e.g., corneal and lens opacities, and vitreous blood), but it can also be due to unusual refractive errors. One tip for better viewing is to have the patient wear his or her corrective lenses while undergoing this test. It is expected that the refractive correction has made the patient "normal-sighted." If the examiner and patient are "normal-sighted, generally a –3 or –4 lens (the red 3 or 4) allows a comfortable view of the fundus.

The *optic nerve head* should be evaluated for margins, shape, and cup. The examiner should be aware of anomalies, such as small disks with little or no cup and central vessels with multiple early bifurcations. Note the presence or absence of spontaneous venous pulsations. Hemorrhages and blurred margins can be critical findings, and should be compared with findings in the other eye. The *macula* should be examined with attention to the presence of hemorrhages, exudates, and edema. It is important to note if these findings are generalized (diabetic or hypertensive retinopathy) or localized (any vascular retinopathy, especially occlusive disease). It is difficult to determine the layer of retinal bleeding, especially when the bleeding is subretinal. Deep retinal hemorrhages tend to be small (dot and blot). Superficial hemorrhages are flame-shaped. Edema makes the retina look gray-white. In central retinal artery occlusion and other causes of a thickened nerve fiber layer of the central retina (e.g., Tay-Sachs disease), one will see a distinctive, central red area called the *cherry-red spot*. This represents the visualization of the normal choroidal circulation through the one area of the retina where the nerve fiber layer is absent (fovea centralis).

Recognition of vascular retinopathies has important implications. The *retinal vessels* are a mirror of the body's microcirculation in a host of systemic processes.

CRITICAL INTERVENTIONS

- Measure the vital sign of the eye, visual acuity
- Take a "step back and look" approach to get the big picture
- Perform a slit-lamp exam to examine the anterior structures
- Measure intraocular pressure to rule out glaucoma

DISPOSITION

Role of the Consultant

The urgency of referral depends on multiple factors, and is detailed further in other chapters. Through a careful history and physical examination, the emergency physician should be able to arrive at a diagnosis. One can never be faulted with a phone consult with the ophthalmologist, documenting the details. Providing the necessary information to the ophthalmologist is the key to an effective consultation. The minimum information the consultant needs includes the patient's age, chief complaint, ocular history (and any pertinent medical history), and visual acuity in both eyes, as well as any other pertinent findings.

COMMON PITFALLS

✔ Failure to consider the possibility of ocular penetration in the setting of a high-velocity or potentially lacerating object (e.g., glass, metal)

✔ Lack of documentation of the patient's *visual acuity*. Each eye must be assessed while occluding the other

✔ Underestimation of the importance of horizontal diplopia, motility disturbance, and ptosis of the lid, which suggest more serious neuroophthalmic etiologies

✔ Excess fluorescein should be avoided when evaluating ocular surface problems or checking intraocular pressure

✔ Discharging a patient with a topical anesthetic, which retards corneal epithelial wound healing

References

1. Colenbrander A. Principles of ophthalmology. In: Tasman W, Jaeger EA, eds. *Duane's clinical ophthalmology*. Philadelphia: Lippincott Williams & Wilkins, 2002.
2. Langston DP. *Manual of ocular diagnosis and therapy*, 5th ed. New York: Lippincott-Raven, 2002.
3. Palay A, Krachmer J. *Ophthalmology for the primary care physician*. St. Louis: Mosby-Year Book, 1997.
4. Patel KH, Javitt JC, et al. Incidence of acute angle closure glaucoma after pharmacologic mydriasis. *Am J Ophthalmol* 1995;120:709–717.
5. Skarf B, Glaser J. Neuro-ophthalmic examination: general consideration and special techniques. In: Tasman W, Jaeger EA, eds. *Duane's clinical ophthalmology*. Philadelphia: Lippincott Williams & Wilkins, 1999.
6. Tate GW Jr, Safir A. The slit lamp: history, principles, and practice. In: Tasman W, Jaeger EA, eds. *Duane's clinical ophthalmology*. Philadelphia: Lippincott Williams & Wilkins, 1998.
7. Vaughan D. *General ophthalmology*, 15th ed. Stamford, CT: McGraw-Hill/Appleton & Lange, 1998.

CHAPTER 16
Common Ophthalmic Medications

Geoffrey Broocker

The information provided here describes representative therapeutic preparations for many ocular conditions. Please refer to compendiums such as the *Physician's Desk Reference for Ophthalmology* for a thorough listing with pharmaceutical manufacturers' specifications. Frequency of medication applications depends on the agent used and the severity of the condition being managed.

DIAGNOSTIC MEDICATIONS

These agents facilitate the ability to examine the eye.

Stains

These are topical solutions that highlight epithelial abnormalities of the cornea and conjunctiva.

Fluorescein: Sterile paper strips are preferred to the 2% solutions, owing to ease of contamination of the latter. This stains areas where epithelium is missing (corneal and conjunctival).

Rose bengal: This 1% solution stains devitalized corneal–conjunctival epithelium; it is helpful in differentiating a herpetic corneal ulcer from a healing abrasion.

Anesthetics

These are topical solutions that promote patient cooperation for the examination; they are also used in conjunction with the aforementioned stains. Anesthetics are usually required for determining intraocular pressure and help facilitate penetration of diagnostic drops.

  Tetracaine hydrochloride (Pontocaine): 0.5% to 1.0% solution, lasts for 15 minutes; may sting

  Proparacaine hydrochloride (Ophthetic, Ophthaine): 0.5% solution, less irritating

  Cocaine (0.25% to 0.5%): Effective but highly toxic to the corneal epithelium

Mydriatics and Cycloplegics

These are used diagnostically or therapeutically to dilate the pupil (mydriasis) and/or paralyze the ciliary body (cycloplegia). This permits evaluation of the internal ocular structures and gauges the baseline refractive error of the eye by blocking accommodation. In addition, these agents prevent synechiae formation (adhesions of the iris to lens and cornea) by reducing intraocular inflammation through stabilization of the blood–aqueous barrier and physically pulling the pupil away from greater contact with the anterior lens surface. These agents are capped in *red*. Duration of mydriasis and/or cycloplegic effects listed below are for normal, uninflamed eyes.

Phenylephrine hydrochloride (Neo-Synephrine, Mydfrin): Vasoconstricts the surface vessels and dilates the pupil without cycloplegia; 2.5% solution is the strength recommended because of a higher incidence of cardiovascular side effects with 10%. Dilation capability varies, used alone, and may last up to 4 hours, depending on the amount of pigmentation of the iris

Tropicamide (Mydriacyl 0.5% and 1.0%): Provides an excellent short-term dilation of the pupil, plus cycloplegia (4 to 6 hours). Relatively easy to reverse (if concerned about potential angle-closure glaucoma); used most often by ophthalmologists

Cyclopentolate hydrochloride (Cyclogyl 0.5%, 1.0%, and 2.0%): Best short-term cycloplegic for determining refractive error, may last for 6 hours up to a day!

Homatropine hydrobromide (1%, 2%, and 5%): Lasts for a few days and is useful for short-term on low-level inflammation (iritis) caused by trauma or abrasions

Scopolamine hydrobromide (Hyoscine 0.25%): Lasts for 3 to 5 days and is more effective for long-term inflammation seen postoperatively or in severe uveitis

Atropine sulfate (0.25% to 2.0% solution, 0.5% and 1.0% ointment): Lasts for 10 to 14 days; most commonly used postoperatively and in severe uveitis. Corneal epithelial and systemic toxicities are important to note

THERAPEUTIC AGENTS

Lubricants

The precorneal tear film is the most important layer of the eye with regard to comfort and vision. Abnormalities of this complex multilayered film are responsible for a large percentage of surface complaints (burning, itching, foreign-body sensation, epiphora, and blurred vision that vacillates with blinking). Artificial lubricants are an effective but temporary treatment for any condition that causes this "dry-eye syndrome."

1. *Artificial tears:* These agents (Table 16.1) usually contain various methylcellulose compounds, but synthetics are available.

TABLE 16.1. Artificial Tear Preparations

Agent in Solution	Trade Name Concentration	Preservative
Carboxymethylcellulose	*Refresh tears* (0.5%)	Purite
	Refresh plus (0.5%)	Preservative-free
	Theratears (0.25%)	Preservative-free
Hydroxypropylmethylcellulose	*Bion tears* (0.3%)	Preservative-free
	Lacritears	Benzalkonium chloride
	Tears naturale free	Preservative-free
	Visine tears	Benzalkonium chloride
Polyvinyl alcohol	*Akwa tears* (1.4%)	Benzalkonium chloride
	HypoTears (1%)	Benzalkonium chloride
	Murine (0.5%)	Benzalkonium chloride
Glycerin	*Moisture eyes* (0.3%)	Benzalkonium chloride
	Computer eye drops	Benzalkonium chloride
Polycarbophil	*AquaSite*	Preservative-free

Trends toward successful use involve the "thickness" of the solution and single-use, nonpreserved packets. Frequency of use, especially when preserved, multiuse bottles are selected, can have limited return on symptoms. Overall, these agents not only are benign, but also relieve most anterior surface irritation from any cause. *Be liberal in dispensing these agents!*

2. *Bland lubricating ointments* (Hypotears, Refresh P.M., others): Especially helpful for lubrication during sleep or conditions with incomplete lid closure (e.g., general anesthesia, seventh-nerve palsies). Nonpreserved varieties without lanolin are preferable (Hypotears Ointment) when prolonged contact time is necessary (e.g., critical care patients).

Antibiotics

See Table 16.2.

Antiinflammatories

These agents are used most often to suppress allergic/inflammatory (i.e., immunologic) reactions of the eye of all types, both externally and internally. It may be necessary to suppress severe external inflammation to avoid corneal scarring or permanent tear-film abnormalities. Within the eye, these agents help to prevent scarring (synechiae) and subsequent development of glaucoma. Topical application often allows excellent penetration into the anterior chamber. This category is divided into steroid and nonsteroid (NSAID) varieties.

Steroid Antiinflammatory Agents

These are very effective in blocking pathways of inflammation. A significant portion of the population will raise their intraocular pressure in response to prolonged use of these agents (generally 2 weeks or more). Because of this and infectious concerns, ophthalmic initiation and follow up may be necessary.

Medrysone 1% (HMS): Mild steroid, few side effects. Used for surface allergy problems

Fluorometholone 0.1% (FML, others): Slightly more potent, with fewer side effects than prednisolone and dexamethasone. As fluorometholone acetate 0.1% (Flarex, Eflone), potency comparable to prednisolone acetate 1% due to better penetration

Rimexolone 1% (Vexol): Similar profile to that of fluorometholone, but with a lower propensity to raise intraocular pressure

Loteprednol etabonate 0.5% (Lotemax), 0.2% (Alrex): Relatively new preparations with high potency and lower propensity to raise intraocular pressure.

TABLE 16.2. Antibiotics for Topical Use

GENERAL PRINCIPLES OF ADMINISTRATION

Administer topical antibiotics 4–6 times daily for simple infections, more frequently for more serious infections (corneal ulcers, gonorrhea). Most common infectious pathogens: *Staphylococcus aureus*, *Haemophilus* species, *Pneumococcus*, *Staphylococcus epidermidis*.

ANTIBACTERIAL AGENTS

Bacitracin: Effective against gram-positive organisms, diphtheroids, *Haemophilus*, *Actinomyces*. Ointment, or mixture with polymyxin B (Polysporin, AK-Poly-Bac).

Chloramphenicol: Effective against many gram-positive and gram-negative organisms. Solution (0.5%) and ointment (1%) (Chloroptic, Chloromycetin). Low allergy index. Usage diminished due to concern for aplastic anemia.

Ciprofloxacin: Fluoroquinolone, with broad-spectrum activity, including *Pseudomonas aeruginosa*. Allows for ambulatory treatment of most corneal ulcers. Low allergy index. Solution (0.3%) (Ciloxan).

Erythromycin: Effective against gram-positive organisms, especially *Staphylococcus* species. Ointment (0.5%) (generic).

Gatifloxacin: Fourth-generation quinolone with enhanced gram-positive coverage (Zymar 0.3%).

Gentamicin: Effective against gram-negative organisms, especially *Pseudomonas*, and gram-positive organisms, including *Staphylococcus* species. Effective, but fairly high sensitizing and potentially toxic corneal epithelial effects. Solution and ointment (Genoptic, Gentacidin, Gentak 0.3%).

Levofloxacin: Approved for treatment of bacterial conjunctivitis with efficacy that parallels ciprofloxacin (Quixin 0.5%).

Moxifloxacin: Fourth-generation quinolone with improved gram-positive coverage (Vigamox 0.5%).

Neomycin: Broad-spectrum, but highly sensitizing and potentially toxic to corneal epithelium. Mixtures in solution or ointment (Neosporin, Ocutricin).

Norfloxacin: Approved for treatment of bacterial conjunctivitis with efficacy that parallels ciprofloxacin (Chibroxin 0.3%).

Olfloxacin: Similar indications and coverage as ciprofloxacin (Ocuflox 0.3%).

Polymyxin B sulfate: Fairly effective against most gram-negative organisms (except *Proteus* or *Neisseria*). Ointment mixtures (Neosporin, Polysporin, others). Solution with trimethoprim (Polytrim).

Sulfacetamide sodium: Broad spectrum. Solution (10%, 15%, and 30%). Ointment (10%) (Bleph-10, Sulf-10, others). Potential for allergy is fairly high.

Tobramycin sulfate: Similar to gentamicin (Tobrex, AK-Tob, others 0.3%).

Trimethoprim sulfate: Effective against some staphylococcal and streptococcal strains, as well as *Haemophilus* species. In combination with polymyxin B (Polytrim), it has a wide range of effectiveness. Its safety and effectiveness has not been determined under 2 months of age. Very low allergy index.

ANTIFUNGAL AGENTS

Natamycin: Effective against many filamentary and yeast forms. Drug of choice for most mycotic corneal injuries (and only ocular formulation commercially available) (Natacyn, 5% suspension).

ANTIVIRALS

Trifluridine (trifluorothymidine): Indicated for corneal herpetic disease, and penetrates cornea fairly well. Toxic to epithelium, like others. 1% solution (Viroptic) must be initiated at an every-2-hour dosage until ulcer is healing.

Prednisolone acetate and phosphate 0.125% and 1.0% (Pred Mild, Pred Forte, Inflamase Forte, others): Potent and highly effective for anterior segment inflammation. High risk for side effects (intraocular pressure and infection, especially herpes simplex facilitation)

Dexamethasone 0.1% (Decadron solution), 0.05% (Ointment): Potent and highly effective. Very high risk for side effects

Nonsteroidal Antiinflammatory Agents

Recent emphasis on these agents used topically has paralleled their systemic usefulness. Although there is therapeutic overlap, the Food and Drug Administration has recommended indications for each of these agents.

Flurbiprofen 0.03% (Ocufen): Used to keep the pupil dilated during cataract surgery

Diclofenac 0.1% (Voltaren): Used for postoperative inflammation after cataract surgery

Ketorolac 0.5% (Acular): A product developed for allergic conjunctivitis

Antibiotic–Steroid Combinations

A number of products are available with broad-spectrum antibiotics combined with varying concentrations of potent topical corticosteroids (e.g., TobraDex *tobramycin/dexamethasone*; Cortisporin *hydrocortisone/neomycin/polymyxin-B*; Blephamide *prednisolone acetate/sulfacetamide*) both in drop and ointment forms. These formulations may be helpful in postoperative circumstances, but they should be reserved for other conditions, with ophthalmic consultation.

Antiglaucoma Agents

These either suppress aqueous production, increase outflow facility, or both. Because the ciliary body and muscle are critical determinants of the intraocular pressure (with regard to aqueous production and outflow), autonomic agents and their blockers may affect the intraocular pressure. Carbonic anhydrase inhibitors block aqueous production because this enzyme is essential in the active production of aqueous humor. The most recent addition to the management regimen includes topical prostaglandins, which act in a different manner by increasing outflow through a uveoscleral route.

(1) *Cholinergic agonists.* Rarely cause systemic problems. Miotics make the pupils small; usually capped in *green*: *Pilocarpine* 0.5% to 10%; *Carbachol* 0.75%, 1.5%, and 3.0%.

(2) *Adrenergic agents.* Tolerance develops commonly, and the eyes turn red! These products have *white* caps: *Epinephrine* compounds 0.5% to 2.0% (Epifrin, others); *Dipivalyl epinephrine* 0.1% (Propine).

(3) *Alpha-2 agonists.* Reduce aqueous production and may increase uveoscleral outflow. Alphagan has fewer side effects. As with most adrenergic agents, ensure that the patient does not have a problem with cardiovascular sensitivity. Beware of use with MAO inhibitors: *Apraclonidine* 0.5% and 1.0% (Iopidine); *Brimonide tartrate* (generic 0.2%) and 0.15% (Alphagan-P).

(4) *Beta-blockers.* Most have *yellow* caps and may cause beta-blocker side effects (heart and lung). Betoptic is cardioselective (beta-1) and has fewer side effects, but also has less ocular efficacy. Cardiac sensitivity and adverse effects on libido and serum cholesterol are reasons to swing toward use of newer agents: *Timolol* 0.25% and 0.5% (Timoptic, others); *Betaxolol* 0.25% (Betoptic-S); *Levobunolol* 0.5% (Betagan); *Metipranolol* 0.3% (OptiPranolol); *Carteolol* 1% (Ocupress).

(5) *Carbonic anhydrase inhibitors.* Mild diuretics, may deplete potassium or precipitate renal stones. Increased side effects with systemic administration. Sulfa-related compounds which may cause allergic reactions: *Oral: Acetazolamide* (Diamox 250-mg tablets, 500-mg extended-release capsules); *Methazolamide* (Neptazane 25 & 50 mg, others). *Topical: Dorzolamide hydrochloride* 2% (Trusopt); *Brinzolamide* 1% (Azopt). Fewer side effects, but less efficacious in reducing the intraocular pressure as are the oral agents. Dorzolamide also comes in combination with the beta-blocker timolol, as Cosopt.

(6) *Prostaglandin analogs.* May increase iris and lash pigmentation, lash growth: *Bimatoprost* 0.03% (Lumigan); *Latanoprost* 0.005% (Xalatan); *Travoprost* 0.004% (Travatan); *Unoprostone* 0.15% (Rescula).

(7) *Osmotic agents.* Shrink the vitreous and lower intraocular pressure. It is essential to know the patient's fluid, renal, and cardiovascular status before using these compounds:

Oral: Glycerin (Osmoglyn) 50% to 75% (1.0 to 1.5 g/kg) over ice, frequently produces nausea and vomiting; be cautious of using in diabetic patients. IV: Mannitol (Osmitrol) 20%, 1 to 2 g/kg IV over 30 to 45 minutes.

OCULAR ALLERGIC CONDITIONS

Surface reactions to a host of airborne agents (e.g., pollen, dust) and irritants can cause conjunctival swelling (chemosis), redness, itching, and tearing. Management of these reactions should start conservatively with cool compresses and decongestant–antihistamine combinations. More aggressive therapy can involve more potent topical antihistamines, mast-cell inhibitors, topical NSAIDs (see previous discussion), and corticosteroids.

Ocular Decongestants

These agents, many of which are available over the counter, are topical solutions used to whiten the eye. Although overtly effective, the utilization of these agents often hinders timely diagnosis and treatment of the condition that presents as "the red eye." Chronic use of these agents causes tolerance and eventual worsening of the vascular dilatation. A few of these agents may also include a mild topical antihistamine, which may be a useful way to initiate therapy for mild allergic phenomena. When an antihistamine is present (antazoline or pheniramine), the decongestant product will usually include the suffix "-A" to indicate such.

Naphazoline hydrochloride (Naphcon, Vasocon, others).

Phenylephrine hydrochloride (AK-Nefrin).

Tetrahydrozoline hydrochloride (Murine, Visine, others). Available over the counter.

Oxymetazoline hydrochloride (Visine L.R.). Similar to, but more potent than tetrahydrozoline.

Antihistamines

Along with the combination antihistamines used with the previously noted decongestants, these agents have been marketed specifically for ocular allergy management as H$_1$-antagonists.

Levocabastine hydrochloride 0.05% (Livostin). Very effective, but does sting on administration.

Emedastine difumarate 0.05% (Emadine).

Azelastine hydrochloride 0.05% (Optivar). Also available in a nasal preparation.

Mast-cell Stabilizers

Seasonal allergy disorders usually revolve around IgE-mediated (Type I) hypersensitivity reactions. This involves the release of histamine and many vasoactive substances that create the signs and symptoms of allergy. By blocking the mast-cell release of these vasoactive substances, symptomatology is relieved. Because these stabilizers affect unsensitized mast cells, the effects of these agents may take days to weeks to work properly.

Cromolyn sodium 4% (Crolom, Opticrom); *Nedocromil* sodium 2% (Alocril); *Lodoxamide tromethamine* 0.1% (Alomide); *Olopatadine hydrochloride* 0.1% (Patanol); *Ketotifin fumarate* 0.025% (Zaditor)

COMMON PITFALLS

✔ Topical corticosteroids, used alone or in combination with other topical medications, should be used only after discussion with an ophthalmologist
✔ Even though ocular medications are most often delivered topically, there are significant systemic side effects seen with certain agents, especially those that treat glaucoma (e.g., beta-blockers)
✔ Discharging a patient with topical anesthetics should be avoided because these agents retard corneal epithelial wound healing

References

1. Bartlett J, et al. *Ophthalmic drug facts 2003.* St. Louis: Facts & Comparisons, Wolters Kluwer Co., September 2002.
2. Langston DP. *Manual of ocular diagnosis and therapy,* 5th ed. New York: Lippincott, Williams & Wilkins, 2002.
3. Patel KH, Javitt JC, et al. Incidence of acute angle closure glaucoma after pharmacologic mydriasis. *Am J Ophthalmol* 1995;120:709–717.
4. *Physician's desk reference for ophthalmology,* 31st ed. Montvale, NJ: Thomson Medical Economics Data Production Company, 2002.

CHAPTER 17

The Red Eye

Robert S. Porter

The red eye is a common emergency department (ED) problem that may present in isolation, or in combination with other ocular or systemic disorders. The causes range from benign to severe, and this chapter addresses the diagnostic approach to, and ED management of the patient with a red eye.

CLINICAL PRESENTATION

A red eye is produced by dilated, inflamed, superficial ocular vessels, which can result from infection, allergy, inflammation, or elevated intraocular pressure. Several ocular components may be involved, most commonly the conjunctiva, but also the uveal tract, episclera, and sclera. Other features such as discharge, blurred vision, pain, tearing, and photophobia are more variable, and depend upon the etiology.

Conjunctivitis and Keratitis

The conjunctiva covers the inner aspect of the lids (tarsal or palpebral conjunctiva) and reflects back on itself to cover the sclera of the anterior globe (bulbar conjunctiva), stopping at the cornea. An acute episode of conjunctivitis rarely has long-term consequences, but chronic inflammation may lead to symblepharon (adhesions between the tarsal and bulbar conjunctiva at the fornices), and sometimes ectropion or entropion with subsequent corneal scarring and visual impairment. Infection, allergy, and irritation are the most common causes of conjunctivitis.

Infectious conjunctivitis is typically viral, and sometimes bacterial (see Chapter 20, Diplopia). Conjunctival inflammation also may accompany corneal infection (keratitis). Patients with infectious conjunctivitis often present with discharge from the eye, with crusting in the morning. Those with herpes keratitis may have intense pain with a corneal dendritic lesion. *Allergic conjunctivitis* (2) may occur seasonally, year-round (perennial conjunctivitis), or as an isolated reaction to material in the eye (often ophthalmic medications, particularly those containing neomycin). Seasonal conjunctivitis is usually caused by airborne pollens and follows the growth cycle of the responsible plant, with peak symptoms in the spring and/or fall. Perennial conjunctivitis is usually caused by allergens present in the home, particularly dust mites and animal dander. Vernal conjunctivitis is a severe conjunctivitis that is probably allergic. It is most common in pre-adolescent and adolescent males with other atopic disorders (e.g., eczema, asthma), waxing in the spring and waning in the winter. Most outgrow the condition. Numerous irritants may also affect the conjunctiva. Common examples include foreign bodies, dust, smoke, and chemical fumes (e.g., ammonia, chlorine).

Symptoms are generally mild irritation, itching, which may be severe in allergic conjunctivitis, and discharge, which is typically watery except in bacterial conjunctivitis in which it is mucopurulent. Vision is not intrinsically affected, but may be blurred by copious or thick discharge. Patients with *infectious conjunctivitis* usually have diffuse hyperemia, while *allergic conjunctivitis* may produce significant conjunctival edema, termed chemosis, which appears as a marked bulging of the conjunctiva. In chronic allergic conjunctivitis, fine papillae may develop on the tarsal surface, giving a velvety appearance. Follicular hyperplasia occurs in viral or chlamydial conjunctivitis, giving a "cobblestone" appearance to the tarsal conjunctiva.

Uveitis

The uveal tract consists of the iris, ciliary body and choroid. Uveitis is classified as anterior, intermediate and posterior. Only anterior uveitis typically produces a visibly red eye; it includes iritis and iridocyclitis (inflammation involving the iris, ciliary body and sometimes anterior vitreous). Intermediate and posterior uveitis typically present with floaters and impaired vision.

Perhaps one-half of cases are idiopathic, most of the remainder are immune-mediated (4,6) and a few are infectious. The seronegative spondyloarthropathies (particularly ankylosing spondylitis, but also reactive arthritis, and the enteropathic arthritis associated with inflammatory bowel disease, Whipple disease, and other chronic gastrointestinal inflammation) are the most common immune-mediated causes (1). In children, juvenile rheumatoid arthritis predominates. Other causes include sarcoidosis, and, in patients from the Middle or Far East, Behçet syndrome. The main infectious cause is herpes virus, both simplex and, in older patients, zoster.

Typical symptoms include pain, photophobia, consensual photophobia (light in the unaffected eye produces pain in the red eye), and decreased vision. Physical findings include decreased visual acuity, pupillary constriction, along with fine vascular dilation concentrated in the area around the cornea (peri-limbal flush). The large, dilated vessels typical of conjunctivitis are absent. On slit-lamp examination, there are cells and flare in the aqueous humor, which in severe cases may contain fibrin clot or even pus (hypopyon).

Episcleritis

The episclera is a thin, membranous layer between the conjunctiva and sclera. Inflammation (5) is usually idiopathic, but is sometimes associated with immune-mediated disorders. It occurs mainly in young adults, more commonly women. Patients have mild discomfort, tearing, and an erythematous, injected patch on the globe. The injected area is usually localized, occupying a quarter or half of the visible globe. Sometimes a small nodule is present. Episcleritis poses no threat to vision and is self-limited.

Scleritis

The sclera is the thick, white connective tissue comprising the protective layer of the globe of the eye. Inflammation (5) is often idiopathic, but about 50% are associated with certain systemic diseases, often immune-mediated disorders (particularly rheumatoid arthritis, systemic lupus erythematosus, polyarteritis nodosa, and Wegener's Granulomatosis). Rarely, scleral bacterial infection occurs (panophthalmitis, see Chapter 21). Scleritis is most common between age 30 and 60, and is somewhat more common in women. Within several years of an acute attack, up to one-third of patients suffer significant loss of visual acuity.

Pain is severe, deep, and typically described as "boring." The pain often interferes with sleep and may radiate to the forehead or jaw. The eye appears diffusely hyperemic, often violaceous, although sometimes only one quadrant is involved. The palpebral conjunctiva is not inflamed. An identifying feature of scleritis is tenderness of the globe to palpation. An avascular-appearing area amidst the hyperemia suggests *necrotizing scleritis*, which can ultimately progress to globe perforation. Necrotizing scleritis in patients with known immune-mediated disorders is often an indication of severe systemic vasculitis.

Acute Angle-Closure Glaucoma

The "angle" is the junction of the cornea and iris, where much of the aqueous humor drains from the anterior chamber. Factors that narrow this angle can impair aqueous outflow, causing a rapid increase in intraocular pressure, with severe pain, hyperemia, and impaired vision often described as "steamy" (see Chapter 21, Acute Eye Infections). Headache, nausea and vomiting may be prominent, perhaps causing the condition to be mistaken for a neurologic emergency. Patients often have decreased visual acuity, as well as a pupil that is mid-position and poorly reactive, and a cloudy cornea. Intraocular pressure is between 40 and 80 mm Hg. If untreated, optic nerve damage occurs quickly, with permanent vision loss.

Corneal Abrasion and Foreign Body

Significant eye trauma typically produces ocular erythema or hemorrhage, but is clinically obvious; patients present with complaint of injury rather than red eye. However, minor corneal abrasions and foreign bodies may be present without recognized trauma, particularly in young children and infants. Conversely, the sensation of an ocular foreign body is nonspecific and may occur with corneal irritation of any cause. Vision is generally unimpaired unless the abrasion or foreign body occupies a central location.

DIFFERENTIAL DIAGNOSIS

The differential for the red eye is broad, and may be best summarized in tabular form (see Table 17.1). Other disorders that might produce scleral injection include chemical irritation, or infections of the surrounding structures, such as blepharitis, periorbital and orbital cellulitis (discussed in Chapter 21, Acute Eye Infections).

EMERGENCY DEPARTMENT EVALUATION

A systematic approach to the red eye should lead one to the correct diagnosis (see Chapter 15 for details of a thorough, systematic examination). Key symptoms and findings that are helpful in discriminating one cause from another are listed in Table 17.1.

History should focus on the eye and relevant systemic complaints, including the type of pain/discomfort, quality of vision, presence and type of discharge, and previous occurrences including timing and relation to activity and location. Autoimmune or rheumatologic diseases or symptoms should also be carefully elicited.

Physical examination of the eye (see Chapter 15, The Ophthalmic Examination) includes visual acuity, delineation of the nature and location of vascular dilation, slit-lamp examination including fluorescein staining, lid eversion for foreign body detection, and in most cases, ocular tonometry. A drop of topical anesthetic (e.g., proparacaine 0.5%) can provide important diagnostic information. Typically, discomfort from conjunctivitis, foreign body or corneal abrasion is relieved, but the pain of uveitis, scleritis, or glaucoma is unaffected. Similarly, drops of phenylephrine 2.5% will not affect the hyperemia of scleritis, but will cause blanching in other causes of red eye (phenylephrine will also cause pupillary dilation, and is contraindicated in patients with a history of glaucoma or if acute glaucoma is suspected).

Laboratory testing is usually not helpful. Serologic tests are sometimes useful when immune-mediated disease is suspected, but may be coordinated with the ophthalmologist and primary care physician. Cultures are rarely indicated on initial presentation, but are useful in cases with severe inflammation, and in patients who present having failed empiric antibiotic treatment.

EMERGENCY DEPARTMENT MANAGEMENT

The treatment options vary widely, depending upon etiology. Ocular infections, closed-angle glaucoma, foreign bodies, and trauma are discussed in detail in Chapters 18, 21, 22, and 176, respectively.

Allergic conjunctivitis should initially be treated with either a nonprescription topical antihistamine/vasoconstrictor such as naphazoline/pheniramine, or prescription agents with combination antihistamine and mast-cell stabilizing activity such as

TABLE 17.1.   Differential Diagnosis of Red Eye

Factor	Infectious conjunctivitis	Allergic conjunctivitis	Anterior Uveitis	Episcleritis	Scleritis	Angle-Closure Glaucoma	Foreign body, Corneal abrasion
Injection	Diffuse bulbar and palpebral	Diffuse bulbar and palpebral	Diffuse ciliary flush	Focal erythema	Diffuse erythema or violaceous hue	Diffuse bulbar	Diffuse bulbar
Discharge	Viral: watery Bacterial: purulent	Copious, watery	Watery	Watery	Watery	Watery	Watery
Pain	Mainly irritation	None	Photophobia	Mild	Severe pain, tender to palpation	Usually severe, but can be minimal	Moderate irritation
Itching	Minimal	Moderate	None	None	None	None	None
Systemic symptoms	Occasional URI symptoms, preauricular nodes	Sneezing, rhinorrhea	Occasional rheumatologic or gastrointestinal	Usually none. Occasional rheumatologic	Usually none. Occasional rheumatologic	Headache, nausea, vomiting	None
Visual acuity	Usually normal, may be decreased in keratitis	Normal	Decreased	Normal	Initially normal, may become abnormal	Decreased	Normal. Decreased with central abrasion
Pupils	Normal	Normal	Constricted, poorly reactive	Normal	Normal	Mid-position, poorly reactive	Normal
Cornea	Normal in conjunctivitis, punctate lesions in keratitis	Normal	Normal. Anterior chamber with cells and flare	Normal	Normal	Hazy or cloudy appearance	Abrasion visible
Intraocular pressure	Normal	Normal	Usually normal	Normal	Usually normal	Elevated	Normal

olopatadine 0.1% 1 drop twice a day at an interval of 6 to 8 hrs, or ketotifen 0.025% 1 drop q 8 to 12 hr. Topical pure mast-cell stabilizers (e.g., pemirolast, nedocromil), NSAIDS, and corticosteroids may subsequently be added as needed by consultants.

Patients with *anterior uveitis* may get relief from photophobia with a topical cycloplegic, pending ophthalmology evaluation. Definitive treatment usually involves corticosteroids (topical, periocular, or systemic) and sometimes immunosuppressives (3). These should be managed by consultants.

Episcleritis is self-limited and generally requires no specific treatment. However, the duration may be shortened by oral NSAIDs or topical prednisolone acetate 1%, 2 drops qid for 5 days, and then tapered over 3 weeks.

The discomfort of *scleritis* may be reduced by oral NSAIDs. Definitive treatment should be initiated by consultants and involves systemic corticosteroids, with immunosuppressives (such as cyclophosphamide or azathioprine) for necrotizing scleritis or unresponsive disease.

CRITICAL INTERVENTIONS

- Record visual acuity in all cases
- Measure intraocular pressure to exclude acute closed-angle glaucoma
- Carefully evert lids to search for a foreign body
- Perform slit-lamp examination with fluorescein staining

DISPOSITION

Acute closed-angle glaucoma requires immediate ophthalmologic consultation and usually admission for frequent medication administration and intraocular pressure measurement. Bacterial corneal ulcers require similarly urgent consultation and admission. Patients with suspected uveitis or scleritis, and other corneal infections should be evaluated by an ophthalmologist within 24 hours. Patients with allergic or infectious conjunctivitis or simple abrasions may have either ophthalmologic or primary care follow up within 2 to 4 days.

COMMON PITFALLS

- ✔ Failing to adequately explain eye pain and decreased vision; these findings almost always indicate a serious disorder
- ✔ Assuming that all causes of red eye are infectious
- ✔ Failing to consider closed-angle glaucoma and measure intraocular pressure
- ✔ Misdiagnosing herpes simplex or other keratitis as simple conjunctivitis
- ✔ Failing to detect a foreign body

References

1. Bañares A, Hernández-García C, Fernández-Gutiérrez B, Jover JA. Eye involvement in the spondyloarthropathies. *Rheum Dis Clin North Am* 1998;24:771–784.
2. Bielory L. Allergic and immunologic disorders of the eye. Part II: ocular allergy. *J Allergy Clin Immunol* 2000;106:1019–1032.

3. Djalilian AR, Nussenblatt RB. Immunosuppression in uveitis. *Ophthalmol Clin N Am* 2002;15:395–404.
4. Harper SL, Foster CS. The ocular manifestations of rheumatoid disease. *Int Ophthalmol Clin* 1998;38:1–19.
5. Jabs DA, Mudun A, Dunn JP, Marsh MJ. Episcleritis and scleritis: clinical features and treatment results. *Am J Ophthalmol* 2000;130:469–476.
6. Patel SJ, Lundy DC. Ocular manifestations of autoimmune disease. *Am Fam Physician* 2002;66:991–998.

CHAPTER 18
Corneal Abrasion and Foreign Bodies

Lori Weichenthal

Corneal abrasions and foreign bodies are among the most frequent ocular conditions that present to the emergency department. It is estimated that the incidence of nonenetrating injuries to the eye is 15.7 per 100,000 persons per year (7). Although a corneal abrasion is usually a self-limited process, a persistent corneal foreign body or undiagnosed intraocular foreign body can cause unnecessary morbidity.

The emergency physician (EP) must be able to accurately diagnose and treat corneal abrasions and foreign bodies in order to reduce pain and prevent complications such as infection, ulceration and vision loss. It is also important that the EP be aware of the potential for intraocular foreign body and be attentive to the historical and physical clues that suggest ocular penetration. This chapter will provide an overview of the evaluation and management of corneal abrasions, corneal foreign bodies and intraocular foreign bodies in the emergency department (ED).

CLINICAL PRESENTATION

Corneal abrasions and corneal foreign bodies often present with a similar history. The patient may relate that something struck or flew into the eye, and pain soon followed. At times, the patient doesn't recall feeling an object entering the eye, but reports being in a situation where such a possibility exists (using a leaf blower, working in an environment with sawdust, etc.) Contact lenses may also cause corneal abrasions, due to prolonged wear, an improper fit, foreign material under the lenses, or trauma associated with the placement or removal of the lenses.

Whether a foreign body is present or not, the patient often complains of a persistent foreign body sensation. With this sensation, there is usually pain, tearing, photophobia, blepharospasm, and a minimal decrease in visual acuity. A headache may also be present but is usually mild. Recurrent erosions may present weeks or months after an initial corneal abrasion, and frequently occur upon awakening from sleep.

An intraocular foreign body should be suspected when the history is of a high velocity injury to the eye. This may be due to a blast effect or due to activities such as grinding metal or jack hammering cement without the use of protective eyewear. Patients with intraocular foreign bodies usually present with similar symptoms as patients with corneal abrasions or foreign bodies, although they frequently describe more visual disturbances. Rarely, they may present without pain or other related symptoms. In these instances, the history alone of a high velocity injury should be enough to alert the EP to the possibility of an intraocular foreign body.

DIFFERENTIAL DIAGNOSIS

The differential diagnosis of corneal abrasion, corneal foreign body and intraocular foreign body should include all the disease processes that come to mind with the acute red eye. For a complete discussion of the red eye, please refer to Chapter 17. When there is no history of a foreign body or trauma, the concern for an infection, autoimmune reaction, or acute angle-closure glaucoma should be heightened.

Infections of the conjunctiva and the cornea (keratitis) are most common and are usually viral or bacterial. Patients with eye infections will have symptoms similar to those described for corneal abrasions and foreign body. However, they may also describe mucopurulent discharge and other symptoms of infection (cough, congestion, etc). The pain associated with eye infections also tends to be more gradual in onset or is first noticed upon awakening (11).

Autoimmune disorders can also cause symptoms similar to those experienced with corneal abrasions and foreign bodies. Anterior uveitis and scleritis are two examples. Patients with these disorders often have other systemic complaints that will help the EP in differentiating them from simple abrasions and foreign bodies.

Acute angle-closure glaucoma can also present with a painful, red eye. This disease process, however, is usually associated with a severe, unilateral headache and decreased visual acuity, which differs from abrasions and foreign bodies.

In contact lens wearers, although corneal abrasions are common, concern for more serious injury and infection should be heightened. Corneal ulcers can occur, as can infectious keratitis. The offending agent is often a gram negative organism, especially *Pseudomonas*, and protozoa, such as *Acanthamoeba*. An ulcer due to *Pseudomonas* can destroy the cornea in as little as 24 hours. Thus, a corneal ulcer in a patient who wears contact lenses requires emergency ophthalmology consultation. Chemical irritation due to the preservatives in contact lens solutions or due to the enzymes used to clean some contact lenses can also lead to symptoms similar to corneal abrasions or foreign bodies.

In the setting of trauma, the differential should include corneal or scleral lacerations, hyphema, globe rupture and traumatic iritis (see Chapter 176, Eye Trauma). Corneal or scleral lacerations range from simple partial-thickness lacerations to injuries that penetrate the eye. When the laceration is extensive and deep enough, the injury is considered a ruptured globe, which is an ophthalmic emergency. Traumatic iritis can present with symptoms very similar to corneal abrasion and foreign body, however, it usually occurs after significant blunt trauma and is associated with a significant headache, photophobia, and decreased vision. If the history is of a high velocity impact to the eye, intraocular foreign body should always be suspected.

If a patient presents with the story of multiple episodes of corneal abrasions, the diagnosis of recurrent corneal erosions should be entertained. Recurrent corneal erosions often occur in people with epithelial basement membrane dystrophy and/or a history of trauma (8).

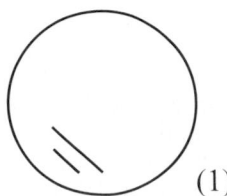 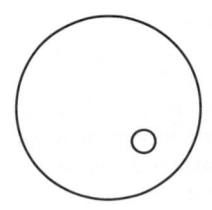 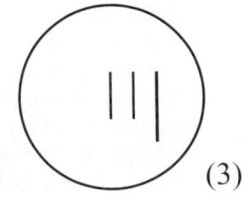 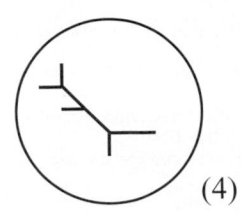

Figure 18.1. Corneal fluorescein uptake patterns for particular injuries. 1. Typical abrasion. 2. Abrasion around a corneal foreign body. 3. Abrasion from a foreign body under the lid. 4. Herpetic dendritic lesion.

EMERGENCY DEPARTMENT EVALUATION

When a patient presents to the ED with the complaint of a foreign body sensation to the eye, the history should focus upon the preceding events and a description of all symptoms, including pain, redness, visual changes, or discharge. The time of onset and progressions of symptoms should also be elicited. If the history suggests an actual foreign body, the suspected type of foreign body (wood, metal, organic material, etc.) as well as the setting (high velocity versus low velocity) should be determined. Previous injuries or surgeries to the eye should be documented, as should the use of glasses or contact lenses. A through review of systems should be obtained to evaluate for systemic illness, as should a general medical history. If nothing in the history suggests a possible systemic problem or multisystem trauma, the physical examination can be focused to the eye.

A visual acuity should be obtained as soon as possible. In patients with corneal abrasions and foreign bodies, the visual acuity is frequently normal or mildly decreased. When an intraocular foreign body is present the visual loss can be significant. The use of a topical anesthetic (proparacaine 0.5 percent solution or tetracaine 0.5 percent solution), one to two drops in the affected eye, will make the patient more comfortable and aid the EP in the examination. The use of topical anesthetic can also be helpful in making the correct diagnosis. If the anesthetic does not relieve the patient's pain, it suggests that the pathology is deeper than the corneal epithelium.

A complete examination of the eye should follow instillation of the topical anesthetic. For a detailed discussion of the eye examination, please refer to Chapter 15. Patients with a corneal abrasion or foreign body often have a slightly swollen eyelid, and the conjunctiva and sclera will be hyperemic. It is particularly important to search the corneal and conjunctival surfaces for a foreign body. This examination should be done under magnification and with a bright light or with a slit lamp. As the superior tarsal plate is a common place for foreign bodies to lodge, lid eversion should be performed in all patients where suspicion of a foreign body exists. To perform lid eversion: Ask the patient to look down; grasp the eyelashes of the upper lid and pull the lid down and out; place a cotton-tipped applicator horizontally above the tarsal plate; fold the upper lid over the applicator to expose the underlying conjunctival surface (2).

Also of importance in evaluation of the patient with a suspected corneal abrasion or foreign body is an examination with fluorescein. It should be noted that fluorescein will permanently stain soft contacts, thus they should be removed prior to instilling fluorescein and the patient should be advised to refrain from wearing contacts for several hours. Fluorescein should be instilled in the eye and the patient asked to blink several times. The eye should then be examined with a cobalt-blue light or a wood's lamp. Defects of the corneal epithelium will appear green. Particular patterns of uptake can suggest specific injuries. A simple abrasion from a low impact foreign body will often appear as a single linear uptake. Uptake of multiple linear markings perpendicular to the eye lid suggest a retained foreign body in the superior tarsal plate. A dendritic lesion viewed on fluorescein examination should suggest herpes keratitis. Corneal ulcers and infectious keratitis may appear on fluorescein examination as corneal staining with surrounding opacification (Fig. 18.1).

The eye examination should be completed with examination of the anterior segment and fundus. The anterior segment is best examined using a slit lamp and is usually normal with abrasions and corneal foreign bodies. The fundiscopic examination is done with an indirect ophthalmoscope and should also be normal.

The measurement of intraocular pressure (IOP) may not be indicated in simple corneal abrasions and foreign bodies due to small and low-speed particles. In fact, some argue that the use of a tonometer on an abraded cornea is a bad idea due to the potential for further injury. However, in abrasions due to larger objects such as a finger, a branch, a ball or a fist, IOP should be measured. IOP should not be measured in a suspected penetrating ocular injury. Pressure on the globe may result in extrusion of intraocular contents (2).

Some of the findings on examination of the eye that are suggestive of an intraocular foreign body or globe penetration include: an irregular pupil; a prolapsed iris; a laceration to the sclera or cornea; hyphema; absence of a red reflex; and/or a positive Seidel test. The Seidel test involves flooding the eye with fluorescein and looking for a small stream of green using the cobalt-blue light or wood's lamp, suggesting that fluid is leaking from the globe.

EMERGENCY DEPARTMENT MANAGEMENT

The management of the patient with suspected corneal abrasion or foreign body will be dictated by the findings on the eye examination. If a corneal, scleral, or conjunctival *foreign body* is found, it must be removed. Frequently, this is as easy as brushing the foreign body with a moistened cotton-tip applicator. Saline irrigation can also be used to rinse foreign bodies out of the eye. This technique is especially useful if there are multiple, small foreign bodies that are difficult to see.

If irrigation is needed, the eye should be well anesthetized. The lids should be held open with gauze pads or by the use of lid retractors. A saline stream can then be instilled in the eye. This can be done by using regular IV tubing attached to a bag of normal saline or a Morgan Lens. The volume and duration of irrigation depends on the suspected foreign body but at least a full liter is recommended (2).

If the foreign body is embedded in the sclera or cornea, it is best removed with a needle (25- to 27-gauge) attached to a syringe or with a commercial stud device (burr). For this to be done, the eye must be well anesthetized. The patient's head should be stabilized and the procedure should be performed under magnification, preferably with a slit lamp. The patient is asked to focus on a distant spot. The stud device or needle is then held tangentially to the globe and the foreign body is gently picked off. If the embedded foreign body is metallic, a rust ring may remain after removal of the metal object. The EP can attempt to remove this ring at the same time that the foreign body is removed by repeatedly picking away with a stud device or needle. However, it is frequently easier to remove the rust ring 24 to 48 hours later when it has had a chance to mature or soften.

TABLE 18.1. Topical Ophthalmic Antibiotics

Aminoglycoside
  Gentamicin 0.3% solution, 0.3% ointment
  Tobramycin 0.3% solution, 0.3% ointment
Fluoroquinolones
  Ciprofloxacin 0.3% solution, 0.3% ointment
  Levofloxacin 0.5% solution
  Norfloxacin 0.3% solution
  Ofloxacin 0.3% solution
Others
  Polysporin ointment
  Sulfacetamide 1, 10, 15, 30% solution, 10% ointment

If a patient has multiple embedded foreign bodies, as if from an explosion, they should be referred emergently to an ophthalmologist.

If anything on history or physical examination suggests the possibility of an *intraocular foreign body*, further studies will be necessary to help in detection. Although plain films and ultrasonography have been used, computer tomography of the orbit is the best test. MRI should not be considered if the foreign body could be metallic. Patients with suspected intraocular foreign body require immediate ophthalmologic consultation.

Once an extraocular foreign body has been removed, the treatment is the same as for a simple corneal abrasion. Treatment for a *corneal abrasion* consists of an antibiotic ointment or drops, and oral analgesics as needed (Table 18.1). Though there is little support in the literature for topical antibiotics in this setting, it remains the standard of care in many institutions. Cycloplegics (1% cyclopentolate or 5% homatropine) have been recommended in the past because they were thought to relieve some of the pain of corneal abrasions by relaxing ciliary body spasm. However, a recent literature review revealed that there is no evidence to support this practice (4). Similarly, patching of the affected eye has been recommended in the past, but studies in adults and children have failed to show any difference in the rate of healing or in the degree of pain between groups with or without a patch (6,7). Some studies even suggest that patching delays healing of corneal abrasions (3,5).

Topical anesthetics, such as tetracaine or proparacaine, should never be prescribed, as prolonged use can cause corneal breakdown and ulceration. However, recent studies have shown that topical nonsteroidal antiinflammatory drug (NSAID) drops may be useful to treat the pain of corneal abrasions (Table 18.2). Three studies showed a greater reduction of pain in patients using a topical NSAID versus those receiving no topical analgesia (1,10,12). Topical NSAIDs, however, can be expensive, and have not been adequately tested against oral analgesics for controlling eye pain due to corneal abrasions and foreign bodies.

For *corneal ulcers*, the use of topical fluoroquinolones and topical steroids are recommended. However, this should be done in consultation with an ophthalmologist and requires urgent follow up. *Recurrent erosions* should be treated with topical lubricants, particularly at bedtime.

TABLE 18.2. Topical Ophthalmic NSAIDS

Ketorolac 0.5% solution
Diclofenac 0.1% solution
Indomethacin 0.1% solution

CRITICAL INTERVENTIONS

- Remove any extraocular foreign body
- Have a high suspicion for intraocular foreign body
- Provide adequate analgesia and close follow up

DISPOSITION

It is rare that patients with corneal abrasions or foreign bodies need admission. Patients with simple *corneal abrasions, recurrent erosions,* or corneal defects following foreign body removal should be followed up within 24 to 36 hours, either in the ED, by primary care, or by an ophthalmologist. Patients with a *corneal ulcer,* especially due to contact lens use, need emergent ophthalmologic consultation. Patients with multiple extraocular foreign bodies or a suspected *intraocular foreign body* also need emergent ophthalmologic involvement. If an ophthalmologist is not available, a transfer should be arranged to a hospital that has an ophthalmologist on call.

Return precautions should be given to all patients who are discharged to home. Patients should be urged to return for any evidence of infection (drainage from the eye, increased redness or pain) or any changes in vision. If a foreign body was the source of the patient's complaint, the use of eye protection should be urged when engaging in future activities that create the risk for injury to the eyes.

COMMON PITFALLS

- ✔ Failure to detect an extraocular foreign body
- ✔ Failure to suspect an intraocular foreign body
- ✔ Failure to provide adequate analgesia
- ✔ Prescribing topical anesthetics

Acknowledgments

Thanks to the previous edition's authors William H. Shoff and Suzanne Moore Shepherd.

References

1. Alberti MM, Bouat CG, Allaire CM, et al. Combined indomethacin/gentamicin eyedrops to reduce pain after traumatic corneal abrasion. *Eur J Ophthalmol* 2001;11:233–239.
2. Barr DH, Samples JH, Hedges JR. Ophthalmologic procedures. In: Roberts JR, Hedges JR, eds. *Clinical prodedures in emergency medicine.* Philadelphia: W.B. Saunders Company, 1991:995–1019.
3. Campanile TM, St Clair DA, Benaim M. The evaluation of eye patching in the treatment of traumatic corneal epithelial defects. *J Emerg Med* 1997;15:769–774.
4. Carley F, Carley S. Toward evidence based emergency medicine: best BETs from the Manchester Royal Infirmary. Mydriatics in corneal abrasion. *Emerg Med J* 2001;18:273.
5. Kaiser PK. A comparison of pressure patching versus no patching for corneal abrasions due to trauma or foreign body removal. *Ophthalmology* 1995;102:1936–1942.
6. Le Sage N, Verreault R, Rochette L. Efficacy of eye patching for traumatic corneal abrasions: a controlled clinical trial. *Ann Emerg Med* 2001;38:129–134.
7. Michael JG, Hug D, Dowd MD. Management of corneal abrasion in children: a randomized clinical trial. *Ann Emerg Med* 2002;40:67–72.
8. Reidy JJ, Paulsu MP, Gona S. Recurrent erosions of the cornea: epidemiology and treatment. *Cornea* 2000;19:767–771.
9. Shingleton BJ, Hersh PS, Kenyon DR, eds. *Eye trauma.* St. Louis: Mosby, 1991.
10. Szucs PA, Nashed AH, Allegra JR, et al. Safety and efficacy of diclofenac ophthalmic solution in the treatment of corneal abrasions. *Ann Emerg Med* 2000;35:131–137.
11. Trobe JD. *The physicians guide to eye care.* San Francisco: American Academy of Ophthalmology, 1993.
12. Weaver CS, Terrell KM. Evidence-based emergency medicine. Update: do ophthalmic nonsteroidal anti-inflammatory drugs reduce the pain associated with simple corneal abrasion without delaying healing? *Ann Emerg Med* 2003;41:134–140.

CHAPTER 19
Acute Vision Loss

Catherine A. Marco

Loss of vision, whether unilateral or bilateral, partial or complete, is an emergent ophthalmologic complaint, and requires rapid and thorough evaluation and management. Major eye diseases are particularly common among the geriatric population, with the predominant disease entities affecting this group including diabetic retinopathy, glaucoma, and macular degeneration; approximately 50% of patients older than age 65 have a major eye disease (15). Emergent evaluation includes taking the relevant ocular history, examination of the eyes and other relevant systems, pertinent laboratory evaluation, determination of the differential diagnosis, and rapid institution of appropriate therapy. Consultation with an ophthalmologist and/or other appropriate specialists is often indicated.

CLINICAL PRESENTATION

Patients may present with complete or partial vision loss, with or without a variety of associated symptoms. Typically, any degree of visual loss is disturbing to the patient and may lead to early evaluation; however, some patients may procrastinate and not seek medical evaluation. A thorough history can be crucial and the most efficient approach to the wide differential diagnosis of visual disturbances.

Several historic points may be particularly useful in determining the etiology of symptoms. The onset of symptoms, whether gradual or abrupt, transient or persistent, constant or waxing and waning, may be of importance. The unilateral or bilateral nature of the disturbance, and association of pain, may be valuable in the differentiation of certain disorders. Associated symptoms, including systemic symptoms (fever, weakness, rash, etc.), previous history of similar symptoms, history of trauma, and other ocular symptoms, including eye pain, redness, discharge, and so forth, should be sought when obtaining historical information from the patient. Following is a discussion of many conditions that cause vision loss.

Inflammatory Processes

Giant-cell Arteritis

Giant-cell arteritis (GCA), an inflammatory disease of medium and large arteries, typically affects patients over the age of 60, with a female predominance of 3:1. Peak incidence occurs between the ages of 70 and 80. GCA is often associated with polymylagia rheumatica. Patients may present with malaise, headache, fever, anorexia, jaw claudication, pain over the temporal or occipital arteries, visual hallucinations, or painless visual loss secondary to ischemic optic neuropathy, retinal artery occlusion (see below), or cranial nerve palsies. Helpful diagnostic tests include an elevated erythrocyte sedimentation rate (ESR) (typically 80 to 100 mm within the first hour; elevated in 98% of documented cases) and an abnormal temporal artery biopsy. Findings and symptoms may be atypical (ESR may be normal and there may be no visual involvement, etc.).

Optic Neuritis

Optic neuritis is an inflammatory disorder from varying etiologies, including multiple sclerosis, sarcoidosis, systemic lupus erythematosus, leukemia, syphilis, collagen vascular diseases, alcohol abuse (23), idiopathic, or other causes (11). It commonly occurs in young or middle-aged females. Acute visual loss, often occurring within 1 week, is typical. Most patients (65%) have pain with eye movement. Typically, there is unilateral involvement, and an afferent pupillary defect, and elevation of the optic disc may be seen on funduscopic examination. Visual field defects may be noted. Optic neuritis often resolves spontaneously over weeks to months.

Uveitis

Uveitis, inflammation of the iris, ciliary body, or choroid, may cause visual impairment. Uveitis may be caused by Reiter syndrome, ankylosing spondylitis, sarcoidosis, tuberculosis, collagen vascular disorders, and other diseases. It may also present as an inflammatory response to corneal abrasion, ulcer, infection, or trauma. The presentation generally includes conjunctival injection, pain, photophobia, and blurred vision.

Vascular Events

Central Retinal Artery Occlusion

Central retinal artery occlusion (CRAO) often presents with sudden, painless visual loss (Fig. 19.1). There may be a history of transient visual loss prior to this event. The cause is often due to emboli from carotid plaques, cardiac valves, fat emboli, arteriosclerosis, or a host of other underlying disorders, including such entities as collagen vascular disease, hypotension, coagulopathy, migraine, procedures such as cardiac catheterization, sickle cell disease, cocaine, certain medications (sildenafil, oral contraceptives, epinephrine, etc.), amniotic fluid embolism, and GCA. Elderly patients are more commonly affected, and men are more commonly affected than are women. Visual loss is typically profound, with 90% of patients sustaining losses that range from counting fingers to light perception. An afferent pupillary defect may be present. Physical findings include pallor of the involved retina, "cherry-red spot" of the fovea, "boxcars" of the arterioles, and opacification of the superficial retina. Ultrasound, including color Doppler imaging, may be helpful in elucidating the diagnosis (24). Echocardiography and carotid artery studies may reveal sources of emboli. Branch RAO may occur and may present with sudden loss of visual field and reduction in visual acuity. The long-term prognosis is related to the duration of symptoms prior to resolution. Full vision may be restored if resolved within 1 to 2 hours (22).

Central Retinal Vein Occlusion

Patients with central retinal vein occlusion (CRVO) typically present with painless, sudden loss of vision (Fig. 19.2). Most patients are older than age 50, and many also have significant cardiovascular disease. CRVO is the second leading cause of visual loss due to retinal vascular disease (second only to diabetic retinopathy). Other associated disorders include hypertension, glaucoma, venous stasis, diabetes mellitus, tobacco use, vasculitis, and collagen vascular disorders. Physical findings may include retinal hemorrhage, which may be pronounced and diffuse, venous dilatation, cotton-wool spots, and optic disc edema. Branch RVO may occur, and may have segments of intraretinal hemorrhage. Complications may include macular edema, ischemia, and neovascularization with associated vitreous hemorrhage.

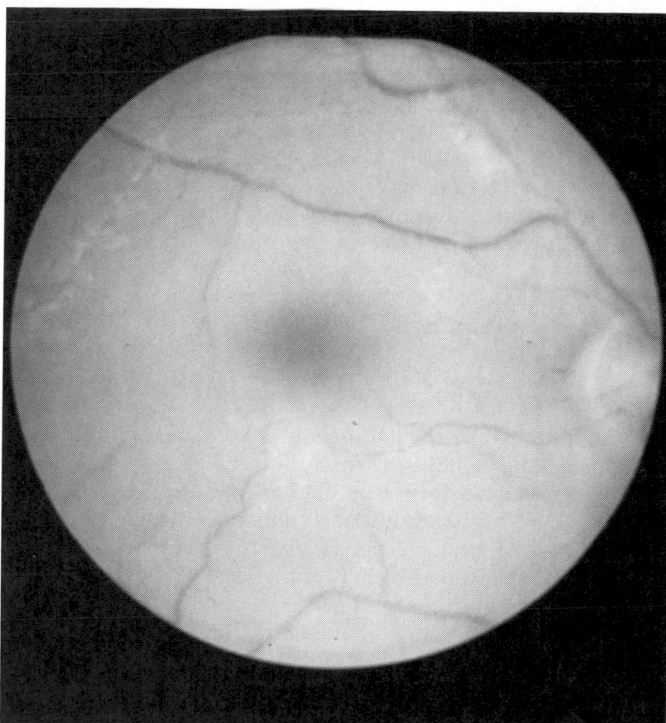

Figure 19.1. Central retinal artery occlusion.

Amaurosis Fugax

Amaurosis fugax, a unilateral transient obstruction of a retinal artery, may cause temporary loss of vision (up to 15 minutes). The visual loss is often described by the patient as a curtain being drawn across the visual field. Amaurosis fugax is usually caused by cholesterol emboli or fibrin–platelet emboli, and may

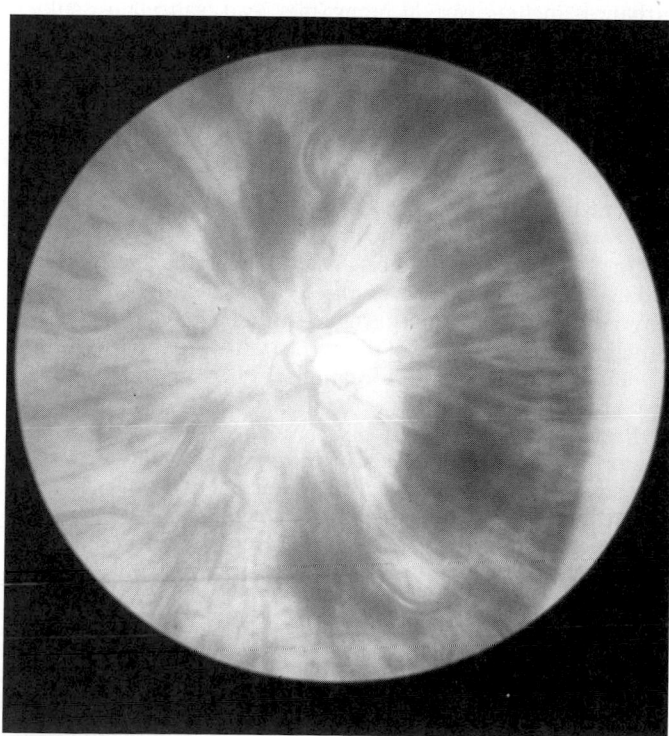

Figure 19.2. Central retinal vein occlusion.

be associated with carotid artery disease, cardiac arrhythmias, anemia, sickle cell disease, hypertension, or episodic hypotension. Carotid and cardiac studies may be indicated to determine the source of the emboli.

Ischemic Optic Neuropathy

Ischemic optic neuropathy is typically found in patients over the age of 50, and often presents with painless decreased visual acuity. This disorder may result from an infarction of the optic nerve (90% of cases), or from GCA (10% of cases). An afferent pupillary defect may be found, as well as a pale, elevated optic disc.

Vitreous and Retinal Disorders

Vitreous Hemorrhage

Vitreous hemorrhage typically presents with acute unilateral painless loss of vision, and may be accompanied by symptoms of "floaters" or "cobwebs." Associated visual disturbances may be mild or severe, depending on the extent of the hemorrhage. The normal red reflex of the fundus is absent. Diffuse, dark, particulate opacities may be seen, or if severe, a black uniform reflex ("eight ball hemorrhage") will be seen instead of the normal retinal red reflex. Vitreous hemorrhage may be associated with numerous disorders, including diabetes, trauma, malignancy, CRVO, leukemia, anemia, and thrombocytopenia.

Diabetic Retinopathy

Diabetic retinopathy is the leading cause of visual loss among retinal vascular disorders, and may be divided into proliferative and nonproliferative disorders. It may occur in Type I or Type II diabetes mellitus. Nonproliferative diabetic retinopathy is a progressive microangiopathy. Symptoms may be mild or nonexistent, and may include hue discrimination abnormalities, scotomas, contrast sensitivity, or a variety of other visual complaints. Physical findings include multiple hemorrhages throughout the retina and macular edema. Proliferative retinopathy refers to ischemia as a result of microvascular occlusions, and may present with cotton-wool spots, retinal vein beading, and irregular dilation of the retinal capillary bed. Sudden visual loss may occur with massive vitreous hemorrhage from fragile neovascularization or from retinal detachment. Progressive loss of vision may be slowed or prevented by laser photocoagulation.

Retinal Detachment

Retinal detachment refers to a separation of the two layers of the retina: the pigment epithelium and neurosensory retina (Fig. 19.3). The most common type, rhegmatogenous, occurs as a result of tears, holes, or breaks in the sensory layer of the retina. It may be associated with advancing age, male gender, significant myopia, diabetes mellitus, sickle cell disease, or ocular contusion or penetrating injury, or it may be idiopathic. Additionally, exudative or traction types of retinal detachment may be seen. Symptoms include photopsia (light flashes), floaters, or a shower of black dots in the periphery secondary to hemorrhage into vitreous humor, or a sensation of a shadow or curtain obscuring the visual field. Visual acuity may be normal if the macula is unaffected, or severely impaired if involved. On examination, the detached area may appear gray, opaque, or translucent. Retinal folds may be seen, and vessels may appear dark red. Symptoms often resolve within 1 week.

Macular Degeneration

Age-related macular degeneration (ARMD) is the most common cause of permanent blindness among older patients, and has an estimated incidence of up to 11.4 per 1,000 (10). The disease can be

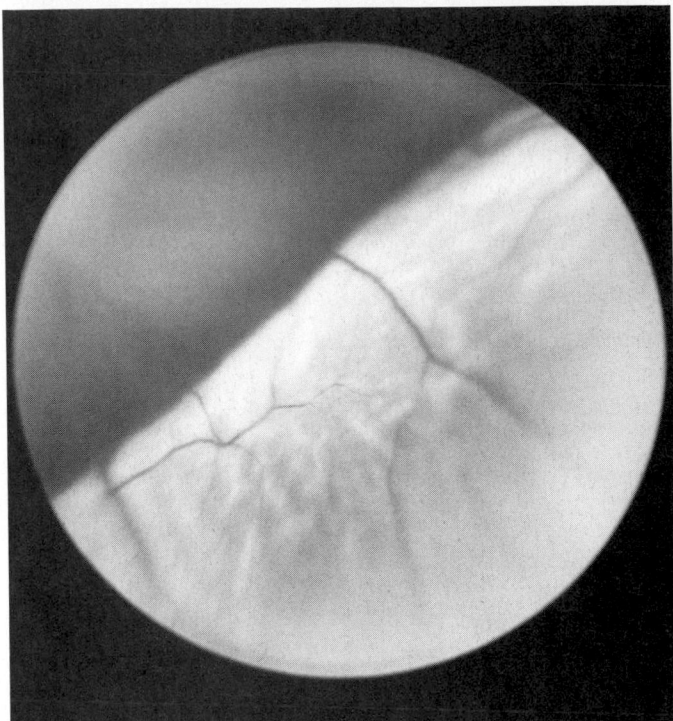

Figure 19.3.   Retinal detachment.

divided into nonexudative (dry) macular degeneration, characterized by drusen (yellowish subretinal deposits) and exudative (wet) macular degeneration, characterized by submacular hemorrhage, yellowish exudates or serous fluid. The incidence is associated with advanced age, family history, tobacco history, race (Caucasian), and gender (slight female predominance). The etiology is unknown. Symptoms include blurred vision, visual distortion, scotoma, or central visual loss. Physical findings include impaired visual acuity, drusen (yellow-white deposits beneath the pigment epithelium) and clumps of pigment throughout the macula.

Neurologic Disorders

Cerebrovascular accidents and *transient ischemic attacks* may be associated with visual loss. A bilateral homonymous hemianopsia may result from involvement of the optic tract or occipital lobes. Involvement of both occipital lobes may produce complete blindness ("cortical blindness").

Cortical blindness may be caused by such entities as ischemia, mass lesions, hydrocephalus, anoxia, encephalitis, meningitis, edema, or hemorrhage into the occipital lobe(s) (4,19). Evaluation should be conducted promptly, and may include CT, MRI, and lumbar puncture.

The optic chiasm may be compressed by mass lesions such as pituitary adenomas, meningiomas, craniopharyngiomas, or aneurysms. These patients may present with bitemporal hemianopia, and advanced imaging is warranted.

Other Causes of Vision Loss

Cytomegalovirus Retinitis

Cytomegalovirus (CMV) retinitis may present with sudden or gradual visual loss when the infection invades the macula. It is seen primarily in immunocompromised patients, such as those with AIDS, or those on chemotherapy, or after organ trans-

plantation. Symptoms include blurred vision, floaters, flashes of light, eye pain, and scotomata (27). Findings include retinal hemorrhagic areas combined with zones of white retinal necrosis ("tomato and cheese pizza" appearance).

Glaucoma

Patients with glaucoma may present with acute or chronic visual loss. Visual field testing may indicate a diminished perception in the nasal region. Optic nerve pallor and cupping is seen on examination. Elevated intraocular pressure (often 50 to 70 mm Hg) is typically found. Associated symptoms often include eye pain, headache, nausea, and vomiting (see Chapter 21, Acute Eye Infections).

Malignancies of the Eye

Although space does not permit a detailed study of ophthalmologic malignancies, it is prudent for the emergency physician to have an awareness of the spectrum of malignancies that may affect vision. Benign intraocular tumors may include retinal angiomas or astrocytic hamartomas. Malignant intraocular tumors include retinoblastoma (usually under age 1, presenting with leukocoria or strabismus) and malignant melanoma. Metastatic tumors may involve the eye, most often with choroidal metastasis (17). Complications of intraocular malignancies that affect vision include hemorrhage from tumor vascularization, retinal detachment, retinal degeneration, and retinopathy. Abnormal physical findings should alert the physician to the importance of timely ophthalmologic follow up.

Methanol Toxicity

Methanol toxicity is associated with transient visual disturbances. Symptoms and signs usually occur within 18 to 48 hours of the ingestion. Associated symptoms include nausea, vomiting, headache, or abdominal pain. Findings include hyperemic, swollen optic discs, with retinal edema. A cherry-red spot may be observed (7).

Other Toxins

Numerous other toxins that may be associated with visual disturbances include carbon monoxide, lead, salicylates, sulfonamides, ergots, tin, quinine, barbiturates, chemotherapy, and nitroglycerin. Visual loss is usually bilateral, and therapy consists of the appropriate treatment of the underlying condition (25).

DIFFERENTIAL DIAGNOSIS

Vision loss may be caused by a variety of ophthalmologic conditions, or in association with other diseases. Some of the more common ophthalmologic causes are summarized in Table 19.1. In general, any abnormality of the cornea, lens, vitreous, retina, optic nerve, optic tract, optic radiations, or occipital cortex should be considered.

Patients with vascular disease may develop vision loss due to hemorrhages of various types, including preretinal, linear, punctate, subretinal, and white central hemorrhages (Roth spots). Additionally, there may be acute ocular ischemia due to infarction of the optic disc (ischemic optic neuropathy), which presents with sudden visual loss, and a pale, swollen optic disc. Causes of ocular ischemia include hypertension, atherosclerosis, choroidal infarction, retinal infarction, and transient retinal ischemia (amaurosis fugax). Patients with AIDS may present with toxoplasmosis, candidal endophthalmitis, herpes zoster ophthalmicus, or optic neuropathy.

The diagnosis of *functional visual loss*, as seen in conversion disorder, should always be one of exclusion. There may be a

TABLE 19.1.   Differential Diagnosis of Selected Causes of Visual Disturbance

Disease Process	Symptoms	Clinical Findings	Ancillary Tests	Management
Giant-cell arteritis	Painless visual loss, sudden or gradual, headache, myalgias	Optic nerve edema, temporal artery tenderness	Elevated ESR	Steroids, ophthalmologic consultation
Optic neuritis	Painful visual loss, pain with EOM	APD, elevation of optic disc		Consider steroids in patients with MS; ophthalmologic consultation
Uveitis	Eye pain, blurred vision, photophobia	Cells in anterior or posterior chamber, flare in aqueous humor		Topical steroids, cycloplegics, ophthalmologic consultation
Central retinal artery occlusion	Sudden, painless, profound visual loss	APD, pallor of retina, cherry red fovea		Globe massage, paracentesis, acetazolamide, inhaled carbogen, ophthalmologic consultation
Central retinal vein occlusion	Sudden, painless visual loss	Retinal hemorrhages, venous dilation, optic disc edema		Ophthalmologic consultation
Amaurosis fugax	Monocular visual loss (transient)		Carotid and cardiac studies	ASA, neurologic consultation
Vitreous hemorrhage	Visual floaters, cobwebs, or severe visual loss	Diminished or absent red reflex ("eight ball" hemorrhage)		Treatment of underlying condition; ophthalmologic consultation
Retinal detachment	Acute, painless visual disturbance; filmy, cloudy vision; peripheral monocular visual loss ("veil")	Gray/translucent detached area with folds, bulging appearance		Ophthalmologic consultation
Macular degeneration	Gradual, painless disturbances; spots in visual field; distortion of straight lines	Drusen, macular pigment clumps		Ophthalmologic consultation
Diabetic retinopathy	Gradual visual disturbances, scotomas	Multiple retinal hemorrhages, macular edema		Ophthalmologic consultation
Ischemic optic neuropathy	Painless, diminished visual acuity	APD, pale, elevated optic disc		Ophthalmologic consultation
TIA	Transient binocular visual loss	Normal	Carotid, cardiac studies	Neurologic consultation, ASA
Cortical blindness	Sudden or gradual, complete visual loss or homonymous hemianopia, HA	Papilledema, other neurologic findings	CT, MRI LP	Neurologic consultation, therapy of underlying disorder
Migraine HA	Transient visual loss	Normal		Neurologic consultation; see Chapter 110
Glaucoma	Sudden, painful visual disturbance, ABD pain, N/V	Optic nerve pallor and cupping	Elevated IOP	Topical beta-blocker; miotic, carbonic anhydrase inhibitor; ophthalmologic consultation; see Chapter 22
CMV retinitis	Sudden or gradual visual disturbance	Retinal hemorrhages, areas of pale retinal necrosis ("tomato and cheese pizza" appearance)	Consider CT/MRI	Foscarnet or ganciclovir, ophthalmologic consultation
Methanol	Transient visual disturbance, N/V, HA	Hyperemic, swollen optic discs, cherry-red spot		ETOH, see Chapter 275
Functional visual loss	Variable symptoms	Normal	Optokinetic nystagmus	Psychiatric consultation

This table represents only a summary of certain disorders, and is not an exhaustive information source for the above disease states.

ESR, erythrocyte sedimentation rate; EOM, external otitis media; APD, afferent pupillary defect; MS, multiple sclerosis; TIA, transient ischemic attack; CT, computed tomography; MRI, magnetic resonance imaging; LP, lumbar puncture; IOP, intraocular pressure; CMV, cytomegalovirus.

variety of complaints, but no abnormalities are seen on examination. The swinging flashlight test, IOP, and external and funduscopic examinations are normal. Optokinetic responses may be tested in a cursory fashion in the emergency department by passing a tape measure, or sheet of paper with prominent vertical lines, rapidly before the affected eye(s). Another simple test involves placing a mirror before the patient's face and rocking the mirror from side to side. The presence of optokinetic nystagmus (following movements with rapid returns to the primary position of the eye) indicates that vision is present. Additionally, patients feigning blindness may demonstrate an inability to oppose outstretched forefingers while bringing outstretched arms together; this ability would not ordinarily be affected by blindness. Additional tests to differentiate organic from functional visual loss may be suggested by ophthalmologic or psychiatric evaluation.

EMERGENCY DEPARTMENT EVALUATION

Complete details of the ophthalmologic examination are included in Chapter 15. Specifically, when evaluating the patient with loss of vision, of primary importance are visual acuity and visual field testing.

Visual acuity is an *essential* element of the physical examination, and can be measured with a Snellen eye chart. The acuity of each eye should be tested independently, with the patient's usual visual correction, if available. For patients who normally wear corrective lenses, but which are unavailable for testing, pinhole testing can be easily performed by creating a device with paper and "pinholes" created with an 18-gauge needle. For patients unable to adequately read from the eye chart, their ability to count fingers, detect movement, and perceive light and dark should be evaluated.

Visual field testing can be useful in determining the extent of visual loss and in developing the appropriate differential diagnosis. Eyes should be tested independently. The confrontation technique may be employed, in which the examiner presents variable numbers of fingers in various visual fields, and asks the patient to count the fingers, while maintaining a forward gaze. Each quadrant should be tested for both eyes. More advanced visual field testing can be performed by an ophthalmologist.

Additionally, the examination should evaluate the external and slit-lamp appearance of the cornea and conjunctiva, and trauma, foreign bodies, hyphema, infection, corneal opacities, and other abnormalities should be ruled out. Intraocular pressure (IOP) should be measured, using a hand-held tonometer, applanation tonometry, or Schiøtz tonometer. Glaucoma is discussed in greater detail in Chapter 22.

Pupils should be evaluated, utilizing the swinging flashlight test. Pupillary response can be valuable in differentiating afferent from efferent defects. The normal response is bilateral pupillary constriction in response to bright light in either pupil.

Funduscopic examination should be performed using a hand-held ophthalmoscope. Pupillary dilation may be required to perform an adequate examination of the retina. In particular, the optic disc, macula, and retina should be evaluated for any abnormalities.

Ultrasound of the eye may be helpful in elucidating certain diagnoses. Radiographic evaluation (including magnetic resonance imaging or computed tomography) may be indicated in cases in which intracranial pathology or mass lesions involving the optic nerve or globe are suspected. Patients presenting with complaints related to loss of vision require a complete ophthalmologic examination, which should include measurement of visual acuity, visual field testing, tonometry, and slit-lamp examination.

EMERGENCY DEPARTMENT MANAGEMENT

Many of the diseases that produce acute vision loss mandate emergent ophthalmologic consultation, intervention, or admission. The unique features of some of the causes are discussed below. It is not meant to be an exhaustive review of the treatment of ophthalmologic disorders, but a summary of salient points relevant to the emergency physician.

For patients with *giant cell arteritis (GCA)*, early administration of corticosteroids (80 to 120 mg of prednisone per day, or intravenous methylprednisolone, 1 g per day) may prevent blindness and other long-term visual defects, as well as contralateral eye involvement (common within 10 days without treatment), and may provide dramatic pain relief (6,7,21). Patients may have a 34% chance of improvement in visual function after steroid therapy (16). Aspirin may have additional protective effects when instituted in conjunction with steroid therapy (28). A biopsy should be performed within 7 to 10 days of steroid initiation, although most biopsies will remain positive up to 4 weeks after initiation of therapy (20). A negative biopsy does not exclude GCA (25,29).

Although the treatment of *optic neuritis* with steroids is not universally beneficial, intravenous methylprednisolone is indicated for patients with suspected multiple sclerosis (8). Investigation for an underlying predisposing condition, in consultation with the primary care physician, is essential. Consultation with an ophthalmologist is indicated for patients with suspected optic neuritis (11).

Uveitis may be treated effectively with topical corticosteroids and cycloplegic agents. Systemic steroids may be indicated in severe cases. Therapy of the underlying disorder should be undertaken (11,12).

Treatment for *central retinal artery occlusion (CRAO)* is often unsatisfactory, but should be attempted, and it may include intermittent globe massage in an attempt to dislodge an embolus (moderate pressure for 5 seconds and release for 5 seconds), anterior chamber paracentesis (to decrease IOP and increase retinal perfusion), intravenous acetazolamide (to decrease IOP), topical timolol 0.5% or topical levobunolol 0.5%, inhaled carbogen (oxygen–carbon dioxide mixture of 95%/5%) to induce retinal vasodilation and increase retinal pO_2 (26). Hyperbaric oxygen and nifedipine have also been reported as successful therapies (1,2). Other treatment offered by an ophthalmologist may include ophthalmic artery infusion of urokinase or tissue plasminogen activator (18).

Central retinal vein occlusion (CRVO) is difficult to treat successfully, but should include a careful evaluation of the probable etiology in order to prevent contralateral eye involvement. Spontaneous resolution may occur in some cases. Treatment offered by an ophthalmologist may include panretinal laser photocoagulation (19). Laser photocoagulation has an important role in the treatment of branch RVO, which has a better prognosis (9).

Amaurosis fugax should be treated with aspirin, and ophthalmologic consultation obtained. *Ischemic optic neuropathy* should be treated with systemic steroids (methylprednisolone, 250 mg IV q 6 h) to prevent contralateral eye involvement.

Retinal detachment should be treated by an ophthalmologist, with options including diathermy, laser photocoagulation, or other intraocular surgical therapies. Treatment for m*acular degeneration* includes laser photocoagulation and the use of low-vision aids (3,10,30).

CMV retinitis may be treated with intravenous or intravitreous antiviral therapy (fomivirsen, foscarnet or ganciclovir) in consultation with an ophthalmologist (13,31).

Glaucoma may be treated with a miotic (e.g., pilocarpine), topical beta-blocker (e.g., timolol), a carbonic anhydrase inhibitor (e.g., acetazolamide), mannitol or glycerin, and topical steroids. A more detailed discussion of glaucoma is found in Chapter 22.

Methanol toxicity may be treated with ethanol or dialysis, and is discussed in Chapter 275.

CRITICAL INTERVENTIONS

- Rapidly recognize and obtain ophthalmologic consultation for patients with CRAO and Amaurosis fugax
- Initiate steroids for patients with giant cell arteritis

DISPOSITION

For the majority of patients with acute visual loss, consultation with an ophthalmologist is indicated. The severity and nature of the disease process will dictate whether emergent or urgent consultation is necessary. Patients considered for hospital admission should be those who require intravenous medications, surgery, or other invasive procedures, or for whom serious worsening of vision is imminent.

COMMON PITFALLS

- ✔ Failure to measure visual acuity
- ✔ Failure to consider the diagnosis of glaucoma in atypical presentations
- ✔ Failure to measure intraocular pressure
- ✔ Failure to test visual fields adequately
- ✔ Failure to administer steroids rapidly to patients with giant cell arteritis
- ✔ Delay in treatment of central retinal artery occlusion

References

1. Alexander LJ. Age-related macular degeneration: the current understanding of the status of clinicopathology, diagnosis and management. *J Am Optom Assoc* 1993;64:822–837.
2. Beiran I, Goldenberg I, Adir Y, et al. Early hyperbaric oxygen therapy for retinal artery occlusion. *Eur J Ophthalmol* 2001;11:345–350.
3. Beiran I, Reissman P, Scharf J, et al. Hyperbaric oxygenation combined with nifedipine treatment for recent-onset retinal artery occlusion. *Eur J Ophthalmol* 1993;3:89–94.
4. Forrester JV. Uveitis: pathogenesis. *Lancet* 1991;338:1498–1501.
5. Hayreh SS. Management of central retinal vein occlusion. *Ophthalmologica* 2003;217:167–188.
6. Hayreh SS, Zimmerman B. Management of giant cell arteritis. Our 27-year clinical study: new light on old controversies. *Ophthalmologica* 2003;217:239–259.
7. Hayreh SS, Zimmerman B. Visual deterioration in giant cell arteritis patients while on high doses of corticosteroid therapy. *Ophthalmology* 2003;110:1204–1215.
8. Hickman SJ, Dalton CM, Miller DH, et al. Management of acute optic neuritis. *Lancet* 2002;360:1953–1962.
9. Hoover BW, Stack LB. Acute bilateral blindness. *Acad Emerg Med* 1996;3:1056–1059.
10. Javitt JC, Zhou Z, Maguire MG, et al. Incidence of exudative age-related macular degeneration among elderly Americans. *Ophthalmology* 2003;110:1534–1539.
11. Janda AM. Sudden nontraumatic visual loss. *Postgrad Med* 1992;91:111–125.
12. Keltner JL, Johnson CA, Spurr JO, et al. Visual field profile of optic neuritis. *Arch Ophthalmol* 1994;112:946–953.
13. Kuo IC, Imai Y, Shum C, et al. Genotypic analysis of cytomegalovirus retinitis poorly responsive to intravenous ganciclovir but responsive to the ganciclovir implant. *Am J Ophthalmol* 2003;135:20–25.
14. La Vene D, Halpern J, Jagoda A. Loss of vision. *Emerg Med Clin North Am* 1995;13:539–561.
15. Lee PP, Feldman ZW, Ostermann J, et al. Longitudinal prevalence of major eye diseases. *Arch Ophthalmol* 2003;121:1303–1310.
16. Liu GT, Glaser JS, Schatz NJ, et al. Visual morbidity in giant cell arteritis. *Ophthalmology* 1994;101:1779–1785.
17. McKellar MJ, Hidajat RR, Elder MJ. Acute ocular methanol toxicity: clinical and electrophysiological features. *Aust N Z J Ophthalmol* 1997;25:225–230.
18. Makino A, Soga T, Obayashi M, et al. Cortical blindness caused by acute general cerebral swelling. *Surg Neurol* 1988;29:393–400.
19. Newell FW. *Ophthalmology: principles and concepts,* 8th ed. St. Louis: Mosby Year Book, 1996:305–308.
20. Ray-Chaudhuri N, Kine DA, Tijani SO, et al. Effect of prior steroid treatment on temporal artery biopsy findings in giant cell arteritis. *Br J Ophthalmol* 2002;86:530–532.
21. Salvarani C, Cantini F, Boiardi L. Polymyalgia rheumatica and giant-cell arteritis. *N Engl J Med* 2002;347:261–271.
22. Schumacher M, Schmidt D, Wakhloo AK. Intra-arterial fibrinolytic therapy in central retinal artery occlusion. *Neuroradiology* 1993;35:600–605.
23. Shimozono M, Townsend JC, Ilsen PF, et al. Acute vision loss resulting from complications of ethanol abuse. *J Am Optom Assoc* 1998;69:293–303.
24. Tranquart F, Berges O, Koskas P, et al. Color Doppler imaging of orbital vessels: personal experience and literature review. *J Clin Ultrasound* 2003;31:258–273.
25. Varma R. *Essentials of eye care: the Johns Hopkins Wilmer handbook.* Philadelphia: Lippincott-Raven Publishers, 1997:357–380.
26. Vaughan DG, Asbury T, Riordan Eva P. *General ophthalmology.* East Norwalk, CT: Appleton & Lange, 1995:187–188.
27. Wei LL, Park SS, Skiest DJ. Prevalence of visual symptoms among patients with newly diagnosed cytomegalovirus retinitis. *Retina* 2002;22:278–282.
28. Weyand CM, Kaiser M, Yang H, et al. Therapeutic effects of acetylsalicylic acid in giant cell arteritis. *Arthritis Rheum* 2002;46:457–466.
29. Weinberg DA, Savino PJ, Sergott RC, et al. Giant cell arteritis: corticosteroids, temporal artery biopsy, and blindness. *Arch Fam Med* 1994;3:623–627.
30. Wormald R, Evans J, Smeeth L, et al. Photodynamic therapy for neovascular age-related macular degeneration. *Cochrane Database Syst Rev* 2003;2:CD002030.
31. Zun LS. Acute visual loss. *Emerg Med Clin North Am* 1988;6:57–72.

CHAPTER 20
Diplopia

James A. Comes

Diplopia is an uncommon yet serious symptom among patients presenting to the emergency department. The differential diagnosis includes ocular and neurologic problems requiring thorough investigation and timely intervention. It may represent the initial symptom of systemic disease. Initial evaluation involves a history of present illness, including an ocular history, a thorough eye exam, pertinent physical and neurologic exam, generation of a focused differential diagnosis, relevant laboratory testing and, frequently, emergent neuroimaging.

Emergency physicians are often expected to act and stabilize patients with an incomplete data base. Definitive management in emergent neurologic and eye disease rests upon making the diagnosis or localizing the site of the lesion. Management decisions after acute stabilization will invariably involve input from ophthalmology, neurology, or neurosurgery.

CLINICAL PRESENTATION

Diplopia is the perception of one object seen as two at different points in space. Acting as yoked pairs, the eyes are normally positioned so that the image falls on the same spot on each retina. Any slight displacement of either image causes diplopia.

While patients commonly use the term double vision in their description of the problem, they may also complain of seeing multiple ghost-like images, blurry vision, or dizziness. The two images may be separated vertically, horizontally or obliquely. Diplopia may vary with the direction of gaze or be equally present in all. It may be monocular or binocular (10).

Monocular diplopia can be distinguished from binocular diplopia when the patient's diplopia persists upon covering the unaffected eye. In binocular diplopia, the relationship of the images to one another should be elicited. Medial or lateral rectus muscle pathology will result in a pure horizontal diplopia, while the other extraocular muscles will result in a vertical and torsional component that may vary with abduction or adduction. Diplopia from extraocular muscle weakness worsens when patients look toward the field of gaze of the affected muscle. Vertical diplopia may be from a brainstem lesion or optic chiasmal compression (10).

Table 20.1 highlights several important features of binocular diplopia that can help to narrow the differential diagnosis. While most diplopia is abrupt in onset or suddenly noticed, a gradual progression suggests a lesion infiltrating the nerve or displacing the globe. If the symptoms are episodic, ocular myasthenia should be considered. Complete, unilateral ptosis is a 3rd cranial nerve (CN) palsy until proven otherwise. Horner syndrome must be considered in patients with a mild ptosis.

Associated pain is concerning for an expanding or ruptured mass lesion. Headache, vertigo, weakness or vomiting may suggest a serious neurologic emergency such as a cerebellar bleed. Proptosis of the globe, particularly if it is associated with swelling or injection of the bulbar conjunctiva, suggests an aneurysm or thrombosis of the cavernous sinus. The most common cause of exophthalmos is thyrotoxicosis. Thyroid eye disease, while commonly bilateral, may be unilateral.

Patients should be asked about using a device whereby the other eye remains closed for periods of time (e.g. telescope, microscope). Other pertinent history includes the presence of hypertension, diabetes or thyroid disease. An ocular history should address the need for corrective lenses, a recent change in refraction or eye surgery. All medications should be reviewed.

DIFFERENTIAL DIAGNOSIS

Monocular diplopia is rare. It usually results from optical disturbances within the refractory medium and does not require emergency diagnosis or management. Monocular diplopia may be external, optic, neurologic, neuromuscular or psychogenic (Table 20.2). The most frequent causes are early cataract, severe astigmatism, and lens abnormalities (10). There are case reports of patients with lesions in the occipital cortex or pituitary gland causing monocular diplopia, but these are invariably associated with visual field defects (9).

Binocular diplopia generally indicates ocular misalignment. The anatomic locations for diplopia include the following: supranuclear (skew deviation-one eye appears higher than another); ocular motor nuclei and infranuclear segment (CN 3,4, or 6); medial longitudinal fasciculus [internuclear ophthalmoplegia (INO)]; neuromuscular junction; muscle (1). Most

TABLE 20.1.   Initial Approach to Binocular Diplopia

Onset and progression
Variability or remission
Presence or absence of ptosis
Associated pain
Presence of exophthalmos or proptosis

TABLE 20.2.   Differential Diagnosis of Diplopia

CONVERGENCE/ACCOMMODATION PROBLEMS

Bifocals/reading glasses

EXTRAOCULAR MUSCLES

Thyroid disease
Trauma
Orbital fractures
Space occupying lesions
Metabolic, inflammatory, infectious causes of muscle weakness

NEUROMUSCULAR JUNCTION

Ocular myasthenia

CRANIAL NERVE NEUROPATHIES

Posterior communicating aneurysm
Multiple sclerosis
Brainstem ischemia/infarct
Cavernous sinus thrombosis
Cavernous sinus IC artery aneurysm
Neoplastic
Vascular
Inflammatory/Infectious
Trauma
Intracranial hypertension
Botulism
Meningitis
Miller-Fisher Variant of AIDP (Guillain-Barre)
Wernicke syndrome
Diphtheria
Alcohol
Arsenic
Lead
Carbon tetrachloride
Phenytoin
Isoniazid
Nitrofurantoin

INTERNUCLEAR OPHTHALMOPLEGIAS

Brain stem ischemia/stroke
Multiple sclerosis
Midbrain syndromes (Parinaud syndrome)

MONOCULAR DIPLOPIA

Corneal disease (astigmatism, dry eye)
Iris (polycoria, trauma)
Lens (cataracts, subluxation)
Foreign body in aqueous or vitreous humor
Retinal disease (rare)
Monocular oscillopsia (nystagmus)
Occipital cortex disease (migraine, epilepsy, tumor, trauma, vascular)
Equipment failure (poor fitting contact lens, ill fitting bifocals in a dementia pt)
Psychogenic

Modified from Richardson LD, Joyce DM. Diplopia in the emergency department. *Emerg Med Clin No Am* 1997;15:649–659.

supranuclear lesions cause conjugate gaze palsies without diplopia (1). Most binocular diplopia is from ocular motor nerve palsies (CN palsy) or disease of the neuromuscular junction (Table 20.2). INOs occur in the elderly with vascular disease affecting the brainstem, but the disease is classically found in those patients with multiple sclerosis (11). With the exception of thyroid eye disease, myopathies are an uncommon cause of diplopia. Direct trauma (blunt or penetrating) or eye surgery may affect the eye muscles. Migraines can be associated with diplopia and cranial nerve palsies; however, new onset migraines are often clinically indistinguishable from serious intracranial pathology(8).

EMERGENCY DEPARTMENT EVALUATION

The complaint of diplopia should prompt a thorough ocular and neurologic examination. Emergency physicians should have a working knowledge of basic neuroanatomy in order to localize the site of the lesion and thereby determine the optimal work up and appropriate consultation.

During the history, inspection of the head and its posture may be a clue to a CN palsy. Patients with a 6th nerve palsy may turn their head in the direction of the palsy to compensate for the weak muscle. This is also true for 4th nerve palsy; the head will be tilted down and to the opposite side of the affected superior oblique (14). Inspection of the external ocular structures should focus on asymmetry of the periorbital and orbital structures including signs of inflammation, injection, ptosis, proptosis or lid retraction.

Patients should have a visual acuity examination performed. A slit-lamp examination with corneal staining should be performed in patients with monocular diplopia. Pupillary size, symmetry, reactivity and the presence of an afferent pupillary defect provide much pivotal information.

Extraocular movements are essential in examining the patient with diplopia. First note any nystagmus at rest (1st degree nystagmus). Test movement in all of the nine cardinal directions of gaze, about 18 inches from the patient to prevent convergence, noting any worsening of diplopia or nystagmus. Nystagmoid movements at the extreme of gaze are more representative of the examiner's technique and are a result of moving too fast and too far in one direction. Elderly patients often have limited ability to look upward. Skew deviation suggests supranuclear pathology, either in the brainstem or cerebellum. Monocular nystagmus can

be seen in acquired blindness in one eye. In ocular myasthenia, nystagmus in the unaffected eye is the rule. Patients with INO have transient diplopia on lateral gaze due to dysconjugate eye movement. When the patient looks to the right, abduction is normal in the right eye with marked nystagmus and adduction fails in the left eye with little or no nystagmus. When the patient looks left, the exact opposite occurs, the left eye abducts normally yet with nystagmus, the right eye has little or no nystagmus yet does not adduct. In the case of nerve lesions, the weak muscles can be detected by observing eye movements. The 3rd, 4th, and 6th CNs control eye movement, upper eyelids and pupils. Since each has a long intracranial course, they are subject to a myriad of insults (8) (Table 20.3).

The 3rd CN innervates the muscles of the eyelid and all external ocular muscles excluding the superior oblique and lateral rectus. It also carries parasympathetic fibers on the external surface of the 3rd CN. Since a complete 3rd nerve palsy paralyzes the eyelid, diplopia only occurs when the lid is held up. The eyelid can still be tightly shut via the 7th CN. Diplopia occurs in all directions of gaze except for lateral gaze of the affected side since the lateral rectus is intact.

Isolated 4th nerve palsies are uncommon, frequently misdiagnosed and produce a very subtle diplopia. The diplopia occurs when the patient looks down and away from the affected eye. Patients may describe difficulty descending stairs or reading a book.

The 6th nerve can be easily tested with lateral gaze. This palsy causes the greatest difficulty for the patient, as there is no ptosis to obliterate the false image. Diplopia occurs in all directions of visual gaze except away from the affected side. Patients often attempt to keep the affected eye shut to reduce the symptoms. If the examiner holds the unaffected eyelid shut, the eye on the side of the "pseudoptosis" will open.

In attempting to localize the lesion, it is important to distinguish an isolated CN palsy from multiple. In the presence of a 3rd nerve palsy, the 6th can be easily tested with lateral gaze.

TABLE 20.3.   Extraocular Nerve Lesions

Location	Symptoms	Diagnoses
Brainstem	Evidence of BS dysfunction	Vascular disease, multiple sclerosis, pontine glioma, extrinsic compression, wernickes encephalopathy
Basilar	Multiple CN palsies, meningeal disease	Tuberculous, fungal, bacterial meningitis, malignancies (carcinomatous or direct invasion from sinuses & nasopharynx), herpes zoster, AIDP (MFS variant) aneurysmal dilatation of basilar artery
	3rd nerve palsy	Posterior communicating aneurysm, infarction (diabetes)
	6th nerve palsy, signs of intracranial HTN	Posterior fossa tumors, pseudotumor cerebri (IIH)
Lesions at the petrous tip of the bone	Ear pain with 6th, 7th, & 8th	Mastoiditis or OM causing inflammation of petrous bone & thrombosis of petrous sinus, lateral sinus thrombosis secondary to mastoiditis
	Nerve lesions	
	Painless 6th nerve palsy	Carcinoma of nasopharynx or paranasal sinuses extending into skull fissures
Cavernous sinus	6th nerve palsy with severe pain, exophthalmos, edema of eyelids, 3rd, 4th, 5th(V1 & V2) CN also may be affected	Cavernous sinus thrombosis, Carotid artery aneurysm
Supraorbital fissure and orbit	Various combinations of 3rd, 4th, and 6th CN palsies with proptosis	Malignant and benign tumors of the orbit, thyrotoxicosis

AIDP, acute inflammatory demyelinating polyneuropathy; BS, brainstem; CN, cranial nerve; HTN, hypertension; IIH, idiopathic intracranial hypertension; MFS, Miller-Fisher syndrome; OM, otitis media; OMN, oculomotor nerve.

However, testing the 4th nerve is difficult since the paralyzed medial rectus does not permit the eye to adduct. The secondary action of the 4th can be observed. The affected eye is usually depressed downward, and if the patient attempts to look further downward, the eye will rotate inward as the superior oblique pulls sideways around the eye.

In addition to the oculomotor CNs and pupillary response, other CN lesions may provide valuable information in localizing the lesion, particularly CN 5, 7, and 8 (Table 20.3).

Emergent neuroimaging often provides diagnostic and pivotal information. MRI has many benefits over CT. It better identifies posterior fossa, brainstem and skull based pathology. Major intracranial vessels can be identified without contrast, and sagittal views are available. It also distinguishes grey/white matter disease more clearly. However, for many institutions, it is not always immediately available. It also requires more patient cooperation and often an inappropriate study for the critically ill. Emergent brain CT scanning remains as the most widely available and rapidly obtainable imaging study in the ED that can guide initial management or consultation decisions. Additionally, patients with suspected CNS infections should have a lumbar puncture performed.

EMERGENCY DEPARTMENT MANAGEMENT

Certain patterns of signs and symptoms require emergent neuroimaging, timely consultation and critical interventions. This section will highlight a selected group of emergent presentations of diplopia and vision disturbances along with relevant ED management. With the exception of clearly identifiable thyroid eye disease, all of the presentations below require neuroimaging and specialty consultation.

3rd Nerve Palsy

The two most common causes of an acute 3rd nerve palsy are an aneurysm of the posterior communicating artery and diabetes. A 3rd nerve palsy with any degree of pupillary involvement is usually due to a space occupying lesion (mass or aneurysm). Most present with a ptosis, diplopia and a headache. The headache is not necessarily abrupt or severe as in subarachnoid hemorrhages. Ischemia from diabetes is the second most common cause of a 3rd nerve palsy. Since the pupillary-constrictor fibers have a dual blood supply from the core and sheath of the 3rd CN, ischemic lesions usually, but not always, spare the pupils.

There has been much classical teaching on distinguishing a surgical 3rd nerve palsy (pupillary involvement) from a medical 3rd nerve palsy (pupillary sparing). While pupillary involvement points to an aneurysm of the posterior communicating artery, it does not rule out an ischemic cause. In 14% to 32% of cases, microvascular infarction affects the pupil. Conversely, 3% to 5% of 3rd nerve palsies associated with aneurysms have pupillary sparing (9). Patients should have emergent CT or MR imaging to rule out other space-occupying lesions, followed by MRA or cerebral angiography in consultation with neurology and neurosurgery.

4th Nerve Palsy

It can be the result of DM or in rare instances a medulloblastoma in children. Trauma is the most common cause of a trochlear nerve palsy; the nerve is damaged by the free edge of the tentorium (2). Aneurysms presenting as a trochlear palsy are extremely rare.

6th Nerve Palsy

Unlike 3rd nerve palsies, isolated 6th nerve palsies are extremely unlikely to be from aneurysmal disease. Since they are often a surrogate marker for intracranial hypertension, emergent neuroimaging is always indicated.

Multiple Cranial Nerve Palsies

Cavernous sinus thrombosis is a serious condition that occurs as a complication of an infection of the skin over the upper face or paranasal sinuses. Multiple CNs pass through the cavernous sinus including 3, 4, 5 (V1 and V2 branches), and 6. The 6th nerve is most vulnerable to disease since it lies free within the sinus. Patients present with severe pain, an eye that is often fixed in gaze, exophthalmos and edema of the eyelids. Extension of the thrombosis to the opposite sinus frequently occurs. These patients often appear ill and require resuscitation, emergent neuroimaging, antibiotics and critical care.

Aneurysmal dilation or rupture of the internal carotid artery in the cavernous sinus usually presents in the elderly female with severe vascular disease. On examination, the eye is injected, proptotic and may be pulsatile (caroticocavernous fistula). If the aneurysm is anterior, exophthalmos, blindness with a 3rd and 4th nerve palsy may occur. If posterior, V1 irritation coupled with a 6th nerve palsy may occur. The palsy may be simultaneous with the onset of severe pain. If the aneurysm ruptures in the cavernous sinus, it is rarely fatal as the sinus contains the hemorrhage. There are case reports of this occurring from a basilar skull fracture (14).

Miller-Fisher Syndrome (MFS) is a monophasic polyneuropathy characterized by ataxia, areflexia, ophthalmoplegia, and sometimes other craniobulbar deficits. The initial symptom is usually diplopia followed by gait ataxia, then days later areflexia. Half of patients will complain of paresthesias. 30% will have proximal muscle weakness and are considered an overlap between MFS and acute inflammatory demyelinating polyneuropathy (AIDP) (12). These patients require urgent neuroimaging and neurologic consultation.

Wernicke syndrome presents similarly to MFS. The syndrome is classically found in alcoholics and is characterized by nystagmus which precedes ophthalmoplegia, gait ataxia and confusion. Although it is a nutritional deficiency of thiamine found predominantly in alcoholics, it also may occur in patients on fad diets. Initial therapy should be with parenteral thiamine. Recovery of neurologic deficits can be dramatic and rapid within hours.

Conditions Mimicking Nerve Lesions

Since extraocular nerve lesions are usually all or nothing, it follows then that all of the muscles supplied by the nerve are affected by nerve lesions. If two muscles supplied by different extraocular nerves are affected, one has to consider thyrotoxicosis, ocular myasthenia or an INO.

Thyroid eye disease is one of the most common causes of binocular diplopia in middle-aged adults (11). Diplopia occurs because of lymphocytic infiltration and inflammation of the extraocular muscles, fat, and proximal structures causing a restrictive myopathy. Other signs include exophthalmos, ptosis, periocular inflammation, lid retraction, and lid lag on downward gaze (2). Weakness of any of the extraocular muscles may cause diplopia in the thyrotoxic patient regardless of whether exophthalmos is present. Patients may be clinically hypothyroid, euthyroid, or hyperthyroid. They need followup care with the appropriate specialist, outpatient thyroid testing, and rarely require emergent neuroimaging unless there is a potential threat to vision or a possibility of intracranial or cavernous sinus disease.

Diplopia and ptosis are common symptoms of ocular myasthenia. Key features of myasthenia gravis (MG) are episodic weakness and fatigability of voluntary muscles with repeat use. In ocular myasthenia, any extraocular muscle can be involved, resulting in diplopia. Weakness solely confined to the extraocular muscles and eyelid muscles is seen in only 15% of patients with myasthenia gravis (4). Nevertheless, ocular symptoms are the presenting symptom in nearly half of patients with MG. Patients with ocular myasthenia may present with a pseudo-INO (decreased adduction of one eye and nystagmoid movements of the abducting eye on lateral gaze) (6). The pupils are unaffected. When there is bedside observation of fatigability of the eyelid or eye movement, the possibility of myasthenia rises. Improvement of eye movements and ptosis can improve with cold packs applied to the eyelids. In consultation with neurology, tensilon testing may be performed in the ED, especially if there is a rapidly quantifiable endpoint (e.g., significant ptosis). Since electrodiagnostic testing is more sensitive, tensilon testing is used less frequently (1).

Patients with multiple sclerosis may present with extraocular nerve palsies (usually 6th). More commonly, they have difficulty with conjugate eye movement (INO) and complain of diplopia without clinical evidence of individual eye movement weakness.

Idiopathic Intracranial Hypertension (Pseudotumor cerebri)

Idiopathic intracranial hypertension (IIH) is a chronic vision threatening disease that classically affects obese women in their child-bearing years. It is eight times more common in women (6). Risk factors are obesity and recent weight gain. Many medications have been linked to IIH (7). Patients may present with any combination of the following complaints: headache, diplopia, nausea and vomiting, blurry vision or vision loss, dizziness. They often have visual field defects; however, the pattern is nonspecific. Exam of the retina demonstrates papilledema, characterized by swollen, hyperemic disc and a blurred disc margin. It may be asymmetrical. Patients may present with a unilateral or bilateral 6th nerve palsy which is suggestive of intracranial hypertension. Emergent brain CT or MR imaging is mandatory to rule out mass lesions, venous sinus thrombosis or hydrocephalus. If the imaging studies are normal, a lumbar puncture is indicated with measurement of the opening pressure and CSF fluid analysis. Since treatment decisions are under the province of neurology, consultation is required, but these patients are often discharged home from the ED.

CRITICAL INTERVENTIONS

- Emergent neuroimaging and consultation in patients with oculomotor CN palsies
- Administration of parenteral thiamine to patients with unexplained ophthalmoplegias

DISPOSITION

Admission decisions often rest with arriving at a preliminary diagnosis in the ED. Patients with a proven nonsurgical 3rd nerve palsy can be safely discharged home with neurology or neurophthalmology follow up. Patients with a 6th nerve palsy, no evidence of intracranial hypertension and normal imaging studies can have further evaluation arranged as outpatients. Because of the frequency of critical illness, patients with ophthalmoplegias

or multiple CN palsies should be admitted. Many disposition decisions will be specialty dependent.

COMMON PITFALLS

✔ Failure to obtain emergent brain imaging in patients with diplopia
✔ Failure to measure opening pressure during a lumbar puncture
✔ Falsely attributing a 3rd nerve palsy to ischemia after inadequate neuroimaging
✔ Delay or failure to consult neurology, ophthalmology or neurosurgery

References

1. Bhatti TM. Double trouble. *Surv Ophthalmol* 2003;48(3):347–355.
2. Brazis PW, Lee AG. Binocular vertical diplopia. *Mayo Clin Proc* 1998;73:55–66.
3. Brazis PW, Lee AG. Elevated intracranial pressure and pseudotumor cerebri. *Curr Opin Ophthalmol* 1998;9:27–32.
4. Heitmiller RF. Myasthenia gravis: Clinical features, pathogenesis, evaluation and medical management. *Semin Thorac Cardiovasc Surg* 1999;11:41–46.
5. Mark AS: Oculomotor motion disorders: Current imaging of cranial nerves 3, 4, and 6. *Semin Ultrasound CT MR* 1998;19:240–256.
6. Massey JM. Acquired myasthenia gravis. *Neurol Clin* 1999;15:577–595.
7. Mousas TZ, Liu GT, Galetta SL, Balcer LJ, Volpe NJ. Current Neuro-ophthalmic therapies. *Neurol Clin* 2000;19:145–172.
8. Patten JP. The third, fourth, and sixth cranial nerves. In: Patten JP, ed. *Neurologic differential diagnosis,* 2nd ed. London: Springer-Verlag Limited, 2001;47–60.
9. Records RE. Monocular diplopia. *Surv Ophthalmol* 1980;24:303–306.
10. Richardson LD, Joyce DM. Diplopia in the emergency department. *Emerg Med Clin No Am* 1997;15:649–659.
11. Ruff RL, Wiener SN, Leigh RJ. Magnetic resonance imaging in patients with diplopia. *Invest Radiol* 1986;21:311–319.
12. Vaphiades MS. The double vision decision. *Surv Ophthalmol* 2003;48:85–91.

CHAPTER 21
Acute Eye Infections

David A. Kramer and Michael A. Bohrn

Eye infections comprise a large percentage of causes of the red eye (Chapter 17, The Red Eye) and clinical judgment must dictate pursuit of noninfectious etiologies. This chapter addresses a variety of eye-related infections, including conjunctivitis, keratitis, keratoconjunctivitis, endophthalmitis, and orbital and periorbital cellulitis (also see Eye Disorders, Chapter 245). The importance of eye infections to the emergency physician is obvious, as vision is a vital sense and any compromise of visual function would be devastating.

Conjunctivitis refers to inflammation of the mucus membranes that line the eyelids and sclera. Viral and bacterial infections are common causes of this disorder. Most patients presenting to the emergency department (ED) with conjunctivitis have a self-limited disease process, although the emergency physician must be wary for complications or alternative diagnoses. *Keratitis* refers to inflammation of the cornea. Infectious keratitis frequently involves the conjunctiva as well and is referred to as *keratoconjunctivitis*. This condition usually causes significant pain for the patient and may have viral or bacterial etiologies as well. *Endophthalmitis* refers to inflammation of the intraocular structures. This condition is frequently infectious in etiology and often represents a significant infection which requires aggressive antibiotic therapy and ophthalmology consultation. *Blepharitis* is a group of inflammatory conditions of the eyelid, and may involve the area nearest the eyelashes and follicles, or may be related to the meibomian glands. A *hordeolum* or *stye* is closely related to blepharitis and signifies local inflammation at the lid margin. A hordeolum typically involves the follicles and eyelashes, or it may represent acute inflammation or infection near the meibomian glands. A *chalazion* is not truly an infection, but rather a chronic inflammatory process leading to granuloma formation surrounding blocked sebaceous or meibomian glands.

Orbital and periorbital infections are relatively uncommon and affect children more frequently than adults. When they do occur, they can be life threatening. The terms *orbital cellulitis* and *periorbital cellulitis* are too often used interchangeably, since the single most important step in managing these diseases is to differentiate the two. Orbital (postseptal) cellulitis is anatomically defined as inflammation of any of the tissues within the orbit posterior to the orbital septum. A more anatomically correct term than periorbital cellulitis is *preseptal cellulitis*. This term includes any inflammation anterior to the orbital septum, a sheet-like layer of fascia that separates the orbit from the eyelids (Fig. 21.1). Preseptal cellulitis is invariably present in orbital infection, as are chemosis and proptosis.

CLINICAL PRESENTATION

Patients with ocular surface infections typically will present with complaints of eye pain, redness, and/or discharge. In general, more significant symptoms such as vision change, photophobia, or headache often signify more serious causes in patients with eye complaints. One or both eyes may be initially or sequentially involved. The quality of discharge or associated findings such as an enlarged ipsilateral preauricular lymph node, are commonly used to differentiate between viral and bacterial conjunctivitis, but there appears to be little evidence of these associations, or of any specific factors aiding this differentiation (10). Crusting and sticking of the eyelids often occurs, and is especially notable after sleep, and mild visual changes may be seen when a discharge is present. Typically, other systemic signs such as fever or other abnormal vital signs are absent. Patients with keratitis usually present with eye pain, and may have other symptoms if keratoconjunctivitis is present. *Herpes keratitis* in particular may also produce a corneal dendritic lesion. Patients with endophthalmitis often exhibit more significant clinical findings. Periorbital cellulitis typically involves erythema, edema, and warmth of the periorbital tissues, and also may involve closure of the palpebral fissures. Fever may be present. However, there should be no complaints of ocular pain, pain with movement of the globe, nor any limitation of globe mobility, all of which suggest the more serious diagnosis of orbital (postseptal) cellulitis. Patients with blepharitis may present with red, swollen eyelids, a foreign body sensation, tearing, crusting of the eyelid margins, or simply eye pain or photophobia. With hordeolum, similar symptoms are often present, but typically a focal area of erythema and swelling of the eyelid is noticed. Similarly, a chalazion usually causes a focal area of inflammation, but this is usually subacute in onset, and most times occurs proximal to the eyelid margin.

DIFFERENTIAL DIAGNOSIS

The differential diagnosis of the red or painful eye is broad (Chapter 17). Infection is a relatively common cause of these symptoms, but a variety of other causes must be considered, including: allergic reactions, irritant causes, foreign body, chemical or thermal burns, trauma, medication reactions, orbital disease related to other medical problems (e.g., thyroid disorders), glaucoma, uveitis, mucocutaneous syndromes (e.g., Kawasaki disease, Stevens-Johnson syndrome, etc.), and cancer. Differential diagnosis of orbital or periorbital cellulitis includes: allergic periorbital swelling, cavernous sinus thrombosis, and subperiosteal or orbital abscess.

EMERGENCY DEPARTMENT EVALUATION

A thorough but focused history and a careful ocular examination are the keys to ED management of the painful or red eye. The

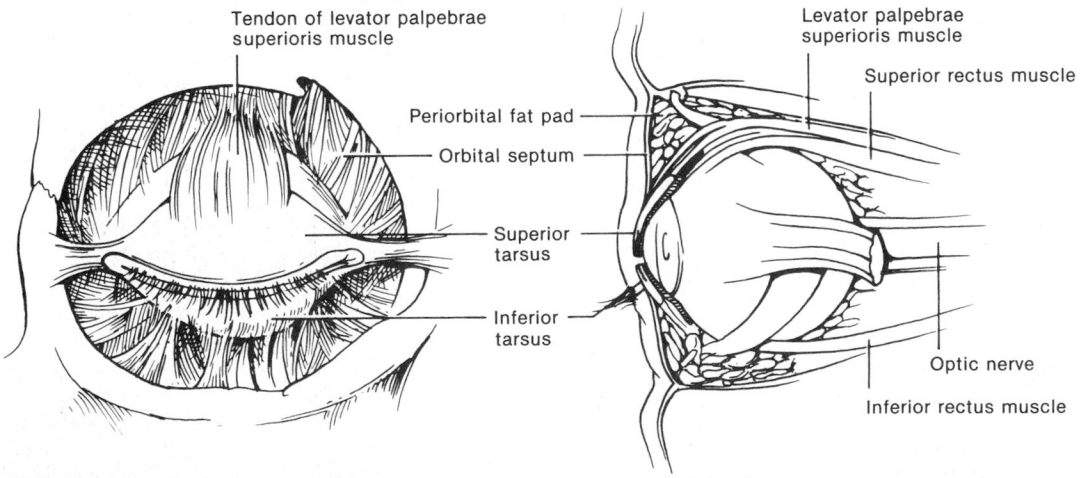

Figure 21.1.   View of orbit–orbital septum.

relevant physical exam is described in more detail in Chapters 15 and 17. History should include documentation of previous visual problems, current vision complaints, use of glasses or contact lenses, use of general or ophthalmic medications, other general medical problems, trauma, contact with other people who may have ocular infections, contact with or exposure to chemicals or toxins, symptoms of systemic illness (e.g., fever, tachycardia, etc.), history of immunocompromised state from medical conditions or medications, and the pattern of development of symptoms (one eye, both eyes, etc.). Visual acuity should always be documented, as visual acuity is the "vital sign" of the eye. This examination should take place before use of any ophthalmologic medications (e.g., topical anesthetics, mydriatics, etc.). Focused examination of the eye and periorbital areas should then be performed.

Lids

Examination of the eyelids is important to evaluate for crusting or other signs of infectious or dermatologic conditions. Any general or focal erythema or swelling of the lids should be noted. Eversion of the lids and inspection of the fornices for foreign body should also be performed.

Conjunctiva

Examination should identify chemosis or discharge. Membranes may be present in infections involving adenovirus, but may be due to *Streptococcus pneumoniae*, diphtheria, or rarely, herpetic disease. Conjunctival hemorrhage may be present and is often petechial when caused by adenovirus. Copious discharge may be present in gonococcal conjunctivitis. Hemorrhage may also be secondary to other organisms such as *Streptococcus pneumoniae*. Follicular reaction, creating a "cobblestone" appearance in the lower palpebral conjunctiva, is typically seen with adenovirus infection, but may be secondary to allergic or toxic causes (15).

Cornea

The cornea should be specifically examined for signs of ulceration. Most ulcers are centrally located, and fluoroscein staining may reveal spots or specks of increased uptake over areas of corneal epithelial damage. Larger areas of corneal epithelial injury signify ulceration and require ophthalmologic consultation for further management because the possible complications include corneal scarring and vision loss. Fluoroscein staining may also reveal the typical dendritic pattern associated with herpes simplex virus (HSV) infections. Varicella-zoster virus (VZV) may also cause corneal ulcers. Care must be taken to examine the nose for involvement with the typical zoster lesions. Herpetic eruptions involving the nose signify that the nasociliary branch of the ophthalmic nerve is involved. Corneal involvement is likely in this scenario and is referred to as Hutchinson sign. Corneal ulcers associated with blue or greenish discharge are often associated with *Pseudomonas aeruginosa* infection. Urgent (next day) ophthalmology referral is often adequate for small corneal ulcerations, but larger or more extensive ulcerations require ophthalmologic consultation in the ED. Fungal ulcers are often caused by *Candida*, *Aspergillus*, or *Fusarium* species. The incidence of fungal infections is increasing secondary to the increasing number of patients with AIDS and also because of the increasing use of immunosuppressive medications. Contact lens use also predisposes to corneal ulceration.

Anterior Chamber

Slit-lamp examination for evaluation of the anterior chamber is important to evaluate for signs of iritis (uveitis). White blood cells ("cells and flare") visualized in the anterior chamber are the key finding with iritis. Iritis may be related to significant corneal surface infections or ulcerations. A *hypopyon*, or layering of the white blood cells in the anterior chamber may be seen, and this represents a true ocular emergency. Presence of a hypopyon requires immediate ophthalmology consultation.

Periorbital Areas and Skin

Erythema and swelling in the periorbital area may be secondary to local inflammatory causes or infection but underlying periorbital or orbital cellulites should be considered. Key points to remember when performing the physical examination of this area include:

Preseptal (periorbital) cellulitis may present with sufficient swelling to affect visual acuity and ocular motility.

1. Fever is absent in as many as 24% of all patients with periorbital and orbital infections.
2. Unilateral involvement is the rule rather than the exception for both periorbital and orbital cellulitis.

Examination should be performed with the assumption that the patient has orbital cellulitis until proven otherwise. Proptosis and painful eye movements or extraocular movement impairment are more often associated with orbital cellulitis, although subperiosteal or orbital abscesses may cause similar findings (6).

The bacterial pathogens in orbital and periorbital cellulitis are typically the same organisms causing the predisposing condition: sinusitis, upper respiratory infection, local skin infection, dental infections, or postsurgical infections. Most commonly *Staphylococcus aureus*, *Staphylococcus epidermidis*, *Streptococcus pneumoniae*, or other streptococcal species are causative agents, but many others have been implicated. *Haemophilus influenzae* type b vaccine has dramatically decreased this organism's role as a pathogen in children with periorbital or orbital cellulitis. *Streptococcus* species are now seen most commonly in children with these infections (13).

When periorbital or orbital cellulitis is considered, further diagnostic testing may be indicated. For the systemically ill patient, particularly pediatric patients, blood cultures may be useful. However, with orbital cellulitis, blood cultures are negative in two-thirds of children and 90% to 95% of adults (11). Cultures of eyelid aspirates and eye secretions are rarely helpful and are not recommended unless there is a clear source of cutaneous infection. Cultures of cerebrospinal fluid are recommended only for infants in whom meningeal signs are evident.

Computed tomography (CT) scanning of the orbit is the preferred method of imaging for orbital infections. CT scanning of the orbit is advocated in all children in whom orbital cellulitis cannot be clearly ruled out by examination. Many authors recommend obtaining axial and coronal CT views to improve diagnostic yield in regard to subperiosteal or orbital abscesses that may be missed if only axial views are obtained (1,3,5). There is no advantage to using contrast-enhanced versus noncontrast CT scans. Orbital or subperiosteal abscesses are identified on CT scans in only 80% of cases and diagnosis of orbital infection remains primarily a clinical one. Ultrasound has been used in some centers for diagnosis and magnetic resonance imaging (MRI) may be a useful alternative for patients requiring surgical treatment.

TABLE 21.1. Common Parenteral Antibiotic Doses for Orbital or Periorbital Infections

Ceftazidime: 1–2 grams IV every 8 hours (30–50 mg/kg IV every 8 hours for children)
Cefuroxime: 750–1500 mg IV every 8 hours (75–100 mg/kg/day IV divided into every 8 hour dose for children)
Chloramphenicol: 50–100 mg/kg/day divided into every 6 hour dose
Clindamycin: 600–900 mg IV every 8 hours (20–40 mg/kg/day divided into every 6 hour dose for children)
Metronidazole: 500 mg IV every 8 hours (7.5 mg/kg IV every 8 hours for children)
Nafcillin: 500 mg-1 gram IV every 6 hours (150 mg/kg/day IV divided into every 6 hour dose for children)
Vancomycin: 500 mg IV every 6 hours or 1 gram IV every 12 hours (40 mg/kg/day IV divided into every 6 hour dose for children)

EMERGENCY DEPARTMENT MANAGEMENT

Examination and other testing should allow somewhat focused treatment of eye infections. If corneal or conjunctival bacterial infections are suspected, topical antibiotics are generally appropriate, although there does not appear to be definitive clinical evidence for their use in conjunctivitis (12).

Table 16-2 (from Chapter 16, Common Ophthalmic Medications) lists topical antibiotics.

Treatment of Ocular Surface and Lid Infections

Recent reviews have evaluated the antibiotic resistance of commonly used ophthalmic antibiotic preparations (4). In general, the narrow-spectrum antibiotics, bacitracin, vancomycin, and cefazolin have retained their effectiveness for gram-positive infections. The broad-spectrum antibiotics include the aminoglycosides gentamicin, tobramycin, neomycin, trimethoprim, and the sulfacetamides. The aminoglycosides continue to have excellent activity against gram-negative bacteria and good activity against *Staphylococcus* species, but are less effective for *Streptococcus* species. Trimethoprim provides excellent coverage for *Haemophilus* species but poor coverage against *Moraxella* and other gram-negative bacteria. The sulfacetamides have excellent efficacy against *Streptococcus* and *Staphylococcus aureus* conjunctival infections, but less activity in cases of *Staphylococcus aureus* keratitis.

Erythromycin has exhibited increased bacterial resistance rates, particularly with *Staphylococcus* infections. Ciprofloxacin and ofloxacin have good activity against most gram-negative organisms and *Streptococcus pneumoniae,* but increased resistance has been seen for *Pseudomonas aeruginosa* and *Staphylococcus aureus.* Failing to reach adequate concentrations of fluoroquinolones will inadequately treat infections and likely will increase bacterial resistance, thus frequent topical dosing is recommended.

Ophthalmic drops are generally well tolerated by adults, but ointment may be useful at bedtime. Ointments may be useful in children due to inherent difficulties in instilling ophthalmic drops in children. Care must be used to avoid complications caused by the topical antibiotics themselves. Neomycin is very sensitizing and can cause reactions with symptoms similar to the patients initial presenting complaints, thus confusing further management. Aminoglycosides, sulfa agents, and bacitracin may also cause similar reactions, although less often. Cross-contamination of ophthalmologic medications also occurs frequently during patients' use of these medications, and highlights the importance of appropriate hand-washing practices for the patient and for health care personnel. This should decrease the possibility of contracting or spreading the infectious agent.

Patients with herpetic corneal lesions may be treated with both a topical antiviral agent such as Trifluridine (Viroptic 1%) and an oral antiviral (acyclovir, famciclovir, valacyclovir) with ophthalmologic consultation and follow up. Gonococcal conjunctivitis should be treated with IM Ceftriaxone. If the infection involves the cornea or deep structures, ophthalmologic consultation and admission are recommended.

Some infections of the corneal surface may be complicated by iritis, and may require treatment with cycloplegics for symptomatic relief. Steroid medications may also be indicated for patients with iritis, but use of these medications is generally deferred to the treating ophthalmologist. *Topical steroids are usually not prescribed by emergency physicians without consultation with an ophthalmologist.*

Initial treatment of uncomplicated blepharitis and hordeolum usually involves use of warm compresses several times daily. Typically, this is the only treatment required for hordeolum, although topical antibiotics may be indicated if there are signs of infection spreading from the area involving the hordeolum, and systemic antibiotics may be needed if there is evidence of a more significant infection.

The key to treatment of blepharitis is an adequate regimen of cleansing the eyelid margins. Topical combination preparations containing an antibiotic and a steroid (e.g., sulfacetamide and prednisolone) may also be useful, but only for a short duration of treatment. Conservative management predominates in the early treatment of chalazion, but surgical excision by an ophthalmologist may be necessary if improvement does not occur with initial treatment.

Treatment of Periorbital and Orbital Cellulitis

Oral antibiotics in the outpatient setting may be acceptable for management of periorbital cellulitis in adults if there is no evidence of orbital infection and the infection is not severe. Antibiotics should cover *Staphylococcus aureus,* group A *Steptococcus,* and Enterobacteriaceae. First generalization cephalosporins (Cephalexin) or penicillinase-resistant synthetic penicillins (Dicloxacillin) are appropriate choices for initial treatment. Treatment should generally continue for 7 to 10 days, unless the infection is suspected to be secondary to sinusitis. In these cases, treatment should continue for 2 to 3 weeks and antibiotics should be targeted at typical organisms associated with sinusitis. Next-day ophthalmology follow up should be arranged in patients for whom outpatient therapy is chosen. Also see Chapter 245 for orbital and periorbital cellulitis in children.

For orbital cellulitis and most cases of periorbital cellulitis, inpatient treatment with parenteral antibiotics is indicated. Common intravenous antibiotic doses are listed in Table 21.1. Combination therapy with beta-lactamase resistant penicillin such as nafcillin, and second or third generation cephalosporin (Cefuroxime, Cefotaxime, Ceftriaxone, Ceftazidime) is recommended. Ticarcillin/clavulanate (Timentin) and ampicillin/sulbactam (Unasyn) are also reasonable choices. For patients with penicillin allergy, vancomycin or clindamycin, plus chloramphenicol, is recommended, though aplastic anemia is a serious complication of chloramphenicol therapy. For infections obviously related to associated skin lesions, beta-lactamase-resistant penicillins such as nafcillin are recommended with vancomycin as an alternative in patients with penicillin allergy.

Several newer antibiotics are gaining use for ophthalmologic infections. Oritavancin is a new glycopeptide antibiotic with activity similar to that of vancomycin, and it is also active against glycopeptide-resistant bacteria, including vancomycin-resistant enterococci (VRE). This agent may be a future weapon in the battle against resistant bacteria (7). Clarithromycin and azithromycin have also been used for ophthalmologic infections, and clarithromycin has been used frequently to prevent post-operative LASIK-related Mycobacterial keratitis in combination therapy with amikacin. Newer fluoroquinolones, such as moxifloxacin and gaitifloxacin, may provide a broader spectrum of antibacterial coverage.

CRITICAL INTERVENTIONS

- Document visual acuity in all patients
- Practice strict hand washing policies to prevent the spread of ocular surface infections
- Seek ophthalmology consultation for hypopyon, endophthalmitis, significant corneal ulcers, or orbital cellulitis
- Initiate intravenous antibiotics for infections of the orbit

DISPOSITION

Role of the Consultant

Patients with signs of severe conjunctivitis and associated corneal ulcer or infiltrate, or hypopyon require immediate ophthalmologic consultation. Other cases necessitating immediate consultation include severe conjunctivitis with history, culture, or gram stain results suggesting a gonococcal source or patients with membranous conjunctivitis. Referral for early ophthalmologic consultation within 24 to 48 hours should be made for patients with conjunctivitis that does not improve within 24 to 48 hours and for patients with findings suggestive of herpetic disease. Patients with signs of true orbital infection require admission for intravenous antibiotics and also urgent ophthalmologic consultation. Surgical exploration and drainage may be required if no improvement occurs within 24 to 48 hours, or if visual acuity worsens.

Indications for Admission

Deeper ocular infections, including endophthalmitis, severe corneal ulcers, or gonococcal conjunctivitis with corneal infiltrates, typically require hospital admission. It is uncommon for a patient with herpes simplex or herpes zoster infection to require admission. In-hospital care is primarily geared toward providing intravenous antibiotics or intravitreal injections, or for very frequent topical antibiotic administration (8).

Patients with orbital cellulitis require admission. Mild cases of periorbital cellulitis may be managed in the outpatient setting in adults if appropriate follow up within 24 hours is available. Intravenous antibiotics should be started in the emergency department when hospital admission is indicated.

Transfer Considerations

Transfer to an inpatient facility is rarely indicated in cases of ocular surface infection. Indications for transfer for deeper or more severe infections such as endophthalmitis or hypopyon parallel those for admission, and transfer should be completed if an ophthalmologist is not available at the treating emergency department's facility. Similarly, orbital infections require transfer if no ophthalmologist is available at the treating facility. In these cases, intravenous antibiotics should be initiated in the ED while transfer arrangements are being made. Advanced life support care is only required in severe infections, such as patients with associated cavernous sinus thrombosis.

COMMON PITFALLS

✔ Physical findings alone are not sufficient to clearly identify the etiology of conjunctivitis
✔ Culture of conjunctival or ocular secretions is not clinically useful for emergency physicians
✔ Failure to recognize the distinction between periorbital (preseptal) and orbital (postseptal) cellulitis
✔ Over-reliance upon tests that are of *little value* in differentiating periorbital from orbital cellulitis, such as: white blood cell count, sinus films, cultures of eyelid aspirates or eye secretions, cerebrospinal fluid cultures (in the absence of meningeal signs), and blood cultures in adults
✔ Failure to use CT scanning as the diagnostic test of choice for differentiating orbital and periorbital cellulitis and abscesses

References

1. Andrews TM, Myer CM. The role of CT in the diagnosis of subperiosteal abscesses of the orbit. *Clin Pediatr* 1992;31:1.
2. Barone SR, Aiuto LT. Periorbital and orbital cellulitis in the *Hemophilus influenzae* era. *J Pediatr Ophthalmol Strabismus* 1997;34:293.
3. Handler LC, et al. The acute orbit: differentiation of orbital cellulitis from subperiosteal abscess by CT. *Neuroradiology* 1991;33:1.
4. Kowalski, RP, et al. Infectious disease: changing antibiotic susceptibility. *Ophthalmol Clin North Am* 2003;16:1.
5. Lahgam-Brown JJ, Rhys-Williams S. CT of acute orbital infection: the importance of coronal sections. *Clin Radiol* 1989;40:5.
6. Lessner A, Stern GA. Preseptal and orbital cellulitis. *Infect Dis Clin North Am* 1992;6:4.
7. Mah, FS. New antibiotics for bacterial infections. *Ophthalmol Clin North Am* 2003;16:11.
8. Montan P. Endophthalmitis. *Curr Opin Ophthalmol* 2001;12:75.
9. Paerregaard A, Lund I. Periorbital and orbital cellulitis in children. *Ugeskr Laeger* 1995;157:6576.
10. Rieveld RP, et al. Diagnostic impact of signs and symptoms in acute infectious conjunctivitis: systemic literature search. *BMJ* 2003;327:789.
11. Sadow KB, Chamberlain JM. Blood cultures in the evaluation of children with cellulitis. *Pediatrics* 1998;101:E4.
12. Schiebel NE. Antibiotics for acute bacterial conjunctivitis (commentary on Cochrane review). *Ann Emerg Med* 2003;41:407.
13. Schwartz GR, Wright SW. Changing bacteriology of periorbital cellulitis. *Ann Emerg Med* 1996;28:617.
14. Skedros, DG, et al. Subperiosteal orbital abscess in children: diagnosis, microbiology, and management. *Laryngoscope* 1993;103(Pt 1):1.
15. Tech DL, Reynolds S. Diagnosis and management of pediatric conjunctivitis. *Pediatr Emerg Care* 2003;19:48.

CHAPTER 22
Acute Angle-Closure Glaucoma

William Bozeman

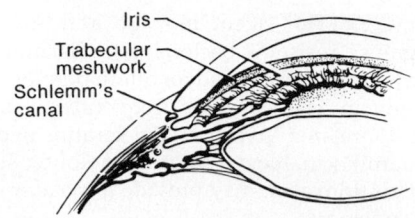

Figure 22.2.   Normal appearance of anterior chamber angle.

Glaucoma is a group of disorders characterized by an intraocular pressure (IOP) elevated to a degree sufficient to result in loss of vision. The clinical presentations and underlying pathologic mechanisms within this group of disorders are diverse. The two common classifications of primary glaucoma, angle closure glaucoma and open-angle glaucoma, occur in about 1 of 50 Americans over age 35, and represent overall the second leading cause of blindness in the United States (22).

Primary angle-closure glaucoma accounts for 6% of all patients with glaucoma, and occurs in 0.6% of the general population. Primary acute angle-closure glaucoma is less common among Blacks than among Whites; however, the chronic form is more common in Blacks, Eskimos, and Southeast Asians. Women are affected three times more often than are men.

There are three clinical types of primary angle-closure glaucoma. The chronic form is often subtle and difficult to diagnose, with a gradual visual loss over a prolonged period. The subacute, or intermittent, form is characterized by periodic episodes of mild pain, blurred vision, and halos. In contrast, the acute form of angle-closure glaucoma typically manifests dramatically with the sudden onset of unilateral ocular pain and decreased visual acuity. Without appropriate therapy, acute angle-closure glaucoma is devastating and can result in blindness within a few days. A high index of suspicion by the astute emergency physician will lead to prompt diagnosis and treatment of acute angle-closure glaucoma.

AQUEOUS HUMOR DYNAMICS AND THE ANTERIOR CHAMBER ANGLE

Aqueous humor is produced by the ciliary body. In the normal eye, the aqueous humor first fills the posterior chamber and then passes between the posterior surface of the iris and the lens to enter the anterior chamber (Fig. 22.1). The iris touches the lens only at the pupillary margin (2). Once the aqueous humor circulates within the anterior chamber, it leaves through the trabecular meshwork of the anterior chamber angle and enters Schlemm canal (Fig. 22.2). The aqueous then passes from Schlemm canal

to episcleral vessels by way of collector channels in the sclera (Fig. 22.3). The level of IOP at any time represents a balance between the rate of formation of aqueous humor and the resistance to outflow from the anterior chamber. In glaucoma, the elevated IOP is due to an obstruction to outflow from the anterior chamber, rather than to higher-than-normal rates of aqueous production.

Obstruction to outflow from the anterior chamber occurs in both open-angle and angle-closure glaucoma. The location and mechanism of the resistance to outflow distinguish these two conditions. In open-angle glaucoma, the angle is open, and the aqueous has access to the trabecular meshwork to exit the anterior chamber. Although the exact nature of the resistance to outflow is not completely understood, the obstruction to outflow is located in the tissue between the trabecular meshwork and Schlemm canal. In angle-closure glaucoma, the peripheral iris touches the trabecular meshwork and blocks the flow of aqueous to the trabecular meshwork. This apposition between the iris and the trabecular meshwork may be temporary or may become permanent if pathologic adhesions develop. These adhesions, known as peripheral anterior synechiae, can occur in eyes with narrow angles, inflammation, fibrovascular proliferation, and previous surgical intervention (Fig. 22.4).

Predisposition and Pathophysiology

Several anatomic features predispose an eye to angle-closure glaucoma. A shallow anterior chamber, which results in excessive narrowing of the entrance to the angle, can be occluded more easily than an anterior chamber of normal depth. In a shallow anterior chamber, the area of lens–iris contact is greater than normal. This lens-to-iris apposition impedes the flow of aqueous from the posterior chamber to the anterior chamber through the pupil. A pressure differential results between the posterior and anterior chambers, with a slightly higher pressure in the posterior chamber. This condition, known as relative pupillary block, produces a forward bowing of the peripheral iris and results in contact between the iris and the trabecular meshwork, thereby closing the angle (Fig. 22.5).

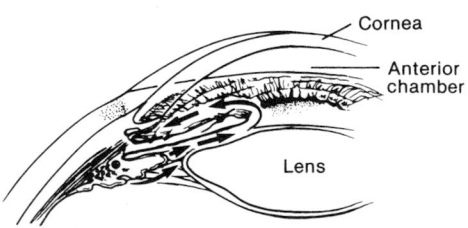

Figure 22.1.   Normal anterior chamber angle. Aqueous passes from the posterior chamber through the pupil into the anterior chamber and out through the trabecular meshwork.

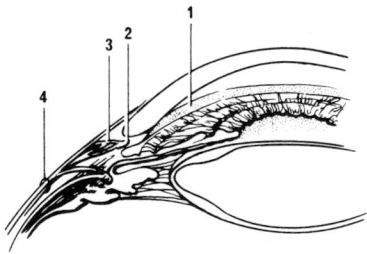

Figure 22.3.   Pathway of aqueous out of the anterior chamber is through *(1)* the trabecular meshwork, *(2)* Schlemm's canal, and by way of *(3)* collector channels to *(4)* the episcleral vessels.

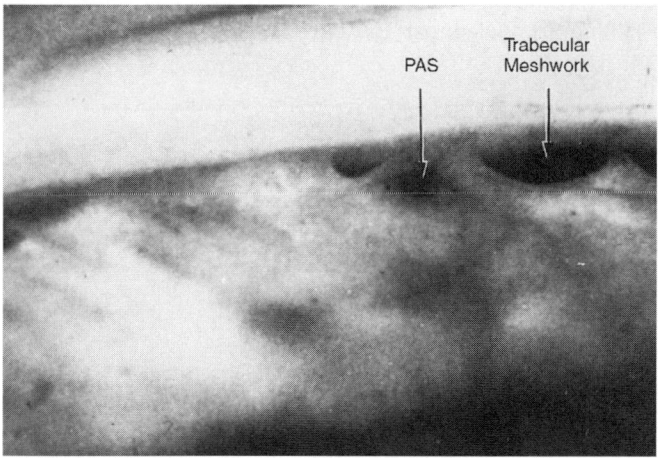

Figure 22.4. Peripheral anterior synechiae *(PAS)*. These abnormal adhesions of the iris to the trabecular meshwork are seen in angle-closure glaucoma.

Eyes prone to develop greater-than-usual degrees of pupillary block are at risk to develop angle-closure glaucoma. Hyperopic (farsighted) eyes are smaller than average (shorter anterior-to-posterior length). These eyes have greater iris-to-lens contact and an increased risk for angle-closure glaucoma. In addition, the lens size and position are major factors in the degree of relative pupillary block. For example, the development of a cataract may thicken the lens and increase the contact of the posterior surface of the iris to the lens, resulting in an increase in pupillary block. These anatomic relations—the size of the eye and the position of the lens—predispose to angle closure. The actual event that triggers an attack of acute angle closure is often identified as a pharmacologic or physiologic event that alters the balance between the aqueous humor dynamics and the pathologic anatomic relations.

In predisposed eyes, pupillary dilatation is the most significant event that can precipitate an acute angle-closure attack. During dilatation, the peripheral iris becomes more flaccid and may be pushed against the trabecular meshwork, closing the angle. There is usually sudden and complete blockage to aqueous outflow. When the pupil is mid-dilated, 5 to 7 mm, both relative pupillary block and peripheral laxness of the iris are greatest (15). If the pupil continues to dilate beyond the mid-position, the peripheral chamber angle deepens as pupillary block is reduced. Such a widely dilated pupil may be at risk to develop angle closure if it assumes the precarious mid-dilated position during constriction.

Pupillary dilatation may occur in response to pharmacologic agents or physiologic situations, such as low illumination, stress, and fatigue (9,20). Two general classifications of topical and systemic medications most often implicated in precipitating acute angle-closure glaucoma are the parasympatholytics and the sympathomimetics. Parasympatholytics, such as atropine, and sympathomimetics, such as 10% phenylephrine, as well as many over-the-counter medications with anticholinergic or sympathomimetic activity, can produce pupillary dilatation and precipitate angle closure (Table 22.1) (5,11,18).

Paradoxically topical parasympathomimetics such as pilocarpine, which produce miosis and are used to treat angle closure, have occasionally been reported to precipitate angle closure by another mechanism. In general, miotics tend to make the peripheral iris more taut and decrease the forward bowing into the peripheral angle. However, in rare cases, they have been reported to aggravate relative pupillary block by increasing the area of surface contact between the iris and the lens.

CLINICAL PRESENTATION

Symptoms

In acute angle-closure glaucoma, outflow of aqueous is suddenly and completely halted. This cessation is associated with a marked elevation of IOP, which can occur within 30 to 60 minutes (17). This acute pressure rise with distention of the ocular coats causes a sudden onset of severe pain that may be either localized to the eye, orbit, or brow, or generalized, as a severe headache. Vagal stimulation with the onset of sudden, severe pain often results in nausea and vomiting. On occasion, the gastrointestinal distress dominates the presenting clinical picture, leading to an erroneous diagnosis of a gastrointestinal illness or an acute surgical abdomen. Blurred vision or the onset of rainbow-colored halos may occur simultaneously or shortly after the onset of pain (Table 22.2).

Clinical Signs and Clinical Course

On presentation, the patient with acute angle-closure glaucoma has a unilateral red eye with congested episcleral and conjunctival blood vessels, nonreactive mid-dilated pupil, corneal edema, shallow anterior chamber, and high IOP (Fig. 22.6). Although mild anterior chamber inflammation is common, keratic precipitates (aggregates of white blood cells) on the corneal endothelium are not a typical finding.

The IOP is usually high, 60 to 90 mm Hg (less than 21 mm Hg is considered normal). However, if the attack has been prolonged, and the ciliary body becomes ischemic and aqueous production is reduced, the IOP may be low. The anterior chamber appearance is shallow. Corneal involvement varies with the duration of the attack. The cornea is usually hazy or steamy-appearing with epithelial edema. Diffuse stromal edema ensues after prolonged exposure to elevated IOP.

The untreated course of acute angle-closure glaucoma is varied. An attack damages the corneal endothelium, the lens, the retinal ganglion cell layer, and the optic nerve. The amount of damage depends more on the duration of an attack than on the degree of pressure elevation (3). The lens may develop *glaukomflecken* (tiny, white focal opacities beneath the lens capsule) as a result of lenticular ischemia. A generalized cataract may occur months to years after the attack. Optic nerve damage is often generalized (10). In some patients, the attack will continue and, if untreated, will result in pain and permanent blindness within 2 to 3 days. Visual prognosis improves with the initiation of prompt, effective treatment (6).

DIFFERENTIAL DIAGNOSIS

The differential diagnosis of the acutely painful red eye includes corneal disease such as keratitis, ulcer, erosion, foreign body,

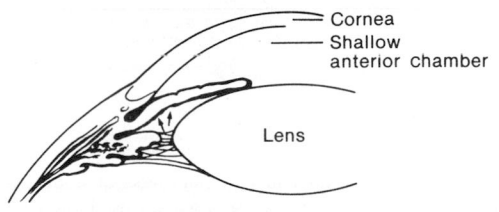

Figure 22.5. Angle closure with pupillary block. The angle is closed as the iris is pushed up against the trabecular meshwork.

TABLE 22.1. Common Pharmacologic Preparations That May Precipitate Angle-Closure Glaucoma

Nonproprietary Name	Trade Name
SYMPATHOMIMETIC ACTIVITY	
Prescription Sympathomimetics	
Epinephrine compounds	
Epinephrine bitartrate	Primatene mist, Bronkaid
Epinephrine hydrochloride	Epifrin drops
Norepinephrine	
Levarterenol	
Norepinephrine bitartrate	Levophed-bitartrate
Terbutaline	Brethaire, brethine
Amphetamine compounds	
Dextroamphetamine sulfate	Dexedrine, obetrol
Hydroxyamphetamine	Paredrine drops
Nonprescription Sympathomimetics	
Propylhexedrine	Benzedrex (nasal inhaler)
Naphazoline hydrochloride	Privine (nasal inhaler)
Tetrahydrozoline hydrochloride	Visine drops
	Tyzine (nasal inhaler)
Oxymetazoline hydrochloride	Afrin
Pseudoephedrine hydrochloride	Actifed, sudafed, afrinol
Monoamine Oxidase Inhibitors	
Tranylcypromine sulfate	Parnate
Phenelzine sulfate	Nardil
Isocarboxazid	Marplan
ANTICHOLINERGIC ACTIVITY	
Mydriatic and Cycloplegic Agents	
Atropine sulfate	
Scopolamine hydrobromide	
Homatropine hydrobromide	
Cyclopentolate hydrochloride	
Tropicamide	
Antispasmodics	
Dicyclomine hydrochloride	Bentyl
Oxyphencyclimine HCl	Daricon
Antipsychotics	
Chlorpromazine hydrochloride	Thorazine
Thioridazine hydrochloride	Mellaril
Trifluoperazine hydrochloride	Stelazine
Haloperidol	Haldol
Antiemetics	
Chlorpromazine	Thorazine
Perphenazine	Trilafon
Prochlorperazine	Compazine
Promethazine	Phenergan
Antihistamines	
Diphenhydramine	Benadryl
Dimenhydrinate	Dramamine
Chlorpheniramine maleate	Chlor-trimeton, dristan
Brompheniramine maleate	Dimetane
Hydroxyzine hydrochloride	Atarax
Hydroxyzine pamoate	Vistaril
Meclizine hydrochloride	Antivert
Tricyclic Antidepressants	
Imipramine	Tofranil
Amitriptyline	Elavil, limbatrol, triavil
Doxepin	Adapin, sinequan
Nortriptyline	Pamelor
Protriptyline	Vivactil
Desipramine	Norpramin, pertofrane
Miscellaneous Agents	
Trihexyphenidyl hydrochloride	Artane
Benztropine mesylate	Cogentin
Ethopropazine hydrochloride	Parsidol

TABLE 22.2. Diagnosis of Acute Angle-Closure Glaucoma

HISTORY

Acute onset of pain
Exposure to dim illumination (i.e., movie theater)
Emotional upset or fatigue
Precipitating medications (anticholinergics, sympathomimetics)

SYMPTOMS

Pain
Blurred vision/halos around lights
Decreased vision
Nausea
Vomiting

SIGNS

Conjunctival injection
Corneal edema (light reflex irregular or steamy appearance)
Mid-dilated, nonreactive pupil
Evidence of a narrow angle (fellow eye should also appear narrow)
Anterior chamber cells—no keratic precipitates

and keratoconjunctivitis and is described in detail in Chapter 17. Causes not related to the corneal surface include acute iritis or anterior uveitis, acute angle-closure glaucoma, episcleritis, scleritis, orbital cellulitis, periorbital cellulitis, and septic cavernous sinus thrombosis. Because headache, nausea, and vomiting may be dominant symptoms in glaucoma, the differential should also include CNS and gastrointestinal disorders. Most conditions are readily distinguished by a careful history and examination. Other ophthalmic disorders that more closely mimic acute angle-closure glaucoma are glaucomatocyclitic crisis, neovascular glaucoma, glaucoma secondary to iritis or uveitis, and the lens-induced glaucoma.

Glaucomatocyclitic crisis produces recurrent attacks of visual blurring and halos. In contrast to acute angle-closure glaucoma, pain is not a prominent feature. Additionally, the anterior chamber is deep, few cells are present in the anterior chamber, and keratic precipitates are on the corneal endothelium.

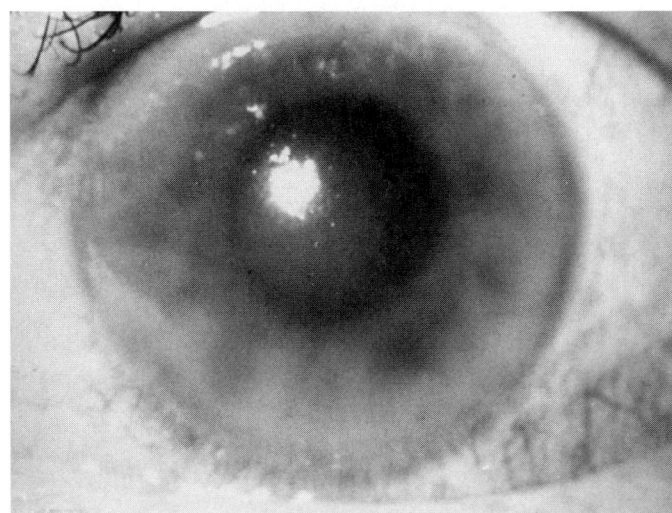

Figure 22.6. This eye demonstrates the hallmarks of acute angle-closure glaucoma: perilimbal injection, corneal edema, and a mid-dilated nonreactive pupil.

Neovascular glaucoma presents with a chief complaint of a painful red eye associated with vision loss occurring months before inflammation of the eye. It is usually associated with other disorders, such as proliferative retinopathy of diabetes mellitus and retinal vascular occlusion. The underlying stimulus for neovascularization is hypoxia. The neovascularization of the iris, known as rubeosis iridis, can be seen on slit-lamp exam as randomly oriented vessels on the surface of the iris (23). These vessels typically progress to the anterior chamber angle, where a fibrovascular membrane covers the trabecular meshwork, preventing outflow of aqueous (21). If the neovascularization is progressive, a secondary form of angle closure develops as the fibrovascular membrane contracts, pulling the iris to the trabecular meshwork, which leads to the development of peripheral anterior synechiae. To distinguish neovascular glaucoma from acute angle-closure glaucoma, a history of diabetes mellitus or previous severe loss of vision before the acute attack is helpful. Also, the pupil is often miotic, and tufts of neovascular vessels may be evident.

Acute iritis with secondary glaucoma presents with moderate pain, photophobia, and blurred vision. The onset is gradual, in contrast to acute angle-closure glaucoma. Clinical findings may mimic angle closure, with conjunctival perilimbal injection (the conjunctiva adjacent to the cornea) and corneal edema. Distinguishing characteristics include miotic pupil, keratic precipitates, and a normal anterior chamber depth (Fig. 22.7).

Phacolytic glaucoma presents with the acute onset of a unilateral painful red eye. Examination reveals a high IOP and conjunctival injection. In contrast to acute angle-closure glaucoma, the anterior chamber depth appears normal, there is moderate-to-marked anterior chamber cell reaction, keratic precipitates are present, and a mature or hypermature (liquid cortex) cataract can be seen (Fig. 22.8). The cause of phacolytic glaucoma is the release of soluble lens protein into the aqueous, which leads to elevated IOP. With the availability of modern cataract surgery, phacolytic glaucoma is a rare cause of acutely elevated IOP.

Lens particle glaucoma is associated with either spontaneous or traumatic disruption of the lens capsule. The presentation in the setting of spontaneous disruption is the acute onset of a unilateral painful red eye. In the case of trauma, either surgical or

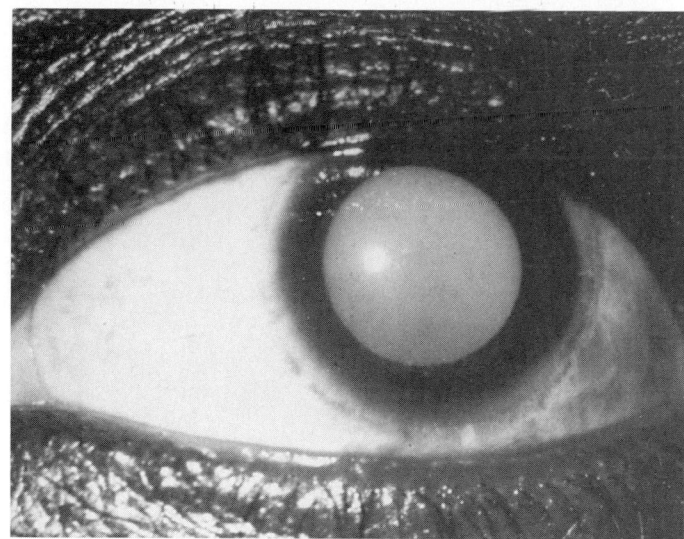

Figure 22.8.   Phacolytic glaucoma. This eye demonstrates the milky-white lens of a hypermature cataract.

accidental, the onset is soon after the inciting event. The IOP is elevated, the conjunctiva injected. In contrast to angle-closure glaucoma, the anterior chamber is of normal depth, the pupil is often miotic, and lens cortical material is present in the anterior chamber (Fig. 22.9). The particulate lens material reduces outflow in the trabecular meshwork, with resultant increased IOP (4).

Intumescent lens associated with the development of an advanced cataract, and is characterized by a gradual, painless loss of vision in the involved eye over many years. The patient presents to an emergency department when secondary angle closure occurs as the cataract changes configuration by absorbing water and swelling. In contrast to acute angle-closure glaucoma, the intumescent (swollen, mature) lens is readily evident (Fig. 22.10) (16). This is a rare cause of secondary angle closure.

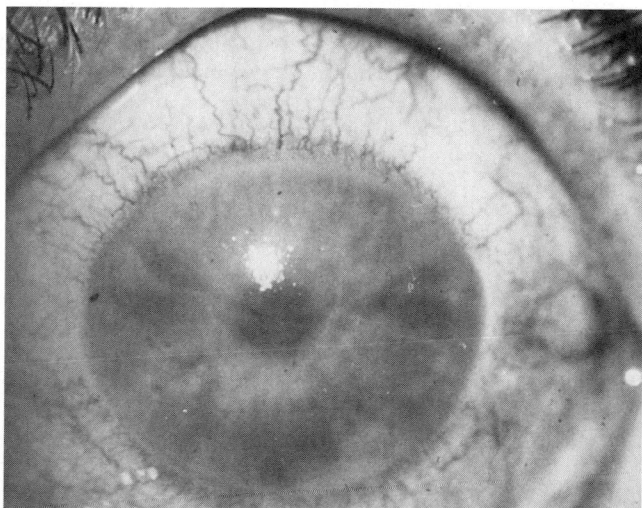

Figure 22.7.   Acute iritis. This eye demonstrates the perilimbal injection and corneal edema that is common to both acute iritis and acute angle-closure glaucoma. The constricted miotic pupil seen here is characteristic of acute iritis.

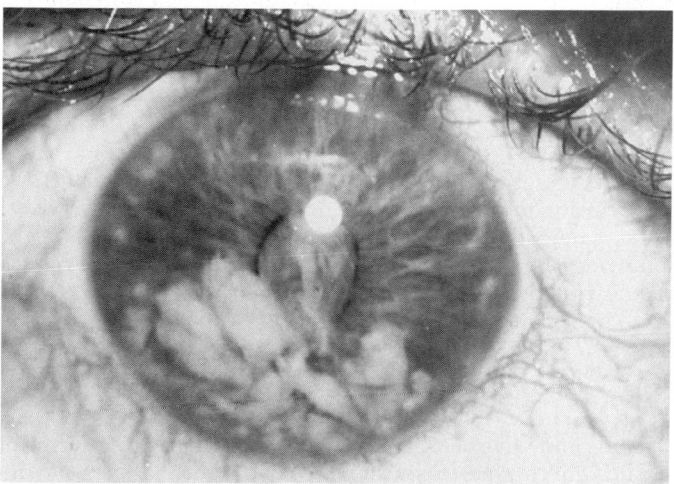

Figure 22.9.   Lens particle glaucoma. The fluffy white material seen here in the anterior chamber is lens cortex. This eye had a spontaneous rupture of the lens capsule in a mature cataract.

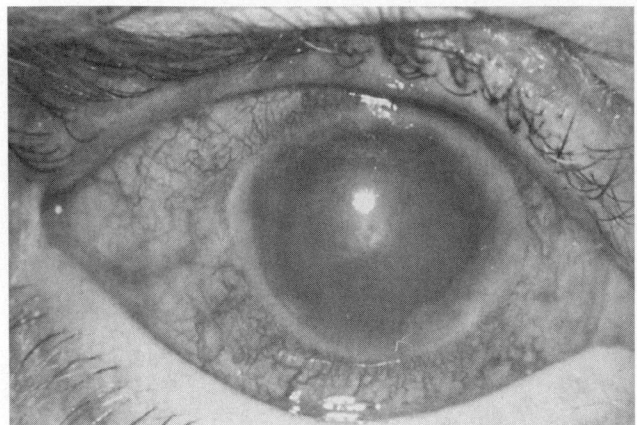

Figure 22.10. Intumescent lens. The large opaque cataract is associated with acute-onset glaucoma.

EMERGENCY DEPARTMENT EVALUATION

History

A careful history is an essential part of the emergency department evaluation of acute angle-closure glaucoma, to establish the diagnosis and plan appropriate therapy. Question the patient about the following factors:

Onset of symptoms (sudden, gradual, subsequent to accidental or surgical trauma)
Previous symptoms similar to those of the current complaint (brief episodes of pain, blurred vision, and halos around lights)
Visual acuity in the affected eye as well as in the other eye
Pain in or around the eye
Discharge or secretions from the eye (tearing is common with ocular pain; however, a purulent discharge may indicate an infectious cause)
Medical history of asthma or congestive heart failure and history of drug allergies (particularly sulfa drugs).

Physical Examination

The detailed ocular exam is described in Chapter 15. Following are aspects of the ocular exam that deserve special emphasis in relation to acute angle closure glaucoma.

Visual Acuity

Visual acuity is probably one of the most important evaluations done during the ocular examination. If a distance or near visual acuity cannot be recorded due to inability to read the chart, the following should be recorded, including the distance at which each is tested: finger counting, hand motions, light perception, or no light perception.

Lids and Adnexa

The lids and adnexa are first observed. Edema and erythema of the lids are common to most of the conditions that present with a painful red eye. Decreased visual acuity associated with lid edema and erythema should prompt the physician to consider acute angle-closure glaucoma, neovascular glaucoma, and lens-induced glaucoma.

Conjunctiva

The conjunctiva is often nonspecifically injected; however, observation of the pattern of injection may be of some assistance. Perilimbal injection may indicate acute iritis or angle closure. Segmental injection characterizes episcleritis, and diffuse injection more commonly typifies keratoconjunctivitis. The presence of purulent discharge should alert the physician to a possible infectious cause.

Cornea

A slit-lamp examination, using a small quantity of fluorescein, helps identify corneal disease such as keratitis, ulcer, erosion, or foreign body as a possible cause of the painful red eye. Corneal edema, either epithelial (hazy) or diffuse stromal (steamy), should be noted. The rapid elevation of IOP is often associated with corneal decompensation.

Anterior Chamber

Assessment of the anterior chamber depth is essential in the evaluation of the painful red eye and the diagnosis of acute angle-closure glaucoma. An accurate determination can be done with gonioscopy, a technique performed by an ophthalmologist. In the emergency department, an adequate estimation of the anterior chamber depth can be accomplished with an oblique flashlight and a slit-lamp examination.

Oblique Flashlight Test. To perform the oblique flashlight test (Fig. 22.11), a penlight is directed to the temporal side of each eye, perpendicular to the corneal limbus. The examiner shines the light across the eye from the temporal side. In an eye with a normal-depth anterior chamber, the entire iris is illuminated. In an eye with a narrow angle or shallow anterior chamber depth, a shadow is cast on the nasal side of the iris (22).

Slit-Lamp Examination. The central and peripheral anterior chamber depth can be estimated during the slit-lamp examination. Van Herick and associates developed a technique for making this estimate. A narrow slit beam of light is directed obliquely to allow an estimate of corneal thickness and of the distance between the corneal beam to the beam on the surface of the iris. The anterior chamber depth is measured and expressed in terms of corneal thickness (Fig. 22.12). When the depth is less than one-fourth of the corneal thickness, the anterior chamber angle is extremely narrow. If the angle is closed, the iris will be seen in contact with the cornea. Both the affected and the nonaffected eye are evaluated. The fellow eye in acute angle-closure glaucoma may vary slightly but will have similar anatomic relations and appear narrow. If a unilateral shallow chamber is detected, the diagnosis of acute angle-closure glaucoma is doubtful.

Pupils

The size and shape of the pupil and its reaction to light are recorded for each eye. Unequal pupil size (anisocoria) is noted, specifically with respect to the involved, red, painful eye. A mid-dilated nonreactive pupil is characteristic of acute angle-closure glaucoma. In contrast, the pupil in acute iritis is miotic and poorly reactive (see Fig. 22.7).

Lens

A mature (opaque) or hypermature (liquid cortex) lens may be associated with lens-induced glaucoma (see Figs. 22.8 to 22.10). Phacodonesis, movement of the lens, indicates a dislocated or subluxed lens. This may occur secondary to trauma (7), or it may

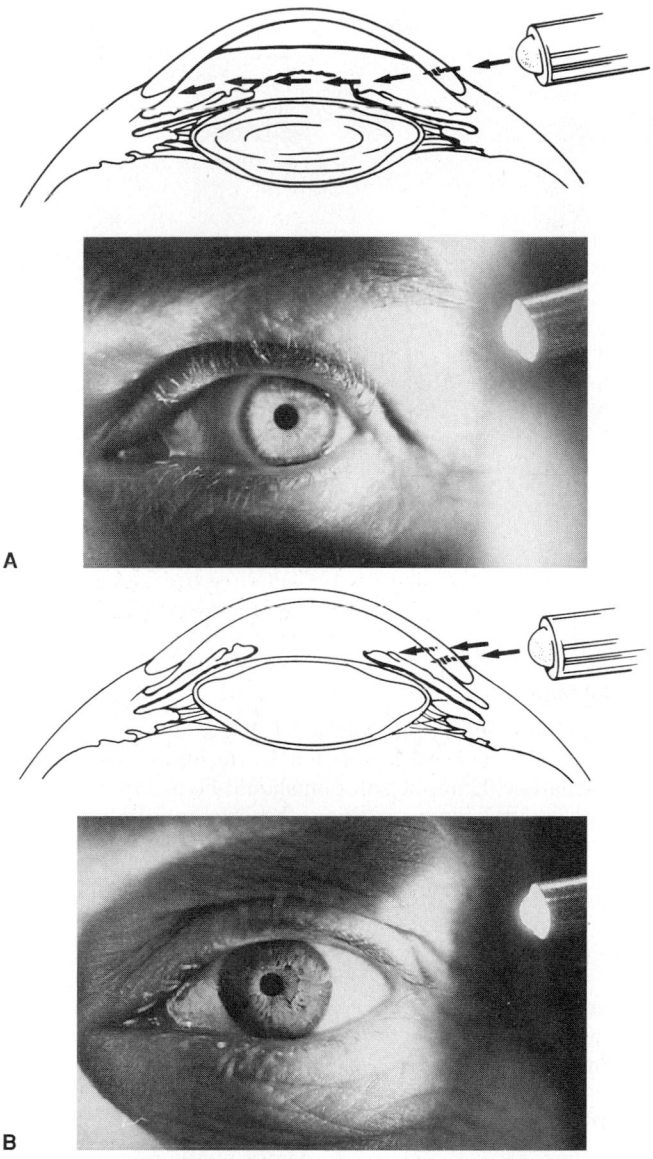

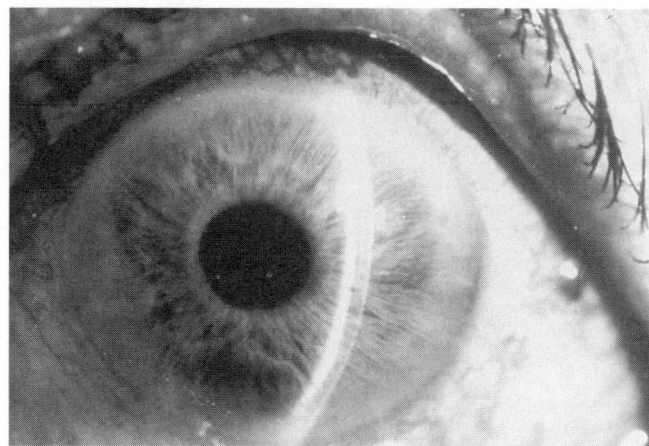

Figure 22.12. Shallow anterior chamber estimation using narrow slit beam on slit-lamp examination.

Figure 22.11. Flashlight test for wide and narrow angles. **(A)** Wide angle: Entire iris is illuminated. **(B)** Narrow angle: Only temporal half of iris is illuminated. (Photo courtesy of D.R. Anderson, M.D.)

be part of a systemic syndrome, most notably Marfan syndrome. The dislocated lens may increase pupillary block and result in a secondary angle-closure glaucoma.

Intraocular Pressure

The range of IOP considered normal is from about 10 to 21 mm Hg (mean, 16 ± 2.5 mm Hg) (20). Three commonly used tonometers available in the emergency department are the air-puff noncontact tonometer, the Schiøtz tonometer, the applanation tonometer, and the Tonopen.

Air-Puff Noncontact Tonometer. The air-puff tonometer measures the IOP without the application of topical anesthesia and without contact between the instrument and the eye. A 3-millisecond puff of air is blown against the cornea. The pressure is calculated by the amount of corneal flattening. This tonometer is not as accurate as the Schiøtz or applanation tonometer, but it has the advantage of use without contact with the eye.

Schiøtz Tonometry. Schiøtz, or indentation, tonometry determines IOP by measuring the indentation of the cornea produced by a known weight. Each instrument is accompanied by a graph that expresses the scale readings in millimeters of mercury. To perform Schiøtz tonometry, the patient is placed in a supine position and a drop of a local anesthetic, such as proparacaine hydrochloride or tetracaine hydrochloride, is instilled. The patient is asked to look upward and fix on some object in the distance. While separating the lids, the instrument is gently placed in a vertical position directly over the cornea, and the plunger is allowed to rest completely on the eye. With the instrument held steady, the pointer will stay fixed at a value on the scale. Readings between 3 and 6 with a 5.5-g weight will be accurate. Readings below 3 are inaccurate, and a 7.5-g weight should be added. Falsely elevated IOPs are associated with excessive lid squeezing or inadvertent pressure on the globe. Falsely low IOPs are associated with high myopia (nearsightedness), thyroid disease, and previous ocular surgery.

Applanation Tonometry. In applanation tonometry, the cornea is flattened, and the IOP determined by measuring the applanating force and the area flattened. To perform standard applanation tonometry, a local anesthetic and fluorescein are instilled into the lower cul-de-sac. Correctly positioned at the slit lamp, with the chin in the chin rest and the forehead firmly against the headband, the patient is asked to look straight ahead. Using the cobalt blue light, the examiner gently contacts the anterior corneal surface with the tip of the Goldmann tonometer (Fig. 22.13). On contact, two fluorescein semicircles are seen. The semicircles are aligned by turning the calibrated dial until the inner borders of each semicircle are aligned. This reading is multiplied by 10 and is the measurement of the IOP in millimeters of mercury.

Tonopen. A hand held electronic applanation tonometer, the Tonopen XL, is frequently used in emergency departments. After initial calibration, the tip of the tonopen is repeatedly tapped on the anesthetized cornea. The instrument calculates and displays the average and standard deviation of several measurements on a small liquid crystal display screen.

Laboratory Studies

Due to vagal stimulation with the sudden increase in IOP, patients with acute angle-closure glaucoma frequently present with nausea and vomiting. The duration and severity of these symptoms may necessitate obtaining appropriate studies to assess metabolic imbalance and dehydration. In elderly patients on

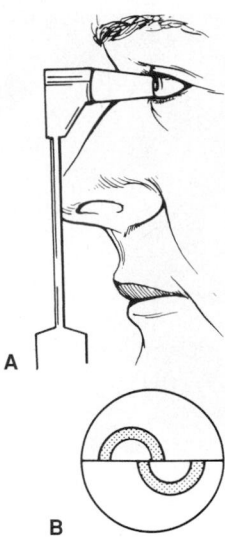

Figure 22.13.   Applanation tonometry. **(A)** The tonometer tip should just contact the patient's cornea. **(B)** Viewed through the slit lamp are two fluorescent semicircles aligned edge to edge.

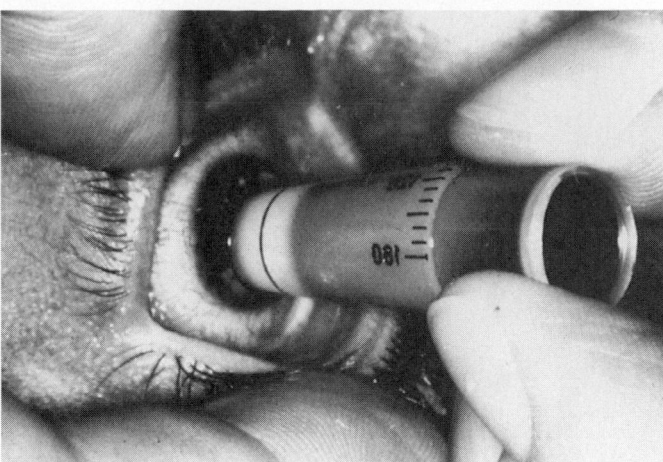

Figure 22.14.   Corneal indentation with applanation prism. (From Anderson DR. Corneal indentation to relieve acute angle-closure glaucoma. *Am J Ophthalmol* 1979;88:1091, with permission.)

multiple medications, including diuretics, serum electrolyte levels should be measured before initiating medical treatment with carbonic anhydrase inhibitors or hyperosmotics.

EMERGENCY DEPARTMENT MANAGEMENT

Acute angle-closure glaucoma is an ophthalmic emergency. Once the diagnosis has been established in the emergency department, the immediate goal is twofold: to obtain appropriate consultation with an ophthalmologist and to decrease the elevated IOP. If examination by an ophthalmologist is imminent, therapy may be delayed. However, if prompt consultation is unavailable, therapy to decrease IOP should be immediately initiated.

Therapy to reduce IOP is directed at decreasing aqueous production, increasing aqueous outflow, and reducing vitreous volume by dehydrating agents. A combination of topical agents and systemic medications directed toward these three goals is often effective in reducing IOP. The therapeutic options used in the medical management of acute angle-closure glaucoma are discussed next. The exact therapy used should be tailored to each patient's medical status.

Corneal Indentation

When IOP is 50 mm Hg or greater, topical miotics are ineffective due to ischemia of the iris constrictors. In this situation, a quick maneuver to lower IOP is corneal indentation (1). As the cornea is indented, the aqueous is displaced and forced into the peripheral anterior chamber, which temporarily opens the angle. This results in an immediate decrease in IOP and, on occasion, can abort an attack. If, however, the attack is long-standing, it is unlikely that the aqueous can be forced through regions of iris to the trabecular meshwork adhesions (peripheral anterior synechiae). Corneal indentation is rapid and may abort an attack without additional medical intervention, but the corneal epithelium may be disrupted, which can complicate further therapy. Any smooth instrument can be used, but a Goldmann applanation prism is readily available, easily held, and frequently used. After application of a topical anesthetic, the prism is held with the fingers to the patient's cornea and firm pressure applied for about 30 seconds (Fig. 22.14).

Topical Therapy

Timolol Maleate

Timolol maleate (Timoptic solution, 0.25% and 0.5%) is a nonselective beta-blocker that lowers IOP by decreasing aqueous humor formation. Timoptic solution should be used with caution in patients with known conditions that are contraindications for the use of systemic beta-blockers, such as asthma, heart block, and heart failure, since systemic absorption may occur. Side effects include decreased pulse rate, bronchial spasm, and altered mental state. The recommended dosage for treating acute angle-closure glaucoma is:

> Timolol 0.5% solution, one or two drops at 10- to 15-minute intervals initially for three doses, and then one drop every 12 hours.

Pilocarpine Hydrochloride 1% and 2%

Pilocarpine is a direct-acting parasympathomimetic miotic agent. The mechanism of action in acute angle-closure glaucoma is mechanical. With miosis, the peripheral iris is pulled taut and away from the trabecular meshwork. Ocular side effects include a brow ache and diminished night vision. As noted previously, in rare cases pilocarpine use may precipitate or worsen an acute angle closure glaucoma attack by increasing the area of surface contact between the iris and the pupil, aggravating a relative pupillary block. Systemic side effects, such as sweating, tremors, bradycardia, and hypotension, are uncommon, but have been observed as a result of too frequent administration of pilocarpine. The recommended dosage is:

> Pilocarpine 2%, one drop every 30 minutes until the pupil constricts, and then one drop every 6 hours.

Miotics cause congestion of the iris stroma and aggravate inflammation; for this reason, concentrations higher than 2% are seldom used in an acute attack. Pilocarpine is not recommended if the diagnosis of acute angle-closure is unclear, or if the patient presents with a unilateral shallow anterior chamber.

Prednisolone Acetate

Topical corticosteroids reduce inflammation. The complications of long-term steroid use are not seen in the acute situation. The recommended dosage is:

Prednisolone acetate 1% (PredForte), one drop every 30 to 60 minutes until surgical treatment is completed.

Apraclonidine

Apraclonidine is a topical alpha-2 agonist used in chronic glaucoma that lowers IOP by reduction of aqueous humor production, and effects are additive to those of topical beta-blockers (9). Success in acute angle-closure glaucoma treatment has also been reported, and its use should be considered (8). The recommended dosage is:

Apraclonidine 0.5% solution, two drops (single administration).

Topical Prostaglandins

Topical prostaglandin drops are thought to decrease pressure by increasing outflow.

Latanoprost (Xalatan) 0.005% solution.

Systemic Therapy

Acetazolamide

Acetazolamide is a carbonic anhydrase inhibitor that inhibits aqueous humor formation. Similar to sulfonamides, it must be given with caution in patients who have a history of allergy to sulfa drugs. Metabolic and, possibly, respiratory acidosis can occur with the use of carbonic anhydrase inhibitors; this medication should be avoided in patients with significant respiratory disease. Hypokalemia can be seen with acute therapy. The recommended dosage for treating acute angle-closure glaucoma is:

Acetazolamide (Diamox), 500 mg i.v. every 12 hours; or if a patient can tolerate oral administration, acetazolamide (250-mg tablets), 500 mg PO every 6 hours.

Mannitol

Mannitol is a hyperosmotic agent that lowers IOP by increasing the serum osmolality. This creates a gradient between the blood and the vitreous and draws water from the vitreous cavity. Side effects include headache, confusion, and dehydration. It can aggravate or precipitate congestive heart failure and should be used cautiously in patients at risk for this problem. Mannitol lowers IOP by increasing the blood osmolality. The recommended dosage for treating acute angle-closure glaucoma is:

Mannitol 20%, 1 to 2 g/kg i.v. over 30 to 60 minutes.

Glycerin and Isosorbide

These hyperosmotic agents can be administered by mouth in patients able to tolerate oral medications. Glycerin should be avoided in diabetic patients because it can produce hyperglycemia and ketosis. Isosorbide is not metabolized to sugar and is a useful oral hyperosmotic in diabetics. The recommended dosage is:

Glycerin 75% (Glyrol), 1.0 to 1.5 g/kg PO (on ice with juice), or Isosorbide 45% (Ismotic), 1.5 g/kg PO.

The hyperosmotic agents (mannitol, glycerin, and isosorbide) should not be used simultaneously.

Surgical Therapy

The definitive treatment of angle-closure glaucoma is release of pupillary block by an iridectomy. Laser iridectomies have now replaced incisional iridectomies (13). Laser surgery is usually completed after the resolution of acute angle-closure glaucoma. At times it is necessary to perform an iridectomy emergently in an eye that is medically unresponsive (12). These cases generally involve patients who have delayed medical attention longer than 24 hours.

CRITICAL INTERVENTIONS

- Measure the visual acuity in all patients with a painful, red eye
- Consider the possibility of glaucoma and measure the intraocular pressure
- Consult an ophthalmologist in all cases of acute angle-closure glaucoma, and initiate therapy to reduce the intraocular pressure

DISPOSITION

Role of the Consultant

Acute angle-closure glaucoma is an ophthalmic emergency. Consultation with an ophthalmologist should occur immediately.

Indications for Admission

Intractable Pain, Nausea, and Vomiting

Due to vagal stimulation as a consequence of the rapid and severe elevation of IOP, patients who present with acute angle-closure glaucoma are often systemically ill and require admission. Analgesic and antiemetic agents may be given if the patient is having severe pain, nausea, or vomiting.

Intensive Medical Therapy and Monitoring

Parenteral administration of medications should be done in the hospital so that the patient can be closely observed for possible untoward reactions. IOP should be monitored every 2 to 3 hours to monitor and assess response to medical therapy. If the eye is responding and IOP is decreasing, then therapy should be continued. If the eye is not responding well to medical maneuvers and the IOP remains elevated, laser surgery (either iridectomy or iridoplasty) should be done within 2 to 4 hours (17).

Transfer Considerations

If the initial receiving hospital cannot obtain an ophthalmology consult, therapy should be initiated and the patient transferred. This should be conducted expeditiously, because delay in treatment is detrimental to the visual prognosis (6).

COMMON PITFALLS

✔ Failure to consider the diagnosis and check intraocular pressures

✔ Failure to obtain specialty consultation

Any patient with a painful red eye and decreased vision is considered an ophthalmic emergency and requires prompt consultation with an ophthalmologist.

Acknowledgments

The author gratefully acknowledges the contribution of Alana L. Grajewski and Richard K. Parrish II who authored previous versions of this chapter.

References

1. Anderson DR. Corneal indentation to relieve acute angle-closure glaucoma. *Am J Ophthalmol* 1979;88:1091.

2. Chandler PA, Grant WM. *Glaucoma,* 2nd ed. Philadelphia: Lea & Febiger, 1979:132.

3. David R, Tessler Z, Yassar T. Long-term outcome of primary acute angle-closure glaucoma. *Br J Ophthalmol* 1985;69:261.

4. Epstein DL, Jedziniak JA, Grant WM. Obstruction of aqueous outflow by lens particles and by heavy-molecular-weight soluble lens proteins. *Invest Ophthalmol Vis Sci* 1978;17:272.

5. Hall SK. Acute angle-closure glaucoma as a complication of combined beta-agonist and ipratropium bromide therapy in the emergency department. *Ann Emerg Med* 1994;23:884.

6. Hillman JS. Acute closed-angle glaucoma: an investigation into the effect of delay in treatment. *Br J Ophthalmol* 1979;63:817.

7. Jarrett WH. Dislocation of the lens: a study of 166 hospitalized cases. *Arch Ophthalmol* 1967;78:289.

8. Krawitz PL, Podis SM. Use of apraclonidine in the treatment of acute angle closure glaucoma. *Arch Ophthalmol* 1990;108:1208.

9. Morrison JC, Robin AL. Adjunctive glaucoma therapy: a comparison of apraclonidine to dipivefrin when added to timolol maleate. *Ophthalmology* 1989;96:3.

10. Murphy MB, Spaeth GL. Iridectomy and primary angle-closure glaucoma. *Arch Ophthalmol Vis Sci* 1974;91:114.

11. Reuser T, Flanagan DW, Borland C, Bannerjee DK. Acute angle-closure glaucoma occurring after nebulized bronchodilator treatment with ipratropium bromide and salbutamol. *J R Soc Med* 1992;85:499.

12. Rich R. Argon laser treatment for medically unresponsive attacks of angle-closure glaucoma. *Am J Ophthalmol* 1982;94:197.

13. Rivera AH, Brown RH, Anderson DR. Laser iridotomy vs. surgical iridectomy: have the indications changed? *Arch Ophthalmol Vis Sci* 1985;103:1350.

14. Roden DR. The prevalence and cost of glaucoma. In: *Glaucoma detection and treatment: proceedings of the First National Glaucoma Conference.* Sponsored by the National Society to Prevent Blindness, Tarpon Springs, FL, 1980: 20.

15. Rutkowski PC, Thompson HS. Mydriasis and increased intraocular pressure. *Arch Ophthalmol* 1972;87:21.

16. Shields MB. Disorders of the lens. In: *A study guide to glaucoma.* Baltimore: Williams & Wilkins, 1982:271.

17. Simmons JR, Belcher CD III, Dallow RL. Primary angle-closure glaucoma. In: Duane TD, Jaeger EA, eds. *Clinical ophthalmology,* 3rd ed. New York: Harper & Row, 1987:1.

18. Singh J, O'Brien C, Wright M. Nebulized bronchodilator therapy causes acute angle-closure glaucoma in predisposed individuals [Letter]. *Respir Med* 1993;87:559.

19. Spaeth GL. The normal development of the human anterior chamber angle: a new system of descriptive grading. *Trans Ophthalmol Soc UK* 1971;91: 709.

20. Stamper RL, Bellows AR. Angle-closure glaucoma. In: Stamper RL, Bellows AR, eds. *Basic and clinical science course of the American Academy of Ophthalmology.* Section 8:72. San Francisco: American Academy of Ophthalmology, 1986–1987.

21. Tasman W, Margargal LE, Augsburger JJ. Effects of argon laser photocoagulation on rubeosis iridis and angle neovascularization. *Ophthalmology* 1980;87:400.

22. Vargas E, Drance SM. Anterior chamber depth in angle-closure glaucoma. Clinical methods of depth determination in people with and without the disease. *Arch Ophthalmol Vis Sci* 1973;90:438.

23. Wand M, Dueker DK, Avello LM, et al. Effects of panretinal photocoagulation on rubeosis iridis, angle neovascularization, and neovascular glaucoma. *Am J Ophthalmol* 1978;86:332.

24. Zimmerman TJ, Wheeler TM. Miotics: side effects and ways to avoid them. *Ophthalmology* 1982;89:76–80.

ENT and Dental Emergencies

CHAPTER 23
Dental Emergencies

Gregory T. Guldner

Dental emergencies prompt almost 3 million emergency department (ED) visits nationally, accounting for 0.7% of all ED patients (7). Factors such as a lack of dental insurance, insufficient funds, lack of a primary care dentist, and few "off-hours" dental clinics have contributed to an increasing number of patients with dental-related complaints presenting to emergency physicians (3,5,12). Despite the common nature of dental-related complaints, many physicians receive little training on dental emergencies (9).

This chapter addresses the common nontraumatic dental emergencies. Dental trauma is addressed in Chapter 175, and odontogenic infections of the face are covered in Chapter 24.

DENTAL ANATOMY

Human teeth are composed of three layers. The outermost layer, enamel, is an extremely hard protective cover that contains no nerve fibers. Enamel covers the visible part, or crown of the tooth. The corresponding outer layer in the portion of the tooth embedded in the gum (the root), is known as cementum, and is much softer than enamel. Under the enamel and cementum is dentin, and at the center of the tooth is the pulp chamber through which the nerves and blood supply connect to the alveolar bone. The tooth sits in a socket with relatively long apices extending into the bone. It is anchored to the bone by the periodontal ligament.

The first set of teeth, known as primary or deciduous dentition, should be completely erupted by 3 years of age. This set consists of 10 maxillary and 10 mandibular teeth. The permanent teeth begin erupting at around 5 years of age. This set consists of 32 teeth divided equally into four quadrants (right upper, right lower, left upper, left lower). In each quadrant there is a central incisor, a lateral incisor, a canine, two premolars, and three molars. The third molar is also called the "wisdom tooth" and may not be visible if it failed to erupt or has been therapeutically removed. To identify a specific tooth, several numbering systems have developed. The most commonly used system numbers the permanent teeth consecutively beginning with the upper right third molar (tooth 1), to the upper left third molar (tooth 16), then down to the lower left third molar (tooth 17), and across to the lower right third molar (tooth 32). However, other numbering systems exist and some patients will have teeth missing, which may make numbering difficult. Generally, physicians should simply describe the tooth involved – for example, the left upper second premolar.

The biting area of a tooth is the occlusal surface for molars or incisal surface for the incisors. In the direction of the occlusal or incisal surface is coronal and in the direction of the root is apical. The medial or mesial aspect faces toward the midline of the jaw, while the distal surface faces the ramus of the mandible. The portion of the tooth facing the tongue or palate is the lingual or palatal surface. That portion facing away from the tongue is the labial or buccal surface. Finally, the portion of the tooth in contact with an adjacent tooth is the interproximal surface.

THE DENTAL EXAMINATION

Patients with dental complaints should first be examined for possible nondental causes of their symptoms. Dental pain can result from sinus infections, temporomandibular joint dysfunction, otitis media, migraine headaches, neuritis, or myocardial ischemia. An examination of the external facial structures and neck can detect swelling, cellulitis, or odontogenic fistulae. Once these conditions are excluded the intraoral examination can begin. This is usually best accomplished with the patient in a semi-reclined position. Look first for trismus (restricted opening of the mouth) and for swelling of the tongue or lips. Using an adequate light source, a tongue depressor, and gloved hands examine the mouth for asymmetry, swelling, or signs of cellulitis. Determine that the uvula is midline and not shifted due to abscess formation. Confirm that the tongue is not elevated and that the floor of the mouth is not tender or indurated (signs of Ludwig angina). Examine the teeth looking for signs of caries (cavities). Pay particular attention to the junction of the tooth and the socket, where foreign bodies can be lodged. The tissue adjacent to the tooth along the alveolar bone should be examined carefully, as odontogenic abscesses typically form in this area. The area overlying the molars should be examined for evidence of erupting teeth (usually the "wisdom tooth"). Each tooth can be gently percussed, preferably with the end of a dental mirror, though a tongue depressor will suffice. The exam of the teeth should focus on determining the presence of cellulitis, abscess, or trapped foreign bodies.

DENTAL ANESTHESIA

Patients with severe dental pain may require anesthesia for either temporary pain relief or for painful procedures such as incision and drainage of a periodontal abscess. Topical anesthesia of the mucosa can be achieved within 2 to 3 minutes by the application of a cotton swab soaked in 20% benzocaine or 10% lidocaine. This can lessen the pain of needle injection for further anesthesia and, in some cases, may provide adequate anesthesia for incision and drainage of a superficial abscess. An individual tooth may be anesthetized by infiltration of lidocaine (2% with 1:100,000 epinephrine) or bupivocaine (0.5% with 1:200,000 epinephrine) at the root of the tooth, using a supraperiosteal injection. Mandibular teeth may be anesthetized by blocking the inferior alveolar nerve as it enters the lower mandible. Dental blocks generally last between 1 and 7 hours depending on the anesthetic and choice of procedure (1). Following is a discussion of common dental disorders and postoperative complications.

CLINICAL PRESENTATION

Caries and Pulpitis

Among the most common dental conditions is dental caries, or "cavities." As oral bacteria ferment dietary carbohydrates, an acid is formed, which demineralizes the tooth enamel. This initially is asymptomatic until the erosion intrudes on the tooth pulp, resulting in inflammation (pulpitis). Caries appear as either a whitish-gray discoloration of the enamel or as a brownish visible defect of the enamel surface. Pulpitis, or inflammation of the pulp of the tooth, causes significant pain, which depends upon the extent of inflammation. Early or reversible pulpitis causes relatively well-localized pain that is usually triggered by hot, cold, or sweet stimuli, usually lasts only a few seconds, and resolves spontaneously. Late or irreversible pulpitis results in poorly localized, severe, and persistent pain.

Periodontitis

If the inflammation of the pulp goes unabated, it will extend to the tooth apices, expand outward from the pulp and cause apical periodontitis. The pain of periodontitis is severe, persistent and localized to a particular tooth (unlike irreversible pulpitis which is usually poorly localized). Periodontitis usually results in a tooth sensitive to percussion.

Abscess and Cellulitis

Should periodontitis progress unchecked the inflammation may extend laterally from the tooth apex to cause an apical abscess. Alternatively, an abscess can form in the absence of dental caries when inflammation begins at the junction of the tooth and gum line, extends down the tooth apices and involves the periodontal ligament and adjacent alveolar bone. This is termed a "periodontal abscess" and results from either chronic bacterial plaque (periodontal disease) or a foreign body lodged between the tooth and gum. Clinically, both abscesses appear as a small fluctuant swelling located adjacent to the involved tooth. It may appear tense and painful or it may be draining pus. Periodontal abscesses may result in teeth that are somewhat mobile due to bone destruction. The area surrounding the abscess should be examined for evidence of cellulitis.

Pericoronitis

A partially erupted molar creates a potential space between the occlusal surface of the tooth and the gingiva through which the tooth protrudes. If plaque or food particles become lodged in this space, the overlying mucosal flap will become inflamed. This presents as a painful, tender area over a partially erupted tooth, often accompanied by a foul taste or odor due to extruded pus.

Gingivitis

Gingivitis is inflammation of the gingiva, usually due to bacterial plaque on the tooth. Simple gingivitis does not typically prompt an ED visit, as it is painless. It appears as redness, swelling, and pocket formation of the gingiva. If the inflammation is significant it can produce some bleeding from the gums after brushing the teeth. Referral to a dentist is indicated.

Acute Necrotizing Ulcerative Gingivitis (ANUG)

If bacteria actively invade the gingiva the inflammation may produce painful, swollen gums, often accompanied by fever, malaise, grayish pseudomembranes, lymphadenopathy, a foul odor, and a metallic taste. This disorder is commonly called "trench mouth."

Gum Hyperplasia

Unusual gum swelling may rarely prompt an ED visit. In addition to gingivitis and ANUG, other conditions that may cause generalized gingival hyperplasia or swelling include acute leukemic infiltration and drug-induced hyperplasia (most commonly phenytoin and nifedipine).

COMMON POSTOPERATIVE COMPLAINTS

Postextraction Bleeding

Teeth are commonly removed for therapeutic reasons and postextraction bleeding is a frequent complication. While life-threatening hemorrhage may occur, most patients present with persistent oozing from the extraction site. In patients with acquired or congenital bleeding disorders, bleeding may be persistent and difficult to stop.

Alveolar Osteitis ("Dry Socket")

Following a tooth extraction, some sockets may lose the protective clot prematurely, exposing the socket down to the bone. Typically, patients present 3 to 5 days following the extraction with severe localized pain. Some patients complain of a foul odor or taste. Physical exam shows a nontoxic appearing patient without signs of infection. The extraction site usually is unimpressive. In contrast, postextraction osteomyelitis often is associated with fever, malaise, and leukocytosis and the surrounding teeth and bone may be sensitive to palpation. A radiograph is usually indicated to rule out retained roots or foreign bodies.

LESIONS OF THE MOUTH

Several systemic diseases can present with oral lesions, though most are nonspecific. Systemic lupus erythematosus, scleroderma, Wegener granulomatosis, pemphigus, Stevens-Johnson syndrome, Behçet, Varicella-Zoster, and several neoplasms all can present with oral manifestations.

Oral Candidiasis

Candidal infections of the mouth are relatively common, especially among children and the immunocompromised. Painful white plaques are present that typically can be easily scraped off to show an erythematous underlying mucosa.

Apthous Stomatitis

Many individuals will experience painful, recurrent oral ulcers. Apthous stomatitis is a common cause, though ulcers from hand-foot-mouth disease, herpangina, and herpetic gingivostomatitis may appear similar. While most apthous ulcers are less than 5 mm they may coalesce to form large lesions. These ulcers are self-limited, and rarely are complicated by a localized cellulitis requiring antibiotic therapy.

Herpetic Gingivostomatitis

In children under 5 years old, a primary herpes virus infection (Herpes Simplex type 1) may present with multiple painful, ulcerated vesicles in the oropharynx. Often there is accompanying fever, lymphadenopathy, erythema, and edema. While the primary infection lasts about 2 weeks, recurrences are common, though these usually present with a lesion at the border of the lip. Eruptions are generally self-limited.

DIFFERENTIAL DIAGNOSIS

While most patients with apparent dental complaints ultimately are diagnosed with relatively minor conditions, a few will have serious illnesses that must be detected by the emergency physician. Rarely, the pain from a myocardial infarction will present with isolated jaw pain, mistaken for a "tooth ache" by the patient and physician. Likewise, pain from the sinuses and ears may radiate to the teeth, mimicking odontalgia. A dental infection can occasionally spread to the face, mouth, or throat causing a potentially life-threatening complication.

EMERGENCY DEPARTMENT EVALUATION

The evaluation of the patient with dental pain begins with a relevant history and physical to determine that the complaint is truly odontogenic in nature. Recent dental procedures, medication allergies, and anticoagulant medications are particularly important. Radiographs may be helpful in the evaluation of some patients, in a search for retained roots or foreign body after a dental procedure. Plain films or CT scanning are indicated if one suspects the extension of an infection to the neck or deep spaces.

EMERGENCY DEPARTMENT MANAGEMENT

The treatment of asymptomatic *dental caries* and reversible *pulpitis* is a dental filling, while irreversible pulpitis requires root canal therapy. In the ED, patients with dental pain due to pulpitis should receive pain medications and a referral to a dentist. Pain medications may include an NSAID, acetaminophen, or a mild narcotic. Antibiotics are not necessary for pulpitis or dental caries. Treatment for *periodontitis* consists of analgesics and referral to a dentist for root canal treatment or extraction of the tooth. Antibiotics are not needed.

An *apical abscess* should be incised and drained following appropriate anesthesia of the area, usually accomplished with a dental block or topical anesthesia. As with other abscesses, treatment with antibiotics alone, without incision and drainage, is not recommended. The use of antibiotics for drained abscesses, without accompanying cellulitis, is controversial. Some authorities recommend antibiotics (11,6) and others do not (4). However, as many as two-thirds of dentists in one study prescribed antibiotics liberally (2). If the cellulitis is relatively minor and localized then oral medications are appropriate:

> Penicillin VK 500 mg qid (Peds: 10 mg/kg/dose qid) for 7 days
> (penicillin allergy: Erythromycin 500 mg qid (Peds: 20 mg/kg/dose qid))

Patients not responding to penicillin or erythromycin within 3 days should be switched to:

> Clindamycin 300 mg qid (Peds: 5 mg/kg tid) for 7 days.

Patients with apical abscesses or cellulitis treated as an outpatient should be referred to a dentist within 1 to 2 days. For cellulitis that is severe, has spread into the deep spaces of the face or neck, or is associated with a toxic appearance or an immunocompromised patient, hospital admission and parenteral antibiotics are recommended:

> Penicillin G 4 million units IV (Peds: 25,000 to 100,000 units/kg every 6 hours)
> Metronidazole 15 mg/kg IV for the first dose, then 7.5 mg/kg every 6 hours

CT scanning of the involved areas to rule out deep space infection should be performed if significant cellulitis is present. It is also important to remember that incision and drainage of a dental abscess may lead to transient bacteremia that could result in endocarditis in susceptible individuals, if not correctly treated with prophylactic antibiotics.

Pericoronitis should be treated with mechanical irrigation under the flap following appropriate anesthesia. Some sources recommend antibiotic treatment with penicillin, erythromycin or clindamycin in the same dosing regimens as noted above. Patients should receive pain medications, and follow up with

a dentist within 48 hours. Cellulitis or abscess accompanying pericoronitis should be evaluated and treated as discussed above.

Acute necrotizing ulcerative gingivitis (ANUG) is treated with systemic antibiotics and rinses with warm saline or 3% hydrogen peroxide. Improved oral hygiene is mandatory and may require prescription analgesics to alleviate the pain. Viscous lidocaine may also assist with pain relief and improve oral hygiene. ANUG requires referral to a dentist.

Postextraction bleeding can usually be stopped by having the patient bite down for 10 to 15 minutes on gauze placed over the site. Arterial bleeding may require ligation of the artery, a procedure that can be difficult without proper dental equipment. Patients taking oral anticoagulants may require reversal with fresh frozen plasma, depending on the initial indication for anticoagulation and the extent of bleeding. Oozing that does not stop with direct pressure may require the topical application of pro-coagulant agents including Gelfoam, Oxycel, Surgicel, or Thrombogen (8).

For *alveolar osteitis*, the socket should be irrigated with warmed saline, dried thoroughly, and packed with eugenol soaked Gelfoam. The patient should be referred to an orthodontist promptly as the packing will usually need to be replaced within 24 hours.

Oral candidiasis may be treated with an oral antifungal agent such as nystatin suspension (100,000 units/mL). Five mL is rinsed in the mouth and held as long as possible prior to swallowing or spitting. *Aphthous stomatitis* should be treated symptomatically with hydrogen peroxide rinses, or benadryl syrup mixed 50/50 with kaopectate (2 teaspoons as a rinse, prn). Oral corticosteroids such as Kenalog in Orobase (dispense 5 mg and apply in a thin layer to the ulcer, tid) may speed healing. *Herpes gingivostomatitis* may also be treated with analgesics, such as acetaminophen or ibuprofen, adequate hydration, and oral application of agents such as "magic mouthwash," variably described as a mixture of equal portions of:

> Diphenhydramine elixir (12.5 mg/5 mL)
> 2% lidocaine hydrochloride, and
> Magnesium aluminum hydroxide (Maalox), or
> Kaolin and pectin mixture (Kaopectate)

For adults with a prodrome of burning or tingling, antiviral therapy may reduce the duration or severity of the oubreak:

> Acyclovir 200 mg five times a day, or
> Valacyclovir 500 mg bid for 5 days

CRITICAL INTERVENTIONS

- Recognize and treat dental infections and abscesses with incision and drainage, and antibiotics when appropriate
- Image a patient when a deep space or neck abscess is suspected
- Provide adequate analgesia for painful dental conditions by using medications and/or dental blocks

DISPOSITION

Most patients with dental disorders may be successfully treated and discharged home from the ED, with appropriate dental follow up. However, as discussed above, some disorders may necessitate emergent dental consultation or hospital admission, such as abscesses that are large or extending over the face and neck, or postextraction bleeding that cannot be controlled by simple measures.

COMMON PITFALLS

✔ Failing to identify a systemic cause, such as myocardial infarction, for face or jaw pain
✔ Failing to recognize the spread of an odontogenic infection to the face or neck
✔ Failing to ascertain antibiotic allergies prior to prescribing penicillin or other common dental antibiotics
✔ Performing dental procedures prior to antibiotic prophylaxis in a patient with risks for endocarditis

Acknowledgment

Thanks to the previous edition's author Alan Hodgdon.

References

1. Arizona Department of Health Services. *Physician's Guide to Dental Emergencies.* Phoenix, AZ: Arizona Department of Health Services, 1998.
2. Dailey YM, Martin MV. Are antibiotics being used appropriately for emergency dental treatment? *Br Dental J* 2001;191:391–393.
3. Dorfman DH, Kastner B, Vinci RJ. Dental concerns unrelated to trauma in the pediatric emergency department: barriers to care. *Arch Pediatr Adolesc Med* 2001;155:699–703.
4. Douglass AB, Douglass JM. Common dental emergencies. *Am Fam Phys* 2003;67:511–516.
5. Graham DB, Webb MD, Seale NS. Pediatric emergency room visits for nontraumatic dental disease. *Pediatr Dent* 2000;22:134–140.
6. Beaudreau RW. Acute nontraumatic dental emergencies. In: Tintinalli JE, Kelen GD, Stapczynski JS, eds. *Emergency Medicine: A Comprehensive Study Guide.* 5th ed. New York, NY: McGraw-Hill; 2000:1539–1556.
7. Lewis C, Lynch H, Johnston B. Dental complaints in emergency departments: A national perspective. *Ann Emerg Med* 2003;42:93–99.
8. Matocha DL. Postsurgical complications. *Emerg Med Clinics* 2000;18:549–564.
9. Patel KK, Driscoll P. Dental knowledge of accident and emergency senior house officers. *Merg Med J* 2002;19:539–541.
10. Roberts G, Scully C, Shotts R. Dental emergencies. *BMJ* 2000;321:559–562.
11. Von Kaenel D. Social factors associated with pediatric emergency department visits for caries-related dental pain. *Pediatr Dent* 2001;23:56–60.

CHAPTER 24
Oral and Maxillofacial Disorders

James T. Amsterdam and William G. Langston, II

POSTOPERATIVE COMPLICATIONS

Oral and maxillofacial disorders (OMFS) procedures involve major facial surgery done in the hospital (e.g., osteotomies of facial bones) and minor procedures done in the office (e.g., removal of teeth). Patients may be referred to the emergency department directly from the surgeon's office after an intraoperative complication, or may have developed a problem several hours or days after hospital discharge or completion of office surgery.

OMFS postoperative complications are unique for two reasons: First, the airway may be compromised, and second, the patient may be in intermaxillary fixation (maxillary and mandibular teeth wired together or secured with elastics). OMFS postoperative complications fall into the following general categories (19):

Intermaxillary fixation (teeth/jaws "wired" closed or secured with elastics):

    Airway concerns
    Vomiting
Bleeding:
    After tooth extraction and alveolar bone surgery
    After periodontal surgery
    After midface osteotomy
Swelling:
    Postextraction infection
    Surgical edema and hematoma
    Salivary gland obstruction
    Fracture of mandible during tooth extraction
Sudden change in occlusion (bite)
Office anesthesia complications
Aspiration versus swallowed instrument, packing, or tooth

The three steps for initial evaluation are the following:

1. Ensure an adequate airway.
2. Control bleeding.
3. Obtain a history of the surgical procedure (what, when, and by whom).

After initial evaluation and stabilization, contact the treating OMF surgeon or the ear, nose, and throat (ENT) consultant.

INTERMAXILLARY FIXATION

Intermaxillary fixation (IMF) consists of tying the upper and lower teeth together with stainless steel wires or elastics. This is a common method of stabilizing the upper and lower jaws to allow for healing of jaw-osteotomy procedures, jaw fractures, and jaw reconstruction procedures. Complications are rare, and the need to release the IMF on an emergency basis is infrequent. The critical reason to cut the fixation is vomiting. If release of IMF during the first 4 weeks after surgery is necessary, reoperation may be necessary or the surgical result will be compromised. The typical duration of this method of fixation is 4 to 8 weeks, during which time the patient must consume only liquids. Speech is usually difficult to understand, and most patients lose 10% to 20% of their weight while the jaws are wired together. If an acrylic surgical bite splint is interposed between the teeth, the oral airway can be greatly restricted. Edema can further restrict the oral airway. If, in addition to a restricted oral airway, the patient has a restricted nasal airway, then breathing becomes difficult. During the first 2 weeks after surgery when IMF is used and some surgical edema remains, some patients become anxious about breathing and adequate nutrition, and may present to the emergency department. Usually, reassurance and possibly a nasopharyngeal airway are all that are needed for treatment. Vomiting while in IMF is frightening to the patient but should not require release of IMF, unless the emesis cannot be cleared.

Release of IMF can be done on an emergency basis when access to the airway is mandatory. Examples of such situations are trauma, significant airway restriction due to acute infection or surgical edema, and a severe medical emergency, such as status epilepticus, septic shock, or cardiac arrest.

Release of IMF is accomplished by using small wire cutters to cut all the wires that cross from one dental arch to the other (all wires traversing from the upper teeth to the lower teeth). There may be 3 to 8 wire loops (6 to 16 wires) to cut. Occasionally, rubber bands are used to hold the teeth together, and these can be cut with a scalpel or scissors. Release of IMF with wires may be time consuming to those untrained in placing IMF. Consider emergency blind nasotracheal intubation or cricothyroidotomy in extremely acute situations. If wires are cut and not removed, small loose wires will remain in the mouth. All patients with IMF should have wire cutters or scissors with them.

MANAGEMENT

Assess the work of breathing and the possibility of fatigue. Consider pulse oximetry, arterial blood gas levels, or capnometry to aid in the determination of the adequacy of ventilation. If ventilation is impaired, a nasopharyngeal airway may be an effective airway adjunct to improve the situation.

In extreme cases, release the IMF by cutting the vertical wires between dental arches with wire cutters or by cutting the elastic bands with a scalpel or scissors. Consider cricothyroidotomy or nasotracheal intubation when immediate airway access is necessary and no experienced person is available to release the wire IMF.

BLEEDING

Bleeding (from the mouth, nose, or both) is one of the more common postoperative complications. Normally, a small amount of bleeding mixes with saliva during the first 12 hours after many intraoral procedures. Significant hemorrhage must be differentiated from this type of bleeding. Problematic hemorrhage is usually apparent during an office procedure or within the first 12 hours. It is important to obtain a history of aspirin or nonsteroidal-antiinflammatory drug (NSAID) use.

Prolonged bleeding from a simple tooth extraction in the absence of a coagulopathy is usually minor and can be controlled with oral gauze packs. For removal of lower wisdom teeth, the incidence of problem bleeding is 0.5% to 1.1% intraoperatively and 0.5% to 0.8% postoperatively (21). Possible sources of bleeding include the extraction socket, inferior alveolar artery, posterior superior alveolar artery, long buccal artery, facial artery, palatine artery, lingual artery, and maxillary artery.

Bleeding after Tooth Extraction or Alveolar Bone Surgery

The most significant hemorrhage related to alveolar bone surgery in the mandible is from damage to the inferior alveolar neurovascular bundle that runs in a bony canal below the roots of the posterior teeth. Damage to this structure can occur during (15) surgical removal of teeth, odontogenic tumors, and cysts and the placement of endosseous dental implants (15).

MANAGEMENT

Reassure the patient, and keep the patient's head elevated 45 degrees. In the case of postextraction bleeding, simply biting on gauze may not be sufficient to stop the bleeding. The gingiva around the extraction site should be infiltrated with 1% or 2% lidocaine with epinephrine. The anesthesia helps the patient to bite with more force, and the vasoconstriction decreases oozing.

If bleeding persists, the socket should be packed with Gelfoam, Surgicel, or Avitene. The packing usually must be se-

cured with a black silk suture. Decide whether the cause is an anatomic problem or a coagulopathy (by history and laboratory evaluation). Consult OMFS or ENT for persistent or severe hemorrhage for possible suturing, electrocautery, or extraoral cutdown on facial, lingual, or external carotid arteries.

Delayed Bleeding after Midface Osteotomy

Delayed bleeding after midface osteotomy involves bleeding from the nose and nasopharynx, or acute swelling of the upper cheeks (unilaterally or bilaterally) within 2 weeks after surgery. Many patients have a small amount of bleeding from the nose after midface osteotomy procedures (e.g., segmental osteotomy and Le Fort I, II, III) due to disruption of the nasal mucosa and pooling of blood in the maxillary sinuses. This minor nasal bleeding must be differentiated from significant hemorrhage. The incidence of severe postoperative bleeding after Le Fort I osteotomy is 0.75% (16,17).

MANAGEMENT

Consider a balloon nasal pack as the first option in significant bleeding, because it simultaneously occludes the posterior, middle, and anterior nasal cavities. For serious or persistent bleeding, consider arteriography to rule out an arteriovenous fistula or a pseudoaneurysm.

Notify the OMFS or ENT surgeon immediately, as hospital admission is often necessary for observation, reoperation, or embolization.

SWELLING

Patients may present with acute swelling after OMFS procedures because of concern over the airway or swallowing, or for an explanation. The swelling may be from a hematoma, surgical edema, acute cellulitis, or abscess.

Hematoma and Surgical Edema

Office procedures that may result in hematoma or surgical edema significant enough to warrant an emergency department visit are procedures in the floor of the mouth (e.g., excision of mandibular tori, excision of the sublingual gland, and removal of a stone from the salivary gland duct).

MANAGEMENT

The airway is the primary concern. Instruct the patient to sit up and lean forward. Perform appropriate monitoring (e.g., pulse oximetry), and consider admission for observation.

In patients with obvious airway compromise, consider the following interventions, in order of preference: nasopharyngeal airway, oral, or nasal endotracheal intubation, cricothyroidotomy, or tracheostomy. Also consider prophylactic antibiotics for patients with hematoma and postsurgical edema in the floor of the mouth, to avoid development of a deep space infection, or Ludwig angina.

Postextraction Infection

A common reason for an emergency department visit is the rapid progression of an infection after removal of an impacted mandibular third molar (wisdom tooth). This can involve several tissue spaces, including the parapharyngeal space. Edema and infection in the masticator space cause trismus (limited mouth opening due to muscle spasm), making examination of the oropharynx difficult. The incidence of infection is 0.6% to 2.5% (14).

MANAGEMENT

Determine if there is significant limitation of mouth opening, and whether it involves parapharyngeal, submandibular, or submental spaces, or extends across the midline. If the airway is compromised, consider inserting a nasopharyngeal airway. If a definitive airway is necessary, nasotracheal intubation is preferred if trismus is present. Cricothyroidostomy or tracheostomy are seldom necessary but are options in severe cases.

Consult the OMF or ENT surgeon, and consider admission for intravenous antibiotics and surgical incision and drainage in the operating room. If trismus and swelling are minimal, oral antibiotics and daily outpatient follow up for 3 or 4 days are essential.

Swelling of Salivary Glands Due to Obstruction of Ducts

Acute swelling of the submandibular glands and, occasionally, the parotid can occur. Surgical edema or a suture obstructing the opening can result from intraoral surgery or placement of intraoral acrylic surgical stents. Swelling typically is mildly tender, without signs of infection. The patient may present hours to 3 days postoperatively.

MANAGEMENT

Examine the salivary ducts for any obstruction that can be eliminated (e.g., sutures or acrylic stents) and consult the OMF surgeon. If edema is the only cause of the obstruction, the swelling will resolve in 3 to 4 days. Antibiotics may be important, especially if the surgery was for removal of a salivary duct stone (*sialolithiasis*) that was causing chronic partial obstruction.

Fracture of the Mandible from Extraction of Teeth

Fracture of the mandible typically results from removal of impacted lower wisdom teeth. Evaluation and treatment are the same as for any jaw fracture. Application of a Barton's bandage to immobilize the jaw is seldom necessary, as prompt OMFS or ENT consultation is required.

Sudden Change in Occlusion

A sudden change in occlusion (bite) during the postoperative period (after jaw osteotomy, fracture repair, or mandibular reconstruction in which rigid internal fixation was used without IMF) can occur due to failure of the internal fixation. Failure of external fixation devices (transcutaneous pins and bars) is readily apparent. The patient will present with a malocclusion (shifting of the bite) that occurred suddenly. There may be mild-to-moderate pain aggravated by jaw movement.

MANAGEMENT

Evaluation is the same as for fractures of the mandible. Treatment is usually reoperation, although emergency admission is typically unnecessary. Notify the OMF surgeon, as it may be desirable to stabilize the mandible immediately by IMF.

Complications from Outpatient Sedation and Anesthesia

Drugs used for office sedation are narcotics, benzodiazepines, barbiturates, and occasionally ketamine. A patient may be transported to the emergency department from a doctor's office because of complications related to such sedation. The most frequent event is loss of an adequate airway, or prolonged hypoventilation, which leads to cardiovascular complications.

MANAGEMENT

Complications from outpatient office sedation are treated according to the patient's condition, and may range from simple observation after a minor reaction to airway management and resuscitation for cardiovascular collapse.

Aspiration or Swallowed Foreign Bodies

Teeth, dental restorations, bone, drill bit, packing, or dental instruments may all be swallowed or aspirated. Usually, the situation is not life threatening. Evaluation includes the probable location of the object and whether arrangements need to be made to remove it. Packing aspiration is the most serious, as it can drape over the carina.

MANAGEMENT

Obtain a description of the object and the events surrounding the aspiration or swallowing. Order a chest x-ray or abdominal radiograph to determine whether the object is in the lungs, stomach, or bowel.

It may be necessary to consult a pulmonologist or gastroenterologist to remove the object by flexible fiberoptic endoscopy. Small, blunt objects may be allowed to pass, without intervention, through the gastrointestinal tract. Sharp or pointed objects in the gastrointestinal tract and objects in the lungs should be removed as quickly as possible. Deeply aspirated surgical packing at the level of the carina is devastating, because both bronchi may be obstructed.

CRITICAL INTERVENTIONS

- Be prepared to utilize techniques other than orotracheal intubation (such as nasotracheal intubation, cricothyroidotomy) in patients with significant edema or obstruction of the oropharynx
- Reverse coagulopathy and consult the OMF or ENT surgeon early for patients with significant postoperative bleeding, as reoperation may be needed

DISPOSITION

If postextraction bleeding can be controlled by the aforementioned measures, the patient can be safely discharged. The patient needs to be instructed not to smoke, use straws, or spit. These actions all create a negative pressure in the mouth, which leads to clot dislodgment and rebleeding. Patients should be instructed to refrain from aspirin- and NSAID-containing products. Persistent bleeding requires OMFS or ENT consultation.

Patients with bleeding after midface osteotomy generally require OMFS or ENT consultation and admission to the hospital.

Disposition in the case of postoperative swelling or infection is based on the severity. Mild postoperative swelling that is not compromising the airway can be managed on an outpatient basis. If there is any doubt, the OMFS or ENT consultant should see the patient. Some postoperative infections can be managed as outpatients. However, because fascial planes of the head and neck can be violated during surgery, a very high index of suspicion is necessary since the infection may spread.

A mandible fracture secondary to an extraction or the disruption of occlusion is a major problem. The OMFS or ENT consultant should be notified immediately. Nondisplaced fractures can be treated with antibiotics, analgesia, soft diet, and referral to the office the next day. Such fractures are normally treated with IMF that is placed in the office. Displaced fractures require immediate consultation and admission.

Aspirated foreign bodies that appear to be in the gastrointestinal tract can generally be managed on an outpatient basis if there is no potential for perforation. If the potential for perforation exists, the gastrointestinal endoscopist should be called. Tracheobronchial aspiration requires immediate pulmonary consultation.

COMMON PITFALLS

✔ Failure to recognize that the IMF can result in aspiration if the patient is unable to clear the airway by expelling vomitus between the teeth
✔ Being too quick to cut the IMF when it may not be necessary, or hesitant when it is
✔ Failure to use local anesthesia and a vasoconstrictor for pain and hemorrhage control
✔ Failure to obtain OMFS or ENT consultation when revision of the surgical area may be required for hemorrhage control
✔ Failure to recognize the potential for airway compromise from swelling or postoperative infection
✔ Failure to recognize tracheobronchial aspiration

TEMPOROMANDIBULAR JOINT (TMJ) SYNDROME

The temporomandibular joint (TMJ) consists of the mandibular condyle (the posterior extension of the mandible covered by the meniscus or articular disk) that articulates in the temporal fossa (23). The temporal fossa is bordered anteriorly by the articular eminence. When the mandible closes, the condyle moves posteriorly and superiorly in the temporal fossa. Therefore, on opening, the condyle moves anteriorly and inferiorly, guided by the articular eminence.

Temporomandibular joint disorders include those with pathology of the joint itself and those involving the muscles of mastication (myofascial pain dysfunction). Disorders of the TMJ involve the trigeminal nerve and its three branches that have sensory synapses in the trigeminal ganglion. The ophthalmic (V1), maxillary (V2) and mandibular (V3) divisions also contain motor fibers innervating the muscles of mastication. The trigeminal nerve also innervates the dura, orbit, paranasal sinuses, tympanic membrane, oral cavity and teeth which help to understand the patterns of pain referral from dysfunction.

Temporomandibular myofascial pain dysfunction syndrome, or simply TMJ syndrome, is a complex neuromuscular disturbance, possibly resulting from and definitely aggravated by occlusal disturbances and the anatomy of the TMJ. Other entities, such as trauma, psychological tension, and neuromuscular habits (e.g., bruxism and clenching), contribute to the problem (20). Patients who present to the emergency department frequently complain of nonspecific unilateral facial pain generalized to the region of the TMJ. The pain is dull, and increases throughout the day with continued jaw motion. Clinical examination frequently reveals spasm of the masseter muscle externally and the internal pterygoid intraorally. There is usually limitation of opening, with deviation toward the affected side.

The TMJ is vulnerable to all conditions that can affect other joints in the body. These include arthritis, dislocations, trauma, ankylosis, and neoplasms. Myofascial pain often has complex symtomatology and psychosocial stressors contribute to and complicate treatment (20). The muscles of mastication are primarily involved and there is usually a unilateral dull aching that increases with muscle use. Common referred areas of pain include headache, otalgia, tinnitus, and rarely decreased hearing.

CLINICAL PRESENTATION

Physical examination findings that support a diagnosis of TMJ arthralgia include the absence of molar teeth in any quadrant, deviation of the jaw to the painful side on wide opening, reproducible pain by pressure below the ear and forward in the direction of the mandibular condyle, or tenderness of the muscles of mastication to palpation.

The term *internal derangement* of the TMJ alludes to any disturbance between the articular components within the joint. It implies a localized structural derangement that interferes with the smooth function of the joint. The patient should be questioned about the presence or history of joint noises. Patients with internal derangement almost always have or have had joint noises. The noise is usually described as either clicking or crepitus. Crepitus is considered to represent advanced disease and occurs as a result of movement across irregular surfaces. This may also indicate a perforation of the disk or its attachments.

Typically, the patient with internal derangement reports a clicking TMJ followed by a period of no joint noise. This click may or may not be associated with pain and can often be palpated over the TMJ or by placing a finger in the patient's external auditory meatus. When the disk is anteriorly displaced and does not reduce to a normal position during opening, the patient will have limited opening, or a "closed-lock" condition. This condition may be either intermittent or persistent. The emergency physician can measure the inter-incisal maximum opening, which is usually limited to 20 mm (normal, 35 to 50 mm).

Arthritic TMJ may present with pain and crepitus. There may be periods of pain exacerbation and remission. As in other arthritides, there is often morning stiffness that wears off with function during the day, as opposed to the TMJ syndrome, which worsens as the day progresses. Degenerative arthritis of the TMJ can be primary as seen in elderly patients, or secondary to trauma or chronic bruxism. Secondary arthritis is seen in younger patients who often have more severe symptoms. They often show osteophyte formation and joint erosion on of the articular surface of the condyle on radiographic studies.

DIFFERENTIAL DIAGNOSIS

When the diagnosis of TMJ dysfunction is considered, the emergency physician should rule out pain of odontogenic origin. Tooth pain or sore teeth, in the absence of odontogenic pathology, may indicate bruxism. Headaches are a common complaint of patients with a TMJ disorder. Patients with an internal derangement frequently complain of headaches on the affected side, but no specific diagnostic pattern has been documented. Because headaches are such a common complaint, one should not assume that an internal derangement is the cause unless more specific diagnostic evidence is present. Headaches associated with internal derangement frequently emanate from the TMJ and radiate to temporal-orbital-occipital areas. This frequently follows jaw function and may be relieved with an occlusal splint or other therapies directed toward internal derangement.

Earache is a common complaint. Tinnitus and occasional dizziness may also be noted. Ear pathology should be considered and ruled out before assuming that an earache is due to TMJ disease.

Neck ache and shoulder pain are often reported by patients with TMJ disorders. These complaints are not specifically diagnostic, but may reflect a more generalized muscle disorder. In general, all pain is exacerbated by chewing.

EMERGENCY DEPARTMENT EVALUATION

Radiographic evaluation of the TMJ should include a panoramic view, which is the easiest to read and requires the least sophisticated technique. The emergency physician can also order a TMJ series or tomograms of the joints, taken in both open and closed positions. Tomograms avoid superimposition of other anatomic structures that make a regular TMJ series difficult to read. The panoramic survey and tomograms are necessary to distinguish arthritis, TMJ pain dysfunction syndrome, or internal derangement. Degenerative joint disease (osteoarthritis) may show flattening of the condylar head, erosions, or osteophyte formation. When any type of internal derangement is suspected, a computed tomography scan of the joints should be ordered to assess bony architecture (22). Magnetic resonance imaging and arthrography may further delineate the pathology, but these studies are best left to the specialist providing definitive care.

EMERGENCY DEPARTMENT MANAGEMENT

TMJ pain or dysfunction, regardless of cause, is treated initially by a combination of physiotherapy (moist heat for 15 minutes four times a day) and a soft diet for 2 weeks. Analgesics such as nonsteroidal-antiinflammatory agents or aspirin–codeine combinations are effective in addition to muscle relaxants such as diazepam (18).

Bite planes (occlusal splints) are used to reposition the mandible to relieve spasm, correct oral habits, and "recapture" a displaced disk. The emergency physician can refer the patient for occlusal therapy to the general dentist, periodontist, or perioprosthedontist.

CRITICAL INTERVENTIONS

- Provide adequate analgesia and appropriate referral

DISPOSITION

A documented internal derangement is usually referred to an oral and maxillofacial surgeon, who may perform arthroscopy or arthroplasty to correct disk position permanently or to reconstruct arthritic joints.

COMMON PITFALLS

✔ TMJ dysfunction is often called the "great impostor" because it mimics so many other facial pain syndromes
✔ The physician who fails to understand disk displacement may confuse it with muscle spasm. A history of joint noise is critical in this regard

TEMPOROMANDIBULAR JOINT DISLOCATION

In acute dislocation of the mandible, the condyle moves too far anteriorly in relation to the eminence and becomes locked. The mouth is in open position as opposed to "closed-lock" position (Fig. 24.1). Subsequent muscular trismus prevents the condyles from moving back into the temporal fossa. The spasm of the external pterygoid, masseter, and internal pterygoid muscles, and associated edema, result in extreme discomfort and anxiety. Predisposing factors include anatomic disharmony between the fossa and the anterior articular eminence, weakness of the capsule forming the TMJ ligaments, and torn ligaments.

CLINICAL PRESENTATION

TMJ dislocation is likely to occur during maximum opening (yawning or laughing), rendering the patient unable to close the mouth. Although the TMJ is a double joint, the dislocation may be bilateral or unilateral. Palpation of the TMJs may reveal them to be anterior to the articular eminence. Patients may experience substantial discomfort or pain.

DIFFERENTIAL DIAGNOSIS

While most cases of TMJ dislocation are clinically obvious, some may be confused initially with fracture of the mandible or acute dystonia.

EMERGENCY DEPARTMENT EVALUATION

Radiographs should be taken to rule out a fracture, as the clinical picture and occlusal disturbances of both fracture and dislocation are similar. Films should also help determine whether the dislocation is unilateral or bilateral.

EMERGENCY DEPARTMENT MANAGEMENT

An understanding of TMJ anatomy is important for proper manual reduction. It may be helpful to relieve the patient's anxiety and intense muscle spasm with intravenous diazepam, 5 to 10 mg or midazolam 1 to 2 mg, titrated by slow injection. When the patient is sufficiently relaxed, the physician should face the patient

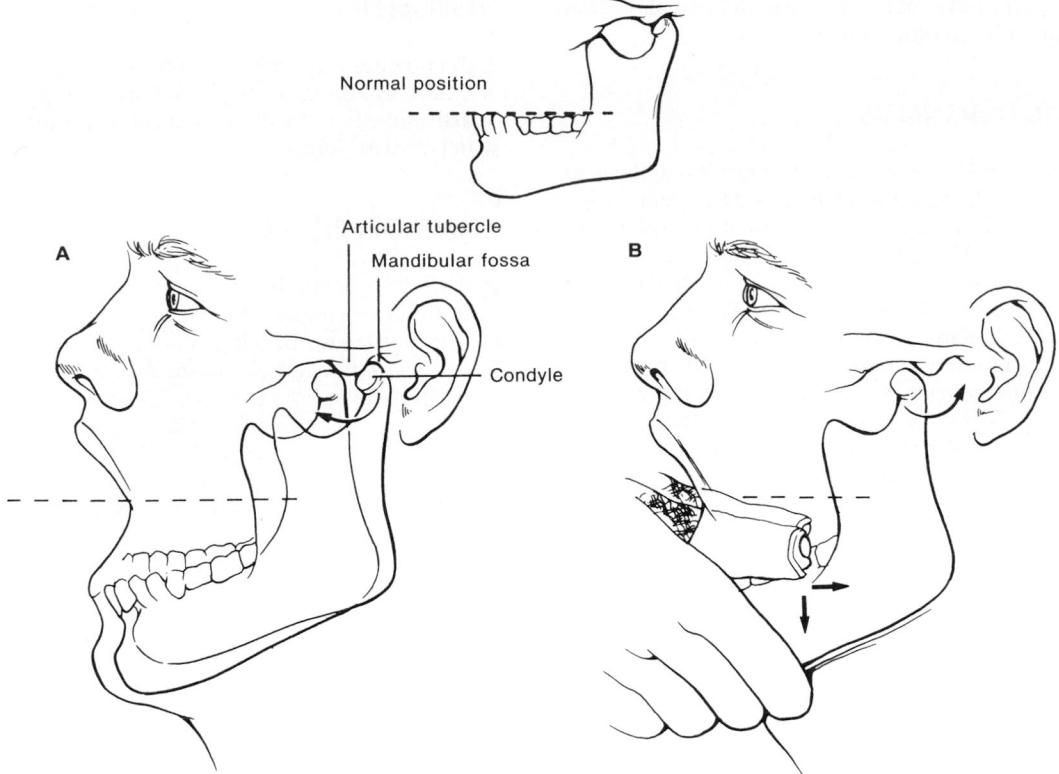

Figure 24.1.   **(A)** Temporomandibular joint dislocation and **(B)** reduction.

and grasp the mandible with both hands, one hand on each side, with the thumbs (wrapped with gauze) placed on the occlusal surfaces of the posterior teeth (see Fig. 24.1). The fingertips are placed around the inferior border of the mandible in the region of the angle. Downward pressure is applied to free the condyles from their position anterior to the eminence. The chin is then pressed backward after the jaw has been forced downward. The mouth closes and the condyle returns to its position in the fossa. Because of severe muscle spasm, the jaw may snap back quickly, so the physician must be aware.

CRITICAL INTERVENTIONS

- Order radiographs to rule out mandible fracture
- Provide adequate sedation and analgesia to facilitate reduction

DISPOSITION

Patients may be safely discharged home after reduction. Postreduction instructions include a soft diet for 1 to 2 weeks, avoidance of wide opening of the mandible, and the use of analgesics and muscle relaxants. Patients who chronically dislocate the TMJ and those who suffer acute recurrences may be helped by a Barton bandage or elastic and Velcro jaw "bra" applied around the head to prevent maximum opening for 2 weeks, but this is seldom done. Severe cases may require intermaxillary wiring and fixation for added control. Patients who have suffered dislocation of the TMJ should be referred to an oral and maxillofacial surgeon for follow up because surgical alteration of the eminence may be necessary.

COMMON PITFALLS

✔ Failure to obtain radiographs to exclude a mandibular fracture
✔ Failure to provide adequate sedation and analgesia to facilitate reduction

PARAPHARYNGEAL SPACE INFECTIONS

The presentation of dental, oral, and salivary gland infections in the emergency department can vary from a patient with a simple complaint of pain or gingival swelling to a toxic patient with massive facial swelling and a compromised airway. Variable factors include the origin and location of the infection and the degree to which the infection has been contained or has spread to the deep spaces of the head and neck. The most common focus of infection is odontogenic, in addition to exposure to trauma or surgery that may violate the natural anatomic barriers of the fascial planes of the head and neck, resulting in deep-space infection (4,3,0).

The key to diagnosis and management of dental infections and space infections of the head and neck is an understanding of the fascial planes of the head and neck (Fig. 24.2). Cellulitis of odontogenic origin usually involves the middle and lower part of the face and neck. Although such infections are generally well contained, in a debilitated host or in the case of a virulent organism, rapid spread of infection may be fatal (1,2,3,5,10,11,12).

The fascial spaces of the head and neck are potential spaces filled with loose areolar tissue that can rapidly break down when subjected to infection. In the case of oral infection, the deep cervical fascia is the most important. The deep cervical fascia consists of several layers that surround the neck, including the superficial and investing layer that attaches to the inferior border of the mandible and splits to form the masticator space. Other

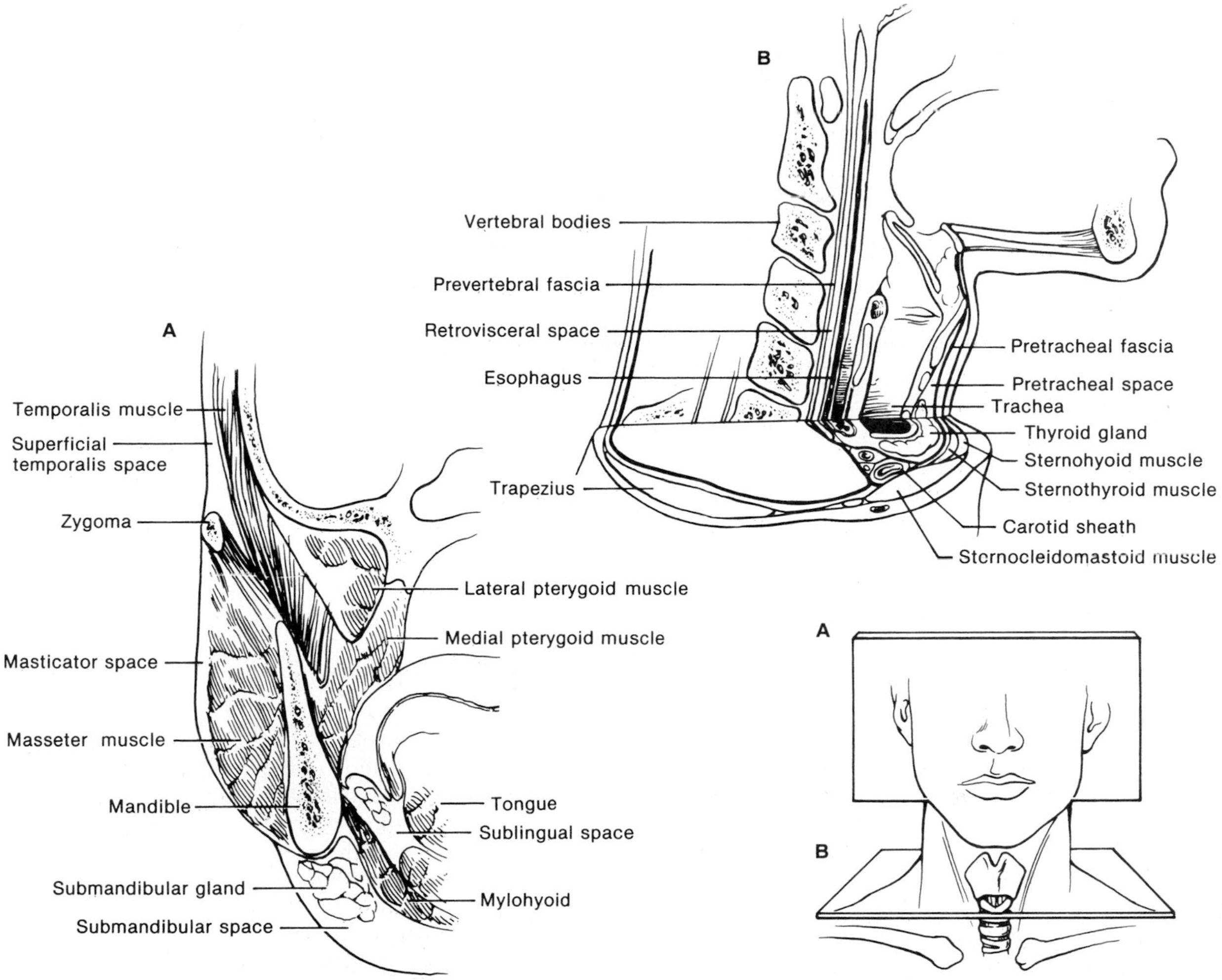

Figure 24.2.   Fascial planes of the head and neck. **(A)** Coronal section of the head. **(B)** Cross section of the fascial planes of the neck.

important spaces include the lateral pharyngeal space (lateral to the pharynx and medial to the masticator space), the retropharyngeal space (between the deep cervical and prevertebral fascia), and the pharyngomaxillary space (from the base of the skull to the hyoid bone), which communicates with all deep spaces (see Fig. 24.2) (1,3).

The mylohyoid muscle of the mandible divides the sublingual (superior) and submaxillary (inferior) spaces. The submental space is anterior to the sublingual space. Infection involving the submaxillary, sublingual, and submental spaces with elevation of the tongue is *Ludwig angina,* a serious infection with a potential for airway obstruction (Fig. 24.3) (1,3,9).

Infections that affect the midface involve the canine space, which is commonly infected by abscessed anterior maxillary teeth, and the buccal space, which is superficial to the buccinator and frequently infected by the molar teeth. Infections in these areas are especially important because of the possibility of cavernous sinus thrombosis due to the fascial venous system (8).

DIFFERENTIAL DIAGNOSIS

Before attributing any swelling of the face or the head and neck to dental infection, other entities should be considered. Tumors may present as nonspecific swellings and may be hard to distinguish from advanced primary infections if secondary infection

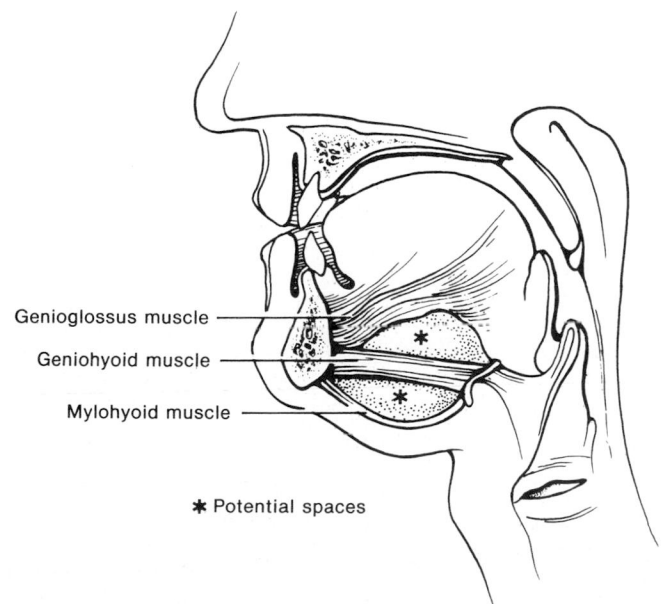

★ Potential spaces

Figure 24.3.   Ludwig angina.

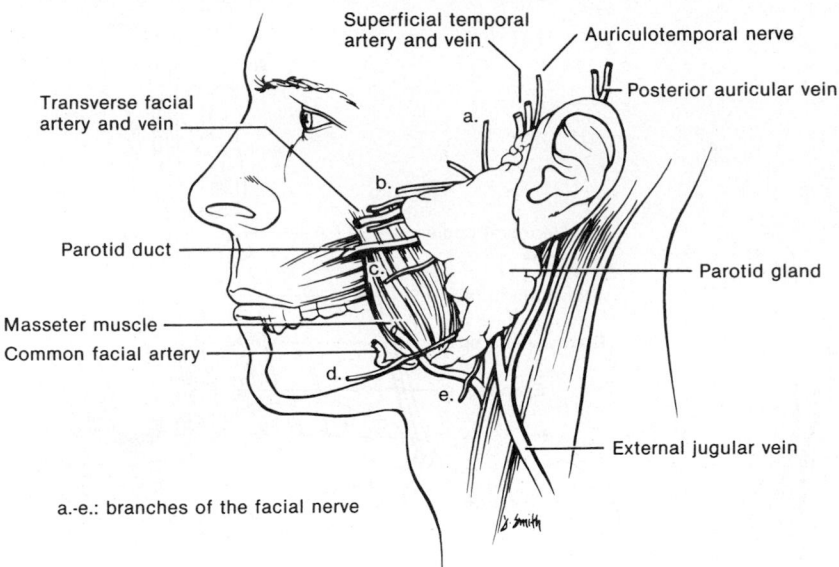

Figure 24.4. Normal anatomy of the parotid gland.

is present. Viral infections, especially those that involve the salivary glands (e.g., mumps), can present as swellings. Less common infections are scrofula (tuberculous cervical lymphadenitis) and actinomycosis. Failure to respond to conventional therapy should lead the clinician to suspect some complication (tumor or uncommon infection). Certain fungal infections, although rare, are more common in the head and neck regions, such as mucormycosis. Fungal infections should be considered in immunocompromised patients (3).

Submaxillary and parotid gland disease is not uncommon. Submandibular gland infection is generally caused by *Streptococcus,* and may be secondary to obstruction caused by a stone (*sialolithiasis*). Patients with inflammation or infection of a salivary gland (*sialoadenitis)* have a history of increasing pain when eating, and they are especially affected by sour foods. Frequently, pus may be expressed from meatus of the salivary duct in the mouth, by applying gentle pressure to the gland or along the duct. *Staphylococcus* is more commonly involved in parotid gland infections. Infectious parotitis is seen in the elderly and especially in diabetics. This entity is usually bilateral and associated with fever and toxicity. Autoimmune diseases, such as Sjögren syndrome and Mikulicz disease, can also cause facial swelling due to enlargement of the salivary glands (Figs. 24.4 and 24.5) (3).

EMERGENCY DEPARTMENT EVALUATION

Initial management of oral, dental, and salivary gland infections begins with localization of the infection. Most infections are of odontogenic origin and localized to a specific tooth. Patients with dental pain should be examined for the presence of infection. Pain to percussion with a tongue blade indicates involvement at the apex of the tooth (periapical abscess). Tender swelling over the gingiva adjacent to a tooth may indicate either a periodontal abscess or extension of a periapical abscess through the cortex of bone into the subperiosteal space. Differentiating these entities without a dental radiograph can be difficult.

The presence of cellulitis indicates that there has been spread of infection. The emergency physician must then determine the following: (1) the extent of involvement of contiguous spaces, (2) the potential for spread of infection to the fascial planes of the head and neck, and (3) potential for airway compromise. Advanced imaging with CT scanning is helpful in this assessment. Once extensive involvement is recognized, it is the role of the oral and maxillofacial surgeon to compartmentalize the spread of infection and determine the site of the initial focus, so that pus can be evacuated under controlled conditions in the operating room (1). Table 24.1 summarizes the essential features of odontogenic and parapharyngeal space infections.

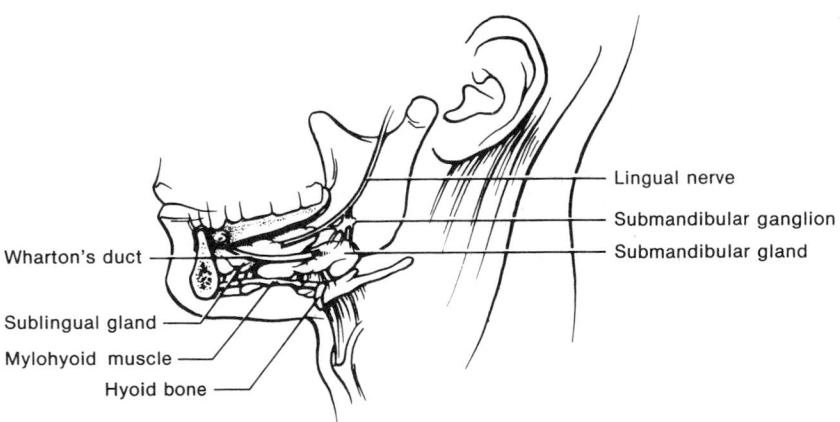

Figure 24.5. Normal anatomy of the submandibular gland.

TABLE 24.1. Essential Features of Odontogenic and Parapharyngeal Space Infections

Fascial Space/ Anatomic Area	Pathophysiology	Clinical Presentation	Diagnosis/Treatment	Disposition	Pitfalls
Periapical abscess	Local confinement may occur, or extension through cortex	Acute or chronic odontalgia Pain with percussion No visible swelling	Periapical lucency on Panorex; analgesics/ABX	Dental referral	Consider extension to deeper space
Subperiosteal	Contained by periosteum of local alveolar bone	Vestibular, palatal, or sublingual swelling/fluctuance	Stab incision to alveolar bone, irrigation ± drain, analgesics/ABX	Dental/oral surgery f/u 24-48 h	Failure to penetrate periosteum with incision; failure to avoid palatine vessels; failure to provide SBE prophylaxis, if indicated
Canine space	Anterior maxillary teeth origin with perforation above levator oris m.	Obliteration of nasolabial groove; may spontaneously drain near medial canthus	Analgesics/ABX; needle aspiration if unsure of abscess (intraoral approach)	OMFS consult if fluctuant/extensive; 24 h f/u for local cellulitis	May produce periorbital cellulitis if untreated; patient must return if eye closes
Buccal space	Premolar/molar teeth origin with perforation beyond buccinator m.	Massive cheek swelling	Analgesics/ABX; fluctuance usually easy to palpate	OMFS consult for abscess drainage; 24 h f/u for cellulitis	May be confused with erysipelas; in child, consider buccal cellulitis (*H. influenzae*)
Masticator spaces: Submasseteric Pterygomandibular Temporal	Mandibular molar origin. These 3 spaces freely communicate and are bound by fascia around the muscles of mastication	Trismus is the clinical hallmark Extraoral swelling may be absent with deep temporal or pterygomandibular space infection	Patients are often dehydrated and may require fluid resuscitation; CT scan may confirm diagnosis	OMFS consult; hospitalize for trismus, toxicity, or severe dehydration	Failure to document trismus (<1 cm intercanine opening); pterygomandibular space swelling may mimic a peritonsillar abscess
Sublingual space	Anterior mandibular teeth with perforation above the mylohyoid line; communicates posteriorly with submandibular space	Sublingual edema, (tongue elevation; minimal extraoral swelling; often crosses midline with bilateral swelling	Airway assessment; i.v. antibiotics; fluid resuscitation if dehydrated	OMFS consult; strongly consider hospitalization unless well localized with close f/u	Failure to recognize threat to airway; failure to involve consultant early
Submandibular space	Mandibular molar origin with perforation below the mylohyoid line; communicates anteriorly with submental and posteriorly with sublingual spaces	Prominent extraoral swelling beneath the mandible	Airway assessment; i.v. antibiotics	OMFS consult; see "sublingual"	Often the precursor of Ludwig's angina
Submental space	Anterior mandibular teeth with perforation below the mentalis m.	Prominent chin swelling extending back to the hyoid bone	Airway, i.v. antibiotics	OMFS consult; see "sublingual"	Communication with submandibular space may lead to Ludwig angina.
Ludwig's angina	Bilateral sublingual, submandibular, and submental space involvement	"Brawny edema" of the neck; upper airway obstruction with stridor	Airway stabilization; broad-spectrum antibiotics	Immediate OMFS or ENT consult; prepare for OR	Failure to be prepared for a surgical airway; almost 100% mortality if untreated (most from airway compromise)
Parapharyngeal infections: Lateral space and retropharyngeal space	Multiple etiologies: Odontogenic, tonsillitis, pharyngitis, foreign body	Pharyngeal bulging, dysphagia, trismus; posterior compartment of lateral space may not produce intraoral swelling; nuchal rigidity with prevertebral involvement	CT scan defines location and extent of abscess; lateral neck x-ray may show retropharyngeal abscess	OMFS consult (if felt odontogenic); ENT consult for peritonsillar or pharyngeal origin.	Differentiating from peritonsillar abscess may be quite difficult
Mediastinitis	Two routes of spread: deep cervical planes, carotid sheath	Chest pain, severe dyspnea, systemic toxicity	Mainly clinical Dx; widened mediastinum on CXR possible	Intravenous antibiotics; hospitalize	Failure to consider Dx, even when odontogenic source may have cleared
Cavernous sinus thrombosis	Thrombophlebitis or septic emboli spread via facial veins	Ocular pain, orbital edema, retinal hemorrhages early; CN III, IV, V, VI deficits; commonly spreads to contralateral side	Usually dramatic findings; CT scan or MRI may confirm Dx	Hospitalize	Failure to consider Dx

ABX, antibiotics; DX, diagnosis; f/u, follow up; m., muscle; OMFS, oral/maxillofacial surgeon; CT, computed tomography; i.v, intravenous; ENT, ear, nose, and throat; OR, operating room; CN, cranial nerve; MRI, magnetic resonance imaging.

The presence of more serious infections is determined by common physical signs such as fever and swelling. Any involvement of the internal pterygoid or the masseter muscle will result in trismus (muscle spasm causing inability to open the mandible). The presence of trismus limits visibility of the oropharynx and makes the clinical diagnosis of retropharyngeal involvement difficult. If a toxic patient with trismus should vomit, the danger of aspiration is high because the emesis cannot be quickly evacuated. Therefore, patients with severe trismus need an aggressive work up (including a CT scan of the retropharyngeal space) and admission for hydration and parenteral antibiotics.

EMERGENCY DEPARTMENT MANAGEMENT

Treatment of patients with a periapical or periodontal abscess consists of a conservative incision and drainage (if fluctuant), and antibiotic therapy (penicillin or erythromycin 250 mg four times a day) (1,2). The gingiva should be anesthetized superficially with 2% lidocaine with epinephrine. A stab incision is made toward the alveolar bone and must extend through the periosteum if no pus is initially encountered; blunt dissection is performed with a mosquito hemostat. The area is irrigated, and, if there is room, a Penrose or iodoform drain can be placed. The drain should be secured with a black silk suture. In the case of these localized infections, there is no need to open the abscess beyond a stab incision. The drain will allow for continued drainage and the source of the infection will be eliminated with extraction of the tooth, root canal (endodontic) therapy, or periodontal therapy (5).

Treatment of odontogenic infections must always begin with the offending tooth. Incision and drainage of swelling addresses the acute situation but the pulp must be removed or the source of infection remains. Despite the increasing emergence of beta-lactamase producing bacteria these antibiotics remain the group of choice in odontogenic infections. Penicillin V (phenoxymethyl penicillin) is an effective, inexpensive first-line choice and unless penicillin allergy exist should be prescribed for outpatient therapy. Penicillin G is a suitable parenteral choice. Extended half-life products should be considered when compliance is a concern. Macrolide antibiotics are not typically first-choice drugs in dental infections but are indicated when patients have a history of adverse reactions to the penicillins. Clindamycin has become a favorite in dentistry. It exhibits bactericidal activity by binding to the same ribosome as erythromycin. It has a small structure that diffuses extremely well into bone with a spectrum that includes oral pathogens and can be used for endocarditis prophylaxis in penicillin-sensitive patients. The initial drug of choice remains penicillin for odontogenic infections but options for patients with a history of adverse reactions to beta-lactams are many.

Odontogenic infections are caused by dissemination of oral flora. Penicillin is the antibiotic of choice for the treatment of most orofacial infections, with the exception of some *Bacteroides* species. High-dose penicillin G (12 million U/d) is required for Ludwig angina. Second- or third-generation cephalosporins are useful in cases that involve *Bacteroides* or penicillin allergy, although cross-over sensitivity must be considered. Ampicillin/sulbactam (Unasyn) also provides excellent anaerobic coverage. Clindamycin is a useful alternative, Chloramphenicol is reserved for extreme situations in which there is no alternative therapy (1,3,12). Failure of an oral infection to respond within 24 hours of penicillin therapy suggests infection with an anaerobic bacteria (*Bacteroides fragilis*).

Patients with mild sialoadenitis may be treated on an outpatient basis with an antibiotic with Gram positive coverage (Cephalexin, Dicloxacillin), and a sialagogue (lemon juice) to stimulate salivary flow.

Parapharyngeal space infections (sublingual, submandibular, submaxillary, lateral pharyngeal, retropharyngeal, and pretracheal) are polymicrobial. Appropriate antibiotic therapy includes penicillin G (high-dose) and metronidazole or cefoxitin. Alternative therapy may include clindamycin or ticarcillin/clavulanate (Timentin). The presence of *Ludwig angina* requires aggressive attention to the airway. This may include nasotracheal intubation, tracheostomy, or observation in an intensive care environment where such procedures can be rapidly undertaken (1,3).

CRITICAL INTERVENTIONS

- Order a CT scan in the patient with a suspected parapharyngeal infection, and initiate early parenteral antibiotic coverage
- Be prepared to manage the airway in the patient with Ludwig angina, and this serious deep space infection has the potential for airway compromise

DISPOSITION

Role of the Consultant

Patients with a simple periapical abscess can be managed with the institution of intraoral saline rinses, analgesia, and oral antibiotics. As discussed, a simple incision and drainage may be indicated. Follow up should be arranged the next day with the oral and maxillofacial surgeon or the family dentist (1,5).

Indications for Admission

All patients with suspicion of extension of infection to the fascial spaces of the head and neck should be admitted. Facial cellulitis with closure of the eye indicates potential spread of infection to the periorbital spaces and increased potential for cavernous sinus thrombosis. Patients with extensive trismus cannot be adequately evaluated by clinical examination.

Patients with Ludwig angina or impending Ludwig angina (i.e., involvement of the three spaces without elevation of the tongue) are at risk for immediate airway obstruction and should be admitted. Such airway obstruction can occur precipitously and without warning, so anticipation is necessary. In most cases, the patient is admitted to the oral and maxillofacial surgeon. When the cause of the infection is unclear, the patient may be managed by an otorhinolaryngologist. Many cases are managed jointly by both services.

Transfer Considerations

If the initial receiving hospital has no surgical backup in the area of the head and neck, the patient should be transferred expeditiously to an appropriate facility. Blood cultures should be obtained and antibiotics instituted after consultation with the receiving physician. Special attention should be given to the airway. Advanced life-support personnel should be used. In the case of Ludwig angina, it may be necessary to establish a definite airway before transfer in order to adequately stabilize the patient.

COMMON PITFALLS

✔ Failure to carefully examine patients with orofacial swelling for an infection extending along fascial planes

✔ Underestimation of the potential for infectious spread to the mediastinum or around the airway, both of which can be fatal

Acknowledgments

The author gratefully acknowledges the contributions of Barry Hendler, Byron Thompson and R. Gregory Smith to the content of this chapter.

References

1. Amsterdam J. Dental Emergencies. In: Mark J, ed. *Rosen's Emergency Medicine: concepts and clinical practice,* 5th ed., C.V. Mosby, 2002.
2. Amsterdam JT, Hendler BH, Rose LF. Dental emergencies. In: Schwartz G, et al, eds. *Principles and practice of emergency medicine,* 2nd ed. Philadelphia: WB Saunders, 1986.
3. Amsterdam JT, Hendler BH. Deep space infections of the head and neck. In: Callaham ML, ed. *Current practice of emergency medicine,* 2nd ed. Philadelphia: BC Decker, 1991.
4. Amsterdam JT. Dental caries. In: Honigman B, ed. *Emergindex.* Denver: Emergency Information Center, 1993.
5. Amsterdam JT. Emergency dental procedures. In: Roberts J, Hedges J, eds. *Clinical procedures in emergency medicine,* 4th ed. Philadelphia: WB Saunders, 2003.
6. Bronstein SL, Tomasetti BJ, Ryan DE. Internal derangements of the TMJ: correlation of arthrography with surgical findings. *J Oral Surg* 1981;39:572.
7. Chase DC, Dolwick MF, Hendler BH, et al. TMJ disorders—treatment. *Patient Care* 1984;18:1.
8. Dice WH, Pryor GJ, Kilpatrick WR. Facial cellulitis following dental injury in a child. *Ann Emerg Med* 1985;11:541.
9. Fonseca R (ed.). *Oral and Maxillofacial Surgery.* Philadelphia: W.B. Saunders, 2000.
10. Hendler BH, Amsterdam JT. Infection of dental origin. *Curr Top Emerg Med* 1981;2:1.
11. Hendler BH, Quinn PD. Fatal mediastinitis secondary to odontogenic infection. *J Oral Surg* 1978;36:308.
12. Hendler BH. Maxillofacial fractures. In: Tintinalli JE, Ruiz E, Krome R, et al., eds. *Emergency medicine—a comprehensive study guide,* 4th ed, chapter 204. New York: McGraw-Hill, 1996.
13. Kaplan A. *Temporomandibular disorders.* Philadelphia: WB Saunders, 1991.
14. Lanigan DT, Hey JH, West RA. Aseptic necrosis following maxillary osteotomies: report of 36 cases. *J Oral Maxillofac Surg* 1990;48:142.
15. Lanigan DT, Hey JH, West RA. Hemorrhage following mandibular osteotomies: a report of 21 cases. *J Oral Maxillofac Surg* 1991;49:713.
16. Lanigan DT, Hey JH, West RA. Major vascular complications of orthognathic surgery: hemorrhage associated with LeFort I osteotomies. *J Oral Maxillofac Surg* 1990;48:561.
17. Lanigan DT, West RA. Management of postoperative hemorrhage following the Le Fort I maxillary osteotomy. *J Oral Maxillofac Surg* 1984;42:367.
18. Laskin D. Medical management of TMJ disorders. *Oral Maxillofac Surg Clin North Am* 1995;7.
19. Peterson LJ. Prevention and management of surgical complications. In: Peterson LJ, Ellis E, Hupp JR, et al., eds. *Contemporary oral and maxillofacial surgery.* St. Louis: Mosby, 1988.
20. Rantala MA, Ahlberg J, Suvinen TI, Nissinen M, et al. Temporomandibular joint related painless symptoms, orofacial pain, neck pain, headache, and psychosocial factors among non-patients. *Acta Ondontol Scand;* 2003;217–222.
21. Sisk AL, Hammer WB, Shelton DW, et al. Complications after removal of impacted third molars. *J Oral Maxillofac Surg* 1986;44:855.
22. Swartz JD, Hendler BH. High-resolution CT in evaluation of TMJ disease. *Head Neck Surg* 1985;7:409.
23. Taro A.*TMJ arthroscopy: a diagnostic and surgical atlas.* Philadelphia: JB Lippincott Co, 1993.

CHAPTER 25
Nontraumatic Upper Airway Obstruction

Joseph E. Clinton

The physician who faces a terrified patient experiencing rapidly progressive airway obstruction knows the meaning of apprehension. Evaluation, differential diagnosis, and emergency intervention all must occur simultaneously. The window of time for solution before irreversible injury occurs is so small that there is no margin for error. Progressive airway compromise exemplifies our need to anticipate, prepare, and practice to deal with the responsibility of emergency airway management.

Effective emergency management requires early recognition of a high-risk clinical situation and anticipation of further deterioration in the airway status. This approach allows intervention to occur at the proper time, before the situation becomes desperate. The necessary therapy is likely to be less traumatic to the patient if given early in a controlled manner. Preparation of equipment, drills of the emergency team, and practice of technique all contribute to lessen risk and improve patient outcome.

This chapter presents an overview of nontraumatic conditions that affect upper airway patency. The focus here is on the development of the airway obstruction, its recognition, and early management.

CLINICAL PRESENTATION

Nontraumatic airway obstruction is often insidious in onset. Once begun, the process may deteriorate gradually or decompensate suddenly without warning. Neither the person eating a large piece of steak nor the adult with epiglottitis expects to soon be suffocating. Obstruction occurs abruptly in the first case; hours may pass during the obstructive process in the second. The emergency physician must understand the disease processes at work and be prepared to intervene quickly.

Several factors may affect individual manifestations of the process. The site of the obstruction, the size of the obstructing agent, and associated spasm and edema are important determinants of the presentation. Historical factors may simplify the diagnosis. Physical findings may be nonspecific, or simply serve to separate patients into a category of obstruction.

In 2000, 160 children in the USA ages 14 years or younger died from an obstruction of the respiratory tract due to inhaled or ingested foreign bodies. Of these, 41% were caused by food items and 59% by nonfood objects (CDC, unpublished data) (17). The well-known "café coronary" syndrome effects adults and usually occurs without warning (11,16).

Airway obstruction can proceed from apparent normalcy to obvious distress with a patient in an agonal state. The pattern of increasing obstruction is first evidenced by some subjective findings of respiratory distress by the patient. The initial subjective finding may appear as "wheezing" with both an inspiratory and an expiratory component. Further obstruction alters the finding to stridor. Next, the airway obstructs completely and the patient struggles, loses consciousness, and will die without effective intervention to restore airway patency.

Apprehension and agitation develop as the obstruction increases. Fear exists in the eyes of a conscious patient experiencing airway obstruction, and all who are present can sense the patient's discomfort. An atmosphere of near hysteria can develop in the absence of an organized approach to relieve the obstruction. One of the benefits of public education on the choking victim has been to provide instruction that channels energies from useless activity into airway-clearing maneuvers.

Although airway obstruction by a foreign body, such as food, occurs suddenly, obstruction by an expanding mass effect within the upper airway is more insidious. Abscesses may obstruct the airway by their location. Expanding hematomas behave similarly. Edema and soft-tissue swelling owing to infection or allergy behave slightly differently because of a more diffuse mass effect.

Signs to anticipate in the patient suspected of developing airway obstruction vary slightly, depending on the cause, but some generalization can be made. The habitus of the patient is important to note. An upright posture with the neck extended in the sniffing position is characteristic in the patient with supraglottic obstruction, such as epiglottitis. Forcing a supine position in such a patient for the convenience of the medical team is disastrous. Pursing of the lips is commonly noted in patients who are struggling for air. An asymmetrical mass may increase in size during the observation period.

DIFFERENTIAL DIAGNOSIS

The differential diagnosis of upper airway obstruction includes several causes for the obstruction. Foreign body obstruction, infection, hypersensitivity, hemorrhagic disorders, extrinsic mass, and neoplasia all may result in the syndrome of upper airway obstruction. The patient's presentation may quickly narrow the diagnosis, or the diagnosis may remain a mystery until late in the patient's course.

Foreign Body Obstruction

The classic example of upper airway obstruction by a foreign body is the "cafe coronary." Food that causes an obstruction has often been poorly masticated. The victim may have painful or poorly fitting dentures or otherwise poor dentition that hampers chewing. Alcohol consumption is often implicated in the condition. This type of obstruction usually occurs in the supraglottic area and responds to the airway maneuvers prescribed by the American Heart Association (2).

Aspirated toys or smaller pieces of food may pass the vocal cords and produce obstruction in the subglottic area. These obstructions may be intermittent and aggravated by the head-down position, which allows gravitational movement of the object to an obstructive position. Back, blows and the head-down position may actually worsen these obstructions. The clinical presentation of a subglottic foreign body may be one of localized wheezing and atelectasis of obstructed pulmonary segments as the foreign body becomes lodged in a bronchus (18).

Any object that can fit in the mouth may produce airway obstruction given proper circumstances. The broad range of possibilities is best approached by attempts to differentiate supraglottic and subglottic obstructions. The site of the obstruction affects management decisions. A supraglottic obstruction that is not removable may be bypassed by tracheal intubation or surgical airway placement. A subglottic obstruction may require a more difficult airway decision, depending on its location. Magill or spongestick forceps may allow removal of foreign bodies under direct vision (9). An aspiration technique devised by Ernest Ruiz, MD (described in abstract form only) uses a blunted (tip cut off) endotracheal tube, wall suction and a meconium aspirator or "Y" connector to the tube. Animal experience demonstrates greatly facilitated removal of subglottic foreign bodies such as balloons and steak (19).

Infection

Cellulitis of oropharyngeal structures produces a treacherous setting in which airway compromise develops with little notice in a patient who has dysphonia and limited communication capacity. *Ludwig angina* (cellulitis of the sublingual space) can quickly obstruct the airway. The condition is a true otolaryngologic emergency that requires airway maintenance and antibiotic therapy (21). *Retropharyngeal* or *parapharyngeal abscess* can cause gradual obstruction owing to expansion and catastrophic deterioration through sudden rupture into the airway (18). *Epiglottitis* may produce sufficient swelling to produce airway obstruction in the adult or child. The natural history of these conditions needs to be kept clearly in mind when evaluating the emergency patient.

Hypersensitivity

Anaphylaxis can present suddenly after exposure to a known or unrecognized antigenic stimulus. When its representation is in the form of laryngeal edema, prompt intervention is needed to interrupt the obstructing process (see Chapter 131). A delay in the initiation of medical therapy may force surgical intervention in order to save the patient's life. Food, drug, and insect sting allergies are commonly encountered causes of anaphylactic airway emergencies. A history of exposure may depend on the patient's ability to communicate, which is directly related to the degree of airway compromise that is present.

Hereditary angioneurotic edema (HANE) is an autosomal dominant-inherited condition that is manifested by sudden edema of the face, hands, abdominal viscera, and airway. Airway obstruction is the most dramatic and life-threatening complication of the disease (4). Episodes may be triggered by minor trauma, emotional distress, and surgery. No race or sex predilection exists, and family history may be negative. HANE is most commonly characterized by a complement deficiency of C1 esterase inhibitor (C1 INH). The postulation is that the excess of a C2 kinin develops because of the inhibitor deficiency, and the C2 kinin is responsible for the increased capillary permeability seen in HANE.

Angiotensin-converting enzyme (ACE) inhibitor agents for control of hypertension have become a new cause of angioedema in patients previously free of the condition (6,24). Moderate to complete airway obstruction may occur. The drugs must be discontinued in patients experiencing this adverse reaction to prevent recurrence.

Hemorrhagic Disorders

The widespread use of anticoagulants for the treatment of cardiac and cerebrovascular disease has increased the population at risk for spontaneous hematoma formation. Spontaneous hematomas may develop throughout the body without any special predilection to one area. When the pharynx, tongue, or soft tissues surrounding these structures are involved, airway compromise is a predictable consequence.

Warfarin-treated patients have been reported with airway compromise owing to hematoma of the sublingual space, retropharynx and hypopharynx (3,5). The syndrome is marked by rapid, unexpected deterioration of a person who, in most cases, was previously healthy. Pain is often noted early, frequently preceding other symptoms. Signs of airway obstruction may develop before the examiner's eyes. Physical examination often reveals an area of swelling, frequently without ecchymosis. Soft-tissue radiography of the neck, computerized tomography, and indirect laryngoscopy are often useful. Close observation during the evaluation period is essential to avoid unrecognized abrupt deterioration with adverse outcome.

Extrinsic Mass

Unusual causes of airway obstruction owing to an extrinsic mass are occasionally seen. An example is the development of an obstruction in the esophagus caused by achalasia (23). The distended esophagus impinges on the airway in the neck and produces recurrent airway obstruction that disappears when the esophageal obstruction is cleared. Cystic lesions of various types may produce a similar syndrome that may require temporary airway support until the lesion is removed.

Neoplasia

Direct or indirect airway obstruction may result from neoplastic disorders. Laryngeal carcinoma and intrinsic airway tumors produce a gradually developing obstruction that may be mistaken for bronchospastic disease. Bypass of the laryngeal lesion by intubation or cricothyrotomy reveals an abrupt decrease in airway resistance. The abrupt resistance change localizes the disease to a site above the distal end of the tracheal tube. Tumor masses extrinsic to the airway may impinge on its lumen in a manner similar to that described for cystic lesions (8). Mediastinal tumors may produce a superior vena caval syndrome leading to airway obstruction (22).

Congenital tumors of the oropharynx or neck may present immediate and unexpected airway emergencies at birth. Such a condition requires immediate availability of neonatal resuscitation capabilities and surgical readiness (10).

Kaposi sarcoma of the larynx is an increasingly occurring cause of emergent airway obstruction. The airway must be carefully managed to avoid hemorrhagic complications (1,20).

EMERGENCY DEPARTMENT EVALUATION

Regardless of the cause of the obstruction, the emergency physician must first gauge its severity by quickly placing the patient in one of four categories:

1. Stable, deterioration risk low
2. Stable, deterioration risk high
3. Compromised respiration
4. Agonal respirations

Once this immediate classification has been made, the evaluation and therapy process can proceed with the appropriate degree of urgency.

A patient in the first category has been determined to be stable and at low risk of deterioration. This categorization is the most hazardous for the emergency physician to make. It implies that the patient can be evaluated at a leisurely pace with a minimal degree of observation. However, airway-obstructing lesions notoriously deteriorate unexpectedly in patients who looked well minutes before the decompensation. Classification of a patient in the first category implies a certainty of diagnosis that is usually absent during initial evaluation. Although the patient may be placed in this category after an observation and data collection period, it is seldom appropriate to place a patient with suspected airway compromise in this category early in the evaluation period.

The second category reflects the appropriate degree of concern during initial evaluation of any patient in whom airway obstruction is suspected. The risk of deterioration calls for con-

stant observation with equipment in readiness to intervene if necessary. Measures intended to arrest the underlying obstructive process should be instituted as soon as possible. Laboratory studies may be helpful in confirming an infectious or hemorrhagic etiology. A lateral cervical spine radiograph may reveal a thick epiglottis or signs of a retropharyngeal abscess, such as prevertebral thickening or gas. CT scan may further delineate a mass or abscess impinging upon the airway, but must be used carefully in the patient who may not tolerate the time and positioning necessary to obtain such studies (see Chapter 25).

The third category, with established airway compromise, calls for immediate decision on airway intervention. The emergency physician must quickly assess the likelihood of success with a medical approach before airway establishment by intubation or surgical approach is required. The judgment must be made using clinical experience. An arterial blood gas analysis may help with the decision when it can be obtained immediately, but often such testing only delays needed therapy.

The last category, with the patient in an agonal state, represents the most straightforward, immediate evaluation and therapy situation. The airway must be established immediately.

EMERGENCY DEPARTMENT MANAGEMENT

Airway management is the second part of the evaluation and therapeutic tightrope that must be walked when dealing with upper airway obstruction. The differential diagnosis coupled with the severity assessment will guide the therapeutic approach.

General Therapy

The patient who is presently stable is a candidate for therapy that might obviate the need for airway intervention. Medical interventions are most effective when directed at a specific cause, but a few nonspecific interventions may be of benefit early. Oxygen supplementation should be initiated in all cases. Consideration needs to be given to nebulization therapy with racemic epinephrine or beta-2 agents and steroids to decrease edema in hypersensitivity or croup syndromes. If infection is a possibility, then appropriate antibiotic therapy should be considered. Bleeding disorders need supplementation of coagulation factors to arrest the process.

A mixture of 80% helium and 20% oxygen (Heliox) has been suggested as a temporizing measure in patients with airway obstruction caused by tumors (14). The density of the mixture is one third that of air. The increased flow of gas allowed by the decreased density may improve oxygenation in selected patients with narrowed upper airways. Application of the gas mixture in other types of airway obstruction has been limited. Care should be exercised when withdrawing Heliox to avoid the abrupt deterioration associated with increased work of respiration.

Specific Therapy

The likelihood that foreign body obstruction exists should prompt airway-clearing maneuvers to be implemented according to widely accepted protocols described by the American Heart Association (2). Failure to clear the airway should lead to more aggressive airway establishment maneuvers.

The incidence of *acute epiglottis* in children under age 5 has dramatically decreased with Hemophilus influenza type B vaccine from 43 per 100,000 in 1987 to 1.3 per 100,000 in 1997 (18). The disease continues to exist with lower frequency due to Hemophilus and other infectious agents. Careful controlled airway establishment is the airway approach preferred by most authors. The disease continues to occur in both children and adults. Either group may deteriorate unexpectedly. They need to be monitored constantly until the infection recedes. Preparation for surgical airway placement must be constant.

The patient with a hemorrhagic disorder with associated warfarin therapy requires some medical therapy to reverse the coagulopathy. The most rapid correction of the clotting abnormality is by administration of fresh frozen plasma (FFP) or prothrombin complex concentrates. Airway obstruction is an indication for rapid reversal with fresh frozen plasma (3,5). Vitamin K enhances clotting factor synthesis in the liver. Levels of dependent factors II, VII, IX, and X begin to increase 2 hours after vitamin K, administration with significant elevation in 6 to 8 hours, and are frequently normal in 24 hours.

The patient with hypersensitivity or anaphylaxis should be treated emergently with epinephrine, diphenhydramine, and steroids (see Chapter 131).

Airway-opening Maneuvers

Airway-opening maneuvers such as chin lift, head tilt, and oral and nasal airways are most useful in patients with a decreased level of consciousness (2). The situation is quite different if the comatose state is a result of hypoxia owing to airway obstruction. Patients who are suffering from an airway obstructive process need more than these devices provide. Specific medical therapy and more aggressive airway intervention therapy are usually indicated.

Nonsurgical Management

A patient with significant airway compromise who does not improve with medical intervention will often require tracheal intubation. Blind nasotracheal or orotracheal intubation will suffice in many cases in which the decision is made before the airway is completely obstructed. Rapid sequence orotracheal intubation will often facilitate intubation. Whether it will facilitate removal of the airway obstruction depends on its etiology and location. The physician must weigh the risks of paralysis against its potential benefit in each case (see Chapters 1 and 2).

Useful adjuncts for difficult intubation include the gum elastic bougie, the lighted stylet, the intubating laryngeal mask airway (ILMA), and the combitube. Inability to remove an obstructive agent or to secure the airway with tracheal intubation is an indication to pursue surgical approaches to the airway.

Surgical Management

Transtracheal needle ventilation using a high-pressure oxygen source temporarily provides oxygenation, and minimal ventilation when exhalation can still occur through the upper airway. The presence of a ball-valve mechanism of the obstruction will allow exhalation to occur. The technique is a temporizing measure that allows time to secure the airway by other, more definitive means. Cricothyrotomy is the emergency surgical airway of choice for most airway-obstructing lesions. If the offending lesion is subglottic, such as a laryngeal abscess, hematoma, or tumor, then tracheostomy is preferred (15).

CRITICAL INTERVENTIONS

- Plan and prepare for airway management in the patient with impending airway obstruction before it occurs
- Rapidly assess and treat the patient simultaneously
- Administer appropriate specific therapies (epinephrine, FFP, antibiotics) in order to potentially avoid the need for airway management

DISPOSITION

Role of the Consultant

The development of protocols for treatment of the wide variety of obstructive conditions needs to be begun by the emergency physician. Cooperative team effort needs to be organized between the emergency, anesthesia, otolaryngology, pediatric, and medicine department personnel who will be dealing with the patients, depending on the cause. Treatment of pediatric epiglottitis is an excellent example of the type of cooperative efforts that can optimize results. Communication and agreement on management should occur in advance for the common, recurrent clinical problems, such as epiglottitis. The cooperative approach developed with these cases will carry over to optimize management of the more unusual causes of airway obstruction.

Indications for Admission

The patient with airway obstruction needs to be under constant observation in an intensive care unit until the risk of airway obstruction has passed. Whenever doubt exists as to the immediate future course of a patient with airway obstruction, intensive care unit admission is mandatory.

COMMON PITFALLS

- ✔ Underestimation of the potential for sudden deterioration
- ✔ Inadequate preparation of equipment and personnel
- ✔ Failure to monitor for the development of pulmonary edema after the airway obstruction has been relieved. The mechanism is unclear but is presumably related to the sudden decrease in hydrostatic pressure (12,13)

References

1. Alkhuja S, Menkel R, Patel B, Ibrahimbacha A. Stridor and difficult airway in an AIDS patient. *AIDS Patient Care STDS* 2001;15:293–295.
2. Association AH. *BLS for healthcare providers*. Dallas, TX: American Heart Association, 2001.
3. Bloom DC, Haegen T, Keefe MA. Anticoagulation and spontaneous retropharyngeal hematoma. *J Emerg Med* 2003;24:389–394.
4. Bork K, Hardt J, Schicketanz KH, Ressel N. Clinical studies of sudden upper airway obstruction in patients with hereditary angioedema due to C1 esterase inhibitor deficiency. *Arch Intern Med* 2003;163:1229–1235.
5. Boster SR, Bergin JJ. Upper airway obstruction complicating warfarin therapy–with a note on reversal of warfarin toxicity. *Ann Emerg Med* 1983;12:711–715.
6. Chiu AG, Newkirk KA, Davidson BJ, et al. Angiotensin-converting enzyme inhibitor-induced angioedema: a multicenter review and an algorithm for airway management. *Ann Otol Rhinol Laryngol* 2001;110:834–840.
7. Clinton JE, Mcgill JW. Basic emergency airway management and decision-making. In: Roberts JR, Hedges JR, eds. *Clinical Procedures in Emergency Medicine*. Philadelphia: W.B. Saunders Co., 1998:1–15.
8. Hasan R, Marshall MC, Jr., Medhi M, et al. Meningioma metastatic to thyroid gland. *Endocr Pract* 2001;7:370–374.
9. Higgins GL, 3rd, Burton JH, Carter WP, Floor AE. Comparison of extraction devices for the removal of supraglottic foreign bodies. *Prehosp Emerg Care* 2003;7:316–321.
10. Holinger LD, Birnholz JC. Management of infants with prenatal ultrasound diagnosis of airway obstruction by teratoma. *Ann Otol Rhinol Laryngol* 1987;96:61–64.
11. Jacob B, Wiedbrauck C, Lamprecht J, Bonte W. Laryngologic aspects of bolus asphyxiation-bolus death. *Dysphagia* 1992;7:31–35.
12. Lim KA. Post-laryngospasm pulmonary oedema in oral & maxillofacial surgery. *Singapore Dent J* 2000;23:38–41.
13. Maroof M, Khan RM, Ryley BG, Cooper T. Post-anaesthetic pulmonary oedema following upper airway obstruction. *J Pak Med Assoc* 1994;44:244–247.
14. McGee DL, Wald DA, Hinchliffe S. Helium-oxygen therapy in the emergency department. *J Emerg Med* 1997;15:291–296.
15. Mcgill JW, Clinton JE. Tracheal Intubation. In: Roberts JR, Hedges JR, eds. *Clinical Procedures in Emergency Medicine*. Philadelphia: W.B. Saunders Co. 1998:15–44.
16. Mittleman RE, Wetli CV. The fatal cafe coronary. Foreign-body airway obstruction. *JAMA* 1982;247:1285–1288.

17. Nonfatal choking-related episodes among children–United States, 2001. *MMWR Morb Mortal Wkly Rep* 2002;51:945–948.
18. Rotta AT, Wiryawan B. Respiratory emergencies in children. *Respir Care* 2003;48:248–258; discussion 258–260.
19. Ruiz E, Stolzenberg BT, Bowker DB. Total obstruction of the trachea by foreign bodies: a practical solution to a rapidly fatal problem. *J Emerg Med* 1998;16(Suppl2):81S.
20. Schiff NF, Annino DJ, Woo P, Shapshay SM. Kaposi's sarcoma of the larynx. *Ann Otol Rhinol Laryngol* 1997;106:563–567.
21. Srirompotong S, Art-Smart T. Ludwig's angina: a clinical review. *Eur Arch Otorhinolaryngol* 2003;260:401–403.
22. Szokol JW, Alspach D, Mehta MK, Parilla BV, Liptay MJ. Intermittent airway obstruction and superior vena cava syndrome in a patient with an undiagnosed mediastinal mass after cesarean delivery. *Anesth Analg* 2003;97:883–884.
23. Turkot S, Golzman B, Kogan J, et al. Acute upper-airway obstruction in a patient with achalasia. *Ann Emerg Med* 1997;29:687–689.
24. Zanoletti E, Bertino G, Malvezzi L, Benazzo M, Mira E. Angioneurotic edema of the upper airways and antihypertensive therapy. *Acta Otolaryngol* 2003;123:960–964.

CHAPTER 26
Sore Throat

Michael F. Murphy

Sore throat is a common presenting complaint in emergency medicine, particularly the acute variety. In Australia, it is the second most common illness for which medical attention is sought (4).

Most causes of sore throat are nonlife threatening. However, life-threatening causes of sore throat do exist. As with all of medicine, pattern recognition and the avoidance of error prone methods of decision-making are keys to identifying the life-threatening causes of sore throat.

Patients ordinarily associate the term 'throat' with what medical professionals term the 'pharynx'. The pharynx is a U-shaped fibromuscular tube extending from the base of the skull to the lower border of the cricoid cartilage where, at the level of the sixth cervical vertebra, it is continuous with the esophagus. Posteriorly it rests against the fascia covering the prevertebral muscles and the cervical spine. Anteriorly it opens into the nasal cavity (the nasopharynx), the mouth (the oropharynx) and the larynx (the laryngo- or hypopharynx).

The oropharyngeal musculature has a normal tone, like any other skeletal musculature, and this tone serves to keep the upper airway open during quiet respiration. Respiratory distress is associated with pharyngeal muscular activity that attempts to open the airway further. Benzodiazepines and other sedative hypnotic agents may attenuate some of this tone. This explains why sedation may lead to total airway obstruction in patients presenting with partial airway obstruction.

The glossopharyngeal nerve supplies sensation to the posterior one third of the tongue, lingual and faucial tonsils, the valleculae, the superior surface of the epiglottis and most of the posterior pharynx. This nerve also supplies sensation to a portion of the tympanic membrane, the carotid sheath, sinus and body, and the stylopharyngeus muscle. The innervation patterns as they relate to the carotid sheath and the epiglottis are important in identifying occult, but potentially lethal causes of sore throat.

Stimulation of the glossopharyngeal nerve at any of these locations may be interpreted by the patient as a "sore throat" (i.e., referred pain).

CLINICAL PRESENTATION

Most patients with sore throat are nontoxic appearing, have a clear voice, and no difficulty with respirations. Patients with streptococcal pharyngitis, however, may experience fever, significant pain, and become dehydrated. The challenge for the clinician is to provide symptomatic relief, and to identify those patients with serious pathology requiring specific treatment.

The patient with a retropharyngeal abscess presents with fever, neck pain, and sore throat out of proportion to the oropharyngeal findings. Other possible findings include odynophagia, neck swelling, drooling, torticollis, meningismus, cervical adenopathy, and stridor. The voice may be normal, though if the abscess is high in the neck, nasal obstruction and a hyponasal voice result, and a *"hot potato"* voice may be present if the swelling is above the level of the larynx. Chest pain associated with these symptoms strongly suggests mediastinal extension.

Peritonsillar abscess is part of a larger continuum of illness from tonsillitis through peritonsillar cellulitis to peritonsillar abscess. The patient may present at any point along this continuum, and symptoms and treatment vary accordingly. Peritonsillar cellulitis consists of inflammation without fluid collection. Patients generally complain of severe, unilateral throat pain.

Supraglottitis (epiglottitis), because of its occult nature, potential lethality and incidence in the population merits special discussion. For purposes of discussion, the clinical presentation may be categorized into a spectrum that varies from a fulminating course developing over hours to a subacute form smoldering for days to weeks:

Category 1: Severe respiratory distress, imminent, or actual respiratory arrest. Patients in category 1 typically report a history of a brief but rapidly progressive illness. Blood culture often reveals *H. influenzae* type B.

Category 2: Intermediate condition with moderate-to-severe symptoms and signs of potential airway compromise. Symptoms and signs include: inability to swallow or lie supine, dyspnea, severe sore throat, muffled voice, stridor, and the use of accessory muscles. The emergency physician should prepare to intervene if the airway should suddenly deteriorate, and then undertake further evaluation of the airway.

Category 3: Mild-to-moderate illness without indications of potential airway compromise. Patients may report a 3- to 14-day history of a sore throat and pain on swallowing, with minimal physical findings on examination. A patient can rapidly worsen with little warning.

DIFFERENTIAL DIAGNOSIS

Pain in the throat, or pharyngalgia, has many causes, and may be acute, subacute or chronic. The most common cause of all forms of sore throat is pharyngitis, meaning "inflammation of the pharyngeal mucous membrane," but "sore throat" and "pharyngitis" are not identical, since many noninflammatory disorders (e.g., oropharyngeal carcinomas) can also cause pharyngeal pain. However, local infection is the most common cause of inflammation of pharyngeal structures, or acute pharyngitis. While a variety of causes may be encountered (see

TABLE 26.1. Differential Diagnosis of Sore Throat

ACUTE PHARYNGITIS

- Bacterial infections:
  - Group A beta hemolytic streptococcus (GABHS)
  - Neisseria gonorrhea
  - Corynebacterium diphtheriae
- Viral infections:
  - Epstein Barr virus
  - Herpesvirus
  - Influenza virus
  - Rhinovirus
  - Coxsackievirus A
- Noninfectious
  - Stevens-Johnson syndrome:
  - Pemphigus
  - Angioedema

CHRONIC PHARYNGITIS

- gastroesophageal reflux disease (GERD)
- obstructive sleep apnea
- Fungal infections (e.g. Candida albicans)
- chronic sinusitis with postnasal drip
- inhalation of irritants (pyrethrins, chlorine gas, heavy smoking)
- breathing dry air
- Glossopharyngeal neuralgia
- Carcinomas: pharyngeal, lingual and tonsillar
- Monomyelocytic leukemia
- Thyroiditis

Retropharyngeal abscess
Peritonsillar cellulitis
Peritonsillar abscess
Supraglottitis/Epiglottitis

Table 26.1). The most common and serious are discussed in more detail below.

Acute Pharyngitis

Acute pharyngitis and tonsillopharyngitis are the most common causes of sore throat. Acute pharyngitis usually presents as the rather abrupt onset of pharyngeal pain particularly with swallowing (odynophagia). The severity of the pain is variable, usually being worse in the morning. Odynophagia that is so severe as to preclude swallowing is decidedly uncommon and should prompt one to consider conditions such as mononucleosis, epiglottitis, and complications of pharyngitis such as retropharyngeal or peritonsillar abscess. Important causes of acute pharyngitis include:

Bacterial infections

Group A beta hemolytic streptococcus (GABHS) is the most common cause of bacterial pharyngitis in children (see Chapter 260). The patient is typically between the ages of 3 and 25, though sore throat can occur at all ages. Over the years it has been felt that a number of historical and physical features favored a diagnosis of GABHS over viral etiologies of acute pharyngitis including younger age, higher fever, absence of a cough, anterior cervical adenitis and palatal petechiae. However, weighted scoring systems utilizing these criteria have not been sensitive or specific (2).

Neisseria gonorrhea: This sexually transmitted disorder may occur independent of a genital infection and is of variable severity. Gonococcal pharyngitis is an important source of gonococcemia (10).

Corynebacterium diphtheriae: This is a potentially lethal cause of pharyngitis. Sore throat and dysphagia are prominent symptoms, and patients exhibit a grey white pharyngeal mucosal membrane of varying size. Airway obstruction may follow. Despite immunization, large portions of the adult population in the United States lack immunity to the diphtheria toxin.

Viral infections: Viruses are the most common infectious causes of pharyngitis in adults and children (see Table 26.1).

Noninfectious causes of acute pharyngitis

Stevens-Johnson syndrome (SJS): an immune-mediated hypersensitivity disorder that is a severe expression of erythema multiforme. It usually involves the skin and the mucous membranes, and may cause severe erythema, edema, sloughing, blistering, ulceration, and necrosis of the oropharyngeal mucous membrane. Four etiologic categories have been identified: infectious (e.g., HSV and mycoplasma), drug-induced (e.g., sulfonamides and phenytoin), malignancy related, and idiopathic. SJS may be fatal.

Pemphigus: a group of rare autoimmune blistering diseases of the skin and/or mucous membranes. Pemphigus vulgaris is characterized by sores and blisters that almost always start in the mouth and carries a moderate to high mortality rate if unrecognized and untreated.

Retropharyngeal Abscess

Retropharyngeal abscess is more often a disease of young children and occurs when lymph nodes in the retropharyngeal space become infected. These lymph nodes involute by puberty. In adults, retropharyngeal abscess is predominantly caused by pharyngeal trauma and ingested foreign bodies, such as fishbones that penetrate the posterior pharyngeal wall (5,10). Traumatic causes include blunt and penetrating neck wounds, which have the potential to develop the delayed complication of an abscess, and iatrogenic injuries secondary to intubation or endoscopy. Uncommon causes include Pott disease (cervical tuberculosis), sinusitis, and otitis media. Retropharyngeal abscesses tend to be polymicrobial, with streptococcus, staphylococcus, and anaerobes most commonly recovered when cultured.

Peritonsillar Cellulitis and Abscess

Peritonsillar abscess is a complication of tonsillitis, whether from group A streptococcus or infectious mononucleosis (15). It occurs more frequently in teenagers and younger adults, but it can present at any age, especially in immunocompromised or diabetic patients. The abscess forms in the potential space between the lateral aspect of the tonsillar capsule and the superior constrictor muscle of the pharynx. When tonsillitis spreads beyond the tonsil capsule, inflammation in this space results in cellulitis and then abscess if left untreated. Abscess cultures tend to be polymicrobial, with the frequent presence of group A beta-hemolytic streptococci and anaerobes such as *Bacteroides*.

Supraglottitis/Epiglottitis

Supraglottitis is an acute disorder that usually produces substantial throat pain but is not generally considered a variant or a complication of acute pharyngitis. Strictly speaking, the term supraglottitis more appropriately defines the condition because the pathologic changes involve not only the epiglottis, but also the aryepiglottic folds and false cords. *Haemophilus influenzae* type B is the most common bacterium found in blood cultures, but *S. pneumoniae* and many others have also been isolated.

EMERGENCY DEPARTMENT EVALUATION

History

As with any presenting complaint the onset, location, radiation, duration, quality, timing and exacerbating and remitting factors of the pain or discomfort ought to be elicited. Throat pain of acute onset is far and away the commonest variety of sore throat encountered in the ED and most of the time a diagnosis of acute infectious pharyngitis is obvious so one needn't spend excessive time pursuing a detailed history or physical examination. However, if the etiology of the throat pain is not obvious, a more complete evaluation is indicated.

Has trauma been involved? Is a foreign body such as an impaled fishbone suspected? Has a caustic, irritative or thermal agent been inhaled or ingested? Is this a single episode of throat pain? Is it recurrent day to day; morning or evening; weekday versus weekend, or is it seasonal. How long has it persisted? Is it positional (erect versus flat)? Does mouth opening or closing affect it? Is it associated with meals, or certain types of foods (spicy or tart)?

The patient is often able to localize the pharyngeal site where the pain is originating i.e. the nasopharynx, the oropharynx, the hypopharynx; or the fauces. The radiation of pain pattern may indicate the location of a lesion; ordinarily, the association with swallowing is associated with faucial, lingual, oropharyngeal or hypopharyngeal disorders. Pain in the throat brought on by exertion and relieved by rest is particularly sinister.

Associated symptoms such as the presence or absence of cough, fever, and coryza should be noted. Additional historical features such as earache, stiff neck, hoarseness, odynophagia, pain on protruding the tongue, trismus, facial pain, perversions of taste, or a bad taste or oral odor may be helpful. Have any masses been noted by the patient? A history of contact with sources of infection is important, particularly in domiciliary and close social settings.

The functional inquiry (review of systems) is rarely helpful in cases of isolated sore throat. The past history may elicit temporal (e.g., seasonal) or situational (e.g., at work) patterns of symptomatology.

Physical Examination

The initial attention is directed to the general appearance of the patient and the vital signs, including oxygen saturation. Signs suggestive of upper airway obstruction are specifically noted. Systemic signs of sepsis should not be missed.

Patients with deep space neck infections and epiglottitis may be much sicker and appear toxic, dehydrated, and febrile. The patient with a retropharyngeal abscess may hold the head stiff, or lean it to one side in the case of a peritonsillar abscess; passive or active motion of the head and neck elicits pain. Inspection of the neck in these patients does not usually reveal any redness or swelling, although anterior displacement of the larynx may be appreciated in a retropharyngeal abscess or lateral displacement in a lateralized deep space infection.

Subsequently, an external examination of the face, mandibular space, and anterior neck is done first looking for:

- Sinus tenderness; parotid tenderness or induration
- Fullness, tenderness or masses in the mandibular space
- Masses (particularly pulsatile ones) and lymphadenopathy
- Tenderness along the carotid sheath and pain on laryngeal manipulation; deep tenderness and pain on laryngeal motion is seen with epiglottitis and low parapharyngeal abscesses

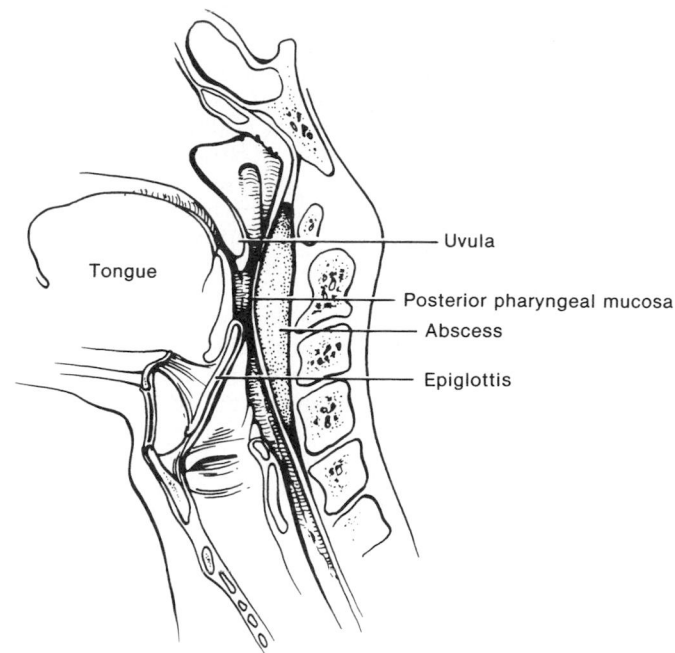

Figure 26.1.   Retropharyngeal abscess.

- Thyroid tenderness
- Cervical spine mobility

The carotids should be auscultated for bruits, and the oral cavity inspected. Trismus is often present with peritonsillar abscess, but not with uncomplicated retropharyngeal abscess or epiglottitis. Inflammation, mucosal ulcerations, purulence, and masses ought to be noted. The area of deep space abscess may appear erythematous, boggy. Displacement of structures (e.g., palatopharyngeal arches, soft palate, posterior pharyngeal wall) is also noted. In the case of a retropharyngeal abscess the posterior pharyngeal wall may be displaced forward toward the uvula (Fig. 26.1); a peritonsillar abscess displaces the tonsil downward and medially and deviates the uvula to the opposite side (Fig. 26.2). A process more caudal in the neck may show no abnormalities on oral examination.

The use of a tongue depressor to facilitate the exposure of oral and pharyngeal structures has generated some controversy due to the prohibition placed on such a maneuver in evaluating the pediatric patient with suspected epiglottitis. With this exception, there ought to be no reluctance to utilize this maneuver. The patient is asked to protrude their tongue as part of this examination and the presence of pain noted.

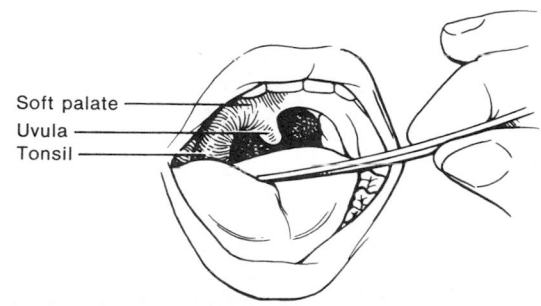

Figure 26.2.   Peritonsillar abscess.

Palpation presents the risk of being bitten or provoking the gag reflex, but it may be necessary particularly if an abscess or a lingual, tonsillar or base of tonsil lesion is suspected. The patient ought to be given lidocaine 4% to gargle and spit out, and gentle palpation undertaken. Additional intravenous moderate sedation and analgesia may be required to undertake this examination. While palpation of the posterior pharyngeal wall may confirm the diagnosis of a retropharyngeal abscess, *this maneuver is not recommended* but because of the risk of rupturing the abscess into an already compromised airway (7).

If a nasopharyngeal (e.g., carcinoma) or hypopharyngeal (e.g., epiglottitis) lesion is suspected but not visible on direct examination of the mouth and oropharynx flexible fiberoptic nasopharyngoscopy may be undertaken following the administration of a vasoconstrictor nasal spray (e.g., 0.25% phenylephrine nasal spray), topicalization of the nasal mucosa (e.g., lidocaine 4% atomized or by pledgets) and lidocaine 4% to gargle and spit out. The procedure is easily learned and performed by emergency practitioners.

Diagnostic Imaging

Radiologic studies are seldom indicated in the evaluation of a patient with sore throat. However, when one suspects the presence of retropharyngeal abscess or supraglottitis, the following studies may be useful:

Lateral soft tissue airway x-ray: this study may be indicated in patients exhibiting signs of upper airway obstruction that in the estimation of the emergency physician need to be retained in a resuscitation area. While this study is moderately highly sensitive (90%) in establishing a diagnosis of supraglottitis, a negative study does not exclude it. Findings that point toward a diagnosis of supraglottitis include enlargement of the epiglottis (*thumb sign*) and aryepiglottic folds, and ballooning of the hypopharynx. One study suggested that epiglottic and aryepiglottic widths greater than 8 mm and 7 mm, respectively, indicated acute epiglottitis (16). However, a 10% to 20% false-negative rate exists. Another study indexed both epiglottic and aryepiglottic width to third cervical vertebral body width and epiglottic width to epiglottic height and found that ratios greater than 0.5, 0.35, and 0.6, respectively, were 100% sensitive for epiglottitis (15). These results were derived from 33 patients, of which only 6 were adults. More recently, the qualitative evaluation of the presence or absence of a deep, well-defined vallecular air space (*vallecula sign*) running parallel to the pharyngotracheal air column that approaches the level of the hyoid bone in lateral soft-tissue neck radiographs was evaluated. This well-defined space was absent in all 26 consecutive confirmed cases of adult epiglottitis. Additionally, the investigators found a 98.2% sensitivity and 99.5% specificity in correctly identifying adult epiglottitis when random case controlled radiographs were examined by blinded participants. The authors suggest that this may be a useful diagnostic screen in patients who *do not require* immediate airway intervention (3).

CT scanning: Contrast enhanced CT scanning may be useful and is the imaging study of choice in defining the extent of deep space neck infection in peritonsillar, retropharyngeal and parapharyngeal abscesses if the patient is cooperative and sufficiently stable to lay flat and permit the study. The same can be said of ultrasound and MRI scanning (17,18).

Laboratory

General studies such as CBC, coagulation profiles, electrolyte studies, renal and hepatic function and others are usually not useful unless otherwise indicated. A blood sugar determination may be useful in diagnosing an occult diabetic.

GABHS studies: The Infectious Disease Society of America published guidelines for the diagnosis of GABHS pharyngitis (1). It recommends that unless the physician is able to confidently exclude the diagnosis of streptococcal pharyngitis on clinical grounds, either a throat culture or a rapid antigen detection test (RADT) should be done. A positive result of either test establishes the diagnosis of "strep throat." However, because of the insensitivity of the RADT, a negative test should be followed by a throat culture. The cost effectiveness of this strategy has been questioned (1). Others support making the decision on a clinical basis, with or without supplemental RADT testing, using clinical criteria such as the *Centor criteria* (fever, tonsillar exudates, cervical adenopathy, absence of cough) (19,20).

Neisseria gonorrhoea and Corynebacterium diphtheriae require specific collection techniques and culture media.

EMERGENCY DEPARTMENT MANAGEMENT

As with all patients that present to the emergency department, initial attention is directed to the ABCs and immediate life threats. The patient is observed for signs of airway compromise, respiratory distress and the vital signs are perused for evidence of cardiovascular compromise. The three cardinal signs of upper airway obstruction are: muffled voice (hot potato voice), difficulty swallowing secretions (either because of pain or obstruction), and stridor. The first two signs do not ordinarily herald imminent total upper airway obstruction, but stridor does. The presence of stridor is generally considered to indicate that the airway has been reduced to roughly 10% of its normal caliber. Any of these findings, along with the patient that insists on sitting erect and refusing to lay flat ought to prompt an immediate upgrade to an acute resuscitation locale in the ED and preparations for rapid evaluation and active airway intervention.

The treatment of sore throat without airway compromise is mostly symptomatic, utilizing gargles and mild analgesics. Ulcerated, extremely painful lesions may be dabbed with a cotton tipped swab containing a solution of 4% lidocaine and kaopectate (to make it adhere), though the efficacy of this therapy in relieving pain is anecdotal and unproven. Some have reported that adults with moderate/severe pharyngitis obtain relief of symptoms sooner if treated with dexamethasone (21,22). Specific management strategies include:

GABHS: A number of antibiotics have been shown to be effective in treating group A beta hemolytic streptococcal pharyngitis including penicillin and its congeners (such as ampicillin, amoxicillin, and the semisynthetic penicillins), as well as numerous cephalosporins, macrolides and clindamycin. Penicillin, however, remains the agent of choice because of its proven efficacy, safety, narrow spectrum, and its low cost (1,4). Patients with acute infectious mononucleosis treated with ampicillin or amoxicillin may develop a rash.

Supraglottitis: Patients with severe airway compromise or obstruction must receive definitive airway management in the emergency department. Patients with mild dyspnea or respiratory complaints may be observed and monitored in the intensive care setting. The remainder should undergo definitive airway management in the controlled setting of the operating room, and subsequently be admitted to the intensive care unit. The antibiotic of choice on empiric grounds is cefuroxime, cefotaxime, ceftriaxone, or ampicillin-sulbactam (Unasyn). Though some recommend the use of steroids, scientific evidence is lacking. Aerosolized epinephrine is not thought to be useful.

Retropharyngeal abscess: Intravenous fluids and intravenous antibiotics—high-dose penicillin (6 million U every 6 hours) and metronidazole (500 mg every 6 hours after a 1-g loading dose), or cefoxitin (2 g every 8 hours)—should be started immediately. An otolaryngology consult should be obtained early. Patients will likely be admitted to the intensive care unit or directly to the operating room. Definitive management includes incision and drainage under carefully controlled circumstances. The presence of mediastinitis mandates a significantly more extensive debridement by a thoracic surgeon (8). Incision and debridement for retropharyngeal cellulitis is at the discretion of the otolaryngologist.

Peritonsillar cellulitis: Intravenous fluids should be started to correct the dehydration that is usually present, and intravenous antibiotics initiated. Penicillin (1 to 2 million U every 4 hours) or clindamycin (600 mg every 8 hours) are good choices (13). Early cellulitis may be treated with hydration and antibiotics alone, though it may be difficult to differentiate from abscess. Needle aspiration may provide both diagnostic information and therapeutic benefit if abscess is present.

Peritonsillar abscess: In addition to the antibiotic regimen described for peritonsillar cellulitis, diagnostic and therapeutic needle aspiration is indicated (13). With patients in the sitting position, hunched slightly forward, apply topical anesthetic to the posterior pharynx. Instruct patients that although they will feel an initial puncture, the procedure will likely reduce their pain significantly. Aiming posteriorly toward the medial aspect of the enlarged tonsil, insert an 18- or 20-gauge needle to a depth of 2 cm, aspirating during insertion. Insertion of the needle more than two cm runs the risk of puncturing the internal carotid artery.

CRITICAL INTERVENTIONS

- Provide emergency airway management for patients with impending airway obstruction, such as severe supraglottitis or retropharyngeal abscess
- Rapidly initiate antibiotic therapy for serious throat infections
- Utilize diagnostic imaging studies as needed to identify patients with supraglottitis or retropharyngeal abscess

DISPOSITION

All patients with signs of upper airway obstruction should to be admitted. Immunocompromised patients may need to be admitted to hospital for aggressive intravenous antibiotic and fluid management and continuous observation.

All patients with epiglottitis or retropharyngeal abscess, whether or not they are intubated, should be admitted to an intensive care unit.

Nonimmunocompromised patients with uncomplicated, peritonsillar cellulitis that can maintain their hydration and take their medications orally may be discharged, provided they are in the company of a reliable caretaker and close follow up is arranged.

Patients with peritonsillar abscess that has been aspirated can be discharged on appropriate antibiotic therapy. If the aspiration does not relieve severe symptoms or if there is any suspicion of spread of infection beyond the peritonsillar area admission for incision and drainage and more intensive care will be required.

COMMON PITFALLS

- ✔ Overtreatment of pharyngitis, most of which is viral in etiology, with antibiotics
- ✔ Excluding the diagnosis of supraglottitis without visualization of the epiglottis and surrounding structures
- ✔ Underestimating the severity or potential for airway compromise in patients with retropharyngeal or peritonsillar abscess

References

1. Bisno AL, Gerber MA, Gwaltney JM Jr, et al. Infectious Diseases Society of America. Practice guidelines for the diagnosis and management of group A streptococcal pharyngitis. Infectious Diseases Society of America. *Clin Infect Dis* 2002;35:113–125.
2. Bisno AL, Peter GS, Kaplan EL. Diagnosis of strep throat in adults: are clinical criteria really good enough? *Clin Infect Dis* 2002;35:126–129.
3. Carey MJ. Epiglottitis in adults [Review]. *Am J Emerg Med* 1996;14:421.
4. Danchin MH, Curtis N, Nolan TM, et al. Treatment of sore throat in light of the Cochrane verdict: is the jury still out? *MJA* 2002;177:512–515.
5. Ducic Y, Hébert PC, MacLachlan L, et al. Description and evaluation of the vallecula sign: a new radiological sign in the diagnosis of adult epiglottitis. *Ann Emerg Med* 1997;30:1.
6. Golding–Wood DG, Whittet HB. The lingual tonsil: a neglected symptomatic structure. *J Laryngol Otol* 1989;103:922.
7. Herzon FS. Peritonsillar abscess: incidence, current management practices, and a proposal for treatment guidelines. *Laryngoscope* 1995;105:1.
8. Kieff DA, Bhattacharyua N, Siegel NS. Selection of antibiotics after incision and drainage. *Otolaryngol Head Neck Surg* 1999;120:57–61.
9. Kline JA, et al. Streptococcal pharyngitis: a review of pathophysiology, diagnosis, and management. *J Emerg Med* 1994;12:665.
10. Melio FR. Upper respiratory tract infections. In: Marx JA, Hockberger RS, Walls RM, et al. eds. *Rosen's Emergency Medicine, Fifth Edition.* Philadelphia: Mosby, 2002;969–985.
11. Neuner JM, Hamel MB, Phillips RS, et al. Diagnosis and management of adults with pharyngitis. A cost effectiveness analysis. *Arch Intern Med* 2003;139:113–122.
12. Ovassapian A, Glassenberg R, Randel GI, et al. The unexpected difficult airway and lingual tonsil hyperplasia: a case series and a review of the literature. *Anesthesiology* 2002;97:124–132.
13. Pichichero ME. Group A streptococcal tonsillopharyngitis: cost-effective diagnosis and treatment. *Ann Emerg Med* 1995;25:390.
14. Postma GN, et al. The professional voice. *Otolaryngol Head Neck Surg* 1998;000:00.
15. Rothrock SG, Pignatello GA, Howard RM. Radiologic diagnosis of epiglottitis: objective criteria for all ages. *Ann Emerg Med* 1990;19:978.
16. Schumaker HM, Doris PE, Birnbaum G. Radiologic parameters in adult epiglottitis. *Ann Emerg Med* 1984;13:588.
17. Scott PM, Loftus WK, Kew J, et al. Diagnosis of peritonsillar infections: a prospective study of ultrasound, computerized tomography and clinical diagnosis. *J Laryngol Otol* 1999;113:229–232.
18. Sethi DS, Stanley RE. Parapharyngeal abscesses. *J Laryngol Otol* 1991;105:1025–1030.
19. Centor RM, Witherspoon JM, Dalton HP, Brody CE, Link K. The diagnosis of strep throat in adults in the emergency room. *Med Decis Making* 1981;1(3):239–246.
20. Cooper RJ, Hoffman JR, Bartlett JG, et al. Principles of appropriate antibiotic use for acute pharyngitis in adults: background. *Arch Intern Med* 2001;134(6):509–517.
21. Marvez-Valls EG, Stuckey A, Ernst AA. A randomized clinical trial of oral versus intramuscular delivery of steroids in acute exudative pharyngitis. *Acad Emerg Med* 2002;9:9 14.
22. O'Brien JF, Meade JL, Falk JL. Dexamethasone as adjuvant therapy for severe acute pharyngitis. *Ann Emerg Med* 1993;22:212–215.

CHAPTER 27
Complications of Tracheostomies

Valerie Ann Dobiesz and Scott Andrew Miller

Tracheostomy is a mainstay in airway management of critically ill patients. A tracheostomy tube is placed because of mechanical obstruction, inability to clear secretions, or need for prolonged ventilation. A tracheostomy provides access for mechanical ventilation, clearance of secretions, and protection of the airway. This procedure may be done in the operating room using an open technique or at the bedside in the intensive care unit using a percutaneous dilation technique (PDT). This surgical procedure has been known for centuries, with references to this practice in Eber's Papyrus (1550 BC) and the ancient Rig Veda texts (two of the three oldest known medical works) (2,6).

Complications of these devices range from minor inconveniences for the patient to life-threatening emergencies and may occur immediately postoperatively or may be delayed in nature. Complications include local bleeding, obstruction, infection, stenosis, tracheoesophageal fistula, as well as pneumothorax, pneumomediastinum, air leaks, dislodgement, false passage, tracheostomy tube fractures, and decannulation. The overall mortality rate is <1% with a total complication rate of up to 65% (7). A greater mortality rate and complication rate is seen in emergency situations, ICU patients, and pediatrics. Because the tracheostomy tube is frequently encountered in the emergency department, emergency physicians must be aware of the purpose, structure, and proper maintenance of these devices so they will be prepared for complications.

HEMORRHAGE

Major hemorrhage during and soon after tracheostomy is rare, but can be life threatening. Bleeding complications account for 20% of ED tracheostomy visits (3). There are numerous vessels in the vicinity that can bleed and cause problems including the superficial blood vessels, thyroid vessels, carotid arteries, anterior jugular veins, and the innominate (bracheocephalic) artery. The lacerated thyroid gland can bleed, as can granulation tissue. Incisional or stomal bleeding may be controlled with cauterization or packing the wound with petroleum jelly gauze.

Of particular concern is the potential for a *tracheoarterial fistula* typically caused by erosion of the tip of the tracheostomy tube into the innominate artery producing massive bleeding that is universally fatal if not recognized and treated immediately. Tracheoinnominate artery fistula occurs in approximately 2% of tracheostomy patients and has a mortality rate of 50% to 75% despite emergent management (3). Patients may experience a sentinel bleed that may present as hemoptysis or mild bleeding at the site hours or days before massive bleeding occurs.

Management

Vigorous resuscitation with fluid and possibly blood transfusion should be started for any brisk bleeding while emergent surgical consultation is obtained for definitive management. Temporizing measures should be attempted to control the bleeding such as hyperinflation of the tracheostomy cuff to compress the artery against the sternal wall. If unsuccessful digital pressure should be applied to the anterior tracheal wall through the tracheostomy, compressing the anterior tracheal wall against the sternum (4).

OBSTRUCTION

A tracheostomy patient that presents with respiratory distress must first be assessed for either a partial or complete obstruction of the tracheostomy tube. Patients with tracheostomies lack the humidification of inspired air by nasal passages and this often results in thick dry secretions. Improper care and maintenance of tracheostomy tubes in the outpatient setting is common. Mucus, inspissated secretions, blood, or dislodgement of the tracheostomy tube may cause life-threatening obstruction. Secretions may act as a ball valve allowing air in but restricting outward ventilation (8).

Management

Proper placement should be confirmed and the tube repositioned if necessary. Treatment with high flow oxygen should be initiated. Saline or N-acetyl cysteine may be used to help loosen secretions, followed by suction with an endotracheal suction catheter.

The inner canula should be removed and cleaned, and if still problematic the outer cannula should be removed and replaced with a new tracheostomy tube. Mechanical problems with the tube such as cuff leak or tube fracture may also necessitate tube replacement or consultation for bronchoscopy (1,8).

INFECTION

Serious infection of the stomal site is rare, even though most fresh wounds are colonized by nosocomial organisms (9). The patient's underlying medical condition as well as the presence of an indwelling device and exposure to flora colonizing ventilator tubing predisposes to infection. Antibiotics should be given for obvious infections and should cover the common respiratory flora. Prophylactic antibiotics are not indicated and should not be given. Tracheostomies predispose the patient to cellulitis, tracheitis, bronchitis, and pneumonia.

Management

Peristomal cellulitis may be treated with outpatient antibiotics. Rarely the infection at the wound site spreads downward and causes the serious complication of mediastinitis, mediastinal abscess, and paratracheal abscess. Patients with signs or symptoms of systemic infection and pain with breathing and swallowing should be evaluated for these complications, usually imaging with computed tomography (CT) scan, and given intravenous antibiotics.

STENOSIS

Constant pressure from the cuff may cause pressure necrosis, ulceration, and formation of granulation tissue that subsequently causes tracheal stenosis (5). This is a late complication presenting weeks to months after decanulation. Typically patients do not become symptomatic until the endotracheal lumen has been reduced by 50% to 75% at which point they may complain of cough, dyspnea, and inability to clear secretions. Diagnosis of stenosis is typically made with bronchoscopy and once identified is treated with operative dilation or resection of granulation tissue.

TRACHEOESOPHAGEAL FISTULA

Tracheoesophageal fistula is a rare but potentially life-threatening complication. It is caused either by perforation of the posterior wall of the trachea during the tracheotomy, or erosion into the esophagus by the tracheostomy tube. Patients may present with cuff-leak, aspiration of food contents, abdominal distention, or copious secretions (7). The diagnosis may be made with bronchoscopy or swallowing studies.

REPLACEMENT OF TRACHEOSTOMY CANNULA

Tracheostomy tubes may be cuffed or uncuffed and may come with an inner cannula that can be removed for cleaning (see Table 27.1). Indications in the ED for replacement of the tracheostomy tube include cuff rupture or leak and complete or partial obstruction. A replacement tube should be the same type and size as the original. In an emergency, however, replacement with a smaller size is preferred if maintaining a patent airway depends on it. If the appropriate size tracheostomy tube is unavailable in an emergency situation, a standard endotracheal tube may serve as a temporary replacement typically size 6 to 7.5 in an adult.

If the tracheostomy tube cannot be replaced and the airway is in jeopardy, the physician should consider oral endotracheal intubation. The original indication for the tracheostomy, however,

may hamper attempts at endotracheal intubation (e.g., laryngeal malignancy). If respiratory distress persists after adequate tube replacement, the physician must not overlook other causes (pneumothorax, pulmonary embolus, or cardiac pathology).

CRITICAL INTERVENTIONS

- Gain rapid control of hemorrhage, and consult a surgeon for definitive care
- Obstruction of a tracheostomy tube can be life-threatening. Remove the inner cannula and clear the obstruction to restore airway patency

DISPOSITION

Patients with minor bleeding or infection around a tracheostomy tube site may be treated and discharged with appropriate follow up. Those with partial obstruction due to deposits or secretion build-up on the tracheostomy tube may also be discharged after the tube is cleaned or changed, and the symptoms resolved.

Patients with persistent bleeding, more serious infection, or difficulty breathing mandate consultation and admission. Those with suspected tracheoesophageal fistula or early stenosis may be further evaluated on an inpatient or outpatient basis, depending upon the severity of symptoms.

COMMON PITFALLS

✔ Failure to rapidly clear an obstructed tracheostomy tube
✔ Inadequate control of hemorrhage around a tracheostomy tube. A tracheoarterial fistula should be suspected if a patient presents with brisk bleeding from the tracheostomy tube site
✔ Overly aggressive application of force when replacing a tracheostomy tube must be avoided, to prevent formation of a false tract

Acknowledgments

Thanks to Karen DeFazio and Brian Mongillo upon whose previous edition's chapter this content was based.

References

1. Feller-Kopman D. Acute complications of artificial airways. *Clin Chest Med* 2003;24:445–455.
2. Frost EA. Tracing the tracheostomy. *Ann Otol Rhinol Laryngo* 1976;85:618–624.
3. Hackeling T, Triana R, Ma O, et al. Emergency care of patients with tracheostomies. A seven year review. *Am J Emerg Med* 1998;16:681.
4. Mirza S, Cameron DS. The tracheostomy tube change: a review of techniques. *Hospital Medicine* 2001;62:158–163.
5. Stauffer JL, Olson DE, Petty TL. Complications and consequences of endotracheal intubation and tracheotomy. A prospective study of 150 critically ill adult patients. *Am J Med* 1981;70:65–76.
6. Stoller JK. The history of intubation, tracheotomy, and artificial airways. *Respir Care* 1999;44:595–601.
7. Sue RD, Susanto I. Long-term complications of artificial airways. *Clin Chest Med* 2003;24:457–471.
8. Tayal V. Tracheostomies. *Emer Med Clin* 1994;12:707–727.
9. van Heurn LW, Brink PR. The history of percutaneous tracheotomy. *J Laryngo Otol* 1996;110:723–726.

TABLE 27.1. Replacement of the Tracheostomy Cannula

1) Pre-oxygenate the patient, and extend the head slightly to facilitate placement. Removal and replacement of tracheostomy tubes should follow the curved path of the tube itself.
2) Lubricate the new tube with a water-soluble lubricant, and place the obturator inside the tube to facilitate insertion. This will be removed after tube placement.
3) A well-positioned tube can be advanced gently with little resistance. Tracheal hooks or a dilator may be used to hold the stoma open.
4) If force is necessary to place the tube, efforts should cease because of the possibility of creating false passages, bleeding, and edema.
5) A safe method to ensure proper placement of a tracheostomy tube is to use a thin red rubber catheter as a guide. The catheter can be placed through the existing tracheostomy before removal. If the tracheostomy tube has accidentally fallen out, the catheter may be placed directly through the stoma. Once the old tracheostomy tube is removed, the new tube without the obturator can be passed over the catheter into place. The red rubber catheter can then be removed (9).
6) Secure the tube with tracheal tube ties tightened enough such that only one finger can fit between the patient's neck and the tube tie.
7) Correct tube placement may be confirmed clinically, radiographically, or using end tidal CO_2 detection.

CHAPTER 28
Sinusitis and Rhinitis

Luis H. Haro and Eric T. Boie

Upper respiratory complaints, including sinusitis, are among the most common disorders encountered by the emergency physician. It is estimated that 14% of the United States population, approximately 30 million people, are treated annually for diseases of the paranasal sinuses (15). Billions of dollars are spent on physician visits, prescription and over-the-counter medications, and workdays lost secondary to sinus disease. Sinus disease is usually a harmless inconvenience; however, it occasionally presents as a fulminant, life-threatening entity in the emergency department (ED).

Sinusitis is an inflammatory disease of the paranasal sinuses resulting from infectious, allergic, or autoimmune processes (21). *Rhinitis* strictly means inflammation of the nasal mucous membranes. Rhinitis may be caused by allergic, nonallergic, infectious, hormonal, occupational, and other factors (6). Allergic rhinitis is the most common type. It is relevant to emergency medicine mostly as a manifestation of a broader spectrum of disease. When present as an isolated complaint, symptomatic treatment and referral to a primary care physician is warranted. This chapter will focus on rhinitis as part of a broader infectious disease spectrum. *Rhinosinusitis* has been proposed as a more precise definition, as inflammation frequently involves the nasal passages, and sinusitis without rhinitis is rare (14). Sinusitis can be further classified as acute, subacute, or chronic based on the duration of symptoms. Acute sinusitis lasts 3 to 4 weeks with complete resolution of symptoms either spontaneously or with treatment. Chronic sinusitis is defined by persistent symptoms lasting more than 3 months despite therapy. In subacute sinusitis, symptoms last from 3 weeks to 3 months (2).

The exact incidence and prevalence of sinusitis is difficult to determine due to a lack of rigid criteria defining sinus disease. Occurrence among men equals that of women. Children are more often affected than adults. Between 0.5% to 2% of upper respiratory infections (URIs) in adults and 5% to 10% of URIs in children are complicated by acute bacterial sinusitis (11,12). Sinus disease in the United States is more prevalent in the Midwest and South compared to the Northeast and West (14). Chronic sinusitis affects 5% to 15% of urban dwellers, and the prevalence of chronic sinusitis is increasing (2).

The human sinuses are composed of four paired, sterile cavities lined with ciliated epithelium. Maxillary and ethmoid sinuses are present at birth. Frontal and sphenoid sinuses develop in the 7th and 10th year of life respectively (13). Individual sinus anatomy is highly variable, with frontal sinuses absent in 2% to 5% of the population (16). The posterior ethmoid and sphenoid sinuses empty into the superior meatus. The frontal, anterior ethmoid, and maxillary sinuses empty into the ostiomeatal complex within the middle meatus. Obstruction of the ostiomeatal complex (OMC) due to inflammation, anatomic abnormality, or other pathology is the critical event in the development of acute sinusitis (13). Maxillary sinusitis is most common, followed by ethmoid, frontal, and sphenoid in descending order of frequency (15).

Most cases of sinusitis follow a viral URI. Viruses injure the sinus epithelium, resulting in ciliary dysfunction and a massive inflammatory cascade. Ciliary dysfunction results in mucostasis, and the damaged epithelium is highly susceptible to secondary bacterial invasion from the contiguous nasal passages. Inflammation results in occlusion of the OMC, obstructing sinus drainage and creating a hypoxic, hypercarbic, acidic environment which is ideal for bacterial growth (11). Multiple factors contribute to the development of sinusitis which does not follow a URI including: dental infection, ciliary dysfunction, occlusion of the OMC, and immunodeficiency. 5% to 10% of acute maxillary sinusitis occurs due to contiguous spread of dental infection (2). Ciliary motility disorders, both congenital (Kartagener syndrome) and acquired, predispose to sinusitis. Inflammatory changes of allergic or infectious origin can result in OMC occlusion. Anatomic abnormalities such as polyps, enlarged adenoids, or malignancies can do likewise. Nasal foreign bodies also result in OMC obstruction and can lead to sinusitis; 95% of nasally intubated patients develop sinusitis (2). Immunecompromised patients, including those with steroid dependence, cystic fibrosis, HIV, diabetes, neutropenia, cancer, chronic renal disease, and organ transplants, are all more susceptible to the development of sinusitis and are more likely to have severe disease (2).

Infectious sinusitis can be of viral, bacterial, or fungal origin. Viral rhinosinusitis is 20 to 200 times more common than bacterial sinusitis (1). Over 200 viruses have been implicated in acute sinusitis, with subtypes of rhinovirus, parainfluenza, and influenza virus being the most common (8). Streptococcus pneumonia (30%), nontypeable Haemophilus influenza (20%), Moraxella catarrhalis, Staphylococcus aureus, other streptococcal species, and anaerobes of dental origin compose the primary pathogens in acute bacterial sinusitis (11). Antibiotic resistance is a growing concern. One-third of Haemophilus isolates and nearly all of Moraxella strains are beta-lactamase producing, and up to half of Pneumococcal strains display penicillin resistance (15). Pseudomonas is an important pathogen in patients with cystic fibrosis and HIV. The bacteriology of chronic sinusitis is not as well defined; however, anaerobes, gram negatives, and staphylococcal species are most frequently implicated (13). Fungal sinusitis presents either as an acute fulminant or a chronic indolent process. The former occurs in those who are significantly immunocompromised. Mucoraceae species including Rhizopus, Mucor, and Absida cause necrotizing invasive disease, most often in patients with diabetic ketoacidosis (7). Aspergillus species are becoming a more common pathogen, manifesting in one of three chronic forms in immunocompetent adults: indolent invasive, mycetoma ("fungus ball"), and allergic fungal sinusitis. The latter is the most recently described and frequent form of fungal sinusitis in the United States (18).

CLINICAL PRESENTATION

The clinical presentation of acute sinusitis is highly variable. Most of the presenting chief complaints are nonspecific and may include: purulent nasal discharge, nasal congestion, facial pressure, dental pain, fever, headache, cough, fatigue, halitosis, or a diminished sense of smell. Such symptoms are almost indistinguishable from those of a viral URI, thus duration of symptoms becomes critical in diagnosis. A patient with cold symptoms which do not resolve after 7 to 10 days has a high likelihood of having acute bacterial sinusitis (1). Criteria have been established to aid in the diagnosis of acute bacterial sinusitis as outlined in Table 28.1. In patients with more than 7 days of symptoms, acute bacterial sinusitis is probable if 2 major factors or 1 major and 2 minor factors are present (15). The presentation of acute

TABLE 28.1.   Major and Minor Factors for Diagnosis
of Acute Sinusitis*

Major**	Minor
Facial pain or pressure	Headache
Purulent nasal discharge	Cough
Fever	Fatigue
Nasal congestion	Halitosis
Nasal obstruction	Dental pain
Hyposmia or anosmia	Ear pain/pressure

**Diagnosis requires 2 major OR 1 major and 2 minor factors in a
patient with symptoms for more than 7 days
*From the Task Force on Rhinosinusitis[1]

sinusitis in children differs from adults. Children with sinusitis most commonly present with rhinorrhea and cough, and
there is often coexistent otitis (11). Children under the age of
five are less likely to complain of facial pain, dental pain, and
headache (12). Periorbital edema occasionally is the presenting sign in a child with ethmoid sinusitis (11). Unilateral sinus
drainage in a child should alert the astute emergency physician to the possibility of a nasal foreign body (12). Chronic sinusitis in adults and children may present similarly to acute
sinusitis, but symptoms tend to be more vague and less severe
(13).

Systemic toxicity, mental status changes, severe headache,
and fever are signs and symptoms indicative of a more serious sinus disease or its complications (16). Periorbital cellulitis is the most common complication of sinusitis, usually originating from the ethmoid sinuses (22). It must be differentiated
from orbital cellulitis (see Chapter 21). Intracranial complications of sinusitis include: meningitis, osteomyelitis, cavernous
sinus thrombosis, and intracranial abscesses (epidural, subdural,
and intracerebral). Meningitis is the most common intracranial
complication of sinusitis, as it is estimated that 15% of meningitis cases may be of paranasal sinus origin (16). Extension of
acute frontal sinusitis with suppurative inflammation of cortical bone results in the *Pott's puffy tumor*, a condition requiring
aggressive surgical and antimicrobial therapy (22). *Cavernous
sinus thrombosis* presents with periorbital edema, exophthalmos,
papilledema, and cranial nerve III, IV, and VI palsies. Intracranial abscesses will usually present with fever and acute neurologic signs. Fortunately, such severe complications of sinusitis
are rare. However, long-term morbidity approaches 33% with
blindness, hemiparesis, seizure disorders, and cognitive impairment as some of the more common postmorbid states (16). A
much less severe complication of sinus disease is asthma instability. Although no cause and effect relationship has been definitively established, it is widely believed that sinusitis exacerbates
asthma (19).

Special consideration must be given to the immunocompromised host with sinus complaints, as invasive fungal sinusitis
is much more common in this population. Patients are typically
toxic and may present with moldy smelling, thick, brown or
black nasal discharge. Nasal crusting is prominent and perforation of the palate, nasal septum, or cribriform plate may be
apparent (18). The invasive organisms cause ischemic necrosis
of the bone and mucosa with hematogenous invasion of the orbit,
skin, and brain. Progression to coma and death can occur within
hours. Interestingly, acute fungal sinusitis is relatively rare in acquired immune deficiency syndrome (AIDS) patients, presenting as a late-stage phenomenon when CD4+ counts drop below
50/mm3 (18). Aspergillus is the most common fungal pathogen
in this group.

DIFFERENTIAL DIAGNOSIS

The differential diagnosis for sinusitis is broad as the signs and
symptoms of sinus disease are neither sensitive nor specific. Viral URI, nasal polyps, cocaine abuse, allergic rhinitis, vasomotor
rhinitis, and rhinitis medicamentosa all may present with symptoms of nasal discharge and congestion. Cerebral spinal fluid
rhinorrhea should be considered in a patient with a history of
head trauma. Persistent unilateral nasal discharge with epistaxis
is concerning for neoplasm or nasal foreign body (15). Tension,
cluster, and migraine headaches, as well as dental disease, are alternative diagnoses in the patient whose sinus disease manifests
as cephalgia or facial pain.

EMERGENCY DEPARTMENT EVALUATION

Acute sinusitis is a diagnosis based primarily on clinical history
and physical findings (Table 28.1). Unfortunately, physical examination findings may not prove helpful, as none are specific
for acute sinusitis (8). Findings in a patient with sinusitis may
include mucosal hyperemia, purulent rhinorrhea, nasal airway
congestion, crusting of the anterior nares, and facial pain. However, palpable facial tenderness is a poor indicator of underlying
sinus infection, and "purulent" discharge is not a reliable indicator of bacterial sinusitis (11). Transillumination has poor correlation with the presence of fluid, poor intraobserver consistency,
and poor specificity. Thus, it is of little use in the diagnosis of
acute sinus disease (8,11).

Radiographic imaging has little role in the diagnosis of acute
sinus disease in the emergency department. Abnormal findings
are common in a large proportion of asymptomatic individuals,
and findings of air-fluid levels, sinus opacification, or mucosal
thickening are insensitive and rarely lead to a change in management (8). Plain radiographs both underestimate and overestimate disease (8,11). Unfortunately, they are often utilized to
support or exclude a diagnosis of sinusitis in children and adolescents. Studies of the sensitivity and specificity of plain films
in these patients have yielded conflicting results. In one study,
pre- and post-treatment pairs of plain maxillary sinus x-rays
(including Caldwell and Waters' views) obtained in 101 symptomatic patients aged 1 to 15 years were independently interpreted by three experienced radiologists and three pediatricians.
The general rate of agreement in plain film interpretation was
18%, and the Kappa value was 0.37–0.39 (consistent with only
fair agreement). Moderate agreement (kappa = 0.46–0.51) was
noted for interpretation of the maxillary sinus findings by radiologists, while only fair agreement was noted among pediatricians
(kappa = 0.33–0.37) (9).

CT scan has become the modality of choice for sinus imaging, but also may be oversensitive in detecting "disease" (10).
Eighty-seven percent of patients with viral URIs have abnormalities consistent with sinusitis on CT (2). In a study of healthy,
asymptomatic children aged 1 to 2, 69% had abnormal sinus
CT scans (11). It is neither medically necessary nor economically
feasible to CT scan every patient with symptoms of sinusitis. Use
of CT in the emergency department should be limited to those
patients in which serious complications of sinusitis are suspected
(10).

Nasal cultures are not helpful in the diagnosis of acute sinusitis, as growth correlates poorly with cultures from sinus aspirates (2). Sinus aspiration is neither practical nor routinely
performed in the emergency department. Blood tests are necessary only in patients who show signs of systemic toxicity,
CNS involvement, or who have significant comorbid disease or
immunosuppression.

The lack of a simple diagnostic test makes the diagnosis of sinusitis challenging, but also creates a tendency to label many common colds as sinusitis (15). Duration and severity of symptoms may provide clues in the diagnosis. In acute bacterial sinusitis, symptoms generally worsen after 5 days, persist for at least 10 days, and are much more severe than those associated with a viral URI (1).

EMERGENCY DEPARTMENT MANAGEMENT

The goal of therapeutic intervention in acute sinusitis is threefold: to relieve obstruction of the ostiomeatal complex, to restore mucociliary clearance, and to re-establish sinus sterility through eradication of infection (13). As acute sinusitis is not purely an infectious process, antimicrobial therapy alone will likely fail (15). Combination treatment with antibiotics, topical steroids, nasal decongestants, muco-evacuents, anticholinergics, antihistamines, and nonpharmacologic measures may provide the best symptomatic and therapeutic outcome.

Antibiotics are frequently used in the treatment of acute sinusitis, but great controversy exists regarding indications for use, choice of antimicrobial agent, and duration of therapy (17,3,4). Mild cases of rhinosinusitis with symptoms lasting less than 7 days are most likely viral in etiology, and the temptation to prescribe antibiotics for these patients should be resisted (1,25). A 48% increase in antibiotic prescribing for children visiting physicians' offices in the United States from 1980 through 1992 coincided with the emergence of antibiotic-resistant bacteria. During the 1990s, multiple national campaigns were implemented to promote appropriate use of antibiotics. Since then, rates of office-based antibiotic prescribing for children below the age of 15 have declined substantially. Analysis of average annual visit-based rates demonstrated a 29% decrease in overall antibiotic prescribing (from 330 per 1,000 visits in 1989–90 to 234 per 1,000 in 1999–2000, $p < 0.001$), and a 14% decrease in antibiotic prescribing for the targeted respiratory infections (from 715 to 613 per 1,000 visits, $p < 0.001$) (17).

In patients meeting the diagnostic criteria for sinusitis with progressive or nonresolving symptoms for more than 7 days, use of a first-line antimicrobial agent can be considered (1). Table 28.2 lists the commonly used first- and second-line antimicrobials for acute sinusitis. Amoxicillin is still highly effective and is the first-line agent of choice in acute sinusitis (11,25). Newer, more expensive antibiotics do not appear to be more effective than amoxicillin or trimethoprim plus sulfamethoxazole (TMP-SMX) in patients with uncomplicated sinusitis (5,25). Most studies suggest that almost any antibiotic results in clinical improvement greater than 85% of the time (21). Although no prospective study has established the optimum duration of therapy, a 10- to 14-day course is generally accepted as adequate (12,15). A small number of studies have shown 3 days of therapy as equally effective, but this is not yet an accepted practice (20). Second-line agents should be initiated if there is progression of symptoms after 2 to 3 days of initial therapy (1,11). The natural course of untreated acute sinusitis is unknown, but, it is estimated that 40% to 50% of cases will resolve spontaneously (11,21). One must remember not to be distracted in the antibiotic controversy and pay close attention to appropriate analgesia. Combination treatment with antibiotics, topical steroids, nasal decongestants, muco-evacuents, anticholinergics, antihistamines, and nonpharmacologic measures may provide the best symptomatic and therapeutic outcome.

The use of topical steroids in acute sinusitis is attractive as they are a potent antiinflammatory agent with few side effects. Studies have demonstrated improved symptom relief, but the clinical efficacy of topical steroids is uncertain (2,8). Steroids are generally well tolerated, with local irritation and bleeding as the most common side effects (8).

Topical alpha-adrenergic agonists, such as oxymetazoline, 3 sprays or drops of 0.05% nasal solution in each nostril twice daily has been used to decrease mucosal edema, promoting sinus drainage and ventilation. These agents should not be used for more than 3 days as this may elicit rhinitis medicamentosa due to rebound vasodilation. Oral systemic decongestants (ephedrine, pseudoephedrine, phenylephrine, phenylpropanolamine, etc.) can also be taken, but side effects including nervousness,

TABLE 28.2. Antibiotic Therapy Alternatives in Acute Sinusitis[3]

Drug	Dose (Adult)	Dose (Pediatric)
FIRST-LINE THERAPY		
Amoxicillin	500 mg PO TID × 7–10 days (high-dose 1 g po TID if *S.pneumoniae* resistance likely)	45 mg/kg/d (high-dose 90 mg/kg/d max. of 3 g/day) PO divided BID × 10–14 days
Trimethoprim-Sulfamethoxazole (TMP-SMX)	160 mg/800 mg PO BID × 10–14 days	>2 months 8 mg/kg TMP component/day PO divided every BID 10 days
SECOND-LINE THERAPY		
Cefprozil	500 mg PO BID × 7–14 days	7.5–15 mg/kg PO divided BID 10–14 days
Cefuroxime axetil	500 mg PO BID × 7–14 days	30 mg/kg/day PO divided BID for 10 days, max 1 g/day
Cefpodoxime proxetil	400 mg PO BID × 7–14 days	15 mg/kg PO divided BID × 10–14 days
Amoxicillin/Clavulanate	875/125 mg PO BID × 7–10 days	80–90 mg/kg/d Amox + 6.4 mg/kg/d Clav PO div BID × 10–14 d
Azithromycin	500 mg PO QD day 1 then 250 mg/day on days 2–5	10 mg/kg PO QD on day 1 followed by 5 mg/kg PO QD days 2–5
Clarithromycin	500 mg PO BID for 14 days	6 mo. & older 15 mg/kg/DAILY (divided BID) for 10 days, MAX 1 g/day
THIRD-LINE THERAPY		
Levofloxacin	500 mg PO QD × 10 days	Safety and efficacy in children under 18 years of age have not been established
Moxifloxacin	400 mg PO QD × 10 days	

insomnia, hypertension, and tachycardia may limit their use. Despite the extensive use of these agents, their efficacy remains unclear (14).

The muco-evacuent *guaifenesin* can be used to increase mucous flow and decrease mucous viscosity (2). Side effects are minimal but may include abdominal discomfort and emesis (8).

Topical anticholinergics like ipratropium bromide may reduce rhinorrhea and thus can also be used as adjunctive therapy (2). Antihistamine use in acute sinusitis remains controversial. While antihistamines may decrease rhinorrhea, some argue their use is contraindicated as they increase mucous viscosity, leading to inspissation and outflow obstruction (12). Nonpharmacologic therapy such as steam inhalation and saline douching provide symptomatic relief by softening crusts and moisturizing dry mucosa.

All of the adjunctive therapies mentioned above are largely based on anecdote and personal preference, as there is little evidence that these additions make a great impact on clinical outcome (12,14). It is likely that the longer acute sinusitis is treated, the more the natural course of infection is seen; that is, spontaneous resolution occurs regardless of what is done (15).

Special consideration is needed for managing sinusitis in children, the elderly, and immune-compromised patients. Although debated, since children experience more URIs than adults, the incidence of acute sinusitis in children may be higher. Sinusitis should be considered in any child with respiratory symptoms not improving after 10 days (12). Any child with recurrent acute sinusitis or chronic sinusitis, despite aggressive therapy, should be referred for evaluation for cystic fibrosis or underlying immune dysfunction (13,19). In elderly patients, the threshold to treat acute sinusitis should be lower, as aggressive medical intervention may be important in reducing morbidity in this group (8). In immunocompromised patients, increased alertness for fulminant sinusitis and its complications is necessary. Sinusitis is one of the most common problems affecting HIV+ patients (23). The treatment of acute sinusitis is essentially the same regardless of HIV status, except for duration of antimicrobial therapy where 21 days is standard (24). When CD4+ counts fall below 200, opportunistic sinus infections become more common and more resistant to standard therapy (23).

CRITICAL INTERVENTIONS

- Obtain imaging and initiate parenteral antibiotics early in a patient with a suspected intracranial complication of sinusitis

DISPOSITION

Most patients with acute, uncomplicated sinusitis or rhinitis can be safely discharged with instructions to return to the emergency department or follow up with their regular doctor if symptoms are worsening or not improving within 2 to 3 days. Patients should be educated on the signs of potential intracranial extension (severe headache, vomiting, and confusion) and advised to return to the ED immediately. Patients with sinus symptoms lasting longer than 1 month despite a complete course of therapy should be referred to an otolaryngologist for CT imaging and further evaluation (15).

Any patient with severe headache, altered mental status, systemic toxicity, meningeal signs, or visual complaints suggestive of intraorbital or intracranial extension requires aggressive management to prevent the significant morbidity and mortality associated with complicated sinus disease. Administration of broad spectrum antibiotic therapy, most appropriately a third-generation cephalosporin plus vancomycin, should not be de-

layed by diagnostic procedures (21). Early antibiotics followed by CT, lumbar puncture, and consultation of ENT, neurosurgery, and ophthalmology where appropriate is critical (15). The majority of these patients will require intensive care unit admission.

Transfer to a referral center is necessary if specialist consultation is not readily available for patients with serious complications of sinus disease. Appropriate stabilization efforts and intravenous antibiotic therapy should be initiated prior to transfer. Advanced cardiac life support–capable transport by ground or air is necessary for patients with intracranial complications.

COMMON PITFALLS

✔ Obtaining radiographic imaging in the setting of acute, uncomplicated sinusitis adds little to the work up except cost. There is rarely a role for imaging in acute sinusitis, unless complications are suspected (10)

✔ Overuse of antibiotics. Using antibiotics in patients with symptoms consistent with rhinitis or sinusitis of less than 7 days duration should be avoided. Antibiotics are often inappropriately dispensed for viral rhinosinusitis which is 20 to 200 times more common than acute bacterial sinusitis (1)

✔ Failure to recognize signs of a serious complication. Patients with sinusitis and marked headache and fever must be carefully evaluated to avoid missing early indicators of intracranial extension of acute sinus disease. The elderly, diabetic, HIV+, and other immune-suppressed patients demand a keen awareness as they are at greater risk for more severe sinusitis and its complications

✔ Remember that despite its prevalence, the classifications, diagnostic criteria, clinical management, and ideal treatment options of acute sinusitis are largely anecdotal and without a prospective, evidence-based foundation

Acknowledgments

Thanks to the previous edition's authors Michael J. Foley and Gregory P. Moore for their contributions to this chapter.

References

1. Ahuja GS, Thompson J. What role for antibiotics in otitis media and sinusitis? *Postgrad Med* 1998;104:93–99, 103–104.
2. Anonymous. Infectious rhinosinusitis in adults: classification, etiology and management. International Rhinosinusitis Advisory Board. *Ear, Nose and Throat* 1997;76:1–22.
3. Anon. Antimicrobial treatment guidelines for acute bacterial rhinosinusitis. Sinus and Allergy Health Partnership. *Otolaryngol Head Neck Surg* 2000;123:5–31.
4. Bucher HC, Tschudi P, Youing J, et al. C. BASINUS (Basel Sinusitis Study) investigators. *Arch Intern Med* 2003;163:1793–1798.
5. de Ferranti SD, et al. Are amoxicillin and folate inhibitors as effective as other antibiotics for acute sinusitis? A meta-analysis. *BMJ* 1998;317:632.
6. Dykewicz Mark S. Rhinitis and sinusitis. *J Allerg Clin Immunol* 2003;111:S520–S529.
7. Eloy P, Bertrand B, et al. Mycotic sinusitis. *Acta Oto-Rhino-Laryngologica Belgica* 1997;51:339–352.
8. Evans KL. Recognition and management of sinusitis. *Drugs* 1998;56:59–71.
9. Fonseca, MTM, et al. Interobserver agreement in assessing plain radiographs of maxillary sinus. *Internat J Ped Otorhinolaryngol* 1998;45:41.
10. Hudgins PA, Mukundan S. Screening sinus CT: a good idea gone bad? *Am J Neur* 1997;18:1850–1854.
11. Incaudo GA, Wooding LG. Diagnosis and treatment of acute and subacute sinusitis in children and adults. *Clin Rev in Allerg and Immunol* 1998;16:157–204.
12. Isaacson G. Sinusitis in childhood. *Pediatr Clin North Am* 1996;43:1297–1318.
13. Josephson GD, Gross CW. Diagnosis and management of acute and chronic sinusitis. *Comprehensive Therapy* 1997;23:708–714.
14. Kaliner MA, Osguthorpe JD, et al. Sinusitis: bench to bedside. Current findings, future directions. *J Allerg and Clin Immunol* 1997;99:S829–S848.
15. Maltinski G. Nasal disorders and sinusitis. *Primary Care; Clinics in Office Practice* 1998;25:663–683.
16. Mansfield EL, Gianola GJ. Intracranial complications of sinusitis. *Journal of the Louisiana State Medical Society* 1994;146:287–290.
17. McCaig LF, et al. Trends in antimicrobial prescribing rates for children and adolescents. *JAMA* 2002;287:3096.

18. Morpeth JF, Rupp NT, et al. Fungal sinusitis: an update. *Ann Allerg, Asthma and Immunol* 1996;76:128–139, 139–140.
19. Nishioka GJ, Cook PR. Paranasal sinus disease in patients with cystic fibrosis. *Otolaryngol Clin North Am* 1996;29:193–205.
20. Pichichero ME, Cohen R. Shortened course of antibiotic therapy for acute otitis media, sinusitis and tonsillopharyngitis. *Pediatr Infect Dis J* 1997;16:680–695.
21. Poole MD. Antimicrobial therapy for sinusitis. *Otolaryngol Clin North Am* 1997;30:331–339.
22. Rao VM, el-Noueam KI. Sinonasal imaging. Anatomy and pathology. *Radiol Clin North Am* 1998;36:921–939.
23. Rombaux P, Bertrand B, et al. Sinusitis in the immunocompromised host. *Acta Oto-Rhino-Laryngologica Belgica* 1997;51:305–313.
24. Tami TA. The management of sinusitis in patients infected with the human immunodeficiency virus (HIV). *Ear, Nose, and Throat Journal* 1995;74:360–363.
25. Werk LN, Bauchner H. Practical considerations when treating children with antimicrobials in the outpatient setting. *Drugs* 1998;55:779–790.

CHAPTER 29
Acute Ear Infections in Adults

Harry W. Severance

ACUTE OTITIS MEDIA

Acute otitis media (AOM) is a well-recognized disease, but there has been disagreement over its definition and classification. International symposia have attempted to develop a uniform system of classification, though some controversy is noted to still exist (1).

AOM is defined as a rapid, short course of signs and symptoms of inflammation of the middle ear without reference to etiology or pathogenesis (1). Figures 29.1 and 29.2 show the anatomy

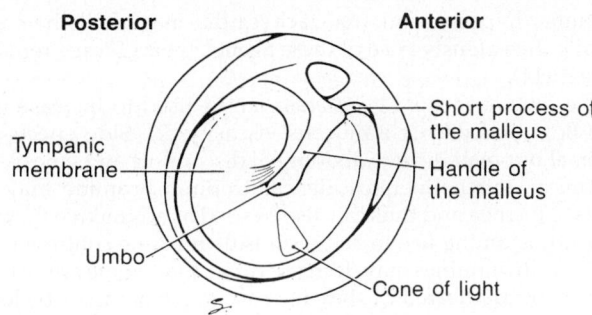

Figure 29.2.   Anatomy of the tympanic membrane.

of the middle ear. An effusion is almost always present in the middle ear space, and is usually assumed to be suppurative. Terms such as *nonsuppurative, serous,* or *secretory* are used for effusions that do not appear to be suppurative. Although AOM is one of the most common and well-reported diseases of children (2–4,14–16,18), it is infrequently reported in adults (2,4,17–19). However, in a 1980 survey by the U.S. National Center for Health Statistics, 20% (2.4 million) of the 11.7 million reported visits for otitis media were in patients older than 15 years. There is little other epidemiologic information on adults in the current literature. However, the epidemiology of pediatric disease has been studied intensively, and adult disease has been assumed to follow similar patterns.

The most frequent organism implicated in AOM is *Streptococcus pneumoniae,* which is found in 30% to 39% of cases. The relative incidence of pneumococcal infection is thought to rise with increasing age into adulthood. Other common organisms include *Haemophilus influenzae, Moraxella* (formerly *Branhamella) catarrhalis, Chlamydia* and *Mycoplasma* species, and many respiratory viruses (7,8,11,12,15). Viruses have an important role in the etiology of AOM (6–8,11,12). They may predispose patients to bacterial infections, or may be the primary causative agent, and may hinder the response to antimicrobial therapy (9,11). The most common species are respiratory syncytial virus (RSV), influenza A and B virus, parainfluenza virus types 1, 2, and 3, rhinovirus, adenovirus, coronavirus, and enterovirus (8,9,11).

The pathogenesis of AOM in adults is thought to be similar to that in children. The onset of symptoms usually follows an upper respiratory infection, or rarely, barotrauma. The precipitating factor is obstruction or dysfunction of the eustachian tube (2,3,12,15,16). Colonizing microbes may proliferate within the middle ear space, thus activating the host's inflammatory defense system. Cytokines such as interleukin-1 and tumor necrosis factor are activated. Secondary mediators are, in turn, produced, and leukocytes migrate to the site of infection and release proteolytic enzymes. The local damage may result in viscous effusions and chronic histologic changes, resulting in hearing impairment (9).

Other predisposing factors include previous otitis infection; congenital, traumatic, or infectious damage to the eustachian tube; and damage to the tympanic membrane (TM). Other obstructive processes, such as nasopharyngeal tumors, can give rise to AOM. Researchers are exploring a possible link between exposure to cigarette smoke and AOM in children and adults (9).

Barotrauma or aerotitis is a subset of eustachian tube dysfunction induced chiefly by air travel, although other causes include rapid elevator descents, or scuba diving, or driving over mountains. Rapid descent produces an increase in ambient atmospheric pressure that is significantly greater than middle ear pressure. Such rapid changes necessitate an active opening of the eustachian tube through contraction of the levator and tensor veli palatini muscles, allowing ambient air to be drawn into

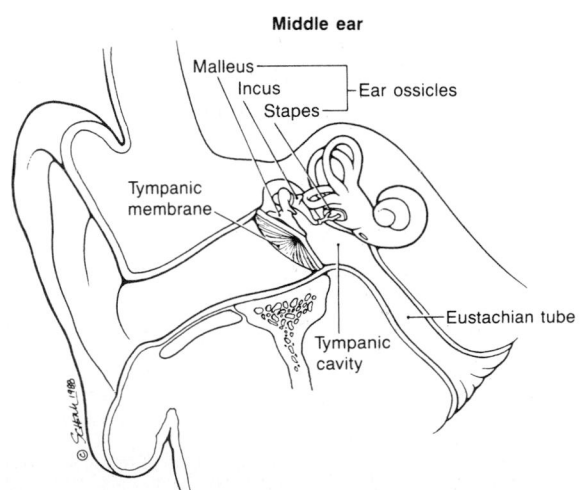

Figure 29.1.   Anatomy of the middle ear.

the middle ear space, thereby equalizing pressure. If the pressure change is too rapid for active middle ear air exchange, or dysfunction of the eustachian tube prevents this exchange, barotrauma results. Uncorrected negative pressure in the middle ear space causes retraction of the TM, immobility of the TM and ossicles, conductive hearing loss, and, if middle ear pressure is not equalized, transudation of serum and blood, or TM rupture.

The natural history of AOM is to resolve without sequelae. The most common acute complication in adults is TM perforation and drainage of the effusion. Rare complications are secondary to local spread of infection and include mastoiditis, facial paralysis, subdural empyema, brain abscess, and meningitis. Chronic, untreated otitis media can lead to such local complications as nonhealing TM perforations, cholesteatomas, and chronic hearing loss.

CLINICAL PRESENTATION

In adults, the usual presenting complaint is ear pain or discomfort (4). Often, only one ear is affected, and the ear may have been the site of previous infection. There is usually a history of concurrent or recent upper respiratory tract infection (4). Other presenting complaints may include hearing difficulty, tinnitus, and vertigo. Fever is variable. In one prospective study, a symptomatic triad of otalgia, impaired hearing, and upper respiratory tract infection was present in almost 100% of patients, with elevated temperature in only 9% (4).

Adults present more commonly than children with spontaneous TM rupture and serosanguineous or purulent discharge from the affected ear. Although the incidence of systemic spread from adult AOM is unknown, high fever and signs of systemic toxicity in the adult with ear pain should cause the examiner to consider a diffuse process and compromised immune system.

In one study in which adults delayed seeking initial evaluation, significant complications were present at the initial presentation. Therefore, the initial examination should include a search for potential complications.

There are two major categories of complications resulting from otitis media: extracranial and intracranial (1). Extracranial complications include TM perforation, mastoiditis, petrositis, facial nerve paralysis, and labyrinthitis. Intracranial complications include extradural abscess, subdural abscess, brain abscess, meningitis, lateral sinus thrombosis, and otic hydrocephalus. Many of these complications used to occur in untreated suppurative otitis media and are now rare. Systemic complications from otitis media, such as bacteremia, pneumonia, and meningitis, are infrequent in adults.

DIFFERENTIAL DIAGNOSIS

Almost any disease process of the head and neck can refer pain to the ear. Dental caries or abscesses commonly refer pain to the ear, as does sialoadenitis or temporomandibular joint syndrome. Sinusitis and pharyngitis can present as ear pain. Acute glaucoma and other optic diseases are occasionally referred to the ear. Otitis externa and soft-tissue infection in proximity to the auricle must be differentiated from otitis media. In most cases, a careful evaluation should produce the correct diagnosis.

EMERGENCY DEPARTMENT EVALUATION

The evaluation of ear pain should include a thorough examination of the head and neck to rule out other causes. Teeth and gums should be examined, and the oral cavity and nasopharynx are inspected for inflammation, sinusitis, and other diseases. The salivary glands and temporomandibular joints should be examined, as well as the auricle, tragus, and surrounding soft tissues. The neck should be inspected, and the carotids auscultated for bruits.

The hallmark of the middle ear examination is otoscopic visualization of the TM. Wax, debris, and discharge that obstruct visualization must be removed. The TM is noted for appearance, landmarks, and light reflex. Signs suggestive of otitis media are loss of normal concavity of the membrane, bulging or retraction, loss of the bony landmarks, a fluid level, bubbles behind the TM, erythema, or an opaque or bluish appearance of the membrane. Barotrauma-induced otitis media may also show hemotympanum or membrane rupture.

Pneumatic otoscopy has classically been the most sensitive and simple bedside test for the presence of effusion behind the TM and should be part of the routine examination. Pneumatic otoscopy does not define whether the effusion is suppurative or nonsuppurative.

The hand-held acoustic otoscope reportedly is a reliable test for the presence of middle ear effusions (3,10,15). In one study, the acoustic otoscope was shown to detect effusions with equal facility in adults and children (10).

EMERGENCY DEPARTMENT MANAGEMENT

Antimicrobial Therapy

Uncomplicated otitis media is usually assumed to be suppurative. Amoxicillin (500 mg orally three times a day for 10 days) or trimethoprim-sulfamethoxazole (TMP-SMX) (double strength twice a day for 10 days) remain the first-line drugs of choice for adult populations, though resistance to these drugs is increasing.

Patients whose signs and symptoms continue after initial antibiotic therapy or those who are allergic to penicillins or TMP-SMX should receive alternative antibiotics, such as a newer macrolide (azithromycin or clarithromycin), an oral cephalosporins, or penicillin-combination such as amoxicillin-potassium clavulanate (2,5,9,12). Quinolones may be effective as possible second-line antimicrobials for AOM in adults (5). A parenteral third-generation cephalosporin or vancomycin is recommended for highly resistant or serious infections (5,12). Extended spectrum antibiotics should also be considered in patients at high risk for complications, such as those with diabetes or the immunocompromized.

Supportive Therapy

Supportive therapy includes fever control, relief of otalgia, and treatment of associated upper respiratory symptoms (3). Acetaminophen or ibuprofen treat pyrexia and otalgia in most adults, though narcotics may be appropriate for some. Otalgia should improve significantly over the first 24 to 48 hours of treatment. Patients who experience continued otalgia or other symptoms should be instructed to return for further evaluation.

Decongestants and antihistamines are effective in reducing the symptoms of an upper respiratory infection, and should also be considered, especially for barotrauma-induced AOM.

Myringotomy has been recommended for adults with severe otalgia and a bulging TM. This technique allows almost instantaneous pain relief and provides material for culture, and should be considered.

TM perforations associated with AOM usually resolve spontaneously without sequelae. Purulent discharge through the perforation may result in an eczematoid external otitis, which may be treated with topical ear drops consisting of a steroid–antibiotic mixture. However, if such drops enter the middle ear space through the perforation, they may cause a chemical ototoxicity (3).

CRITICAL INTERVENTIONS

- Examine the head and neck for alternative origins of symptoms
- Visualize and insuflate the tympanic membrane

DISPOSITION

Adults with uncomplicated AOM can be safely discharged on antibiotics and symptomatic therapy. Patients should be instructed to seek follow up for worsening symptoms or for symptoms of systemic illness. Routine follow-up examination of the ear after completion of therapy has not been evaluated in adults, but those with perforation should receive a follow up to confirm healing of the membrane. Patients with known immunocompromise or other disabling illness should have early referral.

Patients with persistent otorrhea secondary to TM rupture that continues after initial antibiotic therapy should be referred to an otolaryngologist (3). Those whose symptoms persist after the second course of antibiotics also should be referred to an otolaryngologist.

Myringotomy should be considered in patients with worsening symptoms, especially if the diagnosis is in question, severe pain is present, or infectious complications occur.

COMMON PITFALLS

✔ Failure to visualize the TM
✔ Failure to test the mobility of the TM
✔ Confusing a ruptured TM with drainage with otitis externa

ACUTE MASTOIDITIS

Mastoiditis is best defined as an inflammatory process of the pneumatic spaces of the mastoid process, most commonly occurring with acute or subacute otitis media (33). The mastoid is the portion of the temporal bone posterior to the ear that contains a honeycomb of air cells lined with respiratory epithelium (25). These air cells connect with the middle ear (25). Mastoiditis can be divided into acute, subacute or chronic (22,24,38). Acute mastoiditis is considered by many authors to be a continuum of otitis media (OM) as the effusion and inflammation of OM is almost always accompanied by fluid and inflammation in the mastoid (25,31,33,38). In the pre-antibiotic era, coalescent mastoiditis was a complication of acute otitis media in 5%–50% of cases (23,24,40). Currently mastoiditis is relatively rare, though there have been recent reports suggesting an increased frequency of this disease (21,24,30). While uncommon, mastoiditis can result in significant and even life-threatening complications (31,38).

There are slight differences in the bacteriology of acute mastoiditis as compared to AOM (21,24). Most studies report pneumococci and group A streptococci as the most frequently isolated pathogens in mastoiditis (21,22,24,41). Other organisms isolated in acute disease include *Staphylococcus aureus, Pseudomonas aeruginosa, Proteus,* and anaerobes. In immunocompromised patients, *Aspergillus, Mycobacterium tuberculosis,* other atypical *Mycobacterium* sp., and *Pneumocystis carinii* have all been described (32).

CLINICAL PRESENTATION

The most common presenting sign, postauricular tenderness, is seen in over 80% of cases (29). The hallmark triad of symptoms is comprised of otalgia, postauricular pain, and fever (29). Otorrhea and hearing loss are less frequently reported. Protrusion or proptosis of the auricle, and postauricular erythema and swelling are common findings (41). Induration over the mastoid is thought to be a harbinger of impending subperiosteal abscess (29). The auricle may be displaced forward and laterally in adults and older children. On otoscopic examination, the TM is abnormal in 88% of patients (39). The disease should be considered in the case of otitis media that is not resolving.

Increasing headache, otalgia, fever, postauricular pain, swelling, or change in the consistency of the otorrhea in patients with ongoing or evolving chronic otitis media should alert the emergency physician to the possibility of mastoiditis.

DIFFERENTIAL DIAGNOSIS

Localized scalp infections such as furuncles or local trauma, including bites and stings, can present with postauricular swelling. Reactive lymphadenopathy from systemic infections of the head and neck region can also be easily mistaken for mastoiditis. Severe otitis externa with auricular inflammation might be mistaken for acute mastoiditis (21). Systemic lymph node disorders from viral infections or neoplastic disease can present with postauricular swelling. If there is swelling of this area in an adult with a history of tobacco use, a neoplastic source should be considered.

EMERGENCY DEPARTMENT EVALUATION

Laboratory testing of the disease is not useful. While leukocytosis and an increased erythrocyte sedimentation rate are often present, they are neither sensitive nor specific for the disease. Blood cultures are generally not positive. A lumbar puncture should be performed in all patients manifesting signs and symptoms of meningitis.

Plain radiographs may reveal clouding of the mastoid space and bony abnormalities (28,31). However, plain films have been noted to often be unhelpful and/or misleading (22). CT scan or possibly MRI may be more useful in defining the extent of the disease, as well as intratemporal and intracranial complications (22,31,36,38).

EMERGENCY DEPARTMENT MANAGEMENT

All patients with the diagnosis of mastoiditis require otolaryngologic consultation. Intravenous antibiotic therapy should be instituted in the emergency department. The antibiotics selected should be effective for *S. pneumoniae*, the most commonly isolated pathogen. They also should be able to penetrate the blood–brain barrier. Initial selections may include:

Ceftriaxone 1 g IV, or
Cefotaxime 1 g IV
(or a combination of a semi-synthetic penicillin and chloramphenicol) (37).

Concern for anaerobic bacteria may result in the addition of Metronidazole (35).

Immunocompromised patients may require antifungal or antituberculous agents; the use of these should be made in conjunction with otolaryngology and infectious disease specialists.

The need for surgical treatment, such as myringotomy, tympanostomy tubes, and mastoidectomy, may be required if acute disease does not resolve, or progresses. Risk factors for possible early surgical intervention include the presence of fever, leukocytosis, and proptosis of the auricle. A therapeutic mastoidectomy may be required (27). Patients who fail to improve within 24 to 72 hours and have evidence of coalescent disease, a subperiosteal abscess, or intracranial disease are candidates for mastoidectomy.

CRITICAL INTERVENTIONS

- Begin appropriate antibiotics when acute mastoiditis is first suspected
- Immediate emergency department otolaryngology consultation is warranted if acute mastoiditis is suspected

DISPOSITION

Generally, patients with acute mastoiditis require admission for IV antibiotic therapy and possible surgical intervention. Toxic-appearing patients or those with intracranial complications may require intensive care admission and probable neurosurgical referral. The possible use of daily parenteral antibiotics for ambulatory patients has been proposed, if there is close follow up by an otolaryngologist and an infectious disease specialist (26). Transfer to an alternative facility, after intravenous antibiotic therapy has begun, should be sought if no specialty consultation is locally available.

COMMON PITFALLS

✔ Failure to consider mastoiditis in a patient with otitis media that has not resolved in a timely manner
✔ Failure to recognize the significant intracranial or intratemporal complications that can still occur in patients with middle ear disease

ACUTE OTITIS EXTERNA

Otitis externa (OE) is a general term encompassing all of the irritative and infective processes that involve the skin of the external auditory canal (43,57,62). One system of classification divides it into three major groups: *inflammatory OE,* in which the etiology is infectious, *eczematoid (allergic) OE,* and *seborrheic OE* (43). Inflammatory OE can be further subdivided into the acute form, in which the predominant pathogens are bacterial, and chronic, in which fungal organisms predominate.

Acute inflammatory OE is by far the most common type presenting to emergency physicians. It can be further subdivided into diffuse and localized forms (43,54,57). Acute diffuse OE ("swimmer's ear") is the most common of all external ear infections (43,54,57,62). Acute localized OE is often an infection involving a hair follicle in the area of the ear canal (furuncle) (43,54). The initial presentations of these two processes are similar.

Acute Otitis Externa (OE) is found in all age groups, in all climates, and in all seasons. However, the incidence is greatly in-

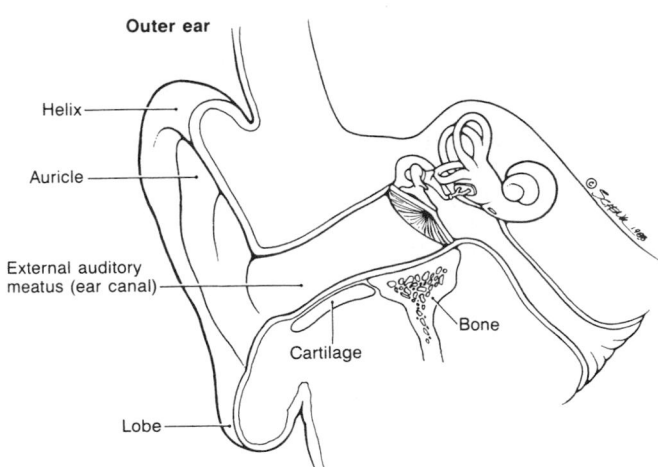

Figure 29.3. Anatomy of the external ear.

creased during the summer, especially among swimmers (hence the term *swimmer's ear*) (43,62). The spectrum of disease produced by this entity ranges from mild itching and irritation of the ear to excruciating pain, swelling, purulent discharge, and systemic illness (62).

Excessive wetness or dryness of the canal, trauma, or a change in the canal environment makes the ear canal epithelium vulnerable to infection by endogenous bacteria, virulent exogenous bacteria, or other microbial pathogens (51). Common pathogenic bacteria include *Pseudomonas aeruginosa, Enterobacter aerogenes, Proteus vulgaris, Klebsiella pneumoniae, S. aureus,* and non–group-A streptococci (47,51,52,54,58,59,62). Commonly cultured fungal organisms are *Aspergillus niger, Candida* sp., *Actinomyces,* or yeasts (43,45,48,59,62). Herpesvirus hominis and varicella-zoster also may cause external otitis (48,51).

Figure 29.3 shows the anatomy of the external ear. The adult external auditory canal is about 24 to 35 mm long and ends medially at the TM (53,54,57,58). In the adult, the distal third of the canal is supported by the cartilaginous base of the auricle; the proximal two-thirds of the canal passes through the temporal bone. The juncture of the cartilaginous and osseous portions of the canal (isthmus) limits the entry of wax and foreign bodies to the area near the TM (54,57). The canal forms an S shape with a slight upward and backward orientation; this likewise discourages foreign-body entry (57). The skin lining the osseous portion of the canal is thin and firmly attached to the periosteum, lacking dermal papilla and subcutaneous tissue (53). Hair follicles are numerous in the outer third and sparse in the inner two-thirds of the canal (54).

The external canal is equipped with barriers to prevent contamination of the canal and injury to the tympanic membrane TM (58,60). The outward movement of keratinized epithelium, along with the normal mandibular chewing motion, propels keratinized debris and cerumen outward, while the S-shape and isthmus of the canal discourage entry of foreign objects (45,57,58). The waxy, water-repellent cerumen is a mixture of secretions from the sebaceous and apocrine glands in this area and the desquamated keratin layer from the stratum corneum. It protects by its stickiness, bacteriostatic effects, and the presence of lysozyme and immunoglobulins (53,56–58). Its acidic pH and the presence of trace metals may also play a protective role (57,58).

The usual precipitating factor in acute OE is the introduction of infectious organisms into the epithelium of a previously traumatized ear canal in which protective defenses have been disrupted (58). Usual traumatic mechanisms are foreign bodies (cotton-tipped applicators, pencils), prolonged wetness (water sports, bathing, increased environmental humidity), or excessive dryness (previous infection, dermatoses, insufficient cerumen). Predisposing factors include previous ear surgery or TM rupture, a narrow or abnormally angled canal, and abnormal cerumen production (45,61).

Malignant OE (necrotizing, invasive) is usually caused by *Pseudomonas*, and is seen almost exclusively in diabetics and other immunocompromised patients. It carries a high incidence of complications, neurologic sequelae, or death (45–47,49,61).

Acute localized OE (aural furunculosis) is usually caused by an infected hair follicle in the cartilaginous ear canal, which, in adults, consists of the outer third of the canal (43,54,58). More rarely, eczema, seborrhea, impetigo, warts, or herpetic eruptions can produce localized OE (57). In most cases the infecting organism is *S. aureus* (43,52). Most cases are caused by direct trauma to the ear canal, although occasionally they are secondary to a blocked sebaceous gland (43).

CLINICAL PRESENTATION

Patients presenting with mild-to-moderate acute OE may complain only of itching or irritation in the affected ear, often heightened by manipulation of the auricle or tragus (43,51,57,62). In more severe presentations, the severity of pain and tenderness may seem disproportionate to the degree of inflammation, probably due to compression of nerve fibers. Edema and erythema are present and the canal may be closed. There is usually a discharge described as yellowish, greenish, or watery. Fungal infections produce a dark or cheesy discharge. Frequently, the canal is so tender and swollen that the entire ear canal and TM cannot be adequately visualized. The canal appears pale, soggy, and edematous, occluded by cerumen and desquamated epithelium (62). The TM, if visualized, may appear normal, opaque, or erythematous. It may have normal mobility or, if the drum is thickened, reduced response to insufflation.

In more severe infections, there can be periauricular inflammation, cellulitis, lymphadenitis, and erythema (51,58,62). Fever is variably present (62) and pain can be intensified by any manipulation of the jaw or the affected side of the face (62). Such presentations often result from combined infections with *Pseudomonas* sp. and *Streptococcus pyogenes* or from *S. aureus*.

DIFFERENTIAL DIAGNOSIS

The differential for acute OE is similar to that of otitis media. Other diagnoses in the differential include parotitis, periauricular adenitis or cellulitis, mastoiditis, dental abscess, temporomandibular joint pain, sinusitis, tonsillitis, or pharyngitis (57,58,62). Acute mastoiditis can be confused with AOE in cases where periauricular edema is extensive.

EMERGENCY DEPARTMENT EVALUATION

The examination should include manipulation of the auricle and tragus, and inspection of the periauricular area. The canal is inspected and if possible, the TM should be visualized. In elderly patients with diabetes and other immunocompromised patients with otorrhea and intense ear pain, the possibility of malignant OE must be considered. A white blood cell count (WBC) and erythrocyte sedimentation rate (ESR) are obtained in these patients, and cultures of the exudates may be helpful (60). Signs of systemic toxicity, local extension of infection to periauricular areas, nuchal rigidity, or facial nerve palsy are sought. CT scanning is the current modality of choice for defining the anatomic extent of disease in suspected malignant OE or mastoiditis (55,60).

EMERGENCY DEPARTMENT MANAGEMENT

Basic management of acute OE includes aural hygiene, elimination of microbes, and analgesics. Hygiene involves cleansing of the ear canal and is considered by many to be the single most important part of therapy (43,57,58). For mild infections, dry-mopping with a small tuft of cotton attached to a wire applicator may be sufficient; sometimes it is even curative (57). In more severe infections, with an inflamed, edematous canal with cheesy secretions and debris, removal by suctioning is recommended (45,57,58). After all major debris and exudate are removed, careful irrigation with warm, sterile saline or a 2% acetic acid solution is recommended to complete the cleansing. Forceful irrigation is contraindicated, as it could traumatize further the macerated epithelium of the canal and actually promote suprainfection. After irrigation is complete, the canal must be dried. Several techniques have been used, including suction or instillation of a drying solution of dilute alcohol. Some authors suggest using a hair dryer (57,58).

Topical otic solutions are recommended by many for eliminating microbes and acidifying the canal in most cases of acute inflammatory OE. There is no consensus, however, on a solution of choice. Many are recommended and available, ranging from acetic acid preparation (2%) and half-strength Burow's solution (aluminum acetate, 1:20) to topical antibiotic preparations containing neomycin (active against gram-positive organisms and also against some gram-negative organisms, notably *Proteus* sp.) with either colistin or polymyxin (active against gram-negative bacilli, notably *Pseudomonas* sp.). Some of these commercially available solutions contain other ingredients, such as corticosteroids, to reduce inflammation (54). Most solutions seem to be effective if used in conjunction with the other recommended treatment measures. Otic solutions are preferable to suspensions, except in TM perforation or the presence of a ventilation tube. Two to four drops, applied three or four times daily for 7 to 10 days should be adequate (45,53).

In canals that are severely inflamed and edematous, an ear wick may be necessary for the application of otic solutions (62). Expandable ear wicks of hydroxycellulose or similar materials are available and are reported by some to be preferable to cotton or gauze, although the latter are still recommended (57). The wick is placed about 10 to 12 mm into the outer third of the canal, and otic drops are placed directly on the wick (51,57). If wicks are required, steroid-containing solutions may have an advantage in hastening the reduction of inflammation. Ear wicks are usually used for 24 to 48 hours and then removed. Often they spontaneously fall out as inflammation subsides.

Pain from OE can be intense, and some patients may require narcotic analgesia during the initial evaluation, cleaning, and wick insertion and during the first 24 to 48 hours of treatment. (43,51,53,57). Mild, locally applied dry heat often helps in pain management (43).

During treatment, introduction of water into the ear canal must be avoided. Swimming is prohibited. Showers should be brief and hair-washing infrequent and followed by instillation of otic drops (58). When bathing, shower caps, ear plugs, or other devices to prevent entry of water into the ear canal can be considered.

Oral antibiotics are generally unnecessary for mild-to-moderate cases of acute diffuse OE. In the vast majority of uncomplicated cases, these local measures should bring about resolution of symptoms. Oral antibiotics have been recommended in patients with more severe presentations, such as intense pain, fever, or lymphadenitis, or in patients who require ear wick insertion (45,54). Cultures of ear aspirates should be obtained in all such patients. Oral antibiotics are also recommended for patients with occluded ear canals who have symptoms, signs, or history suggestive of otitis media.

Parenteral antibiotics are occasionally required in the rare patient with symptoms of systemic toxicity or malignant OE. A combination of an aminoglycoside and an antipseudomonal penicillin should be started (54,57). If *S. aureus* infection is suspected, a cephalosporin or penicillinase-resistant penicillin is the initial therapy. Cultures of ear aspirates may help in treatment decisions. The usual parenteral treatment period for malignant OE has been 4 to 6 weeks (43,53,54) with oral ciprofloxacin after about 1 week in responding cases (49,53). Management of a localized OE (furuncle) is similar to diffuse OE, but if a discrete, painful lesion is identified, incision and drainage may be necessary. If localized cellulitis is present, an oral systemic antibiotic active against *S. aureus* (dicloxacillin or a cephalosporin) should be instituted for 10 days.

CRITICAL INTERVENTIONS

- Fully examine the ear and periauricular structures
- Provide adequate pain control especially if cleaning or examining the ear canal or adjacent structures

DISPOSITION

Most patients with acute diffuse OE may be discharged home with instructions for good aural hygiene, topical antibiotic drops, and symptomatic therapy, including analgesia. Discharge instructions should include avoiding water sports during therapy and for up to 2 to 4 weeks after resolution of symptoms. A 10-day follow up is encouraged. Patients with worsening of symptoms or failure to respond to initial management should be evaluated by an otolaryngologist.

Elderly patients with diabetes or other immunocompromising diseases that are seen for OE should receive close follow-up and monitoring to prevent the rapid onset of malignant OE.

Patients with obstructed canals, with ear wicks inserted, or with severe pain (especially those whose initial otoscopic examination was limited due to pain and swelling), and patients on oral antibiotics or narcotic analgesics should be reevaluated in 12 to 24 hours to ensure that symptoms are resolving and to allow completion of a thorough otoscopic examination.

Admission and parenteral antibiotic therapy are required for patients with systemic toxicity, meningeal signs, facial palsy, or malignant OE.

COMMON PITFALLS

✔ Confusing OE with otitis media
✔ Misdiagnosis of a ruptured TM with purulent drainage as OE
✔ Underdiagnosing OE when symptoms of toxicity or malignant OE are present

AURICULAR CELLULITIS AND PERICHONDRITIS

Auricular cellulitis is an infection of the epidermis and subcutaneous tissue of the auricle, often secondary to minor trauma such as scratching, bites and stings, earring insertion or piercing, cotton swab use or contact dermatitis (65,67,69). Otitis externa is also noted as causative of auricular cellulitis (70). Perichondritis is inflammation or infection of the perichondrium (a dense, fibrous connective tissue surrounding and providing nourishment to underlying cartilaginous areas), most commonly of the external ear (63,65). Auricular perichondritis is usually caused by trauma to the ear, such as from contact sports, accidental trauma, penetrating injuries including bites or stings, burns, and surgeries of the ear (63,65,68). Blood or serum from trauma can collect between the perichondrium and the auricular cartilage and become secondarily infected (63). Progression from an antecedent auricular cellulitis evolving from acute otitis externa can be the etiology (68). Once there is fluctuance with abscess formation and involvement of the cartilage, some define the condition as chondritis (64). The most common risk factor today is ear piercing, especially when piercing involves the cartilage (66,67,71–73). Predisposing factors include diabetes or other immunocompromising diseases. The most common organisms involved in auricular cellulitis include S. aureus and streptococci, while perichondritis is most often caused by Pseudomonas, S. aureus, and streptococcus species (63,65,68,69,72,73).

CLINICAL PRESENTATION

Patients usually present with a painful, erythematous ear (67). There may be a localized area of trauma such as an abrasion or contusion surrounded by erythema. There is often a history of penetrating or blunt trauma; often minor, including bites or stings or a recent episode of ear piercing. There may be an antecedent or concurrent local infection such as acute otitis externa. The auricular infection initially appears as and in fact initially may begin as an auricular cellulitis, but if it progresses to involve the perichondrium it becomes perichondritis. In perichondritis other symptoms may include profound tenderness to touch, induration, and possibly fluctuance, or localized drainage from the initial wound site. In perichondritis the lobule is often spared (65). There may be swelling, deformity, or localized abscess formation, which suggests progression to chondritis. Cellulitis and perichondritis may present with constitutional symptoms such as fever, chills, or malaise (68).

DIFFERENTIAL DIAGNOSIS

The major effort in differential diagnosis is the differentiation of auricular cellulitis from auricular perichondritis. In general as described above, perichondritis should have increased pain, alteration in appearance of the external ear, and more systemic findings such as fever. Severe otitis externa could appear as perichondritis, and in fact can progress to this disorder. Other diagnoses which cause erythema and discomfort to the ear such as contact dermatitis or insect bites may be confused with cellulitis or early perichondritis. Relapsing polychondritis, an episodic, inflammatory disease of the connective tissues and various cartilages in head and neck and upper respiratory tract, can present in similar fashion (65,70).

EMERGENCY DEPARTMENT EVALUATION

Diagnosis of auricular cellulitis or perichondritis is usually made by history, often including a history of antecedent trauma, and physical exam findings as noted above. The traumatic event might be minor such as insect bite or sting, or secondary to an earring or other piercing event, especially if involving the cartilaginous areas of the ear.

Laboratory evaluation may demonstrate leukocytosis (66). Culture of any local drainage may be helpful in defining the infective agent, though cultures from incision and drainage will be more accurate. Imaging procedures have not been generally described in the initial work up of auricular perichondritis, but may be helpful if disease extension or abscess is suspected.

EMERGENCY DEPARTMENT MANAGEMENT

Initial management of *auricular cellulitis* includes local care such as warm compresses, analgesics and antibiotic therapy. Initial antibiotic therapy can be oral or intravenous:

Nafcillin 2 gm IV, or
Cefazolin 1 gm IV, or
Cephalexin 500 mg po qid (65,69).

Otolaryngology consultation should be obtained if perichondritis cannot be ruled out or if the patient condition warrants admission.

Initial ED management of *perichondritis* includes antibiotics, pain control, and consultation by an otolaryngologist. Initial antibiotic therapy includes:

Ticarcillin/clavulonic acid (Timentin) 3.1 gm IV, or
Nafcillin 2 gm IV,
-PLUS-
Ciprofloxacin (500 po or 400 IV) (65,67).

Antibiotic therapy may be required for several weeks (65). Incision and drainage will be required if there is a localized abscess, or to hasten resolution of infection (65). If chondritis is present, intraoperative debridement and removal of infected, necrotic cartilage will usually be part of the initial management (72).

CRITICAL INTERVENTIONS

- Initiate early antibiotic therapy for suspected cases of auricular cellulitis or perichondritis
- Obtain immediate otolaryngology consult if perichondritis is suspected

DISPOSITION

Disposition for patients with auricular cellulitis is individualized based on severity of presenting symptoms, general physical condition, and co-morbidities. Otherwise generally healthy patients with minimal symptoms can be potentially discharged home after initial antibiotic therapy if they have good follow up. Other patients may benefit from admission or observation in a "short-stay" unit for further intravenous antibiotic therapy and consultation if not improving. Patients with significant systemic symptoms, such as significant fever and rigorous chills, should receive consultation and be considered for admission.

For perichondritis, admission for intravenous antibiotics and surgical incision and drainage is generally required (67). Surgical

debridement and removal of necrotic cartilage and tissue is a major part of the management of chondritis (63). As surgery is often part of management, transfer to an alternative facility which offers otolaryngology services might be considered.

COMMON PITFALLS

✔ Not starting appropriate antibiotics once the diagnosis of auricular cellulitis or perichondritis is suspected
✔ Not suspecting the diagnosis of perichondritis

References

Acute Otitis Media

1. Bluestone CD, Gates GA, Klein JO, et al. Definitions, terminology, and classification of otitis media. *Ann Otol Rhinol Laryngol* 2002;111:8–18.
2. Bluestone CD. Otitis media. In: Johnson JT, Yu VL, eds. *Infectious Diseases and Antimicrobial Therapy of the Ears, Nose and Throat.* Philadelphia: WB Saunders, 1997:273–291.
3. Cahill L, Jehle D. Otitis. In: Reisdorff EJ, Roberts MR, Wiegenstein JG, eds. *Pediatric Emergency Medicine.* Philadelphia: WB Saunders, 1993:617–623.
4. Celin SE, Bluestone CD, Stephenson J, et al. Bacteriology of acute otitis media in adults. *JAMA* 1991;266:2249–2252.
5. Durand M, Joseph M. Infections of the upper respiratory tract. In: Braunwald E, Hauser SL, Fauci AS, Longo DL, Kasper DL, Jameson JL, eds. *Harrison's Principles of Internal Medicine,* 15th edition. New York: McGraw-Hill, 2001;187–193.
6. Eskola J, Kilpi T. Potential of bacterial vaccines in the prevention of acute otitis media, *Pediatr Infect Dis J.* 2000;19:72–78.
7. Giebink GS, Bakaletz LO, Barenkamp SJ, et al. Vaccine. *Ann Otol Rhinol Laryngol* 2002;111:82–94.
8. Giebink GS. Otitis media update: pathogenesis and treatment. *Ann Otol Rhinol Laryngol Suppl* 1992;155:21–23.
9. Hoppe HL, Johnson CE. Otitis media: focus on antimicrobial resistance and new treatment options. *Am J Health Syst Pharm* 1998;55:1881–1897.
10. Jehle D, Cottington E. Acoustic otoscopy in the diagnosis of otitis media. *Ann Emerg Med* 1989;18:396–400.
11. Klein JO, Chonmaitree T, Loosmore S, Marchant CD, Ruuskanen O, Shinefield HR, Otitis media: a preventable disease? Proceedings of an international symposium organized by the Marcel Merieux Foundation, Veyrier-du-lac, Farance, February 13 to 16, 2000. *Pediatr Infect Dis J* 2001;20:473–481.
12. Klein JO. Otitis externa, otitis media, mastoiditis. In: Mandell GL, Bennett JE, Dolin R, eds. *Principles and Practice of Infectious Disease,* 5th ed. Philadelphia: Churchill Livingstone, 2000:669–675.
13. Kovatch AL, Wald ER, Michaels RH. Beta-lactamase-producing *Branhamella catarrhalis* causing otitis media in children. *J Pediatr* 1983;102:261–264.
14. McFadden DM, Berwick DM, Feldstein ML, Marter SS. Age-specific patterns of diagnosis of acute otitis media. *Clin Pediatr* 1985;24:571–575.
15. Paradise JL. Otitis media. In: Behrman RE, Kliegman RM, Jenson HB, eds. *Nelson Textbook of Pediatrics,* 17th edition. Philadelphia: Saunders, 2004;2138–2149.
16. Schnore SK, Sangster JF, Gerace TM, Bass MJ. Are antihistamine decongestants of value in the treatment of acute otitis media in children? *J Fam Pract* 1986;22:39–43.
17. Schwartz LE, Brown RB. Purulent otitis media in adults. *Arch Intern Med* 1992;152:2301–2304.
18. Severance HW. Acute otitis media in adults; appropriate diagnosis coding and methods of diagnosis in E. M. populations. *South Med J* 1990;83:2S–20.
19. Sugita R, Fujimaki Y, Deguchi K. Bacteriological features and chemotherapy of adult acute purulent otitis media. *J Laryngol Otol* 1985;99:629–635.
20. Wuorimaa T, Kayhty H. Current state of pneumococcal vaccines. *Scand J Immunol* 2002;56:111–129.

Mastoiditis

21. Bahadori RS, Schwartz RH, Ziai M. Acute mastoiditis in children: an increase in frequency in northern Virginia. *Pediatr Infec Dis J* 2000;19:212–215.
22. Bitar CN, Luka EA, Steele RW. Mastoiditis in children. *Clin Pediatr* 1996;35:391–395.
23. Bluestone CD. Clinical course, complications and sequelae of acute otitis media. *Pediatr Infect Dis J* 2000;19:S37–S46.
24. Dew LA, Shelton C. Complications of temporal bone infections. In: Cummings CW, Fredrickson JM, Harker LA, Krause CJ, Schuller DE, Richardson MA. *Otolaryngology Head & Neck Surgery,* 3rd edition. St. Louis: Mosby, 1998;3047–3075.
25. Durand M, Joseph M. Infections of the upper respiratory tract. In: Braunwald E, Fauci AS, Kasper DL, Hauser SL, Longo DL, Jameson JL, eds. *Harrison's Principles of Internal Medicine,* 15th edition. New York: McGraw-Hill, 2001;187–193.
26. Einhorn M, Fliss DM, Leiberman A, Dagan R. Otolaryngology and infectious disease team approach for outpatient management of serious pediatric

infections requiring parenteral antibiotic therapy. *Int Pediatr Otorhinolaryngol* 1992;24:245–251.

27. Gliklich RE, Eavers RD, Iannuzi RA, Camacho AE. A contemporary analysis of acute mastoiditis. *Arch Otolaryngol Head Neck Surg* 1996;122:135–139.

28. Goycoolea MV, Jung TT. Complications of suppurative otitis media. In: Paparella MM, Shumrick DA, eds. *Otolaryngology*, 3rd edition. Philadelphia: W. B. Saunders Company, 1991;1381–1392.

29. Gross ND, McMenomey SO. Aural complications of otitis media. In: Glasscock ME, Gulya AJ, eds. *Surgery of the Ear*, 5th edition. Hamilton, Ontario: B C Decker, 2003;435–441.

30. Hoppe JE, Koster S, Bootz F, Niethammer D. Acute mastoiditis relevant once again. *Infection* 1994;22:178–182.

31. Klein JO. Otitis externa, otitis media, and mastoiditis. In: Mandell GL, Bennett JE, Dolin R, eds. *Principles and Practice of Infectious Disease*, 5th edition. Philadelphia: Churchill Livingstone, 2000;669–675.

32. Lalwani AK, Sooy CD. Otologic and neurotologic manifestations of acquired immunodeficiency syndrome. *Otolaryngol Clin North Am* 1992;25:1183.

33. Lee E, Chae S, Lim H, Hwang S, Suh H. Clinical experiences with acute mastoiditis–1988 through 1998. ENT–Ear, Nose & Throat J 2000;79:884–892.

34. Luntz M, Keren G, Nusen S, Kronenberg J. Acute mastoiditis revised. *Ear Nose Throat J* 1994;73:648–654.

35. Maharaj D, Jadvat A, Fernandes CM, Williams B. Bacteriology in acute mastoiditis. *Arch Otolaryngol Head Neck Surg* 1987;113:514–515.

36. Migirov L. Computed tomographic versus surgical findings in complicated acute otomastoiditis. *Ann Otol Rhinol Laryngol* 2003;112:675–677.

37. Nadol JB, Eavery RD. Acute and chronic mastoiditis: clinical presentation, diagnosis and management. *Curr Clin Top Infect Dis* 1995;15:204–229.

38. Paradise JL, Otitis media. In: Behrman RE, Kliegman RM, Jenson HB, eds. *Nelson Textbook of Pediatrics*, 17th edition. Philadelphia: Saunders, 2004:2138–2149.

39. Pfaltz CR, Griesmer C. Complications of acute middle ear infections. *Ann Otol Rhinol Laryngol* 1984;112:133–137.

40. Speigel JH, Lustig LR, Lee DC, Murr AH, Schindler RA. Contemporary presentation and management of a spectrum of mastoid abscesses. *Laryngoscope* 1998;108:822–828.

41. Vassbotn FS, Klausen OG, Lind O, Moller P. Acute mastoiditis in a Norwegian population: a 20 year retrospective study. *Int J Pediatr Otorhinolaryngol* 2002;62:237–242.

Acute Otitis Externa

42. Alberti PWRM. Epithelial migration on the Tympanic Membrane. *J Laryngol Otol* 1964;78:808–830.

43. Austin DF. Diseases of the external ear. In: Ballenger JJ, Snow JB, eds. *Diseases of the nose, throat, ear, head and neck*, 15th ed. Baltimore: Williams & Wilkins, 1996:974–988.

44. Babiatzki A, Sade J. Malignant external otitis. *J Laryngol Otol* 1987;101:205.

45. Bell DN. Otitis externa. *Postgrad Med* 1985;78:101–106.

46. Cohen D, Friedman P. The diagnostic criteria of malignant external otitis. *J Laryngol Otol* 1987;101:216–221.

47. Cohen D, Friedman P, Eilmon A. Malignant external otitis versus acute external otitis. *J Laryngol Otol* 1987;101:211–215.

48. Fairbanks D. Otic topical agents. *Otolaryngol Head Neck Surg* 1980;88:327–331.

49. Giamarellou H. Malignant OE. The therapeutic evolution of a lethal infection. *J Antimicrob Chemother* 1992;30:745–751.

50. Goldenberg D, Golz A, Netzer A, Joachims Z. The use of otic powder in the treatment of acute otitis externa. *Am J Otalaryngol* 2002;23:142–147.

51. Haddad J. Diseases of the external ear. In: Behrman RE, Kliegman RM, Jenson HB, eds. *Nelson Textbook of Pediatrics*, 17th edition. Philadelphia: Saunders, 2004;2136–2152.

52. Havelaar AH, Bosman M, Borst J. Otitis Externa by *Pseudomonas aeruginosa* associated with whirlpools. *J Hyg (Lond)* 1983;90:489–498.

53. Hirsch BE. Infections of the external ear. *Am J Otolaryngol* 1992;13:145–155.

54. Klein JO. Otitis Externa, otitis media, mastoiditis. In: Mandell GL, Bennett JE, Dolin R, eds. *Principles and practice of infectious diseases*, 5th edition. Philadelphia: Churchill Livingstone, 2000:669–675.

55. Kraus DH, Rehm SJ, Kinney SE. The evolving treatment of necrotizing external otitis. *Laryngoscope* 1988;98:934–939.

56. Main T, Lim D. The human external auditory canal secretory system—an ultrastructural study. *Laryngoscope* 1976;86:1164–1176.

57. Marcy SM. Infections of the external ear. *Pediatr Infect Dis* 1985;4:192–201.

58. Marcy SM. External otitis due to infection. *Pediatr Infect Dis* 1985;4(Suppl 3):S27–S30.

59. Roland PS, Stroman DW. Microbiology of acute otitis externa. *Laryngoscope* 2002;112:1166–1177.

60. Rubin J, Yu VL. Malignant external otitis: insights into pathogenesis, clinical manifestations, diagnosis, and therapy. *Am J Med* 1988;85:391–398.

61. Salit IE, McNeely DJ, Chait G. Invasive external otitis: review of 12 cases. *Can Med Assoc J* 1985;132:381–384.

62. Schuller DE, Schleuning AJ. Infection and inflammation of the ear. In: Schullers DE, Schleuning AJ, eds. *DeWeese and Saunders' textbook of otolaryngology*, 8th ed. St. Louis: Mosby, 1994:403–433.

Perichondritis

63. Balkany TJ, Ress BD. Infections of the external ear. In: Cummings CW, Fredrickson JM, Harker LA, Krause CJ, Schuller DE, Richardson MA, eds.

Otolaryngology Head & Neck Surgery, 3rd edition. St. Louis: Mosby, 1998;2979–2986.

64. Clemons JE, Severeid LR. Trauma to the auricle. In: Cummings CW, Fredrickson JM, Harker LA, Krause CJ, Schuller DE, Richardson MA, eds. *Otolaryngology Head & Neck Surgery*, 3rd edition. St. Louis: Mosby, 1998;2987–2994.

65. Durand M, Joseph M. Infections of the upper respiratory tract. In: Braunwald E, Fauci AS, Kasper DL, Hauser SL, Longo DL, Jameson JL, eds. *Harrison's Principles of Internal Medicine*, 15th edition. New York: McGraw-Hill, 2001;187–193.

66. Folz BJ, Lippert BM, Kuelkens C, Werner JA. Hazards of piercing and facial body art: a report of three patients and literature review. *Ann Plast Surg* 2000;45:374–381.

67. Hanif J, Frosh A, Marnane C, Ghufoor K, Rivron R, Sandhu G. "High" ear piercing and the rising incidence of perichondritis of the pinna. *BMJ* 2001;322:906–907.

68. Kroon DF, Strasnick B. Diseases of the auricle, external auditory canal, and tympmanic membrane. In: Glasscock ME, Gulya AJ. *Surgery of the Middle Ear*, 5th edition. Hamilton, Ontario: B.C. Decker, 2003;345–367.

69. Metts J. Common complications of body piercing. *West J Med* 2002;176:85–86.

70. Meyerhoff WL, Caruso VG. Trauma and infections of the external ear. In: Paparella MM, Shumick DA, eds. *Otolaryngology*, 3rd edition. Philadelphia: W.B. Saunders, 1991;1227–1235.

71. Simplot TC, Hoffman HT. Comparison between cartilage and soft tissue ear piercing complications. *Am J Otolarngol* 1998;19:305–310.

72. Wu J, Collins NP, Wilson SF. Perils of pinna piercing and pseudomonas perichondritis. *Aust Fam Physician* 2003;32:516–517.

73. Yahalom S, Eliashar R. Perichondritis: a complication of piercing auricular cartilage. *Postgrad Med J* 2003;79:29.

CHAPTER 30
Epistaxis

Jeffrey A. Evans and Todd C. Rothenhaus

Epistaxis is a frequent problem seen by the emergency physician. It is estimated that up to one in seven people will have at least one episode of epistaxis in their lifetime. The incidence is bimodal, with a peak from the ages of 2 to 10, and a broader peak between the ages of 50 and 80 (7). Nasal hemorrhage occurs most commonly in the dry and colder months (10,16,24), and most cases are minor. Of patients presenting to the emergency department (ED), more than 90% can be definitively managed by the emergency physician. While many patients require follow up with an otolaryngologist, only a minority of cases should require an ED consultation for management or admission.

Blood is supplied to the nasal mucosa from terminal branches of both the internal and external carotid arteries (1,5). The anterior and posterior ethmoidal arteries, branches of the internal carotid system, supply both the septum and lateral aspect of the nose superiorly. The sphenopalatine artery, part of the external carotid system, supplies the turbinates and meati posteriorly and the inferoposterior portion of the nasal septum. The superior labial artery and greater palatine artery, also branches of the external carotid, supply the anterior portions of the septum and floor of the nasal cavity.

CLINICAL PRESENTATION

Epistaxis may present in a number of ways. Approximately 90% of nosebleeds are considered anterior, which means the bleeding can be visualized in the anterior portion of the nasopharynx.

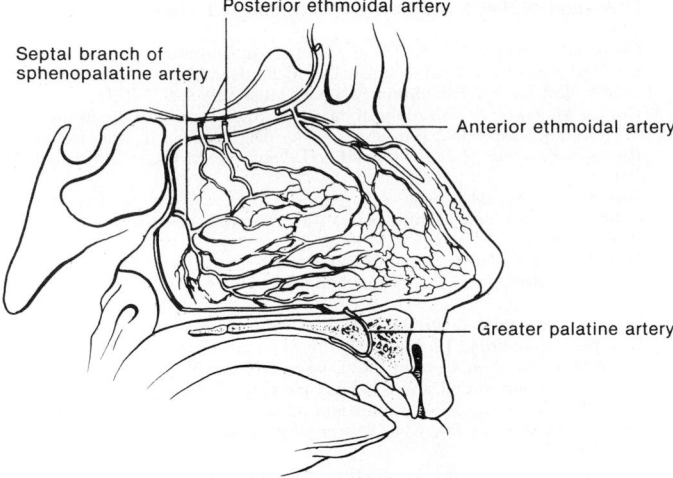

Figure 30.1.   Blood supply to Kiesselbach plexus.

TABLE 30.1.   Causes of Epistaxis
Spontaneous or idiopathic
Trauma
Digital trauma
Facial fractures
Foreign body
Infection
Bacterial rhinitis or sinusitis
Nasal diphtheria
Tumors
Juvenile angiofibroma
Paranasal sinus tumors
Surgery
Chemical irritants
Systemic toxins
Medications
Aspirin
Nonsteroidal antiinflammatory drugs
Warfarin
Heparin
Dipyridamole
Clopidogrel, Ticlopidine
Thrombolytics
Coagulopathy
Thrombocytopenia
Disseminated intravascular coagulation
Hemophilia
von Willebrand disease
Hepatic failure
Leukemia
Venous congestion
Congestive heart failure
Mitral stenosis
Forceful coughing or nose-blowing
Other
Osler-Weber-Rendu syndrome
Barotrauma
Endometriosis
Allergic rhinitis

Anterior hemorrhage most frequently arises from Kiesselbach plexus, also known as Little area, an anastomotic network of vessels on the anterior portion of the nasal septum (Fig. 30.1). Posterior hemorrhage cannot be visualized directly, tends to be more severe, and is not amenable to simple outpatient therapy. Except in cases of trauma, epistaxis is typically localized to one side of the nose, and the source is frequently a single bleeding point.

Patients with an underlying coagulopathy may present with other manifestations of bleeding such as bruising, petechiae, bleeding gums, hematuria, or gastrointestinal bleeding. Patients with a significant amount of blood loss may present with signs and symptoms of hypovolemia such as lightheadedness, fatigue, tachycardia, or hypotension.

DIFFERENTIAL DIAGNOSIS

Most cases of epistaxis are spontaneous and idiopathic. Other causes include facial trauma, nose-picking (epistaxis digitorum), foreign bodies (especially in children, the mentally retarded, and elderly institutionalized patients), and nasal or sinus infections (7). Iatrogenic causes include nasogastric and nasotracheal intubation, surgical complications, and overzealous treatment of self-limited hemorrhage. Hypertension has long been thought to be associated with epistaxis. However, whether hypertension predisposes to epistaxis remains controversial. A deviated septum is a risk factor for recurrent epistaxis, as drying and cracking of the superficial nasal mucosa occurs at sites of turbulent airflow. Use of topical nasal steroid sprays may produce epistaxis through irritation of the nasal mucosa by the propellant.

Children with epistaxis nearly always present with an anterior source associated with local irritation or recent respiratory infection (7). Allergic rhinitis has been implicated as a common cause of recurrent epistaxis in children (15).

Posterior hemorrhage should raise suspicion for juvenile nasopharyngeal angiofibroma in young males, or squamous cell carcinoma in the Asian population. Osler-Weber-Rendu syndrome is characterized by a lack of contractile elements in the muscular wall of vessels, leading to arteriovenous malformations. Patients with acquired immunodeficiency syndrome (AIDS) may have thrombocytopenia from idiopathic thrombocytopenic purpura (ITP), splenomegaly, or drug use, or may present with a qualitative platelet disorder that may predispose

to bleeding (19). Table 30.1 lists some of the many causes of epistaxis.

Occasionally, patients present with massive epistaxis that is initially confused with hemoptysis or hematemesis. If fresh blood is not clearly dripping out of the nose, have the patient sit upright, rinse out their mouth with water if possible, and examine the oropharynx under suitable light. Blood dripping from the posterior nasopharynx confirms nasal hemorrhage.

EMERGENCY DEPARTMENT EVALUATION

A thorough, directed history and physical examination allows the physician to determine the etiology and site of the bleeding. However, if the patient is bleeding profusely, is hemodynamically unstable, or is extremely apprehensive, an initial attempt should be made to control or slow the bleeding before a lengthy history is obtained. The patient's vital signs, as well as extent, duration, and initial side of hemorrhage, should be noted.

Questions concerning past episodes of epistaxis or the presence of systemic diseases are appropriate. Easy bruising or prolonged bleeding after minor surgical procedures suggests the possibility of coagulopathy, and recurrent episodes of epistaxis, even if self limited, should raise suspicion for nasal pathology. Use of alcohol and medications, especially aspirin, nonsteroidal antiinflammatory agents, warfarin, or other antithrombotic or antiplatelet agents, should be noted, as these not only predispose to epistaxis, but also make treatment more difficult (10).

If the nasal hemorrhage is severe enough to produce signs and symptoms of hypovolemia, blood should be sent for hematocrit and type and cross-match. If the patient relays a history of easy bruising, recurrent frequent epistaxis, a history of platelet disorders, neoplasia, or recent administration of chemotherapy (10), a complete blood count is warranted. An international normalized ratio (INR) and partial thromboplastin time (PTT) are generally not indicated unless warfarin use or liver disease is suspected (10).

EMERGENCY DEPARTMENT MANAGEMENT

As with all patients presenting to the ED, attention should first be directed toward the ABCs. Massive hemorrhage may require endotracheal intubation and aggressive resuscitation. Rapid control of epistaxis associated with multiple trauma or significant facial injuries is best secured with epistaxis balloons (11), with consideration given to immediate otolaryngology consultation and angiography to rule out internal carotid artery injury (6). Nontrauma patients with massive epistaxis should be spared lengthy attempts at locating a bleeding source and also be managed with nasal balloons or Foley catheter balloon and anterior packing. Patients with severe hemorrhage should receive intravenous crystalloid infusion, as well as continuous cardiac monitoring and pulse-oximetry.

Most cases of epistaxis, however, are minor, and the episode frequently terminates in the triage area with the proper application of pressure. Although patients may attempt a number of unusual and unfounded techniques to arrest epistaxis, once in the ED, they should be instructed to firmly grasp and pinch the entire, soft, anterior portion of the nose and hold pressure for 10 to 15 minutes (22). If bleeding is not easily controlled, or there is any suspicion of airway compromise or hemodynamic instability, the patient should be brought directly to the treatment area.

Excessively high blood pressure may contribute to hemorrhage and make the bleeding more difficult to control, but should be managed carefully (8,9). Control of bleeding reduces patients' anxiety, and is frequently all that is necessary to reduce blood pressure.

Treatments at the disposal of the emergency physician include topical vasoconstrictors, chemical or electrical cautery, nasal packing using prefabricated nasal tampons or epistaxis balloons, or traditional nasal packing. Every ED should have a prepackaged epistaxis tray or have key materials readily available (Table 30.2).

Preparation is the key to successful management of epistaxis. Both the patient and physician should be adequately gowned. Droplet spread of blood occurs with sneezing and coughing, so gloves and protective eyewear should be worn (1,19). Adequate light should be provided by a headlamp with an adjustable, narrow beam.

Position the patient upright or leaning slightly forward. Adjust the chair so that the patient is just below eye level. The patient's head should be comfortably positioned against the headrest to prevent sudden movements during treatment. Have the patient hold a kidney or emesis basin under the chin to catch blood running from the nose or mouth.

Instruct the patient to blow the nose to clear the nasopharynx, even if bleeding has ceased, as local fibrinolysis of clots can result in recurrence of epistaxis or persistent oozing. An initial attempt to locate the bleeding site should then be undertaken. The nasal speculum is used to spread the nares vertically, with the instrument held in such a manner that the index finger rests on the bridge of the nose for stabilization. Begin the examination at Kiesselbach plexus, moving superiorly and posteriorly along the nasal septum, and conclude with the turbinates and

TABLE 30.2. Equipment Used for Management of Nasal Hemorrhage
ENT chair
Headlamp
Nasal speculum (short and long)
Bayonet forceps
Frazier suction tips (No. 7 and 9)
Yankauer suction tip
Emesis or kidney basin
Gowns
Rubber gloves
Silver nitrate sticks
Electrocautery (optional)
Cotton balls
Dental roll
4×4-inch gauze
Facial tissue
0.5×72.0-in. petrolatum gauze
Antibacterial ointment (Neosporin, Polysporin, or Bacitracin)
0-silk sutures (straight needle)
Silk tape
Tongue depressors
Small plastic cups
Foley catheters (16Fr or 18Fr with 30-mL balloon)
Red rubber catheters (two 8Fr)
Umbilical clamps
Cocaine 4% topical
Pontocaine 2%–4% or lidocaine 2%–4% topical
Phenylephrine 0.25% solution
Epinephrine 1:1,000 for topical use
Prepackaged nasal balloons
Merocel nasal sponges
Avitene, Fibrin Glue, Surgicel, Oxycel, or Gelfoam

ENT, ear, nose, and throat.

lateral wall. Particular attention should be directed to Kiesselbach plexus, the posterior floor of the nasal cavity, the junction of the anterior third and posterior two-thirds of the nasal septum, and the high anterior septum (10). With a well-illuminated and thorough examination, a bleeding point can almost always be identified.

If the point of bleeding is identified and is not bleeding too briskly, application of oxymetazoline (Afrin) alone, or in combination with chemical cautery, has been shown to be effective in the management of anterior epistaxis (12). Electrical cautery has little advantage over silver nitrate (23). Cautery should be performed properly to avoid complications. The tip of the applicator should be rolled gently over the mucosa until a grey eschar forms. If bleeding is very light or has stopped and the mucosa is dry, wetting the tip of the applicator may be necessary. Brisk bleeding may be slowed by cauterizing the four quadrants around the bleeding site or any identifiable vessel just proximal to the area. Diffuse or extensive cautery should be avoided, and only one side of the septum should be cauterized at one time, to avoid septal necrosis or perforation.

If bleeding is brisk, pledgets soaked with an anesthetic–vasoconstrictor solution should be inserted into the nose on the side of the bleeding to provide hemostasis and anesthesia. Dental roll is particularly unsuited for this purpose, as it does not conform to the contours of the nasal cavity, and once impregnated, tends to hold solutions tenaciously. An acceptable pledget can be fashioned by winding a piece of cotton tightly around the bayonet forceps. The cotton is pulled off the forceps and soaked in 4% cocaine or a 1:1 solution of 4% topical lidocaine and epinephrine (1:1,000) or phenylephrine. Multiple pledgets may be placed, one above the other, onto the floor of the nasal cavity, and allowed to remain in place for 10 to 15 minutes. Alternatively, if accessible, the point of bleeding can be injected with 0.5 to 1.0 mL of 1%

lidocaine with epinephrine 1:100,000 using a 27-gauge needle. If application of vasoconstriction alone fails to stop the bleeding, then cautery should still be attempted over the now well anesthetized area.

If a bleeding point cannot be localized, yet bleeding continues, the approximate depth of the bleeding site can be localized using a small Frazier suction catheter. Place the catheter at the nares and tilt the patient's head slightly forward so that the suction captures all bleeding. Gently advance the catheter posteriorly along the floor of the nose until blood returns from the nares. Once the approximate depth of the bleeding site is localized, another attempt can be made at slowing or arresting the bleeding using soaked pledgets.

If direct attempts to cauterize a bleeding point fail, anterior nasal packing should be performed. At this point, it may be a good idea to reconsider whether bleeding is posterior, because placing a posterior pack will necessitate first removing any anterior packing. Furthermore, if the site of bleeding is from the meatus, or from the medial surface of a turbinate, packing may prove to be of little value, and attempts to arrest the bleeding with other methods will be needed.

Traditional anterior nasal packing has been supplanted by preformed nasal tampons or epistaxis balloons. Merocel nasal packing is an effective and quick method to control epistaxis (1,17). After sufficient anesthesia is obtained, lubricate the tip of the Merocel with antibiotic ointment (5,20), or surgical lubricant, hold the Merocel at a 45-degree angle and insert it into the nasal cavity for a distance of 1 to 2 cm. Firmly grasp the length of the Merocel with bayonet forceps, rotate the long axis of the Merocel into the horizontal plane and with firm pressure push the Merocel straight backward into the nasal cavity. Merocel is supplied in different lengths that may be trimmed with scissors for both anterior or anterior–posterior hemorrhage. If an anterior–posterior sponge is employed, it should be inserted until it touches the back wall of the posterior nasal space. If the pack does not fully rehydrate with blood, then saline should be applied. Secure the drawstring to the cheek. Traditional anterior nasal packing should be used if a septal deformity precludes the use of Merocel (17).

Epistaxis balloons (intranasal balloon catheters) are particularly useful in cases of intractable or posterior hemorrhage. Radiographic evidence has shown that these catheters work through multiple mechanisms, including direct tamponade of the bleeding vessel, tamponade of supplying vessels, occlusion of the posterior choana, and pressure on the inferior and middle turbinate arteries. Balloons are available in either anterior (single-balloon) or anterior–posterior (double-balloon) models. A valve affords access to each balloon. After checking the integrity of the balloons, the catheter is copiously covered with water-based lubricant or viscous lidocaine (petroleum-based materials may cause delayed rupture of the balloon) and the catheter is inserted along the floor of the nose. The balloon should be inflated slowly to minimize pain. Air may be used initially, but saline or sterile water should be used in patients in whom the balloon will remain for more than a few hours.

Traditional anterior nasal packing is more difficult, but may be considered if the above measures are unavailable or unsuccessful. The nose should be packed with sterile petrolatum ribbon (0.5 to 1.0 in. wide) gauze, to which is added an antibacterial ointment to prevent the possibility of toxic shock syndrome. Soaking the packing material in topical vasoconstrictors may lead to prolonged absorption and is contraindicated (18). Packing begins by grasping the ribbon about 6 in. from its end with the bayonet forceps. The ribbon is then placed in the nasal cavity as far back as possible ensuring that the free end still protrudes from the nose. This first pass is then pressed onto the floor of the nasopharynx with the closed forceps. The ribbon is then grasped about 4 to 5 in. from the nasal alae, the nasal speculum is repositioned so that the lower blade holds the ribbon against the lower border of the nasal alae, and a second strip is brought into the nose and pressed downward. This process is continued superiorly in a stair-step fashion until there is no room left in the nose. Both ends of the ribbon must protrude from the anterior end of the nose, and the nare is covered with a piece of gauze and secured with tape.

Other alternatives to the traditional anterior nasal pack include fibrin glue, calcium sodium alginate (Kaltostat), Oxycel, Avitene, and balloon tamponade. Topical thrombogenic agents such as fibrin glue, gelatin sponge (Gelfoam), and microfibrillar collagen powder (Avitene) are useful in cases of epistaxis associated with coagulopathy when applied directly to the bleeding area.

Control of Posterior Epistaxis

Bleeding that begins with the sensation of blood in the posterior pharynx, bleeding that cannot be localized anteriorly, or bleeding that fails to arrest with anterior packing is considered posterior and will need to be managed in consultation with an otolaryngologist. However, bleeding should be initially controlled by the emergency physician using one of a number of available techniques.

The traditional method of posterior packing with gauze rolls attached to strings is cumbersome and should be replaced with the use of an epistaxis balloon or inflatable Foley catheter. Balloon catheters are easier to install and just as effective as traditional posterior nasal packs (2). Regardless of technique, posterior packing occludes the posterior choanae only, and requires some form of anterior pack. Once both the posterior choana and the anterior nares are occluded, the entire nasopharynx fills with blood. Hence, if the posterior pack dislodges, a large amount of blood can be aspirated (3). Posterior packs are uncomfortable and fraught with complications, including hypoxia, hypercarbia, exacerbation of obstructive sleep apnea, aspiration, hypertension, bradycardia, arrhythmias, myocardial infarction, and death (4,25). Inflatable balloon catheters designed with a central airway may limit or reduce hypoxia.

If an epistaxis balloon is used, the catheter is first placed as far into the nose as is possible. Next, the posterior balloon is inflated slowly with 4 to 5 mL of water or saline and the catheter is pulled gently forward to fit snugly in the posterior choana. Finally, the anterior balloon is filled with saline until the bleeding stops, the pain is too great, or bowing of the septum is noted. Pressure necrosis and adhesions may result from over inflation, and the amount of fluid placed in each balloon should be recorded.

If a Foley catheter is to be used, a 12 Fr to 16 Fr catheter with 30-cc balloon is placed into the nose along the floor of the nasopharynx until the tip is visible through the mouth in the posterior pharynx. It is then slowly inflated with 15 mL of saline, pulled anteriorly until it is firmly set against the posterior choanae, and secured into place with an umbilical clamp wrapped around a dental roll or matted 4×4-inch gauze to avoid direct pressure necrosis of the ala or columnella.

A traditional posterior pack is fashioned from 4×4-inch gauze rolled into a 1-inch roll and secured with three silk sutures or umbilical tapes. This pack is brought into position in the posterior choana by passing two small, red rubber catheters through each nostril and back out of the mouth, securing each of the two outer sutures to the catheters and pulling the catheters out of the nose again, drawing the pack through the mouth and into position. Each of the sutures is tied together over a gauze buttress to prevent pressure necrosis of the columnella. The third suture is brought out through the mouth and taped to the cheek to facilitate removal.

CRITICAL INTERVENTIONS

- Aggressively resuscitate patients with significant hemorrhage and signs of hypovolemia
- Instruct patients who present to triage with epistaxis to apply squeezing pressure to the nose, since most nosebleeds are anterior and will terminate with this maneuver
- For posterior epistaxis, control the hemorrhage with a balloon catheter, consult an otolaryngologist, and admit to the hospital

DISPOSITION

Because of the number of serious causes of epistaxis, including tumors in the elderly and foreign bodies in children, all patients who present to the ED with epistaxis should be referred for follow up for a complete nasal examination.

Patients with anterior packing should receive follow up with an otolaryngologist in 48 to 72 hours. Anterior nasal packing prevents normal surgical drainage of the sinuses (and frequently the eustachian tubes), and patients should be placed on a penicillin or first-generation cephalosporin. An oral analgesic should also be prescribed.

All patients with posterior packing should to be admitted. Clinicians should also strongly consider admitting elderly, cardiac, or chronic obstructive pulmonary disease (COPD) patients who require anterior packing. Many consulting otolaryngologists are opting for early management of posterior bleeds with endoscopic cautery under direct visualization in the operating suite, early surgical control using arterial ligation, or referral to invasive radiology for selective arterial embolization (14). If time permits and bleeding is not severe, early consultation may spare patients with posterior nasal hemorrhage the discomfort of posterior packing altogether.

Patients who are discharged from the ED should be instructed to avoid blowing the nose, straining, bending over, and participating in sports or other strenuous activity, and to sneeze with their mouth open. Home humidifiers and saline nasal sprays may be helpful in drier, colder months, and patients should avoid any manipulation of the nose. Discontinuation of offending drugs should be individualized and based on the particular indications for each. In most cases, anticoagulated patients with an international normalized ration (INR) in the therapeutic range can continue warfarin without interruption (21). Twice daily application of antibiotic ointment reduces the incidence of recurrent epistaxis (13). Children with frequent nosebleeds and no known bleeding disorder should be referred for coagulation studies (13).

COMMON PITFALLS

✔ Failure to prepare the necessary equipment for control of epistaxis leads to unnecessary inconvenience and delays
✔ Epistaxis in young children is rare and should prompt a search for a foreign body

✔ Failure to identify the source of bleeding or to place an anterior pack properly leads to re-bleeding and necessitates a return to the ED for repacking
✔ Failure to prescribe antibiotics for patients discharged with an anterior pack can lead to sinusitis or toxic shock syndrome
✔ Failure to identify posterior epistaxis until after an anterior pack has been placed necessitates completely unpacking the nose so a posterior pack can be placed

Acknowledgment

The authors gratefully acknowledge the work of Drs. D. Michael Hunt and Ian Paul, who contributed significantly to this chapter in previous editions.

References

1. Alvi A, Joyner-Triplett N. Acute epistaxis. *Postgrad Med* 1996;99:83–96.
2. Cook PR, Renner G, Williams F. A comparison of nasal balloons and posterior gauze packs for posterior epistaxis. *Ear Nose Throat J* 1985;64:446–449.
3. Davis JP. Respiratory obstruction associated with use of the Brighton epistaxis balloon. *J Laryngol Otol* 1993;107:140–141.
4. Fairbanks DN. Complications of nasal packing. *Otolaryngol Head Neck Surg* 1986;94:412–415.
5. Frazee TA, Hauser MS. Nonsurgical management of epistaxis. *J Oral Maxillofac Surg* 2000;59:419–424.
6. Ghorayeb BY, Kopaniky DR, Yeakley JW. Massive posterior epistaxis. *Arch Otolaryngol Head Neck Surg* 1988;114:1033–1037.
7. Guarisco JL, Graham HD. Epistaxis in children: causes, diagnosis, and treatment. *Ear Nose Throat J* 1989;68:522–538.
8. Herkner H, Havel C, Müllner M, et al. Active epistaxis at ED presentation is associated with arterial hypertension. *Amer J Emerg Med* 2002;20:92–95.
9. Herkner H, Laggner AN, Müllner M, et al. Hypertension in patients presenting with epistaxis. *Ann Emerg Med* 2000;35:126–130.
10. Jackson KR, Jackson RT. Factors associated with active, refractory epistaxis. *Arch Otolaryngol Head Neck Surg* 1988;114:862–865.
11. Keen MS, Moran WJ. Control of epistaxis in the multiple trauma patient. *Laryngoscope* 1985;95:874–875.
12. Krempl GA, Noorily AD. Use of oxymetazoline in the management of epistaxis. *Ann Otol Rhinol Laryngol* 1995;104:704–706.
13. Kubba H, MacAndie C, Botma M, et al. A prospective, single-blind, randomized controlled trial of antiseptic cream for recurrent epistaxis in childhood. *Clin Otolaryng* 2001;26:465–468.
14. Moreau S, Valdazo A. Supraselective embolization in intractable epistaxis: review of 45 cases. *Laryngoscope* 1998;108:887.
15. Murray B, Milner R. Allergic rhinitis and epistaxis in children. *Ann Allergy Asthma Immunol* 1995;74:30–33.
16. Nunez DA, McClymont LG, Evans RA. Epistaxis: a study of the relationship with weather. *Clin Otolaryngol* 1990;15:49–51.
17. Pringle MB, Brightwell AP. The use of Merocel nasal packs in the treatment of epistaxis. *J Laryngol Otol* 1996;110:543.
18. Ross GS, Bell J. Myocardial infarction associated with inappropriate use of topical cocaine as treatment for epistaxis. *Am J Emerg Med* 1992;10:219–222.
19. Rothstein SG, Schneider KL, Kohan D, et al. Emergencies in AIDS patients: the otolaryngologic perspective. *Otolaryngol Head Neck Surg* 1991;104:545–548.
20. Shikani AH. Use of antibiotics for expansion of the Merocel packing following endoscopic sinus surgery. *Ear Nose Throat J* 1996;75:524–528.
21. Srinivasan V, Patel H, John DG, Worsley A. Warfarin and epistaxis: should warfarin always be discontinued? *Clin Otolaryngol* 1997;22:542–544.
22. Strachan D, England J. First-aid treatment of epistaxis–confirmation of widespread ignorance. *Postgrad Med J* 1998;74:113–114.
23. Toner JG, Walby AP. Comparison of electro and chemical cautery in the treatment of anterior epistaxis. *J Laryngol Otol* 1990;104:617–618.
24. Viducich R, Gerson L. Posterior epistaxis: clinical features and acute complications. *Ann Emerg Med* 1995;25:592–596.
25. Wetmore SJ, Scrima L, Hiller FC. Sleep apnea in epistaxis patients treated with nasal packs. *Otolaryngol Head Neck Surg* 1988;98:596–599.

TABLE 31.4. Characteristics of Peripheral and Central Vertigo

	Peripheral	Central
Intensity	Moderate to intense	Mild to moderate
Temporal pattern	Brief, episodic	Chronic, continuous
Onset	Abrupt	Gradual
Nystagmus	Rotatory/horizontal	Any kind, including bizarre vertical
Nausea/vomiting	Common	Uncommon
Hearing loss	Possible	Unlikely
Neurologic deficits	Otherwise none	Often present

(*From* Edwards FJ. *Overcoming the diagnostic challenges of dizziness, vertigo, and syncope, Emergency Medicine Reports.* Atlanta: American Health Consultants, Jan. 10, 1994.)

involvement), or recurrent vestibulopathy. Vertigo lasting days and associated with severe nausea and occasional hearing changes is most likely labyrinthitis (vestibular neuritis), although migraine vestibulopathy is also a possibility (3,6).

Physical Examination

Orthostatic hypotension, carotid sinus hypersensitivity, and dysrhythmia can cause vertigo (3,11). Lying and standing vital signs are desirable, but many patients either refuse to move or are too unsteady to stand. A directed physical examination should focus on the cranial nerves (especially hearing), cerebellar function, nystagmus, and positional testing. Painful vesicles on the auricle suggest *Ramsay Hunt syndrome* (herpes zoster oticus) as a central cause of vertigo. The external auditory canal and tympanic membrane should be examined for any abnormality, as cholesteatoma, acute otitis media, tympanic membrane perforation, and even cerumen impactions may cause vertigo. Cholesteatoma will appear as squamous debris in the external auditory canal or in a pocket superior to the short process of the malleus in the tympanic membrane.

Any cranial nerve abnormality strongly suggests a central process. Most commonly, a lesion of the seventh cranial nerve results in facial nerve paresis; a central seventh lesion is suggested by unilaterally decreased eye closing and smiling with

TABLE 31.5. Miscellaneous Causes of Vertigo or Dizziness

Hyperventilation syndrome: A noncentral and nonperipheral cause of vertigo reported in up to 23% of patients with dizziness (21,22). Vertigo follows hyperventilation, sometimes during a panic attack. Typically, the patient has perioral and extremity numbness and dizziness. While usually associated with lightheadedness, hyperventilation has been shown to precede true vertigo in some patients (21). An evaluation may be indicated based on clinical judgment, especially for the patient with true vertigo.

Motion sickness: A perceptual disorientation in healthy people due to rapid changes in position. A sensation of lightheadedness or impending faint without vertigo (often with dimming of vision) suggests a transient decrease of blood to the brain.

Impending faint: Caused by conditions that cause true syncope—vasovagal near-syncope, orthostatic hypotension, blood hyperviscosity syndromes, cardiac dysrhythmia, or cardiac valvular abnormality.

Nonvertiginous "dizziness": May be due to stumbling or falling that is without any head sensation (21). The workup should be directed toward evaluating sensory neuropathy, or poor vision that causes falls.

intact forehead wrinkling due to crossover innervation (1,16). Loss of cranial nerves III, IV, and VI is revealed by a dysconjugate gaze in a particular direction; all directions should be tested (see Chapter 60).

Lesions of the eighth nerve often result in decreased hearing. Sensorineural hearing loss should be ruled out by testing hearing to whispered voice or to rubbing fingers, or with a portable hearing screener. Decreased hearing in one ear requires further evaluation, as it may be sensorineural and signify asymmetry of function of the eighth cranial nerve (9,10). Because most sensorineural loss reduces high-frequency tones, with tinnitus frequently present, a portable hearing screener that tests different frequencies is useful (2).

Tuning fork tests may be helpful in identifying a unilateral sensorineural hearing loss or a conductive hearing loss. If the patient has bilateral sensorineural hearing losses, the tuning fork test will be equivocal. The base of a vibrating tuning fork placed on the midline of the forehead (the *Weber test*) relies on bone conduction; it is normally heard equally in both ears. Decreased sound in one ear implies either a sensorineural loss in that ear or a conductive hearing loss in the other ear. A vibrating tuning fork should be heard longer in air than through bone. In the *Rinne test*, the base of a vibrating tuning fork is applied on the mastoid bone. When the patient no longer feels it vibrating, it is quickly moved in front of the ear. Patients with normal conductive and sensorineural systems will still hear it vibrating. Sensorineural hearing loss is suspected if the hearing is equally reduced by both routes, but air conduction is still better than bone conduction (14). In contrast, in conductive hearing loss, the sound is felt longer by bone than through air.

Cerebellar function is tested by finger-to-nose testing, rapidly alternating hand movements, and the heel-to-shin test. Past pointing or poor coordination suggest central pathology such as multiple sclerosis, cerebellar hemorrhage, or infarction. Station and gait are usually abnormal during acute vertigo and have little discriminatory value. The *Fakuda test* involves marching in place with the eyes closed, and is considered positive for a peripheral lesion when the patient leans or falls to the affected side.

The most helpful physical findings are nystagmus and positional testing. Nystagmus can be characterized as peripheral or central by observing it in a darkened room. Peripheral nystagmus is suppressed with fixation of gaze (opened eyes in a lit room) and is enhanced when the patient looks in the direction of the fast component. Peripheral nystagmus is typically horizontal or rotatory and is worsened with head movement (4,6). Central nystagmus may be of any type; however, nystagmus that is vertical, dysconjugate, direction-changing, or not suppressed by visual fixation is always central (4,6) (Table 31.6).

If nystagmus is subtle or absent, the patient should undergo the *Dix-Hallpike (or Nylen-Barany) maneuver* (Table 31.7). The patient is asked to sit near the top of the gurney in a room with the lights dimmed, with enough room to hang the head off the end of the gurney. He or she is brought rapidly from sitting to lying,

TABLE 31.6. Nystagmus from Central and Peripheral Lesions

	Central	Peripheral
Direction	Any direction	Usually rotatory or horizontal
Laterality	May be one eye	Both eyes
Visual fixation	Enhances nystagmus	Suppresses nystagmus
Effect of gaze toward side of fast component	Does not enhance nystagmus	Enhances nystagmus

TABLE 31.7. Dix-Hallpike Maneuver—Central vs. Peripheral Vertigo

	Central	Peripheral
Negative test	Does not help localize the lesion	5–30 s
Latency	None	
Fatigability	None	Yes
Duration	Sustained	Transient

with the head tilted backward 45 degrees below the horizontal and to the left 45 degrees from midline, with eyes open. A positive test is defined as either the onset of nystagmus, reproduction of the vertigo, or both. After 30 seconds, the patient is brought to the upright position and the test repeated with the patient's head turned to the right. Any positive test should be repeated after a few minutes to see if either the nystagmus or vertigo is less pronounced or "fatigable."

DIFFERENTIAL DIAGNOSIS

Many causes of peripheral and central vertigo are listed in Tables 31.2 and 31.3. Patients, however, complain of "dizziness," which must be further differentiated and identified as vertigo, lightheadedness, loss of balance, or nonspecific dizziness. The differential for lightheadedness is extensive and markedly different from that of vertigo. It includes dehydration, hypovolemia, anemia, dysrhythmia, hypoxia, and other causes.

EMERGENCY DEPARTMENT EVALUATION

Laboratory Testing

Significant electrolyte abnormalities are confined largely to patients taking diuretic medications or those who have a history of electrolyte abnormalities (3,4). Occult metabolic causes of central vertigo are unlikely, but routine glucose measurement should be done to screen for hypoglycemia. Unsuspected significant hypoglycemia is found in about 3% of patients. A complete blood count will identify patients with anemia or polycythemia and an elevated SED rate may point to rheumatoid arthritis or systemic lupus erythematosus. Otosyphilis will be identified with a positive FTA-ABS or MHA-TP serologic test.

Radiologic Imaging

If central vertigo is suspected, further evaluation is needed. Structural CNS lesions should be sought by either emergent head computed tomography (CT) or magnetic resonance imaging (MRI) with gadolinium scanning. These should be selected with regard to whether suspicion tilts toward intracranial tumor, cerebellar infarction or hemorrhage, acoustic neuroma, or multiple sclerosis (12).

Other Studies

Electronystagmography (ENG) is a noninvasive means of detecting eye movements by recording corneoretinal potentials on a moving strip recorder. The eletronystamography is also acutely useful. ENG can often distinguish central from peripheral vertigo as well as identify which ear is the affected side (10,13). This test is usually performed by an audiologist. An audiogram should also be done to evaluate whether there is a hearing loss related to the disorder. These tests are usually done outside of the emergency department, however, a portable audiometer can be a useful screen.

Routine electrocardiograms are abnormal in 20% of dizzy patients older than age 45 (8). Significant findings occur in 3%; these are mostly predicted by a history of cardiac disease (11). The vestibular labyrinth is particularly vulnerable to ischemia and infarction in patients with a history of atherosclerosis (see Table 31.2 (12)).

EMERGENCY DEPARTMENT MANAGEMENT

After the ABCs have been addressed, the patient older than age 45 should have an intravenous line, oxygen, and heart monitor until a cardiovascular cause of vertigo can be reasonably excluded. Symptomatic treatment should begin immediately. Intravenous boluses of isotonic crystalloid should be given to the orthostatic patient, unless a history of congestive heart failure requires a more judicious hydration regimen. Because many dehydrated patients do not manifest orthostatic changes, fluid should also be given to the patient who is vomiting or having prolonged nausea.

Drug overdose or drug toxicity should be managed according to the ingestant, time since ingestion, and overall condition of the patient.

Central vertigo should be managed as a priority. Acute onset of a structural CNS abnormality, manifested by an abnormal neurologic examination, requires that neurology or neurosurgery consultation be obtained. Head CT scanning is usually done, but its inability to see the posterior fossa often requires either clinical diagnosis or referral for MRI.

The patient with labyrinthitis will probably feel better with hydration and time. All unnecessary movement should be avoided. The patient who is vomiting might benefit from intravenous droperidol (2.5 to 5.0 mg). There is no evidence as to the superiority of any one antivertigo medication, but antihistaminic and anticholinergic medications seem to help. Choices include:

Meclizine (Antivert) 25 mg po tid
Diazepam (Valium) 5 mg po qd
Diphenhydramine (Benadryl) 25 mg po qid
Scopolamine 0.5-mg transdermal disc q3 days

Because the elderly are likely to become confused after using scopolamine, it should be avoided in these patients (3,15).

BPV or BPPV is easily managed with the *Epley maneuver*. This series of maneuvers is similar to the Dix-Hallpike (or Nylen-Barany), and begins with the patient sitting up, then laying him or her back, with the affected ear held at a 45-degree angle and the head extended until the vertigo resolves. The head is then turned to the opposite side and held at a 45-degree angle with extension. The patient is then rotated up on that side, with the head looking down at about 135 degrees; once the vertigo is resolved, the patient is seated upright, with the head sideways. The head is then turned forward. This procedure is repeated until there is no nystagmus or vertigo in any of the positions. The patient is then told to stay in an upright position for 24 to 48 hours. A soft cervical collar may be beneficial as well (5,7) (Fig. 31.1). This procedure should not be performed in patients with cervical spine injuries or degenerative joint disease.

An acute attack of Ménière disease may be managed as labyrinthitis, but the patient should be referred to an otolaryngologist for follow up.

Perhaps as valuable as medication is performing Cawthorne head exercises each morning and afternoon (Table 31.8). They worsen the vertigo while they are being performed, but they

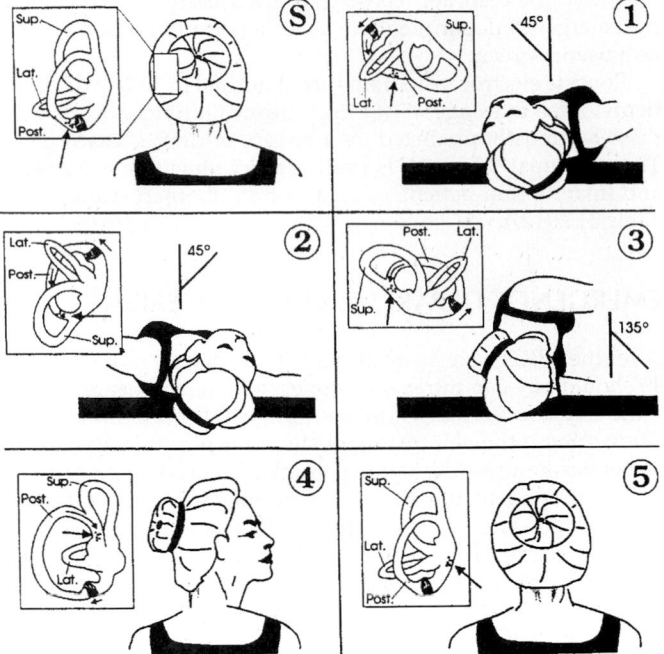

Figure 31.1. Epley Maneuver. Positioning sequence for left posterior semicircular canal as viewed by operator (behind patient). *(Box)* Exposed view of labyrinth, showing migration of particles *(large arrow)*. *(S)* Start—patient seated (oscillator applied). *(1)* Place head over end of table, 45 degrees to left. *(2)* Keeping head tilted downward, rotate to 45 degrees right. *(3)* Rotate head and body until facing downward 135 degrees from supine. *(4)* Keeping head turned right, bring patient to sitting position. *(5)* Turn head forward, chin down 20 degrees. Pause at each position until induced nystagmus approaches termination, or for T (latency + duration) seconds if no nystagmus. Keep repeating entire series (1–5) until no nystagmus in any position.

TABLE 31.8.	Cawthorne's Balance Exercises
1. Eye Exercises	Looking up, then down—at first slowly, then quickly. 20 times.
	Looking from one side to the other—at first slowly, then quickly. 20 times.
	Focus on finger at arm's length, moving it 1 ft in each direction and back again. 20 times.
2. Head Exercises	Bend head forward, then backward with eyes open—slowly, later quickly. 20 times.
	Turn head from side to other side—slowly, then quickly. 20 times.
	As dizziness improves, head exercises should be done with eyes closed.
3. Sitting	While sitting, shrug shoulders. 20 times.
	Turn shoulders to right, then to left. 20 times.
	Bend forward and pick up objects from ground and sit up. 20 times.
4. Standing	Change from sitting to standing and back again. 20 times with eyes open. Repeat with eyes closed.
	Throw a small rubber ball from hand to hand above eye level. 20 times.
	Throw ball from hand to hand under one knee. 20 times.
5. Moving About	Walk across room with eyes open, then closed. 10 times.
	Walk up and down a slope with eyes open, then closed. 10 times.
	Walk up and down steps with eyes open, then closed. 10 times.
	Any game involving stooping or turning is good.

Exercises are to be done for 15 to 30 minutes twice a day.

These exercises help your central nervous system adjust to the current function of your inner ear balance mechanism and will lead to a decrease in your symptoms of positional dizziness. You may omit any exercises that do not cause dizziness.

habituate the vestibular system, thereby allowing the vertigo to improve over time, often long enough to perform a required task.

CRITICAL INTERVENTIONS

- Obtain an imaging study (CT or MRI) for patients with suspected central vertigo
- Provide appropriate medications or maneuvers for patients with peripheral vertigo

DISPOSITION

The patient with vertigo should be given time off from work or school. Patients should be cautioned, in writing, to avoid driving, working at heights, or operating heavy equipment until episodes have resolved completely.

Patients discharged with peripheral vertigo should be told that recurrence is likely, and that they should return for any symptoms of central dizziness. The symptoms appearing on the head injury checklist are useful, except that "dizziness or staggering while walking" is crossed off. Outpatient referral is indicated either to the primary provider for follow up or to an otolaryngologist for further evaluation and management.

In the elderly, falls are especially dangerous, due to decreased strength and bone mass. Such patients should be discharged only if they are steady on their feet. Order a walker and encourage its use to prevent a fall if and when the dizziness recurs (15).

Immediate consultation with a neurologist is indicated for the patient with signs of a new CNS abnormality. Immediate consultation with an otolaryngologist is indicated for the following: sudden sensorineural hearing loss with or without vertigo, signs of otitis media in an immunocompromised patient, malignant external otitis, signs of perilymphatic fistula or cholesteatoma. Consultation with either a specialist or a neurologist should be considered for patients with vertigo of unknown etiology, in those with a history of cardiovascular disease, or those whose vertigo does not improve in the emergency department. Patients with a history of atherosclerosis and suspected labyrinthine ischemia should be seen by an otolaryngologist if attacks continue (6,8).

Admission is indicated for signs of central vertigo, vertigo caused by dysrhythmia, and vertigo that is disabling or associated with persistent vomiting, and for patients who cannot be safely discharged because they lack household help. Admission to a bed with continuous cardiac monitoring is indicated for patients with suspected vertigo from dysrhythmia.

Transfer is indicated for emergent neurologic or neurosurgical consultation or monitoring that is unavailable locally. In most cases, advanced cardiac life-support transport is indicated, owing to possible progression of a CNS lesion or need to treat a symptomatic dysrhythmia.

COMMON PITFALLS

✔ Most, but not all, young vertiginous patients have a peripheral vestibular disorder
✔ Failure to consider a medication as the cause of vertigo

✔ Failure to initiate intravenous hydration in hopes that the nauseated patient will be able to drink

✔ Over-reliance on orthostatic vital signs, which are difficult to define and interpret in vertiginous patients

✔ Failure to recognize neurologic signs and symptoms in association with the vertigo

✔ Discharging an elderly vertiginous patient to home alone. Falls in the elderly may cause hip fractures. Consider admission for all elderly patients who are unsteady

References

1. Adams RD, Victor M. *Principles of neurology.* 7th ed. New York: McGraw-Hill, 2001;318–326.
2. Alvord LS. Handheld screening audiometers: reliability factors of a new screening tool. *Hear Instr* 1991;42:49.
3. Baloh RW. Vertigo. *Lancet* 1998;352:1841–1846.
4. Baloh RW. Differentiating between peripheral and central causes of vertigo. *Otolaryngol Head Neck Surg* 1998;119:55–59.
5. Bernard ME, Bachenberg TC, Brey RH. Benign paroxysmal positional vertigo: the canalith repositioning procedure. *Am Fam Physician* 1996;53(8):2613–2616.
6. Buttner U, Helmchen C, Brandt T. Diagnostic criteria for central versus peripheral positioning nystagmus and vertigo: a review. *Acta Otoluryngol* 1999;119:1–5.
7. Epley JM. Particle repositioning for benign paroxysmal positional vertigo. *Otolaryngol Clin North Am* 1996;29.
8. Gomez CR, Cruz-Flores S, Malkoff MD, et al. Isolated vertigo as a manifestation of vertebrobasilar ischemia. *Neurology* 1996;47:94–97.
9. LaRouere MJ, Seidman MD, Kartush JM. Medical and surgical treatment of vertigo. In: Jacobson GP, Newman CW, Kartush JM, eds. *Handbook of balance function testing.* St. Louis: Mosby, 1993:338.
10. Kentala E. Characteristics of six otologic diseases involving vertigo. *Am J Otolaryngol* 1996;17:883–892.
11. Kinney EL, Wright RJ. Should echocardiography be used to screen dizzy patients? *Angiology* 1988;10:902–906.
12. Kim GW, Heo JH. Vertigo of cerebrovascular origin proven by CT scan or MRI: pitfalls in clinical differentiation from vertigo of aural origin. *Yonsei Med J* 1996;37:47–51.
13. Shi M, Yu X, Niu H, et al. The value of electronystagmography in differential diagnosis of vertigo. *Hunan I Ko Ta Hsueh Hsueh Pao* 1997;22:156–158.
14. Sloane PD. Dizziness in primary care: results from the National Ambulatory Medical Care Survey. *J Fam Pract* 1989;1:33.
15. Sloane PD. Evaluation and management of dizziness in the older patient. *Clin Geriatr Med* 1996;12(4):785–801.
16. Turbiak TW, Reich JJ. Ear emergencies. In: Stair TO, ed. *Practical management of eye, ear, nose, mouth, and throat emergencies.* Rockville, MD: Aspen Systems, 1986:68.
17. Turbiak TW, Miller G. Vertigo and labyrinthine disorders. In: Harwood-Nuss A, ed. *Emergency medicine.* Philadelphia: JB Lippincott Co, 1991:91.
18. Grad A, Baloh RW. Vertigo of vascular origin: clinical and nystagmographic features in 84 cases. *Arch Neurol* 1989;46:281.
19. Gleitman RM, Ballachanda BB, Goldstein DP. Incidence of cerumen impaction in the general adult population. *Hear J* 1992;45:28.
20. Evans RW. Postconcussive syndrome: an overview. *Tex Med* 1987;83:49.
21. Drachman DA, Hart CW. An approach to the dizzy patient. *Neurology* 1972;22:323.
22. Herr RD, Zun L, Mathews JJ. A directed approach to the dizzy patient. *Ann Emerg Med* 1989;18:664.

SECTION V

Section Editor: Jeffrey Schaider

Pulmonary Emergencies

CHAPTER 32
Respiratory Failure

Robert Sigillito and Peter M. C. DeBlieux

Respiratory distress is a combination of multiple signs and symptoms rather than a specific disease process or syndrome. Respiratory complaints account for 11.8% of emergency department visits (11). Congestive heart failure, asthma, chronic obstructive pulmonary disease, and pneumonia are among the most common causes of severe respiratory complaints. Between 1992 and 1999, the rates of ED visits for asthma rose 26%, for pneumonia 12%, for chest pain 50%, and for nonischemic coronary disease 2%. The rate of visits for ischemic heart disease, in contrast fell 25% (4). A large number of patients with longstanding severe respiratory disease use the emergency department as a primary source of health care. In a prospective study, 23% of patients requiring intubation for asthma cited the ED as their usual source of health care (12).

CLINICAL PRESENTATION

Definition of Respiratory Distress and Respiratory Failure

Signs of respiratory distress and failure include tachypnea, hypertension, dysrhythmias, dyspnea, stridor, wheezing, accessory muscle recruitment, abdominal paradox, intercostal retractions, diaphoresis, alteration of mentation, hypoxemia, and hypercapnea.

The degree of deviation from normal that defines respiratory distress depends on the patient's age, comorbid illness, and the ability to perform increased work of breathing. *Respiratory distress* implies that the work of breathing is increased such that the patient experiences or displays signs of difficulty breathing. *Respiratory failure* implies that the patient is not able to maintain adequate oxygenation and ventilation. The specific arterial blood gas criteria for respiratory failure have varied slightly between authors (17). The central concept is that disturbances in arterial PO_2 and PCO_2 are the defining parameters. In general, acute hypercapnea ($PCO_2 > 45$), acute respiratory acidosis (pH < 7.34), or acute hypoxemia ($SaO_2 < 90\%$ or $PO2 < 60$) while breathing room air define acute respiratory failure.

DIFFERENTIAL DIAGNOSIS

The diseases that cause respiratory failure are divided into four general categories based on origin: (1) pulmonary, (2) cardiovascular, (3) neuromuscular and (4) systemic (Table 32.1). Alternatively, the differential diagnosis can be narrowed based on the primary blood gas abnormality into 2 categories: hypoxic respiratory failure (HRF), and hypercapneic/hypoxic respiratory failure (HHRF). This expedient characterization of the type of respiratory failure allows the clinician to focus on common etiologies, a diagnostic plan, and appropriate management strategy.

EMERGENCY DEPARTMENT EVALUATION

The goals of the initial evaluation of a patient in respiratory distress are:

1. Detection of life-threatening gas exchange abnormalities, hypoxemia or hypercapnea.
2. Decision regarding need and candidacy for use of noninvasive positive pressure ventilation (NPPV).
3. Decision regarding need for endotracheal intubation and institution of invasive mechanical ventilation (IPPV).
4. Targeted but thorough physical examination directed at establishing a differential diagnosis list.
5. Formulation of an initial diagnostic plan when the etiology is not clearly evident.
6. Initiation of a treatment strategy based on the most likely diagnoses.

Assessment of Adequacy of Oxygenation

Maintenance of O_2 delivery to the vital tissues is the cornerstone of management of respiratory failure. Determination of the state of hemoglobin saturation with O_2 can be accomplished by three means. The gold standard technique is the use of arterial blood gas cooximetry. The percentage of hemoglobin in the oxyhemoglobin state is directly measured by light absorption and is termed the SaO_2. A second method, employed by common arterial blood gas analyzers, measures the partial pressure of O_2 in the blood sample. The measured PO_2 is then used to determine the SaO_2 using a standardized temperature and pH adjusted O_2-hemoglobin association curve. The third most commonly used method involves noninvasively measuring light transmission of two wavelengths differentially absorbed by oxyhemoglobin and deoxyhemoglobin through a cutaneous vascular bed. The pulse oximeter extracts the signals that are pulsatile from those that are nonpulsatile, thus distinguishing between absorption by arterial blood and absorption by tissue or venous blood. The ratio of transmission of the two wavelengths is compared to a nomogram (derived from healthy volunteers with induced hypoxia) to determine the SpO_2, an estimate of the SaO_2. Advantages of this technique include its rapid availability, low cost, and noninvasive nature.

In healthy individuals, pulse oximetry has been demonstrated to accurately reflect the degree of hemoglobin saturation ($+/-4\%$) when compared with results of cooximetry over a wide range of saturations (60%–100%). In the emergency department, pulse oximetry was found to have a sensitivity and specificity for detection of hypoxemia (defined as $SaO_2 < 90\%$ by co-oximetry) of 92% and 90% respectively when SpO_2 cutoff value of 92% was utilized, in patients with carboxyhemoglobin levels <2% (9). Continuous pulse oximetry, rather than single measurements, is recommended in patients with respiratory distress. Trends in SpO_2 have a high degree of correlation with SaO_2, and are useful in guiding therapeutic decisions (8). Pulse oximetry is not reliable in the presence of carboxyhemoglobin or methemoglobinemia.

Assessment of the Adequacy of Ventilation

Unlike noninvasive measures of oxygenation, noninvasive measures of ventilation have not gained widespread popularity. There are two methods of noninvasive determination of PCO_2. The first is analysis of exhaled gas, using the end exhalation CO_2 tension as an index of average alveolar CO_2 tension. Exhaled capnography does not appear to have diagnostic value in discerning the cause of respiratory failure. The second method involves a heated skin probe, coupled with a thin electrolyte layer separated from the skin by a permeable membrane. CO_2 reaches

TABLE 32.1. Differential Diagnosis of Respiratory Distress and Failure

PULMONARY DISEASES

Diseases of the airway
  Acute foreign body obstruction
  Epiglottitis/ Epiglottic abscess
  Obstructive tumors
  Airway trauma
  Acute laryngotracheitis
  Angioedema
  Vocal cord paralysis
Obstructive Diseases
  Asthma
  COPD
    Chronic bronchitis
    Emphysema
    Cystic fibrosis
    Alpha-1 antitrypsin deficiency
Restrictive Diseases
  Idiopathic pulmonary fibrosis
  Interstitial lung diseases
  Pneumonicoses
  Sarcoidosis
Infectious Diseases
  Pneumonia
  Bronchitis
  Bronchiolitis
Inflammatory Diseases
  Acute lung injury/ARDS
  Pulmonary vasculitides
  Hypersensitivity pneumonitis
  Autoimmune related lung disease
    Rheumatoid arthritis
    Systemic lupus erythematosis
    Scleroderma
Thromboembolic disease
Lung Cancer
Pleural diseases
  Pleural effusion
  Empyema
  Hemothorax
  Pneumothorax
  Malignancy
  Traumatic Injury
  Pulmonary contusion
  Flail Chest
  Hemothorax
  Pneumothorax
  Diaphragmatic rupture

CARDIOVASCULAR DISEASES

Ischemic heart disease
Congestive heart failure
Pericardial disease
Cardiac valvular disease
Congenital heart disease
Dysrhythmias
Aortic dissection

NEUROMUSCULAR DISEASES

Guillain-Barré syndrome
Myasthenia Gravis
Muscular Dystrophy
Spinal Cord Injury
Botulism
Tetanus

SYSTEMIC DISEASES

Sepsis
Hypovolemia
Shock
Toxic exposures
Metabolic and acid-base disturbances
Electrolyte disturbances

equilibrium across this membrane, and alters the pH in the electrolyte layer, which is then measured. No data has been reported about use of this modality in emergency medicine, although its use in combination with pulse oximetry has been initially reported in the perioperative setting.

In contrast to pulse oximetry, arterial blood gas (ABG) analysis has not been proven to affect the diagnosis, treatment, or outcome of patients with respiratory failure. Nonetheless, it remains a time-honored gold standard against which other methods are compared. ABG can be used to assess the adequacy of oxygenation, ventilation, and to evaluate acid-base homeostasis. The chronicity of primary respiratory acid-base disturbance can be determined using formulae listed in Table 32.2. See Chapter 158, Acid-Base Disturbances, for a more detailed discussion of acid-base disturbances. In the setting of respiratory distress, severe hypoxemia unresponsive to supplemental O_2, or respiratory acidosis, whether chronic or acute should lead one to consider institution of NPPV or IPPV.

Noninvasive Ventilation

Evaluation of every patient in respiratory distress should include an early determination of candidacy for institution of (NPPV). Criteria for selection of patients in the acute care setting have been suggested by consensus committee (1) (Table 32.3). In addition to the proven efficacy in avoidance of intubation and the consequent complications, NPPV also allows the emergency physician to continue collecting further medical history and other information from the patient after initiation of ventilatory support. This is a task made difficult, if not impossible, by endotracheal intubation.

Noninvasive ventilation has been shown to be a feasible support modality in a variety of disease states (10). There is convincing data demonstrating the efficacy of NPPV in patients with acute exacerbation of COPD, and an evolving literature base supporting its use in asthma, cardiogenic pulmonary edema, community acquired and nosocomial pneumonias,

TABLE 32.2. Formulae to Predict Acid-Base Compensation

ACUTE RESPIRATORY ACIDOSIS

pH will change 0.08 for each 10 mm Hg change in PCO_2
Predicted pH = 7.40 − 0.008 (change in PCO_2)
HCO_3^- will rise 1 meq/l for each 10 mm Hg rise in PCO_2
Predicted HCO_3^- = 24 + 0.1 (change in PCO_2) +/− 3 meq/l

ACUTE RESPIRATORY ALKALOSIS

pH will change 0.08 for each 10 mm Hg change in PCO_2
Predicted pH = 7.40 + 0.008 (change in PCO_2)
HCO_3^- will decrease 2 meq/l for each 10 mm Hg decrement in PCO_2
Predicted HCO_3^- = 24 − 0.2 (change in PCO_2) +/− 3 meq/l

CHRONIC RESPIRATORY ACIDOSIS

pH will decrease 0.03 for each 10 mm Hg increase in PCO_2
Predicted pH = 7.40 − 0.003 (change in PCO_2)
HCO_3^- will rise 3.5 meq/l per 10 mm Hg increment in PCO_2
Predicted HCO_3^- = 24 + 0.35 (change in PCO_2) +/− 4 meq/l

CHRONIC RESPIRATORY ALKALOSIS

pH will increase 0.02 for each 10 mm Hg decrease in PCO_2
Predicted pH = 7.40 + 0.002 (change in PCO_2)
HCO_3^- will fall 5 meq/l per 10 mm Hg decrement in PCO_2
Predicted HCO_3^- = 24 + 0.5 (change in PCO_2) +/− 4 meq/l

TABLE 32.3. Selection Criteria for Use of NPPV

INCLUSION CRITERIA

At least 2 of the following:
Respiratory distress
  Moderate to severe dyspnea
  Accessory respiratory muscle recruitment
  Paradoxical abdominal movements
Respiratory rate > 25
Acute respiratory acidosis
  pH < 7.35 and PCO_2 > 45
Hypoxemia unresponsive to supplemental O_2

EXCLUSION CRITERIA

Any of the following:
Severe cardiopulmonary instability
  Respiratory arrest
  Hypotension or shock
Serious dysrhythmia
Acute myocardial infarction*
Anatomic problems
  Recent facial, esophageal, or gastric surgery
  Craniofacial trauma or burns
  Chronic anatomic abnormalities of the upper airway,
  nasopharynx, oropharynx
Inability to clear or maintain a patent airway and prevent aspiration
  Impaired protective reflexes

RELATIVE EXCLUSION CRITERIA

Extreme Anxiety
Copious Secretions
ARDS

  *This contraindication is considered relative by some authors.
  ARDS, adult respiratory distress syndrome.

---

neuromuscular disease, trauma and burns, upper airway obstruction, post extubation respiratory distress, and obesity hypoventilation syndrome. Potential benefits of NPPV over IPPV include decreased incidence of ventilator-associated pneumonia, shorter duration of assisted ventilation and ICU stay, lower cost of treatment, increased patient comfort, and lower mortality. The use of NPPV in the emergency department is supported by several studies; however, there has been a single report of increased mortality in a prospective randomized trial in a mixed group of patients with respiratory distress. This study has been criticized, and further supportive evidence is lacking (18).

Endotracheal Intubation

Specific criteria that indicate endotracheal intubation have never been validated. As the evidence of efficacy of NPPV for avoidance of intubation accumulates, it is suggested that failure of a NPPV trial in selected disease processes should be considered one of the criteria for endotracheal intubation. Pierson has reviewed the literature, and concluded that selection of patients for endotracheal intubation should not rest solely on ABG criteria or pulmonary mechanical parameters. Rather, the decision to intubate should begin with consideration of the patient's underlying disease process and cardiopulmonary reserve (17) (Table 32.4). The emergency physician must synthesize a vast amount of data to decide whether a patient will require intubation. Indications for intubation depend upon the patient's lack of rapid improvement after initiation of therapy. Hemodynamic instability, serious dysrhythmias, patient fatigue, acute progressive respiratory acidosis, hypoxemia not responsive to supplemental O_2, loss of airway protective reflexes, alteration in level of consciousness, and lack of response to NPPV should prompt the physician to consider intubation (see Chapter 1, Airway Management).

Physical Examination: Evaluation of the Airway

As with all patients in extremis, evaluation begins with the patient's airway, except when emergent defibrillation or cardioversion is indicated. Compromise of the airway should be suspected whenever the patient has difficulty phonating, displays stridor, or has difficulty clearing secretions. Injury or evidence of swelling in the anterior neck, larynx, or pharynx should lead to suspicion of impending airway compromise. In preparation for intubation, an attempt should be made to obtain an airway history. The risk for encountering a difficult airway should be assessed. A rapid, simple predictor of difficult intubation for use by emergency physicians that is both highly sensitive and specific has not been identified. The Mallampati scale (see Chapter 1, Airway Management), sternomental distance, thyromental distance, or a combination of these indices should aid in the detection of some difficult intubations, and prompt planning of an alternate airway management strategy. Use of neuromuscular blocking agents in a patient with a difficult airway may be fraught with hazard.

Physical Examination: Evaluation of the Cardiopulmonary System

Studies have not been published that focus on the diagnostic accuracy of the physical examination in the evaluation of the undifferentiated patient presenting in respiratory distress. There have been a number of studies that address distinct disease entities or physical findings and their predictive value. Traditionally, respiratory rate (RR) has been thought to be a good index of respiratory compromise. However RR has been shown to be an imprecise measurement (6), with significant interobserver variability, and independent measurements differing by 35%. Respiratory rate has also been demonstrated to be a poor index of hypoxia. In a large prospective trial, 19% of emergency department patients at triage with hemoglobin saturation less than 90% as detected by pulse oximetry exhibited a RR below average for their age (13).

TABLE 32.4. Indications for Initiation of Invasive Mechanical Ventilation in Adults with Respiratory Failure

---

Apnea or impending respiratory arrest
Cardiovascular hemodynamic instability
Altered mental status with need to protect the airway for:
  Patency
  To reduce risk of aspiration
  To manage or control secretions
Acute ventilatory insufficiency in neuromuscular disease with one of the following:
  Acute respiratory acidosis
  Progressive decline in vital capacity to < 10–15 cc/kg
  Progressive decline in maximum inspiratory pressure to < 20–30 cm H_2O
Failure of intensive therapy, possibly including NPPV, in these states:
  Acute exacerbation of COPD or asthma
  Acute hypoxemic respiratory failure
  Acute traumatic brain injury
  Traumatic thoracic injury
  Acute respiratory distress, any cause

Diagnostic Studies: Chest Radiography

The utility of chest radiography in emergency department patients with symptoms referred to the chest has been prospectively studied. In a sample of over 1,000 patients during the winter, it was found that among patients over 40 years old, physical examination alone would have missed 37% of patients with a variety of illnesses including congestive heart failure, pneumonia, pleural effusion, masses, pneumothorax, rib fracture, and vascular abnormalities. Overall, 47% of patients in this group had an acute abnormality demonstrated by CXR. Chest radiography is more sensitive than physical examination in high-risk patients as well as in patients presenting to a walk-in clinic (3,5).

In contrast, another study found that 14% of patients age 18 to 40 had an acute abnormality on CXR. Of those, the majority were predicted by physical examination. Thirty percent of patients with abnormal physical examination and 5% of patients with a normal physical examination were found to have acute abnormalities on CXR. Symptoms that were sensitive for predicting an abnormal CXR included cough and hemoptysis. Sixty-five percent of patients with cough alone had a normal CXR, limiting this symptom as an indication for CXR. When hemoptysis and abnormal physical exam were taken together as an indication for CXR, three fewer patients would have been missed. This group included 7 patients (of a population of 325 patients under age 40), 5 with pneumonia and 2 with masses. Other symptoms including fever, dyspnea, sputum production, and chest pain did not predict radiographic abnormalities in the under-40 age group. The authors concluded that CXR is indicated for all patients with chest symptoms over age 40, and in those under 40 with hemoptysis or an abnormal physical examination (3).

Other Diagnostic Studies

Laboratory Studies: A CBC, electrolytes, glucose, and renal indices should be obtained on patients with respiratory failure. Other studies that may be indicated when specific diseases are suspected include cardiac enzymes (acute coronary syndromes), brain natriuretic peptide (congestive heart failure), D-dimer assay (thromboembolic disease), coagulation profile, liver enzymes (multisystem involvement), erythrocyte sedimentation rate (autoimmune diseases, pericarditis, myocarditis), and LDH (Pneumocystis Carinii pneumonia.)

Electrocardiogram: An initial electrocardiogram should be obtained in any adult with risk factors for coronary disease, or cardiac symptoms. Since shortness of breath is a cardiac symptom, this includes the majority of adult patients. An ECG is of limited value in the pediatric population, except when congenital heart disease is suspected.

Computed Tomography: Chest CT should be ordered in patients with respiratory failure and suspicion of pulmonary emboli, or when plain radiography reveals pathology that requires this imaging modality. In addition to detecting pulmonary emboli, CT is useful in identifying lung parenchymal or pleural disease that may not be evident on plain radiographs.

Ventilation Perfusion Imaging: V:Q scanning is appropriate when pulmonary embolism is considered. The choice between V:Q scanning and CT to establish the diagnosis of pulmonary thromboembolism is controversial. While V:Q scan may offer a slightly higher sensitivity than CT, specificity of V:Q scans is limited in the presence of pulmonary masses, infiltrates, pulmonary edema, pleural effusions, and other processes. While CT may be slightly less sensitive, it is highly specific and may reveal alternative diagnoses.

Peak Expiratory Flow Rate: Measurement of peak expiratory flow rate (PEFR) as a surrogate index for forced expiratory volumes should be standard practice in management of patients with exacerbation of asthma and COPD. Flow rates lower than 50% of personal best or baseline baseline indicate a severe exacerbation. Fluctuation of greater than 10% between readings taken before and after, or during the period between bronchodilator treatments indicates that the patient's distal airway reactivity is unstable and warrants continued therapy. Inpatient therapy is usually required if PEFR remains < 50% of expected PEFR after treatment. Discharge is safe if PEFR is >70% of baseline and symptoms are minimal or resolved. The decision to admit or discharge patients with PEFR 50% and 70% must be individualized (7,15).

EMERGENCY DEPARTMENT MANAGEMENT

Oxygen Supplementation

Simple means of delivering supplemental O_2 include nasal canula, venturi mask, and O_2 reservoir nonrebreathing apparatus. Oxygen delivered via nasal canula is appropriate only when low O_2 flow is required. It is impossible to precisely determine the fraction of inspired O_2 (FiO_2) that is being delivered to any given patient because it varies with RR, the degree of nasal versus mouth breathing, and the O_2 flow rate. In general, if more than 5 LPM of O_2 flow is required to achieve adequate O_2 saturation, then an alternative device should be employed.

A venturi mask produces increasing O_2 supplementation by using various O_2 flow rates combined with various venturi apertures. A higher FiO_2 can be delivered with venturi masks than nasal canula. Although each venturi mask lists specific FiO_2 ratings from 0.28-0.50, these are rough estimates at best. If the highest listed FiO_2 does not provide enough supplemental O_2, then a nonrebreather mask is required.

A nonrebreather apparatus combines a collapsible bag reservoir with high flow O_2 and an exhalation valve so that higher FiO_2 can be delivered. When used optimally, the delivered FiO_2 range may approach 0.8. This is the highest level of supplementation that can be delivered without assisted ventilation.

Initiation of NPPV

Current noninvasive ventilators have characteristics that distinguish them from conventional critical care ventilators. Noninvasive ventilators are more portable. This is accomplished by use of a smaller blower capable of delivering lower pressures than a larger ventilator. Typically a noninvasive ventilator can provide up to 40 cm H_2O of air pressure, compared to critical care ventilators capable of delivering over 100 cm H_2O of air pressure.

Noninvasive ventilators have a single tubing circuit limb through which the patient both receives an O_2 mixture and exhales. To prevent rebreathing of exhaled gases, the tubing is continuously flushed with fresh O_2-air mixture during the expiratory phase. Exhaled gas is released through a small exhalation port near the mask. The machine continuously monitors inhaled and exhaled volumes to determine the degree of air leak and to compensate for the lost volume. The ventilator is designed to allow air escape and leak while maintaining airway pressure.

Noninvasive modes of ventilation differ from invasive modes. The key to understanding the differences in the degree of support that each mode will provide lies in three variables: the trigger, limit, and cycle. The trigger is the event that begins inspiration, either patient-initiated respiratory effort or machine-initiated positive pressure. The limit refers to the parameter that limits airflow during inspiration, either a flow rate or a set pressure. The cycle ends inspiration, either when a set volume is delivered (volume controlled ventilation), a pressure is delivered for a set period of time (pressure controlled ventilation), or the

TABLE 32.5.   Modes of Invasive and Noninvasive Mechanical Ventilation

Mode	Trigger, Mandatory Breaths	Trigger, Spontaneous Breaths	Limit	Cycle, Mandatory Breaths	Cycle, Spontaneous Breaths
Continuous Positive Airway Pressure	N/A	N/A	N/A	N/A	N/A
Synchronized Intermittent Mandatory Ventilation	Time interval*	Patient effort if RR ≤ set RR No trigger for breaths > set RR	Inspiratory flow rate	Delivered tidal volume	Delivered tidal volume for breaths ≤ set RR, flow stops with cessation of patient inspiratory effort for breaths > set RR
Assist Control Ventilation	Time interval*	Patient effort	Inspiratory flow rate	Delivered tidal volume	Delivered tidal volume
Pressure Support Ventilation	N/A	Patient effort	Airway pressure	N/A	Decrease in inspiratory flow (cessation of patient inspiratory effort)
Pressure controlled ventilation	Time interval*	Patient effort	Airway pressure	Time interval**	Time interval**
Spontaneous/timed ventilation	Time interval*	Patient effort	Airway pressure	Time interval**	Decrease in inspiratory flow (cessation of patient inspiratory effort)

* Time interval calculated from set minimum respiratory rate
** Time interval = set inspiratory time, or calculated from respiratory rate and I:E ratio

patient ceases inspiratory effort (pressure support ventilation) (Table 32.5).

Continuous Positive Airway Pressure

Continuous positive airway pressure (CPAP) is not a true form of assisted mechanical ventilation, because additional inspiratory pressure is not provided. Pressure above the ambient atmospheric pressure is supplied, and held constant throughout the respiratory cycle (Fig. 32.1A). During inhalation, the gradient between the airway and pleural pressures is higher than it would be if breathing ambient air. Conversely, the gradient is lower during exhalation. The result is that inhalation requires less effort than breathing without CPAP, and the airways are held open during exhalation, conceptually similar to extrinsic PEEP.

Spontaneous Mode

In spontaneous mode, the airway pressure is cycled between an inspiratory (IPAP) and expiratory (EPAP) pressure. This is commonly referred to as bilevel positive airway pressure (BiPAP). The trigger to switch from EPAP to IPAP is patient inspiratory effort, detected by either a drop in airway pressure, measured inspired volume (usually 5-6cc), or an increase in airflow rate. The limited variable during inspiration is the set level of IPAP. The inspiratory phase cycles off when the machine senses cessation of patient effort, indicated by decrease in inspiratory flow below a set threshold, or a maximum inspiratory time is reached, usually 3 seconds. Tidal volume (Vt) varies from breath to breath, dependent on magnitude and duration of patient effort, and lung compliance. Work of breathing (WOB) is related to initiating and maintaining airflow throughout the inspiratory phase.

Spontaneous-Timed Mode

Spontaneous mode is dependent upon patient effort to trigger inhalation. A patient who is breathing at an inadequately low rate will develop respiratory acidosis. To prevent this occurrence, spontaneous/timed (ST) mode allows the machine to trigger based on a time interval determined by a set minimum respi-ratory rate (RR). If the patient does not initiate respiration during the set interval, IPAP is triggered. The machine cycles back to EPAP based upon a set inspiratory time. Most currently produced ventilators provide only CPAP and ST modes.

Suggested Protocol for Initiation of NPPV

NPPV should be introduced to the patient in a planned, reassuring manner. First, the type of interface must be selected. Nasal mask, oronasal mask, full face mask, and helmets are the interfaces applicable to ED use. With the ventilator set in CPAP mode, the mask should be held to the face, allowing a brief period of acclimatization. The mask should then be secured with straps. If indicated, the ventilator mode should be switched to BiPAP, with IPAP of 8–10 and EPAP of 3–5 cm H_2O. IPAP is then incrementally adjusted to obtain exhaled Vt of 8 to 10 ml/kg ideal body weight, and RR < 30. EPAP is adjusted to maintain adequate oxygenation with FiO2 < 0.6, and to eliminate difficulty triggering the ventilator.

Predicting Failure in NPPV

NPPV fails in 10% to 50% of patients, depending in part on the underlying disease. It is not possible to reliably predict which patients will fail to respond to NPPV. Some predictors of failure include adult respiratory distress syndrome (ARDS), pneumonia, and failure to achieve PaO2:FiO2 ratio >150 after 1 hour of treatment (2).

Initiation of IPPV

Control Mode

Control mode ventilation (CMV) is used almost exclusively in delivery of anesthesia, but knowledge of this mode's limitations aids in the comprehension of other modes' features. In CMV, all breaths are triggered, limited, and cycled by the ventilator. The physician selects Vt, RR, inspiratory flow rate (IFR), FiO$_2$, and positive end expiratory pressure (PEEP). The machine then

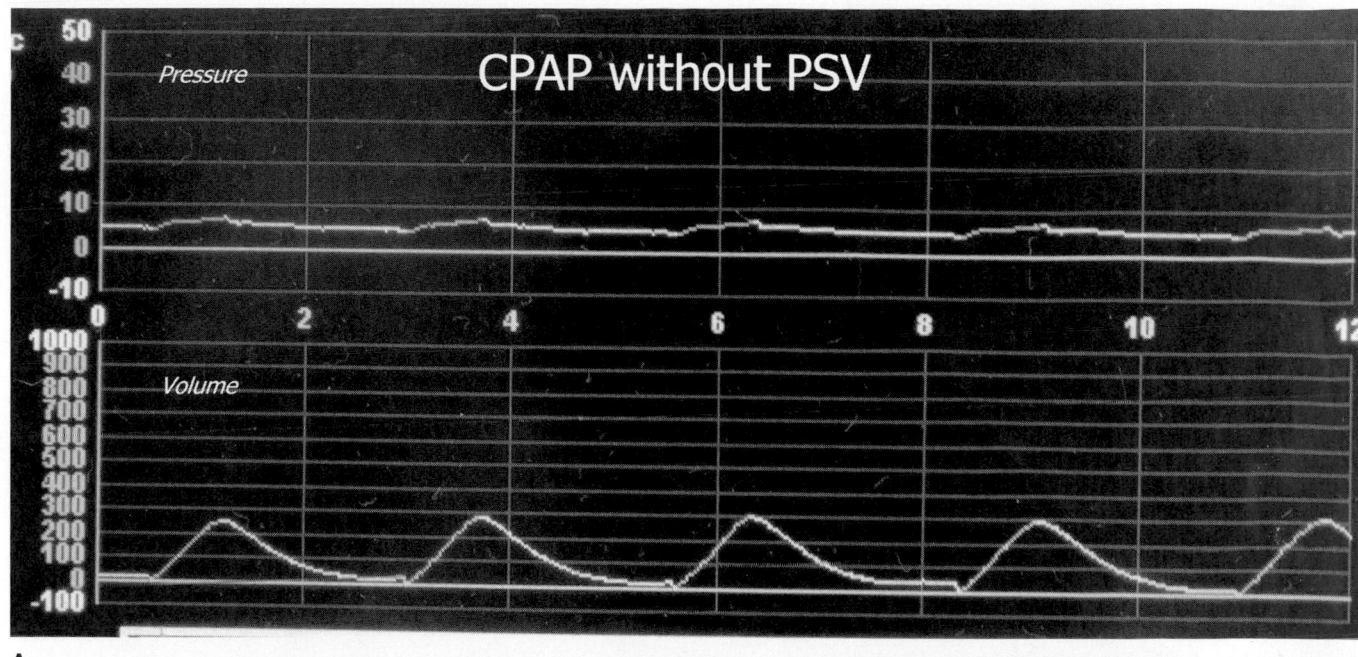

A

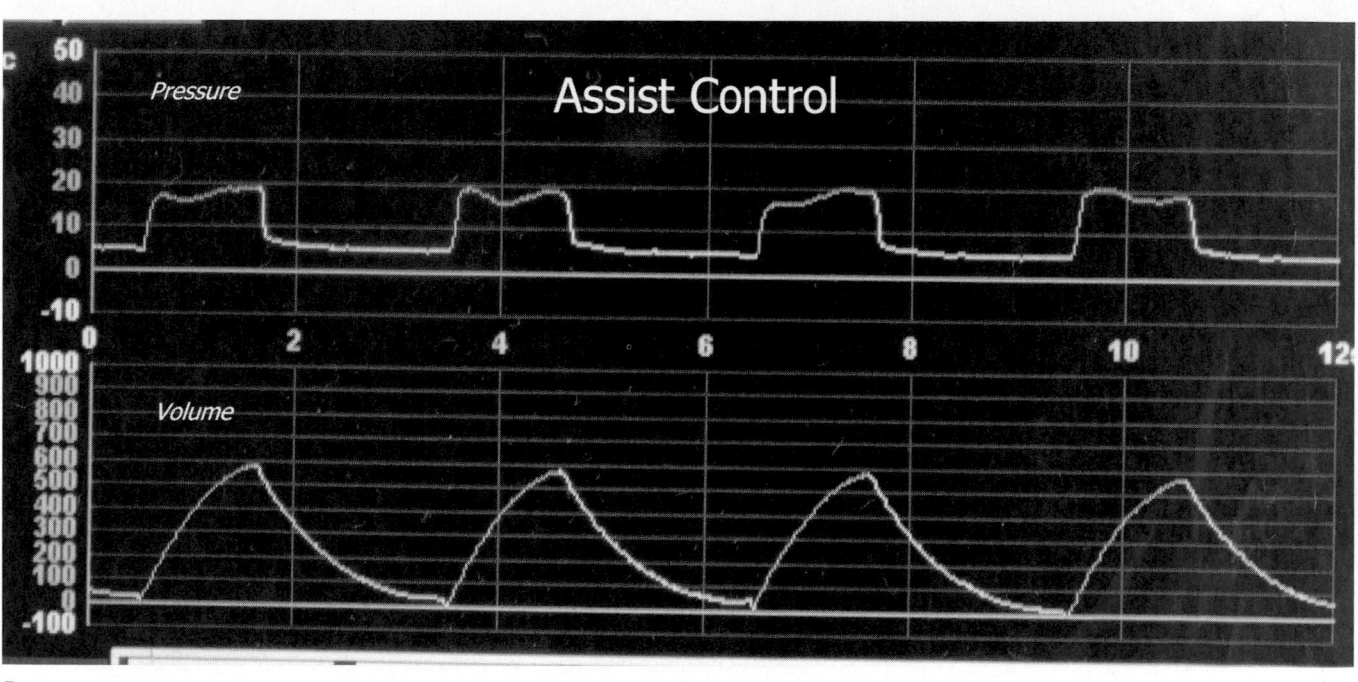

B

Figure 32.1.   Pressure volume relationships with ventilatory support. **(A)** Continuous positive airway pressure. (PSV = pressure support ventilation). **(B)** Assist control mode, volume controlled.

delivers positive pressure based on a time interval, using as much pressure as is required to deliver the set Vt (the cycle) at the set IFR (the limit). The patient is unable to initiate or terminate a breath. If inspiratory effort is initiated before the machine is triggered to deliver a breath, then regardless of the patient's inspiratory force, airflow does not occur. For these reasons, CMV is never used except in apneic, paralyzed, anesthetized patients.

Assist Control Mode

Assist control (AC) mode provides the highest level of ventilatory assistance. The physician sets Vt, RR, IFR, FiO$_2$, and PEEP. In contrast to all other modes, the trigger that initiates inspira-

tion can be either the patient's inspiratory effort or a time interval based on the set RR. When either event occurs, the machine cycles on and delivers the set Vt (Fig. 32.1B). The ventilator follows a time algorithm that synchronizes mandatory breaths with patient-initiated breaths. If the patient is breathing at or above the set RR, then all breaths are patient initiated. If the patient's respiratory efforts are below the set RR, then mandatory breaths are interspersed among the patient's breaths. The WOB is primarily the effort the patient produces to trigger the ventilator.

The majority of the time, AC is used as described above, termed volume controlled ventilation (VCV). As an alternative, some ventilators allow pressure controlled ventilation (PCV)

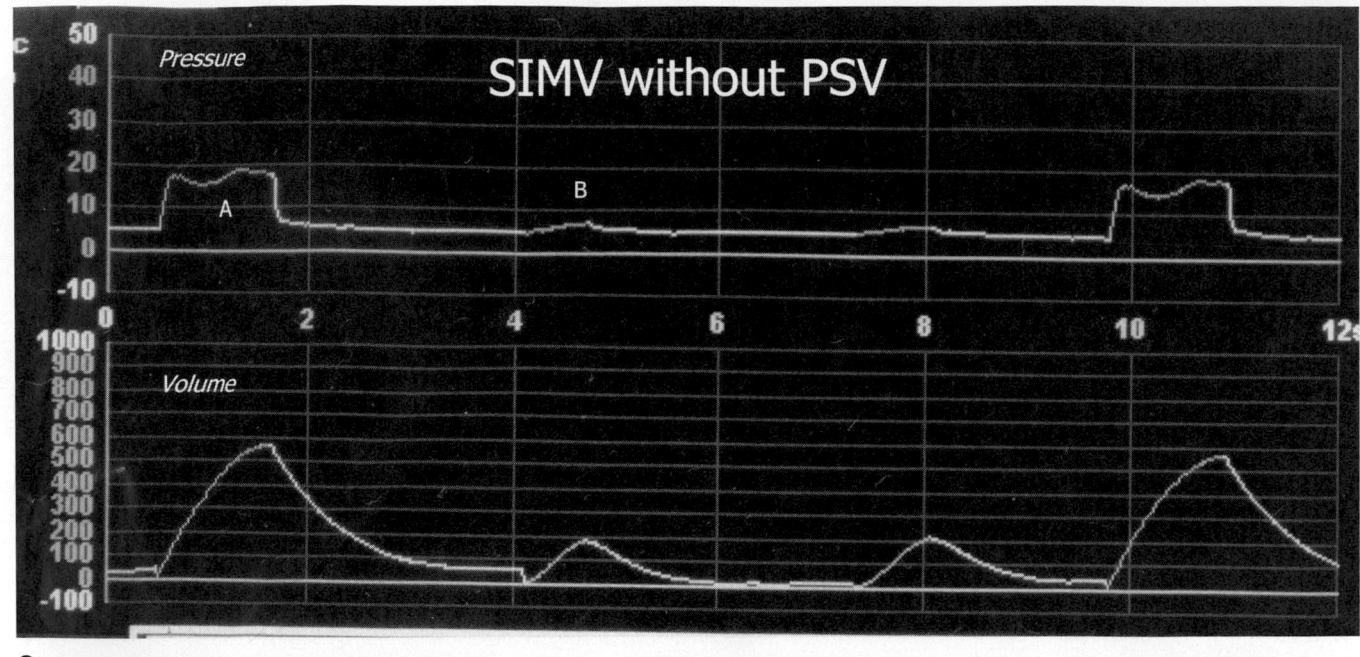

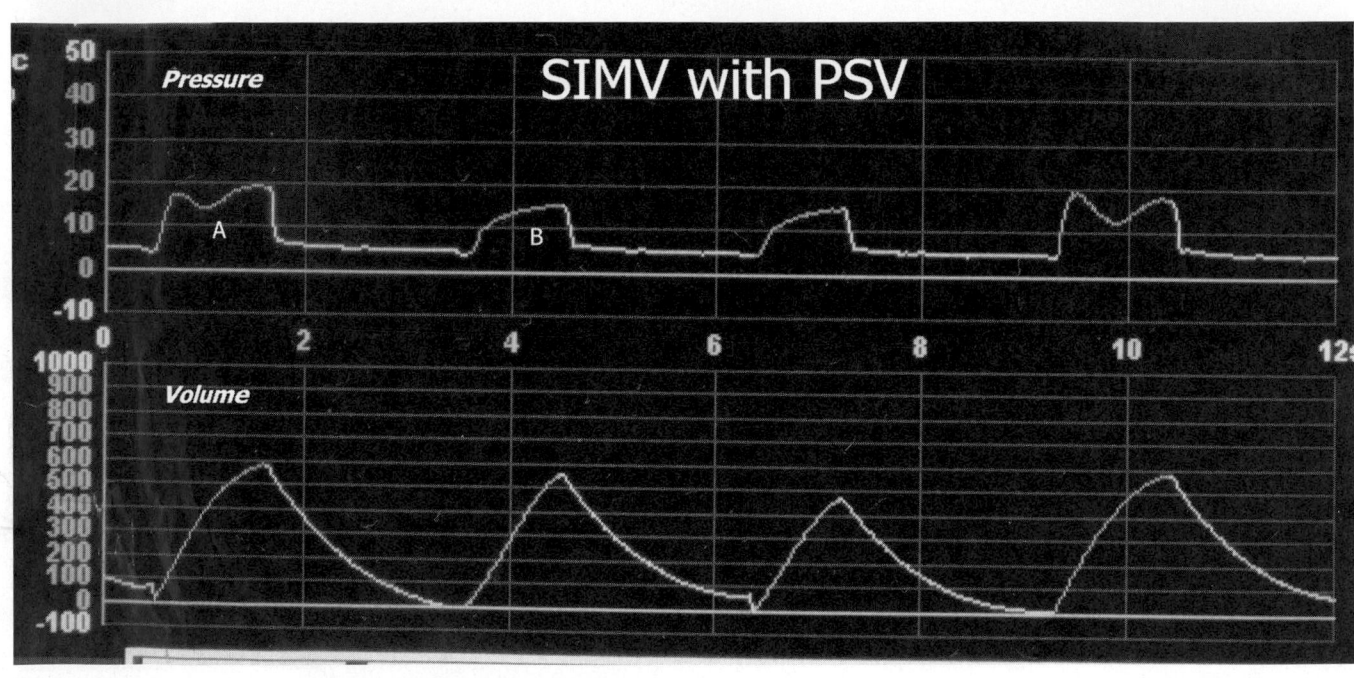

Figure 32.1. *(Continued)* **(C)** Synchronized intermittent mandatory ventilation. A- mandatory breath, B-patient triggered breath. **(D)** Synchronized intermittent mandatory ventilation with added pressure support. A- mandatory breath, B- patient triggered breath.

(not to be confused with pressure support ventilation, described later). Instead of IFR, the limit in PCV is a set inspiratory pressure. Instead of Vt, the cycle is a set inspiratory time (Ti). PCV is sometimes used in neonates and infants.

Synchronized Intermittent Mandatory Ventilation

Synchronized intermittent mandatory ventilation (SIMV) is commonly misunderstood. The physician sets Vt, RR, IFR, FiO_2, and PEEP, as in AC. In contrast, the trigger depends upon the patient's RR relative to the set RR. When the patient breathes at or below the set RR, mandatory breaths are synchronized with patient initiated breaths. In this example, the work of breathing

(WOB) is equivalent to AC. In contrast, if the patient breathes above the set RR, the ventilator does not trigger to assist the spontaneous breaths in excess of the set RR (Fig. 32.1C). In fact, the WOB associated with such breaths is increased. In order to draw a breath, the patient must generate enough negative force to pull air through the ventilator; to overcome the resistance to airflow due to the ventilator circuit tubing, the endotracheal tube, and the patient's airways; and to expand the chest cavity against the elastic recoil of the lungs. WOB may be elevated enough to cause respiratory or metabolic acidosis.

This limitation of SIMV can be diminished by the addition of pressure support ventilation (PSV). PSV is positive pressure

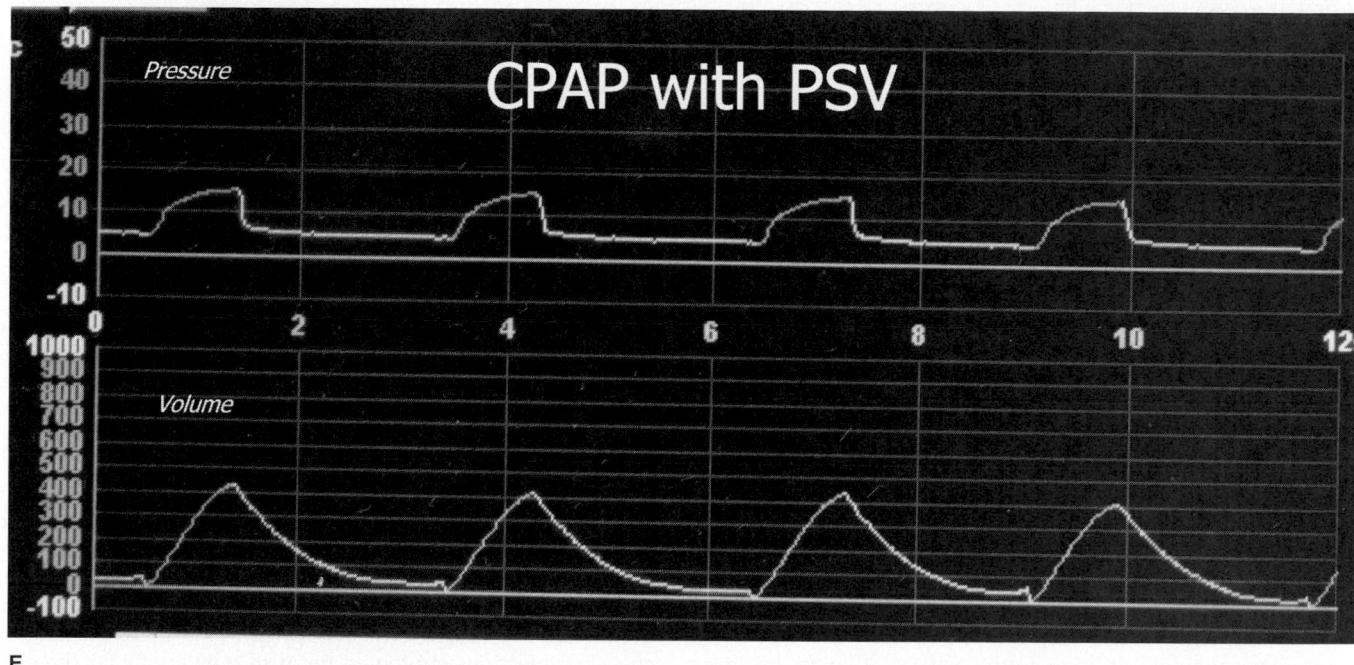

E

Figure 32.1. *(Continued)* **(E)** Continuous positive airway pressure with added pressure support.

added during patient-initiated breaths that exceed the set RR. The patient initiates and terminates inspiration, thereby determining Vt. Once the patient triggers pressure support, it is maintained until the machine senses cessation of patient effort, indicated by a fall in IFR (Fig. 32.1D). Vt, IFR, and Ti are not controlled, but are determined by patient effort. The WOB that a patient performs during PSV involves triggering the ventilator to deliver the pressure and maintaining inspiratory effort throughout inhalation. Contrast this with machine-assisted ventilation in AC or SIMV, where WOB involves triggering the ventilator, with inhalation continuing regardless of whether or not the patient maintains inspiratory effort. The amount of WOB performed is also inversely proportional to the set level of pressure support. Adequate pressure support reduces WOB, and improves Vt and RR. RR seems to be the best index of the adequacy of the level of pressure support, which should be adjusted to maintain RR less than 24 to 30.

Continuous Positive Airway Pressure

As is the case with NPPV, continuous positive airway pressure (CPAP) may be applied via an endotracheal tube. As in SIMV, PSV may be added to CPAP (Fig. 32.1E) Positive pressure is provided during inhalation. The patient initiates and terminates each breath. WOB is performed as the patient initiates each breath and maintains inspiratory effort throughout inhalation. In effect, this is analogous to NPPV in spontaneous mode. The terminology applied is different, however. The values of CPAP and EPAP are equivalent. The value of IPAP is equivalent to the sum of CPAP + PSV. CPAP with PSV cannot be applied in a timed mode, as it can with NPPV.

Selection of a Ventilator Mode

The vast majority of patients who require intubation in the emergency department have respiratory failure, hemodynamic instability, altered level of consciousness, or a combination of the three. The goal of mechanical ventilation is to take over the WOB. The ventilator mode that accomplishes this most effectively is AC, and is the initial mode of choice in most emergency depart-

ment scenarios. In selected cases, when the reason for intubation is protection of the airway, and the patient's drive to breath is intact, CPAP or CPAP with PSV may be appropriate. When set in AC mode, the initial Vt should be 6 to 8ml/kg ideal body weight, RR 14-20 BPM, FiO_2 1.0, and IFR 60 LPM. These settings must be tailored to the individual patient to avoid iatrogenic lung injury.

Monitoring Ventilator Pressures

Mechanical ventilation can cause damage to the lungs on an organ and microscopic level. The concept of ventilator-induced lung injury (VALI) encompasses all forms of injury, including pneumothorax, pneumomediastinum, bronchial rupture, and alveolar damage. Monitoring and controlling pressure delivered to the alveolar level may help prevent VALI. Peak inspiratory airway pressure (P_{peak}) is the highest pressure that is generated during inflation of the lung. P_{peak} is highly variable, dependent on lung compliance and airway resistance. Plateau pressure (P_{plat}) is the end inspiratory airway pressure, measured just after airflow has ceased. P_{plat} in an adult with normal lung compliance is usually in the range of 5 to 15 cm H_2O. Patients with parenchymal lung disease or over-distention have higher P_{plat}. P_{plat} should be maintained below 30 cm H_2O. Intrinsic positive end expiratory pressure ($PEEP_I$) arises when exhalation is incomplete, leading to lung over-distention. To reduce P_{plat} or $PEEP_I$, incrementally reduce Vt and RR, and increase IFR. These measures often lead to respiratory acidosis, but this is considered safer than lung over-distention and damage.

CRITICAL INTERVENTIONS

- Anticipate difficult intubations to avoid unexpected failed airways
- Use the AC ventilator mode as the initial mode post intubation
- Monitor and control pressure delivered to the alveolar level may help prevent ventilator-induced lung injury

DISPOSITION

The overwhelming majority of patients who present with acute respiratory failure will require admission to the hospital. Indications for admission to the ICU include hemodynamic instability, respiratory failure requiring mechanical ventilation, need for frequent respiratory therapy and monitoring, rapid progression of respiratory failure, and failure to respond to intervention. Patients who improve with therapy and become stable may be managed on observation units or inpatient wards. Occasionally, a patient with asthma or mild CHF will respond rapidly to treatment. After a period of stability during observation in the ED, these patients may be safely discharged with close outpatient follow up. This plan should be agreed upon with the patient's primary care physician.

COMMON PITFALLS

✔ Failure to recognize respiratory failure in a patient who does not display tachypnea or other vital sign abnormalities

✔ Failure to consider alternative etiologies of respiratory failure in a patient with chronic respiratory disease

✔ Failure to consider initiating noninvasive ventilation, leading to endotracheal intubation that might be avoided

✔ Over reliance on pulse oximetry to predict adequacy of oxygenation when limitations to interpretation are present

✔ Failure to monitor airway pressures after initiation of IPPV, or failure to individualize ventilator settings, with consequent ventilator induced lung injury

✔ Use of CPAP or SIMV modes without sufficient pressure support, causing increased work of breathing

References

1. American Respiratory Care Foundation. Consensus conference: noninvasive positive pressure ventilation. *Respir Care* 1997;42:364–369.
2. Antonelli M, Conti G, Moro ML, et al. Predictors of failure of noninvasive positive pressure ventilation in patients with acute hypoxemic respiratory failure: a multi-center study. *Intensive Care Med* 2001;27:1718–1728.
3. Benacerraf BR, McLoud TC, Rhea JT, Tritschler V, Libby P. An assessment of the contribution of chest radiography in outpatients with acute chest complaints: a prospective study. *Radiology* 1981;138:293–299.
4. Burt CW, McCaig LF. Trends in hospital emergency department utilization: United States, 1992–99. *Vital Health Stat* 2001;150:1–34.
5. Butcher BL, Nichol KL, Parenti CM. High yield of chest radiography in walk-in clinic patients with chest symptoms. *J Gen Intern Med* 1993;8:115–119.
6. Edmonds ZV, Mower WR, Lovato LM, Lomeli R. The reliability of vital sign measurements. *Ann Emerg Med* 2002;39:233–237.
7. Emerman CL, Cydulka RK. Use of peak expiratory flow rate in emergency department evaluation of acute exacerbation of chronic obstructive pulmonary disease. *Ann Emerg Med* 1996;27:159–163.
8. Jones J, Heiselman D, Cannon L, Gradisek R. Continuous emergency department monitoring of arterial saturation in adult patients with respiratory distress. *Ann Emerg Med* 1988;17:463–468.
9. Lee WW, Mayberry K, Crapo R, Jensen RL. The accuracy of pulse oximetry in the emergency department. *Am J Emerg Med* 2000;18:427–431.
10. Liesching T, Kwok H, Hill NS. Acute applications of noninvasive positive pressure ventilation. *Chest* 2003;124:699–713.
11. Ly N, McCaig LF. National Hospital Ambulatory Medical Care Survey: 2000 outpatient department summary. *Adv Data* 2002;327:1–27.
12. Moore BB, Wagner R, Weiss KB. A community-based study of near-fatal asthma. *Ann Allergy Asthma Immunol* 2001;86:190–195.
13. Mower WR, Sachs C, Nicklin EL, Safa P, Baraff LJ. A comparison of pulse oximetry and respiratory rate in patient screening. *Respir Med* 1996;90;10:593–599.
14. Mower WR, Sachs C, Nicklin EL, Safa P, Baraff LJ. Effect of routine emergency department triage pulse oximetry screening on medical management. *Chest* 1995;108:1297–302.
15. Murphy S. Guidelines for the diagnosis and management of asthma: National Institute of Health National Heart, Lung, and Blood Institute; 1997.
16. Narins RG, Emmett M. Simple and mixed acid-base disorders: a practical approach. *Medicine (Baltimore)* 1980;59:161–187.
17. Pierson DJ. Indications for mechanical ventilation in adults with acute respiratory failure. *Respir Care* 2002;47:249–262, discussion 262–265.
18. Sigillito RJ, DeBlieux PM. Evaluation and initial management of the patient in respiratory distress. *Emerg Med Clin North Am* 2003;21:239–258.

CHAPTER 33
Pneumonia

Gregory J. Moran and David A. Talan

In the United States, more than 3 million persons contract community-acquired pneumonia annually, resulting in about 500,000 hospital admissions. Pneumonia is the sixth leading cause of death in the United States, and the most common infectious cause. Most deaths occur in the elderly or immunosuppressed, but pneumonia occurs in otherwise healthy persons as well. To manage patients with pneumonia successfully, the emergency physician must be knowledgeable about a number of constantly changing factors, including an expanding spectrum of pathogens, changing antibiotic-resistance patterns, and the availability of newer antimicrobial agents. Although several noninfectious diseases may cause pneumonia, this discussion focuses on infectious etiologies, because they are by far the most common in emergency medicine practice.

Traditional pathogens such as *Streptococcus pneumoniae*, *Haemophilus influenzae*, *Mycoplasma pneumoniae*, and viruses continue to be important causes of community-acquired pneumonia. Less common etiologies include *Staphylococcus aureus*, gram-negative bacilli, and oral anaerobes. Organisms such as *Legionella* species and *Chlamydia pneumoniae* are being increasingly recognized as pathogens in a significant number of cases of community-acquired pneumonia. *Pneumocystis carinii* and *Mycobacterium tuberculosis* are important as pathogens related to pulmonary infections in acquired immunodeficiency disease (AIDS) patients. Knowledge of local prevalence patterns for pathogens of community-acquired pneumonia is important to make appropriate choices regarding evaluation and treatment.

CLINICAL PRESENTATION

"Typical" and "Atypical" Pneumonias

Pneumonia is often divided into "typical" (pyogenic bacterial) and "atypical" categories, but this division is somewhat artificial. Prediction of these etiologies based on clinical and radiographic findings is inaccurate (6). The classic presentation of typical pyogenic bacterial pneumonia is the abrupt onset of fever and chills, followed by development of cough that is productive of purulent sputum, and pleuritic chest pain. Elderly or debilitated patients may present with nonspecific complaints, such as altered mental status. Tachypnea and tachycardia are usually present. Examination of the chest may reveal signs of consolidation, such as dullness to percussion, coarse rales, bronchial breath sounds, or increased tactile fremitus.

The atypical pneumonia syndrome is caused by organisms such as *M. pneumoniae*, *C. pneumoniae*, viruses, *Legionella*, or rickettsial organisms such as *Coxiella burnetii*. Patients with this type of pneumonia generally present with a subacute onset of systemic complaints, such as fever, headache, malaise, and myalgias, associated with cough that is often nonproductive. Although mucopurulent sputum generally indicates the presence of pyogenic bacterial pneumonia or bronchitis, it may also be present with mycoplasmal or viral pneumonia. Chest examination often reveals scattered rhonchi or rales. Signs of consolidation are less common.

The high degree of overlap between the clinical and radiographic features of typical pyogenic and atypical pneumonia makes it impossible to definitively identify a specific type of pneumonia without the results of microbiologic or serologic tests. Typical and atypical pathogens sometimes coexist in the same patient, and bacterial infections often follow viral respiratory infections. Although one may not be able to determine with certainty the specific etiology of pneumonia within the time frame of an emergency department evaluation, certain clinical factors may suggest a likely etiology and can help guide empiric therapy. The clinical characteristics of several types of pneumonia are noted next.

Common Etiologies

S. pneumoniae is the single most common identified etiologic agent among adults with community-acquired pneumonia. About 40% of healthy adults carry this organism in the nasopharynx. Patients with a history of diabetes, cardiovascular disease, alcoholism, or malignancy, or with other immunosuppressing illness, are at increased risk of pneumococcal infection. The classic presentation of pneumococcal pneumonia is the abrupt onset of a single shaking chill, followed by fever, cough productive of rust-colored sputum, and pleuritic chest pain. Not all patients exhibit this pattern. Many have had a preceding upper respiratory illness, and the onset of pneumonia may be insidious, especially among the elderly or those with underlying lung disease. Patients with a history of asplenia, sickle cell disease, AIDS, multiple myeloma, or agammaglobulinemia are at increased risk of pneumococcal bacteremia and sepsis. Extrapulmonary complications such as meningitis, endocarditis, or arthritis occasionally develop.

H. influenzae is a common pathogen in adults with chronic obstructive pulmonary disease (COPD), alcoholism, malnutrition, malignancy, or diabetes. The organism is a pleomorphic gram-negative rod that can be encapsulated; among serotypes a through f, type b most commonly leads to serious illness with bacteremia. In several studies, *H. influenzae* has been found to be the second most frequently isolated organism in community-acquired pneumonia among adults. Nontypeable strains (once thought to be benign) are a frequent cause of lower respiratory tract infection in patients with chronic lung disease. Such patients typically present with an insidious worsening of baseline cough and sputum production, and bacteremia is rare. *Moraxella catarrhalis* is another gram-negative rod that can be found in patients with COPD, but it appears to be associated with exacerbations of chronic bronchitis much more frequently than it is associated with pneumonia.

Intravenous (i.v.) drug users may develop hematogenous spread of *S. aureus* that involves both lungs and presents as multiple small infiltrates. This type of pneumonia is often associated with tricuspid valve staphylococcal endocarditis. *S. aureus* may also cause a primary bacterial pneumonia that may be clinically indistinguishable from other bacterial pneumonias. Staphylococcal pneumonias are often necrotizing, with cavitation and pneumatocele formation. An increased incidence of staphylococcal pneumonia has been noted during epidemics of influenza.

Klebsiella pneumoniae rarely causes disease in the normal host and accounts for a very small percentage of community-acquired pneumonias, but it may cause severe pneumonia in debilitated patients with alcoholism, diabetes, or other chronic illness. Sputum is often described as resembling currant jelly because of the necrotizing, hemorrhagic nature of the infection. Abscess formation, empyema, and bacteremia are common, and mortality is high. A chest radiograph characteristically demonstrates a dense lobar infiltrate with a bulging appearance of the fissure, but this finding is nonspecific and most cases present as a more subtle bronchopneumonia. Because the organism is often hospital-acquired, there is a high incidence of antibiotic resistance. *Pseudomonas aeruginosa* is also uncommon as an etiology of community-acquired pneumonia, but it may be present in patients with underlying lung disease, such as bronchiectasis or cystic fibrosis, or in patients who have recently been in a hospital or nursing home.

Seroprevalence studies demonstrate that virtually everyone is infected with *C. pneumoniae* at some time, and that reinfection is common. Most infections in young adults cause a minor, self-limited upper respiratory illness that is subacute in onset. This organism has also been associated with bronchitis, wheezing, sinusitis, pharyngitis, and atherosclerosis. Development of radiographically evident pneumonia is more common in the elderly, in contrast to the common perception that atypical pneumonias occur in the young (9). *C. pneumoniae* is a relatively common etiology of community-acquired pneumonia, accounting for at least 8% of cases in adults; however, this is probably an underestimate, due to the difficulty in diagnosing infection with this organism.

M. pneumoniae is regarded as one of the most common causes of community-acquired pneumonia in previously healthy patients less than 40 years of age. Although most studies have found it to be uncommon among hospitalized pneumonia patients, one study found it to be a common etiology among hospitalized older adults (14). Infection usually begins as a flu-like illness with headache, malaise, and fever. Cough is usually nonproductive, but may sometimes produce clear or even purulent sputum. Skin lesions, including maculopapular, vesicular, urticarial, or erythema multiforme-type rashes, are not uncommon, especially in younger patients. Many patients complain of sore throat or ear pain, but the classic finding of bullous myringitis is less common and is also nonspecific. Common physical findings include pharyngeal erythema, cervical adenopathy, and scattered rales and rhonchi. Rare extrapulmonary manifestations include pericarditis, glomerulonephritis, aseptic meningitis, and Guillain-Barré syndrome. Patients generally do not appear toxic, and the vast majority can be treated as outpatients.

At least 30 species of *Legionella* have been isolated since the 1976 outbreak in Philadelphia from which the organism derives its name. Up to 20% of community-acquired pneumonia cases may be due to this organism (1). *Legionella* is an intracellular organism that lives in aquatic environments. There is no person-to-person transmission. Although it has often been implicated in point-source outbreaks related to cooling towers and similar aquatic sources, the organism also lives in ordinary tap water and has probably been under diagnosed as an etiology of community-acquired pneumonia. Some patients present with a mild, self-limited atypical pneumonia, but older patients, smokers, and those with chronic disease or immunosuppression are at risk for developing the more acute manifestations of a severe systemic illness, with malaise, lethargy, and high fever. There is usually a dry cough, which is accompanied by pleuritic chest pain in 25% to 30% of patients. Purulent sputum often develops later. Gastrointestinal symptoms such as diarrhea and abdominal cramping are often prominent. Patients may appear toxic, with high fever and altered mental status.

Viral pneumonia is common in infants and young children, and has been recognized as an important cause of pneumonia in adults as well. Respiratory syncytial virus (RSV) and parainfluenza viruses are the most common seasonal causes of pneumonia in small children. Influenza viruses are the most common cause of viral pneumonia in adults. Winter influenza outbreaks, usually due to influenza type A, cause an average of 20,000 deaths yearly in the United States, mostly among persons age 65 or older (3). Symptoms of upper respiratory infection, such as rhinitis or sore throat, usually precede the onset of viral pneumonia in adults. The onset of pneumonia may be insidious. Cough is usually nonproductive, and pleuritic chest pain is less common than with bacterial pneumonia. Cytomegalovirus (CMV) can cause pneumonia in persons with severe immunosuppression (e.g., transplant recipients). Varicella zoster virus (chickenpox) may cause pneumonia; this appears to be more common in adults, and factors such as smoking or pregnancy are predisposing conditions. Severe acute respiratory syndrome (SARS) is a respiratory illness due to a coronavirus that was recently identified in southeast Asia. SARS is associated with high a case-fatality rate (approximately 10%–15% overall), which is even greater in the elderly.

Although *P. carinii* does not cause pulmonary disease in normal hosts, the possibility of opportunistic infection and unrecognized AIDS must always be considered. *P. carinii* pneumonia (PCP) is the most common presentation leading to a diagnosis of AIDS, and many patients who present with this pneumonia are unaware of their human immunodeficiency virus (HIV) status. *All* patients who present with pulmonary complaints should be questioned about HIV risk factors, and clinicians should search for signs of HIV-related immunosuppression, such as weight loss, lymphadenopathy, and oral thrush. PCP typically presents subacutely with fatigue, exertional dyspnea, nonproductive cough, pleuritic chest pain, and fever.

Lower respiratory infection due to anaerobic organisms generally results from the aspiration of oropharyngeal contents. These infections are typically polymicrobial, including *Peptostreptococcus* spp., *Bacteroides* spp., *Fusobacterium* spp., *Prevotella* spp., and several other organisms. Presentation is often subacute or chronic, and may be difficult to distinguish clinically from other etiologies of pneumonia. Clinical factors that suggest an anaerobic infection include risk factors for aspiration (e.g., central nervous system depression or swallowing dysfunction), severe periodontal disease, fetid sputum, and radiographic appearance (e.g., location in posterior segment of right upper lobe or superior segment of lower lobe, lung abscess).

Fungal infections due to organisms such as *Histoplasma capsulatum*, *Blastomyces dermatitides*, and *Coccidioides immitis* commonly present as pulmonary disease. These organisms are present in the soil in various geographic areas of the United States: *H. capsulatum* in the Mississippi and Ohio river valleys, *B. dermatitides* in a poorly defined area extending beyond that of *H. capsulatum*, and *C. immitis* in desert areas of the Southwest. These infections should be considered in persons in appropriate geographic areas, especially in persons who are near activities that disturb the soil (e.g., construction, dirtbike riding). The clinical presentation ranges from an acute or chronic pneumonia to an incidental finding of asymptomatic granulomas on chest radiography.

Unusual Causes of Pneumonia

Q fever is an acute febrile illness caused by the rickettsial organism *C. burnetii* that may present as pneumonia. It is most common in persons with occupational exposure to animals. Fever is present in all patients, and a severe headache occurs in about 75% of cases. This infection is rarely fatal.

Plague (caused by *Yersinia pestis*) is endemic in many parts of the world and has been implicated as an organism that could be used in biologic terrorism. It occurs in the southwestern states of the United States in persons bitten by fleas from infected rodents or carnivores. Hematogenous spread may lead to pneumonia that is highly contagious and has a high mortality. It typically presents with cough, chest pain, purulent sputum, and hemoptysis, and is associated with fever and adenopathy.

Hantaviruses have been associated with a syndrome of severe respiratory distress (Hantavirus Pulmonary Syndrome) and shock that has occurred in persons in several areas of the United States. Infection appears to occur from inhalation of aerosols of material contaminated with rodent urine and feces. Patients typically present with a prodrome of fever, myalgia, and malaise, followed in several days by the onset of respiratory distress. Characteristic laboratory findings include thrombocytopenia, hemoconcentration, leukocytosis, and mild elevation of hepatic transaminases. Hypoxia may progress rapidly, requiring ventilatory support. Chest radiographs demonstrate bilateral interstitial lung infiltrates that are more pronounced in dependent areas. If the patient can be supported (there is no known effective antiviral therapy), including the use of extracorporeal membrane oxygenation (ECMO), recovery is usually complete.

Tularemia is a febrile illness, caused by the bacterium *Francisella tularensis* that is spread by contact with body fluids of infected mammals (especially rabbits) or the bite of an infected arthropod. The illness usually begins with an ulcerated skin lesion and painful regional lymphadenopathy. Some patients have a typhoidal form, with only fever, malaise, and weight loss. Pneumonia may occur with either form, presenting as a nonproductive cough and patchy infiltrates on the chest radiograph.

Psittacosis is a chlamydial infection that can be spread to humans from infected birds. It may occur in owners of pet birds, pet shop employees, or others exposed to birds, or workers in poultry-processing plants. Illness often begins rapidly with chills, high fever, myalgias, and malaise; severe headache is often the major complaint. Cough is usually nonproductive. Splenomegaly is often present. Radiographic findings are variable, but patchy perihilar or lower lung field infiltrates are most common.

Anthrax (due to *Bacillus anthracis*) has been used as an agent of biologic terrorism. Inhalation of anthrax spores can cause a syndrome that presents as severe pneumonia, though the more common presentation is severe sepsis without apparent pneumonia. Many patients will have a wide mediastinum on chest x-ray due to swelling of mediastinal nodes. Patients may have concurrent meningitis.

DIFFERENTIAL DIAGNOSIS

Several noninfectious etiologies may result in inflammatory lung processes. These include exposure to mineral dusts (e.g., silicosis), chemical fumes (e.g., chlorine, ammonia), toxic drugs (e.g., bleomycin), radiation, thermal injury, or oxygen toxicity. Immunologic diseases such as sarcoidosis, Goodpasture syndrome, Wegener granulomatosis, collagen vascular disease, or hypersensitivity to environmental agents (e.g., farmer's lung) may also result in pneumonia. Tumors may sometimes be confused with pneumonia radiographically, or may present initially as a postobstructive infection or adenopathy with peripheral infiltrates. Pulmonary emboli must be considered in patients who present with tachypnea, hypoxia, tachycardia, or chest pain in the appropriate clinical setting. Cardiac illness often presents with respiratory complaints such as dyspnea. Aspiration of a foreign body must also be considered as an etiology of pulmonary infiltrates, especially in younger children.

In many studies of community-acquired pneumonia, no microbial etiology can be determined in one-third to one-half of cases, even after thorough investigation. To a great extent, the likely etiologies must be predicted based on epidemiologic considerations and prevalence of pathogens in careful research studies. In general, the likelihood of *S. pneumoniae* is related to the severity of illness, having been identified in as many as 50% of intensive care unit (ICU)–admitted and fatal cases. In studies of adults with community-acquired pneumonia who were hospitalized, traditional pathogens such as *S. pneumoniae* and

H. influenzae accounted for about one-fourth of cases. *Legionella, M. pneumoniae,* and *C. pneumoniae* together accounted for 15% to 40% (6,14). Another large study, in which serologic testing was done for common viral agents, revealed a viral etiology in about 17% of cases, with influenza and parainfluenza viruses, that are the most common (12). Studies of patients with more severe illness who required intensive care unit (ICU) admission have shown the prevalence of *S. pneumoniae* to be as high as 38% and that of *Legionella* to be as high as 22%, although the "unknown" category still accounts for 30% to 50% of cases (18,20). Atypical organisms such as *Mycoplasma* appear to account for a relatively higher proportion of pneumonias in those who have milder illness amenable to outpatient therapy. Nevertheless, it is important to be aware of how frequently atypical organisms are identified in patients with severe illness requiring hospitalization.

EMERGENCY DEPARTMENT EVALUATION

The emergency department evaluation should focus on establishing the diagnosis of pneumonia, determining the presence of clinical features associated with specific infectious etiologies, and identifying host factors that will influence decisions regarding the need for hospitalization and choice of antibiotics.

Chest Radiograph

The chest radiograph is generally the most important test to determine the presence of pneumonia. A number of predictive models have been developed to optimize chest x-ray use in patients with cough in whom pneumonia is suspected. Factors found to be associated with a positive chest x-ray are fever, tachycardia, and tachypnea; rales or decreased breath sounds, sputum production, and absence of rhinorrhea or sore throat have also been predictive in some models. Although use of predictive models may reduce the number of unnecessary chest x-rays, they appear to be less sensitive than physician judgment (5). Because of its relatively low cost and risk, chest x-ray is appropriate when management will be affected by the result (e.g., hospital admission, antimicrobial use, exclusion of other diagnoses). Chest x-ray may be particularly useful in groups such as the elderly (who may have subtle clinical signs of pneumonia), patients with serious underlying disease or severe illness, or those at risk for tuberculosis (TB) (to quickly establish the need for isolation). Young healthy adults who will receive outpatient treatment with empirical antimicrobials may have the chest radiograph deferred unless there is suspicion of immunosuppression or other unusual features of disease. Routine chest radiography for patients with exacerbation of chronic bronchitis or COPD has been shown to be of low yield and can be limited to those with other signs of infection or congestive heart failure (22). Computed tomography of the chest appears to be more sensitive than plain radiographs for detecting the presence of pulmonary consolidation although the natural history of CT-positive, plain radiograph-negative pneumonia is not clear (23).

Although the causative agent cannot be determined solely by the results of chest radiography, certain radiographic patterns tend to be associated with specific pathogens. In pyogenic bacterial pneumonias, radiographs usually show an area of segmental or subsegmental infiltration and air bronchograms. Lobar consolidation is present in a minority of cases of bacterial pneumonia, and is often due to pneumococcus or *Klebsiella.* Bronchopneumonia resulting from spread of infection along the intralobular airway causes fluffy or patchy infiltrates in the involved areas of the lung. A wide variety of bacteria may cause this pattern, as well as agents such as *C. pneumoniae, M. pneumoniae, Legionella,*

and even viruses. An interstitial pattern on the chest radiograph is typically caused by *M. pneumoniae,* viruses, or *P. carinii.* Tiny nodules disseminated throughout both lungs represent a miliary pattern typical of granulomatous pneumonias such as TB or fungal disease. The location of infiltrates may also give a clue to the etiology. Aspiration pneumonia occurs in dependent areas of the lung, most commonly the superior segments of the lower lobes or the posterior segments of the upper lobes. Pneumonia produced by hematogenous spread (such as staphylococcal) tends to be multifocal and peripheral. Apical infiltrates suggest TB.

Additional radiographic features associated with infiltrates may suggest specific etiologies. An infiltrate associated with hilar or mediastinal adenopathy suggests the presence of TB or fungal disease, or may indicate pneumonia associated with a neoplasm. Cavitation is most commonly present with infections caused by anaerobes, gram-negative organisms, fungi, or *S. aureus;* cavitation may also be present in fungal disease or TB. Pneumatoceles or spontaneous pneumothorax may be seen in AIDS patients with PCP. Pleural effusions can be seen with a wide variety of organisms, including many types of pyogenic bacterial pneumonia, *C. pneumoniae, Legionella,* and TB. Anaerobic infections associated with an effusion are especially prone to the development of empyema.

Radiographic findings are nonspecific for a particular infectious etiology. For example, *M. pneumoniae* pneumonia may present with a dense infiltrate, and pneumococcal pneumonia with diffuse interstitial infiltrates. Immunocompromised patients are particularly likely to have atypical radiographic appearances. Occasionally, patients with a clinical picture strongly suggestive of pneumonia have a normal chest radiograph. The absence of findings on the chest radiograph should not preclude the use of antimicrobial therapy in patients thought to have pneumonia on clinical grounds (16).

Other Tests

Laboratory studies are also nonspecific for identifying the etiology of pneumonia. Although an elevated peripheral white blood cell (WBC) count may increase the likelihood of a pyogenic bacterial etiology, this finding is of limited value in making decisions regarding therapy in an individual patient and must be considered in light of other clinical and epidemiologic features (i.e., the pretest probability of various etiologies). A WBC count may be helpful if it yields evidence of immunosuppression, such as neutropenia, or if it reveals lymphopenia that may indicate immunosuppression from HIV infection (2). Serum chemistry studies may be helpful in identifying patients with metabolic acidosis or renal–hepatic dysfunction associated with sepsis or with underlying disease. Such findings may be helpful in predicting a complicated course and may influence decisions regarding disposition, choice of antimicrobial agents, and dosages. These ancillary tests are not necessary in patients with mild illness. In cases in which congestive heart failure is a consideration, B-type natriuretic peptide (BNP) or echocardiography may be helpful.

Assessment of respiratory function with arterial blood gas measurements or pulse oximetry must also be part of the evaluation. Hypoxia is a clear indication for hospital admission.

Although a Gram stain of the sputum is often recommended as a means to identify a bacterial pathogen, the use of the Gram stain as a basis for empiric therapy in the emergency department can be problematic for several reasons. Many patients cannot provide an adequate sputum specimen. Induction of sputum without adequate isolation facilities can put patients and staff at risk if sputum is induced from persons with unrecognized TB. Moreover, the correlation between the identification of pneumococcus on Gram stain and by sputum culture is often poor, even when commonly used criteria for an adequate sputum specimen are applied (fewer than five squamous epithelial cells and more than 25 WBCs per high-power field) (21). The Gram stain is even less likely to demonstrate gram-negative pathogens such as *H. influenzae,* and should not be relied on to rule out a gram-negative etiology. Sputum Gram stains are less accurate when done by less experienced physicians outside the microbiology laboratory and may lead to erroneous conclusions regarding which pathogens are present. Effective empiric antimicrobial therapy can be selected on the basis of clinical information, even if a sputum Gram stain is not done.

The utility of routine blood cultures has been questioned, because studies of nonimmunocompromised adults with pneumonia have demonstrated a low prevalence of noncontaminant bacteremia, and management is rarely changed based on the results (4). Blood cultures should be obtained from immunocompromised patients, those with severe sepsis or shock, or those with risk factors for endovascular infection (e.g., prosthetic valves or intravenous drug use). When positive, blood cultures reflect the etiologic agent more accurately than do sputum cultures. Bacteremia occurs in about 25% to 30% of cases of pneumococcal pneumonia. Routine blood cultures are not indicated for outpatients.

Serologic tests are available for the diagnosis of a number of organisms, including *C. pneumoniae, Legionella,* SARS, and fungi. Serologic tests to determine the etiology of pneumonia may be helpful retrospectively, but both acute and convalescent serum titers are usually required, and are therefore of little use to the emergency physician. *M. pneumoniae* pneumonia is associated with the presence of serum cold hemagglutinins in up to 60% of cases, but they may also be present in a number of viral infections. The diagnosis of the exact etiology of viral pneumonia is made difficult by the nonspecific nature of the presentation and the lack of widely available rapid tests. Rapid diagnostic tests for viral antigens are available for several viruses, including RSV and influenza. Improvements in therapy for specific viral pneumonias (such as newly developed neuraminidase inhibitors for influenza) are likely to make these tests more useful. In the future, rapid testing, using technology such as the polymerase chain reaction, may provide emergency physicians with a reliable method for determining the specific etiology of pneumonia.

EMERGENCY DEPARTMENT MANAGEMENT

As with any seriously ill patient in the emergency department, initial attention should focus on ensuring adequate ventilation, oxygenation, and perfusion. Hypoxic patients with pneumonia should receive supplemental oxygen. Those with severe respiratory compromise may require endotracheal intubation. Patients with underlying asthma or COPD who present with wheezing may benefit from bronchodilator therapy. Seriously ill patients who present with volume depletion or septic shock will require fluid resuscitation and may require vasopressors.

It is usually necessary to begin empiric antimicrobial therapy for pneumonia before a definite microbiologic etiology is established. Antimicrobials should be started in the emergency department for patients who are being admitted to the hospital; deferring treatment until arrival on the ward can sometimes cause significant delays. Mortality has been shown to be reduced among elderly pneumonia patients who receive initial antimicrobials within 8 hours of presentation, as compared with later (15). The antibiotics chosen must provide coverage of the likely etiologies based on clinical, laboratory, radiologic, and epidemiologic information. Though care must be taken not to miss possibly dangerous pathogens, the regimen should be as selective as possible to avoid problems with drug toxicity, emergence of resistance to broad-spectrum agents, and excessive cost.

The prevalence of drug-resistant *S. pneumoniae* (DRSP) has increased steadily over the past decade. In the United States, among outpatient pneumococcal sputum isolates collected between 2001 and 2002, 18.4% had high-level resistance to penicillin (10). Isolates that are resistant to penicillin are also very likely to be resistant to other β-lactams as well as macrolides, tetracyclines, and trimethoprim–sulfamethoxazole (TMP/SMX). A number of respiratory fluoroquinolones have been introduced, such as levofloxacin, moxifloxacin, gatifloxacin and gemifloxacin. These agents have enhanced activity against DRSP as well as other typical and atypical organisms that commonly cause pneumonia, and may offer additional alternatives to vancomycin if DRSP is a concern. Telithromycin, a new antibiotic in the ketolide class (similar to macrolides), also has enhanced activity against DRSP, without the broader gram-negative activity of the quinolones. However, it is not clear that *in vitro* resistance is related to adverse clinical outcome; some studies show increased mortality associated with DRSP, others do not (7,19). Most cephalosporins and macrolides will achieve adequate levels in serum and tissues to successfully treat *S. pneumoniae* respiratory tract infections, even if the laboratory reports that the organism is resistant.

Guidelines have been issued for empirical antibiotics for patients with community-acquired pneumonia (11,17). For patients whose illness is severe enough to require hospital admission and parenteral antibiotics, options include a combination of a third-generation cephalosporin and a macrolide (e.g., i.v. erythromycin or azithromycin, or oral azithromycin), or an extended-spectrum fluoroquinolone alone. These regimens will treat the most common bacterial pathogens, such as *S. pneumoniae, M. catarrhalis,* and *H. influenzae,* as well as atypical pathogens such as *Mycoplasma, Chlamydia,* and *Legionella.* Intravenous azithromycin alone is an option for mild to moderately severe pneumonia in patients without significant comorbidities, though this drug does not achieve significant serum levels and has limited activity against many aerobic gram-negative bacilli and DRSP. If anaerobic organisms are suspected (e.g., aspiration), clindamycin or metronidazole could be added to the regimen, or a β-lactam–β-lactamase inhibitor antibiotic such as ampicillin–sulbactam or piperacillin–tazobactam could be used. Some of the newer quinolones, such as moxifloxacin and gatifloxacin, are also active against anaerobes.

Severely ill and compromised patients are at relatively greater risk of infection due to *S. pneumoniae,* aerobic gram-negative bacilli, *S. aureus,* and, in some areas, *Legionella* spp. Because antimicrobial resistance is more likely to impact the outcome in these patients, it is important to include agents with activity against DRSP. Appropriate empirical therapy could include a combination of a third generation cephalosporin or a β-lactam–β-lactamase inhibitor antibiotic plus a fluoroquinolone. Outcomes with severe pneumococcal pneumonia appear to be better with combination therapy when compared with a single agent such as a fluoroquinolone alone (24). For those patients at risk of infection with *P. aeruginosa* due to neutropenia, bronchiectasis, or recent stay in a hospital or nursing home, drugs such as ceftazidime, piperacillin–tazobactam, ciprofloxacin, or an aminoglycoside would be appropriate. For life-threatening pneumonia in populations in which MRSA is a concern, and patients recently exposed to fluoroquinolones who may have fluoroquinolone-resistant *S. pneumoniae,* vancomycin in addition to a regimen that covers atypical pathogens and gram-negative bacilli may be appropriate.

For patients with AIDS, it is important to treat *P. carinii* as well as bacterial pathogens such as *S. pneumoniae.* TMP/SMX is the treatment of choice; the usual regimen is 20 mg/kg of TMP and 100 mg/kg of SMX in four divided doses (3 amps i.v. q6h for most adults), to be continued for 21 days. For patients allergic to sulfa, pentamidine can be given in a dose of 4 mg/kg over 1 hour.

Because pentamidine has no activity against *S. pneumoniae* or other bacterial pathogens, it is important to add a cephalosporin or other antibacterial agent to the initial empiric regimen. Other options include clindamycin 900 mg i.v. q8h plus primaquine 15 mg PO qd, TMP plus dapsone, atovaquone, or trimetrexate. The addition of steroids (prednisone 40 mg PO b.i.d.) has been shown to reduce mortality and clinical deterioration in patients with PaO_2 less than 70 or A-a gradient greater than 35.

A number of antimicrobials are available for outpatient therapy of community-acquired pneumonia. Appropriate agents for outpatient treatment of adults include macrolides (erythromycin, clarithromycin, azithromycin), fluoroquinolones with enhanced activity against *S. pneumoniae,* or doxycycline. Alternative options that would be appropriate in those patients with a higher likelihood of a "typical" bacterial etiology include amoxicillin–clavulanate or a second-generation cephalosporin such as cefuroxime axetil, cefpodoxime, or cefprozil. These β-lactam agents do not have activity against atypical pathogens. In patients properly identified as low risk for complications and who are evaluated for careful outpatient follow up, use of a macrolide or doxycycline is reasonable, even when there is concern over DRSP. Use of more expensive and more broad-spectrum agents, such as the newer fluoroquinolones, may be justified based on convenience, avoidance of side effects and drug interactions, or concern over DRSP in patients with a higher likelihood of bacterial etiology. Some agents, including azithromycin, levofloxacin (750 mg daily), or moxifloxacin, can be given as a 5-day course. Use of ampicillin or amoxicillin is not generally recommended due to the high incidence of β-lactamase production in pneumonia pathogens, although these have been used successfully in higher doses (e.g., amoxicillin 1 g t.i.d.) in other conditions with a high prevalence of DRSP. TMP/SMX has also been largely abandoned for treatment of pneumonia because of concern about increasing resistance. Except for the administration of fluoroquinolones, these recommendations also apply to school-aged children and adolescents, in whom *Mycoplasma* is common.

Antiviral agents can decrease the duration and severity of influenza if started within 48 hours of symptom onset (3). They are also useful as prophylaxis to control outbreaks within families or group settings such as nursing homes. Because they are not effective against other respiratory viruses, they should be used only if influenza virus is confirmed with a rapid test or is highly likely based on the season and epidemiology. Amantadine and rimantadine are active against influenza A. Dosage should be reduced for debilitated or elderly patients to reduce side effects such as confusion (less common with rimantadine). Zanamavir and oseltamavir are neuraminidase inhibitors that have been shown to be effective against both influenza A and B viruses and appear to have fewer side effects. Zanamavir is given by inhalation and is not recommended for patients with underlying reactive airway disease because of concern about induced bronchospasm. Antiinfluenza virus therapy appears to reduce the duration of symptoms 1 to 2 days and is relatively more effective in patients with fever, comorbidities, and confirmed influenza. Rapid influenza tests, some of which can distinguish influenza A and B, are relatively nonsensitive but may be useful to identify the onset of disease in a community, justify less expensive therapy with amantidine or rimantidine for influenza A, or neuraminidase inhibitors for influenza B.

Many emergency departments initiate outpatient therapy in moderately ill patients, who previously might have been hospitalized, with an initial parenteral dose of a long-acting antibiotic such as ceftriaxone, and employ extended observation (i.e., 12 to 24 hours) while administering supportive care such as hydration, antipyretics, and bronchodilators before discharge on an oral regimen. Certain patients may also be brought back to the emergency department for follow up in 24 hours and receive a second parenteral or observed oral dose of antibiotics. Extended-spectrum fluoroquinolones are another option that may be employed in this strategy, and they have additional activity against atypical pathogens and DRSP. Oral administration of these agents results in blood and tissue levels similar to those with i.v. therapy, provided that normal intestinal absorption exists. Empiric therapy for pneumonia is summarized in Table 33.1.

CRITICAL INTERVENTIONS

- Treat pneumonia based on clinical grounds rather than relying only on radiographic evidence on the chest radiograph
- Obtain blood cultures from immunocompromised patients, those with severe sepsis or shock, or those with risk factors for endovascular infection (e.g., prosthetic valves or intravenous drug use)
- Initiate antimicrobials in the emergency department for patients who are being admitted to the hospital
- Isolate any patient with possible communicable illness. All HIV-infected patients with pneumonia should be isolated until tuberculosis is ruled out

DISPOSITION

The disposition of patients with pneumonia is dictated by the patient's underlying medical conditions, the severity of illness and likelihood of clinical deterioration, and the feasibility of home care and outpatient follow up. Outpatient treatment is 15 to 20 times less expensive than inpatient treatment, and most patients prefer the home environment. The decision to hospitalize a patient with pneumonia is not necessarily a commitment to prolonged inpatient care. Twelve- to 24-hour emergency department or hospital ward observation may allow the early discharge of certain moderate-risk patients.

A prospectively validated prediction rule for mortality among immunocompetent adults with community-acquired pneumonia suggests a two-step approach to assess risk (8). Patients in the lowest risk class are those less than age 50, without significant comorbid conditions (neoplasm, congestive heart failure, cerebrovascular disease, renal disease, liver disease, or HIV), and without the following findings on physical examination: altered mental status, pulse greater than or equal to 125 beats per minute, respiratory rate greater than or equal to 30, systolic blood pressure less than 90, and temperature less than 35°C or greater than or equal to 40°C. Patients who do not fit the lowest risk category are classified into categories based on a scoring system that accounts for age, comorbid illness, physical examination findings, and laboratory abnormalities. Hospitalization is recommended for those in moderate- to high-risk categories. A controlled trial compared education regarding this clinical prediction rule (allowing also independent physician judgment) to conventional management and found that this intervention was associated with a significantly decreased hospital admission rate with no difference in quality-of-life scores, readmission or mortality rates (13). Additional discharge criteria could include improving and stable vital signs over a several-hour observation period, ability to take oral medications, an ambulatory pulse oximetry greater than 90%, home support, and ability to follow up.

Most patients with community-acquired pneumonia do not need respiratory isolation. Those who are suspected of having an etiology of pneumonia that could pose a threat of transmission to other patients (e.g., influenza, varicella, TB, plague) should be isolated. Because the SARS virus appears to be well-adapted to nosocomial transmission, persons with fever and respiratory symptoms who have been in an area with possible exposure to SARS should be immediately isolated. Frequent handwashing

TABLE 33.1. Empiric Therapy for Pneumonia

Clinical Setting	Antibiotic Regimen	Comments
PARENTERAL REGIMENS		
Community-acquired, nonimmunocompromised	3rd generation cephalosporin + macrolide	Add macrolide to treat atypical pathogens.
	Respiratory fluoroquinolone	Treats most common bacterial as well as atypical pathogens. Active vs. DRSP.
	Azithromycin (alone)	Treats most common typical as well as atypical pathogens. High tissue levels, but low serum levels and poor CSF penetration.
	β-lactam/β-lactamase inhibitor (e.g., ampicillin-sulbactam) + macrolide	Superior activity vs. anaerobes. Piperacillin-tazobactam more active vs. Gram negative pathogens, including P. aeruginosa.
Suspected aspiration	β-lactam/β-lactamase inhibitor Clindamycin ± aminoglycoside Metronidazole + 3rd gen. cephalosporin	
Severe pneumonia (ICU)	Cefotaxime, ceftriaxone, cefepime, or β-lactam/β-lactamase inhibitor plus respiratory fluoroquinolone	Consider adding aminoglycoside if septic shock is present. Vancomycin if MRSA is present.
Neutropenic, bronchiectasis, recent hospitalization	Antipseudomonal β-lactam (e.g., piperacillin, ceftazidime, cefepime, imipenem) + fluoroquinolone ± aminoglycoside	Add aminoglycoside if neutropenic or in septic shock. Choice of antipseudomonal aminoglycoside is based on local antibiotic resistance patterns.
ORAL REGIMENS		
Age < 60, otherwise healthy (atypical pathogens likely)	Erythromycin	Poor activity vs. H. influenzae, GI upset common.
	Doxycycline	Preferred for adolescent/young adult when likelihood of mycoplasma is high; variable activity vs. S. pneumoniae.
	Clarithromycin	Treats common typical bacterial and atypical pathogens.
	Azithromycin	Treats common typical bacterial and atypical pathogens.
	Telithromycin	Treats common typical bacterial and atypical pathogens; active vs. DSRP.
	Respiratory fluoroquinolone	Treats common typical bacterial and atypical pathogens; active vs. DRSP.
Age ≥ 60, comorbidities	2nd or 3rd generation cephalosporin (e.g., cefuroxime axetil, cefpodoxime, cefprozil)	No activity vs. atypical pathogens (add macrolide) or some resistant S. pneumoniae.
	Amoxicillin/clavulanate	Better activity vs. anaerobes; frequent diarrhea. No activity vs. atypical pathogens (add macrolide). Better activity vs. DRSP with higher dose (2 gm po bid).
	Respiratory fluoroquinolone	Treats common typical bacterial and atypical pathogens; active vs. DRSP.

CSF, cerebrospinal fluid; DRSP, drug-resistant Streptococcus pneumoniae; GI, gastrointestinal; ICU, intensive care unit.

and use of masks to prevent droplet exposure are also helpful to prevent transmission of SARS and other pathogens. Neutropenic patients are generally placed in reverse isolation. HIV-infected patients who present with any form of pneumonia ideally should be isolated until TB can be ruled out by sputum AFB smears, since delayed diagnosis of TB in these patients is a well-recognized cause of nosocomial TB outbreaks. The chest radiograph cannot be relied on to rule out TB in AIDS patients, because it often does not have the typical appearance of TB. Isolation should be strongly considered for others at high risk for TB, such as inner-city homeless persons or intravenous drug users.

COMMON PITFALLS

✔ Failure to recognize pneumonia in a patient with exacerbation of underlying lung disease, such as asthma or COPD
✔ Delaying initiation of antibiotics for seriously ill patients
✔ Failure to question patients who present with respiratory complaints about HIV risk factors

✔ Failure to consider other possible etiologies of lung infiltrates, such as aspiration of foreign body
✔ Failure to recognize TB and initiate respiratory isolation in a patient with HIV infection or other TB risk factors

References

1. Bates JH, Campbell GD, Barron AL, et al. Microbial etiology of acute pneumonia in hospitalized patients. *Chest* 1992;101:1005–1012.
2. Blatt SP, Lucey CR, Butzin CA, et al. Total lymphocyte count as a predictor of absolute CD4+ count and CD4+ percentage in HIV-infected persons. *JAMA* 1993;269:622–626.
3. Centers for Disease Control and Prevention. Prevention and control of influenza: recommendations of the Immunization Practices Advisory Committee (ACIP). *MMWR* 2003;52(RR-8):1–34.
4. Chalasani NP, Valdecanas MA, Gopal AK, et al. Clinical utility of routine blood cultures in adult patients with community-acquired pneumonia without underlying risks. *Chest* 1995;108:891–936.
5. Emerman CL, Dawson N, Speroff T, et al. comparison of physician judgment and decision aids for ordering chest radiographs for pneumonia in outpatients. *Ann Emerg Med* 1991;20:1215–1219.
6. Fang GD, Fine M, Orloff J, et al. New and emerging etiologies for community-acquired pneumonia with implications for therapy: a prospective multicenter study of 359 cases. *Medicine* 1990;69:307–316.

7. Feikin DR, Schuchat A, Kolczak M, et al. Mortality from invasive pneumococcal pneumonia in the era of antibiotic resistance, 1995–1997. *Am J Public Health.* 2000;90(2):223–9.
8. Fine MJ, Auble TE, Yealy DM, et al. A prediction rule to identify low-risk patients with community-acquired pneumonia. *N Engl J Med* 1997;336:243–250.
9. Grayston JT. Infections caused by Chlamydia pneumoniae strain TWAR. *Clin Infect Dis* 1992;15:757–763.
10. Karlowsky JA, Thornsberry C, Jones ME, et al. Factors associated with relative rates of antimicrobial resistance among *Streptococcus pneumoniae* in the United States: results from the TRUST Surveillance Program (1998–2002). *Clin Infect Dis* 2003;36:963–70.
11. Mandell LA, Bartlett JG, Dowell SF, et al. Update of practice guidelines for the management of community-acquired pneumonia in immunocompetent adults. *Clin Infect Dis* 2003;37:1405–33.
12. Marrie TJ, Durant H, Yates L. Community-acquired pneumonia requiring hospitalization: 5-year prospective study. *Rev Infect Dis* 1989;11:586–599.
13. Marrie TJ, Lau CY, Wheeler SL, et al. A controlled trial of a critical pathway for treatment of community-acquired pneumonia. *JAMA.* 2000;283:749–755.
14. Marston BJ, Plouffe JF, File TM Jr, et al. Incidence of community-acquired pneumonia requiring hospitalization: results of a population-based active surveillance study in Ohio. *Arch Intern Med* 1997;157:1709–1718.
15. Meehan TP, Fine MJ, Krumholz HM, et al. Quality of care, process, and outcomes in elderly patients with pneumonia. *JAMA* 1997;278:891–936.
16. Melbye H, Berdal BP, Straume B, et al. Pneumonia—a clinical or radiographic diagnosis? *Scand J Infect Dis* 1992;24:647–655.
17. Niederman MS, Mandell LA, Anzueto A, et al. Guidelines for the initial management of adults with community-acquired pneumonia: diagnosis, assessment of severity, antimicrobial therapy, and prevention. American Thoracic Society. *Am J Respir Crit Care Med* 2001;163:1730–1754.
18. Pachon J, Prados MD, Capote F, et al. Severe community-acquired pneumonia: etiology, prognosis, and treatment. *Am Rev Respir Dis* 1990;142:369–373.
19. Pallares R, Linares J, Vadillo M, et al. Resistance to penicillin and cephalosporin and mortality from severe pneumococcal pneumonia in Barcelona, Spain. *N Engl J Med* 1995;333:474–480.
20. Potgieter PD, Hammond JM. Etiology and diagnosis of pneumonia requiring ICU admission. *Chest* 1992;101:199–203.
21. Reed WW, Byrd GS, Gates RH, et al. Sputum Gram's stain in community-acquired pneumococcal pneumonia: a meta-analysis. *West J Med* 1996;165:197–204.
22. Sherman S, Skoney JA, Ravikrishnan KP. Routine chest radiographs in exacerbations of chronic obstructive pulmonary disease: diagnostic value. *Arch Intern Med* 1989;149:2493–2496.
23. Syrjala H, Broas M, Suramo I, Ojala A, Lahde S. High-resolution computed tomography for the diagnosis of community-acquired pneumonia. *Clin Infect Dis.* 1998;27:358–363.
24. Waterer GW, Somes GW, Wunderink RG. Monotherapy may be suboptimal for severe bacteremic pneumococcal pneumonia. *Arch Intern Med* 2001;161(15):1837–1842.

CHAPTER 34
Pleural Effusion

Robert Sigillito and Peter M. C. DeBlieux

A pleural effusion is an abnormal collection of fluid within the pleural space. An acute or previously undiagnosed effusion presents the emergency physician with a diagnostic challenge. A pleural effusion that is chronic or has a previously established diagnosis presents therapeutic considerations.

The pleural space is bordered by the visceral pleura that lines the lung and by the parietal pleura that lines the mediastinum, diaphragm, and inner surface of the thoracic wall. A small amount of fluid (a few milliliters) is normally present in this space. As with all capillary beds in the body, there is a dynamic balance between fluid production and absorption in both the parietal and visceral pleura. Only at the parietal pleura, however, do the net forces favor accumulation of fluid, accounting for physiologic

TABLE 34.1.   Causes of Pleural Fluid Accumulation

INCREASED PLEURAL FLUID PRODUCTION

1. Diffusion of fluid across the visceral pleura owing to increased pulmonary interstitial fluid (e.g., secondary to ventricular failure, pneumonia, hypoalbuminemia, or pulmonary embolus)
2. Increased hydrostatic pressure gradient across the parietal and visceral pleural capillary membranes owing to diminished pleural pressure (e.g., with postobstructive pulmonary atelectasis)
3. Increased hydrostatic pressure gradient across the parietal and visceral pleural capillary membranes caused by to increased capillary pressure (right ventricular failure, left ventricular failure, and superior vena cava syndrome)
4. Increased oncotic pressure gradient across the pleural capillary membranes secondary to increased pleural fluid protein concentration (malignancy)
5. Increased peritoneal fluid with transit across the diaphragm (ascites, and peritoneal dialysis)
6. Hemorrhage into the pleural space (malignancy, trauma, and iatrogenic)
7. Disruption of the thoracic duct (trauma, and iatrogenic)
8. Urine diffusion from the retroperitoneum into the pleural space (a rare condition resulting from trauma, urinary obstruction, or disruption of the collecting system)

IMPAIRED PLEURAL FLUID CLEARANCE

1. Obstruction of the lymphatic system, which drains the parietal pleura (malignancy)
2. Elevation of the systemic venous pressure (right ventricular failure, superior vena cava syndrome)

pleural fluid, which is normally cleared from the pleural space via the lymphatic vessels of the parietal pleura (1,12). Pathologic amounts of pleural fluid accumulate when pleural fluid formation increases beyond the capacity of lymphatic clearance, or when the lymphatic clearance is impaired (Table 34.1).

CLINICAL PRESENTATION

Patients with a pleural effusion commonly present with complaints related to the underlying disease process rather than to the pleural effusion itself. Small effusions are often asymptomatic. Symptoms directly attributable to an effusion result from pleural inflammation or infection (pain and fever), compromised pulmonary mechanics (dyspnea, tachypnea, and respiratory distress), impaired gas exchange (hypoxia, hypercapnia, and altered mental status), or compression of the lung with collapse of bronchial structures (cough).

Parietal pleural inflammation causes somatic pain referred to the overlying chest wall. Central diaphragmatic irritation causes pain referred to the ipsilateral shoulder. The visceral pleura is not innervated; therefore, inflammation of visceral pleura does not result in pain.

The predominant findings on physical examination likewise often reflect the underlying disease process. Vital sign abnormalities and hemodynamic instability may be consequences of the underlying disease or the result of compromised cardiopulmonary function. In the latter case, the cardiac chambers may collapse during diastole because of elevated pleural pressure ("effusion under tension"), physiologically mimicking cardiac tamponade (10,27,30,33). Although not all such patients progress to develop instability, as many as 18% of patients with pleural effusion have echocardiographic evidence of right atrial diastolic collapse (30). Oxygen saturation obtained by pulse oximetry may detect significant hypoxemia that would not be demonstrated by other vital sign abnormalities or physical findings (22,25).

The chest should be inspected for asymmetry. As the pleural space fills with fluid, the involved hemithorax increases in total volume, and the lung decreases in volume. Markedly elevated or negative pleural pressure may manifest as bulging or retraction of the intercostal spaces, tracheal deviation, or displacement of the cardiac apical pulse. Percussion of the chest may reveal dullness over the involved hemithorax. Auscultatory percussion, a technique that involves listening for a change in the percussion sound heard at the upper limit of a pleural effusion, has been shown to be both sensitive and specific for the presence of pleural effusion (8). Diminished tactile fremitus may also be easier to detect. Auscultation of the chest may reveal the presence of a pleural rub indicating an irregular pleural surface caused by either a mass or inflammation. An audible rub suggests that the effusion is small or loculated, because a rub will disappear as an enlarging effusion separates the visceral and parietal pleura. Diminished breath sounds are frequently appreciated. Abnormalities of the character of the breath sounds reflect pulmonary parenchymal disease. The remainder of the physical examination should include a meticulous search for clues to the underlying disease process.

DIFFERENTIAL DIAGNOSIS

The most common causes of pleural effusion in adults, in order of decreasing approximate frequency, are congestive heart failure (CHF) (37%), pneumonia (22%), malignancy (15%), pulmonary embolus (11%), viral disease (7%), and ascites (3.5%). Collagen vascular disease, tuberculosis, and other diseases account for a minority of cases (12). In contrast, the relative frequencies of causes of pleural effusion in children are pneumonia (50%), postoperative with congenital heart disease (14%), malignancy (10%), renal disease (9%), trauma (7%), and CHF secondary to congenital heart disease (3%) (2). The differential diagnosis of pleural effusion is narrowed by defining the fluid as transudate or exudate (Table 34.2).

CHF may lead to the development of a pleural effusion in several ways. Increased pulmonary interstitial fluid may diffuse directly into the pleural space. Concomitantly, right and left ventricular failures elevate the hydrostatic pressures within the pleural capillaries of the parietal and visceral pleura, respectively. When the hydrostatic pressures exceed the opposing oncotic pressures, there is net pleural fluid production. Right ventricular failure also leads to elevation of the pressure within the lymphatic vessels, thereby impeding drainage of the pleural space. The combined effect of these mechanisms is the accumulation of pleural fluid.

There are three stages in the development of a parapneumonic effusion and empyema. First, there is an accumulation of sterile pleural fluid characterized by low lactate dehydrogenase (LDH) level, normal pH, normal glucose level, and low white blood cell (WBC) count. If not treated, or if therapy fails, bacteria invade the pleural space. Bacteria, WBCs, debris, and large pleural effusions accumulate. Fibrin sheets line the pleural surfaces, with a tendency to form loculations. The pleural fluid LDH concentration and WBC count rise, while the pH and glucose level fall. Finally, fibroblasts grow into the exudate to form an inelastic pleural coating, or peel, encasing the lung and causing pulmonary restriction (12,17).

Various authors have developed criteria for the definition of *empyema*. Light suggests that the term *complicated parapneumonic effusion* be used to designate those effusions that do not resolve without tube thoracostomy. *Empyema* is reserved for describing those effusions that have the gross appearance of pus (12,17).

Young, otherwise healthy patients with parapneumonic effusion or empyema most often have *Staphylococcus aureus*, *Strep-*

TABLE 34.2. Etiology of Pleural Effusion

Transudate	Exudate
Congestive heart failure	Asbestosis
Cirrhosis with ascites	Chylothorax
Glomerulonephritis	Collagen vascular diseases
Meigs syndrome	Rheumatoid arthritis
Myxedema	Systemic lupus erythematosus
Nephrotic syndrome	Drug-induced pleural disease
Peritoneal dialysis	Esophageal rupture
Pulmonary atelectasis	Hemothorax
Pulmonary embolus	Chest trauma
Sarcoidosis	Aortic dissection
Superior vena cava obstruction	Iatrogenic
Urinothorax	Intraabdominal inflammatory processes
	Cholecystitis
	Hepatitis
	Pancreatitis
	Perihepatitis
	Peritonitis
	Pyelonephritis
	Splenic abscess
	Subphrenic abscess
	Pulmonary or pleural infection
	Empyema
	Parapneumonic effusion
	Tuberculosis
	Viral
	Fungal
	Parasitic
	Neoplasm
	Pericarditis
	Pleuritis
	Pulmonary embolus
	Uremia

tococcus pneumoniae, or *Streptococcus pyogenes* infections. Elderly and infirm individuals with aspiration pneumonia are at higher risk for anaerobic infection. After thoracotomy, postoperative patients are more likely to be infected with *S. aureus* (4). *Klebsiella* pneumonia has a strong association with alcoholism or diabetes mellitus. In a large series, *Klebsiella* were the bacteria most often recovered from patients with empyema thoracis.

In children, the etiology of parapneumonic effusion has changed over the last several decades. *S. aureus*, *S. pneumoniae*, *S. pyogenes*, and *Haemophilus influenzae* were the most common isolated bacteria, although the relative frequency of each species varied across studies (5). The microbiology has been influenced by the introduction of routine childhood vaccination. Previously, *H. influenzae* was one of the most common agents but has decreased in incidence since the introduction of routine vaccination during infancy (2,5,7). It is now rarely encountered. Recent data demonstrate that *S. pneumoniae* is the most common isolate, with the incidence of penicillin- and cephalosporin-resistant strains increasing. The incidence of *S. aureus*, particularly methicillin-resistant strains, is increasing (5). The proportion of parapneumonic effusions that progress to empyema has decreased until 1996. More recent data are not available. The proportion of parapneumonic effusions attributed to respiratory viruses is as high 14%, higher than that in adults (2).

Pleural effusion is a common finding in patients infected with human immunodeficiency virus (HIV). The differential diagnosis includes parapneumonic effusion, malignancy, CHF, hypoalbuminemia, nephrosis, and ascites. In addition to the bacteria encountered in the general population, *Mycobacterium tuberculosis*, *Pneumocystis carinii*, *Cryptococcus neoformans*, and *Histoplasmosis species* must be considered. The most common malignancies encountered are lymphoma and Kaposi sarcoma.

HIV-related dilated cardiomyopathy and nephropathy are both potential causes of transudative effusions (3).

In all demographic groups, other pathogens occur with lower frequency, including enteric Gram-negative organisms, *Enterococcus, Pseudomonas, Legionella, M. tuberculosis, Chlamydia, Mycoplasma,* viruses, rickettsiae, and fungi. Other infectious processes may also lead to pleural effusion. Virtually any abdominal infection or inflammatory process may lead to a sympathetic effusion. Such processes include pancreatitis, hepatitis, perihepatitis, cholecystitis, hepatic amebiasis, splenic abscess, pyelonephritis, glomerulonephritis, peritonitis, pelvic inflammatory disease, and abdominal abscess.

The most common types of malignant effusions are those resulting from lung, breast, lymphoma, ovarian, and gastric tumors (9,31). This type of effusion may be secondary to lymphatic obstruction, superior vena cava syndrome, postobstructive atelectasis, or pleural metastases. In children, the most common malignancy is lymphoma, although pleural effusion is rarely the initial presentation.

A pulmonary embolus may produce either a transudative or an exudative effusion. The mechanism is probably infarction of a portion of lung and visceral pleura, with resultant loss of interstitial fluid across the membrane. This process is unusual in children, but may occur in patients with sickle cell disease and pulmonary infarct.

EMERGENCY DEPARTMENT EVALUATION

Effusions are most frequently identified initially by chest radiography. Because free-flowing fluid follows gravity to the most dependent region of the thorax, small effusions manifest as blunting of the costophrenic angle or elevation of a hemidiaphragm on the upright posteroanterior (PA) film (Figs. 34.1A, B). Experimentally, as little as 25 mL of fluid injected into a cadaver produced hemidiaphragm elevation, and 175 mL of fluid was required to produce blunting of the angle (6). Larger effusions appear to assume a meniscus configuration, suggested by some to be a purely radiographic phenomenon (12). Loculated effusions will not follow gravity to the most dependent part of the hemithorax (Fig. 34.2). The lateral upright radiograph will reveal a smaller effusion than will the PA film, with an air–lung interface evident in the posterior costophrenic recess. Effusion is more difficult to detect on supine anteroposterior (AP) films. The only evidence that fluid is present may be a diffuse homogeneous density of the affected hemithorax, compared with the contralateral side. Bilateral lateral decubitus films should be a routine part of the evaluation of every patient with newly diagnosed, or suspected, effusion (Figs. 34.1C, D). This view allows visualization of as little as 5 mL of pleural fluid (21), and aids in differentiation among effusion, pulmonary infiltrate, tumor, pleural thickening, diaphragmatic abnormalities, and other parenchymal processes. With the affected side down, fluid layers along the lateral wall of the thorax. More than 10 mm of fluid thickness in this view is considered clinically significant and is sufficient to allow thoracentesis (12). With the unaffected side dependent, the fluid layers along the mediastinum allow improved visualization of the underlying lung parenchyma on the affected side.

Ultrasonography has been shown to have sensitivity for small effusions comparable to that of lateral decubitus films (11) but does not demonstrate parenchymal diseases (Fig. 34.3). The procedure is of great utility in guiding thoracentesis with a small or loculated collection of fluid. Computed tomographic (CT) scan is sensitive for detection of pleural fluid, allows for clear characterization of parenchymal abnormalities, and may help identify an effusion as malignant on the basis of features of pleural lesions (19, 32) (Fig. 34.4).

Once the presence of a pleural effusion is confirmed, further emergency department (ED) evaluation should be directed at answering the following questions:

1. Is the effusion new or previously diagnosed?
2. If new, is the effusion a transudate or an exudate?
3. Is the effusion causing respiratory compromise such that therapeutic thoracentesis is indicated?
4. Is chest tube thoracostomy indicated?

In general, a previously diagnosed effusion does not require a new diagnostic workup, unless there is evidence that a complication has arisen (e.g., a patient with a known effusion who presents with sepsis and is suspected of having an infected effusion or empyema).

To narrow the differential diagnosis, it is necessary for a patient with a new effusion to undergo thoracentesis so that the fluid may be characterized as a transudate or an exudate. The exception to this rule is effusion in the setting of acute CHF exacerbation. In that scenario, treatment should be initiated and thoracentesis performed only if the effusion does not resolve with therapy.

Although several sets of criteria have been proposed to identify an exudate, Light's criteria are the most widely accepted and include the following criteria that are considered exudates (16):

1. Pleural fluid-serum protein ratio greater than 0.5
2. Pleural fluid-serum LDH ratio greater than 0.6
3. Pleural fluid LDH greater than two thirds of the upper limit of normal for serum LDH

Other criteria that have been proposed include elevated pleural fluid cholesterol, elevated fluid-serum albumin ratio, and physician clinical impression (29).

If the effusion proves to be a transudate, the differential diagnosis is narrowed to a small list. Exudates, in contrast, require further fluid analysis, including determination of pH, glucose, amylase, fluid hematocrit, cell count with differential, Gram stain, culture, and cytology, and studies to exclude pleural tuberculosis (acid-fast bacillus [AFB] smear and culture, polymerase chain reaction [PCR], adenosine deaminase activity, and pleural biopsy) (26,34) (Table 34.3).

The greatest utility of the pH of pleural fluid lies in aiding the determination of whether a chest tube is required in the management of parapneumonic effusion. Fluid pH of less than 7.0 indicates that the patient has a complicated parapneumonic effusion or empyema, and chest tube thoracostomy is indicated. Fluid pH of greater than 7.2 suggests that the effusion is simple and not likely to require a chest tube for drainage. Patients with a fluid pH between 7.0 and 7.2 fall within an indeterminate range. Management of the effusion must be individualized according to the patient's clinical condition. A few patients will require chest tube thoracostomy, some will require serial thoracentesis, and some will improve and not require further diagnostic procedures (12,14,17).

Pleural fluid glucose level has both diagnostic implications and therapeutic indications. A level of less than 60 mg/dL, although not a sensitive indicator of any particular etiology, suggests that the patient has parapneumonic effusion, empyema, malignancy, rheumatoid disease, or tuberculosis (12,13). Chest tube thoracostomy is indicated when the glucose level is less than 40 mg/dL, if the patient has a parapneumonic effusion or empyema. Higher levels of glucose do not aid in narrowing the differential diagnosis.

Pleural fluid amylase level of greater than 200 IU/L narrows the differential diagnosis. Among transudates, elevated amylase is found in less than 5% of patients, and has been reported in association with CHF and cirrhosis. Among exudates, amylase-rich pleural fluid is most often associated with malignancy (65%),

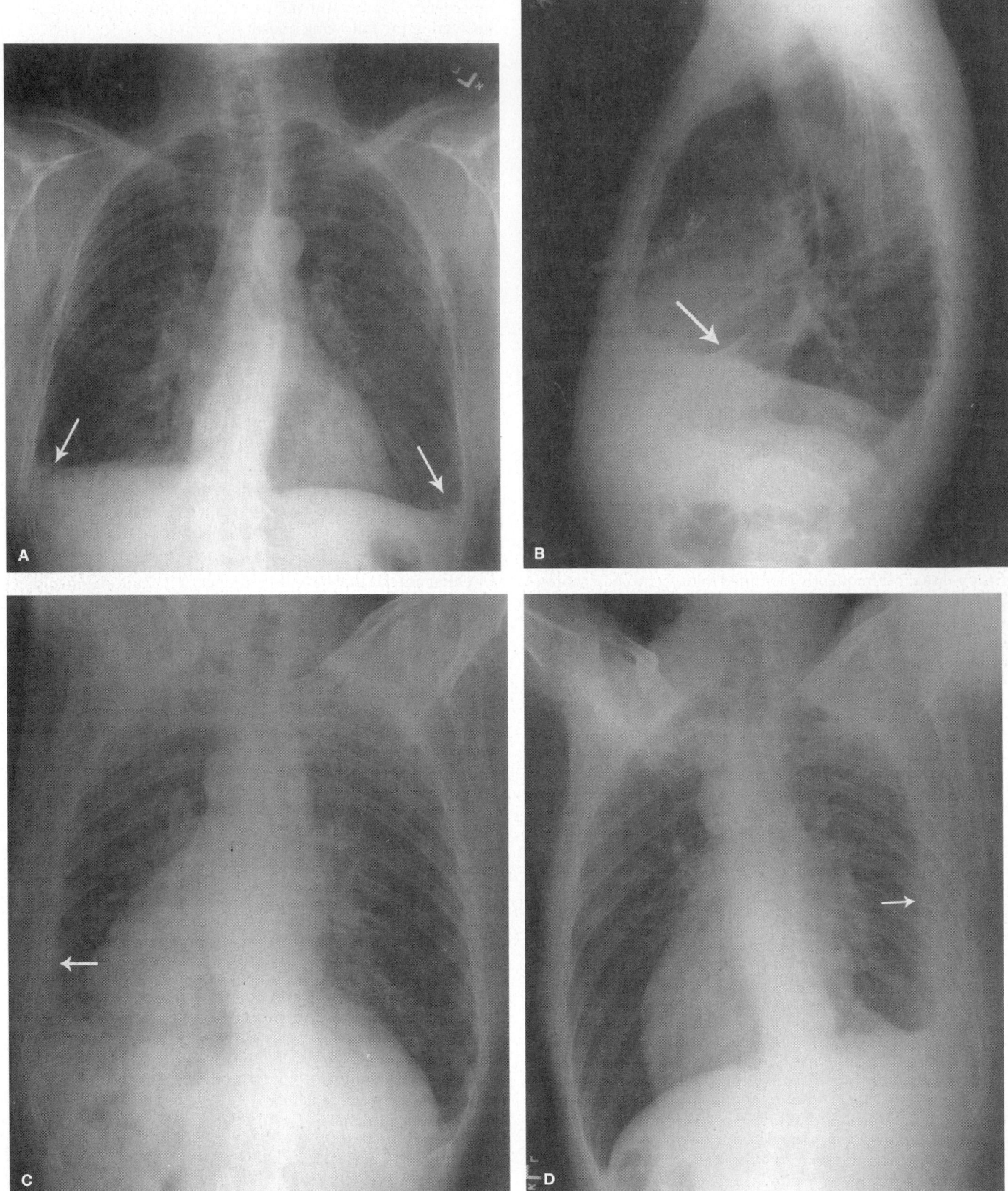

Figure 34.1.   A: Bilateral blunting of the costophrenic angles. **B**: Elevated, flattened right hemidiaphragm shadow suggesting subpulmonic effusion. Note fluid in the major fissure. **C**: Left lateral decubitus film demonstrating small left effusion. **D**: Right lateral decubitus film demonstrating moderate right effusion.

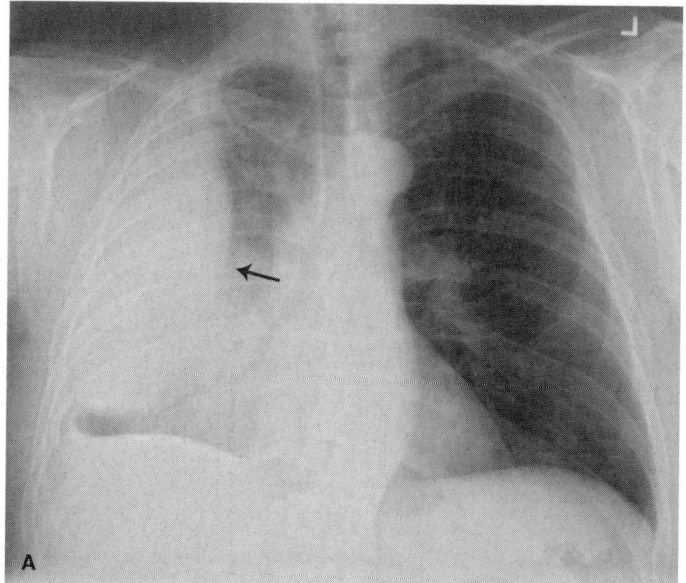

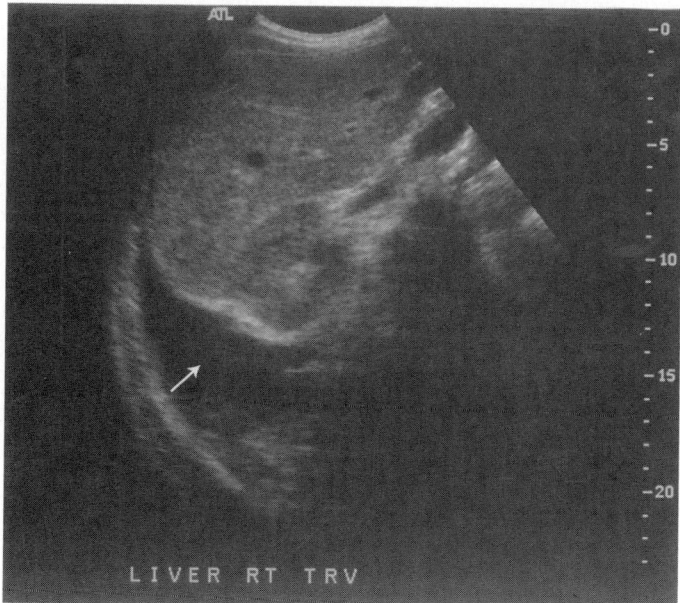

Figure 34.3.   Ultrasonographic image demonstrating pleural effusion behind liver and kidney in posterior costophrenic recess.

Bloody pleural fluid in the absence of trauma suggests the presence of malignancy, but is also found in vascular catastrophes such as aortic rupture, and in some patients with tuberculosis. A pleural fluid hematocrit or red blood cell (RBC) count of greater than half that of the blood defines the effusion as a hemothorax and indicates the need for a chest tube.

The size of an effusion also gives clues to its cause. Large (occupying more than two thirds of a hemithorax) or massive (complete opacification of a hemithorax) effusions are strongly associated with malignancy, tuberculosis, and bacterial parapneumonic effusion (28). Other causes include traumatic hemothorax and complete pneumonectomy.

Additional routine workup should include complete blood count, urinalysis, and levels of serum electrolyte, blood urea nitrogen (BUN), creatinine, and liver and pancreatic enzymes. If there is a history of liver disease or coagulopathy, a prothrombin time can help to assess the risk associated with invasive procedure. Continuous pulse oximetry should be used to monitor

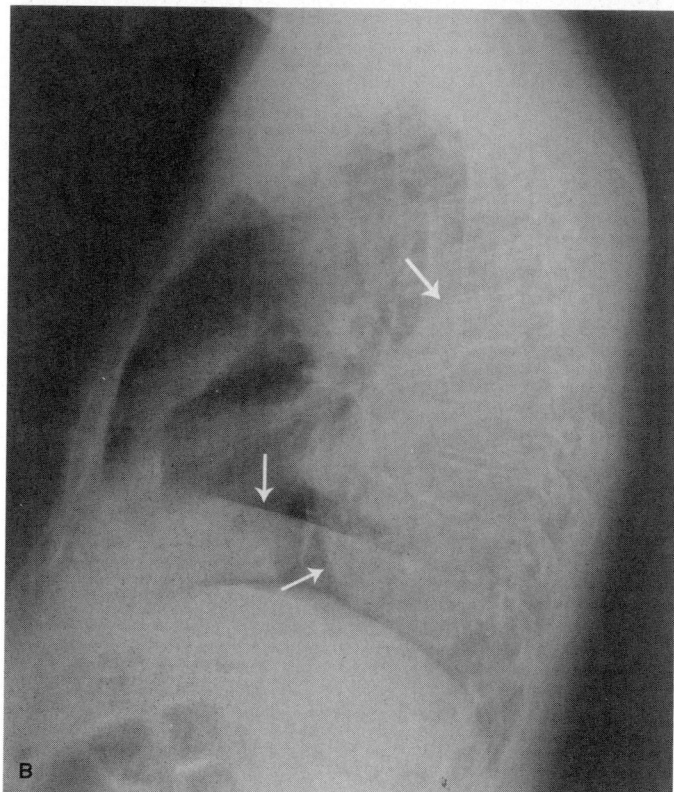

Figure 34.2.   A: Large loculated right effusion with blunted costophrenic angle. B: Linear opacity from free-flowing effusion. Loculated effusion is seen posteriorly.

tuberculosis (18%), acute or chronic pancreatitis (5%), and parapneumonic effusion (3%). Less common disorders include uremic pleuritis, pancreatic trauma, and esophageal rupture (13,35). The use of an assay for pancreatic amylase fractions has not been reported.

Pleural biopsy is usually necessary to establish the diagnosis of malignancy or pleural tuberculosis. Because pleural biopsy is more likely to be complicated by lung perforation and pneumothorax when only a small amount of pleural fluid is present, biopsy should be considered at the time of initial thoracentesis, particularly if the goal is complete evacuation of the pleural fluid.

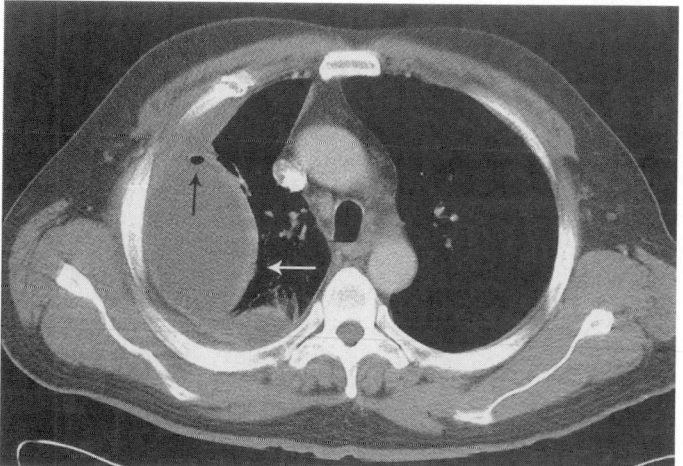

Figure 34.4.   Computed tomographic (CT) image of loculated and free pleural effusion. Note air pocket in loculation suggestive of gas-producing organisms in empyema.

TABLE 34.3. Interpretation of Pleural Fluid Analysis

Cause	Appearance	WBC count	Glucose	pH	Comments
Asbestosis	Serous or serosanguineous	Elevated (may be >25,000)	Normal	7.4	Chronic/recurrent, 25% to 50% have eosinophilia
Chylothorax	Milky	Variable	Normal	—	Centrifuged specimen, supernatant cloudy with elevated triglycerides, lymphoma in 75% of nontraumatic cases
Empyema	Purulent	High	<40 mg/dL	<7.0	Centrifuged specimen, supernatant clear, chest tube indicated
Hemothorax	Bloody	—	—	—	Pleural fluid/whole blood hematocrit >0.5
Neoplasm	Serous to bloody	Variable (1,000–10,000)	Variable	Variable	Low pH and glucose suggest high tumor load, cytology more reliable than pleural biopsy
Pancreatitis	Serosanguineous to bloody	Highly variable (1,000–50,000)	Equal to serum		Elevated fluid amylase
Parapneumonic effusion	Variable clear to turbid	Variable	>40 mg/dL	>7.2	pH 7.0 to 7.2, may require repeat thoracentesis
Pulmonary embolus	—	—	—	—	All indices highly variable, thoracentesis used to exclude other diagnoses
Rheumatoid arthritis	Green	Variable	<60 mg/dL	<7.2	Pleural fluid LDH and rheumatoid factor titer high
SLE	Yellow or serosanguineous	Variable	>80 mg/dL	>7.2	Pleural fluid ANA titer >1:320
Tuberculosis	Yellow or serosanguineous	<10,000	Variable	Variable	Cell differential >50% lymphocytes, protein often >5.0 g/dL, pleural biopsy 90% sensitive
Uremia	Serosanguineous to bloody	Variable	Normal	Normal	Cell differential lymphocyte predominance

ANA, antinuclear antibody; LDH, lactate dehydrogenase; SLE, systemic lupus erythematosus; WBC, white blood cell.

oxygenation status, particularly during thoracentesis. Arterial blood gas determination may be needed on an individual basis to assess the degree of impairment of oxygenation and ventilation. An electrocardiogram (ECG) may reveal associated pericarditis, manifestations of underlying heart disease, or may suggest pulmonary embolus. Additional diagnostic tests (e.g., thyroid function tests, tests for collagen vascular disease, ventilation perfusion scan, CT, or arteriography) may be ordered as indicated by findings on the history, physical examination, and initial laboratory evaluation.

EMERGENCY DEPARTMENT MANAGEMENT

As for all patients who present with acute signs or symptoms, the first priority is evaluation and stabilization of the airway, optimization of oxygenation and ventilation, and circulatory support. Treatment of life-threatening conditions such as pulmonary edema should be initiated.

Diagnostic evaluation of a pleural effusion, as described, is often undertaken on an inpatient basis. For some patients (e.g., those who are likely to have parapneumonic effusion–empyema, esophageal rupture, or sepsis), ED thoracentesis may be indicated for rapid diagnosis, drainage, and institution of specific treatment. Patients with chronic pulmonary disease and the elderly may have diminished cardiopulmonary reserve, and are likely to require urgent therapeutic thoracentesis. It is wise to obtain specialty consultation early in the course, to determine whether thoracentesis is best performed in the ED or after admission to the hospital.

A number of techniques for thoracentesis have been described. The size and location of the effusion should be determined by radiography and by physical examination. Examination for tactile fremitus and percussion of the chest determine

the upper limit of the fluid level. For this evaluation, the patient is usually placed in a seated position, leaning slightly forward. For small effusions, or if the patient cannot tolerate sitting, the lateral decubitus position may be used. A small or loculated effusion is best evacuated under fluoroscopic or ultrasonographic guidance. If a difficult thoracentesis is anticipated, early consultation with an invasive radiologist or pulmonologist may be the most appropriate course of action.

Clotting abnormalities and anticoagulant therapy represent relative contraindications to thoracentesis, although safe thoracentesis is reported with thrombocytopenia (platelet count as low as 50,000/μL), or prolonged prothrombin time and partial thromboplastin time (up to twice the midrange of control) in the absence of active bleeding (20). Likewise, chest-wall infection is contraindicated unless the infected site can be avoided. Thoracentesis should also be avoided when there is diaphragmatic rupture on the side of effusion.

After sterile preparation of the aspiration site, local anesthesia is injected. A small-gauge needle, a catheter and needle, a commercial thoracentesis apparatus, or a pigtail catheter using the Seldinger technique may be used. The usual site for the insertion of the needle is in the posterior midscapular line, in the highest appropriate intercostal space. The needle is directed over the superior part of the rib to avoid the intercostal vessels. The catheter is advanced into the chest, and the fluid is removed under sterile conditions. In most cases, removal of the largest possible amount of fluid until respiratory distress is alleviated or a limit of 1,500 mL is reached, is advisable. Removing larger amounts of fluid may increase the likelihood of developing postexpansion pulmonary edema (15), a syndrome associated with a mortality rate as high as 20% (18). Less fluid should be withdrawn in the hypoalbuminemic patient.

After evacuation of the effusion, the catheter is removed and a chest radiograph is obtained to rule out iatrogenic pneumothorax. If a moderate or large pneumothorax has been inadvertently created, a thoracostomy tube is usually necessary. Other complications of thoracentesis include hemothorax, hemoperitoneum, shearing of the catheter tip, and infection.

CRITICAL INTERVENTIONS

- Obtain bilateral lateral decubitus films in the evaluation of every patient with newly diagnosed, or suspected effusion
- Perform ED thoracentesis for rapid diagnosis, drainage, and institution of specific treatment in patients in respiratory distress or in those who are likely to have parapneumonic effusion–empyema, esophageal rupture, or sepsis

DISPOSITION

The presence of a pleural effusion, in and of itself, does not necessitate admission. A patient with a stable effusion of known etiology may be sent home if the clinical situation allows. When a new effusion is discovered, discussion with the primary care physician or pulmonologist regarding the timing and setting of thoracentesis is appropriate. Clear exceptions are the presence of sepsis, shock, and respiratory distress or failure. These conditions indicate the need for emergent evacuation. If thoracentesis is performed, hospital admission is usually indicated for further treatment of the underlying disease and for observation for procedural complications, although the occasional patient with an uncomplicated course might be discharged after a period of observation. In all other cases, the patient's condition and underlying disease process dictate the need for admission. Patients may be admitted to a bed on a regular floor or observation unit, unless cardiovascular or respiratory instability warrants admission to a monitored bed. When definitive care is available only at another institution, patient transfer may be indicated. If thoracentesis was performed, transfer can be accomplished safely once a follow-up chest radiograph reveals no complications and provided the usual criteria for stability are satisfied.

COMMON PITFALLS

- Failure to recognize the presence of an effusion by failing to order a chest radiograph or, once taken, by misinterpretation of subtle findings. Effusion may be misdiagnosed as thickened pleura or infiltrate. This leads to inadequate or delayed evaluation and treatment, which might be particularly critical in cases of sepsis, empyema, esophageal rupture, or intrathoracic hemorrhage
- An incorrect presumptive diagnosis of the cause of the effusion or an incorrect presumption that an effusion is old and unchanged can likewise result in an inadequate evaluation or treatment. Comparison with old radiographs is essential
- A misdiagnosis of pleural effusion may lead to inappropriate attempts at thoracentesis, with complications such as puncture of an intrathoracic mass (e.g., malignancy) or abdominal contents (in diaphragmatic rupture)
- Failure to recognize the potential need for pleural biopsy before thoracentesis. This makes subsequent biopsy more difficult if only a small effusion remains
- Complications such as pneumothorax (from piercing the lung parenchyma or from leaving the needle or catheter hub exposed to the air); laceration of the liver, spleen, or intercostal vessels; and shearing of the catheter tip by withdrawing it incorrectly through the needle may be best avoided by careful attention to technique

- The risk of postexpansion pulmonary edema is diminished by avoiding removal of very large quantities (e.g., more than 1,500 mL) of pleural fluid and by using very low negative evacuation pressures
- Transient hypoxia during thoracentesis may be avoided by the routine administration of oxygen and by continuous pulse oximetry
- Delay in thoracentesis in the setting of parapneumonic effusion or empyema may lead to longer hospitalization and increased cost of care

References

1. Agostoni E, Zocchi L. Mechanical coupling and liquid exchanges in the pleural space. *Clin Chest Med* 1998;9:241–260.
2. Alkrinawi S, Chernick V. Pleural fluid in hospitalized pediatric patients. *Clin Pediatr (Phila)* 1996;35:5–9.
3. Beck JM. Pleural disease in patients with acquired immune deficiency syndrome. *Clin Chest Med* 1998;19:341–349.
4. Bryant RE, Salmon CJ. Pleural empyema. *Clin Infect Dis* 1996;22:747–762; quiz 763–764.
5. Buckingham SC, King MD, Miller ML. Incidence and etiologies of complicated parapneumonic effusions in children, 1996 to 2001. *Pediatr Infect Dis J* 2003;22:499–504.
6. Colins JD, Burwell D, Furmanski S, et al. Minimal detectable pleural effusions. A roentgen pathology model. *Radiology* 1972;105:51–53.
7. Givan DC, Eigen H. Common pleural effusions in children. *Clin Chest Med* 1998;19:363–371.
8. Guarino JR, Guarino JC. Auscultatory percussion: a simple method to detect pleural effusion. *J Gen Intern Med* 1994;9:71–74.
9. Johnston WW. The malignant pleural effusion. A review of cytopathologic diagnoses of 584 specimens from 472 consecutive patients. *Cancer* 1985;56:905–909.
10. Kisanuki A, Shono H, Kiyonaga K, et al. Two-dimensional echocardiographic demonstration of left ventricular diastolic collapse due to compression by pleural effusion. *Am Heart J* 1991;122;4[Pt 1]:1173–1175.
11. Kocijancic I, Vidmar K, Ivanovi-Herceg Z. Chest sonography versus lateral decubitus radiography in the diagnosis of small pleural effusions. *J Clin Ultrasound* 2003;31:69–74.
12. Light R.*Pleural Diseases*, 3rd ed. Baltimore: Williams & Wilkins, 1995.
13. Light RW, Ball WC, Jr. Glucose and amylase in pleural effusions. *JAMA* 1973;225:257–9.
14. Light RW, Girard WM, Jenkinson SG, et al. Parapneumonic effusions. *Am J Med* 1980;69:507–512.
15. Light RW, Jenkinson SG, Minh VD, et al. Observations on pleural fluid pressures as fluid is withdrawn during thoracentesis. *Am Rev Respir Dis* 1980;121:799–804.
16. Light RW, Macgregor MI, Luchsinger PC, et al. Pleural effusions: the diagnostic separation of transudates and exudates. *Ann Intern Med* 1972;77:507–513.
17. Light RW, Rodriguez RM. Management of parapneumonic effusions. *Clin Chest Med* 1998;19:373–382.
18. Mahfood S, Hix WR, Aaron BL, et al. Reexpansion pulmonary edema. *Ann Thorac Surg* 1988;45:340–345.
19. McLoud TC. CT and MR in pleural disease. *Clin Chest Med* 1998;19:261–276.
20. McVay PA, Toy PT. Lack of increased bleeding after paracentesis and thoracentesis in patients with mild coagulation abnormalities. *Transfusion* 1991;31:164–171.
21. Moskowitz H, Platt RT, Schachar R, et al. Roentgen visualization of minute pleural effusion. An experimental study to determine the minimum amount of pleural fluid visible on a radiograph. *Radiology* 1973;109:33–35.
22. Mower WR, Myers G, Nicklin EL, et al. Pulse oximetry as a fifth vital sign in emergency geriatric assessment. *Acad Emerg Med* 1998;5:858–865.
23. Mower WR, Sachs C, Nicklin EL, et al. Pulse oximetry as a fifth pediatric vital sign. *Pediatrics* 1997;99:681–686.
24. Mower WR, Sachs C, Nicklin EL, et al. A comparison of pulse oximetry and respiratory rate in patient screening. *Respir Med* 1996;90:593–599.
25. Mower WR, Sachs C, Nicklin EL, et al. Effect of routine emergency department triage pulse oximetry screening on medical management. *Chest* 1995;108:1297–1302.
26. Nagesh BS, Sehgal S, Jindal SK, et al. Evaluation of polymerase chain reaction for detection of Mycobacterium tuberculosis in pleural fluid. *Chest* 2001;119:1737–1741.
27. Negus RA, Chachkes JS, Wrenn K. Tension hydrothorax and shock in a patient with a malignant pleural effusion. *Am J Emerg Med* 1990;8:205–207.
28. Porcel JM, Vives M. Etiology and pleural fluid characteristics of large and massive effusions. *Chest* 2003;124:978–983.
29. Romero-Candeira S, Hernandez L, Romero-Brufao S, et al. Is it meaningful to use biochemical parameters to discriminate between transudative and exudative pleural effusions? *Chest* 2002;122:1524–1529.
30. Sadaniantz A, Anastacio R, Verma V, et al. The incidence of diastolic right atrial collapse in patients with pleural effusion in the absence of pericardial effusion. *Echocardiography* 2003;20:211–215.

31. Sahn SA. Malignancy metastatic to the pleura. *Clin Chest Med* 1998;19:351–361.
32. Traill ZC, Davies RJ, Gleeson FV. Thoracic computed tomography in patients with suspected malignant pleural effusions. *Clin Radiol* 2001;56:193–196.
33. Vaska K, Wann LS, Sagar K, et al. Pleural effusion as a cause of right ventricular diastolic collapse. *Circulation* 1992;86:609–617.
34. Villegas MV, Labrada LA, Saravia NG. Evaluation of polymerase chain reaction, adenosine deaminase, and interferon-gamma in pleural fluid for the differential diagnosis of pleural tuberculosis. *Chest* 2000;118:1355–1364.
35. Villena V, Perez V, Pozo F, et al. Amylase levels in pleural effusions: a consecutive unselected series of 841 patients. *Chest* 2002;121:470–474.

CHAPTER 35
Asthma

Rita K. Cydulka

Asthma is characterized by increased airway responsiveness to various stimuli. It is manifested by bronchoconstriction, widespread bronchial wall edema, and thick, tenacious secretions. Although the reversibility of airflow obstruction was once considered a cornerstone of the diagnosis, it is now recognized that reversibility may be incomplete in some patients owing to airway remodeling (2). For the most part, however, acute exacerbations of asthma are interspersed with symptom-free intervals.

Asthma affects about 5% of adults in the United States. About one half of all cases are diagnosed before the patient reaches age 10, and another one third are detected before age 40. The male-to-female ratio of this disease is 2:1 in childhood but equalizes during early adulthood.

The natural course of asthma has not been investigated thoroughly, but studies suggest that 50% to 80% of patients have a good prognosis, especially those with mild disease or disease that develops in childhood. Nevertheless, asthma has a high morbidity rate. The average patient with asthma has 15 days of restricted activity each year and spends 5.8 days in bed. In the United States, more than 4,000 deaths per year are attributable to asthma.

Asthma is a heterogeneous disease. Clinically, it can be separated into two groups: allergic or extrinsic asthma, and nonallergic or intrinsic asthma. Many patients have components of both types. *Extrinsic asthma* accounts for less than 10% of patients with asthma and tends to develop early in life. It is associated with a well-defined sensitivity to inhaled allergens, a family history of allergic diseases, increased serum levels of immunoglobulin (Ig) E, positive immediate skin tests, and blood eosinophilia. It may be seasonal (trees, grasses, and spores) or perennial (animals, gardens, and house dust). A good response to bronchodilator therapy is usually observed.

Intrinsic asthma is the more common type of the disease. An inciting allergen cannot be identified, a family history of allergies is less common, IgE levels may be normal or low, and skin tests are negative. Intrinsic asthma is perennial, tends to be more severe than extrinsic asthma, and has a limited response to bronchodilator therapy.

All individuals with asthma have hyperresponsive airways that narrow when exposed to various stimuli: allergic, infectious, pharmacologic, environmental, occupational, exercise-related, and emotional.

Allergic asthma occurs when inhaled allergens bind to IgE molecules that are bound to mast cells in the lining of the tracheobronchial tree. During the early response, various mediators are released, causing increased vascular permeability, mucosal edema, and bronchial smooth-muscle contraction. A second wave of reaction, the late response, is seen hours to days later and involves the accumulation of inflammatory cells in the bronchial mucosa, thereby perpetuating the reaction.

Although several theories attempt to explain the pathophysiologic changes that occur in nonallergic asthma, none adequately explains all clinically observed phenomena. Research suggests that even patients without atopy have the same pathophysiologic basis for the disease as atopic patients do.

Respiratory infections, particularly viral infections, commonly precipitate bronchospasm. Viruses cause mucosal inflammation and lower the firing threshold of the subendothelial vagal receptors, resulting in enhanced airway reactivity. This hyperactivity may last up to 8 weeks, even in nonasthmatic persons.

Pharmacologic agents also may induce acute asthma. The agents most frequently implicated are aspirin and nonsteroidal antiinflammatory compounds, coloring agents, and β-adrenergic antagonists.

Up to 10% of adults with asthma experience the triad of aspirin-induced bronchospasm, nasal polyps, and eosinophilia. Ingestion of aspirin, nonsteroidal antiinflammatory compounds, and tartrazine (FDC yellow dye no. 5) and other dyes may induce severe asthma in these patients, possibly by diverting arachidonic acid metabolism toward the lipoxygenase pathway and causing the production of leukotrienes, which are potent bronchoconstrictors.

Sulfating agents are used widely as food preservatives and antioxidants in pharmaceutical products. Exacerbation of asthma has been reported after food ingestion and after the use of sulfite-containing drugs, including some inhalation bronchodilators.

A large variety of occupational dusts and fumes may provoke acute airway obstruction. Patients with occupational asthma typically give a cyclic history. They are symptom-free during weekends, vacations, and on arrival at work. As the workday progresses, wheezing develops. A history of similar symptoms in fellow employees may be noted. Three mechanisms are involved in occupational asthma: immunologic reactions (e.g., animal handlers), direct liberation of bronchoconstrictors (e.g., cotton workers), and direct irritant effects (e.g., meat wrappers).

Exercise also may stimulate an asthma attack. Exercise-induced bronchospasm is usually noted within 5 to 20 minutes after the completion of exercise and is related to thermal changes in the respiratory tree. Exercising in a cold, dry environment causes a more marked response than exercising in a warm, humid environment.

Endocrine factors have been recognized as yet another cause of airway hyperresponsiveness. Normal variations in progesterone and estradiol levels are believed to modulate airway reactivity.

Psychological factors also influence asthma exacerbations, probably through modification of vagal efferent activity. The extent to which psychological factors participate in the induction and continuation of an asthma attack is unknown but probably varies from patient to patient and from episode to episode.

Regardless of the underlying precipitant, airway narrowing, bronchial wall edema, bronchial smooth muscle contraction, and mucosal plugging ensue. These changes result in increased airway resistance, decreased forced expiratory volumes and flow rates, lung hyperinflation, increased work of breathing, and ventilation–perfusion mismatch.

CLINICAL PRESENTATION

The classic triad of symptoms during an asthma attack is cough, dyspnea, and wheezing. Chest tightness and nonproductive cough may precede dyspnea and wheezing. As airway obstruction worsens, the expiratory phase becomes prolonged. Asthmatic patients coming to the emergency department are frequently anxious, tachypneic, tachycardic, and mildly hypertensive. Lung hyperinflation, accessory respiratory muscle use, muscle retraction, and pulsus paradoxus may be noted.

Patients may attempt to sit upright or lean forward in an effort to ease the work of breathing. These signs may be absent despite severe airway obstruction, however (16). A silent chest indicates insufficient air movement or extensive mucous plugging and is an ominous sign. Cyanosis may appear only immediately before respiratory arrest and should not be relied on as an indication of the severity of the attack. The termination of an exacerbation is often marked by a cough productive of thick mucous plugs and bronchial casts (Curschmann spirals).

A subset of asthmatic patients experiences the sudden onset of severe symptoms. These individuals tend to respond rapidly to treatment but appear to be at significant risk for a fatal outcome.

Occasionally, an asthmatic patient may complain of intermittent dyspnea or cough on exertion. Patients with cough-equivalent asthma tend to have normal breath sounds on examination, even during an exacerbation, but reversible bronchospasm may be demonstrated on pulmonary function testing.

Complications of asthma include pneumothorax, pneumomediastinum, and subcutaneous emphysema. These may require insertion of a chest tube for evacuation. Mild atelectasis may occur as a result of bronchial mucous plugging, but rarely requires intervention other than conventional bronchodilator therapy. In addition, rib fractures and costochondral strain may occur as a result of excessive coughing. Cough syncope, a rare complication of asthma, is noted most frequently in moderately obese, middle-aged asthmatic men. Finally, dysrhythmias may occur as a result of hypoxia, especially in patients who have received oral adrenergic agents.

DIFFERENTIAL DIAGNOSIS

Wheezing, coughing, and dyspnea are present in many conditions. Common problems include pneumonia, bronchitis, croup, bronchiolitis, chronic obstructive lung disease, congestive heart failure, pulmonary embolism, allergic reactions, and upper airway obstruction from edema or a foreign body. Less common problems include cystic fibrosis, hypersensitivity pneumonitis, carcinoid syndrome, and exposure to odors, dust, and gas. A careful history and physical examination should help differentiate asthma from these other conditions.

EMERGENCY DEPARTMENT EVALUATION

The ability to perform a thorough history and physical examination before initiating treatment is often limited by the patient's dyspnea. Aggressive therapy directed at relieving airway obstruction begins as soon as a diagnosis of asthma is established. Meanwhile, an attempt is made to obtain a history from family members or the patient. Important points to establish include the following (1,17):

- Duration and onset of the current attack
- Identification of precipitating causes
- Type and amount of medications used before arrival in the emergency department
- Response to prior therapy, including current or previous use of steroids
- Frequency of emergency department visits and hospitalizations
- Previous need for intubation or ventilation
- History of concurrent medications and allergies
- History of concurrent medical problems

Immediate attention is also directed to the patient's appearance, vital signs, chest examination, and heart examination. The presence of a pulsus paradoxus is noted.

Judging the state of a patient's ventilatory status and pulmonary function on clinical grounds alone can be misleading. The degree of tachycardia and tachypnea often do not correlate well with the degree of airway obstruction. Pulsus paradoxus may be absent in up to one third of severe asthmatics (6). Furthermore, wheezing is absent if airflow is minimal. To complicate matters, all of the aforementioned clinical parameters can normalize with even minimal improvement in pulmonary function (6,16). Therefore, quantification of airway changes must be assessed by using either the forced expiratory volume in 1 second (FEV_1) or the peak expiratory flow rate (PEFR). An initial FEV_1 of less than 1 L (less than 30% predicted) or a PEFR of less than 100 L/minute (less than 20% predicted) indicates severe obstruction (1,17).

Hypoxemia is not common during most acute exacerbations (16). Pulse oximetry may be useful in assessing and following oxygenation. A saturation of less than 91% generally correlates with severe hypoxemia. Arterial blood gas (ABG) measurements need to be obtained only in patients experiencing severe or prolonged attacks. In general, hypercapnia, severe hypoxemia, or metabolic acidosis does not occur until the PEFR or FEV_1 is less than 25% of predicted values (15), but young children and elderly patients commonly present exceptions to this rule. The degree of hypoxemia determined by ABG generally reflects the extent of ventilation–perfusion mismatch. A normal or increased $PaCO_2$ indicates severe airway obstruction and impending ventilatory failure.

Expectorated sputum may appear purulent because of the presence of eosinophils, but this finding may not reflect infection. A wet preparation of sputum may contain Charcot-Leyden crystals (eosinophilic granules), Curschmann spirals (mucous casts), and bacteria.

Chest radiographs may demonstrate hyperinflation and atelectasis but are usually nondiagnostic. A chest radiograph is necessary only if pneumonia, pneumothorax, or pneumomediastinum is suspected or if the patient fails to respond to aggressive bronchodilator therapy (26,28).

Although electrocardiography occasionally reveals evidence of right ventricular strain, it is generally not helpful, except to rule out concurrent cardiac problems. All older patients, especially those with cardiac disease, should be monitored during therapy.

Blood tests, including a complete blood count, are unlikely to help guide the acute management of an asthma attack. A theophylline level, however, should be obtained to guide therapy if theophylline is used.

Asthma scores that incorporate subjective and objective criteria (pulse, respiratory rate, pulsus paradoxus, subjective dyspnea, accessory muscle use, wheezing, and PEFR) should not be relied on for predicting emergency treatment or disposition (20,24).

EMERGENCY DEPARTMENT MANAGEMENT

Emergency department interventions are guided by pulmonary function tests (FEV$_1$, PEFR), vital signs, chest and heart examinations, and the patient's subjective assessment of dyspnea. The goal of emergency treatment is to ensure adequate oxygenation and to relieve airflow obstruction.

Unfortunately, no ideal therapy is available, and the use of multidrug regimens is common. Supplemental humidified oxygen, inhaled β-adrenergic agonists, oral or intravenous corticosteroids, and, to a lesser extent, inhaled anticholinergic agents are the mainstays of asthma treatment in the emergency department. Although one recent study demonstrated additional bronchodilation when intravenous montelukast was added to inhaled β-adrenergic agonists, their role remains to be further defined (5). The methylxanthines (e.g., theophylline) have fallen out of favor as a routine component of emergency care (19). The benefits of ketamine and halothane remain largely anecdotal and have not been substantiated in controlled trials (12,14,18). Guidelines for the diagnosis and management of acute exacerbations of asthma have been established by the National Asthma Education and Prevention Program (NAEPP) Expert Panel (Fig. 35.1) (1,17). Acute pharmacologic therapy can be divided into three categories: β-adrenergic agonists, glucocorticoids, and anticholinergics. A fourth category of drugs, the methylxanthines, has only a minor role in the emergency department. The role of a

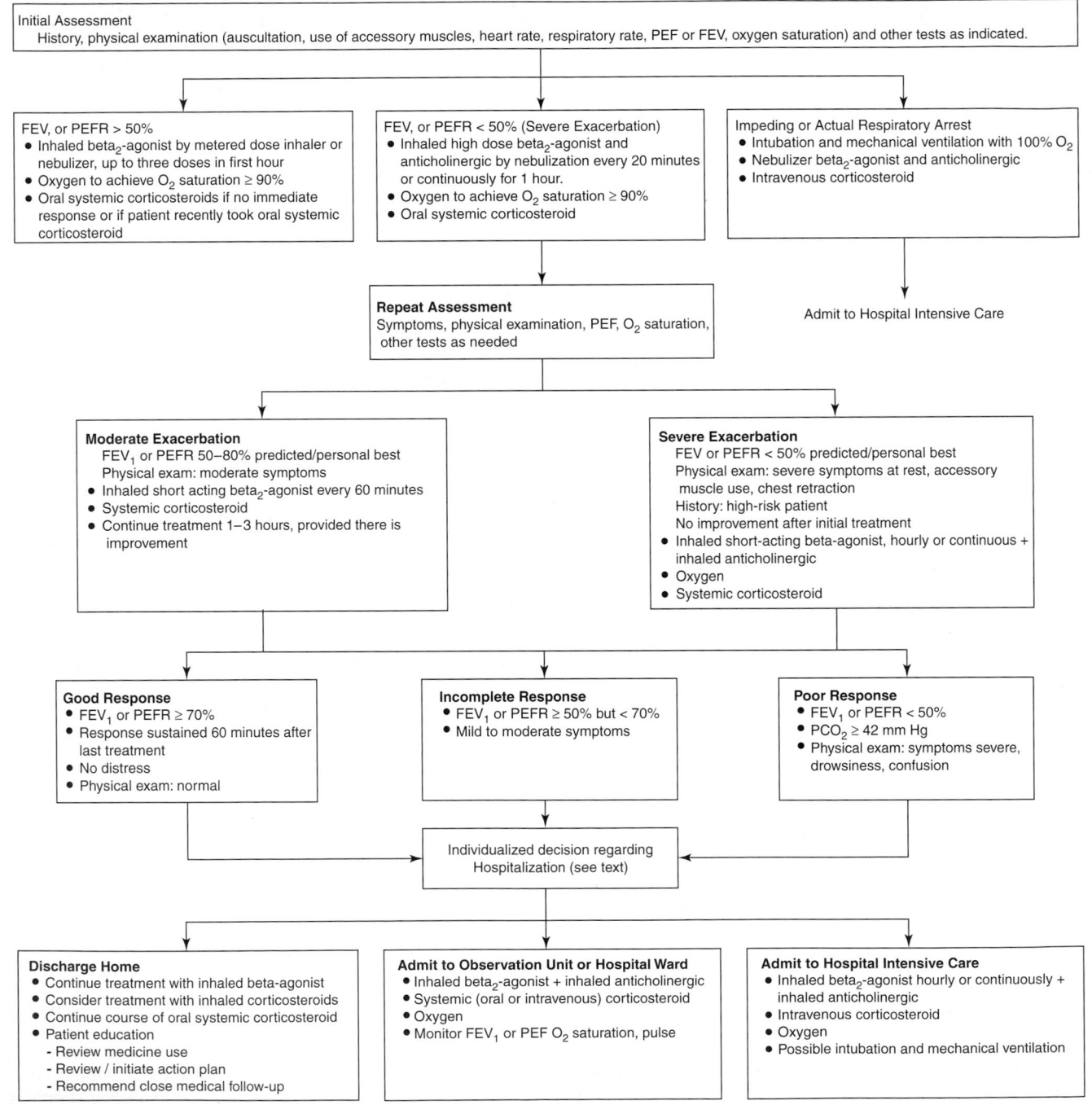

Figure 35.1. Management of asthma exacerbations: Emergency department and hospital-based care. (Adapted from *Expert Panel Report 2: Guidelines for the diagnosis and management of asthma, April 1997*; NIH Publication No. 97-4051. Bethesda, MD: Department of Health and Human Services, 1997.)

fifth category of drugs, the leukotriene antagonists–inhibitors, is still under investigation. A sixth category of drugs used to treat asthma, the chromones (e.g., cromolyn sodium), has no place in emergency treatment. A seventh and new category of drugs, recombinant humanized monoclonal antibody directed against IgE, is indicated for maintenance therapy and has no place in emergency treatment (25). Table 35.1. outlines the preferred treatments recommended by the NAEPP Expert Panel (1,17).

β-Adrenergic Agonists

Short-acting β-adrenergic agonists are the drugs of choice for the management of acute bronchospasm. They produce bronchodilation by stimulating beta receptors, resulting in the formation of cyclic adenosine monophosphate (cAMP), which results in relaxation of bronchial smooth muscle, inhibition of mediator release, and increase in mucociliary clearance. Drugs in this category include resorcinols, saligenins, and catecholamines (Table 35.1).

Resorcinols and saligenins available in the United States include albuterol (salbutamol), levalbuterol, pirbuterol, formoterol metaproterenol, and terbutaline. Aerosol forms are available for albuterol, levalbuterol, and metaproterenol. All are available in metered-dose inhalers (MDIs). Aerosol agents and MDIs are rapid-acting, are theoretically long-lasting, and may be repeated every 20 to 30 minutes in an acute situation. Levalbuterol is the R-isomer of albuterol. Salmeterol is a chemical derivative of albuterol with an extended duration of action and a bronchodilator effect ten times that of albuterol. Formoterol is similar, but is even longer acting than salmeterol. Neither is appropriate for use in acute exacerbations of asthma. Albuterol, metaproterenol, and terbutaline are also available in oral form. Terbutaline and epinephrine are available for subcutaneous injection.

The resorcinols and saligenins are highly β_2-selective and are virtually devoid of cardiac side effects when given in inhaled or aerosol form. A frequent noncardiac side effect is tremor. Inhaled or aerosolized β-agonists rapidly promote bronchodilation comparable with that produced by parenteral agents, appear to be longer lasting, and cause fewer side effects. Treatments given every 20 to 30 minutes or in a continuous fashion result in more effective and sustained improvement of pulmonary function than treatments given less frequently (4). Recent evidence suggests that aerosolized β-agonist treatments may also be administered as a single bolus (8). The use of spacer devices improves drug delivery when patient technique is suboptimal.

Subcutaneous administration of β-agonists (epinephrine or terbutaline) may be of use in the treatment of asthmatics who cannot use inhalation devices effectively, in patients in extremis, in patients for whom initial treatment with aerosol β-adrenergic agents fails, or when preparation of aerosol or metered-dose agents for acute use risks delaying the initiation of therapy (7).

The catecholamines (epinephrine, isoproterenol, and isoetharine) have largely been supplanted by their more selective and longer-acting derivatives. Epinephrine, a nonselective α- and β-adrenergic agonist, may be given by oral inhalation (in a nonprescription preparation) or subcutaneously. The usual subcutaneous dose in adults is 0.3 to 0.5 mL of a 1:1,000 solution, which may be repeated every 20 minutes to a total of three doses. Epinephrine reaches peak blood levels 20 to 40 minutes after injection, and its bronchodilating effects last up to 4 hours. Side effects include increased myocardial irritability, dysrhythmias, and nervousness. Although some studies suggest that epinephrine may be safely used in asthmatics older than 40 years of age, extreme caution should be used in patients with coronary artery disease (7).

Isoetharine is more β_2-selective than epinephrine and is as effective a bronchodilator as albuterol (10). It is supplied as a 1%

aerosol solution or in an MDI preparation. Its duration of action is 30 to 90 minutes. Doses may be repeated every 20 to 30 minutes during an acute attack.

Isoproterenol is a potent selective β-adrenergic agent. It is available in aerosol form, in a new MDI, and as an intravenous solution. The duration of action of the inhaled form is 3 hours, and inhalations may be repeated every 3 hours. Use of isoproterenol inhalants was associated with a number of asthmatic deaths in England and Wales in the 1960s, suggesting that the agent should be used cautiously, although a cause-and-effect relationship was not demonstrated. In addition, inhaled isoproterenol may cause paradoxical bronchospasm. Intravenous isoproterenol should be reserved for dire emergencies, and strict monitoring of heart rate, rhythm, and blood pressure is required.

Glucocorticoids

Glucocorticoids should be administered to any patient whose acute airway obstruction is not promptly relieved by an inhaled β-adrenergic agent. Patients who receive glucocorticoids early require fewer hospital admissions and sustain fewer relapses after discharge from the emergency department (21). Corticosteroids are thought to exert their effect on acute asthma by reducing airway inflammation. The initial dose is 60 to 125 mg of intravenous methylprednisolone or 40 to 80 mg of oral prednisone (27). Doses of 60 to 80 mg intravenous or oral prednisone (or the equivalent dose of prednisone) every 6 to 8 hours should follow. Oral administration of corticosteroids is equivalent to intravenous administration. Data on the use of inhaled corticosteroids during emergency department treatment of asthma has yet to be clearly defined (9). Because the effects of steroids are not noted for 4 or more hours, vigorous concomitant bronchodilator therapy must be continued.

Anticholinergic Agents

There has been a resurgence of enthusiasm for the use of anticholinergic agents to treat acute bronchoconstriction. These medications, including ipratropium bromide and glycopyrrolate, antagonize the neuromuscular transmitter acetylcholine at the postganglionic parasympathetic receptor, reducing vagally mediated bronchoconstriction in the larger central airways. There seems to be an additive effect when β-adrenergic agents and anticholinergic agents are used together, although this effect is not dramatic (23). Peak anticholinergic bronchodilation is achieved within 1 to 2 hours. Aerosolized atropine sulfate and glycopyrrolate, although effective, have fallen out of favor because of the high incidence of anticholinergic side effects (tachycardia, restlessness, irritability, dry mouth, thirst, and difficulty swallowing).

Methylxanthines

Theophylline and its salts have been used to treat acute bronchospasm for more than 50 years. Studies suggest that the methylxanthines, when used alone or in combination with β agonists during an acute episode, are associated with an increased incidence of side effects but do little to relieve bronchospasm. Methylxanthines have a narrow therapeutic–toxic window and are subject to many interactions with other drugs. Toxicity may result in life-threatening cardiac dysrhythmias or seizures.

Patients receiving chronic theophylline therapy who present with acute bronchospasm and a subtherapeutic theophylline level may benefit from oral theophylline or intravenous aminophylline, but methylxanthines otherwise should play no significant role in the acute treatment of airflow obstruction. There is

TABLE 35.1. Dosages of Drugs for Asthma Exacerbations in Emergency Medical Care or Hospital

Medication	Adult	Child*	Comments
Short-Acting Inhaled β_2-Agonists			
Albuterol			
Nebulizer solution (5.0 mg/mL, 2.5 mg/3 mL, 1.25 mg/3 mL, 0.63 mg/3 mL)	2.5–5 mg every 20 minutes for 3 doses, then 2.5–10 mg every 1–4 hours as needed, or 10–15 mg/hr continuously	0.15 mg/kg (minimum dose 2.5 mg) every 20 minutes for 3 doses, then 0.15–0.3 mg/kg up to 10 mg every 1–4 hr as needed, or 0.5 mg/kg/hr by continuous nebulization	Only selective β_2-agonists are recommended. For optimal delivery, dilute aerosols to a minimum of 3 mL, as gas flow of 6–8 L/min
MDI (90 µg/puff)	4–8 puffs every 20 minutes up to 4 hr, then every 1–4 hr as needed	4–8 puffs every 20 minutes for 3 doses, then 1–4 hr inhalation maneuver; use spacer/holding chamber	As effective as nebulized therapy if patient is able to coordinate
Bitolterol			
Nebulizer solution (2 mg/mL)	See albuterol dose	See albuterol dose; thought to be half as potent as albuterol on a milligram basis	Has not been studied in severe asthma exacerbations; do not mix with other drugs
MDI (370 µg/puff)	See albuterol dose	See albuterol dose	Has not been studied in severe asthma exacerbations
Levalbuterol (R-albuterol)			
Nebulizer solution (0.63 mg/3 mL, 1.25 mg/3 mL)	1.25–2.5 mg every 20 min for 3 doses, then 1.25–5 mg every 1–4 hours as needed, or 5–7.5 mg/hour continuously	0.075 mg/kg (maximum dose 1.25 mg) every 20 min for 3 doses, then 0.075–0.15 mg/kg up to 5 mg every 1–4 hr as needed, or 0.25 mg/kg/hour by continuous nebulization	0.63 mg of levalbuterol is equivalent to 1.25 mg of racemic albuterol for both efficacy and side effects
Pirbuterol			
MDI (200 µg/puff)	See albuterol dose	See albuterol dose; thought to be half as potent as albuterol on a milligram basis	Has not been studied in severe asthma exacerbations
SYSTEMIC (INJECTED) β_2-AGONISTS			
Epinephrine 1:1,000 (1 mg/mL)	0.3–0.5 mg every 20 min for 3 doses subcutaneously	0.01 mg/kg up to 0.3–0.5 mg every 20 min for 3 doses subcutaneously	No proven advantage of systemic therapy over aerosol
Terbutaline (1 mg/mL)	0.25 mg every 20 min for 3 doses subcutaneously	0.01 mg/kg every 20 min for 3 doses then every 2–6 hr as needed subcutaneously	No proven advantage of systemic therapy over aerosol
ANTICHOLINERGICS			
Ipratropium bromide			
Nebulizer solution (0.25 mg/mL)	0.5 mg every 30 min for 3 doses then every 2–4 hr as needed	0.25 mg every 20 min for 3 doses, then every 2–4 hr	May mix in same nebulizer with albuterol; should not be used as first-line therapy; should be added to β_2-agonist therapy
MDI (18 µg/puff)	4–8 puffs as needed	4–8 puffs as needed	Dose delivered from MDI is low and has not been studied in asthma exacerbations
Ipratropium with albuterol			
Nebulizer solution (each 3 mL vial contains 0.5 mg ipratropium bromide and 90 µg of albuterol)	3 mL every 30 min for 3 doses, then every 2–4 hours as needed	1.5 mL every 20 min for 3 doses, then every 2–4 hours	Contains EDTA to prevent discoloration. This additive does not induce bronchospasm
MDI (each puff contains 18 µg ipratropium bromide and 90 µg of albuterol)	4–8 puffs as needed	4–8 puffs as needed	
SYSTEMATIC CORTICOSTEROIDS			
	(Applies to the first three corticosteroids)		
Prednisone Methylprednisolone Prednisolone	60 mg initially 120–180 mg/day in 3 or 4 divided doses for 48 hours, then 60–80 mg/day until PEF reaches 70% of predicted or personal best	1 mg/kg every 6 hours for 48 hours then 1–2 mg/kg/day (maximum = 60 mg/day) in 2 divided doses until PEF 70% of predicted or personal best	For outpatient "burst" use 40–60 mg in single or 2 divided doses for adults (children: 1–2 mg/kg/day, maximum 60 mg/day) for 3–10 days

Note: No advantage has been found for higher dose corticosteroids in severe asthma exacerbations, nor is there any advantage for intravenous administration over oral therapy, provided that gastrointestinal transit time or absorption is not impaired. The usual regimen is to continue the frequent multiple daily dose until the patient achieves an FEV, or PEF of 50% of predicted or personal best, and then lower the dose to twise daily; this usually occurs within 48 hours. Therapy following a hospitalization or emergency department visit may last from 3 to 10 days. If patients are then started on inhaled corticosteroids, studies indicate there is no need to taper the systemic corticosteroid dose. If the followup systemic corticosteroid therapy is to be given once daily, one study indicates that it may be more clinically effective to give the dose in the afternoon at 3 p.m., with no increase in adrenal suppression (Beam et al. 1992).

*Children = 12 years of age.

EDTA, ethylenediaminetetraacetate; FEV, forced expiratory volume; MDT, metered-dose inhaler; PEF, peak expiratory flow.

(From *National Asthma Education and Prevention Program Expert Panel Report: Guidelines for the Diagnosis and Management of Asthma*: Update on Selected Topics—2000. *J Allergy Clin Immunol* 2002;110:SI–S209, with permission.)

controversy about the utility of aminophylline in patients requiring hospitalization (23).

Other Agents

Magnesium sulfate, a physiologic regulator of intracellular calcium flux, is an effective bronchodilator. In addition to preventing histamine release from mast cells and opposing the action of acetylcholine, magnesium directly inhibits bronchial smooth-muscle contraction. Both aerosolized magnesium (0.66 g in 10 mL of saline) and intravenous magnesium solutions (1.2 g over 20 minutes) have been used investigationally to treat patients with asthma for whom maximal standard therapy has failed, although neither form is currently approved for this indication in the United States. Bronchodilation is observed within 2 to 5 minutes after administration, but it disappears rapidly after treatment is discontinued; therefore, additional bronchodilator therapy must accompany the use of magnesium. Side effects include hypotension, malaise, and a warm sensation. Cardiac rhythm, blood pressure, pulse, neurologic status, and renal function must be monitored closely.

Nedocromil and cromolyn inhibit the release of inflammatory cytokines from mast cells, but they have no role in acute management. Likewise, leukotriene inhibitors, although useful in long-term management, are not indicated for emergency department treatment.

Heliox, an 80:20 mixture of helium and oxygen, is sometimes considered for treatment in patients with respiratory acidosis who fail conventional therapy. Helium is a low-density, biologically inert gas that lowers airway resistance and decreases respiratory work. Significant improvement may be noted within 10 to 20 minutes of initiating therapy but there are currently insufficient data on whether heliox can avert tracheal intubation, or change intensive care and hospital admission rates and duration, or mortality (11,13).

If the patient's condition deteriorates or fails to improve despite intensive therapy, use of intubation and mechanical ventilation must be considered. Although there are no absolute criteria other than respiratory arrest and coma, the following patients should be considered for intubation and mechanical ventilation:

- Those with worsening pulmonary function tests despite vigorous bronchodilator therapy
- Those with decreasing PaO_2, increasing $PaCO_2$, or progressive respiratory acidosis
- Those with declining mental status or increasing fatigue.

Noninvasive respiratory therapies such as continuous positive airway pressure (CPAP) and biphasic positive airway pressure (BiPAP) have been shown to reduce the work of breathing and to improve oxygenation in some causes of respiratory failure. At this time, there have been no clinical trials performed to evaluate these therapies in the treatment of acute asthma.

Expiratory airflow obstruction can result in air-trapping and higher lung volumes in mechanically ventilated asthmatics. This condition may result in "auto-PEEP," a continuously increased intrathoracic pressure that may decrease venous return and cause hypotension. Auto-PEEP may be avoided by using a rapid inspiratory flow rate, a reduced respiratory frequency, and a prolonged expiratory phase. This type of mechanical ventilation is commonly referred to as "permissive hypercapnia." An acute deterioration can be treated by simply disconnecting the patient from the ventilator and allowing the lungs to deflate completely before reconnecting.

The anesthetic agent halothane is a potent bronchodilator. It has a rapid onset of action and a rapid decay of effects. Side effects of 1% halothane include cardiac dysrhythmias and increased in-

trapulmonary shunting. Close monitoring of heart rate, ABGs, and blood pressure is essential when using either agent.

Narcotics, sedatives, and tranquilizers should be avoided in acute asthma, because respiratory arrest may occur after their use. Mucolytics, expectorants, and hydration do not aid in the treatment of asthma. Antibiotics are advisable only for those patients with fever and purulent sputum, evidence of pneumonia, or suspected bacterial sinusitis (1).

Asthma in Pregnancy

About 0.4% to 1.3% of pregnant women have asthma. One third of pregnant patients with asthma improve during pregnancy, one third of patients remain unchanged, and one third becomes worse. Asthma therapy during pregnancy is directed at providing adequate oxygenation for both mother and fetus. The management of pregnant asthmatics is essentially the same as that for nonasthmatics. The use of subcutaneous or inhaled β-adrenergic agents, theophylline, and corticosteroids appears to be safe during pregnancy (3,22).

CRITICAL INTERVENTIONS

- Perform either the forced expiratory volume in 1 second (FEV_1) or the peak expiratory flow rate (PEFR) to quantify the degree of airway obstruction
- Administer glucocorticoids to patients whose acute airway obstruction is not promptly relieved by an inhaled β-adrenergic agent or those who have recently taken glucocorticoids
- Prescribe oral corticosteroids to patients who receive glucocorticoids in the emergency department
- Avoid auto-PEEP by using a rapid inspiratory flow rate, a reduced respiratory frequency, and a prolonged expiratory phase

DISPOSITION

Several asthma-scoring indices have been proposed to predict the need for hospitalization, but all have proven disappointing (20). The following patients should be considered for hospital admission:

- Those whose condition deteriorates in the emergency department
- Those who return for further therapy within several days after emergency department discharge
- Dyspneic patients with significant hypoxemia (PaO_2 of less than 60), hypercapnia, or acidosis
- Patients with a pretreatment FEV_1 of less than 1.0 L (less than 30% predicted) or a PEFR of less than 100 L/min (less than 20% predicted), and a posttreatment FEV_1 less than 2.1 L (less than 60% predicted) or a PEFR less than 300 L/min (less than 60% predicted)
- Patients who remain subjectively dyspneic after aggressive therapy
- Patients with continued abnormal vital signs after therapy
- Unreliable patients

Even patients who improve enough to be discharged from the emergency department have residual airway obstruction for up to several weeks after the acute episode subsides. Therefore, arrangements must be made for ongoing treatment and early follow-up. A nontapering 3- to 10-day course of oral corticosteroids (40 to 60 mg/d of prednisone) and a 5- to 10-day treatment regimen of a $β_2$-adrenergic MDI (two puffs as needed, up to every 4 to 6 hours) should be prescribed. In addition, a chronic regimen of inhaled corticosteroids (preferred) or leukotriene modifier–inhibitor should be prescribed for all patients who have persistent asthma in accordance with NAEPP guidelines (1,17). Instruction in the proper use of the inhaler is essential, as is a brief educational intervention. Patients receiving chronic theophylline therapy should be continued on a long-acting preparation pending followup with their physician.

COMMON PITFALLS

✔ Failure to recognize that a silent chest or a normal $PaCO_2$ is a sign of severe obstructive disease may result in respiratory arrest

✔ Withholding β-agonist therapy in the emergency department because of β-agonist use at home. This approach has no scientific basis and is extremely dangerous

✔ Failure to use measurements of pulmonary function, in addition to clinical and subjective parameters of dyspnea, when judging the adequacy of bronchodilator therapy

✔ Failure to give glucocorticoids to all but the mildest asthmatics, especially those who fail to respond to one or two doses of β agonists

✔ Failure to consider chronic asthma management in discharge planning

Acknowledgments

Thanks to previous edition author Michael A. Kaufman.

References

1. National Asthma Education and Prevention Program Expert Panel Report: Guidelines for the Diagnosis and Management of Asthma: Update on Selected Topics- 2002. *J Allergy Clin Immunol* 2002;110:S1–S209.
2. Bousquet J. The use of biopsy to study airway inflammation. *Respir Med* 2000;94(Suppl F):S1–S2.
3. Bracken MB, Triche EW, Belanger K, et al. Asthma symptoms, severity, and drug therapy: a prospective study of effects on 2205 pregnancies. *Obstet Gynecol* 2003;102:739–752.
4. Camargo C Jr., Spooner C, Rowe B. Continuous versus intermittent beta-agonists in the treatment of acute asthma. *Cochrane Database Syst Rev* 2003;4:CD001115.
5. Camargo CA Jr., Smithline HA, Malice MP, et al. A randomized controlled trial of intravenous montelukast in acute asthma. *Am J Respir Crit Care Med* 2003;167:528–533.
6. Carden DL, Nowak RM, Sarkar D, Tomlanovich MC. Vital signs including pulsus paradoxus in the assessment of acute bronchial asthma. *Ann Emerg Med* 1983;12:80–83.
7. Cydulka R, Davison R, Grammer L, Parker M, Mathews JT. The use of epinephrine in the treatment of older adult asthmatics. *Ann Emerg Med* 1988;17:322–326.
8. Cydulka RK, McFadden ER, Sarver JH, Emerman CL. Comparison of single 7.5-mg dose treatment vs. sequential multidose 2.5-mg treatments with nebulized albuterol in the treatment of acute asthma. *Chest* 2002;122:1982–1987.
9. Edmonds ML, Camargo CA, Jr., Brenner BE, Rowe BH. Replacement of oral corticosteroids with inhaled corticosteroids in the treatment of acute asthma following emergency department discharge(*): a meta-analysis. *Chest* 2002;121:1798–1805.
10. Emerman CL, Cydulka RK, Effron D, et al. A randomized, controlled comparison of isoetharine and albuterol in the treatment of acute asthma. *Ann Emerg Med* 1991;20:1090–1093.
11. Ho AM, Lee A, Karmakar MK, et al. Heliox vs air-oxygen mixtures for the treatment of patients with acute asthma: a systematic overview. *Chest* 2003;123:882–890.
12. Howton JC. Randomized, double-blind, placebo-controlled trial of intravenous ketamine in acute asthma. *Ann Emerg Med* 1996.
13. Johnson KH. Heliox of minimal benefit in acute asthma. *J Fam Pract* 2003;52:520–522.
14. Lau TT, Zed PJ. Does ketamine have a role in managing severe exacerbation of asthma in adults? *Pharmacotherapy* 2001;21:1100–1106.
15. Martin TG, Elenbaas RM, Pingleton SH. Use of peak expiratory flow rates to eliminate unnecessary arterial blood gases in acute asthma. *Ann Emerg Med* 1982;11:70–73.
16. McFadden ER Jr. Acute severe asthma. *Am J Respir Crit Care Med* 2003;168:740–759.
17. National Asthma Education and Prevention Program. *Expert Panel Report II: Guidelines for the Diagnosis and Management of Asthma.* Baltimore: National Institutes of Health, 1997.
18. Padkin AJ, Baigel G, Morgan GA. Halothane treatment of severe asthma to avoid mechanical ventilation. *Anaesthesia* 1997;52:994–997.
19. Parameswaran K, Belda J, Rowe BH. Addition of intravenous aminophylline to beta2-agonists in adults with acute asthma. *Cochrane Database Syst Rev* 2000;4:CD002742.
20. Rose CC, Murphy JG, Schwartz JS. Performance of an index predicting the response of patients with acute bronchial asthma to intensive emergency department treatment. *N Engl J Med* 1984;310:573–580.
21. Rowe BH, Spooner CH, Ducharme FM, et al. Early use of inhaled corticosteroids in the emergency department treatment of acute asthma. *Cochrane Database Syst Rev* 2001;1:CD002308. Update in *Cochrane Database Syst Rev* 2003;3:CD002308.
22. Schatz M, Dombrowski MP, Wise R, et al. Asthma morbidity during pregnancy can be predicted by severity classification. *J Allergy Clin Immunol* 2003;112:283–288.
23. Stoodley RG, Aaron SD, Dales RE. The role of ipratropium bromide in the emergency management of acute asthma exacerbation: a metaanalysis of randomized clinical trials. *Ann Emerg Med* 1999;34:8–18.
24. van der Windt D. Promises and pitfalls in the evaluation of pediatric asthma scores. *J Pediatr* 2000;137:744–746.
25. Walker S, Monteil M, Phelan K, Lasserton TJ, Walters EH. Anti-IgE for chronic asthma in adults and children. *Cochrane Database Syst Rev* 2004;3:CD003559. Review.
26. Walsh-Kelly CM. Chest radiography in the initial episode of bronchospasm in children: can clinical variables predict pathologic findings? *Ann Emerg Med* 1996;28:4:391–395.
27. Webb JR. Dose response of patients to oral corticosteroid treatment during exacerbations of asthma. *Br Med J* 1986;292:1045–1047.
28. White CS. Acute asthma: admission chest radiography in hospitalized adult patients. *Chest* 1991;100(1):14–16.

CHAPTER 36

Chronic Obstructive Pulmonary Disease

David S. Howes and Marc A. Bellazzini

Chronic obstructive pulmonary disease (COPD) comprises a spectrum of chronic respiratory illnesses characterized by cough, sputum production, dyspnea, airflow limitation, and impaired gas exchange. More recently, the term *COPD* has expanded to include an abnormal inflammatory response in the small airways and lung parenchyma to noxious particles and gases (6,17). The mortality rate is greater than 50% within 10 years of diagnosis (11). COPD is the fourth leading cause of death, costing more than $15 billion dollars for treatment annually and affects at least 15 million Americans (10,11).

The term *COPD* includes conditions, other than asthma, that have the common feature of airflow obstruction and inflammation. The inflammatory response in COPD is different than that seen in asthma and involves the recruitment of neutrophils, macrophages, and cytotoxic T lymphocytes. Inflammation of the small airways leads to fibrosis and narrowing resulting in chronic obstructive bronchitis (6). *Chronic bronchitis* is characterized clinically by a productive cough caused by excessive production of bronchial mucus that must be present for 3 months in a year in at least 2 successive years. *Pulmonary emphysema*, in contrast, is defined from a pathologic standpoint by an irreversible enlargement of the alveolar air spaces with destruction of the alveolar wall and pulmonary capillary bed, mediated by proteases such as matrix metalloproteinases and neutrophil elastase (6). Patients who have pure forms of each condition are the exception, as most patients exhibit characteristics of both.

The predominant risk factor for COPD is tobacco use (9,21). However, 5% to 10% of patients with COPD have never smoked, implicating other causal factors (5). Other risk factors include environmental pollution, passive smoke inhalation, occupational exposure, and repeated respiratory infections (9,21). There may also be genetic factors, the best defined being α_1-antitrypsin deficiency (21). Regardless of etiology, the ultimate outcome is irreversible airflow limitation.

The natural course of COPD is one of progressively worsening dyspnea, hypoxemia, and diminished exercise tolerance, with recurrent exacerbations. Most patients with COPD have modest reversible airway obstruction, and although the forced expiratory volume in 1 second (FEV_1) is classically considered the best single prognostic indicator of disability and death, current investigators prefer to assess disease severity by considering FEV_1, body mass index (BMI), and exercise performance (17). The onset of chronic hypoxemia leads to progressive clinical deterioration owing to cor pulmonale, which worsens already diminished lung function. Recurrent episodes of infection and respiratory failure ultimately result in death. Long-term ambulatory oxygen therapy is the only treatment that has been demonstrated to prolong life in patients with advanced COPD (10)

CLINICAL PRESENTATION

All patients with COPD exhibit airflow obstruction, but the pure forms of emphysema and chronic bronchitis have distinctive clinical features. Patients with emphysema tend to hyperventilate to compensate for the decreased ability of the lungs to oxygenate the blood. These classic "pink puffers" work hard to establish a near-normal PaO_2, and they appear barrel-chested, dyspneic, and tachypneic. They use pursed-lip breathing to create positive end-expiratory pressure (PEEP) in order to prevent early airway closure. Breath sounds are markedly diminished, with a prolonged expiratory phase.

In contrast, patients with chronic bronchitis tolerate hypoxemia well and make no effort to hyperventilate. Chronic hypoxia induces a secondary polycythemia that, combined with the cyanosis of marked desaturation of hemoglobin, produces a plethoric appearance. These patients tolerate an elevated $PaCO_2$ and have a less labored respiratory pattern. With the decreased work of breathing, the patient with chronic bronchitis does not experience muscle wasting like the emphysematous patient. These features produce the picture of the "blue bloater." Lung examination reveals rhonchi, rales, and variable wheezing.

Most patients who present with an acute exacerbation of COPD do not fit either picture precisely. Patients typically complain of dyspnea and chest tightness and often note a change in the character of their sputum. Physical examination may reveal tachypnea and a variable degree of respiratory distress, as evidenced by accessory muscle use, retractions, and cyanosis. On auscultation, one may hear diminished breath sounds, a prolonged expiratory phase, wheezing, rales, or rhonchi. Signs of cor pulmonale should be sought: a centrally displaced point of maximal impulse, heart gallop, tricuspid murmur, peripheral edema, jugular venous distention, or hepatojugular reflux, and hepatomegaly. This complication of long-standing hypoxemia is associated with substantial mortality.

The causes of exacerbation include respiratory infection, noncompliance with (or underdosing of) medications, changes in weather, exposure to certain drugs (e.g., sedatives or β-blockers), cardiac dysrhythmias, left ventricular dysfunction, and environmental exposure to allergens or other irritants. Patients typically present with a gradual, but progressive, deterioration over hours to days.

Acute decompensation may be the result of a number of other conditions. Spontaneous pneumothorax in COPD carries a significantly higher complication and mortality rate than in patients with a normal cardiorespiratory status. The patient with chronic bronchitis is predisposed to embolic and thrombotic phenomena owing to the hyperviscosity associated with polycythemia. Other disorders, such as congestive heart failure (CHF), pneumonia, acidosis, or renal or hepatic failure, may also overwhelm the COPD patient's limited reserves, resulting in respiratory failure.

DIFFERENTIAL DIAGNOSIS

COPD is a clinical diagnosis; it is usually made after extended observation of a patient at risk who demonstrates progressive lung dysfunction. Because those at risk are likely to have sedentary lifestyles, they may present only when an acute event precipitates dyspnea at rest, unmasking previously undiagnosed lung disease.

Other conditions must also be considered in the patient who presents to the emergency department with wheezing, cough, dyspnea, or respiratory failure. Pneumonia or acute bronchitis may present with varying degrees of shortness of breath, cough, and bronchospasm, and previously undiagnosed COPD may be discovered after an acute pneumonic process has resolved. The onset of respiratory symptoms, in the presence of absence of chest pain, when associated with risk factors such as recent surgery, malignancy, immobility, or extended travel, or leg findings consistent with deep venous thrombosis, strongly suggest pulmonary embolism.

Acute left ventricular dysfunction may mimic many findings of COPD including cough, dyspnea, and hypoxemia, and patients may exhibit wheezing, referred to as "cardiac asthma." Orthopnea, paroxysmal nocturnal dyspnea, and cardiomegaly favor CHF, but COPD patients with cor pulmonale may well demonstrate jugular venous distention and peripheral edema. Classically, chest radiography helped distinguish between these entities with a lack of cardiomegaly, and pulmonary venous redistribution and the presence of bullae and hyperinflation of the lungs suggesting COPD. However, patients with both CHF and COPD who present with dyspnea can present a diagnostic challenge. The rapid laboratory quantification of B-type natriuretic peptide (BNP) may allow more accurate distinction between an acute exacerbation of COPD versus CHF. BNP is secreted from ventricles in response to pressure and volume expansion. Low levels of BNP are consistent with exacerbations of COPD, asthma, bronchitis, or pneumonia, whereas a BNP level of 100 pg/mL or greater has been shown to be a strong predictor of CHF. Pulmonary embolism or COPD triggering cor-pulmonale may also produce elevated BNP levels of 200 to 600 pg/mL (4,7,18); therefore, it is best to use the patient's physical examination, history, and ancillary studies together with the BNP level to make the most informed clinical diagnosis and therapeutic decisions.

EMERGENCY DEPARTMENT EVALUATION

If the patient's respiratory status allows a brief history to be taken, attention should be directed to the rapidity of onset, duration of symptoms, precipitating factors, the dosage of medications and when medications were last taken. Information should be sought regarding the character of the sputum, the course of previous exacerbations, and any history of concomitant disease processes.

The physical examination focuses on the patient's mental status and the degree of respiratory distress. Hypercapnia and hypoxia can cause confusion, somnolence, and irritability. The cardiac and pulmonary examinations are vital, and repeated examinations are mandatory after therapeutic interventions in order to monitor the response to treatment.

Pulse oximetry is useful in monitoring oxygen saturation and the effectiveness of oxygen supplementation. Arterial blood gas (ABG) analysis provides information on the $PaCO_2$ and pH, reflecting adequacy of ventilation. The pH is the best single laboratory marker for gauging the severity of acute respiratory insufficiency, since it reflects the speed and degree of change in $PaCO_2$ (19). Baseline or prior ABG results may be useful for comparison; in general, hypercapnia with acidemia suggests acute respiratory failure.

The chest radiograph (CXR) is usually done at the bedside, unless the patient is stable and can tolerate being transported to the radiology suite for posteroanterior (PA) and lateral films. The CXR is useful when findings of COPD are present, but it is even more helpful in ruling out other disease processes, such as pneumothorax, atelectasis, infiltrate, lung mass, or CHF.

Measurements of airflow do not always yield accurate assessments of the severity of illness but may be useful in judging the response to therapy. The peak expiratory flow rate (PEFR) is most commonly used in the emergency department setting, but, in contrast to the asthmatic patient's response, it does not typically demonstrate a marked change in COPD.

Laboratory studies are generally of limited value. A serum theophylline level should be obtained in patients who are taking the medication, as it has a narrow therapeutic window and myriad drug interactions. β-agonists may cause hypokalemia, although this is rarely clinically significant. A complete blood count may reveal anemia, which can compound the problem of hypoxemia, or a high white blood cell count, which may be a clue to pneumonia or other systemic infections. Other tests, for example, the BNP for evaluation of CHF, may be indicated if other disease processes are being investigated.

A 12-lead electrocardiogram (ECG) may suggest right atrial enlargement, low voltage, or right ventricular hypertrophy, or strain (cor pulmonale). Acute ischemic patterns must be appreciated to identify an acute coronary event that may be triggering or complicating the acute COPD attack. Continuous ECG monitoring may be useful in revealing dysrhythmias that may aggravate an acute exacerbation.

EMERGENCY DEPARTMENT MANAGEMENT

The effective management of the COPD patient with an acute decompensation includes rapid estimation of severity, prompt therapy, frequent re-evaluation, and recognition of treatable entities that may have precipitated the emergency department visit or that complicate the patient's course. The patient should be placed on a cardiac monitor and intravenous access should be established. Dysrhythmias such as rapid atrial fibrillation usually reflect coexisting heart disease that is worsened by acute hypoxemia; current evidence suggests that most patients with a COPD exacerbation who exhibit ventricular dysrhythmias have underlying left ventricular diastolic dysfunction (12).

Treatment with oxygen is critical because hypoxemia is the major immediate threat to life. The goal is to maintain a PaO_2 greater than 60 mm Hg or a pulse oximetry reading of 90% to 92% to minimize further risk of hypercapnea and respiratory acidosis (19). A controlled oxygen delivery system is preferable; a Venturi mask system can deliver a precise oxygen concentration ranging from 24% to 50%. Adjustments in oxygen delivery should be guided by continuous pulse oximetry and ABG determinations as needed. In the acutely hypoxemic patient, the administration of oxygen is paramount and far outweighs the risk of hypercarbia

caused by blunting of the hypoxemic drive in a chronic CO_2 retainer.

Sympathomimetics, specifically β_2 agonists, are the initial pharmacologic agents of choice for acute COPD exacerbations. Effectiveness is dependent in part on the reversible component of the patient's obstructive lung disease (9,11,13,14,24); however, a significant benefit of bronchodilator therapy is to decrease dynamic hyperinflation by improving lung emptying during expiration (17). Side effects include tremor, agitation, insomnia, headache, cardiac tachyarrhythmias, and mild hypokalemia (24). Although a metered-dose inhaler (MDI) coupled with a spacer device has been reported to be as effective as treatment delivered by nebulizer aerosolization, the latter delivery method is preferred in the emergency department setting because dyspneic patients may have difficulty effectively performing the MDI procedure (14,21). Although there are many β_2 agonists available, albuterol, 2.5 mg, is the most widely used agent. It is used either in repeated treatments every 20 to 60 minutes or by continuous nebulization, in severe cases. Levalbuterol, the active (R) isomer of racemic albuterol, is available for treatment of COPD by nebulizer; the "on label" dosage is 1.25 mg every 6 to 8 hours, although dosages of up to 1.25 mg every 30 minutes have been reported in clinical studies (3). The inactive (S) isomer found in racemic albuterol is thought to promote hypersensitivity and bronchospasm in susceptible individuals. Patients treated with levalbuterol have been shown to require less medication and experience a longer therapeutic duration of action compared with racemic albuterol (23).

The slower onset of action renders anticholinergic agents to second-line treatment in the acute setting (14,16). Ipratropium bromide, a congener of atropine, has little systemic absorption when inhaled, thus minimizing undesirable anticholinergic effects, and has been shown to have an additive effect when combined with a β_2 agonist (1,11,14). This agent may be administered at a dose of 500 μg per nebulizer treatment. Anticholinergics are considered by some investigators to be the bronchodilators of choice in the management of chronic disease (5,16). A newer long-acting anticholinergic agent, tiotropium bromide, can be given once daily and is reported to be as or more effective than ipratropium bromide given four times a day (6).

Corticosteroids are considered useful in acute exacerbations of COPD (9,11,14). Even patients who do not respond to steroids, when stable, may still benefit from them during acute attacks (9,21). Because steroid use may suppress the adrenal–pituitary axis, patients with current or recent use may require steroids for the stress of any acute illness. Intravenous methylprednisolone at a dose of 125 mg or oral prednisone 60–80 mg are commonly used in the treatment of exacerbations of COPD.

Before the widespread availability of oral or inhaled β_2 agonists, methylxanthines, most commonly theophylline preparations, were used as monotherapy for COPD. Symptomatic improvement of dyspnea and exercise tolerance is presumed to result at least partially from mild bronchodilatation and positive inotropic effects on the diaphragm. However, theophylline has a narrow therapeutic window and is associated with adverse effects including nausea, cardiac dysrhythmias, and, rarely, seizures. Although current recommendations do not support instituting methylxanthine therapy in acute exacerbations, if a patient is maintained on theophylline, one might continue intravenous therapy as guided by drug levels. The therapeutic range of theophylline is 10–20 mcg/ml. Drug levels should be interpreted carefully with special attention given to the time the drug was last administered.

Other medications may be utilized in the management of acute COPD. Magnesium sulfate has modest bronchodilatory effects, and may be given a trial as adjunctive therapy to patients with severe exacerbations who have normal renal function

(22,25). There is no compelling evidence that mucolytics such as acetylcysteine are efficacious in the acute setting (9). Inhibitors of neutrophilic inflammation, protease, leukotriene B4, chemokine, inducible nitric oxide synthase (iNOS), tumor necrosis factor α (TNF-α), and prostaglandins are currently under investigation, but there are, as yet, no data suggesting their practical clinical utility in COPD (5,6).

Cessation of tobacco use may well be the most important intervention for COPD (10,21). Brief counseling can be effective, and an effort should be made to advise the patient to stop smoking and seek further counseling from a primary care physician (6,17). Bupropion and nicotine replacement therapy may be very useful in assisting patients to stop smoking (5). COPD patients in the emergency department are also candidates to receive polyvalent pneumococcal and influenza vaccines in order to decrease the risk of future exacerbations.

It is estimated that only half of acute COPD exacerbations are caused by bacterial infection, with the predominant species being *Haemophilus influenzae, Moraxella catarrhalis,* and *Streptococcus pneumoniae* (20). If dyspnea is associated with a change in the volume or purulence of sputum, or if a new infiltrate is noted on CXR, antibiotic therapy should be instituted (10,21). Gram staining of the sputum may aid in the selection of an antimicrobial, and adjustments may be needed according to geographic location and local resistance patterns. For less severe cases, oral therapy with tetracycline or doxycycline, a second- or third-generation cephalosporin, trimethoprim–sulfamethoxazole, or a β-lactam–β-lactamase inhibitor combination, with or without a macrolide, is appropriate (10). In hospitalized patients with pneumonia or toxicity, parenteral therapy should be instituted with a second- or third-generation cephalosporin, or a β-lactam–β-lactamase inhibitor in conjunction with a macrolide (10). Several of the newer fluoroquinolones such as gatifloxacin, levofloxacin, or moxifloxacin can be started as monotherapy. The choice of antibiotic should be based on local resistance patterns with newer agents and those with broad-spectrum coverage, used only when necessary in order to reduce the incidence of antibiotic resistance.

For patients who do not respond to acute interventions and who begin to show signs of respiratory failure, such as deterioration of mental status, worsening hypoxemia (PaO_2 of less than 50 mm Hg), or worsening respiratory acidosis (pH less than 7.25), assisted ventilation is indicated (14,16). Noninvasive positive pressure ventilation (NIPPV) should be considered for patients who present with moderate exacerbations of COPD and should be instituted for patients with severe exacerbations of COPD who have a relatively normal mental status and who do not require immediate endotracheal intubation. NIPPV will decrease the work of breathing and has been shown to decrease the rate of endotracheal intubation, to decrease hospital mortality, and to shorten hospital stay in patients with severe exacerbations of COPD (15,25). However, for patients who are not candidates for these modalities, or for whom noninvasive ventilation has failed, endotracheal intubation with mechanical ventilation is the treatment of choice.

Those performing endotracheal intubation should be aware of the potential complications associated with positive pressure ventilation in COPD. Hypotension or cardiovascular collapse may result from decreased venous return or reduced sympathetic tone from the administration of sedative agents. If hypotension does not resolve with administration of intravenous fluids, the patient's endotracheal tube should be temporarily disconnected from the ventilator to relieve excess positive intrathoracic pressure (8). Mechanical ventilation should be adjusted to allow for a short inspiratory and long expiratory time with a low tidal volume of 5 to 7 mL/kg (2,8). The frequency of ventilation may be gradually increased to allow for resolution of the acute respiratory acidosis and gradual normalization of pH. Extrinsic PEEP may be added to nearly equal intrinsic or auto-PEEP in order to stent open the airways and reduce gas trapping. Short-term administration of paralytics will eliminate patient-ventilator dyssynchrony and reduce the risk of hyperinflation (8). Proper sedation is imperative if paralytics are administered.

CRITICAL INTERVENTIONS

- The arterial pH is the best single laboratory marker for gauging the severity of acute respiratory insufficiency, since it reflects the speed and degree of change in $PaCO_2$. Hypercapnia with acidemia suggests acute respiratory failure
- In the acutely hypoxemic patient, the administration of oxygen far outweighs the risk of hypercarbia owing to blunting of the hypoxemic drive in a chronic CO_2 retainer
- Use a controlled oxygen delivery system (Venturi mask) to maintain a PaO_2 greater than 60 mm Hg or a pulse oximetry reading of 90% to 92% to minimize further risk of hypercapnia and respiratory acidosis
- Adjust oxygen delivery based on continuous pulse oximetry and serial ABGs

DISPOSITION

Many patients who present with an acute exacerbation of COPD require admission to the hospital. However, if the patient responds to therapy and the vital signs and pulmonary function tests approach baseline, discharge may be considered if good followup is assured. The bronchodilator regimen should be maximized, and steroids should be continued for a short course. Antibiotics should be prescribed for exacerbations of chronic bronchitis. It should be recognized that approximately 15% of patients with COPD who are discharged from the emergency department require readmission (25).

Accepted criteria for hospitalization of patients with COPD include poor response to outpatient therapy, severe limitation of function, inability to eat or sleep owing to dyspnea, presence of significant comorbid conditions, worsening respiratory failure, new or progressive cor pulmonale, and the need for invasive procedures, especially those requiring analgesics or sedatives (25). Guidelines for admission to the intensive care unit are not as well defined. Treatment in an intensive care unit is indicated when the close observation, monitoring, and therapeutic interventions (including assisted ventilation) required by these patients cannot be provided elsewhere.

If transfer to another institution is required, it must be done carefully because transfer is often associated with an interruption in treatment and increased patient fatigue. The transport team must be capable of managing the airway if decompensation occurs.

COMMON PITFALLS

✔ The COPD patient should not be expected to have disease that reverses as rapidly as the asthmatic patient. Look for a slower course of improvement, and have a lower threshold for admission
✔ If the patient has not slept well in the last 2 days, he is tired and the risk of respiratory failure is high, admit the patient
✔ Precipitating or complicating conditions may be overlooked when treating only the exacerbation of COPD. For example, if CHF is complicating the picture, a BNP may be helpful
✔ Oxygen should never be withheld owing to concern about respiratory depression. If inadequate ventilation occurs, ventilatory support should be provided

✔ It is easy to underestimate the severity of illness in patients with chronic dysfunction. Utilize radiography, pulse oximetry, ABG analyses, and pulmonary function tests liberally. Respect the patient's estimation of severity of their illness

Acknowledgments

Thanks to previous edition author Erica E. Remer.

References

1. The COMBIVENT Inhalation Solution Study Group. Routine nebulized ipratropium and albuterol together are better than either alone in COPD. *Chest* 1997;112:1514–1521.
2. The Acute Respiratory Distress Syndrome Network. Ventilation with lower tidal volumes as compared with traditional tidal volumes for acute lung injury and the acute respiratory distress syndrome. *N Engl J Med* 2000;342:1301–1308.
3. Xopenex Full Prescribing Information. 2003, www.xopenex.com. Accessed 10/28/03 Sepracor.
4. Ando T, Ogawa K, Yamaki K, et al. Plasma concentrations of atrial, brain, and C-type natriuretic peptides and endothelin-1 in patients with chronic respiratory diseases. *Chest* 1996;110:462–468.
5. Barnes PJ. New therapies for chronic obstructive pulmonary disease. *Thorax* 1998;53:137–147.
6. Barnes PJ. Chronic obstructive pulmonary disease: 12. New treatments for COPD. *Thorax* 2003;58:803–808.
7. Collins SP, Ronan-Bentle S, Storrow AB. Diagnostic and prognostic usefulness of natriuretic peptides in emergency department patients with dyspnea. *Ann Emerg Med* 2003;41:532–545.
8. Davidson AC. The pulmonary physician in critical care: 11. Critical care management of respiratory failure resulting from COPD. *Thorax* 2002;57:1079–1084.
9. Ferguson GT. Management of COPD. Early identification and active intervention are crucial. *Postgrad Med* 1998;103:129–134, 136–141.
10. Fiel SB. Chronic obstructive pulmonary disease. Mortality and mortality reduction. *Drugs* 1996;52[Suppl 2]:55–60; discussion 60–61.
11. Friedman M. Changing practices in COPD. A new pharmacologic treatment algorithm. *Chest* 1995;107[Suppl 5]:194S–197S.
12. Fuso L, Incalzi RA, Pistelli R, et al. Predicting mortality of patients hospitalized for acutely exacerbated chronic obstructive pulmonary disease. *Am J Med* 1995;98:272–277.
13. Hoyt JW. Debunking myths of chronic obstructive lung disease. *Crit Care Med* 1997;25:1450–1451.
14. Ikeda A, Nishimura K, Izumi T. Pharmacological treatment in acute exacerbations of chronic obstructive pulmonary disease. *Drugs Aging* 1998;12:129–137.
15. Keenan SP, Sinuff T, Cook DJ, Hill NS. Which patients with acute exacerbation of chronic obstructive pulmonary disease benefit from noninvasive positive-pressure ventilation? A systematic review of the literature. *Ann Intern Med* 2003;138:861–870.
16. Levin DC, Little KS, Laughlin KR, et al., Addition of anticholinergic solution prolongs bronchodilator effect of beta 2 agonists in patients with chronic obstructive pulmonary disease. *Am J Med* 1996;100:40S–48S.
17. MacNee W, Calverley PM. Chronic obstructive pulmonary disease: 7. Management of COPD. *Thorax* 2003;58:261–265.
18. Maisel AS, Krishnaswamy P, Nowak RM, et al. Rapid measurement of B-type natriuretic peptide in the emergency diagnosis of heart failure. *N Engl J Med* 2002;347:161–167.
19. Plant PK, Elliott MW. Chronic obstructive pulmonary disease: 9. management of ventilatory failure in COPD. *Thorax* 2003;58:537–542.
20. Schentag JJ, Tillotson GS. Antibiotic selection and dosing for the treatment of acute exacerbations of COPD. *Chest* 1997;112[Suppl 6]:314S–319S.
21. Senior RM, Anthonisen NR. Chronic obstructive pulmonary disease (COPD). *Am J Respir Crit Care Med* 1998;157:S139–S147.
22. Skorodin MS, Tenholder MF, Yetter B, et al. Magnesium sulfate in exacerbations of chronic obstructive pulmonary disease. *Arch Intern Med* 1995;155:496–500.
23. Truitt T, Witko J, Halpern M. Levalbuterol compared to racemic albuterol: Efficacy and outcomes in patients hospitalized with COPD or asthma. *Chest* 2003;123:128–135.
24. Ziment I. The beta-agonist controversy: impact in COPD. *Chest* 1995; 107[Suppl 5]:198S–205S.
25. Zuege DJ, Whitelaw WA. Management of acute respiratory failure in chronic obstructive pulmonary disease. *Curr Opin Pulm Med* 1997;3:190–197.

CHAPTER 37
Spontaneous Pneumothorax and Pneumomediastinum

Susan M. Dunmire

Spontaneous pneumothorax and pneumomediastinum are relatively uncommon entities in emergency medicine; however, it is important for the emergency department physician to be familiar with the presentation and management of these conditions.

A pneumothorax is defined by the presence of gas within the pleural space. A pneumothorax occurring in the absence of penetrating or blunt injury to the chest wall is termed a spontaneous pneumothorax. This can be classified either as *primary*, occurring in patient without known pulmonary disease, or as *secondary*, occurring in the setting of underlying lung disease. A tension pneumothorax occurs when a large accumulation of air in the pleural space impairs venous return, thereby resulting in hypotension.

Although most authorities agree that a spontaneous pneumothorax is the result of rupture of small subpleural cysts or blebs, the etiology of these structural abnormalities (congenital versus acquired) is still controversial. In individuals with a primary spontaneous pneumothorax, computed tomographic (CT) scan demonstrates ipsilateral bullae in 89% of patients compared with 20% of controls matched for age and smoking history (11,14). In a review of 11 studies, the average recurrence rate of a spontaneous pneumothorax is 30% (range, 16% to 52%) (19).

A primary spontaneous pneumothorax typically occurs in tall, thin individuals younger than the age of 40 years, with a male-to-female ratio of 5:1 (15,17). The incidence of primary spontaneous pneumothorax is between 7.4 and 18 cases in 100,000 for male patients and between 1.2 and 6 cases per 100,000 for female patients (3,13). Cigarette smoking significantly increases the risk of a primary spontaneous pneumothorax by as much as 20-fold (3,8).

The incidence of secondary spontaneous pneumothorax in individuals with known chronic obstructive pulmonary disease (COPD) is approximately 26 in 100,000 (7). The peak age for occurrence of a secondary pneumothorax is 60 to 65 years, and the most common underlying risk factor is COPD. Secondary spontaneous pneumothorax occurs in 2% to 6% of patients with human immunodeficiency virus (HIV) and concurrent *Pneumocystis carinii* pneumonia (2,4,12,18). Other less common causes of secondary pneumothorax include malignancy, asthma (sometimes presenting as sudden severe respiratory compromise), pulmonary infarction, histiocytosis X, and Hamman-Rich syndrome (acute interstitial pulmonary fibrosis).

Another less common but interesting entity is *catamenial pneumothorax*. This is a spontaneous pneumothorax occurring in women at the time of menstruation. This entity typically affects women in the age range of 30 to 40 years and occurs within 72 hours of the onset of menses (10). A catamenial pneumothorax is frequently right-sided and has a 50% recurrence rate within the first year. Although its etiology is multifactorial, in some patients the condition results from small implants of endometrial tissue in the pleural lining (5,9,21).

Spontaneous *pneumomediastinum* is the result of alveolar rupture with dissection of air along the bronchus and into the mediastinum. The cause of pneumomediastinum often cannot be identified. Although it is usually a benign entity, more serious causes such as esophageal rupture must be ruled out. A pneumomediastinum can occur in patients with a history of vigorous vomiting or in those who use repetitive and prolonged Valsalva maneuvers to enhance the effects of inhaled pipe-smoked cocaine (20).

CLINICAL PRESENTATION

Patients with spontaneous pneumothorax typically present with the sudden onset of constant, ipsilateral chest or shoulder pain that may or may not increase with inspiration. The majority of patients complain of dyspnea, although the severity depends on the size of the pneumothorax. Patients with a secondary spontaneous pneumothorax will often present with severe dyspnea, even with a small pneumothorax, owing to the degree of underlying pulmonary disease. The onset of symptoms usually occurs at rest or during sleep. Rarely, spontaneous pneumothorax can present as a tension pneumothorax with severe cardiopulmonary compromise.

Symptoms in adults with spontaneous pneumomediastinum include retrosternal chest pain and, less frequently, subcutaneous emphysema caused by tracking of air into the chest wall, neck, face, abdominal wall, and scrotum. If enough air accumulates in the mediastinum, the pleura can rupture, resulting in an associated pneumothorax. Spontaneous pneumomediastinum in infants is a much more serious entity and can cause cardiopulmonary compromise by compression of the hilum (23).

DIFFERENTIAL DIAGNOSIS

Pulmonary embolism, exacerbation of COPD or asthma, pneumonia, and myocardial ischemia should all be in the differential diagnosis of a patient with shortness of breath and chest pain. Often the entity of spontaneous pneumothorax is not considered until the chest radiograph is obtained.

Once the diagnosis of pneumothorax has been made, the physician is obligated to search for the underlying cause. In the case of spontaneous pneumothorax, it is important to reevaluate the history and physical examination to ensure that there is no sign of blunt or penetrating trauma. An elderly person may have forgotten a recent fall, resulting in rib fractures and an underlying pneumothorax. A puncture site in the neck or supraclavicular area can easily be missed in a patient who is an unsuspected drug abuser who has penetrated the pleural space.

Spontaneous pneumomediastinum usually presents as substernal chest pain. The differential diagnosis includes myocardial ischemia, gastroesophageal reflux, pulmonary embolism, and pneumonia.

EMERGENCY DEPARTMENT EVALUATION

Physical examination is often not very helpful in making the diagnosis of spontaneous pneumothorax. Patients often exhibit mild resting tachycardia and tachypnea. Depending on the extent of the pneumothorax, breath sounds may be diminished unilaterally. The presence of hypotension and tachycardia (>140 beats per minute) in combination with jugular venous distention or tracheal deviation should immediately alert the emergency physician to the possibility of a tension pneumothorax requiring emergent decompression.

The diagnosis of pneumothorax is usually made by chest radiography (CXR), which reveals a peripheral lucent area containing no lung markings. Films taken in maximal expiration with the patient in an upright position optimize visualization of small pneumothoraces. The size of a pneumothorax may be roughly gauged from the plain chest film, but such estimates are notoriously unreliable. Algorithms that yield more accurate estimates of size are available but are relatively complicated to apply (16).

Patients with a significant (>25%) pneumothorax have an increase in the alveolar—arterial oxygen gradient. Although hypercapnia is rare with a primary spontaneous pneumothorax, it can become quite severe in the setting of a secondary spontaneous pneumothorax.

The electrocardiogram is not helpful for diagnosis. Nonspecific changes, including T-wave inversion in the precordial leads, decreased amplitude of the R wave, and left axis deviation, are often noted.

The diagnosis of a spontaneous pneumomediastinum is often overlooked and requires a thorough examination and a high index of suspicion. On physical examination, auscultation of the heart may reveal a crunching sound during systole (Hamman sign) (6). Rarely, subcutaneous air may be present. On CXR, a very thin lucent stripe can be seen outlining the heart and mediastinum. A lateral neck radiograph may reveal subcutaneous air. The electrocardiogram is useful only in helping to rule out ischemia in the patient who presents with substernal chest pain.

EMERGENCY DEPARTMENT MANAGEMENT AND DISPOSITION

Most patients with primary spontaneous pneumothorax do not have significant respiratory or cardiac compromise. Any hemodynamic instability should suggest the presence of tension pneumothorax requiring immediate needle decompression followed by tube thoracostomy.

Prospective studies evaluating management of spontaneous pneumothorax have significant limitations. In 2001, the American College of Chest Physicians produced a Consensus Statement regarding the management of spontaneous pneumothoraces. This consensus was reached by combining evidence from these studies as well as a consensus of expert opinion. The following represents their treatment recommendations (1).

Clinically stable patients with a small (<20%) *primary pneumothorax* may be observed 3 to 6 hours in the emergency department. If a repeat CXR does not show any progression of the pneumothorax, these patients may be discharged to home. Follow up CXRs should be performed within 48 hours and again in 7 to 10 days. It is estimated that pleural air is spontaneously reabsorbed at a rate of 1.0% to 1.5% of the volume of the hemithorax per day. Therefore, a small pneumothorax (<15%) would be expected to be reabsorbed within 10 to 15 days. Patients should be instructed to return for any increase in shortness of breath or chest pain or for the development of fever. Admission is recommended if the patient lives a long distance from the treating facility or is considered at risk for not complying with appropriate followup.

Clinically stable patients with a larger (>20%) *primary pneumothorax* should have the affected lung re-expanded by insertion of a small-bore catheter. A pigtail catheter or small-bore chest tube (16–18 French) is recommended. By using the Seldinger technique, one can insert a pigtail catheter at the anterior axillary line between the fourth and fifth ribs (nipple line). Care should be taken when the wire is introduced into the pleural space, and the clinician must be certain that all side holes of the catheter are within the pleural space. The pigtail catheter is then attached to suction. All of these patients should be hospitalized for observation following re-expansion of the pneumothorax.

Clinically stable patients with a small (<20%) *secondary pneumothorax* should be admitted for observation. The coexistent underlying lung disease can result in decompensation with a very small pneumothorax. Some thoracic surgeons advocate placement of a small-bore catheter to evacuate even small collections of air, but the majority recommend invasive management only if decompensation occurs.

Clinically stable patients with a large (>20%) *secondary pneumothorax* should undergo placement of a chest tube (24–28 French). Many of these patients will experience a persistent air leak owing to a fistula. All of these patients will require admission.

Clinically unstable patients with a large pneumothorax require immediate needle decompression. A large-bore intravenous catheter (14 or 16 gauge) should be inserted over the third rib at the midaxillary line on the affected side. The needle should be removed, leaving the plastic catheter in place. This is a temporary treatment and immediate insertion of a chest tube is essential.

A pneumothorax that occurs in the setting of chest wall trauma should be treated with a tube thoracostomy to drain a possible coexisting hemothorax. These patients require admission to the hospital and close monitoring.

Management of pneumomediastinum is conservative. It is essential, however, to exclude potentially catastrophic causes such as Boerhaave syndrome (esophageal rupture), which is associated with a high mortality. A contrast medium—enhanced esophagram is usually recommended in all patients who are at risk for esophageal rupture (post vomiting) with spontaneous pneumomediastinum (22). Patients with spontaneous pneumomediastinum and a negative contrast medium—enhanced esophagram may be discharged as long as they are highly reliable and have close outpatient followup arranged. Antibiotics are unnecessary if the esophagram is normal.

CRITICAL INTERVENTIONS

- Perform immediate needle decompression on patients with suspected tension pneumothorax
- Insert chest tube for patients with large pneumothorax (>20%)
- Perform an esophagram on patients with pneumomediastinum and suspected esophageal rupture

---

COMMON PITFALLS

✔ Spontaneous pneumothorax and spontaneous pneumomediastinum are diagnoses of exclusion. It is essential to consider other causes, including trauma, underlying pulmonary disease, infection, and malignancy

✔ Management of spontaneous pneumothorax by observation alone can save hospitalization and health care costs only if used in the appropriate circumstances and only if the patient is compliant with treatment and receives appropriate discharge instructions

References

1. Baumann MH, Strange C, Heffner JE, et al. Management of spontaneous pneumothorax: an American College of Chest Physicians Consensus Statement. *Chest* 2001;119:590.
2. Beers MF, Sohn M, Swartz M. Recurrent pneumothorax in AIDS patients with *Pneumocystis* pneumonia: a clinicopathologic report of three cases and review of the literature. *Chest* 1990;98:266.
3. Bense L, Eklund G, Odont D, et al. Smoking and the increased risk of contracting spontaneous pneumothorax. *Chest* 1987;9:1009.
4. Byrnes TA, Brevig JK, Yeoh CB. Pneumothorax in patients with acquired immunodeficiency syndrome. *J Thorac Cardiovasc Surg* 1989;98:546.
5. Carter EJ, Ettensohn DB. Catamenial pneumothorax. *Chest* 1990;98:713.
6. Collins RK. Hammans crunch: an adventitious sound. *J Fam Pract* 1994;38:284.
7. Dines DE, Clagett OT, Payne WS. Spontaneous pneumothorax in emphysema. *Mayo Clin Proc* 1970;45:481.
8. Gobbel WG, Rhea WG, Nelson IA, et al. Spontaneous pneumothorax. *J Thorac Cardiovasc Surg* 1963;46:331.
9. Gray R, Cormier M, Yedlicka J, et al. Catamenial pneumothorax: case report and literature review. *J Thorac Imaging* 1987;2:72.
10. Joseph J, Sahn SA. Thoracic endometriosis syndrome: new observations from an analysis of 110 cases. *Am J Med* 1996;100:164.
11. Lesur O, Delorme N, Fromaget JM, et al. Computed tomography in the etiologic assessment of idiopathic spontaneous pneumothorax. *Chest* 1990;98:341.
12. McClellan MD, Miller SB, Parsons PE, et al. Pneumothorax with *Pneumocystis carinii* pneumonia in AIDS: incidence and clinical characteristics. *Chest* 1991;100:1224.
13. Melton LJ, Hepper NG, Offord KP. Incidence of spontaneous pneumothorax in Olmstead County, Minnesota: 1950 to 1974. *Am Rev Respir Dis* 1979;120:1379.
14. Mitlehner W, Friedrich M, Dissmann W. Value of computer tomography in the detection of bullae and blebs in patients with primary spontaneous pneumothorax. *Respiration* 1992;59:221.
15. Primrose WR. Spontaneous pneumothorax: a retrospective review of aetiology, pathogenesis and management. *Scott Med J* 1984;29:15.
16. Rhea JT, Deluca SA, Greene RE. Determining the size of pneumothorax in the upright patient. *Radiology* 1982;144:733.
17. Saha S, Arrants JE, Kossa A, et al. Management of spontaneous pneumothorax. *Ann Thorac Surg* 1975;91:561.
18. Sepkowitz KA, Telzak EE, Gold JWM, et al. Pneumothorax in AIDS. *Ann Intern Med* 1991;114:455.
19. Schramel FM, Postmus PE, Vanderschueren RG. Current aspects of spontaneous pneumothorax. *Eur Respir J* 1997;10:1372.
20. Shesser R, David C, Edelstein S. Pneumomediastinum and pneumothorax after inhaling alkaloidal cocaine. *Ann Emerg Med* 1981;10:213.
21. Shiraishi T. Catamenial pneumothorax: a report of a case and review of the Japanese and non-Japanese literature. *Thorac Cardiovasc Surg* 1991;39:304.
22. Smith BA, Ferguson DB. Disposition of spontaneous pneumomediastinum. *Am J Emerg Med* 1991;9:256.
23. Versteegh FG, Broeders JA. Spontaneous pneumomediastinum in children. *Eur J Pediatr* 1991;150:304.

CHAPTER 38

Pulmonary Embolism

Jeffrey A. Tabas and Erin McNutt

Pulmonary embolism (PE) is a relatively common, life-threatening condition that presents a diagnostic dilemma for the emergency practitioner. The incidence in the United States is estimated at 600,000 patients/year, resulting in 60,000 to 100,000 deaths/year, and PE is the third leading cause of cardiovascular death. Correct diagnosis and treatment reduces mortality from 18% to 30% to 2% to 9% (5,6). Because a missed diagnosis subjects a patient to the consequent risks of recurrence, and overdiagnosis subjects a patient to the risks of unnecessary anticoagulation as well as to the psychologic and financial implications of carrying such a diagnostic label, accurate diagnosis is essential.

CLINICAL PRESENTATION

Pulmonary emboli may result from a myriad of causes. Most commonly, emboli arise from thrombi in the legs, but they may also originate from anywhere in the venous system proximal to the pulmonary arteries, such as pelvic veins, nonportal abdominal veins, upper extremity veins, or right-sided heart valves. Other sources include fat emboli, usually in association with long-bone fractures, amniotic fluid emboli (in the setting of labor and delivery), air emboli, and septic emboli.

The signs and symptoms of pulmonary emboli result from the effects of obstructed pulmonary vasculature. This may result in local tissue ischemia or infarct, increased ventilation-perfusion mismatch that can cause increased alveolar dead space or increased alveolar—arterial oxygen gradient, and increased pulmonary vascular resistance that can cause right heart strain or failure. The spectrum of presentation varies from asymptomatic patients with only subjective complaints to hemodynamically unstable patients with severe hypotension, respiratory failure, or pulseless electrical activity. Differences in size, quantity, and location of emboli, as well as underlying patient characteristics (such as cardiopulmonary reserve) contribute to the wide spectrum of presentation.

The most common signs and symptoms associated with the presence of PE are listed in Table 38.1 (4,21). These include the symptoms of shortness of breath, pleuritic chest pain, cough, and symptoms of deep vein thrombosis such as leg pain or swelling. Clinical signs include tachypnea, rales, and tachycardia. Although low-grade fever is not infrequent, temperatures higher than 38.5°C are less common and suggest other causes. Unfortunately, many of these signs and symptoms are manifestations of other conditions, and there is no combination of clinical findings that has been shown to be diagnostic for PE. In addition, the "classic" triad of hemoptysis, pleuritic chest pain, and tachypnea is uncommon. There is some evidence that the presence of dyspnea, tachypnea, or pleuritic chest pain in a patient without an adequate explanatory diagnosis should suggest PE. This is based on a retrospective analysis of the Prospective Investigation of Pulmonary Embolism Diagnosis (PIOPED) study (2), which revealed that 97% of patients presented with at least one of these signs or symptoms (23).

Any patient with suspected PE should be assessed for risk factors (Table 38.2). Classic risk factors for thrombosis include Virchow's triad of hypercoagulability, venous stasis, and endothelial injury. Commonly acquired hypercoagulable states include cancer, pregnancy, and estrogen therapy. Increasing understanding and discovery of heritable thrombophilias constitute risk factors that may exist but remain unknown at the time of presentation. Venous stasis may result from prolonged immobilization, recent surgery, extended travel, or medical conditions such as paraplegia or previous stroke. Damage to the vascular endothelium may result from fractures, surgery, catheter placement, or other forms of trauma. Demographic factors, such as advanced age, should also be taken into consideration. However, up to 30% of patients with a diagnosed pulmonary embolism have no known risk factors (8). In summary, although the presence of

TABLE 38.2.   Risk Factors for PE
Prior thrombus or thromboembolism
Family history of thrombosis
Cancer
Prolonged immobilization—paralysis, lower extremity cast, travel
Pelvic or lower abdominal surgery, < 6 months
Cerebral vascular accident
Congestive heart failure
Lower extremity or pelvic trauma/fractures/surgery
Obesity
Estrogen therapy–oral contraceptives, hormone replacements
Pregnancy or post-partum
Inflammatory bowel disease
Age, >40 years
Thrombophilias
• Factor V Leiden
• Protein C deficiency
• Protein S deficiency
• Antithrombin III deficiency
• *PT20210A* mutation
• Anticardiolipin antibody syndrome
• Lupus anticoagulant
• Hyperhomocysteinemia
• Thombomodulin
• Plasminogen deficiency

PE, pulmonary embolism.

risk factors increases suspicion for PE, lack of known risk factors does not exclude the diagnosis.

DIFFERENTIAL DIAGNOSIS

Given the wide spectrum of signs and symptoms associated with PE, the differential diagnosis in most presentations is extensive. Other causes of dyspnea or chest pain include pulmonary and cardiac causes such as chronic obstructive pulmonary disease (COPD) or asthma, congestive heart failure, pulmonary infections, pericarditis, acute coronary syndrome, aortic dissection, pneumothorax, trauma, or musculoskeletal pain. Abdominal sources such as biliary colic or pancreatitis may mimic a PE. The evaluation can be complicated by the fact that conditions such as congestive heart failure can both mimic signs and symptoms of PE, as well as be a risk factor for pulmonary embolism. Musculoskeletal pain and anxiety are always diagnoses of exclusion, and should be made only after more life-threatening causes have been confidently eliminated.

EMERGENCY DEPARTMENT EVALUATION

Initial management of PE consists of rapid assessment and stabilization for immediate life-threatening conditions. When appropriate, intravenous access should be established and cardiac and pulse oximetry monitors should be placed. Laboratory testing, electrocardiography, and chest radiography, should be expedited. The emergency department physician should determine a probability of disease (see subsequent text) based on the patient's signs, symptoms, identifiable risk factors, and the presence of an acceptable an alternate diagnosis.

A complete blood count and serum chemistry panel is usually indicated in the general assessment of any patient with chest pain or shortness of breath. A creatinine level is helpful if contrast administration is planned. All patients suspected of having a PE should undergo an electrocardiogram. The electrocardiogram is a nonspecific test for PE, and the primary purpose is to detect

---

TABLE 38.1.   Relative Frequency of Presenting Symptoms and Signs in Patients with PE

Symptom	Sign
Dyspnea, 73%	RR > 20/min, 70%
Pleuritic pain, 66%	Rales, 51%
Cough, 37%	Tachycardia, 30%
Leg swelling, 28%	Loud P$_2$, 23%
Leg pain, 26%	Temp. >38.5°C, 7%
Hemoptysis, 13%	Wheezes, 5%

PE, pulmonary embolism; RR, respiratory rate; Temp., temperature.

other disease processes such as pericarditis or acute coronary syndrome. The most common electrocardiographic findings in patients with PE are nonspecific ST and T-wave abnormalities. Other common findings include tachycardia and T-wave inversion in the anterior precordial leads (V1-V4) (18). The classic electrocardiographic (ECG) finding of S1Q3T3, consisting of an S wave in lead 1, and a Q wave with a flipped T wave in lead 3, is neither sensitive nor specific for PE.

A chest radiograph should be obtained for patients with suspected PE. Given the lack of specific findings for PE, the primary purpose is again to detect other disease processes, such as a pneumothorax, pulmonary edema, malignancy, or pneumonia. More often than not, chest radiographs in patients with pulmonary emboli show nonspecific findings such as atelectasis, small effusions, an elevated hemidiaphragm, or mild infiltrates. Cardiomegaly is a common associated finding with PE, given that congestive heart failure (CHF) is a risk factor (7). Classic radiographic findings, which occur infrequently, include Westermark sign (a prominent central pulmonary artery with decreased pulmonary vasculature distally) and Hampton Hump (a wedge-shaped, pleural based opacity representing pulmonary infarct).

Arterial blood gases are rarely helpful in the evaluation of PE. One analysis of greater than 100 patients with PE who lacked prior cardiopulmonary disease revealed that 38% had a normal Alveolar–arterial (A–a) gradient. Patients with prior cardiopulmonary disease who proved not to have PE, had an elevated A–a gradient 24% of the time (22). One potentially useful scenario may occur when a patient is found to have a large, unexplained A–a gradient. However, these authors rarely obtain arterial blood gases for suspected PE alone.

Based upon the history, physical examination, and preliminary laboratory evaluation, the clinician should categorize a patient into low, moderate, or high probability for PE. Several clinical decision rules have been developed in an attempt to improve implicit clinician judgment. Although these rules appear to improve risk stratification, further validation is needed. The Canadian decision rule (24) is the most extensively tested and is included in Table 38.3 (4).

D-dimer testing is assuming an increasing role in the assessment of patients with suspected PE. D-dimers are degradation products of cross-linked fibrin, and are therefore elevated in the setting of pulmonary embolism. Because of their nonspecific nature, D-dimers are also elevated in other conditions such as

TABLE 38.4.   [11] Sensitivity and Specificity of D-dimer Tests for PE

Screening Test	Sensitivity	Specificity
Conventional ELISA	97%	42%
Latex agglutination	70%	76%
Erythrocyte agglutination	89%	59%
Immunofiltration	95%	33%
Rapid ELISA	93%	30%
Turbidimetric	98%	43%

ELISA, enzyme-linked immunosorbent assay; PE, Pulmonary embolism.

cancer, pregnancy, recent trauma, and even CHF. Assay of the D-dimer level has been shown to be extremely sensitive for PE. However, the sensitivity varies greatly depending on the type of assay selected. Traditional hospital assays utilizing the standard latex agglutination test are only 40% to 70% sensitive, and therefore are inadequate for screening. Research laboratory enzyme-linked immunosorbent assay (ELISA) tests are 94% to 97% sensitive but are not practical for clinical use (14). Several new, rapid assay systems have been developed with much higher sensitivities that are suitable for testing in hospital and emergency department settings (9,14). Some of these show sensitivities as high as 90% to 95% (Table 38.4). Therefore, before using the D-dimer test in the evaluation of PE, it is essential to determine which laboratory test is being used. With a rapid, sensitive D-dimer assay, a negative result is adequate to exclude PE in a patient with low pretest probability for PE. If a patient's pretest probability is moderate to high, a negative test result does not exclude PE, but it significantly lowers the risk that the patient has PE, thereby influencing interpretation of further imaging.

When discussing the diagnostic accuracy of radiographic imaging of patients with suspected PE, it is important to remember that the goal of imaging is to detect the presence of any venous thromboembolism in order to guide the initiation of treatment. The primary aim of treatment is prevention of recurrence. Although patients with small or subsegmental pulmonary emboli may present with milder signs and symptoms, there is no evidence that patients with "clinically insignificant" presentations are at a lower risk of recurrence than those with more clinically evident presentations.

Ventilation/perfusion (V/Q) scanning has been evaluated extensively, and has the benefit of low radiation exposure and high sensitivity. Administration of an intravenous radioactive isotope is used to measure perfusion of the pulmonary vasculature, whereas administration of an inhaled radioactive isotope is used to measure pulmonary ventilation. A normal or near normal result is 98% sensitive for the exclusion of PE. As with most tests, the V/Q scan should be interpreted within the context of pretest probability (Table 38.5). A low pretest probability with a low probability V/Q scan makes pulmonary embolism unlikely, and a high probability scan with a high pretest probability is considered diagnostic for PE. However, discordant results or intermediate probability scans, which account for up to 75% of results, mandate further studies. An indeterminate result is most common in patients with COPD, preexisting cardiopulmonary disease, or markedly abnormal chest radiographs. V/Q scanning for assessment of suspected PE is appropriate in the following circumstance: when it is the only imaging modality available; in patients with a reasonable probability of a diagnostic test result; or in patients who have contraindications to other imaging studies, such as contrast allergy or renal insufficiency. V/Q scanning is most likely to be diagnostic in patients with normal chest radiographs.

TABLE 38.3.   Criteria of Wells et al. for Assessment of Pretest Probability for PE (24)

Criteria	Points
Suspected DVT	3.0
An alternative diagnosis less likely than PE	3.0
Heart rate, >100 beats/min	1.5
Immobilization or surgery in the previous 4 weeks	1.5
Previous DVT/PE	1.5
Hemoptysis	1.0
Malignancy (on treatment, treated in the past 6 mo. or palliative)	1.0

SCORE RANGE (POINTS)	INTERPRETATION OF RISK
0–2	Low
3–6	Moderate
>6	High

DVT, deep venous thrombosis; PE, pulmonary embolism.

TABLE 38.5. Probability of Pulmonary Embolism Based on Clinical Suspicion and Results of Ventilation Perfusion (V/Q) Scan

Clinical Suspicion	V/Q Results			
	High	Interm.	Low	Normal or Near-Normal
High	96%	66%	40%	N/A
Intermediate	88%	28%	16%	6%
Low	56%	16%	4%	2%
All patients	87%	30%	14%	4%

NA, not applicable.
Adapted from The PIOPED Investigators. Value of the ventilation perfusion scan in acute pulmonary embolism: results of the prospective investigation of pulmonary embolism diagnosis (PIOPED). *JAMA* 1990;263:2753–2759.

Spiral computed tomography pulmonary angiography (CTPA) has received widespread acceptance for the assessment of suspected PE. It demonstrates high sensitivity and specificity for PE, and in about one third of cases, provides an alternate diagnosis, such as pneumonia, cancer, or aortic dissection. It is not particularly invasive, and requires only a single breath hold. Reported sensitivities for CTPA vary depending on scanner technology. Sensitivity for single-detector CTPA is 77%, and specificity is 89% based on a recent meta-analysis of nine prospective CTPA studies (14). There are some reports of higher sensitivity for CTPA that arose from studies that reported only on the presence of segmental or larger PEs. Multidetector scanners can obtain images more rapidly with less motion artifact, allowing for greater resolution with thinner image reconstructions. Their sensitivities and specificities are significantly higher than that of single-detector scanners, but have yet to be determined precisely. PIOPED II is a prospective multicenter study designed to assess the efficacy of spiral CTPA and should clarify many of these questions (11).

Lower extremity imaging for deep venous thrombosis in the assessment of suspected PE is most useful when there are clinical signs and symptoms in that extremity. Fifteen to twenty-five percent of patients with PE have clinically evident deep venous thrombosis (DVT). Bilateral lower extremity imaging in a patient without clinical findings of DVT may be useful when PE has not been adequately excluded after V/Q or CTPA evaluation. This may occur in the patient with V/Q scan or CTPA results that are indeterminate or discordant with prior probability. Lower extremity ultrasonographic testing is 93% sensitive and 98% specific for proximal DVT of the lower extremities in symptomatic patients. Sensitivity and specificity are probably somewhat lower in patients with asymptomatic DVT.

Another option for assessment of DVT includes computed tomography venography, which images the pelvis and lower extremities during the venous return phase of the contrast bolus. Computed tomography venography can be performed after CTPA without additional contrast injection and is relatively rapid. It has been shown to have comparable sensitivity to ultrasonography for the lower extremities, with the additional benefit of detecting pelvic and abdominal vessel thrombosis (3). If lower extremity imaging reveals DVT, patients should be treated for PE.

Pulmonary angiography is the traditional gold standard for the diagnosis of PE. It has a false negative rate of 1% to 2% and an indeterminate study rate of 3%. Significant complications include death in 0.5%, major nonfatal complications in 1%, and minor complications in up to 5%.

Transthoracic or transesophageal echo may be helpful in the assessment of pulmonary embolism, especially in the unstable patient. Echocardiographic findings in patients with PE include right ventricular dilatation and hypokinesis, septal flattening and paradoxical motion, failure of the inferior vena cava to collapse during inspiration and, rarely, direct visualization of the thrombus.

Evaluation of the pregnant patient poses a particular challenge for the emergency department practitioner. Pregnancy increases risk of venous thrombosis up to five-fold. For women whose pregnancies result in a live birth, thrombotic pulmonary embolism is the leading cause of death. Although exposure of the fetus to radiation is clearly undesirable, the safety of the mother takes priority. Evaluation of the stable pregnant patient with symptoms of pulmonary embolism may include a rapid sensitive D-dimer test in a low or moderate suspicion patient (although specificity in pregnancy will be decreased), ultrasonographic evaluation of the lower extremities (which if positive, will allow initiation of anticoagulation and deferral of further evaluation), and V/Q scanning or CTPA. Traditionally, V/Q scanning has been the imaging modality of choice. However, recent literature indicates that radiation exposure from CTPA to the fetus, especially in the first or second trimester, is equivalent to or lower than radiation exposure from V/Q scanning (25).

The results of diagnostic testing should be used to determine sequentially what further evaluation is needed to exclude or confirm the presence of PE. A posttest probability of 1% to 2% is a generally accepted risk level (12). This would presumably lead to a subsequent complication rate of <0.7%. Some patients and physicians may be willing to accept more or less risk.

EMERGENCY DEPARTMENT MANAGEMENT

As with any critically ill patient, the emergency physician should start with the "ABCs." Intravenous access, cardiopulmonary monitoring, and oxygen therapy should be initiated. The patient's airway should be maintained, and, if severely hypoxic, the patient should be emergently intubated. Hypotensive patients should be fluid resuscitated while more definitive treatments are being considered.

Anticoagulation remains the primary treatment for patients with PE. Patients who have a moderate-to-high pretest probability for PE should be considered for anticoagulation, even before more definitive studies have been completed. Intravenous unfractionated heparin or low-molecular-weight heparin have been shown to be equally effective in the treatment of pulmonary emboli (15,18). The advantages of low-molecular-weight heparin include its ease of use and lack of need for laboratory monitoring. The U.S. Food and Drug Administration (FDA) has approved two low-molecular-weight heparins in the United States for treating PE with documented deep vein thrombosis: enoxaparin and tinzaparin. The dosing for enoxaparin is 1 mg/kg subcutaneously every 12 hours and for tinzaparin 175 anti-Xa IU/kg subcutaneously once daily. Contraindications include renal insufficiency, obesity, or weight <40 kg. If intravenous unfractionated heparin is used, weight-based dosing has been shown to be superior to standard dosing, with more rapid time to therapeutic levels and decreased rates of recurrence and complications. Patients should receive an initial bolus of 80 U/kg and then an infusion of 18 U/kg/hour (19). The activated partial thromboplastin time is measured every 4 to 6 hours and should be maintained at 1.5 to 2.3 times the control, with adjustment based on an established nomogram.

For patients with hemodynamic instability resulting from PE, thrombolytic therapy is considered the treatment of choice. Although large, randomized, controlled trials are lacking, several previous smaller trials have suggested mortality benefit (1,13). Thrombolytics rapidly improve hemodynamic status by acutely reducing clot burden, whereas heparin only inhibits clot propagation. The FDA has approved streptokinase, urokinase, and recombinant tissue plasminogen activator (r-TPA) for the treatment of massive PE (10). The dosage used for r-TPA is 100 mg over 2 hours. If streptokinase is used, the dosage is 250,000 IU over 30 minutes and then 100,000 IU an hour for 24 hours. Urokinase dosage is 4,400 IU over 10 minutes followed by 4,400 IU an hour for 12 to 24 hours. Unlike for acute myocardial infarction (MI), heparin is not given simultaneously with thrombolytics for pulmonary embolism, but started after thrombolytics have been given and the partial thromboplastin time (PTT) is <80 seconds. A recent analysis suggests that thrombolytics may also improve clinical outcomes in patients with ventricular dysfunction or pulmonary hypertension (16).

Pulmonary embolectomy is an uncommon procedure, but it may be used as treatment for hemodynamically unstable patients with contraindications to thrombolytics or when thrombolytics are not available.

New anticoagulants are currently being developed, which may show improvement over unfractionated heparin and low-molecular-weight heparin. These new agents include direct thrombin inhibitors (DTIs), direct and indirect factor Xa inhibitors, activated protein C, and tissue factor pathway inhibitor. Some of their superior properties include once daily dosing without monitoring, oral administration, and improved pharmacodynamic profiles.

CRITICAL INTERVENTIONS

- Risk stratify patients into low, moderate, or high probability for PE based upon the history, physical examination, and preliminary laboratory evaluation
- Anticoagulate patients with a high clinical suspicion for thromboembolism before definitive studies are performed
- Administer thrombolytic therapy for patients with hemodynamic instability caused by PE

DISPOSITION

Patients diagnosed with PE are admitted to the hospital. If they are hemodynamically stable they may go to a nonmonitored setting. Otherwise, patients should be observed in the intensive care unit or a telemetry bed, depending on their hemodynamic status. If a patient requires transfer to another facility, for higher level of care, and the patient is hemodynamically unstable, anticoagulation and thrombolytics should be administered before transfer.

Patients diagnosed with DVT who show no evidence of pulmonary embolism are routinely treated as outpatients with low-molecular-weight-heparin (see Chapter 52, "Deep Venous Thrombosis and Thrombophlebitis"). These patients transition to oral warfarin in the outpatient setting. Given that up to 50% of patients diagnosed with DVTs have clinically "silent" PE (12),

outpatient treatment for stable pulmonary emboli may become acceptable in the future if prospective trials demonstrate its safety and efficaciousness. Enoxaparin and tinzaparin are currently FDA approved only for inpatient treatment of PE with DVT.

COMMON PITFALLS

✔ Failing to consider PE in a patient presenting with pleuritic chest pain or dyspnea or tachypnea who lacks a convincing alternate diagnosis

✔ Failing to recognize that lack of risk factors does not exclude PE

✔ Failing to recognize atypical presentations, such as syncope, in the elderly

✔ Mistaking nonspecific physical findings of PE for an alternate diagnosis such as costochondritis in a patient with mild chest wall tenderness

✔ Mistaking nonspecific radiographic findings of PE for an alternate diagnosis such as pneumonia in a patient with atelectasis on chest radiography

✔ Assuming that a normal A–a gradient or O_2 saturation excludes PE

✔ Failing to pursue further imaging in a patient with an indeterminate V/Q scan or high clinical probability and a negative CTPA

✔ Failing to recognize that PE can recur in a patient who is adequately anticoagulated

References

1. The urokinase pulmonary embolism trial. A national cooperative study. *Circulation* 1973;47:II1–108.
2. Value of the ventilation/perfusion scan in acute pulmonary embolism. Results of the prospective investigation of pulmonary embolism diagnosis (PIOPED). The PIOPED Investigators [see comments]. *JAMA* 1990;263:2753–2759.
3. Clinical policy: critical issues in the evaluation and management of adult patients presenting with suspected pulmonary embolism. *Ann Emerg Med* 2003;41:257–270.
4. Chunilal SD, Eikelboom JW, Attia J, et al. Does this patient have pulmonary embolism? *JAMA* 2003;290:2849–2858.
5. Coon WW, Willis PW 3rd, Symons MJ. Assessment of anticoagulant treatment of venous thromboembolism. *Ann Surg* 1969;170:559–568.
6. Dalen JE, Alpert JS. Natural history of pulmonary embolism. *Prog Cardiovasc Dis* 1975;17:259–270.
7. Elliott CG, Goldhaber SZ, Visani L, DeRosa M. Chest radiographs in acute pulmonary embolism. Results from the International Cooperative Pulmonary Embolism Registry. *Chest* 2000;118:33–38.
8. Ferrari E, Baudouy M, Cerboni P, et al. Clinical epidemiology of venous thromboembolic disease. Results of a French Multicentre Registry. *Eur Heart J* 1997;18:685–691.
9. Ginsberg JS, Wells PS, Kearon C, et al. Sensitivity and specificity of a rapid whole-blood assay for D-dimer in the diagnosis of pulmonary embolism [see comments]. *Ann Intern Med* 1998;129:1006–1011.
10. Goldhaber SZ, Kessler CM, Heit J, et al. Randomised controlled trial of recombinant tissue plasminogen activator versus urokinase in the treatment of acute pulmonary embolism. *Lancet* 1988;2:293–298.
11. Gottschalk A, Stein PD, Goodman LR, Sostman HD. Overview of prospective investigation of pulmonary embolism diagnosis II. *Semin Nucl Med* 2002;32:173–182.
12. Huisman MV, Buller HK, ten Cate JW, et al. Unexpected high prevalence of silent pulmonary embolism in patients with deep venous thrombosis. *Chest* 1989;95(3):498–502.
13. Jerjes-Sanchez C, Ramirez-Rivera A, deLourdes Garcia M, et al. Streptokinase and heparin versus heparin alone in massive pulmonary embolism: a randomized controlled trial. *J Thromb Thrombolysis* 1995;2:227–229.
14. Kline JA, Johns KL, Coluciello SA, Israel EG. New diagnostic tests for pulmonary embolism. *Ann Emerg Med* 2000;35:168–180.
15. Kline JA, Wells PS. Methodology for a rapid protocol to rule out pulmonary embolism in the emergency department. *Ann Emerg Med* 2003;42:266–275.
16. Konstantinides S, Geibel A, Halsel G, Heinrich F, Kasper W. Heparin plus alteplase compared with heparin alone in patients with submassive pulmonary embolism. *N Engl J Med* 2002;347:1143–1150.
17. Mayo JR, Remy-Jardin M, Muller NL, et al. Pulmonary embolism: prospective comparison of spiral CT with ventilation-perfusion scintigraphy. *Radiology* 1997;205:447–452.
18. Miniati M, Monti S, Bottai M. A structured clinical model for predicting the probability of pulmonary embolism. *Am J Med* 2003;114:173–179.

19. Raschke RA, Reilly BM, Guidry JR, Fontana JR, Srinivas S. The weight-based heparin dosing nomogram compared with a "standard care" nomogram. A randomized controlled trial. *Ann Intern Med* 1993;119:874–881.
20. Simonneau G, Sors H, Charbonnier B, et al. A comparison of low-molecular-weight heparin with unfractionated heparin for acute pulmonary embolism. The THESEE Study Group. Tinzaparine ou Heparine Standard: Evaluations dans l'Embolie Pulmonaire. *N Engl J Med* 1997;337:663–669.
21. Stein PD, Coleman RE, Gottschalk A, Saltzman HA, Tenin ML, Weg JG. Diagnostic utility of ventilation/perfusion lung scans in acute pulmonary embolism is not diminished by pre-existing cardiac or pulmonary disease. *Chest* 1991;100:604–606.
22. Stein PD, Goldhaber SZ, Henry JW, Miller AC. Arterial blood gas analysis in the assessment of suspected acute pulmonary embolism. *Chest* 1996;109:78–81.
23. Stein PD, Terrin ML, Hales CA, et al. Clinical, laboratory, roentgenographic, and electrocardiographic findings in patients with acute pulmonary embolism and no pre-existing cardiac or pulmonary disease [see comments]. *Chest* 1991;100:598–603.
24. Wells PS, Anderson DR, Rodger M, et al. Derivation of a simple clinical model to categorize patient's probability of pulmonary embolism: increasing the models utility with the SimpliRED D-dimer. *Thromb Haemost* 2000;83:416–420.
25. Winer-Muram HT, Boone JM, Brown HL, Jennings SG, Mabie WC, Lombardo GT. Pulmonary embolism in pregnant patients: fetal radiation dose with helical CT. *Radiology* 2002;224:487–492.

TABLE 39.1.   Mechanisms of Bleeding in Hemoptysis

Malignancies: invade vessels, or the tumor itself may become necrotic

Inflammatory and infectious problems: vascular engorgement of the tracheobronchial mucosa

Bronchiectasis: associated with abnormal vascular anastomoses between bronchial and pulmonary arteries

Lung abscesses: bronchial ulceration and necrosis

Mycetomas of cavitary TB: rupture and cause life-threatening hemorrhage

Left ventricular failure or mitral stenosis: increased intravascular pressure with capillary and venous rupture

Pulmonary embolism: infarction of lung parenchyma

Goodpasture syndrome: breakdown of the alveolocapillary basement membrane

Aortic aneurysm: erosion into adjacent vascular structures

Coagulopathy: exacerbation of an underlying reason for bleeding

Cocaine: intense vasoconstriction with cell injury

TB, tuberculosis.

CHAPTER 39
Hemoptysis

Steven J. Parrillo

Few complaints bring a patient to seek medical attention as readily as the coughing up of blood. Hemoptysis is a common symptom in adults, but it is quite uncommon in children, with exceptions noted in subsequent text. Etiologies and presentations are diverse. Adding to the diagnostic challenge is the fact that many cases of presumed hemoptysis are actually caused by ear, nose, and throat (ENT) or gastrointestinal bleeding, so-called pseudohemoptysis. Although typically indicative of primary pulmonary pathology, hemoptysis can also result from numerous systemic illnesses. The severity of bleeding often does not correlate with the gravity of the underlying disease.

Many pathophysiologic mechanisms account for the bleeding. Bleeding sources include bronchial (high pressure) and pulmonary (low pressure) arteries. Massive bleeding—only 1.5% of all cases—almost always arises from bronchial arteries (7,13). The direct cause of bleeding varies greatly depending on underlying etiology. Table 39.1 lists the cause or causes of bleeding for common problems. Several mechanisms may be responsible for bleeding in any given patient. Exsanguination is rarely the ultimate cause of death in hemoptysis. Rather, blood fills alveoli, thereby impairing gas exchange. Clots may occlude the airway before hemoptysis has been identified. Death is secondary to hypoxemia.

CLINICAL PRESENTATION

The overall picture of hemoptysis has changed in the past 2 decades in terms of etiology, diagnosis, and treatment. The most common causes are infections, malignancy, bronchiectasis, bronchitis, and cardiovascular disorders (8,12,17,21). Although tuberculosis (TB) was once a leading infectious cause (and is still the most common cause worldwide), it is now much less common in the United States than pneumonia and bronchitis. The excep-

tion is in regions of high TB prevalence, such as New York City (12,16).

Although uncommon, there have been several reports of hemoptysis secondary to alveolar hemorrhage in patients with systemic lupus erythematosus (20). Travelers or immigrants from Asia, the Middle, East and South America may have parasitic infections (13). Catamenial hemoptysis (hemoptysis occurring at the time of menstruation) may occur in women with thoracic endometriosis (14).

The prevalence of immunocompromised patients has prompted study of common causes in that population. Although many of the data come from hospitalized patients, it appears that the majority of cases are infectious, mostly resulting from bacterial pneumonias. Even in that group, TB is not a common cause of respiratory tract bleeding (18,19).

With the advent of thrombolytic therapy, researchers have sought to determine whether hemoptysis is a common problem. It appears that it is not (6). There have been reports of hemoptysis after glycoprotein IIb/IIIa (abciximab) infusion (15). There has also been a report of early onset amiodarone toxicity presenting with hemoptysis (11).

Lung transplant recipients are at higher risk for hemoptysis after bronchoscopy, independent of coagulation parameters, immunosuppressive medications, or performance of transbronchial biopsy (9).

Goodpasture syndrome may present with hematuria and hemoptysis, as may vasculitis. Occult malignancy should always be considered in a cigarette smoker, even with a normal physical examination and chest radiograph (7,13).

The combination of high resolution CT scanning and bronchoscopy has become the standard to establish the diagnosis in those patients who appear to have anything more than a trivial case of bleeding (7,13). Most patients with significant bleeding—regardless of etiology—were once treated surgically; however, the majority are now managed medically. Surgery is still preferred when massive bleeding is caused by arteriovenous malformations (AVMs), aortic aneurysms, bronchial adenomas, and fungal lesions that do not respond to medical therapy (7).

Three potential biologic weapons of mass destruction cause hemoptysis: plague, tularemia, and T2 mycotoxin (7). Table 39.2 lists the common causes of hemoptysis by category.

Pediatric Presentation

In children, lower respiratory tract infection accounts for 40% of all cases. Cystic fibrosis (CF), foreign body aspiration, bronchial adenomas, and trauma are also common causes of hemoptysis.

TABLE 39.2.   Common Causes of Hemoptysis

INFLAMMATORY

Bronchitis
Bronchiectasis
Lung abscess
Pneumonia (viral, bacterial, and fungal)
Tuberculosis
Parasites (e.g., ascariasis, and schistosomiasis)

NEOPLASTIC

Bronchial adenoma
Bronchogenic carcinoma

CARDIOVASCULAR

Arteriovenous malformation
Arteriovenous fistula
Congestive heart failure
Aneurysm
Pulmonary thromboembolism
Primary pulmonary hypertension
Mitral stenosis
Vascular injury (e.g., foreign body)

CONGENITAL

Cystic fibrosis

IMMUNOLOGIC

Collagen vascular disease
Vasculitis
Goodpasture syndrome

EXTRAPULMONARY DISEASE

Thrombocytopenia
Coagulopathies
Trauma

DRUGS

Anticoagulants
Cocaine
Thrombolytics

CF may be associated with recurrent, severe bleeding in both children and young adults. Hemoptysis in children with CF occurs primarily with increasing age and advancing disease. The majority (60%) will have at least one episode, most of which are not life-threatening (19). Although congenital heart disease and mitral stenosis following rheumatic fever are still reported causes of hemoptysis, corrective surgery for the former and decreasing incidence of the latter make them less frequent causes of bleeding (19). Numerous uncommon causes include bronchiolitis obliterans organizing pneumonia (17), pulmonary embolism, Wegener granuloma, primary pulmonary hemosiderosis, and AVMs (8,19).

DIFFERENTIAL DIAGNOSIS

Hemoptysis must be confirmed before the broad differential diagnosis can be considered. An appropriate, focused history and physical examination should eliminate gastrointestinal and otolaryngologic sources. Gastrointestinal bleeding can usually be identified by its dark red color, the presence of clots and food particles, and an acid pH. True hemoptysis is typically bright red, frothy, and normal to alkaline in pH. Mouth, throat, and nasopharyngeal sources of bleeding can usually be visualized, sometimes with direct, indirect, or fiberoptic laryngoscopy.

EMERGENCY DEPARTMENT EVALUATION

Whenever bleeding is an issue, hemodynamic stabilization takes precedence over efforts to make a definitive diagnosis. For that reason, the first questions that need to be answered concern the status of the airway and rate and quantity of bleeding.

"Massive" hemoptysis (only 1.5% of the total cases) accounts for most of the mortality. As much as 50% of this group will die (12). This condition is usually defined as bleeding of 600 mL within 24 to 48 hours, or at a rate of 100 mL or more per hour. The definition of massive bleeding in children is 8mL/kg/24 hours (19). The differentiation of massive from "submassive" or minor bleeding carries both diagnostic and prognostic implications, but may not be easy to do in the emergency department (ED). Causes of mortality include asphyxiation (owing to airway obstruction with blood) and exsanguination. Most series list TB and bronchiectasis as the most common causes of massive hemoptysis in adults. Other diseases associated with massive bleeding include lung abscess, malignancy, Goodpasture syndrome, Behçet disease, AVMs, trauma, coagulopathies, and aspergilloma (13). In children, massive bleeding is a predictor of mortality in congenital heart disease (8).

Next, the baseline cardiopulmonary status and overall physical condition must be determined. History, physical examination, and laboratory studies can help evaluate the patient's ability to respond to the physiologic stress of hemoptysis and the therapy it necessitates. Almost any amount of bleeding may prove detrimental to the patient who has limited cardiopulmonary reserve or significant underlying disease.

Finally, efforts to determine the cause should begin. "Baseline" ED evaluation includes history, physical examination, pulse oximetry, and chest radiograph. Depending on the clinical scenario, many clinicians would also do a complete blood count, urinalysis, arterial blood gas analysis, coagulation studies, an electrocardiogram, and a sputum evaluation (Gram staining, acid-fast bacillus (AFB), and cultures). Definitive diagnosis may require a ventilation–perfusion scan, high-resolution (12) or standard computed tomographic scans, bronchoscopy, bronchography, sputum cytology, pulmonary function testing, angiography, or specialized sputum studies. Most of those tests will not be done in the ED. Aggressive management must occur at the same time as evaluation. Some diagnostic modalities, most notably bronchial artery embolization, are both diagnostic and therapeutic (5,10,22). Some centers are now using a new technique of bronchoscopic endobronchial sealing with cyanoacrylate (3).

Up to 10% of cases will have no identifiable etiology, even after exhaustive study (13). These patients are classified as having idiopathic or cryptogenic hemoptysis. It is presumed that subtle airway or parenchymal disease is responsible for bleeding.

EMERGENCY DEPARTMENT MANAGEMENT

The primary goals of therapy are prevention of asphyxia and exsanguination, termination of bleeding, and treatment of the underlying cause.

Airway control and adequate oxygenation are the first priorities. Endotracheal intubation, which may be technically challenging, is the procedure of choice. Large tubes (an 8 in the average adult) facilitate suctioning and passage of a fiberoptic laryngoscope. Bag-valve-mask ventilation may be problematic in the patient who is bleeding briskly, because it may spread blood further through the tracheobronchial tree. Separate intubation of left and right main-stem bronchi may be achieved by someone skilled in the use of either the Carlen or Robertshaw tube. Intubation over a fiberoptic laryngoscope may allow selective intubation of one bronchus, but requires skills that many emergency department physicians have not mastered. Empiric intubation of the main-stem bronchus of the involved lung will probably be necessary in that uncommon patient with severe hemorrhage.

In cases involving significant hemoptysis, the patient is placed in the Trendelenburg position, with the suspected bleeding source dependent. This position may protect the uninvolved lung from filling with blood and, in so doing, maximize gas exchange.

Blood should be sent for hematocrit, type and cross-match, coagulation studies, renal and liver function studies, and arterial gases. Significant coughing that may be exacerbating the bleeding should be reduced with small doses (2 mg) of intravenous morphine. Infuse isotonic fluids and blood products as indicated, through large-bore intravenous lines, recognizing that some investigators question the wisdom of initiating infusion before bleeding has been controlled. Place all patients with significant hemoptysis on a cardiac monitor. Some will require continuous hemodynamic monitoring.

Although most causes of bleeding require definitive therapy beyond the scope of emergency medical practice, there are times when treatment should begin in the ED. Examples include coagulopathies and some infectious etiologies.

Pulmonary, ENT, and surgical consultants will soon attempt to localize the bleeding site, especially if surgery is being considered. Techniques including bronchoscopy and angiography may be both diagnostic and therapeutic. Consultants may employ topical vasoconstrictors and catheter tamponade to control bleeding. Intravenous pitressin therapy and bronchial artery embolization have been used successfully in patients with CF (4,10). Selective bronchial artery embolization is currently the most effective nonsurgical treatment for massive hemoptysis but carries the risk of systemic and spinal artery embolization (13). Although success rates of 80% are frequently cited, spontaneous recanalization may occur and may cause more bleeding. Flexible endoscopy may be done at bedside. Rigid endoscopy is usually performed in the operating room (OR).

Hemoptysis may be best controlled by dealing with the source of the problem: mitral valve surgery for stenosis or nephrectomy plus steroids in Goodpasture syndrome. Bleeding associated with CF may respond to intravenous pitressin therapy (4). Bronchial artery embolization has also been used to treat nonmassive bleeding in CF (1).

There are times when surgery is the only way to control bleeding. The patient and the operating surgeon will benefit from accurate localization, identification of cause, and preoperative stabilization. Commonly quoted indications for surgery include leaking aortic aneurysm, AVMs, iatrogenic pulmonary rupture, chest trauma, bronchial adenoma, and fungal lesions resistant to medical therapy (13). Surgical mortality may be as high as 50%.

CRITICAL INTERVENTIONS

- For significant hemoptysis, protect the uninvolved lung from filling with blood and maximize gas exchange by placing patient in the Trendelenburg position, with the suspected bleeding source dependent
- Use large endotracheal tubes when intubating to (8.0 in average adult) to facilitate suctioning and passage of a fiberoptic laryngoscope
- Separate intubation of left and right main-stem bronchi may be achieved by someone skilled in the use of either the Carlen or Robertshaw tube

DISPOSITION

The largest majority of patients with hemoptysis will be treated medically. Admit patients with significant bleeding to an intensive care unit setting, preferably to a pulmonary/critical service or to the service of the surgeon who will go to the operating room. As in all situations of potentially exsanguinating hemorrhage, the OR must be readily available. Transfer to an appropriate facility must be arranged when definitive care is not available at the presenting institution. Stabilization must address airway control and hemodynamic needs. Given the difficulties of trying to establish an airway in a bleeding patient, strong consideration should be given to prophylactic intubation before transfer. Personnel effecting the transfer must be competent in emergency airway management.

Patients at high risk for deterioration—those with limited pulmonary reserves or respiratory compromise—should be hospitalized. Those with mycetomas or cavitary TB are also at high risk (2). Patients with significant underlying disease should be admitted. Immunocompromised patients may need to be admitted if the cause of bleeding is infectious. The possible public health risk of blood-borne diseases may also be a factor in the disposition decision.

Patients in the "submassive" group require an individualized approach. Many can be referred to an appropriate physician after the initial ED evaluation and institution of therapy when appropriate. Followup bronchoscopy is indicated as part of the diagnostic process, especially in men, smokers, patients older than 40 years, patients with a localized abnormality on chest radiography, and those in whom bleeding has lasted more than 7 days. Hemoptysis is a frightening symptom that requires patient reassurance.

Followup instructions must be specific. They should include the name of the physician and the time-frame required. Patients must be reliable and hemodynamically stable.

COMMON PITFALLS

✔ Hemoptysis must be recognized and differentiated from nasopharyngeal or gastrointestinal bleeding

✔ The bleeding rate must be estimated as accurately as possible. Dismissing a few ounces of hemoptysis as trivial during a brief evaluation is a potentially lethal error

✔ Each patient's cardiopulmonary reserve and overall clinical status must be evaluated. Even a small amount of hemoptysis may have potentially devastating consequences for a patient with significant underlying disease

✔ The patient must be closely monitored. Clinical deterioration may respond to such simple measures as repositioning the patient or performing endotracheal intubation, thereby preventing the further spread of blood through the lungs

✔ In situations requiring transfer to a higher level of care, patient stability may require attention not only to hemodynamic status, but also to the airway. Prophylactic intubation should be considered

✔ Radiographic lesions may be subtle. The emergency department physician must obtain the radiologist's final report on all patients with hemoptysis and relay that report to the patient or consulting physician

References

1. Antonelli M. Bronchial artery embolization for the management of nonmassive hemoptysis in cystic fibrosis. *Chest* 2002;121:796.
2. Athayde J, Shore E. Invasive pulmonary *Aspergillosis* presenting as massive hemoptysis in a nonimmunocompromised host. *Chest* 1993;103:961.
3. Bhattacharyya P. New procedure: bronchoscopic endobronchial sealing; a new mode of managing hemoptysis. *Chest* 2002;121:2066.

4. Bilton D, Webb A, Foster H, et al. Life-threatening hemoptysis in cystic fibrosis: an alternative therapeutic approach. *Thorax* 1990;45:976.

5. Brinson G, Noone P, Mauro M, et al. Bronchial artery embolization for the treatment of hemoptysis in patients with cystic fibrosis. *Am J Respir Crit Care Med* 1998;157:1951.

6. Chang YC, Patz EF, Goodman PC, et al. Significance of hemoptysis following thrombolytic therapy for myocardial infarction. *Chest* 1996;109:727.

7. Corder R. Hemoptysis. *Emerg Med Clin North Am* 2003;21:421.

8. Coss-Bu JA, Sachdeva RC, Bricker JT, et al. Hemoptysis: a 10 year retrospective study. *Pediatrics* 1997;100:E7.

9. Diette GB. The higher risk of bleeding in lung transplant recipients from bronchoscopy is independent of traditional bleeding risks: results of a prospective cohort study. *Chest* 1999;115:397.

10. Fernando H, Stein M, Benfield J, et al. Role of bronchial artery embolization in the management of hemoptysis. *Arch Surg* 1998;133:862.

11. Goldstein I. Very early onset of acute amiodarone pulmonary toxicity presenting with hemoptysis. *Chest* 1997;111:1446.

12. Hirshberg B, Biran I, Glazer M, et al. Hemoptysis: etiology, evaluation and outcome in a tertiary referral hospital. *Chest* 1997;112:440.

13. Jean-Baptiste E. Clinical assessment and management of massive hemoptysis. *Crit Care Med* 2000;28:1642.

14. Joseph J, Sahn SA. Thoracic endometrial syndrome: New observations from an analysis of 110 cases. *Am J Med* 1996;100:164.

15. Kalra S. Alveolar hemorrhage as a complication of treatment with abciximab. *Chest* 2001;120:126.

16. McGuiness G, Beacher J, Harkin T, et al. Hemoptysis: prospective high resolution CT/bronchoscopic correlation. *Chest* 1994;105:1155.

17. Mroz B, Sexauer W, Meade W, et al. Hemoptysis as the presenting symptom in bronchiolitis obliterans organizing pneumonia. *Chest* 1997;111(6):1775.

18. Nelson J, Fornan M. Hemoptysis in HIV-infected patients. *Chest* 1996;110:737.

19. Pianosi P, Al-sadoon H. Hemoptysis in children. *Pediatrics in Review* 1996;17:344.

20. Santos-Ocampo AS, Mandell BF, Fessler BJ. Alveolar hemorrhage in systemic lupus erythematosus—presentation and management. *Chest* 2000;118:1083–1090.

21. Santiago S, Tobias J, Williams A. A reappraisal of the causes of hemoptysis. *Arch Intern Med* 1991;151:2449.

22. Swanson KL. Bronchial artery embolization: experience with 54 patients. *Chest* 2002;121:789.

CHAPTER 40

Sarcoidosis

Steven J. Parrillo

Sarcoidosis is a multisystem, chronic granulomatous disease with diverse manifestations and a variable clinical course. It is characterized by a heightened cellular immune response at sites of disease activity; the lungs are the primary target organ and are involved in most cases (11,21). A number of etiologies have been postulated, including exposure to infectious agents (especially *Mycobacterium tuberculosis and Propionibacterium acnes*) (7,23), noninfectious environmental agents (especially beryllium), and autoantigens (11). It is curious that until 1995 only nine human immunodeficiency virus (HIV)–infected patients had been reported to have coexistent sarcoidosis (5,9). Some investigators now postulate that a low CD4 count is "protective" against granuloma formation (8).

In the United States, the prevalence of sarcoidosis is about 5 per 100,000 in whites and about 40 per 100,000 in Blacks. Among Black patients, women usually outnumber men 2 to 1. Curiously, sarcoidosis is virtually unknown on the continent of Africa, raising the issue of environmental influence in the etiology. Although the peak incidence is in the middle years of life (20 to 40 years

of age), the disease has been reported in children and the elderly. Sarcoidosis has also been identified in twins (monozygotic more commonly than dizygotic), in husband–wife pairs, and in firefighters who trained together (3,12). Most cases resolve spontaneously, with or without treatment. Indicators of a favorable prognosis include acute manifestations of inflammation, such as erythema nodosum, polyarthritis, fever, and bilateral lymphadenopathy. Poor prognostic indicators include Black race; lupus pernio; and chronic bone, lung, or nasopharyngeal involvement (10,21).

CLINICAL PRESENTATION

In the United States, approximately 30% to 50% of patients with sarcoidosis are asymptomatic (14), the diagnosis being suspected only because hilar adenopathy is seen on a chest film (Table 40.1). This group may need only to be referred to confirm the diagnosis. For the emergency department physician, however, the more important issue is when to suspect and treat active disease.

In 20% to 40% of cases, acute sarcoidosis develops over a period of several weeks. The symptoms are usually mild and may include fever, malaise, anorexia, and weight loss (3,14). Those with chronic sarcoidosis develop a more indolent form over months. Most have vague respiratory complaints and are likely to have symptomatic relapses. Unfortunately, it is this group that is more likely to develop chronic disease with significant organ damage.

As a multisystem disease, sarcoidosis can present with symptoms referable to a variety of organ systems. The lungs, however, are almost always (90%) involved, and the clinical presentation is often dominated by the presence of interstitial lung disease. These patients are dyspneic, especially on exertion, and have a dry cough. Physical examination may reveal nothing more than dry rales, but wheezing suggestive of reactive airway disease may be heard. Airway hyperreactivity appears to be especially prominent in those patients with endobronchial involvement (19). Ninety percent have an abnormal chest radiograph.

The radiographic findings of sarcoidosis are characteristic, with bilateral hilar lymphadenopathy being the classic, as well as the most common, finding (Fig. 40.1).

Radiographic evaluation is helpful to define pulmonary involvement, rather than to stage the disease, although the American Thoracic Society (ATS) calls the changes "stages." There are four types of involvement shown on chest films (Table 40.2). The ATS lists them as (i) no radiographic abnormality (stage 0); (ii) bilateral hilar adenopathy (stage I); (iii) bilateral hilar

TABLE 40.1.   Characteristics at Clinical Presentation (3)

Characteristic	Incidence (%)
Age (yr)	
<40	75
>40	25
May occur in children and the elderly	
Gender	
Male	60
Female	40
Race	
Black	90
Caucasian	10
Asymptomatic	10–20
Acute/subacute (fever, fatigue, malaise, anorexia, weight loss, respiratory symptoms)	20–40
Insidious (respiratory complaints without constitutional symptoms)	40–70

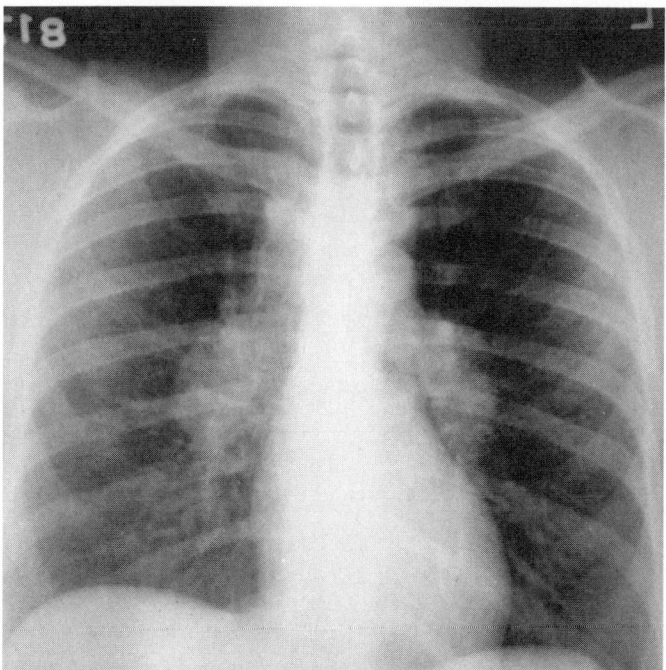

Figure 40.1.   Typical type I radiograph. (Courtesy of Murray K. Dalinka, M.D., Department of Radiology, Hospital of the University of Pennsylvania, Philadelphia.)

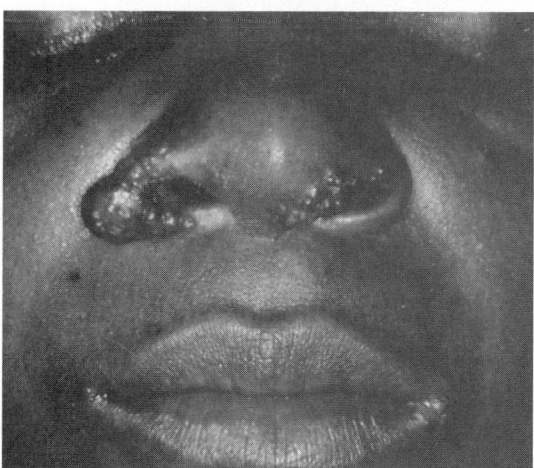

Figure 40.2.   Lupus pernio. (Courtesy of Gerald S. Lazarus, MD, Department of Dermatology, Hospital of the University of Pennsylvania, Philadelphia.)

adenopathy and parenchymal infiltration (stage II); (iv) parenchymal infiltration without hilar adenopathy (stage III); and (v) advanced fibrosis with honey-combing, hilar retraction, bullae, cysts, and emphysema (stage IV) (12,21).

Radiographic staging has some limited prognostic significance, in that stage I changes usually resolve, whereas changes in the other types are chronic. It is important to recognize that these are not stages of the disease, but represent different radiographic manifestations (3).

Although myocardial sarcoidosis is found in 25% of autopsied cases, only 10% of those patients without cardiac symptoms have an abnormal electrocardiogram. Conduction disturbances, including complete heart block, are the most common cardiac presentations and may be the cause of death. Life-threatening ventricular dysrhythmias also may be seen. As many as 25% of those with cardiac dysfunction die of congestive heart failure (3). Myocardial magnetic resonance (MR) imaging appears to be a useful modality for tracking the clinical course of cardiac sarcoidosis (22).

Both hypercalciuria (30%) and hypercalcemia (10%) are common and may lead to nephrocalcinosis and nephrolithiasis. Glomerular disease and renal arteritis may occur. Hypertension is common. Primary renal infiltration with sarcoid granulomas is rare (3).

Hypercalcemia may arise from increased intestinal calcium absorption owing to overproduction of 1,25-dihydroxyvitamin

D_3 by activated macrophages. Corticosteroids can control hypercalcemia by inhibiting the action of this hormone, but severe hypercalcemia is unusual. Hypercalcemia needs to be corrected. Before corticosteroids are considered, treatment begins with conservative measures such as decreasing oral calcium intake (16).

Approximately 25% of patients have eye involvement, most commonly anterior uveitis. Uveitis may develop rapidly and may become chronic, leading eventually to glaucoma, cataracts, and blindness (14). Other lesions include posterior uveitis, conjunctivitis, cataracts, and retinal hemorrhages.

Superficial lymphadenopathy is a frequent finding. Only 20% to 40% of patients have hepatomegaly. Most of those with liver involvement will have elevated enzymes. Portal hypertension is rare. Splenomegaly is seen in only 10%. Clinical disease is uncommon.

Skin lesions occur in about one fourth of patients. Specific lesions include lupus pernio (Fig. 40.2), plaques, and symmetric maculopapular eruptions. The most common lesion is erythema nodosum, a hypersensitivity reaction most commonly seen in women of childbearing age but not specific to sarcoidosis (3,12). This lesion is considered the hallmark of the disease (12).

Joint involvement is very common, with 25% to 50% of patients experiencing arthralgias or true arthritis, mostly in larger joints. Both can be migratory and are usually transient. The arthritis associated with erythema nodosum can be incapacitating and may require corticosteroid therapy. Chronic arthritis is associated with chronic persistent disease and is most frequently seen in Black patients with skin involvement (3).

Nasal and laryngeal involvement occurs in up to 16% of patients with sarcoidosis and may cause severe airway compromise (14).

Less than 10% of patients have neural involvement, with cranial neuropathy (e.g., peripheral seventh nerve palsy), pituitary and hypothalamic lesions being most frequent. Aseptic meningitis and peripheral neuropathy occur occasionally. Seizures are infrequent. Neurologic symptoms usually improve with corticosteroid therapy (6,10,24).

Two other syndromes have been described. Lofgren syndrome includes erythema nodosum and radiographic findings of bilateral hilar adenopathy, and may also be associated with arthritis of small and medium joints especially the ankles. Patients with the Heerfordt-Waldenström syndrome (uveoparotid fever) have fever, anterior uveitis, facial nerve palsy, and parotid enlargement (3,14).

TABLE 40.2.   Radiographic Stage and Prognosis in Sarcoidosis

Stage	% of Patients	Prognosis (Likelihood of Resolution) (%)
0	5–10	—
I	50	60
II	25–30	46
III	15	12

There are two distinct forms of pediatric sarcoidosis. Children under the age of 4 years—early onset disease—are likely to present with the triad of rash, uveitis, and arthritis. Older children and adolescents usually have multisystem disease with lymphadenopathy, pulmonary involvement, and the typical generalized signs and symptoms of fever and malaise (17).

Overall mortality is from 1% to 5% and results from pulmonary, cardiac, or neurologic involvement (14). Sarcoidosis usually improves during pregnancy (3).

DIFFERENTIAL DIAGNOSIS

If there were to be a "classic" presentation of sarcoidosis, it would be of a young adult with a combination of fever, dyspnea, blurred vision, and erythema nodosum, with a chest radiograph showing bilateral hilar adenopathy. Most cases of course are not that typical. Virtually all of the diseases to be considered in the differential diagnosis have the propensity to occur in almost any anatomic location. Sarcoidosis is most likely to be confused with tuberculosis (or other mycobacterial infections), lymphoma, and some fungal disorders (e.g., coccidioidomycosis). Other diseases to be considered include leprosy, berylliosis, and hypersensitivity pneumonitis.

HIV infection must also be considered in patients suspected of having sarcoidosis. Patients with HIV commonly have several of the features found in sarcoidosis, including chest radiograph abnormalities, lymphocytopenia, and a positive gallium-67 chest scan (9). Only a small number of cases of coexisting HIV disease and sarcoidosis has been recorded. Some postulate that since CD4 cells are required for clinical expression of sarcoidosis, their paucity in some with HIV disease may be "protective." That theory is enhanced by the development of sarcoidosis in a few patients who responded to highly active antiretroviral therapy with an increase in CD4 count (8).

A definitive diagnosis of sarcoidosis cannot be made with certainty on initial clinical presentation in an emergency setting, although the clinical suspicion may be high. The patient who already carries the diagnosis of sarcoidosis, however, may present with a complication of the disease or a concurrent, perhaps unrelated, illness and should be evaluated accordingly.

EMERGENCY DEPARTMENT EVALUATION

The initial history should be directed to determine the duration and severity of symptoms, a previous diagnosis of sarcoidosis, and any previous need for corticosteroid therapy.

The major complications of systemic sarcoidosis include upper airway obstruction from laryngeal involvement; cardiac dysrhythmias and conduction disturbances (especially heart block); congestive heart failure; advanced pulmonary fibrosis with cor pulmonale, superimposed tuberculosis, or bacterial infection; sudden loss of vision from ocular complications; incapacitating arthritis or arthralgias; space-occupying lesions of the brain and hydrocephalus; and hypercalcemia with its attendant cardiac, neurologic, and renal sequelae. Severe thrombocytopenia may occur. Abrupt corticosteroid withdrawal may cause the signs and symptoms of adrenal insufficiency (2,15,16).

Physical examination should focus first on the airway and cardiopulmonary systems, but attention should be given to all organ systems that potentially may be involved, as well as to the possibility of relative adrenal insufficiency secondary to rapid withdrawal of corticosteroid therapy.

Ocular, neurologic, skin, or joint complaints dictate the need for more specialized testing or examination. Funduscopic examination is essential in patients with altered mental status or abnormal neurologic findings.

Diagnostic studies in the emergency department should be directed toward detecting the potential problems associated with sarcoidosis. All patients should have a 12-lead electrocardiogram. Consideration should be given to ordering Holter monitoring for discharged patients. Chest radiography, pulse oximetry, and arterial blood gas analysis may be indicated in those who have respiratory complaints. Renal function studies, electrolytes, and calcium and platelet counts should be routine.

Strict criteria must be satisfied to make the diagnosis of sarcoidosis. They include (i) compatible clinical and radiographic findings, (ii) histologic finding of noncaseating granulomas, and (iii) exclusion of other diseases with similar findings (4,21). The emergency physician must establish that the patient meets those exacting criteria. A diagnosis based on only one of these features may be misleading.

Outpatient evaluation often includes serum and cerebrospinal fluid (CSF) studies, isotopic imaging studies, biopsy, and bronchoalveolar lavage. The ATS Sarcoidosis Consensus Group believes that transbronchial biopsy should be done on most patients suspected of having the disease (21). Fine needle biopsy is becoming an important diagnostic tool as well (4). Bronchoalveolar lavage may be performed at the same time as biopsy. An elevated CD4–CD8 ratio in the fluid confirms the diagnosis and occurs in the majority of those with pulmonary sarcoid (4,15,21). Advances in gallium scanning have improved diagnostic accuracy, but this test is not diagnostic of sarcoidosis (20). The Kveim-Siltzbach skin test is also helpful but requires a biopsy at 6 weeks. Most patients will eventually have a 24-hour urinary calcium determination (3). Serum and CSF angiotensin-converting enzyme (ACE) levels are elevated in up to 50% of patients. The use of D-dimer assay has been suggested, but it is not as useful as had been hoped (18).

EMERGENCY DEPARTMENT MANAGEMENT

Incapacitating disease interfering with normal life activities merits serious consideration for corticosteroid therapy. Conversely, relatively asymptomatic disease warrants an optimistic outlook and conservative management without corticosteroids. Causes of symptoms or signs other than progression of sarcoidosis must be excluded to avoid inappropriate management. Systemic corticosteroids (e.g., prednisone 40 mg/day) remain the safest and best form of treatment (1,24).

Strong indications for steroid treatment include significant pulmonary parenchymal disease, hepatic disease, hypercalcemia, myocardial disease, incapacitating arthritis, severe thrombocytopenia, posterior ocular disease, laryngeal involvement, or any other vital organ impairment (1,13). White recommends prednisone at 1 mg/kg/day followed by a taper for patients with neurosarcoidosis because of the high mortality rate (10%) in that group. For severe or fulminant cases, he uses high dose intravenous (i.v.) steroids (1 g/day methylprednisolone) for 2 to 3 days (24). Weaker indications are persistent constitutional symptoms and abnormal results of liver function tests (13,25). Topical corticosteroids are used for anterior ocular and skin disease (1,2,3,16,19).·

Patients with cardiac conduction abnormalities resulting from granulomatous infiltration are usually refractory to conventional pharmacotherapy and often need to be admitted to the hospital to determine the most appropriate pharmacologic or electrical therapy. Cardiac transplantation has been performed successfully in younger patients with severe heart failure. Ventricular aneurysm resection may be required to eliminate refractory dysrhythmias (1,10). Lung transplantation has been performed for end-stage pulmonary disease (10).

Hypercalcemia, if severe or symptomatic, may be treated in the normal fashion, high-dose corticosteroid therapy is initiated. Milder elevations of serum calcium levels may be treated with corticosteroids alone, with frequent monitoring (1,16).

Although corticosteroids remain the mainstay of treatment, a number of other agents have also been used. They include methotrexate, azathioprine, cyclophosphamide, chlorambucil, cyclosporine, nonsteroidal antiinflammatory agents, chloroquine, and hydroxychloroquine.

Sarcoidosis clears spontaneously in one half of patients (3).

CRITICAL INTERVENTIONS

- Obtain a serum calcium level in all patients with suspected or previously diagnosed sarcoidosis
- Do not treat hypercalcemia on an outpatient basis
- Obtain an electrocardiogram on patients with sarcoidosis for cardiac conduction abnormalities

DISPOSITION

The emergency department physician may require the advice and assistance of a variety of specialty consultants in diagnosing and managing the patient with suspected sarcoidosis. Pulmonary, ophthalmologic, dermatologic, and neurologic consultation may be necessary before any definitive therapy is undertaken.

Hospital admission is indicated for patients with cardiac or neurologic symptoms, hypercalcemia, severe thrombocytopenia, or any degree of airway compromise. Admission should be considered for diagnostic purposes at initial presentation.

Because frequent and long-term care is usually required, the family physician, internist, or pulmonary specialist is most commonly called on to provide primary outpatient therapy for sarcoidosis.

COMMON PITFALLS

✔ Sarcoidosis is frequently asymptomatic and should be included in the differential diagnosis of patients with eye findings, suggestive skin lesions, hypercalcemia, persistent cough, or unexplained fever and weight loss
✔ The emergency physician should resist the temptation to announce a firm diagnosis or prognosis to the patient, yet it is essential that followup be arranged so that a definitive diagnosis can be made and appropriate treatment begun

✔ Most cases of sarcoidosis resolve without treatment. Specialty consultation should be obtained before treating with systemic corticosteroids and when dealing with cardiac, neurologic, or ocular disease
✔ Children can and do develop sarcoidosis
✔ The presence of wheezing may incorrectly suggest reactive airway disease. Corticosteroids may not be indicated in this setting

Acknowledgments

Thanks to previous edition author Christopher C. Rose.

References

1. Baughman RP. Therapeutic options for sarcoidosis: new and old. *Curr Opin Pulm Med* 2002;8:464–9.
2. Berkman YM. Radiologic aspects of intrathoracic sarcoidosis. *Semin Roentgenol* 1985;4:356.
3. Crystal RG. Sarcoidosis. In: *Harrison's Principles of internal medicine,* 14th ed., Philadelphia: W. B. Saunders, 1998:1922.
4. Fritscher-Ravens A. Diagnosing sarcoidosis using endosonography-guided fine needle aspiration. *Chest* 2000;118:928.
5. Graniem J. Sarcoid myopathy in a patient with HIV infection. *South Med J* 1995;88:591.
6. Gullapalli D. Neurologic manifestations of sarcoidosis. *Neurol Clin* 2002;20:59.
7. Judson M. The etiologic agent of sarcoidosis. What if there isn't one? *Chest* 2003;124:6–8.
8. Lenner R. Recurrent pulmonary sarcoidosis in HIV-infected patients receiving highly active antiretroviral therapy. *Chest* 2001;119:978.
9. Lowery WS, Whitlock WL, Dietrich RA, et al. Sarcoidosis complicated by HIV infection: three case reports and a review of the literature. *Am Rev Respir Dis* 1990;142:887.
10. Lynch JP, Kazerooni EA, Gay SE. Pulmonary sarcoidosis. *Clin Chest Med* 1997;18:755.
11. Moller DR. Etiology of sarcoidosis. *Clin Chest Med* 1997;18:695.
12. Morey SS. American Thoracic Society issues consensus statement on sarcoidosis. *Am Fam Phys* 2000;61:553–554.
13. Paramothayan NS, Jones PW. Corticosteroids for pulmonary sarcoidosis. *Cochrane Database Syst Rev* 2000;9:CD 001114.
14. Schwartzbauer HR, Tami TA. Ear, nose and throat manifestation of sarcoidosis. *Otolaryngol Clin North Am* 2003;36:673–684.
15. Sharma OP. Sarcoidosis: clinical, laboratory and immunologic aspects. *Semin Roentgenol* 1985;4:340.
16. Sharma OP. Vitamin D, calcium, and sarcoidosis. *Chest* 1996;109:535.
17. Shetty AK, Gedalia A. Sarcoidosis in children. *Curr Probl Pediatr* 2000;30:149.
18. Shorr AF. Circulating D-dimer in patients with sarcoidosis. *Chest* 2000;117:1012.
19. Shorr AF, Torrington KG, Hnatiuk OW. Endobronchial involvement and airway hyperreactivity in patients with sarcoidosis. *Chest* 2001;120:881.
20. Slovik SB, Spencer RP, Palestro CJ, et al. Specificity and sensitivity of distinctive chest radiographs and/or ^{67}Ga images in the noninvasive diagnosis of sarcoidosis. *Chest* 1993;103:403.
21. Statement on sarcoidosis. Joint statement of the American Thoracic Society (ATS), the European Respiratory Society (ERS) and the World Association of Sarcoidosis and Other Granulomatous Disorders (WASOG). *Am J Respir Crit Care Med* 1999;160:736.
22. Vignaux O. Significance of myocardial magnetic resonance abnormalities in patients with sarcoidosis: A 1 year follow-up study. *Chest* 2002;122:1895.
23. Vourlekis JS, Sawyer RT, Newman LS. Sarcoidosis: developments in etiology, immunology and therapeutics. *Adv Intern Med* 2000;45:209.
24. White ES, Lynch JP. Sarcoidosis involving multiple systems—diagnostic and therapeutic challenges. *Chest* 2001;119:1593–1597.
25. Winterbauer RH, Kirtland SH, Corley DE. Treatment with corticosteroids. *Clin Chest Med* 1997;18:843.

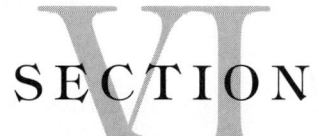

Section Editor: Jeffrey Schaider

Cardiovascular Emergencies

CHAPTER 41
Acute Coronary Syndromes

James T. Niemann

The term "acute coronary syndrome" encompasses three presentations of coronary artery disease (CAD), namely, non-ST-segment elevation myocardial infarction (NSTEMI, previously termed subendocardial or non-Q-wave infarction), ST-segment elevation myocardial infarction (STEMI, previously called transmural infarction or Q-wave infarction), and unstable angina pectoris (UAP) (9). NSTEMI and STEMI are characterized by electrocardiographic abnormalities and elevations of serum markers of myocardial injury, for example, troponin or the MB fraction of creatine kinase (CK-MB) (29). UAP is defined by its clinical presentation, usually a change in angina class as defined by the Canadian Cardiovascular Society (Table 41.1) (10,11). UAP is an uncommon initial manifestation of CAD and typically occurs in patients with known CAD and a history of stable angina pectoris. Acute MI often cannot be differentiated from UAP at the time of initial presentation.

The coronary arterial lesion most commonly encountered in the patient with typical, stable angina pectoris is a smooth-surfaced atherosclerotic plaque that may permit sufficient coronary arterial flow at rest or with minimal exercise to meet the metabolic demands of the myocardium. During physical exertion or emotional stress, myocardial oxygen demand increases owing to an increase in heart rate and blood pressure (the double product). To meet an increase in oxygen demand, either coronary arterial flow or myocardial oxygen extraction must increase. Because myocardial oxygen extraction is near maximal under normal circumstances, the only way to balance myocardial oxygen supply and demand is to increase coronary flow. If a fixed obstructive lesion is present, flow cannot increase sufficiently to meet augmented demands. Supply–demand imbalance ensues, with the development of ischemia, contractile dysfunction, and the classic symptoms of angina. When supply and demand is equalized, the supply–demand imbalance ceases and symptoms subside. Optimization of the supply–demand relationship serves as the foundation for the medical management of chronic stable angina. Nitroglycerin preparations, β-blockers, and calcium channel blockers either increase myocardial oxygen supply or decrease demand.

In contrast, the pathologic substrate for the acute coronary syndrome (ACS) is a complex, irregular, and atherosclerotic plaque. Under many circumstances, this irregular plaque may not be flow-limiting, even during activities that increase the double product. ACS, usually manifested as chest pain, typically follows plaque rupture with hemorrhage beneath the plaque (22,24,33). This unstable plaque is thrombogenic, and complete or nearly complete occlusion of a coronary artery ensues. Myocardial supply–demand imbalance, therefore, occurs because of a decrease in oxygen supply rather than an increase in demand, as in the stable coronary syndrome. Myocardial ischemia can also occur in the absence of coronary atherosclerosis. Common causes of nonatherosclerotic myocardial ischemia are listed in Table 41.2.

CLINICAL PRESENTATION

History of Present Illness

Chest pain or chest discomfort is the most common chief complaint. The chest pain or discomfort in patients with ACS is typically described as chest heaviness, tightness, squeezing, or burning. It is usually retrosternal and may radiate to the left shoulder or to the arm, neck, or jaw because of convergence of sympathetic and somatic afferent pathways at the spinal level. Chest pain caused by ACS is of visceral origin and is poorly localized. Patients with ACS may complain of epigastric abdominal discomfort, which is usually, but not always, accompanied by chest discomfort. Frequent associated symptoms include dyspnea, nausea (sometimes with vomiting), and diaphoresis.

Chest pain associated with ACS usually occurs abruptly, increases in intensity over time, and reaches peak intensity within 2 to 5 minutes of onset. If the pain occurs during or immediately after exertion, it may resolve gradually within minutes of cessation of physical activity. Some characteristics of ACS chest discomfort have been called "typical" or probably of myocardial ischemic origin. Other chest pain characteristics are less likely to be of ischemic origin (Table 41.3). Certain chest pain characteristics have a low likelihood of representing myocardial ischemia and ACS. For instance, chest pain that lasts only seconds or that is constant, unremitting, and lasts for hours to days is not consistent with ACS, especially if the electrocardiogram (ECG) is normal. Similarly, chest pain that is pleuritic; reproduced by palpation;

TABLE 41.1.   Clinical Presentations of Unstable Angina

Angina at rest (usually >20 min) within 1 wk of presentation
New-onset angina of Canadian Cardiovascular Society Classification (CCSC) class III or IV within 2 months of presentation
  • Class III angina: pain when walking less than two blocks or climbing less than one flight of stairs
  • Class IV angina: inability to carryout any physical activity without discomfort
Angina increasing in CCSC class to at least class III or IV

TABLE 41.2.   Causes of Nonatherosclerotic Myocardial Ischemia

VALVULAR HEART DISEASE

Aortic stenosis
Aortic regurgitation
Pulmonary stenosis (right ventricular ischemia)
Mitral stenosis with pulmonary hypertension (right ventricular ischemia)

CONGENITAL HEART DISEASE

Congenital valvular disease
Coarctation of the aorta
Cyanotic heart disease

NONATHEROSCLEROTIC CORONARY DISEASE

Coronary artery spasm, spontaneous or drug-induced (e.g., from cocaine use)
Coronary artery embolus
Congenital coronary disease (anomalous anatomic origin)
Coronary dissection
Coronary artery vasculitis

TABLE 41.3.   Characteristics of Chest Pain for Ischemic Heart Disease

Typical
Substernal in location
Squeezing, heavy, or burning sensation
Precipitated by exertion
Promptly (within 2–3 min) relieved by nitroglycerin
Lasting minutes (typically 5–15 min; longer with acute infarction)

Atypical
Pain described as sharp or stabbing
Fleeting (lasting seconds) or prolonged (>24 h)
Unrelated to exercise
Not relieved by rest or nitroglycerin
Positional or related to respiration ("pleuritic")
Characterized by palpitations without chest pain
Well-localized to a specific point or coin-shaped area on chest wall

---

or that is sharp, stabbing, or positional has a low likelihood of being caused by ACS (9,25).

Some patients with ACS, usually the elderly or those who also have diabetes mellitus or hypertension, may present with symptoms other than chest pain during acute ischemia. Abrupt onset of dyspnea is the most common atypical presentation and is caused by diastolic myocardial dysfunction during ischemia. Decreased ventricular compliance leads to an increase in left ventricular (LV) end-diastolic pressure and pulmonary artery pressure, resulting in an increase in pulmonary interstitial fluid and the sensation of dyspnea.

Patients with a history of chest pain or with known medically controlled angina pectoris may present with new symptoms. Such symptoms would include chest pain at rest (typically of >20 minutes in duration); chest pain associated with previously tolerated levels of exertion; chest pain unrelieved by a previously effective dose of a nitrate preparation; or chest pain of increasing severity, duration, or frequency. These patients usually meet accepted criteria for UAP (Table 41.1). Symptoms of an acute infarction may not be distinguishable from those of a severe stable anginal episode or of UAP, although patients with acute infarction usually have chest pain of typical ischemic quality for at least 30 minutes.

On the basis of a number of studies, major and minor risk factors for CAD have been defined and their presence or absence is usually determined when the medical history is obtained. Major risk factors include family history (MI in a first-degree relative of age less than 55 years), smoking, hypertension, hypercholesterolemia, diabetes mellitus, and male sex. However, risk factors are epidemiologically derived statements about the likelihood of developing CAD over time and have not been demonstrated to be of use in deciding whether a discrete episode of chest pain has been caused by CAD.

Physical Examination

Most patients with chest pain associated with ACS have one or more abnormal physical findings, but these are not specific for ACS and may occur in patients with valvular or congenital heart disease, cardiomyopathy, or chronic ischemic heart disease. If the finding of an S_4 is excluded, about 25% of patients with ACS have a normal cardiac examination.

Common physical findings during myocardial ischemia are noted in Table 41.4 with their respective pathophysiologic explanations. Some physical findings play an important in short-term risk stratification (see subsequent text). The clinician should also seek evidence of risk factors for CAD, for example, hypercholesterolemia (xanthomas and arcus senilis) and hypertension (elevated arterial blood pressure and funduscopic changes).

DIFFERENTIAL DIAGNOSIS

A detailed discussion of the differential diagnosis of chest pain is included elsewhere in this volume (see Chapter 6, "Chest Pain"). Life-threatening diseases, which may be confused with ACS, include aortic dissection, pulmonary thromboembolism, pneumothorax, and esophageal rupture. Pneumonia, valvular heart disease, pericarditis, gastroesophageal reflux disease (GERD), peptic ulcer disease, and chest wall pain should also be included in the differential diagnosis. Particular attention to the character of the pain, precipitating factors, associated symptoms, and the physical examination usually allows the clinician to rule out a number of these other causes for chest pain.

EMERGENCY DEPARTMENT EVALUATION

The emergency department evaluation, management, and triage of patients suspected of having chest pain caused by myocardial ischemia have changed dramatically in the past decade. These changes are the result of cost-containment concerns as well as the demonstration that early reperfusion for STEMI and early administration of antiplatelet and antithrombin agents in the setting of NSTEMI and UAP decrease mortality.

Annually, approximately 3.6 million patients are hospitalized in the United States for chest pain suspected to be related to CAD. However, approximately 70% of these patients are subsequently discharged with a noncardiac diagnosis. Large-scale studies have shown that emergency department chest pain units (CPUs) can quickly identify and stratify patients with chest pain of suspected ischemic origin into low- and high-risk groups to more effectively use the resources uniquely available in the cardiac care unit (CCU) setting (16). Diagnostic efforts in the emergency department should be directed not only toward ACS diagnosis but also toward risk stratification. For these reasons, guidelines for the evaluation and stratification of chest pain patients with suspected ACS have been developed (Tables 41.5 and 41.6) (9). Stratification is based upon short-term risk, generally defined as death, myocardial infarction, reinfarction, or revascularization within 30 days. These guidelines rely strongly on diagnostic aids available to the emergency department physician.

Electrocardiography

An ECG should be obtained and interpreted as early as possible in patients with suspected ACS. Only about 50% of patients eventually discharged with a diagnosis of acute MI will have an initial ECG that is diagnostic for STEMI or NSTEMI. "Nonspecific" or "nondiagnostic" findings are frequent in this group

---

TABLE 41.4.   Physical Signs That Occur During Ischemia

Physical Sign	Underlying Pathophysiology
Soft S_1	Decreased LV dp/dt or first-degree AV block
Paradoxically split S_2	Prolonged LV ejection time
S_3 and/or S_4	Decreased LV compliance
Mitral regurgitation	Papillary muscle ischemia
Palpable precordial systolic bulge	Anterior or lateral dyskinesis
Bibasilar rales	Increased preload

LV, left ventricular; dp/dt, rate of pressure rise; AV, atrioventricular.

TABLE 41.5. Likelihood That Signs and Symptoms Represent an ACS Secondary to CAD

Feature	High Likelihood *Any of the Following:*	Intermediate Likelihood *Absence of High-Likelihood Features and Presence of Any of the Following:*	Low Likelihood *Absence of High- or Intermediate-Likelihood Features But May have:*
History	Chest or left arm pain or discomfort as chief symptom reproducing prior documented angina Known history of CAD, including MI	Chest or left arm pain or discomfort as chief symptom Age >70 years Male sex Diabetes mellitus	Probable ischemic symptoms in absence of any of the intermediate likelihood characteristics Recent cocaine use
Examination	Transient MR, hypotension, diaphoresis, pulmonary edema, or rales	Extracardiac vascular disease	Chest discomfort reproduced by palpation
ECG	New, or presumably new, transient ST-segment deviation ($\geq$0.05 mV) or T-wave inversion ($\geq$0.2 mV) with symptoms	Fixed Q waves Abnormal ST segments or T waves not documented to be new	T-wave flattening or inversion in leads with dominant R waves Normal
Cardiac markers	Elevated cardiac TnI, TnT, or CK-MB	Normal	Normal

CAD, coronary artery disease; MI, myocardial infarction; MR, mitral regurgitation; CK-MB, MB fraction of creatine Kinase; Tn, troponin.
(From Braunwald E, Mark DR, Jones RH, et al. Unstable angina: diagnosis and management. Rockville, MD: Agency for Health Care Policy and Research and the National Heart, Lung and Blood Institute, U.S. Public Health Service, U.S. Department of Health and Human Services; 1994; AHCPR Publication No. 94-0602.)

of patients. A second ECG recorded 30 to 60 minutes after the first emergency department ECG, for instance, is recommended for patients with intermediate or high likelihood of CAD with chest pain likely to be of ischemic origin (Table 41.5) and at intermediate or high short-term risk (Table 41.6). The optimal time-interval at which to perform a repeated emergency department ECG in patients with initial nondiagnostic findings has not been determined.

The earliest electrocardiographic finding resulting from acute MI occurring minutes after interruption of blood flow is the hyperacute T wave, which is often asymmetric with a broad base and is associated with reciprocal ST depression. The hyperacute T wave evolves rapidly to ST-segment elevation over a 5- to 30-minute period.

Additional early electrocardiographic signs of myocardial injury are ST-segment and T-wave changes that may also be seen

TABLE 41.6. Short-Term Risk of Death or Nonfatal MI in Patients with Unstable Angina*

Feature	High Risk *At Least 1 of the Following Features Must be Present:*	Intermediate Risk *No High-Risk Feature But Must have 1 of the Following:*	Low Risk *No High- or Intermediate-Risk Feature But May have Any of the Following Features:*
History	Accelerating tempo of ischemic symptoms in preceding 48 h	Prior MI, peripheral or cerebrovascular disease, or CABG Prior aspirin use	
Character of pain	Prolonged ongoing (>20 min) rest pain	Prolonged (>20 min) rest angina, now resolved, with moderate or high likelihood of CAD Rest angina (<20 min) or relieved with rest or sublingual nitroglycerin	New-onset or progressive CCCS class III or IV angina of the past 2 weeks without prolonged (>20 min) rest pain but with moderate or high likelihood of CAD (see Table 41.5)
Clinical findings	Pulmonary edema, most likely due to ischemia New or worsening MR murmur, S_3 or new or worsening rales Hypotension, bradycardia, tachycardia Age >75 years	Age >70 years	
ECG	Angina at rest with transient ST-segment changes >0.05 mV Bundle-branch block, new or presumed new Sustained ventricular tachycardia	T-wave inversions >0.2 mV Pathological Q waves	Normal or unchanged ECG during an episode of chest discomfort
Cardiac markers	Elevated (e.g., TnT or TnI >0.1 ng/mL)	Slightly elevated (e.g., TnT >0.01 but <0.1 ng/mL)	Normal

MR, mitral regurgitation; MI, myocardial infarction; CABG, coronary artery bypass grafting; CAD, coronary artery disease; CCCS, Cauadian Cardiovascular Society Classification; ECG, eletrocardiogram; Tn, troponin.
*Estimation of the short-term risks of deaths and nonfatal cardiac ischemic events in Unstable Angina is a complex multivariable problem that cannot be fully specified in a table such as this; therefore, this table is meant to offer general guidance and illustration rather than rigid algorithms.
(Adapted from AHCPR Clinical Practice Guideline No. 10, unstable angina: Diagnosis and Management, May 1994. Braunwald E, Mark DR, Jones RH, et al. Unstable angina: diagnosis and management. Rockville, MD: Agency for Health Care Policy and Research and the National Heart, Lung and Blood Institute, U.S. Public Health Service, U.S. Department of Health and Human Services; 1994; AHCPR Publication No. 94-0602.)

TABLE 41.7.   Nonischemic Causes of ECG Changes

Precordial ST-Segment Elevation	ST-Segment Depression	T-Wave Inversion
Left bundle-branch block	LVH	Intracranial event
Left ventricular hypertrophy	Left BBB	Strain pattern
	Digoxin effect	Myocarditis
Pericarditis		
Paced ventricular rhythm	Hypokalemia	Early repolarization
Hypothermia (Osborne J waves)	Hypomagnesemia	Normal variant
Hyperkalemia		
Drug-induced (e.g., tricyclic antidepressants)		
Left ventricular aneurysm		

ECG, electrocardiogram; LVH, left ventricular hypertrophy; BBB, bundle-branch block.

with early or transient reversible ischemia. Although nondiagnostic, new, or presumably new, ST-segment elevation or depression of ≥ 0.5 mm (.05 mV) or T-wave inversion of ≥ 0.2 mm (.02 mV) observed during symptoms may indicate ACS. The presence of new nonspecific ECG changes increases the likelihood that chest pain is caused by myocardial ischemia; however, the predictive value of such a finding is only about 50%. New, or presumably new, ST-segment deviations of ≥ 1 mm or 0.1 mV are more consistent with STEMI or NSTEMI and should prompt therapeutic intervention (30). Patients with ST-segment elevation resulting from acute MI have either obliquely flat or convex waveforms, whereas patients with noninfarctional ST-segment elevation (i.e., early repolarization or left ventricular hypertrophic [LVH] changes) tend to have a concave waveform. ST-segment and T-wave changes are not always caused by ACS. Common nonischemic causes for ST-segment elevation or depression and T-wave inversions suggestive of ACS are listed in Table 41.7. Although a nonconcave ST-segment elevation pattern is more commonly encountered in acute STEMI than in other nonischemic causes of ST elevation, the sensitivity of this morphologic pattern, approximately 75%, precludes absolute diagnostic reliance on its presence or absence.

Nonconventional surface electrocardiographic recordings are of value in some patients with STEMI. The right coronary artery supplies the inferior wall of the left ventricle as well as the right ventricle in 90% of patients. In the setting of inferior MI, a right precordial ECG should be recorded to detect right ventricular (RV) infarction. The right precordial ECG is obtained by placing the V leads over the anterior right chest in a pattern that is the mirror image of the standard left-sided placement. RV infarction occurs in about 60% of patients who have an inferior MI and is detected by ST-segment elevation of >1 mm in lead V_{3R} or V_{4R}, or both. Although RV infarction commonly accompanies infarction of the inferior wall of the left ventricle, RV contractile dysfunction becomes hemodynamically significant in only about 10% of patients. Patients with hemodynamically significant RV infarction typically present with arterial hypotension and jugular venous distention, but with clear lung fields. Arterial hypotension is more likely to occur after nitroglycerin administration in the patient with RV dysfunction owing to decreased RV preload. A posterior wall infarction is reflected by ST-segment depression in the anterior precordial leads. ST-segment depression in these leads may also be a result of reciprocal changes, which occur with an inferior wall infarction. ST-segment elevation of >1 mm recorded in posterior ECG leads (V_7–V_9) is suggestive of posterior wall injury.

Chest Radiography

The most common chest film abnormality in patients with ACS is cardiomegaly, usually the result of a prior infarction or chronic arterial hypertension. Additional radiographic signs of LV dysfunction may also be found (e.g., pulmonary venous hypertension, Kerley B lines, and chronic pleural effusions).

The primary value of the chest radiograph in the evaluation of the patient with chest pain and suspected ACS is in the detection of other causes of chest pain (e.g., pneumothorax, pneumonia, or a widened mediastinum suggesting aortic dissection).

Biochemical Markers

After the clinical history and 12-lead ECG, the third tool readily available to assist in the diagnosis of ACS and stratification is the serial measurement of enzymes and proteins released into the blood during myocardial ischemia. When myocytes are damaged, there is loss of cell membrane integrity, and these macromolecules diffuse into the interstitium and subsequently into the intravascular space and lymphatics. Their patterns of appearance in blood depend on the intracellular location, molecular weight (heavier molecules diffuse more slowly), local blood and lymph flow, and rate of elimination from the blood. The enzyme creatine kinase (CK), its myocardial subunit (CK-MB), and the proteins troponin (Tn) I and T are the most readily available and most commonly used biochemical markers of cardiac ischemia.

Elevations of total CK and CK-MB mass are detectable 4 to 6 hours after acute infarction. Peak CK-MB mass is typically observed 12 to 18 hours after ischemia, whereas the peak of total CK occurs slightly later (12 to 24 hours). Both measurements return to normal levels 24 to 36 hours after the ischemic event; a secondary rise suggests reinfarction. Time to peak levels of total CK and CK-MB mass vary depending on the extent of myocardial injury. Elevations above the reference range or normal value for total CK and CK-MB mass are not specific for myocardial injury. CK and CK-MB are also present in skeletal muscle, and elevations may be seen after vigorous exercise, rhabdomyolysis, skeletal muscle trauma, dermatomyositis or polymyositis, renal failure, and cardiac contusion. Interpretation of total CK and CK-MB mass values must take this nonspecificity into consideration.

The troponins (TnI and TnT) are proteins that regulate calcium-dependent interactions between myosin and actin. The cardiac troponins (cTnI, cTnT) are highly specific for myocardial tissue and are immunologically distinct from the skeletal muscle troponins. Because of this specificity, the concomitant use of a Tn measurement and CK-MB mass assists in differentiating myocardial from skeletal muscle injury in the presence of an elevated CK-MB measurement. Elevated cardiac Tn levels are detectable in serum within 4 to 6 hours following acute cardiac ischemia, reach peak concentrations in approximately 12 hours, and remain elevated after an ischemic event for 3 to 10 days. This temporal pattern allows detection of an acute cardiac event days after it has occurred. Because of its lower molecular weight, TnT appears earlier in the plasma than TnI. This advantage may be offset by the fact that TnT can be artificially elevated in stable renal failure patients, whereas TnI is typically not.

At present, there is an indeterminate range of Tn values (typically dependent upon the manufacturer of the assay) that are not normal yet are below the levels accepted for the diagnosis of acute MI. Such values may be seen in the clinical settings of unstable angina (presumably because of "microinfarction"), chronic congestive heart failure, and myocarditis, and after cardiac surgery. In the setting of suspect ACS, indeterminate values should be interpreted as abnormal until further workup determines otherwise.

A single measurement of total CK, CK-MB mass, and Tn has a low sensitivity (30% to 40%) in ruling out a STEMI or an NSTEMI, despite a specificity of 80% to 99%. Because of this low sensitivity, single normal values usually cannot be relied on to eliminate acute infarction as a diagnostic possibility in a patient with chest pain. It is currently recommended that patients with suspected ACS and negative cardiac markers within 6 hours of symptom onset have a second marker determination 6 to 12 hours after the first. The reported sensitivities, specificities, and positive and negative predictive values for the various biochemical markers vary considerably in the literature (12,34). This variation results from the reported timing of blood sampling (from onset of symptoms or from time of emergency department arrival), the use of one marker or a panel of markers, and the populations studied (e.g., patients with diagnostic vs.nondiagnostic ECGs). In general, sensitivity increases over this period (0 to 6 hours), whereas specificity remains relatively constant (greater than 90%). Within 8 to 10 hours after the ischemic event, the sensitivity of CK-MB mass and the troponins is approximately 90%. Negative serum markers do not rule out a diagnosis of UAP.

Other biochemical markers for acute MI may facilitate the earlier diagnosis of acute infarction, particularly in the patient with a nondiagnostic ECG. Myoglobin is released from the myocardium within 2 to 4 hours of the onset of ischemia and appears earlier in the plasma than CK-MB does. Serial measurements of myoglobin using newer rapid assays have been shown to be 100% sensitive, but with a specificity of approximately 80%, in detecting acute MI within 6 hours of symptom onset. Similarly, measurement of CK-MB isoforms (MB1 and MB2) has a sensitivity and specificity of greater than 90% for detecting acute MI within 6 hours of onset of symptoms. These latter markers are currently not widely used.

EMERGENCY DEPARTMENT MANAGEMENT

The initial management of all patients with chest pain and suspected acute ischemic heart disease (IHD) should include administration of low-flow oxygen, establishment of vascular access, and continuous cardiac rhythm monitoring combined with frequent blood pressure determinations. Continuous pulse oximetry should also be employed.

Interventions in the Patient with Chest Pain and Suspected Unstable Angina Pectoris (UAP) or Non-ST-Segment Elevation Myocardial Infarction (NSTEMI)

The emergency department management of intermediate- and high-risk patients with UAP and patients with NSTEMI are similar. Therapeutic interventions in these clinical setting are directed toward decreasing myocardial oxygen demand and stabilizing thrombogenic atherosclerotic plaques. The American Heart Association (AHA) and the American College of Cardiology (ACC) have made specific recommendations regarding the management of UAP and NSTEMI (9). Because the strength of evidence supporting these recommendations is variable, the AHA and ACC have provided three classes of recommendations. Class I recommendations, that is, those supported by evidence and general agreement that an intervention is useful and effective, applicable to emergency department management are summarized below:

Antiischemic Therapy

1. Sublingual followed by intravenous (i.v.) nitroglycerin for relief of chest pain and associated symptoms.

2. Intravenous morphine sulfate if symptoms are not relieved by nitroglycerin or for pulmonary edema.
3. Intravenous β-blocker followed by oral therapy in absence of contraindications.
4. A calcium antagonist (verapamil or diltiazem) in the absence of severe LV dysfunction or other contraindications in patients with continuing or recurring chest pain when β-blockers are contraindicated.

Sublingual nitroglycerin decreases myocardial oxygen demand by decreasing ventricular preload, improves myocardial perfusion by dilating the coronary vascular bed, and has antiplatelet properties. This combination of pharmacologic effects often results in relief of chest pain. The usual starting dose is 0.3 to 0.4 mg of nitroglycerin sublingually via a tablet or spray. If chest pain persists, this dose may be repeated every 5 minutes if the systolic blood pressure remains greater than 100 mm Hg. If chest pain persists after three to five sublingual doses, the administration of intravenous nitroglycerin should be initiated (50 mg of nitroglycerin in 250 mL of dextrose 5% in water). The initial infusion rate is 10 to 20 μg/minute and can be increased in increments of 5 to 10 μg/minute at 5- to 10-minute intervals until chest discomfort resolves or mean arterial pressure decreases by 10%. Most patients respond to infusion rates of 50 to 200 μg/minute. At low doses, nitroglycerin acts principally as a venous and coronary vasodilator. At high doses it acts as an arterial vasodilator as well, thereby affecting an additional component of myocardial oxygen demand. The major complication of nitrate therapy, whether sublingual or intravenous, is hypotension. This is most likely to occur in patients who are hypovolemic at the time of emergency department presentation or in those who have sustained an RV infarction complicating inferior wall infarction. If hypotension occurs, nitrate therapy should be discontinued and intravenous normal saline administered, with careful monitoring of vital signs and lung sounds. Hemodynamically significant bradydysrhythmias have been reported during nitrate therapy; these should be treated with atropine.

Intravenous morphine may be administered if chest pain is not relieved with sublingual or intravenous nitroglycerin. The usual dose is 2 to 4 mg administered every 5 to 30 minutes if systolic blood pressure remains greater than 100 mm Hg. Morphine may decrease venous tone and decrease ventricular preload, but the required dose for these desired pharmacologic effects may produce respiratory depression. In addition, morphine may relieve pain but not necessarily reverse or modify the pathophysiologic processes involved in acute myocardial ischemia. Other potential complications of morphine therapy are hypotension and bradycardia, which may be treated with normal saline and atropine, respectively.

β-Blockers reduce myocardial oxygen demand by decreasing ventricular contractility (dP/dt), heart rate, and afterload (blood pressure). These agents also have antidysrhythmic properties and may counteract the effects of catecholamines on the myocardium. These agents should be administered in the setting of suspected unstable angina or acute MI if contraindications to their use are not present. There have been a number of randomized trials of intravenous β-blockade initiated early in the course of acute MI (18). Early intravenous β-blockade can reduce mortality by 13% by day 7 of treatment. Continued chronic oral therapy decreases long-term mortality. β-Blockers are contraindicated in the setting of obstructive airway disease (asthma or chronic obstructive pulmonary disease), atrioventricular (AV) block, hypotension, congestive heart failure, or known allergy. Esmolol, a β-blocker with an ultrashort half-life, may be administered by infusion and titrated to effect if β-blockade is necessary in patients with airways disease or depressed MI. Typical dosing schedules are shown in Table 41.8.

TABLE 41.8. Dosing of β-Blockers

ATENOLOL

Administer 5 mg i.v. and repeat in 10 min. After 15 min, give 50 mg orally.

METOPROLOL

Administer 5 mg i.v. every 5 to 10 min to a total dose of 15 mg. After 15 min, give 100 mg orally.

i.v., intravenously.

Antiplatelet and Anticoagulation Therapy

1. Aspirin should be administered as soon as possible.
2. Clopidogrel (Plavix) should be administered to hospitalized patients who are unable to take aspirin because of hypersensitivity or major gastrointestinal intolerance.
3. Clopidogrel should be added to aspirin in hospitalized patients for whom an early noninterventional approach is planned.
4. Clopidogrel should be started in patients for whom a percutaneous coronary intervention (PCI) is planned.
5. Anticoagulation with subcutaneous low-molecular-weight heparin or intravenous unfractionated heparin should be initiated for patients at intermediate or high risk for adverse events (Table 41.6).
6. A platelet glycoprotein IIb/IIIa antagonist should be administered, in addition to aspirin and heparin, to patients for whom PCI is planned. It may also be administered just before PCI.

Aspirin prevents platelet aggregation and platelet-induced coronary vasoconstriction via acetylation of platelet cyclooxygenase and prevention of the formation of thromboxane A_2. The usual initial dose is 162 to 325 mg of a nonenteric formulation. Clopidogrel is a platelet adenosine diphosphate (ADP) receptor antagonist. Its platelet effects are irreversible but take several days to become completely manifest. A loading dose of 300 to 600 mg can be used when rapid onset of action is required. The usual maintenance dosage is 75 mg/day (26).

Unfractionated heparin is a heterogeneous mixture of polysaccharides, which activates antithrombin III, which in turn inhibits thrombin and coagulation factors X to XII. It also inhibits platelet aggregation, platelet vascular adhesion, and leukocyte chemotaxis (19). Heparin should be administered intravenously as a 60 to 70 U/kg bolus (maximum 5,000 U), followed by an infusion of 12 to 15 U/kg/hour (maximum of 1,000 U/hour). The infusion rate should be adjusted according to periodic measurement of the partial thromboplastin time (PTT) (goal, 1.5 to 2.5 times control).

Low-molecular-weight heparin can also be used and is preferred (class IIa recommendation) in the absence of renal failure and when coronary bypass surgery is not planned within 24 hours of administration. The usual dose is 1 mg/kg given subcutaneously every 12 hours. It does not require monitoring of coagulation times, is associated with fewer clinically significant bleeding complications, and may be more effective than unfractionated heparin in preventing infarction, recurrent pain, and the need for early revascularization. The incidence of clinically significant bleeding complications is similar to that for unfractionated heparin (19).

When platelets are activated, the glycoprotein IIb/IIIa receptor undergoes a configuration change that facilitates the binding of fibrinogen to platelet receptors, thereby resulting in platelet aggregation. Glycoprotein IIb/IIIa antagonists prevent this interaction, the final common pathway for platelet aggregation, and

improve short- and long-term outcome (7,8). Eptifibatide (Integrilin, 180 μg/kg bolus [with a serum creatinine <2.0 mg/dL] followed by an infusion of 2.0 μg/kg/minute for 72 to 96 hours) and tirofiban (Aggrastat, 0.4 μg/kg/minute for 30 minutes followed by an infusion of 0.1 μg/kg/minute [half rate of infusion for creatinine clearance <30 mL/minute] for 48 to 96 hours) are the two glycoprotein IIb/IIIa antagonists most commonly used in the emergency department. Heparin at the previously noted dosage should be administered with these two glycoprotein IIb/IIIa antagonists. Preliminary evidence suggests that low-molecular-weight heparin may be as effective as unfractionated heparin (15).

Among patients with UAP or NSTEMI, the benefit of newer therapies, for example, glycoprotein IIb/IIIa antagonists or an early invasive management strategy, increases with increasing short-term risk (9).

Specific Interventions in Patients with ST-Segment Elevation Acute Myocardial Infarction (STEMI)

Acute MI is most commonly caused by abrupt thrombotic occlusion of a coronary artery at the site of a "thrombogenic" atheromatous plaque (i.e., one that is ulcerated or fissured). Therapeutic interventions in this setting are directed toward reopening the occluded coronary artery (recanalization) as well as decreasing myocardial oxygen demand and stabilizing thrombogenic atherosclerotic plaques. As with UAP and NSTEMI, the AHA and ACC have made recommendations regarding the management of STEMI (28). Class I recommendations applicable to emergency department management are summarized:

1. Thrombolysis is recommended for ST elevation (>1 mm in two or more contiguous leads) in patients younger than 75 years of age when time to therapy is 12 hours or less. Thrombolysis is recommended in the setting of bundle-branch block (obscuring ST-segment analysis) and history suggesting acute MI.
2. Primary percutaneous transluminal coronary angioplasty (PTCA) is preferred as an alternative to thrombolytic therapy in patients with acute MI and ST-segment elevation or new or presumed new left bundle-branch block (LBBB), who can undergo angioplasty of the infarct-related artery within 12 hours of symptom onset if performed in a timely fashion by persons skilled in the procedure.
3. Administration of aspirin, clopidogrel, nitroglycerin, morphine, and β-blockers as for UAP or NSTEMI.

Clot dissolution using thrombolytic agents in STEMI is safe and effective. A number of large prospective, controlled clinical trials comparing an intravenous thrombolytic agent with placebo have shown significant reductions in mortality with minimal risk (25% to 30% mortality reduction when used early) (2–4,14). Other trials have compared thrombolytic agents with and without other adjunctive interventions (e.g., aspirin and β-blockers). The latter studies have resulted in controversies regarding the thrombolytic agent of choice and the timing or method of administration. However, it is generally agreed that (i) the promptness of administration of a thrombolytic agent after the onset of symptoms is more important than the choice of agent and (ii) adjunctive drugs add to the mortality reduction observed with thrombolysis alone. Contraindications to the use of thrombolytic agents are enumerated in Table 41.9.

The generally accepted electrocardiographic criteria for thrombolytic therapy are ST-segment elevation of <1 mm in two or more contiguous leads. It is well recognized that LBBB may obscure the diagnosis of acute MI because of the secondary ST-segment and T-wave changes that accompany altered

TABLE 41.9.   Contraindications to Thrombolytic Therapy in ST-Segment Elevation Myocardial Infarction (28)

ABSOLUTE (CONSIDER FOR IMMEDIATE PTCA OR CABG)

Suspected aortic dissection
Previous hemorrhagic stroke at any time; other strokes or CVAs within 1 year
Known intracranial neoplasm
Active internal bleeding (does not include menses)

RELATIVE

Uncontrolled hypertension on presentation (systolic >180 mm Hg, diastolic >110 mm Hg)
Trauma within 2–4 wk, including head trauma or prolonged (>10 min) CPR, or major surgery (<3 wk)
History of prior CVA or known intracerebral pathology not covered in contraindications
Known bleeding disorder
Pregnancy
Allergy to streptokinase (not a contraindication to use of other agents)
Active peptic ulcer; recent (within 2–4 wk) internal bleeding
Current use of oral anticoagulants in therapeutic doses (INR 2–3)
Noncompressible vascular punctures
History of chronic severe hypertension

PTCA, percutaneous transluminal coronary angioplasty; CABG, coronary artery bypass grafting; CPR, cardiopulmonary resuscitation; CVA, cerebrovascular accident; INR, international normalized ratio.

ventricular depolarization. Criteria have been reported to identify acute MI in the presence of an LBBB, but although generally highly specific, they are insensitive in making this diagnosis (31). Because of this problem with recognition of acute MI in the setting of LBBB (either old or new) and the high mortality encountered when LBBB develops during the course of acute infarction, thrombolytic administration is recommended in patients with a history suggestive of acute cardiac ischemia and LBBB, regardless of whether it is new or old.

The time to administration of thrombolytic therapy is critical for achieving maximum benefit. The best outcomes have been observed when the thrombolytic agent is administered within 4 to 6 hours of symptom onset. There still may be some benefit if the agent is given later (up to 12 hours), especially if symptoms have had a "stuttering" character (i.e., an intermittent resolution and recurrence of chest pain).

Patients 75 years of age and older have a higher incidence of intracranial hemorrhage with thrombolytic therapy than do younger patients. However, mortality with acute MI increases with age, and it can be reduced significantly with thrombolytic therapy.

Although thrombolytic agents have been shown unequivocally to reduce mortality from acute MI when compared with placebo or therapy previously considered "standard," the best agent to use in the setting of STEMI continues to evolve. The choice usually remains with each practitioner and is often determined by local practice and experience (Table 41.10). A single-dose regimen of TNKase (tenecteplase) (5,23) is routinely used in most centers. Approximately 25% of patients who are receiving a thrombolytic agent will not recanalize the obstructed coronary artery, and approximately 20% will re-occlude after successful reperfusion. Electrocardiographic and biochemical marker changes after thrombolytic administration have been shown to be relatively reliable noninvasive markers of thrombolytic effect (13,27).

Although a class IIa recommendation, i.v. heparin is recommended in patients undergoing reperfusion therapy with al-

teplase. The recommended dose is 60 U/kg as a bolus at the initiation of alteplase therapy, then an initial maintenance dose of 12 U/kg/hour (with a maximum of 4,000 U bolus and 1,000 U/hour infusion for patients weighing >70 kg). The maintenance dose should be adjusted to a PTT of 1.5 to 2.0 normal. Recent data indicate that enoxaparin (30 mg i.v., and 1 mg/kg subcutaneously) can be used in place of unfractionated heparin when TNKase is used as the thrombolytic agent (6).

Primary PTCA (i.e., used as the initial intervention to achieve coronary reperfusion) has been the subject of much recent investigation and appears to be superior to thrombolytic therapy when performed early (1,17). It is the reperfusion method of choice when acute MI is complicated by cardiogenic shock.

Complications of Acute Ischemia or Infarction

Dysrhythmias

Cardiac rhythm disturbances are common during unstable angina or acute infarction. The most common dysrhythmias are of ventricular origin. Premature ventricular contractions (PVCs) are noted in 80% to 100% of patients who experience an acute MI. Symptomatic ventricular ectopy should be treated with intravenous lidocaine or amiodarone. Lidocaine can be administered with an initial bolus of 1 mg/kg followed by an infusion of 1 to 4 mg/minute. The major side effect of lidocaine is neurotoxicity, typically manifested as altered mental status, slurred speech, and seizures. In low cardiac output states, lidocaine metabolism is decreased and usual therapeutic doses may be toxic. Thus, in this setting, the initial intravenous loading dose should be halved and the continuous infusion should be started at 1 mg/minute. Intravenous amiodarone is administered as 150 mg over 10 minutes, followed by 1 mg/minute for 6 hours, then 0.5 mg/minute. Supplementary infusions of 150 mg may be repeated as necessary for recurrent or resistant dysrhythmias to maximum total daily dose of 2 g.

TABLE 41.10.   Thrombolytic Agents

TPA (ALTEPLASE)

Standard regimen
  Administer 10-mg i.v. bolus, then 90 mg over 3 h. Administer heparin 60 U/kg as a bolus, then an initial maintenance dose of approximately 12 U/kg/h (with a maximum of 4,000-U bolus and 1,000 U/h infusion for patients weighing >70 kg) adjusted to maintain a PTT of 1.5 to 2.0 times control for 48 h.
Accelerated regimen
  Administer 15-mg bolus, then 0.75 mg/kg (up to 50 mg) over 30 min, then 0.5 mg/kg (up to 35 mg) over 60 min. Administer heparin as described previously.

TNKase (TENECTEPLASE)

Administer as a bolus over 5 sec. Dose is body-weight based.

Patient weight (kg)	TNKase (mg)
<60	30
≥60 to <70	35
≥70 to <80	40
≥80 to <90	45
≥90	50

Administer heparin as for alteplase, or, if creatinine level <2.5 mg/dL, consider enoxaparin 30 mg i.v. followed by first subcutaneous dose of 1 mg/kg to be given every 12 hr.

i.v., intravenous; PTT, partial thromboplastin time; TPA, tissue plasminogen activator.

TABLE 41.11. Indications for Temporary Pacing in Acute Myocardial Infarction (28)

CLASS I

Asystole
Complete heart block
Mobitz II second-degree AVB
Bilateral BBB (alternating BBB or RBBB with alternating LAFB/LPFB)
New or indeterminate-age bifascicular block with first-degree AVB
Symptomatic bradycardia (sinus bradycardia or Mobitz I
  second-degree AVB with hypotension not responsive to atropine)

CLASS II

RBBB and LAFB or LPFB (new or age-indeterminate)
RBBB with first-degree AVB
LBBB (new or age-indeterminate)
For overdrive pacing of ventricular tachycardia or treatment of
  sinus pauses >3 sec not responsive to atropine
Bifascular block of indeterminate age
New or age-indeterminate isolated RBBB

AVB, atrioventricular block; LBBB, left bundle-branch block; RBBB, right bundle-branch block; LAFB, left anterior fascicular block; LPFB, left posterior fascicular block; MI, myocardial infarction.

Bradydysrhythmias or tachydysrhythmias that compromise systemic or myocardial perfusion require immediate therapy (see Chapters 43 and 44, "Bradydysrhythmias" and "Tachydysrhythmias").

Conduction Disturbances

Second- and third-degree AV block may occur during either inferior or anterior infarction. In the setting of inferior MI, these conduction disturbances are normally associated with an increase in vagal tone and are usually transient and responsive to atropine. With inferior MIs, the abrupt occurrence of complete heart block is rare. In anterior MI, high-degree AV block is caused by ischemia of the conduction pathways, and complete heart block may occur abruptly. Bundle-branch blocks are usually associated with anterior infarction. The indications for temporary artificial pacing in the setting of acute ischemia are listed in Table 41.11.

Cardiogenic Shock

LV pump failure begins to occur when approximately 40% of the ventricular muscle mass has been lost. Severe contractile dysfunction results and necessitates the use of a number of therapeutic interventions (see Chapter 4, "Shock"). Studies suggest that PTCA may improve both short- and long-term outcomes; this intervention should be considered early in the course of management in selected patients.

Management of Patients with Low-Risk ACS

Not all patients with chest pain of presumed ischemic origin require hospital admission. A low-risk group of patients has been defined (Table 41.6), who are good candidates for an accelerated observation admission. Such patients are typically those that present with chest pain suggestive of cardiac ischemia, have a normal or nondiagnostic ECG, and normal cardiac markers in the absence of recurrent chest pain. Patients who remain pain free, have a normal and nondiagnostic or unchanged ECG, and negative cardiac serum marker measurements at 6 to 12 hours after symptom onset are candidates for an early stress test to provoke ischemia. These patients require a stress or imaging study to detect the presence of CAD. Such testing can be per-

formed before discharge or on an outpatient basis, usually within 72 hours of emergency department discharge (9). Standard treadmill exercise stress testing (EST), myocardial scintigraphy at rest and during exercise, and stress echocardiography are standard diagnostic tests performed in patients with suspected CAD. The sensitivities, specificities, and positive and negative predictive values of these tests have been defined largely in the population of patients with a moderate-to-high probability of CAD.

Standard treadmill EST has been used for evaluation of low-risk patients in the emergency department. On the basis of limited studies, EST in the emergency department assessment of chest pain has a sensitivity ranging from 29% to 90% for detecting CAD, with a specificity of 50% to 99%. In the population with a low prevalence of disease, EST has a negative predictive value of >98% (32).

Acute myocardial ischemia depletes ATP stores, resulting in ventricular contractile dysfunction and ventricular wall motion abnormalities that may occur in the absence of diagnostic electrocardiographic changes. Two-dimensional echocardiography with the patient at rest is sensitive in detecting regional wall-motion abnormalities that accompany acute ischemia, and has been used in the screening of patients with chest pain and suspected acute ischemia. However, echocardiography cannot reliably differentiate prior infarction (with myocardial scarring) from a new ischemic event. The sensitivity and specificity of the test is higher when performed during chest pain rather than after its resolution. On the basis of the results of limited studies, it is estimated that the sensitivity of standard echocardiography in the emergency department for acute cardiac ischemia or infarction is approximately 50% to 90%, with a specificity of 50% to 100% (20,21). Echocardiography with pharmacologically induced stress (dobutamine stress echo) is more predictive of inducible ischemia and is preferred for patients who are unable to exercise.

Technetium-99m–labeled sestamibi is a radionuclide agent that is taken up by the myocardium in proportion to regional blood flow and is therefore capable of demonstrating myocardial perfusion defects. With electrographic-gating, the technique can also detect wall-motion abnormalities. Limited studies indicate that this method of perfusion imaging is >90% sensitive for detecting CAD in an emergency department population, with a specificity of approximately 70% (20,21). The accuracy of the test does not appear to be affected by the presence or absence of chest pain at the time of imaging. It is preferred in patients with resting electrocardiographic abnormalities that might obscure interpretation of the exercise ECG.

DISPOSITION

Patients with suspected ACS who meet criteria for intermediate or high risk should be admitted to the hospital, typically to an intensive care unit or CCU. When acute MI or refractory anginal symptoms are suspected, the consulting cardiologist should be contacted as soon as possible to facilitate interventional therapy if indicated. Patients with low risk criteria are candidates for observation admission with early provocative testing as indicated previously.

Patients in the acute phase of infarction or with unstable angina should not be transferred to another facility unless definitive care cannot be given at the institution where the initial evaluation is performed. In such an instance, transfer in an appropriately equipped vehicle is justified after initial treatment and stabilization. The transport team should include personnel trained in advanced cardiac life support. It has been demonstrated that patients having an acute MI can be safely transported to a referral center for thrombolytic or interventional therapy.

Patients discharged from the emergency department with a diagnosis of stable angina, low risk ACS, or atypical chest pain should be referred to a cardiologist for further evaluation (e.g., EST).

CRITICAL INTERVENTIONS

- Obtain ECG quickly for patients presenting with chest pain to expedite therapeutic interventions
- Unless contraindicated, administer aspirin to all patients with suspected ACS
- Tailor treatment to patient risk stratification
- Expedite "door to needle or angioplasty balloon" time for appropriate patients undergoing an acute myocardial infarction

COMMON PITFALLS

✔ Not maintaining a low admission threshold for patients for whom the diagnosis is uncertain. Because of the limited diagnostic tools available in the emergency setting, only a minority of patients admitted to the hospital with suspected ACS actually has an acute infarct

✔ Negative serum markers do not exclude a diagnosis of UAP

✔ Comparison of a current ECG to a prior or baseline ECG should not be solely relied on to exclude ACS

✔ If the patient meets appropriate criteria, reperfusion therapy (PTCA or thrombolytic agents) should be initiated as soon as possible. Every institution needs to address the issues of appropriate early triage of ambulatory patients with chest pain and rapid access to 12-lead electrocardiography

✔ If thrombolytic therapy is determined to be appropriate, the patient should always be informed of the risks and benefits of these agents

✔ The diagnosis of ACS is often downplayed in women. It should be remembered that CAD is among the leading causes of death in women

References

1. Andersen HR, Nielsen TT, Rasmussen K, et al. A comparison of coronary angioplasty with fibrinolytic therapy in acute myocardial infarction. *N Engl J Med* 2003;349:733–742.
2. Armstrong PW, Collen D. Fibrinolysis for acute myocardial infarction. Current status and new horizons for pharmacological reperfusion, Part 1. *Circulation* 2001;103:2862–2866.
3. Armstrong PW, Collen D. Fibrinolysis for acute myocardial infarction. Current status and new horizons for pharmacological reperfusion, Part 2. *Circulation* 2001;103:2987–2992.
4. Armstrong PW, Collen D, Antman E. Fibrinolysis for acute myocardial infarction. The future is here and now. *Circulation* 2003;107:2533–2537.
5. ASSENT-2 Investigators. Single-bolus tenecteplase compared with front-loaded alteplase in acute myocardial infarction: the ASSENT-2 double blind randomized trial. *Lancet* 1999;354:716–722.
6. ASSENT-3 Investigators. Efficacy and safety of tenecteplase in combination with enoxaparin, abciximab, or unfractionated heparin: the ASSENT-3 randomized trial in acute myocardial infarction. *Lancet* 2001;358:605–613.
7. Bhatt DL, Topol EJ. Current role of platelet glycoprotein IIb/IIIa inhibitors in acute coronary syndromes. *JAMA* 2000;284:1549–1558.
8. Boersma E, Harrington RA, Moliterno DJ, et al. Platelet glycoprotein IIb/IIIa inhibitors in acute coronary syndromes: a meta-analysis of all major randomized clinical trials. *Lancet* 2003;359:189–198.
9. Braunwald E, Antman EM, Beasley JW, et al. ACC/AHA 2002 guideline update for the management of patients with unstable angina and non-ST-segment elevation myocardial infarction. Available at *www.acc.org*.
10. Braunwald E, Jones RH, Mark DB, et al. Diagnosing and managing unstable angina. *Circulation* 1994;90:613–622.
11. Campeau L. Grading of angina pectoris. *Circulation* 1976;54:522–523. Available at *www.ccs.ca/society/position/grading_angina*.
12. Char DM, Israel E, Ladenson J. Early laboratory indicators of acute myocardial infarction. *Emerg Med Clin North Am* 1998;16:1998.
13. Christenson RH, Ohman EM, Topol EJ, et al. Assessment of coronary reperfusion after thrombolysis with a model combining myoglobin, creatine kinase-MB, and clinical variables. *Circulation* 1997;96:1776.
14. Fibrinolytic Therapy Trialists' (FTT) Collaborative Group. Indications for fibrinolytic therapy in suspected acute myocardial infarction: collaborative overview of early mortality and major morbidity results from all randomized trials of more than 1000 patients. *Lancet* 1994;343:311.
15. Goodman SG, Fitchett D, Armstrong PW, et al. Randomized evaluation of the safety and efficacy of enoxaparin versus unfractionated heparin in high-risk patients with non-ST-segment elevation acute coronary syndrome receiving the glycoprotein IIb/IIIa inhibitor eptifibatide. *Circulation* 2003;107:238–244.
16. Graff LG, Dallara J, Ross MA, et al. Impact of the care of the emergency department chest pain patient from the Chest Pain Evaluation Registry (CHEPER) study. *Am J Cardiol* 1997;80:563–568.
17. Grines CL, Serruys P, O'Neill WW. Fibrinolytic therapy. Is it a treatment of the past? *Circulation* 2003;107:2538–2542.
18. Hennekens CH, Albert CM, Godried SL, et al. Adjunctive therapy of acute myocardial infarction—evidence from clinical trials. *N Engl J Med* 1996;335:1660–1667.
19. Hirsh J, Warkentin TE, Shaughnessy SG, et al. Heparin and low-molecular-weight heparin. Mechanisms of action, pharmacokinetics, dosing, monitoring, efficacy, and safety. *Chest* 2001;119:64S–94S.
20. Ioannidis JPA, Salem D, Chew PW, et al. Accuracy of imaging technologies in the diagnosis of acute cardiac ischemia in the emergency department: A meta-analysis. *Ann Emerg Med* 2001;37:471–477.
21. Lau J, Ioannidis JPA, Balk EM, et al. Diagnosing acute cardiac ischemia in the emergency department: A systematic review of the accuracy and clinical effect of current technologies. *Ann Emerg Med* 2001;37:453–460.
22. Libby P. Current concepts of the pathogenesis of the acute coronary syndromes. *Circulation* 2001;104:365–372.
23. Llevadot J, Giugliano RP, Antman EM: Bolus fibrinolytic therapy in acute myocardial infarction. *JAMA* 2001;286:442–449.
24. Maseri A, Fuster V: Is there a vulnerable plaque? *Circulation* 2003;107:2068–2071.
25. Panju AA, Hemmelgarn BR, Guyatt GH, et al. Is this patient having a myocardial infarction? *JAMA* 1998;280:1256.
26. Patrono C, Coller B, Dalen JE, et al. Platelet-active drugs. The relationships among dose, effectiveness, and side effects. *Chest* 2001;119:39S–63S.
27. Purcell IF, Newall N, Farrer M. Change in ST segment elevation 60 minutes after thrombolytic initiation predicts clinical outcome as accurately as later electrocardiographic changes. *Heart* 1997;78:465.
28. Ryan TJ, Antman EM, Brooks NH, et al. ACC/AHA Guidelines for the management of patients with acute myocardial infarction. Available at *www.americanheart.org/Scientific/statements/1999/AMI*.
29. The Joint European Society of Cardiology/American College of Cardiology Committee. Myocardial infarction redefined-a consensus document of The Joint European Society of Cardiology/American College of Cardiology Committee for the Redefinition of Myocardial Infarction. *J Am Coll Cardiol* 2000;36:959–969.
30. Sgarbossa EB, Birnbaum Y, Parrillo JE. Electrocardiographic diagnosis of acute myocardial infarction: current concepts for the clinician. *Am Heart J* 2001;141:507–517.
31. Sgarbossa EB, Pinski SL, Barbagelata A, et al. Electrocardiographic diagnosis of evolving acute myocardial infarction in the presence of left bundle-branch block. *N Engl J Med* 1996;334:481.
32. Stein RA, Chaitman BR, Balady GJ, et al. Safety and utility of exercise testing in emergency room chest pain centers. An advisory from the Committee on Exercise, Rehabilitation, and Prevention, Council on Clinical Cardiology, American Heart Association. *Circulation* 2000;102:1463–1467.
33. Yeghiazarians Y, Braunstein JB, Askari A, et al. Unstable angina pectoris. *N Eng J Med* 2000;342:101–114.
34. Zimmerman J, Fromm R, Meyer D, et al. Diagnostic Marker Cooperative Study for the diagnosis of myocardial infarction. *Circulation* 1999;99:1671.
35. Gerschutz GP, Bhatt DL. The Clopidogrel in Unstable Angina to Prevent Recurrent Events (CURE) study: to what extent should the results be generalizable? *Am Heart J* 2003;145:595–601.

CHAPTER 42
Congestive Heart Failure and Cor Pulmonale

James T. Niemann

CONGESTIVE HEART FAILURE (LEFT HEART FAILURE)

Congestive heart failure (CHF) is not a single disease but a symptom complex (8). The *pathophysiologic definition* of heart failure is "that condition or state in which an abnormality of cardiac function is responsible for failure of the heart to pump blood at a rate commensurate to meet the requirements of the metabolizing tissues." The *clinical definition* is broader in its scope; that is, it is "a condition in which ventricular dysfunction is accompanied by reduced exercise capacity." The latter definition incorporates less severe forms of ventricular dysfunction that are manifest only during exercise.

The incidence and prevalence of CHF have increased in recent years, despite an overall decrease in cardiovascular mortality in the United States. It has been estimated that nearly 5 million Americans have CHF. Approximately 30% to 40% of patients with CHF are hospitalized every year, and CHF is the leading diagnostic-related group among hospitalized patients older than age 65. CHF is associated with increasing age, and these numbers are likely to increase as the number of elderly persons in the United States continues to increase. Prognosis after onset of clinical symptoms and signs of CHF has not changed substantially over the last 15 years and the 1-year mortality rate for severely symptomatic CHF (class III or IV) is about 45% (3,9). The cause of death may be the result of disease progression or may be the sudden result of ventricular dysrhythmias. In most of these studies, CHF was attributed to left heart failure (LHF). In this section only LHF is discussed.

The symptoms and signs of LHF are produced by a variety of primary heart diseases as well as systemic diseases that alter left ventricular (LV) anatomy and result in mechanical dysfunction, myocardial contractile failure, or impaired LV filling. The causes of LHF are listed in Table 42.1. Systolic dysfunction, characterized by a low ejection fraction, is the most common form of CHF. Diastolic dysfunction with impaired LV filling has been increasingly recognized as a cause of LHF and is present in 30% to 40% of patients with CHF (19).

With the advent of early and effective therapy for hypertension in the 1970s, coronary artery disease (CAD) has become the major cause of acute or chronic LHF in the United States. LHF caused by CAD may have multiple causes, such as loss of ventricular muscle, intermittent ischemia and contractile dysfunction (e.g., papillary muscle dysfunction), ventricular aneurysm formation with paradoxical expansion and increased wall stress, and decreased ventricular diastolic compliance (8). The cardiomyopathies (dilated, hypertrophic, and restrictive) of both primary (idiopathic) and secondary origins are also becoming an increasingly more frequent cause of heart failure, especially among younger patients (5).

TABLE 42.1.   Functional Classification and Causes of Left Heart Failure

CONTRACTILE DYSFUNCTION

Ischemic heart disease
Idiopathic cardiomyopathy
Myocarditis

SYSTOLIC PRESSURE OVERLOAD

Aortic stenosis
Systemic hypertension

SYSTOLIC VOLUME OVERLOAD

Aortic regurgitation
Mitral regurgitation

RESTRICTED DIASTOLIC FILLING

Mitral stenosis
Left atrial myxoma
Hypertrophic cardiomyopathy

HIGH-OUTPUT STATES

Hyperthyroidism
Anemia
Arteriovenous fistula

A decrease in effective cardiac output (CO) at normal LV filling pressures is the hemodynamic hallmark of LHF. When CO falls because of such factors as loss of muscle and obstruction to outflow, there are three principal compensatory mechanisms that maintain systemic perfusion: (i) the Frank-Starling principal relating preload to contractile force or CO, (ii) ventricular hypertrophy, and (iii) central neural and peripheral neurohumoral responses to maintain systemic perfusion pressure and effective intravascular volume.

An increase in systemic vascular resistance and maintenance of effective intravascular volume are accomplished by means of complex neurohumoral compensatory mechanisms. Hormonal changes that occur during LHF are summarized in Table 42.2. On the basis of measurements of neurohumoral agents in LHF, hemodynamic profiles of patients with LHF, and the response to pharmacologic agents that attenuate neurohumoral responses to a decrease in CO, it has become evident that compensatory mechanisms may be maladaptive; that is, reflex responses further impede ejection of blood from the compromised ventricle. Manipulating the compensatory response to a fall in CO (e.g., use of β-blockers, angiotensin-converting enzyme inhibitors) has become a therapeutic focus in the management of chronic CHF (7,13).

TABLE 42.2.   Neuroendocrine Changes in Left Heart Failure

Increased circulating catecholamines
Increased angiotensin
Increased aldosterone
Increased arginine vasopressin
Increased B-type natriuretic peptide (BNP)
Increased prostaglandin E2 and prostacyclin

CLINICAL PRESENTATION

The typical patient with LHF presents with dyspnea at rest, decreased exercise tolerance, shortness of breath when supine (orthopnea or paroxysmal nocturnal dyspnea), and ankle swelling and weight gain. In acute LHF (acute pulmonary edema), shortness of breath is the major presenting symptom. Clinical findings usually include (i) rales, caused by pulmonary venous hypertension and extravasation of fluid into the pulmonary interstitium and alveoli; (ii) a third heart sound, caused by decreased LV compliance; (iii) a fourth heart sound, caused by forceful atrial contraction to overcome the rise in LV diastolic pressure (not heard in atrial fibrillation); (iv) peripheral edema, the consequence of renal sodium and water retention initiated by hormonal responses; and (v) jugular venous distention (JVD), owing to pulmonary venous hypertension, restricted right ventricular (RV) output, and fluid retention.

No single feature or physical examination finding reliably distinguishes patients with CHF resulting from systolic dysfunction (decreased ejection fraction, typically <40%) from those with diastolic dysfunction (increased left heart filling pressures, pulmonary capillary wedge pressure [PCWP] typically >18 mm Hg) (19). Patients with systolic dysfunction often have increased filling pressures owing to a decrease in compliance as well as a decrease in ejection fraction. In addition, many of the clinical symptoms of LHF (e.g., exercise intolerance and pedal edema) may be caused by isolated right heart failure, primary pulmonary disease, obesity, or poor physical conditioning (1).

Four highly specific clinical findings suggesting a cardiac cause for dyspnea and pedal edema are pulsus alternans (characterized by a regular rhythm with alternating strong and weak ventricular contractions); reduced proportional blood pressure (BP) (defined as [systolic BP – diastolic BP]/systolic BP <0.25); abnormal BP response to the Valsalva maneuver; and JVD at rest or during the hepatojugular reflex test (1).

DIFFERENTIAL DIAGNOSIS

Common causes of LHF are listed in Table 42.1. Constrictive pericarditis and cardiac tamponade are also characterized by impaired diastolic filling and can mimic LHF.

Although systemic hypertension and CAD are the major causes of LHF in the United States, valvular heart disease (see Chapter 46, "Valvular Heart Disease"), especially aortic and mitral valve disease, should be considered in the elderly (aortic sclerosis) and immigrant populations (rheumatic heart disease).

Cardiomyopathies are becoming an increasingly recognized cause of LHF (5). Patients with a dilated or restrictive cardiomyopathy most commonly present with progressive symptoms. An enlarged cardiac silhouette on chest radiograph, and electrocardiographic findings of four-chamber enlargement and intraventricular conduction defects are commonly seen. Only about 10% of patients with dilated cardiomyopathy have an underlying cause determined after extensive evaluation. Most patients are classified as idiopathic; secondary causes of dilated cardiomyopathy are listed in Table 42.3. Common causes for restrictive cardiomyopathy are listed in Table 42.4; this entity is also commonly idiopathic in origin. Patients with hypertrophic cardiomyopathy rarely present with LHF. Dyspnea on exertion, chest pain that may be anginal in character, palpitations, and syncope are the major symptoms and are caused by a combination of diastolic dysfunction, functional outflow obstruction, and a propensity to dysrhythmias.

Myocarditis is an uncommon cause for LHF but should be considered in the patient who presents with subacute signs and symptoms of heart failure and who relates a history of an an-

---

TABLE 42.3.   Causes of Dilated Cardiomyopathy

Idiopathic
Connective tissue disease (e.g., systemic lupus erythematosus, scleroderma)
Neuromuscular disorders (muscular dystrophies)
Infection (viral, parasitic, bacterial)
Metabolic (e.g., beriberi, hyperthyroidism, or hypothyroidism)
Toxic (alcohol, daunorubicin, cocaine)
Miscellaneous (postpartum)

---

tecedent "viral infection." Coxsackievirus A and B are most commonly implicated. These patients often have elevated serum creatine kinase MB fraction (CK-MB) and troponin levels owing to active myocardial inflammation and necrosis (4).

Common causes of sudden worsening of symptoms in patients with chronic stable CHF are listed in Table 42.5 (17).

EMERGENCY DEPARTMENT EVALUATION

Other than a carefully obtained history and physical examination, there are few other diagnostic aids available to the emergency department physician. The posteroanterior chest radiograph is a readily available and often useful ancillary test (1). Radiographic stages that reflect the severity of LHF have been described, but the classic radiographic progression is not always seen. In addition, the chest radiograph may not correlate temporally with the patient's immediate condition; that is, there may be as long as a 12-hour diagnostic lag from the onset of LHF, and a posttherapeutic lag of up to 4 days after clinical resolution.

The earliest radiographic finding is redistribution or "cephalization" of flow. Normally, more blood flow occurs to the dependent portions of the lungs. When PCWP increases to 12 to 18 mm Hg, flow to the lower lung fields is reduced because of the vasoconstriction, and flow to the upper lung fields increases. Redistribution is best detected on an upright film and is most commonly seen in the setting of chronic LHF. When the PCWP is 18 to 25 mm Hg, fluid accumulates in the interstitial spaces, producing Kerley B lines, and the pulmonary vessels are enlarged and their radiographic shadows become blurred. Alveolar edema occurs when the PCWP acutely rises above 25 mm Hg and is recognized by the classic butterfly pattern of bilateral perihilar infiltrates. In all stages, the cardiac silhouette is typically enlarged (cardiothoracic ratio >50%), and, in chronic LHF, pleural effusions are common.

The electrocardiogram (ECG) is of limited diagnostic value. In chronic LHF, the ECG usually shows enlargement or hypertrophy of one or more chambers. An ECG should be performed in patients who present with chest pain to rule out an acute coronary syndrome (ACS). However, intraventricular conduction defects are frequent, and secondary ST-T wave changes caused by ventricular hypertrophy or bundle-branch blocks often preclude accurate diagnosis of acute ischemia or infarction.

TABLE 42.4.   Causes of Restrictive Cardiomyopathy

Idiopathic
Amyloidosis
Hemachromatosis
Sarcoidosis
Scleroderma
Metastatic malignancy
Hypereosinophilic syndrome

TABLE 42.5. Exacerbation of Chronic Congestive Heart Failure: Precipitating Factors

Lack of medications (noncompliance)
Dietary indiscretion (increased sodium intake)
Dysrrhythmias
Myocardial infarction
Infection (increased metabolic demand)
Pulmonary embolism
Anemia
Thyroid disease

Arterial blood gas analysis predictably shows hypoxemia caused by ventilation–perfusion mismatch, but it is of no value in diagnosis and of limited use in guiding therapy. Other blood tests show typical but nondiagnostic abnormalities (e.g., abnormal liver function tests caused by passive hepatic congestion, and hyponatremia caused by retention of excess free water).

B-type natriuretic peptide (BNP) is secreted by the myocardium in response to increased wall stretch and volume overload (an increase in LV end-diastolic pressure), both of which are hallmarks of LHF. BNP is a compensatory peptide with venous, arterial, and coronary vasodilator properties without direct inotropic or chronotropic effects. A rapid BNP immunoassay test is currently available and has been shown to be better than the clinical examination in detecting CHF in emergency department patients and identifying CHF as the etiology of dyspnea of unclear etiology (12).

EMERGENCY DEPARTMENT MANAGEMENT

All patients with LHF should receive supplemental oxygen; an intravenous (i.v.) line should be placed, heart rate and rhythm should be continuously monitored, and the head of the bed should be elevated. Continuous pulse oximetry should also be used, if available. Treatment is directed primarily toward reducing LV preload or filling pressure, and secondarily toward improving myocardial contractility or decreasing afterload. The sequence of drug therapy and the pace of acute intervention depend on the severity of symptoms (7).

Patients with mild-to-moderate LHF usually have typical symptoms of varying duration. On examination, patients are normotensive or hypertensive and have bibasilar rales, JVD, third and fourth heart sounds, and pedal edema. Murmurs caused by underlying valvular disease may also be heard. Emergency department therapy includes i.v. furosemide (80 mg) to induce diuresis and sublingual (0.8 to 1.2 mg), oral (20 to 40 mg), or transdermal nitroglycerin (1–2 inches) to increase venous capacitance and lower preload. Urine output and BP should be monitored to detect the response to diuresis as well as any complications of excessive preload reduction (e.g., hypotension). Because of the renal vasoconstriction caused by decreased CO, an increase in urine output after diuretic administration may not be immediate and may be delayed for 30 to 60 minutes. If a supraventricular tachydysrhythmia other than sinus tachycardia is present, controlling the ventricular response rate to facilitate ventricular filling also decreases preload and improves CO. The most common supraventricular tachydysrhythmia (excluding sinus tachycardia) encountered in LHF is atrial fibrillation, owing to atrial injury or atrial distention. It is usually chronic in duration, and urgent cardioversion is neither necessary nor likely to be effective. The ventricular response rate, if uncontrolled, can be slowed quickly with an i.v. calcium channel blocker (e.g., diltiazem), amiodarone, or a β-blocker if not contraindicated (6). Mild hypertension caused by neural and hormonal compensatory responses is common in the mildly to moderately symptomatic patient and usually responds to diuresis and preload reduction alone. Aggressive afterload reduction (e.g., nitroprusside infusion) is usually required only when acute CHF is the result of a hypertensive crisis.

Acute pulmonary edema is LHF in its most extreme form and is a life-threatening emergency. The typical patient is anxious, severely dyspneic, diaphoretic, pale, cool, and clammy. Inspiratory rales and wheezes may be heard over all lung fields. A summation gallop may be heard on cardiac auscultation, and JVD is common. Hypertension is usual and is caused by the intense vasoconstriction. Other peripheral signs (e.g., pedal edema and hepatomegaly) may be present if acute decompensation is superimposed on chronic LHF.

Immediate therapy in the normotensive or hypertensive patient with acute pulmonary edema should include furosemide (80 mg i.v.) and i.v. nitroglycerin (5 to 200 μg/minute) (7,16). The transdermal route (e.g., nitroglycerin paste or patch) should not be used, because there is limited skin perfusion in acute pulmonary edema. Nesiritide is a recombinant BNP that is identical to the endogenous hormone produced in the ventricles with identical hemodynamic effects. BNP binds to the guanylate cyclase receptor of vascular smooth muscle and endothelial cells, leading to increased intracellular concentrations of cyclic guanosine monophosphate (cGMP) and smooth muscle cell relaxation. cGMP serves as a second messenger to dilate veins and arteries. Clinical trials have not demonstrated a conclusive benefit of nesiritide greater than that of nitroglycerin in patients with acutely decompensated LHF (2,15). It may be of value in patients who fail to respond to conventional therapy. Nesiritide is administered as an i.v. bolus of 2 μg/kg, followed by a continuous infusion of 0.01 μg/kg/minute. Depending upon the clinical or hemodynamic response, the infusion rate can be increased by 0.005 μg/kg/minute every 3 hours, preceded by a bolus of 1 μg/kg. The maximum dosage is 0.03 μg/kg/minute.

Morphine sulfate administered in small i.v. doses (2-mg increments) is a time-honored therapeutic agent in acute pulmonary edema. Although morphine is a venodilator, its effects on venous capacitance have not been well-established in the setting of acute pulmonary edema caused by LHF, and respiratory depression may occur at doses that do not affect hemodynamic variables. An inhaled selective β-agonist can be used if severe bronchospasm is present. Theophylline preparations should be avoided because of their dysrhythenogenicity. If BP remains severely elevated after initial improvement in symptoms, afterload reduction with nitroprusside, infused at a rate titrated to desired response, or enalaprilat, 1.25 mg every 6 hours, can be used. If the patient is hypotensive at the time of presentation, inotropic agents should precede the use of venodilators and diuretics (7). Dopamine (initial infusion rate of 5 to 10 μg/kg/minute) or a combination of dopamine and dobutamine (each infused at an initial rate of 5 to 10 μg/kg/minute) can be used.

Endotracheal intubation may be required if pulmonary edema is accompanied by severe hypoxemia that does not improve during early treatment. The most reliable indication of life-threatening hypoxemia is a decreasing level of consciousness, although it is a relatively insensitive sign. Noninvasive ventilation may reduce the need for intubation (14). Continuous positive airway pressure (CPAP) at 5 to 10 cm H_2O has been shown to decrease the intubation rate and decrease mortality in hypoxic respiratory failure caused by acute pulmonary edema. Benefit presumably results from recruitment of atelectatic alveoli, thereby increasing pulmonary compliance and decreasing the work of breathing. The use of bilevel positive airway pressure (BiPAP) has been associated with a higher incidence of acute myocardial infarction in patients with pulmonary edema.

CRITICAL INTERVENTIONS

- A rapid BNP immunoassay has been shown to be better than the clinical examination in detecting CHF in emergency department patients and identifying CHF as the etiology of dyspnea of unclear etiology
- Aggressive and early administration of nitroglycerin and diuretics in normotensive and hypertensive patients with pulmonary edema often rapidly reverses the clinical course
- CPAP at 5 to 10 cm H_2O decreases the intubation rate and mortality in hypoxic respiratory failure caused by acute pulmonary edema

DISPOSITION

All patients with acute pulmonary edema should be admitted to an intensive care unit. Invasive hemodynamic monitoring may be required in patients who do not respond to emergency department therapy. Patients with chronic LHF and a mild worsening of symptoms who respond to i.v. diuretics may be discharged after adjustments in the chronic drug regimen (e.g., an increase in the furosemide dose), consultation with the patient's physician regarding medication changes, and assurance of followup within 24 to 48 hours. Patients with more severe symptoms or other complicating factors (e.g., new rhythm disturbances, poorly controlled hypertension, or a suspected acute myocardial ischemic event) should be admitted for observation, evaluation, and optimization of drug therapy. Typical indications for admission are listed in Table 42.6 (10). If an interfacility transfer is required, the patient should be stabilized first.

COMMON PITFALLS

- ✔ The signs and symptoms of cor pulmonale and acute respiratory failure are similar to those of LHF, and, in some cases, it may not be possible to distinguish between these conditions by physical examination alone
- ✔ In the patient with CHF and atrial fibrillation with a rapid ventricular response, digoxin alone should not be used. Slowing of the ventricular response rate is usually not seen for approximately 8 hours after administration
- ✔ RV infarction should always be considered in the patient with an acute inferior wall infarction who has clear lung sounds, JVD, hypotension, and a normal heart rate and rhythm. Increasing venous capacitance in this setting decreases RV filling pressures and further decreases CO. RV infarction can be diagnosed with a right precordial ECG. ST-segment elevation is typically seen in leads V_{3R} and V_{4R} (see Chapter 41, "Acute Coronary Syndromes")
- ✔ If the cardiac silhouette is not enlarged, but other radiographic findings of LHF are seen, the failure is most likely to be of acute onset and caused by valvular disease (e.g., aortic insufficiency resulting from endocarditis, papillary muscle rupture in patients with mitral valve prolapse, valvular dysfunction in patients with prosthetic valves, or acute myocardial infarction). Noncardiogenic pulmonary edema should also be considered

- ✔ CHF is a complex physiologic state. There are a number of drugs that can alleviate symptoms, improve quality of life, and increase long-term survival. However, these drugs have well-described complications. Altering a patient's medical regimen by adding a new medication prior to discharge from the emergency department should not be undertaken without consultation with the patient's primary physician, in order to assure followup monitoring of drug effect

CHRONIC COR PULMONALE (PULMONARY HEART DISEASE)

Chronic cor pulmonale has been defined as a combination of RV hypertrophy and dilatation caused by increased resistance of the pulmonary circulation (pulmonary hypertension) (18) owing to intrinsic pulmonary disease, inadequate function of the chest bellows, or inadequate ventilatory drive from the respiratory centers. Implicit in this definition is the exclusion of congenital heart disease and LHF as causes. Although cor pulmonale may be acute (most commonly caused by pulmonary thromboembolism), only the chronic form is discussed herein. Causes of chronic cor pulmonale are listed in Table 42.7. In the United States, chronic bronchitis and emphysema are the major causes of chronic cor pulmonale, and the yearly incidence of these diseases is approximately ten per 1 million persons. At autopsy, cor pulmonale is estimated to occur in 40% of patients with emphysema or bronchitis. Cor pulmonale is estimated to account for 7% to 10% of all heart disease.

The hemodynamic hallmark of cor pulmonale is pulmonary hypertension (elevated pulmonary artery pressure), which may either manifest at rest and worsen with exercise or occur only during exercise. Increased pulmonary vascular resistance is the result of a reduction in the size of the effective cross-sectional area of the pulmonary vascular bed because of obstruction or

TABLE 42.6.   Acute Exacerbation of CHF: Admission Criteria

Clinical or ECG evidence of acute myocardial ischemia
Pulmonary edema or severe respiratory distress
Oxygen saturation <90% (not caused by pulmonary disease)
Severe complicating medical illness (e.g., pneumonia)
Anasarca
Symptomatic hypotension or syncope
Heart failure refractory to outpatient therapy
Inadequate social support for safe outpatient management

CHF, congestive heart failure; ECG, electrocardiographic.

TABLE 42.7.   Causes of Chronic Cor Pulmonale

DISEASES THAT PRIMARILY AFFECT AIR PASSAGES

Chronic bronchitis/emphysema
Bronchial asthma
Pulmonary fibrosis (e.g., pneumoconiosis)
Granulomas and infiltrates (e.g., sarcoid)
Pulmonary resection
Congenital cystic disease
High-altitude hypoxia

DISEASES THAT PRIMARILY AFFECT CHEST BELLOWS

Kyphoscoliosis
Thoracoplasty
Pleural fibrosis
Chronic neuromuscular weakness
Obesity

DISEASES THAT PRIMARILY AFFECT PULMONARY VASCULATURE

Primary pulmonary hypertension
Pulmonary embolism
Polyarteritis nodosa
Other arterites

destruction and is usually combined with active vasoconstriction. Hypoxemia is a potent pulmonary vasoconstrictor, and concurrent hypercapnia and acidemia are synergistic. Most causes of cor pulmonale are accompanied by these gas exchange and acid–base abnormalities. The rise in pulmonary vascular resistance impedes RV ejection, and a compensatory response results in hypertrophy or dilatation and increased preload.

CLINICAL PRESENTATION

The underlying disease process largely determines the clinical manifestations of cor pulmonale, and symptoms of pulmonary dysfunction most often precede manifestations of right heart failure.

Common symptoms include dyspnea at rest or with minimal exertion, weight gain, ankle swelling, and, in severe cases, abdominal swelling caused by ascites. Physical signs usually include bibasilar crackles and scattered wheezes (caused by lung disease, not interstitial fluid accumulation) on auscultation. The pulmonic component of the second heart sound may be palpable, and the jugular vein may fill paradoxically during inspiration or exhibit no respiratory fluctuations. Tricuspid insufficiency may be present, manifested by a systolic murmur heard best at the lower left sternal border and increasing with inspiration; this is often accompanied by the finding of a pulsatile liver edge.

DIFFERENTIAL DIAGNOSIS

The signs and symptoms of cor pulmonale may mimic those of LHF, constrictive pericarditis, and cardiac tamponade. Severe and advanced mitral stenosis may present with predominant right heart failure or "silent mitral stenosis." When signs and symptoms of cor pulmonale are of abrupt onset, acute pulmonary thromboembolism should be considered.

EMERGENCY DEPARTMENT EVALUATION

The chest radiograph usually shows only evidence of the underlying pulmonary disorder, but it may be helpful in diagnosing the cause of an acute exacerbation (e.g., pulmonary infiltrate). The ECG is not a sensitive test for detecting RV hypertrophy or dilatation, but some findings are reasonably specific. These include a P-pulmonale pattern (P-wave amplitude of at least 2.5 mm in lead II), right-axis deviation, R/S amplitude ratio in V_1 of greater than 1, low-voltage QRS, and right bundle-branch block pattern (10). Failure to detect radiographic or electrocardiographic evidence of RV hypertrophy or dilatation does not rule out the diagnosis. Arterial blood gas analysis usually shows some combination of hypoxemia, hypercapnia, and acidemia. Liver function tests may be abnormal because of passive hepatic congestion. Pulmonary function tests are always abnormal, and the typical patient has a forced expiratory volume in 1 second of less than 1 L. BNP may also be elevated.

EMERGENCY DEPARTMENT MANAGEMENT

Most patients who present with an acute exacerbation of chronic cor pulmonale have acute respiratory failure caused by the worsening or progression of the underlying lung disease. Therapeutic efforts should be directed toward reversing reactive pulmonary vasoconstriction (i.e., improving oxygenation, decreasing hypercarbia, and normalizing pH) (11). Therapy is usually the same as that employed in acute respiratory failure resulting from emphy-

sema or chronic bronchitis. Such therapy should include administration of low-flow oxygen, corticosteroids, and antibiotics and inhaled and systemic bronchodilation (see Chapter 36, "Chronic Obstructive Pulmonary Disease").

DISPOSITION

Role of the Consultant

An acute worsening of chronic cor pulmonale is usually caused by acute respiratory failure. Acute respiratory failure is a life-threatening emergency, and immediate treatment should be instituted before consultation.

Indications for Admission

Indications for admission for an exacerbation of chronic cor pulmonale are usually the same as for acute respiratory failure (see Chapter 33).

COMMON PITFALLS

✔ Clinical symptoms and signs of LHF and cor pulmonale overlap. Administering high-flow oxygen to a patient with suspected LHF who has cor pulmonale may result in worsening of clinical status, because the hypoxic drive is suppressed and hypercapnia worsens

✔ Diagnosis of cor pulmonale cannot be excluded simply by the absence of electrocardiographic or radiographic findings of RV hypertrophy or dilatation

✔ Emergency treatment should be directed toward improving pulmonary function and decreasing pulmonary vascular resistance, rather than toward alleviating signs of right heart failure (e.g., aggressive diuresis, which may decrease RV preload and worsen left heart outflow)

✔ Patients with obstructive sleep apnea typically present with manifestations similar to those of chronic cor pulmonale. A careful history is helpful in suggesting the diagnosis and appropriate referral

References

1. Badgett RG, Lucey CR, Mulrow CD. Can the clinical examination diagnose left-sided heart failure in adults? *JAMA* 1997;277:1712.
2. Colucci WS, Elkayam U, Horton DP, et al, for the Nesiritide Study Group. Intravenous nesiritide, a natriuretic peptide, in the treatment of decompensated congestive heart failure. *N Engl J Med* 2000;343:246–253.
3. Deedwania PC. The key to unraveling the mystery of mortality in heart failure. An integrated approach. *Circulation* 2003;107:1719–1721.
4. Feldman AM, McNamara D. Myocarditis. *N Engl J Med* 2000;343;1388–1398.
5. Franz W, Muller OJ, Katus HA. Cardiomyopathies: from genetics to the prospect of treatment. *Lancet* 2001;358:1627–1637.
6. Fuster V, Ryden LE, Asinger RW, et al. ACC/AHA/ESC guidelines for the management of patients with atrial fibrillation. 2001. Available at: http://www.acc.org.
7. Hunt SA, Baker DW, Chin MH, et al. ACC/AHA guidelines for the evaluation and management of chronic heart failure in the adult. 2001. Available at: http://www.acc.org.
8. Jessup M, Brozena S. Heart failure. *N Engl J Med* 2003;348:2007–2018.
9. Khand A, Gemmel I, Clark AL, et al. Is the prognosis of heart failure improving? *J Am Coll Cardiol* 2000;36:2284–2286.
10. Hunt SA, Baker DW, Chin MH, et al. ACC/AHA guidelines for the evaluation and management of chronic heart failure in the adult: a report of the American College of Cardiology/American Heart Association Task Force on Practice Guidelines (Committee to Revise the 1995 guidelines for the evaluation and management of heart failure), 2001. Available at: http://www.acc.org/clinical/guidelines/failure/hf_index.htm.
11. Langford NJ, Kendall MJ. Pulmonary heart disease–the need for evidence-based management. *J Clin Pharm Ther* 2000;25:157–159.
12. Maisel AS, Krishnaswamy P, Nowak RM, et al, for the Breathing Not Properly Multinational Study Investigators. Rapid measurement of B-type natriuretic peptide in the emergency diagnosis of heart failure. *N Engl J Med* 2002;347:161–167.

13. McMurray J, Pfeffer MA. New therapeutic options in congestive heart failure: Part I. *Circulation* 2002;105:2099–2106. Part II. *Circulation* 2002;105:2223–2228.

14. Pang D, Keenan SP, Cook DJ, et al. The effect of positive pressure airway support on mortality and the need for intubation in cardiogenic pulmonary edema. A systematic review. *Chest* 1998;114:1185.

15. Publication Committee for the VMAC Investigators. Intravenous nesiritide vs nitroglycerin for treatment of decompensated congestive heart failure. A randomized controlled trial. *JAMA* 2002;287:1531–1540.

16. Sacchetti AD, Harris RH. Acute cardiogenic pulmonary edema. *Postgrad Med* 1998;103:145.

17. Schiff GD, Fung S, Speroff T, et al. Decompensated heart failure: symptoms, patterns of onset, and contributing factors. *Am J Med* 2003;114:625–630.

18. Weitzenblum E. Chronic cor pulmonale. *Heart* 2003;89:225–230.

19. Zile MR, Brutsaert DL. New concepts in diastolic dysfunction and diastolic heart failure: Part I. Diagnosis, prognosis, and measurements of diastolic function. *Circulation* 2002;105:1387–1393. Part II. Causal mechanisms and treatment. *Circulation* 2002;105:1503–1508.

CHAPTER 43
Bradydysrhythmias

David Hartman and David T. Overton

The cardiac conduction system consists of pacemaker cells, conducting cells, and contractile cells. *Pacemaker cells* possess the capacity to spontaneously depolarize (termed *automaticity*). The *sinoatrial* (S-A or sinus node), normally the predominant pacemaker of the heart, is located at the junction of the right atrium and the superior vena cava and has an intrinsic basal rate of 60 to 100 bpm. The S-A node is innervated by both sympathetic and parasympathetic nerves, which alter its discharge rate. Its arterial blood supply is either from the right coronary artery (55%) or the left circumflex artery (45%).

The atrioventricular (AV) node, located beneath the right atrial endocardium superior to the insertion of the septal leaflet of the tricuspid valve, can also function as a pacemaker, with an intrinsic rate of 45 to 60 beats per minute. The arterial blood supply of the AV node is from the posterior descending artery of the right coronary artery (90%) or the left circumflex artery (10%). This becomes clinically relevant in the AV nodal dysrhythmias associated with acute inferior myocardial infarction. The AV node fires in the absence of sinus node impulses, or it may itself usurp control from the sinus node. Other cells in the bundle branches and Purkinje network can function as pacemakers as well, but their intrinsic rate is quite low, approximately 30 to 40 bpm.

Electrical impulses in the heart travel over a network of *conducting cells*. Impulses normally originate in the sinus node. Passage through the AV node is relatively slow, accounting for a normal physiologic delay in ventricular depolarization. The AV node blends into the bundle of His, which divides into bundle branches. They, in turn, arborize into a network of Purkinje fibers that transmit impulses to the ventricular myocardial *contractile cells*. Contractile cells in the atria and the ventricles do not depolarize spontaneously.

The electrocardiographic P wave represents atrial depolarization. The P-R interval (normally 0.12 to 0.20 seconds in the adult) reflects intraatrial, AV nodal, and His–Purkinje conduction. The QRS complex, representing ventricular depolarization, has a normal duration of 0.04 to 0.10 seconds, and the following T wave represents ventricular repolarization. The U wave is seen in a variety of circumstances, such as hypokalemia. Its electrophysiologic basis is uncertain. Two basic pathophysiologic mechanisms underlie the production of both tachydysrhythmias and bradydysrhythmias: *disorders of impulse formation* and *disorders of impulse conduction*. Depressed *automaticity* may result in bradydysrhythmias, such as sinus bradycardia or sinus arrest. If S-A node automaticity is sufficiently depressed, escape rhythms originating elsewhere in the heart may assume control. Depressed *impulse conduction* may lead to AV or fascicular blocks.

EMERGENCY DEPARTMENT EVALUATION AND MANAGEMENT

When approaching patients with bradydysrhythmias, as with any patient, the priorities of airway, breathing, and circulation must be addressed first. The urgency and means of treating bradydysrhythmias depend on how symptomatic the dysrhythmia is, the clinical setting in which the dysrhythmia occurs, the propensity for the dysrhythmia to progress, and concurrent drug therapy. Bradydysrhythmias may produce hypotension, lightheadedness, dizziness, fatigue, mental status changes, angina, congestive heart failure, syncope, or even convulsions. Prompt therapy using electronic pacing or intravenous medications is required for these symptoms, which are caused by hypoperfusion of the end-organs affected. However, many dysrhythmias are asymptomatic and require no treatment. A dysrhythmia that occurs during an acute myocardial infarction often mandates a different treatment approach than a dysrhythmia incidentally discovered during a routine physical examination. Electrolyte imbalances and many drugs (e.g., digitalis, β-blockers, calcium channel blockers, gatifloxacin [9], and amiodarone [5]) may cause bradydysrhythmias, and each has its own implications for treatment (1,3,4,8,10). Sleep apnea may also be a cause of bradycardia (6). Symptomatic bradycardias are increasingly common with advancing age. General supportive measures such as oxygenation, ventilation, and correction of electrolyte abnormalities are usually the first step. Specific drug therapy or artificial cardiac pacing may also be required.

Among drug therapies, the cornerstone is atropine sulfate, a vagolytic agent that enhances sinus node automaticity and AV nodal conduction. The usual adult dose is 0.5 to 1.0 mg intravenous push every 3 to 5 minutes to a total maximum dose of 0.04 mg/kg (3 mg) in the adult. Atropine is effective when administered via the endotracheal route; the suggested dose is 2.0 to 2.5 times the recommended intravenous dose diluted in 10 mL of normal saline. Because atropine can increase myocardial oxygen consumption, it should be used with caution in the presence of myocardial ischemia. Adverse effects include sinus tachycardia, ventricular tachycardia, or ventricular fibrillation, as well as manifestations of anticholinergic toxicity. In the patient with high-degree AV block, one may also see, in rare instances, a marked reduction in the heart rate after atropine use.

Isoproterenol, a β-adrenergic sympathomimetic drug with potent inotropic and chronotropic effects, is only used rarely currently, having been largely supplanted by the widespread availability of transcutaneous pacing. Still, isoproterenol may be useful as a temporary measure when other options fail. It is administered as an infusion at a rate of 2 to 10 mg/minute. Isoproterenol markedly increases myocardial oxygen demand and may cause significant adverse effects, including ventricular tachycardia or fibrillation.

Glucagon has been found to be beneficial in treating bradydysrhythmias secondary to β-adrenergic blocking agents and calcium channel blockers. The drug appears to be effective in both toxic and nontoxic patients. Glucagon stimulates the S-A node, resulting in a modest increase in the heart rate. It increases automaticity at the AV node, which may be helpful in slow junctional rhythms. Glucagon has also been shown to increase cardiac contractility, thereby increasing coronary perfusion. The peak action of glucagon occurs approximately 5 to 10 minutes after intravenous administration. Suggested initial dosing ranges are 0.05 to 0.10 mg/kg in children and 0.05 to 0.15 mg/kg in adults. This may be repeated based on the clinical situation and the characteristics of the offending medication.

If drug therapy is ineffective, artificial pacing may be instituted. Transcutaneous pacing is more easily performed than internal pacing, and should be attempted first. Emergent temporary pacing may improve organ perfusion and cognitive function (7).

DISORDERS OF IMPLUSE FORMATION

Atrial Bradydysrhythmias

Sinus dysrhythmia is a physiologic finding commonly seen in healthy young people in which the sinus discharge rate decreases with expiration and increases with inspiration. It is thought to be caused by changes in vagal tone during respiration. P-wave morphology and P-R intervals are usually constant. No treatment is indicated.

Sinus bradycardia, arbitrarily defined as a sinus rhythm of less than 60 bpm, may be the result of organic heart disease, and may cause symptoms, but it is also a common finding in healthy patients and particularly in conditioned athletes. Studies have found that 50% to 85% of conditioned athletes have benign sinus bradycardia, compared to 23% of the general population (2). The significance of sinus bradycardia depends on the clinical setting. It is common during therapy with digitalis and β-blockers, and may not warrant intervention. The following findings should suggest nonphysiologic sinus bradycardia: (i) profound bradycardia in an individual not engaged in strenuous endurance training, (ii) sinus pauses longer than 3 seconds on a Holter monitor, or (iii) syncope or near-syncope at rest or after strenuous exercise (2). When sinus bradycardia is symptomatic, treatment with atropine is usually successful. Cardiac pacing and other drug therapies are sometimes necessary.

The *sick sinus syndrome* encompasses a spectrum of conditions, including severe sinus bradycardia, sinoatrial block, sinus arrest, and the bradycardia–tachycardia syndrome. The latter refers to the intermittent occurrence of bradydysrhythmias and tachydysrhythmias (e.g., atrial fibrillation, flutter, or paroxysmal supraventricular tachycardia) in the same patient. The bradydysrhythmia typically occurs immediately after resolution of an episode of tachycardia. Symptoms such as syncope or chest pain may result from either the tachycardia or the bradycardia. Effective pharmacologic therapy for tachycardia can exacerbate the bradycardia, so cardiac pacing must often be initiated before pharmacologic therapy.

Atrioventricular Nodal Bradydysrhythmias

An AV *junctional rhythm* may be a physiologic rhythm initiated by the AV node in the absence of an adequate sinus stimulus, or may result from an abnormally rapid AV junctional focus that usurps control from the sinus node (e.g., accelerated junctional rhythm). Junctional rhythms usually exhibit a QRS morphology that is the same as the patient's sinus rhythm. The P waves are usually inverted if they are conducted in a retrograde manner, and can fall before, during, or after the QRS complex, depending on the location of the focus within the AV junction and the degree of retrograde AV block. When the P wave occurs before the QRS complex, the P-R interval is usually less than 0.12 second. The absence of P waves may be caused by obliteration by the QRS complex or by retrograde block.

AV *junctional escape* beats occur singly or multiply in the absence of stimuli arriving at the AV node (Fig. 43.1). Their hallmark is occurrence after an interval longer than the dominant cycle. The underlying disorder may be sinus bradycardia, sinus arrest, sinus exit block, or AV block. Digitalis or β-blocker therapy may also be responsible. Junctional escape rhythms may also be incidental findings in otherwise healthy people with increased vagal tone. Treatment is not indicated for asymptomatic patients with infrequent escape beats. If symptoms occur, the clinician should treat the underlying rhythm rather than attempt to obliterate the escape beats, as pharmacotherapy to obliterate the AV nodal escape beats could lead to asystole. Treatment involves withholding offending drugs or using atropine or artificial pacing.

Ventricular Bradydysrhythmias

A ventricular rhythm with a rate of less than 50 bpm is termed a *ventricular escape rhythm*, or idioventricular rhythm. Ventricular escape rhythm represents a physiologic safety mechanism that arises in the absence of stimuli from above, as in sinus bradycardia, sinus arrest, or, more commonly, AV block. Most patients with ventricular escape are symptomatic because the heart rate is low. Treatment is directed at the underlying dysrhythmia (i.e., atropine, or most often, cardiac pacing). Lidocaine, which may abolish the ventricular rhythm, is contraindicated, because it has the potential for causing cardiac standstill.

Also known as idioventricular tachycardia or slow ventricular tachycardia, *accelerated idioventricular rhythm* has a rate of 50 to 100 bpm. It is one cause of isorhythmic dissociation, with occasional fusion beats demonstrating the continued presence of an intact AV node (Fig. 43.2). It may be associated with acute myocardial infarction (particularly after thrombolysis), but it may also be seen in otherwise healthy patients. In the absence of symptoms, specific therapy is not warranted.

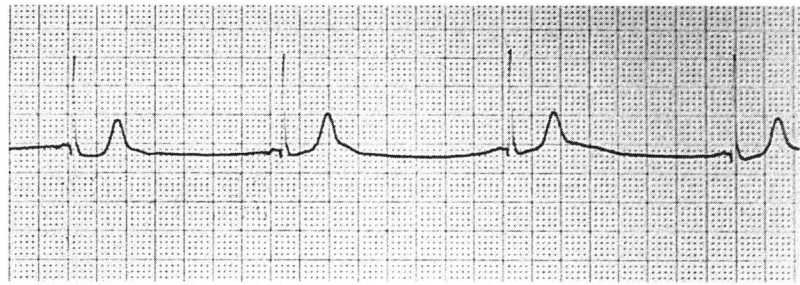

Figure 43.1. Junctional escape rhythm.

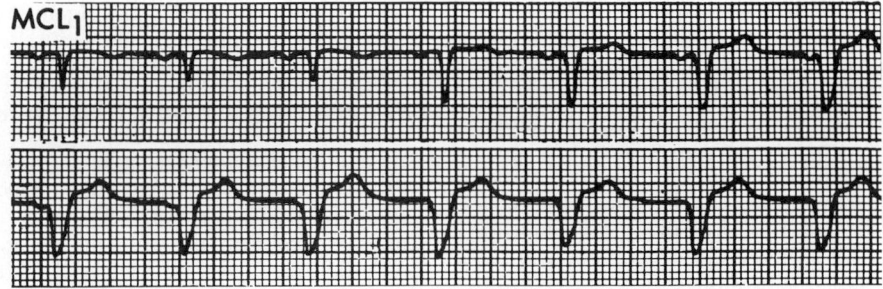

Figure 43.2.   Idioventricular rhythm, with isorhythmic dissociation and fusion beats.

DISTURBANCES OF CONDUCTION

Disorders of Sinoatrial Conduction

The tissue surrounding the sinus node may delay or prevent conduction of sinus node impulses to the atria and AV node. Such conduction disorders are termed *sinoatrial blocks* and are classified in a manner analogous to AV block. However, because of the limitations of the surface electrocardiogram (ECG), their precise diagnosis is more difficult than the varieties of AV block.

In *first-degree sinoatrial block*, there is a delay in the propagation of the sinus node impulse out to the atrial myocardium. However, every beat is transmitted, and no abnormality is detected on the surface ECG.

Similar to AV block, second-degree sinoatrial block may be divided into types I and II. In *type I* (Wenckebach), there is, with each succeeding beat, a progressive delay in conduction from the sinus node to the atria, until conduction in totally blocked and a P wave is dropped (Fig. 43.3). The P-P interval shortens progressively before the dropped P wave, analogous to the situation in second-degree AV block, in which the R-R interval shortens before the dropped QRS complex.

In *type II* second-degree sinoatrial block, there is intermittent failure of the sinus impulse to reach the atria, resulting in a missing P wave and a sudden lengthening of the P-P interval. The resulting P-P interval is usually a multiple of the previous one, which is doubled in the case of 2:1 block (Fig. 43.4). This disorder can be mimicked by blocked premature atrial contractions, in which the P wave is obscured by the preceding T wave (Fig. 43.5).

Third-degree sinoatrial block, in which there is a failure of any sinus node impulses to be conducted to the atria (Fig. 43.6), is usually indistinguishable from sinus arrest, in which there is a failure of impulses to arise from the sinus node.

Disorders of Atrioventricular Conduction

Traditionally, AV blocks have been divided into first, second, and third degree. However, AV block is a relative phenomenon, and the physiologic delay normally present in the AV node is one end of a continuum. For example, in the patient with atrial flutter, "normal" AV conduction usually results in 2:1 block. In addition, the degree of block is rate-dependent. One patient with mild AV disease may exhibit second-degree block at a particularly fast supraventricular rate, whereas another patient with more advanced AV nodal disease may exhibit 1:1 conduction if the supraventricular rate is lower.

A P-R interval of more than 0.20 second defines *first-degree* AV block. All P waves are conducted, 1:1 AV conduction in maintained, and the P-P and R-R intervals are consistent. Most commonly, the delay in AV conduction is within the AV node, and the QRS complex is of normal duration. Delays within the His bundle or His–Purkinje system are less common and are usually associated with widened bundle-branch block QRS patterns.

First-degree AV block may be associated with electrolyte disturbances or the use of digitalis, β-blockers, or calcium channel blockers. It may be seen during acute myocardial infarction, particularly inferior myocardial infarction. Treatment includes correction of electrolyte abnormalities or removal of the responsible drug. During acute myocardial infarction, close observation is warranted to detect progression to higher degrees of block. Otherwise, specific treatment is not indicated.

Second-degree AV block can be divided into Mobitz types I and II. Wenckebach distinguished between these two in the pre-ECG era, by using only physical observation (11).

Mobitz type I (Wenckebach) second-degree AV block is characterized by repeated cycles of progressively slowing AV conduction until conduction is totally blocked. This pattern is manifested electrocardiographically by progressive prolongation of successive P-R intervals until there is a nonconducted P wave,

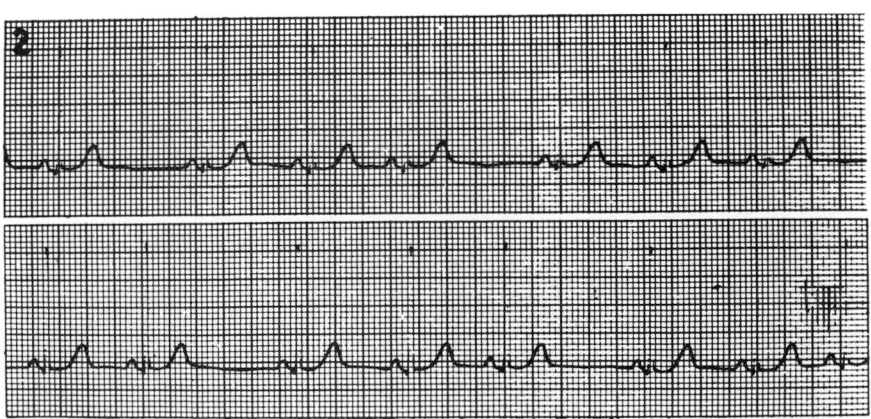

Figure 43.3.   Type I (Wenckebach) sinoatrial block.

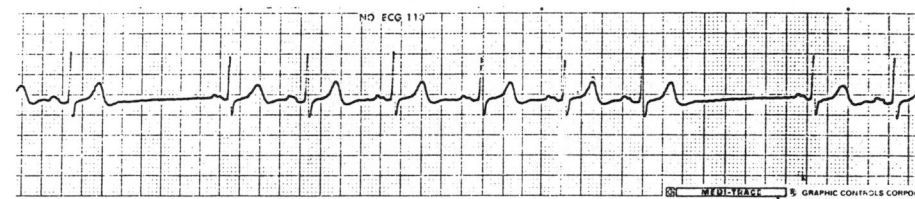

Figure 43.4.   Type II sinoatrial block 2:1.

after which the cycle repeats itself (Fig. 43.7). The cycle is referred to by the ratio of P waves to QRS complexes (i.e., 4:3. 3:2, and so on). Classically the R-R interval shortness as the P-R interval lengthens.

Type I block usually results from conduction delay in the AV node, although delays may occur in the bundle of His, bundle branches, or Purkinje system. For this reason, the QRS complex in Type I block is most often of normal duration. It may be associated with inferior myocardial infarction or the use of digitalis, β-blockers, and calcium channel blockers. Mobitz type I AV block is usually transient and asymptomatic and has a good prognosis. If it is symptomatic, atropine can be given to enhance AV nodule conduction, and pacing is usually not necessary. Offending drugs may need to be withheld.

Mobitz type II second-degree AV block is less common. The site of block is usually within the His–Purkinje system, and, thus a bundle-branch block QRS pattern is usually seen. In type II block, the P-R intervals are constant until single or multiple beats are suddenly dropped (Fig. 43.8). Type II block is usually symptomatic and has a higher likelihood of progressing to complete AV block. If associated with acute anterior myocardial infarction, it carries an ominous prognosis. Most authorities agree that Mobitz type II second-degree AV block requires permanent cardiac pacing. Because emergency drug treatment is often ineffective, temporary pacing may be necessary as a stabilizing measure.

A particular clinical problem is presented by the patient with 2:1 AV block. Although it is often assumed that such patients have type II block, type I block often presents as 2:1 block. The distinction is important, given the difference in prognosis and treatment between the two entities. Although definitive proof may require intracardiac recordings, the following principles may aid in the clinical distinction:

- Type I block is more common than type II.
- A narrow QRS complex usually reflects a type I block (although not all type I blocks have a narrow QRS complex). Type II block usually has a wide QRS complex.
- Coexistent acute inferior myocardial infarction suggests type I block, whereas anterior myocardial infarction suggests type II block.

- Digitalis, β-blocker, or calcium channel blocker therapy tends to be associated with type I block.
- Other areas of the rhythm strip may reflect other patterns of type I conduction, such as 3:2 or 4:3.

In *third-degree (complete) AV block,* no atrial impulses reach the ventricles, and a subsidiary, escape pacemaker usually emerges. AV dissociation results, with constant but independent P-P intervals and R-R intervals. The P-R intervals are variable, and P waves have no discernible relation to QRS complexes (Fig. 43.9). The site of block may be within the AV node, His bundle, bundle branches, or Purkinje system. In general, the lower the site of the block, the more severe the symptoms.

Third-degree AV block may be intermittent or self-limited. If it complicates drug therapy, it usually resolves on withdrawal of the offending agent. It may be associated with acute myocardial infarction, but occasionally it is an asymptomatic finding in an otherwise healthy person.

Like other bradydysrhythmias, the emergent treatment of third-degree AV block depends on symptomatology and clinical setting. Symptomatic patients may improve with atropine, particularly if the block is within the AV node. Symptomatic patients who are unresponsive to pharmacologic therapy require emergent pacing. Stable patients with acute inferior infarction may require only a prophylactic pacemaker. Acute anterior infarction complicated by third-degree AV block is more ominous and requires emergent pacing.

The term *AV dissociation,* although commonly used interchangeably with the term *third-degree AV block,* actually encompasses a much broader range of rhythms. AV dissociation implies that the atria and ventricles are beating independently, a situation that includes not only complete AV block, but also accelerated junctional and idioventricular rhythms (including ventricular tachycardia). In *isorhythmic dissociation* (Fig. 43.10), the sinus rate and the escape or ectopic rate are nearly identical, producing an electrocardiographic pattern characterized by varying P-R intervals as the sinus and ectopic foci slowly change their relative firing rates. Occasional fusion beats are an indication that the cause is not complete AV block.

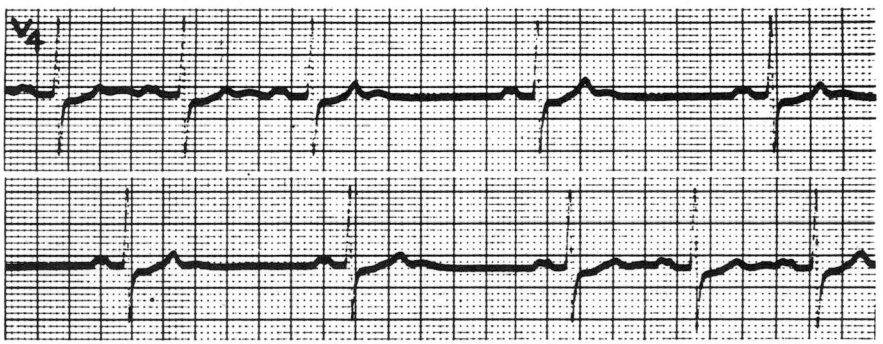

Figure 43.5.   Blocked premature atrial contractions mimicking AV or sinoatrial block.

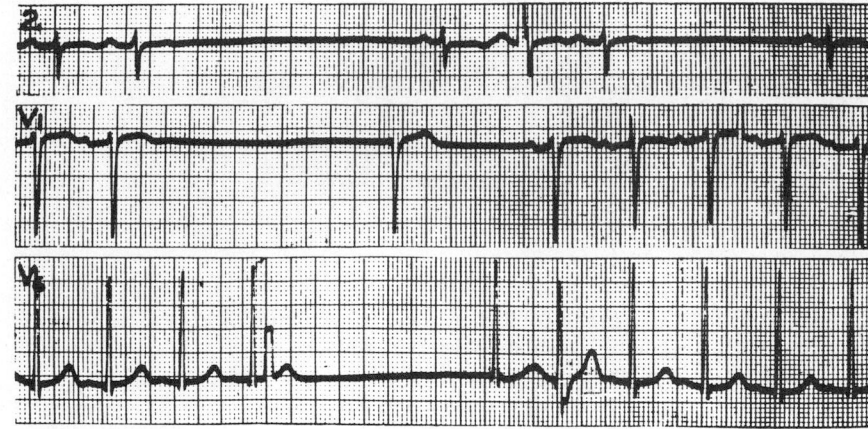

Figure 43.6. Third-degree sinoatrial block, with escape rhythm.

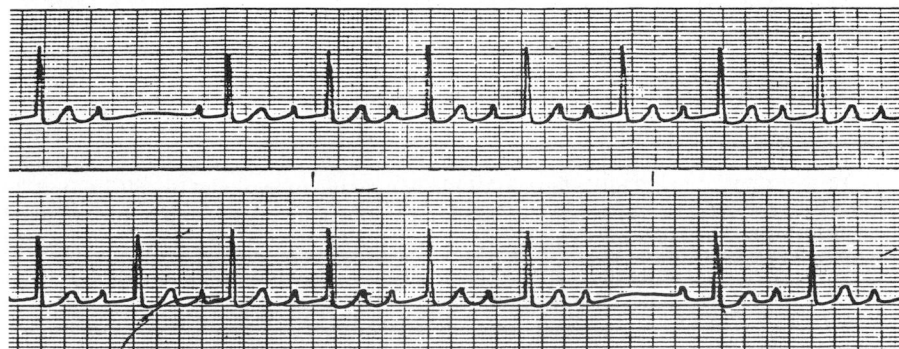

Figure 43.7. Mobitz type I (Wenckebach) second-degree AV block.

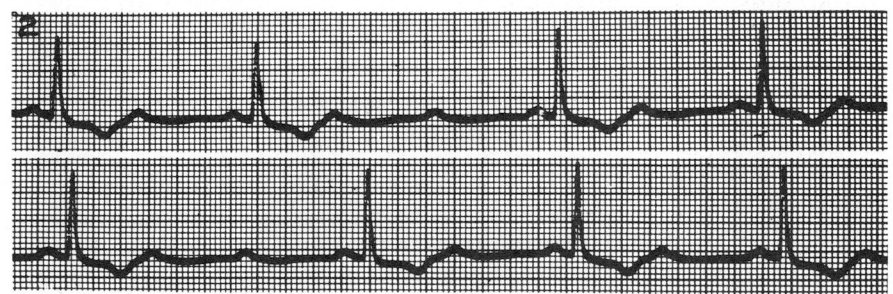

Figure 43.8. Mobitz type II second-degree AV block.

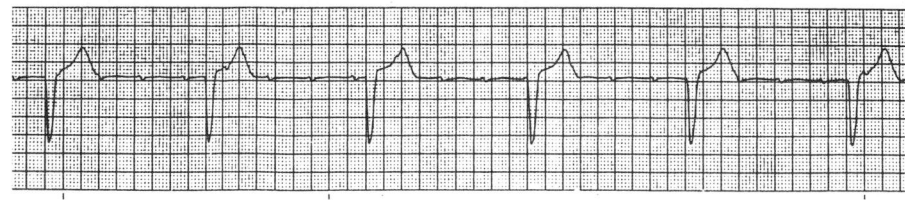

Figure 43.9. Third-degree AV block.

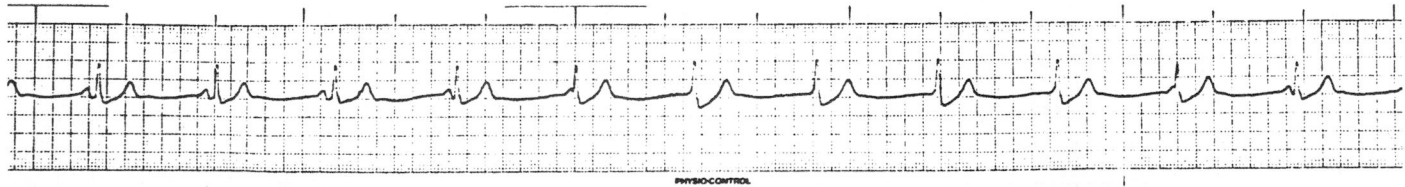

Figure 43.10. AV dissociation with isorhythmic dissociation owing to a junctional focus.

ARTIFICIAL PACEMAKERS

Temporary cardiac pacemakers are normally used in emergent or urgent circumstances, whereas most permanent pacemakers are placed electively. The emergency physician should be familiar with the indications and use of temporary pacemakers, and with the principles of permanent pacemakers and their complications (see Chapter 45, "The Patient with a Pacemaker or Implantable Cardioverter–Defibrillator").

Temporary Pacemakers

Therapeutic emergency cardiac pacing is indicated in any hemodynamically unstable bradycardia that fails to respond to pharmacologic therapy. In addition, prophylactic emergent cardiac pacing may be indicated, even in the absence of symptoms, for patients with acute myocardial infarction in the following circumstances:

- First-degree AV block with new-onset bundle-branch block
- Second-degree AV block Type II
- Third-degree AV block
- Right bundle-branch block with left anterior fascicular block or left posterior fascicular block (either old or new)
- Left bundle-branch block (old or new) and placement of a Swan-Ganz catheter (because of the risk of inducing iatrogenic right bundle-branch block, and hence complete block)

Transcutaneous cardiac pacing involves the application of cutaneous electrodes to the chest and delivery of electrical impulses through the chest wall to the myocardium. Transcutaneous pacing is the technique of choice for emergent pacing in the emergency department, and is the only option available for prehospital use.

The advantages of transcutaneous pacing are its ease and speed of use and the absence of serious side effects. Its disadvantages include an inability to capture in some patients and the discomfort experienced by conscious patients because of chest wall contractions. The latter can usually be treated satisfactorily with analgesics or sedation. Transcutaneous pacers should be considered stabilizing devices, to be replaced by other pacing techniques when possible.

Transvenous cardiac pacing involves the placement of the pacing electrode into the right ventricle by way of central vein, often the subclavian or internal jugular. Therefore, it carries the risk of central venous catheterization, but is the temporary modality that most closely approximates the function of a permanent pacemaker. It does not involve painful muscle contractions or the hazard of direct cardiac puncture, and can be used for relatively prolonged periods. Unfortunately, emergent transvenous pacemaker placement in the emergency department setting is often a lengthy and unsuccessful procedure associated with a high incidence of noncapture. Ideally, placement is performed under fluoroscopic guidance. With the advent of transcutaneous pacing, transvenous pacing has been relegated to those situations in which fluoroscopy is available, in which stabilization has been achieved by another modality, or in which attempts at transcutaneous pacing have been unsuccessful.

Transthoracic cardiac pacing involves the placement of a pacing wire through the skin directly into the right ventricular cavity. Because of significant complications, such as pericardial tamponade, pneumothorax, and coronary vessel injury, transthoracic pacing should usually be considered only when other options are unsuccessful or unavailable.

Once capture has been achieved, regardless of the device used, the pacemaker settings will be dependent on the clinical situation. An initial rate of 80 to 100 bpm is appropriate for the majority of the patients. The initial output setting should be at maximum and then decreased once capture is achieved. The mode should initially be asynchronous (sensitivity off) in those patients requiring emergency pacing for cardiac arrest. However, the mode should be set to synchronous in patients with bradydysrhythmias, as ventricular fibrillation may occur if the pacemaker fires during the vulnerable period (T wave).

CRITICAL INTERVENTION

- Initiate artificial pacing in unstable patients if drug therapy is ineffective

DISPOSITION

Virtually all patients with symptomatic bradydysrhythmia require admission to the hospital. Patients with type II second-degree AV block and complete AV block warrant admission even if asymptomatic. Admission should be to a monitored bed in a unit with the capability of initiating emergent pacing.

If transfer to another facility is necessary, pacing should first be initiated, if indicated and available. En route, the patient should have continuous cardiac monitoring and access to advanced cardiac life support. Transcutaneous pacing capability en route is also desirable.

COMMON PITFALLS

✔ Automatically assuming that a 2:1 second-degree AV block is of the Mobitz type II variety, possibly leading to unnecessary treatment and intervention
✔ Not taking rate into account when evaluating AV and fascicular blocks
✔ Misdiagnosing blocked premature atrial contractions as significant AV block, possibly leading to unnecessary treatment and intervention
✔ Mistakenly blocking an escape rhythm, with the potential for causing cardiac standstill

Acknowledgments

Thanks to previous edition chapter author Mary B. Staten-McCormick.

References

1. Arima H, Sobue K, Tanaka S, et al. Profound sinus bradycardia after intravenous nicardipine. *Anesth Analg* 2002;95:53–55.
2. Bryan G, Ward A, Rippe JM. Athletic heart syndrome. *Clin Sports Med* 1992;11:259.
3. Calvo-Romero JM, Lima-Rodriguez EM. Bradycardia associated with ophthalmic beta-blockers. *J Postgrad Med* 2003;49:186.
4. Castro VJ, Nacht R. Cocaine-induced bradyarrhythmia: an unsuspected cause of syncope. *Chest* 2000;117:275–277.
5. Essebag V, Hadjis T, Platt RW, Pilote L. Amiodarone and the risk of bradyarrhythmia requiring permanent pacemaker in elderly patients with atrial fibrillation and prior myocardial infarction. *J Am Coll Cardiol* 2003;41:249–254.
6. Grimm W, Koehler U, Fus E, et al. Outcome of patients with sleep apnea-associated severe bradyarrhythmias after continuous positive airway pressure therapy. *Am J Cardiol* 2000;86:688–692.
7. Inoue T, Takayanagi K, Sakai Y, et al. Cardiac pacing as emergency care for serious bradyarrhythmias with circulatory shock. *J Med* 2001;32:321–331.
8. Kaur A, Yu SS, Lee AJ, Chiao TB. Thalidomide-included sinus bradycardia. *Ann Pharmacother* 2003;37:1040–1043.
9. Nicholson WJ, Buxton AE, Tammaro D. Bradycardic syncope in two patients who recently began gatifloxacin treatment. *Clin Infect Dis* 2003;36:35–39.
10. Pudil R. Hrncir Z. Severe bradycardia after a methylprednisolone "mini pulse" treatment. *Arch Intern Med* 2001;161:1778–1779.
11. Wenckebach KF. Zur analyse des unregelmassigen Pulses. *Z Klin Med* 1899;37:475.

CHAPTER 44
Tachydysrhythmias

Mel Herbert and Scott R. Votey

The truism that we must treat patients and not electrocardiograms (ECGs) or laboratory results is perhaps nowhere more relevant than in the emergency management of tachydysrhythmias. Decisions must be guided principally by the clinical presentation, and exact rhythm interpretation should be subservient to the goal of prompt appropriate management. Hemodynamic abnormalities are more typically dependent on the heart rate produced by any dysrhythmia than they are on the source of dysrhythmia. Ventricular tachycardia (VT), for example, conjures up images of imminent catastrophe, and supraventricular tachycardia (SVT) is usually assumed to be benign. However, some patients with VT are relatively stable, at least in the short run, whereas, in other patients, SVT can be acutely life-threatening.

TACHYDYSRHYTHMIA PATHOPHYSIOLOGY

Under normal circumstances, the sinoatrial (S-A) node is the pacemaker for the heart. Depolarization is initiated in the S-A node, and the impulse is conducted down the atrium to the atrioventricular (AV) node. Atrial depolarization corresponds to the P wave on the ECG. Conduction is slowed in the AV node, which provides a measure of protection against hemodynamically unstable tachycardias, because even in the presence of atrial tachycardias, ventricular rates will remain relatively slow. The normal slowing in the AV node is seen on the ECG as the PR interval. After the impulse traverses the AV node, it is conducted first down the His bundle, followed by the left and right bundle branches, and is then dispersed to the ventricular myocardium via the Purkinje fibers. Ventricular depolarization corresponds to the QRS wave on the ECG. The His–Purkinje system is made up of specialized myocardial cells that conduct impulses very rapidly. Normal impulse conduction thus produces a narrow QRS complex. Disease of the AV node causes heart blocks; disease of the His–Purkinje system produces bundle-branch blocks.

Tachycardias can be generated from any focus in the heart, because essentially all myocardial tissue has intrinsic pacemaker activity. There are two principal mechanisms by which tachydysrhythmias arise: reentry and enhanced automaticity. *Reentry* is a phenomenon in which an initial depolarizing impulse travels a closed-loop path that returns cyclically to its point of origin, and, in doing so, generates a regular sustained tachydysrhythmia. Dysrhythmias produced by reentry are extremely regular.

The requirements for a reentrant tachydysrhythmia are (i) a closed-loop conduction path; (ii) slower conduction and prolonged refractoriness in one limb of the loop; (iii) propagation of the initiating impulse down the faster limb of the loop, with antegrade conduction down the slower limb blocked; and (iv) retrograde excitation of the initially blocked slower limb, returning the impulse to its point of origin, where depolarization is reinitiated. Repetition of this cycle sustains the dysrhythmia. A premature beat is the typical precipitant. Reentry can occur at a microscopic or a macroscopic level. Most reentry circuits occur with both limbs within the AV node, producing an

AV nodal reentrant tachycardia (AVNRT). Tachycardias generated by reentry circuits that involve a bypass tract are generally called AV reentrant tachycardias (AVRTs). Both of these rhythms, which may be indistinguishable clinically or even on an ECG, are also commonly referred to as paroxysmal supraventricular tachycardias (PSVTs), emphasizing that the nomenclature of SVTs is confusing and not standardized. Reentry is a common mechanism in VT as well, with the reentrant circuit typically contained entirely in a local area of abnormal ventricular tissue.

Enhanced automaticity is an increase in the rate of the spontaneous depolarization of myocardial cells above their electrical threshold. Sinus tachycardia is the physiologic response to enhanced automaticity of the S-A node. When enhanced automaticity results in more rapid depolarization of extranodal myocardial cells, these foci can produce ectopic tachydysrhythmias. Examples include paroxysmal atrial tachycardia (PAT) and junctional tachycardia. Enhanced automaticity often occurs as a result of increased sympathetic tone (e.g., with fever, thyrotoxicosis, or sympathomimetic overdose). Treatment of these dysrhythmias generally should be directed at removing the underlying stressor.

In adults, an AV nodal reentrant tachycardia (i.e., one that does not involve a bypass tract) generally does not generate a ventricular response of more than 180 bpm because of the damping effect of the AV node. In the presence of a bypass tract, however (e.g., the atrial tissue bundle of Kent found in Wolff-Parkinson-White [WPW] syndrome), rates of greater than equal 200 bpm may be reached. VT, on the other hand, particularly when caused by a reentry mechanism, may reach rates as high as 250 to 300 bpm, but is usually less than 220 bpm.

Tachycardias that originate below the AV node produce wide QRS complexes; therefore, any tachycardia with a narrow QRS complex can be presumed to originate from the AV node or above. On the other hand, SVTs and nodal tachycardias can produce wide QRS complexes in several circumstances: underlying bundle-branch block, rate-related bundle-branch block induced by the tachycardia itself, and anterograde conduction from the atrium to the ventricle through a bypass tract that circumvents the AV node. Thus, wide-complex tachycardias can be of either ventricular or supraventricular origin.

Although VT is more likely than SVT to produce hemodynamic decompensation, and thus more likely to initiate an episode of ventricular fibrillation (VF), VT is not always immediately life-threatening, and not every episode of SVT is benign (21). VT tends to be more worrisome, because of the lack of atrial systole and, more important, the generally faster ventricular rate it produces. However, very rapid atrial or junctional tachycardias can produce hemodynamic instability, and results of efforts to distinguish between SVT and VT based purely on symptomatic effects produced by the dysrhythmia are frequently inaccurate (21). The configuration of the QRS complexes seen during an episode of tachycardia is less important as a clue to the origin of the rhythm disturbance than as a guide to choosing between several possible therapeutic approaches.

PRESENTATION AND EMERGENCY DEPARTMENT MANAGEMENT

In the emergency department (ED), where diagnostic data are often limited and the patient's condition warrants prompt action, tachydysrhythmias are most successfully managed using an algorithmic diagnostic and therapeutic schema that is easily remembered and applied. The following approach is broadly applicable to the emergency management of tachydysrhythmias.

Step 1. Be Prepared for a Cardiopulmonary Arrest

Any patient with a tachydysrhythmia is at risk for deterioration, owing to either the dysrhythmia or its treatment. Being prepared for a cardiopulmonary resuscitation by having advanced airway equipment and a defibrillator at the bedside minimizes the patient's risk.

Step 2. Determine Stability

Determine what hemodynamic effect the rhythm is having on the patient. In this context, *unstable* is defined as a heart rate and blood pressure inadequate to maintain vital organ perfusion and function, manifested clinically by significant chest pain, pulmonary edema, altered mental status, syncope, or severe hypotension. Categorizing a patient as stable or unstable is complicated by the innumerable gradations on the continuum from asymptomatic health to cardiopulmonary arrest. The most important feature in determining a patient's stability is the state of perfusion. Altered mental status and ischemic chest pain with electrocardiographic changes of ischemia are convincing evidence of instability. Electrical cardioversion should be used to treat unstable patients with any tachydysrhythmia except sinus tachycardia and multifocal atrial tachycardia (MFAT).

It is important to note that although up to 70% of patients with a tachydysrhythmia complain of chest pain, the majority do not have myocardial ischemia and are not unstable. Chest pain associated with a tachydysrhythmia in a young healthy patient, in the absence of other evidence of hypoperfusion, is rarely clinically important. On the other hand, if the patient has a reasonable chance of underlying coronary artery disease, the chest pain must be taken seriously. Similarly, arbitrary blood pressure cutoffs for defining stable or unstable do not take into account the patient's baseline blood pressure. A systolic blood pressure of 80 mm Hg is of far more concern in a hypertensive elderly patient than in a young and healthy 20-year-old. It should be emphasized that stability is subject to change on a minute-to-minute basis, and therapy must be adjusted accordingly.

After clinical stability is assessed, the ECG should be rapidly and systematically evaluated. Although most therapeutic decisions can be made on the basis of a rhythm strip it is prudent to obtain a 12-lead ECG as soon as it is feasible. A 12-lead ECG can help determine if myocardial ischemia is present, and can aid in differentiating among tachydysrhythmias, especially between sinus tachycardia and other regular supraventricular tachycardias.

Step 3. Determine the Rate

The more extreme the ventricular rate, the more likely the patient is to become unstable. Sinus tachycardia rarely reaches 160 to 180 bpm in adults. Although SVTs typically have rates slower than 180 beats per minute, they can be faster in the presence of a bypass tract. VT is not slowed by passage through the AV node and can thus be much faster (250 to 300 bpm), but is usually less than 220 bpm.

Step 4. Determine the QRS Complex Width

When emergent cardioversion is not required, subsequent decisions can be based on the duration of the QRS complex. In an adult, a QRS width of greater than 0.12 ms is considered "wide." In many adults with a wide-complex tachydysrhythmia, the QRS duration is substantially greater than 0.12 ms. In children, the QRS duration is age-dependent, but any QRS duration over 0.10 ms is considered prolonged (1). It is usually possible to de-termine if a rhythm is wide or narrow from a rhythm strip alone, but if there is uncertainty, the widest QRS complex in the 12-lead ECG should be used as the measure.

Narrow-complex tachycardias can be assumed to be supraventricular. Wide-complex tachycardias are the result of any of three distinct pathophysiologic processes:

1. The rhythm originates in the ventricle and does not use the normal conduction pathway.
2. There is a block of the normal conduction pathway below the AV node (bundle-branch block).
3. The origin of the tachycardia is supraventricular, but there is an accessory conduction pathway that bypasses the normal conduction pathway.

With rare exceptions, a wide-complex tachycardia should be treated as VT for three reasons: (i) VT is the most common cause of a wide-complex tachycardia; (ii) despite the existence of diagnostic criteria, VT cannot be reliably distinguished from SVT with aberrancy in the clinical setting, and treating VT as SVT can be fatal (while treating SVT as VT is not harmful); and (iii) even if the tachycardia has a supraventricular origin, there may be an associated bypass tract, in which case, standard SVT treatment (e.g., verapamil) is contraindicated. It is never safe to assume that a wide-complex tachycardia is caused by aberrancy.

Step 5. Assess the Regularity of the RR Intervals

An irregular narrow-complex tachycardia is usually caused by atrial fibrillation (AF), although it can occasionally be caused by MFAT. Because VT is usually regular except during the first few beats, an irregular wide-complex tachycardia should also raise the suspicion of AF with a bundle-branch block (AF-BBB) or a bypass tract. Distinguishing which patients have AF with a bypass tract is important, because the treatment of choice for these patients is cardioversion, even if they are stable. Although this differentiation can be difficult, two characteristics are helpful. In contrast to patients with AF-BBB, patients with AF with a bypass tract may have (i) very rapid conduction, with some R-R complexes intervals equivalent to >250 bpm, and (ii) bizarre morphology QRS complexes resulting from fusion and partial fusion of beats form normal AV and bypass tract conduction.

Step 6. Determine the Presence or Absence of P Waves

Determine whether P waves are present, their morphologic characteristics, whether they are regular, and how they are related to the QRS complexes. Regular uniform P waves preceding the QRS complex help distinguish sinus tachycardia from other SVTs. A normal P wave axis is one with an upright P wave in lead II and negative in aVR. This axis strongly suggests the atrial activity is coming from the S-A node and is indeed sinus in nature. Although similar P waves may be present with the much rarer PAT, an abnormal P-wave axis or morphology should alert one to the ectopic origin of that rhythm. An irregular narrow QRS complex rhythm with more than three P-wave morphologies is indicative of MFAT. One should, in addition, look for the regular sawtooth deflections of the electrocardiographic baseline that characterize atrial flutter waves.

Application of this scheme organizes dysrhythmias into four major categories based on the electrocardiographic appearance, with the additional distinction of clinically stable or unstable. The four categories are (i) narrow complex, regular, P waves present or absent; (ii) narrow complex, irregular, P waves present or absent; (iii) wide complex regular, no P waves; and (iv) wide complex, irregular, no P waves. Generally, each of the specific dysrhythmias that fall into each of these categories is treated in the same fashion, thus the simplicity of the approach. Occasionally, unstable patients need treatment initiated before analysis of the rhythm can be completed. In addition, once the rhythm is stabilized, the patient may require additional pharmacologic treatment to prevent recurrent dysrhythmias.

NARROW-COMPLEX TACHYCARDIAS

Narrow Complex, Regular, P Waves Present

Sinus tachycardia makes up the vast majority of these cases. PAT is a rare alternative diagnosis. Therapy for sinus tachycardia is directed at the rhythm's underlying cause rather than at the rhythm itself. However, there are exceptions. In the setting of acute myocardial ischemia, slowing the heart rate with β-blockers diminishes myocardial oxygen demand and improves mortality (25). β-Blockers are also important in thyroid storm to counteract the adverse consequences of extraordinary increases in sympathetic drive. In cocaine overdose, β-blockade may be appropriate for control of heart rate, but only once simultaneous α-blockade has been begun to avoid the greater danger of unopposed α-adrenergic stimulation.

Narrow Complex, Regular, No P Waves

The differential diagnosis includes AVNRT-type and AVRT-type PSVT, and atrial flutter with a consistent block. Generally all these rhythms are treated in the same way, blockade of the AV node.

PSVT (AVNRT) (Fig. 44.1) makes up the majority of cases in this category, but it also includes atrial flutter with a consistent block and AVRT. Although the rhythm strips of patients having atrial flutter with a consistent degree of AV nodal block can appear similar, careful inspection of a 12-lead ECG usually reveals flutter waves. Patients with PSVT who have severe signs of end-organ hypoperfusion should be cardioverted; more than 90% convert with small doses of electrical energy (10 to 50 J).

Treatment of PSVT, typically a reentrant tachycardia in which the AV node is part of the circuit, is directed at blockade of the AV node. Vagal maneuvers may be tried first: carotid massage, the Valsalva maneuver, and ice-water immersion work well in many patients. However, because many patients with recurrent PSVT are familiar with vagal maneuvers, they often present for treatment only when these maneuvers have failed; therefore, these maneuvers are often not useful in the ED.

Pharmacotherapy for stable patients with PSVT involves blockade of the AV node. Treatment options include adenosine, verapamil, diltiazem, and β-blockers. Adenosine, owing to its brief duration of action and its resultant lack of sustained hemodynamic effect, has become the drug of choice. The recommended initial dosage of adenosine is a 6-mg bolus over 1 to 3 seconds, followed by a 20-mg flush of normal saline. If there is no response in 1 to 2 minutes, a 12-mg dose can be administered in the same manner. The use of doses of adenosine upward of 24 mg as a bolus have been reported in the literature, but are only marginally more effective than 12 mg. It is important that the drug be given as a rapid bolus, so as to achieve high levels in the heart.

In the absence of any of the standard contraindications to calcium channel blockers (hypotension, congestive heart failure, S-A or AV nodal disease, or the previous use of i.v. β-blockers), verapamil is a safe and effective alternative. The standard initial dose is 0.075 to 0.150 mg/kg. In adults, an initial dose of 5 mg is usually appropriate. Most patients convert to sinus rhythm within about 2 minutes, and incremental doses to a maximum of 15 to 20 mg are usually successful in those who do not. Diltiazem is also effective in a dose of 10 mg i.v., repeated up to a total of 50 mg in the first 30 minutes. Calcium may be used to prevent or treat the hypotensive effects of verapamil and probably diltiazem.

Verapamil is safe when used in patients with narrow QRS complex tachycardias, particularly when calcium is used to prevent or treat transient hypotension. Nevertheless, there is a substantial incidence of adverse effects when contraindications are present, so they should not be ignored (13). Many pediatric cardiologists consider it unsafe to use verapamil in children under 1 year of age, and so use adenosine exclusively in this age group.

Esmolol, an extremely short-acting β-blocking agent with a half-life of less than 10 minutes, is moderately effective in treating PSVT, although success rates are significantly lower than with either adenosine or verapamil and the incidence of hypotension is higher. Esmolol is, therefore, a secondary drug in the treatment of PSVT (23).

Atrial Flutter

Atrial flutter is the most electrosensitive tachycardia, and electrocardioversion is therefore advocated by many authorities. The calcium channel blockers (verapamil and diltiazem), as well as digitalis, are capable of slowing the ventricular response in atrial flutter, and verapamil will convert perhaps 15% to 20% of cases to sinus rhythm (2). Adenosine, although capable of slowing conduction for a few seconds, rarely results in cardioversion and has no role in the management of atrial flutter; however, it can occasionally be of diagnostic value in distinguishing atrial flutter and PSVT. Cardioversion, which occasionally results in AF rather than sinus rhythm, can be done semi-electively in most patients in atrial flutter. Given the small amount of current needed and the availability of excellent sedative agents, cardioversion should be possible with minimal discomfort.

Although the diagnosis of atrial flutter is often fairly easy, some patients with flutter at first glance appear to be in other rhythms. Therefore, it is important to consider and exclude flutter before using any drug (such as procainamide) that speeds conduction through the AV node. This is because atrial activity in flutter is typically much faster than ventricular response, and such drugs can change the conduction from 2 : 1 or 3 : 1 to 1 : 1, with serious hemodynamic consequences. Vagal maneuvers can sometimes slow the ventricular rate enough to bring out flutter waves (if they are present), but adenosine is particularly effective in this regard.

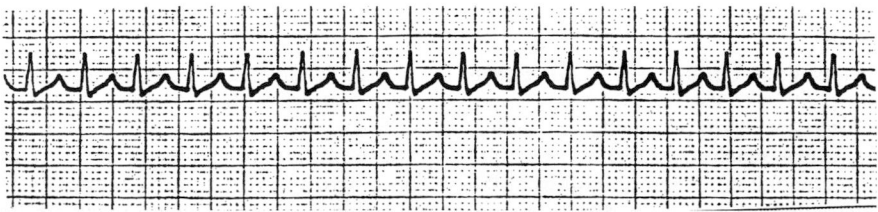

Figure 44.1. Paroxysmal supraventricular tachycardia.

Narrow Complex, Irregular, P Waves Present

Multifocal Atrial Tachycardia (MFAT)

MFAT is characterized by P waves of varying morphologies and by changing PR intervals. Because MFAT originates in the atria, it is associated with narrow QRS complexes, except in the presence of underlying bundle-branch block. MFAT occurs primarily in patients with chronic lung disease, and within this group it is most common in patients with high or toxic levels of theophylline.

Because MFAT has been thought to occur as a result of the hypoxic effects of the underlying lung disease, treatment has been considered futile. The recognition that theophylline toxicity may contribute to this dysrhythmia (14), and several small series demonstrating slowing or conversion of MFAT with magnesium or verapamil, suggest that a nihilistic approach is inappropriate. Although MFAT is seldom life-threatening, the ability to control it can provide symptomatic benefit.

Narrow Complex, Irregular, No P Waves

An irregular narrow-complex tachycardia is almost invariably AF or atrial flutter with variable block (Fig. 44.2). Occasionally, the P waves of MFAT are overlooked and that rhythm is confused with AF.

Atrial Fibrillation (AF)

Although many patients with AF are seen in the ED, not all require emergency therapy. For example, those with chronic AF whose ventricular response rate is well controlled do not require immediate treatment. At the other extreme are patients with extremely rapid heart rates associated with hemodynamic deterioration; these patients require emergent cardioversion regardless of whether the AF is new or old. Because chronic AF is much less likely to convert to (or remain in) sinus rhythm regardless of the therapy used (15), pharmacologic intervention to control the ventricular response rate is extremely important. Nevertheless, if there is evidence of severe end-organ hypoperfusion, cardioversion should always be tried.

For patients presenting with AF and a rapid ventricular response, treatment is directed at slowing the ventricular rate, and conversion to sinus rhythm is, at best, a secondary consideration. In the majority of these patients, the tachycardia itself (which profoundly decreases the time available for diastolic filling of the ventricles as well as coronary artery perfusion), rather than the loss of atrial systole, is responsible for the hemodynamic consequences. Patients with hypertrophic cardiomyopathy, as well as other patients with significant diastolic dysfunction of the heart, are an exception, because their stiff ventricles fill slowly and poorly during the passive phase of early diastole, and they thus rely on active atrial systole for an inordinate proportion of their end-diastolic ventricular volume.

At the other extreme, a slow ventricular response in new-onset AF is worrisome (unless the patient is already taking medications that slow conduction in the AV node), because it implies AV node dysfunction. Such patients are rarely acutely unstable and may not require immediate treatment at all. In fact, attempted cardioversion may lead to asystole or prolonged bradycardia, and even if successful, it is typically followed by early reversion to AF (4). Patients with spontaneously slow ventricular response to new-onset AF generally need to be admitted for consideration of long-term measures, including, in some cases, insertion of a permanent pacemaker.

Calcium channel blockers, in particular diltiazem, have supplanted digoxin as the drug of choice for AF with a rapid ventricular response in stable patients. This change in practice is the result of evidence that, although digoxin is no more effective than placebo in slowing ventricular response (18) in the first few hours, calcium channel blockers slow ventricular response within the first few minutes of i.v. administration. Neither digoxin nor calcium channel blockers are particularly effective at producing cardioversion to sinus rhythm. In stable patients, diltiazem can be given at a dose of 5 to 10 mg i.v. over 2 minutes, repeated as necessary every 5 minutes to a total dose of 50 to 60 mg in the first 30 minutes. To reduce hypotension, patients can be pretreated with calcium as described earlier. Following bolus injection, rate control can be maintained with an i.v. infusion of 5 to 15 mg per hour.

Alternative agents include verapamil, magnesium, β-blockers, and digoxin. Verapamil and magnesium are given in the same doses as those for regular tachydysrhythmias. β-Blockers such as atenolol or metoprolol can be given in doses of 5 mg intravenously, repeated up to a total of 10 mg and 15 mg, respectively. β-Blockers are about as effective as calcium channel blockers for rate control, but are seldom used because of a higher incidence of hypotension. β-Blockers are indicated for rapid AF associated with thyrotoxicosis, a catecholamine excess state for which calcium channel blockers are minimally effective. Digoxin may be given as 0.5 mg i.v. or orally, followed by 0.25 mg, 4 and 8 hours later. Even when using these loading regimens, rate control is no better than with placebo for at least several hours. Diltiazem or verapamil may be given i.v. at the same time as digoxin, in the absence of other contraindications. There may be some advantage to diltiazem in patients with mild hypotension or congestive heart failure, because of its less pronounced negative inotropic effect (11). Calcium channel blockers should be avoided in the presence of digitalis toxicity.

The therapy for unstable patients with narrow-complex AF is one of the most challenging situations in all of dysrhythmia management. Many AF patients have dilated atria and decreased ejection fractions. These patients do not easily cardiovert to sinus rhythm or remain in sinus rhythm if converted. In addition, cardioversion to sinus rhythm does not produce mechanical atrial contraction for hours to days. For this reason, cardioversion should be considered a form of rapid rate control and not a therapy that immediately restores atrial systole. Finally, if the patient has been in AF for more than 2 to 3 days, intraatrial thrombus may have formed and may embolize following cardioversion. For these reasons, cardioversion is considered by many a therapy of last resort.

If the patient is truly unstable, however, electrical cardioversion is required. Although some authorities suggest higher levels, 100 J is the usual starting dose, increasing to 200 J and 300 J as required. For unstable patients in whom electrical cardioversion fails and for somewhat more stable patients, rate control can be achieved by using repeated small boluses of diltiazem following pretreatment with calcium. Intravenous magnesium is a

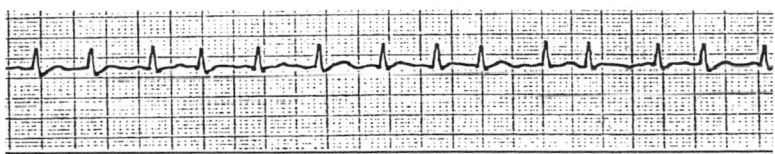

Figure 44.2.   AF or atrial flutter with variable block.

reasonable alternative. Amiodarone has been used in unstable AF in a number of small case series and in one randomized trial in which it was found to be inferior to magnesium (17). Amiodarone slows ventricular rate and increases the frequency of conversion to sinus rhythm. In rare cases, the cautious use of dopamine may be required to maintain blood pressure. The seriousness of this clinical situation cannot be overemphasized, and no therapy is without significant risk.

New-onset AF has many causes, from the benign to the extremely serious. It has long been standard practice to admit almost all patients with new-onset AF in order to evaluate the possibility of serious underlying disease (e.g., acute myocardial infarction, mitral valve disease, pulmonary embolism, thyrotoxicosis, or drug effect) as its cause. However, 80% to 95% of stable patients with new-onset AF do not prove to have an acutely critical etiology, and those who do almost always have other worrisome clinical findings in addition to the dysrhythmia itself (20). Thus, the traditional policy is being questioned. Nevertheless, given the limited data on this subject to date, it remains reasonable to discharge only those patients with new-onset AF who do not have evidence of underlying heart disease or other acute instability, who convert readily or spontaneously in the ED back to sinus rhythm, and who are reliable and have good follow-up. Patients with chronic AF should be admitted to the hospital if they have signs of hemodynamic decompensation that requires cardioversion, or if hemodynamic effects and rapid ventricular response are not easily controlled.

Several agents have been the subject of limited testing in the pharmacologic cardioversion of new-onset AF. These include flecainide, amiodarone, sotalol, clonidine, ibutilide, dofetilide, propafenone, and magnesium. The possible benefits of higher rates of earlier conversion using these drugs are offset by prodysrhythmic effects, a higher incidence of hypotension, and the fact that by 8 hours there is little difference from placebo in conversion rates (6). For these reasons, the chemical conversion of recent-onset AF in the ED remains controversial. The fact that risks and benefits must be carefully explained to the patient, and that a trial of "time" may be very effective by itself, has led some authorities to suggest that attempts at chemical conversion should be performed only in the inpatient setting.

The concept of ED cardioversion of AF can now be seriously challenged owing to the findings of the AFFIRM (Atrial Fibrillation Follow-up Investigation of Rhythm Management) trial (26). In this large randomized trial, long-term rate control and anticoagulation was found to be superior on a number of measures to attempts at long-term rhythm control. If long-term attempts at maintaining sinus rhythm fail, the argument for short-term ED conversion loses most of its merit. When the known adverse effects of drugs like flecainide, amiodarone, and ibutilide are considered as well, it is difficult to recommend conversion as a standard ED practice.

Anticoagulation is an important management issue for patients with AF. Not only are patients with AF that lasts more than several days at risk for systemic embolization, but recent evidence suggests that even shorter periods of AF may carry a risk of embolization, particularly following conversion to sinus rhythm. Even if accurate, a history of a brief duration of AF may fail to preclude the possibility of embolization owing to intraatrial clot formation during the period of atrial stand-still that follows conversion to sinus rhythm. For this reason, some authorities suggest that all patients with acute AF be anticoagulated at the time of diagnosis and for 12 to 24 hours after conversion to sinus rhythm.

On the other hand, recent studies of transesophageal echocardiography (TEE) in ruling out an intraatrial thrombus prior to conversion of AF suggest that a negative TEE reduces the risk of embolization enough to obviate the need for anticoagulation. However, until additional studies more fully define the risks and benefits of these new management strategies, the standard of care is to anticoagulate all patients with AF of more than 72 hours' duration prior to elective electrical or chemical cardioversion. Of course, if it is necessary because of hemodynamic instability, cardioversion should never be withheld. In addition, all patients with chronic AF, except, perhaps, those less than 60 years old who have no other evidence of heart disease, should be on maintenance anticoagulant therapy unless there are substantial contraindications (22).

Patients with chronic AF are usually taking antiarrhythmic medications. Digitalis has long been used for chronic rate control. Cardioversion in patients taking digoxin is a risk because of the potential for asystole. If cardioversion is required because of extreme hemodynamic compromise, it should initially be attempted at lower energy levels, such as 50 J. Many experts now prefer calcium channel blockers to digoxin for chronic rate control, because calcium channel blockers control rate not only at rest, but also during exercise. There are also several recent reports suggesting a role for other drugs, including, particularly, amiodarone and sotalol, in chronic AF, although the overall safety of long-term therapy has been questioned.

WIDE-COMPLEX TACHYCARDIAS

As with narrow-complex tachycardias, tachycardias manifesting wide QRS complexes must be managed primarily according to their hemodynamic effects. Patients with wide-complex tachycardias are more likely to require cardioversion, because most have VT, which is more likely to be associated with end-organ hypoperfusion. Nevertheless, many such patients are relatively stable at presentation and respond to pharmacologic therapy (21).

Wide Complex, Regular, No P Waves

Diagnostic possibilities include VT, PSVT with aberrancy (bundle-branch block), and antidromic WPW syndrome. Several clinical and electrocardiographic criteria have been devised to enable clinicians to distinguish between VT and SVT when the QRS complex is wide. Useful indictors that make VT more likely include a history of heart disease, fusion and capture beats, and the presence of AV dissociation. Although such criteria are relatively accurate in predicting the source of tachycardia in series of patients, no single sign or combination of signs can definitively identify the origin of tachycardia (10). For this reason, wide-complex tachycardia should virtually always be treated as VT. Thus, drugs contraindicated in VT (e.g., verapamil) are almost never used to treat wide-complex tachycardia (16,21). Adenosine may be used to treat regular wide-complex tachycardia of uncertain etiology, because it is probably safe (if only very rarely effective) in VT and will convert most episodes of PSVT, including antidromic WPW syndrome.

Ventricular Tachycardia (VT)

VT is usually a life-threatening medical emergency. Although some patients have intermittent asymptomatic bouts of VT (usually episodes of less than 10 beats), patients who present to an ED with VT are usually either suffering from significant hemodynamic effects or experiencing other acute cardiac problems—including, particularly, myocardial ischemia—that require emergent treatment. Essentially, all patients with VT require consultation with a cardiologist and admission after ED therapy for the dysrhythmia.

The typically very rapid heart rate of sustained VT usually causes hemodynamic deterioration (16). Such patients require emergent electrical cardioversion. Fifty joules is a reasonable initial energy, because about 90% of episodes of VT respond to

10 to 50 watt-seconds of energy. Cardioversion is performed in the synchronized mode to avoid precipitating VF. Lidocaine, procainamide, magnesium, and amiodarone are standard agents used to prevent recurrence of VT after successful cardioversion or to treat patients with recurrent VT. Recent evidence suggests lidocaine is of limited utility, but it is still frequently used because of tradition and a very acceptable side-effect profile in the doses employed.

Sometimes, patients with sustained VT show no signs of hemodynamic instability in the short term. These patients can be treated with lidocaine, procainamide, magnesium, or amiodarone. The medical literature does not provide a clear basis for preferring one agent over another. Lidocaine, which is at best only moderately effective for VT, is given as an initial 100-mg i.v. bolus and may be repeated in 75-mg boluses up to 3 mg/kg. Procainamide, an effective therapy for both VT and PSVT, is given as a 17-mg/kg i.v. bolus at a rate of not more than 50 mg/minute. Procainamide can cause QRS widening and hypotension. Magnesium is effective for VT and moderately effective for PSVT. Usual doses of magnesium are 2 to 4 g i.v. over 5 minutes, followed by an infusion of 1 g per hour. Amiodarone can be given as 150 mg i.v. over 10 minutes, followed by an infusion of 1 mg/minute over the next 6 hours. An additional 150-mg i.v. bolus can be given for breakthrough VT. Amiodarone can cause hypotension (treated with fluid bolus), AV nodal block, and QT prolongation leading to torsade de pointes.

Wide-Complex Paroxysmal Supraventricular Tachycardia (PSVT)

PSVT can manifest with wide QRS complexes when bundle-branch block (either underlying or rate-related) is present (Fig. 44.3). The duration of the QRS complex in this circumstance is not likely to exceed 0.14 second, and heart rates usually range between 130 and 200 bpm. Nevertheless, it is virtually impossible to be certain that a wide-complex tachycardia represents PSVT with bundle-branch block, rather than VT; therefore, treatment should almost never be based on this assumption (10).

Wide QRS complexes are also seen in PSVT in association with the WPW syndrome when anterograde conduction occurs down the bundle of Kent and retrograde conduction occurs through the AV node. It may be possible to make this diagnosis from the ECG in patients with known WPW syndrome, although confusion with VT may still occur. When faced with a stable patient with a regular wide-complex tachycardia of uncertain etiology, adenosine is the preferred antiarrhythmic agent. Neither verapamil nor digoxin is recommended in this circumstance.

When adenosine fails to convert regular wide-complex tachycardia or when VT is considered more likely, procainamide is a rational choice. Procainamide has antiarrhythmic effects on both atrial and ventricular tissue, and it is safe and useful in most cases of wide-complex tachycardia, whether VT or PSVT with anterograde conduction through the bundle of Kent. Wide-complex tachycardia in the setting of possible drug overdose, however, suggests cyclic antidepressant toxicity, in which case, procainamide is absolutely contraindicated. Lidocaine, the first-line pharmacologic agent for treatment of known VT (in the absence of hemodynamic consequences) can occasionally speed conduction through bypass tracts in experimental models;

therefore, lidocaine is less attractive than procainamide when wide-complex tachycardia is suspected to result from WPW syndrome–related PSVT.

Wide Complex, Irregular, No P Waves

Diagnostic possibilities include AF with bundle-branch block, AF with the WPW syndrome, torsade de pointes, and VF.

Wide-Complex AF

A few patients with AF present with wide QRS complexes, owing to an underlying or rate-related bundle-branch block or to the WPW syndrome. In the presence of known underlying bundle-branch block, treatment can be similar to that for routine narrow-complex AF (i.e., cardioversion for unstable patients and a calcium channel blocker for rate control in stable patients).

Patients with rate-related bundle-branch block often demonstrate both wide complexes (in beats that follow short RR intervals) and narrow complexes (in beats that follow longer RR intervals), but patients with AF and the WPW syndrome may also have both wide and narrow QRS complexes, depending on the conduction path followed by each depolarization. It is critical to recognize this latter entity, because agents that slow conduction through the AV node are absolutely contraindicated (9).

WPW is a relatively rare syndrome that involves accessory pathway connections between the atrium and the ventricles. The presence of these rapidly conducting pathways predisposes to a number of dysrhythmias, of which AF is the most dangerous. AF generates impulses at 300 to 600 per minute. The accessory pathways of WPW syndrome, which bypass the AV node and its protective slowing, conduct impulses to the ventricle at rates exceeding 250 bpm. The ventricle will fail or undergo fibrillation if these excessively rapid atrial impulses are conducted for more than a short period. Many patients are aware that they have WPW syndrome. Among patients who give no history of WPW syndrome, the possibility should be considered when the irregular rhythm is wide and very fast, and the QRS complexes are variable and bizarre.

Drugs such as verapamil, diltiazem, and digitalis are contraindicated in WPW syndrome with wide-complex AF, because they can actually increase the speed of conduction through the bypass tract. More importantly, relative blockade of the AV node causes preferential conduction through the bypass tract, thereby resulting in much higher ventricular response rates; an extremely rapid ventricular response to AF can then deteriorate into VF. With calcium channel blockers, other hemodynamic effects, such as decreased inotropy and vasodilation, in the absence of any therapeutic effect, can add to the potentially catastrophic consequences of such therapy.

Although procainamide is unlikely to be harmful in WPW syndrome–related AF, it may not be particularly effective in the acute setting. Therefore, even in the absence of acute hemodynamic deterioration, patients with WPW syndrome–related AF are best treated with electrical cardioversion. After cardioversion, procainamide is given to prolong the refractoriness of the accessory pathway and to prevent recurrence of AF. Because

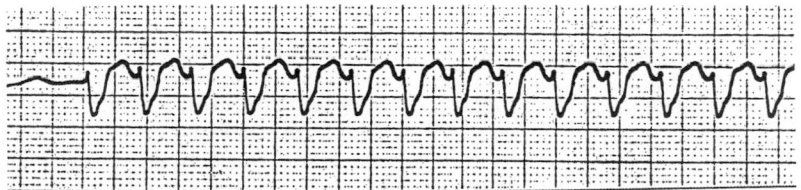

Figure 44.3.   Wide-complex paroxysmal supraventricular tachycardia.

procainamide can increase AV nodal conduction, some authorities suggest the addition of an AV node blocking agent.

Torsade de Pointes

Torsade de pointes is an unusual form of polymorphic VT characterized by the peculiar spiral pattern it produces on the surface ECG. The most common cause is the use of type IA antiarrhythmic agents (e.g., quinidine, procainamide, and disopyramide) that prolong the QT interval, a factor central to the development of this dysrhythmia. Other drugs (most prominently, the phenothiazines), drug interactions, and many other conditions (especially hypocalcemia and hypokalemia) are also associated with torsade de pointes.

Although most episodes of torsade de pointes are self-limited, they are nevertheless life-threatening, because any episode can precipitate VF. Because torsade de pointes usually converts spontaneously to sinus rhythm but then recurs, treatment is directed at preventing recurrences rather than terminating a given episode. In the long term, this often requires only withdrawal of the offending agent. In the ED, however, antiarrhythmic therapy is mandatory.

Magnesium, given as an i.v. infusion of 2 to 4 g over 5 to 10 minutes, is highly effective and is the treatment of choice for torsade de pointes. Alternately, overdrive electrical pacing can be used to speed the heart rate and thereby decrease the dispersion of refractoriness that is the underlying basis for this dysrhythmia. Infusions of isoproterenol have also been used with the same goal, although the prodysrhythmic effect of isoproterenol is worrisome.

Ventricular Fibrillation

VF is the chaotic firing of the ventricle from multiple foci and never results in effective myocardial contraction. It is the most common rhythm found early in cardiac arrest. The only therapy proven to improve the outcome of patients with VF is electrical defibrillation. When a defibrillator is available, no other activity should take precedence. No time should be spent starting i.v. lines, securing an airway, performing cardiopulmonary resuscitation, or giving drugs, as these delay the performance of electrical defibrillation. Immediate defibrillation in the nonsynchronized mode with a dose of 200 J provides the greatest likelihood of success. Increasing of the energy level probably does not improve the likelihood of defibrillation and may, in fact, be detrimental. Good contact with the chest, use of conduction gel, and firm pressure are all important to reduce transthoracic impedance and improve energy transfer to the heart.

Several adjunctive drugs are widely used when initial defibrillation is not successful. Although these drugs are considered standard therapy in this situation, it is important to remember that none of them has been definitively shown to increase the success of defibrillation or to improve long-term outcomes in humans with cardiac arrest. Thus, administration of these agents should never interfere with the rapid use of electrical defibrillation, the only intervention that has been definitively shown to affect outcome.

Specifically, no study has confirmed a positive effect of epinephrine use at either standard or high doses. Indeed high-dose epinephrine use is associated with increased costs from the small but significant increase in severely neurologically impaired survivors. Similarly, there is little evidence that lidocaine or amiodarone significantly improves outcomes in refractory VF. Amiodarone has supplanted lidocaine as the drug of choice in the current American Heart Association (AHA) advance cardiac life support guidelines, based on evidence suggesting that it is marginally more effective.

Intravenous lidocaine or amiodarone is used, however, to help prevent recurrence of VF after successful defibrillation.

Amiodarone in dysrhythmia prophylaxis following successful cardioversion is possibly more effective than lidocaine.

Although sodium bicarbonate and calcium chloride may worsen outcomes if used routinely in cardiac arrest, they still have a role in specific circumstances. Sodium bicarbonate may be lifesaving in tricyclic antidepressant overdose, and i.v. calcium is often an effective antidote for calcium channel blocker overdose.

EMERGENCY DEPARTMENT MANAGEMENT

Electrical Cardioversion

With the exceptions of sinus tachycardia and multifocal atrial tachycardia (MFAT), any tachycardia that produces significant end-organ hypoperfusion can be treated in the same manner, regardless of its mechanism. Patients with tachydysrhythmia and hypotension, altered mental status, significant chest pain, or significant congestive heart failure generally require emergency electrical cardioversion. Expeditious sedation and analgesia should precede electrical cardioversion in awake patients.

The amount of electrical energy required depends on the mechanism of the tachycardia. Fibrillatory rhythms, including both AF and VF, normally require significantly more energy than tachycardias such as PSVT or VT. Atrial flutter is the most electrosensitive rhythm and usually responds to energies in the range of 10 to 50 J. PSVT and VT both respond in at least 80% of cases to energies of 10 to 20 J; an initial energy of 50 J achieves successful conversion in more than 90% of cases. By contrast, AF and VF often require 100 to 200 J, or more. Initial doses should be as low as can reasonably be expected to succeed in converting the rhythm. If conversion fails on the initial attempt, energy levels can be serially increased until cardioversion is achieved.

Antidysrhythmic Agents

Drug therapy (Table 44.1) is reserved for patients who are clinically stable despite the tachydysrhythmia (or for whom cardioversion is either not indicated [MFAT, torsade de pointes] or has been tried unsuccessfully). The standard classification of antidysrhythmic agents provides a useful scheme for the treatment of tachycardias. Class I agents stabilize cell membranes and decrease the slope of phase zero of the action potential. Class II agents, the β-adrenergic blockers, depress the S-A and AV nodes. Class III agents decrease the entire duration of the action potential in all cardiac tissues, and thus have effects on all types of dysrhythmias. Class IV agents, the calcium channel blockers, affect primarily the S-A and AV nodes.

Three subclasses of class I are distinguished by their independent effects on repolarization. Although all of these drugs slow phase zero of the action potential, and thus indirectly lengthen repolarization, the clinical effects of the various subclasses differ because they each have separate direct effects on repolarization. Class IA drugs directly prolong repolarization, class IB drugs independently shorten it, and class IC drugs have little independent effect on repolarization. The total effect on repolarization is thus minimal for class IB drugs, whereas prolongation of repolarization is moderate for class IC agents and pronounced for class IA drugs.

These properties are clinically important, because delayed repolarization (which is reflected on the ECG as a prolonged QT interval) can result in reentrant-type ventricular dysrhythmias. This is of particular concern in the presence of ischemia, when the difference between the refractory periods of normal and ischemic cells is enhanced. Clinically, prolonged QT intervals

TABLE 44.1.   Drugs for Tachydysrhythmias

Drug	Dosage	Contraindications	Side Effects	Comments
Adenosine	6 mg i.v. rapid push Repeated doses of 12 or 18 mg may be used	• Known VT • AV node block • AF with WPW syndrome	Hypotension: transient Prolonged AV block: rare Chest pain Flushing	Reduce dose in patients taking carbamazepine or dipyridamole (start at 3 mg) or heart transplant patients (start at 1–2 mg) or administration via central line (start at 1–2 mg)
Amiodarone	150 mg over 10 min 1 mg/min for 6 h 0.5-mg/min maintenance infusion 150-mg boluses for breakthrough VT/VF	• AV block • Renal failure	Hypotension: Rx fluid bolus AV block: Rx decrease dosage	Amiodarone has many side effects when given chronically, but not acutely. Amiodarone should be considered in stable VT, because it is probably much more effective than lidocaine. Amiodarone is expensive.
Atenolol/ metoprolol	5 mg i.v. over 1–2 min; repeated up to 15 mg if required	• Asthma/COPD • Hypotension • AF with WPW syndrome	Hypotension: Rx with fluids, glucagon 1 mg i.v.; if severe, 1 mg and repeated	Secondary choice for most tachydysrhythmias owing to negative inotropic effects
Diltiazem	5–10 mg i.v. slowly for AF Repeated to total of 50 mg in first 30 min, if required Influsion; 5–15 mg/min	• Regular wide-complex tachycardias • AV node block • Hypotension • Digoxin toxicity • AF in WPW syndrome • Age <2 yr	Hypotension: Rx with fluid and calcium High-degree AV block: Rx with calcium or atropine. May require temporary pacing	Consider calcium pretreatment Studies in class IV heart failure in patients with AF and noted to be safe in small series
Esmolol	500-μg/kg/min bolus 50–300-μg/kg/min influsion	• As for other β-blockers	Hypotension: Rx with fluids, glucagon 1 mg i.v.; if severe, 1 mg and repeated	A very short half-life makes this a good choice when one is unclear whether the patient can tolerate beta blockers. May be particularly useful in AF in patients with thyrotoxicosis.
Lidocaine	1 mg/kg i.v., repeated at 0.5–0.75 mg/kg, i.v. to a total of 3 mg/kg, if required. Infusion of 1–4 mg/h	• AF (increases AV conduction)	Seizures, confusion, lethargy, but only in overdose	Used for stable VT but only 20% effective. May reduce recurrent VT/VF but not helpful for primary prophylaxis
Magnesium	2–4 g i.v. over 5 min Infusion of 1–2 g/h	• AV block • AF with WPW syndrome • Renal failure (infusion)	Hypotension Flushing Respiratory and muscle weakness at high dose	Patients with infusions running should be checked every few hours to determine respiratory status and reflexes. Decreasing reflexes suggest magnesium toxicity, and infusion should be stopped
Procainamide	17 mg/kg loading at no more than 50 mg/min	• Hypotension (relative contraindication)	Hypotension: Rx with fluids QRS widening: If >50% widening, stop infusion, as torsade des pointes may result	More effective than lidocaine for VT. Effective in SVT with aberrancy. Reduces conduction though accessory pathways but may increase conduction through the AV node.
Verapamil	5–10 mg i.v. at 2 mg/min for PSVT	• As for diltiazem	As for diltiazem	May cause more hypotension than diltiazem. Not extensively studied in patients with congestive heart failure

i.v., intravenous; VT, ventricular tachycardia; AV, atrioventricular; AF, atrial fibrillation; WPW, Wolff-Parkinson-White; COPD, chronic obstructive pulmonary disease; SVT, supraventricular tachycardia; PSVT, paroxysmal supraventricular tachycardia.

associated with class IA antiarrhythmic agents are linked to the development of VT of the torsade de pointes variety. Class IA agents are contraindicated if the tachycardia manifests a prolonged QT interval.

The most important class IA agent is *procainamide*. Procainamide is probably more effective for the treatment of VT than is lidocaine, and it is also effective for treating many SVTs. In cases of regular wide-complex tachycardias of uncertain type, it is particularly useful because it treats both VT and SVT with aberrancy. It is also of use in patients with WPW syndrome and AF because it reduces conduction speed in the accessory pathway. It does, however, increase conduction through the AV node, so it should be used in conjunction with an AV node–blocking agent in these cases. It is given in a dose of 17 mg/kg at not more than 50 mg/minutes. Procainamide may cause hypotension and

QRS widening, particularly if given rapidly, and serial assessment of the ECG is required. Long-term therapy is associated with a lupus-like syndrome.

Quinidine and *disopyramide* are class IA agents seldom used in the ED. Tricyclic antidepressants share the same electrophysiologic properties, and tricyclic antidepressant poisoning is associated with prolonged QT intervals (as well as prolonged QRS complexes). Emergency physicians should be familiar with these drugs because in some patients, tachydysrhythmias may result from their proarrhythmic effects (19). *Lidocaine*, the prototype parenteral class IB agent, has long been considered the drug of first choice in the acute treatment of ventricular dysrhythmias. More recent studies suggest that it is not as effective in this role as previously believed; conversion rates for VT may be as low as 30% (8). It continues to be used, however, in the

ED in the treatment of VT in clinically stable patients (i.e., those without signs of end-organ hypoperfusion), to protect against recurrent VF after resuscitation from cardiac arrest, and to treat significant ventricular ectopy in acute ischemia. However, there is no evidence that lidocaine is valuable in the primary prophylaxis of ventricular dysrhythmias in acute myocardial infarction, and its utilization in this manner is widely discouraged (3). Lidocaine is safe when used appropriately. Toxicity, which is primarily related to the central nervous system, can be avoided if appropriate total doses (typically less than 225 mg in adults) are given at rates no faster than 50 mg/minute for the initial 1-mg/kg bolus and 50 mg/5 minutes for further loading doses.

Phenytoin is another class IB drug, but like several newer oral lidocaine analogs, such as mexiletine and tocainide, it is seldom used in the ED as an antiarrhythmic agent.

Class IC agents, including *encainide* and *flecainide*, effectively suppress premature ventricular complexes (PVCs). They are not as effective at preventing propagation of whatever ectopic beats continue to occur, and thus are not useful in the suppression of ventricular tachydysrhythmias. They have powerful proarrhythmic effects and actually increase mortality when given chronically to patients who have sustained a myocardial infarction (7). Although class IC agents have little current role in the ED, there have been sporadic reports of utility in the initial treatment of AF.

Class II agents (β-blockers) play only a secondary role in the acute treatment of tachycardias. They have negative dromotropic and chronotropic effects, and thus are sometimes used to treat sinus tachycardia when the elevated heart rate is associated with significant hemodynamic consequences. They are also occasionally used as adjunctive therapy for tachycardias involving the AV node (23). Because of the superior efficacy and safety of adenosine and calcium channel blockers, however, even esmolol, a very short acting β-blocker, is, in most cases, only a second-line agent in this circumstance. A possible exception to this general rule is the presence of an acute coronary syndrome, in which the use of β-blockers is generally beneficial, and for which there are concerns about the overall effects of calcium channel blocking agents. Although these concerns probably do not apply to the long-acting nondihydropyridine agents such as verapamil and diltiazem, some experts believe that β-blockers should be preferred over calcium channel blockers in this setting.

Sotalol is a noncardioselective β-adrenergic blocker that, unlike other β-blockers, prolongs the duration of the action potential, increases the refractory period, and lengthens the QT interval. As a result, sotalol is an effective antiarrhythmic agent and has been marketed for the treatment of life-threatening ventricular dysrhythmias. Although sotalol also has demonstrated efficacy in the prophylaxis and treatment of AF and PSVT, its role in the emergency management of these conditions remains poorly defined.

Class III agents include *amiodarone* and *bretylium*, as well as *ibutilide*. Amiodarone is a complex antidysrhythmic with multiple effects. Intravenous amiodarone is probably superior to lidocaine and bretylium for treatment of VF and unstable VT, as well as for the treatment of stable VT. Amiodarone has also been moderately effective in the treatment of AF for rate control and conversion to sinus rhythm. Amiodarone can cause hypotension, heart block, and QT prolongation leading to torsade de pointes. Usual doses for VT and VF are 150 mg intravenously over 10 minutes, followed by 1 mg/minute for 6 hours and then 0.5 mg/minute. An additional bolus of 150 mg can be given for breakthrough dysrhythmias. Similar doses can be used for unstable AF (17).

In the past, bretylium was widely used in emergency medicine, particularly in the setting of cardiac arrest. However, in light of the greater safety and efficacy of other agents, bretylium should be considered, at best, a second- or third-line option.

Calcium channel blockers, particularly *diltiazem* and *verapamil*, continue to have a role in the therapy for tachycardias that involve the AV node. These drugs, which constitute class IV, dramatically decrease conduction through the AV node, thereby slowing the ventricular response in conditions such as AF and interrupting reentry in PSVT (both when the circuit is contained entirely in the AV node and when one of its limbs is in the AV node and the other is in a bypass tract, such as occurs in WPW syndrome). Despite the popularity of adenosine, verapamil remains an excellent choice for the treatment of stable patients with regular narrow QRS complex tachycardia (usually PSVT), although it is contraindicated when the QRS complex is wide (13). VT is the most common cause of a regular wide-complex tachycardia, and it cannot be ruled out with certainty on clinical or electrocardiographic grounds; calcium channel blockers may cause fatal degeneration to VF if given to patients with VT. Diltiazem has effects on the AV node similar to those of verapamil, but it has fewer vasodilatory and negative inotropic effects. The primary indication for intravenous i.v. diltiazem is for prompt control of the ventricular response rate in patients with rapid AF, particularly in the presence of mild-to-moderate congestive heart failure (11).

Because of their vasodilatory and negative inotropic effects, calcium channel blocking agents can cause significant hypotension. They are contraindicated in the presence of severe hypotension and should also be used with caution in the presence of significant congestive heart failure. They are contraindicated in the presence of S-A and AV nodal disease. Intravenous calcium blocking agents should be used cautiously in the presence of oral β-blockade, and are relatively contraindicated when β-blockers have recently been used. They are also relatively contraindicated in the presence of digitalis toxicity (but not merely because a patient is on digitalis) because of their effect on the AV node. Calcium, in doses as low as 100 mg of calcium chloride, can ameliorate the vasodilatory and negative inotropic effects of verapamil without diminishing its negative dromotropic effects on the AV node (12).

Several drugs with important antidysrhythmic effects do not fit easily into this classification scheme. *Adenosine* is a naturally occurring nucleotide, which, like verapamil and diltiazem, exerts its principal antidysrhythmic effects by slowing conduction at the AV node. Adenosine also shares the potentially adverse cardiovascular effects of vasodilation, negative inotropy, and potentially excessive blockade of the AV node. The unique pharmacokinetic properties of adenosine, however, which has a serum half-life of less than 10 seconds, set it apart from the calcium channel blockers. In the treatment of AVNRT (which makes up most cases of PSVT), in which only a transient slowing of AV nodal conduction is necessary to interrupt the reentrant impulse and thus effect conversion to sinus rhythm, the shorter duration of action is particularly attractive, because side effects, even when momentarily severe, resolve so quickly that they are typically of minimal clinical consequence. On the other hand, the short half-life may also be responsible for the higher rate of recurrence of PSVT that is seen following conversion with adenosine than with verapamil (5). The ultrashort duration of action also precludes the use of adenosine for control of the ventricular response in AF or atrial flutter.

In addition to its use in the termination of PSVT, adenosine is probably safe in regular wide-complex tachycardias of uncertain origin, and has been used diagnostically in this patient group. This practice should not be routine in patients with a high likelihood of VT (known coronary artery disease, ECG with evidence of AV dissociation) in whom benefit is unlikely. Adenosine is contraindicated in patients with an irregular wide-complex tachycardia (often caused by AF with WPW) in whom VF may be induced.

Although the side effects of adenosine are generally too transient (less than 10 to 30 seconds) to be clinically significant, the drug is uniquely capable of causing brief but sometimes severe chest pain. The cause of this pain, which mimics myocardial ischemia, is uncertain, but it may be related to cardiac afferent innervation. It is not a sign of myocardial ischemia. Reassuring the patient of the benign nature of the pain is the only treatment necessary.

Because of its rapid degradation, adenosine must be given by rapid bolus injection, preferably in a more proximal venous access site (e.g., antecubital fossa), followed by a flush of normal saline. In the treatment of PSVT, an initial dose of 6 mg (0.01 mg/kg) can be followed by a 12-mg dose if the first dose is ineffective. Heart transplant patients are very sensitive to adenosine and require reduced doses, starting at 1 to 2 mg. Adenosine is potentiated by carbamazepine and dipyridamole and is antagonized by the methylxanthines (theophylline and caffeine). Contraindications include AV block, significant hypotension, and known WPW syndrome with AF.

Digoxin slows conduction through the AV node and has long been used for the control of the ventricular response in acute and chronic AF. Although digoxin may still have a role in the long-term management of AF, it has largely been supplanted by diltiazem for acute rate control. Digoxin is no more effective than placebo in converting AF to sinus rhythm, and it is less effective in this regard than are a number of other drugs. Digoxin has a low toxic–therapeutic index and can induce dysrhythmias at concentrations only minimally above therapeutic.

Magnesium appears to be an effective antiarrhythmic agent, although clinical and research experience with it is relatively limited. Magnesium is a necessary cofactor in the energy-dependent transmembrane sodium–potassium ATP pump, and it is important in correcting intracellular hypokalemia (which greatly increases the risk of serious dysrhythmias in the setting of acute ischemia). It also has antiarrhythmic effects in a variety of circumstances in which repolarization abnormalities exist. Clinically, magnesium has been demonstrated to be effective in the treatment of ventricular dysrhythmias, particularly torsade de pointes, for which it is the drug of choice, and stable monomorphic VT.

Magnesium slows the ventricular rate in AF by blocking the AV node and may increase the rate of conversion to sinus rhythm. Magnesium can terminate MFAT and is marginally effective in treating PSVT. Usual doses of magnesium are 2 to 4 g i.v. over 5 minutes, followed by an infusion of 1 g per hour. At these dosages, magnesium is a safe agent that produces few side effects. At excessive doses or rates of administration, hypotension, loss of reflexes, and respiratory depression can occur. Infusions should be avoided in patients with renal failure, as accumulation can result in respiratory failure.

Automated Implantable Cardioverter–Defibrillators

Automated implantable cardioverter-defibrillators (AICDs) (see Chapter 45, "The Patient with a Pacemaker or Implantable Cardioverter–Defibrillator") are being used in a growing number of patients with recurrent ventricular tachydysrhythmias who are at increased risk of sudden death. These devices have a computerized pulse generator, typically implanted in the abdominal wall, and both afferent and efferent cardiac leads. They are de-signed to recognize malignant rhythms and deliver a counter-shock to the heart (24).

AICD failure can take several forms, each of which may result in emergent problems. The device may fail to fire when necessary, or may fire inappropriately (randomly, or in response to a nonmalignant tachycardia). When the AICD fails to fire, a patient can present in cardiac arrest (in VT or VF) or with recurrent bouts of tachycardia-related symptoms (palpitations, light-headedness, or syncope). During an arrest, the AICD should be deactivated by placing a standard pacemaker magnet over the upper right corner of the pulse generator for at least 30 seconds, until the QRS-synchronous beeps are replaced by a single continuous tone. Although the AICD poses no threat to the resuscitation team, it can interfere with the resuscitation. A cardiologist expert in the use of these devices should analyze the reason for AICD failure (sensing problems, lead problems, or pulse generator failure) in an intensive care unit.

Patients may present because the AICD has fired. This could represent an appropriate (and lifesaving) response to a malignant dysrhythmia, or an inappropriate shock due to device malfunction. These patients should be seen by their cardiologist in the ED, and almost all (even those in whom the shock was ostensibly appropriate) should be admitted to a monitored setting to evaluate the underlying dysrhythmia, to monitor antiarrhythmic drug therapy, and to ensure that the AICD is working properly. If the device continues to fire intermittently in the ED in the absence of malignant arrhythmic stimuli, it must be deactivated. This should be done only after ensuring that appropriate resuscitation equipment is immediately available; all such patients require admission to an intensive care unit.

CRITICAL INTERVENTIONS

- Be prepared for clinical deterioration in any patient presenting with an acute tachydysrhythmia. A defibrillator and advanced airway equipment should be ready at the bedside
- Perform defibrillation for patients in ventricular fibrillation before any other intervention
- Perform electrical cardioversion for patients who are unstable in the face of any very rapid tachycardia
- Use a systematic approach to tachydysrhythmias based on the clinical status at presentation

DISPOSITION

In most cases, the disposition of patients with tachydysrhythmia is obvious. The patient resuscitated from cardiac arrest resulting from VF obviously must be admitted to the intensive care unit. Similarly, there should be little controversy about discharging a healthy young patient with a brief, minimally symptomatic episode of PSVT that readily converted to sinus rhythm. In the few patients with a problematic disposition, the physician should remember that ED care involves only initial therapy and not definitive management of the tachydysrhythmia. Several categories of patients should be admitted:

- Patients who are symptomatic after acute onset of tachycardia and who have failed appropriate therapy or responded only transiently.
- Patients who were clinically unstable as a result of a tachycardia, including all patients who require cardioversion because of end-organ hypoperfusion.

• Patients who were treated successfully before the development of serious symptoms but who have the potential for decompensation if the tachydysrhythmia recurs.

The basis of the dysrhythmia also plays a role in disposition decisions: Any patient with a realistic likelihood of a dangerous etiology (e.g., possible acute myocardial infarction) should be admitted, even if the dysrhythmia itself was benign. Finally, it may be appropriate to admit a stable patient for continuous electrocardiographic monitoring during initiation of chronic drug therapy.

COMMON PITFALLS

✔ Being overly concerned with "diagnosis." One should concentrate more on the hemodynamic effects of the rhythm than on its origin. An apparently benign narrow-complex rhythm should not be treated conservatively in the face of end-organ hypoperfusion. Conversely, stable patients can often be managed without electrical cardioversion, even if their tachycardia appears ominous from the standpoint of its cause or morphology

✔ Reliance on electrocardiographic and clinical findings to identify the likely source of an dysrhythmia. Electrocardiographic and clinical findings are suggestive but not infallible guides

✔ The use of a calcium channel blocker to treat a wide-complex tachycardia. Calcium channel blockers are appropriate for many narrow-complex tachycardias but can precipitate VF in wide-complex tachycardias. This is true not only when the rhythm is VT, but also for other wide-complex tachycardias originating above the AV node, such as AF with anterograde conduction down a bypass tract in WPW syndrome

✔ Treatment of symptoms rather than the tachydysrhythmia precipitating those symptoms. In patients having symptoms related to a very rapid tachycardia, controlling the ventricular rate usually ameliorates the symptoms

✔ Failure to seek and, if possible, correct the factors that precipitated a tachydysrhythmia. Examples of specific precipitants include hypoxemia, infectious or inflammatory processes (e.g., endocarditis, myocarditis, and pericarditis), and endocrine or metabolic abnormalities (e.g., thyrotoxicosis, hypokalemia, hyperkalemia, or hypomagnesemia). Dysrhythmias can also be caused by intoxications, such as intentional overdose (e.g., tricyclic antidepressants), drug abuse (e.g., cocaine or alcohol), or therapeutic misadventure with prescribed medications (e.g., digoxin or theophylline). In patients taking antiarrhythmic agents, an acute dysrhythmia may be the result of subtherapeutic drug levels, a dysrhythmogenic effect of the drug at therapeutic or toxic levels, or simply a failure of the drug to prevent a preexisting dysrhythmia

✔ Failure to consider myocardial ischemia in all patients. Myocardial infarction must be ruled out whenever it seems a reasonably likely cause of the dysrhythmia, or when the dysrhythmia has itself produced a substantial period of ischemia as suggested by electrocardiographic changes or symptoms

References

1. Alander SW, Hulse JE. Pediatric ECGs and rhythm disturbances. *Pediatr Emerg Med Rep* 1999;4:63.
2. Aronow WS, et al. Verapamil in atrial fibrillation and atrial flutter. *Clin Pharmacol Ther* 1979;26:578.
3. Berntsen RF, Rasmussen K. Lidocaine to prevent ventricular fibrillation in the pre-hospital phase of suspected acute myocardial infarction: The North Norwegian Lidocaine Intervention Trial. *Am Heart J* 1992;124:1478.
4. Bigger JT Jr. Management of arrhythmias. In: Braunwald E, ed. *Heart disease. A textbook of cardiovascular medicine*. Philadelphia: WB Saunders, 1980:724.
5. Cairns CB, Niemann JT. Intravenous adenosine in the emergency department treatment of paroxysmal supraventricular tachycardia. *Ann Emerg Med* 1991;20:717.
6. Donovan KD, Power B, Hockings EF, et al. Intravenous flecainide versus amiodarone for recent onset atrial fibrillation. *Am J Cardiol* 1995;75:693.
7. Echt DS, Liebson PR, Mitchell LB, et al. Morbidity and mortality in patients receiving encainide, flecainide, or placebo. The Cardiac Arrhythmia Suppression Trial. *N Engl J Med* 1991;324:781.
8. Griffith MJ, Linker NJ, Garratt CJ, et al. Relative efficacy and safety of intravenous drugs of the termination of sustained ventricular tachycardia. *Lancet* 1990;336:670.
9. Gulamhusein S, Ko P, Carruthers SG, et al. Acceleration of the ventricular response during atrial fibrillation in the Wolff-Parkinson-White syndrome after verapamil. *Circulation* 1982;65:348.
10. Herbert ME, Votey SR, Morgan MT, et al. Failure to agree on the ECG diagnosis of VT. *Ann Emerg Med* 1996;27:35–38.
11. Heywood JT, Graham B, Marais GE, et al. Effect of intravenous diltiazem on rapid atrial fibrillation accompanied by congestive heart failure. *Am J Cardiol* 1991;67:1150.
12. Kuhn M, Schriger DL. Low-dose calcium pretreatment to prevent verapamil-induced hypotension. *Am Heart J* 1992;124:231.
13. Kuhn M, Schriger DL. Verapamil administration to patients with contraindications: is it associated with adverse outcomes? *Ann Emerg Med* 1991;20:1094.
14. Levine JH, Michael JR, Guarnieri T. Multifocal atrial tachycardia: a toxic effect of theophylline. *Lancet* 1985;1:12.
15. Mancini GBJ, Goldberger AL. Cardioversion of atrial fibrillation: consideration of embolization, anticoagulation, prophylactic pacemaker, and long term success. *Am Heart J* 1982;104:617.
16. Morady F, Shen EN, Bhandari A, et al. Clinical symptoms in patients with sustained ventricular tachycardia. *West J Med* 1985;142:341.
17. Moran JL, Gallagher J, Peake SI, et al. Parenteral magnesium sulfate versus amiodarone in the therapy of atrial tachyrhythmias: a prospective, randomized study. *Crit Care Med* 1995;23:1816.
18. Roberts SA, Diaz C, Nolan PE, et al. Effectiveness and costs of digoxin therapy for atrial fibrillation. *Am J Cardiol* 1993;72:567.
19. Ruskin JN, McGovern B, Garan H, et al. Antiarrhythmic drugs: a possible cause of out of hospital cardiac arrest. *N Engl J Med* 1983;309:1302.
20. Shlofmitz RA, Hirsch BE, Meyer BR. New onset atrial fibrillation: is there a need for emergent hospitalization? *J Gen Intern Med* 1986;1:139.
21. Stewart RB, Bardy GH, Greene H. Wide complex tachycardia. Misdiagnosis and outcome after emergent therapy. *Ann Intern Med* 1986;104:766.
22. Stroke Prevention in Atrial Fibrillation Investigators. Preliminary report of the Stroke Prevention in Atrial Fibrillation Study. *N Engl J Med* 1990;322:863.
23. Sung RJ, Blanski L, Kirshenbaum J, MacCosbe P, et al. Clinical experience with esmolol, a short acting beta adrenergic blocker in cardiac arrhythmias and myocardial ischemia. *Clin Pharmacol* 1986;26[Suppl A]:A15.
24. Winkle RA. State-of-the-art of the AICD. *Pacing Clin Electrophysiol* 1991;14:961–966.
25. Yusuf S, Sleight P, Rossi P, et al. Reduction in infarct size, arrhythmias, and chest pain by early intravenous beta blockade in suspected acute myocardial infarction. *Circulation* 1983;67[Suppl 1]:132.
26. The AFFIRM Investigators. Survival in patients presenting with atrial fibrillation in the Atrial Fibrillation Follow-up Investigation of Rhythm Management (AFFIRM) Study. *N Engl J Med* 2002;347:1825–1833.

CHAPTER 45
The Patient with a Pacemaker or Implantable Cardioverter–Defibrillator

Robert M. Rodriguez

THE PATIENT WITH A PACEMAKER

The first permanent cardiac pacemakers were implanted in the late 1950s; since that time, advances in microprocessor technology have led to the production of compact pacemakers that adapt to changes in patient physiology (14). Although the earliest models had only single-chamber, asynchronous pacing capability, with less than a 2-year battery life, current dual-chamber pacemakers are rate-responsive to increased patient activity and are powered by lithium batteries that may last longer than 10 years (4). The proven utility of pacemakers has grown over the years. Recent trials have demonstrated the efficacy of pacemakers in the prevention and treatment of atrial fibrillation and as adjunctive therapy for patients with congestive heart failure and ventricular dyssynchrony—manifested by a prolonged QRS interval (1,5,8).

Given that more than 1 million Americans currently have pacemakers (14), the emergency department (ED) physician will undoubtedly care for many patients with these devices. Although detailed knowledge of the myriad complexities of pacemaker programming and operation is unnecessary, the emergency physician must understand the basics of pacemaker terminology and function and must be familiar with the presentation, evaluation, and treatment of common pacemaker-related problems.

Central to the understanding of basic pacemaker function are the five-letter codes used by the North American Society of Pacing and Electrophysiology–British Pacing and Electrophysiology Group (NASPE/BPEG) to characterize the modes of operation of current pacemakers (Table 45.1). In everyday practice, description of the mode of pacing is limited to use of the first three code letters: position I, chamber(s) paced; position II, chamber(s) sensed; and position III, pacemaker response to sensing. A VVI pacemaker thus paces the ventricle only, senses only ventricular depolarizations, and inhibits pacemaker output in response to a sensed ventricular depolarization. The more versatile DDD pacemaker, which is currently the most frequently implanted type of pacemaker (14), may pace the atria, the ventricles, or both; may sense atrial depolarizations, ventricular depolarizations, or both; and may either inhibit or trigger pacemaker output to the atria and ventricles in response to sensed depolarizations. Intrinsic ventricular depolarizations will inhibit both atrial and ventricular output; intrinsic atrial depolarizations will inhibit atrial pacemaker output and will trigger ventricular output if the ventricle itself does not respond after a programmed time interval.

TABLE 45.1. NASPE/BPEG (NBG) Codes

1st position indicates the chamber paced
  V = ventricle
  A = atrium
  D = dual
  O = no pacing
2nd position indicates the chamber sensed
  V = ventricle
  A = atrium
  D = dual
  O = no sensing
3rd position indicates the response to a sensed event
  I = inhibited
  T = triggered/tracking
  D = dual
  O = no response
4th position indicates programmability and rate response
  O = not programmable
  P = simple programming (three functions or less)
  M = multiprogrammable (more than three functions)
  C = communicating (M + telemetry capabilities)
  R = rate responsive
5th position indicates antitachydysrhythmia functions
  O = none
  P = pacing
  S = shock
  D = dual (shock and pacing)

(From Love C, ed. Handbook of Cardiac Pacing. Georgetown, TX: Landes Bioscience, 1998, with permission.)

CLINICAL PRESENTATION AND DIFFERENTIAL DIAGNOSIS

Syndromes of pacemaker malfunction can generally be divided into those that cause underpacing, with associated bradycardia, hypotension, light-headedness, and syncope; and those that produce overpacing, manifested by tachycardia and palpitations with or without ischemia or hypotension symptoms. The differential diagnosis of these nonspecific presenting complaints is broad, however, encompassing multiple other disorders, including dysrhythmias, vasovagal phenomena, anemia, hypovolemia, and non–rate-related syndromes of low cardiac output. These common disorders must be considered, and before attributing presenting symptoms to less common pacemaker malfunction, the physician must first determine whether the device is truly malfunctioning. Patient history, electrocardiographic (ECG) analysis, and determination of the current programming and specifications of the pacemaker are the keys to making this evaluation.

EMERGENCY DEPARTMENT EVALUATION

In addition to elucidating standard history about the symptoms, time course, and precipitants related to the presenting complaint(s), the physician should also seek the following information regarding the pacemaker: pacemaker model, current programming, date of implantation, indication for implantation, history of pacemaker malfunction, and dates of last interrogation and battery check. Some of this vital information may be obtained from the pacemaker identification card, which the patient should carry at all times. If this card is unavailable, a chest radiograph may reveal the pacemaker's identifying serial number or code (15). For technical support or to find out other information about the pacemaker, the physician may call the pacemaker manufacturer's assistance department.

The emergency physician should also ask about exposure to potential sources of environmental electromagnetic interference with pacemaker function. Although most everyday appliances and devices pose virtually no risk to current pacemakers—electric toothbrushes, cellular telephones, induction ovens, and stove plates can markedly alter their operation. Most modern airport security gates pose minimal risk, but antitheft systems in stores emit signals of variable intensity, with unpredictable effects on pacemaker function (11).

Because right ventricular (RV) pacemakers produce left bundle-branch block (LBBB) patterns of depolarization, the ECG diagnosis of myocardial ischemia or myocardial infarction (MI) may be difficult. Discordant T waves after paced beats are the norm; minor ST-segment evaluations inferiorly and anteriorly (leads V_1 to V_3) and ST-segment depression (leads 1, V_1, V_5, and V_6) also commonly occur in the absence of ischemia (3). Pacing may even induce marked ST-segment and T-wave abnormalities when the patient's native, spontaneous rhythm emerges (3).

Applying the criteria used in the evaluation of patients with intrinsic LBBB, however, the physician may still occasionally diagnose MI in the patient with a pacemaker (3). Concordant ST-segment elevations and markedly elevated (greater than 5 mm) discordant ST-segments are highly indicative of MI, especially when the T waves associated with these segments are of opposite polarity (3,21). ST-segment depression in leads V_1, V_2, and V_3 also suggests ischemia or infarction, as does late notching of the ascending QRS limb in the left precordial leads (3,21). A qR pattern after the pacemaker spike in leads 1, V_1, and V_5 has low sensitivity but very high specificity for anteroseptal MI (3). Finally, serial electrocardiograms may demonstrate progressive ST-segment and T-wave changes that lead to the diagnosis of MI. The emergency physician should certainly look for these patterns, but given their low sensitivity, their absence does not at all rule out ischemia or infarction.

Evaluating the utility of an ECG algorithm based on these patterns for the detection of MI in patients with intrinsic LBBB, investigators found that the algorithm had poor sensitivity (less than 10%) for MI prediction (23). If the results of this study can be generalized to pacemaker patients with LBBB depolarization patterns, then the emergency physician must not base decisions about thrombolysis and other coronary vasculature interventions for pacemaker patients with suspected ischemia or infarction solely or even primarily on the electrocardiogram.

Pacemaker Malfunction and Pacemaker-Associated Disorders

Malfunction Associated with Bradycardia

Pacemaker malfunction leading to a slow pulse arises from noncapture, pacemaker output failure, or pacemaker oversensing. Noncapture refers to an absence of ventricular or atrial depolarization after a pacemaker spike (Fig. 45.1). The most common cause of this condition is pacemaker lead dislodgement, which typically occurs within a few weeks of implantation (11). Other mechanical causes include insulation breaks, lead fracture, and inflammatory reaction at the lead tip (11). Reversible metabolic abnormalities, such as hyperkalemia, and drug effects should also be considered. Of note, if a pacemaker spike occurs within 300 milliseconds of a prior ventricular depolarization, the ventricle may be in its refractory period and therefore lack of capture is expected (9). The pacemaker may be firing inappropriately early because of undersensing of the prior depolarization, but it is not truly malfunctioning with regard to pacing (Fig. 45.2).

Absent or inappropriately delayed ventricular pacemaker spikes on the electrocardiogram of a patient with a bradycardic

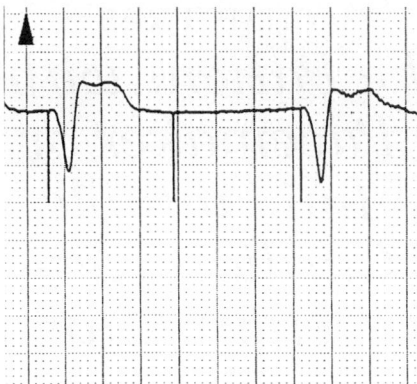

Figure 45.1. Noncaptured pacemaker spike between two captured spikes.

pacemaker indicate primary pacemaker output failure, battery depletion, or output failure secondary to oversensing (reading other signals as true ventricular depolarizations) (11). Causes of primary output failure include lead fracture or disconnection and various pulse generator component failures. Oversensed signals may be of cardiac (P and T waves) or extracardiac (myopotentials) origin and lead to inappropriate inhibition of pacemaker ventricular output (11).

These causes of absent or delayed pacemaker spikes may be distinguished by performing a magnet test of the pacemaker. Application of a ring magnet over a normally functioning pacemaker disables sensing and induces asynchronous pacing at model-specific rates, which may be determined by checking the patient's records or calling the pacemaker manufacturer (11,15). If the problem is oversensing, the magnet will induce asynchronous pacing at that model's characteristic rate. If battery depletion is the cause, asynchronous pacing will occur at a different, generally slower rate (11). If the malfunction is a result of lead displacement or some other primary disconnection, no pacing response to the magnet will be seen.

Malfunction Associated with Tachycardia

Pacemakers may produce inappropriate tachycardia by several mechanisms. When a pacemaker fails to sense intrinsic ventricular depolarizations, it will fail to inhibit pacemaker output, potentially causing a pacemaker-driven tachycardia; that is, "undersensing leads to overpacing" (15). In dual-chamber

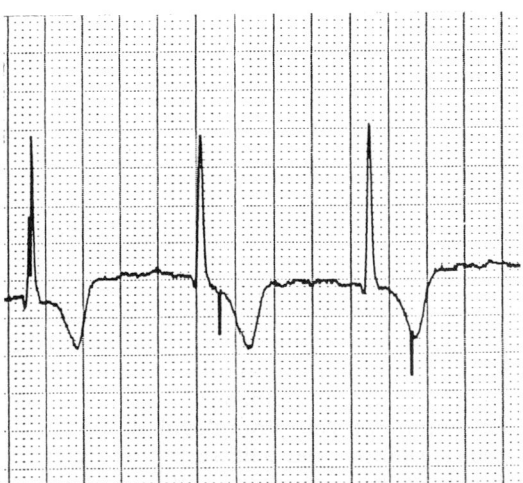

Figure 45.2. Pacemaker undersensing.

systems, the pacemaker circuit may act like an accessory pathway similar to those seen in Wolff-Parkinson-White (WPW) syndrome, thereby propagating a reentrant tachycardia known as pacemaker-mediated tachycardia or "endless-loop tachycardia" (15). This dysrhythmia may be terminated by vagal maneuvers, external magnet induction of asynchronous pacing, intravenous adenosine, or external cardiac pacing with 10 to 20 mA of output (9,15).

A final pacemaker-related tachycardia that occurs only rarely with current pulse generators is "runaway pacemaker," a potentially lethal disorder in which battery depletion or other component failure causes extremely rapid pacing, with rates restricted only by the pacemaker's upper rate limit (12). This disorder generally does not respond to conservative treatment measures, and, in the setting of hemodynamic instability, the emergency physician should attempt to disable the runaway pacemaker by incising over the pacemaker pocket and disconnecting the pulse generator leads (9,12).

Pacemaker syndrome, a classic example of a pacemaker operating correctly according to its programming yet still causing bothersome symptoms, results from a loss of atrioventricular synchrony in the VVI pacing mode (15). Fatigue, lightheadedness, and syncope owing to decreased cardiac output (loss of atrial kick), and disturbing neck pulsations related to regurgitant cannon A waves (atria contracting against closed atrioventricular valves) are the predominant symptoms. Although this disorder is largely limited to patients with VVI pacemakers and is usually ameliorated with a change to synchronized dual-chamber pacing, it can occasionally occur in patients who have DDD pacemakers (22).

Infectious and Mechanical Complications of Pacemakers

In addition to rhythm and hemodynamic problems associated with pacemakers, foreign-body–related complications also occur. Infections of pacemakers and associated hardware occur in approximately 6% to 15% of patients, with staphylococcal species being the most common pathogens (9). In the patient presenting with fever and redness and tenderness over the pulse generator pocket, the diagnosis of pacemaker infection is obvious.

Subtler presentations are common, however, and the emergency physician should consider pacemaker-related infection as a potential cause of unexplained fever in any patient with a pacemaker. Notably, without superimposed endocarditis, embolic phenomena and murmurs are generally absent. Nuclear medicine scans may provide ancillary evidence of infected pacemaker hardware. Confirmed pacemaker infection mandates a course of parenteral antibiotics, and most authorities agree that removal of the device is indicated (17).

Pacemaker-associated thrombosis of the upper extremity vessels is uncommon (less than 5% by venography), but it should be considered in the patient with unilateral arm swelling, erythema, or pain (7). Ultrasound or venography may be used to distinguish this entity from similar-appearing arm cellulitis. Anticoagulation without pacemaker removal has been reported to successfully treat the thrombosis (7).

EMERGENCY DEPARTMENT MANAGEMENT

As with other ED problems, patient stability determines the urgency of intervention in the patient with a pacemaker. The cardiac arrest patient should receive standard advanced cardiac life support (ACLS)–guided resuscitation. During defibrillation or cardioversion, however, the physician should avoid placing pads or paddles directly over the pulse generator (10). Pacemakers of resuscitation survivors should be evaluated for damage or reprogramming arising from countershocks. In nonsurvivors, the pacemaker may continue to produce ECG spikes without associated ventricular capture, which represents isolated pacemaker activity and not true pulseless electrical activity.

The pacemaker patient with hypotensive bradycardia requires the usual emergent therapeutic measures (chronotropic support with medications, external pacing, or transvenous pacing). The physician may attempt to temporarily asynchronously pace the patient's rate with higher current by placing a ring magnet over the pacemaker, as described earlier in this chapter (11). This maneuver may be helpful if the pacemaker is oversensing, and thereby suppressing output (absent or inappropriately slow rate of pacemaker spikes on electrocardiogram), or if low pacemaker current is leading to noncapture.

During the ED management of pacemaker patients, the physician must recognize the multiple potential sources of electromagnetic interference with pacemaker function, especially magnetic resonance imaging (MRI) and electrocautery. Given that MRI may induce complete block of pacemaker output, severe pacemaker-driven tachycardias, and other potentially disastrous pacemaker malfunction, MRI is contraindicated for patients with pacemakers (11). If MRI is absolutely essential to patient management, some authorities have suggested switching the pacemaker to its "off" mode, turning pacemaker output down so that it will not capture, or surgically removing the device (2,4). These maneuvers must be undertaken with the help of an electrophysiologist, and patient informed consent should be obtained. Electrocautery may also induce a number of hazardous abnormalities in pacemaker function; precautions and steps to minimize risk during surgical procedures are described in other reference texts (4).

DISPOSITION

Disposition of the patient with a pacemaker-related problem largely depends on the severity of signs and symptoms, and should be determined collaboratively with the patient's electrophysiologist. Patients with pacing malfunction, such as failure to capture or battery depletion, should be admitted to monitored settings. Patients requiring a higher level of care may occasionally need interhospital transfer. ACLS units should be used, and the patient's rhythm and hemodynamics must be stabilized prior to transfer; backup pacing modalities (transthoracic or transvenous) should be in place during transit.

THE PATIENT WITH AN IMPLANTABLE CARDIOVERTER–DEFIBRILLATOR

The first implantable cardioverter–defibrillator (ICD) was placed in 1980, and, as with pacemakers, technologic improvements have produced smaller, "smarter" defibrillators that are more easily implanted (6). Early models were nonprogrammable shock or no-shock devices that required open thoracotomy for epicardial patch placement. Current programmable devices have defibrillator leads that are inserted transvenously and utilize improved rhythm analysis algorithms to deliver tiered therapy. For example, slow ventricular tachycardia (VT) may be first treated with overdrive pacing; if it fails to convert the VT, low-energy shocks are delivered. If they also fail, higher energy shocks are given (15). Many new ICDs also incorporate antibradycardia (pacing) functions that may be activated if cardioversion or defibrillation results in a bradycardic or asystolic rhythm.

As with pacemakers, the indications for ICD implantation have also expanded. Major trials examining the treatment of patients with frequent ventricular dysrhythmias have demonstrated increased mortality with pharmacologic dysrhythmic

TABLE 45.2.   NBD Codes (for Implantable–Defibrillators)

1st position indicates the chamber shocked
V = ventricle
A = atrium
D = dual
O = no shock therapy
2nd position indicates the chamber for antitachycardia pacing
V = ventricle
A = atrium
D = dual
O = no antitachycardia pacing
3rd position indicates the method of tachycardia detection
E = electrogram
H = hemodynamic
4th position indicates chambers for bradycardia pacing*
V = ventricle
A = atrium
D = dual
O = no bradycardia pacing.

*Alternatively the three or four letter NBG pacing code may be used following the first three letters of the NBD code (e.g., VVE-VVIR indicating ventricular shock, ventricular ATP, electrogram detection and VVIR pacing capability).
(From Love C, ed. Handbook of Cardiac Pacing. Georgetown, TX: Landes Bioscience, 1998, with permission.)

therapy but markedly decreased mortality with ICDs (6). Prophylactic placement of an ICD has also been demonstrated to increase survival in patients who have post-MI low ejection fractions even without electrophysiologic evidence of sustained dysrhythmias (18). Currently, there are approximately 400,000 ICDs in operation worldwide (20).

NASPE/BPEG descriptive codes also characterize the types and functions of ICDs (15): position I, chamber(s) shocked; position II, chamber(s) for antitachycardia pacing; position III, method of tachycardia detection; and position IV, chamber(s) for bradycardia pacing (Table 45.2). However, in everyday practice, these codes are less commonly used than are pacemaker codes.

CLINICAL PRESENTATION AND DIFFERENTIAL DIAGNOSIS

Patients with ICD malfunction generally present with either defibrillation–cardioversion failure or frequent ICD discharge. Defibrillation–cardioversion failure may result from failure to deliver a shock, analogous to pacemaker output failure, or from failure of delivered shock(s) to convert the dysrhythmia, analogous to pacemaker noncapture. ICD discharge for rhythms other than ventricular fibrillation (VF) or VT is common, occurring in 22% of patients over 2 years of follow-up in one case series (13). Although the potential lethality of inappropriate ICD discharge is lower than that of ICD failure to discharge, repeated shocks may cause myocardial injury, temporary ventricular dysfunction, and rapid battery depletion (19). Furthermore, they may be very painful and anxiety-provoking. The most common causes of recurrent discharges are dysrhythmias (supraventricular tachycardias and nonsustained VT) that meet the ICD's threshold heart rates for ICD activation (15).

EMERGENCY DEPARTMENT EVALUATION AND MANAGEMENT

In a study of the mechanisms of sudden death of patients with ICDs, the most common causes were electromechanical dissocia-

tion (EMD) after ICD conversion of VF or VT (29%), shock failure defined as VT or VF that was not terminated by the full complement of 4 to 6 ICD shocks (26%), primary EMD not involving VT or VF (16%), and VT/VF that was successfully converted but recurred over and over (13%) (16). When treating the ICD patient in cardiac arrest, therefore, the physician should focus on treating potentially reversible causes of EMD and on further attempts to convert persistent or recurrent VT/VF. Resuscitation should generally follow ACLS protocols (19). Most ICDs analyze and shock VF or VT within 30 seconds; therefore, if a patient presents in these rhythms, the physician should assume that ICD defibrillation–cardioversion has been unsuccessful and should immediately proceed with external countershocks (10). However, to prevent ICD absorption of current, defibrillator pads or paddles should not be placed directly over the device and, when feasible, should be positioned anteroposteriorly (10). Chest compressions should be given in the standard fashion. Without rubber gloves, the rescuer may feel a slight, harmless shock if an ICD discharges during compressions (10).

After successful resuscitation, the emergency physician should investigate the events surrounding the arrest, focusing on the few causes of ICD failure (electrolyte imbalance, myocardial ischemia or MI, and drug effects) that may be treated without ICD reprogramming or surgery. When feasible, the physician should ask the patient if he or she recalls chest pain, palpitations, or ICD discharges. As with the pacemaker patient, the emergency physician should use direct history, the patient's ICD card, medical records and telephone calls to the ICD manufacturer to gather information about reasons for and date of ICD implantation, most recent ICD interrogation, and prior ICD malfunction. The emergency physician should ask about exposures to the sources of environmental electromagnetic interference described earlier in regard to pacemakers. There are many etiologies of ICD malfunction, and these may be explored later by the electrophysiologist, who may interrogate the ICD for detailed analysis of dysrhythmias and ICD response. In addition, referral to an electrophysiologist is essential to evaluate the ICD for lead fracture or displacement caused by chest compressions and for pulse generator damage or reprogramming arising from external countershocks (19).

When rapid atrial fibrillation triggers frequent ICD discharge, the physician should attempt to slow the ventricular rate with the usual pharmacologic agents (19). If, after a period of close monitoring, it is determined that frequent ICD discharges are not occurring as appropriate responses to significant dysrhythmias, or if frequent ineffective ICD discharges are interfering with resuscitation, the physician may disable the ICD by applying a ring magnet to the chest wall over the device (19). Occasionally, two magnets, stacked one on top of the other, are required to deactivate the ICD in markedly obese patients (19). Although the magnet suspends all antitachycardia functions (i.e., the ICD will not deliver a shock for VT), back-up pacing functions of the ICD may persist. Attention to hemodynamics, close monitoring, and sedation or analgesia for the anxious patient are other keys to ED management of frequent ICD discharges. The emergency physician must understand that although a ring magnet generally causes changes in pacemaker function only during application of the magnet (i.e., the pacemaker resumes its normal function after removal of the magnet), a magnet may reset some ICD models to the "off" mode indefinitely (19). Therefore, if a magnet is either intentionally or inadvertently applied to an ICD, the physician should assume the device has been deactivated and should arrange for ICD interrogation and reprogramming.

The presentation and management of infectious and thrombotic complications of ICDs parallel those of pacemakers, except that ICD infections may be more serious and difficult to treat (17). Hospital admission for administration of parenteral antibiotics and hardware removal is recommended for all infected ICDs

(17). If the patient has an older model with epicardial patches, computed tomographic imaging of the heart and mediastinum is warranted to determine the extent of mediastinal involvement.

CRITICAL INTERVENTIONS

- Distinguish between causes of absent or delayed pacemaker spikes by performing a magnet test of the pacemaker, which in a normally functioning pacemaker disables sensing and induces asynchronous pacing at model-specific rates
- Avoid placing pads or paddles directly over the pulse generator during defibrillation or cardioversion
- Disable the ICD by applying a ring magnet to the chest wall over the device if frequent, inappropriate ICD discharges are causing substantial patient discomfort or are interfering with resuscitation. However, since this action may re-set the ICD to "off" even after removal of the magnet, the ICD must subsequently be interrogated or reprogrammed

DISPOSITION

Given the potentially catastrophic consequences of ICD failure, urgent referral to an electrophysiologist is recommended for essentially all types of ICD malfunction. ICD patients should be observed in or admitted to monitored settings until specialist evaluations are completed. If specialist evaluation or higher level of care issues mandate transfer to another facility, ACLS units should be used, and transthoracic (anteroposterior) defibrillation/pacing pads should be applied to the patient prior to transit.

COMMON PITFALLS

✔ Misdiagnosing pacemaker or ICD malfunction because of inadequate information about the current programming and operation of the device. The physician should gather as much information about the pacemaker or ICD as possible from patient history, device identification cards, pacemaker or ICD registration departments, and patients' cardiologists or electrophysiologists
✔ When evaluating the pacemaker patient for MI, failing to understand both the utility and the limits of 12-lead ECG interpretation. Several ECG patterns are reliable indicators of ischemia or infarction during RV pacing, but a normal LBBB pattern of pacing does not rule out infarction or ischemia
✔ In a patient with cardiac arrest, allowing the presence of a pacemaker or ICD to change resuscitation procedures. Other than anteroposterior positioning of paddles and avoiding shocks over the devices, resuscitation should generally follow the usual ACLS protocols
✔ Assuming that—after magnet application over an ICD or after cardioversion or resuscitation of a patient with an ICD or a pacemaker—the device has reverted to its normal programming and operation. The ICD or pacemaker must be reevaluated after these procedures
✔ Failing to make disposition decisions for most pacemaker problems and for essentially all cases of ICD malfunction in collaboration with an electrophysiologist

References

1. Abraham WT, Fisher WG, Smith AL, et al. Cardiac resynchronization in chronic heart failure. *N Engl J Med* 2002;346:1845–1853.
2. Atlee JL, ed. *Arrhythmias and pacemakers: practical management for anesthesia and critical care medicine.* Philadelphia: WB Saunders, 1996.
3. Barold SS, Zipes DP. Cardiac pacemakers and antiarrhythmic devices. In: Braunwald E, ed. *Heart disease.* Philadelphia: WB Saunders, 1997:705–738.
4. Bourke ME. The patient with a pacemaker or related device. *Can J Anaesth* 1996;43:R24–R32.
5. Bradley DJ, Bradley DA, Baughman KL, et al. Cardiac resynchronization and death from progressive heart failure. *JAMA* 2003;289:730–740.
6. Cannom DS, Prystowsky EN. Management of ventricular arrhythmias: detection, drugs and devices. *JAMA* 1999;281:172–179.
7. Ciocon JO, Galindo-Ciocon D. Arm edema, subclavian thrombosis, and pacemakers. *Angiol J Vasc Dis* 1998;49:315–319.
8. Cooper JM, Katcher MS, Orlov MV. Implantable devices for the treatment of atrial fibrillation. *N Engl J Med* 2002;346:2062.
9. Coppola M, Yealy DM. Transvenous pacemakers. *Emerg Med Clin North Am* 1994;12:633–643.
10. Cummins RO, ed. *Advanced cardiac life support.* Dallas: American Heart Association, 1997.
11. Fischer W, Ritter PH, eds. *Cardiac pacing in clinical practice.* Berlin: Springer-Verlag, 1998.
12. Hayes DL, Vlietstra RE. Pacemaker malfunction. *Ann Intern Med* 1993;119:828–835.
13. Grimm W, Flores BF, Marchlinski FE. Complications of implantable cardioverter defibrillator therapy: follow up of 241 patients. *PACE* 1993;16:218–222.
14. Kusumoto FM, Goldschlager N. Cardiac pacing. *N Engl J Med* 1996;334:89–97.
15. Love C, ed. *Handbook of cardiac pacing.* Georgetown, TX: Landes Bioscience, 1998.
16. Mitchell LB, Pineda EA, Titus JL, et al. Sudden death in patients with implantable cardioverter defibrillators. *J Am Coll Cardiol* 2002;39:1323–1328.
17. Molina JE. Undertreatment and overtreatment of patients with infected antiarrhythmic implantable devices. *Ann Thorac Surg* 1997;63:504–509.
18. Moss AJ, Zareba W, Hall J, et al. Prophylactic implantation of a defibrillator in patients with myocardial infarction and reduced ejection fraction. *N Engl J Med* 2002;346:877–883.
19. Pinski SL, Trohman RG. Implantable cardioverter-defibrillators: implications for the nonelectrophysiologist. *Ann Intern Med* 1995;122:770–777.
20. Santucci PA, Haw J, Trohman RG, et al. Interference with an implantable defibrillator by an electronic antitheft-surveillance device. *N Engl J Med* 1998;339:1371–1374.
21. Sgarbossa EB, Pinski SL, Barbagelata A, et al. Electrocardiographic diagnosis of evolving acute myocardial infarction in the presence of left bundle-branch block. *N Engl J Med* 1996;334:481–530.
22. Schuller H, Brandt J. The pacemaker syndrome: old and new causes. *Clin Cardiol* 1991;14:336–340.
23. Shlipak MG, Lyns WL, Go AS, et al. Should the electrocardiogram be used to guide therapy for patients with left bundle-branch block and suspected myocardial infarction? *JAMA* 1999;281:714–719.

CHAPTER 46
Valvular Heart Disease

Joseph P. Ornato

A wide variety of common diseases and conditions can affect the heart valves (Table 46.1). In the 1950s, virtually all patients with clinically significant valvular disease had complications of acute rheumatic fever or syphilis, or congenital heart disease. Since then, the pattern of disease responsible for valvular dysfunction in adults has changed dramatically (1,2,24). The major reasons for this shift are a marked decline in the incidence and better early treatment of acute rheumatic fever and syphilis; the wide availability of invasive and noninvasive testing to detect valvular heart disease; the development and perfection of surgical techniques for the repair or replacement of diseased valves; the increased longevity of the general population, allowing even normal valves to be subjected to more years of wear and tear; and sociocultural changes in our society (e.g., intravenous drug abuse).

TABLE 46.1. The Most Common Causes of Valvular Heart Disease in Adults

Cause	Specific Disease	Valves Affected	Murmur
Congenital	Bicuspid value	A	S, R
Rheumatic	Rheumatic fever	M>A>T>P	S, R
Infectious	Endocarditis	A, M (rheumatic)	R
		A, M, T, P (i.v. drugs)	
Myxomatous degeneration	Prolapse	M:T	R
	Aortic root dilatation	A	R
Degenerative aging	Sclerosis	A	S

A, aortic; M, mitral; P, pulmonic; T, tricuspid; S, stenotic; R, regurgitant; i.v., intravenous.

TABLE 46.2. Common Complications of Left Heart Valvular Disease in Adults

Valvular Lesion	Common Complications(s)
Mitral stenosis	Pulmonary edema, atrial fibrillation, systemic embolism
Mitral regurgitation	Heart failure, endocarditis
Aortic stenosis	Angina, syncope, heart failure, dysrhythmias, sudden death, endocarditis
Aortic regurgitation	Heart failure, endocarditis

Regardless of the cause, significant acute or chronic valvular dysfunction has predictable hemodynamic consequences. Regurgitant lesions (e.g., mitral or aortic regurgitation) cause volume overload of the affected atrium or ventricle. Although massive acute regurgitation can lead to shock and pulmonary edema rapidly, mild-to-moderate volume overload is usually well tolerated until after months or years, when the ventricle will often dilate and fail, leading to signs and symptoms of heart failure. Stenotic lesions above, at, or below the valve can cause pressure overload of the affected atrium or ventricle. Pressure overload is metabolically more costly to the myocardium than volume overload, and leads to myocardial hypertrophy and eventual heart failure.

The combined hemodynamic effect of multiple valvular lesions is often complex (16). Some compound lesions (e.g., combined aortic regurgitation and stenosis) impose a tremendous burden on the myocardium by producing both volume and pressure overload of a single chamber (in this example, the left ventricle). Other combination lesions may be "protective" of a given chamber (e.g., in aortic stenosis combined with mitral stenosis, the volume of blood reaching the left ventricle is decreased, thereby "protecting" it from heart failure). However, the net effect may be to decrease forward, and thus net, cardiac output.

Some valvular lesions produce a rapidly downhill course. For example, acute, severe mitral or aortic regurgitation can lead rapidly to pulmonary edema, shock, or both, which can usually be remedied only by immediate valve replacement (6,8,17,28). Other lesions, such as chronic mitral or aortic regurgitation, can be tolerated well for decades (1,15,17). A structurally abnormal valve puts the patient at increased risk of developing infective endocarditis, which can further impair valvular function. Other concomitant diseases (e.g., coronary atherosclerosis, myocarditis), dysrhythmias (e.g., atrial fibrillation), or valvular calcification can also unfavorably influence the patient's symptoms and length of survival.

CLINICAL PRESENTATION

Patients with valvular heart disease may present to the emergency department (ED) with a complication of previously known disease, or they may challenge the emergency physician to evaluate a previously undetected and undiagnosed heart murmur. If complex congenital heart disease, such as tetralogy of Fallot, is excluded, complications of adult valvular heart disease are most often the result of left heart lesions (Table 46.2).

When a patient with a heart murmur presents to the ED with symptoms that could be caused by valvular heart disease, an immediate question is whether the heart murmur is *causing, unrelated to,* or *caused by* the symptom complex. For example, if a 70-year-old man with dyspnea and moderate pulmonary edema on chest radiograph has a grade 3/6 systolic ejection murmur at the left upper sternal border and cardiac apex, the murmur may be caused by aortic stenosis or mitral regurgitation, either of which could cause heart failure. The patient's heart failure could be caused by an unrelated problem, such as ischemic heart disease, cardiomyopathy, myocarditis, or a congenital shunt lesion (e.g., atrial septal defect). Finally, left ventricular (LV) failure and dilatation could be causing a "functional" murmur owing to dilatation of the mitral valve and its supporting structures (papillary muscle dysfunction).

Myocardial ischemia (e.g., during angina) can also increase the murmur of papillary muscle dysfunction. "Functional" tricuspid regurgitation can be caused by right ventricular dilatation secondary to left heart failure. In practice, it is sometimes impossible to determine the relationship between the murmur and the patient's symptoms without further diagnostic evaluation, such as echocardiography or cardiac catheterization.

The most frequent pathologic conditions affecting the heart valves in adults presenting to the ED are (i) mitral valve prolapse (MVP); (ii) aortic valve sclerosis in the elderly, with or (more typically) without significant stenosis; (iii) valvular aortic stenosis resulting from congenital bicuspid aortic valve; (iv) mitral regurgitation caused by papillary muscle dysfunction, rheumatic heart disease, infectious endocarditis, or ruptured chordae tendineae; (v) aortic regurgitation caused by rheumatic fever, infectious endocarditis, bicuspid aortic valve, or aortic root disease; and (vi) mitral stenosis resulting from rheumatic fever.

EMERGENCY DEPARTMENT EVALUATION

A careful cardiovascular physical examination, beginning with the pulse and blood pressure, often identifies the cause of a heart murmur (4). A wide pulse pressure accompanied by a brisk (often bifid) carotid upstroke and a bounding ("water-hammer") peripheral pulse is common in moderate-to-severe aortic regurgitation; a narrow pulse pressure with a slow, delayed carotid upstroke ("pulsus parvus et tardus") is found in severe aortic stenosis. When a harsh systolic murmur suggesting valvular aortic stenosis is accompanied by a brisk carotid upstroke (and *no* aortic regurgitation), idiopathic hypertrophic subaortic stenosis (IHSS) should be suspected. In a young person (especially male), hypertension in the upper extremities and a *lower* arterial pressure in the legs with a weak femoral pulse and a basal systolic murmur suggests coarctation of the aorta (which is associated with congenital bicuspid aortic valve in 40% to 80% of cases).

All normal and abnormal heart sounds should be noted carefully. A loud first heart sound (S_1) at the apex and/or an opening snap after the second heart sound halfway between the left sternal border and apex are clues to the presence of mitral stenosis with a mobile valve. Paradoxical splitting of the second heart sound (S_2) (i.e., widening of the split on *expiration*) is seen in moderate-to-severe aortic stenosis. A widely ("fixed") split S_2 that fails to close fully during normal expiration in the upright position suggests atrial septal defect.

A high-pitched, early systolic click that is heard best along the left sternal border and that is followed by a systolic murmur usually signifies valvular pulmonic or aortic stenosis with a pliable, noncalcified valve. Systolic clicks heard later than the carotid upstroke or multiple systolic ("machine gun") clicks suggest mitral valve prolapse.

A third heart sound (S_3) is often heard in healthy children, adolescents, and young adults without heart or valvular disease. When the heart rate is rapid, the third heart sound is usually termed an S_3 gallop. In a person with heart disease, it usually indicates left ventricular failure. Chronic or acute mitral regurgitation is often accompanied by an S_3 (6), but its presence in this condition does *not necessarily* indicate heart failure, because its presence may indicate only the torrential inflow of blood from the left atrium into the left ventricle in early diastole.

A fourth heart sound (S_4) is abnormal in a young person; it can occur with hypertension or aortic stenosis (4,18). A loud S_4 accompanying mitral regurgitation indicates that the lesion is acute and substantial, the sound being caused by the valiant attempt of the left atrium to cope with overwhelming volume overload. With time, the left atrium dilates and the S_4 disappears.

Both an S_3 and S_4 can occur simultaneously, causing a quadruple cadence. Patients with severe, particularly acute, heart failure can have a mild sinus tachycardia (typically in the range of 110 to 120 beats/min) that shortens diastole, allowing an S_3 and S_4 gallop to superimpose into a loud "summation" gallop. Always suspect a summation gallop when a loud triple cadence is heard in the presence of a mild tachycardia. A few seconds of gentle carotid sinus massage during auscultation will usually slow the heart rate slightly, allowing the superimposed S_3 and S_4 sounds to separate into a quadruple cadence, thereby confirming the presence of a summation gallop.

The timing of heart murmurs should be studied carefully and characterized as systolic, diastolic, or continuous (Table 46.3). Innocent murmurs are virtually *never* accompanied by a thrill. In an older individual, a harsh, musical, vibratory murmur with a thrill at the base is usually caused by valvular aortic stenosis. A similar murmur with the thrill at the apex can be heard with mitral regurgitation. A new-onset musical "cooing-dove" murmur at the apex is almost always caused by rupture of the mitral valve chordae tendineae owing to underlying mitral valve prolapse, Marfan syndrome, or trauma (4). It is interesting that, although mitral valve prolapse occurs slightly more often in young women than in men, most complications (infective endocarditis, mitral regurgitation, and ruptured chordae) although unusual, occur disproportionately more often in men (7).

The response of murmurs to "provocative" maneuvers, spontaneously occurring extrasystoles, changes in body position, brief exercise, and pharmacologic intervention can help emergency physicians to differentiate among causative entities (4). Virtually all systolic murmurs—except that caused by IHSS—get softer or disappear during the strain phase of the Valsalva maneuver (Table 46.4). After the Valsalva strain is released, right-sided systolic heart murmurs (such as pulmonic stenosis and many innocent murmurs) usually return during the next 1 to 4 beats as blood rushes back into the right side of the heart. Left-sided systolic heart murmurs (mitral regurgitation, valvular aortic stenosis) are usually not heard well for 8 to 10 heartbeats, until the right heart and pulmonary circulation have refilled.

The isometric handgrip (squeezing two of the examiner's fingers tightly for 30 to 60 seconds), increases the systemic vascular resistance and typically increases the intensity and duration of

TABLE 46.3. Classification of Common Murmurs by Timing

SYSTOLIC MURMURS

Aortic stenosis (valvular, supravalvular, and subvalvular)
Mitral regurgitation, including MVP
Tricuspid regurgitation
Pulmonic stenosis
IHSS
Coarctation of the aorta
Ventricular septal defect
Atrial septal defect
Innocent systolic murmur

DIASTOLIC MURMURS

Mitral stenosis
Tricuspid stenosis
Aortic regurgitation
Pulmonic regurgitation

CONTINUOUS MURMURS (EXTENDING THROUGH S_2 WITHOUT RELATIONSHIP TO AORTIC OR PULMONIC VALVE CLOSURE)

Patent ductus arteriosus
Mammary souffle
Ruptured sinus of Valsalva aneurysm

IHSS, idiopathic hypertrophic subaortic stenosis; MVP, mitral valve prolapse.

mitral or aortic regurgitation. If the patient has extrasystoles or an irregular rhythm, as in atrial fibrillation, the murmur of valvular aortic stenosis usually becomes much louder in the beat following a long pause because of increased LV stroke volume and flow across the valve. In contrast, the murmur of mitral insufficiency generally does not change in intensity with the change in cardiac cycle length.

Listening to murmurs with the patient in different body positions may also be helpful. For example, most innocent systolic murmurs decrease or disappear in the sitting or standing position. These murmurs are often soft and blowing in quality, are heard best along the left sternal border without radiation, and are unaccompanied by any other abnormal clinical findings or symptoms. The diastolic rumble of mitral stenosis is heard best in the left lateral decubitus position with the bell of the stethoscope placed lightly over the apex (see Table 46.4). The high-pitched, early diastolic decrescendo murmur of aortic insufficiency is heard best along the left sternal border with the patient leaning forward and holding a maximal expiration. This murmur is almost always louder to the left of the sternum when aortic regurgitation is caused by rheumatic heart disease or a bicuspid valve. If the murmur is louder to the right of the sternum, one should suspect that aortic regurgitation results from aortic root dilatation caused by aortic dissection, hypertension, syphilis, ruptured sinus of Valsalva aneurysm, or Marfan syndrome.

Catheter balloon valvuloplasty (20) is now being performed for pulmonary, mitral, and aortic valve stenosis. Following a successful procedure, it is common to have a persistent stenotic murmur or a new murmur owing to valve regurgitation. Complications of this procedure include valve regurgitation, inadequate opening of the stenosis, endocarditis, arrhythmias, embolization, or atrial septal defect (mitral valvuloplasty only).

Prosthetic Valves

Surgically implanted prosthetic valves present special diagnostic problems in the ED (23,26). Patients with such devices are at risk

TABLE 46.4.   Differentiation of Common Heart Murmurs in Adults

Valve Lesion	Timing	Pattern	Pitch	Location	Valsalva Strain	Other
AS	Systolic	CD	High	Base, neck	Decr	Slow carotid
IHSS	Systolic	CD	High	Base	Incr	Bifid carotid with rapid upstroke
AR	Diastolic	D	High	LSB	Decr	Water hammer pulse
MS	Diastolic	Rumble	Low	Apex	Decr	OS
MR, rheumatic	Systolic	CD or Pan	High	Apex, axilla	Decr	Increase
MR, MV prolapse	Systolic	CD or Pan	High	Apex, axilla	Decr	Systolic click(s)
PS	Systolic	CD	Med or high	Pulmonic area	Decr	May have systolic ejection click
PR	Diastolic	D	High	Base, LSB	Decr	Slight delay from S_2 to murmur
TS	Diastolic	Rumble	Low	LSB or RSB	Decr	Increase on inspiration
TR	Systolic	CD or Pan	High	LSB	Decr	Systolic pulsation of jugular pulse

A, aortic; M, mitral; T, tricuspid; P, pulmonic; V, valve; S, stenosis; R, regurgitation; Med, medium; C, crescendo; D, decrescendo; Pan, pansystolic; Decr, decrease; Incr, increase; LSB, left sternal border; RSB, right sternal border; OS, opening snap; IHSS, idiopathic hypertrophic subaortic stenosis.

for (i) endocarditis (which may present with fever, chills, or peripheral embolic complications, including stroke [12,13,27]); (ii) embolization resulting from clot formation (which may present as a new stroke, transient ischemic attack, or occluded peripheral artery); and (iii) prosthetic valve dysfunction caused by dehiscence of suture lines, thrombosis of the valve, valve degeneration (porcine heterografts or human homografts), hemolysis, or structural failure (disc devices). Patients with prosthetic valve dysfunction may develop heart failure or fatigue gradually, or may present suddenly with syncope or pulmonary edema.

The sounds and murmurs that should be heard after valve replacement vary from device to device (13,14,23,26). Mechanical disc valves should produce clicking or metallic opening and/or closing sounds. Most implanted mechanical valves are relatively stenotic compared with native valves, so it is common and permissible to have a short systolic murmur with a prosthetic aortic valve or a short diastolic rumble with a prosthetic mitral valve. Short whiffs of aortic regurgitation, common after aortic valve replacement, are often caused by a small periprosthetic leak at the suture line. Prominent mitral regurgitant murmurs are usually not present following mitral valve replacement unless there is a mechanical problem with the valve.

Because severe mitral or aortic regurgitation resulting from prosthetic valve dysfunction occasionally produces no audible murmur, the development of heart failure or the appearance of other potential indicators of valve failure always warrants immediate investigation as to the valve's integrity, even in the absence of a murmur. Fibrinolysis is a highly effective treatment in resolving prosthetic thrombosis. However, because it carries a significant risk of embolization, it should be limited to patients with hemodynamic deterioration in whom surgery could also entail a significant risk of death (25).

EMERGENCY DEPARTMENT MANAGEMENT

All patients with a previously undiagnosed heart murmur should, of course, receive a thorough cardiovascular physical assessment, as described previously. A high-quality posteroanterior and lateral chest X-ray and an electrocardiogram (ECG) complement the physical examination. Specific chamber enlargement (e.g., LV dilatation owing to aortic or mitral regurgitation, or left atrial enlargement resulting from mitral stenosis, regurgitation, or both) or poststenotic dilatation of the aorta or pulmonary artery on X-ray, or chamber hypertrophy on ECG (LV hypertrophy in aortic stenosis, left atrial enlarge-

ment in mitral stenosis, right ventricular hypertrophy in pulmonic stenosis) can help to disclose the cause of a murmur. Cardiomegaly, pulmonary vascular congestion, pulmonary edema, or pleural effusions on chest X-ray can detect or confirm heart failure.

Two-dimensional (2D) echocardiography with Doppler is a sensitive and precise means of detecting and evaluating the severity of valvular lesions noninvasively (2,3,19). It should be performed in the ED or ordered electively for any patient who is being referred to a cardiologist for followup evaluation of a murmur that is suspected to result from valvular disease. This technique can often detect vegetations or intracardiac thrombi in patients with suspected endocarditis or evidence of systemic embolization (12,13,26,27) and can be used to evaluate prosthetic valve motion and function (12–14,23,26). If transthoracic echocardiography cannot provide sufficient resolution to adequately define the anatomy, transesophageal echocardiography can be performed. The latter technique can produce spectacular images of the heart and great vessels.

Specific complications of valvular heart disease, such as heart failure, cardiogenic shock, embolization, or dysrhythmias, should be managed in the normal fashion (1,6,8,16,17). Severe heart failure, hypotension, and shock resulting from massive acute aortic or mitral regurgitation may be refractory to medical therapy (1,6). In such cases, it is often preferable to use dobutamine or low-to-medium doses (5 to 15 μg/kg/minute) of dopamine, or both, rather than potent alpha vasoconstrictors (e.g., high-dose dopamine or norepinephrine), because increases in afterload will only worsen valvular regurgitation. Intraaortic balloon counterpulsation or other LV mechanical assist devices may be required for stabilization prior to cardiac catheterization or surgery.

In general, antibiotic prophylaxis against infective endocarditis should be offered to all patients with significant valvular lesions who are about to undergo procedures that may result in bacteremia (10). It is not clear whether all patients with MVP, which occurs in approximately 5% of the population, require such prophylaxis (9), but those patients who have a systolic murmur or echocardiographic evidence of mitral regurgitation are 35 times more likely to develop endocarditis than are those who have no systolic murmur or other evidence of mitral regurgitation (11). Therefore, all patients with prolapsing and leaking mitral valves, evidenced by audible clicks and murmurs of mitral regurgitation or by Doppler-demonstrated mitral insufficiency, should receive prophylactic antibiotics (5). Whether to provide coverage to other MVP patients is a decision that should be made, in most cases, by each patient's cardiologist.

CRITICAL INTERVENTIONS

- Investigate for prosthetic valve dysfunction when heart failure develops in the absence of a murmur because severe mitral or aortic regurgitation due to prosthetic valve dysfunction occasionally produces no audible murmur
- Initiate antibiotic prophylaxis against infective endocarditis for all patients with significant valvular lesions who are about to undergo procedures that may result in bacteremia
- Listen to murmurs with the patient in different body positions to distinguish the etiology of murmurs

DISPOSITION

Absolute indications for immediate ED consultation by a cardiologist while hospital admission is being arranged include (i) known or suspected valvular lesions that are accompanied by hemodynamic instability (heart failure or shock), fever, dysrhythmia, or embolization; and (ii) new onset or progression of these symptoms; or (iii) significant hemolysis following valve surgery or valvuloplasty. Admission to the intensive care unit is usually indicated for significant dysrhythmia (particularly in new-onset cases or those causing hemodynamic compromise), pulmonary edema, hypotension, or when there are other concomitant life-threatening medical problems. Immediate cardiac catheterization and surgical intervention are indicated for new-onset severe valvular regurgitation, prosthetic valve malfunction, systemic embolization in the face of adequate anticoagulation, valve ring abscess, intractable heart failure, or shock.

If transfer to another facility is required, the emergency physician should consult by telephone with the receiving cardiologist to discuss the initial treatment and stabilization and the appropriate means of transportation. If available, an advanced cardiac life-support team with monitoring and resuscitation equipment should always accompany the patient. Air transport by helicopter or pressurized fixed-wing aircraft may be indicated if the patient is in need of urgent cardiac catheterization and operative intervention.

Most asymptomatic patients in whom a previously undetected heart murmur is found incidentally should be referred electively to a cardiologist for further evaluation. Pregnant patients with newly detected murmurs or abnormal heart sounds should also be referred for further cardiac evaluation if there is any question of the finding not being physiologic during pregnancy, or if there is the slightest possibility that the patient may have structural heart disease.

COMMON PITFALLS

- It is easy to be misled by the physical findings when a patient is seen for the first time. For example, the severity of valvular disease is always underestimated during periods of severe heart failure, shock, or tachycardia because the decreased cardiac output leads to a decrease in the intensity of heart murmurs under such conditions (8,15,16,18). The elderly patient presents a special problem because the presence of concomitant atherosclerosis with rigid vessels may either mask or amplify pulse or blood pressure changes resulting from valvular disease. In addition, the location and radiation of murmurs are notoriously unreliable diagnostic indicators in older patients
- A common error is to mistake a normal heart sound or an innocent murmur in a young person for the presence of structural heart disease. Children or young adults may have a cervical venous hum, heard best in the upright position, at the base of the neck and occasionally in the upper chest. The murmur is continuous, extending throughout the second heart sound, and can mimic a patent ductus arteriosus murmur. It can be correctly diagnosed by proving that it can be obliterated by having the patient lie down, applying pressure at the base of the neck with the stethoscope while listening, and by turning the patient's head away from the examiner
- Murmurs are difficult to evaluate during pregnancy (4,21). They may suddenly appear or disappear as the cardiac output, blood volume, and vascular resistance change during each trimester and in the postpartum period. A continuous, innocent "mammary souffle" murmur can often be heard along the right or left chest during late pregnancy or during lactation following delivery. This murmur is caused by the increased flow of blood through the mammary arteries owing to the hypertrophied breast tissue. It can often be eliminated by direct chest wall pressure or with changes in body position
- The physical examination is often unreliable for detecting the presence of heart failure. For example, almost 60% of chronic heart failure patients with an elevated pulmonary capillary wedge pressure will not have jugular venous distension, rales, or peripheral edema on physical examination. In such cases, a chest X-ray or brain natriuretic peptide (BNP) level may be more helpful for determining whether heart failure is present
- Finally, perhaps the most important pitfall is the failure to consider infectious endocarditis as a possibility in a patient with known or suspected heart valve pathology who presents with suspicious signs or symptoms (e.g., unexplained fever, anemia, heart failure, hypotension, or signs of systemic embolization). Emergency physicians should maintain a relatively high index of suspicion in such cases. When in doubt, consider infectious endocarditis to be present until proven otherwise

References

1. Alpert JS, Dalen JE. Changing concepts in the diagnosis and management of patients with valvular heart disease. *Kardiologia* 1987;76:81–84.
2. Borow KM. The need for an integrated noninvasive approach to valvular heart disease. *Am Heart J* 1983;106:1177–1180.
3. Carabello BA. Assessment of cardiac hemodynamics and valvular function by Doppler echocardiography. *Bull N Y Acad Med* 1987;63:762–796.
4. Constant J. *Bedside cardiology*, 2nd ed. Boston: Little, Brown and Company, 1976.
5. Dajani AS, Taubert KA, Wilson W, et al. Prevention of bacterial endocarditis: recommendations by the American Heart Association. *Circulation* 1997;96:358–366.
6. DePace NL, Nestico PF, Morganroth J. Acute severe mitral regurgitation: pathophysiology, clinical recognition, and management. *Am J Med* 1985;78:293–306.
7. Devereux RB, Hawkins I, Kramer-Fox R, et al. Complications of mitral valve prolapse: disproportionate occurrence in men and older patients. *Am J Med* 1986;81:751–758.
8. Janz TG. Valvular heart disease: clinical approach to acute decompensation of left-sided lesions. *Ann Emerg Med* 1988;17:201–208.
9. Jeresaty RM. Mitral valve prolapse: an update. *JAMA* 1985;254:793–795.
10. Kaye D. Prophylaxis for infective endocarditis: an update. *Ann Intern Med* 1986;104:419–423.
11. MacMahon SW, Hickey AJ, Wilcken DEL, et al. Risk of infective endocarditis in mitral valve prolapse with and without precordial systolic murmurs. *Am J Cardiol* 1986;58:105–108.
12. Mayer KH, Schoenbaum SC. Evaluation and management of prosthetic valve endocarditis. *Prog Cardiovasc Dis* 1982;25:43–54.
13. McClung JA, Stein JH, Ambrose JA, et al. Prosthetic heart valves: a review. *Prog Cardiovasc Dis* 1983;26:237–270.
14. McGoon DC, Fuster V. Prosthetic valves. In: Brandenburg RO, Fuster V, Giuliani ER, et al., eds. *Cardiology: fundamentals and practice*. Chicago: Mosby-Year Book, 1987.
15. Nishimura RA, McGoon MD, Schaff HV, et al. Chronic aortic regurgitation: indications for operation—1988. *Mayo Clin Proc* 1988;63:270–280.
16. Nitter-Hauge S, Horstkotte D. Management of multivalvular heart disease. *Eur Heart J* 1987;8:643–646.
17. O'Rourke RA, Crawford MH. Mitral valve regurgitation. *Curr Probl Cardiol* 1984;9:1–52.
18. Olson LJ, Edwards WD, Tajik AJ. Aortic valve stenosis: etiology, pathophysiology, evaluation, and management. *Curr Probl Cardiol* 1987;12:455–508.

19. Pearlman AS, Scoblionko DP, Saal AK. Assessment of valvular heart disease by Doppler echocardiography. *Clin Cardiol* 1983;6:573–587.
20. Rahimtoola SH. Catheter balloon valvuloplasty of aortic and mitral stenosis in adults: 1987. *Circulation* 1987;75:895–901.
21. Raymond R, Underwood DA, Moodie DS. Cardiovascular problems in pregnancy. *Cleve Clin J Med* 1987;54:95–104.
22. Rose AG. Etiology of acquired valvular heart disease in adults. *Arch Pathol Lab Med* 1986;110:385–388.
23. Schoen FJ, Kujovich JL, Levy RJ, et al. Bioprosthetic valve failure. *Cardiovasc Clin* 1988;18:289–317.
24. Selzer A. Changing aspects of the natural history of valvular aortic stenosis. *N Engl J Med* 1987;317:91–98.
25. Serafini O, Bisignani G, Plastina F. Acute disfunction from thrombosis of a prosthetic mitral valve: thrombolysis with rt-PA in the clinical emergency phase. *G Ital Cardiol* 1998;28:387–391.
26. Silver MD, Butany J. Complications of mechanical heart valve prostheses. *Cardiovasc Clin* 1988;18:273–288.
27. Sugarman B. Infections and prosthetic devices. *Am J Med* 1986;81:78–84.
28. Weinstein L. Life-threatening complications of infective endocarditis and their management. *Arch Intern Med* 1986;146:953–957.

CHAPTER 47
Infectious Endocarditis

Ian D. Jones and Corey M. Slovis

INTRODUCTION

Infective endocarditis (IE) is an infection of the endothelial lining of the heart usually involving the heart valves. The first reported autopsy evidence of the disease dates to 1647. In 1885, Sir William Osler further reported on the autopsy and clinical findings of the disease in a series of classic papers published in the *British Medical Journal*.

Traditionally, IE has been divided into two forms: (i) a relatively insidious, chronic disease—subacute bacterial endocarditis (SBE); and (ii) a more abrupt-onset, fulminant form—acute bacterial endocarditis (ABE).

Although there is broad geographic variation in the incidence of IE, recent studies have shown that the total incidence of the disease is relatively stable (11). Despite a stable number of overall cases of IE, there have been overall trends toward increasing patient age, increasing numbers of prosthetic valve infections, and increasing nosocomial infections. Additionally, there has been an increase in the number of infections from *Staphlococcus aureus* and in the number of patients without predisposing heart disease (4,11,15,17).

The incidence of infective endocarditis is highly variable depending on predisposing risk factors such as prosthetic valves, anatomic valve abnormalities, and intravenous (i.v.) drug use. Reviews of multiple studies have shown that IE is a disease that is rarely seen in patients with healthy valves.

Despite considerable advances in detection and therapy, the disease still continues to be a challenge to diagnose, and morbidity and mortality continue to be high. Once most commonly seen in patients with rheumatic heart disease, IE is now more likely to be encountered in patients with prosthetic heart valves, mechanical intracardiac devices such as pacemakers and implanted defibrillators; patients who are intravenous drug abusers and the

TABLE 47.1.   Emergency Department Patients at Highest Risk for Endocarditis

Patients with valvular or structural heart disease
Intravenous drug abusers
Patients with prosthetic heart valves
Patients with indwelling devices, especially hemodialysis shunts
Elderly patients who have recently undergone an invasive procedure

elderly (11,13,15) (Table 47.1). The organisms most commonly causing IE have also changed. As IE has evolved, the frequency of *Viridans streptocci* as the causative agent has decreased, whereas the incidence of *Staphylococcus* species has risen (3,4,11,15). *S. aureus* is now one of the most common causes of IE and the incidence of methicillin resistant *S. aureus* (MRSA) in these isolates has risen dramatically (3,15,17). *S. aureus* endocarditis also appears to confer a higher risk of mortality than does infection caused by other organisms (15). This is especially true in patients with methicillin-resistant *S. aureus* (MRSA) endocarditis (15). In addition to the changing spectrum of infection, methods for elucidating the causative organism in endocarditis have been improved: better culture techniques, serologic testing, and the use of the polymerase chain reaction (PCR).

There are four steps in the development of SBE: (i) a hemodynamically defective valve produces turbulent blood flow and endothelial disruption; (ii) a sterile platelet–fibrin thrombus forms on the damaged valve lining; (iii) transient bacteremia infects the thrombus; and (iv) high titers of antibodies to the infecting organism are produced. Bacterial endocarditis may also develop on previously normal native and prosthetic heart valves. In these cases, the only necessary measure is an inoculum of a highly invasive organism.

Once endocarditis develops on a valve, the clinical manifestations are attributable to the following series of events: (i) local destruction and malfunction of the cardiac valve; (ii) invasive infection of contiguous structures of the heart; (iii) continuous bacteremia, leading to distant infections; (iv) embolization of vegetations that break off from the valve; and (v) an antigen–antibody response, leading to immune-mediated complications.

IE is often classified into one of four distinct clinical groups: (i) patients with a damaged native valve; (ii) intravenous drug abusers (IVDAs); (iii) patients with prosthetic valves who develop early-onset prosthetic valve infectious endocarditis (PVIE); and (iv) patients with late-onset PVIE (7). Early-onset PVIE is defined as infection that presents less than 2 months after valve replacement surgery; late-onset PVIE presents more than 2 months or more after surgery (8).

DAMAGED NATIVE VALVE

Any condition causing cardiac valve damage (e.g., rheumatic, degenerative, and congenital cardiac abnormalities) can predispose the patient to IE (4). Patients with rheumatic valvular disease, congenital valvular abnormalities, mitral valve prolapse, and degenerative valvular disease are, by far, the highest risk groups for native valve IE (4,15). Patients with native valve IE are most likely to develop a syndrome similar to the classic SBE, a relatively chronic infection with only left-sided cardiac involvement, often with a streptococcal organism. The mitral valve is the most common valve to be infected in the native valve group. Isolated mitral involvement occurs in 35% to 45% of cases, isolated aortic valve involvement in 15% to 35%, and involvement of both valves in 15% to 30% (7). Tricuspid valve IE is unusual in this group and accounts for only 1% to 5% of cases

TABLE 47.2.   Most Common Causes of Infectious Endocarditis

NATIVE VALVE INFECTIOUS ENDOCARDITIS

	Percentages[a]
Streptococcus all species	45–65
S. viridans	25–43
S. bovis	7–15
S. faecalis	10–16
Staphylococcus all species	35–50
Coagulase-positive	20–40
Coagulase-negative	5
Gram-negative rods	<5
Fungi	<5
Culture negative	3–15

INTRAVENOUS DRUG ABUSER

Streptococcus	
S. viridans	5
S. faecalis	8
Staphylococcus	
Coagulase-positive	50
Coagulase-negative	<5
Gram-negative rods	5
Fungi	5
Culture negative	<5

EARLY ONSET PROSTHETIC VALVE INFECTIOUS ENDOCARDITIS

Streptococcus (all groups)	<10
Staphylococcus	
Coagulase-positive	20
Coagulase-negative	25–35
Gram-negative rods	10–15
Fungi	5–10
Diphtheroids	5–10
Culture negative	<5

LATE-ONSET PROSTHETIC VALVE INFECTIOUS ENDOCARDITIS

Viridans streptococci	25–41
Staphylococcus	
Coagulase-positive	10–20
Coagulase-negative	10–20
Gram-negative rods	10
Fungi	<5
Culture negative	<5

[a]Approximations based on multiple studies: references 7,11,15,18. Bayer AS. Infective Endocarditis. *Clin Infect Dis* 1993;17:313; King JW, Shehane RR, Leirl J. Infectious endocarditis at three hospitals in the same city: two study periods a decade apart. *South Med J* 1986;79:151; Molavi A. Endocarditis: recognition, management and prophylaxis. *Cardiovasc Clin* 1993;23:139; Robbins MJ, Soeiro R, Frishman WH, et al. Right-sided valvular endocarditis: etiology, diagnosis and approach to therapy. *Am Heart J* 1986;111:12; Robbins N, DeMaria A, Miller MH. Infective endocarditis in the elderly. *South Med J* 1980;73:1336; and Terpenning MS, Buggy BP, Kauffman CA. Endocarditis: clinical features in young and elderly patients. *Am J Med* 1987;83:626.

(7). Pulmonic involvement is rare in native valve IE, occurring in less than 1% of cases (7).

Native valve IE is caused by streptococcal pathogens in approximately 50% of cases (Table 47.2) (4,15). *S. viridans* is by far the most common *Streptococcus* species causing IE (4,11). *S. viridans* bacteremia and subsequent valvular seeding traditionally have been attributed to dental procedures in patients with preexisting valvular heart disease. This presumed cause-and-effect relationship has been questioned, and there is not compelling evidence that dental procedures are the cause of a significant number of cases of IE (23). *Streptococcus bovis* (up to 15% of cases of native valve IE) and *Streptococcus faecalis* (more than 10%) are

more commonly introduced by bowel and urologic infections or procedures, especially in the elderly (9). Coagulase-positive *Staphylococcus* (up to one third of all cases of native valve IE) and coagulase-negative *Staphylococcus* (less than 5%) are probably introduced via the skin and are most likely to cause infection in patients who have diabetes or chronic obstructive pulmonary disease, and in those who are elderly or are otherwise debilitated (15). Central venous and arterial catheterizations are relatively high-risk procedures for causing IE. Indwelling devices, especially hemodialysis shunts, also increase the risk for IE (23). Gram-negative organisms, fungi, polymicrobial infections, and diphtheroids are seldom contributors to native valve IE (15).

INTRAVENOUS DRUG ABUSERS

Intravenous drug abusers are one of the leading groups at high risk for developing IE. Between 5% and 8% of hospital admissions in IVDAs are because of endocarditis (3,18). Because cocaine abusers inject themselves so frequently, as compared with other IVDA groups, they appear to have the highest risk of developing IE. Their increased relative risk may also be a result of such factors as lack of heating of the drug before injection, needle sharing, immunosuppression from the drug, or direct valvular damage caused by cocaine (11). There are conflicting data in the literature regarding the predominance of right-sided versus left-sided endocarditis in IVDAs. Although left-sided endocarditis is seen in all patient populations, right-sided endocarditis is rarely seen outside of the i.v. drug-abusing population. Thirty-two percent of IE caused by i.v. drug abuse involves the mitral valve, 19% the aortic valve, and almost all of the remaining cases involve the tricuspid valve (3). In right-sided endocarditis, pulmonic valve involvement is rare and is seen in less than 1% of patients (3).

Patients who inject illicit drugs often are infected with organisms that are normal skin flora. *S. aureus* is the most common causative agent in this group of patients, accounting for approximately 50% to 80% of cases (3); *Streptococcus* species are the next most common. Interestingly, coagulase-negative staphylococci are rarely isolated from this patient population. Gram-negative bacilli, fungi, and diphtheroids are seen only slightly more often in IVDA-associated IE than in native valve IE (18).

EARLY-ONSET PROSTHETIC VALVE INFECTIOUS ENDOCARDITIS

Patients with early onset PVIE either are contaminated intraoperatively or develop infection in the perioperative period (7,13). The rate of infection is highest in the first 3 months after surgery and diminishes to between .3 to .6% per year thereafter (13). Early prosthetic valve infections are predominantly nosocomial in etiology. The most common pathogens encountered in the first 2 months after surgery are *Staphylococcus* species (coagulase-negative staphylococci and *S. aureus*). As many as 85% of the coagulase-negative staphylococci are methicillin resistant (17). Other organisms encountered less frequently include gram-negative organisms, *Enterococcus* species, and fungi.

LATE-ONSET PROSTHETIC VALVE INFECTIOUS ENDOCARDITIS

Late PVIE shares characteristics with nosocomial infection and native valve IE. The organisms responsible for late PVIE fall midway between those seen in early PVIE and those common in native valve IE (7). *Viridans streptococci* and staphylococci, both coagulase-positive and coagulase-negative, are most frequent, but gram-negative bacteria and fungi also cause a significant number of infections (2).

Mechanical valves and tissue valves have an approximately equal incidence of infection (overall incidence, 2.2% to 4.4%), but mechanical valves are more likely to develop early onset PVIE (7). Mechanical valves tend to develop perivalvular abscesses, myocardial abscesses with conduction delays, pericarditis, and regurgitation caused by perivalvular leaks (7). An acute regurgitant murmur caused by partial dehiscence of the valve is an emergency because severe heart failure can develop rapidly or the valve can undergo total dehiscence (7). Tissue valves, however, are more likely to develop leaflet tears, also resulting in new regurgitant murmurs and heart failure (7). Valvular stenosis is also a potential complication with tissue valves.

CLINICAL PRESENTATION

Patients with IE may present acutely with fulminant heart failure and sepsis; with a chronic, indolent, nonspecific disease process; or with a syndrome intermediate between the two extremes. Because of the overlap, the artificial separation of ABE and SBE is usually not clinically helpful. Table 47.3 lists the historical and physical findings seen most often in IE.

Complications

Cardiac

Cardiac complications of IE may involve any of the three layers of the heart. Endocardial damage of the valve may result in valvular destruction and variable degrees of congestive heart failure (CHF). CHF is the most common cause of death in patients with IE (22). Severe failure is usually a result of aortic insufficiency and if not promptly amenable to medical intervention is an indication for emergent valve replacement surgery (22). Myocarditis or perivalvular abscess results when the infecting organism invades the contiguous myocardium.

Electrocardiographic abnormalities in cases of IE are much more likely to be seen with perivalvular spread of infection and confer a significant increase in mortality (14). Mortality is significantly higher if there is the presence of infranodal block (14,22). The majority of electrocardiographic abnormalities are conduction abnormalities. The infection involving the conduction system results in conduction delays, bundle-branch block, or complete heart block. Intracranial catastrophes may occur if thrombolytics are used in cases in which complications of IE cause electrocardiographic changes that mimic those of acute ischemia resulting from coronary artery disease (CAD).

Additional complications include aortocardiac fistula, perforated valves, or perforation of the myocardium (22). A perforated myocardial abscess may result in a purulent pericarditis. Large emboli to the coronary arteries can cause acute myocardial infarction or sudden death (8).

Central Nervous System

Central nervous system complications occur not only in 20% to 40% of patients with IE, but also may be the presenting complaints in a significant number of cases (15). Mortality is significantly higher in patients with IE and neurologic manifestations (10). Embolic cerebral infarction or stroke is the most common event and usually involves the middle cerebral artery or its branches (21). Intracerebral hemorrhage, isolated seizures, and transient ischemic attacks are also reported complications (6,10). Cerebral mycotic aneurysms, resulting from septic emboli, may remain asymptomatic or may enlarge, leak or rupture, and present as subarachnoid hemorrhage. Septic emboli give rise to cerebral abscesses or, if meningeal or cortical vessels are involved, produce signs and symptoms consistent with classic bacterial meningitis (19). A syndrome consisting of lethargy, delirium, hallucinations, and psychosis (i.e., toxic encephalopathy) may occur (8). When these findings are accompanied by a stiff neck and cerebrospinal fluid consistent with aseptic meningitis, the patient has meningoencephalitis. The cause is not clear, but multiple microinfarcts or microabscesses may be responsible. The likelihood of an embolic event decreases markedly after the initiation of antibiotics (10).

Emboli and Immunologic Responses

Peripheral embolization can occur anywhere in the body. In addition to the brain and heart, other important areas of embolization are the splenic, renal, mesenteric, and extremity vasculature. The emboli result in endarteritis, mycotic aneurysm, local infection, and distal infarction. Studies have shown that patients with large valve vegetations have a worse prognosis, most likely because of a higher likelihood of embolic sequelae (8). It is not clear how many of the signs and complications of IE are immune complex–mediated. It is thought that glomerulonephritis, aseptic arthritis, and most of the classic skin manifestations are immune-related. Prosthetic joint infections and vertebral osteomyelitis may also be seen likely, a result of bacteremia during the acute phase of the infection (22).

EMERGENCY DEPARTMENT EVALUATION

Patients with IE often have numerous nonspecific complaints. The classic patient presenting with persistent fever of unknown

TABLE 47.3.   Historical and Physical Findings Suggestive of Endocarditis

	History	Physical Examination
General	Fever, chills, malaise, weakness, anorexia, weight loss, back pain, myalgia, arthralgia	Acute or chronically ill appearance, fever, diaphoresis pallor, splenomegaly, arthritis
Cardiopulmonary	Chest pain, dyspnea, edema	Murmurs, especially valvular insufficiency; signs of congestive heart failure
Neurologic	Headache, stiff neck, mental status changes, focal neurologic complaints, extremity pain or paresthesia	Meningismus, abnormal mental status, focal deficits
Other	Hematuria, abdominal pain	Skin: petechiae, Osler nodes, Janeway lesions, splinter hermorrhages
Risk factors	Intravenous drug abuse; heart disease; recent gastrointestinal, genitourinary, or dental procedure; poor dental hygiene	Embolic: mycotic aneurysm, visceral or extremity infarct or ischemia
		Other: pneumonia, skin abscess, urinary tract infection

origin represents only a fraction of endocarditis cases (8). Most patients have nonspecific extracardiac complaints including fever, malaise, anorexia, and weakness (8,15). Approximately one half of patients report headache, weight loss, night sweats, arthralgias, and myalgias (8,15). A history of back pain, rash, dyspnea, or a spectrum of neuropsychiatric symptoms is not uncommon in IE (8,15). Clinicians, however, seldom initially attribute these less common symptoms to IE. Physicians should also be aware of patients at higher risk for IE such as patients with diabetes, immunocompromised patients, IVDAs, patients with poor dentition, and patients receiving chronic hemodialysis (15,24). Patients should be asked about recent dental, gastrointestinal, and urologic procedures. Elderly patients, in particular, may not volunteer or may forget to relate these high-risk procedures. Young patients who are being evaluated "for the flu" seldom provide information about i.v. drug use unless specifically questioned.

Physical findings suggestive of endocarditis are listed in Table 47.3. Patients with IE may appear acutely or chronically ill. Nearly all nonimmunocompromised patients have fever. The presence of unexplained fever that has been present for more than 1 week should raise the clinician's suspicion for endocarditis (8). Other abnormal vital signs, especially tachycardia, are relatively common. It is important for the clinician to be vigilant because many of the symptoms of endocarditis are nonspecific and the classic findings of endocarditis are not commonly seen.

A careful cardiac examination is important in patients suspected of having IE. The majority of patients with IE will have a murmur and many of these will be preexisting (15). Patients most likely to lack murmurs are those with acute IE. Therefore, lack of a murmur in an IVDA should never decrease the suspicion for IE. On the other hand, a new aortic or mitral regurgitant murmur in a febrile patient is very strong evidence for the disease (8). The cardiac examination should also seek any findings suggestive of heart failure. Findings of new-onset heart failure, especially in younger patients without a history of cardiac disease, should prompt a high index of suspicion for endocarditis. Rarely, a large (usually fungal) vegetation may block the outflow tract, resulting in a new stenotic murmur.

A variety of skin lesions are considered classic for IE, but these are relatively uncommon. Petechial lesions may be found in different locations. Splinter hemorrhages are tiny red, purple, brown, or black splinter-like lesions that appear under the fingernails. They are seen in up to 20% of patients with IE, but they are also found in approximately 8% of all hospitalized patients. Osler nodes are small, painful, tender erythematous nodules that are most commonly seen in the distal finger pads; they occur in 5% to 20% of patients. Janeway lesions are small, flat, nontender red spots on the palms and soles; they occur in only about 10% of patients with IE. Conjunctival petechiae may occur in approximately 10% of patients. Roth spots are retinal petechial hemorrhages with central pallor, which may be seen in 10% to 25% of patients with IE. The remainder of the physical examination may reveal abnormal abdominal or neurologic findings. Splenomegaly is a common finding, and a tender, enlarged liver is often noted. Neurologic examination may reveal signs consistent with meningitis, encephalitis, embolic stroke, or a leaking aneurysm. Some patients present with subtle mental status changes or behavioral symptoms that appear to be psychiatric in nature (8).

There are numerous nonspecific laboratory findings in IE (Table 47.4). Normochromic, normocytic anemia occurs in up to 75% of patients, and microscopic hematuria occurs in nearly 50%. Leukocytosis is seen in about one half of cases, and, thus, its absence should not be used to rule out the diagnosis. Studies differ in regard to the value of the erythrocyte sedimentation

TABLE 47.4. Laboratory Findings in Endocarditis

BLOOD	ECHOCARDIOGRAM
Positive blood cultures	Vegetations
Anemia	Valve dysfunction
Microscopic or gross hematuria	Perivalvular abscess
Leukocytosis	Aortic Root aneurysm
Uremia	Chamber enlargement
Elevated ESR or C-reactive protein	Pericardial effusion
	V/Q SCAN
CHEST RADIOGRAPH	Multiple pulmonary infarcts
Cardiomegaly	**CEREBROSPINAL FLUID**
Congestive heart failure	
Pulmonary infiltrates	Purulent meningitis
Pulmonary infarcts	Aseptic meningitis
Pulmonary effusions	Bloody leaking aneurysm
Chamber enlargement	
Abnormal movement of prosthetic valve	**COMPUTED TOMOGRAPHY**
Stimson sign	Mycotic aneurysm
	Cerebral abscess
ELECTROCARDIOGRAM	Subarachnoid hemorrhage
Conduction defect	
Acute myocardial infarction	
Pericarditis	

ESR, erythrocyte sedimentation rate; V/Q, ventilation/perfusion.

rate (ESR) in IE. A recent study indicated 100% sensitivity for an elevated ESR in patients ultimately diagnosed with IE (5). The same study indicated 100% sensitivity for C-reactive protein. Both tests lacked high specificity, but if results are normal, could be helpful in ruling out the disease.

The most important part of the laboratory evaluation is the blood culture. Approximately 20 mL of blood (not 5 to 10 mL) should be drawn for each set of blood cultures and sent for aerobic and anaerobic cultures. The diagnosis of possible endocarditis should appear on the specimen label so that the laboratory will hold the specimen for at least 3 weeks to ensure detection of slow-growing organisms. If at all possible, blood cultures should be from three separate sites and should be drawn over a period of approximately 1 hour.

Blood cultures may be positive in the majority of patients with IE. Even in cases where the blood cultures are negative, other tests can be obtained which may aid in a definitive diagnosis. If the cultures are sterile in cases of proven endocarditis—*Coxiella*, *Bartonella*, and *Chlamydia* species may be identified by the use of serology, immunohistochemical staining, and PCR (15). To maximize the chances of a positive culture and to minimize the confusion caused by contaminants, three to five sets of cultures drawn at least 1 hour apart should be obtained before antibiotic therapy is initiated. Recent antibiotic use by the patient and infection with fastidious or slow-growing organisms are the two major reasons for negative cultures in the context of IE. The patients that most commonly have negative cultures are drug abusers, patients with prosthetic valves, and those who have recently received antibiotics.

Although usually normal, the electrocardiogram (ECG) should always be carefully examined for evidence of pericarditis, ischemia, infarction, conduction delay, or any degree of heart block. These changes may be indirect evidence for the coexistence of myocarditis, myocardial abscess, pericarditis, or coronary artery embolism (14).

The chest radiograph of patients with IE is usually normal. Signs of congestive heart failure, including cardiomegaly, isolated chamber enlargement, and abnormal vascular patterns, provide valuable information regarding abnormal valvular or cardiac function. The chest radiograph may also reveal pneumonia, especially in patients who are IVDAs. Multiple pulmonary infarcts or nodular infiltrates suggest right-sided disease, usually tricuspid valve endocarditis. In PVIE, a double shadow of a mechanical valve, known as Stimson sign, indicates movement of a valve that has undergone partial dehiscence (7). Computed tomographic (CT) scanning and cardiac magnetic resonance imaging (MRI) may have future roles in the evaluation of endocarditis, especially as spatial resolution continues to improve and as improved gating techniques eliminate the inherent motion artifacts seen with imaging of the heart. There are limited data on these modalities in the literature, and their current role in IE continues to be primarily in the research arena (20).

Echocardiograms are almost always performed in patients who are suspected of having IE. The finding of a vegetation is very strong evidence for the diagnosis of IE. However, a negative echocardiogram should never be used as the definitive test to rule out IE, as up to one third of patients with IE have nondiagnostic echocardiograms (12). Although it is probably more appropriate to begin with transthoracic echocardiography (TTE), transesophageal echocardiography (TEE) should be performed in all patients in whom there is strong suspicion for IE (12,20). The greater value of TEE lies in its ability to provide greater spatial resolution of cardiac anatomy and the fact that by placing the probe in the esophagus, limitations from overlying structures and chest wall structures are eliminated (20). Various studies have shown sensitivities for TTE in diagnosing IE at between 18% and 63%. This compares to 48% to 100% sensitivity for TEE in diagnosing IE. Furthermore, TEE is far more sensitive in diagnosing accompanying pathology such as perivalvular abscess. Although, because of their anterior location, aortic root abscesses may be better visualized with TTE (12). Echocardiographic detection of valve malfunction, chamber enlargement, or an associated pericardial effusion may also be helpful in the clinical management of IE. Mechanical valves are too echo-dense for TTE to be of significant value, and valvular function should instead be evaluated by either TEE or cinefluoroscopy (7).

EMERGENCY DEPARTMENT MANAGEMENT

Definitive therapy for IE is guided by the infecting organism's sensitivity to specific antimicrobial agents. Once blood culture and sensitivity data are available, optimal therapy can usually be decided on easily. The choice of optimal empiric therapy for presumed IE prior to culture results is guided by the expected sensitivity of bacteria that cause infection in a specific type of patient.

Antibiotics Based on Known Organism

Most experts recommend a combination of ceftriaxone, or aqueous penicillin (12 to 18 million U/day) combined with gentamicin (1 mg/kg i.v. q8h) for IE in native valve endocarditis caused by *Viridans streptococci* or *S. bovis* (2,25). Single daily dosing of gentamicin is not appropriate for treating IE (25). A combination of high-dose penicillin and gentamicin is also recommended for enterococcal IE (25). Nafcillin (2 g i.v. q4h) and gentamicin are often recommended for *S. aureus* infections on native valves (25). Vancomycin is recommended when *Staphylococcus* species are methicillin-resistant (15,25). Because *Staphylococcus* is the single most common organism in IVDAs, broad-spectrum

antistaphylococcal coverage is essential in this population. Routine antipseudomonal coverage is not typically recommended in IVDAs because of the rarity of this once more-common organism (25).

PVIE occurring within 1 to 2 months of valve surgery is caused by *S. aureus* in approximately 50% of cases and by *Staphylococcus epidermidis* in another 20% (7). Gram-negative organisms and fungi are also common in patients who develop IE soon after surgery. Therefore, antimicrobial coverage usually includes vancomycin, gentamicin, and rifampin (25). PVIE occurring more than 2 months after valve replacement is similar to native value IE, in that *Viridans streptococci, S. bovis*, and *S. aureus* are the most common organisms. Most experts recommend the same initial coverage for early and late PVIE, as coagulase-negative *Staphylococcus* species and gram-negative organisms may also be the causative agents (25).

If a stable patient presents to the emergency department (ED) with the possibility of IE, it is best to obtain at least three sets of blood cultures from separate sites over a period of 1 hour. The patient should then be admitted to an inpatient area and subsequent care and additional culturing should be provided at the direction of the patient's physician or infectious diseases consultant. Antibiotics should, however, be started in the ED if the patient appears septic; is elderly, debilitated, or immunocompromised; has concomitant pneumonia; is in heart failure; or is hemodynamically unstable.

Empiric Antibiotic Coverage

There is no universal agreement on optimal therapy. However, ED physicians can begin therapy by choosing an antibiotic regimen that provides broad-spectrum bactericidal coverage for the most common organisms causing IE. The authors' recommendations for empiric therapy to be begun in the ED appear in Table 47.5.

The recommendations attempt to provide broad coverage divided into two regimens: one for presumed IE in a seriously ill patient with native valves, and a second for presumed IE in a patient with one or more prosthetic valves. The regimens are designed to be easily remembered, and do not address whether the patient may have developed IE in association with i.v. drug abuse or how long ago the prosthetic valve was implanted. In addition, with the increasing frequency of infection caused by methicillin-resistant organisms, *Staphylococcus* should be assumed to be methicillin-resistant until culture data are available.. Consequently, patients with the possibility of IE should receive nafcillin, gentamicin, and vancomycin. Patients with prosthetic valves who require that therapy be initiated on an emergent basis should receive rifampin, gentamicin, and vancomycin. The regimen should be adjusted after the patient is admitted to the hospital, on the basis of inpatient physician preference and culture and sensitivity data. Consultation with the patient's physician should be accomplished at the earliest possible time.

Anticoagulants

Anticoagulation is contraindicated in patients with native valve IE because of the greatly increased risk of intracranial bleeding that occurs in patients with IE who have cerebral emboli. The exception is the patient who develops massive life-threatening pulmonary emboli. Patients with PVIE who are already maintained on anticoagulation should probably continue the medication and be closely monitored for complications (7).

TABLE 47.5.   Empiric Emergency Department Therapy for Presumed Endocarditis Prior to Culture Results

Patients with Native Valves (Including Intravenous Drug Abusers)		Patients with Prosthetic Valves	
Nafcillin[a] and	2 g i.v. q4h	Rifampin and	300 mg po q8h
Gentamicin[b] and	1 mg/kg i.v. q8h	Gentamicin[b] and	1 mg/kg i.v. q8h
Vancomycin	1 g i.v. q12h (or 15 mg/kg)	Vancomycin	1 g i.v. q8h

[a]Consider ceftriaxone 2 g i.v. in penicillin-allergic patients.
[b]Use q8h dosing and not single-daily dosing in infective endocarditis.

Surgery

Valve replacement has become much more widely accepted as a therapy for complicated IE (7). Although there is agreement on the indications for surgery—the timing and specific details are being debated. The following are general indications for valve replacement: heart failure as a result of new valve malfunction, major embolic complications, continued infection despite administration of appropriate antibiotics, dysrhythmia or new conduction defect, or a fungal cause (7,16). Indications for emergent surgical intervention include acute aortic regurgitation with early closure of the mitral valve, rupture of the pericardium, and rupture of a sinus of Valsalva aneurysm into the right heart chamber (16). Further more, certain infections such as those caused by *Brucella* species, *Coxiella burnetii*, *Pseudomonas aeruginosa*, *Staphylococcus lugdunensis*, and Candida species are difficult to manage medically and are best managed by surgery (15,25).

Traditionally, surgical management has been considered superior to medical management alone with regard to the treatment of PVIE. This continues to be true in the case of patients with hemodynamic instability or perivalvular abscess. There is emerging evidence that in a subset of stable patients, medical management with antibiotics alone may suffice (1). It is not clear to what extent the size of the vegetations seen on the echocardiogram determines the prognosis and need for valve replacement.

DISPOSITION

Because of the frequency of serious complications and the need for parenteral antibiotic therapy, all patients who are strongly suspected of having IE should be admitted to the hospital. Patients with overwhelming sepsis, serious embolic complications, or any degree of heart failure or conduction block require admission to an intensive care setting. In addition, intensive care unit admission is mandatory for PVIE patients with any evidence of perivalvular leak.

Two to three sets of blood cultures (20 mL of blood for each set) should be obtained in patients suspected of having IE, but in whom the diagnosis is thought to be unlikely. Outpatient followup for these patients is appropriate if the patient is reliable and can be readily contacted, and if the patient's private physician agrees.

When IE is strongly suspected, a cardiologist should be consulted for possible echocardiographic examination. TEE must be done as soon as possible in any patient with a prosthetic valve in whom the possibility of IE is considered. Patients with PVIE or those who may need valve replacement should have a cardiac surgeon involved early to ensure that the timing of surgery is optimal. For patients with possible brain abscess or aneurysm, a neurosurgeon should be consulted promptly.

ANTIBIOTIC PROPHYLAXIS AGAINST IE

The aim of antibiotic prophylaxis is to prevent bacteremia from occurring during procedures in patients who have conditions that predispose them to IE. Decisions regarding appropriate prophylaxis depend on knowing which patients are at risk, which procedures predictably cause bacteremia, and which are the most common organisms involved in each organ system (Tables 47.6 and 47.7) (8).

There is increasing debate over the efficacy of prophylactic antibiotics in preventing IE caused by instrumentation or other outpatient procedures. Prophylactic antibiotics may, in fact, not confer any significant protection from IE. More importantly, dental procedures and perhaps most other outpatient procedures may not be significant causes of IE.

TABLE 47.6.   Prophylaxis in Certain Cardiac Conditions

HIGH RISK

Prosthetic valves: all types
History of infectious endocarditis
Complex cyanotic heart disease
Surgically constructed pulmonary vasculature

MODERATE RISK

Most other congenital cardiac malformations
Acquired valvular dysfunction, including rheumatic heart disease
Hypertrophic cardiomyopathy
Mitral valve prolapse *with* regurgitation

PROPHYLAXIS NOT RECOMMENDED

Prior coronary artery bypass surgery
Mitral valve prolapse *without* valvular regurgitation
Cardiac pacemakers
Physiologic murmurs
History of rheumatic fever without valvular dysfunction
History of Kawasaki disease without valvular dysfunction
Surgically repaired ASD, VSD, or PDA
Isolated secundum-type ASD

ASD, atrial septal defect; VSD, ventricular septal defect; PDA, patent ductus arteriosus.
(From Dajani AS, Taubert KA, Wilson W, et al. Prevention of bacterial endocarditis: recommendations by the American Heart Association. JAMA 1997;277:1794–1801.)

TABLE 47.7.   Prophylaxis for Dental, Oral, Respiratory, and Esophageal Procedures

	Antibiotic	Dose	Timing
Oral	Amoxicillin	2 g po (50 mg/kg po in children)	1 h before procedure
	or		
Intravenous	Ampicillin	2 g i.v. or i.m. (50 mg/kg i.v. in children)	30 min before procedure
IF PENICILLIN-ALLERGIC			
Oral	Clindamycin	600 mg po (20 mg/kg po in children)	1 h before procedure
	or		
	Azithromycin	500 mg po (15 mg/kg in children)	1 h before procedure
Intravenous	*or*		
	Clindamycin	600 mg i.v. (20 mg/kg i.v. in children)	30 min before procedure

From Dajani AS, Taubert KA, Wilson W, et al. Prevention of bacterial endocarditis: recommendations by the American Heart Association. JAMA 1997;277:1794–1801.

The American Heart Association (AHA) has revised its recommendations for prophylactic antibiotic administration. The 1997 recommendations are simpler and much easier to follow. Now, only a single oral dose of amoxicillin is recommended 60 minutes prior to dental procedures. For patients who cannot take oral medications, a single i.v. dose of antibiotics within 30 minutes of the procedure is recommended. Previous, more complicated, regimens were followed by only about one of four physicians. Despite simplifications in the guidelines, physicians continue to fail to instruct patients regarding the need to

TABLE 47.8.   Prophylaxis for Genitourinary and Nonesophageal Gastrointestinal Procedures

Antibiotic	Dose	Timing
ANTIBIOTICS FOR HIGH-RISK PATIENTS		
Ampicillin plus Gentamicin	2 g i.m. or i.v. (50 mg/kg up to 2 g in children) 1.5 mg/kg i.m. or i.v. (Max, 120 mg)	Within 30 min of procedure
And 6 h Later Ampicillin or Amoxicillin	1 g i.m. or i.v. (25 mg/kg in children) 1 g po (25 mg/kg in children)	6 hours later
ANTIBIOTICS FOR MODERATE-RISK PATIENTS		
Amoxicillin or	2 g po (50 mg/kg in children)	1 h prior to procedure
Ampicillin	2 g i.v. or i.m. (50 mg/kg in children)	Within 30 min of procedure
HIGH-RISK PATIENTS ALLERGIC TO PENICILLIN		
Vancomycin plus Gentamicin	1 g i.v., over 1–2 h (20 mg/kg in children) 1.5 mg/kg i.v. or i.m. (Max, 120 mg)	Complete infusion/injection within 30 min of procedure
MODERATE-RISK PATIENTS ALLERGIC TO PENICILLIN		
Vancomycin	1 g i.v., over 1–2 h (20 mg/kg in children)	Complete infusion/injection within 30 min of procedure

[a]See Table 6 for risk class.
(From Dajani AS, Taubert KA, Wilson W, et al. Prevention of bacterial endocarditis: recommendations by the American Heart Association. JAMA 1997;277:1794–1801.)

take antimicrobial prophylaxis, especially in moderate-risk patients. Specifically, in one study of 108 patients judged to have echocardiographic findings indicating a need for prophylactic antibiotics, 89% of those determined to be at highest risk were given instructions, whereas only 61% of those determined to be at moderate risk were given instructions about antimicrobial prophylaxis (21).

Patients with heart disease at highest risk for developing IE are listed in Table 47.6. Table 47.7 lists the prophylactic regimen required for these patients for dental, oral, and upper respiratory procedures. Guidelines for pre-procedure prophylaxis for gastrointestinal and genitourinary tract procedures are provided in Table 47.8 (9).

CRITICAL INTERVENTIONS

> - Obtain 3 sets of blood cultures from separate sites over a period of 1 hour in stable patients suspected of having endocarditis
> - Initiate antibiotics if the patient appears septic; is elderly, debilitated, or immunocompromised; has concomitant pneumonia; is in heart failure; or is unstable
> - Administer prophylactic antibiotics to at-risk patients undergoing dental, oral, upper respiratory, gastrointestinal, or genitourinary tract procedures

COMMON PITFALLS

✔ Not asking about risk factors in patients who present with nonspecific symptoms consistent with IE

✔ Missing the diagnosis in the elderly by attributing a cardiac murmur to chronic heart disease

✔ Failing to remember that IVDAs are at high risk for endocarditis

✔ Not asking specifically about i.v. drug use in patients who present with nonspecific symptoms consistent with endocarditis

✔ Failing to remember that IE in drug abusers often presents without a murmur

✔ Failing to consider the embolic and immune-mediated complications of IE as the underlying cause of stroke, meningitis, myocardial infarction, septic arthritis, or renal failure

✔ Failing to recognize that, in patients with a mechanical valve, a regurgitant murmur is a sign of impending heart failure or valve dehiscence

✔ Failing to consult a cardiac surgeon in cases of IE that have only mild-to-moderate heart failure

✔ Forgetting that mild degrees of heart block and conduction delays are signs highly suggestive of myocardial abscess or myocarditis

✔ Not asking about risk factors for IE in patients about to undergo a procedure prone to cause bacteremia

✔ Failing to learn the new, simplified single-dose amoxicillin regimen for prophylaxis prior to dental procedures

Acknowledgments

Thanks to previous edition chapter author Rebecca R. Roberts.

References

1. Akowah EF, Davies W, Oliver F, et al. Prosthetic valve endocarditis: early and late outcome following medical or surgical treatment. *Heart* 2003;89:269–272.
2. Berbari EF, Cockerill FR III, Steckelberg JM. Infective endocarditis due to unusual or fastidious microorganisms. *Mayo Clin Proc* 1997;72:532–542.
3. Brown PD, Levine DP. Infective endocarditis in the injection drug user. *Infect Dis Clin North Am* 2002;16:645–665.
4. Castillo JC, Anguita MP, Torres F, et al. Comparison of features of active infective endocarditis involving native cardiac valves in nonintravenous drug users with and without predisposing cardiac disease. *Am J Cardiol* 2002;90: 1266–1269.
5. Chuang R, Olshaker J, Robinson D. The analysis of erythrocyte sedimentation rate, C-reactive protein, white blood cell count, and temperature in the diagnosis of acute endocarditis. *Ann Emerg Med* 2000;35:S34.
6. Chukwudelunzu FE, Brown RD. Neurologic complications of infectious endocarditis: Mayo Clinic Experience, 1980–1996. *Neurology* 1998;50: A213–A214.
7. Cowgil LD, Addonzio VP, Hopeman AR, et al. Prosthetic valve endocarditis. *Curr Probl Cardiol* 1986;11:617.
8. Crawford MH, Durack MB. Clinical presentation of infectious endocarditis. *Cardiol Clin* 2003;21:159–166.
9. Dajani AS, Taubert KA, Wilson W, et al. Prevention of bacterial endocarditis: recommendations by the American Heart Association. *JAMA* 1997;277:1794–1801.
10. Heiro M, Nikoskeilanen J, Engblom E, et al. Neurologic manifestations of infectious endocarditis: a17-year experience in a teaching hospital in Finland. *Arch Intern Med* 2000;160:2781–2787.
11. Hoen B, Alla F, Selton-Suty C, et al. Changing profile of endocarditis: results of a 1-year survey in France. *JAMA* 2002;288:75–81.
12. Jacob S, Tong A. Role of echocardiography in the diagnosis and management of infective endocarditis. *Curr Opin Cardiol* 2002;17:478–485.
13. Karchner AW, Longworth DL. Infections of intracardiac devices. *Cardiol Clin* 2003;21(2):253–271.
14. Meine TJ, Nettles RE, Anderson TJ, et al. Cardiac conduction abnormalities in endocarditis defined by the duke criteria. *Am Heart J* 2001;142:280–285.
15. Mylonakis E, Calderwood SB. Infective Endocarditis in Adults. *N Engl J Med* 2001;345:1318–1330.
16. Olaison L, Pettersson G. Current best practice and guidelines: indications for surgical intervention in infective endocarditis. *Infect Dis Clin North Am* 2002;16:453–475.
17. Petti CA, Fowler VG. *Staphylococcus aureus* bacteremia and endocarditis. *Infect Dis Clin North Am* 2002;16:413–435.
18. Roberts RR, Slovis CM. Infectious endocarditis in the intravenous drug abuser. *Emerg Med Clin North Am* 1990;8:665.
19. Roder BL, Wandall DA, Espersen F, et al. Neurologic manifestations in *Staphylococcus aureus* endocarditis: a review of 260 bacteremic cases in nondrug addicts. *Am J Med* 1997;102:379–386.
20. Sachdev M, Peterson G, Jollis J. Imaging Techniques for Diagnosis of Infective Endocarditis. *Cardiol Clin* 2003;21.
21. Seto TB, Kwiat D, Taira D, et al. Physicians recommendations to patients for use of antibiotic prophylaxis to prevent endocarditis. *JAMA* 2000;284:68–71.
22. Sexton DJ, Spelman D. Current best practice and guidelines: assessment and management of complications in infective endocarditis. *Cardiol Clin* 2003;21.
23. Strom BL, Abrutyn E, Berlin JA, et al. Risk factors of infective endocarditis: oral hygiene and nondental exposure. *Circulation* 2000;102:2842–2848.
24. Strom BL, Abrutyn E, Berlin JA, et al. Dental and cardiac risk factors for infective endocarditis. *Ann Intern Med* 1998;129:761–769.
25. Wilson WR, Karchmer AW, Dajani AS, et al. Antibiotic treatment of adults with infective endocarditis due to streptococci, enterococci, staphylococci, and HACEK microorganisms. *JAMA* 1995;274:1706–1713.

CHAPTER 48
Acute Pericarditis and Cardiac Tamponade

Howard A. Bessen and Richard Byyny

Acute pericarditis is a diagnostic challenge because its presentation is similar to that of several other disorders, and it may have life-threatening complications. Management ranges from symptomatic treatment to lifesaving invasive procedures.

The common causes of acute pericarditis are listed in Table 48.1. In many cases, the cause is unclear (idiopathic pericarditis). Viral pericarditis is frequently diagnosed presumptively in a patient who presents with pericarditis after a viral prodrome. Other infectious causes (bacterial, fungal, and parasitic) are less common, but pericarditis may occur as a complication of another systemic or intrathoracic infection. Patients with human immunodeficiency virus (HIV) infection may develop pericarditis and pericardial effusions (3), caused by a wide variety of infections and acquired immunodeficiency syndrome (AIDS)–related malignancies.

Pericarditis is the most prominent cardiac complication of neoplastic disease, and nontraumatic pericardial tamponade is usually of metastatic origin (9,15). Lymphoma, leukemia, melanoma, and breast or lung carcinoma cause most pericardial metastases. Patients receiving radiation treatment may develop postirradiation pericarditis.

Pericarditis may occur as a complication of chronic renal failure, or of connective tissue diseases such as systemic lupus erythematosus, scleroderma, or rheumatoid arthritis. Medications, including anticoagulants and those associated with a drug-induced lupus syndrome (e.g., hydralazine, methyldopa, and procainamide) may also be implicated.

Pericarditis frequently occurs during the first few days after acute myocardial infarction (4,23) and may also present as a late-onset postinfarction pericarditis (Dressler syndrome) (13). Aortic dissection, cardiac trauma, invasive procedures that involve the great vessels and the heart (central venous pressure catheter insertion and cardiac catheterization), and intrathoracic surgery may also cause pericarditis and pericardial tamponade within hours to weeks.

CLINICAL PRESENTATION

Chest pain is the most common presenting complaint with acute pericarditis. The pain is usually sharp and often pleuritic, but it may also be dull, constrictive, or aching. It may radiate to any part of the chest and back and to the trapezius ridge (11). Typically, the chest discomfort is eased by sitting up and leaning forward and increased with recumbency. The pain is frequently associated with shortness of breath, which may be caused by coexisting pleuritis or by cardiac tamponade. Patients may also present with hypotension and other signs and symptoms of tamponade.

The classic diagnostic physical finding is the pericardial friction rub, which may consist of one, two, or three components and is nearly 100% specific for pericarditis (22). It is important for the clinician to recognize that the rub is often transient and may not be present on the first evaluation; however, frequent careful auscultation allows recognition of a rub in most patients with pericarditis (21). Typically the rub is heard best along the left sternal border and is increased by having the patient sit or lean forward. The rub may be transient or intermittent, and it can be confused with a heart murmur.

DIFFERENTIAL DIAGNOSIS

The differential diagnosis includes other conditions that cause chest pain and dyspnea, such as acute myocardial infarction (MI), congestive heart failure (CHF), pulmonary embolism, pneumonia, pneumothorax, pneumomediastinum, pleuritis, and aortic dissection. Cardiac tamponade may be confused with CHF and cardiogenic shock.

Acute pericarditis is frequently mistaken for acute MI. Both cause chest pain and electrocardiographic abnormalities, and can cause elevations of cardiac enzymes. In contrast to patients with MI, patients with pericarditis may present with fever and typically have sharper pain that increases with body motion and varies with position. The ST-segment elevation in patients with acute MI is typically focal (in the distribution of a coronary artery), with ST-segment depression in reciprocal leads. In pericarditis, ST-segment elevation is more diffuse, without reciprocal ST depression (2), and the Q waves often seen in acute infarction do not develop. Patients with pericarditis (even with tamponade) have clear lung fields, unlike patients with CHF or pneumonia.

On the electrocardiogram (ECG), a normal early repolarization variant may mimic pericarditis (discussion in subsequent text).

EMERGENCY DEPARTMENT EVALUATION

Initial assessment and therapy consist of measures appropriate for any patient who presents with shortness of breath and chest pain: supplemental oxygen administration, intravenous access placement, cardiac monitoring, and a 12-lead ECG.

TABLE 48.1. Causes of Acute Pericarditis

Idiopathic
Infectious
  Viral
  Bacterial
  Tuberculosis
  Fungal
  Parasitic
Malignancy
  Metastatic disease
  Radiation-induced
Uremia
Connective tissue disease
  Rheumatoid arthritis
  Systemic lupus erythematosus
  Scleroderma
Drug-related
  Anticoagulants
  Procainamide
  Hydralazine
  Methyldopa
Cardiac injury
  Postmyocardial infarction
  Postsurgical
  Postinstrumentation
  Cardiac trauma
  Aortic dissection

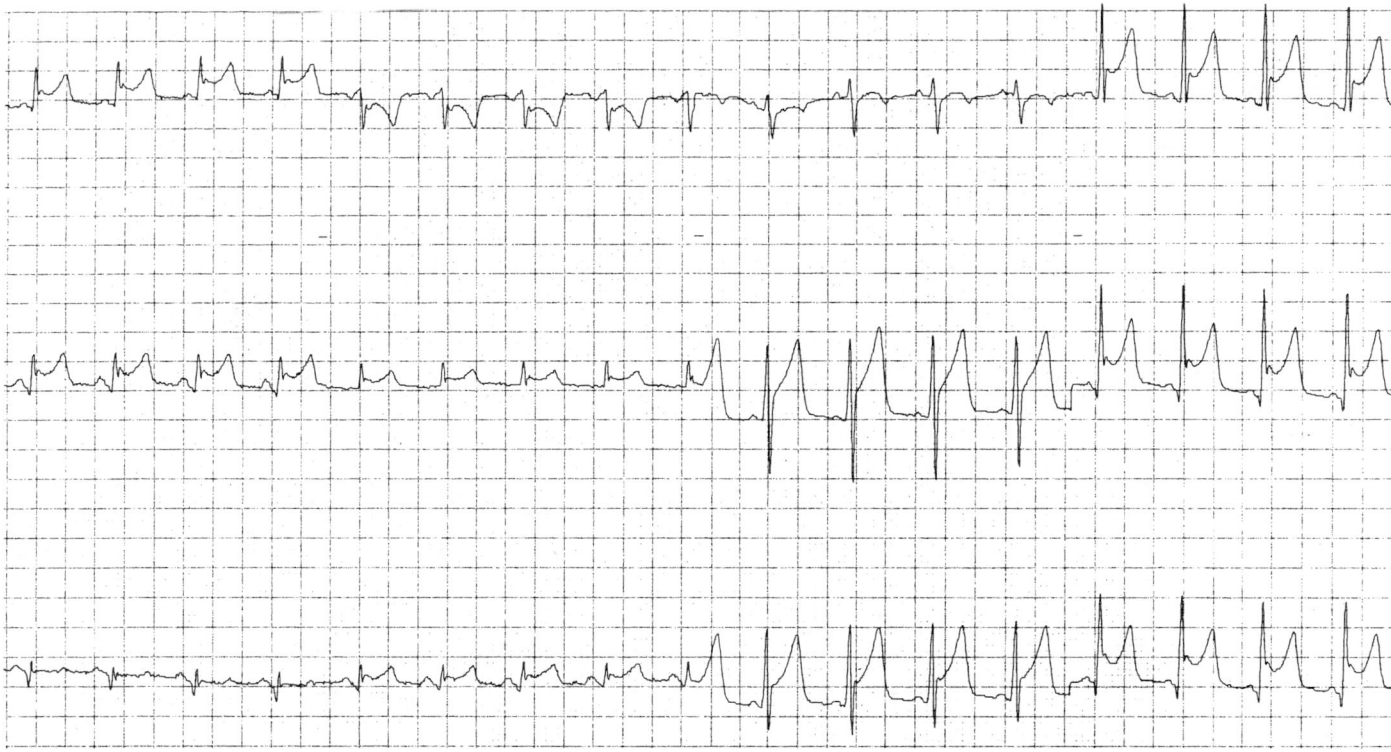

Figure 48.1.   Electrocardiogram of a 35-year-old man with acute (Stage 1) pericarditis. Note the diffuse, concave–upward ST-segment elevation.

The ECG can be diagnostic. Typically, the electrocardiographic changes of acute pericarditis evolve through four stages (2,20):

- Stage 1
  - Most characteristic and will probably be seen when the patient presents with acute symptoms
  - Concave-upward ST-segment elevation is seen in most of the leads; PR segment depression may also be seen (Fig. 48.1)
- Stage 2
  - ST segments return to baseline
  - T-wave amplitude decreases
  - PR segment may be depressed
- Stage 3
  - T-wave flattening and then inversion in the leads with previous ST-segment elevation
- Stage 4
  - ECG normalizes

The ECG findings in acute pericarditis are diffuse changes that are seen in most leads, rather than the focal abnormalities seen in acute MI (2,20).

Although the ECG is usually abnormal, diagnostic changes may be absent in patients with clinically evident pericarditis (14,20). Patients with post-MI pericarditis (diagnosed by the presence of a pericardial friction rub) frequently have no electrocardiographic changes (14).

Early repolarization, a normal electrocardiographic variant characterized by ST-segment elevation, can be difficult to distinguish from pericarditis (2,18). If the clinical presentation suggests pericarditis, serial ECGs may be required to differentiate pericarditis from the benign early repolarization variant. On a single ECG, an ST/T ratio (the amount of ST-segment elevation divided by the height of the T wave) of 0.25 or more in lead V_6 suggests pericarditis, not early repolarization (8).

The chest radiograph is often normal. The cardiac silhouette may be enlarged secondary to a pericardial effusion, but the heart size may be normal, even if an effusion is present (6). In addition, radiographic cardiomegaly is a nonspecific finding and may represent significant myocarditis or many other types of heart disease.

The white blood cell count can range from normal to markedly elevated, and is usually not helpful in making or excluding the diagnosis. Similarly, the erythrocyte sedimentation rate is usually elevated, but this is a nonspecific finding. Cardiac enzyme levels may be significantly elevated because of associated myocarditis (12).

Echocardiography can provide useful information in suspected pericarditis. In the absence of significant associated myocarditis, most patients with pericarditis have normal cardiac wall motion. In contrast, patients with chest pain caused by cardiac ischemia often have focal wall motion abnormalities. Echocardiography is also the best method for detecting and monitoring pericardial effusions (discussion follows).

COMPLICATIONS

The major complications of acute pericarditis are pericardial effusion (potentially leading to cardiac tamponade), recurrent pericarditis, and chronic constrictive pericarditis. Dysrhythmias are unusual in pericarditis but may occur in patients with associated myocarditis or other underlying heart disease.

Cardiac tamponade is an acutely life-threatening complication. The presentation may be subtle, potentially leading to a delayed or missed diagnosis and a poor outcome. Close attention to physical findings is essential to make the diagnosis.

Cardiac tamponade results from the accumulation of fluid within the pericardial space, causing an impairment of cardiac filling and thus a decrease in cardiac output. Tamponade is often mistaken for CHF because patients present with dyspnea, orthopnea, jugular venous distention, and hepatic enlargement.

The classic findings of cardiac tamponade are muffled heart sounds, diminished arterial pressure, and elevated venous pressure. However, these findings are seen only with fully developed tamponade and are much more likely to occur when pericardial fluid accumulates quickly, precluding pericardial distention (7,9).

An important clue to the diagnosis is the presence of pulsus paradoxus, an inspiratory decrease in systolic blood pressure of greater than 10 mm Hg (5,16). Other clinical entities associated with pulsus paradoxus include emphysema, asthma, obesity, pulmonary embolism, cardiogenic shock, right ventricular infarction, and restrictive cardiomyopathy. Patients with acute traumatic tamponade may not have a pulsus paradoxus.

Patients with tamponade may have relatively normal ECGs. With large effusions, reduction of the QRS amplitude or electrical alternans (alternating beat-to-beat variation in QRS amplitude) may be seen. Central venous pressure measurements reveal an elevation of right-sided pressures and help confirm the diagnosis.

Clinical decompensation can be rapid. If time allows, definitive diagnosis using echocardiography is indicated. Echocardiography can detect small amounts of pericardial fluid; in cardiac tamponade, it may demonstrate diffuse hypokinesis, right atrial collapse, and right ventricular diastolic collapse (7,11,19). If possible, echocardiography should be performed emergently in any patient with suspected tamponade, because results of delays in evaluating the presence and size of a pericardial effusion can be disastrous (15).

The diagnosis of tamponade can also be definitively established by measuring pressures in the cardiac chambers. Right atrial, right ventricular diastolic, pulmonary artery diastolic, and pulmonary capillary wedge pressures are equalized in this condition.

Occasionally, after recovering from the acute illness, patients have one or several episodes of recurrent pericarditis, weeks to months after the initial episode (1). Evaluation and management of recurrences are, for the most part, the same as for a first presentation of acute pericarditis.

Constrictive pericarditis, an uncommon complication of acute pericarditis, results when healing of acute pericarditis leads to encasement of the heart in fibrous tissue, impeding ventricular filling (11,17). Patients often present with dyspnea on exertion, ascites, peripheral edema, and hepatic enlargement. The lung fields are clear in these patient, in contrast to patients with CHF. The presence of distended neck veins in constrictive pericarditis helps to separate these patients from those with severe liver disease, who may appear clinically similar. Pericardial calcification on the chest radiograph and pericardial thickening on echocardiography may also provide clues to this diagnosis. The definitive treatment is resection of the pericardium.

EMERGENCY DEPARTMENT MANAGEMENT

The therapy for uncomplicated pericarditis is largely symptomatic, but specific therapy is available for a few causes of pericarditis. Although no controlled trials have been performed, colchicine in combination with ibuprofen reduces the duration of symptoms and reduces the recurrence rate in patients with idiopathic or viral pericarditis (22). Bacterial pericarditis must be treated with drainage and appropriate antimicrobial therapy. Uremic pericarditis is usually an indication for dialysis.

The definitive treatment for pericardial tamponade is pericardiocentesis. However, to "buy time" until pericardiocentesis can be performed, volume infusion is the treatment of choice.

Ideally, pericardiocentesis should be done with echocardiographic or fluoroscopic guidance (often in the cardiac catheterization laboratory), but emergent "blind" pericardiocentesis may be necessary for hypotensive patients who do not respond to volume infusion.

The procedure for emergent pericardiocentesis is fully described elsewhere (10). The pericardium may be approached by a left parasternal or subxiphoid puncture. In the parasternal approach, the needle is inserted perpendicular to the skin in the fifth intercostal space, just lateral to the sternum. In the subxiphoid approach, the puncture is made about 2 cm below and 1 cm to the left of the xiphoid process; the needle enters the skin at a 30-degree to 45-degree angle and is aimed toward the sternal notch or the left shoulder. The needle is advanced with constant syringe aspiration. As much fluid is aspirated as is needed to improve the clinical condition or to obtain specimens for diagnostic use.

After completing the procedure, a chest radiograph is obtained to look for complications such as pneumothorax or pleural effusion secondary to laceration of the lung or myocardium. Serial physical examinations and central venous pressure monitoring are done to detect reaccumulation of fluid. The admitting consultant may choose to observe the patient for fluid reaccumulation, place a soft catheter in the pericardial space for continued drainage, or perform surgical drainage in the operating room.

CRITICAL INTERVENTIONS

- Perform pericardiocentesis (with echocardiographic or fluoroscopic guidance if possible) to treat pericardial tamponade
- Obtain an echocardiogram to exclude pericardial effusion before discharging patients with pericarditis

DISPOSITION

Once the diagnosis of acute pericarditis is made or strongly suspected, most patients should be admitted. The admitting consultant can coordinate the diagnostic evaluation, perform echocardiography and pericardiocentesis as needed, and arrange proper followup care.

Whether all patients with acute pericarditis require admission is controversial. Some young patients with uncomplicated idiopathic or viral pericarditis may be appropriately managed as outpatients. However, pericarditis may occur as a complication of MI, and, in any patient with pericarditis, development of a pericardial effusion and cardiac tamponade may be subtle. Obtaining an echocardiogram before discharge ensures that a pericardial effusion is not missed. Patients who are not admitted require close, careful follow-up.

COMMON PITFALLS

✔ Failing to consider pericarditis in the differential diagnosis of chest pain
✔ Mistakenly diagnosing pericarditis in patients with other causes of chest pain, such as MI, pulmonary embolism, or aortic dissection
✔ Misdiagnosing acute pericarditis as acute MI, potentially leading to the inappropriate administration of thrombolytics
✔ Failing to consider the etiology of pericarditis. Many of the causes listed in Table 48.1 require specific therapy
✔ Failing to consider cardiac tamponade in the differential diagnosis of hypotension, especially in patients with cancer

Acknowledgments

Thanks to previous edition chapter author Franklin D. Pratt.

References

1. Adler Y, Finkelstein Y, Guindo J, et al. Colchicine treatment for recurrent pericarditis: a decade of experience. *Circulation* 1998;97:2183.
2. Chan TC, Brady WJ, Pollack M. Electrocardiographic manifestations: acute myopericarditis. *J Emerg Med* 1999;17:865.
3. Chen Y, Brennessel D, Walters J, et al. Human immunodeficiency virus–associated pericardial effusion: report of 40 cases and review of the literature. *Am Heart J* 1999;137:516.
4. Correale E, Maggioni AP, Romano S, et al. Pericardial involvement in acute myocardial infarction in the post-thrombolytic era: clinical meaning and value. *Clin Cardiol* 1997;20:327.
5. Curtiss EI, Reddy PS, Uretsky BF, et al. Pulsus paradoxus: definition and relation to the severity of cardiac tamponade. *Am Heart J* 1988;115:391.
6. Eisenberg MJ, Dunn MM, Kanth N, et al. Diagnostic value of chest radiography for pericardial effusion. *J Am Coll Cardiol* 1993;22:588.
7. Fowler NO. Cardiac tamponade: a clinical or an echocardiographic diagnosis? *Circulation* 1993;87:1738.
8. Ginzton LE, Laks MM. The differential diagnosis of acute pericarditis from the normal variant: new ECG criteria. *Circulation* 1982;65:1004.
9. Guberman BA, Fowler NO, Engel PJ, et al. Cardiac tamponade in medical patients. *Circulation* 1981;64:633.
10. Harper RJ, Callaham ML.Pericardiocentesis. In: Roberts JR, Hedges JR, eds. *Clinical procedures in emergency medicine*, 3rd ed. Philadelphia: WB Saunders, 1998:231.
11. Hoit BD. Pericardial heart disease. *Curr Probl Cardiol* 1997;22:357.
12. Karjalainen J, Heikkila J. "Acute pericarditis": myocardial enzyme release as evidence for myocarditis. *Am Heart J* 1986;111:546.
13. Kossowsky WA, Lyon AF, Spain DM. Reappraisal of the postmyocardial infarction Dressler's syndrome. *Am Heart J* 1986;102:954.
14. Krainin FM, Flessas AP, Spodick DH. Infarction-associated pericarditis: rarity of diagnostic ECG. *N Engl J Med* 1984;311:1211.
15. Markiewicz W, Borovik R, Ecker S. Cardiac tamponade in medical patients: treatment and prognosis in the echocardiographic era. *Am Heart J* 1986;111:1138.
16. McGregor M. Pulsus paradoxus. *N Engl J Med* 1979;301:480.
17. Mehta A, Mehta M, Jain AC. Constrictive pericarditis. *Clin Cardiol* 1999;22:334.
18. Mehta M, Jain AC, Mehta A. Early repolarization. *Clin Cardiol* 1999;22:59.
19. Reydel B, Spodick DH. Frequency and significance of chamber collapses during cardiac tamponade. *Am Heart J* 1990;119:1160.
20. Spodick DH. Electrocardiogram in acute pericarditis: distributions of morphologic and axial changes by stages. *Am J Cardiol* 1974;33:470.
21. Spodick DH. Pericardial rub: prospective, multiple observer investigation of pericardial friction in 100 patients. *Am J Cardiol* 1975;35:357.
22. Spodick DH. Acute pericarditis: current concepts and practice. *JAMA* 2003;289:1150.
23. Sugiura T, Iwasaka T, Takehana K, et al. Clinical significance of pericardial effusion associated with pericarditis in acute Q-wave anterior myocardial infarction. *Chest* 1993;104:415.

CHAPTER 49
Hypertension

Philip Shayne

When does an elevated blood pressure become an emergency? The World Health Organization (WHO) has established that hypertension contributes to one in every eight deaths worldwide. One quarter of all Americans have hypertension, yet only one half of those individuals receive treatment and less than one third of cases are adequately controlled (9). National treatment guidelines exist, based on large studies involving tens of thousands of patients (6). However, there is a dearth of evidence available to guide the acute management of severely elevated blood pressure (3,5,8,11,16,18,21,22,24,25). As many as one third of all patients in the emergency department (ED) with markedly elevated blood pressure have been referred there for blood pressure evaluation from some other clinical setting, making the emergency physician the recognized expert. Yet few of these patients are in crisis or require immediate intervention. In most cases this leaves the emergency physician to figure out what to do with the incidental finding of an elevated blood pressure in the patient with no symptoms or with nonspecific complaints. The broad spectrum of disease, from the asymptomatic to the critically ill patient, creates the dilemma for the emergency physician in deciding how and when in the process to intervene.

A *hypertensive emergency* involves rapid and progressive decompensation or damage of vital organ function resulting from severely elevated blood pressure. These patients need careful evaluation and monitoring; many, but not all cases need immediate parenteral blood pressure control. There is no evidence to suggest that the severe, but asymptomatic hypertensive patient requires emergent care. Each patient does require a careful and specific evaluation for signs of critical organ compromise. A rational approach to the elevated blood pressure can be formulated on the basis of the patient's history and presentation.

CLINICAL PRESENTATION

The presence or risk of target organ deterioration determines the urgency with which a patient with blood pressure must be treated. A hypertensive emergency is defined as the acute and progressive decompensation or damage of vital organ function caused by an elevated blood pressure. The major organs affected by hypertension are the brain, kidney, heart, and vascular system. Patients with a hypertensive emergency need to be carefully evaluated, monitored, and have their blood pressure controlled. The treatment should be dictated by the clinical situation, not the severity of blood pressure elevation. No degree of hypertension in and of itself defines an emergency.

Many patients present with an elevated blood pressure and with nonspecific symptoms. The emergency physician needs to make a decision as to the etiology of the symptoms to determine how the blood pressure must be managed. If a hypertensive patient's chest pain is possibly anginal, immediate parenteral control might be necessary. However, if that pain is determined not to be cardiovascular in origin, the same patient might need no immediate treatment for the blood pressure. The assessment of the patient determines the need to treat.

The concept of the hypertensive urgency, usually referring to markedly elevated, *asymptomatic* blood pressures requiring rapid intervention, is no longer widely used. Most patients without acute and progressive target organ disease can usually have their severely elevated blood pressure managed on an outpatient basis (22). This approach de-emphasizes the degree to which the blood pressure is elevated. However, the clinician should be aware that certain patients are at higher risk of near-term complications from their uncontrolled hypertension, especially those patients with a history of previous end-organ disease. These patients do require increased vigilance.

Hypertensive Encephalopathy

The triad of severe hypertension, altered mental status, and, often, papilledema characterizes *hypertensive encephalopathy*. It may be accompanied by the acute or subacute onset of lethargy, confusion, headache, visual disturbances, and seizures. Retinopathy may or may not be present. The diagnosis is confirmed if cerebral function improves with lowering of the blood pressure. The mechanism is cerebral overperfusion—in effect the pressure overwhelms the brain's ability to autoregulate cerebral blood flow. Overperfusion results in vasodilation and increased permeability of cerebral blood vessels, leading in turn to the development of cerebral edema. If not adequately treated, hypertensive encephalopathy can progress to cerebral hemorrhage, coma, and death (3).

Hypertensive encephalopathy is most likely to occur in previously normotensive individuals who experience a rapid rise in blood pressure, such as children with acute glomerulonephritis and young women with preeclampsia or eclampsia. Patients with chronic hypertension usually experience a more gradual rise in blood pressure and therefore develop a right shift in their pressure–perfusion autoregulation curve that makes cerebral decompensation less likely. Hypertensive encephalopathy produces characteristic findings on computed tomography (CT), a posterior leukoencephalopathy that predominantly affects the white matter of the parieto-occipital regions bilaterally (20). CT is useful in excluding other causes of altered mental status such as intracranial bleeding.

Accelerated-Malignant Hypertension

Accelerated-malignant hypertension occurs most commonly in young African American men with underlying renal parenchymal disease or renovascular disease. When endothelial vasodilator responses are overwhelmed, endothelial decompensation causes further hypertension and endothelial damage, resulting in an inflammatory vasculopathy (25). The diagnosis is based on marked elevation of blood pressure and characteristic eyeground findings. Flame-shaped hemorrhages occur around the optic disk owing to high intravascular pressures and "soft" exudates are caused by ischemic infarction of the nerve fibers secondary to occlusion of supplying arterioles. Papilledema is considered by many to be the sine qua non of "malignant hypertension." For this reason, the term "accelerated hypertension" has been used to describe the same condition (hemorrhages and exudates) without papilledema. Because absence of papilledema does not connote different clinical features or a better prognosis, the term "accelerated-malignant hypertension" is now recommended (12).

Common symptoms include headache (85%), visual blurring (55%), nocturia (38%), and weakness (30%). Laboratory evidence includes azotemia, proteinuria, hematuria, hypokalemia, and metabolic alkalosis. Accelerated-malignant hypertension is most commonly found in patients with long-standing hypertension and usually occurs without encephalopathy. Since the 1950s, the long-term prognosis of accelerated-malignant hypertension has improved from a 1-year survival rate of 10% to a 5-year survival rate of greater than 75% (13).

Cerebrovascular Crisis

Hypertension frequently complicates the presentation of cerebrovascular ischemia and hemorrhage. An understanding of cerebrovascular physiology is helpful in determining the best treatment strategy (3,12). Cerebral blood flow (CBF) is a function of the cerebral perfusion pressure (CPP), which is equal to the mean arterial pressure (MAP) minus the intracranial pressure (ICP); CPP = MAP–ICP. CBF is maintained by vasoconstriction and vasodilation of the cerebral vasculature. However, cerebral autoregulation fails at about 25% higher or lower than the MAP. In addition, changes in ICP or brain injury can result in loss of the brain's ability to autoregulate blood flow. Increased ICP, commonly seen with hemorrhage or edema, decreases the CPP, making the brain more vulnerable to changes in MAP.

Cardiovascular Crisis

Hypertensive emergencies involving the heart and great vessels include congestive heart failure, acute coronary syndromes, and dissecting aortic aneurysm. Blood pressure is frequently elevated in patients with *acute pulmonary edema*, particularly when a high output state is the cause, as in volume-overloaded patients with renal failure, patients with thyrotoxicosis, or those with severe anemia. Acute pulmonary edema with hypertension and congestive heart failure may be due to transient diastolic dysfunction, which may or may not be a direct result of the elevated blood pressure (7).

Acute coronary syndromes are also frequently accompanied by hypertension. The reduction of myocardial work by lowering the blood pressure and heart rate has been demonstrated to reduce infarct size in patients not receiving thrombolytic therapy.

Acute aortic dissection is thought to occur via aortic dilatation or high blood pressures superimposed on a structural weakness of the arterial wall. The result is a tear of the intimal layer of the aorta. Pulsatile pressure extends the dissection by separating the layers of the arterial wall. Historical series report a mortality of 1% to 2% per hour. The stresses that extend the dissection are related as much to the pulse pressure (dp/dt or difference between systolic and diastolic blood pressure over time) as it is to MAP. Factors that contribute to increased pulse pressure include the heart rate, myocardial contractility and the MAP (15).

Renovascular Crisis

The kidney is unique in being both a target organ as well as the cause of many hypertensive emergencies. Chronic hypertension causes 30% of cases of end-stage renal disease (ESRD), making it the second most common cause after diabetes. Chronic hypertensive patients may develop nephrosclerosis after 10 to 15 years, which is manifested by damage to the medial layer of capillaries, reduced kidney size, and nonnephrotic levels of proteinuria without hematuria. In contrast, malignant hypertension damages the intimal layer of the renal capillary bed and may result in enlarged kidneys, a cellular urinary sediment, hematuria, and severe proteinuria.

Severe hypertension in a young patient should raise the possibility of intrinsic acute renal disease, such as glomerulonephritis. Immunoglobulin (Ig)A nephropathy has surpassed poststreptococcal glomerulonephritis in frequency, and Henoch-Schönlein purpura is the most likely cause of acute glomerular disease among children.

Stenosis of the renal arteries is present in only 1% of unselected hypertensives, but it is present in 4% of blacks and 32% of whites who have severe hypertension (DBP>125 with retinopathy). It is also more common among patients who have a rapidly progressive course. Most patients have atherosclerosis, but a minority of patients are young women with medial fibroplasia of the renal arteries. An abdominal bruit is present in 46% of patients, and these patients are more likely to have the onset of hypertension after age 50. Occasionally a rare but devastating acute renal failure may occur owing to intrarenal vasculitis. This is common in the setting of scleroderma, and may be responsive to ACEIs.

Catecholamine Excess

The most familiar drugs that cause hypertension in emergency departments today are sympathomimetic drugs such as phenylephrine, cocaine, and methamphetamine. Tyramine can induce a hypertensive crisis in patients who are taking a monoamine oxidase inhibitor (MAOI) drug, and hypertension can complicate withdrawal syndromes from alcohol, clonidine, and, less frequently, β-blockers. Pheochromocytomas can cause intermittent hypertensive crises, usually accompanied by headache.

Patients with a pheochromocytoma can secrete a bewildering variety of catecholamines and even peptide hormones in either a constant or wildly intermittent pattern. They can produce many clinical findings other than hypertension, such as headache, sweating, palpitations, pallor, nausea, and, rarely, seizures. Some patients with pheochromocytomas have paroxysms of low blood pressure instead.

Hypertension in Pregnancy

Hypertension in pregnancy is addressed separately in Chapter 97, "Hypertensive Orders of Pregnancy." Emergencies include eclampsia and preeclampsia. Pregnant women between 20 weeks of gestation and two weeks postpartum, and who have any degree of hypertension ($\geq$140/90 mm Hg), or an increase of more than 30/15 mm Hg above their baseline, accompanied by peripheral edema and proteinuria, should be considered to have preeclampsia. Hypertension is important mainly as a symptom of the underlying disorder, rather than a cause. Preeclampsia is important to recognize, since it can progress suddenly to eclampsia, defined by the occurrence of convulsions, and can rapidly progress to coma or death. Magnesium infusion is more effective than other anticonvulsants in this setting (14). Definitive treatment consists of delivery of the fetus, so the emergency physician usually collaborates with an obstetrician early in the patient's progress through the department.

DIFFERENTIAL DIAGNOSIS

There are two entities that are specific complications of uncontrolled hypertension: hypertensive encephalopathy and malignant-accelerated hypertension (12). The other hypertensive emergencies are primary crises of the brain, heart, kidneys, and vasculature, and are thought to be precipitated or exacerbated by the stress of an elevated blood pressure (Table 49.1). For example, a myocardial infarction may occur in a normotensive as well as hypertensive patient. If the blood pressure is elevated in

TABLE 49.1.   Hypertensive Emergencies

PRIMARY

Hypertensive encephalopathy
Accelerated-malignant hypertension

SECONDARY

Cerebrovascular accidents
   Thromboembolic stroke
   Hemorrhagic stroke
   Subarachnoid hemorrhage
Cardiovascular crises
   Myocardial infarction
   Acute coronary syndromes
   Cardiogenic pulmonary edema
   Aortic dissection
   Uncontrollable arterial bleeding
Renal crises
   Acute renal failure
   Glomerular nephritis
   Severe hypertension after kidney transplant
Other emergencies
   Preeclampsia/eclampsia
   Perioperative hypertension
   Catecholamine excess

TABLE 49.2.   Drugs That can Elevate Blood Pressure or Interfere with the Effectiveness of Antihypertensive Agents

Oral contraceptives
Steroids
NSAIDs
Nasal decongestants
Cold remedies
Appetite suppressants
Tricyclic antidepressants
Monoamine oxidase inhibitors

NSAIDs, nonsteroidal antiinflammatory drugs.

the setting of an infarct then it must be managed, but the therapy must be decided primarily in the context of treating the coronary ischemia.

EMERGENCY DEPARTMENT EVALUATION

The clinical evaluation should determine the nature, severity, and management of patients in hypertensive crisis. When a patient with markedly elevated blood pressure presents to the ED, accurate measurement of blood pressure is the first step. Initially elevated ED blood pressures frequently decrease spontaneously by the time a second reading is obtained (17). For this reason alone, interventions should be based on the composite of several separate blood pressure determinations in the ED. For an accurate measurement to be obtained, the patient should be seated with the arm at the level of the heart, and the cuff bladder should cover at least 80% of the arm circumference. Blood pressure should be evaluated in both arms. Blood pressure measurement with an automated cuff is inaccurate in patients with atrial fibrillation and other heart rhythm irregularities. Appropriate pain management and relief of underlying causes (e.g., hypoxia, bladder distention) may resolve hypertension (6). Other medications, over-the-counter preparations, or illicit drugs may exacerbate or mitigate blood pressure (Table 49.2).

If the patient's blood pressure is persistently elevated, the history should start with an assessment of symptoms that might be consistent with target organ compromise. Details include the duration and severity of preexisting hypertension, the degree of previous success with blood pressure control, and the presence of target organ disease (cardiovascular, cerebrovascular, renovascular, and great vessel). The physical examination should be directed toward identifying signs of target organ damage. A funduscopic examination demonstrating the presence of retinal hemorrhage or papilledema is sufficient to diagnose accelerated-malignant hypertension. The cardiovascular examination should focus on identifying signs of heart failure (e.g., increased jugular venous pressure, pulmonary rales, and an S_3) and asymetric pulses. The neurologic examination should assess the level of consciousness, visual fields, and the presence of focal motor and sensory deficits.

Diagnostic studies should be based primarily on the patient's symptoms. A chest X-ray is indicated for patients with dyspnea and a head computed tomographic scan for abnormal neurologic findings. Few studies have assessed the prognostic value of abnormal laboratory findings in patients with severe asymptomatic hypertension (21). If a patient's blood pressure remains persistently over 180/110 mm Hg after treatment of aggravating symptoms, there should be a brief assessment of target organ function. Because renal failure is silent, the measurement of the serum creatinine and a urinalysis is used for evidence of renal failure or nephritis. An ECG is useful in assessing the baseline level of left ventricular hypertrophy, which carries a poor

TABLE 49.3.   Parenteral Drugs for Treatment of Hypertensive Emergencies

Drug	Dose[a]	Onset of Action	Duration of Action	Adverse Effects[b]	Special Indications
VASODILATORS					
Sodium nitroprusside	0.25–10 μg/kg per min as i.v. infusion (maximal dose for 10 min only)	Immediate	1–2 min	Nausea, vomiting, muscle twitching, sweating, thiocyanate and cyanide intoxication	Most hypertensive emergencies; caution with high intracranial pressure or azotemia
Nicardipine hydrochloride	5–15 mg/h i.v.	5–10 min	1–4 h	Tachycardia, headache, flushing, local phlebitis	Most hypertensive emergencies except acute heart failure; caution with coronary ischemia
Fenoldopam mesylate	0.1–0.3 μg/kg per min i.v. infusion	<5 min	30 min	Tachycardia, headache, nausea, flushing	Most hypertensive emergencies; caution with glaucoma
Nitroglycerin	5–100 μg/min as i.v. infusion[c]	2–5 min	3–5 min	Headache, vomiting methemoglobine-mia, tolerance with prolonged use	Coronary ischemia
Enalaprilat	1.25–5 mg every 6 h i.v.	15–30 min	6 h	Precipitous fall in pressure in high-renin states; response variable	Acute left ventricular failure; avoid in acute myocardial infarction
Hydralazine hydrochloride	10–20 mg i.v. 10–50 mg i.m.	10–20 min 20–30 min	3–8 h	Tachycardia, flushing, headache, vomiting, aggravation of angina	Eclampsia
Diazoxide	50–100 mg i.v. bolus repeated, or 15–30 mg/min infusion	2–4 min	6–12 h	Nausea, flushing, tachycardia, chest pain	Now obsolete: when no intensive monitoring available
ADRENERGIC INHIBITORS					
Labetalol hydrochloride	20–80 mg i.v. bolus every 10 min 0.5–2.0 mg/min i.v. infusion	5–10 min	3–6 h	Vomiting, scalp tingling, burning in throat, dizziness, nausea, heart block, orthostatic hypotension	Most hypertensive emergencies except acute heart failure
Esmolol hydrochloride	250–500 μg/kg/min for 1 min, then 50–100 μg/kg/min for 4 min; may repeat sequence	1–2 min	10–20 min	Hypotension, nausea	Aortic dissection, perioperative
Phentolamine	5–15 mg i.v.	1–2 min	3–10 min	Tachycardia, flushing, headache	Catecholamine excess

*These doses may vary from those in the *Physicians' Desk Reference* (51st edition).
[a]i.v., intravenous; i.m., intramuscular.
[b]Hypotension may occur with all agents.
[c]Require special delivery system.
From the National High Blood Pressure Education Program (JNC-VI) [10].

prognosis and will indicate more vigilant followup. When renovascular disease or hypercortisolism are suspected causes of hypertension, a serum tube for plasma renin activity and aldosterone should be drawn before medications are administered. A urine screen for cocaine and amphetamines may help confirm common causes of hypertension. The incremental value of obtaining a chest X-ray or complete blood count in the ED patient without relevant symptoms is generally likely to be low.

EMERGENCY DEPARTMENT MANAGEMENT

The goal of therapy in a hypertensive crisis is a reduction in the mean MAP by 20% to 25% over 1 to 2 hours. Although not evidence-based, this therapeutic guideline is supported by shared practice experience in patients doing poorly with more aggressive blood pressure reduction. The ideal drug for treating hypertensive emergencies has a rapid onset, rapid maximal effect, and rapid offset for easy titration of blood pressure. These characteristics are found only in parenteral agents. The most common of this group are summarized in Table 49.3 from the Sixth Report of the Joint National Committee on Prevention, Detection, Evaluation, and Treatment of High Blood Pressure (JNC-VI) (10).

Nitroprusside remains the classic treatment for patients with hypertensive emergencies (1,10). Nitroprusside is a direct arteriovenous vasodilator that decreases both preload and afterload without significant reflex tachycardia. It is quick in onset of action, and its effect lasts for only 2 to 5 minutes after the drug is discontinued. Nitroprusside should be given with close hemodynamic monitoring to prevent inadvertent hypotension. Thiocyanate toxicity may occur if the drug is used over a period of days, particularly in patients with renal failure. It is contraindicated in pregnancy. Because there is no oral form, the patient must be switched to another antihypertensive once control is achieved. Despite the many benefits of nitroprusside, there are often agents better suited for individual hypertensive crises.

Nicardipine is a rapid-acting parenteral calcium channel blocker. It has a predictable and smooth onset of action, but is relatively long acting. Esmolol is a β-blocking agent that is both rapid in onset and of short duration, making it easy to titrate. Labetalol is a combined α- and β-blocker that is more potent than esmolol, and is perhaps better at maintaining a consistent cerebral perfusion pressure. Unlike esmolol, labetalol has a long half-life, making it possible to administer in mini-boluses rather than a constant perfusion, but it is more difficult to titrate down. β-Blockers should not be used in patients with asthma, chronic obstructive pulmonary disease (COPD), acute congestive heart failure, cocaine abuse, or other contraindications to β blockade. Fenoldopam is a parenteral dopaminergic receptor-blocking agent with an excellent efficacy and safety profile. Fenoldopam holds some promise as being equivalent to nitroprusside in efficacy, without the rare side effects associated with the nitroprusside cyanide moiety and perhaps with less overshoot hypotension, but at present its cost is often prohibitive. Enalaprilat is a parenteral angiotensin-converting enzyme (ACE) inhibitor, and phentolamine is a pure α-blocking agent.

Cerebrovascular Crisis

Blood pressure control in *cerebrovascular hypertensive emergencies* should be undertaken with parenteral drugs that have a short half-life and that are easily titrated with minimal effect on cerebral vasculature. Because labetalol does not dilate cerebral capacitance vessels, it is theoretically attractive for use intracerebral disorders. Direct vasodilators, such as nitroprusside, should be used with caution in the setting of focal brain injury, as they can extend an area of ischemia. Some calcium channel blockers have been linked to a rise in the ICP and therefore are not favored in patients with brain injury, although nicardipine is safe and widely used (23).

The treatment of elevated blood pressure in the setting of *ischemic cerebrovascular accidents* is controversial. When systemic blood pressure is reduced, cerebral autoregulation may fail, thereby producing an ischemic penumbra surrounding the infarct, leading to stroke extension. Alternatively, infarction can lead to edema, which will elevate ICP and reduce CBF further. The current American Heart Association (AHA) guidelines recommend lowering the blood pressure with stroke only when the MAP is greater than 130 mm Hg, or the systolic blood pressure is greater than 220 mm Hg (2).

Theoretically, treatment for elevated blood pressure in *hemorrhagic cerebrovascular accidents and subarachnoid hemorrhage* should be more aggressive than for patients with ischemic strokes. The rationale is to decrease the risk of ongoing bleeding from ruptured small arteries and arterioles; however, the relationship between rebleeding and systemic blood pressure is unproven. As with an ischemic cardiovascular accident, overly aggressive treatment of hypertension may worsen brain injury by decreasing CPP, especially when ICP is increased. The AHA guidelines for blood pressure control with hemorrhagic stroke are similar to those with ischemic stroke: lowering the blood pressure only when the MAP is greater than 130 mm Hg or the systolic blood pressure is greater than 220 mm Hg (4). Nimodipine may be given to decrease the incidence of vasospasm and rebleeding after *subarachnoid hemorrhages,* but the drug is not recommended for blood pressure control (23).

Cardiovascular Crisis

Nitroglycerin (NTG) is favored in the treatment of severe hypertension complicating *cardiac ischemia*. NTG is a direct vasodilator that affects the venous vasculature more than the arterial. NTG dilates the coronary arteries and, in contrast to nitroprusside, promotes a favorable redistribution of blood flow to ischemic areas. β-Blockers are also effective and recommended therapy for acute coronary syndromes. The goal of treatment *for patients with acute coronary syndromes* is reduction of blood pressure to normal, or even lower if evidence of ischemia persists. However, this reduction should occur carefully with the patient monitored intensively. Overly vigorous blood pressure lowering may worsen ischemia, since coronary perfusion depends on diastolic blood pressure.

Most critical cases of *congestive heart failure* are treated with a combination of NTG, furosemide, and an ACE inhibitor (ACEI). For patients with pulmonary edema and hypertension, initiate sublingual NTG while preparing intravenous NTG. An ACEI is helpful whenever there is pulmonary congestion and hypertension; captopril may be given orally or sublingually, or enalaprilat can be given intravenously if the patient cannot take oral medications. If systemic fluid overload is present then administer intravenous furosemide. However, some patients with congestive heart failure will not have signs of right-sided heart failure (e.g., jugular venous congestion, peripheral edema, and hepatomegaly) and will in fact be volume depleted owing to a pressure diuresis, despite the presence of pulmonary edema. In these patients with "dry failure," diuresis may initially exacerbate the underlying pressure natriuresis and further stimulate the renin–angiotensin axis (7). The decision is based on a clinical judgment of whole-body fluid status. β-blockers have been found to improve survival in patients with chronic congestive heart failure; however, this observation should not be extended to patients with acute pulmonary edema because the negative inotropic effects and bradycardia of β-blockade may precipitate immediate worsening. Intravenous nesiritide improves hemodynamic function and symptoms in decompensated heart failure and has a modest antihypertensive effect.

In *aortic dissection*, β-blockers should be initiated before starting nitroprusside to avoid the potential adverse effects of reflex tachycardia. Labetalol is a unique parenteral agent that achieves its maximal effect within minutes and then remains effective for several hours. This allows titration with small boluses, thereby avoiding the constant monitoring required and increased cost incurred with use of nitroprusside (15).

Renovascular Crisis

Compared to nitroprusside, fenoldopam may improve outcomes in patients with hypertension and *acute renal failure*. Although malignant hypertension may precipitate acute renal failure by injuring the kidney's microvasculature, this causal chain is often reversed, with hypertension instead a manifestation of renal failure. Because this distinction cannot be made in the ED, these patients should have their blood pressure lowered. Both nitroprusside and labetalol are excellent choices in this setting. ACEI drugs definitely improve prognosis among chronic hypertensives with mild proteinuria; however, they should be used cautiously in hyperkalemic patients with acute uremia. Nitroprusside cause thiocyanate poisoning over several days in patients with renal failure and should be used only briefly or if the patient is to have dialysis soon.

Treatment with an ACEI may reverse high blood pressure dramatically in patients with unilateral stenosis, but it may provoke acute renal failure and severe hyperkalemia in patients with bilateral stenosis, particularly if these patients are taking supplemental potassium or a potassium-sparing diuretic. This complication can be completely reversed by discontinuing the ACEI (19).

Catecholamine Excess

Patients with severe hypertension resulting from *pheochromocytoma* are commonly treated with the pure α-blocker phentolamine, given intravenously. This may be accompanied by a β-blocker if needed for tachycardia. Administration of beta-blockers alone in the setting of any sympathomimetic (e.g., cocaine) may leave the α receptors "open," with subsequent worsening of hypertension. Therefore, an attractive alternative to β-blockers is labetalol, a β-blocker with some α-antagonist properties. However, the α and β blockade with labetalol may not be equally effective. Although several studies report reductions in blood pressure and heart rate when labetalol is given to patients with cocaine toxicity, case reports indicate that some individuals may get worse. The clinical importance of the "unopposed alpha" effect of labetalol increasing blood pressure requires better evidence.

Hypertension in Pregnancy

The mainstay of antihypertensive treatment for hypertensive crisis in pregnancy in many institutions is hydralazine administered intravenously in boluses of 5 to 10 mg every 20 to 30 minutes. This is in addition to magnesium therapy for seizure control. If treatment is refractory to hydralazine, second-line agents are diazoxide and β-blockers. Calcium channel blockers have been studied in chronic hypertension among pregnant patients, but they may not be effective with proteinuric hypertension.

CRITICAL INTERVENTIONS

- Base clinical decisions on correctly measured and repeated blood pressure
- Search for and correct underlying causes of an elevated blood pressure (e.g., pain, hypoxia, bladder distention)
- Investigate complaints carefully for evidence of target organ disease
- Treat the blood pressure according to specific indications (e.g., ischemia)
- Avoid relative hypotension or dropping blood pressure in the absence of an indication

DISPOSITION

All hypertensive emergencies require admission to a monitored setting. These patients generally require emergent involvement of an appropriate specialist for management of a neurologic, cardiovascular, or renovascular crisis. Close blood pressure monitoring, preferably with an arterial line, is indicated. Patients with preeclampsia/eclampsia require emergent obstetric consultation.

Most patients presenting with elevated blood pressures are not in crisis. In the patient with asymptomatic, elevated blood pressure with no evidence of target organ disease, the most important intervention is to ensure proper followup (6,21). The goal should be life-long control of the blood pressure. When the elevated blood pressure may be the artifact of a systemic process such as pain or infection, the best strategy is to refer the patient for reevaluation of the blood pressure once the primary problem has resolved. If the patient has discontinued their blood pressure medications, the regimen should be restarted, barriers to

TABLE 49.4.   Compelling Indications for Individual Drug Classes for Hypertension Therapy

Compelling Indication[a]	Recommended Drugs[b]					
	Diuretic	BB	ACEI	ARB	CCB	Aldo ANT
Heart failure	X	X	X	X		X
Postmyocardial infarction		X	X			X
High coronary disease risk	X	X	X		X	
Diabetes	X	X	X	X	X	
Chronic kidney disease			X	X		
Recurrent stroke prevention	X		X			

[a]Compelling indications for antihypertensive drugs are based on benefits from outcomes studies or existing clinical guidelines; the compelling indication is managed in parallel with the blood pressure.
[b]Drug abbreviations: ACEI, angiotensin-converting enzyme inhibitor; ARB, angiotensin receptor blockers; Aldo ANT, aldosterone antagonist; BB, β-blocker; CCB, calcium channel blocker.
From the National High Blood Pressure Education Program (JNC-VII) (6).

compliance evaluated, and a primary care physician contacted to ensure reevaluation in a week. The JNC-VII guidelines recommend a thiazide-type diuretic as an initial agent, usually in combination with drugs from other classes (6). The second agent may be from a number of categories and is best chosen in relation to any compelling indications in the patient's history (Table 49.4).

In principle, if there has never been a previous measurement of elevated blood pressure, the blood pressure needs to be rechecked on another visit before the diagnosis of hypertension can be made. However, in individuals with readings persistently greater than 180/110 mm Hg in the ED, the latest national guidelines recommend that they be immediately started on combination therapy (6). Ideally, the physician who will provide ongoing supervision should be the one to pick the initial agents with which they are comfortable. The best role of the emergency physician is to identify a primary physician for the patient and encourage that physician to select an initial antihypertensive agent and provide a followup appointment within the week.

There is an intermediate group of patients with a severely elevated blood pressure and with known target organ disease, but without active decompensation. Examples include a severely hypertensive patient with a previous history of myocardial infarction or stroke. The immediacy arises because the patient with known target organ disease may be considered at higher risk for a hypertension-related adverse event in the short term. There is no good evidence basis for how these patients should best be managed. They should have a treatment strategy initiated from the ED, although the blood pressure does not necessarily need to be lowered during the visit. These patients do require an increased level of vigilance. It may be reasonable to treat these patients as outpatients, although some may need to be held for short-term observation if there is question as to medication compliance or blood pressure monitoring. The decision depends on the clinical judgment of the physician.

COMMON PITFALLS

✔ Diagnosing a hypertensive emergency when one does not exist. Patients with hypertensive emergencies have evidence of acute end-organ dysfunction

✔ Reducing the blood pressure too quickly or to too low a level. In patients with chronic hypertension whose autoregulation curve has been reset, this can lead to cerebral or cardiac ischemia

✔ Lowering a patient's blood pressure acutely without an urgent indication

✔ Failing to diagnose hypertension or preeclampsia in pregnant patients with blood pressures greater than 140/90 mm Hg, or with an increase in blood pressure of more than 30/15 mm Hg

✔ Neglecting to match the antihypertensive agent to the clinical scenario

Acknowledgments

Thank you to previous edition authors Katerina T. Parmele and Alison J. McDonald.

References

1. Abdelwahab W, Frishman W, Landau A. Management of hypertensive urgencies and emergencies. *J Clin Pharm* 1995;35:747–762.
2. Adams HP, Brott TG, Crowell RM, et al. Guidelines for the management of patients with acute ischemic stroke. A statement for healthcare professionals from a special writing group of the Stroke Council, American Heart Association. *Stroke* 1994;25:1901–1914.
3. Blumenfeld JD, Laragh JH. Management of hypertensive crises: the scientific basis for treatment decisions. *Am J Hypertens* 2001;14:1154–1167.
4. Broderick JP, Adams HP Jr., Barsan W, et al. Guidelines for the management of spontaneous intracerebral hemorrhage: a statement for healthcare professionals from a special writing group of the Stroke Council, American Heart Association. *Stroke* 1999;30:905–915.
5. Calhoun DA, Oparil S: Treatment of hypertensive crisis. *N Engl J Med* 1990; 323:1177–1183.
6. Chobanian AV, Bakris GL, Black HR, et al. The Seventh Report of the Joint National Committee on Prevention, Detection, Evaluation, and Treatment of High Blood Pressure. The JNC 7 Report. *JAMA* 2003; May 21, 289, 19, 2560–2572.
7. Gandhi SK, Powers JC, Nomeir AM, et al. The pathogenesis of acute pulmonary edema associated with hypertension. *N Engl J Med* 2001;344:17–22.
8. Gifford RW. Management of hypertensive crises. *JAMA* 1991;266:829–835.
9. Hyman DJ, Pavlik VN. Characteristics of patients with uncontrolled hypertension in the United States. *N Engl J Med* 2001;345:479–486.
10. Joint National Committee on Prevention, Detection, and Treatment of High Blood Pressure. The Sixth Report of the Joint National Committee on Prevention, Detection, Evaluation, and Treatment of High Blood Pressure. *Arch Intern Med* 1997;157:2413–2446.
11. Kaplan NM. Management of hypertensive emergencies. *Lancet* 1994;344:1335–1338.
12. Kaplan NM: *Clinical Hypertension.* 7th ed. Baltimore, MD: Williams & Wilkins, 1998.
13. Lip GY, Beevers M, Beevers DG. Complications and survival of 315 patients with malignant-phase hypertension. *J Hypertens* 1995;13:915–924.
14. Lucas MJ, Leveno KJ, Cunningham FG. A comparison of magnesium sulfate with phenytoin for the prevention of eclampsia. *N Engl J Med* 1995;333:201–205.
15. Pretre R, Von Segesser LK. Aortic dissection. *Lancet* 1997;349:1461–1464.
16. Murphy C. Hypertensive emergencies. *Emerg Med Clinics of N Am* 1995;13:973–1007.
17. Pitts SR, Adams RP. Emergency department hypertension and regression to the mean. *Ann Emerg Med* 1998;31:214–218.
18. Ram CV. Immediate management of severe hypertension. *Cardiol Clin* 1995; 13:579–591.
19. Safian RD, Textor SC: Renal-artery stenosis. *N Engl J Med* 2001;344:431–442.
20. Schwartz RB, Jones KM, Kalina P, et al. Hypertensive encephalopathy: findings on CT, MR imaging, and SPECT imaging in 14 cases. *Am J Roentgenol* 1992;159:379–383.
21. Shayne P, Pitts S. Severe hypertension in the emergency department: a state of the art review. *Ann Emerg Med* 2003;41:513–529.
22. Thach AM, Schultz PJ. Nonemergent hypertension. New perspectives for the emergency medicine physician. *Emerg Med Clinics N Am* 1995;13:1009–1035.
23. Tietjen CS, Hurn PD, Ulatowski JA, et al. Treatment modalities for hypertensive patients with intracranial pathology: options and risks. *Crit Care Med* 1996;24:311–322.
24. Varon J, Marik PE. The diagnosis and management of hypertensive crises. *Chest* 2000;118:214–227.
25. Vaughan CJ, Delanty N. Hypertensive emergencies. *Lancet* 2000;356:411–417.

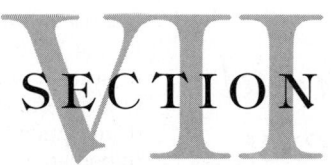

SECTION

VII

Section Editor: Gregory W. Hendey

Vascular Emergencies

CHAPTER 50
Nontraumatic Carotid and Vertebral Artery Disorders

Brian Chinnock

INTERNAL CAROTID AND VERTEBRAL ARTERY DISSECTION

Internal carotid artery (ICA) or vertebral artery (VA) dissection results from an intimal tear. Following the tear, blood under pressure enters the wall of the artery within the tunica media, forming an intramural hematoma. The hematoma, while contained within the tunica media, may press toward either the intima, causing vessel stenosis (Fig. 50.1A), or toward the adventitia (Fig. 50.1B), causing aneurysmal dilation. In addition, in the intracranial portion of the artery, dissection may result in subarachnoid hemorrhage.

The extracranial ICA and VA are much more vulnerable to dissection than are the intracranial segments. This is likely because of the mobility of the vessels extracranially. The ICA is mobile in its entire course from its starting point, the bifurcation of the common carotid artery, to its entry into the skull. The VA is mobile at its proximal and distal segments. Thus, the start site of the ICA dissection is typically just distal to the carotid bulb (which lies within the first 2 cm after the bifurcation) and does not extend past the entry of the artery into the temporal bone. VA dissection most commonly begins at the artery's distal segment, between the first and second cervical vertebrae, at its exit point from the transverse foramen of the axis. Unlike the ICA, which enters the skull through a narrow canal, the VA enters through the much larger foramen magnum, which is why a much higher percentage (approximately 10%) of VA dissections can extend intracranially (17).

Together, ICA and VA dissections cause about 20% of strokes in patients younger than 45 years of age, compared to causing only 2.5% of strokes in elderly patients (1). ICA dissection occurs approximately twice as frequently as VA dissection. Common carotid artery dissection has also been described, but is rarer. Bilateral dissections of the ICA and VA have been described. In addition, simultaneous dissection of the ICA and VA has been described.

ICA or VA dissections that occur in the absence of high-energy blunt or penetrating trauma are termed "spontaneous" dissections. Most of these spontaneous dissections are believed to result from some form of structural wall defect, which can commonly occur with connective tissue disorders. Of these identifiable etiologies for dissection, the most common is Ehlers-Danlos syndrome type IV. Less commonly, osteogenesis imperfecta, Marfan syndrome and autosomal dominant polycystic kidney disease are causative factors (16). Angiographic changes consistent with fibromuscular dysplasia, an arterial disease of unknown etiology affecting mainly the renal, carotid, and vertebral arteries, can be seen in up to 15% of patients. Migraine headache history has also been described as a risk factor. Family history is important in that 5% of patients with a spontaneous ICA or VA dissection will have a family member who has had a dissection of the aorta or one of its main branches. It is important to note that the common predisposing risk factors for the development of carotid and VA stenosis, such as hypertension, hypercholesterolemia, diabetes, or tobacco use, have not been found to be risk factors for artery dissection.

Spontaneous dissection of the ICA or VA is often associated with commonplace events that cause sudden neck movement or sustained positioning of the neck in a position that may predispose to vessel damage. Some of the reported events include (i) forceful flexion-extension movements of the neck, as occur in coughing, vomiting, sneezing, nose-blowing, trampoline use, and roller coaster riding; (ii) prolonged extension of the neck as occurs with painting a ceiling or "beauty-parlor" syndrome in which the neck is extended over the sink; or (iii) prolonged lateral bending of the neck as occurs with propping a phone between the neck and shoulder (14,17,18). Chiropractic treatment involving rapid rotation of the neck, while also being described as a possible precipitant of ICA dissection, is more commonly associated with VA dissection. This is likely because of the rapid rotation of C1 on C2 causing stretch of the VA as it exits the foramen between the vertebrae.

CLINICAL PRESENTATION

The median age of patients presenting with extracranial ICA dissection is 44 years, and for extracranial VA dissection it is 41 years (20). Intracranial dissection of either artery reportedly occurs in younger patients, 20 to 30 years of age (14).

The clinical effects from arterial dissection generally result from the local effects of the dissection itself, which causes pain, and the distal embolization from the dissection site, which causes ischemic symptoms.

ICA Dissection

Table 50.1 illustrates the differences in the clinical presentation of ICA versus VA dissection. Headache is the most prominent initial complaint of the patient with ICA dissection. It is typically frontotemporal and unilateral. The onset is usually gradual, but "thunderclap" headaches have been described. Facial, eye or ear pain, without headache, is described in 10% of patients (20). The unilateral neck pain is typically over the area of the carotid artery itself, and has also been mistaken for a peritonsillar abscess. Oculosympathetic palsy is classically associated with ICA dissection, but only half of patients will have it. It is characterized by ipsilateral miosis and ptosis. Oculosympathetic palsy can be differentiated from Horner syndrome in that there is no facial anhidrosis, since facial sweat glands are innervated by the sympathetic plexus surrounding the external, not internal, carotid artery. The focal cerebral and retinal ischemic symptoms are similar to those described for ICA-territory strokes, and are described in Chapter 112, "Cerebrovascular Disease." They begin a median of 4 days after the onset of pain in extracranial ICA dissection (20). By contrast, in intracranial ICA dissection, the neurologic symptoms begin only a few hours after the onset of the pain (4). Most commonly the neurologic findings are unilateral, but in 15% of cases they can be bilateral. The lower cranial nerves are commonly affected, particularly the hypoglossal nerve. Impairment of taste is noted in 10% of patients. The cranial nerve impairment is thought to be caused by either compression or stretching of the nerve by the enlarged ICA, or by interruption of nutrient vessels of the nerves (14,17,18).

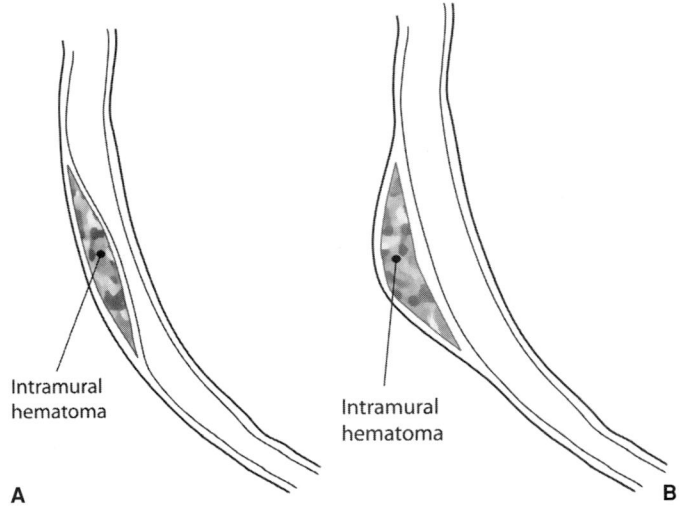

Figure 50.1. **A:** Intramural hematoma producing vessel stenosis. **B:** Intramural hematoma causing aneurysmal dilation without vessel stenosis.

Vertebral Artery Dissection

Headache is the most common presenting complaint of the patient with VA dissection, as it is with ICA dissection. The headache is almost always occipital, but may also involve the frontal area, and may be intermittent. Neck pain is more commonly noted in VA dissection than in ICA dissection, and is more commonly described as posterior. The unilateral arm pain that can occur is caused by dissection that involves the VA within the cervical spine, with local compression on a cervical nerve root, most commonly at the C5-C6 level (3,17).

The focal ischemic neurologic symptoms are typically those of vertebrobasilar insufficiency, as described in Chapter 112. The classic finding is involvement of the posterolateral medulla and cerebellum, termed *Wallenberg syndrome*. The thalamus and cerebral hemispheres may also be affected, although less commonly than the cerebellum and brainstem. Importantly, neck pain has been described as beginning a median of about 2 weeks before the development of neurologic findings like these, whereas headache begins only hours before (15).

TABLE 50.1. Symptoms and Physical Examination Findings of ICA versus VA Dissection

Clinical Presentation of Dissection (% Incidence of Finding)	
Carotid	Vertebral
Unilateral headache (67–90)	Occipital headache (66–83)
Unilateral facial/orbital pain (50)	Posterior neck pain (50)
Unilateral anterior neck pain (25)	Unilateral arm pain
Oculosympathetic palsy (50)	Isolated cervical cord ischemia
Pulsatile tinnitus (25)	Nausea, vomiting
Syncope	
Cerebral or retinal ischemic symptoms (50–95)	Vertebrobasilar ischemic symptoms (70–90)
Cranial nerve palsies (12)	Wallenberg syndrome
More likely to have preceding TIA	Less likely to have preceding TIA
Neurologic findings begin days after headache	Neurologic findings begin hours after headache

ICA, interval carotid artery; VA; vertebral artery; TIA, transient ischemic syndrome.

DIFFERENTIAL DIAGNOSIS

The main differential diagnoses for carotid and VA dissection, before the development of focal neurologic symptoms are meningitis, subarachnoid hemorrhage, subdural or epidural hematoma, migraine or tension headache, and cervical strain, fracture, or radiculopathy. When it has progressed to neurologic symptoms from distal embolization, the differential is similar to that of ischemic stroke. One of the main ways to differentiate ICA or VA dissection from these other disorders is by the history of head or neck pain, followed hours to days later by ICA or VA-territory neurologic symptoms. The ideal situation, however, is to diagnose and treat dissection before the development of neurologic symptoms. This is why it is most important to consider ICA and VA dissection in the differential diagnosis for more benign disorders such as tension headache and cervical strain.

EMERGENCY DEPARTMENT EVALUATION

When ICA or VA dissection is suspected by history and physical examination findings, the most important consideration is which imaging modality is best to evaluate for dissection. The gold standard by which other radiologic tests are measured is four-vessel contrast angiography. The disadvantages of this procedure include its invasiveness and the need to use contrast dye. The most commonly used alternative radiologic tests are duplex ultrasound, magnetic resonance imaging (MRI), and magnetic resonance angioplasty (MRA).

Duplex Ultrasound

Extracranial duplex ultrasound can identify intimal defects and aneurismal dilation. In addition, color-flow duplex ultrasound is useful for identifying the true and false lumens seen in dissection. The true lumen typically has antegrade flow, whereas the false lumen has high-resistance flow that is forward, reversed, or bidirectional. Ultrasound is limited by its inability to visualize intracranial dissection.

The ICA can be easily visualized by duplex ultrasound in all but its most distal extracranial portion. Two prospective studies have compared ultrasound to the gold standard of conventional angiography or MRA in the evaluation of ICA dissection. In the studies, the sensitivity of Doppler to detect flow abnormalities was 93% to 96%. Standard duplex scanning had a sensitivity of 72% to 79%, and color-flow scanning had a sensitivity of 82% (5,21). The sensitivity of ultrasound for diagnosing ICA dissection has likely improved in the last decade owing to substantial technological improvements.

The use of ultrasound in the diagnosis of VA dissection is less clear. It is a technically more difficult study than in the ICA. Most VA dissections show abnormal flow patterns, but no finding is characteristic for VA dissection. Small case series have shown promise, but the current practice is to not rely on ultrasound alone in the initial diagnosis.

Magnetic Resonance Imaging/Magnetic Resonance Angioplasty

MRI can visualize the intramural hematoma itself, usually as a crescent-shaped signal on cross-section of the artery. It can also show aneurysmal dilation. MRA can show luminal irregularities and stenosis without the need for contrast injection, although contrast-enhanced methods are also described. The combination of MRI with MRA demonstrates a sensitivity of 84% to 100% and specificity of 95% to 100% when compared against conventional angiography in small studies (9). One study that examined ICA dissection demonstrated a better sensitivity of the MRI–MRA combination than with conventional angiography (19). This results from contrast angiography being unable to detect an abnormality if there is no lumenal irregularity (Fig. 50.1B). MRI can also show cerebral parenchyma abnormalities in the affected vascular area. The MRI–MRA combination has largely replaced contrast angiography in the evaluation of ICA and VA dissection.

EMERGENCY DEPARTMENT MANAGEMENT

The treatment for an extracranial ICA or VA dissection is anticoagulation with heparin followed by coumadin. The goal is to reduce the risk of distal embolization, the most common cause of neurologic insult. If there is intracranial dissection, there is theoretic concern for hemorrhagic transformation. Despite its wide acceptance, there is no controlled study comparing anticoagulation to placebo in the treatment of dissection. Antiplatelet agents such as aspirin, and less commonly ticlopidine and clopidogrel, have been described as treatment options. There are no randomized trials comparing anticoagulant with antiplatelet drugs, and nonrandomized studies did not demonstrate any difference. Antiplatelet agents are often considered as first-line treatment in patients who are poor candidates for anticoagulation and in those who have a dissection with no ischemic symptoms. Thrombolytics have been used safely in one small study, but in 9 of 11 treated patients, the vessel remained occluded (6). Blood pressure control to a normotensive level has a theoretical benefit in preventing extension of the dissection, but no studies have examined this.

CRITICAL INTERVENTIONS

- Consider ICA and VA dissection in patients with headache and/or neck pain. Early diagnosis may prevent neurologic insult
- Ensure that a head CT scan is done in the patient with a dissection, as subarachnoid hemorrhage is a known complication, and can be worsened significantly with anticoagulation

DISPOSITION

Patients diagnosed with ICA or VA dissection are admitted to the hospital to monitor for further progression of neurologic injury and to establish anticoagulation with heparin. Depending on institutional differences, neurosurgery or vascular surgery services will need to be consulted.

The prognosis for neurologic recovery is good. Approximately 70% of extracranial ICA dissection patients have full neurologic recovery, 14% have a mild deficit, and 16% have a moderate-to-severe deficit or death (18). One long-term followup study of extracranial VA dissection patients showed 88% with good or excellent recovery and 12% with moderate or severe disability (12). Intracranial dissection patients have significantly higher morbidity and mortality rates, as do those with bilateral extracranial dissections. Regarding the dissection itself, 90% of stenoses resolve, 66% of occlusions recanalize, and 33% of aneurysms decrease in size. This resolution almost always occurs within 2 to 3 months. In the patient with a dissection, it will very rarely recur in the same artery, but, in the first month, there is a 2% risk of dissection in a previously unaffected artery. This risk decreases to 1% per year and persists for at least a decade (17). Surgery for ICA or VA dissection may be considered in the patient with deteriorating neurologic symptoms, despite adequate

anticoagulation, or in the patient who demonstrates persistent aneurysm after 6 months of anticoagulation. Surgial treatment may be through an open procedure, or, increasingly, may consist of endovascular treatment with stent angioplasty across the dissection.

COMMON PITFALLS

✔ Failure to consider the diagnosis in a patient with headache or neck pain associated with minor trauma, particularly if neurologic symptoms are present
✔ Failure to consider the diagnosis in a relatively young patient with stroke symptoms

INTERNAL CAROTID AND VERTEBRAL ARTERY STENOSES

Stenosis or occlusion of the ICA or VA is most commonly caused by atherosclerosis. There is a 2% to 5% annual ipsilateral stroke risk for people with ICA stenosis of greater than 50% reduction in diameter. Although there are fewer data on stroke risk in patients with VA stenosis, symptomatic patients with greater than 50% stenosis have a 1-year stroke risk of as high as 22% (22). ICA stenosis is responsible for approximately 30% of all anterior circulation strokes and transient ischemic attacks (TIAs). Cerebral ischemia resulting from the atherosclerotic lesion is either hemodynamic, in which the stenosis causes a low flow state to the brain, or embolic, in which there is distal embolization from the plaque. Embolization is the most common mechanism causing a stroke or TIA. Because of collateral circulation, stroke is less often a result of stenosis and low flow, and when it does occur, the neurologic deficits are less severe. For VA stenosis to cause ischemia because of a low-flow state, significant blockage of both vertebral arteries, along with lack of collateral circulation from the anterior circulation via the circle of Willis, must be present.

Risk factors for the development of ICA or VA atherosclerosis are similar to those for coronary artery atherosclerosis, and include hypertension, tobacco use, hypercholesterolemia, and obesity. Other less common causes of stenosis include fibromuscular dysplasia, radiation and arteritis (i.e. Takayasu arteritis).

The most common location for extracranial ICA stenosis is at the carotid bulb. Extracranial VA stenosis most commonly occurs at the origin of the artery from the aorta or brachiocephalic trunk.

ICA kinking and VA occlusion resulting from rotation (*bow hunter syndrome*) deserve special mention as they are causes of vessel occlusion without, necessarily, any stenosis or dissection (7). ICA tortuosity with kinking is a common finding on ultrasound or angiography that, in the great majority of cases, represents no increased long-term risk of stroke. In some patients the site of kinking can be caused by atherosclerosis and stenosis. However, even if nonstenotic, this kinking can be considered a source of potential embolization in symptomatic patient in which no other abnormality is found. It may also cause reversible cerebral ischemia during head or neck rotation.

The VA may also be occluded because of head or neck rotation. Unlike the ICA, in which the vessel itself is abnormal and becomes occluded, it is usually the structures around the VA that are responsible for occlusion during neck rotation. *Os odontoideum*, a condition in which the dens is hypoplastic, absent, or incompletely fused to the body of C2 with subsequent atlantoaxial instability and bony impingement on the VA during movement, is described as a cause. Other neck rotation-induced occlusions include nerve fibers of the stellate ganglion impinging

TABLE 50.2. Findings in ICA- Versus VA-Territory Strokes or TIAs

ICA Territory	VA Territory
Weakness and/or numbness Contralateral face and extremities	Weakness and/or numbness Ipsilateral face, contralateral extremities
Vision loss Ipsilateral, monocular (*amaurosis fugax*)	Vision loss Bilateral homonymous hemianopia
Aphasia	Ataxia
	Vertigo
	Diplopia

ICA, internal carotid artery; VA, vertebral artery; TIA, transient ischemic attack.

on the VA origin, and lateral cervical disk herniation impinging on the VA as it courses in the foraminal canal.

CLINICAL PRESENTATION

The patient with symptomatic ICA or VA stenosis will usually present to the emergency department with symptoms related to stroke or TIA of the affected vascular area (see Chapter 112). Table 50.2 contrasts the neurologic findings associated with ICA versus VA stenosis, although there can be considerable overlap between the two.

DIFFERENTIAL DIAGNOSIS

As noted previously, TIA and stroke are the most common events bringing the patient with ICA or VA stenosis to the ED. (See Chapter 112 for a more complete discussion the differential for stroke and TIA.)

EMERGENCY DEPARTMENT EVALUATION

In addition to evaluating the patients for history and physical examination findings of stroke (detailed in Chapter 112), imaging can be an important part of the evaluation for ICA or VA stenosis.

Internal Carotid Artery Stenosis

The degree of extracranial ICA stenosis can be used to predict which patients are at the highest risk for stroke, and will get the most benefit from surgery. The North American Symptomatic Carotid Enderarterectomy Trial (NASCET) demonstrated that in patients with 70% to 99% stenosis, carotid enderarterectomy is superior to medical therapy in preventing stroke (11). A systematic review of trials done between 1994 and 2001 compared imaging modalities to the gold standard of conventional angiography in detecting 70% to 99% stenosis and gave the following pooled test characteristics: Duplex ultrasound, sensitivity 86% and specificity 87%; MRA–MRI, 95% and 90%, respectively; and the combination of MRA + duplex ultrasound, 95% and 95%, respectively. Duplex ultrasound is highly operator dependent, and at centers with expertise, it is often used as the sole test in determining degree of stenosis.

Patients with 100% ICA occlusion are not likely to benefit from surgical intervention. Both duplex ultrasound alone and MRA have sensitivities and specificities near 100% in detecting occlusion in most studies.

Vertebral Artery Stenosis

Unlike ICA stenosis, the degree of VA stenosis that is most clinically important is not well defined, although 50% to 99% stenosis is the range that is usually cited as significant. Duplex ultrasound and MRA have difficulty in visualizing the VA origin, the site where approximately 90% of VA stenoses occur. By using colorflow Doppler on other parts of the VA, however, sensitivities near 100% have been reported.

EMERGENCY DEPARTMENT MANAGEMENT

Acute treatment of stroke caused by ICA or VA stenosis is described in detail in Chapter 112, and includes prevention of hyperglycemia and hyperthermia, and monitoring of volume status and blood pressure. An important intervention is to start the patient on antiplatelet therapy, after ruling out hemorrhagic stroke with a CT scan. Aspirin, at a dose of 160 to 300 mg, has been shown to significantly decrease death and disability in acute ischemic stroke. Clopidogrel and ticlopidine are alternatives for patients unable to take aspirin. Knowledge of the degree of ICA or VA stenosis and/or occlusion is not a factor in deciding if the patient is a candidate for thrombolytic treatment.

Patients with 70% to 99% symptomatic ICA stenosis are likely to benefit from carotid enderarterectomy, whereas in those with 50% to 69% stenosis, only certain subgroups, such as those with large hemispheric TIAs, may benefit from surgery (11). The CAVATAS study compared endovascular therapy with balloon or stent angioplasty to enderarterectomy, and found no difference in stroke or death rate in an 8-year followup (2).

The optimal treatment strategies for extracranial VA stenosis are more poorly understood. Surgical options include enderarterectomy or reconstruction (often done by transposing the VA to the common carotid artery). Endovascular therapy with stent angioplasty is largely replacing surgery in the treatment of VA stenosis. Surgery is recommended for patients with symptomatic ICA kinking. Correction of the process that causes extrinsic VA compression during neck rotation (i.e., atlantoaxial stability or cervical disk protrusion) is also necessary to prevent further cerebral ischemia.

CRITICAL INTERVENTIONS

- Aspirin 160 to 325 mg is recommended for patients with symptomatic ICA or VA stenosis, or clopidogrel or ticlopidine for those who cannot take aspirin
- Obtain imaging studies of patients with stroke or TIA to determine whether they may be candidates for carotid endarterectomy

DISPOSITION

Stroke resulting from significant ICA or VA stenosis mandates admission to the hospital to monitor for deterioration, cerebral edema, or hemorrhagic transformation. Cardiac monitoring, swallowing studies, and aggressive rehabilitation are also commonly needed.

Patients with TIAs that are not crescendo or recurrent, and that are unlikely to have an embolic source, may be candidates for outpatient care with urgent imaging and rapid followup. However, one study demonstrated that 5% of patients presenting to an ED with a TIA will have a stroke within 2 days after presentation (8). Consultation should involve the patient's primary care doctor and/or a neurologist. Patients who are found to have significant ICA or VA stenosis as an acute cause of TIA or stroke are candidates for inpatient evaluation for endarterectomy or angioplasty.

COMMON PITFALLS

✔ Failure to recognize the difference between ICA and VA territory neurologic symptoms. A normal carotid duplex ultrasound study is irrelevant when the symptomatology suggests VA stenosis

✔ Failure to consider ICA kinking or "bow hunter syndrome" in the patient with stroke/TIA symptoms with head/neck rotation

Acknowledgments

Thanks to previous edition chapter author James W. Dennis upon whose chapter some of this chapter text may have been based.

References

1. Bogousslavsky J, Pierre P. Ischemic stroke in patients under age 45. *Neurol Clin* 1992;10:113–124.
2. CAVATAS investigators. Endovascular versus surgical treatment in patients with carotid stenosis in the Carotid and Vertebral Artery Transluminal Angioplasty Study (CAVATAS): a randomized trial. *Lancet* 2001;357:1729–1737.
3. Chang AJ, Mylonakis E, Karanasias P, Orchis DF, Gold R. Spontaneous bilateral vertebral artery dissections: case report and literature review. *Mayo Clin Proc* 1999;74:893–896.
4. Chavez C, Estol C, Esnaola MM, et al. Spontaneous intracranial internal carotid artery dissection. *Arch Neurol* 2002;15:977–981.
5. De Bray JM, Lhoste P, Dubas F, et al.Ultrasonic features of extracranial carotid dissections: 47 cases studied by angiography.
6. Derex L, Nighoghossian N, Turjman F, et al. Intravenous tPA in acute ischemic stroke related to internal carotid artery dissection. *Neurology* 2000;54:2159–2161.
7. Horowitz M, Jovin T, Balzar J, et al. Bow hunter's syndrome in the setting of contralateral vertebral artery stenosis: evaluation and treatment options. *Spine* 2002;27:E495–498.
8. Johnston SC, Gress DR, Browner WS, Sidney S. Short-term prognosis after emergency department diagnosis of TIA. *JAMA* 2000;284:2901–2906.
9. Levy C, Laissy JP, Raveau V. Carotid and vertebral artery dissections: Three-dimensional time-of-flight MR angiography and MR imaging versus conventional angiography. *Radiology* 1994;190:97–103.
10. Nadgir RN, Loevner LA, Ahmed T, et al. Simultaneous bilateral internal carotid and vertebral artery dissection following chiropractic manipulation: case report and review of the literature. *Neuroradiology* 2003;45:311–314.
11. NASCET investigators. Clinical alert: benefit of carotid endarterectomy for patients with high-grade stenosis of the internal carotid artery. *Stroke* 1991;22:816–817.
12. Nakagawa K, Touho H, Morisako T, et al. Long-term follow-up study of unruptured vertebral artery dissection: clinical outcomes and serial angiographic findings. *J Neurosurg* 2000;93:19–25.
13. Nederkoorn PJ, van der Graaf Y, Hunink M. Duplex ultrasound and magnetic resonance angiography compared with digital subtraction angiography in carotid artery stenosis: a systematic review. *Stroke* 2003;34:1324–1332.
14. Norris JW, Beletsky V. Cervical arterial dissection. *Adv Neurol* 2003;92:119–125.
15. Saeed AB, Shuaib A, Al-Sulaiti G, Emery D. Vertebral artery dissection: warning symptoms, clinical features and prognosis in 26 patients. *Can J Neurol Sci* 2000;27:292–296.
16. Schievink WI, Michels VV, Piepgras DG. Neurovascular manifestations of heritable connective tissue disorders: a review. *Stroke* 1994;25:889–903.
17. Schievink WI. Spontaneous dissection of the carotid and vertebral arteries. *N Engl J Med* 2001;344:898–906.
18. Scovell SD, Masaryk T. Carotid artery dissection. *Semin Vasc Surg* 2002;15:137–144.
19. Stringaris K, Liberopoulos K, Giaka E, et al. Three-dimensional time-of-flight MR angiography and MR imaging versus conventional angiography in carotid artery dissections. *Int Angiol* 1996;15:20–25.
20. Sturnezegger M. Spontaneous internal carotid artery dissection: early diagnosis and management in 44 patients. *J Neurol* 1995;242:231–238.
21. Sturnezegger M, Mattle HP, Rivoir A, Baumgartner RW. Ultrasound findings in carotid artery dissection: analysis of 43 patients. *Neurology* 1995;45:691–698.
22. WASID Study Group. Prognosis of patients with symptomatic vertebral or basilar artery stenosis. The Warfarin-Aspirin Symptomatic Intracranial Disease (WASID) study group. *Stroke* 1998;29:1389–1392.

CHAPTER 51
Peripheral Arterial Disease

Darren Braude

Peripheral arterial disease (PAD) is usually secondary to atherosclerosis and occurs most frequently in the lower extremities. Venous insufficiency, which usually presents as varicose veins, thrombophlebitis, or deep-venous thrombosis is discussed in Chapter 52. "Deep Venous Thrombosis and Thrombophlebitis" (1).

Asymptomatic PAD is common among emergency department (ED) patients with cardiovascular disease and risk factors, but the acutely ischemic limb must be promptly recognized and treated. Irreversible damage to nerves and muscle may develop within 6 hours (4).

Peripheral arterial disease is analogous to acute coronary syndrome. Stable angina equates to noncritical ischemia presenting as predictable claudication. Unstable angina equates to the progression of chronic disease to critical limb ischemia presenting as rest pain, ulceration, or gangrene. Myocardial infarction equates to acute, critical limb ischemia caused by thrombus or embolism.

CLINICAL PRESENTATION

Peripheral arterial disease may be categorized as acute or chronic, critical or noncritical, and limb-threatening or not. Acute ischemia most often occurs secondary to in situ expansion of an atherosclerotic thrombus or the lodging of an embolus from a more proximal source. Chronic noncritical ischemia includes intermittent claudication and asymptomatic arterial insufficiency. Chronic critical ischemia includes rest pain and/or skin ulcerations, infections, or necrosis. Limb-threatening ischemia includes both acute ischemia of a lower extremity and chronic critical ischemia (Table 51.1).

Because most PAD in developed countries is related to underlying atherosclerosis, the typical patient will have known atherosclerotic disease or obvious risk factors including advanced age, diabetes, obesity, smoking history, hypertension, and/or hyperlipidemia (7).

Acute Ischemia

Patients with acute ischemia usually present to the ED because of persistent, severe pain in a lower extremity. Pain is usually not well defined and in most cases, depending on the location of the obstruction and the degree of collateral flow, it extends above the ankle. Patients with coexisting diabetic neuropathy may not have typical pain. Patients may also complain of paresthesias, weakness or numbness, and/or that their leg is white or blue.

Acute ischemia is usually caused by an arterial embolism or thrombus of a native artery or bypass graft. Thrombosis is much more common than embolism (4). Patients with an arterial thrombosis become symptomatic from extension and subsequent arterial occlusion. Most patients will have had prior chronic arterial insufficiency with claudication, rest pain, typical trophic skin changes, and/or prior bypass grafting.

TABLE 51.1. Classification of Peripheral Arterial Disease

Limb-threatening ischemia
  Acute thrombus or embolism
  Chronic critical ischemia
    Rest pain
    Ischemic skin changes—ulcers or gangrene
Non–limb-threatening ischemia
  Chronic noncritical ischemia
    Asymptomatic
    Intermittent claudication

Because long-standing disease has led to the development of collateral circulation, symptoms and physical findings may not be as dramatic as with embolism.

Arterial embolism arises from the heart in 80% to 90% of cases (4,8); usually from a ventricular thrombus in a postmyocardial infarction ventricular aneurysm or an atrial thrombus in the setting of mitral valve disease and/or atrial fibrillation (4). Unless the patient has significant coexisting lower extremity atherosclerosis, they will not have established collateral circulation to circumvent the occlusion. Arterial embolism, therefore, usually presents in a more dramatic fashion than thrombosis does. The hallmarks are sudden onset of symptoms without preceding symptoms of chronic PAD, an identifiable embolic source, and a normal circulatory examination of the unaffected leg (7).

Chronic Critical

Patients with chronic critical ischemia usually present to the ED because of new or worsening rest pain or skin changes. As circulation is affected by gravity, rest pain typically occurs while the patient is sleeping or whenever the patient is supine. Pain occurs distally, in the forefoot or toes, but not in the calves. Because the pain is exacerbated by leg elevation and improved with dependency, many patients will sleep in a chair or hang their leg over the side of the bed to keep them dependent. Symptoms worsen in the cold, and the pain is vague but severe. Associated ischemic peripheral neuropathy may cause sharp shooting pains and sensations of heat and cold.

Chronic Noncritical

Patients with chronic noncritical ischemia usually present to the ED because of new or worsening intermittent claudication (IC), which is angina of the legs. Patients will report leg cramping or aching after a consistently reproducible amount of activity, which prompts the patient to stop activity. The pain is relieved by a consistently reproducible short period of rest. Therefore the ability to ambulate sufficiently far to produce ischemia is prerequisite. Depending on the site of the occlusion, claudication may occur in the calf, hip, buttock, or thigh. Foot claudication is rare with atherosclerosis but may be seen in Buerger disease.

DIFFERENTIAL DIAGNOSIS

Acute Ischemia

If both legs are involved, the clinician should consider a low cardiac output state or an aortic dissection tracking into both iliac arteries. If only one leg is involved the differential includes conditions that mimic ischemia such as phlegmasia cerulea dolens and acute compressive neuropathy as well as nonatherosclerotic causes of true ischemia such as phlegmasia alba dolens, arterial trauma, aortic dissection, arteritis, and spontaneous thrombosis from hypercoagulable states, and vasospasm.

Chronic Ischemia

Rest Pain

Any distal sensory neuropathy may also present with pain primarily at night. This pain tends to be symmetric foot-based shooting pains that are neither exacerbated by elevation nor relieved with dependency, except ischemic neuropathy associated with chronic arterial ischemia. The most common type is diabetic neuropathy; other causes include vitamin deficiency and alcohol abuse. Gout may cause extremity pain at rest, although this pain persists with dependency, is localized to a joint, and is almost always associated with visible findings. Compressive neuropathies such as disc herniation of the lumbosacral nerve roots may produce pain at rest, although this pain usually persists with dependency, follows a dermatomal pattern, is associated with back complaints, and presents with a normal vascular examination. Some confusion may arise with straight-leg raising, which causes pain in both conditions. Reflex sympathetic dystrophy, a poorly understood condition, often presents with burning pain and skin changes. Pain is not exacerbated by elevation and pulses should be normal. Finally, simple night cramps cause calf rather than foot pain that is not exacerbated by elevation, relieved with massage, and not associated with pulse changes.

Ulcers

Ulcers secondary to arterial ischemia must be differentiated from ulcers secondary to venous stasis and diabetes. Ulcers related to venous insufficiency are the most common. The ulcers associated with venous stasis tend to occur more proximally, produce less pain that is relieved with elevation, be found in the setting of edema and stasis dermatitis, and have a wet base with lots of granulation tissue. The ulcers of diabetes may occur in the same distal pressure point locations as PAD-associated ulcers but tend to be painless, deep, and surrounded by much callus and/or inflammation (4).

Gangrene

The primary differential of dry gangrene is frostbite. Wet gangrene may originate in other skin ulcers or wounds.

Intermittent Claudication

Calf claudication in patients with atherosclerotic risk factors may be confused with venous claudication, compressive neuropathy, calf spasms, or symptomatic Baker cyst. Venous claudication follows treatment for deep venous thrombosis, resolves slowly when exercise stops, gets better with limb elevation, and is usually associated with edema. Compressive neuropathy usually produces distinctly dermatomal sharp pain that is usually associated with back pain and does not resolve immediately when activity stops. Baker cyst discomfort persists at rest.

Hip, thigh, or buttock claudication may be confused with arthritis of the hip and spinal stenosis. Pain from arthritis is not consistently reproduced with activity, is often present at rest, and is not relieved quickly with rest. Spinal stenosis symptoms are dermatomal, are usually associated with back pain, and are relieved more by bending forward than by stopping activity.

Foot claudication is rare from atherosclerosis but it common with Buerger disease. Foot pain may also be confused with arthritis but the pain in this case is not consistently reproducible with activity, is often present at rest and is not rapidly relieved when activity ceases.

EMERGENCY DEPARTMENT EVALUATION

Peripheral arterial disease is primarily a clinical diagnosis based upon history and physical examination, including the ankle-brachial pressure index. In patients with evidence of acute ischemia, vascular surgery consultation should precede diagnostic studies. This may require transfer prior to definitive diagnosis. The ED physician may consider ordering a Doppler ultrasound prior to consultation in the patient with previously undiagnosed PAD without evidence of critical ischemia or in very unclear cases. Definitive diagnostic testing, such as arteriogram (or possibly magnetic resonance angioplasty (MRA)), should be at the discretion of the vascular surgery consultant given the associated potential delays and adverse effects. There is no major role for computed tomographic (CT) scanning, expect perhaps for the confirmation of an arterial aneurysm.

Physical Examination

Examination of the lower extremities should include bilateral inspection for sores, edema, dermatitis, and signs of infection; palpation of skin temperature; assessment of capillary refill time; palpation of the femoral, popliteal, dorsalis pedis, and posterior tibial pulses; auscultation of the femoral artery; and the motor and sensory examination. Capillary refill has not been found to be useful in assessing chronic peripheral vascular disease (3). The abdomen should be examined for masses or bruits suggestive of abdominal aortic aneurysm.

The signs and symptoms in acute arterial occlusion resulting from an embolus can be dramatic and reflect the "six Ps" of ischemia (3):

- Pain
- Pallor
- Pulselessness
- Poikilothermia
- Paralysis
- Paresthesias

Because these patients usually do not have preexisting PAD, the unaffected extremity should have a normal examination and forms the basis for comparison. The affected extremity is white or cyanotic and cool to the touch; pulses are absent. There is no appreciable swelling except that which may have preexisted. There will usually be some component of neuropathy as well with weakness and sensory deficits. Sensory deficits begin with diminished light touch, two-point discrimination, and proprioception. Loss of deep pain and pressure sensation and motor deficits reflect more advanced ischemia (4,7). The intrinsic muscles of the feet are the most sensitive and may be tested by having the patient spread their toes.

In arterial thrombosis, findings may be more subtle than with embolus owing to collateral blood flow and/or slower onset, although by definition the major pulses distal to the obstruction will still be absent. Unfortunately there is variability in the presence of peripheral pulses and their detection (4,7). Comparison with the unaffected extremity and the use of a Doppler are very helpful. The presence of pulses detected on Doppler pulses indicates blood flow but does not exclude ischemia, given the extreme sensitivity of the Doppler. Both the affected and the unaffected extremity should show findings of chronic PAD including: atrophy of calf muscles, loss of hair over the dorsum of the foot, thickened toenails, shiny skin, diminished pulses (unaffected limb), and possibly skin ulcers. Some edema may be noted, as patients reflexively keep their extremities dependent at all times.

TABLE 51.2.   Technique for the Measurement of Ankle-Brachial Index

Place patient supine
Measure systolic pressure at the anterior and posterior tibial arteries of affected leg by using Doppler.
- If neither is obtainable, limb is immediately threatened
- Select higher value of the two
Measure systolic pressure at brachial artery of both arms
- Select higher of the two
Divide higher tibial pressure by higher brachial pressure

ABI, ankle-brachial index.
[2,5].

Patients with rest pain secondary to PAD will show many of the changes noted previously for chronic PAD. These patients, however, do not have complete occlusion, and, therefore, capillary refill should be present, although delayed, and pulses will be present, at least by Doppler. Another useful finding of severe ischemia is Buerger sign. A positive test is the observation of pallor with foot elevation of at least 12 inches. Exaggerated delayed erythema with subsequent dependency should also be seen.

Skin ulcerations from arterial insufficiency tend to occur distally at pressure points, including the tips of the toes, between the toes, on the heel, or at over the malleoli. These ulcers often have an irregular border and a pale base, and show signs of infection (4,7). Plain radiography is appropriate to screen for underlying osteomyelitis when the ulcer appears sufficiently deep or infected.

Gangrene is rarely missed when the distal extremities are examined. Uninfected gangrene is dry. Discharge, weeping, crepitance, lymphangitis, and proximal cellulitis suggest infection.

Patients with intermittent claudication will likely have a normal examination at rest, although they may have some subtle findings of chronic ischemia as noted previously.

Ankle-Brachial Pressure Index

The ankle-brachial pressure index (ABPI or ABI) is a rapid objective measurement of arterial insufficiency. ABI should be assessed in any patient in whom you arterial insufficiency is suspected. If the ABI can be measured, the limb is not immediately threatened but may still be ischemic as Doppler signals are very sensitive. If arterial signals are absent, limb loss is likely without emergent revascularization (4). Absent venous pulsations indicate even more severe ischemia (4). It is helpful to check the ABI in the nonaffected leg to ascertain whether the patient has underlying arterial disease or noncompressible vessels. The technique for determining the ABI and its interpretation are included in the figures. Some sources consider the upper limit of normal as 1.0, 1.1, or 1.2 (4,5,7) (Tables 51.2 and 51.3).

TABLE 51.3.   Interpretation of ABI Results

ABI	Interpretation
>1.3	Noncompressible vessel (nondiagnostic)
0.91–1.3	Normal
0.4–0.9	Mild-to-moderate disease
<0.4	Severe disease

ABI, ankle-brachial index.

EMERGENCY DEPARTMENT MANAGEMENT

Supportive care for all patients includes keeping the affected limb dependent and warm, appropriate analgesia, and maximization of cardiac output. Aspirin and/or clopidogrel should be considered in all patients, although their role in the acute setting has not been adequately investigated (7).

Acute Ischemia

In the absence of contraindications, all patients with acute critical ischemia should receive anticoagulation, despite little objective evidence. Weight-based unfractionated heparin is still the standard therapy. Supplemental oxygen may be helpful and should be provided when acute ischemia is considered. Options for definitive therapy include surgical or interventional radiology procedures. The choice of therapy will be at the discretion of the vascular surgeon. Considerations will include degree and duration of ischemia, contraindications, local resources, and results of arteriography. In patients with severe ischemia, angiography may be performed interoperatively to minimize delays. Surgical options include direct removal of the occlusion (most common with established thrombi), bypass grafting, primary amputation, and Fogarty catheter embolectomy (most common with emboli or suspected new thrombi). Interventional radiology options include the direct interthrombus (interarterial) administration of thrombolytics and angioplasty. There is currently no accepted role for intravenous thrombolytics.

Chronic Critical Ischemia with Rest Pain

Those patients with rest pain even in the dependent position should be treated as for acute ischemia. Patients with rest pain only while the foot is elevated represent an intermediate group. Definitive therapy for this group may involve pharmacotherapy, endovascular procedures, and/or surgery, but these measures do not need to be started immediately. At a minimum, phone consultation with the patient's primary care physician, cardiologist, or vascular surgeon is appropriate. These patients may be discharged home after consultation with an adequate followup plan and return precautions.

Chronic Critical Ischemia with Ulcerations or Gangrene

Patients with uninfected ulcerations require wound debridement and dressing, close monitoring for the development of infection, analgesia and at a minimum, phone consultation with a vascular surgeon. Admission should be considered but is not mandatory when adequate followup is assured.

Patients with infected ulcerations will need supportive care, aggressive wound management, systemic antibiotics, admission, and vascular surgery consultation. Appropriate antibiotic choices include: nafcillin 2 g q4hr, or cefazolin 1 g q8hr, or clindamycin (600 mg q8hr).

Patients with diabetes or recent hospitalization, nursing home patients, or patients with more serious infections should receive antibiotic coverage for gram-negative organisms as well: ampicillin/sulbactam (Unasyn) 1.5 to 3 g q6hr.

Patients with dry-gangrene will require supportive care and timely surgery consultation. Patients with evidence of gas gangrene, wet gangrene, or sepsis may require intensive care unit (ICU) admission and immediate surgical consultation, as well as antibiotics with anaerobic coverage (1,4,6): clindamycin 900 mg q8h plus penicillin G, 4 million U q4h.

Chronic Noncritical Ischemia = Intermittent Claudication

Once identified, IC is not an emergency. These patients should be reassured that walking, despite causing pain, is not harmful. No medications, including aspirin, have been shown to be of acute benefit. These patients will require close followup with their primary care physician, cardiologist, or vascular surgeon.

CRITICAL INTERVENTIONS

- Recognition of potentially limb-threatening ischemia: rest pain, skin loss, or any acute ischemia, particularly with sensory loss, muscle weakness, or absent arterial Doppler pulses
- Weight-based heparin (80 mg/kg bolus followed by 18 mg/kg/hour drip) for acute ischemia and rest pain that persists in the dependent position if not contraindicated
- Emergent vascular surgery consultation (including transfer as necessary) for limb-threatening ischemia or infection
- Supportive care: keep affected extremity warm and dependent, maximize cardiac output, and provide supplemental oxygen
- Early initiation of antibiotics for patients with signs of infection

DISPOSITION

All patients with PAD will require vascular surgery consultation. The emergency physician must decide according to the acuity of the situation, whether that consultation must take place emergently in the ED, or on an out-patient basis. In some situations it may also be acceptable to admit the patient to their primary care provider, hospitalist, or cardiologist with urgent vascular surgery consultation as an inpatient.

Obtain emergent vascular surgery consultation on all patients with acute ischemia or evidence of serious infection in an ischemic extremity. If vascular surgery consultation is not available, the patient should be transferred expeditiously. Air medical transport is appropriate if ground transportation is delayed or prolonged. The goal should be to get the patient to a vascular surgeon as quickly and safely as possible.

Patients with chronic critical ischemia will also require emergent vascular surgery consultation in most cases. Patients with rest pain that is well controlled with supportive measures and patients with uninfected ulcers without gangrene might be candidates for admission with urgent vascular surgery consultation as an inpatient.

Patients with newly diagnosed noncritical ischemia may be discharged home with close outpatient followup. Consultation with a vascular surgeon before discharge is recommended when possible.

COMMON PITFALLS

✔ Delaying consultation or transfer for definitive diagnosis
✔ Falsely elevated ABI or neuropathy masking pain in diabetics
✔ Congenital absence of pedal pulses, particularly the dorsalis pedis
✔ Claudication history not obtained as individual's activity is too limited
✔ Failure to recognize that intermittent claudication can occur in the hip, buttock, or thigh

Acknowledgment

Thank you to previous edition author Henry C. Veldenz.

References

1. Baddour LM. Treatment of cellulitis. *UpToDate* 2003.
2. Hiatt WR. Medical treatment of peripheral arterial disease and claudication. *N Engl J Med* 2001;344:1608–1621.
3. McGee SR, Boyko EJ. Physical examination and chronic lower-extremity ischemia: a critical review. *Arch Intern Med* 1998;158:1357–1364.
4. Rutherford RB (ed). *Vascular surgery*, 5th ed. Philadelphia: WB Saunders, 2000.
5. Sacks D, et al. Position statement on the use of the ankle-brachial index in the evaluation of patients with peripheral vascular disease. *J Vasc Interv Radiol* 2003 Sept.;14(9 Pt 2):S389.
6. Stevens DL. Clostridial myonecrosis. *J Vasc Interv Radiol* 2003 Sept.;14(9 Pt 2):S389.
7. The TASC Working Group. Management of peripheral vascular disease (PAD): TransAtlantic Inter-Society Consensus (TASC). *J Vasc Surg* 2000;31[Suppl 1]:S1–S288.
8. Way LW, Doherty GM. *Current surgical diagnosis and treatment*, 11th ed. New York: McGraw-Hill, 2003.

CHAPTER 52

Deep Venous Thrombosis and Thrombophlebitis

Edward A. Panacek and J. Douglas Kirk

Deep venous thrombosis (DVT) of the lower extremity is a relatively common diagnosis made in the emergency department (ED), and up to 600,000 Americans are hospitalized with this diagnosis each year. However, because DVT is often occult, the true incidence is unknown (2). Thromboembolic disease is responsible for an estimated 200,000 deaths annually in the United States, and millions more experience sequelae such as stasis dermatitis and venous ulcers. The elderly are at highest risk, and DVT is associated with a 21% mortality rate in this age group (11). Subsets of children are also at risk, particularly those with spinal cord injuries or hypercoagulable conditions.

The risks for development of DVT were first described by Virchow in his description of the famous triad that includes stasis, hypercoagulability, and endothelial injury. It is now known that there are other conditions that either cross categories or separately place patients at risk (Table 52.1). Increased estrogen causes a fall in protein S level (and cigarette smoking increases this tendency), yet the risk of DVT is only slightly increased with use of low-estrogen contraceptives, progesterone-only pills, or Norplant (8). These risk factors are additive in nature, and it is important to be familiar with them in order to evaluate patients appropriately. However, 25% to 50% of patients with DVT do not have obvious risk factors (3) and a substantial proportion of them have been found to have the Leiden variant of factor V or other hypercoagulable disorders. The proportion appears to be even higher in patients with recurrent DVT.

The initiating stimulus for thrombus formation is often an intimal defect. The dynamic interplay of coagulation and fibrinolytic forces then results in clot propagation or dissolution. Conditions affecting the balance of these forces are what place patients at increased risk for symptomatic thrombus formation.

If the process is of sufficient severity or duration, the associated vein can become inflamed; the condition is then referred to as thrombophlebitis.

The vast majority of significant DVTs develop in the deep iliofemoral system. Although isolated superficial thrombophlebitis generally does not pose a significant risk for embolization, 25% of patients with symptoms of superficial thrombophlebitis have been shown to have involvement of the deep system as well (10). In addition, patients with a first episode of DVT complicated by superficial thrombophlebitis have a two-fold increased risk of recurrent DVT compared to patients without superficial thrombophlebitis (17). Patients with isolated calf vein involvement are also at increased risk. In up to 20%, these thrombi have been shown to propagate proximally above the popliteal fossa and embolize (14).

Although embolization to the lung is the most serious complication of DVT, it can also result in other complicating conditions. Venous hypertension and persistent clot can destroy valves, thereby leading to a postphlebitic syndrome (chronic leg pain and venous stasis) in perhaps half of patients. Other patients develop only recurrent edema. Occasionally, acute cases

---

TABLE 52.1.   Risk Factors for Deep Venous Thrombosis

STASIS

Immobility
  Bed rest (≥3 d)
  Prolonged sitting owing to long rides (plane, car, or train)
Paralysis
  CNS injury
  Cast

ENDOTHELIAL INJURY

Intravenous drug abuse
Vascular trauma
Recent surgery
Central lines

HYPERCOAGULABILITY

Malignancy
Previous thromboembolic disease
Inflammatory conditions (e.g., SLE)
Nephrotic syndrome (loss of antithrombin III)
Coagulation disorders
  Protein S deficiency or resistance
  Protein C deficiency
  Antithrombin III deficiency
  Factor V Leiden
Increased estrogen
  Pregnancy
  Postpartum <3 mo
  Oral contraceptives
Disorders of fibrinogen or plasminogen
  Antiphospholipid antibodies (lupus anticoagulant and
    anticardiolipin)

MULTIFACTORIAL

Recent trauma
Recent surgery
Age >60 yr
Cardiac disease (especially CHF)
Obesity
Venous insufficiency
Smoking

CNS, central nervous system; SLE, systemic lupus erythematosus; CHF, congestive heart failure.

can even develop a compartment syndrome of the thigh or lower leg. Most importantly, up to 40% of patients with DVT have clinically silent pulmonary emboli (PEs) (15).

CLINICAL PRESENTATION

Patients with DVT can present with a symptom complex that ranges from completely occult to obvious (2). Most commonly, they present with lower extremity pain or swelling that may worsen with standing or walking. Manifestations are almost always unilateral, except in the rare and life-threatening case of inferior vena cava (IVC) involvement. Generally, DVT symptoms develop over a period of several days, whereas sudden severe pain is more likely related to an injury. Associated symptoms, such as chest pain or dyspnea, may also be present, particularly as they relate to the presence of PE. Risk factors can be identified in the majority of patients.

DIFFERENTIAL DIAGNOSIS

Several medical conditions can present with symptoms suggestive of DVT (Table 52.2). Many of these conditions generally cause bilateral leg swelling resulting from either increased production of edema fluid or an IVC obstructive process. However, if prior DVT has resulted in damage to the venous valves, these conditions can exacerbate asymmetric swelling. In addition, abdominal masses (e.g., a gravid uterus) can occasionally compress a single iliac vein, resulting in unilateral venous stasis. One of the most difficult conditions to distinguish from DVT is the postphlebitic syndrome. Patients with prior DVT can develop recurrent unilateral pain and swelling that is clinically indistinguishable from acute DVT. Other conditions that are most often confused with DVT are cellulitis, *superficial thrombophlebitis*, and *septic thrombophlebitis*. There is much clinical overlap among these conditions, and a low threshold for objective diagnostic testing is required.

EMERGENCY DEPARTMENT EVALUATION

The clinical evaluation of the patient with possible DVT focuses both on identifying findings consistent with DVT and on diagnosing alternative conditions that may explain the patient's presentation. It is important to question the patient about risk

---

TABLE 52.2. Differential Diagnosis of Deep Venous Thrombosis

Postphlebitic syndrome
Cellulitis/abscess
Muscle injury/hematoma
Popliteal cyst (Baker cyst)
Superficial thrombophlebitis
Septic thrombophlebitis
Congestive heart failure
Lymphedema
Malignancy (obstructive)
Capillary leak syndrome
Fracture
Sciatica
Acute arthritis
Myositis
Pregnancy
Superior vena cava syndrome (upper extremity DVT)

DVT, deep venous thrombosis.

TABLE 52.3. Clinical Probability Scoring for DVT

CLINICAL FEATURE	SCORE
Active cancer (treatment within 6 mo)	1
Paralysis, paresis, or recent cast immobilization of lower extremity	1
Recent bedridden (>3 d) or surgery within 4 w	1
Localized tenderness along deep venous system	1
Entire leg swollen	1
Calf swelling >3 cm compared to unaffected extemity	1
Greater pitting edema in the affected leg	1
Collateral superficial veins (nonvaricose)	1
Alternative diagnosis as likely or more than that of DVT	−2

High probability	$= \geq 3$
Moderate probability	**= 1 or 2**
Low probability	**= 0 or less**

DVT, deep venous thrombosis.
Adapted from Wells PS, Anderson DR, Bormanis J, et al. Value assessment of pretest probability of deep-vein thrombosis in clinical management. *Lancet* 1997;350:1795.

---

factors for DVT (Table 52.1) including a family history. As many as one fourth of patients with acute DVT have a history of prior DVT (2).

Assessment of risk factors can be subjective, but there are commonly used scoring systems (22). These have been validated for use in the ED setting (18). Those with one or two factors are considered medium risk, and those with no factors are considered low risk (Table 52.3). Bed rest is generally considered to be "prolonged" if it occurs for 3 or more days. Immobility or prolonged sitting from long rides is considered to be significant if it is of at least 12 hours' duration. The period of risk after surgery and trauma (incriminated in up to 40% of cases of DVT) probably extends for a few weeks. Patients with three or more risk factors or specific examination findings are generally considered high risk (22).

The physical examination can provide useful findings but must be interpreted with caution. Although patients with cellulitis and other infections usually have a fever, DVT can also result in temperature elevations, although often only low grade. Unilateral warmth and erythema are common with both DVT and cellulitis. The presence of an abscess, enlarged lymph nodes, and ulcerations can be important clues for distinguishing an infectious etiology. A difference of 3 cm in the circumference of the calves, measured 10 cm below the tibial tuberosity, or 3 cm in the circumference of the thighs, measured equally from the patella, is clinically significant and one of the most specific findings for DVT. The presence of palpable "cords" in the thigh is considered fairly specific but quite insensitive for thrombosis. In the popliteal fossa, they can easily be confused with a Baker cyst. Homan sign was classically taught as being important in the evaluation of DVT, but it is now well known that its sensitivity and specificity are only about 50%.

DVT is a difficult diagnosis to make clinically; between 50% and 75% of patients suspected of having DVT will not have the diagnosis confirmed by objective tests (2). Therefore, patients in whom the diagnosis is suspected must undergo further diagnostic studies. The D-dimer assay, which is abnormally elevated in the presence of acute thrombus degradation, can be a useful laboratory marker in excluding patients with suspected DVT. Early enthusiasm as a result of the assay's high sensitivity (93% to 98%) was somewhat tempered by its poor specificity (40% to 80%) (1). False negatives are particularly common in chronic or subacute DVT or other inflammatory disorders. D-dimer testing should not replace imaging studies altogether as first line testing in high-risk patients but its discriminate use in low-risk patients can be advocated. Wells et al. described a clinical predictive model with a relatively simple scoring system that accurately identified patients at low, intermediate, or high risk of DVT (18). This model has been subsequently combined with D-dimer testing to further stratify patients' risk of DVT (18,22). Low-risk patients (0 points) can be assessed solely with D-dimer testing, which if negative, warrants no additional imaging. It must be emphasized that only the more sensitive enzyme-linked immunosorbent assay (ELISA), and Simpli-Red and turbidimetric assays should be used, not the early generation latex agglutination methods, which have lower sensitivity. [Gosselin] The results of small studies also suggest that using D-dimer testing may also be reliable in patients with intermediate pre-test risk, correctly identifying those without DVT, but this is controversial. Larger, randomized, controlled clinicaltrials are needed before the latter application can be fully endorsed for widespread use.

The primary imaging study to identify patients with DVT is now ultrasonography. It is relatively inexpensive, noninvasive, and widely available (12). Although a number of techniques are used, looking at compressibility of the vein with B mode is the standard for confirming the diagnosis. Ultrasound is considered 95% to 99% sensitive for acute thrombi above the knee and it can also occasionally identify other conditions such as tumor, cysts, or aneurysms. However, scans can be reader-dependent, and some institutions lack individuals with sufficient expertise or experience. In addition, the test is less accurate in the second half of pregnancy and for pelvic vein thrombus, for which the Doppler mode of the duplex ultrasound scan can be more helpful. In these situations, or in patients felt to be at very high risk for DVT, it may not be appropriate to end the evaluation with a single negative ultrasound examination. Use of additional tests such as venography or close outpatient follow-up with serial ultrasound examinations is recommended (4).

Although venography has historically been considered the gold standard for the diagnosis of DVT, it has a number of problems that have led to its limited use. Approximately 10% of the studies are technically inadequate and radiologists often disagree on interpretation. Some patients develop phlebitis from the procedure, and there are occasional cases of anaphylaxis from the contrast material. Patients also report the procedure to be painful. For all of these reasons, the role of venography has largely been supplanted by ultrasound (12). The main role of venography is in patients with a history of prior DVT in whom ultrasound is equivocal. It can better distinguish between acute and chronic changes.

Impedance plethysmography (IPG) measures changes in lower extremity venous volume in response to selected maneuvers and draws comparisons between the two lower extremities. Although relatively inexpensive and noninvasive, IPG has been shown to be operator-dependent, and its sensitivity is only 65% to 85% (12). therefore, it is not recommended for use in ED patients. Likewise, radiolabeled fibrinogen studies, which are designed to identify growing thrombus, are relatively insensitive, take prolonged periods to perform, and are not useful in ED patients.

Magnetic resonance imaging (MRI) is developing a growing role in the evaluation of DVT. Its sensitivity (97%) and specificity (95%) are the equal of ultrasound (20). In addition, this technique is particularly useful for identifying thrombus in the pelvis, an area where ultrasound has limitations. It is also approved as safe for use during pregnancy and is the test of choice in that patient population (20). MRI can distinguish mature from recent clot and also has applications for identifying PEs. However, it is relatively expensive, not consistently available, and requires greater patient cooperation, thereby limiting its use.

Although much less common, DVT can also develop in the upper extremities, usually in the subclavian or axillary veins (5). The use of diagnostic imaging studies in such cases is not well studied. Because of differences in the anatomy, ultrasound may not be as sensitive as in the lower extremity, but it is still recommended as the first-line diagnostic test. However, inadequate or negative examinations in high-risk patients should be followed with contrast venography.

EMERGENCY DEPARTMENT MANAGEMENT

Patients with isolated DVT rarely require immediate lifesaving interventions. However, many of these patients have occult PEs and all are at risk for new emboli. When a PE is strongly suspected, starting heparin prior to imaging studies is appropriate. In addition, occasional patients can present with complete venous obstruction, a condition referred to as "phlegmasia dolens." These patients should also undergo immediate heparinization and fluid resuscitation prior to imaging studies when the diagnosis is suspected. They may also require thrombolytics and occasionally, urgent thrombectomy (Table 52.4).

For most patients, the initial treatment for DVT is anticoagulation with heparin. Those patients with absolute contraindications to anticoagulation require inferior vena caval interruption with a filter (6). These devices are approximately 95% effective in preventing further PEs, but have a 10% complication rate on insertion. However, this rate is not appreciably higher than that of full anticoagulation.

Heparin blocks extension of thrombus and reduces the risk of further emboli. It does not actively lyse clot, but allows the body's own fibrinolytic mechanism to operate over a period of several days to weeks (9). Heparin has a relatively narrow therapeutic

---

TABLE 52.4.   Disposition and Treatment

DEEP VENOUS THROMBOSIS (PROXIMAL DVT)

Heparin bolus 2,500 U and infusion (18 U/kg/h); decrease for older patients
Warfarin on first day
Admit to hospital (floor bed) or consider outpatient protocol using LMWH in selected patients
IVC filter if heparin contraindicated or fails anticoagulation therapy

SUPERFICIAL THROMBOPHLEBITIS

Ultrasound to exclude DVT
Outpatient care with elevation, NSAIDS; consider compression bandages

CALF THROMBI (DISTAL DVT)

Same as proximal DVT
Or treat like superficial thrombophlebitis, but with serial outpatient studies to detect propagation

PHLEGMASIA DOLENS

Immediately heparinize
Fluid resuscitate
Admit to Intensive care unit
Consider thrombolysis
Vascular surgery consult (consider thrombectomy)

DVT, deep venous thrombosis; LMWH, low-molecular-weight heparin; NSAIDs, nonsteroidal autiinflammatory drugs.

index and is noteworthy as the most common cause of drug-related deaths in the hospital. Significant bleeding occurs in up to one fourth of patients; the elderly and those on aspirin are at greatest risk. However, these complications rarely occur during the first few hours of treatment or during the time the patient is in the ED.

Unfractionated heparin is commonly given as a 5,000-U bolus (often 10,000 U if PE is expected), followed by 1,000 U per hour (7). However, this "standard dosing regimen" often results in inadequate anticoagulation at 24 hours secondary to an excessive bolus dose and an inadequate infusion dose (23). It has been shown that more accurate dosing occurs when the heparin regimen is weight-based. One of the most commonly used regimens is an 80 U/kg bolus followed by an 18 U/kg per hour infusion (16). However, bolus doses of as little as 1,600 to 2,500 U have been shown to be adequate to reach an initial therapeutic activated partial thromboplastin time (aPTT) (23). Overshooting the therapeutic target with a large bolus often leads to an inappropriate lowering of the infusion dose within the first few hours when the first aPTT measurement returns supratherapeutic. Complex nomograms utilizing weight, age, sex, and clinical diagnosis have been developed and are reliable at attaining therapeutic anticoagulation. They are available in some hospital pharmacy departments. Short of using one of these nomograms, a reasonable approach would be a 2,500-U bolus followed by an 18 U/kg per hour infusion. Consideration should be given to lowering the infusion rate in older patients (23). The rate is then titrated, with the goal of prolonging the aPTT time by 1.5 to 2.5 times above control or the upper limits of normal. Contraindications to heparin include active internal bleeding, malignant hypertension, central nervous system neoplasm, very recent surgery or significant trauma, or a history of heparin-induced thrombocytopenia. Relative contraindications include gastrointestinal bleeding or prior hemorrhagic stroke. Once heparin has been initiated, warfarin (10 mg orally) may be begun, although this is generally not administered in the ED. *Low-molecular-weight heparins (LMWHs)* have gained popularity in recent years for the treatment of DVT. These are fractionated versions of standard heparin that have a more predictable effect (and therefore do not require close monitoring) and fewer side effects or complications. Most studies comparing these with standard heparin show that LMWHs have significant advantages but higher drug costs (13). However, because they can be given subcutaneously once a day and do not require repeated blood tests, outpatient treatment of DVT is feasible and reduced hospitalization cost could more than offset the additional cost of the drug (13,19). Some health systems have protocols for discharge from the ED of selected stable patients with DVT for home LMWH therapy while transitioning to warfarin therapy. Compared to controls treated with unfractionated heparin in the inpatient setting, these outpatient protocols have demonstrated very favorable outcomes with respect to short-term (2 weeks) events such as PEs, propagation of thrombus, and minor bleeding (21).

Although occasionally recommended, there is no clear role for thrombolytic therapy in patients with isolated DVT, and the emergency physician should not initiate it independently. There is some weak evidence that thrombolytics may decrease the incidence of subsequent complications, but these are balanced by an increased rate of acute complications. Therefore, its routine use is not recommended (7).

There is controversy regarding recommended management of DVT below the knee. Historically, most of these cases have been treated conservatively, with elevation and antiinflammatory drugs. More recently, however, it has been recognized that these DVTs often propagate, and, in as many as one third of patients, eventually embolize. Therefore, it is generally recommended that these DVTs be treated in a manner similar to that for iliofemoral DVTs (14). For those patients in whom the decision is not to acutely anticoagulate, there should be close followup and serial noninvasive studies to document clot regression, generally with ultrasound.

Similarly, there has been controversy regarding the ideal treatment of *superficial thrombophlebitis* of the leg. Here, the danger of acute embolism may be less than for calf DVT but it must be confirmed that propagation to the deep system has not occurred at the time of the ED visit and, again, close followup must be arranged. Compression bandages, antiinflammatory drugs, and elevation are standard recommendations but anticoagulation should be considered in patients with a prior history of DVT (17). If the patient is an intravenous drug user or appears toxic, *septic thrombophlebitis* must be ruled out. Septic thrombophlebitis most commonly occurs at a site of intravenous (i.v.) catheter placement, and because the most common causative organism is *Staphylococcus aureus*, appropriate antibiotic therapy should be administered.

CRITICAL INTERVENTIONS

- Traditional loading doses of heparin result in inconsistent anticoagulation of many patients. Weight-based dosing is more effective
- Isolated DVT distal to the knee is not as benign as previously thought. It should be treated more like proximal DVT in terms of therapeutic aggressiveness

DISPOSITION

Historically, all patients with proximal lower extremity or upper extremity DVT required admission to the hospital. However, many institutions have now initiated protocols by which a select subset of patients (with stable symptoms, no comorbid diseases, and who are reliable) are being discharged directly home from the ED on a subcutaneous LMWH protocol with close outpatient followup. The emergency physician should not independently initiate this, other than as part of a hospital or health-care system protocol.

Conversely, the treatment of patients with DVT distal to the knee was historically similar to that of superficial thrombophlebitis. Now, with increasing concerns that these patients have risks for embolization that are only modestly lower than those patients with proximal DVT, it is recommended they be treated as those with proximal DVT, or entered into a close outpatient followup protocol.

There is one group of patients that requires a more aggressive approach, namely those patients with *phlegmasia dolens*. This condition represents a life-threatening emergency and requires admission to an intensive care unit. These patients also require vascular surgery consultation for consideration of thrombectomy when there is risk of loss of the limb without urgent intervention. Fortunately, phlegmasia dolens is very uncommon, but, in this situation, the lack of vascular surgery capability would be an indication for transport to a higher level of care.

COMMON PITFALLS

✔ Patients with a painful or swollen leg should be considered to have DVT until proven otherwise. Clinical evaluation alone is not sufficient to rule out the diagnosis

✔ The traditional physical examination findings of DVT are notoriously inaccurate. The Homan test should be abandoned, and the presence of a palpable cord should not be relied on

✔ A negative highly sensitive D-dimer test is useful only in patients with a low clinical risk of DVT. It should not be used to exclude the diagnosis in high-risk patients

✔ Although ultrasound examination is generally an excellent test for DVT, it can be operator-dependent, and there are false negatives. Patients with a very high clinical suspicion for DVT but a negative ultrasound should either undergo additional diagnostic testing or be admitted for serial evaluations

Acknowledgment

Thanks to previous edition chapter author Timothy C. Flynn.

References

1. Bounameaux H, de Moerloose P, Perrier A, et al. Plasma measurement of D-dimer as diagnostic aid in suspected venous thromboembolism. An overview. *Thromb Haemost* 1994;72:488–490.
2. Carter CJ. The natural history and epidemiology of venous thrombosis. *Prog Cardiovasc Dis* 1994;36:423–438.
3. Cogo A, Bernardi E, Prandoni P, et al. Acquired risk factors for deep-vein thrombosis in symptomatic outpatients. *Arch Intern Med* 1994;151:164–168.
4. Cronan JJ. Venous thromboembolic disease: the role of US. *Radiology* 1993;186:619–630.
5. Ellis MH, Manor Y, Witz M. Risk factors and management of patients with upper limb deep vein thrombosis. *Chest* 2000;117:43–46.
6. Ferris EJ, McCowan TC, Carver DK, et al. Percutaneous inferior vena caval filters: follow-up of seven designs in 320 patients. *Radiology* 1993;188:851–856.
7. Ginsberg JS. Management of venous thromboembolism. *N Engl J Med* 1996;335:1816–1828.
8. Hewitt G, Cromer B. Update on adolescent contraception. *Obstet Gynecol Clin North Am* 2000;27:143–162.
9. Hirsh J, Dalen JE, Deyken D, et al. Heparin: mechanism of action, pharmacokinetics, dosing considerations, monitoring, efficacy and safety. *Chest* 1992;104:337S–3351S.
10. Jorgensen JO, Hanel KC, Morgan AM, et al. The incidence of deep venous thrombosis in patients with superficial thrombophlebitis of the lower limbs. *J Vasc Surg* 1993;18:70–73.
11. Kniffin WD Jr, Baron JA, Barrett J, et al. The epidemiology of diagnosed pulmonary embolism and deep venous thrombosis in the elderly. *Arch Intern Med* 1994;154:861–866.
12. Kristo DA, Perry ME, Kollef MH. Comparison of venography, duplex imaging, and bilateral impedance plethysmography for diagnosis of lower extremity deep vein thrombosis. *South Med J* 1994;87:55–60.
13. Lensing AW, Prins MH, Davidson BL, et al. Treatment of deep venous thrombosis with low-molecular-weight heparins: a meta-analysis. *Arch Intern Med* 1995;155:601–607.
14. Lohr JM, Kerr TM, Lutter KS, et al. Lower extremity calf thrombosis: to treat or not to treat? *J Vasc Surg* 1991;14:618–623.
15. Moser KM, Fedullo PF, LitteJohn JK, et al. Frequent asymptomatic pulmonary embolism in patients with deep venous thrombosis. *JAMA* 1994;271:223–225.
16. Raschke RA, Reilly BM, Guidry JR. Weight-based heparin dosing nomogram compared with a standard care nomogram: a randomized controlled trial. *Ann Intern Med* 1993;119:874–881.
17. Schonauer V, Kryle PA, Weltermann A, et al. Superficial thrombophlebitis and risk for recurrent venous thromboembolism. *J Vasc Surg* 2003;37:834–838.
18. Shields GP, Turnipseed S, Panacek EA, Melnikoff N, Gosselin R, White RH. Validation of the Canadian probability model for acute venous thrombosis. *Acad Emerg Med* 2002;9:561–566.
19. Smith BJ, Weekley JS, Pilotto L, et al. Cost comparison of at-home treatment of deep venous thrombosis with low molecular weight heparin to inpatient treatment with unfractionated heparin. *Intern Med J* 2002;32:29–34.
20. Spritzer CE, Evans AC, Kay HH. Magnetic resonance imaging of deep venous thrombosis in pregnant women with lower extremity edema. *Obstet Gynecol* 1995;85:603–607.
21. Vinson DR, Berman DA. Outpatient treatment of deep venous thrombosis: a clinical care pathway managed by the emergency department. *Ann Emerg Med* 2001;37:251–258.
22. Wells PS, Anderson DR, Bormanis J, et al. Value of assessment of pretest probability of deep-vein thrombosis in clinical management. *Lancet* 1997;350:1795–1798.
23. White RH, Zhou H, Woo L, Mungall D. Effect of weight, sex, age, clinical diagnosis and thromboplastin reagent on steady-state intravenous heparin requirements. *Arch Intern Med* 1997;157:2468–2472.

CHAPTER 53
Complications of Vascular Grafts

Hoori Hovanessian

Vascular disease is a progressive, degenerative condition that disproportionately affects a subset of patients with other comorbid conditions such as diabetes and hypertension. When vascular disease progresses despite medical management, surgical treatment often becomes necessary. Although surgery significantly improves quality of life, it is important to realize that the underlying disease continues to progress. These patients are frequent consumers of the healthcare system whether because of early or late postoperative complications, natural progression of their disease process, or seemingly nonspecific or unrelated complaints. They pose a challenge in both diagnosis and management to even seasoned clinicians. Knowledge of the pathologic processes that affect the vascular system as well as potential accompanying postoperative complications is essential for emergency physicians.

VASCULAR GRAFTS

Vascular pathology can be subdivided into aneurysmal and occlusive diseases. Aortic aneurysm (a ballooning out of part of the wall of the aorta resulting in the formation of a sac) and aortic dissection (an intimal tear in the wall of the aorta causing blood to dissect into the wall of the aorta) are pathologic processes with potential life-threatening consequences. When an aortic aneurysm becomes symptomatic or reaches a predetermined size, aneurysm repair is undertaken with graft replacement. Conventional treatment of aortic dissection involves resection of the damaged segment of the aorta, preferably with removal of the part at which the intimal tear originates, and closure of the entrance into the false lumen. Closure of the lumen can be accomplished by placing sutures or by using biologic glue to seal the layers of the dissected part of the aortic wall. The diseased section of the aorta that is removed is replaced by a prosthetic graft.

Patients with occlusive disease of the vasculature may undergo extraanatomic and infrainguinal procedures. Extraanatomic bypasses are performed in patients with complications following aortoiliac surgery or in patients with intraabdominal infections or high-risk comorbidities (2). Extraanatomic procedures include femoral–femoral, axillofemoral (or bifemoral), and iliofemoral bypasses. Prosthetic grafts are preferred in extraanatomic reconstruction. Infrainguinal arterial occlusive disease can affect the femoral, popliteal, or tibial arteries. Autogenous veins are used in below-the-knee reconstructions. Both autogenous and prosthetic grafts are used in above-the-knee repairs (2). Polytetrafluoroethylene (PTFE) is the most commonly used synthetic graft. Tissue can grow through the interstices of the graft, incorporating the graft into tissue. This theoretically decreases the chance of thrombosis and infection.

Endovascular repair of aortic aneurysms and dissection is a newer, less invasive approach to the management of these diseases in selected patients. Endovascular repair has been making steady gains in popularity over the last decade. This method allows for transfemoral placement of stent grafts over a catheter or guidewire. Placement of an endovascular graft can completely obliterate the site of leakage into the aneurysm. Placement of stent-grafts in aortic dissection closes the intimal tear (site of entry into the false lumen), allows for thrombosis of the false lumen, and helps eliminate obstruction of branch vessels caused by the dissection.

Endovascular grafts have been used to treat a variety of vascular pathologies, including abdominal aortic aneurysms, thoracic aortic aneurysms, iliac artery aneurysms, and occlusive disease, with promising short-term and mid-term results.

DIALYSIS ACCESS GRAFTS

Adequate and reliable long-term access to the circulatory system is crucial in the management of chronic renal failure patients who require dialysis. Such access (dialysis shunts) can be obtained through the formation of an *arteriovenous fistula (AVF)*, whereby an artery and vein are anastomosed. Alternatively, a *prosthetic graft* can be used to join an artery and vein. AVFs are currently preferred over prosthetic grafts because of their lower complication rates (less potential for thrombosis and lower infection rate). Prosthetic grafts may be the only option for patients with failed AVFs, those with poor peripheral veins, or for patients in whom dialysis will become necessary before an AVF has time to mature.

GRAFT COMPLICATIONS

The complications of vascular grafts range in presentation from relatively straightforward to subtle and complex. They can be divided into the following categories:

1. Stenosis, thrombosis and occlusion
2. Infection
3. Erosion into contiguous structures with fistulization
4. Pseudoaneurysm formation
5. Hemodynamic complications (vascular access grafts)
6. Complications associated with endovascular grafts

CLINICAL PRESENTATION

Stenosis, Thrombosis and Occlusion

There is a 12% to 80% rate of graft failure within 5 years depending on the procedure as well as graft characteristics (2). Early failure of vein grafts (within the first 30 days) generally indicates a technical problem such as a kink or twist within the graft or incompletely lysed valves when autogenous grafts are used. Failures occurring 30 days to 2 years postoperatively are usually a result of intimal hyperplasia at the anastomotic sites. Failures that occur beyond 2 years are generally a result of progressive atherosclerosis (2).

Graft thrombosis may result in a relatively sudden return of the patient's previous symptoms. These may include claudication or ischemic rest pain that is localized to the forefoot. Pain caused by arterial insufficiency is usually severe unless it is masked by neuropathy. Signs may include skin breakdown with the formation of nonhealing ulcers. Such ulcers may also form between adjacent toes as a result of mild friction. Superinfection of these ulcers as well as osteomyelitis is a well-documented resultant complication. Painful toes that have a cyanotic appearance are suggestive of microemboli.

Dialysis access graft thrombosis is common despite the fact that heparin is used routinely during dialysis and despite the increased bleeding tendency in uremic patients. Complication-free graft use of 51% at 2 years and 39% at 3 years has been reported with PTFE grafts (5). Thrombosis and occlusion occur secondary to intimal hyperplasia. Thrombosis and occlusion can be accelerated by hypotension, dehydration, and by excess pressure applied to the graft site either because of occlusive bandages or perigraft hematomas. Patients may complain of a sensation of coldness, tingling, or numbness and weakness to the involved extremity.

Infection

The incidence of infection after arterial reconstructive surgery with the use of synthetic grafts ranges from 1% (aortic and iliac artery repair) to as high as 5% (in situations where the graft is placed in the inguinal area) (9). Infection is a significant problem in patients with prosthetic dialysis access grafts with the incidence approaching 11% to 20% (3). The incidence of infection is higher in patients with similar grafts who have acquired immunodeficiency syndrome (AIDS) or in those with a history of intravenous drug abuse.

Intraoperative contamination is likely the most common mechanism for early graft infection. Spread of pathogens from contiguous infected or colonized tissue may explain the relatively higher rate of infection in the groin. Other mechanisms contributing to graft infection include hematogenous spread of microorganisms as well as erosion of the graft into contiguous bowel lumen, resulting in direct graft contamination.

Patients with graft infections may present with frank sepsis, with an infected wound, or with cellulitic changes adjacent to the involved graft. More subtle presentations may include low-grade fever, vague abdominal discomfort, or malaise. Still more complicated presentations may include bleeding, evidence of distal emboli, or the presence of an abdominal mass as a consequence of a false aneurysm. Graft infection can also contribute to graft thrombosis, therefore, graft infection should be in the differential diagnosis when patients present with signs and symptoms that are more traditionally associated with graft thrombosis.

Erosions into Contiguous Structures with Fistulization

Erosions of the prosthetic graft into the bowel can result in the formation of an aortoenteric fistula (AEF). Most commonly these occur between an aortic prosthetic graft and the distal duodenum. However, such fistulization has been reported after aortoiliac and aortofemoral procedures as well as after renal vascular graft placement. Fistulization to the bowel at sites other than the duodenum may also occur. Mechanical trauma, prosthetic graft or perigraft infection, and pressure necrosis all contribute to fistulization.

The time-frame for AEF development is wide. Fistulization may occur several days to many years after the initial surgery (4). Clinical presentation is commonly that of gastrointestinal bleeding: hematemesis, hematochezia, melena, or occult blood loss. Patients may present with self-limited herald bleeding several hours to days before exsanguinating hemorrhage ensues. Some patients may have nonspecific symptoms of back or abdominal pain. Because fistulization may be secondary to graft infection, other signs and symptoms may include fatigue and malaise, low-grade fevers, and leukocytosis.

Pseudoaneurysms

Disruption of the suture line (dehiscence) at the site of an anastomotic junction may give rise to a false aneurysm (pseudoaneurysm). False aneurysms most commonly occur in femoral artery graft anastomoses. Leaking blood is contained by the adjoining tissues as well as by fibrous scar formation. Infection is an important cause of pseudoaneurysm formation.

Patients with pseudoaneurysms may complain of pain in the groin, back, or abdomen. They may harbor a pulsatile mass in these locations. Other presentations may include hemorrhage (ranging from occult to life-threatening) caused by rupture of the false aneurysm or signs and symptoms associated with distal emboli. False aneurysms occur most commonly in the groin.

Repeated needle puncture for dialysis access can weaken the vessel wall, thereby leading to aneurysm formation. Pseudoaneurysms can form when the graft material is lacerated with the dialysis needle. In both cases, a pulsatile mass may be present. Pseudoaneurysms will expand and eventually rupture, resulting in a potentially significant degree of hemorrhage. Pseudoaneurysm expansion can also threaten the viability of the overlying skin, thereby exposing the underlying graft to infection.

Hemodynamic Complications (Vascular Access Grafts)

Patients with borderline cardiac reserve and an excessive flow rate through their shunt (greater than 500 mL/minute) may exhibit signs and symptoms of congestive heart failure (7). An arterial steal syndrome with resultant distal ischemia may occur in patients with shunts. The incidence is somewhat higher in patients with proximal than those with distal access sites. The steal syndrome occurs when the blood flows from the artery into the low-resistance vein with less arterial blood available distal to the site of the shunt (7). An alternate complication can occur with high-pressure arterial flow into the low-pressure venous system: venous hypertension distal to the shunt ensues with swelling of the distal tissue and eventual skin induration and hyperpigmentation (7). Shunt repair may be necessary if the steal syndrome and venous hypertension cause clinical symptoms.

Neurovascular problems associated with vascular access include pain, weakness, muscle atrophy, and paresthesias. These hemodynamic and neurovascular complications are more problematic with fistulas but do occur with prosthetic grafts as well.

Complications Associated with Endovascular Grafts

Given that endovascular repair is a new technique, data on long-term complication rates are sparse. However, some short-term and mid-term complications have been delineated: Limb complications such as ischemia or occlusion may require subsequent extraanatomic (femoral–femoral) bypass, thrombectomy and angioplasty, or thrombolysis. These complications may occur intraoperatively (during endovascular graft placement) or as late as 490 days postprocedure in one study of mid-term results of patients undergoing endovascular aortic aneurysm repair (14). These complications are a result of vascular trauma as well as underlying peripheral vascular disease, which many of these patients harbor. Endoleaks, which complicate 10% to 20% of repairs, are defined as incomplete exclusion of the aneurysm with persistent leakage of blood into the aneurysmal sac (13). This can potentially result in enlargement of the sac and/or increased pressure in the sac, ultimately leading to aneurysmal rupture. Several types of endoleaks have been defined including those that occur at the site of attachment of the graft to the aorta (from

incomplete seal of the endograft) or through the stent graft itself (via a tear or fracture) (12). Other potential complications include distal embolization, graft occlusion, kinking, migration or prolapse into the aneurysm, and infection. Migration of the stent-graft may present as an endoleak. Stent-graft erosion into the esophagus has also been reported (6).

DIFFERENTIAL DIAGNOSIS

Because the signs and symptoms associated with vascular graft complications can be either vague and nonspecific or can overlap with other more common medical problems, the differential diagnosis is vast. Limb weakness may result from a cerebrovascular accident or a nerve compression syndrome. In patients with fever or a septic appearance, other sources of infection should be evaluated. Embolic events may be caused by atrial fibrillation. Gastrointestinal bleeding will require extensive evaluation to rule out sources that are much more common than an aortoenteric fistula. Complaints of back and abdominal pain should prompt standard evaluation for these complaints in addition to evaluation for possible graft complications.

In general, although other causes of abdominal pain, gastrointestinal hemorrhage, fever, and weakness are much more common, in a patient with a history of a vascular graft, the graft should be thoroughly evaluated as the potential cause for the patient's symptoms.

EMERGENCY DEPARTMENT EVALUATION

Stenosis, Thrombosis, and Occlusion

Examination of distal pulses via palpation and Doppler is mandatory. Neurosensory examination is less useful in patients with neuropathy, but should be attempted. Skin temperature and the color of the affected limb should also be evaluated. The limb may become pale on elevation with a dusky or cyanotic rubor with dependency. Findings in the affected extremity should be compared to findings on the contralateral side. An ankle-brachial index (ABI) measurement can also provide important information. The technique and interpretation are described in Chapter 51, "Peripheral Arterial Disease." If the patient's old chart is available, comparison of the current ABI with previous ABIs will be important. A loss of a previously palpable pulse or a change of 0.15 from a previous ABI requires further evaluation with duplex ultrasonography or angiography. Finally, low cardiac output (hypovolemic or cardiogenic) may enhance thrombosis and accelerate occlusion resulting in acute limb ischemia. The patient needs to be evaluated for evidence of intravascular fluid depletion (blood loss, dehydration, and sepsis) or cardiac insufficiency (myocardial infarction or decompensated congestive heart failure).

Infection

Because graft infection can be the causative factor of graft thrombosis, aortoenteric fistula, and false aneurysm formation, it is necessary to exclude infection when evaluating a patient for any type of graft complication. The most common causative organism of graft infection is Staphylococcus aureus. Other implicated agents include coagulase-negative staphylococci, enterococci, Pseudomonas aeruginosa, Enterobacteriaceae, and Bacteroides species. Polymicrobial infections occur in 12% to 37% of patients (9). Blood cultures should be obtained, although they may be negative because the infection does not involve the graft lumen. CT scanning may reveal perigraft inflammation or fluid collection, or air adjacent to the graft. In the case of grafts that are located close to the skin, the diagnosis is relatively easy in the presence of cellulitic changes, fluctuance, or obvious drainage of pus from the vicinity of the graft site. However, local signs of infection may be absent initially. Patients may present with fever of unclear etiology or with nonspecific malaise and fatigue. Graft infection should be considered in any febrile patient, even in the absence of any local findings. Finally, occult infection may be present in old, nonfunctioning dialysis access grafts. The graft may have become seeded from a previous episode of bacteremia or may have become directly inoculated from needle puncture at the time the graft was in use. This source of potential infection should be considered in dialysis as well as in renal transplantation patients with fever of unclear etiology (1,11). The diagnosis can be established on an inpatient basis by using indium-111 scanning, which has a greater than 90% sensitivity and specificity when used in the evaluation of vascular graft infection (1).

Erosions into Contiguous Structures with Fistulization

AEF should be considered in any patient with gastrointestinal bleeding and a history of aortic repair with graft placement. In the stable patient, workup for other sources of bleeding should be initiated, as other sources of bleeding are more common than bleeding through an AEF. Endoscopy (upper and lower) is important primarily in evaluating other, more common causes of gastrointestinal bleeding. If endoscopy does not yield a clearcut answer, abdominal CT with oral and intravenous (i.v.) contrast should be obtained to evaluate for inflammatory changes around the anastomotic sites (4,10).

Pseudoaneurysms

A high index of clinical suspicion is needed to make this diagnosis. The clinical suspicion can then be further evaluated via duplex ultrasound, computed tomography (CT), or magnetic resonance imaging (MRI). By using ultrasonography, a skilled operator can gauge the size of the pseudoaneurysm, and determine the presence of any hematoma and the status of the surrounding vasculature. In situations in which other methods of evaluation are inconclusive or not feasible, angiography is an alternate option.

EMERGENCY DEPARTMENT MANAGEMENT

Stenosis, Thrombosis, and Occlusion

The patient's fluid status should be optimized if this is found to be a factor contributing to his or her symptoms. Heparinization to prevent further thrombosis should be counterbalanced against the timing of angiography and the possible use of thrombolytic agents. This decision will obviously need to be made in conjunction with the vascular surgeon, so surgical consultation should be obtained early.

Infection

As with graft thrombosis, the patient's fluid status should be evaluated and optimized to prevent accelerated graft thrombosis and occlusion secondary to poor perfusion through the graft site. Emergency department incision and drainage of suspected abscesses in the vicinity of a graft should not be attempted as it can result in catastrophic hemorrhage. Empiric antibiotic ther-

apy should be initiated in the emergency department. Definitive treatment consists of surgical excision of the infected graft as well as debridement of the surrounding infected tissues. Four to 6 weeks of antibiotic therapy, guided by results obtained from culture of the infected tissue at surgery, should follow the surgical repair (9).

In suspected infections of vascular access grafts, broad-spectrum antibiotic therapy should be initiated pending blood culture results, even though *S. aureus* is the most common culprit in vascular access infections. Although some investigators recommend the empiric use of vancomycin and aminoglycosides owing to convenience in the dosage schedule, others caution against indiscriminate use of these drugs given the significant numbers of negative blood cultures as well as the emergence of vancomycin-resistant organisms (3,8).

Erosions into Contiguous Structures with Fistulization

Unstable patients with suspected AEF require emergency laparotomy to control the bleeding. Diagnostic studies in these patients should be limited to the essential minimum. Studies should include a complete blood count, type and cross, coagulation factors, electrolytes, blood urea nitrogen (BUN), creatinine, and glucose. The patient's hemodynamic status should be evaluated and blood loss replaced prior to surgery. Even in stable patients with an AEF, surgical consultation should be obtained early as the treatment is invariably surgical.

Occasionally, grafts erode through the skin. These grafts should be considered infected. The patient should receive antibiotics, and a vascular surgeon should be consulted for urgent repair.

Pseudoaneurysms

Surgical consultation is essential, although other management options such as thrombin injection and embolization procedures are currently being evaluated. In addition, antibiotics should be considered if the pseudoaneurysm is thought to have an infectious etiology. Treatment of vascular access graft aneurysms and pseudoaneurysms involves surgical repair.

CRITICAL INTERVENTIONS

- The patient's hemodynamic status should be evaluated and fluid losses should be replenished
- In patients with massive gastrointestinal hemorrhage and the presence of an intraabdominal graft, emergent vascular consultation should be obtained and the patient readied for surgery expeditiously
- Empiric antibiotic therapy should be initiated in any febrile or septic-appearing patient with a fever of unknown etiology and the presence of a vascular graft (functional or nonfunctional)

DISPOSITION

Graft complications will need surgical consultation and management in a hospital setting. After diagnosis and initial management measures such as the initiation of antibiotic therapy and replenishment of fluid and blood losses are undertaken, stable patients should be admitted and managed by a vascular surgeon. Unstable patients will require a more focused and expedited workup prior to emergent surgical intervention.

Should patients with suspected endovascular graft–associated complications present to the emergency department, diagnostic and management decisions should ideally be made in conjunction with a vascular surgeon as well as an interventional radiologist skilled in these relatively novel procedures.

COMMON PITFALLS

✔ Failure to consider graft thrombosis when a patient with a vascular graft has a recurrence of claudication, rest pain, skin breakdown, or nonhealing ulcers

✔ Failure to exclude infection when evaluating patients for any type of graft complication

✔ Failure to evaluate the ABI and compare it to previously obtained values

✔ Failure to consider AEF in any patient with gastrointestinal bleeding and a history of aortic repair

✔ Failure to consider a false aneurysm in patients with a history of vascular repair and complaints of abdominal or groin pain, hemorrhage, or pulsatile mass

✔ Failure to appreciate that low flow states may contribute to vascular access site thrombosis

Acknowledgment

Thanks to previous edition chapter author Timothy C. Flynn.

References

1. Ayus JC, Sheikh-Hamad D. Silent infection in clotted hemodialysis access grafts. *J Am Soc Nephrol* 1998;9:1314–1317.
2. Belkin M, Whittemore AD, Donaldson MC, et al.Peripheral arterial occlusive disease. In: Townsend CM, ed. *Townsend: Sabiston Textbook of Surgery*, 16th ed. Philadelphia: WB Saunders, 2001:1373–1402.
3. Cheung AH, Wong LM. Surgical infections in patients with chronic renal failure. *Infect Dis Clin North Am* 2001;15:775–796.
4. Christodoulou D, Tang S, Ottaway C. GI hemorrhage caused by renal vascular graft-enteric fistula: case report and review. *Gastrointest Endosc* 2003;58:137–139.
5. Feldman HI, Kobrin S, Wasserstein A. Hemodialysis vascular access morbidity. *J Am Soc Nephrol* 1996;7:523–535.
6. Gowda RM, Misra D, Tranbaugh RF, et al. Endovascular stent grafting of descending thoracic aortic aneurysms. *Chest* 2003;124:714–719.
7. Haisch CE, Atkinson CK.Access and Ports. In: Townsend CM, ed. *Townsend: Sabiston Textbook of Surgery*, 16th ed. Philadelphia: WB Saunders, 2001:1453–1459.
8. Ifudu O. Care of patients undergoing hemodialysis. *N Engl J Med* 1998; 339:1054–1062.
9. Karchmer AD.Infections of prosthetic valves and intravascular devices. In: Mandell GL, Bennet JE, Dolin R, eds. *Mandell: Principles and practice of infectious diseases*, 5th ed. Philadelphia: Churchill Livingstone, 2000:913–915.
10. Kovacs TO. Recent advances in the endoscopic diagnosis and therapy of upper gastrointestinal, small intestinal, and colonic bleeding. *Med Clin North Am* 2002;86:1319–1356.
11. Nassar GM, Ayus, JC. Infectious complications of old nonfunctioning arteriovenous grafts in renal transplant recipients: a case series. *Am J Kidney Dis* 2002;40:832–836.
12. Ouriel K. Endovascular therapies: an update on aortic aneurysm repair and carotid endarterectomy. *J Am Coll Surg* 2002;195:549–552.
13. Powell JT, Greenhalgh RM. Small abdominal aortic aneurysms. *N Engl J Med* 2003;348:1895–1901.
14. Tonnessen BH, Conners MS, Sternbergh WC III, et al. Mid-term results of patients undergoing endovascular aortic aneurysm repair. *Am J Surgery* 2002;184:561–566.

CHAPTER 54
Venous Gas Embolism

Christopher H. Linden

Venous gas embolism may occur whenever the integrity of a vein is violated and its lumen is exposed to air or any gas (e.g., carbon dioxide, helium, or oxygen). A pressure gradient is also required. Gas may be forced into an open vein by positive external pressure, it may be drawn in by negative intravascular pressure, or it may passively enter any open vein (e.g., in a surgical field or traumatic injury) above the level of the heart. Inspiration, which augments venous return and decreases central venous pressure, facilitates aspiration of air into exposed veins, particularly central ones.

Small venous air emboli (a few milliliters) are common during intravenous infusion but are clinically insignificant. They are frequently unrecognized or ignored and are rarely reported. Significant amounts of air may sometimes enter a vein during gravity infusion as a result of tubing defects, an obstructed filter, or the presence of air in a collapsible infusion bag (10). Large air emboli are rare but quickly fatal, and they often remain undiagnosed until autopsy (17,19,20,24,25). Estimates of the fatal volume range from 100 to 500 mL, depending on the rate of infusion and underlying disease. Slow infusions are better tolerated than rapid ones. Emboli of intermediate size result in significant respiratory, cardiovascular, and neurologic dysfunction. Because signs and symptoms are nonspecific, knowledge of the clinical settings in which venous air embolism may occur will aid in the proper diagnosis.

Physiologically significant venous air emboli are most commonly reported after surgical procedures such as craniotomy (particularly posterior fossa surgery), sinus and neck surgery, central venous or pulmonary artery catheterization, cervical laminectomy, hemodialysis, lung biopsy, cardiothoracic and hepatic surgery, invasive cardiopulmonary support procedures, hip and shoulder arthroplasty, thoracentesis, thyroidectomy, and tracheostomy (6,8,17,19–21,24,25). The sitting (Fowler) position and the noncollapsibility of intracranial veins account for the relatively high incidence during craniotomy. Air may be rapidly aspirated into cervical or thoracic veins via central venous catheters that become disconnected, particularly when the patient assumes an upright position or inspires (6,22). Central venous catheter air emboli may be prevented by Trendelenburg positioning, Valsalva maneuver, covering the catheter hub with a finger during placement, and securing the catheter and its connections with sutures or tape. Because air embolism can also enter through the catheter tract, applying pressure to the venipuncture site after catheter removal is also important.

Blunt or penetrating chest trauma with concomitant airway and venous disruption may result in either insidious or acute air embolism (8,11,19–21,24,25). The same is true when veins of the head or neck are exposed to air as a result of blunt or penetrating head trauma and penetrating neck trauma (1,8,19–21,24,25). With head trauma, air can enter the venous circulation via open skull fractures, basilar fractures crossing the cavernous sinus, and those involving dural venous (petrosal, sigmoid, sphenoparietal, or transverse) sinuses and paranasal air (usually ethmoid) sinuses.

Serious emboli may also occur as a complication of any diagnostic or therapeutic procedure that uses air or another gas under pressure. Examples include pneumoarthrography, pneumoencephalography, pneumourethrocystography, presacral or retroperitoneal pneumography, Rubin test (vaginal insufflation), nasal sinus irrigation, positive-pressure ventilation, pressurized intravenous infusions, spinal epidural catheterization (using air rather than liquid as a guide to catheter placement), gas-cooled laser surgery, laparoscopy, wound irrigation with hydrogen peroxide (which generates oxygen), vacuum abortion with accidental reversal (i.e., pressurization) of the suction catheter, and improper ventilation of a phlebotomy collection bottle (3,8,17,19–21,24,25). Embolization of air to vertebral veins, an unusual form of venous air embolism, is a rare complication of epidural catheter placement and diagnostic or therapeutic endoscopy of the upper or lower gastrointestinal tract (in patients with preexisting or iatrogenic bowel perforation) (4).

In the nonmedical setting, pressure-induced gas embolism may result from attempted criminal abortion, vaginal douching, insufflation of the vagina during cunnilingus (in pregnant women), recreational inhalation of helium or nitrous oxide from pressurized tanks, and the self-injection (usually suicidal) of air into the scrotum, urethra, or a peripheral vein (5,10,17,19–21,24,25). Attempted suicide by blowing air into a heparin lock has also been reported.

Venous gas embolism results in gas-bubble obstruction of the right ventricular pulmonary outflow tract and consequent pulmonary vasoconstriction, pulmonary hypertension, hypoxemia, systemic hypotension, and arterial ischemia (9,13,15,16,19–21,24,25). The whipping or churning of blood and gas by ventricular contractions also causes platelet and red blood cell aggregation and fibrin and fat globule formation, with deposition in, and obstruction of, pulmonary arterioles. Secondary effects include decreased lung compliance, increased airway resistance, ventilation–perfusion mismatching, and pulmonary edema leading to additional hypoxia and hemodynamic compromise. A systemic inflammatory response can also occur. In patients with atrial or ventricular septal defects, paradoxical embolization of venous gas to the left side of the heart may result in gas-bubble occlusion of the arterial circulation, with symptoms identical to those of direct arterial gas embolism (see Chapter 354, High-Altitude Illness). Although pulmonary capillaries effectively filter small or slowly infused volumes of gas, large boluses can overwhelm the filtering capacity of the lung or reach the arterial circulation through pulmonary arteriovenous anastomoses, thereby leading to paradoxical embolization in the absence of demonstrable intracardiac shunts.

CLINICAL PRESENTATION

Patients with large venous gas emboli that develop over a short period often experience sudden dyspnea or gasping, chest pain, loss of consciousness, and cardiovascular collapse. In severe cases, there may be an immediate cardiac arrest (5,9,11,17,19–21,24,25). Cyanosis, wheezing, rales, hypotension, coma, tachycardia, hemoptysis, and tachypnea are typical physical findings. Auscultation of the heart may reveal a characteristic loud churning sound or "millwheel" murmur. This coarse, continuous (systolic and diastolic), metallic or machine-like murmur is transient and may be preceded or followed by tympanic, resonant, or drum-like valvular sounds, gallop rhythms, and a softer systolic murmur. Jugular venous distention may be present.

Patients with smaller gas emboli may complain of faintness, dizziness, shortness of breath, weakness, palpitations, and chest pain. Lesser degrees of hypotension, tachycardia, tachypnea, and central nervous system dysfunction (e.g., anxiety and confusion) may be noted on physical examination. Abnormal cardiopulmonary findings and increased central venous pressure may sometimes be present. Manifestations of vertebral air emboli include numbness, sensory deficits, weakness, and loss of sphincter control and tone below the level of spinal cord involvement. In paradoxical embolization, the patient may present with manifestations of cerebral, cardiac, limb, or intraabdominal organ ischemia or infarction (see Chapter 354) as well as signs and symptoms of venous gas embolism.

DIFFERENTIAL DIAGNOSIS

Venous air embolism should be suspected in any patient who develops acute respiratory, neurologic, or cardiovascular decompensation following a diagnostic, therapeutic, or traumatic event involving the insufflation or use of pressurized air or other gas or potential venous disruption with a communication with an external or internal gaseous atmosphere. It is most often confused with pulmonary thromboembolism and acute myocardial infarction. Without prior monitoring, the clinical setting and characteristic murmur are the primary diagnostic clues. In pregnant patients, amniotic fluid embolism should also be considered in the differential diagnosis (7). Signs and symptoms are similar, but amniotic fluid embolism occurs almost exclusively at or about the time of delivery and is usually associated with a coagulopathy.

In patients with multiple trauma, conditions such as hemothorax, pneumothorax, hypovolemia, cardiac tamponade, tracheobronchial disruption, and aortic transection are more common causes of cardiovascular collapse. Fat embolism should also be considered. Hemoptysis and unexpected deterioration or arrest, especially if occurring immediately after intubation and positive-pressure ventilation in a patient with lung trauma, are suggestive of venous air embolism.

Paradoxical arterial embolization and venous air embolism alone both cause central nervous system and cardiac dysfunction. Although headache, seizures, respiratory arrest, focal neurological signs and symptoms, and focal myocardial ischemia or infarction on electrocardiogram suggest paradoxical embolization, focal abnormalities can also result from venous air embolism in patients with underlying cerebrovascular and coronary artery disease. Signs and symptoms of vertebral air embolism are similar to those of spinal cord ischemia, infarction, and trauma.

EMERGENCY DEPARTMENT EVALUATION

The history should include details of the precipitant circumstances and the nature and timing of symptoms. If known, the site and volume of air or other gas involved should be documented. The physical examination should focus on the vital signs and the cardiovascular, neurologic, and respiratory status, paying particular attention to cardiac auscultation for murmurs and abnormal heart sounds. Although the correct diagnosis is usually suggested by the clinical setting, it should be confirmed by ancillary testing and radiographic imaging.

Ancillary evaluation of patients with suspected venous air embolism should include arterial blood gas measurements, cardiac monitoring, a 12-lead electrocardiogram, and a chest radiograph. Hypoxemia, metabolic acidosis, and an increased or decreased $PaCO_2$ may be noted on arterial blood gas analysis. If continuously monitored, the end-expiratory CO_2 concentration (a reflection of the alveolar PCO_2) will show an abrupt decrease. Thrombocytopenia is relatively common but disseminated intravascular coagulation is rare. The electrocardiogram may reveal evidence of ischemia (e.g., right ventricular ST-T wave changes), dysrhythmias, or acute cor pulmonale (e.g., right axis deviation, P pulmonale, and right bundle-branch block).

In patients with esophageal or precordial Doppler ultrasound monitoring during surgery, an abrupt change in heart sounds may be noted when air enters the right ventricle (24). The chest radiograph may show pulmonary edema without cardiomegaly (12,14). Rarely, it may show intracardiac or pulmonary arterial air and thus confirm the diagnosis (14). Air in the heart, or pulmonary and coronary arteries, or vertebral veins can sometimes be seen on CT.

In stable patients, transesophageal echocardiography should also be performed. Transesophageal echocardiography is the most sensitive test for visualizing intracardiac air (24). Inferior wall akinesis on echocardiography is suggestive but not diagnostic of venous air embolism. The sensitivity of transthoracic echocardiography is unknown. All reports to date involve the transesophageal approach. Central venous, intracardiac, and pulmonary artery pressures may be elevated. Aspiration of air from a central venous, right atrial, right ventricular, or pulmonary artery catheter also confirms the diagnosis (13,16,19–21,23–25).

In unstable patients, a central venous or, preferably, a right-sided heart (Swan-Ganz) catheter should be inserted and aspiration of air should be attempted, both for diagnostic and therapeutic purposes. Measurement of the end-expiratory CO_2 concentration and evaluation of heart sounds by Doppler flow-meter are useful only if baseline parameters are known. Patients with suspected vertebral air embolism should have CT or MRI imaging of the spinal cord at the level involved. The absence of air does not exclude air embolism because small amounts of air may not be visible. In some cases, angiography may be necessary to clarify the diagnosis. Because spontaneous thrombolysis occurs more slowly than the dissipation of gas, the absence of thrombus supports a diagnosis of air embolism even if air is not visualized.

EMERGENCY DEPARTMENT MANAGEMENT

Advanced life-support measures should be instituted as necessary. Initial treatment should include prevention of further air embolization by manually sealing, if possible, the portal of air entry and termination of any insufflation procedure. When venous air embolism occurs during surgery, the surgical field should be flooded with saline (24). If possible, the patient should be positioned so that the surgical field is below the level of the right atrium. All patients should be given 100% oxygen to hasten the absorption of embolized air. Because air is 80% nitrogen, decreasing the partial pressure of nitrogen in the blood by giving oxygen will result in the diffusion of nitrogen from the embolus into the blood, thereby decreasing the size of the air bubble (8,19–21,24,25). Conversely, nitrous oxide diffuses into and increases the size of air bubbles. Hence, the inhalation of nitrous oxide, if used for anesthesia, should be discontinued (18,21,24). If vital signs remain or become stable, supportive care is all that is necessary. Small amounts of air will eventually dissolve in the blood.

Unstable patients should be placed in a head-down (Trendelenburg) or head-down, left lateral (Durant) position so that the air present in the heart can be displaced from the pulmonary outflow tracts and rise toward the apex (2,6,8,17,19–21,24,25). Closed-chest cardiac massage may be effective in forcing air out of pulmonary arteries and into smaller vessels. In patients with profound shock or cardiac arrest due to nontraumatic venous air embolism, transthoracic aspiration of air from the heart may be lifesaving (8,17,19–21,24,25). To accomplish a right ventricular puncture, an 18-gauge, 3.5-in or larger needle, with or without a catheter, is inserted into the fourth or fifth intercostal space at the left sternal border perpendicular to the chest wall. Alternatively,

the needle can be inserted just to the left of the xiphoid process and directed toward the inferior tip of the left scapula. Because transthoracic cardiac puncture may result in coronary artery or myocardial laceration and pericardial tamponade, the preferred treatment for patients who are not in extremis is transvenous aspiration of the air embolus. This is performed through a central venous or Swan-Ganz catheter, with the catheter tip placed at the junction of the superior vena cava and right atrium (2,16,19–21,22–25). When blunt or penetrating chest trauma is the underlying etiology, thoracotomy is indicated. Hilar cross-clamping is performed for initial control of bronchovenous communications. Intubation of the right or left mainstem bronchus and ventilation of the uninvolved lung can reduce the flow of air into the venous circulation, facilitate resuscitation, and obviate the need for thoracotomy in some trauma patients (11).

The management of patients with paradoxical (arterial) gas embolism is described in Chapter 354. The use of hyperbaric oxygen therapy in the treatment of venous gas embolism without paradoxical arterial embolization has not been reported. It might be of value in patients with vertebral air embolism who fail to improve with supportive care.

CRITICAL INTERVENTIONS

- Prevent further entry of air by sealing the site of entry, stopping insufflation, or flooding the surgical field with saline
- Place the patient in a head-down, left lateral decubitus position, and give 100% oxygen
- In unstable patients, perform right ventricular cardiac puncture or insert a central venous or pulmonary artery catheter and aspirate for gas

DISPOSITION

Symptomatic patients with documented or suspected venous air embolism should be admitted. The level of care should be based on the degree of hemodynamic compromise and respiratory dysfunction. Depending on the circumstances, consultation with a cardiothoracic or trauma surgeon or a hyperbaric medicine specialist may be indicated. In patients who survive the acute event, the long-term outcome depends on the degree of anoxic injury and associated illnesses or trauma.

COMMON PITFALLS

✔ Failure to consider venous air embolism as a cause of acute hemodynamic, respiratory, or neurological decompensation
✔ Failure to recognize that venous air embolism is a complication of head, neck, and chest trauma and of many diagnostic and therapeutic procedures
✔ Failure to recognize and follow measures designed to avoid iatrogenic air embolism
✔ Failure to consider and to treat concomitant arterial embolization (paradoxical embolization)

References

1. Adams VI, Hirsch CS. Venous air embolism from head and neck wounds. *Arch Pathol Lab Med* 1989;113:498.
2. Alvaran SB, Toung JK, Graff TE, et al. Venous air embolism: comparative merits of external massage, intracardiac aspiration and left lateral decubitus position. *Anesth Analg* 1978;57:166.
3. Banagale RC. Massive intracranial air embolism: a complication of mechanical ventilation. *Am J Dis Child* 1980;134:799.
4. Chorost MI, Wu JT, Webb H, et al. Vertebral venous air embolism: an unusual complication following colonoscopy. *Dis Colon Rectum* 2003;46:1138.

5. Doostan DK, Steffenson SL, Snoey ER. Cerebral and coronary air embolism: an intradepartmental suicide attempt. *J Emerg Med* 2003;25:20.

6. Feliciano DV, Mattox KL, Graham JM, et al. Major complications of percutaneous subclavian vein catheters. *Am J Surg* 1974;138:869.

7. Gei AF, Vadhera RB, Hankins GD. Embolism during pregnancy: thrombus, air, and amniotic fluid. *Anesthesiol Clin North Am* 2003;21:165.

8. Gottlieb JD, Ericsson JA, Sweet RS. Venous air embolism: a review. *Anesth Analg* 1965;44:773.

9. Hartveit F, Lystad H, Minken A. The pathology of venous air embolism. *Br J Exp Pathol* 1968;49:81.

10. Hill BF, Jones JS. Venous air embolism following orogenital sex during pregnancy. *Am J Emerg Med* 1993;11:155.

11. Ho AM-H, Ling E. Systemic air embolism after lung trauma. *Anesthesiology* 1999;90:564.

12. Ishak BA, Seleny FL, Noah ZL. Venous air embolism: a possible cause of acute pulmonary edema. *Anesthesiology* 1976;45:453.

13. Khan MA, Alkalay I, Suetsugu S, et al. Acute changes in lung mechanics following pulmonary emboli of various gases in dogs. *J Appl Physiol* 1972;33:774.

14. Kizer KW, Goodman PC. Radiographic manifestations of venous air embolism. *Radiology* 1989;144:35.

15. Liu FC, Tsao CM, Lui PW: Hemodynamic changes caused by venous gas embolism in dogs: comparisons among air, carbon dioxide, and oxygen. *Acta Anaesthesiol Sin* 2001;39:71.

16. Marshall WK, Bedford RF. Use of a pulmonary artery catheter for detection and treatment of venous air embolism. *Anesthesiology* 1980;52:131.

17. Michenfelder JD. Air embolism. In: Orkin FK, Cooperman LH, eds. *Complications in anesthesiology*. Philadelphia: JB Lippincott Co, 1982:268.

18. Munson ES. Effect of nitrous oxide on the pulmonary circulation during venous air embolism. *Anesth Analg* 1971;50:785.

19. Muth C. Gas Embolism. *N Engl J Med* 2000;342:476.

20. O'Quin RJ, Lakshminarayan S. Venous air embolism. *Arch Intern Med* 1982;142:2173.

21. Orebaugh SL. Venous air embolism: clinical and experimental considerations. *Crit Care Med* 1992;20:1169.

22. Roberts S, Johnson M, Davies S. Near-fatal air embolism: fibrin sheath as the portal of air entry. *South Med J* 2003;96:1036.

23. Sink JD, Corner PB, James PM, et al. Evaluation of catheter placement in the treatment of venous air embolism. *Ann Surg* 1976;183:58.

24. Souders JE. Pulmonary air embolism. *J Clin Monit Comput* 2000;16:375.

25. Van Hulst RA, Klein J, Lachmann B. Gas embolism: pathophysiology and treatment. *Clin Physiol Funct Imaging* 2003;32:237.

CHAPTER 55

Aortic Dissection and Thoracic Aortic Aneurysms

Shawna J. Perry

AORTIC DISSECTION

Aortic dissection is the most frequent catastrophic event involving the aorta. First recognized postmortem by Morgagni in 1761, aortic dissection remains a diagnostic challenge to the emergency physician because of its nonspecific presentation, variable population at risk, and time pressure for diagnosis. Delays or errors in diagnosis can have devastating consequences.

Dissection of the aorta begins with a tear in the inner most layer of the vessel, the intima. This tear occurs most commonly in the proximal ascending portion of the thoracic aorta. It may begin in the aortic root or between the origin of the left subclavian artery and the ligamentum arteriosum. These two areas of the aorta are relatively fixed and it is believed that maximum stress is applied to these areas during systole, thereby initiating the tear. The intimal tear allows blood to penetrate down into the middle layer of the vessel (the media), causing separation of the intima from the outer most layer of the vessel, the adventitia. The length of time required to dissect the entire aorta can be seconds, with the dissection proceeding either distally or proximally. *Reentry tears* occur distal to the initial site, creating an alternate path for aortic blood flow, called the *false lumen*. An intramural hematoma can develop within this false lumen, minimizing flow and occasionally causing dilation. A small number of patients develop an intramural hematoma with no evidence of a re-entry tear (9). The dissection may dilate as the flow of blood increases through the false lumen or as an intramural hematoma organizes. The term *dissecting aneurysm* is frequently used because of this pathologic finding, but it is done so incorrectly, as this is not a true aneurysm (see later discussion in this chapter of thoracic aortic aneurysms). Spontaneous rupture is common and is most often into the pericardium. Dissections with a tear beginning high in the aorta and an open false lumen have a poor prognosis.

The cause of the intimal tear is unknown, and the role of a structural defect of the aortic wall remains unclear. Histologic changes of recurrent injury and repair of the aorta in patients with Marfan syndrome and within the wall of a dissection may contribute to the process. Hypertension is the most common predisposing factor to dissection and is seen in up to 78% of descending aortic dissections (24). Smoking, cocaine use, and dyslipidemia may also be contributing factors. *Marfan syndrome* is a widely recognized risk factor that carries a mortality rate of greater than 90% in the event of dissection or aneurysm rupture. Other risk factors for aortic dissection are congenital abnormalities of the aorta, such as bicuspid valve and coarctation. Connective tissue diseases such as *Turner syndrome, Ehlers-Danlos syndrome,* and systemic lupus erythematosus, as well as cocaine use and blunt trauma have all been associated with aortic dissection (20). Iatrogenic aortic dissection can result from invasive vascular procedures (i.e., cardiac catheterization) or cardiac surgery such as a valve replacement (11). Dissection has also been reported in the third trimester of pregnancy, with most cases having evidence of systemic hypertension and/or connective tissue abnormalities as seen with Marfan syndrome. Aortic dissection is not caused by atherosclerotic disease. Dissection is most likely a multifactorial disease, with hypertension being the principal risk factor.

DeBakey originally classified aortic dissections into three categories according to the origin of the dissection: type I, involving the entire length of the aorta; type II, beginning in the ascending aorta (the aortic root to the left subclavian); and type III, originating from the area distal to the left subclavian (2).

The *Stanford* classification is a simpler scheme that divides dissections into type A, involving the ascending aorta, and type B, confined to the descending aorta and beginning after the left subclavian (Fig. 55.1). This more widely used nomenclature aids in determining treatment options and prognosis.

Type A dissections are more common (80%) and are considered surgical emergencies. Possible complications at presentation of type A dissections may include aortic rupture, cardiac tamponade, aortic valve insufficiency, involvement of coronary arteries resulting in acute myocardial infarction, stroke, and shock. Type B dissections are predominantly managed medically, unless they are complicated by rupture, vascular occlusion, acute expansion, or impending rupture. Up to one fourth of patients with type B dissection require urgent operation for hemorrhage, limb or organ ischemia, intractable pain, or progression of dissection. Paraplegia is a significant complication of surgical intervention for type B dissections.

The most common cause of death for untreated type A dissections is rupture of the aortic wall into the pericardial sac at

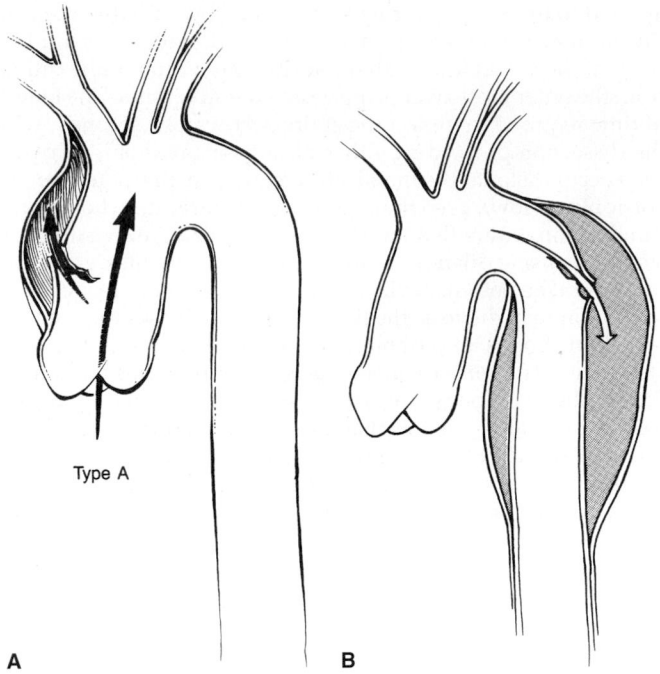

Type A

A   B

Figure 55.1.   Classification of aortic dissections. **A:** Dissection of ascending aorta. **B:** Dissection of descending aorta.

the level of the right lateral wall of the aorta, where the adventitia is thinnest. Rupture may also occur into the pleural space or the mediastinum. Death may also occur as a result of congestive heart failure, myocardial infarction, or cerebral vascular accident.

The mortality rate of patients with untreated type A dissection is 52% to 75%. The rate for surgically treated type A dissection ranges from 15% to 26% with a marked increase to 40% to 62% for patients older than 75 years of age (5). Risk factors for death are (i) older age (≥ 70 years), (ii) history of hypertension, (iii) preoperative cardiopulmonary resuscitation, (iv) preoperative hemodynamic instability or shock, (v) lack of cerebral perfusion, (vi) syncope with residual neurologic dysfunction, and (vii) cardiac tamponade (5,9,17). Mortality postoperatively ranges from 16% to 35%, with a 10-year survival of 55% to 80% (6,8,19). Reoperation, however, after initial surgery is a very poor prognostic sign.

CLINICAL PRESENTATION

To make the diagnosis of aortic dissection, the emergency physician must include it in the differential diagnosis at presentation. The pain of aortic dissection is classically described as "ripping" or "tearing," although these symptoms are not specific for dissection (1). The pain is severe and is frequently described as dull and pressure-like. A study of 464 patients with aortic dissection found that patients reported the classic tearing or ripping in only 51% of cases (1,8). The majority of patients reported abrupt onset with a pain of sharp, severe quality, located in anterior or posterior chest (73%). Back pain was experienced in more than one half (53%) with 30% reporting abdominal pain (1,8,21). With this presentation, history should focus on identifying risk factors for aortic dissection, especially hypertension, Marfan syndrome and prior cardiac surgery (i.e., valve replacement and cardiac catheterization). In addition to pain in the chest and back,

accompanying locations for discomfort included the neck, throat, mandible, abdomen, and leg. Patients may also complain of pain in the lower back, pelvis, and a lower extremity. Study of emergency physicians has demonstrated a high index of suspicion (86%) in patients with dissection who presented with both chest and back pain, with lower levels of suspicion in patients who presented with only chest pain (45%) or abdominal pain (8%) (22). A total of 15% to 20% of dissections are painless at onset, and a history of initial pain, followed by a pain-free interval, is most ominous and highly indicative of an impending rupture (15,24).

On examination, the patient may clinically appear to be in shock, exhibiting cool and diaphoretic skin, yet paradoxically the patient may have a normal or elevated blood pressure. The majority of patients present this way, but nearly one fourth will present hypotensive because of leaking at the dissection site or rupture. A variety of signs and symptoms can result owing to vascular compromise from the dissection or proximity to the dissection site. The majority of signs are neurologic (33%): syncope, altered mental status, cerebrovascular accident, paraplegia, or visual disturbances (1). Syncope is the initial complaint in 13% of patients, but decreased level of consciousness occurs more frequently. Syncope may be a sign of the development of hemopericardium or stroke, and is associated with increased mortality (17). Other associated findings with dissection are cardiac tamponade and congestive heart failure.

Cardiovascular collapse is seen most often with type A dissection. Proximity to the dissection site or developing hematoma can cause hoarseness (laryngeal nerve compression), dyspnea, or stridor with wheezing (tracheal compression) and dysphagia (esophageal compression). Despite initial hypertension on examination, the patient may show clinical signs of shock, with end-organ hypoperfusion. The presence of hypotension strongly suggests a type A dissection, a rupture of either type of dissection, or a dissection into the mesenteric or brachiocephalic artery. Gastrointestinal symptoms include mid-epigastric pain, hemorrhage, or melena secondary to splanchnic vessel infarctions, and these symptoms are frequently misdiagnosed as primary abdominal pathology. Renal artery involvement may lead to hematuria, flank pain, oliguria, or uncontrollable hypertension resulting from excess renin release.

Head and neck examination may reveal the presence of jugular venous distension secondary to congestive heart failure, cardiac tamponade, or an expanding hematoma around the aorta causing outflow obstruction. Aortic insufficiency murmur occurs in 16% to 20% of patients, resulting from proximal dissection causing dilation of the aortic valve ring and loss of commissural support of the aortic valve.

Poor prognostic factors include pleural effusion, cardiac tamponade, and pericardial friction rub. The presence of these signs implies leakage of the dissection into the pericardial space. The abdominal examination may reveal tenderness to palpation or rigidity. Rarely, a pulsatile mass is palpable (9). Examination of the limbs may reveal unequal, decreased, or absent peripheral pulses in 50% of cases, with these findings less likely to be present in the elderly (14). A complete deficit of pulse is found in 8% to 10% of patients (24). Differential blood flow to the extremities is often manifested by a marked discrepancy in blood pressure between arms and between the arms and legs, should dissection extend the entire length of the aorta. Rare but reported initial presentations of dissection have included hemoptysis, superior vena cava syndrome, dysphagia, acute arterial occlusion, right atrium or ventricular rupture, and deep vein thrombosis (9). Cranial nerve deficits secondary to dissection into the carotid arteries, or motor deficits secondary to distal dissection of spinal arteries, may also be present.

DIFFERENTIAL DIAGNOSIS

Chest pain with associated back pain is the most prevalent symptom of aortic dissection; therefore, the differential diagnosis is broad and contains numerous other life-threatening conditions. Myocardial infarction is the principal diagnosis of exclusion, as well as cerebrovascular accident in patients with neurologic symptoms. Misdiagnosis of either could result in the use of anticoagulation or thrombolytic therapy, consequently increasing the risk of death from exsanguination. Other diagnoses to exclude are hypertensive crisis, pulmonary embolism, thoracic aneurysm, pneumothorax, multilobar pneumonia, mediastinal cyst or tumor, pericarditis, pancreatitis, cholelithiasis, cholecystitis, perforated viscus, esophagitis, peptic ulcer disease, gastritis, and peripheral vascular disease.

The diagnosis of aortic dissection should be considered in the presence of the following clinical features: history of hypertension, connective tissue disease, or congenital aortic abnormalities; aortic insufficiency with chest or back pain; atypical chest or back pain; chest pain plus acute neurologic symptoms (rare with myocardial infarction); diminished or absent peripheral pulses; syncope; chest pain in the third trimester of pregnancy; acute unexplained left ventricular failure; flank pain and hematuria without an obvious source; and multiple sites of ischemia.

EMERGENCY DEPARTMENT EVALUATION

Patients suspected of aortic dissection should be managed aggressively in anticipation of impending leak or rupture. The patient should be placed on a cardiac monitor, and intravascular access should be established with at least two large-bore catheters (16-gauge or larger). A blood specimen should be obtained and sent for type and crossmatch. Initial laboratory studies should include a complete blood cell count; determination of serum levels of electrolytes, amylase, and cardiac enzymes; urinalysis; and a 12-lead electrocardiogram (ECG). Although routine laboratory studies are not usually helpful in the diagnosis of aortic dissection, they may rule out other causes. The complete blood cell count often reveals leukocytosis. If a sufficient amount of blood has accumulated in the false lumen, the hematocrit may be low. Renal artery involvement may result in increased blood urea nitrogen and creatinine levels, as well as hematuria, indicating ischemia or infarction of the kidney. An elevated lactic acid may point to the presence of ischemic bowel secondary to dissection. A normal creatinine phosphokinase level is useful in distinguishing dissection from myocardial infarction. In a small number of patients, however, the dissection occurs proximally into the right coronary artery and they sustain a myocardial infarction. Electrocardiographic changes compatible with myocardial infarction and pericarditis can be seen in approximately 25% of patients with dissection. The role of the biochemical marker, serum smooth-muscle myosin heavy chain (liberated from the smooth muscle cells of the media of the aorta), in the diagnosis of aortic dissection of is yet to be determined (23).

The most readily available imaging study to assist in the diagnosis of aortic dissection is the chest radiograph, which demonstrates some abnormality in 65% to 85% of cases (1). A widened mediastinum is the most common finding, but a left-sided pleural effusion or an indistinct aortic knob may also be seen (Fig. 55.2). The deviation of a calcified aortic intima by greater than 6 mm from the outer wall of the aorta is considered pathognomonic of dissection. Other findings suggestive of dissection are the double density sign (a false lumen that is less radiopaque than the true lumen), tracheal deviation, and an irregular aortic contour. Unfortunately, a normal chest radiograph does not exclude the diagnosis. If the diagnosis of dissection is considered despite a negative or equivocal chest radiograph, further evaluation is required by either aortography, computed tomography

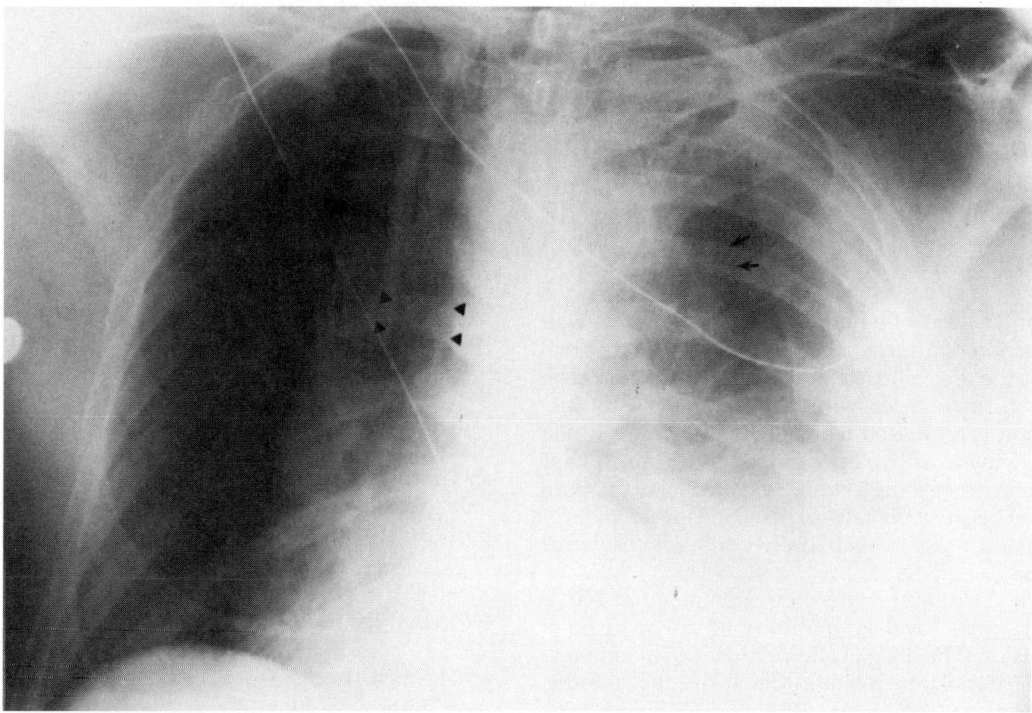

Figure 55.2.   Chest radiograph of a 65-year-old woman with type A dissection. Note the widened mediastinum, indistinct aortic knob *(arrows)*, tracheal deviation *(triangles)*, and left pleural effusion.

(CT), or transesophageal echocardiography (TEE) (13). These more definitive tests are also useful in confirming the diagnosis in those with suspicious findings on chest radiography.

The *aortogram* is still considered the "gold standard" for diagnosis of aortic dissection (sensitivity and specificity greater than 90%), but it has the disadvantages of a large contrast dye load, of being a time-consuming procedure, and of having a significant false-negative rate if the false lumen is thrombosed. In addition to confirming the diagnosis, the aortogram reveals the extent of dissection, the condition and patency of the distal vessels, and the pattern of blood flow in the true and false lumens. False-positive results are seen in any process that causes thickening of the aortic wall, such as a clotted aneurysm, mediastinal hematoma, neoplasms, or periaortic fat.

CT scan is used as a supplement to aortography and in some institutions has replaced it for making the diagnosis of dissection. The advantages of CT are (i) superior visualization of fluid collection in the pericardium, pleura, and mediastinum; (ii) demonstration of distal vessel patency; (iii) noninvasiveness; and (iv) sensitivity and specificity equal to aortography. Its main disadvantages are the necessary exposure to contrast dye for the examination and its inability to localize the site of the intimal tear. Spiral CT, with its three-dimensional reconstruction feature, is more expedient and has demonstrated improved delineation of the intimal tear and assessment of the great vessels (18). Spiral CT does not show greater sensitivity or specificity than TEE or magnetic resonance imaging (MRI) (21).

TEE is frequently used as the first diagnostic study in suspected dissection, if it is available. It has a sensitivity and specificity of 99% and 98%, respectively. The goals of TEE in aortic dissection are (i) to confirm the diagnosis, (ii) differentiate true and false lumens, (iii) localize the intimal tear, (iv) evaluate left ventricular wall motion, (v) determine the presence of fluid collections, and (vi) detect aortic insufficiency. It demonstrates a diagnostic accuracy of 100% for aortic insufficiency and cardiac tamponade. TEE provides limited ability to evaluate the great vessels and coronary vessels. Complications of transient atrioventricular (AV) block, bradycardia, and asthma can occur during introduction of the probe (4). Images may be limited in obese or emphysematous patients. TEE is often combined with CT.

MRI has a sensitivity and specificity no better than those of TEE or CT, and it is seldom used in the emergent setting because of cost, length of time needed for the study, and relative unavailability. MRI and TEE combined have the same sensitivity and specificity as TEE and CT (21).

EMERGENCY DEPARTMENT MANAGEMENT

The most important aspects of emergency department management are the reduction of arterial blood pressure and the forceful contractility of the left ventricle. These measures should be initiated before confirmatory tests are performed if clinical suspicion for dissection is high. Reductions in these aspects of the cardiovascular system have developed empirically in an attempt to limit the propagation of a dissection. Systolic blood pressure control is important because the rate of dissection is directly proportional to the blood pressure, especially to the rate of rise of arterial blood pressure.

The systolic blood pressure should be maintained at 100 to 110 mm Hg or the lowest level compatible with adequate renal and cerebral perfusion. The drug of choice to control blood pressure is *nitroprusside* (initial infusion rate 0.5 to 1.0 μg/kg/minute, titrate).

Intravenous β-antagonist therapy should also be used in order to suppress the reflex tachycardia from the initiation of nitroprusside and concomitant rise in arterial pressure. The target heart rate is between 60 and 80 bpm. Appropriate β-antagonists include *esmolol* (0.5 mg/kg loading dose, 0.05 mg/kg/minute infusion, titrate) or *propranolol* (0.5 to 1.0 mg i.v., at 5-minute intervals). Congestive heart failure, heart block, and bradycardia are contraindications for propranolol use.

An alternative to the combination of nitroprusside and β-antagonist therapy for patients with mild hypertension and no contraindications of chronic obstructive pulmonary disease or asthma is the mixed a- and β-blocker, *labetalol* (10 to 20 mg i.v., every 10 minutes, or initial infusion rate 2 mg/minute, titrate).

Intravenous verapamil or diltiazem may also be used if β-blockers are contraindicated. Morphine may also be helpful in reducing blood pressure via treatment of pain associated with the dissection. Oral agents should never be used at any time in patients for whom there is a suspicion of aortic dissection.

The medical therapy and surgical mortality rates for uncomplicated type B dissections remain the same; therefore, medical therapy is used first-line in uncomplicated patients (16,25). The use of β-blockers and afterload-reducing medication appears to decrease the risk of extension or dilation of the dissection. It does not stop the progression of the disease indefinitely, and aortic replacement will eventually be needed. The 30-day mortality rate of uncomplicated type B dissection is 10% with aggressive medical management and 45% to 60% at 5 years (6,8,12). Complicated type B dissections, with rupture or impending rupture, vascular occlusion, or acute expansion, have a high surgical mortality, with death almost certain in the presence of mesenteric, renal, or peripheral vascular ischemia (25). Ongoing research suggests that percutaneous stent-graft placement may provide better results than surgery (10).

CRITICAL INTERVENTIONS

- The most important intervention for the emergency physician is to suspect the disease and make the diagnosis
- Initiate aggressive control of the blood pressure and heart rate with short-acting parenteral agents
- Arrange immediate transport to the nearest appropriate hospital if your facility has inadequate resources for diagnosis and management of dissection

DISPOSITION

Management of the patient with aortic dissection requires urgent multispecialty involvement. The radiologist should be consulted emergently to obtain the appropriate diagnostic procedures. The cardiothoracic surgeon should also be notified. Once the diagnosis of dissection has been made, an internist may need to be consulted for medical management if a stable type B dissection if found. All patients suspected of having acute aortic dissection should be admitted to an intensive care unit. Indications for transfer include inadequate facilities or personnel to definitively make the diagnosis or treat the condition. If transfer is indicated, air transport should be used to minimize the time required. If only ground transport is available, an advanced cardiac life support (ACLS) unit should be used.

COMMON PITFALLS

- ✔ The most common mistake is failure to consider the diagnosis of aortic dissection
- ✔ Unexplained, severe, and sustained chest pain (especially with associated back pain) must be evaluated with aortography, CT, or TEE to rule out dissection

TABLE 55.1.   Diseases Contributing to Thoracic
Aortic Aneurysms

Atherosclerosis
Coarction of the aorta
Cystic medial necrosis
Giant cell arteritis
Marfan syndrome
Mycotic aneurysms
Seronegative spondyloarthropathies
Syphilis
Tuberculosis
Takayasu arteritis

THORACIC AORTIC ANEURYSM

Thoracic aortic aneurysm is very insidious in onset and presentation. It is defined as a localized or diffuse dilation of the aorta to a diameter of greater than 6 cm. Dilation is the result of an undermining of the overall strength of the aortic wall by direct loss of supportive proteins such as elastin and collagen. Once the wall of the aorta is weakened, there is progressive alteration in anatomy, with the growing diameter and thinning wall that lead to dilation and rupture. Turbulent flow can lead to thrombus formation. Causes for the undermining of the aortic wall are listed in Table 55.1.

The prevalence of thoracic aortic aneurysm is 5.9 new aneurysms per 100,000 person-years according to retrospective studies. The incidence is equal between men and women, with an increasing prevalence with advancing age. Risk factors are hypertension, advanced atherosclerotic disease, and smoking. The natural history of thoracic aneurysms is progressive dilation and rupture, with a 76% mortality rate at 2 years in untreated patients and a rate after surgical repair of 2.5% for ascending and 8% for descending aneurysm at experienced centers (3).

Aneurysm diameter is a significant risk factor for rupture. The median size at time of rupture is 6.0 cm for ascending aneurysms and 7.0 cm for descending aneurysms. The risk of rupture increases 31% for ascending diameters greater than 6.0 cm, with a 43% increase in risk for descending diameters greater than 7.0 cm (3). The average increase in diameter is 0.1 cm per year (0.7 cm ascending and 0.19 cm descending) (3). In patients with Marfan syndrome, rupture occurs at smaller diameters. Surgical intervention is, therefore, planned according to the patient's stability at time of diagnosis and diameter of the aneurysm as monitored over time, with annual calculation of risk of rupture (7).

CLINICAL PRESENTATION

The most common scenario for diagnosis of thoracic aneurysm is as an incidental finding on chest X-ray. Occasionally, patients will present with aortic regurgitation murmurs or with symptoms related directly to impingement of thoracic structures by the aneurysm. In cases of rupture or impending rupture, the patient will present with deep, aching, or throbbing chest or back pain. A sudden escalation of pain and hypotension are signs of aneurysm rupture. Rupture may also present as cardiopulmonary arrest secondary to intrathoracic or intraabdominal hemorrhage, should the aneurysm extend beyond the diaphragm.

DIFFERENTIAL DIAGNOSIS

Because most thoracic aortic aneurysms are discovered incidentally on a chest radiograph, the differential diagnosis includes tumors and cysts of the mediastinum and surrounding structures. Lung, thymus, or neurogenic tumors, lymphoma, mediastinal adenopathy, and bronchogenic or pleuropericardial cysts may all produce a mediastinal mass that must be differentiated from thoracic aortic aneurysm. For symptomatic patients, the differential is broad, and includes disorders such as myocardial infarction, pulmonary embolus, aortic dissection, and superior vena cava syndrome.

EMERGENCY DEPARTMENT EVALUATION

Aortography, CT, and TEE can be used to evaluate suspected aneurysms. If the diagnosis has not been made previously, aneurysms suspected in the emergency department should be evaluated at the time of presentation, even if asymptomatic. CT scan is the preferred study, owing to its ability to differentiate aortic aneurysm from the many other causes of a mediastinal mass. Because 21% of first-order relatives of patients with known thoracic aneurysms are likely to also have an aneurysm, they should be referred for screening.

Bedside transthoracic and transabdominal echo can be of assistance in locating large collections of fluid in patients with suspected rupture.

EMERGENCY DEPARTMENT MANAGEMENT

Consultation with a thoracic surgeon is recommended to determine the treatment plan. Those patients not needing immediate surgical repair should have periodic outpatient diagnostic tests to monitor the aneurysm diameter. Patients with suspected rupture require aggressive supportive care (including airway management, transfusion, correction of coagulopathy, and pressors as needed) and immediate involvement of a thoracic surgeon.

CRITICAL INTERVENTIONS

- Initiate aggressive supportive care for the patient with suspected rupture
- Arrange an expeditious evaluation for the patient with an asymptomatic aneurysm

DISPOSITION

Disposition is based on the aneurysm diameter, risk of rupture, and surgical risk to the patient.

COMMON PITFALLS

✔ Failure to consider the diagnosis in a patient with nonspecific chest symptoms and a mediastinal mass

References

1. Armstrong WF, Bach D. Clinical and echocardiographic findings in patients with suspected acute aortic dissection. *Am Heart J* 1998;136:1051.
2. DeBakey M, Henley W. Surgical management of dissecting aneurysms of the aorta. *J Thorac Cardiovasc Surg* 1965;49:130.
3. Elefteriades, J. Natural history of thoracic aortic aneurysms: indications for surgery, and surgical versus nonsurgical risks. *Ann Thorac Surg* 2002;74:S1877.
4. Erbel R, Hellmut O. Effect of medical and surgical therapy on aortic dissections evaluated by transesophageal echocardiography: implications for prognosis and therapy. *Circulation* 1993;87:1604.
5. Erlich M, Fang C. Perioperative risk factors for mortality in patients with acute type A dissection. *Circulation* 1998;98[Suppl II]:II–294.

6. Fann J, Smith J. Surgical management of aortic dissection during a 30-year period. *Circulation* 1995;92[Suppl II]:II–113.
7. Griepp R, Ergin M. Natural history of descending thoracic and thoracoabdominal aneurysms. *Ann Thorac Surg* 1999;67:1927.
8. Hagan P, Nienaber C. The international registry of acute aortic dissection (IRAD): new insights into an old disease. *JAMA* 2000;283:897.
9. Hirst A, Varner J. Dissecting aneurysm of the aorta: a review of 505 cases. *Medicine* 1958;37:217.
10. Ince H, Nienbauer C. The concept of interventional therapy in acute aortic syndrome. *J Cardiol Surg* 2002;17:135.
11. Januzzi J, Sabatine M. Iatrogenic aortic dissections. *Am J Cardiology* 2002;89:623.
12. Juvonen T, Ergin M. Risk factors for rupture of chronic type B dissections. *J Thorac Cardiovasc Surg* 1999;117:776.
13. Keren A, Kim C. Accuracy of biplane and multiplane transesophageal echocardiography in diagnosis of typical acute aortic dissection and intramural hematoma. *J Am Coll Cardiol* 1996;28:627.
14. Mehta R, O'Gara P. Acute type A dissection in the elderly: clinical characteristics, management and outcomes in the current era. *J Am Coll Cardiol* 2002;40:685.
15. Meszaros I, Morocz J. Epidemiology and clinicopathology of aortic dissection. *Chest* 2000;117:1271.
16. Miller DC. The continuing dilemma concerning medical versus surgical management of patients with acute type B dissections. *Semin Thorac Cardiovasc Surg* 1993;60:33.
17. Nallamothu B, Mehta R. Syncope in acute aortic dissection: diagnostic, prognostic and clinical implications. *Am J Med* 2002;113:468.
18. Oliver T, Murchison J. Spiral CT in acute non-cardiac chest pain. *Clin Radiol* 1999;54:38.
19. Pansini S. Early and late risk factors in surgical treatment of acute type A dissection. *Ann Thorac Surg* 1998;66:779.
20. Perron AD, Gibb M. Thoracic aortic dissection secondary to crack cocaine ingestion. *Am J Emerg Med* 1997;15:507.
21. Sommer T, Fehske W. Aortic dissection: a comparative study of diagnosis with spiral CT, multiplane transesophageal echocardiology and MR imaging. *Radiology* 1996;199:347.
22. Sullivan PR, W. Diagnosis of acute thoracic aortic dissection in the emergency department. *Am J Emerg Med* 2000;18:46.
23. Suzuki T, Katoh H. Diagnostic implications of elevated levels of smooth-muscle myosin heavy chains in acute aortic dissection: smooth muscle myosin heavy chain study. *Ann Intern Med* 2000;133:537.
24. Torossov M, Singh A. Clinical presentation, diagnosis and hospital outcome of patients with documented aortic dissection: The Albany Medical Center experience 1986–1996. *Am Heart J* 1999;137:154.
25. Umana JP, Miller DC. What is the best treatment for patients with acute type B aortic dissections–medical, surgical or endovascular stent grafting? *Ann Thorac Surg* 2002;74:S1840.

CHAPTER 56
Abdominal Aortic Aneurysm

Matthew R. Lewin and Robert L. Wears

A 71-year-old man presents with right lower quadrant abdominal pain and syncope. A 75-year-old woman presents with back pain and radiculopathy (23). A 65-year-old man presents with right flank pain and hematuria (30). An 86-year-old woman presents with diffuse abdominal pain and left leg swelling, and a 68-year-old man presents with abdominal pain, hypotension, and a pulsatile abdominal mass. These are just a few presentations of a diagnosis which should be feared—especially if missed.

The timely recognition of an abdominal aortic aneurysm (AAA or "triple A") is a major challenge to the emergency physi-cian. The presentation may be confusing and accurate diagnosis difficult, and the cost of delay or misdiagnosis devastating (3,25). AAA is one of the most common causes of unexpected death following discharge from the emergency department (ED) (17), and is one of the highest risk areas for medical malpractice litigation in emergency medicine (15).

AAAs (defined as a 50% or greater increase in aortic diameter or an infrarenal aortic diameter greater than or equal to 3 cm (14)) are present in nearly 2% of the elderly (9). The prevalence is increasing (5,26), even after adjusting for improved methods of detection. As the proportion of the population older than 60 years of age grows, emergency physicians can expect to encounter patients with AAAs more frequently.

The etiology of AAA remains obscure. A variety of evidence suggests that atherosclerosis alone is not the principal cause; smoking is the strongest independent risk factor for AAA (20), but familial, biochemical, and hemodynamic factors have all been implicated (9,14,16). New evidence suggests that up to 20% of AAAs have a dominant genetic component with incomplete penetrance (37). Most patients are male, but the prevalence of AAA increases with increasing age in both sexes (33); it is roughly as common (approximately 5%) in 90-year-old women as it is in 80-year-old men (9).

The natural history of the AAA is one of gradual expansion (although sudden changes in size may occur) followed by rupture, exsanguination, and death (34). Most AAAs are asymptomatic until rapid expansion or leakage occurs. In addition, 80% of patients with untreated, symptomatic AAAs will be dead within 1 year of the onset of symptoms (33% in 1 month and 74% in 6 months) (32).

The risk of rupture and death depends on the size of the aneurysm. Aneurysms less than 4.0 cm in diameter are at low risk for rupture (8). For diameters between 4.0 and 5.0 cm, the 5-year risk is between 3% and 12%, and for diameters greater than 5.0 cm that risk is between 25% and 41% (9). However, there is considerable difference of opinion among vascular surgeons about the risk of rupture, and better data are needed (19).

Early detection and elective repair of AAAs lead to increased life expectancy, even for elderly patients (34,10). Operative mortality for elective surgery is roughly 2% to 7% in all age groups (29). However, mortality in the setting of rupture approaches 90% (9,32). Because rupture of an AAA is inevitable given enough time, elective resection is generally recommended for aneurysms of 5.0 cm or more (9). Although some researchers have repaired AAAs as small as 4.0 cm (13,16), two randomized, controlled trials of active ultrasonic (28) and computed tomographic (CT) scan (22) surveillance versus immediate repair of small aneurysms have showed no evidence favoring early operation.

CLINICAL PRESENTATION

AAAs typically present in three ways: asymptomatic, symptomatic, and ruptured. Physical examination is the key to recognition, because about one half of asymptomatic AAAs are palpable (31). The sensitivity of physical examination depends on the size of the aneurysm, ranging from about 50% for aneurysms between 4 and 5 cm to 76% for those between 5 and 6 cm (21). Unfortunately, this sensitivity is not sufficient to confidently rule out an aneurysm based on a negative physical examination. Most palpable aneurysms are found in the epigastrium, extending to the paraumbilical areas on both sides of the midline. False-positive physical findings are common, illustrating the difficulty of the diagnosis (2).

Asymptomatic Aneurysm

Occasionally, an AAA is discovered on routine examination for another, clearly unrelated problem. Frequently, the aneurysm is noted on abdominal plain films or CT scan (24). The emergency physician's task in this setting is to confirm that the aneurysm is truly asymptomatic.

Symptomatic Aneurysm

Patients who are hemodynamically stable but who have symptoms referable to an AAA can present in a variety of ways, and are therefore easily misdiagnosed. In fact, almost one half of all AAAs are misdiagnosed on their initial presentation (3,25). Abdominal, low-back, or flank pain is the cardinal symptom of AAA, but it is nonspecific. The pain may be associated with syncope at the time of onset. The discomfort occasionally radiates to the testis or leg, causing the symptoms to be attributed to renal colic, inguinal hernia, or lumbar spine disease. The pain is usually not much affected by movement and can vary considerably in location (27). Radicular findings (23) or hematuria (30) may be present, falsely reassuring the physician.

Less common presentations of symptomatic AAA include hydronephrosis or leg swelling (usually left) from compression, new onset or worsening of hypertension (secondary to renal artery compression), testicular swelling, or evidence of peripheral embolization. Aortovenous or aortocaval fistulas are uncommon, and usually present as high-output failure with marked distention of the lower abdominal and leg veins, accompanied by more typical evidence of AAA, such as abdominal mass and back pain (6).

About 10% of patients with symptomatic AAAs present with severe pain and marked abdominal tenderness (32). Because these patients have the appearance of an acute abdomen, identifying them as "emergent" cases is not as much of a problem as in other symptomatic patients, even though the presumptive diagnosis may be erroneous (e.g., perforated viscus). Symptomatic AAA may present acutely as complete aortic occlusion with a clinical picture similar to that of a saddle embolus or acute Leriche syndrome (aortoiliac compression causing impotence). This complication requires prompt surgery and still carries an approximate 50% mortality (32).

An uncommon, acute presentation of a symptomatic AAA is gastrointestinal bleeding secondary to an aortoenteric fistula (11). Such bleeding may be massive and can distract the emergency physician from suspecting vascular disease. In particular, aortoenteric fistula should be assumed whenever a patient who has had a previous repair of an AAA presents with gastrointestinal bleeding. Endovascular repair is becoming more common (1). Because an abdominal incision is not required, postoperative abdominal complications are lower. Nevertheless, aneurysm remodeling and shortening can cause stent-graft dislodgement or kinking, and progression of underlying atherosclerotic disease can cause compression of the lower extremity limbs of the graft (4). Post AAA endograft complications include pelvic ischemia, impotence, buttock claudication, and colonic ischemia (1). Fortunately, it is rare for an AAA to rupture following endovascular repair. Emergency physicians need to be familiar with identification and management of postoperative complications of the traditional and endovascular AAA repair.

Ruptured Aneurysm

The classic triad of findings in ruptured AAA is back pain, hypotension, and a pulsatile abdominal mass, but all three findings are present in only about one half of the patients who survive to reach the ED (18). Therefore, the presence of any one of these findings in a patient with a known AAA is sufficient to make the diagnosis of rupture without confirmatory testing (9). Unfortunately, most patients presenting with ruptured AAAs have no prior knowledge of their aneurysm (31). Rupture of an AAA is correctly diagnosed preoperatively in about 70% of patients (25); mortality increases dramatically with misdiagnosis (12).

DIFFERENTIAL DIAGNOSIS

The differential diagnosis of AAA includes the differentials of shock, abdominal pain, and back pain. If shock is present, the differential also includes acute myocardial infarction, hemorrhagic pancreatitis, perforated viscus, and mesenteric infarction. In patients whose presentation is less severe—renal or biliary colic, diverticulitis, and lumbosacral disc disease also need to be considered. Because these conditions are more common than AAA, it is useful to consider the differential diagnosis in reverse; for example, when entertaining a diagnosis of renal colic in a patient over age 60, AAA should be considered.

EMERGENCY DEPARTMENT EVALUATION

Laboratory studies are rarely helpful in the diagnosis of AAA, but should be obtained in the symptomatic patient to evaluate the status of other comorbid conditions (diabetes and renal insufficiency, among others) or to investigate other possibilities in the differential. Blood cell counts and coagulation studies should be evaluated in patients with suspected hemorrhage or coagulopathy, and blood should be made available in the blood bank in such cases.

Radiographic Imaging

Plain films of the abdomen are occasionally helpful in the diagnosis of AAA, in that calcified walls are visible in about one half of cases (24). Fusiform calcifications show the presence of an aneurysm, but not whether the aneurysm is enlarging or leaking. Absent or "normal" aortic calcifications are of no value in ruling out the diagnosis. Therefore, plain films should not be ordered to evaluate the presence of an AAA or its complications.

Abdominal ultrasonography is useful in quickly and accurately establishing the presence of an aneurysm with almost 100% sensitivity (9) (Fig. 56.1). However, this technique is NOT reliable in determining whether rupture has occurred or in estimating the proximal and distal extent of the aneurysm. Its role in the ED lies in rapidly establishing the presence of AAA at the bedside when there is doubt. The detection of a saccular aneurysm of any size warrants the immediate attention of a vascular surgeon. It is also useful to remember that AAA compressing a ureter can cause hydronephrosis. Unexplained hydronephrosis warrants further ultrasonographic examination of the aorta.

Computed tomography provides greater detail than ultrasound does and a more accurate measure of size. It is particularly useful in identifying leakage, rupture, or complications of AAA (38). Because computed tomography takes more time and requires intravenous contrast and removal of the patient from the ED, it should be limited to stable patients in whom precise information is required. Magnetic resonance imaging also provides detailed images but it is expensive, not widely available, and contraindicated in patients with pacemakers or metallic implants or clips; therefore, it currently offers no substantive advantage over ultrasound or computed tomography (9).

Aortography is useful in selected cases in planning the operative repair of AAAs, but should not be used for diagnosis

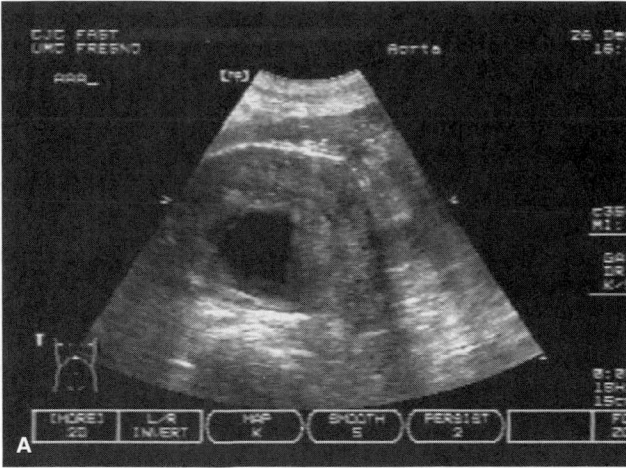
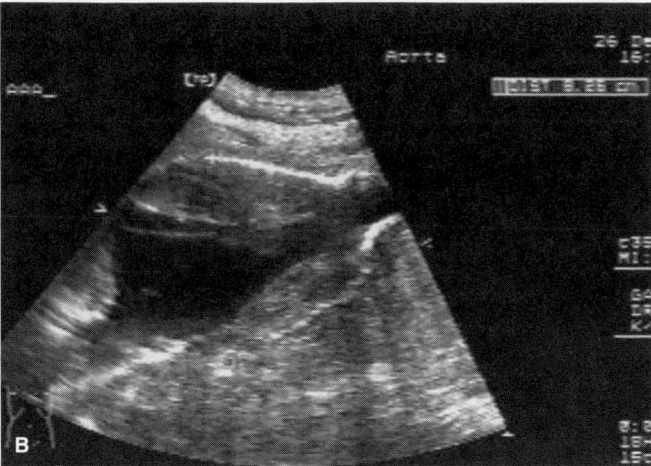

Figure 56.1.   **(A)** Transverse view reveals an abdominal aortic aneurysm (AAA) with mural thrombus. **(B)** Longitudinal view of the same patient who presented with abdominal pain and a pulsatile abdominal mass (courtesy of Dr. Carolyn Chooljian, Fresno, California).

or to establish size. The decision to use angiography should be left to the surgical consultant, who may need information about renal or iliofemoral involvement, mesenteric artery stenosis, or suspected visceral lesions (e.g., horseshoe kidney) (7).

High speed MRI, 3-dimensional reconstruction vascular CTs, and sensitive and specific biochemical markers of aneurysm and dissection are exciting and promising areas of vascular research. Soon, rapid visualization techniques and proteomic approaches may be able to diagnose and track the progression of aneurysms and dissection, even in the emergency department setting. Ultrasound by ED physicians is already a routine and reliable way to detect and measure aneurysms in the acute care setting (35).

EMERGENCY DEPARTMENT MANAGEMENT

The ED management of a patient with a suspected AAA must be tailored to the patient's presentation. The use of fluid resuscitation and appropriate blood pressure maintenance are arbitrary. Large volumes of blood or crystalloid may dislodge a metastable clot or cause coagulopathy. Conversely, older patients (the demographic most commonly presenting with symptomatic AAA) do not tolerate hypotension and its sequelae well, especially in the setting of common comorbidities. All patients with suspected ruptured, or symptomatic AAA should have cardiac monitoring, be on oxygen, and have two large-bore i.v. catheters securely in place and at least 6 units of packed, red blood cells typed and crossed, along with at least 4 units of fresh frozen plasma and platelets available for emergency transfusion. There have been no formal studies of blood pressure optimization in the setting of symptomatic or ruptured AAA. Pharmacological and fluid management to maintain low, but end-organ perfusing blood pressures (e.g., mean arterial pressures [MAPs] between 60 and 80 mm Hg) will likely be helpful. The use of medical anti-shock trousers (MAST) and aortic cross-clamping has been reported in the setting of profound hypotension. If possible, the patient's resuscitation and emergency surgery preferences should be established as early as possible and discussed with the surgical consultant. Some patients may wish to decline surgery. A notable example was Albert Einstein, whose original diagnosis was "cholecystitis" and who refused a second surgery after becoming symptomatic following the first repair.

Asymptomatic Aneurysm

If the AAA is clearly unrelated to the patient's symptoms, the patient should be referred promptly to a vascular surgeon for further evaluation and possible elective repair. An abdominal ultrasound examination may be useful in establishing the presence or absence of AAA, but it *cannot* provide evidence that the AAA is NOT ruptured, leaking, or expanding.

Symptomatic Aneurysm

An aneurysm producing symptoms should be assumed to be ruptured, rapidly expanding, or otherwise complicated (infected, dissecting). Therefore, although these patients may appear hemodynamically stable, prompt surgical consultation should be obtained, and preparations for fluid resuscitation and operative repair should be made by placing several large-bore intravenous lines and sending blood for type and crossmatch, hemoglobin, renal function, and coagulation studies. Vigorous fluid resuscitation should not be started unless there is evidence of peripheral hypoperfusion (9), and hypertension should be controlled if present (31). Patients presenting as an acute abdomen or patients with known AAA and any one of the findings in the classic triad require immediate surgery without the usual preoperative evaluation and preparation, as rupture is either imminent or has already occurred but has been temporarily confined to the retroperitoneum (9). In less acute presentations, radiologic imaging may be helpful but should be ordered with the greatest of caution.

Ruptured Aneurysm

Patients in shock from a ruptured AAA need rapid resuscitation and prompt surgical intervention. Except in unusual circumstances, these patients should be transported to the operating room as quickly as possible without waiting for diagnostic testing or stabilization. A policy of immediate operation in such circumstances maximizes the patient's chances of survival. Even if it is discovered that a ruptured AAA is not present, many of these patients will have another surgical condition requiring operation, so the risk of unnecessary laparotomy is not great (36).

CRITICAL INTERVENTIONS

- Rapid diagnosis of a patient with a symptomatic or ruptured AAA, with emergent consultation for operative repair
- Aggressive resuscitation of shock with fluids and blood products as necessary

DISPOSITION

Any asymptomatic patient with an aortic diameter equal to or greater than 3.0 cm should be referred to a vascular surgeon for further evaluation for elective resection. Patients with a symptomatic AAA, regardless of size, should be admitted for close observation. These patients will require prompt surgery if it becomes clear that the aneurysm is the source of their symptoms. Patients who present with rupture of their AAA should go straight to the operating room.

Role of the Consultant

All patients with suspected symptomatic or ruptured AAAs should have a prompt surgical consultation, preferably with a vascular surgeon. Patients in whom the AAA is truly an incidental finding may be referred for later consultation if otherwise appropriate. Patients with a history of AAA repair, whether open or endovascular, are still at risk for rupture, infection, occlusion, and other vascular catastrophes. Graft clots may require thrombolysis, thrombectomy, or emergent surgical revision. Therefore, an emergency physician should have a low threshold for vascular surgery consultation even long after AAA repair. In referral centers, a large percentage of AAA patients may already have one or more aneurysm repairs.

Indications for Admission

All patients with symptomatic AAAs should be admitted to the hospital for close observation and further investigation. One should assume that abdominal or back pain in the presence of AAA is caused by sudden expansion or rupture.

Transfer Considerations

If the initial hospital does not have sufficient surgical capability to treat an AAA, transfer to a more appropriate institution may be indicated. The decision to transfer may be a difficult one for patients who present with cardiovascular instability. The current hospital's capabilities, the length of time in transit, and the likelihood of survival to the second hospital must be considered.

COMMON PITFALLS

✔ AAAs are frequently misdiagnosed, especially in obese patients. Any palpable abdominal pulsation in an obese patient should be suspected of being an AAA, even if a mass cannot be clearly discerned. Back pain is a common symptom, and because peritoneal signs may not be present unless free rupture into the abdominal cavity has occurred, the emergency physician may be misled to one of the common misdiagnoses of AAA, such as renal colic or lumbosacral disease. Falsely reassuring symptom complexes and laboratories (e.g., flank pain and hematuria mistaken for "renal colic," or left lower quadrant pain and guaiac-positive stool mistaken for "diverticulosis") may result in deadly delays in care

✔ Assuming that an aneurysm discovered on physical examination is incidental and not the source of the patient's symptoms. Any back or abdominal pain in the presence of a pulsatile abdominal mass should be considered to be a result of an expanding or leaking aneurysm unless there is overwhelming evidence to the contrary

✔ Abbreviating the ED evaluation due to "gatekeeping" or managed care concerns. AAAs are often a surprise for both doctor and patient, and difficulties with preauthorization by medical plans may arise. These factors should not be allowed to prevent a thorough assessment of the older patient with back or abdominal pain (39)

References

1. Aquino Rand et al. *Quality of life assessment in patients undergoing endovascular or conventional AAA repair. J Endovasc Ther* 2001;8:521.
2. Beede S, Ballard D, James E, et al. Positive predictive value of clinical suspicion of abdominal aortic aneurysm: implications for efficient use of abdominal ultrasonography. *Arch Intern Med* 1990;150:549–551.
3. Bengtsson H, Bergqvist D. Ruptured abdominal aortic aneurysm: a population-based study. *J Vasc Surg* 1993;18:74–80.
4. Berry A, et al. Age versus comorbidities as risk factors for complications after elective abdominal reconstructive surgery . *J Vasc Surg* 2001;33:345.
5. Bickerstaff L, Hollier L, Van Peenen H, et al. Abdominal aortic aneurysms: the changing natural history. *J Vasc Surg* 1984;1:6–12.
6. Calligaro K, Savarese R, DeLaurentis D. Unusual aspects of aortovenous fistulas associated with ruptured abdominal aortic aneurysms. *J Vasc Surg* 1990;12:586–590.
7. Campbell J, Bell D, Gaspar M. Selective use of arteriography in the assessment of aortic aneurysm repair. *Ann Vasc Surg* 1990;4:419–423.
8. Cronenwett J, Murphy T, Zelenock G, et al. Actuarial analysis of variables associated with rupture of small abdominal aortic aneurysms. *Surgery* 1985;98:472–483.
9. Ernst C. Abdominal aortic aneurysm. *N Engl J Med* 1993;328:1167–1172.
10. Goldstone J. Aneurysms of the aorta and iliac arteries In: Moore WE, ed. *Vascular surgery: a comprehensive review.* Philadelphia: WB Saunders, 1993:401–421.
11. Grigsby W, Eitzen E, Boyle D. Aortoenteric fistula: a catastrophe waiting to happen. *Ann Emerg Med* 1986;15:731.
12. Hoffman M, Avellone J, FR P, et al. Operation for ruptured abdominal aortic aneurysms: a community-wide experience. *Surgery* 1982;91.
13. Hollier L, Taylor L, Ochsner J. Recommended indication for operative treatment of abdominal aortic aneurysms. *Vasc Surg* 1992;5:1046–1056.
14. Johnston K, Rutherford R, Tilson M, et al. Suggested standards for reporting on arterial aneurysms. *J Vasc Surg* 1991;13:452–458.
15. Karcz A, Holbrook J, Burke M, et al. Massachusetts emergency medicine closed malpractice claims. *Ann Emerg Med* 1993;22:553–559.
16. Katz D, Littenberg B, Cronenwett J. Management of small abdominal aortic aneurysms: early surgery vs watchful waiting. *JAMA* 1992;268:2678–2686.
17. Kefer M, Hargarten S, Jentzen J. Death after discharge from the emergency department. *Ann Emerg Med* 1994;24:1102–1107.
18. Kiel C, Ernst C. Advances in management of abdominal aortic aneurysm. *Adv Surg* 1993;26:73–98.
19. Lederle F. Risk of rupture of large abdominal aortic aneurysm. Disagreement among vascular surgeons. *Arch Intern Med* 1996;156:1007–1009.
20. Lederle F, Johnson G, Wilson S, et al. Prevalence and associations of abdominal aortic aneurysm detected through screening. Aneurysm Detection and Management (ADAM) Veterans Affairs Cooperative Study Group. *Ann Intern Med* 1997;126:441–449.
21. Lederle F, Simel D. Does this patient have abdominal aortic aneurysm? *JAMA* 1999;281:77–82.
22. Lederle F, Wilson S, Johnson G, et al. Immediate repair compared with surveillance of small abdominal aortic aneurysms. *N Engl J Med* 2002;346:1437–1444.
23. Lodder J, Cheriex E, Oostenbroek R, et al. Ruptured abdominal aortic aneurysms presenting as radicular compression syndromes. *J Neurol* 1982;227:121–124.
24. Loughran C. A review of the plain abdominal radiograph in acute rupture of abdominal aortic aneurysms. *Clin Radiol* 1986;37:383–387.
25. Marston W, Ahlquist R, Johnson G, et al. Misdiagnosis of ruptured abdominal aneurysms. *J Vasc Surg* 1992;16:17–22.
26. Melton LI, Bickerstaff L, Hollier L, et al, Changing incidence of abdominal aortic aneurysm. *Am J Epidemiol* 1984;120:379–386.
27. Merchant R, Cafferata H, DePalma R. Pitfalls in the diagnosis of abdominal aortic aneurysm. 1981;142:756–758.
28. Participants T. U. K. S. A. Long-term outcomes of immediate repair compared with surveillance for small abdominal aortic aneurysms. *N Engl J Med* 2002;346:1445–1452.
29. Paty P, Lloyd W, Chang B, et al. Aortic replacement for abdominal aortic aneurysm in elderly patients. *Am J Surg* 1993;166:191–193.

30. Phillips S, King D. The role of ultrasound to detect aortic aneurysms in "urological" patients. *Eur J Vasc Surg* 1993;7:298–300.
31. Rothrock S, Green S. Abdominal aortic aneurysms: current clinical strategies for avoiding disaster. *Emerg Med Rep* 1994;15:125–136.
32. Scobie T. Abdominal aortic aneurysms: how can we improve their treatment? *Can Med Assoc J* 1980;123:725–729.
33. Scott R, Ashton H, Kay D. Abdominal aortic aneurysm in 4237 screened patients: prevalence, development and management over 6 years. *Br J Surg* 1991;78:1122–1125.
34. Szilagyi D, Smith R, DeRusso F, et al. Contribution of abdominal aortic aneurysmectomy to prolongation of life. *Ann Surg* 1966;164:678–699.
35. Tayal V, Graf C, Gibbs M. Prospective study of accuracy and outcome of emergency department ultrasound for abdominal aortic aneurysms over two years. *Acad Emerg Med* 2003;10:867–961.
36. Valentine R, Barth M, Myers S, et al. Nonvascular emergencies presenting as ruptured abdominal aortic aneurysms. *Surgery* 1993;113:286–289.
37. Verloes A, Sakalihasan N, Koulischer L, et al. Aneurysms of the abdominal aorta: familial and genetic aspects in three hundred thirteen pedigrees. *J Vasc Surg* 1995;21:646–655.
38. Weinbaum F, Dubner S, Turner J, et al. The accuracy of computed tomography in the diagnosis of retroperitoneal blood in the presence of abdominal aortic aneurysm. *J Vasc Surg* 1987;6:11–16.
39. Young G, Lowe R. Adverse outcomes of managed care gatekeeping. *Acad Emerg Med* 1997;4:1129–1136.

CHAPTER 57
Mesenteric Ischemia and Infarction

Kendall Ho

Mesenteric ischemia is the failure of normal oxygenation of the small or large intestine resulting from interruption of vascular flow (Fig. 57.1). The consequences of this failure of oxygenation occupy a spectrum that ranges from intermittent, nonspecific intestinal symptoms to frank gut infarction with death of the patient (24). Despite the increasing volume literature and medical familiarity with the lethal nature of the condition, mortality remains greater than 50%, and is primarily attributable to delay in diagnosis (7,24,25). Mortality rates can be significantly reduced with aggressive diagnostic and therapeutic approaches.

Acute mesenteric ischemia (AMI) is much more common than chronic mesenteric insufficiency. The vascular interruption in AMI can be divided into three categories: arterial occlusion, venous occlusion, and nonocclusive mesenteric ischemia (NOMI). Embolus to the superior mesenteric artery (SMA) accounts for approximately 50% of the cases, and SMA thrombosis accounts for an additional 25% (18). An estimated 5% to 15% of AMI cases are caused by venous thrombosis (2,21,24). NOMI, accounts for approximately 20% of all AMI cases and occurs mostly in systemically and critically ill patients, with periods of markedly reduced blood flow (16,18,20). Strangulated small or large bowel caused by herniation, adhesions, or volvulus is another cause of acute vascular occlusion (19). A chronic syndrome of inadequate mesenteric blood flow without complete vascular occlusion or bowel infraction, also termed *intestinal angina*, may occur but is uncommon (19,24).

Once ischemia is established, the pathologic sequence is identical, regardless of the causative mechanism. Four major factors contribute to the extent and severity of ischemia: hypoxic injury, reperfusion injury, toxic luminal factors, and bacteria and toxins (19). Hypoxia initially causes epithelial and submucosal damage, followed by full-thickness involvement and eventual loss of bowel integrity with continuing oxygenation failure. Should perfusion be restored in ischemic regions, generation of superoxides and free radicals could add further insult to already damaged tissues. Toxic luminal substances, such as hydrochloric acid and digestive enzymes, penetrate the edematous and porous intestinal mucosal barrier to cause further cellular damage. Bacterial invasion and toxin excretion lead to systemic sepsis (19). Hypotension resulting from blood and fluid losses and exacerbated by sepsis, leads to further compromise of vascular flow to the gut, and the process becomes self-propagating. In the most severe cases, AMI can lead to the development of multiorgan dysfunction syndrome (MODS) (15,19).

This disorder has a distinct epidemiologic preference for the elderly (15,19,20,27). Many patients have evidence of significant preexisting cardiac diseases, especially congestive heart failure (19,27). Postoperative and critically ill patients, and those exposed to vasospastic substances such as norepinephrine, cocaine, or digoxin are at an increased risk of developing NOMI (11,15,16,19,20). If AMI occurs in young adults (18 to 40 years of age), hypercoagulable states should be suspected (22,24).

CLINICAL PRESENTATION

It is highly difficult to establish reliable diagnostic criteria for AMI because the symptoms are nonspecific and the presentation is often unremarkable until the compromised gut (and often the patient) is not salvageable. Therefore, high vigilance for the possibility of this diagnosis and prompt investigations once the condition is suspected or recognized remain the best defense against high mortality in this population (5,18,24).

History

Historical features are highly variable. Characteristically, abrupt onset of severe abdominal pain disproportionate to physical findings mandates consideration of AMI (8,18,19,24). The character of abdominal pain may be localized or diffuse, and may be either colicky or constant (11,19,24,27). Suddenness of onset is a useful, but not completely reliable symptom, because pain may develop over seconds, minutes, hours, or even days or weeks, depending on the underlying process (8,16,19,24). Fever, nausea, anorexia, vomiting, and diarrhea are all frequently reported or observed, and in approximately 15% of cases melena or hematochezia occurs (11,19,24,27). Weight loss is invariably present in chronic mesenteric ischemia (19). Nausea, anorexia, and sitophobia (fear of eating) often longstanding, will be reported in some cases (24).

Historically, the patient will usually have a combination of the following: advanced age, a history of significant cardiovascular disease, a history of thromboembolic events, and concurrent medication with digitalis and a diuretic (16,19,24,25,27). The patient may report episodes of vague abdominal fullness or discomfort after meals, and a history of unexplained weight loss is often present, if sought. However, most patients will present with AMI without a preceding history of intermittent or chronic symptoms.

Physical Examination

The physical examination may be normal. The patient may appear completely well, apart from the presenting pain. Twenty percent to 40% of patients will appear dehydrated, some to the

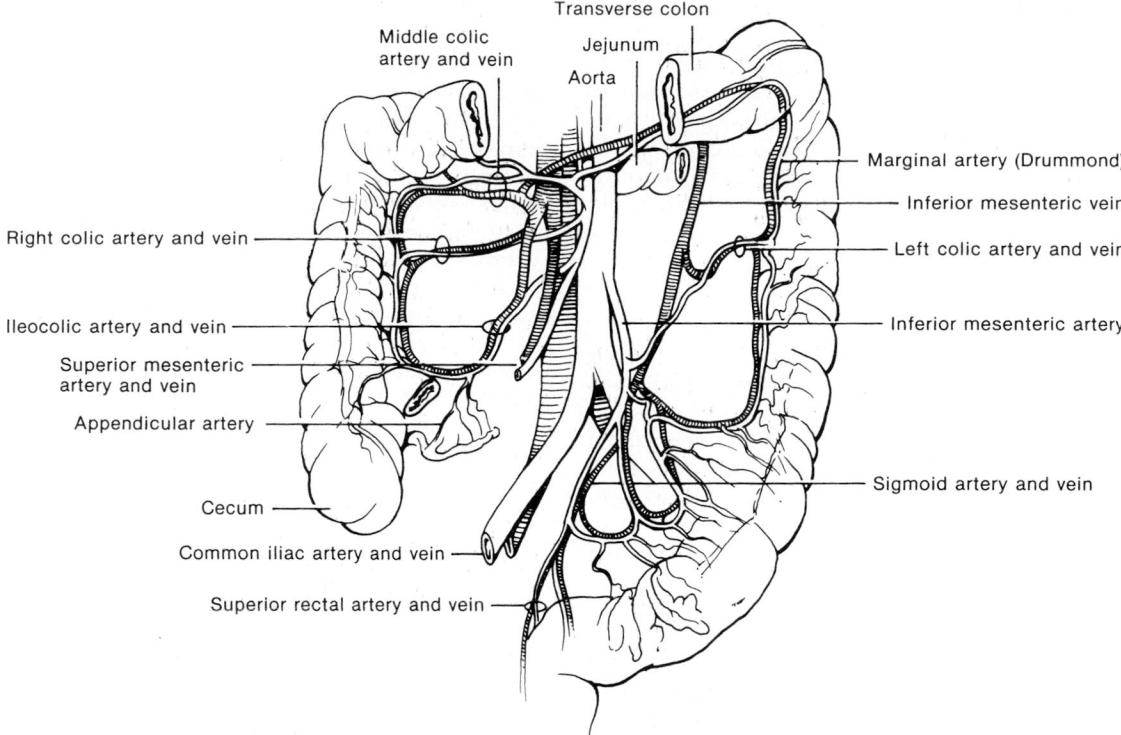

Figure 57.1.   Vascular supply to the colon.

point of frank circulatory shock (16,18,24). Fever and modest tachycardia are often, but not invariably, present (18,24). Abdominal examination is completely normal in only a very few cases. However, abnormalities, when noted, are often mild and belie the catastrophic nature of the disease. Signs of peritoneal irritation are present to some degree in some but not all cases (18,24). Less urgent abdominal findings, such as increased or decreased bowel sounds, localized or diffuse tenderness, distention, bruit, or mass, are present in almost all cases. Most patients have occult blood in the stool, especially later in the course of the process (19).

Approximately 10% of patients present are in crisis, with catastrophic hemodynamic collapse, signs of severe systemic toxicity, altered mental status, and signs of frank peritonitis. Although the need for operative intervention is immediately obvious in this type of presentation, the outcome is universally fatal.

DIFFERENTIAL DIAGNOSIS

The differential diagnosis of abdominal pain in the elderly is notoriously difficult. Symptoms are often vague or poorly represented. The patient may have other serious medical illness or dementia that interferes with the history taking and physical examination. Physical examination is unreliable in the elderly and may be falsely reassuring.

Nevertheless, abdominal pain in a patient older than 50 years of age must be considered representative of an ominous process until thorough medical evaluation proves this not to be the case. The differential diagnosis is myriad and mirrors that of abdominal pain in any other age group with one exception: As the patient ages, the likelihood of vascular disease increases. This introduces the entire spectrum of vascular disorders to the differential diagnostic list: aneurysm, dissection, renal vascular disease, mesenteric vascular disease, myocardial infarction, and systemic embolization. Other considerations, such as diverticuli-

tis, appendicitis, volvulus, obstruction, perforation, peptic ulcer disease, gallbladder disease, pancreatitis, splenic infarction, inflammatory disease, malignancy, gastrointestinal hemorrhage, and functional bowel disease, are discussed elsewhere in this text.

The principal diagnostic approach is the determination of whether a surgical condition is present, and if so, whether the situation is urgent. In mesenteric ischemia, although both of these criteria are present, they are rarely appreciated.

EMERGENCY DEPARTMENT EVALUATION

Patients older than 50 years of age who present with abdominal pain should undergo a timely diagnostic workup to ensure that serious conditions, especially mesenteric ischemia, are not missed. More than 80% of patients presenting to emergency departments with mesenteric ischemia will be misdiagnosed or will undergo extensive and time-consuming evaluations, thereby increasing their risk of mortality (2,7). Even when the condition is suspected, the patient may have a bad outcome. The value of an aggressive approach to the diagnosis and management of AMI is emphasized in the literature (8,9,11,19,24,25).

The ED evaluation is dictated by the patient's condition. When the patient presents in hemodynamic or septic crisis, immediate therapeutic measures must precede definitive diagnosis. Initial resuscitation is described in subsequent text, and should include sending blood to the laboratory and blood bank. Additional studies may be indicated, such as continuous electrocardiographic monitoring and a 12-lead electrocardiogram. The ultimate diagnosis in these cases may be obscured by the systemic nature of the presentation, and the prognosis is grim.

In patients with no hemodynamic compromise, the presentation most suggestive of ischemia is that of *abdominal pain that is disproportionate to physical findings*. Aggressive, early investigation of ischemia should be undertaken in these patients, especially if they are elderly and have risk factors for AMI and if there is not another satisfactory explanation for the pain. Delaying investigation of suspected AMI until more prominent abdominal findings are present will substantially increase mortality (8,19,24,25). In all cases, it is advisable to establish intravenous access, because the patient's condition may deteriorate rapidly, especially if the presenting problem is vascular. After a thorough history and physical examination, laboratory specimens should be obtained, as indicated earlier.

Laboratory Studies

Unfortunately, because laboratory studies are nonspecific their results are little help. Although it has been said that the principal use of the laboratory in mesenteric ischemia is to exclude other entities (19), this is often not possible. In fact, misdiagnosis often follows erroneous interpretation of the laboratory results, such as when a modest elevation of the serum amylase value leads to an incorrect attribution of the patient's condition to acute pancreatitis. Nevertheless, laboratory studies should be performed and carefully interpreted.

The hemoglobin value is almost universally elevated owing to hemoconcentration late in the course of the disease, but it may be normal earlier. Leukocytosis is present in almost all cases and is often marked. Approximately 25% of patients will have white blood cell (WBC) counts of 10,000 to 15,000/μL, 50% will have WBC counts of 15,000 to 30,000/μL, and 25% will exceed 30,000/μL (10). Serum amylase determination will show a modest elevation, in the range from the upper limit of normal to twice normal, about half the time (19). Occasionally, profound elevations are seen. Metabolic acidosis, presumably on the basis of the anaerobic metabolism initiated by the ischemic process, may be present but is not universally so (19,24). Other laboratory findings, such as azotemia, hyperbilirubinemia, elevated enzyme and inorganic phosphate levels, and other, more exotic determinations are of no diagnostic value (8,19,27). In the end, none of these laboratory tests have been shown to be sensitive or specific in discriminating mesenteric ischemia from other intraabdominal pathologic processes (15,19,20,24).

Imaging

Plain radiography is likewise nonspecific. Abdominal gas may be absent, sparse, or normal or may demonstrate an ileus pattern (9,14,19,24). In the majority of cases, the films will be normal or not suggestive of any particular pathologic process (14,19,24). The finding of gas in the intestine wall or in the portal venous system invariably occurs only late in the process (19,24). Thumbprinting of the intestinal mucosa, shown in relief against air or barium, is strongly suggestive but not specific (19,24).

The gold standard in the evaluation of a patient with suspected mesenteric ischemia is aortic and mesenteric biplanar angiography (1,8,9,12,19,24,28). In cases of vascular occlusion, this modality can accurately identify the location of the occlusion and scrutinize atherosclerotic changes in all vessels. Angiography also allows the selective infusion of vasodilating or thrombolytic agents directly into the affected vessels as a therapeutic maneuver (3,23,24).

Computed tomography (CT) scanning is emerging as a reasonable and noninvasive imaging technique to consider in AMI (13,24,28). Intraperitoneal free fluid, visualization of thrombus in splanchnic arteries or veins, and abnormal bowel wall characteristics such as wall thickening, pneumatosis, or streaky mesentery are highly suggestive findings (12,21,28). One series of 54 cases suggested that CT might be as sensitive as angiography in detecting mesenteric infarction (14). In addition, CT has some advantages over angiography in evaluating other possible causes of the abdominal process. CT angiography can increase diagnostic accuracy in demonstrating venous thrombosis, nonenhancement of arteries, or signs of intestinal necrosis, including pneumatosis or portal vein gas (8,13). However, if mesenteric ischemia is strongly suspected, angiography should still be the first-line diagnostic procedure over CT.

Early experience with duplex ultrasound with Doppler signal analysis shows that it has promise as a screening tool for mesenteric ischemia (6,9,10,15). This modality demonstrates low-flow states by estimating splanchnic arterial and venous flow (6,10,15). However, its utility is limited, as there is a great variation in vascular flow between normal and affected subjects. Furthermore, duplex ultrasound cannot demonstrate anatomy to assist in surgical planning, and its image quality can be easily affected by patient movement and bowel gases (14).

Magnetic resonance (MR) and MR angiography are potential imaging techniques for noninvasive screening of mesenteric ischemia (3,4,9). However, limited experience with this modality and its infrequency of emergent availability in most institutions limit the consideration of MR in the diagnosis and management of AMI at this time.

The advantages of using laparoscopy to diagnose mesenteric ischemia include bedside performance in unstable patients, direct visualization of bowel appearance, and serial performances or a second look in following patients' progress (29). Its disadvantages include visualization of the serosal surface only and inability to detect mucosal ischemia, the induction of pneumoperitoneum that may further impair splanchnic blood flow, and inability to detect pulses of the bowel vasculature (29). The concomitant use of pulse oximetry, measurement of intraluminal $PaCO_2$, together with laparoscopy, may enhance diagnostic accuracy, as there is a strong association between gastrointestinal ischemia and an increased intraluminal $PaCO_2$ in animal and human models (15,26).

EMERGENCY DEPARTMENT MANAGEMENT

In the acutely ill patient, resuscitation should be initiated. Patency of the upper airway must be ensured, and the ability of the patient to maintain the airway and to ventilate and oxygenate adequately must be assessed. High-flow oxygen, preferably by mask, should be administered. Examination of the airway and chest, supplemented by determination of arterial blood gases, will determine the need for immediate intubation. Two intravenous lines should be established and crystalloid solution should be administered to replenish intravascular volume. The degree of volume depletion should be determined and, although patients are elderly, crystalloid should be rapidly administered, because the hypovolemia is known to aggravate the mesenteric hypoperfusion. Rapid bedside determination of serum glucose level should be undertaken, with intravenous glucose administered as indicated. Blood samples should be obtained, and laboratory blood tests, including complete blood cell count, and levels of electrolytes, amylase, urea, creatinine, glucose, coagulation parameters, and crossmatch, should be ordered.

Because definitive care for mesenteric ischemia cannot be provided in the ED, the most important aspects of emergency management include a rapid diagnosis or suspicion, aggressive resuscitation, and early surgical consultation.

CRITICAL INTERVENTIONS

- Ultimately, only extreme vigilance will lead to the diagnosis
- Elderly patients who present with abdominal pain, especially those with risk factors for mesenteric ischemia, must undergo a rapid diagnostic sequence leading to a sound provisional diagnosis
- Patients with suspected mesenteric ischemia mandate consideration of early CT angiography or biplanar angiography to confirm or exclude the diagnosis
- Early surgical consultation must be sought in cases of suspected mesenteric ischemia because delay may prove fatal. Waiting for "confirmation" of the diagnosis by development of significant metabolic acidosis, circulatory collapse, frank peritoneal signs, or definitive findings on imaging studies places the patient in profound jeopardy

DISPOSITION

Role of the Consultant

Mesenteric ischemia is a surgical disease. Measures such as thrombolytic agent infusion during angiography should be used only in selective cases in the presence of the surgeon, whereas in most cases revascularization or resection is the mainstay of therapy (1,9,11,19,20,24,27). Surgical and radiographic consultation should be sought early.

Indications for Admission

The decision to admit an elderly patient with undiagnosed abdominal pain should not be difficult. The list of serious causes of abdominal pain in the undiagnosed elderly patient significantly outweighs the list of trivial or benign conditions. In addition, elderly patients with "benign" conditions, such as biliary colic, often fare poorly and deteriorate precipitously. In patients with a clear diagnosis that is not believed to require hospitalization, close consultation with the patient's primary physician and early follow-up examination are mandatory. When the diagnosis is in doubt, or when the patient carries an established prior diagnosis such as "diverticulosis" but appears to be developing another acute process, admission and early surgical consultation are indicated.

Transfer Considerations

If facilities for vascular surgery or invasive radiography are not present in the institution of presentation, immediate general surgical consultation should be sought. The advisability of transfer of the patient versus laparotomy without preceding angiography depends on local circumstances and the patient's condition.

COMMON PITFALLS

✔ Failure to make the diagnosis while the patient is still salvageable. Extreme vigilance, appropriate selection and interpretation of the diagnostic imaging, and institution of an aggressive therapeutic approach improve diagnostic accuracy and decrease morbidity. Admission of a patient with suspicion of

mesenteric ischemia to a hospital mandates immediate surgical consultation
✔ Reluctance to obtain CT angiography or biplanar angiography. Early radiographic consultation and refusal to "wait until morning" are essential to early diagnosis and a good outcome

Acknowledgment

Thank you to previous edition author Ron M. Walls.

References

1. Batellier J, Kieny R. Superior mesenteric artery embolism: eighty-two cases. *Ann Vasc Surg* 1990;4:112–116.
2. Boley SJ, Kaleya RN, Brandt LJ. Mesenteric venous thrombosis. *Surg Clin North Am* 1992;72:183–201.
3. Bull PG, Hagmuller GW, Kreuzer W. New aspects in the diagnosis and management of acute mesenteric infarction. *Int J Angiol* 1993;2:51–60.
4. Burkart DJ, Johnson CD, Reading CC, Ehman RL. MR measurements of mesenteric venous flow: prospective evaluation in healthy volunteers and patients with suspected chronic mesenteric ischemia. *Radiology* 1995;194:801–806.
5. Cleveland TJ, Nawaz S, Gaines PA. Mesenteric arterial ischaemia: diagnosis and therapeutic options. *Vasc Med* 2002;7:311–321.
6. Danse EM, Laterre PF, Van Beers BE, et al. Early diagnosis of acute intestinal ischaemia: contribution of colour Doppler sonography. *Acta Chir Belg* 1997;97:173–176.
7. Edwards MS, Cherr GS, Craven TE, et al. Acute occlusive mesenteric ischemia: surgical management and outcomes. *Ann Vasc Surg* 2003;17:72–79.
8. Eldrup-Jorgensen J, Hawkins RE, Bredenberg CE. Abdominal vascular catastrophes. *Surg Clin North Am* 1997;77:1305–1320.
9. Geelkerken RH, van Bockel JH. Mesenteric vascular disease: a review of diagnostic methods and therapies. *Cardiovasc Surg* 1995;3:247–260.
10. Gentile AT, Moneta GL, Lee RW, et al. Usefulness of fasting and postprandial duplex ultrasound examinations for predicting high-grade superior mesenteric artery stenosis. *Am J Surg* 1995;169:476–479.
11. Kaleya RN, Boley SJ. Acute mesenteric ischemia. *Crit Care Clin* 1995;11:479–512.
12. Kim AY, Ha HK. Evaluate of suspected mesenteric ischemia: efficacy of radiologic studies. *Radiol Clin North Am* 2003;41:327–342.
13. Kirkpatrick ID, Kroeker MA, Greenberg HM. Biphasic CT with mesenteric CT angiography in the evaluation of acute mesenteric ischemia: initial experience. *Radiology* 2003;229:91–98.
14. Klein HM, Lensing R, Klosterhalfen B, et al. Diagnostic imaging of mesenteric infarction. *Radiology* 1995;197:79–82.
15. Kolkman JJ, Groeneveld ABJ. Occlusive and non-occlusive gastrointestinal ischaemia: a clinical review with special emphasis on the diagnostic value of tonometry. *Scand J Gastroenterol Suppl* 1998;225:3–12.
16. Kolkman JJ, Mensink PBF. Non-occlusive mesenteric ischaemia: a common disorder in gastroenterology and intensive care. *Best Pract Res Clin Gastroenterol* 2003;17:457–473.
17. Li KL. Mesenteric occlusive disease. *MRI Clin North Am* 1998;6:331–338.
18. Lock G. Acute mesenteric ischaemia: classification, evaluation and therapy. *Acta Gastroenterol Belg* 2002;65:220–225.
19. Montgomery RA, Venbrux AB, Bulkley GB. Mesenteric vascular insufficiency. *Curr Probl Surg* 1997;34:941–1025.
20. Newman TS, Magnuson TH, Ahrendt SA, et al. The changing face of mesenteric infarction. *Am Surg* 1998;64:611–616.
21. Rhee RY, Gloviczki MD. Mesenteric venous thrombosis. *Surg Clin North Am* 1997;77:327–338.
22. Sanders BM, Dalsing MC. Mesenteric ischemia affects young adults with predisposition. *Ann Vasc Surg* 2003;17:270–276.
23. Savassi-Rocha PR, Veloso LF. Treatment of superior mesenteric artery embolism with a fibrinolytic agent: case report and literature review. *Hepatogastroenterology* 2002;49:1307–1310.
24. Sreenarasimhaiah J. Diagnosis and management of intestinal ischaemic disorders. *BMJ* 2003;326:1372–1376.
25. Tendler DA. Acute intestinal ischemia and infarction. *Semin Gastrointest Dis* 2003;14:66–76.
26. Tollefson DFJ, Wright DJ, Reddy DJ, Kintanar EB. Intraoperative determination of intestinal viability by pulse oximetry. *Ann Vasc Surg* 1995;9:357–360.
27. Urayama H, Ohtake H, Kawakami T, et al. Acute mesenteric vascular occlusion: analysis of 39 patients. *Eur J Surg* 1998;164:195–200.
28. Wiesner W, Khurana B, Ji H, Ros PR. CT of acute bowel ischemia. *Radiology* 2003;226:635–650.
29. Zamir G, Reissman P. Diagnostic laparoscopy in mesenteric ischemia. *Surg Endosc* 1998;12:309.

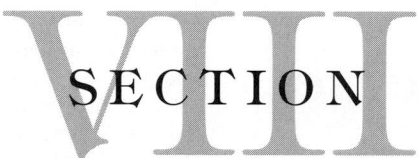

SECTION

VIII

Section Editor: Gregory W. Hendey

Gastrointestinal Emergencies

CHAPTER 58
Esophageal Disease

Charles M. Seamens and Marc Mickiewicz

Patients with esophageal disease generally present to the emergency department in one of four ways: (i) odynophagia, (ii) heartburn or chest pain, (iii) dysphagia, or (iv) gastrointestinal (GI) bleeding. There is often a great deal of overlap in these symptoms, however. For example, disorders causing mucosal destruction may result not only in odynophagia, but also in dysphagia, whereas certain motor disorders may cause both dysphagia and chest pain. Esophageal disease that causes bleeding is usually due to varices, and is discussed in Chapters 59, "Upper Gastrointestinal Bleeding" and 65, "Hepatic Failure and Cirrhosis."

ODYNOPHAGIA

Clinical Presentation

Odynophagia refers to pain on swallowing and implies mucosal disease of the oropharynx or esophagus. Inflammation of adjacent structures may produce symptoms indistinguishable from mucosal inflammation. The pain may be described as a retrosternal ache, a burning sensation, or a stabbing pain with radiation to the back. Esophagitis typically presents as odynophagia, with or without dysphagia. Other common complaints include atypical chest pain, a sensation of feeling each bolus of food as it passes down, heartburn, or, occasionally, anorexia and weight loss. The most important immediate consequences of esophagitis are local pain and impaired oral alimentation. Rarely, the initial manifestation of esophageal disease is GI bleeding.

Infectious esophagitis should always be a consideration in immunocompromised individuals. In esophageal candidiasis, odynophagia is usually relatively mild. If symptoms are so severe that the patient consciously limits oral intake, ulcerative esophagitis of some other etiology is likely. Oropharyngeal candidiasis is noted in many patients with *candidal esophagitis*, but it is not a very good predictor of its presence. About 25% of patients with candidal esophagitis will not have oral *thrush*, so its absence does not rule out this entity (21).

Herpetic esophagitis is the most common viral infection affecting the esophagus, and presents with odynophagia that is typically abrupt in onset. It is also suspected when symptoms of dysphagia or odynophagia do not improve with typical antifungal medications in immunocompromised patients (8). Immunocompetent patients often give a history of an upper respiratory tract infection before the onset of swallowing problems, and most have skin or oral lesions of herpes simplex virus (HSV) infection. In contrast, oropharyngeal and perioral lesions are frequently absent in immunosuppressed patients.

Cytomegalovirus (CMV) esophagitis presents in a similar fashion, with odynophagia, dysphagia, and variable degrees of substernal chest pain, but nausea and vomiting seem to be more common in CMV esophagitis.

Complications of candidal or viral esophagitis are uncommon; they include hemorrhage, perforation, esophageal narrowing with stricture formation, and dissemination of infection.

The true incidence of *medication-induced* esophageal injury is unknown because many cases are not reported in the literature and many more go unrecognized. Tablets and capsules can adhere to the esophageal wall and dissolve locally despite normal esophageal function. Although patients with structural abnormalities and motility disorders are more likely to develop medication-induced esophagitis, most patients have normal esophageal motility. The elderly are at increased risk.

Patients with pill esophagitis typically report retrosternal pain, odynophagia, and dysphagia that are temporally related to ingestion of medication. A significant proportion gives a history of taking the medication with little or no water. Symptoms generally improve within a couple of days, provided the medication is discontinued, but complete resolution may take several weeks, and there are no sequelae. Pill esophagitis may affect the proximal esophagus, usually at the level of the aortic arch or left atrium, in contrast to reflux esophagitis, which affects the distal esophagus. The most common complication is stricture formation.

Odynophagia is usually not a prominent component of *reflux esophagitis*, which is discussed elsewhere in this chapter.

Differential Diagnosis

The differential diagnosis of odynophagia includes diffuse infectious causes and localized trauma or inflammation. Candidal esophagitis is increasing in incidence, probably because of aggressive immunosuppressive therapy in patients with cancer and the emergence of acquired immunodeficiency syndrome (AIDS). HSV esophagitis is less common, and CMV is another important cause of infectious esophagitis in patients with AIDS as well as in patients who have undergone bone marrow transplantation.

Pill-induced esophagitis may be confused with other causes of esophagitis if the patient does not relate the ingestion of medication with symptoms. As with other causes of esophageal pain, cardiac disease must be excluded. The age and sex of patients with drug-induced esophagitis reflects the population group most likely to receive commonly prescribed drugs. Doxycycline and tetracycline are more commonly prescribed in younger patients for sexually transmitted diseases and respiratory infections. Potassium chloride and quinidine tablets, which also cause a large number of cases of pill-induced esophagitis, are more frequently used in elderly patients. Alendronate (Fosamax) is an agent used to treat osteoporosis, and it can cause severe esophageal injury (7). Ferrous sulfate, aspirin, and nonsteroidal antiinflammatory drugs (NSAIDs)are used by patients of all ages.

Odynophagia localized to the posterior pharynx may be caused by a pharyngitis or abscess. Epiglottitis is another potential concern. The patient should also be asked about the possibility of ingestion of foreign bodies or food impaction (see Chapter 75, "Gastrointestinal Foreign Bodies").

EMERGENCY DEPARTMENT EVALUATION

The initial history should focus first on the duration and severity of the symptoms and on the patient's ability to maintain normal oral intake. The patient should be asked about a history of diagnosed human immunodeficiency virus (HIV) infection, risk factors for HIV, or other conditions associated with an immunocompromised state. Patients should be further questioned about a possible association of symptoms with pill ingestion or possible foreign bodies, as well as any symptoms suggestive of esophageal reflux.

Esophageal candidiasis is common in patients with AIDS and other immunocompromised individuals, but severe odynophagia that results in diminished oral intake or dehydration is uncommon in patients with candidal esophagitis alone. More than one potential pathogen may be identified in severely symptomatic patients.

The physical examination should concentrate initially on the patient's state of hydration. Blood pressure, pulse, and orthostatic changes should be noted, as well as skin turgor and the condition of the mucous membranes.

The oropharynx should be examined for oral candidal or herpetic lesions, and signs of cancer or AIDS or other possible opportunistic infections should be sought. A soft-tissue lateral neck radiograph should be obtained if a retropharyngeal or prevertebral abscess or epiglottitis is a consideration. If hydration is adequate and the patient does not otherwise appear ill, evaluation may continue on an outpatient basis.

Two options are available for further evaluation of odynophagia: barium swallow and esophagoscopy. The advantages of the barium swallow are its lower cost, lesser degree of invasiveness, and decreased risk to health-care workers and other patients. However, findings on barium swallow are often nonspecific, making endoscopy necessary. Air-contrast barium studies also provide more sensitivity, but patients with severe odynophagia are often unable to perform these tests. Endoscopy allows one to obtain tissue samples for cytology or culture and is thus usually more useful in making a specific diagnosis. Other parts of the upper GI tract can be examined at the same time, increasing diagnostic ability without adding much to the cost, duration, or risk of the procedure.

Serologic tests for CMV and HSV, although commercially available, play little role in the diagnosis of acute esophageal disease.

EMERGENCY DEPARTMENT MANAGEMENT

A number of antifungal agents have been used to treat oral and esophageal candidiasis in patients with AIDS. Fluconazole is now the drug of choice. Clinical experience with local therapy, such as nystatin and clotrimazole lozenges, suggests some efficacy against oropharyngeal candidiasis, but these are generally considered inadequate for esophageal candidiasis. Symptoms may clear and oropharyngeal candidiasis may be eradicated, even in the presence of persistent endoscopically visible esophageal disease. Fluconazole is also associated with a higher cure rate than other antifungal agents, such as itraconazole (2). The usual dose is 200 mg the first day, followed by 100 mg daily for 14 to 21 days. Other antifungal options exist, but they are generally tolerated less well and have more undesirable side effects. The combination of itraconazole and flucytosine may be an effective alternative if fluconazole cannot be used (3). Patients who are granulocytopenic or who are otherwise at high risk for disseminated candidiasis are candidates for intravenous amphotericin B, as are those who are not at high risk but cannot take oral medications. Caspofungin is a newer agent that compares well with amphotericin B and had fewer side effects in a recent clinical trial (1). All systemic antifungal prescriptions should be written with care and checked against the patient's other medications, for many can cause potentially serious drug–drug interactions.

Foscarnet and ganciclovir appear to be similarly effective and safe in the treatment of AIDS-related CMV esophagitis. Consequently, the choice of the anti-CMV agent should be tailored to the individual patient according to side-effect profiles (17). HSV esophagitis may be self-limited in the immunocompetent host, but therapy with oral or intravenous acyclovir should be instituted in immunocompromised patients.

In patients presenting with mild esophageal symptoms that do not limit oral intake, an empiric trial of antifungal therapy with fluconazole is reasonable regardless of the presence or absence of oral candidiasis. If symptoms improve after 7 to 10 days of treatment, a presumptive diagnosis of esophageal candidiasis may be made and the patient is continued on chronic suppressive therapy. If symptoms have not responded to a short course of empiric therapy, the patient should proceed to endoscopy to investigate the possibility of other causes.

If *pill-induced esophagitis* is recognized early and is treated appropriately, it is generally reversible. The offending medication should be discontinued or changed to liquid form when possible. Because swallowing and salivation occur less during sleep, patients should be instructed not to take medications immediately before bedtime. Other commonsense caveats apply: Small tablets are swallowed more quickly than larger ones, oval pills better than round ones, and coated pills faster than uncoated pills. Patients should also be instructed to take medications with plenty of water and to avoid lying down shortly after ingesting their pills. Symptomatic resolution and endoscopic healing of pill esophagitis is usually evident in 3 days to 6 weeks (20).

CRITICAL INTERVENTION

- Identify immunocompromised patients at risk for candida and herpes esophagitis

DISPOSITION

Immunocompetent patients with mild symptoms may be treated as outpatients. Referral and followup are appropriate for these patients, as well as for those who do not respond to initial therapy.

Patients who are experiencing severe difficulty with swallowing and who are unable to maintain hydration require hospital admission. Patients at risk for disseminated infection should be admitted for intravenous therapy.

Patients with pill esophagitis should be referred to their primary care physician to ensure that timely resolution of symptoms occurs.

COMMON PITFALLS

✔ Pain on swallowing is not always caused by pharyngitis. Immunocompromised patients at risk for infectious esophagitis should be identified
✔ Foreign bodies and food impaction are not uncommon, especially in the elderly and the alcoholic, whose oropharyngeal tactile sense is blunted. Pill esophagitis is likewise an underappreciated problem

ESOPHAGEAL CHEST PAIN

Clinical Presentation

The two most common esophageal disorders in patients presenting with angina-like chest pain are *gastroesophageal reflux* and esophageal motility disorders such as *achalasia* and *esophageal spasm*.

Symptomatic gastroesophageal reflux disease (GERD) is common. It is estimated that 10% of the general population has daily heartburn and that at least one third of the population experiences heartburn once a month. Acid reflux can be detected in the distal esophagus for up to 75 minutes a day in healthy individuals, and many patients who suffer complications of acid reflux never experience heartburn or reflux (19). It has been widely held that nocturnal reflux is the most important factor in the pathogenesis of reflux disease. Twenty-four-hour esophageal pH has shown, however, that, in the majority of patients (those who have mild erosive esophagitis or no endoscopic abnormality), most reflux occurs in the daytime postprandial periods, and especially in the early evening, with relatively little reflux during the night. More severe esophagitis, which is caused by greater acid exposure, is, however, associated with an increase in nocturnal reflux.

There has also been much debate about the relationship between the presence of hiatal hernia and GERD. Hiatal hernias seen on routine chest radiography do not correlate well with clinical reflux disease. However, approximately 80% of patients with hiatal hernia have an abnormal reflux frequency (as measured with 24-hour pH monitoring), compared with only about 40% of those without hernias.

The primary determinant of GERD is the structural and functional integrity of the lower esophageal sphincter (LES). The most important factor contributing to GERD is transient relaxation of the esophagogastric junction (8,24). The incidence of GERD rises dramatically after age 40. Factors that influence the degree of reflux injury include the volume and pH of the gastric refluxate, the efficiency of gastroesophageal clearance, and the resistance and restorative repair capabilities of the esophageal epithelium. Patients with severe complications of GERD generally have an incompetent LES (24). Esophagitis results from excessive reflux of gastric juice (12).

Patients typically suffer from GERD for years before seeking medical assistance. The predominant complaint is that of pyrosis, or "heartburn," which results from mucosal irritation caused by refluxed gastric contents. The discomfort is usually described as a burning pain felt behind the sternum, often seeming to ascend from the epigastrium toward the throat, where a bitter taste may be sensed, and sometimes radiating to the back. There may be radiation of the discomfort to the neck or left arm. The intensity is variable, ranging from a dull ache to severe pain; the duration of discomfort may be minutes or hours. Symptoms may occur spontaneously and are rarely precipitated by swallowing, although they may also seem to be brought on by exercise, bending, or lying down. A large meal, as well as certain foods, such as chocolate, peppermint, alcohol, onions, and fat, increase esophageal acid exposure, whereas cola, beer, and milk increase gastric acid secretion. Orange juice, tomato juice, and coffee have a direct irritative effect on the esophagus (24). Heartburn often disappears quickly on drinking liquids or antacids. It is of interest that only 30% to 40% of patients who complain of heartburn have demonstrable mucosal injury of the esophagus, and, conversely, reflux disease can occur without heartburn. Strictures, manifested clinically by dysphagia, are the most common complication of reflux esophagitis. They appear to be caused by a combination of deep esophageal mural inflammation, fibrosis, spasm, and edema.

Motility disorders comprise the second group of esophageal disorders and present predominantly as chest pain. *Achalasia* means "failure to relax" and is a disorder characterized by the absence of peristalsis throughout the esophagus and, usually, deficient LES relaxation during swallowing. It is associated with chest pain in about one half of patients with the condition, although the pain is rarely severe and may vary in quality. Chest pressure may be caused by esophageal dilation from delayed emptying of food; heartburn or odynophagia may result from stasis esophagitis and bacterial overgrowth or esophageal pill retention. Achalasia is eventually diagnosed in up to 10% of patients with noncardiac chest pain.

The primary neurologic defect responsible for achalasia remains unknown. The most consistent pathologic finding is a decrease of ganglion cells in the myenteric plexus at the LES. The disorder may occur at any age, but its exact incidence and prevalence are unknown. The disease typically follows an indolent course; at the time of presentation, symptoms have usually been present for an average of about 7 years. Longitudinal population studies of patients with achalasia suggest that the disease does not affect life expectancy.

Diffuse esophageal spasm is characterized by simultaneous contractions in the body of the esophagus occurring with at least 30% of swallows. The contractions are frequently repetitive, spontaneous, of prolonged duration, or of high amplitude. Patients present with dysphagia or intermittent chest pain. The chest pain is not necessarily related to eating, although it may be triggered by the ingestion of very hot or very cold liquids. The diagnosis of diffuse esophageal spasm requires that both clinical and manometric criteria be fulfilled, because asymptomatic individuals can display similar manometric features. No organic lesion is demonstrable radiographically, endoscopically, or histologically. In *nutcracker esophagus*, motility is ordered and peristaltic, but the waves are of longer duration and of higher amplitude than normal.

Differential Diagnosis

A cardiac etiology must always be excluded when a patient presents with burning substernal chest pain. Chest pain of esophageal origin may be impossible to distinguish from angina by history alone. One must remember that the administration of an antacid or "GI cocktail" is a therapeutic intervention and not a diagnostic procedure. It has been documented that cardiac chest pain can respond to these preparations, for reasons that are open to speculation.

Even among patients with a history that is classic for cardiac ischemia, a significant percentage (approaching 30% in some studies) who undergo cardiac catheterization have normal or clinically nonsignificant occlusions (5,8). Unfortunately, there are no characteristic features of chest pain that are pathognomonic of esophageal disorders, including response to antacids, nitroglycerin, or calcium channel blockers. Even pain that is associated with dysphagia and is unrelated to exertion may be ischemic in origin.

EMERGENCY DEPARTMENT EVALUATION

If a cardiac cause can be excluded and the patient gives a history of heartburn without dysphagia, weight loss, or GI bleeding, no laboratory or imaging studies are needed in the emergency department.

Further evaluation is needed if heartburn persists after treatment or if it recurs when treatment is stopped. Heartburn refractory to treatment, or heartburn accompanied by dysphagia, odynophagia, or GI bleeding, requires endoscopy to exclude other causes (12). However, endoscopy shows no evidence of ulcerations in most patients who seek treatment for uncomplicated reflux symptoms (19). The most useful tests for diagnosing reflux disease are barium swallow, endoscopy, and 24-hour gastric pH monitoring, all of which are performed on an outpatient basis.

Evaluation of esophageal motility disorders usually employs esophageal manometry and is also carried out on an outpatient basis.

EMERGENCY DEPARTMENT MANAGEMENT

Mild symptomatic esophagitis can usually be managed empirically with lifestyle and dietary modifications, antacids, and non-prescription H_2-antagonists (12,16).

Lifestyle modifications alone are rarely sufficient to relieve symptoms of mild GERD, but they can be an adjunct to pharmacologic management (4). Patients are often advised to raise the head of the bed approximately 6 inches or to elevate their shoulders with a wedge. The effects of these maneuvers on esophageal acid exposure are modest and appear to be greater when the patient has severe disease. This is consistent with pH monitoring studies that show that, in the majority of patients, most acid exposure occurs during the daytime. The nonpharmacologic measures most likely to benefit the patient are a reduction in fat intake, elimination of tobacco use, and elevation of the head of the bed (19).

Antacids provide rapid relief and are useful in controlling daytime symptoms, but they are inadequate for patients with moderate-to-severe symptoms, who require around-the-clock therapy. For mild reflux esophagitis, H_2-antagonists, prokinetic agents, or sucralfate may be used initially. Superior healing rates of erosive esophagitis have been noted with H_2-blockers, and they are generally considered the first line initial therapy for patients with symptomatic reflux. However, because H_2-antagonists at higher doses than those used in peptic ulcer disease are needed for more severe esophagitis, proton pump inhibitors (PPIs) may be a more cost-effective alternative for long-term therapy in patients. In general, they result in faster healing rates and greater symptom relief than H_2-antagonists, and are employed whenever H_2-antagonists fail to completely alleviate symptoms (9,13,19,24). There are a number of PPIs now on the market: omeprazole (now available over the counter), lansoprazole, pantoprazole, rabeprazole, and esomeprazole. All likely have similar efficacy for the treatment of reflux esophagitis (11).

Therapy is usually continued for 6 to 8 weeks. All patients who do not respond to a 4-week trial of PPIs for typical GERD symptoms should be considered for endoscopy to establish a diagnosis (14,24). These patients may also require higher dosages of PPIs than previously were recommended for acid control and symptom relief (13).

Sucralfate, which inhibits pepsin, as well as absorbs and inactivates bile salts, has been shown to be superior to placebo and comparable to antacids and H_2 blockers. Metoclopramide increases LES pressure and accelerates gastric emptying in retention states. Its effectiveness is not clearcut, and it has a relatively high side-effect profile; it is not recommended as first-line therapy.

The treatment of esophageal motility disorders is discussed in the next section.

CRITICAL INTERVENTION

- Consider cardiac ischemia in the differential of patients with symptoms of GERD
- Initiate treatment of GERD with antacids, H_2-antagonists, or PPIs, depending upon the severity of symptoms

DISPOSITION

If the diagnosis of GI chest pain is not in doubt, the patient can be discharged and referred to the primary care physician. For resistant symptoms or suspected complications of reflux esophagitis, the patient may be referred to a gastroenterologist for endoscopy or 24-hour pH monitoring.

COMMON PITFALL

✔ Attributing the pain of cardiac ischemia to a GI source, especially when substernal burning or atypical chest pain appears to be relieved by antacids or a "GI cocktail"

DYSPHAGIA

Clinical Presentation

Dysphagia refers to difficulty or impairment in swallowing. Difficulty in moving a food bolus from the mouth to the upper part of the esophagus is termed *oropharyngeal* dysphagia, whereas a problem with the passage of food or liquid down the esophagus to the stomach is referred to as *esophageal* dysphagia. Oropharyngeal dysphagia is often accompanied by drooling, nasal regurgitation, inability to initiate swallowing, coughing during swallowing, aspiration pneumonia, and dysarthria or nasal speech. There may be weight loss owing to fear of eating (15).

In esophageal dysphagia, when the esophagus does not empty in a coordinated, sequential manner, dysphagia may be accompanied by odynophagia, heartburn, GI chest pain, or nausea and vomiting. *Globus hystericus* is the constant sensation of a lump in the throat, associated with the need to swallow with no identifiable cause. In contrast to true dysphagia, there is no difficulty when swallowing is actually performed (25).

Dysphagia is often the principal presenting symptom of esophageal motility disorders, which usually present during middle age and are more common in women (20). These include primary esophageal disorders, such as achalasia, diffuse esophageal spasm, and nutcracker esophagus, as well as esophageal dysfunction secondary to other conditions, most notably scleroderma. Although patients with these disorders frequently experience dysphagia, not all patients with abnormal motility have symptoms.

Achalasia, discussed previously and characterized by deficient peristalsis and failure of the LES to relax on swallowing, is the best studied disorder of esophageal motility. Dysphagia to both liquids and solids is present in nearly all patients with achalasia, but is usually intermittent at first and typically worsens with time. The site of obstruction is often correctly located by the patient in the xiphoid area. Patients with achalasia learn maneuvers to assist esophageal emptying, such as throwing the shoulders back, extending the neck, or performing a Valsalva maneuver (20).

Food eventually empties into the stomach as gravity aids in its passage through the nonrelaxing sphincter, but stagnant undigested food may also be regurgitated. This occurs most commonly at night because of the recumbent position; vomitus may be noted on the pillow on awakening in the morning. Not surprisingly, aspiration is a complication of achalasia and may present as cough, pneumonia, or lung abscess. Weight loss is also a feature of the motility disorders and is results not only from the physical difficulty of swallowing, but also from decreased oral intake because of fear of dysphagia and chest pain.

Nutcracker esophagus and diffuse esophageal spasm, also discussed previously, are also characterized by dysphagia and intermittent chest pain but are much less well studied than achalasia.

Obstructive dysphagia may be caused by *benign* structural lesions of the esophagus, including *esophageal webs* and *rings* and intramural hematomas and dissections (23). Webs are squamous mucosal protuberances that are either congenital or acquired, usually single, and are located in the proximal 2 to 4 cm of the esophagus. Rings could easily be called distal esophageal webs; however, these terms are entrenched in the literature. The typical ring lies within the LES at the squamocolumnar junction. Like a web, it is a mucosal lesion. Its cause is unknown, but a hiatal hernia is usually present. Rings greater than 20 mm in diameter are rarely symptomatic; those less than 13 mm in diameter almost always cause dysphagia (20,25). Rings are probably congenital, but the elasticity of the ring decreases with age, explaining why symptoms rarely occur before age 40 (10).

Intramural hematomas and dissections are rare submucosal lesions of the esophagus. Esophageal hematomas and dissections present in much the same manner as esophageal perforations. Nonbloody emesis followed acutely by chest pain, often radiating to the back, dominates the clinical picture of both conditions. Patients with perforations, however, appear more toxic, and their condition deteriorates rapidly. *Esophageal carcinoma* is a very important cause of dysphagia and is important to recognize early in its course, because the prognosis is dismal by the time a patient presents with progressive dysphagia. Squamous cell carcinoma accounts for most malignant lesions of the esophagus; adenocarcinoma arising from *Barrett esophagus* comprises the remainder. Squamous cell tumors are equally distributed among the upper, middle, and lower thirds of the esophagus. Heavy alcohol intake and smoking significantly increase the likelihood of squamous cell carcinoma of the esophagus, whereas adenocarcinoma tends to occur in patients with a long history of GERD (25).

The symptoms of esophageal carcinoma are usually insidious in onset. Initially, substernal discomfort and slight alterations in eating habits may go unrecognized. Patients may complain of substernal burning that mimics reflux esophagitis. Carcinoma should be suspected if reflux esophagitis is refractory to therapy or if symptoms change. In addition to dysphagia, anorexia and weight loss are other common manifestations. As the esophageal lumen progressively narrows, clearance of liquids and, eventually, even secretions becomes difficult, leading to recurrent aspiration pneumonia. As with other esophageal disorders, physical examination is unrevealing except for signs of malnutrition. Laboratory evaluation may reveal anemia secondary to blood loss from the tumor.

Differential Diagnosis

In 80% of cases of *oropharyngeal dysphagia*, the underlying cause is neuromuscular, including central, peripheral, and motor endplate disorders. Central neuromuscular causes include cerebrovascular accidents or tumors (usually in the region of the brainstem), Parkinson disease, multiple sclerosis, and amyotrophic lateral sclerosis.

If the history suggests *esophageal dysphagia*, the distinction must be made between motor disorders and obstructive lesions. The history is often helpful, because chest pain is a more significant and more frequent complaint in patients with motility disorders. The dysphagia associated with achalasia tends to occur with solids and liquids from the outset, whereas progressive, obstructive lesions present as difficulty swallowing solids, which then progresses to difficulty swallowing solids, liquids, and secretions.

EMERGENCY DEPARTMENT EVALUATION

The evaluation of dysphagia should begin, as always, with attention to the airway, breathing, and circulation and particularly to

hydration status. A basic history should be obtained and physical examination should be performed. As in evaluating patients with symptoms suggestive of reflux, a cardiac cause of chest pain should first be considered before implicating the esophagus. If, after initial questioning, esophageal dysphagia is suspected, a chest radiograph should be obtained once the patient's condition has been stabilized. Radiographic hints that achalasia may be present include a widened mediastinum (caused by a dilated esophagus), the presence of an air-fluid level in the posterior mediastinum (caused by the dilated, fluid-filled esophagus), and the absence of a gastric air bubble (because swallowed air cannot get into the stomach). A chest radiograph may also reveal an extrinsic mass causing compression of the esophagus.

The remainder of the diagnostic evaluation can generally take place on an outpatient basis. Double-contrast barium esophagography provides excellent visualization of structural lesions and should be the initial test performed in patients with esophageal dysphagia or odynophagia (22). An upper GI series is not a suitable substitute for a barium esophagram, because this study focuses on the stomach (20,25).

Patients with suspected motility disorders are better studied with dynamic techniques or cinefluorography. In achalasia, results of these studies reveal a paucity of peristaltic movements and a dilated, fluid-filled esophagus tapering to a characteristic "bird's beak" narrowing at the LES. Patients with diffuse esophageal spasm demonstrate diffuse, powerful contractions, appearing as "curling," that obliterate normal peristaltic contractions (14).

Esophageal manometry is the gold standard for diagnosing motility disorders. However, it will provide a diagnosis in only 25% of patients and findings are normal in half of those patients referred for dysphagia. Provocative testing during manometry, using edrophonium, esophageal balloon distention, or acid perfusion, may further clarify the diagnosis (25).

Obstructive lesions can be further evaluated by barium swallow under fluoroscopy, which can usually be performed on an outpatient basis. Esophageal rings, webs, and carcinoma may be seen; occasionally, some findings, such as proximal dilation with rapid tapering at the LES, may mimic achalasia. More typical findings of mass lesions are asymmetric stenosis, distinct mucosal irregularities, strictures, and masses. If any suspicious abnormality is seen after the barium study, the patient should undergo upper GI endoscopy for biopsy and cytologic brushings.

Endoscopy is indicated in all patients with food impaction, whether the food bolus is eventually passed or not, because this may be the first sign of an obstructive lesion.

EMERGENCY DEPARTMENT MANAGEMENT

In patients in whom normal alimentary intake has been prevented, attention should initially focus on hydration and nutritional status.

Pharmacologic options for managing painful motility disorders are directed principally at reducing smooth muscle spasm or decreasing LES pressure. Treatment of diffuse esophageal spasm is aimed at decreasing the amplitude of esophageal contractions by the use of nitrates and calcium channel blockers. Patients for whom medical therapy fails can be treated with myotomy or dilations (15,21). Treatments for achalasia include sublingual isosorbide dinitrate and calcium channel blockers with meals or as needed. Other useful medications include anticholinergics, psychotropics, and analgesics (5,6,8,20). Botulinum toxin administered by endoscopic injection may give relief of dysphagia (8,18,20). Pneumatic dilation is a final therapeutic avenue.

Although some squamous cell carcinomas are responsive to chemotherapy, most esophageal cancers are incurable. Esophageal dilation is an integral part of most palliative treatment programs. A small amount of bleeding is commonly seen after dilation, but massive bleeding is unusual. The major risk of esophageal dilation is perforation, which occurs at a rate of one in every 400 to 1,000 dilations.

CRITICAL INTERVENTIONS

- Hospitalize patients with severe dysphagia that prevents adequate intake of food and liquids

DISPOSITION

Patients with dysphagia whose hydration and nutritional status are adequate may be discharged home and should be referred to their primary care physician or gastroenterologist for further evaluation and treatment. If coronary artery disease cannot be ruled out, the patient should be admitted to a monitored bed; a cardiac evaluation must be undertaken before a GI workup is launched.

COMMON PITFALLS

✔ Failure to consider cardiac ischemia in patients who describe chronic, intermittent, nonspecific chest discomfort
✔ Failure to evaluate and refer patients with mild dysphagia, in whom a potentially treatable obstructive lesion may be the cause
✔ Attribution of persistent symptoms of dysphagia to "globus hystericus" or anxiety without referring the patient for further testing

Acknowledgment

Thank you to previous edition chapter author Allan B. Wolfson.

References

1. Arathoon EG, Gotuzzo B, Noriega LM. Randomized, double-blind, multicenter study of caspofungin versus amphotericin B for treatment of oropharyngeal and esophageal candidiases. *Antimicrob Agents Chemother* 2002;46:451–457.
2. Barbaro G, Barbarini G, Calderon W. Fluconazole vs itraconazole for candida esophagitis in acquired immunodeficiency syndrome. *Gastroenterology* 1996;111:1169–1177.
3. Barbaro G, Barbarini G, DiLorenzo G. Fluconazole vs itraconazole-flucytosine association in the treatment of esophageal candidiasis in AIDS patients: a double blind, multi-center placebo-controlled study. *Chest* 1996;110:1507–1514.
4. Boyce HW. Therapeutic approaches to healing esophagus. *Am J Gastroenterol* 1997;92[Suppl 4]:S22–S27.
5. Bremner RM, DeMeester TR. Current management of patients with esophageal motor abnormalities. *Adv Surg* 1996;30:349–384.
6. Clement DJ. Achalasia management: difficult no matter how you slice it [letter]. *Am J Gastroenterol* 1998;93:478–480.
7. de Groen PC, Lubbe DF, Hirsch U, et al. Esophagitis associated with the use of alendronate. *N Engl J Med* 1996;335:1016–1021.
8. Domenech B, Kelly J. Swallowing disorders. *Med Gun North Am* 1999;83:97–113.
9. Franko TG, Richter JE. Proton-pump inhibitors for gastric acid-related disease. *Cleve Clin J Med* 1998;65:27–34.
10. Johnson DA. Medical therapy for gastroesophageal reflux disease. *Am J Med* 1992;92[Suppl 5A]:885.
11. Johnson MC. The esophagus. *Prim Care* 2001;28:459–485.
12. Kahrilas PJ. Gastrocsophageal reflux disease. *JAMA* 1996;276:983–988.
13. Katzka DA, Rustgi AK. Gastroesophageal reflux disease and Barrett's esophagus. *Med Clin North Am* 2000;84:1137–1161.
14. Malagelada JR, Distrutti E. Management of gastrointestinal motility disorders. *Drugs* 1996;52:494–506.
15. Mathog RH, Reming SM. A clinical approach to dysphagia. *Am J Otolaryngol* 1992;13:133.
16. Minocha A, Joseph AS. Pathophysiology and management of noncardiac chest pain. *Korean Med Assoc J* 1995;93:196–201.
17. Parente F, Bianchi PG. Treatment of cytomegalovirus esophagitis in patients with acquired immune deficiency syndrome: a randomized controlled study of foscarnet versus ganciclovir. *Am J Gastroenterol* 1998;93:317–322.
18. Patti MG, Way LW. Evaluation and treatment of primary esophageal motility disorders. *West J Med* 1997;166:263–269.
19. Reynolds JC. Influence of pathophysiology, severity, and cost on the medical management of gastroesophageal reflux disease. *Am Health Syst Pharm* 1996;53:S5–S12.
20. Richter JE. Practical approach to the diagnosis and treatment of esophageal dysphagia. *Compr Ther* 1998;24:446–453.
21. Shaker R, Staff D. Esophageal disorders in the elderly. *Gastroenterol Clin North Am* 2001;30:335–361.
22. Shapiro J. Evaluation and treatment of swallowing disorders. *Compr Ther* 1992;18:1721.
23. Shay SS. Benign structural lesions of the esophagus. *Gastroenterol Clin North Am* 1991;20:673.
24. Steele GH. Cost-effective management of dyspepsia and gastroesophageal reflux disease. *Gastroenterology* 1996;23:561–576.
25. Trate DM, Parkman HP, Fishr RS. Dysphagia. *Gastroenterology* 1996;23:417–441.

CHAPTER 59
Upper Gastrointestinal Bleeding

Edward A. Panacek and Deborah Diercks

More than 2% of all hospital admissions in the United States, and 5% of admissions from emergency departments, are related to acute gastrointestinal bleeding. In the vast majority of these patients, the bleeding source is in the upper gastrointestinal tract (10). Although bleeding stops spontaneously in up to 80% of patients, approximately 10% of those admitted require intervention to control their hemorrhage. Despite advances in diagnostic and therapeutic care, the overall mortality of admitted patients is 8% to 10% and has remained relatively unchanged for the past 40 years (10,13,16). For this reason, gastrointestinal bleeding should always be considered potentially life-threatening until proven otherwise.

The source of gastrointestinal bleeding is generally divided into three anatomic regions. *Upper gastrointestinal bleeding* (UGIB) is defined as occurring proximal to the ligament of Treitz. This anatomic site is important, in that bleeding distal to the ligament of Treitz rarely regurgitates back into the duodenum or stomach. *Middle gastrointestinal tract bleeding* is from the ligament of Treitz to the ileocecal valve (i.e., the jejunum and the ileum). *Lower gastrointestinal tract bleeding* is that which occurs in the colon or rectum.

The most common causes of UGIB are listed in Table 59.1; up to 30% of patients may have multiple causes or numerous anatomic sites involved. UGIB can occur in people of any age but is most common in adults older than 40 years of age, and it is more common in males than in females (2:1 ratio). Elderly patients have less ability to compensate for acute hemorrhage, and the majority of deaths occurs in elderly patients (4,5,13).

TABLE 59.1. Causes of Upper Gastrointestinal Tract Bleeding

MOST COMMON (90%)

Peptic ulcer (duodenal two thirds, gastric one third)	40%
Erosive gastritis	25%
Varices (esophageal and gastric)	20%
Mallory-Weiss tear	5%

UNCOMMON (10%)

Epistaxis, hemoptysis
Aortoenteric fistula
Boerhaave syndrome
Carcinoma
Vascular anomalies
Caustic ingestion
Anastomotic ulcer

CLINICAL PRESENTATION

Most patients with acute UGIB have obvious related signs or symptoms, but the presentation can be subtle. Patients may present primarily with severe tachycardia, angina, acute myocardial infarction, hypotension, syncope, weakness, confusion, or even full cardiac arrest. The classic presentation, however, is with hematemesis and/or melena. Another common presentation is with abdominal pain or cramps, usually with a change in bowel habits. The character of the pain can vary, but it is most often described as "burning" or "sharp" and located in the epigastrium. Although it is often assumed that hematochezia is a result of lower gastrointestinal hemorrhage, a massive UGIB is the cause in up to 11% (10). Maroon, burgundy, currant-jelly, and melenic stools differ from each other by containing varying amounts of metabolized hemoglobin. Stool appearance alone generally does not help to localize the site of hemorrhage and is more dependent on the volume and timing of the bleeding. However, the black, tarry stool of melena requires substantial digestion of the blood within the gastrointestinal tract, and, therefore, almost always represents a bleeding source proximal to the right colon.

When severe, UGIB can result in varying degrees of hemodynamic compromise. An acute blood loss of 10% of normal volume can usually be compensated for, with minimal physiologic change. Greater degrees of blood loss (10% to 20%) initiate reflex sympathetic mechanisms, resulting in peripheral vasoconstriction, tachycardia, widened pulse pressure, and orthostatic hypotension. Such patients often complain of thirst, apprehension, weakness, or light-headedness. When blood loss exceeds 20%, reflex mechanisms can no longer fully compensate; hypotension develops and organ perfusion is impaired. This can result in oliguria, mental confusion or coma, metabolic acidosis, and dyspnea.

DIFFERENTIAL DIAGNOSIS

The exact anatomic site or cause for bleeding in the upper gastrointestinal tract cannot always be determined in the emergency department, but the differential diagnosis can usually be shortened. Importantly, 90% of UGIBs are the result of only four causes (see Table 59.1).

The single most common cause is *peptic ulcer disease* involving the duodenum or stomach. The usual history is that of persistent burning, sharp, or aching pain in the epigastrium that develops 1 to 2 hours after eating. However, bleeding peptic ulcers are sometimes painless, and melena can be the sole presentation. Predisposing factors for peptic ulcers include cigarette smoking,

ingestion of alcohol, and hereditary factors. It is now also felt that many ulcers are related to infections with *Helicobacter pylori* (23).

Erosive gastritis is also a common cause of UGIB. The resultant bleeding can range from minimal to massive. The clinical presentation is often indistinguishable from that of peptic ulcer, and suspicion of the diagnosis is generally based on the clinical setting and history. The most common predisposing factor is the use of nonsteroidal anti-inflammatory drugs. Other risk factors include use of alcohol, prolonged corticosteroid use, and major trauma, burns, or head injury.

Patients with bleeding esophageal or gastric *varices* can be among the most difficult to manage. Because varices result from portal hypertension, this diagnosis should be suspected in patients with a history of cirrhosis or other stigmata of severe hepatic dysfunction. Bleeding can be sudden and massive. Complicating the evaluation, however, is the fact that up to 50% of episodes of UGIB in patients with known varices is not caused by to the varices (i.e., results from gastritis or peptic ulcer disease). Patients with variceal hemorrhage have poor prognosis, with a projected 1-year mortality of 70%. They account for one third of all deaths from UGIB.

Mallory-Weiss tears are longitudinal ruptures of the gastroesophageal junction, usually caused by recurrent forceful vomiting or retching. The history of sudden hematemesis of bright red blood after retching is characteristic, but it is present in only one half of patients. Risk factors include alcohol abuse, hiatal hernia, and underlying esophagitis. The amount of bleeding can range from mild to massive, but, in the absence of complicating medical conditions, the course is usually benign.

Other, less common, conditions account for the remaining 10% of episodes of UGIB (see Table 59.1). *Aortoenteric fistula* has a high mortality rate, with patients generally presenting with extremely massive bleeding resulting from erosion of an aortic aneurysm or a synthetic aortic graft into the distal duodenum. There is usually no time for diagnostic studies, and the patient must be moved rapidly to the operating room. Some patients experience a "herald" bleed of smaller volume within a week before the massive hemorrhage, but this is not usual.

EMERGENCY DEPARTMENT EVALUATION

Stabilization takes precedence over comprehensive evaluation in patients with potential UGIB. Patients who are hemodynamically or otherwise unstable must undergo rapid resuscitation and initial treatment concurrent with a focused clinical evaluation.

The history and physical examination often help to localize the bleeding source and indicate the severity of hemorrhage, but they have their limitations. Food products or medications that look very much like blood can mislead patients. Estimates regarding the amount of blood lost are notoriously inaccurate, whether reported by patients or prehospital personnel. The history should focus initially on selected items; the onset of bleeding (specifically, was the onset before or after vomiting?), the amount of blood loss, any related medical history (e.g., prior bleeding episodes, history of hepatic disease, aortic graft repair or known aneurysm, alcohol use, use of NSAIDs), associated symptoms (e.g., abdominal pain, peritoneal symptoms, or change in bowel habits), and complicating symptoms (e.g., chest pain, dyspnea, light-headedness, or syncope).

The goals of the initial examination are to assess the patient's hemodynamic status, estimate the severity of bleeding, search for clues to the bleeding source, and identify evidence of other complications. A supine systolic blood pressure of less than 100 mm Hg or an orthostatic pulse increase of more than 20 to 30 beats per minute suggests an acute blood loss of at least 1 L in an adult. However, changes in vital signs are not reliable, especially at the extremes of age. Findings of flat neck veins; cold, mottled extremities; altered mental status; or diaphoresis can contribute to the clinical assessment, but they are too subjective to be relied on primarily. Evidence of hepatic disease (especially portal hypertension) or an underlying coagulopathy, should be sought. The nose and oropharynx should also be examined for potential bleeding sources, particularly in atypical or confusing cases.

Stool appearance can be misleading, so it should be tested to confirm the presence of blood. Stools can test positive for occult blood for 2 weeks after a single episode of bleeding. False-positive results can be caused by iron preparations, heavy ingestion of red meats, and bromide preparations. Magnesium-containing antacids, ascorbic acid, and activated charcoal, as well as a number of other medications and food substances can cause false-negative results.

A nasogastric tube should be placed in patients with suspected gastrointestinal bleeding. There is no evidence that passage of a nasogastric tube in a patient with esophageal varices results in variceal trauma or increases bleeding (2). Even if the patient has obvious hematemesis, a tube should be placed to assess ongoing bleeding and to decrease the risk of aspiration. Flecks of red blood that accompany initial gastric intubation can be ignored. Testing of nonbloody aspirates for occult blood is of little clinical use. If blood is found, the nasogastric tube should be capable of fully evacuating the stomach; a large evacuator tube may be necessary when large amounts of blood or clots are present. Lavage should be carried out, ideally with the patient in the left lateral decubitus position, using normal saline, until the gastric contents become clear. Large volumes of tap water lavage should be avoided, as they can induce hyponatremia. Iced fluids should be avoided because they can interfere with normal coagulation function and can induce hypothermia. There is no advantage to the addition of vasoconstrictors or antacids to the lavage fluid. A negative nasogastric tube aspirate will miss up to 25% of bleeding duodenal ulcers, because it does not reliably sample material past the pylorus, unless bile is present in the aspirate.

Initial laboratory evaluations should include a complete blood cell count; determination of electrolyte, blood urea nitrogen, and creatinine levels; and tests of coagulation. An elevated blood urea nitrogen value is often seen in the setting of an UGIB and the blood urea nitrogen to creatinine ratio has been shown to be a sensitive, but not specific, marker of UGIB (7). A chest radiograph is indicated in patients in whom aspiration is clinically suspected. Abdominal films are indicated in the subset of patients in whom there is concern about perforation, obstruction, or intestinal dilatation. Barium contrast studies are rarely indicated in the emergency setting and can interfere with subsequent endoscopy and angiographic studies.

EMERGENCY DEPARTMENT MANAGEMENT

Once the patient reaches the emergency department, acute resuscitative interventions and stabilization assume the highest priority. Definitive localization of the bleeding site and identification of the cause are neither always possible nor necessary in the emergency department.

If not already initiated by prehospital personnel, patients with any degree of compromise should be immediately placed on a cardiac monitor and be given supplemental oxygen. Intravenous access should be established with a large-bore (14- to 18-gauge) catheter. Hypotensive patients should have at least two large-bore intravenous catheters, or a central line placed depending on the severity of the patient's condition or the presence of active

bleeding. Initial laboratory studies should be sent immediately, including a sample for type and screen of blood. One or 2 L of crystalloid is infused initially, or until the patient is stable. The hematocrit is rechecked after each 2 L of intravenous fluid or every 2 to 4 hours. If the clinical condition has not substantially improved after 2 L of fluid, and there is clinical evidence of ongoing hemorrhage or severe anemia, blood product transfusions should be ordered. The hemoglobin values can be misleading in the setting of acute bleeding, because compensatory hemodilution may not occur fully for several hours. Therefore, a normal blood cell count does not rule out an acute massive hemorrhage.

When active bleeding continues, or the patient's condition remains unstable, other diagnostic options must be considered. These include acute endoscopy, radionuclide imaging, and arteriography. Of these, endoscopy is the most valuable and the most available (4,19). Studies suggest that patients can be risk-stratified for the need for emergent endoscopy based on selected factors; that is, the presence of fresh blood in the nasogastric tube, hemoglobin level of <8 g/dL, and elevated white blood cell count of >12,000/μL. The presence of any two of these factors identified a group at moderate to high risk for active bleeding (1). Urgent endoscopy may also be indicated in patients with liver disease or when an aortoenteric fistula is suspected, although the patient's clinical condition in such cases may not allow time for endoscopy (5,22). In preparation for endoscopy, the patient's stomach must be fully evacuated to allow for optimal visualization. This is best performed with a large gastric lavage tube.

Emergent endoscopy provides potential therapeutic options for treatment of persistent UGIB in addition to therapeutic guidance and prognostic information. Stigmata found on endoscopy can predict recurrent bleeding. The main endoscopic techniques to manage UGIB are thermocoagulation and injection therapy, which can significantly reduce further bleeding, the need for surgery, and subsequent mortality (4,9). Sclerosis of visible vessels is also an option (9).

The administration of histamine-2 (H$_2$) antagonists and similar medications has been shown to prevent bleeding from stress ulcers in high-risk patients in the intensive care unit (ICU) and to speed the healing of peptic ulcers. However, they have not shown benefit in controlling bleeding in the acute setting (10). In contrast, intravenous use of proton pump inhibitors (PPIs) has been shown to decrease the rate of re-bleeding, but have no proven effect on mortality (14). Nonetheless, unless there is a specific contraindication, it is recommended to initiate therapy with an H$_2$ antagonist or a PPI by giving an initial bolus dose in the emergency department (e.g., cimetidine 300 mg, ranitidine 50 mg, or omeprazole 40 to 80 mg intravenously). Cost-effective analyses from Canada suggest that routine use of intravenous PPIs in all patients who present to the emergency department with UGIB is cost-effective (6). If early endoscopy is indicated, antacids and sucralfate should be withheld to avoid interfering with endoscopic visualization.

The therapeutic approach to patients with acute hemorrhage from esophageal varices differs substantially from that employed for other types of UGIB. The presence of prior variceal hemorrhage does not reliably predict a variceal source for the current bleeding. For this reason, emergent endoscopy is important, both diagnostically and therapeutically, in these patients (8). In the acute setting, emergent endoscopic therapy is often used in combination with pharmacologic agents, and the rate of initial control of bleeding is 90% to 95% (8,12).

Endoscopic therapy is divided into two types: endoscopic variceal sclerotherapy and band ligation. With the first, sclerosing agents are injected into the esophageal vessels, causing thrombosis and eventual necrosis. Up to 30% of patients can have complications, including ulcerations and fibrosis (19). Band ligation involves endoscopic placement of a rubber band around the varix, inducing obstruction and eventual tissue necrosis that obliterates the varix. This has recently become the preferred endoscopic approach, owing to lower complication rates (22). However, the technique is more difficult technically, and active bleeding can preclude adequate visualization. For these reasons, medical therapy is generally the favored initial approach in such patients.

Somatostatin, or its synthetic analog, octreotide (25 to 50 μg/hour infusion) have both shown benefit in terms of bleeding control, incidence of rebleeding, and in-hospital mortality for variceal bleeds (3,8,12). They may also reduce the risk of bleeding resulting from nonvariceal causes (11).

Another therapeutic option for variceal hemorrhage is intravenous vasopressin (0.2 to 0.4 U/minute infusion), a potent nonselective vasoconstrictor, which can be used in conjunction with endoscopic therapy or as the sole therapy when sclerotherapy is unsuccessful or unavailable. Vasopressin must be used with caution in patients with coronary artery or other vascular disease; a reduction in dosage or the concurrent use of nitroglycerin decreases the risk of adverse effects such as myocardial or extremity ischemia (8).

When sclerotherapy and vasoconstrictor therapy have been unsuccessful, balloon tamponade is the next therapeutic option. The *Sengstaken-Blakemore tube* (with three lumens) and the *Minnesota tube* (with four lumens) are most commonly used. They are less successful than sclerotherapy or medical therapy but can temporarily control bleeding acutely in up to 80% of cases (8). However, the use of these tubes is associated with a number of major complications, including esophageal necrosis and rupture, pulmonary aspiration, and airway compromise. The tubes come with an explicit list of instructions that should be reviewed in detail before their use, and they are best placed by an experienced practitioner.

Although most patients with UGIB never require surgery, early surgical consultation is advisable for any patient who has been hemodynamically unstable or who requires early blood transfusions. Most of the indications for surgical intervention are defined by the patient's clinical course during the initial 24 hours of hospitalization. However, for patients who present with hypotension or shock and massive uncontrollable hemorrhage that is not from varices, immediate surgery should be considered (5). For variceal bleeding, acute endoscopic therapies and balloon tamponade should be considered before turning to surgical intervention (8).

CRITICAL INTERVENTIONS

- Aggressively resuscitate patients with UGIB and clinical signs of shock
- Arrange emergent endoscopy for those with persistent bleeding

DISPOSITION

Historically, all patients with UGIB were admitted to the hospital, but it is now accepted that there is a subset of patients who can be safely discharged from the emergency department with close followup (5,18,20,21). Of patients requiring hospitalization, about one half meet high-risk criteria for rebleeding or other complications that necessitate admission to a monitored ICU or telemetry bed (15,20).

Although each study has used different thresholds or predictive factors, the general criteria for outpatient management are listed in Table 59.2. Some investigators recommend an age cutoff of 60 years, but the majority use an age of 65 or 75 years (13,15).

TABLE 59.2.   Criteria for Outpatient Management of Acute UGIB

Age younger than 65 years
No unstable comorbid illness
No evidence of portal hypertension or ascites on examination
Normal coagulation function
Systolic blood pressure >100 mm Hg, no orthostatic changes within 1 hour of presentation to ED
Nasogastric aspirate free of fresh blood after initial lavage
Hemoglobin ≥10 g/dL
Patient compliant with reliable access to close followup

ED, emergency department; UGIB, upper gastrointestinal bleeding.

Candidates for outpatient management must have reliable access to close outpatient followup and a demonstrated history of compliance with medical instructions, and they must have remained stable during at least 4 hours of emergency department observation. The specific criteria for admission to an ICU are listed in Table 59.3. In general, patients should be admitted to an ICU or monitored bed if their condition is unstable in the emergency department, if bleeding persists, or if they are at high risk for rebleeding or associated complications. Other patients with UGIB are appropriately admitted to a nonmonitored ward bed. In addition to the criteria in Table 59.2, early endoscopy, performed in the emergency department, can identify a subset of at least 25% of patients who would otherwise be admitted, who can be managed safely as outpatients. This aggressive approach could provide overall cost savings (17,18,21).

Those who are discharged with outpatient followup should be placed on a PPI as the first choice (e.g. omeprazole 20 mg twice a day or lansoprazole 30 mg twice a day), or an H_2 blocker (e.g., cimetidine 300 mg four times a day or 800 mg two times a day). They should also be prescribed liquid antacids as needed. The advantages of a bland diet are controversial, but known gastric stimulants such as alcohol, tobacco, and caffeine are best avoided. Frequent small meals may also be beneficial. Followup should be arranged within 3 to 7 days, with instructions to return earlier for recurrence of bleeding, worsening of pain, or orthostatic symptoms (23).

Patients who require ICU admission or emergency consultation should be considered for transfer to a referral hospital if either general surgery or endoscopy consultants are not available. Because UGIB patients often have encephalopathy and recurrent vomiting, transport personnel must be skilled in airway

TABLE 59.3.   Intensive Care Unit Admission Guidelines for Patients with UGIB

UNSTABLE VITAL SIGNS IN THE ED

Persistent bleeding that does not clear with lavage
Advanced age (older than 75 years)
Presence of coagulopathy
Portal hypertension or ascites
Severe anemia (e.g., hematocrit <20%)
Large drop in hematocrit (>8%)
Unstable comorbid disease (e.g., unstable coronary artery disease, chronic obstructive pulmonary disease, renal insufficiency, peripheral vascular disease, cerebrovascular disease)
Endoscopic findings of a "visible vessel" or an "overlying clot" or a variceal source
Use of vasopressin drip or esophageal tamponade balloon

UGIB, upper gastrointestinal bleeding; ED, emergency department.

management and resuscitation. The patient must have multiple large-caliber intravenous lines in place, and crossmatched blood should be sent with the patient, if available.

COMMON PITFALLS

✔ Because a number of foods, medications, or other substances can be mistaken for blood, the presence of blood in the gastrointestinal tract should be confirmed by testing

✔ Although uncommon, patients may exsanguinate into the gastrointestinal tract, with no acute external evidence of blood

✔ Underestimation of blood loss. Some patients can lose up to 20% to 30% of their blood volume and still maintain a relatively normal blood pressure in a supine position

✔ Over-reliance on negative nasogastric aspirates, as occurs in up to 25% of patients with acute UGIB. These are usually patients with a duodenal bleeding source and a closed pylorus

✔ Failure to recognize aortoenteric fistula as a cause of sudden massive hematemesis

References

1. Adamopoulos AB, Baibas NM, Efstathiuo SP, et al. Differentiation between patients with acute upper gastrointestinal bleeding who need early urgent gastrointestinal endoscopy and those who do not. A prospective study. *Eur J Gastroenterol Hepatol* 2003;15:381–387.
2. Ahmed A, Aggarwal M, Watson E. Esophageal perforation: a complication of nasogastric tube placement. *Am J Emerg Med* 1998;16:1.
3. Avgerinos A, Armonis A, Raptis S. Somatostatin or octreotide versus endoscopic sclerotherapy in acute variceal hemorrhage: a meta-analysis. *J Hepatol* 1995;22:247–251.
4. Cook DJ, Guyatt GH, Salena BJ, Laine LA. Endoscopic therapy for acute non-variceal upper intestinal hemorrhage. A meta-analysis. *Gastroenterology* 1992;102:139–148.
5. Corley DA, Stefan AM, Wolf M, et al. Early indicators of prognosis in upper gastrointestinal hemorrhage. *Am J Gastroenterol* 1998;93:336–340.
6. Enns RA, Gagnon YN, Rioux KP, Levy AR. Cost-effectiveness in Canada of intravenous proton pump inhibitors for all patients presenting with acute upper gastrointestinal bleeding. *Aliment Pharmacol Ther* 2003;17:225–233.
7. Ernst AA, Haynes ML, Nick TG, Weis SJ. Usefulness of the blood urea nitrogen/creatinine ratio in gastrointestinal bleeding. *Am J Emerg Med* 1999;17:70–72.
8. Grace ND. Diagnosis and treatment of gastrointestinal bleeding secondary to portal hypertension. *Am J Gastroenterol* 1997;92:1082–1090.
9. Gralnek IM, Jensen DM, Kovacs TO, et al. An economic analysis of patients with active arterial peptic ulcer hemorrhage treated with endoscopic heater probe, injection sclerosis, or surgery in a prospective, randomized trial. *Gastrointest Endosc* 1997;46:105–112.
10. Gupta PK, Fleischer DE. Nonvariceal upper gastrointestinal bleeding. *Med Clin North Am* 1993;77:973–992.
11. Imperiale TF, Birgisson S. Somatostatin or octreotide compared with H2 antagonist and placebo in the management of acute nonvariceal upper gastrointestinal hemorrhage: A meta-analysis. *Ann Intern Med* 1997;127:1062–1066.
12. Jenkins SA, Shields R, Davies M, et al. A multicenter randomized trial comparing octreotide and injection sclerotherapy in the management and outcome of acute variceal haemorrhage. *Gut* 1997;41:526–533.
13. Katschinski B, Logan R, Davies J, et al. Prognostic factors in upper gastrointestinal bleeding. *Dig Dis Sci* 1994;39:706–712.
14. Khuroo MS, Yattoo GN, Javid G, et al. A comparison of omeprazole and placebo for bleeding peptic ulcer. *N Engl J Med* 1997;336:1054–1058.
15. Kollef MH, O'Brien JD, Zuckerman GR, et al. BLEED: a classification tool to predict outcomes in patients with acute upper and lower gastrointestinal hemorrhage. *Crit Care Med* 1997;25:1125–1132.
16. Laine L, Peterson WL. Bleeding peptic ulcer. *N Engl J Med* 1994;331:717–727.
17. Lee JG, Turnipseed S, Romano PS, et al. Endoscopy-based triage significantly reduces hospitalization rates and costs of treating upper GI bleeding: a randomized controlled trial. *Gastrointest Endosc* 1999;50:755–761.
18. Longstreth GF, Feitelberg SP. Successful outpatient management of acute upper gastrointestinal hemorrhage: use of practice guidelines in a large patient series. *Gastrointest Endosc* 1998;47:219–222.
19. Roberts LR, Kamath PS. Pathophysiology and treatment of variceal hemorrhage. *Mayo Clin Proc* 1996;71:973–983.
20. Rockall TA, Logan RFA, Devlin HB, et al. Risk assessment after acute upper gastrointestinal hemorrhage. *Gut* 1996;38:316–321.
21. Rockall TA, Logan RF, Devlin HB, et al. Selection of patients for early discharge or outpatient care after acute upper gastrointestinal hemorrhage. *Lancet* 1996;347:1138–1140.
22. Schoenfeld PS, Butler JA. An evidence-based approach to the treatment of esophageal variceal bleeding. *Crit Care Clin* 1998;14:441–455.
23. Soll AH. Consensus conference. Medical treatment of peptic ulcer disease. Practice guidelines. Practice Parameters Committee of the American College of Gastroenterology. *JAMA* 1996;275:622–629.

CHAPTER 60
Lower Gastrointestinal Bleeding

Catherine B. Custalow

Lower gastrointestinal bleeding (LGIB) is a common complaint of patients who present to the emergency department (ED). It is less common than upper gastrointestinal bleeding (UGIB), with an estimated annual incidence of 20 to 27 cases per 100,000 adults, compared to 100 to 200 cases per 100,000 for UGIB (6). The mortality rate for LGIB ranges from 2% to 4% (6).

The spectrum of illness is clinically broad, ranging from minor anorectal disorders to severe and life-threatening bleeding that results in hypovolemic shock and death. Depending upon the volume and rate of bleeding, patients can rapidly deteriorate in the emergency department. Therefore the clinician and ED staff must remain vigilant in the monitoring and care of these patients.

CLINICAL PRESENTATION

Lower GI bleeding is defined as arising distal to the ligament of Treitz, which is the suspensory muscle of the duodenum. This includes bleeding from the distal one fourth of the duodenum and from the jejunum, ileum, colon, rectum, and anus.

The appearance of the stool may provide a suggestion as to the location of the bleed, but is not an absolute indicator of the anatomic origin of the bleed. The terms melena and hematochezia are common descriptors of gastrointestinal bleeding. Melena appears as black, tarry stool and usually reflects the presence of blood that has remained in the gastrointestinal tract for longer than 8 hours. Melena is approximately four times more likely to reflect an UGIB (10); therefore, although melena most commonly originates from the duodenum or jejunum, it can occasionally come from the lower portions of the small intestine and proximal colon. *Hematochezia*, described as bright red or maroon stool, usually indicates an LGIB. It is about six times more likely to be caused by a lower gastrointestinal source than an upper source (10). However, 10% to 15% of patients with UGIB present with bright red blood coming from the rectum, as may occur with brisk bleeding and rapid transit of blood. Small amounts of bright red blood may come from minor anorectal sources and may be noticed on the outside of the stools or toilet paper following a bowel movement. Occasionally, drops of blood from an anorectal source, when diffused in the toilet water, will cause patients to overestimate the volume and severity of the bleed.

Because patients are not always aware of GI bleeding, clinicians should consider this diagnosis in patients who present with other concerning symptoms and signs such as hypotension, tachycardia, angina, syncope, weakness, confusion, stroke, myocardial infarction, shock or cardiac arrest.

DIFFERENTIAL DIAGNOSIS

Hemorrhoids are dilated anorectal veins. They are quite common, but rarely result in massive hemorrhage. Hemorrhoids are associated with chronic constipation, straining, low fiber diet, and pregnancy. Patients may describe small amounts of bright red blood, pruritus ani, a protruding mass, pain with defecation, or pain when sitting on a hard surface. Hemorrhoids are divided into two major types. External hemorrhoids are found below the dentate line in well-innervated squamous epithelium and present with pain. Internal hemorrhoids originate above the dentate line and are most commonly located at 2, 5, and 9 o'clock on anoscopy.

Anal fissures are usually associated with hard stools, but may also be seen with diarrhea. They present with extremely painful defecation; 90% are located in the posterior midline (4).

Anorectal varices are caused by portal hypertension of chronic liver disease and appear as discrete, bluish-gray submucosal veins. They are usually more compressible and serpiginous than internal hemorrhoids and extend below the dentate line (4). Anorectal varices may cause severe rectal bleeding.

Rectal foreign bodies that cause tears should be seen immediately by a surgeon. Improper technique or delay in removal of a retained rectal foreign body may cause perforation with subsequent infection and bleeding. Broken glass from a retained foreign body may tear the rectum and cause bleeding (11).

Ulcerative colitis affects the colon and rectum, and presents with bloody stools, crampy abdominal pain, and tenesmus. Lesions involve both the mucosa and the submucosa. Distal disease is usually more severe.

Crohn's disease has a bimodal distribution of age of onset with peaks occurring in the 20s and at around age 70. Crohn's disease involves all layers of the bowel and lymph nodes. Any section of the gastrointestinal tract is vulnerable, but the distal ileum is the most commonly affected site. When present, colonic involvement is usually patchy with rectal sparing (4). During flares, patients describe bloody diarrhea, abdominal pain, fever, and weight loss.

Pseudomembranous colitis usually presents after the patient has been taking broad-spectrum antibiotics and is caused by the subsequent overgrowth of *Clostridium difficile*. Patients present with fever, crampy abdominal pain, and watery or bloody diarrhea, usually 7 to 10 days after a course of antibiotics. Pseudomembranous colitis rarely causes severe bleeding. The diagnosis can be confirmed by sending stool for *C. difficile* toxin or by finding the characteristic pseudomembranes on colonoscopy (4).

Infectious diarrhea, most commonly bacterial, may be associated with a significant inflammatory response and blood and mucus in the stool ("dysentery"). There is typically an abrupt onset with cramping abdominal pain.

Human immunodeficiency virus (HIV)–related causes of gastrointestinal bleeding include cytomegalovirus colitis, Kaposi sarcoma, and gastrointestinal lymphoma (4).

Radiation colitis or proctitis most commonly occurs after radiation for cervical or prostate cancer. The onset of bleeding usually occurs between 9 and 15 months following radiotherapy, but it may occur as far out as 41 months (6). Acute radiation colitis presents with rectal pain, diarrhea, and rectal bleeding.

Diverticulosis is described as the most common cause of severe lower gastrointestinal bleeding in adults. In adults, diverticulosis and angiodysplasia together account for nearly 80% of significant lower gastrointestinal bleeds (7). Patients usually present with painless bleeding, which may be of a large volume. Diverticula are sac-like herniations (2–5 mm in greatest dimension) of the colonic mucosa and are most common in the sigmoid colon.

The diagnosis should be considered in all patients older than 40 years of age. The prevalence increases with each decade of life, and more than 50% of patients have diverticula by age 60 (3). Other risk factors include living in industrialized countries, and a diet that is deficient in fiber, high in fat, and high in red meat.

Angiodysplasias often bleed chronically and may present with occult fecal blood or iron-deficiency anemia. Angiodysplasias may also present as acute bleeding with hematochezia. This disease is more common in the elderly, in patients with renal failure, and in those with hereditary hemorrhagic telangiectasia (*Osler-Weber-Rendu* syndrome) (4).

Mesenteric ischemia most commonly presents in patients older than 50 years of age, especially in those with underlying cardiovascular disease. Risk factors also include atrial fibrillation, coronary artery disease (CAD), congestive heart failure (CHF), recent myocardial infarction (MI), valvular heart disease, hypercoagulable states, and hypotension. Specific causes are arterial embolus (most common), venous thrombosis, atherosclerosis, external compression of vessels, and low flow states. Mesenteric ischemia commonly presents with sudden onset of abdominal pain (if arterial embolus), pain out of proportion to examination findings, and heme-positive stools.

Colonic polyps may cause LGIB and can be diagnosed and removed at colonoscopy. Post-polypectomy bleeding, although not common (up to 0.4%) (2), may be quite severe. Early bleeding most likely occurs because there is inadequate hemostasis of the blood vessel in the stalk of the polyp. Later bleeding (up to 15 days following the procedure) may occur as a result of sloughing of the clot (6).

Colon cancer accounts for approximately 10% of major intestinal bleeding and 20% of minor bleeding in the elderly (6). Advanced colon cancer presents with altered bowel patterns, abdominal pain, involuntary weight loss, rectal bleeding, and anemia. Distal colon or rectal cancer may also cause a change in the caliber of the stools.

Aortoenteric fistula must be considered in patients who have abdominal aortic grafts and develop gastrointestinal bleeding.

EMERGENCY DEPARTMENT EVALUATION

The initial assessment should include the patient's general appearance, vital signs, and mental status. Relevant questions include a history of colonic polyps, cancer, inflammatory bowel disease, or recent travel with bloody diarrhea. Medication use is also important, since there is an association between aspirin or nonsteroidal antiinflammatory drug (NSAID) use and LGIB (6).

Orthostatic vital signs may be helpful in some cases. If the patient has significant postural changes or is hypotensive lying down, assume that blood loss is significant. One should endeavor to estimate the amount of blood loss but should keep in mind that estimates are frequently inaccurate. Other clues that may be helpful in establishing a diagnosis include skin lesions such as telangiectasia, bruises, or petechiae. Hyperpigmentation of the lower abdomen may suggest previous radiation therapy. Diverticulosis, angiodysplasia, and cancer are unusual before the age of 40. Likewise, Meckel's diverticulum rarely presents after adolescence (1). Stigmata of liver disease (ascites, jaundice, spider angiomata, and caput medusae) suggest the possibility of anorectal varices.

The perianal region and rectum should be carefully examined, both externally and by digital rectal examination, to check for masses, strictures, hemorrhoids, and blood. Stool should be tested for the presence of occult blood using the guaiac (Hemoccult) test. False-positive results may be seen with ingestion of red fruits, red meat, iron, and bismuth.

Laboratory testing may be helpful, including measurement of hemoglobin, hematocrit, platelets, prothrombin (international normalized ratio [INR]), and partial thromboplastin time (PTT). A type-and-screen or crossmatch is recommended if blood loss is significant or ongoing. Other laboratory studies which may be useful include a liver profile, blood urea nitrogen (BUN), creatinine, and electrolytes. Lactate and anion gap should be measured if mesenteric ischemia is suspected, but these tests may be normal early in the course of the disease. Likewise, the initial hematocrit may not accurately reflect the amount of acute blood loss. Cardiac ischemia can occur in gastrointestinal bleeding because of decreased oxygen delivery; therefore, an electrocardiogram should be performed and supplemental oxygen should be administered if ischemia is suspected.

It is important to determine whether the bleeding is a result of LGIB or UGIB. Aspiration of the gastric contents with a nasogastric tube is helpful in this assessment. Should the initial aspirate be negative, the clinician should lavage with saline or tap water to rule out the presence of blood in the stomach. If the lavage is positive for red blood or "coffee grounds" (suggestive of partially digested blood), note the volume of lavage it takes to clear the stomach or whether the blood cannot be cleared with lavage. The results of this examination may be falsely positive if the nasogastric tube insertion was traumatic (causing nasal trauma). Conversely, one should remember that nasogastric lavage is often negative in the presence of an UGIB when the source is distal to the pylorus.

EMERGENCY DEPARTMENT MANAGEMENT

Adherence to a systematic approach to LGIB will help the clinician to be adequately prepared for sudden clinical deterioration. With any suspicion of significant blood loss, the patient should be placed on a monitor, oxygen should be administered and intravenous access should be obtained with two large-bore intravenous (i.v.) catheters. Crystalloid solutions should be administered, and the fluid status should be evaluated frequently. Blood products should be transfused as needed.

Surgical consultation should be considered when the patient is persistently unstable despite treatment, when there has been massive initial bleeding, when the source of bleeding has been detected and is amenable to surgery, or when perforation is identified or strongly suspected. Older patients usually need more aggressive surgical management. Patients with a history of anorectal varices, persistent postural changes in the vital signs, or significant volumes of bright red blood per rectum are more likely to require surgery than patients without these findings. Patients presenting with gastrointestinal bleeding who have abdominal aortic grafts should have urgent vascular surgery consultation because of the possibility of an aortoenteric fistula.

Anoscopy may reveal an anorectal source of bleeding or may show bleeding from above the reach of the anoscope suggesting a more proximal cause of bleeding. To perform this examination, place the patient in the lateral decubitus or knee-chest position. Lubricate the anoscope and insert it (with obturator) until the flange rests at the anal verge, and remove the obturator. Shine a bright light (e.g., an otoscope, penlight, or flashlight) into the center of the anoscope and visualize the rectal mucosa and stool above the opening to look for bleeding coming from above the anoscope. Finally, withdraw the anoscope slowly to look for anorectal disorders such as bleeding hemorrhoids, proctitis, or fissures. Although the presence of blood proximal to the anoscope may be seen with retrograde passage of blood, it usually indicates a more proximal bleed and should be further investigated.

Abdominal X-rays are rarely indicated in LGIBs unless perforation or bowel obstruction is suspected.

Angiography is more commonly used in the evaluation of LGIB than in UGIB. The procedure is invasive and should be done in consultation with a surgeon and an interventional radiologist. A fairly brisk bleeding rate of 0.5 to 2.0 mL/minute is required in order for angiography to be diagnostic. Although angiography rarely identifies the specific cause of the bleeding, it can help to identify the location, which can facilitate limited bowel resection during surgery (9). Available catheter-based interventional angiography techniques include intra-arterial infusion of vasopressin and arterial embolization. For intraarterial vasopressin, a 20-minute infusion at a rate of 0.2 U/minute is given first. The infusion rate may be increased subsequently to 0.3 and then 0.4 U/minute if bleeding continues. Unfortunately, when the infusion is stopped the vasoconstrictive effects of vasopressin dissipate rapidly, so a stable clot must be formed and retained in order to prevent rebleeding. Recurrent hemorrhage is relatively common and occurs in 36% to 43% (5).

Arterial embolization used to be reserved for UGIB, because bowel infarction was a frequent complication of embolization in LGIB. However, with modern embolization techniques, clinically significant bowel ischemia has become an uncommon complication (5). Angiography is associated with a combined complication rate of 2% to 9%. These include hematomas, arterial dissection, renal failure, contrast allergy, and bowel ischemia and infarction.

Technetium-labeled red cell scans provide a rough localization of bleeding. This test can detect bleeding rates as low as 0.1 mL/minute, and, therefore, appears to be more sensitive than angiography. It may be particularly useful in patients who cannot tolerate angiography or other procedures. It is important to note that this diagnostic test should not delay definitive treatment of massive bleeding.

Colonoscopy, in addition to identifying anorectal disorders, can diagnose many causes of lower gastrointestinal hemorrhage, including diverticulosis and angiodysplasia. Unfortunately, in emergent cases, the bowel is not adequately prepared and the presence of stool can obscure lesions. Emergency colonoscopy in acute LGIB can miss the diagnosis in 40% of cases, especially in small bowel bleeding below the ligament of Treitz (9). Colonoscopy can also be used therapeutically to ablate bleeding sites, but fails to stop the bleeding in about 20% of cases (9).

The initial diagnostic procedure of choice (colonoscopy, angiography, or scintography) is controversial. These decisions are commonly dependent upon the institution and the preferences of the consultant.

Thrombosed external hemorrhoids can be excised under local anesthesia if pain is severe (see Chapter 74, "Perianal, Rectal, and Anal Diseases"). Hemorrhoids and anal fissures are best treated with stool softeners, increased fiber, sitz baths, and external analgesics (see Chapter 74). Treatment for ulcerative colitis and Crohn's disease include analgesia, corticosteroids, sulfasalazine, and metronidazole (see Chapter 71, "Inflammatory Bowel Disease"). Pseudomembranous colitis is treated with oral vancomycin or metronidazole. Infectious diarrhea is treated with appropriate antibiotics to which the pathogen is sensitive (see Chapter 72, "Diarrhea and Proctitis").

CRITICAL INTERVENTIONS

- Initiate aggressive resuscitation in hypovolemic patients with LGIB, using crystalloid and blood as needed
- Obtain emergent surgical consultation for unstable patients

DISPOSITION

Optimizing the management of patients with gastrointestinal bleeding involves stratification of the risk of rebleeding and mortality. Evaluating these criteria can help the clinician to make management decisions such as (i) hospitalization versus outpatient treatment; (ii) admission to an unmonitored bed, a monitored bed, or an intensive care unit bed; (iii) emergency versus elective endoscopy; (iv) timing and number of packed red blood cell transfusions; and (v) diagnostic angiography versus conservative therapy (8).

Factors predicting rebleeding and mortality include age older than 60 years, comorbidity (particularly liver disease, renal disease, pulmonary disease, encephalopathy, cancer, recent major surgery, trauma, or coexisting disease in three-organ systems), low hematocrit, melena, hematochezia, or prolonged PT. Other factors include requiring more than 5 U of packed red blood cells, tachycardia, hypotension, shock, elevated serum transaminases, and elevated serum creatinine (8). Mortality in elderly patients has been shown to be 16% to 25% higher than in younger patients. Mortality increases by 25% to 70% in patients who require transfusion of more than 5 U of packed red blood cells. Patients with high risk criteria should be admitted to the intensive care unit. Patients who are at low risk can be admitted to the floor and have arrangements made for colonoscopy.

If bleeding hemorrhoids, proctitis, or fissures are found on anoscopy and there is no evidence of portal hypertension, the patient may be discharged home with treatment and followup.

COMMON PITFALLS

✔ Failure to appreciate the significance and volume of lower gastrointestinal bleeding or to anticipate the possibility of rapid clinical deterioration
✔ Failure to adequately resuscitate the patient with crystalloid fluids and blood
✔ Failure to consider gastrointestinal bleeding in patients who present with other seemingly unrelated complaints such as syncope, angina, myocardial infarction, weakness, dyspnea, altered mental status or shock

Acknowledgments

Thank you to previous edition chapter authors Daniel T. Schelble and David J. Peter.

References

1. Beckman JW, Tedesco FJ. Acute management of lower GI bleeding. *J Crit Illn* 1986;1:14–20.
2. Billingham RP. The conundrum of lower gastrointestinal bleeding. *Surg Clin North Am* 1997;77:241–52.
3. Bokhari M, Vernava AM, Ure T, Longo WE. Diverticular hemorrhage in the elderly-is it well tolerated? *Dis Colon Rectum* 1996;39:191.
4. Cappell MS, Friedel D. The role of sigmoidoscopy and colonoscopy in the diagnosis and management of lower gastrointestinal disorders: endoscopic findings, therapy and complications. *Med Clin North Am* 2002;86:1253–1288.
5. Darcy M. Treatment of lower gastrointestinal bleeding: vasopressin infusion versus embolization. *J Vasc Interv Radiol* 2003;14:535–543.
6. Farrell JJ, Friedman LS. Gastrointestinal bleeding in the elderly. *Gastroenterol Clin North Am* 2001;30:377–407.
7. Henneman PL. Gastrointestinal bleeding. In: Marx JA, et al. eds. *Emergency Medicine: Concepts and Clinical Practice*, 5th ed. Philadelphia: Mosby, 2002:194–200.
8. Hussein H, Lapin S, Cappell MS. Clinical scoring systems for determining the prognosis of gastrointestinal bleeding. *Gastroenterol Clin North Am* 2000;29:445–464.
9. Lefkovitz Zvi, Cappell MS, Kaplan M, et al. Radiology in the diagnosis and therapy of gastrointestinal bleeding. *Gastroenterol Clin North Am* 2000;29:489–512.
10. Peura DA, Lanza FL, Goustout CJ, et al. The American College of Gastroenterology Bleeding Registry: preliminary findings. *Am J Gastroenterol* 1997;92:924.
11. Strear CM, Coates WC. Anorectal Procedures. In: Roberts JR, Hedges JR, Chanmugan AS, Chudnofsky C, Custalow CB, Dronen SC, eds. *Clinical Procedures in Emergency Medicine*. Philadelphia: WB Saunders, 2004:868–880.
12. Wilcox CM, Alexander LN, Cotsonis G. A prospective characterization of upper gastrointestinal hemorrhage presenting with hematochezia. *Am J Gastroenterol* 1997;92:231.

CHAPTER 61
Peptic Ulcer Disease

Dale S. Birenbaum

Peptic ulcer disease (PUD) eventually affects one of every 10 Americans. The prevalence of PUD in the population, between 1.7% and 2.9%, implies that there are 4 to 8 million active cases at any given time (10). Despite these disconcerting numbers, there has been a significant decline in the total number of cases since the 1960s. Interestingly, the disease is becoming less common in developed countries and more common in developing nations (12).

It is estimated that in the United States peptic ulcer disease accounts for 20 billion dollars per year of economic losses and health care expenditures resulting from lost worker productivity, restricted activity, physician visits, and hospitalizations (19). The management and treatment of this common disease has changed significantly over the last 25 years. Treatment of peptic ulcer disease has evolved from dietary modifications and antacids to gastric acid suppression with H_2 receptor antagonist and proton pump inhibitors. Eradication of *Helicobacter pylori* infection and gastroprotective therapy with cyclooxygenase 2 (COX-2) inhibitors and prostaglandin congeners have reshaped modern therapy (20,22).

Duodenal ulcer is more common than gastric ulcer (5:1), and men are afflicted more commonly than women (1.8:1). The incidence is increased in patients with renal failure and transplants, alcoholic cirrhosis, and chronic obstructive pulmonary disease (COPD). Among the elderly, gastric or duodenal ulceration is an increasing problem. Although mortality rates for PUD have generally declined over the past 30 years, they remain amazingly high for the elderly—50 to 100 times greater at age 75 than at age 35 years (12,21).

PATHOPHYSIOLOGY

The mechanisms of peptic ulcer formation in the stomach and in the duodenum are not thought to be the same, but they do share some elements. There appears to be an imbalance between the production of acid and the ability of the mucosa to prevent itself from being damaged (Table 61.1). Acid secretion has been considered the key to ulcer formation, and indeed, ulcers will not form without it. Furthermore, reduction of acid secretion or acid neutralization promotes ulcer healing.

Because duodenal and gastric ulcers develop in patients who are not acid hypersecretors, acid production is not the sole

TABLE 61.1. Factors Acting on or in Gastric Mucosa

Endogenous Aggressive Factors	Endogenous Defensive Factors
Acid	Mucosal barrier
Pepsin	Mucus
Bile	Bicarbonate
Lysolecithin	Cell renewal
	Mucosal blood flow
	Prostaglandins

(From Emas S. Medical principles for treatment of peptic ulcer. *Scand J Gastroenterol* 1987;137:28–32.)

TABLE 61.2. Risk Factors for Peptic Ulcer

Helicobacter Pylori
Nonsteroidal antiinflammatory drugs (NSAIDs)
Acid hypersecretory conditions (Zollinger-Ellison)
Aspirin
Associated disease (COPD, cirrhosis, chronic renal failure)
Male gender
Advanced age

COPD, chronic obstructive pulmonary disease.

factor involved; weakened defensive factors also play a role in ulcerogenesis. Healthy gastric or duodenal mucosa is an impressive barrier to the diffusion of hydrogen ions and can maintain a gradient of 3 million to 1 between lumen and blood. It also secretes bicarbonate and mucus, which form a buffering gel over the mucosa. Mucosal gel thickness is increased by the E prostaglandins and diminished by aspirin and nonsteroidal antiinflammatory drugs (NSAIDs). Maintenance of normal blood flow to the mucosa is an essential component of resistance to injury. When ulceration does occur, pain results from direct chemical irritation by hydrochloric acid and disordered motor activity of the stomach and duodenum.

Research has focused on the small microaerophilic gram-negative spiral bacterium *Helicobacter pylori*, which is strongly linked to the formation of duodenal ulcers. This agent increases antral gastrin production, causes chronic gastric metaplasia and duodenitis, and decreases mucosal integrity. The most compelling evidence for the role of *H. pylori* in peptic ulcer disease is that the 1-year relapse rate for duodenal ulcers is less than 15% following eradication therapy but 70% to 80% after H_2-receptor antagonist therapy alone. The eradication of this microorganism from the gastrointestinal (GI) tract on first presentation has been routinely advocated; this search and treat strategy has been associated with accelerated ulcer healing, a reduced rate of ulcer recurrence, and cure of the disease (3).

In some patients with duodenal ulcer, there is an increase in the number of acid-producing gastric parietal cells and a direct relation between acid hypersecretion and the severity of ulcer disease. However, 50% of ulcer patients have normal acid secretion and show no relation between the severity of illness and the level of acid secretion. Other explanations of duodenal ulcer formation involve the delivery of a large, unbuffered acid load to the duodenum with subsequent mucosal damage, as occurs, for example, in the Zollinger-Ellison syndrome, in which serum gastrin levels are astronomic and normal feedback inhibition does not occur. More than 90% of duodenal ulcers occur within 3 cm of the junction of the pyloric and duodenal mucosa, and most are small (less than 1 cm).

Gastric ulcers are larger and more extensive, and the majority are found on the lesser curvature of the stomach at the junction of the body and antral mucosa. Formation is probably related to an abnormality of the gastric mucosal barrier. Although their role in ulcer formation is yet to be proved, human bile, aspirin, and ethanol increase the permeability of the gastric mucosa to hydrogen ions. Pyloric dysfunction, bile reflux, and gastritis have been proposed to lead to gastric ulceration by weakening the normal mucosal defense mechanisms. Many factors predispose to the development of ulcers (Table 61.2). Despite popular opinion, alcohol and caffeine ingestion have not been conclusively linked to ulcer disease. Diet also is not clearly related to PUD, and, at present, the only reasonable dietary recommendation for ulcer patients is to avoid foods that produce symptoms (10).

COMPLICATIONS

PUD continues to produce major complications despite the introduction of several apparently effective pharmacologic agents. However, the type of surgical procedure performed for complications of PUD has changed since the introduction of H_2 blockers. Fewer elective procedures are performed in the relatively fit, younger population, and more emergent operations are performed on older and sicker patients who are less able to tolerate surgery (6,18).

Perforation continues to occur in peptic ulcer patients despite the availability of reasonably effective medical treatment (18). Perforation is heralded by a dramatic change in the pain pattern. Either severe pain and a surgical abdomen develop rapidly secondary to release of air and secretions into the peritoneal cavity, or a constant, deeper pain increases gradually with the slower development of surgical signs as a result of posterior penetration or a partially occluded perforation. Whether presenting suddenly or gradually, perforation is a surgical emergency requiring rapid diagnosis, resuscitation, and operation.

Hemorrhage from peptic ulcers is usually self-limited but is occasionally massive and life-threatening; it accounts for 20% to 30% of patients who require surgery for PUD (7). It is a common complication of PUD, with presentations ranging from melena alone to frank hypovolemic shock. Upper GI bleeding should be anticipated in any ulcer patient.

Gastric outlet obstruction, the result of scarring from repeated episodes of ulceration and fibrous healing, is usually associated with duodenal ulcer. It may also be caused by edema from an active ulcer. Fluid and gas accumulate in the stomach, causing fullness or distress that is often relieved by vomiting. Massive distention of the stomach can occur; volume depletion and electrolyte disturbances may be dramatic. In the emergency department, fluid resuscitation should be undertaken and the stomach should be decompressed by means of a nasogastric tube, but surgery may be necessary for definitive treatment. Gastric outlet obstruction may be the indication for as many as 30% of ulcer operations (7).

Nonhealing, the failure of a gastric ulcer to improve with medical treatment, is suggestive of malignancy.

CLINICAL PRESENTATION

Peptic ulcer is a chronic but not necessarily life-long disease, frequently running a course of 10 to 15 years and marked by periods of acute exacerbation and remission. Pain may develop without obvious cause and persist for several days or weeks, but rarely longer. Because these episodes sometimes resolve with over-the-counter preparations, many patients do not seek medical assistance. Most ulcer patients experience a benign course, except for occasional symptomatic periods, but 10% to 20% develop some complication of the disease.

Most patients present to the emergency department for relief from a constant burning, gnawing, or aching pain. The pain of PUD is primarily epigastric, but it can be localized anywhere in the upper abdomen. With perforation of a posterior duodenal ulcer, pain often begins in the epigastrium and moves to the back. If pneumoperitoneum develops, pain may be referred to the shoulder as well.

The description and location of the pain is not as important in diagnosis as is its timing and any exacerbating and ameliorating factors. Gastric ulcer usually produces pain immediately after eating, when acid production increases in response to food. The pain of duodenal ulcer is most common between or just before meals and at night, when the upper GI tract is empty. Ingestion of food or antacids may bring rapid relief. Pain at 2 or 3 a.m. is classic for duodenal ulcer, probably because acid production is high and unbuffered by food. Acid production is at its lowest later in the morning, and pain is rarely present at this time. The classic history of a repetitive pain–food–relief sequence remains one of the better clinical diagnostic clues to PUD.

Asymptomatic peptic ulcer is not uncommon; an estimated 20% to 25% of all ulcers may be silent (9). In fact, nearly one third of patients with ulcer perforation and one fifth of those with upper GI hemorrhage have no previous symptoms of ulcer disease.

Uncomplicated PUD does not produce remarkable physical findings. Epigastric tenderness may be noted, but guarding and rebound are not present. Bowel sounds are most often normal, and there is no organomegaly. Rectal examination may show guaiac-positive stool if there has been unrecognized bleeding. The purpose of the physical examination is to exclude complications and other diseases, rather than to confirm the presence of peptic ulcer. Therefore, examination of the heart and lungs is indicated to help rule out cardiac or pulmonary disease masquerading as an abdominal process.

Guarding, rebound, and a tense abdomen signal perforation of an ulcer. There may be slight improvement immediately following perforation, but, within hours, shock ensues. Patients with perforation usually lie perfectly still, because the slightest movement produces intense peritoneal pain. In the elderly, findings may be minimal or absent, tending to delay the diagnosis in the group least able to tolerate delay.

Hemorrhage from PUD may cause surprisingly few physical findings on examination. A history of melenic stools should be sought, and orthostatic vital signs may help uncover occult but clinically important bleeding. Frequently, significant bleeding presents with hematemesis.

Gastric outlet obstruction usually produces some degree of bloating and a tympanitic epigastrium or succussion splash secondary to a distended stomach.

DIFFERENTIAL DIAGNOSIS

Myocardial infarction and angina are perhaps the most important diagnoses to consider in the differential diagnosis. They may present atypically as midepigastric pain, with complaints of nausea, bloating, and burning surprisingly similar to those of PUD, but without the typical periodicity and ameliorating factors. Moreover, many ulcer patients also have coronary artery disease. A careful history and electrocardiographic examination can usually differentiate heart disease, however.

Gastritis usually produces a constant feeling of bloating and may not be relieved by antacids. Gastroenteritis produces colicky or crampy abdominal pain associated with diarrhea and vomiting. Biliary tract disease causes upper abdominal pain (classically after ingestion of fatty foods), but typically there is no history of early morning pain or improvement with antacids. Esophagi-

tis as a complication of hiatal hernia may be associated with intense pain immediately or shortly after swallowing. The constant, boring pain of pancreatitis frequently radiates to the back and is associated with elevated serum amylase and lipase levels.

A host of other conditions can produce pain in the upper abdomen, but, for the most part, these conditions are readily ruled out by history and physical examination.

EMERGENCY DEPARTMENT EVALUATION

A careful history and physical examination remain the most important methods for evaluating uncomplicated peptic ulcer. However, because other diseases may also present with epigastric distress, and because some complications of PUD may not be immediately apparent, additional diagnostic interventions are recommended.

For any patient in the age group at risk for coronary artery disease, an electrocardiogram should be performed and cardiac monitoring used, at least initially. A nasogastric tube should be passed if bleeding or obstruction is suspected, but routine use is not necessary. Chemical tests for the presence of occult gastric blood are available if doubt exists.

The abdominal series, including an upright chest X-ray, is a useful adjunct for detecting free air from perforation and for ruling out thoracic disease. The patient is placed in an upright sitting position for 10 to 15 minutes before the X-ray to allow time for any free air to rise to the diaphragm; insufflating 100 to 200 mL of air through the nasogastric tube may enhance the chances of detecting free air radiographically. Unfortunately, pneumoperitoneum is seen on X-ray in less than 50% of patients with perforation, and the absence of this finding is often associated with delayed diagnosis and significantly increased mortality.

A complete blood count is justified in most emergency department patients in whom a bleeding ulcer is suspected. Low red blood cell cat and hematocrit values may reveal significant recent blood loss, and the red cell indices can suggest that anemia is from chronic blood loss. The white blood cell count is usually normal in uncomplicated PUD, but it may help to differentiate upper abdominal pain of other causes. The white blood cell count rises with perforation. Serum amylase or lipase determinations are helpful if pancreatitis is a possibility, but they are not of much value for uncomplicated PUD. Liver function tests, including alkaline phosphatase and bilirubin levels, may be useful when a hepatobiliary process remains in the differential diagnosis.

Electrolytes, blood urea nitrogen, and serum creatinine levels, and type and screen are useful for critically ill patients and those who are bleeding, vomiting, or "third-spacing" fluids. Hypochloremic hypokalemic metabolic alkalosis may be noted with intractable vomiting or gastric outlet obstruction.

Relief with antacids is a strong part of the classic peptic ulcer history and can be a helpful indicator, but it is not diagnostic of PUD. As many as one fourth of ulcer patients may have concomitant coronary artery disease; therefore, it is often difficult to ascribe symptoms or relief of symptoms to one or the other (18). The indiscriminate use of "GI cocktails" consisting of various combinations of antacids, anticholinergics, barbiturates, and viscous lidocaine, particularly as a diagnostic maneuver, should be discouraged.

EMERGENCY DEPARTMENT MANAGEMENT

Most patients with PUD have normal vital signs, are in minimal distress, and do not require any major intervention. These patients may be given antacids to help relieve pain. Because

TABLE 61.3.   Therapeutic Regimens for *Helicobacter pylori* Infection

ANTIMICROBIAL REGIMENS[a]	DURATION
Bismuth subsalicylate (Pepto Bismol) 525 mg (2 tabs) q.i.d. + metronidazole 250 mg q.i.d. + tetracycline 500 mg q.i.d. + H$_2$-receptor antagonist[b]	Antibiotics for 2 weeks H$_2$antagonist for 4 weeks
Lansoprazole 30 mg or omeprazole 20 mg b.i.d. + clarithromycin 500 mg b.i.d. + metronidazole 500 mg b.i.d.	2 weeks
Lansoprazole 30 mg or omeprazole 20 mg b.i.d. + clarithromycin 500 mg b.i.d. + amoxicillin 1 g b.i.d.	2 weeks
Bismuth subsalicylate (Pepto Bismol) 525 mg (2 tabs) q.i.d. + metronidazole 500 mg q.i.d. + tetracycline 500 mg q.i.d. + omeprazole 20 mg or lansoprazole 30 mg q. a.m.	2 weeks

[a]Antibiotics are felt to work best when taken with food; proton pump inhibitors work best when taken before breakfast.
[b]To be taken in the dosage and frequency indicated by manufacturer for the treatment of ulcers.
b.i.d., twice a day; q.i.d., four times a day.
(Adapted from Smoot DT, Go MF, Cryer B. Peptic ulcer disease. *Primary Care; Clin in Office Practice* 2001;28:487–503, with permission.)

salicylates and other NSAIDs are associated with the development of peptic ulcer, these agents should be discontinued if in use.

With the recognition that *H. pylori* plays a central role in the pathogenesis of peptic ulcer, the objective of therapy is now eradication and cure. Thus, patients with documented peptic ulcer disease by upper GI contrast radiography or endoscopy should be treated for *H. pylori*. This should be done with appropriate consultation to guide the decision on the most effective antibiotic regimen. Detection of *H. pylori* can be confirmed on histologic mucosal biopsies, by culture, serologically by enzyme-linked immunosorbent assay (ELISA), and urea breath test (19). Serology is now widely used for routine detection and to monitor treatment. Caution should be used for those patients who display signs and symptoms of gastric hypersecretory state, recent antibiotic therapy, and recent use of NSAIDs. If there is nothing to suggest that complications have occurred, specific diagnostic testing for *H. pylori* may be unnecessary, and treatment for eradication may begin as discussed (2–4,8,11–17,19,20). Treatment regimens in current use are listed in Table 61.3 (2–4,8,11–17,19,20). Traditional agents for PUD are used in an adjunctive role and for symptomatic relief of peptic ulcer. In addition, these agents neutralize or reduce acid secretion, accelerate the rate of ulcer healing, and prevent recurrence and complications.

H$_2$-receptor antagonists competitively inhibit the action of histamine on H$_2$ receptors located in gastric parietal cells and dramatically reduce basal acid secretion as well as secretion in response to feeding, gastrin, hypoglycemia, and vagal stimulation. They are generally safe and effective. Currently, four H$_2$ antagonists are available in the United States: cimetidine, 800 mg p.o. q.h.s; ranitidine, 150 mg p.o. b.i.d. (or 300 mg q.h.s.); famotidine, 40 mg p.o. q.h.s.; and nizatidine, 300 mg p.o. q.h.s.

A single bedtime dose of any of these medications appears to be roughly as effective as several doses given throughout the day. When used primarily for exacerbations of PUD, low-dose maintenance therapy with H$_2$-receptor antagonists may also be safe and effective.

Sucralfate is an aluminum salt of sucrose that forms a polymer in the acid environment of the stomach. This polymer adheres selectively to the ulcer crater, forming a physiologic dressing for the damaged mucosa and protecting it from acid; other mechanisms may be at work as well. Sucralfate appears to heal ulcers as effectively as do H$_2$ blockers. It is nonabsorbable and has a very low incidence of side effects. The usual initial dose is sucralfate 1 g p.o. q.i.d., or 2 g b.i.d.

Anticholinergics have been used to treat patients with PUD for many years and are available in a number of formulations. They decrease acid production, but they also produce dry mouth, urinary retention, and other anticholinergic side effects.

Other agents now available have been found to be at least as efficacious as the H$_2$ blockers. These include the prostaglandin congeners, such as misoprostol, which increase the cytoprotective properties of the gastric mucosa, and proton pump inhibitors, which effectively reduce gastric acid secretion (1,5): omeprazole, 40 mg p.o. q.d.; lansoprazole 15 to 30 mg p.o. q.d.; rabeprazole 20 mg p.o. q.d.; esomeprazole 40 mg p.o. q.d.; pantoprazole 40 mg p.o. q.d.

Patients with complications of PUD require more intensive management, including intravenous infusion of crystalloid or blood, supplemental oxygen, cardiac monitoring, and more specific endoscopic or surgical intervention.

Transfusion is indicated for bleeding patients who fail to stabilize after receiving 2 L of crystalloid, have known coronary artery disease, or who are experiencing angina. Trends in hemoglobin and hematocrit values are more useful than a single value; any significant decrease should be considered an indication for transfusion.

CRITICAL INTERVENTION

- Be vigilant for serious complications of PUD, such as significant GI bleeding or perforation

DISPOSITION

Patients who are obviously critically ill, have unstable vital signs, or who are suffering from a complication of PUD require hospital admission and prompt consultation with a specialist. Other patients may need admission for pain control, gastric decompression, or fluid resuscitation, and do not necessarily require monitoring. Cases of apparently uncomplicated PUD may be referred to a family physician or internist. Initiation of PUD therapy in the emergency department does not obviate the need for outpatient referral, because for a subset of patients therapy will fail and these patients may be candidates for endoscopy.

Ulcer patients who require admission may need to be transferred to another institution for endoscopy, critical care services, or surgery. Potentially unstable patients should be transported by an advanced life support unit.

COMMON PITFALLS

✔ Failure to consider other life-threatening etiologies for epigastric pain, especially myocardial infarction or abdominal aortic aneurysm

✔ Failure to recognize sudden changes in symptomatology that herald the onset of a serious complication

✔ Failure to refer the patient to an appropriate specialist for evaluation of response to therapy and the need for further diagnostic workup

Acknowledgment

Thank you to previous edition chapter author David J. Vukich.

References

1. Ballinger A. Cytoprotection with misoprostol: use in the treatment and prevention of ulcers. *Dig Dis* 1994;12:37.
2. Cotton P. NIH consensus panel urges antimicrobials for ulcer patients, skeptics concern with caveats. *JAMA* 1994;271:808.
3. De Boer WA, Tytgat GN. Search and treat strategy to eliminate *Helicobacter pylori* associated ulcer disease. *Gut* 2001;48:567–570.
4. Fennerty MB. *Helicobacter pylori. Arch Intern Med* 1994;154:721.
5. Florent C. Progress with proton pump inhibitors in acid peptic disease: treatment of duodenal and gastric ulcer. *Clin Ther* 1993;15[Suppl B]:14.
6. Fowler SF, Khoubian JF, et al. Peptic ulcers in the elderly is a surgical disease. *Am J Surgery* 2001;182:733–737.
7. Hermann RE. Obstructing duodenal ulcer. *Surg Clin North Am* 1976;56:1403.
8. Howden CW, Hunt RH. Guidelines for the management of *Helicobacter pylori* infection. *Am J Gastroenterol* 1998;93:2330.
9. Jorde R, Burhol PG. Asymptomatic peptic ulcer disease. *Scand J Gastroenterol* 1987;22:129.
10. Kurata JH, Haile BM. Epidemiology of peptic ulcer disease. *Clin Gastroenterol* 1984;13:289.
11. Labenz J, Ruhl GH, Bertrams J, et al. Medium or high-dose omeprazole plus amoxicillin eradicates *Helicobacter pylori* in gastric ulcer disease. *Am J Gastroenterol* 1994;89:726.
12. Langman MJS. Peptic ulcer treatment now and tomorrow. *J Clin Gastroenterol* 1987;9[Suppl 2]:2.
13. Maniatis AG, Brazer SR. Omeprazole/amoxicillin versus ranitidine/triple therapy for duodenal ulcer: when is the same the same? *Am J Gastroenterol* 1994;89:947.
14. Meurer LN, Bower DJ. Management of *Helicobacter pylori* infection. *Am Fam Physician* 2002;65:1327–1336.
15. NIH Consensus Conference. *Helicobacter pylori* in peptic ulcer disease. *JAMA* 1994;272:65.
16. Peura D. The report of the Digestive Health Initiative International Update Conference in *Helicobacter pylori. Gastroenterology* 1997;113:S4–S8.
17. Peura D. *Helicobacter pylori*: rational management options. *Am J Med* 1998;105:424–430.
18. Scheeres DE, DeKryger LL, Dean RE. Surgical treatment of peptic ulcer disease before and after introduction of H₂ blockers. *Ann Surg* 1987;53:392.
19. Shiotani A, Graham DY. Pathogenesis and therapy of gastric and duodenal ulcer disease. *Med Clin North Am* 2002;86:1447–1466.
20. Smoot DT, Go MF, Cryer B. Peptic ulcer disease. *Primary Care Clin Office Pract* 2001;28:487–503.
21. Walt RP, Katschinski B, Logan R, et al. Rising frequency of ulcer perforation in elderly people in the United Kingdom. *Lancet* 1986;i:489.
22. Wolfe F, Anderson J, et al. Gastroprotective therapy and risk of gastrointestinal ulcers: risk reduction by COX-2 therapy. *J Rheumatol* 2002;29:467–473.

CHAPTER 62
Approach to Jaundice

Tobias D. Barker and Gus M. Garmel

Jaundice may be defined as a yellowing of the skin, sclera, and other tissues owing to excess circulating bilirubin. The challenge comes not with the identification of jaundice, but with the workup to delineate which pathological process is responsible. This chapter will discuss an approach to the jaundiced patient, with particular attention to understanding bilirubin metabolism. It also includes historical, physical examination, laboratory, and imaging findings that clinicians will find useful in developing a differential and establishing a diagnosis.

BILIRUBIN METABOLISM

Bilirubin is one end product of heme metabolism. Approximately 75% of bilirubin is derived from the hemoglobin of senescent red blood cells; the remainder comes from myoglobin and respiratory enzymes with structures similar to that of heme (8). Initially, all bilirubin produced in the body is unconjugated. This unconjugated bilirubin is actively transported from albumin into liver cells. Here, bilirubin is combined with glucuronic acid in the smooth endoplasmic reticulum to become conjugated bilirubin. Conjugated bilirubin is then excreted from the hepatocyte to the biliary tract, where it eventually reaches the intestines and is excreted from the body (Fig. 62.1A).

CLINICAL PRESENTATION

The jaundiced patient typically presents with one of several complaints. Skin color changes may occur in isolation, or with nausea, vomiting, abdominal pain, pruritus, and/or fever. Although rarely a true medical emergency, physicians must quickly assess for possible life-threatening conditions, such as hypotension, sepsis, or alterations in mental status. Sir William Osler stated "Jaundice is the disease your friends diagnose"(1). Regardless of who identifies these color changes, patients are likely to be concerned about the underlying cause.

DIFFERENTIAL DIAGNOSIS

The differential diagnosis for the patient presenting with jaundice is extensive. Jaundice has many possible etiologies, including hemolysis, hereditary disorders of bilirubin metabolism, hepatocellular dysfunction, and biliary obstruction. Certain epidemiologic factors may provide clues to the cause of a patient's jaundice. In general, younger patients are more likely to have parenchymal liver disease, whereas older patients are more likely to have biliary stones or malignant disease. Table 62.1 suggests common causes of jaundice grouped by age.

Causes of yellow skin in the absence of hyperbilirubinemia include carotenemia, quinacrine ingestion, and occupational exposure to chemicals used in the manufacturing of explosives such as dinitrophenol and tetryl (3). One feature that differentiates jaundice from other causes of yellow skin is that only bilirubin stains the sclera. Other areas where jaundice may be identified

Normal Bilirubin Metabolism

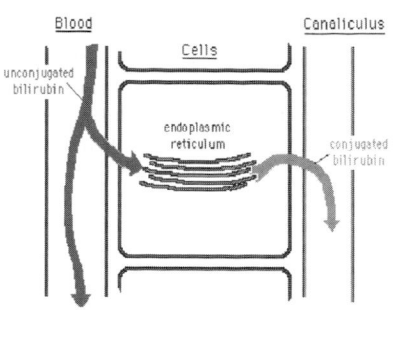

A

Decreased Bilirubin Uptake by Hepatocytes

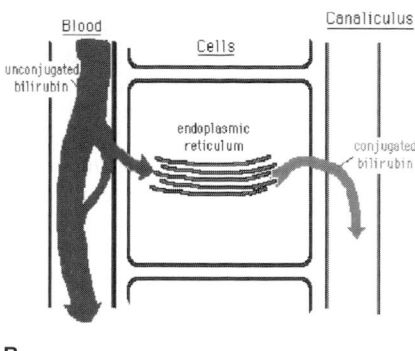

B

Impaired Bilirubin Conjugation

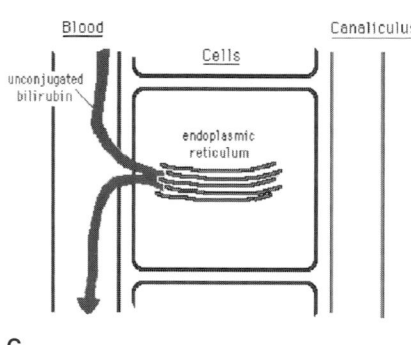

C

Bilirubin Production Beyond the Liver's Ability to Conjugate

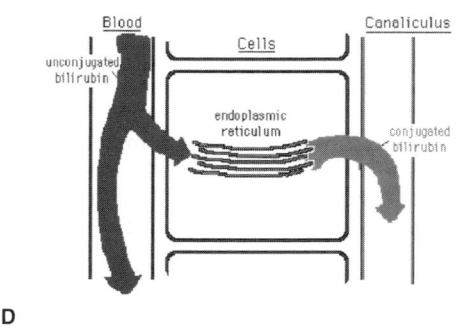

D

Defective Secretion of Conjugated Bilirubin from Hepatocytes

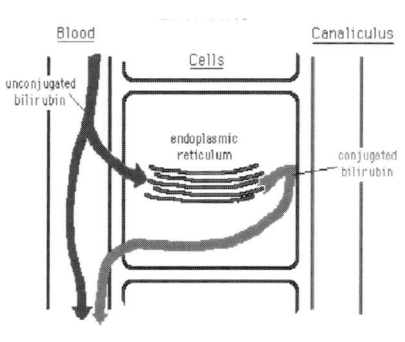

E

Obstruction in the Biliary Network

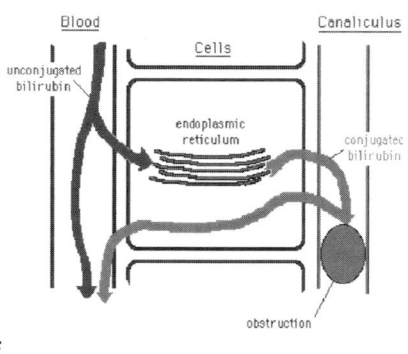

F

Figure 62.1.   Mechanisms of hyperbilirubinemia. **(A)** Normal bilirubin metabolism. **(B)** Gilbert disease and certain drugs: defective bilirubin uptake from the blood, resulting in unconjugated hyperbilirubinemia. **(C)** Physiologic jaundice of the newborn, and Crigler-Najjar syndrome: inability to conjugate bilirubin. **(D)** Hemolytic anemia: the capacity of the hepatocytes is overwhelmed, resulting in an unconjugated hyperbilirubinemia. **(E)** Dubin-Johnson syndrome: hepatocytes are unable to secrete conjugated bilirubin into the biliary system. **(F)** Obstruction in the biliary outflow tract (e.g., gallstones, tumor, mass) results in backup and reabsorption of conjugated bilirubin. (Modified from Baggott J, Dennis SE. Diseases associated with hyperbilirubinemia. http://www.mcphu.edu/netbiochem/hi7d.htm.)

are those regions relatively free of melanin, such as the palms, soles, and the undersurface of the tongue.

EMERGENCY DEPARTMENT EVALUATION

The underlying pathology behind a patient's jaundice can often be uncovered with a thorough history, physical examination, and selected laboratory and imaging tests. In one study, these were successful in delineating the cause of jaundice as obstructive or nonobstructive in 75% of cases (9). One approach to the jaundiced patient is provided in Figure 62.2. History, physical examination, and testing will be discussed in the following sections.

History

As always, a good history can help delineate possible etiologies responsible for a patient's presentation. Important historical points in a jaundiced patient include:

New-onset dark urine indicates a conjugated hyperbilirubinemia, since unconjugated bilirubin is not filtered into the urine. Patients often notice dark urine before skin discoloration. Thus, the onset of dark urine may be the first indication of hyperbilirubinemia.

Clay-colored stool indicates bilirubin is not leaving the biliary ducts because of obstruction, resulting in a conjugated hyperbilirubinemia.

Medications, alcohol, and a number of *environmental hepatotoxins* such as phosphorus, petrochemicals, organic solvents, or toxic mushrooms may result in jaundice. Medications such as acetaminophen, anabolic steroids, and sulfonamides can cause jaundice through direct cellular damage or by interfering with biliary secretion.

Nausea and vomiting preceding jaundice most often indicates acute hepatitis or common duct obstruction by a stone. Abdominal pain, chills, or rigors favor the latter. Recent flu-like symptoms and aspirin use raises the possibility of Reye's syndrome in younger patients. Anorexia and malaise, especially long-standing, suggest alcoholic liver disease, chronic hepatitis, or pancreatic cancer.

Infectious exposures, intravenous drug use, or blood transfusions increase the possibility of viral hepatitis.

Pregnancy suggests benign recurrent cholestasis or acute fatty liver of pregnancy.

TABLE 63.2.   Differential Diagnosis of Acute Diseases of the Gallbladder

Complications of gallstones
Acute cholecystitis
Hepatitis
Pancreatitis
Peptic ulcer disease
Esophageal disease, with or without perforation
Appendicitis
Bowel obstruction
Colonic pathology
Pelvic inflammatory disease
Fitz-Hugh–Curtis syndrome/perihepatitis
Renal colic
Pyelonephritis
Pneumonia
Pulmonary embolism
Acute myocardial infarction
Aortic dissection
HELLP syndrome

HELLP, hemolytic anemia, elevated liver enzymes, low platelet count.

with nonspecific symptoms of biliary disease, with 50% of patients having no pain and 45% presenting with jaundice (14).

DIFFERENTIAL DIAGNOSIS

When patients present with complaints attributable to gallbladder disease, a wide range of both intraabdominal and extraabdominal processes must be considered (Table 63.2). Failing to consider biliary tract pathology in the differential diagnosis of nonspecific abdominal pain, fever, or sepsis in some special populations can be problematic. Elderly or debilitated patients are often difficult to assess and require ancillary studies to rule out life-threatening disease. Because pregnancy is associated with increased incidence of biliary sludge and cholesterol stone formation (8), biliary disease must be considered in the differential diagnosis of the pregnant patient with abdominal pain. In children, biliary disease, although uncommon, is increasing in frequency. Children with cholelithiasis typically have underlying risk factors for the development of stones and biliary disease, such as sickle cell disease or other hemolytic anemias, total parenteral nutrition, infection, and, particularly in neonates, dehydration and sepsis (15).

EMERGENCY DEPARTMENT EVALUATION

Despite the diversity in acute gallbladder pathology, evaluation should follow a relatively straightforward sequence based on the patient's clinical status (Table 63.1). The goal of the emergency physician is to rule out life-threatening problems and, if gallbladder pathology is suspected, to rule out acute cholecystitis and other complicated acute gallbladder disease. If the patient presents with pain or other symptoms attributable to gallstones, but is otherwise well, referral for outpatient ultrasound and follow-up is appropriate. No further emergency department workup is necessary. In the patient with more severe symptoms or dehydration, further workup is indicated, including a complete blood count, electrolytes, liver function tests, bilirubin, amylase, lipase, urinalysis, and possibly diagnostic imaging.

Diagnostic Imaging

Confirmation of acute cholecystitis and its complications is primarily radiographic. Plain radiographs are helpful only for diag-

nosing associated bowel obstruction or ileus, although gallstones are visible on plain radiographs in approximately 10% of cases.

Because of its ease of use and low risk, ultrasound is the first-line method for evaluating the gallbladder and biliary tree. Gallstones alone do not make the diagnosis of acute cholecystitis. The best indicator of acute cholecystics includes the triad of a thickened gallbladder wall (>3 mm), a sonographic Murphy sign, and presence of gallstones. Gallbladder wall thickening is nonspecific and can occur in chronic cholecystitis, CHF, cirrhosis, hepatitis, and many other conditions (9). Other relevant findings include sludge in the gallbladder, gallbladder distention, and pericholecystic fluid. Ultrasound is also helpful in making the diagnosis of complications of acute cholecystitis. A dilated CBD or intraluminal stone is diagnostic of choledocholithiasis. Free fluid suggests gallbladder perforation. Ultrasound can also assess other extrabiliary causes of RUQ pain involving liver, kidney, or pancreas (21,24).

Cholescintigraphy tests the patency of the cystic duct. Failure to visualize the gallbladder is highly sensitive for acute cholecystitis. Hepatobiliary scanning is usually used when there is a high suspicion for acute cholecystitis, with an equivocal or negative ultrasound examination, particularly if acalculous cholecystitis is suspected (24).

Computed tomographic (CT) scanning is reserved for patients with atypical presentations in whom other intraabdominal pathology is a consideration. It is most useful in evaluating complications of gallstones and acute cholecystitis, including gallbladder perforation, pericholecystic abscess, and gangrenous and emphysematous cholecystitis (9).

EMERGENCY DEPARTMENT MANAGEMENT

Emergency department management of symptomatic cholelithiasis includes hydration, antiemetics, and analgesia. These patients can usually be sent home with appropriate followup. If acute cholecystitis or another complicated presentation of gallbladder disease is considered, prompt consultation with a general surgeon is mandatory. Attention to the patient's fluid volume and electrolyte status, antiemetics and analgesia, typically with nonsteroidal antiinflammatory drugs or narcotics, is appropriate (3).

If the patient is febrile and acute cholecystitis is suspected, antibiotics are typically indicated, but this should be discussed with the consultant. The patient who is septic or is suspected of having ascending cholangitis, perforation, or emphysematous cholecystitis should be given antibiotics promptly. Typical biliary pathogens include enteric gram-negative bacteria and gram-positive species such as enterococcus or streptococci. Anaerobic species, particularly *Clostridium* and *Bacteroides fragilis*, occur in approximately 10% to 15% of cases, usually in the elderly or in those patients with obstructive disease. Appropriate coverage includes a parenteral antipseudomonal penicillin such as ticarcillin/clavulanate 3.1 g q.6.h. or piperacillin/tazobactam 3.375 g q.6.h. Alternative regimens, especially if anaerobes are suspected, include a second- or third-generation cephalosporin or an aminoglycoside plus clindamycin or metronidazole (6).

Definitive treatment for symptomatic gallstones is usually surgical, with laparoscopic cholecystectomy or open cholecystectomy (24). Oral dissolution therapy for gallstones, occasionally in conjunction with extracorporeal shock-wave lithotripsy, is used in patients who are substantial surgical risks or do not want surgery (11).

In patients who present with pain, fever, or jaundice after laparoscopic cholecystectomy, one must consider the increasingly recognized complications of the procedure, including biliary injury and fistulas, wound infections, and intraabdominal abscesses, which may present weeks to months after surgery (24).

Definitive treatment for acute cholecystitis and complicated gallstone disease is almost always surgical. Currently, urgent cholecystectomy, typically laparoscopic, within a few days of presentation, is preferred over delayed surgery (23). Percutaneous cholecystostomy followed by cholecystectomy is an option for patients with significant comorbidities who are expected to develop complications from urgent cholecystectomy (17). In patients with CBD stones, endoscopic sphincterotomy or dilatation to relieve obstruction followed by elective cholecystectomy is typically performed, rather than open cholecystectomy with CBD exploration (23). Almost all patients with ascending cholangitis require urgent biliary decompression. Typically this is performed by using endoscopic sphincterotomy, rather than surgical approaches (10). All patients with gallbladder perforation, emphysematous cholecystitis, or gallbladder empyema need emergent surgery (20).

CRITICAL INTERVENTIONS

- Confirmatory imaging studies in all cases of suspected acute cholecystitis or its complications
- Surgical consultation in all cases of acute cholecystitis or acute biliary disease
- Early surgical or gastroenterology consultation if biliary decompression is indicated
- Antibiotics in suspected acute cholecystitis or cholangitis

DISPOSITION

Most patients with symptomatic cholelithiasis may be managed as outpatients, with analgesics, antiemetics, and followup with a general surgeon. Those with more severe symptoms refractory to emergency department treatment should be admitted to the hospital.

Patients with acute cholecystitis, choledocholithiasis, ascending cholangitis, or complications of chronic cholelithiasis such as gallstone ileus must be admitted to the hospital for antibiotics and/or surgical care.

COMMON PITFALLS

✔ Acute complications of gallstone disease must be considered and recognized, particularly in the elderly and debilitated
✔ Remember to consider cholecystitis or cholangitis in the elderly, diabetic, or debilitated patient who presents with fever of unknown origin, change in mental status, or other nonspecific complaints
✔ Symptomatic gallstones should be considered in patients with mild or atypical presentations, such as nausea, dyspepsia, or vague abdominal pain
✔ Always consider acute gallbladder disease in the pregnant woman with abdominal pain
✔ Always obtain timely surgical consultation when complications of gallstone disease are considered

References

1. Abou-Saif A, Al-Kawas FH. Complications of gallstone disease: Mirizzi syndrome, cholecystocholedochal fistula and gallstone ileus. *Am J Gastroenterol* 2002;97:249–254.
2. Agrawal S, Jonnalagadda S. Gallstones, from gallbladder to gut. *Postgrad Med* 2000;143–153.
3. Akriviadis EA, Hazigavriel M, Kapnias D, et al. Treatment of biliary colic with diclofenac: a randomized, double-blind, placebo-controlled study. *Gastroenterology* 1997;113:225.
4. Barie PS, Eachempati SR. Acute Acalculous Cholecystitis. *Curr Gastroenterol Rep* 2003;5:302–309.
5. Diehl A. Epidemiology and natural history of gallstone disease. *Gastroenterol Clin North Am* 1991;20:1.
6. Elsakr R, Johnson DA, Younes Z, et al. Antimicrobial treatment of intra-abdominal infections. *Dig Dis* 1998;16:46.
7. Gandolfi L, Torresan F, Solmi L, et al. The role of ultrasound in biliary and pancreatic diseases. *Eur J Ultrasound* 2003;16:141–159.
8. Gilar T, Knoikoff F. Pregnancy and the biliary tract. *Can J Gastroenterol* 2000;14:55–59.
9. Gore RM, Yaghmai V, Newmark GM, et al. Imaging benign and malignant disease of the gallbladder. *Radiol Clin North Am* 2002;40:1307–1323.
10. Gouma DJ. Management of acute cholangitis. *Dig Dis* 2003;21:25–29.
11. Kalser S. National Institutes of Health Consensus Development Conference statement on gallstones and laparoscopic cholecystectomy. *Am J Surg* 1993;165:390.
12. Lee BY, Morilla C. Acute emphysematous cholecystitis: a case report and review of the literature. *N Y State J Med* 1992;92:406.
13. Leiva JI, Etter El, Gathe J, et al. Surgical therapy for 101 patients with acquired immunodeficiency syndrome and symptomatic cholecystitis. *Am J Surg* 1997;174:414.
14. Levin B. Gallbladder carcinoma. *Ann Oncol* 1999;4:129–130.
15. Lobe TE. Cholelithiasis and cholecystitis in children. *Semin Pediatr Surg* 2000;9:170–176.
16. O'Brien PE, Dixon JB. A rational approach to cholelithiasis in bariatric surgery: its application to the laparoscopically placed adjustable gastric band. *Arch Surg* 2003;138:908–912.
17. Patino JF, Quintero GA. Asymptomatic cholelithiasis revisited. *World J Surg* 1998;22:1119.
18. Pellegrini C. Surgery for gallstone pancreatitis. *Am J Surg* 1993;165:515.
19. Portincasa P, Moschetta A, van Erpecum KJ, et al. Pathways of cholesterol crystallization in model bile and native bile. *Dig Liver Dis* 2003;35:118–126.
20. Reiss R, Deutsch AA. State of the art in diagnosis and management of acute cholecystitis. *Dig Dis* 1993;11:55.
21. Saini S. Imaging of the hepatobiliary tract. *N Engl J Med* 1997;336:1889.
22. Savoca P. The increasing prevalence of acalculous cholecystitis in outpatients. *Ann Surg* 1990;211:433.
23. Schwesinger WH, Sirinek KR, Strodel WE. Laparoscopic cholecystectomy for biliary tract emergencies: state of the art. *World J Surg* 1999;23:334–342.
24. Strasberg S. Cholelithiasis and acute cholecystitis. *Baillieres Clin Gastroenterol* 1997;11:643.
25. Trowbridge RL, Rutkowski NK, Shojania KG: Does this patient have acute cholecystitis? *JAMA* 2003;289:80–86.

CHAPTER 64
Hepatitis

Mark J. Ault and Joel M. Geiderman

Viruses are responsible for the majority of cases of acute hepatitis. The primary hepatotropic viruses include hepatitis A virus (HAV), hepatitis B virus (HBV), hepatitis C virus (HCV), hepatitis D virus (HDV, also called the delta agent), hepatitis E virus (HEV), and the non–A through E hepatitis viruses. In addition, Epstein-Barr virus (EBV), cytomegalovirus (CMV), and other viruses are known to cause hepatitis as part of a systemic infection, as are a variety of bacteria, rickettsiae, and protozoal organisms (Table 64.1). A similar histopathologic picture can result from a variety of toxic and anoxic processes.

CLINICAL PRESENTATION

The clinical manifestations of hepatitis, regardless of cause, are protean and vary from individual to individual with respect to severity of symptoms, duration of illness, and outcome. The ultimate course of the illness is thought to depend on the nature

TABLE 64.1. Infectious Agents Known to Cause Hepatitis

PRIMARY HEPATITIS VIRUSES

Hepatitis A (HAV)
Hepatitis B (HBV)
Hepatitis C (HCV)
Hepatitis D (HDV)
Hepatitis E (HEV)
Non–A through E

SECONDARY HEPATITIS VIRUSES

Epstein-Barr
Cytomegalovirus
Herpes simplex
Varicella-zoster
Rubella
Rubeola
Mumps
Adenovirus
Coxsackievirus B
Yellow fever

NONVIRAL INFECTIOUS AGENTS

Brucellosis
Ehrlichiosis
Gram-negative sepsis
Gram-positive toxic shock syndromes
Legionellosis
Leptospirosis
Malaria
Mycoplasma disease
Plague
Q fever
Salmonellosis
Syphilis
Toxoplasmosis
Tularemia
Tuberculosis

of the etiologic agent, the extent of preexisting or underlying liver disease, and, with infectious causes, the interaction between host factors and the pathogen.

In its classic presentation, viral hepatitis has a highly characteristic clinical picture that is easily recognizable in its various stages. After a variable incubation period, a *prodromal phase* of illness occurs, with symptoms such as anorexia, low-grade fever, malaise, and lassitude. Often characterized as *flu-like* symptoms, they are nonspecific constitutional complaints typical of a variety of viral illnesses. Gastrointestinal symptoms may predominate, particularly in the adult patient, and abdominal discomfort representing hepatic, and occasionally splenic, enlargement may be reported. Within days to weeks after the onset of symptoms, the patient who enters the *icteric phase* of the illness first notes discoloration of the urine, representing the early rise of direct-reacting bilirubin and the spillage of bilirubin pigment into the urine. Subsequently, light (clay-colored) stools develop, scleral icterus may be noted, and clinical jaundice may become evident both to the patient and to the clinician as the serum bilirubin level exceeds 3 to 4 mg/dL. At this point, particularly in hepatitis A, symptoms may begin to resolve, heralding the convalescent phase of the illness.

Physical findings are highly variable in that the examination findings may be completely normal or may reveal frank jaundice and evidence of hepatic dysfunction. Liver enlargement and tenderness are common, and splenomegaly and lymphadenopathy may be present in 15% to 20% of cases.

Hampered frequently by unfamiliarity with the patient; by misleading, confusing, vague, or nonspecific historical details; and by multiple etiologic possibilities, the emergency physician may not recognize hepatitis when it does not present as the classic textbook picture. This may occur, for example, when surreptitious toxin ingestion is involved or when the patient is reluctant to reveal specific risk factors for viral hepatitis.

If the patient is frankly jaundiced, hepatitis is usually readily considered. Recognition of the more subtle findings of scleral discoloration, sublingual yellowing, or evidence of excoriations, which may be evident only on careful head-to-toe examination, also may lead to the discovery of hepatic disease.

When frank jaundice is absent, however—the rule rather than the exception in viral hepatitis—a higher index of suspicion is necessary. When present, constitutional symptoms alone are not at all specific for hepatitis but nonetheless are usually a sensitive marker for active hepatic disease and may provoke initial preliminary laboratory screening.

Extrahepatic manifestations are particularly prevalent in hepatitis B and are generally considered to result from formation of immune complexes, with deposition in various extrahepatic sites. They include urticaria and morbilliform rashes, arthralgias and frank arthritis, hematuria and proteinuria, and, less commonly, vasculitis of the mixed cryoglobulinemia or polyarteritis nodosa types (7). Other extrahepatic manifestations are not believed to be immunologically mediated. Pancreatitis, pneumonitis, and myocarditis are thought to be caused by direct viral involvement.

Occasionally, a patient presents with advanced hepatic failure and no history of previous hepatitis. This may occur in the context of progressive chronic hepatitis, a toxic insult, or acute-on-chronic hepatitis. Unexplained encephalopathy (which may be as subtle as a personality change) coagulopathy, hypoglycemia, or respiratory alkalosis should prompt consideration of a hepatic disorder and a diligent search for confirmatory evidence. Following is a discussion of the many causes of hepatitis.

Viral Hepatitis

Acute viral hepatitis is characterized by four stages: the incubation period, the preicteric phase, the icteric phase, and convalescence. During the incubation period, there are no clinical manifestations of disease, but viral replication is occurring, and serologic and chemical markers of this activity and the host response to it can be measured. Clinical manifestations appear only if and when enough hepatocytes are invaded. The etiologic agent causing hepatitis cannot be determined from the clinical presentation; all of the hepatotropic viruses are capable of producing a similar clinical picture. Therefore, in evaluating the patient with presumed viral hepatitis and attempting to determine the cause, it is imperative to understand the significance of the serologic markers associated with the various types.

Hepatitis A virus (HAV) is spread primarily by the fecal–oral route, although the virus can be found in the blood as well as in the liver, bile, and stool during the latter part of the incubation period. The 2-week period before the onset of jaundice is the time of greatest infectivity; viremia, fecal shedding in the stool, and infectivity diminish markedly by the time the icteric phase begins (Fig. 64.1). Source outbreaks are the result of fecal contamination of water supplies (e.g., with poor sanitation or during disasters), or when food becomes contaminated. The disease may also be spread by oral–anal contact. The incubation period is short: 2 to 7 weeks. The *preicteric* phase of hepatitis A, usually lasting 4 to 14 days, presents nonspecifically with weakness, malaise, anorexia, nausea, and vomiting. There may be pain in the right upper quadrant and a characteristic loss of taste for cigarettes. Rash, urticaria, and joint pain occur infrequently, but the diagnosis

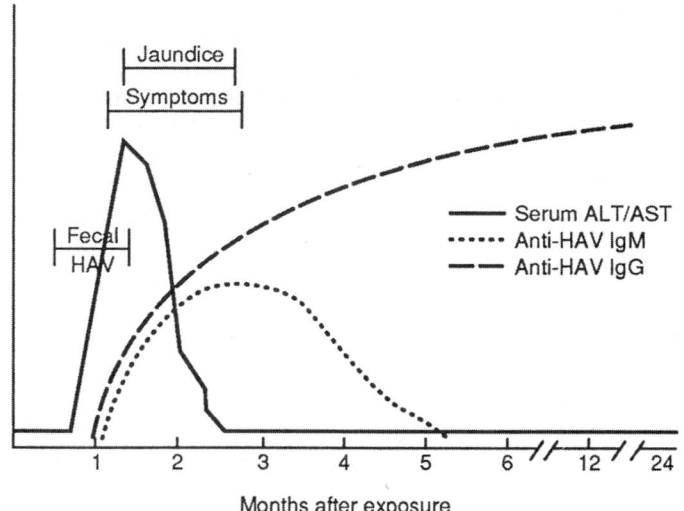

Figure 64.1.   Serologic course of viral hepatitis A. Children usually have only mild symptoms with no jaundice. Adults more often develop jaundice. (Adapted from Hoofnagle JH. Serologic diagnosis of acute and chronic hepatitis. In: Hepatology update/portal hypertension: viral hepatitis [postgraduate course of the American Association for the Study of Liver Diseases]. *Hosp Med* 1988;6:26.)

Acute type B hepatitis

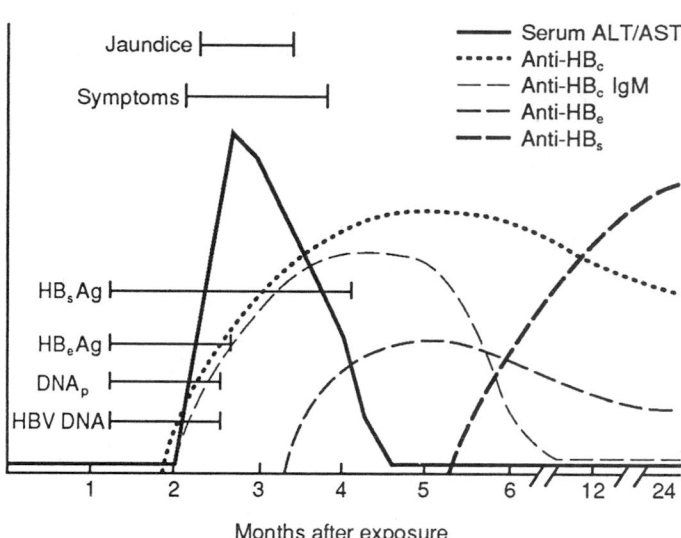

Figure 64.2.   Serologic course of acute hepatitis B. This is more likely to cause jaundice than type A or non-A/non-B types. (Adapted from Hoofnagle JH. Serologic diagnosis of acute and chronic hepatitis. In: Hepatitis update/portal hypertension: viral hepatitis [postgraduate course of the American Association for the Study of Liver Diseases]. *Hosp Med* 1988;6:33.)

of acute hepatitis should be considered in patients with these complaints. The term *preicteric* is presumptive, because not all patients go on to have clinically evident jaundice. Children with hepatitis A typically present with gastroenteritis and commonly do not develop jaundice.

The presence of dark urine frequently heralds the onset of the icteric phase and is often what prompts the patient to seek medical attention. Most of the other symptoms, with the exception of malaise, resolve shortly after the appearance of jaundice, which may persist for up to a month. However, jaundice appears in the minority of patients infected with HAV. The convalescent period is variable; weakness and malaise may last for months. This tends to be true less often with hepatitis A than with the other viral hepatitides, but such an observation is of little use in making the initial diagnosis. The onset of hepatitis A is usually more abrupt and less insidious than that of the other types of viral hepatitis, but this observation is not useful in the individual case. Figure 64.1 depicts the usual serologic and biochemical course of hepatitis A. The alanine aminotransferase (ALT, formerly serum glutamic pyruvic transaminase [SGPT]) level begins to rise late in the incubation phase, just before the onset of symptoms. Fecal shedding has peaked before this time and is abating. During the symptomatic period, about 4 to 5 weeks after exposure, immunoglobulin M (IgM) antibodies to HAV (anti-HAV IgM) begin to rise. Because this antibody usually becomes undetectable after 4 to 5 months, its presence implies recent infection; HAV itself is not measured. Antibodies of the IgG variety (anti-HAV IgG) rise a little later and remain detectable for life. The presence of such antibodies in the serum of at least 50% of adults reflects the high incidence of asymptomatic or unrecognized disease early in life, and is responsible for the effectiveness of pooled serum in preventing disease in exposed individuals.

Hepatitis B virus (HBV) is spread by the parenteral route, including exposure to blood or certain blood products, contaminated needles and syringes (both in drug abusers and accidentally in health-care workers), infected excretions or saliva, sexual contact, and perinatal contact. Its prevalence is high among homosexual men, intravenous drug abusers, dialysis patients, and patients and staff of institutions for the mentally retarded, and in certain endemic regions of the world. HBV has an

incubation period of 45 to 160 days. During this phase, the virus is actively replicating and is present not only in the hepatocyte, but also in virtually all body fluids, including blood, saliva, semen, and vaginal secretions. The implications of this fact are important: Patients can transmit disease during this incubation period, biochemical and serologic markers can be measured before disease becomes clinically apparent, and appropriate immunoprophylactic measures given after exposure, but before the onset of symptoms, may prevent or ameliorate the disease.

Acute hepatitis B usually follows a course similar to that of hepatitis A. Infrequently, a serum sickness–like illness occurs with the onset of symptoms. Jaundice is more likely to occur in hepatitis B than in hepatitis A, but still occurs in a minority of cases. Eighty percent to 85% of cases resolve completely, leaving the patient immune to hepatitis B. One percent to 3% of cases evolve into fulminant hepatitis, with a mortality rate of 90%; the remaining 5% to 10% of cases become chronic.

The serologic and biochemical courses of acute hepatitis B are depicted in Fig. 64.2. The first marker to appear in the serum is the hepatitis B surface antigen (HBsAg), indicating infection with hepatitis B. Next, DNA polymerase, HBV DNA, and the hepatitis B e antigen (HBeAg) appear in the serum. These reflect active HBV replication and infectivity and appear well before the onset of biochemical damage to the liver. Of this group, only HBeAg can be measured easily; the presence of antibody to the HBeAg (anti-HBe) suggests low infectivity. In patients who become symptomatic, the ALT level rises and, in some, jaundice appears. Most patients seen at this time will still be HBsAg-positive.

It is important to understand the significance of the next immunologic event—the appearance of antibody to the hepatitis B core antigen (anti-HBc), first of the IgM class and then IgG. This rise precedes the rise in antibodies to the surface antigen (anti-HBs). (In Fig. 64.2, note the gap between the box labeled *HBsAg* and the line labeled *anti-HBs*.) Therefore, in some patients recently infected with HBV who are seen during this gap or, "window," the sole specific marker of recent infection with HBV is the presence of anti-HBc IgM.

Chronic type B hepatitis

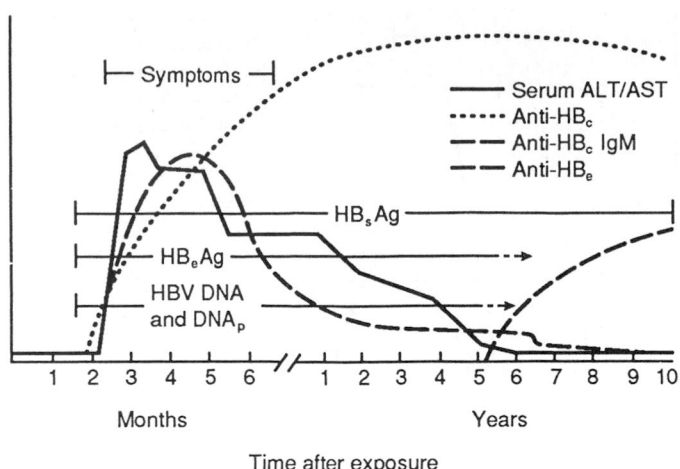

Figure 64.3.   Serologic course of chronic hepatitis B virus (HBV) disease. (Adapted from Hoofnagle JH. Serologic diagnosis of acute and chronic hepatitis. In: Hepatitis update/portal hypertension: viral hepatitis [postgraduate course of the American Association for the Study of Liver Diseases]. *Hosp Med* 1988;6:33.)

Anti-HBsAg is a neutralizing antibody; therefore, its rise correlates with abatement of symptoms and the return of ALT to normal levels and signifies immunity to HBV. Thereafter, the patient will test positive only for Anti-HBs, Anti-HBc IgG, and Anti-HBe.

When hepatitis B fails to resolve a chronic carrier state occurs. This is characterized by the persistence of HBsAg for a period exceeding 6 months and may be associated with the presence of either HBeAg or the antibodies to HBeAg. The former is associated with more active inflammation (the presence of a higher viral load), is considered more infectious, and portends a more aggressive clinical course. The latter signifies clearance of the HBeAg and is associated with less infectivity and a more favorable prognosis. The carriage rate in United States is only 0.1% to 0.5% but may be as high as 5% to 20% in some demographic groups. Figure 64.3 depicts the typical serologic course of chronic HBV disease. Note that the HBsAg remains positive, antibodies (anti-HBs) are lacking, and the patient remains susceptible to further liver damage or to superinfection with hepatitis D.

Two variants of chronic hepatitis B disease are worthy of mention as they may be associated with presentations that mimic acute illness. The first of these is seroconversion from HBeAg to anti-HBeAg. The key determinant of the natural history of chronic hepatitis B involves this spontaneous immunologic resolution of the chronic carrier state. Longitudinal studies have documented the likelihood of clearing HBeAg to be between 50% and 70%. Associated with seroconversion is a marked reduction in HBV replication and biologic and histologic remission of the inflammatory activity in majority of patients.

Occasionally, spontaneous HBeAg seroconversion may be associated clinically with acute exacerbation of hepatitis, with transaminases elevated to levels generally associated with acute hepatitis. This is believed to represent immune-mediated lysis of HBV-infected hepatocytes and may last for 2 to 4 months. The flares are frequently asymptomatic; however, symptoms of acute hepatitis or hepatic decompensation may occur.

The second serologic variant to be considered is HBeAg-negative chronic hepatitis. Patients with this serologic variant will have HBsAg present, undetectable HBeAg, absent anti-HBe, and detectable HBV DNA. ALT levels will be elevated and his-

tologic evaluation will demonstrate significant necroinflammation. Patients with HBeAg-negative chronic hepatitis tend to be older, and severe necroinflammation is seen in more than 50% of cases. Patients may present initially with severe advanced liver disease. Fluctuations in viremia and aminotransferases are common, may be severe and recurrent, and may correlate with an increased risk of progression to cirrhosis. Although this variant may be more common than initially suspected, the complexity of the serologic profile will not generally lend itself to emergency department evaluation. Nevertheless, consideration of this possibility, appropriate serologic evaluation, and exclusion of concurrent hepatitis or exposure to hepatotoxic agents is an important evaluation strategy.

Hepatitis C virus (HCV) is an RNA virus of the Flaviviridae family. After the introduction of donor screening for HBV infection, posttransfusion hepatitis continued to be a significant problem. This led to the conclusion that most posttransfusion hepatitis was caused by another blood-borne pathogen, which was designated non-A, non-B (NANB) hepatitis. After the discovery of HCV in 1989 and the routine screening of the blood supply in the United States since 1990, it became clear that 80% to 90% of parenterally transmitted NANB hepatitis was caused by HCV. Extensive genetic heterogeneity of this virus may explain variations in clinical course, difficulties in vaccine development, and variations in response to therapy (1). It may also explain why the virus so frequently escapes immunosurveillance, leading to chronic infection.

The incidence of newly acquired HCV infection has fallen dramatically since 1989 owing to the effectiveness of blood donor screening (1). Currently, since the advent of genomic testing, the risk of transfusion-related hepatitis C is in the range of one in 1,000,000 units transfused. Aside from blood transfusion, other parenteral sources of HCV infection include intravenous drug use, noninjection illegal drug use (sharing instruments for intranasal cocaine use), hemodialysis, organ transplantation, and occupational exposure. Low levels of transmission occur in sexual and household contacts and perinatally (i.e., vertical transmission). There is no evidence that breast feeding transmits HCV from mother to baby. Sporadic cases also occur.

Hepatitis C viral RNA can be detected in blood within 1 to 3 weeks of exposure. Anti-HCV can be detected in 50% to 70% of patients at the onset of symptoms and in approximately 90% of patients 3 months after the onset of infection. However, the majority of infected patients are asymptomatic and anicteric.

The symptoms of HCV—malaise, weakness, and anorexia—are similar to those seen with other types of hepatitis; however, compared with hepatitis B, the acute disease is usually milder, the peak ALT level lower, and the patient less likely to be icteric. Serum transaminase levels fluctuate and may even normalize during the course of both acute and chronic disease, and they may not indicate resolution of disease. Acute HCV infection rarely causes fulminant disease.

Chronic disease, with persistent although sometimes intermittent viremia, occurs in 85% of infected patients (10). Most patients with chronic disease are clinically well, with a small minority (20% or fewer) experiencing mild intermittent fatigue and malaise. Unfortunately, although the natural history of HCV infection is somewhat unclear, most researchers would agree that the disease causes progression to clinically significant liver disease in a large portion of infected patients. Important factors leading to more accelerated progression of hepatic fibrosis include coinfection with HIV, infection with other hepatotropic viruses, alcohol use, and young age of acquisition.

Hepatitis C is the leading reason for liver transplantation in the United States, owing to the high prevalence rate estimated to be approximately 4 million (3). Chronic HCV infection also leads to an incidence of hepatocellular carcinoma of 1% to 5%

after 20 years. In the presence of cirrhosis, the rate of acquiring hepatocellular carcinoma rises to 1% to 4% per year.

A commercially available enzyme immunoassay (EIA) is routinely used to detect antibodies to regions of the HCV genome. The test detects anti-HCV in approximately 90% of infected patients. Antibody is detectable 5 to 6 weeks after the onset of clinical hepatitis in 80% of patients, but seroconversion may take as long as 32 weeks in some individuals. The limitations of anti-HCV screening are that (i) anti-HCV is not detected in 10% of infected persons; (ii) assays do not distinguish among acute, chronic, and past infection (i.e., positive titers do not reflect either infectivity or immunity); (iii) there is a prolonged interval between onset of illness and seroconversion in some cases; and (iv) positive tests are frequently falsely positive in populations with a low prevalence of infection.

The more specific recombinant immunoblot assay (RIBA) may be used to screen out false-positive results. Future development of a test for IgM would help in determining the time of onset of disease. Polymerase chain reaction (PCR)–band assays have been developed to detect the RNA virus directly, but these are mainly of research interest.

Additional testing should include determination of HCV genotype. Hepatitis C virus has 6 major genotypes and more than 50 subtypes. Among patients in the United States, approximately 70% have genotype 1 and 25% have genotype 2 or 3. Although genotype does not correlate with severity of illness or rate of disease progression, it does correlate with response to therapy. Response rates are significantly higher and duration of therapy necessary is significantly shorter with genotypes 2 and 3. Therefore it is recommended that HCV genotype be determined one time prior to therapy to guide subsequent antiviral treatment (12).

It appears that passive immunization with immune serum globulin derived from patients with previous HCV infection is unlikely to prevent disease, and no active vaccine is presently on the horizon. Treatment now includes combination therapy with recombinant α-interferon and ribavirin. This has resulted in a two- to three-fold improvement in virologic response rates over the prior α-interferon monotherapy regimens. Multicenter trials have determined the overall virologic response rates of 54%, with 42% response rates in patients infected with genotype 1 and 82% in patients infected with genotype 2 or 3. It is not known whether combination treatment with α-interferon can prevent the development of cirrhosis and hepatocellular carcinoma.

Side effects of therapy are frequent and may prompt emergency department evaluation. Side effects of interferon include fever, nausea, irritability, and depression. Hemolytic anemia with subsequent decrease in the hematocrit is a nearly ubiquitous side effect of ribavirin and may require dose reduction.

Hepatitis D, or delta hepatitis, is caused by a defective virus, the replication of which is dependent on the presence of HBsAg synthesis. The virus consists of the delta-antigen–bearing core encapsulated by an HBsAg coat. It should not be surprising that a virus that requires HBV for its replication follows a similar transmission pattern. The clinical course of HDV infection depends on whether the virus is acquired at the same time as HBV (coinfection) or whether HDV infects a patient with chronic HBV infection (superinfection).

In coinfection, the fate of HDV parallels that of HBV. Because most cases of acute HBV are subsequently cleared, HDV, which requires the presence of HBV for replication, is also cleared. The clinical course of HDV is similar to that described for hepatitis B, although it is often more severe.

Because patients with HDV superinfection, by definition, have not been able to mount an immunologic response sufficient to clear their HBV infection, in these individuals, HDV replication may go unchecked, resulting in fulminant hepatitis in a large proportion. Rarely, acute delta superinfection results in clearance of HBV in a chronically infected patient, a phenomenon attributed to nonspecific stimulation of the immune system by a new antigen. This apparently occurs in only about 3% of patients (4). It is important to remember that immunity to hepatitis B renders one immune to hepatitis D infection.

Bearing in mind the serologic courses of acute and chronic HBV infection, it is simple to predict the serologic courses of HDV coinfection and superinfection. Table 64.2 lists the serologic features of HBV/HDV coinfection and HBV/HDV superinfection. The anti-delta IgM rises within 5 weeks of HDV infection and then persists in low titer, whereas the anti-delta IgG continues to rise as long as HBV infection persists. Therefore, IgG antibody to delta does not indicate immunity, but it is consistent with ongoing infection if associated with the presence of HBsAg (7).

Hepatitis E, formerly called enterically transmitted non-A, non-B hepatitis (ET-NANB), is responsible for more than 50% of acute viral hepatitis occurring in some developing countries. More recently, large outbreaks have occurred in Sudan and Iraq (5). It is generally of little concern in the United States, although "imported" cases have occurred in patients who have traveled to endemic areas, such as India, Nepal, Pakistan, and parts of the former Soviet Union and Mexico.

As its former name suggests, hepatitis E is enterically spread. The incubation period is 2 to 9 weeks (average, 6 weeks), with an icteric phase that lasts 3 to 8 weeks. Nausea, vomiting, and diarrhea, which are frequent, usually resolve with the onset of jaundice. Fulminant disease occurs in 5% of cases, with a predilection for pregnant women. A carrier state has not been demonstrated.

A fluorescent antibody–blocking assay to detect hepatitis E infection is available experimentally through the Centers for Disease Control and Prevention. Patients who receive pooled immune globin in the United States before travel to endemic areas are unlikely to be protected against hepatitis E because anti-HEV antibodies are not present in the American population. Travelers to endemic areas should be advised as to enteric precautions, whether they are immunized or not.

Non–A through E Hepatitis refers to the small population of patients with clinical hepatitis in whom all serologic studies on both the donor and the recipient patients are negative. Acute or chronic hepatitis in which both nonviral causes and infection

TABLE 64.2. Serologic Factors in HBV/HDV Coinfection and HBV/HDV Superinfection

HBV/HDV Coinfection		HBV/HDV Superinfection	
HbsAg + [a] anti-HBcIgM +	Implies recent HBV infection	Anti–HBc IgM − Anti–HBc IgG +	Implies chronic HBV infection
Anti–delta IgM +	Implies recent HDV infection	Anti–delta IgM +	Implies recent HDV infection

[a] Unless in window period.

with any of the five hepatitis viruses have been excluded is de-scribed as non–A through E hepatitis (2). With the discovery of new viruses and the development of new serologic tests, these patients will undoubtedly be further differentiated.

One of these, independently discovered and named hepatitis G virus (HGV) and hepatitis GB virus C (HGBV-C), is an RNA virus of the Flaviviridae family. It appears to be blood-borne and has been found in as many as 10% of patients with non–A through E hepatitis. Its role has been questioned, and its defi-nition as a true hepatotropic cause of acute or chronic hepatitis is yet to be determined (6). Similarly, hepatitis F virus has been isolated from the stool of a patient with hepatitis and transmit-ted to primates. As with hepatitis G, the role of this virus as a significant cause of non–A through E hepatitis is unclear.

Infectious, Nonviral Hepatitis

Although uncommon, hepatitis can accompany a wide variety of bacterial, rickettsial, and protozoal diseases. Included in this list are legionellosis, salmonellosis, tularemia, leptospirosis, brucel-losis, plague, syphilis, gram-negative sepsis, gram-positive toxic shock syndromes, Q fever, mycoplasmal disease, tuberculosis, toxoplasmosis, ehrlichiosis, and malaria (see Table 64.1).

Autoimmune Hepatitis

Autoimmune hepatitis is a chronic inflammatory liver disorder of uncertain etiology. A standardized definition and diagnostic criteria have been developed (8). The diagnosis relies heavily on the exclusion of viral etiologies, lack of exposure to alcohol and other hepatotoxic agents, and hypergammaglobulinemia with gamma globulin levels greater than 1.5 times the upper limits of normal. A scoring system for the quantitative diagnosis of autoimmune hepatitis has been proposed by the International Autoimmune Hepatitis Group. With a sensitivity of 97% to 100% and a specificity of 66% to 92%, it has utility in clinical practice es-pecially for atypical or overlapping cases. Liver biopsy remains essential to the diagnosis and evaluation of disease severity in patients with autoimmune hepatitis. Compounding the diag-nostic clarity of this illness is the recognition that the overlap syndrome, the simultaneous presence of autoimmune hepatitis and another liver disease seems to occur more frequently than expected (9).

Clinically, the presentation may be extremely variable and dif-ficult to differentiate from viral hepatitis. Two types have been described based on the presence of circulating autoantibodies. Type I (classic) autoimmune hepatitis has been associated with antinuclear and anti–smooth muscle antibodies, and type II has been characterized by the presence of autoantibodies against liver–kidney microsome type I (anti-L K M-1). Both types are more prevalent in young females, and appropriate diagnosis is crucial, as they may be treated with prednisone and immuno-suppressive therapy.

Toxic Hepatitis

Liver injury may result from direct hepatocellular toxicity or from idiosyncratic injury caused by a hypersensitivity-type re-action (10). Toxic exposures also may manifest as cholestasis, in which elevations of alkaline phosphatase and bilirubin lev-els predominate. Pharmacologic and chemical agents produce a diverse spectrum of hepatic insults, including both acute and chronic liver disease (Table 64.3). Drug-induced hepatic injury is the most frequent reason cited for withdrawal from the market of a U.S. Food and Drug Adminstration (FDA)–approved drug and it accounts for more than 50% of cases of acute liver failure in the United States. Although any evidence of hepatic dysfunc-tion should prompt a diligent search for both intentional and

TABLE 64.3.   Drug-Induced Hepatitis

Clinical/Morphologic Presentation	Examples
Hepatitis (acute)	α-Methyldopa Isoniazid Phenytoin Chlorothiazide Nonsteroidal antiinflammatory agents Statins
Cholestasis	Anabolic steroids Flutamide Oral contraceptive agents Erythromycin estolate Methimazole Chlorpropamide Chlorpromazine
Hepatic necrosis	Carbon tetrachloride *Amanita phalloides* mushrooms Acetaminophen Yellow phosphorus
Hepatitis (chronic)	α-Methyldopa Arsenic Isoniazid Halothane

inadvertent exposure to any of a number of chemical agents, several agents deserve specific mention because of the inherent likelihood of hepatocellular injury, because of their widespread use, or because of their particular relevance to the practice of emergency medicine.

Acetaminophen is one of the most common agents encountered in the acute setting that is responsible for striking liver enzyme elevations (see Chapter 280, "Acetaminophen"). Toxicity is dose-dependent, but several factors have been shown to contribute in a synergistic way to toxicity even at relatively low doses. These in-clude concomitant alcohol ingestion, chronic phenobarbital use, or chronic exposure to moderately large doses of acetaminophen.

Hepatitis caused by *isoniazid* clinically resembles acute viral hepatitis and may occur in as many as 20% of patients taking the drug, with the risk and severity of injury increasing with the age of the patient. Clinical toxicity generally occurs in the first few months of therapy, but transaminase elevations greater than 2 to 3 times normal at any time must be considered potentially serious, because progression to fulminant hepatitis may occur.

Statins are generally well tolerated but have been associated with severe hepatocellular injury. Moreover, there is concern that concomitant use of nicotinic acid for the treatment of hyper-cholesterolemia may promote additional toxicity.

Although overt hepatotoxicity to *phenytoin* is unusual, use of the drug is particularly common, and prevention of serious toxic-ity requires an awareness of the nature and mechanisms of injury. Hepatic injury is believed to be caused by toxic metabolites; cur-rent evidence has implicated a heritable metabolic defect that may predispose to a viral hepatitis–like hypersensitivity reac-tion within weeks of starting therapy at usual therapeutic doses. Like the other toxic exposures, early detection and interruption of therapy can result in complete resolution and the avoidance of serious hepatic injury.

Troglitazone (Rezulin) was the first of a new class of oral agents used for the treatment of type II diabetes. The agent was originally approved by the FDA in 1997, and the recognition of significant hepatotoxicity appeared to outweigh the benefits of therapy, thereby leading to the withdrawal of troglitazone from the market. Two new agents of the same class have been available since 1999, rosiglitazone (Avandia) and pioglitazone

(Actos). They do not appear to have the same degree of hepatic toxicity, although liver injury has been reported. Recognition of potential severe liver injury, monitoring of liver enzymes, and early discontinuation of therapy are important to maintain the safety of these agents (11).

Flutamide is an antiandrogen drug used in the treatment of metastatic prostate cancer. Well-documented cases of serious hepatotoxicity have been reported. Although the toxicity appeared to be reversible, several patients have died of massive hepatic necrosis, emphasizing the need for prompt consideration and diagnosis.

Hepatitis has been reported to be associated with the use of several of the *nonsteroidal antiinflammatory drugs* (NSAIDs). Because of the frequency with which NSAIDs are used, emergency physicians should be aware of their potential for causing hepatic toxicity. Sulindac has received special attention because it has been well established as a cause of hepatitis, including fatal hepatic necrosis. Similarly, bromfenac was introduced for short-term use for the treatment of orthopedic pain. Reports of severe liver injury led to withdrawal of this agent.

Well described as causes of fulminant hepatic failure, *halothane* and *methoxyflurane* are unusual causes of hepatitis. Patients may present with fevers and jaundice 1 to 2 weeks postoperatively. Specific risk factors may include obesity, multiple exposures to halothane over a brief period, and previous untoward reactions to halothane. Although no specific therapy is indicated, the emergency physician may be in the position of evaluating the postoperative patient who returns to the emergency department after discharge from the hospital. Recognition of this entity may avoid a fruitless search for other causes and, more importantly, will prevent reexposure.

A careful medication history should include an inventory of complementary and alternative medications. Studies have demonstrated that use of these modalities is common but volunteer reporting of their use to the physician is limited. Often referred to as simply "Chinese herbs," specific compounds of interest include germander, chaparral leaf, and weight loss preparations containing usnic acid.

It is worth mentioning that alcohol is probably the most common chemical to result in liver injury; this is covered in depth in Chapters 273 ("Ethanol") and 279 ("Other Complications of Chronic Ethanol Abuse").

Metabolic Causes of Hepatitis

Although the metabolic causes of liver disease are numerous, several are notable for the potential for acute presentations. *Wilson disease* is a disorder of copper excretion. Patients generally present in adolescence when copper has had sufficient time to accumulate to excess. Liver involvement is common, but occasionally in younger patients the illness will present as fulminant hepatitis. Prompt recognition and treatment are necessary to limit end-organ damage (13).

Microvesicular fatty liver is a histologic abnormality associated with acute fatty liver of pregnancy. This abnormality occurs late in pregnancy, presents with jaundice and hepatic failure, and resolves with termination of pregnancy. Other disorders leading to similar presentations in the absence of pregnancy include toxic reactions to valproic acid, excessive doses of tetracycline, and Jamaican vomiting sickness caused by the unripened *Ackee fruit*.

Reye syndrome presents almost exclusively in children younger than 15 years of age. While an association with salicylate use has been noted, it can be seen in the absence of salicylates. It is generally seen after upper respiratory illness, especially influenza and chickenpox, and is characterized by hepatic injury, hypoglycemia, and encephalopathy. Care is supportive, and chronic liver disease has not been reported when recovery occurs.

Another cause of elevated transaminase levels (transaminitis) that should be considered in the differential diagnosis is *hepatobiliary disease*. Elevated ALT and aspartate amino transferase (AST, formerly serum glutamic oxaloacetic transaminase [SGOT]) levels should not lead one on a fruitless search for infection or toxic causes of hepatitis when the chemistry patterns suggest hepatobiliary obstruction (i.e., elevated serum bilirubin, alkaline phosphatase, and γ-glutamyl transpeptidase levels [GGTP]).

DIFFERENTIAL DIAGNOSIS

The differential diagnosis for the patient with right upper quadrant abdominal pain is extensive, and includes hepatitis, biliary colic, peptic ulcer disease, renal colic, cardiac ischemia, and right lower lobe pneumonia. The differential for jaundice includes many other possibilities, and is discussed further in Chapter 62, "Approach to Jaundice." Once the differential has been narrowed to hepatitis, the next task is to determine the specific etiologic agent, whether infectious, toxic, metabolic, or autoimmune. Eliciting a history of risk factors, medications, exposures, and clinical course as described previously, combined with laboratory testing, will help in determining the specific cause.

EMERGENCY DEPARTMENT EVALUATION

Evaluation of suspected hepatitis may be divided into several steps. The first step is to make the diagnosis, which, in light of the previous discussion, may not be entirely straightforward. Clearly, a reasonable index of suspicion is necessary in most cases, and the physician must consider the relative likelihood of illness in each particular patient compared with the risk of excessive testing in the many patients with nonspecific symptomatology.

If the likelihood of hepatitis is present but low, as in a patient followed serially for development of hepatocellular disease after a needlestick, a reasonable approach initially is to order a serum AST level as a preliminary screen. AST is a cytoplasmic enzyme that is released with hepatocellular injury. Although nonspecific, this is a sensitive screen, and a normal AST value virtually excludes hepatocellular disease.

In the patient in whom hepatic disease is believed to be more likely or who has an abnormal AST level on the preliminary screen, more extensive laboratory testing is necessary. This should consist of indices of necrosis (AST and ALT) as well as indices of cholestasis (alkaline phosphatase, total bilirubin, or GGTP). Although these values lack diagnostic specificity, certain patterns may be helpful in limiting the differential diagnosis and in directing further evaluation. For instance, a transaminase elevation of greater than 10 times normal strongly suggests acute viral or toxic injury and essentially excludes chronic hepatitis. Elevation of alkaline phosphatase and bilirubin values suggests intrahepatic or extrahepatic obstruction. Transaminase elevations of 2 to 3 times normal, with the AST higher than the ALT, suggest alcoholic injury.

In the second step of the workup, after the diagnosis of liver disease has been made, specific tests of hepatic synthetic function are necessary. Tests of serum protein, albumin, and glucose levels should be ordered routinely and can be used in conjunction with the serum bilirubin level to assess the extent of hepatocellular dysfunction. If central nervous system involvement is suspected, or if unexplained lethargy, psychiatric symptoms, or other indicators of encephalopathy are present, a serum ammonia level may be obtained, which can serve as a useful baseline for further serial evaluations.

At the third step, other evaluations are performed to define more specifically the cause of the illness. If hepatocellular necrosis is the dominant picture, detailed serologic studies

TABLE 64.4.   Immunoprophylaxis of Viral Hepatitis

Type	Persons at Risk	Immunoprophylaxis
A	Household and sexual contacts[a] Staff and attendees of daycare centers Staff and residents of custodial institutions	Immune globulin, 0.02 mL/kg i.m.
B	Sexual contacts	Hepatitis B immune globulin, 0.06 mg/kg i.m.
	Percutaneous or transmucosal exposure	Begin active immunization (Heptavax or Recombivax)
C	Intravenous drug abusers, intranasal cocaine abusers, homosexuals, multiple sexual partners, perinatal exposure, household contacts	None
D	Same as B	Protection against hepatitis B
E	Travelers to endemic areas	None in serum pooled from U.S. donors
Non–A through E	Percutaneous exposure to blood or certain products of patients with no serologic evidence or HAV, HBV, or HCV	None

[a] Residents of dormitories and barracks are frequently included in this group.
HAV, hepatitis A virus; HBV, hepatitis B virus; HCV, hepatitis C virus.

(anti-HAV IgM, HBsAg, anti-HBs, anti-HBc, anti-HCV, and Monospot test) are warranted, as well as a diligent historical search for foreign travel to HEV-endemic regions and drug or toxic exposures. If cholestasis is the dominant picture, ultrasound examination should be performed to exclude mechanical obstruction.

EMERGENCY DEPARTMENT MANAGEMENT

Patients with acute viral hepatitis may present to the emergency department because of signs and symptoms typical of a viral syndrome that may include prostration, nausea, vomiting, and dehydration. Treatment for these patients is symptomatic and is usually limited to intravenous fluids, acetaminophen, and antiemetics. Metoclopramide (Reglan) or ondansetron (Zofran) are the antiemetic agents of choice, because phenothiazines can impair hepatic excretory function and may produce cholestasis. Patients who present without symptoms or present because they have noticed jaundice require no specific therapy.

For patients with diagnosed viral hepatitis, there is no specific therapy indicated beyond supportive care and symptomatic treatment. If the prothrombin time is prolonged, the patient should receive vitamin K. Immune globulin is of no use for the patient who has already contracted hepatitis. Corticosteroids are probably harmful rather than beneficial.

Patients who present because they have been exposed, or think they have been exposed, to hepatitis present a different management problem. (For needlestick patients, see Chapter 150, "Blood and Body Fluid Exposures in the Health-Care Worker.)" Immunoprophylaxis is highly effective if given under the proper circumstances. Because this treatment should be guided in part by serologic studies, it is often not initiated in the emergency department.

If results of serologic testing are not available, or not available in a timely fashion, therapy must be empiric and, as such, must be based on probabilities. The discussion that follows and the material in Table 64.4 should help guide immunoprophylactic therapy.

Patients considered at risk for contracting hepatitis A include household and sexual contacts of persons with hepatitis A; staff and attendees at daycare centers; and staff and residents in close contact at custodial care institutions. Immune globulin, which is derived from pooled human serum but treated so as not to be capable of transmitting HIV infection or other diseases, is given as a single intramuscular dose of 0.02 mL/kg as soon as possible within the first 2 weeks after exposure. Casual contacts need not be treated; such patients need little more than education and reassurance.

Postexposure prophylaxis for hepatitis B is indicated for sexual contacts of persons with hepatitis B, or after percutaneous or transmucosal exposure to HBsAg-positive blood. For nonimmunized patients, treatment is with hepatitis B immune globulin, 0.06 mL/kg intramuscularly; active immunization is begun at the same time. This recommendation assumes that serologic data are available on the index patient with hepatitis and that the immune status of the exposed patient is known. If the data are not available but can be obtained within 5 to 7 days, it is reasonable to wait. If not, one must make a decision on the basis of lifestyle and risk factors; the history should include information about sexual contacts and intravenous drug use. See Chapter 150 for more information on postexposure prophylaxis.

Immunoprophylaxis has not proven useful in patients who have been exposed to hepatitis C or in those suspected of being exposed to non–A through E hepatitis.

CRITICAL INTERVENTION

- Hospitalize patients with evidence of fulminant hepatitis (significantly impaired synthetic function, encephalopathy)

DISPOSITION

Most patients with hepatitis do not require hospital admission, but it is recommended under the circumstances—intractable nausea and vomiting; dehydration, or electrolyte imbalance—that cannot be reasonably corrected in the emergency department, or for signs of hepatic deterioration, as evidenced by changes in sensorium or increased international normalized ratio (INR). Obviously, patients with signs or symptoms suggesting a fulminant course of hepatic failure require admission. The absolute levels of serum transaminase values should not be a criterion for admission.

Patients with acute viral hepatitis who are discharged should be prescribed antiemetic agents and instructed to ensure adequate caloric intake. It is best to allow patients to eat small meals of foods of their choice rather than insist they follow some of the high-calorie or high-protein dietary regimens that have been proposed. Prolonged bed rest, once a staple of care, has been shown to be of no value and has its own risks (6). Most patients will limit their physical activities as needed. Alcohol consumption should be avoided during the acute illness. After complete recovery, alcohol consumption has not been shown to be any more harmful for these patients than for the general population. (4) Estrogen-based oral contraceptives may be continued during hepatitis.

Patients with acute hepatitis should be seen by an internist or gastroenterologist for followup within a few days; it is prudent to wait for the results of serologic tests before this visit. Patients with any prolongation of the prothrombin time are often admitted to the hospital, but those who are not should probably be seen the next day. Instructions should include an admonition to return if food and fluids cannot be kept down or if there is any change in sensorium.

Finally, it is the duty of the emergency physician in many locales to notify public health authorities of cases of acute hepatitis. Patients and their close contacts should be counseled with regard to preventing the spread of hepatitis.

COMMON PITFALLS

✔ Missed toxic ingestion or exposure, with continued exposure
✔ Failure to recognize hepatitis B or hepatitis C by performing serologic tests during "window periods" between infection and seroconversion
✔ Missed hepatobiliary disease, with failure to diagnose surgically correctable lesions
✔ Failure to recognize the distinction between liver tests and liver function (e.g., patients with cirrhosis may have nearly normal enzyme levels; patients with "sky high" transaminase levels may have reasonably intact synthetic capability)
✔ Inappropriate admission of patients with uncomplicated hepatitis and markedly elevated ALT or AST levels without consideration of synthetic factors or clinical status
✔ Inappropriate discharge of patients with early evidence of synthetic failure
✔ Failure to followup contacts for recommended prophylaxis
✔ Inappropriate restrictions: patients with hepatitis need not be excluded from school or work; education regarding precautions is indicated
✔ Failure to consider the effects of hepatitis on drugs with hepatic clearance, resulting in high serum levels or long duration of action

References

1. Alter M. Epidemiology of hepatitis C. *Hepatology* 1997;62S–65S.
2. Alter M, Gallagher M, Morris TT, Moyer LA, et al. Acute non-A-E hepatitis in the United States and the role of hepatitis G virus infection. Sentinel Counties Viral Hepatitis Study Team. *N Engl J Med* 1997;336:741–754.
3. Alter MJ, Kruszon-Moran D, Nainan OV, McQuillan GM, et al. The prevalence of hepatitis C virus infection in the United States, 1988 through 1994. *N Engl J Med* 1999;341:556–562.
4. DeCock KM, Govindarajan S, Chin KP, Rededcer AG, et al. Delta hepatitis in the Los Angeles area: a report of 126 cases. *Ann Int Med* 1986:108–114.
5. Emerson SU, Purcell RH. Running like water–the omnipresence of hepatitis E. *N Engl J Med* 2004;351:2367–2368.
6. Herrera JL. Hepatitis E as a cause of acute non-A, non-B hepatitis. *Arch Intern Med* 1993;153:773.
7. Schiff ER. Viral hepatitis. In: Schiff ER, Sorrell MF, Maddrey WC, eds. Diseases of the liver, 9th ed. Philadelphia: Lippincott Williams & Wilkins, 2003:741.
8. Krawitt EL. Autoimmune hepatitis. *N Engl J Med* 1996;334:897–903.
9. Durazzo M, Premoli A, Fagoonee S, Pellicano R. Overlap syndromes of autoimmune hepatitis: what is known so far. *Dig Dis Sci* 2003;48:423–430.
10. Lee WM. Drug-induced hepatotoxicity. *N Engl J Med* 2003;474–486.
11. Misbin RI. Troglitazone-associated hepatic failure. *Ann Intern Med* 1999;330.
12. Herrine S. Approach to the patient with chronic hepatitis C infection. *Ann Intern Med* 2002;136:747–75713.
13. Podalsky DK. Infiltrative, genetic, and metabolic diseases of the liver. In: Kasper DL, Fauci AS, Longo DL, Braunwald E, et al. *Harrison's principles of internal medicine.* 16th ed. New York: McGraw–Hill, 2002:1869.

CHAPTER 65
Hepatic Failure and Cirrhosis

David M. Cline

Acute hepatic failure differs clinically, prognostically, and therapeutically from an exacerbation of chronic liver failure, but the priorities for the management of both entities are similar. The exact mechanism for the widespread neural inhibition seen in this condition continues to elude investigators. Ammonia, a substance liberated from the intestinal flora and known to accumulate in hepatic failure, is a key factor in the development of hepatic encephalopathy (23). However, ammonia accumulation causes an excitable state rather than neural inhibition, and the severity of hepatic coma does not always correlate with blood ammonia levels (1). No single mechanism has explained all the features of this disorder. Recently it has been shown that a systemic inflammatory response is an essential component initiating hepatic encephalopathy (17). Infection generally plays a role in this inflammatory response (24).

Viral hepatitis has traditionally been regarded as the most common cause of fulminant hepatic failure (FHF) worldwide (18). In the United States, drug-related hepatotoxicity accounts for greater than 50% of acute liver failure, including that from acetaminophen (40%) and idiosyncratic drugs (12%) (13). Cocaine and ecstasy are two important drugs in this later category. In 20% of cases, the cause cannot be determined. Less common causes include fatty degeneration of pregnancy, Reye syndrome, heat stroke, *Amanita phalloides* mushroom poisoning, and metastatic cancer to the liver.

Hepatic cirrhosis most commonly is caused by alcoholism; chronic active hepatitis is the second most common cause. Typically, there is progressive destruction over several years of the normal sinusoidal architecture with resulting fibrosis. Progressive hepatocellular dysfunction results in impaired glycogen storage, coagulopathy, and loss of detoxifying capability. Continued fibrosis shunts blood away from the hepatic artery directly into the portal vein, resulting in secondary portal hypertension and esophageal varices.

TABLE 66.4.   Time of Occurrence and Management of Infections in OLT Recipients

Infectious Disease	Time of Presentation after OLT	Diagnostic Evaluation	Treatment[a]
Bacterial infections	Peak in months 1–2, progressive decline in incidence. Rare after 12 months, unless patient is still taking high-dose immunosuppressive regimen, or has indwelling venous catheter.	Blood, urine, and sputum cultures.[b] Culture all indwelling venous catheter and biliary tube fluid if T-tube still present.	Empiric broad-spectrum antibiotic coverage pending culture results (e.g., ceftazidime 1 g i.v. q8h and ampicillin/sulbactam 3 g i.v. q6h)
Fungal infections	Peak in months 1–2. Rare after 2 mo, unless patient is still taking high-dose immunosuppressive regimen.	Blood, urine, and indwelling venous catheter cultures.	Amphotericin B or fluconazole[c]
Viral infections	Most common in month 2 after OLT; rare after 2 months. Cytomegalovirus is most common infection.	Blood, urine, and indwelling venous catheter cultures.[d]	Ganciclovir or foscarnet
Protozoal infections	Rare, but occasionally occur months 1–6. *Pneumocystis carinii* pneumonia is the most common pathogen.	Chest radiograph and sputum culture. Most require bronchoalveolar lavage; diagnosis is not usually made in emergency department.	Trimethoprim-sulfamethoxazole, 20 mg/kg i.v. divided q.i.d. for 14–21 days.

[a] Medication dosages must be adjusted on the basis of patient's renal function.

[b] Obtain sputum cultures and chest radiograph when clinically appropriate (e.g., patient with fever and cough). Consider stool cultures and *Clostridium difficile* toxin assay if infectious colitis is suspected.

[c] Antifungal and antiviral therapy are not routinely indicated in the emergency department. They are usually reserved for the hospital course of patients with orthotopic liver transplant when fungal infection has been documented or the patient's condition fails to improve with antibacterial therapy.

[d] Definitive diagnosis of clinically significant viral disease is difficult. Further diagnostic testing, such as polymerase chain reaction, serologic studies, and tissue histologic analysis, is performed later in the hospital course and is not an immediate priority during the emergency department visit.

Because the presentations of many important complications of OLT are nonspecific, patients presenting to the ED generally require extensive laboratory testing (15). Laboratory tests should include a complete blood count and platelet count to screen for leukopenia or thrombocytopenia related to medications. Electrolytes and serum creatinine concentrations are useful to detect the nephrotoxic effects of either tacrolimus or cyclosporine. Total bilirubin, AST, ALT, and alkaline phosphatase levels, and prothrombin time or INR are used to evaluate graft function. Patients presenting with a fever should have blood and urine cultures and a urinalysis (Table 66.4).

When suspicion of vascular complications arises, several diagnostic modalities may be useful. Duplex ultrasonography and spiral computed tomography (spiral CT) are noninvasive modalities that have a reported sensitivity of greater than 90% for detecting vascular complications. Angiography is helpful in equivocal cases. Emergency physicians should have a low threshold for using ultrasonography or spiral CT to evaluate OLT patients for vascular complications in the presence of abdominal complaints or laboratory evidence of graft dysfunction. Although ultrasound or CT imaging may suggest biliary complications, definitive diagnosis is made by visualization of the biliary tract with T-tube cholangiography, endoscopic retrograde cholangiopancreatography, percutaneous transhepatic cholangiography, or operative exploration.

Rejection is definitively diagnosed by liver biopsy. The histologic triad of portal tract inflammation and mononuclear cell involvement of portal vein branches and small bile ducts is diagnostic for acute rejection. Liver biopsy in chronic rejection reveals destruction and loss of interlobular bile ducts, mononuclear portal inflammation, arteriopathy, centrilobular cholestasis, and varying degrees of hepatocellular damage.

EMERGENCY DEPARTMENT MANAGEMENT

Emergency physicians should remember that rapid deterioration may occur in clinically stable OLT patients with acute infections, particularly during times of peak immunosuppression.

High-risk OLT patients presenting with fever, including recipients within 6 months of transplantation, should receive empiric broad-spectrum antibiotic therapy pending definitive culture results. Antibiotic coverage should include gram-positive organisms, gram-negative organisms (including *Pseudomonas aeruginosa*), and anaerobic organisms. Specific therapy against fungal, viral, and protozoal pathogens is rarely instituted in the ED.

A majority of OLT patients with vascular complications require surgical intervention for definitive therapy, and management of their cases should be done in concert with the liver transplantation team.

Patients diagnosed with bile leaks require parenteral antibiotics, percutaneous drainage of any abscess, and, occasionally, surgical intervention for refractory cases. Bile leaks occurring earlier in the post-OLT period tend to be more severe and are often unresponsive to conventional therapy, probably because the higher initial level of immunosuppression renders patients incapable of eradicating infection. Infections tend to be polymicrobial and include the typical biliary tract bacterial pathogens (*Enterobacter, Enterococcus, Bacteroides,* and *Clostridium* species). Broad-spectrum gram-positive, gram-negative (including *P. aeruginosa*), and anaerobic coverage is recommended pending culture results. Many patients diagnosed with biliary strictures may be nonoperatively managed with stents or balloon dilatation of their strictures.

Treatment of acute rejection involves the administration of high-dose intravenous methylprednisolone. Therapy is rarely initiated in the ED, because the definitive diagnosis of rejection is usually made later in the patient's hospital course by liver biopsy. Corticosteroids are effective in reversing 65% to 80% of acute rejection episodes. Patients who do not respond to glucocorticosteroids are treated with regimens using muromonab-CD3 (Orthoclone OKT3), with an 85% salvage rate. Chronic rejection does not respond to immunosuppressive regimens as uniformly as do acute rejection episodes. OLT recipients in whom chronic rejection is suspected should be referred to a liver transplantation center for evaluation because many patients with chronic rejection will suffer eventual graft failure and require retransplantation.

CRITICAL INTERVENTIONS

- Initiate broad spectrum antibiotic coverage for febrile, immunocompromised OLT patients
- Involve the liver transplantation team early in the care of OLT patients

DISPOSITION

Serious illness is common in OLT patients who present to the ED. Not surprisingly, OLT recipients typically undergo extensive diagnostic evaluations and are frequently hospitalized. Much of the definitive diagnostic testing that patients with OLT require is beyond the scope of typical emergency medicine practice. Appropriate ED goals are assessing the severity and possible causes of an acute illness, stabilization, and transfer of care to the primary liver transplantation team. Emergency physicians should involve the liver transplantation team early in the decision-making process to help coordinate the timing and location of the evaluation, especially if transfer to a tertiary care center is necessary.

New-onset graft failure mandates admission. The causes of graft failure are diverse, and their evaluation is best performed in the inpatient setting.

In general, febrile OLT patients who are less than 1 year post-transplantation and who are without an obvious source of infection are admitted. Febrile patients that are more than 1 year posttransplantation but who are still maintained at a high level of immunosuppression (e.g., chronic rejection patients) should also be hospitalized. Well-appearing, febrile patients who are more than 1 year posttransplantation, with an uncomplicated post-OLT course, and whose immunosuppressives have been tapered, may be managed on an individual basis. Because maintaining a desired level of immunosuppression is vital in preventing rejection episodes, admission is mandatory if compliance with the immunosuppressive regimen is in doubt (e.g., because of intractable vomiting).

COMMON PITFALLS

- ✔ Failure to appreciate the complex nature of OLT patients resulting from the balance between allograft rejection and adequate immunosuppressive therapy
- ✔ Failure to coordinate the ED evaluation of OLT recipients with the primary liver transplantation team
- ✔ Failure to manage fever aggressively in OLT recipients, especially early in the posttransplantation period when immunosuppression is at its peak
- ✔ Using the leukocyte count as a marker for severity of infection. More than 50% of OLT patients with serious bacterial infections have a normal leukocyte count

- ✔ Assuming that a soft and nontender abdominal examination excludes hepatobiliary complications
- ✔ Prescribing medications to patients with OLT without careful consideration for potential drug interactions or adverse effects of medications

Acknowledgment

Thank you to previous edition chapter author Don Mebust.

References

1. Asfar S, Metrakos P, Fryer J, et al. An analysis of late deaths after liver transplantation. *Transplantation* 1996;61:1377–1381.
2. Broelsch CE, Frilling A, Testa G, et al. Early and late complications in the recipient of an adult living donor liver. *Liver Transpl* 2003;9:S50–53.
3. Brown RS, Russo MW, Lai ML, et al. A survey of liver transplantation from living adult donors in the United States. *N Engl J Med* 2003;348:818–825.
4. Chang FY, Singh N, Gayowski T, et al. Fever in liver transplant recipients: changing spectrum of etiologic agents. *Clin Infect Dis* 1998;26:59–65.
5. Egawa H, Inomata Y, Uemoto S, et al. Biliary anastomotic complications in 400 living related liver transplantations. *World J Surg* 2001;25:1300–1307.
6. Gunsar F, Rolando N, Pastacaldi S, et al. Late hepatic artery thrombosis after orthotopic liver transplantation. *Liver Transpl* 2003;9:605–611.
7. Langnas AN, Marujo W, Stratta RJ, et al. Vascular complications after orthotopic liver transplantation. *Am J Surg* 1991;161:76–83.
8. McDiarmid SV. Current status of liver transplantation in children. *Ped Clin North Am* 2003;50:1335–1374.
9. Organ Procurement and Transplantation Network, http://www.optn.org on April 5, 2004.
10. Quirós-Tejeira RE, Ament ME, McDiarmid SV, et al. Late-onset bacteremia in uncomplicated pediatric liver-transplant recipients after a febrile episode. *Transpl Int* 2002;15:502–507.
11. Rabkin JM, Orloff SL, Reed MH, et al. Biliary tract complications of side-to-side without T tube versus end-to-end with or without T tube choledochocholedochostomy in liver transplant recipients. *Transplantation* 1998;65:193–199.
12. Rand EB, Olthoff KM. Overview of pediatric liver transplantation. *Gastroenterol Clin North Am* 2003;32:913–929.
13. Rodino MA, Shane E. Osteoporosis after organ transplantation. *Am J Med* 1998;104:450–469.
14. Savitsky EA, Uner AB, Votey SR. Evaluation of orthotopic liver transplant recipients presenting to the emergency department. *Ann Emerg Med* 1998;31:507–517.
15. Savitsky EA, Votey SR, Mebust DP, et al. A descriptive analysis of 290 orthotopic liver transplant patient visits to an emergency department. *Acad Emerg Med* 2000;7:898–905.
16. Singh N, Gayowski T, Wagener MM, et al. Predictors and outcome of early- versus late-onset major bacterial infections in liver transplant recipients receiving tacrolimus (FK506) as primary immunosuppression. *Eur J Clin Microbiol Infect Dis* 1997;16:821–826.
17. Smith DM, Agura E, Netto G, et al. Liver transplant-associated graft-versus-host disease. *Transplantation* 2003;75:118–126.
18. Starzl TE, Demetris AJ, Van Thiel D. Liver transplantation—first of two parts. *N Engl J Med* 1989;321:1014–1022.
19. Starzl TE, Demetris AJ, Van Thiel D. Liver transplantation—second of two parts. *N Engl J Med* 1989;321:1092–1099.
20. Stratta RJ, Wood RP, Langnas AN, et al. Diagnosis and treatment of biliary tract complications after orthotopic liver transplantation. *Surgery* 1989;106:675–684.
21. Van Thiel DH, Iqbal M, Jain A, et al. Gastrointestinal and metabolic problems associated with immunosuppression with either CyA or FK506 in liver transplantation. *Transplant Proc* 1990;22:37–40.
22. Walker RW, Brochstein JA. Neurologic complications of immunosuppressive agents. *Neurol Clin* 1988;6:261–278.
23. Wiesner RH, Rakela J, Ishitani MB, et al. Recent advances in liver transplantation. *Mayo Clin Proc* 2003;78:197–210.

CHAPTER 67
Pancreatitis

David C. Seaberg and Allan B. Wolfson

Pancreatitis is a problem frequently encountered in most emergency departments. Its incidence varies with patient population and geographic location, but it has been estimated to affect up to 0.5% of the general population in the United States. Pancreatitis can be divided somewhat arbitrarily into two types: acute and chronic. Acute pancreatitis, although commonly a relatively mild disease, may be a life-threatening illness characterized by infection and necrosis of pancreatic tissue and potentially lethal manifestations in other organ systems. The mortality associated with acute pancreatitis may be as high as 5% (4). Chronic pancreatitis, typically manifested by recurrent episodes of acute pancreatitis superimposed on a chronically damaged pancreas, is fatal only rarely.

The major causes of acute pancreatitis are shown in Table 67.1. In the United States alcoholism and cholelithiasis account for 80% to 90% of all cases (11). Alcohol-associated acute pancreatitis is clinically recognized in 1% to 10% of alcoholics; episodes usually occur only after a prolonged period (generally at least 6 to 8 years) of heavy alcohol abuse. In nonalcoholic patients which acute pancreatitis, gallstones can be demonstrated in 60%. Pancreatitis is a rare cause of abdominal pain in pediatric patients. An analysis of the literature found that idiopathic and traumatic etiologies accounted for 45% of the cases, with the remainder attributed to structural anomalies, multisystem diseases, viral infections, drugs and toxins (6). Recurrence occurred in 9% of the children, with a mortality rate of 9.7%.

In 15% to 20% of cases of acute pancreatitis, no underlying cause can be identified. Studies have found, however, that occult biliary microlithiasis and biliary sludge may be the cause of perhaps two thirds of cases of "idiopathic" acute pancreatitis (17).

The pathologic mechanism responsible for the development of acute pancreatitis is believed to be autodigestion by inappropriate intrapancreatic activation of proteolytic enzymes (primarily trypsin) and release of other substances such as elastase, phospholipase A, lipase, and vasoactive polypeptide (11). These events result in coagulation necrosis and vascular injury, thereby causing hemorrhage, edema, and pain. Severe cases of acute pancreatitis are associated with systemic effects in a wide variety of organ systems, presumably because of the release of vasoactive factors into the circulation. These systemic manifestations can include cardiac dysfunction, acute renal failure, central nervous system dysfunction, and disseminated intravascular coagulation (Table 67.2) (30). Significant pulmonary complications such as pleural effusion, hypoxemia, and the adult respiratory distress syndrome occur in an appreciable proportion of patients (30).

Subcutaneous fat necrosis occurs in some individuals. Severe hypocalcemia is another systemic effect; although it has been attributed to the formation of soaps by necrotic pancreatic tissue, other factors such as hypoalbuminemia appear to be at least as important (11). As acute pancreatitis resolves, it may be complicated by the development of pancreatic pseudocyst or pancreatic abscess.

Chronic pancreatitis is a destructive inflammatory disorder commonly characterized by recurrent attacks of acute pancreatitis and often leading to pancreatic exocrine and endocrine dysfunction. The development of an enlargement of the pancreatic

TABLE 67.1. Causes of Acute Pancreatitis

METABOLIC

Ethyl alcohol and methyl alcohol
Hyperlipoproteinemias
Medications (azathioprine, estrogens, metronidazole, pentamidine, tetracycline, diuretics, sulfonamides, valproic acid, didanosine)[13]
Hypercalcemia
Scorpion envenomation
Amanita phalloides ingestion
Cystic fibrosis
Pregnancy
Hereditary

MECHANICAL

Biliary tract disease
Abdominal surgery
Trauma
Iatrogenic (e.g., endoscopic retrograde cholangiopancreatography, upper gastrointestinal endoscopy)
Sphincter of Oddi dysfunction
Carcinoma of the pancreas
Duodenal obstruction
Posterior penetrating ulcer

VASCULAR

Vasculitis
Thrombosis
Atheroembolism
Surgery
Ischemia or shock

INFECTIOUS

Coxsackievirus
Mumps
Mycoplasma
Legionella
Campylobacter

IDIOPATHIC

(Adapted from Geokas MC, Baltaxe HA, Banks PA, et al. Acute pancreatitis. Ann Intern Med 1985;103:86; and Ranson JHC. Etiologic and prognostic factors in human acute pancreatitis: a review. Am J Gastroenterol 1982;77:633.)

TABLE 67.2. Complications of Acute Pancreatitis

Local	Systemic
Necrosis	Shock
Sterile tissue	Coagulopathy
Infected tissue	Respiratory failure
Pancreatic fluid collections	Acute renal failure
Pseudocyst	Hyperglycemia
Abscesses	Hypocalcemia
Necrotizing obstruction or	Subcutaneous nodules
fistulization of colon	Retinopathy
Gastrointestinal hemorrhage	Psychosis
Ulceration	
Gastric varices	
Rupture of pseudoaneurysm	
Right-sided hydronephrosis	
Splenic rupture or hematoma	

head, the "pacemaker of the disease," parallels pain and potential organ complications such as common bile duct stenosis or portal hypertension (27). Excessive alcohol consumption is by far the most common cause, accounting for 75% of cases (19). The remaining cases are attributed to idiopathic causes, congenital anatomic predispositions, neoplasia, trauma, or metabolic disease such as hyperlipidemia, cystic fibrosis, or hyperparathyroidism. Gallstones are believed not to play a major etiologic role in chronic pancreatitis.

CLINICAL PRESENTATION

Although no clinical finding is pathognomonic of acute pancreatitis, abdominal pain is its most striking clinical feature. The pain is usually severe and constant; it may be diffuse but is commonly localized to the epigastrium or left upper quadrant and often radiates through to the back, presumably because of retroperitoneal irritation. The pain is typically exacerbated by recumbency and relieved by sitting up and flexing forward. Nausea and vomiting are noted in the majority of cases. On physical examination, there is usually abdominal tenderness and guarding, often with signs of peritoneal irritation. Fever, tachycardia, and diaphoresis may also be noted, depending on the severity of the case.

Necrotizing acute pancreatitis is a systemic disease. Intravascular volume loss due to massive edema and exudation of fluid into the peritoneal cavity, to systemic effects of released vasoactive substances, or to pancreatic hemorrhage may lead to frank hypovolemic shock (5). Two classic signs of retroperitoneal hemorrhage are the Cullen sign (periumbilical ecchymosis) and the Grey Turner sign (flank ecchymosis), but these are uncommon. In fact, the term *hemorrhagic pancreatitis* has been abandoned because hemorrhage is not usually a major component of acute pancreatitis (4). In some cases the clinical picture is dominated by manifestations of remote organ system dysfunction or by the systemic effects of pancreatic abscess.

The hallmarks of *chronic pancreatitis* include abdominal pain, weight loss, steatorrhea, exocrine and endocrine dysfunction, and pancreatic calcification. Two distinct patterns of painful episodes can occur. The first is characterized by brief painful episodes (usually less than 10 days' duration) separated by longer pain-free intervals. The second pattern consists of long periods of daily pain necessitating repeated hospitalizations (1).

Patients with chronic pancreatitis often present to the emergency department with recurrent attacks of abdominal pain, although in some patients pain is overshadowed by weight loss and the effects of pancreatic endocrine or exocrine dysfunction (i.e., diabetes mellitus or malabsoprtion and steatorrhea). In fact, up to 20% of patients with chronic pancreatitis may initially present with symptoms of pancreatic dysfunction without pain (16). More than 90% of the gland must be destroyed before exocrine insufficiency results in clinically significant malabsorption of protein, fat, and fat-soluble vitamins. Pancreatic endocrine dysfunction, with deficient insulin and glucagon secretion, may result in diabetes mellitus that is occasionally "brittle" and associated with frequent episodes of hypoglycemia.

DIFFERENTIAL DIAGNOSIS

The most common conditions confused with acute pancreatitis are acute cholecystitis and peptic ulcer disease, but essentially any intraabdominal emergency may be mimicked. The pain of cholecystitis is located more often in the right upper quadrant, tends to be more gradual in onset, and is not always constant.

Ultrasound examination and radionuclide scanning are useful in establishing the diagnosis of biliary tract disease. An elevation of the alkaline phosphatase level in the absence of a comparable elevation in serum transaminase levels is also suggestive. Although simple acute cholecystitis may be complicated by acute pancreatitis, the serum amylase value may be elevated in both conditions. Gallstones should be excluded early in all patients with acute pancreatitis because their presence is associated with increased morbidity and mortality (8).

Alcoholic gastritis is commonly present in association with alcohol-induced pancreatitis, and distinguishing between the two entities clinically is often difficult or impossible. Tenderness and peritoneal signs are more likely to represent pancreatitis, but a posterior penetrating ulcer may produce features of both illnesses. Other serious disorders may be responsible for significant abdominal pain in association with elevated serum amylase levels, and failure to recognize this fact may lead to dangerous misdiagnosis. These disorders include intestinal obstruction, ruptured ectopic pregnancy, mesenteric infarction, leaking aortic aneurysm, peritonitis, acute appendicitis, and diabetic ketoacidosis. The differential diagnosis of upper abdominal pain must also include myocardial infarction, pneumonia, and renal colic.

The diagnosis of chronic relapsing pancreatitis is primarily a clinical one. Calcific deposits on radiographs are fairly specific for chronic pancreatitis, however, whereas jaundice is much more common with carcinoma of the head of the pancreas. Endoscopic retrograde cholangiopancreatography (ERCP) is often useful in differentiating pancreatitis from cancer, although an identical picture can be seen in both entities (10). ERCP also allows for the collection of pancreatic secretions for cytologic examination (18).

EMERGENCY DEPARTMENT EVALUATION

The challenge of the emergency department evaluation of suspected pancreatitis is to make the diagnosis and to exclude other causes of abdominal distress, yet to keep in mind the fact that other serious illness may occur in combination with pancreatitis. Once the diagnosis is made, one must assess the severity of the pancreatitis to make an appropriate disposition.

The diagnosis of pancreatitis is based primarily on the history and physical examination and is supported by laboratory studies, most notably the serum amylase and lipase levels. The "gold standard" of diagnosis is direct inspection or pathologic examination of the pancreas; all other diagnostic modalities are indirect. Therefore, it is often stated that pancreatitis should remain a "working diagnosis" that one should feel free to modify in the face of a changing clinical picture.

An elevation of the serum *amylase* is often incorrectly considered to be diagnostic of acute pancreatitis. Because amylase is found in a variety of extrapancreatic locations (including the salivary glands, the small intestine, and the female genital tract), reliance on the amylase level alone may be misleading. The serum amylase value is a reasonably sensitive test, so the diagnosis should be questioned if the level is normal. Nevertheless, a normal amylase value was found in about one third of patients with clinical pancreatitis in one series, and there is no correlation between the severity of pancreatitis and the degree of amylase elevation (32). There are several possible reasons for this. Renal clearance of amylase is rapid, and the serum amylase level in pancreatitis may remain elevated for only up to 72 hours; therefore, in a patient who presents a few days after the onset of symptoms, the level may be only minimally elevated or normal (32). Moreover, in some individuals who have had many episodes of acute pancreatitis, extensive scarring may result in a "burned out" pancreas that releases little amylase. One other cause for spuriously low serum amylase measurements is severe hypertriglyceridemia, in which there may be a circulating amylase inhibitor; this laboratory artifact may be corrected for by measuring the serum amylase activity in serial dilutions of plasma.

Despite the reasonably good sensitivity of the serum amylase test, it is nonspecific, at least when the conventional upper limit of normal is employed (28). Interestingly, elevated serum total amylase in patients with clinical pancreatitis was noted in one series to be caused by the salivary isoenzyme in 26% of individuals (29). Using a higher cutoff level greatly increases the specificity of the total amylase determination, whereas sensitivity appears to be maintained (25). The urinary amylase/creatinine clearance, although recommended as a more specific test for acute pancreatitis, particularly to distinguish it from biliary tract disease, appears to offer no advantage (32).

Because of its availability and high specificity (99%), the serum *lipase* level is the confirmatory test that is most widely used when the diagnosis of pancreatitis is in doubt (25). Because the pancreas is the only major source of lipase, an increased level, particularly more than 3 times the upper limit of normal, is very specific for acute pancreatic inflammation. Other confirmatory tests, such as measurements of amylase isoenzymes (pancreatic and salivary), and levels of C-reactive protein, trypsinogen, serum elastase, interleukins, procalcitonin, serum amylase A, and phospholipase A_2, have been investigated, but they are less widely available for use in emergency department patients (25,30,32). A number of these tests are not only more specific (about 85%) than the total amylase, but also are reported to remain abnormal for significantly longer (7 to 14 days) than does the total serum amylase level (15,25).

Plain radiographs of the chest and abdomen should be considered, primarily to rule out other entities, such as pneumoperitoneum or small bowel obstruction. The abdominal radiograph in acute pancreatitis may show regional or localized ileus ("sentinel loop"), gallstones, widening of the duodenal sweep, blurring of the left renal outline and psoas margin, elevation of one or both hemidiaphragms, or pleural or pericardial effusion (11). These radiographic findings are caused initially by motility disturbances in the surrounding bowel and later by pancreatic edema and peripancreatic fluid collections. The finding of pan-

creatic calcifications is an indication that previous episodes of acute pancreatitis have occurred and is essentially diagnostic of chronic pancreatitis.

Other diagnostic imaging studies sometimes are extremely helpful. Ultrasonography can identify pancreatic edema as well as such complications as pancreatic pseudocyst or abscess. It is also useful in identifying the presence of gallstones or dilatation of the biliary tree, findings that have important diagnostic and therapeutic implications (24). A recent practice guideline for acute pancreatitis recommends that an abdominal ultrasound should be part of the evaluation of the initial episode of acute pancreatitis and should be performed in the initial 24 to 48 hours of hospitalization (4). Its most important use among patients with subsequent episodes of pancreatitis is to determine whether the cause is gallstones. Ultrasound visualization is difficult, however, if the pancreas is surrounded by large amounts of adipose tissue or if there are overlying distended loops of bowel.

In recent years, dynamic contrast-enhanced computed tomography (CECT) has become the imaging gold standard for evaluating the presence and extent of pancreatic necrosis and other local anatomic sequelae of acute pancreatitis, and has become a routine part of the diagnostic work-up of most patients (2). CECT assessment of disease severity has been based on semi-quantitative estimation of pancreatic and peripancreatic inflammation, presence and degree of necrosis, and associated abnormalities such as pleural effusion or ascites (9). Table 67.3 lists the CT severity index developed by Balthazar and Ranson (3,22). This index assigns points on the basis of CT grade and amount of necrosis. The practice guideline for acute pancreatitis by the American College of Gastroenterology recommends that CECT be performed in patients who are clinically demonstrated to have severe pancreatitis. Magnetic resonance imaging has not been shown to be superior to CT for diagnosing pancreatitis (26). A new modality, magnetic resonance cholangiopancreatography (MRCP) may better visualize intrahepatic and intraductal stones and thus may have a role in defining the etiology of acute pancreatitis (12,14). This test is usually not available to most emergency departments.

ERCP should be considered for patients in whom the cause of pancreatitis remains unclear after initial evaluation. ERCP may be helpful in elucidating the cause of pancreatitis in up to one

TABLE 67.3. Balthazar CECT Scoring System

CT Grade	Grade Score	Definition
A	0	Normal pancreas
B	1	Focal or diffuse pancreatic enlargement
C	2	Intrinsic pancreatic abnormality + haziness/streaky densities in peripancreatic fat
D	3	Single, ill-defined fluid collection
E	4	Multiple ill-defined fluid collections or pancreatic or peripancreatic gas
Gland necrosis (%)	**Necrosis score**	
None	0	Uniform pancreatic enhancement
<30	2	Nonenhancement of region(s) of gland equivalent in size to the pancreatic head
30–50	4	Nonenhancement of 30% to 50% of the gland
>50	6	Nonenhancement of over 50% of the gland

Severity index = Necrosis score + Grade score. Mild pancreatitis = severity index 1–3; moderate pancreatitis = severity index 4–6; severe pancreatitis = severity index 7–10.
CECT, contrast enhanced computed tomography.
(Adapted from Balthazar EJ, Freeny PC, van Sonnenberg E. Imaging and intervention in acute pancreatitis. Radiology 1994;193:297.)

TABLE 67.4. Prognostic Factors for Severe Pancreatitis

Early prognostic signs
- Ranson signs ≥3
- APACHE-II score ≥8

Organ failure
- Shock: systolic BP <90 mm Hg
- Pulmonary insufficiency: PaO$_2$ ≥60 mm Hg
- Renal failure: creatinine >2 mg/dL
- GI bleeding: >500 mL/24 h

Local complications
- Necrosis
- Abscess
- Pseudocyst

(Adapted from Banks PA. Practice guidelines in acute pancreatitis. Am J Gastroenterol 1997;92:377.)

drogenase and aspartate aminotransferase levels (suggesting hepatic and other tissue injury or necrosis); marked hyperglycemia (reflecting possible pancreatic endocrine dysfunction); hypocalcemia (from the formation of soaps by necrotic pancreatic tissue or other poorly defined mechanisms); rising blood urea nitrogen levels (secondary to third-space fluid losses or renal impairment); a falling hematocrit (reflecting both initial hemoconcentration and hemorrhagic necrosis); arterial hypoxemia (owing to pleural effusion or adult respiratory distress syndrome from systemic effects of severe pancreatic damage); and the development of metabolic acidosis or marked fluid retention.

The APACHE-II score is based on 12 physiologic variables, the patient's age, and any history of severe organ-system insufficiency or immunocompromised state. Recent studies have indicated that measurement of APACHE-II score on the day of admission has a high sensitivity and specificity in distinguishing mild from severe pancreatitis, and is superior to other grading systems for this purpose (4). The value of the APACHE-II system is that it allows measurement of severity at presentation and can be measured daily, whereas other systems (including Ranson criteria) require data at 48 hours. In general, when the APACHE-II score is less than 8 during the first 24 to 48 hours, the patient usually survives. A recent study found the APACHE-II score to be superior to CT grading in the initial evaluation of the severity of acute pancreatitis (9).

Emergency department evaluation of chronic pancreatic disease should evaluate both functional and structural components. Clinical examination should seek evidence of endocrine and exocrine manifestations such as hyperglycemia or hypoglycemia, hyperlipidemia, steatorrhea, and nutritional deficiencies. Structural abnormalities in chronic pancreatitis or cancer can be identified by imaging or endoscopy. Plain abdominal radiographs show diffuse calcification of the pancreas in about 20% of cases of chronic pancreatitis. Ultrasonography, CT, and ERCP can all be used to diagnose ductal abnormalities, pancreatic tumors, pseudocyst, abscess, or phlegmon.

half of such individuals (28), revealing small pancreatic tumors, pancreatic ductal stricture, gallstones, pancreas divisum, choledochocele, or sphincter of Oddi dysfunction.

After establishing the diagnosis of acute pancreatitis, the second priority is to determine its severity. Five percent to 10% of patients develop serious complications or die of the disease. Severe cases are indicated by the presence of organ failure (including shock, pulmonary insufficiency, and renal failure) and/or the presence of local complications (especially pancreatic necrosis) (4,7). Early predictors of severity within the first 48 hours of hospitalization, including Ranson criteria and the Acute Physiology and Chronic Health Evaluation (APACHE-II) score, serve as an early warning sign that an episode is likely to be severe (Table 67.4) (22). The practice guideline for acute pancreatitis recommends that a formalized system of scoring should be generated for each patient. The APACHE-II and/or Ranson criteria score should be generated on the day of admission to help identify patients with severe pancreatitis (4,5).

An increased risk of major complications has been associated with a number of clinical features, the so-called Ranson criteria or their modifications (Table 67.5) (3,22). Among them are age greater than 55 years; leukocytosis (reflecting the degree of inflammatory response); elevated serum lactate dehy-

EMERGENCY DEPARTMENT MANAGEMENT

Ninety percent of all cases of acute pancreatitis may be treated with supportive measures only. The aim of medical therapy is generally held to be "to place the pancreas at rest." Although it is commonly recommended that oral intake be withheld, it appears that the oral intake of clear liquids is not harmful, at least in mild to moderately severe cases. Intravenous fluids should be administered as needed, and electrolyte abnormalities such as hypokalemia, hypocalcemia, and hypomagnesemia corrected. In patients with moderate-to-severe pain, meperidine has traditionally been recommended because it is thought to cause less spasm of the ampulla of Vater than morphine. Antiemetics such as prochlorperazine or hydroxyzine may be given to control vomiting. Nasogastric suction, long thought to be a necessary component of management, has not been shown to offer any additional benefit in mild-to-moderate pancreatitis if ileus is not present (20). In patients with ileus or intractable vomiting, however, a nasogastric tube may be helpful. Anticholinergics are not thought to be of value. Although it was speculated that cimetidine might decrease the severity or the duration of episodes of acute pancreatitis by decreasing the acid stimulus to pancreatic secretion, several studies have shown it to have no benefit (20).

About 5% of cases of acute pancreatitis result in serious complications or death (see Table 67.2). These patients commonly require large amounts of fluid replacement because of retroperitoneal sequestration of pancreatic exudate and remote systemic

TABLE 67.5. Ranson Criteria for Predicting the Severity of Acute Pancreatitis

ON ADMISSION

Age >55 years
WBC>16,000/mm^3
Blood glucose >200 mg/dL
Lactate dehydrogenase>350 IU/L
Aspartate transaminase >250 U/L

WITHIN 48 HOURS

BUN >5 mg/dL
PaO$_2$ <60 mm Hg
Serum calcium <8 mg/dL
Hematocrit decrease >10%
Base deficit >4 mEq/L
Fluid sequestration >6 L

Mortality is based on the number of prognostic signs as follows: 0–2, 1%; 3–4, 15%, 5–6, 40%; >6, 100%.
(Adapted from Ranson JHC. Etiologic and prognostic factors in human acute pancreatitis: a review. Am J Gastroenterol 1982;77:663.)

effects of released vasoactive substances. A central venous or Swan-Ganz catheter and an indwelling urinary catheter may be needed to monitor intravascular volume status and to guide fluid replacement. Antibiotic administration should generally be reserved for those patients with evidence of established infection. However, several metaanalyses have concluded that early prophylactic use of antibiotics in severe acute necrotizing pancreatitis decreases the incidence of sepsis and mortality (21,23).

In patients with chronic pancreatitis the overall goals of therapy are symptom relief and prevention or correction of local and systemic complications. Pancreatic enzyme supplementation and balanced nutritional intake are the basics of therapy for pancreatic exocrine insufficiency (13). Provision of adequate amounts of supplemental oral pancreatic enzymes (pancreatin or pancrelipase) can lead to relief of pain, presumably by a process of negative feedback inhibition (13). Diabetes mellitus as a consequence of endocrine insufficiency requires close attention to insulin administration and diet to avoid ketoacidosis and other complications.

Control of chronic abdominal pain is also of prime importance. Impaired absorption of orally administered medications because of pancreatic disease may necessitate the use of parenteral analgesics. Surgery may be necessary for the treatment of regional complications of chronic pancreatitis (e.g., drainage of a pseudocyst, decompression of the biliary tree, or alleviation of duodenal obstruction) (33).

CRITICAL INTERVENTIONS

- Aggressive fluid resuscitation in patients with acute pancreatitis, who often have substantial retroperitoneal sequestration of fluids
- Adequate analgesia for patients with severe pain

DISPOSITION

Patients with mild pancreatitis in whom the likelihood of biliary tract disease is believed to be low may be managed on an outpatient basis if they are able to tolerate clear liquids in the emergency department and have no evidence of systemic complications. For these individuals a clear liquid diet and oral analgesics should be prescribed and close followup should be arranged. Patients with alcohol-associated pancreatitis should be encouraged to stop drinking.

All other patients must be admitted to the hospital. If severe or necrotizing acute pancreatitis is suspected, admission to an intensive care unit is mandatory for critical care monitoring of cardiac, pulmonary, and renal function. Surgical consultation is indicated for patients with clinically severe pancreatitis or evidence of large peripancreatic fluid collections, abscess, or pancreatic necrosis on CT. In the patient with unremitting fulminant or infected pancreatitis, laparotomy may be necessary to débride the necrotic pancreas and to ensure that there is no other cause amenable to surgical treatment. Prompt surgery is indicated when there are signs of sepsis or pancreatic abscess (11). For patients who do not respond to initial supportive measures, peritoneal lavage has been recommended to help remove the toxic pancreatic exudate from the abdominal cavity. Individuals with gallstone-induced pancreatitis may benefit from early endoscopic papillotomy.

For patients with chronic pancreatitis, indications for hospital admission include uncontrollable pain, intractable vomiting, severe nutritional deficiencies, or complications requiring surgery. Any adjustments in the regimen for analgesia or pancreatic enzyme supplementation should be carried out in consultation with the patient's primary care physician.

COMMON PITFALLS

✔ No clinical or laboratory finding is pathognomonic of pancreatitis. The serum amylase value is not a specific test, and an elevated serum amylase value is not pathognomonic

✔ Underestimating the severity of an attack. Measurements of APACHE-II and/or Ranson criteria should be made to estimate severity. The criteria in Tables 67.4 and 67.5 are helpful in providing objective guidelines by which the clinician can identify patients with a high likelihood of clinical deterioration

References

1. Ammann RW, Muellhaupt B. The natural history of pain in alcoholic chronic pancreatitis. *Gastroenterology* 1999;116:1132.
2. Balthazar EJ, Freeny PC, van Sonnenberg E. Imaging and intervention in acute pancreatitis. *Radiology* 1994;193:297.
3. Balthazar EJ. Acute pancreatitis: assessment of severity with clinical and CT evaluation. *Radiology* 2002;223:603.
4. Banks PA. Practice guidelines in acute pancreatitis. *Am J Gastroenterol* 1997; 92:377.
5. Baron TH, Morgan DE. Acute necrotizing pancreatitis. *N Engl J Med* 1999; 340:1412.
6. Benifla M, Weizman Z. Acute pancreatitis in childhood: analysis of literature data. *J Clin Gastroenterol* 2003;37:169.
7. Blamey ST. Imrie CW, O'Neill J, et al. Prognostic factors in acute pancreatitis. *Gut* 1984;25:1340.
8. Blamey SL, Osborne DH, Gilmour WH, et al. The early identification of patients with gallstone-associated pancreatitis using clinical and biochemical factors only. *Ann Surg* 1983;198:574.
9. DeSantis JT, Lee MJ, Gazelle GS, et al. Prognostic indicators in acute pancreatitis: CT vs. APACHE II. *Clin Radiol* 1997;52:842.
10. Fernandez-del Castillo C, Warshaw AL. Diagnosis and preoperative evaluation of pancreatic cancer, with implications for management. *Gastroenterol Clin North Am* 1990;19:915.
11. Geokas MC, Baltaxe HA, Banks PA, et al. Acute pancreatitis. *Ann Intern Med* 1985;103:86.
12. Gore RM, Yaghmai V, Newmark GM, et al. Imaging benign and malignant disease of the gallbladder. *Radiol Clin North Am* 2002;40:1307.
13. Isaksson G, Ihse I. Pain reduction by an oral pancreatic enzyme preparation in chronic pancreatitis. *Dig Dis Sci* 1988;28:97.
14. Kim TK, Kim BS, Kim JH, et al. Diagnosis of intrahepatic stones: superiority of MR cholangiopancreatography over endoscopic retrograde cholangiopancreatography. *AJR Am J Roentgenol* 2002;179:429.
15. Kolars JC, Ellis CJ, Levitt MD. Comparison of serum amylase, pancreatic isoamylase and lipase in patients with hyperamylasemia. *Dig Dis Sci* 1984;29:289.
16. Layer P, Yamamoto H, Kalthoff L, et al. The different courses of early- and late-onset idiopathic and alcoholic pancreatitis. *Gastroenterology* 1994;107: 1481.
17. Lee SP, Nicholls JF, Park HZ. Biliary sludge as a cause of acute pancreatitis. *N Engl J Med* 1992;326:589.
18. Lowenfels AB, Misonneuve P, Cavallini G, et al. Pancreatitis and the risk of pancreatic cancer. *N Engl J Med* 1993;328:1433.
19. Mergener K, Baillie J. Chronic pancreatitis. *Lancet* 1997;350:1379.
20. Navarro S, Ros E, Aused R, et al. Comparison of fasting, nasogastric suction and cimetidine in the treatment of acute pancreatitis. *Digestion* 1984;30: 224.
21. Powell JJ, Miles R, Siriwardena AK. Antibiotic prophylaxis in the initial management of severe acute pancreatitis. *Br J Surg* 1998;5:582.
22. Ranson JHC. Etiologic and prognostic factors in human acute pancreatitis: a review. *Am J Gastroenterol* 1982;77:633.
23. Sharma VK, Howden CW. Prophylactic antibiotic administration reduces sepsis and mortality in acute necrotizing pancreatitis: a metaanalysis. *Pancreas* 2001;22:28.
24. Silverstein W, Isikoff MB, Hill MC. Diagnostic imaging of acute pancreatitis: prospective study using CT and sonography. *Am J Radiol* 1981;137:497.
25. Smotkin J, Tenner S. Laboratory diagnostic tests in acute pancreatitis. *J Clin Gastroenterol* 2002;34:459.
26. Stark DD, Moss AA, Goldberg HI, et al. Magnetic resonance and CT of the normal and diseased pancreas: a comparative study. *Radiology* 1984;150: 153.
27. Strate T, Knoefel WT, Yekebas E, et al. Chronic pancreatitis: etiology, pathogenesis, diagnosis and treatment. *Int J Colorectal Dis* 2003;18:97.
28. Steinberg WM, Tenner S. Acute pancreatitis. *N Engl J Med* 1994;330:1199.
29. Swensson EE, King ME, Malkpour A, et al. Serum amylase isoenzyme alterations in acute abdominal conditions. *Ann Emerg Med* 1985;14:421.

30. Tenner S, Banks PA. Acute pancreatitis: Nonsurgical management. *World J Surg* 1997;21:143.
31. Wanebo HJ, Verzeridis MP. Pancreatic carcinoma in perspective. *Cancer* 1996; 78:580.
32. Werner J, Hartwig W, Uhl W, et al. Useful markers for predicting severity and monitoring progression of acute pancreatitis. *Pancreatology* 2003;3:115.
33. Werner, Uhl W, Buchler MW. Surgical treatment of acute pancreatitis. *Curr Treat Options Gastroenterol* 2003;6:359.

CHAPTER 68
Acute Appendicitis

Brian K. Snyder

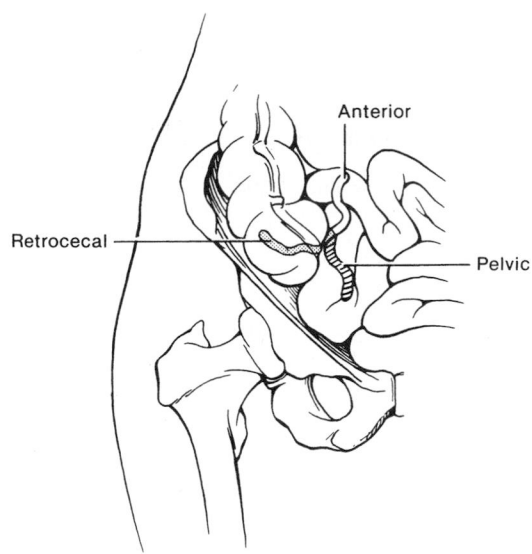

Figure 68.1. Various anatomic positions of acute appendix.

Acute appendicitis can mimic virtually any intraabdominal process; therefore, to know acute appendicitis is to know well the diagnosis of acute abdominal pain.—Zachary Cope

Appendicitis is an acute inflammatory process of the appendix resulting from obstruction of the lumen with subsequent bacterial invasion, distention, ischemia, and ultimate rupture. As traditionally taught, appendicitis presents with initial periumbilical pain, which later migrates to the right lower quadrant (RLQ). Anorexia, nausea, and vomiting are associated symptoms. Physical examination reveals a low-grade fever and RLQ tenderness, with guarding and rebound as the process progresses. Laboratory evaluation reveals a leukocytosis with neutrophilia. Unfortunately, this classic presentation occurs in only a minority of cases and the diagnosis may be difficult to make. In one large series, diagnostic accuracy averaged only 85%, with a 19% perforation rate. A percentage of the perforation rate surely results from delayed diagnosis. Incidence of perforation increases with the extremes of age, and perforation is associated with greater morbidity and mortality (1).

The lifetime risk of appendicitis is 8.6% for males and 6.7% for females, with an annual incidence of 1.1 : 1,000. The male-to-female ratio for appendicitis is 1.4 : 1, although females have a higher rate of negative appendectomies. The peak incidence for males is between 10 and 14 years, and for females, between 14 and 19 years. Appendicitis rates are 1.5 times higher for whites than for non-whites, and are higher in summer (1). The cause of these differences is unknown, but temporospatial clustering and outbreaks of appendicitis point to an infectious agent as a cause of some cases of appendicitis.

The normal, uninflamed appendix is a hollow visceral structure with a closed distal end arising from the cecum; on average, it is 9.5 to 10.0 cm in length. Although the density of immune cells in lymphoid follicles in the appendix suggests an immunologic role, the function of the appendix is unknown. Its anatomic position can be anterior (post-ilial, pre-ilial, and pelvic) or posterior (retrocecal and subcecal), and many appendices are mobile (Fig. 68.1). The traditional surface landmark for the location of the appendix is McBurney point, which is located 1.5 to 2.0 inches from the inferior aspect of a line drawn from the anterior superior iliac spine point to the umbilicus. However, barium studies reveal that most appendices lie inferior to this point; therefore, making clinical decisions based on the presence or absence of pain or tenderness at exactly McBurney point is unjustified (10).

PATHOPHYSIOLOGY

The common pathophysiologic event in appendicitis is obstruction of the lumen. Obstruction can be from lymphoid hyperplasia, intraluminal objects (fecaliths, foreign bodies, or parasites) or tumors (carcinoid, adenocarcinoma, or metastatic tumors). A variety of inflammatory conditions can result in hyperplasia of appendiceal lymphoid follicles that progresses until the appendiceal wall itself obstructs the lumen. Conditions noted for this process include respiratory infections, mumps, mononucleosis, amoebiasis, and bacterial gastroenteritis.

Crohn disease can affect the appendix (21). Patients with the acquired immunodeficiency syndrome (AIDS) can have other processes of the appendix, including Kaposi sarcoma, lymphoma, or opportunistic infections (e.g., cytomegalovirus) (19).

Once the appendiceal lumen is obstructed, secretion of mucus within the appendix raises intraluminal pressures until lymphatic and venous return is impaired. Ischemic injury to the mucosa results, followed by bacterial invasion of the appendiceal mucosa and submucosa. Continued inflammation and bacterial proliferation result in perforation of the appendix and spillage of inflammatory cells and bacteria into the peritoneum, resulting in peritonitis. At times, the peritoneal infection is contained by the omentum and a periappendiceal abscess forms (21).

CLINICAL PRESENTATION

History

The characteristic clinical presentation of acute appendicitis is abdominal pain in association with anorexia, nausea, and vomiting (Table 68.1). Approximately 50% of patients present within 24 hours of the onset of symptoms, 33% between 24 and 48 hours, and the remainder thereafter. Abdominal pain occurs in nearly 100% of patients, is epigastric in onset in 74%, and migrates to the RLQ in 50%. Anorexia is present in 92% of patients, accompanied by nausea and vomiting in 78% and 54% of patients, respectively.

TABLE 68.1.   Signs and Symptoms of Acute Appendicitis

	Nonperforated (%)	Perforated (%)	All Cases (%)
SYMPTOMS			
Abdominal pain	99.6	99.3	99.6
Epigastric at onset	74.4	70.1	73.5
Constant RLQ	25.5	29.1	26.0
Anorexia			92
Nausea	78.0	79.8	78.3
Vomiting	51.8	64.2	54.2
Migration of pain	52.3	38.0	49.6
Fever	16.3	39.6	20.8
Diarrhea	15.0	22.4	16.4
Constipation	8.3	14.2	9.4
Lucid interval[a]	3.2	11.2	4.8
SIGNS			
Abdominal tenderness			
Direct RLQ	99.6	99.3	99.6
Referred RLQ	26.3	18.6	24.9
Lower abdominal	7.8	21.6	10.6
Generalized	9.6	21.6	11.9
Right-sided rectal tenderness	48.7	41.8	47.4
Local rigidity over RLQ	26.3	45.5	30.1
Generalized rectal tenderness	11.4	19.4	12.9
Rebound tenderness	4.8	4.5	4.8
Positive psoas test	4.8	3.7	4.7
Generalized rigidity	0.7	12.7	3.1
Palpable mass in RLQ	0.5	3.7	1.2

RLQ, right lower quadrant.
[a] *Lucid interval* refers to a period after perforation in which pain is temporarily lessened; some authorities do not consider this a legitimate phenomenon.
(Data from Lewis FH, Holcroft JW, Boey J, et al. Appendicitis: a critical review of diagnosis and treatment in 1,000 cases. Arch Surg 1975;110:677; and Pieper R, Kager L, Näsman P. Acute appendicitis: a clinical study of 1018 cases of emergency appendectomy. Acta Chir Scand 1982;148:51.)

Physical Examination

Although often regarded as a reliable clinical feature of appendicitis, fever is reported in only one fifth of all cases and in only 16% of cases of appendicitis uncomplicated by perforation. The most reliable sign of acute appendicitis is RLQ tenderness, present in nearly 100% of patients. Twenty-five percent of patients demonstrate referred RLQ tenderness under remote palpation (*Rovsing sign*); rigidity in the RLQ is present in 30% of patients. Nearly one half of patients demonstrate right-sided rectal tenderness.

The most significant complication of acute appendicitis is perforation, which either leads to generalized peritonitis and sepsis or is contained as an intraabdominal abscess. The mortality rate of perforated appendicitis is 1.66%, 7 times greater than that of patients undergoing appendectomy for simple, acute appendicitis (0.24%) and 12 times greater than that of appendectomy for a normal appendix (0.14%) (25). It is clear that the clinician must try to diagnose cases of simple acute appendicitis before perforation occurs.

There are few reliable clinical features that distinguish nonperforated from perforated appendicitis (see Table 68.1). The duration of symptoms tends to be longer in patients with perforation (greater than 48 hours). Signs that suggest perforation include lower or generalized abdominal tenderness, local or generalized rigidity over the RLQ, the presence of a palpable RLQ mass, and generalized rectal tenderness.

Pediatric, geriatric, and pregnant patients deserve special mention. Because diagnosis often is more difficult in these groups, their morbidity and mortality is greater.

Pediatric Patients

Appendices in children have a much thinner wall than those in the adult, allowing more rapid mucosal penetration and subsequent perforation. Perforation rates average 37% to 59% in children younger than age 13. In children who are younger than age 3, the perforation rate increases to 67% to 79%. The inability of the very young to verbalize their symptoms contributes to the difficulty in diagnosis (4,16). Diarrhea is a presenting complaint in about one third of appendicitis patients who are younger than the age of 3 (4,9) (see Chapter 256, "Newborn Problems").

Geriatric Patients

Only 20% of patients over age 60 who are diagnosed with appendicitis present with the classic nausea, vomiting, RLQ tenderness, and elevated white blood count or shift. Consequently, the perforation rate is 67% to 90%. The mortality rate is 4.6%, 23 times greater than that of patients younger than age 60 (1,8) (see Chapter 7, "Abdominal Pain").

Pregnant Patients

The physiologic changes of pregnancy, especially during the second and third trimesters, impede the diagnosis and create a physiologic environment that suppresses the normal host response to inflammation. As the uterus enlarges, the appendix rotates in a counterclockwise direction out of the pelvis. In addition, as the expanding uterus lifts the abdominal wall away from the appendix, the omentum is less available to wall off the infectious process following perforation. Diffuse peritonitis develops preferentially over a periappendiceal abscess. The increase in serum steroids during pregnancy diminishes the inflammatory response and facilitates a more rapid and overwhelming peritonitis. These physiologic and anatomic processes result in a perforation rate of 43%. The maternal mortality rate remains low at 0.7%, but fetal mortality may approach 8.5% (14).

DIFFERENTIAL DIAGNOSIS

A variety of conditions mimic appendiceal inflammation (1) (Table 68.2); the diagnostic accuracy of appendectomy for suspected acute appendicitis is only 85%. Disorders most commonly associated with removal of a normal appendix despite clinical suspicion of acute appendicitis include mesenteric lymphadenitis, other diseases of the appendix, and gynecologic ailments. The greatest diagnostic difficulties are encountered in women of childbearing age. The overall diagnostic accuracy for females is 77%; in contrast, the diagnostic accuracy for males is 91% (1).

EMERGENCY DEPARTMENT EVALUATION

Despite the widespread use of radiologic studies and other diagnostic aides in the evaluation of appendicitis, the diagnosis can still remain elusive. Appendicitis should be suspected on the basis of history and physical examination. The emergency physician should be particularly aggressive in evaluating the very young, the elderly, and the pregnant patient, as the morbidity and mortality rates of acute appendicitis in these subpopulations exceed those of others. No laboratory or radiographic study is completely sensitive for acute appendicitis, but several are commonly relied on for their supportive value.

TABLE 68.2.   Differential Diagnosis of Acute Appendicitis

Discharge Diagnoses Most Commonly Recorded after Negative Appendectomy	Percentage
Other diseases of the appendix (colic, concretion, Meckel diverticulum, fecalith, fistula, intussusception, mucocele)	19.4
Other appendicitis (chronic, recurrent, relapsing, or subacute)	16.5
Mesenteric lymphadenitis	22.0
Abdominal pain	12.2
Gastroenteritis, noninfectious	6.4
Cholelithiasis	4.1
Ovarian cyst	5.5
Uterine leiomyoma	4.3
Endometriosis	4.0
Lymphoid hyperplasia of the appendix	3.1
Cervicitis, endocervicitis	2.7

Other considerations in the differential diagnosis include regional enteritis, perforated peptic ulcer, diverticulitis, carcinoma of the bowel, ureteral calculi, pelvic inflammatory disease, and Mittelschmerz.

(Data from Addis DG, Shaffer N, Fowler S, et al. The epidemiology of appendicitis and appendectomy in the United States. Am J Epidemiol 1990;132:910.)

Laboratory Studies

Acute appendicitis is classically associated with leukocytosis with a left shift. In one large study, 88% of adult patients with acute appendicitis had a white blood cell count of great than 10,000 cells/μL, and 94% had a leukocytosis *or* a neutrophilia of greater than 75%. Specificity was only 76% and 62%, respectively. Approximately 10% of patients with acute appendicitis have normal leukocyte and neutrophil counts (12). Unfortunately, an elevated leukocyte count is nonspecific, the specificity being reported as low as 38%. Further complicating matters, the normal range for the leukocyte count changes with age. By calculating likelihood ratios, one finds that the leukocyte count has minimal effect on the probability of disease, except for the extremes of the leukocyte count. However, only a small minority of patients will have such leukocyte values (22). Some authors advocate serial leukocyte counts and progressive leukocytosis as being suggestive of acute appendicitis. Studies regarding the clinical utility of sequential leukocyte counts are inconclusive, and it appears that utility, if any, is limited to a small percentage of the total patient population (5).

Other serum markers of inflammation, such as the C-reactive protein, have also been evaluated as an aid in diagnosis of acute appendicitis but generally demonstrate the same limitations as the leukocyte count.

Urinalysis, often obtained in the evaluation of abdominal pain, cannot be relied on to distinguish disease of the urinary tract from that of the appendix. In one study of patients with histologically confirmed acute appendicitis, 30% had an abnormal urinalysis, regardless of the position of the appendix. In those patients with either a ruptured or an inflamed appendix in the retrocecal or pelvic position, abnormal urinalysis was detected in 50%. Diagnostic decisions should not be based on the presence of pyuria or bacteriuria (20).

Imaging Studies

Radiologic studies should be reserved for those with equivocal symptoms and physical findings. In cases of strongly suspected appendicitis, time-consuming diagnostic procedures should not be used. Because the incidence of perforation is related directly to the interval between symptom onset and surgery, tests that may delay definitive therapy should be used cautiously.

Plain radiographs sometimes yield findings consistent with appendicitis, including a fecalith, localized ileus, or obscuration of fat–tissue interfaces (7). These findings are nonspecific and the diagnostic yield is low (2). Plain radiographs should be obtained only when other diagnoses are high in the differential (e.g., bowel obstruction).

A barium enema can used to evaluate potential appendicitis on the basis of the premise that a normal appendix can be filled with barium but an obstructed appendix will not allow the passage of barium. Generally, a barium enema is highly accurate in the diagnosis of appendicitis, although false-positive examinations occur and there is a relatively high incidence of technical failure (7).

Labeled white blood cell scanning provides good sensitivity (90% to 97%) and specificity (89% to 97%). A major disadvantage of such nuclear medicine studies is that although early positive studies are possible, the procedure can take up to 4 hours to complete (18).

Abdominal ultrasonography is often used in the evaluation of appendicitis. When obstructed, the appendix appears as a blind-ended, immobile, noncompressible structure that cannot be displaced under direct pressure from the ultrasound probe. An appendix that is visualized on ultrasound examination is

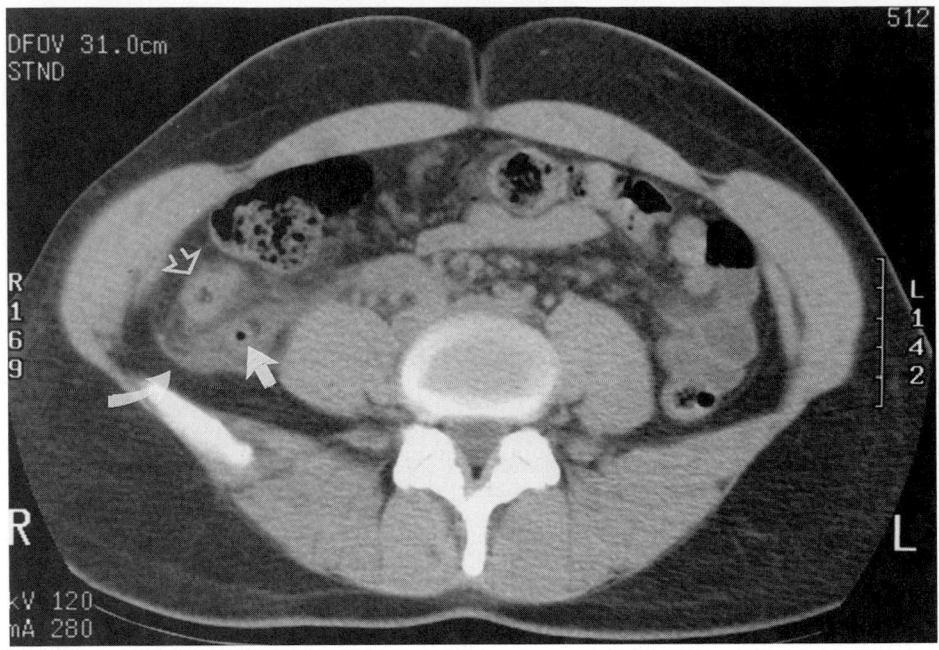

Figure 68.2. Computed tomographic appearance of appendicitis. Note the enlarged, thickened appendix (*open arrow*), surrounding fat stranding and inflammation (*curved arrow*) and extraluminal air, implying perforation (*closed arrow*).

considered diagnostic of appendicitis. If the appendix cannot be seen, appendicitis is excluded. Unfortunately, ultrasonography is nondiagnostic in 3% to 11% of cases owing to pain, guarding, obesity, or overlying gas. Sensitivity ranges from 75% to 89% and specificity from 86% to 100%. Poorer results are obtained in early appendicitis, perforation, and retrocecal appendicitis (7). Ultrasound is the preferred modality in pregnant patients, since it does not involve contrast or radiation (13).

Helical computed tomographic scanning of the abdomen is fast and highly accurate in the evaluation of acute appendicitis. The sensitivity of unenhanced helical computed tomography (CT) is approximately 90%; with the addition of oral, rectal, or intravenous contrast, the sensitivity increases up to 97% to 98% (11,17). Specificity is equally high at 94% to 97%. Findings include a fecalith, an inflamed appendix, stranding in the surrounding fat or periappendicular fluid, phlegmon, or abscess (Fig. 68.2). Helical CT in the evaluation of appendicitis appears to be cost-effective, and its use may decrease the negative laparotomy and perforation rates (17). Furthermore, CT often provides an alternative diagnosis, and may decrease the time to operative intervention for female patients (24). In addition, it is useful in the assessment of cases of suspected perforated appendicitis with periappendiceal abscess formation, which may be treated conservatively or with percutaneous drainage and interval appendectomy (15). Diagnostic laparoscopy has advocates, especially for women of childbearing age. It is highly accurate and safe (3).

EMERGENCY DEPARTMENT MANAGEMENT

The patient suspected of having acute appendicitis should be given nothing by mouth. Intravenous fluid is indicated to ensure hydration. Surgical consultation should be obtained promptly, as timely appendectomy of an inflamed but nonperforated appendix is of paramount importance. If acute appendicitis is suspected but in doubt, radiologic study, emergency department observation, or admission for inpatient observation with sequential examination are reasonable alternatives. Observation is a safe and effective way to distinguish patients with appendicitis from those without (6).

Although traditional edict warns that analgesia will obscure the diagnosis in acute abdominal pain, the use of narcotics has not been shown to increase the number of delayed or missed diagnoses (23). The judicious use of short-acting narcotics is reasonable in patients with acute abdominal pain while evaluation is in progress, especially those in which a radiologic procedure is to be performed or surgical consultation is delayed.

When perforation is highly suspected, intravenous antibiotics should be administered. Antibiotics that cover typical intestinal flora such as "triple antibiotics" (ampicillin 2 g, gentamicin 2 mg/kg, and metronidazole 500 mg) or a second-generation cephalosporin (cefotetan 1–2 g) or a quinolone (ciprofloxacin 500 mg or levofloxacin 500 mg) with metronidazole are appropriate.

CRITICAL INTERVENTIONS

- Obtain immediate surgical consultation for patients with a high likelihood of appendicitis, to reduce delay to the operating room and subsequently, the perforation rate
- When in doubt, admit the patient for observation to an emergency department observation area or surgical service for sequential physical examinations
- Administer intravenous antibiotics when perforation is highly suspected

DISPOSITION

Patients in whom the clinical suspicion of appendicitis is moderate or high, and those with a positive imaging study should be admitted to the hospital for further evaluation or surgery. For patients being discharged without definitive diagnoses, who have low likelihood of appendicitis or other significant intraabdominal process, it is important to provide clear, legible instructions explicitly detailing conditions meriting a return visit for further evaluation. (e.g., continued or worsening pain, new symptoms). Advising a scheduled return visit in 6 to 8 hours for reassessment is good practice. In addition, when the diagnosis is uncertain, refrain from documenting a definitive diagnosis (e.g., gastroenteritis), rather refer to the process as "abdominal pain of undetermined origin."

COMMON PITFALLS

✔ Abdominal pain and tenderness are present in nearly 100% of patients with appendicitis; other clinical features are less reliable

✔ Caution is advised in evaluating the young, the elderly, pregnant women, and women of childbearing age. The diagnosis is often elusive, and many patients in these groups proceed to perforation

✔ Reliance on the leukocyte count is unwarranted and usually leads to false reassurance

References

1. Addiss DG, Shaffer N, Fowler S, et al. The epidemiology of appendicitis and appendectomy in the United States. *Am J Epidemiol* 1990;132:910–925.
2. Boleslawksi E, Panis Y, Benoist S. Plain abdominal radiography as a routine procedure for acute abdominal pain of the right lower quadrant: prospective evaluation. *World J Surg* 1999;23:262–264.
3. Borgstein PJ, Gordijn RV, Eijsbouts QAJ, et al. Acute appendicitis—a clear-cut case in men, a guessing game in women: a prospective study on the role of laparoscopy. *Surg Endosc* 1997;11:923–927.
4. Daehlin L. Acute appendicitis during the first three years of life. *Acta Chir Scand* 1982;148:291–294.
5. Errikson S, Granstrom L, Carlstrom A. The diagnostic value of repetitive preoperative analyses of C-reactive protein and total leukocyte count in patients with suspected acute appendicitis. *Scand J Gastroenterol* 1994;29:1145–1149.
6. Graff L, Radford MJ, Werne C. Probability of appendicitis before and after observation. *Ann Emerg Med* 1991;20:503–507.
7. Hoffmann J, Rasmussen O. Aids in the diagnosis of acute appendicitis. *Br J Surg* 1989;76:774–779.
8. Horattas MC, Guyton DP, Wu D. A reappraisal of appendicitis in the elderly. *Am J Surg* 1990;160:291–293.
9. Horwitz JR, Gursoy M, Jaksic T, et al. Importance of diarrhea as a presenting symptom of appendicitis in very young children. *Am J Surg* 1997;173:80–82.
10. Karim OM, Boothroyd AE, Wyllie JH. McBurney's point—fact or fiction? *Ann R Coll Surg Engl* 1990;72:304–308.
11. Lane MJ, Katz DS, Ross BA, et al. Unenhanced helical CT for suspected appendicitis. *AJR Am J Roentgenol* 1997;168:405–409.
12. Lau WY, Ho YC, Chu KW, et al. Leukocyte count and neutrophil percentage in appendectomy for suspected appendicitis. *Aust N Z J Surg* 1989;59:395–398.
13. Lim HK, Bae SH, Geo GS. Diagnosis of acute appendicitis in pregnant women: value of sonography. *AJR Am J Roentgenol* 1992;159:539–542.
14. Mahmoodian S. Appendicitis complicating pregnancy. *South Med J* 1992;85:19–24.
15. Oliak D, Yamini D, Udani VM, et al. Nonoperative management of perforated appendicitis without periappendiceal mass. *Am J Surg* 2000 Mar;179:177–181.
16. Putnam TC, Gagliano N, Emmens RW. Appendicitis in children. *Surg Gynecol Obstet* 1990;170:527–532.
17. Rao PM, Rhea JT, Rattner DW, et al. Introduction of appendiceal CT; impact on negative appendectomy and appendiceal perforation rates. *Ann Surg* 1999;229:344–349.
18. Rypins EB, Kipper SL. 99mTc-hexamethylpropyleneamine oxime (Tc-WBC) scan for diagnosing acute appendicitis in children. *Am Surg* 1997;63:878–881.
19. Savioz D, Lirionia A, Zurbuchen P, et al. Acute right iliac fossa pain in acquired immunodeficiency: a comparison between patients with and without acquired immunodeficiency syndrome. *Br J Surg* 1996;83:644–646.
20. Scott JH, Amin M, Harty JI. Abnormal urinalysis in appendicitis. *J Urol* 1983;129:1015.
21. Silen ML, Tracy TF. The right lower quadrant "revisited." *Pediatr Clin North Am* 1993;40:1201–1211.
22. Snyder BK, Hayden SR. Accuracy of the leukocyte count in the diagnosis of acute appendicitis. *Ann Emerg Med* 1999;33:565–574.
23. Thomas, SH, Silen W, Cheema F, et al. Effects of morphine administration analgesia on diagnostic accuracy in emergency department patients with abdominal pain, a prospective, randomized trial. *J Am Coll Surg* 2003;96:18–31.
24. Torbati SS, Guss DA. Impact of helical computed tomography on the outcomes of emergency department patients with suspected appendicitis. *Acad Emerg Med* 2003;10:823–829.
25. Velanovich V, Satava R. Balancing the normal appendectomy rate with the perforated appendicitis rate: implications for quality assurance. *Am Surg* 1992;58:264–269.

Philip L. Henneman and Susan P. Torrey

Intestinal obstruction is a common disorder that has been recognized by physicians for centuries. It accounts for approximately 4% of patients presenting to an emergency department with nontraumatic abdominal pain of less than 7 days' duration. The challenge to the emergency physician is to promptly identify the patients with bowel obstruction from the many patients presenting to an emergency department with abdominal pain and vomiting, without doing multiple tests and without delaying initial treatment, surgical consultation, and admission.

Intestinal obstruction was associated with a 60% mortality in 1900. This has decreased to approximately 5% owing to early recognition, aggressive stabilization with fluid resuscitation, simple nasogastric decompression, and, in most cases, surgical intervention. Mortality can still result from strangulation leading to bowel infarction and subsequent sepsis. Early recognition and initiation of treatment are the only way for the emergency physician to minimize major morbidity or mortality.

Intestinal obstruction accounts for about 20% of all acute surgical admissions. The obstruction most commonly affects the small intestine but involves the colon in up to 20% of patients. The vast majority of bowel obstructions are caused by postoperative adhesions, accounting for 50% of small bowel obstructions. Other common causes include inflammatory bowel disease (especially Crohn's disease), hernias and neoplasm in adults and intussusception, hernias, and congenital abnormalities in children (6). Feces, foreign bodies, strictures, abscesses, trauma, and volvulus are other less common causes (4,6).

The stomach, small bowel, biliary tract, and pancreas collectively secrete 8 to 10 L of fluid daily. Almost all of this volume is reabsorbed in the large bowel. Obstruction prevents the flow of fluid and other intraluminal contents to the colon, resulting in accumulation in the more proximal sections of the bowel. This causes a gradual distention of the bowel proximal to the obstruction, and increasing intraluminal pressure. As pressure increases within the bowel, hypersecretion of fluid into the bowel develops, and absorption from the bowel is retarded. Volume losses into the intraluminal space are variable but can be up to 9 L in 24 hours, causing significant depletion of intravascular volume. Further increases in intraluminal pressure result in capillary and lymphatic obstruction with resulting edema of the bowel wall. Retrograde peristalsis eventually develops, resulting in vomiting by the patient. If allowed to progress, venous and finally arterial obstruction will occur. Bacterial overgrowth occurs in the stagnant bowel contents. Hemorrhagic necrosis, gangrene of the bowel, and leakage of contaminated contents finally develop, resulting in bacterial peritonitis and sepsis. It is the goal of therapy to prevent these life-threatening complications (8).

CLINICAL PRESENTATION

Bowel obstruction should be considered in all patients with abdominal pain and vomiting, especially if they have a history of previous abdominal surgery or colorectal cancer. Pain is the initial and primary complaint, although it may be poorly appreciated or communicated in patients with altered mental status. The pain is usually intermittent and colicky, with cramps occurring every 3 to 10 minutes, depending on the location of obstruction. Vomiting generally follows the development of abdominal pain. The more proximal the obstruction, the earlier vomiting develops; in obstruction of the colon, vomiting may not develop for 24 to 48 hours. Although obstipation (i.e., no passage of feces or flatus) is the rule once obstruction is complete, the passage of stool and flatus may continue until the distal bowel is evacuated. Diarrhea may even occur when there is partial obstruction. Late in the course, abdominal distention may develop. This may be subtle to the physician, but the patient is often aware of this change.

The patient's vital signs, including postural changes, may reflect the degree of volume depletion and in general are only modestly altered until late in the disease process. Hypotension and tachycardia imply advanced disease. Gangrenous bowel, however, may be present without fever or tachycardia.

A helpful sign in diagnosing early small bowel obstruction is the auscultatory finding of crescendo–decrescendo rushes of high-pitched peristalsis sounds coincident with the patient's crampy abdominal pain. Bowel sounds eventually decrease and disappear with overdistention and infarction of the bowel.

Abdominal tenderness is present in most patients. The determination of rebound tenderness is often complicated by the presence of distended bowel, which may give a false-positive result of increased pain with rapid decompression of the abdominal wall. The absence of percussion tenderness (tapping on the abdomen) or pain with jostling of the patient's gurney or bed implies that peritoneal signs are not present. The absence of local tenderness or rebound, however, does not exclude the possibility of vascular compromise or infarction.

It is important to evaluate for the presence of an external hernia. An incarcerated hernia may be easily reducible with immediate relief of the intestinal obstruction.

In the 1998 prospective study of Bohner et al. of 48 patients with bowel obstruction, the clinical variables most useful in diagnosing bowel obstruction were history of previous surgery, history of constipation, age over 50, vomiting, distended abdomen, and increased bowel sounds (2). Variables not classified as helpful in this study included sex, progress of complaint in relation to the onset of pain, nausea, history of similar complaints, guarding, and the severity of pain.

DIFFERENTIAL DIAGNOSIS

There are multiple reasons for abdominal pain and vomiting, including cholecystitis, hepatitis, pancreatitis, peptic ulcer disease, appendicitis, myocardial infarction, nonspecific abdominal pain, and pregnancy, to name a few. The presence of right upper quadrant tenderness should help to differentiate hepatobiliary disease. Elevated lipase or amylase will identify pancreatitis. Patients with peptic ulcer disease may have heme-positive stool. Appendicitis usually presents with right lower quadrant tenderness. The absence of abdominal tenderness may imply cardiac etiology in an elderly patient with risk factors. Patients with kidney stones may complain of abdominal pain but do not usually have abdominal tenderness. An electrocardiogram (ECG) may help diagnose myocardial ischemia, and patients with kidney stones usually have hematuria. A pelvic examination and pregnancy test will identify the pregnant patient. Colicky pain can be associated with appendicitis, cholelithiasis, kidney stones, or gastroenteritis. Diarrhea occurs in all patients with gastroenteritis but is an uncommon complaint in patients with bowel obstruction. Uremia and hepatitis can be associated with abdominal distention (ascites) and vomiting. Ascites and periph-

eral edema do not occur with bowel obstruction. The presence of jaundice should direct the emergency physician to the diagnosis of liver disease. Finally, air–fluid levels on abdominal X-rays are a common finding in patients with gastroenteritis, but frequent diarrhea, lack of distended loops of bowel, and fecal leukocytes or heme-positive stool will help in making the correct diagnosis.

EMERGENCY DEPARTMENT EVALUATION

The general appearance of the patient will help determine the overall degree of illness. A complete history and physical examination are critical in making the diagnosis of bowel obstruction. Ill-appearing patients require supportive treatment (e.g., monitor, intravenous fluid, etc.) before a complete history can be obtained. Inspection of the patient's vital signs is critical to determine the patient's volume status and risk of infection. Tachycardia and hypotension should prompt the emergency physician to provide immediate fluid resuscitation. The presence of fever indicates an infectious etiology to the patient's symptoms and implies bowel infarction if bowel obstruction is diagnosed. Evaluation of the skin will help to identify jaundice in the patient with hepatobiliary disease or poor capillary refill in a patient in shock. Auscultation of the lungs may reveal a pulmonary cause of the patient's symptoms. Inspection of the abdomen may reveal distention or surgical scars. Auscultation of the abdomen may reveal crescendo–decrescendo, decreased, or absent bowel sounds. Gentle palpation of the abdomen demonstrates areas of tenderness, the presence of ascites or a mass, and the presence of guarding or rebound tenderness. Gentle tapping of the patient's costovertebral angle should be undertaken to determine the presence or absence of tenderness, which would imply renal disease. Pelvic examination is appropriate in all women with abdominal pain, looking for discharge, cervical motion or adnexal tenderness, or masses—none of which are usually present in patients with bowel obstruction. Rectal examination and testing of stool for occult blood, although important in the evaluation of patients with abdominal pain, should be delayed until an upright abdominal X-ray is obtained in patients for whom there is a high clinical suspicion of bowel obstruction. Digital examination may introduce air into the rectum, confusing the determination of complete bowel obstruction. Inspection and examination for an external hernia may identify the cause of a patient's complaints and lead to early reduction and relief of an obstruction.

The most important diagnostic test for bowel obstruction is the upright abdominal X-ray. Patients who are too ill to stand can undergo a left lateral decubitus abdominal X-ray, which will reveal the same findings. X-ray findings in bowel obstruction include dilated loops of bowel, air–fluid levels, and strings of air pockets called the "string of beads" sign (Figs. 69.1 and 69.2). In approximately 5% of patients with bowel obstruction, the abdominal X-ray is normal; if the bowel lumen is completely filled with fluid, it will not show the characteristic interface of air and fluid. Absence of air in the rectum may be a sign of obstruction unless the rectal examination was performed before the abdominal X-ray. Air within the distal portions of the bowel may occur if the obstruction is only partial. In general, the diagnosis of bowel obstruction is made with plain films. However, if plain radiographic findings are negative and clinical suspicion is high, abdominal computed tomography (CT) should be utilized, as it is superior to ultrasound and plain films in determining the level and cause of obstruction (7). In most cases, abdominal CT is not necessary from the emergency physician's perspective, although it may help the surgeon decide the cause of the obstruction (3,5).

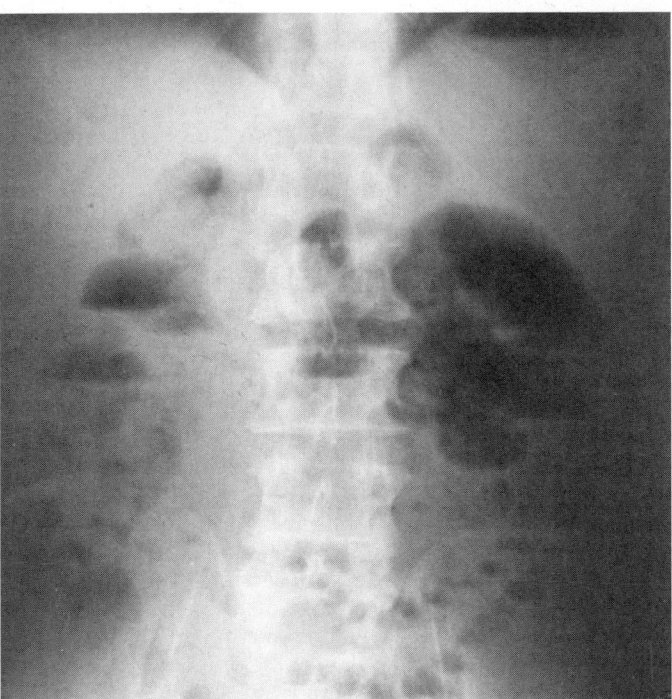

Figure 69.1. "Stepladder" pattern of air–fluid levels on upright view in patient with small bowel obstruction.

Patients with bowel obstruction may have metabolic abnormalities from profuse vomiting, third spacing of fluid into the lumen of the bowel, and resulting dehydration. Once the diagnosis of bowel obstruction is made, electrolytes, blood urea nitrogen, and creatinine results should be obtained and abnormalities corrected. A complete blood count may reveal an elevated white blood cell count in an elderly patient without other signs of early sepsis, but this finding is nonspecific. A hemoglobin or hematocrit may be elevated from hemoconcentration or decreased from hemorrhagic complications of bowel necrosis or chronic blood loss from a malignancy.

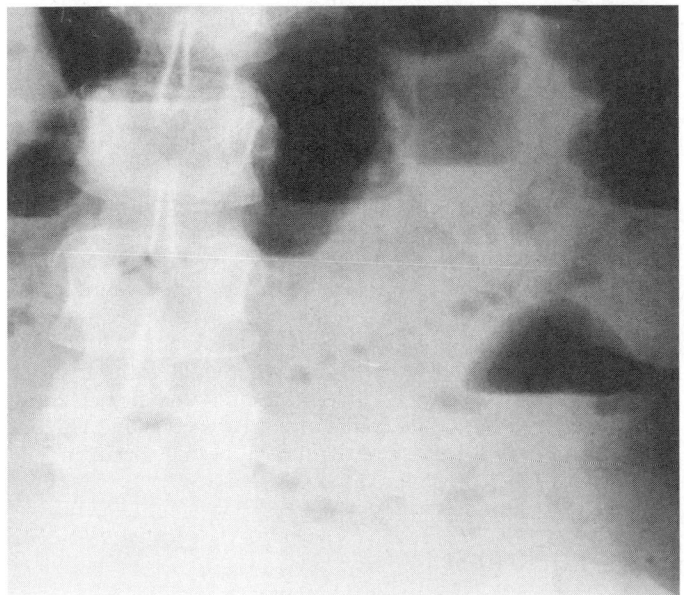

Figure 69.2. "String of pearls" sign on upright view in patient with small bowel obstruction.

EMERGENCY DEPARTMENT MANAGEMENT

An intravenous line should be started, and signs of hypovolemia should initiate prompt fluid resuscitation with normal saline. Patients who are vomiting or nauseated should be treated with an antiemetic (e.g., promethazine) to make them more comfortable.

On confirmation of the diagnosis and after discussing the planned clinical course with the patient, a nasogastric tube should be inserted, after anesthetizing the nasal passage and posterior pharynx, and attached to intermittent suction. The gastric contents should be visualized to determine the presence or absence of blood. The patient should be given intravenous narcotic analgesics for relief of abdominal discomfort. Surgical consultation should be obtained and the patient admitted to the hospital. Febrile patients or those with evidence of peritonitis should also be given antibiotics as soon as possible to cover bowel flora (1,8).

CRITICAL INTERVENTIONS

- Initiate fluid resuscitation, as many patients with bowel obstruction are hypovolemic
- Administer antiemetics and narcotic analgesics for patient comfort
- Obtain upright abdominal X-ray
- Place a nasogastric tube to allow decompression and reduce the pain and distention
- Facilitate surgical consultation and hospital admission

DISPOSITION

Patients with bowel obstruction should be admitted to the hospital. Determining the appropriate hospital bed depends on the patient's condition and comorbid illnesses. Surgical consultation should be obtained promptly, with direct communication by the emergency physician. The challenge for the surgeon is to determine whether strangulation has occurred and whether the patient requires acute operative management or whether a trial of observation (12 to 24 hours) and bowel rest can be attempted.

Stable patients may be transferred if the patient requests it or requires resources available at another facility.

COMMON PITFALLS

✔ Delay in promptly and adequately treating a patient's hypovolemia
✔ Delay or failure to treat a patient's symptoms with antiemetics and narcotic analgesics
✔ Extensive laboratory and radiographic testing that delays the diagnosis and early consultation with a surgeon
✔ Delay or failure to place a nasogastric tube after making the diagnosis of obstruction

References

1. Bass KN, Jones B, Bulkley GB. Current management of small-bowel obstruction. *Adv Surg* 1997;31:1.
2. Bohner H, Yang Q, Franke C, et al. Simple data from history and physical examination help to exclude bowel obstruction and to avoid radiographic studies in patients with acute abdominal pain. *Eur J Surg* 1998;164:777.
3. Frager D. Intestinal obstruction: role of CT. *Gastroenterol Clin North Am* 2002; 31:779.
4. Lopez-Kostner F, Hool GR, Lavery IC. Management and causes of acute large-bowel obstruction. *Surg Clin North Am* 1997;77:1265.
5. Maglinte DD, Heitkamp DE, Howard TJ, et al. Current concepts in imaging of small bowel obstruction. *Radiol Clin North Am* 2003;41:263.

6. Miller G, Boman J, Shrier I, et al. Etiology of small bowel obstruction. *Am J Surg* 2000;180:33.
7. Suri S, Gupta S, Sudhakar PJ, et al. Comparative evaluation of plain films, ultrasound and CT in the diagnosis of intestinal obstruction. *Acta Radiol* 1999;40:422.
8. Torrey SP, Henneman PL. Small intestine. In: Marx JA, Hockberger RS, Walls RM, et al., eds. *Rosen's emergency medicine: concepts and clinical practice*, 5th ed. St. Louis: CV Mosby, 2002:1283.

CHAPTER 70
Hernias

Sharon Elizabeth Mace

A hernia is the protrusion of a structure or organ through the tissues that normally contain it. This all-inclusive definition would include abdominal wall hernias as well as internal hernias. External hernias are, by far, the most common types of hernia and will be the focus of this chapter. Hernias are commonly encountered in clinical practice. It is estimated that 5% of the population has a hernia (4). *Herniorrhaphy* accounts for 10% to 15% of all the procedures in a general surgical practice (4), with about 1 million such operations performed in the United States each year (6). Herniorrhaphy is the most common operation in general surgical practice (5).

CLASSIFICATION

Hernias can be classified as an external, internal, or interparietal hernia. An external hernia protrudes completely through the abdominal wall to the outside and, therefore, can be seen and palpated. Examples of external hernias include incisional, umbilical, inguinal, and femoral hernias. An interparietal hernia is a rare hernia in which the hernial sac is contained within the abdominal wall. An internal hernia is a hernia in which the herniated part or organ occurs within the confines of a body cavity. Internal hernias include diaphragmatic hernias, hernias through a tear in the mesentery or omentum, and hernias through the foramen of Winslow into the lesser sac. Internal hernias are much less common than external hernias and can be very difficult to diagnose.

Hernias of the abdominal wall involve protrusion of part of the abdominal contents beyond the normal confines of the abdominal wall. Hernias can occur wherever there is a weakness in the abdominal wall. The weakness or defect allows protrusion of peritoneum and abdominal contents. The abdominal wall contains various fascial and muscular layers that are designed to contain the contents of the abdomen. Thus, the abdominal wall generally consists of a multilayered arrangement of peritoneum, muscle, aponeuroses of the muscles, fascia, fat, and skin. Hernias occur where there is a weakness in the abdominal wall so that peritoneum and other internal abdominal structures or organs can protrude through the abdominal wall defect or weak area. Therefore, hernias represent a failure of the abdominal wall to contain the enclosed peritoneum and other abdominal structures or viscera. The intestines are the most common structure that undergo herniation but all intraperitoneal structures can herniate, from a tiny piece of omentum to part of or an entire organ such as the bowel, bladder, kidney, or liver.

DEFINITIONS

A *reducible hernia* is a hernia in which the protruding or herniated structures can be returned through the abdominal wall defect back into the abdominal cavity. An *irreducible hernia* is a hernia in which the protruding or herniated structures cannot be returned through the abdominal wall defect back into the abdominal cavity. Another term for an irreducible hernia is an *incarcerated hernia*, which is sometimes mistakenly used to imply an irreducible hernia about to become strangulated.

A *strangulated hernia* is a hernia in which the blood supply to the herniated structures or viscus is compromised. Gangrene will occur in the strangulated viscus if the vascular compromise is not relieved. Strangulation of a hernia is a life-threatening situation, with significant associated morbidity and mortality, which requires emergency treatment and surgical intervention. Hernias that have a small neck or opening and a fairly large sac have a tendency to strangulate. As the size of the hernial orifice increases, the likelihood of strangulation decreases. All strangulated hernias are irreducible or incarcerated but not all irreducible or incarcerated hernias are strangulated.

Groin hernias, which include inguinal hernias (both direct and indirect) and femoral hernias, are the most common, accounting for 85% of all hernias (80% groin, 5% femoral). Adding umbilical and incisional hernias to groin hernias would comprise 95% to 98% of all hernias.

Other much rarer abdominal wall hernias include epigastric, pelvic, lumbar, and spigelian hernias (3). *Epigastric hernias* are hernias that occur in the midline of the abdominal wall between the umbilicus and the xiphoid. *Pelvic hernias*, which are rare, involve the protrusion of abdominal contents through areas in the floor of the abdominal cavity. The obturator hernia, which is the most common of the pelvic hernias, involves herniation through the obturator foramen, and generally occurs in elderly females. *Lumbar hernias* occur in the superior and inferior lumbar triangles, which are two naturally weak regions of the posterior abdominal wall. *Spigelian hernias* are protrusions of abdominal contents lateral to the rectus abdominis muscle through the external oblique fascia.

Ventral hernias include umbilical, epigastric, and spigelian hernias. Incisional hernias can be another type of ventral (anterior) hernia (2). Incisional hernias constitute about 10% of all hernias and result from postincisional weakness of the anterior abdominal wall.

Umbilical hernias are very common in infants, occurring in up to 65% of African American infants versus 10% of Caucasian infants. The majority of umbilical hernias in infants close spontaneously, usually by age 2 years, and rarely incarcerate or strangulate. Conversely, umbilical hernias in adults often incarcerate, with strangulation occurring in 20% to 30% of adult umbilical hernias. Ulceration and perforation can also occur in adults with umbilical hernias, complications that are associated with a high morbidity and mortality, especially in patients with cirrhosis. Patients with increased intraabdominal pressure, such as those with ascites, or during pregnancy, or with obesity; have a higher incidence of umbilical hernias. Umbilical hernias occur in 20% of patients with cirrhosis and ascites.

GROIN HERNIAS

The *inguinal hernias* (direct and indirect) and the *femoral hernia* are the three types of groin hernias (1). Anatomic location distinguishes the inguinal hernias from the femoral hernia. The inguinal hernias are above, or superior to, the inguinal ligament, whereas the femoral hernia is below, or inferior to, the inguinal ligament. The two types of inguinal hernias, direct and indirect, are also differentiated on the basis of anatomy. The protruding abdominal contents pass through the internal (or deep) inguinal ring and into the inguinal canal and lie lateral to the inferior epigastric vessels with an indirect hernia. The protruding abdominal contents with a direct hernia lies medial to the inferior epigastric vessels and protrudes through a weak area in the aponeurosis of the transversus abdominal muscle in Hesselbach triangle (or the inguinal triangle). Hesselbach triangle is an area bounded by the inferior epigastric artery (on the lateral aspect), the lateral border of the rectus abdominis muscle (on the medial aspect), and the inguinal ligament (on the inferior border). Of all inguinal hernias, about two thirds are indirect inguinal hernias and one third are direct inguinal hernias.

An indirect inguinal hernia transverses the deep inguinal ring into the inguinal canal and follows the path of a patent processus vaginalis. The processus vaginalis is formed during fetal development in order to allow the descent of the testes in the male from their original retroperitoneal site into the scrotum. If the processus vaginalis fails to close off after birth, an indirect hernia may occur which could allow abdominal contents to progress down the inguinal canal, even into the scrotum. In females, the processus vaginalis follows the round ligament, whereas in males the processus vaginalis follows the spermatic cord.

Inguinal hernias are much more frequent in males than in females because there is a much smaller aperture for the round ligament compared to the spermatic cord. Because of this embryology, childhood hernias are usually indirect hernias. Indirect inguinal hernias commonly incarcerate, whereas direct inguinal hernias almost never incarcerate.

A femoral hernia is the protrusion of abdominal contents between the femoral vessels (artery and vein) and the lacunar ligament in the femoral canal. Because of the narrow neck or opening, femoral hernias frequently incarcerate. Because of differences in the structure of the pelvis, femoral hernias occur almost exclusively in women. However, because of the rarity of femoral hernias, the most common hernia in a female is an indirect inguinal hernia not a femoral hernia.

CLINICAL PRESENTATION

Most hernias are asymptomatic and are usually found, by chance, by the patient or by the physician on a routine physical examination. The most common presenting complaints of a hernia are swelling and/or pain and discomfort. Reducible hernias usually present with minimal pain and tenderness and no induration.

In patients with an incarcerated hernia, the swelling is tender and often indurated. There may be the sudden onset of severe pain with nausea and vomiting. The pain occurring with an acute incarcerated hernia is caused by edema and inflammation of the herniated structures and the surrounding tissues. Some patients also have a low-grade fever, tachycardia, and signs and symptoms of bowel obstruction. Incarcerated hernias are the second most common cause of bowel obstruction in the United States, with postoperative adhesions being the most common cause of bowel obstruction.

If strangulation is present, the patient may present with signs and symptoms of bowel obstruction, perforation, peritonitis, abscess, and even septic shock. Occasionally, the initial symptoms may be somewhat misleading. In some patients, the pain from an incarcerated groin hernia may be located in the epigastrium because of traction on the abdominal contents from the hernia. In other patients, strangulation can occur without any symptoms and signs of bowel obstruction when only part of the bowel wall is herniated. This occurs with a *Richter hernia*, a hernia where only one side of the intestinal wall is within the hernia sac.

Pain and/or hypesthesia located along the medical aspect of the thigh radiating to the knee owing to irritation of the obturator nerve (*Howship-Romberg sign*) occurs in half of patients with an obturator hernia.

DIFFERENTIAL DIAGNOSIS

The most common diagnoses to consider in a patient presenting with a groin mass are an inguinal hernia, enlarged inguinal lymph node(s), and a hydrocele of the spermatic cord. Other less common etiologies include a lipoma, a saphenous vein varix, a psoas abscess, and an incarcerated ovary. When the hernia sac lies within the scrotum, the presentation may be confused with that of testicular torsion, epididymitis, hydrocele, or varicocele (see Chapter 77, "Acute Scrotal Pain").

EMERGENCY DEPARTMENT EVALUATION

Physical examination should include inspection and gentle palpation for any bulges or masses. Cooperative patients may be asked to cough or strain, which increases intraabdominal pressure, in an attempt to demonstrate the hernia. Palpation of the external inguinal ring in a male patient may also be helpful in detecting an inguinal hernia.

Patients with a reducible hernia and no sign of incarceration or strangulation usually require no further testing in the ED.

Those with an incarcerated hernia may present with obstruction, dehydration, and may require surgery. Therefore, laboratory testing and radiographs are often indicated.

Patients with a strangulated hernia may be seriously ill and should be evaluated with laboratory and imaging studies. Leukocytosis with a left shift is usually present, although these findings may not occur in geriatric patients. Dehydration with electrolyte abnormalities and elevated blood urea nitrogen (BUN) often occurs. Acute abdominal series radiographs are indicated in patients with a suspected strangulated hernia or obstruction. The upright chest X-ray is necessary to rule out free air under the diaphragm resulting from perforation or dead bowel. Flat plate and upright abdominal films may demonstrate bowel obstruction and occasionally a hernial sac.

Ultrasound is useful in differentiating hernia from testicular torsion or epididymitis in patients with a scrotal mass.

EMERGENCY DEPARTMENT MANAGEMENT

Patients with hernias can be grouped into three categories: (i) asymptomatic or minimal symptoms (swelling or mild discomfort) with a reducible hernia, (ii) irreducible but not strangulated hernia, and (iii) strangulated hernia.

Patients in category 1 usually require no specific ED management and may be referred to a general surgeon on an outpatient basis.

If the patient has an acute, irreducible hernia without evidence of strangulation (category 2), nonsurgical reduction should be attempted. Cool compresses may be placed over the hernia site to diminish local blood flow and decrease intraluminal gas pressure. Appropriate sedation is given. If the patient has a groin hernia, the patient is placed in a 20-degree Trendelenburg position. The hernia may spontaneously reduce. If not, gentle manipulation may be attempted. Slow, steady compression should be used, rather than sudden, forceful attempts.

If the hernia cannot be reduced, then emergency surgery is done as soon as fluid and electrolyte abnormalities are corrected.

Complications of nonsurgical or manual hernia reduction include partial reduction and hernia reduction in masse. Hernia reduction en masse is a rare complication in which the hernia sac is manipulated into the preperitoneal space. This gives the false impression that the hernia has been reduced although it is still incarcerated and at risk of strangulation.

Patients with a strangulated hernia (category 3) represent a true emergency. Aggressive fluid resuscitation, correction of electrolyte abnormalities, and broad-spectrum antibiotics are indicated. Surgical management is mandatory for all incarcerated hernias that can not be reduced and for all strangulated hernias.

CRITICAL INTERVENTIONS

- Quickly recognize the patient with a strangulated hernia
- Initiate emergent surgical consultation and aggressive fluid resuscitation

DISPOSITION

Patients with a reducible hernia should be given discharge instructions, which include the warning signs of incarceration and strangulation, and to avoid exercise and straining. They need referral to general surgery for evaluation for elective herniorrhaphy.

Patients who present with an incarcerated hernia that is subsequently reduced in the ED may be referred for outpatient management, provided there are no signs of obstruction or strangulation. Herniorrhaphy within a few days is ideal. This allows local edema to resolve. Because the incidence of recurrence is high, urgent surgery is recommended. If reduction attempts are unsuccessful, admission and surgery are warranted. A strangulated hernia mandates admission and emergent surgery.

COMMON PITFALLS

✔ Confusing a hernia with other causes of a groin or scrotal mass
✔ Failure to identify an incarcerated or strangulated hernia
✔ Failure to rapidly diagnose and aggressively resuscitate a patient with a strangulated hernia

References

1. Avisse C, Delattre JF, Flament JB. The inguinal rings. *Surg Clin North Am* 2000;80:49–69.
2. Eubanks WS. Hernias. In: Townsend CM Jr., Beauchamp RD, Evers BM, et al., eds. *Sabiston textbook of surgery*, 16th ed. Philadelphia: WB Saunders, 2001:783.
3. Hanford W, Geyarajah R. Abdominal hernias and their complications, including gastric volvulus. In: Feldman M, Friedman LS, Sleisinger MH, eds. *Gastrointestinal and liver disease pathophysiology/diagnosis/management*, vol. 1, 7th ed. Philadelphia: Saunders, 2002:375.
4. Parangi S, Hodin R. Abdominal cavity: anatomy, structural anomalies and hernias. In: Yamada T, Alpers DH, Kaplowitz N, et al., eds. *Textbook of gastroenterology*, 4th ed. Philadelphia: Lippincott, Williams and Wilkins, 2003:2526.
5. Read RC. Recent advances in the repair of groin herniation. *Curr Prob Surg* 2003;40:13–79.
6. Richards AT, Quinn TH, Fitzgibbons RJ Jr. Abdominal wall hernias, In: Greenfield LJ, Mulholland MW, Oldham KT, et al., eds. *Surgery—scientific principles and practice*, 3rd ed. Philadelphia: Lippincott, Williams and Wilkins, 2001:1185.

CHAPTER 71
Inflammatory Bowel Disease

Howard A. Werman

Inflammatory bowel disease (IBD) comprises two chronic intestinal disorders: *ulcerative colitis* and regional enteritis or *Crohn's disease*. Both are characterized by recurrent episodes of gastrointestinal disturbances separated by periods of remission, and both are associated with a variety of systemic manifestations. The emergency physician must be familiar with IBD for two reasons. First, these disorders must be considered in the differential diagnosis of patients with gastrointestinal complaints, particularly if they are recurrent. Second, patients with well-established diagnoses of IBD often present to the emergency department (ED) for management of acute exacerbations and complications of their disease.

The causes of both disorders remain unknown. Immunologic, infectious, genetic, dietary, and psychologic factors have all been implicated. The role of steroids and immunosuppressive agents in ulcerative colitis and the efficacy of agents such as antitumor necrosis factor in Crohn's disease suggest that immunologic factors play a prominent role in IBD (11). For both diseases, there is a bimodal distribution in the age at onset, with peaks at 15 to 25 years and at 55 to 60 years (10). Ten percent to 15% of patients with IBD have relatives who are also affected, particularly those with early onset of disease. The incidence of Crohn's disease and ulcerative colitis, which had been rising in recent years, has recently stabilized in the United States (8).

Ulcerative colitis tends to remain localized to the colon; in the majority of patients, the disease is found in the rectum and left colon only. The entire colon is affected (pancolitis) in the most severe cases. Ulcerative colitis is usually limited to the intestinal mucosa and submucosa. In the most severe cases, oozing ulcerations and pseudopolyps are seen. Diffuse involvement producing a finely granular, friable mucosa explains the propensity for bloody diarrhea noted in these patients. Crohn's disease can be found along the entire gastrointestinal tract; involvement is often discontinuous ("skip areas"). In 30% of cases, only the terminal ileum is involved; 20% of patients have colonic disease only. Both small and large bowels are affected in the remaining 50%. Disease of the mouth, esophagus, and stomach is found in less than 1% of patients. The lesions of Crohn's disease tend to involve all of the bowel wall layers and extend into the mesentery. Deep ulcerations, which often penetrate the bowel wall, are common and account for the development of fissures, fistulas, and abscesses. About one third of patients with Crohn's disease will manifest perianal complications such as abscesses, fistulas, fissures, and skin tags.

CLINICAL PRESENTATION

The most common signs and symptoms in patients with Crohn's disease are chronic diarrhea, abdominal pain, fever, anorexia, and weight loss. The presentation characterizes 75% to 80% of patients with this disease, but the symptoms are sufficiently nonspecific that there is typically a long delay (weeks to months) in establishing the diagnosis. The presentation of cases seen in the ED varies, depending on the site of involvement of Crohn's disease. Patients with primary ileal disease present with right lower quadrant abdominal pain that is associated with fever, abdominal distention, vomiting, and either profuse watery diarrhea or decreased output of stool and gas. Severe cases of Crohn colitis are characterized by abdominal pain associated with fever and massive diarrhea. Less common causes of emergent presentations include severe epigastric pain similar to peptic ulcer disease, acute pancreatitis, and large aphthous ulcers of the mouth.

There is commonly a delay of several months from the onset of symptoms of IBD to the time the diagnosis is established. Therefore, failure to suspect IBD and refer patients appropriately is not uncommon. Patients with previous episodes of similar symptoms, with a family history of IBD, with perirectal disease, or with any extraintestinal manifestations (rashes, back pain, arthritis, or iritis) that might suggest the diagnosis should be referred to an appropriate specialist for endoscopic evaluation or barium examination.

As in Crohn's disease, the presentation of ulcerative colitis is quite variable, and often depends on the anatomical distribution of disease. In fact, separation of these disorders on the basis of clinical findings alone can be very difficult. In mild cases, occasional constipation and rectal bleeding may be the only complaints. In the more severe forms, patients have more than six to eight bloody diarrheal stools per day, as well as crampy abdominal pain, tenesmus, fever, tachycardia, and anemia. Ulcerative colitis is more commonly associated with rectal bleeding, whereas abdominal pain, abdominal masses, and perianal lesions are more common in patients with Crohn's disease.

A common reason for patients with well-established IBD to present to the ED is complications of their underlying disease (2). The major intestinal complications of Crohn's disease and ulcerative colitis include intraabdominal abscess formation, bowel perforation, massive hemorrhage, intestinal obstruction, dehydration, perianal complications (fissures, fistulas, and perirectal abscesses), and toxic megacolon. Complications such as massive hemorrhage and toxic megacolon are more commonly seen in ulcerative colitis, whereas abscesses, obstruction, and perianal complications are far more common in Crohn's disease.

In addition to recognizing these complications, the emergency physician must also be aware that medications taken by patients with IBD, particularly corticosteroids and immunosuppressive agents, may mask the findings typically associated with complications. Other drug-associated complications include leukopenia, thrombocytopenia, fever, infection, diarrhea, and pancreatitis, as well as renal and liver insufficiency.

Toxic megacolon is perhaps the most significant complication seen in patients with IBD. This process is the result of a loss of muscular tone in the patient with advanced disease. Toxic megacolon should be suspected in patients with active colitis who report a decrease in stool output, particularly if they are on antidiarrheal agents, narcotics, or cathartics, or have undergone a recent colonoscopy. Affected patients appear toxic; the abdomen is distended, tender, and tympanitic. Fever, tachycardia, and signs of volume depletion are noted. Other findings include leukocytosis, anemia, and electrolyte disturbances. Abdominal radiographs demonstrate a long, continuous dilated segment of bowel (greater than 6 cm in width), loss of haustra and "thumbprinting," as the result of bowel wall edema. Abdominal CT findings in toxic megacolon include thinning of the colonic wall, distention of the bowel lumen, intramural gas, and, in extreme cases, evidence of perforation. The mortality associated with this complication can be as high as 50% if perforation occurs.

Twenty-one percent to 36% of patients with IBD have extraintestinal manifestations of their disease (13). Occasionally, these symptoms actually appear before gastrointestinal ones, particularly in children. The most common of these manifestations are polyarthritis, ankylosing spondylitis, erythema nodosum, pyoderma gangrenosum, nongranulomatous anterior uveitis, and hepatobiliary disease (1) (cholelithiasis, fatty liver, pericholangitis, chronic active hepatitis, and primary sclerosing cholangitis). In Crohn's disease with small bowel involvement, malabsorption syndromes as well as fluid and electrolyte disturbances can occur. Gallstones are found in up to 33% of patients with Crohn's disease. Calcium oxalate nephrolithiasis is also common. Patients with IBD may also develop a hypercoagulable state, resulting in deep venous thrombosis, pulmonary embolus, and, occasionally, arterial occlusion. Patients with thromboembolic complications have a mortality rate of approximately 25%. Pneumaturia and recurrent urinary tract infection occasionally occur with Crohn's disease because of enterovesical fistulae.

A long-term complication, particularly of patients with ulcerative colitis, is colon carcinoma. Patients with ulcerative colitis have 10 to 30 times the risk of developing colon cancer when compared with the general population, and patients with Crohn's disease have a threefold increase in risk. Symptoms of a new colon cancer may overlap considerably with those of IBD, often making diagnosis difficult.

DIFFERENTIAL DIAGNOSIS

The major challenge for the emergency physician is to differentiate IBD as a cause of diarrhea, vague abdominal pain, malaise, and low-grade fever from other treatable causes of these symptoms. Several other entities present with similar complaints. Acute infectious diarrheal illness due to *Shigella*, *Salmonella*, *Campylobacter jejuni*, cytomegalovirus, or *Yersinia* species must be considered. Parasitic disease such as amoebiasis can also masquerade as IBD. Stool cultures and examination of stool for ova and parasites are necessary to identify an infectious cause of the patient's symptoms. In addition, serologic tests can be used to rule out invasive amoebiasis, but in up to 50% of cases of infectious diarrhea, no pathogen can be identified. When the symptoms primarily involve the rectum, anal intercourse–associated bowel syndrome should be considered. Symptoms of chronic diarrhea, low-grade fever, and cachexia are also consistent with human immunodeficiency virus (HIV) infection.

Antibiotic-induced colitis attributable to the overgrowth of *Clostridium difficile* must also be considered. Ischemic colitis and diverticulitis, generally seen in older patients, and radiation colitis may present, with a clinical and pathologic pattern similar to that of IBD.

When abdominal pain is the major complaint, IBD must be distinguished from other causes of the acute abdomen, including appendicitis, cholecystitis, intestinal obstruction, abdominal aortic aneurysm, and mesenteric ischemia. These entities can often be distinguished from IBD on the basis of history and physical examination. Abdominal radiographs including CT scanning, a complete blood cell count, serum amylase and lipase determination, and urinalysis can also be helpful. The emergency physician should consider IBD as a cause of abdominal complaints only after these other potentially serious causes of abdominal pain have been excluded.

EMERGENCY DEPARTMENT EVALUATION

Patients with an acute or subacute exacerbation of their IBD may present to the ED without any evidence of an emergent complication requiring surgical intervention, although the physician must first be concerned with identifying any significant complications of IBD, particularly gastrointestinal hemorrhage, intestinal obstruction, bowel perforation, and toxic megacolon. A careful history should ascertain the frequency of bowel movements, associated symptoms, severity of abdominal pain, and history of hospitalizations. The physical examination should assess signs of toxicity, dehydration, and metabolic imbalance and should include a careful abdominal examination. The stool should be examined for the presence of blood.

Laboratory evaluation should include a complete blood cell count, blood chemistry profile, urinalysis, and type and screen if bleeding is significant. If there is suspicion of liver involvement, liver function studies should be ordered. Erythrocyte sedimentation rate and serum albumin may be followed to determine disease activity. Abdominal radiographs are useful to detect clinically inapparent intestinal perforation, obstruction, or toxic megacolon. An abdominal computed tomographic scan may be helpful in identifying intraabdominal abscesses, mesenteric inflammation, and fistulas (15).

EMERGENCY DEPARTMENT MANAGEMENT

Patients with significant hemorrhage, obstruction, or perforation as a result of IBD are managed in the same manner as other patients with these conditions. Aggressive fluid management, nasogastric decompression, blood product administration as necessary, and surgical consultation are indicated. Antibiotic coverage of gram-negative and anaerobic bacteria is appropriate in cases of suspected perforation. In patients chronically maintained on corticosteroids, stress doses of intravenous corticosteroids (hydrocortisone 300 mg/day) should also be administered to prevent symptoms of adrenal insufficiency.

Patients with toxic megacolon are given a 24- to 48-hour trial of intensive medical therapy for the disease before surgical intervention is undertaken. Such therapy includes aggressive fluid and electrolyte replacement, nasogastric decompression, and antibiotic coverage for bowel pathogens (enteric bacilli and anaerobes). Intravenous methylprednisolone (60 mg/day) or hydrocortisone (300 mg/day) is routinely administered. Early surgical consultation is necessary should the patient's condition fail medical management.

For patients who do not require hospital admission, arrangements should be made for followup with a gastroenterologist or internist. Continuing management, which usually includes dietary adjustment, bowel rest, antibiotics, and medications such as sulfasalazine and steroids, should be planned in discussion with the consulting physician (5,7). Typical outpatient medications include oral prednisone, 40 to 60 mg/day; sulfasalazine, 4 to 6 g/day; or its alternative oral or topical derivatives such as mesalamine, olsalazine, and balsalazide; and antidiarrheal agents such as loperamide (Imodium) 4 to 16 mg/day or diphenoxylate (Lomotil) 5 to 20 mg/day. Metronidazole (10 to 20 mg/kg per day) is useful for perianal complications and fistulas in patients with Crohn's disease (6,12).

Patients admitted to the hospital usually require intravenous fluids, corticosteroids, and sulfasalazine. Patients with severe IBD typically require intravenous steroids; budesonide, a controlled-ileal released derivative may also added in patients with Crohn's disease with ileal involvement. Patients with medically resistant Crohn's disease may respond to antitumor necrosis factor antibody infliximab 5 mg/kg (Remicade) (14). Azathiaprine, 6-mercaptopurine, and thioguanine may be added later to reduce steroid dependence, in patients with fistulae and those with contraindications to surgery (4,9). Cyclosporine

4 mg/kg/day has been advocated for fulminant cases of ulcerative colitis (3).

CRITICAL INTERVENTIONS

> - Recognize serious complications of IBD, such as hemorrhage, obstruction, perforation, and toxic megacolon
> - Initiate aggressive supportive care (including fluid resuscitation, antibiotics, and steroids) for patients with serious complications of IBD

DISPOSITION

Fortunately, most cases of IBD can be managed in an outpatient setting. Patients who should be considered for hospital admission include those with severe manifestations (more than six bowel movements daily, severe abdominal pain, or grossly bloody stool); those with systemic toxicity (fever, tachycardia, weight loss, and cachexia); those with dehydration or metabolic disturbances; those with acute complications (intestinal obstruction, bowel perforation, gastrointestinal hemorrhage, and toxic megacolon); and those who are refractory to outpatient therapy. Surgical consultation is indicated in those patients with complications of the disease, including intestinal obstruction or hemorrhage, perforation, abscess or fistula formation, toxic megacolon, and perianal disease.

COMMON PITFALLS

✔ Mistaking one of the serious complications of IBD (such as abscess, perforation, obstruction, and toxic megacolon) with an exacerbation of chronic symptoms
✔ Failure to refer a patient with recurrent abdominal symptoms that is consistent with IBD for further diagnostic evaluation
✔ Failure to administer intravenous fluids, analgesics, and steroids to patients with an acute exacerbation of IBD

References

1. Balan V, LaRusso NF. Hepatobiliary disease in inflammatory bowel disease. *Gastroenterol Clin North Am* 1995;24:647–669.
2. Bitton A, Peppercorn MA. Emergencies in inflammatory bowel disease. *Crit Care Clin* 1995;11:513–529.
3. Cohen R, Stein R, Hanauer S: Intravenous cyclosporin in ulcerative colitis; a five-year experience. *Am J Gastroenterol* 1999;94:1587–1592.
4. Dubinsky MC, Feldman EJ, Abreu MT, et al. Thioguanine: a potential alternate thiopurine for IBD patients allergic to 6-mercaptopurine or azathioprine. *Am J Gastroenterol* 2003;98:1058–1063.
5. Hanauer SB, Sandborn W. Management of Crohn's disease in adults. *Am J Gastroenterol* 2001;96:635–643.
6. Harrison J, Hanauer SB. Medical treatment of Crohn's disease. *Gastroenterol Clin North Am* 2002;31:167–184.
7. Kornbluth A, Sachar DB. Ulcerative colitis practice guidelines in adults. *Am J Gastroenterol* 1997;92.
8. Loftus Jr. KV, Sandborn WJ. Epidemiology of inflammatory bowel disease. *Gastroenterol Clin North Am* 2002;31:1–20.
9. Robinson M. Optimizing therapy for inflammatory bowel disease. *Am J Gastroenterol* 1997;92:12S–17S.
10. Russell MGVM, Stockbrugger RW. Epidemiology of inflammatory bowel disease: an update. *Scand J Gastroenterol* 1996;31:417–427.
11. Rutgeerts P. Modern therapy for inflammatory bowel disease. *Scand J Gastroenterol Suppl* 2003;237:30–33.
12. Scribano ML, Pantera C. Review article: medical treatment of active Crohn's disease. *Aliment Pharmacol Ther* 2000;16[Suppl 4]:35–39.
13. Su CG, Judge TA, Lichtenstein GR. Extraintestinal manifestations of inflammatory bowel disease. *Gastroenterol Clin North Am* 2002;31:307–327.
14. Targan SR, Hanauer SB, Ven Deventer SJH, et al. A short-term study of chimeric monoclonal antibody CA2 to tumor necrosis factor α for Crohn's disease. *N Engl J Med* 1997;337:1029–1035.
15. Wills JS, Lobis IF, Denstman FJ. Crohn's disease: state of the art. *Radiology* 1997;202:597–610.

Diarrhea and Proctitis

Philip Salen and Michael Heller

DIARRHEA

The patient with diarrhea presents emergency physicians with a problem that is not only physical but also social and personal. Acute diarrhea is defined as the passage of a greater number of stools of decreased form than usual, lasting less than 14 days (3). Many restrict the term chronic diarrhea to indicate diarrheal illness lasting at least 1 month. The term gastroenteritis should be reserved for those diarrheal diseases in which the patient also exhibits nausea and vomiting. Dysentery refers to diarrhea containing blood and pus. The annual rate of diarrheal illness in the United States among adults averages about one episode per person per year. Physicians are consulted in 8.2 million cases and 250,000 people require hospitalization (6). In the United States, mortality is rare and occurs mainly in the elderly and in young children (12).

Patients may present to the emergency department (ED) with an acute onset of diarrhea, or an acute exacerbation of chronic diarrhea. The most common causes of acute diarrhea are infectious agents; however, less commonly implicated causes are drugs and toxins, chemotherapy, fecal impaction (overflow diarrhea), and psychosocial stress. Among infectious causes of diarrhea, viruses account for 50% to 70% of all cases, bacteria for 15% to 20%, and parasites for 10% to 15%. Diarrhea is especially problematic in particular settings: for children in day care settings, travelers to tropical and semitropical regions, homosexual males, immunocompromised individuals, people living in an unhygienic environments, and those with exposure to contaminated water or foods (6).

Although an enormous number of stimuli may produce diarrhea, the four basic pathophysiologic mechanisms are alterations in mucosal morphology, alterations in ion secretion from the intestinal villi, alterations in intestinal motility, and osmotic diarrhea. The majority of diarrheal illnesses are noninflammatory, usually arising in the upper small bowel from the action of an enterotoxin or other process that specifically alters the absorptive function of the villus tip. Dysentery usually arises in the colon from an invasive process that causes inflammation (3). In addition to treating patients symptomatically and stabilizing patients hemodynamically, the goal of the emergency physician is to determine whether the patient's diarrhea is inflammatory, which usually signifies a more severe diarrheal illness, and whether specific therapy is warranted.

CLINICAL PRESENTATION

Diarrhea is both a symptom and a sign. As a symptom, diarrhea can be described as an increase in stool frequency, an increase in stool volume, and a decrease in stool consistency. Associated gastrointestinal symptoms are nausea, vomiting, abdominal discomfort, abdominal cramps, bloating, tenesmus (constant urge to defecate), rectal urgency, perianal discomfort, intestinal gas-related complaints, and incontinence. As a sign, diarrhea is defined objectively as an increase in watery stool excretion to an amount greater than 200 mL every 24 hours (3). Depending on the etiology, the diarrhea may be liquid or soft, nonbloody or bloody, mucoid, voluminous, or scant. Physical examination can reveal fever, tachycardia, abdominal tenderness, and dehydration. When fever and bloody stool are present, the patient characteristically has intestinal inflammation owing to invasive bacteria. From the standpoint of functional impairment from the illness, diarrhea may be categorized as mild (no change in normal activities), moderate (forced change in activities), or severe (disability with confinement to bed) (6).

When evaluating complaints of diarrhea, the physician should first distinguish whether the diarrhea is truly diarrhea or nondiarrheal rectal discharge, rectal bleeding, or abnormally colored stools. Once the diagnosis of diarrhea is confirmed, the clinician must decide whether (i) the patient is seriously ill, (ii) a diagnostic workup is necessary, (iii) an etiology can be identified, (iv) specific treatment is necessary, and (v) if there are social and community health implications. The severity of illness is directly correlated to the fluid and electrolyte status of the patient and whether the diarrhea has an inflammatory component.

DIFFERENTIAL DIAGNOSIS

Although there are hundreds of causes of acute diarrhea, most cases presenting to the emergency physician will be infectious and are transmitted by significant ingestion of the organism.

Viral Diarrhea

The most common cause of diarrhea, viral enteritis, is characterized by destruction of villus mucosa. Shortened villi decrease the intestinal surface area available for fluid absorption and alter ion secretion (19). The noroviruses and rotavirus are responsible for more than 50% of viral enteric infections (11). Rotavirus is an important diarrheal agent that causes a significant amount of morbidity in developed as well as developing nations, predominantly affecting infants between 3 to 15 months. Enteric adenoviruses are the second most common viral pathogen in young children. Hallmarks of viral diarrhea are the absence of high fever, nausea, and the occurrence of many nonbloody stools per day. Concomitant vomiting is common, but severe abdominal pain is uncharacteristic. Although improved hygiene has reduced bacterial diarrheal illness in the developed world, it has had less effect in preventing spread of viral gastroenteritis, in particular rotavirus (11).

Bacterial Diarrhea

Bacterial enteritis alters mucosal morphology by invasion of mucosa and submucosa of the terminal ileum and colon, thereby resulting in inflammation. Edema, bleeding, and leukocyte infiltration of the colonic wall typically occurs, which results in the appearance of red and white blood cells in the stool. Common etiologies are *Salmonella, Shigella, Escherichia coli, Yersinia,* and *Campylobacter*. Fever is a characteristic feature, which may be quite marked, especially in the pediatric patient (6). Passage of many stools per day, particularly when they are bloody and explosive in character, suggests bacterial enteritis. Special care must be taken when evaluating patients with suspected dysentery to eliminate the possibility that there may be an anatomic cause, such as a bowel obstruction or ischemic colitis, for their diarrhea, abdominal pain, and toxic appearance.

Enterohemorrhagic *E. coli* O157:H7 is a common cause of bloody and nonbloody diarrhea and is estimated to cause more than 20,000 infections each year. The organism produces a Shiga-like toxin, which causes colonic vasculitis and allows inflammatory mediators to gain access to the circulation at times initiating the hemolytic-uremic syndrome (4). Transmission is typically from ingestion of contaminated beef, or from person to person. Symptoms and signs that distinguish *E. coli* O157:H7 from other bacterial enteric diseases are the absence of fever in the presence of other symptoms and signs of inflammatory colitis, such as abdominal pain and bloody stool. Hemolytic uremic syndrome occurs in 6% of affected patients, usually 6 days after onset of the diarrhea, and is the most common cause of acute renal failure in children. Clinical features of hemolytic uremic syndrome include hemolytic anemia, thrombocytopenia, and acute renal failure. Once an isolate has been identified, the local health department should be notified so that if the infected child attends daycare the facility can increase its surveillance for and prevent epidemics of diarrheal illness.

Infectious diarrhea may be associated with systemic manifestations. Both enterohemorrhagic *E. coli* O157:H7 and *Shigella* can cause hemolytic anemia, thrombotic thrombocytopenic purpura, and renal failure with associated high mortality rate. Immune-mediated extraintestinal manifestations such as reactive arthritis or Reiter syndrome can occur after diarrheal illness from *Salmonella, Shigella, Yersinia, and Campylobacter*. Persistent abdominal pain, fever, mesenteric adenitis, erythema nodosum, or other immunologic manifestations may suggest *Yersinia enterocolitica* or *Yersinia Pseudotuberculosis* (18). *Yersiniosis* may also lead to an autoimmune-type thyroiditis, pericarditis, and glomerulonephritis.

Food Poisoning

Although any toxin-produced gastrointestinal syndrome can be called food poisoning, this term is most commonly applied to gastroenteritis syndromes in which upper gastrointestinal symptoms predominate. Food poisoning occurs when infectious agents within the gut produce enterotoxin or the enteroxin is ingested from contaminated food. Depending on the type of organism that produces it, the enterotoxin can cause upper or lower gastrointestinal symptoms. Concurrent illness in other persons exposed to the same food strongly suggests food poisoning. Staphylococcal food poisoning is the most common form and typically occurs when contaminated food is not cooked at temperatures sufficient to kill the bacteria. It is manifested by nausea, vomiting, abdominal cramps, and diarrhea 2 to 6 hours after ingestion of food contaminated by the enterotoxin. *Bacillus cereus* causes two distinct food-poisoning syndromes: (i) an enterotoxin induces vomiting and abdominal cramping 2 hours after eating contaminated rice, (ii) an enterotoxin from ingestion of contaminated meat products results in a diarrheal syndrome.

Scombroid is a food poisoning that causes a histamine-like reaction after ingestion of heat-stable toxins produced by bacterial action on dark-meat fish such as tuna and mackerel. Ciguatera food poisoning results from the ingestion of a neurotoxin, which accumulates in fish species that frequent coral reefs, such as red snapper and sea bass. Affected patients develop gastroenteritis and a potpourri of neurologic symptoms such as paresthesias, dysesthesias, weakness, and even altered mental status. *Clostridium botulinum* diarrheal illness can result in hypotonia and descending muscle weakness.

Protozoan Diarrhea

Giardia lamblia is neither rare nor exotic. *G. lamblia* has been shown to be the most frequently identified intestinal parasite in the United States (5). Travel history, sexual history, pregnancy, and drinking well water are important risk factors. It has been documented that children with undiagnosed giardiasis may transmit symptomatic disease to family members. When evaluating patients who have persistent, nonspecific complaints of persistent diarrhea such as bloating and excessive flatulence, it is important to consider *G. lamblia* as the cause. Typically, the diarrhea will be noninflammatory and will not contain blood or pus.

Bloody diarrhea in recent immigrants or travelers returning from regions where *Entamoeba histolytica*, amoebiasis, is endemic (such as tropical Africa, Asia, or Latin America) should prompt fecal testing for that pathogen (18). Genital–anal sexual contact makes homosexuals at particular risk for this organism. Ingestion of *E. histolytica* cysts, an enteric protozoan, causes infection (13). Numerous fecal leukocytes are not common in patients with intestinal amoebiasis. Therefore, when a patient with diarrhea is passing bloody stools and there are few leukocytes, amoebiasis should be considered (6). Hepatic involvement results from the organism ascending the portal venous system, which can cause hepatic necrosis from obstruction of portal vessels. The diagnosis remains dependent on the morphologic identification of cysts in the affected patient's diarrhea (13).

Traveler's Diarrhea

Traveler's diarrhea is a self-limited illness that usually resolves spontaneously within a few days, but it has the potential for wrecking a meticulously planned vacation. Traveler's diarrhea is usually defined as the passage of at least three unformed stools in a 24-hour period, together with nausea, vomiting, abdominal pain or cramps, fecal urgency, tenesmus, or the passage of bloody or mucoid stools in a person who lives in an industrialized region and who has traveled to a developing semitropical or tropical country (17). Among the 35 million people who travel from industrialized countries to a developing country annually, traveler's diarrhea has an incidence rate of 20% to 50% per 2-week stay. Although different organisms predominate in different regions, the principal agents in most of the high-risk areas are enterotoxigenic *E. coli*, Rotavirus, noroviruses, *Salmonella, Campylobacter*, and *Giardia* (17). The most common sources of traveler's diarrhea are contaminated food and water.

Antibiotic-Associated Diarrhea

The spectrum of findings in antibiotic-associated diarrhea ranges from colitis, which is a potential source of serious progressive disease, to "nuisance diarrhea," which is defined as frequent loose and watery stools with no other complications. Although infections caused by *Clostridium difficile* account for only 10% to 20% of the cases of antibiotic-associated diarrhea, the organism accounts for the majority of cases of inflammatory colitis associated with antibiotic therapy. An overgrowth of *C. difficile*, which occurs when native bowel flora is killed by antibiotics, is responsible for elaborating the enterotoxin. The enterotoxin induces a pseudomembranous colitis. Major risk factors for *C. difficile* infection include advanced age, hospitalization, and exposure to antibiotics. Hospitalized adults have rates of colonization of 20% to 30%, as compared with a rate of 3% in outpatients. Relapse with *C. difficile* colitis is common after therapeutic resolution and occurs in about 25% of cases. Antibiotic-associated diarrhea may also be caused by other enteric pathogens, by the direct effects of antimicrobial agents on the intestinal mucosa, and by the metabolic consequences of reduced concentrations of fecal flora (2).

Diarrhea in the Immunocompromised Hosts

Individuals at pronounced risk for diarrhea include those with either primary immunodeficiency (e.g., immunoglobulin (Ig)A deficiency and hypogammaglobulinemia) or secondary immunodeficiency states (e.g., AIDS and pharmacologic immunosuppression). Diarrhea is a common and distressing symptom in patients with AIDS, occurring in more than 90% of individuals at some time during the course of their illness. AIDS patients are at risk from all the infectious causes of diarrhea that occurs in the immunocompetent population and are also at risk from other pathogens as well. A significant amount of morbidity and mortality of late AIDS is associated with gastrointestinal disease (14). Enteric protozoa infections are the most common causes of diarrhea in AIDS patients followed by cytomegalovirus and *Mycobacterium avium intracellulare. Microsporidia, Isospora belli* and *Cryptosporidia parvum*, common causes of protozoal diarrheal illness in AIDS patients, cause disruption of small intestinal villi architecture and severe malabsorption, maldigestion, and diarrhea (14). Cytomegalovirus-induced colitis produces diarrhea that can be persistent or intermittent, as well as lower abdominal pain, fever, and weight loss. *Mycobacterium avium intracellulare* infects the small intestine and is characterized by diarrhea, abdominal pain, fever, nausea, weight loss, and malabsorption (16). The frequency of unexplained diarrhea in AIDS patients remains approximately 20% even after extensive evaluations are performed. Many factors have been implicated in this idiopathic diarrhea such as alteration in intestinal villi architecture, undetectable infections, and HIV-induced cellular infection.

Other Causes of Diarrhea

Many other diseases present with diarrhea as a primary or secondary manifestation. Viral hepatitis, malaria, and toxic shock syndrome can cause severe diarrhea, and can additionally affect hepatic, hematogenous, and central nervous system functions.

Noninfectious and extraintestinal processes may present as acute diarrhea. In patients with persistent or chronic diarrhea, a noninfectious cause of the illness should be considered. Some of the important diagnoses to consider include irritable bowel syndrome, inflammatory bowel disease, ischemic bowel disease (particularly in patients older than 50 years with other evidence of peripheral vascular disease), bowel obstruction, volvulus, and intussusception. Pernicious anemia, pellagra, Whipple disease, diabetes mellitus, small bowel scleroderma, and various malabsorption syndromes may present as acute or persistent diarrhea that resembles infectious diarrhea.

EMERGENCY DEPARTMENT EVALUATION

Most cases of diarrhea are managed without need for medical attention. Medical evaluation should be initiated for a subset of patients with more severe illness. Assessment of the severity of illness, presence of dehydration, character of stool patterns, presence of fever, vomiting, or dysentery will help to focus the evaluation to determine the likely cause of the illness. Detailed history including travel, sexual practices, or immunocompromised status is crucial because it will often point to an etiology. Noninflammatory enteritis typically presents with emesis; minimal or absence of fever; mild crampy pain; and watery diarrhea; all of which reflect upper intestinal involvement. Inflammatory enteritis presents with fever, significant abdominal pain, tenesmus, and bloody diarrhea, which indicate invasive colonic involvement. Seasonal occurrence plays a role as well; that is, rotavirus and the noroviruses have winter peaks and *G. lamblia* has a spring peak (5). Bacterial causes of diarrhea are more common in summer. On physical examination, special attention should focus on the abdomen, which may be notable for generalized tenderness and increased bowel sounds but lacking peritoneal signs. Specific indications for further medical evaluation of patients with

diarrhea are dehydration; dysentery; significant abdominal pain and tenderness; suspicion of a concurrent systemic illness; and disease in the very young, the elderly, and in immunocompromised patients.

Normal feces should have few or no white blood cells. Table 72.1 documents infectious agents that produce fecal leukocytes. The fecal sample can be examined for fecal leukocytes as a wet preparation under the high dry lens or as a Wright stain or gram stain under the oil lens. Identification of fecal polymorphonuclear leukocytes can quickly provide additional laboratory evidence to support a presumptive diagnosis of inflammatory diarrhea. The sensitivity and specificity of fecal leukocytes for inflammatory diarrhea are 0.73 and 0.84, respectively (18). Some authorities consider hemoccult-positive diarrhea in patients with acute enteric illness to be clinically equivalent to having fecal leukocytes (18,21). The most commonly identified bacterial pathogens in patients with fecal leukocytes include *Shigella, Salmonella, Campylobacter, E. coli, Aeromonas, Yersinia, Vibrio parahaemolyticus*, and *C. difficile*. Fecal leukocytes can also be seen in nonenteritis conditions, such as appendicitis and inflammatory bowel disease.

Relatively well-appearing patients presenting with signs and symptoms of bacterial enteritis can be treated empirically with antibiotics, and stool cultures need not be sent. In the patient with symptoms of hypovolemia, red or white blood cells in the stool, or an abnormal abdominal examination, further investigation may be warranted. Table 72.2 lists specific indications for sending diarrhea for culture. Clinicians should be wary of resistant infections because of the recent emergence of multidrug-resistant bacterial diarrheal illnesses (20). If the patient has been taking antibiotics antecedent to onset of diarrhea, *C. difficile* must be considered and stool should be sent for the *C. difficile* toxin assay. It is rarely necessary to send stool for ova and parasites for laboratory analysis after initial evaluation for diarrhea in the emergency department. However, illnesses lasting longer than 14 days should prompt consideration of parasites, most notably *Giardia*, particularly in travelers who have returned from areas where untreated water is consumed and for immunocompromised patients. For immunocompromised patients, endoscopy and biopsy are indicated when the diarrheal illness persists, routine stool cultures are unrevealing, and courses of empiric antibiotics and antihelminthics do not lead to resolution (13).

EMERGENCY DEPARTMENT MANAGEMENT

The assessment and treatment of dehydration and the relief of symptoms remain the cornerstones of emergency department care. The main objectives in the evaluation of diarrhea are to (i) assess the degree of dehydration and provide fluid and electrolyte replacement, (ii) prevent spread of the enteropathogen, and (iii) provide specific therapy if indicated.

Fluid and Electrolyte Therapy

Regardless of the causative agent, initial therapy should include rehydration. Unless the patient is comatose or severely dehydrated, oral rehydration with a glucose-based electrolyte solution is preferred. The standard formulation recommended by the World Health Organization or a newer reduced-osmolarity formula for children can be life-saving in resource-poor regions and is valuable in the industrialized world for infants, the elderly, immunocompromised patients, and anyone with profuse watery diarrhea (18). Sport drinks, diluted fruit juices, flavored soft drinks augmented with saltine crackers, broths, and soups can meet the fluid and salt needs in nearly all cases in nondehydrated otherwise healthy persons with acute diarrhea.

TABLE 72.1. Clinical Features of Infection with Selected Diarrheal Pathogens[18]

Infectious Agent	Common Epidemiologic Setting	Fever	Abd Pain	Vomit	Bloody Stool	FL	Therapy	Clinical Pearls
Norovirus (e.g. Norwalk virus)	Epidemic winter outbreaks in nursing homes, cruise ships; foodborne transmission	+/−	+	+	−	−	Symptomatic therapy	Vomiting more common in children; diarrhea more common in adults
Rotavirus	Infants and young children	−	−	+	−	−	Oral rehydration solution	Early caloric refeeding
Vibrio parahaemolyticus, Vibrio vulnificus	Seafood ingestion	+/−	+/−	+/−	+	+	Symptomatic	Antibiotic therapy does not shorten course
Campylobacter	Undercooked poultry	+	+	+	+	+	Macrolides	Resistance to fluoroquinolones ⇑
Yersinia	Pork, raw milk	+	+	+	+	+	Fluoroquinolones	Appendicitis mimic
Shigella	Contaminated food	+	+	+	+	+	Fluoroquinolones	Can also cause hemolytic uremic syndrome
Salmonella	Foodborne transmission	+	+	+	+	+	Fluoroquinolones	Healthy host with mild illness—no therapy necessary
Escheridria coli O157:H7	Ground beef; sprouts	−	+	+/−	+	−	None	Antibiotic and antimotility therapy ⇑⇑ risk of hemolytic uremic syndrome
E. coli (enterotoxigenic, enteropathogenic, enteroinvasive)	Contaminated uncooked vegetables, fruits	+	+	+	+	+	Fluoroquinolones	Most common cause of traveler's diarrhea
Staphylococcus aureus	Undercooked meat	+	+	+	−	−	Symptomatic therapy	Reheated, undercooked foods
Clostridium botulinum	Preserved meat, fish, vegetables	+	+	−		−	None	Very difficult to culture organism
Clostridium difficile	Nosocomial; post–antibiotic complication	+	+	+	+	+	Metronidazole; Oral Vancomycin	Cause of pseudomembranous colitis
Clostridium perfringens	Incompletely cooked meat	+	+	+	−	−	Metronidazole	Reheated, undercooked foods
Vibrio cholerae	Waterborne transmission	−	+/−	+/−	−	−	Doxycycline	Primary therapy is rehydration
Bacillus cereus	Rice	−	+	+		−	Symptomatic therapy	Primarily an emetic syndrome
B. cereus	Meat products; vegetables	−	+	+/−	−	−	Symptomatic therapy	Primarily a diarrheal syndrome
Giardia	Fecally contaminated water	−	+	+/−	−	−	Metronidazole	Common cause of persistent diarrhea
Erotamoeba histolytica	Travel to tropics	+	+	+/−	+	−	Metronidazole	Consider if there are bloody stools with few fecal leukocytes
Cryptosporidium	Contaminated water	+/−	+/−	+/−	−	−	Paromomycin with azithromycin	Prevalent in AIDS patients
Cyclospora	Foodborne transmission	+/−	+/−	+	−	−	TMP-SMX	Fatigue, which may be profound, is present in ≥90% of patients with cyclospora
Isospora	Fecal–oral, contaminated water	+/−	+/−	+/−	−	−	TMP-SMX	Prevalent in AIDS patients

TMP-SMZ, trimethoprim sulfamethoxazole; + Common; − not Common; +/− occasional; FL, fecal leukocytes; Abd, abdominal.

TABLE 72.2. Indications for Stool Culture in Patients with Acute Diarrhea

Immunocompromised hosts
Travel history to third world
Homosexual activity
Failure to respond to empiric antibiotic therapy
Individuals with close contact to others where fecal oral spread can occur (daycare workers, health care workers, food handlers)
"Toxic" clinical appearance
Persistent diarrhea (≥7 days), with suspicion of protozoal cause
Severe, bloody, inflammatory diarrheal illness
Suspicion of antibiotic-resistant bacteria
Recent antibiotic use–related
Bloody diarrhea with suspicion of hemolytic uremic syndrome

Dietary Advice

Fatty foods or foods high in simple sugars, including juices and carbonated sodas, should be avoided because they can exacerbate diarrheal illness. Caloric intake facilitates enterocyte renewal during a bout of acute diarrhea. Complex carbohydrates such as rice, wheat, potatoes, bread, and cereals, lean meats, yogurt, fruits, and vegetables are recommended as soon as the patient can tolerate feeding. Although clinical lactose intolerance is uncommon in cases of acute diarrhea, many authorities recommend dairy product avoidance in the first few days of illness (6).

Antimotility Agents

Codeine, diphenoxylate with atropine, and loperamide reduce urgency, bowel movement frequency, and stool volume in diarrheal illness. They work by slowing the intraluminal flow of liquid, thereby facilitating intestinal absorption (8). Loperamide is generally the recommended agent when antimotility agents are prescribed because of its safety and expected efficacy in which stool quantity is reduced by approximately 80% (7). Loperamide is the recommended treatment for patients with AIDS in the absence of inflammatory disease of the colon and when the diarrhea persists in the face of empiric antimicrobial and antihelminthic therapy. Antimotility agents may be used in patients with infectious enteritis of mild-to-moderate severity but must be used judiciously in the setting of dysentery, as they can inhibit clearance of the offending organism.

Bismuth and Attapulgate

Bismuth subsalicylate is effective therapy for acute diarrhea, reducing the number of stools passed by approximately 50% (7). The antisecretory salicylate effect is responsible for its antidiarrheal effect. It is highly effective in relieving the vomiting associated with enteric viral infections (7). In addition, it has antibacterial properties that may explain its value in prevention of traveler's diarrhea and has been shown to prevent infection caused by enterotoxigenic E. coli. A typical dose for adults is 2 tablets every 6 hours for 2 to 3 days. An important caveat is to warn patients that this medication will turn their feces black. Furthermore to prevent the occurrence of salicylism, which may result from excessive dosing, bismuth subsalicylate should not be given to immunocompromised patients and others with chronic diarrhea (6). Attapulgite (Kaopectate), a clay-like material, absorbs water and makes stools more formed. It is not absorbed and can be used safely in most diarrheal illnesses.

Antibiotics

There are patients who are candidates for empiric antimicrobial therapy without additional evaluation. For patients with fever plus either leukocyte- or hemoccult-positive diarrhea, or for patients with moderate-to-severe traveler's diarrhea, antimicrobial therapy may be given empirically. Generally, a fluoroquinolone antimicrobial is recommended for 3 to 5 days as empiric therapy unless diarrheal culture results are available to tailor therapy. Table 72.1 refers to antimicrobial therapy of choice for specific pathogens. Patients with traveler's diarrhea are characteristically infected with bacterial pathogens and their illness is shortened by antimicrobial therapy. After appropriate evaluation, AIDS patients can be started on empiric therapy with fluoroquinolone for 10 days for acute onset diarrhea. As in infections outside the gut in immunocompromised patients, curative treatment requires prolonged therapy. Physicians must be wary about the dramatic increases in the rate of fluoroquinolone resistance, contemporaneous with the widespread use of fluoroquinolones in poultry feeds, which now limit the usefulness of these agents for certain enteric pathogens, most notably *Campylobacter* and *Salmonella species* (18,20).

Patients with diarrhea lasting 2 to 4 weeks without systemic symptoms or dysentery may be treated empirically with metronidazole, since *Giardia* is such a common cause of persistent diarrhea and testing often fails to reveal the organism (6). Metronidazole is also effective against small bowel bacterial overgrowth syndrome that is associated with persistent diarrhea, *C. difficile* colitis, and intestinal amoebiasis.

Special Advice to Travelers

Educating travelers about prevention and treatment of diarrhea is important because it is estimated that 25% to 40% of travelers in the developing world will develop diarrhea (17). Traveler instruction should consist of (i) methods of diarrhea prevention, (ii) use of prophylactic agents, and (iii) how to replete fluid and electrolytes. Travelers trying to avoid diarrhea should be advised to follow the old British colonial axiom "cook it, boil it, peel it–or forget it." Bismuth subsalicylate, fluoroquinolone antimicrobials, and doxycycline are effective prophylactically and as pharmacologic self-therapy for traveler's diarrhea.

Special Advice for Caring for Infants and Children

Children who require hydration should be fed age-appropriate diets as soon as they have been rehydrated (1). More than 80% of children with diarrhea can tolerate undiluted milk. Infants fed human milk can be nursed safely during episodes of diarrhea (1). Antimotility agents should be used with caution in children and should not be used in infants. In patients with enterohemorrhagic *E. coli* O157:H7 infection, the hemolytic uremic syndrome may be facilitated by administering antimotility agents.

CRITICAL INTERVENTIONS

- Recognize gastroenteritis-induced dehydration and institute appropriate fluid, salt, and caloric repletion
- Consider systemic processes that may be causing diarrhea, that is, bowel obstructions or bowel ischemia

DISPOSITION

The emergency physician can manage almost all cases of diarrhea presenting to the ED. Patients with diarrhea who are significantly dehydrated and who remain unable to tolerate oral fluids should be considered for admission. Situations in which there is a possible pathologic process such as inflammatory bowel disease or ischemic bowel will require medical or surgical consultation.

Moderately ill patients who are sent home, patients with traveler's diarrhea, and patients with AIDS should have followup arranged with their primary care provider.

COMMON PITFALLS

✔ Overdiagnosing viral gastroenteritis. There is a temptation to label all diarrheal illnesses of uncertain cause as viral. Particularly in older patients, the diagnosis of viral gastroenteritis is less likely and bacterial causes are more likely. If there are white blood cells or red blood cells in the stool or if the abdominal examination is abnormal, diarrhea should not be attributed to a viral cause

✔ Failing to examine the stool. Examination of the stool for blood and WBCs is one of the most useful tests in guiding therapy

✔ Many medical and surgical problems can manifest with diarrhea as a cardinal complaint, notably hepatitis, small bowel obstruction, inflammatory bowel disease, mesenteric infarction, and cancer. The emergency physician must be vigilant to distinguish between these diseases and infectious diarrhea

PROCTITIS

Proctitis is formally defined as inflammation of the rectal mucosa. Alternatively, it can be defined as anorectal symptoms associated with sigmoidoscopic findings limited to the distal 15 cm of the rectum. Proctitis should be distinguished from *proctocolitis*, which has different infectious etiologies. *Acute proctitis* is a nonspecific term that refers to several specific disease conditions that include inflammatory bowel disease, infections, venereal disease, antibiotics, radiation, and chemotherapy (22).

The epidemiology of proctitis in ED patients varies with demographics. In urban areas with large populations of homosexual males, high rates of sexually transmitted infectious proctitis are seen; in facilities treating more elderly populations, proctitis is more frequently the sequela of other gastrointestinal disorders, exemplified by radiation proctitis or ulcerative proctitis.

CLINICAL PRESENTATION

Most patients have similar nonspecific symptoms of rectal discomfort, tenesmus (urge to defecate), and hematochezia. Other symptoms are pain with defecation, disordered bowel function (typically constipation), lower abdominal pain and pelvic pain, mucopurulent rectal discharge, and feelings of incomplete evacuation. Infectious and inflammatory conditions that involve the anal mucosa are typically very painful. Rectal mucosal erythema, friability, and a mucopurulent discharge are noted on physical examination. Patients with proctitis attempt frequent fecal evacuation that typically produces bloody mucus and little fecal matter (23). Symptoms of fever, weight loss, abdominal pain, nausea, and vomiting indicate that proctitis may be manifestation of a more generalized process.

DIFFERENTIAL DIAGNOSIS

Before diagnosing symptoms of rectal pain and discharge as proctitis, the clinician must first exclude other entities that can cause these symptoms, such as perirectal abscess, rectal polyps, and anal fissures. The causes of proctitis are divided into infectious causes (most typically venereal diseases) and noninfectious causes.

Infectious Proctitis

Both homosexual and heterosexual anal intercourse have the potential for transmitting enteric pathogens and venereal infections, especially when people have multiple sexual partners and fail to use condoms. The most common infectious cause, and by far the most common cause in sexually active homosexual men, is gonorrhea (24). In symptomatic gonococcal proctitis, the usual presenting complaint is rectal discharge, often noted as staining of the underwear. Additionally, scant bloody discharge and rectal pain may be noted spontaneously or with rectal intercourse. Gonococcal infection of the rectum occurs commonly in conjunction with gonococcal urethritis. Gonococcal infection of the female rectum is most commonly the result of anal intercourse, but may be caused by the spread of the organisms through vaginal secretions. Perhaps 10% to 20% of all patients with genital gonorrhea have positive rectal cultures for the organism.

Along with gonorrhea, chlamydia should be considered in patients with proctitis that appears to be sexually transmitted (24,27). Infections with lymphogranuloma venereum (LGV) types are more severe but much less frequent than those caused by other strains of chlamydia. Although some patients are asymptomatic, anorectal pain, tenesmus, left lower quadrant abdominal tenderness, constipation, and a bloody mucopurulent discharge can be noted. Chlamydial proctitis may have a subacute or even chronic presentation, with regional adenopathy and fibrosis and stricture of the rectum. Granulomatous rectal changes with LGV chlamydial strains resemble Crohn disease, especially when perirectal abscesses and fistulas are present (24).

Proctitis caused by herpes simplex virus (HSV) infection, either type 1 or 2, is a common cause of proctitis; however, HSV-2 infections are more severe and recur more frequently. The predominant complaints are severe anorectal pain, discharge, and change in bowel habits (constipation being more frequent than diarrhea). Systemic symptoms are fever, chills, and malaise. Vesicles, in clusters surrounded by an erythematous base, hemorrhage, vascular congestion, and pus may extend as high as 15 cm up the rectal mucosa. With severe HSV proctitis, urinary dysfunction, impotence, neuralgia, and paresthesias in the buttocks and thighs may occur secondary to viral infection of the sacral plexus. Persistent herpes proctitis is seen almost exclusively in AIDS patients.

Noninfectious Proctitis

Patients who have signs and symptoms of rectal disease and histories of anal erotic activity may manifest primarily noninfectious consequences of their sexual behavior. Foreign objects inserted into the anus may cause mucosal damage and allow penetration by normal colonic organisms, with secondary inflammation. Anal and lower rectal mucosal inflammation caused by the trauma of sexual activity may be extremely difficult to differentiate from inflammatory changes secondary to infectious agents.

Allergic proctitis occurs when substances used as lubricants during anal intercourse sensitize through abraded anal skin or intact mucosa. When used as lubricants, soaps, shampoos, cooking oil, suntan preparations, or medicinal creams may be directly irritating and can reduce the protective effectiveness of condoms. Even lubricating jelly has been associated with allergic contact sensitivity owing to the propylene glycol vehicle.

Ulcerative colitis is a chronic inflammatory bowel disorder of unknown origin that is characterized by inflammation of the bowel. The proximal extent of the colonic mucosal inflammation varies among individuals, but the rectum is almost always involved. With predominantly rectal involvement, constipation and tenesmus are typical complaints. Patients with ulcerative proctitis usually have milder manifestations of inflammatory bowel disease and typically do not have the systemic manifestations of the disease.

Radiation proctitis is caused by pelvic irradiation for gynecologic or prostatic malignancies. Symptoms of anorectal pain and bloody discharge can be severe. Proctoscopic findings are erythematous and edematous mucosa in the acute phase and characteristic telangiectasias and ulcerations in the chronic phase. Large ulcerations can result in distal rectal strictures or rectovaginal fistulas (25).

EMERGENCY DEPARTMENT EVALUATION

An accurate diagnosis can be made by use of a careful history, anoscopy, culture, rectal biopsy, and stool analysis (22). A sexual history is important in the evaluation of anorectal complaints. The patient may not volunteer a sexual history because of embarrassment or fear of a hostile response from health-care personnel. Patients with a history of receptive anal sex are at risk for a variety of sexually transmitted infections, including HIV infection (26). Also important to obtain is a history of previous treatment for sexually transmitted disease, because it may have been ineffective in eradicating unrecognized rectal infection. Anoscopy with appropriate cultures identifies most sexually transmissible intestinal infections and should be carried out in all those who practice receptive anal intercourse who present with symptoms suggestive of proctitis.

Although specimens can be obtained with a pledget blindly inserted 2 cm into the canal and rotated, swabbing under direct anoscopic visualization raises the positive yield on gram staining from 34% to 79% (26). Cultures for sexually transmitted disease should be obtained not only from the rectum, but also from the urethra and the cervix. Immunofluorescence stains and viral cultures for HSV should be carried out, even when no lesions are grossly visible. Whenever patients have proctitis secondary to sexually transmitted disease, they should also be tested for concomitant infections such as syphilis and AIDS.

EMERGENCY DEPARTMENT MANAGEMENT

The ED management of infectious proctitis is analogous to that of urethritis. When sexually transmitted disease is suspected based on patient history, empiric therapy for gonorrhea and chlamydia is recommended (27). Third-generation cephalosporins and quinolones are the preferred treatment for gonococcal infections. Doxycycline or macrolide antibiotics should be prescribed to treat chlamydial infections. Occasionally, rectal LGV requires several courses of antibiotic therapy.

Systemic therapy of herpetic proctitis with acyclovir is indicated when the diagnosis is suspected (27). Oral acyclovir effectively reduces the duration of symptomatic lesions, rectal pain, discharge, and the period of viral shedding. In immunocompetent hosts, the dosage is 400 mg, 5 times daily for 10 days. AIDS patients require intravenous acyclovir for longer courses of therapy (26). Patients with symptoms or signs of severe herpes proctitis, such as severe pain or urinary retention, should be admitted for aggressive pain control and intravenous acyclovir.

Even when a new presentation of proctitis does not appear to be caused by infection, it is wise to treat empirically for common infectious etiologies. Pseudoinfectious and allergic proctitis are best treated by removal of the agents causing the disease. Ulcerative proctitis is responsive to oral, parenteral, and rectal administration of corticosteroids. Treatment should also be aimed at treating the perianal discomfort, which can be severe. Sitz baths for 20 minutes 3 to 4 times daily are helpful.

CRITICAL INTERVENTIONS

- Differentiate proctitis from surgical disease, such as perirectal abscess
- Initiate antibiotic coverage appropriate for sexually transmitted diseases

DISPOSITION

Most patients with proctitis can be managed in the ED without consultation or admission. Consultation is advisable when there is a problem with the diagnosis of an unusual mucosal appearance, a question of perirectal infection, systemic symptoms or local signs suggesting malignancy, or a suspicion of inflammatory bowel disease. If outpatient therapy is elected, these patients require close followup. Worsening of symptoms or failure to improve in response to antibiotic therapy and Sitz baths within 48 hours necessitates admission and further endoscopic evaluation. All patients should be referred to an appropriate physician for followup endoscopy and evaluation of culture results.

COMMON PITFALLS

- ✔ Failure to elicit a sexual history and consider a sexually transmitted disease
- ✔ Failure to question a sexual history once elicited; many patients do not at first admit to rectal intercourse
- ✔ Failure to visualize the mucosa by anoscopy and to examine and culture any exudate
- ✔ Failure to arrange for proper identification and treatment of contacts
- ✔ Failure to consider or identify other rectal lesions that mimic proctitis, such as anal fissure, anal fistula, and perirectal abscess

References

1. American Academy of Pediatrics. The management of acute gastroenteritis in young children. *Pediatrics* 1996;97(3):1–23.
2. Bartlett JG. Antibiotic associated diarrhea. *N Engl J Med* 2002;346:334–339.
3. Binder HJ. Pathophysiology of acute diarrhea. *Am J Med* 1990;88:6A–25.3.
4. Boyce JH, Swerdlow DL, Griffin PM. *Escherichia coli* and the hemolytic-uremic syndrome. *N Engl J Med* 1995;333:364.
5. Caeiro JP, Mathewson JJ, Smith MA, et al. Etiology of outpatient pediatric nondysenteric diarrhea: a multicenter study in the United States. *J Pediatr Infect Dis* 1999;18:94–97.
6. Dupont HL. Guidelines on acute infectious diarrhea in adults. *Am J Gastroenterol* 1997;92:1962.
7. Dupont HL, Sanchez JT, Ericsson CD. Comparative efficacy of loperamide hydrochloride and bismuth subsalicylate in the management of acute diarrhea. *Am J Med* 1990;88:6a–15s.
8. Ericsson CD, Johnson PC. Safety and efficacy of loperamide. *Am J Med* 1990; 88:6A–10S.
9. Garthright WE, Archer DL, Kvenberg JE. Estimate of incidence and costs of intestinal infectious diseases in the United States. *Pub Health Rep* 1988;103:107.
10. Hanauer SB. Inflammatory bowel disease. *N Engl J Med* 1996;334(13):841–848.
11. Kapikian AZ. Viral gastroenteritis. *JAMA* 1993;269:627.
12. Lew JF, Glass RI, Gangarosa RE, et al. Diarrheal deaths in the United States; 1979 through 1987. *JAMA* 1991;265:3280.
13. Ravdin JI. Amebiasis. *Clin Infect Dis* 1995;20:1453.
14. Sharpstone D, Gazzard B. Gastrointestinal manifestation of HIV infection. *Lancet* 1996;348:379.
15. Siegel D, Edelstein PH, Nachamkin I. Inappropriate testing for diarrheal disease in the hospital. *JAMA* 1990;263:979.
16. Simon D, Brandt LJ. Diarrhea in patients with the acquired immunodeficiency syndrome. *Gastroenterology* 1993;105:1238.
17. Steffen R, Collard O, Tornieporth N, et al. Epidemiology, etiology and impact of traveler's diarrhea in Jamaica. *JAMA* 1999;281:811.
18. Thielman NM, Guerrant RL. Acute infectious diarrhea. *N Engl J Med* 2004;350: 38–47.
19. Vesikari J. Rotavirus vaccines against diarrhoeal disease. *Lancet* 1997;350:1538.

20. Villar RG, Macek MD, Simons S, et al. Investigation of multidrug-resistant *Salmonella* serotype typhimurium DT104 infections linked to raw-milk cheese in Washington State. *JAMA* 1999;281:1811–1816.
21. Vogtlin J. Stalder H. Hurzeler L, et al. Modified guaiac test may replace search for faecal leukocytes in acute infectious diarrhea [letter]. *Lancet* 1983;2:1204.
22. Babb RR. Evaluation of acute proctitis. *JAMA* 1980;244:358.
23. Tytgat GNJ, Fookens RH, Schotborgh RH, et al. Proctitis. *Neth J Med* 1990;37:537.
24. Quinn TC, et al. *Chlamydia trachomatis* proctitis. *N Engl J Med* 1981;305:195–200.
25. Bartelsman JF, Tytgal GN. Extra-ordinary forms of proctitis. *Neth J Med* 1990; 37:552.
26. Bassford J. Treatment of common anorectal disorders. *Am Fam Physician* 1992;45:1788.
27. Klausner JD, Kohn R, Kent C. Etiology of clinical proctitis among men who have sex with men. *Clin Infect Dis* 2004;15;38:300–302.

CHAPTER 73
Diverticular Disease

Michael D. Witting

In the industrialized world, the increasing prevalence of diverticular disease parallels the advancing age of the population. The prevalence of diverticular disease increases from 5% in persons younger than age 40 years, to 30% in those older than age 50, to 50% in those older than age 70, and to 66% in those older than age 85 years (3). Diverticulosis is equally common among men and women. The disease has widely differing prevalence rates in various geographic areas and ethnic groups (3).

The key factor in the development of diverticulosis appears to be a reduction in dietary fiber content. The pathophysiology is related to a pressure gradient between the colonic lumen and the serosa and areas of relative weakness in the bowel wall. Very high intraluminal pressure can develop within short segments of the colon. According to Laplace law of pressures within a cylinder, pressure equals tension divided by radius. Accordingly, the descending and sigmoid colons, which have narrow lumens, have the greatest intraluminal pressures. This pressure causes herniation of diverticula at the points where the intramural vessels penetrate the circular muscle layer, usually between the mesenteric and antimesenteric taenia. Increased fiber enlarges the lumen size, thereby decreasing the intraluminal pressure.

The sigmoid colon is involved in more than 90% of patients with the disease, and in approximately one half of the patients it is the only segment of the bowel involved. The cecum is involved in 2%, the ascending colon and rectum in 4% each, and the transverse colon in 10%. Most individuals with diverticulosis remain asymptomatic throughout their lives. The longer a patient has diverticulosis, the greater is the probability of complications, primarily diverticulitis and bleeding. There is no relationship, however, between the number and size of diverticula and the incidence of complications or probability of recurrent disease. The use of nonsteroidal antiinflammatory drugs is an etiologic factor in the development of diverticulitis (3). Diverticulitis results from inflammation of diverticula, resulting in microperforation or macroperforation (abscess, fistula, peritonitis, or obstruction). Diverticular bleeding results from an arterial lesion in the vasa recta, characterized by eccentric intimal thickening, altered internal elastic lamina, and focal medial thinning (6). A disproportionately high tendency exists for diverticula on the right side of the colon to hemorrhage. One theory holds that the wider necks and domes of right-sided diverticula cause greater exposure to injurious factors than in left-sided diverticula (6). Bleeding from diverticulosis is massive in about one fourth of patients in whom it occurs and mandates transfusion in approximately one third (11). Fortunately, the vast majority of diverticular bleeding ceases spontaneously.

CLINICAL PRESENTATION

Patients with diverticulosis present to the emergency physician with three common clinical presentations: (i) acute diverticulitis, (ii) lower gastrointestinal (GI) bleeding, and (iii) painful diverticular disease, with mild lower left quadrant pain.

Acute Diverticulitis

Patients with acute diverticulitis classically present with abrupt onset, severe, constant left lower quadrant pain; localized tenderness; and fever, leukocytosis, or other signs of systemic toxicity. Occasionally, the pain and tenderness occur in the left upper quadrant. Patients may present with a picture of a ruptured viscus with diffuse tenderness, rebound, guarding, and diminished or absent bowel sounds. Rarely, diverticulitis may present with signs of fistulization, such as pneumaturia and draining infections of the lower abdomen or medial aspect of the upper thigh. Diverticulitis often presents atypically in immunocompromised patients, such as those with acquired immunodeficiency syndrome (AIDS), renal failure, or diabetes, and those receiving immunosuppressive therapy. In these patients, fever, abdominal pain, or abdominal tenderness may be absent (8). In addition, the incidence of free perforation, a rare complication in the immunocompetent, is much higher among immunocompromised patients (4,8,10).

Lower Gastrointestinal Bleeding

Patients with diverticulosis may present with painless, massive rectal bleeding. Such bleeding is characteristically sudden, often profuse from the onset, and more frequent in older persons. The blood is usually bright or dark red, and although the patient may feel faint, initial hypotension is not common.

Painful Diverticular Disease

Although most patients with diverticulosis are asymptomatic, some develop recurrent episodes of left lower quadrant abdominal pain. The pain is usually dull, crampy, and intermittent and is often alleviated by the passage of flatus or stool. Signs of infection are absent.

DIFFERENTIAL DIAGNOSIS

Diverticulosis

Painless diverticular bleeding must be distinguished from other causes of lower GI bleeding, such as angiodysplasia, ischemic colitis, ulcerative colitis, hemorrhoids, polyps, and colonic or rectal cancer. Upper GI hemorrhage may present with rectal bleeding.

When diverticulosis presents as mild, left lower quadrant pain, it must be differentiated from irritable bowel syndrome,

Crohn disease, colon cancer, and nephrolithiasis, which may present with pain radiating to the left lower quadrant.

Acute Diverticulitis

Acute diverticulitis must be distinguished from more severe presentations of Crohn disease, ulcerative colitis, and ischemic colitis, although diverticulitis and inflammatory bowel disease may coexist. Vascular catastrophe, such as from aortic rupture or dissection or mesenteric ischemia, is generally distinguished by pain out of proportion to physical findings. In women, diverticulitis that presents as a left lower quadrant mass has been misdiagnosed as a gynecologic mass (8). High fever, leukocytosis, and left lower quadrant mass should suggest perforation and abscess. These findings may also be caused by inflammatory bowel disease, colon cancer, sigmoid volvulus, iatrogenic perforation of the rectosigmoid, or a tuboovarian abscess (7). Right-sided diverticulitis, a rare disease seen primarily in Asian populations, may mimic acute appendicitis (12).

EMERGENCY DEPARTMENT EVALUATION

Left Lower Quadrant Pain

Historical information should focus on GI symptoms, previous similar attacks, prior diagnostic studies, and change in bowel habits. The duration of the attack, characteristics of the pain, and history of fever should also be elicited. With diverticulitis, the pain may be intermittent, crampy, and associated with nausea and vomiting. The attack may be associated with either constipation or diarrhea.

The physical examination should take careful note of the patient's temperature, pulse rate, and blood pressure. Complete abdominal, pelvic, and rectal examinations are necessary. In rare cases, tenderness may be found only on rectal examination. Palpation may reveal the outline of the sigmoid colon as a rope-like mass. Minimal tenderness and mobility point to an irritable colon; a large, sausage-like, markedly tender, fixed mass points to diverticulitis. Signs of peritonitis and the presence of a mass on pelvic and rectal examinations are important to note. A complete blood cell count (CBC) may be helpful, in that leukocytosis with a left shift is often noted in patients with diverticulitis.

Although acute diverticulitis can be diagnosed solely on clinical grounds, confirmatory imaging is necessary for all but mild, recurrent cases. Abdominal and chest X-ray films may show obstruction or free air, but computed tomography (CT) is the most cost-effective test in the evaluation of diverticulitis (4). CT allows evaluation of vascular structures, estimates the extent of diverticulitis, allows possible percutaneous drainage, and is less invasive than traditional contrast enema evaluation (5) (Fig. 73.1). The method also has greater sensitivity than contrast enema (1). If CT is unavailable, contrast enema remains a safe and effective option (10,11). A few centers have reported high accuracy in diagnosing diverticulitis with ultrasonography (9–11). Ultrasonographic findings seen in diverticulitis include the following: hypoechoic, tender, thickened colonic segment; visible diverticula; and increased echogenicity surrounding the diseased colon (4). Sigmoidoscopy should be avoided in patients with acute diverticulitis.

Lower Gastrointestinal Bleeding

The history should focus on the onset, color, amount, and frequency of bloody bowel movements. A history of previous attacks, bleeding tendencies, and bowel habits is important. Hemodynamic instability should be assessed (blood pressure, pulse,

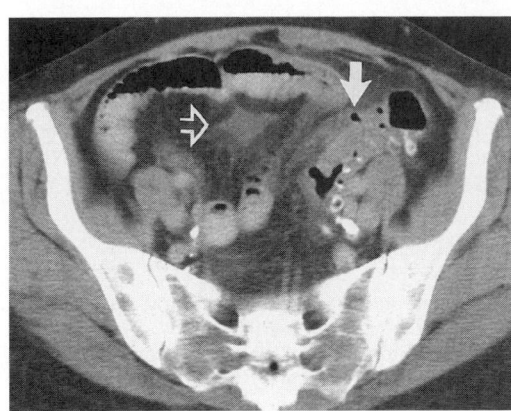

Figure 73.1.   Sigmoid diverticulitis. CT scan shows multiple sigmoid diverticula, inflammatory stranding (*arrow*), and a small amount of free fluid (*open arrow*). From Harris and Harris, eds. *The Radiology of Emergency Medicine*, 4th ed. New York: Lippincott, 2000:651.

and orthostatic changes). Orthostatic changes in systolic blood pressure and pulse may indicate hypovolemia; one study found these to have a specificity of 95% to 98% (13). The abdominal examination should focus on areas of tenderness and the presence or absence of a mass. The rectum should be palpated for masses, and the color of the blood in the rectal vault should be examined. Nasogastric intubation may indicate upper GI hemorrhage, particularly if the source is proximal to the duodenum. If there is brisk, bright red bleeding, anoscopy can exclude anorectal causes such as internal hemorrhoids. Laboratory studies should include a CBC to help estimate the amount of blood loss, and a type and screen if transfusion is considered.

EMERGENCY DEPARTMENT MANAGEMENT

Diverticulitis

For the patient in whom the diagnosis of severe diverticulitis is likely, an intravenous line should be started, blood and urine specimens should be collected, and intravenous antibiotics begun. For both complicated and uncomplicated diverticulitis, antibiotics should target gram-negative rods and anaerobic bacteria. Effective single agents include cefoxitin (1 to 2 g), imipenem/cilastatin (0.5 to 1 g), ampicillin/sulbactam (3 g), piperacillin/tazobactam (3.375 g), and an effective traditional triple-therapy regimen consists of ampicillin (0.5 g), gentamycin (1.5 mg/kg), and metronidazole (0.5 to 1 g) (3,4). Outpatient management for mild cases may include a combination of metronidazole and either trimethoprim–sulfamethoxazole or ciprofloxacin, or monotherapy with amoxicillin/clavulanate.

Diverticular Bleeding

For the patient with massive lower GI bleeding, two large-bore intravenous lines (16-gauge or larger) should be inserted. A blood specimen should be obtained and sent for type and crossmatch for 4 to 6 U of blood. A Foley catheter should be placed. Lactated Ringer solution or normal saline should then be infused at a rate determined according to the patient's vital signs and cardiac status. If the patient is not stabilized after 2 L of crystalloid infusion, blood transfusion should be considered. Fluid resuscitation should be aimed at restoring urine output to a rate of approximately 1 mL/kg/hour. Patients with only minor bleeding may require no specific treatment.

Painful Diverticular Disease

For the patient with left lower quadrant pain with no mass or signs of infection, institution of a high-fiber diet is effective in relieving pain. Anticholinergic agents have long been used, but their efficacy remains unproved. A followup flexible sigmoidoscopy should be done to rule out rectal cancer.

CRITICAL INTERVENTIONS

- Administer parenteral antibiotic therapy and analgesics for those with acute, severe diverticulitis
- Provide adequate fluid and blood component therapy for patients with significant lower GI bleeding

DISPOSITION

A surgical consultation should be requested for admitted patients in whom the diagnosis of acute diverticulitis is suspected and in patients with massive lower GI bleeding.

Indications for Admission

Patients with diverticulitis complicated by abscess or fistula formation, obstruction, or free perforation should be admitted to a surgical service. Patients suspected of having severe acute diverticulitis and those with gross lower GI bleeding must be admitted. Septic patients, those with severe concomitant diseases, and those with massive GI bleeding should be admitted to an intensive care unit.

Outpatient management should be limited to immunocompetent patients with mild uncomplicated diverticulitis, or diverticulosis with minimal bleeding. Immunocompromised patients with diverticulitis should be admitted, even those with benign-appearing presentations.

COMMON PITFALLS

✔ Although less frequently encountered in patients younger than age 40 years, diverticulosis is relatively more likely to be complicated and require surgery in younger patients than in older patients (2)
✔ The classic signs and symptoms of diverticulitis are often absent in immunocompromised patients. These patients have a higher incidence of free perforation, failure of medical therapy, and postoperative morbidity and mortality (8,10)

Acknowledgments

The author acknowledges the substantial contributions of Dr. C. Gene Cayton and Dr. Annie T. Sadosty to earlier versions of this chapter.

References

1. Ambrosetti P, Jenny A, Becker C, et al. Acute left colonic diverticulitis—compared performance of computed tomography and water-soluble contrast enema: prospective evaluation of 420 patients. *Dis. Colon Rectum* 2000;43:1363–1367.
2. Cunningham MA, Davis JW, Kaup KL. Medical versus surgical management of diverticulitis in patients under age 40. *Am J Surge* 1997;174:735–736.
3. Dickman RC, Checking LJ. Diverticular disease in the elderly. *J Am Geriatr Soc* 1993;40:986–993.
4. Ferzoco LB, Raptopoulos V, Silen W. Acute diverticulitis. *N Engl J Med* 1998;338:1521–1526.
5. Hulnick DH, Megibow AJ, Balthazar EJ, et al. Computed tomography in the evaluation of diverticulitis. *Radiology* 1984;152:491–495.
6. Meyers MD, Alonso DR, Gray GF, et al. Pathogenesis of bleeding colonic diverticulosis. *Gastroenterology* 1976;71:577–583.
7. Naliboff JA, Jongmire-Cook SJ. Diverticulitis mimicking a tuboovarian abscess. *J Reprod Med* 1996;41:921–923.
8. Perkins JK, Shield CF, Chang FC, et al. Acute diverticulitis. *Am J Surg* 1984;148:745–748.
9. Pradel JA, Adell J, Taourel P. Acute colonic diverticulitis: prospective comparative evaluation with US and CT. *Radiology* 1997;205:503–512.
10. Roberts P, Abel M, Rosen L, et al. Practice parameters for sigmoid diverticulitis—supporting documentation. *Dis Colon Rectum* 1995;38:125–132.
11. Vernava AM, Moore BA, Longo WE, et al. Lower gastrointestinal bleeding. *Dis Colon Rectum* 1997;40:846–858.
12. Wong SK, Ho YH, Leong AP, et al. Clinical behavior of complicated right-sided and left-sided diverticulosis. *Dis Colon Rectum* 1997;40:344–348.
13. Witting MD, Gallagher K. Unique cutpoints for sitting-to-standing orthostatic vital signs. *Am J Emerg Med* 2003;21:45–57.

CHAPTER 74

Perianal, Rectal, and Anal Diseases

Wendy C. Coates

A variety of anorectal conditions can prompt a visit to the emergency department. These conditions may be isolated and temporary or may signal an underlying systemic disease. Great sensitivity is required in dealing with patients who have problems in this area, as they may be embarrassed to share details with the health care provider.

The rectum originates at the end of the sigmoid colon and stores stool until a convenient time for defecation. The anal canal is the terminal portion of the digestive system and is approximately 4 cm in length. At the dentate line of the anal canal, the epithelium changes from the columnar epithelium of the intestine to a modified squamous epithelium. Several glands reside in this area to provide lubrication for the easy passage of stool. Fecal continence is maintained by a cooperation of both voluntary and involuntary muscle groups called sphincters.

CLINICAL PRESENTATION

A thorough history and physical examination are important in distinguishing common anorectal complaints (3) (Fig. 74.1). Local symptoms such as pain, bleeding, discharge, and itching are the foundation for the history. Questions about underlying gastrointestinal [GI] conditions (e.g., Crohn disease, inflammatory bowel disease, and GI cancer); systemic illnesses (e.g., diabetes mellitus, AIDS, and cancer); and trauma provide clues about the etiology of the symptoms. Some people use the rectum during intercourse and others introduce foreign objects that they cannot retrieve.

The physical examination should begin with an observation of hygiene, structural integrity, and the presence of lesions, blood, or discharge. A digital rectal examination (DRE)

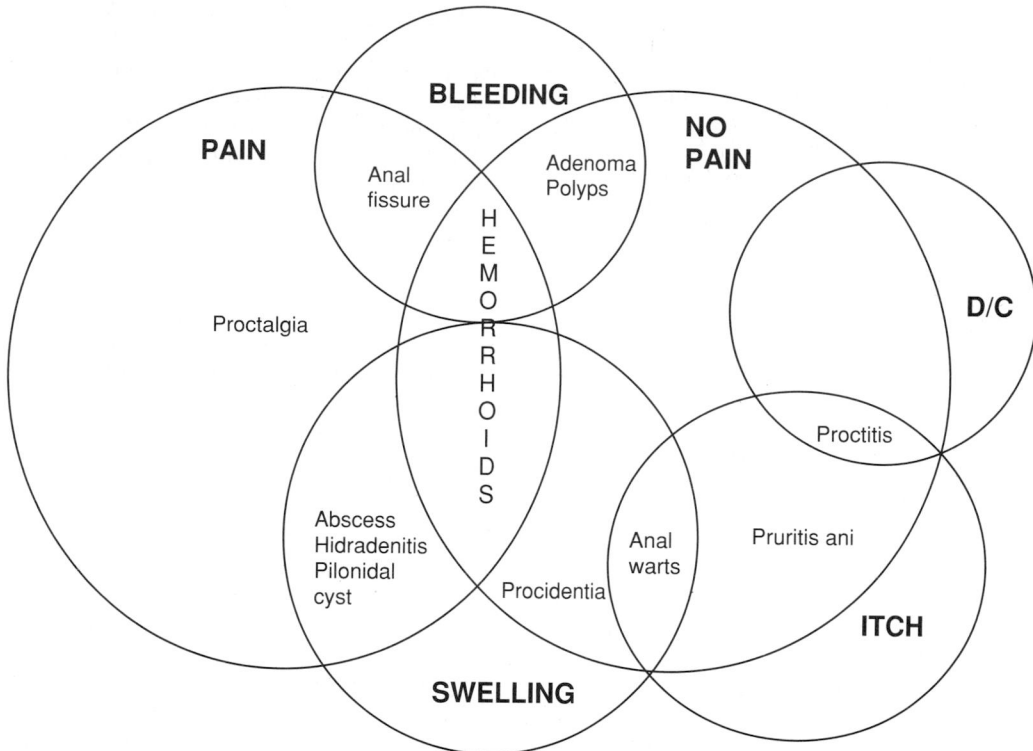

Figure 74.1.   Anorectal complaints algorithm. Venn diagram.

can be used to assess sphincter tone and can reveal masses in the anorectum or adjacent structures. Any stool remaining on the examiner's glove can be used to check for occult blood. Finally, anoscopy can be performed to identify lesions in the anal canal.

Painful Swelling

Anorectal abscess is a common acute infection involving the anorectum. The etiology may be the entrapment of mucous and bacteria in the glands of the anal crypts. When deep abscesses rupture, a fistulous tract may form. A complex network of abscesses and fistulas may evolve if the condition goes untreated. Abscesses are named according to their location (Fig. 74.2).

Symptoms and sequelae vary depending on the depth and natural ability of the abscess to drain. The clinical presentation depends on the depth and location of the abscess. Superficial

(*perianal*) abscesses usually present as tender swellings near the anus. People may presuppose that they have hemorrhoids and report this as their chief complaint. Foul smelling pus may drain from spontaneously rupturing abscesses. Deep abscesses may cause pain within the rectal cavity or pelvis and progress to a systemic infection. Fistulous tracts that open directly into the anorectum or through the skin of the buttocks may develop from abscesses near the rectum or the skin surface (5,12).

A *pilonidal abscess* (cyst) is a painful, indurated swelling that occurs in the presacral midline (6). Sinus tracts may develop and open into the surrounding skin of the buttocks. Many patients also demonstrate hair in the midline in other locations of their bodies, such as the eyebrows.

Hidradenitis suppurativa is caused by an infection to the apocrine glands and is related to poor hygiene or an underlying disease, such as diabetes mellitus. Patients frequently have fever and leukocytosis and may have similar lesions in the axilla or sternum (16).

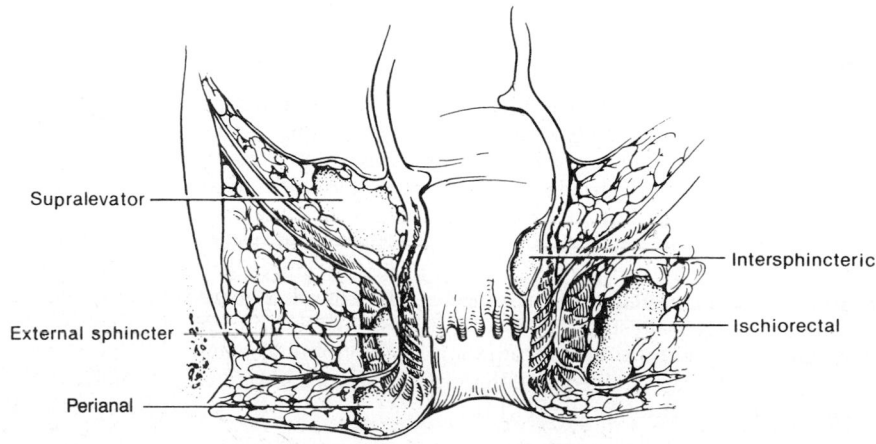

Figure 74.2.   Anorectal abscesses.

Painful Bleeding

Anal fissures produce sudden, sharp, tearing pain at the anal orifice during defecation. The patient generally reports seeing bright red blood on the tissue. It is the most common pediatric anorectal complaint. *Hemorrhoids* can present in a variety of ways, but the classic presentation is painful bright red blood that coats the stool. A variety of factors predispose patients to develop hemorrhoids. Most often, the condition is self-limited and is caused by frequent diarrhea, prolonged sitting, low fiber diet, pregnancy, and may be exacerbated by underlying medical conditions such as obesity, portal hypertension, or bleeding disorders. Patients may complain of anorectal swelling with moist discharge, or intense, unbearable pain and swelling 1,5,15).

Pain without Bleeding or Swelling

Some patients have rectal pain that does not have any of the pathophysiologic mechanisms described. Their pain may be of sudden or gradual onset and takes on different characteristics depending on the cause. Before making a diagnosis of the two common entities, *levator syndrome* or *proctalgia fugax*, it is important to exclude other causes of pain.

Painless Conditions

Patients with *rectal prolapse (procidentia)* present with a large externally protruding mass. The presentation may be preceded by defecation, sneezing, or coughing. Most patients are in the extremes of age. A foul odor may be present (2,8).

Anal warts (condylomata acuminata) may also present as a painless swelling at the anal opening. Patients generally report concurrent itching and often have had contact with another individual with a similar condition. Genital warts are caused by the human papilloma virus (HPV). A sexual history highlighting the role of the anus in intercourse is essential. Children with genital warts may have contracted them as a result of sexual assault or simply by the transmission of the virus on the hands of the person changing their diaper (17). Other causes of perianal itching (*pruritus ani*) range from dietary habits (caffeine, citrus, and spicy foods) or drugs (steroids, tetracycline, and colchicine) to hygiene and underlying skin conditions (pinworms and psoriasis). Patients frequently complain of an insurmountable urge to scratch, and the symptoms typically are worse in the warm months. Underlying anorectal disease (fistula, fissures, proctitis, and prolapsed hemorrhoids) may present as pruritus ani.

Foreign Bodies

People who have inserted foreign objects into their rectums for sexual purposes occasionally find that the object cannot be retrieved easily. When they present to the emergency department, it is likely that they have tried every maneuver at their disposal to remove the object, but have not been successful. They may be reluctant to share the details of their condition with triage personnel, and may be inventive about the circumstances surrounding the introduction of the object. Chief complaints are varied, but range from straightforward admission of the foreign body in their rectum to vague complaints of abdominal pain. In those who have sustained an enteric perforation, symptoms typical to this condition prevail (4,14).

DIFFERENTIAL DIAGNOSIS

Painful swellings of the anorectum include hemorrhoids, abscesses, pilonidal disease, and hidradenitis suppurativa (Fig. 74.1). The presence of pus or fever suggests an abscess. For many patients with abscesses and fistulas, their problem is recurrent. A specialized abscess that is lined with epithelium and is found in the presacral area is a pilonidal cyst. This condition occurs more frequently in young men and reflects a midline defect in which debris from hair follicles and glandular secretions collects and becomes indurated.

Patients who present with painful bleeding are likely to have hemorrhoids or an anal fissure. Fissures tend to present as sudden, sharp, and tearing pain with subsequent burning, whereas hemorrhoids generally have a more gradual onset and a more varied course. Hemorrhoids can mimic any anorectal condition. A thorough history and physical examination can confirm an ultimate diagnosis of hemorrhoids.

Rectal pain that occurs from a cause other than those already mentioned may be of neuromuscular etiology. Levator ani syndrome is distinguished by its gradual onset and persistence as a dull pain that is exacerbated by defecation. Patients with sudden, intense spasmodic pain in the rectal area may have proctalgia fugax. This condition is frequently associated with the "type A" personality, but may occur in any patient. Its onset is often during intercourse, urination, defecation, or sleep (3,19).

Patients who present with rectal bleeding that is unaccompanied by pain may have internal or external hemorrhoids that are neither thrombosed nor lodged in the sphincter to produce pain. These patients typically have bright red blood that coats the stool. Patients with bright red blood mixed in with the stool should be evaluated for brisk upper or lower GI bleeding (see Chapter 60, "Lower Gastrointestinal Bleeding"). Patients whose source of bleeding is of uncertain etiology should be evaluated for rectal cancer or polyps.

Procidentia may be complete (all layers of the rectum protrude) or incomplete (mucosal layer only). In young children, the diagnosis of cystic fibrosis is suspected. It is important to distinguish this from prolapsed internal hemorrhoids and rectal masses (2).

Patients with pruritus ani should be examined closely and questioned about potential sources of their condition. Those with condylomata acuminata may falsely complain of a "hemorrhoid." Other diseases to consider in the differential diagnosis of condylomata acuminata are squamous cell carcinoma or secondary syphilis (condyloma latum), which is flatter.

Foreign bodies should be sought when a patient admits this or if one's presence is suspected. Patients whose clinical presentation is suggestive of bowel perforation may have a foreign body. The presence of a foreign body may produce bleeding or a discharge depending on the characteristics of the object and the duration of its presence (14).

EMERGENCY DEPARTMENT EVALUATION

Abscesses are defined by their location. *Perianal abscesses* are adjacent to the anal outlet and are superficial in nature. Most patients are afebrile. Visual inspection of perianal area may reveal pus or a fluctuant mass with or without surrounding erythema. *Ischiorectal abscesses* are exterior to the sphincter muscles and form in the buttocks. Patients frequently cite severe buttock pain. Deeper ischiorectal abscesses may cause fever and leukocytosis. *Intersphincteric abscesses* form above the external sphincter and below the levator ani muscles. They may appear as a protrusion into the rectum and may be confused with inflamed hemorrhoids upon anoscopy. *Supralevator abscesses* are uncommon and are located deep to the levator ani muscles. There is an increased predominance in patients who are immunocompromised and in those with associated conditions (e.g., Crohn disease, pelvic inflammatory disease, or diverticulitis). Diagnosis relies on a high index of suspicion in patients with pelvic pain, fever and leukocytosis. DRE may reveal a fistulous outflow track in the anal canal that may be palpable (5,12).

Patients with a painful swelling in the presacral area that has associated openings from sinus tracts have pilonidal disease. They are usually fluctuant and tender and may spontaneously begin to drain hairy pus. Extension of the disease to the entire presacrum is common (6). Multiple infected openings that are not limited to the presacral area may indicate hidradenitis suppurativa. Local lymphadenopathy is a common finding, and many patients are febrile and have an elevated white blood cell count (16).

Anal fissures are suspected when there is a sudden pain near the anus and bright red blood on the tissue. Most benign fissures are located in the anoderm at the posterior midline. Although women may have fissures in the anterior midline, fissures in other locations often herald a serious underlying disease (e.g., Crohn, leukemia, tuberculosis, or human immunodeficiency virus [HIV]). The acute appearance of the fissure is similar to that of a laceration of the anoderm. Chronic changes may occur if a fissure is left untreated and include the development of tissue edema, a sentinel pile (hypertrophic and edematous skin), and skin tags upon resolution (10).

Hemorrhoids may be classified as external or internal. External hemorrhoids are close to the anal orifice and are covered with the same anoderm epithelium. Careful inspection reveals a coloring of the epithelium that is similar to that of surrounding tissue. Patients may have perianal skin tags that have resulted from prior episodes of external hemorrhoids. A hard, bluish mass in the location of an external hemorrhoid denotes a thrombosed external hemorrhoid (1,13).

Internal hemorrhoids originate superior to the dentate line and are supplied by the superior hemorrhoidal vessels. Their covering appears mucosal in nature and does not resemble skin at all. A classification system of four grades has been developed. Grade I internal hemorrhoids produce symptoms of fullness and pain with bleeding, but do not exit the anus at any time. Grade II internal hemorrhoids prolapse during defecation but spontaneously retract when straining is stopped. Grade III internal hemorrhoids prolapse during defecation and require manual replacement. Grade IV internal hemorrhoids prolapse at any time, cannot be reduced, and may thrombose or become gangrenous (1,13).

To delineate the cause of rectal pain that does not fit into one of the categories described previously, one must first rule out a serious underlying condition, including cauda equina syndrome, cancer, or endometriosis. The diagnosis of proctalgia fugax or levator ani syndrome is typically based on historical findings. If the patient tolerates a rectal examination, the levator ani muscles may be tender to palpation in levator ani syndrome (19).

Evaluation of patients with painless rectal bleeding includes DRE with subsequent hemoccult testing and anoscopy to view hemorrhoids or potential erosions in the mucosal wall. Procidentia may be identified by noting concentric rings of mucosal tissue that is ulcerated and is associated with a mucoid discharge or is covered with stool. If all layers are involved in the prolapse, they can be identified as well (9).

Anal warts appear as papilliform lesions that often coalesce at the anus and may extend to the anal canal. Direct irritation to the warts may induce minimal bleeding. A detailed sexual history

may reveal that the patient is HIV-positive or has concurrent STDs. Evaluation of pruritus ani begins with a detailed history and physical examination.

Evaluation for foreign bodies begins with a thorough history and physical examination. Objects found in the rectum range from household objects and food products to small animals. It is possible to feel an anal canal foreign body, but it is unlikely that a rectal foreign body will be palpable on DRE. Abdominal examination may reveal a mass or abnormal bowel sounds. Abdominal radiographs or ultrasound may demonstrate the foreign body and highlight the extent of injury. Ileus or perforation may be seen on plain radiographs.

EMERGENCY DEPARTMENT MANAGEMENT

General treatment of most anorectal conditions focuses on maintaining good hygiene and producing stool that is easy to pass. This can be accomplished by following the WASH regimen (Fig. 74.3).

Perianal abscesses can usually be incised and drained in the ED with good local anesthesia. Exceptions include abscesses in children and in patients who are immunocompromised (11). Superficial ischiorectal abscesses may be incised and drained via a skin incision on the buttocks. However, deeper abscesses generally require drainage in the operating room (OR) under anesthesia. Once the pus is evacuated, antibiotics are unnecessary unless there is surrounding cellulitis or fever. Drainage of intersphincteric and supralevator abscesses must take place in the OR. Antibiotics are helpful when fever and leukocytosis are present. If a fistula is palpated in the anorectum or along the surface of the buttocks, it should be left intact to prevent the inadvertent puncture and subsequent extension of the fistulous network. Definitive treatment is a fistulectomy in the OR, although fibrin glue has been tried successfully as a less-invasive management strategy (10,18). Patients with a fistula without evidence of an abscess may have Crohn disease, cancer, or tuberculosis. These patients should be referred appropriately when a fistula is detected.

The ED treatment of an isolated pilonidal cyst begins with its identification in the presacrum. Incision and drainage should be done lateral to the midline to prevent further scarring and worsening of the disease. Antibiotics may be used as an adjunct to incision and drainage in patients who have accompanying cellulitis. Patients with extensive spread of pilonidal disease may be referred to surgery for wide excision (6).

Treatment of hidradenitis suppurativa begins with attention to improved hygiene. Incision and drainage of pustules may provide symptomatic relief, but a broad-spectrum antibiotic may be necessary to diminish the severity of the exacerbation of this condition (16).

Anal fissures should be treated acutely by following the WASH regimen so that the stool is easier to pass. Application of topical nitroglycerin ointment (0.4%) twice daily may alleviate symptoms. Topical nifedipine gel (0.2%) with lidocaine (1.5%) alleviates symptoms and may promote healing. Finally, the

W	Warm water	Promotes anal sphincter relaxation and good hygiene
A	Analgesics	Provides symptomatic relief from pain
S	Stool softener	Makes stool easier to traverse anal opening
H	High fiber diet	Produces stool with bulk and air and reduces transit time

Figure 74.3. The WASH regimen.

injection of botulinum toxin (2.5 to 5.0 million units) into the muscular anal sphincter produces rapid relief from the fissure, but may cause temporary fecal incontinence (10). ED management of external hemorrhoids is to follow the WASH regimen. Topical creams available over the counter may provide symptomatic relief, but do not alter the course of the disease. Prolonged use of local anesthetic or steroid creams can lead to local skin irritation and breakdown. Thrombosed external hemorrhoids may be excised in the ED by anesthetizing the skin and completely excising the clot and its overlying tissue. The use of excision rather than incision and drainage prevents the formation of perianal skin tags. It is critical to distinguish between external and internal thrombosed hemorrhoids before attempting an excision (7).

Internal hemorrhoids should be managed with the WASH regimen. Warm water may produce enough anal dilatation to reduce prolapsed internal hemorrhoids. Pain medications can be administered, but care should be taken to prevent constipation. Thrombosed fourth-degree internal hemorrhoids should not be managed in the ED. If they progress to a gangrenous state, the patient should be referred for immediate surgical repair (13,15). If a benign source of rectal bleeding (e.g., internal hemorrhoid) cannot be identified, the patient should be referred to a specialist for endoscopic evaluation of the rectum and colon (3).

Treatment of levator ani syndrome focuses on the relaxation of the involved muscles using benzodiazepines, topical nitrates, or warm water baths (19). In addition to these regimens, patients who have proctalgia fugax have reported relief when applying upward pressure with their fist against the anus.

Procidentia can be managed in the ED or the OR by attempting reduction. Gauze moistened with saline can be applied to the protruding rectum, which can be reinserted through the anal verge. In most cases, sedation is required. If the reduction is successful, conservative management using the WASH regimen may prevent recurrence, especially in children (2). However, it is likely that a more permanent cure is surgical to strengthen the muscles that enabled the rectum to prolapse through the anus (8,9).

Once anal warts have been diagnosed, the cause should be identified. A full sexual history should be taken and the patient should be referred for HIV testing. Children should be referred for testing for sexual abuse if there is not a credible source for inadvertent transmission of the virus during routine care. Treatment can be done as an outpatient with 0.5% podofilox gel for isolated condylomas. Diffuse disease requires frequent visits to the physician for application of podophyllin resin, excision, or other removal techniques (17).

Treatment of pruritus ani is directed at the cause. It may include advice on how to maintain proper hygiene or alter the diet to reduce intake of the offending food or beverage. If an anorectal problem is the cause, treating the underlying condition is likely to improve the symptoms. Medical conditions, both dermatologic and systemic, should be treated appropriately.

Evaluation of foreign bodies for possible ED extraction should focus on the potential hazards that may be encountered upon removal. For example, glass or metal objects with sharp edges can cause bowel injury and necessitate surgical intervention. Large objects may be difficult to remove without general anesthesia. Deep sedation in the ED may facilitate removal of some items. Several maneuvers can be attempted with a cooperative patient who has received enough sedation in the ED. For example, large forceps may be inserted and affixed to the edge of an object that can be guided through the anus with the patient performing the Valsalva maneuver. Insertion of a Foley catheter past the retained foreign body with subsequent inflation of the balloon can sometimes be effective. Following the removal, a full evaluation of the patient's anorectum should take place. This should include visual inspection, a DRE to assess sphincter integrity, and

anoscopy. Postremoval radiographs may indicate injury to the bowel wall (4,14).

CRITICAL INTERVENTIONS

- Initiate antibiotics and surgical consultation for patients with a suspected deep abscess and systemic signs of infection
- Stabilize patients with acute blood loss of anorectal origin
- Search for signs of complications (hemorrhage and perforation) in patients with rectal foreign bodies

DISPOSITION

Most patients with limited anorectal complaints can be discharged safely from the ED and told to follow the WASH regimen (Fig. 74.3). For abscesses that cannot be drained easily in the ED, operative management is indicated. Those who display signs of systemic infection, such as fever and leukocytosis, should receive prompt surgical intervention. Several surgical options are available for repair of hemorrhoids, and an appropriate referral should be made. Immediate referral for emergency hemorrhoidectomy should be made for gangrenous fourth-degree internal hemorrhoids. For patients whose genital warts are widespread, referral for repetitive topical treatment or surgical management can be made. Patients with rectal foreign bodies can be discharged if the removal was routine and uncomplicated. Many require admission for surgical intervention.

COMMON PITFALLS

✔ Do not assume that a patient complaining of "hemorrhoids" actually has them–consider underlying disease with an anorectal component that may be described as hemorrhoids by the patient
✔ Mistaking a thrombosed internal hemorrhoid for an external one and excising it
✔ Do not probe anorectal fistulas in the ED
✔ Do not attempt the removal of broken glass foreign bodies in the ED. If foreign body removal is contemplated, adequate sedation is necessary

Acknowledgment

The author would like to thank Nancy C. Schneider for her assistance in graphic design and preparation of this chapter.

References

1. Alonso-Coello P, Castillejo MM. Office evaluation and treatment of hemorrhoids. *J Fam Pract* 2003;52:366–374.
2. Corman ML. Rectal prolapse in children. *Dis Colon Rectum* 1985;28:535–539.
3. Gopal DV. Diseases of the rectum and anus: a clinical approach to common disorders. *Clin Cornerstone* 2002;4:34–48.
4. Hellinger MD. Anal trauma and foreign bodies. *Surg Clin North Am* 2002; 82:1253–1260.
5. Helton WS. 2001 Consensus Statement on Benign Anorectal Disease 1. *J Gastrointest Surg* 2002;6:302–303.
6. Hull TL, Wu J. Pilonidal disease. *Surg Clin North Am* 2002;82:1169–1185.
7. Jongen J, et al. Excision of thrombosed external hemorrhoid under local anesthesia: a retrospective evaluation of 340 patients. *Dis Colon Rectum* 2003; 46:1226–1231.
8. Karulf RE, Madoff RD, Goldberg SM. Rectal prolapse. *Curr Probl Surg* 2001; 38:771–832.
9. Madbouly KM, et al. Clinically based management of rectal prolapse. *Surg Endosc* 2003;17:99–103.
10. Maria G, Brisinda G. Chronic anal fissure: advances and insights in pathophysiology and treatment. *Gastroenterology* 2003;125:995–996.
11. Murthi GV, et al. Perianal abscess in childhood. *Pediatr Surg Int* 2002;18:689–691.

12. Nelson R. Anorectal abscess fistula: what do we know? *Surg Clin North Am* 2002;86:1139–1151, v–vi.
13. Nisar PJ, Scholefield JH. Managing haemorrhoids. *BMJ* 2003;327:847–851.
14. Ooi BS, et al. Management of anorectal foreign bodies: a cause of obscure anal pain. *Aust NZ J Surg* 1998;68:852–855.
15. Sardinha TC, Corman ML. Hemorrhoids. *Surg Clin North Am* 2002;82:vi,1153–1167.
16. Slade DEM, Powell BW, Mortimer PS. Hidradenitis suppurativa: pathogenesis and management. *Br J Plast Surg* 2003;56:451–461.
17. Trombetta LJ, Place RJ. Giant condyloma acuminatum of the anorectum: trends in epidemiology and management: report of a case and review of the literature. *Dis Colon Rectum* 2001;44:1878–1886.
18. Venkatesh KS, Ramanujam P. Fibrin glue application in the treatment of recurrent anorectal fistulas. *Dis Colon Rectum* 1999;42:1136–1139.
19. Wald A. Functional anorectal and pelvic pain. *Gastroenterol Clin North Am* 2001;30:243–251, viii–ix.

CHAPTER 75
Gastrointestinal Foreign Bodies

Valerie C. Norton

Gastrointestinal (GI) foreign bodies present a diverse set of challenges to the emergency physician. Presentations range from the obvious to the occult, from the mundane to the bizarre, and from the benign to the life-threatening. Management options are accordingly diverse as well, ranging from watchful waiting to emergent endoscopy or surgery.

Physicians must be familiar with the signs and symptoms of ingested foreign bodies, especially in small children or psychiatric patients who have no obvious history of ingestion. They must have a good understanding of various removal techniques for foreign bodies in the esophagus or rectum. They must also know which situations require emergent intervention and whom to consult when intervention is necessary.

Children account for about 80% of cases of ingested foreign bodies (see Chapter 246, "Foreign Bodies"), and tend to ingest coins, toys, and other small objects left within their reach. Adult patients at highest risk include psychiatric patients, prisoners, those with impaired mental status or intoxication, those with underlying esophageal abnormalities such as strictures, and denture wearers, who have reduced sensation of the palate (4). Adults most commonly have trouble with boluses of meat and animal bones, although psychiatric patients and prisoners may intentionally ingest unusual objects such as razor blades or open safety pins.

Ingested foreign bodies frequently become lodged in the esophagus, often requiring urgent removal. Much more rarely, objects fail to pass the pylorus or the ileocecal valve. More than 80% of ingested foreign bodies that pass into the stomach will traverse the rest of the gut uneventfully (19). Objects that are less likely to pass spontaneously are those longer than 6 cm, sharp objects such as pins and toothpicks, and blunt objects greater than 2.5 cm wide, though many of these will still pass without sequelae (4,11).

Of primary concern are objects lodged in the esophagus, since these are at highest risk for complications such as mu-

cosal erosions, perforation, or airway compromise. Objects typically lodge at the level of the cricopharyngeus muscle, the level of the aortic arch, or the lower esophageal sphincter. High esophageal impactions are most common in children; adults most often have obstructions at the lower esophageal sphincter (19). Food boluses, particularly meat, are the most common cause of esophageal impaction in adults, and often result from underlying esophageal pathology (4). Foreign bodies with toxic contents, such as button batteries and packages of cocaine, represent special cases (discussed in Chapter 324, "Cocaine,"). A button battery lodged in the esophagus is a true emergency requiring immediate endoscopic removal.

Rectal foreign bodies are usually the result of sexual misadventure or assault, although occasionally a patient will present with an ingested foreign body, such as an animal bone, that passes through the entire gut only to become lodged in the rectum (2,21). Men are at least 28 times more likely than women to present with rectal foreign bodies (19). Objects inserted into the rectum include vibrators, vegetables, broomsticks, drugs or other contraband, and even live animals such as gerbils. Many objects are not visible on X-rays, although most are low-lying and palpable on rectal examination. Mucosal lacerations and rectal perforations are fairly common, especially in assault victims, and may result in life-threatening sepsis.

CLINICAL PRESENTATION

Healthy adults with ingested foreign bodies often give a clear history of the inciting incident and may report a foreign body sensation if the object is lodged in the upper esophagus where somatic nerve endings are present. If a meat bolus or other object is impacted in the lower esophagus, they usually complain of more visceral-type chest pain, odynophagia, and difficulty handling secretions. Objects that have passed into the stomach or beyond frequently cause no symptoms, unless obstruction or perforation has ensued.

Small children and adults with impaired mentation may not give a clear history of foreign body ingestion. Clinicians may have to rely on symptoms of obstruction, such as drooling if the object is in the esophagus, or vomiting and distention if it is impacted below the stomach. Patients may also present with GI bleeding or signs and symptoms of peritonitis owing to perforation. Small children often display indirect symptoms such as gagging and choking, refusal to eat, irritability, or respiratory distress if the object is compressing the trachea or causing aspiration of saliva. The possibility of foreign body ingestion should always be considered in small children with new-onset wheezing, especially if it does not respond to bronchodilators (1).

Patients with rectal foreign bodies usually state clearly that something is in the rectum, although they may be very vague as to how it got there. These patients or their partners have often made multiple attempts to remove the object (19). Occasional patients may be unaware of the object if intoxicated at the time of insertion, or may be too embarrassed to admit to it, complaining instead of rectal pain or bleeding. Patients with extraperitoneal rectal perforation may present with sepsis, whereas those with intraperitoneal perforation present with peritonitis.

DIFFERENTIAL DIAGNOSIS

In the absence of a history of ingestion or insertion of a foreign body, the differential diagnosis is difficult. It should include all processes that can obstruct, irritate, erode, or perforate the GI tract. Other organ systems may initially be the focus of concern, since esophageal pain can mimic cardiac angina, and children with esophageal obstruction may present with stridor or other respiratory symptoms that may be mistaken for croup, asthma, or allergic reaction.

Subacute and chronic presentations do not rule out foreign bodies. A wealth of literature has reported objects dwelling in the stomach or intestines for years before causing symptoms. Esophageal foreign bodies have been impacted for a month or more in some children without serious sequelae (6,9). Clinicians should also be aware that even when there is a clearcut history of foreign body ingestion or insertion, other unsuspected pathology may be present, such as a second foreign body, a mucosal laceration, or underlying esophageal disease (1,2).

EMERGENCY DEPARTMENT EVALUATION

Initial assessment should aim at immediate detection and treatment of those with frank airway compromise, sepsis, or perforation. In more stable patients, the physical examination may find signs of esophageal obstruction such as drooling or gagging, signs of lower intestinal obstruction, or evidence of GI bleeding. In the majority of patients with upper GI foreign bodies, the physical examination will be unrevealing. By contrast, rectal foreign bodies are usually palpable on rectal examination. Some authors advise against a digital rectal examination prior to obtaining radiographs, since the examiners may injure themselves if an unexpectedly sharp object is present (19).

Imaging studies are often helpful, although a negative study does not rule out a radiolucent foreign body. For suspected esophageal foreign bodies, both anteroposterior and lateral radiographs of the neck and chest are recommended in order to avoid missing a second foreign body located behind the first or lower in the esophagus (4,8,19,20). Both views also help to rule out a tracheobronchial foreign body. Flat objects in the esophagus, such as coins, typically appear "en face" on anteroposterior views and "on end" on lateral views, since the easily compressible esophagus typically lies somewhat flattened between the trachea and the spine. Tracheal coins, by contrast, typically appear "on end" on anteroposterior views, since the more rigid tracheal rings have their widest diameter in the sagittal plane (19). Radiographic evidence of esophageal edema on a lateral view indicates a prolonged impaction and the need for urgent endoscopic evaluation (1,6,8,17).

Occasionally a contrast study of the esophagus is contemplated when a radiolucent foreign body is suspected, such as in a child with refractory drooling, dysphagia, or wheezing, and negative plain films (1). However, several authors have suggested that in symptomatic cases with high clinical suspicion, the patient should go straight to endoscopy, as barium can obscure endoscopic visualization of the object and carries the risk of aspiration (4,14).

Some investigators have advocated the use of a hand-held metal detector in lieu of plain films to evaluate the presence and location of metal foreign bodies (3,15,16,18). However, studies published to date indicate that hand-held metal detectors are not as sensitive as radiographs. Small objects with low metallic mass can be missed, and even coins are occasionally missed or incorrectly localized. More importantly, it appears that metal detectors cannot reliably make the crucial distinction between the lower esophagus and the stomach when localizing an object (3,15,16,18).

One advantage of a metal detector as a supplement to plain films is that it can identify aluminum foreign bodies, such as soda can pull tabs, which can be radiolucent on plain films (3). However, the routine use of metal detectors in place of radiographs is ill-advised, since failure to detect an esophageal foreign body can have serious consequences. One exception to this may be in the case of prisoners or psychiatric patients who falsely claim to have ingested large objects such as spoons, since a negative metal detector scan in these patients would reliably prove the absence of a foreign body, thereby eliminating the need for radiographs. This potential application has not yet been adequately studied.

Objects below the esophagus may be evaluated with standard plain films or contrast radiography if necessary. In most cases the primary reasons to obtain radiographs are to determine whether an ingested object has passed beyond the esophagus, and whether the object has any physical characteristics that will make passage or extraction more difficult, such as a sharp edge.

EMERGENCY DEPARTMENT MANAGEMENT

Patients with signs of airway compromise require definitive airway management and emergent endoscopic consultation to remove the foreign body. Those with signs of hollow viscus perforation, massive bleeding, or sepsis require immediate resuscitation, intravenous antibiotics, and emergent surgical consultation.

The management of stable patients depends on the type, location, and duration of impaction of the foreign body. Management guidelines are summarized in Figure 75.1. In the esophagus, sharp objects and button batteries mandate immediate endoscopic removal. Patients with respiratory symptoms or high-grade obstruction with inability to swallow secretions also require emergent endoscopy.

All other blunt esophageal foreign bodies can be divided into objects in the mid-to-upper esophagus and objects at the lower esophageal sphincter. Objects in the upper half of the esophagus are unlikely to pass spontaneously, thereby mandating intervention. The standard of care at most large institutions is prompt

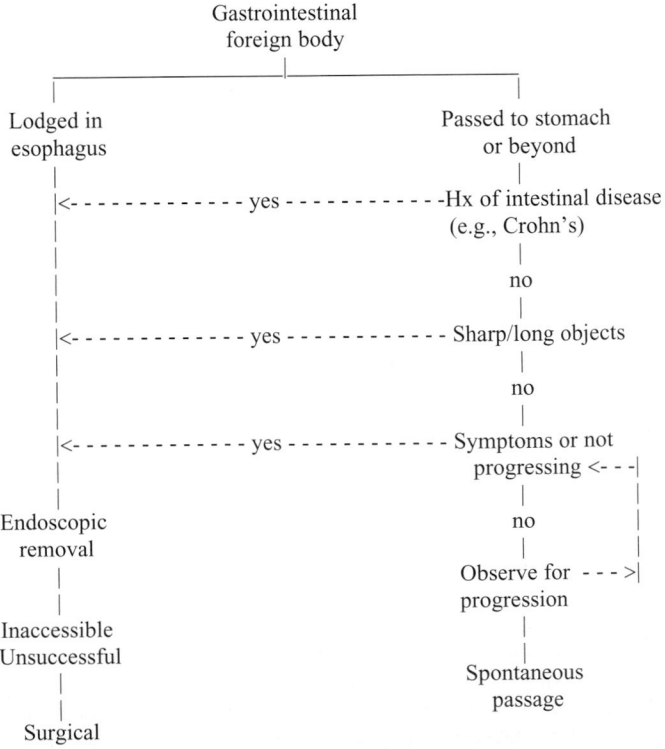

Figure 75.1.   Guidelines for the management of stable patients with no signs of airway compromise.

endoscopic removal (4,14,19,20). If the patient has a full stomach or if endoscopy is not readily available, it may be postponed briefly as long as the patient is able to handle secretions. Most experts recommend removal within 12 to 24 hours (4,20).

Objects lodged at the lower esophageal sphincter are often managed with a trial of watchful waiting with or without measures to relax the sphincter, since many of these objects will pass spontaneously. Glucagon may be given to help relax the lower esophageal sphincter: glucagon 1–2 mg i.v. However, its use is controversial and may cause vomiting (19). This dose may be repeated once in 20 to 30 minutes if unsuccessful. If passage has not resulted in 12 to 24 hours, most authors recommend endoscopic removal (4,20).

The management of impacted esophageal food boluses generally follows the guidelines described previously. Most authors recommend prompt endoscopic removal of boluses causing high-grade obstruction or of those that are seen radiographically to contain sharp bones, since these are more likely to cause esophageal perforation. Other boluses may be managed by watchful waiting with or without glucagon, with removal in less than 24 hours if passage does not occur (4). The use of gas-producing liquids such as carbonated beverages to aid in break-up and passage of the bolus has been reported (7) but remains controversial. Proteolytic enzymes (such as meat tenderizers) are contraindicated, as they can cause severe damage to the esophageal mucosa.

Although endoscopic removal of esophageal foreign bodies is standard at many institutions, the choice of technique is controversial in some areas given concerns about cost. A number of authors have advocated the alternative, less costly techniques of fluoroscopic Foley catheter extraction and esophageal bougienage (advancement of the foreign body with an esophageal dilator) (5,6,9,17). In experienced hands and in selected patients, these techniques have success and complication rates comparable to endoscopy. However, in patients with a history of prolonged impaction or a sharp-edged foreign body, the object may become embedded in the esophageal mucosa and be very difficult to remove (1). These alternative techniques should, therefore, be limited to patients with a blunt foreign body (usually a coin), impaction of less than 24 hours duration, no history of esophageal disease, no radiographic evidence of esophageal edema, and no signs of respiratory distress or airway compromise (5,6,8,9,17). Advanced airway management should be immediately available at all times. The procedure should be terminated if resistance is met or multiple attempts are needed, as serious complications have occurred in these settings (17).

Cost has become less of an issue, as flexible endoscopy under conscious sedation in the emergency department (ED) has increasingly replaced rigid endoscopy under general anesthesia in the operating room, thereby resulting in lower charges and shorter recovery times. In many institutions flexible endoscopy is now comparable to catheter extraction or bougienage in terms of cost and convenience.

Objects in the stomach and small intestine are much less problematic than those in the esophagus, since most will pass spontaneously. The exceptions are sharp objects, which may cause perforation in up to 35% of patients; they should be removed endoscopically if still in the stomach or duodenum (4,13,14,19). Some authors also recommend endoscopic removal of objects more than 6 cm long or 2.5 cm wide that are found in the stomach or duodenum (4), although one study of adults found that gastric foreign bodies as long as 13 cm passed into the stool without problem (11). Two special cases that usually require urgent laparotomy are magnetic jewelry beads, which can trap bowel wall between them with resultant erosion and perforation (12), and metal "crosses" ingested by prisoners (13). "Crosses" are made from two thin pieces of metal, such as pieces of paper clip,

which are formed into a cross with a rubber band, then twisted into parallel and wrapped in paper to permit swallowing. Once the paper degrades in the stomach, the cross opens up and nearly always causes perforation.

Small, blunt objects that pass into the stomach can be followed clinically, with repeat X-rays in 3 to 4 weeks if passage in the stool is not noted. A high-fiber diet may aid passage of the foreign body. Blunt objects should be given 3 to 6 weeks to pass out of the stomach before resorting to endoscopic removal (4,20). Objects may be given 2 to 3 weeks to traverse the rest of the gut. The development of symptoms or the failure of the object to progress mandates surgical consultation.

Rectal foreign bodies frequently require surgical consultation to bring about removal, although various authors report being able to remove 20% to 60% of objects in the ED (2,21). Removal in the ED is dependent on the ability to achieve adequate relaxation of the anal sphincter and the ability to locate and retrieve the foreign body. Many patients with long histories of rectal stimulation will have lax anal tone and may require only lidocaine gel with or without conscious sedation to relax the sphincter. Other patients may require infiltrative local anesthesia, and some may only achieve adequate relaxation with spinal or general anesthesia in the operating room.

Soft, low-lying objects with an edge can often be grasped and removed manually or with forceps. Some objects create suction on the rectal mucosa with downward traction; this can be overcome by passing a Foley catheter beyond the object and insufflating air into the rectum (10,19). Sigmoidoscopy after removal is mandatory to look for complications such as abscesses or mucosal lacerations, as these are very common (2,19,21). Hard, smooth-edged, or high-lying objects usually cannot be removed manually and require surgical consultation for removal by flexible sigmoidoscopy in the operating room or endoscopy suite (21). Laparotomy is a last resort for foreign bodies in which sigmoidoscopy is unsuccessful.

CRITICAL INTERVENTIONS

- Immediate airway management and endoscopic intervention in patients with respiratory compromise resulting from an esophageal foreign body
- Immediate stabilization, antibiotics, and surgical consultation in patients with sepsis, massive GI bleeding, or perforation caused by a foreign body anywhere in the GI tract
- Emergent endoscopic removal of all sharp objects, button batteries, and objects causing high-grade obstruction in the esophagus
- Prompt surgical consultation for rectal foreign bodies that are not amenable to removal in the ED

DISPOSITION

Asymptomatic patients with uncomplicated, blunt foreign bodies in the stomach or small intestine can be discharged from the ED with observation of the stools or radiographic followup at appropriate intervals to ensure progress of the object through the gut. All other patients require consultation with an endoscopist or a surgeon, depending on the type and location of the foreign body and the presence of any complications. Following the uncomplicated removal of a foreign body in the ED, asymptomatic patients who have fully recovered from any sedation can be sent home with close followup by their primary care provider or an appropriate consultant. Patients who remain symptomatic or who develop complications after a procedure require admission.

COMMON PITFALLS

✔ Failure to consider an esophageal foreign body in patients without a foreign body history but with suggestive symptoms such as gagging, drooling, wheezing, or refusal to eat

✔ Failure to obtain immediate endoscopy for patients with high-grade esophageal obstruction, sharp esophageal foreign bodies, or button batteries in the esophagus

✔ Inappropriate use of Foley catheter or other removal techniques in patients with sharp or irregularly shaped esophageal foreign bodies, prolonged impactions, esophageal edema, signs of respiratory compromise, or when initial attempts meet resistance—all of these may lead to serious complications

✔ Failure to obtain X-rays to rule out sharp objects prior to digital examination in patients with rectal foreign bodies

✔ Inappropriate, repeated attempts to remove hard, smooth, or high-lying rectal foreign bodies in the ED—this may lead to further mucosal damage or even rectal perforation

✔ Failure to obtain sigmoidoscopy after removal of rectal foreign bodies to rule out mucosal lacerations

References

1. Chen MK, Beierle EA. Gastrointestinal foreign bodies. *Pediatr Ann* 2001;30:736–742.
2. Cohen JS, Sackier JM. Management of colorectal foreign bodies. *J R Coll Surg Edinb* 1996;41:312–315.
3. Doraiswamy NV, Baig H, Hallam L. Metal detector and swallowed metal foreign bodies in children. *J Accid Emerg Med* 1999;16:23–125.
4. Eisen GM, Baron TH, Dominitz JA, et al. Guideline for the management of ingested foreign bodies. American Society for Gastrointestinal Endoscopy. *Gastrointest Endosc* 2002;55:802–806.
5. Emslander HC, Bonadio W, Klatzo M. Efficacy of esophageal bougienage by emergency physicians in pediatric coin ingestion. *Ann Emerg Med* 1996;27:726–729.
6. Harned RK, Strain JD, Hay TC, et al. Esophageal foreign bodies: safety and efficacy of Foley catheter extraction of coins. *AJR Am J Roentgenol* 1997;168:443–446.
7. Karanjia ND, Rees M. The Use of Coca-Cola in the management of bolus obstruction in benign oesophageal stricture. *Ann R Coll Surg Engl* 1993;75:94–95.
8. Kaye RD, Tobin RB. Interventional procedures in the gastrointestinal tract in children. *Radiol Clin North Am* 1996;34:903–917.
9. Kelley JE, Leech MH, Carr MG. A safe and cost-effective protocol for the management of esophageal coins in children. *J Pediatr Surg* 1993;28:898–900.
10. Kouraklis G, Misiakos E, Dovas N, et al. Management of foreign bodies of the rectum. *J R Coll Surg Edinb* 1997;42:246–247.
11. Kurkciyan I, Frossard M, Kettenbach J, et al. Conservative management of foreign bodies in the gastrointestinal tract. *Z Gastroenterol* 1996;34:173–177.
12. Lee SK, Beck NS, Kim HH. Mischievous magnets: unexpected health hazard in children. *J Pediatr Surg* 1996;31:1694–1695.
13. Losanoff JE, Kjossev KT. Gastrointestinal "crosses": an indication for surgery. *J Clin Gastroenterol* 2001;33:310–314.
14. Mosca S. Management and endoscopic techniques in cases of ingestion of foreign bodies. *Endoscopy* 2000;32:272–273.
15. Ros S, Cetta F. Detection of ingested foreign bodies with a metal detector. *J Pediatr* 1992;121:837–838.
16. Sacchetti A, Carraccio C, Lichenstein R. Hand-held metal detector identification of ingested foreign bodies. *Pediatr Emerg Care* 1994;10:204–207.
17. Schunk JE, Harrison AM, Corneli HM, et al. Fluoroscopic Foley catheter removal of esophageal foreign bodies in children: experience with 415 episodes. *Pediatrics* 1994;94:709–714.
18. Seikel K, Primm PA, Elizondo BJ, et al. Handheld metal detector localization of ingested metallic foreign bodies: accurate in any hands? *Arch Pediatr Adolesc Med* 1999;153:853–857.
19. Stack LB, Munter DW. Foreign bodies in the gastrointestinal tract. *Emerg Med Clin North Am* 1996;14:493–521.
20. Wahbeh G, Wyllie R, Kay M. Foreign body ingestion in infants and children: location, location, location. *Clin Pediatr* 2002;41:633–640.
21. Yaman M, Deitel M, Burul CJ, et al. Foreign bodies in the rectum. *Can J Surg* 1993;36:173–177.

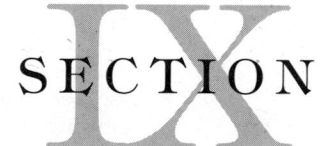

SECTION

LX

Section Editor: Gregory W. Hendey

Renal and Urologic Emergencies

CHAPTER 76
Hematuria

H. Gene Hern, Jr.

There are many causes of nontraumatic hematuria, and the emergency physician must be able to differentiate between the serious and nonserious etiologies. Hematuria may be a chief complaint or an incidental finding. In either case, the physician must be able to proceed through a logical system of evaluation. Such a system should be simple enough to remember, but should provide the clinician with a framework to determine if more testing is required, either in the emergency department (ED) or in the outpatient clinic.

Evaluation of hematuria begins with a classification of the hematuria as either gross or microscopic. The clinician then proceeds to evaluate historical and symptomatic clues to the etiology. If none are found, the clinician should attempt to classify the source of the hematuria as glomerular or nonglomerular and the duration as transient or persistent.

CLINICAL PRESENTATION

Hematuria distresses patients but in most cases does not represent a true emergency. The color of the urine does not correlate with the amount of blood loss. As little as 1 mL of blood in 1 L of urine is enough to discolor the urine (15). However, hematuria alerts the clinician to the need to evaluate the patient for potential dangerous underlying conditions.

Nontraumatic hematuria occurs surprisingly frequently; the prevalence in the general population ranges between 3% and 4% (17). One study reported that among men over 50 years of age, 10% tested positive for hematuria over the course of 3 months (9).

Hematuria is defined as an abnormally high number of red blood cells in the urine. Gross hematuria frequently prompts the patient's ED visit, whereas microscopic hematuria is often found incidentally. Although both forms of hematuria may be caused by similar conditions, in most cases (trauma being the notable exception) there is little correlation between the amount of blood and the seriousness of the cause.

Gross hematuria refers to visibly bloody urine. A variety of disorders can, however, cause red urine. The clinician must first centrifuge the urine and examine the sediment and supernatant. If only the sediment is red and the supernatant is clear, hematuria is present. If the supernatant is red and a urine dipstick registers a positive reaction for heme, hemoglobin or myoglobin is present in the supernatant. If the dipstick does not register a positive heme reaction, the patient may have another, nonheme, cause of the red supernatant. This condition, or *pseudohematuria*, occurs in a variety of conditions, including porphyria, the use of phenazopyridine, and, occasionally, the ingestion of beets.

Blood in the urine not visible to the clinician defines *microscopic hematuria*. It is often discovered incidentally when a urinalysis is performed for other purposes. Although the gold standard for microscopic hematuria is microscopic examination of the urine sediment, the urine dipstick frequently replaces the time-intensive microscopic examination. Urine dipsticks accurately detect hemoglobin in very small quantities, with reported sensitivities from 86% to 100%; The specificity ranges from 65% to 99% (5,19). The high sensitivity results in more false positive results but fewer false negative results. More importantly, however, the high sensitivity provides the clinician with an earlier chance to evaluate potentially serious causes of the hematuria. A negative urine dipstick reliably excludes the presence of myoglobin or hemoglobin in the urine.

DIFFERENTIAL DIAGNOSIS

Historical features of the patient's presentation provide clues to the underlying diagnosis (Table 76.1). Hematuria in a patient with dysuria and pyuria indicates cystitis as a likely cause. Unilateral flank pain that radiates to the groin or testicle may indicate a renal calculus. Of note, up to 15% to 17% of patients with renal calculi do not have hematuria, making it an unreliable predictor (7,13). Vigorous exercise occasionally produces hematuria (1); whether from direct contact sports (football, boxing) or other aerobic exercise (biking, long distance running), exercise-induced hematuria is usually short lived and benign.

Symptoms of *benign prostatic hypertrophy (BPH)* such as dribbling, hesitancy, and poor stream may also suggest the cause of hematuria; new vessels in the proliferative tissue may be fragile and prone to disruption. Some controversy exists as to whether there is a higher incidence of hematuria in patients with PBH than in controls (4,11), but the presence of BPH should not deter the clinician from further evaluating hematuria, since older men have a higher incidence of cancers of the genitourinary tract. Similarly, hematuria in patients who are taking anticoagulants may originate from a potentially serious lesion, not merely from the anticoagulated state itself. Results of ontrolled studies show rates of hematuria in anticoagulated patients similar to those in patients who are not taking anticoagulants (3), but a significant proportion of patients were found to have serious underlying conditions, including bladder cancer.

Hematuria in women that occurs during menstruation may be caused by contamination of the urine specimen during collection or by endometriosis of the urinary tract. If contamination is suspected, a tampon can be inserted, the perineum thoroughly cleaned and a catheterized specimen obtained.

The clinician should also seek clues suggestive of intrinsic renal disease. A family history of polycystic kidney disease or hereditary nephritis suggests a possible explanation of hematuria. Patients with a recent upper respiratory infection may have postinfectious glomerulonephritis (poststreptococcal or nonspecific mesangioproliferative) or immunoglobulin (Ig)A

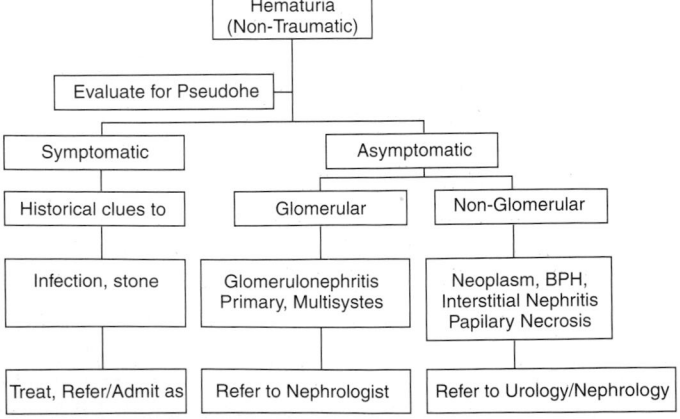

Figure 76.1. Approach to nontraumatic hematuria.

TABLE 76.1. Causes of Hematuria

PSEUDOHEMATURIA

Pigmenturia—myoglobinuria, hemoglobinuria, porphyria
Foods—beets, blackberries, rhubarb
Drugs—phenazopyridine, rifampin
Vaginal/perineal bleeding
Automanipulation—foreign body insertion, addition of blood to urine

SYSTEMIC MANIFESTATION OF DISEASE

Sickle cell disease
Coagulopathy—ITP, hemophilia, anticoagulation
Autoimmune disease—SLE, scleroderma

RENAL (GLOMERULAR)

Glomerulonephritis—Primary: Poststreptococcal GN, IgA
  Nephropathy
—Multisystem: SLE, HSP, PAN, HUS, Goodpasture

RENAL (NONGLOMERULAR)

Pyelonephritis
Infarction
Trauma
Interstitial nephritis
Papillary necrosis
Malignancy
Vascular malformation

POSTRENAL

Infection—cystitis, prostatitis, urethritis
Calculi
Trauma—blunt trauma, exercise, Foley catheter placement
Malignancy

ITP, idiopathic turombocytopeuk purpura; SLE, systemic lupus erythematosus; GN, gonorrhea; HUS, hemolytic uremic syndrome; Ig, immunoglobulin.

nephropathy. These episodes of hematuria can range from mild asymptomatic microscopic hematuria to a full-blown nephritic syndrome and renal failure. Recent use of medications known to cause nephritis (e.g., penicillins, sulfonamides, cimetidine, and allopurinol) may be helpful in suggesting the etiology for hematuria. Finally, patients with sickle cell trait or disease occasionally have papillary necrosis and resultant hematuria.

EMERGENCY DEPARTMENT EVALUATION

Once hematuria is identified, if the etiology is unclear from historical clues, the clinician should determine the source within the genitourinary tract. The main distinction is between hematuria into glomerular and nonglomerular bleeding. A glomerular source is suspected when red blood cell casts (pathognomonic for a glomerular source) are seen on urine microscopy or, secondarily, dysmorphic red blood cells. Urinary protein excretion greater than 500 mg/day (on a specimen without gross blood) also indicates glomerular involvement. If none of these signs are present, the bleeding is likely of nonglomerular origin. In addition, the presence of clots suggests that the blood is from a more distal urologic source, as tissue plasminogen activators and urokinase in the renal tubules prevent clot formation (15). Patients with a glomerular source of bleeding do not require further ED workup for a urologic source and, if clinically stable, may be referred to a nephrologist for further evaluation.

If the hematuria is urologic in origin, the three-tube test helps to identify potential sources. This test involves examining small amounts of urine from different parts of the urinary stream: the first few milliliters, a specimen from midstream, and a specimen from the last few milliliters. When blood is seen predominantly in the first sample a urethral source is likely, and blood in the last sample suggests a lesion near the bladder trigone. Equivalent amounts of blood in each sample suggest a diffuse bladder, ureteral, or renal source.

Hematuria associated with the clinical symptoms of renal colic should prompt evaluation with imaging studies to identify a stone and to gauge its location and size. The traditional method of evaluation, the intravenous pyelogram (IVP), has been superseded by the noncontrast enhanced computed tomographic (CT) scan, which is less invasive (no intravenous line is required); does not subject the patient to the risks of intravenous contrast; and has excellent sensitivity for the presence, size, and location of stones. The size of the stone helps to predict whether it will ultimately pass. Finally, computed tomography also provides information about other potentially lethal causes of hematuria such as an abdominal aortic aneurysm (12) or neoplasms of the kidney, ureter, or bladder.

EMERGENCY DEPARTMENT MANAGEMENT

The clinically stable patient with nontraumatic hematuria rarely requires urgent or emergent ED management. As always, patients with significant pain and discomfort should be given parenteral analgesics. Further management is determined by the individual clinical situation.

Patients with uncomplicated nephrolithiasis should be given outpatient pain medications, a strainer, and referred for followup with a urologist as an outpatient. Admission and urologic consultation are indicated if there is protracted vomiting, unremitting pain, or evidence of concomitant infection. Consultation should also be made for large calculi that are unlikely to pass, for high-grade obstruction, and for patients with a solitary kidney (see Chapter 81, "Urolithiasis").

For uncomplicated urinary tract infection (symptoms of dysuria and hesitancy as well as white blood cells or bacteria in the urine), outpatient management with oral antibiotics is appropriate. Outpatient management is also possible in patients with uncomplicated pyelonephritis. However, if the patient appears ill, has uncontrolled nausea and vomiting, or has a social situation not amenable to outpatient therapy, admission and intravenous antibiotics are appropriate. High-risk patients with diabetes mellitus, pregnancy, concomitant calculi, malignancy, or other immunocompromised state should also be admitted (see Chapter 78, "Urinary Tract Infections").

The risk of complications associated with the glomerulonephritis (e.g., volume overload, pulmonary edema, electrolyte imbalance, and oliguria) is significant and requires consultation with a nephrologist.

CRITICAL INTERVENTIONS

- Provide volume resuscitation for the rare patient with hemodynamic compromise caused by severe hematuria
- Exclude rhabdomyolysis and renal failure during the evaluation

DISPOSITION

Most patients with nontraumatic hematuria are managed as outpatients, regardless of cause. Admission is required for

TABLE 76.2. Frequent Causes of Hematuria According to Age

AGE 0–20 Y

Acute glomerulonephritis
Infection
Congenital abnormalities with obstruction

AGE 20–40 Y

Infection
Urolithiasis
Bladder malignancy

AGE 40–60 Y

Infection
Urolithiasis
Bladder malignancy

AGE 60 YEARS AND OLDER

Infection
Bladder malignancy
Benign prostatic hypertrophy (men)

(Adapted From Restrepo NC, Carey PO. Evaluating hematuria in adults. Am Fam Physician 1989;40:149–156.)

those with complicated etiologies of their hematuria (e.g., pyelonephritis with uncontrolled pain or vomiting). Other patients may have a clinical presentation that requires admission (e.g., nephritis with volume overload and acute renal failure with complications), but hematuria alone is generally not the reason for admission.

Asymptomatic nonglomerular hematuria requires outpatient referral to the primary care physician, urologist, or nephrologist, but not admission or emergent consultation. Young patients with asymptomatic hematuria should have a repeat urinalysis in 1 to 2 weeks to determine whether hematuria is persistent. Up to age 40 years the most common causes of hematuria are urinary tract infection and glomerulonephritis (Table 76.2). In patients older than age 40 years, however, more serious causes must be considered. Results of population-based studies suggest that asymptomatic patients older than 40 years of age are at a much higher risk of bladder and other urologic malignancies and should thus be referred for further evaluation. A number of screening studies in asymptomatic men with hematuria show a risk of urinary tract malignancy of 8% to 9% (2,8,10).

COMMON PITFALLS

✔ Mistaking a life-threatening condition such as abdominal aortic aneurysm for a renal calculus. Both can present with flank pain and hematuria
✔ Using a negative urinalysis for heme to eliminate renal stone as a diagnosis
✔ Failing to provide adequate followup for asymptomatic patients with hematuria, especially those older than age 40 years who have a high risk of malignancy

Acknowledgments

Thank you to previous edition chapter authors James P. d'Etienne and Steven A. Godwin.

References

1. Abarbanel J, Benet AE, Lask D, Kimche D. Sports hematuria. *J Urol* 1990; 143:887–990.
2. Britton JP, Dowell AC, Whelan P. Dipstick haematuria and bladder cancer in men over 60: results of a community study. *BMJ* 1989;299:1010–1012.
3. Culclasure TF, Bray VJ, Hasbargen JA. The significance of hematuria in the anticoagulated patient. *Arch Intern Med* 1994;154:649–652.
4. Ezz el Din K, Koch WF, de Wildt MJ, et al. The predictive value of microscopic haematuria in patients with lower urinary tract symptoms and benign prostatic hyperplasia. *Eur Urol* 1996;30:409–413.
5. Gleeson MJ, Connolly J, Grainger R, et al. Comparison of reagent strip (dipstick) and microscopic haematuria in urological out-patients. *Br J Urol* 1993;72:594–596.
6. Knudson MM, McAninch JW, Gomez R, et al. Hematuria as a predictor of abdominal injury after blunt trauma. *Am J Surg* 1992;164:482–485.
7. Luchs JS, Katz DS, Lane MJ, et al. Utility of hematuria testing in patients with suspected renal colic: correlation with unenhanced helical CT results. *Urology* 2002;59:839–842.
8. Mariani AJ, Mariani MC, Macchioni C, et al. The significance of adult hematuria: 1,000 hematuria evaluations including a risk-benefit and cost-effectiveness analysis. *J Urol* 1989;141:350–355.
9. Messing EM, Young TB, Hunt VB, et al. The significance of asymptomatic microhematuria in men 50 or more years old: findings of a home screening study using urinary dipsticks. *J Urol* 1987;137:919–922.
10. Messing EM, Young TB, Hunt VB, et al. Home screening for hematuria: results of a multiclinic study. *J Urol* 1992;148:289–292.
11. Mohr DN, Offord KP, Melton LJ 3rd. Isolated asymptomatic microhematuria: a cross-sectional analysis of test-positive and test-negative patients. *J Gen Intern Med* 1987;2:318–324.
12. Pomper SR, Fiorillo MA, Anderson CW, Kopatsis A. Hematuria associated with ruptured abdominal aortic aneurysms. *Int Surg* 1995;80:261–263.
13. Press SM, Smith AD. Incidence of negative hematuria in patients with acute urinary lithiasis presenting to the emergency room with flank pain. *Urology* 1995;45:753–757.
14. Restrepo NC, Carey PO. Evaluating hematuria in adults. *Am Fam Physician* 1989;40:149–156.
15. Rose B, Fletcher R. Evaluation of hematuria. *UpToDate* Online version 11.2. www.uptodate.com, 2003 April.
16. Saunders F, Argall J. Towards evidence based emergency medicine: best BETs from the Manchester Royal Infirmary. Investigating microscopic haematuria in blunt abdominal trauma. *Emerg Med J* 2002;19:322–323.
17. Schoolwerth AC. Hematuria and proteinuria: their causes and consequences. *Hosp Pract (Off Ed)* 1987;22:45–52, 55–6, 58–62.
18. Stalker HP, Kaufman RA, Stedje K. The significance of hematuria in children after blunt abdominal trauma. *AJR Am J Roentgenol* 1990;154:569–571.
19. Sutton JM. Evaluation of hematuria in adults. *JAMA* 1990;263:2475–2480.

CHAPTER 77
Acute Scrotal Pain

Robert E. Schneider

The acute scrotal mass can be a challenging differential diagnosis. The three most common diagnoses are torsion of the testis and spermatic cord, acute epididymitis, and torsion of the appendix testis or epididymis. Less-frequent diagnoses include orchitis, acute hydrocele, spermatocele, varicocele, spermatic granuloma, and inguinal hernia. The ischemic insult from testicular torsion makes acute scrotal pain a true surgical emergency. The evaluation is most often difficult, even though a careful history and physical examination narrow the possibilities.

The male external genitalia must be examined systematically in both the supine and standing positions. The former prevents

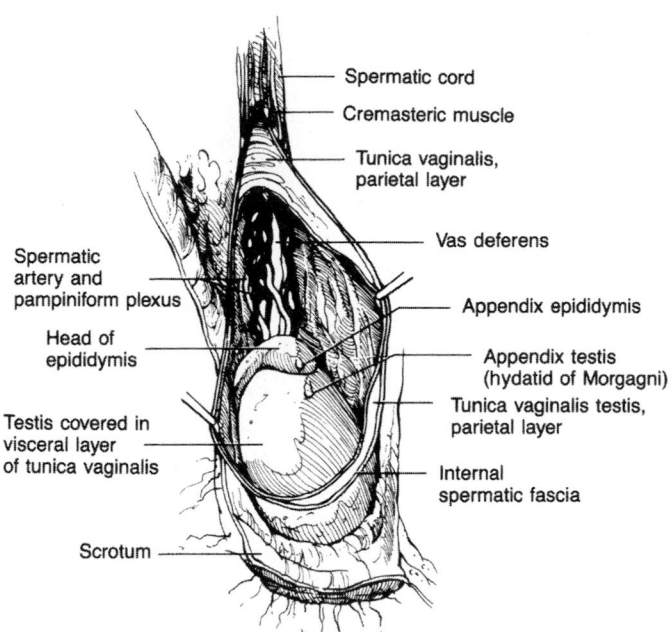

Figure 77.1.   Normal anatomy of the scrotum.

the patient from retreating during the examination, whereas the latter provides optimum positioning to evaluate the lie of each testis, the presence or absence of a varicocele or an inguinal hernia. After quickly assessing the penis and retracting the foreskin to expose the glans, both testes are compared for size and consistency. A testis is best examined with two hands, one palpating and assessing the testicular consistency while the other evaluates the epididymis. The normal testis should be examined first to provide a baseline. The testes normally are oriented vertically with a slight and variable forward tilt. The rubbery consistency should be homogeneous and similar to the thenar eminence of the thumb. The surface is smooth. A normal testicle is 6.0 cm long by 4.0 cm wide by 2.5 cm thick. The testes should be freely mobile within the scrotum (Fig. 77.1). Any palpable mass is described in relationship to the testis, epididymis, spermatic cord, or as a separate entity. All masses should be transilluminated with a penlight or flashlight placed in contact with the posterior scrotal wall and the findings described as positive (does transilluminate) or negative (does not transilluminate).

The epididymis is a 1-cm thick, discrete, sausage-shaped structure, usually located on and firmly attached to the posterior wall of the testicle. In 7% of patients it is anteriorly oriented. The epididymal head, or globus major, is the thickest portion and lies on the top of the testis. The body of the epididymis is a continuation of the head and tapers to the tail, or globus minor, which is contiguous with the vas deferens. The 1 × 3-mm testicular and epididymal appendages are not normally palpable, but are most commonly located anteriorly, near the upper pole of the testis and the head of the epididymis.

From the testis, the spermatic cord can be palpated ascending into the fascial cleft of the subcutaneous external inguinal ring. The vas deferens is a firm tubular structure lying within the 1.5- to 2.0-cm-diameter cord. The spermatic arteries are not palpable and the veins are palpable only when enlarged (varicocele). With the patient in a standing position, a cough or Valsalva maneuver may elicit an overt hernia or, most often, an impulse consistent with an early tear in the fascial ring while the external inguinal ring is palpated. This maneuver also may elicit or accentuate a varicocele.

TESTICULAR TORSION

Torsion of the testis has an incidence of one in 4,000 males. It can occur at any age but is most common between the ages of 12 and 18 years (27,34). Testes predisposed to torsion lack posterior fixation to the scrotal wall and have an abnormally high attachment of a voluminous tunica vaginalis (Fig. 77.2). The tunica vaginalis normally fixes the testis and epididymis to the posterolateral surface of the scrotum (Fig. 77.1). However, complete envelopment of the testis by the tunica vaginalis permits rotation of the testis (clapper) within the tunica (bell), resulting in the classic "bellclapper" deformity (23).

The resultant ischemic event is an emergency. Initially, the testis and cord twist within the tunica vaginalis, thereby causing occlusion of the venous system (31). Arterial flow is subsequently decreased by both the twisting mechanism and the secondary edema consequent to venous occlusion. The degree of testicular damage is related to the duration and extent of vascular occlusion. There are no serum markers to identify the ischemic process. Partial arterial flow may persist with less than 540 degrees to 720 degrees of rotation until edema results in complete occlusion. The variable degree of testicular ischemia makes the absolute window for testicular viability unknown. Testicular salvage times emanate from animal data and show that damage occurs after 2 hours of complete cessation of blood flow. A history of continuous pain for 24 hours is usually associated with an infarcting testis. A salvage rate of 100% following manual or surgical detorsion within 6 hours of ischemic onset is often quoted (4,5,32). However, following acute detorsion, nearly half of the involved testes atrophy by more than 20% (1). An atrophic testicle may have impaired fertility. Significant preexisting testicular histologic abnormalities have been shown to antedate the acute ischemic event (16). Therefore, consequent fertility damage to a contralateral testicle from ipsilateral torsion is unlikely (15).

CLINICAL PRESENTATION

Sudden onset of testicular pain and swelling is the classic presentation for testicular torsion. Unfortunately, in the majority of cases, the history is nonspecific and misleading and should not be used alone to diagnose the acute scrotal mass (18). Pain is most often present or is a significant part of the event (27). Pain can be acute or insidious in onset and mild to excruciating in intensity.

Often, the pain is abdominal and may mimic acute gastroenteritis. In one study, scrotal pain with radiation to the abdomen or inguinal region occurred in 50% of patients with testicular torsion, whereas abdominal or inguinal pain without scrotal pain occurred in 12.5% (14).

A history of a similar event can be elicited in one half of the patients and results from previous episodes of torsion followed by spontaneous detorsion. Approximately one half of patients report the onset of pain during sleep. Cold weather, sexual arousal, and scrotal trauma are often important inciting events. Nausea, vomiting, and low-grade fever are common clinical findings. Voiding symptoms such as dysuria, urgency, and hesitancy are rarely described (12).

Physical examination reveals either a painful or often nonpalpable testis that has elevated cephalad in the hemiscrotum owing to the twisting and foreshortening of the spermatic cord. Engorgement of the testicle and secondary swelling of the scrotum are usually present. Instead of lying in the usual vertical orientation, the affected testis is often found lying horizontally in the scrotum because of its abnormal mobility within the tunica vaginalis.

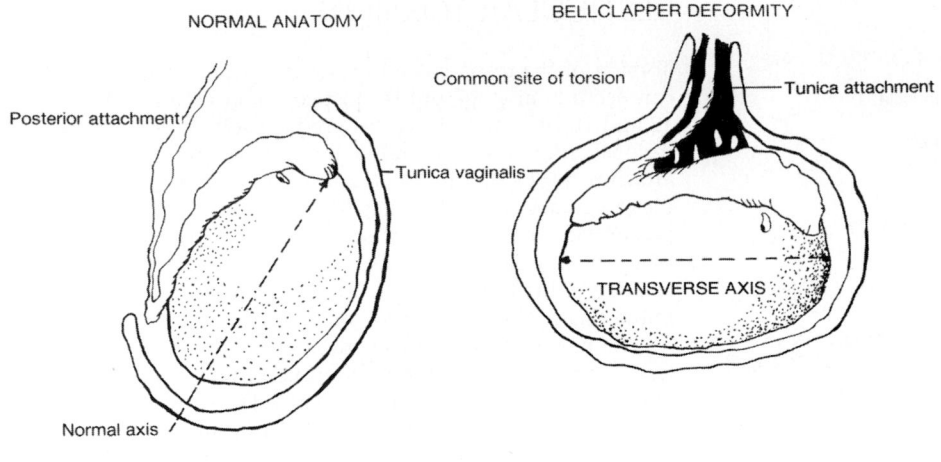

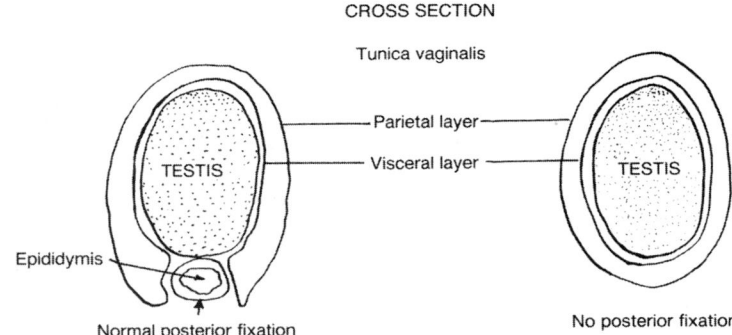

Figure 77.2.   Bellclapper deformity.

The epididymis may be malrotated anteriorly but is usually nontender when palpated. Chronicity of the event usually results in the epididymis becoming globally enlarged and sausage-shaped anatomically. The spermatic cord tends to become thickened in the area of torsion. Elevation of the testis does not relieve the discomfort (Prehn sign) as it does in epididymitis, because torsion is primarily an ischemic event, not an inflammatory process. With the passage of time, however, testicular torsion evolves into a secondary inflammatory process. Laboratory data are nonspecific and not helpful. One third of patients have a nonspecific leukocytosis of more than 10,000 white blood cells per cubic millimeter, and almost all patients have a normal urinalysis (14,20).

When these classic findings are absent, the entire hemiscrotum is usually swollen, tender, and firm. A reactive hydrocele may have developed (11). The overlying scrotal skin rapidly develops redness and edema, and within a few hours, the testis and epididymis are no longer anatomically separable. In a series of 206 patients with torsion, 42% presented with swelling and precluded palpation of the intrascrotal contents (20). Finally, the hemiscrotum becomes an amorphous, painful scrotal mass referred to as "missed torsion."

The ipsilateral loss of the cremasteric reflex with testicular torsion and its preservation in most cases of epididymitis is a soft finding and certainly not diagnostic of one event or the other (26). The cremasteric reflex is a superficial skin reflex mediated by spinal nerves T-12 to L-2, elicited by stroking the skin of the inner aspect of the ipsilateral thigh in an upward motion, resulting in contraction of the cremasteric muscle and elevation of the testis by at least 0.5 cm. This is best demonstrated with the patient in the supine, frogleg position and requires the absence of any inflammatory process in the overlying scrotal skin. Occasionally, the cremasteric findings are equivocal and unre-

liable in severe epididymitis associated with marked overlying scrotal skin inflammation.

DIFFERENTIAL DIAGNOSIS

In an adolescent, acute scrotal swelling is torsion until proven otherwise. The differential diagnosis includes acute epididymitis, torsion of the testicular or epididymal appendices, orchitis, testicular tumor, inguinal hernia, and traumatic hydrocele or hematocele. Age does not preclude the diagnosis of testicular torsion. A series of 243 patients with testicular torsion revealed that 31% were prepubertal, 60% were 12 to 18 years old, 5% were older than 30 years, and isolated case reports in the elderly continue to be reported (10).

Acute *epididymitis*, the most common entity mistaken for testicular torsion, is rare before puberty. Sixty percent of patients with epididymitis are older than 30 years. Epididymitis classically has a more gradual onset than testicular torsion. The diagnosis of epididymitis is in the history and must be pursued compulsively. Usually, a history of urinary tract infection, painful voiding, urethral discharge, or an indwelling urethral catheter suggests the diagnosis of epididymitis. A work or exercise history consistent with a lot of lifting, straining, or events that increase intrapelvic pressure favors epididymitis (roofer, construction worker, weight lifter). A history of previous episodes of testicular pain suggests testicular torsion. Nausea with vomiting is more common in testicular torsion. The physical examination may not be helpful, and often times is confusing.

A thorough understanding of the pathophysiology of epididymitis is imperative when examining the scrotal contents. The retrograde development of epididymitis dictates that the pain often originates in either abdominal lower quadrant and then migrates down into the scrotum. Initially, the testicular pain is felt in the globus minor or the tail of the epididymis. This is usually disclosed as a firm, hard mass at the inferior portion of the normally smooth testis. If the diagnosis is missed or delayed, the inflammatory process will ascend into the body, then to the head, or globus major, of the epididymis, producing the large sausage-shaped mass often found on the posterior surface of the testis. In the late stages of either disease process, the tenderness and diffuse swelling that often accompany torsion and epididymitis can obscure any discernible physical findings.

Primary *orchitis* is very rare. In fact, if this is your diagnosis, consultation with a colleague is recommended for confirmation. A history of mumps orchitis and manifestations of a systemic illness should be present. Otherwise, orchitis seldom occurs unless it represents contiguous spread of infection from the epididymis to the testis (epididymoorchitis). In primary orchitis, the onset of testicular pain and swelling is more gradual and global. The epididymis is normal. The spermatic cord may be tender but is not indurated or thickened.

Torsion of a testicular or epididymal appendage can cause venous engorgement with subsequent arterial occlusion and infarction. The appendix testis is the most common appendage to twist (14). It is usually located anteriorly, near the upper pole of the testis. Appendiceal testicular torsion occurs in the same age group as testicular torsion. Sudden onset of scrotal pain without radiation is the most common presentation. The onset of pain may not be as rapid as that of testicular torsion and may occur intermittently and then progress over 3 to 5 days. The symptoms are usually less severe than in testicular torsion. Nausea and vomiting occur more often in testicular torsion than in appendiceal torsion. Diagnostically, early in the process, the testicular appendage may be palpated separately as a tender mass at the head of the testis. The often-referenced "blue dot" sign refers to a small, tender, infarcted (blue), pea-like structure seen through the hormonally unstimulated, prepubertal scrotal skin held taught over the head of the testis (14). Localized tenderness in the head of the testis without comparable mass or erythema of the scrotal skin, however, is more commonly found in appendiceal torsion (18). Excision of the twisted appendage is the standard treatment, although nonsurgical observation has been successful because autoinfarction is the consequence. Surgical exploration is often required in delayed cases to confirm the diagnosis of appendiceal torsion and to exclude testicular torsion.

Carcinoma of the testis is the most common cancer in males age 15 to 35 years, a similar age range for the occurrence of testicular torsion (28). The initial diagnosis is incorrect 25% of the time; the most common misdiagnosis is epididymitis. Symptoms from testicular tumors normally have a more gradual onset. Pain is not generally a major complaint for testicular tumor, although 10% of patients with intratesticular tumor hemorrhage can experience the sudden onset of pain. On examination, the affected testicle is characteristically nontender. The testis may be generally enlarged and feel heavy to the patient, but, more often, a distinct, firm, intratesticular mass is palpated by the examiner. The scrotum usually has less erythema and edema than in testicular torsion, and, on palpation, the affected testicle can be separated from the other normal intrascrotal structures. In a delayed presentation, a testicular tumor can appear similar to missed testicular torsion. Ten percent of testicular tumors have a reactive hydrocele, which can obscure palpation. Signs of metastatic disease, such as an abdominal mass, lower extremity edema, neurologic abnormalities, lumbar back pain, or weight loss, may be present in up to 10% of patients with testicular tumors. The urinalysis is usually normal.

Incarcerated scrotal *hernias* account for less than 2% of acute scrotal masses, but may present with a history similar to that of testicular torsion. The young age of the patient and the associated unrelenting nausea and vomiting tend to support this diagnosis. Abdominal pain and groin pain are usually present. The scrotal hernia can usually be palpated extending into the groin, and the testis may be displaced lower in the scrotum.

A traumatic *hydrocele* and hematocele are included in the differential diagnosis because a trauma history also accompanies 5% to 10% of cases of testicular torsion. The testis is usually not as painful as in testicular torsion, and the epididymis and spermatic cord, if palpable, are in their normal positions. Swelling often obscures the examination, and ancillary tests are recommended to confirm the diagnosis.

EMERGENCY DEPARTMENT EVALUATION

A rapid presumptive diagnosis of testicular torsion should be suspected on the basis of the history and physical examination findings. Because the presentation most often is variable and the scrotum develops erythema from many causes, testicular torsion must be the primary consideration for any scrotal complaint in the young and the adolescent.

Diagnostic tests, such as color Doppler ultrasound or radionuclide testicular scintigraphy, are always adjunctive and should never delay urologic consultation, attempted manual detorsion, and scrotal exploration (33). These adjunctive tests are not required to make the diagnosis.

Radionuclide imaging assesses testicular perfusion with a sensitivity that approaches that of color Doppler ultrasound (6,33). Despite a 90% to 100% accuracy rate in defining testicular blood flow, testicular scintigraphy provides little anatomic information, is labor intensive, and is often unavailable in the middle of the night. Testicular scintigraphy is radiologist-reader–dependent. In early testicular torsion, the scan demonstrates relatively decreased or absent testicular blood flow to the affected testis, and a "cold spot" on delayed images corresponds to the nonperfused testis. After 7 hours of relatively continuous ischemia, the nonperfused testis develops a reactive edema and hyperemia. The scan may display a halo of increased tracer activity (i.e., the rim sign) around the cold testis, often confused with and appearing quite similar to acute epididymitis. In acute epididymitis, relatively increased global perfusion to the affected hemiscrotum is seen. A nuclear scan cannot reliably differentiate torsion of a testicular or epididymal appendage from epididymitis, but it is helpful in confirming testicular blood flow and eliminating testicular torsion as the cause of the patient's pain.

A normally perfused testis with a surrounding lucency from accumulated fluid is seen with a hydrocele. A testicular tumor usually demonstrates increased radioisotope uptake in comparison with its contralateral mate. A color Doppler ultrasound is the preferred diagnostic modality for suspected testicular tumor (19).

Color Doppler ultrasound yields the most information in evaluation of the acute scrotum because it provides information about both anatomy and arterial perfusion. It can determine whether a mass is intratesticular or extratesticular and is particularly applicable when swelling or a reactive hydrocele has made physical examination difficult or impossible. The normal testis has characteristic echoes that are homogeneous and finely granular, whereas the epididymis is distinguished by its coarser texture. A typical testicular tumor is detected as a hypoechoic, inhomogeneous mass within the testis. Epididymitis displays a thickened and enlarged epididymis. Abscess cavities may be apparent within both the testes and epididymis.

Although color Doppler ultrasound and radionuclide scans are helpful, an aggregate clinical impression derived from a thorough history and physical examination is more important. The imaging test used often depends on the consultant, the availability of the examination, the quality of the equipment, and the experience of the technician and radiologist-reader. Adjunctive tests should never delay operative exploration. Imaging may be obtained while waiting for an operating suite, but it is imperative that the examining physician remember that testicular torsion is diagnosed at surgical exploration. Once the diagnosis of testicular torsion is suspected, immediate urologic consultation is initiated. Meticulous charting and documentation of the history and physical examination, the suspected diagnosis and need for scrotal exploration, as well as the time-course for all of these events, is imperative (5,22).

If the urologist requests adjunctive testing, this must be documented in the emergency department record. The urologist should be informed that an attempt at manual detorsion will be made while awaiting the patient's transfer to the operating room or the radiology suite, and documentation carried out should the urologist discourage or request that detorsion not be attempted.

EMERGENCY DEPARTMENT MANAGEMENT

Manual detorsion is successful in 30% to 70% of patients (8,13). Spontaneous or successful manipulative preoperative testicular detorsion results in a 100% testicular salvage rate (5). Manual detorsion can be attempted with the patient standing or supine, but most often is done with the patient supine, in bed, or on a stretcher, with the physician standing on the patient's right side (29). Classically, the patient is placed in the frogleg lithotomy position to allow total access to his scrotum and testis. The patient must be informed that manual detorsion is a painful maneuver. Light sedation or spermatic cord block may be done to lessen the patient's discomfort. A spermatic cord block allows multiple detorsion attempts and experimentation with direction, but it eliminates pain relief as an end point to judge successful detorsion. Most testes twist in a lateral-to-medial direction, so manual detorsion is initially attempted from medial to lateral, similar to opening a book; that is, the patient's right testis is detorsed in a counterclockwise direction, and the left testis in a clockwise direction. The testis is rotated 180 degrees in one direction and maintained in position. Further rotation is continued as necessary (25).

If the initial detorsion increases the pain, the detorsion should be attempted in the opposite direction. One to three turns is usually sufficient. The detorsion is stopped when either the anatomy is restored or the testicular pain is relieved. Both should occur promptly. Significant swelling makes the initial detorsion maneuver more difficult and there is much less chance of success.

Ideally, manual detorsion should be followed by surgical exploration to confirm success and fixate both testes, because torsion is an anatomic abnormality and tends to be bilateral. There have not been any reported cases of recurrent ischemia in the interval between successful manual detorsion and orchiopexy.

The technique of spermatic cord block is simple (33). The spermatic cord is palpated and encircled with the nondominant hand at the scrotal inguinal junction. Three to four injections with 1% plain lidocaine are made at different angled approaches with a 25-gauge, 1.5-inch needle.

An alternative method can be instituted if the cord cannot be palpated because of severe pain or pronounced swelling. After palpating the pubic tubercle, a needle is inserted vertically downward, 1 cm below and medial to the pubic tubercle onto the anterior aspect of the pubic bone. Repeated slow injections should be made at different angles, attempting to infiltrate the area around the ilioinguinal nerve and genital branch of the gen-

itofemoral nerve. The duration of a successful lidocaine spermatic cord block is about 1 to 3 hours.

CRITICAL INTERVENTIONS

- Consult a urologist immediately for a high suspicion case of testicular torsion, without adding the delay of diagnostic studies
- Perform manual detorsion while the patient awaits the operating room, in order to reduce the ischemic time to the testicle

DISPOSITION

The urologist or general surgeon is obligated to establish a final diagnosis and perform definitive *orchiopexy* or *orchiectomy*, depending on the operative findings. Selected ancillary tests must not delay surgical exploration. When securing written informed operative consent, the consultant should explain the need for bilateral orchiopexy, the possibility of orchiectomy, and the option for placement of a testicular prosthesis. An unequivocally infarcted testis is usually removed at exploration to lessen the chance for persistent pain and promote resolution of the inflammatory process. Bilateral orchiopexy is always required, because the anatomic defect is present bilaterally.

All patients for whom testicular torsion is suspected should be admitted and taken to the operating suite. Observation and serial examinations are not useful in the management of suspected testicular torsion. Preoperative emergency department laboratory studies should be completed quickly to expedite surgery. If preoperative manual detorsion successfully reestablishes testicular blood flow, arrangements for delayed orchiopexy can be made by the consultant. The urologist or general surgeon is ultimately responsible for any planned or self-directed delay in scrotal exploration and orchiopexy.

The unavailability of a urologist, general surgeon, or immediate operating room facilities warrants prompt transfer. The lack of radionuclide scanning or color Doppler ultrasonography does not affect the treatment; that is, the patient needs to undergo attempted manual detorsion and surgical exploration.

COMMON PITFALLS

✔ Misdiagnosis and delays in attempted testicular detorsion are common pitfalls in the evaluation of acute scrotal pain
✔ Fifty percent of testes lost because of testicular torsion are associated with initial misdiagnosis. The history and physical examination are often misleading. An antecedent history of trauma most often misleads the examiner
✔ Reliance on a single "classic" differentiating parameter, such as age, onset of pain, or physical examination findings, can erroneously convince the examiner that testicular torsion is not present
✔ Scrotal erythema and swelling tend to promote a diagnosis of infection, rather than initial ischemia with subsequent inflammatory sequelae
✔ Unnecessary delays in consulting with a urologist or general surgeon may result while awaiting ancillary tests. The examiner should not delay consultation to obtain adjunctive tests
✔ If testicular torsion is a consideration, the emergency physician cannot accept an alternative diagnosis by the consultant over the telephone
✔ Manual detorsion by the emergency physician is the most rapid means of reestablishing blood flow to an ischemic testis. However, the ultimate responsibility for confirming

detorsion, testicular viability, and definitive fixation to the scrotal wall rests with the urologist or general surgeon

ACUTE EPIDIDYMITIS AND ORCHITIS

Inflammation or infection that is limited to the epididymis and causes acute pain and swelling of gradual onset is termed *acute epididymitis* (21). Epididymoorchitis implies extension of the inflammation or infection onto the adjacent testis. Epididymitis occurs in less than one in 1,000 men per year and is the most common cause of acute scrotal pain (24). It is primarily a disease of adults and seldom occurs before puberty unless there is an associated anatomic abnormality of the lower urinary tract that promotes urinary tract infection. Epididymitis most often results from retrograde spread of infected urine down the vas deferens into the globus minor, or tail, of the epididymis. Occasionally, reflux of sterile urine causes the same inflammatory process (i.e., chemical epididymitis) (3).

In men younger than age 35 years, the organisms most often responsible are those that cause urethritis: *Chlamydia trachomatis* and *Neisseria gonorrhoeae* (17,24,30). In men older than age 35 years, bacteriuria caused by obstructive urinary disease is more common, and *Escherichia coli*, enterococci, *Pseudomonas*, and *Proteus* predominate. Tuberculous epididymitis is rare. Any organism may invade the epididymis in association with a systemic infection, such as blastomycosis and meningococcus. *Candida* and *E. coli* epididymitis have been seen in patients with acquired immune deficiency syndrome (AIDS). Amiodarone (Cordarone) has been associated with drug-induced epididymitis confined to the globus major, or head, of the epididymis.

In the prepubertal patient, coliform bacteria predominate. Nongonococcal bacterial epididymitis in a boy younger than age 10 years should prompt a thorough diagnostic evaluation for genitourinary anomalies or neurogenic bladder disease, as underlying urogenital abnormalities exist in 47% of prepubertal patients with bacterial epididymitis (2,3,7). A negative urine culture is evidence against an anatomic anomaly.

Initially, gradual development of scrotal pain, swelling, and inflammation occurs when only a small portion of the epididymis or vas deferens is involved. With progression, the globus minor of the epididymis becomes involved and extends superiorly into the body, then into the globus major, or head, of the epididymis if the condition is not diagnosed and treated appropriately. The eventual large, red, hot, swollen scrotal mass of epididymoorchitis may indirectly compress the terminal branches of the spermatic artery and vein, causing testicular ischemia—hence, the importance of early diagnosis and aggressive management. Bacteria can also invade an ischemic testis, leading to testicular and epididymal abscesses.

Acute orchitis, by definition, is a primary infection of the testis and, as such, is rare. Most often, orchitis is seen as a secondary infection related to an initial epididymal infection. Orchitis may occur during a systemic illness in which systemic seeding of the testis occurs with *E. coli, and Klebsiella, Pseudomonas, Staphylococcus,* and *Streptococcus species*. Most commonly, influenza, infectious mononucleosis, tuberculosis, syphilis, and amoebiasis cause orchitis. The latter pathogens occur most often in immunocompromised patients.

Mumps orchitis occurs in males who are systemically infected with the virus, but seldom before puberty. About 15% to 20% of postpubertal males with mumps develop orchitis. The onset of the testicular swelling normally occurs 3 to 7 days after the development of parotitis. One third of men with mumps orchitis, however, do not have parotitis. One third of cases may be bilateral. Atrophy results in about 50% of involved testes.

CLINICAL PRESENTATION

The gradual onset of scrotal pain and swelling peaks over a period of 3 to 24 hours. The pain can be sharp and often radiates to the groin and either lower abdominal quadrant, simulating appendicitis or diverticulitis, but, commonly, the only complaint is a dull ache in the scrotum.

Irritative voiding symptoms, such as frequency, dysuria, and urgency, occur in 10% to 20% of patients (18,30). A history of fever is not common. On occasion, a debilitated or immunocompromised patient may present with bacteremia. A history of recent cystoscopy, an indwelling urethral catheter, urinary tract infection, or genitourinary surgery should be sought, especially in older men. Similarly, a thorough history of sexual relationships, previous exposures to sexually transmitted disease, work-out routines, and job-related duties (any activity that promotes a Valsalva maneuver or increases intrapelvic pressure and promotes retrograde flow of sterile or infected urine) must be evaluated. Body builders who lift a lot of weight, and roofers and construction workers who climb and do a lot of heavy lifting, are prototypes for the development of epididymitis.

Nausea occurs in 15% of patients (11). Bilateral epididymal involvement occurs in 10% of cases. Rarely, abdominal pain attributed to infection involving the vas deferens and spermatic cord is the sole initial and presenting symptom. This has been mistaken for appendicitis or diverticulitis (12,30).

On examination, a localized, indurated, tender portion of the epididymis may be palpated inferiorly and separate from a less painful testis. Eventually, the entire epididymis becomes involved, and the distinction between the testis and epididymis is less evident. The involved testis hangs low in an erythematous and edematous scrotum. Most often, testicular discomfort can be relieved by scrotal elevation and support (a positive Prehn sign), as epididymitis is an inflammatory process. A urethral discharge is present in 10% of patients (12,30).

Progression of the infection can result in scrotal wall fixation to the underlying testis and epididymis and epididymal abscess formation. More commonly, an erythematous, edematous scrotum overlies an amorphous, tender mass.

The usual presentation of orchitis is high fever, nausea, vomiting, and gradual onset of testicular pain radiating to the groin. There are usually no urinary or urethral symptoms. The testis is uniformly enlarged and tense and tender to palpation, whereas the epididymis is normal. A reactive hydrocele, cutaneous erythema, and scrotal enlargement are common and may make palpation of the testis difficult.

DIFFERENTIAL DIAGNOSIS

The differential diagnosis of epididymitis is the same as that discussed previously. Testicular torsion is the most important disorder in the differential that also includes tumor, inguinal hernia, and hydrocele or hematocele.

EMERGENCY DEPARTMENT EVALUATION

After the history and physical examination, a urinalysis and urine culture should be obtained. A properly collected urinalysis shows pyuria or bacteriuria in 50% of patients (20). A small number of patients have a urethral discharge that can be gram-stained. The white blood cell count is commonly elevated, nonspecific, and not helpful in the differential diagnosis. Color Doppler ultrasound can confirm testicular blood flow and help differentiate epididymitis from testicular torsion. It can also aid in the evaluation of the epididymis for enlargement and abscess formation. If gram-negative bacteremia is suspected, blood cultures should be obtained and intravenous fluids and broad-spectrum antibiotic therapy initiated as quickly as possible.

EMERGENCY DEPARTMENT MANAGEMENT

Aggressive initial management of acute epididymitis is crucial to reduce the potential morbidity associated with this disease process. Complete bedrest, scrotal elevation with ice applied to the affected epididymis for 10 minutes 3 times per day, organism-specific antibiotic therapy, nonsteroidal antiinflammatory drugs, narcotic pain medication, and stool softeners are the initial treatment modalities recommended for acute epididymitis. Patients are instructed to observe strict bedrest, getting up only to eat or go to the bathroom. Once pain-free in bed, they are encouraged to be ambulatory with a scrotal supporter and are instructed emphatically not to lift or strain, especially when having a bowel movement, as this will promote a recurrence of the pathophysiologic inflammatory process.

Antibiotics are prescribed in all cases. Despite an infectious cause, cultures of the urine and urethral discharge may be negative. If there is a history of sexually transmitted disease or if the causative organism is not known, a single 250-mg intramuscular dose of ceftriaxone (Rocephin) is administered in the emergency department. This is followed by a 10-day course of doxycycline 100 mg orally every 12 hours, ofloxacin (Floxin) 400 mg orally every 12 hours for 10 days, levofloxacin (Levaquin) 500 mg orally daily for 10 days, or alternatively, azithromycin (Zithromax) 1 g orally as a single dose in the emergency department prior to discharge (9). Men older than 35 years who are suspected of having a urinary tract infection caused by enteric gram-negative bacilli or *Pseudomonas* should be initially treated based on the suspected organism, with their treatment altered, if necessary, based on the results of the emergency department urine culture. Empiric treatment for gram-negative rods and gram-positive cocci should be initiated with ciprofloxacin 500 mg orally every 12 hours for 7 to 10 days. Therapy with trimethoprim–sulfamethoxazole (TMP-SMX) (Septra or Bactrim) 1 tablet every 12 hours or ofloxacin (Floxin) 400 mg every 12 hours is an excellent alternative. Urology followup is encouraged within 5 to 7 days.

Treatment for mumps orchitis is generally supportive with bedrest, scrotal elevation, and analgesics. Resolution requires 1 to 3 weeks. Steroid therapy is probably not helpful. Making incisions in the testicular tunica albuginea early in the course of the disease has been tried as a means of reducing intratubular pressure but has shown no appreciable benefit. Atrophy occurs in about 50% of affected testes, regardless of treatment.

CRITICAL INTERVENTIONS

- Provide antibiotics and analgesics for patients with acute epididymitis or orchitis
- If suspicion exists, testicular torsion must be excluded by Doppler ultrasound

DISPOSITION

Immediate urologic consultation should be obtained if testicular torsion is considered. Outpatient management of epididymitis is appropriate in most cases. Urologic followup should be arranged for 5 to 7 days, unless worsening of the patient's condition necessitates an earlier visit. All pediatric cases of epididymitis require urologic consultation to evaluate the potential for lower urinary tract anomalies and urinary obstruction as the cause of the epididymitis.

Adult patients with suspected bacteremia or severe constitutional symptoms, including intractable pain or nausea and vomiting, require hospitalization and parenteral antibiotics. Patients in whom the physical examination and ultrasonography are equivocal for abscess formation should also be admitted for antibiotic therapy and serial ultrasound examinations.

Hospitalization is required for severe cases of epididymitis or when an epididymal or testicular abscess is suspected. Selected epididymotomy or epididymectomy may prevent testicular damage when an abscess is diagnosed. Occasionally, orchiectomy may be the most time-efficient and definitive treatment option.

The unavailability of a urologist may necessitate transfer if operative intervention is necessary. Most cases of epididymitis can be treated initially by emergency physicians.

COMMON PITFALLS

- ✔ Epididymitis is the most common misdiagnosis in cases of testicular tumor and testicular torsion
- ✔ Bladder outlet obstruction and urinary retention must be considered in the older patient with epididymitis

HYDROCELE AND OTHER DISORDERS OF THE SPERMATIC CORD

A hydrocele is the most common cause of nonacute intrascrotal swelling. It is an accumulation of serous fluid in the potential space between the visceral and parietal layers of the tunica vaginalis that normally envelops and fixes the anterolateral aspect of the testis and epididymis to the posterior scrotal wall, thereby preventing testicular torsion. Most hydroceles are found in older patients, and an underlying cause is not identified. A sudden onset of a symptomatic hydrocele can occur secondary to epididymitis, trauma, or tumor.

Approximately 10% of testicular tumors have a reactive hydrocele as the presenting complaint (14). In pediatric hydroceles, congenital failure of the tunica vaginalis to obliterate after birth allows communication between the scrotum and the peritoneum, creating a hydrocele or hernia. These "communicating hydroceles" acutely enlarge and shrink depending on patient activity, as peritoneal fluid and occasionally a loop of intestine fill the scrotum when the patient is in the upright position and spontaneously decompress when the patient is supine. This is the classic history of scrotal swelling that vanishes when the child sleeps.

CLINICAL PRESENTATION

Most hydroceles in adults develop gradually and are asymptomatic. A chronically enlarging hydrocele may present as scrotal enlargement associated with a heavy sensation, occasionally radiating to the groin. An acute hydrocele may present with pain, depending on the inciting event.

The classic hydrocele is a cystic, pear-shaped mass located anterior to the testis and epididymis. It often obscures definitive palpation of the testis. Transillumination most often reveals a translucent mass surrounding an opaque testicular shadow. A hydrocele should be confined to the scrotum, with a normal spermatic cord above it. Rarely, a hydrocele of the spermatic cord can be palpated in the region of the external inguinal canal.

DIFFERENTIAL DIAGNOSIS

The most common disorders to consider in the differential diagnosis include spermatocele, varicocele, traumatic hematocele, and inguinal hernia.

A *hematocele* is blood or a blood clot within the potential space between the two leaves of the tunica vaginalis. It occurs most often after needle aspiration of a hydrocele, but it can accompany testicular torsion or trauma. A cyst-like mass, similar to a hydrocele, can be felt on examination. However, the mass does not transilluminate. Following trauma, this type of swelling may become quite large. Ultrasonography can differentiate blood from less echogenic hydrocele fluid and reveal a ruptured testis or testicular tumor. In the absence of a reasonable history or diagnostic ultrasonography, a hematocele should be explored.

A *spermatocele* is a common cystic mass lying above and posterior to the testis. Spermatoceles are retention cysts arising from the epididymis and contain spermatozoa (14). Usually painless, these masses may alarm the patient about a possible testicular tumor. A spermatocele is usually soft, freely mobile, and lucent on transillumination, but may become firm in a chronic state. Most spermatoceles are less than 1 cm in greatest dimension, but can become as large as 10 cm. It is not possible to differentiate a spermatocele from a lipoma or other adnexal mass by palpation alone. Combining the examination with ultrasonography can usually confirm the diagnosis. Excision is required only when the size of the spermatocele causes pain or there is a question regarding the diagnosis.

A *varicocele* is a dilatation of the testicular pampiniform venous plexus (2). A varicocele is usually a chronic condition, but the acute appearance of a varicocele, especially on the right side, can herald a retroperitoneal tumor, tumor adenopathy, renal cell carcinoma, or renal vein thrombosis. Varicoceles are more common on the left than on the right and usually present as a mass above the testis, often referred to as a "bag of worms" because of the multiple torturous vessels imprinting the scrotal skin. Nearly 20% of men have a left varicocele of some degree (29). The left side predominates because the left testicular vein drains perpendicularly into the left renal vein without valves to reduce hydrostatic pressure, as compared with the right testicular vein, which drains obliquely into the inferior vena cava. Right-sided varicoceles are only seldom seen without a concomitant left varicocele.

Most varicoceles are asymptomatic, but if symptoms occur, they are usually limited to the upright position (increased gravity) and include heaviness on the affected side that is usually relieved by assuming a supine position. Most often, reassurance suffices.

An *inguinal hernia* may present as an acute swelling in the scrotum. The clinical history is variable and not helpful. The exception is an incarcerated hernia that occurs most commonly during the first year of life and is accompanied by signs of peritoneal irritation or obstruction (i.e., nausea and/or vomiting). Most hernias may be palpated in the superior scrotal and inguinal regions (14). Transillumination is usually not helpful. The auscultation of bowel sounds in the hemiscrotum may help to identify a hernia. Uncomplicated reduction of bowel through the inguinal defect into the abdominal cavity confirms the diagnosis.

A *sperm granuloma* is an inflammatory response to sperm that have entered the interstitium; it can occur in the epididymis, vas deferens, or testis. A sperm granuloma is most commonly found at the site of a previous vasectomy or in the epididymis following an epididymotomy. A sperm granuloma is generally small and asymptomatic, but, at times, presents as a palpable, painful intrascrotal mass. This creates a problem only in differentiating the granuloma from a testicular tumor. The physical and ultrasound examinations demonstrate an extratesticular mass that is usually confluent with the epididymis or vas deferens. Rarely, testicular granulomas require diagnostic exploration. Emergency department treatment consists of antiinflammatory agents and pain medication.

EMERGENCY DEPARTMENT EVALUATION

Many hydroceles preclude palpation of the testis. Transillumination is insensitive in eliminating tumor as the inciting cause. Often, the history suggests epididymitis as the cause, but the epididymis is hidden by the hydrocele. Epididymitis should be suspected if the urinalysis discloses pyuria. Scrotal ultrasonography is the diagnostic test of choice for detecting masses within the testis; it is the best modality to image the epididymis through a hydrocele.

EMERGENCY DEPARTMENT MANAGEMENT

The priority in emergency department evaluation of hydroceles is disclosing the etiology. Underlying reversible causes should be treated. Very infrequently, aspiration of the hydrocele is required to permit adequate examination and provide relief from painful swelling. The technique involves anterior aspiration through an 18-gauge, pliable venous catheter inserted over a needle cannula.

The indwelling, flexible, atraumatic tip prevents damage to the opposing testicle during collapse of the hydrocele and can be positioned in the most dependent area of the scrotum to ensure adequate drainage. The maneuver is not definitive because recurrence is guaranteed. Surgical exploration is necessary if a palpable mass remains poorly defined. Otherwise, the treatment of hydroceles is elective, being indicated when the size of the scrotum is unacceptable cosmetically or interferes with physical activity.

CRITICAL INTERVENTION

- In many cases, the diagnosis must be clarified by ultrasound

DISPOSITION

The acute development of a hydrocele requires referral based on the suspected underlying cause.

COMMON PITFALL

✔ Dismissal of a newly developed hydrocele as a benign process may delay diagnosis of an underlying testicular malignancy

References

1. Anderson JB, Williamson RLN. The fate of the human testes following unilateral torsion of the spermatic cord. *Br J Urol* 1986;58:698.
2. Bar-Charma N, Palmer LS, Cohen S, et al. The adolescent varicocele: when to treat. *Emerg Med* 1993;73.
3. Bennett RT, Bhagwant G, Kogan SJ. Epididymitis in children: the circumcision factor. *J Urol* 1998;160:1842.
4. Bird S. Failure to diagnose—testicular torsion. *Austral Fam Physician* 2003;32:527–528, 2003 Jul.
5. Boyarsky S, Steinhardt GF, Onder R. Medical aspects of testicular torsion. *Mo Med* 1990;87:359.

6. Burks DD, Markey BJ, Burkland TK, et al. Suspected testicular torsion and ischemia: evaluation with color Doppler sonography. *Radiology* 1990;175: 815.

7. Cappele O, Liard A, Barret E, et al. Epididymitis in children: is further investigation necessary after the first episode? *Eur Urol* 2000;38:627–630.

8. Cattolica EV. Preoperative manual detorsion of the torsed spermatic cord. *J Urol* 1985;133:803.

9. Centers for Disease Control and Prevention. 2002 Guidelines for treatment of sexually transmitted diseases. *MMWR Morb Mortal Wkly Rep* 2002;51(RR-6):1.

10. Cummings JM, Boullier JA, Sekhon D, Bose K. Adult testicular torsion. *J Urol* 2002;167:2109–2110.

11. Escobar JI, Eastman ER, Harwood Nuss AL. Genitourinary disease. In: Rosen P, ed. *Emergency medicine*, 5th ed. St. Louis: CV Mosby, 2002:1422.

12. Friedman SC, Sheynkin YR. Acute scrotal symptoms due to perforated appendix in children: case report and review of literature. *Pediatr Emerg Care* 1995;181.

13. Garel L, Dubois J, Azzie G, et al. Preoperative manual detorsion of the spermatic cord with Doppler ultrasound monitoring in patients with intravaginal acute testicular torsion. *Pediatr Radiol* 2000;30:41–44.

14. Gilchrist BF, Lobe TE. The acute groin in pediatrics. *Clin Pediatr* 1992;31:488.

15. Gold SJ. *Physicians medical law letter* [monograph]. New York: Prof Liability Pub, 1987.

16. Hagen P, Buchholz MM, Eigenmann J, et al. Testicular dysplasia causing disturbance of spermiogenesis in patient with unilateral torsion of the testis. *Urol Int* 1992;49:154.

17. Hagley M. Epididymo-orchitis and epididymitis: a review of causes and management of unusual forms. *Int J STD AIDS* 2003;14:372–377; quiz 378.

18. Knight PJ, Vassy LE. The diagnosis and treatment of the acute scrotum in children and adolescents. *Ann Surg* 1984;200:664.

19. Kravchick S, Cytron S, Leibovici O, et al. Color Doppler sonography: its real role in the evaluation of children with highly suspected testicular torsion. *Eur Radiol* 2001;11:1000–1005.

20. Lee LM, Wright JE, McLaughlin MG. Testicular torsion in the adult. *J Urol* 1983;130:93.

21. Luzzi GA, O'Brien TS. Acute epididymitis. *BJU Int* 2001;87:747–755.

22. Matteson JR, Stock JA, Hanna MK, et al. Medicolegal aspects of testicular torsion. *Urology* 2001;57:783–786; discussion 786–787.

23. Muschat M. The pathological anatomy of testicular torsion, an explanation of its mechanism. *Surg Gynecol Obstet* 1932;54:758.

24. Prater JM, Overdorf BS. Testicular torsion: a surgical emergency. *Am Fam Physician* 1991;44:834.

25. Procedures for your practice—testicular detorsion. *Patient Care* 1991;143.

26. Rabinowitz R. The importance of the cremasteric reflex in acute scrotal swelling in children. *J Urol* 1984;131:89.

27. Rabinowitz R, Hulbert WC. Acute scrotal swelling. *Urol Clin North Am* 1995; 22:101.

28. Rowland G, Donohue JP. Scrotum and testis. In: Gillenwater JY, Grayhack JT, Howards SS, Duckett JW, eds. *Adult and pediatric urology*, 2nd ed. Chicago: Year Book, 1991:1565.

29. Schneider RE. Urologic procedures. In: Roberts JR, Hedges JR, eds. *Clinical procedures in emergency medicine*, 4th ed. Philadelphia: WB Saunders, 2004.

30. Schwab R. Acute scrotal pain requires quick thinking and plan of action. *Emerg Med Rep* 1992;13:11.

31. Sessions AE, Rabinowitz R, Hulbert WC, et al. Testicular torsion: direction, degree, duration and disinformation. *J Urol* 2003;169:663–665.

32. Smith RD. Testicular torsion: time is the enemy. *ANZ J Surg* 2003;72:316.

33. Wilbert DM, Schaerfe CW, Stern WD, et al. Evaluation of the acute scrotum by color-coded Doppler ultrasonography. *Urology* 1993;149:1475.

34. Williams CR, Heaven KJ, Joseph DB. Testicular torsion: is there a seasonal predilection for occurrence? *Urology* 2003;61:638–641; discussion 641.

CHAPTER 78
Urinary Tract Infections

Eric T. Boie, Deepi G. Goyal, and
Annie T. Sadosty

Urinary tract infections (UTIs) are among the most common infections encountered by the emergency physician. Complaints related to the urinary tract account for 7 million annual outpatient visits (1.5 million emergency department [ED] visits), 1 million hospitalizations, and billions of dollars in health care costs annually (12,27). Although most UTIs are benign, limited-duration infections of healthy hosts, the spectrum of disease includes aggressive infections with significant morbidity and mortality in both competent and compromised hosts. UTI is a leading cause of bacteremia in the elderly (27). Women are affected disproportionately to men prior to age 50 years; young, sexually active women are 30 times more likely than their male contemporaries to have a UTI (27). Fifty percent to 70% of women will have a UTI sometime in their lifetime, placing annual incidence of infection between 3% and 10%. (7,27) Of those women affected, 20% to 30% have more than three UTIs per year (3,7). Although UTIs are reported in 15% of men prior to age 35 years, they are much more common later in life as disorders of the prostate become more prevalent (3). The overall incidence of UTI increases with age, affecting elderly men and women with nearly equal frequency (26).

Urinary tract infections comprise a collection of diseases that can be classified on the basis of both the anatomy and the complexity of the disease. Anatomically, upper urinary tract infections involve the kidney, thereby resulting in pyelonephritis. Pyelonephritis may be chronic, subclinical, or acute; this chapter focuses on management of the latter. Lower UTIs involve the urethra and bladder and result in acute urethritis and acute cystitis respectively.

Urinary tract infections can be further classified as complicated or uncomplicated. A UTI is complicated when associated with a condition that increases risk for acquiring infection, failing therapy, or increased morbidity (28). These associated conditions may be structural (obstruction, catheterization, and renal calculi), metabolic (diabetes, pregnancy, and chronic renal failure), functional (impaired host, acquired immunodeficiency syndrome [AIDS], and neutropenia) or pathogen related. Table 78.1 lists factors that place a patient at risk for a complicated urinary tract infection. Complicated UTIs can range in severity from simple cystitis to urosepsis with shock, therefore it is the associated conditions, not severity of disease, which make a UTI "complicated." It is generally held that all UTIs in males are complicated; many authors argue that true uncomplicated UTIs occur only in nonpregnant, healthy adult females with no neurologic, metabolic, or structural dysfunction (21). Eighty percent of UTIs fall into this group (30).

The urinary tract is normally an enclosed, protected, and sterile mucosal surface. Wash out of bacteria by urine flow is the primary host defense against infection (28). This process is nearly continuous in the upper tract, but only intermittent in the lower. Any interference with normal urine flow and wash out predisposes to UTI (28). The relative virulence of uropathogens differs

TABLE 78.1. Risk Factors for Development
of Complicated UTI

Anatomic/obstruction
  Bladder diverticuli
  Nephrolithiasis
  Other renal structural abnormality
  Polycystic kidney disease
  Prostatic hypertrophy
  Solitary kidney
  Urethral/ureteric stricture
Epidemiologic
  Age >55 years
  Childhood UTI (Prior to age 12 years)
  Hospitalization
  Male
  Pregnancy
Functional
  Incontinence
  Neurogenic bladder
  Urinary retention/increased postvoid residual
Immunosuppression
  Chronic renal failure
  Diabetes mellitus
  Drug or alcohol abuse
  HIV/AIDS
  Organ transplantation
  Sickle cell anemia and trait
  Steroids/Immunosuppressant drugs
Instrumentation
  Indwelling catheter
  Intermittent catheterization
  Ureteric stent
Other
  Prolonged symptoms prior to treatment (>7 days)
  Resistant etiologic organisms
  Treatment failure

UTI, urinary tract infection; HIV, human immunodeficiency virus; AIDS, acquired immunodeficiency syndrome.

Developed for information in articles by Bass PF III et al.,[3] Miller O II and Krieger,[27] and Nicolle LE.[26]

between complicated and uncomplicated UTIs. Bacterial virulence is crucial for overcoming defenses in a normal host (19). Uropathogenic bacteria are highly adapted to ascend, colonize, and grow in the urinary tract, subsequently causing cell damage and infection (35). In contrast, in complicated UTIs bacterial virulence is less important, as host factors largely determine the risk of UTI acquisition, clinical course, and outcome (19). Organisms that rarely cause disease in healthy patients can cause significant disease in hosts with anatomic, metabolic, or immunologic abnormalities (32).

Most uropathogens reside in the colon, with 95% of UTIs resulting from enteric bacteria ascending the urinary tract (27). However, the pathogenesis of UTI differs for men and women. The female urinary tract is prone to colonization with enteric bacteria, owing to the close proximity of the urethra to the rectum, the moist mucosa surrounding the introitus, and the relatively short (3 to 4 cm) female urethra. Although the exact process of infection is unknown, bacteria colonize the vagina and periurethral area, ascend the urethra into the bladder, multiply in the urine, reflux into the ureters, and ultimately colonize and invade the renal parenchyma. The primary risk factors in young healthy women for development of a UTI are recent sexual intercourse, spermicide use, diaphragm or cervical cap use with spermicide, and prior UTI (11,15,19,27). Much traditional teaching that emphasizes behavioral modification to reduce risk of UTI has not been supported in studies. Specifically, volume of water intake, timing of voiding relative to intercourse, direction of wiping, and consumption of cranberry juice or lactobacillus

(yogurt) do not affect risk for development of UTI (19,26). In contrast to that of women, the male genitourinary tract is less conducive to uropathogens. The male urethra is approximately 5 times longer, is distant from the perineum, and is surrounded by dry squamous epithelium rather than by moist mucosa (20). Because most UTIs occur in older men, they are hypothesized to result from bladder obstruction secondary to prostate enlargement, thereby resulting in postresidual urine. Surprisingly, little evidence exists to support this theory (20,21). Instrumentation of the genitourinary tract is a frequent means by which young men develop UTI (21). Risk factors for development of UTI in healthy men include insertive anal intercourse, a sexual partner with the same uropathogen, and lack of circumcision (20,21). Only 5% of UTIs result from hematogenous spread during septicemia, most often in immunocompromised hosts (27). These organisms tend to be more aggressive, thereby causing severe pyelonephritis or even microabscesses within the kidney (2).

The most common uropathogens responsible for development of UTI are enteric gram-negative bacilli of the class Enterobacteriaceae. *Escherichia Coli* is responsible for 80% to 90% of UTIs in reproductive-aged females. *Staphylococcus saprophyticus* causes an additional 5% to 20% of UTIs in this group. Other Enterobacteriaceae and *Enterococcus* are responsible for the balance of UTIs in women (30). In men, *E. Coli* is responsible for approximately one half of all cases of cystitis. *Proteus* and *Providencia* are frequent isolates, with *Klebsiella, Citrobacter, Pseudomonas,* and *Enterobacter* being less common. Gram-positive cocci, including *Enterococcus faecalis, Staphylococcus epidermidis,* and *Staphylococcus aureus* cause about one fifth of UTIs in men (3,21). Causative organisms for urethritis include *Chlamydia trachomatis* (25% to 40%), Neisseria gonorrhoeae (20%), *Ureaplasma, Mycoplasma, Haemophilus,* adenovirus, and herpes simplex virus. Institutionalized, catheterized, and immunosuppressed patients tend to experience UTIs caused by gram-positive cocci, other Enterobacteriaceae, and *Candida* (3). *E. Coli* is less common in these populations, causing less than 40% of infections (30).

CLINICAL PRESENTATION

Asymptomatic Bacteriuria

Asymptomatic bacteriuria (ASB) is simply the presence of bacteriuria in a patient with no symptoms of cystitis or pyelonephritis. ASB is most common in the elderly. Although ASB occurs in only 5% of healthy young women, incidence increases with age to as high as 40% in women older than 60 years (3,30). Rates of ASB in elderly men are similar. Thirty percent of individuals with ASB develop symptomatic UTI within 1 year (30). However, identification of ASB in the elderly is of questionable benefit, as no association with excess morbidity and mortality has been demonstrated. In contrast, the identification of ASB in pregnant women is critical. Although only 4% to 7% of pregnant women will have ASB, if untreated, 30% of these will subsequently develop pyelonephritis, thereby increasing the risk of premature delivery, fetal mortality, or pregnancy-induced hypertension (27,34).

Acute Cystitis

Acute cystitis is most commonly seen in reproductive-aged women and men older than 50. The most typical symptoms include dysuria, frequency, urgency, and suprapubic or abdominal discomfort. Hematuria occurs in up to 40% of women with acute cystitis (16). More general complaints may also be described such as fatigue, malaise, irritability, and diaphoresis (23). Fever (>38°C) and severe abdominal pain are rare and in these cases

TABLE 79.2.   Two glass urine test

| | PRE MASSAGE URINALYSIS | | | POST MASSAGE URINALYSIS | | |
Category	WBC Count	Bacteria	Cultures	WBC Count	Bacteria	Cultures
1	++	+	+	Not Indicated		
II	+ −	+ −	+ −	+	+	+
III A	−	−	−	+	−	−
III B	−	−	−	−	−	−

WBC, white blood cell.

Other than to establish a diagnosis of prostatic abscess, there is little reason to image the prostate in the emergency department.

The diagnosis of chronic bacterial prostatitis should be considered in men with recurrent urinary tract infections, asymptomatic bacteriuria, as well as with perineal discomfort and other urinary tract symptoms. Traditionally the diagnosis has been confirmed by results of the Meares-Stamey 4 glass urine test. In patients with a 10-fold higher concentration of the uropathogen in the prostatic secretions or urine obtained after digital massage of the prostate the diagnosis is definitively established (16).

Distinguishing between the subtypes of CP/CPPS requires pre- and postmassage urinalysis, or expressed prostatic secretions, and urine culture. The inflammatory subtype (IIIA) will have a white blood cell count of greater than 10/hpf, no bacteria, and a negative urine culture. Although the urine white blood cell count may fluctuate over time, less than 10/hpf is normal (16).

The practicality of the 4 glass urine test in the emergency department is debatable. A survey of urologists revealed that 34% of respondents never used the test and 47% rarely did. Treatment of chronic prostatitis did not differ between those who used the 4 glass test and those who did not (15). It has also been shown that prostatic tissue cultures may be positive in the setting of negative urine culture and there may be no difference of bacterial localization rates in prostatic specific specimens in men with CP/CPPS and controls (18,22). Although it is not the gold standard, a 2 glass urine test has been recommended as a cost-effective simple replacement to the 4 glass test. A midstream premassage urine and postmassage initial 10 mL urine samples are obtained. Microscopy and cultures categorize the majority of chronic prostatitis patients almost as accurately (91% sensitivity and specificity) as do prostatic secretions (21) (Table 79.2).

EMERGENCY DEPARTMENT MANAGEMENT

Acute bacterial prostatitis is a serious and potentially severe disease. Because there is little evidence-based literature on management of prostatitis syndromes, treatment is largely empiric. The toxic patient requires parenteral antibiotics, adequate hydration, analgesics, and rest. Drug penetration of the normal prostate is complex and dependent on lipid solubility, degree of protein binding and ionization, size and shape of the molecule, and pH. With acute inflammation there is an increase in prostatic permeability; therefore, acute bacterial prostatitis is generally responsive to a wide variety of antibiotic agents. A urine gram stain may be helpful in guiding the initial therapy but the usual causes of infection are the Enterobacteriaceae gram-negative bacteria. *Escherichia coli* accounts for 65% to 85% of infections, and *Pseudomonas, Klebsiella, Proteus, and Serratia* account for 10% to 15%. Enterococcus and other gram-positive organisms may account

for 5% to 10% of acute infections (20). In sexually active young men, *Neisseria gonorrhoeae* and *Chlamydia trachomatis* should be considered. *Mycoplasma* and *Ureaplasma* have also been implicated as causes of prostatitis (1).

Selection of antibiotics should take into consideration not only the most likely organism but the antibiotic susceptibility data available for the gram-negative uropathogens. The Infectious Diseases Society of America (IDSA) recommends that alternative antibiotics be selected when the resistant rates exceed 10% to 20% (24). The most commonly used oral antimicrobials for bacterial prostatitis have been trimethoprim–sulfamethoxazole (TMP–SMX) and the fluoroquinolones (20). In many areas of the United States the resistance of *E. coli* to TMP–SMX is greater than 25% (23). Fluoroquinolones have been shown to be superior to TMP–SMX, and levofloxacin once a day (500 mg) for 28 days is as effective as ciprofloxacin (500 mg) twice a day for 28 days (16). A total of 4 to 6 weeks of antibiotics may be required owing to difficulty in tissue penetration of the prostate as the inflammation resolves. Patients who cannot tolerate oral medications, appear toxic, are immunocompromised, have urinary retention, or for whom outpatient therapy has failed should be admitted and treated with parenteral broad-spectrum antibiotics. A cephalosporin or aminoglycoside should be given along with a fluoroquinolone or ampicillin. Outpatient therapy for acute bacterial prostatitis should include a fluoroquinolone or TMP–SMX (20) (Table 79.3). Although most patients respond to therapy, complications may include chronic bacterial prostatitis, epididymitis, bacteremia, prostatic abscess, and metastatic spread of the infection.

TABLE 79.3.   Treatment Recommendations

NIH Consensus Category	Antibiotic/Dosage
Category I parenteral cephalosporin+ quinolone or aminoglycoside+ampicillins continue therapy with oral antibiotics on the basis of culture results for 4 weeks	Ceftriaxone 1–2 g i.v. q.d. Cefoxamine 1–2 g i.v. q.6.h.–q.8.h. Gentamycin or tobramycin 3–5 mg/kg/day q.6.h. Ampicillin 1–2 g i.v. q.6.h. Levofloxacin 500 mg i.v./p.o. q.d.
Category II oral fluroquinolone or TMP–SMX (based on resistance rate of gram-negative rods) for 4–12 weeks	Levofloxacin 500 mg p.o. q.d. Ciprofloxacin 500 mg p.o. q.d. TMP–SMX 1 p.o. b.i.d. (160 mg/ 800 mg b.i.d.)
Category III treat symptomatically with sitz baths and analgesics; consider antibiotics as in Category II if timely referral is unavailable	

TMP–SMX, trimetuoprim–sulfamethoxazole.

Chronic bacterial prostatitis is usually caused by the same bacterial flora that causes acute bacterial infection, and recurrent infections are generally caused by the same organism that caused the prior infection. Treatment strategies for chronic bacterial prostatitis include both full-dose prolonged antibiotic therapy for 4 to 12 weeks or daily suppressive therapy (8). The decision to place the patient on suppressive therapy is best left to the urologist or primary care physician.

Management of CP/CPPS is often difficult for the physician and frustrating for the patient. Although this condition may be noninfectious, some clinicians will treat the inflammatory subtype with a trial of antibiotics for the possibility of infections caused by *Chlamydia, Mycoplasma,* or *Ureaplasma* (1). A recent study that compared tissue cultures from prostate biopsy of asymptomatic controls to patients with CP/CPPS demonstrated that patients in category IIIA had more positive cultures than patients in category IIIB, but there was no statistical difference between cultures in controls compared to those in category III (11). One Canadian multicenter, randomized, placebo-controlled study demonstrated no difference in symptom improvement after 6 weeks of levofloxacin compared to placebo (19). Symptomatic treatment with sitz baths and nonsteroidal antiinflammatory medications may be helpful. α-Blockers, allopurinol, hormones, muscle relaxants, and a variety of nontraditional therapies have been recommended for CP/CPPS, but there is insufficient evidence to justify their routine use in the emergency department (20).

CRITICAL INTERVENTION

- Initiate parenteral antibiotic therapy for toxic patients with acute bacterial prostatitis

DISPOSITION

Toxic patients with acute bacterial prostatitis should be admitted to the hospital for parenteral antibiotics. Because outpatient treatment of both acute and chronic bacterial prostatitis is prolonged and based on urinalysis, culture results, and, in many cases, biopsy, it is important to involve the patient's urologist or primary care physician in management and followup decisions. Performing a 2 glass urine test may be a cost-effective, simple method for categorizing prostatitis. Because the etiology of CP/CPPS may be multifactorial, treatment is difficult. Patients with CP/CPPS should be treated symptomatically and referred to a urologist. If subspecialty referral is not easily obtainable, a trial of antibiotics for patients with CP/CPPS is reasonable.

COMMON PITFALLS

✔ Digital massage of the prostate and urethral catheterization should be avoided in bacterial acute prostatitis
✔ Failure to place a suprapubic catheter in the setting of bladder outlet obstruction from acutely inflamed prostate
✔ Empiric treatment of acute bacterial prostatitis should be as if the patient had gram-negative rods
✔ Imaging of the prostate in the emergency department is unnecessary except for the suspicion of an abscess

Acknowledgments

Thank you to previous edition chapter authors David S. Howes and Erica E. Remer.

References

1. Brunner H, Weidner W, Schiefer HG. Studies on the role of Ureaplasma and Mycoplasma in prostatitis. *J Infect Dis* 1983;147:507–513.
2. Bundrick W, Heron SP, Ray P, et al. Levofloxacin vs. ciprofloxacin in the treatment of chronic bacterial prostatitis in a randomized double-blind multicenter study. *Urology* 2003;62:537–541.
3. Chia JK, Longield RN. Computerized axial tomography in the early diagnosis of prostatic abscess. *Am J Med* 1986;81:942–944.
4. Clairmont GJ, Zon L, et al. Haemophilus parainfluenzae prostatitis in a homosexual man *Am J Med* 1987;82:175.
5. Collins M, Stafford RS, O'Leary MP, Barry MJ. How common is prostatitis? A National Survey of Physician Visits. *J Urology* 1998;159:1224–1228.
6. Gibly RL. Infections of the urinary tract and male genitalia. In: Brillman JC, Quenzer RW, eds. *Infectious disease in emergency medicine,* 2nd ed. New York: Lippincott-Raven, 1998:601–627.
7. Hircahada JP, Vilana R. Transrectal Prostatic ultrasonography in acute bacterial prostatitis: findings and clinical implications. *Scand J Infect Dis* 2003;35:114–120.
8. Krieger JN. *Infect Dis Clin North Am* 2003;17:395–409.
9. Krieger J, Nyberg L Jr., Nickel JC. NIH Consensus definition and classification of prostatitis. *JAMA* 1999;282:236–237.
10. Krieger JN, Egan KJ, Ross SO, et al. Chronic pelvic pain represent the most prominent urogenital symptom of chronic prostatitis. *Urology* 1996;48:715–721.
11. Lee JC, Muller CH, Rothman I, et al. Prostate biopsy culture findings of men with chronic pelvic pain syndrome do not differ from those of healthy controls. *J Urol* 2003;169:584–587.
12. Leporte C, Rousseau F, et al. Bacterial Prostatitis in patients infected with HIV. *J Urol* 1989;141:334–336.
13. Lipsky BA. Prostatitis and urinary tract infections in men: what's new; what's true? *Am J Med* 1999;106:327–334.
14. Ludwig M, Schroeder-Printzou I. Comparison of expressed prostatic secretions with urine after prostatic massage. *Urology* 2000;90:24–32.
15. McNaughton-Collins M, Fowler FJ, Elliot DB, et al. Diagnosing and treating chronic prostatitis, do urologists use the 4 glass test? *Urology* 2000;55:403–407.
16. Meares EM Jr., Stamey TA. Bacteriologic localization patterns in bacterial prostatitis and urethritis. *Invest Urol* 1968;5:492–518.
17. Moon TD, Hagen L, Heisey DM. Urinary Symptomatology in younger men. *Urology* 1997;50:700–703.
18. Nickel JC, Alexander RB, Schaeffer AJ. Leukocytes and bacteria in men with chronic prostatitis/chronic pelvic pain syndrome compared to asymptomatic controls. *J Urol* 2003;170:818–822.
19. Nickel JC, Downey J, Clark J. Levofloxacin for chronic prostatitis/pelvic pain syndrome. *Urology* 2003;62:614–617.
20. Nickel JC. Prostatitis and related conditions. In: Walsh PC, ed. *Campbell's urology.* Philadelphia: Saunders, 2002:603–630.
21. Nickel JC. The pre and post massage test: a simple screen for prostatitis. *Tech Urol* 1997;3:38–43.
22. Nickel JC, Costerton JW. Bacterial localization in antibiotic-refractory chronic bacterial prostatitis. *Prostate* 1993;23:107–114.
23. Sahm DF, Thornsberry C, Mayfield DC, et al. Multidrug resistant urinary tract isolates of *Escherichia coli. Antimicrob Agents Chemother* 2001;45:1402–1406.
24. Warren JW, Abrutyn E, Hebel JR, et al. Guidelines for antimicrobial treatment of uncomplicated acute bacterial cystitis and acute pyelonephritis in women. *Clin Infect Dis* 1999;29:745.

CHAPTER 80
Fournier's Gangrene

Gregory W. Hendey and Robert E. Schneider

Originally described in 1764 by Baurienne, perineal gangrene today bears the name of Jean-Alfred Fournier, a French dermatologist, who described a case in 1883 (4). Fournier's gangrene is the most severe end of a spectrum of scrotal and perineal infections, ranging from cellulitis to abscesses to necrotizing gangrene. Primary abscesses of the scrotal skin may originate from

but they usually signify other causes of abdominal pain such as appendicitis, pelvic inflammatory disease, diverticulitis, or a perforated viscus. The testes should be examined to evaluate for other causes of testicular pain.

Typical symptoms of *vesical calculi* are pain on voiding and hematuria. The pain, which may be dull or sharp, is often severe, with exercise or sudden movement, at the end of micturition. Hematuria often occurs at the end of voiding. Interruption of the urinary stream from impaction of the stone at the bladder neck may occur. Frequency, urgency, and dysuria are present in up to 50% of patients. Urinary tract infection is common, especially if an indwelling catheter is present. Some patients, especially those with prostatic enlargement, have no symptoms directly referable to the calculi but present only with symptoms of outflow obstruction.

DIFFERENTIAL DIAGNOSIS

The differential diagnosis of a patient with suspected urinary calculus is sizable (Table 81.2). Urologic diseases that simulate urolithiasis may be divided according to anatomic site. Upper tract diseases include renal infarct, which results in sudden pain, hematuria, and leukocytosis, and produces a characteristic rise in serum transaminase levels, especially serum lactate dehydrogenase. Renal tumors may present as acute hemorrhage into the tumor, producing symptoms that are similar to those of a renal stone. The upper ureter may be obstructed by urethral tumors, blood clots (especially in anticoagulated patients), and sloughed renal papillae. Sloughed renal papillae are seen in patients with sickle cell disease, analgesic abuse, and diabetes mellitus. Ureteral obstruction may be secondary to prior urologic instrumentation, tuberculosis, ureteral strictures, surgery, intrinsic urothelial tumors, or metastasis from tumors such as breast cancer.

Nonurologic causes of diseases that may simulate urolithiasis are commonly a result of intraabdominal or retroperitoneal conditions such as peritonitis, abdominal aortic aneurysm, appendicitis, diverticulitis, biliary colic, ovarian cyst, retroperitoneal lymphadenopathy from tumors (the most common of which is lymphoma), and retroperitoneal fibrosis.

A Münchhausen-like syndrome is sometimes seen in the ED evaluation of suspected urolithiasis. These patients are typically itinerant and quite knowledgeable about urolithiasis. They often give a history of uric acid urolithiasis and a contrast medium allergy, usually of an anaphylactic nature. The hematuria usually resolves when the urine is collected in the presence of a nurse or physician. These patients typically require large doses of intravenous or intramuscular narcotics to alleviate pain. This group of patients poses a significant management problem for the physician, and the burden of proof is on the physician to rule out a true pathologic process.

EMERGENCY DEPARTMENT EVALUATION

It is important to be certain that an *obstructive* calculus does not coexist with urinary infection, because such patients are at significant risk for the development of urosepsis. The ED evaluation of patients with suspected renal stone should reflect these concerns.

The most important initial laboratory test is the urinalysis. Most patients with urolithiasis have hematuria, but 10% to 15% do not. The urinalysis may reveal the presence of crystalluria. Crystals of calcium oxalate, the coffin lids of struvite, and the hexagonal crystals of cystine are easily recognized. A pH greater than 7.5 in a fresh urine specimen suggests infection with urea-splitting organisms. Culture is helpful in such cases.

Serum electrolyte levels are usually normal; however, prolonged vomiting may lead to metabolic alkalosis. Hyperchloremic metabolic acidosis occurs with renal insufficiency or distal renal tubular acidosis. Serum creatinine levels are usually normal but can be elevated in cases of prolonged, high-grade obstruction. Hypercalcemia (calcium level greater than 10.2 mg/dL) in a patient with nephrolithiasis often signals the presence of primary hyperparathyroidism. Leukocytosis is common owing to demargination of white blood cells caused by the stress of renal colic and does not necessarily suggest infection alone.

Radiologic studies are essential in establishing the diagnosis of urolithiasis. Approximately 90% of urinary calculi contain calcium, but most studies report that less than one half are actually visualized on plain radiographs. An imaging study such as helical abdominal computed tomography (CT) or intravenous pyelography (IVP) is necessary for the initial diagnosis of urolithiasis. Most investigators recommend that plain films are unnecessary. Spiral or helical CT has emerged as the diagnostic procedure of choice in many EDs for the evaluation of patients with suspected urolithiasis.

With sensitivity and specificity ranging from 96% to 100%, no other noninvasive diagnostic procedure can equal non–contrast-enhanced spiral CT (7). Furthermore, non–contrast-enhanced spiral CT is a more rapid test than IVP and is without the risks associated with intravenous contrast administration. Spiral computed tomographic scanning is also useful for the accurate prediction of ureteral obstruction (8). Spiral computed tomographic scanning has even been used experimentally to predict stone composition *in vitro*, but it has yet to be proven in human studies (1,16). CT provides excellent demonstration of renal and ureteral calculi, including radiolucent calculi, and gives information regarding the presence or absence of hydronephrosis and the degree of obstruction (Fig. 81.1). In addition, CT may provide useful information about other retroperitoneal and intraabdominal conditions in approximately 16% of cases (4). The main disadvantage of CT is its greater expense compared with that of IVP, but this difference has been decreasing over time.

IVP is an alternative that is less often used now in the ED, although it still remains a viable diagnostic modality if CT is unavailable. Findings on a positive study include a delayed nephrogram, columnization, dilation of the kidney and collecting system, and visualization of the stone (Fig. 81.2). Extravasation occasionally occurs with complete obstruction and subsequent

---

TABLE 81.2. Diseases that Simulate Urolithiasis

Urologic Disease
  Renal infarct
  Renal parenchymal tumors
  Papillary necrosis
  Pyelonephritis
  Hematoma
  Ureteral stricture
  Urinary retention
Non-Urologic Disease
  Appendicitis
  Diverticulitis
  Biliary colic
  Intestinal obstruction
  Abdominal aortic aneurysm
  Retroperitoneal adenopathy
  Tumor
  Ovarian cyst
  Endometriosis
  Musculoskeletal back pain

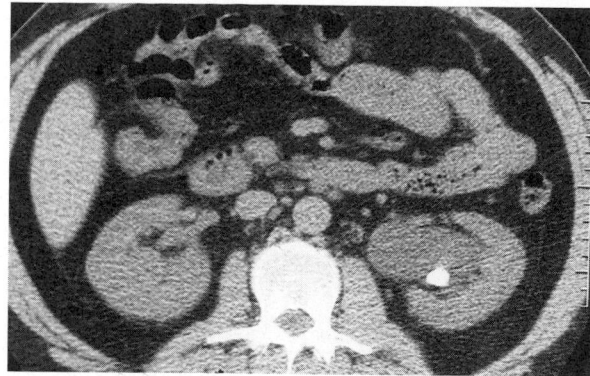
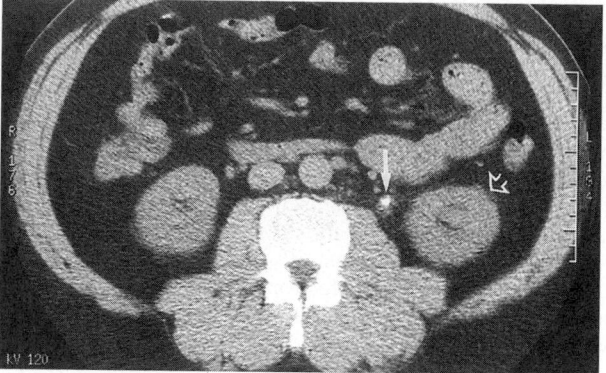

Figure 81.1.   Noncontrast spiral computed tomography (CT). **A:** Large stone in the hydronephrotic left kidney. **B:** A 5-mm stone in the ureter, surrounded by soft tissue—the "soft tissue rim" sign (*solid arrow*). Also note minimal left perinephric stranding near inferior pole of kidney (*open arrow*). (From [West OC, Tamm EP, Kawashima A, Jarolimek AM. Nontraumatic emergencies. In: Harris JH Jr, ed. *The radiology of emergency medicine,* 4th edition. Philadelphia: Lippincott Williams & Wilkins, 2000:622] with permission.)

rupture of a calyceal fornix, but it is usually self-limited and benign if the duration of obstruction is short and infection is absent. It is important to identify patients with prior contrast medium reactions and preexisting renal insufficiency before using IVP.

In some cases, it is desirable to avoid both contrast and radiation (i.e., pregnancy). Ultrasound emerges as a third alternative in the diagnosis of urolithiasis. Ultrasonography may detect lucent or opaque renal stones, as well as hydronephrosis. However, most ureteral stones cannot be identified by using ultrasonography, and the reported sensitivity is lower than that of either CT scan or IVP.

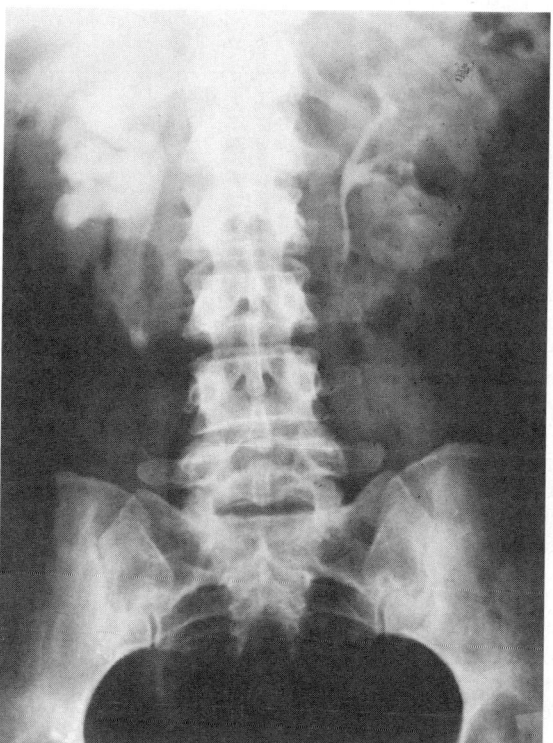

Figure 81.2.   Intravenous pyelogram demonstrating marked dilation of the renal collecting system and ureter proximal to the calculus. A stone of this size has a less than 10% chance of spontaneous passage, and, therefore, immediate urologic intervention is appropriate.

EMERGENCY DEPARTMENT MANAGEMENT

The therapeutic goals in the ED are to make the proper diagnosis and provide relief of the pain. If the pain is typical colic, or if the patient has had similar pain with previous stones, then pain medication should be administered immediately without waiting for the results of diagnostic tests. If the pain is atypical and an intraabdominal process is suspected, judicious pain medication may be administered and appropriate workup for the etiology of abdominal pain initiated. Morphine and meperidine (Demerol) are common parenteral narcotics used in treating colic, and large and repeated doses of either may be necessary to relieve the initial pain. Once the initial ureteral spasm is relieved, however, the patient's pain often will be quite mild, if it returns at all. Anticholinergic, spasmolytic, or antiinflammatory medications, commonly used in Europe, have not been found to be uniformly useful in the United States.

The pain of ureteral colic is mediated by prostaglandins released by the ureter in response to dilation. Prostaglandins act to increase peristaltic action of the ureter to aid in passage of the stone, but they also sensitize nociceptors to stimuli such as bradykinin, thereby inducing pain and visceral responses to prostaglandins (nausea and vomiting) (19). Nonsteroidal antiinflammatory drugs (NSAIDs) inhibit the prostaglandin synthesis pathways and decrease glomerular filtration. Ketorolac (Toradol) is the only parenteral NSAID available in the United States, and when given parenterally, it is as effective as narcotics in relieving the pain of ureteral obstruction (3). Maximal pain relief using ketorolac has been shown to occur approximately 45 to 60 minutes after a parenteral dose. It would seem reasonable for treatment of severe pain to use a narcotic analgesic with a fast onset (i.e., Fentanyl) given simultaneously with the initial dose of a NSAID such as ketorolac.

Ketorolac should be used with caution in patients with a history of gastrointestinal bleeding, renal insufficiency, cardiovascular disease, or recent regular NSAID use. Acute decreases in renal blood flow (35%) were noted after acute infusion of ketorolac in a unilateral ureteral obstruction dog model (14). Acute, transient renal failure occurred in six patients with cardiovascular disease when given ketorolac (6).

Nausea and vomiting are common with ureteral colic and can be exacerbated by narcotics. In such patients, administration of an antiemetic agent is appropriate. Intravenous fluid therapy has not been clearly demonstrated to improve outcome in acute urolithiasis, but in patients that are volume depleted, intravenous fluid therapy is reasonable. Current stone-dissolving agents play a limited role in active renal stone treatment, and the main options are either conservative or surgical (22).

Infected stones, or calculus pyelonephritis, can be associated with significant morbidity, especially in the setting of high-grade urinary obstruction (8). The common organisms in urine and blood cultures are *E. coli*, and *Proteus* and *Klebsiella* species. Bacteremia is seen in 70%, and septic shock occurs in approximately 20% (9). Antimicrobial coverage, usually with fluoroquinolones, is directed at these organisms. Infection in the setting of high-grade obstructive uropathy often requires emergent decompression, or drainage of the kidney.

Urologic Interventions

The acute management of urinary tract stones is dependent on the presence of related complications, namely renal impairment secondary to an obstructing calculus (acute obstruction alone is not a primary indication for intervention) (15). In these cases, emergency drainage is required and can be achieved either by placement of a nephrostomy catheter or a retrograde stent. Neither method is of proven superiority, and often the choice between nephrostomy and retrograde stent is based on local experience and resources. In the presence of significant sepsis and thick pus, a nephrostomy may be preferable (15).

Several technologic advancements have revolutionized the treatment of symptomatic urolithiasis in the last several decades (Table 81.3). The most important of these advancements has been the development of extracorporeal shock wave lithotripsy (ESWL). This technology has proven effective in the management of 85% to 90% of urolithiasis cases that require intervention. Patients with large stones (i.e., greater than 2 cm in diameter), cystine stones, and staghorn calculi are much less likely to become stone-free with ESWL monotherapy (Fig. 81.3).

Another important technologic advance is percutaneous nephrostolithotomy (PCNL), which involves the establishment of a tract from the skin into the renal collecting system through which stones can be fragmented with ultrasonic, laser, electrohydraulic, or pneumatic devices and removed by using various endoscopes, grasping forceps, and stone baskets.

Ureteral calculi can also be managed effectively with ureteroscopy with or without stenting. This allows visualization of the entire ureter from the bladder to renal pelvis and removal of ureteral calculi under direct visualization. Various energy sources (ultrasound, laser, electrohydraulic, and pneumatic) can be used through the ureteroscope to fragment stones if necessary. Ureterorenoscopy is most successful when applied to stones in the distal ureter. In general, upper ureteral calculi tend to be managed with ESWL or nephroscopy, whereas ureteroscopy is commonly used for distal ureteral stones (17).

In addition to the treatment of existing symptomatic stones, an important goal is to prevent further stone formation. Medical therapy based on a careful metabolic stone evaluation can dramatically reduce the incidence of recurrent stone formation

TABLE 81.3.   Current Options for Urolithiasis Management (in Decreasing Order of Invasiveness)

1. Open surgery
2. Percutaneous nephrostolithotomy
3. Ureteroscopy
4. Extracorporeal shock wave lithotripsy
5. Observation

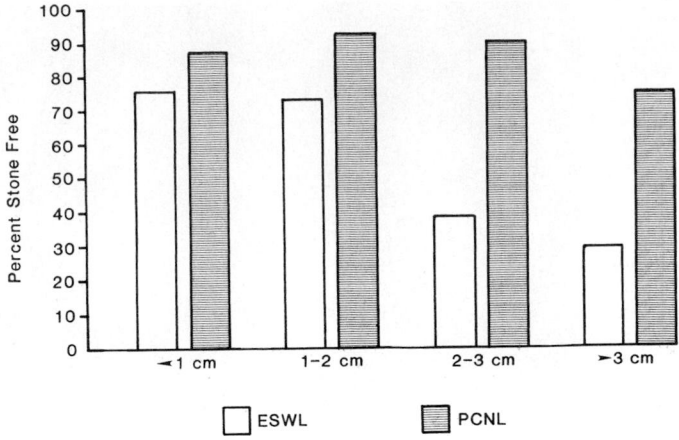

Figure 81.3.   Percentage of patients who are stone-free after extracorporeal shock wave lithotripsy (ESWL) and percutaneous nephrostolithotomy (PCNL), stratified by initial stone size. Most ureteral calculi are less than 2 cm in diameter.

(12,13). This evaluation may be initiated in the ED or during followup evaluation, by checking serum electrolyte levels (looking for distal or type I renal tubular acidosis) and serum calcium level (hypercalcemia usually indicates primary hyperparathyroidism). More detailed studies (i.e., 24-hour urine collections) should be delayed for 2 to 4 weeks after resolution of an acute stone event.

CRITICAL INTERVENTIONS

- Search for evidence of concomitant urine infection
- Use helical CT to establish the correct diagnosis of urolithiasis, evaluate for alternate diagnoses, and to assess for high-grade obstructive uropathy
- Provide adequate analgesia with a combination of opiate and NSAID medications.

DISPOSITION

Once the diagnosis of a stone has been made and the patient has been made comfortable, disposition of the case should be made in conjunction with the consulting urologist who will be responsible for the patient's ongoing care. The most common factor that necessitates patient admission is pain that is refractory to oral pain medications. Once the patient has been made comfortable with parenteral medications, an oral narcotic or NSAID should be prescribed for continued pain. If pain relief is inadequate, admission will be necessary for pain control. Persistent nausea and vomiting, obstruction with infection, and urinary extravasation are other indications for admission (Table 81.4).

Infection in the presence of high-grade obstruction from a stone is a urologic emergency that necessitates not only admission, but also immediate urologic intervention. This situation essentially represents an abscess with ready vascular access by way of the renal circulation. The appropriate therapy for this, as with any abscess, is drainage. The obstructed kidney can be drained either by cystoscopy and passage of a ureteral catheter or by placement of a percutaneous nephrostomy tube. Both procedures can be readily accomplished under local anesthesia. Antibiotics alone are not adequate therapy in these circumstances, because the patient can experience continued bacteremic

TABLE 81.4. Indications for Admission

Obstruction with infection
Pain not controlled by oral analgesics
Persistent nausea and vomiting
Urinary extravasation
Hypercalcemic crisis

RELATIVE INDICATIONS FOR ADMISSION

High-grade obstruction
Solitary kidney
Intrinsic renal disease
Size of obstructing stone
Duration of symptoms
Social situation

showering, progression to frank urosepsis, and rapid destruction of the involved kidney until drainage is achieved. Stabilization of ongoing sepsis and vascular instability should not take precedence over drainage in these patients, because improvement may not occur until the septic source is removed. Effective drainage can be achieved rapidly, and delay in drainage can lead to significant mortality.

Other factors deserve consideration in determining the disposition of the patient. The likelihood that the patient will be able to pass the calculus without intervention should be considered. Factors to weigh in this regard include the duration of symptoms and the size of the obstructing stone. Ureteral calculi less than 5 mm in greatest dimension usually pass spontaneously, whereas those greater than 8 mm rarely do (21). Patients with high-grade obstruction according to CT or IVP are more likely to require intervention and admission. Patients with a solitary kidney or underlying intrinsic renal disease are more likely to experience significant decrease in overall renal function with any degree of obstruction; therefore, the threshold for admission of such patients is lower. In addition, calculi that develop in renal transplantation patients most often should be managed in the inpatient setting to best preserve the graft.

Most patients who present to an ED with renal calculi may be discharged. Sufficient oral narcotic agents, NSAID, and an antiemetic agent should be prescribed. Prophylactic antibiotics are not necessary. Patients should be instructed to strain their urine and save any solid material for analysis. They should be told to return to the ED immediately or seek medical attention for recurrent severe pain, persistent vomiting, or the onset of fever. Outpatient urologic followup should be arranged within 1 to 2 weeks.

COMMON PITFALLS

✔ The most common misdiagnosis in patients ultimately found to have abdominal aortic aneurysm is kidney stone. Helical CT can evaluate for both conditions
✔ Pain not responding to appropriate pain control measures is often associated with high-grade obstruction

References

1. Bartfield JM, Kern AM, Raccio-Robak N, et al. Ketorolac tromethamine use in a university-based emergency department. *Acad Emerg Med* 1994;1.532–538.
2. Boyce WH, Garvey FK, Strawcutter HE. Incidence of urinary calculi among patients in general hospitals: 1948–1952. *JAMA* 1956;161:1427.
3. Colistro R, Torreggiani WC, Lyburn ID, et al. Unenhanced helical CT in the investigation of acute flank pain. *Clin Radiol* 2002;57:435–441.
4. Cordell WH, Wright SW, Wolfson AB, et al. Comparison of intravenous ketorolac, meperidine, and both (balanced analgesia) for renal colic. *Ann Emerg Med* 1996;28:151–158.
5. Corelli RL, Gericke KR. Renal insufficiency associated with intramuscular administration of ketorolac tromethamine. *Ann Pharmacother* 1993;27:1055–1057.
6. Elton TJ, Roth CS, Berquist TH, et al. A clinical prediction rule for the diagnosis of ureteral calculi in emergency departments. *J Gen Intern Med* 1993;8:57–62.
7. Fielding JR, Fox LA, Heller H, et al. Spiral CT in the evaluation of flank pain: overall accuracy and feature analysis. *J Comput Assist Tomogr* 1997;21:635–638.
8. Koga S, Arakaki Y, Matsuoka M, Ohyama C. Calculous pyelonephritis. *Int Urol Nephrol* 1992;24:109–112.
9. Lingeman JE, Coury TA, Newman DM, et al. Comparison of results and morbidity of percutaneous nephrostolithotomy and extracorporeal shock wave lithotripsy. *J Urol* 1987;138:485–490.
10. Mostafavi MR, Ernst RD, Saltzman B. Accurate determination of chemical composition of urinary calculi by spiral computerized tomography. *J Urol* 1998;159:673–675.
11. Pak CY, Britton F, Peterson R, et al. Ambulatory evaluation of nephrolithiasis. classification, clinical presentation and diagnostic criteria. *Am J Med* 1980;69:19–30.
12. Perlmutter A, Miller L, Trimble LA, et al. Toradol, an NSAID used for renal colic, decreases renal perfusion and ureteral pressure in a canine model of unilateral ureteral obstruction. *J Urol* 1993;149:926–930.
13. Richards JR, Christman CA. Intravenous urography in the emergency department: when do we need it? *Eur J Emerg Med* 1999;6:129–133.
14. Sandhu C, Anson KM, Patel U. Urinary tract stones—Part II: current status of treatment. *Clin Radiol* 2003;58:422–433.
15. Saw KC, Lingeman JE, McAteer JA, et al. Spiral CT scan for predicting stone composition: the effect of CT collimation and stone size. In: *American Urological Association national meeting,* vol. 1. Dallas: AUA Press, 1999.
16. Segura JW, Preminger GM, Assimos DG, et al. Ureteral Stones Clinical Guidelines Panel summary report on the management of ureteral calculi. *J Urol* 1997;158:1915–1921.
17. Selmy GI, Hassouna MM, Khalaf IM, et al. Effects of verapamil, prostaglandin F2 alpha, phenylephrine, and noradrenaline on upper respiratory tract dynamics. *Urology* 1994;43:31–35.
18. Shuster J, Schaeffer RL. Economic impact of kidney stones in white male adults. *Urology* 1984;24:327–331.
19. Ueno A, Kawamura T, Ogawa A, et al. Relation of spontaneous passage of ureteral calculi to size. *Urology* 1977;10:544–546.
20. Vieweg C, Teh C, Freed K, et al. Unenhanced helical computerized tomography for the evaluation of patients with acute flank pain. *J Urol* 1998;160:679–684.
21. Westenberg A, Harper M, Zafirakis H, Shah PJ. Bladder and renal stones: management and treatment. *Hosp Med* 2002;63:34–41.

CHAPTER 82
Urinary Incontinence and Retention

Stephen J. Wolf

Micturition is a process that relies on the nervous, musculoskeletal, and genitourinary systems. Disruption of the physiologic "flow" of any of these systems can potentially lead to urinary dysfunction, be it incontinence or retention. Urinary dysfunction in and of itself, following bladder decompression in urinary retention, is not an emergency. The key aspect for an emergency physician in treating patients with incontinence or retention is ruling out emergent causes or complications of the urinary dysfunction (e.g., spinal cord compression or acute postobstructive nephropathy). Often times in doing this, the emergency physician is able to identify key contributing pathology. Once the emergency issues are ruled out, most patients can be referred for an outpatient workup of their urinary complaints.

CLINICAL PRESENTATION

Urinary incontinence is the involuntary loss of urine, often associated with social embarrassment, isolation, depression, and hygienic complications. It can be attributed to a sudden increase in intraabdominal pressure (stress incontinence), involuntary bladder contractions (urge incontinence), a mixture of the two (mixed incontinence), overflow in the setting of urinary retention (overflow incontinence), complete disruption of the continence apparatus (true incontinence), or nonpathologic causes (functional incontinence).

Urinary retention is the inability to void voluntarily, resulting in painful or nonpainful bladder distention, depending on the duration of onset. With this distention, symptoms of prostatism often develop, including frequency, urgency, hesitancy, dribbling, decrease in voiding stream, and a sense of incomplete emptying. This can further progress to acute or chronic postobstructive nephropathy. These symptoms may be exacerbated with the application of suprapubic pressure (the *Credé maneuver*). In the past this maneuver has been used to initiate voiding in patients with retention; however, it is not recommended because of high complication rates and poor efficiency.

Although urinary retention is often considered a disorder of elderly men with enlarged prostates, it can affect men and women of all ages and even is seen in children. Often the retention is insidious in its onset, resulting from chronic progressive obstructive or neurosensory causes (e.g., diabetes); however, acute presentations do occur, especially in the setting of urologic infections, certain medications, or neurologically related insults.

DIFFERENTIAL DIAGNOSIS

Urinary Incontinence

Stress urinary incontinence (SUI) results when a rapid rise in intraabdominal pressure is transmitted to the bladder, thereby causing a leakage of urine. This can be from sneezing, coughing, laughing, exercise, and so forth. Normally the vesiculourethral anatomy is such that this transmitted abdominal pressure results in a narrowing of the posterior ureterovesical angle, making leakage of urine more difficult. However, this is not the case if there is hypermobility of the urethra or a laxity in the intrinsic urethral sphincter. There are several risk factors to these physiologic abnormalities. Nearly 85% of SUI occurs in women who have given birth, which can cause a laxity of the anterior vaginal wall and pelvic floor musculature. This results in urethral hypermobility. Other risk factors include obesity and previous urinary incontinence surgery. The intrinsic urethral sphincter deficiency can result from mechanical issues (trauma, surgery, and chronic bladder overdistention) or from neurophysiologic issues (estrogen deficiency, diabetes, corticosteroid therapy, and radiation therapy). Although the majority of SUI occurs in women, transurethral resection of the prostate (TURP) is a particular risk factor in men, and structural abnormalities should be considered as a cause for SUI in children.

Urge incontinence occurs when there is uninhibited involuntary contraction of the detrusor muscle and bladder wall (*detrusor instability*). This is often called a "spastic bladder" or an "overactive bladder." Detrusor instability is the most common cause

of urinary incontinence among the elderly, with a prevalence of 40% to 70%. Urinary frequency and urgency are often associated, whereas dysuria is not in the absence of a urinary tract infection. Up to 90% of these cases are considered to be idiopathic. The remaining 10% result from bladder wall irritation/inflammation, urethral syndrome, and neurologic causes.

Bladder wall irritation and inflammation are usually caused by urinary infections. Treatment often results in resolution of the urge incontinence. Cystitis can, however, also be caused by calculi, radiation, medications (cyclophosphamide, bacille Calmette-Guérin (BCG) vaccine), or carcinoma in situ. *Interstitial cystitis* is an idiopathic, noninfectious, inflammatory cystitis involving the muscular layers of the bladder wall. It usually affects women in their third decade of life and results in progressive vesicular fibrosis, resulting in eventual decreased bladder compliance and capacity.

Urethral Syndrome, a disorder that commonly affects women, is a syndrome that consists of urgency, frequency, and dysuria. It is often clinically misdiagnosed as infectious cystitis, however; urine cultures are negative and the urinary sediment is noninflammatory, showing squamous epithelial cells regardless of estrogen status.

Neurologic causes of urge incontinence include, but are not limited to, stroke, multiple sclerosis, hydrocephalus, and supra sacral spinal cord lesions (acute cord compression or cauda equina syndrome). In these instances the normal physiologic relations between the detrusor-sphincter reflexes, pontine micturition center, and sacral micturition center can be disturbed resulting in detrusor hyperreflexia as opposed to instability.

Often the diagnosis of stress versus urge incontinence is not straight forward, and the clinical pictures overlap yielding a mixed incontinence diagnosis. Fifty percent to 60% of patients presenting for evaluation of SUI also have an urgency component.

Overflow incontinence is a form of incontinence that occurs in the setting of obstructive urinary retention. Obstruction can result in constant dribbling, frequency, and an urge incontinence pattern with detrusor instability.

True incontinence occurs in the absence of stress or urge and is usually a result of complete disruption of the continence apparatus or fistula formation, functionally producing a "'drainspout urethra.'" This can result from trauma, prolonged third stage of parturition, vaginal or cesarean deliveries, surgeries (TURP or previous urethral surgeries), or malignant erosion or ischemic disease from operative, chemical, or radiation factors. Congenital abnormalities are also a cause for true incontinence in children.

Finally, functional or nonpathologic incontinence needs to be considered in the differential diagnosis. Functional incontinence is not caused by pathology in the continence anatomy and physiology but rather by an inability to appropriately void because of physical or psychologic constraints on making it to the bathroom on time. Such constraints would include altered mental status, ethanol intoxication, isolated urinary tract infection, medication use, depression, excessive urine production, or restricted mobility. Other nonpathologic causes of incontinence include enuresis in the pediatric population and incontinence for other psychologic gains. The latter is associated with a sparing of nighttime incontinence while the patient sleeps.

Medications often contribute to urinary incontinence through causing detrusor instability, decreasing sphincter tone, causing urinary retention with subsequent overflow incontinence, and altering the patient's sensorium resulting in a functional incontinence. Table 82.1 lists classes of medications that may contribute to urinary incontinence. An often referred to mnemonic for transient causes of urinary incontinence can be found in Table 82.2.

TABLE 82.1.   Medication Classes Contributing to Voiding Dysfunction*

Drug classes that can contribute to urinary retention[†]
  α-Adrenergic agents
  Antiarrhythmic
  Anticholinergics[‡]
    Antidepressants
  Antihistamines[‡]
    Antiparkinsonian agents
    Antipsychotics[‡]
    Antispasmodics
    β-Adrenergic agents
    Calcium channel blockers
    Opioids[‡]
Drug classes that can contribute to urinary incontinence
  Alcohol[‡]
    α-Adrenergic antagonists
    Caffeine
    Diuretics
    Sedative–hypnotics[‡]
  Sympatholytics

*Prescription and over-the-counter.
[†]Medications that contribute to urinary retention can also contribute to overflow urinary incontinence.
[‡]Medications that can alter sensorium can also contribute to urinary incontinence.

Urinary Retention

Urinary retention is most often the result of obstruction; however, it can also result from neuropathologic disease, pharmacologic side effects, or psychogenic causes. Special congenital considerations also arise when considering the etiology of urinary retention in the pediatric population (see Table 82.3). Urinary retention needs to be delineated from anuria and oliguria, which is a lack or decrease of urine production from the kidneys, and not an issue of voiding dysfunction.

Obstructive urinary retention can be a result of multiple etiologies and occurs much more frequently in men. Benign prostatic hypertrophy is the most common etiology, usually occurring in their sixth decade of life. The enlarged prostate is appreciated on the rectal examination as being smooth and symmetric. Prostate cancer is a much more rare cause of obstruction, where the prostate is irregular and firmer on examination, and the prostate specific antigen level (PSA) is markedly elevated. Fibromuscular contracture of the bladder outlet can occur in the younger male, with a normal prostate also resulting in obstruction. At the level of the bladder outflow tract, large bladder calculi or blood clots caused by hemorrhagic cystitis, cancerous hemorrhage, or calculi can all cause obstruction. At the level of the urethra, obstruction can be secondary to inflammation or stricture. Inflammatory causes can include purulent urethritis, prostatitis, tuberculosis, echinococcosis, and herpes simplex. Strictures can result from gonococcal urethritis, trauma, surgery,

TABLE 82.2.   DIAPPERS Mnemonic for Causes of Transient Urinary Incontinence

Delirium/confusional state
Infectious
Atrophic urethritis/vaginitis
Pharmacologic agents
Psychologic
Excessive urine output
Restricted mobility
Stool impaction

TABLE 82.3.   Obstructive Causes of Urinary Retention

Functional
  Benign prostate hypertrophy (BPH)
  Bladder calculi
  Bladder neck stenosis
  Blood clot
  Cancer (e.g., prostate, bladder, urethral, cervical, and colon)
  Cystocele
  Iatrogenic (e.g., previous antiincontinence procedures)
  Meatal stenosis
  Phimosis/paraphimosis
  Pregnant uterus
  Prolapsed uterus
  Rectocele
  Trauma
  Urethral obstruction (e.g., calculi, inflammation, trauma, and tumor)
  Urethral diverticulum
  Urethra stricture (male predominance)
Infections/inflammatory
  Cystitis
  Genital herpes
  Periurethral abscesses
  Prostatitis
  Sexually transmitted diseases
  Tuberculosis
  Urethritis
  Vesicoureteral reflux (female predominance)
Additional pediatric causes
  Benign hyperplasia of the prostatic utricle
  Congenital obstructed duplications of the urinary system
  Constipation
  Cystic enlargement of the posterior urethra
  Foreign bodies
  Hydrocolpos (from an imperforated hymen)
  Urethral valves (posterior or anterior)
  Ureterocele
  Ureteropelvic junction narrowing
  Ureterovesical junction narrowing
  Vaginal atresia/vaginal stenosis

or radiation, and they tend not to result from nongonococcal urethritis. Although many of these obstructive causes can occur in women, a higher incidence of psychogenic urinary retention tends to be found in women. Table 82.3 includes a list of causes of obstructive urinary retention.

Neuropathologic causes of urinary retention deserve special attention. Voiding and continence is neurologically mediated, both at the level of the spine and the level of the central nervous system. Motor nuclei of sacral nerves S2 through S4 control the detrusor muscles and the sphincteric muscles via a parasympathetic *spinal reflex arc* involving the pudendal nerve. Parasympathetic stimulation results in detrusor contraction and internal sphincteric relaxation. Parasympathetic inhibition results in detrusor relaxation. In addition, β-adrenergic sympathetic innervation from levels T10 to T12 allow for detrusor and bladder relaxation, thereby promoting urine storage, whereas α-adrenergic innervation of the internal vesicular sphincter results in its resting tone. Cortical and subcortical centers are responsible for further controlling the micturition process with subconscious relaxation of the bladder muscles and conscious retention or voiding when needed.

Neurologic lesions (e.g., trauma, mass lesions, and infections) at the level of the sacral nuclei, the second lumbar vertebra, can result in disruption of this spinal reflex arc, thereby causing a flaccid paralysis of the bladder and an inability to void. *Suprasacral lesions* of the spinal cord or CNS may initially result in spinal shock–type physiology with urinary retention but usually progress to overflow and urge incontinence with

TABLE 82.4.   Neuropathologic Causes of Urinary Retention

Suprasacral pathology resulting in DSD
  Encephalitis
  Hydrocephalus
  Meningitis
  Parkinson disease
  Shy-Drager syndrome
  Spinal cord trauma
  Spinal cord tumors (benign, primary, malignant)
  Spinal/paraspinal infections (abscesses, osteomyelitis, discitis)
  Stroke
  Tabes dorsalis
Sacral pathology resulting in the disruption of the reflex arc
  Inflammatory polyradiculopathy
  Sacral spinal/parasacral infections
  Sacral dysgenesis
  Sacral trauma
Supra sacral or sacral pathology resulting in an impaired spinal
    reflex arc
  Diabetes mellitus
  Landry-Guillain-Barré syndrome
  Multiple sclerosis
  Pernicious anemia
  Poliomyelitis
  Syringomyelia
  Transverse myelitis
  Isolated bladder atony and urinary retention

DSD = detrusor-sphincter dyssynergy.

detrusor hyperreflexia owing to the lack of upper motor neuron control. However, a complication to suprasacral injuries can be *detrusor-sphincter dyssynergy (DSD)*, in which there is external sphincter spasm during bladder contraction. This can occur to varying degrees and results in urinary retention. A list of neuropathologic causes of urinary retention can be found in Table 82.4.

Lastly, various medications, both prescription and over-the-counter, can precipitate urinary retention. This risk is even greater in the setting of other risk factors, for example, a male patient with benign prostatic hypertrophy (BPH) taking an over-the-counter cold medicine with diphenhydramine. Table 82.1 lists some of the more common medications that can cause urinary retention.

EMERGENCY DEPARTMENT EVALUATION

Urinary Incontinence

The emergency department evaluation of urinary incontinence should be focused on identifying acute emergent or correctable causes. Most emergent causes tend to be the neurologic causes resulting in detrusor hyperreflexia, whereas most correctable causes are often infectious, overflow, or medication-induced incontinence where treatment can be initiated in the emergency department. For the most part, evaluation should focus on a thorough history covering past medical, surgical, psychosocial, and a medication history. Any of these elements may yield clues to the patient's etiology. The physical examination should be comprehensive; including an extensive neurological examination, when indicated, evaluating mental status, gait, deep tendon reflexes, saddle sensation of the perineum, rectal tone, and the bulbocavernosus reflex. An absent bulbocavernosus reflex in male patients is almost always associated with a neurologic lesion. In women it can be absent up to 30% of the time.

SUI is often implied by the history and is accompanied by a normal physical examination. If needed, a provocation test for SUI can be performed by instilling 200 to 300 mL of sterile saline into the bladder following the measurement of a postvoid residual (PVR). The patient can then be asked to sneeze, cough, or strain. Isolated, leakage suggests SUI. Furthermore, if the *Marshall test*, digital urethral support during a provocation test, prevents the incontinence, the diagnosis is confirmed. Leakage with an inability to stop further urine flow during a provocation test suggests urge incontinence with detrusor instability. Urge incontinence may require investigation into associated signs and symptoms (e.g., back pain) for inflammatory etiologies and/or neurologic etiologies. Associated back pain or an abnormal neurologic examination warrants evaluation of the patient's PVR. It should be no more that 100 mL or 20% of the voided sample. The PVR can also be used to diagnosis overflow incontinence associated with an obstructive urinary retention.

Urinalysis and urine cultures should also be sent for all of these patients. This may assist in the diagnosis of infection and noninfectious inflammatory causes, thereby allowing for immediate treatment with antibiotics or aiding of the outpatient workup when the patient is discharged.

Emergent urology consultation is not indicated in the emergency department, and extensive urography and urodynamic evaluation is reserved for the outpatient urologic evaluation. Appropriate radiographic evaluation of the spine or brain and neurosurgical or neurologic consultation should be obtained, when indicated, to evaluate for potential emergent neurologic causes.

Urinary Retention

Evaluation of acute or chronic urinary retention in the emergency department should be directed at identifying the cause, when possible, and evaluating for the sequela of renal parenchymal damage. For the majority of cases of retention, the etiology will be recognized through a thorough history and physical examination. Special attention should be paid to the review of the patient's medication history, the rectal examination, and a thorough neurologic examination. These can provide significant information as to the potential life-threatening etiologies of the urinary retention. It should be noted that a normal prostate on examination does not exclude prostatic cause from the differential diagnosis.

There are two adjunctive tests that can be used to help confirm the diagnosis of retention. A PVR of greater than 100 mL of urine or greater than 20% of the voided volume suggests retention. An emergency department bedside ultrasound can document bladder distention suggestive of outlet or urethral obstruction. This may be especially useful if symptoms persist in the setting of perceived adequate drainage.

Laboratory evaluation of patients found to have urinary retention should include a urinalysis with culture, blood urea nitrogen (BUN), and serum creatinine. The urinalysis can provide clues to infectious etiologies, calculi, or tumors, whereas the culture is necessary for detecting potential subclinical infections. Postobstructive nephropathy will be evident by an elevated BUN/creatine (Cr), often with a ratio of greater than 10. If new or previously undiagnosed renal insufficiency is present, a more complete workup with electrolytes and a renal ultrasound looking for hydronephrosis, hydroureter, or renal parenchymal damage is suggested prior to the patient being discharged.

EMERGENCY DEPARTMENT MANAGEMENT

Urinary Incontinence

Management of urinary incontinence is directed at the suspected cause. Emergent neurologic causes should be addressed as dictated in the emergency department, such as ordering emergency magnetic resonance imaging (MRI) in cases of suspected spinal cord compression. Transient causes (Table 82.2) should also be addressed in the emergency department when possible: antibiotics for infectious cystitis, changing or holding offending medications when not contraindicated by issues of continuing patient care and follow-up evaluation. Overflow incontinence requires its own appropriate evaluation and management as discussed later in this chapter.

Further management of stress, urge, true, functional, and nonpathologic incontinence falls into the realm of outpatient urologic consultation. The management of SUI and true incontinence is often surgical, with repositioning of vesicourethral angle (e.g., bladder neck suspensions and pubovaginal slings). Alternatives for SUI include Kegel exercises, weight reduction, estrogen replacement, electrostimulation methods, and α-agonists (pseudoephedrine, phenylpropanolamine) for increasing bladder neck and urethral tone. Periurethral collagen injection therapy and urethral occlusion devices have also been used with moderate success for treating SUI. Urge incontinence management is directed at its individual cause. Behavioral modification also plays a significant role by way of urination schedules. Pharmacologic intervention can be added, but generally it will not abolish detrusor instability. Anticholinergics (propantheline, hyoscyamine) increase the tolerable bladder volume and decrease involuntary bladder contractions. Tricyclic antidepressants (doxepin, imipramine) can also be used owing to their central and peripheral anticholinergic effect and because they increase bladder outlet tone. Oxybutynin and dicyclomine inhibit involuntary bladder contraction through anticholinergic effects and cause smooth muscle relaxation in the bladder wall. Tolterodine has similar effect as oxybutynin via antimuscarinic activity.

Urinary Retention

Initial management of urinary retention should focus on identifying serious neurologic causes and obtaining symptom relief through bladder decompression. The former requires both an understanding of the pathophysiologic characteristics and the differential diagnosis and a complete history and physical examination, as discussed previously.

Decompression can be done with a well-lubricated 16 to 18 French Foley catheter and should be done in a timely manner. If this is unsuccessful, attempts can be made with an angulated Coudé catheter. Its angulated tip can facilitate catheter passage beyond the median lobe of the prostate. If this fails, further attempts should be made through consultation with urology.

When urologic consultation is not readily available, temporary relief may be provided by suprapubic trocar cystostomy or insertion of a small drainage tube into the bladder through a large-bore needle. These procedures require a palpable bladder and the absence of prior suprapubic surgery. If there is doubt about bladder distention (as in the obese patient), ultrasound confirmation is advisable. For these percutaneous drainage techniques, make a simple midline puncture one fingerbreadth above the symphysis pubis, with the trocar or needle directed slightly caudally and then advanced until urine is returned. The catheter or tubing is then advanced, the needle is withdrawn, and drainage is secured in position.

A single straight catheterization of patients with ongoing or undiagnosed causes of urinary retention is not recommended, since recurrence of symptoms is very likely and the risk of infection is high. A noteworthy exception to indication for prompt urethral catheterization pertains to the patient with pelvic fracture, prostate displacement on rectal examination, or blood at the urethral meatus. Suspected urethral trauma should be investigated initially by retrograde ureterography. Confirmation of urethral injury mandates urologic consultation and manage-

ment. Catheterization should be deferred and drainage established otherwise.

Bladder mucosal hemorrhage and postobstructive diuresis are two complications of bladder decompression, particularly in the patient with chronic urinary retention. Bladder mucosal hemorrhage is thought to be the result of sudden expansion of bladder wall veins following decompression. In the past, clamping of the catheter following a certain amount of drainage was recommended in an attempt to avoid this complication. However, it has been shown that the hydrostatic pressure in the bladder begins to fall immediately with catheter placement and falls markedly within the first 100 mL of urine drained. Therefore, clamping of the catheter does not affect the risk of mucosal hemorrhage and is not indicated.

Postobstructive diuresis may occur following the decompression of obstructive urinary retention at a rate up to or greater than 1 per hour. However, it is believed that this diuresis is an appropriate correction of volume overload. Therefore, milliliter-for-milliliter replacement of this diuresed fluid is not indicated. What is indicated is replacement of the concomitant electrolyte loss that goes along with the diuresis. This can often be done through administering a maintenance rate of one half isotonic saline during the diuresis.

CRITICAL INTERVENTIONS

- Exclude serious neurologic disease (such as spinal cord compression) as the cause of acute urinary incontinence or retention
- Quickly place a bladder catheter to relieve the severe discomfort of bladder distention in patients with acute urinary retention

DISPOSITION

Patients with an obstructive uropathy usually require continuous urinary drainage. The patient in otherwise good health with no ancillary requirements for hospital care may be discharged from the emergency department with Foley catheter drainage collected into a leg bag. Followup should be arranged prior to discharge and include a thorough discussion with understanding of events that require a prompt medical response. Urinary retention related to drugs or medication requires referral to the prescribing physician for recommended adjustment or substitution therapy.

For patients in whom an acute neurogenic cause of retention is suspected neurologic consultation, emergent imaging, and admission is required.

COMMON PITFALLS

✔ Failure to diagnose a true neurologic emergency such as cord compression or cauda equina in the patient with urinary retention or incontinence
✔ Patients with voiding dysfunction should always be asked about their over-the-counter medication use
✔ The most important axiom to remember in the effort to relieve urinary retention is "do no harm"; overly aggressive catheter insertion can result in urethral injury
✔ Inadequate emergency department evaluation of the elderly male patient with urinary retention, neglecting to test for concomitant infection and postobstructive nephropathy
✔ In woman with urinary retention, multiple sclerosis and diabetes should be considered as underlying causes

Acknowledgments

Thank you to previous edition chapter author Norman E. Peterson.

References

1. Arya LA, Myers DL, Jackson ND. Dietary caffeine intake and the risk for detrusor instability: a case-control study. *Obstet Gynecol* 2000;96:85–89.
2. Barbalias GA, Klauber GT, Blaivas JG. Critical evaluation of the Crede maneuver: a urodynamic study of 207 patients. *J Urol* 1983;130:720–723.
3. Burgio KL, Goode PS, Locher JL, et al. Behavioral training with and without biofeedback in the treatment of urge incontinence in older women: a randomized controlled trial. *JAMA* 2002;288:2293–2299.
4. Burgio KL, Locher JL, Goode PS, et al. Behavioral vs drug treatment for urge urinary incontinence in older women: a randomized controlled trial. *JAMA* 1998;280:1995–2000.
5. Chang SM, Hou CL, Dong DQ, Zhang H. Urologic status of 74 spinal cord patients from the 1976 Tangshan earthquake, and managed for over 20 years using the Crede maneuver. *Spinal Cord* 2000;38:552–554.
6. Chutka DS, Fleming KC, Evans MP, et al. Urinary incontinence in the elderly population. *Mayo Clin Proc* 1996;71:93–101.
7. Curtis LA, Dolan TS, Cespedes RD. Acute urinary retention and urinary incontinence. *Emerg Med Clin North Am* 2001;19:591–619.
8. Foster MC, Upsdell SM, O'Reilly PH. Urological myths. *BMJ* 1990;301:1421–1423.
9. Higgins PM, French ME, Chadalavada VS. Management of acute retention of urine: a reappraisal. *Br J Urol* 1991;67:365–368.
10. Howards SS. Postobstructive diuresis: a misunderstood phenomenon. *J Urol* 1973;110:537–540.
11. Kobashi KC, Leach GE. Stress urinary incontinence. *Curr Opin Urol* 1999;9:285–290.
12. Kogan BA, Solomon MH, Diokno AC. Urinary retention secondary to Landry-Guillain-Barre syndrome. *J Urol* 1981;12
13. Lockhart JL, Webster GD, Sheremata W, et al. Neurogenic bladder dysfunction in the Shy-Drager syndrome. *J Urol* 1981;126:119–121.6:643–644.
14. McGuire EJ, Savastano JA. Urodynamic findings and long-term outcome management of patients with multiple sclerosis-induced lower urinary tract dysfunction. *J Urol* 1984;132:713–715.
15. Rackley RR, Appell RA. Evaluation and medical management of female urinary incontinence. *Cleve Clin J Med* 1997;64:83–92.
16. Resnick NM. Urinary incontinence. *Lancet* 1995;346:94–99.
17. Rortveit G, Daltveit AK, Hannestad YS, Hunskaar S. Urinary incontinence after vaginal delivery or cesarean section. *N Engl J Med* 2003;348:900–907.

CHAPTER 83

Genitourinary Stents and Catheters

Paul Phrampus and Benjamin Davies

URETHRAL CATHETERS

Placement of urinary catheters is a common procedure in the emergency department. Indications include the relief of urinary retention, monitoring urinary output during resuscitation, treatment of gross hematuria, and urine cultures. Although ordinarily a simple task, urethral catheter placement can sometimes be challenging. As with any other procedure, there are associated risks and complications. Emergency physicians should be able to utilize different types of catheters, overcome the common difficulties encountered in placing them, and be aware of the acute and chronic complications of urethral catheters.

The tortuous anatomy and common anatomic pathologic conditions of the male urethra can make urinary catheter placement difficult. In each section of the urethra there are specific problems that can be encountered. Meatal stenosis, either from prior infections or from congenital malformation, can be diagnosed when the meatus of the penis is fibrotic and nondistensible. A dilation procedure performed by a urologist may be necessary for catheter placement. Hypospadias, a congenital condition in which the true urethral lumen is on the ventrum of the penis, can make placement difficult. Often there is a blind-ended false lumen on the glans penis and the health provider need only look at the ventral aspect of the penis to find the true lumen. The patient can generally tell the clinician which lumen is the true one. Once the lumen is located, it is usually easily catheterized.

The penile and bulbar urethra are the most common sites of urethral strictures. Strictures are usually noticed when the catheter cannot be advanced more than half way into the bladder. An attempt to force the catheter through a stricture often leads to the creation of false passages in the urethra, which can cause urethral diverticula, infection, and the development of fistulas. If this situation is encountered, further attempts to place the catheter should be discontinued until a urology consultation can be obtained. The stricture may require a dilatation procedure or urethroplasty.

In the prostatic urethra, the lobes of the prostate project centrally, making this the site of the most common problem encountered in the placement of urinary catheters. The incidence of benign prostatic hypertrophy (BPH) increases dramatically with advancing years, and,most men older than age 70 have anatomic changes as well as signs and symptoms of BPH. There are a few easy "tricks" that can help negotiate the tip of the catheter around an enlarged prostate. The coudé (elbowed) catheter has an upturned end that slips over the swollen gland. Other techniques include placing a finger in the rectum and applying gentle pressure to the prostate as the catheter is passed. In addition, injecting a water-soluble lubricant retrograde into the urethra to decrease friction will often help.

Patients with a history of a radical or simple prostatectomy commonly have bladder neck contractures (2). Coudé catheters are similarly helpful with these patients. In all instances when the emergency department placement of a catheter has been unsuccessful, the urologist should be consulted.

Although most difficult catheterizations are in men, difficulties can at times arise in the catheterization of women. Women have short and discrete urethras that are usually less than 2 cm in length, which makes them generally easy to traverse with a standard urethral catheter. At times finding the meatus can be problematic. Some obese women have redundant labia majora, which can make visualization of the urethral meatus difficult. In these cases placing the patient in the frog-leg position, using proper lighting, and having someone retract redundant tissue will aid in the location of the urethra and subsequent placement of the catheter.

Prolapse of the pelvic organs (cystocele, enterocele, rectocele, or uterocele) can sometimes obscure the view of the female meatus, but applying gentle pressure to the offending organ generally brings the meatus into view. Some women have a partially prolapsed urethra called a caruncle which can distort the normal anatomy, but a standard urethral catheter can usually be placed around the caruncle without difficulty.

Complications from the placement of urinary catheters occur, but are uncommon. Applying too much pressure to a catheter that is being impeded by a stricture or large prostate can lead to creation of a false passage by undermining the urethral mucosa. This can cause significant hematuria, promote stricture formation, and lead to infection and sepsis. It is thus best to avoid applying significant force when placing a urethral catheter. In patients with pelvic trauma, urethral patency should be assured via a retrograde urethrogram prior to the placement of a catheter. Multiple attempts at urethral catheter placement should be avoided to lessen the chance of causing or exacerbating urethral injury.

Occasionally a urethral catheter cannot be removed from a patient because the balloon will not deflate. The easiest maneuver is to cut the valve from the end of the catheter, which often facilitates removal. If that does not relieve the obstruction, a guidewire can be introduced into the balloon lumen of the catheter to attempt to relieve the obstruction. If this fails and the catheter needs to be removed emergently, a urologist may have to perform invasive maneuvers for catheter removal. Puncturing the balloon via the perineum is one such technique, but cystoscopy will also be needed to ensure that fragments of the balloon have not been left in the bladder. Fragments left in the bladder put the patient at risk for bladder stone formation.

Patients with alteration in mental status often pull catheters out of their bladder. Replacing the catheter is usually not difficult. However, consideration must be given to the indication for catheter placement. Repeatedly pulling out a urinary catheter puts the patient in jeopardy of developing incontinence secondary to external sphincter damage and can cause significant blood loss.

Chronic complications seen in long-term urethral catheter placement are urinary tract infections and concomitant bacteremia. Sepsis resulting from a chronic indwelling catheter is thought to be rare (5). When a patient presents with signs and symptoms of a urinary tract infection, the catheter should be changed, since bacteria easily colonize catheters after only several days. Patients who have long-term urethral catheterization should have their catheters changed once a month. It should be noted that chronic catheters are almost universally colonized. As such, antibiotic treatment is usually not started for asymptomatic patients. Many studies have documented the overuse of urethral catheters. Probably the best prevention strategy for catheter-related infection is therefore to limit the use of urethral catheterization to cases in which there is a clear indication (4).

Other problems from long-term indwelling catheters include local infections (orchitis, balanitis, and prostatitis), erosive hypospadias, and bladder stone formation (1). In general, urethral catheters are not the treatment of choice for debilitated or incontinent patients. These patients should be managed either with intermittent catheterization or suprapubic catheters.

THREE-WAY IRRIGATION CATHETERS

Placement of a three-way irrigation catheter may be required in the emergency department patient with gross hematuria who complains of symptoms of bladder obstruction. Significant gross hematuria, particularly when clots are present, should be treated aggressively with placement of a three-way catheter and continuous bladder irrigation. Three-way irrigating catheters, as the name implies, have three ports. One port is for saline or sterile water to be dripped in by passive means such as a "Kelly" bag, a 3 L bag of saline that can be attached to the catheter, or a normal 1 L bag if Kelly bags are not available. The second port is for usual urine drainage, and the third port is to inflate the balloon. There are several types of three-way catheters, ranging from a soft plastic coudé-type to others with large holes at the distal end to help the passage of large clots. When there is significant bleeding and clot formation, one should use a three-way catheter with the largest tolerated diameter.

SUPRAPUBIC CATHETERS

Patients with a suprapubic tube to drain the bladder are not uncommon in the emergency Department. Suprapubic tubes often become clogged with mucus or debris. Suprapubic tubes require routine replacement every 4 to 6 weeks as a result. The tube can be flushed to attempt to relieve the obstruction, as with a standard urinary catheter. If the suprapubic tube has been in place for longer than a month, it can readily be removed without fear of losing the tract. If the SP catheter needs to be changed, the bladder should be filled with water or normal saline before the tube is removed, thereby providing a method of confirmation to ensure correct placement of the new tube.

It is occasionally necessary to place a suprapubic tube on an emergency basis. This will usually be accomplished by a consulting urologist. Although there are various ways to place a suprapubic tube, most urologists use the percutaneous Selinger technique. Patients who are significantly obese, who have had prior abdominal or genitourinary surgery, or who have had multiple prior suprapubic tubes are not candidates for percutaneous tube placement and will require an open procedure to avoid significant complications.

URETERAL STENTS

Ureteral stents are commonly used in urology to facilitate urine flow. The most common indication is for stone disease. These are usually double J stents that have curls both in the bladder and in the renal pelvis. They can readily be seen on X-ray and fluoroscopic examination. Emergency physicians should be aware of their indications, complications, and side effects.

Placement of a stent allows the unimpeded passage of urine and helps the passage of renal lithiasis by passively dilating the ureter. In addition, the stents allow edematous ureters to heal. They can allow small stones to pass without any invasive treatment at all. Patients who have signs and symptoms of infected urine and also have an obstructed kidney (either by stones or strictures, or by other entities) often will be stented emergently to prevent septic sequelae.

Common complications from ureteral stents include infection, migration, obstruction, and encrustation. Bacterial colonization of ureteral stents is common. Should the patient with a ureteral stent manifest symptoms of urinary infection or pyelonephritis, therapy with antibiotics that provide adequate coverage for *Pseudomonas aeruginosa* should be started promptly (3).

Sometimes the patient's anatomy does not allow for perfect alignment of the ureteral stent either in the bladder or the renal pelvis. When this happens the stent can migrate either up proximally into the ureter or distally toward the bladder. Stent migration manifests with patient discomfort either from hydronephrosis (flank pain) because the stent is not draining correctly or with irritative voiding symptoms. A simple kidney, ureter, and bladder (KUB) X-ray study can verify the placement of the stent (Fig. 83.1).

Other common complications include stent encrustation and obstruction. If ureteral stents are not removed or changed in 3 months, many patients develop encrustation around the stent, and hydronephrosis or renal failure can result. Urgent consultation for removal or changing of the stent is indicated.

The side effects of ureteral stents are a product of irritating the mucosa of either the renal pelvis or the bladder. Patients commonly complain of flank pain, dysuria, frequency, gross hematuria, and urgency. The symptoms usually abate over time and can be controlled with anti-cholinergics such as tolterodine or

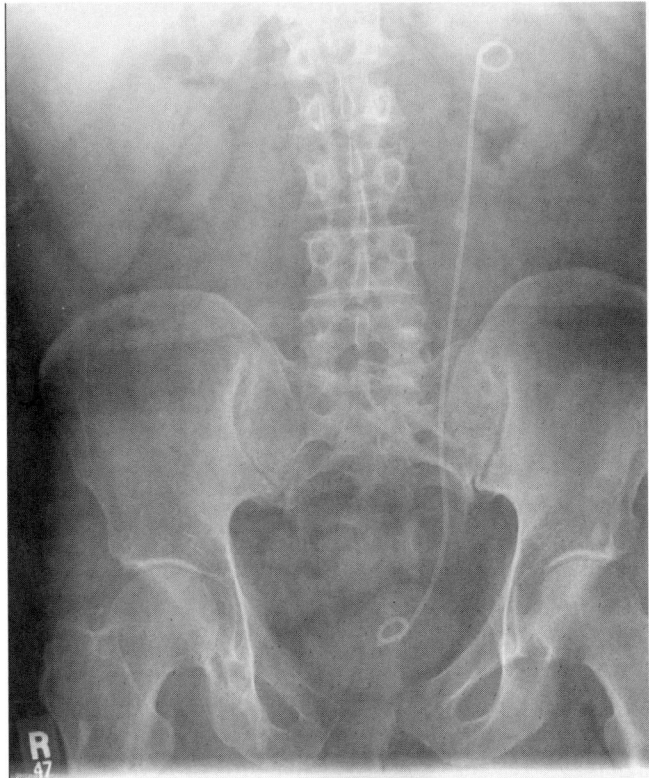

Figure 83.1.   A KUB showing a stent in proper placement.

oxybutynin, which may be started in consultation with the patient's urologist.

URINARY CONDUITS

The use of a loop of bowel to serve as a conduit for urine is a common urologic practice. Radical cystectomy (removal of the bladder) with urinary diversion to a segment of bowel is used for muscle-invasive bladder cancer and other entities. The majority of patients have an ileal conduit, a short piece of ileum that has been removed from the normal fecal stream and has had the ureters attached to it. The distal end is made into a stoma, and urine is collected via an external urostomy bag. Alternative procedures form neobladders that are orthotopically placed; these patients void in the normal fashion. Still other procedures form catheterizable stomas, usually through the umbilicus, which the patient drains with a straight catheter. Emergency physicians should be aware of the common complications—metabolic and mechanical—that occur, primarily of the ileal conduit. Urologic consultation is usually required, since patients often have complicated urologic histories.

As is the case after any large abdominal or pelvic operation, these patients can develop small bowel obstruction. The most common site is around the mesentery of the ileal loop. Hernias can develop around the stoma (parastomal hernias), and incisional hernias are also possible. Because the ureter is sutured to

the bowel, strictures commonly occur at the anastomosis, potentially resulting in hydronephrosis, insidious renal failure, or pyelonephritis and urosepsis. Given that most of the ureteroileal anastomosis are freely refluxing, pyelonephritis is common in these patients; chronic pyelonephritis associated with a conduit can result in renal failure. Conduits are chronically colonized with fecal flora, and, therefore, positive urine culture findings should be treated only if the patient is symptomatic.

The use of a loop of ileum or colon for urinary conduits frequently causes a mild hyperchloremic metabolic acidosis, and some patients require chronic alkali supplementation.

Dehydration may exacerbate this chronic acidosis. If it becomes necessary to monitor the urinary output of a patient with an ileal conduit, the emergency physician can insert a small red-rubber catheter in the stoma to drain and monitor the output. Hydrating the patient with normal fluid that is high in bicarbonate and low in chloride is advisable.

CRITICAL INTERVENTION

- Use a coudé-type catheter for difficult placement of the catheter if the prostate or bladder neck is the area of obstruction

DISPOSITION

Most patients may be discharged home after successful placement or replacement of a urinary catheter. Patients with infected or obstructed ureteral stents usually require urologic consultation and admission.

PITFALLS

✔ Overzealous attempts by staff to place a urinary catheter leading to the formation of a false passage
✔ Failure to consult urology after the unsuccessful attempts at catheter placement
✔ Failure to ensure urethral patency prior to placing a catheter in a trauma patient to avoid further urethral injury

Acknowledgments

Thank you to previous edition chapter authors Karen DeFazio and Brian Mongillo.

References

1. Bregenzer T, Frei R, Widmer AF, et al. Low risk of bacteremia during catheter replacement in patients with long-term urinary catheters. *Arch Intern Med* 1997;157:521–525.
2. Farsi HM, Mosli HA, Al-Zemaity MF, et al. Bacteriuria and colonization of double-pigtail ureteral stents: long-term experience with 237 patients. *J Endourol* 1995;9:469–472.
3. McDowell G, Hayden L, Wise H. Penile necrosis secondary to an indwelling Foley catheter. *J Urol* 1987;138:1243.
4. Patrick C, Walsh MD et al. ed. *Campbell's Urology.* 8th ed. St. Louis: Saunders, 2002.
5. Saint S, Lipsky B. Preventing catheter-related bacteriuria: Should we? Can we? How? [Review] *Arch Intern Med* 1999;159:800–808.

CHAPTER 84
Penile Disorders

Douglas McGee

BALANOPOSTHITIS, PHIMOSIS, AND PARAPHIMOSIS

Clinical Presentation

Balanitis describes inflammation of the glans penis. *Posthitis* describes inflammation of the prepuce of the penis. Because balanitis and posthitis usually occur together, *balanoposthitis* correctly describes a male with inflammation of the glans and prepuce. Balanitis is more common in uncircumcised men who exercise poor hygiene, but it may affect young boys. Patients with balanoposthitis have an edematous, erythematous, fissured, and painful prepuce and glans. A variety of skin changes are possible based on the etiology.

When the foreskin is not retractable behind the glans penis, the condition is termed *phimosis*. Physiologic phimosis is present until normal adhesions between the foreskin and glans have separated. Although most young boys are able to retract the foreskin by puberty, retraction is usually possible at an earlier age (4,6). As normal secretions accumulate and epithelial sloughing occurs, smegma is formed. Smegma assists in the separation of the foreskin from the glans and is normal. Parents may confuse smegma with infectious penile discharge if expressed from the penis. Pathologic phimosis, or simply phimosis, occurs when retraction of the foreskin is not possible after puberty or when the foreskin was previously retractable.

Paraphimosis occurs when the retracted foreskin is not replaced, usually after cleansing or catheter insertion. After foreskin retraction, the constricting phimotic ring causes progressive edema and impairs venous return, threatening the viability of the glans. Most patients complain of pain and usually provide a history of foreskin retraction; however, debilitated, uncircumcised patients may not provide this history. Do not confuse paraphimosis with balanitis in these patients.

Differential Diagnosis

The differential diagnosis may be divided into infectious and noninfectious causes. Fungal infections resulting from *Candida albicans* cause itching and burning of the penis and are accompanied by white discharge, discrete ulcerated papules, and white and cheesy plaques. Group B streptococci, *Gardnerella vaginalis*, and mixed anaerobes have been isolated from men with balanoposthitis. Secondary syphilis and condyloma latum may infect the glans. Protozoal infections with *Trichomonas vaginalis* and amoebiasis have been reported. Genital herpes may cause necrotizing balanoposthitis, and human papillomavirus (HPV) can induce genital warts on the glans or foreskin.

Noninfectious causes of balanoposthitis include trauma, latex allergy, and various dermatoses. Dermatologic lesions include psoriasis, lichen planus, erythema multiforme, and a variety of premalignant and malignant lesions. When balanoposthitis is severe, phimosis may occur and precipitate urinary retention.

Emergency Department Evaluation

The emergency department evaluation is usually limited to the history and physical examination. Test the patient's blood glucose when infection caused by *C. albicans* is suspected, and perform serologic testing for syphilis when this organism is suspected. Acetic acid whitens the superficial epithelial skin layer when applied to lesions infected with HPV.

Emergency Department Management

Meticulous hygiene, including retraction of the foreskin and cleansing of the glans penis and prepuce, is the mainstay of treatment. Direct the treatment of infectious balanoposthitis toward the offending organism. Treat fungal infections of the glans with topical antifungal agents. Use metronidazole to treat *Gardnerella*, anaerobic infection, and *Trichomonas* infections. Treat secondary syphilis according to established guidelines.

Asymptomatic phimosis does not require emergent treatment. Reassure concerned parents when physiologic phimosis is present and discourage them from attempting forceful retraction. Several recent studies have demonstrated that topical steroids applied to the foreskin for a month are 90% effective in young boys with childhood phimosis when retraction is desired (1,15,17,24). When severe phimosis causes urinary retention or interferes with placement of a urinary catheter, a slit made in the dorsal aspect of the foreskin facilitates access to the urethral meatus (12,20). After achieving adequate local anesthesia of the penis with a dorsal nerve block or ring block placed at the base of the penis, gently separate adhesions between the foreskin and glans with a hemostat. Place one jaw of the hemostat inside the dorsal foreskin, taking care not to include the urethral meatus or glans. Crush the foreskin for 3 to 5 minutes by closing the hemostat and incise the crushed foreskin with straight scissors. The crushed edges rarely bleed but may require absorbable suture for hemostasis if they separate. Although some patients are satisfied with the cosmetic appearance of the foreskin after the dorsal slit procedure, the urologist may perform elective circumcision.

Paraphimosis requires definitive treatment in the emergency department. After adequate sedation or penile anesthesia, attempt manual reduction. Place the fingers of both hands behind the phimotic ring and foreskin and apply gentle, steady pressure on the glans with the thumbs (4,2,20). Gauze placed under the fingers may improve traction on the foreskin while bringing it over the glans, but lubricants are rarely helpful. Several other techniques are described to treat paraphimosis; application of these techniques should be guided by the physician's skill and training in the maneuvers. Use a 21-gauge needle to puncture the edematous foreskin; manual compression after puncture may allow the escape of enough edema fluid to facilitate reduction (2,12). Repeated punctures or blood aspirated from the engorged glans after a tourniquet is placed at the base of the penis may allow reduction (10,19). Subdermal hyaluronidase injected into the edematous foreskin facilitates dispersion of edema fluid and may make reduction possible (5). Granulated sugar has been applied to the edematous glans and foreskin to extract tissue water and ease reduction (11). When less aggressive methods fail, the phimotic ring is incised with a scalpel to facilitate foreskin reduction (20). Prevention is key; emergency department personnel must replace the foreskin after urinary catheter placement.

CRITICAL INTERVENTION

- Reduce a paraphimosis in the emergency department; it cannot be referred for outpatient management

Disposition

Treat patients who have balanoposthitis as outpatients except when they have associated medical conditions, such as diabetes. This group of patients require hospital treatment if the diabetes is poorly controlled, complicating outpatient treatment. When phimosis is present and causes urinary retention, consultation in the emergency department with a urologist may be required to relieve the phimosis to allow free drainage of urine if the emergency physician cannot place a urinary catheter. All patients with balanoposthitis require followup with their primary physician and may benefit from urologic evaluation for circumcision. Refer patients with skin lesions suspicious for precancerous changes or malignancy to a dermatologist for evaluation.

Common Pitfalls

✔ Phimosis is normal in young boys and does not require treatment in asymptomatic adults
✔ Paraphimosis can look like balanitis unless the emergency physician recognizes that the foreskin is retracted
✔ Failure to return the foreskin to its anatomic location after retraction

PRIAPISM

Clinical Presentation

Priapism is characterized by a prolonged, painful, unwanted penile erection, usually in the absence of sexual stimulation. The physiologic balance achieved between venous outflow and arterial dilation of the corpora cavernosa controls erectile function. Priapism occurs when normal physiologic blood flow is altered and this balance is disrupted. Today, medications used to treat erectile dysfunction in men (sildenafil, papaverine, prostaglandin E1, among others) cause most cases of priapism (3,8,21). It is uncommon in boys, unless sickle cell disease is present, and it is rare in neonates (22). Henoch-Schönlein purpura has caused priapism (13). Patients with priapism complain of penile pain and persistent erection, even after ejaculation. The mean time to presentation in one series of 34 patients was 30 hours (8). The penis is erect and painful to palpation. The corpora cavernosa are engorged, but in contrast to normal erections, the corpus spongiosum and glans penis are flaccid.

Differential Diagnosis

The differential diagnosis is divided into "low-flow" and "high-flow" priapism (8). Simply stated, low-flow priapism results from abnormally venous outflow; high-flow priapism results from abnormally increased arterial inflow.

Low-flow priapism is far more common than high-flow priapism and is often caused by vasoactive drugs that cause engorgement of the corpora cavernosa. Impaired venous outflow causes sludging, thrombosis, acidosis, and decreased oxygen tension within the corporal bodies. This pathophysiologic cascade causes the irreversible cellular damage and corporal fibrosis responsible for the long-term complications of low-flow priapism. Oral and intracavernosal agents used for erectile dysfunction, antihypertensive agents, psychotropic drugs, cocaine, and ethanol are among the drugs that have been implicated. Leukemia, sickle cell anemia, and a variety of neoplastic etiologies are also responsible for priapism (8,18).

High-flow priapism is uncommon and usually results from trauma to the penis or perineum (9). Arterial fistula formation between the cavernosal artery and the corporal bodies increases arterial flow into the penis that exceeds venous outflow.

Emergency Department Evaluation

The history usually suggests the etiology of the patient's priapism. Careful attention to prescription or illicit drug use may help determine whether these agents are responsible. Suspect sickle cell disease among patients at risk when the history of sickle cell disease is unknown. Record the onset of erection and elicit the history of prior episodes of priapism. The penis is painful to palpation and the corporal bodies are engorged, but the glans and the corpus spongiosum are soft. Some authors recommend blood gas analysis of blood aspirated from the corporal bodies to assist in differentiating between low and high flow states (8,20). Low pH, low oxygen tension, and high carbon dioxide levels suggest low-flow, venous obstruction. Blood gas parameters similar to arterial blood suggest high-flow priapism, a condition usually seen after trauma. Order Doppler flow ultrasonography of the penis and perineum to document arteriovenous fistulas when high-flow priapism is suspected (9).

Emergency Department Management

Most cases of priapism encountered in the emergency department treatment will be low-flow priapism. There is conflicting literature describing the efficacy of terbutaline in priapism. The results of some small clinical trials demonstrate that oral terbutaline is more effective than placebo in achieving detumescence (14); others have shown no benefit (7). Because of its relative safety in patients without hypertension or coronary artery disease, a trial of subcutaneous terbutaline (0.25 to 0.5 mL injected subcutaneously, repeated in 20 minutes if needed), or 5 mg of oral terbutaline, repeated in 15 minutes, may be attempted (20). When sedation, analgesia, or terbutaline do not result in detumescence, corporal aspiration and irrigation are indicated (8,20). Anesthetize the penis and aspirate 30 to 60 mL of blood from a single corporal body at the 10 o'clock or 2 o'clock positions. Do not puncture the glans; anastomoses between the corporal bodies obviate the need for bilateral aspiration. When the erection persists after aspiration, carefully inject phenylephrine into the punctured corpus cavernosum. Dilute 1 mg of phenylephrine in 9 mL of sterile saline to achieve a concentration of $100\,\mu g/mL$. Inject 200-μg aliquots of phenylephrine up to 3 times to achieve detumescence. Monitor the blood pressure and cardiac rhythm when repeated injections are required.

Sickle cell patients with priapism require analgesia, hydration, and supplemental oxygen. Although one study challenged its efficacy, red blood cell exchange transfusion may be employed when traditional anti-sickling measures fail (16,18). Emergent therapy in the emergency department is not required for high-flow priapism because it does not cause the ischemic injury seen in low-flow priapism.

CRITICAL INTERVENTIONS

- Priapism is a urologic emergency that requires rapid ED treatment in coordination with the consulting urologist
- Red cell exchange therapy may be necessary when priapism occurs in a patient with sickle cell disease

Disposition

When detumescence is accomplished in the emergency department, the patient is usually discharged and instructed to followup with the urologist. When emergency department treatment fails to relieve the erection or when high flow priapism is suspected, a urologic evaluation is indicated. If the urologist is unavailable, transfer the patient to definitive care.

Common Pitfalls

✔ Failure to achieve detumescence of priapism in the emergency department

✔ Failure to consider the underlying diagnosis of sickle cell disease

References

1. Ashfield JE, Nickel KR, Siemans DR, et al. Treatment of phimosis with topical steroids in 194 children. *J Urol* 2003;169:1106–1108.
2. Barone JG, Fleisher MH. Treatment of paraphimosis using the "puncture" technique. *Pediatr Emerg Care* 1993;9:298–299.
3. Broderick GA. Intracavernous pharmacotherapy. *Urol Clin North Am* 1996; 23:111–126.
4. Brown MR, Cartwright PC, Snow BW. Common office problems in pediatric urology and gynecology. *Pediatr Clin North Am* 1997;44:1091–1115.
5. DeVries CR, Miller AK, Packer MG. Reduction of paraphimosis with hyaluronidase. *Urology* 1996;48:464–465.
6. Golubovic Z, Milanovic D, Vukadinovic V, et al. The conservative treatment of phimosis in boys. *Br J Urol* 1996;78:786–788.
7. Govier FE, Jonsson E, Kramer-Levien D. Oral terbutaline for the treatment of priapism. *J Urol* 1994;151:878–879.
8. Harmon WJ, Nehra A. Priapism: diagnosis and management. *Mayo Clin Proc* 1997;72:350–355.
9. Ilkay AK, Levine LA. Conservative management of high flow priapism. *Urology* 1995;46:419–424.
10. Kumar V, Javle P. Modified puncture technique for reduction of paraphimosis. *Ann R Coll Surg Engl* 2001;83:126–127.
11. Kerwat AS, Stephenson B. Reduction of paraphimosis using granulated sugar. *Br J Urol* 1998;82:755.
12. Langer JC, Coplen DE. Circumcision and pediatric disorders of the penis. *Pediatr Clin North Am* 1998;45:801–812.
13. Lind J, Mackay A, Withers SJ. *J Pediatr Child Health* 2002;38:526–527.
14. Low FC, Jarow JP. Placebo-controlled study of oral terbutaline and pseudoepinephrine in management of prostaglandin E1-induced prolonged erections. *Urology* 1993;42:51–53.
15. Lund L, Wai KH, Mui LM, Yeung CK. Effect of topical steroid on non-retractile prepubertal foreskin by a prospective, randomized, double blind study. *Scand J Urol Nephrol* 2000;34:267–269.
16. McCarthy LJ, Vattuone J, Weidner J, et al. *Ther Apher* 2000;4:256–258.
17. Orsola A, Caffaratti J, Garat JM. Conservative treatment of phimosis in children using topical steroid. *Urology* 2000;56:307–310.
18. Powars DR, Johnson CS. Priapism. *Hematol Oncol Clin North Am* 1996;10:1363–1372.
19. Raveenthiran V. Reduction of paraphimosis: a technique based on pathophysiology. *Br J Surg* 1996;83:1247.
20. Scheinder RE. Urologic procedures. In: Roberts JR, Hedges JR, eds. *Clinical procedures in emergency medicine.* Philadelphia: WB Saunders, 2004:1075.
21. Sur RL, Kane CJ. Sildenafil citrate-associated priapism. *Urology* 2000;55:950.
22. Walker JR, Casale AJ. Prolonged penile erection in the newborn. *Urology* 1997; 50:796–799.
23. Waugh MA. Balanitis. *Dermatol Clin* 1998;16:757–762.
24. Webster TM, Leonard MP. Topical steroid therapy for phimosis. *Can J Urol* 2002;9:1492–1495.

CHAPTER 85
Azotemia and Acute Renal Failure

Todd C. Rothenhaus and Deborah R. Wong

Normal kidney function depends on adequate renal perfusion, efficient filtration of plasma at the glomeruli, nearly complete reabsorption of filtered solutes by the renal tubules, and the unhampered passage of formed urine from the body. In addition to the elimination of wastes, the kidney is also involved in maintaining volume status and electrolyte balance.

Acute renal failure (ARF) is defined as a recent (over hours to days) decline in renal function and accounts for about 1% of hospital admissions (21). The hallmark of ARF is azotemia, in which nitrogenous wastes such as creatinine and urea accumulate in the blood. A decrease in urine output may or may not accompany ARF. Because about 400 to 600 mOsmol of solute is created by the body every 24 hours, and because maximum urine osmolality is approximately 1200 mOsmol/L, urine output must be at least 300 to 500 mL per day to maintain adequate solute clearance from the body. Oliguria is thus defined as urine output less than 400 mL per day and anuria as urine output less than 100 mL per day.

Renal function is most often measured by determining the clearance of creatinine (C_{cr}), a clinical estimate of the glomerular filtration rate (GFR). Creatinine is released continuously from skeletal muscle as a byproduct of the metabolism of creatine, and is completely filtered at the glomerulus. Blood creatinine concentration is proportional to muscle mass and inversely proportional to GFR (13). The Cockroft-Gault formula provides an estimate of creatinine clearance from a single measurement of serum creatinine (S_{cr}) (4):

$$C_{cr} \text{ (mL/min)} = (140 \text{ age})(\text{lean body weight in kg})/72 \times S_{cr} \text{ (mg/dL)}$$

The result is multiplied by 0.85 in women, to correct for approximately 15% less muscle mass in proportion to body weight. These calculated results are accurate only in the steady state. For example, sudden bilateral ureteral obstruction would cause true GFR to fall to zero, but GFR calculated from the previous equation would only slowly decline, as serum creatinine increased at the rate of 1 to 3 mg/dL per day, as expected from ongoing endogenous production.

ARF can lead to life-threatening complications such as pulmonary edema, hyperkalemia, acidemia, severe hypertension, and uremic pericarditis with effusion and tamponade. The goal of the emergency physician is to recognize these complications and to halt any further decline in renal function by correcting any reversible underlying cause.

CLINICAL PRESENTATION

No presenting symptom or sign is pathognomonic of ARF, which most often occurs in the setting of other illness (19). Patients may present in critical condition, or asymptomatic azotemia may be discovered on routine blood screening. Most symptoms, such as fatigue, weakness, shortness of breath, or peripheral edema, are nonspecific. The diagnosis is thus established only after

TABLE 86.2.   Major Manifestations of Uremia

DERANGEMENTS OF HOMEOSTASIS

Sodium balance
Water balance
Hyperkalemia
Metabolic acidosis
Hypocalcemia
Hyperphosphatemia
Hypermagnesemia

DERANGEMENTS OF METABOLISM

Azotemia
Decreased glucose tolerance
Hyperlipidemia

SPECIFIC ORGAN SYSTEM EFFECTS

Cardiovascular
Hypertension, volume overload, pericarditis
Pulmonary
Pulmonary edema, pleuritis
Neurologic
Lethargy, difficulty concentrating, altered mental status, seizures, myoclonic twitching, asterixis, hiccups, cramps, peripheral neuropathy
Gastrointestinal
Anorexia, nausea, vomiting, gastrointestinal ulceration, pancreatitis
Musculoskeletal
Secondary hyperparathyroidism, renal osteodystrophy, crystal-induced arthritis, myopathy, spontaneous tendon rupture, carpal tunnel syndrome
Hematologic
Anemia, altered immunity, qualitative platelet abnormality

TABLE 86.3.   Reversible Factors and Treatable Causes of Chronic Renal Failure

REVERSIBLE FACTORS

Hypovolemia
Congestive heart failure
Pericardial tamponade
Severe hypertension
Catabolic state/protein loads
Nephrotoxic agents
Obstructive disease
Reflux disease

TREATABLE CAUSES

Renal artery stenosis
Malignant hypertension
Acute interstitial nephritis
Hypercalcemic nephropathy
Multiple myeloma
Vasculitis (e.g., systemic lupus erythematosus, Wegener granulomatosis, periarteritis nodosa)
Obstructive nephropathy
Reflux nephropathy

nephropathy accounting for the largest single group. Hypertensive nephrosclerosis is another major cause, particularly among blacks. The history, physical examination, and laboratory and imaging studies may provide clues to other specific etiologies. Although determining the exact etiology of chronic renal failure allows the underlying cause to be treated in some cases, this is the exception rather than the rule.

Progressive loss of renal function eventually results in a syndrome termed *uremia*. Especially in younger patients, clinical manifestations are not always evident even when the GFR has decreased to approximately 25% of normal. This occurs despite the fact that laboratory abnormalities may be impressive, because the remaining functioning nephrons are able to compensate reasonably well for those that have been lost. Beyond a certain point, however, significant amounts of metabolic byproducts are retained. These poorly defined substances appear to be responsible for many of the clinical manifestations of uremia.

Uremia is associated with derangements in homeostasis and metabolism and results in specific defects in multiple organ systems (Table 86.2). Many of these manifestations are corrected or relieved by dialysis, but others are not. All tend to develop gradually in patients with chronic renal failure, although some result in dysfunction that may present acutely.

APPROACH TO THE PATIENT

Patients with chronic renal failure, particularly if they are not yet on dialysis, most commonly present to the emergency department with nonspecific complaints such as generalized weakness, poor appetite, or increasing confusion. These symptoms are typ-

ically of insidious onset. The first clue to the diagnosis may be a laboratory finding of a reasonably well tolerated but rather severe anemia. Elevated blood urea nitrogen and serum creatinine levels can then confirm the diagnosis.

Once it has been ascertained that the patient is in no immediate danger (e.g., from life-threatening hyperkalemia), the next step is to establish that renal failure is indeed chronic rather than acute. A well-documented history of chronic renal disease, either from medical records or from the patient or family, may provide the most reliable confirmation, but one should consider the possibility of a previously overlooked correctable cause. A finding of bilaterally small kidneys on plain radiography or ultrasonography is good evidence for chronic renal disease, although the presence of normal-sized or large kidneys does not rule out chronic renal failure. Ascertaining a history of familial kidney disease, such as polycystic kidney disease or Alport syndrome, may also be helpful.

Laboratory abnormalities such as anemia, acidosis, hyperkalemia, hypocalcemia, and hyperphosphatemia can occur with *acute* renal failure as early as 10 days after its onset, but they tend to be better tolerated in patients with chronic renal disease. Findings on urinalysis are usually not helpful. Attention must be directed toward potentially reversible factors (e.g., volume depletion or obstruction), as they may represent the only opportunity to reverse the patient's disease rather than simply to manage its effects (Table 86.3).

DIALYSIS

Patients with chronic kidney failure are often sustained on chronic hemodialysis or peritoneal dialysis (PD). Although usually seen regularly by their nephrologists and nurse specialists, they continue to be relatively frequent visitors to emergency departments, being subject to those complications of chronic renal failure that are not corrected by dialysis, to the manifestations of underlying systemic diseases, and to complications of the dialytic therapy itself (8,22,23).

Compared with other patients, dialysis patients are less able to tolerate the stresses of intercurrent illness or trauma. Moreover, there is a significant potential for iatrogenic illness owing to inappropriate fluid or drug administration. Even apparently innocuous agents, such as antacids and enemas, can cause serious problems. Physicians caring for patients with chronic kidney failure should thus have ready access to a reference compendium containing guidelines for the adjustment of drug dosages in renal failure (2).

A number of serious problems are commonly encountered both in dialysis patients and in those with chronic renal failure who have not yet undergone dialytic therapy. The approach is similar in the two patient groups. The two major dialysis modalities, hemodialysis and PD, are themselves associated with specific complications with which the emergency physician should be familiar (9,17).

Hemodialysis

In hemodialysis, the patient's heparinized blood passes through an extracorporeal dialyzer circuit in which it is in contact with an artificial dialysis membrane. Water and solutes from the blood diffuse across this membrane to normalize blood volume and correct metabolic abnormalities. The amount of fluid transferred depends on the pressure under which blood is pumped through the dialyzer. Hemodialysis is usually performed several times a week for 3 to 5 hours per treatment. The high blood-flow rates that are necessary to make this an efficient process necessitate special access to the patient's circulation, generally through a surgically created arteriovenous fistula or through an artificial vascular graft, both of which are usually placed in the arm. For temporary hemodialysis access, a surgically placed, tunneled subclavian catheter is often used.

The vascular access device must be treated with care to avoid causing thrombosis or bleeding or introducing infection. The blood pressure should never be taken in the involved arm, and a tourniquet should never be applied. Unless absolutely essential, one should avoid drawing blood from the access or placing an intravenous line in it. In an emergency, if no other site is available and it is essential to obtain blood samples (e.g., if blood is needed immediately for crossmatch in a patient with serious bleeding), the fistula or graft can be used. A hemodialysis nurse should be called to access these sites whenever possible, however. Careful skin cleansing and sterile technique are mandatory, and firm but nonocclusive pressure should be applied to the site for 10 minutes after the puncture. The presence of a thrill both before and after the procedure should be documented.

Likewise, if intravenous access is critical but otherwise impossible, an intravenous line may be placed in the access, but with similar infection precautions and continuous observation during the infusion. Special care should be taken not to puncture the back wall of the access. An automated infusion pump is necessary to control the infusion rate, particularly when using the relatively high-pressure vessels in artificial arteriovenous grafts. With the low pressure typical of mature dilated fistulas, an infusion pump is still advisable.

Hemodialysis patients may present to the emergency department with a variety of complaints relating to the vascular access. Hemorrhage from a recent puncture site is usually easily managed with continuous, firm, but nonocclusive pressure over the site. Thrombosis, signaled by the loss of the thrill in the access, requires immediate consultation with a vascular surgeon, who may elect to perform a radiocontrast fistulogram, to infuse a thrombolytic agent, or to revise the access surgically. Forceful irrigation attempts are inadvisable.

The most common access-related problem is access infection, which is a serious concern in these patients because of the associated risk of bacteremia and metastatic infection, as well as the risk that the access may have to be removed because of persistent infection or impaired function. Infection is more likely to occur in an artificial graft than in a native fistula.

Most access infections are staphylococcal; contamination with skin flora at the time of puncture is believed to be the most likely cause. The diagnosis of access infection is not always obvious. When there is warmth, redness, tenderness, or local induration over the area and the patient is febrile, there is little cause for confusion, but some patients lack definite local signs and may present with repeated episodes of bacteremia or with fever and no obvious source of infection. In this situation, one should suspect access infection, draw blood cultures, and begin antibiotic therapy promptly.

A commonly used regimen is vancomycin 1 g, given intravenously as a single loading dose. Vancomycin is minimally hemodialyzable and needs to be given only once every 5 to 7 days, making it an attractive choice for staphylococcal coverage. A third-generation cephalosporin or an aminoglycoside can be added to this regimen for additional coverage, particularly if infection with a gram-negative organism is suspected. Local practice may vary, however, and emergency physicians should be familiar with the regimens in common use in their own institutions. Although a febrile illness may prove to be of viral etiology, it is prudent to treat such patients on the presumption of bacterial illness, because they can deteriorate rapidly and do have a high risk of access infection.

Not all febrile dialysis patients need to be admitted to the hospital. After intravenous antibiotic loading, a reliable patient who otherwise feels and looks relatively well may be sent home with careful instructions to return if there is any clinical deterioration. This decision is best reached in conjunction with the consulting nephrologist.

Peritoneal Dialysis

In PD, the patient's own peritoneum serves as the membrane across which diffusion of water and solutes occurs. Sterile dialysis fluid is infused into the peritoneal cavity through a surgically implanted Tenckhoff catheter. There are two types of PD: chronic ambulatory peritoneal dialysis (CAPD) and continuous cycling peritoneal dialysis (CCPD). In CAPD, after a dwell period dialysate is exchanged for fresh fluid, either manually or by an automated cycler machine. Exchanges are performed by the patient at home, usually four times a day, 7 days a week, using a sterile exchange technique. In CCPD, the exchanges are done automatically by a machine at night and once or twice during the day by the patient. Osmotic forces generated by high concentrations of glucose in the dialysis fluid ensure adequate removal of fluid volume from the blood; this is in contrast to hemodialysis, in which the amount of fluid removed is controlled by adjusting the pressure difference across the dialyzer membrane. PD offers several advantages over hemodialysis: greater patient independence, smoother control of excess volume and hypertension, and avoidance of rapid solute shifts and intermittent anticoagulation.

As with hemodialysis, many of the emergency problems encountered by the patient on PD are related to access devices, in this case the peritoneal catheter. By far the most common problem is peritonitis, caused by inadvertent contamination of the peritoneal cavity when exchanges are performed or by direct invasion of organisms from an infected catheter exit site. Peritonitis in these patients is, as a rule, less severe than other types of peritonitis. In fact, many of these infections can be treated on an outpatient basis, despite the fact that they involve the presence of a foreign body. Occasionally, if infection cannot be eradicated with antibiotic therapy, the catheter must be removed surgically and hemodialysis initiated pending placement of a new catheter after the infection has cleared.

About 75% of episodes of peritonitis are caused by gram-positive organisms, predominantly staphylococci. In most of the remainder, assorted gram-negative organisms are responsible; a small percentage are caused by fungal infection, which is usually considered an indication for catheter removal. Polymicrobial infection suggests a communication with the bowel or genitourinary tract.

The diagnosis of peritonitis is usually based on the patient's observation of cloudiness in the dialysate effluent at the time an exchange is performed. This is generally the earliest sign of peritonitis; therefore, patients are instructed to seek medical attention immediately when they notice it. Abdominal pain and fever often develop if treatment is not initiated promptly. Hospital admission becomes necessary if there is high fever, hypotension, severe abdominal pain, or nausea and vomiting, or if the patient cannot continue to carry out exchanges at home.

In the emergency department, the diagnosis of peritonitis is confirmed by the finding of organisms on Gram stain of the peritoneal fluid or of a cell count of more than 100 white blood cells per μL (with more than 50% neutrophils). This cell count corresponds approximately to the level at which cloudiness begins to be grossly detectable. Even in patients who have not noted cloudiness of the peritoneal effluent but who have fever, abdominal pain, or vague malaise, it is advisable to obtain a sample of fluid for examination, because the presentation of peritonitis can initially be subtle.

The fluid is obtained using meticulous sterile technique, and preferably by a dialysis nurse when possible. Fluid is sent for cell count and differential and for Gram stain and culture.

PD-related peritonitis can usually be treated on an outpatient basis (10). In general, treatment decisions should be made in conjunction with the patient's nephrologist or the PD nurse specialist, because these individuals usually are aware of the patient's overall medical condition, the types of infection recently experienced, and any psychosocial considerations that might affect outpatient management.

A common treatment regimen is vancomycin 30 mg/kg intraperitoneally at the time of diagnosis, followed by once-weekly intraperitoneal dosing. Intraperitoneal cefazolin, with or without gentamicin, is another commonly chosen regimen. Heparin 1,000 U may be added to each bag for the first few days of treatment in an effort to decrease the risk of fibrin's obstructing the catheter. A third-generation cephalosporin or an aminoglycoside can be added to the regimen for gram-positive coverage if there is reason to suspect infection with gram-negative organisms (e.g., positive Gram stain, recent gram-negative infection). These are typically given as an intraperitoneal loading dose, followed by a once-daily intraperitoneal maintenance dose. Arrangements should be made for the patient to be seen within 2 days to make sure the infection is responding to treatment and to check culture results and adjust therapy accordingly. Again, because practice may vary in different settings, emergency physicians should be familiar with the regimens in common use in their own institutions.

Several important caveats should be noted regarding the diagnosis of peritonitis. Other acute abdominal processes, such as pancreatitis, diverticulitis, or ruptured viscus, may present with a picture similar to that expected for peritonitis, and thus may not be diagnosed if the physician's suspicion is not aroused (19). To confuse the picture further, the finding of intraabdominal free air on radiographs may be the result of its inadvertent introduction during dialysis exchanges and does not necessarily indicate perforation (11). (The finding of brownish or fecal material in the dialysate mandates immediate surgical consultation.)

Several other problems related to the peritoneal dialysis procedure occasionally bring the PD patient to the emergency department. An exit site infection or an infection of the subcutaneous catheter tunnel may present as tenderness, warmth, or induration, or simply as a painless purulent exudate. Any exudate should have gram staining and culture. Treatment can be started with an oral antibiotic active against skin flora, but intensive local cleansing and skin care are also a critical part of management. Closed infections of the subcutaneous tunnel may be difficult to appreciate, and these infections respond poorly to medical therapy unless they are drained. If the patient should develop a leak of dialysis fluid from the tubing, bag, or catheter, or from around the catheter, evaluation and treatment should proceed as with peritonitis. The leaking elements must be replaced, if possible. A switch to low-volume exchanges may be helpful for leaks around the catheter, but surgical intervention may be necessary.

Difficulties with inflow or outflow of the dialysis fluid also occur occasionally. After ruling out straightforward problems such as kinked tubing or closed clamps, the physician must consider more troublesome mechanical causes, including obstruction of the catheter lumen, in which case surgical or nephrologic consultation is necessary. The most common cause of poor inflow or outflow is constipation. Catheter position is usually evaluated with plain abdominal X-rays. A contrast catheterogram may help to direct specific intervention. Fibrinolytic agents are sometimes helpful with obstructed catheters, but catheter replacement is often required.

CLINICAL PRESENTATION

Infection

Infections are a major cause of death in dialysis patients, and vascular access infection and peritonitis are the most common infections in hemodialysis patients and patients with PD, respectively (9,17). Most infections are caused by the usual pathogens rather than by opportunistic organisms. The challenge for the clinician arises from the fact that classic findings may not be obvious.

Dialysis patients commonly do not present with high fever in response to infection. Rather, they are likely to have nonspecific constitutional complaints such as fatigue, malaise, decreased appetite, or generalized weakness. Some manifestations of infections may be attributed to chronic renal failure per se, to the effects of dialysis, or to other underlying medical illness. For instance, pneumonia may present as dyspnea alone, which is easily attributed to volume overload or to the effects of chronic anemia. Urinary tract infection can occur even in patients who are essentially anuric (4); upper urinary tract infection, presenting as renal colic or with symptoms typical of pyelonephritis, is most common in patients with polycystic kidney disease. These and other infections are generally treated as in any other patient, but antibiotic doses must be adjusted for chronic kidney failure and the type of dialysis being used.

Hypotension

Hypotension commonly occurs in hemodialysis patients during or immediately after the dialysis procedure, but it usually resolves spontaneously or responds readily to fluid infusion. It is usually the result of rapid fluid and electrolyte shifts. Patients with PD are not subject to this cause of hypotension, but they too can become volume depleted if intake does not keep up with fluid losses that occur through dialysis. Other potentially lethal causes of hypotension must also be considered. Sepsis, drug effects, myocardial dysfunction, dysrhythmia, myocardial infarction, and pericardial tamponade are important considerations in patients treated by either dialysis modality; acute electrolyte disturbances, vascular instability, anaphylactoid reaction, and air embolism are considerations primarily in hemodialysis patients.

Pericardial tamponade may develop acutely when there is bleeding into the pericardial sac or when volume depletion allows a previously subclinical effusion to produce significant circulatory compromise. Although tamponade in this setting generally presents with the expected physical findings, coexistent cardiac or pulmonary disease may make the diagnosis difficult. Echocardiography is useful in detecting pericardial fluid; the size of an effusion does not correlate well with the presence of tamponade, however.

Many dialysis patients have effusions (of varying size) that do not appear to cause clinical difficulties. Echocardiographic demonstration of right ventricular collapse is a much better indicator of tamponade. Emergency pericardiocentesis may be necessary if the patient's condition deteriorates rapidly and tamponade is thought likely; it can establish the diagnosis and buy time until definitive surgical therapy can be undertaken. Another temporizing measure that is useful when tamponade has been precipitated by volume depletion is intravenous saline infusion to raise filling pressures.

Dyspnea and Volume Overload

Dyspnea in the dialysis patient is most commonly caused by volume overload. In the hemodialysis patient, it usually develops during the interval between dialyses. Physical examination is not always reliable in detecting volume overload in these patients; even chest radiographic findings may be misleading (12). The most reliable clue is a history of recent weight gain.

The definitive treatment of volume overload is dialysis, but several temporizing measures are available (Table 86.4) (6,18). Oxygen should be administered and the patient kept in the sitting position. Sublingual nitroglycerin can be administered quickly and does not require intravenous access; it often provides very rapid relief by reducing preload and afterload. Obviously, it should not be used if the patient is hypotensive. Intravenous nitroglycerin and nitroprusside are additional useful options and can be titrated to blood pressure and clinical effect; thiocyanate toxicity can result from prolonged use of nitroprusside in patients with renal failure, however.

Morphine can also be given, as in nondialysis patients, but may increase the need for intubation. Intravenous furosemide has a minimal diuretic effect in most dialysis patients. Finally, the use of continuous positive airway pressure devices may make it possible to avoid intubation in some patients who would otherwise require it.

Although volume overload is the most likely cause of shortness of breath in the dialysis patient, dyspnea can also be the result of cardiac impairment of any cause, hypotension, infection, pleural or pericardial effusion, or any of the other causes of dyspnea in nondialysis patients.

TABLE 86.4. Treatment of Pulmonary Edema in Renal Failure

Dialysis
  Hemodialysis
  Hemofiltration
  Peritoneal dialysis
Oxygen
Nitroglycerin (sublingual or intravenous)
Nitroprusside (if there is severe hypertension)
Morphine (but may increase the need for intubation)
Loop diuretics (if there is residual renal function)

Another potentially adverse effect of volume overload is severe hypertension, because, in most dialysis patients, blood pressure is at least partly volume dependent. For hypertensive crisis (i.e., hypertension, usually severe, with evidence of acute end-organ dysfunction), therapy should include not only sodium nitroprusside by intravenous infusion, or intravenous labetalol, but also prompt initiation or intensification of dialysis to lower blood volume.

Chest Pain

Chest pain in a dialysis patient should always suggest coronary artery disease. A significant proportion of dialysis patients die of cardiovascular causes (3,7). Chronic kidney failure itself appears to be a risk factor for coronary artery disease (16), and most patients have other risk factors such as hypertension, hyperlipidemia, and carbohydrate intolerance. Added to this are the effects of chronic anemia and intermittent or chronic volume overload. The hemodialysis procedure itself is often the occasion for additional ischemic stress to the myocardium because of transient hypoxemia and hypotension.

Initial interventions for suspected ischemic chest pain are similar to those for other patients, but particular attention should be directed toward such correctable factors as volume overload, hypertension, and anemia. The diagnosis of myocardial infarction by standard electrocardiographic and enzyme criteria is generally not affected by the abnormalities of kidney failure (14,15,21). Although baseline cardiac enzyme levels may be somewhat higher than in the nondialysis population, when infarction occurs, the pattern of enzyme changes is not affected. Troponin I appears to be the most reliable serum marker of infarction in these patients (15,21). Decisions as to the most appropriate reperfusion therapy for dialysis patients with acute coronary syndromes should be made in concert with a cardiologist and the patient's nephrologist.

Chest pain may, of course, result from any of the other commonly incriminated causes, but pericarditis should always be a consideration in the dialysis patient once myocardial ischemia has been excluded. Pericarditis (and tamponade) may occur even in well-dialyzed patients. The signs and symptoms are the same as those noted in nondialysis patients. Based on experience in undialyzed uremic patients, it has traditionally been taught that increased or intensified dialysis, without heparin anticoagulation, hastens resolution of pericarditis or prevents the development of tamponade or pericardial constriction, although this remains an open question. For many patients with pericarditis, indomethacin may provide prompt relief of pain. Intrapericardial instillation of corticosteroids, or pericardial stripping, is ultimately necessary in other patients.

Bleeding

Bleeding is relatively common in dialysis patients; it is, at least in part, related to platelet dysfunction (which is not completely corrected by dialysis) and, in hemodialysis patients, to transient anticoagulation. It is important to ascertain what the bleeding patient's usual hemoglobin level has been. Epoetin or darbepoetin are now administered routinely to almost all dialysis patients, but untreated, the baseline hemoglobin level may be 6 to 7 g/dL. Moderately severe anemia may present with increased angina or dyspnea. Other symptoms, sometimes life-threatening ones, may be caused by occult bleeding into particular anatomic sites; spontaneous intracranial, intraocular, pericardial, and retroperitoneal bleeding have been reported.

Treatment of acute bleeding episodes follows standard principles. It should also be established that dialysis has been adequate. Because correction of severe anemia (hematocrit less than

25%) improves bleeding time (probably by a rheologic effect), red blood cell transfusion should be considered, and additional acute treatment with desmopressin (0.3 μg/kg intravenously or subcutaneously) or conjugated estrogens (0.6 mg/kg intravenously) should be begun (9). For life-threatening bleeding, cryoprecipitate infusion and platelet transfusions are recommended (5).

Neurologic Dysfunction

Neurologic dysfunction in the form of *disequilibrium syndrome* can occur during and just after the hemodialysis procedure, although usually only in patients with high BUNs who are just initiating dialytic therapy. Typical mild manifestations are headache, nausea, and muscle cramps; more severe cases may cause altered mental status and grand mal seizures. Disequilibrium is presumed to be caused by the rapid changes in intracellular composition and osmolality that occure with the removal of large volumes of fluid or the correction of marked metabolic and electrolyte abnormalities with hemodialysis (it does not occur with PD). It usually resolves within a few hours after the treatment is completed; symptoms often respond promptly to intravenous infusion of mannitol or hypertonic saline during dialysis.

However, because there are many other potential causes for neurologic dysfunction in these patients (not the least of which are intracranial bleeding, hypertensive encephalopathy, infection, and untoward drug effects), it is unwise to attribute any acute neurologic abnormality to the disequilibrium syndrome without carefully considering other causes. If findings are focal, appear suddenly, or fluctuate or become worse after a reasonable period of observation, attention should be directed to all of the other potential causes. Similarly, the presence of fever, papilledema, or severe hypertension should suggest more serious etiologies.

Electrolyte Abnormalities

Hyperkalemia is a common life-threatening emergency in undialyzed patients with acute or chronic renal failure, but it is seldom a serious problem in the dialyzed patient. When hyperkalemia does occur, it usually results from noncompliance with dietary restrictions or dialysis treatments. On occasion, it may also be the result of intercurrent disorders such as rhabdomyolysis, sepsis, or severe acidosis. Hyperkalemia is particularly dangerous because it is generally completely asymptomatic until dangerous cardiac effects develop. Although many dialysis patients chronically tolerate moderate hyperkalemia (6 to 7 mEq/L) with no apparent problem, a potassium level in this range must still be considered potentially dangerous because severe effects can develop fairly rapidly. Moreover, the electrocardiogram is occasionally completely normal even when hyperkalemia is severe (20), and it cannot be relied on to exclude any danger of serious hyperkalemic complications developing. Thus, the serum potassium level should always be checked.

The treatment of hyperkalemia is outlined in Chapter 166. The guidelines for treatment in dialysis patients follow those for treatment in other patients, but particular attention must be directed to avoiding volume overload, symptomatic hypocalcemia, or other potential complications of therapy. These interventions are temporizing measures only, and dialysis should be instituted or reinstituted as promptly as possible. A particularly convenient and effective method of decreasing the serum potassium level is by the administration of nebulized albuterol in a dose 4 to 8 times as great as that used in the typical patient with asthma. This intervention provides rapid and sustained improvement in the serum potassium concentration for at least

several hours and appears to be associated with few side effects (1).

A dialysis patient in cardiac arrest should be presumed to be hyperkalemic and should receive intravenous calcium and intravenous bicarbonate (through separate lines to prevent precipitation). This is one group of patients to whom these two drugs should still be administered routinely despite the recent revisions of advanced cardiac life-support guidelines.

Other electrolyte abnormalities can occur in patients with kidney failure under a variety of conditions, but the most important and the most common are hypocalcemia and hypermagnesemia. Hypocalcemic symptoms are uncommon in dialyzed patients, but may occur in patients who have not been treated with vitamin D and calcium supplementation, particularly when intravenous bicarbonate is given to treat hyperkalemia or severe acidosis. Symptomatic hypocalcemia should be treated with intravenous calcium gluconate or calcium chloride.

Mild hypermagnesemia is common in chronic kidney failure, but symptoms do not usually occur until magnesium levels are high, generally greater than 4 mg/dL. Symptomatic hypermagnesemia is almost always a result of inadvertent ingestion of magnesium-containing antacids or laxatives. Intravenous calcium acts as a direct antagonist to the neuromuscular effects of hypermagnesemia, but in the absence of the renal route of excretion, removal of excess magnesium from the body requires emergent dialysis.

CRITICAL INTERVENTIONS

- Quickly diagnose and initiate treatment for severe complications of chronic renal failure, such as hyperkalemia, fluid overload, and pericardial effusion
- Initiate antibiotic treatment for patients with infected dialysis catheters or peritonitis

DISPOSITION

A critical decision commonly facing the emergency physician is whether emergency dialysis is necessary for patients presenting to the emergency department with acute clinical problems. Some patients may have deteriorated between hemodialysis treatments or despite continuing PD; others may have failed to undergo scheduled dialyses. The most common indication for emergency dialysis (Table 86.5) is severe volume overload or pulmonary edema; available temporizing measures for managing the patient until dialysis can be effective have already been described. Appropriate temporizing measures also may be employed to manage malignant hypertension, severe electrolyte disturbances, or severe acidosis while awaiting the definitive treatment afforded by dialysis.

Uremic symptoms (e.g., lethargy, confusion, asterixis, nausea, and vomiting) indicate that dialysis is needed but are not, in and of themselves, indications for *emergency* dialysis unless they are severe. Similarly, serum creatinine and blood urea nitrogen levels correlate only roughly with uremic symptoms or life-threatening

---

TABLE 86.5.   Indications for Emergency Dialysis

Pulmonary edema
Severe uncontrollable hypertension with volume overload
Severe or uncontrolled hyperkalemia
Other severe electrolyte or acid–base disturbances
Some overdoses
? Pericarditis

metabolic disturbances and do not, in and of themselves, indicate an urgent need for dialysis. The appearance of pericarditis, with or without pericardial tamponade, is often considered an indication for urgent or intensified dialysis, but pericarditis can occur even in well-dialyzed patients, and it is not clear that there is an increased risk of clinical deterioration if it is not treated aggressively.

A key component of the emergency department management of all types of problems in the dialysis patient must always be consultation with the patient's nephrologist or dialysis nurse, both to take advantage of the expertise of these specialists in caring for these patients' complicated problems and to ensure optimal continuity of care. However, the emergency physician has a responsibility to be familiar with the evaluation of and therapy for acute problems in dialysis patients so that emergency interventions can be performed promptly when necessary.

COMMON PITFALLS

✔ Failing to identify treatable factors in patients who may have a reversible component of their chronic renal insufficiency (especially obstruction)
✔ Causing iatrogenic illness through inappropriate fluid or drug administration
✔ Allowing the vascular access to be used for taking blood pressure or drawing blood, or for intravenous infusion
✔ Failing to consider vascular access infection in hemodialysis patients, or peritonitis in PD patients, because of lack of specific findings on history and physical examination
✔ Failing to consider the diagnosis of tamponade because the patient does not demonstrate all of the classic signs and symptoms
✔ Failing to treat volume overload because of a lack of specific findings
✔ Overlooking anemia as a cause of increased angina or shortness of breath
✔ Inappropriately attributing any neurologic dysfunction to disequilibrium syndrome
✔ Failing to seek evidence of hyperkalemia by blood test or electrocardiogram
✔ Inducing symptomatic hypocalcemia by ill-advised bicarbonate therapy

References

1. Allon M, Dunlay R, Copkney C. Nebulized albuterol for acute hyperkalemia in patients on hemodialysis. *Ann Intern Med* 1989;110:426.
2. Aronoff GR, Berns JS, Brier ME, et al. *Drug prescribing in renal failure: dosing guidelines for adults.* Philadelphia: American College of Physicians, 2002.
3. Bleyer AJ, Russell GB, Satko SG. Sudden and cardiac death rates in hemodialysis patients. *Kidney Int* 1999;55:1553.
4. Chaudhry A, Stone WJ, Breyer JA. Occurrence of pyuria and bacteriuria in asymptomatic hemodialysis patients. *Am J Kidney Dis* 1993;21:180.
5. Eberst ME, Berkowitz LR. Hemostasis in renal disease: pathophysiology and management. *Am J Med* 1994;96:168.
6. Gehm L, Propp DA. Pulmonary edema in the renal failure patient. *Am J Emerg Med* 1989;7:336.
7. Herzog CA. Acute myocardial infarction in patients with end-stage renal disease. *Kidney Int* 1999;56:S130–S133.
8. Hodde LA, Sandroni S. Emergency department evaluation and management of dialysis patient complications. *Am J Emerg Med* 1992;10:317.
9. Ifudu O. Care of patients undergoing hemodialysis. *N Engl J Med* 1998; 339:1054–1062.
10. Keane WF, Bailie GR, Boeschoten E, et al. Adult peritoneal dialysis-related peritonitis treatment recommendations: 2000 update. http:// www.ispd.org/2000_treatment_recommendations.html. Accessed January 3, 2005.
11. Kiefer T, Schenk U, Weber J, et al. Incidence and significance of pneumoperitoneum in continuous ambulatory peritoneal dialysis. *Am J Kidney Dis* 1993;22:30.
12. Kohen JA, Opsahl JA, Kjellstrand CM. Deceptive patterns of uremic pulmonary edema. *Am J Kidney Dis* 1986;7:456.
13. Levey AS, Coresh J, Balk E, et al. National Kidney Foundation practice guide-

lines for chronic kidney disease: evaluation, classification, and stratification. *Ann Intern Med* 2003;139:137–147.
14. Martin GS, Becker BN, Schulman G. Cardiac troponin-I accurately predicts myocardial injury in renal failure. *Nephrol Dial Transplant* 1998;13:1709.
15. McCullough PA, Nowak RM, Foreback C, et al. Performance of multiple cardiac biomarkers measured in the emergency department in patients with chronic kidney disease and chest pain. *Acad Emerg Med* 2002;9:1389–1396.
16. Muntner P, Hamm LL, Kusek JW, et al. The prevalence of nontraditional risk factors for coronary heart disease in patients with chronic kidney disease. *Ann Intern Med* 2004;140:9–17.
17. Pastan S, Bailey J. Dialysis therapy. *N Engl J Med* 1998;338:1428–1437.
18. Sacchetti A, McCabe J, Torres M, et al. ED management of acute congestive heart failure in renal dialysis patients. *Am J Emerg Med* 1993;11:644.
19. Steiner RW, Halasz NA. Abdominal catastrophes and other unusual events in continuous ambulatory dialysis patients. *Am J Kidney Dis* 1990;15:1.
20. Szerlip HM, Weiss J, Singer I. Profound hyperkalemia without electrocardiographic manifestations. *Am J Kidney Dis* 1986;7:461.
21. Watnick S, Perazella MA. Cardiac troponins: utility in renal insufficiency and end-stage renal disease. *Semin Dialysis* 2002;15:66–70.
22. Wolfson AB, Singer I. Hemodialysis-related emergencies: I. *J Emerg Med* 1987;5:533.
23. Wolfson AB, Singer I. Hemodialysis-related emergencies: II. *J Emerg Med* 1988;6:61.

CHAPTER 87

The Patient with a Renal Transplant

Louis G. Graff

The kidney is the most commonly transplanted organ in the United States: More than 10,000 are transplanted each year (19). In contrast to dialysis, transplantation allows the patient to live a normal life. Transplant patients do not need a treatment (dialysis) 3 times a week, do not need to restrict their diets (potassium, sodium, and fluid intake), and can have children (6,20). Therefore, transplantation is the preferred treatment for patients with end-stage renal disease.

Kidneys have been successfully transplanted for more than 40 years (9,14). The transplanted kidney is obtained from a living-related donor or from a cadaver. At surgery, it is connected to the common iliac vein and artery in the pelvic fossa, and the ureter is anastomosed to the bladder. The transplanted kidney is placed in the pelvic area not only because it is anatomically convenient for anastomosis to the vasculature and the bladder, but also because it is accessible for direct palpation, biopsy, or removal. The patient and transplanted organ are matched for the human leukocyte antigen (HLA) major histocompatibility complex (MHC) gene to minimize the risk of transplant rejection. Initially the patient is inducted with a few day treatment with a T-cell depleting agent such as antilymphocyte antibody or basiliximab (9,14,21). Then the patient is maintained on a combination of immunosuppressive drugs such as corticosteroids, mycophenolate mofetil, cyclosporine, or tacrolimus (3,9,14). Graft survival is 98% at 1 year for properly matched, living-related donors, and 91% for cadaveric donors (10,14). Patient survival is higher (greater than 98% at 1 year for living-related donors and 95% for cadaveric donors), as the patient can go back on dialysis if the transplant fails.

The unique aspects of caring for the patient with a transplanted kidney must be considered when such a patient presents to the emergency department. Evaluation and management of even minor problems is often complicated by the patient's immunosuppressed state and the presence of a transplant. Transplant patients often have a limited ability to tolerate intercurrent illness, trauma, or other physiologic stresses. Moreover, chronic immunosuppression places them at increased risk for severe infectious disease, and often makes it difficult to evaluate emergent problems such as abdominal pain or fever. The status of the transplanted kidney must always be a concern as well. Patients may present with complications of the transplant surgery or with subtle signs and symptoms of graft rejection.

MEDICATIONS

Treatment is often more complicated in the transplant patient because certain medications may have adverse effects or be frankly contraindicated in these patients (Table 87.1). For example, potassium-sparing diuretics can cause severe hyperkalemia in patients who are taking cyclosporine. Nephrotoxic drugs can act synergistically with cyclosporine and contribute to renal dysfunction. Lovastatin can cause a severe myopathy in patients taking cyclosporine. Also, a number of medications can increase or decrease cyclosporine, tacrolimus, and sirolimus levels (2) and thus affect drug effectiveness and toxicity (see Table 87.1).

Emergency physicians should be familiar with the adverse effects of medications routinely prescribed to the transplant patient (see Table 87.2). Induction agents such as antilymphocyte antibodies or Daclizumab cause leukopenia and thrombocytopenia and may lead to infections or bleeding. Maintenance agents such as cyclosporine, tacrolimus, and azathioprine increase the patient's susceptibility to infection, particularly by opportunistic organisms. The patient's risk of cancer (especially lymphoma, cervical cancer, and skin cancer) is 3% or 4% (8). Because azathioprine causes leukopenia in more than 50% of patients, close monitoring of the blood count is necessary. These drugs can also cause hepatotoxicity, so liver enzymes should be checked in patients with symptoms consistent with hepatitis. In addition, liver failure can decrease the metabolism of cyclosporine and cause cyclosporine nephrotoxicity. Corticosteroids can contribute to the development of peptic ulcer disease, hypertension, accelerated coronary artery disease, diabetes, osteoporosis, aseptic necrosis of the hip, impaired healing, cataract, hemorrhagic pancreatitis, and candidal pharyngitis. Mycophenolate mofetil and sirolimus are newer immunosuppressive agents are being developed and brought into clinical practice. These agents have their own side effects and adverse interactions with other medications (27).

EARLY COMPLICATIONS OF TRANSPLANTATION SURGERY

Early after transplantation, complications of the surgery may bring patients to the emergency department. There may be acute tubular necrosis, especially if the graft preservation time before surgery was prolonged. Vascular complications, such as renal artery stenosis or thrombosis or renal vein thrombosis, can cause graft dysfunction or localized pain. Ureteral stenosis can cause decreased graft function as well. Clarification of the cause of the patient's problem may be evident on examination of the urinalysis or with CT imaging of the kidney or evaluation of renal artery flow with Doppler ultrasound (18).

TABLE 87.1.   Some Drugs to Avoid in the Renal Transplantation Patient

NEPHROTOXINS

Gentamicin, tobramycin, vancomycin, cimetidine, ranitidine, diclofenac, amphotericin B, ketoconazole, melphalan, trimethoprim-sulfamethoxazole, azapropazone

DRUGS THAT DECREASE CYCLOSPORINE EFFECTIVENESS

Rifampin, phenobarbital, phenytoin, carbamazepine, isoniazid, nafcillin, octreotide, ticlopidine

DRUGS THAT INCREASE CYCLOSPORINE EFFECTIVENESS AND TOXICITY

Diltiazem, nicardipine, verapamil, danazol, bromocriptine, metoclopramide, ketoconazole, fluconazole, itraconazole, erythromycin, clarithromycin, doxycycline, methylprednisolone, oral contraceptives, allopurinol

DRUGS THAT INCREASE TACROLIMUS EFFECTIVENESS AND TOXICITY

Diltiazem, nicardipine, nifedipine, verapamil, clotrimazole, fluconazole, itraconazole, ketoconazole, clarithromycin, erythromycin, imipenem, cisapride, metoclopramide, bromocriptine, cimetidine, cyclosporine, danazol, methylprednisolone, protease inhibitors, nephrotoxins (aminoglycosides, amphotericin B, cisplatin)

DRUGS THAT DECREASE TACROLIMUS EFFECTIVENESS

Carbamazepine, phenobarbital, phenytoin, rifabutin, rifampin, nafcillin, valproic acid

DRUGS THAT INHIBIT AZATHIOPRINE METABOLISM

Allopurinol

DRUGS THAT INCREASE SIROLIMUS EFFECTIVENESS

Diltiazem, ketoconazole, cyclosporine, nicardipine, verapamil, clotrimazole, fluconazole, itraconazole, clarithromycin, erythromycin, troleandomicin, cisapride, metoclopramide, bromocriptine, cimetidine, danazol, ritonavir, indinavir

DRUGS THAT DECREASE SIROLIMUS EFFECTIVENESS

Rifampin, carbamazepine, phenobarbital, phenytoin, rifabutin, rifapentine, St. John's Wort

POTASSIUM-SPARING DIURETICS

Amiloride, spironolactone, triamterene

LOVASTATIN

May cause myopathy

Local hematoma or lymphocele can cause pain or compromise graft function by mass effect. The immunosuppressive drugs given to prevent graft rejection also inhibit wound healing and the normal response to infection. At least 20% of patients develop a wound infection, and many others develop other infections. Most patients with surgical complications present within days or weeks of transplantation, although some complications (e.g., ureteral stenosis and smoldering infection) may have a delayed presentation.

TABLE 87.2. Adverse Effects of Renal Transplantation Medications

INDUCTION AGENTS

Antilymphocyte antibody (category C in pregnancy, may be excreted in milk)—fever, chills, leukopenia, dizziness

Basiliximab (category B in pregnancy, may be excreted in milk)—nausea, vomiting, headache, dizziness, bleeding, leukopenia

Daclizumab (category C in pregnancy, may be excreted in milk)—nausea, vomiting, headache, dizziness, bleeding, leukopenia

MAINTENANCE IMMUNOSUPPRESSIVE AGENTS

Azathioprine (category D in pregnancy, some excretion in milk)—serious infections, leukopenia, thrombocytopenia, lymphoma, skin malignancies, alopecia, nausea and vomiting, hepatotoxicity, gingival hyperplasia

Tacrolimus (category C in pregnancy, excreted in milk)—precipitation of diabetes mellitus, hypertension, lymphoma, skin malignancies, nephrotoxicity, neurotoxicity (tremor, headache, mental status change, sensory function change, insomnia), hepatotoxicity, hyperkalemia, serious infections

Cyclosporine (category C in pregnancy, excreted in milk)—serious infections, nephrotoxicity, hyperkalemia, neurotoxicity (tremor, seizure, headaches), hypertension, lymphoma, hepatotoxicity, hyperuricemia, cosmetic side effects (gingival hyperplasia, hypertrichosis)

Sirolimus (category C in pregnancy, may be excreted in milk)—anemia, leukopenia, thrombocytopenia, hypokalemia, hyperlipidemia, nephrotoxicity, hepatotoxicity

Mycophenolate mofetil (category C in pregnancy, may be excreted in milk)—serious infections, neutropenia, gastrointestinal hemorrhage, pulmonary edema, lymphoma, hypertension

Corticosteroids—adrenal insufficiency, osteoporosis, hypertension, hyperglycemia, cataracts, avascular necrosis, peptic ulcer disease, Cushing syndrome, congestive heart failure, seizure, headaches, papilledema, glaucoma

TABLE 87.3. Differential Diagnosis of Renal Failure in the Patient with a Renal Transplant

PRERENAL

Hypovolemia
Renal artery stenosis
Renal artery thrombosis
Renal vein thrombosis

RENAL (INTRINSIC DISEASE)

Recurrence of disease (e.g., diabetes mellitus, systemic lupus erythematosus, focal glomerulosclerosis, Goodpasture syndrome, Wegener granulomatosis, glomerulonephritis)
Acute rejection
Chronic rejection
Acute tubular necrosis
Cyclosporine toxicity

POSTRENAL (OBSTRUCTION)

Prostate
Abscess
Urinoma
Lymphocele
Ureteral stenosis at the anastomosis

RENAL DYSFUNCTION

Evidence of renal dysfunction should always be sought in the patient with a renal transplant, and any reversible cause of renal failure must be identified and treated promptly (Table 87.3). Small changes in the serum creatinine level may indicate important changes in renal function. For example, an increase in the serum creatinine level from 1 to 2 mg/dL represents a 50% decrease in renal function. During the first days after transplantation surgery, the most common causes of renal failure are acute tubular necrosis, hyperacute rejection, urinary tract obstruction, urine leak, compression of the graft or renal artery by hematoma, and hypovolemia. During the first 12 weeks after transplantation surgery, the patient may experience acute rejection, renal artery stenosis, or urinary tract obstruction. Renal failure more than 3 months after surgery is usually a result of acute rejection, chronic rejection, recurrence of underlying renal disease, or new renal disease.

All patients with renal dysfunction must be evaluated for obstruction. There are often no clues to this; the urinalysis is negative and urine output may be unchanged. Ultrasound, however, can show hydronephrosis and confirm the diagnosis of obstruction.

Prerenal causes are often responsible for decreased renal function in transplantation patients (see Table 87.3). The patient may be volume-depleted or have widespread arteriosclerotic disease.

The anastomosis to the native artery may be a site of particular vulnerability to stenosis. A high blood urea nitrogen (BUN)–

creatinine ratio and a low urine sodium are consistent with this cause of renal failure. If the stenosis is not severe, the only sign or symptom may be severe hypertension. Percutaneous transluminal angioplasty has been successful in reversing hypertension and renal failure (25), but surgical reconstruction may be necessary. Radioisotope scanning using technetium or hippuran or Doppler ultrasound evaluation (18) can identify renal artery stenosis; complete occlusion can result in irreversible infarction unless blood flow is restored within 2 hours.

Renal vein thrombosis can also occur. Patients may present with graft pain and tenderness, fever, hypertension, and proteinuria. The treatment is long-term anticoagulation.

Clues to the presence of intrinsic renal disease (see Table 87.3) may be found in the urinalysis. Red blood cell casts or proteinuria is seen in glomerulonephritis and vasculitis. Consideration should be given to recurrence of the disease that originally caused renal failure (30), especially with systemic diseases such as diabetes mellitus or vasculitis. Glomerulonephritis may recur in the graft if the disease is still active in the original kidneys at the time of transplantation.

REJECTION

Patients with kidney transplants are always at risk for transplant rejection. Acute rejection usually occurs within 4 weeks of transplantation but can occur many months later, and can result in complete loss of graft function. The precipitant is usually unknown, but the clinician should be circumspect in exposing the transplant patient to antigens, whether in the form of drugs or blood transfusions (4). The clinical findings are often those of prerenal or intrinsic renal disease (i.e., low urine sodium level and high BUN–creatinine ratio). The kidney is enlarged and tender, and there may be fever, hypertension, or oliguria. An increased serum level of β_2-microglobulin supports the diagnosis of acute rejection, but the diagnosis must usually be confirmed by percutaneous renal biopsy (29). The prognosis is poor when acute rejection occurs more than 6 months after transplantation or shows evidence of increased severity (by histologic grade or change in the serum creatinine) (16).

Treatment is hospitalization and administration of a combination of immunosuppressive drugs, including high-dose corticosteroids (e.g., methylprednisolone 500 to 1,000 mg/day). Chronic rejection, which cannot be treated, occurs months to years after transplantation and is manifested by a gradual deterioration of renal function.

Cyclosporine and tacrolimus are low-molecular-weight fungal metabolites that are very effective at preventing transplant rejection by depleting circulating T lymphocytes. Unfortunately, they produce nephrotoxicity in up to 50% of patients (27), which usually occurs more than 6 weeks after transplantation. Some centers change from these drugs to azathioprine at 4 to 6 months after transplantation to avoid the risk of nephrotoxicity. The BUN–creatinine ratio tends to reflect a prerenal process. The graft is not tender or swollen, and ultrasound examination is normal. A reduction in the dose of immunosuppressives can lead to return of renal function. In practice, the question often is whether a decrease in renal function is caused by transplant rejection, thereby requiring an increase in the dose of drug, or to drug nephrotoxicity, requiring a decrease in the dose. Assays for blood drug levels can help differentiate rejection from drug nephrotoxicity (1).

FEVER OR INFECTION

Kidney transplantation patients are at increased risk of infection (Fig. 87.1). Organ transplantation became possible because of the development of immunosuppressive agents to prevent organ rejection, but at the cost of greatly increased infectious complications. An aggressive approach to identifying and treating infection has been the primary factor responsible for today's high survival rates for transplant patients.

As is the case with other immunosuppressed patients, the signs and symptoms of infection in renal transplant patients may be masked, and opportunistic infections may require specialized diagnostic and treatment modalities (26). In contrast to the usual approach to the non-immunosuppressed patient with fever, in whom treatment can generally be instituted on the basis of clinical criteria, aggressive efforts to identify a responsible organism are usually justified in transplantation patients. Twenty percent of transplantation patients develop urinary tract infections that are readily diagnosed on urinalysis. Ten percent develop clearcut surgical wound infection. Sepsis, which may be evidenced only by positive blood cultures, occurs in 5%; occult abscess is found in another 5% (7). Two percent to 4% develop systemic fungal infections, and 9% to 10% develop local fungal infections.

Because the signs and symptoms of serious infection may be masked, blood cultures should be undertaken for any transplantation patient with fever, and hospital admission should be considered when the source of infection cannot be identified. Uncomplicated urinary tract infections and wound infections may be treated with conventional antibiotics on an outpatient basis.

Five percent to 12% of renal transplantation patients develop cytomegalovirus (CMV) infection, which includes symptoms of fever, adenopathy, leukopenia, and myalgias. Complications include retinitis, pneumonitis, hepatitis, fungal and parasitic superinfection, and transplant rejection. Preoperative administration of CMV immunoglobulin or ganciclovir significantly reduces the risk of postoperative CMV infection (23,28).

Meningitis can present very subtly in the transplantation patient. Classic signs of meningitis (e.g., fever or meningismus) may not be present. Headache, which may suggest other serious disease, such as temporal arteritis or subarachnoid hemorrhage (12), is the most common symptom. Opportunistic organisms such as *Cryptococcus* species are more likely to cause disease than are the usual pathogens (17). The emergency physician must have a high level of suspicion and a low threshold for performing a diagnostic lumbar puncture.

Trimethoprim–sulfamethoxazole prophylaxis has become the standard treatment in renal transplantation patients because of the high risk of infections (11). *Pneumocystis carinii* pneumonia ordinarily develops in up to 12% of patients, but it is eliminated with prophylaxis. In addition, prophylaxis with trimethoprim–sulfamethoxazole for the first 6 months reduces the risk of urinary tract infection from greater than 50% to 5% (11).

ABDOMINAL PAIN

Evaluation of abdominal pain in the transplantation patient is challenging because immunosuppressive medications can mask the signs and symptoms of disease. In one series of transplantation patients with abdominal pain, 10% developed an acute abdomen, and one half of them required surgery for perforation or bowel obstruction (15). Of those who required surgery, only 29% had fever and only 29% had leukocytosis. Because of the subtle presentation and difficulty in diagnosis, delays before surgery were substantial (ranging from 18 to 96 hours), and 71% of patients had sustained perforation by the time of surgery. Notably, 43% had signs of perforation on plain abdominal radiographs.

The most common causes of an acute abdomen in transplantation patients are similar to those in the general population: gastroduodenal bleeding or perforation, colonic bleeding or perforation, bowel obstruction, appendicitis, cholecystitis, volvulus, and ovarian torsion (5,15). Patients with polycystic kidney disease may have abdominal pain because of hemorrhage or infection in the cysts, if their own kidneys have not been

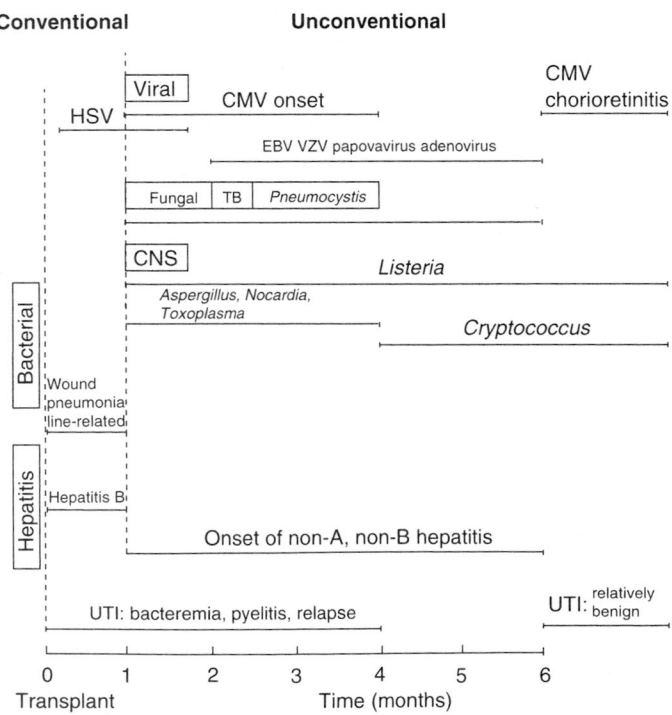

Figure 87.1. Timetable for the occurrence of infection in renal transplant recipients. HSV, herpes simplex virus; CMV, cytomegalovirus; EBV, Epstein-Barr virus; VZV, varicella zoster virus; TB, tuberculosis; CNS, central nervous system; UTI, urinary tract infection. (Redrawn after Rubin RH. Infectious disease complications of renal transplantation. *Kidney Int* 1993;44:224.)

removed. Ultrasound testing can evaluate these patients. Because both azathioprine and cyclosporine can cause hepatitis with abdominal pain, liver enzymes should be measured in transplant patients with abdominal pain. The transplant patient has an increased risk of developing lymphoma, probably because of chronic immunosuppression (24). Abdominal computed tomographic scanning can identify enlarged retroperitoneal nodes or tumor mass.

Pancreatitis occurs infrequently (1%) in renal transplantation patients. When it does occur, it is quite serious, with 80% to 100% mortality (22).

IMMUNIZATIONS

Killed and antigen-based vaccines (tetanus, diphtheria, rabies, influenza, and pneumococcal vaccines) can be safely used in patients who have undergone transplantation. There is no contraindication to treatment with immunoglobulin. Live or attenuated vaccines (measles, mumps, rubella, oral polio, bacille Calmette-Guérin (BCG), yellow fever, and typhoid) are contraindicated in the immunosuppressed patient, because they can cause serious infection.

CRITICAL INTERVENTIONS

- Recognize and admit patients with acute rejection to the hospital
- Order an ultrasound to rule out obstruction in patients with renal dysfunction
- Aggressively seek the source of fever in immunosuppressed patients

DISPOSITION

The threshold for hospitalizing the transplantation patient should be very low. One must always suspect a pathologic process, even in patients who seem to have only minor complaints. When a transplant-related problem is identified, the emergency physician should not hesitate to seek appropriate consultation or to arrange transfer of the patient to a facility with the resources to manage transplant patients. Nevertheless, the emergency physician can manage most acute problems in renal transplant patients if a thorough and meticulous approach is used.

COMMON PITFALLS

✔ Prescribing potentially nephrotoxic drugs in the renal transplant patient

✔ Failing to realize that a small rise in the transplant patient's creatinine level may represent a relatively large decrement in renal function, necessitating aggressive evaluation

✔ Assuming that a normal urine output excludes obstruction as the cause of acute renal failure

✔ Failing to remember that the immunosuppressed transplant patient often does not show classic signs or laboratory findings of infection

✔ Failing to remember that certain drugs may decrease cyclosporine or tacrolimus levels and lead to transplant rejection; likewise, certain drugs may increase these drug levels and lead to toxicity

✔ Failing to provide increased doses of steroids when transplant

patients taking corticosteroids undergo major stress, such as surgery, myocardial infarction, major trauma, or sepsis

✔ Giving a blood transfusion without a clear indication, because stimulation by exogenous antigens may lead to rejection

✔ Overlooking the fact that the transplant patient may have three kidneys (two original, one transplanted), all of which may become infected or be injured

References

1. Beutler D, Molteni S, Zeugin T, et al. Evaluation of instrumental, nonisotopic immunoassays (fluorescence polarization immunoassay and enzyme-multiplied immunoassay technique) for cyclosporine monitoring in whole blood after kidney and liver transplantation. *Ther Drug Monit* 1992;14:424.
2. Bottiger Y, Brattstrom C, Tyden G, et al. Tacrolimus whole blood concentrations correlate closely to side-effects in renal transplant recipients. *Br J Clin Pharmacol* 1999;48:445–448.
3. Bunnapradist S, Daswani A, Takemoto SK. Graft survival following living donor renal transplantation: a comparison of tacrolimus and cyclosporine microemulsion with mycophenolate mofetil and steroids. *Transplantation* 2003;76:10–15.
4. Burlingham WJ, Stratta R, Mason B, et al. Risk factors for sensitization by blood transfusions. *Transplantation* 1989;47:140.
5. Chan MK, Wilcox DT, Trompeter RS. Acute appendicitis in children after renal transplantation. *Arch Dis Child* 1999;81:372.
6. Davison JM, Bailey DJ. Pregnancy following renal transplantation. *J Obstet Gynaecol Res* 2003;29:227–233.
7. Dempsey J, Scott R. Duplex Doppler examination of a perinephric abscess in a renal transplant. *South Med J* 1990;83:1213.
8. Feczko BJ, Mezwa DC. Gastrointestinal carcinomas in renal transplant recipients. *Gastrointest Radiol* 1991;16:351.
9. Ferguson RM, Henry M, Elkhammas E, et al. Twenty years of renal transplantation at Ohio State University: the results of five eras of immunosuppression. *Am J Surgery* 2003;186:306–311.
10. Fischel RJ, Payne WD, Gillingham KJ, et al. Long-term outlook for renal transplant recipients with 1-year function. *Transplantation* 1991;51:118.
11. Fishman JA, Rubin RH. Infection in organ-transplant recipients. *N Engl J Med* 1998;338:1741–1751.
12. Fontanarosa PB. Recognition of subarachnoid hemorrhage. *Ann Emerg Med* 1989;18:1199.
13. Gentil MA, Rocha JL, Rodriguez-Algarra G, et al. Impaired kidney transplant survival in patients with antibodies to hepatitis C virus. *Nephrol Dial Transplant* 1999;14:2455–2460.
14. Gritsch HA, Smith CV, Rajfer J, et al. Kidney transplantation at UCLA. *Clinical Transpl* 2002;137–142.
15. Hubbard SG, Bivins BA, Lucas BA, et al. Acute abdomen in the transplant patient. *Am Surg* 1980;46:116.
16. Humar A, Kerr S, Gillingham KJ, et al. Features of acute rejection that increase risk for chronic rejection. *Transplantation* 1999;68:1200–1203.
17. Kong NC, Shaariah W, Morad Z, et al. Cryptococcosis in a renal unit. *Aust N Z J Med* 1990;20:645.
18. Patel U, Khaw KK, Hughes NC. Doppler ultrasound for detection of renal transplant artery stenosis-threshold peak systolic velocity needs to be higher in a low risk or surveillance population. *Clin Radiol* 2003;58:772–777.
19. Renal Data System. *USRDS 1999 annual report*. Bethesda, MD: National Institute of Diabetes and Digestive and Kidney Diseases, 1999.
20. Robinson TW, Wilkerson SA, Joyce MR. Pregnancy in renal transplant recipients: case report. *Am J Perinatal* 1992;9:52.
21. Sheashaa HA, Bakr MA, Ismail AM, et al. Basiliximab reduces the incidence of acute cellular rejection in live-related donor kidney transplantation: a three year prospective randomized trial. *J Nephrol* 2003;16:393–398.
22. Slakey DP, Johnson CO, Cziperle DJ, et al. Management of severe pancreatitis in renal transplant recipients. *Ann Surg* 1997;225:217–222.
23. Snydman DR, Wemer BG, Heinze-Lacey B, et al. Use of cytomegalovirus immune globulin to prevent cytomegalovirus disease in renal transplant recipients. *N Engl J Med* 1987;317:1049.
24. Soler MJ, Puig JM, Mir M, et al. Posttransplant lymphoproliferative disease: treatment and outcome in renal transplant recipient. *Transplant Proc* 2003;35:1709–1713.
25. Thomas CP, Riad H, Johnson BF, et al. Percutaneous transluminal angioplasty in transplant renal artery stenosis: a long-term follow-up. *Transpl Int* 1992;5:129.
26. Tilney NL, Storn TB, Vineyard GC, et al. Factors contributing to the declining mortality rate in renal transplantation. *N Engl J Med* 1978;299:1321.
27. VanBuskirk AM, Pidwell DJ, Adams PW, et al. Transplantation immunology. *JAMA* 1997;278:1993–1999.
28. Walton T, Kankari B, Wyner L. Comparison of ganciclovir and immune globulin containing regimens in preventing cytomegalovirus infection in patients with renal transplants. *Am J Health Syst Pharm* 1999;56:1831–1834.
29. Wilczek HE. Percutaneous needle biopsy of the renal allograft: a clinical safety evaluation of 1129 biopsies. *Transplantation* 1990;50:790.
30. Ylinen K, Gronhagen-Riska C, Honkancn E, et al. Outcome of patients with secondary amyloidosis in dialysis treatment. *Nephrol Dial Transplant* 1992;7:908.

Section Editor: Gregory W. Hendey

Gynecologic Emergencies

CHAPTER 88
Pelvic Pain

Joseph Schmidt

CLINICAL PRESENTATION

Pelvic pain is a common emergency department presentation. The practitioner must rapidly differentiate among etiologies that range from benign to life-threatening. This requires a complete but focused history and physical examination combined with a broad knowledge of potential disease processes to generate a differential diagnosis. This differential diagnosis can then be tested by using appropriate diagnostic studies and generating an assessment and plan that will allow for the timely treatment and disposition of the patient.

DIFFERENTIAL DIAGNOSIS

The differential diagnosis of pelvic pain is broad and falls into two main categories. This discussion is focused on the presentation of acute pelvic pain, which by definition is pain of less than 6 months in duration. Chronic pelvic pain is an enormous topic and will be mentioned only in the context that a diligent evaluation of the patient with chronic pain must be accomplished to avoid missing a more worrisome complication or new diagnosis.

The differential diagnosis of acute pelvic pain encompasses multiple organ systems (Table 88.1). A useful organizational strategy is to divide the patients into functional categories according to reproductive status. This approach highlights the special consideration of each group. Children and adolescents who are prepubertal have a number of concerns that are unique to that group (Table 88.2). Likewise women who are postmenopausal are at risk for conditions that are uncommon in other age groups (Table 88.3). The remainder of the section highlights the most common and important etiologies in each category. It is important to remember that significant overlap between these categories does occur.

Prepubertal

The approach to pelvic pain in the prepubertal patient requires attention to a broad spectrum of organ systems. Gastrointestinal and urologic causes are the most common etiologies in this group. Significant gynecologic pathology is rare but does occur. Pelvic pain related to accidental perineal trauma is not uncommon; however, a high index of suspicion should be maintained for possible sexual abuse. Any suspicion of abuse warrants a complete investigation (see Chapters 93 and 234, "Sexual Assault" and "Abuse: Sexual," respectively). In the peripubertal age group, complications of sexual activity should be part of the differential diagnosis. In this age group symptoms surrounding menarche are also common. In younger children, vulvovaginitis can arise from chemical irritation (i.e., bubble bath) or a vaginal foreign body.

Reproductive Age

Gynecologic and obstetric etiologies of pelvic pain increase in frequency as women enter reproductive age.

TABLE 88.1. Differential Diagnosis of Acute Pelvic Pain

Gynecologic/Obstetric

1. Pregnancy-related
   a. Ectopic pregnancy
   b. Abortion, threatened or incomplete
   c. Septic abortion
2. Acute infections
   a. Endometritis
   b. Pelvic inflammatory disease (PID)
   c. Tuboovarian abscess
3. Adnexal disorders
   a. Hemorrhage/rupture of ovarian cyst
   b. Torsion of adnexa
   c. Twisted paraovarian cyst
4. Recurrent
   a. Mittelschmerz (midcycle pain)
   b. Primary/secondary dysmenorrheal
   c. Endometriosis

Gastrointestinal

1. Gastroenteritis
2. Appendicitis
3. Bowel obstruction
4. Perirectal abscess
5. Diverticulitis
6. Inflammatory bowel disease
7. Irritable bowel syndrome

Genitourinary

1. Cystitis
2. Pyelonephritis
3. Ureteral lithiasis

Musculoskeletal

1. Abdominal wall hematoma
2. Psoas hematoma
3. Hernia

Vascular

1. Pelvic thromboplebitis
2. Aneurysm
3. Ischemic bowel

PID, pelvic inflammatory disease.
(Modified from Jolin JA, Rapkin A. (11))

Ectopic pregnancy (EP) is more fully discussed in Chapter 95, "Ectopic Pregnancy." The classic presentation of EP is catastrophic pain in association with missed menses and vaginal bleeding. Multiple variations of this presentation are common. Early stretch and growth of the ectopic gestation in the fallopian tube can result in mild pain caused by tubal distention and contraction. Intermittent leaking of blood, which often precedes rupture by several days, will cause mild, focal, and intermittent peritoneal irritation, which is often poorly characterized by the patient.

In one study of 441 patients, in which 13% were diagnosed with an EP, the signs and symptoms that were most predictive of EP were pain reported as moderate to severe, lateral, or sharp; peritoneal signs; cervical motion tenderness; or lateral or bilateral abdominal or pelvic tenderness. Risk factors predictive of EP included a history of infertility or use of an intrauterine device, prior tubal ligation, or other pelvic surgery (4). Because of the diversity of presentations, almost one half of ectopic pregnancies are missed on initial physician contact (1).

Miscarriage in any of its forms can cause pelvic pain. Examination of the cervical os may differentiate a threatened abortion (closed os) from an abortion in progress, with products of conception in the cervix or vagina. *Septic abortion* presents with a tender, boggy, palpable uterus and fever. Traction on the *round*

TABLE 88.2.   Differential Diagnosis of Prepubertal Pelvic Pain

Reproductive

1. Trauma
   a. Laceration
   b. Hematoma
   c. Sexual abuse
2. Vaginal foreign body
3. Vaginal infection
4. Vulvar dermatitis
   a. Chemicals
   b. Poor hygiene
   c. Allergic dermatitis
   d. Parasitic infestation (pinworms)
5. Outflow tract obstruction
   a. Imperforate hymen
   b. Labial adhesions
   c. Congenital abnormalities
6. Dysmenorrhea

Gastrointestinal

1. Appendicitis
2. Gastroenteritis
3. Obstruction
4. Constipation
5. Volvulus

Musculoskeletal

1. Muscle–tendon injury
2. Growth-plate injury
3. Ligamentous injury
4. Avulsion fracture
5. Inguinal hernia
6. Intervertebral disc herniation

Urologic

1. Nephrolithiasis
2. Cystitis
3. Pyelonephritis
4. Urethritis

Other

1. Diabetic ketoacidosis
2. Sickle cell crisis
3. Neoplasms

(Modified from Wheeler and Sornsin (19) and Schroeder and Sanfilippo (16).)

ligament and other pelvic structures as the uterus grows during pregnancy can cause significant but transient pain.

Torsion of the ovary or other adnexal structures is a gynecologic emergency. The pain associated with torsion is generally intense, severe, and unilateral, with frequent radiation to the back or thigh. The pain may be intermittent and associated with nausea and vomiting. An adnexal mass is often palpable. Common predisposing factors include pregnancy, ovarian hyperstimulation syndrome, and ovarian or paraovarian cyst disease. The ovary is usually enlarged. Because the ovary and the kidney have the same innervation (T10-11), the clinical picture may mimic renal colic.

Pelvic Inflammatory Disease (PID) is discussed more fully in Chapter 89 ("Pelvic Inflammatory Disease"). A dull lower abdominal pain, most often bilateral, characterizes uncomplicated

TABLE 88.3.   Differential Diagnosis of Postmenopausal Pelvic Pain

Gynecologic

1. Vaginitis
   a. Atrophic
   b. Infectious
   c. Allergic
2. Uterine prolapse
3. Cervical polyps
4. Uterine fibroids
5. Endometrial hyperplasia
6. Neoplasm
   a. Uterine
   b. Ovarian

Gastrointestinal

1. Rectocele
2. Diverticulitis
3. Neoplasm
4. Appendicitis
5. Ischemic bowel

Urologic

1. Infection
   a. Cystitis
   b. Urethritis
   c. Pyelonephritis
2. Cystourethrocele

(Modified from Wheeler SJ, Sornsin SM. Pelvic pain in women. In: Schwartz GR, Cayten CG, Mangelsen MA, et al., eds. Principles and practice of emergency medicine. Philadelphia: Lea and Febiger, 1992:535–546, with permission.)

PID. Onset is more frequent within 1 week of menses, but the pain may be subacute and develop over several days. If infection extends beyond the endometrium and tubes, pain can become more severe and peritoneal irritation is seen. Clinical signs and laboratory parameters tend to be nonspecific and can include fever, vaginal discharge, cervical motion tenderness, uterine or adnexal tenderness, and, rarely, a mass. Risk factors include multiple sex partners, prior PID, young age, and either no contraception or the use of an intrauterine device (3,21). Mild symptoms of low abdominal pain and uterine tenderness may be the only signs of PID, although pathologic changes may still be significant with clinically mild disease.

Tuboovarian abscess (TOA) may occur with severe PID, particularly when caused by or associated with anaerobic organisms. TOA is the most common intraabdominal abscess in premenopausal women. TOAs represent the most serious and dangerous complication of adnexitis. The mortality of PID has been reported to be as high as 8.6% when associated with rupture (12). Some TOAs are detected when PID fails to resolve with appropriate antibiotic treatment. In other cases, sterile hydrocele or pyosalpinx results from a remote acute infection. Risk factors for TOA include PID risk factors as well as recent surgery or instrumentation (20). The most common signs and symptoms include abdominal pain, fever, and a palpable pelvic mass (14). Rupture of an abscess causes sudden, frank pain resulting from peritoneal contamination, and it is a gynecologic emergency.

Primary *dysmenorrhea* occurs in adolescents, usually within 1 to 2 years of menarche. Pain caused by myometrial contractions occurs just before or coincident with menstruation, and it is described as severe, crampy, and suprapubic. It tends to occur with every menstrual period and may be incapacitating, particularly for the first 1 to 2 days of menses. Physical examination shows midline tenderness over the uterus with otherwise normal findings. Secondary dysmenorrhea can occur at any age in a menstruating woman and is most often associated with endometriosis. The rate of dysmenorrhea decreases with increasing age. In a study of 165 university students aged 17 to 19, dysmenorrhea caused absenteeism or loss of activity at least once for 42% of the women studied. The most significant associated risk factors were early age at menarche, long menstrual periods, smoking, alcohol intake, and weight (greater than the 90th percentile) (8).

Sexual abuse has also been strongly associated with dysmenorrhea and chronic pelvic pain. In a study of 581 nonpregnant women ages 18 to 45 with complaints of dysmenorrhea and chronic pelvic pain, there was a childhood incidence of sexual abuse of 26% and an adult incidence of 28% (10).

Uterine myomata, or fibroid tumors, of the uterus are common, particularly during later reproductive years. Myomata often cause heavy, irregular, and crampy menses. These tumors may undergo ischemia, necrosis, hemorrhage, or torsion. Torsion of the fibroid causes a sharp increase in severity of pain. Physical examination in a patient with fibroids reveals a tender, enlarged, and often irregular uterus. Myomata may also interfere with fertility, increasing the risk of spontaneous abortions (7).

Mittelschmerz is unilateral adnexal pain at the time of ovulation, resulting from leakage of blood or fluid from the Graafian follicle. Sudden, sharp, well-localized peritoneal irritation is usually found without fever, hypotension, or signs of inflammation or infection. An adnexal mass is infrequent. Occasionally, symptoms can be severe and generalized, but they classically decrescendo and resolve within 24 to 48 hours. In some patients, midcycle pain is recurrent and predictable.

Ovarian cyst disease may occur at any age. There are several types of cysts, including simple, functional cysts, which may contain follicular fluid or blood; corpus luteal cysts; and benign or malignant cysts, including dermoids, endometriomas, and serous and mucinous cysts. *Corpus luteum cysts* are extremely vascular. Ruptured corpus luteum cysts are common in pregnancy, presenting with sudden unilateral pain that is usually mild and localized. In rare cases, pain may be diffuse if cyst fluid or blood contaminates the entire abdominal cavity. Rupture of a cyst may lead to a significant and life-threatening amount of hemoperitoneum (18). With cyst rupture, rapid onset of pain is characteristic and local peritoneal irritation is common, but fever or systemic signs are rare. On physical examination, there is often a tender, unilateral, adnexal mass and focal peritonitis. Cervical motion tenderness caused by adjacent pelvic irritation is also common. Ovarian cysts may also cause pain if the cyst distends rapidly, or cause severe ischemic pain if torsion occurs.

Appendicitis is the most common nonobstetric surgical emergency in pregnancy. It is particularly difficult to diagnose in women, reflected by the 35% false-negative appendectomy rate for women in reproductive years. Diagnosis of many diseases such as appendicitis becomes more difficult as pregnancy progresses because the uterus obscures the examination and distorts the location of the affected organ. Delays in surgical management in pregnancy result in increased morbidity for both the mother and the fetus (1). Cervical motion tenderness may occur in either PID or appendicitis, and pyuria occurs in 10% to 20% because of the proximity of the ureters to the adnexa and appendix. The presence of significant bilateral adnexal tenderness and longer symptom duration (greater than 3 days) may suggest PID, but laparoscopy may be required to differentiate the two.

Urologic causes of pelvic pain include cystitis, pyelonephritis, and renal calculi. *Pyelonephritis* usually causes unilateral pain in the lower abdomen and flank and is common in pregnancy. Suprapubic tenderness and costovertebral angle tenderness are frequently elicited. Evaluation of the urine specimen for bacteria and leukocytes is supportive. Renal calculi typically cause severe unilateral, colicky pain. The patient may have a history of renal calculi, and hematuria is frequently present. An intravenous pyelogram, helical CT, or ultrasound can usually confirm the diagnosis.

A *Bartholin gland cyst or abscess* can cause incapacitating pelvic pain. The glands are located in the labia minora at approximately the four and eight o'clock positions. Simple incision and drainage, with or without antibiotics, is rarely successful. Two potential emergency department treatment strategies are placement of a Word catheter or marsupialization of the cyst. Details of these procedures can be found in a number of sources (9).

Postmenopausal

Pelvic pain in the postmenopausal patient adds a unique set of concerns to those already mentioned. In this age group, *atrophic vaginitis* is a common problem but should be a diagnosis of exclusion. Malignancies of both the reproductive and gastrointestinal systems increase with age. *Urinary tract infections* also increase in frequency; however, caution must be used in attributing symptoms to a questionable urinalysis. *Diverticulitis* can occur in younger women but is most common in this age group. Finally, *ischemic bowel* must be considered especially, when pain is out of proportion to the physical examination findings.

EMERGENCY DEPARTMENT EVALUATION

An appropriate history includes a description of the pain—onset, progression, quality, character, intensity, and radiation—as well as the reason for the emergency department presentation. The menstrual history includes gravidity, parity, date, and duration of the last two menstrual periods; regularity; any recent menstrual abnormalities; as well as time of menarche and menopause, when applicable. A history of sexually transmitted diseases (STDs), use and type of contraceptives, recent vaginal discharge, breast symptoms, dyspareunia, and urinary complaints should be obtained. Gastrointestinal complaints must also be evaluated, including nausea, vomiting, diarrhea, or constipation. A history of fever and chills should be noted.

The physical examination should be directed but complete. General appearance may be helpful, although individual pain thresholds vary greatly. The patient who avoids movement may have peritoneal irritation, whereas the patient rocking in distress suggests a viscus under pressure. Alterations in vital signs may help identify systemic infection, sepsis, or significant hypovolemia. Abdominal, pelvic, and rectal examinations are mandatory in all women with pelvic pain.

The abdominal examination should focus on a search for masses or palpable organs, localizing areas of tenderness, and demonstrating peritonitis. Peritonitis is detected by performing maneuvers that move the peritoneum but do not put pressure on visceral organs (heel tap, cough, light percussion, pelvic jarring, and general patient movement). "Rebound" tenderness has been the classic procedure for demonstrating peritoneal irritation, yet it is probably the least accurate for diagnosing peritonitis. Interobserver variability is substantial, and the test causes unnecessary pain in patients with potentially surgical disease (13).

The pelvic examination should include inspection of the external genitalia as well as the introitus and cervix. The bimanual examination assesses uterine size, palpable masses, and cervical motion tenderness (CMT). CMT is often considered a sign of PID. However, other diseases such as appendicitis, cyst rupture, and EP, also produce pelvic peritoneal irritation and may cause significant cervical motion tenderness, whereas patients with mild PID may have minimal pain. A uterus that is fixed and poorly mobile often indicates adhesions secondary to endometriosis, tumor, or prior infection. Rectal examination involves palpation for masses, induration, nodularity, or blood.

A qualitative, sensitive pregnancy test (urine or serum) for the beta subunit of human chorionic gonadotropin (β-HCG) is essential for evaluation in all women of childbearing age. With a low threshold (less than 50 mIU/mL International Reference Preparation), false-negative pregnancy tests occur in less than 1% of patients, even with an abnormal pregnancy (ectopic or miscarriage). A quantitative serum β-HCG will assist in the interpretation of ultrasound results in first trimester pregnancies and allow tracking of pregnancy progression at follow-up. Significant pelvic pathology may exist despite a normal complete blood count. However, an increased white blood cell count may reflect systemic infection, whereas chronic blood loss may be suspected if a low hematocrit is obtained.

An uncontaminated (usually catheterized) urinalysis is needed to diagnose a urinary tract infection and may assist in differentiating renal colic from ovarian torsion. Vaginal wet mount suspension can indicate various causes of vaginitis (rarely a cause of pelvic pain, but possibly a marker for STD exposure). Cervical cultures or tests to detect *Neisseria gonorrhoeae* and *Chlamydia trachomatis* may assist in the diagnosis of PID.

Plain radiography in the evaluation of pelvic pain is largely relegated to the exclusion of alternative diagnoses such as bowel obstruction or perforated viscous.

Pelvic ultrasound is the primary imaging modality if the suspected etiology involves the reproductive tract. Emergency physicians increasingly perform these tests, and several studies have suggested that this practice is safe, accurate, and efficient (5,6,17). Transvaginal ultrasound can reliably identify intrauterine pregnancy in the first trimester. A gestational sac and fetal pole should be seen by 5 weeks and fetal heart beat by approximately 8 weeks. Pelvic ultrasound is also adept at identifying adnexal masses, and with the use of flow technology can confirm perfusion of the ovaries.

Computed tomography (CT) may be useful in the diagnosis of pelvic pain of otherwise unclear etiology. Helical CT is rapidly becoming the primary imaging modality for renal colic. Abdominal CT with oral or rectal contrast is an appropriate study when appendicitis or other bowel pathology leads the differential diagnosis.

Laparoscopy is the gold standard study in the diagnosis of pelvic pain. It remains the procedure of choice to confirm the diagnosis for the patient who is acutely ill or for whom surgical disease (e.g., appendicitis) cannot be excluded. In a study of laparoscopic examination of 316 women with acute pelvic pain, more than 76% had an abnormal laparoscopic examination, and 45% of those with abnormal laparoscopic examinations had ectopic pregnancy (15).

Culdocentesis may be helpful in rapidly diagnosing hemoperitoneum or serious infection, but is rarely necessary. Aspiration of nonclotting blood suggests a ruptured EP or other source of bleeding in the pelvis or abdomen; purulent fluid may be indicative of PID or ruptured TOA; a normal culdocentesis yields straw-colored fluid. A dry tap occurs in 10% to 20% and is nondiagnostic.

EMERGENCY DEPARTMENT MANAGEMENT

The emergency department treatment of the patient with pelvic pain can be broken down into several critical questions.

Is the Patient Hemodynamically Stable?

Large-bore intravenous access, monitoring, and crystalloid fluid resuscitation are the first steps in managing the unstable pelvic pain patient. Early operative intervention is indicated when patients are persistently unstable. When multiple etiologies are being considered it is reasonable to simultaneously consult the respective services.

Is the Patient Pregnant?

Early establishment of pregnancy status is critical. It should occur as early as possible and concurrent with resuscitation when necessary. A positive pregnancy test requires effort to be focused first on confirming or excluding ectopic pregnancy.

Does the Patient Have Severe Pain or Peritoneal Signs?

The presence of peritonitis requires a diligent search for surgically correctable etiologies. Early consultation for consideration of direct operative evaluation is prudent. Atypical presentations or severe pain without evidence of peritoneal irritation may require appropriate imaging studies to further focus the differential diagnosis. Pain control should be a primary goal and evidence suggests analgesia may improve diagnostic accuracy (2).

Does the Pelvic Examination Reveal Evidence of Infection?

Pelvic examination findings suggestive of pelvic inflammatory disease in the absence of severe pain or peritonitis can be treated by a number of approved regimens (see Chapter 89, "Pelvic Inflammatory Disease"). Imaging in PID is limited to the evaluation of possible complications such as TOA.

Does the Patient Have an Alternative Diagnosis?

An alternative diagnosis should be considered in the stable, nonpregnant patient with mild-to-moderate symptoms and no evidence of PID. Urologic and gastrointestinal etiologies are most common. If other diagnoses are reasonable excluded, symptom control and outpatient referral are indicated.

CRITICAL INTERVENTIONS

- Provide aggressive resuscitation and monitoring of unstable pelvic pain patients
- Obtain pregnancy status for all patients with pelvic pain

DISPOSITION

Admission is necessary for potential surgical disease, including appendicitis, selected cases of PID, and ectopic pregnancy associated with significant symptoms.

Observation may be necessary if a surgical etiology is possible, pain remains severe, or vomiting and other signs of systemic toxicity are worrisome to the clinician. Observation is appropriate for patients with focal peritonitis secondary to presumed cystic rupture or for suspected early appendicitis. Patients observed in the emergency department should have serial examinations and clear criteria for admission.

If a patient is discharged from the ED with pelvic pain in which the etiology is uncertain but the patient is stable, instructions for appropriate and early followup are imperative. Any woman with abdominal pain who is discharged from the ED must be instructed to obtain a repeat evaluation if her pain continues or worsens. Because many causes of pelvic pain, particularly when the pain is chronic, are not amenable to ED diagnosis, there will exist a population of patients for whom exclusion of surgical disease, short-term pain relief, and referral for definitive diagnosis are the appropriate actions in the ED.

COMMON PITFALLS

✔ Failure to recognize the severity of illness by underestimating abnormal vital signs
✔ Failure to obtain pregnancy status particularly around the time of menarche and menopause
✔ Failure to obtain pregnancy status in patients who report birth control use or history of sterilization procedures
✔ Attributing pelvic pain to a diagnosis of urinary tract infection based on a questionable urinalysis
✔ Failing to recognize that cervical motion tenderness is neither specific nor sensitive for PID

Acknowledgment

The author gratefully acknowledges the contribution of Patrice Ringo, who wrote the previous version of this chapter.

References

1. Abbot J, Emmams LS, Lowenstein S. Ectopic pregnancy: ten common pitfalls in diagnosis. *Am J Emerg Med* 1990;8:515–522.
2. Attard A, Corlett MJ, Kidner NJ, et al. Safety of early pain relief for acute abdominal pain. *Br Med J* 1992;305:554.
3. Baines, PA, Allen GW. Pelvic pain and menstrual related illnesses *Emerg Med Clin North Am* 2001;19:763–781.
4. Dart RG, Kaplan B, Veraklis K. Predictive value of history and physical examination in patients with suspected ectopic pregnancy. *Ann Emerg Med* 1999;33:283–290.

5. Durham B, Lane B, Burbridge L, Balasubramaniam S. Pelvic ultrasound performed by emergency physicians for the detection of ectopic pregnancy in complicated first-trimester pregnancies. *Ann Emerg Med* 1997;29:338–347.

6. Durston W, Carl ML, Guerra W. Patient satisfaction and diagnostic accuracy with ultrasound by emergency physicians. *Am J Emerg Med* 1999;17:642–646.

7. Grabo T, Fahs PS, Nataupsky LG, et al. Uterine myomas: treatment options. *J Obstet Gynecol Neonatal Nurs* 1999;28:23.

8. Harlow DS, Park M. Longitudinal study of risk factors for occurrence, duration and severity of menstrual cramps in a cohort of college women. *Br J Obstet Gynecol* 1996;103:1134–1142.

9. Hill DA, Lense JJ. Office management of Bartholin gland cysts and abscesses. *Am Fam Physician* 1998;57:1611–1616.

10. Jamieson DJ, Steege JF. The association of sexual abuse with pelvic pain complaints in a primary care population. *Am J Obstet Gynecol* 1997;177:1408–1412.

11. Jolin JA, Rapkin A. Pelvic pain and dysmenorrhea. In: Berek JS, eds. *Novak's Gynecology*. Philadelphia: Lippincott Williams and Wilkins, 2002:421–452.

12. Krivak T, Propst A, Horowitz G. Tobo-ovarian abscess; principles of contemporary management. *The Female Patient* 1997;22:27–44.

13. Liddington MI, Thompson WHF. Rebound tenderness test. *Br J Surg* 1991;78:795–796.

14. McNeeley SG, Hendrix SL, Mazzoni MM, Kmak DC, Ransom SB. Medically sound, cost-effective treatment for pelvic inflammatory disease and tuboovarian abscess. *Am J Obstet Gynecol* 1998;178:1272–1276.

15. Mikkelson A, Felding C. Laparoscopic and ultrasound examination in women with acute pelvic pain. *Gynecol Obstet Invest* 1990;30:162.

16. Schroeder B, Sanfilippo JS. Pelvic pain in children and adolescents. In: Carpenter SEK, Rock JA, eds. *Pediatric and Adolescent Gynecology*. Philadelphia: Lippincott Williams and Wilkins, 2000:281–292.

17. Shih CHY. Effect of emergency physician-performed pelvic sonography on length of stay in the emergency department. *Ann Emerg Med* 1997;29:348–351.

18. Tarraza HM, Moore RD. Gynecologic causes of the acute abdomen in pregnancy. *Surg Clin North Am* 1997;77:1371–1394.

19. Wheeler SJ, Sornsin SM. Pelvic pain in women. In: Schwartz GR, Cayten CG, Mangelsen MA, Mayer TA, Hanke BK, eds. *Principles and Practice of Emergency Medicine*. Philadelphia: Lea and Febiger, 1992:535–546.

20. Wiesenfeld HC, Sweet RL. Progress in the Management of tuboovarian abscess. *Clin Obstet Gynecol* 1993;36:433–444.

21. Zeger W, Holt K. Gynecologic infections *Emerg Med Clin North Am* 2003;21:631–665.

CHAPTER 89
Pelvic Inflammatory Disease

Alfred Sacchetti

Pelvic inflammatory disease (PID) comprises a spectrum of inflammatory diseases of the upper genital tract in women. PID may include any combination of endometritis, salpingitis, tuboovarian abscess, or pelvic peritonitis (2,5,10,19). In the majority of cases, sexually transmitted pathogens (*Neisseria gonorrhoeae* and *Chlamydia trachomatis*) are implicated. However, PID may also be caused by other organisms, including anaerobic bacteria, *Gardnerella vaginalis*, *Haemophilus influenzae*, enteric gram-negative rods, *Streptococcus agalactiae*, *Mycoplasma*, and *Ureaplasma urealyticum* (5,27). More than 100 aerobic and anaerobic bacterial strains have been recovered from the pouch of Douglas or high cervical cultures in patients with PID (8). The peak incidence of gonorrhea occurs between the ages of 15 and 19 years with a second peak between 20 and 24 years of age (9). Child abuse must be suspected in any prepubertal female with the diagnosis of salpingitis.

Most pelvic infections originate from colonization of the vagina or cervix. From this site, the pathogens ascend through the cervical os into the lower uterine segment and uterine cavity. Normal cervical mucus presents a natural barrier to vaginal organisms; however, both *N. gonorrhoeae* and *C. trachomatis* appear able to produce uterine infections despite this protection. Certain cervical conditions, including recent menses, surgical cervical procedures, foreign bodies (intrauterine devices), and various hormonal changes during a menstrual cycle, decrease the defensive ability of the cervix. The hormonal changes induced by oral contraceptive agents enhance rather than reduce the bacteriostatic properties of the cervix if administered prior to colonization. There is recent evidence that indicates that oral contraceptives may mask the symptoms of chlamydial infection once it does become established (5,17).

Once entry into the uterus has been gained, the uterine lining becomes inflamed. In postpartum patients, the myometrium becomes infected, but in other patients, this inflammation is seldom invasive and is limited to the endometrium. The inflammation may produce uterine bleeding, but in the nongravid uterus, the infection is seldom clinically significant. The pathogens then continue their migration through the fallopian tubes. In the case of mycoplasmal infection, ascension may occur by way of parametrial structures rather than through the uterine cavity.

Initial tubal infection is limited to the mucosa of the lumen, but the inflammation rapidly extends through the full thickness of the tubes. This transmural reaction of the fallopian tubes often causes the early pain of pelvic infection. In severe cases, the purulent material from the fallopian lumens exudes through the open fimbriae into the abdominal cavity, thereby producing peritonitis (5,10,15).

The infection of the endometrium and fallopian tubes results in an inflammation of the surrounding parametrial structures. Although these structures may not undergo actual infection by the invading pathogens, their proximity to the true infection produces a severe parametritis in many patients.

The inflammation initiated by *N. gonorrhoeae* or *C. trachomatis* frequently overwhelms the normal uterine defense mechanisms and results in infections from opportunistic pathogens, particularly *Bacteroides* species (5,6).

Inflammation and stagnation of host defenses, particularly in the fallopian tubes, allow for the possibility of unchecked bacterial growth. A tuboovarian abscess may develop; originating in the fallopian tube, the abscess may extend to involve the fimbriae and ovary as well. The bacterial content of a tuboovarian abscess is mixed, with a preponderance of anaerobes (5,20).

Localized pelvic infection is not the only result of infection caused by *N. gonorrhoeae* and *C. trachomatis*. Escape through the end of the right fallopian tube and ascent to the right colic gutter may result in inflammation around the liver. The *Fitz-Hugh-Curtis syndrome* (*perihepatitis*) is usually associated with *C. trachomatis* but may occur in 8% to 10% of all cases of salpingitis.

CLINICAL PRESENTATION

A clinical diagnosis of PID may be difficult owing to the wide variation in signs and symptoms. Some authorities believe that the examination is notoriously inaccurate in the diagnosis of pelvic infections. No single historical, physical, or laboratory finding is both sensitive and specific for the diagnosis of acute PID. The Centers for Disease Control and Prevention (CDC) estimate that a clinical diagnosis of PID has a positive predictive rate of 65% to 90% for salpingitis (5). In a separate study, clinicians failed to recognize *N. gonorrhoeae* or *C. trachomatis* in 38% of infected women and overtreated 88% of woman with no infection

TABLE 89.1.   Diagnosis of Pelvic Inflammatory Disease (PID)

MINIMUM CRITERIA FOR THE DIAGNOSIS OF PID

Empiric treatment of PID should be instituted in sexually active females considered at risk on the basis of the presence of the following three clinical criteria for PID and in the absence of an established cause other than PID
- Lower abdominal tenderness
- Bilateral adnexal tenderness
- Cervical motion tenderness

ROUTINE CRITERIA

For women with severe clinical signs, more elaborate diagnostic evaluation is warranted because incorrect diagnosis and management may cause unnecessary morbidity. These additional criteria may be used to increase the specificity of diagnosis
- Oral temperature >38.3°C (101°F)
- Abnormal cervical or vaginal mucopurulent discharge
- Presence of white blood cells on saline microscopy or vaginal secretions
- Elevated erythrocyte sedimentation rate
- Elevated C-reactive protein
- Laboratory documentation of cervical infection with *Neisseria gonorrhoeae* or *Chlamydia trachomatis*

ELABORATE CRITERIA FOR DIAGNOSING PID

Histopathologic evidence of endometritis on endometrial biopsy
Tuboovarian abscess, thickened or fluid-filled tubes on transvaginal sonography, magnetic resonance imaging (MRI) or other radiologic tests
Laparoscopic abnormalities consistent with PID

(Adapted from Centers for Disease Control and Prevention. Sexually Transmitted Disease Guidelines 2002, MMWR, Morb Mortal Wkly Rep 2002;51 (RR-6), also available at http://www.cdc.gov/std/treatment/5-2002TG.htm.)

from these pathogens (15). Mild or nonspecific complaints may go unrecognized by the clinician (e.g., abnormal bleeding, dyspareunia, or vaginal discharge). Most authorities recommend a low threshold for diagnosis of PID because of the long-term effects and potential damage to the reproductive system of women. Criteria for diagnosis have been published (5) and appear in Table 89.1.

Although attempts have been made to distinguish between features of infection caused by *N. gonorrhoeae* and *C. trachomatis*, they have not been consistent or reliable. *N. gonorrhoeae* salpingitis develops in the first few days after menses, producing a purulent vaginal discharge and severe pelvic pain. *C. trachomatis* infection may occur at any point in the menstrual cycle, and results in less cervical discharge and milder symptoms. More important, however, is that both of these infections frequently coexist in 35% to 42% of patients (16).

The patient with pelvic infection almost invariably presents to the emergency department with a complaint of lower abdominal pain. Inflammation of the endometrium, fallopian tubes, and parametrial structures usually produces diffuse bilateral pelvic pain. When questioned, most women describe a dull, constant, poorly localized pain, although almost any characterization of the pain has been reported. Because of the sensitive nature and social stigma of sexually transmitted diseases, physicians should be empathetic and tactful in eliciting the patient's history (5). Pelvic pain is seldom the only presenting complaint. *N. gonorrhoeae* or *C. trachomatis* cervicitis results in a vaginal discharge in greater than 50% of patients, whereas abnormal vaginal bleeding is seen in 30%. Gastrointestinal complaints, including nausea and vomiting, are less common but may be present.

Urinary tract symptoms are common, with 20% of laparoscopically proven pelvic infections associated with irritative voiding symptoms (10). Pelvic infection should be suspected in patients who complain of dysuria or suprapubic pain that occurs only during micturition and is unaccompanied by frequency and urgency. The urinalysis is normal because the bladder is not infected.

A temperature greater than 38°C (100.4°F) is found in only 33% of patients; fever supports the diagnosis but does not confirm it; nor does its absence preclude the diagnosis of PID. The abdominal examination commonly reveals tenderness in both lower quadrants, although one side may be more tender. Peritoneal signs indicate a more severe infection, with free exudate in the pelvis or abdomen (10), and intraperitoneal extension should be considered. If perihepatitis is also present, there may be tenderness in the right upper quadrant.

Pelvic examination must be approached carefully if meaningful information is to be gained. Because of pain or previous experience, this examination may be very difficult for many patients (4). Speculum examination may reveal a vaginal discharge. A markedly inflamed purulent cervix is indicative of an acute cervicitis and is supportive of some degree of pelvic infection. Bimanual examination begins with very careful testing for cervical motion tenderness. Gentle motion of the cervix should be attempted initially. Too aggressive performance of this maneuver to begin the bimanual examination may produce reflexive guarding by the patient and severely limit the remainder of the examination. Elicitation of pain with either lateral or anteroposterior motion of the cervix is sensitive but not specific for pelvic infection. The emergency physician must remember that other causes of pelvic irritation: fluid from ruptured cysts, appendicitis, and blood from ectopic pregnancies can also produce this sign. The uterus is frequently firm but tender. *Bilateral adnexal tenderness is one of the most consistent physical findings in studies evaluating diagnostic criteria for salpingitis* (1,5,10,24). An adnexal mass may be appreciated but is not a consistent finding in the absence of a tuboovarian abscess. Findings on pelvic examination may be atypical in patients who have had multiple prior infections or tubal ligation. Obstruction of the fallopian tube may prevent extension of the infection beyond the proximal tube, limiting the degree of adnexal tenderness.

DIFFERENTIAL DIAGNOSIS

The differential diagnosis of lower abdominal pain in women should include at least three possibilities: (i) ectopic pregnancy, (ii) PID, and (iii) appendicitis. Ovarian cyst, urinary tract infection, hernia, and ovarian torsion should also be considered. Ectopic pregnancy is addressed in Chapter 94 ("Emergencies in Early Pregnancy"), and the approach to pelvic pain is described in Chapter 88 ("Pelvic Pain"). All women with pelvic pain, regardless of their menstrual history, should have a pregnancy test; the only exception is the woman who has had a hysterectomy (23). *Salpingitis* is the most common incorrect diagnosis in missed ectopic pregnancy and should be considered only after ectopic pregnancy has been ruled out (1). The coexistence of infection and pregnancy is possible but unusual, because, after implantation, a mucous plug forms, preventing the spread of lower genital infections into the upper genital system. However, there is a brief window between insemination and mucous plug formation during which infection may occur. *Appendicitis* may be differentiated from PID by its unilateral nature, but this is by no means diagnostic. Between 65% and 90% of patients with clinical presentations consistent with PID actually have pelvic infections on laparoscopic examination (5,10,21).

EMERGENCY DEPARTMENT EVALUATION

When PID is suspected, additional support for the diagnosis may be obtained through laboratory analysis. Although results are not immediately available, cervical cultures for *Chlamydia* and *N. gonorrhoeae* should be done during the speculum examination. A system must exist for followup of patients whose positive-culture results return to the emergency department after the patient has been discharged (12).

Gonorrhea cultures are obtained by placement of a sterile swab 1 to 2 cm into the endocervical canal, with rotation of the swab for 10 to 30 seconds (1). Following collection, the swab should be immediately plated on either chocolate agar or Thayer-Martin agar (4). The presence of white blood cells in a gram stain or saline mount of vaginal secretions is suggestive of a pelvic infection but is neither sensitive nor specific (5).

Chlamydia detection techniques include culture, antibody detection (enzyme-linked immunosorbent assay [ELISA] and fluorescent), and nucleic acid probes (22,26). In contrast to gonorrhea testing, nonculture techniques are the preferred detection procedures for the diagnosis of *C. trachomatis*. Both direct fluorescent antibody tests and ELISA-type antibody tests have been shown to be 70% to 90% sensitive and more than 90% specific in *Chlamydia* infections in women (4).

Nucleic acid probe tests that appear to be highly sensitive and specific have been developed for both of these organisms. These tests are very sensitive and specific and may be applied not only to cervical specimens but also to urine and vaginal swabs (7,8,14,22,26).

Additional laboratory studies should include urinalysis to rule out urinary tract infection and a urine or serum pregnancy test (23). A complete blood count may be obtained for use in some disposition decisions, but the clinician should recognize that the test has limited usefulness. In toxic patients with severe unilateral symptoms, pelvic ultrasonography is indicated to rule out a tuboovarian abscess, although laparoscopy is more accurate (24). Serology for syphilis and counseling for HIV testing should be considered in patients with clinical PID or arranged at followup for those with laboratory-proven infections.

EMERGENCY DEPARTMENT MANAGEMENT

Treatment regimens for PID are summarized in Table 89.2. The management of acute pelvic infection centers on prompt antibiotic therapy toward both *N. gonorrhea* and *C. trachomatis*. The goal of treatment is to prevent continued or worsened infection and limit the complications of PID, including chronic pain, ectopic pregnancy, infertility, and chronic infection (5,11). Selection of the appropriate antimicrobial combination depends on the current recommendations of the local public health department and the CDC.

Single-dose treatments with azithromycin and ciprofloxacin have been described for the treatment of cervicitis and urethritis. The clinician may consider such therapies more convenient; however, none of these have been endorsed by the CDC for upper tract or established pelvic infections (13,18,28).

Because of the potential for changes in antimicrobial sensitivities, practitioners should monitor public health service publications concerning recommendations for treatment of sexually transmitted diseases in their areas. Resistance of *N. gonorrhoeae* to ciprofloxacin and other antibiotics has increasingly been reported in both the United States and other countries (3,11,25,29).

Patients coinfected with human immunodeficiency virus (HIV) do not require any significant modifications in their treatment regiments for PID. These patients are more likely to have infections with *Mycoplasma hominis, Candida* and *streptococcal*

TABLE 89.2. Antibiotic Therapy of PID

ORAL REGIMEN

Regimen A
  Ofloxacin 400 mg orally twice a day for 14 days,
    or
  Levofloxacin 500 mg orally once daily for 14 days,
    with or without
  Metronidazole 500 mg orally twice a day for 14 days

Regimen B
  Ceftriaxone 250 mg IM in a single dose
    or
  Cefoxitin 2 g i.m. in a single dose and probenecid 1 g orally administered concurrently in a single dose,
    or
  Other parenteral third-generation cephalosporin (e.g., ceftizoxime or cefotaxime)
    plus
  Doxycycline 100 mg orally twice a day for 14 days
    with or without
  Metronidazole 500 mg orally twice a day for 14 days

PARENTERAL TREATMENT

Regimen A
  Cefotetan 2 g i.v. q12h
    or
  Cefoxitin 2 g i.v. q6h
    plus
  Doxycycline 100 mg i.v. or orally q12h

Regimen B
  Clindamycin 900 mg i.v. q8h
    plus
  Gentamicin (load, 2 mg/kg i.v., maintenance 1.5 mg/kg q8h; single daily dosing may be substituted)

Alternate Parenteral Regimens
  Ofloxacin 400 mg i.v. q12h
    or
  Levofloxacin 500 mg i.v. once daily
    with or without
  Metronidazole 500 mg i.v. q8h
    or
  Ampicillin/sulbactam 3 g i.v. q6h
    plus
  Doxycycline 100 mg i.v. or orally q12h

Note: All patients with PID, gonorrhea, or chlamydial infection should have serologic testing for syphilis and should be offered confidential counseling and testing for HIV infection.
(Centers for Disease Control and Prevention. Sexually Transmitted Disease Guidelines 2002, MMWR Morb Mortal Wkly Rep, 2002; 51 (RR-6), also available at http://www.cdc.gov/std/treatment/5-2002TG.htm.)

---

species, and human papilloma virus. However, disposition and determination of the need for hospitalization should be based on the patient's overall clinical condition and not the presence of both PID and HIV.

CRITICAL INTERVENTIONS

- Rule out tuboovarian abscess in patients with PID and severe unilateral pelvic tenderness
- Initiate parenteral antibiotics for toxic patients with PID and for those with tuboovarian abscess

DISPOSITION

Suggested criteria for admission are listed in Table 89.3. Hospitalization is frequently indicated for pregnant patients. A combination of ceftriaxone and erythromycin is considered safe in

TABLE 89.3.   Criteria for Which Hospitalization Should be Considered in Patients with PID

1. Surgical emergencies (e.g., appendicitis) cannot be excluded
2. Pregnancy
3. Patient does not respond clinically to oral antimicrobial therapy
4. Patient unable to follow or tolerate an outpatient oral regimen
5. Patient has severe illness, nausea and vomiting, or high fever
6. Patient has tuboovarian abscess

Note: None of these criteria is absolute; all should be applied on an individual basis.
Clinical criteria for improvement within 72 hours consist of defervescence, reduction in direct or rebound abdominal tenderness, and reduction in uterine, adnexal, and cervical motion tenderness within 3–5 days of initiation of therapy.
(Adapted from Centers for Disease Control and Prevention. Sexually Transmitted Disease Guidelines 2002, MMWR, 2002; 51 (RR-6), also available at http://www.cdc.gov/std/treatment/5-2002TG.htm.)

these patients, although the estolate form of the erythromycin must be avoided because it may produce hepatitis.

Outpatient management is appropriate for those patients not meeting criteria for admission shown in Table 89.3. All discharged patients should receive followup care to ensure response to treatment. If cultures are obtained, a mechanism should be in place to ensure that patients and their physicians or the public health department is notified of positive results (12).

COMMON PITFALLS

✔ All women with abdominal pain do not have PID; a differential diagnosis must be maintained, particularly in regard to ectopic pregnancy and appendicitis
✔ The clinician should question the diagnosis of PID in any patient with unilateral pelvic pain
✔ Pregnancy must be ruled out
✔ Urinary tract irritative voiding symptoms may confuse the picture in PID; a pelvic examination is mandatory to rule out PID
✔ Serologic testing for syphilis and HIV testing counseling are indicated for most women with a documented sexually transmitted disease

References

1. Abbott J, Emmans L, Lowenstein R. Ectopic pregnancy: 10 common pitfalls in diagnosis. *Am J Emerg Med* 1991;8:515.
2. American College of Obstetricians and Gynecologists. Gonorrhea and chlamydia infections. Technical Bulletin no. 190. Washington, DC: American College of Obstetrics and Gynecology, 1994.
3. Arredondo JL, Diaz V, Gaitan H, et al. Oral clindamycin and ciprofloxacin versus intramuscular ceftriaxone and oral doxycycline in the treatment of mild-to-moderate pelvic inflammatory disease in outpatients. *Clin Infect Dis* 1997;24:170.
4. Birnbaumer D. Diagnosis and management of sexually transmitted diseases, Part 1. *Crit Decis Emerg Med* 1993;7:256.
5. Centers for Disease Control and Prevention. Sexually Transmitted Disease Guidelines 2002, *MMWR Morb Mortal Wkly Rep* 2002;51 (RR-6). Also available at http://www.cdc.gov/std/treatment/5-2002TG.htm7. Centers for Disease Control and Prevention. Chlamydia trachomatis genital infections-United States, 1995. *MMWR Morb Mortal Wkly Rep* 1997;46:193.
6. Chaudhry R, Thakur R, Talwar V, et al. Anaerobic and aerobic microflora of pouch of Douglas aspirate vs. high vaginal swab in cases of pelvic inflammatory disease. *Ind J Pathol Microbiol* 1996;39:115.
7. Cosentino LA, Landers, DB, Hillier SL. Detection of Chlamydia trachomatis and Neisseria gonorrhoeae by strand displacement amplification and relevance of the amplification control for use with vaginal swab specimens. *J Clin Microbiol* 2003;41:3592.
8. Culler EE, Caliendo AM, Nolte FS. Reproducibility of positive test results in the BDProbeTec ET system for detection of Chlamydia trachomatis and Neisseria gonorrhoeae. *J Clin Microbiol* 2003;41:3911.
9. Dicker LW, Mosure DJ, Berman SM, Levine WC. Gonorrhea prevalence and coinfection with Chlamydia in women in the United States 2000. *Sex Transm Dis* 2003;30:472.
10. Eschenbach DA, Wolner-Hanseen P, Hawes DE, et al. Acute pelvic inflammatory disease: associates of clinical and laboratory findings with laparoscopic findings. *Obstet Gynecol* 1997;16:157.
11. Fenton KA, Ison C, Johnson AP, et al. Ciprofloxacin resistance in Neisseria gonorrhoeae in England and Wales in 2002. *Lancet* 2003;361:1867.
12. Kuhn GJ, Campbell A, Merline J, et al. Diagnosis and follow-up of Chlamydia trachomatis infections in the ED. *Am J Emerg Med* 1998;16:157.
13. Lea AP, Lamb HM: Azithromycin. A pharmacoeconomic review of its use as a single-dose regimen in the treatment of uncomplicated *Chlamydia trachomatis* infections in women. *Pharmacoeconomics* 1997;13:596.
14. Leslie DE, Azzato F, Ryan N, et al. An assessment of the Roche Amplicor Chlamydia trachomatis/Neisseria gonorrhoeae multiplex PCR assay in routine diagnostic use on a variety of specimen types. *Commun Dis Intell* 2003;27:373.
15. Levitt MA, Johnson S, Engelstad L, et al. Clinical management of Chlamydia and gonorrhea infection in a county teaching emergency department-concerns in overtreatment, undertreatment and follow-up treatment success. *J Emerg Med* 2003;25:7–11.
16. Lyss SB, Kamb ML, Peterman TA, et al. Chlamydia trachomatis among patients infected with and treated for Neisseria gonorrhoeae in sexually transmitted disease clinics in the United States. *Ann Intern Med* 2003;139:178.
17. Mardh PA, Hoff V. Are oral contraceptives masking symptoms of chlamydial cervicitis and pelvic inflammatory disease? *Eur J Contracept Reprod Health Care* 1998;3:41.
18. Martin DH, Mroczkowski TF, Dalu ZA, et al. A controlled trial of a single dose of azithromycin for the treatment of chlamydial urethritis and cervicitis. *N Engl J Med* 1992;327:921.
19. McCormack WM. Pelvic inflammatory disease. *N Engl J Med* 1994;330:115.
20. McNeeley SG, Hendrix SL, Mazzoni MM, et al. Medically sound, cost-effective treatment for pelvic inflammatory disease and tuboovarian abscess. *Am J Obstet Gynecol* 1998;178:1272.
21. Morcos R, Frost N, Hnat M, et al. Laparoscopic versus clinical diagnosis of acute pelvic inflammatory disease. *J Reprod Med* 1993;38:53.
22. Paavonen J, Lehtinen M. Chlamydial pelvic inflammatory disease. *Hum Reprod Update* 1996;2:519.
23. Ramoska EA, Sacchetti AD, Nepp M. Reliability of patient history in determining the possibility of pregnancy. *Ann Emerg Med* 1989;18:48.
24. Sellors J, Mahony J, Goldsmith C, et al. The accuracy of clinical findings and laparoscopy in pelvic inflammatory disease. *Am J Obstet Gynecol* 1991;164:113.
25. Sosa J, Ramierz-Arcos S, Ruben M, et al. High percentages of resistance to tetracycline and penicillin and reduced susceptibility to azithromycin characterize the majority of strain types of Neisseria gonorrhoeae isolates in Cuba, 1995-1998. *Sex Transm Dis* 2003;30:443.
26. Takahashi S, Shimizu T, Takeyama K, et al. Efficacy of an RNA detection test kit in the diagnosis of genital chlamydial infection. *J Infect Chemother* 2003;9:90.
27. Taylor-Robinson D, Furr PM. Genital mycoplasma infections. *Wien Klin Wochenschr* 1997;109:578.
28. Treatment of sexually transmitted diseases. *Med Lett Drugs Ther* 1999;36:913.
29. Veitch MG, Griffith JM, Morgan ML. Ciprofloxacin resistance emerges in Neisseria gonorrhoeae in Victoria, 1998 to 2001. *Commun Dis Intell* 2003;27[Suppl]:S75–9.

CHAPTER 90
Vaginal Bleeding in the Nonpregnant Patient

Eric Anderson

Abnormal vaginal bleeding is a common complaint in Emergency Medicine. It is one of the ten most frequent complaints for which patients seek emergency department (ED) care (1). Life-threatening bleeding must be quickly distinguished from bleeding that is abnormal but not of hemodynamic consequence. It is incumbent upon the emergency physician to promptly rule out a pregnancy-related cause of vaginal bleeding.

TABLE 90.1. Causes of Anovulation

Endocrine disorders (also see Table 90.2)
Inflammatory bowel disease
Cystic fibrosis
Poor nutritional status
Emotional distress

CLINICAL PRESENTATION

Menorrhagia is increased volume or duration of bleeding at the normal time of menstruation. Menorrhagia often represents a disorder of ovulation; however, it may represent a disorder of hemostasis. *Metrorrhagia* is bleeding at irregular intervals other than the usual time of menstruation. Metrorrhagia usually represents an anovulatory disorder. Various causes of anovulation are listed in Tables 90.1 and 90.2. This bleeding varies from spotting to heavy menstrual flow. Anovulatory dysfunctional uterine bleeding is more common at the extremes of the reproductive years; that is, postmenarchal and premenopausal years (2). *Menometrorrhagia* is frequent irregular bleeding that may be excessive in flow and duration. *Dysfunctional uterine bleeding* typically is defined as abnormal endometrial bleeding in the absence of pelvic pathology (19). Dysfunctional uterine bleeding is typically painless, irregular vaginal bleeding of endometrial origin that may be excessive, prolonged or unpatterned (10).

Common categories of nonpregnancy-related abnormal vaginal bleeding include dysfunctional uterine bleeding, endocrine causes, trauma, infection, neoplasm, coagulopathy, medication, foreign body, and anatomic anomalies (Table 90.3). Normal menstrual cycle values are outlined in Table 90.4.

Many of these conditions will not represent a true emergency; however, these symptoms are often distressing to the patient and her family. Anxiety about the etiology of the bleeding may precipitate an emergency department visit.

The emergency physician should determine if this vaginal bleeding is imminently life-threatening. If the vaginal bleeding is life-threatening, resuscitative efforts should begin immediately. If the patient is stable, diagnostic efforts should be initiated to determine which category of vaginal bleeding is the cause (Table 90.3). Always consider the possibility of occult pregnancy (1).

DIFFERENTIAL DIAGNOSIS

Premenarchal Patients

Neonates may experience withdrawal bleeding usually within the first 2 weeks of birth (18). Toddlers may present with bleeding secondary to a foreign body in the vagina, often toilet paper

TABLE 90.2. Endocrine Disorders Associated with Anovulation

Poorly controlled diabetes
Primary ovarian dysfunction
Hypothyroidism
Hyperprolactinemia
Cushing syndrome
Addison disease
Congenital adrenal hyperplasia
Polycystic ovarian syndrome

TABLE 90.3. Causes of Nonpregnancy-Related Vaginal Bleeding

Anatomic	Cervical or uterine polyps
	Uterine fibroids
	Congenital anomalies
	Urethral prolapse
Coagulopathy	DIC
	Von Willebrand Disease
	Leukemia
	Thrombocytopenia
Endocrine	Postnatal withdrawal from maternal hormonal milieu
	Congenital adrenal hyperplasia
	Cushing syndrome
	Polycystic ovary disease
	Hypothyroidism
Foreign Bodies	IUD, sexual devices, toys, retained condoms, tampons, cotton balls, tissue
Hormonal	Anovulatory cycle
	Administration of exogenous sex steroids
Infections	Gonorrhea
	Chlamydia
	Trichomonas
	Cervicitis
	Nonspecific vaginitis
	Condyloma acuminatum
	Urinary tract infection
	Erosion of abdominal infection into the genitourinary tract
Medicines	Birth control pills
	Coumadin
	Phenytoin
	Phenobarbital
	Heparin
Neoplasm	Vaginal neoplasm
	Cervical neoplasm
	Uterine neoplasm
	Erosion of an abdominal neoplastic process into the genitourinary tract
Trauma	Sharp
	Blunt
	Sexual
Other	Stress
	Excessive dieting
	Excessive exercising
	Crohn disease of the vulva
	Premature menarche (children)

DIC, disseminated intravascular coagulopathy; IUD, intrauterine device.

(17). School age children may present with vulvar or perineal trauma secondary to a straddle injury. Sexual abuse should be considered in children with vulvar and perineal injuries. Sexually transmitted diseases in children are consistent with sexual child abuse or rape. Urethral prolapse, urinary tract infections, and gastrointestinal causes should also be considered. The most common cause of malignancy in the lower genital tract of young girls is tumor-embryonal rhabdomyosarcoma (sarcoma

TABLE 90.4. Menstrual Cycle Normal Values

	Normal	Abnormal
Cycle length	28 Days ± 7	<21 or >35 Days
Duration	4 Days ± 3	>8 Days
Blood loss	30–35 mL (range, 5–60 mL)	>80 mL
Menarche onset	9–14 yr (mean, 12.88 yr)	<8 y.o. >14 y.o.

References 19 and 20.

botryoides) (17). Sarcoma botryoides is a rare cause of bleeding in this age group (20). These conditions can be differentiated by history and physical examination. Information about acuity of onset, amount of bleeding, recent trauma or known sexual activity will help differentiate these conditions.

Perimenarchal Patients

By far the usual cause of bleeding in these adolescent-age patients is immaturity of the hypothalamic-pituitary-ovarian axis (5). Anovulatory cycles occur in approximately 55% to 82% of girls during the first 2 years of menstruation. After 5 years, 20% of cycles may remain anovulatory (19). The earlier the onset of menarche, the shorter the duration of anovulatory cycles. If menarche occurs before the age of 12 years, by 1 year later 50% of cycles are ovulatory (19). If menarche occurs after age 13, then 50% of cycles may become ovulatory by 4.5 years later (19).

Less common causes of prolonged or excessive bleeding may be the first manifestation of a bleeding disorder. Von Willebrand disease is the most common of the hereditary conditions, affecting 1% of the world wide population. Von Willebrand factor is a platelet adhesion molecule (6). There are three subtypes of von Willebrand disease: type 1 affects 80% of von Willebrand patients and is the most amenable to treatment, type 2 affects up to 19%, and type 3 affects 1% to 3% (13). Other causes of bleeding in this age group include idiopathic thrombocytopenia purpura, prothrombin deficiency, Glanzmann disease, Fanconi anemia, and thalassemia major (19).

Childbearing-Age Patients

The possibility of pregnancy and the consequences of an ectopic pregnancy must be considered. Pelvic infections should be considered, especially in patients who present with low abdominal pain in addition to their abnormal vaginal bleeding. These patients may or may not have a fever and a purulent vaginal discharge. Recent gynecologic surgeries, unprotected sex with multiple partners, and an intrauterine device (IUD) use are risk factors for pelvic infections. Retained vaginal or uterine foreign bodies should also be suspected. Patients who are obese may present with disordered menstruation secondary to exogenous estrogen production in adipose tissue.

The patient's memory of the amount of bleeding has been known to be inaccurate and unreliable (12). The number of tampons or pads used over the preceding several hours may provide more objective evidence of the amount of bleeding; however, the accuracy of these methods is dubious.

Systemic illnesses that can manifest as vaginal bleeding include marked obesity, hypothyroidism, liver cirrhosis, and coagulation disorders (2,22). Iatrogenic causes of uterine bleeding include oral, subdermal, or injectable sex steroids used for contraception, hormone replacement therapy, treatment for hirsutism, dysmenorrhea, premenstrual syndrome, acne, or endometriosis (1).

A variety of uterine, cervical, and vaginal lesions should be considered. These include cervicitis, vaginitis, endometrial and cervical polyps, cervical erosions and submucosal leiomyomas, and cervical tears or vaginal perforations. Vulvar, vaginal, and cervical lesions can be detected by a pelvic examination. Malignancy (vagina, cervix, or uterus), fibroids, or adenomyosis can cause significant bleeding in patients in this age group.

Postmenopausal Patients

Menopause is defined as the period after one full year of amenorrhea if a woman is not receiving hormone replacement therapy. Patients receiving hormone replacement therapy (HRT) may experience breakthrough bleeding or withdrawal bleeding. Generally these patients will not present with a life-threatening bleed. They will complain of abnormal bleeding and some degree of anxiety about the etiology of the bleeding, and they want to know when the bleeding will stop.

Bleeding in this age group is usually anovulatory. Malignancy should be suspected in postmenopausal patients who present with vaginal bleeding (2,4). Up to 10% of these patients will be found to have carcinoma, and 80% to 90% of women with endometrial cancer present with vaginal bleeding (20,9,7,4).

Dysfunctional uterine bleeding is considered when other diagnostic possibilities can reasonably be ruled out. It is characterized by painless irregular uterine bleeding that may be excessive or prolonged and not from any other identifiable cause (5).

Other causes of bleeding in this age group include atrophic vaginitis, vaginal infection, urinary tract infection, or gastrointestinal tract bleeding. Other hormonal, coagulation, anatomic, infectious, medication, and other causes are outlined in Tables 90.1, 90.2, and 90.3 and also apply to this age group.

EMERGENCY DEPARTMENT EVALUATION

During the history and physical examination, particular attention should be paid to the patient's usual menstrual pattern and duration of menses. The history of the last "normal" menstrual period should be obtained. A history of any other abnormal bleeding should also be obtained. If there is a recent history of abnormal menstrual bleeding, it is important to ask what is different about today's bleeding that brings the patient into the emergency department. Explore with the patient the possibility of pregnancy, sexually transmitted disease, or genital trauma. Physicians should question adolescents about sexual activity, without parents present, to evaluate for the possibility of sexual trauma, sexually transmitted disease, or pregnancy.

Physical examination should include abdominal, pelvic, and rectal examinations. If no blood is seen in the vaginal vault of a patient who insists that she has had recent copious vaginal bleeding, then place a urinary catheter to assess for a possible urinary source of the bleeding. Perform a rectal examination with hemoccult testing to assess for a gastrointestinal source. Abnormal vital signs in a patient who appears pale and complains of weakness or lightheadedness indicate significant blood loss.

Emergency laboratory assessment includes pregnancy test to rule out the bleeding as a complication of pregnancy. Urinalysis or urine Chemstrip® results are easily obtainable when urine is being used for pregnancy testing. Obtain a complete blood count (CBC) in ill-appearing or hemodynamically unstable patients, and when the diagnosis and disposition are in doubt. Clotting studies, bleeding time, and liver and thyroid function tests are reserved for unusual cases in which these etiologies of bleeding are seriously considered.

Ultrasonography is very useful in diagnosing a variety of gynecologic conditions in nonpregnant patients (1). It is helpful in the evaluation of patients with menorrhagia, amenorrhea, oligomenorrhea, postmenopausal bleeding, lost IUD, pelvic mass, intrauterine and ectopic pregnancies, pelvic inflammatory disease, or tuboovarian abscess (22). Ultrasonography is also used to evaluate anatomic sources of the vaginal bleeding such as cervical and endometrial polyps, and myomas (7). Patients who are stable with spotting or minimal or moderate bleeding can have the ultrasound evaluation as an outpatient. Those who are hemodynamically compromised should have the ultrasound during their emergency department evaluation, after fluid resuscitation.

EMERGENCY DEPARTMENT MANAGEMENT

The unusual patient who presents as hemodynamically unstable requires simultaneous evaluation and resuscitation. If the physical examination reveals the genital tract as the source of the bleeding, then further assessment about the specific source of the bleeding is required. It should be stressed that further emergency department diagnostic workup should not delay the resuscitation; both activities should occur simultaneously. Blood is drawn for evaluation while intravenous lines are started for fluid administration.

Patients who remain unstable and continue to bleed should have an immediate gynecologic consultation during the resuscitation. Unstable patient should receive blood products if the bleeding is so copious that they do not respond to crystalloid boluses by rapid i.v. infusion. Blood products to be considered include packed red blood cells (RBCs), platelets, and fresh-frozen plasma. Specific blood products can be administered for a known specific bleeding diathesis. In hypovolemic patients with menorrhagia, curettage is the fastest method to stop the bleeding (3). A neoplastic process is often the cause of copious vaginal bleeding in postmenopausal patients.

Medical therapy is recommended for patients with vaginal bleeding not secondary to causes listed in Table 90.1 (i.e., dysfunctional uterine bleeding). Bleeding caused by trauma, infection, medications, cancer, or structural anomalies of the uterus should be treated according to the underlying pathology. Other sections of this textbook address these other causes of bleeding. A variety of medications are available for treatment of dysfunctional uterine bleeding including nonsteroidal antiinflammatory drugs (NSAIDs), conjugated estrogens, and progesterones. Estrogen or estrogen–progestin therapy may be initiated in the emergency department. Initiation of sex steroid therapy is usually done in consultation with the patient's primary physician or with a gynecologist, since there are many treatment options and various cocktails for ovulatory and anovulatory bleeding.

High-dose estrogen therapy is the treatment of choice to control acute bleeding episodes (3). *Conjugated equine estrogens (Provera)* 2.5 mg orally 4 times per day or 25 mg i.v. every 2 to 4 hours for 24 hours. Either route will rapidly reduce the bleeding within 24 hours (3). When bleeding is controlled, patients are switched to an oral estrogen, 10 mg per day. This is continued for 21 to 35 days. Oral *medroxyprogesterone acetate*, 10 mg daily, is given with the estrogen for the last 7 to 10 days. Then medications are withdrawn and the patient will have an episode of withdrawal bleeding. Another option is to use high-dose estrogen progestin therapy by using combination oral contraceptives 3 to 4 tablets daily. Treatment should be continued for at least 1 week after bleeding stops. Then use standard oral contraceptive dose, one tablet daily for 21 days. An alternative to standard oral contraceptive use is to use oral medroxyprogesterone acetate 10 mg per day for 10 days each month for the next two or three menstrual cycles.

To prevent recurrent episodes of anovulatory dysfunctional bleeding, alternatives include (1) *medroxyprogesterone acetate* 10 mg orally daily for days 16 through 25 of each cycle, (2) *norethindrone* 5 to 10 mg 1 to 3 times daily. Prolonged use of high-dose progestins may cause fatigue, mood changes, weight gain, and atherogenic changes in the lipid profile (3). Other medications useful in the prevention of recurrent bleeding episodes include oral contraceptives or IUDs impregnated with a slow-release progesterone or levonorgestrel.

Adolescents often have anovulatory vaginal bleeding secondary to an immature hypothalamic-pituitary-ovary axis. They may respond to progestins for 10 days a month as noted previously, or to standard oral contraceptives. Perimenopausal patients must have more ominous causes (cancer) ruled out, and

can then be managed with *conjugated equine estrogen* 0.625 to 1.25 mg daily for 25 days. *Medroxyprogesterone* 10 mg orally daily is added to the estrogen regimen for days 15 through 25 (3). Alternatively, the perimenopausal patient who is a nonsmoker without a history of vascular disease may be treated with a standard oral contraceptive.

NSAIDs reduce endometrial prostaglandin levels by inhibition of cyclooxygenase, which is the enzyme largely responsible for conversion of arachidonic acid to prostaglandins (16). NSAIDs have been shown to decrease menstrual bleeding by 30% to 50% (11). Efficacious regimens include (1) *mefenamic acid*, 250 to 500 mg, 2 to 4 times per day for 3 to 5 days and (2) *naproxen* 250 mg every 6 to 8 hours (15,16,3).

Iron is considered standard adjuvant therapy for patients with abnormal vaginal bleeding (15). Ferrous sulfate, 325 mg, 2 to 3 times per day or ferrous gluconate, 300 mg, 3 to 4 times per day are standard therapy for iron deficiency often associated with chronic (or profuse intermittent) vaginal bleeding. Iron supplemental therapy consists of one tablet of either ferrous sulfate or ferrous gluconate.

Silver nitrate sticks can be used to stop bleeding secondary to cervical erosions or postoperative oozing.

Surgical treatment is left to the discretion of the gynecologic consultant. Surgical interventions include curettage, polypectomy, hysteroscopic, and laparoscopic procedures, as well as open laparotomy. Other procedures include endometrial ablation (surgical, radiofrequency, local hyperthermia, cryotherapy, microwave, and neodymium aluminum garnet (Nd:YAG) laser (15). Arterial embolization via percutaneous administration of polyvinyl alcohol particles is another method that is under investigation (14).

CRITICAL INTERVENTIONS

- Aggressively resuscitate the "sick patient" who is pale, ill-appearing, and has a history of significant blood loss
- Rule out pregnancy in patients of reproductive age, despite any denials of sexual activity

DISPOSITION

The majority of women who present to the emergency department with a chief complaint of vaginal bleeding can be sent home safely with instructions to followup with their primary physician. All unstable patients require admission. Patients in whom the disposition is uncertain should be admitted to an observation unit where the results of medications can be assessed and gynecologic consultation and repeat blood counts can be obtained when warranted.

COMMON PITFALLS

✔ Failure to always obtain a pregnancy test on women of reproductive age
✔ Failure to consider malignancy in postmenopausal women with vaginal bleeding
✔ Failure to always take the time to obtain a sexual history from adolescents
✔ Failure to obtain a current medication list with particular attention to the compliance and use of sex steroids and anticoagulants

Acknowledgment

Thank you to previous edition chapter author H. Trent MacKay.

References

1. American College of Emergency Physicians. Clinical policy for the initial approach to patients presenting with a chief complaint of vaginal bleeding. *Ann Emerg Med* 1997;29:435–458.
2. Brenner PF. Differential diagnosis of vaginal bleeding. *Am J Obstet Gynecol* 1996;175:766.
3. Chuoung CJ, Brenner BF. Management of abnormal vaginal bleeding. *Am J Obstet Gynecol* 1996;175:787.
4. Davidson KG, Dubinsky TJ. Ultrasonographic evaluation of the endometrium in postmenopausal vaginal bleeding. *Radiol Clin North Am* 2003;41:769–780.
5. Dealy MF. Dysfunctional uterine bleeding in adolescents. *Nurse Pract* 1998; 23:12–13, 16, 18–20.
6. Ewenstein BM. The pathophysiology of bleeding disorders presenting as abnormal uterine bleeding. *Am J Obstet Gynecol* 1996;175:770–777.
7. Goldstein RB, Bree RL, Benson CB, et al. Evaluation of Radiologists in ultrasound-sponsored consensus conference statement. *J Ultrasound Med* 2001; 20:1025–1036.
8. Good AE. Diagnostic options for assessment of postmenopausal bleeding. *Mayo Clinic Proc* 1997;72:345–349.
9. Goodman A. Abnormal genital tract bleeding. *Clin Cornerstone* 2000;3:25–35.
10. Jaffe S, Jewelewicz R. Dysfunctional uterine bleeding in the pediatric and adolescent patient. *Adolesc Pediatr Gynecol* 1991;4:62–69.
11. Jennings JC. Abnormal uterine bleeding. *Med Clin North Am* 1995;79:1357.
12. Livingston M, Fraser IS. Mechanisms of abnormal uterine bleeding. *Hum Reprod Update* 2002;8:60–67.
13. Lusher JM. Systemic causes of excessive uterine bleeding. *Semin Hematol* 1999; 36[Suppl 4]:10–20.
14. Mihmanli I, Cantasdemir M, Kantarci F, et al. Percutaneous embolization in the management of intractable vaginal bleeding. *Arch Gynecol Obstet* 2001;264:211–214.
15. Munro MG. Dysfunctional uterine bleeding: advances in diagnosis and treatment. *Curr Opin Obstet Gynecol* 2001;13:475–489.
16. Munro MG. Medical management of abnormal uterine bleeding. *Obstet Gynecol Clin North Am* 2000;27:287–304.
17. Poirier MP, Friedland LR. Pediatric vaginal bleeding, urethral prolapse. *Acad Emerg Med* 1995;2:527–528,563–565.
18. Quint EH, Perlman SE. Premenarchal vaginal bleeding. *J Pediatr Adolesc Gynecol* 2001;4:135–136.
19. Rimsza M. Dysfunctional uterine bleeding. *Pediatr Rev* 2002;23:227–233.
20. Shwayder JM. Pathophysiology of abnormal uterine bleeding. *Obstet Gynecol Clin North Am* 2000;27:219–234.
21. Thomas AM, Hickey M, Fraser IS. Disturbances of endometrial bleeding with hormone replacement therapy. *Hum Reprod Update* 2000;15:7–17.
22. Weissman AM, Barloon TJ. Transvaginal ultrasonography in nonpregnant and postmenopausal women. *Am Fam Physician* 1996;56:2065–2072.

CHAPTER 91
Vaginitis

Constance S. Greene

Vaginal discharge is the most common gynecologic symptom in women during reproductive years, and many seek emergency care for the discomfort. Other symptoms of vaginal infection are unpleasant odor, pruritus, burning, dyspareunia, and dysuria. In this age group, vaginitis usually results from one of three different causes: a fungus (*Candida albicans*), a protozoan (*Trichomonas vaginalis*), or the replacement of the hydrogen peroxide (H_2O_2)–producing, gram-positive lactobacilli of natural vaginal flora with anaerobic bacteria and *Gardnerella vaginalis* in far greater concentrations than they are normally found (*bacterial vaginosis*). In postmenopausal women, these symptoms are most likely caused by *atrophic vaginitis*. A careful history, pelvic (speculum) examination, with pH determination and microscopic ex-

amination of a wet mount slide of the discharge, will yield a diagnosis in about 80% of cases (Table 91.1). Although cultures were considered the gold standard for diagnosis in the past, polymerase chain reaction identification of the organisms may be more sensitive, but these methods are more suited to the gynecologist's practice than to the emergency department (ED) (3).

Candida vulvovaginitis is caused by an airborne fungus, *C. albicans*. Its filamentous forms penetrate the mucosal surface, thereby causing hyperemia and lysis of tissue locally. This infection occurs predominantly during reproductive years, with 75% of women experiencing at least one episode in their lifetimes. Fungi can be isolated from the vaginas of 10% to 20% of asymptomatic women and need not be treated. It is commensal until the ecosystem of the vagina is disturbed. Predisposing factors include hormonal shifts (pregnancy and just premenstrual), antibiotic or immunosuppressant (e.g., corticosteroid) use, diabetes mellitus, and immune suppression, such as with acquired immunodeficiency syndrome (AIDS). Oral contraceptives, once thought to increase risk, do not in the present low-estrogen dosages. Candidal infections do not occur simultaneously with bacterial vaginosis or *Trichomonas* infection, but may follow treatment.

T. vaginalis, a unicellular protozoon that is sexually transmitted, causes approximately one fourth of vaginal infections. It is found in the vagina and 90% of the time in the lower urethra and Skene ducts. Male partners are usually asymptomatic, but may complain of the symptoms of urethritis. They harbor the organisms in the urethra and paraurethral glands and occasionally in the seminal vesicles, epididymis, and prostate. Trichomoniasis is often concurrent with bacterial vaginosis and gonorrhea, and probably other sexually transmitted diseases as well.

Trichomonads are also suspected of being vectors in pelvic inflammatory disease. In any event, because the epidemiology of all sexually transmitted diseases is similar, the emergency physician should either do appropriate screening for gonorrhea, chlamydia, and syphilis or refer the patient for these and for human immunodeficiency virus (HIV) counseling regarding testing and safe sexual practice.

Bacterial vaginosis (BV) is the most common cause of an abnormal vaginal discharge, and has undergone several name changes as our understanding of the pathogenesis has evolved. High concentrations of anaerobic bacteria replace the normal lactobacilli, especially those species that produce hydrogen peroxide. Anaerobes increase tenfold, and *Gardnerella* species even more. The anaerobic vibrios from the *Mobiluncus* group are seen in about 50% of symptomatic patients. Therefore, bacterial vaginosis is best understood as a syndrome of bacterial synergism in which the vaginal flora become predominantly anaerobic. It does not produce inflammatory changes, hence the term, *vaginosis*, rather than vaginitis.

CLINICAL PRESENTATION

The predominant symptoms in patients with vaginitis depend upon the etiology. Patients with *Candida vulvovaginitis* primarily complain of vulvar itching, burning, external dysuria, and dyspareunia. The quantity of the discharge is variable. It does not have an odor and may not be a presenting symptom. Vulvar signs are erythema, edema, and traumatic excoriation. There may be satellite pustules at the periphery of inflammation. Insert the speculum gently, as the vagina may be very sore. The typically thick, clumpy discharge will be adherent to the walls or may look like thrush patches. The pH of the vagina is less than 4.5.

The primary symptom of acute *Trichomonas* infection is profuse vaginal discharge. Patients often complain of feeling wet.

TABLE 91.1. Features of Vaginal Discharge

Features of Discharge	Normal	Candidiasis	*Trichomonas vaginalis*	Bacterial Vaginosis
Color	Clear, white	White	Gray, green-yellow	Gray, white
Consistency	Floccular	Clumped, adherent to vaginal mucosa	Homogenous, occasionally frothy	Homogenous, occasionally frothy
Quantity	Variable; usually scant	Scant to moderate	Profuse	Moderate
pH	≤4.5	≤4.5	≥5.0	≥4.5
Amine odor with KOH	Negative	Negative	Usually positive	Positive
Wet mount	Epithelial cells, lactobacilli	WBCs, epithelial cells, spores, mycelia or pseudohyphae Recommend KOH to dissolve nonfungal cellular elements	WBC, motile trichomonads	Few WBCs, clue cells

KOH, potassium hydroxide; WBC, white blood cell.

The discharge is thin and may be white, gray, yellow, or green. It has been classically described as "frothy," but this is only present 10% to 20% of the time. It is often malodorous. Dysuria is present 20% of the time. Patients with chronic infection may complain only of a malodorous discharge. The examiner frequently notes the discharge on the vulva, which can also be erythematous and edematous. Unlike candidiasis, which can cause extensive involvement of the vulva and perineum, inflammation caused by *Trichomonas* is usually limited to the vestibule and labia minora. The vaginal walls are inflamed and the discharge is copious in amount.

The most uniform complaint of women with *BV* is an unpleasant vaginal odor, particularly noted after intercourse, when alkaline semen triggers the release of aromatic amines. The odor may be described as "fishy" or "musty." The discharge is most often thin and adherent to the walls of the vagina. There is rarely any pruritus or erythema of the vulva or vagina unless concomitant *Trichomonas* infection is present.

EMERGENCY DEPARTMENT EVALUATION

The most efficient diagnostic test in the ED is to put a small sample of the discharge onto two slides, one with 1 to 2 drops of saline, and another with 1 to 2 drops of a 10% or 20% solution of potassium hydroxide (KOH). The KOH will dissolve the cellular elements (and the microscope lens as well, if a cover slip is not used). Several fields may have to be scrutinized to identify the mycelia or pseudohyphae of *Candida*, which appear as tangled, branching chains, or the oval spores that are about one fourth of the size of a white blood cell (WBC). Although the sensitivity of this method varies widely (from 22% to 80%, averaging 65%), the clinical picture coupled with either the patient's self diagnosis or the absence of a watery discharge or amine odor should prompt the ED physician to treat for *Candida* in most cases (1).

The saline wet mount of the discharge should be viewed under low power first to identify areas of relatively few WBCs. In fresh warm preparations, trichomonads will have a twitchy forward motion. They are slightly larger than WBCs. If the slide has an abundance of WBCs, or the typical movement is not seen, a higher power should be tried, dampening down the condenser to give better contrast. If WBCs are clumped on the protozoa or the preparation is cold, only the beating of the flagella may be seen. The wet mount is diagnostic up to 70% of the time. It is characteristic to see many WBCs (also seen in atrophic vaginitis and sexually transmitted diseases, but not in *Candida* or bacterial vaginosis). The pH, using colorimetric paper, will usually be above 5 and can be as high as 7. If KOH is added to the discharge, a "fishy" or amine odor may be present.

A wet mount classically reveals "clue cells" in patients with *BV*. These are epithelial cells that have bacteria "studded" all over the surface, obscuring the cell wall. Few WBCs or lactobacilli are noted, but clumps of bacteria may be seen. The pH of the discharge is 5 to 6. When KOH is added to the slide, a fishy odor is released, a positive "whiff test."

EMERGENCY DEPARTMENT MANAGEMENT

Candida albicans is almost uniformly sensitive to all azoles. Intravaginal agents are inexpensive, available over the counter, effective, and well tolerated by most women. They may be less acceptable to many women than a single dose (150 mg) of oral fluconazole, which has similar cure rates (13). If fluconazole is used in diabetic patients on oral hypoglycemic agents, there may be significant hypoglycemia caused by drug interaction. Table 91.2 provides a listing of specific preparations and dosing.

For *Trichomonas*, metronidazole 2 g orally in a single dose has been the standard first-line treatment, although 1.5 g has been shown to be equally effective (14), the Centers for Disease Control and Prevention (CDC) has not changed its dosage recommendation as of 2002 (4). A 7-day course of 500 mg daily has similar (95%) cure rates, but compliance is lower. Metronidazole affects the hepatic metabolism of alcohol in the same manner as disulfiram (Antabuse), so patients should abstain from alcohol for 24 hours after the last dose. Metronidazole vaginal gel does not appear to be as effective against *T. vaginalis* (<50%) and is not recommended (6). Patients who are allergic to metronidazole may be treated with topical clotrimazole, but cure rates are low. These patients can be referred for desensitization. Trichomonads are often noted on urine microscopy in asymptomatic women. Since one third of these women will become symptomatic within 3 months, it is prudent to treat them.

Metronidazole 500 mg twice daily for 7 days is the longstanding treatment of choice for *bacterial vaginosis*. It results in 85% to 95% cure and a return of normal lactobacilli. Single-dose therapy is considerably less effective. Topical therapy with either metronidazole gel or clindamycin cream is also recommended

TABLE 91.2. Treatment of Vaginitis

Disorder	First Line	Alternative	Partner	In Pregnancy
T. Vaginalis	*Metronidazole 2 g po single dose	*Metronidazole 500 mg b.i.d. for 7 days	*Metronidazole 2 g po single dose	Treat only if symptomatic but treat partner 1st trimester, clotrimazole 100 mg hs for 7 days After 1st trimester, 2 g *Metronidazole
Bacterial vaginosis	*Oral* *Metronidazole 500 mg b.i.d. for 7 days *or* Clindamycin 300 mg po b.i.d. for 7 days *or* *Intravaginal* 0.75% Metronidazole gel b.i.d. for 5 days *or* 2% clindamycin cream hs for 7 days	*Metronidazole 2 g po single dose *or* Amoxicillin/clavulinic acid 500 mg t.i.d. for 7 days	Exam for STD No Rx if normal	1st trimester, clindamycin vaginal cream 2%, one applicator vaginally for seven days if symptoms are distressing After 1st trimester, 2 g Metronidazole po once *or* 500 mg b.i.d. for 7 days po
Candidiasis	Butoconazole 2% cream 5 g intravaginally for 3 days *or* Fluconazole 150 mg po single dose	Clotrimazole 1% 5 g cream intravaginally for 7–14 days (OTC)	Candicidal cream if dermatitis persent	Avoid fluconazole and ketoconazole. Treat for 7 days

*Patients should be warned to avoid alcohol for 24 hours after last dose.

by the CDC (4). The clindamycin cream is slightly less efficacious. The U.S. Food and Drug Administration (FDA) has approved metronidazole 750 mg extended-release tablets once daily for 7 days, but there are no data on its equivalence to the recommended regimens. Women who are allergic to metronidazole may be treated with clindamycin cream. Alternative therapy is listed in Table 91.2.

Recurrence

Recurrence of symptoms after a "cure" is particularly problematic in *candidal vulvovaginitis*. The cause may be hypersensitivity to the organism or to the vehicle in topical agents, noncompliance (more likely with topical preparations), infection with an uncommon fungus species, true azole resistance, reinfection from a symptomatic partner, or risk factors, possibly unidentified. Patients who report several episodes should have their urine checked for sugar, especially if they present before puberty or after menopause.

Recurrence of *Trichomonas* usually results from reinfection or noncompliance with therapy. There are resistant strains of *Trichomonas*; they usually respond to a 7-day course of metronidazole, 1 to 2 g daily.

Clindamycin 300 mg every 12 hours for 7 days is the standard treatment for recurrent *bacterial vaginosis*. Repeated regimens of metronidazole are not well accepted by patients. In one small study, recurrent infection was successfully (78%) treated with a 3-minute instillation of 3% hydrogen peroxide in the vagina (16).

Treatment of Sexual Partners

Many studies have found no evidence of sexual transmission of Candida, and routine treatment of partners does not reduce the incidence of reinfection; therefore, there is no rationale for treating them. About 10% to 27% of men have a balanoposthitis. They should be treated with either the same topical preparation as the patient or a dermatologic fungicide. Oral treatment has not been evaluated.

It is necessary to treat all sexual partners of women diagnosed with *Trichomonas*. There is a 2.5-fold increase in reinfection rates if the sexual partner is not treated.

Sexual transmission of *bacterial vaginosis* is probable but not certain, and there is no consensus on treatment of partners. The CDC does not recommend routine treatment, and no decrease in recurrence has been shown if partners are treated (5).

Pregnancy

The incidence of vulvovaginal candidal infection is increased 10- to 20-fold in pregnancy. Oral fluconazole is not recommended, but any of the topical agents recommended is effective and safe (12).

Treatment of *T. vaginalis* infection in pregnancy in the past has been controversial. Metronidazole has both mutagenic and carcinogenic effects in animal studies. There is no evidence of either in human studies. A metaanalysis of the literature concluded that there is no relationship between metronidazole use in the first trimester and the incidence of birth defects (3). On that basis, the CDC now recommends the same treatment for symptomatic pregnant patients (4). Patients with incidental findings (such as trichomonads on urinalysis) who are asymptomatic should be referred to their prenatal caregivers. Although vaginal trichomoniasis has been associated with adverse pregnancy outcomes, data do not support treatment in lessening those events (10).

Symptomatic patients with *bacterial vaginosis* should be treated by using either metronidazole 250 mg orally three times a day for 7 days or clindamycin 300 mg orally twice a day for 7 days. BV is associated with premature rupture of membranes, chorioamnionitis, preterm birth, and postpartum infection. Clindamycin cream should not be used during pregnancy, as it has been associated with an increase in adverse outcomes. Treatment of asymptomatic patients with BV in a group at high risk for preterm delivery (previous preterm birth) has been shown to reduce the incidence of preterm delivery in several randomized controlled trials, but other trials have failed to show a reduction (2,11,15). Treatment of asymptomatic pregnant women should be the prerogative of the prenatal caregiver.

CRITICAL INTERVENTIONS

- Recommend treatment for partners of patients with *Trichomonas*
- Instruct patients to avoid alcohol for 24 hours after taking metronidazole

COMMON PITFALLS

✔ The patient with a chief complaint of vaginal discharge is never a high priority in a busy ED

✔ The most common pitfall is failure to do a good history and methodical examination

✔ Misdiagnosing urinary tract infection in patients who complain of dysuria that is actually external and due to *Candida* vulvovaginitis or *Trichomonas*

✔ Overlooking noninfectious causes of vaginal symptoms, such as chemical irritants (bubble bath, topical contraceptive, and feminine hygiene products, scents, deodorants, and soaps) or hormone depletion in postmenopausal women

✔ Failure to provide or refer for counseling regarding behavior risks and testing for HIV and other sexually transmitted diseases for patients with *Trichomonas* infection

References

1. Abbott J. Clinical and microscopic diagnosis of vaginal yeast infection: a prospective analysis. *Ann Emerg Med* 1995;25:587–591.
2. Carey JC, Klebanoff MA. National Institute of Child Health and Human Development Maternal-Fetal Medicine Units Network. What have we learned about vaginal infections and preterm birth? *Semin Perinatol* 2003;27:212–216.
3. Caro-Paton T, Carvajal A, Martin de Diego I, et al. Is metronidazole teratogenic? A meta-analysis. *Br J Clin Pharmacol* 1997;44:179–182.
4. Centers for Disease Control and Prevention. Sexually transmitted diseases—treatment guidelines 2002. *MMWR Morb Mortal Wkly Rep* 2002;51(No. RR-6).
5. Colli E, Landoni M, Parazzini F, et al. Treatment of male partners and recurrence of bacterial vaginosis: a randomized trial. *Genitourin Med* 1997;73:267–270.
6. duBouchet L, Spence MR, Rein MF, et al. Multicenter comparison of clotrimazole vaginal tablets, oral metronidazole, and vaginal suppositories containing sulfanilamide, aminacrine hydrochloride, and allantoin in the treatment of symptomatic trichomoniasis. *Sex Transm Dis* 1997;24:156–160.
7. Eschenbach DA, Edelman R, Carey JC, et al. Trichomonas vaginalis associated with low birth weight and preterm delivery. The Vaginal Infections and Prematurity Study Group. *Sex Transm Dis* 1997;24:353–360.
8. Ferris DG, Litaker MS, Woodward L, et al. Treatment of bacterial vaginosis: a comparison of oral metronidazole, metronidazole vaginal gel and clindamycin vaginal cream. *J Fam Pract* 1995;41:443–449.
9. Forna F, Gulmezoglu AM. Interventions for treating trichomoniasis in women. *Cochrane Database Syst Rev* 2003;2:CD000218.
10. Leitich H, Brunbauer M, Bodner-Adler B, et al. Antibiotic treatment of bacterial vaginosis in pregnancy: a meta-analysis. *Am J Obstet Gynecol* 2003;188:752–758.
11. Klebanoff MA, Carey JC, Hauth JC, et al. Failure of metronidazole to prevent preterm delivery among pregnant women with asymptomatic *Trichomonas vaginalis* infection. *New Engl J Med* 2001;345:487–493.
12. Moudgal VV, Sobel JD. Antifungal drugs in pregnancy: a review. *Expert Opin Drug Saf* 2003;2:475–483.
13. Sobel JD, Brooker D, Stein GE, et al. Single oral dose fluconazole compared with conventional clotrimazole topical therapy of candida vaginitis. Fluconazole Vaginitis Study Group. *Am J Obstet Gynecol* 1995;172[4 Pt 1]:1263–1268.
14. Spence MR, Harwell TS, Davies MC, et al. The minimum single oral metronidazole dose for treating trichomoniasis: a randomized, blinded study. *Obstet Gynecol* 1997;89[5 Pt 1]:699–703.
15. Ugwumadu A, Manyonds I, Reid F, Hay P. Effect of early oral clindamycin on late miscarriage and preterm delivery in asymptomatic women with abnormal vaginal flora and bacterial vaginosis: a randomized controlled trial. *Lancet* 2003;22;361:983–988.
16. Winceslaus SJ, Calver G. Recurrent bacterial vaginosis—an old approach to a new problems. *Int J STD AIDS* 1996;7:284–287.

CHAPTER 92
Breast Masses and Breast Infection

John M. Howell and Ellen M. Dugan

CLINICAL PRESENTATION

Effective emergency department evaluation of a breast mass depends on recognition of two major processes: cancer and infection. A breast abscess usually occurs in lactating women, but it may also represent inflammatory carcinoma in the elderly (8,11,14,16,17). Cancer, on the other hand, may present in a manner similar to that of fulminant mastitis (11,17). Experienced physicians can diagnose only 70% of breast cancers by examination alone (17). The initial evaluation of a breast mass may be difficult, challenging, and highly relevant to ultimate patient outcome.

Masses that are smooth, movable, and firm with distinct margins are usually benign (Table 92.1). Seventy-five percent to 80% of cancerous lesions are hard and cartilaginous with distinct edges that are serrated and irregular (14). However, 20% to 25% of cancerous nodules are less firm and less fibrotic in consistency, making accurate clinical diagnosis more difficult (14).

Cancerous nodules are usually located in the upper outer quadrant (14,17). Associated skin changes range from none to local edema or frank ulceration (14,17). Fibrosis may shorten Cooper ligament and cause skin dimpling, a process also seen in fat necrosis (14,17). Bloody nipple discharge suggests ductal carcinoma, or it may reflect the presence of an intraductal papilloma (17). Lymph nodes involved in the spread of breast cancer are initially rubbery and shotty, but eventually they become hard and matted with progressive infiltration (14). Axillary glands are most commonly involved, although spread to the parasternal and supraclavicular regions may also occur (14,17). Once in the lymphatic system, breast cancer cells disseminate to the lung, liver, and bony skeleton (14).

Erythema, edema, tenderness, and induration are late skin changes in the setting of breast cancer, but they also may be seen in acute mastitis (5,16). Most breast infections occur 1 to 3 months postpartum (8,14,16,17); therefore, mastitis or abscess in a nonlactating woman, as well as delayed resolution of a puerperal infection, is a warning sign of inflammatory cancer (12).

TABLE 92.1. Physical Findings Suggestive of Benign and Malignant Breast Masses

Benign Malignant	Malignant
Soft or firm on palpation	Firm or hard on palpation
Discrete, regular margins	Indistinct margins
No attachments	Attached to skin or deep fascia
More likely to be tender	Less likely to be tender
No discharge	Bloody discharge
No skin changes	Dimpling of overlying skin or nipple retraction
Mobile	Less likely to be mobile

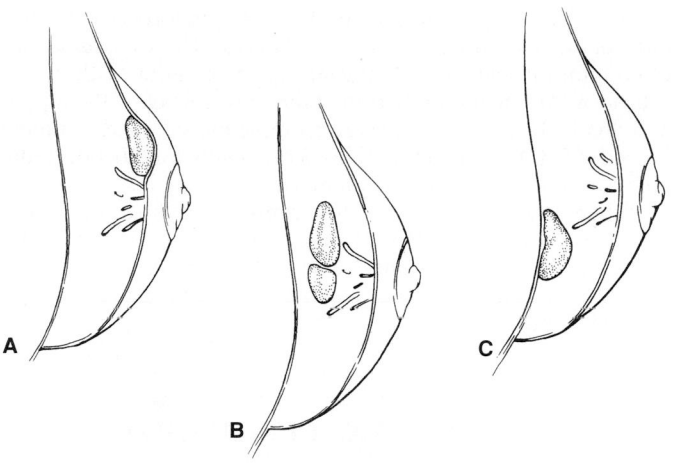

Figure 92.1. Breast abscesses. (**A**) Superficial abscess. (**B**) Intramammary abscess. (**C**) Retromammary abscess.

Mastitis in the lactating breast causes pain, fever, erythema, edema, tenderness, and induration. Fluctuance in a centrifugal location is the hallmark of a superficial abscess. Intramammary and retromammary loculations occur deep in breast tissue and near the pectoralis musculature, respectively (Fig. 92.1) (16). For this reason, fluctuance may not be readily apparent (16). The breast appears indurated, and the patient withdraws in re-

sponse to palpation (14). Paradoxically, decreasing induration and diminished pain may reflect the need for wide incision and drainage (17).

Postmenopausal breast abscesses are commonly subareolar. A mamillary fistula is identified by expressing pus from the nipple or areola (15). Nipple retraction and inversion are also observed (12).

Breast bud enlargement occurs in the first 1 to 2 weeks of life in 60% of neonates. These enlarged breast buds may become infected, usually with either *Staphylococcus aureus* or *Escherichia coli*. The clinical presentation is either simple cellulitis or abscess (18).

Paget disease of the nipple reflects carcinoma of the mammary ducts underlying the areola (14,17). The nipple initially appears dry, scaling, cracked, and eczematoid (14,17). The condition may progress to chronic skin inflammation and a surface crust. Subareolar fullness may or may not be palpable (14).

DIFFERENTIAL DIAGNOSIS

Cancer

One of nine women in the United States develops breast cancer. This disease is diagnosed in 180,000 patients annually (1). Risk factors for breast cancer are listed in Table 92.2. In women who are younger than 25 years of age, fewer than 5% of breast masses

TABLE 92.2. Established and Probable Risk Factors for Breast Cancer

Risk Factor	Comparison Category	Risk Category	Typical Relative Risk
Family history of breast cancer	No first-degree relatives affected	Mother affected before the age of 60	2.0
		Mother affected after the age of 60	1.4
		Two first-degree relatives affected	4.6
Age at menarche	16 yr	11 yr	1.3
		12 yr	1.3
		13 yr	1.3
		14 yr	1.3
		15 yr	1.1
Age at birth of first child	Before 20 yr	20–24 yr	1.3
		25–29 yr	1.6
		≥30 yr	1.9
		Nulliparous	1.9
Age at menopause	45–54 yr	After 55 yr	1.5
		Before 45 yr	0.7
		Oophorectomy before 35 yr	0.4
Benign breast disease	No biopsy or aspiration	Any benign disease	1.5
		Proliferation only	2.0
		Atypical hyperplasia	4.0
Radiation	No special exposure	Atomic bomb (100 rads)	3.0
		Repeated fluoroscopy	1.5–2.0
Obesity	10th Percentile	90th Percentile	
		Age, 30–49 yr	0.8
		Age, ≥50 yr	1.2
Height	10th Percentile	90th Percentile	
		Age, 30–49 yr	1.3
		Age, ≥50 yr	1.4
Oral contraceptive use	Never used	Current use	1.5
	1.5	Past use	1.0
Postmenopausal estrogen-replacement therapy	Never used	Current use all ages	1.4
		Age, <55 yr	1.2
		Age, 50–59 yr	1.5
		Age, ≥60 yr	2.1
Alcohol use	Nondrinker	Past use	1.0
		1 drink/day	1.4
		2 drinks/day	1.7
		3 drinks/day	2.0

are malignant. The incidence of breast cancer rises significantly during childbearing years, and by the age of 70 more than 75% of breast masses are malignant (2,10). Discussions of breast cancer histopathology and staging are beyond the scope of this chapter and are contained elsewhere (14).

Benign Neoplasms

Fibroadenomas are the most common benign neoplasms of the breast (14). They usually present during the third to fourth decades of life and are spherical, firm, mobile, and well defined (14). Fibroadenomas should be removed to rule out cancer and to preclude continued enlargement (14). Fibrocystic disease causes cyclic pain and swelling of one or both breasts just before menses (11). The nodules or cysts range from 2 or 3 mm to several centimeters in diameter (14). They are firm, round, distinct, and rubbery, and they transilluminate (14). Women with fibrocystic disease should be followed longitudinally because their risk of breast cancer is 3 to 5 times that of the general population (17). Conservative treatment includes a well-fitting brassiere, heat, and analgesics (11). Danazol, an androgen derivative, may be effective if hormonal treatment is indicated (16).

Fat Necrosis

Fat necrosis may present as a tender lump in the breast. This follows trauma in 50% of cases (11,14,17). The mass usually does not enlarge (8,10), but nipple retraction may be seen. Excision for definitive diagnosis is indicated (11).

Lipomas

Lipomas are superficial and occur in any quadrant of the breast. Mammography is usually diagnostic.

Mondor Disease

Mondor disease is thrombosis of the lateral thoracic or thoracoepigastric veins as they traverse the breast (11). The inflamed vein is characteristically tubular and may cause retraction of the skin. Mondor disease is self-limited and usually diagnosed with ease (11).

Idiopathic Granulomatous Mastitis

Idiopathic granulomatous mastitis (IGM) is a rare *inflammatory* breast disease of unknown etiology. The clinical presentation is similar to that of mammary carcinoma, and IGM can be misdiagnosed as carcinoma. IGM is associated with women who have experienced childbirth and oral contraceptive use. Treatment consists of resection or corticosteroids. There is a 38% recurrence rate following treatment (7).

Mastitis and Abscess

Most breast abscesses occur 1 to 3 months postpartum, but postmenopausal women may also develop mastitis (8,14,16,17). A postpartum breast abscess is caused by normal skin pathogens that invade through cracks in the nipple (15). Breast milk is an ideal culture medium. Unrecognized infection coalesces into abscesses, usually located away from the areola (17). Staphylococci are the most common causative agents (5,14,15); streptococci are cultured less often (8). Preventive measures include nipple hygiene (cleaning), hand washing, cleansing of the infant's skin, and early recognition (5,14,17).

Postmenopausal breast abscesses are distinct from puerperal forms in cause and presentation. Causative bacteria include *E. coli* (12), group D streptococci (6), staphylococci (12), and anaerobes, including *Bacteroides* species (15). These abscesses are often found in the subareolar region in association with ductal ectasia, a chronic inflammation of major ducts below the nipple and areola. Recurrence rates after simple incision and drainage exceed 39% (3) Mamillary fistulas occasionally form between the areola and infected lactating glands (8,9).

Tuberculosis remains the most common cause of persistent breast abscess (14,17). Chronic infection also occurs after inadequate drainage of partitioned areas within an abscess (17). Untreated chronic infection may result in substantial morbidity and cosmetic deformity (17).

EMERGENCY DEPARTMENT EVALUATION

The evaluation in the emergency department hinges upon the information gathered during the history and physical examination. As noted previously, many features including the size, location, tenderness, skin changes, and rapidity of onset are helpful in narrowing the differential. The important distinction is cancer versus infection. Asymptomatic patients with a mass suspicious for cancer usually require no further emergency department evaluation, but need expeditious outpatient referral. Patients with signs or symptoms of metastatic cancer should have further emergency department evaluation including laboratory and imaging studies to search for complications and the extent of spread. Ultrasound may be helpful in diagnosing a breast abscess if the clinician is uncertain.

EMERGENCY DEPARTMENT MANAGEMENT

Simple mastitis in the lactating woman, without abscess formation, is treated with antimicrobials that are effective against staphylococci and streptococci (5,8). Either cephalexin (250 to 500 mg 4 times a day), dicloxacillin (250 to 500 mg 4 times a day), or erythromycin (250 to 500 mg 4 times a day) in penicillin-allergic patients, is appropriate. Breast milk should be cultured for aerobes and anaerobes (5). Feedings may be discontinued for up to 48 hours if there is concern about infant diarrhea; however, drainage must be accomplished by continued feeding or pump (5,8,16). Local heat should be applied (17). Treat simple, nonlactating breast infections with amoxicillin-clavulanic acid at 875 mg twice a day (18).

Superficial abscesses may be drained and treated in the emergency department if there is no fever or toxicity. Incision and drainage may be performed by an emergency physician or a surgeon who is qualified to perform this procedure. Incision is performed in a curvilinear manner along skin lines (14) or in a radial manner (16). A circumareolar approach may also be used (8,17). Care should be taken to ensure that there are no loculations that might result in a chronic abscess. In superficial abscesses, needle aspiration has been successful in a few patients (C.M. Magnant, personal communication, 1994). Culture (anaerobic and aerobic) and gram staining of the drainage should be performed (8). The patient should be given antimicrobials and instructed in the same local measures as for simple mastitis. Patients should be educated about causal factors, symptoms, and how to avoid recurrent episodes of mastitis (4).

Treat neonatal breast bud infections with parenteral antibiotics (e.g., ampicillin 50 mg/kg and cefotaxime 50 mg/kg) following cultures of the blood and urine. Incision and drainage are frequently required and should be performed peripherally to avoid cosmetic complications (19).

DISPOSITION

Women suspected of having breast cancer should be referred immediately to a consultant who is experienced in the diagnosis and management of breast disorders. Mammography may be used to evaluate suspicious breast masses in women who are not pregnant and are at least age 20 years. Arrangements may be made for mammography to be performed on an outpatient basis. If mammography is performed, a subsequent visit to a specialist is important. About 18% of mammograms show a false-negative result for breast cancer (3), so patients should be counseled that a negative study does not necessarily mean the absence of disease (13).

Nontoxic patients with mastitis or superficial abscess should be reevaluated in 24 hours. Mamillary fistulas should be referred to a surgeon for excision and definitive closure (8,9,12). Postmenopausal intramammary abscesses necessitate surgical consultation because of the high recurrence rate after simple drainage (11,15). Incision and drainage of superficial abscesses may be referred to a surgeon for cosmetic reasons if the emergency physician is not skilled in the procedure.

Patients with suspicious breast masses need not be admitted unless either breast cancer is advanced on presentation, with intractable pain or serious secondary infection, or family or socioeconomic factors place admission in the patient's best interest. In general, the initial evaluation of suspicious breast masses is done on an outpatient basis.

Women with mastitis with marked temperature elevation or toxic appearance should be admitted and placed on intravenous antibiotics that are effective against staphylococci and streptococci. Women with simple infections that do not improve or that worsen after 24 hours should also be admitted. Patients with deep intramammary and retromammary abscesses are hospitalized for operative drainage (16).

Consider transfer or referral when no physician experienced in the management of breast disorders is available. Women transferred for operative care should be stable, without evidence of septic shock. Antimicrobials should be initiated by the referring hospital and pain controlled before transfer.

CRITICAL INTERVENTIONS

- Refer all patients with a suspicious breast mass for expeditious outpatient evaluation
- Incise and drain superficial breast absusses

COMMON PITFALLS

✔ Inflammatory cancer may present with erythema, edema, and tenderness. Infection in a nonlactating breast and failure of a postpartum infection to abate in a timely manner should suggest the possibility of cancer

✔ Inadequate drainage of a breast abscess may lead to chronic infection with substantial morbidity and cosmetic deformity

References

1. Boring CC, Squires TS, Tong T. Cancer statistics. *CA Cancer J Clin* 1992;42:19.
2. Willett WC, et al. Epidemiology and nongenetic causes of breast cancer. In: Harris JR, Lippman ME, Morrow M, et al., eds. *Diseases of the breast.* Philadelphia: Lippincott, Williams and Wilkins, 2000.
3. Donegan WL. Evaluation of a palpable breast mass. *N Engl J Med* 1992;327:937.
4. Fetherston C. Management of lactation mastitis in a western Australian cohort. *Breastfeed Rev* 1997;5:12–19.
5. Fiorica JV. The breast. In: Danforth DN, Scott JR, Di Saia PJ, et al., eds. *Danforth's obstetrics and gynecology,* 8th ed. Philadelphia: Lippincott Williams & Wilkins, 1999.
6. Harris JR, Lippman ME, Veronesi U, et al. Breast cancer. *N Engl J Med* 1992;327:319.
7. Imoto S, Kitaya T, Kotama T, et al. Idiopathic granulomatous mastitis: case report and review of the literature. *Jpn J Clin Oncol* 1997;27:274–277.
8. Clare SE, Morrow M.Management of the palpable breast mass. In: Harris JR, Lippman ME, Morrow M, et al., eds. *Diseases of the breast.* Philadelphia: Lippincott, Williams and Wilkins, 2000.
9. Lambert ME, Bates CD, Sellwood RA. Mamillary fistula. *Br J Surg* 1986;73:367.
10. Ligon RE, Stevenson DR, Diner W, et al. Breast masses in young women. *Am J Surg* 1980;140:779.
11. Magnant CM.Fat necrosis, hematoma and trauma. In: Harris JR, Lippman ME, Morrow M, et al., eds. *Diseases of the breast.* Philadelphia: Lippincott–Raven, 1996.
12. Maier WP, Berger A, Derrick BM. Periareolar abscess in the nonlactating breast. *Am J Surg* 1982;144:359.
13. *Physician Insurers Association of America Cancer Study—March 1990.* Pennington, NJ: Physician Insurers Association of America, 1990.
14. Harris JR. Staging of breast cancer Harris JR, Lippman ME, Morrow M, et al., eds. Diseases of the breast. Philadelphia: Lippincott, Williams and Wilkins, 2000.
15. Scholefield JH, Duncan JL, Rogers K. Review of a hospital experience of breast abscesses. *Br J Surg* 1987;74:469.
16. Warden TM, Fourre MW.Incision and drainage of cutaneous abscesses and soft tissue infections. In: Roberts JR, Hedges JR, eds. *Clinical procedures in emergency medicine,* 2nd ed. Philadelphia: WB Saunders, 1991.
17. Wilson RE.The breast. In: Sabiston DC, ed. *Textbook of surgery,* 13th ed. Philadelphia: WB Saunders, 1986.
18. Nixon JM, Bundred NJ. Management of disorders of the ductal system and infections. In: Harris JR, Lippman ME, Morrow M, et al., eds. *Diseases of the breast.* Philadelphia: Lippincott, Williams and Wilkins, 2000.
19. Melish ME, Campbell KA.Coagulase-positive staphylococcal infections. In: *Textbook of pediatric infectious diseases.* Philadelphia: W.B. Saunders and Co., 1998.

CHAPTER 93
Sexual Assault

Gwendolyn L. Hoffman

An emergency physician confronts a great variety of medical emergencies. One of the more complex of these is sexual assault, or rape. The emergency physician must be adept at meeting the physical, emotional, and judicial needs of these patients. The legal definition of *sexual assault,* which is gender-neutral, requires three key elements: (i) threat or the use of force, (ii) evidence of sexual contact, with or without penetration, and (iii) lack of effective consents (5). Rape, on the other hand, requires forced genital, anal, or oral penetration by the offender in which the force is either physical or psychologic (2). In 2002, the Bureau of Justice Statistics estimated 247,730 rapes and sexual assaults against victims age 12 and older (18,21). This number continues to decline yearly and is down by half over the last decade (21). The number of reported rapes and sexual assaults continue to rise from approximately 31% in 1993 to 1995 to 46.8% in 2000 to 2002 (18,21). Greater societal knowledge and openness along with tough-on-crime policies are factors to the increased willingness to report. In addition, there are approximately 2% to 10% of noninstitutionalized men who are victims of sexual assault (17). This chapter will not specifically deal with men, but much of what is discussed can be extrapolated to the male victim. Information in regards to pediatric sexual abuse can be found in Chapter 234.

CLINICAL PRESENTATION

The sexual assault victim may present to the emergency department immediately after the event. She is often accompanied by friends, family, or the police. She may have visible physical trauma and be emotionally distraught. On the other hand, it may be hours or days later before she presents. The victim may feel guilt, shame, humiliation, and embarrassment. She may not be immediately able to share her experience with anyone and may delay seeking treatment. The victim with physical trauma, such as airway compromise, severe laceration, or fracture, is most likely to obtain early medical intervention.

EMERGENCY DEPARTMENT EVALUATION

The emergency physician's first duty to the rape victim is to evaluate for any life-threatening or serious physical injury. If specific treatment is administered, care must be taken not to destroy or alter any evidence on the patient's person or at the scene. If the patients herself calls the emergency department to say she has been sexually assaulted, she should be advised to come immediately for evaluation and treatment. She should be encouraged not to bathe, shower, douche, gargle, brush her teeth, eat, drink, urinate, defecate, take medications, or change her clothing. If she has already changed clothes, she should be advised to place in a paper bag the clothes she removed and bring them to the hospital. If she has not notified the police, she should be advised to do so, or the emergency physician should offer to do it for her.

At the emergency department, the patient should be ushered into a private room where care can begin. Informed consent must be obtained in writing and witnessed before hospital personnel may perform the medical examination, collect and analyze specimens, take pictures, release information to legal authorities, or render treatment. If the hospital has a special sexual assault team, the team should initiate involvement with the victim at this point. An increasing number of institutions are associated with a sexual assault nurse examiner (SANE) program (10,11).

Once consent has been obtained, the pertinent historical facts can be obtained if the patient is physically able. The history need not be an exhaustive account of the details of the encounter. Information about minute details that the victim provides at a time of acute emotional strain may later prove confusing in court if any discrepancy is noted between the hospital and the police reports. The history should include information necessary for medical treatment and for the collection of evidence, including time, date, and place of the event. The information may be important when trying to relate physical findings, such as a bruise, to the assault, or when looking for corroborating evidence, such as sand if the assault occurred at the beach. Threats of violence or reprisal made by the assailant should be noted. It should be noted if any type of weapon, restraints, foreign bodies, alcohol, or drugs were involved. This determinate may direct the physical examination looking for specific injuries, which when found, have been correlated with successful prosecution (7). The number of assailants should be noted as well as if vaginal, oral, or anal penetration was attempted and also if ejaculation occurred. If ejaculation occurred, seminal deposits must be carefully sought on clothing as well as on the patient's person. The patient should be asked if she has douched, bathed, urinated, or defecated since the assault. If she has, some evidence might have been destroyed.

A pertinent gynecologic history should include gravidity, parity, last menstrual period, contraceptive history, date of last consensual intercourse, history of recent sexually transmitted disease, and any recent gynecologic surgery. If the victim is taking birth control pills, she should be asked if she has missed taking any pills. All of this information will assist in deciding what type of medical treatment is necessary.

The medical history should include current medication, allergies, and tetanus immunization status. In some emergency departments, nurses take the history and collect specimens. It does not matter who gathers this evidence as long as it is done in a caring and professional manner. The important thing is that important information is not omitted and the chain of evidence is not broken. For this reason, most departments have specific protocols and prepared forms that should be used. The physician must be thoroughly familiar with department procedure (2).

It does not matter whether the physical examination is performed by a female or male physician. It is important that the physician be understanding, supportive, and caring. The purposes of the physical examination are to determine the need for medical treatment, to gather specimens for analysis, and to make and document observations for corroboration of the assault. If the police are present and if the victim is wearing the clothes she wore during the attack, the police may want to take photographs before she undresses. In this case, the patient should be asked to place her clothes in a paper bag, or to place each item in a separate bag, depending on protocol. Paper bags are used instead of plastic bags, because plastic bags do not "breathe" and may promote molding of blood and seminal stains. The patient should put the clothes in the bag herself to avoid possible cross-contamination from blood group antigens in the sweat of the hospital personnel.

When the patient has donned a hospital gown and is ready, the physician should thoroughly explain what the physical examination will entail. The skin should be inspected for scratches, lacerations, abrasions, contusions, and bite marks; special attention should be paid to the neck, mouth, breasts, wrists, and thighs. When the mouth is being examined for trauma, a saliva sample should be obtained. The sample can be used to determine the patient's status as a blood group antigen secretor or nonsecretor. The teeth should be swabbed for acid phosphatase and sperm analysis. In addition to noting evidence of trauma, the presence of any foreign material, such as hair, blood, or semen, should also be noted. Foreign material should be scraped from under the fingernails and placed in the appropriate envelope. This material may reveal bits of the assailant's hair, blood, or skin, if the victim was able to actively resist. Semen may appear as lightly crusted areas. A Wood light can help to identify these areas because they fluoresce in ultraviolet light (13). Semen can be removed with a water-moistened swab. Fluorescence is not pathognomonic of semen because other stains and urine may fluoresce, but it may be helpful.

If photographs are not taken, the examiner must be even more careful to document the findings completely and accurately. Documenting thoroughly at the time of the examination makes it easier to recall the examination accurately when called on in a court of law.

The pelvic examination should be performed next. The external genitalia should be checked for trauma and evidence of semen. If semen is present on the upper inner thighs, it can be swabbed as previously described. If it is present on pubic hair, the hairs should be trimmed. The patient's pubic hair should be combed to find strands of the assailant's hair, which can be analyzed to help identify the assailant's race and hair color (6). In order to differentiate it from the victim's hair, some of her hair must be plucked for analysis also. Each specimen should be placed in the appropriate envelope.

Small vaginal lacerations can be identified with the use of toluidine blue (5). A small amount of the blue dye can be applied to the vaginal mucosa at the introitus. A positive test result is indicated by a linear blue stain, because the dye will be taken up by the nuclei of exposed submucosal cells. The dye is applied externally, not intravaginally. Therefore, it should not interfere with the collection of other evidence, but any excess should be wiped off before the speculum is inserted, just to be sure.

The hymen should be inspected to determine if it is present, intact, absent, or traumatized, with bleeding and fresh clots. In adolescent girls with an estrogenized hymen, the examination is more difficult. A Foley catheter (14 French) inserted through the hymen orifice and inflated, using 40 cc of air, has been used successfully to assess the redundant hymen (16). The speculum should be lubricated only with water; other lubricants may affect the acid phosphatase determination and sperm motility. The vaginal wall should be inspected for lacerations and for evidence of the penetration of any foreign objects. Any secretions that have pooled in the posterior fornix should be aspirated and placed in a sterile receptacle. These secretions can be used to determine the presence of sperm, acid phosphatase, and blood group antigens. If no secretions are present, the vagina should be washed with 5 to 10 mL of nonbacteriostatic sterile saline solution and followed with aspiration. If washing is not necessary, the posterior fornix should be swabbed with a cotton-tipped applicators and secretions smeared on two glass slides for later laboratory examination. One more swab should be obtained for wet mount examination. A Papanicolaou smear should be obtained from the cervix to help determine the presence of nonmotile sperm (the smear is useful up to several days after the assault). Cultures for gonorrhea, chlamydial infection, and herpes should be obtained, if indicated. A bimanual examination should be performed, and uterine size, adnexal masses, and tenderness noted. The rectal area should be examined carefully, especially if anal intercourse took place. Signs of trauma, semen stain, blood, and lubricant should be noted. Anal and rectal swabs can be obtained through the lumen of a water-lubricated anoscope; these are used to determine the presence of motile and nonmotile sperm and acid phosphatase. It is often difficult to document genial findings in sexual assault victims by gross visualization alone. Magnification with colposcopic and photography allows the examiner to document and characterize genital findings with more accuracy. Many emergency department have a colposcope readily available (12,19).

Blood should also be drawn for ABO analysis, syphilis serology, drug and alcohol screen, if indicated, and beta human chorionic gonadotropin (β-hCG). Routine testing for hepatitis B virus and human immunodeficiency virus must also be considered. This is especially true in an area of high seropositivity or if the assailant is known to be in a high-risk group (1,3). Pregnancy may be detected as early one week after implantation by using the radioimmunoassay beta subunit of hCG or the Tandem Icon II hCG urine assay. If the test result is negative initially and positive at a followup visit, the pregnancy probably originated at the time of the assault.

The oral, vaginal, and rectal swabs obtained for the identification of sperm must be examined microscopically for motile and nonmotile sperm. Sperm are not usually found motile after 12 hours. The presence of motile sperm is a reliable indication that the assault occurred at some point during the 12 hours preceding the examination, provided consensual intercourse did not also take place during that period. Nonmotile sperm may be present for 72 hours or longer.

The acid phosphatase enzyme may also indicate sexual contact. This enzyme is present in vaginal secretions but is found in much greater quantities in prostatic secretions. A high concentration of acid phosphatase is an excellent indicator of the presence of seminal fluid, even in the absence of sperm. The presence of acid phosphatase may be a more accurate indicator of the postcoital interval than the presence of nonmotile sperm.

A major seminal plasma glycoprotein produced in the prostate, p30, has been identified as another semen-specific marker. This protein is male-specific; therefore, the finding of any p30 in vaginal fluid establishes the presence of semen. p30 is present in men who have had vasectomies as well as in men who have not, and it can be found for approximately 48 hours after the assault.

The forensic laboratory will also develop a specific genetic profile of the assailant to compare with that of the victim. Genetic typing can determine the blood group and type of both parties. Three genetic markers found in semen are phosphoglucomutase (PGM), the peptidase-A (Pep-A) enzyme marker, and the ABO blood group antigens. With electrophoretic analysis, PGM and Pep-A can be further subdivided into a total of 40 possible combinations. Reference markers for the victim must be obtained at the initial evaluation; these markers are also in vaginal secretions but in lower concentrations.

DNA typing or fingerprinting has significant accuracy in identifying the assailant. This method involves the extraction of DNA from a small sample of blood, semen, or other DNA-bearing cells. Through various procedures, a specific "DNA fingerprint" is developed. This "fingerprint" can be analyzed and compared with the assailant's to establish a positive identification. The chance that two unrelated persons having the same DNA fingerprint is one in a quadrillion 4,7,15).

EMERGENCY DEPARTMENT MANAGEMENT

Physical trauma experienced by a sexual assault victim is treated like trauma in any other patient. In addition, the possibilities of psychological trauma, pregnancy, and venereal disease must be addressed.

Efforts to decrease the victim's distress can begin with her arrival at the emergency department. The staff must be attentive and encourage the victim to share her feelings. She has just experienced a threat to her life and must be helped to feel safe and secure. It is often helpful to have a rape crisis volunteer present to provide additional support and to make sure the patient understands the procedures explained to her by the physician and nurse. Her emotional trauma may be significant.

Rape is sudden and does not allow the victim to gather adequate defenses. Also, the victim feels trapped and often cannot fight back. The ability to trust is destroyed when the perpetrator is known (13). Rape also often involves intentional cruelty and physical injury. The victim will feel most comfortable with hospital personnel who are capable of projecting both professional objectivity and person concern.

The possibility of pregnancy should be explained to the patient. It is estimated that the risk of pregnancy without contraception is 1% to 5%. If mid-cycle (days 14 to 16), the risk is higher (2). Pregnancy should be ruled out before prophylactic treatment is considered. If prophylaxis is desired, combination therapy with estrogen and progestin is 75% to 85% effective if given within 72 hours of intercourse (20). Often, this is referred to as the Yuzpe regimen: ethinyl estradiol 100 μg po, plus levonorgestral 0.5 mg po; repeat in 12 hours

An antiemetic should also be prescribed because nausea and vomiting are common side effects (2). A history of pulmonary embolism, thrombophlebitis, estrogen-dependent tumor, or cardiovascular or liver disease is a contraindication to the administration of estrogen. An alternate regimen, "Plan B," has been found to be slightly more effective in preventing pregnancy and much less likely to cause nausea and vomiting than the Yuzpe regimen (8,20). It consists of levonorgestrel 0.75 mg po; repeat in 12 hours. This is becoming the preferred treatment for emergency contraception.

If the initial pregnancy test result is negative and a followup test result is positive, counseling is indicated, after which the patient may decide to have a suction curettage or a therapeutic abortion.

The risk of contracting sexually transmitted disease as the result of sexual assault is difficult to estimate. Risk varies according to geographic area, the populations within that area, and whether the assault is reported. Some reports have indicated that the incidence of acquiring a sexually transmitted disease from a single sexual encounter is 5% to 10% (9). Prophylaxis should be given if the patient requests it, if evidence of infection is present on examination, if followup is questionable, and if the assailant is suspected of being infected. The most frequently diagnosed infections among women who have been sexually assaulted are gonorrhea, chlamydia, trichomoniasis, and bacterial vaginosis (3).

Patients are usually treated by using one of the following regimens. (For gonorrhea) ceftriaxone 125 mg i.m., or ciprofloxacin 500 mg po, or ofloxacin 400 mg po, plus (for chlamydia) azithromycin 1g po, or doxycycline 100 mg po twice a day for 7 days, plus (for trichomoniasis) metronidazole 2 g po (or 500 mg bid x 7 days for bacterial vaginosis).

Ciprofloxacin and ofloxacin are contraindicated in pregnancy. Spectinomycin, 2 g i.m., is recommended only for use during pregnancy in patients allergic to β-lactams. Erythromycin, except for erythromycin estolate (500 mg po 4 times a day for 7 days) can be used in pregnancy. Both doxycycline and erythromycin will cover early syphilis, but the drug of choice remains penicillin G benzathine (2.4 million units i.m. once) (3). Hepatitis B virus vaccine should be considered if the patient was previously unimmunized. A dose of 1.0 mL i.m. should be given acutely and repeated 1 and 6 months later. Hepatitis B immune globulin should be reserved for a high-risk exposure, such as if the assailant is an intravenous drug user or if multiple assailants were involved (3).

Victims may be particularly concerned about the transmission of human immunodeficiency virus (HIV). The risk is felt to be very low, but appropriate counseling should be arranged as well as pretesting if deemed necessary. If high risk for exposure is determined, treatment must be initiated within 72 hours and continue for 28 days. Standard treatment is zidovudine, 300 mg twice a day or 200 mg 3 times a day, and lamivudine, 150 mg twice a day (1,14). The risks and side effects of antiretroviral therapy must be discussed with the patient, and many states have postexposure prophylaxis (PEP) hotlines to assist in such decisions. Repeat HIV antibody testing needs to be done in 6 weeks, 3 months, and 6 months (1).

CRITICAL INTERVENTIONS

- Assess and treat for serious physical injuries
- Carefully collect all specimens and maintain a chain of evidence so that samples will be admissible in court
- Offer prophylaxis for pregnancy and sexually transmitted diseases
- Arrange appropriate counseling and followup care

DISPOSITION

A gynecologist may be called during the initial examination if the emergency physician deems it necessary, especially if an operative intervention is needed. The emergency physician should strongly recommend that the victim seek followup care from a gynecologist or family physician.

Most hospitals have rape crisis volunteers available to consult with the victim during the first 24 hours after the assault. Encourage the patient to talk to the volunteers or to seek counseling with psychologists or psychiatrists, if indicated.

Admission to the hospital may be required in the case of significant physical trauma. As a rule, the sexual assault victim may be discharged from the emergency department in the company of relatives or friends. Followup care for the victim must be arranged before discharge. She will need to return after 2 weeks and after 6 weeks to be reevaluated for pregnancy and venereal disease. Any physical injury, such as a laceration, needs followup care. Psychological trauma may necessitate long-term treatment (9). The short-term phase, characterized by disorganization, may last from a few days to a few weeks. During this time, the victim may exhibit a wide range of emotional behavior, from being quiet and subdued to demonstrating anger and fear. The long-term phase, characterized by reorganization, may last for months or years. Many victims experience depression, flashbacks, anxiety, and sexual dysfunction (5). These experiences may explain why 80% of rape victims end primary relationships within 1 year of the rape (5). Because the rape victim may have a large spectrum of psychological needs and concerns, the emergency physician must be certain that followup evaluation will address them. The patient should be reevaluated psychologically approximately 1 to 2 weeks after the initial medical evaluation. At that visit, the need for further counseling should be discussed. Up to 70% of rape victims do not return for their followup visits (9). Therefore, it is advisable that some member of the medical team, such as a social worker, contact the victim after discharge, to address concerns that arise later and to encourage followup care.

COMMON PITFALLS

✔ Failure to appropriately collect, transfer, and document specimens. This legal protocol is the chain of evidence and safeguards the rights of the accused during the judicial process. All specimens must be correctly collected and labeled. Documentation must be made for each person who takes possession of the evidence—the physician or nurse who gathers the evidence, the police officer who transfers it to forensic laboratory, and laboratory technicians. No break must occur in this process, or the evidence will not be admissible in court
✔ Each institution and state may have some variation in their requirements and protocol, so the emergency physician must be familiar with the local procedures, kits, and forms
✔ Failure to offer appropriate prophylactic therapy for pregnancy and sexually transmitted diseases

References

1. Bamberger JD, Waldo CR, Gerberding JL, Katz MH. Postexposure prophylaxis for human immunodeficiency virus (HIV) infection following sexual assault. *Am J Med* 1999;106:323.
2. Cantu M, Coppola M, Lindner AJ.Evaluation and management of the sexually assaulted woman. In: Coppola M, Della Giurstina D, eds. *Emergency Medicine Clinics of North America: Obstetric and Gynecological Emergencies*. Philadelphia: WB Saunders Co. 2003;21:3.
3. Centers for Disease Control and Prevention. Sexually Transmitted Disease Treatment Guidelines 2002. *MMWR Morb Mortal Wkly Rep* 2002;51 (RR-6).
4. Dawkins R. Arresting evidence. *The Sciences* 1998; Nov-Dec, 20.
5. DeLahunta E, Baram DA. Sexual assault. *Obstet Gynecol* 1997;40:648.
6. Ferris LE, Sandercock J. The sensitivity of forensic tests for rape. *Med Law* 1998;17:333.
7. Gray-Eurom K, Seaburg DC, Wears RL. The prosecution of sexual assault cases: correlation with forensic evidence. *Ann Emerg Med* 2002;39:1.
8. Health   Professionals.   http://www.go2plan-b.com/section/health_professionals
9. Holmes MN, Resnick HS, Frampton D. Follow-up of sexual assault victims. *Am J Obstet Gynecol* 1998;179:336.
10. Houmes BV, Fagan MM, Quintana NM. Establishing a sexual assault nurse examiner (SANE) program in the emergency department. *J Emerg Med* 2003; 25:111.
11. Ledray LE. Sexual assault: clinical issues. *J Emerg Nurs* 1998;24:197.
12. Lenahan LC, Ernst A, Johnson B. Colposcopy in evaluation of the adult sexual assault victim. *Am J Emerg Med* 1998;16:183.
13. Lynnerup N, Hjalgrim H. Routine use of ultraviolet light in medicolegal examinations to evaluate stains and skin trauma. *Med Sci Law* 1995;35:165.
14. Merchant RC, Keshavarz R. HIV postexposure prophylaxis practices by US ED practitioners. *Am J Emerg Med* 2003;21:323.

15. O'Donnell P, Archambault J, Bell K, Turman KM. DNA evidence in sexual assault. In: Giardino AP, Datner EM, Asher JB, eds. *Sexual assault*. St. Louis: GW Medical Publishing, Inc., 2003.
16. Persaud DI, Squires JE, Rubin-Remer O. Use of Foley catheter to examine estrogenized hymens for evidence of sexual abuse. *J Pediatr Adolesc Gynecol* 1997;10:83.
17. Pesola GR, Westfal RE. Kuffer CA. Emergency department characteristics of male sexual assault. *Acad Emerg Med* 1999;6:792.
18. Rape, Abuse, and Incest National Network (RAINN). Washington, DC. http://www.rainn.org
19. Rogers D. Physical aspects of alleged sexual assaults. *Med Sci Law* 1996;36:117.
20. Task Force on Postovulatory Methods of Fertility Regulation. Randomised controlled trial of levonorgestrel versus the Yuzpe regimen of combined oral contraceptives for emergency contraception. *Lancet* 1998;352:428.
21. United States Department of Justice, Bureau of Justice Statistics, Crime and Victim Statistics 2002. http://www.ojp.usdoj.gov/bjs.

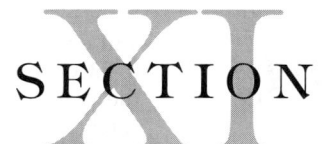

SECTION

XI

Section Editor: Gregory W. Hendey

Obstetric Emergencies

and treat UTIs in pregnant patients to potentially prevent miscarriage.

Routine screening for Rh status in the pregnant patient with vaginal bleeding is controversial (24). It has been well established that completed abortion, ectopic pregnancy, antepartum hemorrhage, and trauma are associated with possible fetomaternal transfusion, and, therefore, potential for Rh isoimmunization if the mother is Rh– and the fetus is Rh+. It is unclear whether the same phenomenon occurs in threatened abortion (21). However, owing partly to poor access to follow-up care of some patients who present to the emergency department, it has become common practice to give Rh immune prophylaxis to Rh– pregnant women with vaginal bleeding (1,14).

A CBC is often obtained in patients with vaginal bleeding to obtain an estimate of the amount of blood loss. A baseline hematocrit may be useful for comparison if serial hematocrits are obtained during that or subsequent visits.

The *quantitative beta human chorionic gonadotropin*, or β-*hCG* is a measure of trophoblastic tissue activity, which is a marker for the volume of living trophoblastic tissue and a function of renal clearance. Both ectopic and intrauterine pregnancies produce β-hCG, although they usually differ in the rate at which the quantitative β-hCG level increases. Patients with ectopic pregnancy tend to have a lower quantitative β-hCG level than those with viable intrauterine pregnancy (IUPs) for the same gestational age (6). In addition, patients with abnormal IUPs may have lower β-hCGs than patients with normal IUPs do (2). Because of the large range of β-hCG for each stage of embryonic development, a single value of β-hCG is not useful for differentiating among normal IUP, abnormal IUP, and ectopic pregnancy. However, a variation in the expected rate of rise of the β-hCG level can be helpful. The β-hCG normally doubles in 1.9 ± 0.5 days when the β-hCG is less than 10,000 mIU/mL (22). Furthermore, an increase of greater than 66% over 48 hours is seen in 85% of patients with normal IUPs. A less than expected increase (less than 66% over 48 hours) is 75% sensitive and 93% specific for an abnormal gestation of some variety (17,22). A total of 85% of ectopic pregnancies and 15% of normal IUPs have an abnormal rate of rise of the β-hCG (17). Declining β-hCG levels indicate nonviability of the pregnancy, either ectopic or intrauterine. The rate of fall of the β-hCG has been found to differ significantly between the two entities. The half life of the β-hCG is greater than 7 days in ectopic pregnancy, whereas it is less than 1.4 days in aborting IUPs (18). It is important to note that a falling β-hCG does not exclude the possibility of tubal rupture. The β-hCG level is usually higher than expected for gestational age (generally greater than 100,000 mIU/mL) in molar pregnancy.

The primary value of *pelvic ultrasonography* in the evaluation of a pregnant vaginal bleeding patient is to confirm the presence of an IUP, which ostensibly rules out ectopic pregnancy. Ultrasound is also useful in evaluating the prognosis for a threatened gestation because there are sonographic findings consistent with normal gestational development at various levels of β-hCG (8). An understanding of what is necessary to make the sonographic diagnosis of an IUP is important for the clinician to optimally use the information. The hormones of pregnancy cause an early uterine decidual reaction that may be seen on ultrasound soon after a missed menses, but this is nonspecific and occurs with both IUPs and ectopic pregnancies. The earliest sonographic landmark consistent with an IUP is the gestational sac. With endovaginal ultrasound, this can be visualized as early as 4.5 weeks after the LMP, and reliably by 5 weeks. The gestational sac lies eccentrically within the decidua of the endometrium, and is seen to have two distinct layers sonographically. These two layers give a sonographic appearance of two rings, thus called the "double ring sign," that is diagnostic of an intrauterine gestational sac (see Fig. 94.1). The yolk sac seen within the gestational sac is the

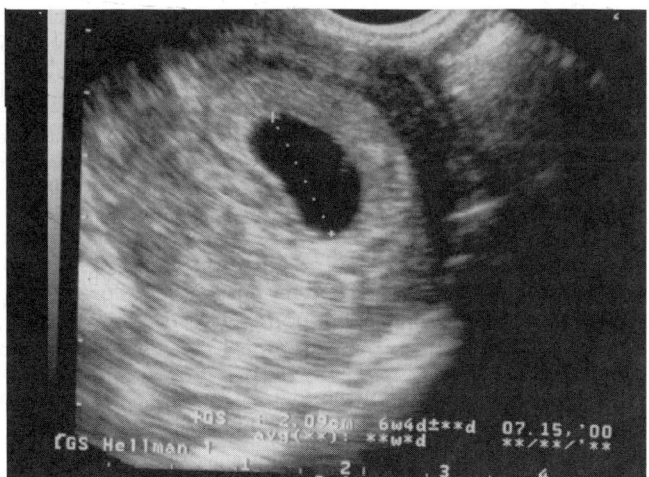

Figure 94.1. Transvaginal ultrasound of a gestational sac, showing the "double ring."

next sonographic landmark of the developing pregnancy, and it is seen reliably by the end of the fifth week. The embryo and cardiac activity are seen concurrently and reliably adjacent to the yolk sac by 6.5 weeks gestation by endovaginal ultrasound (5). Table 94.3 lists the sonographic findings of early pregnancy development with their corresponding discriminatory levels of β-hCG and gestational ages.

The sonographic finding that is most reassuring for a favorable prognosis is the presence of embryonic cardiac activity. For women younger than 35 years of age at 8 weeks estimated gestational age (EGA), the presence of cardiac activity sonographically indicates a spontaneous abortion rate of 3% to 5%. This increases to about 8% for women who are 35 years of age and older. Sonographic findings that foreshadow a poor outcome include a slow embryonic heart rate (less than 90 bpm), a small gestational sac for the size of the embryo, and a large yolk sac (greater than 6 mm) (7). The effects of a subchorionic hematoma, gestational age, and maternal age together on gestational prognosis have been investigated. It was found that gestations with a hematoma greater than two thirds the circumference of the chorion had a twofold increase in their rate of spontaneous abortion (19%) compared to those with a small- or medium-sized hematoma (9%). In addition, the spontaneous abortion rates for women who are 35 years or older was twice that for those younger than 35, 14% versus 7%, respectively (4).

Molar pregnancy has a characteristic but unusual pattern on ultrasound that is referred to as a *snowstorm pattern* (Fig. 94.2).

Emergency Department Management

The first consideration in management of a first trimester patient who has vaginal bleeding is her hemodynamic status. A patient who is bleeding heavily and is symptomatic should

TABLE 94.3. Sonoembryology of Early Pregnancy

Sonographic Landmarks of Early Pregnancy	EGA (wk)	Serum Quantitative β-hCG (mIU/mL)
Gestational sac	4.5	>1500
Yolk sac	5.5	1,000–7,500
Embryo with cardiac activity	6.5	7,000–23,000

EGA, estimated gestational age; β-hCG, beta human chorionic gonadotropin.

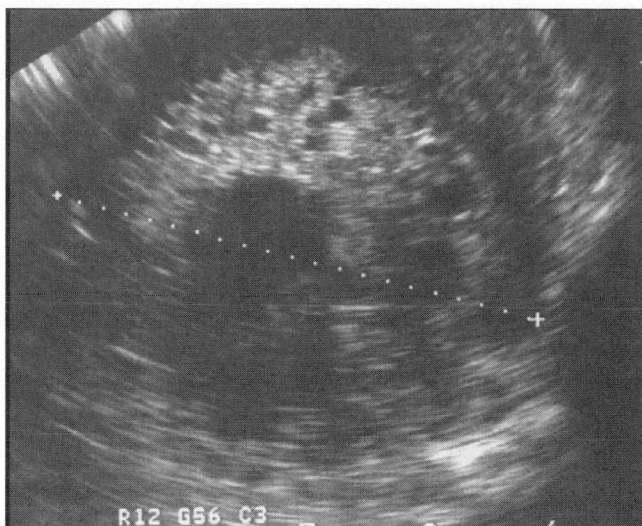

Figure 94.2. Transvaginal ultrasound of a molar pregnancy, with typical "snowstorm" appearance.

be resuscitated with intravenous fluids. Obtain type-specific blood for transfusion if the patient's hemodynamic status does not respond to 2 L of crystalloid. Patients with heavy vaginal bleeding will need an immediate gynecologic consultation regardless of the etiology of the bleeding, as an emergent dilation and curettage (D&C) may be required. The exception to this is the patient who has products of conception in the open cervical os at the time of examination. Such a patient may have her products of conception easily removed manually by *gentle* traction with a ring forceps, thereby completing the spontaneous miscarriage. If more than gentle traction is required, there may be incomplete separation of tissue from the endometrium. Do not simply pull harder, as mechanical separation can result in severe hemorrhage. Rather, obtain gynecologic consultation for assistance in this instance. However, if tissue is removed manually or spontaneously, a rapid decrease in bleeding and pain should follow. After a few hours of observation to ensure continued clinical resolution of their bleeding and cramping, as well as the internal cervical os at least beginning to close, such patients usually can be sent home with routine gynecologic followup. Patients who continue to have an open internal cervical os should receive gynecologic consultation for possible D&C of their presumptively incomplete abortion.

Septic abortion is a polymicrobial infection and should be treated immediately with broad-spectrum intravenous antibiotics, evacuation of the uterus and admission. In addition, blood and cervical discharge should be obtained for culture. Disseminated intravascular coagulation is sometimes seen in this setting, either as a result of prolonged retention of fetal tissue caused by release of necrotic tissue into the bloodstream or in women who have developed frank septic shock.

It is common practice to give Rh immune prophylaxis to Rh– pregnant women with vaginal bleeding (14). If the gestation is less than 12 weeks, a dose of 50 micrograms is sufficient. However, as pregnancy dating is difficult and inaccurate, some recommend that all unsensitized Rh– women with vaginal bleeding receive 300 micrograms of Rh immune globulin in the first or second trimester. This should be given before the patient leaves the emergency department, but protection occurs if it is administered within 72 hours of the bleed. It is not necessary to repeat the dosage at subsequent emergency department or clinic visits for continued or repeat bleeding before 20 weeks of gestation. A subsequent 300 micrograms dose should be administered in the third trimester or prior to delivery.

CRITICAL INTERVENTIONS

> - Evaluate all patients with first trimester vaginal bleeding for ectopic pregnancy, regardless of their clinical complaints or results of physical examination
> - Administer broad-spectrum antibiotics to patients with suspected septic abortion or infected retained products of conception

Disposition

Patients who are hemodynamically stable and who appear nontoxic, with a closed internal cervical os, and reliable access to gynecology followup may be sent home. If a patient is known to not have an ectopic pregnancy, then once the result of the urinalysis and Rh screen have been interpreted and the patient treated accordingly, the patient with either threatened or completed spontaneous abortion may have routine (1–2 week) gynecologic followup. Generally these patients will have serial β-hCG levels followed in order to definitively make their diagnosis, and it should be determined prior to emergency department discharge whether the primary care provider or the emergency department will be doing this. There is no evidence that reduction of activity or medical therapy will affect the outcome of the threatened abortion. Despite this, rest it is often prescribed for social and psychologic reasons. It is important to emphasize to a patient and her partner that normal pregnancies tolerate normal physical activity. Patients with embryonic demise or *blighted ovum* (Table 94.1) may be managed according to the preference of the gynecologist and the patient. Unless there is heavy bleeding or fever, there is no urgency to evacuate the uterus. Patients may be managed expectantly for up to 2 weeks without increased risk of complication. However, many gynecologists prefer to perform a D&C sooner than 2 weeks. Patients will also vary in their preferences, with some insisting on immediate evacuation, and others preferring expectant care.

All patients who are discharged from the emergency department should be encouraged to return immediately if they develop worrisome symptoms or fever. Most importantly, all patients with vaginal bleeding should be reassured that the cause of their bleeding and/or miscarriage is not their fault and that there is nothing they can do to prevent miscarrying an abnormal pregnancy. Patients and family members may have many misconceptions about this, and a physician reinforcing the correct thought process may be very important to the psychologic well-being of these patients. The emotional response to a spontaneous abortion is variable, from relief to overwhelming grief. A sensitive approach to these families is a critical part of treatment and is often the most significant effect a clinician can have. Offering referral to professional counseling or support groups should be a routine part of managing these women, and preprinted discharge instructions with appropriate referral phone numbers may be very useful.

COMMON PITFALLS

✔ Failure to consider ectopic pregnancy in the first trimester of pregnancy
✔ Underestimating the amount of blood loss. Because these patients tend to be healthy young women, they can maintain nearly normal vital signs despite large volume losses, until abrupt decompensation occurs

NAUSEA AND VOMITING OF PREGNANCY

Despite the common nature of nausea and vomiting in pregnancy, most pregnant women will never become sick enough to present to the emergency department, and only 1% to 2% require hospital admission (20). *Hyperemesis gravidarum* is defined as the syndrome of intractable vomiting and weight loss, hypokalemia, or ketonemia. Although the exact etiology of nausea and vomiting of pregnancy and hyperemesis gravidarum are still unknown, hormonal, neurologic, metabolic, toxic, and psychosomatic factors are all described. Most experts consider hCG to be a causative factor (19), although this association remains controversial (25,26).

Clinical Presentation

The usual sequence of events of nausea and vomiting of pregnancy includes loss of appetite at 5 to 6 weeks of gestation, followed by nausea and subsequent vomiting. Typically, eating or drinking quickly exacerbates these symptoms. Pain is uncommon in pregnancy-induced nausea and vomiting and suggests another etiology. Patients with pregnancy-induced nausea and vomiting present with few physical signs other than those of dehydration, with or without associated vital sign changes. Late findings such as dry mucosa or poor skin turgor may be present if symptoms are more severe or longstanding. Generally there are no specific findings on physical examination. Abnormal electrolytes suggest the diagnosis of hyperemesis gravidarum, and these patients will likely require admission to the hospital for continued intravenous hydration (11).

Differential Diagnosis

The differential diagnosis of nausea and vomiting in the pregnant patient is extensive, and includes disorders related to and unrelated to pregnancy (Table 94.4). Nausea and vomiting of pregnancy and hyperemesis gravidarum are common, but the clinician must also consider nonobstetric causes such as infection (pyelonephritis), abdominal disorders (appendicitis, bowel obstruction, cholelithiasis, pancreatitis, and gastritis), central nervous system (CNS), toxic, or metabolic causes.

Emergency Department Evaluation

The history and physical examination obtained in the emergency department should focus on assessing the severity of symptoms and findings, the need for resuscitation, and the exclusion of other more serious causes of these symptoms. A medication history is necessary to identify prescription, over-the-counter, or other drugs that can cause nausea and vomiting.

Assessment for other etiologies in the differential requires focused examination looking specifically for jaundice and costovertebral tenderness. The presence of abdominal tenderness or distention must lead to assessments for gynecologic, surgical, or infectious disorders. Rectal examination may be appropriate to identify stool impaction and should include testing for occult blood. Pelvic examination is generally necessary in the presence of abdominal or pelvic pain, vaginal bleeding, or discharge, as typically ectopic pregnancy or incomplete abortion have not been ruled-out at that point in the patient's evaluation.

Laboratory testing that may be helpful includes a CBC, serum electrolytes and ketone levels, BUN and creatinine, and urinalysis. Elevated hematocrit and BUN may be present because of hemoconcentration. Hyper- or hyponatremia, or hypokalemia may be evident. Urinalysis is important for assessing the degree of dehydration and for evidence of infection. Radiographic

TABLE 94.4.   Differential Diagnosis of Nausea/Vomiting in Pregnancy

Diagnosis	Key Distinguishing Clinical Diagnostic Features
Gastric mucosal irritation: NSAIDs, EtOH	Abd pain ↓ by eating
Appendicitis	Abd pain, tenderness, fever
Cholelithiasis/cholecystitis	Abd pain ↑ with eating, ↑ LFTs
Hepatitis	Abd pain, ↑ LFTs, icterus
Pancreatitis	Abd pain, ↑ lipase
Endocrine disorders: thyrotoxicosis, DKA, hyper or hypoparathyroidism, adrenal insufficiency	History, laboratory abnormalities
Bowel obstruction	Abd pain, vomiting ↑ by eating
Vestibular nerve stimulation	Nystagmus
↑ Intracranial pressure	Headache, papilledema
Meningeal irritation	Headache
Medications: antiseizure agents, theophylline, digitalis, salicylates	History, drug levels
Reflux esophagitis	Retrosternal burning type pain
Diaphragmatic hernia	Similar to bowel obstruction history
Achalasia	Difficulty swallowing
Psychiatric disease	History
Acute gastroenteritis	Diarrhea, fever
Food poisoning	History of very abrupt onset

NSAID, nonsteroidal anti-inflammatory drug; EtOH, ethanol; LFT, liver function test; Abd, abdominal; DKA, diabetic ketoacidosis.

imaging should be obtained as dictated by the clinical picture. In patients who are determined to have hyperemesis gravidarum, pelvic ultrasonography may be helpful to assure the presence of fetal cardiac activity, to identify multiple gestations, or to diagnose molar pregnancies. An abdominal ultrasound should be obtained if the clinical evaluation suggests gallbladder disease, pancreatitis, or liver disease. Unnecessary radiation exposure should be avoided, but in some cases computed tomographic scan may be necessary to rule out appendicitis, diverticulitis, or other intraabdominal pathology.

Emergency Department Management

If the patient appears clinically dehydrated or when ketonuria is present, infusion of 20 mL/kg (usually 1 to 2 L) of D5-lactated Ringers (D5LR) or D5-normal saline (D5NS) should be performed. If laboratory study results are within normal limits, the goal is to correct the dehydration and ensure the patient is able to tolerate oral intake prior to discharge from the emergency department.

When a patient presents to the emergency department with intractable vomiting and weight loss, and laboratory studies reveal hypokalemia or ketonemia, the criteria are met for the diagnosis of *hyperemesis gravidarum*. Initial intravenous rehydration is started with 3 to 5 L of D5LR or D5NS. Because of the potential, although rare, for the complication of Wernicke encephalopathy in these patients, many advocate giving thiamine either as part of the initial intravenous fluid replacement or before administration of dextrose. The patient's symptoms are the primary end point in initial rehydration, although correction of laboratory abnormalities is also a goal of emergency department management. Antiemetics are often necessary in this circumstance and should be administered intravenously. Please see Chapter 101 ("Drugs in Pregnancy and Lactation") for discussion of the relative safety of the various antiemetics. Phenothiazines, (Phenergan, Compazine), metoclopramide (Reglan), and trimethobenzamide (Tigan) are commonly used in this setting with little apparent risk to the fetus. Additional effective modalities for outpatient management include psychotherapy, hypnotherapy, and behavior modification.

CRITICAL INTERVENTIONS

- Provide aggressive fluid resuscitation for dehydrated patients with hyperemesis gravidarum
- Admit patients with persistent vomiting and/or electrolyte abnormalities and/or ketosis despite resuscitation, or weight loss greater than 10% of the prepregnancy weight

Disposition

Admission criteria for patients with hyperemesis gravidarum include persistent vomiting, electrolyte abnormalities, ketosis despite intravenous fluid resuscitation, or weight loss greater than 10% of the pre-pregnancy weight. Readmission for relapse of hyperemesis gravidarum occurs in about 27% of these patients (13).

The most important discharge instruction one can give, after providing rehydration and excluding more serious causes of their symptoms, is reassurance. Teaching the usual expected events of pregnancy is important for the patient's well-being and decreases the likelihood of return visits to the emergency department. The worst symptoms usually occur in weeks 8 through 12, and resolve by 20 weeks (13,28,29). Although this syndrome is typically called "morning sickness," only 50% of pregnant women experience their symptoms in the morning, whereas one third experience them throughout the day and the remainder have symptoms at night (16). Patients should be advised that the recurrence rate in future pregnancies is 60% (12). They generally are happy to learn that a decreased risk of miscarriage (16,28,29), fetal mortality (20,27), and perinatal mortality (28) has been noted for women with nausea and vomiting during pregnancy. Discharge instructions should include followup with their provider, and patients should be instructed to seek care sooner if symptoms are different or severe, such as persistent dizziness, or inability to keep down anything by mouth. Routine bed rest is not generally recommended.

Other recommendations that have been shown to be safe for treatment of mild-to-moderate nausea and vomiting during pregnancy include acupressure, wrist or "sea bands" (available in boating stores, automobile clubs, and some drug stores), ginger ale or ginger root–containing capsules of 250 mg 4 times a day, and phosphorated carbohydrate (Emetrol), 15 to 30 mL po every 15 minutes as needed (3,10).

COMMON PITFALLS

✔ Failure to consider that the female patient with abdominal pain might be pregnant and having a complication of pregnancy
✔ Failure to consider that the patient with a spontaneous or therapeutic abortion who has a tender uterus on examination may have retained products of conception or endometritis with a septic abortion
✔ Failure to consider that a pregnant patient with excessive nausea and vomiting and a tender abdomen on physical examination may have an intraabdominal surgical emergency

Acknowledgments

Thank you to the previous edition chapter authors Edward Newton and Sean O. Henderson.

References

1. American College of Emergency Physicians Clinical Policies Committee and the Clinical Policies Subcommittee on Early Pregnancy: critical issues in the initial management of patients presenting to the emergency department in early pregnancy. *Ann Emerg Med* 2003;41:123–133.
2. Batemen BG, Nunley WC, Kolp LA, et al. Vaginal sonography findings and hCG dynamics of early intrauterine and tubal pregnancies. *Obstet Gynecol* 1990;75:421–427.
3. Belluomini J, Litt RC, Lee KA, Katz M. Acupressure for nausea and vomiting of pregnancy: A randomized blinded study. *Obstet Gynecol* 1994;84:245.
4. Bennett GL, Bromley B, Lieberman E, Benacerraf BR. Subchorionic hemorrhage in first trimester pregnancies: prediction of pregnancy outcome with sonography. *Radiology* 1996;200:803–806.
5. Cacciatore B, Tittinen A, Stenman U, et al. Normal early pregnancy: serum hCG levels and vaginal ultrasound findings. *Br J Obstet Gynaecol* 1990;97:899–903.
6. Cartwright PS, Victory DF, Moore RA. Performance of a new enzyme-linked immunoassay urine pregnancy test for detection of ectopic gestation. *Ann Emerg Med* 1986;15:1198–1199.
7. Chin RKH. Antenatal complications and perinatal outcome in patients with nausea and vomiting-complicated pregnancy. *Eur J Obstet Gynecol Reprod Biol* 1989;33:215.
8. Dart RG, Kaplan B, Cox C. Transvaginal ultrasound in patients with low B-human chorionic gonadotropin values: how often is the study diagnostic? *Ann Emerg Med* 1997;30:135–140.
9. Everett C. Incidence and outcome of bleeding before the 20th week of pregnancy: prospective study from general practice. *BMJ* 1997;315:32–34.
10. Fischer-Rasmussen W, Kjaer SK, Dahl C, et al. Ginger treatment of hyperemesis gravidarum. *Eur J Obstet Gynecol Reprod Biol* 1990;38:19.
11. Fitzgerald C. Nausea and vomiting in pregnancy. *Br J Med Psychol* 1984;57:159.
12. Gadsby R, Barnie-Adshead AM, Jagger C. A prospective study of nausea and vomiting during pregnancy. *Br J Gen Pract* 1993;43:245.
13. Godsey RK, Newman RB, Hyperemesis gravidarum: a comparison of single and multiple admissions. *J Reprod Med* 1991;36:287.
14. Grant J, Hyslop M. Underutilization of Rh prophylaxis in the emergency department: a retrospective survey. *Ann Emerg Med* 1992;21:104–106.
15. Gratacos E, Torres PJ, Vila J, et al. Screening and treatment of asymptomatic bacteruria in pregnancy prevent pyelonephritis. *J Infect Dis* 1994;169:1390–1392.
16. Jarnfelt A, Samsioe G, Velinder GM. Nausea and vomiting in pregnancy: a contribution to its epidemiology. *Gynecol Obstet Invest* 1983;16:221.
17. Kadar N, Romero, R. Observations on the log human chorionic gonadotropin-time relationship in early pregnancy and its practical implications. *Am J Obstet Gynecol* 1987;157:73–78.
18. Kadar N, Romero R. Further observations on serial chorionic gonadotropin patterns in ectopic pregnancies and spontaneous abortions. *Fertil Steril* 1988;50:367–370.
19. Kauppila A, Huhtaniemi I, Ylikorkala O. Raised serum human chorionic gonadotropin concentrations in hyperemesis gravidarum. *Br Med J* 1979;1:1670.
20. Klebanoff M, Koslowe P, Kaslow R, et al. Epidemiology of vomiting in early pregnancy. *Obstet Gynecol* 1985;66:612.
21. Kuller JA, Laifer SA, Portney DL, Rulin MC. The frequency of transplacental hemorrhage in patients with threatened abortions. *Gynecol Obstet Invest* 1994;37:229–231.
22. Pittaway DE. BhCG dynamics in ectopic pregnancy. *Clin Obstet Gynecol* 1987;30:130–135.
23. Ramoska EA, Sacchetti AD, Nepp M. Reliability of patient history in determining the possibility of pregnancy. *Ann Emerg Med* 1989;18:48–50.
24. Sabin N. Underutilization of Rh prophylaxis in the emergency department [letter]. *Ann Emerg Med* 1993;22:867–868.
25. Soules MR, Hughes CL, Garcia JA, et al. Nausea and vomiting in pregnancy: Role of human chorionic gonadotropin and 17-hydroxyprogesterone. *Obstet Gynecol* 1980;55:696.
26. Swaminathan R, Chin RK, Lao TTH, et al. Thyroid function in hyperemesis gravidarum. *Acta Endocrinol* 1989;120:155.
27. Tierson F, Olsen C, Hook EB. Nausea and vomiting of pregnancy and association with pregnancy outcome. *Am J Obstet Gynecol* 1986;155:1017.
28. Weigel MM, Weigel RM. Nausea and vomiting of early pregnancy and pregnancy outcome: a meta-analytical review. *Br J Obstet Gynecol* 1989;96:1312.
29. Weigel MM, Weigel RM. Nausea and vomiting of early pregnancy and pregnancy outcome: an epidemiological study. *Br J Obstet Gynecol* 1989;96:1304.

CHAPTER 95
Ectopic Pregnancy

G. Richard Braen and Richard S. Krause

One of the leading causes of maternal morbidity and mortality in the United States is ectopic pregnancy. It is also a major factor in decreasing the future fertility of the affected woman and is aptly called an unqualified disaster in human reproduction (11). Fetal wastage is virtually 100%. Unfortunately, the frequency of ectopic pregnancies in the United States has increased by fivefold since 1970 (5). Pooled data indicate that the current incidence of ectopic pregnancy is about 19 per 1,000 pregnancies (2% of all pregnancies in women in the United States will be ectopic) (1,33). Furthermore, it is estimated that of 100 women with a history of ectopic pregnancy, approximately 50% will be infertile, 35% to 40% will subsequently have a successful pregnancy, and 10% to 15% will experience a second ectopic pregnancy (25).

Ectopic pregnancy is the result of implantation of a fertilized ovum at a site other than the endometrium of the uterine cavity. The most frequent site of implantation is the lateral two thirds of the fallopian tube (80%) (Fig. 95.1). About 15% implant in the medial one third. Interstitial or cornual implantation occurs in approximately 3% of ectopic gestations. Interstitial and abdominal implantations carry the greatest risk of mortality because of their hemorrhagic tendencies (12). Extratubal ectopic gestations occur in about 5% of cases: in the ovary (3%), within the abdominal cavity (2%), or in the cervix (rare). Interstitial pregnancies (where the fertilized egg implants in the intrauterine portion of the fallopian tube) occur in less than 3% of tubal pregnancies (23). Combined intrauterine and extrauterine gestations (heterotopic pregnancy) were formerly very rare, with an estimated incidence of one in 30,000 pregnancies (38). Combined pregnancies are now estimated to occur in up to one in 3,000 normal patients and 1 in 100 patients being treated with assisted reproductive technologies (14).

The most common predisposing factors include intrinsic or extrinsic abnormalities of the fallopian tube and abnormal development of the embryo itself. Abnormalities of the fallopian tube have been studied extensively and are believed to be the most important cause of ectopic pregnancies. The most common source of tubal pathology is pelvic inflammatory disease (PID). The risk

of ectopic pregnancy is known to be several times more likely among women with a history of salpingitis (36). All pathogens, including *Chlamydia* and gonococci, are believed to cause tubal distortion and scarring, which adversely affect tubal patency and motility. Subacute infection with less virulent organisms may actually increase the amount of residual tubal pathology because diagnosis and treatment may be delayed (15). Up to 64% of fetuses associated with ectopic pregnancy are abnormal (27). However, it is not known whether these abnormalities cause altered transit through the fallopian tube or whether they result from the poor growth environment of the ectopic implantation site (31).

There are multiple risk factors for developing an ectopic pregnancy. Table 95.1 lists several important population characteristics. The numerical risk assigned to each population characteristic applies to a pregnant woman with that particular characteristic. Table 95.1 is most useful in assessing the relative risk a woman has of harboring an ectopic gestation if she is known to be pregnant. However, up to 42% of women with ectopic pregnancy have no historic risks factors (37).

Age at the time of conception is a relative risk factor for developing an ectopic pregnancy. The percentage of pregnancies that are ectopic increases with maternal age and is threefold greater in the older age group than in the younger (29).

Fourteen percent of all pregnancies in women with an intrauterine device (IUD) are ectopic. The IUD does not prevent ovulation, as does the oral contraceptive, but interferes with intrauterine implantation of the ovum. Therefore, a woman wearing an IUD is potentially at risk for tubal implantation if her ovum becomes fertilized. Additionally, IUD wearers are frequently subjected to delayed diagnosis of ectopic pregnancy (31). Health-care providers may confuse the symptoms caused by an ectopic pregnancy with those related to the mechanical or inflammatory response of an IUD (which indeed may be identical) and fail to consider the possibility of an ectopic gestation in an IUD wearer (16).

Ectopic pregnancy must be considered after tubal sterilization procedures. Sixteen percent of women who become pregnant after tubal sterilization have an ectopic gestation. In most cases, this probably represents partial recanalization with access of the sperm to the ovum but impaired passage of the fertilized ovum to the uterine cavity. Like IUD wearers, patients who have had prior tubal sterilization are frequently subjected to a delay in diagnosis of ectopic gestation. Physicians often neglect to consider this diagnosis early in the presentation.

Women who have had an elective abortion within the preceding 2 weeks and who present with symptoms referable to the genital tract are at risk of having an undiagnosed ectopic pregnancy. Confirmation of the products of uterine extraction is

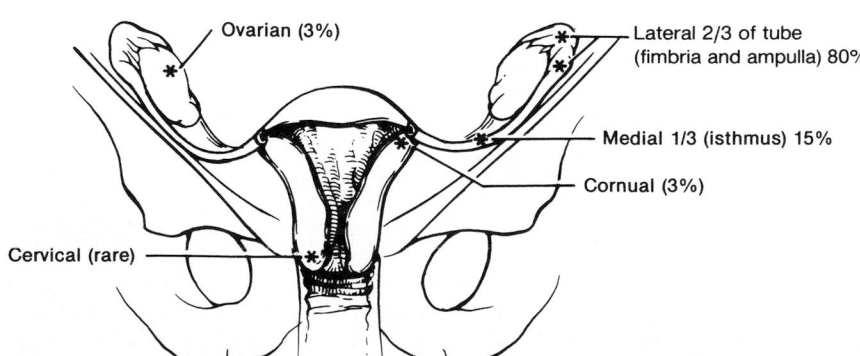

Figure 95.1. Sites of implantation in ectopic pregnancy.

TABLE 95.1. Rates of Ectopic Pregnancy for Various Population Subgroups

Population Characteristic	Ectopic Pregnancies as a Percentage of Total Pregnancies in Each Population Group (%)
Overall	0.94
Age (yr)	
15–19	0.45
20–29	0.82
30–39	1.42
Contraception	
Oral contraceptives	0
Barrier	0.002
IUD	14.0
One or more episodes of salpingitis (by laparoscopy)	6.9
Prior tubal sterilization	16.0
Prior ectopic pregnancy	11.2

IUD, intrauterine device.
(Adapted from Westrom L, Bengtsson L, March PA. Incidence, trends and risks of ectopic pregnancy in a population of women. Br Med J 1981;282:15.)

necessary to exclude the diagnosis of ectopic pregnancy. This is a frequent problem in large urban clinics with a high incidence of therapeutic abortions performed with unreliable followup (32). Although many of the features discussed increase the risk of ectopic pregnancy, no combination of risk factors confirm or exclude the diagnosis with a high degree of certainty (10).

The major life-threatening condition associated with an ectopic pregnancy is intraabdominal hemorrhage with shock. Refractory hemorrhagic shock is the cause of death in approximately 85% of fatalities from ectopic pregnancy (12). Misdiagnosis contributes to one half of the fatalities (12).

CLINICAL PRESENTATION

Any female with lower abdominal pain or vaginal bleeding with a positive pregnancy test should be suspected of having an ectopic pregnancy. The "classic" triad of amenorrhea, vaginal bleeding, and abdominal pain is neither sensitive nor specific for ectopic pregnancy. Of patients with ectopic pregnancies, approximately 15% present with this classic picture, and of patients with the classic constellation of signs and symptoms, only 14% actually have an ectopic gestation (30).

Abdominal pain is the most common symptom and is reported in more than 97% of patients. Abnormal vaginal bleeding is present in 55% to 86% of cases (3,17,26,32). A "normal" menstrual history is obtained in 15% to 30% of patients, and abdominal pain occurs *without* bleeding in up to one third of patients. It should be emphasized that consideration of an ectopic pregnancy is based on a history of abdominal pain and a positive pregnancy test in the first trimester. The quality, character, and location of the pain are highly variable (17). It may be cramping, colicky, steady, or dull. Flank or lower back pain may be noted, or tenesmus may occur from rectal irritation caused by blood in the cul-de-sac (8). The pain may be localized to either lower quadrant or may be generalized, suggesting hemoperitoneum (3,17). Profuse vaginal hemorrhage occurs in the minority of cases and suggests rupture of a cornual implantation (9).

Vital signs are often normal, except in those patients with significant blood loss. This will be manifested by orthostatic hypotension, tachycardia, or frank shock. Paradoxic bradycardia may be seen. Any woman of childbearing age who presents with

signs of hemorrhagic shock without historic or physical evidence of trauma has a ruptured ectopic pregnancy until proved otherwise.

Tenderness on pelvic examination is the most common sign and is present in 83% to 97% of cases (3,17,26,32). The physical findings depend on whether intraperitoneal irritation has occurred from leakage or rupture of the ectopic gestation.

A palpable mass may represent the ectopic gestation or may be felt on the side opposite the ectopic gestation, possibly representing a corpus luteum cyst rather than the ectopic pregnancy (26). Transmigration of the fertilized ovum to the opposite tube is presumed to have occurred in these cases (19).

Patients with ectopic pregnancy are more likely to have moderate-to-severe sharp abdominal pain with abdominal or pelvic tenderness and a small uterus on physical examination. Peritoneal signs are uncommon but highly predictive of ectopic pregnancy.

DIFFERENTIAL DIAGNOSIS

Given the broad spectrum of patient complaints and physical findings, the differential diagnosis of ectopic pregnancy is proportionally broad. The most common pelvic conditions that share clinical aspects of ectopic pregnancy include PID, threatened or incomplete abortion, corpus luteum or follicular cyst, ovarian cyst with a twisted pedicle, endometriosis, gastrointestinal disorders, dysfunctional uterine bleeding, mittelschmerz, and intrauterine pregnancy.

PID is commonly confused with ectopic pregnancy (15). The signs and symptoms may be identical and the same population is at risk. A significant percentage of normal intrauterine pregnancies are associated with pelvic pain and vaginal bleeding in the first trimester, as are almost all cases of nonviable intrauterine pregnancies. Rupture of a corpus luteum cyst of pregnancy is associated with a positive pregnancy test, pain, and a tender pelvic mass—identical symptoms of an ectopic pregnancy. Serous cul-de-sac fluid may help to differentiate the two.

Gastrointestinal disorders to be differentiated include appendicitis, diverticulitis, irritable bowel syndrome, and gastroenteritis. Nephrolithiasis should also be considered.

Patients who merit special consideration are those with a history of PID, tubal ligation or other pelvic surgery, an IUD in place or recently removed, or a recent history of an elective or spontaneous abortion. An especially high risk group includes those undergoing treatment of infertility with embryo transfer procedures or ovulation-inducing agents. These patients are at increased risk of mortality because of the *failure to consider ectopic pregnancy.*

EMERGENCY DEPARTMENT EVALUATION

The evaluation of suspected ectopic pregnancy may be organized into three general categories based on hemodynamic stability (Table 95.2).

The history should emphasize the patient's reproductive past, menstrual history, and risk factors, and a chronologic review of the nature and intensity of the symptoms.

The physical examination should focus on changes associated with normal pregnancy and signs of peritoneal inflammation or significant blood loss. Uterine size, adnexal masses, appearance of cervix and os, and rectal examination should be noted. Serial abdominal examinations may aid in the assessment. A pelvic examination should be repeated only as necessary because of the concern that overly aggressive palpation may precipitate rupture.

TABLE 95.2. Categories for Evaluating Suspected Ectopic Pregnancy Based on Hemodynamic Stability

CATEGORY A

Patients presenting in hypovolemic shock

CATEGORY B

Patients of reproductive age presenting with complaints and physical findings indicative of an acute abdomen but who are hemodynamically stable

CATEGORY C

Patients presenting with abdominopelvic complaints suggestive of an ectopic pregnancy but who are clinically judged to be at low risk of immediate deterioration

Laboratory studies should include a urinalysis and a pregnancy test. For patients in categories A and B (see Table 95.2), a hematocrit and a blood bank specimen are necessary.

Sensitive urine pregnancy tests with a human chorionic gonadotropin (hCG) threshold of 20 mIU/mL should be used as a screening test for possible ectopic gestation. The current generation of urine hCG assays using monoclonally derived, enzyme-tagged antibodies meets this sensitivity requirement. These assays allow detection of pregnancy at 1 week postconception (3 weeks of gestation). Almost all patients with an ectopic pregnancy will have a positive pregnancy test if the threshold for hCG is 20 mIU/mL (6). Up to 1% of ectopic pregnancies will be associated with hCG values of less than 20 mIU/mL (22). The chance for a false-negative result exists when the serum hCG level is low and the urine is dilute (specific gravity less than 1.010) (4). A patient highly suspected of harboring an ectopic gestation with a dilute urine and a negative urine pregnancy test should have a serum β-hCG radioimmunoassay.

Patients in category C (see Table 95.2) may benefit from serial quantitative serum hCG level determinations. Serum β-hCG levels rise exponentially during the first 6 weeks of gestation and peak at approximately 100,000 mIU/mL. A single quantitative serum β-hCG value serves as an objective substitute for a menstrual history (i.e., it dates the pregnancy). This becomes important because one third of patients with an ectopic pregnancy cannot recall the date of their last menstrual period. The irregular bleeding associated with ectopic gestation clouds certainty about the duration of amenorrhea in others. Serial quantitative serum β-hCG levels normally double every 2 days in early normal *intrauterine* pregnancies. Abnormal gestations, both intrauterine and extrauterine, have prolonged doubling times (20). Patients in whom serum β-hCG levels do not increase by more than 66% (1.66-fold increase) in 48 hours are likely to have an abnormal pregnancy and should have further evaluation. Serial serum quantitative β-hCG determinations can be used in stable patients to more accurately detect a nonviable intrauterine or ectopic gestation.

The gestational sac of a normal intrauterine pregnancy becomes visible with transabdominal ultrasonography at 5 to 6 weeks of gestation, corresponding to a quantitative β-hCG of 6,000 to 6,500 mIU/mL (18). With transvaginal sonography, a gestational sac is commonly visualized when the β-hCG level exceeds 1,000 mIU/mL (1).

This level of β-hCG is often referred to as the discriminatory zone (20,21). Intrauterine pregnancy or findings suggestive of an ectopic gestation may be seen with very low β-hCG levels. β-hCG levels should, therefore, not be used as a basis for delaying ultrasonography when ectopic pregnancy is suspected. Ultrasonography results are operator dependent and the technique has a high incidence of nonspecific findings with gestational ages earlier than 5 to 6 weeks. With transvaginal ultrasonography, a gestational sac is identified and localized outside the uterus in about 62% of ectopic pregnancies (37). False-negative and false-positive results occur in up to 25% of patients (7). Although a positive diagnosis of ectopic pregnancy can be made by identifying an extrauterine gestation, in practice, ultrasonography is more helpful in excluding the diagnosis when it demonstrates an intrauterine pregnancy, because simultaneous intrauterine and ectopic gestation is rare.

The correlation of ultrasonographic findings with quantitative serum β-hCG levels increases the accuracy of diagnosis in ectopic pregnancy. This is especially true if the quantitative β-hCG level is above the discriminatory zone (20,21). The absence of a gestational sac with a serum β-hCG titer above the discriminatory zone has a sensitivity of 100%, a specificity of 96%, a positive predictive value of 86%, and a negative predictive value of 100% for the diagnosis of ectopic pregnancy (28). The ultrasonographic absence of an intrauterine sac, with hCG levels below the discriminatory zone, does not allow the definitive diagnosis of an ectopic pregnancy.

In summary, urine hCG testing screens for pregnancy and ultrasonography locates it. A single quantitative serum β-hCG assay is used to date the pregnancy and increase the accuracy of interpreting ultrasonographic results, whereas serial quantitative levels merely tell the clinician whether the pregnancy is behaving in a normal biochemical manner.

Serum progesterone levels are sometimes used to screen for ectopic pregnancies. Only 1% to 2% of cases of ectopic pregnancy will be associated with a progesterone level of greater than 25 ng/mL, and only 0.16% of viable pregnancies will be associated with levels less than 5 ng/mL. Thus, if the progesterone level is abnormally low, and the hCG levels are abnormally or erratically rising, a nonviable pregnancy (possibly ectopic) should be suspected. In emergency department practice, progesterone levels are generally not available, but some patients who come to the emergency department may have had levels determined in an outpatient setting. If these levels are available to the emergency physician, the appropriate diagnosis may be made (24).

Because pregnancy can be biochemically detected at approximately 1 week of gestation but may not be located reliably with ultrasonography until 5 to 6 weeks of gestation, a 4- to 5-week period of uncertainty exists. During this period, a pregnancy can be detected but often cannot be located by noninvasive means. Laparoscopy performed on all patients in the period of uncertainty results in a high incidence of unnecessary diagnostic laparoscopies for normal intrauterine pregnancies (30). Therefore, patients in category C (see Table 95.2) during the period of uncertainty, who are stable and reliable, are best evaluated by serial serum quantitative β-hCG levels, provided that an initial sonogram is nondiagnostic. Failure of β-hCG levels to increase normally suggests an ectopic or other abnormal pregnancy.

Culdocentesis is a simple, rapid, and accurate method of detecting intraperitoneal blood. It may be used when ultrasonography is not immediately available or when ultrasonography results are equivocal. A positive test is one in which nonclotting blood is aspirated from the cul-de-sac with a hematocrit higher than 15%. A "dry tap" is nondiagnostic. A negative tap occurs when clear fluid is obtained. Patients in categories B and C may benefit from either ultrasonography or culdocentesis. However, if either modality delays operative intervention in category A patients, it should not be used, because findings will not alter management, but delay treatment (2,13).

EMERGENCY DEPARTMENT MANAGEMENT

Management is guided by the patient's hemodynamic status, reliability for followup, and the availability of ultrasonography (Fig. 95.2) (37). *Patients in category A* should be treated for hemorrhagic shock: The patient should be placed in the Trendelenburg position and administered high-flow oxygen by nonrebreather mask. Large-bore peripheral venous access should be established and crystalloid infusion begun. Baseline blood samples should be obtained in addition to a clot tube for the blood bank. Transfusion with O-negative, type-specific, or fully crossmatched blood should be considered after crystalloid infusion, depending on the urgency and the response to initial therapy. Immediate gynecologic consultation for laparotomy should be obtained.

Patients in category B are stable but have potential for rapid progression to category A. Anticipation of fluid resuscitation and rapid confirmation of the diagnosis dictate the course of evaluation and management. Large-bore venous access should be established. Baseline blood studies include complete blood cell count, Rh typing, and typing and screening for potential blood replacement. A sensitive urine pregnancy test must also be performed. Ultrasonography should be used if immediately available. Culdocentesis may be used if ultrasonography results are nondiagnostic or if ultrasonography is not available. Patients in category B, by definition, have an acute abdomen, and therefore warrant urgent consultation.

Patients in categories A and B present few problems in evaluation and management. *Patients in category C,* who are stable and ambulatory, pose the greatest diagnostic and management problems. Figure 95.2 provides a useful management scheme. The evaluation of a possible ectopic pregnancy starts with a urine pregnancy test for *all* women of childbearing age who present with abdominopelvic pain. The *only exception* is the woman who

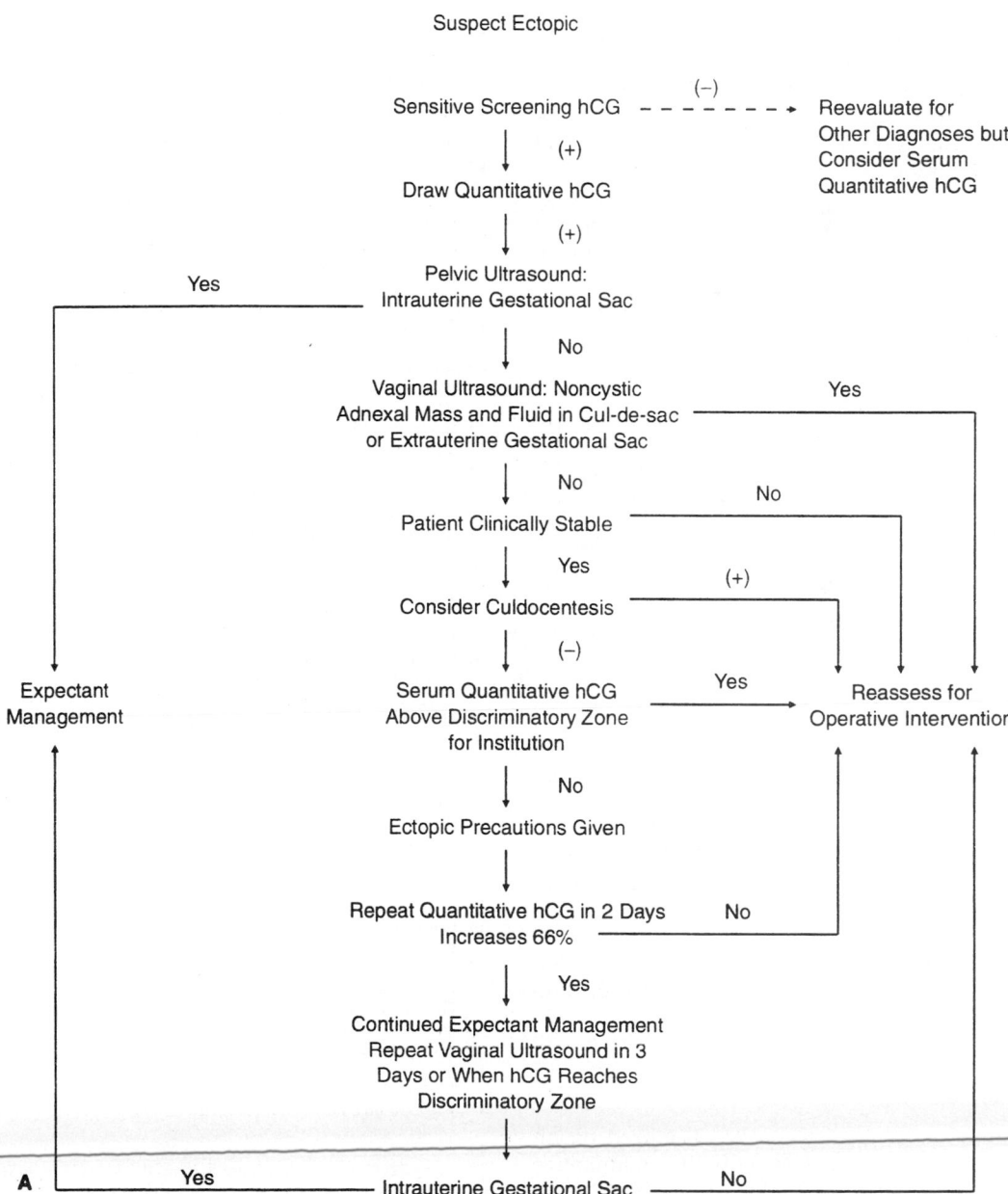

Figure 95.2. Algorithm for evaluation and management of suspected ectopic pregnancy. (Adapted from [Wolcott HD, Stock RJ, Kaunitz AM. Ectopic pregnancy. In: Benrubi G, ed. *Obstetric and gynecologic emergencies.* Philadelphia: JB Lippincott Co, 1994], with permission.)

has had a hysterectomy. The presence of an IUD, tubal ligation, a partner with a vasectomy, or incidental trauma should not deter consideration of an ectopic pregnancy. The diagnosis should be pursued until reasonably eliminated.

Medical Therapy for Unruptured Ectopic Pregnancies

Selected patients with unruptured ectopic pregnancies may be treated nonsurgically by the gynecologist. Methotrexate may be used for these cases when given orally, intramuscularly, or intravenously, along with leucovorin rescue to prevent toxicity to bone marrow. Regimens exist that include single-dose methotrexate/leucovorin with minimal toxicity to the patient.

Patients treated medically for ectopic pregnancy may experience abdominal pain 3 to 7 days after treatment. This is thought to be secondary to methotrexate-induced tubal abortion. It may be difficult to differentiate expected pain from pain due to rupture of a persistent ectopic pregnancy. Patients presenting with abdominal pain in this timeframe following methotrexate administration should have a complete blood count and ultrasound to rule out significant free fluid in the cul-de-sac, and should be evaluated for other causes of abdominal pain. The patient may need consultation and/or admission to the hospital for observation. Hemodynamic instability and/or falling hematocrit would require surgical intervention.

Stable patients with an ectopic pregnancy and no cardiac activity on ultrasound may be followed with serial examination and repeat quantitative β-hCG levels. If the levels continue to fall, no invasive interventions may be necessary. In addition to the repeat β-hCG levels, repeat transvaginal ultrasonic scanning should be considered to ensure reabsorption of the embryo (3).

CRITICAL INTERVENTIONS

- Obtain immediate gynecologic or surgical consultation in patients who are in shock and who have a positive pregnancy test
- Initiate resuscitation with fluids and/or blood as appropriate

DISPOSITION

Given the broad spectrum of presentations and the lack of pathognomonic findings in suspected ectopic pregnancy, there should be a low threshold for requesting consultation from the gynecology, radiology, and surgery services. Consultation should be obtained for patients in category A or B. Early notification of consulting services may allow early mobilization of operating room personnel. The timing for consultation in category C patients is more flexible and dependent on results of emergency department testing, local resources, consultant availability, and whether the patient has a previously established relationship with a gynecologist.

All patients in categories A and B require admission. Category C patients may be discharged with gynecologic followup in 48 hours, except in the following instances:

- When no intrauterine pregnancy can be visualized on ultrasonography in a symptomatic patient with a quantitative serum β-hCG level above the discriminatory zone
- Progressive symptomatology or physical findings
- Patients unreliable for followup
- Positive ultrasound or culdocentesis for blood

The usual timing of followup is 48 hours, the standard sampling interval for quantitative serum β-hCG levels. Most outpatients will be evaluated by this method. A system should be in place to followup on serial hCG levels or on the products of uterine extraction in women who have undergone uterine evacuation procedures in the emergency department for suspected incomplete abortion. If the pathology report shows "no chorionic villi," ectopic pregnancy is the likely diagnosis and the patient should be followed by an obstetrician/gynecologist for further evaluation.

In general, patients should be transferred only if there is no operating facility and an ectopic pregnancy has been diagnosed or if an ectopic pregnancy is strongly suspected but diagnostic resources are unavailable. Stable patients and patients in hypovolemic shock who undergo successful volume resuscitation may be transferred with appropriate personnel.

COMMON PITFALLS

✔ The most common pitfall is failure to consider the diagnosis of ectopic pregnancy, especially in women with few symptoms
✔ In making a diagnostic decision, clinical findings consistent with ectopic pregnancy should outweigh any single negative test result
✔ Delays have been documented in cases that involve women who have undergone tubal sterilization, women with an IUD in place or recently removed, and women who have undergone a recent spontaneous or therapeutic abortion. Ectopic pregnancy does occur in these groups and must be ruled out

References

1. American College of Emergency Physicians. Clinical policy: critical issues in the initial evaluation and management of patients presenting to the emergency department in early pregnancy. *Ann Emerg Med* 2003;41:123.
2. Braen GR. Culdocentesis. In: Roberts JR, Hedges JR, eds. Clinical procedures in emergency medicine, 4th edition. Philadelphia: WB Saunders, 2004:1144–1150.
3. Carson SA, Buster JE. Ectopic pregnancy. *N Engl J Med* 1993;329:1174.
4. Cartwright PS. Performance of a new enzyme linked immunoassay for the detection of ectopic gestation. *Ann Emerg Med* 1986;15:1198.
5. Centers for Disease Control. Ectopic pregnancy surveillance, United States, 1970–1987. *MMWR Morb Mortal Wkly Rep* 1988;39:9.
6. Christensen H, Thyssen H, Schebye O, et al. Three highly sensitive "bedside" serum and urine tests for pregnancy compared. *Clin Chem* 1990;36:1686.
7. Chinn DH, Callen PW. Ultrasound of the acutely ill obstetrics and gynecology patient. *Radiol Clin North Am* 1983;21:585.
8. Cohen AW, ed. *Emergencies in obstetrics and gynecology.* New York: Churchill Livingstone, 1981.
9. Curran JW. Economic consequences of pelvic inflammatory disease in the United States. *Am J Obstet Gynecol* 1980;138:848.
10. Dart R, Kaplan B, Varaklis K. Predictive value of history and physical examination in patients with suspected ectopic pregnancy. *Ann Emerg Med* 1999;283–290.
11. DeCherney AH. Ectopic pregnancy. In: Kase NG, Weingold AB, eds. *Principles and practice of clinical gynecology.* Vol. 2. New York: John Wiley and Sons, 1983:483.
12. Dorfman SF, Grimes DA, Cates W, et al. Ectopic pregnancy mortality, United States, 1979 to 1980: clinical aspects. *Obstet Gynecol* 1984;64:386.
13. Eisinger SH. Culdocentesis. *J Fam Pract* 1981;13:95.
14. Gamberoella FR, Marrs RP. Heterotopic pregnancy associated with assisted reproductive technology. *Am J Obstet Gynecol* 1999;160:1520–1523.
15. Gonzalez FA, Waxman M. Ectopic pregnancy: a prospective study on differential diagnosis. *Diagn Gynecol Obstet* 1981;3:101.
16. Gump DW, Gibson M, Ashikaya T. Evidence of prior pelvic inflammatory disease and its relationship to *Chlamydia trachomatis* antibody and intrauterine contraceptive device use in infertile women. *Am J Obstet Gynecol* 1983;146:153.
17. Helvancioglu A, Long EM, Yang SL. Ectopic pregnancy, an eight-year review. *J Reprod Med* 1979;22:87.
18. Hill LM, Breckle R, Wolfgram KR. An ultrasonic view of the developing fetus. *Obstet Gynecol Surv* 1983;38:375.
19. Iffy L, Gasser RF. Tubal pregnancy. *Obstet Gynecol* 1976;47:380.
20. Kadar N, Caldwell B, Romero R. A method of screening for ectopic pregnancy and its indications. *Obstet Gynecol* 1980;58:162.
21. Kadar N, Devore G, Romero R. Discriminatory HCG zone: its use in the sonographic evaluation for ectopic pregnancy. *Obstet Gynecol* 1981;58:156.
22. Kalinski MA, Guss DA. Hemorrhagic shock from a ruptured ectopic pregnancy in a patient with a negative urine pregnancy result. *Ann Emerg Med* 2002;40:102.

23. Kim SW, Ha YR, Chung SP. Ruptured interstitial pregnancy presenting with negative β-hCG and hypovolemic shock. *Am J Emerg Med* 2003;21:511.

24. Lipscomb GH, Stovall TG, Ling FW. Primary care: nonsurgical treatment of ectopic pregnancy. *N Engl J Med* 2000;343:1325.

25. Metha L, Young ID. Recurrence risk for common complications of pregnancy—a review. *Obstet Gynecol Surv* 1987;42:218.

26. Pagano R. Ectopic pregnancy: a seven year survey. *Med J Aust* 1981;2:586.

27. Poland BJ, Dill FJ, Stylbo C. Embryonic development in ectopic human pregnancy. *Teratology* 1976;14:315.

28. Romero R, Kadar N, Jeanty P, et al. The value of the discriminatory HCG zone in the diagnosis of ectopic pregnancy. *Obstet Gynecol* 1985;66:357.

29. Rubin GL, Peterson HB, Dorfman SF, et al. Ectopic pregnancy in the United States, 1970 through 1978. *JAMA* 1983;249:1725.

30. Schwartz RO, DiPietro DL. Beta HCG as a diagnostic aid for suspected ectopic pregnancy. *Obstet Gynecol* 1980;56:197.

31. Scott J, DiSaia PJ, Hammond C, et al., eds. *Danforth's obstetrics and gynecology*, 7th ed. Philadelphia: JB Lippincott Co, 1994.

32. Tancer ML, Delke I, Veridiano NP. A fifteen year experience with ectopic pregnancy. *Surg Gynecol Obstet* 1981;152:179.

33. Tulandi T, Sammour A. Evidence-based management of ectopic pregnancy. *Curr Opin Obstet Gynecol* 2000;12:289.

34. Westrom L, Bengtsson L, Mardh PA. Incidence, trends and risks of ectopic pregnancy in a population of women. *Br Med J* 1981;282:15.

35. Wolcott HD, Stock RJ, Kaunitz AM. Ectopic pregnancy. In: Benrubi G, ed. *Obstetric and gynecologic emergencies*. Philadelphia: JB Lippincott Co, 1994.

36. Yaghoobian J, Pinck RL, Ramanathan K, et al. Sonographic demonstration of simultaneous intrauterine and extrauterine gestation. *J Ultrasound Med* 1986;5:309.

CHAPTER 96
Complications of Induced Abortion

Lynne McCullough

Following the *Roe v. Wade* decision in 1973, legalized abortions have become one of the most frequently performed surgical procedures in the United States and one of the most prevalent means of fertility control worldwide (8). Since 1990, the number of abortions performed in the United States has declined each year. In 2000, 1.3 million were reported, most within the first trimester, with an overall complication rate of 1 in 100 (4,7). Although the rate of complications increases with advanced gestational age, serious complications are rare at any age.

CLINICAL PRESENTATION

Complications after an induced abortion may be divided into (1) early (immediate, or within 3 hours of the procedure), (2) delayed (after 3 hours to 28 days), and (3) late (more than 28 days after the procedure). Following elective termination of pregnancy, patients may present to the emergency department (ED) complaining of pain, bleeding, or fever. The degree of discomfort, height of the fever, amount and quality of the bleeding, as well as the patient's past medical history are all relevant to the differential diagnosis.

The most commonly encountered complications of induced abortion are delayed: presenting within the first few days following the procedure. Infection is the most common, occurring in 0.1% to 12% of all patients undergoing elective pregnancy termination (1,14). If symptoms occur within 2 to 3 days of the procedure, approximately 70% have retained products of conception (POC) and secondary infection (4). Because infection is the most common complication of abortion worldwide, it is prudent to maintain a high index of suspicion and expedite the administration of antibiotics to avoid complications such as sepsis, or later onset of chronic pelvic pain, dyspareunia, and infertility. Risk factors for infection include age younger than 20 years, previous pelvic inflammatory disease, presence of a pathogen in the cervix at the time of the surgical abortion and nulliparous status (16). However, it is important to note that most infections occur in women with no risk factors for disease (14).

Mild bleeding is to be expected following an induced surgical or medical abortion, but persistent or heavy bleeding is unusual and most commonly a result of retained products of conception (4). Incomplete or failed abortion, as well as missed ectopic pregnancy can also present with pain, bleeding, and/or fever.

Less commonly, patients can present immediately after an abortion procedure with a number of complications, such as uterine perforation, persistent or delayed hemorrhage secondary to uterine atony (more common in multiparous patients), retained products of conception (POCs), previously undiagnosed coagulopathy, cervical lacerations, anesthesia complications, amniotic fluid or pulmonary embolism, as well as disseminated intravascular coagulopathy (DIC) (3).

Late complications such as cervical stenosis and "*Asherman syndrome*," the development of intrauterine adhesions in addition to cervical stenosis, may present to the ED as persistent amenorrhea associated with increasing abdominal distention and cyclical pelvic pain (14). These late complications are relatively uncommon and do not represent true emergencies to be managed in the ED.

DIFFERENTIAL DIAGNOSIS

Because the most common chief complaints include abdominal pain, pelvic pain, vaginal bleeding, and fever, the differential is broad. Symptoms may be related or unrelated to the recent termination procedure. Postprocedural complications include disorders such as uterine perforation, uterine atony, retained products of conception, trauma, undiagnosed ectopic pregnancy, endometritis, peritonitis, delayed hemorrhage, and cervical stenosis.

Uterine perforation occurs in 1 in 1,000 to 1 in 10,000 first trimester procedures, and 3 in 100 to 8 in 100 of those performed in the second trimester. It is likely under diagnosed at the time of the surgical procedure and a rare cause of serious sequelae (9–11). Patients may present with complaints of abdominal pain, referred scapular pain, symptoms consistent with bowel obstruction secondary to entrapped mesentery in the perforation, low-grade temperature, rectal pressure, and excessive or persistent vaginal bleeding.

Cervical laceration is a relatively common complication (1 in 100) that is rarely serious (10).

Disseminated intravascular coagulopathy is the most likely form of coagulopathy in the previously healthy patient in this setting. DIC is more common in second trimester abortions, and in cases of prolonged intrauterine demise and in cases of massive blood loss (4,14).

Incomplete abortion with retained POC is a relatively common complication of suction evacuation (0.03% to 0.5% of first trimester abortions) that is characterized by a slightly tender or enlarged uterus in the setting of excessive bleeding (10,12). This condition should also be considered when heavy bleeding is unresponsive to uterotonic agents.

Acute hematometra/"postabortal syndrome" occurs most commonly in late first trimester or early second trimester abortions (11 to 14 weeks). The overall incidence is less than 5 in 1,000 cases (4,10). Patients typically complain of rapid onset of lower pelvic pain, not associated with increased bleeding or unstable vital signs. They may complain of intermittent expulsion of maroon clots with pelvic pressure and low-grade temperature.

Endometritis has an incidence of 0.46%, and sepsis was identified in 0.028% of patients (10). Infections are typically polymicrobial, including Gram-positive and Gram-negative anaerobes, facultative or obligate anaerobes, *Neisseria gonorrhoeae* and *Chlamydia trachomatis* (17). *Endomyoparametritis* defines spread of the intrauterine infection to the myometrium and or parametrial structures (i.e., the fallopian tubes; the round, uterosacral, and broad ligaments; and the peritoneum covering those structures). Patients will complain of the postabortal triad of symptoms (pain, bleeding, and fever); foul-smelling discharge may be identified and leukocytosis is common.

Septic pelvic thrombophlebitis "right ovarian vein syndrome" occurs in approximately 1 in 10,000 pregnancies, typically from the late first trimester onward and is the result of progression of endomyoparametritis (5). It can also be secondary to damage to the pelvic venous system during surgical abortion leading to the development of a thrombus that becomes secondarily infected.

Similar symptoms of pain, bleeding, and fever may be produced by disorders unrelated to the procedure, such as appendicitis, pyelonephritis, pelvic inflammatory disease, endometriosis, menses, and ovarian cyst rupture.

EMERGENCY DEPARTMENT EVALUATION

Patients who have recently undergone either medical or surgical termination of their pregnancy who present to the emergency department must be rapidly evaluated according to their chief complaint. A focused medical history should be taken to include the number of prior pregnancies; the estimated gestational age of the fetus at the time of the termination; the date, time, and method of the abortion; any prior history of pelvic infection or known coagulopathy; the patient's Rh status; the results of any pre-procedure evaluation as well as any known complications that may have occurred during or immediately following the procedure.

For those patients complaining of significant or increased bleeding with signs of hemorrhagic or septic shock such as tachycardia and hypotension, one to two intravenous (i.v.) lines should be established with normal saline boluses initiated, and blood should be sent for complete blood count. If the bleeding is brisk, signs of shock are present, or a coagulopathy is known, a type and screen or cross should be performed during the initial evaluation. The evaluation of suspected DIC includes checking platelet and fibrinogen levels, prothrombin time/partial thromboplastin time (PT/PTT), and fibrin degradation products. Febrile patients should have blood cultures obtained as well. A quantitative β-hCG level may be helpful in the event that a missed ectopic or failed abortion is in the differential and values from the patient's clinician can be obtained for comparison.

While supportive measures are instituted, the patient should be evaluated according to the chief complaint. The most common presenting complaints include pelvic and/or abdominal pain, increased or excessive bleeding, and fever. A focused physical examination must include a complete pelvic evaluation, including direct visualization with a vaginal speculum and bimanual palpation. Pelvic examination may reveal the source of mechanically induced bleeding, as from a cervical laceration or retained POCs in the cervical os. It also may reveal the source of pain and fever. The presence of a nonfirm, boggy uterus suggests uterine atony. A tender uterus may be consistent with either retained products, continued bleeding into the uterus, or the development of endometritis. Pelvic ultrasound is a very useful adjunct in the evaluation of postabortive patients in the emergency department and can demonstrate retained POCs, uterine abnormalities, which may have led to an incomplete evacuation of the uterus (i.e., an accessory uterine horn or septum), the presence of hemoperitoneum or an unexpected ectopic gestation. A quantitative β-hCG level may also be helpful in diagnosing ectopic pregnancy by demonstrating a persistent level despite anticipated termination of the pregnancy. The β-hCG levels should fall 66% within 48 hours of the abortion procedure, but may decline much more slowly over the next several weeks (14).

EMERGENCY DEPARTMENT MANAGEMENT

The cause of excessive bleeding can usually be identified by visualization of the cervix on vaginal speculum examination or with bimanual palpation. While evaluating a patient for the potential cause of excessive bleeding, consider uterine tamponade with a Foley catheter balloon, the use of uterotonic agents, and the possibility of pelvic vessel embolization for persistent excessive bleeding (2).

Uterine atony, characterized by a soft, nontender uterus and a steady trickle of blood from the cervix, should be treated with manual uterine massage, intramuscular, intravenous or intracervical uterotonic agents (see Table 96.1) (4,14,18).

Uterine perforation should be treated empirically with antibiotics when this diagnosis is being considered (see Table 96.2), and prompt gynecologic consultation should be obtained. Diagnosis and definitive management are accomplished with explorative laparoscopy and laparotomy when indicated.

*Cervical laceration*s are usually minor injuries, with bleeding that can be controlled by the topical application of silver nitrate. If more significant lacerations are identified, they can be repaired in the emergency department with 0-chromic catgut on a CT-1 needle in most cases (4).

TABLE 96.1.   Uterotonic Agents to be Used Sequentially

Methylergonovine maleate (Methergine)	0.2 mg i.m., may repeat and continue oral treatment with 0.2 mg t.i.d. for 3 days
Oxytocin[1]	10 U i.v. bolus or 10 U i.m., consider 40 U in 1,000 mL normal saline to infuse at a rate necessary to control bleeding for persistent and severe hemorrhage[2]
Vasopressin	2.5-4.0 units injected directly into the cervix
Misoprostol	400 μg orally
Carboprost tromethamine 15(s)-methyl PGF2α	200 μg /10 mL saline in a transvaginal intrauterine injection or 250 μg i.m.

[1]Can be given i.m. or i.v. The number of oxytoxin receptors in the uterus rises throughout pregnancy; therefore, a diminished response may be seen in first trimester of pregnancy.

[2]Water intoxication can be seen secondary to the mild antidiuretic properties of oxytocin.

(*Adapted from Stubblefield P, Borgatta L. Complications of induced abortion. In: Pearlman M, Tintinalli J, Dyne P, ed.* Obstetric & gynecologic emergencies. *New York: McGraw-Hill, 2003:65–86.*)

TABLE 96.2.   Antibiotic Regimens for Postabortal Infectious Complications

Uterine perforation (suspected or proven)	Doxycycline 100 mg po (if nonsurgical management) and cefoxitin 1g i.v. before laparotomy[1]
Endometrial infection, mild, oral regimen	Doxycycline 100 mg b.i.d. for 10 days with metronidazole 500 mg t.i.d. for 7 days; amoxicillin and clavulonic acid 500 mg t.i.d. for 7 days[2]
Ascending infection, abscess or sepsis, i.v. regimen indicated	Cefoxitin 2 g q.i.d. or cefotetan 2–3 g with doxycycline 100 mg b.i.d. or clindamycin 600 mg q.i.d.[3] or clindamycin 600 mg/gentamicin 3–5 mg/kg/day[4]

[1–3]Darney PD, Horbach NS, Korn AP. First-trimester abortion. In: *Protocols for office gynecologic surgery.* Massachusetts: Blackwell Science; 158–193.

[4]Reed SD, Landers DV, Sweet RL. Antibiotic treatment of tuboovarian abscess: comparison of broad-spectrum beta-lactam agents versus clindamycin-containing regimens. *Am J Obstet Gynecol* 1991;164:1556–1562.

The treatment of *DIC* includes fluid volume and clotting factor replacement with fresh-frozen plasma (FFP), cryoprecipitate, and in severe cases, packed red blood cells (RBCs). Most important is the attempt to identify and treat any stimulus of DIC, such as retained POCs or infection. Frequent monitoring of coagulation parameters is also indicated. Each unit of FFP (200 to 250 mL) raises fibrinogen levels 25 mg/dL. In early DIC, 4 to 8 units of FFP is usually adequate to restore clotting function (14).

Incomplete abortion with retained POCs is usually treated with dilation and curettage. However, if POCs are identified in the cervical os on speculum examination, they should be removed immediately to reduce the incidence of continued bleeding.

Acute hematometra/"postabortal syndrome" should be treated with prompt suction and evacuation of the uterus, which leads to symptom resolution. A low-grade temperature does not typically indicate infection, and it resolves following reevacuation (14).

Endometritis should be treated with uterine evacuation if retained POCs are suspected, and outpatient antibiotic regimens for PID are appropriate for mild-to-moderate postabortal endometritis (6,17). If there is no improvement or worsening following 2 to 3 days of outpatient therapy, the patient should be admitted for parenteral treatment (14). *Endomyoparametritis* requires parenteral antibiotics, as serious complications such as bacteremia may occur in 5% to 10% of these infections, abscesses may form and the patient may develop a sepsis syndrome (6). In patients presenting with high fever, tachycardia, marked tenderness to palpation, and leukocytosis, a pelvic ultrasound should be performed to evaluate for an abscess (6).

Septic pelvic thrombophlebitis "right ovarian vein syndrome" may be diagnosed by computed tomography or magnetic resonance imaging, as well as by prompt clinical improvement following empiric heparin for patients with septic abortion who are unresponsive to parenteral antibiotic therapy (5,13).

CRITICAL INTERVENTIONS

- Stop any sources of continued bleeding that are accessible to direct pressure or tamponade
- Obtain immediate gynecologic or surgical consultation for patients with persistent bleeding or suspected uterine perforation
- Administer parenteral antibiotics to patients with suspected endomyoparametritis

DISPOSITION

Patients who present complaining of postabortal bleeding can be safely discharged home following an evaluation that demonstrates hemodynamic stability and if the possibility of ectopic pregnancy or retained POCs have been ruled out as the cause. These patients should be reevaluated for persistent bleeding and return to the emergency department for increased bleeding, signs of shock, or the development of fever or increased discomfort. For patients who require uterotonic agents to assist a poorly responsive uterus, cervical repair of a laceration, or in whom a uterine perforation is suspected, gynecologic consultation should be obtained and close followup arranged if the patient is stabilized for disposition to home.

In cases of fever and pelvic pain when the infection is limited to the endometrium, the patient may be discharged on oral antibiotics as listed in Table 96.2. Close followup should be arranged and precautions to return to the emergency department or their doctor should include nonresolution of symptoms in 48 to 72 hours or worsening pain, increased fever, or other systemic signs of illness such as vomiting or lightheadedness. When the infection is found to ascend beyond the endometrium, or when septic symptoms are present, emergent gynecologic evaluation should be obtained in the emergency department following the administration of antibiotics as listed in Table 96.2. These patients must be hospitalized to the level of care warranted by their clinical presentation.

Emergent gynecologic consultation should also be obtained in the following clinical settings: when products of conception are identified in the setting of postabortal bleeding or when infection is present; when the patient presents with DIC; when vaginal bleeding is unresponsive to uterotonic agents; when uterine perforation is suspected; or when an ectopic pregnancy is identified.

COMMON PITFALLS

✔ Failure to identify retained products of conception by using ultrasound in the postabortal patient. This can result in the development of serious infection and uncontrollable bleeding
✔ Failure to identify a failed abortion (i.e., an intact gestation) and providing medications that may be toxic to the developing fetus
✔ Discharge of a patient without considering an ectopic gestation that was unaffected by endometrial dilation and curettage
✔ Inadequate examination of the intravaginal structures to rule out cervical laceration as the source of bleeding
✔ Not assessing and treating the Rh-negative patient with RhoGAM if they have not received treatment in the previous 3 weeks

Acknowledgments

Thank you to previous edition chapter authors James L. Jones and Andrew M. Kaunitz.

References

1. Barclay ML. Septic abortion. In: Sciarra JJ, Watkins TJ, eds. *Gynecology & obstetrics,* volume 2. Philadelphia: Lippincott-Raven, 1997:1–5.
2. Borgatta L, Chen AY, Reid SK, et al. Pelvic embolization for treatment of hemorrhage related to spontaneous and induced abortion. *Am J Obstet Gynecol* 2001;185:530–536.
3. Castadot RG. Pregnancy termination: techniques, risks, and complications and their management. In: Wallach EE, ed. *Modern trends: fertility and sterility,* volume 45. USA: The American Fertility Society, 1986.5–17.
4. Darney PD, Horbach NS, Korn Ap. First-trimester elective abortion. In: *Protocols for office gynecologic survey.* Massachusetts: Blackwell Science, 1996:158–193.

5. Faro S. Septic pelvic vein thrombophlebitis. In: Stenchever MA, ed. *Current topics in obstetrics & gynecology, infections and abortion.* New York: Elsevier, 1992:61–72.

6. Faro S. Treatment of Septic Abortion. In: Stenchever MA, ed. *Current topics in obstetrics & gynecology, infections and abortion.* New York: Elsevier, 1992:73–89.

7. Finer LB, Henshaw SK. Abortion incidence and services in the United States in 2000. *Perspect Sex Reprod Health* 2003;35:6–15.

8. Grimes DA, Cates W. Complications from legally induced abortion: a review. *Obstet Gynecol Surv* 1979;34:177–191.

9. Grimes DA. Sequelae of abortion. In: Baird DT, ed. *Modern methods of inducing abortion.* Oxford: Blackwell Science, 1995:95–111.

10. Hakim-Elahi E, Tovell HMM, Burnhill MS. Complications of first-trimester abortion: a report of 170,000 cases. *Obstet Gynecol* 1990;76:129–135.

11. Kaali SG, Szigetvari IA, Bartfai GS. The frequency and management of uterine perforations during first-trimester abortions. *Am J Obstet Gynecol* 1989;161:406–408.

12. Kaunitz AM, Rovira EZ, Grimes DA, Schultz KF. Abortions that fail. *Obstet Gynecol* 1985;66:533–537.

13. Ledger WJ, Peterson EP. The use of heparin in the management of pelvic thrombophlebitis. *Surg Gynecol Obstet* 1970;1115–1121.

14. Lichtenberg ES, Grimes DA, Paul M. Abortion complications, prevention and management. In: Paul M, Lichtenberg ES, Borgatta L, et al., eds. *A clinician's guide to medical and surgical abortion.* New York: Churchill Livingstone, 1999:197–216.

15. Reed SD, Landers DV, Sweet RL. Antibiotic treatment of tuboovarian abscess: comparison of broad-spectrum beta-lactam agents versus clindamycin-containing regimens. *Am J Obstet Gynecol* 1991;164:1556–1562.

16. Sawaya GF, Grady D, Kerlikowske K, Grimes DA. Antibiotics at the time of induced abortion: the case for universal prophylaxis based on a metaanalysis. *Obstet Gynecol* 1996;87:884–890.

17. Stubblefield PG, Grimes DA. Septic abortion. *N Engl J Med* 1994;331:310–314.

18. Stubblefield P, Borgatta L. Complications of induced abortion. In: Pearlman M, Tintinalli J, Dyne P, eds. *Obstet Gynecol Emerg* New York: McGraw-Hill, 2003:65–86.

CHAPTER 97
Hypertensive Disorders of Pregnancy

Jan Marie Shoenberger and Sean O. Henderson

High blood pressure (BP) complicates 8% to 10% of all pregnancies, 20% of pregnancies in young nulliparas, and 40% to 50% of the pregnancies of women carrying twins (15). Preeclampsia, a hypertensive disorder characterized by vasospasm and coagulation abnormalities, is a leading cause of fetal and maternal morbidity and death, one that increased 40% from 1991 to 1999 (23). This dramatic increase has been attributed to a higher number of multifetal gestations (secondary to in vitro fertilization techniques) and a higher number of older mothers with a higher baseline prevalence of chronic hypertension (16). Eclampsia, the most severe form of hypertension in pregnancy, occurs in approximately one in 2000 (0.05% to 0.2%) deliveries, and the incidence is higher in women who have not received appropriate prenatal care (2,13).

Historically, maternal mortality from eclampsia ranges from 1% to 20% of all deliveries, although most current reports place mortality at approximately 5% (22). In such severe forms of preeclampsia/eclampsia, intracerebral hemorrhage has been identified as the final event in more than 50% of the patients who die. The mother is also at risk from the repeated seizure activity, which may lead to aspiration pneumonia, pulmonary edema, acute renal failure, or hypoxemia and acidemia (22). Abruptio placentae and subsequent maternal disseminated intravascular coagulopathy (DIC) may also be present. Finally, cardiovascular collapse may occur from overaggressive treatment or massive intracerebral hemorrhage.

The effects on the fetus are similarly dramatic. Combined with the compromised uteroplacental perfusion caused by the characteristic vasospasm, the effects of multiple convulsions result in 10% to 28% fetal mortality (2).

Causes of hypertension in pregnancy are multiple. The recently published report of the Working Group on Research on Hypertension During Pregnancy (16) has categorized hypertension during pregnancy as follows:

1. Preeclampsia/eclampsia
2. Gestational or transient hypertension
3. The continued presence of chronic hypertension
4. Superimposed preeclampsia on chronic hypertension

Hypertension is defined as a systolic blood pressure (SBP) of ≥140 mm Hg or a diastolic blood pressure (DBP) of ≥90 mm Hg and *preeclampsia* is present when hypertension is combined with proteinuria exceeding 0.3 g per 24 hour. Because edema is a nonspecific finding, it is no longer included in the diagnostic criteria. Neither is the previous criteria of an increase of 30/15 mm Hg over baseline included in this most recent definition.

PATHOPHYSIOLOGY

The pathophysiology of preeclampsia/eclampsia is unclear. Several theories have been proposed, most of which involve the uteroplacental circulation; that is, reduced perfusion resulting from abnormalities in implantation or vascular remodeling are associated with the development of preeclampsia (16). Normal pregnancy is characterized by an increase in prostaglandin I2 (prostacyclin). In patients with preeclampsia/eclampsia, peripheral vasospasm may be stimulated by an increase in the vasoactive prostaglandin, thromboxane, with a simultaneous lower-than-normal production of prostacyclin (15). The severe vasospasm that occurs exceeds the ability of the cerebral autoregulatory system, and seizure activity results.

Another suggested theory is based on the supposed presence of a single recessive or dominant gene with subsequent inadequate placentation (8). The hypoxia and hypoperfusion that result disturb the functioning of the placental endothelial cells, with changes in circulating vasoactive substances and the sensitivity of the vascular bed to same (8).

It does appear that both mother and fetus contribute to the risk of preeclampsia. There is a higher incidence of preeclampsia in daughters of preeclamptic women. It has also been demonstrated that when a woman becomes pregnant by a man who has been the father of a preeclamptic pregnancy in a different woman, the risk of preeclampsia is 1.8 times that of normal (12).

CLINICAL PRESENTATION

Preeclampsia and Eclampsia

Preeclampsia is a condition of pregnancy that occurs most often after the twentieth week of gestation. In nulliparous patients it occurs most commonly near term. By definition, it is characterized by new-onset hypertension (systolic blood pressure of ≥140 mm Hg or diastolic blood pressure of ≥90 mm Hg) combined with proteinuria, defined as more than 300 mg in

TABLE 97.1. Risk Factors for Preeclampsia

- Nulliparity
- Advanced maternal age
- Multifetal gestation
- Obesity
- Family history of preeclampsia/eclampsia
- Preeclampsia in a previous pregnancy
- Pregestational diabetes mellitus/insulin resistance
- Thrombophilias
- Hypertension or renal disease

24 hours. If 24-hour urine collection data are not available, then a rough estimate of the required amount of proteinuria is defined as a concentration of at least 30 mg/dL ($\geq 1+$ on dipstick) in at least two random urine samples collected at least 6 hours apart (17). Because proteinuria may be a delayed manifestation of preeclampsia, clinicians are advised to be suspicious when new-onset elevated blood pressure is accompanied by any of the following: headache, abdominal pain or abnormal laboratory tests, specifically low platelet counts, and abnormal liver enzymes. These latter elements are the hallmarks of the *HELLP syndrome*, a variant of preeclampsia, which is characterized by hemolytic anemia (H), elevated liver enzymes (EL), and low platelets/thrombocytopenia (LP), as well as by the classic hypertension and proteinuria (2).

Preeclampsia may progress rapidly to the convulsive phase of the disease, *eclampsia* (15). This life-threatening complication is usually preceded by warning signs and symptoms in a patient without previously recognized preeclampsia (2). Factors predisposing to preeclampsia/eclampsia are listed in Table 97.1 (16,17). Preeclampsia regresses rapidly after delivery, and its signs and symptoms usually abate within 48 hours postpartum. The risk of eclampsia does continue postpartum, however, as 13% to 37% of cases have been reported in the postpartum period. The differential diagnosis of altered mental status in a postpartum patient should include eclampsia. Although there have been reported cases of postpartum seizures attributed to eclampsia up to 23 days postpartum, the vast majority occurs within the first 24 hours after delivery. Nevertheless, the differential diagnosis of altered mental status in a postpartum patient should include eclampsia.

A division of preeclampsia into mild and severe forms is useful for both disposition and prognosis. Severe preeclampsia exists when any of the following are present in a patient with a BP $\geq$140/90 mm Hg and proteinuria, greater than 300 mg per 24 hours:

1. BP $\geq$60/110 mm Hg on two occasions 6 hours apart with patient at rest
2. Proteinuria $\geq$5 g per 24 hours
3. Urinary output $\leq$500 mL per 24 hours
4. Persistent central nervous system (CNS) symptoms (altered mental status, headache, blurred vision or blindness)
5. Epigastric or right upper quadrant pain
6. Pulmonary edema
7. Platelet count $<100 \times 10^3/\mu L$

Gestational or Transient Hypertension

Gestational or transient hypertension is defined as the development of hypertension during pregnancy or within the first 24 hours postpartum without other signs of preeclampsia or pre-existing hypertension. The BP usually returns to normal within 10 days after delivery, but elevated BP has a high rate of recur-

rence in later pregnancies. It may also be predictive of eventual chronic hypertension (17).

Chronic Hypertension

BP greater than or equal to 140/90 mm Hg in the period before pregnancy or before the twentieth week of gestation is considered chronic hypertension. Hypertension diagnosed for the first time during pregnancy and persisting beyond the forty-second postpartum day is also classified as chronic hypertension (15). Differentiation of chronic hypertension from preeclampsia is important, as the latter may necessitate inpatient management, whereas the former may be treated on an outpatient basis. Chronic hypertension typically occurs in the older, multiparous woman, often with a history of hypertension in a previous pregnancy. The presence of chronic hypertension increases the risk of developing superimposed preeclampsia, abruptio placenta, fetal growth restriction or intrauterine death, and accelerated or malignant hypertension.

Preeclampsia Superimposed on Chronic Hypertension

Any existing hypertensive disease predisposes the gravid woman to the development of preeclampsia/eclampsia. This diagnosis is usually made if the multisystem disorder that is preeclampsia is superimposed on chronic hypertension. The outcome for mother and child with preeclampsia superimposed on existing hypertension is worse than with de novo preeclampsia (16).

DIFFERENTIAL DIAGNOSIS

The diagnostic dilemma in a gravid patient with hypertension revolves primarily around distinguishing between chronic hypertension, transient hypertension, and preeclampsia. Transient hypertension is characterized by the presence of increased systolic or diastolic pressures in the absence of proteinuria. The patient with chronic hypertension will have a history of hypertension that antedates the twentieth week of pregnancy. Causes of hypertension in this group of patients are similar to those in the nongravid patient population.

Seizures in a woman after 20 weeks of gestation who had not been previously diagnosed with preeclampsia must be accompanied by two of the following within 24 hours of presentation to be considered eclamptic: hypertension, proteinuria, thrombocytopenia, or increased liver enzyme levels (13). Seizures before the twentieth week of gestation or after 48 hours postpartum are generally not considered attributable to eclampsia and should be worked up and treated as in the general population. Some causes to consider include idiopathic epilepsy, trauma, systemic lupus erythematosus, chronic alcohol use, dialysis, electrolyte or metabolic disturbances, ischemic encephalopathy, drug withdrawal, infection, toxin exposure, primary brain or metastatic tumor (6), stroke, intracranial hemorrhage, psychogenic (pseudoseizure), or status post epidural anesthesia (2,7).

EMERGENCY DEPARTMENT EVALUATION

Preeclampsia should be suspected in the presence of headache, blurred vision, scotomata, epigastric pain, diastolic BP $\geq$100 mm Hg, increasing serum creatinine, consumptive coagulopathy, or abnormal transaminases.

Postpartum eclampsia may occur in up to 30% of patients with preeclampsia, usually within the first 12 to 24 hours and rarely beyond the forty-eighth hour. Anecdotal reports of seizures occurring 3 to 23 days postpartum have been attributed to eclampsia, but they are controversial (7). Patients with late postpartum eclampsia frequently present with complaint of headache, visual disturbances of several days' duration, or epigastric discomfort followed by convulsions. Hypertension is present as is the characteristic proteinuria.

Laboratory testing should include an evaluation of electrolytes, including sodium and bicarbonate, as well as liver function tests, to rule out the presence of the HELLP syndrome. A complete blood count with platelets and DIC screen may be indicated. The urine should be screened for protein; an electrocardiogram and a chest radiograph are indicated to search for hypertensive complications, such as ischemia or congestive heart failure. The fetus should be monitored continuously for signs of distress.

Computed tomography of eclamptic encephalopathy shows low attenuation areas in the cortex, with consistent involvement of the posterior areas and occasionally the basal ganglia. In more severe cases, intracerebral hemorrhage may be present (7,14).

EMERGENCY DEPARTMENT MANAGEMENT

Prevention of Preeclampsia and Eclampsia

A number of randomized trials have demonstrated the benefit of low-dose aspirin therapy in reducing the incidence of gestational hypertension in pregnant women at risk for this condition (18). Although more recent trials in larger patient populations show less of a protective effect, the benefit in a high-risk group of patients (previous preeclampsia, chronic hypertension, multiple gestation, and diabetes mellitus) appears to outweigh the small increase in bleeding complications and abruptio placentae associated with salicylate use (5,20).

Magnesium sulfate is well established as prophylaxis for eclampsia (4,19). In patients who are preeclamptic and receiving MgSO$_4$, the incidence of eclampsia falls from 1.2% to 0.3%. Concerns over the delay of spontaneous or induced labor have not been validated (11).

Another suggested prophylactic measure is the use of calcium supplementation during pregnancy. A recent review of randomized trials that compared calcium supplementation of at least 1g daily to placebo showed that there was a reduction in the risk of preeclampsia. The effect was greatest for women at high risk of gestational hypertension and in communities with low dietary calcium intake (9). The mechanism of action is unclear and further research is required to validate this effect on low-risk groups.

Initial Treatment for Preeclampsia and Eclampsia

- Maintain oxygen delivery to both mother and fetus
- Minimize the aspiration risk by placing the mother in the left lateral decubitus position
- Invasive hemodynamic monitoring is indicated only for patients with complications such as pulmonary edema or continued oliguria (15)
- In most cases, volume replacement therapy is not indicated except as needed to maintain urine output of 1 to 2 mL/kg/hour. Overly aggressive fluid therapy may actually precipitate pulmonary or cerebral edema (4)
- Monitor urine output using a Foley catheter
- Treat seizures with magnesium sulfate, as discussed in subsequent text
- Treat blood pressure as discussed in subsequent text

The final step in the treatment of preeclampsia/eclampsia involves delivery or termination of the pregnancy with the least harm to the infant and mother. In cases in which there is evidence of advanced disease or of impending eclampsia, delivery is indicated, regardless of the age of the fetus. In these cases, evacuation of the uterus is the only measure that will halt the advance of the disease. Delivery should also occur if there is evidence of fetal distress (13).

Blood Pressure Management

The goal of antihypertensive therapy is to reduce BP without adverse effects on the fetus. Acute antihypertensive treatment is indicated when the diastolic BP is greater than 105 mm Hg; the goal is to reduce the pressure to 90 to 100 mm Hg. Placental hypoperfusion must be avoided (15). Targets for BP control include a systolic BP of 140 to 150 mm Hg and a diastolic BP between 90 and 100 mm Hg. Specific medications to be used in the treatment of this disorder include the following.

Hydralazine (5 mg i.v., over 1 to 2 minutes) is a vasodilator and the most commonly used agent. It is recommended as the first-line agent. Although it may be used as continuous intravenous medication, intermittent bolus injections are more commonly employed. Doses of 5 to 10 mg may be repeated every 20 to 30 minutes as indicated. Once the desired effect is obtained, additional doses are repeated as necessary to a maximum dose of 80 mg (17). If a total dose of 20 mg is administered without therapeutic response, other hypertensive agents should be considered. Side effects of hydralazine include hypotension (reported more often in preeclamptics than in gravidas with chronic hypertension), headache, tremulousness, nausea, vomiting, and tachycardia. Neonatal thrombocytopenia has also been reported.

Diazoxide, a potent arteriolar vasodilator, is recommended for the occasional patient who is refractory to hydralazine. The use of 30 mg "mini boluses" is recommended. It may be administered every 5 minutes as needed. Diazoxide may cause arrest of labor, which can be overcome by oxytocin. Other effects include maternal and neonatal hyperglycemia caused by suppression of insulin release and displacement of highly protein bound drugs such as phenytoin, resulting in increased toxicity.

Labetalol (20 to 40 mg i.v.) is both an α- β-blocker and appears to have a faster onset of action and an absence of reflex tachycardia when compared with hydralazine. It may be repeated every 10 to 15 minutes until the desired BP is achieved or to a maximum dose of 220 mg (17). Continuous infusion may be started at 1 to 2 mg/minute (no more than 1 mg/kg) to control BP and run at 0.5 mg/minute for maintenance.

Nifedipine (10 to 20 mg), an oral calcium channel blocker, has reemerged as an option for emergency control of hypertension in pregnancy. It may be given every 30 minutes to a maximum dose of 50 mg (17).

Nitroprusside is a potent vasodilator reserved for patients who are unresponsive to more conventional therapy. Nitroprusside has a rapid onset of action and is reversible with discontinuation of therapy. The drug is metabolized to cyanide and thiocyanate, which may cross the placenta. Low doses of nitroprusside have not been associated with clinically evident fetal toxicity.

ACE inhibitors are contraindicated in pregnancy as they have been demonstrated to have adverse effects on the renal perfusion of the fetus. These are thus reserved for postpartum use for the management of hypertension.

Nimodipine has been suggested as both an antihypertensive and an antiseizure medication in the setting of eclampsia (1). It causes a decreased vascular resistance and, therefore, a decreased mean arterial pressure, without affecting peripheral oxygen delivery. Initial reported studies on the use of nimodipine as single-agent therapy for eclampsia are promising but small.

Diuretics are not used as first-line therapy, but should be reserved for those patients with documented congestive heart failure or fluid overload (15). They cause little harm to the fetus.

Seizure Therapy

Magnesium sulfate is the drug of choice for eclampsia in the United States (21). The goal of therapy is to raise the maternal magnesium plasma level to 5 to 8 mg/dL. The most commonly employed protocol in the United States was developed by Zuspan and modified by Sibai and colleagues, and recommends a 6 g i.v. loading dose, then 2 g i.v. per hour (13,15). A commonly used loading dose of 4 g will achieve such a therapeutic maternal plasma level; the effect, however, is transient, and the level will fall within 60 minutes. There also exists an alternative dosing regimen by Pritchard which entails intramuscular loading (19). The specific regimens are outlined in Table 97.2. The side effects of magnesium sulfate treatment range from mild effects such as flushing, loss of deep tendon reflexes, and double vision to life-threatening consequences such as excessive bleeding, respiratory depression, muscle paralysis, and cardiac arrest. When magnesium toxicity is suspected (Table 97.3), calcium gluconate 1 g may be administered slowly. The effect of the calcium is transient and, therefore, continuous monitoring of the patient is warranted.

The magnesium sulfate administration should continue until 24 hours after delivery. Signs of improvement will include a decrease in BP, improvement in sensorium, and an increase in urine output. Magnesium is excreted by the kidney, so in those cases in which urinary output is decreased or in the presence of renal failure, magnesium doses should be adjusted to avoid toxicity. Although there may be an initial decrease in BP for the first 30 to 45 minutes after the initiation of $MgSO_4$ therapy, the drug itself is not an antihypertensive agent. As such, one of the medications detailed below should be added to the treatment regimen to control the BP and minimize further end organ damage.

Postdelivery, fetal magnesium may have equilibrated with the mother's, causing hypotonia, respiratory depression, or hypotension. Calcium gluconate may be administered to the infant in those cases (22).

Phenytoin (Dilantin) has historically been the drug of choice in Europe for the control of eclamptic seizures. It provides prolonged seizure protection and has an antihypoxic effect (10).

TABLE 97.2. Drug Therapy for Eclampsia

Magnesium Sulfate Dosing Regimen

PRITCHARD (INTRAMUSCULAR)

Loading dose	4 g i.v. over 3–5 minutes plus 10 g i.m.
Maintenance dose	5 g i.m. every 4 hours

ZUSPAN

Loading dose	4 g i.v. over 5–10 minutes
Maintenance dose	1–2 g i.v. every hour

TABLE 97.3. Effects of Magnesium Sulfate on the Mother

Serum Level (mg/dL)	Clinical Effects
1.5–2.5	Normal
4–8	Therapeutic for seizure prophylaxis
8–12	Loss of patellar reflexes, double vision, flushing, somnolence, slurred speech
15–17	Muscle paralysis
30–35	Cardiac arrest

Recently, however, phenytoin does not appear to be as effective in controlling eclamptic seizures as magnesium sulfate (13).

In cases in which status epilepticus caused by eclampsia occurs, intubation and muscular paralysis are indicated. Other options include the administration of a short-acting barbiturate such as sodium amobarbital at a dose of 250 mg intravenously, or a benzodiazepine (13).

Chronic Hypertension and Transient Hypertension

In most cases (90%), mild-to-moderate (preexisting) essential hypertension is associated with good outcome for both mother and child (3). Conditions that may prompt pharmacologic management include advanced maternal age (over 40 years of age), evidence of end organ damage, intrauterine growth retardation, history of previous perinatal death, or hypertension of greater than 15 years' duration. The presence of any one of these factors should prompt consideration of pharmacologic intervention, regardless of the BP.

Treatment of the hypertensive disorders of pregnancy varies according to the BP and the presence of other signs and symptoms of preeclampsia/eclampsia. The only definitive care for preeclampsia and eclampsia is delivery of the fetus. Pharmacologic therapy serves as a temporizing measure only.

Women with chronic hypertension who become pregnant are generally treated with α-methyldopa based on a single prospective study performed in the late 1970s that demonstrated safety in the infants. Although some antihypertensive agents such as angiotensin-converting enzyme (ACE) inhibitors are contraindicated in pregnancy, at this time, there are no studies with sufficient numbers of patients to definitively support the use of other drugs in the management of chronic hypertension (16).

CRITICAL INTERVENTIONS

- Early recognition of preeclampsia in symptomatic third trimester or postpartum patients
- Treat the seizures of eclampsia with magnesium sulfate
- Aggressively monitor and treat the hypertension of severe preeclampsia
- Emergently consult an obstetrician for patients with suspected preeclampsia or eclampsia, as delivery is ultimately indicated

DISPOSITION

For patients with chronic or transient hypertension, nonmedical management should be considered for individuals not at high risk for preeclampsia/eclampsia. In certain cases—in which the patient has a history of hypertension preceding the pregnancy and the systolic BP is 140 mm Hg or the diastolic BP is 90 to 99 mm Hg in the appropriate clinical setting (after 20 weeks of gestation)—patients may serve a short stay in the hospital to rule out preeclampsia and be discharged home with close followup.

Role of the Consultant

Because the definitive therapy for eclampsia is delivery of the fetus, an obstetrician should be consulted as soon as the diagnosis is entertained. In cases in which preeclampsia is suspected or newly diagnosed, the need for admission should be determined after discussion with the obstetrician. Discharge should occur only if close followup is feasible.

Indications for Admission

Patients with severe preeclampsia and eclampsia must be admitted to monitored settings after appropriate consultation with the obstetrician. Some cases of early preeclampsia and hypertension in pregnancy may be managed on an outpatient basis if followup is available and the patient is compliant. Such decisions should follow appropriate emergency department interventions, including discussion with the obstetrician.

Transfer

Except in those cases in which a higher level of care is needed, patients experiencing symptomatic preeclampsia or those with eclamptic seizures are not candidates for transfer. The dynamic nature of the disease, the need for continuous monitoring during therapy, and the high fetal and maternal mortality make this disease inappropriate for interfacility transfer.

COMMON PITFALLS

✔ Making the diagnosis of preeclampsia may be difficult for the emergency physician, because the diagnostic elements—hypertension and proteinuria—may not occur simultaneously, may be present as part of another disease process, or may be present as part of a normal pregnancy (18)
✔ The emergency physician must be aware of and monitor the patient's serum magnesium levels during treatment for eclampsia to prevent overtreatment as well as undertreatment
✔ When BP is measured by different observers at different times, the values may vary. Characteristically, the BPs reflect the altering vasospasticity and cardiovascular reactivity of the patient. Higher pressures should not be disregarded in the face of subsequent lower observed pressures (25)
✔ Seizure activity in the third trimester of pregnancy or immediately after delivery that is not responsive to magnesium sulfate mandates immediate computed tomography scan and lumbar puncture to exclude other etiologies of seizures (24)

References

1. Anthony J, Mantel G, Johanson R, et al. The haemodynamic and respiratory effects of intravenous nimodipine used in the treatment of eclampsia. *Br J Obstet Gynecol* 1996;103:518.
2. Brady WJ, Dehnke DJ, Carter CT. Postpartum toxemia: hypertension, edema, proteinuria and unresponsiveness in an unknown female. *J Emerg Med* 1995;13:643.
3. Burrows R, et al. Report of the Canadian Hypertension Society Consensus Conference—2. Nonpharmacologic management and prevention of hypertension disorders in pregnancy. *Can Med Assoc J* 1997;157:907.
4. Coetzee EJ, Dommisse J, Anthony J. A randomized controlled trial of intravenous magnesium sulfate versus placebo in the management of women with severe preeclampsia. *Br J Obstet Gynaecol* 1998;105:300.
5. Coomarasamy A, Honest H, Papaioannou S, et al. Aspirin for prevention of preeclampsia in women with historical risk factors: a systematic review. *Obstet Gynecol* 2003:101:1319–1332.
6. Delanty N, Vaughn CJ, French JA. Medical causes of seizures. *Lancet* 1998;352:383.
7. Druelinger L. Postpartum emergencies. *Emerg Med Clin North Am* 1994;12:219.
8. Erkkola R. Can preeclampsia be predicted and prevented? *Acta Obstet Gynecol Scand* 1997;76:598.
9. Hofmeyr GJ, Roodt A, Atallah AN, Duley L. Calcium supplementation to prevent preeclampsia–a systematic review. *S Afr Med J* 2003;93:224–228.
10. Jagoda A, Riggis S. Emergency department approach to managing seizures in pregnancy. *Ann Emerg Med* 1991;20:80.
11. Leveno KJ, Alexander JM, McIntire DD, et al. Does magnesium sulfate given for prevention of eclampsia affect the outcome of labor? *Am J Obstet Gynecol* 1998;178:707.
12. Lie RT, Rasmussen S, Brunborg H, et al. Fetal and maternal contributions to risk of preeclampsia: population based study. *BMJ* 1998;316:1343.
13. Lipstein H, Lee CC, Crupi RS. A current concept of eclampsia. *Am J Emerg Med* 2003;21:223–226.
14. Manfredi M, Beltramello A, Bongiovanni LG, et al. Eclamptic encephalopathy: imaging and pathogenetic considerations. *Acta Neurol Scand* 1997;96:277.
15. Probst BD. Hypertensive disorders of pregnancy. *Emerg Med Clin North Am* 1994;12:73.
16. Roberts JM, Pearson G, Cutler J, et al. Summary of the NHLBI Working Group on Research on Hypertension During Pregnancy. *Hypertension* 2003;41:437–445.
17. Sibai BM. Diagnosis and management of gestational hypertension and preeclampsia. *Obstet Gynecol* 2003;102:181–192.
18. Sibai BM, Cartis SN, Thom E, et al. Prevention of preeclampsia with low dose aspirin in healthy, nulliparous pregnant women. *N Engl J Med* 1993;329:1213.
19. Sibai BM, Graham JM, McCubbin JH. A comparison of intravenous and intramuscular magnesium sulfate regimens in preeclampsia. *Am J Obstet Gynecol* 1984;150:728.
20. Subtil D, Goeusse P, Puech F, et al. Aspirin (100 mg) used for prevention of preeclampsia in nulliparous women: the Essai Regional Aspirine Mere-Enfant study (Part 1). *Br J Obstet Gynecol* 2003;110:475–484.
21. The Eclampsia Trial Collaborative Group. Which anticonvulsant for women with eclampsia? Evidence from the collaborative eclampsia trial. *Lancet* 1995;345:1455.
22. Usta IM, Sibai BM. Emergent management of puerperal eclampsia. *Obstet Gynecol Clin North Am* 1995;22:315.
23. Ventura SJ, Curtin SC, Menacker F, et al. Births: final data for 1999. *Nat Vital Stat Rep* 2001;49:1–100.
24. Witlin AG, Friedman SA, Egerman RS, et al. Cerebrovascular disorders complicating pregnancy-beyond eclampsia. *Am J Obstet Gynecol* 1997;176:1139.
25. Zuspan FP. Problems encountered in the treatment of pregnancy-induced hypertension. *Am J Obstet Gynecol* 1978;131:591.

CHAPTER 98
Emergencies of Late Pregnancy

Moss H. Mendelson

Although women in the second half of pregnancy (greater than 20 weeks of gestation) commonly have their own physician, some emergent problems require intervention and stabilization by the emergency physician and rapid consultation with an obstetrician. Because a potentially viable second "patient" exists after 23 to 24 weeks, the approach must consider alterations in physiology, differential diagnosis, and medications and doses, as well as the potential need to rescue the fetus to prevent its demise. The most common problems of late pregnancy encountered in the emergency department (ED) are vaginal bleeding, shortness of breath, and coma or seizure.

VAGINAL BLEEDING IN LATE PREGNANCY

Vaginal bleeding after 20 weeks of gestation is not uncommon and can be frightening to the patient as well as to the physician. Definitive treatment, if required, should be performed by an obstetrician. The emergency physician must stabilize the patient hemodynamically and should be aware of the differential diagnosis, the studies necessary to define the problem, as well as the indications for transfer if limited facilities exist for management of the premature or distressed newborn.

Abruptio placentae, premature separation of part of the placenta from the uterine wall, complicates 1% to 2% of all pregnancies. Risk factors include hypertension and maternal tobacco and cocaine use. In addition, abdominal trauma with transmission of forces to the uterus can cause shearing of the placenta from its attachments (6). *Placenta previa,* which accounts for about 20% of third-trimester bleeding, is a placenta that overlaps the cervix to varying degrees. Placenta previa is more common with a uterus scarred from previous cesarean section and with advanced maternal age. Of placentas that overlie the cervix before 20 weeks of gestation (approximately 5% of pregnancies), less than 10% remain so at delivery (10). The other 50% of patients who experience late bleeding often have no definite cause identified. It is believed that most episodes of bleeding represent small marginal separations of the placenta, but this cannot usually be proven. Other causes include vaginal or cervical trauma, lower genital tract infections, polyps, or hemorrhoids.

The pregnant patient undergoes several changes in cardiovascular physiology that are crucial to remember. Maternal blood volume expands by about 1.5 L during a normal pregnancy, resulting in a dilutional anemia that is physiologic (hematocrit 32% to 34%). Pregnant patients also manifest a baseline increase in heart rate (90 to 100 bpm) and stroke volume, resulting in a cardiac output 30% to 40% higher at term than seen in the nonpregnant state. Systematic vascular resistance is decreased, however, and the net hemodynamic result of these changes is a blood pressure lower than that in the nonpregnant state. Finally, the uteroplacental bed does not have any autoregulatory function; placental blood flow is determined strictly by maternal blood pressure and cardiac output. Because of the expanded intravascular volume, signs of extensive blood loss can occur late, and significant fetal hypoperfusion may exist before maternal signs of shock are apparent. Pregnancy is also associated with a rise in concentration of many clotting factors (especially fibrinogen), resulting in a hypercoagulable state.

CLINICAL PRESENTATION

The patient with bleeding after 20 weeks of gestation may present with a spectrum from painless spotting or bloody mucoid discharge to dark or exsanguinating bleeding and severe uterine pain. Placenta previa is most often seen as bright red, painless vaginal spotting. The bleeding is rarely severe (except during labor or after pelvic examination with probing of the cervical os). The patient may be aware of an abnormal placental location. The patient with abruptio placentae more often has dark, variable bleeding, accompanied by uterine tenderness and irritability, manifested by intermittent or steady cramping. Bleeding between the placenta and uterine wall may result in significant occult blood loss, with maternal and fetal compromise, but without evidence of significant external bleeding. Fetal distress (heart rate out of the normal range of 120 to 160 beats per minute) can occur if a significant degree of separation has occurred. Abruptio placentae may also trigger maternal coagulation, thereby resulting in evidence of consumptive coagulopathy, with bleeding from needle sticks, urine, and other sites.

DIFFERENTIAL DIAGNOSIS

The main disorders that must be considered in the third-trimester pregnant patient with vaginal bleeding are abruptio placentae and placenta previa. Other possibilities would include bleeding from a cervical or vaginal lesion, or from a nonvaginal source such as genitourinary (cystitis, urethritis, and nephrolithiasis) or gastrointestinal (hemorrhoids, polyp, and ulcer).

EMERGENCY DEPARTMENT EVALUATION

The patient with vaginal bleeding should first be assessed hemodynamically. With significant maternal blood loss, fluid resuscitation is begun. Blood should be sent for complete blood cell count (CBC), prothrombin time (PT), partial thromboplastin time (PTT), and fibrinogen levels. The patient's blood should be typed and crossmatched, and fresh-frozen plasma or fresh whole blood may be needed. The mother's Rh type should be determined and a Kleihauer-Betke test sent to determine whether significant fetomaternal transfusion has occurred (4). The fetus should be evaluated for signs of distress: bradycardia less than 120 bpm, tachycardia more than 160 bpm, decelerations after uterine irritability, or loss of beat-to-beat variability during continuous fetal monitoring.

History should include known obstetric problems or ultrasonographic diagnoses. Other historical information includes amount of bleeding, passage of clots, character of blood (bright red or dark, older blood), presence of uterine cramping or pain, prior cervical or vaginal lesions or infection, drug use, and history or evidence of abdominal trauma (including domestic violence). The abdominal examination should confirm uterine size as well as the presence of contractions or tenderness to palpation. Vaginal examination *should not be performed* in the ED if adequate obstetric backup is available, and should be preceded by ultrasonography whenever possible to diagnose or exclude placenta previa.

Ultrasonography remains the diagnostic modality of choice for late-pregnancy bleeding. The major purpose of ultrasonography is to locate the placenta and its relationship to the cervix. In addition, information regarding gestational age and general fetal well-being may be obtained (2). Transabdominal ultrasound (TAS) is usually performed first but is noted to have a false-positive rate of 2% to 6% for placenta previa. False positives can be caused by obesity, a posterior placenta, a full bladder, or a focal myometrial contraction. Endovaginal sonography (EVS) eliminates many of these false positives and has been proven safe in many studies. Although TAS is easily performed in the ED, the role of EVS in the ED assessment of vaginal bleeding in late pregnancy is less well defined (11,13).

On the other hand, ultrasonography is insensitive for abruption. Findings in abruption are variable and are affected by the type of abruption (retroplacental or subchorionic) and the timing of the study in relationship to the onset of bleeding. Retroplacental bleeding may have a sonographic appearance very similar to that of a normal placenta, creating an area of thickened placenta or an area mistaken for a fibroid or contraction. Marginal bleeding may be recognized sonographically as a hematoma, although the amount of apparent blood collection seen may significantly underestimate true losses. Evidence of abruption by ultrasound is helpful to the obstetrician in developing a care plan for the patient, and can be followed with serial examinations. A negative study does not eliminate abruption from the differential, and, in fact, a patient with late pregnancy bleeding and an ultrasound negative for placenta previa is often assumed to have abruption. With abruption, fetal monitoring becomes the primary tool for management decisions (2,6).

A vaginal examination is ideally performed after ultrasonography in an operating suite capable of converting to an emergent surgical delivery with fetal resuscitation, in the event that severe bleeding is triggered. If immediate obstetric consultation is not available, patients with significant bleeding should be prepared for transport to a facility that is able to provide a wide range of resuscitative services. If the bleeding is not severe, a cautious vaginal examination in the ED is rational, preferably after placenta previa has been excluded with ultrasonography. The purpose of the examination is to exclude hemorrhoidal bleeding or vaginal or cervical lesions that cause bleeding. Neither fingers nor instruments should be placed in the cervical os, because uncontrolled bleeding from a placenta previa can be triggered by such manipulation.

EMERGENCY DEPARTMENT MANAGEMENT

Prehospital triage of the woman with bleeding after 24 weeks of gestation (a uterus above the umbilicus provides a rough measure) should be to a facility that can manage a potentially high-risk or premature delivery. Management consists of assessment of the amount of bleeding from evidence at the scene and degree of bleeding at the perineum (if a private evaluation of this can be made), administration of maternal supplemental oxygen, positioning of the patient on her left side, and intravenous administration of fluids en route.

The ED should ideally be a place of cardiovascular stabilization and triage only. If the mother has hemodynamic compromise secondary to hemorrhage, fluid resuscitation should be initiated rapidly with crystalloid. Appropriate blood work is initiated, including coagulation tests, as noted earlier. In the mother with rapid exsanguination, O-negative blood transfusion may be required. Fresh whole blood or packed cells with fresh-frozen plasma may be needed if an abruptio placentae is suspected, because this can cause consumption of clotting factors. Fetal heart rate should be quickly measured, with initiation of continuous monitoring if possible. Rapid transport to the obstetric suite is the goal.

In the patient with less emergent bleeding, referral to the obstetric unit is preferred for definitive diagnosis. The standard method of evaluation is ultrasonography followed by vaginal examination in a delivery suite, where the discovery of a fetus-threatening placenta previa can be treated with rapid delivery. In the patient with presumed or visible abruptio placentae, admission to a high-risk prepartum unit for continuous monitoring is appropriate. A cautious vaginal examination in the ED may be appropriate, particularly in a hospital where transfer will be needed if no simple bleeding source is found. Continued fetal well-being should always be documented if the patient spends any significant time in the ED, because hypovolemia is frequently detected by signs of fetal distress before maternal vital sign changes. If the mother is Rh-negative (with an unknown or Rh-positive father) or if a positive Kleihauer-Betke test is positive for fetomaternal hemorrhage, RhoGAM should be administered. If fetomaternal hemorrhage in excess of 15 mL of fetal RBCs has occurred, additional RhoGAM will be necessary (consider 10 μg for every additional 0.5 mL fetal RBCs) (4).

CRITICAL INTERVENTIONS

- Do not perform an internal vaginal examination in the ED for third-trimester pregnant patients with vaginal bleeding
- Provide aggressive volume resuscitation as appropriate
- Immediately consult an obstetrician, or arrange transfer to a suitable facility if necessary

DISPOSITION

All patients with third-trimester vaginal bleeding require obstetric consultation. The only exception is the patient who is discovered to have bleeding from a nonvaginal source, such as external hemorrhoids. Interfacility transfer to a high-risk unit should be accomplished after initial diagnosis or assessment by an obstetrician and is usually performed by specialized obstetric or high-risk neonatal transport units. In general, predelivery transport is safest and is associated with the best outcome, but it must be accomplished in a controlled fashion, with personnel capable of supporting the mother and managing fetal distress or a premature delivery en route.

COMMON PITFALLS

✔ Vaginal examinations should be limited to visual inspection of the perineum and vaginal vault to look for obvious noncervical bleeding sources. Fingers or instruments should *never* be placed in or near the cervix, because uncontrolled bleeding from a placenta previa can result

✔ Coagulopathy should be considered in patients with severe hemorrhage because clotting factors are consumed when significant bleeding occurs with abruptio placentae, and coagulopathy can seriously compromise the mother's ability to limit uterine bleeding

SHORTNESS OF BREATH

Breathlessness is a common symptom in pregnancy. A respiratory alkalosis is common, with normal PCO_2 levels in pregnancy of 27 to 32 mm Hg. "Dyspnea," the sensation of increased breathing effort, is likewise common, particularly in the first two trimesters. It usually improves after about 28 weeks and is thought to be related in some women to progesterone-induced stimulation of the respiratory center. The alveolar–arterial PCO_2 gradient increases to a mean of about 14 mm Hg near term in the sitting position and may be as high as 20 mm Hg in the supine position. Arteriolar–alveolar gradients greater than 20 mm Hg are clearly abnormal, but those between 10 and 20 mm Hg are difficult to interpret (5).

Respiratory physiology in pregnancy shows important changes in response to the stress of illness or injury. Oxygen consumption normally increases by 25%, and residual volume is impaired, particularly in late pregnancy, resulting in poor reserve when a pulmonary insult occurs. The fetus is more sensitive than the mother to a hypoxic insult, because fetal hemoglobin is "left shifted." Tachypnea causes an alkalosis that leads to constriction of the uteroplacental vascular bed and decreased fetal blood flow (5).

CLINICAL PRESENTATION

Respiratory distress presents in pregnancy much as it does in the nonpregnant patient. Predominant signs include increased rate or depth of breathing, use of accessory muscles or other evidence of increased work of breathing, and cyanosis if oxygenation is significantly impaired. Increased respiratory effort may be combined with other clinical evidence of infection in the patient with sepsis or another infectious cause. Wheezing may be caused by asthma, but amniotic fluid embolus, pulmonary embolus (PE), or simple pneumonia must also be considered.

DIFFERENTIAL DIAGNOSIS

Differentiating normal pulmonary changes of pregnancy from respiratory distress caused by illnesses requiring treatment may be difficult. *Pulmonary embolus* occurs with increased frequency in pregnancy because of hypercoagulability and stasis induced by pregnancy, as well as the vessel trauma that occurs at delivery. *Amniotic fluid embolus* is a rare but frequently fatal cause of respiratory distress and cardiovascular collapse that results from amniotic fluid (with antigenic foreign debris) entering the maternal circulation and being filtered in the pulmonary vascular bed. Other potential causes of respiratory distress include asthma, respiratory insufficiency from systemic infection or sepsis, pneumonia, or other etiologies as in nonpregnant patients (see Chapter 8, "Shortness of Breath") (12).

EMERGENCY DEPARTMENT EVALUATION

Assessment of the pregnant patient with respiratory distress is similar to that of nonpregnant patients. A pertinent history includes prior respiratory risk factors such as asthma, smoking, or hypercoagulability independent of pregnancy itself. Proximate symptoms should be sought, such as fever, sputum production, and the nature and location of associated chest pain. Physical examination focuses on the lungs and clues to bronchospasm, local or diffuse consolidation, or fluid overload. Vital signs include an accurate respiratory rate, temperature, and pulse oximetry as an initial screen. In any patient with increased work of breathing, arterial blood gases (ABGs) should be considered to assess oxygenation (PO_2) and ventilation (PCO_2). Chest radiography is safe and usually necessary in the pregnant patient with respiratory symptoms of significance. X-ray beams with a margin greater than 10 cm from the fetus give a negligible radiation exposure, and abdominal/pelvic shielding can be done in pregnant patients to minimize exposure and reassure the patient.

Pulmonary embolism (PE) remains a significant cause of maternal morbidity and mortality in pregnancy. The period of highest risk for thromboembolism remains unsettled in the literature. Studies suggest that most deep venous thromboses associated with pregnancy occur in the antepartum period, although two thirds of PEs are noted in the postpartum period. Increased venous stasis in combination with increases in coagulation factor levels are the most important risk factors. Other factors, such as prolonged bedrest, prior thrombotic disease, and intercurrent illness, also contribute. The clinical presentation can be confusing, as many normal, near-term patients give a history of dyspnea and leg discomfort and have tachypnea and lower extremity swelling on examination. Because of the immediate morbidity and mortality associated with PE and the longer term implications of having the disease (prolonged heparin therapy, prophylaxis during subsequent pregnancies, future use of contraceptives), the emergency physician treating pregnant patients with significant respiratory complaints should be aggressive in pursuing the diagnosis (15).

The workup for PE in pregnancy proceeds in a stepwise fashion, and does not deviate much from the evaluation in nonpregnant patients. (See Chapter 38, "Pulmonary Embolism" for further details.) Assessment of pretest probability is key, and the ideal algorithm for diagnosis remains elusive. Chest radiography is indicated, and ABGs are often assessed, although results of the latter can be difficult to interpret, as outlined earlier. The use of D-dimer studies in pregnancy is not well studied, and may be associated with many false-positive results. The total amount of radiation exposure during workup for PE is small if shielding is used and should never be a barrier to making a diagnosis. Some authors favor lower extremity ultrasound studies first, since a positive study ends the workup, and the patient is treated for DVT and PE. However, a normal lower extremity study is inconclusive and requires further evaluation (8).

EMERGENCY DEPARTMENT MANAGEMENT

The pregnant patient with respiratory distress requires supplemental oxygen, adequate fluids, and positioning on her left side to maximize uterine perfusion. This can be initiated in the prehospital phase. Respiratory support and control of ventilation should be prompt if it is indicated, because the fetus is disproportionately affected by respiratory acidosis or hypoxia. Conservative and prompt therapy for hypoxia and increased work of breathing is recommended, because pregnancy impairs normal maternal compensatory mechanisms and reserve. The threshold for admission or intubation of pregnant patients with respiratory distress is *much lower* than in nonpregnancy.

Treatment of asthma in pregnancy is similar to that in nonpregnancy (see Chapters 35, "Asthma," and 101, "Drugs in Pregnancy and Lactation"). Inhaled β-agonists are the mainstay of acute therapy. Epinephrine can be used if these fail, but it has the theoretic disadvantage of α-stimulation (which causes uterine contraction). Steroids are safe, and their use should be encouraged (12).

Treatment of PE is problematic because warfarin is contraindicated in pregnancy. In the ED, intravenous heparin (large molecule which does not cross the placenta) should be started when the diagnosis of PE is made. Low-molecular-weight heparin (LMWH) is an acceptable alternative (1). Because warfarin (Coumadin) causes a multitude of fetal abnormalities, anticoagulation is maintained with ongoing use of heparin or LMWH for 2 to 6 weeks postpartum. Patients who have received thrombolytic treatment for massive pulmonary embolism without adverse fetal outcome have been reported (15).

CRITICAL INTERVENTIONS

- Anticoagulate the patient with a PE with heparin
- Maximize maternal oxygenation with airway support as needed in order to prevent fetal hypoxia

DISPOSITION

Whether the etiology is PE, pneumonia, asthma, or congestive heart failure (CHF), patients with significant respiratory impairment requiring hospitalization should usually be managed jointly by an obstetrician and an internist. Fetal well-being is optimized by maintaining maternal oxygenation and acid–base balance aggressively and by minimizing the work of breathing.

Those with dyspnea that has been adequately treated in the ED (such as an asthma exacerbation) may be discharged home with appropriate followup.

COMMON PITFALLS

✔ Failure to appreciate the lack of respiratory reserve in late pregnancy
✔ Failure to aggressively treat asthma because of fear of harming the fetus
✔ Reluctance to pursue all ancillary studies that are appropriate in the pregnant woman with possible PE because of concerns about fetal radiation exposure

SEIZURES AND ALTERED LEVEL OF CONSCIOUSNESS

CLINICAL PRESENTATION

Central nervous system problems such as seizure and coma have a wide differential diagnosis in pregnancy. The most common cause of seizures in pregnancy is epilepsy. In about 40% of women with epilepsy, seizure frequency increases in pregnancy; this is particularly common in patients with poor prior control (5). Several factors can affect anticonvulsant levels, including decreased drug bioavailability owing to physiologic changes in pregnancy and decreased medication intake because of nausea and maternal concerns about teratogenicity of antiseizure medicines. Indeed, the risk of congenital defects is increased two- to threefold in patients with epilepsy. The relative contribution of drugs needed to manage seizures, epilepsy itself, or prolonged acidosis from maternal seizures is unknown (14).

DIFFERENTIAL DIAGNOSIS

The differential diagnosis of seizures in a pregnant patient should include eclampsia, preexisting seizure disorder, thrombotic or hemorrhagic stroke, subarachnoid hemorrhage, CNS tumor, metabolic causes, and drug toxicity (cocaine and cyclic antidepressants). Rarely, an amniotic fluid embolus or a PE can present with seizure. See Chapter 113 ("Seizures") for the approach to the seizure patient.

Coma has a similar differential diagnosis, with a postictal state caused by seizure from epilepsy or eclampsia as the most common consideration. The differential and ED evaluation are similar to that of the nonpregnant patient (see Chapter 11, "Altered Mental Status and Coma"). Stroke must be considered in the patient whose condition does not reverse rapidly or who has a focal deficit (7). Pregnant patients with diabetes have increased metabolic demands as well as peripheral insulin resistance, and they may be more prone to either hyperglycemia or hypoglycemia. Overdose is not uncommon in pregnancy and should be considered in the patient with a decreased level of consciousness or a picture consistent with a clinical toxidrome.

EMERGENCY DEPARTMENT EVALUATION

Assessment of the seizing patient usually consists of emergent interventions to ensure an adequate airway and oxygenation, stopping the seizure, and then focusing on the potential etiology. Focal signs should be noted. Once the seizure is terminated, clues to eclampsia (hyperreflexia, proteinuria, persistent hypertension, and marked edema) should be sought. Obstetric history (including symptoms of preeclampsia), history of epilepsy or diabetes, compliance with current medications, use of other current medications, including alcohol and antidepressants, and

risk factors for thrombosis are all determined. The physical examination should include a detailed neurologic examination for focal findings and trauma. Evaluation of the comatose patient also includes all of the aforementioned, in addition to a determination of the depth of coma.

Laboratory studies should include rapid glucose determination and measurement of antiseizure medication levels. A toxicology screen may be useful in the patient with suspected overdose, as may be an electrocardiogram (to detect cardiac effects of cyclic toxicity).

Computed tomography is rarely useful in the known epileptic or in the eclamptic whose neurologic examination normalizes with standard therapy. It may be useful to detect intracranial hemorrhage, however, in the patient with focal or persistent deficits or continued coma. In all other patients, it is a standard part of the evaluation of the patient with an otherwise unexplained, sudden central nervous system event.

EMERGENCY DEPARTMENT MANAGEMENT

Airway protection is paramount in the comatose patient and in the patient with seizures. Intubation should be considered early, because the fetus suffers disproportionate injury from hypoxia, hypercarbia, and acidosis. The diagnosis of eclampsia should be strongly considered early in the course of a pregnant patient with seizures, and treated with magnesium. Magnesium is superior to both benzodiazepines and Dilantin in the treatment of eclamptic seizures (3,9) (see Chapter 97, "Hypertensive Disorders of Pregnancy").

Most medications for seizures are rated as U.S. Food and Drug Administration (FDA) category D drugs. Despite this, they are generally accepted as safe for acute use and preferable to the hypoxia and acidosis of persistent seizure activity. If benzodiazepines cause respiratory depression in the mother, intubation should be performed. Because of the changes in phenytoin pharmacokinetics, adjustment of dosing may be necessary in pregnant patients.

CRITICAL INTERVENTIONS

- Correct hypoglycemia and hypoxemia in patients with seizure or altered mental status
- Consider eclampsia as a likely cause of seizure in the third-trimester pregnant patient, and administer magnesium

DISPOSITION

Admission is required for control of persistent seizures and for management of the comatose patient. Early involvement of the obstetric team is desirable, and a neurologist may also need to be involved, unless the patient has clear evidence of eclampsia. Patients with a history of seizure disorder who return to baseline in the ED may be discharged home.

COMMON PITFALLS

✔ Eclampsia should be considered in any comatose patient or patient with seizures in the third trimester, and clues to this systemic disease should be sought
✔ Hypertension and coma may be seen in hemorrhagic central nervous system events, and a computed tomographic scan should be considered if the patient with presumed eclampsia does not respond promptly to magnesium sulfate

References

1. AGOC Committee Opinion: safety of Lovenox in pregnancy. *Obstet Gynecol* 2002;100:845–846.
2. Benedetti TJ. Antepartum hemorrhage. In: Gabbe SG, ed . *Obstetrics—normal and problem pregnancies,* 4th ed. New York: Churchill Livingstone, 2002.
3. Duley L, Gulmezoglu AM, Henderson-Smart DJ. Magnesium sulphate and other anticonvulsants for women with pre-eclampsia. (Cochrane Review). In: The Cochrane Library, Issue 1, 2004. Chidester, UK: John Wiley & Sons, Ltd.
4. Fung KF, Eason E, Crane JA, et al. Prevention of Rh alloimmunization. *J Obstet Gynaecol Can* 2003;25:765–773.
5. Graves CR. Acute pulmonary complications during pregnancy. *Clin Obstet Gynecol* 2002;45:369–376.
6. Hladky K, Yankowitz J, Hansen WF. Placental abruption. *Obstet Gynecol Surv* 2002;57:299–305.
7. Kitner SJ, Stern BJ, Feeser BR, et al. Pregnancy and the risk of stroke. *N Engl J Med* 1996;335:768–774.
8. Kline JA, Johns KL, Colucciello SA, Israel EG. New diagnostic tests for pulmonary embolism. *Ann Emerg Med* 2000;35:168–180.
9. Lipstein H, Lee CC, Crupi RS. A current concept of eclampsia. *Am J Emerg Med* 2003;21:223–226.
10. Neilson JP. Interventions for suspected placenta previa (Cochrane Review). In: The Cochrane Library, Issue 1, 2004. Chidester, UK: John Wiley & Sons, Ltd.
11. Phelan MB, Valley VT, Mateer JR. Pelvic ultrasonography. *Emerg Med Clin North Am* 1997;15:789.
12. Practical Guide for the Diagnosis and Management of Asthma. NIH Publication No. 97-4053 October 1997.
13. Sherer DM, Abulafia O, Anyaegbunam AM. Intra- and early postpartum ultrasonography: a review. Part II. *Obstet Gynecol Surv* 1998;53:181.
14. Tatum WO 4th, Liporace J, Benbadis SR, Kaplan PW. Updates on the treatment of epilepsy in women. *Arch Intern Med* 2004;164:137–145.
15. Toglia MR, Weg JG. Venous thromboembolism during pregnancy. *N Engl J Med* 1996;335:108.

CHAPTER 99
Emergency Delivery

Michael D. Burg and Daan Biesbroeck

Although it is widely recognized that emergency departments (EDs) and the prehospital environment are suboptimal locations for deliveries, they can, and do, occur there (3,7,11,14,15,21,22,24). Exact data on the incidence of ED deliveries are not readily available but two studies suggest that prehospital or ED delivery occurs in 1:160 to 1:695 births (3,24). These births are frequently attended by a high rate of maternal and neonatal complications (3,7,24).

Generally, the ED lacks sophisticated fetal monitoring devices, practiced obstetrical personnel, and advanced delivery technologies that serve to optimize outcomes for mothers and babies. In addition, pregnant women who receive little or no prenatal care, abuse drugs or alcohol, and have limited access to health care are all overly represented in the ED patient population (3,4).

CLINICAL PRESENTATION

Patients present to the ED with a wide variety of delivery and pregnancy-related conditions, such as spontaneous or premature rupture of the membranes (5), preterm labor, shoulder dystocia (17), preeclampsia and eclampsia (6,20), fetal distress, nuchal umbilical cord, breech presentations, postpartum hemorrhage, prolapsed umbilical cord (12,16), and meconium staining. Depending on practice setting and the availability of obstetric consultants, emergency physicians may be called upon to initiate management for these patients. A basic understanding of these conditions and an organized approach to their management is essential for treatment of these often stress-provoking and challenging patients. Patients may present to the ED in the third trimester of pregnancy with symptoms that may represent labor, such as pelvic cramping and low back pain.

The definition of *preterm labor* is uterine contractions with cervical changes occurring prior to a gestational age of 37 weeks. About 8% of infants are born preterm. Complications in preterm neonates result in increased morbidity and more than 70% of neonatal deaths not resulting from congenital or genetic abnormalities (19,20).

DIFFERENTIAL DIAGNOSIS (TRUE VERSUS FALSE LABOR)

All near-term pregnant women presenting to the ED with abdominal pain should be considered to be in labor until proven otherwise.

True labor is defined as a process of regular, rhythmic, progressive uterine contractions that produce effacement and dilation of the cervix (20). False labor (Braxton-Hicks contractions) consists of short irregular uterine contractions without cervical effacement or dilation. Braxton-Hicks contractions do not intensify in strength or frequency and tend to resolve with mild sedation and analgesia. False labor can stop spontaneously or progress to true labor (20). Alternatively, musculoskeletal low back pain may be confused with labor pains, as may other abdominal pathology, such as appendicitis.

EMERGENCY DEPARTMENT EVALUATION

Assessment of the pregnant patient at any gestation age greater than 20 weeks with any complaint possibly referable to the pregnancy should include an evaluation of that patient for possible pregnancy-related problems. Fetal distress, preterm labor, imminent delivery, hemorrhage, severe preeclampsia, eclampsia, and a prolapsed umbilical cord may mandate immediate ED management or transfer to the delivery suite and cut short a more comprehensive assessment.

A focused history and physical examination is performed. Specific historical data to gather include the presence and characteristics of uterine contractions, vaginal fluid leakage, vaginal blood loss, and past medical and surgical history with an emphasis on obstetric and gynecologic history. Vaginal blood loss that is scant and dark generally signals "bloody show" or the passage of the cervical mucus plug. Active, or large-volume vaginal blood (like a normal menses) may indicate placenta previa or placental abruption (9,14,21).

Premature rupture of the membranes (PROM) is defined as membrane rupture prior to labor onset and occurs in up to 8% of pregnancies (20). PROM prior to 37 weeks of gestational is called preterm PROM (20).

Diagnosing *preterm labor* is sometimes difficult because of nonspecific symptoms at presentation (20). In general, a patient who is at less than 37 weeks of gestation with regular contractions and cervical dilation of 3 cm and effacement of 80% should be considered to be in preterm labor. Serial examinations are indicated in patients with contractions and only minimal cervical dilation (20). Ultrasound-aided assessment of fetal breathing may help discriminate between true and false labor, as the fetus usually stops breathing in true labor (20). A high correlation between preterm PROM and preterm labor has been observed (20). Intrauterine death, nonviability of the fetus, and pregnancy-related maternal medical problems, such as severe preeclampsia, requiring early delivery of a viable fetus are contraindications for treating preterm labor (20).

Although most patients in *active labor* present with either abdominal pain, cramps, or back pain, some may display a variety of nonspecific symptoms such as nausea, vomiting, urinary urgency or incontinence, and anxiety (14). Some patients—notably teenagers or obese females—may deny any possibility of pregnancy or missed menses.

The patient's record of prenatal care and any complications associated with the present pregnancy should be reviewed. A history of present illness is detailed as well. Fever and/or chills, headache, visual disturbances, seizures, excessive weight gain and fluid retention, and epigastric or right upper quadrant abdominal pain are important review of system positives.

Maternal vital signs should be within the normal range for the mother's stage of pregnancy and appropriate to the clinical setting. Abnormal values are reassessed. If fever, hypertension, hypotension, tachypnea, or tachycardia is detected, the cause(s) of the abnormal vital sign(s) are sought and treatment begun as needed.

Fetal heart rate, which normally ranges between 120 and 160 bpm during the third trimester, is assessed with either handheld Doppler or ultrasound. The maternal pulse rate is palpated during fetal heart rate determination to avoid confusing the two (20).

A general physical examination should focus on evaluating the airway, the cardiopulmonary systems, neurologic function, and the gravid abdomen. Edema should be noted, particularly of the face and hands. Fluid retention often accompanies normal pregnancy; however, edema or proteinuria with hypertension, headache, or visual changes and right upper quadrant or epigastric discomfort suggest preeclampsia (20).

Abdominal examination, which may be augmented by transabdominal ultrasound, concentrates on approximating fetal age (20). In the hypotensive, tachycardic, or febrile pregnant female important clues to the cause of her condition may be found during the abdominal examination. It is important to realize that rolling the mother from the supine to the left lateral decubitus position can reverse maternal hypotension caused by the gravid uterus resting on the inferior vena cava. However, conditions other than mechanical impedance of maternal cardiac preload can cause maternal hypotension. Blood loss, either frank or occult, sepsis, dehydration, and other possibilities should be considered.

In a normal singleton gestation, the uterus becomes a nonpelvic organ at about 12 weeks and may be palpable above the pelvic brim. By 20 weeks of gestation the uterine fundus generally abuts the umbilicus. From 20 to 34 weeks, the distance from the pubic symphysis to the fundus in centimeters approximates the gestational ages in weeks (20).

If time permits, Leopold maneuvers are used to evaluate fetal position. Information gained during the performance of these maneuvers may also be augmented by transabdominal ultrasound. The uterine fundus is palpated first to determine if the head (round and hard) or the buttocks and legs (irregular and firm) occupy it. Secondly, the uterine sides are palpated to identify the fetal back. Thirdly, one hand palpates just above the pubic symphysis to feel which fetal part is low in the pelvis (20). In a majority of cases the round hard fetal head will be palpable here.

After the completion of the abdominal examination, a sterile digital vaginal examination is done. An exception to this guideline occurs in the case of excessive vaginal bleeding, which should prompt a concern for placenta previa or placental abruption. If either of these two entities is suspected the patient is transferred expeditiously to labor and delivery for further evaluation, without internal vaginal examination in the ED (see Chapter 98, "Emergencies of Late Pregnancy").

Suspected rupture of the membranes is also a contraindication to immediate digital vaginal examination. Spontaneous rupture of the membranes (SROM), which is heralded by leakage of clear or faintly cloudy vaginal fluid, is defined as rupture of the chorionic and amniotic membranes and may be confirmed by a nitrazine paper test or by the presence of ferning (5,9,20). SROM may occur before or during active labor and should be strongly suspected on the basis of patient history or when fluid is observed flowing from the cervical os or is seen pooling in the vagina (9,20). The nitrazine paper test relies on the fact that the pH of amniotic fluid approximates that of serum (7.35 to 7.45) and will turn the normally yellow nitrazine-impregnated paper blue (9,20). Vaginal fluid has a more acidic pH (9,20). Amniotic fluid forms a characteristic fern-like appearance (ferning) when the fluid is allowed to air-dry on a glass microscope slide (9,20).

Diagnosing SROM is an important decision branch-point in the ED for three reasons. First, it may signal the onset of active labor (5,20). Second, prolapse of the umbilical cord through the cervical os may occur as intrauterine fluid volume suddenly decreases (9), and third, the risk of intrauterine infection rises (9,20). To minimize the risk of intrauterine infection (chorioamnionitis or endometritis), a sterile speculum examination is performed if membrane rupture is suspected. During the sterile speculum examination, the cervical length, dilation, and consistency are evaluated visually rather than manually (9,20).

The purpose of the vaginal examination is to evaluate the progression of labor by assessing cervical effacement (thinning), cervical dilation, and fetal station. Cervical effacement is expressed as a percentage from zero to 100, with zero percent representing a completely uneffaced cervix (about 2 cm in length) and 100% representing a maximally thinned cervix. Cervical dilation refers to the diameter of the cervical os. A 10-cm cervical os is completely dilated. Fetal station is determined by comparing the level of the presenting fetal part to the maternal ischial spines, which represent zero station. Negative station indicates that the presenting fetal part is above the level of the spines, and positive station indicates that the presenting part is below the level of the spines (20).

EMERGENCY DEPARTMENT MANAGEMENT

Preterm Labor

The goal of treatment is to prevent or postpone preterm delivery in the critical period from 22 to 32 weeks of gestation. If no contraindications exist and the infant is expected to survive, medical management is indicated, starting with admission for lateral decubitus bed rest and maternal hydration. Rapid hydration is begun in the ED with an i.v. bolus of 500 mL of balanced electrolyte solution over a 30-minute period followed by an infusion of at least 125 mL per hour, taking care to avoid fluid overload (20). Tocolytics can be used to prevent preterm delivery, with the two most common classes being intravenous magnesium sulfate and β-adrenergic agonists. All tocolytic medications have contraindications and possible life-threatening side effects, some of which are mentioned in this text.

Magnesium sulfate is administered initially as 4 to 6 g in 250 mL of solution over a 30-minute period, followed by an infusion rate of 2 to 4 g per hour. Serious side effects are neurologic depression, respiratory compromise, and cardiac dysrhythmias.

For the β-agonist ritodrine, the recommended starting dose is 100 μg per minute i.v., titrated upward in increments of 50 μg per minute every 10 minutes to a maximum of 350 μg per minute. Terbutaline, also a β-agonist, can be given subcutaneously in an initial dose of 0.25 mg, which can be repeated every 20 to 60 minutes or i.v., 2.5 to 5 μg per minute (20). A serious side effect associated with β-agonist use for preterm labor is the development of pulmonary edema.

Although tocolytic therapy fails in about 25% of all patients, it can potentially allow time for transfer of the patient to an appropriate center and the start of fetal lung maturation therapy (20).

Normal Delivery

Childbirth is a physiologic process, not a pathologic one; therefore, physician involvement in a delivery often involves primarily facilitation and support. Normal delivery is the process by which the products of conception (fetus, placenta, and membranes) are expelled from the uterus through involuntary uterine contractions and voluntary abdominal efforts.

Labor is divided into stages as an aid to help follow its progression and to help identify problems requiring physician intervention.

Labor's first stage (cervical stage) starts when contractions become regular and progressively stronger, longer, more frequent, and coordinated (latent phase). This may last from a few hours to several days depending on maternal factors. During this phase, cervical effacement with minimal dilation often occurs. Taking care not to prematurely rupture the membranes, one can identify presenting parts and determine fetal station. Frequent vaginal examinations are unnecessary and increase infection risk (20). The next phase (active phase) is generally shorter, averaging 5 hours in nulliparas and 2 hours in multiparas. The cervix usually dilates fully (20). The deceleration phase marks the end of the first stage of labor and is notable for slowing cervical dilatation.

Depending on local resources and transfer time, patients in the first stage of labor may be considered for transfer to an obstetrician. If transfer is not possible, preparations for the second stage of labor should be made. This involves preparation for delivery, fetal monitoring, and supplying comfort and support to the laboring woman. Laboratory testing (if not documented in the prenatal record) may include CBC, blood typing and Rh status, antibody screen, rubella titer, and tests for syphilis, hepatitis and HIV, among others, depending on clinical considerations (20). An intravenous line should be started if not already in place.

In the absence of more sophisticated methods, fetal monitoring can be performed with ultrasound or a hand-held Doppler and should be done on a regular basis. Ultrasound has also been recommended for determination of position and anatomy of the placenta and umbilical cord.

The second stage of the labor starts with the cervix fully dilated and the woman experiencing an urge to push with contractions, and ends with newborn delivery. Cervical examination is performed to assess whether complete dilation has occurred. During this stage, uterine contractions are strong and regular, lasting 1 to 2 minutes, in cycles of 3 to 5 minutes, and are accompanied by the mother's urge to bear down. During contractions, efforts to push should be encouraged; between contractions the mother should rest. After each contraction the fetal heart rate is monitored. To facilitate physician assessment and intervention some authors recommend the patient assume the dorsal lithotomy position, with or without an inverted bedpan placed under the buttocks, others recommend Sims position (left lateral position) (20). The only position that has been shown to adversely affect fetal outcome is the maternal supine position (20).

Preparation for delivery consists of gentle perineal cleansing, and, time permitting, sterile perineal draping. All involved medical personnel should don universal precautions (goggles, mask, gloves, gown, and shoe covers). Between contractions, sterile digital vaginal examinations should be performed to evaluate labor progression. Coaching of the mother during contractions and calm communication between contractions helps facilitate a coordinated, controlled fetal expulsion. Delivery is imminent when the presenting part begins to distend the perineum. During this critical interval the mother is instructed to pant and not push, allowing slow crowning and controlled delivery of the head.

Episiotomy

Although the use of routine episiotomy in normal delivery has diminished in favor of other strategies, indications including malpresentations, shoulder dystocia, and imminent perineal tear, among others, remain (20). A detailed description of this procedure (and its repair) can be found in any standard obstetrics text.

The modified Ritgen maneuver promotes delivery while minimizing injury to the maternal perineum, and involves applying direct pressure to the perineum with a draped hand (indirectly putting pressure on the fetal chin), so that slight fetal head extension occurs. Simultaneously, the emergency physician's other hand is placed gently on the fetal head positioning it with its smallest diameter as the presenting part and preventing an uncontrolled movement of the head as it clears the perineum (14,20). As the head delivers it will rotate to a transverse position. If a nuchal cord is present it is gently freed by slipping it over the fetal head. Irreducible nuchal cords can be doubly clamped and cut and a rapid delivery performed. The fetal face, nares, and oropharynx can be cleared by means of gentle suctioning with a bulb or DeLee trap to minimize aspiration risk. Generally, gentle bimanual downward and subsequent upward traction on the head in conjunction with controlled, minimal maternal efforts will deliver the anterior and posterior shoulder, respectively. After delivery of the shoulders, the rest of the body will follow easily. The newborn is positioned slightly lower than or even with the perineum until the umbilical cord is clamped and cut. The cord should be incised between two clamps 4 to 5 cm apart with the proximal clamp applied approximately 5 to 10 cm from the newborn's abdomen (20). Care must be taken not to let the baby slip before it is dried, bundled, and given to the mother, Apgar scores permitting.

The second stage of labor averages 50 to 60 minutes in nulliparas and 15 to 20 minutes in multiparas (20). Generally, if it lasts longer than 2 hours, abnormal labor has developed (20).

The third stage begins after the delivery of the baby and ends with the delivery of the placenta, usually within 30 minutes. Signs of imminent placental delivery are umbilical cord lengthening, a gush of uterine blood, and the uterus becoming more globular and rising in the maternal abdomen. Maternal efforts are usually sufficient to deliver the placenta but can be aided by *gentle* traction on the umbilical cord, keeping in mind that uterine inversion is a potentially disastrous complication of pulling on the cord (20). Applying manual pressure just superior to the symphysis pubis can help prevent uterine inversion (14,20). The placenta and membranes are inspected for completeness.

If the placenta is not fully delivered within 30 minutes, manual removal is a consideration (20). After delivery, the uterus is assessed frequently for its usually contracted postdelivery state. Transabdominal uterine massage may be used to maintain uterine tone. In addition, 20 units of oxytocin may be diluted in a liter of intravenous fluid and titrated to effect (usually 2 to

10 mL per minute), to decrease the risk of postpartum hemorrhage caused by uterine atony (20).

Initial newborn assessment is performed and the mother is checked for birth canal and perineal tears. These tears can be a source of significant blood loss and prompt repair is advised (14).

COMPLICATIONS OF DELIVERY

Shoulder Dystocia

Shoulder dystocia is defined as failure of the fetal shoulders to deliver after delivery of the fetal head and complicates up to 2% of all vaginal deliveries (2,9,17). This diagnosis is suspected when not one of the fetal shoulders deliver, or when the fetal head moves back into the introitus after it presents (the *"turtle" sign*) (9). Shoulder dystocia heightens the risk of neonatal mortality and morbidity including aspiration, asphyxia, brachial plexopathies, and humeral and clavicular fractures (2,14). Maternal risk of postpartum hemorrhage is increased as well (2). Consequently, management of this complication focuses on minimizing the time between delivery of the fetal head and body and minimizing traction on the fetal head and neck which can worsen the shoulder impaction or cause fetal injury (14).

A variety of maneuvers have been described to resolve shoulder dystocia. Disagreement exists about which maneuver, or series of maneuvers, is likely to be most successful (17). While calling for obstetrical back-up the emergency physician can drain the maternal bladder to create space anteriorly and perform an episiotomy to allow posterior shoulder delivery (14,17,21). Alternatively, hyperflexion of the maternal thighs onto the abdomen may be attempted (9). Another technique involves an assistant applying suprapubic pressure on the maternal abdomen in an attempt to dislodge the impacted fetal shoulder while the emergency physician applies *gentle* downward traction on the fetal head (9,14,17). The "all-fours" maneuver alone, which involves placing the laboring mother on her hands and knees, resulted in an 83% success rate in one recent study (2). More elaborate techniques involving fetal rotation or "reconstitution" of the fetus into the uterus with subsequent cesarean section have been described and can be found in standard obstetrics texts (9).

Fetal Distress

Fetal heart rate, which normally ranges between 120 and 160 bpm during the third trimester, can be assessed with either hand-held Doppler or ultrasound in the ED, since more sophisticated fetal monitoring devices are frequently unavailable. The maternal pulse rate should be palpated during fetal heart rate determination to avoid confusing the two. It is recommended that fetal heart rate be assessed every 15 minutes during stage one of labor and every 5 minutes during stage two (11). Monitoring is initiated at the end of a contraction and continues for 1 minute (11).

A fetal heart rate greater than 160 bpm defines fetal tachycardia. Brief (less than 20 seconds) fetal heart rate accelerations often occur during labor and are considered normal. The differential diagnosis for sustained fetal tachycardia includes maternal temperature elevation, medications, and fetal distress among other entities (20).

A fetal heart rate less than 120 bpm represents fetal bradycardia. Brief periods of fetal bradycardia, occurring during a contraction and ending shortly after the contraction, are normal, probably resulting from pressure on the fetal head. Fetal heart rate decelerations that persist long after a contraction may signal uteroplacental insufficiency. Decelerations that have no temporal relationship to uterine contractions may indicate umbilical cord compression (20).

Nuchal Umbilical Cord

The incidence of umbilical cord loops encircling the fetal neck approaches 25%. After the fetal head delivers, the clinician should check for a nuchal cord either visually or manually with a finger sweep of the neck. Occasionally two or more loops are found. If a nuchal cord is detected it can be lifted up and over the fetal head. In the case of a tight cord that will not slip easily over the head it may be doubly clamped and cut and delivery completed rapidly (20).

Breech Presentations

Breech presentation, in which the fetal buttocks are the presenting part, is the most common malpresentation, occurring in approximately 4% of all deliveries. It is closely associated with prematurity and more specifically, birth weight, in general, the smaller the fetus the higher the incidence of breech presentation. Predisposing factors to breech are congenital and uterine abnormalities, although in 50% of cases no causative factor is identified. An association between breech and increased perinatal morbidity and mortality exists, although only about one third of perinatal deaths in breech presentations are related to potentially preventable factors, such as trauma and asphyxia during delivery (20). A breech presentation may be suspected after Leopold maneuvers or vaginal examination of the dilated cervix, and confirmed by ultrasound. Breech delivery is difficult because, unlike cephalic presentations, dilation of the cervix by the presenting parts is insufficient while successively larger and less compressible parts, culminating in the fetal head, try to pass. This can cause entrapment of the fetal head and predisposes for umbilical cord prolapse (14,20). Procedures for delivery in various types of breech presentations can be found in obstetrics texts (20).

When a breech presentation is identified or suspected, immediate consultation with an obstetrician should be obtained.

Prolapsed Umbilical Cord

Umbilical cord prolapse occurs when the cord passes through the cervix before the presenting fetal part (12,20). It is a fairly rare but potentially lethal obstetrical complication, which must be promptly recognized and managed (12). Rupture of the amniotic membranes, with a sudden decrease in intrauterine fluid volume, is a risk factor for cord prolapse. Fetal bradycardia may signal that cord prolapse and compression have occurred (14,20).

If fetal distress is present, a prompt vaginal examination is mandatory to check for a cord prolapse. The simplest treatment is elevation of the fetal presenting part off the umbilical cord to restore blood flow to the fetus (14). This elevation must be maintained until delivery, usually by cesarean section, is accomplished (20). Alternatively the mother may be placed in a lateral decubitus, knee-chest, or steep Trendelenburg position to achieve the same end point (9,12,14,20). One study, which examined patients with cord prolapse in whom delivery was *not* imminent, found that bladder filling with 500 to 700 mL of saline and intravenous ritodrine resulted in good fetal outcomes (12).

Resolution of fetal bradycardia after treatment for cord prolapse is a reassuring sign (9). Although one author has suggested that, posttreatment, examiners may gently palpate the umbilical cord for a pulse, another author cautions that cord palpation may compromise blood flow (9,20). Use of a hand-held Doppler or ultrasound may be the safest routine method of monitoring fetal heart rate under these circumstances in the ED.

Meconium Staining of Amniotic Fluid

Meconium is fetal fecal material and contaminates amniotic fluid in up to 20% of deliveries (9,20). Aspirated meconium can cause severe neonatal lung disease and death. When meconium-stained amniotic fluid is passed during delivery, suctioning of the fetal mouth and nose is performed prior to the first breath (20). Endotracheal intubation and endotracheal suctioning is indicated for depressed neonates and those exposed to thick (particulate) meconium (9,20). It is important to realize that unresolved controversies exist for the management of neonates exposed to meconium.

Perimortem Cesarean Section

In cardiac arrest patients suspected of being greater than or equal to 24 weeks pregnant, perimortem cesarean section should be considered as a life-saving intervention for both mother and fetus (9,11). Full cardiopulmonary resuscitative efforts should be continued during and after completion of the procedure, since maternal survival after perimortem cesarean section has been reported (11). Fetal hypoxia is minimized and fetal survival optimized if the procedure is performed within 5 minutes of maternal arrest (11,19). Immediate obstetric and pediatric or neonatal consultations should be requested coincident with performing the procedure (19).

To perform a perimortem cesarean section, a vertical midline incision is created from the maternal epigastrium to the pubic symphysis into the peritoneal cavity. Next the uterus is identified and incised in the midline from the fundus to the bladder reflection (11,18,21). Finally the fetus is removed and the umbilical cord doubly clamped and cut (18,21). Some authors also recommend removal of the placenta at this stage (11). Within reason, sterile surgical technique should be used throughout the procedure and care taken to provide hemostasis and minimize damage to adjacent maternal structures (11,21).

CRITICAL INTERVENTIONS

- If shoulder dystocia is encountered, attempt maneuvers such as bladder emptying, hyperflexion of the hips, and suprapubic pressure
- Consult an obstetrician immediately for any complications of delivery such as breech presentation, shoulder dystocia, or any sign of fetal distress

Disposition

When delivery is not imminent, the patient in preterm labor should be transferred to an obstetrics unit more suited to provide the specialist care that is needed (19). If such facilities are not readily available or the mother is in late stage labor, medical management is initiated in the ED and immediate obstetrical consultation obtained.

Patients who deliver in the ED should be moved to the delivery area for postdelivery obstetrical care. Those with a delivery complication or episiotomy require further postdelivery evaluation and treatment by an obstetrician. Well-appearing, term newborns should be transferred to the nursery. Preterm newborns and those in distress may require ED resuscitation with subsequent transfer to a neonatal intensive care unit (ICU) (see Chapter 205, "Newborn Resuscitation").

COMMON PITFALLS

- ✔ Failure to recognize that fetal distress places the fetus at risk for sustained fetal hypoxia and resultant neonatal complications
- ✔ Failure to diagnose preterm labor may place the newborn at risk of disorders resulting from prematurity
- ✔ Failure to diagnose and prepare for imminent delivery places mother and infant at risk for a wide variety of maternal and neonatal complications
- ✔ Failure to seek and obtain obstetric consultation early can put both maternal and fetal well-being at risk
- ✔ ED deliveries are inherently high risk. Equipment and expertise for critical neonatal and maternal care must be available

Acknowledgment

Thank you to previous edition chapter author Lynnette Doan-Wiggins.

References

1. Centers for Disease Control and Prevention. Achievements in public health, 1900–1999: healthier mothers and babies. *MMWR Morb Mortal Wkly Rep* 1999;48:849–858.
2. Bruner JP, Drummond SB, Meenan AL, Gaskin IM. All-fours maneuver for reducing shoulder dystocia during labor. *J Reprod Med* 1998;43:439–443.
3. Brunette DD, Sterner SP. Prehospital and emergency department delivery: a review of eight years experience. *Ann Emerg Med* 1989;18:1116–1118.
4. Centers for Disease Control and Prevention. Maternal mortality—United States, 1982–1996. *JAMA* 1998;280:1042–1043.
5. Cox SM, Williams M, Leveno KJ. The natural history of preterm ruptured membranes: what to expect of expectant management. *Obstet Gynecol* 1988;71:558–562.
6. Cunningham FG, Lindheimer MD. Hypertension in pregnancy. *N Engl J Med* 1992;326:927–932.
7. Di Benedetto MR, Piazze JJ, Unfer V, et al. An obstetric and neonatal study on unplanned deliveries before arrival at hospital. *Clin Exp Obstet Gynecol* 1996;23:108–111.
8. Doan-Wiggins L. Emergency delivery and related topics. In: Hardwood-Nuss AL, et al., eds. *The clinical practice of emergency medicine.* 3rd ed. Philadelphia: Lippincott, Williams & Wilkins, 2001;367–373.
9. Gianopoulos JG. Emergency complications of labor and delivery. *Emerg Med Clin North Am* 1994;12:201–217.
10. Hansen WF, Hansen AR. Problems in pregnancy. In: Tintinalli JE, Ruiz E, Krome RL, eds. *Emergency medicine: a comprehensive study quide.* 4th ed. New York: McGraw-Hill, 1996;564–575.
11. Higgins SD. Emergency delivery: prehospital care, emergency department delivery, perimortem salvage. *Emerg Med Clin North Am* 1987;5:529–540.
12. Katz Z, Shoham Z, Lancet M, et al. Management of labor with umbilical cord prolapse: a 5-year study. *Obstet Gynecol* 1988;72:278–281.
13. Mallon W, Henderson S. Labor and delivery. In: Marx J, Hockberger R, Walls R, eds. *Rosen's emergency medicine: concepts and clinical practice.* 5th ed. Saint Louis: Mosby, Inc., 2002;2460–2484.
14. Mendelson M, Abbott JT. Emergency delivery and related topics. In: Harwood-Nuss AL, Linden CH, Luten RC, et al., eds. *The clinical practice of emergency medicine,* 2nd ed. Philadelphia: Lippincott-Raven, 1996;326–331.
15. Moscovitz HC, Magriples U, Keissling M, Schriver JA. Care and outcome of out-of-hospital deliveries. *Acad Emerg Med* 2000;7:757–761.
16. Murphy DJ, MacKenzie IZ. The mortality and morbidity associated with umbilical cord prolapse. *Br J Obstet Gynecol* 1995;102:826–830.
17. Naef RW, Morrison JC. Guidelines for management of shoulder dystocia. *J Perinatol* 1994;14:435–441.
18. Neufeld JDG, Moore EE, Marx JA, Rosen P. Trauma in pregnancy. *Emerg Med Clin North Am* 1987;5:623–640.
19. Paneth N, Kiely JL, Wallenstein S, Susser M. The choice of place of delivery. *Am J Dis Child* 1987;141:60–64.
20. Scott JR, Di Saia PJ, Hammond CB, Spellacy WN, eds. *Danforth's obstetrics and gynecology,* 8th ed. Philadelphia: Lippincott Williams & Wilkins, 1999.
21. Stallard TC, Burns B. Emergency delivery and perimortem C-section. *Emerg Med Clin North Am* 2003;21:679–693.
22. Verdile VP, Tutsock G, Paris PM, Kennedy RA. Out-of-hospital deliveries: a five-year experience. *Prehospital Disaster Med* 1995;10:10–13.
23. von Oeyen PT. Emergency delivery. In: Tintinalli JE, Ruiz E, Krome RL, eds. *Emergency medicine: a comprehensive study guide.* 4th ed. New York: McGraw-Hill, 1996;578–582.
24. Weir PE, Beischer NA. Birth before arrival in hospital. *Med J Aust* 1980;2:31–33.

CHAPTER 100
Postpartum Emergencies

Moss H. Mendelson and Joseph Lang

TABLE 100.1.   Causes of Postpartum Hemorrhage
EARLY HEMORRHAGE (<24 Hours)
Uterine atony
Genital tract laceration
Retained placental parts
Placenta accreta
Hematoma
Uterine inversion
Uterine rupture
Coagulopathy
LATE HEMORRHAGE (UP TO 6 WEEKS)
Infection (endometritis)
Retained placental parts
Delayed placental site involution
Sloughing of placental site eschar

Postpartum patients can present to the emergency department with any of a diverse number of diseases that are common in the postpartum period. Anatomic and physiologic changes before, during, and after delivery predispose to most of them. Many of these problems are life-threatening.

In the third trimester, maternal blood volume is 35% to 50% higher than normal, the plasma volume is increased by 1,200 mL, and the red blood cell volume by 250 mL. Cardiac output is increased by about 1.5 L per minute; 600 mL per minute of blood flows through the placental site at term. Consequently, uterine and ovarian veins handle a 60-fold increase in volume during pregnancy. In addition, the hypercoagulable state of pregnancy and the trauma from delivery predispose to disseminated thrombosis in the puerperium, experienced as deep venous thrombosis (DVT) or cerebrovascular accident.

The postpartum uterus returns to its nonpregnant anatomic shape and position by loss of cellular fluid and protein and consequent reduction in cell size. Most involution (about 40%) occurs in the first week postpartum. The uterus resumes its intrapelvic position by 2 weeks and normal size by palpation at 6 weeks postpartum. The mean time to ovulation is 70 to 75 days in nonlactating mothers and 190 days in those who lactate. Vaginal bleeding generally diminishes several hours after delivery to a red-brown discharge, which may last through day 3 or 4 postpartum. A mucopurulent discharge may wax and wane over 4 to 6 weeks. Menstruation resumes by about 12 weeks in most nonlactating women (mean, 7 to 9 weeks) but may be delayed in breastfeeding mothers up to 36 months (8).

POSTPARTUM HEMORRHAGE

CLINICAL PRESENTATION

Postpartum hemorrhage may be divided into early (less than 24 hours) and late (greater than 24 hours, less than 6 weeks) presentations (Table 100.1). Early postpartum hemorrhage is most often due to uterine atony. Bleeding can be brisk, and shock can develop rapidly. Maternal vital signs are often falsely reassuring, and blood loss can be hidden within the uterus and/or pelvis, making recognition of significant bleeding difficult in some cases. Late causes of hemorrhage include infection, delay in placental site involution, and retained placental parts. There may also be a normal, transient increase in bleeding in the second postpartum week due to sloughing of the eschar that covers the placental attachment site (10).

DIFFERENTIAL DIAGNOSIS

Early Postpartum Hemorrhage

Uterine atony is responsible for most cases of early postpartum hemorrhage. Failure of the uterus to contract properly allows continued blood loss from the placental site. Myome-

trial dysfunction occurs more frequently if the uterus has been overdistended (multiple gestations, hydramnios, multiparity, and macrosomia); if there has been precipitous or prolonged labor, general anesthesia, or previous postpartum hemorrhage; if leiomyomas or amnionitis is present; or if fetal demise or amniotic fluid embolus occurs. Adherent fragments of placenta can also interfere with myometrial contractile function.

Minor *pelvic trauma* occurs in almost all deliveries. However, some vaginal and cervical lacerations may lead to severe hemorrhage. Pelvic vessels can be injured in the process of delivery, causing a pelvic hematoma. Vulvar hematomas are the most common; because the bleeding is bounded by superficial fascial planes, the hematoma usually dissects to the skin and is visible. Deeper vaginal hematomas can be occult and accumulate a significant amount of blood, distending into the pelvic space under the peritoneum. Patients may present with complaints of rectal pressure. Retroperitoneal hematomas are the least common but most dangerous type of hemorrhage. They are associated with significant blood loss, usually the result of trauma to a branch of the hypogastric artery, and can present with shock.

Retained placenta is a common cause of both immediate and late postpartum hemorrhage. Premature, assisted delivery of the placenta increases the risk for retained fragments, which can result in impairment of full uterine contraction and failure to develop hemostasis. *Placenta accreta*, an abnormally deep attachment of the placenta to the myometrium, is suspected if placental delivery is difficult and no cleavage plane between placenta and uterus is found at manual exploration (8).

Uterine inversion is uncommon (12). Inversion is usually recognized soon after delivery of the placenta, and is more likely if traction is exerted on the umbilical cord. If the uterine corpus passes through the cervix, the inversion is complete; if not, it is incomplete, and may be occult. The patient presents with acute onset of abdominal pain, hemorrhage (average loss, 2 L), and shock. Often, hypotension occurs before significant visible blood loss (22).

Uterine rupture can be catastrophic and often results in fetal and even maternal demise, although the clinical spectrum of morbidity is broad. Factors associated with a rupture include previous curettage, cesarean section (especially with a high uterine incision) or rupture, hydramnios, multiple fetuses, and placenta accreta. Although more common in a previously scarred uterus, rupture of the nonscarred uterus does occur.

Coagulopathy can complicate postpartum hemorrhage that occurs from any source. In addition, abruption, amniotic fluid embolus, and pregnancy-induced hypertensive disease can cause consumptive coagulopathy, thereby leading to postpartum hemorrhage.

Late Postpartum Hemorrhage

The differential diagnosis of late postpartum hemorrhage includes endometritis, retained placental parts, placental site subinvolution or eschar sloughing, and resumption of menses (10).

EMERGENCY DEPARTMENT EVALUATION

The evaluation of the patient with postpartum bleeding should begin with an assessment of the extent of blood loss and concomitant resuscitation if hypovolemia and/or shock are present. In all cases of significant immediate postpartum bleeding, laboratory studies should include a complete blood count and coagulation studies. Early establishment of vascular access is critical. The patient is typed and crossmatched, and fresh-frozen plasma should be available.

Abdominal and bimanual examinations are necessary to identify the size, position, shape, and tone of the uterus, and the placenta (if available) should be inspected for completeness.

Ultrasonography may aid in narrowing the differential in stable patients with both early and late postpartum hemorrhage. Ultrasound of the uterine cavity can be used to help rule out retained placental tissue by demonstrating a normal uterine stripe. Ultrasound may also be able to distinguish between retained tissue (echogenic mass) and a large intrauterine clot (sonolucent). Occult hematomas can be identified and those patients rapidly triaged to angiography and subsequent embolization. Computed tomography (CT) scanning, although more time-consuming, may also show hematomas that would be amenable to percutaneous drainage (15). It is unclear whether the advent of rapid spiral CT scanning will change imaging algorithms for patients with postpartum hemorrhage.

EMERGENCY DEPARTMENT MANAGEMENT

Patients with significant blood loss require aggressive resuscitation with i.v. fluids and blood as needed. If the uterus feels boggy and *uterine atony* is suspected, manual massage is performed: One hand massages in a circular fashion on the abdomen, with intravaginal fingers massaging the uterus upward. Massage may cause temporary uterine contraction, with recurrent bleeding after relaxation (6). Pharmacologic treatment (Table 100.2), started concomitantly, includes drugs that increase uterine muscular tone (oxytocin, prostaglandins, and ergot alkaloids). Intravenous infusion of oxytocin is first-line treatment.

If bleeding continues, the birth canal should be inspected for trauma. Vaginal or cervical lacerations longer than 2 cm or those that are bleeding are repaired. Adequate exposure is needed, which can require general anesthesia. With persistent bleeding or a placenta that appears incomplete, digital exploration of the uterine cavity may be indicated to look for retained placental fragments or uterine rupture. If placental elements remain, an obstetrician is consulted for uterine cavity curettage (6).

Management of *uterine inversion* includes manual restoration of uterine anatomy, followed by removal of the placenta if it remains attached. Manual replacement through the vagina is usually successful. The uterus is compressed between both hands intravaginally and gradually replaced. General anesthesia or tocolytics may be required to allow adequate uterine relaxation. Only after replacement of the uterus is oxytocin started (22).

Refractory bleeding from any source may require emergent surgical intervention or arterial catheterization and embolization. Uterine rupture, once diagnosed, almost always requires surgery. Retroperitoneal hematomas frequently require surgery or embolization. Increasingly, angiographic embolization is being utilized in refractory cases of bleeding. Very high success rates for embolization have been cited, even cases that have failed traditional surgical intervention. Availability (time to catheter placement) and comfort and skill levels of the personnel involved can influence its use (3).

Traditional therapy of late postpartum hemorrhage has been curettage. However, placental tissue is often not retrieved, and bleeding may worsen after the procedure. With the ability of uterine ultrasound to rule out retained placental parts, initial therapy now relies on pharmacologic management, using the drugs in Table 100.2. If bleeding stops, the patient is observed. Curettage may be indicated if bleeding persists or if retained placenta is seen by ultrasound (6).

CRITICAL INTERVENTIONS

- Initiate uterine massage and oxytocin therapy for suspected uterine atony
- Resuscitate hypovolemic patients with i.v. fluids and blood products as needed

DISPOSITION

Many causes of early postpartum hemorrhage are best treated in the labor and delivery suite, where obstetric surgical facilities, including general anesthesia and skilled personnel, are available. The disposition of a patient with late postpartum hemorrhage depends on the amount of bleeding, the response to initial therapy, and the probable cause of the bleeding. Decisions are best made in consultation with the patient's obstetrician.

TABLE 100.2.   Medical Management of Uterine Atony

Drug	I.M. Dose	I.V. Administration	Side Effects
Oxytocin	10 U	20–30 U in 1 L normal saline at 200 mL/hour	Hypotension if given as bolus; cramping
Ergonovine maleate	0.2 mg		Cramping
Methylergonovine	0.2 mg		Cramping
15-Methyl-prostaglandin	0.25 mg		Nausea and vomiting

I.M., intramuscular; I.V., intravenous.

COMMON PITFALLS

✔ Visually estimating blood loss is not an accurate method; young women may have significant blood loss without developing typical signs of hypovolemia, making recognition of significant bleeding difficult in some cases

✔ Intravenous boluses of oxytocin can cause hypotension

✔ Uterine atony is the most common cause of postpartum hemorrhage; if it responds rapidly to manual massage, oxytocin should be given as well to prevent subsequent relaxation

✔ Genital tract lacerations are the second most common cause of postpartum hemorrhage; blood loss may be excessive if these are not considered and ruled out by visual inspection early on

PUERPERAL FEVER

CLINICAL PRESENTATION

Fever in the postpartum period may be classified as early (less than 48 hours) or late (greater than 48 hours, less than 6 weeks). Patients may present with symptoms and signs that make the diagnosis obvious, such as findings associated with respiratory or urinary tract infection. Many causes of puerperal fever, however, have nonspecific presentations. Lower abdominal pain may be due to persistent contractions or inflammation. Vaginal discharge can be scant or profuse in the face of metritis or normal involution. Abdominal tenderness and foul-smelling lochia are nonspecific signs, as are tachycardia and decreased bowel sounds. Wound sites should always be examined for tenderness, dehiscence, induration, edema, erythema, and discoloration (18). Mastitis presents initially with fever, flu-like symptoms, and, usually, a localized, painful site in the affected breast, with erythema and induration. Septic thrombophlebitis may present with refractory fever or symptoms of pulmonary embolism (PE).

DIFFERENTIAL DIAGNOSIS

Early infections (within 48 hours) most often occur in the uterus and peritoneum following cesarean section (often polymicrobial) or are related to the urinary or respiratory tracts. Late infections (after more than 48 hours) include uterine infection following vaginal delivery (usually the result of ascending endogenous organisms), abdominal and episiotomy wound infections, breast infections, and complications of uterine infection (such as abscess or thrombophlebitis). Table 100.3 outlines common causes of puerperal fever.

Endometritis is infection of the endometrium (the decidua and adjacent myometrium), but often the process extends beyond the uterus into the parametrial tissue, causing a diffuse pelvic cellulitis. The incidence of postpartum uterine infection is 1% to 6% in vaginally delivered women (6). Cesarean section increases both the frequency and the severity of infection: Endometritis occurs in up to 10% to 20% of patients undergoing cesarean section, despite prophylactic antibiotics (16). Other risk factors include premature rupture of membranes, prolonged time from rupture of membranes to delivery, the number of cervical examinations performed, intrauterine manipulation, preterm labor, and low socioeconomic status. Endometritis can lead to sepsis, peritonitis (rare), adnexal infections (most often perisalpingitis), pelvic abscess, septic pelvic thrombophlebitis, parametrial phlegmon, and toxic shock syndrome.

Most endometritis is the result of ascending (polymicrobial) infection of normal cervicovaginal flora or preexisting geni-

TABLE 100.3.   Causes of Puerperal Fever

Site	Examples	Comment
Pelvic	Endometritis	Single most common cause of puerperal fever; suspect especially after cesarean section
	Wound infection	Requires local exploration and opening
	Fasciitis	
	Pelvic abscess	Diagnosed by ultrasound
	Septic thrombophlebitis	Suspect with failure to respond to antibiotics for endometritis
Urinary	Pyelonephritis	Catheterized UA for diagnosis
Pulmonary	Atelectasis	Consider aspiration if general anesthesia
	Pneumonia	
Breast	Engorgement	Within 24–28 hours; diffuse, bilateral erythema and distention
	Milk stasis	
	Mastitis	Fever, flu-like symptoms; focal erythema and tenderness
Other	Breast abscess	
	Bacteremia	
	Sepsis	
	Endocarditis	
	I.V. site	
	Viral syndrome	

UA, urinalysis; I.V., intravenous.

tal tract infection. The placental attachment site and the tissue trauma associated with delivery provide good growth media for bacteria. Infections are often polymicrobial.

Wound infections complicate 1.5% to 13.0% of deliveries. Most infections are caused by skin or genital tract flora. Common pathogens include *Staphylococcus aureus*, groups A and B streptococci, *Escherichia coli*, *Proteus* species, and anaerobes (especially *Clostridium* and *Bacteroides*). If cesarean section is performed emergently or amnionitis is present, a higher rate of wound infection is noted. Many patients initially are diagnosed with endometritis, but despite antibiotic therapy continue to spike temperatures because they require debridement and drainage. Complications of wound infection include synergistic bacterial gangrene (especially with clostridial species), necrotizing fasciitis (most commonly a group A β-hemolytic streptococcal infection), wound dehiscence, and toxic shock syndrome.

Episiotomy and pelvic floor infections complicate less than 1% of deliveries. The fascial anatomy dictates the depth and spread of the infection and may obscure the findings. Causative bacteria include streptococci and staphylococci, gram-negative enterics, and *Bacteroides* species. Most infections are superficial and mild, limited to the skin and superficial fascia in the area adjacent to the episiotomy. More extensive disease can involve Scarpa fascia, causing a potentially life-threatening necrotizing fasciitis (8).

Septic pelvic thrombophlebitis develops from an infection of the placental site and associated thrombosed myometrial veins. Once established, the process can proceed beyond the local venous system to include the vena cava. Most often the process is unilateral, usually right-sided. Septic pelvic thrombophlebitis is most common following cesarean section (6).

One percent to 2% of postpartum women develop mastitis, which is usually seen between weeks 2 and 6 after delivery. *S. aureus* is the most common causative agent.

Engorgement of the breasts consists of distended, firm, nodular breasts in the first 24 to 48 hours postpartum, while lacteal secretion is developing. The condition is painful and often associated with mild transient fever. Milk stasis is the result of incomplete emptying of the milk glands. This noninfectious process can complicate the evaluation of the febrile postpartum patient and can progress to sporadic infectious mastitis.

EMERGENCY DEPARTMENT EVALUATION

After a detailed obstetric history is taken, the examination focuses on the genital tract, wounds, the breasts, and the urinary and respiratory systems. Examination may reveal tenderness of the lower abdomen and a purulent or foul-smelling lochia. The uterus may be tender and boggy, with parametrial thickening. If an adnexal mass is palpable, it might represent an abscess or an infected hematoma. The entire perineum and genital tract are inspected for signs of infection from a laceration or episiotomy. A rectovaginal examination should help identify parametritis or other abscesses or hematomas.

Laboratory evaluation should include blood cultures, a complete blood count, and a urinalysis. Endometrial culture should be considered but may be difficult to interpret because of cervical contamination. Chest X-ray may be indicated; plain films of the pelvis may reveal soft-tissue gas if fasciitis is present.

Imaging studies may be helpful in puerperal fever, particularly when the source is unclear or there is no clinical response to 48 to 72 hours of appropriate antibiotic therapy. CT scanning in endometritis shows intrauterine debris, fluid, and gas in some patients. Ultrasound may reveal endometrial gas, which is sometimes associated with infection but is also seen in clinically well women. Ultrasound, CT scanning, and magnetic resonance imaging can be helpful in the diagnosis of several occult, intrapelvic, infectious sources, such as abscess, infected hematoma, and septic thrombus. Generally, ultrasound is the first-line test of choice; a CT scan can be performed if initial ultrasound is negative. Pelvic venography may be required to diagnose septic thromboses (20,23).

EMERGENCY DEPARTMENT MANAGEMENT

Endometritis is treated empirically. If the patient is toxic or has underlying medical problems (e.g., diabetes) or the clinician suspects anaerobic infection, clindamycin and gentamicin or clindamycin and a third-generation cephalosporin are given. Ampicillin–sulbactam (Unasyn), ticarcillin–clavulanate (Timentin), piperacillin-tazobactam (Zosyn), and imipenem-cilastatin (Primaxin) are all effective single, broad-spectrum antibiotics (7). Data on the outpatient treatment of endometritis are limited. Most patients will require admission, although in some with mild late disease, oral agents can be appropriate. Consultation with an obstetrician is prudent prior to discharge.

Treatment of wound infection may include opening and debriding the area under adequate anesthesia. If more than local cellulitis is suspected, exploration under general anesthesia should be considered (18). Fascial necrosis is a surgical emergency requiring immediate consultation. Mortality approaches 100% in patients treated with antibiotics alone and drops to 50% with combined surgical and pharmacologic treatment. Abscesses and some superficial hematomas can be incised and drained.

If *septic thrombophlebitis* is suspected, anticoagulation and antibiotics for 7 to 10 days are usually necessary. The incidence of heparin-related bleeding in the postpartum state is low (1% to 2%) (8).

Mastitis is usually treated with dicloxacillin or clindamycin orally, along with continued emptying of the breast. With prompt treatment, mastitis usually resolves within 48 hours. Breast feed-

ing can continue unless an abscess has formed. If an abscess has occurred, incision and drainage is necessary and breast feeding should stop. If milk stasis develops without infection, more efficient emptying of the breast is needed. Nursing should continue, and treatment includes breast support, ice, and analgesia. If the patient is not breastfeeding, and conservative methods are not sufficient for relief of pain, suppression of lactation may be helpful. Bromocriptine has been withdrawn for lactation suppression, but other agents are available. Consultation with the obstetric service is indicated.

CRITICAL INTERVENTIONS

- Initiate parenteral broad-spectrum antibiotic therapy for febrile postpartum patients with endometritis
- Order imaging studies such as ultrasound or CT for the patient with a suspected pelvic abscess

DISPOSITION

The disposition varies with the type and severity of illness. If the patient is toxic (from any source), inpatient parenteral antibiotic therapy is indicated. Patients with abscesses, septic thrombophlebitis, or complicated wound infections also require inpatient therapy.

COMMON PITFALLS

✔ Necrotizing fasciitis is life-threatening; it requires emergent surgical consultation, aggressive debridement, and antibiotic therapy. Despite prompt, appropriate treatment, mortality is high

✔ Failing to consider nongynecologic sources of postoperative infections, such as urinary tract infection, may lead to a delay in diagnosis

✔ Do not assume that breast pain and fever in the first 2 to 4 days postpartum are caused by mastitis. Engorgement often causes these symptoms and does not require antimicrobials

HYPERTENSIVE DISEASE

Pregnancy-related hypertension is classified as preeclampsia and eclampsia, chronic hypertension, preeclampsia superimposed on chronic hypertension, and transient hypertension (5). The occurrence of these diseases antepartum is discussed in Chapter 97, "Hypertensive Disorders of Pregnancy." However, it should be noted that preeclampsia and eclampsia can both occur postpartum. Treatment is the same as for antepartum patients. New onset preeclampsia or eclampsia require admission to the hospital and should be managed along with an obstetrician.

NEUROLOGIC AND ENDOCRINE DISEASE

The onset of many diseases occurs during the weeks after delivery, including previously subclinical thyroid disease. Postpartum ischemic necrosis of the anterior pituitary (*Sheehan syndrome*) may develop if severe postpartum hemorrhage with shock has occurred.

In general, the presentation and underlying pathologies of postpartum headache are similar to those in other patients, but the clinician should keep in mind causes that could be related to the recent delivery. Headache can be secondary to elevated blood pressure, and can herald the onset of postpartum preeclampsia. Patients who have had spinal anesthesia during labor can have a persistent cerebrospinal fluid (CSF) leak that requires a blood patch. Patients with migraine headaches prior to pregnancy often note that headaches improve during pregnancy, presumably because of increasing levels of circulating estrogen. Patients with benign postpartum headaches are generally treated in the same manner as other headache patients unless they are breastfeeding: ergot alkaloids are contraindicated in the nursing mother.

The risk of both hemorrhagic and ischemic stroke is at its maximum in the 6 weeks postpartum, and stroke remains responsible for a significant number of maternal deaths. The increased risk of ischemic stroke seems to result from spontaneous thrombosis, possibly related to heightened coagulability. Predisposing factors such as preeclampsia, chronic hypertension, diabetes, and hypotensive episodes are found in about one third of patients. Embolic sources should also be considered in pregnant patients suffering an acute ischemic stroke (11). CT scanning, followed by lumbar puncture if needed, is used to exclude hemorrhage. *Cortical venous thrombosis* is also reported, particularly 1 to 4 weeks postpartum. Initial symptoms are variable and may include headache, lethargy, and vomiting. Seizures are common (up to 30%), and hemiplegia may occur (gradual onset). Care is supportive, although prophylactic anticonvulsant therapy is usually given. Most authors do not recommend anticoagulation, as bleeding frequently follows clot resolution. Mortality may be as high as 20%, despite aggressive supportive treatment (17).

In a distinct syndrome known as *postpartum cerebral angiopathy*, the patient presents with headache, vomiting, seizures, and focal neurologic signs. Angiography shows multiple areas of segmental narrowing in the cerebral arteries; these usually clear spontaneously. Finally, postpartum women also have an increased incidence of idiopathic *Bell palsy*. The course and expression of the disease are unaltered by pregnancy.

THROMBOEMBOLIC DISEASE

The risk of thromboembolic disease in pregnancy is roughly 5 times higher than in the nonpregnant population. Although most thromboses develop in the antepartum period, recent data indicate that two thirds of pulmonary emboli occur in the postpartum period. PE remains a significant cause of maternal death. Diagnosing deep venous thrombosis (DVT) and PE can be difficult in the puerperium. Leg edema and calf soreness are common postpartum. Pelvic thrombosis is often clinically silent until PE occurs. See Chapters 38 ("Pulmonary Embolism") and 98 ("Emergencies of Late Pregnancy") for further discussion of PE.

PERIPARTUM CARDIOMYOPATHY

Peripartum cardiomyopathy is the development of cardiac failure in the last month of pregnancy or in the first 5 postpartum months, in the absence of an identifiable cause for the cardiac failure or of prior demonstrable heart disease. The incidence is reported to be between one in 1,300 and one in 15,000 deliveries. Ninety-seven percent present in the first 2 postpartum months. The disease is more common in older multiparous women and in patients with twin gestations. Patients often have superimposed preeclampsia, obesity, or coexisting obstetric infection or anemia. Clinically, patients present with left ventricular failure. Renal insufficiency can also be seen. Most patients have nonspecific but abnormal electrocardiograms, demonstrating ST-T wave changes, left ventricular hypertrophy or bundle-branch block,

atrial fibrillation, and atrial and ventricular premature contractions. An echocardiogram shows four-chamber enlargement and abnormalities of left ventricular contractility. The workup is directed at excluding other causes of heart failure. Primary therapy is bedrest, sodium restriction, digoxin, and diuretics. Anticoagulation is considered if cardiac dilation is pronounced. Patients can become refractory to medical management, and overall maternal mortality ranges from 25% to 50% in the long term. Ten percent to 20% of patients die during their first hospitalization. If the heart size returns to normal, the prognosis is good; cardiomyopathy that persists after 6 months is a poor prognostic sign. PE is a common complication (9).

POSTPARTUM PSYCHIATRIC DISEASE

A woman's risk of psychiatric admission peaks in the first postpartum year. Fifty percent to 70% of postpartum patients experience "maternity blues." Typically starting on postpartum day 3 or 4, this is a mild depression most prevalent in the first 2 weeks. It is probably a normal reaction to the stresses of childbirth. Common symptoms include tearfulness, irritability, and lability.

Clinical depression occurs in about 7% to 10% of women; in half of these patients, the symptoms were not present during or before the pregnancy. Risk factors include maternal personality traits such as anxiety, neuroticism, and cognitive style; poor marital adjustment; poor social support systems; and an excess of life events. Stresses during the pregnancy and labor may also contribute (4,21).

Postpartum psychosis is rare (0.25% incidence). Usually, the disease has a rapid onset in the first few days postpartum; mania is a common presentation. Postpartum psychosis is thought to represent exacerbation of preexisting disease. The duration of illness is usually 2 to 3 months (8).

References

1. AGOC Committee Opinion: safety of Lovenox in pregnancy. *Obstet Gynecol* 2002;100:845–846.
2. Briggs GG, Freeman RK, Yaffe SJ. *Drugs in pregnancy and lactation*, 6th ed. Baltimore: Lippincott Williams & Wilkins, 2002.
3. Chung JW, Jeong HJ, Joh JH, et al. Percutaneous transcatheter angiographic embolization in the management of obstetric hemorrhage. *J Reprod Med* 2003;48:268.
4. Cox JL, Murray D, Chapman G. A controlled study of the onset, duration and prevalence of postnatal depression. *Br J Psychol* 1993;163:27.
5. Cunningham FG, Lindheimer MD. Hypertension in pregnancy. *N Engl J Med* 1992;326:927.
6. Cunningham FG, MacDonald PC, Gant NF, et al., eds. *Williams' obstetrics*, 19th ed. Norwalk, CT: Appleton & Lange, 1993.
7. French LM, Smaill FM. Antibiotic regimens for endometritis after delivery. *Cochrane Database Syst Rev* 2002;1:CD001067.
8. Gabbe SG, Nielbyl JR, Simpson JL, eds. *Obstetrics: normal and problem pregnancies*. New York: Churchill-Livingstone, 1986.
9. Homans DC. Peripartum cardiomyopathy. *N Engl J Med* 1985;312:1432.
10. Khong TY, Khong TK. Delayed postpartum hemorrhage: a morphological study of causes and their relation to other pregnancy disorders. *Obstet Gynecol* 1993;82:17.
11. Kittner SJ, Stern BJ, Feeser BR, et al. Pregnancy and the risk of stroke. *N Engl J Med* 1996;335:768.
12. Lago J. Presentation of acute uterine inversion in the emergency department. *Am J Emerg Med* 1991;9:239.
13. Marcus DA, Scharff L, Turk D. Longitudinal prospective study of headache during pregnancy and postpartum. *Headache* 1999;39:625.
14. Scharff L, Marcus DA, Turk DC. Headache during pregnancy and postpartum: a prospective study. *Headache* 1997;37:203.
15. Sherer DM, Abulafia O, Anyaegbunam AM. Intra- and early postpartum ultrasonography: a review. Part II. *Obstet Gynecol Surv* 1998;53:181.
16. Smaill F, Hofmeyr GJ. Antibiotic prophylaxis for cesarean section. *Cochrane Database Syst Rev* 2002;3:CD000933.
17. Smolke GA, Cox SM, Cunningham FG. Cerebrovascular accidents complicating pregnancy and the puerperium. *Obstet Gynecol* 1991;78:37.
18. Soper DE, Brockwell NJ, Dalton HP. The importance of wound infection in antibiotic failures in the therapy of postpartum endometritis. *Surg Gynecol Obstet* 1992;174:265.

19. Toglia MR, Weg JG. Venous thromboembolism during pregnancy. *N Engl J Med* 1996;335:108.
20. Urban BA, Pankov BL, Fishman EK. Postpartum complications in the abdomen and pelvis: CT evaluation. *Crit Rev Diagn Imaging* 1999;40:1.
21. Wolman WL, Chalmers B, Hofmeyr GJ, et al. Postpartum depression and companionship in the clinical birth environment: a randomized, controlled study. *Am J Obstet Gynecol* 1993;168:1388.
22. Zahn CM, Yeomans ER. Postpartum hemorrhage: placenta accreta, uterine inversion and puerperal hematomas. *Clin Obstet Gynecol* 1990;33:422.
23. Zuckerman J, Levine D, McNicholas MM, et al. Imaging of pelvic postpartum complications. *AJR Am J Roentgenol* 1997;168:663.

CHAPTER 101
Drugs in Pregnancy and Lactation

David H. Adler and Flavia Nobay

The management of emergency medical conditions in pregnant women requires a thorough understanding of the risks and benefits of the use of pharmacologic agents during all stages of pregnancy. The risk of uncontrolled systemic disease in the pregnant woman must be considered while the emergency physician balances the need to treat with the potential adverse effects on the developing fetus. This chapter will address the relative safety of pharmacologic therapy that the emergency physician is likely to consider using in the pregnant patient and the management of common medical diseases and infections during pregnancy.

TERATOLOGY

Major malformations occur in 2% to 4% of all newborns, 1% of which can be attributed to the adverse effects of medications (47). The period from 4 to 12 weeks after the first day of the last menstrual period is the period of greatest susceptibility of the embryo to organ malformation (47). After this period of organogenesis, teratogens can still adversely affect the growth and function of organs. During the later stages of pregnancy drugs may adversely affect the fetus and newborn, causing complications during delivery or in the post-natal period (Table 101.1).

FDA CLASSIFICATION

In 1979, the U.S. Food and Drug Administration (FDA) developed a five-category classification system for risk of drugs to the developing fetus. These categories, however, are not perfect and have not been consistently updated to reflect advance in knowledge (30).

Category A. Controlled human studies have shown no risk to the fetus.
Category B. Either (1) animal studies have shown no risk and no human studies have been done, or (2) animal studies have

TABLE 101.1. Commonly Used Drugs That Are Contraindicated in Pregnancy

Condition	Drug	Use During Lactation
Analgesia	Salicylates	No
	Ibuprofen	Yes
Cardiac	Captopril	Yes
	Diltiazem	Yes
Infectious	Ciprofloxacin	No
	Fluconazole	Yes
	Sulfonamides*	Yes
	Tetracyclines	Yes
Endocrine	Oral hypoglycemics	Unknown
ENT	Diphenhydramine	No
	Pseudoephedrine	Yes
Psychiatric	Haldol	No
	Diazepam	Yes

*Do not use in third trimester.
ENT, ear nose and throat.

shown no adverse effects, but this has not been confirmed in humans.
Category C. Either (1) animal studies have shown an adverse effect and there are no controlled human studies, or (2) there are no studies in animals or humans.
Category D. There is a demonstrated human fetal risk, but the benefit of use may outweigh the risk.
Category X. Studies have demonstrated human risk and the risk outweighs any possible benefit.

Practically speaking, category B classification reflects the greatest safety we see. It is almost unheard of to have a category A classification, as studies on drug safety rarely are done in pregnant patients (Table 101.2). Drugs may have dual classification that reflects safe use during one period of pregnancy and unsafe use in another. Information services are available to physicians to assist in determining the safety of drugs in pregnancy:

Motherisk program: (416) 813-6780; www.motherisk.org
Organization of Teratology Information Services: (801) 328-2229; www.otispregancy.org

TREATMENT OF COMMON MEDICAL ILLNESSES DURING PREGNANCY

In general, when considering the use of medications in the pregnant patient, the physician should keep the following principles in mind: no drug should be prescribed without a clear indication, drug exposure should be minimized by using the smallest effective dose for the shortest duration possible, and effective drugs that have been in use for a long time and have well-understood safety profiles are preferable to newer medications.

PAIN

Analgesics, along with antibiotics and antiemetics, are the most commonly used drug in pregnancy (36).

Acetaminophen (category B) is the analgesic and antipyretic of choice throughout pregnancy—large population-based studies have demonstrated no increase in congenital malformations with its use (38,45).

Aspirin (category D) is commonly taken during pregnancy and readily crosses the placenta into the fetal circulation. Two large U.S. studies have failed to demonstrate significant fetal

TABLE 101.2.   Commonly Used Drugs Considered Relatively Safe During Pregnancy

Condition	Drug	Use during lactation
Analgesia	Acetaminophen	Yes
	Hydrocodone with acetaminophen	Unknown
		Yes
	Codeine*	Yes (in low doses)
	Meperidine*	Yes
	Methadone*	
Infectious	Penicillins	Unknown
	Cephalosporins	Yes
	Erythromycins (not estolate)	Yes
	Azithromycin	Unknown
	Clindamycin	Yes
	Nystatin	Yes
	Clotrimazole	Yes
	Metronidazole**	No
	Nitrofurantoin***	Yes
	Permetherin	Unknown
Cardiac	Labetalol	Yes
	Methyldopa	Yes
	Hydralazine	Yes
	Digoxin	Yes
	Adenosine	Unknown
	Lidocaine	Yes
ENT	Chlorpheniramine	Unknown
	Guaifenesin	Unknown
	Nasal steroids	Yes
	Nasal cromolyn	Yes
Gastrointestinal	Antacids	Unknown
	Simethicone	Unknown
	Cimetidine, famotidine, ranitidine	Yes
		No
	Metoclopramide	Yes (not salicylate)
	Bisacodyl docusate (not salicylate)	Unknown
		Unknown
	Doxylamine	Unknown
	Meclazine	
	Odansetron	
Pulmonary	See Table 101.1	
Psychiatric	Fluoxetine	No
	Desipramine	No
	Doxepin	No
Other	Heparin	Yes
	Insulin	Yes
	Prednisone	Yes

*Except in long term use or high doses, **Except in first trimester, ***Contraindicated at term and during labor and delivery.

risk from aspirin. The Collaborative Perinatal Project studied over 50,000 pregnancies and found no increase in stillbirth, reduced birth weight, teratology, or perinatal death among pregnant women exposed to low-dose aspirin (49). Likewise, the Michigan Medicaid Surveillance Study investigated 1,709 pregnancies with first trimester exposure to aspirin and found no increase in congenital malformations (43). High-dose aspirin in the second half of pregnancy, however, may be harmful. Given near to delivery, high-dose aspirin has been shown to increase the risk of infant bleeding, in particular central nervous system hemorrhage (43). The use of aspirin near term may also cause constriction or premature closure of the fetal ductus arteriosus owing to prostaglandin inhibition (44).

Nonsteroidal Antiinflammatory Drugs (NSAIDs) are prostaglandin inhibitors and have been associated with premature closure of the ductus, causing infantile pulmonary hypertension (44). Although the Michigan Medicaid Surveillance Study found no teratogenicity among more than 3,000

first-trimester exposures to ibuprofen, a reduction in amniotic fluid volume has been associated with NSAIDs (43). It does appear, however, that the adverse effects of NSAIDs on the ductus and amniotic fluid volume are reversible with discontinuation of the drug when used as a tocolytic (43). Overall the potential toxicity of NSAIDs is the basis for the recommendation that they be used with caution during pregnancy, and not during the third trimester.

Opiates. The use of morphine, meperidine, and oxycodone during pregnancy is considered safe (9), although the use of any opiate can produce respiratory and central nervous system (CNS) depression in the mother and newborn. Naloxone can safely reverse the effects of opiates in the newborn. Neonatal opiate addiction and withdrawal may result from chronic use of opiates during pregnancy (9). Codeine, methadone, and hydrocodone, although commonly prescribed, are all classified as category C drugs during pregnancy. Meperidine has not been reported to cause complications in therapeutic doses unless used during labor. It rapidly crosses the placenta and is found in cord blood within 2 minutes following intravenous administration and 30 minutes after intramuscular administration (21). It is considered risk category D if used for prolonged periods or in high doses at term.

ASTHMA

Asthma complicates 0.4% to 1.3% of pregnancies (24). Pregnancy itself has a variable impact on chronic asthma, although in patients with chronic severe asthma, pregnancy may cause worsening of the disease (23). Although in the past poorly controlled asthma was associated with increased fetal mortality, recent studies have shown that fetal loss can be reduced to that of the general population in asthmatic mothers who are managed with B2 agonists, theophylline, and corticosteroids (24,48) (Table 101.3). Furthermore, congenital malformation rates are not increased among infants of asthmatic mothers. It should be noted that the effects of pregnancy on pulmonary physiology include relative hypocapnia and frequently a slight respiratory alkalosis due to increased tidal volume. Arterial PCO_2 of 27 to 32 mm Hg is considered normal in pregnancy, and a PCO_2 of greater than 40 mm Hg is suggestive of ventilatory failure.

Evaluation of asthma in the pregnant patient is largely the same as that in the nonpregnant patient with two notable exceptions: first, as noted previously, baseline pH and PCO_2 are altered by pregnancy and the interpretation of arterial blood gas (ABG) results must take these effects into consideration; second, the decision of whether to obtain a chest radiograph in a pregnant woman is complicated by the potential adverse effects of

TABLE 101.3.   Medications Used to Treat Asthma During Pregnancy

CONSIDERED SAFE

Aminophylline	Theophylline
β-adrenergic agents	Tertbutaline, albuterol, Metaproterenol
Corticosteroids	Prednisone, prednisolone, Methylprednisolone

CONSIDERED CONTROVERSIAL

Sympathomimetics	Epinephrine

radiation on the developing fetus. Radiation has the potential to lead to birth defects during the first trimester, as well as to fetal growth retardation, microcephaly, and mental retardation (7). A routine single-view chest film exposes the fetus to less than 0.04 rads—an exposure of 5 rads or less is thought to be safe for the developing fetus (7). If the abdomen is appropriately shielded with a lead apron, radiation exposure to the fetus is negligible. It is important to remember that because of the elevation of the diaphragm during pregnancy, the cardiac silhouette may appear enlarged and lung markings increased, making the diagnosis of congestive heart failure more difficult.

β-adrenergic agonists are the initial treatment of choice in pregnancy. Albuterol (category C), metaproterenol, and terbutaline have been used safely in pregnancy and do not increase the risk of congenital malformation (18,47). These medications may cause fetal tachycardia as well as transient fetal hyperglycemia (9).

Epinephrine (category C) may reduce uterine blood flow in humans and has been shown to do so in animal studies (41). It has also been associated with an increase in fetal malformation when used early in pregnancy (27). Although selective B2 agonists are the preferred bronchodilators during pregnancy, epinephrine is only relatively contraindicated and may be used when all other agents fail.

Cromolyn (category B) inhibits histamine release from mast cells and is used as a prophylactic medication. No teratogenic or other adverse effects have been shown in both animal and human studies of cromolyn use throughout pregnancy (18,47,17).

Corticosteroids (category C) are important adjuncts in the management of asthma in the pregnant patient who does not exhibit adequate improvement with bronchodilator therapy and are considered more beneficial than the risk of poorly controlled disease (18,47). Aerosolized corticosteroids are the preferred preparation and are considered safe (18,47). Systemic corticosteroids have been shown to increase the risk of fetal malformations in certain animal species, but have been used extensively in humans during pregnancy and are not considered teratogenic (10). In general, steroids readily cross the placenta where they are rapidly converted to less active forms by the fetoplacental unit, although the active form of prednisone, prednisolone, crosses the placenta poorly and with resulting fetal levels that are lower than maternal levels.

DIABETES

Despite advances in the management of diabetes, perinatal mortality among infants of diabetic mothers remains 15% to 25% above that seen in the general population (1). Pregnancies among diabetic women are 3 to 5 times more likely to be complicated by preeclampsia (53). Likewise, the incidence of major malformations is three to four times higher in these infants. These anomalies are thought to be secondary to hyperglycemia during embryogenesis (26); therefore, maintaining a euglycemic state in pregnant diabetic women is of the utmost importance. Maternal glucose readily crosses into fetal circulation where it can result in fetal hyperinsulinemia (beginning late in the first trimester, fetal insulin production begins). Insulin acts as a potent fetal growth stimulus, and excessive fetal growth (macrosomia) may result in its attendant hazards of injury to the fetus or mother during delivery (34).

The developing fetus depends primarily on glucose for energy requirements and amino acids for protein synthesis. Fetal glucose levels are only 10 to 20 mg/dL less than maternal levels. In part owing to the siphoning of glucose by the fetus, maternal glucose levels after a 12 to 14 hour fast are 15 to 20 mg/dL lower during pregnancy. This results in a decreased maternal insulin release with a resulting elevated ketonemia. Even overnight fasting can result in maternal ketoacid levels that are up to 4 times higher than in the general population. This *accelerated starvation ketosis* is characterized by fasting hypoglycemia, decreased insulin concentration, and ketonemia and explains why pregnant women should have some caloric intake in the early mornings. This physiologic principle explains the increased risk of diabetic ketoacidosis (DKA) in pregnancy (13). During pregnancy, DKA often develops rapidly and can occur with relatively low serum glucose levels of 200 to 300 mg/dL. DKA during pregnancy is associated with a 50% fetal loss rate (13). The gravid patient with DKA generally presents with a fluid deficiency of 3 to 6 L, and correction of this profound hypovolemia is important to help reverse DKA. Rapid correction of acidosis in the pregnant woman is important because of the tremendous fetal risk from acidemia. Usually, bicarbonate is not given unless the pH is less than 7.10 and with values higher than this, *in utero* fetal resuscitation is done by correction of the hyperglycemia and fluid deficits.

Potassium deficits are similar to those of nongravid patients. Urine testing for glucose is not useful during pregnancy, since benign glucosuria is frequently found among nondiabetic pregnant patients. Therefore, capillary glucose testing is mandatory in the pregnant diabetic patient. Diabetes in pregnancy is, by definition, a high-risk situation. Optimal prenatal care requires the involvement of an obstetrician experienced in the management of diabetes in pregnancy or a maternal-fetal medicine specialist.

Gestational diabetes affects approximately 3% of pregnant women. Most patients with gestational diabetes do well with diet modifications and only 15% will require insulin therapy (28). In this pregnancy-related medical condition, patients cannot increase their insulin secretion to meet the demand of higher glucose concentrations compared to the nonpregnant state. Human placental lactogen production (HPL) is thought to cause insulin resistance in this condition, and, since HPL production is a reflection of placental mass, carbohydrate intolerance in gestational diabetes is generally not present until after 26 to 28 weeks of gestation. There is a low risk of fetal malformations because most of these women are euglycemic during early pregnancy—fetal macrosomia with resulting birth trauma is the major risk. Approximately 60% of patients with gestational diabetes develop overt diabetes later in life.

Oral hypoglycemic agents are contraindicated in pregnancy because they cross the placenta and may cause fetal hypoglycemia (9) and excessive fetal insulin secretion. Fetal hyperinsulinemia is associated with macrosomia, myocardial hyperplasia, stillbirth, and delayed lung maturation.

Insulin (category B) is safe in pregnancy (including long-acting preparations). Perinatal morbidity and mortality are related to the degree of glycemic control, and most diabetic women will require multiple daily injections of insulin to achieve this.

HYPERTENSION

Hypertension must be carefully managed during pregnancy. Although even mild chronic hypertension that is untreated increases the risk of fetal wastage, care must be taken not to overtreat the condition and cause maternal hypotension and resultant placental hypoperfusion (8,18). Fetal wastage in untreated severe hypertension (greater than 160/100 mm Hg) is as high as 40%. See Chapter 97, "Hypertensive Disorders of Pregnancy."

ACE Inhibitors (category C first trimester; category D second and third trimesters) should be avoided in pregnancy owing to the risk of fetal renal toxicity (8). Oligohydramnios, renal and cranial structural defects, and neonatal anuria have all been associated with angiotensin-converting enzyme (ACE) inhibitors.

β-**Blockers** (atenolol, category D; labetalol, metoprolol, category C) are sometimes used during pregnancy but do have associated risks. Atenolol may increase the risk of intrauterine growth retardation when started in the first trimester (18). Labetalol is not known to be teratogenic and has been shown to increase fetal pulmonary surfactant, which may be advantageous among premature infants (8,18). Newborns of mothers taking β-blockers should be monitored closely for neonatal bradycardia, respiratory depression, and hypoglycemia (16).

Calcium channel blockers (category C) should be used only as a last resort during pregnancy. Nifedipine has been shown to be teratogenic in animal models and intrauterine growth restriction (IUGR) and fetal death have been reported. Likewise, diltiazem has been associated with skeletal deformities in animal studies. Verapamil is considered the drug of choice within this category, but is still associated with the risk of maternal hypotension and placental hypoperfusion.

Thiazide diuretics (hydrochlorothiazide, category B) and **Furosemide** (category C) are not teratogenic but should be used with caution in pregnancy. An increased risk of perinatal mortality and congenital defects has been associated with these drugs, most likely a result of decreased maternal plasma volume and placental hypoperfusion (8,18).

Methyldopa (category B) is a commonly used antihypertensive medication during pregnancy and has not been shown to have any adverse fetal or neonatal effects. It is the drug of choice for managing chronic hypertension among pregnant women (18).

Hydralazine (category C) is the drug of choice for managing acute exacerbations of hypertension in pregnant women (8,18) (see Chapter 97, "Hypertensive Disorders of Pregnancy"). It is not associated with teratogenicity or IUGR. It is clear that the fetus has equal concentrations if not greater than the mother (35).

DYSRHYTHMIAS

All antidysrhythmic drugs cross the placenta (16). Still, several of these agents have long histories of safe use during pregnancy.

Digoxin (category C) is considered safe during pregnancy when given in appropriate doses, although digoxin toxicity has been associated with fetal death and miscarriage (16).

Adenosine (category C) is not associated with adverse fetal effects and is effective in terminating atrioventricular (AV) node–dependent tachydysrhythmias during pregnancy.

Amiodarone (category D) only crosses the placenta to a limited extent; however, it should only be used in pregnancy when absolutely necessary owing to several associated risks (16). The high iodine content of amiodarone is thought to be responsible for an association with neonatal goiter, hypothyroidism, and IUGR. Fetal bradydysrhythmias have also been associated with amiodarone use.

The Class 1A agents **Quinidine** and **procainamide** (category C) are considered safe in pregnancy (16). **Lidocaine** is thought to be safe in appropriate doses (category C), although large doses have been associated with low APGAR scores and neonatal lidocaine toxicity. **Ibutilide** has been demonstrated to be teratogenic in animal studies and is not recommended in pregnancy (16). Little information is available regarding the effects of **mexiletine**, **flecainide**, **propafenone**, and **sotalol**

during pregnancy, although none are known to be teratogens (16).

THROMBOEMBOLIC DISEASE

Pregnant women are at increased risk of deep venous thrombosis and pulmonary embolism.

Heparin (category C) is the anticoagulant of choice in pregnant patients (9). It does not cross the placenta and probably causes no direct risk to the fetus.

Warfarin (category X) is absolutely contraindicated in pregnancy because of its significant association with congenital malformations. The approximate risk of malformation caused by warfarin use is 30% (9). The highest risk occurs during the third month of gestation, although CNS malformations may result from exposure to warfarin during any stage of pregnancy.

Thrombolytics (category C) are relatively contraindicated in the pregnant patient. Although there are successful case reports, the risk of antepartum hemorrhage is considered to be significant.

SEIZURE DISORDERS

The treatment of seizure disorders during pregnancy requires a particularly nuanced risk–benefit analysis. Although seizures increase the risk of miscarriage and hypoxic injury to the fetus (there are case reports of fetal demise after a single maternal seizure) (54), the risk of birth defects in women taking a single antiepileptic medication is double that of the general population (15). This teratogenic risk is increased with the use of multiple antiepileptic medications (15). For these reasons, women who require pharmacologic management of seizure disorders are best treated with a single agent at the lowest effective dose.

Phenytoin is a human teratogen and is categorized as category D. Fetal exposure to phenytoin is associated with a 7% to 10% risk of IUGR, motor and developmental delays, facial dysmorphia, and limb abnormalities (18). Up to 3% may have major craniofacial abnormalities such as cleft lip, cleft palate, and microcephaly (18). Pregnant women who require treatment with phenytoin are generally also treated with vitamin K and folic acid to decrease the respective risks of neonatal coagulopathy, and neural cord defects (15,18) resulting from the decrease in these substances that is associated with phenytoin.

Phenobarbital may also contribute to folic acid deficiency and neonatal coagulopathy (18). Although categorized as a category D agent, no conclusive evidence of teratogenicity has been demonstrated (18). Still, respiratory depression and barbiturate withdrawal symptoms may be seen in the neonate exposed to phenobarbital during late gestation.

Carbamazepine (category C) has been associated with craniofacial defects and developmental delays in infants exposed to it during gestation (15,18). As with phenytoin and phenobarbital, folic acid deficiency may develop and lead to neural tube defects.

Valproic Acid (category D) is teratogenic in humans (9,15,18). Neural tube defects occur in approximately 2.5% of infants exposed to valproate in utero (18). In general, valproate should not be used in women of childbearing age (18).

Benzodiazepines (category D) easily cross the placenta and concentrate in fetal tissues. A 1998 review of the literature on the subject of anticonvulsants in pregnancy reported no increase in the prevalence of congenital malformations in infants exposed to benzodiazepines (54). Nonetheless, among women treated chronically or in large perinatal doses, newborn apnea, hypotonia, hypothermia, and withdrawal symptoms may be seen (54).

Trimethadione (category X) is associated with a 80% rate of malformation and is absolutely contraindicated during pregnancy. Little information is available regarding the safety of the newer agents, **felbamate**, **gabapentin**, **lamotrigine**, and **topiramate**, during pregnancy.

PSYCHIATRIC DISORDERS

Tricyclic antidepressants (TCAs) (category C) and **selective serotonin reuptake inhibitors** (SSRIs) are widely prescribed among women of childbearing age and have not been demonstrated to have teratogenic effects (4,31,32).

Lithium (category D) is associated with the "floppy-baby" syndrome, characterized by neonatal hypotonia, cyanosis, and poor sucking. It also increases the risk of cardiovascular abnormalities (4,31) and may affect neonatal thyroid function (4).

Several large prospective trials have failed to demonstrate any teratogenic effects from **Phenothiazines** and **haloperidol** (category C) (31). It has been recommended that these antipsychotics be discontinued 5 to 10 days prior to delivery to decrease the risk of neonatal extrapyramidal symptoms (31). Although there is no current evidence of teratogenicity among the newer antipsychotics, **clozapine** (category B), **risperidone** (category C), and **olanzapine** (category C), little information is available regarding their safety in pregnancy.

GASTROINTESTINAL DISORDERS

During pregnancy, the lower esophageal sphincter is relatively relaxed and pressure on the abdominal contents from the uterus increases the frequency of heartburn symptoms. Similarly, nausea and vomiting are well known features of early pregnancy and often require treatment.

Antacids containing aluminum, magnesium, and calcium are considered safe during pregnancy, and no teratogenicity has been reported from animal studies (11). **Sucralfate** (category B) is not systemically absorbed and, therefore, is known to be safe in pregnancy.

H2 Receptor antagonists appear to be well-tolerated during pregnancy. **Cimetidine** (category B) was not demonstrated to be associated with congenital defects among the 460 newborns studied in the Michigan Medicaid Surveillance Study (11). Animal studies did not demonstrate teratogenic or fetotoxic effects of **famotidine** (category B) (11). There have been reports of IUGR and malformations in association with high dose **nizatidine**.

Omeprazole (category C), a proton pump inhibitor, was not found to increase the risk of fetal malformation in a Swedish cohort study (29), although it does cross the placenta (33).

Prochlorperazine and **promethazine** (category C) are commonly used antiemetics and have not been shown to be teratogenic (9,18). The Collaborative Perinatal Project (CPP) monitored 50,282 mother child pairs; 877 had first-trimester prochlorperazine exposures and 2,023 anytime during pregnancy exposures, and there was no evidence to suggest malformations or perinatal adverse events outside the expected for the general populations (50). The CPP also evaluated promethazine among 114 first-time exposures and 746 anytime exposures and found no evidence to suggest a relationship to large categories of major or minor malformations (50).

Metoclopramide (category B) was evaluated in the Michigan Medicaid Surveillance Study. Ten major malformations were observed among the 192 newborns exposed to the drug, whereas eight malformations were expected given the background rate in the population. This was not found to be a statistically significant finding (11).

Odansetron is a potent and expensive antiemetic that works well in hyperemesis and early pregnancy-induced nausea. It is a category B drug that is gaining widespread popularity in obstetrics.

Laxatives, which act locally in the gastrointestinal tract such as castor oil, senna, milk of magnesia, and the docusates, are safe for use in pregnancy (14).

Metronidazole can be used to treat *Giardia* and is considered safe in the second and third trimesters (category B). Some investigations have found an increased risk when the agent was used in early pregnancy (5). However, one study reviewed 20 years of experience with the drug and involved 1,469 pregnant women, 206 who were treated in the first trimester. No associations with congenital malformations, abortions, or stillbirths were found (6). The CPP, which studied 50,282 pregnant women, found a possible risk of malformation based on four birth defects. The statistical significance of this is unclear. The manufacturer considers the drug unsafe in the first trimester and a reasonable alternative in the second and third trimesters.

URINARY TRACT INFECTIONS

Urinary tract infection (UTI) is among the most common complications in pregnancy. Pregnancy increases the risk of UTI and also renders the upper urinary tract more vulnerable to infection. Asymptomatic bacteriuria is present in 2% to 10% of all pregnant women, and 20% to 40% of these patients will go on to develop pyelonephritis if they are not treated (37). The bacteria responsible for UTI among pregnant women are the same as those in the general population, with *Escherichia coli* accounting for more than 75% of cases. Other microbes, such as *Klebsiella*, *Proteus*, group B *streptococcus*, *Staphylococcus Saprophyticus*, and enterococci, may also be causative agents.

Cystitis and asymptomatic bacteriuria should both be aggressively treated in the pregnant patient. Single-dose regimens are not recommended, although 3-day courses of antibiotics have been shown to be effective in otherwise healthy women (51). Longer courses should be considered in diabetic patients.

Pyelonephritis is a very serious condition in the pregnant patient. Preterm labor and premature delivery have been associated with pyelonephritis, although the physiologic mechanism for this phenomenon is not clear. Approximately 15% of pregnant women with pyelonephritis will be bacteremic (39). With rare exceptions, the pregnant patient with pyelonephritis should be admitted and initially treated with an aminoglycoside or cephalosporin.

Cephalosporins are considered safe during pregnancy and are all listed as category B drugs (9, 22).

Aminoglycosides are listed as category C drugs and may be used to treat gram-negative infections in pregnant women with infections that are resistant to less toxic alternatives (22). Aminoglycosides have been associated with a high prevalence of transient renal dysfunction in the pregnant patient. If an aminoglycoside is needed, **gentamicin** is the aminoglycoside of choice during pregnancy.

Fluoroquinolone therapy for UTI is contraindicated during pregnancy due to well recognized teratogenic effects.

Ampicillin, amoxicillin (category B), and all other β-**lactam antibiotics** are considered safe in pregnancy (36). Although often considered first-line agents for UTI in pregnant patients, up to 30% or more of *E. coli* may be resistant (20).

Sulfonamides cross the placenta but are considered safe during early pregnancy. However, during the third trimester they are contraindicated because they compete with bilirubin for albumin binding sites and may cause kernicterus (9,22). **Trimethoprim** is a folate agonist and is not recommended during pregnancy so combination agents should be avoided (22).

Nitrofurantoin (category B) is commonly used during pregnancy but may cause neonatal hyperbilirubinemia and should be avoided during the third trimester.

RESPIRATORY TRACT INFECTIONS

There is no evidence that pregnant women are at higher risk for pneumonia than the general population. However, functional residual lung capacity is reduced in the pregnant patient, leaving her with less respiratory reserve. For this reason, pregnant women with pneumonia are generally treated initially as inpatients.

Erythromycin and **azithromycin** are both listed as category B agents and are commonly used in pregnancy to treat pneumonia (9,22). As previously mentioned, **cephalosporins** are also considered safe in pregnancy, and **fluoroquinolones** are contraindicated.

Tetracycline and **doxycycline** should be avoided during pregnancy (9,22). They are listed as category D agents owing to their association with genitourinary and limb malformations. Tetracyclines also chelate calcium and may stain teeth and bones (9,22).

The pregnant patient with tuberculosis or streptococcal pharyngitis can be treated with the same agents as the general population.

Isoniazid is a first-line antituberculous agent in pregnant women, although it is category C (9,22). **Rifampin** (category C) crosses the placenta and is associated with neonatal coagulopathy. Still, the benefit of use outweighs the risk of untreated disease. Prophylactic administration of vitamin K along with rifampin during the third trimester is recommended. **Ethambutol** (category B) is considered safe in pregnancy. **Streptomycin** is associated with fetal ototoxicity and should be avoided during pregnancy.

Penicillin (category B) and its derivatives are considered safe in pregnancy. In the penicillin allergic patient **erythromycin** can be considered. **Clindamycin** (category B) may be used in pregnant women who are allergic to penicillin and erythromycin. There is no evidence of associated teratogenicity in animal studies (8).

Most pregnant women will have at least one viral upper respiratory infection during their pregnancy. However, many of the medications commonly used for symptomatic relief of these infections are not recommended during pregnancy. **Diphenhydramine** has been associated with a number of malformations and is not recommended (9). Likewise, **brompheniramine** is a well-known teratogen and is contraindicated in the pregnant patient. The antihistamines **chlorpheniramine** (category B), **pheniramine**, and **tripelennamine** are not known to be teratogenic (9). **Astemizole** was not found to be fetotoxic in initial studies (40). Decongestant medications such as **phenylephrine**, **pseudoephedrine**, and **phenylpropanolamine** should be used with great caution during pregnancy. Pseudoephedrine is known to be teratogenic in animals (9). All sympathomimetics have been shown to be associated with minor malformations such as clubfoot and hernias (42). **Dextromethorphan** (category C) is considered safe for use as an antitussive during pregnancy.

GENITAL TRACT AND SEXUALLY TRANSMITTED INFECTIONS

Vaginitis can be categorized as secondary to yeast (*Candida*), *Trichomonas vaginalis*, or bacterial vaginosis (BV).

Antifungal vaginal creams (including clotrimazole, miconazole, and nystatin) for yeast vaginitis are considered safe during pregnancy (9). However, oral **fluconazole**, **ketoconazole**, and **itraconazole** are associated with fetal malformations and should be avoided during pregnancy.

Metronidazole is considered safe after the first trimester of pregnancy for the treatment of *Trichomonas* infection. It has been suggested that *Trichomonas* infection may increase the risk of premature rupture of membranes (PROM) and preterm labor.

Clindamycin or **metronidazole** (after the first trimester) may be used to treat bacterial vaginosis in the pregnant patient. BV increases the risk of PROM, preterm labor, and intraamniotic infection, and should, therefore, be aggressively treated.

The common causes of cervicitis, *Neisseria gonorrhoeae* and *Chlamydia*, are both associated with obstetric complications. Infection with *N. gonorrhoeae* may lead to PROM, preterm labor, and chorioamnionitis. Concern regarding chlamydial infection during pregnancy is more related to neonatal transmission than to obstetric complications per se. **Cephalosporins** such as **ceftriaxone** or **cefixime** are safe for the treatment of *N. gonorrhoeae* infection during pregnancy. **Spectinomycin** may be used for patients who are allergic to cephalosporins. **Macrolide** therapy (especially **azithromycin**) can be used to treat *Chlamydia* during pregnancy. **Fluoroquinolones** and **tetracyclines** are contraindicated during pregnancy.

Syphilis can be transplacentally transmitted at any stage of pregnancy with potentially devastating fetal effects. Treatment with **benzathine penicillin** is recommended.

There are no current recommendations for the treatment of human papilloma virus infection during pregnancy. The cytotoxins, **podophyllin** and **5-fluorouracil** are contraindicated.

Herpes virus infection during pregnancy raises concern for perinatal transmission. The neonatal infection rate is nearly 50% with vaginal delivery during a primary maternal outbreak (20). **Acyclovir** (category B) use in pregnant women has been reported hundreds of times (2) and there is no indication of associated fetal toxicity.

Most women who are infected with HIV are of reproductive age and are susceptible to the same spectrum of opportunistic infections as nonpregnant patients. There have been numerous reports of safety and improved fetal outcome among HIV-positive pregnant women who are treated with **zidovudine**. Primarily, zidovudine has been shown to have a substantial reduction in the perinatal transmission of HIV (19). Pregnant patients with HIV infection can be treated with multidrug regimens of antiretrovirals and protease inhibitors, and these regimens are well established.

OTHER SELECTED INFECTIONS

Clearly, pregnant women are as susceptible as the general population to countless infectious diseases, in addition to certain infections that are specific to pregnancy. The following text details acceptable treatments for a selection of other infectious diseases that may be encountered in the pregnant patient.

Scabies during pregnancy can be treated with **pyrethroids**. Lindane is potentially neurotoxic (25) and was found to be possibly associated with hypospadias in the Michigan Medicaid Surveillance Study (9).

Varicella has a potentially lethal course in pregnancy. Pregnant woman, being relatively immunocompromised, are prone to varicella pneumonia and this increases the risk of maternal complication and death by 40%. Fetuses exposed to varicella in the first trimester are prone to limb and digit abnormalities, microphthalmos, and microcephaly. Infection in the last two trimesters is less threatening. Peripartum varicella infection (from 5 days before delivery to 2 days after delivery) places the fetus at high risk for morbidity and mortality (20). Varicella immune globulin should be given within 96 hours to an exposed pregnant patient with no history of chicken pox and a negative antibody titer (12).

IMMUNIZATIONS DURING PREGNANCY

Few vaccines have been formally tested among pregnant women. Live vaccines should be avoided during pregnancy because of the theoretical risk of infection (46). Because high fevers during the first trimester have been associated with neural tube defects and fevers may result from immunizations, it is generally recommended to avoid any form of immunization during the first trimester (46). Commonly used immunizations that are safe to administer during pregnancy include **tetanus toxoid**, **tetanus-diphtheria toxoid**, **tetanus immune globulin**, **rabies human diploid cell vaccine**, **rabies immune globulin**, **hepatitis B vaccine**, **hepatitis B immune globulin**, **varicella zoster immune globulin**, and **pooled immune globulins**. The **hepatitis A vaccine** is listed by the FDA as category C because of the risk of febrile response (46). The influenza vaccine may be given after the first trimester (46).

COMMON PITFALLS

- ✔ Given the importance of minimizing risk to the fetus, no drug should be prescribed unless clearly indicated
- ✔ Drug exposure should be minimized by using the smallest effective dose for the shortest duration possible
- ✔ Drugs that have been in use for long periods and that have well-understood safety profiles are preferable to newer medications
- ✔ Many drugs may be safely used during one portion of pregnancy and not during another
- ✔ Caution against herbal supplements that have not been well studied

Acknowledgments

Thank you to previous edition chapter authors Mary H. Stewart, John F. Huddleston, Donald C. Willis and Carol C. Coulson.

References

1. American College of Obstetricians and Gynecologists. *Diabetes and pregnancy.* ACOG technical bulletin no. 200. Washington, DC: ACOG, 1994.
2. Andrews EB, Yankaskas BC, Cordero JF, et al. Acyclovir in pregnancy registry: six years' experience. *Obstet Gynecol* 1992;79:7.
3. Arwood LL, Dasta JF, Friedman C. Placental transfer of theophylline: two case reports. *Pediatrics* 1979;63:844.
4. Austin MP, Mitchell PB. Psychotropic medications in pregnant women: treatment dilemmas. *Med J Aust* 1998;169:428–431.
5. Beard CM, Noller KL, O'Fallon WM, et al. Lack of evidence for cancer due to metronidazole. *N Engl J Med* 1979;301:519–522.
6. Berget A, Weber T. Metronidazole and pregnancy. *Ugeskr Laeger* 1972;134:2085–2089.
7. Brent RL. The effects of embryonic and fetal exposure to x-ray, microwaves, and ultrasound. *Clin Obstet Gynecol* 1983;26:484.
8. Briggs GG. Medication use during the perinatal period. *J Am Pharm Assoc* 1998;38:717–726, 726–727.
9. Briggs GG, Freeman RK, Yaffee SJ. *Drugs in pregnancy and lactation*, 5th ed. Baltimore: Williams & Wilkins, 1998.
10. Briggs GG, Freeman RK, Yaffe SJ. *Drugs in pregnancy and lactation*, 2nd ed. Baltimore: Williams & Wilkins, 1986;366, 422.
11. Broussard CN, Richter JE. Treating gastro-oesophageal reflux disease during pregnancy and lactation; what are the safest options? *Drug Saf* 1998;19:325–337.
12. Brown JS, Crombleholme WR. *Handbook of gynecology and obstetrics.* Norwalk: Appleton & Lange, 1993.
13. Brumfield CG, Huddleston JF. The management of diabetic ketoacidosis in pregnancy. *Clin Obstet Gynecol* 1984;27:50.
14. Carpenter CC, Fischl MA, Hammer SM. Antiretroviral therapy for HIV infection in 1998. *JAMA* 1998;280:78–86.
15. Chang SI, McAuley JW. Pharmacotherapeutic issues for women of childbearing age with epilepsy. *Ann Pharmacother* 1998;32:794–801.
16. Chow T, Galvin J, McGovern B. Antiarrhythmic drug therapy in pregnancy and lactation. *Am J Cardiol* 1998;82:581–621.
17. Chung KF, Barnes PJ. Prescribing in pregnancy: treatment of asthma. *BMJ* 1987;294:103.
18. Colie CF. Medications in pregnancy. *Curr Opin Obstet Gynecol* 1996;8:398–402.
19. Connor EM, Sperling RS, Gelber R, et al. Reduction of maternal-infant transmission of human immunodeficiency virus type I with Zidovudine treatment. Pediatric AIDS Clinical Trial Group Protocol 076 Study Group. *N Engl J Med* 1994;331:1173.
20. Coulson CC. Infections in Pregnancy. In: Harwood-Nuss A, Wolfson AB, Linden CM, et al., eds. *The clinical practice of emergency medicine*, 3rd ed. Philadelphia: Lippincott Williams & Wilkins, 2001.
21. Crawford JS, Rudofsky S. The placental transmission of pethidine. *Br J Anaesth* 1965;37:929–933.
22. Dashe JS, Gilstrap LC. Antibiotic use in pregnancy. *Obstet Gynecol Clin* 1997;24:617–629.
23. Gluck JC, Gluck PA. The effects of pregnancy on asthma: a prospective study. *Ann Allergy* 1976;37:164.
24. Greenberger PA, Patterson R. Management of asthma during pregnancy. *N Engl J Med* 1985;312:897.
25. Guenther L. Skin drugs in pregnancy—which ones to use. *Derm Nsg* 1997;9:233–236, 265.
26. Hagay Z, Reece EA. Diabetes mellitus in pregnancy and periconceptional genetic counseling. *Am J Perinatol* 1992;9:87.
27. Heinonen OP, Slone D, Shapiro S. *Birth defects and drugs in pregnancy.* Littleton, MA: Publishing Sciences Group, 1977;345.
28. Huddleston JF, Willis DC. Common Medical Diseases in Pregnancy. In: Harwood-Nuss A, Wolfson AB, Linden CM, et al, eds. *The clinical practice of emergency medicine*, 3rd ed. Philadelphia: Lippincott Williams & Wilkins, 2001.
29. Kallen B. Delivery outcome after the use of acid-suppressing drugs in early pregnancy with special reference to omeprazole. *Br J Obstet Gynaecol* 1998;105:877–881.
30. Koren G, Pastuszak A, Ito S. Drugs in pregnancy. *N Engl J Med* 1998;338:1128–1136.
31. Kuller JA, Katz VL, McMahon MJ, et al. Pharmacologic treatment of psychiatric disease in pregnancy and lactation: fetal and neonatal effects. *Obstet Gynecol* 1996;87:789–794.
32. Kulin NA, Pastuszak A, Koren G. Are the new SSRIs safe for pregnant women?. *Can Fam Physician* 1998;44:2081–2083.
33. Lalkin A, Magee L, Addis A, et al. Acid-suppressing drugs in pregnancy. *Can Fam Physician* 1997;43:1923–1924.
34. Landon MB, Gabbe SG. Fetal surveillance in the pregnancy complicated by diabetes mellitus. *Clin Perinatol* 1993;20:549.
35. Liedholm H, Wahlin-Boll E, Ingemarsson I, Melander A. Transplacental passage and breast milk concentrations of hydralazine. *Eur J Clin Pharm* 1982;21:417–419.
36. Loebstein R, Lalkin A, Koren G. Pharmacokinetic changes during pregnancy and their clinical relevance. *Clin Pharmacokinet* 1997;33:328–343.
37. Lucas MJ, Cunningham FB. Urinary infection in pregnancy. *Clin Obstet Gynecol* 1993;36:821.
38. McElhatton PR, Sullivan FM, Volans GN, et al. Paracetamol poisoning in pregnancy: an analysis of outcomes of cases referred to the teratology information service of the National Poison Information Service. *Hum Exp Toxicol* 1990;9:147.
39. Mabie WC, Barton JR, Sibai B. Septic shock in pregnancy. *Obstet Gynecol* 1997;90:553.
40. Mazzotta P, Koren G. Nonsedating antihistamines in pregnancy considering astemizole. *Can Fam Physician* 1997;43:1509–1511.
41. Misenhimer HR, Margulies SI, Panigel M, et al. Effects of vasoconstrictive drugs on the placental circulation of the rhesus monkey. *Invest Radiol* 1972;7:496.
42. Onuigbo M, Alikhan M. Over-the-counter sympathomimetics: a risk factor for cardiac arrhythmias during pregnancy. *South Med J* 1998;91:1153–1155.
43. Ostensen M, Ramsey-Goldman R. Treatment of inflammatory rheumatic disorders in pregnancy: what are the safest treatment options? *Drug Saf* 1998;19:389–410.
44. Rayburn WF. Connective tissue disorders and pregnancy. Recommendations for prescribing. *J Reprod Med* 1998;43:341–349.
45. Rudolf AM. Effects of aspirin and acetaminophen in pregnancy and in the newborn. *Arch Intern Med* 1981;141:358.
46. Samuel BU, Barry M. The pregnant traveler. *Infect Dis Clin North Am* 1998;12:325–354.
47. Schatz M. Asthma treatment during pregnancy. What can be safely taken? *Drug Saf* 1997;16:342–350.

48. Schatz
    munol
49. Slone I
    tions. /
50. Slone I
    iazines
    weigh
    488.

CHAPTER 102
Painful Syndromes of the Hand and Wrist

Gary M. Vilke

Repetitive motion disorders are a group of musculotendinous maladies that are typically associated with occupational activities. Injuries caused by repetitive motions are quite common, increasing in incidence, and have a tremendous economic impact on the workforce. *Carpal tunnel syndrome, Guyon canal (ulnar tunnel) syndrome, hypothenar hammer syndrome*, and *De Quervain tenosynovitis* are discussed in detail in this chapter.

CLINICAL PRESENTATION

Carpal Tunnel Syndrome

Carpal tunnel syndrome (CTS) involves the median nerve at the wrist and is the most commonly encountered compressive peripheral neuropathy. At the wrist, the median nerve along with the flexor tendons and their sheaths, pass through an anatomic tunnel that is formed dorsally by the carpal bones and volarly by the fibrous, but rigid, transverse carpal ligament. Any condition that decreases the internal area of the canal or increases the volume of the contents within the canal can potentially reduce capillary blood flow rates below that which is essential for the maintenance of median nerve and induce carpal tunnel syndrome. Numerous clinical conditions have been causally associated with the development of carpal tunnel syndrome, but the disorder is most commonly idiopathic. Other occupational causes include typing and key entry jobs, repetitive use of tools, and repetitive grasping motions.

Females account for more than 78% of all cases of CTS with the typical age range at diagnosis being between 40 and 60 years. The clinical presentation is often a bilateral condition with the patient typically complaining of numbness, tingling, burning, or paresthesias in the hand along the thumb, index, middle, and radial aspect of the ring fingers. These symptoms characteristically awaken the patient from sleep and may be relieved by shaking the hand and wrist. A nocturnal pain pattern is considered the hallmark of CTS and as the syndrome progresses, the frequency and intensity of symptoms increase. The symptoms are often exacerbated by activities that maintain the wrist flexed, and patients may also complain of weakness or clumsiness in the hand manifested by difficulty with fine motor functions such as picking up objects, holding things, and buttoning clothing.

Guyon Canal Syndrome

Guyon Canal (Ulnar Tunnel) Syndrome: The ulnar nerve provides the primary motor innervation to the intrinsic muscles of the hand as well as supplying sensation for a significant portion of the hand, including the skin over the hypothenar eminence, the little finger and the ulnar side of the ring finger. The ulnar nerve and artery pass together into the wrist on the radial side of the pisiform bone via an anatomic space called the canal of Guyon,

a 4-cm-long channel located between the pisiform bone and the hook of the hamate (20).

Patients with ulnar nerve compression at the wrist typically present with wrist pain that radiates into the ulnar two digits. Patients should be asked about a history of previous falls onto an outstretched hand, that may have resulted in an occult hamate fracture, that can impinge on the nerve as it passes through Guyon canal. Fractures of the hook of the hamate have been reported to account for 14% of all cases of ulnar nerve compression in the wrist (2). Patients should also be asked about repetitive trauma, as repeated blows to the ulnar side of the hand have been implicated as a cause of ulnar neuropathy at the wrist.

Hypothenar Hammer Syndrome

Hypothenar Hammer Syndrome (HHS): The distal ulnar artery is most exposed to potential trauma at the base of the hypothenar eminence, just distal to the volar carpal ligament, where it is no longer protected within Guyon's canal and is covered only by skin, subcutaneous fat, and in 85% of the population, the palmaris brevis muscle (1). Given its susceptible position, the ulnar artery is easily compressed between hard objects and the hook of the hamate (6). Repetitive ulnar artery injury can result in traumatic vasospasm, thrombosis, or aneurysm formation (6,13). These can occur any time the hypothenar aspect of the base of the palm is subjected to trauma and thus, HHS is most commonly seen in those individuals who use the palms of their hands to push, pound, or hammer as part of their daily work activities (6,13). Table 102.1 lists activities that have been implicated as causes of HHS.

Hypothenar Hammer Syndrome is a treatable syndrome that should be considered in patients presenting with complaints of symptomatic digital ischemia (4). Clinical findings in HHS include a male predominance, unilateral hand involvement, and acute onset of pain, followed by the more gradual development of a severe Raynaud's phenomenon, defined as increased sensitivity of the digits with exposure to cold, and a lack of thumb involvement (1,7). At presentation, a patient may complain of one or more episodes of acute, lancinating pain over the hypothenar eminence that occur after striking a blow with the palm of the hand (22). This pain typically radiates into the fourth and fifth fingers, and a dull, aching hypothenar pain may then ensue. Other patients describe an immediate pain episode that resolves completely over time. Then, days to weeks to months afterward, ischemic finger symptoms develop as a consequence of a slowly progressing thrombosis of the ulnar artery (13). More severe trauma to the ulnar artery can damage the internal elastic lamella, leading to formation of intraarterial thrombi (1).

TABLE 102.1.   Activities Reported to Cause Hypothenar Hammer Syndrome

Automobile mechanics
Badminton/Tennis
Baseball/Softball
Carpentry
Football
Frisbee
Handball
High-speed hand-held vibratory tools use
Hockey
Machine or lathe operating
Martial arts
Metal working
Mountain biking
Weight lifting

Use of keyboard or adding machine
Excessive writing
Washing or wringing clothes
Chopping wood
Cutting cloth with heavy scissors
Sewing, knitting, weaving
Operating lathes, drills, presses, grinders, buffing machines
Piano playing
Playing an instrument and supporting its weight with the thumb

Embolization of traumatized intima and thrombus cause digital ischemia by occluding the end arterial supply to the fingers (6,13). Thrombosis involving the adventitia may affect periarterial sympathetic fibers, resulting in vasospasm that limits surrounding collateral circulation (13).

De Quervain's Tenosynovitis

De Quervain's Tenosynovitis (DQT) is the most common tendonitis of the extensor tendons of the hand and wrist. It is a nonsuppurative tenosynovitis of the first dorsal compartment, or "tunnel" of the wrist through which the tendons of the hand's extrinsic extensor muscles pass (10,12,15,22). This compartment overlies the styloid process of the radius and contains the tendons of the abductor pollicis longus (APL) and the extensor pollicis brevis (EPB) (12). The APL tendon inserts at the base of the dorsum of the thumb's metacarpal, and the EPB tendon inserts at the base of the thumb's proximal phalanx. At the wrist, these tendons and their synovial sheaths lie between the carpal bones and a fibrous band called the dorsal retinaculum. Tasks involving repeated pronation and supination of the forearm combined with forceful exertion of the thumb beyond the point of fatigue are commonly implicated in DQT, which represents a derangement in the normal gliding of the APL and/or the EPB tendons (12). Table 102.2 lists activities reported to cause DQT. Other reported activities that can lead to a tenosynovitis of the first dorsal compartment include performing tasks that may be new or unfamiliar to the patient, with many patients beginning to have symptoms within days of starting a new job or resuming an old one after a holiday (9,12).

Pain at the radial styloid is a classic and defining symptom of DQT, with a history of gradual onset of pain and the absence of fracture or acute trauma being another hallmark of the syndrome (1). It typically affects women more than men, approximately 10:1, and presents between the ages of 35 and 55 years. The pain is more or less constant, is exacerbated by thumb abduction, ulnar deviation of the wrist, and simple grasping, and is usually described by patients as severe in quality, with advanced cases having swelling and crepitus noted at the site of maximal pain. The pain may radiate proximally into the forearm or distally to the thumb and occasionally may be so intense that sleep is disturbed. Some patients may complain of weakness or an inability to use the affected hand secondary to the pain, and holding the thumb at rest offers only minimal relief.

DIFFERENTIAL DIAGNOSIS

Carpal Tunnel Syndrome (CTS): Cervical root irritation, especially at the C6 and C7 levels, secondary to either a herniated cervical disc or osteoarthritis with neural foramina encroachment, may produce numbness in the median-innervated fingers, with pain radiating to the shoulder. However, cervical root pathology usually causes radicular symptoms that are seldom bilateral or worse at night.

Pronator syndrome, which is compression of the median nerve in the proximal forearm, can present similar to CTS. However, Phalen's test should be negative and Tinel sign should be negative as well. There would, however, be positive findings with percussion performed at the level of the forearm.

Guyon Canal Syndrome: Lesions at any location along the length of the ulnar nerve or the nerve roots from which it arises can cause symptoms of wrist or hand pain. Proximal lesions, such as cervical disc disease affecting the C8 or T1 nerve roots, can cause similar symptoms. Brachial plexus pathology may also be responsible for symptoms in the distribution of the ulnar nerve. Pancoast's tumor, an apical tumor of the lung, can exert pressure on or grow into the brachial plexus, resulting in symptoms distant from the primary site (11). Thoracic outlet syndrome can also result in a brachial plexopathy.

The most common location of ulnar nerve compression is in the cubital tunnel of the elbow. Most patients presenting with a combined ulnar motor and sensory finding have compression from a ganglion. Anomalous muscle bellies, lipomas, giant cell tumors, schwannomas, thickened ligaments, bipartite hamuli, and pisiform-hamate coalitions are also responsible for ulnar nerve compression at the wrist (2,3). Hamate fractures, ulnar artery thrombosis, hypothenar hammer syndrome, and rheumatoid tenosynovitis are other causes of ulnar nerve symptoms.

Hypothenar Hammer Syndrome: Collagen vascular diseases and various vasculitides and coagulopathies may all cause poor perfusion of the hands and fingers (9). These disorders, however, tend to be more systemic and typically have generalized findings. Buerger disease, also known as thromboangiitis obliterans, affects primarily young males, and presents with Raynaud phenomenon; the upper extremity examination may be indistinguishable from that of HHS, including an absent or diminished ulnar pulse. Buerger disease is found almost exclusively in cigarette smokers and is often a systemic condition involving both upper and lower extremities, while HHS is confined to the upper extremity only and is most often unilateral.

De Quervain tenosynovitis: As the anterior terminal branch of the radial nerve, which provides sensation to the dorsum of the thumb, passes into the hand almost directly over the extensor retinaculum of the first dorsal compartment, radial nerve entrapment can present similarly to DQT (12). Arthritis at the carpal–metacarpal joint of the thumb as well as fractures of the radial styloid, scaphoid, or trapezium can also present with similar symptoms (10). Intersection syndrome, another tenosynovitis of the radial extensor tendons, may be confused with DQT. Patients with this disorder typically have pain, swelling and crepitus in a more proximal, ulnar distribution in the region where the radial wrist extensors of the second dorsal compartment and the tendons of the first dorsal compartment intersect, rather that at the radial styloid as seen in DQT (9,10,22).

EMERGENCY DEPARTMENT EVALUATION

Carpal tunnel syndrome: Physical examination may reveal decreased sensation to light touch or decreased two-point discrimination in the median nerve distribution. Phalen's wrist-flexion test and Tinel's sign are frequently found to be positive in carpal tunnel syndrome, but are neither sensitive nor specific (14,19). Phalen test is considered to be positive if holding the wrist in complete, but unforced, flexion for 30 to 60 seconds reproduces or exaggerates the numbness and paresthesias in the median nerve distribution. Tinel sign is positive if light tapping over the median nerve at the wrist causes a tingling sensation distally along the

suspected in any patient with a neutrophil count as low as 1,500 per μl, but an even lower WBC count in bursal fluid does not rule out infection (37). Gram stains of culture-proven septic bursitis have been reported as negative in about 30% of cases and hence cannot be used alone to exclude a septic bursitis.

Routine cultures should be done of the aspirate. Some series indicate that *Staphylococcus aureus* is found in 80% to 100% of positive cultures; streptococcus (Group A beta-hemolytic strep most commonly) is seen in less than 10%. *S. epidermidis* has been cultured as well. Anaerobes, mycobacteria, fungi, Haemophilus influenza and other gram positive and gram negative organisms have been found infrequently (18,30,31,37).

Crystal-induced bursitis, most commonly associated with gout, should reveal negatively birefringent urate crystals. Olecranon bursitis caused by calcium pyrophosphate dihydrate crystals has been reported as well. The appearance of the fluid may range from straw colored to bloody. Cell counts overlap septic and other nonseptic etiologies, ranging from 1,000 to 6,000 per μl, and concomitant gouty and septic bursitis have been reported (18). A recently injected bursal sac may contain the birefringent crystals of a long-acting steroid preparation (37).

Depending upon the history, radiographs may be indicated. Soft tissue abnormalities, such as calcifications, swelling or gas, may be seen. Bony disruption as a result of trauma, foreign body, and other possible etiologies or associated abnormalities should be considered. Although not common, an associated osteomyelitis has been described, and was associated with a longer delay to diagnosis from onset of symptoms (> 3 weeks). Ultrasonography, computed tomography (CT), or magnetic resonance imaging (MRI) may also be indicated in specific circumstances (9,37).

EMERGENCY DEPARTMENT MANAGEMENT

An inflamed olecranon or prepatellar bursa associated with a positive aspirate warrants appropriate antibiotic treatment. Penicillin antibiotics have been shown to achieve effective bursal concentrations when given either intravenously or orally. A 14-day course should be given. The presence of a bursal infection for more than two weeks before the initiation of antibiotic treatment is associated with persistently positive cultures on serial aspirations and thus may require more prolonged therapy. Patients with a history of bursitis (septic or nonseptic), rheumatoid nodules, gouty tophi, immunocompromised with severe infection, or septic bursitis due to unusual organisms also may require a prolonged course of antibiotics (18). Empiric antibiotic therapy should include coverage for both *Staphylococcus aureus* and Streptococcus species. There have been apparent treatment failures with erythromycin; close follow-up and possible repeated aspiration may thus be necessary (18).

Supportive measures such as warm soaks, wound care for associated lesions, and protection of the bursa from further trauma are important. Some cases of bursitis may require surgical excision and drainage, and recovery from septic bursitis may take months (27,29).

Treatment of acute nonseptic bursitis (traumatic or idiopathic), beyond initial aspiration, has included the utilization of compression dressings and administration of nonsteroidal anti-inflammatory agents (18). Although steroid injections into the nonseptic bursa has been suggested by some (18), it seems prudent in the emergency department to await the results of cultures and arrange for follow-up rather than to initiate such long-term therapy in the ED, especially in the face of a possible septic bursitis. In one series, complications of intrabursal steroid injections included skin atrophy over the bursa (20%), chronic pain associated with pressure applied to the elbow (30%), and the development of a septic bursitis (10%) (18,34).

DISPOSITION

As oral antibiotics seem to provide good bursal coverage in septic bursitis, patients with a noncomplicated olecranon or prepatellar bursitis, and without significant co-morbidity, may be discharged with appropriate follow-up. It has been recommended that those with a purulent aspirate should be aspirated at one to three day intervals as long as the effusion persists (18).

Those with severe bursitis, purulent drainage, or other underlying medical problems should be considered for hospital admission and treatment with intravenous antibiotics. Indications for inpatient therapy include the presence of a high fever, severe bursal infection (intense peribursal cellulitis or wound infection), or systemic toxicity (18). As noted above, there have been reports of treatment failure with the use of erythromycin on an outpatient basis.

COMMON PITFALLS

✔ Failure to distinguish between a septic and nonseptic bursitis
✔ Failure to distinguish between a septic arthritis and a septic bursitis
✔ Failure to discern underlying bony or soft tissue pathology causing persistent symptoms
✔ Failure to arrange appropriate follow up

TENDINOPATHY

Tendons are structures that connect muscle and bone, hence enabling joint movement (14). They consist of collagen bundles that provide tensile strength and an extracellular matrix that, among other duties, provides structural support. The tendon is covered by the epitenon, a loose connective tissue that contains the blood, lymphatic, and nerve supply. The epitenon is surrounded by the paratenon, and the two are sometimes called the peritendon (14).

Tendinopathies have commonly been referred to as "tendonitis" (17). Many understand that when the term is used in a clinical context, it refers to a clinical syndrome and not a histopathologic diagnosis (17). However the term "tendinosis" is becoming more frequently used as a result of histopathologic findings of "angiofibroblastic tendinosis" in the injured tendon, with the etiology presumed to be a degenerative process (20,22). Although the term "tendinitis" has been used to describe theoretical chronic inflammatory changes in the painful, overused tendon, (15,22) an increasing body of evidence suggests that such overuse tendinopathies may not involve inflammatory changes (1,15). Hence, the inclusive term "tendinopathy" will be used to refer to the clinical presentations involving tendons in this discussion. It is important to consider that the natural history of a tendinopathy is often to take weeks to months for improvement (17).

As a rule, a history of overuse is common in many tendinopathies (22). Cumulative, repetitive microtrauma may cause tissue damage (23). Participation in athletics and occupational duties that require repetitive motions have been implicated in overuse syndromes. Some relatively common tendinopathies discussed that may present to the ED include those of the *rotator cuff* (both noncalcific and calcific), the *biceps tendon*, the *lateral elbow (tennis elbow)*, and the *patellar tendon* (14).

CLINICAL PRESENTATION

The classic presentation of a patient presenting with a painful tendon is one of increasing pain at the site of the tendon, and often a history of an increase in the use (hence, "overuse") of the attached muscle. The pain is often related to the load. An early tendinopathy may be noted to cause discomfort early in the activity, diminish with continued activity, and then recur after the activity if it has been prolonged. Subsequent episodes may be of increased severity (14).

The pain is usually well localized and has been described as "sharp" or "severe" during the early stages, progressing to a "dull ache" in some patients. The pain usually does not radiate. Exacerbation is caused by activity that increases the load on the tendon, and factors that relieve the discomfort may include relative rest, ice, NSAIDs or other analgesic medications (14).

Associated systemic diseases that may prompt consideration of an etiology may not be caused by mechanical stressors, but rather a secondary tendinopathy, include an underlying spondyloarthropathy (e.g., psoriasis), as well as a tendinopathy related to a sexually transmitted disease (e.g., gonococcemia) or treatment with a fluoroquinolone (13,14).

Rotator Cuff Tendinopathy

Rotator cuff tendinopathy is the most common manifestation of what has been described as the Subacromial Pain Syndrome (SPS) (35). The rotator cuff consists of a set of four muscles (supraspinatus, infraspinatus, teres minor, and subscapularis) which, with the deltoid muscle, enable the arm to be positioned in the overhead position. The rotator cuff muscles, anchored on the scapula, pass beneath the coracoacromial arch. Diminished space as a result of anatomy, swelling, or trauma may cause the classic presentation of rotator cuff tendinopathy by causing impingement of the supraspinatus against the anterior inferior aspect of the acromion or the coracoacromial ligament. An external rotator of the humerus as well, the supraspinatus tendon assists the deltoid in abducting the arm, with its greatest contribution being the initiation of abduction (36). The impingement injury has three stages. The first is edema and hemorrhage. As impingement becomes repetitive, fibrosis and thickening of the subacromial bursa with tendinopathy in the supraspinatus occurs. The third stage represents a tear of the tendon, either partial or complete (36).

The clinical presentation of rotator cuff tendinopathy (or tear) includes pain, weakness, and decreased range of motion. Pain is noted in the anterior, superior, and lateral aspects of the shoulder. Acute tendinopathy may be associated with mild pain when attempting to do overhead activities. As the tendinopathy becomes more persistent, the pain may occur at rest and increase with overhead activities. As there is progression to a partial- or full-thickness tear, there may be persistent pain at rest and pain at night. There may be weakness and limited active range of motion (36).

With *calcific tendinopathy*, deposition of calcium hydroxyapatite crystals in the tendon is seen radiographically. Bilateral involvement is not uncommon (28). However, up to 20% of adults with no shoulder pain may have evidence of calcification of the rotator cuff tendon (12,28). Patients may complain of variable degrees of pain, either at rest or on movement. Discomfort at night, and a "catching" on movement have been described (28). Pathophysiologically, the rotator cuff tendon goes through several stages, beginning with an asymptomatic fibrocartilaginous

transformation, which is followed by the development of calcification within the cuff. The next stage (resorptive) is described as the most incapacitating as there is formation of crystals that may cause severe pain and restriction of movement. Some patients may have systemic symptoms including fever and malaise, and may have an elevated erythrocyte sedimentation rate and neutrophilia. In such cases, the differential diagnosis includes gout and a septic joint. This stage may last for 2 weeks. The final stage involves healing and repair of the rotator cuff, associated with some residual pain and restriction of movement. Specific tenderness over the greater tuberosity and symptoms similar to the impingement syndrome may be seen (12).

Biceps Tendinopathy

A similar tendinopathy to that of the rotator cuff, especially seen in those with overhead activities and impingement, is that of the biceps tendon. It may occur either with rotator cuff symptoms or independently. Most cases of bicipital tendinopathy are believed to be secondary to impingement (24). Patients may have anterior shoulder pain (at the bicipital groove) that is exacerbated with supination and pronation, and on palpation have pain at the bicipital groove.

Lateral Elbow Tendinopathy (Tennis Elbow)

Tennis elbow is reflective of tendon overuse and failed healing. Initial signs and symptoms include activity-related discomfort followed by pain at rest after pathologic changes become more extensive (22). Palpable tenderness over the lateral elbow (lateral epicondyle) may be present in the early stages. Pain of the lateral elbow caused by extensor involvement is not uncommon, often seen in those who play racquet sports ("tennis elbow"). This is seen with eccentric overuse of the forearm extensors (e.g., backhand) (21). Pain with manual stress testing (i.e., extension/supination of the elbow) usually confirms the site of the lesion (22). Tennis elbow has been described as primarily involving the extensor carpi radialis brevis (ECRB) and secondarily the extensor digitorum communis (20,22). Pain with extension of the middle finger against resistance may cause pain over the insertion of the ECRB over the lateral elbow.

Patellar Tendinopathy

The knee pain of patellar tendinopathy may have an insidious onset, and is often ascribed to an activity involving jumping, or an episode of exercise that is related to a heavy training session. The patient complains of pain usually localized to an area over the anterior knee region, often complaining of tenderness at the inferior pole of the patella. As is not uncommon early in the course of a tendinopathy, discomfort may ease completely with exercise, progressing to the point of discomfort at rest (6).

DIFFERENTIAL DIAGNOSIS

Depending upon the location of pain, the differential diagnosis of various tendinopathies should include fracture, bursitis, arthritis, muscle strain, ligamentous sprains, and referred pain. Apparent rotator cuff symptoms may represent pain referred from the cervical spine, pain from the AC joint, osteolysis of the distal clavicle, or other shoulder pathology (e.g., instability, labral tear etc.). Another potential etiology to be considered is referred cardiac pain.

The differential diagnosis of *tennis elbow* also includes posterior interosseus nerve entrapment (motor component of the radial nerve in the forearm). The clinical manifestations of this neuropraxia includes diffuse pain and tenderness along the track of the radial nerve in the extensor mass of the proximal forearm (22). Synovitis, plica, chondromalacia, and adolescent osteochondral defect (OCD) are also in the differential diagnosis. Lateral elbow discomfort may also be associated with referred pain from the cervical spine (14,22).

Patellar tendinopathy must be differentiated from patellofemoral pain syndrome, especially in the athlete who participates in jumping sports. However, the clinical features are generally distinctive (6). Lesions of the quadriceps (e.g., tear), patellar lesions, and the possibility of rupture may also be considered.

EMERGENCY DEPARTMENT EVALUATION

A thorough history and directed physical examination is important in the evaluation of the patient who presents to the emergency department with a tendinopathy. Although not routinely performed in the emergency department setting, imaging of tendinopathies, may be accomplished with the use of diagnostic ultrasound and magnetic resonance imaging (MRI) (14,15). These may be helpful in confirming the clinical diagnosis. Other imaging techniques as indicated (e.g., radiography, CT, bone scan) may be useful in ruling out other possibilities in the differential diagnosis.

In *rotator cuff tendinopathy*, physical examination may reveal signs of impingement or a tear. The supraspinatus, the most common rotator cuff component exhibiting a tendinopathy, may be examined by resistance testing. In an attempt to isolate the supraspinatus, the arms are abducted 90° in the scapular plane (30° anterior to the coronal plane). The arms are internally rotated so that the thumbs point downward. A downward force is placed on the arms, while the patient attempts to resist by maintaining the arms parallel to the floor. An inability to resist the force is an indication of isolated supraspinatus weakness (36). With advanced impingement and a full thickness rotator cuff tear, the patient may be unable to abduct the arm, and on examination may be unable to maintain the arm in an abducted position after the examiner places it there. This is the drop arm sign (35).

The impingement sign described by Neer consists of forward flexing the arm, causing the greater tuberosity of the humerus to impinge upon the anterior and inferior surface of the acromium. An abnormal test is indicated by pain. The examiner should fully flex the patient's shoulder to 180°. If pain is produced at the end range of the arc, it is considered to be positive. Testing of the infraspinatus and teres minor is done by having the patient place the arms to the side, flex the elbow, and attempt to externally rotate against resistance (19,36). With longstanding disease, range of motion may be limited. The subsequent development of adhesive capsulitis may make the diagnosis of impingement more difficult (35).

In patients with suspected *bicipital tendinopathy*, *Speed test* is performed by having the elbow extended and the forearm supinated. The examiner then resists forward flexion of the adducted shoulder pain that radiates to the bicipital groove is a positive test (24). *Yergason test* is performed by having the patient flex the elbow to 90° with the arm at the side. The patient is asked to supinate forcefully against resistance. Pain referred to the bicipital groove with resisted supination of the forearm is a positive test (24).

Patients with *patellar tendinopathy* are often tender to palpation of the patellar tendon attachment at the inferior pole of the patella. Tenderness is generally elicited on the deep surface of the proximal attachment of the patellar tendon when the knee is flexed at 30 degrees with the quadriceps muscle in total relaxation (5). Depending upon the chronicity of the condition,

quadriceps wasting may be seen (6). Although mild tenderness may be a normal finding in active athletes, moderate and severe tenderness have been noted to be associated with ultrasonographic evidence of tendinopathy. Pain may also be reproduced with the decline squat test, which places a greater load on the patellar tendon than does a squat on level ground (6).

Diagnostic imaging in the ED, if indicated, may include radiographs of the affected location. A routine shoulder series should include an anteroposterior (AP) view with both internal and external rotation of the humerus. An axillary view will permit better visualization of the glenohumeral joint, the glenoid margin, and the acromion. A scapular Y-view assesses the anterior slope of the acromion (36). Although generally not emergent, diagnostic modalities in the acute evaluation of shoulder pain, ultrasonography and MRI have been utilized in the evaluation of the rotator cuff (36). The diagnosis of *calcific tendinopathy* is confirmed by radiographs that show calcium restricted to the tendon without affecting the bone. Patients with *bicipital tendinopathy* may show signs of impingement or spurs in the bicipital groove (24). Up to 20% of patients with *lateral elbow tendinopathy* may exhibit tendon calcification or a reactive exostosis at the tip of the lateral epicondyle (20).

EMERGENCY DEPARTMENT MANAGEMENT

Treatment of the tendinopathy necessitates a long term plan, and most important, including a supervised program of physical therapy. A tendinopathy may take from weeks to months to heal. Depending upon the circumstances, protection, rest, ice, compression, elevation, and medication have been advised (21). In the ED, along with rest from the inciting activity, the patient may be prescribed an NSAID for pain relief. The efficacy of NSAIDs as a treatment for "inflammation" in the tendinopathies has been questioned, given the paucity of data for the occurrence of inflammation seen. In fact, the analgesic effect of NSAIDs may permit patients to ignore the early symptoms of tendinopathy (14,32). Cryotherapy has also been suggested as an effective modality (15,21).

Some have advocated injection of a corticosteroid. However, given the potential complications of steroid injections (including the possible injection of steroid into the tendon and hence a loss of tensile strength and spontaneous rupture), it seems prudent to pursue conservative therapy in the ED and arrange for appropriate follow up. Should nonoperative treatment fail, surgical options may be indicated (35,36).

Treatment of *calcific tendinopathy* includes control of pain and maintenance of function. The acute phase may require rest of the affected arm in a sling (beware, however, of adhesive capsulitis, i.e., "frozen shoulder"). Pain may be controlled with aspirin, NSAIDs, acetaminophen or ice (28). Corticosteroid injection is controversial in the acute phase, as it has been argued that it may inhibit the resorptive process. Others have advocated its use, especially when the rotator cuff impinges on the undersurface of the acromium as a result of inflammation (28). Fluoroscopically guided needle lavage in the resorptive phase, performed in the operating room or radiology suite, has been noted to be effective (12). The use of ultrasound as well as extracorporeal shock wave therapy have also been studied as therapeutic modalities (12,28). Arthroscopic surgery may also be required (12).

Load reduction and relative rest are key to management of a *patellar tendinopathy*. Complete immobilization is contraindicated as the tensile load stimulates collagen production and directs the alignment. Cryotherapy (i.e., ice) may decrease blood and protein extravasation from new capillaries seen in the tendinopathy as well as decreasing the metabolic rate of the tendon (6).

CRITICAL INTERVENTIONS

- Advise initial conservative therapy for patients with a tendinopathy, including rest, ice, and an NSAID
- Identify patients with calcific tendinopathy, as they are at risk for capsulitis

DISPOSITION

Given the potential chronicity of a tendinopathy, the need for appropriate patient education, physical therapy, and the potential need for surgical intervention, it is important to arrange appropriate outpatient follow up.

COMMON PITFALLS

✔ Underestimation of the potential extended time for healing
✔ Failure to consider other entities in the differential diagnosis that may present with similar findings (e.g., underlying stress fracture as a cause of pain)
✔ Discharge without an appropriate followup plan

References

1. Almekinders LC, Temple JD. Etiology, diagnosis, and treatment of tendonitis: an analysis of the literature. *Med Sci Sports Exerc* 1998;30:1183–1190.
2. Bywaters EGL. The bursae of the body. *Ann Rheum Dis* 1965;24:215–218.
3. Canoso JJ, Yood RA. Acute gouty bursitis: Report of 15 cases. *Ann Rheum Dis* 1979;38:326–328.
4. Canoso JJ, Yood RA. Reaction of superficial bursae in response to specific disease stimuli. *Arthritis Rheum* 1979;22:1361–1364.
5. Cook JL, Khan KM, Kiss ZS, , et al. Reproducibility and clinical utility of tendon palpation to detect patellar tendinopathy in young basketball players. *Br J Sports Med* 2001;35:65–69.
6. Cook JL, Khan KM, Maffulli N, Purdam C: Overuse tendinosis, not tendonitis. Part 2: Applying the new approach to patellar tendinopathy. *Phys Sportsmed* 2000;28:31–32, 35–36, 39–41, 45–46.
7. Dye SF, van Dam BE, Westin GW. Eponyms and etymons in orthopaedics. *Contemp Ortho* 1985;10:83–85.
8. Fullerton A. The surgical anatomy of the synovial membrane of the knee-joint. *Br J Surg* 1917;4:191–200.
9. García-Porra C, González-Gay MA, Ibañez D, García-País MJ. The clinical spectrum of severe septic bursitis in Northwestern Spain: A 10 year study. *J Rheumatol* 1999;26:663–667.
10. Ho G Jr, Tice AD, Kaplan SR. Septic bursitis in the prepatellar and olecranon bursae. An analysis of 25 cases. *Ann Intern Med* 1978;89:21–27
11. Ho G Jr. Tice AD. Comparison of nonseptic and septic bursitis. Further observations on the treatment of septic bursitis. *Arch Intern Med* 1979;139:1269–S1273.
12. Hurt G, Baker CL Jr. Calcific tendinitis of the shoulder. *Ortho Clin N Am* 2003;34:567–575.
13. Khaliq Y, Zhanel GG. Fluoroquinolone-associated tendinopathy: A critical review of the literature. *Clin Inf Dis* 2003;36:1404–1410.
14. Khan K, Cook J. The painful nonruptured tendon: clinical aspects. *Clin Sports Med* 2003;711–725.
15. Khan KM, Cook JL, Taunton JE, Bonar F. Overuse tendinosis, not tendonitis. *Phys Sportsmed* 2000;28:38–43,47–48.
16. Larsson, L-G, Baum J. The syndromes of bursitis. *Bull Rheum Dis* 1986;36:1–8.
17. Maffuli N, Wong J, Almekinders LC. Types and etiologies of tendinopathy. *Clin Sports Med* 2003;22:675–692.
18. McAfee JH, Smith DL. Olecranon and prepatellar bursitis: diagnosis and treatment. *West J Med* 1988;149:607–610.
19. Neer CS II. Anterior acromioplasty for the chronic impingement syndrome in the shoulder: a preliminary report. *J Bone Joint Surgery (Am)* 1972;54:41–50.
20. Nirschl R, Pettrone F. Tennis elbow: the surgical treatment of lateral epicondylitis. *J Bone Joint Surg* 1979;61A:832–841.
21. Nirschl RP, Kraushaar BS. Assessment and treatment guidelines for elbow injuries. *Phys Sportsmed* 1996;24:42–44,47–50,55,56,60.
22. Nirschl RP, Ashman ES. Elbow tendinopathy: tennis elbow. *Clin Sports Med* 2003;22:813–836.
23. O'Connor FG, Howard TM, Fieseler CM, Nirschl RP : Managing overuse injuries: A systemic approach. *Phys Sportsmed* 1997;25:88–90,99, 102–106, 112–113.
24. Patton WC, McCluskey GM III. Biceps tendinitis and subluxation. *Clin Sports Med* 2001;20:505–529.
25. Raddatz DA, Hoffman GS, Franck WA. Septic bursitis: presentation, treatment, and prognosis. *J Rheumatol* 1987;14:1160–1163.
26. Richards CF, Koutouzis TK.Tendonitis and Bursitis. In: Marx JA, ed. *Rosen's Emergency Medicine. Concepts and Clinical Practice.* Volume Two. 5th ed. St. Louis: Mosby, Inc. 2002;1599–1607.
27. Shell D, Perkins R, Cosgarea A. Septic olecranon bursitis: recognition and treatment. Jnl *Amer Board Fam Pract* 1995;8:217–220.
28. Speed CA, Hazleman BL. Calcific tendinitis of the shoulder. *N Engl J Med* 1999;340:1582–1584.
29. Stell IM. Septic and non-septic olecranon bursitis in the accident and emergency department–an approach to management. *Jnl Accident & Emerg Med* 1996;13:351–353.
30. Stell IM. Management of acute bursitis: outcome study of a structured approach. *J R Soc Med* 1999;92:516–521.
31. Stell IM, Grandsen WR. Simple tests for septic bursitis: comparative study. *BMJ* 1998;316:1877.
32. Stovitz SD, Johnson RJ. NSAIDs and musculoskeletal Treatment. What is the clinical evidence? *Phys Sportsmed* 2003;31:35–40,52.
33. Thompson GR, Manshady BM, Weiss JJ. Septic bursitis. *JAMA* 1978;240:2280–2281.
34. Weinstein PS, Canoso JJ, Wohlgethan JR. Long-term followup of corticosteroid injection for traumatic olecranon bursitis. *Ann Rheum Dis* 1984;43:44–46.
35. Wolf WB III. Shoulder tendinoses. *Clin Sports Med* 1992;11:871–890.
36. Wolin PM, Tarbet JA. Rotator cuff injury: Addressing overhead overuse. *Phys Sportsmed* 1997;25:54–56,59–60,66–70,72,74.
37. Zimmerman B III, Mikolich DJ, Ho G Jr. Septic Bursitis. *Sem Arthrit Rheum* 1995;24:391–410.

CHAPTER 104
Hand Infections

Carl R. Chudnofsky and Paul B. Vanderbeek

ESSENTIAL ANATOMY

The nail plate inserts into a depression on the dorsum of the finger called the proximal nail fold, which divides the proximal nail fold into superficial and deep epithelial surfaces called the dorsal roof and ventral floor, respectively. The eponychium, commonly called the cuticle, is a horny layer extension of the proximal nail fold that extends a short distance onto the dorsum of the nail. It seals the potential space between the nail plate and the proximal nail fold. Laterally, the proximal nail fold is continuous on either side with the lateral nail folds or paronychium. The soft tissue under the distal free edge of the nail is called the hyponychium (Fig. 104.1) (3).

The distal pulp space of a finger or thumb is composed of fat globules that are divided into small fascial compartments by 15 to 20 vertical fibrous septa (see Fig. 104.1). The presence of these compartments has a substantial impact on the pathophysiology and management of pulp space infections.

The flexor tendons are surrounded by a tendon sheath that is composed of an outer fibrous sheath and an inner synovial sheath. The inner synovial sheath has a visceral and parietal layer with a potential space between them. The tendon sheaths of the index, middle, and ring fingers extend from the midpalmar crease to just beyond the distal interphalangeal joints. The tendon sheath of the flexor pollicis longus tendon begins at the base of the distal phalanx of the thumb and extends to the pronator quadratus muscle in the wrist. Between the base of the thumb metacarpal and the wrist, the tendon sheath of the flexor pollicis longus tendon is called the radial bursa. The tendon sheath surrounding the flexor tendons of the little finger begin just distal

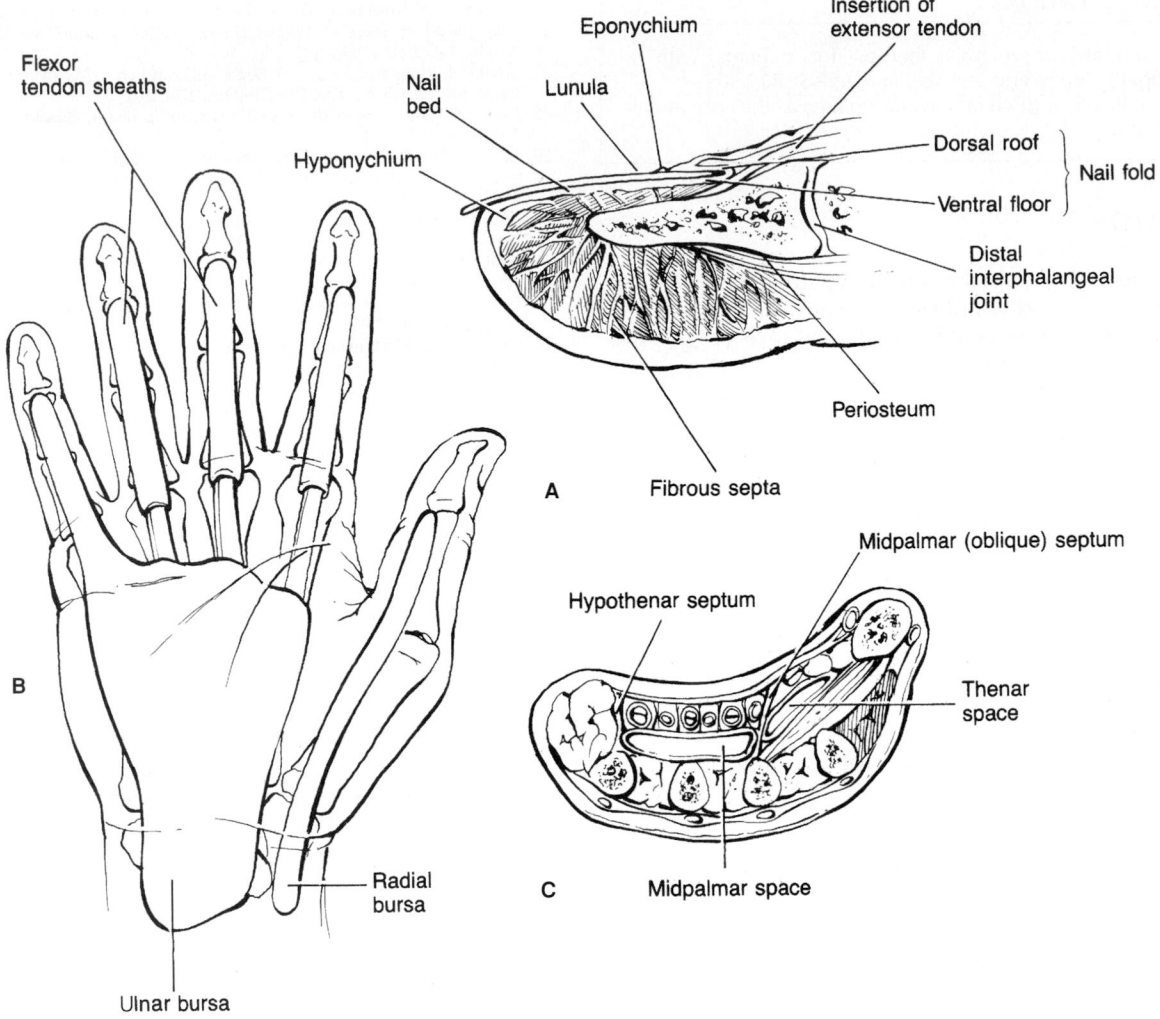

Figure 104.1.   Anatomy. **(A)** Fingertip and nail bed. **(B)** Flexor tendon sheaths. **(C)** Deep palmar spaces.

to the distal interphalangeal joint and, like the tendon sheath of the flexor pollicis longus tendon, ends at the pronator quadratus muscle in the wrist. The ulnar bursa is that part of the tendon sheath between the fifth metacarpal and the pronator quadratus muscle (see Fig. 104.1). The radial and ulnar bursas communicate with each other in 50% to 80% of patients (2,25). The hand contains several fascial spaces that are potential sites of infection. The most frequently infected spaces are the deep palmar spaces, which include the thenar space, midpalmar space, hypothenar space, and Parona's space, and the web spaces (see Fig. 104.1). The thenar space is bounded on its ulnar side by the vertical septum between the third metacarpal and the long finger profundus and radially by the lateral edge of the adductor pollicis. The adductor pollicis also forms the dorsal roof of the compartment. The midpalmar space lies deep into the flexor tendons. Radially it is bordered by the vertical septum between the third metacarpal and the long finger profundus and ulnarly by the hypothenar muscles. The dorsal roof is formed by the fascia over the second and the third palmar interossei and the third and fourth metacarpals (12). The hypothenar space contains the hypothenar muscles. It is bordered radially by a fibrous septum from the fifth metacarpal to the palmar fascia (23). Parona space communicates with the hand via the carpal tunnel, and is responsible for allowing infections of the hand to propagate into the forearm. This space is bordered palmarly by the flexor tendons, dorsally by the fascia overlying the pronator quadratus,

radially by the flexor carpi radialis, and ulnarly by the flexor carpi ulnaris (35).

MICROBIOLOGY

The majority of hand infections are caused by *Staphylococcus aureus* and *Streptococcus* species. Anaerobes, alone or in combination with aerobic bacteria, are seen in approximately 30% of all hand infections, and in 40% of infections secondary to human bite or clenched-fist injury and intravenous drug abuse (26). Gram-negative organisms are rare in normal hosts but are common in patients with diabetes mellitus or a depressed immune system (20). In the past, methicillin-resistant *S. aureus* (MRSA) was predominantly found in intravenous drug users (12); however, recent reports indicate that MRSA is increasingly the cause of hand infections in immunocompetent nonintravenous drug users as well (2,5,22). Polymicrobial infections are relatively common, particularly with infections caused by bite wounds and intravenous drug abuse (26). Chronic hand infections may be caused by atypical mycobacteria, particularly *Mycobacterium marinum*, a common cause of hand infections occurring in aquatic environments (13). Sporotrichosis is a subcutaneous infection caused by *Sporothrix schenckii*. It usually involves the upper extremity, and is the most common subcutaneous fungal infection (15). Immunocompromised patients may be infected with a

Nature and setting of any preceding trauma
Progression of symptoms
Nature and location of local symptoms
Duration of symptoms before arrival
Associated extraextremity symptoms
Underlying medical problems
History of intravenous drug abuse
Current medications

variety of fungi, including *Candida albicans* (27), *Coccidioides immitis* (15), *cryptococcus* (1,36), *and Aspergillus flavus* (16).

HISTORY AND PHYSICAL EXAMINATION

A careful and detailed history and physical examination are essential in the diagnosis and management of hand infections. Important historical information is listed in Table 104.1.

A history of trauma, especially penetrating trauma, is frequently obtained from patients with a hand infection. The type of trauma and the setting in which it has occurred can provide valuable clues to the causative organism. For example, infections from injuries occurring at home or in industry are caused predominantly by gram-positive organisms (12). Cat bites are commonly infected with *Pasteurella multocida*, while infected human bite wounds or clenched-fist injuries are frequently caused by *Eikenella corrodens* and other oral flora (12). The progression of symptoms may also be helpful in determining the type of bacteria present. Streptococcal infections evolve over 24 to 48 hours and are more often associated with cellulitis and lymphangitis. In contrast, *Staphylococcus aureus* is more likely to cause a suppurative infection that develops over 3 to 6 days. Chronic infections are more often due to fungi or atypical mycobacteria (12). The nature and location of pain and swelling may be helpful in determining the location and severity of infection, while the duration of symptoms can be an important determinant of the need for surgical intervention. Associated symptoms may aid in gauging the severity of infection and the choice of initial antimicrobial therapy. For example, a urethral or endocervical discharge in a patient with a suspected flexor tenosynovitis suggests the possibility of disseminated gonorrhea (24). Finally, the presence of underlying medical problems (e.g., diabetes mellitus, cancer, and acquired immunodeficiency syndrome [AIDS]), intravenous drug abuse, and the use of certain medications, particularly immunosuppressive agents, frequently have a significant impact on the diagnosis, treatment, and microbiology of hand infections.

On physical examination, the position of the hand and fingers at rest and the presence of any wounds or breaks in the continuity of the skin should be noted. The location and nature of any swelling, fluctuance, erythema, warmth, or tenderness should be carefully documented. The hand and individual digits should be put through a full range of motion. Any limitation or pain with movement should be clearly described. A thorough and well-documented neurovascular assessment is mandatory.

PARONYCHIA

Paronychia is an infection involving the lateral nail fold (paronychium). It is the most common infection of the hand (23,29). It results from mechanical separation of the eponychium from the nail plate with subsequent invasion of bacteria or fungi (20).

Common causes of a paronychia include hangnails, manicuring, and nail biting (12,25). Individuals whose hands are repeatedly submerged in water (e.g., dishwashers) seem to be particularly susceptible (20). Extension of the infection to involve the adjacent eponychium and proximal nail fold is called an eponychia (4,23).

CLINICAL PRESENTATION

Pain, swelling, and redness usually begin in the proximal portion of the lateral nail fold in the area adjacent to the eponychium. If ignored or untreated, it may extend to involve the onychium and proximal nail fold (i.e., eponychia) or, rarely, to the lateral nail fold on the opposite side (i.e., run-around infection) (4,23,25). The involved tissue is usually very tender. Fluctuance is generally present but may be absent early in the course of the infection. In severe infections, pus may extend beneath the nail. Large amounts of subungual pus may result in a floating nail. Systemic signs and symptoms such as fever or tachycardia are unusual.

DIFFERENTIAL DIAGNOSIS

The differential diagnosis of an acute paronychia includes herpetic whitlow, a chronic paronychia, and a felon. Herpetic whitlow is a viral infection caused by the herpes simplex virus. It can usually be differentiated from a paronychia by careful history and physical examination (see the section on herpetic whitlow). A chronic paronychia is a smoldering infection frequently associated with *C. albicans*. It is not clear whether candida plays an infectious role or is a frequent colonizer in an inflammatory process (34). It is most common in diabetics and in middle-aged women whose hands are frequently exposed to water containing irritants or alkali (23). Patients usually complain of a waxing and waning infection. Pain and tenderness are less severe in comparison to an acute paronychia (21). A severe infection may be confused with a felon. However, rather than subungual pus or fluctuance of the nail folds, patients with a felon have tense swelling of the distal pulp space.

EMERGENCY DEPARTMENT EVALUATION

The diagnosis of a paronychia is made by history and physical examination. Radiographs may be useful in selected situations (e.g., trauma, suspicion of a foreign body) but are generally not helpful, and laboratory testing is unnecessary in the majority of patients.

EMERGENCY DEPARTMENT MANAGEMENT

If the diagnosis is made before the accumulation of pus, management is nonsurgical and includes an oral antimicrobial agent effective against *Staphylococcus* and *Streptococcus* species (Table 104.2) and warm soaks. Rest and elevation of the affected part are helpful adjuncts. Once fluctuance has been identified, however, surgical drainage must be performed. The method of drainage depends on the severity of the infection.

A digital block provides anesthesia for drainage. Local preparation includes cleansing the digit with povidone–iodine or a similar agent. Hemostasis is obtained by placing a 1-in. Penrose drain securely around the proximal portion of the affected digit.

Superficial infections are drained by inserting a no. 11 blade between the nail and eponychium. The eponychium is lifted

TABLE 104.2.   Recommendations for Initial Antimicrobial Therapy of Hand Infections[a]

Infection	Initial Antimicrobial Therapy[b]	Comments
Felon/paronychia	Cephalexin 500 mg PO q.1.d. for 7 days	Cefazolin should be used for admitted patients.
Severe Infections[c]	Cefazolin 1 g i.v., and penicillin G 2 million units i.v.	Ceftriaxone 1 g i.v. is given for flexor tenosynovitis due to disseminated gonorrhea.
Diabetic/immuno-compromised patients	Cefazolin 1 g i.v., and pencillin G 2 million units i.v., and gentamicin 1.0 mg/kg i.v., or aztreonam 12 g i.v.	High incidence of gram-negative organisms
Intravenous drug abuser	Cefazolin 1 g i.v., and vancomycin 1 g i.v.	High incidence of methicillin-resistant *Staphylococcus aureus*
Herpetic whitlow	None	Consider acyclovir for suppression of recurrent attacks and for severe infection in immunocompromised patients.

[a] Agents or a combination of agents with similar coverage may be substituted. Alternatives for penicillin- and/or cephalosporin-allergic patients are discussed in the text.
[b] Initial antimicrobial therapy should be adjusted as the results of culture and sensitivity tests become available.
[c] Flexor tenosynovitis, web space abscess, and palmer space infection.

away from the nail to drain the pus (Fig. 104.2). If necessary, the blade can then be swept around to incise the lateral nail fold. The incision should be made tangential to the dorsolateral curve of the nail, with the blade directed away from the nail bed and nail matrix to avoid injury to these structures. After drainage, a small gauze wick should be inserted between the eponychium and nail to facilitate continued drainage.

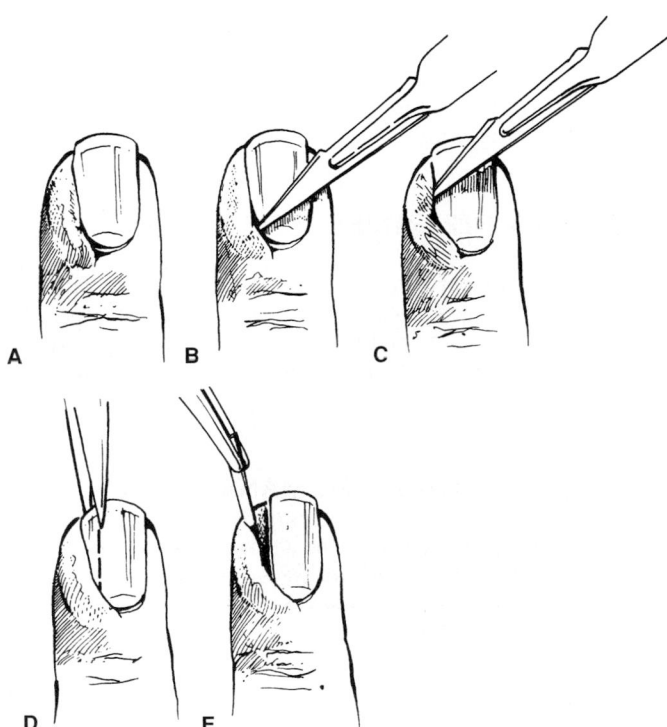

Figure 104.2.   Drainage of a paronychia. **(A)** Superficial paronychia. **(B)** Elevation of the eponychia using a no. 11 blade. **(C)** If necessary, the lateral nail fold may be incised to achieve adequate drainage. **(D)** A more extensive paronychia with pus extending under the adjacent portion of the nail. **(E)** Removal of the adjacent one-fourth of the nail to drain the subungual pus. If removal of the nail does not allow complete drainage, the lateral nail fold may be incised as in **(C)**.

If pus is present under the adjacent portion of the nail, one-fourth of the nail on that side should be removed for adequate drainage to occur (see Fig. 104.2) (12,25,29). The portion of nail to be removed is first separated from the underlying nail bed by inserting a small hemostat or iris scissors beneath the distal free edge of the nail and gently opening and closing the instrument as it is worked proximally toward the eponychium. Once separated, an iris scissors is used to cut longitudinally along the nail from the distal edge to the eponychium. The nail is then gently removed with the aid of a Kelly clamp. If this does not allow complete drainage of pus, an incision can be made into the lateral nail fold as previously described. A gauze wick is inserted to promote drainage.

If pus is discovered under the dorsal roof of the proximal nail fold or beneath the nail in the nail fold, or if the patient presents with a floating nail, drainage requires removal of the proximal one-third of the nail (12,23,25,29). However, controversy exists as to whether incision of the eponychial tissue is necessary for adequate drainage.

If the infection involves the eponychium and one lateral nail fold (in addition to pus under the dorsal roof or nail root), some authors recommend making a single incision starting at the mid-point of the lateral nail fold and extending it proximally to the base of the nail (21.23). The eponychial tissue and lateral nail fold are bluntly elevated from the nail, and the proximal one-third of the nail is removed (Fig. 104.3). If a run-around infection is present, Neviaser (31) and Siegel and Gelberman (33) recommend making an incision in each lateral nail fold as just described. The entire eponychium is gently elevated as a flap to expose the underlying nail root, and the proximal one-third of the nail is excised using iris scissors (see Fig. 104.3) (23,25). In contrast, Zook (37) maintains that it is not necessary to make incisions in the eponychium. He agrees that the proximal portion of the nail must be removed, but argues that an incision in the eponychium will frequently not heal primarily in the face of infection and may result in a notch or square corner in the eponychium. Unfortunately, there are few scientific data regarding the optimal approach. If a floating nail is present, incision of the eponychia tissue is probably unnecessary because removal of the nail can be easily performed by pushing back the lateral nail fold and excising the loose nail (see Fig. 104.3). However, if the nail is partially adherent it may be difficult to remove the

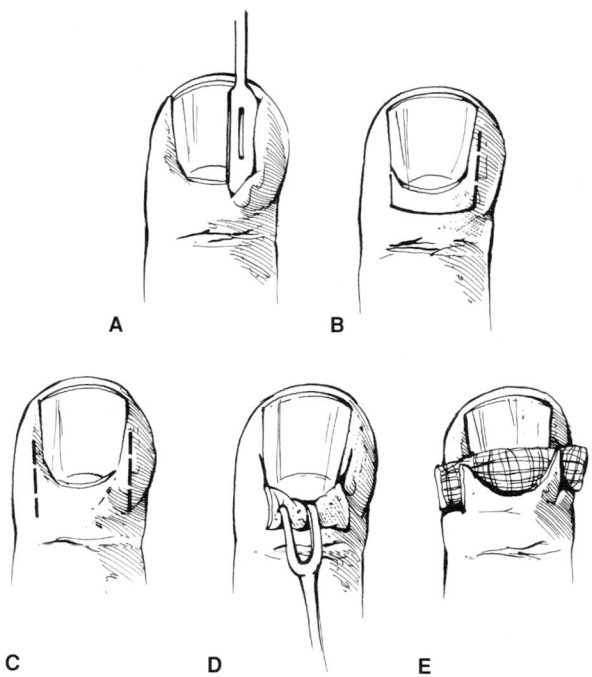

Figure 104.3. Drainage of a paronychia associated with a floating nail, or with pus beneath either the dorsal roof of the proximal nail fold or the nail within the proximal nail fold. **(A)** Elevation of the eponychial fold with a flat probe to expose the base of the nail for excision of a floating nail. **(B)** Placement of an incision to drain the eponychium and lateral nail fold and to elevate the eponychial fold for excision of the proximal one-third of the nail. **(C–E)** Incisions and procedure for elevating the entire eponychial fold for excision of the proximal one-third of the nail. A gauze pack prevents premature closure of the cavity. (Redrawn from Neviaser RJ. Infections. In: Green DP, ed. *Operative Hand Surgery,* 3rd ed. New York: Churchill Livingstone, 1993: 1023.)

proximal portion without incising one or both sides of the eponychium. Regardless of which technique is used, after removal of the proximal portion of the nail, a gauze wick should be placed between the eponychium and exposed nail to prevent adhesion of the eponychium to the nail bed and to facilitate continued drainage.

Treatment of chronic paronychias remains controversial. Reducing chronic exposure to irritating agents is clearly beneficial. In addition, a recent prospective, randomized, double-blinded study demonstrated a small benefit of topical methylprednisolone over systemic antifungals (34). Unfortunately, the numbers in this study were too small to make any firm recommendations regarding the use of methylprednisolone for chronic paronychias.

DISPOSITION

The majority of patients with a paronychia may be discharged from the emergency department. The affected digit should be kept clean and dry. Elevation should be stressed to help diminish pain and swelling. Patients with a small superficial paronychia should be rechecked at 24 hours. At this time, the gauze wick is removed and the patient is started on warm soaks. For larger, more extensive infections, the drain should remain in place for 48 to 72 hours before beginning warm soaks (23). An oral antimicrobial agent effective against *Staphylococcus aureus* and *Streptococcus* species is indicated if there is surrounding cellulitis (see Table 104.2). The need for admission is rare, but it should be considered for those patients who have an extensive surrounding cellulitis or lymphangitis, particularly in high-risk individuals

such as diabetics, those on immunosuppressive agents, and patients with AIDS. Consultation with a hand surgeon is recommended for all high-risk patients presenting with a severe infection.

COMMON PITFALLS

✔ Failure to recognize the need for surgical drainage. If the presence of pus is suspected, drainage should be performed
✔ Failure to remove the adjacent portion of the nail when subungual pus is present. If this is not done, adequate drainage may not occur
✔ Failure to place a wick between the eponychium and nail plate after drainage. This may result in reaccumulation of pus and, if the proximal portion of the nail was removed, adhesions between the aponychium and underlying nail bed

FELON

A felon is an infection of the distal pulp space of a finger or thumb. It occurs more commonly in the right hand, with the thumb and index finger most frequently affected (20). The infection frequently results from a puncture wound to the tip of the digit. A subcutaneous abscess rapidly forms in the pulp space, breaking down the fibrous septa as it expands. If left untreated, the infection may extend to the distal phalanx, causing osteomyelitis, or to the skin, resulting in necrosis and a draining sinus on the volar surface of the fingertip (23). Moreover, because the fibrous septa create a closed space within the fingertip, pressure from the expanding abscess and associated edema can lead to ischemia of the pulp space and, ultimately, slough of the tactile portion of the finger pad.

CLINICAL PRESENTATION

The patient with a felon typically presents with a red, swollen, and painful fingertip. There is a history of penetrating trauma in approximately two-thirds of cases, but this is not necessary to make the diagnosis (21). Early in the course of the infection, the patient usually complains of an aching pain that increases when pressure is applied to the fingertip. The pain rapidly becomes severe and throbbing. Systemic signs and symptoms are rare. On examination, the fingertip is extremely tender and there is erythema and swelling of the distal pulp space. As a rule, the swelling does not extend proximal to the distal interphalangeal joint (12). Fluctuance is generally present within 48 hours (23). In some cases, the abscess will point, while in others there will be a more diffuse collection of pus. If the infection has spread toward the skin, a draining sinus may be visible on the volar surface of the fingertip. In advanced cases, there may be necrosis of the tactile portion of the finger pad. Other complications of an untreated felon include necrosis of the distal phalanx secondary to osteomyelitis, pyogenic arthritis of the distal interphalangeal joint, and, rarely, a flexor tenosynovitis from proximal extension (4,12,23).

DIFFERENTIAL DIAGNOSIS

The differential diagnosis of a felon includes herpetic whitlow, cellulitis of the fingertip, and a severe run-around infection (Herpetic whitlow is discussed later in this chapter). In cellulitis of the fingertip, fluctuance is usually absent, and pain, tenderness, and swelling are less severe. In addition, unlike a felon, cellulitis will often spread proximal to the distal interphalangeal joint. Patients with a severe run-around infection have fluctuance of the eponychium and both lateral nail folds. In contrast, the fluctuance associated with a felon is much greater in the distal pulp space.

EMERGENCY DEPARTMENT EVALUATION

The diagnosis of a felon is made by history and physical examination. Radiographs of the affected digit are recommended to assess for osteomyelitis. Gram stain and culture and sensitivity testing of spontaneous or surgically obtained drainage will aid in making a bacteriologic diagnosis and help guide the choice of antimicrobial agent. Other laboratory tests (e.g., complete blood cell count, electrolytes, glucose) may be helpful in certain patients, such as those with a complication of an untreated felon (e.g., pyogenic arthritis, flexor tenosynovitis, osteomyelitis) or those with significant underlying medical disorders (e.g., diabetes mellitus, AIDS, cancer). In general, however, laboratory testing is unnecessary.

EMERGENCY DEPARTMENT MANAGEMENT

If the patient presents in the early stages of the infection (i.e., before the onset of fluctuance), management includes an oral antimicrobial agent and supportive care. The antimicrobial agent chosen should be effective against *Staphylococcus* and *Streptococcus* species (see Table 104.2). Supportive measures include rest, immobilization, and elevation of the affected extremity. Surgical drainage is indicated when there is fluctuance present or if associated swelling threatens to interrupt blood flow to the distal pulp space. Although the presence of pus may be difficult to assess in some patients, it is usually present if the process has been going on for more than 48 hours (23).

The basic goal of surgical intervention is to provide adequate drainage without creating a disabling scar or unstable fat pad, injuring the digital artery and nerve, or violating the flexor tendon sheath, causing an iatrogenic flexor tenosynovitis (23). In the past, several surgical approaches have been recommended (Fig. 104.4). Many of them, however, are associated with a high incidence of unacceptable complications and are therefore no longer recommended (Table 104.3). At the present time, the unilateral longitudinal approach is the technique most often employed (12,23,25).

Before drainage, a tourniquet (sterile Penrose drain) should be placed around the proximal portion of the digit, as described

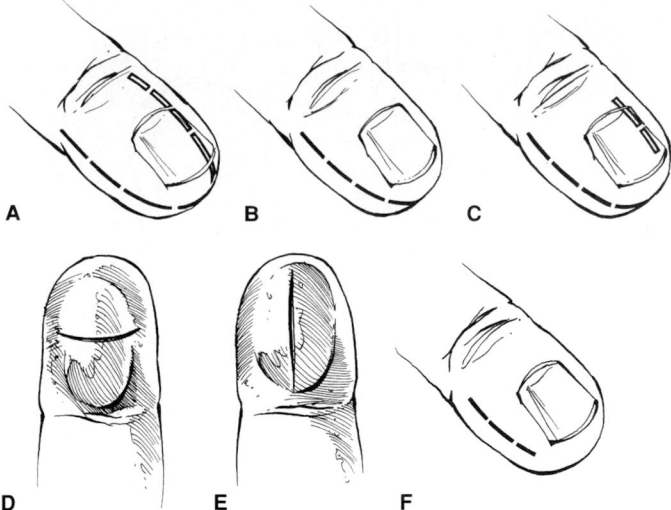

Figure 104.4. Incisions for drainage of felons. **(A)** Fish-mouth incision. This approach has significant complications and should be avoided. **(B)** Hockey stick or J incision. This should be reserved for an extensive or severe abscess or felon. Its routine use is no longer recommended. The incision should be more dorsal at the tip than shown (i.e., at the junction of the skin and nail bed). **(C)** Incision for through-and-through drainage of a felon is rarely, if ever, necessary. Again, the distal incision should be at the junction of the skin and the nail bed. **(D)** Volar drainage. Useful if the abscess points volarward, but this incision risks injury to digital nerves. **(E)** Alternative volar approach. Less risk to digital nerves but should not touch or cross the distal interphalangeal flexion crease. **(F)** Unilateral longitudinal approach. (Redrawn from Neviaser RJ. Infections. In: Green DP, ed. *Operative hand surgery*, 3rd ed. New York: Churchill Livingstone, 1993: 1025.)

previously. The unilateral longitudinal incision is made dorsal to the neurovascular bundle on the ulnar side of the index, long, and ring fingers or on the radial side of the thumb and little finger. The incision starts approximately 0.5 cm distal to the distal flexion crease and extends in a straight line to a point in line with the beginning of the hyponychium (see Fig.104. 4). The blade is carefully inserted deeper and deeper until the abscess is entered. The opening of the cavity is enlarged using a small Kelly clamp until complete evacuation is achieved. Blunt rupture of all the fibrous septa should be avoided because it frequently results in an unstable fat pad. The cavity is irrigated with saline, and the wound is packed with 0.25-inch gauze packing. The hand is splinted and elevated, and the patient is started on an oral antimicrobial agent effective against *Staphylococcus* and *Streptococcus*

TABLE 104.3. Surgical Approaches for Draining a Felon

Surgical Approach	Indications	Complications	Comments
Unilateral longitudinal incision	All felons	Injury to the neurovascular bundle	Technique of choice for most felons; incision should be made dorsal to the neurovascular bundle.
Longitudinal volar incision	Presence of a draining sinus or pointing on the volar fat pad	Sensitive scar on the tactile surface of the digit	Incision should not cross the distal flexion crease; if a sinus is present, necrotic skin edges should be debrided.
Transverse volar incision	Pointing in the center of the volar fat pad	Sensitive scar on the tactile surface of the digit; injury to the neurovascular bundle	Offers no advantage over the longitudinal volar incision
Through-and-through incision	All felons	Injury to the neurovascular bundle; potential for an unstable fat pad	Rarely, if ever, necessary for adequate drainage
Hockey stick or J incision	Severe infections	Unsightly, tender scar; unstable fat pad; rare skin slough	Not recommended for routine use
Fish-mouth incision	Severe infections	Unsightly, tender scar; unstable fat pad; rare skin slough	No longer recommended

species (see Table 104.2). The gauze pack is removed in 48 hours, at which time the patient is started on warm soaks.

For patients with a draining sinus or pointing abscess on the volar surface of the fingertip a midline longitudinal incision is recommended (18,23). Because the abscess cavity lies directly under the draining sinus or area of pointing, a midline longitudinal incision made directly through this area produces excellent drainage with few complications. The incision is made through the sinus (or over the area of pointing), starting 0.5 cm distal to the distal flexion crease, and extends to the beginning of the hyponychium (see Fig. 104.4). Care should be taken not to cross the distal flexion crease because this may result in a disabling scar. The incision is deepened until the abscess cavity is entered. A small Kelly clamp is used to gently widen the opening and ensure complete drainage. After drainage, the cavity is irrigated with saline; but in contrast to the unilateral longitudinal approach, no packing is necessary. Instead, the application of a thick coat of zinc oxide (or similar agent) will keep the exudate from drying up and closing the wound, and it will enhance sequestration of the necrotic core (18). A bulky dressing is applied, and the distal extremity is immobilized and elevated.

DISPOSITION

Most patients with a felon may be discharged from the emergency department. Patients should be encouraged to keep the affected digit clean and dry. Elevation of the involved extremity will help decrease pain and swelling and facilitate healing. The patient should be reevaluated in 48 hours, at which time the gauze wick is removed and warm soaks initiated. If a zinc oxide dressing is used, it should be changed every 2 days. An oral antimicrobial agent effective against *Staphylococcus* and *Streptococcus* species is also recommended (see Table 104.2). In addition, a few days of an oral narcotic analgesic (e.g., oxycodone or hydrocodone with acetaminophen) will be appreciated by most patients. The need for admission is rare but should be considered for a severe infection in high-risk individuals such as immunocompromised patients and diabetics. Consultation is recommended for these patients before making a final disposition. Moreover, patients who develop a pyogenic arthritis, flexor tenosynovitis, osteomyelitis, or an ischemic digit will require immediate consultation and admission.

COMMON PITFALLS

✔ Failure to recognize the need for surgical drainage. If the patient has been symptomatic for 48 hours or more, the presence of pus is highly likely and the pulp space should be surgically drained. Moreover, if swelling is so severe that it could compromise distal blood flow, the finger should be opened regardless of whether pus is present

✔ Improperly placed incisions. For example, a volar incision that crosses the distal flexion crease may cause a disabling scar, while a lateral incision not made dorsal to the neurovascular bundle may result in permanent sensory loss or ischemia of the distal fat pad

✔ Blunt rupture of all the fibrous septa. This is no longer recommended because it frequently results in an unstable fat pad

HERPETIC WHITLOW

Herpetic whitlow is a viral infection of the fingertip caused by type 1 and type 2 herpes simplex viruses. In the past, the disease was thought to be most common in medical and health-care professionals. However, researchers in one study found that individuals most often affected are adults with genital herpes and patients of all ages with herpetic gingivostomatitis (7). In addition, several case reports of AIDS patients with whitlow describe a very aggressive and destructive form of the disease (8,32). The infection most often affects the distal pulp space and, occasionally, the proximal and lateral nail folds (7). The fingers are affected more often than the thumb. Herpetic whitlow is self-limited and usually resolves in 3 to 4 weeks. About 20% of patients experience recurrent infections that tend to be less severe than the original (6).

CLINICAL PRESENTATION

Patients initially have pain and dysesthesia or burning of the distal phalanx. This is usually followed by swelling and erythema. Despite associated swelling, however, the distal pulp space usually remains soft (21). This helps to differentiate herpetic whitlow from a felon, in which there is tense swelling of the distal pulp space. One or more small vesicles then appear and often coalesce to form bullae. On examination, tenderness is present, but usually much less severe than that seen with bacterial infections (23). Some patients may have associated fever, lymphadenopathy, lymphangitis, and constitutional symptoms (6). The vesicles may contain fluid that is clear, turbid, or occasionally hemorrhagic but not purulent. If purulence is present, it suggests a secondary bacterial infection (14,17). After 10 days, the vesicles or bullae will begin to crust over and, shortly after this, the area peels to reveal normal skin.

DIFFERENTIAL DIAGNOSIS

The differential diagnosis of herpetic whitlow includes a felon and a paronychia. The features differentiating these conditions have been described previously in this chapter.

EMERGENCY DEPARTMENT EVALUATION

The diagnosis of herpetic whitlow is usually clinical. It can often be confirmed in the emergency department by a Tzanck smear. This is performed by first unroofing a vesicle and scraping the base with a wooden applicator. The scrapings are spread on a slide and allowed to air dry or are fixed with ethyl alcohol. The slide is stained with Giemsa or Wright stain or with methylene blue and examined for the presence of multinucleated giant cells (6). If the Tzanck smear is negative or unable to be performed, a culture can be obtained. This is more sensitive than a Tzanck smear, but results take up to 48 hours. Electron microscopy and the fluorescent antibody test are complicated by both false-positive and false-negative results, and serologic tests often require more than a week to become positive (6).

EMERGENCY DEPARTMENT MANAGEMENT

Management of herpetic whitlow is symptomatic. The digit is covered with a dry dressing to reduce the spread of infection. An oral analgesic and aspiration of tense vesicles may be helpful in relieving pain. The use of acyclovir has not been evaluated in a large, prospective-controlled trial, but several anecdotal reports have documented suppression of recurrent attacks with oral acyclovir (9,19). More recently, famcyclovir and valacyclovir at doses recommended for the treatment of primary genital herpes have also been reported to be effective in suppressing recurrent attacks (11,28). Topical acyclovir has not been shown to be effective in the treatment of herpetic whitlow. Incision and drainage is contraindicated because it can result in secondary bacterial infection.

DISPOSITION

Patients with herpetic whitlow may be discharged from the emergency department. A followup visit is arranged in 7 to 10 days with the primary care physician or a hand specialist. Discharge instructions should include signs of secondary bacterial infection. If there is a suspicion of an associated bacterial infection (i.e., a paronychia or felon), consultation with a hand surgeon is highly recommended.

COMMON PITFALL

✔ Misdiagnosing herpetic whitlow as a felon or paronychia requiring incision and drainage. Surgical intervention causes unnecessary discomfort and may lead to secondary bacterial infection

FLEXOR TENOSYNOVITIS

Infection of a flexor tendon sheath can be one of the most devastating hand infections encountered in clinical practice. It is most commonly caused by a penetrating injury, particularly at the distal and proximal flexion creases where the tendon sheaths are more superficial. It may also result from direct extension of a neighboring infection and, rarely, by hematogenous or lymphatic spread. The thumb, index finger, and middle fingers are the digits most commonly involved, and the right hand is affected about twice as often as the left hand (21). If not recognized and treated early, purulence within the tendon sheath can destroy the delicate gliding mechanism. Persistent infection leads to the formation of adhesions, resulting in severe limitation of movement. If allowed to continue, the infection will eventually destroy the blood supply to the tendon, producing tendon necrosis.

CLINICAL PRESENTATION

Patients with flexor tenosynovitis complain of severe pain, swelling, and limited motion of the affected digit. There is a history of penetrating trauma in approximately 90% of cases (21). Kanavel (21) described four cardinal signs of flexor tenosynovitis: (1) excessive tenderness over the course of the sheath but limited to the sheath, (2) symmetric enlargement (edema) of the whole finger, (3) a flexed position of the finger at rest, and (4) excruciating pain on passive extension of the finger, most marked at the proximal end. The latter is the most valuable of these signs and may be the only one present very early in the disease process (23). In established infections, swelling frequently involves the dorsum of the hand. This is most commonly due to lymphatic drainage from the affected digit, rather than from extension of infection. Dorsal swelling is usually less than that seen with a thenar or midpalmar space infection. If the patient does not seek medical treatment early, the infection may spread to one of the deep palmar spaces, especially the thenar space and midpalmar space, or to adjacent bone or joints, causing an associated osteomyelitis or septic arthritis, respectively.

Infection of the tendon sheath of the little finger or thumb may extend to involve the ulnar bursa and radial bursa, respectively. Patients with involvement of the ulnar bursa will develop severe pain and tenderness in the palm and wrist. There is usually swelling of the entire hand, and dorsal edema becomes more pronounced. The other fingers become sensitive to touch and assume a semiflexed position. Any attempt at passive extension of the fingers is resisted because of severe pain. Similarly, patients with involvement of the radial bursa will develop severe pain and tenderness over the thenar eminence and radial aspect of the wrist. The thenar eminence becomes swollen, but usually not to the degree of a thenar space infection. Swelling over the dorsum of the hand also becomes more prominent. The hand is usually held in moderate flexion and radial deviation. In contrast to patients with infection of the ulnar bursa, patients with infection of the radial bursa do not have pain or limitation of movement of the other fingers. If this occurs, it usually means the infection has spread from the radial bursa to the ulnar bursa, causing a "horseshoe abscess."

DIFFERENTIAL DIAGNOSIS

The differential diagnosis of flexor tenosynovitis includes a palmar space infection, cellulitis, osteomyelitis, and septic arthritis. However, the diagnosis of flexor tenosynovitis can usually be made if a detailed physical examination is performed, with emphasis on the four cardinal signs described by Kanavel (21). The finding of excruciating pain on passive extension of the digit is particularly helpful because it is often present early in patients with flexor tenosynovitis and is generally not seen with other hand infections (palmar space infections are discussed later in this chapter). Patients with a cellulitis of the digit have symptoms and physical findings that are usually less severe than those associated with flexor tenosynovitis. In particular, tenderness is localized to the area affected with cellulitis, the digit is not held flexed, and severe pain with passive extension of the digit is generally lacking. Likewise, patients with osteomyelitis and septic arthritis tend to have findings that are more localized to the infected bone or joint, respectively.

EMERGENCY DEPARTMENT EVALUATION

The diagnosis of flexor tenosynovitis is made by history and physical examination. Radiographs of the affected digit are recommended to look for a foreign body and osteomyelitis. A complete blood cell count and blood cultures may be helpful in those individuals with systemic involvement. Urethral or endocervical cultures for *Neisseria gonorrhoeae* may be useful in the appropriate clinical setting. Other tests should be based on the patient's presenting complaints, underlying medical problems, and the need for operative drainage.

EMERGENCY DEPARTMENT MANAGEMENT

Emergency department management of suspected flexor tenosynovitis includes elevation and immobilization of the affected hand, intravenous antimicrobial therapy, and relief of pain. Antimicrobial therapy should be undertaken on a broad spectrum, aimed at both gram-positive aerobic bacteria as well as anaerobic organisms (see Table 104.2). Intravenous cefazolin and penicillin G are initially recommended (26). Gentamicin or aztreonam should be added for suspected gram-negative infection (i.e., infection in a diabetic or immunocompromised patient). Nafcillin can be used in place of cefazolin for gram-positive coverage, but, unlike cefazolin, it does not have activity against gram-negative organisms. Both lack anaerobic coverage. In patients with a nonanaphylactic allergy to penicillin (i.e., patients who can safely be given a cephalosporin), cefoxitin provides coverage for common gram-negative and gram-positive bacteria, as well as many anaerobic organisms (26). Vancomycin and clindamycin may be used in patients with a cephalosporin or severe penicillin allergy. Patients who present with tenosynovitis secondary to a human bite need coverage for *Eikenella*, which is resistant to clindamycin, cephalexin, metronidazole and erythromycin. Fortunately, penicillin G, ampicillin, amoxicillin/clavulanate, trimethoprim/sulfamethoxazole and most floroquinolones provide acceptable coverage for *Eikenella* (11). Patients who present with infections following a cat bite have a high incidence of Pasteurella multocida, which is generally sensitive to amoxicillin/clavulanate (this also covers *Staphylococcus aureus)*, cefuroxime axetil, doxycycline, and penicillin G (11). Patients with evidence of disseminated gonorrhea should receive intravenous ceftriaxone. Finally, patients with severe pain will benefit from a parenteral narcotic while awaiting surgical consultation.

DISPOSITION

All patients with suspected flexor tenosynovitis require immediate consultation with a hand surgeon and admission to the hospital. Patients presenting greater than 48 hours after the onset of symptoms require drainage in the operating suite. If the patient presents within the first 24 to 48 hours, conservative therapy with continued elevation and immobilization, intravenous antimicrobial agents, and close observation may be attempted. If the patient's condition is not markedly improved within 24 hours or if physical findings are not resolved within 2 days, surgical drainage is indicated (12,23). The choice of conservative versus operative management is best left to the consulting surgeon.

COMMON PITFALLS

✔ Failure to make the diagnosis on initial presentation. A careful history and physical examination, with close attention to the cardinal signs of flexor tenosynovitis and a low threshold for consultation and admission, will help avoid a late diagnosis
✔ Sending the patient with equivocal findings home without having been seen by the consulting surgeon. The emergency physician should stand firm on admitting all patients with suspected cases of flexor tenosynovitis and should be adamant that the consulting hand surgeon see the patient in the emergency department or shortly after admission. This request should be clearly documented in the emergency department record

WEB SPACE (COLLAR BUTTON) ABSCESS

An infection of a web space usually results from a break in the skin surrounding an infected palmar blister. Consequently, it is seen most often in individuals who do manual labor. If left untreated, the infection spreads dorsally to the dorsal subcutaneous space and deep into the palmar web space. This creates an hourglass configuration to the abscess, hence the term *collar button abscess*. Rarely, an untreated infection in the web space between the index and middle fingers will spread medially to involve the other two web spaces (4).

CLINICAL PRESENTATION

Patients usually complain of pain and swelling of the involved web space and surrounding palm. Systemic signs and symptoms are unusual in uncomplicated infections. Examination reveals tenderness and swelling of the affected web space. Anteroposterior pressure over the web space elicits severe discomfort (4). Swelling may be more prominent on either the palmar or the dorsal aspect, depending on the nature of the infection (23).

Because of pus and swelling, the fingers adjacent to the affected web space are held abducted at rest. Patients with a neglected web space abscess may present with signs of tendon sheath or palmar space involvement. Untreated infections may also dissect distally along the course of the lumbricals, leading to tissue slough (4). Rarely, the infection will spread to involve the dorsal subaponeurotic space (4). If this occurs, patients will have pain, tenderness, and fluctuance involving the dorsum of the hand.

DIFFERENTIAL DIAGNOSIS

The differential diagnosis of a web space abscess includes a dorsal subcutaneous space infection, an infected palmar blister, and a deep palmar space infection. As with other infections of the hand, a careful history and physical examination will lead to the appropriate diagnosis. In a dorsal subcutaneous space infection, the fingers are not held abducted at rest and palmar tenderness is minimal or absent. Although infection of a palmar blister usually precedes a web space abscess, pain and tenderness are mild in comparison and are localized over the blister, not the web space. Furthermore, swelling is usually minimal and, when present, does not involve the dorsum of the hand. The findings associated with a deep palmar space infection vary with the involved space. (Palmar space infections are discussed later in this chapter.)

EMERGENCY DEPARTMENT EVALUATION

The diagnosis of a web space infection is made by history and physical examination. Radiographs of the affected hand are recommended if a foreign body or osteomyelitis is suspected. Gram stain and culture and sensitivity testing of spontaneous drainage may aid in making a bacteriologic diagnosis and help guide the choice of antimicrobial agent. A complete blood cell count and blood cultures may be helpful in those individuals with systemic involvement. Additional tests should be based on the patients' presenting complaints, their underlying medical problems, and institutional requirements for drainage in the operating suite.

EMERGENCY DEPARTMENT MANAGEMENT

Emergency department management includes elevation of the affected hand, antimicrobial therapy, and pain control. Initial antimicrobial therapy is the same as described for flexor tenosynovitis (see Table 104.2). Pain should be treated with a parental analgesic.

DISPOSITION

All patients with a suspected web space infection require immediate consultation with a hand surgeon and admission to the hospital. Definitive management requires drainage in the operating suite.

COMMON PITFALLS

✔ Diagnosing a primary dorsal space infection because of the presence of dorsal edema
✔ Failure to recognize palmar involvement when dorsal edema is more prominent
✔ Failure to obtain consultation early in the evaluation process

PALMAR SPACE INFECTIONS

The palm of the hand contains four fascial spaces that are important sites of infection: the thenar space, the midpalmar space, the hypothenar space and Parona's space. The compartments may become infected from direct penetrating trauma; from contiguous infection, such as a tenosynovitis or osteomyelitis; or, rarely, from hematogenous seeding. Deep space infections may be associated with significant morbidity and permanent loss of function; thus, prompt diagnosis and treatment are essential.

CLINICAL PRESENTATION

The clinical presentation of patients with a palmar space infection depends on which space is involved. However, any patient may present with fever, chills, and other manifestations of a serious infection. A thenar space infection causes severe pain and tenderness and tense swelling of the thenar eminence. Because lymphatic drainage from the palm is directed dorsally, there is usually marked dorsal edema as well. However, there is little, if any, tenderness over the dorsum of the hand. Fluctuance is often present in the web space between the thumb and index finger. The thumb is held abducted and flexed; passive adduction produces severe pain. In contrast, patients with a midpalmar space infection have pain and tenderness over the central palm. There is marked fluctuance and swelling of the midpalmar space, resulting in a loss of normal palm concavity. In severe infections, there is frequently a bulge or convexity of the palm, a finding considered by Mann (30) to be almost pathognomonic of a midpalmar space infection. As with other serious hand infections, there is also edema over the dorsum of the hand, but no tenderness, erythema, or fluctuance. Motion of the middle and ring fingers is painful and limited (23). Infection of the hypothenar space is rare. There is pain and fullness over the hypothenar eminence, with a noticeable lack of swelling in the palm and fingers. Isolated infections in Parona's space are rare; infections here are usually associated with tenosynovitis or other deep space infections that have propagated into the forearm.

DIFFERENTIAL DIAGNOSIS

The differential diagnosis of a palmar space infection includes a cellulitis or superficial abscess of the palm, a web space infection, and flexor tenosynovitis. Once again, the history and physical examination are the keys to the correct diagnosis. Both a cellulitis and a superficial (subcutaneous) abscess of the palm produce pain and tenderness that may not be localized to a particular space. In addition, they cause far less palmar swelling, and dorsal edema is minimal or absent. Moreover, unless there is digital involvement, movement of the fingers or thumb causes little, if any, discomfort. The findings associated with a web space abscess and flexor tenosynovitis have already been described.

EMERGENCY DEPARTMENT EVALUATION

The diagnosis of a palmar space infection is made by history and physical examination. Radiographs of the affected hand are recommended to look for a suspected foreign body, osteomyelitis, or gas in the tissues. A complete blood cell count and blood cultures may be helpful in those individuals with systemic involvement. Additional tests should be based on the patients' presenting complaints and underlying medical problems and on institutional requirements for admission and drainage in the operating suite.

EMERGENCY DEPARTMENT MANAGEMENT

Emergency department management of a palmar space infection includes elevation and immobilization of the affected hand, broad-spectrum intravenous antimicrobial therapy, and pain control. Once again, antimicrobial therapy is the same as for other serious hand infections (see Table 104.2). A parenteral analgesic such as morphine or meperidine is indicated for patients with severe discomfort.

DISPOSITION

All patients with a suspected palmar space infection require immediate consultation with a hand surgeon and admission to the hospital. Definitive management requires drainage in the operating suite.

COMMON PITFALLS

✔ Failure to appreciate the presence of a palmar space infection, particularly early in the disease process. Therefore, it is essential to maintain a high index of suspicion and consider the possibility of a palmar space infection in any patient who presents with erythema, swelling, and tenderness of the palm
✔ Misinterpreting the presence of dorsal edema as a dorsal hand infection
✔ Sending home patients who have an equivocal examination, without their having been examined by the consulting surgeon. Thus, evaluation in the emergency department by the consulting hand surgeon is mandatory before releasing any patient with a suspected palmar space infection

Acknowledgment

Thanks to the previous edition's chapter author Paul Blackburn who wrote a chapter upon which this chapter was based.

References

1. Abraham KA, Little MA, Casey R, et al. A novel presentation of cryptococcal infection in a renal allograft recipient. *Ir Med J* 2000;93:82.
2. Berlet G, Richards RS, Roth JH. Clentched-fist injury complicated by methicillin-resistant Staphylococcus aureus. *Can J Surg* 1997;40:313.
3. Boles SD, Schmidt CC. Pyogenic flexor tenosynovitis. *Hand Clin* 1998;14:567.
4. Chudnofsky CR, Sebastian S. Special wounds: nail bed, plantar puncture, and cartilage. *Emerg Med Clin North Am* 1992;10:801.
5. Connolly B, Johnstone F, Gerlinger T, et al. Methicillin-resistant Staphylococcus aureus in a finger felon. *Am J Hand Surg* 2000;25:173.
6. Crandon JH.Common infections of the hand. In: Grayson TH, ed. *Flynn's hand surgery*, 4th ed. Baltimore: Williams & Wilkins, 1991:762.
7. Feder HM, Long SS. Herpetic whitlow: epidemiology, clinical characteristics, diagnosis, and treatment. *Am J Dis Child* 1983;137:861.
8. Garcia-Plata MD, Moreno-Gimenez JC, Velez GA, et al. Herpetic whitlow in an AIDS patient. *J Eu Acad Dermatol Venereol* 1999;12:241.
9. Gill MJ, Arlette J, Buchan K. Herpes simplex virus infection of the hand: a profile of 79 cases. *Am J Med* 1988;84:89.
10. Gill M, Buchan K, Arlette J, et al. Acyclovir therapy for herpetic whitlow [Letter]. *Ann Intern Med* 1986;105:631.
11. Gilbert DN, Moellering RC Jr., Sande MA. Hand infections. In: *The Sanford Guide to Antimicrobial Therapy* 31st ed. Vermont: Antimicrobial Therapy, Inc, 2001:19.
12. Goldstein EJC, Barones MF, Miller TA. *Eikenella corrodens* in hand infections. *J Hand Surg* 1983;8:563.
13. Gunther SF, Gunther SB. Diabetic hand infections. *Hand Clin* 1998;14:647.
14. Hausman MR, Lisser SP. Hand infections. *Orthop Clin North Am* 1992;23:171.
15. Hoyen HA, Lacey SH, Graham TJ. Atypical hand infections. *Hand Clin* 1998;14:613.
16. Hurst LC, Amadio PC, Badalamente MA, et al. *Myobacterium marinum*infection of the hand. *J Hand Surg* 1987;12:428.
17. Hurst LC, Gluck R, Sampson ST, et al. Herpetic whitlow with bacterial abscess. *J Hand Surg* 1991;16:311.
18. Iverson RE, Vistnes LM. Coccidioidomycosis tenosynovitis in the hand. *J Bone Joint Surg* 1973;55:413.

19. Jebson PJL. Infections of the fingertip—paronychias and felons. *Hand Clin* 1998;14:547.
20. Jones NF, Conklin WT, Albo VC. Primary invasive aspergillosis of the hand. *J Hand Surg* 1986;11:425.
21. Kanavel AB. *Infections of the hand.* Philadelphia: Lea & Febiger, 1939:17.
22. Karanas YL, Bogdan MA, Chang J. Community acquired methicillin-resistant Staphylococcus aureus hand infections: case reports and clinical implications. *Am J Hand Surg* 2000;25:760.
23. Kilgore ES, Brown LG, Newmeyer WL, et al. Treatment of felons. *Am J Surg* 1975;130:194.
24. Kono M, Stern PJ. The history of hand infections. *Hand Clin* 1998;14:511.
25. Kour AK, Looi KP, Pho RWH. Hand infections in patients with diabetes. *Clin Orthop Rel Res* 1996;331:238.
26. Laskin OL. Acyclovir and suppression of frequently recurring herpetic whitlow. *Ann Intern Med* 1985;102:494.
27. Louis DS, Jebson PJL. Mimickers of hand infections. *Hand Clin* 1998;14:519.
28. Manian FA. Potential role of famciclovir for prevention of herpetic whitlow in the health setting. *Clin Infect Dis* 2000;31:E18.
29. Mann RJ, Peacock JM. Hand infections in patients with diabetes mellitus. *J Trauma* 1977;17:376.
30. Mann RJ. *Infections of the hand.* Philadelphia: Lea & Febiger, 1988.
31. Neviaser RJ.Infections. In: Green DP, ed. *Operative Hand Surgery,* 3rd ed. New York: Churchill Livingstone, 1993:1021.
32. Robayana MG, Herranz P, Rubio FA, et al. Destructive herpetic whitlow in AIDS: report of three cases. *Br J Eu Acad Dermatol* 1997;137:812.
33. Siegel DB, Gelberman RH. Infections of the hand. *Orthop Clin North Am* 1988;19:779.
34. Tosti A, Piraccini BM, Ghetti E, et al. Topical steroids versus systemic antifungals in the treatment of chronic paronychia: an open, randomized, double-blind and double dummy study. *J Am Acad Dermatol* 2002;47:73.
35. Tsai E, Failla JM. Hand infections in the trauma patient. *Hand Clinics* 1999;15:373.
36. Vandermissen G, Meuleman L, Tits G, et al. Cutaneous cryptococcosis in corticosteroid-treated patients with AIDS. *Acta Clin Belg* 1996;51:111.
37. Zook EG.The perionychium. In: Green DP, ed. *Operative hand surgery,* 3rd ed. New York: Churchill Livingstone, 1993:1303.

CHAPTER 105
Low Back Pain

David Della-Giustina

Back pain is a complaint that is commonly seen in the emergency department (ED), affecting up to 90% of the population at some point in their lives. With an annual incidence of 5% (10), back pain is second only to upper respiratory illness as a reason for physician visits (9,13). Up to 85% of patients with low back pain will have no definite etiology determined for their symptoms (9,17). Fortunately, despite the lack of a definite etiology, almost 90% of patients will have resolution of their symptoms within 1 month (1). In the approach to the patient with back pain, patients may be categorized into three groups: (1) back pain in adults, (2) back pain with sciatica, and (3) back pain in children. By far, the majority of patients with back pain presenting in the ED fall into the first category.

CLINICAL PRESENTATION

The clinical presentation of the patient with back pain ranges from the patient with mild pain who requires a work excuse to the patient with the severe, unrelenting pain of an epidural abscess. More important than recognizing a particular "classic" presentation for the various diseases is the thorough evaluation

TABLE 105.1. Red Flags in the History and Physical Exam

HISTORY

Pain greater than 6 weeks
Age less than 18 or over 50
History of trauma
Sciatica
Neurological complaints (paresthesias, anesthesia, weakness)
Incontinence of bowel or bladder
Night pain
Unrelenting pain despite rest and analgesics
Fever, chills, and night sweats
History of injection drug use
History of cancer

PHYSICAL EXAM

Fever
Patient writhing in pain
Point vertebral tenderness
Neurological deficits
Positive straight leg raise

of each patient, with a focus on the *red flags* found in the history and physical examination that raise suspicion for serious disease (Table 105.1).

Sciatica is defined as a radicular pain into the leg in the distribution of a lumbosacral nerve root; it is often accompanied by a neurosensory or motor deficit (10). Back pain with sciatica is much less common than back pain without sciatica, afflicting only 1% of patients with low back pain (10). There are many etiologies for sciatica, but most commonly it is due to a herniated disc. Generally, patients with sciatica have a more protracted course than routine back pain patients, with only 50% of patients with sciatica recovering within 1 month. However, of all patients with sciatica, only 5% to 10% will require surgery (9,10).

Children are a separate category, because back pain is a rare condition in children and is more likely to be caused by a serious diagnosable etiology. The differential diagnosis for the child with back pain is different from that of the adult, and it varies further based on the age of the child. Due to the higher potential for serious disease, one should approach the child with back pain more aggressively than the adult.

DIFFERENTIAL DIAGNOSIS

Adults with Nonspecific Back Pain

The majority of patients seen in the ED for acute low back pain have symptoms that fall into the category of nonspecific back pain (Fig. 105.1). This syndrome is known by many other names, such as mechanical back pain, back sprain/strain, and lumbago, but it is essentially an episode of acute low back pain without associated sciatica or neurologic deficits.

The patient typically complains of mild-to-moderate pain in the lumbar area that may radiate to the buttocks or thigh, and is worsened by activity and relieved with rest. The inciting incident is usually unremarkable, varying from an unusual posture for a period of time to lifting a heavy object. Physical examination typically reveals mild paraspinal tenderness, negative straight-leg raise testing, normal neurologic examination, and no other significant findings. The investigation of red flags, if any, from the history and physical examination is negative. Because 90% of the patients will see spontaneous resolution of their symptoms within 4 weeks, there is no need to perform diagnostic testing

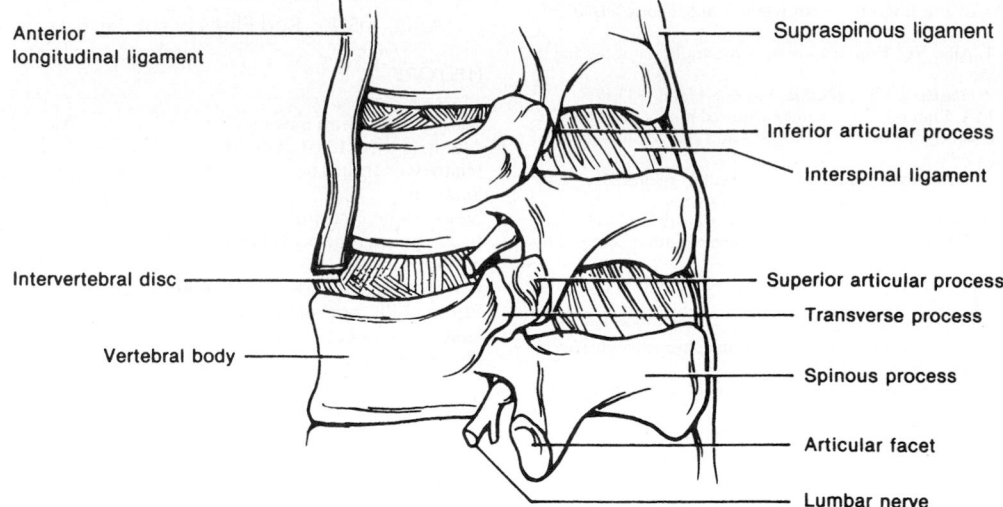

Figure 105.1. Normal anatomy of the lumbar spine.

unless red flags are uncovered. This saves the patient unnecessary pain, expense, and radiation exposure.

Spinal Infections

Vertebral osteomyelitis and spinal epidural abscess are uncommon etiologies for back pain. However, due to the potential morbidity and mortality that result from missed infection, one must remain vigilant concerning these possibilities. These infections occur more commonly in injection drug users, the immunocompromised, diabetics, and the elderly. These infections frequently occur secondary to hematogenous spread of *Staphylococcal aureus*. Patients with spinal infection usually present with moderate-to-severe back pain accompanied by fever, chills, unrelenting pain, night sweats, and weight loss. With epidural abscess, the patient may have concomitant sciatica and neurologic symptoms. Additionally, some patients with epidural abscess may present with sepsis. The peripheral white blood cell (WBC) count may be elevated or normal, but the erythrocyte sedimentation rate (ESR) is almost always elevated (11). One should always consider back pain in a patient who is an injection drug user as a spinal infection until proven otherwise.

Sciatica

The differential diagnosis for sciatica includes all etiologies that cause compression or inflammation of the spinal nerve roots, cauda equina, and spinal cord (Table 105.2). The major cause of sciatica is herniated disc. However, in the ED one should consider other etiologies, including spinal stenosis and compression of the cauda equina or spinal cord by tumor, infection, or hematoma.

Herniated Disc

Although sciatica affects only 1% of patients with low back pain, it is present in almost all patients with a symptomatic herniated disc. Ninety-eight percent of herniated discs involve either the L4-5 or L5-S1 intervertebral discs (9,10). Herniated disc most commonly occurs in patients during the fourth or fifth decades of life. Patients often complain of weeks of nonradicular low back pain preceding the onset of the radicular symptoms. The radicular symptoms are the hallmark of the nerve root compression and usually become the prominent symptom, with a diminution

of the back pain. Clinically, the diagnosis of herniated disc is made by localizing the pain to an isolated nerve root and demonstrating neurologic dysfunction in the distribution of that nerve root. Positive straight-leg raise testing increases the probability of herniated disc, especially if the crossed straight-leg raise test

TABLE 105.2. Differential Diagnosis of Sciatica

LUMBOSACRAL NERVE ROOT LESION

Disc herniation
Neoplasm
Infection (bone, disc, epidural space, nerve)
Spondylosis
Spondylolisthesis
Spinal stenosis
Subarachnoid hemorrhage
Arachnoiditis
Arachnoid cyst
Paget's disease

LUMBOSACRAL PLEXUS LESION

Hematoma
Pregnancy
Pelvic tumors (uterine, bladder, prostate)
Endometriosis
Aneurysm of common iliac or hypogastric artery
Endometriosis

SCIATIC NERVE LESION

Trauma
Entrapment
Ischemia
Tumor

REFERRED LEG PAIN

Degenerative disc
Facet joint disease
Bone tumor
Osteoarthritis of the hip
Sacroiliac joint disease
Spinothalamic tract lesion

(Modified from Bay JW. Other causes of low back pain and sciatica. In: Hardy RW, ed. *Lumbar disc disease*, 2nd ed. New York: Raven Press, 1993, with permission.)

is positive (9). If a diagnosis of herniated disc is entertained, one should ensure that only one nerve root is involved. The involvement of multiple nerve roots is cause for concern for a larger central disc herniation or a spinal mass.

Epidural Compression Syndrome

Epidural compression syndrome is a collective term encompassing spinal cord compression, cauda equina syndrome, and conus medullaris syndrome. This term is commonly used to group these syndromes together for two reasons. First, the presentation for these syndromes is similar, except for the level of the neurologic deficit. Secondly, the initial evaluation and management of these syndromes is similar, until the actual diagnosis is known. This syndrome is due to compression of the cauda equina or spinal cord by tumor, large central disc herniation, infection, or hematoma. The patient usually presents with minimal to moderate back pain and sciatica in association with bilateral neurologic deficits and incontinence. The physical examination will demonstrate evidence of bilateral nerve root involvement. The most common sensory deficit found in cauda equina syndrome occurs over the buttocks, perineum, and posterior–superior thighs in the "saddle" distribution (8). Urinary retention is the most consistent finding in cauda equina syndrome (sensitivity 90%) (8). This proves useful in the patient with a benign history and physical examination but who complains of urinary incontinence. By evaluating a postvoid residual, a negative test (no urinary retention) makes it extremely unlikely that the patient has incontinence due to epidural compression (8). All patients with suspected epidural compression require emergency neurosurgery consultation, high-dose steroid therapy, and emergent magnetic resonance imaging (MRI) to determine the etiology.

Spinal Stenosis

Spinal stenosis is a narrowing of the spinal canal that may occur at single or multiple spinal levels and is associated with radiculopathy or claudication (15). Generally, it is a cause of chronic back pain, but it has associated flares of acute pain. The symptoms, which usually begin in the sixth decade, include low back pain aggravated by prolonged standing and spinal extension, and relieved by rest and forward flexion. The classic symptom for spinal stenosis is *pseudoclaudication*, although this is seen in only 60% of patients. Pseudoclaudication is pain of the lateral legs that occurs with walking, and is relieved with rest. It is termed pseudoclaudication because it is caused by neurologic compression, not arterial insufficiency (6).

Back Pain in Children

Children rarely present to the ED with complaints of back pain. When they do, however, one must perform a more thorough diagnostic evaluation, as there is a much higher probability of a serious treatable etiology. The history should be directed toward those questions asked of the adult. Additionally, one must ask about a recent increase in physical activity or involvement in sports such as football, dance, and gymnastics. These activities are associated with an increased likelihood of spondylolysis or spondylolisthesis. The physical examination should specifically evaluate for the presence of birthmarks, such as café au lait spots (indicative of neurofibromatosis), as well as midline skin abnormalities of the back that may indicate underlying developmental spinal abnormalities. Etiologies to consider in the child under age 10 are discitis, tumor, and osteomyelitis. Etiologies for children age 10 and older include spondylolysis, spondylolis-

thesis, Scheuermann's disease, tumor, vertebral osteomyelitis, herniated disc, and ankylosing spondylitis.

EMERGENCY DEPARTMENT EVALUATION

The ED evaluation must concentrate on the identification of red flags in the history and physical examination (see Table 105.1). The presence of red flags will direct the diagnostic evaluation and treatment regimens. The absence of red flags means that it is unlikely that the patient has significant disease, and, thus, no diagnostic tests are required.

All children without an obvious etiology for their back pain should be evaluated with a complete blood count (CBC), ESR, urinalysis (UA), and plain spinal radiography.

History

Back pain is differentiated into three categories based on the duration of the symptoms: acute (<6 weeks), subacute (between 6 and 12 weeks), and chronic (>12 weeks). Pain that is subacute or chronic is a red flag because 90% of back pain episodes resolve within 4 to 6 weeks. Patients who have had back pain for greater than 6 weeks require further diagnostic evaluation.

Patients older than 50 or younger than 18 years also raise a red flag due to the higher probability of pathology, such as tumor or infection. Furthermore, those patients under age 18 have a higher likelihood of congenital and bony abnormalities, such as spondylolysis and spondylolisthesis. In patients older than age 50, causes such as fracture, vascular disease, pancreatitis, and other intraabdominal or retroperitoneal processes are more common.

A history of trauma suggests fracture and is usually a readily available historical clue. In an otherwise healthy patient, a major mechanism (motor vehicle crash or a fall from a significant height) is required to cause vertebral fracture. However, one must realize that the patient with osteoporosis may sustain a vertebral fracture from even minor trauma.

A history of radicular pain (sciatica) suggests nerve root compression or irritation. Patients with sciatica commonly complain more of the leg symptoms than the back pain. In addition to the radicular symptoms, one must inquire about neurologic deficits such as weakness, paresthesias, anesthesia, gait disturbances, and bowel and bladder incontinence. Any neurologic deficit raises a red flag for compression of at least a single spinal nerve root, but may signal compression of the cauda equina or spinal cord. Bilateral or rapidly progressive symptoms, or urinary or fecal incontinence, are very worrisome and suggest an epidural compression syndrome such as cauda equina syndrome or spinal cord compression.

The typical description for a benign etiology of back pain is that of a dull, aching pain that usually worsens with movement but improves with rest and lying still. Atypical pain features, such as night pain and unrelenting pain despite rest and appropriate or even supernormal analgesic use, raise red flags for infection and tumor. Other atypical features suggestive of disc herniation include pain that is worsened with prolonged sitting, sneezing, coughing, or the performance of the Valsalva maneuver (7,9). Finally, bilateral sciatica pain that worsens with activities such as prolonged standing, walking, and back extension, and is relieved by rest and forward flexion is consistent with spinal stenosis.

Constitutional symptoms, such as fever, chills, night sweats, malaise, and an undesired weight loss, are all red flags that suggest infection or malignancy. The significance of these symptoms is increased if the patient has additional infectious risk factors, such as injection drug use, is immunocompromised, experienced recent bacterial infection, or recent genitourinary or gastrointestinal procedure.

A history of cancer or a history suggestive of undiagnosed cancer raises the suspicion for spinal metastases. Back pain is the initial symptom of spinal metastases in 96% of these cases (14). Malignancies at a high risk to metastasize to the spine include breast, lung, thyroid, kidney, prostate, myeloma, lymphoma, and sarcoma.

Physical Examination

The physical examination is directed toward verifying neurologic complaints, identifying neurologic deficits, and uncovering red flags (see Table 105.1). The presence of fever raises a concern for spinal infection. However, it is insensitive, ranging from 27% for tuberculosis osteomyelitis to 50% for pyogenic osteomyelitis and 83% for spinal epidural abscess (8).

The patient who is writhing in pain suggests a serious etiology, because, most often, patients with a benign etiology for back pain find more relief lying still. In evaluating the writhing patient, one should consider etiologies such as a rupturing abdominal aortic aneurysm, nephrolithiasis, vertebral osteomyelitis, and epidural abscess. All patients with back pain require an abdominal examination to evaluate for bruits, masses, tenderness, and an enlarged, pulsatile aorta consistent with an aortic aneurysm.

Examination of the back should include a search for evidence of underlying infection or trauma. Inspect the back, looking for contusion or swelling consistent with trauma, and erythema, warmth, or drainage consistent with infection. Point tenderness to percussion of the vertebral bodies is found with bacterial infection with a sensitivity of 86%, but is nonspecific (8). Straight-leg testing is performed to evaluate for evidence of a herniated disc with nerve root compression. A positive test is a reproducible radicular pain that radiates below the knee. This pain is usually relieved by decreasing the elevation, and is worsened by ankle dorsiflexion. Reproduction of the patient's back, buttock, hamstring, or thigh pain is not a positive test (8,9). A positive straight-leg raise test is 80% sensitive for a L4-5 or L5-S1 herniated disc (Fig. 105.2). Radicular pain in the affected leg when elevating the asymptomatic leg (positive crossed straight-leg raise test) is highly specific, yet insensitive, for nerve root compression by a herniated disc (8,9).

The neurologic examination is the most important part of the physical examination. The examination should evaluate lower extremity strength, sensation, and reflexes. Rectal examination does not need to be performed on all patients with back pain; however, it should be performed in those patients with red flags and neurologic signs or symptoms; in men in whom prostatic disease is probable; and in those with severe pain. On rectal examination, one is evaluating for sensation, tone, masses, and evidence of perirectal abscess.

Laboratory Testing

If the patient has red flags raised for infection or tumor, one should obtain a CBC, a UA, and an ESR. With infection, the WBC count may be normal or elevated, but the ESR is usually increased, though it is nonspecific. One would expect that the C-reactive protein (CRP) should follow the changes seen with the ESR, but its utility in this setting has not been studied. The UA can be positive in infection if it is the source of hematogenous spread, but it is otherwise normal.

In patients with cancer, the CBC and UA are usually normal unless there is specific involvement of the hematologic or urinary system. The ESR is commonly elevated in cancer patients, and is sometimes recommended as a screening test in this setting.

Imaging Studies

Plain spinal radiographs should always be obtained in children or in adults when there is concern of fracture, spinal infection, or tumor, or if neurologic dysfunction is present. In adults, only anteroposterior (AP) and lateral views of the lumbar spine are necessary. Oblique views and a cone-down view of L5-S1 add minimal information and more than double the radiation exposure (10). In children, the oblique views should be obtained after reviewing the AP and lateral views because these additional views may demonstrate spondylolysis or spondylolisthesis, which are common problems in children. It is not necessary to obtain initial plain radiographs in suspected disc herniation. However, they may be obtained to rule out other etiologies for the radicular symptoms, such as fracture, tumor, or infection.

MRI is the imaging study of choice for most emergent indications relevant to the lumbar spine. It is the gold standard test for suspected epidural compression syndrome, spinal infection, herniated disc, and spinal hematoma. MRI provides the best resolution of the spinal cord and spinal canal as well as disc disease. In cases of suspected cauda equina syndrome, obtain an MRI of the lumbosacral spine only, especially if a midline herniated disc is suspected as the etiology. In cases of suspected spinal cord compression, one should obtain an MRI of the entire spine for two reasons. First, there is a risk of false localization to a spinal level on physical examination. Second, in metastatic spinal cord compression there is a 10% risk of asymptomatic metastases distant from the affected site that may alter the treatment regimen. Although it is the gold standard for disc herniation, MRI should very rarely be ordered from the ED to evaluate for a herniated disc in the absence of signs or symptoms of cord compression. For suspected herniated disc, a spinal MRI is ordered on a routine basis after the patient fails to respond to 4 to 6 weeks of conservative management.

Computed tomography (CT) scanning is superior to MRI in evaluating the bony architecture of the spine, especially in the assessment of a vertebral fracture. However, it provides less resolution of the spinal cord and spinal canal than does MRI. When used in conjunction with myelography (CT-myelogram), CT scanning approaches MRI and should be considered the imaging method of choice in the patient who is unable to undergo an MRI (4).

EMERGENCY DEPARTMENT MANAGEMENT

The treatment of patients with *nonspecific low back pain* should focus on the areas of activity modification, analgesia, manipulation, and other modalities. In terms of activity modification, patients should continue their routine daily activities as tolerated, using pain as the limiting factor. Routine activity has been demonstrated to allow more rapid recovery than either bed rest or back-mobilizing exercise (11). Appropriate analgesia is paramount in treating the patient with nonspecific back pain. The primary treatment regimen should involve acetaminophen alone or in combination with a nonsteroidal antiinflammatory drug (NSAID). When employing NSAIDs, one must consider that no single NSAID has been shown as being most effective (5,9). Thus, one should initiate therapy with a less expensive agent such as ibuprofen, naproxen, or indomethacin. The use of the injectable NSAID ketorolac should be reserved for the patient who is unable to tolerate an oral NSAID. Additionally, NSAIDs should be used with caution in patients at risk of adverse effects, such as the elderly and those with peptic ulcer disease or renal disease. Muscle relaxants have been proven to be efficacious in treating nonspecific

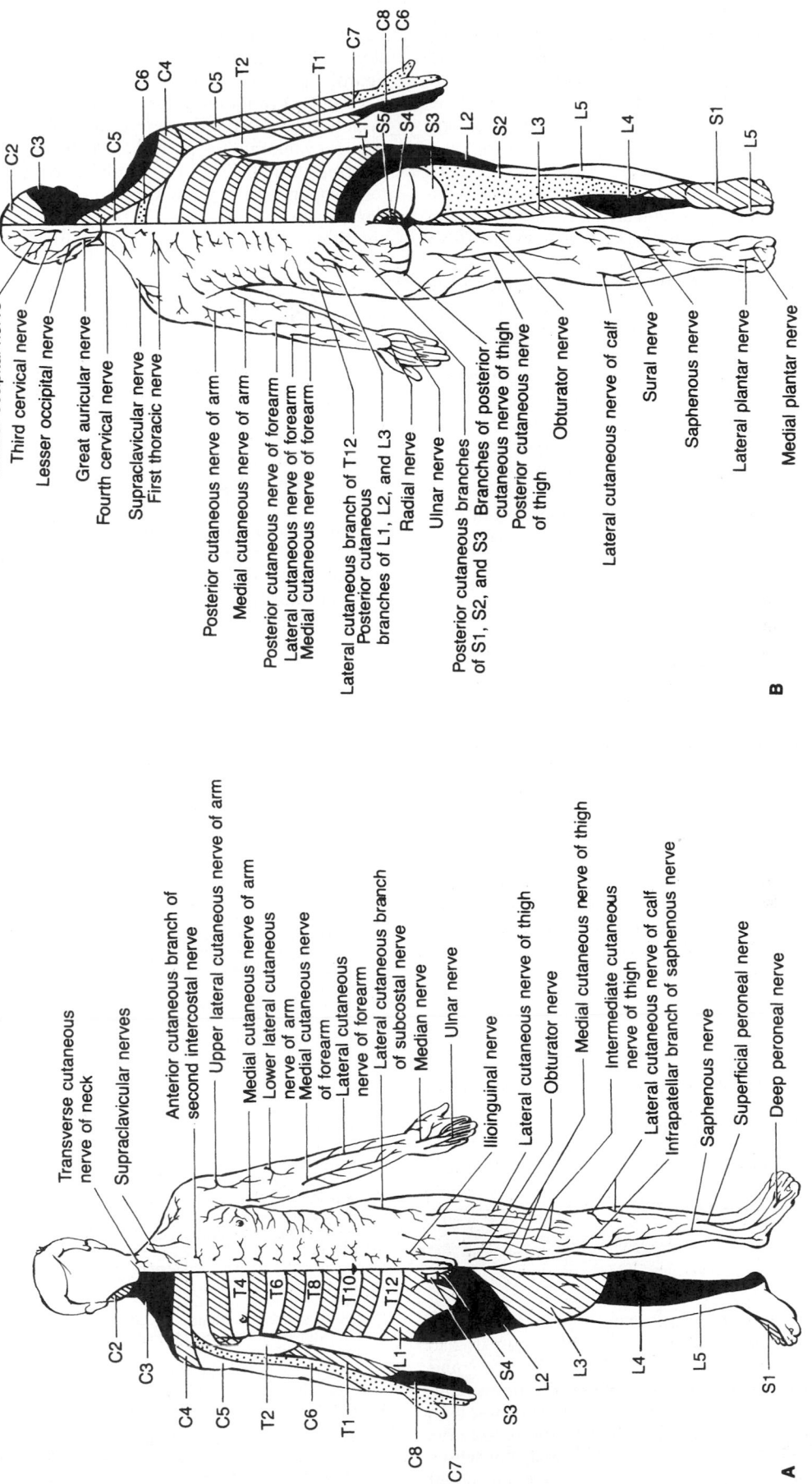

Figure 105.2.   Sensory dermatomal segments. **(A)** Anterior view. **(B)** Posterior view.

back pain. However, clinical trials have not clearly identified which patients benefit from them, and the side effects, especially sedation, are common (5,9). Opiate analgesics should also be prescribed for patients with moderate-to-severe back pain. The prescriptions for these medications are best limited to 1 to 2 weeks' duration due to the risk of sedation, addiction, and constipation. Manipulation is a controversial area of treatment. Although safe and recommended as effective by the 1995 AHCPR guidelines, more recent literature shows it is no more effective than exercises and only minimally more effective in improving patient satisfaction with care than giving the patient an instructional booklet (3). The use of other physical modalities, such as traction, TENS units, diathermy, and ultrasound, is ineffective (1).

The treatment regimen for *herniated disc* mirrors that for acute lumbosacral strain, including the use of routine activity as opposed to bed rest (14), with the exception that manipulation should be used with extreme caution.

The patient with suspected *epidural compression* due to tumor or disc herniation requires treatment with high-dose dexamethasone though the use of steroids in the patient with spinal epidural abscess is controversial. The exact dexamethasone dose is controversial and ranges from 10 mg to 100 mg intravenously (3). A rational approach is to administer 10 mg to the patient with equivocal signs of compression and 100 mg to the patient who has more significant findings, such as partial or complete paraplegia, saddle anesthesia, or incontinence with poor rectal tone (2). Regardless of the exact dose given, one should not delay steroid administration in order to get the definitive confirmation by imaging studies. The MRI should be obtained emergently and not delayed until the next day. For patients with spinal cord compression due to neoplasm, emergent radiation therapy is also recommended.

In the patient with suspected *spinal infection*, obtain at least two sets of blood cultures, as these are frequently positive. One should discuss the need for antibiotics in the ED with the consultant prior to their administration, because these patients may require open biopsy with culture of the site, and the administration of antibiotics may obscure the culture results. Patients with paralysis or sepsis due to infection require antibiotics and one should not delay their administration. Empiric antibiotic therapy should be directed against *Staphylococcus aureus*, such as parenteral Vancomycin, Nafcillin, or Cefazolin. If a source for the infection is found, such as the urinary tract, antibiotics should be appropriate for that source.

CRITICAL INTERVENTIONS

- Order emergent imaging (MRI) for patients with suspected cord compression
- Administer dexamethasone to patients with suspected cord compression
- Administer antistaphylococcal antibiotics for suspected spinal infection

DISPOSITION

Patients with acute lumbosacral strain and sciatica can be discharged home with primary care physician follow up in 2 to 4 weeks. They should be treated with acetaminophen and NSAIDs, such as ibuprofen 800 mg three times daily, unless contraindicated. Most patients may benefit from a short course (1 to 2 weeks) of opiate analgesia, such as hydrocodone or oxycodone. If patients have a deficit in a single nerve root consistent with a herniated disc, the primary care physician should see the patient within 7 to 10 days. All patients suspected of having an epidural compression syndrome require emergent MRI and consultation

in the ED by a spine surgeon. If known or suspected metastatic disease is present, an oncologist should also be consulted. All patients with suspected spinal infection require hospital admission and spinal MRI within 24 hours or earlier if there is any neurologic involvement.

Transfer to another facility is necessary in the patient with suspected spinal infection or epidural compression syndrome, if the facility evaluating the patient is unable to obtain an appropriate imaging study (MRI or CT-myelogram). These patients are safe to transport utilizing a BLS ground transport unit, unless they have unstable vital signs. In patients with suspected epidural compression syndrome, steroids should be administered before the transfer.

COMMON PITFALLS

✔ Failure to consider a rupturing abdominal aortic aneurysm in the patient over age 55 with acute low back pain
✔ Overutilization of diagnostic tests in the patient with low back pain and no "red flags"
✔ Underutilization of testing in children with back pain, who have a much higher incidence of serious diagnosable etiologies
✔ Failure to consider a spinal infection in the immunocompromised patient or the injection drug user with back pain, especially when fever is present
✔ Overutilization of MRI in patients with suspected herniated disc. Such patients do not require imaging with MRI unless they fail to improve within 4 to 6 weeks
✔ Failure to administer dexamethasone and order emergent imaging and consultation in patients with suspected epidural compression syndrome

Acknowledgments

Thanks to previous edition chapter authors Ellen H. Taliaferro and Allan B. Wolfson.

References

1. Bigos S, Bowyer O, Braen G, et al.Acute low back problems in adults. Clinical practice guideline. *Quick reference guide number 14.* Rockville, MD: U.S. Department of Health and Human Services, Public Health Service, Agency for Health Care Policy and Research, AHCPR Pub. No. 95-0643, December 1994.
2. Byrne T. Spinal cord compression from epidural metastases. *N Engl J Med* 1992;327:614–619.
3. Cherkin D, Deyo R, Battie M, et al. A comparison of physical therapy, chiropractic manipulation, and provision of an educational booklet for the treatment of patients with low back pain. *N Engl J Med* 1998;339:1021–1029.
4. Deen HG. Diagnosis and management of lumbar disk disease. *Mayo Clin Proc* 1996;71:283–287.
5. Deyo R. Drug therapy for back pain: which drugs help which patients. *Spine* 1996;21:2840–2850.
6. Deyo R. Rethinking strategies for acute low back pain. *Emerg Med* 1995;28:38–56.
7. Deyo R, Loeser J, Bigos S. Herniated lumbar intervertebral disc. *Ann Intern Med* 1990;112:598–603.
8. Deyo R, Rainville J, Kent D. What can the history and physical examination tell us about low back pain. *JAMA* 1992;286:760–765.
9. Deyo R, Weinstein J. Primary Care: Low Back Pain. *N Engl J Med*. 2001;344:363–370.
10. Frymoyer J. Back pain and sciatica. *N Engl J Med* 1988;318:291–300.
11. Malmivaara A, Hakkinen U, Aro T, et al. The treatment of acute low back pain-bed rest, exercise, or ordinary activity. *N Engl J Med* 1995;332:321–325.
12. Martin R, Yuan H. Neurosurgical care of spinal epidural, subdural and intramedullary abscesses and arachnoiditis. *Orthop Clin North Am* 1996;27:125–136.
13. Mazanec D. Back pain: medical evaluation and therapy. *Cleve Clin J Med* 1995;62:163–168.
14. Schmidt R, Markovchick V. Nontraumatic spinal cord compression. *J Emerg Med* 1992;10:189–199.
15. Sengupta D, Herkowitz H. Lumbar Spinal Stenosis: Treatment Strategies and Indications for Surgery. *Orthop Clin N Amer* 2003;34:281–295.
16. Vroomen P, de Krom M, Wilmink J, et al. Lack of effectiveness of bed rest for sciatica. *N Engl J Med* 1999;340:418–423.
17. White A, Gordon S. Synopsis: Workshop on idiopathic low-back pain. *Spine* 1982;7:141–149.

CHAPTER 106
Common Foot Disorders

Valerie Dobiesz and Louis G. Poulos[†]
([†]deceased)

Foot pain is a common complaint in the emergency department and foot disorders can be extremely debilitating. Foot injuries rank second only to knee injuries as the most common injuries associated with sports. Nontraumatic causes of foot pain are usually chronic or subacute in nature. In the vast majority of cases, overuse conditions or improperly fitting shoes are the cause. The emergency physician can often provide symptomatic relief as well as definitive care. Special attention needs to be given to diabetic patients with foot disorders, as they are at high risk for serious complications.

The vast majority of foot disorders can be diagnosed easily without further testing, and can be successfully treated on an outpatient basis. Patients should be referred to a primary care physician, a podiatrist, or an orthopaedic surgeon for definitive care and follow up.

SUBUNGUAL HEMORRHAGE (BLUE OR BLACK TOENAIL SYNDROME)

Painful and black toenails are often a result of improper footwear, resulting from the toenails' rubbing on the undersurface of the shoe or the foot sliding forward to jam the toes. If the symptoms are acute, the treatment is to drain the hematoma with nail trephination, which can be done using a heated paper clip or an electrocautery device. To prevent recurrence, the patient can be instructed to use a metatarsal pad under the metatarsal heads or a tongue pad underneath the tongue of the shoe.

ONYCHOCRYPTOSIS (INGROWN TOENAIL)

Ingrown toenails are often the result of poorly fitting shoes, abnormal nail growth, or poor nail cutting. A sharp edge of the nail pierces the epidermis of the sulcus and penetrates the dermal tissues. The hallux or great toe of male adolescents is most often involved. Symptoms include pain, swelling, erythema, and purulent drainage of the affected toe.

Warm soaks are helpful in the treatment of mild-to-moderate cases. If a paronychia is present, partial nail resection and nail bed ablation is indicated. Utilizing a digital nerve block and local anesthetic, an oblique wedge of nail should be dissected free of the sulcus and inflamed tissue with a scalpel. Phenol or a cotton pledget can be applied to the nail edge. If pus is present, oral or topical antibiotics are indicated. A nonsteroidal antiinflammatory agent is appropriate for pain. Definitive treatment should be with a podiatrist or orthopaedic surgeon (7,10).

MORTON'S INTERDIGITAL NEUROMA

Morton's neuroma is a degenerative neuropathy caused by repetitive trauma compressing the interdigital nerve most often between the third and fourth metatarsal heads. It is seen in patients who are runners, dancers, and basketball players, and in those who have to stand for long periods of time or wear high-heeled shoes. Symptoms are sharp, stabbing pain and paresthesia between the toes.

Diagnosis is made clinically by pinching between the metatarsal heads and simultaneously using the other hand to compress the forefoot with pressure on the first and fifth metatarsal heads. This maneuver will elicit pain and possibly a palpable mass or an audible click, known as Mulder's click. Treatment includes ice in acute cases, orthotics, rest, steroid injections, and possible surgical excision (12).

METATARSAL STRESS FRACTURES

Stress fractures are the result of repetitive loading forces, causing the bone to fatigue, rather than of an acute event. Metatarsal bones are a common site of stress fractures. The most common metatarsal stress fracture occurs at the neck of the second metatarsal. This injury is more common in patients with Morton syndrome (the first ray shorter than the second) (1).

Symptoms include localized pain that is worsened by activity or weight bearing and is relieved with rest. Plain x-rays typically do not reveal stress fractures until 10 to 14 days after they occur. Bone scans are helpful but not practical in the emergency department setting. The condition is treated conservatively by having the patient avoid weight bearing on the site for 4 to 6 weeks, applying ice, and administering nonsteroidal antiinflammatory drugs.

BUNIONS (HALLUX VALGUS)

Bunions are inflammation at the first metatarsophalangeal (MTP) joint. Inflammation at the base of the little toe is called a bunionette (tailor's bunion). This condition is more common in females at a 10:1 ratio. The hallux valgus deformity consists of lateral deviation of the hallux and medial deviation of the first metatarsal. The etiology of both is unclear but may be hereditary biomechanical abnormalities and improperly fitting shoes. Symptoms of bunions are pain and erythema at the MTP joint. Treatment in the emergency department is focused on analgesia with nonsteroidal antiinflammatory drugs, bunion pads, ice and patient education on proper shoes with a wide toe box and no high heels. In severe cases, surgical correction is indicated.

BLISTERS, CALLUSES, AND CORNS

Excessive localized pressure or friction between the foot and improperly fitted shoes or from constant sliding of the foot inside a shoe can result in blisters, calluses, and corns. *Blisters* result from shearing forces, causing fluid to accumulate within the layers of the skin. There is some controversy regarding the treatment of blisters. Several options exist in management, including leaving the blister intact, debridement, and aspiration.

Calluses develop from excessive pressure, causing hypertrophy of the squamous cell layer of the epidermis on skin that is normally thick, such as the sole. A callus is painless and may be diffuse or localized. Treatment includes regular debridement with a callus file, pumice stone, or scalpel.

A *corn* is a painful conical thickening of skin with recurrent pressure; the apex of the cone points inward and causes pain. Corns usually occur over bony prominences such as the fourth or fifth toe. When they occur in moist areas, such as between the toes, they are called soft corns. Treatment is aimed at prevention with appropriate footwear and padding proximal to the lesions to relieve pressure. These lesions should be aggressively pursued and treated in diabetic patients because of the risk of infection and long-term sequelae.

PLANTAR WARTS (VERRUCA VULGARIS)

Plantar warts are caused by the human papillomavirus and are painful when the patient puts weight on them. Children, especially teens, are more susceptible to infection than adults. Warts are hard and flat with well defined boundaries and may be brown or gray with the center containing one or more pinpoints of black. Callus formation over the wart is common. Distinguishing warts from calluses may be difficult. Warts occur at any site, whereas calluses appear only on pressure areas. Pinching around the lesion and producing pain, supports an underlying wart. If the hyperkeratotic area is scraped, the underlying wart typically bleeds and has a spotted appearance, representing thrombosed vessels.

Treatment in the emergency department consists of application of pressure-relieving dressing and administration of analgesics, topical solutions containing salicylic acid, or duct tape occlusion therapy for a maximum of 2 months. Refractory warts may require cryotherapy with liquid nitrogen, laser or surgical excision (3).

PLANTAR FASCIITIS

The plantar fascia is a band of connective tissue on the plantar surface of the foot that extends from the calcaneal tuberosity to the metatarsal heads. Irritation and micro tears due to overuse and repetitive heel strikes cause degeneration of the fascia, resulting in heel pain. The pain is often in the morning or with prolonged sitting. It is believed to be a degenerative process without inflammation. This entity accounts for 10% of running injuries and primarily afflicts the middle-aged, the elderly, and athletes. Physical examination findings include: (1) point tenderness over the medial calcaneal tuberosity, (2) reproduction of pain with passive dorsiflexion of the ankle or toes, or (3) heel pain with standing on the toes. Treatment is focused on relaxing the tension on the fascia and includes rest, ice, stretching the gastrocnemius muscle, arch taping, use of orthotics, administration of nonsteroidal antiinflammatory drugs, dorsiflexion night splints, advising the patient to wear proper shoes, and surgery (2,6,13).

CALCANEAL STRESS FRACTURES

The cause of calcaneal stress fractures is repetitive stresses. Patients typically present with insidious onset of heel pain aggravated by weight-bearing activities. On examination, there is localized tenderness over the medial or lateral aspects of the calcaneus, and pain is elicited by squeezing the calcaneus from both sides; the heel "squeeze" test. Radiographs are typically normal initially or show a typical sclerotic appearance on the lateral view parallel with the posterior margin of the calcaneus. Treatment is conservative with rest, administration of nonsteroidal antiinflammatory drugs, and advising the patient not to put weight on the site.

ACHILLES TENDONITIS

Achilles tendonitis is caused by overuse and is seen most commonly in middle-aged or older adult distance runners. Inflammation of the tendon results in pain 3 to 6 cm above the tendon insertion. Tenderness anterior to the tendon is more consistent with retrocalcaneal bursitis. Treatment includes rest, ice, heel lifts, nonsteroidal antiinflammatory drugs, ultrasound, stretching of the gastrocnemius and soleus muscles, and, rarely, surgery (5,8).

RETROCALCANEAL BURSITIS

Retrocalcaneal bursitis is an inflammation of the bursa that lies between the Achilles tendon and the posterior border of the calcaneus. Symptoms begin early in activity and are exacerbated by dorsiflexion of the foot. Tenderness is just anterior to the Achilles tendon (deep) and posterior to the calcaneus. Hind foot swelling is often present. The treatment is rest and administration of nonsteroidal antiinflammatory medications. The patient is instructed on stretching exercises and use of a heel lift. This condition also may be treated with steroid and local anesthetic injections.

BROMHIDROSIS

Malodor of the feet is caused by keratin decomposition in the presence of hyperhidrosis or excessive production of sweat. A corynebacterial overgrowth or fungal colonization may occur, worsening the condition. Treatment includes measures to reduce sweat production and to control secondary infection. Use of talcum powder, spray deodorants, and absorbent insoles may be helpful.

TINEA PEDIS

The most common fungal infections of the skin are on the feet. Males are more commonly affected and the incidence increases with age. Occlusive footwear, because it causes moisture and warmth between the toes, and hyperhydrosis predisposes to this condition; communal activity such as swimming and bathing promotes its spread. The most frequent dermatophyte involved is *Trichophyton rubrum.*

There are four types of tinea pedis. The interdigital type involves maceration and desquamation in the lateral toe spaces, the vesicular type manifests as episodes of unilateral acute vesiculation on the soles, the chronic hyperkeratotic or moccasin type causes dry pruritic erythema with diffuse scaling over the soles, and the ulcerative type presents with vesiculopustular lesions and secondary bacterial infection. Symptoms are extreme itching, burning, and irritation on the soles of the foot and between the toes. Treatment includes a variety of topical antimycotic agents, such as imidazoles, pyridones, allylamines and benzylamines. These agents should be used twice daily from 1-6 weeks depending on the agent used. Widespread infections, cases involving the nails (onychomycosis), cases in patients with immunocompromised states or diabetes, or failed topical therapy are treated with systemic antimycotics such as itraconazole, terbinafine, fluconazole or the imidazoles.

COMMON PITFALLS

✔ Failure to aggressively manage diabetic patients with foot disorders; the risk of complications is high if such patients are inadequately treated

✔ Failure to recognize metatarsal stress fractures, which are common and may not be visualized radiographically. If a stress fracture is suspected, treat it conservatively with avoidance of weight bearing

✔ Failure to distinguish between plantar warts and calluses. Accurate diagnosis is important, because management and treatment are different for the two conditions

References

1. Caillet R.*Foot and ankle pain,* 3rd Ed. New York: F.A. Davis, 1997.
2. Cornwall, MW, et al. Plantar fasciitis: etiology and treatment. *J Orthop Sports Phys Ther* 1999;29:756–760.
3. Focht DR III, et al. The efficacy of duct tape versus cryotherapy in the treatment of verruca vulgaris (the common wart). *Arch Pediatr Adolesc Med* 2002;156:971–974.
4. Freedberg IM, Eisen AZ, Wolff K, et al.*Fitzpatrick's Dermatology in General Medicine,* 5th Edition. New York: McGraw-Hill. 1999:2349–2351.
5. Galloway MT, Jokl P, Dayton OW. Achilles tendon overuse injuries. *Clin Sports Med* 1992;11:771.
6. Lemont H, et al. Plantar fasciitis: a degenerative process (fasciosis) without inflammation. *J Am Podiatr Med Assoc* 2003;93:234–237.
7. Lorimer DL. *Neale's Disorders of the Foot Diagnosis & Management,* 6th ed. Philadelphia: Harcourt Publishers, 2001.
8. Mazzone MF, et al. Common conditions of the Achilles tendon. *Am Fam Physician* 2002;65:1805–1810.
9. Myerson MS.*Foot and Ankle Disorders,* vol 2. Philadelphia: WB Saunders, 2000.
10. Roberts JR, Hedges JR. *Clinical procedures in emergency medicine,* 4th ed. Philadelphia: Saunders, 2004.
11. Van Wyngarden TM. The painful foot, part I: common forefoot deformities. *Am Fam Physician* 1997;55:2207.
12. Wu KK. Morton neuroma and metatarsalgia. *Curr Opin Rheumatol* 2000;12:131–142.
13. Young CC, et al. Treatment of plantar fasciitis. *Am Fam Physician* 2001;63:467–474, 477–478.

CHAPTER 107
Monoarticular Arthritis

Alan C. Heffner

Monoarticular arthritis is a common emergency condition and carries a broad differential diagnosis. Trauma and crystal disease are the most common causes of acute joint pain while bacterial infection carries the greatest potential for morbidity (2,18). The most important steps in the emergent evaluation of acute monoarticular arthritis are arthrocentesis and synovial fluid analysis.

CLINICAL PRESENTATION

Acute arthritis typically presents with joint pain and swelling. The onset and severity of inflammation varies greatly depending on the etiology and host factors such as age, comorbid disease, and immunocompetence. Septic arthritis is traditionally divided into gonococcal and nongonococcal disease, reflecting the variant pathogenesis and management of these entities.

Gonococcal Arthritis

Neisseria gonorrhoeae remains the most common cause of septic arthritis in young, healthy, sexually-active adults in the U.S. (5). Disseminated gonococcal infection (DGI) should be suspected in any sexually active patient with joint complaints. Women are more frequently affected than men; and are predisposed to systemic spread as a result of pregnancy and the peri-menstrual interval (4). DGI presents in two distinct patterns. Forty percent of patients manifest acute suppurative monoarthritis involving the knee, wrist, or ankle. Polyarthralgias may precede localization to a single joint. The remaining cases present with the arthritis-dermatitis syndrome (4,20). Hematogenous spread of bacteria and immune complexes underlie the triad of *dermatitis, tenosynovitis, and migratory polyarthritis.* The classic skin lesions are scattered small painless erythematous macules or petechiae, which evolve into pustular to necrotic lesions on an erythematous base. Transient painful extensor tenosynovitis may involve the wrists, hands, and ankles while asymmetric migratory polyarthralgia of the extremity joints are the most common symptom. Toxicity varies greatly in DGI. Most patients experience only mild constitutional symptoms and low-grade fever. Symptoms of primary genital infection may be mild or completely absent (20).

Nongonococcal Septic Arthritis

Nongonococcal septic arthritis is a medical emergency that can lead to rapid joint destruction and death. Permanent joint damage complicates 40% of septic joints (8,20). Overall mortality is 15% but reaches as high as 50% in some subgroups (8,9). Large weight-bearing joints such as the knee and hip are most commonly involved with the shoulder, ankle, elbow, and wrist occurring with decreasing frequency. Intravenous drug use can result in seeding of atypical sites such as the sternoclavicular, costochondral, and sacroiliac joints.

Nongonococcal septic arthritis classically presents in fulminant fashion with abrupt onset, progressive joint pain and swelling, marked toxicity and fever. Chronic illness increases the risk of septic arthritis but may mute the presenting symptoms. Elderly patients with underlying medical conditions often have insidious clinical progression with little or no fever (8). Polyarticular involvement occurs in 10% to 20% of patients (8,9).

Local factors such as antecedent arthritic conditions, prior joint trauma, and intra-articular steroid injections predisposes patients to septic arthritis. The pathogenesis involves one of four mechanisms: hematogenous seeding, contiguous spread, direct traumatic implantation, or postoperative invasion of prosthetic hardware (9). Hematogenous seeding of the vascular synovium is the most common cause of septic arthritis (20). Bacteremia related to intravenous drug use, indwelling vascular access, invasive procedures, and distant infection are risks for joint seeding. Contiguous spread into a joint may occur from adjacent cellulitis, tenosynovitis, osteomyelitis, or abscess. This is most commonly seen in diabetic foot infections and pediatric metaphyseal osteomyelitis. Direct joint inoculation may occur via iatrogenic endeavors or traumatic penetration; the clenched fist "fight bite" injury and cat bites to the hand and wrist are commonly overlooked injuries. Infections complicate up to 2% of prosthetic joint procedures with revision arthroplasty carrying even greater risk (9). Pain localized to a prosthetic joint may signify mechanical loosening, prosthesis failure, or joint infection. Crystal-induced arthritis is rare in prosthetic joints (2).

Gram-positive cocci remain the major nongonococcal pathogens in adults. *Staphylococcus aureus* accounts for 60% of non-gonococcal infections, followed by streptococci including *Streptococcus pneumoniae* (5,20). Gram negative bacilli including *Escherichia coli* and *Pseudomonas aeruginosa* account for 20% of infections and occur predominantly in immunocompromised patients and intravenous drugs users (20). Anaerobes are isolated in a minority of cases (6,20). Inoculation of oral flora occurs in penetrating bite wounds. Mycobacterial and fungal arthritis are uncommon but are important considerations in immunocompromised patients presenting with subacute progressive joint pain of the spine or weight-bearing joints.

Crystal-Induced Monoarthritis

Crystal-induced acute arthropathy is more common than septic arthritis and represents the most important mimic of infection. Gout and pseudogout may be clinically indistinguishable from septic arthritis. In both disorders, patients may demonstrate systemic symptoms such as fever and confusion (2).

Gout develops when monosodium urate crystals precipitate within joints and trigger an acute inflammatory reaction. The typical presentation is a middle-aged man with severe joint pain, swelling, redness, and warmth that evolves rapidly over hours to days. Most cases of acute gout affect a single joint but attacks may be polyarticular. While any joint may be affected, the first metatarsophalangeal (MTP) joint is involved in 60% of cases (podagra) followed by the ankle, midfoot, and knee. The initial attack is monoarticular in 85% of cases. Constitutional complaints including fever may be present (2). If left untreated, gout follows a course of increasingly frequent attacks separated by shorter intercritical periods. Recurrent exacerbations eventually result in chronic arthritic changes with bony erosions resembling rheumatoid arthritis or degenerative joint disease. Noninflammatory soft tissue tophaceous deposits may develop in the Achilles' tendon or extensor surface of the fingers, forearms, or elbows. Common precipitants of acute attacks include increased purine intake, enhanced cellular breakdown (i.e., chemotherapy), alcohol, and joint trauma. In contrast to the classic gout presentation, older men and postmenopausal women may present with subacute to chronic polyarticular synovitis involving the small joints of the fingers. This presentation resembling rheumatoid arthritis is strongly associated with diuretic use and renal insufficiency (1).

Pseudogout is the result of calcium pyrophosphate dihydrate (CPPD) crystal deposition, and manifests three common clinical courses: (1) asymptomatic radiographic stippling of articular cartilage (chondrocalcinosis), (2) acute attacks of mono or oligoarticular inflammatory arthritis (pseudogout), and (3) progressive degenerative joint changes similar to osteoarthritis. Pseudogout usually develops after age 50, and may involve single or multiple joints, especially the knees, wrists, ankles, and elbows. Acute attacks exhibit an abrupt onset and marked discomfort, clinically indistinguishable from gout or septic arthritis (17). More commonly, the exacerbations evolve over days. Attacks may be triggered by systemic illness, surgery, or trauma. Most cases are idiopathic, but CPPD deposition is associated with hyperparathyroidism and hemochromatosis (1,17).

DIFFERENTIAL DIAGNOSIS

Monoarticular arthritis may result from inflammatory, infectious, ischemic, neoplastic, traumatic, mechanical, or hemorrhagic causes (Table107.1). The major disorders to consider in the differential include septic arthritis, gout, and pseudogout, but many other disorders produce pain, swelling, and erythema in or around a joint.

Periarticular conditions such as cellulitis, tendonitis, and bursitis may be mistaken for intraarticular pathology. Bursitis results in pain and swelling directly overlying bony prominences. Most cases are noninfectious but septic bursitis may occur in the setting of local trauma; the olecranon and prepatellar bursas are the most commonly infected.

A variety of classically polyarticular inflammatory conditions including *rheumatoid arthritis, seronegative spondyloarthropa-*

TABLE 107.1.   Differential Diagnosis of Acute Monoarticular Arthritis

Infectious
Bacterial
Gonococcal
Nongonococcal
Mycobacterial (*M.tb* and atypical)
Spirochete (Lyme, syphilis)
Fungal
Viral (HIV, Hep B, Rubella, others)
Postinfectious

Crystal-Induced
Gout (monosodium urate)
Pseudogout (CPPD)
Calcium apatite

Traumatic
Fracture
Ligamentous injury
Overuse injury

Ischemic
Avascular necrosis
Vasoocclusive crisis
Decompression illness
Spontaneous osteonecrosis

Hemorrhagic
Posttraumatic
Hemophilia
Systemic anticoagulation

Neoplastic
Metastasis
Osteochondroma
Osteoid osteoma
Pigmented villonodular synovitis

Systemic disease
Remote infection, infectious endocarditis
Rheumatic fever
Seronegative spondyloarthropathies (AS, IBS, psoriatic, reactive)
Reiter syndrome, Bechet disease
Rheumatoid arthritis, SLE
Sarcoidosis, amyloidosis

thy, systemic lupus erythematosus, and *postinfectious arthritis* may present with acute monoarticular symptoms. The seronegative arthritides, characterized by the absence of rheumatoid factor, include *ankylosing spondylitis, psoriatic arthritis, enteropathic arthritis* (associated with inflammatory bowel disease), and reactive arthritis (such as *Reiter syndrome*). Sterile postinfectious arthritis may be triggered by preceding or coincident infection with a variety of agents including Group A streptococci, HIV, Parvovirus, Hepatitis B and C, and Rubella.

Lyme disease may present with musculoskeletal features ranging from acute episodic arthralgias to chronic mono or oligoarticular arthritis. Knee involvement is common. A history of tick exposure, travel to an endemic region, or erythema migrans rash is helpful but not always present.

Vascular compromise may lead to bone infarction and osteonecrosis. The weight-bearing surface of the femoral head and medial condyle of the knee are common locations. Patients complain of severe pain in the absence of trauma. Precipitants include sickle cell vasoocclusive disease, vasculitis, decompression illness, posttraumatic injury (i.e., hip dislocation), and corticosteroid-induced avascular necrosis.

Traumatic joint injuries are common. Development of an immediate joint effusion after injury suggests hemarthrosis due to ligamentous disruption or osteochondral fracture. Hemarthrosis may occur spontaneously or after minor trauma in the setting of coagulopathy due to anticoagulation or hemophilia.

Osteoarthritis is a chronic slowly progressive disease affecting weight-bearing joints. Acute exacerbations may coincide with new or worsening effusion following overuse or minor trauma. Neoplastic lesions often present with pain or pathologic fracture.

Children who present with a limp or refusal to walk may have septic arthritis or *acute transient synovitis*. Transient synovitis is the most common cause of hip pain in children 3 to 10 years of age. This self-limited inflammatory condition typically presents one to three weeks after a viral illness. There is considerable overlap in the clinical presentation of septic arthritis and transient synovitis. Consider *slipped capital femoral epiphysis (SCFE)* in a portly pubescent child and *Legg-Calve-Perthes disease* (aseptic necrosis of the femoral head) in young school-age children. See Chapter 229 for more information on the evaluation of the child with a limp.

EMERGENCY DEPARTMENT EVALUATION

Septic arthritis poses risk of joint destruction and even death if treatment is delayed. For this reason, the emergency department evaluation of any joint complaint should focus on excluding infection. Assessment centers on history, physical exam, and arthrocentesis when indicated. Serum analysis of peripheral WBC count, uric acid level, and acute phase reactants rarely confirm or exclude a diagnosis. These studies may mislead the physician if used as a substitute for arthrocentesis.

The temporal course, duration of symptoms, and history of similar joint symptoms should be clarified; acute and acute-on-chronic presentations deserve special attention. A history of recurrent monoarthritis or typical podagra suggests crystal-induced or other noninfectious arthritis. However, patients presenting with a marked exacerbation of chronic arthritis, especially rheumatoid arthritis, mandate exclusion of a superimposed infection (5). Recent trauma suggests a fracture or musculotendinous injury but even minimal trauma may precipitate gout. Penetrating injuries may introduce infection. Constitutional symptoms and diffuse morning stiffness are classically associated with rheumatic diseases. The degree and distribution of joint involvement enables separation of arthritides into mono, oligo (less than 3 joints), and polyarthritis patterns. Patient with oligo or polyarticular disease may complain of a single painful joint to the exclusion of other symptoms unless prompted.

Helpful aspects of the history also include a review of comorbid diseases, especially immunosuppression. Potential septic sources include recent infection, invasive procedures, intravenous drug use, sexually transmitted diseases, and tick exposure. Genital ulcerations or discharge may occur in gonococcal disease or Reiter's syndrome. Rash, oral ulcers, uveitis, urethritis, and diarrhea suggest reactive arthritis. Medications should be reviewed with attention to potential precipitants of crystal arthropathy, such as diuretics. Immunomodulating drugs and antibiotics may blunt the clinical presentation of acute infection. Infection resulting from intraarticular injections is possible but uncommon (5,16).

Patients with acute worsening of a preexisting arthritic condition deserve special attention. Antecedent joint pathology predisposes to infection (9). Acute worsening of chronic arthritis cannot be attributed to progression of disease until superimposed infection is excluded. Rheumatoid arthritis carries a 10-fold higher incidence of septic arthritis and greater mortality compared to the general population; delayed diagnosis contributes to this poor outcome (8,20).

Examination begins with general assessment of toxicity and hemodynamic stability. Systemic findings including fever and tachycardia are more common in patients with septic arthritis but are not specific. Fever is absent in more than 20% of pa-

tients with septic arthritis (8). Extraarticular sources of infection are identified in 50% of cases of septic arthritis. Cellulitis, pneumonia, and genitourinary infections are frequent sources (5,9). The skin examination may provide important clues; oral ulcers may be present in Behcet syndrome, Reiter syndrome, and systemic lupus erythematosus. Oral thrush suggests immune suppression. Infectious endocarditis commonly manifests musculoskeletal symptoms and should be considered in any patient with a murmur and concomitant arthritis (20). Acute rheumatic fever and systemic lupus may also present this clinical picture.

Examine all joints to classify the degree, number, and symmetry of joint involvement. Testing active and passive range of motion distinguishes intraarticular from periarticular conditions such as bursitis, tendonitis, strain/sprain, and cellulitis. Pain on gentle motion, whether active or passive, is the hallmark of joint inflammation. *Patients with intraarticular pathology have significant pain with any range of motion.* Refusal to actively move the joint is common. In contrast, periarticular conditions produce focal inflammation and localized tenderness; they do *not* produce marked pain with passive movement.

Resting position provides important clues to intraarticular pathology. The inflamed hip is often flexed and externally rotated. An irritable knee is commonly held in mild flexion. Deep axial joints are difficult to evaluate. Pain localized to the sacroiliac joint may be exacerbated with the FABER maneuver (placing the hip into forced *F*lexion, *AB*duction, and *E*xternal *R*otation).

Synovial fluid analysis is the diagnostic cornerstone for acute arthritis. Arthrocentesis should be performed in all cases of monoarticular arthritis, with the possible exception of classic recurrent gout. The emergency physician can safely aspirate most peripheral joints; deep joints such as the hip and sacroiliac require specialist consultation and fluoroscopic or ultrasound guidance. Orthopaedic consultation is advisable before arthrocentesis of prosthetic joints.

All synovial fluid samples should be analyzed for total leukocyte count with differential, Gram stain, culture, and light microscopy for crystals. These tests generally require 1–2 mL of fluid. Culture remains the single most informative test if fluid is limited. Synovial fluid chemistries including LDH, glucose, protein, and lactate provide little additional information and may be misleading (21). Normal synovial fluid is clear, straw colored, and highly viscous.

Synovial fluid leukocyte count distinguishes inflammatory versus noninflammatory effusions. Normal fluid contains less than 200 WBC/mm^3. Leukocyte counts less than 2,000 WBC/mm^3 are considered noninflammatory and occur in osteoarthritis and chronic or inactive inflammatory diseases. Greater than 2,000 WBC/mm^3 indicates an inflammatory process (10,13). The synovial fluid of septic arthritis is typically opaque to purulent with leukocyte counts of 50,000 to 150,000 WBC/mm^3. However, an elevated leukocyte count is not specific for infection; rheumatoid and crystal arthropathy may induce vigorous inflammatory responses. Early infection, prior antibiotics, and immunocompromise may manifest lower leukocyte counts in the setting of infection. A predominance of polymorphonuclear cells (especially greater than 90%) also suggests infection (2).

Gram stain and culture should be performed on every diagnostic specimen. The gram stain is diagnostic in 80% of Gram-positive infections, but the sensitivity is much lower for Gram-negative organisms (2,16). This mandates routine culture of all diagnostic synovial fluid aspirates, including those yielding crystals. Unfortunately, synovial fluid culture may also be falsely negative (20). Direct inoculation of joint fluid into blood culture bottles and onto chocolate agar medium may enhance the yield of organisms (11,19). If suspicion for septic arthritis is high, all potential sources of infection should be cultured including blood, urine, genital tract, oropharynx, rectum, and skin lesions, since infection in these locations may be asymptomatic (19,20). Fungal and mycobacterial cultures should not be ordered routinely but are warranted in high-risk patients.

Polarized light microscopy is the gold standard for crystal identification. Monosodium urate appears as needle-shaped or elongated crystals exhibiting brilliant negative birefringence. The rhomboid or rod-shaped crystals of CPPD are more difficult to visualize under white light, and display weak positive birefringence. Differentiating intracellular and extracellular crystal formations is not diagnostically helpful. Because of interobserver variability, repeat examination is warranted when initial microscopy is inconclusive and the clinical suspicion of crystal disease is high (23).

Although commonly ordered, blood tests rarely identify the etiology of acute monoarthritis. Peripheral WBC counts greater than 10,000 cells/mm^3 are present in only half of patients with septic arthritis, while patients with acute gout can have significant leukocytosis (6,11). Elevated acute phase reactants such as erythrocyte sedimentation rate (ESR) and C-reactive protein (CRP) are common in bacterial arthritis but also rise in noninfectious disease. A normal ESR makes bacterial arthritis less likely but does not exclude infection (3,15). Once the diagnosis of septic arthritis has been established, serial acute phase reactants are sometimes utilized to follow therapeutic response. Serum uric acid levels are likewise discouraged, as they do not correlate with acute gout symptoms (22). *In short, blood tests are often unhelpful or misleading in attempts to exclude septic arthritis.*

Radiography is of limited utility in the evaluation of acute monoarticular arthritis. Plain films commonly reveal nonspecific soft tissue swelling and joint effusion in the setting of inflammation. Joint space narrowing, periarticular osteoporosis, and erosive osteomyelitis caused by infection typically take weeks to develop. Neonates may rarely manifest joint dislocations or subluxation in the setting of septic arthritis (14,19). Chronic or recurrent gout may induce joint space narrowing and juxta-articular bony erosions with overhanging edges. Linear stippling and punctate densities of articular cartilage such as the menisci or triangular ligament of the radioulnar joint identifies chondrocalcinosis of CPPD but does not exclude other disease. Prosthetic loosening may be evident on plain films but does not differentiate mechanical failure from infection. In patients with subacute to chronic symptoms, x-rays may identify fractures, foreign bodies, avascular necrosis, loose joint bodies, chronic joint changes, osteomyelitis, tumors, Paget disease, and osteochondritis desiccans among other processes.

Advanced imaging such as ultrasound, computed tomography (CT), and magnetic resonance imaging (MRI) can differentiate articular from periarticular soft tissue processes and are sensitive for joint effusions. This is particularly helpful in difficult-to-examine joints such as the hip, sternoclavicular, and sacroiliac joints (9). Unfortunately, these techniques cannot distinguish infected from noninfected joint fluid. Radionuclide scintigraphy scanning has limited specificity but is used to identify infection at prosthetic joint sites.

EMERGENCY DEPARTMENT MANAGEMENT

Septic Arthritis

Rapid diagnosis and therapy is paramount in preventing the morbidity and mortality of septic arthritis. Treatment requires appropriate antibiotics and surgical drainage in most cases. As with any infectious process, begin antibiotics immediately after appropriate culture collection if the diagnosis is highly sus-

pected. Antibiotic selection is based on the clinical probability of a specific pathogen as determined by patient presentation, age, comorbid risks, and Gram stain. Empiric broad-spectrum parenteral antibiotics are indicated in most situations (Table 107.2). Combination therapy with a penicillinase-resistant synthetic penicillin (nafcillin 1–2 gm q6h) *and* a third-generation cephalosporin (ceftriaxone 1 gm qd, cefotaxime 1 gm q8h, or ceftizoxime 1 gm q8h) are excellent choices in adults. Although the pathogens are somewhat dissimilar, empiric pediatric antibiotic selection parallels coverage in adults (synthetic penicillin: nafcillin 50 mg/kg q6h *and* third generation cephalosporin: ceftriaxone 50 mg/kg qd, cefotaxime 50 mg/kg q6h, or ceftizoxime 50 mg/kg q6–8h). Penicillin allergic individuals and those at risk for methicillin-resistant *S. aureus* (high MRSA prevalence and nosocomial, prosthetic joint, or post-operative infection) warrant vancomycin pending culture and sensitivity results. Patients with Gram-negative bacilli identified on initial stain and those at risk for such organisms demand additional coverage via an antipseudomonal penicillin, aminoglycoside, or fluoroquinolone. Initial therapy for disseminated gonococcal disease is a parenteral third generation cephalosporin (ceftriaxone 1 gm qd, cefotaxime 1 gm q8h, or ceftizoxime 1 gm q8h). Alternative regimens include spectinomycin 2 gm IM q12 hours or IV floroquinolone (levofloxacin 500 mg daily, or ciprofloxacin 400 mg q12h). Patients with gonococcal infection also require empiric therapy for concurrent chlamydial infection.

Crystal-Induced Arthritis

Although acute crystal induced arthritis is generally self-limited, treatment relieves discomfort and prevents progressive joint changes. Nonsteroidal antiinflammatory drugs (NSAIDs) are the treatment of choice for most patients (22). Naproxen (750–1000 mg per day for 3 days with subsequent taper) and Indomethacin (150–300 mg per day for 3 days with subsequent taper) provide marked relief within 24 hours (7). The usefulness of NSAIDs is limited by their side effects including gastropathy and renal dysfunction.

Intraarticular steroids are very effective for crystal disease but their use requires confident exclusion of infection (17,22). The appropriate intraarticular steroid dose is dependent on joint size; 20–60 mg of methylprednisolone acetate is adequate for larger joints such as the knee, while 5–10 mg is appropriate for smaller joints. Alternatively, systemic steroids may be utilized. Oral prednisone (40–60 mg daily for 3 days followed by a 7-day taper) and intramuscular triamcinolone acetonide (60 mg single dose) or corticotropin (25–40 units) are typical regimens (7,22).

The leukocyte inhibitor colchicine provides dramatic relief if utilized within 24 hours of gout onset but carries a higher risk of adverse effects (22). Traditional oral dosing is 1 mg followed by 0.5 mg every two hours to a maximum of 8 mg or bothersome gastrointestinal side effects (7). An abbreviated regimen of 0.6 mg every hour for up to three hours is also described (22). A single 1–2 mg dose of intravenous colchicine may provide prompt relief with fewer gastrointestinal effects but increases the risk of systemic toxicity (7). Patients should not take additional colchicine for seven days following an oral or intravenous load. Elderly patients and those with renal and hepatic dysfunction are not candidates for colchicine.

Serum urate lowering agents such as allopurinol and probenecid are contraindicated in the setting of acute or resolving gout. The resultant change in serum urate may exacerbate or prolong an attack. Joint rest and cold applications provide symptomatic relief. Warm compresses exacerbate joint inflammation and should be avoided (22). Narcotic analgesics (hydrocodone or oxycodone with or without acetaminophen) provide further relief.

TABLE 107.2.   Treatment of Monoarticular Arthritis*

	Example Regimen	Alternative Regimen
Infectious Empiric and Non-GC (Pediatric dose)	PCN-ase resistant synthetic PCN: Nafcillin 1–2 gm (50 mg/kg) Cefazolin 1–2 gm (25 mg/kg) *And* 3rd generation cephalosporin Ceftriaxone 1 gm qd (50mg/kg qd) Cefotaxime 1 gm q8h (50mg/kg) Ceftizoxime 1 gm q8h (50mg/kg)	Vancomycin 1 gm (15 mg/kg) Levofloxacin 500 mg qd Ciprofloxacin 400 mg BID
Isolated GC	Ceftriaxone 1 gm qd Cefotaxime 1 gm q8h Ceftizoxime 1 gm q8h *Treat empirically for concurrent chlamydia	Spectinomycin 2 gm IV q12h Levofloxacin 500 mg qd Ciprofloxacin 400 mg BID

Crystal-induced	NSAID:
	Indomethacin 50 mg PO TID for 3 days and
	   taper over 4–7 days
	Naproxen 500 mg PO BID for 3 days and taper
	   over 4–7 days
	
	Narcotic analgesics as needed
		Corticosteroids:
		Prednisone 40–60 mg PO QD for 3d and taper
		   over 7 days
		Triamcinolone acetonide 60 mg IM
		Corticotropin 25–40 USP units IM
		Methlyprednisolone 5–60 mg IA
		
		Colchicine:
		0.6 mg PO each hour for up to 3 doses
		1 mg PO followed by 0.5 mg q1h until relief, GI
		   upset, or 8 mg max
		1–2 mg IV over 30 minutes
		*No further doses after initial load

Traumatic	Joint aspiration for tense effusion Rest, Ice, Compression, Elevation (RICE) Orthopaedic f/u as needed	
Hemorrhagic	Correct coagulopathy RICE	
Inflammatory	Indomethacin 50 mg PO TID with taper (or comparable NSAID) High dose ASA for RA Narcotic analgesics as needed	

*See text for details. ASA, aspirin (acetylsalicyclic acid); IM, intramuscular; RA, rheumatoid arthritis.

CRITICAL INTERVENTIONS

- Perform arthrocentesis in patients with suspected septic arthritis. No radiographic or blood tests can rule out septic arthritis
- Rapidly initiate parenteral antibiotic therapy for patients with septic arthritis

DISPOSITION

Patients with nongonococcal septic arthritis require hospitalization. Daily aspiration versus open surgical drainage of septic joints is controversial and should be left to the discretion of the orthopaedic consultant. Gonococcal arthritis is typically responsive to antibiotics and may not require surgical drainage. Intraarticular antibiotics provide no additional value and may result in chemical synovitis (16,20). Reliable nontoxic patients with gonococcal disease of nonweight bearing joints may be treated as outpatients with daily parenteral therapy (ceftriaxone 1 gm daily) and close monitoring. Clinical improvement should occur within 48 hours at which time patients may be transitioned to oral therapy (floroquinolone or cefixime 400 mg BID). Counseling includes discussion of sexually transmitted diseases, birth control, partner information, and referral for HIV and syphilis testing.

Most patients with acute gouty attacks are successfully treated as outpatients. Factors that may have precipitated the episode, such as alcohol, purine-rich foods, and diuretics should be addressed.

COMMON PITFALLS

- ✔ Failure to obtain synovial fluid for analysis
- ✔ Excluding septic arthritis based on a normal peripheral WBC count or the absence of fever
- ✔ Failure to consider infection in patients with acute worsening of preexisting arthritis
- ✔ Forgetting that gonococcal arthritis commonly presents with migratory polyarthritis and tenosynovitis rather than acute monoarthritis
- ✔ Failure to search for a distant infection in a patient diagnosed with septic arthritis
- ✔ Diagnosing or excluding gout based on a serum urate level
- ✔ Ordering protein and glucose on synovial fluid
- ✔ Failure to perform routine culture on all diagnostic synovial fluid specimens
- ✔ Prescribing serum urate lowering agents at the time of an acute gouty attack

Acknowledgment

Thanks to previous edition chapter author Stephen A. Coluciello.

References

1. Agudelo CA, Wise CM. Crystal-associated arthritis. *Clin Geriatr Med* 1998;14:495–512.
2. Baker DG, Schumacher HR. Acute monoarthritis. *N Engl J Med* 1993;329:1013–1020.

AIDS Arthritis

Several polyarthritic syndromes have been described in association with HIV infection (2,4,13). A painful, asymmetric, oligoarticular arthritis affecting the knees and ankles has been widely reported. Also seen are seronegative spondyloarthritis (particularly Reiter syndrome and psoriatic arthritis) and lupus-like syndromes. These polyarthritides may occur at any stage of HIV infection and have been reported to develop months or years before the actual diagnosis of HIV. Due to impaired immunity, HIV patients are at risk for pyogenic infections of joints. Streptococcus and Staphylococcus species predominate but opportunistic pathogens may be involved. All HIV patients should undergo arthrocentesis of a newly inflamed joint.

DIFFERENTIAL DIAGNOSIS

There are a number of disorders that may produce polyarticular arthritis, including rheumatoid arthritis, acute rheumatic fever, gonococcal arthritis, Lyme disease, Reiter syndrome, postviral arthritis, serum sickness, systemic lupus erythematosus, osteoarthritis, ankylosing spondylitis, ulcerative colitis, regional enteritis (Crohn disease), and psoriatic arthritis. Clinical features that may be helpful in distinguishing between the disorders are listed in Tables 108.1 and 108.2.

Inflammation in the periarticular soft tissues (tendons, bursae) can cause swelling and limitation of motion simulating joint disease. Arthritis generally affects both active and passive motion equally, whereas acute tendinitis or bursitis limits active motion significantly more than passive motion. Synovitis, manifested by swelling, warmth, effusion and tenderness of the joint is indicative of joint inflammation. A diagnosis of polyarthritis demands objective evidence of inflammation in at least two joints.

EMERGENCY DEPARTMENT EVALUATION

In an undiagnosed patient, sudden onset of joint pain (developing over several hours, rather than days) strongly suggests gout (almost always monoarticular) or infection. The most important joint disorder to diagnose accurately and early is infectious arthritis. The persistence of symptoms for over 4 to 6 weeks suggests a systemic rheumatologic disease.

Symmetric joint involvement is seen in RA or SLE. Asymmetric joint involvement is seen in the seronegative arthritides (e.g., Reiter syndrome and psoriatic arthritis). Migratory involvement (leaving one joint before involving another) is typical of acute rheumatic fever (ARF). A family history of arthritis supports a diagnosis of RA or one of the seronegative spondyloarthropathies. Thiazides are known to increase the serum uric acid level and may precipitate gout. Hydralazine, procainamide, isoniazid, and phenytoin can induce a lupus-like reaction.

To assess patterns of involvement and chronicity, all joints should be examined not just those that are symptomatic. Several acute polyarthritides are associated with a characteristic rash. Subcutaneous nodules are seen in 35% of patients with RA and less than 10% of those with ARF. Psoriatic arthritis is usually associated with pitting of the nails and the typical papulosquamous eruption. A general physical examination may note such important findings as a pleural effusion in SLE and RA or clinical signs of liver dysfunction in arthritis associated with hepatitis. A pelvic examination should be performed on all women with unexplained arthritis to rule out *Neisseria gonorrhoeae*. Generalized lymphadenopathy or oral thrush may suggest the human immunodeficiency virus (HIV).

For either the previously undiagnosed patient or the patient with diagnosed disease and a new acute complaint, the most important laboratory test is examination of the joint fluid. Usual fluid studies to obtain include white cell count with differential, Gram stain, culture and crystal analysis. Specific diagnostic tests (e.g., antinuclear antibody, rheumatoid factor, Lyme titer, HIV, hepatitis screen) are seldom available on an emergency basis. They should be ordered in appropriate patients for use in subsequent evaluation. The erythrocyte sedimentation rate (ESR) and C-Reactive Protein (CRP) can be elevated in any inflammatory condition and although of only marginal assistance in the differential diagnosis may be useful to monitor the activity of a chronic arthritis. The diagnosis of ARF requires laboratory confirmation of recent group A streptococcal pharyngitis. An elevated antistreptolysin-O (ASO) titer is seen in most patients. In patients with gonoccoccal arthritis, arthrocentesis cultures are positive in only half of affected joints. One is significantly more likely to obtain a positive culture from the mucosal surface of initial infectious contact (throat, cervix, urethra, or rectum). Polymerase chain reaction (PCR) may be useful in identifying gonococcal infection from a joint that is culture-negative.

Radiographs are of limited utility in the evaluation of the patient with nontraumatic joint pain. Radiographically visible inflammatory changes (such as symmetric erosions of the wrist and metacarpophalangeal joints in RA) occur late in the course of disease, and a normal radiograph does not rule out a diagnosis of arthritis. The main use of radiographs in the emergency department is to exclude complications in patients with chronic arthritis.

The diagnosis of RA is based largely on observation of the clinical course over a period of months to years. Rheumatoid factor, although not a specific marker for RA, is present in the serum of 75% of patients. Clinical criteria to consider as established by the American Rheumatism Association include prolonged morning stiffness, symmetry of joint involvement particularly in the wrist metacarpophalangeal and hand proximal interphalangeal joints, chronicity, rheumatoid nodules and radiographs revealing erosions. Recent studies reveal the characteristic bone erosions may be visualized by ultrasound and magnetic resonance imaging (MRI) significantly earlier than by conventional radiography (9,16).

EMERGENCY DEPARTMENT MANAGEMENT

The mainstay of treatment for polyarthritis is nonsteroidal anti-inflammatory drugs (NSAIDs). These agents control both pain and inflammation. A common error is to prematurely conclude that a particular NSAID is ineffective or to advance hastily to more potent agents, such as corticosteroids. If one NSAID fails to control symptoms, another in a different class may work well.

Recent research into the etiology of the inflammatory process has revealed that two enzymes, cyclooxygenase 1 and 2 (COX-1, COX-2), are fundamental. Aside from mediating inflammation, COX-1 plays a cytoprotective role in the gastrointestinal (GI) tract. Typical NSAIDs inhibit COX-1 and thus place the GI tract at risk for erosive damage. COX-2 is also instrumental in the inflammatory process but has no demonstrated GI cytoprotection. Recently developed COX-2 blocking agents appear to have a lower likelihood of causing gastric erosions while still inhibiting the inflammatory process.

Several disorders require more specific treatment. Patients with a first attack of ARF should be hospitalized and closely monitored for worsening carditis and arrhythmias. High-dose salicylates may be useful. A course of penicillin is recommended to eradicate any remaining streptococci and the patient may be kept on low-dose penicillin prophylaxis indefinitely thereafter.

Most patients with gonococcal arthritis should be hospitalized. Therapy is initiated with a parenteral third-generation cephalosporin, or spectinomycin. Repeated joint aspirations, arthroscopy or surgery may be required. In most cases, dramatic clinical improvement is noted in several days and the patient may transition to oral antibiotics. Patients should be treated concurrently for chlamydia.

Lyme disease in early stages is generally treated with doxycycline. Advanced cases may require treatment with ceftriaxone. Reiter syndrome is not curable, but treatment of the initial urethritis may prevent development of the full-blown disease. Arthritic inflammation is treated symptomatically.

RA and psoriatic arthritis may initially respond to NSAIDs but treatment with "disease-modifying agents" including antimalarials, gold salts, penicillamine, methotrexate, cytotoxic agents, prednisone and antitumor necrosis factors may significantly retard disease progression.

Complications of Rheumatoid Arthritis

RA is the most common and most serious of the chronic polyarthritides and may be associated with a number of emergent complications (Table 108.3). In addition to suffering direct complications of the disease, patients are also subject to the potential toxic effects of treatment. The emergency physician should be aware of the potential for acute problems in patients with well-established RA.

Radiographic abnormalities of the cervical spine are common, particularly subluxation of C-1 on C-2. Usually these abnormalities are asymptomatic but the appearance of neurologic symptoms or signs necessitate neurosurgical consultation. Patients may note a peculiar slipping sensation with neck movements that is associated with either exacerbation or relief of symptoms. Flexion and extension views of the cervical spine may aid in the diagnosis. A patient with RA who sustains even minor cervical trauma is at risk for serious injury. The potential for cervical spine instability should be considered when intubating a patient with chronic RA.

Various entrapment neuropathies occur in RA, carpal tunnel syndrome is the most common. Patients initially complain of sensory changes over the distribution of the median nerve and a "toothache-like" pain at the wrist. Tinel sign, the induction of a tingling sensation in the same distribution upon tapping over the median nerve with a reflex hammer, is a useful physical finding.

TABLE 108.3. Complications of Rheumatoid Arthritis

Organ	Manifestations
Neurologic	Subluxation C-1, C-2 (cord compression); entrapment neuropathy (carpal tunnel); peripheral neuropathy; myositis; necrotizing vasculitis (central nervous system)
Musculoskeletal	Septic arthritis; tendon rupture; synovial cyst knee (pseudophlebitis); rheumatoid nodules
Larynx	Cricoarytenoid arthritis (airway)
Lung	Pleurisy; effusion; fibrosis
Cardiac	Pericarditis; tamponade; conduction defects; valvular (nodules); myocardial infarction (coronary arteritis)
Hematologic	Anemia; leukopenia; hyperviscosity; Felty syndrome (splenomegaly, neutropenia)
Ocular	Sjögren syndrome; episcleritis; scleritis
Blood vessels	Vasculitis (usually dermal, can be widespread)

The diagnosis is confirmed with electromyography and nerve conduction studies. Treatment consists of splinting the wrist and arranging consultation with a rheumatologist, orthopaedist or neurologist. Local corticosteroid injection is occasionally useful. Surgical release of median nerve entrapment is sometimes necessary. Generalized muscle wasting, weakness, and peripheral neuropathy in RA patients may also be manifestations of systemic vasculitis.

Rupture of the extensor tendons of the hand is not uncommon in advanced RA. Once one tendon ruptures, the increased strain on the remaining tendons may lead to rupture of others. Patients cannot extend the fingers actively at the metacarpophalangeal joints but passive extension is still possible. The treatment is elective surgical repair.

The development of a synovial cyst behind the knee is common in RA. Synovial inflammation may result in large knee effusions and high pressure generated during flexion of the knee may cause cyst formation in the popliteal fossa. The diagnosis is confirmed by an arthrogram or ultrasound of the knee joint. Curative treatment is difficult. Joint aspiration and local corticosteroid injection may be temporarily helpful. These cysts may rupture, dissecting into the calf. The resulting calf pain, swelling, and redness may suggest the presence of deep vein thrombosis. Duplex sonography is helpful in distinguishing these clinical entities.

The cricoarytenoid joint is a synovial articulation and can be involved in RA (7). Patients may present with stridor and significant airway obstruction or with less severe involvement, dyspnea, dysphagia, painful speech, foreign-body sensation, or hoarseness (12). There may be tenderness over the thyroid cartilage. Laryngoscopy reveals redness and edema over the arytenoids and abnormal bowing of the vocal cords during inspiration. Intubation may be difficult (5). Cricothyrotomy or tracheostomy may be necessary to secure the airway. Corticosteroids and cool humidification are useful for milder cases. Extubation has been associated with acute airway obstruction.

The most common type of *vasculitis* associated with RA involves small dermal vessels, causing relatively benign infarctions in the periungual areas of the fingers. Occasionally patients develop a necrotizing vasculitis which can follow a fulminant course. The presenting manifestations may be large ulcerations, digital gangrene, neuropathies, mesenteric ischemia or coronary arteritis. Patients with systemic vasculitis usually have fever, leukocytosis, high titers of rheumatoid factor, an elevated ESR and antinuclear antibodies. They should be admitted to the hospital for initiation of high-dose corticosteroids. At times cytotoxic agents or apheresis is useful. The prognosis in patients with extensive vasculitic involvement is poor.

Sjögren syndrome (keratoconjunctivitis sicca), not uncommonly associated with RA, is characterized by dry eyes and dry mouth and is caused by decreased lacrimal and salivary gland function. Patients complain of grittiness in the eyes and thick mucus beneath the eyelids. The diagnosis is made by the Schirmer test which measures tear production. Treatment consists of artificial tears, humidified air, and eye goggles to minimize tear evaporation.

Episcleritis, also associated with RA, is usually benign but should be followed by an ophthalmologist because it can lead to *scleritis*. A brief course of topical corticosteroids as prescribed by an ophthalmologist is usually beneficial. Scleritis is a more diffuse process and can cause uveitis, glaucoma, and rupture of the globe. Patients complain of a deep aching sensation and tenderness on gentle palpation of the globe. Slit-lamp examination reveals cellular exudate in the anterior chamber. Prompt ophthalmologic consultation is indicated.

Hematologic problems, including anemia, leukopenia, and hyperviscosity occur in RA. Felty syndrome (triad of RA, splenomegaly, and neutropenia) is associated with severe disease. These patients are prone to recurrent infections and have hepatic dysfunction and recurring cutaneous ulcers. Splenectomy is occasionally beneficial.

Pleurisy and pleural effusions are common in RA but are not usually life-threatening. Pericarditis is also common but only rarely does pericardial tamponade or constrictive pericarditis occurs. Rheumatoid nodules may affect the heart valves or cardiac conduction system. Myocardial infarction secondary to vasculitis involving the coronary arteries has been reported.

CRITICAL INTERVENTIONS

- Perform arthrocentesis to establish a diagnosis, or to exclude infectious complications in patients with preexisting arthritis
- Administer antibiotics to patients with an infectious source, and an NSAID to patients with painful, inflammatory arthritis

DISPOSITION

Patients with a first attack of ARF should be hospitalized. Most patients with gonococcal arthritis should also be hospitalized for initial therapy. Lyme disease in early stages is generally treated with doxycycline on an outpatient basis. Advanced cases may require hospitalization.

Patients with RA or SLE may present with severe pain or complications requiring admission, but isolated exacerbations of joint pain are often managed successfully on an outpatient basis. Admission decisions for other causes of polyarticular arthritis are often dependent upon the certainty of diagnosis, the adequacy of pain control, and the presence of absence of other disease complications.

COMMON PITFALLS

✔ Failure to analyze synovial fluid in a patient with undiagnosed arthritis or in one with new joint tenderness, warmth, and swelling
✔ Failure to recognize an acute septic joint in a patient with underlying polyarthritis
✔ Failure to recognize rheumatic fever and initiate appropriate therapy
✔ Failure to recognize symptoms due to therapy rather than to underlying disease
✔ Failure to appreciate extraarticular manifestations of chronic polyarthritis
✔ Failure to consider underlying HIV infection in a person with a newly diagnosed, seronegative spondyloarthropathy or lupus-like syndrome

References

1. Cucurull E, Espinoza JLR. Gonococcal arthritis. 1998;24:305.
2. Cuellar M. HIV infection associated inflammatory musculoskeletal disorders. *Rheum Dis Clin North Am* 1998;24:403.
3. Firestein, G. Rheumatic arthritis. *Sci Am* 1998;3:15.
4. Golbus J. Rheumatic disease and AIDS. *Postgrad Med* 1992;92:1233.
5. Hakala P, Randell T. Intubation difficulties in patients with rheumatoid arthritis. A retrospective analysis. *Acta Anaesthesiol Scand* 1998;42:195–198.
6. Kaye B. Rheumatologic manifestations of infection with human immunodeficiency virus. *Ann Intern Med* 1989;111:158.
7. Leicht Ng, Harrington TM, David DE, et al. Cricoarytenoid arthritis: a cause of laryngeal obstruction. *Ann Emerg Med* 1987;16:885.
8. Levine M, Siegel LB. A swollen joint: why all the fuss? *Am J Ther* 2003;10:219–24.
9. Lopez-Ben R, Bernreuter WK, Moreland LW, Alarcon GS. Ultrasound detection of bone erosions in rheumatoid arthritis: a comparison to routine radiographs of the hands and feet. *Skeletal Radiol* 2004;33(2):80–84.
10. Masferrer JL, Isakson PC, Seibert K. NSAIDs, eicosanoids and the gastroenteric tract. *Gastroenterol Clin* 1996;25:363.
11. Massell BF, Chute CG, Walker AM, et al. Penicillin and the marked decrease in morbidity and mortality from rheumatic fever in the United States. *N Engl J Med* 1988;318:280.
12. McGeehan DF, Crinnnion JN, Strachan DR. Life-threatening stridor presenting in a patient with rheumatoid involvement of the larynx. *Arch Emerg Med* 1989;6:274–276.
13. Mody GM, Parke FA, Reveille JD. Articular manifestations of HIV infection. *Best Pract Res Clin Rheumatol* 2003;17:265–287.
14. Moore TL. Parvovirus-associated arthhritis. *Curr Opin Rheumatol* 2000;12:289–294.
15. Moreland LW, Bridges SL Jr. Early rheumatoid arthritis: a medical emergency? *Am J Med* 2001;111:498–500.
16. Ostergaard M, Hansen M, Stolenberg M, Jensen KE, Szkudlarek M, Pedersen-Zbinden B, Lorenzen I. New radiographic bone erosions in the wrists of RA, MRI results. *Arthritis Rheum* 2003;48(8):2128–2131.
17. Rose CD, Eppes SC. Infection related arthritis. *Rheum Dis Clin North Am* 1997;23,3:677.
18. Sigal LH. Pitfalls in the diagnosis and management of Lyme disease. *Arthritis Rheum* 1998;41:195.
19. Snyderman R, Haynes BF. The Medical Clinics of North America. *Adv Rheumatol* 1997;81:57.
20. Spiegel BM, Targownik L, Dulai GS, Gralnek IM. *Ann Intern Med* 2003;138:795–806.
21. Stanley KL, Weaver JE. Pharmacologic management of pain and inflammation in athletes. *Clin Sports Med* 1998;17:375.
22. Tutar E, Atalay S, Yilmaz E, Ucar T, Kocak G, Imamoglu A. Poststreptococcal reactive arthritis in children. *Rheumatol Int* 2002;22(2):80–83.
23. Vassilopoulos D, Calabrese LH. Rheumatologic manifestations of hepatitis C infection. *Curr Rheumatol Rep* 2003;5200–5204.
24. Veasy LG, Tani LY, Hill HR. Persistence of acute rheumatic fever in the intermountain area of the United States. *J Pediatr* 1994;124(1):9.
25. Weiner SR. Emergencies in rheumatoid arthritis. *Am Fam Physician* 1984;29:127.
26. Winchester R. The co-occurrence of Reiter's syndrome and acquired immunodeficiency. *Ann Intern Med* 1987;106:19.

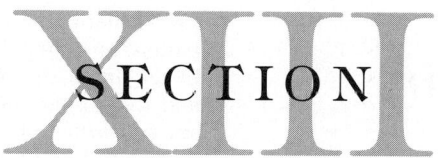

SECTION XIII

Section Editor: Jeffrey Schaider

Neurologic Emergencies

CHAPTER 109
Organic Brain Syndrome

Rebecca R. Roberts, MD

Often, patients in acute distress from mental health causes seek treatment in the emergency department (ED) (26). Emergency Departments also provide comprehensive medical evaluations prior to civil commitment for many patients in psychiatric crisis (13,26). The purpose of these evaluations is to detect the presence of medical illness complicating or even causing the psychiatric symptoms. Differentiating between functional (psychiatric) and organic (medical) causes of behavioral abnormalities may seem somewhat arbitrary (5,16). However, arranging the proper tests, treatments, consultants, and site of care depends on accurately making this determination. Several studies have documented high rates of patients receiving treatment for psychiatric illnesses that are caused by undetected and treatable medical illness (11,12,22,24).

CLINICAL PRESENTATION

The term organic brain syndrome (OBS) covers a wide range of clinical manifestations. The first two, delirium and dementia, are always presumed to be due to an organic cause (Table 109.1) *Delirium* is often due to a life-threatening medical cause (4,15,18). Delirium, especially common in the elderly, is characterized by recent abrupt onset with rapid progression and wide fluctuations in symptoms. There is always disturbance of consciousness; patients may not be aware of their surroundings and may be overly responsive to hallucinations and delusions. They may be hyper-alert to external stimuli, but respond inappropriately, often with anxiety or fear. There are also changes in cognition, especially orientation, language, and memory. Delirious patients often do not have the attention span, concentration, or understanding of their surroundings to participate in any further testing of cognition or memory (15). One of the hallmarks of delirium is the speed of onset and rapidly fluctuating mental status (15). Delirium is also likely to be transient with the patient recovering with treatment or resolution of the underlying cause (18).

Dementia is the more gradual development of intellectual impairment sufficient to interfere with social and physical functioning (15,18). The hallmark finding is memory impairment. Memory deficits can be remarkable in patients who appear to function well otherwise. In addition, there must be at least one other cognitive function alteration such as loss of language, visual-spatial, abstraction ability, judgment, a personality change or reduced organizational skills. In contrast to delirium, consciousness is not clouded (15,18). In addition, dementia develops over a more prolonged time course. The maintenance of normal consciousness, self-awareness, and slow progression can result in severe loss of function before family or providers detect the problem. In fact, frequently an acute precipitant such as medical illness or change in living situation calls attention to the long-term decline. Sometimes, it is not clear what precipitated the ED visit for a patient with chronic dementia. Sensitive questioning will sometimes reveal that the family feels no longer able to safely care for the patient and they desire help or even nursing home placement. Other times, the patient has had a catastrophic anger reaction and the family was not aware of this as part of the syndrome and so did not mention it.

In addition to delirium and dementia, all of the major psychiatric diagnostic groups can be mimicked by new medications, medical or surgical illnesses (4,25). Underlying medical diseases can cause presentations similar to psychosis, mania, depression, anxiety disorders, or even personality disorders. For some illnesses, a neuropsychiatric manifestation can be the first symptom prompting treatment (25). Lastly, development of serious medical illnesses can cause an acute worsening of behavioral symptoms in patients with chronic dementia or preexisting psychiatric diseases (21). Vigilance is required to avoid missing psychiatric patients suffering from new unrelated medical illness.

DIFFERENTIAL DIAGNOSIS

The first challenge is to distinguish between functional psychiatric illness and OBS (4). One of the most important features in OBS is cognitive dysfunction (3,4,7,10). This may be undetectable

---

TABLE 109.1.   Diagnostic Criteria for Delirium and Dementia*

DELIRIUM

Definition: Disturbance of consciousness accompanied by change in cognition; not due to a preexisting dementia.
A. Disturbance of consciousness:
  Alterations or lack of clarity awareness of the environment
  Reduced ability to concentrate
  Attention: inability to focus, sustain, or shift attention
B. At least 2 cognitive deficits:
  Memory deficit
  Disorientation
  Language disturbance
  Perception alteration (i.e.: hallucination or illusions)
C. Rapid, abrupt onset over hours or days
D. Organic cause
  Clinical evidence by history, physical, or testing, that the disturbance is due to the physiologic manifestations of a general medical condition or substance abuse or both

DEMENTIA

Definition: Multiple cognitive deficits (especially memory) that are not due to delirium; consciousness is not necessarily clouded
A. Memory impairment
  Impaired ability to learn new information
  Impaired ability to recall previously learned information
B. At least one cognitive deficit
  Aphasia (language disturbance)
  Apraxia (decreased ability to carry out motor activities despite intact motor function)
  Agnosia (not recognizing or identifying objects despite intact sensory function)
  Disturbed executive function (planning, organizing, sequencing, abstracting)
C. The intellectual impairments interfere with normal social or occupational function
D. Organic cause
  The defects are caused by an underlying medical condition
  The specific causes are important as some are correctable and some are not

*References: 2,15,18,23

unless specifically sought (8,26). Most patients with functional psychiatric disease, even psychotic schizophrenic patients, have normal vital signs, motor and speech function, cognitive function, and memory (25). Therefore, abnormalities in these areas cannot be assumed to reflect chronic psychiatric illness. Another technique for distinguishing OBS from functional disorders such as mania or depression is to compare the patient's syndrome to the standard psychiatric definition. The presence of atypical psychiatric features point to an organic cause (25). Next, it is useful to note similarities between the presentation of delirium and dementia and the more standard psychiatric diagnoses. Delirium shares clinical features with anxiety disorders, acute psychosis, or mania (18). Severe alcohol withdrawal is also a form of delirium (19). Dementia can appear similar to depression, chronic schizophrenia, or personality disorders. This same overlap occurs in the medical causes of these problems and can assist in working through the differential diagnosis.

Nearly any medical problem can at times result in compromised mental functioning and psychiatric clinical manifestations (4,12,21,23). Table 109.2 lists the most common causes by clinical syndrome. Medications are by far the most common causes of OBS (1,4). Common culprits are medicines with any anticholinergic activity, narcotics, histamine blockers, corticosteroids, antihypertensives such as beta-blockers or clonidine, and sedative-hypnotics. The major life-threatening causes can be summarized as any profound disruption in blood or nutrient supply to the brain: shock, hypoxia, sepsis, anemia, hypoglycemia, hypertensive encephalopathy, hyperthermia, fluid, electrolyte or acid-base imbalance, carbon monoxide, intracranial infection, mass, subdural hematoma, or stroke (4,8,12). In addition, alcohol withdrawal and Wernicke's require emergent recognition and treatment. Infections, both neurological as well as systemic, are important causes of OBS. Some neurologic infections, such as West Nile Virus encephalitis or other viral causes of encephalitis, are seasonal. The most common nonneurologic infections are pulmonary, urinary, bloodstream, and rarely endocarditis. Metabolic derangements with behavioral symptoms are common in liver, renal, pulmonary, thyroid, and adrenal diseases (4,8,12,22). Trauma, illicit drugs, toxins, and HIV infection are common causes in the young (9,20,22). Altered behavior in patients with cancer, heart disease, collagen vascular disease, or HIV infection should prompt consideration of organic causes.

EMERGENCY DEPARTMENT EVALUATION

Any patient with neuropsychiatric symptoms should receive a thorough history and physical examination (26). This includes a mental status exam to detect cognitive deficits (3,7,10,22,26). Often, the history must be obtained from family or paramedics. Sometimes family members can only articulate that the patient has changed or worsened in some indefinite way. A frequent complaint for the elderly is a sudden refusal or inability to eat (13).

The history should include information on medications, alcohol and drug use, including over-the-counter and herbal preparations, recent hospitalizations, surgeries, or trauma (1,6,18,19,21,25). Specifically ask about past psychiatric, endocrine, pulmonary, cardiac, renal, hepatic, malignant, and collagen vascular diseases, as well as potential exposure to toxins and possible HIV infection (4,6,12,20,26). Complaints such as headache, focal neurologic deficits, abdominal pain, dyspnea, fever, incontinence, nonauditory hallucinations, weight loss, cough, vomiting or diarrhea also point to organic causes (13). The patient's normal level of functioning and the pattern and rate of behavioral change must be ascertained. Recent, abrupt onset of change in a previously normal patient or new onset of psychiatric manifestations in older patients is a key sign of organic cause (4). Visual hallucinations, distortions, or illusions are also important clues to an organic etiology (25). Sometimes an elderly patient with chronic, mild dementia will develop an acute delirium due to a new or worsening medical condition (21). Acute worsening of chronic dementia will occur with new stroke, sepsis, pneumonia, myocardial infarction, metabolic or endocrine derangements, and new medications.

The physical exam findings indicative of an organic cause are abnormal vital signs, diaphoretic skin, jaundice, or pallor. Note any motor disturbance such as tremor, or partial seizure activity (25). Either increased or decreased psychomotor activity levels may be seen (23). Pay special attention to the ear, nose, and throat exam. Look for signs of thyroid or adrenal disease. The heart, liver, kidney and lung exam may reveal signs of infection or disease. A complete neurologic exam, including gait and tests of cognitive function, is required (3,4,7,10,23).

The following findings in the mental status exam indicate an organic cause for behavioral changes (6). A neat, well-groomed appearance in a patient who is now disorganized indicates a very abrupt onset (6,26). Altered awareness of the environment, anxiety, labile mood or rapid changes in mental status are also associated with OBS. Language abnormalities, altered speech quality, or disordered visual-spatial abilities are further signs of OBS.

The specific changes in cognitive function can help distinguish between delirium and dementia (8,18). Delirium is defined first by disturbed consciousness. Patients have altered awareness of the environment, difficulty in focusing, sustaining, or shifting their attention, and reduced ability to concentrate. Delirious patients may be hyperalert, but have inappropriately fearful responses to normal stimuli. There must also be disturbances in at least two of the following: perception, language, sleep cycles, memory, or psychomotor activity. However, frequently the limited awareness and inability to concentrate make testing these functions impossible (15). The patient may be hallucinating, very hyperactive, or combative; delirium is recent and abrupt in onset with rapid fluctuation in the clinical picture.

In dementia, the major finding is intellectual impairment that interferes with social and physical functioning. Progressive short-term memory loss is the lead finding. In addition, at least one of the following must be present: personality change, poor judgment, or reduced ability in language, visual-cortical function, or abstraction. In contrast to delirium, the consciousness is not clouded, the pattern is usually gradually progressive rather than abrupt and fluctuating, and some patients can adapt and function for a long time before deficits are detected.

A host of medical illnesses can also cause organic syndromes that closely mimic the traditional functional psychiatric illnesses such as psychosis, mania, depression, and anxiety disorders. In addition to the clues mentioned above, new onset of mania in a patient over the age of 30 and psychosis in patients over 40 is unusual and should prompt testing for organic causes.

When deciding what tests will detect the underlying cause of OBS in a specific patient, it helps to categorize those causes as: medication related, toxicologic, neurologic, endocrine, metabolic, infectious, hepatic, renal, cardiac, and pulmonary (24). The specific evaluation should be guided by findings in the history, physical and mental status examinations (4,24). All patients should receive glucose, electrolytes, complete blood count, and renal function tests (25). If no clear cause such as a medication side effect or drug intoxication is discovered, additional testing should include electrocardiogram (ECG), liver and thyroid function tests, toxicology, arterial blood gases for hypoxia, CO_2

TABLE 109.2. Causes of Organic Brain Syndrome by Manifestation*

Organic Brain Syndrome	Causes	Organic Brain Syndrome	Causes
DELIRIUM		**ANXIETY DISORDERS**	
Emergency Causes	Shock from any cause	Medications/Toxins	Any drug with anticholinergic properties
	Hypoxia from any cause		Bronchodilators
	Hypoglycemia		Decongestants
	Electrolyte/Acid-base imbalance		Diet pills & stimulants
	Acute thiamine deficiency (Wernicke)		Digitalis toxicity
	Hyperthermia		Hallucinogens
	Thyroid storm		Hypotensive agents
	Intracranial catastrophe (mass, blood,	Neurologic	Seizure disorder
	trauma, ischemia, abscess)		Vertigo from another cause
	Carbon monoxide poisoning		Essential tremor
	Alcohol withdrawal		Intracranial mass, blood, trauma, abscess
Medications/Toxins	Any drug with anticholinergic properties		Stroke, TIA
	Clonidine		Postconcussion syndrome
	Lidocaine		Cerebritis: Systemic lupus erythematosus
	Antabuse	Endocrine	Cushing disease
	Caffeine, Ergot		Hyperthyroidism
Neurologic	Subarachnoid hemorrhage		Menopause
	Status seizure (petit mal, partial)		Hypoglycemia
	Postictal syndrome	Metabolic/Dietary	Hyperkalemia
	Hypertensive encephalopathy		Hypocalcemia
Endocrine	Diabetes		Hyponatremia
	Hyperthyroidism		Hyperthermia
	Cushing disease (exogenous)		Vitamin B_{12} and folate deficiency
	Addison disease		Secreting tumors: Carcinoid, insulinoma,
Metabolic/Dietary	Hepatic encephalopathy		Pheochromocytoma
	Renal failure		Porphyria
	Hypomagnesemia		Caffeine
Infectious	Encephalitis/Meningitis/brain abscess		Monosodium glutamate
	Sepsis	Infectious	Pneumonia
	Infective Endocarditis		Encephalitis/meningitis
	Neurosyphilis		Sepsis
	Tuberculosis	Miscellaneous	Any hypoxia, hypovolemia
	Typhoid fever		Anemia
	Rheumatic fever		Myocardial infarction, arrhythmias
Miscellaneous	Alcohol or drug withdrawal syndromes		Pulmonary edema, congestive heart failure
	Congestive heart failure		Hypertension
	Anemia		Valvular disease
	Illicit drug intoxication		Anaphylaxis
			Asthma, chronic obstructive pulmonary
DEMENTIA			disease
Medications	Beta-blockers		Pneumothorax
	Any drug with anticholinergic properties		Pulmonary embolism
	Methyldopa		Alcohol or drug withdrawal
	Clonidine		Illicit drug intoxication
	Sedatives		
Neurologic	Intracranial mass, blood, trauma, abscess	**MANIA**	
	Stroke, TIA	Medications	Any drug with anticholinergic properties
	Multiinfarct dementia		Corticosteroids
	Normal pressure hydrocephalus		Isoniazid
	Chronic subdural hematoma		Histamine blockers
Endocrine	Addison Disease		Cocaine/amphetamines
	Cushing Disease (endogenous)		Phencyclidine
	Diabetes		Flexeril
	Hyperparathyroidism		Bromides
Metabolic/Dietary	Vitamin B_{12} deficiency		Levodopa
	Chronic liver disease	Neurologic	Intracranial mass, blood, trauma, abscess
	Hypercalcemia		Stroke, TIA
	Chronic electrolyte imbalance		Temporal lobe seizure
	Pernicious anemia		Multiple Sclerosis
	Uremia		Wilson Disease
	Thiamine deficiency (Korsakoff)	Endocrine	Hyperthyroid
Infectious	Neurosyphilis		Cushing disease (exogenous)
	Tuberculosis (meningitis, military)		Addison Disease
	HIV/AIDS	Metabolic	Hepatic encephalopathy; early
Miscellaneous	Chronic anemia		Hemodialysis
	Hypoxia	Infectious	Encephalitis
	Hypercarbia		Meningitis
	Depression		Sepsis
			Neurosyphilis

TABLE 109.2. (Continued)

Organic Brain Syndrome	Causes		Organic Brain Syndrome	Causes	
Miscellaneous	Alcohol or drug withdrawal		DEPRESSION		
	Illicit drug intoxication		Medications/Toxins	Beta-blockers	
				Oral contraceptives	
PSYCHOSIS				Steroids	
Medications/Toxins	Any drug with anticholinergic			Neuroleptics	
	properties			Ranitidine	
	Corticosteroids			Anticholinesterases	
	Histamine blockers			Benzodiazepines	
	Dilantin			Efaviren 2	
	Efaviren 2			Propanolol	
	Alprazolam			Alpha methyldopa	
	Stimulants/diet pills		Neurologic	Stroke	
	Isoniazid			Multiple sclerosis	
	Antihypertensives			Early dementia	
Neurologic	Intracranial mass, blood, trauma,			Frontal brain mass	
	abscess			Epilepsy	
	Stroke, TIA			Tumors—pancreas, lung, prostate,	
	Cerebritis: Systemic lupus			brain	
	erythematosus		Endocrine	Hypothyroidism	
	Complex partial seizure			Hyperthyroidism	
Endocrine	Cushing disease (exogenous)			Cushing disease (endogenous)	
	Addison disease			Addison disease	
	Hyperthyroidism			Diabetes	
	Diabetes mellitus		Metabolic/Dietary	Hyperparathyroidism	
Metabolic/Dietary	Hypercalcemia			Hyponatremia	
	Hypomagnesemia			Hypokalemia	
	Hypoglycemia			Hypocalcemia	
	B_{12} deficiency			B_{12} deficiency	
	Thiamine deficiency (Wernicke and			Folate deficiency	
	Korsakoff)			Chronic hepatic encephalopathy	
	Acute hepatic encephalopathy			Uremia	
Infectious	Encephalitis			Neurosyphilis	
	Meningitis		Infectious	Mononucleosis	
	Neurosyphilis			Hepatitis	
	Pancreatitis			Influenza	
	HIV/AIDS				
Miscellaneous	Alcohol or drug withdrawal				
	Illicit drug intoxication				

*References: 1,4,6,8,9,12,15,19,20,21,22,23,25,26. TIA, transient ischemic attack.

retention, and carbon monoxide exposure. A chest x-ray, urinalysis, urine and blood cultures should be done when infection or sepsis is suspected. Most would recommend computerized tomography of the head and lumbar puncture with cerebrospinal fluid (CSF) cultures including tests for tuberculosis and viral encephalitis (25). In patients with dementia, additional testing for correctable causes should include vitamin B_{12}, folate, and rapid plasma reagent (RPR) levels.

EMERGENCY DEPARTMENT MANAGEMENT

In general, the ED management will depend on the underlying cause of the OBS findings. The first and foremost task is to rapidly identify and treat life threats. This may mean rapid airway control and circulatory support for a patient with hypoxia or shock. Take action to prevent injury from falling out of bed, or wandering away. Since unsuspected alcoholism is common, and the diagnosis of Wernicke or withdrawal can be difficult, give thiamine empirically and check the glucose level early and frequently (25). Be cautious when initiating early behavioral control with sedatives, unless you are certain the patient is suffering from alcohol withdrawal and does not have a life-threatening condition causing global brain dysfunction (23). Frequent reassessment is especially critical in those with delirium, since the underlying causes are so seri-

ous and the acute condition can change rapidly. Talk to the family about the need for patient safety while in the ED and the possible need for one-to-one observation, sedatives, or even restraints to provide safety during the evaluation and treatment (23).

CRITICAL INTERVENTIONS

- Treat the following life threats: poor perfusion or shock from any cause, hypoxia, hypoglycemia, severe anemia, thyroid storm, adrenal crisis, sepsis, central nervous system (CNS) infection, mass, bleeding, or ischemia, alcohol withdrawal and toxins such as acetaminophen and carbon monoxide
- Distinguish between functional psychiatric illness and OBS
- Search for new medical illness superimposed upon a chronic dementia that can cause an acute but reversible decline or change

DISPOSITION

Nearly all patients suffering from acute organic brain syndrome need to be hospitalized for continued diagnostic evaluation, treatment, and safety (18). The most common exception is a patient with chronic dementia from past infarcts or newly suspected, but chronic Alzheimer disease. Often the patient has been slowly drifting and the family has not noticed. Frequently such patients are brought to emergency departments during holidays. Any new medical illness superimposed upon a chronic dementia can cause an acute but reversible decline or change (8). Therefore, those with acute dementia or previous dementia and new acute worsening or change also need admission (8). The other exception is someone suffering from a recreational drug or alcohol intoxication that clears in the ED. Patients with chronic dementia or those who have recovered from acute intoxication must go home with responsible family or friends to watch them. In addition, families caring for patients with progressive dementia need to be warned about the dangers of driving, cooking, or starting fires. They also need to know that patients can wander away, or if under stress, can exhibit catastrophic anger reactions. It helps families to know that these reactions can be a normal consequence of dementia. Ensure that good ambulatory care follow up is available. Social services may also be helpful in arranging nursing care in the home.

The majority of patients with OBS will require hospital admission. In some hospitals, psychiatry consult is necessary to determine patient competency if the patient's judgment is in question. Some patients may want to leave once they go to the hospital ward and an existing psychologic evaluation is helpful to hospital staff unfamiliar with the patient. In general, patients with acute judgment, consciousness and cognitive defects do not have sufficient decision-making capacity to sign themselves out of the hospital against medical advice (17).

COMMON PITFALLS

✔ Assuming all psychiatric symptoms are due to functional psychiatric disorders (4,22)
✔ Failing to do a complete history, physical, and mental status exam in all patients with psychiatric symptoms (3,4,10,22)
✔ Ignoring abnormal vital signs
✔ Assuming all physical complaints in a psychiatric patient are due to functional causes (13)
✔ Not detecting a mild early cognitive deficit, or assuming it is due to chronic functional illness
✔ Missing acute delirium that is newly occurring in patients with chronic dementia (8)
✔ Becoming distracted by combative or abnormal behavior and failing to follow through in performing a complete history, physical, and frequent reassessments

Acknowledgment

Thanks to the previous edition's chapter author Sandra M. Schneider.

References

1. Drugs That May Cause Psychiatric Symptoms. *The Medical Letter* 2002;1134:59–62.
2. American Psychiatric Association, American Psychiatric Association, Task Force on DSM-IV. *Diagnostic and statistical manual of mental disorders DSM-IV-TR.* 4th ed. Washington, DC: American Psychiatric Association, 2000.
3. Crum RM, Anthony JC, Bassett SS, Folstein MF. Population-based norms for the Mini-Mental State Examination by age and educational level. *JAMA* 1993;269:2386–2391.
4. Dorsey ST, Bazarian JJ. Medical conditions that mimic psychiatric approach for evaluation of patients who present with psychiatric symptomatology. *Emergency Medicine Reports* 2002;23:233–243.
5. Eisenberg L. Psychiatry and society: a sociobiologic synthesis. *N Engl J Med* 1977;296:903–910.
6. Fauman MA, Fauman BJ. The differential diagnosis of organic based psychiatric disturbance in the emergency department. *JACEP* 1977;7:315–323.
7. Folstein MF, Folstein SE, McHugh PR. "Mini-mental state." A practical method for grading the cognitive state of patients for the clinician. *J Psychiatr Res* 1975;12:189–198.
8. Francis J, Martin D, Kapoor WN. A prospective study of delirium in hospitalized elderly. *JAMA* 1990;263:1097–1101.
9. Horwath E. Psychiatric and neuropsychiatric manifestations of HIV infection. *J Int Assoc Physicians AIDS Care (Chic Ill)* 2002;(1 Suppl 1):S1–15.
10. Irons MJ, Farace E, Brady WJ, Huff JS. Mental status screening of emergency department patients: normative study of the quick confusion scale. *Acad Emerg Med* 2002;9:989–994.
11. Koenig HG, Pappas P, Holsinger T, Bachar JR. Assessing diagnostic approaches to depression in medically ill older adults: how reliably can mental health professionals make judgments about the cause of symptoms? *J Am Geriatr Soc* 1995;43:472–478.
12. Koranyi EK. Undiagnosed physical illness in psychiatric patients. *Ann Rev Med* 1982;33:309–316.
13. Korn CS, Currier GW, Henderson SO. "Medical clearance" of psychiatric patients without medical complaints in the Emergency Department. *J Emerg Med* 2000;18:173–176.
14. Lishman WA. *Organic psychiatry: the psychological consequences of cerebral disorder.* 3rd ed. Oxford: Blackwell Science, 1998.
15. Meyers J, Stein S. The psychiatric interview in the emergency department. *Emerg Med Clin North Am* 2000;18:173–83.
16. Miller H. Fifty years after Flexner. *Lancet* 1966;2(7465):647–654.
17. Miller SS, Marin DB. Assessing capacity. *Emerg Med Clin North Am* 2000;18:233–242.
18. Murphy BA. Delirium. *Emerg Med Clin North Am* 2000;18:243–252.
19. Olmedo R, Hoffman RS. Withdrawal syndromes. *Emerg Med Clin North Am* 2000;18:273–288.
20. Perry SW. Organic mental disorders caused by HIV: update on early diagnosis and treatment. *Am J Psychiatry* 1990;147:696–710.
21. Purdie FR, Honigman B, Rosen P. Acute organic brain syndrome: a review of 100 cases. *Ann Emerg Med* 1981;10:455–461.
22. Reeves RR, Pendarvis EJ, Kimble R. Unrecognized medical emergencies admitted to psychiatric units. *Am J Emerg Med* 2000;18:390–393.
23. Samuels SC, Evers MM. Delirium. Pragmatic guidance for managing a common, confounding, and sometimes lethal condition. *Geriatrics* 2002;57:33–38.
24. Sox HC, Jr. Koran LM, Sox CH, Marton KI, Dugger F, Smith T. A medical algorithm for detecting physical disease in psychiatric patients. *Hosp Community Psychiatry* 1989;40:1270–1276.
25. Talbot-Stern JK, Green T, Royle TJ. Psychiatric manifestations of systemic illness. *Emerg Med Clin North Am* 2000;18:199.
26. Williams ER, Shepherd SM. Medical clearance of psychiatric patients. *Emerg Med Clin North Am* 2000;18:185–98.

CHAPTER 110
Headache

E. John Gallagher and Adrienne J. Birnbaum

Head pain accounts for nearly 1 million emergency department (ED) visits annually in the United States. Fortunately, the vast majority of headaches presenting to the ED do not represent serious underlying disease. The goal in managing the patient with headache in the ED is to distinguish the small fraction of patients with serious illness who require immediate diagnosis and hospitalization from the great majority in whom the clinical focus is directed toward headache-specific, short-term pain management, prophylaxis against recurrence, as indicated, explanation, reassurance, and careful follow up.

CLASSIFICATION OF HEAD PAIN

The simplest means of categorizing headaches is to dichotomize them into primary headaches (e.g., migraine) versus secondary (or "organic") headaches. The latter are so named because they are "secondary" to some underlying cause (e.g., subarachnoid hemorrhage [SAH]).

TABLE 110.1. Differential Diagnosis of Headache

Acute Single Headache (presenting within hours of onset)	Acute Recurrent Headache (presenting within days to weeks of onset)	Subacute Headache (presenting within weeks to months of onset)	Chronic Headache (presenting within months to years of onset)
Bacterial meningitis	Migraine	Chronic subdural hematoma	Chronic tension-type headache
Subarachnoid hemorrhage	Cluster	Brain tumor	Transformational migraine
Cerebral ischemia	Episodic tension-type headache	Brain abscess	Analgesic abuse/rebound
Hypertension	Trigeminal neuralgia	Subacute/chronic sinusitis	Depression
Narrow-angle glaucoma	Postherpetic neuralgia	Temporomandibular joint	
Optic/retrobulbar neuritis	Coital headache	syndrome	
Acute sinusitis		Chronic posttraumatic headache	
Spontaneous dissection of cranial arteries		Headache associated with low CSF pressure	
Acute posttraumatic headache		Idiopathic Intracranial hypertension	
Acute headache associated with metabolic disorder		Temporal arteritis	
Acute headache associated with substances or withdrawal		Headache in HIV-positive patients	

The pain-sensitive structures of the head include the blood vessels and all extracranial structures of the head and neck. The only intracranial structures sensitive to pain are the arteries at the base of the brain, their major branches, the periarterial dura mater, and the venous sinuses. The parenchyma of the brain itself and most of its meningeal coverings are not pain-sensitive.

For many years, traditional teaching held that there were three major mechanisms of head pain: vasodilatation within the cranial vasculature, causing a "vascular" headache; spasm of the neck and scalp muscles, causing a "muscle contraction" headache; and traction on blood vessels or inflammation around or within these and other pain-sensitive structures, causing a "traction–inflammatory" headache.

In light of more recent evidence, traditional concepts of the etiology of headache, particularly of migraine, have given way to more evidence-based explanations in which neuropeptides, most notably serotonin, and their many central nervous system (CNS) receptors play an important role. Experimental observations of the relationship between these neural transmitters and alterations in CNS vascular tone suggest that an exclusively neurogenic or vasogenic etiology is unlikely to provide a unifying theory of migrainous and other headaches (9).

TABLE 110.2. Ten Headaches to Worry About

1. Single acute headache, characterized as "first or worst" of the patient's life
2. Single acute or subacute headache with fever unexplained by other systemic illness
3. Single acute or subacute headache with vomiting unexplained by other systemic illness
4. Any headache associated with focal findings, unless focality is known to be chronic and unchanged from baseline
5. Any headache associated with abnormal mental status, unless cognitive changes are known to be chronic and unaltered from baseline
6. Any headache associated with papilledema (specific, not sensitive for increased ICP)
7. Single acute headache with pain on neck flexion, but absent on rotation
8. Subacute headache, unremitting or progressively worsening
9. Acute or subacute headache in the elderly
10. Any headache in the immunocompromised host, especially if HIV-positive or with risk factors for HIV

ICP, intracranial pressure.

Perhaps the most useful categorization scheme for the emergency physician is to classify headache into one of four groups based on the temporal profile of the pain pattern: acute single headache; acute recurrent headache; subacute headache; and chronic headache (Table 110.1) (24).

Ten worrisome headache patterns are listed in Table 110.2. Only about 1% to 3% of headaches seen in the ED will fit any of these patterns, but they are among the most important headaches to diagnose.

CLINICAL PRESENTATION AND DIFFERENTIAL DIAGNOSIS

Acute Single Headache

Bacterial Meningitis

Diffuse headache is a characteristic but not invariable feature of meningitis. Although only about two-thirds of community-acquired cases of bacterial meningitis have the triad of fever, nuchal rigidity, and altered mental status, all patients appear to demonstrate at least one of these features. Among these, fever ($\geq 37.7°$C or $100°$F) is present in 95%, neck stiffness in nearly 90%, and altered mental status in about 80% (6).

Subarachnoid Hemorrhage

Headache of subarachnoid hemorrhage (SAH) is the prototypic "first or worst" headache of one's life, of sudden onset, often associated with nausea, vomiting, neck stiffness, and a transient alteration of consciousness. In patients with focal findings or sustained abnormalities of consciousness, the need for a neuroimaging study is apparent. However, in the many patients without neurologic findings, this entity may be clinically indistinguishable from a first attack of migraine, particularly in the case of SAH due to bleeding from an arteriovenous malformation, which may be considerably less dramatic than that of a ruptured aneurysm.

An especially difficult challenge for the emergency physician is identification of the "sentinel leak" that precedes major hemorrhage in more than one-third of patients. Detection of this premonitory bleed presents an opportunity to prevent a neurologic catastrophe.

Cerebral Ischemia

Although about 35% of stroke patients and about 25% of patients with transient ischemic attacks experience headache, the diagnosis is usually evident because the clinical picture is dominated by focal findings. It is not possible to distinguish hemorrhagic from nonhemorrhagic causes of stroke on clinical grounds alone.

Hypertension

Most headaches in hypertensive patients are either migrainous or tension-type, and only rarely are due to elevated blood pressure. In general, hypertensive headache requires an acute elevation of diastolic pressure by about 25% above baseline or sustained diastolic elevations in excess of 130 mm Hg.

Narrow-Angle Glaucoma

Ocular or periorbital pain characterizes headache caused by narrow-angle glaucoma. Because many migrainous headaches are periorbital, the diagnosis of acute glaucoma also requires diminished visual acuity, a pupil that is typically fixed in mid-position, an edematous ("steamy") cornea, perilimbal injection, and increased intraocular pressure. Vomiting may be the dominant feature, especially in the elderly, who may also present with altered mentation.

Optic or Retrobulbar Neuritis

In optic or retrobulbar neuritis, the characteristic feature of this ocular–periorbital headache is the "deafferented" pupil, which paradoxically dilates when a bright light is moved from the contralateral to the involved eye. In optic neuritis, there is evidence of inflammation of the disc, but in retrobulbar neuritis, the fundus may appear normal. In contrast to acute papilledema, in which vision is not impaired, visual acuity is usually diminished in both optic and retrobulbar neuritis.

Acute Sinusitis

Although acute sinusitis is said to be characterized by local pain and tenderness over the involved sinuses, it remains a poorly defined and difficult clinical diagnosis.

Spontaneous Dissection of the Cranial Arteries

Spontaneous dissection of the cranial arteries is an uncommon syndrome, often associated with surprisingly minor trauma. It is marked by sudden onset of headache associated with neck pain and focal ischemic symptoms. The pain and its location are determined by the location of the dissection in the carotid or vertebrobasilar system. In the carotid system, the pain is anterior and often accompanied by monocular symptoms, Horner's syndrome, and other focal findings. With dissection in the posterior circulation, the pain is occipital and brainstem findings predominate.

Acute Headache Associated with Metabolic Disorders

Most metabolic disorders produce acute single or acute recurrent headache. Of all patients presenting to the ED with headache, just over one-third have a systemic illness, usually associated with fever, causing their head pain. Other metabolic causes of headache include hypoglycemia, hypoxia, and hypercarbia.

Acute Headache Associated with Substances or Their Withdrawal

Among substance-related headaches, the single most important entity is carbon monoxide poisoning, which is the leading toxicologic cause of accidental death in the United States. Because the temporal profile of the headache associated with chemicals, drugs, and toxins depends on the pattern of exposure and withdrawal, substance-related head pain can fit any of the four categories of headache in Table 110.1.

Acute Recurrent Headache

The differential diagnosis of acute recurrent headache includes some of the serious entities discussed previously under "Acute Single Headache": SAH presenting as recurrent sentinel bleeds; repeated transient ischemic attacks; substance-related headache, varying as a function of exposure to toxins; and, rarely, severe hypertension, if the elevations are episodic. Tumors, brain abscesses, subdural hematomas, and idiopathic intracranial hypertension (pseudotumor cerebri) can present as acute recurrent headache, but these are more commonly subacute or chronic.

The differential diagnosis of acute recurrent headache centers about the two most common primary ("nonorganic") headache syndromes seen in emergency practice: migraine and episodic tension-type headache. However, this differential may represent a distinction without a meaningful clinical difference, because there is increasing evidence that tension-type headache may be related to migraines (3).

Migraine

The definition of *migraine* has been broadened in recent years. Although migraine is classically defined as a throbbing, unilateral headache, neither the quality of the pain nor its location offers as much clinical discrimination between migraine and other causes of headache as do the associated symptoms and signs (7). During the headache, most patients complain of photophobia, phonophobia, or gastrointestinal symptoms such as nausea (90%), anorexia (75%), vomiting (60%), and diarrhea (15%). *Constitutional symptoms* occur primarily during the prodrome (which precedes the aura) and the "postdrome." These include mood changes, fatigue, myalgias, food cravings, and irritability. *Neurologic symptoms* occur mainly during the migrainous aura (which occurs in a minority of patients), and include visual phenomena such as bright sparkling lights (scintillating scotomata), jagged lines (fortification spectra), and geometric figures. A unique characteristic of migrainous visual auras is their propensity to move across the visual field and to vary in color or intensity, sometimes shifting from positive to negative phenomena (scotomata). Less common migrainous auras include motor abnormalities (hemiparesis, ophthalmoplegia, aphasia), sensory dysesthesias, and brainstem disturbances (vertigo, ataxia).

Cluster Headache

In contrast to migraine, cluster headache is uncommon, affecting about 0.1% of the population, predominantly middle-aged men. Characteristic features are listed in Table 110.3. The first episode of cluster headache may be indistinguishable from SAH or from acute orbital, periorbital, or ocular disease. Usually, however, the short-lived, self-limited nature of the headache, accompanied by the findings in Table 110.3, clarify the diagnosis before further workup is necessary.

Episodic Tension-type Headache

Formerly known as muscle contraction headache, episodic tension-type headache may represent a migraine variant (3,20). It is usually bilateral and dull, often bandlike, and occurs without nausea or vomiting. Tenderness of the pericranial musculature may be a feature of one form of this headache, although electromyographic studies have shown that muscle contraction is also associated with typical migraines (19).

Trigeminal Neuralgia

Trigeminal neuralgia is the prototypic form of facial neuralgia, characterized by repetitive, unilateral, lancinating pain in the distribution of at least one branch of the trigeminal nerve. Attacks may be triggered by some minor stimulus, such as a light touch on the face.

TABLE 110.3. Principal Distinguishing Features of Cluster and Migraine Headache

Feature	Cluster	Migraine
Location of pain	Always unilateral, periorbital	Unilateral (60%) or bilateral (40%)
Age at onset	20–50 yr	10–40 yr
Sex incidence	90% male	70% female
Occurrence of attacks	Daily for several weeks to several months with headache-free intervals	Intermittent
Time of day	Often nocturnal, same time each night	Anytime
Seasonal occurrence	More common in spring and fall	No variation
Duration of pain	10 min to 3 h	4–48 h
Aura	Absent	30% of cases
Nausea or vomiting	5%	90%
Lacrimation	Frequent, unilateral	Infrequent
Nasal congestion	70% unilateral	Uncommon
Ptosis	30%	1% to 2%
Polyuria	2%	40%
Family history of vascular headaches	7%	90%
Miosis	50%	Absent
General appearance	Agitation, pacing	Lying immobile

Adapted from Diamond S, Dalessio DJ, eds. *The practicing physician's approach to headache*, 5th ed. Baltimore: William & Wilkins, 1992:90.

Postherpetic Neuralgia

The syndrome of postherpetic neuralgia results from a prior attack of herpes zoster. It is characterized by dermatomal hyperesthesia and pain that is often severe.

Coital Headache

Headache that occurs immediately before, during, or shortly after orgasm is termed *coital* or *orgasmic headache*. The pain is often severe and may persist for several hours. If there is no prior history of coital headache, SAH must be excluded (17).

Subacute Headache

A new and unremitting headache that is present for weeks warrants a complete neurologic investigation, particularly in patients who do not usually suffer from headache. There are only a few entities that conform to the temporal profile of subacute headache, but most of them are worrisome.

Chronic Subdural Hematoma

Chronic subdurals may be produced by minor trauma, especially in the elderly. As many as half the patients have no recollection of head trauma. Focal findings are often minimal and therefore undetected about half the time. Alterations in mental status are often subtle and may require knowledge of the patient's baseline level of cognition to be appreciated. In elderly patients with subdurals, a gradual deterioration in mental status may be misdiagnosed as dementia.

Brain Tumor

Headache is the presenting symptom of brain tumor in about 40% of cases. Like that of other space-occupying lesions, the headache is usually mild to moderate, diffuse, and often relieved by over-the-counter analgesics, at least initially. In approximately 90% of patients who can adequately describe their symptoms, the headache is intermittent, dull, rarely throbbing, and sometimes worse in the morning. Nausea and vomiting occur in about half the patients. In approximately 25%, the headache is worsened by Valsalva maneuvers (e.g., coughing or straining). It is exceedingly rare for a patient to have the diagnosis of brain tumor made on the basis of headache alone.

Brain Abscess

The headache of brain abscess is similar to that of brain tumor, but it is typically accompanied by fever and other evidence of infection. Often, it is associated with a chronic focus of infection in the ears or sinuses, a cerebrospinal fluid (CSF) leak from a basilar skull fracture, or an embolic cardiac or pulmonary source.

Subacute and Chronic Sinusitis

Subacute and chronic sinusitis is more poorly defined than is acute sinusitis, and are accordingly even more challenging to diagnose. Pain, if present, is said to be dull and pressure-like, and is usually associated with nasal congestion or rhinorrhea.

Temporomandibular Joint Syndrome

Temporomandibular joint syndrome (TMJ) is another poorly defined syndrome that may be caused by malocclusion, which produces masseter spasm. Features of tension-type headache and depression have also been reported in association with TMJ syndrome.

Posttraumatic Headache

Although it may present acutely, posttraumatic headache is more commonly subacute. It is no longer classified as postconcussion syndrome because loss of consciousness is not a prerequisite for its development. Symptoms are usually present within the first 24 to 48 hours postinjury and are marked by a postural component to the head pain and associated postural dizziness. Typically, symptoms are improved by lying down. Transient neurocognitive impairment, depression, irritability, and emotional lability are common. The syndrome persists for more than 2 months in 60% of patients and can cause major disruptions in patient's personal and professional lives.

Headache Associated with Low Cerebrospinal Fluid Pressure

Headache after a lumbar puncture (LP) is thought to be due to low CSF pressure resulting from a post-LP CSF leak. It has some of the orthostatic features of the posttraumatic headache: worsening of pain, dizziness, and nausea when upright, and improvement on lying down. Usually, the history is diagnostic. If a repeat LP is performed to exclude arachnoiditis or infection, an opening CSF pressure of less than 30 mm H_2O strongly suggests this diagnosis.

Idiopathic Intracranial Hypertension (Pseudotumor Cerebri)

Headache in idiopathic intracranial hypertension is associated with high CSF pressures in the absence of intracranial structural disease. Pain is often postural and associated with pulsatile tinnitus, nausea, vomiting, and progressive visual loss. Papilledema is present in about 90% of patients. The diagnosis is confirmed by CSF pressures greater than 250 mm H_2O and no mass on computed tomography (CT).

Temporal (Cranial) Arteritis

Headache is the dominant complaint in this progressive, systemic, inflammatory disorder. It may occur anywhere in the scalp, and is localized to the temporal area in only half the cases. The syndrome tends to occur in patients older than 50 years of age and is accompanied by constitutional symptoms such as anorexia and weight loss. The onset is gradual, with polymyalgia, proximal weakness, masseter claudication, and periocular discomfort developing over months to years. The diagnosis is suggested by a firm, tender, nonpulsatile cranial artery and an elevated erythrocyte sedimentation rate (>50 mm/h), although about 25% of cases have only mild elevations of the sedimentation rate. Major complications include monocular blindness and stroke.

Headache in HIV-Positive and AIDS Patients

Headache in this group of patients is usually subacute, and is often associated with positive clinical findings. The list of possible opportunistic CNS infections includes mycobacteria (*Mycobacterium tuberculosis* and *Mycobacterium avium-intracellulare*), spirochetes (*Treponema pallidum*), viruses (herpes simplex, herpes zoster, cytomegalovirus, and HIV-1), fungi (*Cryptococcus*), protozoa (*Toxoplasma*), and actinomycetes (*Nocardia*). Noninfectious causes of headache include CNS lymphoma (primary and secondary) and Kaposi sarcoma.

Chronic Headache

Patients presenting to the ED with chronic headache (i.e., headache that has been present for months to years) are part of what has been called the "last straw" syndrome (7). Most of the serious entities included in this category have been discussed previously under subacute headache, and usually conform to a similar temporal profile.

Chronic headaches can be divided clinically into several different groups, each requiring a different diagnostic and therapeutic strategy. These include patients with features of chronic tension-type headache, so-called transformational migraine (transformed from an episodic pattern to a chronic daily pattern), analgesic abuse, depression, and, rarely, tumor, subdural hematoma, idiopathic intracranial hypertension, and posttraumatic headache.

Most patients with chronic tension-type headache have mild-to-moderate pain, rarely see a doctor, and only occasionally come to the ED. Fewer still see neurologists. Consequently, little is known about these patients other than the fact that, on the basis of anonymous prevalence surveys, they seem to exist in large numbers. The existence of transformational migraine supports the theory that migraine and many of the more severe tension-type headaches are related. Among a large cohort of migraineurs, 80% of whom had their first headache before the age of 26, 90% had developed chronic daily headache by age 45 (22). Many of these patients also suffered from superimposed periodic episodes of typical migraine.

Some patients with severe tension-type headache or frequent migraines overuse nonnarcotic analgesics or ergotamines, resulting in worsening of their headache. Gradual withdrawal provides relief, but it may require hospitalization for supervised detoxification (11).

As noted previously, depression is a frequent concomitant of chronic headaches of all varieties. This relationship may simply represent a response to living with constant pain, or it may reflect the central role of serotonin in both headache and depression.

Although chronic headache is rarely a presentation of a space-occupying lesion or increased intracranial pressure (ICP), most of these patients warrant a CT at some point in their work up.

EMERGENCY DEPARTMENT EVALUATION

A meticulous history is the key to headache diagnosis. Only in unusual circumstances does the neurologic examination, laboratory testing, or a neuroimaging procedure reveal an abnormality that was completely unsuspected following a careful history.

Headache History

Temporal Profile

Because this is the primary axis along which headaches can be classified in the ED, this information should be obtained first in order to place the patient into one of the four groups shown in Table 110.1.

1. Single acute: Is this a "first/worst" headache of sudden onset?
2. Recurrent acute: What are the frequency, pattern, and duration of individual headache episodes?
3. Subacute: Is the headache progressively worsening?
4. Chronic: Has there been a pattern break or is this a "last straw" visit to the ED?

Associated Symptoms

In particular, look for transient loss of consciousness at onset, nausea, vomiting, neck stiffness, unilateral lacrimation or rhinorrhea, photophobia, and phonophobia.

Circumstances of Onset

For single acute headaches, determine exactly what the patient was doing when the headache began. For recurrent headache, identify any usual precipitants.

Prodromes and Aura

Prodromes such as a shift in appetite or mood suggest migraine. Characteristic visual aura essentially defines a subtype of migraine.

Location of Pain

Hemicranial, hemifacial, and unilateral ocular and periorbital pain have greater discriminating value than holocranial or bilateral pain.

Quality and Severity of Pain

This has limited value in identifying the type of headache, and correlates poorly with the seriousness of underlying disease.

Age at Onset

New-onset headache in the elderly is worrisome.

Recent Trauma

This is relevant to chronic subdural hematomas and posttraumatic headaches, although trauma may also precipitate a migraine or cluster headache.

Relief Measures

Headaches that are substantially relieved by lying down are usually posttraumatic or low CSF pressure (post-LP) headaches.

Family History

Migraine, depression, and, to a lesser extent, a predisposition to SAH are inherited.

Medical History

Ask about concurrent illnesses, medications (including oral contraceptives), hospitalizations, allergies, smoking, alcohol, drug use, and risk factors for HIV.

Occupational History

Note exposure to carbon monoxide, fumes, solvents, and other toxins.

Psychosocial History

Search especially for signs and symptoms of depression, anxiety, and stress.

Multiplicity

Many patients suffer from different kinds of headaches. To minimize confusion, it is important to determine this early and to obtain parallel but distinct histories of each headache type.

Physical Examination

General Examination

After obtaining vital signs, the remainder of the nonneurologic examination should be goal-directed, including the eyes, neck, face, and scalp. Visual acuity should be checked with a pinhole and the eye examined for ptosis, conjunctival injection (perilimbal vs. diffuse), corneal clouding, and pupillary size, reactivity, and equality. Any suggestion of acute glaucoma mandates measurement of intraocular pressure. The swinging flashlight test should be performed as described earlier to detect optic or retrobulbar neuritis.

A funduscopic examination is essential, looking specifically for signs of increased ICP, severe hypertension, optic neuritis, or subhyaloid hemorrhage (preretinal hemorrhages obscuring retinal vessels due to overlying blood in the subarachnoid space). Spontaneous venous pulsations (SVPs) are lost when the ICP exceeds about 200 mm H_2O. However, monitoring has shown enormous pressure fluctuations in patients with increased ICP, ranging from 50 to 500 mm over a 24-hour period. Thus, a patient with increased ICP might have SVPs if examined during a transient trough in intracranial pressure. In addition to the problem of false negatives (presence of SVPs in patients with increased ICP), there is the problem of false positives (absence of SVPs in patients with normal ICP), which is seen in about 20% of the normal population. Bilateral papilledema is a highly specific indicator of increased ICP, but, because it may lag behind acute elevations of ICP by several hours, this finding lacks sensitivity.

The neck should be examined for pain with flexion, which indicates meningeal irritation secondary to chemical or infectious meningitis. Tension-type headache also characteristically produces tightness in the paracervical muscles with discomfort on flexion. Unlike the nuchal rigidity of meningitis, tension-type headache causes pain with chin to shoulder rotation of the head. Because it may take several hours for subarachnoid blood to reach the cervical area of the meninges, and several more hours for it to produce a chemical meningitis, absence of nuchal rigidity early in the course of an SAH does not reliably exclude this entity.

The sinuses, temporomandibular joints, and scalp should be palpated for tenderness, paying special attention to the temporal arteries in older patients. In posttraumatic headache, hemotympanum, CSF otorrhea, infraorbital ecchymoses, posterior auricular ecchymoses, and CSF rhinorrhea indicate basilar skull fracture.

Neurologic Examination

Mental status assessment is a critically important feature of the neurologic examination that is commonly overlooked. Focality is detected most readily by pronator drift, asymmetry of cranial nerves II to VIII, and abnormalities of gait and station. In general, sensory examination (other than cranial nerve V), assessment of reflexes, and motor testing of individual muscle groups are not efficient use of the emergency physician's time in the evaluation of the patient with headache.

Laboratory Testing

As with the physical examination, laboratory tests are usually normal. In patients with a history strongly suggestive of a particular kind of headache (e.g., migraine), no laboratory tests are necessary. The erythrocyte sedimentation rate in patients suspected of having cranial arteritis is an exception to this rule. Other tests of occasional value include hemoglobin, leukocyte count, glucose, pulse oximetry, arterial blood gas, and carboxyhemoglobin level.

Imaging

When a diagnosis can be made on the basis of the history and a normal clinical exam, no imaging is needed. Other patients with acute single or recurrent headache should probably have a CT or magnetic resonance imaging (MRI) at the time of their ED visit. Those with subacute and chronic headache may have an imaging procedure scheduled electively.

CT is preferred for the detection of acute intracranial bleeding, idiopathic intracranial hypertension, and hydrocephalus. Noncontrast CT, followed by a contrast CT, is useful in HIV-positive patients, in whom a ring-enhancing lesion suggests toxoplasmosis. Patients with suspected spontaneous SAH constitute a special case. Fourth generation CT scans obtained within 12 hours of the onset of headache in suspected SAH have a sensitivity of 98% (95% CI, 94% to 100%), a specificity of 100% (95% CI, 94% to 100%), a negative likelihood ratio of 0.02 (95% CI, 0.005 to 0.06), and a positive likelihood ratio of at least 33 (95% CI, 11 to 316) (29).

Because a negative CT cannot completely exclude the diagnosis of SAH, the lumbar puncture (LP) remains the criterion standard for this diagnosis (31). As shown by the likelihood ratios, a negative CT markedly reduces the probability of this entity by decreasing the odds of SAH by about 50-fold from the clinician's pretest estimates. Thus, the pretest probability of SAH would have to exceed 33% in order for the posttest probability of SAH to remain above 1% following a negative CT. The sensitivity of CT drops off as the time from headache onset increases. The sensitivity of MRI is inferior to that of CT during the first 24 hours following a SAH, becomes slightly superior between 24 and 72 hours, and exceeds that of CT thereafter (18).

The choice of CT versus MRI depends on the clinical picture, cost, and availability. In addition to late identification of SAH, MRI is preferred for imaging the posterior fossa (cerebellum and brainstem), detecting nonhemorrhagic strokes less than 2 days old, and visualizing transient ischemic attack, tumor, localized infection, or chronic subdural hematoma.

Finally, magnetic resonance angiography (MRA) promises to replace traditional angiography as the imaging modality of choice for aneurysms, arteriovenous malformations, and dissection of the cranial arteries.

Lumbar Puncture

There are two primary indications for an emergency LP in a patient with headache: suspicion of CNS infection (e.g., meningitis) or a substantial suspicion of SAH despite a normal CT. The other two circumstances in which an LP is the diagnostic standard in headache due either to high (idiopathic intracranial hypertension) or low (post-LP) CSF pressure. In the first instance, the LP is clearly indicated and often therapeutic. In the case of a post-LP headache, another LP should be done only if the diagnosis is in serious doubt.

The risk of herniation after LP in patients with increased ICP or a mass lesion is low but has not been precisely quantified. Proponents of LP without prior CT argue that an association between herniation and LP has not been causally established. Proponents of CT prior to LP cite a small number of instances in which herniation has been temporally associated with LP. Two recent studies sought to identify a subset of ED patients that can safely undergo LP without screening CT (10, 12). However, the current absence of validation of these results in large, independent populations, the utility of CT to identify alternate diagnoses, and wide availability and increased speed of CT with newer generation scanners has led many clinicians to perform a CT prior to LP, provided that appropriate time-dependent emergency care (e.g., immediate institution of antibiotics in suspected bacterial meningitis) is not delayed.

Postural headache is a common occurrence following diagnostic lumbar puncture. Despite common teaching, no evidence exists from randomized trials to suggest bed rest is more effective than immediate mobilization after lumbar puncture (1,25). The role of fluid supplementation in the prevention of postural puncture headache remains uncertain (25). Several meta-analyses have found the use of smaller diameter and atraumatic-tip (Sprotte) needles to be associated with a lower incidence of postural puncture headache than larger and bevel-tip needles respectively (26). If a beveled needle is used, the bevel should be aligned parallel to the dural fibers (i.e., longitudinally).

EMERGENCY DEPARTMENT MANAGEMENT AND DISPOSITION

Treatment of the following causes of headache is discussed in the corresponding chapters elsewhere in this text: bacterial meningitis, SAH, stroke, cranial artery dissection, hypertensive encephalopathy, acute glaucoma, optic neuritis, retrobulbar neuritis, sinusitis, temporomandibular joint syndrome, toxic–metabolic disorders, chronic subdural hematoma, brain tumor, and brain abscess.

Migraine

Table 110.4 lists some of the many therapies for treatment of acute migraine in the ED. Identification of optimal migraine abortive agents suffers from a lack of head to head comparison studies, failure of clinical trials to target uniform end points, inconsistent documentation of adverse effects and recurrence rates, variability in methods of pain measurement, and lack of a consistent measure of overall effectiveness and tolerability that corresponds to patient satisfaction.

Dihydroergotamine (DHE-45) is an effective abortive agent for the treatment of moderate to severe migraine (23). Intravenous metoclopramide and intravenous and intramuscular prochlorperazine can be used as monotherapy or as adjunctive therapy in combination with other abortive agents. Results of two randomized, placebo-controlled trials favor intravenous prochlorperazine over metoclopramide, although intravenous prochlorperazine is difficult to obtain in many parts of the United States (4,15). DHE and a dopamine antagonist provide the benefit of two effective abortive agents plus an antiemetic. Proposed doses of prochlorperazine range from 3.5 mg to 10 mg. When used in combination therapy with intravenous DHE, 3.5 mg may be nearly as effective as higher doses, but with fewer adverse effects, such as sedation and akathisia (21). Prochlorperazine suppositories have been shown to be effective in the ED setting, but, like the alternative routes of administration for sumatriptan, do not work as rapidly as parenteral treatment.

Akathisia has been demonstrated to occur in more than one third of patients treated with these agents. Adjuvant intravenous diphenhydramine 50 mg reduces the incidence of akathisia induced by prochlorperazine but is associated with increased sedation (30).

The established efficacy and selective pharmacology of the triptans have earned this group of drugs a central role in the abortive management of migraine over the past decade (9). Sumatriptan, the first drug of its class, is highly effective (76% of patients experience improvement in headache and 48% are pain free 1 hour after subcutaneous administration) (2,27), and provides a more rapid onset of action than DHE. Limitations to triptan use include cost, lack of efficacy in some patients (up to 1/3 in clinical trials), headache recurrence (two and a half times as likely with sumatriptan than dihydroergotamine in one trial) (32), and significant side effects (injection site reaction, chest pressure or heaviness, flushing, weakness, drowsiness, malaise, warmth and paresthesias, and rare reports of myocardial infarction and sudden death).

Newer triptans offer additional dosage forms (Table 110.5) and longer half-lives. Few clinical trials have compared the triptans to one another. A recent large meta-analysis of newer oral formulations found the drugs to be uniformly effective and well tolerated with relatively small differences in efficacy, tolerability and consistency (8). ED use of these drugs may be limited by nausea, vomiting and delayed oral absorption that frequently accompanies attacks. A systematic review of randomized trials of subcutaneous, oral and intranasal administration of sumatriptan concluded that subcutaneous sumatriptan (6 mg) has a higher efficacy and more rapid onset of action than oral and intranasal preparations but is associated with more adverse events (28). Onset of action of the intranasal preparation is intermediate between that of subcutaneous and oral administration (5). Recently published data describing the use of rizatriptan oral wafers in the ED treatment of severe migraine are promising (13). However, lack of controlled randomized trials investigating the use of these newer agents as abortive therapy in the ED precludes recommendation of their use in lieu of other agents at the present time.

At present, for initial ED treatment of migraine, we recommend 10 mg of prochlorperazine (20 mg of metoclopramide may be nearly equivalent and easier to obtain) (4,15), and 50 mg of diphenhydramine (3), administered intravenously (21). Sumatriptan, administered subcutaneously is a reasonable alternative. Although dihydroergotamine has been largely displaced by the triptans, addition of 1 mg of intravenous dhihydroergotamine (DHE-45, given by intravenous Soluset over 30 minutes) to diphenhydramine and prochlorperazine or metoclopramide remains an alternative option for patients who cannot tolerate triptans and have not responded to the agents suggested above.

Neurologic consultation is indicated in the ED if the diagnosis is in doubt, if the attack does not conform to the patient's typical migraine, or if intractable vomiting or unrelenting pain is encountered. Following successful treatment, patients should be referred to a neurologist or headache specialist. Indications for admission are summarized in Table 110.6.

Cluster

High-flow 100% oxygen should be administered as soon as the patient enters the ED. Because many patients with cluster are smokers, they should be observed for carbon dioxide retention while on oxygen. As indicated in Table 110.4, DHE and sumatriptan are effective in the ED management of cluster (sumatriptan has been shown to provide relief in about 10 minutes). However, concerns about coronary vasospasm limit the use of these drugs in patients with any cardiovascular risk factors. On discharge, patients with an exacerbation of cluster should receive a trial of prophylactic verapamil, starting at 80 mg t.i.d., if there are no contraindications. A tapering course of steroids should also be given until the verapamil can be increased to therapeutic levels (about 120 mg t.i.d.). Indications for admission are summarized in Table 110.6.

TABLE 110.4. Emergency Management of Migraine and Related Headache

Drug	Indications	Dose	Route	Repeat Dose	Comments	Evidence[a] (Ref)
NSAID						
Ketorolac (Toradol)	Mild/moderate headache	60 mg	i.m.	30–45 mg i.m. in 6 h	Less effective than DHE + metoclopramide	Level I, Grade A
Indomethacin (Indocin)	Mild/moderate headache	50 mg	PO or PR	q6–8h	Prophylaxis against coital headache	Level I, Grade A
SEROTONIN AGONISTS						
Dihydroergotamine (DHE)	Moderate/severe migraine, cluster, status migrainosis, severe/intractable, tension-type headache	1 mg (0.25-mg test dose + 0.75 mg)	i.m./S.C. or i.v. over 30–60 min	0.5–1.0 mg i.m./s.c. or i.v. over 30–60 min (max 3 mg per attack)	Contraindicated in cardiovascular disease and pregnancy; D/C if chest pain, worsening headache or increased blood pressure	Level I, Grade A
Sumatriptan (Imitrex)	Moderate/severe migraine and cluster	6 mg	s.c.	6 mg s.c. in 1 h (max 12 mg per 24 hrs)	More rapid action than DHE; 50% rebound within 24 h; higher cost	Level I, Grade A
DOPAMINE ANTAGONISTS						
Prochlorperazine (Compazine)	Moderate/severe migraine	10–20 mg	i.v. over 2 min	10–20 mg in 1 h	May cause dystonia (akathesia); PR less effective than i.v.	Level I, Grade A
+ Diphenhydramine	Moderate/severe migraine	25–50 mg				
Metoclopramide (Reglan)	Moderate/severe migraine	10–20 mg	i.v. in 50 mL D5W over 20 min	40 mg in 1 h	Enhances gastric emptying; may cause dystonia	Level I, Grade A
+ Diphenhydramine	Moderate/severe migraine	25–50 mg				
Chlorpromazine (Thorazine)	Moderate/severe migraine	12.5–25 mg	i.v. over 2 min	12.5 mg q20 min × 2 (max 50 mg)	Give 500 mL saline, to offset orthostasis; drowsiness; may cause dystonia	Level I, Grade A
COMBINATION REGIMENS						
DHE + metoclopramide	Same as DHE	1 mg DHE + 10–20 mg metoclopramide	i.v. as above under individual agents	0.5 mg DHE + 10–20 mg metoclopramide in 1 h	Premedication with metoclopramide may reduce emesis from DHE	Level I, Grade A
+ Diphenhydramine		+25–50 mg				
DHE + prochlorperazine+ diphenhydramine	Same as DHE	1 mg DHE + 10–20 mg prochlorperazine + 25–50 mg diphenhydramine	i.v. as above under individual agents; diphenhydramine may be i.v. push	0.5 mg DHE + 10–20 mg prochlorperazine in 1 h	Premedication with prochlorperazine may reduce emesis from DHE; diphenhydramine reduces dystonias	Level I, Grade A
CORTICOSTEROIDS						
	Status migrainosis, intractable episodic, cluster	10–20 mg dexamethasone	i.v.	60 mg prednisone tapering 5 mg/d	May decrease inflammation; interval medication until prophylactic agents take effect	Level II, Grade B
LOCAL ANESTHETICS						
Lidocaine	Moderate/severe migraine, cluster	0.5 mL (4% solution without epinephrine) in one nostril if unilateral, each nostril if bilateral	Intranasal	Repeat same dose after 2 min	Usefulness limited by high early relapse rate; may be useful while instituting other measures	Level II, Grade B
OPIOIDS						
	Last resort	0.1 mg/kg morphine	i.v.	Titrate against pain p/n.	Most of above regimens provide superior pain relief in controlled trials	Level I, Grade A

[a] Level of Evidence
I: Evidence from at least one randomized controlled trial.
II: Evidence from well-designed controlled trials but without randomization; well-designed cohort or case-control studies; or dramatic results from uncontrolled experiments.
Class of recommendation
A: Good evidence to support procedure or treatment.
B: Fair evidence to support procedure or treatment.
(Adapted, with modifications, from Ducharme J. Canadian Association of Emergency Physicians guidelines for the acute management of migraine headache. *J Emerg Med* 1998;17:137.)

significant arthritis predisposing the patient to formation of cervical osteophytes that could mechanically compress the extracranial vessels? This would indicate a need for radiologic evaluation of the cervical spine.

The neurologic examination in patients with TIAs is often unremarkable, but a thorough assessment is essential. Orthostatic blood pressures should be measured in patients with vertebrobasilar TIAs, because symptoms are often related to postural changes. Auscultation for cervical and subclavian bruits should be performed, as well as evaluation for cardiac dysrhythmias, murmurs, and left ventricular dysfunction.

Laboratory evaluation of patients with suspected TIA includes a complete blood cell count to assess hemoglobin and hematocrit (anemia or polycythemia) and a glucose determination. An erythrocyte sedimentation rate is useful for suspected vasculitis, and a serologic test for syphilis should also be obtained if clinically indicated. An electrocardiogram and cranial CT scan should be performed. Transthoracic and/or transesophageal echocardiography is indicated when cardiac emboli are suspected.

Patients with anterior circulation TIAs who have no obvious cardiac etiology and no contraindications for vascular surgery should be screened with duplex ultrasonography for significant carotid artery stenosis. These patients represent a subgroup of TIA patients known to have an improved outcome with carotid endarterectomy; they should be identified as early as possible.

EMERGENCY DEPARTMENT MANAGEMENT

Medical therapy is indicated for patients with posterior circulation TIAs, patients with anterior circulation TIAs who have less than 50% stenosis on carotid duplex scanning, and patients who are not candidates for carotid endarterectomy. Medical treatment options are limited to antiplatelet therapy and anticoagulation.

Antiplatelet therapy with aspirin (50 to 325 mg/d) reduces the incidence of nonfatal stroke, nonfatal myocardial infarction, and death from all vascular causes in patients with TIAs. Because the lower dosages require several days to achieve maximal platelet inhibition, therapy in the early setting should be initiated with 300 to 325 mg/day. The ESPS-2 trial found dipyridamole (200 mg b.i.d.) to have an additive protective effect when used with low-dose (50 mg/d) aspirin, with a combined 37% reduction in recurrent stroke in patients with previous stroke or TIA (9). This is the first study to report an independent effect of dipyridamole when used with aspirin and the combination is marketed commercially as Aggrenox® (1 capsule PO BID).

Clopidogrel (Plavix®, 75 mg PO daily) is a newer ADP-inhibitor and, though structurally similar to the older ticlopidine, does not cause neutropenia. Its role as a primary or secondary agent in the treatment of TIA is debated, given its cost and the small (0.5%) absolute improvement in reducing risk for the combined endpoint of stroke, AMI, and vascular death in patients with atherosclerotic vascular disease compared to aspirin alone (2).

The use of anticoagulation in patients experiencing noncarembolic TIA lacks a rigorous scientific basis. Though heparin has traditionally been used in select patients with TIA, no prospective randomized study of significant size has demonstrated a clear benefit and its use cannot be recommended on the basis of existing data. If used at all, it should be reserved for "high-risk" patients such as those with crescendo TIAs, vertebrobasilar TIA, recurrent TIA while receiving maximum antiplatelet therapy, high-grade carotid stenosis, or a suspected cardiac source for emboli. Neurologic consultation is recommended prior to initiation.

Adjusted-dose oral anticoagulation with warfarin remains the therapy of choice for stroke prevention in patients with a cardioembolic TIA due to atrial fibrillation. A target international normalized ration (INR) of 2.0 to 3.0 is recommended. The efficacy of aspirin is considerably less than warfarin in this population and is recommended as an alternative for those with contraindications to oral anticoagulation. Anticoagulant therapy may be appropriate for patients with other sources of cardiogenic emboli who have a TIA; however, randomized clinical trials have not been performed in these specific patient populations.

A subset of patients with TIA has surgically correctable carotid stenosis and represent an important group for the emergency physician to identify. Those with greater than or equal to 50% carotid stenosis on duplex scanning are potential candidates for endarterectomy and should begin medical therapy in the emergency department pending a decision on vascular intervention.

The North American Symptomatic Carotid Endarterectomy Trial (NASCET) found symptomatic patients with high-grade (70% to 99%) stenosis randomized to carotid endarterectomy had a 17% reduction in the risk of ipsilateral stroke after 2 years, compared with the optimal medical treatment group. The surgical data for patients with moderate (50% to 69% stenosis) found a smaller risk reduction of 10.1% at 5 years; no benefit was identified for those with less than 50% stenosis (7). The beneficial effect of endarterectomy for high-grade stenosis is further supported by the European Carotid Surgery Trial (16).

Transluminal angioplasty with intravascular stent placement for carotid and intracranial stenosis is currently being evaluated as an alternative to surgical approaches and prospective randomized trials are underway. Until the results of these studies are available, angioplasty for carotid and intracranial stenosis should be considered investigational.

CRITICAL INTERVENTIONS

- Initiate antiplatelet therapy for patients with TIA
- Identify and refer patients with surgically correctable carotid stenosis

DISPOSITION

Patients who have a new anterior circulation TIA, and are potential surgical candidates, should not be discharged without arranging expeditious evaluation of the carotid arteries. If duplex scanning is not immediately available, the patient should be started on antiplatelet therapy and carotid duplex scanning performed as soon as possible, with subsequent vascular consultation for patients determined to have greater than or equal to 50% stenosis.

Patients with an anterior circulation TIA, who are not defined as "high risk" (crescendo TIAs, vertebrobasilar TIA, recurrent TIA on maximal antiplatelet therapy, high-grade carotid artery stenosis, or presumed cardioembolic source), and have less than 50% carotid stenosis on duplex scanning may be discharged home on antiplatelet therapy, with close follow up. Clear instructions on stroke signs and symptoms should be given to ensure rapid return. Patients with suspected dysrhythmias require a monitored bed and evaluation for ischemic heart disease, as appropriate.

Because of the increased short-term risk of stroke, it may be optimal to admit patients with TIA to an inpatient or observation bed. Admission and neurologic consultation should be considered for high-risk patients. Standard protocols for patients with TIAs should be jointly developed with neurologic specialists in each institution. Active collaboration can ensure the provision of efficient and consistent patient care and facilitate future modifications as new data becomes available.

COMMON PITFALLS

✔ Failing to recognize a TIA when the symptoms are remote in time from the emergency department presentation. Establishing the diagnosis becomes more difficult when the patient is unable to recall the specific events surrounding the TIA

✔ Discharging patients with anterior circulation TIAs before determining whether there is a potentially surgically correctable carotid lesion. This carries a high medicolegal risk

✔ Failure to obtain consultation in high-risk patients: those with crescendo TIAs, vertebrobasilar TIA, recurrent TIA on maximal antiplatelet therapy, high-grade carotid artery stenosis, or presumed cardioembolic source

✔ Failing to discuss signs and symptoms of stroke and the need to immediately return for recurrent symptoms with the patient

ISCHEMIC STROKE

Ischemic strokes have traditionally been classified by clinical presentation, time course of onset, progression of deficits, accompanying symptoms, and risk factor profiles. The clinical description of the deficit identifies the extent and location of the stroke and allows accurate communication regarding patient status. The time course and progression of symptoms suggest certain etiologies; for example, prolonged, "stuttering" deficits indicate a thrombotic phenomenon, while an abrupt onset of the maximal deficit suggests an embolic event. Associated symptoms may suggest other causes for neurologic deficits (e.g., a seizure preceding a Todd paralysis or chest pain preceding an ischemic stroke of cardioembolic origin). Consideration of cerebrovascular risk factors helps to classify the stroke as lacunar, embolic, thrombotic, extracranial, or intracranial.

CLINICAL PRESENTATION

Anterior Cerebral Artery Syndrome

Patients with infarction in the territory of the anterior cerebral artery present with hemiparesis involving the leg more than the face or arm. Urinary incontinence and primitive reflexes (grasp and suck) are often present. The patient may perseverate with speech or motor movements and respond slowly to questions. If both anterior cerebral arteries originate from a common trunk, a bilateral parasagittal infarct may occur, with paraplegia and speechlessness (anarthria).

Middle Cerebral Artery Syndrome

Infarction in the distribution of the middle cerebral artery is the most common of the stroke syndromes. Patients with infarcts of the middle cerebral artery present with weakness of the face and arm greater than that of the leg, often with corresponding cortical sensory loss. The presence of aphasia localizes the lesion to the dominant hemisphere. Inattention, extinction on double simultaneous sensory or visual testing, neglect, or constructional or dressing apraxia indicates nondominant hemisphere involvement. Homonymous hemianopia and conjugate eye deviation toward the side of the infarct may also be found. All of these findings are present in the patient with a proximal trunk occlusion and variably present when branches of the middle cerebral artery are involved.

Posterior Cerebral Artery Syndrome

Infarcts in this territory present with homonymous hemianopia secondary to visual cortex involvement. The patient is often unaware of the deficit until formally tested. Motor involvement is minimal, but sensory loss, including both light touch and pinprick, may be severe. There is no aphasia or disruption of nondominant hemisphere functions. Small branches of the posterior cerebral artery anastomose with branches of the anterior and middle cerebral arteries in border zones between the arterial distributions. These areas are at risk for *watershed infarcts* during periods of decreased blood flow.

Vertebrobasilar Artery Syndrome

The classic sign of brainstem stroke is the presence of crossed symptoms: ipsilateral cranial nerve palsy and contralateral hemiplegia. One of the most common strokes in this region is due to occlusion of the vertebral or posterior inferior cerebellar artery, resulting in the *lateral medullary (Wallenberg) syndrome*. Patients may present with ipsilateral facial pain (described as a sharp or stabbing sensation to the face or eye), vertigo, headache, limb ataxia, Horner syndrome, and weakness of the soft palate, with dysphagia and dysphonia. Contralateral symptoms include loss of pinprick and temperature sensation in the arm and leg. Other brainstem syndromes may result in deafness, nausea, vomiting, vertigo, and diplopia.

Cerebellar Infarction

A subset of posterior circulation strokes involves the cerebellum. The most common initial symptom is the sudden inability to walk or stand. This may be followed by complaints of headache, nausea, vomiting, central vertigo, and, possibly, a stiff neck. Cranial nerve findings may also be present. Although the initial CT scan is often unremarkable, one-third of patients develop significant posterior fossa edema. In this confined space, edema produces pressure on the brainstem, causing a decrease in the level of consciousness, typically after a stable period of 6 to 12 hours. Pathologic respiratory patterns and pupillary dilation are late findings, indicating impending herniation. Recognition of cerebellar infarction is critical, and frequent neurologic assessment imperative. Repeat CT scanning or MRI is indicated for patients with a declining level of consciousness. Surgical decompression and/or medical treatment of elevated ICP may be lifesaving.

Lacunar Syndromes

Lacunar infarcts cause several distinct stroke syndromes. Lacunes are found almost exclusively in the basal ganglia, internal capsule, thalamus, and brainstem and are associated with hypertensive arteriopathy. Approximately 20% of patients with lacunar infarctions have had a prior TIA, and the onset of symptoms is often surprisingly gradual (over 36 hours in up to 30% of patients). Deficits often improve with time, and treatment is aimed at control of hypertension after the acute episode resolves. An evaluation for embolic sources should also be undertaken. Lacunar strokes are classified by clinical presentation.

The most frequent lacunar syndrome, *pure motor stroke*, causes paresis/paralysis of the face, arm, and leg. It is easily diagnosed when the deficit involves all three areas equally, but may also present as a partial deficit. The location of the lacune may be in the internal capsule or pons. Cortical sensory deficits are notably absent.

Pure sensory stroke is the result of infarction of the ventral posterior nuclei of the thalamus and results in sensory loss in the face, arm, and leg. The patient may also complain of paresthesias involving the affected side. There is no hemiplegia or other cortical signs.

Patients with *clumsy hand–dysarthria syndrome* present with slurred speech and weakness and ataxia of the upper limb. Facial weakness may also be present. The syndrome is most commonly associated with lesions of the anterior limb and genu of the internal capsule and typically has a good functional outcome.

Differential Diagnosis

Table 112.1 lists conditions that may mimic ischemic stoke and is divided into structural and nonstructural diseases. CT scanning is used initially to evaluate these possibilities and to rule out structural causes of neurologic deficits.

Diseases presenting with features similar to posterior circulation strokes can be difficult to distinguish from stroke. Wernicke encephalopathy presents as the triad of ophthalmoplegia, ataxia, and confusion and is found typically in chronic alcoholics. Ménière's disease, with its characteristic triad of vertigo, tinnitus, and deafness, occurs in patients between the ages of 30 and 60 and is paroxysmal in nature. Gross ataxia and other cranial nerve deficits should be absent. Multiple sclerosis typically presents in the third to fourth decades of life and has variable symptoms, depending on the location of demyelination. Symptoms of phenytoin and carbamazepine toxicity include sedation, nystagmus, vertigo, ataxia, and nausea. Central nervous system symptoms of acute lithium toxicity include confusion, hyperreflexia, tremors, and cranial nerve deficits; dysarthria also may be a prominent feature.

Special consideration should be given to stroke patients younger than 50 years of age or those who have preexisting heart disease, hematologic disorders, or vasculitis. These patients typically fall into the cardioembolic, other or unknown subtype classifications and may have reversible etiologies or other contributing disease states that should be identified as rapidly as possible. Conditions associated with each of these groups are listed in Table 112.2. An extensive discussion of each of these entities is beyond the scope of this chapter.

TABLE 112.1.   Differential Diagnosis of Ischemic Stroke

Structural Causes	Nonstructural Causes
ACUTE	
Intracerebral hemorrhage	Meningitis
Epidural hematoma	Encephalitis
Subdural hematoma	Hypertensive encephalopathy
	Wernicke's encephalopathy
CHRONIC	Hypoglycemia
Intracranial tumor	Complicated (hemiplegic) migraine
Intracranial abscess	Todd's postictal paralysis
	Peripheral nerve palsy (Bell's palsy)
	Labyrinthitis
	Ménière's disease
	Demyelinating disease (multiple sclerosis)
	Drug toxicity (phenytoin, lithium)

TABLE 112.2.   Differential Diagnosis of Special Patient Groups with Ischemic Stroke

Condition	Comments
YOUNG ADULTS WITH STROKE	
Arterial dissection	Age between 15 and 50
	Accounts for 20% of strokes in the young, often preceded by minor trauma
Cardioembolism	Mitral valve prolapse, patent foramen ovale with paradoxical emboli, rheumatic heart disease
Premature atherosclerosis	Hyperlipidemia
Migrainous stroke	Female predominance
Air embolism	Scuba diving, medical procedures
Substance abuse	Heroin, cocaine, amphetamines, LSD
PREEXISTING CARDIAC DISEASE	
Ischemic heart disease	Peripheral emboli from mural thrombus
Dysrhythmias	Atrial fibrillation, ventricular tachycardia, sick sinus syndrome, etc.
Valvular heart disease	Rheumatic heart disease, prosthetic valves
Dilated cardiomyopathies	Peripheral emboli from mural thrombus
Endocarditis	Associated fever and murmur
HEMATOLOGIC DISORDERS	
Hyperviscosity syndromes	Cancer, myeloproliferative diseases, dysproteinemia, thalassemia, sickle cell disease, polycythemia
Coagulopathies	Disseminated intravascular coagulation, protein C or S deficiencies, antithrombin III deficiency, antiphospholipid antibody syndrome
Thrombotic thrombocytopenic purpura	Rare disorder with fever, microangiopathic hemolytic anemia, thrombocytopenia, neurologic and renal impairment
VASCULAR DISORDERS	
Infectious vasculitis	Herpes zoster, human immunodeficiency virus infection, syphilis, tuberculosis, aspergillosis
Noninfectious vasculitis:	
Necrotizing	Polyarteritis nodosa
Nonnecrotizing	Giant cell arteritis (patients >age 50; females > males), Takayasu's arteritis
Cerebral venous thrombosis	Presents with headache and papilledema; magnetic resonance imaging is diagnostic

EMERGENCY DEPARTMENT EVALUATION

Like myocardial infarction, stroke is an acute disease necessitating early identification and treatment. Prehospital personnel should obtain information surrounding the onset of symptoms, particularly noting the time deficits started. Patients found lying immobile for prolonged periods are at risk for decubitus ulcers, dehydration, hypothermia or hyperthermia, and rhabdomyolysis. Intravenous access should be obtained and a fingerstick glucose level determined when possible. In the prehospital phase, it is unusual for patients with ischemic stroke to have an altered level of consciousness; an altered sensorium suggests the presence of other etiologies. Glucose-containing solutions and routine administration of dextrose (D_{50}) should be avoided unless hypoglycemia is documented or strongly suspected. Narcan is generally not required unless there are historic features or pinpoint pupils, suggesting opiate ingestion.

On arrival in the emergency department, stroke patients require a monitored bed and rapid assessment of airway, breathing, and circulatory status. Complete vital signs should be obtained, including a core temperature. A focused physical examination should be performed, including a search for evidence of head trauma. The neck should be examined for meningeal signs present with either infection or SAH. Auscultation for carotid bruits, particularly on the side opposite a clinical deficit, should be performed. The heart is examined for rate, regularity, and murmurs, searching for conditions predisposing to stroke, such as atrial fibrillation and mitral valvular disease. The extremities should be assessed for evidence of peripheral vascular disease or emboli, and the skin examined for needle tracks or evidence of petechiae or ecchymosis, suggesting endocarditis, sepsis, or coagulopathy.

The neurologic exam should include a brief assessment of mental status, including level of consciousness, language, memory, and interpretation. A careful eye examination should follow, with testing of both visual acuity and visual fields. Pupillary size, reactivity, and extraocular movements provide information on brainstem function and cranial nerves III, IV, and VI. Anisocoria suggests a third-nerve palsy, potentially from elevated intracranial pressure, and should be investigated with a "swinging flashlight" test. Conjugate eye deviation toward the normal arm and leg suggests a hemispheric lesion, while deviation toward the paretic arm or leg suggests a brainstem lesion. Funduscopic examination of the retina may reveal papilledema, hypertensive changes, Hollenhorst plaques, diabetic changes, or Roth spots suggestive of specific stroke etiologies. Cranial nerves V and VII through XII may quickly be assessed by examining facial and corneal sensation; smiling symmetry, eyebrow raising, and forehead wrinkling; gross auditory acuity; gag reflex; shoulder shrug (trapezius strength); head rotation against resistance (sternocleidomastoid strength); and tongue protrusion, respectively.

Motor strength and tone should be assessed in both proximal and distal muscle groups. Pronator drift is a sensitive indicator of upper extremity weakness.

The sensory examination is the most subjective part of the neurologic examination and should be interpreted in view of the patient's ability to cooperate and the overall examination. Double simultaneous extinction is tested at this time, particularly if visual field deficits were identified. The ability of a patient to identify, by touch, common objects such as keys or pens (stereognosis) and to identify a number drawn on the skin surface (graphesthesia) is an easy test of sensory function done in the emergency department.

Cerebellar function can be assessed by finger-to-nose and heel-to-shin tests; these are particularly useful with the bedridden patient. Important reflex arcs to test routinely include the biceps (C-5, C-6), triceps (C-6, C-7, C-8), patellar (L-2, L-3, L-4), and Achilles (L-5, S-1), as well as pathologic reflexes. Asymmetry of deep tendon reflexes or a unilateral Babinski sign may indicate corticospinal tract lesions.

Assessment of station and gait is one of the most revealing parts of the neurologic examination. Subtle weakness, ataxia, rigidity, and sensory defects can be identified by observation of the gait, toe-walking, heel-walking, tandem walking, and Romberg tests.

Further diagnostic evaluation in the emergency department should include a 12-lead electrocardiogram, complete blood cell count, electrolyte and glucose determinations, PT/aPTT/INR and renal function studies. A serum creatine phosphokinase determination should be obtained (along with urine myoglobin) in patients with prolonged immobilization. Arterial blood gases, blood cultures, toxicologic screens, alcohol level, pregnancy test and other laboratory studies are ordered as necessary. A chest x-ray is indicated if lung disease is suspected. Lumbar puncture should be performed if SAH or an infectious etiology is suspected. EEG may be indicated in patients with suspected seizures.

A nonenhanced CT scan of the head should be obtained in all patients to identify intracranial hemorrhage and to evaluate other causes of neurologic deficits. An ischemic stroke does not become hypodense for 6 to 72 hours after vessel occlusion and is often not visible on initial CT evaluation. If CT scanning is unavailable, the patient should be stabilized and transferred as rapidly as possible to a facility with CT capability.

MRI, carotid ultrasonography, echocardiography, and angiography have limited roles in the acute evaluation of most patients with ischemic stroke and are utilized in selected cases after hospital admission. An exception is the patient with a suspected vertebrobasilar or carotid artery dissection. These patients should be considered for emergent ultrasound, angiography, or MR angiogram (MRA), as dissection is commonly treated with anticoagulation.

Advances in the evaluation of acute ischemic stroke continue. As MRI becomes faster and more available, it may become the diagnostic test of choice, allowing earlier assessment of the size of infarction and measurement of tissue perfusion and metabolism. CT angiograms now allow identification of specific vascular occlusions. Transcranial Doppler can noninvasively identify occlusion of the middle cerebral artery. These modalities may prove useful in the future in refining patient selection for thrombolytic therapy.

EMERGENCY DEPARTMENT MANAGEMENT

The goal of acute stroke management in appropriate patients who present within 3 hours of symptom onset is the reversal of clinical deficits by re-establishing cerebral blood flow with intravenous thrombolytic agents.

In patients presenting with major stroke symptoms suggestive of middle cerebral artery involvement, intraarterial thrombolysis represents an option for treatment within 6 hours of onset (10). Case series data support intraarterial thrombolytic use in patients with basilar artery occlusion with longer time windows. However, definitive intraarterial studies with a commercially available agent are lacking. In patients not meeting thrombolytic criteria, no acute intervention has proven effective in improving functional outcome and the objective of treatment is to limit infarct extension and recurrence. Current approaches to preventing or minimizing infarct extension include maintenance of adequate cardiac output to preserve cerebral blood flow, regulation of core temperature, and control of the blood glucose level. Strategies to prevent infarct recurrence focus on antiplatelet and anticoagulation therapy.

Thrombolytic Therapy

Current recommendations by the American Heart Association and American Academy of Neurology support the use of recombinant tissue plasminogen activator (r-TPA, Activase®) in carefully selected patients when the diagnosis has been established by physicians with expertise in stroke and the cranial CT has been interpreted by a qualified individual. These recommendations followed Food and Drug Administration approval for use of r-TPA in acute ischemic stroke and are based primarily on the results of the NIH/NINDS Stroke Study, Parts I and II. These trials found that stroke patients treated with r-TPA were at least 30% more likely to have minimal or no disability 3 months after the event, compared with those who received placebo (absolute increase in favorable outcome, 11% to 13%). Though treated patients had a symptomatic hemorrhage rate of 6.4% (vs. 0.6% for placebo), there was no significant difference in mortality at 3 months (17% r-TPA, 21% placebo) (1). Posthoc analyses do not support withholding therapy from any patient on the basis of suspected stroke subtype, age, clinical deficit, or CT findings of early ischemic changes.

Concern has been raised regarding the fact that only the NINDS trials have shown benefit, while four other trials (ASK, MAST-E, MAST-I, and ECASS) found either no benefit or potential harm. It should be noted there were fundamental differences between the NINDS trials and the other studies, making direct comparison problematic. These differences include thrombolytic agent used, dose, time-to-treatment, blood pressure management, and number of protocol violations. Two subsequent thrombolytic trials (ECASS II and ATLANTIS) specifically evaluated the use of intravenous r-TPA beyond 3 hours and found no benefit.

Other concerns address the reproducibility of the results in the community setting and the delivery of thrombolytic therapy without adequate specialist support. Sixteen post-approval studies have been published involving more than 1500 r-TPA–treated patients worldwide and suggest r-TPA can be delivered both in tertiary centers and smaller community and rural hospitals successfully. The presence of active stroke centers and physician education can have a positive impact on the number and effectiveness of stroke interventions while limited experience and protocol violations may contribute to increased complications and mortality. Emergency physician diagnostic accuracy for identifying strokes for r-TPA treatment appears similar to that of specialized stroke teams (17).

The development of treatment guidelines for stroke may improve patient selection and speed the delivery of thrombolytics to appropriate patients. The National Institutes of Health recommends a target "door-to-needle" time for eligible r-TPA patients of 60 minutes. This target, however, remain elusive. Even in systems with advanced delivery capability the reported "door-to-needle" times typically approach 90 minutes.

Table 112.3 outlines inclusion and exclusion criteria for the use of intravenous r-TPA in acute stroke. Eligible patients should be treated with 0.9 mg/kg of r-TPA (maximum dose, 90 mg), with 10% given as a bolus over 1 to 2 minutes, and the remainder given over 60 minutes via infusion pump. Table 112.4 presents

---

TABLE 112.3.   Intravenous TPA in Ischemic Stroke: Inclusion and Exclusion Criteria[1,5]

	Yes	No
Inclusion Criteria		
1. Age 18 or older		
2. Clinical diagnosis of ischemic stroke		
3. Time of onset well established to be less than 180 minutes before treatment would begin. *"Time of onset" of stroke is defined as that point at which a change in the baseline neurologic function occurred. If that time is not known (e.g., the patient awakens from sleep with new symptoms), the last time the patient was observed to be neurologically intact must be considered to be the time of onset.*		
Medical History Exclusions	Yes	No
1. Current use of oral anticoagulants (e.g., warfarin sodium) AND an INR greater than 1.5?[a]		
2. Use of heparin in the previous 48 hours AND a prolonged aPTT?[a]		
3. History of another stroke (any type) in previous 3 months?		
4. History of a serious head injury in the previous 3 months?		
5. History of major surgery, biopsy of a parenchymal organ, or serious trauma within the preceding 14 days?		
6. History of any prior intracranial hemorrhage (any type)?		
7. History of intracranial neoplasm, arteriovenous malformation, or aneurysm?		
8. History of seizure at the time of stroke onset?[b]		
9. History of gastrointestinal or urinary bleeding within the preceding 21 days?		
10. History of myocardial infarction in the past 3 months?		
11. History of pregnancy or parturition within past 30 days?		
12. History of hereditary or acquired abnormal hemostasis?		
13. History of recent (within 7 days) lumbar puncture?		
14. History of recent (within 30 days) arterial puncture at a noncompressible site?		
Clinical Examination Exclusions	Yes	No
1. Rapidly improving neurologic signs?		
2. Isolated, mild neurologic deficits, such as ataxia alone, sensory loss alone, dysarthria alone, or minimal weakness (NIH stroke scale less than 4 AND normal speech AND visual fields)?		
3. Presentation that suggests SAH, even if CT scan is normal.		
4. Pretreatment hypertension: systolic blood pressure greater than 185 mm Hg OR diastolic blood pressure greater than 110 mm Hg?[c]		
5. Presumed septic embolus (any stroke with a fever)?		
6. Glucose less than 50 mg/dL?		
7. Platelet count less than 100,000/mm?		
8. Clinical presentation suggesting aortic dissection?		
Cerebral CT Exclusions	Yes	No
1. High-density lesion consistent with hemorrhage or possible hemorrhage of any degree or type on CT?		

[a] In patients without recent use of oral anticoagulants or heparin, treatment with r-TPA can be initiated before the availability of coagulation study results, but should be discontinued if either the PT is greater than 15 seconds (INR greater than 1.7) or the PTT is elevated by local laboratory standards.

[b] Patients with a seizure at the time of stroke onset might be eligible for treatment if the clinician is convinced that the residual impairments are due to stroke and not the seizure.

[c] Hypertension may be treated with labetalol 10–20 mg IV over 1–2 minutes (may repeat × 1) or nitroglycerine paste 1–2 inches and TPA initiated if reduction to above levels occurs. More aggressive treatment to reduce blood pressure excludes the patient from treatment with TPA.

TABLE 112.4. Post r-TPA Blood Pressure Management in Acute Stroke[5]

A. Monitor BP every 15 minutes.
B. If systolic BP is > 180 mm Hg or if diastolic BP is 105 to 140: Give labetalol 10 mg intravenously over 1 to 2 minutes. The dose may be repeated or doubled every 10 to 20 minutes, up to 300 mg. Alternatives include an initial labetalol dose followed by an infusion at a rate of 2–8 mg/min. If blood pressure not controlled consider sodium nitroprusside infusion.
C. If diastolic BP is >140 mm Hg: Infuse sodium nitroprusside at a rate of 0.5 mcg/kg/min and titrate to desired pressure.

post-treatment blood pressure control guidelines. An algorithm for the management of suspected intracranial hemorrhage secondary to thrombolytic therapy is shown in Figure 112.1.

The development of institution-specific evaluation and treatment guidelines is recommended to identify local responsibilities concerning thrombolytic delivery and posttreatment care and disposition. A multidisciplinary approach will deliver the highest level of care in a time-critical setting.

Hypertension Management

Acute elevations of blood pressure typically decline, without treatment, within a few days to pre-stroke levels. Because the benefit of blood pressure control is unproved, it is reasonable to avoid treating hypertension in the absence of specific indications such as thrombolytic therapy for acute stroke, AMI, hypertensive encephalopathy, arterial dissection, and hemorrhagic trans-

formation. Although no data exists to define the point of treatment for severe isolated hypertension in stroke, consensus exists that antihypertensive agents should be withheld unless the diastolic blood pressure is >120 mm Hg or unless the systolic blood pressure is >220 mm Hg.

In stroke patients requiring antihypertensive therapy (and not eligible for r-TPA), the goal is a gradual reduction of blood pressure by 15%. For patients with SBP > 220 or DBP 121 to 140 mm Hg, labetalol, 10 to 20 mg IV over 1 to 2 minutes, repeated or doubled every 10 minutes (maximum dose 300 mg) or nicardipine 5 mg/hr IV infusion as initial dose; titrated to desired effect by increasing 2.5 mg/hr every 5 min to maximum of 15 mg/hr, is recommended. For patients with DBP > 140, a sodium nitroprusside infusion, 0.5 mcg/kg/min IV as initial dose with continuous blood pressure monitoring and titration, is recommended. The use of antihypertensive agents requires frequent neurologic checks so that treatment may be discontinued if neurologic deterioration occurs (5).

Volume Management

Maintenance of intravascular volume is important in optimizing cardiac output in stroke patients. These patients are often unable to maintain adequate oral intake, and up to one-third may be significantly hypovolemic. Volume deficits should be corrected as rapidly as possible and followed by maintenance fluids. Avoidance of hypoosmolar solution is recommended to prevent exacerbation of cerebral edema. Patients with underlying cardiac or renal disease may require invasive hemodynamic monitoring to guide fluid management. Aggressive hypervolemic therapy to increase cerebral blood flow should be avoided, because it does

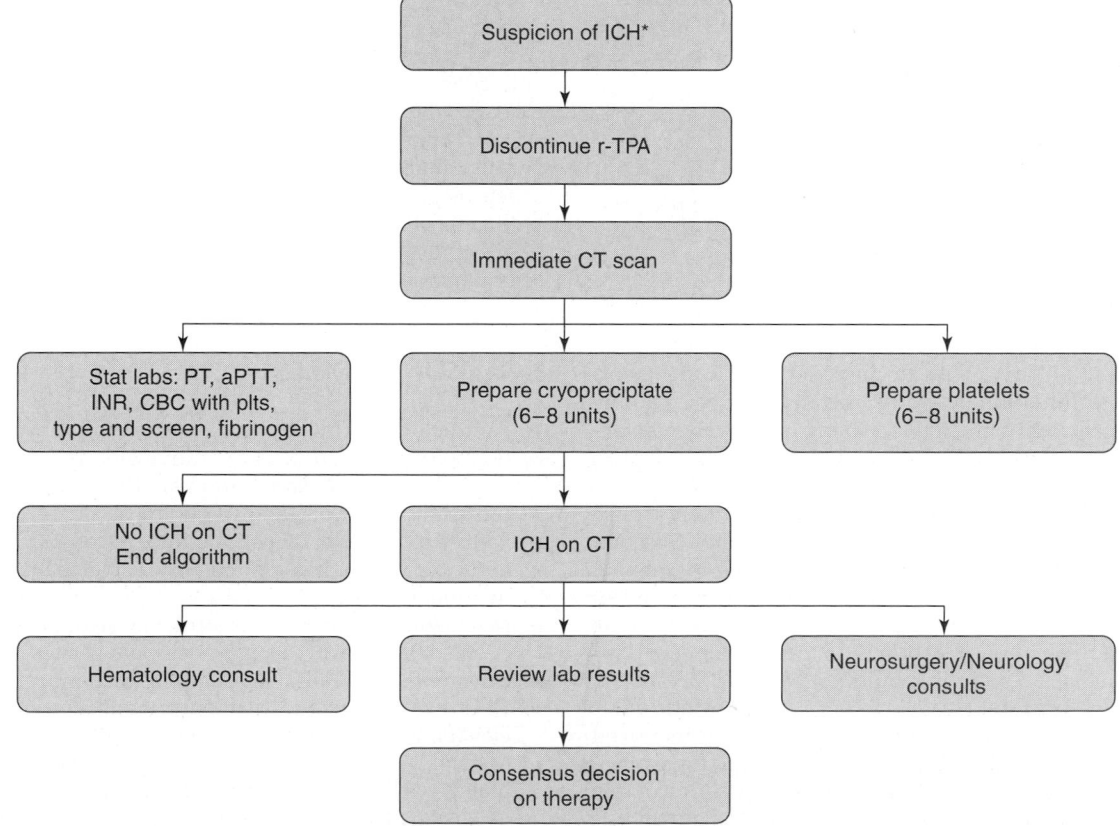

Figure 112.1. Management of suspected intracranial hemorrhage following r-TPA use. * = Symptoms such as neurologic deterioration, new headache, acute hypertension, nausea, vomiting.

not improve outcome and may contribute to cerebral edema. Hemodilution has also not been proven to alter stroke outcome and cannot be recommended.

Temperature Regulation

Temperature regulation of the ischemic stroke patient is often neglected in the emergency department. Experimentally, hypothermia has a protective effect on ischemic neurons, whereas hyperthermia may worsen damage by increasing cellular metabolic demand. Fever is not uncommon in stroke patients and should be promptly treated.

Glucose Regulation

Because the optimal glucose level following stroke is unknown, it is reasonable to treat excessive levels with insulin to maintain a glucose level of less than 300 mg/dL and to avoid the overuse of glucose-containing solutions (5).

Anticoagulation

Although anticoagulation has been used in stroke for more than 50 years, its efficacy is unproved. In patients with ischemic stroke, early anticoagulation has no proven benefit and is associated with an increased risk of serious bleeding complications and hemorrhagic transformation of the infarct. No well-controlled, randomized, clinical trial has demonstrated a benefit from anticoagulation even in potentially high-risk groups: patients with intracardiac or intraarterial thrombi, vertebrobasilar disease or arterial dissection. Therefore, emergent anticoagulation to improve neurologic outcome or prevent early recurrent stroke is not recommended (5). Additional studies are required to determine if certain subgroups may benefit from urgent anticoagulation. Given the lack of evidence and the potential risks, consultation is recommended prior to anticoagulation initiation in stroke. All anticoagulants should be withheld for 24 hours following the use of r-TPA in acute stroke.

Antiplatelet Therapy

Antiplatelet therapy is a cornerstone of stroke management and reflects the central role of platelet activation in clot formation. The use of aspirin in patients with a previous mild stroke or TIA results in a 20% reduction in stroke risk. In patients treated within 48 hours of stroke onset, with 300 mg of aspirin daily, there was a statistically significant reduction in recurrent ischemic stroke at 14 days, with no increase in risk of hemorrhagic stroke (3). Initiation of aspirin therapy may begin in the emergency department with 300 to 325 mg in patients who are not treated with thrombolytic therapy and do not have aspirin sensitivities.

Clopidogrel (Plavix) is slightly more effective than aspirin in preventing a combined endpoint of stroke, AMI, and vascular death (2) while aspirin combined with dipyridamole (Aggrenox) was more effective than aspirin alone in preventing recurrent stroke or death (9). Studies have not evaluated their use in acute stroke, however. The onset of action is delayed for several days with clopidogrel, suggesting it should not be relied on acutely to inhibit platelet function. Headaches are a common side effect with dipyridamole. Given these limitations and their increased cost, the emergent use of these agents is best reserved for aspirin-intolerant patients or those failing aspirin therapy. Glycoprotein IIb/IIIa inhibitors in acute stroke are in clinical trials with one small, randomized, placebo-controlled, dose-escalation study of abciximab reporting relative safety in its use in acute stroke (4).

CRITICAL INTERVENTIONS

- Obtain an emergent CT scan
- Initiate aspirin therapy for nonhemorrhagic ischemic strokes that are not eligible for TPA
- Identify patients eligible for thrombolytic therapy and expedite their diagnostic evaluation
- Correct hyperthermia

DISPOSITION

Factors influencing disposition in the patient with ischemic stroke include infarct location, time of symptom onset, infarct size, stroke etiology, concurrent medical conditions, and social resources available to the patient. The vast majority of stroke patients are admitted to the hospital, often to a specialized unit or floor skilled in the care of patients with neurologic deficits. Cardiac monitoring should be arranged for those with potential dysrhythmias either as an etiology or as a consequence of the infarct.

Patients with minor, completed strokes are potential candidates for evaluation in an emergency department clinical decision unit. Predefined protocols for neurologic consultation, subsequent neurologic and vascular imaging, and initiation of therapy to prevent recurrent stroke in this setting speed patient care and reduce length of hospital stay.

Patients treated with r-TPA and those with impaired gag or swallowing reflexes or mental status changes should be admitted to the intensive care unit. Intensive care unit admission is also indicated for patients with cerebellar strokes and should be considered for patients with large hemispheric strokes who are at risk for the development of cerebral edema.

Stroke patients are often cared for in the inpatient setting without neurologic consultation. Neurologic consultation in the emergency department is indicated when the diagnosis is unclear or when further evaluation is required (e.g., arterial dissection, migrainous infarct, unusual hematologic conditions). Because anticoagulation is not recommended, consultation with a neurologist should occur before initiating heparin. Patients with cerebellar infarction should have neurosurgical consultation, because decompressive craniectomy may be lifesaving in selected patients.

COMMON PITFALLS

✔ Failure to perform a complete history and physical examination, particularly in uncooperative elderly patients. The history and physical examination are the basis for determining the extent of a stroke and its etiology

✔ Failure to consider unusual etiologies of stroke, such as arterial dissection and emboli in younger patients with new neurologic deficits

✔ Misdiagnosis of cerebellar stroke as alcohol or drug intoxication, labyrinthitis, benign positional vertigo, or severe gastroenteritis, and failure to obtain neurosurgical consultation

✔ Failure to optimize cardiac output and to treat temperature elevations in the emergency department

✔ Managing blood pressure too aggressively. Reduction of blood pressure may reduce cerebral blood flow and cause extension of an ischemic stroke

✔ Initiation of anticoagulation in patients with acute stroke prior to consultation

HEMORRHAGIC CEREBROVASCULAR DISEASE

Intracerebral hemorrhage (ICH), defined as hemorrhage directly into the brain parenchyma, affects 10% to 15% of all stroke patients. Major risk factors for intracranial hemorrhage include advanced age, hypertension, and race. Blacks have a higher incidence of ICH than do Whites; Asians have an even higher incidence. Other risk factors include cigarette smoking and alcohol use.

The most common site for ICH is the putamen, which accounts for 35% to 50% of all hemorrhages. Next in frequency are the subcortical white matter (30%), the cerebellum (16%), the thalamus (10% to 15%), and the pons (5% to 12%) (14). Pathologically, these are areas of the brain supplied by small arteries that are 50 to 200 μm in size.

CLINICAL PRESENTATION

The onset of ICH is usually heralded by a sudden headache, vomiting, and neurologic deficit. The majority of patients exhibit a decreased level of consciousness due to elevated intracranial pressure (ICP). ICH often occurs during activity and only rarely has its onset during sleep. In one-third of cases, clinical deficits are maximal at onset. In the remaining two-thirds, the symptoms follow a steadily progressive course over the first 30 minutes. Coma is a poor prognostic sign and is associated with larger hemorrhages and ventricular extension. Headache and vomiting are typically absent in ischemic strokes and thus are of help in identifying patients with ICH. Early seizures are uncommon in ICH involving the putamen, thalamus, and pons but may be present in up to one-third of patients with subcortical white matter ("lobar") hemorrhages. Hypertension is noted in over 90% of patients with ICH.

The clinical deficits are related to the location and size of the hemorrhage. Putaminal hemorrhages cause a dense contralateral hemiplegia with sensory loss and homonymous hemianopia. The eyes show conjugate deviation away from the paralyzed side, which may be overcome with caloric testing or doll's-eye reflex testing. Thalamic hemorrhages cause similar motor and sensory findings but may also cause conjugate downward gaze with pinpoint, unresponsive pupils. Deficits from a lobar hemorrhage depend on the size and location of the hemorrhage. Pontine hemorrhage typically causes a severe occipital headache, followed rapidly by a decreased level of consciousness; coma is present in 80% of patients. Patients may become hyperthermic and may have severe neurologic deficits. These include quadriplegia, loss of corneal reflexes, and pinpoint pupils with absent horizontal eye movements on caloric or doll's-eye reflex testing. Cerebellar hemorrhage causes extremity and truncal ataxia and an inability to walk. These symptoms are commonly accompanied by vomiting, dysequilibrium, and headache. An ipsilateral gaze palsy may also be present. Patients with cerebellar hemorrhage may initially appear stable but can deteriorate rapidly to coma and death.

DIFFERENTIAL DIAGNOSIS

The presence of intracerebral blood on head CT should not automatically be ascribed to a hypertensive hemorrhage. Various nonhypertensive causes of ICH include arteriovenous malformation, berry aneurysm, sympathomimetic drug use, intracranial tumor, anticoagulant and thrombolytic agent use, hematologic disorders (e.g., leukemia, thrombotic thrombocy-topenic purpura, hemophilia), cerebral vasculitis, and mycotic aneurysm.

EMERGENCY DEPARTMENT EVALUATION

The evaluation of patients with suspected ICH is similar to that for ischemic stroke. However, patients with ICH may exhibit rapid neurologic deterioration and a decreased level of consciousness, necessitating acute airway intervention. Vital signs should be monitored closely, and frequent neurologic assessments are required. Laboratory data should be obtained to help identify possible contributing causes, such as coagulopathy, thrombocytopenia, or platelet dysfunction. Toxicologic screening is indicated for patients with atypical presentations and for younger patients without a history of hypertension. Cardiac monitoring is essential, because dysrhythmias are common from either increased sympathetic discharge or impending tonsillar or uncal herniation.

The CT scan typically shows high attenuation in the area of hemorrhage. There is usually a "ring" of low attenuation surrounding the hemorrhage because of edema of the adjacent tissue. Angiography or MRI/MRA should be considered when an aneurysm, arteriovenous malformation, or central nervous system tumor is strongly suspected.

EMERGENCY DEPARTMENT MANAGEMENT

The goals of emergency care for ICH are rapid diagnosis, management of the airway, control of ICP, and early neurosurgical consultation. Oxygen should be administered to all patients. Intubation is indicated for airway protection or hyperventilation to reduce ICP. Rapid-sequence intubation with paralytic agents may be necessary to obtain adequate CT images in a combative patient.

Management of hypertension in the patient with ICH is directed at managing the competing interests of decreasing ongoing hemorrhage against over-reduction of cerebral perfusion pressure. Current recommendations are to maintain a mean arterial pressure below 130 mm Hg in persons with a history of hypertension (8). In patients without a history of hypertension the guidelines for management of hypertension in ischemic stroke may be adapted for use in patients with ICH. In patients with an ICP monitor, cerebral perfusion pressure (mean arterial pressure ICP) should be kept above 70 mm Hg. Useful antihypertensive agents in the setting of ICH include nitroprusside, esmolol, and labetalol.

Intracranial pressure control is important in the patient with ICH. Elevations in ICP, defined as readings ≥ 20 mmHg for 5 minutes, may present as a decreasing level of consciousness and/or neurologic deterioration and is initially managed with (1) elevation of the head (30 degrees), (2) osmotherapy, and (3) hyperventilation. Although there is no universally accepted standard therapy for the management of ICH, current recommendations support the use of a stepwise approach beginning with mannitol (20% solution; 0.25 to 0.5 g/kg every 4 hours) in patients with progressively increasing ICP values or clinical deterioration. Furosemide (10 mg every 2 to 8 hours) may be administered simultaneously with osmotherapy (8).

Reduction of the pCO_2 to 30 to 35 mm Hg lowers ICP by 25% to 30% in most patients, though peak ICP reduction may be delayed up to 30 minutes after the pCO_2 is changed. Because hypocarbia causes cerebral vasoconstriction, overaggressive reduction in pCO_2 may reduce cerebral blood flow below critical values; this should thus be avoided.

In general, ICP monitoring is indicated in patients with a Glasgow Coma Scale score of less than 9 and in those whose condition is thought to be deteriorating due to increases in ICP. Other patients may warrant ICP monitors, however, particularly those with intraventricular hemorrhage. Intraventricular catheter placement offers the potential for direct removal of CSF and reduction of ICP.

Neurosurgical consultation should be obtained early, and, if unavailable, the patient should be stabilized and transferred. The indications for hematoma evacuation depend on many factors, including patient age, hemorrhage location and size, and surgical accessibility. Patients who present initially with coma or loss of brainstem function generally do not benefit from surgical evacuation, whereas those who experience progressive deterioration after a lobar hemorrhage are often operated on. In patients with cerebellar hemorrhage, surgery is recommended for all hematomas exceeding 3 cm in diameter.

CRITICAL INTERVENTIONS

- Protect the airway
- Manage elevated ICP
- Obtain neurosurgical consultation

DISPOSITION

All patients with ICH should be admitted for close observation and monitoring. Typically, intensive care unit monitoring is required. If neurosurgical treatment capabilities are not available locally, arrangements should be made to transfer the patient.

COMMON PITFALLS

✔ Failure to diagnose cerebellar hemorrhage. Patients may be misdiagnosed with acute viral syndrome, labyrinthitis, or intoxication. Surgical intervention may be lifesaving

✔ Delay in transport. Patients with ICH require early neurosurgical consultation and should be transported to an appropriate facility if immediate neurosurgical attention is not otherwise available

Acknowledgments

Thanks to Dr. William Barsan for contributions to this chapter in earlier editions of this book.

References

1. Tissue plasminogen activator for acute ischemic stroke. The National Institute of Neurological Disorders and Stroke rt-PA Stroke Study Group. *N Engl J Med* 1995;333:1581–1587.
2. A randomised, blinded, trial of clopidogrel versus aspirin in patients at risk of ischaemic events (CAPRIE). CAPRIE Steering Committee. *Lancet* 1996;348: 1329–1339.
3. The International Stroke Trial (IST): a randomised trial of aspirin, subcutaneous heparin, both, or neither among 19435 patients with acute ischaemic stroke. International Stroke Trial Collaborative Group. *Lancet* 1997;349:1569–1581.
4. Abciximab in acute ischemic stroke: a randomized, double-blind, placebo-controlled, dose-escalation study. The Abciximab in Ischemic Stroke Investigators. *Stroke* 2000;31:601–609.
5. Adams HP, Jr, Adams RJ, Brott T, et al. Guidelines for the Early Management of Patients With Ischemic Stroke: A Scientific Statement From the Stroke Council of the American Stroke Association. *Stroke* 2003;34:1056–1083.
6. Albers GW, Caplan LR, Easton JD, et al. Transient Ischemic Attack – Proposal for a New Definition. *N Engl J Med* 2002;347:1713–1716.
7. Barnett HJ, Taylor DW, Eliasziw M, et al. Benefit of carotid endarterectomy in patients with symptomatic moderate or severe stenosis. North American Symptomatic Carotid Endarterectomy Trial Collaborators. *N Engl J Med* 1998;339:1415–1425.
8. Broderick JP, Adams HP, Jr, Barsan W, et al. Guidelines for the management of spontaneous intracerebral hemorrhage: A statement for healthcare professionals from a special writing group of the Stroke Council, American Heart Association. *Stroke* 1999;30:905–915.
9. Diener HC, Cunha L, Forbes C, et al. European Stroke Prevention Study. 2. Dipyridamole and acetylsalicylic acid in the secondary prevention of stroke. *J Neurol Sci* 1996;143:1–13.
10. Furlan A, Higashida R, Wechsler L, et al. Intra-arterial prourokinase for acute ischemic stroke. The PROACT II study: a randomized controlled trial. Prolyse in Acute Cerebral Thromboembolism. *JAMA* 1999;282:2003–2011.
11. Gillum RF. Stroke in blacks. *Stroke* 1988;19:1–9.
12. Johnston SC, Gress DR, Browner WS, Sidney S. Short-term prognosis after emergency department diagnosis of TIA. *JAMA* 2000;284:2901–2906.
13. Kappelle LJ, van Latum JC, Koudstaal PJ, van Gijn J. Transient ischaemic attacks and small-vessel disease. Dutch TIA Study Group. *Lancet* 1991;337:339–341.
14. Kase C, Mohr J, Caplan L. Intracerebral hemorrhage. In: Barnett H, Mohr J, Stein B, Yatsu F, eds. *Stroke: Pathophysiology, Diagnosis, and Management*. Second edition. New York: Churchill Livingstone. 1992:561–616.
15. Matsumoto N, Whisnant JP, Kurland LT, Okazaki H. Natural history of stroke in Rochester, Minnesota, 1955 through 1969: an extension of a previous study, 1945 through 1954. *Stroke* 1973;4:20–29.
16. Rothwell PM, Gutnikov SA, Warlow CP. Reanalysis of the final results of the European Carotid Surgery Trial. *Stroke* 2003;34:514–523.
17. Scott PA, Silbergleit R. Misdiagnosis of stroke in tissue plasminogen activator-treated patients: characteristics and outcomes. *Ann Emerg Med* 2003;42:611–618.

CHAPTER 113
Seizures

Peter Shearer and Andy Jagoda

Seizures account for an estimated 1% to 2% of emergency department visits. Two to 4 million Americans have epilepsy, a condition of recurrent unprovoked seizures. A much larger number of people have seizures provoked by an underlying pathologic process.

Seizures result from excessive and disorderly neuronal discharge in the cerebral cortex. Epilepsy is a condition of unprovoked seizures, whereas an underlying pathologic process provokes other seizures. The manifestations of a seizure reflect the area of the brain in which neurons are discharging, and can involve the entire cerebral cortex. Thus some seizure discharges and symptoms may be focal or may be generalized. Consequently, the clinical spectrum of seizures includes focal or generalized motor activity, altered mental status, sensory or psychic experiences, or autonomic disturbances.

Ictus refers to the period during which a seizure occurs. An *aura*, or "warning," represents the beginning of a partial seizure, which can remain focal or can spread into a generalized event; a corollary is that patients with a primary generalized seizure disorder do not have an aura. The period after a seizure but before the patient returns to baseline mental status is called the *postictal* period.

Status epilepticus formerly referred to seizures that last more than 30 minutes or in which there are recurrent seizures without a return to baseline mental status between events. Currently some researchers define status epilepticus as a seizure that lasts 5 to 10 minutes or 2 seizures without full recovery between them (17). There are a projected 126,000 to 195,000 cases of status epilepticus each year in the United States, with an overall mortality of 22%. There is a bimodal distribution of cases, with the highest incidence occurring in the first year of life and after the age of 60. Over one-half of patients presenting to the emergency department in status epilepticus have no prior seizure history.

If the seizure lasts more than 30 minutes, the body's homeostatic regulating mechanisms begin to deteriorate; blood pressure begins to decrease; serum pH and lactate level can normalize if the patient's respiratory status is not compromised. It is hypothesized that even if systemic factors such as acidosis and hypoxia are controlled, prolonged status epilepticus results in neuronal damage secondary to the release of neurotoxic excitatory amino acids and influx of calcium into cells.

CLINICAL PRESENTATION

The classification of seizures (Table 113.1) is based on the behavioral, electrophysiologic and clinical features of the event rather than on pathophysiologic mechanisms or anatomic localization. Seizures can be broadly divided into primary generalized seizures and partial seizures (also called focal seizures). *Primary generalized seizures* do not have an inciting focus, but begin bilaterally in both hemispheres of the cerebral cortex. *Partial seizures* begin in a localized area of the brain; they may remain focal but can also spread to incorporate both hemispheres, in which case, the seizure is termed *secondary generalized*. Among the types of new onset seizures in adults, partial seizures are more common than primary generalized seizures (7).

There are 6 types of generalized seizures (see Table 113.1), which are divided into the 5 with convulsive activity, and 1 with nonconvulsive activity—also known as *absence* seizures. All primary generalized seizures, except myoclonic seizures, are associated with an altered level of consciousness. Generalized convulsive seizures classically begin as myoclonic jerks followed by loss of consciousness and sustained generalized skeletal muscle contractions. The seizure activity lasts 90 to 120 seconds and is associated with urinary incontinence and tongue biting. The convulsive seizure is followed by the postictal state characterized by a brief period of confusion and somnolence. Thus, it is not possible to have a bilateral tonic–clonic event with preservation of mental status, and this criterion can be helpful at times in distinguishing neurogenic seizures from psychogenic seizures.

Absence seizures are primary generalized events characterized by an alteration in mental status without significant motor activity. Patients have short episodes of sudden immobility and a blank stare. They are more frequent in the young, usually beginning between the ages of 5 and 10 years, and are infrequent after the mid-teens. The average duration is 10 seconds, and there is rarely a postictal period.

Partial seizures are subdivided according to associated impairment of consciousness. *Simple partial seizures* have brief sensory or motor manifestations with no impairment of consciousness and are categorized according to clinical presentation (see Table 113.1). Partial seizures that are associated with an impairment of consciousness are termed *complex partial seizures*—also know as temporal lobe or psychomotor seizures and are characterized by mental and psychological symptoms including changes in affect, confusion, or hallucinations. Partial seizures that evolve to generalized seizures are associated with altered consciousness just as other generalized seizures.

TABLE 113.1.   Classification of Seizures

Partial Seizures
  A. Simple partial
    1. Motor
    2. Somatosensory
    3. Autonomic
    4. Psychic
  B. Complex Partial
  C. Secondary Generalized

Generalized Seizures
  A. Nonconvulsive (absence)
  B. Convulsive
    1. Tonic–clonic
    2. Clonic
    3. Tonic
    4. Myoclonic
    5. Atonic

Status Epilepticus
  A. Convulsive generalized
  B. Convulsive focal
  C. Nonconvulsive

Differentiation between primary generalized seizures and secondary generalized partial seizures can be difficult; usually upon arrival to the ED both types of patients have either generalized seizure activity or are postictal. With a careful history clinicians can elicit a preceding symptom such as an aura, abnormal focal movement abnormality, or even staring behavior leading to a diagnosis of partial seizure that has generalized. A focal finding on CT scan suggests a partial seizure that has secondarily generalized.

Aside from the seizure activity itself, seizures may have harmful secondary traumatic or metabolic consequences. They may result in a fall or a motor vehicle accident. The convulsive movements of a seizure may result in injury from direct trauma to head, trunk, or limbs. There is typically a period of transient apnea and hypoxia, the duration of which varies with the duration of seizure activity. There is an increase in blood pressure, serum lactate and serum glucose levels, and white blood cell (WBC) count without a left shift. Body temperature is frequently elevated. (14). Lactic acidosis occurs within 60 seconds of a convulsive event and normalizes within 1 hour after ictus (12). A transient cerebrospinal fluid pleocytosis of up to 20 WBC/μL has been reported to occur in 2% to 23% of seizure patients (Table 113.2).

TABLE 113.2.   Physiologic and Systemic Consequences of Convulsive Seizures

Physiologic
Hyperthermia
Acidosis
Hypoglycemia/hyperglycemia
Hypoxia
Acidosis
Leukocytosis
Cerebrospinal fluid pleocytosis

Systemic
Central nervous system edema
Pulmonary edema
Hypertension followed by hypotension
Dysrhythmias
Rhabdomyolysis
Disseminated intravascular coagulation
Fractures/dislocations

DIFFERENTIAL DIAGNOSIS

Emergency physicians encounter a number of clinical scenarios involving seizures: new onset seizures; patients with known seizures presenting with recurrent seizures; conditions that are not seizures, but can be mistaken for a seizure. Such conditions include syncope, arrhythmia, migraine, vertigo, sleep disorders, decerebrate posturing, drug reactions, tetanus, strychnine poisoning, and psychogenic events. A detailed history and physical can usually differentiate among these.

Syncope can be associated with occasional twitching movements that can be misdiagnosed as a seizure and can be called *convulsive syncope*. Full tonic–clonic movements, tongue biting, and postictal amnesia have not been commonly described in convulsive syncope. When put in the context of when and where the event occurred, length of event, and type of movements, convulsive syncope can usually be reliably differentiated from seizure.

Migraine with an aura can be confused with nonconvulsive seizures. This is compounded by the finding that many migraine patients have abnormal electroencephalograms (EEGs). Basilar migraine can result in loss of consciousness, making the differentiation even more difficult.

Other entities that have been confused with seizures include narcolepsy, hyperventilation syndrome, hypoglycemia, and dystonic reactions. Of note, tonic, clonic, and tonic–clonic seizures are associated with altered consciousness, while dystonic reactions are not.

Psychogenic seizures, also referred to as pseudoseizures, are functional events with a clinical presentation mimicking neurogenic seizures, yet with no corresponding alteration in EEG activity. These events are often conversion reactions and not under the patient's conscious control. It is estimated that 20% of patients followed in epilepsy clinics are misdiagnosed and actually have psychogenic seizures (6).

Psychogenic seizures often last longer than neurogenic events, frequently for more than 5 minutes. There usually is not a postictal period; patients can often recall events during the seizure, have not been incontinent, and do not incur physical injury. However, it must be stressed that exceptions to the aforementioned are commonly found, including incontinence and prolonged postictal periods. Psychogenic seizures are classically manifested by forward-thrusting pelvic movements and head-turning from side to side (6).

Several maneuvers and tests are useful in diagnosing psychogenic seizures. These patients often avoid or resist noxious stimuli. They may display gaze aversion and look away from an examiner, regardless of position. On laboratory testing, psychogenic seizure patients do not have a metabolic acidosis, which is nearly universal with generalized convulsive seizures. Furthermore, there is not a postictal increase in serum prolactin levels.

The medical causes of new seizures may be the result of acute or progressive neurologic insults or systemic stressors, and the evaluation of the patient with seizures must always look for those potentially reversible or treatable causes (Table 113.3). The two most commonly identified etiologic antecedents to seizures are neurologic injury from birth (8%) and cerebrovascular disease (11%) (7). Other identified etiologies of secondary seizures include trauma (5.5%), neoplasm (4%), degenerative disease (3.5%), and infection (2.5%). In the elderly the cause of seizure is more likely to be vascular (stroke), degenerative or neoplastic, than the causes in the young (2).

Metabolic and toxin-related etiologies must always be considered in the differential diagnosis, and are often the most reversible. Hypoglycemia is the most common metabolic cause of seizures; hyponatremia, hypocalcemia, and hypomagnesemia are much less common (18). Interestingly, the metabolic encephalopathies, such as nonketotic hyperglycemia and uremia,

TABLE 113.3. Etiology of Seizures
I. Idiopathic
II. Structural
A. Degenerative disease (e.g., multiple sclerosis, tuberous sclerosis)
B. Neoplasm
C. Scar from birth trauma, other trauma, anoxic damage
III. Infection: Bacterial, Viral, Parasitic, Syphilitic
A. Meningitis
B. Encephalitis
C. Abscess
IV. Metabolic
A. Hypoglycemia
B. Hyperosmolar states
C. Hyponatremia
D. Hypocalcemia
E. Hypomagnesemia
F. Hypoxia
G. Uremia
H. Thyroid disease
I. Nutritional deficiency
V. Toxin
A. Drug withdrawal
1. Alcohol
2. Benzodiazepine
3. Antiepileptic drug
B. Drug overdose
1. Isoniazid
2. Tricyclic antidepressant
3. Anticholinergics, including antihistamines
4. Salicylates
5. Theophylline
6. Gamma-hydroxybutyrate
7. Cocaine and related stimulants
VI. Vascular
A. Subdural hematoma
B. Epidural hematoma
C. Intraparenchymal hemorrhage
D. Stroke
E. Subarachnoid hemorrhage
F. Arteriovenous malformation
VII. Eclampsia

can cause both focal and generalized seizures. Alcohol is the toxin most commonly associated with seizures, followed by tricyclic antidepressants, anticholinergics, cocaine, amphetamines, antihistamines, theophylline, and isoniazid. Drug withdrawal, including noncompliance with anticonvulsant medications in patients with a known seizure disorder, is a leading cause of recurrent seizures (14).

Acute central nervous system (CNS) infections are responsible for 4% to 12% of acute isolated seizures and up to 28% of cases of refractory status epilepticus.

A number of physiologic and psychological stressors can activate seizure disorders. These stressors include fatigue, sleep deprivation, hyperventilation, photic stimulation, emotional stress, and menstruation. In rare cases, seizures can be triggered by colors, objects, music, and voices. Pregnancy can also result in the onset of a seizure disorder, separate from eclamptic seizures.

EMERGENCY DEPARTMENT EVALUATION

History and Physical

The evaluation of the patient who has had a seizure should begin with a careful history that includes a description of the event and an indication of the frequency, pattern, and duration of recent or previous seizures. A history of incontinence, loss of consciousness, and self-injury during the event are important. It should be determined whether there was an aura or a postictal period. Every attempt should be made to interview observers and EMS to obtain a clear description of the seizure to avoid misdiagnosing nonseizure events. Inciting factors such as medication noncompliance, infection, pregnancy, sleep deprivation, alcohol use, or other drug or medication use should be identified. A history of head trauma, headaches, diabetes, cancer, cerebrovascular disease, electrolyte imbalances, or infections can prove vital to making a diagnosis.

The physical examination begins with the vital signs, which can provide important red flags of underlying pathology. Signs of trauma should be sought, and a careful neurologic examination performed. Both unilateral and bilateral pupillary dilatation as a result of seizure has been reported. Postictal patients often have hyperreflexia, upgoing toes, evidence of incontinence, or a tongue laceration. A focal deficit can represent a metabolic derangement such as hypoglycemia, an old lesion, new intracranial pathology, or a Todd paralysis secondary to the seizure. Todd paralysis can be manifested as either a motor or a sensory deficit. Although it typically resolves within hours of seizure, neuroimaging is usually necessary to differentiate a Todd paralysis from other causes of acute focal neurologic dysfunction.

Note should be made of the patient's mental status before and after a seizure. Postictal confusion is common, but almost always resolves over a few hours. Other causes of altered mental status must be strongly considered in patients whose mental status remains impaired, or when family or friends note an abnormally long postictal phase or unusual behavior manifestations. It is estimated that approximately 15% of patients treated for convulsive status epilepticus continue to be in nonconvulsive status after their motor activity is controlled; this unrecognized status may be a factor in the high mortality associated with status epilepticus and suggests the need for EEG monitoring if there is a prolonged "postictal" period (6). Causes of altered mental status in patients who have had a seizure are listed in Table 113.4.

Lab Testing

Patients are often brought to the emergency department after having had an episode of loss of consciousness of unknown

TABLE 113.4.   Causes of Altered Mental Status in Patients Who Have Had a Seizure

Postictal state
Persistent nonconvulsive seizures
Metabolic abnormality
Hyperosmolar state
Central nervous system infection
Central nervous system vascular event
Drug effect
Psychiatric dysfunction

cause. The differential diagnosis in these difficult cases includes seizures, and there are clues that can suggest that a seizure occurred. Laboratory testing in postictal patients often demonstrates a metabolic acidosis or an elevated serum creatine phosphokinase level. These findings can be helpful and should be sought, but, unfortunately, they are time and patient dependent and their absence does not rule out the possibility that a seizure occurred.

The details of the history and physical examination should dictate the urgency and course of any further emergency department evaluation. Of all laboratory tests, serum glucose determination followed by a serum sodium determination has been found to be the most valuable in diagnosing an unsuspected etiology of seizure (1,15). The decision to measure other electrolytes, creatinine, blood urea nitrogen, calcium, and magnesium is based on the individual patient assessment; generally, these tests are of limited value in patients with no underlying medical problems who have returned to baseline. An arterial blood gas analysis is indicated when hypoxia or an underlying acidosis is suspected. A pregnancy test should be obtained in all women of childbearing age (1). Serum antiepileptic drug levels should be checked in patients taking such medications and in those who have had a seizure when a history cannot be obtained (Table 113.5). Such therapeutic levels are available for phenytoin, carbamazepine, valproate and phenobarbital. Serum levels of most of the newer anti-epileptic drugs cannot be measured rapidly in most hospitals.

TABLE 113.5.   Drugs Used in the Treatment of Epilepsy

Drug	Trade Name	Route	Seizure Type	Loading Dose (mg/kg)	Daily Dose for Adults (mg)	Therapeutic Range (μg/mL)
Phenytoin	Dilantin	PO, i.v.	P, GC	20	300–400	10–20
Fosphenytoin	Cerebex	i.v., i.m.	P, GC	20	—	10–20
Carbamazepine[a]	Tegretol	PO	P, GC	—	800–1,600	6–12
Valproate[b]	Depakene	PO	All	—	1,000–3,000	50–120
Divalproex sodium	Depakote	PO	All	—	1,000–4,800	50–120
	Depacon	i.v.	All	10–20	—	50–120
Phenobarbital		PO, i.v., i.m.	P, GC	10–20	90–150	15–35
Primidone	Mysoline	PO	P, GC	—	750–1,250	6–12
Clonazepam	Klonopin	PO	A, M	—	1.5–20.0	0.02–0.08
Ethosuximide[c]	Zarontin	PO	A	—	750–1,250	40–100
Lamotrigine	Lamictal	PO	All	—	200–600	—
Felbamate[d]	Felbatol	PO	P, GC	—	1,800–4,800	—
Gabapentin[e]	Neurontin	PO	P, GC	—	900–3,600	—
Topiramate	Topamax	PO	P, GC	—	200–600	—
Tiagabine		PO	P, GC	—	32–48	—
Diazepam[f]	Diastat	Rectal	All	0.2–0.5	—	—

PO, orally; i.v., intravenous; P, partial seizure; GC, generalized seizure; i.m., intramuscular; A, absence seizure; M, myoclonic seizure.
[a] Drug of choice for partial seizures, with or without secondary generalization.
[b] Drug of choice for primary generalized tonic–clonic seizures.
[c] Drug of choice for absence seizures.
[d] Associated with aplastic anemia in one in 5,000 patients; hepatic failure in one in 30,000.
[e] Only anticonvulsant that is renally metabolized; recommended in patients with multiple medical problems.
[f] Used primarily in children to control clusters of breakthrough seizures.

Alcohol is by far the most common drug of abuse associated with seizures, followed by cocaine. Serum alcohol, salicylate, lithium and theophylline levels and urine drug-screening tests should be ordered based on clinical suspicion. It is worth remembering that patients with epilepsy can have other medical problems (e.g., depression), so other possibilities (e.g., tricyclic overdose) should not be overlooked. An ECG should be done in all cases as a screen for tricyclic overdose.

Patients who have had a seizure but who are not immunocompromised and who do not have an abnormal mental status, fever, or meningeal signs do not require a lumbar puncture as part of their emergency department evaluation (5). However, seizures, especially status epilepticus, are associated with hyperthermia, leukocytosis, and altered mental status, thus often forcing consideration of meningitis. It is also important to note that, as mentioned previously, seizures can cause cerebrospinal fluid pleocytosis, further confusing the issue occasionally. Antibiotics, once started, must be continued until cerebrospinal fluid culture results are available.

Neuroimaging and EEG

Computed tomographic (CT) scanning of the head should be performed in the emergency department when an acute intracranial event, such as subdural or subarachnoid hemorrhage, is suspected. Patients with acute trauma, a past history of malignancy, or with an abnormal neurologic examination, are most likely to have an abnormal imaging study. Special populations should also have a CT scan performed. These include immunocompromised hosts, the elderly who have a higher incidence of focal findings, and immigrants from countries where cysticercosis is endemic.

All patients who have had a first-time seizure will need an imaging study, but not necessarily an emergent CT scan obtained during the emergency department stay. If the patient has a normal mental status and neurologic examination and is judged to be reliable for follow up, it is reasonable, after consultation with a neurologist, to arrange for outpatient magnetic resonance imaging (MRI). MRI is superior to CT scanning in identifying structural epileptogenic abnormalities (2).

EEG monitoring is not a standard practice in the emergency department, yet there are clear indications for its use on an emergent basis. Any patient with altered mental status in whom nonconvulsive status epilepticus is suspected requires an emergent EEG. An emergent EEG is also indicated in patients with refractory status epilepticus who have been managed with paralysis or intravenous anesthetic agents for refractory status epilepticus.

Additional laboratory and radiographic testing may be indicated to identify underlying complicating factors, such as cardiac dysrhythmia, urinary tract infection, sepsis, or pulmonary disease.

EMERGENCY DEPARTMENT MANAGEMENT

Most seizures are self-limited and do not require immediate intervention. If the patient is seen during the seizure, the focus should be on protecting the patient from injury, but objects should not be forced into the patient's mouth. Patients who have experienced a seizure once are at risk for recurrent seizure episodes, so proper precautions should be taken to keep the guard rails on stretchers up and to prevent the patient from ambulating unaccompanied.

First-Time Seizures

Patients who have had a single, unprovoked seizure have about a 35% risk of recurrence within the next 5 years; the risk of recur-

rences increases to approximately 75% after two or three seizures (11). When a cause of the seizure is identified, management is based on the underlying pathology. When no cause can be identified, a risk–benefit analysis regarding initiation of antiepileptic therapy must be performed. There are significant psychological and social consequences of a diagnosis of epilepsy (i.e., individual state limitations on driving cars), as well as potential dangers from the chronic use of antiepileptic medications. Thus, one must be cautious when labeling patients as epileptic and instituting treatment from the emergency department.

For most first-time seizures, if a head CT was not indicated, or if one is done and is negative, the patient can be discharged with very close follow up by a primary care physician or neurologist. If such follow up cannot be assured, a neurologist should see the patient prior to discharge.

If there is a structural cause noted on CT scan that does not need emergent intervention, such as calcification suggestive of cysticercosis or a remote ischemic lesion—the patient should be started on an antiepileptic drug in consultation with a neurologist. Similarly, in the case of a patient who has had prior seizures, but is not on any medications, an antiepileptic drug should be started.

Choice of drug is based upon the type of seizure and ease of achieving therapeutic serum levels. First-line medications that are effective for both primary generalized seizures and partial seizures with or without secondary generalization are carbamazepine, phenytoin and valproate. Of these, phenytoin (and fosphenytoin) are more commonly available for intravenous loading in emergency departments although some may have intravenous valproate. Oral carbamazepine may take days to reach therapeutic levels.

Intravenous phenytoin loading, 15–20 mg/kg, can be accomplished quickly and leads to therapeutic blood levels within 1 hour of the infusion's completion. Intravenous phenytoin loading can be associated with local infusion site irritation and even necrosis if extravasation occurs. Confusion, ataxia and hypotension—due to the diluent propylene glycol—are dose- and rate-related effects and so infusions should not be run faster than 50 mg/min in adults. Fosphenytoin is a water-soluble disodium phosphate ester of phenytoin, which does not need a propylene glycol vehicle and has a more physiologic pH than does phenytoin. It has fewer side effects than phenytoin, though rapid infusion can still cause hypotension, ataxia, and confusion. Fosphenytoin is measured in phenytoin equivalents (PE) and so its dosing is the same 20 mg (PE) as phenytoin though it can be given at up to 150 mg (PE)/min. Fosphenytoin can also be given safely by the intramuscular route, with 100% bioavailability and therapeutic serum levels within 1 hour of a loading dose (7). Oral phenytoin loading is another option; it results in unpredictable absorption, however, with only 60% of patients being therapeutic at 12 hours after a 1-g dose. A daily maintenance dose of 300 mg can be given at bedtime, although, in some patients, divided dosing can provide better seizure control by minimizing variations in the blood level.

Recurrence of Seizures in Patients with Known Seizure Disorder

Noncompliance with anticonvulsant medication is, by far, the most common cause of seizure recurrence in a patient with a known seizure disorder. A patient who has been on phenytoin, but has a subtherapeutic level, should be given supplemental intravenous phenytoin or fosphenytoin to raise serum levels in the therapeutic range. Intramuscular fosphenytoin is another option and eliminates the need for infusion pumps and cardiac monitoring. The patient can then be discharged with instructions to resume oral dosing within 12 hours. Likewise, patients with subtherapeutic valproic acid levels can be supplemented with intravenous valproic acid administered over 1 hour at a rate no faster than 20 mg/min, and discharged on their oral regimen.

Patients managed on carbamazepine that have a seizure due to noncompliance present more of a management problem because this drug cannot be loaded orally or intravenously. In these cases, especially if the level is undetectable, consideration should be given to loading the patient with phenytoin and continuing on this drug until therapeutic levels of carbamazepine are achieved.

Patients who have seizures despite therapeutic anticonvulsant levels must be evaluated carefully for precipitating factors such as infection, new anatomic lesions, or new medications. Decisions to increase the drug dose should be made only after communication with the patient's primary care physician. A second anticonvulsant should be added to the patient's regimen only when seizures are refractory to monotherapy and there are clinical signs of toxicity.

The evaluation of pregnant patients with new-onset seizures should follow the same principle as in other patients. However, if no etiology is identified, anticonvulsants should be withheld and the patient referred for close follow up. Eclampsia is an additional consideration in patients at more than 20 weeks' gestation (see Chapter 97, Hypertensive Disorders of Pregnancy).

Noncompliance and sleep deprivation are the two most common causes of seizure recurrence in pregnant patients with epilepsy (4). Active seizures should be treated pharmacologically just as in the nonpregnant patient because the risks to the fetus of seizure-related hypoxia and acidosis are greater than the potential teratogenicity of anticonvulsant medications. Phenytoin and phenobarbital have similar teratogenetic profiles; carbamazepine is probably the safest of the anticonvulsants to use in pregnancy. Beyond 24 weeks' gestation, fetal monitoring should be provided during and after a seizure.

Alcohol-Related Seizures

Alcohol-related seizures deserve special mention because alcohol use is frequently involved in patients presenting to emergency departments with seizures. Alcohol-withdrawal seizures classically occur 6 to 48 hours after a significant reduction in the serum alcohol level, but they have also been associated with *rising* blood ethanol levels in some patients.

Alcohol-related seizures are temporally associated with alcohol use but are not necessarily solely the result of the alcohol. Alcoholics are susceptible to cerebrovascular insults, trauma, metabolic disorders, and infections, and are thus at increased risk for seizures.

Management of the alcoholic who has had a seizure focuses on determining whether the event was a withdrawal seizure or due to another etiology. Patients with a first-time alcohol-related seizure should be evaluated fully in the same manner as any other patient.

The diagnosis of alcohol-withdrawal seizures is based on the history, and the clinician must always consider the possibility that another etiology is responsible. There is no good evidence to support the use of phenytoin either acutely or chronically in the management of alcohol-withdrawal seizures. Benzodiazepines alone are sufficient to prevent successive withdrawal seizures in the acute setting. Patients who have had one alcohol-withdrawal seizure should be treated with lorazepam 2 mg intravenously. Following this, if they have been observed to remain seizure-free and at baseline mental status for 6 hours with no evidence of withdrawal, they can be discharged if a suitable environment is available (3,25).

Psychogenic Seizures

Psychogenic seizures should be suspected in patients who are refractory to anticonvulsants and whose clinical presentation is atypical. The diagnosis is suspected particularly when a convulsing patient does not have a metabolic acidosis, and it can be confirmed, when possible, by demonstrating that an abnormal EEG does not accompany the clinical convulsion. Management of psychogenic seizures is dependent on making the correct diagnosis; although this sounds obvious, the anxiety associated with evaluating a convulsing patient often leads to the initiation of pharmacologic interventions before an adequate assessment can be performed (8). The key to management is avoiding iatrogenic harm by aggressive pharmacologic interventions or supportive measures such as intubation. Long-term management usually involves a comprehensive evaluation in an epilepsy monitoring unit, with a coordinated approach involving both an epileptologist and a psychiatrist.

Status Epilepticus

The management of convulsive status epilepticus involves simultaneous maintenance of the patient's airway, breathing, and circulation; diagnostic testing; and pharmacologic intervention (Fig. 113.1). Status epilepticus tends to occur more frequently in patients with an underlying neurologic insult, either old or new, and refractory status epilepticus almost always indicates the presence of an underlying CNS disorder. Morbidity and mortality in status epilepticus is related to the etiology, duration, and systemic consequences of the event. First line agents treat status epilepticus with lorazepam and diazepam, and phenytoin or fosphenytoin. Patients who continue to seize despite aggressive use of these are considered to be in *refractory status epilepticus* and need to be treated with intravenous anesthetic dose of midazolam, propofol or pentobarbital.

Airway support should be aggressive, and continuous pulse oximetry should be employed. Patients should be intubated at any sign of hypoxia or loss of protective gag reflex. Intravenous access should be secured using a nondextrose-containing solution, because phenytoin precipitates if it is inadvertently administered with dextrose (dextrose will not precipitate fosphenytoin). Fluids should be run at keep-open rates unless the patient is hypotensive, because status epilepticus can be associated with both cerebral and pulmonary edema (19). When intubated, short-acting paralytic agents should be used as continued motor activity will be masked by long-acting agents lulling a clinician into a false sense of security. If prolonged paralysis is needed to carry out a procedure, a bedside EEG should be arranged.

The blood glucose level should be checked immediately by bedside testing. Blood should be tested for electrolytes, magnesium, phosphate, calcium, liver and renal function, hematocrit, WBC count, platelet count, antiepileptic drug levels, toxic drug screen (particularly salicylates), and alcohol. The urine should be checked for evidence of rhabdomyolysis, and a pregnancy test should be sent on all women of childbearing age. The family should be questioned for possibility of isoniazid (INH) overdose.

Patients in status epilepticus should be placed on a cardiac monitor, and an electrocardiogram should be done. A nasogastric tube should be placed to prevent gastric distention, and a Foley catheter should be placed to help monitor volume status. A head CT scan should be done at some point in all patients. Consideration should be given to performing a lumbar puncture.

The pharmacologic management of status epilepticus begins while the patient is being stabilized and diagnostic testing performed. Hypoglycemia is treated immediately with thiamine and dextrose. Antibiotics should be given very early in the management of any patient in whom meningitis or sepsis is suspected.

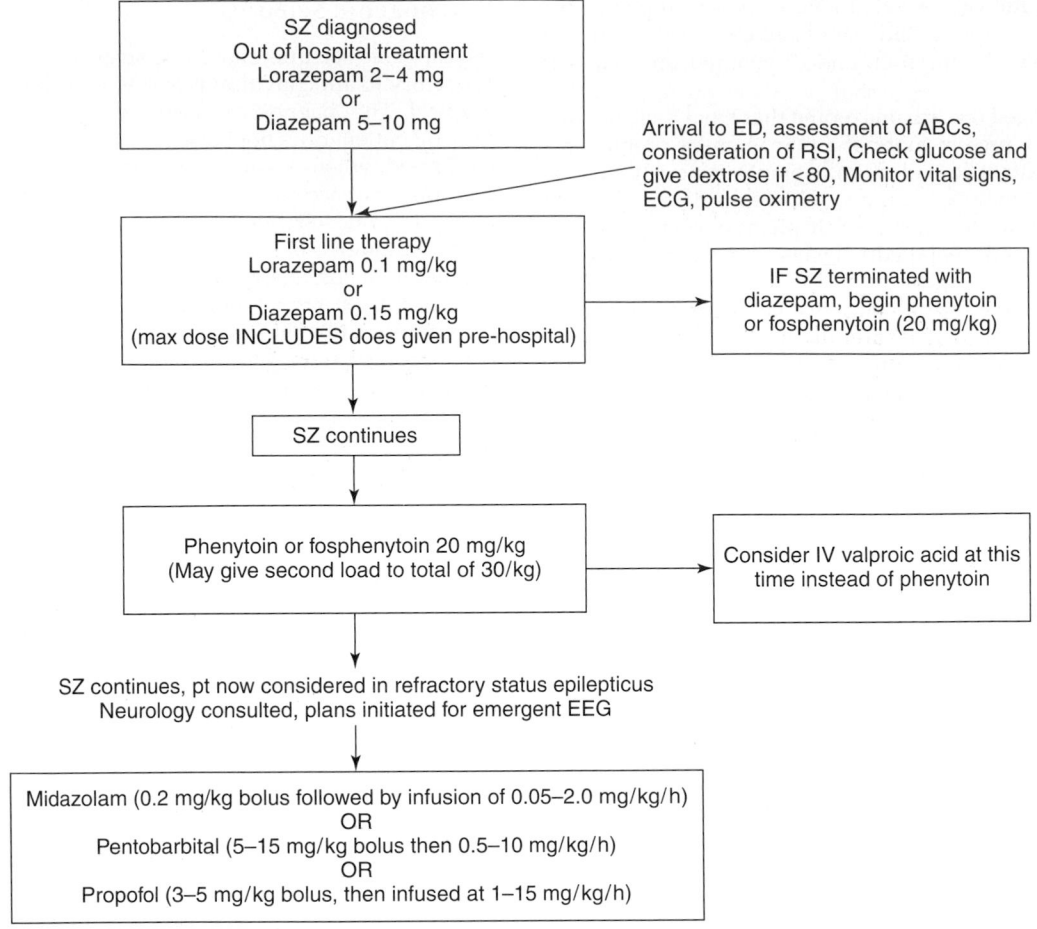

Figure 113.1.   Approach to patient in status epilepticus. (Modified from Shearer P. Status epilepticus. *Ann Emerg Med*)

The benzodiazepines diazepam and lorazepam are considered the first-line drugs in the management of status epilepticus. Lorazepam (0.1 mg/kg IV, up to 10 mg) or diazepam (0.15 mg/kg IV, up to 20 mg) will stop seizures in the majority of cases. Both drugs are efficacious, but lorazepam is preferred because its anticonvulsant action lasts up to 12 hours, compared with 20 minutes for diazepam, which quickly enters but then redistributes out of the CNS. Consequently, if lorazepam terminates the seizure activity, no additional anticonvulsant needs to be immediately given; a long-lasting anticonvulsant such as phenytoin must be added when diazepam is used, otherwise, the patient is at high risk of seizure recurrence (13).

When seizures persist despite a full loading dose of a benzodiazepine, phenytoin or fosphenytoin is added at a rate of 50 mg/min or 150 mg/min, respectively. If seizures persist, the current recommendation is to give additional phenytoin, up to a total dose of 30 mg/kg (13). Consideration may be given to using intravenous valproate instead of phenytoin although it is not as commonly available, and is perhaps best used for patients who are known to have been controlled with it in the past.

Status epilepticus resulting from isoniazid poisoning should be treated with pyridoxine (1 gram IV for each gram of ingested INH). Administer 5 g of pyridoxine if an unknown quantity of INH was ingested.

Status epilepticus that does not terminate at this point is usually the result of some significant underlying CNS lesion. Beyond this, the patients are considered to be in refractory status epilepticus and should be treated with anesthetic doses of midazolam, pentobarbital or propofol. Studies have not shown one to be

better than the other (21). The choice of drug for refractory status epilepticus is made on the basis of accessibility, familiarity with use, the potential role of side effects of each drug, and consideration of the preference of the admitting neurologic service.

Midazolam is given as a loading dose of 0.2 mg/kg and is followed by an infusion of 0.05–2.0 mg/kg/hour (22). Midazolam is often more readily available in an ED than propofol or pentobarbital, and is felt to cause less hypotension.

Pentobarbital is given as 5–15 mg/kg at 25 mg/min, followed by 0.5–10.0 mg/kg/h as an infusion (23). Besides requiring ventilatory support, these patients are at significant risk for hypotension, and therefore require hemodynamic monitoring. Hypotension should be treated with fluids and vasopressors as needed. EEG monitoring should be instituted to evaluate for continued seizure activity (13). Pentobarbital has the longest duration of action of the three agents, making it more difficult to remove when evaluating seizure suppression.

There are limited studies on the efficacy of propofol efficacy in status epilepticus, but there is evidence that it provides almost immediate suppression of seizure activity after a bolus infusion (24). It is rapidly metabolized and can be titrated easily. Propofol is given as a bolus of 3–5 mg/kg followed by an infusion at 1–15 mg/kg/hr. The propofol infusion syndrome of hypotension, lipidemia, rhabdomyolysis, and metabolic acidosis limits the prolonged infusion of propofol in both adults and children (25,26).

Many other intravenous and inhalational drugs have been tried in the management of refractory status epilepticus, but no controlled trials support their use (9). These include continuous infusions of inhalational anesthetics, ketamine, intravenous lidocaine, and rectal chloral hydrate (13,15). Current recommendations would support use of these drugs only if all other measures fail.

Nonconvulsive Status Epilepticus

Nonconvulsive status epilepticus presents as altered mental status ranging from a mild behavioral alteration noticeable only to family or friends to frank coma (10,16). Other manifestations may include speech arrest, cognitive deficits, delusions, paranoia, hallucinations, or psychosis. Because, by definition, there is rarely a significant motor component, the diagnosis is often missed, and there are many case reports of these patients initially being diagnosed with a psychiatric illness. Nonconvulsive status epilepticus has been reported in every age group, can be the initial presentation of a seizure disorder, and has been reported to last as long as 8 weeks.

The diagnosis should be suspected in patients with a seizure history who present with a prolonged postictal period or an unusual behavior pattern. It should also be considered in patients without a seizure history who present with altered mental status of undetermined etiology. The diagnosis is made by electroencephalography. Treatment is the same as for convulsive status epilepticus, beginning with lorazepam, 2 mg/min, until the EEG normalizes or a total of 10 mg is administered. This should be followed by phenytoin loading, although it is questionable whether phenytoin is effective in absence status (17).

CRITICAL INTERVENTIONS

- Check a rapid glucose in patients with seizures or refractory status epilepticus
- Protect actively seizing patients from injury
- Administer rapid, aggressive benzodiazepine therapy for status epilepticus
- Provide aggressive airway for patients in status epilepticus and intubate if signs of hypoxia or loss of protective gag reflex

DISPOSITION

The disposition of patients who have had a seizure depends on the etiology of the event and, often, on the socioeconomic environment to which the patient will return. Of prime importance is communication with the primary care provider who will be responsible for following up on the patient's diagnostic tests and medications.

Hospital admission should be considered when the cause of a seizure is unclear, when seizure recurrence has not been controlled, when the seizure is secondary to a treatable underlying illness, or when there is concern that the patient will not receive timely outpatient evaluation. All patients who have been in status epilepticus should be admitted, usually to an intensive care setting.

COMMON PITFALLS

- ✔ Failure to maintain and protect the airway during the management of status epilepticus
- ✔ Infusion of phenytoin with a dextrose solution
- ✔ Failure to perform a complete secondary survey in postictal patients
- ✔ Assumption that altered mental status is due to a postictal state and failure to consider other possible etiologies
- ✔ Confusion of decerebrate posturing for a tonic seizure
- ✔ Failure to obtain a pregnancy test in women of childbearing age
- ✔ Failure to make a reasonable effort to obtain witnesses' accounts of a seizure
- ✔ Failure to recognize a psychogenic seizure as a nonneurologic event
- ✔ Failure to advise a patient who has had a seizure not to drive or operate dangerous equipment
- ✔ Increasing a patient's anticonvulsant medication dose without obtaining a proper history for precipitating stressors or medication compliance
- ✔ Failure to communicate with the primary care provider

Acknowledgment

Thanks to previous edition's chapter author Silvana Riggio.

References

1. American College of Emergency Physicians. Clinical policy for the initial approach to patients presenting with a chief complaint of seizure, who are not in status epilepticus. *Ann Emerg Med* 1997;29:706.
2. American College of Emergency Physicians, American Academy of Neurology, American Association of Neurological Surgeons, American Society of Neuroradiology. Practice parameter: neuroimaging in the emergency patient presenting with seizure [Summary Statement]. *Ann Emerg Med* 1996;27:113.
3. Chance J. Emergency department treatment of alcohol withdrawal seizures with phenytoin. *Ann Emerg Med* 1991;20:520.
4. Delgado-Escueta A, Janz D. Consensus guidelines: preconception counseling, management, and care of the pregnant woman with epilepsy. *Neurology* 1992;42[Suppl 5]:149–161.
5. Engel J. Diagnostic evaluation. In: Engle J, ed. *Seizures and epilepsy.* Philadelphia: FA Davis Co, 1989:312.
6. Gates J, Ramini V, Whalen S. Ictal characteristics of pseudoseizures. *Epilepsia* 1983;24:246.
7. Hauser W, Anneger J, Kurland L. Incidence of epilepsy and unprovoked seizures in Rochester, Minnesota: 1935–1984. *Epilepsia* 1993;34:453.
8. Howell S, Owen L, Chadwick D. Pseudostatus epilepticus. *Q J Med* 1989;71:507.
9. Jagoda A, Riggio S. Refractory status epilepticus in adults. *Ann Emerg Med* 1993;22:1337.
10. Lee S. Nonconvulsive status epilepticus: ictal confusion in later life. *Arch Neurol* 1985;42:778.
11. Lowenstein D, Alldredge B. Status epilepticus. *N Engl J Med* 1998;338:970.
12. Orringer C, Eustace J, Wunsch C, et al. Natural history of lactic acidosis after grand-mal seizure. *N Engl J Med* 1977;297:796.
13. Osorio I, Reed R. Treatment of refractory generalized tonic clonic status epilepticus with pentobarbital anesthesia after high dose phenytoin. *Epilepsia* 1989;30:464.
14. Simon R. Physiologic consequences of status epilepticus. *Epilepsia* 1985; 26[Suppl 1]:58.
15. Tardy B, LaFond P, Convers P, et al. Adult first generalized seizure: etiology, biological tests, EEG, CT scan, in an ED. *Am J Emerg Med* 1995;13:1.
16. Tomson T, Lindbom U, Nilsson B. Nonconvulsive status epilepticus in adults: thirty-two consecutive patients from a general hospital population. *Epilepsia* 1992;33:829.
17. Treiman D, Meyers P, Walton N, et al. A comparison of four treatments for generalized convulsive status epilepticus. *N Engl J Med* 1998;339:792.
18. Turnbull T, Vanden Hoed T, Howes D, et al. Utility of laboratory studies in the emergency department patient with a new-onset seizure. *Ann Emerg Med* 1990;19:373.
19. Working Group on Status Epilepticus. Treatment of convulsive status epilepticus: recommendations of the Epilepsy Foundation of America's working group on status epilepticus. *JAMA* 1993;270:854.
20. Schold C, Yarnell PR, Earnest MP. Origin of seizures in elderly patients. *JAMA* 1977;238:1177–1178.
21. Claassen J, Hirsch LJ, Emerson RG, Mayer SA. Treatment of refractory status epilepticus with pentobarbital, propofol, or midazolam: a systematic review. *Epilepsia* 2002;43:146–153.
22. Kumar A, Bleck TP. Intravenous midazolam for the treatment of refractory status epilepticus. *Crit Care Med* 1992;20:483–488.
23. Manno EM. New management strategies in the treatment of status epilepticus. *Mayo Clin Proc.* 2003;78:508–518.
24. Brown LA, Levin GM. Role of propofol in refractory status epilepticus. *Annals of Pharmacotherapy,* 1998;32:1053–1059.
25. Bray, RJ. Propofol infusion syndrome in children. *Paed Anesth,* 1998;8:491–499.
26. Vasile B, Rasulo F, Candiani A, Latronico N. The pathophysiology of the propofol infusion syndrome: a simple name for a complex problem. *Intensive Care Med,* 2003;29:1417–1425.
27. D'Onofrio G; Rathlev NK, Ulrich AS, Fish SS, Freedland ES. Lorazepam for the prevention of recurrent seizures related to alcohol. *N Engl J Med* 1999;340:915–919.

CHAPTER 114
Transient Global Amnesia

Lauren Grossman and Richard M. Kaplan

Transient global amnesia (TGA) is a distinct clinical entity characterized by an abrupt, but transient, inability to form new memories and acquire new information. Because TGA is relatively uncommon, its incidence is not well documented; however, it appears to be diagnosed with a frequency of 5 to 32 episodes per 100,000 population annually (11). Three pathophysiologic explanations for TGA have been hypothesized, but none have been proven clinically; these are that TGA represents: (1) a cerebrovascular accident akin to a transient ischemic attack; (2) seizure activity manifesting as a pure amnestic episode; or (3) a migraine-related syndrome. In support of a nonvascular cause for TGA, Lauria performed a case-control study of 170 patients with TGA who were age-matched with first-time transient ischemic attack (TIA) patients and found that TGA patients had a lower incidence of atrial fibrillation and diabetes than TIA patients (10). Also, the normal controls had a higher prevalence of smoking and diabetes than the TGA population (10).

CLINICAL PRESENTATION

Transient global amnesia is characterized by an abrupt onset of anterograde amnesia (difficulty forming memories of the present and immediate past) that usually lasts only several hours but can last up to a day. The patient, typically older than 50 years of age, is disoriented to time and place but not to self. Phrases and questions are commonly repeated and patients have difficulty making sense of their immediate circumstances, which often leads to noticeable anxiety. The patient remains attentive and can follow commands. Patients may be able to perform simple cognitive tests well (i.e., memorizing a list of words, spelling "world" backwards), but they forget their responses moments later and typically forget that the task was performed at all (2). Motor skills, speech, language, personality, alertness and judgment remain intact. The neurologic exam is nonfocal. During the episode the patient may behave in a completely normal fashion, and only directed questioning reveals the disorientation and short-term memory deficit.

It is imperative to obtain an accurate history regarding the specific symptoms that led to the emergency department visit. Patients may complain of symptoms such as hyperventilation, palpitations, dizziness, nausea, presyncope, paresthesias, and a choking sensation that may simply reflect the anxiety caused by their acute sense of disorientation (3). Emotionally intense or stressful events, including sexual activity, physical exertion, and exposure to extremes in temperature or pain have all been temporally related to TGA.

Upon recovery, the patient has complete amnesia to events that occurred during the episode and may complain of a mild headache. In fact, some patients with TGA seek medical attention with a complaint of having "lost" a certain period of time, typically a few hours. There is some evidence that new learning may be impaired for as long as a week following an episode (1).

DIFFERENTIAL DIAGNOSIS

Delirium is defined by the following diagnostic criteria: (1) inattention, (2) an acute onset over hours to days with a fluctuating course, (3) disorganized thinking, and (4) altered level of consciousness (4). In TGA, there is an acute onset but the course is not a fluctuating one. There may appear to be disorganized thinking, but only because the patient is having difficulty connecting one moment to the next. There is no illogical or incoherent conversation. The patient with TGA clearly does not have an altered level of consciousness.

Stressful events and anxiety disorders are sometimes associated with an acute onset of *psychogenic amnesia*. Hysterical amnesia occurs in young females who may or may not have a history of anxiety disorders but who may under emotional stress experience an acute amnesia and may come to medical attention seeking their identity.

The clinical findings in patients with *complex partial seizures* may also mimic those of TGA. TGA differs from any classical definition of a seizure in several important ways. There is no warning or aura related to the onset of TGA and no postictal period. An episode of TGA usually lasts hours, whereas a seizure typically lasts only seconds to minutes. Patients with TGA do not experience incontinence, and the vital signs should remain within normal limits. In patients undergoing EEG testing during an episode of TGA, there have been rare findings of brain wave slowing but no epileptiform patterns (7).

Cerebrovascular insufficiency in memory-related areas of the brain, due to a transient ischemic attack (TIA) or other hemodynamic compromise, could theoretically cause transient memory loss. However, patients diagnosed with an episode of TGA do not have a higher incidence of vascular risk factors than the population at large, unlike those experiencing TIAs. Moreover, patients with TGA have a benign prognosis, in contrast to patients who have had a TIA and frequently go on to have a major stroke (3).

TGA can be confused with migraine since both can be associated with transient behavioral changes or complaints. However, migraine typically presents with a prodrome and unilateral head pain associated with nausea.

Hypoglycemia, hyperglycemia, hyponatremia, uremia and hypocalcemia can be associated with a change in mental status and in some cases, a presyncopal, syncopal or a seizure-like event that may be confused with an episode of TGA. Glucose and electrolyte determinations distinguish these conditions from TGA.

Several cases have been reported of young healthy climbers at very high altitudes who experienced TGA. There were no injuries, signs of neurologic abnormalities, or symptoms related to hypoxia. Upon partial descent from altitude, their symptoms resolved completely and they were later able to tolerate even higher altitudes than those at which they had become confused (6).

Illicit or prescription drugs can cause confusion or delirium. Specifically, there are case reports describing an association between Sildenafil (Viagra) and apparent TGA (12). Toxins such as solvents or heavy metals, as well as drug withdrawal, can cause similar symptoms.

Chronic alcoholism and vitamin B deficiencies can cause an amnestic disorder called Korsakoff syndrome. Patients have chronic memory loss, confusion, peripheral neuropathies, nystagmus and ophthalmoplegia.

Retrograde amnesia (difficulty recalling events from the immediate recent past) and anterograde amnesia (inability to learn new information following the injury) occur with head trauma. This may be confused with TGA which has anterograde amnesia as the prominent feature.

EMERGENCY DEPARTMENT EVALUATION

TGA is a diagnosis that can be made almost entirely by a thorough history and the help of a reliable witness to the events preceding the hospital visit. The physical exam, including a complete neurologic exam, reveals normal findings. Glucose and electrolytes, including calcium should be obtained in patients with amnestic symptoms.

CT scan of the brain is usually obtained on patients with TGA, but is of questionable utility. Pai noted that of 17 patients with TGA, two CT abnormalities were noted, an old left and a right thalamic infarct (8). Zorzon reviewed 50 head CTs on patients diagnosed with TGA and observed one left occipital and one right temporal infarction (9). However, no clear relationship between any head CT findings and TGA has been identified.

EMERGENCY DEPARTMENT MANAGEMENT

TGA is a benign condition with a good prognosis. No particular treatment is recommended, however, some practitioners suggest beginning daily aspirin, despite the fact that no vascular component has been identified.

When the diagnosis is made, the patient and family require reassurance regarding the benign nature of the disease and the excellent prognosis.

CRITICAL INTERVENTIONS

- Obtain an accurate and detailed history reported by reliable observer
- Perform a thorough neurologic exam
- Reassure the patient (this may have to be repeated frequently) and the patient's family or companions

DISPOSITION

The typical patient with TGA has an uncomplicated course and a complete recovery. Recurrences, although reported, are not the rule. If the diagnosis is clear and the episode has resolved, the patient can be discharged, preferably accompanied by family or friends.

If the episode is still in progress or if there is any question about the diagnosis, the patient should be admitted for observation, neurology consultation, and a further work up that may include a diffusion-weighted MRI and an EEG.

COMMON PITFALLS

✔ Failure to consider the diagnosis

References

1. Adams RD, Victor M, Ropper AH. *Principles of Neurology.* New York: McGraw-Hill, 1997;429–430.
2. Brown, J. ED Evaluation of Transient Global Amnesia. *Ann Emerg Med* 1997;30:522–526.
3. Pantoni, L., Lamassa M., Inzitari D. Transient Global Amnesia: A Review Emphasizing Pathogenic Aspects. *Acta Neurol Scand* 2000;102:275–283.
4. Johnson, M. Assessing Confused Patients. *Neurology in Practice* 2001;71:i7–12.
5. Fisher, CM. Unexplained Sudden Amnesia. *Arch Neurol* 2002;59:1310–1313.
6. Litch, JA, Bishop, RA. Transient Global Amnesia at High Altitude. *N Engl J Med* 1999;340:1444–1445.
7. Sirven, JI. Acute and Chronic Seizures in Patients Older Than 60 Years. *Mayo Clin Proc* 2001;76:175–183.
8. Pai, MC, Yang SS. Transient Global Amnesia: A Retrospective Study of 25 Patients. *Chinese Med J* 1999;62:140–145.
9. Zorzon M, Antonutti L, Mase G, et al. Transient Global Amnesia and Transient Ischemic Attack. Natural History, Vascular Risk Factors and Associated Conditions. *Stroke* 1995;26:1536–1542.
10. Lauria G, Gentile M, Fassetta G, Casetta I, Caneve G. Transient Global Amnesia and Transient Ischemic Attack: A Community-Based Case-Control Study. *Acta Neurol Scand* 1998;97:381–385.
11. Pantoni L, Lamassa M, Inzitari D. Transient global amnesia: a review emphasizing pathogenic aspects. *Acta Neurol Scand* 2000;102(5):275–283.
12. Gandolfo C, Sugo A, Del Sette M. Sildenafil and transient global amnesia. *Neurol Sci* 2003;24:145–146.

CHAPTER 115
Peripheral Neuropathies

Phyllis A. Vallee and Christopher A. Lewandowski

Peripheral neuropathies are confusing entities for both emergency physicians and neurologists alike. The types and etiologies of peripheral neuropathy are numerous, and the pathophysiology is not well understood in many cases. Nevertheless, only 15% to 30% of patients undergoing intensive evaluation fail to have a diagnosis made (2,7).

The peripheral nervous system begins within the spinal canal with the ventral and dorsal nerve roots. These merge to form the spinal nerves which then supply the visceral nerves, nerve plexuses and peripheral nerves. Several generalizations can be made about the findings attributed to each of these areas. Lesions affecting the dorsal (afferent) roots produce pain, sensory loss and decreased reflexes while muscle strength is preserved. Ventral (efferent) root lesions produce muscle weakness, spasm, and autonomic symptoms without pain. A combination of all these symptoms occurs when spinal nerves are affected. Disorders affecting the visceral fibers will produce autonomic symptoms, which include extreme fluctuations in cardiac rhythm, blood pressure, gastrointestinal motility, urogenital function, sweating and salivation. When faced with disorders of the peripheral nervous system, emergency physicians should attempt to localize the process and determine the chronicity, pattern, and symmetry of symptoms to establish a working differential diagnosis (2,7,24). In general, peripheral neuropathies can be divided into several basic categories: polyneuropathy, plexopathy, radiculopathy, and mononeuropathy.

ACUTE POLYNEUROPATHY

Polyneuropathy results from the simultaneous dysfunction of multiple peripheral nerves. Symptoms include diffuse motor or sensory loss or both, with variable autonomic nervous system dysfunction. Polyneuropathies that develop over several days to

2 weeks are considered acute. Of these, Guillain-Barré syndrome (GBS) is the most common (9,11,18,20).

CLINICAL PRESENTATION

GBS, also known as acute inflammatory demyelinating polyradiculoneuropathy, is a worldwide, nonseasonal, acute polyneuropathy that affects all ages, with a yearly incidence of 0.4 to 2.4 cases per 100,000 population (20,24). Men are affected slightly more than women by a ratio of 1.25 to 1.5 : 1 (9,11,18,20). The exact etiology is unclear, but pathologic examination reveals inflammation and segmental demyelination as the primary defect in 85% of cases, while primary axonal degeneration occurs in 15% of cases (11). Axonal GBS is associated with a more rapid onset, early muscle atrophy and a worse prognosis (24).

Classically, patients experience a prodromal event such as an upper respiratory tract infection, gastroenteritis (in fact, *Campylobacter jejuni* infection, is the most commonly identified pathogen associated with GBS (11,12,24)), surgery, vaccination, or infection with agents such as *Mycoplasma*, the herpesviruses, CMV and the human immunodeficiency virus (HIV). This is followed in 1 to 3 weeks by the onset of distal paresthesias and a symmetric ascending motor paralysis that progresses to its peak over 10 to 14 days. Motor weakness is both proximal and distal, with legs being involved prior to the arms and trunk. Additional findings include hyporeflexia or areflexia within 1 week of symptom onset, mild sensory losses, cranial nerve palsies (facial diplegia occurs in 50% of cases (24)), and autonomic dysfunction. Bowel and bladder disturbances are uncommon (15%) and brief in duration (24). Patients are afebrile and mental status is unaffected. It is not unusual for patients to initially present with low-back, hip, and thigh pain that is confused with disc disease or lumbar strain.

Several atypical presentations or variants of GBS are described, each with its own differential diagnosis. Variants include pure motor GBS, pure sensory GBS, pure pandysautonomia, the Miller Fisher variant of GBS with ophthalmoplegia, ataxia, and areflexia and the regional variants such as pharyngeal-cervical-brachial GBS, and paraparetic GBS. The former four are associated with global areflexia, while the later two demonstrate only regional areflexia (21). The variants make the diagnosis difficult; however, when considering the differential diagnosis of classic GBS, marked or persistent asymmetry of weakness, lack of facial and respiratory muscle weakness in a patient with generalized paralysis, prolonged incontinence, a sharp sensory level, or fever strongly suggests an alternate diagnosis (20,24).

DIFFERENTIAL DIAGNOSIS

Tick Paralysis

Tick paralysis typically affects children in the spring and summer months. An acute ascending motor paralysis nearly identical to GBS results from a toxin present in the saliva of ticks (usually *Dermacentor* in the U.S.) that have been attached to a human host for a period of 5 to 7 days. Unlike GBS, sensory loss and CSF abnormalities are not seen in tick paralysis (24). The diagnosis is made when the offending tick is located, and treatment consists of its removal and supportive care. Symptoms begin to improve within hours of tick removal, and generally resolve completely within 2 to 3 days. One tick species found in Australia, *Ixodes holocyclus,* is associated with paralysis that can progress despite tick removal. For this species, a hyperimmune serum has been developed (10,15).

Botulism

Exposure to botulinum toxin, which inhibits the release of acetylcholine at neuromuscular junctions, usually results from the ingestion of improperly canned foods, GI tract colonization in young infants fed raw honey or, rarely, from cutaneous infection with *Clostridium botulinum*. The toxin is considered a possible weapon of mass terror and exposure may be via ingestion or inhalation. Initial symptoms of botulism begin hours to several days after exposure and include nausea, vomiting, and dry mouth in patients who have ingested the toxin. Neurologic symptoms begin with cranial nerve palsies with prominent ocular findings (e.g., blurred vision, dilated pupils, diplopia). These are rapidly followed by symmetric, descending motor weakness and autonomic dysfunction. Sensation and mental status are not affected and fever is absent. Treatment consists of antitoxin therapy (available through the Centers for Disease Control [CDC]) and supportive care (15) (see Chapter 335, Botulism).

Poliomyelitis-Like Syndromes

In the United States, poliomyelitis is rare and nearly all cases are related to the use of the live attenuated oral vaccine. Patients with polio first develop an acute viral illness with fever, headache, meningeal signs, muscle pain and tenderness. These symptoms are present 1 to 2 days before weakness develops. Polio paralysis is more proximal than distal; legs are involved more than arms; and, classically, involvement is asymmetric. Sensory loss is extremely rare, and its presence should raise the suspicion of other diagnoses. The most serious complication of polio is respiratory muscle paralysis. Progression of paralysis abates when patients become afebrile. A similar paralytic syndrome may occur following infection with other nonpolio enteroviruses (15).

Since the introduction of the West Nile Virus, a flavivirus, into the United States in 1999, there have been case reports of acute flaccid paralysis associated with infection by this agent. Although some reports present a symptom complex nearly identical to GBS (1), investigation by the CDC has characterized the paralysis as being most similar to poliomyelitis with involvement of the anterior horn cells and motor axons. In the CDC series the acute paralysis tended to be asymmetric and presented with an acute febrile illness and evidence of CSF pleocytosis (4).

Diphtheria

Diphtheria begins as a pharyngeal infection caused by an exotoxin-producing *Corynebacterium diphtheriae*. Subsequent toxicity, both cardiac and neurologic, correlates with the severity of the pharyngeal disease. Paralysis of local pharyngeal muscles, followed by cranial nerve palsies, occurs in the first or second week of infection. Cardiac toxicity begins 1 to 2 weeks after the onset of illness. The polyneuropathy, which is mainly motor, does not develop for 5 to 8 weeks. Weakness may begin in all extremities simultaneously, or it may first appear in proximal muscles and then spread distally. Occasionally, the primary site of infection is a skin wound, in which case sensorimotor changes are first noted near the infected wound. Treatment of diphtheria involves use of antitoxin within the first 48 hours of infection. Treatment of the neuropathy consists of supportive care (15,24).

Acute Intermittent Porphyria

In this disorder, stimulation of an enzymatically deficient heme synthesis pathway results in the buildup of neurotoxic precursors. An acute attack classically begins with severe abdominal pain, which is followed by tachycardia, hypertension, and mental status changes. Seizures may occur. A sensorimotor polyneuropathy that can be symmetric or asymmetric, and ascending or descending, may develop and can progress to respiratory failure and death. Treatment consists of intravenous glucose and hematin to shut down the defective pathway, beta blockers to control hypertension, and supportive care (3,7,24).

Heavy Metals

Most neuropathies due to heavy metal poisoning are subacute or chronic. Acute presentations are associated with thallium exposure and massive arsenic exposure. Thallium ingestion produces abdominal pain, vomiting, and diarrhea, followed by painful paresthesias and the rapid onset of diffuse motor weakness. Differentiation from GBS is often made 1 to 2 weeks after the onset of symptoms, when thallium-induced alopecia becomes apparent. Acute arsenic polyneuropathy, which is also clinically similar to GBS, begins 8 to 20 days after a large exposure and is associated with gastrointestinal symptoms, renal failure, hepatic failure, and mental status changes (24).

Others

Acute polyneuropathy may also develop as a complication of collagen vascular disease, critical illness, uremia and dialysis, malignancy, nutritional deficiencies, infectious agents, or a host of toxins and drugs. Generalized weakness produced by metabolic disorders such as acute hypophosphatemia, hypermagnesemia, hyperkalemia, hypokalemia, and periodic paralysis may mimic GBS. Hysteria and malingering should also be considered.

Neurologic and muscular disorders that produce weakness and must be differentiated from GBS include myelopathy, transverse myelitis, lumbar disc disease, myasthenia gravis, and acute myopathy. Within this category, cervical myelopathy deserves added attention. It presents with an ascending paraplegia or quadriplegia and a sensory level. Unlike GBS it is associated with localized neck pain or tenderness, hyperreflexia (unless spinal shock is present) and loss of sphincter tone. Respiratory compromise is not seen unless the cord is involved above the C5 level. Active or passive neck motion may exacerbate symptoms. Acute myelopathy is usually the result of trauma. Subacute myelopathy is seen with neoplasm, subdural or epidural abscess, disc herniation and hematoma; however, these etiologies may present with acute onset of symptoms, especially if the vascular supply to the cord is compromised. Patients that have symptoms suggestive of a myelopathy must undergo rapid imaging with a MRI or CT myelogram as correct diagnosis and intervention may prevent permanent deficits.

EMERGENCY DEPARTMENT EVALUATION AND MANAGEMENT

Patients presenting with the acute onset of weakness warrant rapid assessment of airway, ventilatory capacity, and cardiovascular status. Following stabilization, history and physical examination, including a detailed neurologic examination, are the principal methods of emergency department evaluation. The emergency physician should obtain a complete blood count, serum electrolytes, calcium, magnesium, phosphate, glucose, blood urea nitrogen, creatinine, liver function tests (23), erythrocyte sedimentation rate, chest radiograph, and electrocardiogram on all patients.

Additional studies may be needed to rule out other causes of acute weakness; they include antinuclear antibodies, rheumatoid factor, thyroid function tests, creatinine phosphokinase, serum and urine protein electrophoresis, cryoglobulins, vitamin B12, heavy-metal screens, urinary porphobilinogens, and serologic tests for HIV, Lyme disease, Epstein-Barr virus, and

West Nile virus (WNV) (2,3,4,6,7,16,18,24). Some of these studies might be obtained by the emergency physician if clinical evaluation raises the suspicion of a specific disease process. Otherwise, additional testing should be left to the consulting neurologist following characterization of the neuropathy by nerve conduction studies and electromyography.

Patients suspected of having GBS should undergo lumbar puncture. The characteristic findings are normal pressure and albuminocytologic dissociation (elevated protein levels with fewer than 10 mononuclear cells/μL). Cerebrospinal fluid changes may be delayed 1 to 2 weeks after the onset of symptoms. An increased cell count should raise the suspicion for HIV, WNV, or Lyme disease as the precipitating event (3,4,16,18,20).

Baseline measurements of pulmonary function are important, because 25% to 33% of patients with GBS eventually require mechanical ventilation (12,18,23). Forced vital capacity (FVC) or inspiratory force (IF) should be tested in the emergency department. A quick bedside test is to have the patient take a deep inspiration and then count as long as possible; the ability to count to 25 correlates with an FVC of 2 L, and a count to only 10 with an FVC of 1 L (18). FVC of less than 12 to 15 mL/kg or an IF of less than 20 cm H_2O are indications of imminent respiratory failure and the need to initiate mechanical ventilation (3,9,13,18,23). Patients who remain in the emergency department for several hours should have serial pulmonary function testing. Bulbar muscle strength should also be followed, as intubation may be required to maintain a patent airway and prevent aspiration. Frequent vital signs and continuous cardiac monitoring are essential to identify life-threatening cardiovascular autonomic dysfunction. Blood pressure fluctuations should be treated, as needed, with fluids and short-acting agents.

DISPOSITION

Every patient with an acute polyneuropathy should be evaluated by a neurologist. Admission to the hospital for further diagnostic studies and continued monitoring of vital signs and respiratory status is required. Whether an intensive care unit is necessary for all patients is controversial. Clearly, any patient with significant respiratory impairment, inability to protect the airway or autonomic instability should be admitted to an intensive care unit. Several recent studies have identified specific criteria associated with a high rate of mechanical ventilation (13,23) the presence of any of these should prompt an ICU admission. The criteria include: FVC less than 20 ml/kg, IF less than 30 cm H_2O, EF (expiratory force) less than 40 cm H_2O, more than a 30% reduction in FVC from baseline, less than 7 days from symptom onset to hospital admission, and the inability to cough, stand, or lift the elbows or head off the bed. For all other patients, the admission destination depends on the adequacy of monitoring in other settings. Patients with severe or rapidly progressive GBS benefit from early plasma exchange or immune globulin therapy; therefore, these patients should be transferred to a facility capable of providing such therapies (9,20,24).

While the vast majority of patients with GBS recover completely or with minimal deficits, it should be noted that GBS has a 3% to 5% mortality. Ten percent of patients will have severe persistent deficits. In addition, 5% to 10% will have recurrent episodes of acute peripheral neuropathy (24).

COMMON PITFALLS

✔ Mistaking the low back pain of GBS for disc disease or back strain
✔ Mistaking the symptoms of cervical myelopathy or other spinal cord pathology for GBS

✔ Failing to admit patients with minimal, but suggestive, symptomatology

✔ Inadequately monitoring for respiratory and autonomic dysfunction

✔ Ascribing the symmetric weakness of GBS or other acute polyneuropathies to a psychiatric disorder

✔ Failing to recognize variant presentations of GBS

SUBACUTE POLYNEUROPATHY

CLINICAL PRESENTATION

Polyneuropathy that develops over a period of several weeks to months is said to be subacute; however, the distinction between subacute and acute polyneuropathy is not always clear. For example, while half of patients with GBS present with symptoms that develop over 10 to 14 days, in the other half, symptoms progress over 3 to 4 weeks (3,7). Subacute polyneuropathy (SPN) may be symmetric or asymmetric. Symmetric disease generally begins with distal sensorimotor losses and tends to produce marked sensory impairment. Asymmetric SPN are frequently the result of neuronal ischemia; nerves are randomly affected, producing patchy sensorimotor losses.

DIFFERENTIAL DIAGNOSIS

The differential diagnosis of SPN includes GBS, chronic inflammatory demyelinating polyneuropathy (CIDP), mononeuritis multiplex, and other neuromuscular diseases that produce subacute weakness such as myelopathy, myasthenia gravis, amyotrophic lateral sclerosis, Parkinson disease, and depression. Perhaps more important with SPN are the numerous underlying etiologies.

The etiologies for *symmetric* SPN include diabetes mellitus, collagen vascular and autoimmune diseases, nutritional deficiencies (e.g., alcoholism), uremia, amyloidosis, heavy-metal intoxication, industrial solvents (e.g., glue sniffing), a multitude of toxins and medications, Lyme disease, and HIV infection.

The etiologies of *asymmetric* SPN include diabetes mellitus (e.g., diabetic amyotrophy), collagen vascular and other autoimmune diseases, peripheral vascular disease, sarcoidosis, neoplastic disease, paraproteinemia, leprosy, Lyme disease, HIV infection, and idiopathic disease.

EMERGENCY DEPARTMENT EVALUATION AND MANAGEMENT

History and physical examination are the principal methods of evaluation. Key historic elements to elicit are a history of neuromuscular or systemic disease, medications (prescription and nonprescription), and potential infectious or toxic exposure. Laboratory studies should include complete blood count, serum electrolytes, calcium, magnesium, phosphate, glucose, blood urea nitrogen, creatinine, and a screening chest radiograph. As with acute neuropathies, further studies should be obtained only if a specific etiology is suspected following evaluation of the patient (6).

DISPOSITION

Most patients with SPN may be referred to their primary care physician for outpatient evaluation and referral to a neurologist.

If a medication is suspected as the etiology, it should be discontinued or changed after consultation with the primary care physician. Short-term follow-up should be arranged.

COMMON PITFALL

✔ Attributing subacute polyneuropathy to a chronic medical condition, thus overlooking potentially treatable causes such as nutritional deficiencies, medication exposure, infections or vasculitis

PLEXOPATHY AND RADICULOPATHY

CLINICAL PRESENTATION

A plexopathy is a disorder that affects the brachial or lumbosacral plexus. Symptoms include pain and mixed motor and sensory deficits in a pattern that cannot be attributed to individual peripheral nerves or nerve roots.

Acute or subacute plexopathies are associated with local trauma (e.g., shoulder dislocation), compression (e.g., retroperitoneal hematoma or abdominal aortic aneurysm), vascular disease (usually due to diabetes or collagen vascular disease), or infection (e.g., Lyme disease), or they may be idiopathic. Idiopathic lumbosacral plexopathy is rare (7), but acute idiopathic brachial plexopathy is well described. It is seen most commonly in men in the third or fourth decade of life (14), and there appears to be some association with recent viral illnesses and immunizations (7,14). Symptoms of brachial plexopathy begin with the sudden onset of severe shoulder pain that may extend into the neck and upper arm. Less commonly, the lower plexus cords may be affected, producing symptoms in the forearm and hand. Within days to weeks, motor weakness and sensory loss develop, usually coinciding with resolution of pain (7,14). About 90% of patients recover good neurologic function by 3 years (14). Chronic plexopathy is associated with infections, vascular disease, collagen vascular disease, tumor, infiltrative processes, and radiation therapy.

In contrast to plexopathy, a radiculopathy affects spinal nerve roots or spinal nerves. Symptoms include pain and sensorimotor deficits in a pattern consistent with the involved nerve root (e.g., lancinating pain along the L-5 nerve root dermatome). Frequently, several adjacent roots are affected, making differentiation from a plexopathy or multiple mononeuropathies clinically impossible. The etiologies of radiculopathy include all those of a plexopathy, as well as specific spinal canal or cord disorders such as herniated disc, spinal stenosis, and epidural tumor, abscess, hematoma, granuloma, and infection (8,24).

DIFFERENTIAL DIAGNOSIS

The differential diagnosis of plexopathy includes polyneuropathy, multiple mononeuropathies, and spinal cord and root disorders. Brachial plexopathy can easily be confused with C-5 root compression, and lumbosacral plexopathy with L-4 compression (8). The pain of idiopathic brachial plexopathy tends to resolve as motor symptoms develop, unlike the persistent pain of C-5 root compression (8). In addition, C-5 root pain increases with neck movement, coughing, and sneezing, while brachial plexopathy pain increases with shoulder movement (7). Pain from both lumbosacral plexopathy and L-4 root compression is persistent. Iliopsoas weakness is common in lumbosacral plexopathy but is not seen with L-4 root lesions.

Thoracic outlet syndrome (TOS) can mimic brachial plexopathy by producing pain and weakness in the arm. Other local joint or tendon disorders, muscular disorders, and amyotrophic lateral sclerosis may also mimic plexopathy, but can usually be differentiated by their lack of sensory abnormalities.

EMERGENCY DEPARTMENT EVALUATION AND MANAGEMENT

The history and physical examination, including a detailed neurologic examination, are essential in management decisions. Motor findings are more reliable than sensory findings when evaluating the upper extremity (19). The pattern of muscle weakness is unique for each nerve root (C5-T1) and peripheral nerve. In the lower extremity, the sensory exam is more reliable than the motor exam when evaluating root disorders (19). The lower extremity sensory exam reveals root dermatomes that run horizontally or diagonally across the anterior leg while the peripheral nerve dermatomes run vertically. A plexopathy will produce a pattern of muscle and sensory deficits that are a blend of both root and peripheral nerve pathology. Patten's *Neurological Differential Diagnosis* provides a detailed review of the complex clinical exam findings that will help differentiate spinal nerve root versus plexus versus peripheral nerve disorders (19).

Patients with symptoms of *acute brachial plexopathy* should have cervical spine, chest, and shoulder radiographs (7,14). Laboratory studies such as complete blood cell count, serum electrolytes, glucose, blood urea nitrogen, creatinine, and sedimentation rate should be obtained if the history or physical examination suggests infection, diabetes, or collagen vascular disease.

Acute lumbosacral plexopathy generally occurs secondary to another disease process. A complete blood cell count, serum electrolytes, glucose, blood urea nitrogen, creatinine, erythrocyte sedimentation rate, and lumbosacral films are appropriate. An abdominal ultrasound or computed tomography is indicated if an aortic aneurysm or other retroperitoneal pathology (e.g., bleed, tumor) is suspected. A determination of postvoid residual urine volume will aid in defining the extent of the neurologic deficit.

The approach to an *acute radiculopathy* is dictated by the history and physical examination. While an evaluation consistent with an acute herniated disc and no objective neurologic deficits may require only conservative management with analgesia, muscle relaxants, limited activity, and close follow up, the presence of objective deficits or another etiology will require an aggressive evaluation, including blood testing, a determination of postvoid residual urine volume, spinal imaging and consultation.

In patients with chronic symptoms, minimal immediate diagnostic work up is necessary. A chest and neck radiograph or lumbosacral films are reasonable screening tools for such patients.

DISPOSITION

Acute symptoms resulting from plexopathies are often difficult to distinguish from root and spinal cord disorders (7,8), therefore, they generally require urgent neurosurgical consultation. Spinal computed tomography, magnetic resonance imaging, or myelography may be required to determine the correct diagnosis, and hospital admission to complete such testing is recommended. Outpatient follow up is appropriate for patients with chronic symptoms.

COMMON PITFALLS

✔ Attribution of symptoms to mononeuropathy, and thereby failing to proceed with the appropriate diagnostic evaluation required for plexopathies and radiculopathies
✔ Failure to consider potentially catastrophic etiologies for acute plexopathies (e.g., abdominal aneurysm)
✔ Failure to consider potentially catastrophic etiologies for acute radiculopathies (e.g., spinal epidural abscess or acute cord compression)

MONONEUROPATHY

CLINICAL PRESENTATION

Mononeuropathies produce variable symptoms of pain and sensorimotor loss in the distribution of a single peripheral nerve. The actual neuronal injury may be classified as neuropraxia (a "stunned" nerve), axonotmesis (damaged axon in an intact nerve trunk), or neurotmesis (disrupted nerve trunk) (14,17). The speed and degree of neurologic recovery are related to the type of injury present.

Nerve compression (e.g., Saturday Night Palsy, usually associated with an intoxicated patient who falls asleep with an arm draped over the back of a chair resulting in compression of the radial nerve against the humerus) and nerve entrapment are the most frequently encountered etiologies for mononeuropathies in the emergency department. Entrapment syndromes (e.g., carpal tunnel syndrome) have been associated with repetitive activity, pregnancy, rheumatoid arthritis, osteoarthritis, gout, hypothyroidism, acromegaly, amyloidosis, multiple myeloma, collagen vascular disease, and local tumors (7,24). Other causes of mononeuropathies are trauma, collagen vascular disease, diabetes mellitus, peripheral vascular disease, infection, granulomatous disease, infiltrative disorders, neoplasia, radiation therapy, and primary nerve tumors.

A unique form of mononeuropathy is mononeuritis multiplex. This entity involves the simultaneous or near-simultaneous dysfunction of two or more peripheral nerves. It may result from multiple pressure palsies, infections (e.g., leprosy, Lyme disease, HIV infection), infiltrative or neoplastic disease, vascular disease, or collagen vascular disease (7). The abrupt onset of mononeuritis multiplex in patients with a collagen vascular disease or other vasculitis is of specific concern, as it generally indicates an acute necrotizing vasculitis that requires aggressive treatment (24).

DIFFERENTIAL DIAGNOSIS

The differential diagnosis of a mononeuropathy includes radiculopathy, plexopathy, polyneuropathy, local joint or muscular disorders, hysteria, and malingering.

EMERGENCY DEPARTMENT EVALUATION AND MANAGEMENT

The evaluation of a mononeuropathy should focus on the nature of the deficit and historical factors such as duration, any traumatic injury, occupational factors (e.g., repetitive activity), or symptoms suggestive of diabetes or collagen vascular disease. The physical examination should determine whether the deficit fits the distribution of a single peripheral nerve. A concise summary of peripheral nerve dermatomes, as opposed to spinal root dermatomes, can be found in Appendix A in *Disorders of Peripheral Nerves*, by Schaumburg et al (22). Provocative symptoms (e.g., Tinel's sign, and Phalen's sign) may help elicit symptoms that are only episodic. Palpation along the course of the nerve may reveal areas of compression. Evidence of systemic disease should also be sought.

Complete blood cell count, electrolytes, blood glucose, erythrocyte sedimentation rate, antinuclear antibody testing, thyroid function tests, and serum protein electrophoresis are indicated only if a systemic disorder is suspected. Radiographs may be helpful in cases associated with trauma or when bone abnormalities are a possible cause of entrapment.

CRITICAL INTERVENTIONS

- Perform rapid assessment of airway and ventilatory capacity including measurements of pulmonary function for patients with suspected Guillain-Barré syndrome
- Perform lumbar puncture on patients suspected of having Guillain-Barré syndrome
- Always consider and evaluate for the catastrophic causes of any acute radiculopathy or plexopathy
- Admit patients with acute mononeuropathy multiplex and known or suspected collagen vascular disease or vasculitis

DISPOSITION

Most patients with a mononeuropathy can be discharged, with a splint, to outpatient follow up. Identified etiologies, such as diabetes or repetitive activities, should be addressed, and patients in whom the etiology is unclear should be referred to their primary care physician or a neurologist for further testing, which may include nerve conduction studies and electromyography.

Urgent evaluation by a plastic surgeon, orthopedic surgeon, or neurosurgeon is indicated for posttraumatic mononeuropathy. Hospital admission is indicated for acute mononeuropathy multiplex in patients with known or suspected collagen vascular disease or vasculitis since this disorder usually indicates an acute necrotizing vasculitis, which requires aggressive steroid or other immunosuppressive therapy (24).

COMMON PITFALLS

✔ Failure to differentiate a mononeuropathy from a polyneuropathy, plexopathy, or radiculopathy
✔ Failure to detect systemic signs of collagen vascular disease or other vasculitis disorder in patients with mononeuropathy multiplex

Acknowledgments

Thanks to the previous edition's chapter author Kevin M. Reilly.

References

1. Ahmed S, Libman R, Wesson K, Ahmed F, Einberg K. Guillain-Barre syndrome: an unusual presentation of West Nile virus infection. *Neurology* 2000;55:144–146.
2. Barohn RJ. Approach to peripheral neuropathy and neuronopathy. *Semin Neurol* 1998;18:7–18
3. Bella I, Chad DA. Neuromuscular disorders and acute respiratory failure. *Neurosurg Clin North Am* 1998;16:391–417.
4. Centers for Disease Control and Prevention. Acute flaccid paralysis syndrome associated with West Nile virus infection—Mississippi and Louisiana, July-August 2002. *MMWR Morb Mortal Wkly Report* 2002;51:825–828.
5. ChioA, Cocito D, Leone M, et al. Guillain-Barre syndrome: a prospective, population-based incidence and outcome survey. *Neurology* 2003;60:1146–1150.
6. Dyck PJ, Dyck JB, Grant IA, et al. Ten steps in characterizing and diagnosing patients with peripheral neuropathy. *Neurology* 1996;47:10–17.
7. Dyck PJ, Thomas PK, eds. *Peripheral neuropathy,* 3rd ed. Philadelphia: WB Saunders, 1993.
8. Fager CA. Identification and management of radiculopathy. *Neurosurg Clin North Am* 1993;4:1–12.
9. Fulgham JR, Wijicks FM. Guillain-Barré syndrome. *Crit Care Clin* 1997;13:1–15.
10. Grattan-Smith PJ, Morris JG, Johnston HM, et al. Clinical and neurophysiological features of tick paralysis. *Brain* 1997;120:1975–1987.
11. Hahn AF. Guillain-Barré syndrome. *Lancet* 1998;352:635–641.
12. Hughes RA, Rees JH. Clinical and epidemiologic features of Guillain-Barré syndrome. *J Infect Dis* 1997;176[Suppl 2]:S92–98.
13. Lawn ND, Fletcher DD, Henderson RD, et al. Anticipating mechanical ventilation in Guillain-Barre syndrome. *Arch Neurol* 2001;58:893–898.
14. Leffert RD. Neurological problems. In: Rockwood CA, Matsen FA, eds. *The shoulder.* Philadelphia: WB Saunders, 1990:750–773.
15. Mandell GL, Bennett JE, Dolin R, eds. *Mandell, Douglas, and Bennett's principles and practice of infectious diseases.* 5th ed. New York: Churchill Livingstone, 2000.
16. McLeod JG. Investigation of peripheral neuropathy. *J Neurol Neurosurg Psychiatry* 1995;58:274–283.
17. Nuber GW, Assenmacher J, Bowen MK. Neurovascular problems in the forearm, wrist, and hand. *Clin Sports Med* 1998;17:585–610.
18. Pascuzzi RM, Fleck JD. Acute peripheral neuropathy in adults: Guillain-Barré syndrome and related disorders. *Neurol Clin* 1997;15:529–547.
19. Patten J. *Neurological differential diagnosis.* 2nd ed. London: Springer-Verlag, 1996.
20. Rees J. Guillain-Barré syndrome: clinical manifestations and directions for treatment. *Drugs* 1995;49:912–920.
21. Ropper AH, Wijdicks EFM, Traux BT. *Guillain-Barré syndrome.* Philadelphia: FA Davis Co, 1991.
22. Schaumburg HH, Berger AR, Thomas PK. *Disorders of peripheral nerves,* 2nd ed. Philadelphia: FA Davis Co, 1992.
23. Sharshar T, Chevret S, Bourdain F, Raphael, J, et al. Early predictors of mechanical ventilation in Guillain-Barre syndrome. *Crit Care Med* 2003;31:278–283.
24. Victor M, Ropper AH. *Adams and Victor's principles of neurology,* 7th ed. New York:McGraw-Hill, 2001.

CHAPTER 116

Bell's Palsy and Trigeminal Neuralgia

Lauren Grossman

The cranial nerves (CN) have central, peripheral, motor and sensory components; CN disorders can thus be responsible for a variety of complaints among emergency department (ED) patients.

BELL'S PALSY

The most common disorder of the facial nerve (cranial nerve VII) is known as Bell's palsy. It is an acute, unilateral, peripheral facial nerve palsy which occurs in approximately 23 (reported range of 13–34) per 100,000 patients annually (1,8,9).

Bell's palsy occurs equally in women and men, most commonly between 10 to 40 years of age (9). Seasonal, geographic or racial predilections have not been identified. Pregnant women, however, are at three times greater risk of developing a Bell palsy, especially during the peripartum phase, compared to nonpregnant women of the same age (5). Additionally, up to 10% of patients with Bell's palsy have diabetes.

While the cause appears to be idiopathic in many patients, herpes simplex virus-1 (HSV-1) has been isolated in the fluid and muscle surrounding the facial nerve in a large percentage of patients with Bell palsy. An inflammatory etiology, either idiopathic or secondary to viral infection, has also been proposed and may account for the increased incidence with pregnancy and diabetes.

CLINICAL PRESENTATION

Patients with Bell's palsy often report a dramatic onset of facial weakness that is noticed upon awakening or progresses over several hours. There may be unilateral facial droop, flattened nasolabial fold, inability to close the eye, difficulty eating, loss of taste in the anterior two-thirds of the tongue, hyperacusis (sound distortion or tinnitus), or decreased production of tears and saliva. Bell's phenomenon occurs when the eye rolls back when the patient attempts to close the lid. The patient may recall a prodrome involving periauricular pain and abnormalities of hearing or taste.

Any other neurologic complaints should prompt a more extensive search for other etiologies of facial weakness. Pertinent past medical history includes similar previous episodes, recent trauma, pregnancy, and diabetes.

On physical exam, a unilateral facial palsy is usually evident on careful physical examination. It is critical, however, to distinguish a central from a peripheral facial nerve deficit. The central 7th nerve palsy spares the forehead, therefore the patient's forehead will still wrinkle when he or she is asked to elevate the brows. With a peripheral facial nerve deficit seen in Bell's palsy, the entire side of the face is weak. If there is any visual deficit, the eye should be completely examined, including an evaluation for corneal abrasions that may have occurred because of difficulty in closing the lid. The external auditory canal should be inspected for vesicles caused by herpes zoster infection; this is a defining feature of the Ramsay-Hunt syndrome (see below).

DIFFERENTIAL DIAGNOSIS

Until the mid to late 1990s, Bell's palsy had been defined, in part, by its idiopathic nature. Given its recently established association with HSV-1 (1), it may currently and more accurately be called herpetic facial paralysis.

Lyme disease (see Chapter 141, Lyme Disease) may also cause a unilateral or bilateral facial nerve palsy. Painless swelling and erythema of the face preceding the palsy is the distinguishing feature. Other manifestations of Lyme disease, such as history of a tick bite, the typical erythema chronicum migrans rash (an expanding erythematous ring-like rash with partial central clearing), arthritis, and vertigo should be sought. Serologic diagnostic tests may be misleading, and in any event results are not generally available during the emergency department visit.

HIV infection may cause facial palsy during the period of seroconversion, when it is associated with cerebrospinal fluid lymphocytosis. After the seroconversion phase, a facial palsy is more likely to have an infectious etiology. Mononeuropathy multiplex is also associated with early HIV infection; it may present with facial palsy, laryngeal palsy, wrist drop, or foot drop. This syndrome usually resolves spontaneously, although more severe cases may be associated with cytomegalovirus infection and require antiviral treatment. The most severe cases may progress to quadriparesis.

The Ramsay-Hunt syndrome, a herpes zoster infection of the geniculate ganglion (the confluence of cranial nerve branches found in the temporal bone just proximal to the internal auditory canal), presents as a peripheral, unilateral facial nerve palsy accompanied by a vesicular rash in the external auditory canal or oropharynx. Cranial nerve VIII may also be involved, causing vertigo and hearing abnormalities.

The 7th and 8th cranial nerves travel together through the internal acoustic meatus. Thus, the facial nerve palsy accompanied by any deficit in hearing, particularly if it develops over months, suggests a diagnosis of acoustic neuroma. Patients may be asked whether they have changed the side they prefer for using a telephone. A contrast-enhanced CT with cerebellopontine angle cuts can be used as an initial screening test; however, MRI is the diagnostic test of choice. In later stages, CNs V, IX, X and XI may be affected.

Other causes of peripheral facial nerve palsies include temporal bone trauma, mononucleosis, tuberculosis, mumps, Mycoplasma pneumoniae infection, Sjögren syndrome, and leprosy (1,4,6,8). Guillain-Barré syndrome and sarcoidosis may also cause a bilateral peripheral facial nerve palsy.

EMERGENCY DEPARTMENT EVALUATION

The patient's history and physical examination can lead to a definitive diagnosis of Bell's palsy, eliminating the need to gather any further diagnostic information.

Diagnostic imaging is indicated only if there are atypical signs or symptoms or if a typical Bell's palsy is not resolving after three or more weeks. A plain head CT scan with temporal bone images should be the initial screening exam. An MRI with and without enhancement may be useful as a subsequent diagnostic modality. However, this is rarely necessary during an emergency department evaluation. Enhancement of the geniculate ganglion is the most common MRI finding in patients with Bell's palsy.

EMERGENCY DEPARTMENT MANAGEMENT

The mainstays of treatment for Bell's palsy include corticosteroids, antiviral therapy, and eye protection. Pharmacologic therapy is recommended if the patient presents within seven days of the onset of symptoms. While evidence regarding drug treatment and its timing is weak, it is commonly thought that earlier treatment is associated with a better outcome (3,7,9). Recommended treatment is prednisone 40 to 60 mg daily for 7 to 14 days, and acyclovir 400 to 800 mg five times daily or valacyclovir 1g three times daily. The eye should be protected by wearing glasses or a patch if there is inadequate closure of the lid. Artificial tears may be helpful for keeping the eye well lubricated, especially when lacrimal gland function is compromised.

CRITICAL INTERVENTIONS

- Differentiate between central versus peripheral cranial nerve VII palsy
- Eliminate other neurologic causes of facial nerve deficit
- Perform a thorough ophthalmologic examination
- Provide eye protection if needed

DISPOSITION

In clear cases of Bell's palsy, the patient should be discharged with close ENT follow up. The vast majority (85%) of patients with Bell's palsy begin to recover within 3 weeks of onset, although complete recovery may take up to 1 year. Patients with incomplete paralysis tend to have a complete recovery, while only 60% of those with complete paralysis regain normal function (8). Resolution of the paralysis may be preceded by a recovery of normal taste.

Ophthalmology follow up is required for patients with extensive corneal abrasions. Neurology or infectious disease consultations may be helpful when other diagnostic possibilities are being considered.

COMMON PITFALLS

✔ Expensive and unnecessary work up for simple case of Bell's palsy
✔ Missed corneal abrasions
✔ Missed comorbidities (e.g., diabetes, HIV) that may have predisposed the patient to the disease process

TRIGEMINAL NEURALGIA

The trigeminal nerve (CN V), with its three anatomic divisions (V1-ophthalmic, V2-maxillary, and V3-mandibular) contains sensory fibers that innervate the face, the mucous membranes of the oral and nasal cavity, and the cornea. V1 supplies the sensory fibers to the cornea; with decreased function, ocular sensation may be affected, predisposing the patient to injury, drying, or ulceration that can lead to loss of vision. The nerve's motor fibers innervate the muscles of mastication.

CLINICAL PRESENTATION

Trigeminal neuralgia (tic douloureux) is characterized by brief, recurrent episodes of excruciating unilateral facial pain usually involving the second (V2) and third (V3) divisions of the trigeminal nerve. The pain occurs more commonly on the right and lasts from a few seconds to less than 2 minutes. The pain has a lightning-like quality and often causes unilateral facial grimacing. The patient may be able to identify a trigger point or event that initiates the episodes, such as chewing gum, applying makeup, or feeling a breeze on the face. The episodes may persist for months, followed by long symptom-free periods.

There is a slight female predominance and most cases occur in those >50 years of age. The annual incidence is 4 per 100,000 individuals. Although previously thought to be idiopathic, trigeminal neuralgia is now believed to be caused in many cases by compression of the trigeminal nerve at its entry into the pons.

DIFFERENTIAL DIAGNOSIS

Other causes of trigeminal neuralgia-like facial pain include traumatic, vascular, or space-occupying lesions (e.g., acoustic neuroma) and demyelinating diseases (e.g., multiple sclerosis). Other causes of facial pain include herpes zoster, sinus infection, odontogenic pathology, migraine, and temporomandibular joint dysfunction.

Herpes zoster (shingles) commonly infects CN V1. Patients often present after the typical rash has appeared, but may notice the pain a day or so beforehand. Postherpetic neuralgia causes severe unilateral facial pain after the typical herpetic rash has resolved. The pain is described as burning, lancinating, electric shock-like, or pruritic, and the affected part of the face may be hyperesthetic. Factors that increase the risk for postherpetic neuralgia include age > 75 and more severe initial episodes of shingles. Aggres-

sive treatment of the initial episode aggressively with acyclovir or related drugs, steroids, and analgesics is believed to diminish the likelihood of postherpetic neuralgia.

Glossopharyngeal neuralgia presents with episodic pain similar to that of trigeminal neuralgia except that it involves the areas innervated by CNs IX and X. Patients complain of severe unilateral pain in the ear, throat, and tongue. Any sensory stimulation to the area, including light touch, taste, coughing, or talking, may trigger the symptoms.

EMERGENCY DEPARTMENT EVALUATION

The diagnosis of trigeminal neuralgia is made primarily on a clinical basis. A thorough history should include a specific description of the pain, what triggers or ameliorates it, and any associated symptoms. There may be associated muscle spasms of the face. Important historical clues include trauma, dental problems or procedures, and depression. The neurologic exam is normal with no objective abnormalities of the motor or sensory functioning of CN V. Special attention should be given to the head and neck, especially the oral cavity.

Diagnostic imaging with MRI and MRA is recommended to eliminate other causes of facial pain such as space-occupying lesions or multiple sclerosis. Those who require emergent imaging include:

1. Any neurologic findings, particularly signs of increased intracranial pressure
2. Sensory deficits of CN V
3. Younger age groups
4. Bilateral symptoms
5. Intractable symptoms

EMERGENCY DEPARTMENT MANAGEMENT

Treatment for trigeminal neuralgia includes analgesics and carbamazepine (Tegretol®), 100-200 mg BID initially, and increased by 200 mg per day until symptoms are controlled. The maximum dose is 1200 mg daily.

Other medications used to control trigeminal neuralgia include phenytoin, baclofen, valproate sodium, lamotrigine, and gabapentin. Surgical management including alcohol or glycerol injection, gamma-knife radiosurgery or microvascular decompression may be indicated for patients with persistent symptoms who fail medical therapy.

CRITICAL INTERVENTIONS

- Exclude masses and vascular lesions, particularly those of the cerebellopontine angle, as cause of pain
- Exclude odontogenic causes of pain
- Provide adequate pain relief

DISPOSITION

If the diagnosis of trigeminal neuralgia as been carefully made on clinical grounds, and the pain has been controlled satisfactorily, the patient may be discharged home. Close follow up for patients on Tegretol® is mandatory to monitor blood levels and liver function tests.

COMMON PITFALL

✔ While the patient may have a convincing history and physical exam that clearly points to a diagnosis of trigeminal neuralgia, this label should be applied as a diagnosis of exclusion, given the potentially life-threatening alternatives to be considered

References

1. Adams RD, Victor M, Ropper AH. *Principles of Neurology*. New York: McGraw-Hill, 1997;187–188, 1376–1377.
2. Cohen Y, Lavie O, Granovsky-Grisaru S, et al. Bell Palsy Complicating Pregnancy: A Review. *Obst and Gynecol Surv,* 2000;55:184–188.
3. Guberman A. *An Introduction to Clinical Neurology*. Boston: Little, Brown and Company, 1994;67.
4. Hadithi M, Stam F, et al. Sjogren's syndrome: an unusual cause of Bell's palsy. *Ann Rheum Dis* 2001;60:724–725.
5. Papaevangelou V, Falaina V, et al. Bell's Palsy Associated With Mycoplasma Pneumoniae Infection. *The Pediat Infect Dis J* 1999;18:1024–1026.
6. Ramsey M, Der Simonian R, et al. Corticosteroid Treatment for Idiopathic Facial Nerve Paralysis: A Meta-analysis. *Laryngoscope* 2000;110:335–341.
7. Salinas R, Alvarez G, et al. Corticosteroids for Bell's palsy (idiopathic facial paralysis) Cochrane Database Systematic Review 2002.
8. Salinas R. Bell's Palsy. Barton S, ed. *Clinical Evidence (7)*. London: BMJ Publishing Group, 2002;1140–1143.
9. Sugiura K, Robinson G, Stuart D. *Illustrated Guide to the Central Nervous System*. St. Louis: Ishiyaku EuroAmerica, Inc. Publishers, 1989.

CHAPTER 117
Myopathies and Disorders of Neuromuscular Transmission

Sharad Pandit

Although weakness is a common complaint of patients presenting to the emergency department, it is uncommonly caused by a primary muscle disorder or a disorder of neuromuscular transmission. Diagnosis and management of these disorders present particular challenges to the emergency physician as these disorders are rare and their clinical presentation is often subtle and variable.

Many neuromuscular disorders can present with rapidly progressive generalized weakness that can potentially cause life-threatening ventilatory compromise. It is therefore important for the emergency physician to have an organized approach, which is safe and quick while simultaneously thorough.

Commonly recognized conditions fall into the categories of myopathies (diseases of the muscle), disorders of the neuromuscular junction (myasthenia gravis) or peripheral neuropathies.

MYOPATHY

Myopathy is a muscle disease unrelated to any disorder of innervation or neuromuscular junction. Primary muscle disease presents with muscle weakness as the predominant symptom.

Impaired function whilst performing activities of daily life and muscle pain may be some of the other symptoms.

CLINICAL PRESENTATION

Weakness is generally progressive, proximal and symmetric in distribution. It typically spares the extraocular, facial and bulbar muscles (distinguishing the myopathies from myasthenia gravis and other disorders of neuromuscular junction). Although myopathic disease is of gradual onset with a slow progression of symptoms, it is important to bear in mind that rapidly progressive generalized weakness can occur. An overview of the spectrum of myopathic disorders is given in Table 117.1.

Hereditary myopathies include the various forms of muscular dystrophy as well as the metabolic myopathies and periodic paralysis. Muscular dystrophies are chronic, progressive, inherited myopathies that present from early childhood to adolescence. The various types are differentiated by mode of inheritance, age at onset, rate of progression, and the selectivity of muscle involvement (9). Duchenne dystrophy, observed in boys younger than 5 years, causes the most severe disease. Cardiomyopathy is common in affected children. Weakness and muscle wasting in a child with elevated CK occurs with Duchenne dystrophy, but other dystrophies (e.g., fascioscapulohumeral,

---

TABLE 117.1. Classification of Myopathies

Inflammatory
- Collagen vascular diseases (polymyositis, dermatomyositis, SLE, RA)
- Idiopathic
- Other (granulomatous, eosinophilic)

Infectious
- Trichinosis
- Cysticercosis (*Taenia solium*)
- Toxoplasmosis
- Human immunodeficiency virus (HIV)
- Coxsackie A and B viruses
- Influenza
- Lyme disease
- Staphylococcus aureus

Endocrine/Metabolic
- Endocrine
  - Addison disease
  - Cushing disease
  - Hypothyroidism (CK may be mildly elevated)
  - Hyperthyroidism (CK may be normal)
  - Hyperparathyroidism
  - Hyperaldosteronism
- Electrolyte abnormality (Na, K, Ca, Mg, Phos)

Drug-Induced
- Myopathy (steroids, AZT, lovastatin, cocaine, colchicine)
- Myositis (procainamide)
- Rhabdomyolysis (alcohol, opiates, barbiturates, phencyclidine, amphetamines)
- Neuroleptic malignant syndrome (neuroleptics)
- Malignant hyperthermia (general anesthetics, depolarizing muscle relaxants)

Hereditary
- Muscular dystrophies
- Periodic paralysis (hyperkalemic, hypokalemic and normokalemic)
- Metabolic

Others
- Trauma
- Ischemia
- Sepsis

AZT, zidovudine; CK, creatinine kinase; RA, rheumatoid arthritis; SLE, systemic lupus erythematoses.

limb-girdle, myotonic) may occur in boys and girls with normal muscle enzyme levels. Patients with mild cases may lead fairly normal lives, but progressive weakness and scoliosis impairing pulmonary function often results in recurrent infections and exacerbation of weakness. Diagnosis of muscular dystrophies is made on the basis of family history, clinical features, and the results of creatine phosphokinase (CK) determination, electromyography, and muscle biopsy.

Metabolic myopathies are disorders of glucose or lipid utilization and energy production in skeletal muscle. They have common abnormalities of muscle energy metabolism that result in skeletal muscle dysfunction. Metabolic myopathies have a wide age range of symptom onset. Most patients, however, present early in life (i.e., infancy, childhood, young adulthood).

Metabolic myopathies present with exercise intolerance, muscle cramps, and myoglobinuria. Cramps and muscle discomfort may occur after brief exercise or after prolonged physical activity. Glycogen is the main source of energy during brief exercise, while free fatty acids are the most important source of fuel during prolonged exercise. Accordingly, cramps are the hallmark of glycogen storage diseases (e.g., Cradle disease). However, in lipid storage disease (e.g., CPT deficiency), muscle cramps and exercise intolerance occur only after prolonged exercise and are worse during fasting.

Metabolic myopathies presenting with progressive muscle weakness may mimic limb-girdle muscular dystrophy or polymyositis and are a common manifestation of deficiencies of acid maltase, debrancher enzyme, and carnitine.

Periodic paralyses are a group of diseases that cause patients to present with acute weakness due to potassium shifts, leading to muscle dysfunction. A genetic defect of the sodium ion channel in muscle cell membranes is responsible for the paralysis, which may last from hours to days. Acute periodic paralysis may be classified as normokalemic, hypokalemic or hyperkalemic.

Normokalemic paralysis causes the most severe and prolonged attacks. Patients usually feel well between attacks, but some have myotonia (i.e., muscle stiffness) or residual weakness after repeated episodes. A genetic defect has been linked to these diseases, but in some instances, hypokalemia may cause acute weakness in healthy individuals.

Acute hypokalemic periodic paralysis may be primary (i.e., familial) or secondary to excessive renal or GI losses or endocrinopathy. In these cases, intracellular shift of potassium depolarizes the cell membrane rendering it inexcitable and no muscle contraction can occur; hence, the patient experiences paralysis. This may occur independent of the sodium-potassium pump. The diagnosis is based on patient history and serum potassium determination (usually 2.5–3.5 mEq/L during attacks) and occasionally on provocative testing with glucose and insulin infusion (performed in a controlled setting by a neurologist). In Asians and Hispanics, hypokalemic periodic paralysis can occur in association with thyrotoxicosis, so thyroid function tests should also be ordered (3). Familial periodic paralysis usually occurs in Caucasian males, is autosomal dominant, and may last as long as 36 hours. Attacks generally occur at night or in early morning upon awakening and can be precipitated by a diet high in carbohydrates, rest following exercise, or glucose and insulin given intravenously.

In the hyperkalemic form of periodic paralysis, attacks are more frequent and of shorter duration (usually less than two hours) and are provoked by rest, exertion, or fasting. During an attack the serum potassium is in the range of 5 to 7 mEq/L.

Polymyositis (PM), an inflammatory disorder of skeletal muscle, is the most common primary myopathy to affect adults. Muscle damage is caused by cell- and antibody-mediated autoimmune attack. Five clinical types have been identified: adult polymyositis; dermatomyositis; myositis associated with malignancy; childhood myositis; and myositis associated with connective tissue disorders. Clinically similar to adult PM, dermatomyositis (DM) is an idiopathic inflammatory myopathy associated with characteristic dermatologic manifestations.

Symptoms of adult PM gradually accrue over a period of 3 to 6 months. Diagnosis is usually delayed because, unlike in DM, no associated rash occurs before onset of muscle disease. Patients usually present with symmetric proximal muscle weakness in the upper and lower extremities. Distal muscle weakness may occur late in the course of the disease. Patients may report muscle pain and tenderness that may be confused with polymyalgia rheumatica. Constitutional symptoms include morning stiffness, fatigue, anorexia, fever (associated with antisynthetase antibodies such as anti-Jo-1) and weight loss. Dysphagia secondary to oropharyngeal and esophageal involvement occurs in about a third of patients and is a poor prognostic sign. Dysphonia is also a poor prognostic sign but is much less common. Ocular muscles are never involved in generalized PM. However, isolated orbital myositis, an inflammatory disorder involving the extraocular muscles is well described. Facial and bulbar muscle weaknesses are extremely rare manifestations. The diagnosis of polymyositis is made on the basis of a combination of proximal muscle weakness, elevated muscle enzymes, characteristic electromyogram and muscle biopsy. The erythrocyte sedimentation rate is often normal or only mildly elevated and is not a reliable indicated of disease severity.

DIFFERENTIAL DIAGNOSIS

Myopathic weakness may be caused by myasthenia gravis, inflammatory polyneuropathy (Guillain-Barré syndrome); neurotoxin exposure (e.g., botulism, tick paralysis, organophosphate poisoning); severe electrolyte abnormalities; drug and alcohol induced myopathy; periodic paralysis; and rarely polymyositis.

The differential diagnosis of subacute or chronically progressive weakness includes polymyositis, the muscular dystrophies, myasthenia gravis, polymyalgia rheumatica and druginduces myopathy. Thyroid or other endocrine myopathy can also present with proximal muscle weakness as can severe hypokalemia, hypophosphatemia or hypomagnesemia (14). Chronic alcohol abuse can produce a syndrome of proximal muscle weakness and wasting, often with coexistent evidence of alcoholic peripheral neuropathy (12).

EMERGENCY DEPARTMENT EVALUATION

In the face of profound weakness, immediate attention to the ventilatory status and airway stabilization are indicated before performing a detailed history and physical. Patient evaluation should focus on distinguishing neurologic from muscular dysfunction. Key components of the history include: onset and time course, symmetry and fluctuation of symptoms; sensory deficits; involvement of proximal or distal muscle groups; association with activity, such as climbing stairs; difficulty swallowing; precipitating factors; associated pain or stiffness; and sensory deficits. Complaints that suggest a central nervous system origin include diplopia, dysphagia, ataxia, or hemiparesis. Information should also be elicited about family history, history of underlying medical illnesses, medication use and exposure to homemade or contaminated food.

On physical examination the patient should be tested for his ability to perform simple tasks (e.g., lifting arms above head, ability to make a tight fist, rising on the toes, rising from the chair). Determine the distribution of muscle involvement including the extraocular, facial or bulbar musculature. Pathologic muscle fatigue may be elicited by having the patient sustain an upward gaze, count loudly, or hold the arms horizontal. The muscles should be inspected for size and irritability and palpated for tenderness. The neurologic exam must include an evaluation of pupillary size and reactivity, sensory function and deep tendon reflexes. Deep tendon reflexes (DTRs) and sensory perception should be normal in myopathies. DTRs may be diminished or absent in hypokalemic paralysis. A careful search for an adherent tick is important when appropriate.

Using the history and physical examination, it is generally possible to exclude disorders of neuromuscular transmission (myasthenia gravis), peripheral neuropathy, lower and upper motor neuron disease from the diagnosis of myopathy. The diagnosis of myasthenia gravis is suspected on the basis of weakness and fatigability in the typical distribution, without loss of reflexes or impairment of sensation or other neurologic function. Peripheral neuropathy is characterized by areflexia, sensory ataxia, varying degree of cutaneous sensory deficit, and variable degrees of motor dysfunction, sometimes severe. Lower motor neuron dysfunction and early denervation, is characterized by insidiously developing asymmetric weakness, progressive muscle wasting and atrophy with loss of deep tendon reflexes. Finally upper motor neuron disease is characterized by spasticity in the extremities (usually legs more than arms), brisk tendon reflexes, up going plantar reflexes and minimal to no sensory deficits.

Essential lab studies should include complete blood count, erythrocyte sedimentation rate, thyroid function tests, CK with isoenzymes, electrolytes, calcium, magnesium, phosphorus, myoglobin, serum creatinine and BUN, urinalysis (looking for myoglobinuria), Chest X-ray and electrocardiogram. Arterial blood gases and bedside spirometry or peak expiratory flow rate should be performed to evaluate for ventilatory compromise.

EMERGENCY DEPARTMENT MANAGEMENT

In patients with neuromuscular disease presenting with *severe and rapidly progressing weakness,* the crisis is usually precipitated by an intercurrent illness, most commonly a respiratory tract infection. These patients often present with ventilatory compromise, ineffective cough, and difficulty handling secretions. Decompensation to respiratory failure can be rapid. Immediate attention should be directed to oxygenation and ventilatory status. Serial physical examination, arterial blood gas determination, and spirometry are essential, and endotracheal intubation should be performed at the earliest sign of difficulty. Normal levels of pCO_2 and pO_2 are often maintained nearly to the point of profound respiratory failure and respiratory arrest.

The need for intubation and mechanical ventilation is best guided by serial measurement of vital capacity. A declining vital capacity or a vital capacity less than 15 mL/kg is an indication for urgent intubation. Patients with severe weakness should be ventilated, at least initially, in the controlled mode.

Attention to hemodynamic stability is the next priority, with continuous electrocardiographic monitoring and evaluation of fluid needs. Creatine phosphokinase determination and urinalysis are mandatory to identify acute rhabdomyolysis.

For *polymyositis,* prednisone is the first-line treatment of choice. Typically, the dose is 1 mg/kg/d, either as a single dose or divided. This high dose is usually continued for 4 to 8 weeks, until the creatine kinase (CK) level returns to normal. Corticosteroid myopathy can occur during the course of treatment and must be distinguished from reactivation of muscle disease. CK level is usually within reference ranges in cases of steroid myopathy. No improvement is observed with higher doses of steroids, and the condition worsens if the dose is increased. Immunosuppressive agents are indicated if patients do not show improvement with steroids within 4 weeks or if adverse effects from corticosteroids develop. Patients with poor prognostic indicators, such as dysphagia or dysphonia, are likely to require immunosuppressive

agents. Despite relapses, most patients improve with therapy, and up to 50% can eventually discontinue steroid treatment.

Acute attacks of the *hyperkalemic form of periodic paralysis* should be treated with calcium gluconate (1 to 2 gm i.v.) or with glucose and insulin (1 amp $D_{50}W$ with 5 units of regular insulin i.v.). To prevent attacks, chronic therapy with a thiazide diuretic or acetazolamide may be given.

Treatment of *acute hypokalemic periodic paralysis* includes intravenous potassium (40 mEq KCl in 250 ml NS at 10 mEq/hr) or oral KCl (40 mEq hourly for two doses) (10). Acetazolamide prophylaxis and avoidance of high-carbohydrate meals are useful in chronic management.

DISPOSITION

Patients with *severe weakness* require admission to an intensive care setting for supportive care, monitoring of cardiorespiratory status, treatment of any underlying illness, and further diagnostic evaluation. Admission is indicated for patients with *slowly progressive neuromuscular weakness* if there is any concern about the patient's respiratory reserve, if the degree of pharyngeal muscle weakness suggests a risk of aspiration, if rhabdomyolysis is suggested by creatine phosphokinase determination and urinalysis, or if the patient cannot function satisfactorily at home. The decision to manage the problem on an outpatient basis must be made after consultation with the primary care physician, internist, or neurologist, and on the condition that follow-up can be reliably arranged.

DISORDERS OF NEUROMUSCULAR TRANSMISSION

The neuromuscular junction is the critical link between the central nervous system and the musculoskeletal system. Maintaining integrity of neuromuscular transmission is essential for effective communication between nerve and muscle and is required for maintaining skeletal muscle function, including the mechanism of breathing. Although disease states associated with malfunction of the neuromuscular junction only rarely present in the emergency department (ED), these conditions are potentially fatal ailments, and, therefore, must be considered in all patients who present with isolated or generalized muscle weakness of unknown etiology (Table 117.2). Alternatively these disorders can be divided according to the site of derangement as seen in Table 117.3.

The hallmark of weakness associated with failure in neuromuscular transmission is fatigability. The patient may present to the ED with complaints of gradual weakness followed by the precipitous onset of muscular exhaustion. Typically, muscle weakness resolves briefly after a short rest and then worsens again. Neuromuscular transmission failure should also be considered in patients who report complaints of more generalized symptoms such as chronic fatigue and shortness of breath, especially when there is no other obvious explanation for the clinical presentation (7).

MYASTHENIA GRAVIS

CLINICAL PRESENTATION

Myaesthenia gravis (MG), the most common disease of the neuromuscular junction, is an autoimmune disorder in which antibodies are directed against the acetylcholine receptor, reducing

TABLE 117.2. Disorders of Neuromuscular Transmission

Congenital
- Congenital myasthenia gravis
- Acetyl-cholinesterase deficiency

Toxin induced
- C. botulinum
- Snake/Scorpion envenomation,
- Paralytic shellfish poisoning

Autoimmune
- Myasthenia gravis
- Eaton-Lambert syndrome

Poisoning
- Organophosphate poisoning, carbamates

Drugs
- Magnesium
- D-penicillamine
- Aminoglycosides
- Chloroquine
- Fluoroquinolones
- Phenytoin
- Beta blockers
- Quinidine
- Procainamide
- Chlorpromazine
- Lidocaine

the number of available receptors and impairing neuromuscular transmission (23). It is almost always associated with an abnormality of the thymus gland, either thymoma (15%) or thymitis (75%). The thymus appears to be the site where B cells are sensitized to the acetylcholine receptors, initiating the disease process. A reduction in the number of acetylcholine receptors results in a characteristic pattern of progressively reduced muscle strength with repeated use of the muscle and recovery of muscle strength following a period of rest.

The incidence of myasthenia is estimated to be about 14 per 100,000 in the general population (18). The disease is most common in women in their mid-twenties although it can occur at all ages. The peak incidence for men is the sixth or seventh decade of life (5).

The hallmark of myasthenia gravis is pathologic fatigue, owing to the loss of the generous physiologic reserve that normally supports transmission across the neuromuscular junction. Muscle weakness worsens with sustained activity and improves with rest; patients commonly report worsening of symptoms as the day progresses.

Myasthenia gravis is a disease of insidious onset, developing over a period of weeks to months. The muscle weakness occurs at first in transient attacks, at times precipitated by in-

TABLE 117.3. Division of Disorders of Neuromuscular Transmission By Categories

Presynaptic
- Eaton-Lambert syndrome
- Botulism
- Hypermagnesemia
- Scorpion toxin

Synaptic
- Organophosphate poisoning
- Acetylcholinesterase deficiency

Postsynaptic
- Myasthenia gravis
- Congenital myasthenia
- Snake venom

fection, stress, or pregnancy. The extraocular muscles are most commonly affected, and the most typical presentation is one of recurring episodes of diplopia and ptosis that are often noticed later in the day. There may also be weakness of eye closure, weakness of the muscles of facial expression, or difficulty chewing. Transient dysarthria and dysphagia are common. Patients may also have involvement of the proximal limb and truncal and respiratory muscles and note difficulty climbing stairs or combing their hair.

The disease is extremely variable in its clinical presentation and may affect diverse muscle groups in an asymmetric, unpredictable manner, fluctuating in intensity over time. Spontaneous remissions and relapses are common, and the ultimate progression of the disease is highly variable. Respiratory crisis requiring mechanical ventilation occurs in up to 20% of patients.

DIFFERENTIAL DIAGNOSIS

The differential diagnosis includes drug-induced myasthenia, Eaton-Lambert myasthenic syndrome, neuroasthenia or psychoneurotic fatigue, botulism, inflammatory polyneuropathy (Guillain-Barré syndrome), periodic paralysis, and other causes of oculomotor paralysis (diabetes, multiple sclerosis, aneurysm). History, physical examination, and simple laboratory investigations should enable the emergency physician to readily distinguish between these entities (see below). It is important for the emergency physician to consider the possibility of one these diagnoses before making a diagnosis of functional or psychiatric illness.

EMERGENCY DEPARTMENT EVALUATION

The clinical evaluation of the patient presenting with a history of episodic weakness and fatigue involving extraocular, facial or bulbar musculature, should focus on obtaining a careful history, ruling out an underlying precipitating illness, demonstrating pathologic fatigue on physical examination, and considering possible etiologies.

On physical examination, the physician can perform provocative maneuvers, the simplest being extraocular movements. Fatigue with repeated muscle contraction supports the diagnosis. Other maneuvers that may be used to unmask underlying neuromuscular fatigability include having the patient count up to 100 or chew for 30 seconds while observing signs of functional deterioration. It is important to remember that the patient with myasthenia gravis has normal pupils, deep tendon reflexes, and sensation. A major focus of evaluation of myasthenia gravis in the ED is ongoing evaluation of the patients' respiratory status and ability to handle secretions. Bedside spirometry is helpful, at the least as a baseline, as is arterial blood gas analysis looking for evidence of CO_2 retention.

The diagnosis of MG is confirmed by noting improved strength in response to a short-acting anticholinesterase agent (edrophonium test) and by electrophysiologic testing. Intravenous edrophonium (Tensilon) is an anticholinesterase inhibitor with rapid onset of action (about 30 seconds) and a short duration of action (about 5 minutes). Administration produces rapid improvement of ocular symptoms in patients with myasthenia gravis. Edrophonium should be used with caution, especially in cardiac patients, because of its potential for causing bradycardia. When this test is performed, the patient should be placed on a monitor and atropine should be available at the bedside. Administer 1 to 2 mg of edrophonium chloride intravenously and re-examine the patient for a resolution of the weakness. Reversal of eyelid ptosis is the most specific sign. If there is no response to the 2-mg dose give 8 mg of edrophonium after 2 minutes, and again test muscle strength. A false-positive response to edrophonium chloride has been reported in amyotrophic lateral sclerosis, Eaton-Lambert myasthenic syndrome, GBS, wound botulism, cavernous sinus lesions, poliomyelitis, and alcoholic myositis (6,19).

A more definitive test is a repetitive nerve stimulation study. In MG, there is a decrement in the amplitude of the evoked muscle action potential when the motor nerve is repetitively stimulated at 3 cycles/sec.

If the diagnosis of MG is confirmed further testing should include an assay for circulating anti-acetylcholine receptor antibodies. A chest x-ray, thyroid function tests and serologic testing for associated autoimmune diseases should also be performed. Thyroid disorders may be seen in as many as 4% of patients with myasthenia, and symptoms of hyperthyroidism or hypothyroidism may be present.

EMERGENCY DEPARTMENT MANAGEMENT

The major focus of ED management of all disorders of neuromuscular transmission is ongoing evaluation of the patients' respiratory status. The maintenance of a patent airway may be difficult because of increased oral secretions, and inadequate protective reflexes. Evidence of respiratory failure may be noted on ABG, pulmonary function tests, or pulse oximetry. Rapid sequence intubation should be modified because depolarizing paralytic agents (e.g., succinylcholine) have less predictable results in patients with myasthenia. The relative lack of acetylcholine receptors makes these patients relatively resistant to succinylcholine; therefore, higher doses must be used to induce paralysis. Once paralysis is achieved, it may be prolonged. A rapid-onset nondepolarizing agent (i.e., rocuronium, vecuronium) is the preferred paralytic agent in this circumstance.

Once the airway is secured, investigation into the cause of the weakness or exacerbation of myasthenia may be undertaken. There are five major therapeutic options in managing patients with MG: anticholinesterases, immunosuppressives, thymectomy, plasmapheresis and intravenous immunoglobulin.

Anticholinesterases are considered first-line agents for treatment of myasthenia gravis. Their primary action is to increase the concentration of acetylcholine at the synapse; pyridostigmine is the most frequently used agent in this class. Although the anticholinesterases provide symptomatic relief they do not influence the progression of the disease. The starting dose of pyridostigmine is 15 to 60 mg q 4 hrs.

Immunosuppressive therapy is added to the medication regimen of patients whose symptoms are inadequately controlled by anticholinesterase drugs. Corticosteroids are the initial agent of choice followed by other agents such as azathioprine, cyclosporine, or cyclophosphamide if steroids are contraindicated or ineffective.

Thymectomy is indicated in selected patients younger than 60 years of age who have the generalized form of MG, as well as in those individuals who have thymoma. Overall, about 59% of patients with myasthenia gravis have sustained improvement after thymectomy (11,16).

Plasmapheresis and IV immunoglobulin are two short-term therapeutic options that are particularly useful when rapid clearance of antibody is required either to improve symptoms in myasthenic crisis or in patients in whom immunosuppressive treatment has been initiated. The recommended dose for immunoglobulin is 400 mg/kg/d for 5 days, and the improvement begins within 4 to 5 days following administration (13,22).

Some medications including anticonvulsants, neuromuscular blockers, some antibiotics, and major analgesics (Table 117.4)

TABLE 117.4. Common Drugs Capable of Impairing Neuromuscular Transmission or Exacerbating Weakness in Patients with Myasthenia

Antibiotics
- Aminoglycosides
- Tetracycline
- Clindamycin
- Sulfonamides

Anticonvulsant
- Phenytoin
- Barbiturates

Cardiovascular
- Beta-blockers
- Lidocaine
- Quinidine
- Procainamide

Hormonal Agents
- Corticosteroids

Psychotropics
- Chlorpromazine
- Lithium

Analgesics/Muscle relaxants
- Morphine
- Meperidine
- Benzodiazepines

---

should not be administered in patients with myasthenia gravis. Acute intercurrent medical and surgical problems in patients with myasthenia gravis should always be managed in consultation with a neurologist (1).

Myasthenic Crisis vs. Cholinergic Crisis

One of the confusing factors in treating patients with MG is that rapid worsening of the disease due to insufficient medication (i.e., myasthenic crisis) and side effects of excessive medication (i.e., cholinergic crisis) can present in similar ways. Cholinergic crisis results from an excess of cholinesterase inhibitors (i.e., neostigmine, pyridostigmine, physostigmine) and resembles organophosphate poisoning. Excessive acetylcholine stimulation of striated muscle at nicotinic junctions produces flaccid muscle paralysis that is clinically indistinguishable from weakness due to MG. As a rule, in cholinergic crisis, worsening muscle weakness should be accompanied by symptoms of cholinergic excess, including salivation, lacrimation, urination, diarrhea, gastric distress (cramps), emesis, miosis, and bradycardia. Edrophonium can be a useful tool; this agent should make myasthenic weakness better and should exacerbate the cholinergic crisis. Unfortunately, edrophonium has limited use in an acutely decompensating, apprehensive patient. Therefore, it is recommended that all anticholinesterase medications be stopped in myasthenic crisis (2,21).

In practice, the distinction between myasthenic crisis and cholinergic crisis may not be very relevant, since even for the patient with myasthenic crisis initial management does not involve the administration of cholinergic agents.

Myasthenic crisis is a true emergency and usually requires respiratory support. Up to 20% of myasthenic patients will experience at least one episode of myasthenic crisis (21). In the majority of patients with myasthenic crisis, an underlying precipitating event can be identified. Infection is the most common risk factor, followed by aspiration pneumonitis and changes in medication (especially initiation or withdrawal of corticosteroid). In up to one-third of the patients with myasthenic crisis, no precipitating factor can be identified (21). Management of the patient with myasthenic crisis requires general supportive measures and rapid reduction in anti-acetylcholine receptor antibody load. Plasmapheresis is beneficial in myasthenic crisis, and improvement in the patient's clinical status can be seen within a few days. Intravenous immunoglobulin (IG) should also be considered. In a critically ill patient with a secured airway, high-dose steroid therapy should be initiated immediately. All medications that may impair neuromuscular transmission should be discontinued.

BOTULISM

Botulism is caused by a neurotoxin produced by the anaerobic organism *Clostridium botulinum*. *C. botulinum* toxin irreversibly binds to the presynaptic membrane and prevents release of ACh. A rapidly progressive descending paralysis follows and is accompanied by prominent, autonomic symptoms and respiratory involvement. Because the disorder is at the neuromuscular junction, there is no sensory deficit and no sense of pain.

Botulism may vary from a mild illness to a fulminant, fatal one. Cranial nerve findings in the presence of GI symptoms should alert the ED physician to the diagnosis of botulism. Prodromal symptoms of nausea, vomiting, diarrhea, and a dry, painful throat develop hours to days after ingestion of contaminated food. Neurologic symptoms are usually noted within 72 hours of ingestion and include anticholinergic effects (dry eyes, dry mouth, dilated pupils, ileus, and urinary retention) and fluctuating but rapidly progressive weakness, with early involvement of the extraocular and bulbar muscles (with ptosis, diplopia, dysphagia, and dysphonia as common early symptoms). The disease then progresses over several days to involve all the muscles of the trunk and extremities. Respiratory compromise can develop rapidly as the symmetric paralysis descends.

See Chapter 335 for detailed information on the clinical presentation and management of botulism.

EATON-LAMBERT SYNDROME

Eaton-Lambert myasthenic syndrome is a rare, autoimmune condition affecting the presynaptic membrane. Failure of neuromuscular transmission in Eaton-Lambert syndrome is due to the insufficient release of a neurotransmitter at the presynaptic terminal. Antibody-mediated blockade of the voltage-gated calcium channel (VGCC) compromises rapid influx of calcium, which, in turn, results in deficient neurotransmitter release.

Eaton-Lambert syndrome exists in a primary form but may be a manifestation of a paraneoplastic disorder. Malignancy is a common cause of rapidly evolving symptomatology in patients with Eaton-Lambert syndrome. The majority of patients with Eaton-Lambert syndrome are older than 60 years of age, but it has been described in all age groups.

The weakness in Eaton-Lambert syndrome is severe at the onset, but improves soon after initiation of activity, and then deteriorates. Muscle weakness in Eaton-Lambert syndrome tends to be symmetrical and is most pronounced in the lower extremities. Altered gait after prolonged walking usually is the initial symptom. This may progress to inability to rise from a chair or walk up stairs. Ocular and bulbar symptoms are not common and are mild in nature when present. Autonomic symptoms are common and occur in more than half of the patients. On physical examination, proximal muscle weakness is the most prominent clinical finding. The peculiar weakness in Eaton-Lambert syndrome patients may be demonstrated during hand grip. The initial grip may be weak but gets stronger only to weaken again.

The treatment for nonneoplastic cases of Lambert-Eaton myasthenic syndrome includes glucocorticoids, immunosuppressants (azathioprine), and plasmapheresis. The neoplastic variant may respond to similar treatment, however, in addition, it requires treatment of the underlying malignancy (8,16).

TICK PARALYSIS

Tick paralysis is the result of envenomation from the gravid female tick and presents as an ascending flaccid paralysis or as an acute ataxia (17). In the United States the disease occurs primarily in children during warmer months and is caused by the common dog tick *(Dermacentor variabilis)* or female wood tick *(Dermacentor andersoni)*. The primary abnormality is in conduction in the peripheral nerves at the neuromuscular junction. The presentation is similar to Guillain-Barré syndrome. The presenting symptoms are ascending symmetric paralysis over 1 to 2 days, eventually involving the bulbar muscles. Ataxia may be present and may be the earliest finding. Sensory changes are rare, and deep tendon reflexes are absent or decreased. The physician should perform a careful physical examination noting the presence and subsequent removal of the tick. The ticks are often found in the scalp, especially at the hairline. The removal is followed by prompt recovery. Unrecognized, the patient may progress to respiratory paralysis with a fatality rate approaching 10% (17).

The definitive treatment for tick paralysis involves a careful examination for detection of the tick and its removal.

CRITICAL INTERVENTIONS

- Determine the need for intubation and mechanical ventilation by serial measurement of vital capacity. A declining vital capacity or a vital capacity less than 15 mL/kg is an indication for urgent intubation
- Use a rapid-onset nondepolarizing agent (i.e., rocuronium, vecuronium) when paralysis is needed for intubating patients with myasthenia gravis
- Perform a thorough search for an underlying precipitating illness in a patient with myopathy or myasthenia gravis who presents with an exacerbation
- Perform a thorough search for a tick in patients presenting with new weakness
- Obtain electrolytes on patients presenting with weakness

COMMON PITFALLS

✔ Attributing a history of episodic weakness to neuroasthenia (psychogenic weakness) without considering the possibility of a neurologic disorder (e.g., periodic paralysis, myasthenia gravis, or multiple sclerosis)

✔ Failing to take a careful focused history in a patient presenting with a possible neurologic complaint

✔ Failing to perform a thorough search for an underlying precipitating illness in a patient with myopathy or myasthenia gravis who presents with an exacerbation

✔ Attempting an edrophonium test or other pharmacologic maneuvers in the acute management of myasthenic patients presenting in crisis. Acute treatment involves attention to airway and ventilatory status, with a low threshold for endotracheal intubation. Management decisions should be made in consultation with a neurologist

✔ Prescribing medications that may exacerbate weakness in myasthenia gravis. Emergency physicians must be aware of drugs that can impair neuromuscular function. Treatment decisions should be made in consultation with a neurologist

Acknowledgments

Thanks to previous edition's chapter author James J. Walter.

References

1. Adams S, Mathews J, Grammer L. Drugs that may exacerbate myasthenia gravis. *Ann Emerg Med* 1984;13:532.
2. Bella I, Chad D. Neuromuscular disorders and acute respiratory failure. *Neurol Clin N Am* 1998;16:391–417.
3. Bergeron L, Sternbach G. Thyrotoxic periodic paralysis. *Ann Emerg Med* 17:843, 1988.
4. Coffield JA, Bakry N, Zang J, et al. In vitro characterization of botulinum toxin types A, C, and D. Action on human Tissue: Combined electrophysiologic, pharmacologic, and molecular biologic approaches. *J Pharmacol Exp Ther* 1997;280:1489–1498.
5. Donaldson DH, Ansher M, Horan S. The relationship of age to outcome in myasthenia gravis. *Neurology* 1990;90:56–66.
6. Drachman D, et al (eds). *Harrison's Principles of Internal Medicine,* 15th ed. New York: McGraw-Hill, 2001:Chapter 380, 2394.
7. Dushay KM, Zibrak JD, Jensen WA. Myasthenia gravis presenting as isolated respiratory failure. *Chest* 1990;97:232–234.
8. Fukuhara N, Takamori M, Gutmann L, et al. Eaton-Lambert syndrome. *Arch Neurol* 1972;27:67.
9. Gardner-Medwin D. Clinical features and classification of the muscular dystrophies. *Brit Med J* 1980;36:109.
10. Griggs R, Resnick J, Engel K. Intravenous treatment of hypokalemic periodic paralysis. *Arch Neurol* 1980;40:539.
11. Grip S, Hilgers K, Wurm R, et al. Thymoma: Prognostic factors and treatment outcomes. *Cancer* 1998;83:1495.
12. Haller R, Knochel J. Skeletal muscle disease in alcoholism. *Med Clin North Am* 1984;68:91.
13. Howard JF, Jr. Intravenous immunoglobulin for the treatment of acquired myasthenia gravis. *Neurology* 1998;51(Supp 5):S30–36.
14. Kendall-Taylor P, Turnbull D. Endocrine myopathies. *Brit Med J* 1983;287:705.
15. Midura TF. Update: Infant botulism. *Clin Microbiol Rev* 1996;9:119–125.
16. O'Neill JH, Murray NMF, Newsom-Davis J. The Lambert-Eaton myasthenic syndrome: A review of 50 cases. *Brain* 1988;111:577–596.
17. Pearn J. Neuromuscular paralysis caused by tick envenomation. *J Neurol Sci* 34:37, 1977.
18. Phillips LH. The epidemiology of myasthenia gravis. *Neurol Clin N Am* 1994;12:264–271.
19. Seybold M. Myasthenia gravis: A clinical and basic science review. *JAMA* 1983;250:2516.
20. Tacket C, Wayne S, Mann J, et al. Equine antitoxin use and other factors that predict outcome in type A food-borne botulism. *Am J Med* 1984;76:794–798.
21. Thomas CE, Mayer SA, Gungor BS. Myasthenic crisis, clinical features, mortality, complications, and risk factors for prolonged intubation. *Neurology* 1997;48:1253.
22. Thornton CC, Griggs R. Plasma exchange and intravenous immunoglobulin treatment in neuromuscular disease. *Ann Nerurol* 1994;35:260–268.
23. Zweiman B, Arnason B. immunologic aspects of neurological and neuromuscular diseases. *JAMA* 1987;258:2970.

CHAPTER 118
Demyelinating Disease

Adrienne J. Birnbaum

Multiple sclerosis (MS) is the most common autoimmune inflammatory disease of the central nervous system (CNS). It is characterized pathologically by multifocal areas of axonal demyelination with relative preservation of axons. Disease pathogenesis is thought to occur as a result of the interaction between undefined environmental factors and genetic susceptibility. An autoimmune response is triggered that results in inflammatory injury and eventual neurodegeneration.

Clinically, MS is characterized by neurologic symptoms and signs that are attributable to lesions in different locations and that appear at different times over the patient's course. Primarily a disease of young adults, MS follows a course that is highly variable and relatively unpredictable. While approximately 25% of patients with the diagnosis of MS never suffer an effect on activities of daily living, up to 15% become severely disabled within a short time (5). Apart from trauma, MS ranks as the most significant cause of neurologic disability afflicting young adults. As such, the disease has major physical, psychological, and economic consequences for patients, families, and society.

The disease occurs with an incidence of about 7 per 100,000 per year and a lifetime risk of 1 in 400 (5). Women are affected approximately twice as often as men. The incidence of the disease varies geographically with white northern European populations disproportionately affected. The majority of patients report their first symptoms between 20 and 45 years of age. The disease course is most often characterized by exacerbations of acute or subacute onset that last for days to months. Exacerbations are more commonly manifested by the reappearance of previous signs and symptoms than by the development of new ones. Recovery between exacerbations may be complete or incomplete. *Relapsing, remitting disease* refers to a situation in which the clinical course between exacerbations is stable. In general, a pattern of intermittent exacerbations is more common in the earlier stages of the disease, while progressive deterioration, with or without superimposed exacerbations, are more common in the later stages (secondary progressive course). A small percentage of patients experience disease progression from the onset, with or without superimposed exacerbations (primary progressive and progressive relapsing disease, respectively) (1).

CLINICAL PRESENTATION

New Patient with Acute Focal Neurologic Deficit

The first diagnosis of MS cannot be appropriately and definitively made in the emergency department (ED). First, no single clinical feature or diagnostic test is sufficient for final diagnosis, although some are relatively characteristic. While criteria and terminology associated with diagnosis have evolved over time, diagnosis continues to focus on objective demonstration of dissemination of lesions in time and space. This temporal perspective is generally unavailable to the emergency physician seeing the patient at only one point in time. Second, diagnostic test results that enhance the confidence of a clinical diagnosis of MS are often not immediately available in the ED. Finally, the diagnosis of MS imposes a significant psychological burden and should therefore not be made without a substantial degree of certainty.

MS will typically enter into the differential diagnosis of a young adult with two or more clinically distinct episodes of CNS dysfunction or the occurrence of highly suggestive lesions such as optic neuritis or internuclear ophthalmoplegia. Symptoms of MS generally develop over hours or days, but may sometimes occur with the suddenness characteristic of strokes. Negative signs or symptoms (e.g., loss of vision, strength, or sensation) are due to slowed or blocked conduction in axons that undergo demyelination. The demyelinating process can also result in the generation of ectopic impulses, abnormal transmission of impulses between neighboring nerve fibers, and increased mechanical sensitivity. These phenomena are the basis for the generation of "positive" symptoms, such as Lhermitte's sign, (an electric shock–like, tingling, or vibrating sensation in the torso or extremities that is produced by flexion of the neck), flashes of light on eye movement (phosphenes) and paroxysmal symptoms such as trigeminal neuralgia, ataxia and dysarthria or painful tetanic posturing of the limbs triggered by touch or movement. Conduction in partially demyelinated axons fails with an increase in temperature, giving rise to a characteristic worsening of symptoms with

TABLE 118.1. Common Initial Symptoms of
Multiple Sclerosis

Visual loss
Paresthesias and numbness
Diplopia and oculomotor dysfunction
Weakness: monoparesis, paraparesis
Lhermitte sign
Incoordination, unsteady gait, abnormal balance
Acute transverse myelopathy
Vertigo
Bladder, bowel dysfunction
Tremor

a rise in temperature as may occur with exercise or a warm bath (Uhthoff phenomenon) (5). Demyelination can occur anywhere within the CNS and the possible clinical manifestations of MS are therefore extremely varied. However, MS lesions have a predilection for certain sites, resulting in a relatively limited distribution of typical initial symptoms (17). While no symptoms or neurologic findings are pathognomonic, some are characteristic and may heighten the clinician's diagnostic suspicions (Table 118.1). The majority of patients present with one or more of these signs and symptoms.

Decreased visual acuity and symptoms related to oculomotor dysfunction (e.g., diplopia) are among the most common initial presenting symptoms of MS. Optic neuritis characteristically presents with subacute monocular loss of vision although simultaneous or sequential loss of vision can occur in both eyes. Visual loss typically progresses over days to 2 weeks and is accompanied by headache or retroorbital or periocular pain in most but not all cases that may be exacerbated by movement of the eye. Maximal loss of visual acuity varies from blurring to absence of light perception in the affected eye. Alteration of color vision and visual field defect may occur. Slit lamp exam is usually normal but occasionally may reveal cells and flare in the anterior chamber. The optic disc appears swollen on initial presentation in 36% to 58% of cases. An afferent pupillary defect (Marcus Gunn pupil), consisting of diminished response to a direct light stimulus and a normal consensual response to a light stimulus in the opposite eye, may be noted (8). Optic nerve involvement may remain as an isolated manifestation, but roughly half of these patients are diagnosed with MS within 15 to 20 years (8,14,18,19).

Neuromyelitis optica or Devic disease, an uncommon disorder, consists of optic neuritis and transverse myelitis.

Nystagmus and diplopia occur commonly in patients with MS. The finding of internuclear ophthalmoplegia, especially in a young adult, is very suggestive. This form of dysconjugate gaze, referable to the medial longitudinal fasciculus of the brainstem, involves limited adduction of one eye and nystagmus in the abducting eye on lateral gaze.

Sensory symptoms are among the most common presenting symptoms in MS and include numbness, tingling, pins and needles, tightness, and coldness of the limbs or trunk. Radicular pain and itching in a dermatomal distribution can occur. Symptoms are variable in distribution and can be referable to spinothalamic, posterior column, and dorsal nerve root or can occur distally in the extremities or in a patchy distribution. Motor weakness may occur as paraparesis, hemiparesis, or monoparesis and is generally accompanied by signs of upper motor neuron dysfunction (e.g., hyperreflexia and positive Babinski sign) (5). Transverse myelitis can be the initial neurologic event. Symptoms include ascending weakness and numbness below the level of the lesion.

Transient attacks of paroxysmal dysarthria and ataxia are also suggestive of demyelinating disease when they occur in a young person without vascular risk factors.

Patients with Known Multiple Sclerosis

In most cases, the natural history of MS is characterized by episodes of neurologic dysfunction alternating with periods of stabilization or remission of symptoms. Common signs and symptoms of chronic disease are listed in Table 118.2. Patients with known MS may present to the ED because of an exacerbation of previous deficits, because of the development of new deficits, or because of medical complications of the disease.

Factors that have been cited as having an association with the occurrence of MS exacerbations are infection (including minor respiratory infections and gastrointestinal infections), and the postpartum period. Pregnancy itself has not been associated with an increase in frequency of attacks (5,10).

Common secondary complications in patients with MS are pneumonia, infections of the urinary tract, septicemia, respiratory failure, pulmonary embolism, bladder and renal calculi, and pressure ulcers of the skin (17). Elevated body temperature, occurring as a result of infection or because of exposure to heat, can be associated with a transient increase in neurologic symptoms.

TABLE 118.2. Common Chronic Problems of Multiple Sclerosis

Problem	Drugs Used in Treatment[15,16]
Weakness: monoparesis, paraparesis, hemiparesis, quadriparesis	Corticosteroids, potassium channel blockers (i.e., 4-aminopyridine, 3,4-diaminopyridine)
Spasticity	Baclofen (oral or intrathecal), benzodiazepines, dantrolene, tizanidine
Paresthesias	Amitriptyline, carbamazepine, gabapentin, corticosteroids if disabling
Bladder dysfunction	Depends on type of impairment
Optic atrophy, blurred vision, central scotomata	Intravenous methylprednisolone for acute optic neuritis
Internuclear ophthalmoplegia, diplopia	Corticosteroids
Loss of balance, incoordination, ataxia, tremor	Clonazepam for tremor; corticosteroids for balance
Cognitive changes	Disease modifying agents (e.g. Interferon beta, glatiramer acetate); assessment for depression
Depression	Antidepressants
Sexual dysfunction	Sildenafil, intracavernosal prostaglandins (for erectile dysfunction)
Fatigue	Amantadine, CNS stimulants
Vertigo	Meclizine, prochlorperazine, diazepam, metoclopramide
Paroxysmal symptoms: itching, burning, twitching, Lhermitte sign	Carbamazepine, phenytoin, tricyclic antidepressants, low-dose antipsychotics, gabapentin
Pseudobulbar palsy	Amitriptyline, levodopa, bromocriptine

Exacerbations that include dysphagia can result in aspiration pneumonia.

Fatigue is a common complaint of patients with MS. It typically increases with exercise, heat exposure, or as the day progresses. Spasticity, a manifestation of upper motor neuron disease, is characterized by increased muscle tone, hyperreflexia, decreased mobility, painful muscle spasms, and weakness. There is conflicting evidence as to whether seizures occur more frequently in MS patients than in the general population. When seizures occur, they should not be attributed to MS until other causes have been ruled out. Similarly, aphasia and dementia should prompt a search for alternate causes.

Major depression has a lifetime occurrence of 50% in patients with MS. A recent critical review did not find adequate evidence to substantiate concerns that newer disease modifying agents for the treatment of MS might be associated with an increase in the incidence of depression or worsening of depressive illness. Treatment of depression with usual psychotherapy and pharmacotherapy are often effective (6).

DIFFERENTIAL DIAGNOSIS

The differential diagnosis of an acute focal neurologic deficit is broad and includes the intracranial and spinal cord processes listed in Table 118.3. Some of the more common diseases capable of causing multifocal CNS lesions disseminated over time are systemic lupus erythematosus, Lyme disease, sarcoidosis, and CNS vasculitis. Because MS is a disease that is confined to the CNS, patients generally lack the rheumatologic and constitutional symptoms and laboratory abnormalities that are present in many of these other disease states. Spinal cord compression by mass lesions or hematomas must be considered in the patient who presents with symptoms referable to the spinal cord. The differential diagnosis of transverse myelitis includes both infectious (e.g., herpes simplex) and postinfectious causes.

EMERGENCY DEPARTMENT EVALUATION

When faced with a patient with one or more focal neurologic deficits in whom MS is suspected, a critical task of the EM provider is the exclusion of other disease entities that may mimic the diagnosis and require specific immediate treatment. The definitive diagnosis of MS is most appropriately left to the neurologist in the non-ED setting. MS remains primarily a clinical diagnosis, requiring the demonstration of focal neurologic signs and symptoms scattered over time and space. Just as no neurologic findings are pathognomonic for MS, no laboratory test is universally diagnostic. Diagnostic evaluations used to confirm the diagnosis or aid in situations in which the diagnosis cannot be made definitively on clinical grounds include visualization of anatomic dissemination of lesions in time and space with MRI of the brain and spinal cord; assessment of inflammation and immunologic dysfunction through cerebrospinal fluid (CSF) examination; and demonstration of alteration of conduction in a pattern consistent with demyelination through the use of evoked potentials (5,12).

Magnetic resonance imaging (MRI) is the most sensitive and specific paraclinical test used to make the diagnosis of MS (12). T2-weighted brain imaging is superior in sensitivity to contrast-enhanced computed tomography (CT). MRI is used to monitor the course of the disease and its response to treatment and is useful in identifying alternate diagnoses such as intracranial neoplasm, vascular abnormalities, and spinal cord lesions. Characteristic lesions observed on MRI are plaques typically found in the periventricular region and juxtacortical white matter. Plaques correspond pathologically to multifocal areas of demyelination and perivascular infiltration of lymphocytes, macrophages and plasma cells. Typical lesions are ovoid and are arranged like fingers radiating away from the walls of the lateral ventricles. In addition, lesions commonly involve the corpus callosum, white matter abutting the temporal horns and trigones of the lateral ventricles, brainstem and cerebellum, and spinal cord (16). Signal enhancement with gadolinium is characteristic of the disruption of the blood–brain barrier that occurs with active inflammatory lesions. The number, size, and distinctive location of areas of increased signal found on MRI help distinguish MS from other neurologic diseases. A negative MRI does not, however, have sufficient sensitivity or negative predictive value to rule out the diagnosis (13). Diseases that may produce similar lesions include ischemia, systemic lupus erythematosus, Behcet disease, other vasculitides, HTLV-1 and sarcoidosis.

Findings on MRI are common in patients with optic neuritis, even when there is no other clinical evidence of MS. MRI has been demonstrated to have prognostic value in predicting conversion from isolated syndromes, such as optic neuritis, myelitis, and internuclear ophthalmoplegia, to MS (2,4,16).

Examination of the CSF can help to confirm the diagnosis by demonstration of immune and inflammatory mediators of disease. For the diagnosis of MS, CSF abnormality is defined as the presence of oligoclonal IgG bands different from bands in the serum and/or the presence of an elevated IgG index (12). Other common CSF findings include elevated total protein and a

---

TABLE 118.3.   Differential Diagnosis of Acute Focal
Neurologic Deficit

BLEEDING (SPONTANEOUS OR TRAUMATIC)

Subdural hematoma
Intraparenchymal hemorrhage
Epidural hematoma
Subarachnoid hemorrhage

INFECTION

Abscess
Brain
Epidural
Subdural
Meningitis/encephalitis

NEOPLASM

Primary
Metastatic

VASCULAR

Thrombosis
Embolism

METABOLIC

Hypoglycemia
Hyperosmolar hyperglycemia
B_{12} deficiency (spinal cord)

MISCELLANEOUS

Postictal
Migraine
Bell palsy
Psychogenic (diagnosis of exclusion)

modestly increased mononuclear cell count (less than 50 cells/μL). In addition, CSF analysis permits the exclusion of infection as the cause of symptoms.

Evoked potentials (EPs) are electrodiagnostic studies that measure the electrical potentials (voltages) that are evoked in response to the application of brief sensory stimuli. Demyelination causes abnormal axonal conduction that can be picked up on EP testing as abnormal potentials. This modality falls into the domain of the neurologist and is not part of the ED evaluation.

EMERGENCY DEPARTMENT MANAGEMENT

Treatment of acute exacerbations of MS is most appropriately undertaken in consultation with a neurologist. The antiinflammatory effects of steroids have traditionally been the primary therapy for relapses in patients with known disease. Corticosteroids shorten the duration of relapses and their short term morbidity but have not been demonstrated to alter the evolution of resulting permanent deficits (5,7). It has been suggested by some that this failure to demonstrate a reduction in disability from relapses may relate to delay in administration (5).

Studies comparing different steroid regimens (e.g., intravenous vs. oral) have failed to demonstrate a clear advantage of one over the other (1,5). An exception is the use of corticosteroids in the treatment of optic neuritis. Current evidence-based recommendations support the use of higher dose oral or parenteral methylprednisolone (usual dose is 1 gram per day of intravenous methylprednisolone for three days with or without an oral taper) but not lower dose (1 mg/kg) oral prednisone in the treatment of optic neuritis (8). Benefit has been demonstrated in speed and degree of recovery of visual function but this benefit diminishes over time and evidence of long-term benefit for visual function is lacking (8). A reduction in the rate of development of MS has been demonstrated at 2 years for short-term treatment of optic neuritis with intravenous methylprednisolone followed by prednisone, but not for prednisone alone (2,3). However, this benefit was not sustained at 5 years (14).

Prevention of the exacerbations associated with MS and alteration of the progression of neurologic disability are the focus of extensive ongoing research. Therapeutic interventions are aimed at limiting demyelination, enhancing remyelination, and improving conduction in demyelinated fibers. Interferon beta and glatiramer acetate are currently the most commonly prescribed disease modifying drugs. The annual relapse rate of patients treated with these drugs is lower than that in those treated with placebo and more treated patients remain relapse free compared with untreated patients (15). Their use may be limited by adverse events (such as flu-like symptoms, depression, injection site necrosis, elevated liver enzymes, leukopenia and anemia), cost, and uncertain long term clinical benefit. Treatments currently under investigation include mitoxantrone, natalizumab, alemtuzumab, statins, and estrogens (15). Administration of disease-altering drugs generally falls under the domain of the neurologist.

In the patient with known disease who presents with fever, sources of infection should be sought and treated aggressively. Patients with bladder dysfunction are particularly susceptible to urinary tract infection; decubitus ulcers and pneumonia are other common sources of infection that should be considered. Antipyretics should be administered. An elevated temperature that is related to heat exposure should be treated by active cooling measures. Table 118.2 lists some of the more common fixed neurologic symptoms of MS along with their treatments.

CRITICAL INTERVENTIONS

- Do not make the initial diagnosis of MS in the emergency department
- Initiate high dose oral or parenteral methylprednisolone in the treatment of optic neuritis
- Diagnose and treat fever in MS patients since elevated body temperature, occurring as a result of infection or exposure to heat, can be associated with a transient increase in neurologic symptoms

---

DISPOSITION

The patient with new onset clinically suspected MS may warrant hospital admission to complete the diagnostic workup, to exclude other causes of signs and symptoms, and to undergo aggressive treatment of debilitating symptoms. For the patient with known MS, determination of the need for hospitalization depends on the general medical condition as well as the neurologic status. Patients may also require hospitalization for medical complications of MS (e.g., infection), for the administration of aggressive treatment of neurologic symptoms, and for the supportive care necessary because of disability during disease exacerbations.

COMMON PITFALLS

✔ Failure to identify and treat other disease entities in the patient with known or suspected MS

✔ Failure to consider the possibility of intercurrent medical illnesses, especially those that commonly affect the chronically ill neurologic patient (e.g., urinary tract infection, pneumonia, decubitus ulcers)

✔ Failure to realize that rheumatologic or constitutional symptoms or abnormal laboratory values should call the diagnosis of MS into question

✔ Allowing the diagnosis of MS in a patient with progressive disease at a single site (e.g. spinal) when other diagnoses have not been adequately excluded

✔ Failure to consider MS in the young patient presenting with focal neurologic signs and symptoms. The presenting symptoms of MS can be vague and transient, and can seem bizarre. A psychogenic etiology remains a diagnosis of exclusion

References

1. Barnes D, Hughes RA, Morris RW, et al. Randomised trial of oral and intravenous methylprednisolone in acute relapses of multiple sclerosis. *Lancet* 1997;349:902.
2. Beck RW, Cleary PA, Trobe JD, et al. The effect of corticosteroids for acute optic neuritis on the subsequent development of multiple sclerosis. *N Engl J Med* 1993;329:1764.
3. Beck RW, Cleary PA, Anderson MM, et al. A randomized controlled trial of corticosteroids in the treatment of acute optic neuritis. *N Engl J Med* 1992;326:581.
4. Beck RW, Arrington J, Murtagh FR, et al. Brain magnetic resonance imaging in acute optic neuritis—experience of the optic neuritis study group. *Arch Neurol* 1993;50:841.
5. Compston A, Coles A. Multiple Sclerosis. *Lancet* 2002;359:1221.
6. Feinstein A. Multiple Sclerosis, disease modifying treatments and depressions: A critical methodological review. *Mult Scler* 2000;5:343.
7. Filippini G, Brusaferri L, Sibley WA, et al. Corticosteroids or ACTH for acute exacerbations in multiple sclerosis (Cochrane Review). In: The Cochrane Library, 1, 1999. Oxford.
8. Hickman SJ, Dalton CM, Miller DH, et al. Management of acute optic neuritis. *Lancet* 2002;360:1953–1962.
9. Kaufman DI, Trobe JD, Eggenberger ER, et al. Practice parameter: The role of corticosteroids in the management of acute monosymptomatic optic neuritis: Report of the quality standards subcommittee of the American College of Neurology. *Neurology* 2000;54:2039.

10. Lynch SG, Rose JW. Multiple sclerosis. *Dis Monogr* 1996;11:10.
11. Lublin FD, Reingold SC, et al. Defining the clinical course of multiple sclerosis: results of an international survey. *Neurology* 1996;46:907.
12. McDonald WI, Compston A, Edan G, et al. Recommended diagnostic criteria for multiple sclerosis: guidelines from the International Panel on the diagnosis of multiple sclerosis. *Ann Neurol* 2001;50:121.
13. Mushlin AI, Detsky AS, Phelps CE, et al. The accuracy of magnetic resonance imaging in patients with suspected multiple sclerosis. *JAMA* 1993;269:3146.
14. Optic Neuritis Study Group. The 5-year risk of MS after optic neuritis: experience of the optic neuritis treatment trial. *Neurology* 1997;49:1404.
15. Polman CH, Uitdehaag MJ. New and emerging treatment options for multiple sclerosis. *Lancet Neurol* 2003;2:563.
16. Pretorius PM, Quaghebeur G. The role of MRI in the diagnosis of MS. *Clinical Radiology* 2003;58:434.
17. Raine CS, McFarland HF, Toutellotte WW, eds. *Multiple sclerosis: clinical and pathogenetic basis.* London: Chapman & Hall, 1997.
18. Rizzo JF, Lessell S. Risk of developing multiple sclerosis after uncomplicated optic neuritis: a long-term prospective study. *Neurology* 1988;38:185.
19. Rodriguez M, Siva A, Cross SA, et al. Optic neuritis: a population-based study in Olmsted County, Minnesota. *Neurology* 1995;45:244.

CHAPTER 119
Parkinsonism and Other Movement Disorders

Brendan R. Furlong

Parkinsonism, or Parkinson syndrome, is a group of progressive degenerative central nervous system disorders characterized by cardinal motor signs of bradykinesia, tremor, rigidity, and postural instability. Idiopathic Parkinson disease (PD) is the most common cause of parkinsonism and accounts for 80% of cases. Secondary parkinsonism, from a host of disparate causes, constitutes the remaining 20% (Table 119.1).

The incidence of parkinsonism and PD is approximately 20 per 100,000 and increases with age (11,15). There does not appear to be a genetic predisposition for PD when the disease begins after age 50, although there may be one for early-onset disease (15). There is no gender difference, but PD appears to be more common in Whites than in other groups (17). The survival rate for appropriately treated PD approximates that of the general population, whereas that of secondary parkinsonism is markedly less and the clinical course more complicated (8).

Although the precise cause and pathophysiology of PD is not known, recent studies suggest inflammation, oxidative stress, and abnormal protein accumulation lead to cell death in the substantia nigra (12,13,17). Profound localized depletion of the neurotransmitter dopamine in the substantia nigra is the biochemical marker for the disease (3,14). The mainstay of therapy for PD is neurotransmitter replacement in the form of levodopa. Infections (von Economo's pandemic of encephalitis lethargica), toxins (the designer drug methylphenyl tetrahydropyridine [MPTP], the pesticide rotenone) (13), and medications (phenothiazines) are known causes of secondary parkinsonism (see Table 119.1).

In practice, the diagnosis of parkinsonism and PD is made on clinical grounds, but the ultimate diagnosis still rests with neuropathologic confirmation at autopsy (4). The various secondary parkinsonian syndromes show etiology-specific pathologic changes in the extrapyramidal system and the cortex of the brain. PD has distinct cellular degeneration of the substantia nigra with characteristic Lewy bodies (5). Precisely how the neurochemical and pathologic changes in parkinsonism result in dysfunction of the regulation of tone and motor activity is not completely understood (8). Advanced imaging techniques such as functional magnetic resonance imaging and positron emission tomography are contributing to a better understanding of functional anatomy (2).

CLINICAL PRESENTATION

Patients can present to the emergency department (ED) with complaints referable to undiagnosed parkinsonism or with complications of previously diagnosed illness. Emergent interventions are rarely needed for the disease itself. However, it is important to make the diagnosis as soon as possible because effective symptomatic treatment is available and there is the possibility of preventing disease progression.

The clinical manifestations of parkinsonism develop insidiously and gradually. Motor deficiencies are usually asymmetric. Rigidity may be present on flexion and extension of the extremities and neck, and "cogwheel" rigidity on passive extension of the elbow or circumduction of the wrist may be noted. Early on, ambulation is generally slow; short or shuffling steps (*march à petits pas*), instability, and falls occur later. The classic tremor of PD is a 3- to 6-Hz distal resting tremor that increases in periods of anxiety and disappears during sleep or voluntary motor activity. Monotonous speech and decreased speech volume are other early features, and there is eventual development of drooling, dysphagia, and masked facies. Sensory findings are generally absent.

The Mini-Mental State Examination is usually normal early in the disease. Depression may occur. The presence of early dementia and psychosis (unrelated to medicines), autonomic dysfunction (orthostasis), cerebellar findings, and supranuclear gaze palsy suggest one of the secondary causes of parkinsonism (4,8).

In patients with known PD, complications of therapy or a worsening of symptoms while on therapy is often the reason for presentation to the ED. The so-called on–off phenomenon, sudden wide fluctuations in motor function, ranging in severity from dyskinesia to freezing, can be particularly troubling to patients. "Wearing off," or loss of therapeutic effect, should prompt a reassessment of the medication regime and also confirmation that secondary parkinsonism has not been erroneously diagnosed as PD. Orthostasis, nausea, vomiting, and acute psychosis can be caused by various dopaminergic and anticholinergic agents.

TABLE 119.1. Causes of Parkinsonism

Parkinson disease (PD)
Neurodegenerative processes
  Multiple system atrophy (MSA)
  Progressive supranuclear palsy (PSP)
  Corticobasal degeneration (CBD)
Drugs—phenothiazines, butyrophenones, anticonvulsants
Toxins—Methylphenyl tetrahydropyridine (MPTP), carbon monoxide, manganese, rotanone
Trauma
Malignancy—lymphoma, glioma
Arteriosclerotic parkinsonism
Infections—epidemic encephalitis, von Economo encephalitis

Differentiating disease progression from medication inadequacy or excess can be difficult, but is an important part of ED management.

Other complications related to general motor disability (e.g., traumatic injuries due to falls) are significant reasons for ED presentation. In addition, many older patients, the cohort most affected by parkinsonism, have multiple medical conditions that can be more difficult to manage in the setting of progressive parkinsonism.

DIFFERENTIAL DIAGNOSIS

The primary entities in the differential diagnosis of parkinsonism are idiopathic PD and secondary parkinsonism. To help distinguish PD from secondary parkinsonism on a clinical basis, Gelb et al (4), have suggested specific diagnostic criteria for PD: bradykinesia, rigidity, and the asymmetric onset of resting tremor, all of which must have a substantial and sustained response to levodopa or dopamine agonist therapy. The presence of postural instability, freezing phenomena, hallucinations, dementia, severe dysautonomia, or supranuclear gaze palsy within the first 3 years of disease presentation suggests a secondary form of parkinsonism (4). PD has a gradually progressive course; rapid progression strongly suggests another form of parkinsonism (4).

EMERGENCY DEPARTMENT EVALUATION

The ED evaluation of a patient with clinical symptoms suggestive of parkinsonism consists primarily of a history and physical examination. For patients with new symptoms, clinical assessment is aimed at identifying parkinsonism and then differentiating between the secondary parkinsonian syndromes and PD. MRI is useful in the comprehensive evaluation of parkinsonism, but rarely indicated in the ED (6).

For patients previously diagnosed with parkinsonism, evaluation should focus on progression of disease, complications of medical treatment, and concomitant medical conditions.

EMERGENCY DEPARTMENT MANAGEMENT

Strategies for the management of parkinsonism in the ED should be coordinated with the physician who will treat the patient for the long term.

For patients who are *newly diagnosed* with PD, treatment includes agents to alleviate disabling symptoms, as well as agents that are potentially neuroprotective. Table 119.2 outlines treatment options. The centrally acting dopamine agonist levodopa is the mainstay of symptomatic treatment. It is desirable to use the minimum amount of levodopa necessary to control symptoms, because the metabolism of levodopa is thought to contribute to an excess of oxyradicals in the substantia nigra, leading to further cell degeneration. Levodopa's peripheral side effects (nausea, vomiting, and orthostasis) are thus limited as well (14). Carbidopa blocks the peripheral metabolism of levodopa, allowing lower doses of levodopa to be effective centrally. For this reason, the levodopa–carbidopa combination drug, Sinemet, has become a mainstay of treatment. Agents with neuroprotective effects (dopamine agonists, MAO-B inhibitors) are used more prominently (12). Agents which control inflammation (NSAIDS, aspirin) are currently under review (17). The anticholinergic drug benztropine is prescribed selectively for patients with tremor predominance. For those with severe disease refractory to medical management, deep-brain stimulation of the subthalamic

TABLE 119.2.   Management of Parkinson Disease

MEDICAL

Dopamine Precursor
Levodopa: precursor of the pathologically deficient dopamine, which is able to cross the blood-brain barrier; improves symptoms; most often used in combination with carbidopa
Side effects: dyskinesia, anorexia, nausea, vomiting, postural hypotension

Peripheral Dopa-decarboxylase Inhibitor
Carbidopa: peripheral dopa-decarboxylase inhibitor; decreases peripheral breakdown of levodopa, allowing lower dose therapy
Side effects: may exacerbate central dopaminergic side effects when levodopa dose not reduced sufficiently

Dopamine Agonist
Bromocriptine: dopamine agonist used as adjuvant to levodopa; decreases the dopamine requirement, thus allowing lower dose levodopa therapy (7); also appears to decrease dyskinesias and "on-off" side effects
Side effects: hypotension, nausea, vomiting, constipation, fatigue, hallucinations
Pergolide: dopamine agonist used as adjuvant to levodopa; also used by some as monotherapy, particularly early in young-onset PD
Side effects: hypotension, nausea, vomiting, constipation, confusion, hallucinations, dyskinesias, dystonias

MAO-B Inhibitor
Selegiline: MAO-B inhibitor thought to reduce the peroxide produced as MAO-B metabolizes dopamine (9); may also have some therapeutic effect
Side effects: sleep disturbances, psychosis, agitation, confusion, dyskinesias

Anticholinergic Drugs
Benztropine: striatal muscarinic blocker; useful in treating the tremor of PD
Side effects: typical anticholinergic symptoms and signs

SURGICAL

Electrical deep-brain stimulation
Posteroventral pallidotomy
Neural cell transplantation

PD, Parkinson disease.

nucleus or the pars interna of the globus pallidus has been shown to significantly improve motor symptoms (9).

For patients with *known* PD, ED management is directed at recognizing the inadequacy or excess of the medication regimen and adjusting dosages accordingly. The "on–off" phenomenon is thought to be due to fluctuations in drug concentrations. Changing doses or dosing intervals and adding other antiparkinsonism agents may be necessary. A sustained-release levodopa–carbidopa combination appears to reduce the total levodopa requirement, as well as variations in drug concentration (1). Medication excess may cause acute psychiatric and cognitive side effects, such as psychosis, hallucinations, delusions, agitation, and confusion. This may require a decrease in dopaminergic and anticholinergic medications and the initiation of clozapine (14). The peripheral side effects of excessive dopamine (nausea, vomiting, and orthostasis) are treated by reducing levodopa doses. Optimizing the balance of various agents can be difficult and should be coordinated with the patient's primary physician.

The management of the parkinsonian syndromes other than PD is generally less effective. Parkinsonism due to prescription medications may improve with cessation of the implicated agent, but parkinsonism associated with prior methylphenyl tetrahydropyridine use is not reversible. Symptoms of neurodegenerative parkinsonism can be managed with the same agents as used for those of PD, but there tends not to be a sustained response to therapy.

For all parkinsonian syndromes, injuries from falls, infections (e.g., aspiration pneumonia), and concomitant medical conditions should be evaluated and managed as with other patients, keeping in mind the limitations imposed by the patient's chronic level of functioning.

CRITICAL INTERVENTIONS

- Direct management at recognizing the inadequacy or excess of the medication regimen for patients with *known* PD
- Coordinate management strategies of parkinsonism with the physician who will treat the patient for the long term

DISPOSITION

Whether the diagnosis of parkinsonism is made in the ED or the patient is being seen for complications of therapy or progression of symptoms, the patient's primary care physician or neurologist should be consulted. This assures continuity of care, which is essential to optimize the management of this chronic condition. Rarely is admission to the hospital or transfer to a tertiary care center indicated for parkinsonism itself. Complications such as sepsis or injuries from falls are more likely to be indications for inpatient management.

COMMON PITFALLS

✔ The diagnosis of parkinsonism may be missed in patients with vague complaints of dizziness, unsteadiness, or inability to walk, unless the signs are specifically sought on careful neurologic examination

✔ The complex medical regimens for PD require precise modifications to maximize clinical benefit while minimizing side effects

References

1. Capildeo R. Implications of the 5-year CR FIRST trial. *Neurology* 1998;50: [Suppl 6]:S15.
2. Cebellos-Baumann, AO. Functional imaging in Parkinson's disease: activation studies with PET, fMRI, and SPECT. *Journal of Neurology* 2003;250 [Suppl 1]:15.
3. Duvoisin RC. A brief history of parkinsonism. *Neurol Clin* 1992;10:301.
4. Gelb DJ, et al. Diagnostic criteria for Parkinson disease. *Arch Neurol* 1999;56:33.
5. Gibb WRG. Neuropathology of Parkinson's disease and related syndromes. *Neurol Clin* 1992;10:361.
6. Lachenmayer L. Differential Diagnosis of parkinsonian syndromes: dynamics of time courses are essential. *Journal of Neurology* 2003;250[Suppl 1]:11.
7. Little NE. Parkinson disease. In: Harwood-Nuss AL, Linden CH, Luten RC, et al, eds. *The clinical practice of emergency medicine*, 2nd ed. Philadelphia: Lippincott–Raven Publishers, 1996:897.
8. Litvan I. Parkinsonian features: when are they Parkinson disease? *JAMA* 1998;280:1654.
9. Obeso JA, et al. Deep-brain stimulation of the subthalamic nucleus or the pars interna of the globus pallidus in Parkinson's disease. *NEJM* 2001;345:956.
10. Olanow CW, Koller WC, et al. An algorithm (decision tree) for the management of Parkinson's disease: treatment guidelines. *Neurology* 1998;50[Suppl 3]: S1.
11. Rajput AH, et al. Epidemiology of parkinsonism: incidence, classification, and mortality. *Ann Neurol* 1984;16:278.
12. Riess O, et al. Therapeutic strategies for Parkinson's disease based on data derived from genetic research. *Journal of Neurology* 2003;250[Suppl 1]:3.
13. Siderowf A, Stern M. Update on Parkinson Disease. *Annals of Internal Medicine* 2003;138:651.
14. Stern MB. Contemporary approaches to the pharmacotherapeutic management of Parkinson's disease: an overview. *Neurology* 1997;49[Suppl 1]:S2.
15. Tanner CM, et al. Parkinson disease in twins: an etiologic study. *JAMA* 1999;281:341.
16. Tanner CM. Epidemiology of Parkinson's disease. *Neurol Clin* 1992;10:317.
17. Wullner U, Klockgether T. *Journal of Neurology* 2003;250[Suppl 1]:35.

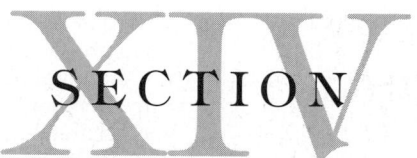

SECTION XIV

Section Editor: Jeffrey Schaider

Psychiatric Emergencies

CHAPTER 120
Medical Clearance

Kerry B. Broderick and Carrie D. Mendoza

One of the more challenging responsibilities for the emergency physician (EP) is the medical clearance of the psychiatric patient. Several studies have estimated that psychiatric complaints account for 2% to 12% of Emergency Department (ED) visits (1,2). Before the patient can be transferred to a psychiatric facility or service, the EP is responsible for identifying any significant medical condition(s). The term 'medical clearance' seems to have developed in the 1970s. Weissberg's 1979 article (3) describes the common scenarios in which EPs apply the concept of medical clearance: (1) the psychiatric patient found to have no physical illness, (2) a psychiatric patient with a known medical condition which is not currently impacting the psychiatric illness, and (3) the psychiatric patient whose acute medical issue has been treated and is now ready for transfer to a psychiatric facility.

There is a lack of standardized nomenclature in this area. The terms *organic disease* and *functional disease* are, perhaps, most frequently used. Organic disease denotes nonpsychiatric causes, and functional disease indicates a psychiatric cause. To define a mental disorder as 'organic', however, implies that a nonorganic or functional mental disorder is unrelated to physical or biologic factors or processes (4,5). In fact, many chemical neurophysiologic and genetic factors, have been documented to be related to psychiatric disease. *The Diagnostic and Statistical Manual of Mental Disorders*, Fourth Edition (DSM-IV), eliminates the terms *organic* and *functional* and distinguishes "mental disorders that are due to a general medical condition" or secondary mental disorders from "primary mental disorders" (6).

Treatment depends on differentiating between predominant psychiatric illness and predominant medical illness in patients who present in these various ways. The prevalence of physical illness among psychiatric patients appears to be dependent upon the population studied. One study specifically reviewing emergency department practice found that 80% of patients in whom medical disease should have been identified in the emergency department were documented as "medically clear" (7). While another study found "medical problems" in only 19% of ED patients (8).

CLINICAL PRESENTATION AND EMERGENCY DEPARTMENT EVALUATION

Patients that require medical clearance may be separated into two general categories: those patients with a known psychiatric illness and those without a prior psychiatric diagnosis but who are presenting with abnormal behavior and thought. The clinical evaluation of these patients includes a focused history and physical exam, individual patient directed laboratory and ancillary tests, and consideration of the care available by the receiving psychiatric facility or service.

History

Approaching patients in a consistent, nonjudgmental manner is less threatening to the patients and maximize the history accuracy. Important questions to ascertain include: the time frame involved in the onset of symptoms, as well as other events leading up to presentation. Obtaining history from the patient and their perception of the current situation as well as using paramedics, caretakers, and caseworkers will assure the most comprehensive and accurate history.

Medication use or noncompliance and substance abuse are important historical factors. Psychiatric patients with substance abuse comorbidity have a significantly higher number of ED visits than those without substance abuse (9). A detailed history on medication use, recent changes, and noncompliance, both prescribed and not prescribed, are important as these frequently cause or contribute to psychiatric complaints, especially in the elderly (10).

Medical problems must be excluded. Infections, particularly CNS, cardiopulmonary, and urinary, can aggravate a patient's underlying illness. Questions regarding fever, weight loss, appetite, recent surgery and trauma should be asked.

When a patient presents with psychiatric symptoms but does not have a known psychiatric disorder, it is critical to differentiate primary psychiatric illness versus secondary psychiatric illness (medical etiology). Factors strongly supporting a medical cause include age greater than 40 years old with no prior psychiatric history, abnormal vital signs, recent memory loss, and clouded consciousness (5,11). Medical conditions may manifest with significant psychiatric symptoms. The differential diagnosis of medical conditions that can present with psychiatric symptoms is broad. Table 120.1 includes some of these conditions.

Physical Examination

Multiple studies have documented that both emergency medicine and psychiatric physicians do a less than optimal job at documenting the physical examination (7,12). Psychiatrists surveyed reported completing a physical in only 13% of their inpatients, citing that they feel incompetent to do so (12). Therefore, it is very important that the Emergency physician perform a thorough search for evidence of medical illness that needs urgent treatment.

Two of the more frequent conditions encountered are delirium and dementia, and distinguishing between these two can be very important. Delirium is most often due to a medical condition and is an acute condition. Dementia is a more chronic condition. See Chapter 109, Organic Brain Syndrome, for additional information on dementia and delirium.

DIFFERENTIAL DIAGNOSIS

Anticholinergics, sympathomimetics, and serotonergics may be the etiology of a patient's altered thoughts. The information about a patient's prescription and over-the-counter medications, use of herbal supplement, drugs purchased on the Internet, and use of other person's medications is critical in the evaluation of the patient. Standard management of the toxidrome in consultation with the local Poison Center, if needed, should be followed.

Patients taking cocaine, methamphetamines, and PCP may exhibit psychosis. Common withdrawal syndromes associated with acute psychiatric features include alcohol withdrawal, particularly delirium tremens.

Medications may be an important source of acute psychiatric symptoms. Elderly patients are particularly susceptible to toxic effects of medications due to polypharmacy, dosing errors, and altered metabolism. If a medication is identified as the precipitant, clear instructions for dosing changes or drug substitution must be communicated with caregivers.

Thyroid diseases may be the etiology of acute psychiatric symptoms. Thyrotoxic patients may appear manic, delusional,

TABLE 120.1.   Treatable Causes of Acute Mental Disorders Due to a General Medical Condition

CARDIAC

Arrhythmias
Congestive heart failure
Myocardial infarction

PULMONARY

Chronic obstructive pulmonary disease
Pulmonary emboli

HEPATIC

Cirrhosis
Hepatitis
Wilson disease

RENAL

Worsening of mild nephritis by urinary tract infection
Dehydration with elevation of BUN >50 mg/dL

VASCULAR

Subdural hematoma
Cerebrovascular accident
Infection

ENDOCRINE DISEASE

Thyroid disease
Cushing disease
Diabetes
Addison disease
Hypoglycemia

ELECTROLYTE IMBALANCE

Hyponatremia
Hypernatremia
Hypercalcemia

VITAMIN DEFICIENCIES

Thiamine
Niacin
Riboflavin
Folate
Ascorbic acid
Vitamin A
Vitamin B_{12}

DRUG-INDUCED

Alcohol
Tranquilizers
Over-the-counter preparations
Any drug used to treat medical illness (e.g., phenytoin, aminophylline, digitalis, steroids)

EXOGENOUS TOXINS

Carbon monoxide
Bromide
Mercury
Lead

TUMORS

NONCONVULSIVE STATUS EPILEPTICUS

NORMAL PRESSURE HYDROCEPHALUS

DEPRESSION

---

or confused. Extremes in glucose can cause profound mental status changes. Those with adrenal disease are also susceptible to profound behavioral changes, which may mimic psychiatric symptoms. See Table 120.1 for additional causes of acute mental disorders.

EMERGENCY DEPARTMENT MANAGEMENT

Extreme agitation is often part of the syndrome of delirium or psychiatric disease and can significantly interfere with evaluation. Rapid tranquilization (RT) is a safe and effective method for controlling agitated or overtly violent patients (13). RT is accomplished by administering a standard dose of a high-potency antipsychotic medication, such as haloperidol® or droperidol®, in 15- to 30-minute intervals. Research indicates that the combination of antipsychotic medication with lorazepam is more effective than either medication alone, though the synergistic effects may cause excessive sedation (14,15). See Chapter 123, The Agitated or Violent Patient.

Ancillary Testing

Ancillary testing is a matter of great debate in the literature. Some facilities require mandatory testing, while others rely on their emergency physician's judgment. Most would agree that a thorough history and physical will guide most clinicians in indicated ancillary testing. Studies have demonstrated that where history is obtainable, patient self-reporting on medical symptoms has a 94% sensitivity of predicting disease (8).

While there is no consensus from the literature on laboratory testing, there are some useful guidelines. New onset psychiatric complaints may signal more extensive testing for a medical etiology (16). Routine testing in patients over the age of 40, especially in the geriatric population may have a higher pretest probability for significant positive results that either demonstrate the etiology of the symptoms to be medical or signal the need for urgent treatment prior to medical clearance (17–19). Alcohol levels and toxicologic screens may be useful in patients in cases where there is uncertainty as to the extent of the role that those substances are impacting the patients altered state.

Transfer of patients to an outside facility is a legitimate area of concern regarding the medical screening exam. Some psychiatric facilities request mandatory toxicologic, alcohol levels or various ancillary tests prior to accepting patients into their facilities. While these levels usually do not impact the ED care, the psychiatrist may find this information useful in their treatment of the patient (20). Zun et al. working with state agencies and other health care facilities developed a protocol to aid the emergency clinician in medical screening and eventual transfer to a state psychiatric facility (21). This protocol addressed some of the controversial areas involved in the psychiatric medical screening exam, including routine ancillary testing. Familiarity with these requirements and developing a regional or local working task force to assure that these protocols and guidelines are routinely reviewed and updated is essential to both patient safety and cost control.

CRITICAL INTERVENTIONS

- Perform a thorough search for evidence of medical illness that needs urgent treatment
- Distinguish between delirium and dementia during the patient evaluation
- Control agitated or overtly violent patients with rapid tranquilization when indicated

DISPOSITION

Identified illnesses associated with a risk of morbidity or mortality warrant hospital admission (2).

The treatment of delirium is based on detection of the underlying cause. Hospital admission is necessary if the patient's behavior jeopardizes further medical evaluation or care. If no specific cause of delirium can be found while in the emergency department, the patient should be admitted for further workup, with psychiatric consultation as needed. A patient should be discharged only after a cause has been identified, treatment has been initiated, and adequate follow up has been ensured.

Upon completion of the medical screening examination and a determination that the patient is medically clear, patient care may be transferred to the psychiatric services.

COMMON PITFALLS

✔ Delirious patients who present to the emergency department are often inappropriately referred to a psychiatrist. This is especially true for those who present with bizarre and agitated behavior

✔ Psychiatric patients who behave in a bizarre, disruptive manner may not be approached with the same sense of urgency or seriousness as are patients with cardiovascular disease or trauma. Out of a sense of discomfort and an urgency to get to the "really sick" patients, the physician may decide that the patient is "medically clear" without conducting a complete and thorough evaluation

✔ A common misunderstanding is that delusions, hallucinations, and disorganized thoughts are diagnostic of primary mental disorders. On the contrary, such symptoms, like fever or pain, are nonspecific and occur in both primary mental disorders and mental disorders caused by a medical condition, as well as in certain personality disorders

✔ There is a tendency to refer violent patients prematurely to a psychiatrist. Yet, like disordered perception, violence is etiologically nonspecific. A significant proportion of violence that occurs in psychiatric settings results from underlying medical illness or drug intoxication (23). Thus, the evaluation of the violent patient must include a search for these conditions

✔ The least tolerated patients are those who are believed to create their own disease (e.g., alcoholic patients, drug abusers, and suicidal patients) (3). Thus, a patient who overdoses on tricyclic antidepressants and is fully alert and clinically stable may be treated with an inappropriate lack of urgency. Similarly, Wernicke encephalopathy is rarely given consideration in confused, belligerent patients who present with chronic alcoholism (24)

✔ Clinicians often fail to take seriously the complaints of elderly patients, commonly attributing their symptoms to "old age" (25). This attitude is particularly unfortunate when the patient suffers from dementia, because 60% of all dementias are treatable or reversible (4,26). For many clinicians, dementia implies a chronic, progressive, irreversible deterioration of higher intellectual functions. Dementia is not etiologically specific, however, and does not imply irreversibility. Premature labeling tends to preclude the exhaustive physical, neurologic, and laboratory evaluation necessary to identify potentially reversible causes of dementia or delirium

Acknowledgments

Thanks to previous edition chapter authors Philliph I. Bialecki, Douglas A. Rund, and William R. Dubin.

References

1. Adityanjee A, et al. Determinants of emergency room visits for psychological problems in a general hospital. Int J Soc Psychiatry 1988;34:25–30.
2. Rund DA, Hutzler JC. Emergency Psychiatry. St. Louis: CV Mosby, 1983.
3. Weissberg MP. Emergency room medical clearance: an educational problem. Am J Psychiatry 1979;136:787.
4. Dubin WR. Assessment and management of psychiatric manifestations of organic brain disease. In: Dubin WR, Hanke N, Nickens HW, eds. Clinics in emergency medicine: psychiatric emergencies. New York: Churchill Livingstone, 1984.
5. Koranyi EK. Physical illness underlying psychiatric symptoms. Psycother Psychosom 1992;58:155–160.
6. American Psychiatric Association. Diagnostic and statistical manual of mental disorders, 4th ed. Washington, DC: American Psychiatric Press, 1994; XXV.
7. Tintinalli JE, Peacock FW, Wright MA. Emergency medical evaluation of psychiatric patients. Ann Emerg Med 1994;23:859.
8. Olshaker JS, Browne B, Jerrard DA. Medical Clearance of the psychiatric patients in the emergency department. Acad Emerg Med 1 Feb, 1997;4(2):124–128.
9. Curran GM, Sullivan G, Williams K. Emergency department use of persons with co morbid psychiatric and substance abuse disorders. Ann Emerg Med 1 May, 2003;41(5):659–667.
10. Drugs that can cause psychiatric symptoms. Med Lett Drugs Ther 1989;31:113–118.
11. Williams ER, Sheperd SM. Psychiatric emergencies. Emergency Med Clinics N. America 2000;18.
12. McIntyre JS, Romano J. Is there a stethoscope in the house (and is it used)?. Arch Gen Psychiatry 1977;34:1147–1151.
13. Dubin WR, Weiss KJ, Dorn JM. Pharmacotherapy of psychiatric emergencies. J Clin Psychopharmacol 1986;6:210.
14. Garza-Trevino ES, Hollister LE, Overall JE, et al. Efficacy of combination of intramuscular antipsychotics and sedative-hypnotics for control of psychotic agitation. Am J Psychiatry 1989;146:1588.
15. Dubin WR. Rapid tranquilization: antipsychotics of benzodiazepines. J Clin Psychiatry 1988;49[Suppl]:5.
16. Henneman PL, Mendoza R, Lewis RJ. Prospective evaluation of emergency department medical clearance. Ann Emerg Med. 1994;24:672–677.
17. Aisen PS. Medical evaluation of the elderly psychiatric patient. Mt Sinai J Med. 1991;58:85–90.
18. Lewis LM, Miller DK, Morley JE. Unrecognized delirium in the ED geriatric patients. Am J Emerg Med, 1995;13:142–145.
19. Lipowski ZJ. Delerium in the elderly patient. N Engl J Med. 1989;320:578–581.
20. Riba M, Hale M. Medical clearance: fact or fiction in the hospital emergency room. Psychosomatics 1990;31:400.
21. Zun LS, Leikin JB, Stotland ND. A tool for the emergency medicine evaluation of psychiatric patients. Am J of Em 1996;14:329–333.
22. Wise MG. Delirium. In: Hales RE, ed. Textbook of neuropsychiatry. Washington, DC: American Psychiatric Press, 1987.
23. Tardiff K, Sweillam A. Assault, suicide, and mental illness. Arch Gen Psychiatry 1980;37:164.
24. Reuler JB, Girard DE, Cooney TG. Wernicke's encephalopathy. N Engl J Med 1985;16:1035.
25. Goodstein RK. Common clinical problems in the elderly, camouflaged by ageism and atypical presentation. Psychiatr Ann 1985;15:299.
26. Dubin WR, Weiss KJ, Zeccardi JA. Organic Brain Syndrome: The psychiatric imposter. JAMA 1983;249:60–62.

CHAPTER 121
Depression and Suicide Ideation

Robert S. Hockberger and Matthew Smith

Depression is the most common psychologic disturbance affecting humankind. Its lifetime prevalence is 10% to 20% in the general population and 20% to 50% in patients seen by physicians in general practice settings (2). Suicide, the most notable sequela of depression, is the eighth most common cause of death in the United States, accounting for approximately 30,000 deaths annually (2,3). The number of annual suicide deaths is likely underestimated with the actual number of suicide deaths thought to approach 100,000 annually (15). The overall incidence of suicide nationwide does not appear to be increasing; however, recent epidemiologic studies have shown an increase among certain groups, including the young (particularly adolescents), inner-city minorities, and patients with AIDS (2,3). Of note, suicide is now the third leading cause of death among adolescents and young adults aged 15 to 24 years, and the relative suicide rate for men with AIDS is 36 times that of men without AIDS (14). This significant loss of life is accompanied by substantial economic loss. In a 2003 productivity audit, United States workers with depression cost employers approximately $44 billion per year in lost productive time (11).

Patients frequently seek nonpsychiatric medical care shortly before committing suicide. Up to 75% of those who commit suicide have visited a physician in the months prior to their death (14). It is sometimes difficult for physicians without formal psychiatric training to recognize and evaluate depression and suicide potential because many of these patients do not specifically complain of depression or readily admit to suicidal ideation unless specifically questioned (16,17). Emergency physicians are further hampered by the hectic environment of an emergency department, constantly changing priorities that limit one's ability to spend significant time with individual patients, and the difficulty in obtaining after-hours psychiatric consultation. Nevertheless, the emergency physician's ability to make these assessments and to decide when to seek urgent psychiatric referral or hospitalization for potentially suicidal patients is a vital link in the effective management of a highly disabling and often fatal affliction. In a 2001 report, the U.S. Public Health Service emphasized this vital role of emergency departments in enhancing suicide prevention efforts, and recommended that, by 2005, guidelines be developed for the assessment of suicide risk among persons receiving care in emergency departments (14). To date however, there are no universally accepted guidelines for the determination of suicide risk.

CLINICAL PRESENTATION

Depressed patients commonly complain of multiple vague, ill-defined somatic symptoms such as weakness, malaise, weight loss, headache, and back pain; however, a thorough medical evaluation should be made before attributing such physical complaints to a psychological cause. Depressed individuals frequently have the following: low self-esteem; loss of interest in or lack of enjoyment of pleasurable activities; depressed mood (irritability in adolescents); loss of energy; poor appetite and weight loss (weight gain less often); sleep disturbances, including insomnia or hypersomnia; decreased attention span and ability to concentrate; decreased productivity at school, work, or home; episodes of tearfulness or crying; irritability or excessive anger; feelings of hopelessness and worthlessness with a pessimistic attitude toward the future; and recurrent thoughts of death (16).

The potential for suicide should be considered in the following groups of patients:

(1) Patients who have made a recent suicide attempt or have experienced recent suicidal ideation. While most completed suicides involve firearms, drug overdose accounts for 70% to 90% of all suicide attempts (3). Major and minor tranquilizers and antidepressants have replaced barbiturates and other sedatives as the major agents involved in intentional overdose.

(2) Patients who state that they are depressed or who complain of symptoms of depression.

(3) Patients who present with problems related to chronic alcoholism, drug withdrawal, or any psychiatric disorder (particularly affective disorders, psychosis, and panic attacks).

(4) Patients who present with apparently unintentional overdoses or self-inflicted gunshot wounds, lacerated wrists, falls from heights, or motor vehicle accidents of unclear cause (i.e., one-car, one-victim accidents in clear weather).

DIFFERENTIAL DIAGNOSIS

A number of psychiatric and medical disorders may present with symptoms of depression. Approximately 80% of people suffering bereavement have one or more symptoms of depression for 1 year or more following the death of a loved one (3). Persons suffering from an adjustment disorder may develop similar symptoms within several months of the onset of psychosocial stresses (e.g., economic loss, physical illness, or troubled interpersonal relationships) with which they are unable to cope. The diagnosis of organic affective syndrome is made when symptoms of depression are found to accompany organic neurologic disease such as organic brain syndrome (i.e., Parkinson Disease), stroke, tumor, or trauma. Symptoms of depression may be exacerbated or even caused by medications, including antihypertensive drugs (beta blockers, clonidine, methyldopa, and reserpine), antidepressants, antihistamines, neuroleptic agents, sedative–hypnotic drugs, cimetidine, and alcohol (12).

When these diagnostic possibilities have been eliminated in a patient exhibiting symptoms of depression, a final diagnosis of dysthymic disorder (depressive neurosis or minor depression) or major affective syndrome (major depressive disorder) should be considered. This difference is one of degree with each of these disorders falling somewhere on the disease spectrum of depressive illness, and the final diagnosis best left to a psychiatrist.

EMERGENCY DEPARTMENT EVALUATION AND MANAGEMENT

The clinical assessment of depression and suicide risk is an art as well as a science. Patients feel more at ease to talk about difficult personal issues when health professionals exhibit a friendly, nonjudgmental, supportive attitude and convey their willingness to listen. However, several studies have shown that this is frequently not the case, particularly among emergency department staff. Reasons cited for this include inadequate time and staffing, patient behavior that is perceived as either abusive or manipulative, value conflicts, and staff frustration regarding ineffective disposition and follow-up options (7,9). Expression of a negative or hostile attitude by a respected authority figure, such as a physician or nurse, reinforces a depressed patient's feeling of diminished self-worth and may actually increase the likelihood of another suicide attempt.

Overtly depressed and suicidal patients are not very diagnostically challenging, while covertly suicidal patients presenting solely with somatic complaints can pose a diagnostic dilemma. Subtle presentations of a psychiatric problem may include midnight visits for minor complaints, multiple nonspecific somatic complaints involving many organ systems, unusual patient requests, indications of difficulties at home, and trauma that might reflect domestic violence. These potentially "silently suicidal" patients should be assessed in a sympathetic but direct manner. First, the presenting complaint should be addressed by asking general questions about the patient's home, work, and social situations. These general questions should then be followed by specific questions regarding the signs and symptoms of depression. Finally, the physician should ask direct questions regarding suicide, such as, "Have you ever felt so bad that you thought about killing yourself?" or "Do you have thoughts of harming yourself now?" and "What plans have you made to do this?" Physicians are occasionally reluctant to ask patients directly about suicidal thoughts, fearing that this line of questioning will bring to the surface subconscious thoughts of suicide and result in suicide attempts. There is no evidence to support this concern; to the contrary, most depressed patients are relieved by the opportunity to openly discuss their problems when the clinician demonstrates an interest and a willingness to listen.

The main objective of the emergency department management of markedly depressed and suicidal patients is protecting the patient from further self-harm. Suicidal patients must be kept under constant observation by a staff member, and should be accompanied at all times including restroom visits. Patients must be searched for medications and weapons, and then placed in a quiet area of the emergency department that is free of potentially harmful objects. No potentially suicidal patient should be allowed to leave the emergency department before an evaluation is completed; all states have statutes permitting physicians to detain individuals deemed to be dangerous to themselves or others. Mechanical restraints should be used only when necessary to protect the patient or health-care providers. The reasons for using restraints and how the patient was restrained must be documented in the medical record. Also, restrained patients must be rigorously monitored and evaluated for complications. Chemical restraints such as intramuscular haloperidol or lorazepam may be required for patients who remain agitated or violent, but these agents can impair psychiatric evaluation and should be avoided when possible.

Following the medical management of a patient's overdose, injury, or associated medical problems, the patient's degree of depression and potential risk for suicide should be assessed. Many studies have attempted to identify patients at high risk for suicide. Although no combination of clinical characteristics has been found that accurately identifies all patients likely to complete suicide, a number of high-risk characteristics have been determined. For example, a young woman who takes a few aspirin as a suicide gesture after fighting with her boyfriend is at less risk for successfully committing suicide than an elderly man who tries to hang himself on the anniversary of his wife's death. Most patients fall somewhere between these two extremes, and estimating a particular individual's risk for suicide is often difficult (13). Adding to this challenge for emergency physicians is the fact that potentially suicidal patients often present at night and on weekends when psychiatrists are not readily available for consultation. Moreover, there are no studies demonstrating that hospitalization of high-risk patients prevents further suicide

TABLE 121.1. Sad Persons Score

	Description	Points
S = Sex	Male	1
A = Age	< 19 or > 45 years old	1
D = Depression or hopelessness	Admits to depression or decreased concentration, appetite, sleep, libido	2
P = Previous attempts or psychiatric care	Previous attempt, or previous inpatient or outpatient psychiatric care	1
E = Excessive alcohol or drug use	Stigmata of chronic addiction or recent frequent use	1
R = Rational thinking loss	Organic brain syndrome or psychosis	2
S = Separated, divorced, or widowed	Recent or on anniversary	1
O = Organized or serious attempt	Well-thought-out plan or life-threatening presentation	2
N = No social supports	No close family, friends, job, or active religious affiliation	1
S = Stated future intent	Determined to repeat attempt, or ambivalent	2
		SCORE

Score	Risk
< 6	Low
6–8	Intermediate
> 8	High

attempts or completed suicides. This lack of evidence, combined with the national push toward more cost-effective outpatient treatment regimens, places the busy emergency physician in the position of making disposition decisions with high medical-legal risk.

Fortunately, the vast majority of patients attempting suicide do not go on to successfully complete suicide, which has led numerous investigators to develop and test more than 20 clinical rating scales to predict suicide risk. Only one such clinical rating scale has been used in the emergency department setting to guide the decision to admit patients based on suicide risk, the modified SAD PERSONS scale (MSPS). The SAD PERSONS mnemonic incorporates several high-risk characteristics which can help the clinician assess potentially suicidal patients (Table 121.1) (4,8). In one study, for nonintoxicated patients whose history can be corroborated by family or friends, the numerical SAD PERSONS score correlated closely with the need for hospitalization as determined by a psychiatrist. In this study, hospitalization was deemed necessary in almost all patients with a high SAD PERSONS score (>8), in approximately half of patients with intermediate scores (6 to 8), and in almost none of the patients with low scores (<6) (4). The authors concluded that patients with a MSPS of <6 can be safely referred for expedited outpatient psychiatric evaluation, while a score of 6 or greater required emergent psychiatric evaluation and likely hospitalization (sensitivity of 94% and specificity of 71%) (4). A more recent study prospectively evaluated six clinical rating scales, including the MSPS. The outcome variable was eventual admission based on assessed suicide risk. In this study, all six scales had 100% sensitivity for identifying patients requiring hospitalization. This confirmed the usefulness of the MSPS in the emergency setting; the remaining five scales were just as sensitive but were more complex and less practical for use in the ED (1). While the modified SAD PERSONS score is a rapid and convenient tool to help organize, document, and communicate the assessment of a patient's suicide potential, a low score (<6) should not preclude emergent psychiatric consultation when the physician is uncomfortable with his or her assessment or when the patient requests to see a psychiatrist. Strict cut-off scores alone should not be used to dictate consultation and admission to the hospital.

DISPOSITION

Potentially suicidal patients generally require hospitalization and admission to an inpatient psychiatric unit. Discharge from the emergency department should not be considered unless the following conditions have been met:

- The patient's injuries or associated medical problems do not necessitate hospitalization.
- The patient states that he or she is no longer suicidal, and is not intoxicated, demented, or psychotic. Patient must be directly asked about the presence of auditory hallucinations, and must be specifically assessed for signs of psychosis.
- The acute precipitant of the crisis has been identified, and addressed and resolved.
- The patient has cooperated with an evaluation and is deemed to be at very low risk for suicide. In general, nonpsychotic younger patients whose attempts involve low risk, high likelihood of rescue, and high manipulative intent can be discharged safely.
- Psychiatric consultation has been obtained (at least by telephone) and hospitalization is judged unnecessary.
- Short-term outpatient follow up (within 1 to 2 days) has been arranged. The reliability of such patients in keeping follow-up appointments is poor. When emergency department personnel demonstrate a positive, supportive attitude and when the patient is given a scheduled outpatient follow-up appointment at the time of emergency department discharge, patient compliance with follow up improves markedly (5,6,10).
- The patient agrees to return to the emergency department immediately if further self-destructive urges arise.
- A positive, supportive environment with family or friends is available into which the patient can be released. Arrangements should be made to ensure removal of all pills, poisons, and weapons, especially guns, from the home.

A potentially suicidal patient should not be transferred to another facility or to a psychiatrist's office unless accompanied by medical personnel or family members who agree to deliver the patient and maintain close observation of the patient during transport.

COMMON PITFALLS

- ✔ "Accidental" trauma may be a manifestation of suicidal behavior. When the stated mechanism of injury is questionable or inconsistent with the injury seen, a more in-depth evaluation of the patient's emotional state and motives is warranted to screen for depression and suicide risk
- ✔ The information obtained from a potentially suicidal patient must be corroborated with family or friends. Patients who vehemently deny suicide intent, refuse to answer questions, give abrupt answers to questions, or appear anxious to leave the emergency department may be committed to finishing the act they began
- ✔ Anxiolytics, antidepressants, or any other potentially lethal medication should not be prescribed to patients who are depressed or potentially suicidal. More than half of patients who die by intentional overdose use a single prescription drug (14)

Acknowledgment

Thanks to previous edition's chapter author Roger Yang.

References

1. Cochrane-Brink KA, Lofchy JS, Sakinofsky I. Clinical rating scales in suicide risk assessment. *General Hospital Psychiatry* 2000;22:445–451.
2. Cooper-Patrick L, Krum RM, Ford DE. Identifying suicidal ideation in general medical patients. *JAMA* 1994;272:1757.
3. Hirschfeld RM, Russell JM. Assessment and treatment of suicidal patients. *N Engl J Med* 1997;337:911.
4. Hockberger RS, Rothstein RJ. Assessment of suicide potential by non psychiatrists using the "SAD PERSONS" score. *J Emerg Med* 1988;6:99.
5. Jellinek M. Referrals from a psychiatric emergency room: relationship of compliance to demographic and interview variables. *Am J Psychiatry* 1978;135:209.
6. Knesper DJ. A study of referral failures for potentially suicidal patients: a method of medical care evaluation. *Hosp Commun Psychiatry* 1982;33:49.
7. Pallikkathayil L, Morgan SA. Emergency department nurses' encounters with suicide attempters: a qualitative investigation. *Scholar Inquiry Nurs Pract* 1988;237:2.
8. Patterson WM, Dohn HH, Brid J, et al. Evaluation of suicidal patients: the SAD PERSONS scale. *Psychosomatics* 1983;24:343.
9. Soukas J, Lonnquist J. Work stress has negative effects on the attitudes of emergency personnel towards patients who attempt suicide. *Acta Psychiatr Scand* 1989;474:79.
10. Spirito A. Emergency department assessment of adolescent suicide attempters: factors related to short-term follow-up outcome. *Pediatr Emerg Care* 1994;10:6.
11. Stewart WF, et al. Cost of lost productive time among US workers with depression. *JAMA* 2003;289:3135–3144.
12. Thienhaus OJ. Assessment of suicide risk. *Psychiatr Serv* 1997;48:293.
13. Tueth NJ. Predicting suicide in the emergency department. *Am J Emerg Med* 1996;14:434.
14. U.S. Public Health Service. National Strategy for Suicide Prevention: Goals and Objectives for Action, 2001. Available at: www.mentalhealth.org/suicideprevention. Accessed September 25, 2003.
15. Vastag B. Suicide prevention plan calls for physicians' help. *JAMA* 2001;285:2701–03.
16. Verdick BM, Homes CB, Waln RF. Recognition of suicide signs by physicians in different areas of specialization. *J Med Educ* 1983;58:716.
17. Weissberg M. The meagerness of physicians' training in emergency psychiatric intervention. *Acad Med* 1990;65:747.

CHAPTER 122
Anxiety Disorders and Panic Attack

Douglas A. Rund, Phillip I. Bialecki,
Radu V. Saveanu, and Anna Kate Corbin

Anxiety is a common complaint of patients who present to emergency departments and other outpatient medical facilities. It is a nonspecific symptom that has diverse causes and clinical manifestations. Anxiety can be the chief complaint of a patient with a primary anxiety disorder, but often it accompanies a comorbid medical disorder. It is important for the emergency medicine physician to recognize an underlying emergent medical disorder in the anxious patient and at the same time be able to diagnose those patients in whom anxiety has become a pathologic condition.

Clinically significant anxiety that is not associated with general medical illness, substance use, or substance withdrawal may warrant diagnosis of a primary anxiety disorder. It is important to remember, however, that anxiety may be a feature of almost any psychiatric condition. In particular, anxiety is often prominent in schizophrenia and other psychotic disorders, and in depression and bipolar disorders. These conditions are discussed elsewhere in this book. The emergency physician should have a general understanding of the clinical characteristics and diagnostic criteria of all major psychiatric disorders, their chronic modes of treatment, and the emergency department assessment and management of acute presentations.

CLINICAL PRESENTATION

Subjectively, the anxious patient feels a sense of worry, apprehension, and nervousness that are often accompanied by physical symptoms that reflect sympathetic activity (e.g., palpitations, dry mouth, dizziness, paresthesia and faintness). Anxiety is a pathologic condition when the patient's physical and emotional responses surpass the normal response to a perceived threat and interfere with optimal functioning. The mental status examination of patients who suffer from a primary anxiety disorder is generally unremarkable.

Panic Attack

Panic attacks are extremely distressing experiences that often lead to emergency department visits. These episodes are abrupt, almost paroxysmal, in onset and progress rapidly to a degree of anxiety grossly disproportionate to any perceived threat or danger. The total duration is usually 10 minutes or less, and almost never as long as 30 minutes. Following cessation of the acute episode, patients typically experience considerable residual anxiety centered on concerns about possibly having life-threatening illness. Some patients describe their first panic attack as the worst experience of their lives.

DSM-IV-TR defines a panic attack as "a discrete period of intense fear or discomfort, in which *at least 4 of the several possible symptoms* developed abruptly and reached peak intensity within 10 minutes." The DSM IV-TR criteria for panic attacks are listed in Table 122.1.

Although only four symptoms are required, a full-blown panic attack may include nearly all of these features. In particular, fear of dying or other impending disaster is almost universal. Episodes having fewer than four symptoms are referred to as *partial symptom attacks.* These may occur in the early stages of a disorder (in which they will later progress to full-blown panic attacks), or as breakthrough episodes in persons already receiving treatment.

Because of their inherently short duration, most panic attacks are clinically evaluated only retrospectively. Patients commonly seek emergency medical care following these very upsetting experiences, especially if the attack was uncued. By the time they are examined, measurable physiologic functioning (e.g., heart rate, cardiac rhythm, blood pressure, respiration) usually has returned to baseline. Even during the actual attacks, objective physiologic changes may be far less impressive than the degree of distress suggests. Panic attacks are brain events, and any peripheral changes are secondary manifestations. They are clinically recognized from the description of the person's internal experience, not from externally observable characteristics.

The differential diagnosis of panic attacks depends on the specific circumstances in which they occur. *Situational or cued*

TABLE 122.1. Criteria for Panic Attack

A discrete period of intense fear or discomfort, in which four (or more) of the following symptoms developed abruptly and reached peak intensity within 10 minutes:

1. palpitations, pounding heart, or accelerated heart rate
2. sweating
3. trembling or shaking
4. sensations of shortness of breath or smothering
5. feeling of choking
6. chest pain or discomfort
7. nausea or abdominal distress
8. feeling dizzy, light-headed, unsteady, or faint
9. derealization (feelings of unreality) or depersonalization (being detached from oneself)
10. fear of losing control or going crazy
11. fear of dying
12. paresthesias (numbness or tingling sensations); and chills or hot flashes

(Used with permission, American Psychiatric Association, Diagnostic and Statistical Manual–IV-TR, American Psychiatric Association, Washington, D.C., 2002.)

panic attacks occur in association with particular experiences or stimuli, which may be internal or external, recognized or unrecognized. *Uncued panic attacks* are experienced as occurring "out of the blue" and are especially frightening because of the assumption that they are a symptom of life-threatening illness.

Before considering psychiatric diagnoses, the emergency physician should keep in mind that uncued or even cued panic attacks may be associated with substance use (e.g., caffeine or stimulants), with substance withdrawal (from alcohol, barbiturate-like sedatives, or benzodiazepines), and with a wide variety of nonpsychiatric conditions (e.g., hyperthyroidism, hypoglycemia, hyperparathyroidism, vestibular dysfunction, seizure disorders). After these conditions have been ruled out, possible psychiatric diagnoses are as follows:

In *phobic disorders,* panic attacks may occur in connection with the unreasonable degree of fear associated with a particular stimulus or situation (e.g., giving a speech or encountering a snake) that the person makes effort to avoid. Uncued attacks never occur.

In *acute and posttraumatic stress disorders,* panic attacks may be triggered by environmental reminders, distressing memories, or flashbacks of the traumatic experience. For example, military veterans may experience panic attacks in response to sudden loud noises that remind them of traumatic combat experiences, or a victim of violent assault may experience a panic attack when returning to the environment in which it happened. Again, uncued attacks never occur.

In *obsessive-compulsive disorder,* panic attacks may be caused by situations in which the person fears being overwhelmed by the obsessional concern. For example, a person who vacuums the floor and dusts furniture excessively because of fear of contamination may experience a panic attack if the vacuum cleaner bag bursts and releases a cloud of dirt.

Panic Disorder

The only psychiatric condition in which uncued panic attacks occur is *panic disorder.* This condition has been described and studied for at least 100 years. In older literature it was referred to by terms such as soldier's heart, neurocirculatory asthenia, cardiac neurosis, and anxiety neurosis. When its psychiatric nature was recognized, it was often trivialized as being a sign of character defect or unconscious conflict.

Panic disorder is now recognized as a cause of serious morbidity, and considerable data support the conclusion that it has a neurobiologic substrate. Recent surveys of the adult U.S. population report an annual prevalence rate of 1% to 2% and a morbid risk (lifetime risk) of 2% to 4%. It also has a very high rate of comorbidity with other psychiatric and general medical conditions. Over 90% of patients with panic disorder also meet DSM-IV criteria for major depressive disorder, another anxiety disorder, a personality disorder, or a substance use disorder. They also have significantly increased prevalence of irritable bowel syndrome, peptic ulcer, asthma, migraines, and mitral valve prolapse (MVP).

DSM-IV criteria for panic disorder include recurrent uncued panic attacks leading to at least one month of significant impairment of functioning. This impairment may include persistent fear of having additional attacks, worry about the implications or possible causes or consequences of the attacks, or significant changes in behavior related to the attacks.

Although uncued panic attacks are necessary for the diagnosis of panic disorder, and are sufficient if they cause significant impairment of functioning over at least one month, most patients also experience cued panic attacks. As the disorder progresses, patients become increasingly fearful and worry about having additional attacks. They often change their behavioral patterns to avoid or minimize situations they consider especially risky. As a result of this anticipatory anxiety, panic attacks actually become more likely in such situations. This often leads to increased avoidance behavior, sometimes as extensive as to constitute *agoraphobia*, and possibly resulting in serious invalidism.

In agoraphobia, fears and avoidance behavior expand and generalize until the patient becomes virtually homebound, or unable to leave home except in the presence of a trusted companion (usually a relative). DSM-IV defines agoraphobia as "anxiety about being in places or situations from which escape might be difficult or embarrassing, or in which help might not be available, in the event of having a panic attack or panic-like symptoms. Agoraphobic fears typically involve clusters of situations with a common theme, such as: being away from home alone; standing in lines and other situations involving crowds; and traveling in a bus, plane, train, or car." When these situations cannot be avoided, anxiety escalates and panic attacks increase, accelerating the vicious cycle. Finally, recent studies have found that patients with panic disorder have increased risk for suicidal ideation, suicide attempts, and successful suicide (5).

Specific Phobia

Specific phobia is a marked and persistent fear that is excessive or unreasonable, cued by the presence of a specific object or situation (e.g., flying, heights, animals, receiving an injection, seeing blood). Exposure to the stimulus almost invariably provokes an immediate anxiety response, which may take the form of a situationally predisposed panic attack. In this disorder, the patient recognizes that the fear is excessive, but feels powerless to prevent it, except by avoiding the trigger. This "phobic avoidance" then significantly interferes with normal, routine occupational, social, or relationship functioning.

Social Phobia

Social phobia is characterized by marked or persistent fear of one or more social or performance situations. Patients fear that they will act in a humiliating or embarrassing manner. The anxiety generated by this fear may lead to a situationally bound or predisposed panic attack. Common social phobias include fear of public speaking, performance anxiety, inability to eat in public

or to use public restrooms. Social phobia is differentiated from "normal" anxiety by the amount and severity of social and professional limitations that it produces. In the case of individuals with social phobia or specific phobias, emergency presentations are unlikely.

Obsessive Compulsive Disorder

Patients with obsessive compulsive disorder (OCD) suffer from obsessions or compulsions (most commonly, both). They usually recognize that their behavior is excessive or unreasonable and are distressed because their behavior causes marked impairment in daily function. Obsessions are recurrent or persistent thoughts, impulses, or images that are experienced as intrusive and inappropriate and cause severe anxiety. These are not excessive worries about real-life problems. Patients recognize that the obsessional thoughts, impulses, or images are products of their own mind. Compulsions are repetitive behaviors (e.g., repetitive hand washing, ordering, or checking) or mental acts (e.g., repetitively praying or counting, or repeating words silently) that the patient feels driven to perform in response to an obsession, or according to rules that must be rigidly applied. This behavior significantly impairs normal functioning. Individuals with OCD do not usually present to the Emergency Department, but when the impairment rises to a severe level, an emergency visit may involve complete loss of control or inability to function.

Posttraumatic Stress Disorder

Patients with Posttraumatic Stress Disorder (PTSD) have usually experienced or witnessed an event that involves actual or threatened serious personal injury, death, or a threat to the physical integrity of self or others. The response to such an event involves intense fear, helplessness, or horror. The traumatic event is typically reexperienced by either recurrent or intrusive recollections of the event or distressing dreams of the event. The patient may act or feel as if the event is recurring, or may experience intense psychological distress at exposure to internal or external cues that resemble some aspect of the event. In order to diminish the intensity of these painful feelings, patients persistently avoid any stimuli associated with the traumatic event, and frequently develop a general numbing of all emotions. Patients often manifest symptoms of increased arousal, with difficulty falling or staying asleep, irritability or outbursts of anger, difficulty concentrating, hypervigilance, or an exaggerated startle response. The diagnosis is made only if the disturbance has persisted for more than 1 month and has caused significant social or occupational dysfunction.

Acute Stress Disorder

Acute stress disorder is similar to PTSD, except that there is a closer temporal association between the traumatic event and the onset of symptoms, typically a period of less than 4 weeks. Patients often experience dissociative symptoms during or immediately following the event. Other symptoms may include subjective numbing, detachment, or absence of emotional responsiveness; a reduction in awareness of the surrounding environment, such as "being in a daze;" feelings of derealization or depersonalization; and dissociative amnesia.

Generalized Anxiety Disorder

Patients presenting with generalized anxiety disorder display excessive anxiety and worry that occur on most days for at least 6 months. Patients have difficulty controlling the worry and have associated symptoms of restlessness or feeling on edge, fatigability, difficulty concentrating, irritability, muscle tension, or sleep disturbances. To classify the anxiety as a disorder, the symptoms should significantly impair daily functioning, and not be due to any specific medical condition.

Anxiety Disorders and Other Cormorbid Psychiatric Disorders

Most patients diagnosed with an anxiety disorder will also have another comorbid psychiatric disorder. Comorbidity usually predicts more severe impairment, a poorer response to treatment, a poorer prognosis, and higher suicide risk. The disorders that are most frequently comorbid with anxiety disorders include depression, substance abuse, and personality disorders.

DIFFERENTIAL DIAGNOSIS

Most medical conditions are associated with some degree of anxiety, but certain conditions can be present with anxiety as a predominant feature. Examples include asthma exacerbation, hypoglycemia, pulmonary embolism, myocardial infarction, drug intoxication or withdrawal, caffeine toxicity, mitral valve prolapse, paroxysmal atrial tachycardia, thyrotoxicosis, pheochromocytoma, and carcinoid syndrome (5). In addition, anxiety itself may exacerbate a medical comorbidity because its associated symptomatic responses create demands on previously impaired organ systems.

EMERGENCY DEPARTMENT EVALUATION

It is important to exclude primary or comorbid medical disorder as an important aspect of the initial and ongoing assessment. A focused history and physical examination initiate the assessment when medical illness or comorbidity is suspected. Screening laboratory tests might include a complete blood count, urinalysis, serum electrolytes, glucose, hepatic function tests, thyroid function tests, toxicology screen, pulse oximetry, and a standard 12-lead EKG. Other tests can be ordered, based on the findings of the initial evaluation.

After excluding other causes for the patient's condition, the diagnosis of anxiety disorders and panic attacks are made when their symptoms fit the clinical presentation or DSM-IV definition.

EMERGENCY DEPARTMENT MANAGEMENT

Reassurance is the first-line intervention in patients with anxiety disorders. Patients should be assured that they are safe and that they are going to receive help. A firm, direct approach in a quiet, comfortable environment helps the patient feel secure and in better control. If a supportive interview is unsuccessful, pharmacologic intervention may be considered.

The benzodiazepines are used to treat acute anxiety. As a group, benzodiazepines are similar in their clinical effect, although they differ in pharmacokinetic properties. Short-acting benzodiazepines (half-life: 5 to 20 hours) include lorazepam (Ativan) and alprazolam (Xanax). The long-acting benzodiazepines (half-life: 20 to 200 hours) include diazepam (Valium), chlordiazepoxide (Librium), and clonazepam (Klonopin). These medications are usually effective for anxiety disorders. In the setting of acute anxiety, a benzodiazepine with a rapid onset is preferred. Lorazepam 1 to 2 mg PO or IM is usually effective in

20 to 30 minutes. Administration of intravenous benzodiazepines (lorazepam 0.5 mg IV q 20 min) is appropriate for patients who are so anxious that a threat is posed to self or others, especially if there is a history of poor impulse control.

When used chronically, however, benzodiazepines can cause physical dependence. Furthermore, when administered acutely in the emergency department, administration of the medication can reinforce the belief that the only way to control anxiety is by the use of a chemical substance. The patient may subsequently turn to alcohol and nonprescription drugs when the prescription medication expires or no longer provides the needed relief. Substance abuse, including alcohol and other sedatives, sometimes occurs in patients with panic disorder as they attempt to self-medicate. Unfortunately, however, these agents can precipitate an exacerbation of anxiety and panic attacks as their blood levels decline in the patient (6). This is often the beginning of a cycle of dependency.

For this reason, pharmacotherapy should be used in conjunction with psychotherapies, biofeedback, and behavior modification in the chronic management of such conditions (7). Although not all forms of anxiety are successfully treated by such techniques, there is a growing attitude that they should be tried, because they often bring partial, if not total, relief of symptoms.

Propanolol and other beta-blockers have been used to control the autonomic symptoms of anxiety, such as tremor, tachycardia, and palpitations. If such symptoms can be relieved, the anxiety itself often abates. Propranolol is frequently used by individuals who have anxiety or stage fright. It is not recommended for the treatment of other anxiety disorders.

In the primary care setting selective serotonin reuptake inhibitors (SSRIs) are used as first-line treatment for panic disorder, as well as other anxiety disorders, even in the absence of depression. SSRIs are generally safe in both therapeutic doses and mild overdoses and are frequently effective in a number of anxiety disorders. They require approximately 1 month to take effect, therefore the more rapidly acting benzodiazepines may be needed concurrently in the short term.

SSRIs should be started at a low dose and the dose needs to be increased slowly over time. These antidepressants may initially worsen anxiety symptoms and restlessness in patients who suffer from an anxiety disorder. Buspirone may be used for patients with generalized anxiety disorder. Unlike benzodiazepines it does not cause dependence, but the need for multiple daily doses and slow onset of action make it problematic. Buspirone is also ineffective against panic attacks.

The high rate of suicidal ideation or suicide attempts among patients with panic disorder must be considered, especially since approximately half of those who attempt suicide by overdose do so by using medication prescribed within the week prior to the attempt. If benzodiazepines are prescribed, only a small quantity should be given, and close follow up and subsequent psychiatric evaluation should be arranged. More importantly, the patient should first be carefully assessed for suicide potential.

CRITICAL INTERVENTIONS

- Assess suicidal and violence potential before discharging the patient with anxiety disorder
- Administer short acting benzodiazepines in the setting of acute anxiety

DISPOSITION

Most patients with anxiety disorders can be discharged from the emergency department with primary care or psychiatric follow up. Patients who are actively suicidal, violent, or significantly disabled by their anxiety should be admitted to the hospital. Likewise, when the cause of acute anxiety is unclear, short-term admission for further medical and psychiatric evaluation should be considered.

COMMON PITFALL

✔ Assuming that an acutely anxious patient who is known to suffer from an anxiety disorder has no medical problem; patients presenting with anxiety must be presumed to have a medical condition as the cause until it is ruled out by an appropriate emergency evaluation

References

1. Bernstein CA (editor), *The Psychiatric Clinics of North America.* W.B. Saunders 1999;22(4).
2. Davies SJ, Ghahramani P, Jackson PR, et al. Association of panic disorder and panic attacks with hypertension. *Am J Med* 1999;107:310.
3. Hyman SE, Tesar GE. *Manual of Psychiatric Emergencies, 3rd Edition.* Boston: Little Brown and Company, 1994.
4. Katon W. Panic disorder and somatization: a review of 55 cases. *Am J Med* 1984;77:101.
5. Kercher E. Anxiety. Psychiatric aspects of emergency medicine. *Emerg Med Clin North Am* 1991;9:161
6. Post RM, Uhde TW, Putnam FW. Kindling and carbamazepine in affective illness. *J Nerv Ment Dis* 1982;170:717
7. Weissman MM. Suicidal ideation and suicide attempts in panic disorders and attacks. *N. Engl J Med* 1989;321:18.
8. Zaubler TS, Katon, W. Panic disorder and medical comorbidity: A review of the medical and psychiatric literature. *Bull Menninger Clin* 1996;60(2):A13.

CHAPTER 123
The Agitated or Violent Patient

Katherine Bakes and Vince Markovchick

CLINICAL PRESENTATION

One of the most common and dramatic patient presentations in the Emergency Department (ED) is the out of control, agitated, and violent patient. Screaming and combative behavior immediately get the attention of staff, patients and visitors. It is important that every ED has a standard approach and protocol in place to effectively and efficiently deal with these patients.

This behavior usually begins in the field and is first encountered by emergency medical technicians (EMTs) and law enforcement. If the system is in place, advanced notification via communications with field personnel should be provided to the ED so as to mobilize the resources and the beds for management of such patients. This will obviate the situation where a patient is held in a public area such as a hallway for a prolonged period of time while the staff scrambles to free up a bed in an appropriate treatment room.

Physical restraint and chemical sedation can and should commence in the field in certain situations. Prehospital care services should have in place appropriate protocols for physical and chemical restraint. EMTs should contact the base station to discuss appropriate treatment of such patients and to give advance notification of patient arrival.

In many instances it is not possible to obtain a coherent history from the patient. Careful questioning of EMTs, family members, bystanders, friends or anyone else who has observed the evolution of this patient's behavior should be undertaken. Members of appropriate personnel, including security, should be mobilized in order to safely transport, and when necessary, physically restrain such patients. The situation must be brought under control expeditiously in order to insure the safety of the ED staff and the patient.

DIFFERENTIAL DIAGNOSIS

The first role of the emergency physician is to rapidly identify reversible causes of acute organic brain syndrome that, if not treated, may caused morbidity and potential mortality. Examples of these are hypoglycemic reactions, severe amphetamine or cocaine toxicity, hypoxia, hyperthermia, anticholinergic toxicity, and alcohol intoxication or withdrawal. In addition, the ultimate role of the emergency physician is to differentiate organic from functional disorders. Refer to the chapter on organic brain syndrome (Chapter 109) for a detailed description of the mental status examination and the differentiation of organic from functional disease state.

Immediately reversible causes of agitated, violent behavior should be identified via a finger stick glucose determination, an oxygen saturation measurement, and a physical examination. Life-threatening sympathomimetic agitated states may be identified by the presence of one or more of the following: significant tachycardia, hypertension, hyperthermia, extreme violent muscular activity and dilated pupils. Violent postictal states may be identified by a history of a seizure and secondary signs on physical examination of major motor seizures (i.e., tongue lacerations and incontinence). When feasible, a mini mental status examination should be performed as well as a complete neurologic examination.

If any focal neurologic deficits are identified, the differential diagnosis should be expanded to include CNS lesions such as brain tumors or intracranial hemorrhage. Specific toxidromes should be identified (i.e., sympathomimetic, anticholinergic and cholinergic presentations), since each requires a specific therapy as is discussed in the toxicology section of this text and in the ED management of such patients. Furthermore, the following should raise a concern that the cause of the patient's agitation may be organic in nature. These include features of delirium, new violent or psychotic behavior in patients over 40 years of age, abnormal autonomic signs, visual hallucinations and an acute time course (4).

EMERGENCY DEPARTMENT MANAGEMENT

While ensuring safety in the Emergency Department is essential (below), it is also critical to recognize and treat any medical condition causing the patient's behavior. All too often, a physician fails to consider an organic etiology for violent behavior in the patient with a psychiatric history. Easily diagnosed and reversible etiologies for agitation should be quickly excluded or treated. A thorough physical exam, including a rectal temperature and pulse oximetry, is mandatory. Fever with agitation or violence, without a clear explanation, necessitates a sepsis work up. If the work up fails to identify an etiology, and the patient has an organic brain syndrome, a head CT and lumbar puncture should be considered to exclude intracranial pathology. Hypoxia must be quickly excluded as a cause of aggressive behavior and treated appropriately. Likewise, hypoglycemia must be diagnosed rapidly either at the time of IV placement or with a finger stick after physical restraints are instituted. A toxidrome-focused exam should be performed, which includes vital signs, pupillary and skin evaluation, lung and bowel sounds and neurologic assessment including mental status. If the history and physical exam do not lead to a clear cause for agitation, lab studies such as a urine toxicology screen and serum electrolytes should be considered.

Control of Violent Patient

Control of the violent patient is paramount to ensure the safety of the ED staff and patients. At times the physician can avoid the need for restraints or chemical sedation by applying some basic principals to establish a trusting relationship with the volatile individual. If possible, the patient should be put in a calm private room with limited external stimuli, placed in a patient gown, thus removing any weapons or medications, and offered items of comfort such as a warm blanket. If possible, the department should have a designated room, with two exits and proper visibility that create a feeling of safety for both patient and provider. Trained security personnel should be notified of the possibility for violence, so that they can be immediately available if the situation escalates (5).

After the patient is accommodated, he can be directly and empathetically questioned about his or her potential for violence. With pointed questioning, one can often quickly establish if the patient is planning on harming himself or others, has a weapon, or has been using drugs or alcohol. While remaining calm and controlled, the physician should relay their concern for the patient, assure the patient that they are in a safe environment, and yet make clear the consequences of violence in the department. This technique of verbal deescalation may obviate the need for further measures (5).

Patient Restraints

Unfortunately, many patients prove too agitated for the aforementioned approach, and either physical or chemical restraints become necessary. For the violent individual, four-point soft leather restraints should be utilized. At least five staff members should restrain the patient, one for each limb and a fifth to stand at the head of the bed to calm and to explain the process to the patient. To avoid undermining a therapeutic relationship with the patient, the physician should not be a member of this team. Restraints should be secured firmly, yet loosely enough to allow a finger to move between the restraint and the extremity. All patients should be assumed to be at risk of aspiration and therefore should be restrained on their side or with the head of the bed slightly elevated (5). Restraint of an upper limb in hyperabduction and extension for a prolonged period of time may cause peripheral nerve injury and thus be repositioned at the patients side as soon as adequate control of the patient is attained.

The Centers for Medicare and Medicaid Services (CMS), which works with the Joint Commission on Healthcare Accreditation (JCAHO), has put forth guidelines on the use of seclusion or restraint (see below). To maintain patient rights and avoid the liability associated with placing a patient in restraints, a hospital protocol should be established. It should include documentation of the following: necessity of restraints, alternative measures

attempted, at least every 4-hour reassessment and orders for the continuation of restraints and decided endpoints for discontinuation of restraints. After placement, nursing should optimally perform frequent neurovascular checks of each limb (2).

Federal directions on the use and standards for seclusion or restraint include:

- Physician or other independent licensed practitioner must see and evaluate patient within 1 hour of initiating intervention.
- Use of seclusion or restraint only when clinically justified and after consideration of alternative treatment options.
- Time-limited orders: 4 hours for adults; 2 hours for adolescents; 1 hour for children (<9 years old).
- Continuous in-person patient monitoring and periodic reevaluation with the intent to discontinue intervention at the earliest possible time; face-to-face reevaluation before each renewal of initial time-limited orders.
- Notification of clinical leadership (i.e., medical director) after 12 hours of continuous seclusion or restraint and every 24 hours thereafter.
- With patient informed consent, prompt family notification when seclusion or restraint is initiated.
- Debriefing with patient and staff after intervention has been discontinued.
- Deaths must be reported to CMS (2).

Patient Sedation

Although the Food and Drug Administration has not approved any medication for the treatment of violence in the ED, the use of chemical sedation can and should be used in order to prevent harm to patients and staff members. The most common drugs used for this purpose include the antipsychotic butyrophenone haloperidol and the benzodiazepines diazepam and lorazepam.

Haloperidol, a high potency antipsychotic, has multiple advantages including the ability to be administered orally, intramuscularly and intravenously. It should be dosed 5 mg to 10 mg intramuscular (IM) or intravenous (IV) every 10 to 30 minutes. Peak serum levels occur approximately 30 minutes after IM, 10 minutes after IV and 3 to 6 hours after oral administration. Most patients respond to 1 to 3 doses given 30 to 60 minutes apart (4). If no response is seen after two doses, a benziodiazepine should be added.

Unlike the phenothiazines, haloperidol has negligible anticholinergic side effects and rarely causes hypotension. Due to the high potency of haloperidol, extrapyramidal side effects (BPS) (dystonia, torticollis, opisthotonos or oculogyric crises) are common and not dose related, occurring in 10% to 20% of people in the first 24 hours. Akathesia, a feeling of uneasy restlessness, has been reported to occur in up to 75% of people receiving 5 mg of haloperidol. Fortunately, both of these side effects are easily treatable in minutes with diphenhydramine 25 mg to 50 mg IM or IV or benztropine 2 mg IM or IV. Prophylactic treatment should be considered in patients with a history of EPS or fear of developing BPS. Since the onset of side effects can be delayed on the order of hours, the patient can be prescribed oral benztropine 2 mg or diphenhydramine 25 mg at discharge and instructed to take them if symptoms develop. Although more common with the low potency antipsychotics, haloperidol also has the theoretical potential to lower the seizure threshold and thus should be avoided with patients who are post-ictal, prone to seizures or experiencing amphetamine or cocaine toxicity (3,4).

Droperidol (2.5–5 mg IM or IV) has recently fallen out of favor due to an FDA "Black Box" warning against the use of droperidol due to apparent association with QTc prolongation and precipitation of "torsades de pointes" arrhythmia.

The two benzodiazepines often used for sedation are lorazepam and diazepam. Although diazepam is often preferred due to its low cost, lorazepam has the advantage of superior intramuscular absorption and bioavailability. Furthermore, lorazepam is preferred in patients with cirrhosis or alcohol dependence, since its inactivation is preserved in the setting of liver disease (6). The side effects of these medications are mainly sedation and respiratory depression (4). The intramuscular combination of low dose haloperidol (5 mg) and lorazepam (2 mg) has been shown to be more effective in control of the agitated patient than higher doses of either alone (1). For acute amphetamine or cocaine toxicity, megadoses of benzodiazapines may be necessary in a closely monitored environment where active airway control may be instituted if respiratory depression ensues.

Other atypical antipsychotics are promising and are being investigated for the use of acute behavioral control. Though more expensive, these agents, which may have a more favorable side effect profile, include risperidone, olanzapine and ziprasidone. However, limited experience exists with these medications in the emergency setting and thus objective data is sparse (2).

CRITICAL INTERVENTIONS

- Approach the volatile patient in a safe environment with verbal deescalation techniques
- Use a documented hospital-based protocol after instituting physical restraints that includes justification for its use and frequent re-assessment of the patient's condition
- Obtain pharmacologic control of the violent patient using the combination of parenteral haloperidol and a benzodiazepine
- Diagnose and treat reversible causes of agitation, such as hypoxia and hypoglycemia
- Apply continuous monitoring of O_2 saturations after benzodiazepine administration

DISPOSITION

Once the patient is under control and an organic etiology has been excluded, disposition will depend on the patient's course in the department. The patient might require psychiatric evaluation for suicidal or homicidal ideation or for being gravely disabled. Alternatively, the patient may be discharged once the acute violent or agitated behavior subsides. This usually requires a short observation until an intoxicant is metabolized. And finally, if the patient has been physically violent toward staff, he may be arrested and discharged to the appropriate authorities.

COMMON PITFALLS

✔ Failure to undress the patient and search for weapons
✔ Failure to take steps to minimize the risk of aspiration and peripheral nerve injury in a restrained patient
✔ Inadequate doses of chemically sedating agents

References

1. Battaglia J, Moss 5, Rush J, Kang J, et al. Haloperidol, lorazepam, or both for psychotic agitation? A multicenter, prospective, double-blind, emergency department study. *Am J Emerg Med* 1997;15:335–340.
2. Buckley PF, Noffsinger SG, Smith D, Hrouda D, Knoll J IV. Treatment of the psychotic patient who is violent. *Psychiatr Clin North Am* 2003;26.
3. Clinton JE, Sterner 5, Steimachers Z, Ruiz E. *Ann of Emerg Med* 1987;16:319–322.
4. Dubin WR, Feld J. Rapid tranquilization of the violent patient. *Am J Emerg Med* 1989;7:313–320.
5. Hill 5, Petit J. The violent patient. *Emerg Med Clin North Am* 2000;18:301–315.
6. Tesar GE. The agitated patient, part II: pharmacologic treatment. *Hosp Community Psychiatry* 1993:44:627–629.

CHAPTER 124
Factitious Illness, Malingering, and Conversion Disorder

Jeffrey Dubin and Mark Smith

Factitious illness, malingering, and conversion disorder constitute a spectrum of medical conditions in which the patient's symptoms are false, pretended, or grossly exaggerated. The patient's symptoms may be voluntary (malingering and factitious illness) or may be an involuntary expression of an underlying psychological conflict (conversion disorder) (2). Distinguishing the physiologic conditions from the functional while addressing the patient's psychological issues is a test of the emergency physician's diagnostic acumen and therapeutic skill.

FACTITIOUS ILLNESS

CLINICAL PRESENTATION

Factitious illness is classified by the American Psychiatric Association according to whether the patient's presenting symptoms are psychological or physical (2). In the syndrome of factitious illness with psychological symptoms, which is not discussed here, the patient presents with imaginary psychological complaints, such as hallucinations, suicidal ideation, memory loss, or dissociative feelings.

The syndrome of factitious illness with physical symptoms is better known as Munchausen syndrome, named by Asher (3) after the character in a book that had a penchant for telling fabricated stories, based on an actual eighteenth-century, retired German cavalry officer. In the novel by Rudolf Raspe, the Baron enjoyed a series of fanciful, fantastic, and fabricated adventures. Like the Baron, the patient with Munchausen syndrome is often a peregrinating impostor, that is, a wanderer and a liar.

Munchausen patients are impostors who invent bizarre and often fantastic stories and accept painful and potentially dangerous procedures (e.g., cardiac catheterization, exploratory laparotomy) to reach their presumed goal: to become a patient admitted to the hospital. There seems to be no other secondary gain, thus distinguishing the Munchausen patient from the malingerer.

Munchausen patients typically present to the emergency department in a dramatic fashion, with a constellation of physical symptoms, plausibly suggesting the presence of substantial pathologic illness that is not present. Munchausen patients may simulate signs of disease (e.g., mixing a drop of their own blood into their urine sample) or actually induce a disease state in themselves (e.g., injecting exogenous material in themselves to produce fever and infection). They are typically young or middle-aged men (although the age range spans the pediatric to the geriatric), have a history of extensive travel, and report a medical history of previous hospitalizations and operations that have usually been performed in other cities. They are knowledgeable about hospital routines, but are often vague or inconsistent about medical details. Although Munchausen patients

a sudden onset. *La belle indifférence,* an attitude of relative unconcern despite the seriousness of the symptom, may be present, but its diagnostic importance is minimal. Patients with conversion disorder may also present with vomiting or symptoms of pregnancy (pseudocyesis).

The diagnosis of conversion disorder depends on demonstrating that the patient's symptoms are not due to organically based malfunction. With most neurologic presentations of conversion disorder, this is not difficult, because the patient's deficits usually do not make neuroanatomic sense. The physician's knowledge of neuroanatomy is usually better than the patient's; moreover, the patient is not consciously trying to fool the physician.

Typical "mistakes" made by the conversion disorder patient with neurologic symptoms include the following:

- Acute onset of sensory loss in a sharp stocking-glove pattern (although this may be mimicked by the peripheral neuropathies of diabetes or alcoholism, and vascular lesions such as aortic dissection or subclavian vein thrombosis)
- Complete paralysis and sensory loss of one leg, with preservation of deep tendon reflexes and antigravity muscle activity
- Hemianesthesia without contralateral pain–temperature loss or with nonanatomic midline splits in vibratory sensation
- Complete loss of motor function on one side of the body, with inability to turn the head to the side of paralysis (indicating contralateral sternocleidomastoid muscle dysfunction)
- Pseudoseizures: seizure-type movements unaccompanied by characteristic electroencephalographic (EEG) patterns. Patients with a true seizure disorder may also experience pseudoseizures. Features suggestive of pseudoseizures include the presence of fluttering eyelids, thrashing of extremities or side-to-side head movement, dramatic vocalizations, and evidence of responsiveness to environmental stimuli during an apparent grand mal seizure. In addition, there is typically absence of tongue biting, incontinence, physical injury, or postictal depression. Differentiating a pseudoseizure from a true seizure can be difficult; for example, a complex partial seizure, with its seemingly purposeful behavior, may be mistakenly identified as a pseudoseizure (20).
- Cogwheel response on manual muscle testing (21).
- Slowness of motion: Patients with nonorganic muscle weakness may exhibit a general slowing of motor movements, not realizing that certain tests require more strength when performed slowly (e.g., deep knee squat) (22).
- Inconsistencies in physical signs during unresponsiveness: The patient with nonorganic unresponsiveness often does not permit an upraised and suspended arm to strike the face when released, but rather allows it to glide harmlessly over the face (note that substantial injury can occur to the nose and mouth if the arm does drop directly onto them). Such a patient often vigorously resists manual eye opening by the physician; if opened, the eyes may be closed actively, in contrast to the smooth, effortless glide seen in the organically unresponsive patient (21).
- Nonorganically unresponsive patients always demonstrate both the fast and slow components of nystagmus on oculovestibular stimulation (cold calorics). Patients with a cortical lesion but an intact brainstem show only tonic deviation of the eyes; patients without either cortical or brainstem function show no deviation of the eyes whatsoever.
- Inconsistencies in blindness: The patient for whom blindness is a conversion symptom demonstrates a remarkable ability to avoid injury and misstep. For patients complaining of tunnel vision, the visual field extending into space may be described as cylindrical rather than cone-shaped.
- Nonneurologic presentations of conversion disorder are uncommon. Persistent unexplained vomiting may be a manifestation of revulsion and disgust; a psychological conflict that triggered the symptom should be sought. False pregnancy can be confirmed with a negative pregnancy test; the task is then to assess the patient's underlying psychiatric diagnosis.

DIFFERENTIAL DIAGNOSIS

Conversion disorder must be distinguished from organic illness, malingering, and Munchausen syndrome, as well as from somatization disorder and hypochondriasis.

The tendency should be strongly resisted to diagnose conversion disorder in any patient with vague symptoms. Up to 30% of patients who, at some time, have been given a diagnosis of conversion disorder are eventually found to have organic disease that could explain these symptoms (11). Illnesses such as systemic lupus erythematosus, multiple sclerosis, and hyperthyroidism may present in the emergency department as subtle perturbations of physical functions; hypoglycemia can present in myriad different guises.

The diagnosis of conversion disorder should not be made solely on the basis of a negative organic work up; the precipitating emotional stress and the unconscious conflict that the symptoms are designed to solve must be identified (11).

Patients with conversion disorder lack the characteristic features of the Munchausen patient: There is no tendency to submit to multiple procedures, and there is a lack of sophistication with respect to medical terminology. Unlike the malingering patient, there is no conscious fabrication of illness or disability.

EMERGENCY DEPARTMENT MANAGEMENT

Patients with conversion disorder must be handled delicately, deftly, and with respect. These patients have usually experienced a recent or remote traumatic experience. It is unacceptable to confront the patient with an assertion or proof that the illness is faked or not real. The patient should be told that, although the symptoms are bothersome, they do not appear to be manifestations of a serious illness. Planting the suggestion that they will improve over the next several hours can sometimes relieve symptoms. Patients with aphonia can be told that they will be able to whisper; patients with paralysis can be told that they will begin to experience movement in their toes.

Simultaneously, the physician can probe for underlying psychosocial conflicts that might have led to the appearance of the symptom. Hypnosis may aid in identifying the underlying emotional conflict. An amobarbital interview may be useful in the management of the psychogenically unresponsive patient and in certain types of discrete conversion disorder (15).

DISPOSITION

The neurologic consultant may assist the physician in differentiating organic from nonorganic illness. If the diagnosis of conversion disorder is secure and the patient's symptoms persist and prevent the patient from carrying out the activities of ordinary living, a psychiatric consultant may assist in the process of symptom resolution in the emergency department, using talk therapy, hypnosis, or amobarbital.

Many patients with conversion disorder experience resolution of their physical symptoms during their emergency department stay, but some require admission to the hospital. If the diagnosis of conversion disorder is uncertain and if the presenting symptom could signify dangerous illness, hospital admission is warranted. Even when the diagnosis of conversion disorder is clear, patients whose manifestations persist and who cannot manage on their own (e.g., psychogenic unresponsiveness or paralysis) require inpatient care.

CRITICAL INTERVENTIONS

> - Treat patients with suspected but not confirmed Munchausen syndrome as if an organically based disease is present until the diagnosis is confirmed
> - Resist diagnosing conversion disorder in any patient with vague symptoms
> - Treat suspected malingering patients with a minimal amount of gratification and invoke general rules or established policies that prevent the provider from filling the patient's demands completely

COMMON PITFALLS

✔ Failing to appreciate that the patient has an unusual presentation of an organic illness

✔ Permitting unpleasant aspects of the patient's personality to result in dismissal of the patient's problem as "psychogenic"

✔ Inadequately distinguishing among malingering, conversion disorder, and Munchausen syndrome

✔ Classifying all patients with symptoms having no discernible anatomic cause as "crocks"

✔ Losing interest in caring for the patient once it has been determined that the patient's symptoms are not organically based

References

1. Aduan RP, Fauci AS, Dale DC, et al. Factitious fever and self-induced infection. *Ann Intern Med* 1979;90:230.
2. American Psychiatric Association. *Diagnostic and statistical manual of mental disorders,* 4th edition. Washington, DC: American Psychiatric Press, 2000.
3. Asher R. Munchausen's syndrome. *Lancet* 1951;1:339.
4. Ben-Chetrit, E, Melmed, R. Recurrent hypoglycaemia in multiple myeloma: a case of Munchausen syndrome by proxy in an elderly patient. *J of Int Med* 1998;244:175.
5. Byard RW, Beal SM. Munchausen syndrome by proxy: repetitive infantile apnoea and homicide. *J Paediatr Child Health* 1993;29:77.
6. Dickson H, Cole A, Engel S, et al. Conversion reaction presenting as acute spinal cord injury. *Med J Aust* 1984;141:428.
7. Duffy TP. The Red Baron. *N Engl J Med* 1992;327:408.
8. Ifudu O, Kolanski SI, Friedman EA. Brief report: kidney-related Munchausen's syndrome. *N Engl J Med* 1992;327:388.
9. Edi-Osagie EC et al. Munchausen's syndrome in obstetrics and gynecology: a review. *Obstetrical and Gynecological Survey* 1998;45.
10. Kounis NG. Munchausen syndrome with cardiac symptoms, cardiopathia fantastica. *Br J Clin Pract* 1979;33:67.
11. Lazare A. Conversion symptoms. *N Engl J Med* 1981;305:745.
12. Manolis AS, Sanjana VM. Cardiopathia fantastica and arteritis factitia as manifestations of Munchausen syndrome. *Crit Care Med* 1987;15:526.
13. Meadow R. Fictitious epilepsy. *Lancet* 1984;2:25.
14. Mendel JG. Munchausen's syndrome: a syndrome of drug abuse. *Compr Psychiatry* 1974;15:69.
15. Perry JC, Jacobs D. Overview: clinical applications of the Amytal interview in psychiatric emergency settings. *Am J Psychiatry* 1982;139:552.
16. Roelofs, K, et al. Childhood abuse in patients with conversion disorder. *Am J Psychiatry* 2002;159:1908.
17. Rose MI, et al. Factitious gastrointestinal bleeding: a case of autophlebotomy and ingestion. *Am J gastroenterol* 1996;91:1457
18. Samuels MP, Southall DP. Munchausen syndrome by proxy. *Br J Hosp Med* 1992;47:759.
19. Swartz MS, McCracken J. Emergency room management of conversion disorders. *Hosp Commun Psychiatry* 1986;37:828.
20. Trimble MR. Pseudoseizures. *Neurol Clin North Am* 1986;4:531.
21. Warden RE, Johnson EW, Burk RD. Diagnosis of hysterical paralysis. *Arch Phys Med* 1961;4:122.
22. Watson CG, Buranen C. The frequency and identification of false-positive conversion reactions. *J Nerv Ment Dis* 1979;167:243.
23. Weintraub MI. Hysteria, a clinical guide to diagnosis. *Clin Symp* 1977;29.
24. Zuger A, O'Dowd MA. The Baron has AIDS: a case of factitious human immunodeficiency virus infection and review. *Clin Infect Dis* 1992;12:211.

CHAPTER 125
Bereavement and Grief Reactions

Kenneth V. Iserson

Death, especially when it is sudden and unexpected as often happens in the emergency department (ED), shocks and devastates patients' family and friends. For them, it is a sentinel and life-changing event, with every nuance burned into their memories. While they may not consciously acknowledge it, these losses may deeply affect emergency department personnel, even those hardened by the almost constant exposure to life's disasters that traverse EDs. This makes death notifications and dealing with the survivors so important and yet so difficult.

INTERACTING WITH SURVIVORS

Even though notifying survivors of a sudden, unexpected death is one of the most difficult parts of the emergency clinician's job, they rarely are taught the skills necessary to perform this delicate and emotion-laden task. Notifying survivors is emotionally draining—70% of emergency physicians find death notifications to be personally difficult. Perhaps this is because only one-half received any type of death-notification education in medical school and only one-third received any such training during residency (22).

TELEPHONE NOTIFICATIONS

The first intervention after a sudden, unexpected death is to contact survivors (12). This must often be done via telephone. Telephone contact, let alone notification, can be problematic.

Because there is no ongoing relationship between the emergency department staff and the survivors, the person designated to call the survivors should identify himself or herself and should establish the identity of the survivor. Talk to an adult, and try to determine whether someone is present to provide emotional or physical support.

The question constantly arises: Should ED personnel notify someone of the death by telephone? Most Americans, especially if they live locally, prefer to only be told that the patient is "critical," and to be told of the death when they arrive. The majority of those who wish to be told immediately are men.

After identifying himself, the caller should initially say that the patient is in critical condition, and that their presence is requested. Be certain that the recipient writes down all necessary contact information; have them repeat it back. If they demand to know whether the person is dead, you must tell them.

When calling relatives outside the local area, tell them of the death. They should never be put in a position to be rushed to the side of a "critical" or "dying" relative's side when they are already dead.

The only information appropriate to leave on a telephone message system is that a specific person, identified by name or position (e.g., son of George White), should return the call as soon as possible. Leave the name of someone who will be

medical examiner completes the necessary postmortem examination. Describe any equipment that remains on the body and explain why it is there. Cover the body with a sheet or blanket, but leave the head and hands exposed for the family to touch, and encourage them to do this. Move the body to a private room, if possible. Let them cut off a lock of hair, if requested. Allow family to be alone with the body, unless there are legal reasons (e.g., ongoing police investigation) for not doing so. Staff should remain nearby outside of the room and should be available for support while the family is viewing the body. Most family members will leave within 15 minutes.

MAKING FINAL ARRANGEMENTS

Part of death notification involves answering survivors' questions in a knowledgeable manner. This means knowing something about body disposition options, medical examiner/coroner laws and procedures, and organ and tissue donation (10). These subjects are rarely discussed in medical or nursing curriculums.

After the family has viewed the body, it is then appropriate to have necessary documents signed (1,12,15). Tell them the cause of death that you will put on the death certificate and offer them the use of a telephone so that they can call a funeral home. Ask again if there are any questions. Generally, no question should remain unanswered, unless the information is unavailable. Tell them how to reach you if they have questions at a later time.

Explain the role of medical examiners and police in cases of sudden, unexpected, or violent deaths and how the decedent's belongings will be handled. If an autopsy is mandatory, explain that fact to the family. If the cause of death is unclear and the physician feels the results will be helpful, inform the family of this and ask them for permission for an elective autopsy.

The issue of organ and tissue donation should be broached before family members leave the hospital; in fact, most states require that this option be addressed. One might ask, "Has your family ever discussed organ or tissue donation?" or "Our hospital offers organ and tissue donation. Would you like to discuss this further with someone from the transplant program?" If the family expresses an interest, contact the appropriate agency immediately.

Have a list of clergy and local accommodations available for out-of-town survivors. Unless necessary for the medical examiner or police investigation, give survivors the decedent's personal effects and any clothing removed from the body. Advise them of the condition of clothing and place it in a paper or plastic belongings bag, not a trash bag. Inform them when everything they need to do is completed and that they may leave whenever they like. The physician or a designated staff member should accompany the survivors to the door.

DEATH-NOTIFICATION EDUCATION

Although rarely and poorly done (12,18), educating emergency department professionals about sudden-death notification is vital, since doing it poorly can adversely affect both the survivors and the healthcare professionals themselves. Resources to do this education and materials to help remind emergency department personnel of the steps involved are available (10–14).

The easiest and most effective way to include this education is to add a module into one of the many resuscitation courses that emergency medicine personnel must take on a periodic basis. Such education can help ED personnel deal with their own emotions (e.g., feelings of defeat, guilt, impotence, and incompetence) and fears of death as well as survivors' reactions. This helps them not to reduce their own stress by delaying the news, thus increasing the family's anxiety, or by rushing in unprepared and presenting the news in an awkward manner (1,19).

A staff that is aware of the dynamics of grieving and survivors' needs can facilitate the grief process, cushion the trauma of loss, and establish a basis for a healthy grief response (5,12).

COMMON PITFALLS

✔ Not communicating well
✔ Making remarks such as, "Everything will be okay" or "It was God's will," which may prematurely seal off the grief response
✔ Failing to use a "D" word (Death, Dead, Died) to clearly indicate that the patient has died
✔ Not allowing and encouraging survivors to express their feelings
✔ Impeding or impairing survivors' ability to grieve, by routinely prescribing medication
✔ Failure to address survivors' support systems
✔ Not offering family members the option of organ and tissue donation

Acknowledgments

The author gratefully acknowledges Christopher H. Linden and William R. Dubin who wrote the previous versions of this chapter, and Galen Press, Ltd., Tucson, AZ, who gave permission for reproduction of much of the material in this chapter.

References

1. Albrizio M. The client who is bereaved. In: Gorton JC, Partridge R, eds. *Practice and management of psychiatric care.* St. Louis: Mosby, 1982:256.
2. Cassem NH. Treating the person confronting death. In: Nicholi AM, ed. *The Harvard guide to modern psychiatry.* Cambridge, MA: Belknap Press of Harvard University Press, 1978:579.
3. Clayton P, Desmaris L, Winokur GA. A study of normal bereavement. *Am J Psychiatry* 1968;125:168.
4. Doyle CJ, Post H, Burney RE, et al. Family participation during resuscitation: an option. *Ann Emerg Med.* 1987;16:673–5.
5. Dubin WR, Sarnoff JR. Sudden unexpected death: intervention with the survivors. *Ann Emerg Med* 1986;15:54.
6. Goodstein RK. Situational emergencies. In: Dubin WR, Hanke N, Nickens HW, eds. *Clinics in emergency medicine: psychiatric emergencies.* New York: Churchill Livingstone, 1984:167.
7. Hanke N. Stress disorders. In: Hanke N, ed. *Handbook of emergency psychiatry.* Lexington, MA: Collamore Press, 1984:200.
8. Honigman B, Armstrong J. Life and death. In: Rosen P, Barkin R, Danzl DF, eds. *Emergency medicine: concepts and clinical practice,* 4th ed. St. Louis: Mosby, 1998, pp. 197–212.
9. Iserson KV. Critical leadership. *J Emerg Med.* 1986;4(4):335–340.
10. Iserson KV. *Death to dust: what happens to dead bodies?* 2nd ed., Tucson, AZ: Galen Press, Ltd., 2001.
11. Iserson KV. *Grave words educational slide sets.* Tucson, AZ: Galen Press, Ltd., 1999.
12. Iserson KV. *Grave words: notifying survivors about sudden, unexpected deaths.* Tucson, AZ: Galen Press, 1999:14, 31–47, 68–76, 76–82, 167–168, 318–332.
13. Iserson KV. *Pocket protocols: notifying survivors about sudden unexpected deaths.* Tucson, AZ: Galen Press, Ltd., 1999.
14. Iserson KV. *The gravest words: notifying survivors about sudden, unexpected deaths* (Video), Tucson, AZ: Galen Press, Ltd., 2000.
15. Jones WH. Emergency room death: what can be done for the survivors?. *Death Educ* 1978;2:231.
16. Lapwood R: Chaplain to casualty. *Br Med J Clin Res.* 1982;285:194–195.
17. Lindeman E. Symptomatology and management of acute grief. *Am J Psychiatry* 1944;101:141.
18. Olsen JC, Buenefe ML, Falco WD. Death in the emergency department. *Ann Emerg Med* 1998;31:758.

19. Robinson MA. Informing the family of sudden death. *Am Fam Physician* 1981;23:115.
20. Robinson S, Mackenzie-Ross S, Hewson GLC, et al. Psychological effect of witnessed resuscitation on bereaved relatives. *Lancet* 1998;352:614–617.
21. Rund DA, Hutzler JC.Psychiatric emergencies associated with death. In: Rund DA, Hutzler JC, eds. *Emergency psychiatry*. St. Louis: Mosby, 1983:213.
22. Schmidt TA, Tolle SW: Emergency physicians' responses to families following patient death. *Ann Emerg Med* 1990;19:125–128.
23. Stussman BJ. National hospital ambulatory medical care survey: 1995 emergency department summary. *Advance Data from Vital & Health Statistics of the National Center for Health Statistics.* 1997;15:285.
24. Swisher LA, Nieman LZ, Nilsen GJ, et al. Death notification in the emergency department: a survey of residents & attending physicians. *Ann Emerg Med* 1993;22:1319–1323.
25. Walters DT, Tupin JP. Family grief in the emergency department. *Emerg Med Clin North Am.* 1991;9:189–206.
26. Weissman AD. Coping with untimely death. *Psychiatry* 1973;36:366.
27. Wright B. Sudden death: aspects which incapacitate the carer. *Nursing (Lond.* 1988;31:12–15.

SECTION XV

Section Editor: Jeffrey Schaider

Dermatologic Emergencies

CHAPTER 126
Life-Threatening Dermatoses

Alan T. Forstater and Kenneth J. Neuburger

Cutaneous lesions are often the first clinical sign of serious systemic disease. In this chapter, the focus is on the recognition and acute management of the common life-threatening dermatoses listed in Table 126.1. These disorders can be conveniently grouped into diffuse red rashes, vesiculobullous eruptions, localized or discrete lesions, and purpuric or hemorrhagic lesions (Table 126.2).

TABLE 126.1. Life-Threatening Dermatoses

DIFFUSE RED RASHES

Urticaria with anaphylaxis
Toxic shock syndrome[a]
Kawasaki disease
Toxic epidermal necrolysis[a]
Staphylococcal scalded skin syndrome[a]
Generalized exfoliative erythroderma[a]
Pustular psoriasis
Cutaneous T-cell lymphoma[a]
Systemic lupus erythematosus

LOCALIZED OR DISCRETE LESIONS

Erysipelas and cellulitis[a]
Gonococcemia[a]
Ecthyma gangrenosum[a]
Brown recluse spider bite
Behçet syndrome
Malignant melanoma[a]
Kaposi's sarcoma and AIDS[a]
Basal Cell Carcinoma[a]
Squamouus Cell Carcinoma[a]

VESICULOBULLOUS DISEASES

Pemphigus[a]
Pemphigoid[a]
Stevens-Johnson syndrome[a]
Toxic epidermal necrolysis[a]
Disseminated zoster
Disseminated herpes simplex

PURPURIC OR HEMORRHAGIC

Meningococcemia[a]
Gonococcemia[a]
Disseminated intravascular coagulation
Palpable purpura[a]
Brown recluse spider bite
Rocky Mountain spotted fever[a]
Miscellaneous hematologic disorders

[a] Discussed in chapter.
Adapted from Krusinski PA, Flowers, FP. Life-threatening dermatoses. In: Flowers FP, Krusinski PA. *Dermatology in ambulatory and emergency medicine, a clinical guide with algorithums.* Chicago: Year Book Medical, 1984.

Several entities are not discussed in detail here but deserve brief mention. *Palpable purpura* is a skin manifestation of vasculitis; it is not a manifestation of thrombocytopenia or clotting disorder. Involvement may be limited to the skin or may be systemic. Treatment is for the underlying vasculitic disorder.

Generalized exfoliative erythroderma (formerly called exfoliative dermatitis) is a diffuse, widespread dermatitis that covers most of the body surface. This condition not only causes pruritus and pain, but also may be complicated by hypothermia; fluid, electrolyte, and protein loss; invasion of bacteria and opportunistic organisms through the skin; and high-output congestive heart failure secondary to severe vasodilatation. The causes of exfoliative erythroderma include previously existing skin diseases (e.g., psoriasis, atopic eczema, contact dermatitis) (50%); drug eruptions (10%); lymphoproliferative disorders (e.g., Hodgkin disease, leukemia, Sézary syndrome) (15%); and idiopathic (25% to 40%). Mortality is less than 5%.

Other potentially life-threatening entities, such as angioedema (see Chapter 132) and disseminated herpetic infection, are discussed in other chapters.

Finally a brief discussion at the end of the chapter will focus on the recognition of the various types of skin cancer.

DIFFUSE RED RASHES

Staphylococcal scalded skin syndrome (SSSS) (Fig. 126.1) occurs in children and, rarely, adults, and is caused by an exotoxin from an infecting strain of coagulase-positive *Staphylococcus aureus*. The disease may present as a prodrome of fever, irritability, malaise, and exquisite skin tenderness; in other cases, the child presents with the sudden onset of generalized erythema. The skin is red, warm, and very tender. Flaccid bullae that are ill defined and hard to see then desquamate in large sheets. Gentle lateral stroking of the skin causes the epidermis to separate (Nikolsky sign).

Therapy consists of systemic antibiotics effective against penicillinase-producing *Staphylococcus*. Children older than 1 year and with mild symptoms may be treated as outpatients. Children who appear toxic and infants should be admitted. Despite proper treatment, most of the superficial body surface will desquamate; but because the site of blister cleavage is in the superficial layer of the dermis, healing occurs rapidly over 10 to 14 days.

Toxic epidermal necrolysis (TEN) (Fig. 126.2) is a disease of adults in which the skin also sloughs in large sheets. Although it is very similar in appearance to SSSS, it is quite different. It may actually represent the most severe form of erythema multiforme and begins, like erythema multiforme, with constitutional symptoms of fever, malaise, and myalgia. The skin is initially diffusely painful, hot, and red. Within 24 hours, blisters and large areas of denuded skin develop; erosive, sloughing lesions of the oral mucosa are common. The Nikolsky sign is positive (9).

The differences between TEN and SSSS are noteworthy. SSSS almost always occurs in children and is secondary to staphylococcal infection. TEN almost always occurs in adults and is precipitated by drugs such as phenytoin, sulfas, penicillins, and some nonsteroidal antiinflammatory agents (17) or by graft-versus-host reactions (e.g., after bone marrow transplantation) or blood product transfusions. Mucous membrane involvement in SSSS is rare and limited to the lips, but, in TEN, erosive oral lesions are common. Although SSSS sloughs only the superficial layers of epidermis, TEN desquamates the entire thickness of the epidermis, accounting for the high associated mortality rate: The mortality rate in SSSS is very low, while that of TEN is more than 50% (9).

TABLE 126.2. Identification of Life-Threatening Diseases Associated with Fever and Rash

Disease	History	Characteristics of Rash	Distribution of Rash	Associated Clinical Findings	Diagnostic AIDS
Rocky Mountain spotted fever (RMSF)	Tick exposure (75%) May-Sept. in temperate zone states Heaviest endemic area: middle Atlantic states and Southeast	Initial maculopapular petechiae appearing on second to sixth febrile day and usually painless.	Begins on wrists, ankles, forearms, spreading within 6–8 hr to palms, soles, trunk	Prodrome of fever, headache, myalgias Hyponatremia, normal to slightly increased WBC, thrombocytopenia, hypoalbuminemia	Biopsy of involved skin with immunofluorescence and other serologic tests. Serology: Complement fixation more sensitive and more specific than Weil-Felix agglutination.
Meningococcemia	Tends to occur in late winter, early spring Outbreaks in military recruits, crowded living conditions	*Acute:* May be maculopapular initially. Small petechiae with irregular borders ("smudging"), at times with vesicular or grayish ulcer. May coalesce. Painful. *Chronic:* Maculopapules, petechial vesicles, or pustules; tender nodules.	*Acute:* Extremities and trunk in random fashion *Chronic:* Extremities, particularly over joints	*Acute:* Meningitis, disseminated intravascular coagulation, shock, acidosis *Chronic:* Rash appears with recurrent cycles of fever over 2–3 mo	*Acute:* Aspiration of center of skin lesions for Gram-stain, culture (up to 60% positive). Blood cultures. Cerebrospinal fluid culture and Gram stain. *Chronic:* Blood culture usually positive during febrile episode. Biopsy findings resemble leukocytoclastic angiitis.
Disseminated gonococcal infection	Incidence higher in women than in men Young, sexually active Onset often related to menstruation	Pustules on erythematous base most characteristic. Also, macules, papules, pustules, and bullae less commonly.	Over extremities, with relative sparing of face and trunk; usually few (5–40) lesions	Migratory polyarthralgia, tenosynovitis, septic arthritis	Gram-stain of lesion. Blood, joint fluid culture (50%) prove diagnosis. Cervical, rectal, throat cultures support diagnosis.
Pseudomonas septicemia	Hospitalized patients, especially with neutropenia or burns	*Vesicles:* Isolated or in small clusters rapidly becoming hemorrhagic. *Ecthyma gangrenosum:* Round, indurated, ulcerated painless lesion with central gray eschar. *Maculopapular lesion:* Small erythematous lesion resembling "rose spots." Gangrenous cellulitis.	Random Axillary or anogenital area, thigh Trunk Localized	Generally extremely toxic, with fever; septic picture	Aspiration of lesions for Gram-stain culture. Cultures of blood, urine, sputum, etc.
Toxic shock syndrome	Young female predominance, esp with menses Rare in men 1–4 days prodrome of fever, myalgias, arthralgias, and diarrhea	*Erythroderma:* Seen at presentation. Diffuse, blanching, macular (deep-red "sunburned" appearance). Resolves within 3 days, followed 5–12 days later by desquamation, most commonly of hands and feet. *Mucosal hyperemia:* Pharynx, conjunctivae, vagina.	Diffuse, hands and feet predominantly	Fever, severe hypotension, multisystem involvement (gastrointestinal, muscular, renal, hepatic, hematologic, CNS)	Clinical criteria. See Chapter 148 Identification of toxin producing strain of *S. aureus*. Negative serology for RMSF, leptospirosis, measles.

From Stein JH (ed): *Internal medicine*, ed 5, St Louis, 1998:1382, Mosby. CNS, Central nervous system.

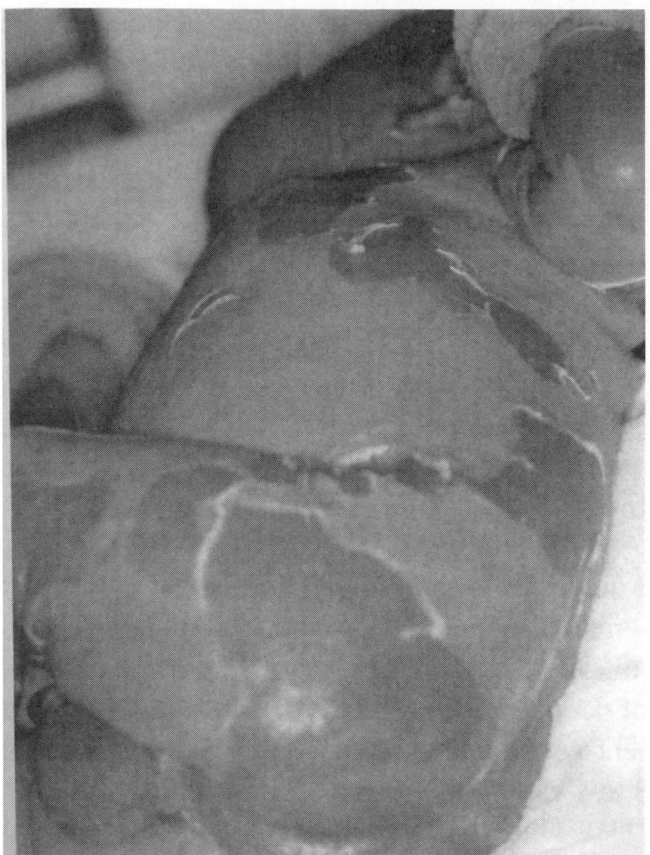

Figure 126.1. Staphylococcal scalded skin syndrome. A 10-day-old Caucasian boy with staphylococcal scalded skin syndrome. He was treated with fluids, oral dicloxacillin, and wound care. His skin healed completely and without scarring within 2 weeks of this photograph being taken. (From Fleisher GR, Ludwig S, Baskin MN, *Atlas of Pediatric Emergency Medicine*, Philadelphia, Lippincott Williams & Wilkins, 2004, with permission.)

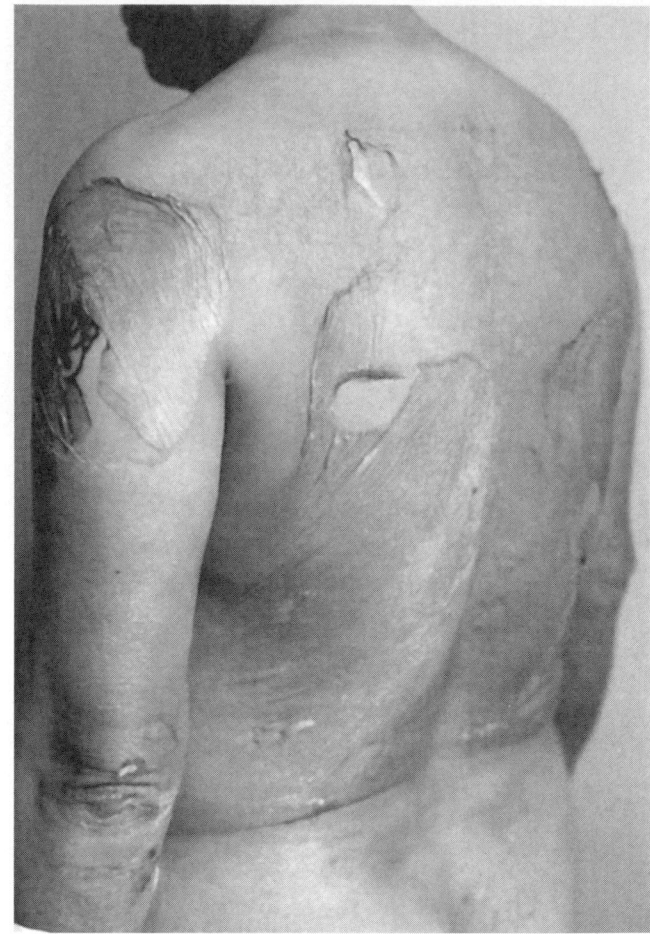

Figure 126.2. Toxic epidermal necrolysis caused by a sulfonamide diuretic showing classic flaccid bullae and denuded skin. Several years after this photograph was taken, the patient was unfortunately reexposed to a sulfonamide medication and despite treatment in a burn unit, died within a week. (From Ostler HB, Maibach HI, Hoke AW, Scwab IR, *Diseases of the Eye & Skin: A Color Atlas*, Philadelphia, Lippincott Williams & Wilkins, 2004, with permission.)

The diagnosis of TEN is made by clinical presentation and confirmed by biopsy. Treatment is removal of the precipitating agent, if possible, and, as in burn patients, judicious fluid and electrolyte therapy and prevention of infection. Early transfer to a burn center is associated with significantly decreased bacteremia and mortality (16). Corticosteroid treatment is controversial because it may not speed recovery, yet may predispose the patient to infectious complications (16). There are recent case reports of rapid improvement with IV N-acetylcysteine (26).

Toxic shock syndrome (TSS) (see Chapter 148, Toxic Shock Syndromes) is an acute, febrile illness associated with localized infection by strains of *S. aureus* that produce an exotoxin (TSST-1) believed to be the cause of the clinical signs and symptoms. Characteristic signs and symptoms include an early macular rash, hypotension, abnormalities in multiple organ systems, and acral desquamation occurring 1 to 2 weeks after the onset of the illness (Fig. 126.3). About 90% of the *S. aureus* isolates from patients with TSS produce the exotoxin. Eighty-five percent to 90% of cases are reported in menstruating women (25). In fact, the disease was originally described in association with the use of highly absorbent vaginal tampons that could be kept in place for many hours before being discarded. Other cases are associated with localized infection in men, children, and nonmenstruating women (4).

The early cutaneous rash is scarlatiniform and blanches with pressure; it can be difficult to appreciate because it is often quite pale. Coincident with the rash, there is often erythema of the mucous membranes of the oropharynx, conjunctivae, and vagina. Desquamation of the skin of the distal extremities occurs 1 to 2 weeks after the onset. Hair and nail loss follows 1 to 2 months later (1).

Strict criteria for the diagnosis of TSS are fever, hypotension or orthostasis, an erythematous macular rash, involvement of at least three organ systems, and the presence of an *Staphylococcus aureus* infection. Most patients have facial and extremity edema. Hypoalbuminemia and hypocalcemia not accounted for by the decreased albumin level have been described (25). The illness can proceed rapidly. Hypotension may appear early; most patients present to the hospital with at least orthostasis.

The differential diagnosis of TSS includes Rocky Mountain spotted fever (RMSF), scarlet fever, sepsis, Kawasaki disease (rare in those older than 8 years), leptospirosis, Colorado tick fever (in which photophobia is common), and other viral infections. Supportive treatment for dehydration and hypotension includes fluid replacement and the use of pressors, if necessary. The adult respiratory distress syndrome is common in serious cases.

Although it has not been proved that antibiotics are always necessary for recovery, provided the site of located staphylococcal infection is drained (e.g., removal of tampons or incision of abscesses), treatment with a penicillinase-resistant penicillin or a first-generation cephalosporin is considered mandatory if the diagnosis cannot be excluded. In the penicillin-allergic

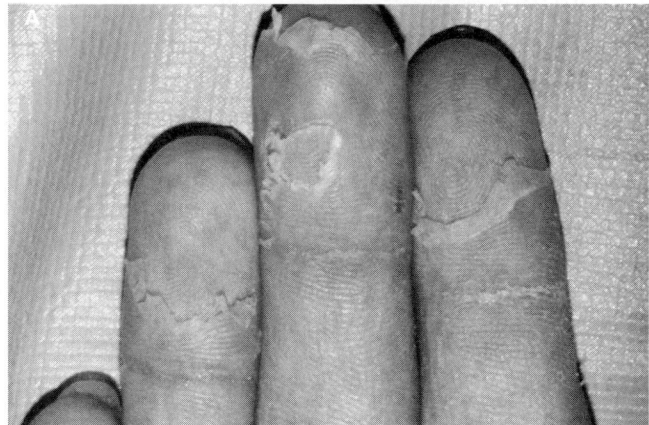
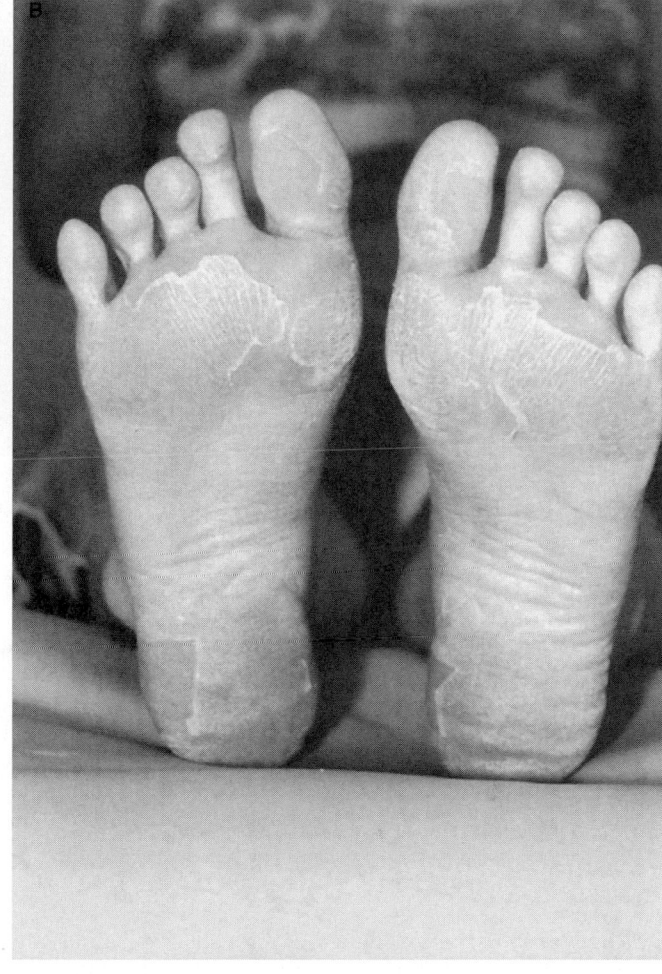

Figure 126.3. Toxic shock syndrome. A. Desquamation of the palmar surface of the fingers. B. Desquamation of the soles. (A&B courtesy of B. Zane Horowitz, MD). (Reprinted with permission from Greenberg MI, Hendrickson RG, Silverberg M, et al., *Greenberg's Text-Atlas of Emergency Medicine,* Philadelphia: Lippincott Williams & Wilkins, 2005: in press.)

patient, vancomycin or clindamycin is an appropriate alternative. Because TSS reoccurs in a large percentage of women with tampon-associated TSS who continue to use tampons, it is recommended that women forgo tampon use. All symptomatic patients suspected of having TSS require admission for vigorous supportive treatment.

The hallmark of streptococcal TSS, first described in the mid 1980s, is a relatively early onset of shock and multiorgan failure. The currently proposed criteria for streptococcal TSS are isolation of group A streptococci from a sterile or nonsterile site, hypotension, and at least two of the following: renal impairment, coagulopathy, liver function test abnormalities, adult respiratory distress syndrome, soft-tissue necrosis, and rash (which may be generalized macular or possibly scarlatiniform and may desquamate) (14). Treatment is with high-dose penicillin (20 to 24 million units/d); cephalosporins, clindamycin, erythromycin, vancomycin, and penicillinase-resistant penicillins are also effective. Aggressive supportive care is mandatory, as is surgical drainage or debridement for abscess, pyonecrosis, or necrotizing fasciitis. Even with prompt treatment, mortality is reported to be between 20% and 30% (28).

VESICOBULLOUS DISEASES

The spectrum of acute, self-limited immunologic reactions causing vesicles includes bullous erythema multiforme, Stevens-Johnson syndrome, and TEN. The causes are the same as those listed in the previous discussion of TEN, although erythema mul-

tiforme is often related to herpes simplex, and Stevens-Johnson syndrome is usually related to drugs. The classic lesion of erythema multiforme is the target lesion, a central gray wheal or bulla surrounded by concentric rings of erythema and normal skin. As the name implies, however, many types of lesions may be present simultaneously: macules, papules, urticaria (though non pruritic), and bullae. The extremities are involved more than the trunk; the palms and soles are often affected. The rash appears abruptly and may be accompanied by fever, malaise, and pruritus.

Further along the spectrum is *Stevens-Johnson syndrome*: bullous erythema multiforme accompanied by constitutional symptoms and involving at least two mucous membranes (9). A prodrome of fever, malaise, and myalgia is followed by the explosive appearance of blisters on mucous membranes and skin. Symmetric blistering begins on the dorsa of the hands and feet and on extensor surfaces. Erosive lesions begin on oral mucosa, lips, and bulbar conjunctiva and can extend to the pharynx, larynx, esophagus, and genital mucosa (Fig. 126.4). Ocular lesions can result in corneal ulceration, panophthalmitis, and even blindness, requiring early recognition and treatment. The prognosis of Stevens-Johnson syndrome is usually excellent (22). However, the disorder may progress to an illness clinically indistinguishable from TEN, with large confluent bullae and sloughing of epidermis in sheets.

Milder cases of Stevens-Johnson syndrome can be treated with oral antihistamines and topical corticosteroids; more severe cases require hospital admission. The use of systemic corticosteroid therapy is controversial (10).

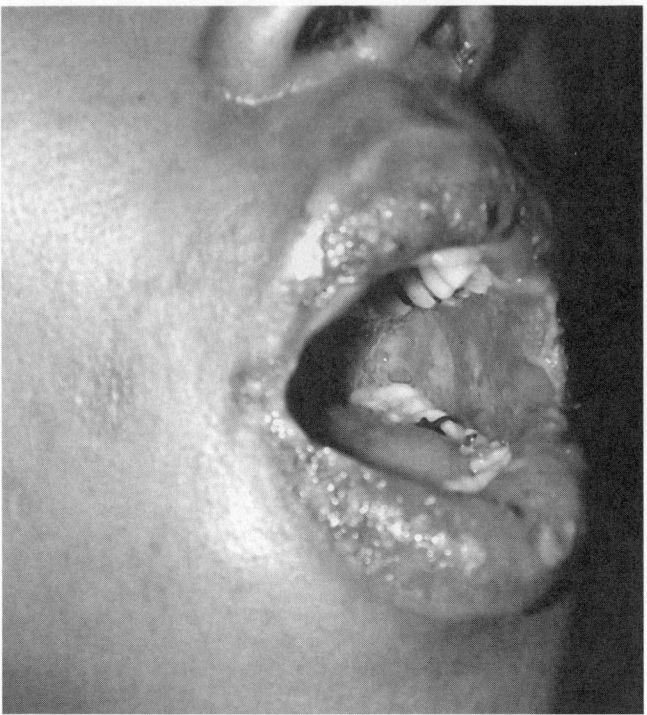

Figure 126.4. Mucosal sloughing in a mild form of Stevens Johnson syndrome. (Courtesy of Robert Hendrickson, MD) (Reprinted with permission from Greenberg MI, Hendrickson RG, Silverberg M, et al., *Greenberg's Text-Atlas of Emergency Medicine*, Philadelphia: Lippincott Williams & Wilkins, 2005: in press.)

Pemphigus vulgaris, a rare disease, occurs mostly in adults 40 to 60 years old and is distinguished from other blistering diseases by its fulminant course. Early identification and aggressive treatment may avert a poor outcome. Initially, blisters may be localized to small areas of the mucous membranes or skin; lesions may be present for months before the blistering becomes generalized. The lesions are typically painful flaccid bullae that may rupture easily or painful erosions where bullae have ruptured (Fig. 126.5). The Nikolsky sign is positive. Half of patients present initially with oral lesions; 90% have oral lesions at some time during the course of the illness. These painful erosions or

collapsed bullae can persist despite successful treatment of skin lesions (9).

The diagnosis of pemphigus is made by biopsy of intact skin adjacent to a bulla. Direct immunofluorescent staining for antiepithelial antibodies localized to the epidermal cell membrane is confirmatory. Indirect immunofluorescence of the patient's serum or blister fluid detects a pemphigus antibody that reacts with epithelial cell membranes of most species. Therapy is with corticosteroids and immunosuppressive agents.

Bullous pemphigoid is an autoimmune blistering disease occurring mostly in the elderly. The bullae of bullous pemphigoid, unlike those of pemphigus vulgaris, are tense rather than flaccid, and oral lesions are less common The Nikolsky sign is positive. Bullous pemphigoid is characterized by spontaneous remissions and exacerbations and a low mortality rate; most patients experience complete remission (9). As with pemphigus vulgaris, the diagnosis is made by biopsy of the skin adjacent to a blister. Direct immunofluorescence studies reveal antibodies bound to the basement membrane; these antibodies can often be found in the serum as well. Mild cases are treated with erythromycin, topical corticosteroids, or intralesional injections; severe cases require systemic corticosteroids with or without immunosuppressive agents (10).

LOCALIZED OR DISCRETE LESIONS

Patients with gram-negative sepsis may manifest the skin lesions known as *ecthyma gangrenosum* (Fig. 126.6). Originally described in *Pseudomonas* septicemia, they may also occur with bacteremia due to *Escherichia coli* or *Klebsiella* and have been reported in the absence of disseminated infection (6). Because the lesions of ecthyma gangrenosum are manifestations of life-threatening illness, the diagnosis must be made early. Ecthyma gangrenosum is a true dermatologic emergency; patients with it are critically ill and usually immunocompromised (e.g., with leukemia or lymphoma).

The appearance of the lesion can vary, depending on the stage of the illness at presentation. Beginning as a painless macule or vesicle, it indurates and assumes the appearance of a pustule or bulla on a blue or red base. The lesion then sloughs, leaving

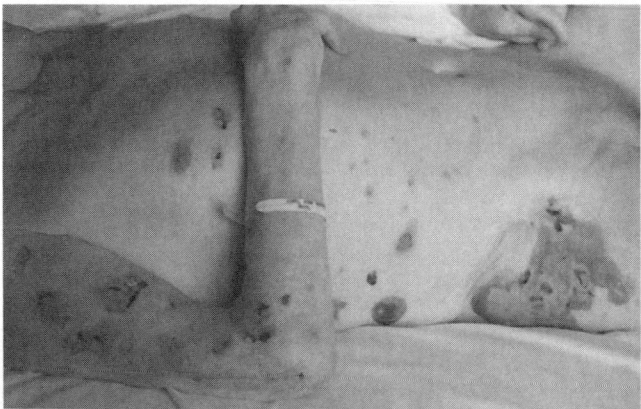

Figure 126.5. Ruptured bullae as seen in pemphigus vulgaris. Note flaccid bullae and erosions typical of pemphigus vulgaris. (From Ostler HB, Maibach HI, Hoke AW, Scwab IR, *Diseases of the Eye & Skin: A Color Atlas*, Philadelphia, Lippincott Williams & Wilkins, 2004, with permission.)

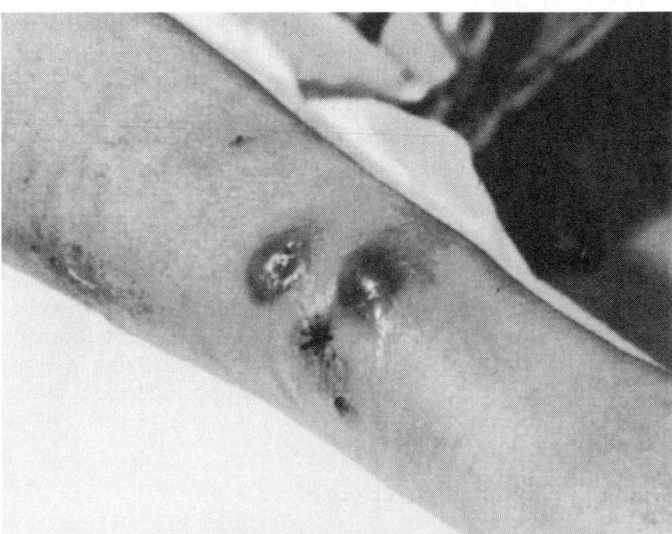

Figure 126.6. Ecthyma gangrenosum. Deep-seated hemorrhagic necrotic nodules on forearm. (From Greene S, et al., Ecthyma gangrenosum: report of clinical histopathologic and bacteriologic aspects of eight cases. *J Am Acad Dermatol* 1984;11:781, with permission.)

a gangrenous ulcer, usually several centimeters in size. These solitary or multiple lesions usually occur mainly in the perineal region or on the extremities.

Disseminated gonococcal infection (DGI) usually occurs in individuals with asymptomatic infection of the pharynx, rectum, or genitalia. The patient commonly presents with fever, skin lesions, arthritis, periarthritis, tenosynovitis, or any combination of these signs. DGI occurs most commonly in women during menstruation or pregnancy, but it can occur in any patient with gonococcal infection.

The skin lesions are pustules or vesicles on an erythematous base about 5 mm in diameter, but they may also be petechial, bullous, papular, or hemorrhagic. There are usually relatively few (fewer than ten to as many as 30), and they typically appear on the extremities and resolve rapidly (usually in less than a week). The periarthritis of DGI presents with joint swelling and tenderness, which are often transient and migratory. Septic arthritis occurs most commonly in the larger joints (knees, hands, ankles, and elbows, in descending order of occurrence). Complications such as endocarditis, meningitis, and sepsis are rare.

The diagnosis of gonococcemia (Fig. 126.7) is a clinical one. Any sexually active person with polyarthritis, tenosynovitis, and typical skin lesions can be given a presumptive diagnosis of gonococcemia with little doubt as to its accuracy. Gonococcal cultures should be performed on specimens obtained from all mucous membrane surfaces, as well as blood and (when appropriate) joint fluid. The diagnosis can also be made on the basis of a response to empiric treatment; DGI responds quite promptly to antibiotic treatment (see Chapter 140).

The differential diagnosis should include Reiter syndrome (a syndrome of urethritis, conjunctivitis, and arthritis that usually occurs after a diarrheal illness, has dissimilar skin lesions, and does not respond to antibiotics), meningococcemia (which has more numerous petechial lesions), immune complex diseases (which may have joint manifestations but a different type of skin lesion), and rheumatic fever.

Admission is indicated only for patients with severe systemic signs and symptoms or severe joint involvement (especially of weight-bearing joints) and those who cannot be followed closely as outpatients.

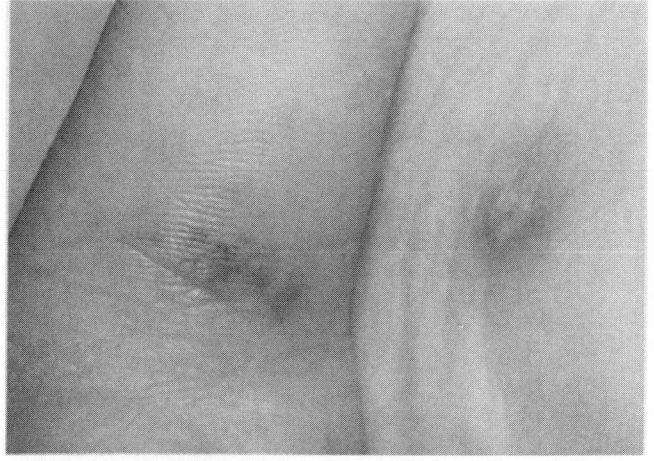

Figure 126.7. Disseminated gonococcemia. Neisseria gonorhoeae may disseminate from mucosal surfaces via the bloodstream and produce arthritis/arthralgia and a rash. The most characteristic lesion is the hemorrhagic vesicopustule seen in the web space of the teenage girl's hand. There is a pustule on the sole of her foot. (From Fleisher GR, Ludwig S, Baskin MN, *Atlas of Pediatric Emergency Medicine,* Philadelphia Lippincott Williams & Wilkins, 2004, with permission.)

Erysipelas is a superficial cellulitis that progresses rapidly in extent and involves the associated lymphatic channels. The classically described offending organism is the group A streptococcus, but groups C and D streptococci and *S. aureus* have also been isolated (26). The infection is most common in infants and children and in the elderly. The source, in most cases, is probably an inapparent wound. Erysipelas may range from a self-limited process that resolves spontaneously, even without antibiotics, to a rapidly progressive and severe infection leading to bacteremia. Admission is indicated for patients with extensive facial or neck involvement or for patients with fever and a toxic appearance.

The involved skin is erythematous, warm, and tender to palpation and has an advancing margin that is slightly elevated. Fever is common. The diagnosis is usually clinical, because local aspiration is rarely positive. Punch biopsy may be useful, but it is usually not readily available. The differential diagnosis includes cellulitis, maxillary or frontal sinus infections (if localized to the face), and erysipeloid (if localized to the hands).

Treatment with penicillin is rapidly effective if erysipelas is due to streptococci, but, because it is rarely easy to identify the causative organism, either a first-generation cephalosporin or a penicillinase-resistant penicillin should be used to cover *Staphylococcus.* Clindamycin or vancomycin may be used in the penicillin-allergic patient. Hospital admission is based on the patient's clinical status. Some affected individuals may be treated as outpatients with close follow up, and admitted if there is no response or any worsening after 1 to 2 days of oral antibiotic therapy.

Cellulitis, an acute, spreading inflammation of the skin and subcutaneous tissue, appears as a warm, tender, erythematous area with indistinct margins. Its differentiation from erysipelas is based on the appearance of the advancing edge of the infection. In cellulitis, the edge is not raised. In practice, the clinical management of patients with erysipelas and with cellulitis is similar. Erysipelas is more likely, however, to require prompt initiation of antibiotic therapy because it can progress so rapidly.

PURPURIC OR HEMORRHAGIC LESIONS

Neisseria meningitidis colonizes the nasal mucosa in humans (5% to 15%) but may invade the bloodstream and cause disease. Most cases occur in children and adolescents, although any age group may be affected. The mortality of meningococcemia is higher than that of meningococcal meningitis.

Meningococcemia usually follows an upper respiratory tract infection with flu-like symptoms of headache, myalgias, nausea, and vomiting. The severity of the disease can range from an indolent, slowly evolving infection to a fulminating illness causing prostration within a few hours after the onset of symptoms. The classic skin lesions can be petechial, macular, or maculopapular with pale gray vesicular centers. All are a few millimeters in size but may progress to a confluent hemorrhagic rash (2). They are most commonly localized to the extremities and trunk but may appear on any part of the body. Meningitis presents with the usual symptoms of meningeal irritation—neck soreness, photophobia, headache—while, in meningococcemia, meningeal signs are typically absent.

Gram stain and culture of scrapings of the skin lesions are positive in only about half of cases. The diagnosis must often rest on clinical findings and is confirmed by positive cultures of blood or cerebrospinal fluid.

One should entertain the diagnosis of meningococcemia in any patient who presents with fever, malaise, and a petechial or maculopapular rash, and include it in the differential diagnosis of other bacteremias (e.g., *H. influenzae, S. pneumoniae,*

S. aureus), subacute bacterial endocarditis, gonococcemia (few distal papular, hemorrhagic lesions), vasculitis (usually distal purpuric lesions), enteroviral exanthems, and RMSF.

The treatment of choice for meningococcemia is high-dose intravenous antibiotics. Penicillin G (2 million units every 2 hours), ampicillin (2 g every 6 hours), chloramphenicol (4 g/d), and ceftriaxone (up to 4 g/d [100 mg/kg] in children) have all been shown to be effective. Complications such as shock, disseminated intravascular coagulation, adult respiratory distress syndrome, or metabolic acidosis require aggressive supportive care. Prophylaxis is recommended for close school and household contacts. Rifampin, 600 mg (10 mg/kg for children, 5 mg/kg for infants younger than 1 month old), is given orally twice daily for 2 days. Single dose therapy of ciprofloxacin 500 mg orally or ceftriaxone 250 mg IM are also alternatives for adults.

A related syndrome, chronic meningococcemia, presents as periodic fever, localized rash, myalgia, and arthralgias lasting for several days. The number of skin lesions is small. Episodes may recur over a period of weeks to months. The diagnosis is established by positive cultures (especially of blood) during the febrile episodes. A fair percentage of patients proceed, if untreated, to an acute phase of disease. The differential diagnosis includes subacute bacterial endocarditis, rheumatic fever, gonococcemia, and Henoch-Schönlein purpura.

Treatment is the same as for acute meningococcal disease, except that lower doses of intravenous antibiotics are generally considered sufficient to eradicate the infection. All patients suspected of having meningococcal disease should be admitted to the hospital for evaluation and treatment, regardless of clinical appearance.

Rocky mountain spotted fever (RMSF) (see Chapter 142, Rocky Mountain Spotted Fever) is an acute infectious disease caused by *Rickettsia rickettsii* and transmitted by the bites of several species of ticks (*Dermacentor andersoni* in the western United States, *Dermacentor variabilis* in the eastern United States, and *Amblyomma americanum* in some southwestern areas). RMSF is not limited to the Rocky Mountain area; in fact, the areas of highest incidence are in the South Atlantic region and western south-central states. The organisms can be introduced directly into the skin by a tick bite or may enter broken skin with the tick's feces. Once the infection is established, the organisms invade vascular endothelial cells, causing localized thrombosis and necrosis. The disease is manifested clinically by fever, rash, myalgia, and headache. It ranges in severity from a mild, self-limited illness to severe, life-threatening disease (19).

RMSF is seen most commonly in the late spring and early summer. The incubation period ranges from 3 to 12 days. There is an abrupt onset of fever, chills, arthralgia, and headache and sometimes nausea, vomiting, and photophobia. The rash appears between the second and sixth days of the illness, beginning peripherally on the wrists, ankles, and forearms as a macular erythematous rash and extending to the palms, soles, and torso. The lesions become maculopapular in a few days in most cases and become petechial shortly thereafter (2 to 4 days after the start of the rash). The rash may be absent in 12% to 17% of cases and may be difficult to appreciate in dark-skinned individuals (30). Areas of decreased circulation, such as the distal extremities, nose, and ear lobes, may develop areas of infarction; finding such lesions on the scrotum or vaginal area can be an additional clue to the diagnosis.

The differential diagnosis of RMSF includes TSS, meningococcal meningitis, Kawasaki disease, measles, leptospirosis, Colorado tick fever, enteroviral infections, any cause of disseminated intravascular coagulation and vasculitis, mononucleosis, rat-bite fever, atypical measles, and other rickettsial diseases. Among the latter are murine typhus and epidemic typhus, which both have rashes that usually begin on the trunk rather than on the distal extremities.

The treatment of choice for RMSF is doxycycline (100 mg every 12 hours) for 7 to 10 days or tetracycline (25 to 50 mg/kg in divided doses four times daily, not to exceed 2 g/d). Because of concern over dental effects of tetracycline, chloramphenicol (50 to 100 mg/kg/d in four divided doses) may be used to treat children. Tetracycline usually does not affect enamel formation in the incisors, canines, and bicuspids after age 7 (11). Moreover, in children younger than 5 years old, it is unlikely to result in any apparent change in tooth color when fewer than five courses of therapy are given in the usual oral dosage (11).

SKIN CANCER

Skin cancers are life-threatening if not diagnosed early. Yet early diagnosis can lead to cure rates in greater than 90% of patients in the most common types of skin cancer. Discussion in this chapter will focus on clinical recognition as described below, illustrated with supplementary photographs. Since management is primarily by the dermatologist, definitive diagnostic points and treatment are discussed only briefly.

Basal Cell Carcinoma (Fig. 126.8) is the most common skin cancer. It is usually found in men over 50 years old. Ninety percent are on the sun-exposed head and neck, with the trunk being the next most common site. There are four types. The *Noduloulcerative* basal cell carcinoma begins as a small pearly papule that enlarges over the years into a nodule with a waxy edge, a few telangiectatic vessels and an ulcer on the surface. The *pigmented type* looks the same with the addition of some black or brown pigment. *Sclerosing basal cell cancer*, usually on the face, looks like a whitish scarred patch without any ulceration or telangiectases. *Superficial basal cell cancer* is the most innocuous looking, resembling a dermatitis. It usually appears on the back and the chest and it looks like a reddish patch with slight scale. The border may have telangiectatic vessels and be slightly raised. The center may be atrophic with superficial ulceration (12).

Squamous cell carcinoma (Fig. 126.9) accounts for 20% of all skin cancer other than melanoma. It occurs most commonly on sun-exposed areas of the face, scalp, lip, ear, and neck as well as the dorsal hand. Scars from radiation or burns may develop

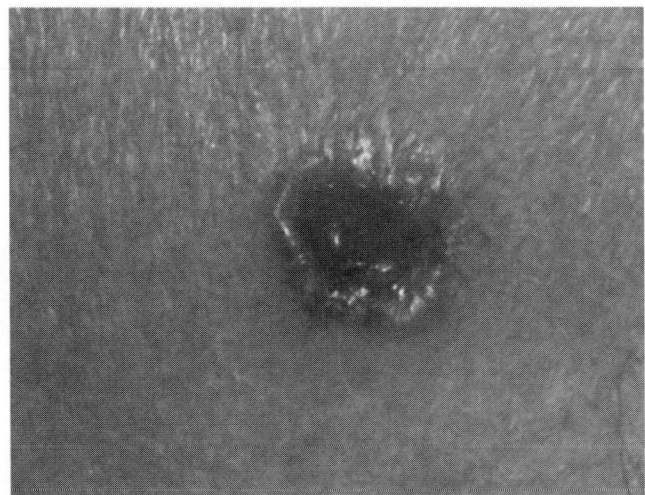

Figure 126.8.   Nodular basal cell carcinoma. This is a close-up showing rolled borders with telangiectasia. (From Goodheart HP. *Goodheart's Photoguide of Common Skin Disorders: Diagnosis and Management.* Philadelphia: Lippincott Williams & Wilkins, 2003, with permission.)

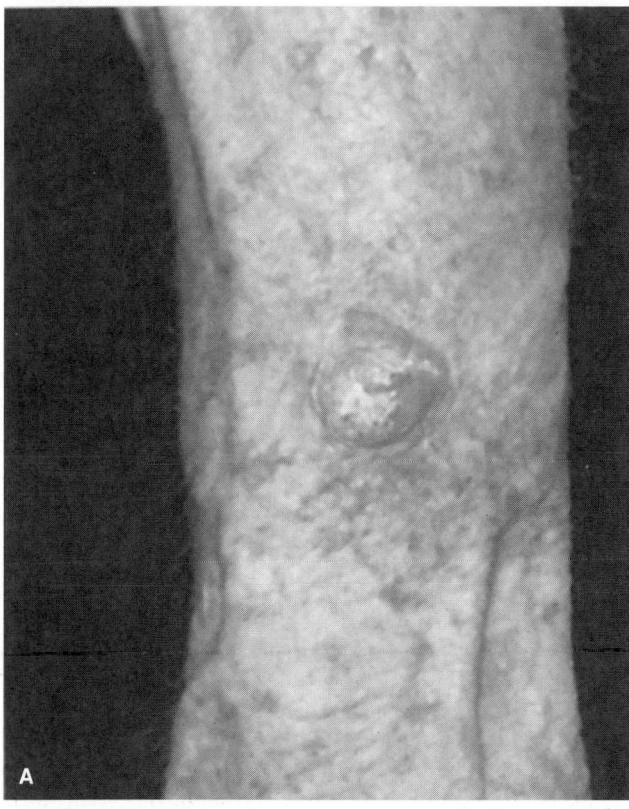
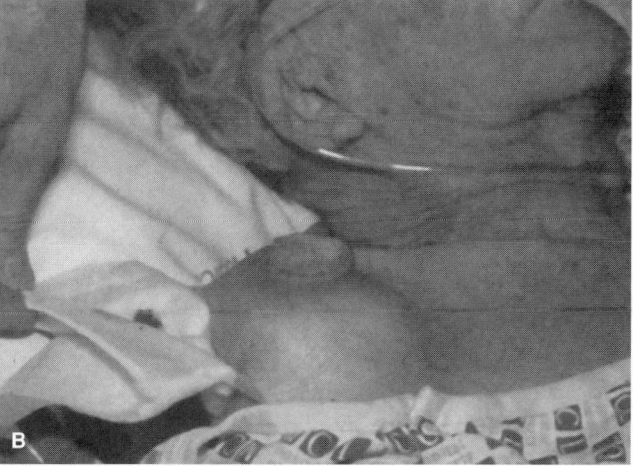

Figure 126.9. (A) Squamous cell carcinoma. This reddish nodule is indistinguishable from basal cell carcinoma. (B) squamous cell carcinoma. This neglected tumor has ulcerated. (From Goodheart HP, *Goodheart's Photoguide of Common Skin Disorders: Diagnosis and Management,* Philadelphia: Lippincott Williams & Wilkins, 2003, with permission.)

squamous cell carcinoma, and are more likely to metastasize (7). The most common lesion is a quickly growing nodule with an ulcerated center and a firm raised border surrounded by redness. Cure rates are 90% and metastasis (4% overall) manifests as regional lymphadenopathy.

Malignant melanoma (Fig. 126.10) is a pigmented skin cancer developing on previous nevi or *de novo* on sun-exposed areas, such as the face and forearms, or on the back of men and the lower legs of women. Amelanotic melanomas are rare and challenging to diagnose. Although melanomas make up only 1% of the skin cancers in the U.S., they account for over 60% of the deaths. Yet, the most common type, the superficial spreading melanoma, has 5-year survival rates of almost 98% when thin and removed early. It has five cardinal features (7):

A = Asymmetry
B = Border is irregular
C = Color is mottled, haphazard display of brown, black, gray, and pink (beware of no color in amelanotic melanoma)
D = Diameter > 6 mm (the size of a pencil eraser).
E = (1) Enlargement growth in size; (2) Elevation, usually with surface distortion

Changes in a recent or longstanding skin lesion that are suspicious include changes in size, shape, pigmentation, surrounding erythema, induration, friability and ulceration (13).

Diagnosis of all the skin cancers relies on early clinical suspicion and referral to a dermatologist for diagnosis by removing the lesion for pathologic diagnosis and staging. Additional chemotherapy or radiation therapy may be indicated for metastasis squamous cell carcinoma or advanced melanoma.

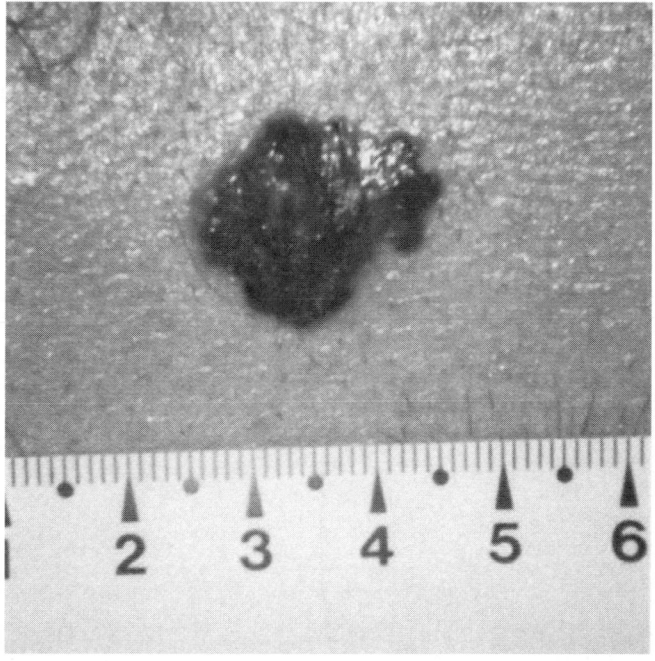

Figure 126.10. Superficial spreading melanoma. Note the "ABCD" features: asymmetry, notched border, varied colors, and diameter of more than 6 mm. (From Goodheart HP, *Goodheart's Photoguide of Common Skin Disorders Diagnosis and Management,* Philadelphia: Lippincott Williams & Wilkins, 2003. Fig. 22-27, p 354, with permission.)

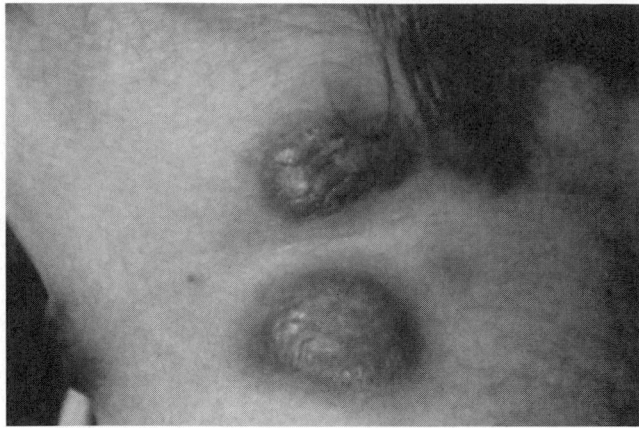

Figure 126.11. Epidemic Kaposi's sarcoma. Violaceous nodules. (From Goodheart HP, *Goodheart's Photoguide of Common Skin Disorders: Diagnosis and Management,* Philadelphia: Lippincott Williams & Wilkins, 2003, with permission.)

Kaposi sarcoma (Fig. 126.11) is a vascular neoplasm seen in the U.S. mostly in patients with AIDS and low CD4 cell counts. With the advent of effective therapy to manage HIV, Kaposi is uncommonly seen now. It can also occur sporadically in elderly men and in Europeans and Africans unrelated to their HIV status.

It appears as red, purple or brown papules or plaques, solitary or multiple, on skin or mucous membrane. Internal organs may be involved as well, including the GI tract and lungs. Diagnosis is made by clinical appearance in the appropriate individual. Management focuses on controlling the underlying disease (8).

Cutaneous T-cell lymphoma (mycosis fungoides) (Fig. 126.12) is a cancer of CD4 cells. It usually affects people in their 40s and 50s; twice as many men than women; twice as many blacks than whites. They report asymptomatic or pruritic patches of abnormal-appearing skin unresponsive to treatment. Occasionally, they may have fever, night sweats and weight loss. Diagnosis is made by multiple lesional biopsies over time. Treatment is with a combination of UV therapy, chemotherapy, and radiation therapy (17).

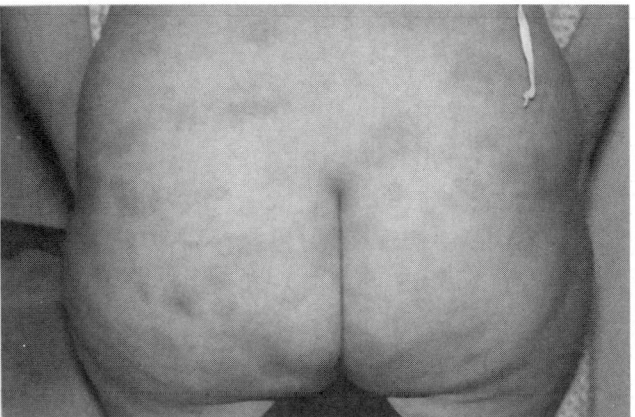

Figure 126.12. Mycosis fungoides (cutaneous T-cell lymphoma). Lesions have characteristic "smudgy," poorly-defined patches and plaques in a typical location. (From Goodheart HP, *Goodheart's Photoguide of Common Skin Disorders: Diagnosis and Management,* Philadelphia: Lippincott Williams & Wilkins, 2003, with permission.)

CRITICAL INTERVENTIONS

- Search for Nikolsky sign in diffuse red skin rashes
- Initiate antibiotics for patients with suspected meningococcemia
- Recognize that most melanomas are pigmented and develop changes in size, shape, and pigmentation

COMMON PITFALLS

✔ TEN can easily be confused with SSSS. TEN requires the removal of any possible precipitating agent, most commonly a drug; SSSS must be treated with appropriate antibiotics. The prognosis of the two diseases is markedly different

✔ The rash of TSS may be indistinct. The diagnosis should be considered in any patient with fever and signs of volume depletion, even in the absence of a history of tampon use. The disease can occur in men and children

✔ Bullous pemphigoid can easily be confused with pemphigus vulgaris. Early consultation with a dermatologist may be necessary to avoid misdiagnosis and inappropriate treatment

✔ In a febrile, seriously ill patient, skin lesions may be a manifestation of sepsis. The lesions should be opened and their contents Gram stained and cultured

✔ Rapid identification and treatment are crucial in ecthyma gangrenosum. The underlying septic process can be fatal if not treated promptly

✔ The diagnosis of gonococcemia is often overlooked in persons presenting with tendonitis without any history of injury

✔ The early rash of meningococcemia may be macular, maculopapular, or petechial

✔ In RMSF, the rash is absent in a significant proportion of cases. An increased index of suspicion is necessary for any patient presenting with a viral-like illness in the late spring or early summer

✔ Although basal cell carcinoma is usually waxy and ulcerative, it may be innocuous-looking, like a dermatitis, at first glance

✔ Asymptomatic or pruritic patches of abnormal skin which are unresponsive to treatment may represent cutaneous T-cell lymphoma

References

1. Bach MC. Dermatologic signs in toxic shock syndrome: clues to diagnosis. *J Am Acad Dermatol* 1983;8:3.
2. Baxter P, Priestly B. Meningococcal rash. *Lancet* 1988;2:1166.
3. Dahl M. The blistering diseases. In: *Common office dermatology.* New York: Grune & Stratton, 1983.
4. Davis JP, et al. Toxic shock syndrome: epidemiologic features, recurrence, risk factors and prevention. *N Engl J Med* 1980;303:1429.
5. Domonkos AN, Arnold HL, Odom RB. *Andrews' diseases of the skin.* Philadelphia: WB Saunders, 1982:311.
6. Fergie J, Patrick C, Lott L. *Pseudomonas aeruginosa* cellulitis and ecthyma gangrenosum in immunocompromised children. *Pediatr Infect Dis J* 1991;10:496.
7. Fitzpatrick TB, Johnson RA, Wolff K, et al. *Color atlas and synopsis of clinical dermatology,* 3rd ed. New York: McGraw-Hill, 1997:180–207.
8. Fitzpatrick TB, Johnson RA, Wolff K, et al. *Color atlas and synopsis of clinical dermatology,* 3rd ed. New York: McGraw-Hill, 1997:926–933.
9. Flowers FP, Krusinski PA. *Dermatology in ambulatory and emergency medicine.* Chicago: Year Book Medical, 1984:813.
10. Fury N. Blistering disorders. In: Roenigk H, ed. *Office dermatology.* Baltimore: Williams & Wilkins, 1981:171.
11. Grossman ER, et al. Tetracyclines and permanent teeth. *Pediatrics* 1971;47:567.
12. Hall JC. *Sauer's Manual of Skin Diseases,* 8th ed. Philadelphia: Lippincott—Raven Publishers, 2000:335–338.
13. Hall JC. *Sauer's Manual of Skin Diseases,* 8th ed. Philadelphia: Lippincott—Raven Publishers, 2000:347–349.
14. Hoge CW, Schwartz B, Talkington DF, et al. The changing epidemiology of invasive group A streptococcal infections and the emergence of streptococcal toxic shock-like syndrome. *JAMA* 1993;269:384.
15. Kaplan JE, Schonberger LB. The sensitivity of various serologic tests in the diagnosis of Rocky Mountain spotted fever. *Am J Trop Med Hyg* 1986;35:840.

16. McGee T, Munster A. Toxic epidermal necrolysis syndrome: mortality rate reduced with early referral to a regional burn center. *Plast Reconstr Surg* 1998;102:1018–1022.
17. Noble J. *Textbook of Primary Care Medicine,* 3rd ed., St. Louis: Mosby, 2001: 774–775.
18. Peters W, Zaidi J, Douglas L. Toxic epidermal necrolysis: a burn center challenge. *Can Med Assoc J* 1991;144:1477.
19. Petri WR. Tick-borne diseases. *Am Fam Physician* 1988;37:95.
20. Raman GV. Meningococcal septicaemia and meningitis: a rising tide. *BMJ* 1988;296:1141.
21. Reingold AL, et al. Toxic shock surveillance in the United States, 1980–1981. *Ann Intern Med* 1982;96:875.
22. Schopf E, et al. Toxic epidermal necrolysis and Stevens-Johnson syndrome. *Arch Dermatol* 1991;127:839.
23. Sexton D, Kaye K. Rocky Mountain Spotted Fever. *Med Clin North Amer* 2002;86:2;351–360.
24. Shands KN. Toxic shock syndrome in menstruating women. *N Engl J Med* 1980;303:1436.
25. Swartz MN, Weinberg AN. Infections due to gram-positive bacteria. In: Fitzpatrick TB, Eisen EZ, Wolff K, et al., eds. *Dermatology in general medicine,* 3rd ed. New York: McGraw-Hill, 1987:2100.
26. Redondo P, De Felipe I, De la Peña A, Aramendia JM, Vanaclocha V. Drug-induced hypersensitivity syndrome and toxic epidermal necrolysis: treatment with N-acetylcysteine. *Br J Dermatol* 1997;136:645.
27. Taylor J, et al. Toxic epidermal necrolysis: a comprehensive approach. *Clin Pediatr* 1989;28:404.
28. The Working Group on Severe Streptococcal Infections. Defining the group A streptococcal toxic shock syndrome: rationale and consensus definition. *JAMA* 1993;269:390.
29. Vélez A, Moreno J. Toxic epidermal necrolysis treated with N-acetylcysteine *J Amer Acad Dermatol* 2002:46.
30. Wright S. North American tick-borne diseases. *Ann Emerg Med* 1988;17;964.

CHAPTER 127
Papulosquamous Eruptions

John J. Kelly and Mark Spektor

Papulosquamous lesions are characterized by papules and scaly desquamation of the skin. The lesions may also be macular and erythematous. Diseases in this group include psoriasis, seborrheic dermatitis, pityriasis rosea, lichen planus, and secondary syphilis. Other diseases that may be part of the differential diagnosis include tinea, discoid lupus erythematosus, mixed connective-tissue diseases, and scabies. Papulosquamous eruptions are the most common cutaneous manifestations of human immunodeficiency virus (HIV) infection, and their appearance may be the first clue of HIV infection in an otherwise asymptomatic host (19). In addition, a large number of drugs are known to cause papulosquamous eruptions.

When evaluating a papulosquamous eruption in the emergency department, the physician should look for clues to help differentiate the possible etiologies. Is the rash disseminated or localized? Does it appear on specific areas of the body, such as the elbows, knees, scalp, palms, soles, web spaces, or sun-exposed areas? Is it a well-marginated, ring-shaped, or isolated lesion (herald patch)? Are the papules pruritic or purple? Answering these basic questions and using the algorithm in Figure 127.1, most papulosquamous diseases are diagnosed without dermatologic consultation.

PSORIASIS

Psoriasis, the most common papulosquamous dermatosis, is found in about 2% to 3% of the general population. The prevalence is equal between males and females, and the disease affects Caucasians twice as frequently as blacks or Asians (9). Although it is more common during the second and third decades, it may manifest itself at any age, and has been reported to be present at birth. The pathogenesis of psoriasis is not completely understood. Cell-mediated immune mechanisms appear to drive development of the plaques and heredity plays a well-demonstrated role in acquiring the disease (14).

CLINICAL PRESENTATION

The most common form of psoriasis, plaque psoriasis, occurs in approximately 80% of patients. In this type of disease presentation, lesions are characterized by well-delineated, salmon-colored papules that are soon covered by silvery-white scales (Fig. 127.2). They involve both the dermis and epidermis; the depth of involvement depends on their age and location. As the lesions age, the epidermal layer thins, exposing underlying capillary beds. These capillary beds may bleed when the overlying keratotic epidermis is sheared away by mechanical force. This phenomenon, known as the Auspitz sign, is diagnostic of psoriasis. Common sites for plaque psoriasis are the scalp, extensor surfaces of the extremities, palms, soles, nails, and the intergluteal cleft. Patients may present with inverse psoriasis in which the lesions affect the flexural sites such as axillae, antecubital and popliteal fossae.

Between 5% and 42% of patients with psoriasis develop psoriatic arthritis, which is seronegative for rheumatoid factor. Cutaneous lesions precede joint disease in 60% to 70% of the cases, but may present simultaneously. In 20% of patients, the onset of arthritis is prior to the skin changes (2).

Nail abnormalities are eventually seen in most patients. The nails are commonly pitted and show a brownish or whitish discoloration and an accumulation of scale on the nail bed (20) (Fig. 127.3).

Pustular psoriasis is characterized by erythematous areas covered with sterile pustules. It may be localized or general, and may affect the hands and feet in addition to the trunk and extremities. In extreme cases, pustules become confluent forming large lakes of pus. Generalized pustular psoriasis has an acute onset associated with malaise, pyrexia, and leukocytosis, and it is potentially fatal if untreated. Factors known to induce generalized pustular psoriasis include a tapering of the dose of systemic corticosteroids, withdrawal of potent topical steroids, nonsteroidal antiinflammatory agents, pregnancy, viral upper respiratory tract infections, and beta-hemolytic streptococcal infections (7).

Guttate psoriasis usually follows streptococcal infections. It is characterized by sudden appearance of lesions on the trunk and extremities.

DIFFERENTIAL DIAGNOSIS

The differential diagnosis of psoriasis includes tinea cruris, candidiasis, secondary syphilis, pityriasis rosea, cutaneous lupus erythematosus, and seborrheic dermatitis (6), as well as intertrigo when the eruption occurs in the intertriginous areas. Seborrheic dermatitis may resemble psoriasis of the scalp, but usually has finer and more widespread yellow scaling. A helpful clue in differentiating psoriasis from other conditions is the presence of psoriatic nail changes: pitting of the nails and separation of

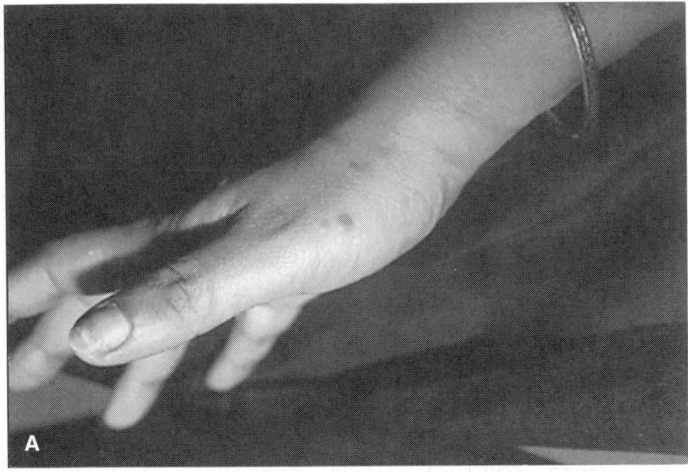
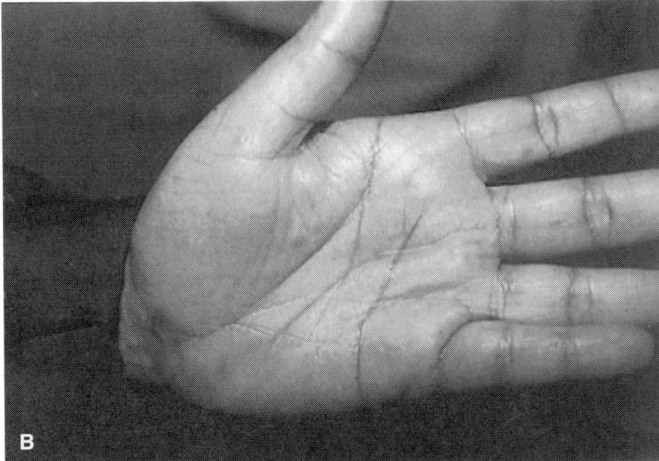
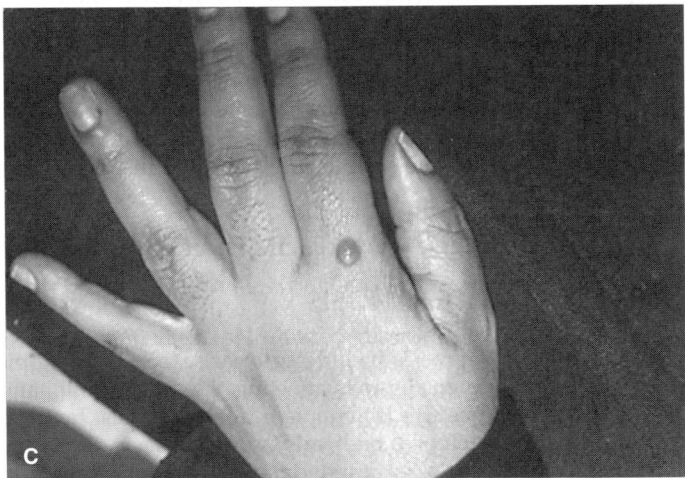

Figure 127.8.   (A–C). Secondary syphilis.

SECONDARY SYPHILIS

Syphilis (see Chapter 140) is a sexually transmitted infectious disease caused by *Treponema pallidum*. The rash of secondary syphilis appears 9 to 90 days after the onset of the chancre; the average is 3 weeks. Most individuals contract the disease from sexual activity with a person in the early stages of syphilis. The risk of transmission ranges from 9% to 63%, and incidence has been reported at a rate of 3.2 cases per 100,000 persons (18).

CLINICAL PRESENTATION

The rash of secondary syphilis is generalized, painless, and nonpruritic. A primary chancre may be present in as many as one-third of patients with secondary syphilis. As many as 60% of patients do not report recall having a chancre (18). The rash involves the skin as well as the mucous membranes in 30% to 50% of the cases. On the skin, it tends to follow the lines of cleavage, especially on the trunk. It has a special predilection for the palms and soles (Figs. 127.8a-c). The lesions are scaling, "raw ham" or copper-colored papules and plaques that are discrete and sharply demarcated rather than confluent (Fig. 127.9). Annular plaques on the mouth, nose, and lip areas are virtually diagnostic. The patient's presenting complaint may be an apparently unrelated other symptom, such as headache, sore throat, malaise, and generalized arthralgia.

DIFFERENTIAL DIAGNOSIS

The differential diagnosis of secondary syphilis includes pityriasis rosea, Rocky Mountain spotted fever, meningococcemia, drug reaction, and lichen planus. Palmar lesions that mimic secondary syphilis may be secondary to drug eruption.

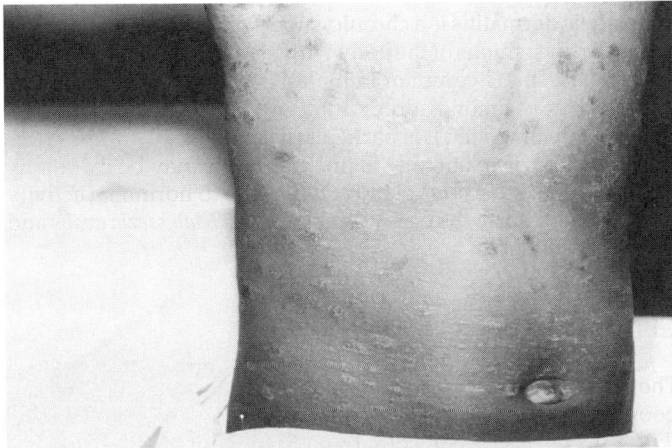

Figure 127.9.   Diffuse erythematous papules and plaques with scaling in a patient with the rash of secondary syphilis.

EMERGENCY DEPARTMENT MANAGEMENT AND DISPOSITION

Diagnostic studies such as VDRL or RPR should be ordered. Dark-field examination of scrapings from lesions may also be performed. If either test is positive, the patient is treated in the emergency department with either benzathine penicillin G (2.4 million units intramuscularly) or aqueous procaine penicillin G (600,000 units intramuscularly daily for 8 days). Patients allergic to penicillin may be treated with tetracycline or erythromycin for 10 days.

If the diagnosis of secondary syphilis cannot be made in the emergency department, the patient should be referred to a private physician or clinic pending the results of VDRL or RPR testing. Hospital admission is unnecessary for secondary syphilis, but the patient should be instructed to abstain from sexual contact until the diagnosis is clear and any necessary treatment has been administered, and to refer all sexual partners to testing and treatment, as indicated.

CRITICAL INTERVENTION

- Obtain a RPR for papulosquamous lesions of unclear etiology

COMMON PITFALLS

✔ Failing to elicit a history of a primary lesion preceding the rash. This history and an adequate sexual history are helpful in the initial diagnosis
✔ Failing to appreciate the typical erythematous, hyperpigmented, scaly papules on the palms and soles may lead to an inappropriate diagnosis
✔ Because of the strong association of HIV and syphilis, patients newly diagnosed with syphilis should be referred for HIV testing

Acknowledgment

The authors thank Howard Goldman, DO, Professor of Dermatology at Philadelphia College of Osteopathic Medicine, for contributing the photographs used in this chapter.

References

1. Bernardin RM, Ritter SE, Murchland MR. Papular pityriasis rosea. *Cutis* 2002;70(1):51–55.
2. Biondi C, Scarpa R, Pucino A. Psoriasis and psoriatic arthritis. *Acta Dermatol Venereol* 1989;146:69–71.
3. Chuh AA, Chan HH. Prospective case-control study of chlamydia, legionella and mycoplasma infections in patients with pityriasis rosea. *Eur J Dermatol* 2002;12(2):170–173.
4. Cribier B, Frances C, Chosidow O. Treatment of lichen planus. An evidence-based medicine analysis of efficacy. *Arch Dermatol* 1998;134:1521–1530.
5. Drago F, Malaguti F, Ranieri E, Losi E, Rebora A. Human herpes virus-like particles in pityriasis rosea lesions: an electron microscopy study. *J Cutan Pathol* 2002;29:359–361.
6. Feldman SR, Clark AR. Psoriasis. *Med Clin North Am* 1998;82:1135–1144.
7. Ferrera PC, Dupree ML, Verdile VP. Dermatologic problems encountered in the emergency department. *Am J Emerg Med* 1996;14:588–601.
8. Goeckerman WH. Treatment of psoriasis. *Northwest Med* 1925;24:15.
9. Green MS, Prystowsky JH, Cohen SR, Cohen JI, Lebwohl MG. Infectious complications of erythrodermic psoriasis. *J Am Acad Dermatol* 1996;34:911–914.
10. Gupta AK, Bluhm R, Cooper EA, Summerbell RC, Batra R. Seborrheic dermatitis. *Dermatol Clin* 2003;21:401–412.
11. Hartley AH. Pityriasis rosea. *Pediatr Rev* 1999;20:266–269.
12. Larsson A, Warfvinge G. Malignant transformation of oral lichen planus. *Oral Oncol* 2003;39:630–631.
13. Lebwohl M, Ast E, Callen JP, et al. Once-daily tazarotene gel versus twice-daily fluocinonide cream in the treatment of plaque psoriasis. *J Am Acad Dermatol* 1998;38:705–711.
14. Mendonca CO, Burden AD. Current concepts in psoriasis and its treatment. *Pharmacol Ther* 2003;99:133–147.
15. Nagpal S, Lu J, Boehm MF. Vitamin D analogs: mechanism of action and therapeutic applications. *Curr Med Chem* 2001;8:1661–1679.
16. Nocente R, Ceccanti M, Bertazzoni G, et al. HCV infection and extrahepatic manifestations. *Hepatogastroenterology* 2003;50:1149–1154.
17. Sharma PK, Yadav TP, Gautam RK, Taneja N, Satyanarayana L. Erythromycin in pityriasis rosea: A double-blind, placebo-controlled clinical trial. *J Am Acad Dermatol* 2000;42:241–244.
18. Singh AE, Romanowski B. Syphilis: review with emphasis on clinical, epidemiologic, and some biologic features. *Clin Microbiol Rev* 1999;12:187–209.
19. Singh F, Rudikoff D. HIV-associated pruritus: etiology and management. *Am J Clin Dermatol* 2003;4:177–188.
20. Tham SN, Lim JJ, Tay SH, et al. Clinical observations on nail changes in psoriasis. *Ann Acad Med Singapore* 1988;17:482–485.
21. van de Kerkhof PC, Franssen ME. Psoriasis of the scalp. Diagnosis and management. *Am J Clin Dermatol* 2001;2:159–165.
22. Vidimos AT, Camisa C. Tongue and cheek: oral lesions in pityriasis rosea. *Cutis* 1992;50:276–280.
23. Zouboulis CC, Xia L, Akamatsu H, et al. The human sebocyte culture model provides new insights into development and management of seborrhoea and acne. *Dermatology* 1998;196:21–31.

CHAPTER 128
Blistering Disorders

Lisa R. Palivos

Vesicular lesions are commonly seen in the emergency department. Like other dermatologic lesions, vesicles can present a challenge in determining their etiology, contagiousness, and proper treatment (2,3,5,6).

Vesicles are circumscribed epidermal elevations 1 to 4 mm in diameter that usually contain clear fluid. Several characteristics help distinguish the lesion from other vesicular disorders, including the nature of the contained fluid (seropurulent, serosanguineous), the shape of the lesion's apex (rounded, acuminate, umbilicated), the pattern of the eruption (discrete, irregularly scattered, grouped, linear), and the distribution over the body and associated mucous membrane involvement.

In this discussion, there are two types of vesicular disorders: those appearing in groups and those that are individual or disseminated.

GROUPED LESIONS

Herpes Simplex

Herpes simplex infections are caused by two different virus types (HSV-1 and HSV-2). Both viruses can infect oral or genital mucosa and are spread by direct contact. The hallmark of herpes simplex virus (HSV) infections is the ability to infect epithelial cells then travel up the peripheral nerve to the dorsal root ganglia where it may remain latent for years followed by reactivation.

CLINICAL PRESENTATION

The lesions of herpes simplex are typically tightly clustered on an erythematous base and evolve into pustules and erosions over 5 to 7 days. Grouped, crusted erosions are the typical presentation. Associated symptoms may include fever, local pain, regional lymphadenopathy, fatigue, and malaise. Urinary retention occasionally occurs with genital lesions and generally requires hospital admission.

Primary lesions are usually more widespread with a bilateral distribution. Recurrent lesions typically are tightly clustered, unilateral, and occur in the same location as previous episodes of infection. Recurrences are usually milder, involve fewer lesions and heal faster. Approximately 50% of patients with recurrent lesions have a 24-hour prodrome of local itching, burning, tingling, and stinging. Precipitating factors for recurrence include stress, fever, infections, sunburn, menstruation, or trauma.

Primary lesions usually resolve in 2 to 3 weeks, but the duration may be longer in immunocompromised patients. Typical sites of involvement are the oral, genital, and periorbital areas and the fingertips (herpetic whitlow), but any body area may be involved. With periorbital lesions, fluorescein staining of the cornea is necessary to rule out herpetic keratitis. Patients with herpetic keratitis should be referred to an ophthalmologist. Herpes gladiatorium is contracted by athletes, especially wrestlers. It is transmitted by direct skin-to-skin contact and usually appears in the head and neck region. With the increasing incidence of the acquired immunodeficiency syndrome and the growing use of bone marrow and solid organ transplantation, more severe manifestations of herpes infections are being seen (10).

DIFFERENTIAL DIAGNOSIS

The differential diagnosis of Herpes simplex includes aphthous stomatitis, tinea cruris, hand-foot-and-mouth disease, herpangina, and primary syphilis. Aphthous stomatitis consists of one or two painful lesions in the mouth but they are not in a circumscribed area. Although, early tinea, which is vesicular, can be difficult to distinguish from herpes, later tinea has central healing. Lesions in hand-foot-and mouth disease are asymptomatic. The chancre in primary syphilis is classically painless and the borders are indurated.

EMERGENCY DEPARTMENT EVALUATION

Diagnosis of Herpes simplex is usually made clinically. Viral cultures of vesicular fluid or direct fluorescent antibody stain of scraped lesions may be helpful for definitive diagnosis. The presence of intranuclear inclusions and multinucleated giant cells on a Tzanck preparation supports a diagnosis of herpes infection but does not distinguish between herpes simplex virus and varicella zoster virus. PCR and serology testing are not widely available, and are expensive.

EMERGENCY DEPARTMENT MANAGEMENT AND DISPOSITION

Acyclovir is the most widely used antiviral agent in clinical use. Treatment with 200 mg of oral acyclovir five times per day for 10 days is indicated for primary genital herpes. However, the duration of symptoms is decreased only minimally with this therapy and only if started within 24 hours after onset of the rash. Time to crusting decreases from 2.7 days to 2.2 days. In immunocompromised patients, a dose of 400 mg is recommended. Other medications that are effective and available for treating herpetic infections are famciclovir and valacyclovir (Table 128.1). Over the counter tetracaine cream (Viractin) may reduce healing time of recurrent herpes labialis by about 2 days. Topical penciclovir 1% cream (Denavir), which is more expensive, can minimally reduce average time to healing of recurrent orolabial herpes simplex virus infections by 0.7 days and the duration of pain by 0.6 days (12). Topical acyclovir is less effective than oral formulation and its use is discouraged. All three oral agents have been shown to reduce the frequency of symptomatic recurrences of genital herpes. Importantly, patients receiving suppressive antiviral medication should be counseled that they may still transmit herpes simplex virus to their sexual partners. Intravenous therapy (5 mg/kg every 8 hours) should be considered for patients with urinary retention, compromised immunity, or life-threatening disseminated infection.

COMMON PITFALLS

✔ Failure to instruct patients about measures to prevent transmission to others
✔ Failure to admit patients with herpes and urinary retention
✔ Failure to admit patients with disseminated infection

Herpes Zoster

Herpes Zoster (shingles) results from the reactivation of a dormant varicella zoster virus that entered the dorsal root ganglia during an earlier episode of chicken pox. Herpes Zoster (HZ) can occur in patients of any age who have had a previous infection of varicella zoster virus. The incidence of HZ increases with age, peaking in the 7th decade. Reactivation factors include fever, wind, U.V. light, illness or stress. An attack of HZ does not confer

TABLE 128.1. Treatment of Herpes Simplex

Treatment of Herpes Simplex	Primary Infection	Recurrent Lesions	Suppressive Therapy
Acyclovir	200 mg 5x/day for 10 days	400 mg 3x/day for 5 days	400 mg 2x/day for 12 months
Famciclovir*	250 mg 3x/day for 10 days	125 mg 2x/day for 5 days	250 mg 2x/day for 12 months
Valacyclovir*	1g 2x/day for 10 days	500 mg 2x/day for 3 days	1 g daily for 6–12 months

* Reduction in dosage is recommended in patients with reduced renal function. Valacyclovir should not be prescribed in patients with HIV or transplant recipients because of the observation of TTP and hemolytic uremic syndrome. Famciclovir is contraindicated with Denavir.

immunity and it is not unusual to have two or three episodes in a lifetime.

CLINICAL PRESENTATION

Herpes Zoster is characterized by unilateral vesicular eruption along one or two adjacent dermatomes that is associated with severe pain. Dermatomes T3-L3 are most frequently involved (Fig. 128.1). Occasionally the lesions may extend beyond the midline. There is usually a prodrome of pain, itching, burning, hyperesthesia in the same dermatome 4 to 7 days before the lesions appear. Fever, headache, malaise along with lymphadenopathy may also precede the eruption. The pain may imitate myocardial infarction, appendicitis, renal colic or migraine headache and may present a diagnostic dilemma until the characteristic rash develops. The eruption begins as an erythematous maculopapular rash that gives rise to vesicles containing purulent fluid. These pustules either umbilicate or rupture before forming crusts. The crusts fall off in 2 to 3 weeks.

When the ophthalmic division of the trigeminal nerve is involved Herpes Zoster ophthalmicus results. Lesions can appear on the forehead, eyelid, and nose. Symptoms include headache, fever, malaise, and eye pain. Ocular involvement is common and each individual should have a thorough eye exam. Hutchinson sign (lesion at the tip of the nose) usually heralds ocular involvement. Urgent (next day) ophthalmology referral is indicated. When the sensory branch of the facial nerve is involved, Herpes Zoster oticus results. Lesions appear in the ear, mouth, face, neck or scalp. Patients can complain of severe otalgia, vertigo, hearing loss or loss of taste in the anterior two-thirds of the tongue. When associated with facial paralysis, the disease is called Ramsay-Hunt syndrome. Treatment consists of acyclovir, corticosteroids, and diazepam for vertigo. Facial paralysis and hearing loss may be permanent. Patients should be referred to ENT urgently. Hospitalization should be considered in severe cases. The severe pain associated with Herpes Zoster is the principal reason that patients seek medical care. Traditionally, pain that is present while the rash persists or in the first thirty days from onset has been termed acute pain. Pain that is present after this period is termed *post herpetic neuralgia (PHN)* and may persist for months to years after lesions have disappeared. As age increases the risk and duration of PHN also rises. Nearly half of

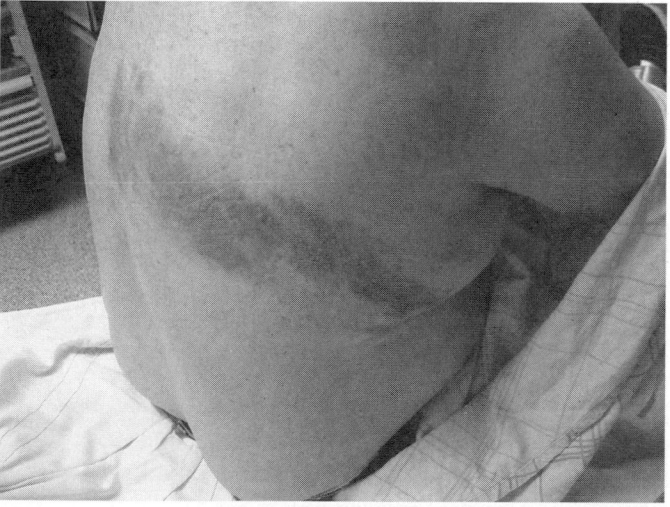

Figure 128.1. Herpes Zoster. Lesions can involve more than one dermatome. (Courtesy of Scott Sherman, MD.)

the patients older than 60 years have this complication. Other complications of HZ include secondary bacterial infections and pneumonitis.

DIFFERENTIAL DIAGNOSIS

The differential diagnosis includes chemical burns, Bell palsy, conjunctivitis, trigeminal neuralgia. The blisters in poison ivy often occur in a linear "dermatomal" but they are painless.

EMERGENCY DEPARTMENT EVALUATION

The diagnosis of HZ is based on history of pain and appearance of the dermatomal rash. Laboratory tests are not necessary. Scraping for a Tzanck smear or viral culture is usually negative and a biopsy is usually required for definitive diagnosis.

EMERGENCY DEPARTMENT MANAGEMENT AND DISPOSITION

A meta-analysis found that acyclovir reduces pain duration and prevalence, especially in patients 50 years of age or older (17). The recommended therapy is acyclovir 800 mg five times a day for 7 days. Famciclovir 500 mg or valacyclovir 1,000 mg t.i.d. for 7 days has also been shown to decrease the median duration of postherpetic neuralgia (1,13). Treatment should be started within 72 hours to be effective. Symptomatic treatment with oral analgesics and Burow solution–soaked compresses three times a day is often helpful as well.

It is unclear whether adding prednisolone is beneficial (16). Corticosteroids do not change the incidence or duration of PHN but they may improve the quality of life (time to return to usual activity, cessation of use of analgesic agents, and time to return to uninterrupted sleep) in patients over 50 years of age with acute herpes zoster (8,15). A tapering dose of 60 mg per day for 7 days, then 30 mg per day for 7 days, then 15 mg per day for 7 days can be used. Relative contraindications to the use of corticosteroids include hypertension, renal insufficiency, diabetes, osteoporosis, and peptic ulcer disease. The incidence of adverse effects is higher in patients treated with corticosteroids.

The treatment of PHN includes capsaicin cream, lidocaine patches, tricyclic antidepressants, neurontin, and sympathetic blocks.

Ophthalmologic consultation is indicated if the ophthalmic division of the trigeminal nerve is involved. Dissemination beyond the original dermatomes should raise the suspicion of immunodeficiency.

Hospital employees who are exposed to patients with herpes zoster should be tested for antibody to the varicella-zoster virus. Isolation for 8 to 21 days after exposure is recommended when antibody is not detected. If antibody is present, isolation is unnecessary (11).

COMMON PITFALLS

- ✔ Failure to instruct patients about measures to prevent transmission. Patients with HZ can transmit the virus as chickenpox to persons who have not already been infected
- ✔ Failure to recognize a central cause of facial paralysis
- ✔ Failure to recognize and treat ocular involvement
- ✔ Failure to recognize or admit immunocompromised individuals

Allergic Contact Dermatitis

Because allergic contact dermatitis is a result of delayed hypersensitivity, skin lesions may appear hours to days after exposure to the offending antigen, and it is often difficult to identify that antigen. Commonly identified etiologic agents include poison ivy, oak, and sumac; soaps; detergents; and perfumes. Pruritus is the initial symptom, which is quickly followed by erythema and vesiculation. Areas with a thin stratum corneum (such as eyelids and genitalia) may swell severely. Without treatment, symptoms may persist for 2 to 3 weeks.

Mild contact dermatitis may be treated with topical corticosteroids. For severe cases, oral prednisone (40 to 60 mg/d for 7 days) accelerates resolution of symptoms (usually within 24 to 48 hours) and poses minimal risks of adverse effects.

Fixed Drug Eruption

Like herpes simplex, fixed drug eruption causes recurrent episodes of skin lesions in one location. Unlike herpes simplex, however, fixed drug eruption generally leaves persistent slate-gray to brown hyperpigmentation after the attack resolves. The most commonly implicated drugs include phenolphthalein (e.g., Ex-Lax, Feen-a-Mint), tetracycline, sulfa, and barbiturates. Symptoms usually arise 1 to 2 days after ingestion. Pruritus generally occurs first, followed by the appearance of clusters of vesicles or bullae in a hyperpigmented macule. The process resolves in 2 to 3 weeks, after discontinuation of the offending agents.

Other Causes of Vesicular Eruptions

Dyshidrotic eczema (pompholyx) usually occurs on the medial and lateral aspects of the fingers and sometimes on the palms and soles. It is intensely pruritic and responds to topical corticosteroids. If severe, oral steroids can be used.

The vesicular eruption of tinea pedis may usually be diagnosed clinically by potassium hydroxide staining of vesicle fluid. Treatment is with a topical antifungal agent such as clotrimazole. Accompanying involvement of the hands is often an eczematous reaction.

Atopic dermatitis is generally accompanied by a personal or family history of eczema, allergic rhinitis, asthma, or urticaria. Nonetheless, the eruption is usually precipitated by physical irritation (wool gloves, soap, and water) or emotional stress. Treatment with topical steroids is effective.

Dermatitis herpetiformis (unrelated to the herpes viruses) may be confused with scabies or neurotic excoriations. It generally presents with broken, excoriated vesicles on an erythematous base. It usually begins on extensor surfaces and is pruritic. Treatment is with dapsone and oral antihistamines.

INDIVIDUAL OR DISSEMINATED VESICLES

Varicella

Varicella (chickenpox) is primarily a disease of childhood but it is not uncommon in adults. It is acquired by direct contact with infected lesions or inhalation of airborne droplets. Varicella begins with replication of the virus at the sites of contact and is followed by the development of a primary viremia, which establishes replication in the reticuloendothelial system. A secondary viremia occurs after one week, which disseminates the infection to the skin. The virus then establishes latency in the sensory ganglion. Reactivation of the latent infection causes Herpes Zoster.

CLINICAL PRESENTATION

Varicella presents with a rash, low-grade fever, and malaise. The lesions start as erythematous macules, progress to vesiculation with the classic "dew drop on a rose petal" appearance, become pustules, and finally crust over (Fig. 128.2). The hallmark of varicella rash is the simultaneous presence of lesions in all stages of development. The lesions usually appear on the trunk and face, and then spread to other areas of the body including scalp, mouth, ears, and genitalia. They are intensely pruritic. There may be a history of exposure 10 to 14 days before the rash. Varicella is highly contagious. Second attack rates for this virus may reach 90% for susceptible household contacts. Patients are considered infectious 2 days before the appearance of the rash until all vesicles have formed crusts, which is usually 5 to 6 days after the first appearance of the eruption. The severity of the illness varies from individual to individual and is inversely related to age. An attack of chickenpox usually confers lifelong immunity, although secondary attacks can happen. Varicella vaccine is now available in the United States and is approved for children and adults.

Varicella is usually a benign illness in immunocompetent patients. Immunocompromised individuals or those using immunosuppressive drugs, especially systemic corticosteroids are at a greater risk for complications (4). The most common complication in children is secondary bacterial skin infections after scratching, leading to a cellulitis. Varicella pneumonitis is rare in children but is the most common serious complication in adults. It can present with tachypnea, cough, fever, and pleuritic chest pain leading to acute respiratory distress syndrome (ARDS). Other complications include hepatitis, nephritis, orchitis, and encephalitis. Encephalitis in children is usually self-limited and includes cerebellar ataxia, nystagmus, and headache. Adult encephalitis has a mortality rate of 35% (9). Reye syndrome is an encephalopathy with fatty liver and is associated with salicylate use. Twenty to 30% of Reye syndrome cases are preceded by varicella (7).

Varicella during pregnancy poses a risk to both mother and child. The highest risk for fetal varicella syndrome is between

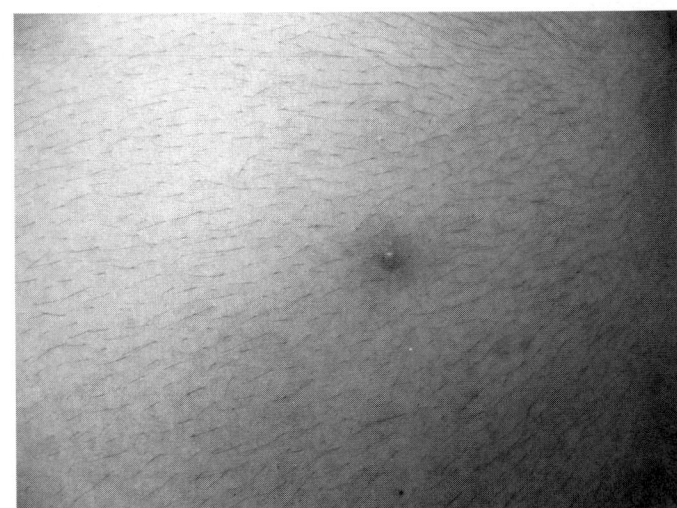

Figure 128.2.   Varicella: The lesion starts as a 2–4-mm red papule then develops into an irregular outline (rose petal) as a thin clear vesicle appears on the surface (dewdrop).

TABLE 128.2. Varicella Zoster Immune Globulin Indications

Immunocompromised children
Newborns whose mother had varicella 5 days before to 2 days post delivery
Infants exposed in nursery
All premature infants less than 28 weeks
Susceptible pregnant women
Healthy or immunocompromised adolescents and adults who are unvaccinated and susceptible postexposure prophylaxis*

*Administration may prevent or reduce intensity of disease. It is not indicated once clinical disease has developed. VZIG may be administered within 96 hours after exposure.

13 to 20 weeks of gestation. It is characterized by small infant size, cicatricial skin lesions, limb hypoplasia and other anomalies. For newborns the risk of infection and complications is greatest when the mother develops chickenpox 5 days before to 2 days post delivery. These infants have an increased chance of dissemination since they lack both maternal antibodies and a mature immune system. They should be given varicella zoster immune globulin (VZIG). VZIG is effective in preventing chickenpox in exposed susceptible, especially immunocompromised individuals (Table 128.2).

DIFFERENTIAL DIAGNOSIS

The differential diagnosis includes disseminated zoster, disseminated herpes simplex, eczema herpeticum, and folliculitis.

EMERGENCY DEPARTMENT EVALUATION

Diagnosis is usually made clinically. A Tzanck smear and viral culture may aid in making the diagnosis. A chest x-ray should be obtained if respiratory symptoms develop.

EMERGENCY DEPARTMENT MANAGEMENT AND DISPOSITION

Treatment of varicella is generally symptomatic and consists of daily baths and soaks to destroy the virus. Close cropping of the fingernails, calamine lotion and antihistamines to avoid excessive excoriations can provide relief. Isolate the patient especially from immunocompromised hosts. Avoid aspirin and Caladryl lotion, which can lead to an anticholinergic response from excessive skin absorption. Acyclovir (800 mg 5 times a day for 5 days) if started within 24 hours of rash development has been shown to reduce the number of lesions, duration of fever, illness and reduce pruritus. Therapy after the first day of illness is of no value in uncomplicated cases of adult varicella (14). All immunocompromised individuals with varicella should be hospitalized for intravenous acyclovir (10 mg/kg every 8 hours for 7 days). Hospitalization is also required for skin sepsis, pneumonitis, dense or hemorrhagic rash, and bleeding.

COMMON PITFALLS

✔ Failure to instruct patients about measures to prevent transmission
✔ Failure to admit patients who are immunocompromised

Coxsackievirus and Echovirus Infections

Coxsackievirus and echovirus infections may cause papulovesicular lesions that are evenly spread across the face and torso. Associated symptoms may include fatigue, malaise, fever, vomiting, and diarrhea. Resolution occurs spontaneously in 10 to 14 days, and treatment is symptomatic.

Hand–foot–mouth disease caused by coxsackieviruses presents with tender, flat-topped, whitish vesicles 3 to 4 mm in diameter on the palms and soles and in the mouth. It is commonly associated with mild systemic complaints. The duration is generally 4 to 5 days, and no treatment is necessary.

Insect Bites

Vesiculobullous skin lesions may occur as hypersensitivity reactions to insect bites, commonly those of fleas, bedbugs, and mites. A clue to the diagnosis is a linear or grouped pattern of lesions; some may have central puncta. Treatment is with topical corticosteroids and oral antihistamines, and avoidance of further contact with the insect.

CRITICAL INTERVENTIONS

- Initiate acyclovir within 24 hours of the onset of rash in adult varicella and within 72 hours of onset of herpes zoster
- Obtain ophthalmology consult for patients with herpetic keratitis due to herpes simplex or with involvement of the ophthalmic division of the trigeminal nerve in herpes zoster

Acknowledgments

Thanks to previous edition's chapter author M. Andrew Levitt for his contribution to this chapter.

References

1. Beutner KR, Friedman DJ, Forszpaniak C, et al. Valaciclovir compared with acyclovir for improved therapy for herpes zoster in immunocompetent adults. *Antimicrob Agents Chemother* 1995;39:1546–1553.
2. Dahl M. The blistering diseases. In: Dahl M. *Common office dermatology.* New York: Grune & Stratton, 1983.
3. Domonkos AN, Arnold HL, Odom RB. *Andrews disease of the skin.* Philadelphia: WB Saunders, 1982.
4. Dowell SF, Bresee JS. Severe varicella associated with steroid use. *Pediatrics* 1993;92:223–228.
5. Flowers FP, Krusinski PA. *Dermatology in ambulatory and emergency medicine.* Chicago: Year Book Medical, 1984.
6. Furey N. Blistering disorders. In: Roenigk H, ed. *Office dermatology.* Baltimore: Williams & Wilkins, 1981.
7. Hurwitz ES, et al. National surveillance for Reye syndrome: a five-year review. *Pediatrics* 1982;70:895–900.
8. Mcfarlane LL, Simmons MM, Hunter MH. The use of corticosteroids in the management of Herpes Zoster. *J Am Board Fam Pract* 1998;11:224–228.
9. Preblud SR. Varicella: complications and costs. *Pediatrics* 1986;78:728–735.
10. Sasadeusz JJ, Sacks SL. Systemic antivirals in herpes virus infections. *Dermatol Clin* 1993;11:171.
11. Sayre MR, Lucid EJ. Management of varicella-zoster-virus exposed hospital employees. *Ann Emerg Med* 1987;16:421.
12. Spruance SL, Rea TL, Thoming C, et al. Penciclovir cream for the treatment of herpes simplex labialis. A randomized, multicenter, double-bind, placebo-controlled trial. *JAMA* 1997;277:1374–1379.
13. Tyring S, Barbarash RA, Nahlik JE, et al. Famciclovir for the treatment of acute herpes zoster: effects on acute disease and postherpetic neuralgia—a randomized, double-blind, placebo-controlled trial. *Ann Intern Med* 1995;123:89–95.
14. Wallace MR, Bowler WA, et al. Treatment of adult varicella with oral acyclovir. A randomized, placebo-controlled trial. *Ann Intern Med* 1992;117:358–363.
15. Whitley RJ, Weiss H, Gnann JW, et al. Acyclovir with and without prednisolone for the treatment of herpes zoster—a randomized, placebo-controlled trial. *Ann Intern Med* 1996;125:376–383.
16. Wood MJ, Johnson RW, McKendrick MW, et al. A randomized trial of acyclovir for 7 days or 21 days with and without prednisolone for treatment of acute herpes zoster. *N Engl J Med* 1994;330:896–900.
17. Wood MJ, Kay R, Dworkin RH, et al. Oral acyclovir therapy accelerates pain resolution in patients with herpes zoster: a meta-analysis of placebo-controlled trials. *Clin Infect Dis* 1996;22:341–347.

CHAPTER 129
Purpuric Eruptions

Stephen C. Hartsell and Steven M. Joyce

The term *purpura* (Latin, meaning "purple") refers to any skin or mucous membrane eruption caused by bleeding into the skin. Purpura is a sign of underlying disease, usually a disorder of platelets or small vessels and only rarely of clotting factors. The cause of purpura varies, ranging from the trivial (e.g., actinic purpura in the elderly) to the life-threatening (e.g., thrombotic thrombocytopenic purpura) (Table 129.1).

The lesions of purpura vary in size, consistency, and distribution. Lesions smaller than 3 mm are called *petechiae* and usually result from platelet or vascular abnormalities, whereas larger lesions are termed *ecchymoses* and generally are secondary to trauma or clotting disorders (10). Lesions vary from red to purple and do not blanch with pressure, because the lesions represent extravasated blood in the dermis rather than erythema due to dilated vessels. Lesions may be flat and nonpalpable when inflammation is absent (as in thrombocytopenic purpura), or palpable papules or macules when inflammation is present (as in septic embolic disease or vasculitis) (Table 129.1) (10). Purpura may appear with a variety of other lesions, again depending on the underlying cause and stage of development (e.g., immune-mediated vasculitis may progress from areas of urticaria to necrotic, confluent ecchymoses). The skin and mucous membrane lesions are the outward signs of a systemic process in most cases, and the effects of visceral bleeding, infection, and inflammation must be considered.

Purpura may occur in any age group, may be rapidly or slowly progressive, and may be accompanied by none, few or many systemic manifestations.

In addition to various medical conditions, purpura may be caused by a variety of drugs, which can cause small vessel or platelet disorders by direct toxicity, inhibition of function, or immune-mediated mechanisms. Almost every class of drug has been implicated as a cause of purpura (Table 129.2).

CLINICAL PRESENTATION

Patients with purpura present to the emergency department for a variety of reasons. Some patients may simply be concerned about the rash itself, whereas others present because of manifestations accompanying the rash (e.g., abnormal bleeding, easy bruising, or constitutional symptoms such as fever, malaise, and arthralgias). Less commonly, patients present due to severe manifestations of the underlying illness, such as spontaneous bleeding or mental status changes (e.g., due to intracranial hemorrhage or meningococcal meningitis).

Regardless of the appearance of the rash or associated symptoms and signs, the presence of spontaneous bleeding ("wet" purpura) is a grave sign requiring immediate intervention (3). Bleeding gums, epistaxis, intraocular hemorrhage, guaiac-positive stool, menorrhagia, or hematuria are all included in this category. The cause is usually thrombocytopenia. The immediate threat to life is intracranial hemorrhage. Severe anemia and shock from blood loss are possible but not common.

In thrombocytopenia, easy bruising may be noted with platelet counts of 30,000 to 50,000/mm^3, while spontaneous ecchymoses or petechiae may not appear until the platelet count

---

TABLE 129.1. Disorders Causing Purpura

EXTRAVASCULAR (NONPALPABLE)—LOSS OF DERMAL VASCULAR CONNECTIVE TISSUE

Actinic disorders (senile purpura)
Scurvy
Corticosteroid therapy
Amyloidosis
Hereditary connective tissue disorders (Ehlers-Danlos syndrome, Marfan syndrome)

VASCULAR—DAMAGE TO VESSEL WALLS

Mechanical (Nonpalpable)—Vessel Walls Normal
Increased intravascular pressure (vomiting, cough, straining at childbirth, Valsalva maneuver)
Suction to skin ("love bites," suction cups, depilatory waxing)
Trauma (bruise, coining)
Factitial (self-induced by various methods, e.g., Gardner-Diamond Syndrome)
Stasis purpura (increased hydrostatic pressure)

Anoxic (Nonpalpable)—Microvascular Obstruction
Consumptive coagulopathies (DIC, TTP, HUS, purpura fulminans)
Fat emboli
Thrombocytosis, polycythemia, myeloproliferative disorders
Dysgammaglobulinemias

Inflammatory Vasculitis (Palpable)
Drug-induced (see Table 129.2)
Hypersensitivity vasculitis—Henoch-Schönlein and other allergic purpuras, collagen–vascular disorders, certain infections (e.g., streptococcus, hepatitis B, cytomegalovirus, Epstein-Barr virus), dysgammaglobulinemias, malignant neoplasms, cryoglobulinemia, serum sickness
Granulomatous vasculitis—Wegener, giant cell
Infectious vasculitis (embolic or dermal Shwartzman reaction)—meningococcus, streptococcus, gonococcus, measles, mumps, smallpox, Rocky Mountain spotted fever

INTRAVASCULAR/HEMATOLOGIC (NONPALPABLE)

Thrombocytopenia
Decreased platelet production (bone marrow disorders)—radiation, chemicals, chemotherapeutic agents and other drugs (see Table 129.2), bone marrow failure, neoplasm, megakaryocyte destruction (as in hemorrhagic smallpox)
Increased platelet destruction—immune-mediated (ITP, SLE, CLL, HIV, drugs [see Table 129.2], posttransfusion, neonatal), nonimmune (artificial surfaces, consumptive coagulopathies DIC, TTP, HUS, purpura fulminans)
Platelet sequestration—hypersplenism, hypothermia
Infections (by above listed mechanisms and others)
Viral (including HIV and Viral Hemorrhagic Fevers), rickettsial, bacterial, mycotic, protozoal

Functional Platelet Disorders
Drug-induced (see Table 129.2)
von Willebrand Disease
Storage pool disorders (rare, inherited)
Other—diabetes, hemachromatosis, liver disease, myeloma, myeloproliferative syndrome, uremia

Coagulopathies
Hemophilias
von Willebrand
Consumptive coagulopathies (DIC, TTP, HUS, purpura fulminans)
Acquired coagulopathies: venom toxicity (snake, scorpion, spider), vitamin K deficiency, liver disease

MIXED MECHANISMS

Many disorders may cause purpura by several different mechanisms. See references 5, 6, 8, 9, 12–15, 17. For example, viral hemorrhagic fevers may cause purpuric eruptions due to direct and inflammatory vascular damage as well as thrombocytopenia, platelet dysfunction and coagulopathy.

DIC, disseminated intravascular coagulation; *TTP*, thrombotic thrombocytopenic purpura; *HUS*, hemolytic–uremic syndrome; *ITP*, immune thrombocytopenic purpura; *SLE*, systemic lupus erythematosus; *CLL*, chronic lymphocytic leukemia; *HIV*, human immunodeficiency virus.

TABLE 129.2.   Common Drugs That May Cause Purpura

ANALGESICS

Acetylsalicylic acid
Acetaminophen
Nonsteroidal antinflammatory drugs (NSAIDs)
Codeine

ANTIBIOTICS

Antituberculous agents
Penicillins
Sulfonamides
Chloramphenicol
Nitrofurantoin
Tetracyclines
Erythromycin
Cephalosporins
Aminoglycosides
Streptomycin

ANTICONVULSANTS

Barbiturates
Carbamazepine
Diphenylhydantoin
Primidone
Valproate sodium

ANTIHYPERTENSIVES

Methyldopa
Reserpine

ANTICOAGULANTS

Coumadin
Heparin
GP IIb/IIIa Inhibitors

CARDIOVASCULAR AGENTS

Atropine
Quinidine
Digitalis
Nitroglycerin
Propranolol

ANTIRHEUMATICS

NSAIDs
Gold
Corticosteroids
Mechanisms include direct or immune-mediated
  thrombocytopenia, vascular injury, platelet
  inhibition, and coagulopathies. Many drugs may
  cause purpura by several of these mechanisms
  (7,16).

DIURETICS

Thiazides
Furosemide
Spironolactone

HYPOGLYCEMICS

Tolbutamide
Chlorpropamide

SEDATIVES, HYPNOTICS

Meprobamate
Phenobarbital
Chlordiazepoxide

ANTIPSYCHOTICS, ANTIDEPRESSANTS

Tricyclics
Phenothiazines

MISCELLANEOUS

Antimetabolites, chemotherapeutic agents
Ethanol
Allopurinol
Serum products, immune globulins
Estrogens, oral contraceptives
Heroin
Quinine
Hydroxychloroquine
Antihistamines
Guaiafenesin
Clofibrate
Chlorpheniramine
Arsenicals
Cimetidine
Griseofulvin
Iodides
Dextroamphetamine
Bismuth
Organic hair dyes
Menthol
Insecticides
Benzene
Metal compounds

---

drops below 30,000/μL. Internal bleeding, including intracranial hemorrhage, rarely occurs with platelet counts above 10,000/μL (1).

Patients without spontaneous bleeding ("dry" purpura) may have extensive petechiae or ecchymoses on the skin and mucous membranes, but are in less immediate danger. However, spontaneous bleeding may develop at any time, so rapid determination of the cause is still indicated.

Any patient presenting with purpura and mental status changes requires immediate evaluation for intracranial hemorrhage or central nervous system (CNS) infection. Empiric treatment (e.g., platelet transfusion or intravenous antibiotics) based on the presumptive diagnosis and preliminary laboratory results

(complete blood count [CBC] with platelets, prothrombin time, partial thromboplastin time [PTT]) may be instituted during such evaluation.

DIFFERENTIAL DIAGNOSIS

The lesions of purpura are characteristic and difficult to mistake for other disorders. Some lesions appear purpuric but do not reflect an underlying illness. Normal bruising resulting from trauma is technically a form of ecchymosis. Ecchymoses may be induced by trauma due to folk remedies such as coining. A rare syndrome of raised, tender ecchymoses which appear spontaneously in young women with psychiatric problems (Gardner Diamond Syndrome) was formerly attributed to "autoerythrocyte sensitization," but is now thought to be due to self-inflicted trauma (12). Purpuric lesions may be created by increased hydrostatic pressure or suction in normal skin. Examples include facial and conjunctival petechiae due to increased venous pressure (as with protracted vomiting or sneezing, or strangulation) or isolated ecchymosis from suction applied to the skin (as with "love bites" or electrocardiographic suction cups). These lesions are classified as mechanical or factitial purpura (12). Other erythematous rashes, such as viral exanthems and urticaria, can be differentiated from purpura by their light red color and in that they blanch with pressure (because they represent hyperemia rather than extravasation of blood). Similarly, telangiectases and hemangiomata are discrete collections of abnormally dilated blood vessels that appear bright red and usually blanch with pressure. Diascopy, the use of a glass slide to apply pressure over a lesion, is a simple visual method to differentiate lesions due to vascular dilation (which blanch with pressure) from those due to purpura (which do not).

The lesions of Kaposi's sarcoma begin as reddish macules and evolve in 1 to 2 weeks into purple or brown rounded lesions measuring from several millimeters to centimeters in size (4).

EMERGENCY DEPARTMENT EVALUATION

The history and physical examination should be directed toward identifying the underlying cause of the purpura. The history should include recent infections, recent medication or drug ingestion, radiation or chemical exposure, and systemic symptoms. A personal or family history of purpura or abnormal bleeding after surgical or dental procedures or trauma should be elicited. History of hepatic, renal, rheumatologic, or hematologic disease, malignancy, immunosuppression or human immunodeficiency virus (HIV) infection is also important.

A complete list of medications and allergies should be obtained. Except for hereditary coagulation disorders, which rarely present as purpura, and rare hereditary thrombocytopenias, the family history is usually unremarkable. The social history should include questions regarding alcohol and drug use and risk factors for HIV infection. Patients may report easy bruising, prolonged bleeding after surgical or dental procedures, or spontaneous bleeding such as epistaxis, menorrhagia, or melena.

The physical examination should allow rapid differentiation between trivial and serious causes of purpura. The distribution of the rash may be an indicator of the cause of the purpura. Senile or actinic purpura occurs on sun-exposed areas, usually the forearms, of elderly patients. Vasculitic purpura is usually symmetric and predominates in the lower extremities (e.g., Henoch-Schönlein purpura) (Fig. 129.1). A more generalized distribution of discrete petechiae may be noted when purpura is associated with bacterial illness such as meningococcemia or subacute bacterial endocarditis. Purpuric lesions in thrombocytopenia tend to occur in areas of minor trauma or areas of pressure, such as the belt line or over bony prominences. The purpura of scurvy classically appears as perifollicular petechiae, whereas that of Rocky Mountain spotted fever begins over the distal joints and spreads centrally. The lesions of purpura fulminans are large, symmetric ecchymoses of the lower extremities and buttocks, often with infarcted areas or bullae.

The morphology of purpuric lesions may likewise suggest their cause. Raised or "palpable" purpura signifies dermal inflammation, usually caused by a vasculitis, whether infectious or immune-mediated (see Table 129.1). When bacterial infections cause purpura, the lesions may have a central purulent papule (e.g., disseminated gonococcemia). Immune-mediated vasculi-

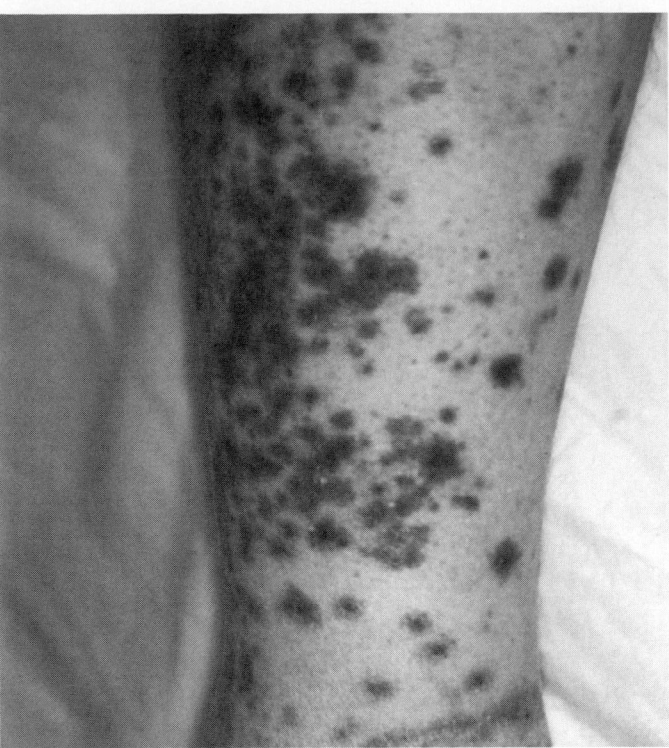

Figure 129.1. Henoch-Schönlein purpura. (From John Zone, MD, with permission.)

tides often have lesions of erythema, bullae, or urticaria in association with palpable purpura. Flat, nonpalpable petechiae or ecchymoses usually indicate thrombocytopenia or coagulation defects. Coumadin-associated vasculopathy results in necrotizing ecchymoses.

The physical examination may further reveal specific abnormalities in certain causes of purpura. In thrombocytopenia, the optic fundi and mucous membranes may show petechiae. Painful joint effusions may accompany various types of immune-mediated purpura, disseminated gonococcemia, and coagulation disorders. Lymphadenopathy or lesions characteristic of Kaposi's sarcoma may be indicators of HIV seropositivity, which may present with purpura in up to 9% of cases (11). Lymphadenopathy may also be found in patients with lymphoma, infectious mononucleosis, and leukemia. Splenomegaly (as well as other forms of hypersplenism) may also be noted in these same illnesses, but is absent in most other types of thrombocytopenic purpura (e.g. ITP) and coagulation defects (10).

All but the trivial causes of purpura (e.g., actinic, mechanical, factitial) require laboratory studies to elucidate the underlying cause. A complete blood count with differential screens for anemias, bone marrow disorders, various malignancies, infection, or hemolysis. A platelet count screens for thrombocytopenia, although purpura is rare with platelet counts over 30,000/μL, and spontaneous bleeding rarely occurs until the platelet count drops below 10,000/μL (1). The peripheral blood smear screens for abnormal red blood cell and platelet morphology (indicative of hemolysis and various platelet abnormalities, respectively). Prothrombin time (PT) and activated partial thromboplastin time (PTT) screen for coagulation or mixed platelet and/or coagulation disorders) (13,17). Determination of bleeding time may be of limited use in the emergency department in confirming platelet dysfunction or vascular disorders. The fibrinogen level, along with fibrin–fibrinogen degradation products (FDP, D-dimer), may also be useful (13). Because therapy with blood products is sometimes necessary and their use may confound subsequent diagnosis, extra tubes for type and screen and for other platelet and coagulation assays should be obtained before treatment.

On subsequent (usually inpatient) evaluation, the following tests may be indicated, depending on the suspected etiology: bone marrow aspiration (frequently necessary in thrombocytopenia), skin biopsy, bleeding time, autoimmune disease screening tests, clotting factor assays, and platelet function tests (17).

EMERGENCY DEPARTMENT MANAGEMENT

First, life-threatening complications of spontaneous bleeding should be stabilized, and efforts should be made to ascertain the cause of purpura. As described, the history, physical examination, and laboratory studies should allow rapid determination of the category of illness causing the purpura and associated symptoms.

When thrombocytopenia is the cause of purpura, platelet transfusion should be considered only when there has been abnormal bleeding. Generally, each unit of platelets may be expected to raise the platelet count by about 5,000 to 10,000/μL (15). Spontaneous mucous membrane or CNS bleeding can usually be controlled when the platelet count is restored to more than 20,000/μL. Platelet transfusion is relatively contraindicated in disorders caused by intravascular thrombosis (such as disseminated intravascular coagulation [DIC] and thrombotic thrombocytopenic purpura [TTP]), because platelets may contribute to further thrombosis.

When immune-mediated thrombocytopenia is likely, as in immune thrombocytopenic purpura (ITP) or posttransfusion purpura, the half-life of transfused platelets is short (in hours) compared with that for other disorders (in days) (3). In these cases, alternative therapy, such as corticosteroids, splenectomy, or plasmapheresis, may eventually be indicated (1).

Coagulopathies presenting with spontaneous bleeding may be treated by replacement of specific coagulation factors (when known). In acquired coagulopathies from coumadin or liver disease, vitamin K is indicated. Fresh frozen plasma may be helpful in a variety of coagulopathies and thrombolytic disorders when specific factor replacement is not available or cannot be determined (2).

If purpura is thought to be due to a drug, regardless of the suspected mechanism, that drug should be discontinued. Anticoagulants or platelet inhibitors (in proper dosages) may be reinstituted, if indicated, when the disorder is controlled.

Specific therapy directed to underlying disorders should be initiated once the etiologic factors have been defined and a diagnosis established. See Chapters 151 "Bleeding Disorders," 152 "Antithrombotic Therapy and Its Complications," and 153 "Disseminated Intravascular Coagulation, Thrombotic Thrombocytopenic Purpura, and Hemolytic-Uremic Syndrome."

CRITICAL INTERVENTIONS

- Intervene immediately with the combination of purpura and spontaneous bleeding ("wet"' purpura)
- Evaluate and treat patients presenting with purpura and mental status changes for intracranial hemorrhage or central nervous system (CNS) infection

DISPOSITION

Because purpura may reflect hematologic, rheumatologic, or infectious disorders, consultation is obtained from appropriate specialists once trivial causes of purpura have been ruled out.

When the diagnosis is unclear, a dermatology consultation can be helpful.

Because the underlying disorders that are responsible for purpura often have the potential for progressing to life-threatening emergencies, patients with purpura are often admitted to the hospital for confirmation of the diagnosis and definitive treatment. For example, patients with thrombocytopenia may require a bone marrow biopsy or aspirate to confirm the exact cause of illness. If vasculitis secondary to penicillin is suspected, however, and signs and laboratory abnormalities are mild, the drug may be withdrawn and outpatient follow up provided. In general, however, the consultant should choose between inpatient and outpatient treatment. Patients presenting with spontaneous bleeding or life-threatening complications, such as CNS hemorrhage or septic shock, require immediate hospital admission, usually to an intensive care unit.

Emergency transfer of patients with life-threatening complications of purpuric illness is indicated when the needed blood products, specialty consultation, or level of care is not available. Stabilization with intravenous fluids and emergently indicated blood products (when available) should be accomplished before transfer, after consultation with the accepting physician. Patients whose illness may progress rapidly (e.g., meningococcemia, DIC) should be considered for air ambulance transfer when ground transport times would be prolonged.

COMMON PITFALLS

✔ Failure to recognize the trivial causes of purpura may result in unnecessary time and expense spent in pursuing a diagnostic workup

✔ Drugs are a common cause of purpura and, unless an adequate history of drug exposure is obtained, the causal agent may initially be missed

✔ When spontaneous bleeding is noted, consultation should be obtained immediately and platelet or coagulation factor transfusion (when indicated) should be initiated to minimize the chance of CNS hemorrhage

✔ Premature administration of drugs or blood products may delay laboratory diagnosis and, in some cases, may worsen the disease process causing purpura

References

1. Cines DB. Immune thrombocytopenic purpura. *NEJM* 2002;346:995–1008.
2. Cohen H. Avoiding the misuse of fresh frozen plasma. *BMJ* 1993;307:395–396.
3. Crosby WH. Wet purpura, dry purpura. *JAMA* 1975;232:744.
4. Friedman-Kien AE, Laurenstein LJ, Rubinstein P, et al. Disseminated Kaposi's sarcoma in homosexual men. *Ann Intern Med* 1982;96:693–700.
5. Gibson LE, Danielson WP. Cutaneous vasculitis. *Rheum Dis Clin North Am* 1995;21:1097–1113.
6. Kitchens CS. Surgery and hemostasis: the influence of one on the other. In: Ratnoff OD, Forbes CD, eds. *Disorders of hemostasis, 3rd Ed.* Orlando, FL: Grune & Stratton, 1996:356.
7. Marcus AJ. Platelets and Their Disorders. In: Ratnoff OD, Forbes CD, eds. *Disorders of hemostasis, 3rd Ed.* Orlando, FL: Grune & Stratton, 1996:79.
8. McGovern TW, Christopher GW, Eitzen EM. Cutaneous manifestations of biological warfare and related threat agents. *Arch Dermatol* 1999;135:311–322.
9. Minton SM. Clinical Hemostatic Disorders Caused by Venoms. In: Ratnoff OD, Forbes CD, eds. *Disorders of hemostasis, 3rd Ed.* Orlando, FL: Grune & Stratton, 1996.
10. Piette WW. Hematologic diseases. In: Freedeberg IM, Eisen AZ, Wolff K, et al., eds. *Dermatology in general medicine*, 6th ed. New York: McGraw-Hill, 2003:1523.
11. Ratner L. Human immunodeficiency virus–associated autoimmune thrombocytopenic purpura: a review. *Am J Med* 1989;86:194.
12. Ratnoff OR. Psychogenic Bleeding. In: Ratnoff OD, Forbes CD, eds. *Disorders of hemostasis, 3rd Ed.* Orlando, FL: Grune & Stratton, 1996:505.
13. Rogers GM, Bithell TC. The diagnostic approach to the bleeding disorders. In: Lee GR, Foerster J, Lukens J, et al., eds. *Wintrobe's clinical hematology*, 10th ed. Baltimore: Williams & Wilkins, 1999:1557.

14. Sauer GC. Vascular dermatoses. In: Hall JC, Saver GC, eds. *Saver's Manual of skin diseases*, 8th ed. Philadelphia: JB Lippincott Williams & Wilkins, 2000.

15. Schafer AI. Acquired disorders of platelet function. In: Loscalzo J, Schafer A, eds. *Thrombosis and hemorrhage*, 2nd ed. Baltimore: Williams & Wilkins, 1998:707.

16. Swinyer LJ. Drug eruptions in an emergency department setting. *Emerg Med Clin North Am* 1985;3:717.

17. Taylor RE, Blatt PM. Clinical evaluation of the patient with bruising and bleeding. *J Am Acad Dermatol* 1981;4:348–368.

CHAPTER 130
Urticaria

Theodore A. Christopher, Richard Bruno, and Joseph D. Kim[a]

Urticarial rash is one of the most common skin lesions seen in emergency medicine. Making the diagnosis is not nearly as challenging to the emergency physician as defining the etiology, which very often remains elusive.

Urticaria, or "hives," is a vascular reaction of skin, resulting in wheals, raised white or red welts that itch and sting. It can occur in any age group, but young adults are most commonly afflicted. An estimated 20% of the population experiences at least one attack of urticaria in a lifetime.

Acute urticaria is characterized by symptomatic attacks lasting 6 weeks or less. It occurs with equal frequency in men and women and is often associated with an atopic history or an allergic etiology. *Chronic* urticaria is characterized by attacks that last longer than 6 weeks and is more common in middle-aged women. These attacks tend to be less frequent and less severe than acute attacks. Half of the patients with chronic urticaria have the disease for 5 years, and 25% have it for 20 years. In 90% of cases, no specific etiology can be identified.

The etiologies of urticaria are extensive and complex in nature. Generally, they may be broken down into several broad categories based on their underlying pathophysiology (see Table 130.1). These categories include immunologic, nonimmunologic, idiopathic, and urticarias associated with chronic diseases.

Histologically, the fact that urticaria involves the superficial dermis only distinguishes it from angioedema, which involves the deeper dermis. Perivascular lymphocytic and mast cell infiltration are also features. Mast cell degranulation, with release of mediators such as histamine, acetylcholine, serotonin, neuropeptides, cytokines, prostaglandins, anaphylatoxins, leukotrienes, eosinophilic chemotactic factor, platelet activating factor, kallikrein, and bradykinin, appears to be responsible for the pathogenesis of urticaria (9,14). Degranulation is initiated by immunologic (type I–IgE mediated; type III–complement mediated) and nonimmunologic (chemicals, foods, drugs) mechanisms, but numerous modulating factors also undoubtedly play significant roles.

More recently, anti-FcεRI autoantibodies have been identified in a number of patients with chronic urticarias. These autoantibodies are thought to activate IgG mediated complement pathways in certain subtypes of chronic urticarias (11). Complement C5a, a component of this pathway and mast cell activator, has been shown to play a role in chronic urticaria as well (12). Complement C5a has no receptors in the lung, which may explain the lack of pulmonary involvement in these chronic urticarias.

CLINICAL PRESENTATION

Urticaria presents as pruritic, edematous, slightly erythematous, raised wheals or papules that usually persist for less than 24 hours on unexposed areas of skin. Urticaria can be circumscribed, annular, or serpiginous; central clearing may or may not be present. The lesions commonly blanch with pressure, reflecting local vasodilatation.

Table 130.2 summarizes types and triggers of urticaria. Foods and drugs are probably the most common causes of both acute and chronic urticaria. They act through both immunologic and nonimmunologic mechanisms. Among foods, nuts, berries, shellfish, chocolate, fish, tomatoes, and eggs are frequent offenders in acute urticaria. In urticarias of chronic duration, milk, cereals, beef, pork, cheese, garlic, onions, and spices may be responsible. Food additives, both natural and synthetic, also appear to be

[a] Deceased

TABLE 130.1. Classification of Urticaria[b]

IMMUNOLOGIC URTICARIAS

Atopic disease history
Physical
  Cholinergic
  Dermatographism
  Pressure
  Cold
  Solar
  Vibratory
  Aquagenic
  Heat
  Adrenergic
Contact
Food
Insects
Inhalants
Drugs

NONIMMUNOLOGIC URTICARIAS

Drugs
  Aspirin/NSAIDs
  Opiates
  Antibiotics
  Antihypertensives
  Curare
  Radiocontrast media
Food additives
PUPP

IDIOPATHIC

URTICARIAS IN CHRONIC DISEASE

Systemic vasculitis/collagen vascular disease/malignancy
Infections
Genetic

[b]Note: This table does not differentiate acute vs. chronic duration of symptoms.

TABLE 130.2.   Precipitants of Urticaria

AGENTS KNOWN TO CAUSE URTICARIA

Medications
  ACEi
  Anesthetics
  Narcotics
  Penicillins
  Cephalosporins
  Sulfas
  Diuretics
  Aspirin
  NSAIDs
  Iodides
  Bromides
  Quinidine
  Chloroquine
  Vancomycin
  Isoniazid
  Antiepileptic Drugs
Infections
  Viral
  Amebiasis
  Malaria
Foods
  Shellfish
  Eggs
  Cheese
  Chocolate
  Nuts
  Berries
Environment
  Extremes of temperature
  Dander
  Dust
  Molds
  Water
Pregnancy
Contact
  Nickel
  Latex
  Nail Polish
  Chemicals
Exercise

important etiologic factors. Acute reactions occur within minutes of ingestion, whereas delayed symptoms may develop several hours later, presumably when a reactive antigen is formed by the digestive actions of proteolytic enzymes.

Antibiotics and analgesics head a lengthy list of common drugs that cause urticaria. Aspirin intolerance has been identified in 20% to 50% of patients with urticaria and is thought to act by a nonimmunologic mechanism (2). Increased prostaglandin levels have been found in affected patients. Urticaria may occur 15 minutes to 20 hours after aspirin ingestion and is often accompanied by wheezing, increased bronchial secretions, rhinorrhea, and flushing.

With physical urticarias, wheals and itching develop at sites of a physical stimulus (8). *Dermatographism* is defined as a whealing reaction of skin within 10 minutes of receiving a moderate stroke stimulus of less than 36 g/mm (2,3). Clinically, dermatographism typically occurs within seconds after stimulation and usually fades within 30 minutes. It is often due to contact with seatbelts, garters, or brassieres. In contrast to dermatographism, pressure urticaria occurs when more sustained physical pressure applied to the skin produces itchy, often painful wheals. These lesions can present as early as 30 minutes after application of pressure, but typically present in 6 hours and often last up to 72 hours

(3). Common causes are tight-fitting garments and prolonged walking (feet) or sitting (buttocks).

Cholinergic urticaria is characterized by pruritic 1- to 4-mm wheals surrounded by a red flare and produced within 15 minutes of any stimulus that causes an increase in core temperature (3). Exercise, hot baths, and emotional stress can precipitate episodes of cholinergic urticaria, which usually begins on the upper thorax and neck before spreading to the entire body, usually sparing the palms and soles. The exact pathophysiology is unclear, but appears to involve the release of acetylcholine and degranulation of histamine from mast cells (16). Clinically, patients can present with varied symptoms, including lacrimation, salivation, diarrhea, abdominal pain, weakness, flushing, and headache. Rarely, severe, life-threatening symptoms (e.g., angioedema, bronchospasm, vascular collapse, and hypotension) can occur (16).

Solar urticarias present as a whealing response within 10 minutes in skin exposed to ultraviolet or visible radiation from any source (3). In addition to hives, symptoms may include wheezing, dizziness, and (rarely) hypotension; all resolve within 1 to 3 hours after the light stimulus is removed. Both histamine and prostaglandins have been implicated (1).

Cold urticaria occurs on exposed areas, such as the face and hands, and is commonly induced by swimming. It occurs within minutes of exposure, usually during rewarming, and can be elicited by placing an ice cube on the skin, holding cold objects in the hand, or drinking cold fluids (leading to lip swelling). It also may be associated with other symptoms, including syncope and shock (17).

Other physical urticarias include generalized aquagenic urticaria, which is induced by contact with water of any temperature; vibratory urticaria, in which localized swelling occurs within minutes of local vibration; and adrenergic urticaria, a variant of stress-related urticaria, characterized by increased blood levels of norepinephrine and epinephrine (10).

Insect bites can cause widespread urticarial lesions that are distinct from the common local erythematous and vesicular reaction. Wasps, hornets, fleas, gnats, mites, mosquitoes, and bedbugs are common offenders.

Urticaria is also associated with infection (bacterial, fungal, viral, and parasitic). In most cases, urticaria does not appear to be related to hypersensitivity to the infectious agent. Many of these infections are thought to be a likely cause for urticarias of chronic duration.

Contact urticaria is whealing of the skin due to exposure to certain substances in susceptible patients. A diverse range of agents has been implicated, including food, metals (nickel, platinum, rhodium), and hair-care products (18). Of particular concern to health-care workers is the emergence of natural rubber latex allergy, which presents as a local or generalized urticaria but can rapidly progress to angioedema and anaphylaxis.

Urticaria pigmentosa, a familial disorder, will cause wheals to form when the underlying plaques of the disease are subjected to physical stimuli.

Pregnancy is thought to be another trigger for urticarial illness. Pruritic Urticarial Papulaes and Plaques of Pregnancy (PUPPP) are often seen in third trimester or early postpartum women. These lesions appear suddenly on the abdomen, and spread symmetrically to include the upper extremities and buttocks. They spare the face and clear within one week of delivery.

Finally, several underlying systemic diseases may be responsible for unexplained chronic duration urticaria. Malignancies (leukemia, lymphoma), collagen vascular disease, serum sickness, C1 esterase inhibitor deficiency, cryoglobulinemia and cryofibrinogenemia are all recognized causes. Hepatitis B and C, Lyme disease, and chronic tinea pedis have also been associated with urticaria (4).

symptoms obscures a cause-and-effect relation or when the syndrome is only partially expressed. Anaphylaxis often presents as the acute development of only one component of the syndrome. Differentiating acute, severe urticaria, for example, from anaphylaxis is a moot point. The greatest confusion may arise when anaphylaxis presents as isolated hypotension; it should therefore be considered in the differential diagnosis of syncope and vascular collapse (18).

The acute development of isolated angioedema of the skin and upper airway is a common presentation of anaphylaxis, but it may also be due to hereditary angioedema. This rare, autosomal dominant disease is characterized by the absence of a functional C1 esterase inhibitor, allowing free activation of the complement cascade. Hereditary angioedema is characterized by repeated episodes of angioedema of the skin, upper airway, and gut. Episodes generally date from adolescence, clustering in the 11 to 45 age range. Episodes may be precipitated by minor trauma or surgery, but most occur without an external trigger. Gastrointestinal involvement is usually very prominent, often mimicking an acute abdomen. Both urticaria and hypotension are absent in hereditary angioedema, and the administration of epinephrine, antihistamines, and steroids is ineffective. A reduction in the C4 level during an attack is diagnostic. Laryngeal edema can cause acute airway obstruction and death, but usually the progression is gradual, peaking in 8 hours. Typically, the edema will plateau for 24 hours, followed by gradual resolution over the next 3 days. C1 esterase inhibitor concentrate is the treatment of choice for potential airway compromise, providing relief of symptoms within 30 to 60 minutes. Fresh-frozen plasma may be substituted but it carries a risk of exacerbating symptoms in some patients. Danazol and aminocaproic acid are only effective as chronic prophylaxis (3).

Rapid development of edema of the upper airway may also result from viral or bacterial infection. However, pain, fever, and findings of erythema and exudate are not present in anaphylaxis.

Angiotensin-converting enzyme inhibitors (ACEI) produce cough in 10% to 20% of patients, but life-threatening tongue and palatal angioedema in 0.1% to 0.2% (favoring African-Americans). Although the appearance is indistinguishable from anaphylactic swelling, its development is more gradual and other features of anaphylaxis are absent. Angiotensin receptor-blockers (ARB) may be substituted, but similar angioedema has been described. Anaphylaxis to any precipitant may manifest accentuated hypotension if the patient is on a preexisting regimen of an ACEI or ARB (22).

Rarely, patients may experience stridor and obstructive airway symptoms secondary to vocal cord dysfunction or as a manifestation of hysteria; indirect laryngoscopy is the only means to verify these suspicions.

Scombroid fish poisoning may mimic anaphylaxis, presenting with acute, severe urticaria, nausea and vomiting, headache, and dysphagia. This syndrome occurs shortly after eating fish with a high histidine content (such as tuna or mahi-mahi) that has spoiled slightly, so that the histidine has been broken down to histamine. A clustering of cases of apparent anaphylaxis is often the clue to this entity (7).

The flushing seen in monosodium glutamate reactions may be confused with anaphylaxis, but the prominence of headache and burning chest discomfort distinguishes it from an allergic reaction.

Systemic mastocytosis and the carcinoid syndrome may present with intense flushing and hypotension, mimicking anaphylaxis; prominent gastrointestinal symptoms, hepatomegaly, and provocation by alcohol help distinguish these entities.

The systemic capillary leak syndrome is a rare disorder characterized by life-threatening episodes of hypovolemic shock, often accompanied by facial and extremity swelling. Transient polycythemia and hypoalbuminemia during attacks are pathognomonic; the presence of a monoclonal gammopathy may provide a clue to the diagnosis between attacks.

EMERGENCY DEPARTMENT EVALUATION AND MANAGEMENT

Evaluation of the upper airway and careful blood pressure monitoring are the immediate priorities in the care of the patient with possible anaphylaxis. Angioedema of the lips, tongue, uvula, and soft palate, as well as symptoms of hoarseness, stridor, dysphagia, or lump in the throat, should alert the physician to progressive airway compromise. Such patients are treated immediately with epinephrine 0.3 mL (1:1000 dilution) intramuscularly (0.01 mL/kg in children) before attempting any further evaluation. For both children and adults, the IM route is preferred, since it has been demonstrated to have a faster onset and significantly higher blood levels than the subcutaneous route. In addition, the lateral thigh is the preferred injection site, demonstrating superior bioavailability compared the deltoid region (1,8). Beta-adrenergic stimulation promotes the synthesis of cyclic AMP in mast cells, which blocks further release of chemical mediators. Epinephrine also exerts a therapeutic benefit by its alpha-adrenergic effect, causing vasoconstriction with resulting improvement in blood pressure and decreased swelling of edematous tissues (13,14).

The patient is placed on a cardiac monitor and given oxygen by cannula, and an intravenous line of normal saline is established. If hypotension is present, saline should be infused wide open until the blood pressure responds (typically 1 to 2 liters in an adult, or one or two 20-mL/kg boluses in a child). If hypotension persists or is profound from the outset, or if airway obstruction appears imminent, intravenous epinephrine may be administered. The most common error made in this situation is to give too much epinephrine too fast, precipitating cardiac dysrhythmias or chest pain. The recommended dose is 1.0 mL of 1 : 10,000 epinephrine diluted in 10 mL of normal saline, and given as a slow intravenous push over 3 to 5 minutes. If life-threatening symptoms persist, the intravenous dose may be repeated as clinically indicated (1,8).

In this dire situation, massive angioedema may preclude orotracheal intubation, such that cricothyroidotomy may have to be performed. Aerosolized epinephrine (racemic 2.25% solution, 0.5 mL in 3.5 mL saline; or levo-epinephrine 1:1000, 5 mL) may decrease supraglottic and laryngeal edema briefly, thereby buying time while preparations are made to establish an airway and parenteral epinephrine administered. In addition, heliox decreases airflow resistance and improves ventilation in upper airway obstruction, providing a very valuable temporizing measure. If intravenous access is unavailable, sublingual or intraosseous injection or endotracheal administration of epinephrine is considered. If symptoms are resolving, epinephrine can be continued in a dose of 0.3 mL intramuscularly at 20-minute intervals, or an epinephrine drip can be considered (1 to 10 μg/min intravenously) (3).

Hypotension generally responds to one or two intramuscular (IM) doses of epinephrine and rapid saline infusion. H₂-histamine blockers given intravenously may have an ameliorating effect on hypotension as well. If airway protection is not an issue, placing the patient in Trendelenburg position is a simple adjunct. If hypotension persists, virtually all patients will respond to intravenous (IV) epinephrine. Patients refractory to IV epinephrine, may respond to methylene blue an inhibitor of nitric oxide production, given as a IV bolus of 1.5–2.0 mg/kg (9). If available, application of a MAST suit has shown benefit as well.

Most patients with anaphylaxis do not require such intensive therapy, however. In general, one or two doses of epinephrine subcutaneously at 15- to 20-minute intervals (based on symptom response) and 1 L of saline intravenously are adequate. Patients with acute, severe urticaria alone may benefit from a single dose of epinephrine, yet it is usually not necessary, because there is no life threat. Bronchospasm in anaphylaxis is responsive to epinephrine alone, but in patients with preexisting asthma, repeated albuterol nebulizations may be necessary.

Corticosteroids are recommended in all patients with anaphylaxis. Although there is no immediate benefit to their administration, steroids speed the resolution of angioedema and urticaria, and are thought to prevent a biphasic course in anaphylaxis (13,15). Dosage recommendations are similar to those for status asthmaticus: methylprednisolone (Solu-Medrol), 125-mg intravenous push, followed by 60 mg, 4 to 6 hours in patients whose symptoms persist despite standard therapy. Milder episodes are often treated with oral prednisone 40 to 60 mg initially.

All patients with anaphylaxis should receive an antihistamine such as diphenhydramine (Benadryl), 25 to 50 mg, to a maximum of 100 mg, in more severe reactions. The route of administration depends on the severity of the reaction. Although less effective for pruritis, H_2 blockers appear equivalent to H_1 blockers in urticaria and anaphylaxis, and they may offer an advantage if hypotension is prominent or if sedation and anticholinergic side affects are undesirable. The combination of H_1- and H_2-blockers are superior to either agent alone, especially in severe anaphylaxis (20). Famotidine 20 mg or ranitidine 50 mg by IV push or Cimetidine 300 mg by IV infusion appear equivalent. Although more evidence exists for cimetidine, its use is discouraged because of infusion-related hypotension and potential for drug interactions. The addition of fexofenadine (Allegra) or cetirizine (Zyrtec) allows more complete histamine blockade without associated sedation or anticholinergic effects (24). Antihistamines should not be relied upon as the sole treatment in anaphylaxis, except perhaps in the most mild, self-limited of cases

Preventing further exposure to the antigen is critical; for instance, a tourniquet can be placed above an injection site, the stinger of a honey bee can be removed, offending chemicals can be washed off, even charcoal could be considered.

Throughout therapy, the vital signs are reassessed frequently and the airway is checked for edema of the uvula or oropharynx. The patient is asked about symptoms of laryngeal edema or bronchospasm and examined for signs of stridor, retractions, or wheezing. These assessments are made at 1- or 2-minute intervals at first, with the intervals lengthened as the patient stabilizes.

With patients over age 50 or those with a cardiac history, saline is given cautiously for hypotension, while monitoring closely for volume overload. Epinephrine should not be withheld in patients with potential upper airway obstruction or in those with hypotension unresponsive to volume loading. A test dose of epinephrine, 0.10 to 0.15 mL (1:1000) subcutaneously or intramuscularly, can generally be given safely. If no chest pain or cardiac dysrhythmias develop, another test dose or a full dose is then given. However, intravenous epinephrine should be avoided in these patients unless death appears imminent without its use.

Another special situation arises when anaphylaxis occurs in a patient who is taking a β-adrenergic blocker, in which case,

epinephrine therapy may have a net α-adrenergic effect only, thereby limiting its efficacy. In this situation glucagon, 1 to 2 mg given intravenously over 5 minutes may be of great benefit. Terbutaline, 0.25 mg subcutaneously or an isoproterenol drip, may also be considered (25). Table 131.3 summarizes treatment guidelines for anaphylaxis.

TABLE 131.3. Treatment of Anaphylaxis

1. Remove antigen, delay absorption.
2. Maintain an adequate airway.
3. Epinephrine (1,8)
   0.3 mL SC 1:1000; given IM in the lateral thigh, repeat at 10- to 20-min intervals.
   If severe may increase dose to 0.5 mL.
   If shock or incipient airway obstruction, give 1 mL of 1:10,000 dilution diluted further in 5–10 mL saline slow IV over 3–5 min, repeating as indicated by clinical response.
   If protracted severe symptoms, start a drip: 1 mg in 250 mL DSW, 1–10 µg/min.
   If patient is >50 yr old or has a cardiac history and life-threatening symptoms exist, give a test dose of 0.1–0.15 mL SC or IM (1:1000).If shock resistant to other measures or imminent airway closure, consider a drip as above.
4. Volume expansion with saline or lactated Ringer
   Shock: 1 L over 15 min, then repeat 1–2 more times if needed
5. Antihistamines (20,24)
   Diphenhydramine: 25–50-mg IM or IV push. May repeat within 15 min to a maximum of 100 mg, then smaller doses q2–4h as needed.
   H2 Blocker: Famotidine 20 mg or Ranitidine 50 mg IV push repeated at 6-h intervals as needed; given as an adjunct to diphenhydramine if refractory to treatment or if sedation and anticholinergic effects are a problem.
6. Methylprednisolone
   125-mg IV push; may repeat 60 mg q4h if persistent symptoms.
7. If resistant hypotension:
   Continue aggressive fluid resuscitation
   Trendelenburg position
   Epinephrine infusion titrated to toxicity
   H2 blocker IV
   MAST suit
   Methylene blue 1.5–2.0-mg/kg IV push (9)
8. If imminent airway obstruction (stridor, drooling, hoarseness):
   Nebulized racemic epinephrine (0.5 mL of 2.25% in 3.5 mL normal saline) or epinephrine (5 mL of 1:1000 dilution)
   Heliox by mask (70/30 or 80/20 with additional O_2 by nasal canula)
   Prepare for intubation or cricothyrotomy
   Consider IV epinephrine
9. If resistant bronchospasm (usually preexistent asthma):
   Albuterol by nebulization (3–6 mL of 0.083% solution) +/− ipratropium; repeat as needed.
10. If beta blocker-accentuated anaphylaxis: (25)
    Glucagon 1 mg IV push over 4–5 min; repeat as needed up to 5 mg, Isoproterenol drip
    Terbutaline 0.25 mg SC
11. Outpatient regimen if stable for discharge:
    Prednisone 40–60 mg/d for 3 d
    Prescribe one to two antihistamines for 3 days (only one per class) (24)

    H₁ blocker (traditional)
       Diphenhydramine 25–50 mg q6h prn
       Hydroxyzine 25 mg q6h prn
    H₁ blocker (non-sedating)
       Cetirizine 10 mg/d
       Fexofenidine 180 mg/d
    H₂ blocker
       Famotidine 40 mg/d
       Ranitidine 300 mg/d
    Prescribe EpiPen or EpiPen 2-Pak and refer to allergist if idiopathic or high risk of recurrence (food, bee sting, idiopathic). Training with placebo trainer recommended.

CRITICAL INTERVENTIONS

- Administer epinephrine intramuscularly immediately for patients presenting with angioedema of the lips, tongue, uvula, and soft palate
- Treat supraglottic and laryngeal edema with aerosolized epinephrine while preparing to establish an airway
- Administer corticosteroids and antihistamines in all patients with anaphylaxis

DISPOSITION

If all symptoms of anaphylaxis resolve rapidly and completely with initial therapy, the patient can be observed in the emergency department without further treatment. If symptoms do not recur in the next 2 to 3 hours, the patient may safely be discharged and should continue on a 3-day course of prednisone (40 mg/d) and one or two antihistamines, such as diphenhydramine (25 mg every 4 hours as needed), famotidine (40 mg/d), fexofenidine (180 mg/d), or cetirizine (10 mg/d). An Epi-Pen should be prescribed for patients with food-related, Hymenoptera, and idiopathic anaphylaxis. The patient should be instructed on the technique of Epi-Pen administration (using a placebo trainer) and the lateral thigh emphasized as the preferred injection site. Since approximately one-third of anaphylactic episodes require two doses of epinephrine, an Epi-Pen 2-Pak, which also contains a trainer device, may be preferable (8). Discharge instructions should caution the patient to avoid any suspected inciting cause, such as medications, foods, chemicals, or even exercise. The patient should be instructed to return to the emergency department immediately if hoarseness, dysphagia, wheezing, dyspnea, dizziness, or worsening rash and swelling develop. Follow up with an allergist should be recommended, particularly if no obvious etiology has been identified in the emergency department or if bee sting desensitization is indicated.

Patients who had a life-threatening manifestation on presentation (shock or upper airway obstruction), even if it resolved with acute therapy, should be admitted. Those who had a slow or incomplete response to therapy or any worsening of symptoms during emergency department evaluation and treatment also require admission, as do elderly or debilitated patients or those with serious underlying cardiac disease. If hypotension or significant airway compromise persist, admission to an ICU is mandatory. For most of the remaining patients, a 12- to 24-hour observation period is indicated, preferably in an ED Observation Unit, if available; otherwise, inpatient admission is advised.

Transfer Considerations

Because anaphylaxis can progress in such a fulminant manner, transfer to another institution is not recommended unless prolonged observation in the emergency department has shown the patient to be stable.

COMMON PITFALLS

- ✔ Giving dangerously large doses or inappropriate concentrations of epinephrine intravenously (1)
- ✔ Withholding epinephrine therapy in the elderly or cardiac patient with imminent airway obstruction or refractory shock

- ✔ Not recognizing the possibility of recrudescence of symptoms 4 to 8 hours after an initial complete response to therapy (15)
- ✔ Not identifying common etiologies of anaphylaxis, such as antiinflammatory drugs (especially over-the-counter preparations), foods (shellfish, nuts), antibiotics (despite the lack of previous reactions and regardless of duration of therapy), antihypertensive drugs (beta-blockers, angiotensin-converting enzyme inhibitors), and exercise
- ✔ Not treating upper airway symptoms, such as hoarseness and dysphagia, with appropriate aggressiveness
- ✔ Not recognizing uvular and pharyngeal angioedema as warning signs of laryngeal involvement
- ✔ Misdiagnosing anaphylaxis as the flushing of a monosodium glutamate reaction or as scombroid fish poisoning (7)
- ✔ Failing to recognize that anaphylaxis can present with shock or acute airway obstruction alone, without any other manifestations of the classic anaphylactic syndrome (18)
- ✔ Failing to prescribe EpiPen and to provide allergy referral to patients with idiopathic anaphylaxis and those at high risk for recurrent episodes (8)

References

1. Barach EM, Nowack RM. Epinephrine for treatment of anaphylactic shock. *JAMA* 1984;25:2118.
2. Bock SA, Munoz-Furlong A, Sampson HA. Fatalities due to anaphylactic reactions to foods. *J Allergy Clin Immunol* 2001;107:191–193.
3. Bork K, Hardt J, Schicketanz KH, et al. Clinical studies of sudden upper airway obstruction in patients with hereditary angioedema due to C1 esterase inhibitor deficiency. *Arch Intern Med* 2003;163:1229–1235.
4. Brown AF, McKinnon D, Chu K. Emergency department anaphylaxis: A review of 142 patients in a single year. *J Allergy Clin Immunol* 2001;108:861–866.
5. Castells MC, Horan RF, Sheffer AL. Exercise-induced anaphylaxis. *Curr Allergy Asthma Rep* 2003;3:15–21.
6. Cianferoni A, Novembre E, Mugnaini L, et al. Clinical features of acute anaphylaxis in patients admitted to a university hospital: an 11 year retrospective review (1985–1996). *Annals Allergy Asthma Immunol* 2001;87:27–32.
7. Eckstein M, Serna M, DelaCruz P, et al. Out-of-hospital and emergency department management of epidemic scombroid poisoning. *Acad Emerg Med* 1999;6:916–920.
8. Ellis AK, Day JH. The role of epinephrine in the treatment of anaphylaxis. *Curr Allergy Asthma Rep* 2003;3:11–14.
9. Evora PR, Oliveira Neto AM, Duarte NM, et al. Methylene blue as treatment for contrast medium-induced anaphylaxis. *J Postgrad Med* 2002;48:327.
10. Golden DB. Stinging insect allergy. *Am Fam Physician* 2003;67:2541–2546.
11. Grattan CEH. Aspirin sensitivity and urticaria. *Clin Exp Derm* 2003;28:123–127.
12. Keldar PS, Li JTC. Cephalosporin allergy. *N Engl J Med* 2001;345(11):804–809.
13. Kemp SF. Current concepts in pathophysiology, diagnosis, and management of anaphylaxis. *Immunol Allergy Clin North Am* 2001;21:611–634.
14. Kemp SF, Lockey RF. Anaphylaxis: a review of causes and mechanisms. *J Allergy Clin Immunol* 2002;110:341–348.
15. Lee JM, Greenes DS. Biphasic anaphylactic reactions in pediatrics. *Pediatrics* 2000;106:762–766.
16. Lenchner K, Grammer LC. A current review of idiopathic anaphylaxis. *Curr Opin Allergy Clin Immunol* 2003;3:305–311.
17. Lieberman P. Anaphylactic reactions during surgical and medical procedures. *J Allergy Clin Immunol* 2002;110(2 Suppl):S64–S69.
18. Lieberman P. Unique clinical presentation of anaphylaxis. *Immunol Allergy Clin North Am* 2001;21:813–825.
19. Lin RY. A perspective on penicillin allergy. *Arch Intern Med* 1992;152:930–936.
20. Lin RY, Curry A, Pesola GR, et al. Improved outcomes in patients with acute allergic syndromes who are treated with combined H1 and H2 antagonists. *Ann Emerg Med* 2000;36:462–468.
21. Maddox TG. Adverse reactions to contrast material: recognition, prevention, and treatment. *Am Fam Physician* 2002;66:1229–1234.
22. Montanaro A, Bardana E. The mechanisms, causes, and treatment of anaphylaxis. *J Invest Allergol Clin Immunol* 2002;12:2–11.
23. Neugut AI, Ghatak AT, Miller RL. Anaphylaxis in the United States: an investigation into its epidemiology. *Arch Intern Med* 2001;161:15–21.
24. Winbery SL, Lieberman PL. Histamine and antihistamines in anaphylaxis. *Clinical Allergy Immunol* 2002;17:287–317.
25. Wyatt R. Anaphylaxis. How to recognize, treat and prevent potentially fatal attacks. *Postgrad Med* 1996;100:87–99.

CHAPTER 132
Angioedema

Susan Mumm Fitzgerald and Eric R. Snoey

Angioedema is well-demarcated, nonpitting edema of deep subcutaneous tissue characteristically localized to the face, intraoral areas, genitals, and distal extremities. It results when fluid extravasates into interstitial tissues via histamine, bradykinin, or complement-mediated vasodilation and increases in vascular permeability. The potential for rapidly life-threatening airway compromise via intraoral and laryngeal edema makes identification and rapid treatment of angioedema of special importance to the emergency physician (3,10,14,16,21).

The most important mechanisms in adults include angiotensin-converting enzyme inhibitor (ACEI) use; IgE-mediated allergic reactions to a food, drug, or environmental trigger; loss of C1 esterase inhibitor, either hereditary or acquired; nonsteroidal antiinflammatory use; chemical histamine release; and idiopathic causes (Table 132.1) (21). Pediatric angioedema (PAE) also occurs but is less common. The predominant mechanism in PAE is thought to be an IgE-mediated allergic reaction (16).

With approximately 35 million people now taking ACEIs worldwide, ACEI angioedema is on the rise (11,18). Angioedema occurs in 0.1% to 0.2% of patients on ACEI, or approximately 1 to 2 out of 1,000 patients (12,13,14,18). Between 20% to 58% of emergency department visits for angioedema are accounted for by ACEI use (1,3,10,18). The pathophysiology of angiotensin-converting enzyme inhibitor (ACEI) angioedema relates to both the inhibition of bradykinin degradation, and the blockage of angiotensin II-mediated vasoconstriction (10,14). African-Americans using ACEIs may be at 5 times higher risk for angioedema presumably due to lower endogenous bradykinin levels and resultant increased sensitivity to ACEI-mediated increases in bradykinin (2,3,6).

Angioedema may occur months or years after starting the drug and is dose-independent (6,10,18). For unclear reasons, ACEI angioedema appears to have a predilection for the head/neck region but has also been associated with angioedema involving the intestinal wall (12,13,21). Angiotensin II inhibitors, while professing a lower overall side-effects profile, are not protective against angioedema, with several case reports implicating these agents as well. Patients with a prior history of ACEI angioedema are thought to be at increased risk (14).

The IgE-mediated angioedema is a Type I hypersensitivity reaction in which mast cell IgE receptors are bound by allergen resulting in degranulation and histamine release. Between 17% to 33% of angioedema cases result from some form of allergen

---

TABLE 132.1. Causes of Angioedema

Angiotensin converting enzyme inhibitors (20%–58%).
IgE-mediated allergic reaction to a food, drug, or environmental trigger (17%–33%).
C1 esterase inhibitor deficiency, either hereditary or acquired (<1%–2%).
Nonsteroidal antiinflammatory drugs.
Chemical histamine release.
Idiopathic causes (21%–59%).

---

exposure (21). Typical triggers are foods, drugs, contrast dye, inhalants, environmental allergens, and insect stings (1,3,14).

Hereditary and acquired C1 esterase inhibitor losses are rare causes of angioedema, accounting for fewer than 1% to 2% of angioedema cases (1,12,14,19). Hereditary angioedema (HAE) is either the result of low levels of functional enzyme (Type 1, 80%) or production of nonfunctional enzyme (Type 2, 20%) (8,12,19,21). The risk of life-threatening angioedema via severe airway obstruction is thought to be increased in HAE, with a mortality rate that approaches 50% without appropriate treatment (10,12,19). Abdominal involvement is also more common in this form of angioedema, with dramatic clinical presentations that may mimic surgical abdominal emergencies (12,13). In contrast, acquired angioedema (AAE) results when C1 inhibitor levels are decreased via increased activation of C1, or when C1 inhibitor is rendered nonfunctional by binding of antibody in B-cell lymphoproliferative or autoimmune disease (8,19,21).

In both HAE and AAE, loss of C1 inhibitor results in complement pathway deregulation, leading to increased vascular permeability, mast cell degranulation as well as increased bradykinin levels (8,11,12,19). Triggers for HAE/AAE attacks include trauma, medical procedures, emotional stress, menstruation, oral contraceptives, infections, and drugs (12). Features that suggest HAE include presentation in the second or third decades of life, recurrent attacks of otherwise unexplained angioedema or abdominal pain, and sometimes rapid progression to airway obstruction. Hereditary angioedema must also be considered in patients with a personal or family history of angioedema, or a history of attacks in the setting of trauma or minor surgery (10). Features that distinguish AAE from HAE include late onset, absent family history, and clinical signs/symptoms that point toward malignancy (5).

Angioedema related to nonsteroidal antiinflammatory use (including aspirin) is less well defined. Patients with single reactions to only one type of NSAID are thought likely to have IgE-mediated reactions. Conversely, repetitive episodes of urticaria/angioedema related to use of a variety of NSAIDs are thought to be mediated by sensitivity to COX-1 inhibition. This type of angioedema appears to be more common in those with atopic disease (8,17,20).

Angioedema may result from a direct chemical-induced release of histamine, similar to anaphylactoid reactions seen with contrast dyes. Agents most commonly associated with this form of reaction are opiates, highly cationic antibiotics, and muscle relaxants (10).

Of note, a significant number of angioedema patients have no clear cause for their symptoms despite all attempts to identify a trigger or precipitating event; numbers as high as 21% to 58% have been reported for idiopathic angioedema (10, 21).

Angioedema in the pediatric population is an uncommon and poorly understood phenomenon. Pediatric angioedema is generally less severe than the adult form, responds more quickly to treatment with intravenous (IV) H_1-blockers and steroids, and is less likely to require airway intervention or intensive care unit (ICU) care. Links to food and other environmental triggers suggest an IgE-mediated mechanism explaining the more benign course. In one study, it was attributed to food in 40%, insect bites in 30%, upper respiratory infection in 20%, and antibiotic use in 10%. Forty percent of children presenting with angioedema have experienced some form of allergic reaction in the past (16).

CLINICAL PRESENTATION

Angioedema patients typically present with complaints of acute (minutes to hours) onset of swelling in the face, lips, distal extremities, or genitals. The swelling may be accompanied by rash and is sometimes referable to a suspected trigger. If airway involvement is present, patients will likely describe difficulty breathing, throat tightness or swelling, dysphagia, drooling, and/or voice changes. If the abdominal wall is involved, complaints may include abdominal pain, nausea, vomiting, or diarrhea (3,11,12,14,15,16,19).

On physical examination, angioedema presents as localized well-demarcated nonpitting edema most commonly involving the lips, tongue, face, and eyelids. Less commonly it may involve the larynx, genitals, and distal extremities (3,14,16,19). It may present with or without urticaria and is frequently nonpruritic (11). Hoarseness, dysphonia, stridor, and respiratory distress indicate significant airway involvement (14). The abdominal exam in abdominal angioedema may mimic a surgical abdomen with significant tenderness and rigidity, sometimes resulting in unnecessary surgical exploration (12,15).

The emergency department course of angioedema and its response to treatment is varied. Clinical evolution may merely reflect the natural course of the disease rather than specific response to treatment. Frequent reevaluation of the angioedema patient is essential because response to treatment is varied and impossible to predict.

There are some important differences between adult and pediatric angioedema. Pediatric patients presented primarily with face (80%) and lip (40%) involvement. Fifty percent had hoarseness, drooling, dysphagia, and dyspnea on emergency department arrival. Concomitant rash was present in 50% of patients. Despite this apparent severity on initial presentation, all patients responded rapidly to intravenous (IV) H_1-blockers and IV corticosteroid treatment.

DIFFERENTIAL DIAGNOSIS

It is important to consider alternative diagnoses, such as infection, local reaction to insect bites, congestive heart failure, renal disease, and liver disease (3). Features that suggest angioedema include a relatively rapid onset, asymmetric distribution in nondependent areas, association of some forms with anaphylaxis, and lack of symptoms that point to other etiologies.

EMERGENCY DEPARTMENT EVALUATION

In the acute setting, the diagnosis of angioedema is established primarily on clinical grounds. As always, initial emergency department evaluation should focus on airway, breathing, and circulation (ABCs.) Rapid assessment of the airway and initiation of immediate and appropriate treatment as indicated is the first priority of the emergency department physician (Fig. 132.1). The anatomic location of the angioedema has important diagnostic, therapeutic, and prognostic implications. In one study, those presenting with voice change, hoarseness, stridor, or dyspnea were more likely to require aggressive airway intervention and ICU care (1). Another study established location of edema in the oral cavity/oropharynx as the most important predictor of need for airway intervention. Increasing age was also determined to be predictive (21). There is also some evidence suggesting laryngeal involvement as diagnosed by fiberoptic nasopharyngoscopy to be predictive (1).

With the airway assessment complete and therapy started, a goal-directed history and physical examination should follow, focusing on potential inciting agents and patterns of prior involvement. A thorough medication, food, and environmental exposure history should be documented. Special attention must be paid to use of ACEIs and NSAIDs since these agents have been clearly associated with angioedema. Other historical features are

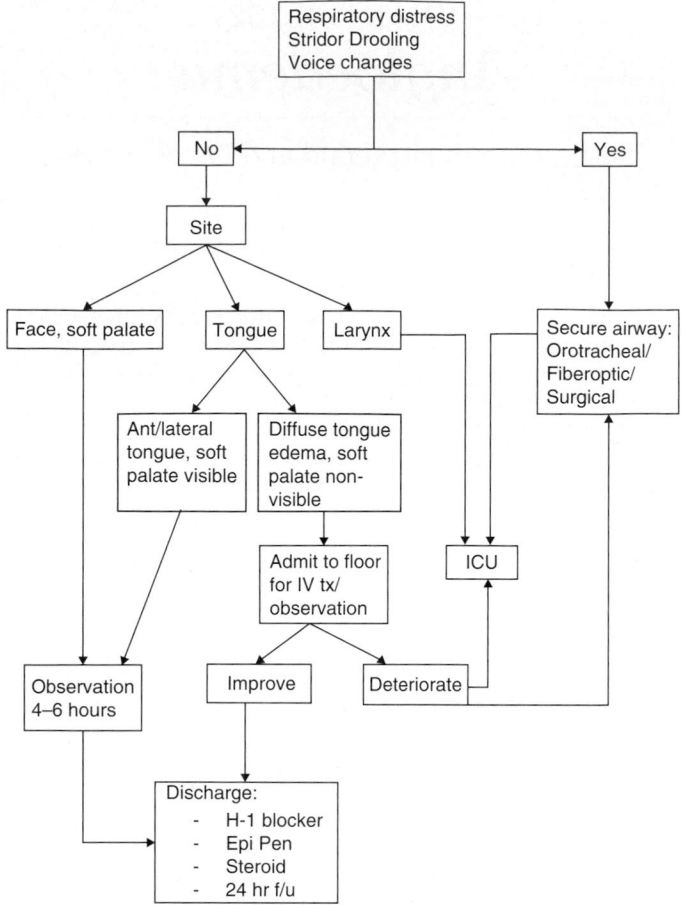

Figure 132.1. Clinical approach to angioedema.

helpful as well. An IgE-mediated mechanism is suggested by the presence of urticaria or pruritus. Likewise, prior episodes of angioedema with exposures to the same allergen also point toward this mechanism (12,21).

Laboratory and radiographic studies are helpful largely in order to exclude competing etiologies of the edema. However, suspected HAE or AAE cases should be evaluated with C1 esterase and C4 levels. There are also case reports describing the use of abdominal ultrasound and abdominal/pelvis CT to help diagnose abdominal angioedema. Findings on ultrasound include bowel wall thickening and ascites. Findings on CT include bowel wall thickening, mucosal hyperemia, and submucosal edema (4,15). In addition, patients suspected of having AAE must ultimately be evaluated for underlying malignancy as well (5,10).

EMERGENCY DEPARTMENT MANAGEMENT

Initial ED treatment assumes an allergic reaction and focuses on relief of upper airway obstruction if present. The mainstays of treatment when the airway is involved are supplemental oxygen, a parenteral H_1-blocker to counteract any allergic component, a parenteral steroid to reduce inflammation, and subcutaneous epinephrine. While most cases respond well to medical management alone (Tables 132.2 and 132.3), up to 22% of patients go on to require aggressive airway management (21).

Angioedema presenting with urticaria, likely an IgE-mediated reaction, usually responds well to epinephrine, antihistamines, and corticosteroids. Likewise, angioedema due to chemical histamine release is likely to respond to these agents

TABLE 132.2.   Medical Treatment of Adult Angioedema

Medication	Dose	Frequency	Route
Epinephrine 1:1000	0.3 mg	q 10–15 min	sq
H1-Blocker			
Diphenhydramine	25–50 mg	q 4–6 hrs	po/im/iv
Hydroxyzine	25–100 mg	q 4–6 hrs	po/im
H2-Blocker			
Cimetidine	300 mg	q 6 hrs	po/im/iv
Ranitidine	50 mg	q 6–8 hrs	im/iv
	150 mg	BID	po
Corticosteroids			
Methylprednisolone	125 mg	qd	im/iv
Prednisone	60 mg	qd	po

(10). There is also some evidence that adding ranitidine, an H_2 blocker, to the more traditional use of H_1 blockers may also improve IgE-mediated angioedema (9). Angioedema without urticaria is more likely bradykinin-mediated and thus less likely to respond to typical allergic reaction therapy (11,12). Standard of care dictates administration of these agents regardless of suspected etiology.

For patients who require definitive airway intervention, intubation by direct laryngoscopy (DL) remains first choice. However, angioedema patients requiring intubation are likely to have distorted anatomy. They may be very difficult or impossible to intubate by DL, making awake fiberoptic a better choice. Concomitant preparation for a surgical airway (i.e. cricothyrotomy or tracheotomy, is essential). These interventions are most safely achieved in the operating room if time permits (21). The best choice will incorporate consideration both of anticipated difficulty and the provider level of comfort with the methods available. The anticipated degree of difficulty in securing the airway also has important implications for the choice of sedation agents and paralytics. Some authors recommend using mild sedation without paralysis in the setting of angioedema in order to preserve respiratory effort should the intubation be difficult or impossible. If rapid sequence intubation technique is used, short-acting agents such as etomidate and succinylcholine are best. A parallel set up for cricothyrotomy should be open and ready.

The treatment of acute attacks of HAE/AAE remains controversial. In the case of HAE, recent evidence suggests an infusion of C1 inhibitor concentrate may be effective in mitigating the severity and progression of an acute attack (19). C1 inhibitor concentrate appears to be less effective in AAE, though it is still considered first-line treatment in countries where routinely used (not yet approved in the United States) (12). Aminocaproic acid, tranexamic acid, and the androgens danazol and stanozol are used prophylactically in the United States with 80% to 90% success rates (19). Additionally, fresh frozen plasma is sometimes used for short-term prophylaxis prior to invasive medical or dental procedures, though use in acute episodes is not recommended because it contains complement substrate and may accelerate the reaction (3,10).

CRITICAL INTERVENTIONS

- Treat all cases of angioedema as if IgE- or histamine-mediated with antihistamines, steroids, and epinephrine if airway compromise is present
- Perform a rapid and accurate assessment of the need for airway intervention
- Recognize and discontinue the suspected inciting agents that cause angioedema

DISPOSITION

The disposition of patients with angioedema is determined by the severity of initial symptoms, the anatomic location of the angioedema, the disease course, and response to therapy. In general, patients with angioedema not involving the head and neck have a universally favorable course. Patients should be started on standard oral therapy (see Tables 132.2 and 132.3) and discharged with appropriate follow up. One exception may be patients with angioedema involving the abdominal wall where complications may arise from delays in diagnosis, unnecessary testing or, in rare cases, operative intervention.

Patients presenting with involvement of the head and neck accompanied by evidence of respiratory distress, drooling, voice changes, or stridor require rapid and definitive airway management. The timing and method used will be determined by the acuity, level of distress, and local practice patterns (Fig. 132.1). In the absence of obvious evidence of airway compromise, patients may be selectively managed based upon the location and degree of swelling. Any involvement of the larynx as determined by indirect or direct laryngoscopy requires ICU admission and parenteral therapy even in the absence of airway symptomatology.

In contrast, patients with angioedema limited to the face and lips may be discharged home on PO therapy following a 4- to 6-hour period of observation in the ED. Similarly, patients with localized tongue edema but a fully visible soft palate may be discharged home after a suitable period of observation documenting no further extension. Patients with diffuse tongue involvement that obscures the soft palate should be admitted to a regular hospital ward for parenteral medications and observation (1,3,7,16,21).

TABLE 132.3.   Medical Treatment of Pediatric Angioedema

Medication	Dose	Frequency	Route
Epinephrine 1:1000	0.01 mg/kg (max 0.3 mg)	q 10–15 min	sq
H1-BLOCKER			
Diphenhydramine	5 mg/kg (max 50 mg)	q 4–6 hrs	po/im/iv
Hydroxyzine	*<6 yo*		
	2 mg/kg	div q 6–8 hrs	po
	0.5–1 mg/kg	q 4–6 hrs	im
	6–12 yo		
	12.5–25 mg	q 6–8 hrs	po
	0.5–1 mg/kg	q 4–6 hrs	im
H2-BLOCKER			
Cimetidine	*infants*		
	10–20 mg/kg/d	div q 12 hrs	po/im/iv
	children		
	20–40 mg/kg/d	div q 6 hrs	po/im/iv
Ranitidine	*>2 weeks of age*		
	4–5 mg/kg/d (max 300 mg)	div q 12 hrs	po
	2–4 mg/kg/d	div q 6–8 hrs	im/iv
Corticosteroids			
Dexamethasone	2 mg/kg	qd	po/im/iv
Prednisone	2 mg/kg	qd	po

COMMON PITFALLS

✔ Failure to adequately assess the airway
✔ Failure to adequately assess the risk of airway deterioration
✔ Failure to recognize that many cases of angioedema will not respond to treatment
✔ Failure to address underlying precipitants and discontinue their use
✔ Failure to initiate appropriate HAE/AAE workups

Acknowledgments

Thanks to the previous edition's chapter author Joyce M. Mitchell-Savinsky.

References

1. Bentsianov BL, Parhiscar A, Azer M, Har-El G. The Role of Fiberoptic Nasopharyngoscopy in the Management of the Acute Airway in Angioneurotic Edema. *The Laryngoscope* 2000;110:2016–2019.
2. Brown NJ, Snowden M, Griffin MR. Recurrent Angiotensin-Converting Enzyme Inhibitor-Associated Angioedema. *JAMA* 1997;278:232–233.
3. Cohen EG, Soliman AMS. Changing Trends in Angioedema. *Ann Otol Rhinol Laryngol* 2001;110:701–706.
4. Dinkel HP, Maroske J, Schrod L. Sonographic appearances of the abdominal manifestations of hereditary angioedema. *Pediatr Radiol* 2001;31:296–298.
5. Dobson G, Edgar D, Trinder J. Angioedema of the Tongue Due to Acquired C1 Esterase Inhibitor Deficiency. *Anaesth Intensive Care* 2003;31:99–102.
6. Gainer JV, Nadeau JH, Ryder D, Brown NJ. Clinical aspects of allergic disease. *J Allergy Clin Immunol* 1996;98:283–287.
7. Ishoo E, Shah UK, Grillone GA, Stram JR, Fuleihan NS. Predicting airway risk in angioedema: Staging system based on presentation. *Otolaryngology—Head and Neck Surgery* 1999;121:263–268.
8. Kulp-Shorten CL, Callen JP. Urticaria, Angioedema, and Rheumatologic Disease. *Rheum Dis Clin North Am* 1996;22:95–115.
9. Lin RY et al. Improved Outcomes in Patients With Acute Allergic Syndromes Who Are Treated With Combined H1 and H2 Antagonists. *Ann Emerg Med* 2000;36:462–468.
10. Megerian CA, Arnold JE, Berger M. Angioedema: 5 Year's Experiences, With a Review of the Disorder's Presentation and Treatment. *Laryngoscope* 1992;102:256–260.
11. Nussberger J, Cugno M, Cicardi M. *N Engl J Med* 2002;347:621–622.
12. Nzeako UC, Frigas E, Tremaine W. Hereditary Angioedema. *Arch Intern Med* 2001;161:2417–2427.
13. Chopra, S. Image of the Month. *Gastroenterology* 2000;119:1190, 1424.
14. van Rijnsoever EW, Kwee-Zuiderwijk WJM, Feenstra J. Angioneurotic Edema Attributed to the Use of Losartan. *Arch Intern Med* 1998;158:2063–2065.
15. Sadeghi N, Van Daele D, Hainaux B, Engelholm L, Michel O. Hereditary angioedema involving the gastrointestinal tract: CT findings. *Eur Radiol* 2001;11:99–101.
16. Shah UK, Jacobs IN. Pediatric Angioedema, Ten Years' Experience. *Arch Otolaryngol Head Neck Surg* 1999;125:791–795.
17. Stevenson DD. Anaphylactic and Anaphylactoid Reactions to Aspirin and Other Nonsteroidal Anti-Inflammatory Drugs. *Immunol and Allergy Clin North Am* 2001;21.
18. Thompson T, Frable MAS. Drug-Induced, Life-Threatening Angioedema Revisited. *Laryngoscope* 1993;103:10–12.
19. Visentin DE, Yang WH, Karsh J. C1-esterase inhibitor transfusions in patients with hereditary angioedema. *Ann Allergy Asthma Immunol* 1998;80:457–461.
20. Wong JT, Nagy CS, Krinzman SJ, Maclean JA, Bloch KJ. Rapid oral challenge-desensitization for patients with aspirin-related urticaria-angioedema. *J Allergy Clin Immunol* 2000;105.
21. Zirkle M, Bhattacharyya N. Predictors of airway intervention in angioedema of the head and neck. *Otolaryngology—Head and Neck Surgery* 2000;123:240–245.

CHAPTER 133
Drug Allergy and Other Drug Reactions

Donna Kinser

Adverse drug effects occur in up to 15% of drug regimens and are said to be the basis of the majority of iatrogenic illness. Patients with acute symptoms are likely to present to the emergency physician for diagnosis and care.

Adverse drug reactions are predictable (80%) or unpredictable (20%). Predictable reactions are those related to known pharmacologic activity; they include side effects of immediate expression, side effects of delayed expression (carcinogenicity, teratogenicity), effects of overdosage or toxicity, secondary or indirect effects, and drug interactions. Unpredictable reactions are those related to individual immunologic response or genetic difference; they include drug intolerance, drug idiosyncrasy, allergic reaction and pseudoallergic reaction, plus psychophysiologic reaction (vasovagal, hyperventilation).

DRUG ALLERGY

Drug allergy or hypersensitivity accounts for 5% to 10% of adverse drug reactions. Allergic reactions manifest signs and symptoms characteristic of an underlying allergic mechanism. They occur in a minority of patients receiving a particular drug. There is typically a history of prior uneventful use of the drug, although allergic reactions can occur during the first course of therapy if continuing for more than about a week. Allergic reactions usually subside soon after discontinuation of the causative agent. There may be rapid reaction on reexposure to a small dose of the same or a related drug.

Risk factors for drug allergy include the degree of host reactivity (genetic predisposition), the characteristics of the drug (chemical properties, molecular weight), the parameters of exposure (high dose, intermittent dosing schedule), and the route of administration (topical and parenteral of greater risk than oral). Some drugs are complete antigens (e.g., insulin, streptokinase, and heterologous antisera), but most are low-molecular-weight incomplete antigens that must form a stable bond with tissue or plasma proteins to become immunogenic. Usually, it is one or more of the drug's metabolites that form the union. Because the metabolites of most drugs are not well identified (the notable exception being penicillin), tests to confirm specific drug sensitivity and to elucidate the mechanism of reactivity are limited.

CLINICAL PRESENTATION

Classification of Reactions

Some drug-induced allergic reactions can be categorized according to the classification system of Gell and Coombs. They include IgE-mediated immediate hypersensitivity (type I), cytotoxic antibody reactions (type II), immune complex-complement reactions (type III), and cell-mediated delayed hypersensitivity (type IV).

Type I reactions are mediated by preformed drug-specific IgE antibodies attached to the surface of tissue mast cells and circulating basophils. Bridging of the IgE antibodies by the drug in antigenic form results in mediator release and clinical sequelae such as urticaria, angioedema, laryngeal edema, bronchospasm, and hypotension. Maculopapular rashes may also be type I reactions. Type II cytotoxic reactions result when IgG or IgM antibodies interact with cell-bound drug and mediate cell injury through complement and mononuclear cell activation. Almost all type II reactions involve formed elements of the blood, for example, manifesting as immune hemolytic anemia or thrombocytopenia. In type III reactions, circulating immune complexes (consisting of drug+IgG or drug+IgM) lodge in blood vessel walls. Tissue injury ensues through activation of the complement cascade. Serum sickness is the prototype of the type III reaction. Penicillins and foreign antisera are among the recognized causes. Clinical presentations include fever, rash (ranging from urticaria to palpable purpura), arthralgias, and lymphadenopathy. Type IV reactions are mediated by sensitized T-lymphocytes that recognize a particular drug antigen and recruit other lymphocytes and mononuclear cells to the site of that antigen. Type IV reactions primarily occur as allergic contact dermatitis, for example to neomycin.

Many drug reactions do not strictly fit the Gell and Coombs classification but are presumed to be immunologic. They include drug-induced fever, fixed drug eruptions, Stevens-Johnson syndrome, exfoliative dermatitis, toxic epidermal necrolysis, the anticonvulsant hypersensitivity syndrome, and certain cases of pulmonary, hepatic, and renal hypersensitivity. They also include vasculitis syndromes such as hypersensitivity angiitis and leukocytoclastic vasculitis.

Reactions that resemble type I IgE-mediated hypersensitivity reactions but do not involve IgE are termed pseudoallergic reactions. They are clinically indistinguishable from true allergic reactions because comparable mediators produce comparable target-organ sequelae. When life-threatening, they are termed anaphylactoid. Commonly used agents that can cause nonspecific mast cell and basophil release of preformed and generated mediators include radiocontrast media (RCM), opiates, muscle-relaxing anesthetic agents, and colloid volume expanders. The "red man" syndrome is a dose-dependent reaction to vancomycin caused by direct stimulation of mast cells to release histamine. The quinolones have been associated with anaphylactoid reactions, often with the first dose. Patients reacting to one quinolone are likely to react to other drugs of this class.

Aspirin and nonsteroidal antiinflammatory drugs (NSAIDs) cause various adverse reactions, most of which are nonimmunologic: anaphylactoid reactions, urticaria, or angioedema, and exacerbation of respiratory symptoms in some patients with asthma and nasal polyps. Some anaphylactoid reactions to aspirin and NSAIDs have features that are consistent with Ig-E-mediated reactions (occurring after two or more exposures to one specific drug in this class), but aspirin-specific Ig-E antibodies have only rarely been demonstrated. Reactions to angiotensin-converting enzyme (ACE) inhibitors include cough and angioedema. These agents promote accumulation of bradykinin and other vasoactive peptides and are not thought to act through a classic immunologic mechanism.

EMERGENCY DEPARTMENT EVALUATION

The diagnosis of adverse drug reaction hinges on the history of drug exposure. Improvement of symptoms after withdrawal of the suspected drug is suggestive information. Confirmatory tests are generally unavailable. Skin testing to detect immediate hypersensitivity has only a limited role for some high-molecular-weight compounds and for penicillin. Patch testing may be performed for drug-induced contact dermatitis. *In vitro* radioallergosorbent or enzyme-linked immunosorbent tests are applicable in special circumstances. The indirect Coombs' test is a diagnostic aid in immune hemolytic anemia. Graded direct challenge is potentially hazardous and rarely indicated, but it occasionally has a role in evaluating local anesthetic reactions.

EMERGENCY DEPARTMENT MANAGEMENT

The standard management of adverse drug reactions includes prompt discontinuation of the medication and provision of supportive care that is specific to the type and severity of manifestations. Mild pruritis, flushing, and rash may be treated with antihistamines. Corticosteroids are usually administered only for more severe systemic reactions. Early epinephrine is the mainstay of treatment for anaphylactic reactions. Oxygen and airway support, inhaled beta agonists, intravenous fluids, and pressors also may be required.

Certain steps can be taken to prevent or minimize drug reactions. Medications should be prescribed only when necessary; in one study of anaphylactic deaths, 40% of the cases involved drugs for which there was no clear indication. The oral route should be used when possible. Preparations that are less sensitizing (e.g., human insulin rather than pork insulin) are preferred when available. Drug history should be carefully elicited. Frequently, information that can prevent an adverse drug reaction is available from the patient, the patient's relatives, or previous medical records. Documentation in the medical record of any apparent reaction may help avert a similar or worse reaction. Finally, when potentially immunogenic parenteral agents are given in the emergency department, patients should be observed for at least 20 minutes after administration. Discharge instruction should include cautions regarding possible reaction.

DISPOSITION

Disposition decisions for patients with drug reactions hinge on the nature and severity of the reaction. Patients who present with mild reactions, respond well to treatment, and are reliable with good support systems may be considered for expedited discharge home. In borderline cases, a period of observation of several hours may be helpful. Patients with persistent or recurring airway edema, bronchospasm, hypotension, cardiovascular complications, or altered mental status require admission to the hospital in an intensive care setting. Patients who receive treatment for an initially severe reaction but who rapidly improve are typically either observed for a period of 6 to 12 hours or admitted to the hospital; in the case of anaphylaxis, this facilitates treatment if a late-phase reaction occurs.

PENICILLIN ALLERGY AND CEPHALOSPORIN ALLERGY

Penicillin and its derivatives are among the most widely prescribed antibiotics and are the most common cause of drug-induced allergic reactions. Penicillin may be responsible for any of the four types of Gell and Coombs reactions, and also may cause other reactions, such as interstitial nephritis, exfoliative dermatitis, and drug fever. The overall incidence of adverse reactions to penicillins is estimated to be 2% (range, 0.7% to 10%). The incidence of anaphylaxis is thought to be 0.015% to 0.04% of treatment courses, and approximately 10% of anaphylactic episodes are fatal. Anaphylaxis is usually an immediate reaction (occurring within 30 minutes of administration), but, in approximately 10% of cases, symptoms begin more than 1 hour after administration.

IgG and IgM antibodies to penicillin–protein complexes are produced on first exposure to penicillins in virtually all individuals, whereas IgE antibodies develop in only a small subset. Sensitization may occur through medical use or through occult food, environmental, or medication exposure. There seems to be a genetic predisposition to formation of IgE antibodies, but atopy is not a risk factor. IgE production usually occurs within 1 to 3 weeks of exposure. Depending on the individual, the half-life varies from days to years.

Early reactions consistent with a generalized systemic response (e.g., generalized urticaria, angioedema, bronchospasm, or hypotension) are usually categorized as anaphylactic, even if they are mild, and these should be treated promptly. Therapy should be tailored to the severity of the reaction, and, after epinephrine, may include antihistamines, corticosteroids, intravenous fluids, and pressors. Penicillin and penicillin derivatives should thereafter be avoided in these patients. Regarding risk of future use of the other beta-lactam antibiotics, cross-reactivity is high with the carbapenems (e.g., imipenem), less with the cephalosporins, and minimal with the monobactams (e.g., aztreonam). If there is not an acceptable or effective alternative to penicillin (e.g., for central nervous system syphilis or gestational syphilis), the patient should be considered for penicillin skin testing and in-hospital desensitization.

When a patient develops a maculopapular rash after receiving a penicillin drug, it may represent an IgE-mediated skin reaction, or one mediated by IgG or IgM. Alternatively, the rash may be an unrelated manifestation of the underlying disease. In some cases, the disease plus the penicillin drug result in the adverse reaction. For example, patients with infectious mononucleosis are likely to develop a morbilliform rash 3 to 8 days after commencing ampicillin or amoxicillin therapy. A similar problem may develop in patients with cytomegalovirus infection, hyperuricemia, or chronic lymphocytic leukemia. When a maculopapular rash occurs and is attributable to a penicillin drug allergy, the antibiotic should be discontinued. Additionally, the patient should be instructed to avoid all penicillins, since the side chain reactions cannot be clinically distinguished from reactions to the beta-lactam structure common to penicillin drugs.

The frequency of cephalosporin-induced skin reactions such as urticaria, rash, exanthem, and pruritus is 1% to 3% and the risk of anaphylactic reactions is 0.0001% to 0.1% with rare reported deaths. Once there has been a reaction to a penicillin drug or to a cephalosporin, whether to use a cephalosporin antibiotic requires consideration of the risks and benefits in the clinical circumstances. The risk of allergic reactions to cephalosporins in patients with positive skin tests to penicillin appears to be less than 2%, with first-generation cephalosporins posing a greater risk than second or third generation cephalosporins. Cross-reactivity among cephalosporins is a complex issue because the number of potential haptens that may participate in the hypersensitivity reaction from the side chain and nuclear components is large. A patient who has an allergic reaction to a cephalosporin should not receive that cephalosporin again. The risk of a drug reaction when a different cephalosporin is administered to a patient with a history of allergy to one cephalosporin is unknown, although it has been suggested that the degree of cross-reactivity is low.

LOCAL ANESTHETIC REACTIONS

Local anesthetics are among the most frequently administered drugs in emergency medicine. They can be divided into two main chemical groups: the esters and the amides (Table 133.1). The

TABLE 133.1. Local Anesthetic Chemical Groups

GROUP I: ESTERS (MAY CROSS-REACT)

Benzocaine (Americaine)
Procaine (Novocain)
Proparacaine (Alcaine, Ophthaine)
Tetracaine (Pontocaine)

GROUP II: AMIDES (UNLIKELY TO CROSS-REACT)

Bupivacaine (Marcaine, Sensorcaine)
Lidocaine (Xylocaine)
Mepivacaine (Carbocaine)
Prilocaine (Citanest)

OTHERS: FOR MUCOUS MEMBRANES

Dibucaine (Nupercainal)
Dyclonine (Dyclone)
Pramoxine (Tronothane)

amides have a longer half-life in tissues and are favored for local anesthesia. Although true allergic reactions are rare, many patients report "allergy to 'caines," because a variety of nonallergic reactions are associated with the administration of local anesthesia. The differential diagnosis includes hyperventilation, vasovagal reaction, sympathetic stimulation, and toxic drug levels.

The approach to the patient who reports allergy to local anesthesia depends on the analysis of the available information. When the history supports prior nonallergic reaction to local anesthesia, any of the standard anesthetic agents may be used. When the suspected drug can be identified, an agent from a structurally unrelated group is preferred. Hypersensitivity and intragroup cross-reactivity occur more prominently with ester anesthetics.

When all local anesthetic agents seem contraindicated, local anesthesia may be provided by the use of diphenhydramine. Diphenhydramine 1% (1.5 to 5.0 mL intradermally) provides effective anesthesia for repair of minor lacerations. Pain during initial administration is greater than with lidocaine, but pain during the procedure is equally well controlled. Sleepiness occasionally occurs after anesthesia with 1% diphenhydramine. Lower concentrations (e.g., 0.5%) seem less effective for anesthesia, and higher concentrations (2% to 5%) have been associated with local irritation, burning, erythema, vesicle formation, skin sloughing, and prolonged anesthesia or paresthesias.

Patients for whom local anesthetics will be needed in the future, but which cannot be ascertained as safe by history, should be referred for allergy testing. There are protocols for testing serial dilutions of the agent in question. Experience has shown that true-positive reactions are rare (less than 1%) and that the sensitivity does not necessarily correlate with the presence of paraben or methylparaben preservatives. Although serial testing could be conducted in the emergency department, time constraints usually make it impractical.

RADIOCONTRAST MEDIA REACTIONS

First-generation radiocontrast agents are ionic monomers that are highly osmolal (1500–1800 mosmol/kg) compared with the osmolality of plasma. Second generation agents, such as iohexol, are nonionic monomers that are categorized as being low-osmolal (600–850 mosmol/kg). The newest agents are nonionic dimers with even lower osmolality. Iodixanol, for example, is iso-osmolal at approximately 290 mosmol/kg. The newer agents are more expensive than the older agents, and this may be a factor in clinical protocols.

Anaphylactoid reactions are one type of significant adverse effect that can follow administration of contrast media. Immediate adverse reactions that are not simply related to the physicochemical chemical properties of the contrast agent are likely anaphylactoid reactions. Anaphylactoid reactions typically follow intravascular injection of radiocontrast media reactions (RCM) but, in rare instances, may occur after contrast is introduced into extravascular structures. The anaphylactoid reactions tend to be more severe and less dose- and concentration-dependent than the physicochemical reactions. Bronchospasm, laryngeal edema, widespread urticaria or angioedema, hypotension, or dysrhythmias manifest within 30 minutes of the infusion. Although the initiating pathophysiology does not seem to be that of an IgE-mediated allergic reaction, there is comparable release of histamine and other mediators from mast cells. Therefore, the treatment is the same as for true anaphylaxis. Estimated rates of incidence are 0.22% for the high-osmolality (ionic) contrast agents versus 0.04% for low-osmolality (nonionic) contrast agents. Deaths have been reported with the use of each type of agent. Patients with a history of contrast reaction have more than five times the incidence of a subsequent reaction in comparison with previous nonreactors. Patients with allergic diathesis, asthma, or cardiac disease are at increased risk for these anaphylactoid reactions, but there is no evidence that sensitivity to seafood or cutaneous iodine sensitivity predispose to reactions to RCM.

Nephrotoxicity is another significant adverse effect that can ensue after administration of RCM. The mechanism is not completely understood (possibly related to renal vasoconstriction or direct toxic effects of the contrast agents), but the clinical picture is that of an increase in the serum creatinine level that begins within 24 hours of exposure to the agent. Risk factors for nephrotoxicity include preexisting renal insufficiency (plasma creatinine exceeding 1.5 mg/dl), diabetes mellitus, multiple myeloma, and causes of reduced renal perfusion such as advanced heart failure and hypovolemia. Also, high total dose of RCM is a factor. Although the degree of protective benefit is not uniform or certain, low osmolality (nonionic) agents are generally recommended for patients with one or more of the risk factors for nephrotoxicity, and the isoosmolal agent iodixanol seems to further decrease risk for diabetic patients with renal insufficiency.

Fever, chills, rash, arthralgias, diarrhea, nausea, vomiting, headache, and other nonspecific symptoms may occur as a delayed reaction 30 minutes to 3 days after contrast media injection in 4% to 8% of patients. Fever typically abates within 8 hours and is speculated to represent a hypothalamic response to RCM injection. Treatment of delayed reactions is supportive.

The risk-to-benefit ratio of a contrast study should be considered before it is ordered and performed. In some situations, a study that does not require contrast (e.g., ultrasound or magnetic resonance imaging) can be substituted. In others, it may be possible to take mitigating steps in addition to selection of the lowest-risk contrast agent available. In the case of prior anaphylactoid reaction, if the radiocontrast test can be delayed for 12 to 36 hours, the patient can be pretreated with corticosteroids and antihistamines to decrease the likelihood of recurrent anaphylactoid reaction. One established protocol is to administer methylprednisolone, 32 mg by mouth, 12 hours and 2 hours before contrast administration, and diphenhydramine, 50 mg by mouth or intramuscularly, 1 hour before contrast administration. Pretreatment can be expected to reduce the incidence of reactions to high-osmolality agents by approximately one-third. Simply using low-osmolality agents alone may reduce risk to a similar level. Combining pretreatment and low-osmolality agents may provide extra protection but extends the time until the test can be performed. Regarding patients with renal insufficiency at risk

for nephrotoxicity, one consideration is saline hydration, for example, 1 ml/kg of 0.45% isotonic saline for 12 hours before and 12 hours after the dye load. Another consideration, particularly in diabetics with renal insufficiency, is the administration of the antioxidant acetylcysteine, 600 mg bid the day before and the day of the scan. Nonsteroidal antiinflammatory drugs should be avoided since they increase renal vasoconstriction.

ANGIOTENSIN-CONVERTING ENZYME INHIBITOR REACTIONS

The propensity of the angiotensin-converting enzyme (ACE) inhibitors to cause cough and angioedema has been increasingly recognized and studied in recent years. These reactions are not allergic in nature and appear to involve the kinin system.

Cough is the more frequent but less serious of the two adverse reactions and occurs in 1% to 20% of patients treated with ACE inhibitors. It occurs more often in females and may be dependent on dose. The onset of cough is typically within 1 week of initiation of therapy, but it may develop up to 6 months later. There is no associated alteration in pulmonary function. The diagnosis is a clinical one. In most cases, management consists simply of withdrawal of the ACE inhibitor, and the diagnosis is confirmed by resolution of the cough within 1 to 3 weeks. Subsequent challenge with the same agent or another ACE inhibitor almost always results in recurrence of cough.

Angioedema, typically of the face, neck, or upper airway, occurs in 0.1% to 0.2% of patients treated with ACE inhibitors (and also has been reported in some patients treated with angiotensin II receptor antagonists). The reaction can progress rapidly to airway obstruction and death. The risk is highest in the first few hours to first week of treatment but can also occur in patients who have been taking the drug uneventfully for months to years. The risk abates within hours of stopping the drug.

When angioedema secondary to an ACE inhibitor occurs, administration of the standard allergic anaphylaxis treatment of subcutaneous epinephrine, diphenhydramine, and corticosteroids cannot be relied on to reverse the process. Furthermore, the progression of the edema is unpredictable, and there may be rebound. Early airway control is therefore recommended, because massive edema of the tongue and pharynx can make orotracheal and nasotracheal intubation difficult, and neck edema may make creation of a surgical airway difficult as well (see Chapter 132 Angioedema). Limited case reports suggest patients refractory to standard treatment may benefit from infusion of fresh frozen plasma.

CRITICAL INTERVENTIONS

- Administer antihistamines for mild reactions, corticosteroids for severe reactions and epinephrine for anaphylactic reactions
- Use diphenhydramine for local anesthesia when the patient is allergic to the typical amide and ester local anesthetics

References

1. Asaverreaza EE. Penicillin allergy: a review. *Tex Med* 1989;85:37.
2. Cohan RH, Leder RA, Ellis JH. Treatment of adverse reactions to radiographic contrast media in adults. *Radiol Clin North Am* 1996;84:1055.
3. deShazo RD, Kemp SF. Allergic reactions to drugs and biologic agents. *JAMA* 1997;278:1895.
4. deShazo RD, Nelson HS. An approach to the patient with a history of local anesthetic hypersensitivity: experience with 90 patients. *J Allergy Clin Immunol* 1979;63:87.
5. Ernst AA, Anand P, Nick T. Lidocaine versus diphenhydramine for anesthesia in the repair of minor lacerations. *J Trauma* 1993;34:354.
6. Greenberger PA, Patterson R. The prevention of immediate generalized reactions to radiocontrast media in high-risk patients. *J Allergy Clin Immunol* 1991;4:867.

7. Gruchalla R, Drug allergy. *J Allergy Clin Immuno* 2003;111:S548.
8. Israili ZH, Hall WD. Cough and angioneurotic edema associated with angiotensin-converting enzyme inhibitor therapy. *Ann Intern Med* 1992;117:234.
9. Kelkar P, Li J. Cephalosporin allergy. *N Engl J Med* 2001;345:804.
10. Kim K, Evans R III, Mahr TA. Drug allergy. *Allergy Proc* 1990;11:299.
11. King BF, Hartman GW, Williamson B. Low-osmolality contrast media: a current perspective. *Mayo Clin Proc* 1989;6:976.
12. Lin RY. A perspective on penicillin allergy. *Arch Intern Med* 1992;152:930.
13. Suresh A, Reisman RE. Risk of administering cephalosporin antibiotics to patients with histories of penicillin allergy. *Ann Allergy Asthma Immunol* 1995;74:167.
14. Westhoff-Bleck M, Bleck JS, Jost S. The adverse effects of angiographic radiocontrast media. *Drug Saf* 1991;6:28.

CHAPTER 134
Multisystem Autoimmune Disease

Theodore I. Benzer

Patients with multisystem autoimmune disorders may present for initial medical evaluation with a bewildering array of symptoms or complaints. Many of the tests needed to diagnose these "rheumatic disorders" cannot be performed during an emergency department visit. However, the emergency physician must recognize that an autoimmune disorder may be responsible for the patient's clinical picture and must decide which patients require admission and which can safely undergo an outpatient evaluation. Likewise, when a patient with known multisystem autoimmune disease presents to the emergency department with new symptoms, the physician must determine whether they represent an exacerbation of known disease, a manifestation of an unrelated disorder, or a complication of therapy.

Evolving therapies and variations in individual response to treatments make rheumatologic consultation appropriate in many cases. Although the ultimate cause of the autoimmune disorders remains a mystery, it is increasingly clear that specific autoantibodies directed against cellular components are markers for, and probable causes of, many of the manifestations. Positive tests for these antibodies not only correlate with current symptoms, but are also predictive of the patient's course. The use of these specific disease markers can improve accuracy in diagnosis and can guide therapy directed at specific pathologic entities.

Despite the fact that definitive therapies for most autoimmune disorders are lacking, there is often much that can be done to alleviate symptoms and prevent progression of tissue damage. Nevertheless, every pharmacologic treatment has a potential for toxicity that must be balanced against the potential benefit it may provide to the patient.

SYSTEMIC LUPUS ERYTHEMATOSUS

Systemic lupus erythematosus (SLE) is the prototypical autoimmune disease. Its prevalence is one in 2,000, with a 10 : 1 predominance of women over men and a predilection for non-Whites.

The prevalence is one in 750 for Black women between the ages of 20 and 64 (6).

The cause of SLE remains unknown; hormonal, metabolic, genetic, environmental, and infectious factors have all been proposed as etiologic agents. The pathophysiology of SLE involves the production of autoantibodies initiated by an unknown stimulus. These antibodies react with cell constituents and initiate an inflammatory response that results in the fixing of complement and the elaboration of chemotactic factors and other inflammatory mediators. Antibody-dependent cytotoxic leukocytes are also activated.

Antinuclear antibodies (ANAs) are almost invariably detected in patients with SLE. Although ANAs are found in low titers in many other autoimmune and nonrheumatologic disorders, high titers are more specific for SLE; high titers of antibodies to double-stranded DNA are seen only in patients with SLE (16). Antibodies to the Smith antigen are also specific for SLE, as well as being associated with more severe symptoms. During active SLE, complement levels are depressed and may be helpful in following the course of disease (6).

CLINICAL PRESENTATION

SLE can affect any tissue or organ and, in fact, has been said to have replaced syphilis as "the great imitator" of other diseases (6). Patients often make multiple visits to physicians before SLE is initially recognized. Some of the more common manifestations are listed in Table 134.1.

The most typical initial complaints are fatigue and arthralgias, but fever, anemia, anorexia, and a malar rash are other common presenting symptoms. The arthralgias are commonly fleeting and migratory, typically appearing in the proximal interphalangeal and metacarpophalangeal joints, the wrists, and the knees, but they may also be due to frank synovial inflammation.

The rash of SLE varies from a slight blush to a well-demarcated and somewhat edematous maculopapular erythematous eruption covering both cheeks and the bridge of the nose. It tends to spare the nasolabial folds, but can cause scarring and atrophy of skin structures. It is characteristically exacerbated by sun exposure and may often cause a patient to seek medical attention before any other symptoms of SLE have developed.

TABLE 134.1. Systemic Lupus Erythematosus: Characteristic Features and Suggestive Signs and Symptoms

System	Presentation
Constitutional	Fever, fatigue, malaise, weight loss
Vascular	Raynaud's phenomenon, arterial occlusion, extremity ulcers
Dermatologic	Diffuse alopecia, malar rash, discoid rash, photosensitivity
Hematologic	Hemolytic anemia, leukopenia, thrombocytopenia, thrombosis
Immunologic	False-positive serologic test for syphillis
Gastrointestinal	Nausea, vomiting, oral ulcers
Cardiac	Pericarditis, myocarditis
Pulmonary	Diffuse interstitial pneumonitis, pleuritis, pleural effusion
Musculoskeletal	Nonerosive arthritis
Renal	Glomerulonephritis, nephrotic syndrome
Reproductive	Spontaneous abortion, preeclampsia
Neurologic	Psychosis, depression, mania, seizures, headache, organic brain syndrome, aseptic meningitis, peripheral neuropathy

Although the kidneys are commonly affected in SLE, nephrotic syndrome and peripheral edema are rarely seen before other manifestations of disease have led to the diagnosis of SLE (12). Patients with SLE frequently present with acute, potentially life-threatening problems. Complaints of chest pain, abdominal pain, and neurologic dysfunction can indicate an acute flare of disease or a serious complication of therapy. Patients with acute chest pain, with or without fever, may have pleuritis, pericarditis, or pneumonitis. Abdominal pain may indicate an acute flare of polyserositis.

Neurologic problems of virtually any type may be seen in SLE. Most common are central disorders ranging from mood disorders to frank psychosis. Seizures are also common, especially in younger patients. SLE should be in the differential diagnosis of new-onset seizures, especially in young women.

The lupus anticoagulant, also called the anticardiolipin antibody or antiphospholipid antibody, is an antibody that produces an artifactually prolonged partial thromboplastin time *in vitro*, but a "paradoxical" procoagulant effect *in vivo*. Although antiphospholipid antibodies are associated with SLE, they may occur as a part of a distinct pathologic entity referred to as the antiphospholipid syndrome (1,8). Both conditions can lead to deep venous thrombi, pulmonary emboli, stroke, chronic ulcers of the extremities, and thrombocytopenia (1,8). Patients with recurrent or unusual thrombosis should be evaluated for antiphospholipid autoantibody and SLE (13).

Patients with *known* SLE may present to the emergency department with either exacerbations of their disease or complications of therapy.

DIFFERENTIAL DIAGNOSIS AND EMERGENCY DEPARTMENT EVALUATION

Given the variety of possible presentations, the differential diagnosis of SLE is exceedingly broad. A thorough history and physical examination are required to identify multisystem involvement and recurrent symptoms. The differentiation of SLE from the other autoimmune syndromes may require repeated rheumatologic evaluation and specific autoantibody testing.

Tan and associates (20) have published a list of 11 criteria diagnostic for SLE (Table 134.2); the diagnosis is established if four or more of these findings are present serially or simultaneously. A medication history must be elicited to rule out drug-induced lupus. Attention to detail in evaluating the patient with nonspecific symptoms may lead one to suspect the diagnosis of SLE. The diagnosis should be particularly entertained in women of childbearing age who have recurrent or vague symptoms that do not clearly point to a discrete disease entity.

Drug-induced SLE is a distinct entity that has been associated with many medications, including procainamide, hydralazine, anticonvulsants, chlorpromazine, isoniazid, methyldopa, penicillamine, quinidine, propylthiouracil, and sulfasalazine. Drug-induced SLE has a milder course than idiopathic SLE and does not cause renal and central nervous system involvement (18). Specialized antinuclear antibody (ANA) testing panels reveal only histone-binding ANAs rather than the multiple varieties characteristic of SLE (6).

The evaluation of patients with established SLE should focus on the presenting complaint. However, attention should also be given to signs and symptoms of the potentially life-threatening complications of SLE, such as thrombotic disease, pleural and pericardial effusions, and infections secondary to immunosuppressive therapy.

Patients presenting with new-onset monoarthritis or oligoarthritis generally require diagnostic arthrocentesis to rule

TABLE 134.2. Diagnostic Criteria for Systemic Lupus Erythematosus[a]	
1. Malar rash	Fixed erythema, flat or raised, over the malar eminences
2. Discoid rash	Erythematous raised patches with adherent keratotic plugging; atrophic scarring may occur
3. Photosensitivity	
4. Oral ulcers	Incudes oral and nasopharyngeal, observed by physician
5. Arthritis	Nonerosive arthritis involving two or more peripheral joints, characterized by tenderness, swelling, or effusion
6. Serositis	Pleuritis or pericarditis documented by electrocardiogram or rub or evidence of pericardial effusion
7. Renal disorder	Proteinuria greater than 0.5 g/d or greater than 3+, or cellular casts
8. Neurologic disorder	Seizures without other cause, or psychosis without other cause
9. Hematologic disorder	Hemolytic anemia or leukopenia (less than 4,000/μL) or lymphopenia (less than 1,500/μL) or thrombocytopenia (less than 100,000/μL) in the absence of offending drugs
10. Immunologic disorder	Positive lupus erythematosus cell preparation or anti-dsDNA or anti-Sm antibodies or false-positive VDRL
11. Antinuclear antibodies	An abnormal titer of ANAs by immunofluorescence or an equivalent assay at any point in time in the absence of drugs known to induce ANAs

[a] If four of these criteria are present at any time during the course of disease, a diagnosis of SLE can be made with 98% specificity and 97% sensitivity.

out infection or crystal-induced arthritis. Fluid should be sent for Gram stain, culture, cell count and differential, and examination for crystals. The synovial fluid in autoimmune arthritis is typically inflammatory, with an elevated white cell count (20,000 to 80,000/μL mixed polymorphonuclear cells and lymphocytes), a negative Gram stain, and no crystals.

The specific organs affected by SLE and the severity of the disease vary widely between individuals and over time in any given individual. Not only does the variability of the disease make diagnosis difficult but, with the exception of the characteristic rash, each of the manifestations of lupus may occur from other causes. Although a presentation of one of these conditions alone would not prompt consideration for autoimmune disease, recurrent symptoms or the sequential development of multiple conditions associated with lupus warrants referral for ANA testing.

EMERGENCY DEPARTMENT MANAGEMENT AND DISPOSITION

The specific clinical presentation dictates the management indicated in the emergency department. Patients presenting with mild symptoms may require nothing more than screening for renal and hematologic involvement with a urinalysis and complete blood cell count. More severe symptoms are managed as in any other disease. For example, a large pleural effusion should be tapped, and anticoagulation should be started for thromboembolic disease.

ST elevations and PR depressions seen on the electrocardiogram that are associated with a pericardial friction rub indicate pericarditis. If pericarditis is suspected, a careful evaluation should be made for signs of pericardial tamponade including a bedside echocardiogram if available. Elevated neck veins, elevated pulsus paradoxus, or hypotension should prompt a formal urgent echocardiogram to rule out tamponade. Infectious complications should be considered in patients with established disease who are taking chronic immunosuppressive medications.

Patients with significant pleural or pericardial effusion, or any thrombotic complication, require hospital admission and rheumatologic consultation. Immunosuppressed patients with documented infection require admission for parenteral antibiotics.

Neuropsychiatric complications are frequent in SLE. Cerebritis, aseptic meningitis, seizures, ischemic strokes, peripheral neuropathy, and acute psychosis are all recognized manifestations of SLE. In addition, corticosteroid treatment and other immunosuppressive agents predispose to infectious meningitis and corticosteroid-induced psychosis.

The acute presentation of an SLE patient with a neuropsychiatric complaint is always a challenge. The diagnosis of lupus flare should be made only after infectious etiologies have been ruled out. Patients presenting with severe disease are often treated with "stress" doses of corticosteroids (hydrocortisone, 100 mg intravenously; or methylprednisolone, 125 mg intravenously) and often receive empiric broad-spectrum antibiotic coverage after samples of blood, urine, sputum and possibly cerebral spinal fluid are obtained for culture.

Patients with established disease who present with a flare of symptoms may require the initiation of corticosteroids or an increase in the dose. When more than 5 to 10 mg of prednisone a day is required, many rheumatologists prescribe combination therapy in an effort to limit adverse effects. Medications commonly used include nonsteroidal antiinflammatory drugs (NSAIDs), antimalarial agents, azathioprine, and cyclophosphamide. Because every therapeutic agent has adverse effects, the risks of medication must be weighed against the morbidity of the clinical presentation. The aggressiveness and urgency of treatment depends on the presence of major organ involvement. Changes in a patient's usual medication regimen are best carried out in conjunction with the patient's rheumatologist.

Patients with suspected or newly diagnosed SLE may be managed as outpatients if the manifestations are mild and a life-threatening pathologic process is absent. An ANA panel should be ordered. Rheumatologic consultation can be obtained by telephone concerning any further studies, initiation of corticosteroid therapy, and appropriate follow up. Newly diagnosed patients with SLE should be educated about the importance of adequate sleep and avoidance of ultraviolet light. Ibuprofen and estrogens may exacerbate disease and should be avoided (12). Hypertension should be controlled rigorously because it appears to have a synergistic effect in exacerbating renal disease. In drug-induced lupus, after the medication is discontinued, symptoms usually resolve within days to weeks (9,18).

COMMON PITFALLS

✔ Failure to recognize vague, atypical complaints as a presentation of SLE or other autoimmune disease
✔ Failure to include SLE in the differential diagnosis of patients with pericarditis, pleuritis, renal dysfunction, neurologic symptoms, or recurrent venous thrombosis
✔ Failure to differentiate disease exacerbation from an adverse effect of therapy
✔ Failure to suspect infection in an immunocompromised patient

RHEUMATOID ARTHRITIS

Rheumatoid arthritis (RA) is a chronic autoimmune disorder characterized by widespread synovial inflammation and, often, progressive destruction of joints. It affects women three times as often as men; its prevalence increases with age and is approximately 1%.

The pathophysiology of RA involves the production of immunoglobulins against native IgG; these are referred to as rheumatoid factor. Helper T cells are also activated and produce lymphokines that promote cellular proliferation (15). Activation of the inflammatory response leads to the elaboration of vasoactive substances, chemotactic factors, and complement in synovial tissues. Mononuclear cells infiltrate the subsynovial stroma, and polymorphonuclear cells appear in the synovial fluid. A "pannus" of inflamed, thickened, redundant synovium invades and replaces cartilage and periarticular bone and tendon. Polymorphonuclear cells in the synovial fluid release lysozymes, which break down hyaluronic acid polymers in the synovial fluid and articular cartilage (6). Although the symptoms and signs are primarily related to the joints, RA is a multisystem autoimmune disease that frequently involves the heart, lungs, and blood.

CLINICAL PRESENTATION

RA typically presents initially as constitutional symptoms such as low-grade fever, weight loss, fatigue, and lymphadenopathy. Stiffness in the morning or after periods of inactivity may also be a complaint.

Articular symptoms initially involve any number or size of joints. Either arthralgia (pain) or arthritis (inflammation) may be present in an unpredictable pattern. Later, in established disease, the typical symmetric pattern of arthritis develops.

The most commonly affected joints are the metacarpophalangeal and proximal interphalangeal joints, wrists, knees, and upper spine. Although some cases of RA remain mild or even resolve, the typical course is one of unpredictable exacerbations and remissions, with progressive deformity and disability.

As tissue damage progresses, typical ulnar deviation of the carpometacarpal joints and valgus deformity of the knees develop. Baker cysts may develop in the popliteal fossa. Of prime importance for the emergency physician is the development of instability of the atlantoaxial joint, with laxity and even rupture of the transverse ligament. The result is an unstable cervical spine, which may lead to spinal cord compression following even apparently trivial injury (13).

RA, however, is a systemic disease. Over time, subcutaneous nodules over the elbows, occiput, and sacrum, thought to be vasculitic in origin, develop in 20% to 25% of patients. Pericarditis, pleuritis, pulmonary fibrosis, scleritis, Sjögren syndrome, nerve entrapment, and vasculitis may also occur. Felty syndrome, consisting of splenomegaly, anemia, thrombocytopenia, and granulocytopenia, sometimes complicates RA.

DIFFERENTIAL DIAGNOSIS AND EMERGENCY DEPARTMENT EVALUATION

RA is rarely misdiagnosed when it reaches the stage of symmetric polyarthritis in characteristic joints. At earlier stages, or with milder involvement, the clinical picture may be suggestive of inflammatory or infectious joint disease or other autoimmune diseases. When joint manifestations become apparent, infectious and crystalline synovitis must be considered.

In practice, most patients presenting to the emergency department with oligoarthropathy should have joint aspiration to

---

TABLE 134.3. Criteria for the Diagnosis of
Rheumatoid Arthritis

1. Morning stiffness[a]
2. Arthritis of three or more joints[a]
3. Swelling of proximal interphalangeal, metacarpophalangeal, or
   wrist joint[a]
4. Symmetric arthritis[a]
5. Rheumatoid nodules
6. Presence of rheumatoid factor
7. Erosions or periarticular osteopenia in radiographs of hands or
   wrists

   [a] Duration of at least 6 weeks required.

---

rule out infection or crystal-induced arthritis. Although RA or another autoimmune disorder may be suspected, the definitive diagnosis is made at follow-up, when further data, such as final culture results, rheumatoid factor tests, and response to antiinflammatory therapy, are available.

The American Rheumatism Association has developed a set of seven criteria, four of which must be present to establish the diagnosis (Table 134.3) (2). In practice, most such patients presenting to the emergency department must have other significant disease ruled out (e.g., infectious arthritis, SLE); and although there may be a suspicion of RA, the definitive diagnosis is usually made on further evaluation at follow up.

Patients with known RA who present with an exacerbation of joint inflammation require evaluation for possible secondary infections or crystalline arthropathy. Others may present with new systemic symptoms. Although the problem may be related to RA, this should not be assumed to be the case until other serious causes have been excluded. Evaluation based on presentation should be pursued as in any patient without RA. Special consideration should be given to complications of therapy; for example, pulmonary interstitial disease may be a result of either RA or treatment.

If a diagnosis of RA is considered, a rheumatoid factor titer should be ordered. If other autoimmune disorders are considered possible, other autoantibody titers, complement levels, and an erythrocyte sedimentation rate (ESR) may be indicated. Monoarticular or oligoarticular arthritis should cause one to consider crystalline and infectious arthritis. Joint aspiration is indicated, as well as oropharyngeal and genital cultures for *Neisseria gonorrhoeae*.

Few laboratory tests results are abnormal in RA, and, in general, the results tend to be nonspecific. The ESR is elevated and parallels disease activity. There may be a mild normocytic anemia. A test for mixed cryoglobulins, reflecting large amounts of circulating immune complexes, may be positive, but complement levels are usually normal. Arthrocentesis of involved joints typically yields sterile fluid with hallmarks of inflammation: decreased mucin clot formation and 20,000 to 80,000 white blood cells per microliter, of which 50% to 70% are polymorphonuclear cells (3). The classic laboratory finding of a positive serum rheumatoid factor is found in 80% of patients, but a positive rheumatoid factor can also be found in 1% to 5% of persons without RA (e.g., patients with other rheumatic disorders, leprosy, tuberculosis, liver disease, or bacterial endocarditis).

EMERGENCY DEPARTMENT MANAGEMENT AND DISPOSITION

NSAIDs are the mainstay of chronic treatment of RA. Patients experiencing a flare of known disease often require therapy in addition to NSAIDs. These include heat modalities, antimalarial agents, sulfasalazine, gold salts, D-penicillamine, azathioprine,

cyclophosphamide, chlorambucil, methotrexate, and surgical replacement of joints. Recently several anticytokine therapies have become available for RA that interfere with the action of tumor necrosis factor. These drugs have been shown to improve symptoms and slow progression of disease in those patients who have had an inadequate response to traditional therapies.

Corticosteroids are usually reserved for the treatment of extraarticular manifestations. Each of the therapeutic agents has associated adverse effects. Sulfasalazine may cause leukopenia. Gold salts and D-penicillamine have renal and myeloid toxicity. Gold may also cause a pruritic rash and mouth ulcers. The antineoplastic agents can all cause myelosuppression and a host of other adverse effects (5). Anticytokine therapy has been associated with severe infection and may be associated with increased incidence of demyelinating disease, lymphoma, and worsening symptoms of congestive heart failure. Second-line agents should be initiated only after discussion with a rheumatologist who will be observing the patient.

Appropriate disposition depends on the severity of the presenting symptoms. Outpatient treatment is appropriate in individuals who do not appear toxic, even those with a new diagnosis of RA. These patients should be started on a standard dose of an NSAID and have rheumatologic follow up arranged. Patients who appear ill require hospital admission for more intensive evaluation, particularly to rule out infectious disorders, and rheumatologic consultation. Hospitalization may be required for social reasons or if disability prevents adequate functioning at home.

COMMON PITFALLS

✔ Prescribing corticosteroids as a first-line therapy for RA
✔ Failure to recognize nonspecific complaints as a manifestation of autoimmune disease
✔ Failure to consider possible C1-C2 instability when intubating an RA patient

SCLERODERMA

Scleroderma (or systemic sclerosis) is an autoimmune disorder characterized by abnormal collagen production that results in pathologic fibrosis of the skin and internal organs. It occurs equally in all races and geographic areas, but it is four times more common in women than in men. In most cases, the onset is during the third decade of life (17). The course is typically progressive over decades, but it may be fulminant and fatal. Collagen accumulation and endothelial cell proliferation in the vascular intima lead to severe narrowing of the arterial lumen.

Scleroderma can be classified according to its predominant manifestations. The CREST syndrome consists of subcutaneous *c*alcinosis, *R*aynaud's phenomenon, *e*sophageal dysmotility, *s*clerodactyly, and *t*elangiectasia and is associated with a specific antibody (14,19). "Diffuse scleroderma" denotes the full systemic disease. A third subset is mixed connective-tissue disease or undifferentiated connective-tissue disorder, which combines features of SLE, scleroderma, and polymyositis (4). Clinical criteria have been developed for the diagnosis of systemic sclerosis (Table 134.4).

CLINICAL PRESENTATION

Patients with scleroderma most commonly present to the emergency department because of painful fingers due to Raynaud phenomenon, dyspnea due to restrictive lung disease, or

TABLE 134.4.   Clinical Criteria for the Diagnosis of Systemic Sclerosis

MAJOR CRITERION

Proximal scleroderma	Typical sclerodermatous skin changes involving areas proximal to the metacarpophalangeal or metatarsophalangeal joints, affecting other parts of the extremities, face, neck, or trunk; usually bilateral, symmetric, and almost always including similar changes in the digits

MINOR CRITERIA

Sclerodactyly	Sclerodermatous skin changes limited to the digits
Digital pitting, scars, or loss of substance from the finger pad	Depressed areas at the tips of digits or loss of digital pad substance from the finger pad tissue as a result of digital ischemia rather than trauma or exogenous causes
Bibasilar pulmonary fibrosis	Bilateral reticular pattern of linear or lineonodular densities that are most pronounced in basilar portions of the lungs on standard chest roentgenogram; may assume appearance of diffuse mottling or "honeycombing lung," and should not be attributable to primary lung disease

Classification as definite systemic sclerosis requires the presence of (1) the major criterion or (2) two or three of the minor criteria.[21]

dysphagia due to esophageal dysfunction. Malignant hypertension due to scleroderma renal disease is a true emergency.

Raynaud phenomenon is present in virtually all cases of scleroderma and is the initial manifestation in 70% of cases. Skin involvement is usually first manifested as edema of the fingers. As the disease progresses, the skin becomes shiny and taut, with loss of the normal skin folds. Joints become immobilized from tight encasement in thickened skin, as well as from contractures of muscles, tendons, and palmar fascia.

DIFFERENTIAL DIAGNOSIS AND EMERGENCY DEPARTMENT EVALUATION

Established scleroderma causes a characteristic taut, smooth appearance of the hands and face. This sign should be apparent to the physician, although the patient may not have noticed the gradual changes.

Early disease may be difficult to recognize, however. The most common early symptom is painful fingers due to Raynaud phenomenon, but this is a nonspecific feature of many autoimmune disorders that may also be due to occlusive arterial disease, repetitive trauma to the fingers, cryoglobulinemia, neurogenic lesions, or vasospastic drugs. In fact, Raynaud phenomenon unassociated with scleroderma is extremely common in women. Specific autoantibody testing may distinguish early cases of scleroderma from other causes of Raynaud phenomenon. Radiography of the hand may also be helpful. Subcutaneous calcinosis and resorption of the tufts of the distal phalanges are pathognomonic findings. More than 90% of patients with scleroderma have a positive ANA test.

An awareness of the systemic manifestations of disease is important in the evaluation of the patient with known scleroderma. Systemic collagen deposition may result in cardiac conduction abnormalities or cardiomyopathy, restrictive lung disease and pulmonary hypertension, gastrointestinal dysmotility and malabsorption, and renal arteriolar necrosis leading to malignant hypertension. Recognition of these manifestations in patients with advanced illness is critical.

EMERGENCY DEPARTMENT MANAGEMENT AND DISPOSITION

The majority of patients with Raynaud syndrome do not have symptoms requiring treatment in an emergency department. Patients with persistent vasospasm may, however, respond to simple interventions, such as warming of the hands or oral administration of nifedipine. Only rarely are more invasive maneuvers, such as interarterial or local phenoxybenzamine or prazosin, required.

Systemic manifestations may require evaluation for dysfunction caused by scarring in many organ systems. Intestinal hypomotility may be treated with metoclopramide. Esophageal reflux should be treated with antireflux maneuvers and medications, as necessary. Patients with increased blood pressure, renal failure, and internal organ involvement are frequently treated with angiotensin-converting enzyme inhibitors.

Most patients with scleroderma do not require hospitalization, but admission may be necessary for dehydration due to gastrointestinal dysfunction or for pulmonary compromise. Patients with hypertensive emergency due to renal crisis should be placed on nitroprusside and admitted to an intensive care unit.

Only those women with severe Raynaud phenomenon and those men without a history of trauma to the hands require periodic monitoring for the development of scleroderma. Patients should be instructed in the importance of keeping the hands warm and avoiding nicotine and caffeine. Suppressive pharmacologic therapy may be necessary if attacks are frequent.

Patients with signs and symptoms beyond Raynaud phenomenon should be referred for diagnostic autoantibody testing, occupational therapy, or orthopedics.

COMMON PITFALLS

✔ Failure to consider the systemic manifestations of scleroderma
✔ Failure to recognize scleroderma as the cause of a hypertensive emergency

GIANT-CELL ARTERITIS

Giant-cell arteritis is characterized by inflammation of branches of the carotid artery (temporal arteritis) or the aortic arch (Takayasu arteritis), and can present with emergent manifestations.

CLINICAL PRESENTATION

Temporal arteritis usually occurs in women over 50 years of age. Symptoms may be nonspecific: fever, headache, myalgias, and fatigue. Patients may have the syndrome of polymyalgia rheumatica, manifested by chronic stiffness and aching of the neck, shoulder, and hip girdle. However, chronic or subacute headache is often the presenting complaint.

The temporal artery may be tender and nodular (7), and there may be jaw claudication. The chief complication of temporal arteritis is monocular visual loss due to ischemic optic neuritis. Visual loss or impairment generally occurs 3 or 4 months after onset of initial symptoms (10).

Takayasu arteritis has a predilection for involvement of branches of the aortic arch. It is a rare disease. Patients are usually young women who present with nonspecific symptoms of fever, night sweats, fatigue, myalgias, and weakness. Signs of large vessel occlusion with decreased peripheral pulses, cerebrovascular accidents, or myocardial ischemia occur only months to years after initial presentation (11).

DIFFERENTIAL DIAGNOSIS AND EMERGENCY DEPARTMENT EVALUATION

The differential diagnosis of patients with temporal arteritis is wide because of the nonspecific symptoms. Mild anemia is typical. A markedly elevated erythrocyte sedimentation rate (ESR) in a patient over 50, with headache and nonspecific symptoms, particularly polymyalgia rheumatica, should prompt further evaluation.

Takayasu arteritis, although rare, should be considered in any young female patient with signs of large vessel ischemia (e.g., cerebrovascular accident, upper extremity ischemia, cardiac ischemia).

EMERGENCY DEPARTMENT MANAGEMENT AND DISPOSITION

Patients with suspected temporal arteritis rarely need admission to the hospital. However, prompt diagnosis and treatment is essential in order to prevent visual impairment. In the emergency department, patients should be started on 40 to 60 mg of prednisone daily. Arrangements should be made for definite follow-up and semi-urgent temporal artery biopsy. Response to corticosteroid treatment is usually dramatic, with relief of systemic symptoms and headaches within days. Treatment is generally continued for 1 to 2 years.

The diagnosis of Takayasu arteritis is not usually made in the emergency department. The diagnosis should be entertained in young women who need admission for large vessel occlusive disease. Angiography of the affected vessels shows narrowing or occlusion of large vessels, with well-developed collateral circulation (21). No treatment has been proven effective, but corticosteroids and cyclophosphamide have been used.

CRITICAL INTERVENTIONS

- Perform a diagnostic arthrocentesis to rule out infection or crystal-induced arthritis in patients presenting with new-onset monoarthritis or oligoarthritis
- Treat cervical spine trauma in the Rheumatoid arthritis patient carefully due to the development of instability of the atlantoaxial joint
- Initiate corticosteroid therapy in the emergency department in a patient suspected of having temporal arteritis

References

1. Alarçon-Segovia D. Clinical manifestations of the antiphospholipid syndrome. *J Rheumatol* 1992;19:1778.
2. Arnett FC, Edworthy SM, Block DA, et al. The American Rheumatism Association 1987 revised criteria for the classification of rheumatoid arthritis. *Arthritis Rheum* 1988;31:315.
3. Benzer TI, Leonard K, Raymond F. Evaluating bodily fluids. In: Flomenbaum N, et al., eds. *Emergency diagnostic testing*, 2nd ed. St. Louis: Mosby, 1995:291–328.
4. Black C, Isenberg DA. Mixed connective tissue disease—goodbye to all that. *Br J Rheumatol* 1992;31:695.
5. Brooks PM. Clinical management of rheumatoid arthritis. *Lancet* 1993;341:286.
6. Condemi JJ. The autoimmune diseases. *JAMA* 1992;268:2882.
7. Fauci AS, Haynes BF, Katz P. The spectrum of vasculitis: clinical, pathologies, immunologic, and therapeutic considerations. *Ann Intern Med* 1978;89:660.
8. Feinstein DI, Francis RB. The lupus anticoagulant and anticardiolipin antibodies. In: Wallace DJ, Hahn BH, eds. *Dubois' lupus erythematous*, 4th ed. Philadelphia: Lea & Febiger, 1993:246–253.
9. Fritzler MG, Rubin RL. Drug induced Lupus. In: Wallace DJ, Hahn BH, eds. *Dubois' lupus erythematous*, 4th ed. Philadelphia: Lea & Febiger, 1993:442–443.
10. Goodman BW. Temporal arteritis. *Am J Med* 1979;67:839.
11. Hall S, et al. Takayasu's arteritis. A study of 32 North American patients. *Medicine (Baltimore)* 1985;64:89.
12. Kotzin BL, O' Dell JR. Systemic lupus erythematous. In: Frank MM, et al., eds. *Sammter's immunologic diseases*, 5th ed. Boston: Little, Brown and Company, 1995:667–697.
13. Kramer J, Jolesz F, Kleefiend J. Rheumatoid arthritis of the cervical spine. *Rheum Dis Clin North Am* 1991;17:757.
14. LeRoy EC, et al. Scleroderma (systemic sclerosis): classification, subsets, and pathogenesis. *J Rheumatol* 1988;15:202.
15. Panayi GS. The immunopathogenesis of rheumatoid arthritis in the thorax. *J Thorac Imaging* 1992;7:19.
16. Pisetsley DS. Antinuclear antibodies. *Rheum Dis Clin North Am* 1992;18:1.
17. Silman AJ. Epidemiology of scleroderma. *Ann Rheum Dis* 1991;50:846.
18. Skaer TL. Medication-induced systemic lupus erythematosus. *Clin Ther* 1992;14:496.
19. Sturgess A. Recently characterized autoantibodies and their clinical significance. *Aust N Z J Med* 1992;22:279.
20. Tan EM, Cohen AS, Fries JF, et al. The 1982 revised criteria for the classification of systemic lupus erythematosus. *Arthritis Rheum* 1982;25:1271.
21. Yamato M, et al. Takayasu's arteritis: radiographic findings in 59 patients. *Radiology* 1986;161:329.

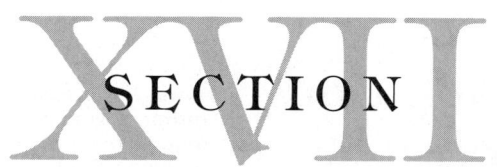

SECTION

XVII

Section Editor: Jeffrey Schaider

Infectious Disease Emergencies

CHAPTER 135

Bacteremia, Sepsis, and Septic Shock

Nathan I. Shapiro and Stephen Trzeciak

Bacteremia is defined as the presence of viable bacteria in the blood (3). Bacteremia can be transient, as is commonly seen after injury to mucosal surfaces (e.g., from tooth brushing, urethral catheterization, sigmoidoscopy, etc), where intact host defenses neutralize the bacteria and their harmful products, preventing clinically significant manifestations of infection. In other instances, bacteremia triggers an activation of the inflammatory cascade causing a condition know as sepsis. *Sepsis* is characterized by a host response to an infectious stimulus via endogenous mediators of systemic inflammation. In sepsis, the host response is as important as the source of infection itself in terms of pathophysiology and disease severity. Historically, definitions of sepsis have been diverse. In order to promote uniformity of inclusion criteria in sepsis clinical trials, consensus conference definitions of sepsis were published by the American College of Chest Physicians and the Society of Critical Care Medicine in 1992 (1) (Table 135.1). The consensus conference definitions introduced the term Systemic Inflammatory Response Syndrome (SIRS). Indicators of systemic inflammation (SIRS criteria) are defined as the presence of two or more of the following conditions: (a) T $>38°C$ or $<36°C$; (b) HR >90/minute; (c) RR >20/minute (or a $PaCO_2$ less than 32 torr); or, (d) WBC count $>12,000$/mm^3 or $<4,000$/mm^3 (or $>10\%$ band forms). The consensus conference also defined the terms sepsis, severe sepsis, and septic shock. *Sepsis* is defined as two or more SIRS criteria in the presence of a known or presumed infection. *Severe sepsis* is defined as sepsis plus acute organ dysfunction attributable to sepsis. *Septic shock* is defined as profound sepsis-induced hypotension (systolic blood pressure <90 mm Hg or a drop of more than 40 mm Hg), accompanied by hypoperfusion abnormalities such as oliguria, acidosis, or alteration of mental status, that is refractory to intravascular volume expansion (1).

Angus and collaborators utilized international classification of diseases (ICD)–9 codes for infection and acute organ dysfunction to estimate that 751,000 severe sepsis cases occur in the United States every year (2). An earlier multicenter study identified a rate of approximately 2 cases per 100 hospital admissions (3). Of these cases, approximately half were diagnosed in the intensive care unit (ICU), 12% in the emergency department (ED), and one-third in a non-ICU patient care unit. The incidence of sepsis cases is projected to increase sharply in the future due to age-based shifts in the demographics of patient populations (2).

In large clinical trials of septic shock, control arm mortality rates have ranged from 33% to 87% (4). Although septic shock mortality was reportedly decreasing from the 1960s to the 1990s (5), an increase in mortality (1.5% per year) has been observed since 1995 (2). This has been attributed to the emergence of multi-drug resistant organisms, increasing numbers of immunosuppressed patients, and an age-based shift in the demographics of sepsis patients. With advances in cardiovascular and respiratory support of high severity patients, it has become increasingly clear that the major threat to survival is not a sudden decompensation

---

TABLE 135.1.   Definitions

Systemic Inflammatory Response Syndrome (**SIRS**): the physiologic response to a variety of severe clinical insults manifested by two or more of the following
  A. Temperature $>38°C$ or $<36°C$
  B. Heart rate >90 beats/min
  C. Respiratory rate >20 breaths/min or a $PaCO_2$ <32 mm Hg
  D. White cell count (WBC) $>12,000$ cells/L, $<4,000$ cells/L, or $>10\%$ immature (band) forms
Sepsis: the systemic response to infection manifested by the presence of SIRS
Severe Sepsis: sepsis associated with organ dysfunction or hypoperfusion. Hypoperfusion and perfusion abnormalities may include, but are not limited to, lactic acidosis, oliguria, or an acute alteration in mental status
Septic Shock: sepsis with hypotension (SBP < 90 mm Hg), despite adequate fluid resuscitation, along with the presence of perfusion abnormalities that may include, but are not limited to, lactic acidosis, oliguria, or an acute alteration in mental status
Multiple Organ Dysfunction Syndrome (**MODS**): presence of altered organ function in an acutely ill patient such that homeostasis cannot be maintained without intervention

Adapted from American College of Chest Physicians, Society of Critical Care Medicine, Consensus Conference. Definitions of sepsis and organ failure and guidelines for the use of innovative therapies in sepsis. *Crit Care Med* 1992;20:864–874.

---

or a specific complication, but a process of progressive failure of multiple organs. This process has been termed *multiple organ dysfunction syndrome* (1) and is the major cause of death in patients with severe sepsis and septic shock.

CLINICAL PRESENTATION

Bacteremia is usually found in association with an acute illness and symptoms of fever, chills, and general illness—the so-called toxic state. Bacteremia and sepsis are dynamic processes in which the observed clinical manifestations depend on when in the disease course the patient presents, and on the degree to which the body's immune system and inflammatory cascade have been activated. Patients who progress to sepsis typically present with signs of systemic inflammation including fever, tachycardia, tachypnea, or elevated white blood cell count. However, not all patients have such a classic presentation or dramatic inflammatory response, particularly the elderly and the immunocompromised. The ED presentation of sepsis is not always clinically apparent in the initial stages. Since sepsis can be devastating, the ED physician must maintain heightened awareness and index of suspicion when evaluating patients with suspected bacteremia or sepsis.

Patients who progress to severe sepsis (sepsis plus organ failure) develop one or more organ dysfunctions including: neurologic, respiratory, renal, hepatic, metabolic (acid-base), hematologic, and cardiovascular. Central nervous system dysfunction typically presents as lethargy or acute alteration of mental status. Respiratory system dysfunction may include acute hypoxemic respiratory failure from acute lung injury/acute respiratory distress syndrome (ALI/ARDS). Acute renal insufficiency is common and may progress to oliguric renal failure. Cholestasis is the most common sign of hepatic dysfunction. Metabolic derangements include hyperglycemia and severe metabolic acidosis (usually from elevated lactate levels). Hematologic manifestations include a consumptive coagulopathy, which is typically subclinical (6), but may present initially with thrombocytopenia, and then progress to disseminated intravascular coagulation (DIC).

The cardiovascular manifestations of sepsis are numerous, as septic shock is the most complex of all shock profiles. What sets sepsis apart from other shock profiles is the fact that three different components of shock etiology may be occurring at the same time, especially during acute phase ED management (4,7). Septic shock may have features of cardiogenic shock (secondary to cytokine-induced myocardial depression), hypovolemic shock (secondary to profound capillary leak), or distributive shock (secondary to vasodilation). Because the pro-inflammatory response in sepsis causes diffuse microvascular injury with capillary leak, the septic shock patient often has a markedly decreased cardiac preload, especially in the initial phases of ED resuscitation. Although septic shock is typically considered a high cardiac output vasodilatory shock ("warm shock"), the combination of myocardial depression and markedly decreased preload in the early hours of disease presentation cause the early stages of sepsis to sometimes display a low cardiac output ("cold shock").

Fluid resuscitation administered in the acute phase of therapy actually modulates the hemodynamic profile of septic shock (4). Only after achieving restoration of cardiac filling pressures with aggressive intravascular volume expansion will a septic shock patient be able to generate a high cardiac output. Despite cytokine-induced depression of the myocardial ejection fraction, a high cardiac output can be generated (after restoration of cardiac filling pressures) because of tachycardia and ventricular dilation. Hypoperfusion abnormalities in septic shock may persist despite a normal or high cardiac output due to marked peripheral vasodilation and alterations in blood flow distribution to the tissues (distributive shock) (7). The hallmark of septic shock is vasodilation (low systemic vascular resistance) causing arterial hypotension that requires vasopressor support (8). At the microcirculatory level, tissue perfusion abnormalities may exist even in the absence of arterial hypotension, and may manifest as lactic acidosis in normotensive sepsis.

DIFFERENTIAL DIAGNOSIS

The clinical signs of bacteremia and sepsis may at times be subtle and difficult to detect. In other instances, infection and systemic inflammation may be obvious, but the source of the infection may be difficult to identify. Although an inflammatory response is often due to a bacterial infection, other possible etiologies must be considered. Acute infections due to viruses, rickettsiae, mycobacteria, and parasites may present as acute "sepsis," but severe infection due to these organisms is less common than that due to bacteria. Early diagnosis of sepsis requires an awareness of specific predisposing host factors.

In addition to identifying the presence of a bacterial infection, one needs to localize the source of infection (i.e., pulmonary, intra-abdominal, skin, urogenital, cerebrospinal fluid) and determine the most likely organism(s). This will help guide therapy, including source control and antibiotic selection. Consideration must be given to a wide variety of host factors that may alter the spectrum of likely organisms such as recent hospitalization or an immunocompromised state (HIV, chemotherapy, elderly, diabetes etc.).

Diagnoses such as pancreatitis, congestive heart failure, adrenal dysfunction, hypothalamic injury, overdose, diabetic ketoacidosis, anaphylaxis, heat exhaustion, and neuroleptic malignant syndrome, may mimic the inflammatory response seen with sepsis.

Although an elevated temperature often represents infection, at times it may be misleading. Hyperthermia and heat stroke may mimic many of the cardiopulmonary and neurologic manifestations of sepsis. Chills, however, are not expected with heat stroke. Identification and confirmation of a source of infection through history, physical exam, laboratory testing, and radiologic studies can help to narrow the differential.

The recognition of the shock state is essential in the approach to the septic patient. Patients with a systolic blood pressure less than 90 mm Hg with accompanying hypoperfusion abnormalities (after an initial fluid challenge) are by convention in shock. This will result in cell dysfunction or death. In septic shock, although initially a low cardiac output "cold shock" state may be observed (see above), the patients are classically in a hyperdynamic state with warm, extremities, and tachycardia. The patient will likely have fever and may have flattened neck veins or a reduced central venous pressure. Cardiogenic shock patients tend to have cool extremities as a result of a compromised cardiac output, and may show signs of cardiac ischemia through complaints of chest pain, shortness of breath, or an acute injury pattern on electrocardiogram. Hemorrhagic shock patients will typically have evidence of low hemoglobin concentrations, a source of blood loss, and will have cold and clammy extremities accompanied by flattened neck veins, tachycardia, and the absence of infectious symptoms. Patients with anaphylactic shock can typically be identified by an urticarial rash, pruritus, bronchospasm, throat tightness, and a history of exposure to a known allergen. Finally, patients with neurogenic shock due to spinal cord injury should be easy to identify by evidence of paralysis. Assessing the etiology of the patient's shock state is critical for guiding clinical management.

In summary, one must consider a broad differential in determining the presence of an infection, whether it is bacterial, viral, parasitic or otherwise. In assessing the response to infection to determine whether it is truly sepsis, many other diagnoses need to be entertained. Finally, once a shock state is reached, assessing for the presence or absence of characteristic findings of the various shock profiles may help to determine the etiology of the shock.

EMERGENCY DEPARTMENT EVALUATION

Because sepsis may progress rapidly, the emergency department evaluation must be expeditious. Appropriate stabilization measures are often carried out simultaneously with assessment. Vital signs must be reviewed. Unexplained tachycardia or tachypnea may be early clues to infection. Oral temperatures do not always accurately reflect core temperature; rectal temperature measurement is recommended in any patient with suspected hypothermia or fever.

The physical examination should concentrate on potential sources for sepsis including lungs, abdomen, urinary system, central nervous system and skin as the most common locations. Violation of a mucosal or cutaneous barrier carries the risk of sepsis; all indwelling catheters and lines are possible sources.

A wide variety of laboratory and ancillary tests are potentially useful in assessing the septic patient, but the following basic tests usually yield the most information: chest radiograph; serum electrolytes, glucose, blood urea nitrogen, and creatinine determinations; complete blood cell count, including white blood cell count and differential; urinalysis; blood cultures; and cultures of overt foci of infection. A serum lactate level helps to assess severity of illness and risk prognostication.

Many of the patients who present to the emergency department with fever and possible sepsis have localizing signs or symptoms, which identify a focal infection. More difficult to assess are those patients without localizing signs or symptoms.

TABLE 135.2. Presence of Bacteremia or Focal Bacterial Infection in Adults Presenting to the Emergency Department with Unexplained Fever

Number of Features Present	Bacteremia	Any Occult Infection
0	0/21 (0%)	1/21 (5%)
1	3/45 (7%)	15/45 (33%)
2	6/38 (16%)	15/38 (39%)
3–5	12/31 (39%)	17/31 (55%)

Features: age greater than 50; presence of diabetes mellitus; Wintrobe erythrocyte sedimentation rate greater than 30 mm/h; white blood cells greater than 15,000/μL; absolute neutrophil count greater than 1500/μL.

Adapted from Mellors JW, Horwitz RI, Harvey MR. A simple index to identify occult bacterial infection in adults with acute unexplained fever. *Arch Intern Med* 1987;147:666–670.

Mellors and coworkers found that five factors (age > 50; diabetes mellitus; ESR > 30 mm/h; WBC > 15,000/μL; absolute neutrophil count > 1500/μL) were useful in predicting the likelihood of bacteremia or occult focal bacterial infection in adults presenting to the emergency department with unexplained fever (9). The risk of bacterial infection increased with the number of factors present (Table 135.2). The presence of high fever (greater than 103°F [39.4°C]) or a "toxic" appearance had no correlation with the presence of bacterial infection.

Bates et al. developed a bacteremia prediction rule in the inpatient population that included temperature > 38.3°C, presence of rapidly (<1 month) or ultimately (<5 years) fatal disease, shaking chills, intravenous drug abuse, acute abdomen on exam and major co-morbidity (10). These factors, combined into a prediction rule, estimated of the prevalence of bacteremia ranging from 1% to 2% for patients at the lowest risk to 15% for those at the highest risk (11).

Assessing patients for severity of illness and risk of mortality is always difficult, especially in the emergency department. A number of scoring systems have been created for this purpose in the intensive care unit patients, including the APACHE-II, SOFA, MODS, MPM-II scores. However, there is one scoring system specifically derived and validated in the ED setting for patients with suspected infection, the Mortality in Emergency Department Sepsis (MEDS) score. The MEDS score was created to identify patients at increased risk of death among ED patients presenting with possible infection. The components of the rule and scoring system are shown in Table 135.3. The different risk factors are "red flags" that should be sought to identify ED patients who are at increased risk of death during their hospital admission.

TABLE 135.3. The Mortality in Emergency Department Sepsis Rule

Variable	Odds Ratio	95% CI	Points
Terminal illness (<30d predicted mortality due to underlying illness – e.g., end stage CA, AIDS)	6.1	(3.6 to 10.2)	6
Tachypnea (RR>20) or hypoxia (pox<90%)	2.7	(1.6 to 4.3)	3
Septic Shock (SBP < 90 mm HG after fluid challenge)	2.7	(1.2 to 5.7)	3
Platelets < 150,000 /mm^3	2.5	(1.5 to 4.3)	3
Bands > 5%	2.3	(1.5 to 3.5)	3
Age > 65	2.2	(1.3 to 3.6)	3
Lower respiratory infection	1.9	(1.2 to 3.0)	2
Nursing home resident	1.9	(1.2 to 3.0)	2
Altered mental status	1.6	(1.0 to 2.6)	2

Mortality Estimates:

Mortality Risk	Points	Mortality
Very Low	0–4	0.9%
Low	5–7	2%
Moderate	8–12	7.9%
High	13–15	20%
Very High	>15	50%

Mortality in Emergency Department Sepsis score used to identify patients ED patients with suspected infection at increased risk of death. Mortality estimates are determined using a point system derived from the clinical variables.

Adapted from reference 27.

EMERGENCY DEPARTMENT MANAGEMENT

Stabilization often begins before assessment is complete. As always, careful attention to the basic principles of the ABCs of Emergency Department resuscitation is essential. In particular, one should have a low threshold for intubation. Wheeler et al. reported that 85% of patients with severe sepsis are ultimately intubated. Early intubation not only protects the airway, it also reduces work of breathing and improves oxygen delivery (12). Adequate intravenous access should be ensured, cardiac monitoring instituted, and fluid resuscitation should begin.

Almost all patients with sepsis require supplemental fluids. The amount and rate of infusion are guided by assessment of the patient's volume and cardiovascular status. Because of peripheral vasodilatation and capillary leakage that are seen with sepsis, large quantities of fluid may be required to support the circulation. Volume administration is best guided by observing the response of the central venous pressure (CVP) or pulmonary artery wedge pressure to aliquots of fluid given over a short period of time. In the absence of CVP monitoring, if there is a concern of causing pulmonary edema with aggressive intravascular volume expansion, fluid administration titrated using continuous pulse oximetry. Fluid administration is continued and then slowed down when the supplemental oxygen requirement begins to increase.

It is important to maintain an aggressive fluid resuscitation even in the elderly or those with a history of congestive heart failure. These patients require very careful monitoring as the fluids are administered. Colloids (albumin, hetastarch) have no proven benefit over crystalloids (normal saline or Ringer's lactate) in resuscitation (13).

Rivers et al. demonstrated the benefits of aggressive and goal-directed resuscitation of the septic patient in a randomized, double blind placebo controlled trial (14). They used a combination of CVP monitoring, arterial blood pressure monitoring, and continuous measurement of mixed venous saturation from the superior vena cava (ScvO$_2$) to guide an aggressive ED resuscitation protocol for patients with septic shock or normotensive patients with a serum lactate level > 4 mmol/dl. By continuously optimizing preload, perfusion, and oxygen delivery in the first 6 hours of a patient's care, mortality was reduced by 16% (absolute risk reduction). This ED-based study was associated with a mortality benefit greater than any other study of sepsis performed in a randomized controlled fashion to date.

The goal-directed protocol brings ICU level care into the emergency department, and mandates an early resuscitation targeted to meet specific endpoints. Figure 135.1 summarizes the protocol. It normalizes preload by mandating a CVP 8–12 mm Hg, and corrects preload with fluid boluses if the CVP is low. Perfusion

1) Supplemental oxygen +/– intubation
2) Central Venous Line Placement

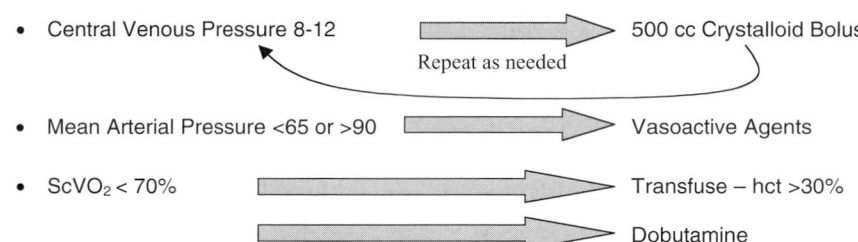

- Central Venous Pressure 8-12 ⟶ 500 cc Crystalloid Bolus
  Repeat as needed

- Mean Arterial Pressure <65 or >90 ⟶ Vasoactive Agents

- $ScVO_2$ < 70% ⟶ Transfuse – hct >30%

⟶ Dobutamine

Figure 135.1.   Summary of goal-directed therapy protocol.

pressure is corrected with vasopressors and afterload reduction to obtain a mean arterial pressure between 65–90 mm Hg. Once preload and perfusion are normalized, the ScvO2 is checked as a marker of tissue hypoxia. If preload and perfusion are normalized, and the Scvo2 < 70%, the patient is considered to be in a state of tissue hypoxia. This is addressed by first assuring that the patient has adequate oxygen carrying capacity (hematocrit > 30%). If the hematocrit is low, the patient should be transfused packed red blood cells. If the patient has adequate oxygen carrying capacity, and the ScvO2 < 70%, then dobutamine should be started to improve cardiac output. Once all goals are met (ideally within the first 6 hours), the patient parameters are continuously monitored to ensure they stay with the normal range. Treatment beyond the airway control and fluid resuscitation has four components: (1) parenteral antibiotics; (2) removal or drainage of infected foci; (3) vasopressors; and (4) adjunctive therapies (i.e., activated protein c and steroids).

Antibiotics

Initial parental antibiotics should be administered early in the emergency department course. Selection of particular agents is empiric, based on assessment of the patient's underlying host defenses, potential sources of infection, and most likely responsible organisms (15). Antibiotics must be "broad spectrum," covering both gram-positive and gram-negative bacteria, because both classes of organisms produce an identical clinical picture (Table 135.4). Immunocompetent patients can usually be treated with a single drug that has broad-spectrum coverage, for example, a third-generation cephalosporin such as cefotaxime, ceftriaxone, or cefuroxime.

Monodrug therapy in the immunocompromised adult is also possible with either an antipseudomonal penicillin (ticarcillin or piperacillin) or a carbapenem (imipenem or meropenem). Alternatives include ceftazidime plus either clindamycin or metronidazole; or a parenteral fluoroquinolone plus clindamycin. However, immunocompromised patients usually require coverage with two broad-spectrum antibiotics with overlapping coverage, such as an aminoglycoside plus either ticarcillin, piperacillin, or ceftazidime. Vancomycin should be administered in patients with a history of recent or multiple hospitalizations.

Antistaphylococcal coverage is recommended for patients with a history of intravenous drug abuse or indwelling intravascular lines or devices. Coverage against anaerobes should be

TABLE 135.4.   Antibiotic Regimens in Patients with Sepsis

	Modifying Factors	Antibiotic
Sepsis unknown source	*Immunocompetent*	Ceftriaxone (2.0 mg q12 iv) or Pipercillin (3.0 g q4 iv) or Imipenem (0.5 g q6 iv) or Meropenem (1.0 g q8 iv)
	For better Pseudomonas coverage	*plus* Gentamicin (2.0 mg/kg load then 1.7 mg/kg q 8 iv)
	Immunocompromised (includes neutropenia and burns)	Pipercillin (3.0 g q4 iv) *plus* Gentamicin (2.0 mg/kg load then 1.7 mg/kg q 8 iv) or Ceftazidime (2.0 g q8 iv) *plus* Vancomycin (1.0 g q12 iv)
	Recent hospitalization or institutionalized	Add Vancomycin (1.0 g q12 iv) to the above regimen
Abdominal infection	*Immunocompetent*	Ampicillin (30 mg/kg iv q4), *plus* Gentamicin (2.0 mg/kg load then 1.7 mg/kg q 8 iv), *plus* Metronidazole (1.0 g iv q12)
IV catheter infection (remove catheter)	*Outpatient acquired MRSA suspected*	Ceftriaxone (2.0 mg q12 iv) *plus* Vancomycin (1.0 g q12 iv)
Intravenous drug abuse	*MRSA not suspected*	Nafcillin (2.0 g q4 iv) *plus* Gentamicin (2.0 mg/kg load then 1.7 mg/kg q 8 iv)
	MRSA suspected	Vancomycin (1.0 g q12 iv) *plus* Gentamicin (2.0 mg/kg load then 1.7 mg/kg q 8 iv)

TABLE 135.5.   Vasoactive Drugs Commonly Used in Septic Shock

Vasoactive Agent	Typical Dose	Vasoconstriction	Inotropy	Chronotropy
Norepinephrine	2–30 µg/min	++	+	+
Dopamine	6–20 µg/kg/min	+ (low dose) ++ (high dose)	++	++
Phenylephrine	20–200 µg/min	++	0	0
Vasopressin	0.01–.04 U/min	++	0	0
Dobutamine	2.5–10 µg/kg/min	0 (mild vasodilation)	++	++

included for patients with intra-abdominal or perineal infections. Antipseudomonal coverage is indicated in patients with neutropenia or burns.

Within these general guidelines, no one combination of antibiotics is clearly superior to another. The early and appropriate use of antibiotics has been repeatedly shown to improve mortality (16–19). Failure to include adequate antibiotic coverage for what is later found to be the causative organism has been associated with an increased mortality risk (20).

Vasoactive Agents

If the patient's blood pressure does not respond to several liters of isotonic crystalloid (usually 4 L or more), despite an adequate preload being achieved (i.e., CVP 8-12), vasopressors are necessary. Several different agents (including norepinephrine, dopamine, phenylephrine, and vasopressin) are used to effectively achieve the blood pressure targets in septic shock (Table 135.5).

The two drugs most commonly used for initial management of septic shock are dopamine and norepinephrine. In the absence of high-level evidence advocating one over the other, either agent is acceptable as a first choice in septic shock. Although both dopamine and norepinephrine raise blood pressure and the cardiac output, dopamine is associated with a greater augmentation of myocardial contractility. However, dopamine may cause or exacerbate tachycardia to such an extent that a decrease in diastolic filling time decreases stroke volume. Norepinephrine is often a more potent drug than dopamine in achieving blood pressure goals, and will produce a mild increase in cardiac output. Although adverse events associated with potent norepinephrine-induced vasoconstriction (i.e., digital ischemia, etc) are possible, the incidence of these events is actually very uncommon in clinical practice (4).

Use of a pure alpha-agonist agent (vasoconstrictor) like phenylephrine will not cause or exacerbate tachycardia and will likely also achieve blood pressure targets. However, the increase in afterload on the heart without any augmentation of cardiac contractility may decrease cardiac output in a patient who already has myocardial depression (either sepsis-induced or pre-existing).

Vasopressin is an agent that is gaining a larger role in management of septic shock. Via vascular smooth muscle receptors, vasopressin is a potent vasoconstrictor. In septic shock, a relative deficiency of endogenous vasopressin may develop, and this is thought to contribute to the pathophysiology of vasodilatory shock in sepsis (22). Low-dose vasopressin infusion can produce a dramatic restoration of blood pressure in septic shock.

Consensus recommendations (23) regarding the use of vasopressin in sepsis advocate that the agent be administered to patients with septic shock refractory to other vasoactive drugs (i.e., when other agents fail to achieve blood pressure targets). The agent should only be administered in low doses

(0.01 to 0.04 U/min), in order to replace a relative deficiency of endogenous vasopressin.

Because of potent vasoconstriction, vasopressin should be avoided in patients with known atherosclerotic heart disease, and should not be administered in high doses. In addition, the vasoconstriction can increase afterload on the heart, which may impair cardiac output, especially if the patient already has poor cardiac contractility. There are multiple trials currently underway to investigate whether or not vasopressin administration in septic shock improves outcome.

Inotropic support may also be required for the patient with septic shock. If septic myocardial depression is identified either by echocardiography or by low-mixed venous oxygen saturation, an inotropic agent may be necessary. Although dobutamine is the most commonly used inotropic agent, it may cause mild vasodilation that could decrease blood pressure slightly. Therefore, administration of dobutamine may require some support from another vasoactive drug in order to safely maintain blood pressure. Like with dopamine, dobutamine may induce or exacerbate tachycardia to such an extent that diastolic filling time and stroke volume decrease. Extreme tachycardia should be avoided if possible.

Adjunctive Therapy

Recombinant activated protein C (APC) is a novel sepsis therapeutic agent that has recently been shown to improve survival by 6.1% (absolute risk reduction) in patients with severe sepsis (24). It is the first such anti-sepsis agent to demonstrate a mortality benefit in a large randomized controlled trial. Activated protein C has a mechanism of action that involves a simultaneous interaction with both the inflammatory and coagulation cascades. It promotes fibrinolysis while inhibiting thrombosis and inflammation. In theory, this decreases the production of microvascular thromboses, which are believed to be a contributing factor to acute sepsis-associated organ dysfunction, as well as decreasing systemic inflammation. The benefit to this therapy primarily occurs in the more severely ill population. The FDA has approved APC for use in the APACHE-II score > 25 group only. Because APACHE II scores are not commonly calculated in clinical practice, a vasopressor requirement could be a good clinical surrogate for the high severity patient who is an APC candidate. APC administration is commonly reserved for seriously ill patients in the ICU. Patients who may be candidates for APC administration should be identified in the ED.

The concept of steroids as a potent mediator of inflammation has been well explored in sepsis. There is theoretical and experimental support for the use of corticosteroids in severe sepsis and septic shock. Initially, a number of randomized human studies found large doses of corticosteroids to not prevent the development of shock, reverse the shock state, or improve the 14-day mortality (25). However, a more recent study was able to demonstrate a benefit to steroid supplementation in patients with adrenal suppression. Annane et al. performed a multicenter randomized, double-blind, placebo-controlled study that demonstrated benefit when steroids (hydrocortisone 50 mg IV every 6 hours, plus fludrocortisone 50 micrograms each day) were given to nonresponders of a corticotropin stimulation test (26). The study enrolled 300 intubated patients with septic shock. In non-responders to the corticotropin stimulation test, those treated with steroids had a 53% mortality compared to 63% in the placebo group for a 10% absolute benefit (p = 0.02). Steroid therapy was not beneficial to those who responded to the corticotropin stimulation test, and in fact showed a trend towards worsening outcome. The results of this trial are currently being validated in large multicenter studies. In the interim, one possible approach is to administer dexamethasone in the ED so a formal corticotropin stimulation test may be done in the inpatient setting. Steroid supplementation therapy should be considered for all patients who are requiring vasopressors, along with a corticotropin stimulation test, to determine whether glucocorticoid therapy should be continued.

CRITICAL INTERVENTIONS

- Proceed with early airway management
- Initiate aggressive fluid resuscitation
- Identify the source of infection
- Administer appropriate broad spectrum antibiotics
- Initiate Goal Directed Therapy
  - fluid resuscitate to a CVP 8–12
  - start vasopressors for MAP < 65 mmHg
  - transfuse to hematocrit > 30 and initiate dobutamine if ScvO2 < 70%

DISPOSITION

The disposition from the emergency department of patients with a fever and no localizing signs of infection presents a dilemma. Otherwise healthy individuals in a stable clinical state and at low risk for occult bacterial infection can be discharged with instructions for fever control, and a warning to return if symptoms persist or worsen.

Patients who are elderly, with underlying immunodeficiency, or with disorders that predispose them to bacterial infection and other sepsis syndromes require a low admission threshold. Patients with a risk for bacteremia above 2% to 5%, even if they appear well, should be admitted because of the difficulties in excluding potentially serious infections and predicting the clinical course. For example, it has been found clinically impossible to determine which febrile intravenous drug users have serious infections and which do not when they present to the emergency department.

Given the 30% to 50% mortality for patients with septic shock, plus the benefit of intensive therapy, all patients with septic shock should be admitted to an ICU. Additionally, patients who are perceived to be at high risk of developing septic shock, including normotensive patients with lactic acidosis, should be admitted to an ICU as well.

COMMON PITFALLS

- ✔ Failure to consider serious bacterial infection as a possibility in the assessment of subtle signs and symptoms
- ✔ Restriction of fluid resuscitation for fear of inducing pulmonary edema, even though large quantities of fluid may be required in patients with sepsis

References

1. American College of Chest Physicians/Society of Critical Care Medicine Consensus Conference: definitions for sepsis and organ failure and guidelines for the use of innovative therapies in sepsis. *Crit Care Med* 1992;20:864–874.
2. Angus DC, et al. Epidemiology of severe sepsis in the United States: analysis of incidence, outcome, and associated costs of care. *Crit Care Med* 2001;29:1303–1310.
3. Sands KE, et al. Epidemiology of sepsis syndrome in 8 academic medical centers. Academic Medical Center Consortium Sepsis Project Working Group. *JAMA* 1997;278:234–240.
4. Dellinger RP. Cardiovascular management of septic shock. *Crit Care Med* 2003;31:946–955.
5. Friedman G, Silva E, Vincent JL. Has the mortality of septic shock changed with time. *Crit Care Med* 1998;26:2078–2086.
6. Yan SB, et al. Low levels of protein C are associated with poor outcome in severe sepsis. *Chest* 2001;120:915–922.
7. Parrillo JE. Pathogenetic mechanisms of septic shock. *N Engl J Med* 1993;328:1471–1477.
8. Landry DW, Oliver JA. The pathogenesis of vasodilatory shock. *N Engl J Med* 2001;345:588–595.
9. Mellors JW, et al. A simple index to identify occult bacterial infection in adults with acute unexplained fever. *Arch Intern Med* 1987;147:666–671.
10. Bates DW, et al. Predicting bacteremia in hospitalized patients. A prospectively validated model. *Ann Intern Med* 1990;113:495–500.
11. Pfitzenmeyer P, et al. Predicting bacteremia in older patients. *J Am Geriatr Soc* 1995;43:230–235.
12. Wheeler AP, Bernard GR. Treating patients with severe sepsis. *N Engl J Med* 1999;340:207–214.
13. Investigators T. S. S. A Comparison of Albumin and Saline for Fluid Resuscitation in the Intensive Care Unit. *N Engl J Med* 2004;350:2247–2256.
14. Rivers E, et al. Early goal-directed therapy in the treatment of severe sepsis and septic shock. *N Engl J Med* 200;345:1368–1377.
15. Astiz ME, Rackow EC. Septic shock. *Lancet* 1998;351:1501–1505.
16. Aube HC, Milan , Blettery B. Risk factors for septic shock in the early management of bacteremia. *Am J Med* 1992;93:283–288.
17. Bates DW, et al. Predicting bacteremia in patients with sepsis syndrome. Academic Medical Center Consortium Sepsis Project Working Group. *J Infect Dis* 1997;176:1538–1551.
18. Opal SM, et al. Confirmatory interleukin-1 receptor antagonist trial in severe sepsis: a phase III, randomized, double-blind, placebo-controlled, multicenter trial. The Interleukin-1 Receptor Antagonist Sepsis Investigator Group. *Crit Care Med* 1997;25:1115–1124.
19. Pittet D, et al. Bedside prediction of mortality from bacteremic sepsis. A dynamic analysis of ICU patients. *Am J Respir Crit Care Med* 1996;153:684–693.
20. Kollef MH, et al. Inadequate antimicrobial treatment of infections: a risk factor for hospital mortality among critically ill patients. *Chest* 1999;115:462–474.
21. Kreger BE, Craven DE, McCabe WR. Gram-negative bacteremia. IV. Re-evaluation of clinical features and treatment in 612 patients. *Am J Med* 1980;68:344–355.
22. Holmes CL, et al. Physiology of vasopressin relevant to management of septic shock. *Chest* 2001;120:989–1002.
23. Dellinger RP, et al. Surviving sepsis campaign guidelines for management of severe sepsis and septic shock. *Crit Care Med* 2004;32:858–873.
24. Bernard, GR, et al. Efficacy and safety of recombinant human activated protein C for severe sepsis. *N Engl J Med* 2001;344:699–709.
25. Cronin L, et al. Corticosteroid treatment for sepsis: a critical appraisal and meta-analysis of the literature. *Crit Care Med* 1995;23:1430–1439.
26. Annane D, et al. Effect of treatment with low doses of hydrocortisone and fludrocortisone on mortality in patients with septic shock. *JAMA* 2002;288:862–871.
27. Shapiro, NI, Wolfe, RE, Moore, RB, et al. Mortality in Emergency Department Sepsis (MEDS) score: a prospectively derived and validated clinical prediction rule. *Critical Care Med* 2003:31:3:670–675.

CHAPTER 136
Skin and Soft-Tissue Infections

Alexander T. Trott

FOLLICULITIS AND CUTANEOUS ABSCESS

CLINICAL PRESENTATION

Folliculitis is an inflammation of hair follicles due to infection, overhydration, chemical irritation, or physical injury of the skin (22). The most common sites of involvement are the apocrine areas of the upper back, chest, buttocks, hips, and axillae. However, folliculitis can occur in any hair-bearing region of the body. The most common infecting organism is *Staphylococcus aureus,* but streptococci and gram-negative organisms are implicated in many cases. *Pseudomonas aeruginosa* has been reported after exposure to hot tubs as well as ordinary baths and showers (6). The individual lesion of folliculitis is a 2- to 5-mm dome-shaped pustule with a central hair shaft surrounded by a rim of erythema. Superficial folliculitis is often primarily pruritic rather than painful, and heals without scarring. If inflammation progresses deeper into the follicle, pain and tenderness develop, and scar formation is more likely to occur with healing.

Pseudofolliculitis is a foreign-body reaction caused by close shaving in persons of African descent. It is a noninfectious, inflammatory condition that can affect both men and women (21). The hair shaft becomes trapped below the follicle exit, and, because of its propensity for tight curling, grows into the follicular wall. Sycosis barbae is a deep infectious progression of pseudofolliculitis that, if untreated, can lead to significant facial scarring.

An untreated follicular infection, or one that does not resolve on its own, can evolve into a *furuncle* or *carbuncle* (13). Furuncles are single, deep cutaneous nodules involving the hair follicle. These nodules often go on to suppurate. The bacteriology is the same as that of folliculitis. Carbuncles are formed by multiple interconnecting furuncles that drain through several skin openings. Common locations of carbuncles include the chin, back of the neck, and scalp.

Cutaneous *abscesses* can originate in any part of the body through local breaks in the skin. Patients with conditions such as diabetes, inflammatory bowel disease, and immune disorders are at greater risk. Involvement of the head and neck is often due to obstruction and infection of a sebaceous gland or cystic acne. Intravenous drug abuse is a common cause of cutaneous abscesses seen in large, urban hospitals. Many of these abscesses are culture-negative (18). Pure *Staphylococcus aureus* is cultured in 25% to 45% of common abscesses; streptococci, gram-negative organisms, and anaerobes are recovered in other cases, often as polymicrobial cultures (6,7).

A recent, and disturbing, trend in the microbiology of abscesses and cellulites is the emergence of methicillin-resistant *Staphylococcus aureus* as a community acquired infection, CA-MRSA (5). These soft-tissue infections are found more commonly in healthy, children and young adults. They can be severe and even life-threatening. While some can be traced back to hospital MRSA (H-MRSA), many infections are arising in the community *de novo*. Fortunately, few strains are multiply resistant to antibiotics. There are no clear clinical characteristics that help differentiate between CA-MRSA and H-MRSA infections. C-MRSA infections tend to occur in clusters, therefore, culture are important to obtain in a suspected outbreak. Incision and drainage is the mainstay of CA-MRSA abscesses. Antibiotics if indicated depend on close follow up and culture results.

A cutaneous abscess presents as a red, painful, usually fluctuant mass. The patient typically experiences discomfort and swelling for several days before presentation for care. Systemic symptoms (fever, chills, tachycardia, malaise) are unusual but can occur if the abscess is extensive, is surrounded by significant cellulitis, or extends along a mucous membrane such as the rectum or oral cavity.

Cutaneous abscesses are frequently associated with other conditions. Hidradenitis suppurativa is a recurrent, suppurative, and scarring disease of the apocrine glands, most commonly involving the axillae and pubic regions of persons of African descent (14). Their greater concentration of apocrine glands leaves these persons more susceptible to infection from chemicals (deodorants, depilatories), trauma (shaving), or poor hygiene. Hidradenitis can be divided into acute and chronic phases. In the acute phase, when burning and itching predominate, single abscesses can develop. In the chronic phase, sinus formation and honeycombed scarring can be seen. Multiple and recurring abscesses are not uncommon.

Abscesses of the buttock and perineum can arise from multiple sources (6). An abscess in the proximal buttock crease is often associated with pilonidal disease. This condition generally afflicts hirsute young males, but its origins are unclear (22). Ingrown hair or, possibly, congenital remnants of hair follicles and squamous epithelium at the sacrococcygeal junction predispose to abscess formation.

When an abscess arises close to the anus, careful differentiation has to be made between a true perianal and a simple buttock lesion. Perianal abscesses originate from anal crypts, are very painful on rectal examination, and are often associated with systemic symptoms such as fever, malaise, and anorexia (1,7). If left untreated, they can dissect proximally into the ischiorectal space and become perirectal abscesses. Recurrent or persistent buttock and perianal abscesses can originate from fistulous tracts created by inflammatory bowel disease.

Bartholin gland abscess is a common problem that can arise from duct obstruction and infection with vaginal flora. The Bartholin glands are located within the vaginal vestibule at the 4 o'clock and 8 o'clock positions. A cyst or infection manifests as a mass medial to and often including the labium minus. The predominant organisms are anaerobic, including *Bacteroides fragilis* and peptostreptococci, and are associated with a variety of gram-negative enteric organisms in mixed culture (1). Of the identified aerobic organisms, *N. gonorrhoeae* is the most important because treatment of these abscesses should include antibiotics for sexually transmitted diseases.

DIFFERENTIAL DIAGNOSIS

When considering folliculitis, the differential diagnosis includes acne vulgaris, impetigo, cutaneous fungal infections, skin infestations (scabies), insect bites, and viral disorders (herpesvirus). The lesions of a systemic bacterial infection (*P. aeruginosa* and *N. gonorrhoeae*) can appear like scattered follicular disease. Abscesses have to be differentiated from other nodular lesions, such as uninfected cutaneous cysts, malignant tumors, nodular fungal lesions, and foreign-body granulomas.

EMERGENCY DEPARTMENT EVALUATION

When assessing a patient for folliculitis, furuncles, or a cutaneous abscess, the most important differentiation is between those lesions that contain pus and those that do not. Folliculitis and early furuncles are nodular, whereas abscesses have a soft or "fluctuant" center. Fluctuance indicates the presence of pus and, therefore, usually the need for incision and drainage. Buttock and breast abscesses are often mistaken for simple cellulitis because the large amount of fibrous tissue can obscure the presence of fluctuance. Whenever there is doubt, the lesion should be aspirated with an 18-gauge needle attached to a small syringe (3 to 10 mL). If pus is discovered, incision and drainage should follow.

An assessment of underlying conditions is necessary to determine the overall risk to the patient. Patients with diabetes, immunosuppression, blood dyscrasia, altered white blood cell function, or valvular heart disease are at greater risk from cutaneous infections. The presence of systemic signs such as malaise, fever, and tachycardia indicates a more widespread involvement of the cutaneous infection and requires a somewhat more extensive emergency department evaluation.

Gram stain and culture are unnecessary in healthy patients with simple cutaneous abscesses. A stain and culture may be useful, however, in managing patients who are at higher risk, who have systemic signs, or to whom systemic antibiotics have been administered. The results can guide future management decisions, particularly if resolution is slow or inadequate.

EMERGENCY DEPARTMENT MANAGEMENT AND DISPOSITION

Treatment for folliculitis depends on the extent and depth of follicular involvement. For uncomplicated common folliculitis and hot tub folliculitis, removing the offending agent and a gentle regimen of once- or twice-daily skin cleansing with mild hand soap often suffices (20). This regimen can be supplemented by topical applications of antibiotics such as bacitracin and polymyxin B (Polysporin) or mupirocin (Bactroban). Pseudofolliculitis is managed by allowing the involved hair areas, usually on the face, to grow at least 2 to 3 mm above the surface. Special commercially available razors (PFB foil-guarded Remington and Norelco electric razors) are designed for people with this condition.

If the folliculitis is painful or more extensive and involves the deep portions of the follicle, a 5- to 7-day course of oral antibiotics is added to the aforementioned measures (Table 136.1). Patients with recurrent folliculitis should seek follow up for consideration of prophylactic measures, such as the prolonged administration of an oral antibiotic or intranasal mupirocin to eliminate an *S. aureus* carrier state (9).

Untreated folliculitis can progress to a furuncle. If the furuncle has yet to suppurate, as demonstrated by the inability to obtain pus on needle aspiration, a regimen of warm soaks and antibiotics is recommended (see Table 136.1). For the buttock and perineal area, warm soaks or sitz baths are recommended at least twice a day. Patients should be seen within 48 to 72 hours for follow up, at which time, surgical drainage can be performed if the furuncle has suppurated. Carbuncles are more likely to present as obvious suppuration that will require surgical drainage.

Incision and drainage is indicated for most cutaneous abscesses. Appropriate analgesia, sedation, and anesthesia should be provided. For most small (less than 5 cm) superficial abscesses, local anesthesia of the skin over the abscess usually suffices. For very small abscesses, ethyl chloride spray can be followed by immediate incision. Local anesthesia can be supplemented by administering a parenteral opioid before intervention. For large or deep abscesses or those located in particularly sensitive areas, such as the perineal region, consideration can be given to intravenous administration of short-acting sedative and analgesic agents with appropriate monitoring.

Before incision, the abscess is cleansed with povidone–iodine or a similar skin cleanser. The incision is made with a no. 11 surgical blade attached to a knife handle. To provide for maximum drainage and access, the length of the incision should be at least two-thirds the diameter of the actual cavity to allow for digital or gentle instrument probing and disruption of loculations and pockets in the irregularly shaped cavity. Probing is followed by saline irrigation with a soft-tipped catheter attached to a syringe. Probing and irrigation are terminated when the effluent is pus free and blood tinged.

The cavity is lightly packed with gauze tape (one-fourth or one-half inch) to encourage further drainage. Excessive packing can result in obstruction of drainage. A bulky dressing is usually necessary to absorb continuing secretions. The packing can most often be removed at follow-up in 48 to 72 hours. This is followed by a regimen of warm soaks or sitz baths at least two times a day until drainage ceases. An abscess cavity takes 10 to 14 days to heal. Large abscesses take longer to heal and may need to be repacked once or twice at 48-hour intervals.

Special considerations apply to the management of Bartholin abscess. The incision is made on the medial portion of the abscess, close to the vaginal introitus, to avoid excessive bleeding. Instead of gauze packing, a small balloon-tipped (Word) catheter is recommended for drainage (24). This is followed by once- or twice-daily sitz baths. The catheter is left in place for 4 to 6 weeks to produce epithelialization of the incision and drainage site and to reduce the risk of abscess recurrence.

Early consultation should be considered for patients with facial, perianal, pilonidal, and Bartholin abscesses, as well as infection secondary to parenteral drug abuse. For cosmetic reasons, the approach to drainage of facial abscesses (e.g., needle aspiration, mucosal approach) should be discussed with a consultant. Perianal abscesses often require general anesthesia in an operative setting. Patients with pilonidal and Bartholin disease require appropriate follow up because of the potential for recurrence. Soft-tissue infections in parenteral drug users can be deceptively extensive and involve the deep soft tissue; these patients are also at risk for systemic and cardiac valvular disease. They often require hospital admission for evaluation and treatment.

Ordinarily, cutaneous abscesses need not be treated with systemic antibiotics (15). Antibiotics are indicated, however, under certain conditions. Relative indications include systemic toxicity as manifested by fever and chills; cellulitis extending well beyond the abscess cavity; underlying comorbid conditions (e.g., diabetes, immunosuppression); and failure to respond to incision and drainage. Table 136.1 lists the possible antibiotic

---

TABLE 136.1. Oral Antibiotic Regimens for Adults with Uncomplicated Cutaneous Infections

Codition	Antibiotic	Dose	Interval
Folliculitis,	Cephalexin	250–500 mg	q6h
furuncles,	Dicloxacillin	250–500 mg	q6h
abscesses,	Erythromycin	250–500 mg	q6h
localized	Azithromycin	500 mg (day 1);	q24h
cellulitis/		250 mg	
erysipelas		(days 2–5)	
Hot tub folliculitis	Ciprofloxacin	250–500 mg	q12h
Bartholin abscess	Ceftriaxone	250 mg IM *plus*	
	Doxycycline	100 mg	b.i.d.

TABLE 136.2. Intravenous Antibiotic Regimens for Adults with Serious or Complicated Cutaneous Infections

Condition	Antibiotic	Dose	Interval
Abscesses	Ampicillin/sulbactam	1.5–3 g	q6h
Cellulitis			
Suspected *Streptococcus/*	Cefazolin	1–2 g	q6h
Staphylococcus	Erythromycin	500–1,000 mg	q6h
Suspected *Haemophilus*	Ampicillin/sulbactam	1.5–3 g	q6h
influenzae	Cefuroxime	0.75–1.5 g	q8h
	Trimethoprim/sulfamethoxazole	8 mg/kg[a]	q8h
Suspected gram-negative	Ticarcillin/clavulanate	3.0 g	q4–6h
bacteria, diabetes	Clindamycin plus	300–900 mg	q8h
	ciprofloxacin	200–400 mg	q12h
Deep cutaneous infections	Ampicillin/sulbactam	1.5–3 g	q6h
(also, clostridial infections,	Ticarcillin/clavulanate	3.0 g	q4–6h
diagnosis unconfirmed)	Clindamycin plus	300–900 mg	q8h
	gentamicin	1–1.7 mg/kg	q8h
Clostridial infections (diagnosis	Penicillin	4 mU	q4h
confirmed)	Clindamycin	900 mg	q8h

[a]Based on trimethoprim content

choices for oral outpatient therapy. Intravenous antibiotic regimens for patients who require hospitalization are summarized in Table 136.2. The duration of treatment is usually 5 to 7 days. Because Bartholin gland abscesses are associated with STD's, after I & D, treatment for *N. gonnorhoeae* and *C. trachomatis* is recommended (1).

Manipulation of an abscess can cause bacteremia in 30% of cases but is most relevant in patients with preexisting cardiac valve disease. These patients must be given adequate antibiotic prophylaxis, as recommended by the American Heart Association guidelines, before intervention (3).

COMMON PITFALLS

✔ Mistaking an abscess for a small area of cellulitis or a furuncle and failing to carry out needle aspiration
✔ Making an abscess incision that is too small to permit adequate drainage
✔ Mistaking a perianal abscess for a buttock abscess
✔ Removal of the catheter prematurely from a Bartholin abscess
✔ Failure to consider the possibility of coexisting cardiac valve disease and to provide antibiotic prophylaxis when draining an abscess
✔ Failure to refer patients with recurrent cutaneous infections for consideration of prophylaxis

CUTANEOUS CELLULITIS

CLINICAL PRESENTATION

Cellulitis is an acute, spreading infection of the skin and subcutaneous tissue characterized by pain, warmth, swelling, and erythema. It is most often caused by group A *Streptococcus* and *S. aureus* (20,22). The first sign of common cellulitis is local skin discomfort, which is rapidly followed by frank tenderness, erythema, and swelling (4). Within 24 hours, there is noticeable expansion of the process, even though the margins themselves are indistinct. In spite of the progression, fever and chills occur in less than 10% of cases (4). Lymphangitic "streaking," that extends from the primary site proximally, is a very specific and reliable diagnostic sign. In the preantibiotic era, this progression was known as "blood poisoning" and not uncommonly led to death.

Erysipelas is a distinctive form of cellulitis caused almost exclusively by group A streptococci, although occasional cases are due to *S. aureus*. Erysipelas is most common in infants and young children, but it occurs in adults as well (23). It can begin as a result of minor skin trauma, surgical intervention, or a preexisting skin condition. In adults, it is likely to occur in the setting of venostasis, lymphedema, diabetes, or alcohol abuse. In contrast to common cellulitis, the lesion of erysipelas is sharply demarcated, indurated, and easily palpable. Characteristically, it is also shiny red. It is usually associated with fever and an elevated white blood cell count. Untreated lesions can form bullae that break down and leave raw, weeping surfaces.

A serious form of cellulitis seen in children, and occasionally in adults, is caused by *Haemophilus influenzae* type B. Although most commonly involving the face and the periorbital tissues, *H. influenzae* cellulitis can also involve the arms and legs. In adults, it may originate as a respiratory infection and then involve the neck and chest. In children, the cellulitis often takes on a blue-red to purple-red appearance. In both adults and children, *H. influenzae* cellulitis is associated with systemic toxicity and a significant risk of sepsis and secondary site involvement.

Aeromonas hydrophila and *Vibrio vulnificus* are two water-related organisms that can cause uncommon forms of cellulitis (8,11). The skin infection of *A. hydrophila* follows local trauma and exposure to fresh water; early infections are indistinguishable from streptococcal cellulitis but often progress to bullae, abscess formation, and foul-smelling exudate. *V. vulnificus* cellulitis occurs after trauma and exposure to salt water. The infection can range from mild cellulitis to an aggressive infection associated with vesicles, bullae, and myositis that can mimic gas gangrene.

DIFFERENTIAL DIAGNOSIS

Cellulitis can be difficult to distinguish from other cutaneous conditions. The most serious condition to be considered is thrombophlebitis, particularly when the lower extremity is involved. Cellulitis can be differentiated by the presence of fever, lymphangitic streaking, an advancing margin, and an elevated white blood cell count, although these findings are not consistently present.

Viral and drug-related exanthems can be localized, but usually are associated with recognizable precipitants and specific syndromes.

Dermatitis can appear red and somewhat warm but is usually associated with considerable itching and scaling. Secondary infection of dermatitic lesions, however, is not uncommon.

Insect stings, particularly due to *Hymenoptera*, can cause significant local reactions that can be confused with cellulitis, and these reactions can persist up to 7 days (25). As compared with cellulitis, insect stings produce more pain than tenderness, cause more edema and less erythema, and are pruritic.

Fungal infections of the skin, particularly with *Candida*, appear in characteristic locations (often intertriginous), have a distinctive appearance (moist, bright red), and can be identified by potassium hydroxide staining.

EMERGENCY DEPARTMENT EVALUATION

Common cellulitis and erysipelas, when localized to a small area in an otherwise healthy patient, need no invasive or laboratory testing. With more extensive cellulitis, a white blood cell count is performed to check for signs of systemic involvement and to gauge the severity of infection. Because of the low bacterial count in the lesions of cellulitis, aspiration of the advancing margin for gram stain and culture is of little value. In any event, these tests do not aid in immediate treatment decisions.

In compromised hosts and in patients in whom *H. influenzae* infection is suspected, a more extensive workup is indicated. The incidence of bacteremia ranges from 5% in toxic streptococcal cellulitis to 90% in *H. influenzae* cellulitis. Gram stain and culture, while of low yield, can be performed in an attempt to identify the causative organism. Older patients and those with underlying conditions such as diabetes or immunocompromised states should be evaluated for metabolic derangements and any evidence of other sites of involvement. Outlining the margins of the cellulitis with a marker can aid in the monitoring and follow up of patients with cellulitis by indicating lesion progression or regression.

EMERGENCY DEPARTMENT MANAGEMENT AND DISPOSITION

Common, localized cellulitis and mild, uncomplicated erysipelas in patients without risk factors can be treated as outpatients. Oral antibiotics (see Table 136.1) are begun, and close (48- to 72-hour) follow up is arranged. Duration of treatment ranges from 7 to 14 days. As a rule, antibiotics are continued for 3 days after the resolution of clinical findings. Resolution of cellulitis of the lower extremities can be slow because of dependency and associated edema (2). For this reason, strict elevation for several days is mandatory. If significant resolution has not occurred within 2 or 3 days, a brief hospitalization might be necessary.

Other indications for hospital admission and infectious disease consultation the presence of signs of systemic toxicity; underlying illnesses such as diabetes; specific involvement of areas such as the face, orbit, hand, perineum, or extensive lower extremity (particularly with preexisting edema); presumed *H. influenzae* infection; or suspected gram-negative organisms or mixed infections. Patients who require admission should be treated with intravenous antibiotics (see Table 136.2).

COMMON PITFALLS

✔ Failure to instruct the patient about elevation and care of the involved area
✔ Misdiagnosing deep vein thrombosis as lower extremity cellulitis

✔ Failure to arrange follow up in 48 to 72 hours for patients with cellulitis
✔ Unnecessarily treating insect stings with antibiotics

DEEP CUTANEOUS AND NECROTIZING SOFT-TISSUE INFECTIONS

Deep cutaneous and necrotizing soft-tissue infections are a group of disorders with many pre-disposing factors and a wide spectrum of bacteria (16). While early recognition and aggressive treatment are important ways to reducing an already high mortality yet, these infections can be deceptively benign in appearance (14). This benign presentation is no better illustrated than in Group A streptococcal infections caused by streptococci, sometime called "super strep," that elaborate highly toxic super antigens (19). Patients with soft-tissue involvement can complain of severe, disabling pain without skin or soft-tissue changes. Early recognition of these infections before they evolve to full blown Streptococcal toxic shock syndrome is important to reducing morbidity and mortality. See Chapter 148 for a more complete discussion.

CLINICAL PRESENTATION

Early in their clinical course, attempts at separating the various types of deep infections into discrete syndromes are made difficult by the fact that they share many characteristics. However, it is recognition of these characteristics that alerts the clinician to a potentially emergent condition:

1. These infections occur in settings that include trauma, foreign-body penetration, contamination with soil, surgical intervention, ischemia, or diabetes.
2. Tissue involvement is extensive, but classic signs of common cellulitis (heat, redness, induration) are often not present.
3. As the infection progresses, blebs, maceration, and exudate appear.
4. The hallmark of these infections, which, however, is not always present, is crepitance secondary to gas formation.

Specific deep cutaneous infections are summarized in Table 136.3.

Crepitant cellulitis occurs most commonly in the setting of pre-existing, lower extremity, peripheral arterial disease; decubitus ulcer; or a moderately severe traumatic wound. Also known as nonclostridial anaerobic cellulitis, this is a gas-forming infection that results from the synergistic interaction of anaerobic bacteria (*Bacteroides* species and peptostreptococci) and of gram-negative bacteria of enteric origin. In spite of its seriousness, it is usually gradual in onset, with mild local tenderness, and is not likely to cause serious systemic toxicity. In the area of involvement, the skin is minimally discolored and may appear grayish to brown, depending on local vascularity. The exudate, if present, is dark and foul smelling. The hallmark of this infection is crepitance and abundant gas formation, as seen on radiographs. The infection remains localized to the skin and subcutaneous tissues without extending to muscle.

Synergistic necrotizing cellulitis has also been called nonclostridial gangrene and nonclostridial anaerobic myonecrosis. Fournier gangrene of the male genitalia and perineum is a variant of this condition. Synergistic necrotizing cellulitis occurs most often in older patients with serious underlying disease, such as diabetes, congestive heart failure, or renal failure, and in the setting of obesity and perirectal infections. Gram-positive streptococci (both aerobic and anaerobic), gram-negative enteric bacilli,

TABLE 136.3.   Deep Cutaneous and Necrotizing Soft-Tissue Infections

Characteristics	Crepitant Cellulitis	Synergistic Necrotizing Cellulitis	Necrotizing Fasciitis	Clostridial Cellulitis	Clostridial Myonecrosis
Predisposing conditions	Wounds, decubiti, peripheral vascular disease, diabetes	Diabetes, obesity, advanced age	Postoperative wounds, perianal infection, chronic cutaneous ulcers, intravenous drug use	Contaminated wound	Devitalized tissue, focal contamination
Onset	Gradual	Subacute, over several days	Variable, indolent to fulminant	Gradual, 4–5 days	Acute, 1–3 days
Pain	Mild	Severe	Minimal, sometimes hypesthesia	Mild	Severe, early
Systemic toxicity	Mild to moderate	Moderate to severe	Marked	Mild to moderate	Marked, early
Overlying skin	Minimal, discoloration brown to gray	Blue-gray, necrosis	Initially spared, then pale followed by gangrene	Minimal change, occasional blebs	Initially normal, then pale bronze discoloration followed by necrosis
Exudate	Minimal, dark	Thin, reddish brown ("dishwater pus")	Rare, serous	Thin, dark	Serosanguinous
Odor	Foul	Foul	Foul	Rarely foul	"Mousy," slightly sweet
Gas formation	Abundant	Mild, up to 25%	Little	Abundant	Initially minimal, eventually moderate
Muscle involvement	No	Prominent feature, moderate spread	Rare, late	No	Prominent
Common pathogens	Anaerobes, Enterobacteriaceae	*Bacteroides fragilis*, streptococci, Enterobacteriaceae	Enterobacteriaceae, streptococci, *Bacteroides*, peptostreptococci	*C. perfringens*, *C. septicum*, *C.novyi*	*C. perfringens*, *C. septicum*, *C. novyi*

From Brillman JC, Quinzer RW, eds. *Infectious disease in emergency medicine.* Boston: Little, Brown and Company. 1992:822–823, with permission.

and anaerobes (*B. fragilis*), interacting synergistically, have been implicated in this infection. The onset can be acute or subacute, but the infection rapidly progresses to severe local and systemic toxicity with high fever. There is often severe pain at the site of infection, and the skin is blue-gray. Necrosis of the fascia and muscle occurs. Twenty-five percent of cases have clinical crepitance and gas evident on radiographs. The exudate is thin and foul smelling and has the appearance of dish water. Bacteremia occurs in 50% of cases, and mortality has been reported to be as high as 75%.

Necrotizing fasciitis is predominantly a disease of the subcutaneous tissue and fascia, with early sparing of the skin and very late involvement of the muscle (23). This condition can occur after trauma or abdominal surgery, or with perirectal infections, cutaneous ulcers, intravenous drug abuse, and infections of the head and neck. A wide range of organisms, including gram-negative enteric bacilli, gram-positive streptococci (aerobic and anaerobic), and other anaerobes, has been implicated. Although the infection is usually mixed, it can also be caused by single organisms, such as group A *Streptococcus*. The onset is acute, and the patient develops severe systemic toxicity. In the early stages, the skin appears erythematous and is minimally painful. Later, as the subcutaneous tissue becomes involved, there is mottling, discoloration, marked edema, and bleb formation as a result of interruption of the blood supply to the skin. The exudate is foul smelling and seropurulent, but not abundant. Although gas can be seen on radiographs, clinical crepitance is unusual.

Clostridial cellulitis, also known as clostridial anaerobic cellulitis, is most commonly a result of traumatic wounds. The presence of foreign debris, soil, and necrotic tissue allows rapid growth of clostridial organisms, including *C. perfringens*, *C. septicum*, and *C. novyi*. It is distinguished from clostridial myonecrosis (gas gangrene) by the lack of muscle involvement. Unlike gas gan-

grene, the onset is gradual, and systemic toxicity is only mild to moderate. Skin changes are minimal, but there is a thin, dark, occasionally foul-smelling exudate at the site of the wound. The most prominent feature of the wound site is crepitance and gas formation that often extends well beyond the actual area of cellulitis. The gas tends to appear on a radiograph as aggregates of bubbles in the subcutaneous tissues.

Clostridial myonecrosis, or gas gangrene, almost always results from a deep injury to skeletal muscle that causes ischemia and tissue necrosis. The same organisms that cause clostridial cellulitis are responsible for this disorder. The incubation period can range from 7 hours to 6 weeks (14), but once symptoms begin, severe deterioration can occur within 6 hours. Muscle swelling and severe pain are prominent features. Systemic toxicity, as a result of the many toxins elaborated by the clostridial organisms, is profound and leads to tachycardia and an altered sensorium, although fever is not a prominent feature. The involved skin has a yellow or bronze appearance, and the skin involvement progresses to bulla formation and green or black patches of necrosis. A serosanguineous discharge can develop with a characteristic "mousy" odor. Gas formation is minimal at the onset but extends throughout the muscle in a feathery pattern as it dissects through muscle fibers and bundles. Intravascular hemolysis, with thrombocytopenia, is often present. *These patients can die within hours.*

DIFFERENTIAL DIAGNOSIS

There is little difficulty in recognizing the picture of full-blown deep cutaneous and necrotizing soft-tissue infections. Occasionally, they can be confused with such conditions as dry ischemic vascular gangrene, pressure necrosis of a limb, acute deep venous thrombosis, and preexisting changes of venous insufficiency. Air can be introduced into the skin by traumatic lacerations and occasionally can cause some diagnostic concern.

It is important to emphasize, however, that these infections can be missed when they are not full blown. This is where difficulty can arise for the patient presenting to the emergency department in the early stages of infection.

EMERGENCY DEPARTMENT EVALUATION

The presence of a suspected deep cutaneous infection mandates an extensive and aggressive evaluation. This must be initiated promptly and carried out while any resuscitative or stabilizing interventions are in progress. Standard hematologic, biochemical, and clotting profiles are obtained, as well as arterial blood gas studies, a chest radiograph, and an electrocardiogram. A type and crossmatch may be indicated to correct blood loss or anemia.

A wound culture is taken and a gram stain performed immediately, particularly if a clostridial etiology is suspected. The presence on gram stain of gram-positive rods with few white blood cells indicates a clostridial infection. A finding of many white blood cells on the smear is more suggestive of a synergistic or mixed bacterial infection. Radiographs of anatomic areas of concern are obtained to look for soft-tissue gas. Because the infection can advance up to 10 cm an hour, the area of involvement should be outlined with a marker and checked at frequent intervals.

EMERGENCY DEPARTMENT MANAGEMENT AND DISPOSITION

Because it can progress so rapidly, clostridial myonecrosis is a true emergency. Concurrent with emergency department evaluation, planning and execution of intervention is carried out in consultation with a surgeon. A combination of hyperbaric oxygen (HBO), surgery, and antibiotics provides optimal treatment (12). HBO can arrest the advance of the hemolytic, necrotizing, and potentially lethal tissue toxins. HBO produces a tissue level of 300 mm Hg, which is 50 mm Hg in excess of that required to cause bacteriostasis and halt production of tissue toxins. HBO significantly reduces the need for extensive debridement and amputation and assists the surgeon in demarcating clearly necrotic from viable tissue. If necessary, however, a fasciotomy can be performed before HBO is done in order to relieve compartmental swelling and pressure.

In clear cases of clostridial myonecrosis or cellulitis, high-dose penicillin is still the antibiotic of first choice. Clindamycin can be used in βlactam–sensitive patients. If the diagnosis is uncertain, the antibiotics listed in Table 136.2 are also appropriate choices. Antitoxin therapy has never proven efficacious.

The primary treatment for other deep cutaneous infections consists of antibiotics and surgical intervention (14). Patients with an immunocompromised state or rapidly spreading infection can significantly benefit from adjunctive HBO; this intervention should be considered for all patients with these infections, especially Fournier gangrene (12). Broad-spectrum antibiotics are usually initiated empirically in the emergency department (see Table 136.2).

COMMON PITFALLS

✔ Failure to recognize a deep cutaneous infection because of a lack of classic skin changes of cellulitis
✔ Failure to perform a Gram stain in the emergency department
✔ Failure to take radiographs and thus missing subcutaneous gas
✔ Initiating only limited-spectrum antibiotics
✔ Delaying surgical consultation

CRITICAL INTERVENTIONS

- When draining an abscess, be sure the incision extends across at least two-thirds the diameter of the actual cavity to allow for digital or gentle instrument probing and disruption of loculations
- Initiate therapy for *N. gonnorhoeae* and *C. trachomatis* when treating Bartholin gland abscesses
- Treat *Clostridial Myonecrosis* with a Combination of Hyperbaric Oxygen (HBO), Surgery, and Antibiotics

References

Brook I. Microbiology and management of polymicrobial female genital tract infections. *J Pediatr Adolesc Gynecol* 2002;15:217.

Cox NH. Management of lower leg cellulitis. *Clin Med* 2002;2:22.

Dajani AS, Taubert KA, Wilson, et al. Prevention of bacterial endocarditis: recommendations by the American Heart Association. *JAMA* 1997;274:1794.

Dong SL, Kelly SD, Oland RC, et al. ED management of cellulitis: a review of 5 urban centers. *Am J Emerg Med* 2001;19:535.

Eady EA, Cove JH. Staphylococci resistance revisited: community-acquired methicillin resistant *Staphylococcus aureus*— an emerging problem for the management of skin and soft tissue infections. *Curr Opin Infect Dis* 2003;16:103.

Feingold FS, Hirschmann JV, Leyden JJ. Bacterial infections of the skin. *J Am Acad Dermatol* 1989;20:469.

Garcea G, Lloyd T, Jacobs M, et al. Role of microbiological investigations in the management of non-perineal cutaneous abscesses. *Postgrad Med J* 2003;79:519.

Gold WL, Salit IE. Aeromonas hydrophila infections of the skin and soft tissue: report of eleven cases. *Clin Infect Dis* 1993;16:69.

Hedstrom SA. Treatment and prevention of recurrent staphylococcal furunculosis: clinical and bacteriologic follow-up. *Scand J Infect Dis* 1985;17:55.

Hepburn MJ, Dooley DP, Ellis MW. Alternative diagnoses that often mimic cellulites. *Am Fam Physician* 2002;16:2471.

Howard RJ, Lieb S. Soft tissue infections caused by halophilic marine vibrios. *Arch Surg* 1988;123:245.

Hyperbaric Oxygen 2003. Indications and Results. The Hyperbaric Oxygen Committee Report. Bethesda, MD: Undersea and Hyperbaric Medicine Society, 2003.

Ko WT, Adal KA, Tomecki KJ. Infectious diseases. *Med Clin North Am* 1998;82:1001.

Lewis RT. Soft tissue infections. *World J Surg* 1998;22:146.

Llera J, Levy RC. Treatment of cutaneous abscesses: a double-blind study. *Ann Emerg Med* 1985;14:57.

Malangoni MA. Necrotizing soft tissue infections: are we making any progress? *Surg Infect* 2001;2:145.

Marcus R, Stine R, Cohen M. Perirectal abscess. *Ann Emerg Med* 1995;25:597.

Meislin HW. Pathogen identification of abscesses and cellulitis. *Ann Emerg Med* 1986;15:329.

Norrby-Teglund A, Norrby R, Low DE. The treatment of severe group A streptococcal infections. *Curr Infect Dis Rep* 2003;5–28.

O'Dell M. Skin and wound infections: an overview. *Am Fam Physician* 1998;57:2424.

Perry PK, Cook-Bolden FE, Rahman Z, et al. Defining psudofolliculitis barbae in 2001: A review of the literature and current trends. *J Am Acad Dermatol* 2002;46:S113.

Sadick NS. Current aspects of bacterial infections of the skin. *Dermatol Clin* 1997;15:341.

Stone DR, Gorbach SL. Necrotizing fascitis: the changing spectrum. *Infect Dis Dermatol* 1997;15:213.

Woodruff JD, Friedrick EG. The vestibule. *Clin Obstet Gynecol* 1985;28:134.

Zuckerberg AL, Schweich PJ. An arm red and hot: infection or not? *Pediatr Emerg Care* 1990;6:275.

CHAPTER 137
Tetanus

Daniel T. Wu

Tetanus is a severe and often fatal disease caused by the gram-positive anaerobic organism *Clostridium Tetani*. The infection has been described in the medical literature as far back as the 5th century B.C. and the organism can be found almost ubiquitously in nature, especially in soil and feces (3). Due to an aggressive vaccination program started in the 1940s, combined with improved sterilization procedures, tetanus has become a rare disease in the United States, with an average of 43 cases reported each year from 1998 to 2000 (2). Unfortunately, despite the availability of an effective vaccine, tetanus still remains prevalent in many Third World countries, with an estimated incidence of 500,000 to 1 million cases per year and a mortality rate as high as 20% to 30% (6,10,12).

The *Clostridium tetani* bacterium is heat-sensitive and cannot survive in the presence of oxygen, but it produces spores, which are heat-resistant and can survive indefinitely until they germinate. This can occur weeks after its entry into a wound, which accounts for many of the infections that occur after a wound has fully healed. Under anaerobic conditions, the spores germinate into mature organisms and release two neurotoxins, tetanolysin and tetanospasmin. Tetanolysin is known to cause tissue damage but is not thought to be a major contributor to the clinical manifestations of tetanus. Tetanospasmin is a very potent neurotoxin, which enters peripheral nerves and travels retrograde to the CNS where it disrupts the release of inhibitory neurotransmitters such as gamma-aminobutyric acid (GABA). This leads to uncontrolled motor nerve activity and the clinical manifestations of muscle spasms and autonomic instability that characterize tetanus infections. The incubation period is approximately 1 week, but can be as short as 2 to 3 days or as long as several weeks (3,2,7). A shorter incubation period is generally associated with more severe disease and an increased risk of death.

CLINICAL PRESENTATION

There are four different types of tetanus infections: generalized, localized, neonatal and cephalic.

Generalized tetanus is the most common type and represents approximately 80% of all tetanus infections in the United States and developed countries. Symptoms usually start with muscle stiffness and pain, most often occurring in the facial and jaw muscles causing trismus, and frequently resulting in the characteristic facial appearance known as risus sardonicus. The symptoms then spread to the neck, torso and extremities. Tetanic spasms of the back muscles produce opisthotonos, in which only the back of the head and the heels rest on the bed. Spasms may involve the muscles of respiration, producing a fixed chest wall and eventual asphyxia.

Systemic symptoms in mild cases are often minimal, but in severe cases marked autonomic disturbances are seen, with tachycardia, wide swings in blood pressure, hyperpyrexia, and cardiac dysrhythmias. These manifestations appear to be due to excessive catecholamine release and are the most common cause of death from tetanus. Trivial stimuli may trigger not only severe spasms, but also wide swings in vital signs.

Localized tetanus is a less common form of the disease, and accounted for 17% of cases in the United States from 1998 to 2000 (2). It manifests as localized spasms around the area of initial infection, and may last for weeks before fully resolving. The prognosis of localized infections is very good with a mortality rate of approximately 1% (2,6). Yet, it is important to note that what may appear to be a localized infection could be the early stages of a generalized infection.

Neonatal tetanus is a generalized form of tetanus that occurs in neonates during the first few weeks of life and is often caused by infection of the umbilical stump. The initial symptoms are spasms, rigidity, and poor feeding. It has become a rare disease in the United States since the introduction of the tetanus vaccine and modern sterilization techniques, but remains a serious problem in many developing countries where babies are born without passive immunity because their mothers have not been vaccinated. Worldwide, the neonatal form of tetanus accounts for over half of all tetanus deaths (11).

Cephalic tetanus is a very rare variant of the disease, which often occurs after head injury or otitis media. Trismus and cranial nerve involvement are characteristic, most commonly the seventh and sixth cranial nerves. Cephalic tetanus can initially be misdiagnosed as Bell Palsy.

DIFFERENTIAL DIAGNOSIS

The only entity with which an established case of tetanus may be confused is strychnine poisoning. Muscle spasms associated with strychnine poisoning may resemble those of tetanus, but there are several important differences. The muscles of the jaw are not involved early in the course of strychnine poisoning or may be spared completely. In tetanus, the jaw muscles are involved early in the course, and trismus is almost always present. Also, in a patient with strychnine poisoning, muscle rigidity disappears completely between spasms.

The early stages of tetanus may be confused with psychoneurotic complaints and with dystonic reactions from such agents as phenothiazines. Dystonic reactions can be rapidly and safely treated, and therefore ruled out, by the administration of benztropine or diphenhydramine. Dental infections may produce trismus, but there is no progression, and signs of local infection are almost always present.

EMERGENCY DEPARTMENT EVALUATION

The diagnosis of tetanus remains a clinical one, and laboratory testing offers little or no benefit. Wound cultures and serum antitoxin antibody levels can be obtained, but neither is available quickly enough to make the diagnosis during the initial presentation of the disease (5). Moreover, wound cultures for tetanus are positive only about 30% of the time. Laboratory studies, although not diagnostic for tetanus infections, should be sent to rule out other etiologies and to assess oxygenation status in severe infections.

The source of the infection should be investigated. Wounds secondary to acute trauma accounts for the majority of cases in the United States, but an acute skin wound is not necessary to contract a tetanus infection, and as mentioned previously, the incubation period can be quite long. More than 25% of the infections from 1998 to 2000 occurred in patients without a history of acute trauma and were attributed to other infections such as abscesses, ulcers, and gangrene.

The majority of cases in the United States have occurred in patients who were inadequately vaccinated or who had an unknown vaccination history. From 1998 to 2000, only 16% of the tetanus cases in the United States took place in individuals who had received 3 or more doses of tetanus toxoid within the previous 10 years (2). Several groups appear to be at risk for developing tetanus. These include the elderly, diabetics, and injection-drug users (IDU) (2,3,4). The elderly comprised over a third of the cases of tetanus infections between 1995 and 2000 in the United States and appear to be at risk because of declining immunity over time (4,8). Protection, as defined by adequate serum antibody levels, decreases with age, and it was found that less than 30% of those over 70 years of age had protective levels of antibodies (4).

EMERGENCY DEPARTMENT MANAGEMENT

The management of tetanus has three goals: stabilizing the patient, neutralizing the toxin, and removing any remaining organisms.

In the initial stages, management is largely supportive, with emphasis on airway control. Patients with severe infections may require ventilatory support to prevent asphyxiation from severe muscle spasms. Airway management may be difficult due to trismus, and may require the use of paralytic agents. Succinylcholine can be used in early tetanus but should be used with caution, if at all, in the later stages of the disease because of the risk of hyperkalemia secondary to the up-regulation of acetylcholine receptors. Prophylactic intubation should be considered in the early stages of cases in which the airway may be threatened. Severe muscle spasms and rigidity can be treated with benzodiazepines but often requires large doses.

The toxin should be neutralized by administration of tetanus immune globulin (TIG). The dose is 3000 to 6000 units IM for both adults and children (3,9). Some authorities have recommended that part of the dose be locally infiltrated around the wound, although this may cause local irritation and has not been proven to be beneficial. TIG does not affect toxin that is already bound to nerve endings, but it can help to remove unbound toxin.

Removal of any remaining tetanus organism is important in limiting the severity of infection. If a wound is identified, it should be cleaned well and débrided to remove any necrotic tissue. Metronidazole is effective eliminating *Clostridium tetani* and has become the antibiotic of choice, with penicillin as an alternative treatment (1,9).

Autonomic instability, which manifests as hypertension and tachycardia, usually occurs days to weeks after the onset of symptoms and is also a major cause of death; fatality rates are as high as 28% (6). There is no universally accepted treatment protocol, but labetalol has been used frequently for its beta and alpha-blocking effects. Other agents that have been used with varying effectiveness include opiates, clonidine, and magnesium.

It is important to note that clinical infection does not confer immunity, so all patients who recover from tetanus must be actively immunized.

CRITICAL INTERVENTIONS

- Administer tetanus toxoid and tetanus immune globulin for tetanus-prone wounds if a patient has not previously completed a full vaccination series
- Administer tetanus toxoid if the patient has not received tetanus toxoid within 5 years for tetanus-prone wounds or within 10 years for nontetanus-prone wounds

DISPOSITION

All patients with clinical tetanus must be admitted to an intensive care setting for observation and management. Since it is difficult to predict the severity and progression of the disease when it is in its early stages, patients should be monitored to ensure maintenance of an airway and to identify and treat autonomic instability and cardiac arrhythmia.

PREVENTION

With the introduction of an effective vaccine in the 1940s and improved sterilization techniques, tetanus has become an almost entirely preventable disease. There has been a steady decline in both the incidence of the disease and mortality rates. Since almost all recent cases of tetanus in the United States have occurred in persons who have never been vaccinated or have not had a recent booster, it is the responsibility of emergency physicians to inquire about the immunization status of all patients and administer the toxoid and/or immune globulin as indicated.

The primary vaccination series should be completed by the age of 18 months. Children should then receive a booster at ages 4 and 11 and every 10 years thereafter. The adult tetanus Td (containing diphtheria and tetanus toxoid) should be used for anyone 7 years of age or older.

For clean minor wounds, tetanus toxoid is indicated if the patient has received fewer than three doses of the vaccine in the past, if the vaccination history is unknown, or if it has been more than 10 years since the last Td booster. For tetanus-prone wounds (those contaminated with feces, dirt, or saliva, as well as burns, crush injuries, and puncture wounds) tetanus toxoid should be administered if the patient has not received it within the last five years; TIG should also be administered if the patient has not previously completed a full vaccination series (Table 137.1).

COMMON PITFALLS

✔ Clinical tetanus infection does not confer immunity, and active immunization should be given to all patients who have infections
✔ The elderly are at particular risk for contracting infections because of their declining immunity
✔ An acute laceration is not required to develop tetanus. Infections can originate from lacerations that have already started healing or from other sources such as abscesses, ulcers, or injection sites in drug users

TABLE 137.1. Tetanus Prophylaxis for Wound Management

Vaccination History (prior Td doses)	Clean, Minor Wounds		All Other Wounds	
	Td	TIG	Td	TIG
Unknown or <3 doses	Yes	No	Yes	Yes
3 or more doses	No*	No	No**	No

*Td should be given if more than 10 years since last booster
**Td should be given if more than 5 years since last booster
Source: CDC - *The Pink Book*, American Academy of Pediatrics—*Red Book: Report of the Committee on Infectious Diseases*.

References

1. Ahmadsyah I, Salim A. Treatment of tetanus: an open study to compare the efficacy of procaine penicillin and metronidazole. *Br J Med* 1985;291:648–650.
2. CDC. Tetanus Surveillance—United States, 1998–2000. *MMWR* 2003;52 (SS-3):1–7.
3. CDC. Tetanus. *Epidemiology and Prevention of Vaccine-Preventable Diseases*, 8th Edition (The Pink Book).
4. Gergen PJ, McQuillan GM, Kiely M, et al. A population-based serologic survey of immunity to tetanus in the United States. *N Engl J Med* 1995;332:761–766.
5. Henderson SO, Mody T, Groth DE, et al. The presentation of tetanus in an emergency department. *J of Emerg Med* 1998;16:705–708.
6. Hsu SS, Groleau G. Tetanus in the emergency department: a current review. *J of Emerg Med* 2001;20:357–365.
7. Loscalzo LI, Ryan J, Loscalzo J, et al. Tetanus: a clinical diagnosis. *J of Emerg Med* 1995;13:4.
8. McQuillan GM, Kruszon-Moran D, Deforest A, et al. Serologic immunity to diptheria and tetanus in the United States. *Ann Intern Med.* 2002;136:660–666.
9. Pickering L, ed. 2000 Red Book: Report of the committee on infectious diseases. 25th ed. *American Academy of Pediatrics*, 2000.
10. Richardson JP, Knight AL. The management and prevention of tetanus. *J of Emerg Med* 1993;11:737–742.
11. Sanford JP. Tetanus—forgotten but not gone. *N Engl J Med* 1995;332:812–813.
12. Thawaites CL, Farrar JJ. Preventing and treating tetanus. *BMJ* 2003;326:188–119.

CHAPTER 138
Meningitis and Encephalitis

Richard Mark Kaplan

Meningitis and encephalitis are infectious and inflammatory processes occurring in the leptomeninges (meningitis), brain structures (encephalitis), or both (leptomeningitis). These disorders are discussed together because of considerable clinical and etiologic overlap. By convention, meningitis is classified as either bacterial or, when due to any other cause, the aseptic meningitis syndrome. During the latter part of the 20th century, the annual incidence of bacterial meningitis in the United States was about 3 cases/100,000 population in the U.S. to 500/100,000 in the "meningitis belt" of Africa, while fatality rates approximated 20% (10,24,26).

Streptococcus pneumoniae and *Neisseria meningitidis* account for approximately three-fourths of all cases of bacterial meningitis (24,26). A recent study observed that *S. pneumoniae* accounted for 47% of meningitis cases, while *N. meningitides* was responsible for about 25% (26). Durand (10) noted that for community-acquired meningitis, *S. pneumoniae* accounted for 38%, *N. meningitides* (14%), Listeria monocytogenes (11%), and Haemophilus influenza (4%). *S. pneumoniae* is the most common agent in adults, while *N. meningitidis* is most frequently noted in children and adolescents. *L. monocytogenes* and *Streptococcus agalactiae* (Group B streptococcus) are generally found in children younger than 3 months of age, the elderly and immunocompromised individuals. Prior to the *H. influenza* vaccine, *H. influenza* meningitis ranged from 4% to 16% (10,24,26). The vaccine has decreased the incidence of *H. influenza* meningitis by more than 90%. Staphylococcal species and gram-negative bacilli are more rare causes of meningitis in adults. There is an increased incidence of gram-negative bacilli in nosocomial meningitis (10).

Risk factors associated with bacterial meningitis include age (the very old and the very young), ear-nose-throat conditions (otitis, mastoiditis, sinusitis), neurosurgical procedures, chronic disease, diabetes mellitus, immunosuppression, alcohol abuse, and tobacco exposure (active and passive). Overcrowded living conditions (e.g., college dormitories, military barracks) and poverty increase the risk of contracting meningococcal meningitis. Risk factors for listeria meningitis include the immunocompromised state and the ingestion of *Listeria*-contaminated foods. Chronic immunosuppression is an increasingly recognized risk factor for fungal meningitis. Following trauma or neurosurgical procedures, there is concern regarding nosocomial and gram-negative organisms (29).

The aseptic meningitis syndrome is primarily of viral etiology and is generally a self-limited symptom complex of fever, headache, and nuchal rigidity with cerebrospinal fluid (CSF) findings of lymphocytosis, variable protein elevation, and normal glucose. Enterovirus is the most common cause of aseptic meningitis (20). Nonbacterial causes of aseptic meningitis include intrathecal injections, nonsteroidal antiinflammatory agents, and antibiotics.

Acute encephalitis is generally a viral-related illness in which the brain matter (cerebral hemispheres, brainstem, or cerebellum) is injured either as a direct result of viral invasion or as a hypersensitivity reaction to a systemic viral illness. Occasionally, encephalitis occurs shortly after vaccination for measles, rubella, chickenpox, or rabies. The diagnosis of encephalitis should be considered in all patients who present with fever, headache, nuchal rigidity, altered mental status (AMS), seizures, or focal neurologic signs. In the United States, the most common causes of acute encephalitis include Herpes simplex virus (HSV), enteroviruses, arboviruses and HIV. The arboviruses include West Nile virus (WNV), St Louis, California, Western and Eastern equine. In 2002, a WNV outbreak of arboviral meningocephalitis resulted in a 9% mortality (17), while mortality due to HSV encephalitis ranges from 30% (if treated with acyclovir) to 60% if untreated (23).

CLINICAL PRESENTATION

Fever, headache, AMS, and nuchal rigidity should prompt serious consideration of the diagnosis of meningitis. Attia (1) reported that the absence of fever, neck stiffness, and AMS virtually eliminated the diagnosis of meningitis. For pooled sensitivity data, fever was noted in 85% of patients, while the sensitivities of neck stiffness and AMS were 70% and 67%, respectively. Sigudardottir (26) reported fever (97%), neck stiffness (88%), AMS (66%), and the triad in 51% of meningitis patients. Durand (10) noted similar results with fever (95%), neck stiffness (83%), AMS (78%) and the triad in about 67%.

Any of the encephalitides may demonstrate hypersomnia as an acute symptom. Fever is commonly noted with meningitis or encephalitis, but is not invariably present, especially in the elderly and the immunocompromised. Headache is occasionally absent early in the course of disease and in elderly patients. Focal findings reflect the portion of the brain that is involved (e.g., hemiparesis, cranial nerve abnormalities, aphasia, ataxia). Nausea and vomiting, reflecting central nervous system (CNS) inflammation and raised intracranial pressure, can be observed in either condition.

Two clinical signs are characteristic of meningeal irritation, but cannot always be elicited. The Brudzinski sign occurs when flexion of the neck results in flexion of the knees and hips. The Kernig sign is elicited by extending the knee with the hip flexed;

stretching of the lumbar roots causes pain in the hamstring and paraspinal muscles. Petechiae, purpura, and morbilliform rash are commonly noted in association with meningococcal meningitis (15). In one study (26), 80% of the patients with *N. meningitides* had a purpuric or petechial rash, while similar findings were noted in 7% of patients with *S. pneumoniae*. Rashes may also be noted in association with meningitis due to *Staphylococcus, H. influenzae,* or viral meningitides.

An in-depth neurologic examination is obviously of paramount importance in the evaluation of any patient thought to harbor a CNS infectious process. Mental status or behavioral changes are commonly noted with encephalitis and occasionally are the only clinical findings that may suggest the diagnosis of meningitis. Seizures are uncommon in meningococcal meningitis, whereas they may be the sole presenting sign of encephalitis. Seizures noted in association with encephalitis are usually focal; while either focal or generalized seizures may be noted in 10% to 30% of patients with meningitis (10,26). Following a WNV outbreak in New York City (16), neurologic abnormalities included abnormal cranial nerve function (22%), diffuse flaccid paralysis (10%), seizure (3%), and muscle weakness (27%)

DIFFERENTIAL DIAGNOSIS

The differential diagnosis of meningitis and encephalitis includes infectious, neurologic, toxicologic, metabolic, environmental, and behavioral disorders. Infectious disorders include encephalopathy without actual invasion of the brain substance, brain abscesses, septic emboli, and cortical septic thrombophlebitis. Various noninfectious neurologic disorders, such as migraine and other vascular headaches, prolonged postictal states, and new-onset seizures, share some features common to both encephalitis and meningitis.

Drug ingestion (e.g., phencyclidine, salicylates) often presents in the form of febrile, mind-altered states and must be considered in the differential diagnosis. Metabolic disturbances (e.g., electrolyte imbalances, hypoglycemia, and hyperglycemia) and acute environmental toxicity (e.g., heat stroke) must also be considered. Behavioral alterations (e.g., psychosis, mania) should never be considered to be purely of psychological origin without an evaluation for the possibility of underlying organic causes such as meningitis and encephalitis.

EMERGENCY DEPARTMENT EVALUATION

The majority of patients with meningitis or encephalitis who present to the emergency department display the classic complaints of severe headache and fever. Nuchal rigidity may be noted with meningitis and meningoencephalitis, and patients with encephalitis generally demonstrate some symptoms and signs of direct brain involvement. The astute emergency physician is aware that up to 20% of cases of meningitis may present in an atypical fashion and that one must have a high index of suspicion for atypical presentations and maintain a low threshold for performing a lumbar puncture. If meningitis is suspected, obtain cultures and appropriate laboratory studies then administer antibiotics without delay.

Identification of risk factors may aid in the diagnosis of meningitis and assist in directing antibiotic therapy. Most risk factors can be identified with a few questions guided by the six I's:

- *I*nfection (e.g., antecedent or concomitant upper or lower respiratory tract infection, sinusitis, otitis)

- *I*mmunosuppression (e.g., splenectomy, sickle cell disease, corticosteroids, Hodgkin disease, myeloma, organ transplant, AIDS)
- *I*njury (head trauma, neurologic, or otolaryngologic procedures)
- *I*ndwelling (catheters, shunts, ventricular reservoirs)
- *I*mbiber (alcoholic)
- *I*dentification (close contacts, such as spouses, roommates, and paramedics)

Many of the more common viruses causing outbreaks of encephalitis demonstrate characteristic seasonal and geographic distributions. For example, arbovirus and enterovirus infections tend to occur in summer and early fall, mumps in winter and spring, and lymphocytic choriomeningitis in fall and winter. Eastern equine encephalitis occurs in the eastern United States, and Venezuelan equine encephalitis is generally found in Florida and the southwestern United States, whereas Herpes simplex encephalitis demonstrates no characteristic geographic pattern. WNV has spread from the East coast to the Pacific coast with about 85% of human infections occurring in August and September (17). Some important data to be elicited in suspected cases of encephalitis can be summarized through the use of the six V's:

- *V*acation/travel (to endemic areas, foreign or domestic)
- *V*eterinary or other animal contact (rabies)
- *V*ectors (recent mosquito or tick bites)
- *V*iral infections (recent or concurrent)
- *V*accinations (recent for measles, varicella, rubella, rabies)
- *V*ital statistics (contact local or national health agencies regarding outbreaks)

The physical examination should focus on possible sources of infection, namely, the oropharynx, ears, and sinuses. Similarly, the chest examination should focus on evidence of pulmonary or cardiac sources of infection. The entire body should be scrutinized for the presence of any rashes. Funduscopy is mandatory to rule out papilledema. The neurologic examination must be performed in a timely, but meticulous, fashion. With encephalitis, only subtle clues of neurologic dysfunction such as inattention or drowsiness may be noted.

CT Scan

There is controversy regarding the need to perform computed tomography (CT) of the head prior to a lumbar puncture. If a patient has a suspected cerebral mass, focal neurologic findings, a prolonged or deteriorating course or papilledema, the patient should undergo CT of the head. Hasbun (12) concluded that at the age of at least 60 years, immunocompromised status, history of CNS disease, seizure within the last week, abnormal language, inability to correctly answer two consecutive questions, and abnormal level of consciousness were among the findings associated with an abnormal head CT.

Lumbar Puncture

Lumbar puncture is the key to confirming the diagnosis of meningitis and encephalitis. Two definite contraindications to lumbar puncture are infection at the site of the puncture and evidence of obstructive (noncommunicating) hydrocephalus. Papilledema, anticoagulant use, and the presence of a space-occupying lesion in the brain are relative contraindications. In the event that lumbar puncture is required in a patient with papilledema, one may consider withdrawing a small amount of fluid with a 22- or 24-gauge needle. Cerebrospinal fluid (CSF) evaluation includes a cell count and differential, gram stain, culture, protein, and glucose. CSF tests may also include bacterial antigens, polymerase chain reaction (PCR), lactate or antibody titers.

Cerebrospinal Fluid Parameters

Gram Stain

The visualization of the responsible organism on a CSF gram stain is pathognomonic of bacterial meningitis. Gram-stained, centrifuged samples of CSF demonstrate bacterial organisms in 80% to 90% of culture-proven cases of bacterial meningitis (2). India ink preparations for the detection of fungal elements in CSF are positive in as few as one-half of cases. Similarly, acid-fast smears of CSF for diagnosing tuberculous meningitis are not consistently sensitive.

Antigen, PCR, and Antibody Detection

Several ancillary CSF tests may identify a bacterial or viral source of CNS infection. CSF antigen studies are available for *H. influenza* type B, *N. meningitides* A, B, C, Y, W-135, *S. agalactiae* (Group B), *S. pneumoniae*, and E. coli. These antigen studies may identify an organism when the gram stain is equivocal or "negative." Following antibiotic therapy, bacterial antigens may persist in the CSF for several days (28). PCR tests may identify serogroup-specific *N. meningitides* DNA (22) or specific viruses (21). Enterovirus may be diagnosed with enterovirus-specific reverse transcriptase chain reaction PCR test (20). IgM antibodies in the CSF may be detected within 8 days of symptoms in patients with WNV meningoencephalitis (17).

Glucose

Normally, the ratio of CSF to serum glucose concentration is 0.60. Hypoglycorrhachia—a CSF glucose level of less than 50 mg/dL, or a CSF/serum glucose ratio of less than 0.50, is noted in more than 50% of cases of bacterial, fungal, and tuberculous meningitis. Normal CSF glucose levels are generally noted in most viral meningitides and encephalitides.

Protein

Normal protein levels in the CSF range from 15 to 45 mg/dL. Subarachnoid space infection results in increased protein permeability of the choroid plexus, ependyma, and pia mater. Marked protein elevations are observed in bacterial, fungal, and tuberculous meningitis. Viral meningitides or encephalitides generally manifest normal or only moderately elevated levels of protein (18). The presence of 1,000 RBCs in the CSF corresponds to a 1 mg increase in CSF protein.

Lactic Acid

CSF lactic acid levels are usually normal in viral meningitis and have been reported to be elevated in bacterial, fungal, and tuberculous meningitis (13). Elevated CSF lactic acid, coupled with other CSF findings and the history and physical examination, may also be of diagnostic utility in partially treated meningitides (11).

Cell Count and Differential

Normal CSF has a white blood cell (WBC) count of less than 5 cells/mm^3 and all of the cells are mononuclear. Following centrifugation, the finding of a single CSF granulocytic cell may be considered normal if the total CSF WBC count is less than 5 cells/mm (3,7). Bacterial meningitis is classically described as having CSF cell counts ranging from 100 to 10,000 cells/mm^3 with polymorphonuclear forms predominating early. In the acute stages of viral encephalitis, a mild-to-moderate rise in mononuclear lymphocytes (e.g., 10 to 250 cells) is noted, with higher cell counts suggestive of concomitant meningeal involve-

ment. In WNV meningoencephalitis, CSF findings include an elevated protein count and pleocytosis with a predominance of lymphocytes.

The normal CSF has no RBCs. The hemorrhagic lesion of herpes encephalitis may lead to an elevated RBC count in the CSF or xanthochromia. A traumatic LP may lead to an increase of one WBC/700-1,000 RBCs.

There is considerable overlap in the CSF findings of bacterial meningitis, the aseptic meningitis syndrome, and encephalitis. It has been reported that as many as 10% of patients with bacterial meningitis initially demonstrate a CSF lymphocytosis (2,18). Viral meningitis characteristically manifests a CSF lymphocytosis with cell counts of 10 to 1000 cells/mm^3. In viral meningitis, there is usually a predominance of mononuclear cells, a normal glucose concentration, and a slightly to moderately increased protein level. Occasionally, in early cases of viral meningitis, the CSF WBC count will exceed 1,000 cells/mm^3 and the neutrophils will predominate. Mononuclear cells usually predominate in cases of tuberculous, fungal or aseptic meningitis syndrome. Tuberculous and fungal meningitis may also present with CSF findings of neutrophilia, a normal to decreased glucose and an elevated protein.

CSF obtained very early in the course of bacterial meningitis may be totally devoid of cells, organisms or abnormalities in glucose or protein levels. Occasionally, the CSF in fulminant meningitis demonstrates no cells but is teeming with bacteria. Although no single CSF laboratory value can, of itself, make the diagnosis of meningitis when the Gram stain is negative, certain patterns are more closely related to certain etiologic agents. A pattern of CSF neutrophilia, very low glucose (5 to 20 mg/dL), and elevated protein (100 mg/dL) strongly suggests bacterial meningitis.

Cultures

The CSF should be cultured in all cases of suspected meningitis. The diagnosis is made only from the culture in about 20% of cases (4,9). One study noted negative blood and CSF cultures in 11% of patients with meningitis (26). Talan's review noted that about 50% of patients with bacterial meningitis had positive blood cultures (28). Cultures take on even more importance in fungal and tuberculous meningitis, in which the India ink or acid-fast preparations are negative in 50% or more of cases (2,27).

EMERGENCY DEPARTMENT MANAGEMENT

The patient who presents to the emergency department with fever, nuchal rigidity, AMS and headache should be considered to have meningitis until proven otherwise. An altered sensorium accompanied by fever and headache should also prompt consideration of encephalitis. If meningitis is suspected, antimicrobial therapy should be promptly administered and not withheld pending lumbar puncture or laboratory results. It is unlikely that antibiotic administration will alter CSF parameters within one to two hours (19,28). A retrospective bacterial meningitis study by Blazer noted that in 65 of 68 children that the cytology and biochemistry of the CSF was not altered by 44 to 68 hours of IV antibiotics (3). Blazer concluded that it was less likely that partial antibiotic treatment would distort a "bacterial" CSF.

Empiric antibiotic therapy for meningitis should be directed against *S. pneumoniae*, *N. meningitiditis* and *H. influenzae* (Table 138.1) Patients should be promptly treated with a 3rd generation cephalosporin (Cefotaxime or Ceftriaxone 2 grams i.v.) and Vancomycin (15 mg/kg, maximum of 1 gram) (19).

There has been controversy regarding the administration of steroids to patients with bacterial meningitis. A recent publication concluded that treatment with dexamethasone (10 mg i.v.)

TABLE 138.1. Empiric Parenteral Antibiotic Therapy for Meningitis

---

Ceftriaxone or Cefotaxime (2 g) and Vancomycin (15 mg/kg, max 1 gram)
If penicillin/cephalosporin allergy:
  Vancomycin (15 mg/kg) and chloramphenicol (25 mg/kg, max 1 gram)
  If chloramphenicol is not available:
    Consider Vancomycin with:
    Ciprofloxacin* (400 mg i.v.) or Levofloxacin* (500 mg i.v.)
Dexamethasone 10 mg i.v. for suspected pneumococcal meningitis
If suspicion of Listeria (adults > 50):
  Ampicillin (2 g i.v.) or
  Trimethoprim-sulfamethoxazole (80 mg TMP/400 mg TMX/5 cc) (15–20 mg/kg/day, Q 6–8 hrs)
  May add gentamicin (2.5 mg/kg i.v.)
If suspicion of Group B Streptococcus:
  Ampicillin (2 g i.v.)
If immunocompromised, recent head trauma or neurosurgical procedure add:
  Ceftazidime (2 g i.v.)

*Quinolones are not promoted for use in bacterial meningitis

---

15 to 20 minutes before or with the antibiotic and then every 6 hours for 4 days, improved outcome in patients with bacterial meningitis; particularly in patients with penicillin-susceptible pneumococcal meningitis (8). There are concerns that steroids may decrease the CNS penetration of vancomycin and decrease its efficacy. For adult patients with pneumococcal meningitis who are treated with dexamethasone, it has been recommended to add rifampin (600 mg i.v.) (19,29).

There are limited antibiotics available for patients with severe allergic reactions to penicillin or 3rd generation cephalosporins. Chloramphenicol may not be available on the hospital formulary. Vancomycin does not provide ideal coverage for empiric treatment of bacterial meningitis. Quinolones have not been promoted for treating bacterial meningitis and there are limited data available regarding CNS penetration and efficacy of selected quinolones (14). As a result, the emergency medicine physician and an infectious disease specialist, may consider treatment with an i.v. quinolone.

For AIDS-associated cryptococcal meningoencephalitis, i.v. amphotericin (0.6 to 0.8 mg/kg/day) and flucytosine (100 mg/kg/day) have been recommended for induction therapy. If the examination suggests the possibility of herpes encephalitis, i.v. acyclovir is instituted at 10 mg/kg over 1 hour. The identification of nonviral agents of encephalitis (e.g., syphilis, toxoplasmosis, tuberculosis) will guide specific therapy. Patients with clinical evaluation suggestive of viral meningitis and equivocal CSF findings should have strong consideration given for a second lumbar puncture in 8 to 24 hours. Cases of uncomplicated viral meningitis may be treated with antipyretics and supportive care and may be discharged from the hospital when the diagnosis is definite. For patients with probable viral meningitis who are admitted to hospital, the decision to institute antibiotic coverage in the ED should be made by the emergency medicine physician on the basis of the patient's clinical picture and associated risk factors.

Chemoprophylaxis

Although no hard and fast rules exist for ascertaining who should receive chemoprophylaxis after exposure to individuals with bacterial meningitis, certain guidelines may be useful. Close contacts (e.g., families, roommates, daycare contacts) of patients with meningococcal meningitis have an increased risk (400-800 fold) of contracting the disease (22). Close contacts with

H. influenzae meningitis also have increased risks of contracting the disease. Clearly, these individuals deserve the benefit of chemoprophylaxis. Paramedics and hospital personnel who have had close contact with the patient should also receive chemoprophylaxis.

Rifampin (20 mg/kg/day for 4 days, maximum of 600 mg/day) is the approved prophylaxis regimen for *H. influenza* meningitis. For *N. meningitidis*, the rifampin dose is 600 mg orally every 12 hours for a total of four doses. Alternative prophylaxis regimens for *N. meningitidis* include ciprofloxacin (500-mg single dose), ceftriaxone (250 mg IM, if pregnant) or a single oral dose of azithromycin (500 mg). Individuals at risk for pneumococcal meningitis (e.g., postsplenectomy) should receive oral penicillin (500 mg every 6 hours for 7 days).

It is important to emphasize that 5% to 10% of adults are asymptomatic nasopharyngeal carriers of *N. meningitides* and most are not pathogenic. Oropharyngeal or nasopharyngeal cultures are not helpful in determining chemoprophylaxis (22). Antibiotics that eliminate nasopharyngeal carriage of *N. meningitides* include rifampin, ciprofloxacin, and cefriaxone.

The quadrivalent meningococcal vaccine (A, C, Y, W-135) has been recommended for outbreaks and military personnel. The American College Health Association recommends that college students consider the meningococcal vaccine (6). The quadrivalent vaccine is ineffective in children less than 2 years of age. As part of a preventive care, the pneumococcal vaccine should be given to patients over the age of 65.

CRITICAL INTERVENTIONS

- Administer antibiotics promptly and before lumbar puncture if meningitis is suspected after obtaining cultures and appropriate laboratory studies Obtain cultures and laboratory studies prior to antibiotic administration
- Perform head CT for suspected cerebral mass, focal neurologic findings, a prolonged or deteriorating course, papilledema, immunocompromised status, history of CNS disease, seizure within the last week, abnormal language, inability to correctly answer two consecutive questions, and abnormal level of consciousness
- Provide prophylaxis to significant contacts of patients with meningococcal or *H. influenzae* meningitis including families, roommates, daycare, paramedics and hospital personnel who have had close contact

DISPOSITION

All patients with bacterial meningitis require IV antibiotics and hospital admission. Patients with clinical evaluation suggestive of viral meningitis and equivocal CSF findings should have strong consideration given for a second lumbar puncture in 8 to 24 hours. Cases of uncomplicated viral meningitis may be treated with antipyretics and supportive care and may be discharged from the hospital when the diagnosis is definite. For patients with probable viral meningitis who are admitted to hospital, the decision to institute antibiotic coverage in the ED should be made by the emergency medicine physician on the basis of the patient's clinical picture and associated risk factors.

COMMON PITFALLS

✔ Relying on classic signs and symptoms alone, which results in some cases of meningitis being missed because of atypical presentations

✔ Failure to appreciate occasional overlap in CSF findings between aseptic and bacterial meningitis
✔ Delay in starting antibiotic therapy when there is a reasonable suspicion of meningitis

Acknowledgments

Thanks to the previous edition's chapter authors Raymond J. Roberge, Ralph J. Riviello and Douglas A. Rund.

References

1. Attia J, Hatala R, Cook DJ, et al. Does this adult patient have acute meningitis? *JAMA* 1999;282:175–181.
2. Benson CA, Harris AA. Acute neurologic infections. *Med Clin North Am* 1986;70:987.
3. Blazer S, Berant M, Alon U. Effect of antibiotic treatment on cerebrospinal fluid. *Am J Clin Pathology* 1983;80:386–397.
4. Bohr V, Paulson CB, Rasmussen N. Pneumococcal meningitis: Late neurological sequelae and features of prognostic impact. *Arch Neurol* 1984;41:1045.
5. Bolan G, Barza M. Acute bacterial meningitis in children and adults: A perspective. *Med Clin North Am* 1985;69:231.
6. Bruce MG, Rosenstein NE, Capparella JM, et al. Risk factors for meningococcal disease in college students. *JAMA* 2001;286:688–693.
7. Conley JM, Ronald AR. Cerebrospinal fluid as a diagnostic body fluid. *Am J Med* 1983;76:102.
8. De Gans JD, De Beek DV, et al. Dexamethasone in adults with bacterial meningitis. *NEJM* 347:1549–1556.
9. Dougherty JM, Jones J. Cerebrospinal fluid cultures and analysis. *Ann Emerg Med* 1986;15:317.
10. Durand ML, Calderwood SB, Weber DJ, et al. Acute bacterial meningitis in adults. A review of 493 episodes. *NEJM* 1993;328:21–28.
11. Genton B, Berger JP. Cerebrospinal fluid lactate in 78 cases of adult meningitis. *Intensive Care Med* 1990;16:196.
12. Hasbun R, Abrahams J, Jekel J, et al. Computed tomography of the head before lumbar puncture in adults with suspected meningitis. *NEJM* 2001;345:1727–1733.
13. Lindquist L, Linne T, Hansson LO, et al. Value of cerebrospinal fluid analysis in the differential diagnosis of meningitis: a study in 710 patients with suspected central nervous system infection. *Eur J Microbiol Infect Dis* 1988;7:374.
14. Lutsar A, McCracken GH, Friedland IR. Antibiotic pharmacokinetics in cerebrospinal fluid. *Clin Infectious Diseases* 1998;27:1117–1129.
15. Mancebo J, Domingo P, Blanch L, et al. The predictive value of petechiae in adults with bacterial meningitis. *JAMA* 1986;156:2820.
16. Nash D, Mostashari F, Fine A, et al. The outbreak of West Nile Virus in the New York City area in 1999. *NEJM* 2001;344:1807–1814.
17. Petersen LR, Marfin AA, Gubler DJ. West Nile Virus. *JAMA* 2003;290:524–528.
18. Powers WJ. Cerebrospinal fluid lymphocytosis in acute bacterial meningitis. *Am J Med* 1985;19:216.
19. Quagliarello VJ, Scheld VM. Treatment of bacterial meningitis. *NEJM* 1997;336:708–716.
20. Ramers C, Billman G, Hartin M, et al. Impact of a diagnostic cerebrospinal fluid enterovirus polymerase chain reaction test on patient management. *JAMA* 2000;283:2680–2685.
21. Read SJ, Jeffery KJM, Bangham CRM. Aseptic meningitis and Encephalitis: The role of PCR in the diagnostic laboratory. *J Clinical Microbiology* 1997;35:691–696.
22. Rosenstein NE, Perkins BA, Stephens DS, et al. Meningococcal Disease. *NEJM* 2001;344:1378–1388.
23. Rowland LP ed. *Merritt's Textbook of Neurology*, 9th Edition. Williams and Wilkins, 1995:107–117.
24. Schuchat A, Robinson K, Wenger JD, et al. Bacterial meningitis is the United States in 1995. *N Engl J Med* 1997;337:970.
25. Seligman S. The rapid differential diagnosis of meningitis. *Med Clin North Am* 1973;57:1417.
26. Sigurdardottir B, Byrnsson OM, Jonsdotter KE, et al. Acute bacterial meningitis in adults. A 20-year overview. *Arch Intern Med* 1997;157:425–431.
27. Stockstill MT, Kauffman CA. Comparison of cryptococcal and tuberculous meningitis. *Arch Neurol* 1983;40:81.
28. Talan DA, Hoffman JR, Yoshikawa TT, et al. Role of empiric antibiotics prior to lumbar puncture in suspected meningitis: State of the art. *Rev of Infect Diseases* 1988;10:365.
29. Williams AJ, Nadel S. Bacterial Meningitis. Current controversies in approaches to treatment. *CNS Drugs* 2001;15:909–919.

CHAPTER 139
Central Nervous System Abscess

E. Bradshaw Bunney

Central nervous system suppurative infections include brain abscess, cranial subdural empyema, cranial epidural abscess, and spinal epidural abscess. Although uncommon, they can produce serious morbidity and mortality if their diagnosis is delayed. The emergency physician must consider these conditions when evaluating patients who present with headache, fever, alteration of consciousness, back pain or new neurologic deficits. Early identification with the administration of antibiotics and immediate neurosurgical consultation can result in an improved outcome.

BRAIN ABSCESS

Brain abscesses can range from microscopic collections of inflammatory cells to necrosis of an entire hemisphere. Brain abscess is the most common intracranial focal suppurative process but only occurs about 2% as commonly as brain tumors. It accounts for 4 to 10 cases per year on a busy neurosurgical service, or for approximately 1 in 10,000 hospital admissions (7,21). The incidence had been declining due to improved therapy for otic and sinus infections; however, an increase in its incidence may be seen due to enhanced use of neurosurgical procedures, improved imaging techniques, and an increasing population of immune-compromised patients (7).

There is a 2 to 3:1 male-to-female predominance. The age distribution relates to the predisposing condition. Abscess from an otic origin usually occurs in those less than 20 years old or more than 40 years old. With a paranasal sinus focus, most patients are 10 to 30 years of age. Approximately 25% of cases occur in children less than 15 years old and are most commonly due to cyanotic congenital heart disease or otic sources. An abscess rarely occurs in those less than 2 years of age, but when it does, it is often secondary to gram-negative bacillary meningitis (7,21).

Brain abscesses arise from either contiguous or hematogenous spread from an infectious source. Contiguous spread from craniofacial sites (middle ear, sinuses, dental) account for about one third of all cases (12,17,21). Otitis media (chronic) and mastoiditis classically spread to the temporal lobe (50% to 75% of cases) and the cerebellum (one-third of cases). Approximately 85% to 99% of cerebellar abscesses are from an otic source. Frontal and ethmoidal sinusitis spread to the frontal lobe. Dental sources also tend to affect the frontal lobe (7,21). Posttraumatic (penetrating) and post neurosurgical procedure abscesses now account for up to 24% of cases (17). These contiguous infections can lead to abscess formation by two mechanisms: by direct extension through infected bone or by retrograde thrombophlebitis from emissary and diploic veins (7,12,21).

About 25% of cases arise from hematogenous spread from a cardiac or pulmonary source, including lung abscess, bronchiectasis, cyanotic congenital heart disease (tetralogy of Fallot), and bacterial endocarditis. It is important to note that most of these sources of hematogenous spread occur from areas of relatively low oxygen tension thus leading to a strong predominance of anaerobic organisms. Hematogenously spread abscesses tend to be multiple and lie in the distribution of the middle cerebral artery at the gray-white junction where microcirculatory flow is poorest. Other causes include hereditary hemorrhagic telangiectasia (Osler-Weber-Rendu disease), dental extractions, abdominal or pelvic infections, and following esophageal stricture dilation and endoscopic sclerosis of esophageal varices (7,21). There is no clearly identifiable cause in the remaining 10% to 15% of cases (21).

The blood-brain barrier (BBB) is quite resistant to penetration of these microorganisms from the blood into the brain, which is why this condition is so rare, despite the frequency of bacteremia. Improved microbiologic culture techniques have yielded a better understanding of the microbiology of brain abscesses. The microbiology is location dependent, and over 50% of abscesses involve mixed flora (8,16,21). Anaerobes play a large role, being isolated in 40% to 60% of cases (7). The most commonly isolated anaerobes are *Bacteroides* species (from ear or sinus infection) and anaerobic streptococci (from dental and chronic pulmonary infections). Aerobic and microaerophilic streptococci (*Streptococcus milleri*, *S. viridans*) are the most common bacteria isolated, being found in up to 70% of abscesses (7). *Staphylococcus aureus* and *S. epidermis* are frequently isolated from posttraumatic or postsurgical abscesses. Gram-negative bacilli, found in 23% to 33% of cases, are associated with chronic otitis, postoperative infections, and abdominopelvic infection (7,21).

Granulocytopenia, cellular and humoral-mediated immune dysfunction are predisposing factors to the development of CNS infections in immune compromised patients. The acquired immunodeficiency syndrome (AIDS) and the increasing use of immunosuppressive drug therapy have lead to more atypical, fungal, and protozoal brain abscesses, such as *Nocardia, Listeria, Cryptococcus, Mycobacterium, Aspergillus,* and *Candida. Toxoplasmosis gondii* is the most common cause of brain abscess in patients with AIDS (6,7,11). However, the recommendations for the management of intracranial mass lesions in human immunodeficiency virus-infected individuals have changed as the incidence of toxoplasmic encephalitis has decreased with the use of trimethoprim-sulfamethoxazole prophylaxis (3). Another important subgroup of patients with a compromised immune system are transplant patients. Brain abscesses occur in approximately 1% of transplant recipients. Fungi, particularly Aspergillus are the most frequent etiological agent (20).

CLINICAL PRESENTATION

The classic triad of fever, headache, and focal neurologic deficit is present in less than half of patients who present with a brain abscess (7). There are no pathognomonic signs for a brain abscess, therefore, history and a high clinical suspicion are important features to proper diagnosis.

Headache, the earliest presenting symptom, is present in 70% of patients and is frequently severe, hemicranial, and persistent. The headache is usually insidious occurring over days to weeks. Abrupt onset of the headache is a poor prognostic indicator. Fever is absent in more than 50% of patients. Alterations in consciousness, ranging from drowsiness to coma, occur in 50% of cases, as do nausea and vomiting. A focal neurologic deficit is seen in 50% to 75% of patients, and can include aphasia, hemiparesis, visual fields deficits, nystagmus, or ataxia. Cerebellar abscesses are usually associated with ataxia and dizziness. Cranial nerve findings are suggestive of a brainstem abscess. These physical findings may be helpful in localizing the abscess. Focal or generalized seizures occur in 30% of cases. These seizures generally respond to benzodiazepines. Unfortunately, papilledema is a late and often absent finding (7,13,21,23).

The patient with a brain abscess is at risk for three major complications producing sudden deterioration: uncal or tonsillar herniation, hemorrhage into an abscess, or rupture of the abscess into the ventricular or subarachnoid space (7,16,24). Severe morbidity and mortality have been associated with abrupt onset of symptoms, depressed mental status at presentation, multiple abscess locations and hematogenous dissemination (4,19).

DIFFERENTIAL DIAGNOSIS

Primary or metastatic brain tumor can mimic cerebral abscess on a computed tomography (CT) scan. History and CT appearance easily differentiate other infectious diseases, such as viral encephalitis, subdural empyema, epidural abscess, and meningitis. Subarachnoid hemorrhage, cerebral infarction, central nervous system (CNS) vasculitis, and migraines can mimic abscesses (7,8,23,24).

Immune compromised patients account for a large proportion of patients presenting to the emergency department (ED) with intracranial mass lesions. Because of the wide variety of pathologic processes involving the CNS of immune-compromised patients, brain biopsy is often needed for definitive diagnosis and treatment. Other considerations include *Cryptococcus, Candida,* lymphoma, Kaposi sarcoma, and progressive multifocal leukoencephalopathy (6,11).

EMERGENCY DEPARTMENT EVALUATION

The history and physical examination should focus on sites of potential infection and the possibility of life-threatening complications. Routine laboratory evaluation is rarely helpful. Leukocytosis may be present, but approximately 30% to 40% of patients will have a normal white blood cell count. An elevated erythrocyte sedimentation rate is seen in only 40% of cases, however, the C-reactive protein may help to distinguish abscess from tumor. Blood cultures are positive in about 10% of cases, but should be obtained even if the patient is afebrile. Lumbar puncture is relatively contraindicated in patients with brain abscess. Chest films may reveal a pulmonic source of infection; sinus or mastoid films may identify infection in these areas.

MRI and CT scan are the studies of choice when evaluating a patient for a brain abscess. Diffusion-weighted MRI provides greater detail but is less readily available in many hospitals. In addition, MRI is not accessible to critically ill patients. Therefore, a CT scan remains a very good alternative. MRI has better sensitivity and specificity than contrast CT. MRI is better at detecting mass effect, edema, petechial hemorrhage, smaller lesions, and multifocal involvement (10).

A CT scan of the brain, with and without contrast, is the most likely study to be obtained. CT has a reported sensitivity of 95% to 99% (7). CT helps to localize the abscess and stage its evolution. During the "early cerebritis" stage (first 3 days), a CT scan reveals an irregular area of low density representing focal inflammation and edema. This area does not enhance with contrast and represents the necrotic center of the abscess. In the late cerebritis stage (days 4–9), patchy enhancement is present and the necrotic center develops. As the abscess evolves into the early capsule stage (days 10–14), a homogenous central area of low density is seen, and a thick, diffuse, ringlike vascular capsule is present. This enhancement correlates with formation of the collagen capsule. During the late capsule stage (after day 14) the ring becomes thinner as the capsular development progresses, and it is narrower on the ventricular surface of the abscess (5). Features that help to identify the mass as an abscess include gas within the center of the mass, a thinner rim (less than 5 mm), and ependymal enhancement. Patients given corticosteroids may have diminished enhancement of the abscess ring (7). If clinical suspicion is high and a CT scan is negative, an MRI should be performed.

EMERGENCY DEPARTMENT MANAGEMENT

Initial management of the patient with a suspected brain abscess includes airway control, intravenous access, and maintenance of adequate ventilation and circulation. If signs of elevated intracranial pressure and/or impending herniation are present, one must act rapidly to reduce the pressure. These are, however, only temporizing measures and include intubating and hyperventilating the patient, elevating the head of the bed 30 degrees, and instituting pharmacologic therapy with mannitol and dexamethasone. Immediate neurosurgical consultation is required.

Definitive management includes antibiotic therapy and surgical decompression. Immediate surgical decompression is indicated if there is a deteriorating level of consciousness, increasing neurologic deficit, or signs of increasing intracranial pressure (8). Surgical options include drainage, aspiration, or excision of the abscess (13). Intravenous antibiotics should be initiated in the ED and should be selected to treat likely pathogens. Table 139.1 outlines the choices of empiric antibiotics based on the suspected source of the abscess and organisms involved (1,7,12,15,21). Pending culture and sensitivity results, one standard regimen includes a third-generation cephalosporin plus metronidazole. In post surgical or posttraumatic abscesses, vancomycin or an antistaphylococcal penicillin should be used to cover *Staphylococcus*. If *Pseudomonas* is thought to be a causative organism, ceftazidime plus an aminoglycoside should be used (23).

Corticosteroids should be reserved specifically for treating any significant cerebral edema associated with the abscess; in other circumstances, the use of steroids is associated with increased mortality. Because corticosteroids may reduce antibiotic penetration into the abscess cavity and may delay encapsulation, they are indicated only when there is evidence of a significant mass effect, with progressive neurologic deficit or changing level of consciousness (7,8,21). The standard regimen is dexamethasone 10 to 12 mg intravenously, followed by 4 mg every 6 hours.

DISPOSITION

All patients diagnosed with a brain abscess in the ED require admission to the hospital and immediate neurosurgical consultation. If a neurosurgeon is not available, arrangements should be made for transfer to a neurosurgical center after stabilization. Young persons, those without underlying disease, and those without neurologic deterioration or mental status changes have a better prognosis. With early diagnosis, advanced neuroradiologic imaging, and rapid treatment, mortality is less than 30%, but in patients presenting with signs of herniation, mortality is greater than 50% (7,16,21). Persistent neurologic deficits, including seizure, intellectual or behavioral impairment, and motor deficits, are seen in 30% to 55% of patients (7).

CRANIAL EPIDURAL AND SUBDURAL SPACE INFECTIONS

Subdural empyema and cranial epidural abscess are rare but life-threatening intracranial suppurative infections. Subdural empyema accounts for 15% to 25% of focal intracranial infections, while cranial epidural abscess is much less common. Subdural empyema is a disease of teen-agers and young adults, with most cases occurring in the 10- to 40-year age group. On the other hand, epidural abscess rarely occurs in young children and has been reported in patients from ages 12 to 68. Both conditions exhibit a 3:1 male-to-female predominance (7).

Subdural empyema forms between the dura mater and arachnoid mater, while cranial epidural abscess forms outside the dura mater. Both entities share a similar pathogenesis and etiology, and the two infections can coexist. The infections are thought to occur through direct extension or by hematogenous spread through the emissary veins (7,21). Paranasal sinus disease, especially frontal and ethmoidal sinusitis, accounts for 60% to 70% of cases. Other causes include cranial osteomyelitis, mastoiditis, otitis media, head trauma, cranial surgery, ventriculoperitoneal shunt, halo traction pins, orbital infections, and chronic subdural hematoma (7,9,12). In children, bacterial meningitis is the most common predisposing condition (21).

TABLE 139.1.   Choices of Empiric Antibiotics Based on the Suspected Source of the Abscess and Pathogens Involved

Source	Anatomic Location	Causative Agent	Treatment*
Penetrating trauma	Depends on site	*St. aureus* *Clostridia sp.* *Enterobacteriacaea*	Nafcillin + Cefotaxime
Postoperative	Variable	*St. epi,* and *aureus* *Enterobacteriacaea* *Pseudomonal sp.*	Vancomycin + Ceftazidime
Paranasal sinuses	Frontal lobe	Aerobic & anaerobic *streptococci* *Hemophilus sp.* Anaerobes (bacteroides, fusobacteria)	Penicillin (or cefotaxime) + Metronidazole
Otogenic	Temporal lobe Cerebellum	*Streptococci* *Enterobacteriacaea* Pseudomonas aeruginosa *Bacteroides sp.*	Penicillin + Metronidazole + Cefotaxime
Hematogenous	Multiple lesions, often in the MCA territory	Depends on source Endocarditis Intraabdominal Lung abscess	Nafcillin + Metronidazole + Cefotaxime

*The IV dosages for adults of these antibiotics are:
Cefotaxime: 1–2 gm q4–8h (max 12gm/d)
Ceftazidime: 1–2 gm q4–8h (max 12gm/d)
Metronidazole: 500 mg q6h
Nafcillin: 2 gm q4h
Penicillin G: 2–4 million units q4h
Vancomycin: 1 gm q12h

The microbiology of these infections can be predicted by the primary source of infection. Aerobic, anaerobic, and microaerophilic streptococci are isolated in the majority of cases due to otorhinogenic origin. *S. aureus* and coagulase-negative staphylococci are found in sinus, otic, postoperative, and posttraumatic cases. Gram-negative bacilli can usually be seen in otic and posttraumatic sources. Polymicrobial infections are common, and a sterile culture may be found in 20% to 30% of cases. In children, the most common causative agents are those responsible for the underlying meningitis (7,9,21).

CLINICAL PRESENTATION

The clinical presentation of subdural empyema is fever, headache, and nuchal rigidity. The nonspecific symptoms of a sinus or ear infection, fever and malaise rapidly progress to severe headache and meningismus. A classic presentation is a young male with frontal sinusitis, who develops progressive obtundation and hemiparesis (12). The headache, present in 90% of cases, is focal but then becomes more generalized. Nausea and vomiting are common. Varying degrees of encephalopathy can be seen, ranging from mild confusion to coma. Focal neurologic signs (including hemiparesis, third and sixth cranial nerve palsies, and focal or generalized seizures) are seen in 75% of patients (7,21). Postoperative and posttraumatic subdural empyema has a very indolent course due to the slow accumulation of fluid. Headache is often absent, and the disease course is more benign (2,7).

The presentation of epidural abscess is more insidious. Symptoms can take weeks to months to develop. Patients often present with a long history of nonspecific symptoms, without focal signs or mental status changes. Once the fluid mass reaches critical size, nausea, vomiting, headache, drowsiness, and lethargy occur. Focal neurologic signs, seizure, and coma do not occur unless the infection spreads to the subdural space or cerebral herniation occurs. A patient with an epidural abscess involving the petrous bone may present with unilateral facial pain and fifth and sixth cranial nerve palsies, leading to lateral rectus weakness (Gradenigo syndrome) (2,7,9).

DIFFERENTIAL DIAGNOSIS

The initial presentation of subdural empyema and epidural abscess is similar to that of other intracranial processes. Meningitis, brain abscess, subdural hematoma, subarachnoid hemorrhage, herpes encephalitis, venous sinus thrombosis, and tumor should be considered (2,7). CT scanning and the more sensitive MRI allows definitive diagnosis in most cases.

EMERGENCY DEPARTMENT EVALUATION

History and physical examination should focus on finding potential sources of infection. A detailed neurologic examination should be performed. Routine laboratory evaluation is of limited value. The white blood cell count may be only mildly elevated and oftentimes is normal. The sedimentation rate may be elevated if osteomyelitis is present (9). CSF analysis is usually not helpful and is relatively contraindicated, due to the risk of herniation (2,7).

CT scanning with intravenous contrast remains the mainstay of ED diagnosis for both subdural empyema and cranial epidural abscess. Subdural empyema reveals a crescent-shaped, hypodense fluid collection in the subdural space, with displacement of the arachnoid. A mass effect is common, and an enhancing rim may be seen. Epidural abscess appears as a poorly defined, lentiform, extraaxial area of low or intermediate density. A hypodense, medial enhancing rim, representing inflamed dura, helps to differentiate it from a subdural collection (22). Cranial osteomyelitis may be detected (7,21).

Diffusion-weighted MRI with gadolinium is more sensitive in detecting these processes, but may not be readily available in most EDs. MRI advantages include increased delineation between bone, CSF, and brain parenchyma; better ability to localize fluid to the epidural or subdural space; ability to characterize fluid type (blood, pus, or sterile effusion) in the collection; and ready detection of subtle edema and parenchymal abnormalities (7,22). MRI should be used when CT scanning is negative in the face of high clinical suspicion.

EMERGENCY DEPARTMENT MANAGEMENT

Once the diagnosis is made, immediate neurosurgical consultation is required. If signs of impending herniation are present, temporizing measures must be employed.

Antibiotic coverage should begin in the ED. The choice of antibiotic should be tailored to the suspected source until culture results are available. A scheme for antibiotic selection is outlined in Table 139.1.

DISPOSITION

All patients require admission. If neurosurgical services are not available, the patient, once stabilized, should be transferred to an appropriate center with available neurosurgical services. Patients with an isolated cranial epidural abscess have an excellent prognosis. Most recover with good neurologic outcome.

The mortality for subdural empyema ranges from 6% to 20%. Of those that survive, 15% to 44% have a persistent neurologic deficit (seizure disorder, hemiparesis, aphasia). Outcome is directly related to advanced patient age, degree of encephalopathy present, and delay to appropriate therapy.

SPINAL EPIDURAL ABSCESS

Spinal epidural abscess (SEA) is a rare disease, accounting for less than 1 case per 10,000 hospital admissions. The major risk factors for SEA are intravenous drug abuse, diabetes, trauma, prior spinal surgery, immunocompromised host, and a history of a spinal nerve block. Males are more commonly affected than females by a 2:1 ratio. Ages range from infancy to elderly, with a peak incidence between ages 40 and 60. The most frequently isolated organism is *Staphylococcus aureus,* with up to 15% being methicillin-resistant strained. *Streptococcus, Escherichia coli, Pseudomonas, Klebsiella, Acinetobacter* and *Mycobacterium tuberculosis* have also been found (18).

CLINICAL PRESENTATION

Back pain is the most common complaint, followed by paresthesia, motor deficit and fever. Nearly all patients with spinal epidural abscess have back or neck pain at the site of the abscess, but fever is noted in less than 50% of patients at the time of presentation. Sensory and motor deficits are also seen in less than 50% of patients. Symptoms can occur within hours, or take weeks to months to develop. If neurologic deficits are present, particularly for greater than 48 hours prior to arrival, the prognosis for a full recovery is worse.

DIFFERENTIAL DIAGNOSIS

The presentation of a spinal epidural abscess is similar to that of many types of back pain. Other diagnoses to keep in mind when evaluating a patient with back pain include intervertebral disc herniation, metastatic epidural spinal cord compression, spinal epidural hematoma and simple back strain. Separating these requires a thorough history and physical exam. MRI and CT scan provide further information as to the cause of the back pain.

EMERGENCY DEPARTMENT EVALUATION

The back pain associated with a spinal epidural abscess is usually radicular. Radicular pain is caused by irritation of the nerve roots, usually caused by compression. Radicular pain usually circumscribes the territory of innervation of the given nerve root. In addition, radicular pain is frequently exacerbated by any maneuver that raises the pressure of cerebrospinal fluid, such as Valsalva or cough. Most patients with radicular back pain will recline on their side with knee and hips flexed to decrease strain on the nerve root. The straight leg raising maneuver is positive if radicular pain is produced before the leg makes a 70-degree angle with the bed. Tension on the inflamed nerve root is what makes this occur. Further evidence of radicular pain is exacerbation of the pain of straight leg raising with dorsiflexion of the foot, and relief of the pain of straight leg raising with flexion of the knee.

A peripheral white blood cell count may be helpful if it is elevated, but it may be elevated in only 60% of patients with SEA. The erythrocyte sedimentation rate may also be elevated; in one study it was elevated in all 50 patients with SEA who were tested (18). Plain spinal radiographs are helpful only if there is vertebral involvement. MRI is the test of choice because of the enhanced definition of soft tissue structures. If MRI is not available, CT scan can allow for detection of a mass within the spinal canal and assess for both spinal cord impingement and vertebral involvement.

EMERGENCY DEPARTMENT MANAGEMENT

Surgery and antibiotics are the mainstays of therapy. Surgery is dependent upon the severity of the neurologic deficits, the extent of the spine involved, and the infecting organism, if known. Patients in whom nonoperative management should be considered include patients with multilevel spinal involvement, patients with lumbosacral SEA with a normal neurologic exam, and patients with neurologic deficits that have been present for more than 48 hours. Antibiotics should be started immediately after the diagnosis is established. Initial therapy should include vancomycin, because of the high incidence of methicillin-resistant organisms, and either an aminoglycoside or a third-generation cephalosporin (14). The antibiotic regimen is adjusted once definitive culture and sensitivities are available. Antibiotic treatment is usually continued for 4 to 6 weeks.

CRITICAL INTERVENTIONS

- Obtain a CT or MRI to detect CNS abscess
- Administer antibiotics in the ED
- Obtain neurosurgical consultation

DISPOSITION

All patients with a spinal epidural abscess require admission usually to a neurosurgical service. If neurosurgery is not available the patient should be stabilized, have antibiotics started and then transferred to an appropriated center with neurosurgical capabilities. Neurologic deficits for greater that 48 hours, immune-compromised patients, involvement of the thoracic spinal cord and methicillin-resistant Staphylococci as the causative organism all worsen the prognosis for a complete recovery.

COMMON PITFALLS

✔ Failure to include a suppurative CNS infection in the differential diagnosis of patients presenting with headache or back pain
✔ Inappropriate antibiotic selection because the likely origin of the infection was not considered
✔ Delay in reducing intracranial pressure and neurosurgical consultation

Acknowledgments

Thanks to the previous edition's chapter authors Ralph J. Riviello and Douglas A. Rund.

References

1. Bamberger DM. Outcome of medical treatment of bacterial abscesses without therapeutic drainage: review of cases reported in the literature. *Clin Infect Dis* 1996;23:592–603
2. Brock DG, Black TP. Extra-axial suppurations of the central nervous system. *Semin Neurol* 1992;12:263.
3. Calfee DP, Wispelwey B. Brain abscess. *Semin Neurol* 2000;20:353–360.
4. Ciurea AV, Stoica F, Vasilescu G, Nuteanu L. Neurosurgical management of brain abscesses in children. *Childs Nerv Syst* 1999;15:309–317.
5. Enzmann DR, Britt DH, Placone R. Staging of human brain abscesses by computed tomography. *Radiology* 1983;146:703.
6. Hall WA. Neurosurgical infections in the compromised host. *Neurosurg Clin North Am* 1992;3:435–442.
7. Heilpern KL, Lorber B. Focal intracranial infections. *Infect Dis Clin North Am* 1996;4:879.
8. Kaplan K. Brain abscess. *Med Clin North Am* 1985;59:345.
9. Krauss WE, McCormick PC. Infections of the dural spaces. *Neurosurg Clin North Am* 1992;3:4.
10. Leuthardt EC, Wippold FJ, Oswood MC, Rich KM. Diffusion-weighted MR imaging in the preoperative assessment of brain abscesses. *Surg.Neurol* 2002;58:395–402.
11. Levy RM, Berger JR. Neurosurgical aspects of human immunodeficiency virus infection. *Neurosurg Clin North Am* 1992;3:443.
12. Luby JP. Southwestern Internal Medicine Conference: infections of the central nervous system. *Am J Med Sci* 1992;6:379.
13. Mampalam TJ, Rosenblum ML. Trends in the management of bacterial brain abscess: a review of 102 cases over 17 years. *Neurosurgery* 1988;23:451.
14. Manfredi PL, Herskovitz S, Folli F, Pigazzi A, Swerdlow ML. Spinal epidural abscess: treatment options. *Eur Neurol* 1998;40:58–60.
15. Mathisen GE, Johnson JP. Brain abscess. *Clinical Infectious Diseases* 1997;25:763–781.
16. Osenbach RK, Loftus CM. Diagnosis and management of brain abscess. *Neurosurg Clin North Am* 1992;3:403.
17. Pruitt AA. Infections of the nervous system. *Neurosurg Clin North Am* 1998;2:419.
18. Rigamonti D, Liem L, Sampath P, et al. Spinal epidural abscess: contemporary trends in etiology, evaluation, and management. *Surg Neurol* 1999;52:189–196.
19. Seydoux C, Francioli P. Bacterial brain abscesses: factors influencing mortality and sequelae. *Clin Infect Dis* 1992;15:394–401.
20. Singh N, Husain S. Infections of the central nervous system in transplant recipients. *Transpl Infect Dis* 2000;2:101–111.
21. Townsend GC, Scheld WM. Infections of the central nervous sytem. *Adv Intern Med* 1998;43:403.
22. Weingarten K, Zimmerman RD, Becker RD, et al. Subdural and epidural empyemas: MR imaging. *AJR* 1989;152:615.
23. Wispelwey B, Scheld WM. Brain abscess. *Semin Neurol* 1992;12:273.
24. Yoshikawa T, Quinn W. The aching head: intracranial suppuration due to head and neck infections. *Infect Dis Clin North Am* 1988;2:265.

CHAPTER 140
Sexually Transmitted Diseases

Christine Anderegg and Diane M. Birnbaumer

Sexually transmitted diseases (STDs) are commonly encountered in the emergency department and primary care settings. The problem is widespread: there are 333 million new cases of curable STDs globally each year. The United States has the highest rates of STDs in the industrialized world, estimated to be 50 to 100 times higher than other nations, with over 12 million new cases per year (5). Patients may present with a broad range of complaints. Diagnosis and treatment is important in order to prevent future complications of untreated disease, such as infertility, and to prevent the further spread of infection.

The history and physical examination are paramount in diagnosing sexually transmitted diseases. Important aspects of the history include symptoms and their duration, history of previously sexually transmitted diseases, timing and occurrence of sexual contacts, use of contraceptive agents or devices, and in women, menstrual history. A thorough exam of the genital area is important, with emphasis on observation for lesions and for the presence of discharge. In addition, examination for lymphadenopathy (local and systemic), a joint examination (if the patient is symptomatic) and examination of the skin for rashes and lesions is critical.

Most sexually transmitted diseases can be easily categorized as those presenting with ulcers and/or inguinal adenopathy, and nonulcerative diseases, which often present with urethral, cervical or vaginal discharge. Tables 140.1 and 140.2 list the differential diagnoses of both ulcerative and nonulcerative genital complaints.

ULCERATIVE STDS

Patients may present with complaints of an ulcer or sore on or adjacent to the genitalia. Diseases presenting with genital lesions may be difficult to distinguish from one another based on exam

---

TABLE 140.1.   Differential Diagnosis of Ulcerative STDs

Herpes
Syphilis (primary)
Chancroid
LGV
Granuloma inguinale (Donovanosis)
Molluscum contagiosum
Genital warts
Pediculosis
Scabies
Pyoderma
Trauma
Excoriations
Behcet disease
Drug reaction
Yeast infection

STDS, sexually transmitted diseases.

TABLE 140.2.   Differential Diagnosis of Nonulcerative STDs

Gonorrhea
Chlamydia
Nongonococcal urethritis
Secondary/tertiary syphilis
Candidal vaginitis
Trichomonas
Bacterial vaginosis
Endometriosis

---

alone, so history is of significant importance in determining the cause of the lesion. Key points in the history include the characteristics of the lesion(s) including type of initial lesion, whether the lesion is single or multiple, painful or nontender, has regular or irregular borders, or is indurated or soft. If adenopathy is part of the presentation, determine whether it is painful or not, whether it is unilateral or bilateral, and if it is fluctuant (see Table 140.3).

Treatment is often necessary before test results are available; treatment decisions should be based on the most likely diagnosis. The most common ulcerative diseases in the United States are herpes, syphilis, and, in rare outbreaks, chancroid (5). Any patient with an ulcerative lesion should have HSV culture and syphilis serology sent, and if possible, a dark field examination of the lesion. Despite this testing, 25% of patients will have no laboratory-confirmed diagnosis (6). As ulcerative diseases increase the risk of HIV infection, all patients should also be referred for HIV testing (11).

HERPES GENITALIS

Genital herpes is a sexually transmitted disease caused by the herpes simplex virus type 2 (HSV-2) and, less commonly, type 1 (HSV-1). Herpes lesions are the most common form of genital ulceration in developed countries, with over 50 million persons infected in the United States (5). Although herpes infection alone does not often produce serious sequelae in nonpregnant patients, HSV-2 plays a major role in the spread of HIV. Persons infected with genital herpes are more susceptible to HIV infection, and herpes infection can make HIV-positive persons more infectious.

CLINICAL PRESENTATION

The presentation of genital herpes is divided into primary herpes infection and recurrences. Primary herpes infection is the initial infection in a patient without circulating antibodies to either HSV-2 or HSV-1. After an incubation period of 2 to 7 days, the primary infection occurs and is usually associated with systemic symptoms, including low-grade fever, malaise, headache and myalgias. Grouped, multiple small vesicles appear on an erythematous base, which after 3 to 5 days develop into painful, shallow ulcers. The severity of local symptoms reaches its peak between 8 to 10 days, gradually receding over the second week of illness. The lesions of the primary episode are generally present for 2 to 4 weeks until complete healing occurs. Patients may also develop adenopathy, most often during the second or third week. The nodes are usually bilateral, slightly enlarged, nonfluctuant and mildly tender. Severe dysuria, another common symptom, is more often seen in women, and may lead to urinary retention. Urinary retention can also occur as a consequence of sacral radiculomyelopathy, which may also cause constipation and sensation changes in the lumbosacral distribution. Other

TABLE 140.3. Characteristics of Ulcerative Sexually Transmitted Diseases

Disease	Nature of Genital Ulcer	Incubation Period	Painful	Inguinal Adenopathy	Diagnostic Tests
Syphilis	Indurated, sharply demarcated, with red, smooth base; heals spontaneously	9–90 days; avg 2–3 weeks	No	Firm rubbery nodes; nontender	Dark field exam; serologic
Herpes Simplex	Multiple, small grouped vesicles on a red base, which form shallow ulcers; may coalesce; resolve spontaneously but recurrence is common	2–7 days	Yes	Bilateral, firm, tender	Culture, serology
Chancroid	Irregular, sharply demarcated borders with undermined edges, shallow, often multiple	3–6 days	Yes	Unilateral most common; overlying erythema, fixed and tender, suppuration may occur	Culture
Lymphogranuloma venereum	Usually single lesion, papule or ulcer, transient, frequently not noticed	5–21 days	No	Unilateral most common; firm, tender, matted fixed. May suppurate or form fistulas	LGV complement fixation (serology)

LGV, lymphogranuloma.

complications of primary herpes infection include aseptic meningitis and transverse myelitis (17,24).

Herpes is a lifelong infection; the virus remains latent, and recurrences occur in 60 to 90 percent of patients. The symptoms of recurrence are distinctly milder than during the primary infection. Systemic symptoms are rare, and patients typically have fewer lesions, with a shorter time to complete healing. Prodromal symptoms occur in more than half of the patients who experience recurrence, including localized paresthesias, itching, burning, or hypersensitive skin at the site of subsequent lesions. Virus is shed from the primary lesion and recurrent lesions for several days after ulcerations or erosions first appear.

Serologic data suggests that many people infected with HSV2 are not aware of their infection (14,15) and may have acquired the infection with minimal to no symptoms.

EMERGENCY DEPARTMENT EVALUATION

The diagnosis is often made clinically, but wherever possible, confirmatory testing is recommended, particularly in women of childbearing age. Definitive diagnosis requires positive culture or detection of virus by direct antigen methods (12). Virus isolation by culture is the gold standard; however, the sensitivity of culture declines rapidly as lesions begin to heal. False negative results are common due to improper collection or transport, and results take 3 to 10 days. Antigen detection tests are also available, but are less sensitive than culture, and do not distinguish between HSV-1 and HSV-2. Cytologic detection of herpes virus is insensitive and nonspecific (Tzanck prep or PAP smear) and should not be used for diagnosis. Serologic testing is available, and can give type-specific results, which are useful in confirming a clinical diagnosis of herpes (12,14,15).

EMERGENCY DEPARTMENT MANAGEMENT

Genital herpes is a lifelong infection without a definitive cure, but skin lesions are self-limited, and heal spontaneously unless secondarily infected. Systemic antiviral drugs (acyclovir, valacyclovir and famciclovir) are the mainstay of therapy (6), as they partially control the symptoms and signs of herpes, shorten the duration of symptoms, decrease duration of shedding and can abort recurrence episodes. Table 140.4 outlines the different treatment regimens for genital herpes. Unfortunately, these drugs neither eradicate latent virus nor affect the risk, frequency or severity of recurrences after the drug is discontinued. Suppressive therapy can reduce the frequency of genital herpes recurrences by 80%. Acyclovir has been shown to be safe for up to 6 years continuous use; the other antivirals are proven safe for one year (6). Other goals of treatment are symptomatic treatment, and include pain control and genital hygiene.

All patients should be counseled to refer partners for evaluation, and counseled that the disease is transmissible even when asymptomatic. Women of childbearing age must inform their doctor of their history of genital herpes when becoming pregnant. Women who acquire herpes during pregnancy have a significantly increased risk of fatal neonatal herpes infections (15,24), and high rates of neonatal morbidity have been reported in association with both symptomatic and asymptomatic primary infections acquired late in pregnancy (3). If active lesions are present at the onset of labor, delivery should be performed via c-section. As the safety of systemic acyclovir, valacyclovir and famciclovir therapy in pregnant women has not been established; consultation with the patient's primary care doctor is recommended before starting any treatment regimen in pregnant patients.

SYPHILIS

Syphilis is a disease caused by the spirochete *Treponema pallidum*, and is capable of involving any organ of the body. Transmission occurs primarily during sexual contact, and exposure to moist skin or mucous membranes is necessary for the infection to occur. In 2001, 6,103 cases of primary and secondary syphilis were reported in the United States (5).

CLINICAL PRESENTATION

Left untreated, the disease progresses through several stages.

1. *Primary*. The incubation period varies from 9 to 90 days, with an average of 2 to 4 weeks. The primary lesion, called the primary chancre, occurs at the point of inoculation. It begins as a small papule, which erodes and becomes ulcerative. The chancre is characteristically painless, usually single, and has

a smooth, slightly raised edge, with sharply defined borders and an indurated base. A few days after appearance of the chancre, if the primary lesion is on the genitalis, patients may develop unilateral or bilateral inguinal lymphadenopathy, which is usually painless. The lesion is indolent, and if not treated, usually persists 2–6 weeks before spontaneously healing, and the infection progresses to the secondary stage (10,17,20,24).

2. *Secondary.* The average interval between the appearance of the primary chancre and secondary lesions is 5 to 8 weeks. Patients typically develop a macular rash, which starts on the trunk and spreads to the abdomen, shoulders and limbs, evolving into a symmetric papulosquamous rash, which may resemble pityriasis rosea. The rash often involves the palms and soles with maculopapular lesions. Patients may also develop condyloma lata; hypertrophic, broad-based papules with flat moist tops, most common on the labia, around the anus and between the buttocks. Constitutional flu-like symptoms are common, including low-grade fever, malaise, headache, sore throat, arthralgias and generalized lymphadenopathy. When adenopathy is present, the nodes are discrete, nontender, and rubbery. If untreated, this stage also resolves spontaneously.

3. *Latent.* This stage begins when secondary symptoms disappear. Patients lack clinical manifestations during the latent phase, and disease is detected solely by serologic testing. Latent syphilis acquired within the preceding year is referred to as early latent syphilis; all other cases of latent syphilis are either late latent syphilis or latent syphilis of unknown duration.

4. *Tertiary.* This stage may appear 3–4 years or later after the primary stage, and is characterized by involvement of the cardiovascular and nervous systems. Specific manifestations include meningitis, peripheral neuropathy (tabes dorsalis), thoracic aortic aneurysms, and gummatous lesions of the mu-

cous membranes. Tertiary syphilis is uncommon in the United States (6,10,20).

EMERGENCY DEPARTMENT EVALUATION

Darkfield examinations and direct fluorescent antibody tests of lesion exudates or tissue are the definitive methods for diagnosing early (primary) syphilis. However, the sensitivity is only approximately 80%, and lack of availability of darkfield microscopy and trained personnel may limit the use of this technique (8). Currently, serologic testing is the mainstay of diagnosis for secondary, latent, and tertiary syphilis. Serologic tests are divided into nontreponemal and treponemal tests, and both are required for definitive diagnosis. Nontreponemal tests measure nonspecific antibodies found in the serum of patients with syphilis. These tests include VDRL and RPR, and they vary in their sensitivity based on the stage of syphilis. Nontreponemal tests are positive about 2 weeks after appearance of the primary lesion, and are quantitative. The antibodies reach their highest levels during secondary syphilis, during which time the sensitivity of nontreponemal tests approach 100%. As they are nonspecific for *T. pallidum*, false positive tests do occur. Treponemal tests (FTA-ABS or MHA-TP) measure specific antibodies formed by the host in response to infection with *T. pallidum*. However, these tests are technically difficult and expensive to perform, and therefore are not used for screening. They are necessary to confirm the diagnosis of syphilis if nontreponemal test results are positive (8,12).

EMERGENCY DEPARTMENT MANAGEMENT

For primary and secondary syphilis, benzathine penicillin G 2.4 million units IM × 1 is the treatment of choice (6) (see Table 140.4 for alternative treatment regimens and for treatment of latent

---

TABLE 140.4.   Treatment Guidelines

Disease	Recommended Treatment Regimen	Alternative(s)
Chlamydia	Azithromycin 1 g PO in a single dose OR Doxycycline 100 mg PO bid × 7 days	Erythromycin base 500 mg PO qid × 7 days OR Ofloxacin 300 mg po bid × 7 days OR Levofloxacin 500 mg po qd × 7 days
Gonorrhea	Cefixime 400 mg po in a single dose OR Ceftriaxone 125 mg IM × 1 OR Ciprofloxacin 500 mg po × 1 OR Ofloxacin 400 mg PO × 1	Spectinomycin 2 g IM × 1
Syphilis, primary or secondary	Benzathine penicillin G 2.4 million units IM × 1	Doxycycline 100 mg po bid × 14 days OR Tetracycline 500 mg po qid × 14 days
Syphilis, late latent	Benzathine penicillin G 2.4 million units IM in 3 doses, 1 week apart	
Herpes simplex, first episode	Acyclovir 400 mg po tid × 7–10 days OR Acyclovir 200 mg po 5× /day × 7–10 days OR Famciclovir 250 mg po tid × 7–10 days OR Valacyclovir 1 g po bid × 7–10 days	
Herpes simplex, recurrent	Acyclovir 400 mg po tid × 5 days OR Acyclovir 200 mg po 5×/day × 5 days OR Acyclovir 800 mg po bid × 5 days OR Famciclovir 125 mg po bid × 5 days OR Valacyclovir 1 g po qd × 5 days OR Valacyclovir 500 mg po bid × 5 days	
Herpes simplex, suppressive	Acyclovir 400 mg po bid OR Famciclovir 250 mg po bid OR Valacyclovir 500 mg po bid OR Valacyclovir 1 g po qd	
Chancroid	Azithromycin 1 go po × 1 OR Ceftriaxone 250 mg IM × 1 OR Ciprofloxacin 500 mg po bid × 3 days OR Erythromycin base 500 mg po tid × 7 days	
Lymphogranuloma venereum	Doxycycline 100 mg po bid × 21 days	Erythromycin base 500 mg po qid × 21 days

and tertiary syphilis). Sexual partners within the last 90 days should be tested but treated presumptively; partners greater than 90 days should be evaluated and treated if indicated. All patients should be referred for HIV testing. Patients should be referred for reexamination clinically and serologically 6 months and 12 months following treatment, as RPR and VDRL should become nonreactive after successful treatment. A four-fold or greater decrease in titers after six months correlates with decreasing antibody levels and successful treatment. Parenteral penicillin G is the only therapy with documented efficacy for syphilis during pregnancy. Because congenital syphilis can be so devastating, pregnant women with syphilis in any stage who report penicillin allergy should be desensitized and treated with penicillin (6,17).

CHANCROID

Chancroid is caused by *Haemophilus ducreyi*, a small gram-negative bacterium. It is characterized by painful genital ulcerations and frequent bubo formation (spontaneous rupture of fluctuant nodes leading to the formation of inguinal ulceration and excavation). While common in developing countries (20), the disease is rare in the United States, with only 38 cases reported to the CDC in 2001 (5); however, outbreaks have been reported. In addition, as *H. ducreyi* is difficult to culture, the condition may be substantially under diagnosed.

CLINICAL PRESENTATION

The incubation period is 3 to 6 days, after which a small, tender red papule or pustule appears at the site of inoculation. The papule rapidly progresses to an ulcer, characterized by sharply demarcated edges and sloughing bases, often with necrotic exudates. Multiple lesions are common, and lesions may coalesce. Lymphadenitis appears in 50% of patients, approximately one week after the ulcer, and is typically unilateral, painful and fluctuant. The overlying skin is often erythematous, and suppuration is common. Buboes may spontaneously rupture.

EMERGENCY DEPARTMENT EVALUATION

Diagnosis is often based on clinical presentation and is often a diagnosis of exclusion, after ruling out other diseases such as herpes and syphilis. Definitive diagnosis requires isolation and identification of *H. ducreyi*. Lesions can be cultured, but *H. ducreyi* requires a special medium for growth, which is not widely available (19). A probable diagnosis can be made if all of the following criteria are met: (1) the patient has one or more painful genital ulcers; (2) the patient has no evidence of *T. pallidum* infection by dark field exam or serologic testing; (3) the clinical presentation, appearance of genital ulcers and regional lymphadenopathy are typical for chancroid; and (4) a test for HSV performed on the ulcer exudates is negative (17,19,24).

EMERGENCY DEPARTMENT MANAGEMENT

Treatment is curative. Recommended regimens (6) include azithromycin 1 g PO × 1 or ceftriaxone 250 mg IM × 1 (see Table 140.4 for more treatment options). About 10% of patients who have chancroid acquired in the United States are coinfected with *T. pallidum* or HSV, and chancroid is a cofactor for HIV transmission. All patients should be referred for HIV and other STD testing. Sex partners of patients with chancroid should be examined and treated if they have had sexual contact with the patient during the ten days preceding the patient's onset of symptoms.

Patients should be referred for reexamination 3 to 7 days after initiation of therapy to confirm response to treatment.

LYMPHOGRANULOMA VENEREUM

Lymphogranuloma venereum (LGV) is a chronic sexually transmitted disease caused by specific serotypes of *Chlamydia trachomatis*, characterized by a transitory genital lesion followed by involvement of the lymphatic channels and nodes of the genitalia, pelvis, and rectum (17,24). The disease is prevalent in many tropical countries, but is rare in the United States.

CLINICAL PRESENTATION

The incubation period is 3 days to 3 weeks. The primary lesion is a small, painless ulcer that is transient and may go unnoticed. The disease usually presents in the secondary stage, when regional lymphadenitis appears, usually 7 to 30 days following the disappearance of the primary lesion. Inguinal lymphadenopathy is most often unilateral, and enlargement of the glands above and below Poupart ligament give the characteristic LGV "groove sign." The enlarged nodes are often painful, with overlying erythema. The nodes either eventually break down, with the formation of multiple draining sinuses, or form a hard inguinal mass without suppuration. Late complications result from the blockage of lymphatic channels by the infection, resulting in distal edema.

EMERGENCY DEPARTMENT EVALUATION AND MANAGEMENT

Diagnosis is based on clinical picture and serologic testing. Other causes of inguinal lymphadenopathy and genital ulcers must be ruled out. Treatment cures infection and prevents ongoing tissue damage. Doxycycline, 100 mg PO bid × 3 weeks is the preferred treatment. Erythromycin 500 mg PO qid × 21 days is an alternate regimen (6). Patients should refer their sexual partners for evaluation and treatment, and all patients should be referred for HIV testing.

NONULCERATIVE STDS

These infections are characterized by urethral or cervical discharge, and lack ulcerations or extensive lymphadenopathy. The two most common nonulcerative STDs are chlamydia and gonorrhea. Clinical manifestations of these two infections closely resemble each other, and the two commonly occur together. Therefore, it is usually not possible to distinguish the two diseases based on signs and symptoms alone (11) and patients are often treated for both infections. Table 140.2 lists the differential diagnosis for nonulcerative STDs.

CHLAMYDIA

In the United States, chlamydia is the most commonly reported sexually transmitted disease, with 3 to 5 million cases estimated annually (5). It is caused by *Chlamydia trachomatis*, an obligate intracellular organism, which infects columnar and pseudostratified columnar epithelial surfaces (8,12,17,24). *C. trachomatis* can cause urethritis, proctitis, epididymitis, prostatitis, cervicitis, and perihepatitis, as well as pelvic inflammatory disease (PID) (see Chapter 89.) (9).

CLINICAL PRESENTATION

The incubation period is 1 to 3 weeks. Males may present with symptoms of urethritis or epididymitis. Females, when symptomatic, may complain of symptoms ranging from dysuria to peritonitis. Frequently, women may have only vague, nonspecific complaints, including vaginal discharge or bleeding, abdominal or pelvic pain. Asymptomatic infection is common among both men and women; it is estimated that 75% of infected women and 50% of infected men will have no symptoms. Sexually active adolescent females have a particularly high rate of infection, and chlamydial infection has been found in up to 10% of asymptomatic young women in family planning clinics. Infection in women can lead to pelvic inflammatory disease (PID), ectopic pregnancy and infertility. It is estimated that 40% of women with untreated chlamydial infections will develop PID.

EMERGENCY DEPARTMENT EVALUATION

Historically, the gold standard for diagnosis was cell culture. However, newer tests have better sensitivity and specificity than culture, and are becoming the new gold standard. Nucleic acid amplification tests (NAATs), which include LCR, PCR, strand displacement amplification and transcript-mediated amplification, amplify nucleic acid sequences that are specific for the organism being tested. They do not require viable organisms. NAATs, including ligase chain reaction (LCR) and polymerase chain reaction (PCR), and nucleic acid hybridization tests, have sensitivities that exceed that of culture (>90% versus 60%–80% respectively), with specificities greater than 99%. In fact, the sensitivity of NAATs exceeds those of other nonculture tests (DNA probe testing, latex agglutination testing) by 17% to 35% (2,7,12,23). NAATs can be performed on both swabs (endocervical or urethral) and urine, although the sensitivities of NAATs are lower when performed on urine than on endocervical swabs (2,18). Endocervical swabs using NAATs are the test of choice in females. Urine screening NAATs is adequate for males, especially when symptomatic; urethral swabs are generally not necessary (7,18,23). Culture is still preferred when an isolate is needed (such as in sexual abuse cases) and should be done in addition to NAATs in these cases (4).

EMERGENCY DEPARTMENT MANAGEMENT

Treatment consists of azithromycin 1 g PO × 1 or doxycycline 100 mg PO bid × 7 days (6). Co-infection with gonococcal infection is common; therefore treating patients with suspected chlamydia for both infections is recommended unless gonorrhea is definitively ruled out (see Table 140.3 for alternative regimens). Patients treated for chlamydia should be instructed to abstain from sexual intercourse for 7 days after single-dose therapy or until completion of 7-day regimen. Patients should be instructed that their partner needs testing and treatment, and should be instructed to abstain from sexual intercourse until all of their sex partners are treated. No follow up for test of cure is required unless symptoms persist or reinfection is suspected.

GONORRHEA

Gonorrhea is a sexually transmitted disease caused by the gram-negative diplococcus *Neisseria gonorrhoeae*. It is the second most frequently reported STD after chlamydia. It is estimated that 600,000 new *N. gonorrhoeae* infections occur in the United States each year (5). Bacterial infection affects columnar or transitional epithelium; it may therefore be found in the urethra, rectum, cervical canal, pharynx, upper female genital tract and the conjunctival sac (11,17).

CLINICAL PRESENTATION

The clinical presentation of localized disease varies based on the sex of the patient and the site of infection. In men, acute urethritis is the most common presentation. Symptoms include dysuria and a penile discharge, starting within 1 to 14 days of exposure. Physical examination findings in symptomatic males include meatal erythema and a purulent urethral discharge. Patients may also complain of testicular pain and swelling, with evidence of epididymitis, although this is an uncommon presentation (epididymitis is discussed in depth elsewhere in this text).

Primary infections in women are often asymptomatic or produce only vague complaints until complications such as PID have occurred. If symptoms do occur, they are usually mild or nonspecific, and can include vaginal discharge, abnormal vaginal bleeding, abdominal or pelvic pain, or urinary symptoms such as dysuria and frequency. Up to 20% of women with gonorrhea develop PID, with symptoms including abnormal uterine bleeding, abdominal pain, and dyspareunia. Both symptomatic and asymptomatic cases of PID can result in tubal scarring that may lead to infertility or ectopic pregnancy (see Chapter 89). Other presenting complaints may include Bartholin abscess or RUQ pain secondary to perihepatitis (Fitz-Hugh Curtis syndrome).

Other sites of primary infection include the oropharynx and anorectal area. Oropharyngeal gonococcal infection is often asymptomatic, but can present with sore throat and exudative tonsillitis, and most cases are self-limited. Anorectal involvement is more common in homosexual men and heterosexual women. It is often asymptomatic; when symptomatic, patients complain of rectal discomfort, anorectal pain, tenesmus, constipation, dyspareunia, pruritus ani, and purulent or mucoid anal discharge or bleeding. Anoscopy may reveal mucopurulent exudate and friable mucosa (11).

Disseminated gonococcal infection results from gonococcal bacteremia. The most common presentation is the arthritis-dermatitis syndrome, which presents with fevers, chills, polyarticular arthritis or arthralgias, a rash, and tenosynovitis. The rash is characterized by petechial or pustular acral skin lesions, which are usually found peripherally on the extremities. Typical lesions are small tender papules that become pustular (described as necrotic pustules on an erythematous base), and most likely represent septic emboli to small blood vessels during episodes of bacteremia. Other manifestations include hepatitis, myocarditis, endocarditis and meningitis (very rare). If disseminated gonorrhea involves the joints, the subsequent arthritis presents with an acute, monoarticular septic arthritis. The involved joint is erythematous, warm, and often has an effusion. The knees are most commonly involved, followed by elbows, ankles, wrists and small bones of the hands and feet. Definitive diagnosis of disseminated gonococcal arthritis is confirmed by isolating gonococci from the blood, synovial fluid, or infected epithelium (11). Presumptive diagnosis is based on the appropriate clinical presentation combined with isolation of gonococci from a source site.

EMERGENCY DEPARTMENT EVALUATION

In symptomatic males or patients with gonococcal conjunctivitis, gram stain of the discharge may have a sensitivity and specificity approaching 100% (4,13). The gram stain is a quick means of diagnosis in these cases, with results returned during the ED visit, and sensitivity and specificity of gram stain is comparable to culture. In females and asymptomatic males, however, the gram stain is less useful, with significantly decreased sensitivity. Culture for gonorrhea is considered the gold standard (4), but accurate results may be limited by improper collection and handling of specimens. To maintain viability of gonococcal organisms, specimens should be inoculated directly onto the appropriate medium. If the specimen is from a sterile site, such as CSF or synovial fluid, nonselective medium such as chocolate agar is best. Specimens from nonsterile sites such as the cervix, urethra, rectum or oropharynx, where normal bacterial flora is present, should be inoculated on selective media such as Martin Lewis agar. Specimens should be incubated at 35 to 36.5 C in carbon dioxide-enriched atmosphere immediately after collection, and transported to the lab in a carbon dioxide-enriched atmosphere (4,12,13).

NAATs have been shown to have good sensitivity and excellent specificity for detection of gonorrhea from endocervical, urethral and urine samples. NAATs have been approved by the FDA for the detection of *C. trachomatis* and *N. gonorrhoeae* in endocervical swabs from women, urethral swabs from men, and urine from both men and women (4). Although sensitivities of NAATs are comparable with culture (95%–99%) (13), selected NAATs may be less sensitive when performed on urine than when performed on endocervical specimens or male urethral swabs. Therefore, NAATs of endocervical swabs in women or urethral swabs in males are good alternatives to gonococcal culture, especially when conditions during holding and transport of culture media are not adequate to maintain viability of organisms (4,13,21).

Culture is required to isolate organisms from sites such as oropharynx, synovial fluid, anorectal area and cerebrospinal fluid. Culture is the test of choice when the results will be used as evidence in legal investigations. Finally, only culture can be used to isolate the organism for antimicrobial testing and determination of antibiotic sensitivities, so this modality may be useful in areas of rapidly emerging resistance.

EMERGENCY DEPARTMENT MANAGEMENT

Recommended single-dose therapy for gonorrhea includes ceftriaxone 125 mg IM × 1 or a single dose of cefixime 400 mg PO (see Table 140.4 for other alternatives) (6). In addition, because patients are often co-infected with chlamydia, treatment for presumptive chlamydia should also be provided unless coinfection can be ruled out (11). Although quinolones are listed as possible choices for treating gonorrhea, there is a growing concern due to the increasing frequency of quinolone-resistant strains. As a result, treatment with a quinolone is not recommended for infections acquired in areas with a high level of resistance such as Asia, Hawaii or California (6). Patients should be instructed that their partners need referral for evaluation, testing and treatment. Patients should be instructed to avoid sexual intercourse until therapy is completed and until they and their sex partners are no longer symptomatic. Referral for HIV testing should be offered.

Because so many patients at risk for sexually transmitted diseases use the emergency department as a primary source of healthcare, the role of emergency departments in screening for and treating STDs has been debated. Although it has been shown that health care providers are significantly over-treating women who are gonorrhea and chlamydia negative (16), one-third of patients who test positive for STDs in the emergency department are not treated during the initial visit, and the majority of untreated patients do not return for subsequent treatment (1,16,22). Unfortunately, many test results are not available during the emergency department visit, and treatment decisions are therefore made on presumptive diagnosis. Providers must weigh the cost of over-treatment against the risk of untreated disease.

It is recommended that patients be treated presumptively in the emergency department unless good follow up for test results can be assured.

NONGONOCOCCAL URETHRITIS (NGU)

Patients with NGU present with urethral discharge and dysuria or urethral pruritus. The etiology in many cases is unknown, although *C. trachomatis* is implicated as the most common cause (9). Diagnosis is made by gram stain (>5 WBC per high power field and no gram-negative diplococci) (4), positive leukocyte esterase test on urinalysis or >10 WBC per high power field on urinalysis. All patients with urethritis should be evaluated for both gonorrhea and chlamydia. Treatment consists of Azithromycin 1 g orally in a single dose or doxycycline 100 mg PO bid for 7 days (6). In women, other causes of vaginal discharge must be ruled out, including chlamydia, trichomoniasis, and candidiasis (causes of vaginitis and dysuria are discussed elsewhere in this text).

CRITICAL INTERVENTIONS

- Obtain HSV culture and syphilis serology on patients with ulcerative lesions
- Refer all patients with STDs for HIV testing
- Emphasize the importance of examination and treatment of sexual partners

COMMON PITFALLS

✔ A significant number of patients with one sexually transmitted disease will also be co-infected with another

✔ Treat the patient with the expectation that they may not get follow up. Observed single-dose therapy is the best guarantee of compliance with treatment

✔ Syphilis, gonorrhea, chlamydia and AIDS are reportable diseases in every state. HIV infection and chancroid are reportable in many states. Clinicians should be familiar with local reporting requirements, and if unsure, should seek advise from local health departments

Acknowledgments

Thanks to the previous edition's chapter authors Rodney Smith, Richard Wolfe, and Stephen W. Bretz.

References

1. Bachmann LH, Richey CM, Waites K, et al. Patterns of chlamydia trachomatis testing and follow-up at a university hospital medical center. *Sex Transm Dis* 1999;26:496–499.
2. Black C, Marrazzo J, Johnson RE, et al. Head to Head multicenter comparison of DNA Probe and Nucleic Acid Amplification Tests for Chlamydia trachomatis infection in women performed with an improved reference standard. *J Clin Microbiol Oct* 2002;40:3757–3763.
3. Brown ZA, Vontver LA, Benedetii J, et al. Effects on infants of a first episode of genital herpes during pregnancy. *N Engl J Med* 1987;317:1246–1251.
4. Centers for Disease Control and Prevention. Screening Tests to Detect *Chlamydia trachomatis* and *Neisseria gonorrhoeae* Infections – 2002. *MMWR* 2002;51.
5. Centers for Disease Control and Prevention. Sexually transmitted Disease Surveillance, 2001. Atlanta, GA: U.S. Department of Health and Human Services, Centers for Disease Control and Prevention, September 2002.
6. Centers for Disease Control and Prevention. Sexually transmitted diseases treatment guidelines 2002. *MMWR* 2002;51(RR-6):1–80.
7. Cheng H, Macaluso M, Vermund S, et al. Relative accuracy of nucleic acid amplification tests and culture in detecting chlamydia in asymptomatic men. *J Clin Microbiol* 2001;39:3927–3937.
8. Clyne B, Jerrard D. Syphilis Testing. *J Emerg Med* 2000;18:361–367.
9. Heller M. Clamydial infections. *Ann Emerg Med* 1984;13:170–174.
10. Hook EW, Marra CM. Acquired syphilis in adults. *N Engl J Med* 992;326:1060–1068.

11. Hook E, Holmes K. Gonococcal infections. *Ann Intern Med* 1985;102:229–243.
12. Judson FN, Ehret J. Laboratory diagnosis of sexually transmitted infections. *Pediatr Ann.* 1994;23:361–369.
13. Koumans E, Johnson RE, Knapp JS, et al. Laboratory testing for neisseria gonorrhoeae by recently introduced nonculture tests: a performance review with clinical and public health considerations. *Clin Infect Dis* 1998;27:1171–1180.
14. Koutsky LA, Stevens CE, Holmes KK, et al. Underdiagnosis of genital herpes by current clinical and viral-isolation procedures. *N Engl J Med* 1992;326:1533–1539.
15. Kulhanjian JA, Soroush V, Au DS, et al. Identification of women at unsuspected risk of primary infection with herpes simplex virus type 2 during pregnancy. *N Engl J Med* 1992;326:916–920.
16. Levitt MA, Johnson S, Engelstad L, et al. Clinical management of chlamydia and gonorrhea infection in a community teaching emergency department – concerns in over treatment, undertreatment, and follow-up treatment success. *J Emerg Med* 2003;25:7–11.
17. Mroczkowski TF. New York: Igaku-shoin Medical Publishers. *Sex Transm Dis* 1990.
18. Schachter J, Moncada J, Whidden R, et al. Noninvasive tests for diagnosis of chlamydia trachomatis infection: application of ligase chain reaction to first-catch urine specimens of women. *J Infect Dis* 1995;172:1411–1414.
19. Schmid GP, Sanders LL, Blount JH, Alexander R. Chancroid in the United States reestablishment of an old disease. *JAMA* 1987;258:3265–3268.
20. Singh AE, Roamnowski B. Syphilis: review with emphasis on clinical, epidemiologic, and some biologic features. *Clin Microbiol Rev* 1999;12:187–209.
21. Smith K, Ching S, Lee H, et al. Evaluation of ligase chain reaction for use with urine for identification of neisseria gonorrhoeae in females attending a sexually transmitted disease clinic. *J Clin Microbiol* 1995;33:455–457.
22. Todd CS, Haase C, Stoner BP. Emergency department screening for asymptomatic sexually transmitted infections. *Am J Public Health* 2001;91:461–465.
23. Toye B, Peeling RW, Jessamine P, Claman P, Gemmill I. Diagnosis of Chlamydia trachomatis infections in asymptomatic men and women by PCR assay. *J Clin Microbiol* 1996;34:1396–1400.
24. Wilson A, Hawkins DA. *Diagnosis in color sexually transmitted diseases.* 2nd ed. London: Mosby-Wolfe, 1997.

CHAPTER 141
Lyme Disease

Edward B. Bolgiano and Robert A. Barish

Lyme disease (LD), a tick-borne illness caused by the spirochete *Borrelia burgdorferi*, is the most common vector-borne disease in the United States. *Ixodes scapularis* (the deer tick, formerly named *I. dammini*) and related tick species are the primary vectors in the transmission of the disease to humans. LD occurs worldwide and has been reported on every continent except Antarctica. The three major epidemiologic foci in the United States are the northeastern coastal, mid-Atlantic, and north-central states (3). Most human infections with *B. burgdorferi* occur during the months of May through August, when *I. scapularis* nymphal-stage activity and human outdoor activity are both at their peak. Early diagnosis and treatment are important to prevent morbidity (and, rarely, mortality) associated with later stages of the illness (20).

CLINICAL PRESENTATION

LD is a complex multisystem disorder with three clinical stages, each having a range of clinical manifestations (Table 141.1). Clinical features may occur alone or recur at intervals, and late symptoms may occur without any preceding early symptoms.

TABLE 141.1.   Clinical Stages of Lyme Disease

Stage	Time	Manifestations
Early localized infection	7–14 days (range, 3–30 days)	Erythema migrans (EM) with or without nonspecific constitutional symptoms (fever, malaise, fatigue, headache, myalgia, and arthralgia) Asymptomatic
Early disseminated infection	Days to weeks	Multiple or secondary EM lesions Nervous system Musculoskeletal system Heart
Late disseminated disease	Weeks to months	Arthritis Chronic neurologic manifestations

LD shares many features with other spirochetal diseases, namely, (1) the skin or mucous membrane is a portal of entry; (2) spirochetemia occurs early in the course of the disease, with wide dissemination; and (3) periods of latency occur, followed by multisystemic involvement.

LD usually begins with localized infection of the skin, manifested by a lesion termed *erythema migrans* (EM), and its associated nonspecific constitutional symptoms. The lesion is followed by dissemination of the spirochete to other organs. Neurologic or cardiac symptoms may occur days to weeks later, and chronic arthritic and neurologic abnormalities may occur weeks to months later.

Early Localized Infection

LD begins with the inoculation of *B. burgdorferi* by the nymphal form of the tick vector during feeding, generally about 2 days after attachment (19). The onset of symptoms is usually about 1 week (range: 3 to 32 days) after the tick bite.

EM, the most characteristic clinical manifestation of LD, is nevertheless absent in about 20% of patients. It usually (but not always) occurs at the site of a tick bite, beginning as red macules that expand centrifugally. There are two general forms: (1) an expanding red patch with varying intensities of redness within the patch (Fig. 141.1A) and (2) a central red patch surrounded by normal-appearing skin, that is, in turn, surrounded by an expanding red band, resembling a target or a ring-within-a-ring configuration (see Fig. 141.1B).

Most lesions are smooth, although scaling may be present, and the involved area is warmer than the surrounding normal-appearing skin. The centers of some lesions may become red and indurated, crusted, or vesicular and necrotic; partial or complete central clearing may occur. Most EM lesions are annular, but triangular and elongated patches may occur. Most demonstrate gradual enlargement, but others expand rapidly, forming a large patch in a relatively short period. Although a rash diameter of at least 5 cm is necessary to satisfy the Centers for Disease Control surveillance criteria, individual patients with LD may not have lesions this size. In patients seen 1 to 7 days after the appearance of lesions, the average size is 8 × 10 cm (ranges from 2 × 3 cm to 25 × 25 cm). Although most lesions are asymptomatic, some patients describe burning, itching, or, rarely, a painful sensation (14).

The EM rash usually fades within several days of antibiotic therapy. Without treatment, primary and secondary lesions

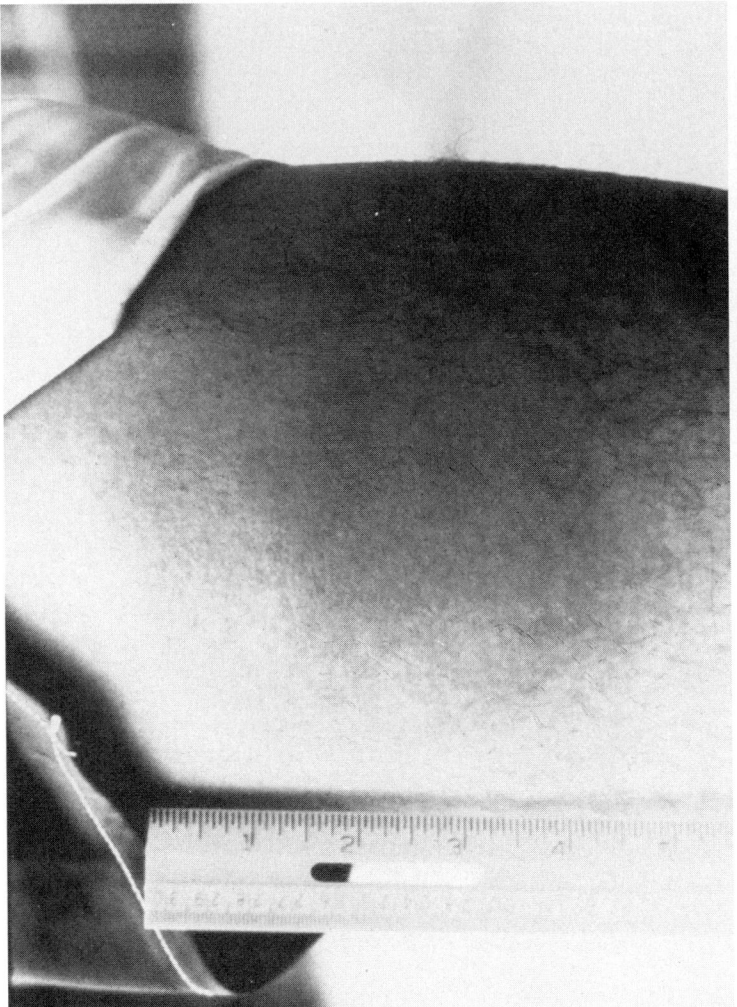

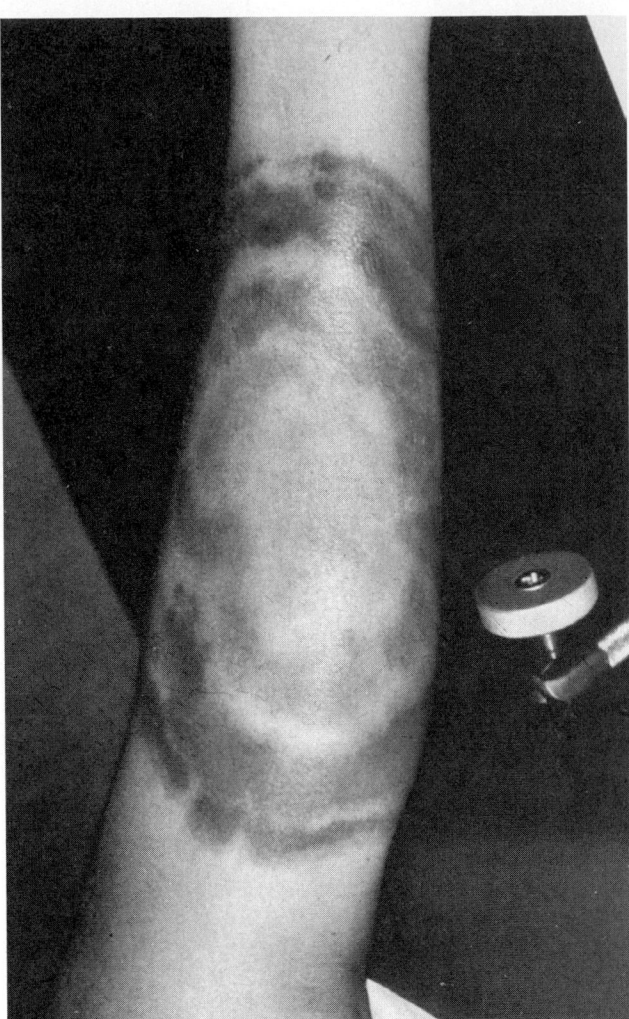

Figure 141.1. Two general forms of erythema migrans. **(A)** Expanding red patch. **(B)** Target configuration. (Courtesy of the Centers for Disease Control and Prevention.)

generally persist for about 28 days (range: 1 week to 14 months). Recurrent lesions may develop in patients who do not receive antibiotics. Untreated, the rash resolves over several weeks.

Minor constitutional symptoms commonly occur in early LD (13,17). Malaise, fatigue, and lethargy are most common (approximately 80% of patients). Fever is typically low grade and intermittent. Regional lymphadenopathy in the distribution of the rash often accompanies EM. General lymphadenopathy and splenomegaly may occur. Musculoskeletal symptoms such as arthralgias and myalgias are common and characterized by a migratory, asymmetric, and evanescent pattern. Often, symptoms last only hours in one location and reappear later in another location. Frank arthritis with joint effusion may occur during this stage, but it is rare.

Upper respiratory symptoms such as sore throat occur less commonly. Signs and symptoms of hepatitis, including anorexia, nausea, vomiting, and abdominal pain, may be noted. Headache is a common complaint and may be accompanied by photophobia, nausea, vomiting, and stiff neck, but Kernig and Brudzinski signs are usually absent. At this stage, the neurologic examination and cerebrospinal fluid (CSF) both yield normal findings.

In the absence of the characteristic rash or a history of a tick bite, the nonspecific nature of the early signs and symptoms can easily result in misdiagnosis of early LD as a viral illness or collagen vascular disorder. Symptoms usually last for several weeks in untreated patients but may persist for months.

Early Disseminated Infection

After a variable latent period, early disseminated symptoms usually occur from days to weeks after the initial infection, but these can overlap with other manifestations. The skin, nervous system, heart, and eyes are the main targets in early disseminated disease.

Within several days to several weeks, 20% to 50% of patients develop multiple annular secondary skin lesions, which are smaller than the initial ones. Usually asymptomatic, they typically spare the palms, soles, and mucous membranes.

Neurologic involvement occurs in approximately 15% of untreated patients. The most common neurologic manifestation is a fluctuating meningoencephalitis. Symptoms of cranial neuropathy, peripheral neuropathy, or radiculopathy may be superimposed, or may each occur alone (11). Headache is usually present, and there may be nausea, vomiting, lethargy, or irritability. As in early LD, Kernig and Brudzinski signs are absent, and results of computed tomography are normal (19,21). By contrast with early findings, however, CSF examination in disseminated disease may reveal a lymphocytic pleocytosis and an elevated protein level; glucose levels are normal.

Cranial neuropathy is seen in approximately 50% of patients with Lyme meningitis. Most commonly it is manifested as a unilateral peripheral seventh-nerve palsy (it may be bilateral in about a third of patients). Peripheral nervous system manifestations may include mononeuritis and motor or sensory radicular involvement or brachial plexitis.

Estimates of the incidence of cardiac involvement in untreated patients with LD range from 4% to 8%. Lyme carditis usually presents as transient myocarditis associated with varying degrees of atrioventricular block (7). The average time from the initial illness to the development of carditis is about 5 weeks (range, 4 days to 7 months) (13). Common presenting symptoms of Lyme carditis are nonspecific, but include syncope, lightheadedness, dyspnea, palpitations, and chest pain. Atrioventricular block of some degree occurs in almost 90% of patients (13). More than half of them have either high-grade or complete block, yet almost all are symptomatic. Left ventricular dysfunction has been documented by two-dimensional echocardiography and radionuclide studies; in most reported cases, it has been mild and transient. Pericarditis is uncommon, and the heart valves are spared.

A variety of ocular manifestations of LD have also been reported. They include conjunctivitis, keratitis, choroiditis, retinal detachment, optic neuritis, and blindness. Papilledema, with or without increased CSF pressure, is associated with Lyme encephalitis.

Late Disseminated Infection

The chronic phase of LD typically occurs months to years after the initial infection and is characterized by arthritic and, less commonly, neurologic symptoms. As with syphilis, chronic manifestations follow a variable latent period.

Before antibiotic therapy for LD became standard, approximately 50% of untreated patients developed arthritis characterized by intermittent attacks of joint swelling and pain developing several weeks to several years after the onset of the illness (21). The typical pattern of joint involvement is a monoarticular or asymmetric oligoarticular arthritis of the large joints. The knee is most often affected, with large, sometimes relatively asymptomatic joint effusions. The shoulder, elbow, temporomandibular joint, ankle, wrist, hip, and small joints of the hands and feet are involved less commonly. Episodes of arthritis are typically brief (weeks to months), separated by variable periods of complete remission.

Exacerbations and remissions often occur over a period of several years, with a gradual tendency toward less frequent and less severe occurrences. In untreated patients, there is a spontaneous long-term remission rate of 10% to 20% per year, but 10% of untreated patients develop chronic synovitis. An autoimmune response that persists after the pathogen has been eradicated may explain the unresponsiveness of some patients with chronic arthritis to antibiotic therapy. Chronic arthritis is much less common now, because most patients with early Lyme symptoms are recognized and treated.

Neurologic manifestations of late disease include a wide variety of abnormalities of the central and peripheral nervous systems, as well as fatigue syndromes (11). The diagnosis is difficult because the symptoms may mimic those of a number of other neurologic conditions and because late neurologic symptoms may be the first symptoms of the disease (17). Subtle encephalopathy with disturbances in mood, memory, or sleep may occur. Cases of cognitive dysfunction ranging from a mild "confusional" state to slowly progressive dementia have also been reported (2,11). Incapacitating fatigue is a widely described late feature.

Late disease may also involve the cranial nerves, spinal roots, plexuses, or peripheral nerves. The neurologic symptoms of late disease commonly manifest as a subtle polyneuropathy, with spinal or radicular pain or numbness and tingling in the hands and feet. A demyelinating condition with multiple sclerosis–like exacerbations and remissions has been described (17).

Acrodermatitis chronica atrophicans is a late cutaneous manifestation of LD that occurs in approximately 10% of European patients but has rarely been reported in North America. It is characterized initially by an edematous infiltration that progresses to an atrophic lesion resembling localized scleroderma.

DIFFERENTIAL DIAGNOSIS

Although LD presents in many ways, each stage has characteristic clinical findings that are helpful in narrowing a differential diagnosis that may, at first, seem rather broad.

Early disease may easily be confused with a variety of other diseases, especially if the rash is absent. Even in endemic areas, most patients who present with "flulike" symptoms during the summer months do not have LD. The principal diagnostic distinction to be made is between LD and the enteroviral diseases and other causes of aseptic meningitis. The enteroviral diseases are frequently accompanied by diarrhea, which is not a feature of LD. Abdominal pain, anorexia, and nausea may suggest hepatitis. Sore throat, adenopathy, and fatigue, as seen in mononucleosis, may occur. When myalgias and arthralgias are the predominant symptoms, connective tissue disease may be considered. A distinctive feature of early LD, however, is that musculoskeletal pain is typically migratory and evanescent, and often occurs in brief attacks in one or a few locations at a time.

The characteristic initial skin lesion, EM, in its classic form is virtually pathognomonic for LD. Secondary skin lesions may, however, be confused with the target lesions of erythema multiforme. The lesions of erythema multiforme are generally smaller and nonexpanding and also involve the mucous membranes and palms and soles; EM does not. Hypersensitivity reactions to insect bites or spider bites may mimic EM, but these reactions usually occur within several hours of exposure, rather than 3 or more days after the exposure. Erythema nodosum has a predilection for the extensor surfaces of the legs and generally causes more painful induration than does EM.

Erythema marginatum secondary to acute rheumatic fever may mimic EM, but the lesions of EM are generally fewer, larger, and less evanescent, and they migrate more slowly. Other common cutaneous entities to be considered in the differential diagnosis of EM include cellulitis and fixed drug-related eruptions. A useful rule is that LD must be considered in a patient with an atypical rash that is accompanied by a flulike or meningitis-like illness during the months of peak incidence.

The cardiac manifestations of LD may suggest coronary artery disease, viral myocarditis, or acute rheumatic fever. As noted previously, varying degrees of heart block are characteristic. As with rheumatic fever, carditis in LD may follow pharyngitis and migratory polyarthritis. Although the clinical aspects of the Jones criteria may be satisfied by some patients with LD, several features serve to distinguish the two illnesses:

1. EM usually precedes the carditis in LD, whereas, in rheumatic fever, skin lesions usually occur with the onset of arthritis.
2. Evidence of a preceding streptococcal infection (elevated antistreptolysin-O titer) is lacking in patients with LD.
3. Valvular involvement is not a feature of Lyme carditis.

The differential diagnosis of the neurologic manifestations of LD is wide and includes aseptic meningitis, herpes simplex encephalitis, Bell palsy, multiple sclerosis, Guillain-Barré syndrome, dementia, primary psychosis, cerebral vasculitis, and brain tumor. Lyme encephalopathy is usually associated with CSF abnormalities such as lymphocytosis, elevated protein, and the presence of antibody to the spirochete. Chronic fatigue syndrome and fibromyalgia are frequently misdiagnosed as LD (23).

In contrast to patients with rheumatoid arthritis, those with Lyme arthritis rarely have symmetric polyarthritis, morning stiffness, positive rheumatoid factor, or subcutaneous nodules. LD is commonly mistaken for seronegative rheumatoid arthritis, but it is most similar to the rheumatoid variants, particularly, Reiter's syndrome. The absence of the extraarticular features of Reiter's syndrome (conjunctivitis, urethritis or cervicitis, balanitis, keratodermia blennorrhagica) at the time of the arthritis helps distinguish LD from Reiter syndrome. In children, LD may mimic juvenile rheumatoid arthritis.

EMERGENCY DEPARTMENT EVALUATION

The diagnosis of LD is primarily clinical, based on the presence of EM and other specific manifestations, as well as a history of exposure in an endemic area. Diagnosis is difficult, however, especially in the early stages. A history of tick bite is present in only about one-third of cases. EM is present in most patients, but isolated late symptoms may appear months after the initial infection, and the patient might not recall having had a rash.

Routine laboratory studies are nonspecific and generally are not helpful in diagnosing LD. Culture of blood, tissue, and bodily fluids for *B. burgdorferi* are generally not clinically useful. Specialized laboratory studies must be cautiously interpreted within the clinical context and should be regarded as only adjuncts in the diagnosis.

Serologic testing for *B. burgdorferi* infection is the most practical and useful means of confirming clinical diagnosis of LD. However, problems with the performance and interpretation of the tests often result in diagnostic confusion. False-negative and especially false-positive results are common.

The antibody response to *B. burgdorferi* develops slowly. Immunoglobulin M (IgM) titers peak between 3 and 6 weeks after the onset of illness, so assays for IgM are often negative during the first several weeks of infection. Moreover, IgM usually returns to nondiagnostic levels 4 to 6 weeks after peak. The IgM response may persist for many months or years despite effective antimicrobial therapy. Thus, the presence of specific IgM antibodies cannot be used as the sole criterion to diagnose a recent infection (9,18). IgG antibody may be detectable 2 months after exposure and peaks approximately 12 months into the illness. Early antibiotic therapy may blunt or even abolish the antibody response. Patients with late disease usually have positive IgG antibody titer results. Nevertheless, a true-positive serologic result merely indicates previous exposure; the symptoms under evaluation may not be related to active LD. Long-term seropositivity may also result from previously treated LD.

Serologic cross-reactivity between *B. burgdorferi* and other spirochetes, most notably *Treponema pallidum*, can cause false-positive test results. Other illnesses known to be associated with false-positive serologic results include infectious mononucleosis, rheumatoid arthritis, and systemic lupus erythematosus.

Testing with the enzyme-linked immunosorbent assay (ELISA) is the cornerstone of the laboratory diagnosis of LD. Although ELISA alone has a sensitivity of 89% and a specificity of 72%, a positive result in patients with a pretest probability of LD of less than 0.20 is more likely to be a false positive than a true positive (2). In patients with a positive or equivocal ELISA, a confirmatory Western blot should be ordered (4). Polymerase chain reaction (PCR) has been used to amplify the genomic DNA of *B. burgdorferi* in skin, blood, CSF, and synovial fluid, and PCR

is superior to culture in the detection of *B. burgdorferi* in joint fluid (15). The Lyme urine antigen test is unreliable and should not be used (10).

In cases of suspected neurologic involvement, CSF should be examined for evidence of meningitis (11). In addition to routine cerebrospinal fluid (CSF) examination, paired serum and CSF serologic tests should be obtained. Intrathecal antibody production is more often positive in patients with acute neuroborreliosis, especially those with meningitis, than in patients with chronic neuroborreliosis (20). The overall sensitivity of cerebrospinal fluid PCR is only in the range of 20% (6); therefore, a negative PCR result does not exclude the diagnosis of Lyme disease.

EMERGENCY DEPARTMENT MANAGEMENT

The emergency management of patients with suspected LD should be focused on recognizing the illness, obtaining appropriate diagnostic studies, delivering supportive care when necessary, and arranging appropriate follow up.

Active *B. burgdorferi* infection is usually amenable to antibiotic therapy, and treatment can begin in the emergency department. In making treatment decisions, however, the clinical findings and the meaning and the reliability of laboratory results must be closely analyzed on an individual basis. For this reason, decisions regarding antibiotic therapy (which are almost invariably nonurgent) are often made in consultation with the patient's primary physician. Table 141.2 is a summary of recommended antibiotic regimens. Treatment recommendations have been developed on the basis of disease stage and clinical manifestations.

Prompt treatment of early disease shortens the duration of symptoms and, more important, prevents progression to later stages in most patients. The decision of whom to treat is often difficult. As noted, early LD is diagnosed by clinical presentation alone, without the luxury of serologic confirmation. Patients are often seronegative at presentation, and curative antibiotic therapy may abort the development of a mature immune response and prevent seroconversion after treatment. Treatment is clearly indicated for a patient who has the characteristic skin lesion and a history of tick bite; there is no reason to wait for a positive antibody assay before beginning therapy. Patients in endemic areas who have a rash that is consistent with EM should be treated for LD without serologic testing.

Oral therapy with doxycycline or amoxicillin is recommended for treatment of early localized or early disseminated LD (see Table 141.2) (13). Amoxicillin is preferred for pregnant or lactating women and for children younger than 8 years old (10). Doxycycline has the advantage of being efficacious for treatment of human granulocytic ehrlichiosis (HGE), which may occur simultaneously with early LD. Jarisch-Herxheimer–like reactions (fever, chills, myalgias, headache, tachycardia, increased respiratory rate, and leukocytosis) may occur in the first 24 hours of treatment. Cefuroxime axetil is as effective as doxycycline (1), but cephalexin is ineffective in LD.

Macrolide antibiotics are not recommended as first-line therapy for early LD. They should be reserved for patients who are intolerant of doxycycline, amoxicillin, and cefuroxine axetil. Adult regimens are as follows: azithromycin, 500 mg orally daily for 7 to 10 days; erythromycin, 500 mg orally 4 times daily for 14 to 21 days; and clarithromycin, 500 mg orally twice daily for 14 to 21 days (24).

The duration of antibiotic therapy should be individualized according to the severity of illness and the rapidity of clinical response. EM and associated constitutional symptoms generally respond within days. Treatment failures or relapses despite recommended courses of antibiotics have been reported.

TABLE 141.2.   Recommended Antibiotic Regimens

Drug	Adult Dosage	Pediatric Dosage*
EARLY LYME DISEASE		
Doxycycline[†]	100 mg PO bid for 14–21 days	Age <8 yr: not recommended Age ≥8 yr: 1–2 mg/kg bid (maximum, 100 mg/dose)
or		
Amoxicillin	250–500 mg PO tid for 21 days	50 mg/kg/day divided tid (maximum, 500 mg/dose)
Alternatives		
Cefuroxime axetil	500 mg PO bid for 21 days	30 mg/kg/day divided into two doses (maximum, 500 mg/dose)
or		
Macrolides (less effective than doxycycline or amoxicillin and not recommended as first-line therapy [see text])		
NEUROLOGIC DISEASE		
Facial nerve paralysis	As an isolated finding, oral regimens for early disease, used for at least 30 days, may suffice. As a finding associated with other neurologic manifestations, intravenous therapy is recommended.	
Lyme meningitis[‡]		
Ceftriaxone	2 g IV by single dose for 14–28 days	75–100 mg/kg/day IV
Alternatives		
Chloramphenicol	1 g IV q6h for 10–21 days	
Penicillin G	18–24 million units IV/day Divided into doses given q4h	200,000–400,000 units/kg/day, divided into doses given q4h
Cefotaxime	2 g IV tid	150–200 mg/kg/day IV Divided into 3 or 4 doses
CARDIAC DISEASE		
Mild[§]		
Doxycycline[†]	100 mg PO bid × 21 days	
or		
Amoxicillin	250–500 mg PO tid × 21 days	50 mg/kg/day divided tid
More severe		
Ceftriaxone	2 g IV daily by single dose for 14–21 days	75–100 mg/kg/day IV
or		
Penicillin G	18–24 million units daily in divided doses for 14–21 days	200,000–400,000 units/kg/day, divided into doses given q4h
ARTHRITIS		
Oral		
Doxycycline[†]	100 mg PO bid for 28 days	
or		
Amoxicillin	500 mg PO tid for 28 days	50 mg/kg/day divided tid
Parenteral		
Ceftriaxone	2 g IV by single dose for 14–28 days	75–100 mg/kg/day IV
or		
Penicillin G	20 million units IV daily in divided doses for 14–28 days	300,000 units/kg/day IV

*Pediatric dosage should not exceed adult dosage.
[†]Tetracycline, 250–500 mg PO qid, may be substituted for doxycycline. Neither doxycycline nor any other tetracycline should be used for children under 8 years old or for pregnant or lactating women.
[‡]Regimens for radiculoneuropathy, peripheral neuropathy, and encephalitis are the same as those for meningitis.
[§]Oral regimens are reserved for mild cardiac involvement (see text).
Adapted from Wormser GP, Nadelman RB, Dattwyler RJ, et al. Practice guidelines for the treatment of Lyme disease. The Infectious Diseases Society of America. *Clin Infect Dis* 2000;3(suppl 1):1–14.

Neurologic Disease

Facial nerve palsy may occur within the first month of illness (mean time from the onset of EM is 20 days). There is controversy regarding the approach to patients with seventh-cranial nerve palsy associated with *B. burgdorferi* infection. Some experts recommend performing a CSF examination on all these patients, whereas others reserve lumbar puncture for patients in whom there is strong clinical suspicion of CNS involvement (e.g., severe headache or nuchal rigidity). Patients with normal CSF may be treated with the same oral regimens used for patients with erythema migrans, whereas patients in whom there is clinical and laboratory evidence of CNS involvement should be treated with parenteral regimens effective against meningitis.

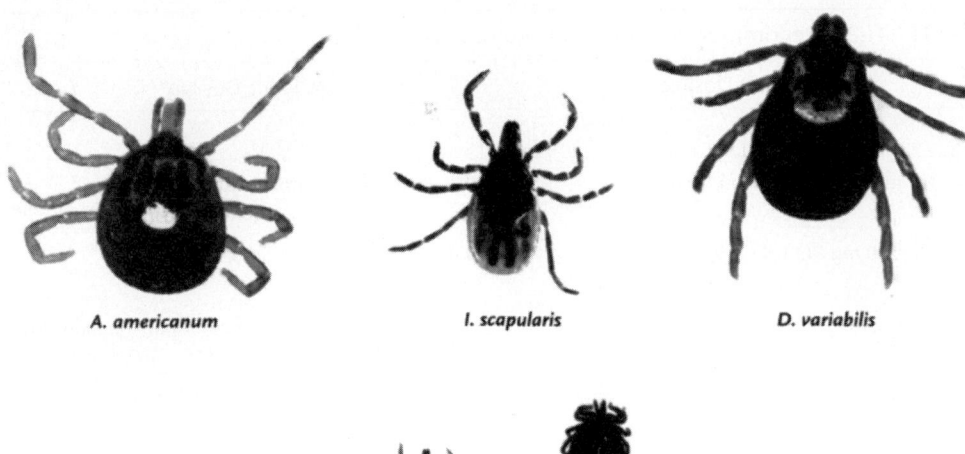

A. americanum   I. scapularis   D. variabilis

1 mm   Unengorged   Engorged

I. scapularis nymph

Figure 141.2.   Adult female *Amblyomma americanum* (Lone Star tick), adult female and nymphal *Ixodes scapularis* (deer ticks), and adult female *Dermacentor variabilis* (dog tick). (From Hayes EB, Piesman J. How can we prevent Lyme disease? *N Engl J Med* 2003;348:2424–2430.)

For patients with more serious complications, such as meningitis, other cranial or peripheral neuropathies, cognitive deficits, or encephalitis, parenteral antibiotic therapy is required.

Cardiac Disease

Recommended antibiotic therapy for patients with cardiac involvement depends on the degree of heart block noted (see Table 141.2). Patients with minor cardiac involvement (first-degree atrioventricular block but a PR interval less than 0.30 second) can usually be treated orally, whereas those with more severe cardiac involvement (high-degree atrioventricular block) require intravenous antibiotics. Temporary cardiac pacing may be necessary in the latter group. Heart block generally resolves completely with antibiotic therapy.

Arthritis

Lyme arthritis usually responds to a 1-month course of oral doxycycline or amoxicillin (see Table 141.2). The response may be delayed for several weeks or months, however, regardless of antibiotic choice or route of administration. Oral regimens appear to be as effective as parenteral penicillin or ceftriaxone.

The diagnosis of LD should be confirmed by serologic testing of synovial fluid when possible. Chronic arthritis may not be responsive to antibiotic therapy (either oral or intravenous) in certain genetically susceptible individuals. Antiinflammatory agents may be useful in the treatment of this presumably immune-mediated syndrome.

Prophylaxis

Although earlier studies of prophylactic treatment of tick bites did not show a protective effect, a recent clinical trial demonstrated that a single 200-mg dose of doxycycline administered within 72 hours after a recognized *I. scapularis* bite had an efficacy of 87% in preventing erythema migrans (12). This strategy is recommended to prevent Lyme disease among adults who live in areas where Lyme disease is endemic and who seek treatment for a bite from a deer tick that is obviously engorged or that was attached more than 72 hours. If the tick was attached less than 36 hours, it is not necessary to treat the bite (8).

Single-dose prophylactic doxycycline is not recommended in patients who present more than 72 hours after removing a tick.

Although the tick specimen usually is not available at presentation, emergency physicians should learn to distinguish among the principal tick species (Fig. 141.2), because bites from *D. variabilis* (dog tick) and *A. americanum* (Lone Star tick) do not require treatment.

The efficacy of doxycycline in the prevention of other infections transmitted by *I. scapularis* (e.g., babesiosis and HGE) is not known and cannot be assumed (12). In addition, it cannot be assumed that other antibiotics that are effective for the treatment of Lyme disease (e.g., amoxicillin) or even other regimens of doxycycline (e.g., 100 mg twice daily) would have efficacy when used for short-term prophylaxis.

Any patient who has been bitten by a tick should be told to seek medical attention if signs of tick-borne illness develop (Table 141.3).

Vaccination

An LD vaccine (LYMErix) directed against the outer-surface protein A of *B. burgdorferi* is available. LYMErix is administered by injection of 0.5 mL (30 µg) into the deltoid muscle. Three doses are required for optimal protection. The first dose is followed by a second dose 1 month later, and a third dose administered 12 months after the first dose. In a randomized, controlled clinical trial involving over 10,000 subjects, the vaccine's efficacy in

---

TABLE 141.3.   Guidelines for Prophylactic Treatment of Tick Bites

---

Within 72 hours after the discovery of a deer tick that is obviously engorged or that was attached more than 72 hours, on an adult from an area where Lyme disease is endemic, administer 200 mg doxycycline as a single dose.

If the tick was attached less than 36 hours and is not engorged, it is not necessary to treat the bite.

Persons who have received Lyme disease vaccine should be at lower risk and probably do not need prophylaxis.

In children, dosing and efficacy of prophylactic treatment have not been evaluated.

Bites from *D. variabilis* (dog tick) and *A. americanum* (Lone Star tick) do not require prophylactic treatment.

Adapted from Hayes EB, Piesman J. How can we prevent Lyme disease? *N Engl J Med* 2003;348:2424–2430 and from Shapiro ED. Doxycycline for tick bites? Not for everyone [editorial]. *N Engl J Med* 2001;345:79–84.

protecting against "definite" LD was 76% (95% CI = 58% to 86%) (22).

Vaccination will cause a positive enzyme-linked immunosorbent assay (ELISA) result but a negative Western blot. LD vaccination should be considered for persons who reside, work, or enjoy recreation in areas of high or moderate risk and who engage in activities that result in frequent or prolonged tick exposure (5).

CRITICAL INTERVENTIONS

- Administer preventive therapy consisting of a single 200-mg dose of doxycycline administered within 72 hours after a recognized *I. scapularis* bite
- Order the ELISA to aid in the diagnosis of Lyme disease
- Base treatment recommendations on the disease stage and clinical manifestations

DISPOSITION

Decisions regarding the disposition of patients with documented or suspected LD are made on the basis of disease stage and severity of clinical manifestations.

Almost all patients with early disease can be appropriately managed as outpatients. Many patients with the chronic neurologic and arthritic manifestations of late disease remain fully ambulatory and can be treated on an outpatient basis, although admission may be necessary for selected patients requiring intravenous antibiotics. Follow-up care by a primary care physician, rheumatologist, or infectious disease specialist should be arranged for patients who are discharged from the emergency department.

Hospital admission for cardiac monitoring is required for patients with Lyme carditis and any manifestation more severe than mild PR prolongation. Patients with prominent neurologic symptoms usually must be treated with intravenous antibiotics and often require a degree of supportive care that warrants hospital admission.

COMMON PITFALLS

✔ Late symptoms of LD may occur without any preceding early symptoms. Because late symptoms usually occur months after the initial tick exposure, there is no constant seasonal incidence suggestive of a tick-borne illness. The diagnosis of LD might therefore not be considered, for example, in a patient who presents during February with an isolated knee effusion
✔ Disorders such as chronic fatigue syndrome and fibromyalgia are commonly misdiagnosed as LD, resulting in inappropriate treatment with antibiotics. Despite LD's variable presentations and the limitations that remain in serologic testing, in most cases, it is possible to distinguish between *B. burgdorferi* infection and these disorders
✔ If an attached tick is removed quickly, no other treatment is usually necessary
✔ Specific diagnostic laboratory tests should not be used in screening, but rather to confirm the clinical diagnosis of LD. Even in endemic areas, most patients with "summer flu" do not have LD. Indiscriminate serologic testing of these patients results in a high rate of false-positive tests

References

1. Abramowitz M, ed. Treatment of Lyme disease. *Med Lett* 2000;42(1077):37.
2. American College of Physicians. Guidelines for laboratory evaluation in the diagnosis of Lyme disease. *Ann Intern Med* 1997;127:1106–1108.
3. Centers for Disease Control and Prevention. Lyme disease—United States, 2000. *MMWR* 2002;51:29–31.
4. Centers for Disease Control. Notice to readers: recommendations for test performance and interpretation from the Second National Conference on Serologic Diagnosis of Lyme Disease. *MMWR* 1995;44:590–591.
5. Centers for Disease Control and Prevention. Recommendations for the use of Lyme disease vaccine: recommendations of the Advisory Committee on Immunization Practices (ACIP). *MMWR* 1999;48(RR07):1–17.
6. Dumler JS. Molecular diagnosis of Lyme disease: review and meta-analysis. *Mol Diagn* 2001;6:1–11.
7. Evans J. Lyme carditis. In: Rahn D, Evans J, eds. *Lyme disease.* Philadelphia: American College of Physicians, 1998:77–88.
8. Hayes EB, Piesman J. How can we prevent Lyme disease? *N Engl J Med* 2003;348:2424–2430.
9. Kalish RA, McHugh G, Granquist J, Shea B, Ruthazer R, Steere AC. Persistence of immunoglobulin M or immunoglobulin G antibody responses to Borrelia burgdorferi 10–20 years after active Lyme disease. *Clin Infect Dis* 2001;33:780–785.
10. Klempner MS, Schmid C, Hu L, et al. Intralaboratory reliability of serologic and urine testing for Lyme disease. *Am J Med* 2001;110:217–219.
11. Logigian E. Neurologic manifestations of Lyme disease. In: Rahn D, Evans J, eds. *Lyme disease.* Philadelphia: American College of Physicians, 1998:89–106.
12. Nadelman RB, Nowakowski J, Fish D, et al. Prophylaxis with single-dose doxycycline for the prevention of Lyme disease after an *Ixodes scapularis* tick bite. *N Engl J Med* 2001;345:79–84.
13. Nadelman RB, Wormser GP. Lyme borreliosis. *Lancet* 1998;352:557–565.
14. Nadelman R, Wormser G. Management of tick bites in early Lyme disease. In: Rahn D, Evans J, eds. *Lyme disease.* Philadelphia: American College of Physicians, 1998:49–76.
15. Nocton JJ, Dressler F, Rutledge BJ, et al. Detection of Borrelia burgdorferi DNA by polymerase chain reaction in synovial fluid from patients with Lyme arthritis. *N Engl J Med* 1994;330:229–234.
16. Pacher AR. *Borrelia burgdorferais* in the nervous system: the new "great imitator." *Ann NY Acad Sci* 1998;539:5b.
17. Rahn DW. Natural history of Lyme disease. In: Rahn D, Evans J, eds. *Lyme disease.* Philadelphia: American College of Physicians, 1998:35–48.
18. Reed KD. Laboratory testing for Lyme disease: possibilities and practicalities. *J Clin Microbiol* 2002;40:319–324.
19. Sood SK, Salzman MB, Johnson BJ, et al. Duration of tick attachment as a predictor of the risk of Lyme disease in an area in which Lyme disease is endemic. *J Infect Dis* 1997;175:996–999.
20. Steere AC. Lyme disease. *N Engl J Med* 2001;345:115–125.
21. Steere AC, Schoen RT, Taylor E. The clinical evolution of Lyme arthritis. *Ann Intern Med* 1987;107:725–731.
22. Steere AC, Sikand VK, Meurice F, et al. Vaccination against Lyme disease with recombinant *Borrelia burgdorferi* outer-surface lipoprotein A with adjuvant: Lyme Disease Vaccination Study Group. *N Engl J Med* 1998;339:209–215.
23. Steere AC, Taylor E, McHugh G, et al. The overdiagnosis of Lyme disease. *JAMA* 1993;269:1812–1816.
24. Wormser GP, Nadelman RB, Dattwyler RJ, et al. Practice guidelines for the treatment of Lyme disease. The Infectious Diseases Society of America. *Clin Infect Dis* 2000;3(suppl 1):1–14.

CHAPTER 142
Rocky Mountain Spotted Fever

Michael A. Gibbs

Rocky Mountain spotted fever (RMSF) is the most common and most lethal tick-borne illness in the United States, and one of the most serious systemic infections seen in clinical practice. Emergency physicians must maintain a high index of suspicion for RMSF and consider early empiric therapy in patients at risks.

Despite significant advances in diagnosis and therapy, the case-fatality rate of RMSF remains between 5% and 10%. The disease continues to confound physicians because of its sporadic occurrence and nonspecific clinical presentation. Difficulties in making the diagnosis are especially relevant, because the prognosis is directly related to the timeliness of appropriate treatment.

In one study, 90% of patients were seen by a physician within 5 days of the onset of symptoms, yet less than half received treatment before day 6. Patients who received antirickettsial therapy within 5 days were significantly less likely to die than were those who received treatment later (6.5% vs. 22.9%). Three independent predictors of a failure to initiate therapy on first presentation to a physician were absence of a rash, presentation between August 1 and April 30, and presentation within the first 3 days of illness (3).

EPIDEMIOLOGY

RMSF is caused by *Rickettsia rickettsii*, an obligate intracellular bacterium. It is transmitted by several species of ticks that also serve as the reservoir or natural host. In the Eastern states, the wood tick, *Dermacentor andersoni*, is the major vector; the dog tick, *Dermacentor variabilis*, is the predominant vector in Western states. More than 95% of cases occur between April 1 and August 31, the incidence corresponding to the seasonal life cycle of the tick.

RMSF has been a reportable disease since the 1920s. Since then, roughly 250 to 1,200 cases are reported annually, although this figure is likely an underestimate. The disease is reported throughout the continental United States, Canada, and Mexico. RMSF tends to be focally endemic, with clustering of cases within larger endemic areas. Although first described in Idaho and Montana, the disease is now infrequent in the Western states. There has been a steady increase in the number of cases in the Southeastern states, particularly North Carolina, Tennessee, and South Carolina.

Centers for Disease Control (CDC) surveillance data from 1981 to 1990 indicate that RMSF is most common among children 5 to 9 years of age and least common among people 10 to 29 years of age. The case fatality rate is highest for people 40 years of age or older (8.2%), compared with 2.3% for those less than 40 years old. The case-fatality rate is also higher for people whose treatment is begun more than 3 days after the onset of symptoms (6.2%) than for those treated within the first 3 days (1.3%). RMSF is more common in men than in women, reflecting a greater potential exposure to the tick vector. Despite the fact that RMSF is more common in Whites than in Blacks, the case-fatality rate is significantly higher in the latter group (16% vs. 3%) (5), a fact most likely related to the difficulty of detecting the characteristic rash on dark skin.

CLINICAL PRESENTATION

RMSF is a systemic vasculitis that may affect any organ system. For this reason, signs and symptoms are varied and nonspecific. A history of tick bite or presence of a tick is elicited in just over half of patients. The onset of illness is usually acute, with fever, headache, nausea, vomiting, abdominal pain, and myalgia, a presentation that is easily confused with a clinically benign viral illness. The clinical findings and their prevalence are summarized in Table 142.1.

A *rash* of one type or another is seen in the majority of patients with RMSF, but "Rocky Mountain spotless fever" has been reported in 5% to 15% of cases (6). When patients present at symptom onset, the rash is typically absent, which is one reason that diagnosis is difficult. Likewise, the rash may be unappreciated in patients with dark skin. This group is at especially high risk for

TABLE 142.1. Clinical Manifestations of Rocky Mountain Spotted Fever

SIGN OR SYMPTOMS	Any Time (%)	First 3 Days (%)
Fever (100°F–102°F)	99	73
Fever (>102°F)	90	63
Fever + rash + tick bite	67	3
DERMATOLOGIC		
Any rash	88	49
Rash, maculopapular	82	46
Rash, petechial or hemorrhagic	49	13
Rash on palms and soles	74	28
Edema	18	3
Conjunctivitis	30	13
NEUROLOGIC		
Headache, mild/moderate	91	71
Headache, severe	57	40
Altered mental status	26	6
Meningeal irritation	18	5
Decreased hearing	7	1
Seizures	8	2
CARDIOPULMONARY		
Pneumonitis	12	2
Dysrhythmias	7	1
Myocarditis	5	0
GASTROINTESTINAL		
Abdominal pain	52	30
Nausea/vomiting	60	38
Diarrhea	19	9
Jaundice	9	2
MUSCULOSKELETAL		
Myalgias, mild/moderate	83	57
Myalgias, severe	47	25

From Helmick CG, et al. Rocky Mountain spotted fever: clinical, laboratory, and epidemiological features of 262 cases. *J Infect Dis* 1984;150:480.

delays in diagnosis and therapy, and thus increased morbidity (5).

The rash usually appears on the third day of illness and is first seen on the palms, soles, wrists, and ankles and progresses centripetally, but the rash may begin on the trunk (approximately 10%) or have a diffuse onset (approximately 10%). Lesions are initially macular and later evolve to become petechial and maculopapular in 50% of cases. Application of a tourniquet or blood pressure cuff causes the appearance of additional lesions distally (Rumpel-Leede sign). In severe cases, there may be extensive purpura, skin sloughing, ulceration, and gangrene. Rarely, an eschar may be seen at the site of the tick bite (7).

The *central nervous system* is perhaps the most crucial target "organ" of RMSF. Varying degrees of meningeal inflammation and cerebral vasculitis cause a wide range of neurologic signs and symptoms. Rickettsial encephalitis, which is manifested by severe headache, confusion, stupor, coma, and seizures, carries a particularly grave prognosis (8). Focal neurologic deficits, deafness, sensory neuropathy, tardive dyskinesia, and Guillain-Barré syndrome have all been described in patients with RMSF (9,10).

Neuroimaging with computed tomography (CT) or magnetic resonance imaging (MRI) may reveal a variety of subtle nonspecific abnormalities, including infarcts, cerebral edema, meningeal enhancement, and increased signal of the perivascular spaces (11). There is some evidence that the presence of these radiographic findings may be associated with a less favorable clinical outcome. In patients with central nervous system involvement, the cerebrospinal fluid is almost always abnormal (discussion follows).

The *cardiovascular* effects of RMSF are the result of myocarditis and myocardial vasculitis (12). Clinical manifestations include varying degrees of atrioventricular (AV) block, dysrhythmias (atrial and ventricular tachycardia, atrial fibrillation), and left ventricular dysfunction. It has been hypothesized that cardiac involvement may play an important role in the cases of fatal RMSF.

Rickettsial *pneumonitis* results from microvascular injury and leakage of fluid into the interstitial tissues and alveolar airspaces. This potentially life-threatening complication occurs in 2% to 17% of patients. Signs and symptoms include cough, dyspnea, pleuritic chest pain, and hypoxemia. Chest radiography typically reveals diffuse patchy infiltrates.

Up to 80% of patients with RMSF have prominent *gastrointestinal* complaints early in the course of disease, including abdominal pain, nausea, vomiting, and diarrhea. This symptom complex may lead the clinician to incorrectly diagnose acute gastroenteritis, or even an acute surgical abdomen. Not surprisingly, patients with RMSF have undergone exploratory laparotomy for suspected appendicitis, cholecystitis, and perforated diverticulitis (13). Acute hepatitis and clinical jaundice have been described in severe cases (14).

Approximately 10% to 15% of patients with RMSF develop significant *renal* dysfunction, the result of systemic hypovolemia and prerenal azotemia, as well as direct injury to the glomerulus. Renal biopsy in these patients demonstrates acute glomerulonephritis with subendothelial immune deposits.

Ocular abnormalities are not uncommon in patients with RMSF. Conjunctivitis occurs in 15% to 60% of patients. Less common findings include anterior uveitis, retinal vasculitis and hemorrhage, papilledema, arterial occlusion, and iris nodules.

Host factors associated with severe or fatal RMSF include: advanced age, male sex, African-American race, chronic ethanol abuse and G6PD deficiency.

DIFFERENTIAL DIAGNOSIS

The clinical diagnosis of RMSF can be difficult despite a careful history and physical examination and appropriate screening laboratory studies. Depending on the constellation of signs and symptoms present, the individual patient with RMSF may be misdiagnosed as having a viral illness (e.g., measles, infectious mononucleosis, or nonspecific viral syndrome), meningococcemia, gastroenteritis, acute surgical abdomen, pneumonia, toxic shock syndrome, ehrlichiosis, or encephalitis. RMSF may also mimic noninfectious entities, including idiopathic thrombocytopenic purpura, thrombotic thrombocytopenic purpura, drug reaction, and immune-complex vasculitis.

As with RMSF, diagnosis must be made quickly and accurately in acute meningococcemia. Both diseases may present with headache, fever, nausea, vomiting, and upper respiratory symptoms. Meningococcemia is typically more abrupt in onset. In contrast to RMSF, the meningococcemic rash appears within 24 hours of symptom onset, is petechial at onset, and lacks a characteristic pattern. Gram stain of cerebrospinal fluid is diagnostic, and the causative organism can also be detected using latex agglutination and counterimmunoelectrophoresis. If either diagnosis is in question, immediate therapy for both RMSF and meningococcemia is mandatory.

Toxic shock syndrome is an acute febrile illness characterized by the appearance of a diffuse desquamating erythroderma. Mucous membrane involvement and conjunctivitis are typical. Headache, myalgias, nausea, vomiting, and diarrhea are often present. Criteria for toxic shock syndrome include (1) fever greater than 38.9°C, (2) the typical rash, (3) hypotension, and (4) involvement of at least three organ systems.

Distinguishing RMSF from an enteroviral infection can also be quite difficult. Fever, headache, aseptic meningitis, and a maculopapular rash are common to both presentations. The rash of enteroviral infections usually starts centrally, but may also involve the palms and soles. Petechial lesions are not uncommon.

Measles (rubeola) occurs most often in unimmunized children during the winter and early spring. A prominent respiratory prodrome (cough, coryza, conjunctivitis), and the presence of Koplik spots are important distinguishing features. The rash of measles typically begins on the face and upper trunk and spreads to the extremities and downward.

Infectious mononucleosis is characterized by fever, fatigue, malaise, sore throat, and prominent lymphadenopathy. A maculopapular rash involving the trunk and extremities is often present, and it may become more prominent if the patient is inadvertently treated with ampicillin. The diagnosis is confirmed by a positive Monospot test, or by detection of antibodies against the Epstein-Barr virus.

EMERGENCY DEPARTMENT EVALUATION

Laboratory studies typically available in the emergency department offer little help in the diagnosis of RMSF. While routine studies may provide subtle clues, these are inconsistent and nonspecific. It must be emphasized that treatment must be based on clinical findings alone, and should never be withheld while waiting for specific serologic confirmation of the disease.

Hematologic findings seen in RMSF include a normal or decreased white blood cell count, anemia, thrombocytopenia, and a high peripheral band count. It has been suggested that the observation of an increased percentage of immature white cells in the absence of leukocytosis can help distinguish RMSF from meningococcemia. Anemia and thrombocytopenia are seen in 30% and in 30% to 50% of patients, respectively. Hyponatremia is seen in roughly one-fourth of cases. Elevation of serum transaminases and bilirubin may be noted in patients with hepatic involvement.

A lumbar puncture is mandatory in all patients with severe headache, fever, or signs of meningeal irritation. Elevated cerebrospinal fluid protein and pleocytosis are the typical finding in RMSF. Differential cell counts may reveal either lymphocytic or polymorphonuclear cell predominance. Of note, a cerebrospinal fluid white blood cell count more than 100 cells/μL is uncommon, occurring in only 11% of cases (15).

Serologic tests are of value in the retrospective confirmation of RMSF, but are not helpful in the acute setting, as results are not reliably positive for 6 to 10 days after the onset of clinical illness. Currently, the most widely used tests, all of which rely on the presence of antibodies to *R. rickettsii* antigens, are the indirect immunofluorescent antibody assay (IFA), indirect hemagglutination assay (IHA), latex agglutination, and polymerase chain reaction (PCR) (16). IFA is generally considered the reference standard for confirming cases of RMSF and is the test currently used by the CDC and most state public health laboratories.

Another approach to RMSF diagnostics involves identification of *R. rickettsii* in skin biopsy specimens. While this probably offers the best option of making a diagnosis in the acute setting, there are important limitations. Tissue immunostaining can only be used when the skin rash is present, and the sample should be obtained from an infected patient prior to therapy or within the first 48 hours after therapy has been initiated. Because rickettsiae are focally distributed in skin lesions, the organism may not be apparent even when an appropriate punch biopsy has been used. For this reason, testing of several samples is recommended. Even in laboratories with expertise in performing this test, the sensitivity is only about 70% on biopsied tissue.

EMERGENCY DEPARTMENT MANAGEMENT

For the majority of the conditions seen in emergency medicine, a diligent search for the cause is undertaken, and specific therapy is initiated based on the findings. This management paradigm is not realistic or acceptable in RMSF for several important reasons: (1) Clinical signs and symptoms are typically nonspecific; (2) the results of specific diagnostic tests are unavailable in a timely fashion; and (3) outcome is directly affected by delays in initiating therapy.

The most important factor contributing to the persistent case-fatality rate of 5% is delayed administration of specific therapy (3). In one series, all patients treated within 5 days of symptom onset survived, whereas the mortality of those treated after the sixth day was 60%. It is not only appropriate, but essential for the clinician practicing in an endemic area to initiate antibiotic therapy in the patient with clinical findings suggestive of, but not necessarily diagnostic of RMSF without the aid of serologic testing.

The tetracyclines and chloramphenicol are both effective in the treatment of RMSF and are considered the drugs of choice for therapy (17). There are no randomized, controlled trials comparing the efficacy of these two agents. The fluoroquinolones have also been demonstrated to possess antirickettsial activity (18). The penicillins, cephalosporins, erythromycin, sulfonamides, clindamycin, and aminoglycosides are ineffective against RMSF. Both the tetracyclines and chloramphenicol have significant adverse side effects; therefore, agent selection should be guided by the characteristics of the individual patient.

Because of a significant risk of thrombophlebitis and hepatotoxicity with the use of intravenous tetracycline, intravenous chloramphenicol is the preferred agent in the severely ill patient who cannot tolerate oral therapy. Chloramphenicol has also been advocated for treatment of RMSF during pregnancy. The recommended dosage is 50 to 100 mg/kg/d. Side effects associated with chloramphenicol include bone marrow depression, hemolytic anemia in patients with the Mediterranean form of glucose-6-phosphate dehydrogenase deficiency, "gray baby" syndrome in premature infants and neonates, and (rarely) aplastic anemia. Because chloramphenicol is metabolized by the liver, drug interactions may occur in patients taking either inhibitors or inducers of hepatic enzymes.

The tetracyclines are considered the drugs of choice for oral therapy in adults. The recommended dosages for tetracycline hydrochloride and doxycycline are 500 mg four times a day, and 100 mg twice a day, respectively. Doxycycline is the most favorable agent for the treatment of RMSF in children less than 9 years of age because of its documented effectiveness, broader margin of safety, and convenient dosing schedule. The recommended dosage is 4.4 mg/kg in divided doses every 12 hours for the first day of therapy, followed by a daily dose of 2.2 mg/kg.

Treatment of the pregnant patient with suspected RMSF poses a unique challenge. Tetracyclines are generally not recommended in the pregnant patient because of the associated risk of malformations of teeth and bones in the fetus. Chloramphenicol is the suggested alternative in this setting, although this drug is also associated with a wide range of side effects.

Prior recommendations discouraged administration of doxycycline to children because of concerns about staining of the teeth. More recent evidence suggests that up to five short courses of doxycycline may be administered with minimal risk of dental staining (19). Adverse effects associated with the use of tetracyclines include hepatitis, diarrhea, rash, thrombophlebitis, and impaired fetal bone formation.

Regardless of the agent selected, patients should be treated for at least 7 to 10 days, and therapy should be continued as necessary until the patient is afebrile and clinically improved for 24 to 48 hours (20).

Successful treatment of the critically ill patient with RMSF requires meticulous attention to fluid and electrolyte balance. Widespread systemic vasculitis and resultant fluid shifts may cause hypotension, oliguric renal failure, disseminated intravascular coagulation, adult respiratory distress syndrome, and shock. In the treatment of these complications, the clinician must maintain a delicate balance between adequate restoration of intravascular volume and overresuscitation with precipitation of pulmonary edema. Isotonic saline should be given in small serial boluses. Vasopressors may be required in patients with impaired tissue perfusion that is unresponsive to fluid therapy. Hemodynamic monitoring with a pulmonary artery catheter may provide the treating physician with an extra margin of safety, and is recommended in the unstable patient.

Prevention

Emergency physicians play an important role in educating the public about disease prevention. People who reside or work in tick-infested areas should be informed about tick-borne diseases and their prevention. The optimal method for preventing RMSF is avoidance of tick-infested areas. People entering these areas should wear protective clothing and use tick repellent. Exposed areas of the body should be examined for tick attachment. Remove ticks by grasping them with fine tweezers at the point of attachment and pulling slowly and steadily.

CRITICAL INTERVENTIONS

- Initiate antibiotic therapy in patients in endemic areas with clinical findings suggestive of, but not necessarily diagnostic of RMSF without the aid of serologic testing
- Administer tetracyclines or chloramphenicol to promptly treat RMSF in order to decrease morbidity and mortality

DISPOSITION

When an otherwise healthy, clinically stable patient presents with one or several clinical findings suggestive of RMSF, it is appropriate to initiate empiric therapy without confirmatory diagnostic testing and discharge the patient with appropriate follow up. In endemic areas, patients presenting with a flu-like illness during the spring or summer months are frequently discharged home on doxycycline. In this situation, contact with a primary care provider, or a return visit to the emergency department in 24 to 72 hours, is a sensible part of the discharge plan.

Patients presenting with more severe disease should be admitted to the hospital. This group includes those with significantly abnormal vital signs, dehydration, or end-organ dysfunction. Patients with severe organ dysfunction (e.g., cerebritis, pneumonitis, myocarditis) or hemodynamic instability should be admitted to an intensive care unit. Prompt administration of antibiotics and early consultation with an intensivist and an infectious disease specialist are also appropriate.

COMMON PITFALLS

✔ A recent review (21) identified the following eight pitfalls in the diagnosis and treatment of RMSF:
   1. Waiting for a petechial rash to develop before diagnosis,
   2. Misdiagnosis as gastroenteritis,
   3. Discounting a diagnosis when there is no history of tick bite,
   4. Using an inappropriate geographic exclusion,
   5. Using an inappropriate seasonal exclusion
   6. Failing to treat on clinical suspicion,
   7. Failing to elicit an appropriate history,
   8. Failing to initiate prompt treatment with doxycyline

✔ Another survey of 148 primary care physicians revealed that while 99% of physicians correctly identified doxycycline as the antibiotic of choice for the treatment of adults with RMSF, only 21% of family practice physicians and 25% of emergency physicians correctly identified doxycycline as the antibiotic of choice for the treatment of children 8 years of age or younger (22). Twenty-three percent of physicians responded that waiting for the development of a rash before prescribing antibiotics is an appropriate treatment strategy. It is important to recognize that roughly 15% patients with RMSF present without a rash ("Rocky Mountain spotless fever"). Among ultimately fatal cases, a rash is absent at the time of first presentation to a physician in more than 80%

References

1. Bonawitz C, et al. Comparison of CT and MR features with clinical outcome in patients with Rocky Mountain spotted fever. *Am J Neuroradiol* 1997;18:459.
2. Cale DF, et al. Treatment of Rocky Mountain spotted fever in children. *Ann Pharmacother* 1997;31:492.
3. Centers for Disease Control. Current trends in Rocky Mountain spotted fever—United States, 1990. *MMWR* 1991;40:451.
4. Dalton MJ, et al. National surveillance for Rocky Mountain spotted fever, 1981–1992: epidemiologic summary and evaluation of risk factors for fatal outcome. *Am J Trop Med Hyg* 1995;52:405.
5. Faham RH, et al. Rocky Mountain spotted (and spotless) fever. *Compr Ther* 1992;18:18.
6. Hall GW, et al. White blood cell count and differential in Rocky Mountain spotted fever. *North Carolina Med J* 1979;40:212.
7. Helmick CG, et al. Rocky Mountain spotted fever: clinical, laboratory, and epidemiological features of 262 cases. *J Infect Dis* 1984;150:480.
8. Horney LF, et al. Meningoencephalitis as a major manifestation of Rocky Mountain spotted fever. *South Med J* 1988;81:915.
9. Kirk JL, et al. Rocky Mountain spotted fever: a clinical review based on 48 confirmed cases: 1943-1986. *Medicine* 1990;69:35.
10. Kirkland KM, et al. Therapeutic delay and mortality in cases of Rocky Mountain spotted fever. *Clin Infect Dis* 1995;20:1118.
11. Lochary ME, et al. Doxycycline and staining of permanent teeth. *Pediatr Infect Dis J* 1998;17:429.
12. Marin-Garcia J, et al. Myocardial function in Rocky Mountain spotted fever: echocardiographic assessment. *Am J Cardiol* 1983;51:341m.
13. Sexton DJ, et al. Rocky Mountain "spotless" and "almost spotless" fever: a world in sheep's clothing. *Clin Infect Dis* 1992;15:439.
14. Shaked Y. Rickettsial infection of the central nervous system: the role of prompt antimicrobial therapy. *Q J Med* 1991;79:301.
15. Trianabos T, et al. Detection of *Rickettsia rickettsii* DNA in clinical specimens by using polymerase chain reaction technology. *J Clin Microbiol* 1989;27:2866.
16. Voggli VL, et al. Pulmonary pathology of Rocky Mountain spotted fever (RMSF) in children. *Pediatr Pathol Lab Med* 1980;104:171.
17. Weber DJ, et al. Rocky Mountain spotted fever. *Infect Dis Clin North Am* 1991;5:19.
18. Wei TY, et al. Acute disseminated encephalomyelitis after Rocky Mountain spotted fever. *Pediatr Neurol* 1999;21:503.
19. Westerman EL. Rocky Mountain spotless fever: a dilemma for the clinician. *Arch Intern Med* 1982;142:1106.
20. Woodard TE, et al. Prompt confirmation of Rocky Mountain spotted fever: identification of rickettsiae in skin tissues. *J Infect Dis* 1976;134:297.
21. Masters EJ, Olson GS, Weiner SJ, et al. Rocky Mountain spotted fever: a clinician's dilemma. *Arch Intern Med* 2003;163:769.
22. O'Reilly M, Paddock C, Elchos B, et al. Physician knowledge of the diagnosis of Rocky Mountain spotted fever: Mississippi, 2002. *Ann New York Acad Sci* 2003;990:295.

CHAPTER 143
Other Tick-Borne Diseases

Ann P. Nguyen

Ticks are blood-feeding arthropods of the class *Arachnidae*, which also includes mites, spiders and scorpions. Ticks are second in importance only to mosquitoes as vectors of human illness, and hundreds of tick-borne diseases occur worldwide (2,10,25). Eight tick-borne diseases are endemic in North America: Lyme disease, Rocky Mountain spotted fever, ehrlichiosis, tularemia, babesiosis, tick-borne relapsing fever, Colorado tick fever and tick paralysis. These diseases peak in incidence in the spring and summer, when the feeding activity of ticks coincides most with the outdoor activity of humans. Lyme disease is discussed in Chapter 141 and Rocky Mountain Spotted Fever in Chapter 142. Due to the protean number of tick-borne diseases, only the most prevalent North American tick-borne illnesses will be discussed here (Table 143.1)

EHRLICHIOSIS

Ehrlichiosis consists of two clinically similar, identically managed diseases: human monocytic ehrlichiosis (HME) and human granulocytic ehrlichiosis (HGE). HME occurs in the Southeastern and South Central United States (primarily Arkansas, Missouri, Oklahoma and Tennessee) while HGE is distributed in the Northeastern and Midwestern states (Connecticut, Minnesota, Rhode Island and New York) and California. The pathogen in HME is *Ehrlichia chaffeensis*, a rickettsia, which infects monocytes. The Lone Star tick (*Amblyomma americanum*) is its main vector, although *Dermacentor* and *Ixodes* species have also been found to transmit this organism (see Fig. 141.2.). The pathogen in HGE is *Anaplasma phagocytophila*, a rickettsia, which infects granulocytes. Deer ticks (*Ixodes* species) transmit HGE. In immunosuppressed patients, HGE has also been found to be caused by *Ehrlichia ewingii* via the *A. americanum* vector, but this is exceedingly rare and fewer than 20 cases have been documented (18,22). The Centers for Disease Control (CDC) consider both HME and HGE to be notifiable diseases. In endemic areas, disease incidence is approximately 14 to 16 cases per 100,000 persons per year for HME and 24 to 51 cases per 100,000 persons per year for HGE (19).

CLINICAL PRESENTATION

HME and HGE present after a 7- to 10-day incubation period, with abrupt onset of symptoms resembling those of an acute viral syndrome: fever, rigors, diffuse myalgias and arthralgias, headache, nausea, vomiting and occasionally diarrhea. Upper respiratory symptoms are uncommon. In HME more often than in HGE, up to 20% of patients will show evidence of central nervous system infection (1,17,19,22). Following roughly 1 week of illness, a nonpruritic, erythematous maculopapular or petechial rash appears on the trunks and extremities of 40% of HME patients and 10% of HGE patients. Rash is more common in children

TABLE 143.1. North American Tick-Borne Diseases

Disease	Causative Agent	Vector	Geographic Distribution	Clinical Features	Treatment
Ehrlichiosis					
Human Monocytic	*Ehrlichia chaffeensis* (Rickettsia)	*Amblyomma*	Southeast South central	Nonspecific febrile syndrome Rash in 10%–40% Elderly and immunosuppressed patients at risk	Doxycyline OR Rifampin
Human Granulocytic	*Anaplasma phagocytophila Ehrlichia ewingii* (Rickettsia)	*Ixodes*	Northeast Midwest California	ARDS, thrombocytopenia, DIC, opportunistic infections	
Tularemia	*Francisella tularensis* (Bacteria)	*Amblyomma* *Dermacentor*	Southeast South central All regions	Nonspecific febrile syndrome Ulceroglandular, glandular, typhoidal, pneumonic, oropharyngeal and oculoglandular forms	Streptomycin OR Gentamicin
Babesiosis	*Babesia microti* (Protozoan)	*Ixodes*	Northeast	Fever, sweats, hemolysis Splenectomized patients at risk	Quinine PLUS Clindamycin
Relapsing fever	*Borrelia* species: *B. hermsii, B. parkerii B. turicatae, B. dugesi*	*Ornithodoros*	Rocky Mountains Texas, Mexico	Multiple remissions and relapses Neonates and pregnant women at risk Jarisch-Herxheimer reaction when treated	Tetracycline OR Erythromycin
Colorado tick fever (CTF)	CTF virus (*Arbovirus*)	*Dermacentor*	Rocky Mountains	Biphasic fever pattern Prolonged convalescence	Supportive
Tick paralysis	Tick neurotoxin	*Ixodes* *Dermacentor* *Amblyomma*	Eastern Rocky Mountains South central	Flaccid symmetric ascending paralysis Affects primarily young children Death due to respiratory muscle paralysis	Tick removal

(66%) than adults. Children have milder disease than adults, although long-term neurologic sequelae have been reported in two children, whereas no post-infectious sequelae have been reported in adults (13,19). Most patients recover spontaneously within 2 weeks.

Host defense against *E. chaffeensis*, *A. phagocytophila* and *E. ewingii* consists of a cellular immune response; patients with impaired cellular immunity are at the highest risk for severe illness. Poor outcome has been associated with age greater than 60, HIV infection or other immunodeficient states, diabetes mellitus, and connective tissue disease (1,17-19). Delayed administration of appropriate antibiotic therapy and recent use of trimethoprim-sulfamethoxazole has also been associated with increased rates of complications. Complications occur in 10% to 20% of patients and include pulmonary edema, acute respiratory distress syndrome (ARDS), thrombocytopenia with life-threatening hemorrhage, disseminated intravascular coagulation (DIC), acute tubular necrosis, cardiomyopathy, encephalopathy and seizures. Opportunistic infections with cytomegalovirus, candida, aspergillus and cryptococcus occur due to a poorly understood ehrlichia-associated immunosuppression, and are a common cause of HGE-related deaths (1,17). Even with appropriate antibiotic treatment, HME carries a 3% mortality rate and HGE, a 1% mortality rate (1,16–19).

DIFFERENTIAL DIAGNOSIS

The nonspecific presentation of HME and HGE lends itself to a broad differential diagnosis: Rocky Mountain spotted fever or other tick-borne illness, viral gastroenteritis, hepatitis,

cytomegalovirus infection (in immunocompromised patients), infectious mononucleosis, endocarditis, Kawasaki disease and collagen vascular disease. The presence of neurologic findings suggests meningococcemia or encephalitis.

EMERGENCY DEPARTMENT EVALUATION AND MANAGEMENT

Physical examination is unrevealing, although some patients may demonstrate hepatomegaly or splenomegaly. The most common findings on routine laboratory testing are lymphopenia, thrombocytopenia and mild-to-moderate elevation of AST and ALT. Serum sodium and hematocrit may be decreased in 50% of cases. When neurologic symptoms are present, CSF shows a lymphocytic pleocytosis with elevated protein but normal glucose. Laboratory derangements normalize with antibiotic therapy, and can be used to monitor treatment efficacy (1,17–19).

HME and HGE can be diagnosed by visualizing rickettsiae on peripheral blood smear, though the poor sensitivity of this test means that a "negative" smear does not rule out ehrlichiosis (22). Serologic testing is the gold standard. Acute sera should be compared with convalescent sera taken 4 to 6 weeks later; a four-fold rise in antiehrlichial antibodies confirms ehrlichial infection, although immunocompromised patients may not seroconvert at all. Acute titers >1:80 for HGE or >1:64 for HME suggests active infection. Recently developed PCR tests are up to 87% sensitive and 100% specific, and have the advantage over serology in that a diagnosis can be made during the acute phase of illness (17). Lyme titers should also be obtained in patients with suspected ehrlichiosis, as both diseases share a vector and cases of ehrlichial and borrelial coinfection have been reported (1,19).

Should any of the complications listed above occur, appropriate resuscitative therapy should be initiated. However, most patients will not be critically ill and management should focus on supportive care. Empiric antibiotics are appropriate in high-risk groups, as confirmatory tests take days to complete and delayed therapy is associated with poor outcome (22). The drug of choice is doxycycline 100 mg PO q12h (children: 3 to 4 mg/kg) for 10 to 14 days. The course should be extended to 21 days when Lyme disease coinfection is detected. Rifampin 300 mg PO q12h × 14 days has been used when doxycycline is contraindicated (e.g., allergy or pregnancy) (3). Failure to improve after 24 to 48 hours of doxycycline or rifampin indicates a diagnosis other than ehrlichiosis.

DISPOSITION

All patients with complications of HME or HGE must be admitted. Admit patients belonging to high-risk groups for 24 to 48 hours of observation. Nontoxic patients may be discharged home, with arrangements made for clinical reevaluation in 48 hours and for follow up of serologic testing.

TULAREMIA

Tularemia is caused by a Gram-negative coccobacillus, *Francisella tularensis*. Two strains of *F. tularensis* infect humans: Type A, which is tick-borne and causes 90% of tularemic disease, and Type B, which is rodent- and water-borne and causes mild to subclinical disease (4). Half of all cases of tularemia are transmitted by tick vectors: the Lone Star tick (*Amblyomma americanum*) (see Fig. 141.2.) in the Southeastern and South Central states, the Rocky Mountain wood tick (*Dermacentor andersoni*) in the Western states and the dog tick (*Dermacentor variabilis*) in all regions of North America (8). Arkansas, Oklahoma, and Missouri account for half of all tick-borne cases. The other half of tularemia cases are transmitted by insect vectors such as biting flies and mosquitoes, and by handling infected animals (primarily rabbits and rodents), ingesting contaminated meat or water, inhaling aerosolized bacteria, or inoculating mucous membranes (e.g., touching one's eyes after handling animals). Tularemia has a nationwide incidence of approximately 300 cases per year, although this figure is declining annually (4,8). The CDC considers tularemia to be a reportable disease.

CLINICAL PRESENTATION

The spectrum of illness ranges from asymptomatic to fatal. Six clinical syndromes are classically described, although overlapping presentations are common. All syndromes begin with an incubation period ranging from 2 to 14 days (3 to 6 days on average) followed by the abrupt onset of fever, chills, headache and generalized myalgias. Cough, vomiting, diarrhea and diffuse arthralgias often occur. A nonspecific, pruritic maculopapular or papulovesicular rash may appear on the extremities of 25% of patients, 2 weeks after symptom onset. Symptoms usually last for 1 to 4 weeks but may persist for months (12).

The most common tularemic syndrome is ulceroglandular tularemia. The ulceroglandular form comprises 66% to 80% of tularemia cases and carries a <3% mortality rate (4,8). It is characterized by a solitary skin ulcer at the tick-bite site, developing 2 weeks after the onset of constitutional symptoms. The ulcer is usually 0.5 to 3.0 cm in diameter with sharply undermined borders and a flat black or red base. It can evolve into an abscess or

necrotic eschar, and is accompanied by regional lymphadenopathy with or without lymphangitis. The next most common syndrome is glandular tularemia, which occurs in 8% to 15% of cases (4,8). This syndrome presents like ulceroglandular tularemia, only without the ulcer. Pronounced, tender, fluctuant regionalized lymphadenopathy is the hallmark of this syndrome, with possible suppuration or necrosis of the lymph nodes.

Typhoidal tularemia comprises <14% of cases but accounts for 30% to 60% of fatalities (4,5,8,12). Patients display the nonspecific febrile syndrome described above, but are toxic in appearance and may progress to overwhelming sepsis. Tularemic pneumonia, which presents with a dry cough, pleuritic chest pain and dyspnea, occurs in 10% to 15% of patients with ulceroglandular tularemia and in 50% of patients with the typhoidal form (4,5,8,12). It is caused by hematogenous spread or direct inhalation of aerosolized *F. tularensis*. Oropharyngeal tularemia occurs in 3% to 5% of cases and is due to ingestion of infected meat or water, rather than from a tick bite (4,5,8,12). It is characterized by exudative pharyngitis, vomiting, diarrhea and abdominal pain with tenderness to palpation. The diarrhea ranges from mild to fatal, with bowel ulceration. The rarest syndrome is oculoglandular tularemia (1% of cases), where pathogens are inoculated into the eye either by a splash of infected blood or by rubbing one's eye after handling infected animals. This syndrome is characterized by a painful, ulcerative conjunctivitis, preauricular lymphadenopathy, and periorbital edema and erythema.

Tularemia carries an overall mortality rate of 2% to 4% (8% if untreated, 1% to 2% if treated early) (4). Persons at highest risk are young children and the elderly. Complications are usually due to the pneumonic or typhoidal forms and include ARDS, meningitis, pericarditis, endocarditis, hepatitis, rhabdomyolysis, peritonitis, osteomyelitis, DIC and septic shock.

DIFFERENTIAL DIAGNOSIS

Ulceroglandular and glandular tularemia may resemble bubonic plague, anthrax, sporotrichosis, cat-scratch disease, lymphogranuloma venereum, mycobacterial infection, streptococcal or staphylococcal skin lymphadenitis or lymphoma. Typhoidal tularemia may resemble Rocky Mountain spotted fever, typhoid fever, brucellosis, tuberculosis, or septic shock from any other pathogen. Tularemic pneumonia may resemble a viral pneumonitis or an atypical or fungal pneumonia. Oropharyngeal tularemia may be mistaken for diphtheria, streptococcal pharyngitis, infectious mononucleosis or inflammatory bowel disease. Oculoglandular tularemia shares its preauricular lymphadenopathy with coccidioidomycosis, although the latter occurs in the Southwest where tularemia is not endemic.

EMERGENCY DEPARTMENT EVALUATION AND MANAGEMENT

It is imperative that the patient be examined thoroughly for the pathognomonic ulcer and regional lymphadenopathy. These findings are present in 60% to 86% of adults but only 45% of children (4,8,12). Lesions are usually found on the lower extremities in cases of tick bite, with corresponding femoral and inguinal lymphadenopathy, and on the upper extremities in cases of animal handling, with epitrochlear and axillary lymph node involvement. The patient's scalp must also be checked or else lesions may be missed, especially in children. A pulse-temperature dissociation (i.e., bradycardia relative to the height of fever) has also been described and is considered pathognomonic. A yellow-white oropharyngeal pseudomembrane may be seen in oropharyngeal tularemia, and corneal nodules and ulcers may be seen in oculoglandular tularemia.

The most common findings on routine laboratory testing are elevated transaminase levels, decreased serum sodium, and normal to mildly elevated leukocyte count with a normal differential cell count. Chest x-ray may show the "classic tularemic triad" of ovoid opacities, pleural effusions and hilar adenopathy, or may show a variety of unilobar, multilobar, patchy, miliary or cavitary infiltrates.

Diagnosis is made by serology. An acute titer of 1:160, or a four-fold rise in the convalescent titer compared to the acute titer, indicates acute tularemia. It is possible to culture *F. tularensis* from various bodily fluids, but this technique is only 10% sensitive, requires specialized culture medium, and requires special precautions to limit the risk of bacterial inhalation by laboratory personnel (8).

Streptomycin 1 g IM q12h (children: 15 mg/kg) or gentamicin 5 mg/kg/day IM or IV (children: 2.5 mg/kg q8h) for 10 to 14 days are the drugs of choice. Alternative regimens are doxycycline 100 mg IV q12h (children: 2.2 mg/kg) or chloramphenicol 15 mg/kg IV q6h for 14–21 days. Chloramphenicol must be added to the aminoglycoside regimen if central nervous system infection is suspected. Ciprofloxacin 400 mg IV q12h × 10 days (children: 15 mg/kg) has also been successfully used (4,5,8,12). Abscesses and infected lymph nodes may need incision and drainage. An emergent ophthalmology consult is indicated in oculoglandular cases as corneal perforation may result if this disease is not properly treated.

DISPOSITION

As parenteral antibiotics are indicated in all cases of tularemia, all patients must be admitted. Patients may be switched to oral antibiotics after a few days and discharged if clinically well (5,12).

BABESIOSIS

The agent of human babesiosis is *Babesia microti*, an intraerythrocytic protozoan. Like the plasmodial agent of malaria, *B. microti* causes red blood cell hemolysis. Babesiosis is mainly reported along the Northeast coast of the United States between Cape Cod and New Jersey, but prevalence is increasing in California, Washington, and the Midwest. The vector is the deer tick, *Ixodes scapularis* (see Fig. 141.2.). Transmission also occurs via transfusion of red blood cells and via transplacental infection in neonates (15). Babesiosis is not a notifiable disease and its true incidence is unknown, but over 300 cases have been documented since 1969 (23).

CLINICAL PRESENTATION

The disease spectrum ranges from asymptomatic infection to mild flu-like illness to moderately severe malaria-like disease to fulminant sepsis resulting in death. Symptom onset follows the tick bite by 1 to 6 weeks, and consists of high fever with drenching sweats, fatigue, malaise, rigors and headache. Myalgias, arthralgias, cough and vomiting are less common and rash is uncommon. Jaundice and hemoglobinuria may result from parasite-induced intravascular hemolysis. Symptoms last from weeks to months, and the majority of patients recover spontaneously although subclinical parasitemia may persist for years and relapse is possible (15,23,24).

A history of splenectomy is a major risk factor for severe babesial infection, as parasitized red blood cells are normally cleared by the spleen. Splenectomized patients have demonstrated burdens of parasitemia as high as 85%, compared to 1% to 20% in immunocompetent patients (15). Babesiosis is also considered a disease of the elderly, as three-quarters of older adults suffer severe disease, whereas only half of infected children will do so. The chief complications are congestive heart failure (11%) and ARDS (8%) (24). The next most common complications are shock, DIC and renal failure. Complications may not occur until days after treatment is started, and the mortality rate is 6% to 9% (15,23,24).

DIFFERENTIAL DIAGNOSIS

Acute babesiosis resembles malaria, any of the viral hemorrhagic fevers, hepatobiliary infection, or other tick-borne illnesses. Milder cases suggest a flu-like syndrome. Meningitis and encephalitis should be in the differential diagnosis if the patient has headache, vomiting, photophobia or an altered mental status.

EMERGENCY DEPARTMENT EVALUATION AND MANAGEMENT

High fever may be the only physical finding, although 11% to 14% of patients have hepatomegaly or splenomegaly and 4% have jaundice (15,24). Routine laboratory tests may show evidence of hemolysis: bilirubinuria; decreased hemoglobin and hematocrit; increased reticulocyte count, LDH, indirect bilirubin, and haptoglobin. Transaminase and alkaline phosphatase levels are elevated in 50% of patients (15).

The gold standard for diagnosis is direct microscopy of peripheral blood smears. This test is rapidly obtained and highly specific, but its sensitivity depends on the patient's parasitemic load. Because of its greater sensitivity and specificity, PCR is becoming the assay of choice (15,23). Acute and convalescent serology can also be compared; a four-fold titer rise or an acute titer of >1:256 indicates active infection. Babesiosis shares the same tick vector and geographic distribution as ehrlichiosis and Lyme disease, so coinfection with 2 or more of these pathogens can occur. Serologic testing for all 3 diseases should be done if babesiosis is suspected (23).

Most patients improve spontaneously and only require supportive care. Pharmacotherapy is reserved for those with severe symptoms and for splenectomized or otherwise immunocompromised individuals (15,23,24). First-line therapy is quinine 650 mg PO q8h (children: 8 mg/kg) plus clindamycin 600–900 mg PO q8h (children: 5 to 10 mg/kg) for 7 to 10 days (23). If no improvement occurs within 72 hours or if these drugs are not tolerated, the patient should be switched to the second-line regimen: atovaquone 750 mg PO q12h (children: 20 mg/kg) plus azithromycin 500 mg PO on the first day (children: 12 mg/kg) then 250 mg PO qd thereafter, for 7 days. The second regimen has not been tested in children, so quinine and clindamycin remain the pediatric treatment of choice (15,23,24). Patients who fail to respond to either regimen, who have >4% parasitemia (>1% in high risk individuals), or who have massive symptomatic hemolysis are candidates for exchange transfusion (15,23,24). Some experts also recommend the addition of doxycycline 100 mg PO bid in endemic Lyme disease areas until the Lyme serology results are known (23).

DISPOSITION

Patients with any of the above complications must be admitted. Other predictors of poor outcome are: age older than 50, splenectomized state, immunocompromised state, history of cardiac disease, parasitemia >4%, alkaline phosphatase level >125 U/L, and leukocytosis $>5 \times 10^9/L$ (15,24). These patients require antibabesial medication and should be admitted to observe their response to treatment. If not toxic, all other patients may be discharged without specific pharmacotherapy and reevaluated as outpatients.

TICK-BORNE RELAPSING FEVER

Relapsing fever is caused by spirochetes of the genus *Borrelia* and may be transmitted via ticks, lice, blood transfusion, percutaneous exposure to infected blood, and transplacental infection of neonates (6,7). The recurring pattern of illness and remission characteristic of this disease is due to the ability of *Borrelia* to vary their surface antigens to evade and restimulate the host's immune system. Tick-borne relapsing fever (TBRF) is endemic in states abutting the Rocky Mountains (pathogens: *B. hermsii*, *B. parkeri*), and in central Texas and Mexico (pathogens: *B. turicatae*, *B. dugesi*) (6,7). Ticks of the genus *Ornithodoros* serve as vectors. Unlike other ticks which attach to passing hosts and feed for days, *Ornithodoros* ticks seek out sleeping humans, feed quickly (15 to 90 minutes), then return to their nests. TBRF is not a notifiable disease and its true incidence is unknown, but over 450 cases have been reported in the United States from 1977 to 2000 (7).

CLINICAL PRESENTATION

Patients occasionally report a pruritic eschar at the tick bite site, which later progresses into an ulcer. Generalized symptoms begin 4 to 18 days (mean 7 days) after the bite and consist of high fever, headache, myalgias, rigors, arthralgias, nausea and vomiting. Up to one-third of patients also complain of abdominal pain, diarrhea, meningismus and photophobia. A nonspecific diffuse maculopapular or petechial rash that spares the palms and soles occurs in 18% of cases and jaundice, hepatomegaly and splenomegaly have been found in 10% (6,7). After 1 to 17 days (mean 3 days), symptoms resolve with a rapid defervescence and drenching sweats. Patients experience an average remission of 1 week's duration (range 3 to 36 days) before symptoms return. The mean number of relapses experienced is 2, although 22% of patients have more than 4 (6,7).

TBRF carries a 0% to 8% mortality, depending on the reporting state (6,7). No adult deaths have been reported. Infants are at highest risk; neonates infected in utero die of overwhelming sepsis. Pregnant women are also high risk, as placental infection frequently results in abortion and fetal demise. Other complications include thrombocytopenia with life-threatening hemorrhage, liver failure, renal failure, encephalitis, meningitis, and iritis or endophthalmitis leading to permanent visual impairment.

DIFFERENTIAL DIAGNOSIS

The nonspecific symptoms of TBRF may resemble any viral syndrome or tick-borne disease (especially tularemia, if the patient develops a bite-site ulcer), malaria, yellow fever, dengue fever or any of the viral hemorrhagic fevers, brucellosis, leptospirosis, or rat bite fever. One should also consider occult malignancy and in children, juvenile rheumatoid arthritis.

EMERGENCY DEPARTMENT EVALUATION AND MANAGEMENT

Suspect TBRF if the patient gives a history of sleeping in a mountain cabin or in a cave in Texas. There are no specific findings on physical exam or laboratory testing, but leukocytes, bilirubin

and transaminases may be mildly elevated and platelets may be decreased. CSF may show a lymphocytic pleocytosis with normal glucose. TBRF is diagnosed by microscopic visualization of spirochetes in peripheral blood smears, or by serology. Neither method is sensitive, as spirochetes only circulate in peripheral blood during febrile episodes, and vary their surface antigens so often that the serologic assay may not react with the antigens on a particular patient's spirochete (6,7).

Tetracycline or erythromycin 500 mg PO q6h (children: 5 to 10 mg/kg) for 10 days eliminates most relapses (6,7). Doxycycline 100 mg PO q12h (children: 3 to 4 mg/kg) for 10 days has also been used. A Jarisch-Herxheimer reaction (JHR) occurs in 40% to 50% of patients, within 4 hours of starting antibiotic therapy (6,7). This syndrome of hypotension, tachycardia, fever, rigors and diaphoresis is due to massive cytokine and endotoxin release as spirochetes are lysed. JHR is a significant cause of TBRF mortality due to cardiovascular collapse. Treatment is supportive. Antipyretics and steroids are not effective, although meptazinol 300 to 500 mg IV has been found to decrease JHR severity in louse-borne relapsing fever (20).

DISPOSITION

All patients must be observed for at least 4 hours following initiation of antibiotics. Patients with severe JHR must be admitted to a critical care unit for hemodynamic monitoring, and pregnant women and neonates should be admitted to observe for septic deterioration. Consider admitting infants and very young children. If not toxic, all other patients may be discharged and reevaluated as outpatients.

COLORADO TICK FEVER

The pathogen in this disease is Colorado tick fever (CTF) virus, a double-stranded RNA arbovirus of the *Reoviridae* family. CTF virus infects hematopoietic cells, causing leukopenia. This virus is spread by the Rocky Mountain wood tick (*Dermacentor andersoni*), although blood transfusion-related infection has also been reported (14,21). The wood tick vector is active in the Rocky Mountain regions of North America, at elevations from 1,200 to 3,300 meters. Two hundred to three hundred cases are reported annually in the United States (14,21). CTF is not a CDC notifiable disease.

CLINICAL PRESENTATION

CTF is also called saddleback fever, for the pathognomonic biphasic fever pattern that occurs in 50% of cases. Following a 3- to 14-day incubation period (mean 5 days), patients present with an abrupt onset of high fever, myalgias, rigors and headache. Abdominal pain, nausea, vomiting, diarrhea, meningismus, photophobia and pharyngitis appear in approximately one-quarter of patients (14,21). A single painless target lesion may be seen, or less commonly, a fine maculopapular or petechial rash. The fever persists for 2 to 3 days, remits for 2 to 3 days, recurs for 2 to 3 days, then finally resolves. Although CTF is benign and self-limiting, patients often report a prolonged convalescence featuring lethargy, fatigue, malaise and myalgias that may last for months.

Complications primarily occur in children and include meningitis and encephalitis (5% to 10%), pneumonitis, myocarditis, hepatitis, epididymoorchitis, DIC and gastrointestinal hemorrhage (14,21).

DIFFERENTIAL DIAGNOSIS

The nonspecific, self-limiting symptoms of CTF are suggestive of any other viral syndrome, though in particular the leukopenia and thrombocytopenia are also found in dengue fever. The prolonged recovery phase may be confused with chronic fatigue syndrome, fibromyalgia, polymyalgia rheumatica or other rheumatologic or connective tissue diseases.

EMERGENCY DEPARTMENT EVALUATION AND MANAGEMENT

A complete blood count should be obtained. The hallmark of CTF is a leukocyte count less than $4000/mm^3$, with neutropenia more pronounced than lymphopenia (14,21). Thrombocytopenia is occasionally seen. Direct microscopy of peripheral blood smears is the quickest diagnostic test for CTF; immunofluorescent staining reveals viral antigen on erythrocyte membranes. Serologic and PCR assays are also available.

Should any of the complications listed above occur, appropriate resuscitative therapy should be initiated. However, most patients will not be critically ill and treatment is purely supportive.

DISPOSITION

The majority of patients will be nontoxic and safe for discharge. All patients with complications of CTF must be admitted.

TICK PARALYSIS

Tick paralysis is caused by a neurotoxin in the saliva of female *Ixodes* ticks: *Dermacentor variabilis* and *Ixodes scapularis* in the Eastern United States, *Dermacentor andersoni* in the Rocky Mountain states and *Amblyomma americanum* in the South Central states. This uncommon disease primarily affects young children (ages 1 to 5) (11).

CLINICAL PRESENTATION

Twelve hours to 7 days following a tick bite (mean 5 days), children complain of general irritability, fatigue and myalgias. Some also report paresthesiae of the hands and feet. Within 2 days of the initial complaints, the patient is noted to be ataxic or refusing to walk. Physical exam reveals a symmetric ascending motor weakness, proximal greater than distal, with flaccid tone and diminished or absent deep tendon reflexes. Sensation, anal sphincter tone and sensorium are normal. Temporal disease progression leads to paralysis of muscles innervated by cranial nerves, causing facial droop, diplopia, dysarthria, and dysphagia. Pupillary reaction is spared. Fever and rash are not part of this disease; consider other concurrent tick-borne illnesses if fever or rash are present (10,11).

Tick paralysis carries a 10% mortality rate. Deaths are secondary to ventilatory failure from respiratory muscle paralysis. Hypoxic seizures have been reported, as have myocarditis and myositis (10,11). The treatment is simply tick removal. Recovery begins within 1 hour of tick removal and is usually complete, with no residual deficits, 24 hours postremoval (10,11). The exception to this course is in cases of envenomation by the Australian scrub tick, *Ixodes holocyclus*. These patients may have worsened symptoms immediately after tick removal, and take days to weeks for full recovery (10,11).

DIFFERENTIAL DIAGNOSIS

Tick paralysis is most commonly mistaken for Guillain-Barré syndrome, which may present identically except that progression usually occurs over weeks rather than days. Also on the differential diagnosis are acute cerebellar ataxia, transverse myelitis, poliomyelitis, myasthenia gravis, serum electrolyte abnormalities, metabolic encephalopathies, familial periodic paralysis, diphtheria, organophosphate toxicity, heavy metal toxicity, porphyria-related polyneuropathy and botulism.

EMERGENCY DEPARTMENT EVALUATION AND MANAGEMENT

Patients with impending respiratory muscle fatigue should be intubated and mechanically ventilated while awaiting definitive evaluation. An Australian canine antitoxin is available but not recommended because of the risk of anaphylaxis and serum sickness (10,11).

No derangements are expected on routine blood or CSF testing. Brain CT and MRI are also unrevealing. Electromyography (EMG) shows decreased motor neuron conduction velocity and decreased amplitude of the muscle's action potential, findings which are also present in Guillain-Barré syndrome (10). The diagnosis is achieved by a thorough physical exam, keeping in mind that ticks range in size from 2 to 30 mm and that multiple ticks may be attached. It is imperative that all body areas be checked, including the scalp, ear canal, nares, umbilicus, perineum and axillae (10). Once a tick is found, it should be pulled out with blunt forceps, grasping as close to the patient's skin as possible and taking care not to disrupt the tick's abdomen. Ticks should never be handled with bare hands.

CRITICAL INTERVENTIONS

- Examine patients thoroughly for the pathognomonic ulcer and regional lymphadenopathy found in tularemia. Lesions are usually found on the lower extremities in cases of tick bite, with corresponding femoral and inguinal lymphadenopathy, and on the upper extremities in cases of animal handling, with epitrochlear and axillary lymph node involvement
- Observe patients treated for tick-borne relapsing fever for at least 4 hours following initiation of antibiotics since 40% to 50% of patients develop a Jarisch-Herxheimer reaction
- Perform a careful search for a tick and remove it to cure tick paralysis
- Evaluate patients with suspected ehrlichiosis, babesiosis, or Lyme Disease for all three diseases, as these diseases share the same tick vector and coinfection has been reported
- Admit all patients with tularemia for parenteral antibiotics

DISPOSITION

All patients should be admitted for observation of symptom progression and for further work up if necessary.

COMMON PITFALLS

✔ Failure to consider tick-borne illness in the differential diagnosis of patients with fever and headache, fever and rash, fever and body aches, fever and abdominal pain, or fever and jaundice

✔ Failure to consider tick-borne illness when evaluating patients with neurologic deficits

✔ Failure to obtain an occupational, recreational, residential, and travel history in patients presenting with febrile syndromes

✔ Failure to obtain a history of symptom patterns in patients presenting with febrile syndromes

References

1. Bakken JS, Dumler JS. Human granulocytic ehrlichiosis. *Clin Infect Dis* 2000;31:554–560.
2. Bratu S, Lutwick LI. Active immunization against human tick-borne diseases. *Expert Opin Biol Ther* 2002;2:187–195.
3. Buitrago MI, Ijdo JW, Rinaudo P, et al. Human granulocytic ehrlichiosis during pregnancy treated successfully with rifampin. *Clin Infect Dis* 1998;27:213–215.
4. Choi E. Tularemia and Q Fever. *Med Clin N Am* 2002;86:393–416.
5. Dennis DT, Inglesby TV, Henderson DA, et al. Tularemia as a biological weapon: medical and public health management. *JAMA* 2001;285:2763–2773.
6. Dworkin MS, Schwan TG, Anderson DE. Tick-borne relapsing fever in North America. *Med Clin N Am* 2002;86:417–433.
7. Dworkin MS, Shoemaker PC, Fritz CL, Dowell ME, Anderson DE. The epidemiology of tick-borne relapsing fever in the United States. *Am J Trop Med Hyg* 2002;66:753–758.
8. Ellis P, Oyston PCF, Green M, Titball RW. Tularemia. *Clin Microbiol Rev* 2002;15:631–646.
9. Gardner SL, Holman RC, Krebs JW, Berkelman R, Childs JE. National surveillance for the human ehrlichioses in the United States, 1997–2001, and proposed methods for evaluation of data quality. *Ann N Y Acad Sci* 2003;990:80–89.
10. Grattan-Smith PJ, Morris JG, Johnston HM, et al. Clinical and neurophysiologic features of tick paralysis. *Brain* 1997;120:1975–1987.
11. Greenstein P. Tick paralysis. *Med Clin N Am* 2002;86:441–446.
12. Jacobs RF. Tularemia. *Pediatr Infect Dis* 1997;12:55–68.
13. Jacobs RF. Human monocytic ehrlichiosis: similar to Rocky Mountain spotted fever but different. *Pediatr Ann* 2002;31:180–184.
14. Klasco R. Colorado tick fever. *Med Clin N Am* 2002;86:435–440.
15. Krause PJ. Babesiosis. *Med Clin N Am* 2002;86:361–373.
16. McQuiston JH, Paddock CD, Holman RC, Childs JE. The human ehrlichioses in the United States. *Emerg Infect Dis* 1999;5:635–642.
17. Olano JP, Walker DH. Human ehrlichioses. *Med Clin N Am* 2002;86:375–392.
18. Paddock CD, Folk SM, Shore GM, et al. Infections with Ehrlichia chaffeensis and Ehrlichia ewingii in persons coinfected with human immunodeficiency virus. *Clin Infect Dis* 2001;33:1586–1594.
19. Paddock CD, Childs JE. Ehrlichia chaffeensis: a prototypical emerging pathogen. *Clin Microbiol Rev* 2003;16:37–64.
20. Tekku B, Habte-Michael A, Warrell DA, White NJ, Wright DJ. Meptazinol diminishes the Jarisch-Herxheimer reaction of relapsing fever. *Lancet* 1983;8329:835–839.
21. Tsai TF. Arboviral infections in the United States. *Infect Dis Clin N Am* 1991;5:73–102.
22. Walker DH and the Task Force on Consensus Approach for Ehrlichiosis. Diagnosing human ehrlichioses: current status and recommendations. *ASM News* 2000;66:287–290.
23. Weiss LM. Babesiosis in humans: a treatment review. *Expert Opin Pharmacother* 2002;3:1109–1115.
24. White DJ, Talarico J, Chang HG, Birkhead GS, Heimberger T, Morse DL. Human babesiosis in New York State: review of 139 cases and analysis of prognostic factors. *Arch Intern Med* 1998;158:2149–2154.
25. Wilson ME. Prevention of tick-borne diseases. *Med Clin N Am* 2002;86:219–238.

CHAPTER 144
Tuberculosis

Gregory J. Moran and David A. Talan

Tuberculosis (TB) causes more deaths worldwide than any other single infectious disease (3). Approximately one third of all humans are infected with *Mycobacterium tuberculosis*. Eight million new cases of active disease develop annually, resulting in about 3 million deaths worldwide (1). An estimated 10 to 15 million persons in the United States (4% to 6% of the population) are infected with *M. tuberculosis*.

The incidence of TB in the United States had been decreasing since the 1950s due to the introduction of better public health measures and effective anti-TB drugs. In the mid-1980s, however, that trend reversed itself and an increase in TB cases was noted. The resurgence of TB has disproportionately affected the poor, ethnic minorities, immigrants, and prison and homeless populations. Multidrug-resistant strains of *M. tuberculosis* have also been found in increasing numbers, especially among immigrants and patients with the acquired immunodeficiency syndrome (AIDS). Increased efforts to control the disease in the United States have led to a decrease in TB cases in recent years (4).

M. tuberculosis is a slow-growing bacterium transmitted between persons by droplet nuclei produced from coughing and sneezing. The small size of the droplets allows them to remain suspended in the air for long periods of time. Infection may occur if contaminated droplets are inhaled and reach the alveoli. The risk of infection is a function of the level of contamination of the air and the length of time the air is breathed. Small, enclosed areas with poor ventilation are more likely to promote the spread of TB.

The small size of airborne droplet nuclei containing infectious organisms allows them to enter the alveoli of the lung. *M. tuberculosis* infection usually begins in the alveoli, where bacilli are able to multiply. Infection may spread through the lymphatics to regional lymph nodes, and subsequently to the bloodstream. In most persons, cell-mediated immunity will develop over 2 to 10 weeks and is adequate to contain the infection. The TB skin test usually becomes positive during this period. In this situation, in which the immune system prevents further spread, the person is said to have *M. tuberculosis* infection without disease. These people have no clinical symptoms of TB and cannot infect others.

M. tuberculosis survives within macrophages as a facultative intracellular parasite, and thus may remain dormant in the body for many years. Active TB develops within 2 years in about 5% of patients, and another 5% will develop reactivation disease at some later point in life. Reactivation is more likely to occur in people with impaired cell-mediated immunity, such as those with diabetes, renal failure, immunosuppressive therapy, and malnutrition.

AIDS patients lack the ability to mount an effective cell-mediated immune response and are thus much more likely to progress to active disease. The incidence of TB in AIDS patients is almost 500 times that in the general population. The risk of developing active TB in human immunodeficiency virus (HIV)–infected persons with a positive tuberculin skin test is estimated to be 5% to 10% per year, compared with the 5% to 10% lifetime risk for people not infected with HIV (13).

Multidrug-resistant TB (MDR-TB) is defined as that due to an organism with in vitro resistance to two or more first-line anti-TB drugs (currently, isoniazid [INH], rifampin, rifapentine, rifabutin, pyrazinamide [PZA], and ethambutol). Factors associated with the presence of MDR-TB include previous treatment (especially patients who were given an inadequate regimen or were not fully compliant), exposure to a known case of MDR-TB, birth or residence in an area of high MDR-TB incidence (e.g., Asia, South and Central America, and Africa), and living in environments such as homeless shelters and prisons, where there may be a high risk of MDR-TB transmission. HIV-infected patients who are exposed to MDR-TB are at especially high risk of developing disease.

Several factors contribute to the development and spread of MDR-TB. One of the most important is incomplete compliance with medications. Failure to take medication as prescribed may allow drug-resistant organisms to develop. The prescribed regimen must contain at least two drugs to which the organism is susceptible. Because susceptibility testing takes several weeks to complete, some patients receive inadequate treatment regimens while susceptibility results are pending. With ineffective therapy, the patient remains infectious and can spread the resistant organism to others.

Because patients on inadequate therapy are infectious for longer periods of time, MDR-TB may have a selective advantage over susceptible strains, which may lead to an increasing frequency of MDR-TB. Until more effective therapies or vaccines are available, the best weapon against TB is an aggressive infection control program focusing on early diagnosis, isolation, and directly observed therapy for TB patients.

CLINICAL PRESENTATION

The symptoms of TB vary dramatically, depending on the site and stage of infection and the overall health and immune status of the host. Some patients have mild symptoms that go unnoticed; some may be truly asymptomatic. Such patients may be identified only through exposure history, an abnormal chest radiograph, a positive TB skin test, or a positive TB culture.

Early pulmonary TB often causes no symptoms. As the disease progresses, patients may develop insidious constitutional symptoms such as fatigue, anorexia, weight loss, fevers, and night sweats. Cough may progress slowly over weeks to months, becoming productive of mucopurulent sputum. TB must be considered in any patient at risk who has a cough of more than 2 to 3 weeks' duration. Hemoptysis due to endobronchial erosion may be present, usually indicating more advanced disease. Some patients present with a more acute onset of fever, chills, cough, and myalgias, similar to an episode of acute bronchitis or pneumonia. Chest findings of rales or consolidation may be present. Patients may have a dull ache or tightness in the chest, or they may have pleuritic pain related to tuberculous pleuritis. Signs of pleural effusion may indicate a tuberculous empyema.

Most cases of disseminated TB have a subacute presentation with systemic symptoms. However, some patients with hematogenous dissemination of TB may present with an acute illness of fever, dyspnea, and cyanosis, mimicking bacterial sepsis. Physical findings may include hepatosplenomegaly, lymphadenopathy, erythema nodosum, and tuberculous lesions visible on examination of the optic fundi. Elderly patients are particularly prone to presenting with unexplained fever and hematologic abnormalities such as pancytopenia or leukemoid reaction.

TB may involve virtually any structure in the body and produce symptoms and signs related to the affected organs as well as systemic symptoms. In about 15% of TB cases, major involvement is seen at an extrapulmonary site. Granulomatous lymphadenitis is usually caused by *M. tuberculosis* in adults, but nontuberculous mycobacteria are a more common cause in children. The cervical and supraclavicular nodes are the most common sites of infection, but any nodes may be involved. Genitourinary TB may present as recurrent urinary tract infections without the growth of the usual bacterial pathogens (i.e., pyuria without bacteriuria) or simply recurrent fever. Skeletal tuberculosis is most common in the spine (Pott disease) and weight-bearing joints and usually presents as fever and localized pain.

Tuberculous meningitis is more common in small children as a complication of initial infection, but it can occur in any age group. TB meningitis typically has a subacute onset and may present as headache, altered mental status, or seizures. Cranial nerve signs attributable to involvement of the basilar meninges may be present. Some patients may have new psychiatric symptoms. The cerebrospinal fluid characteristically shows a moderate lymphocytic pleocytosis (usually 100 to 500 cells/mm^2), elevated protein, and low glucose.

HIV-infected patients are especially prone to having atypical presentations of TB. TB usually causes disease at an earlier stage of HIV infection than opportunistic pathogens such as *Pneumocystis carinii*, presumably because TB is more virulent than these other pathogens. Extrapulmonary involvement is much more common in HIV-infected patients with TB, occurring in 40% to 75% of cases, usually with concomitant pulmonary disease. In patients with advanced HIV infection, cavitary lung disease and localized extrapulmonary disease are relatively less common; diffuse interstitial pneumonia (mimicking *P. carinii* pneumonia) and disseminated infection are more typical (21).

DIFFERENTIAL DIAGNOSIS

Pulmonary TB can potentially mimic many other diseases, including pneumoconiosis, bacterial pneumonia, bronchiectasis, sarcoidosis, lung abscess, neoplasm, and fungal infections such as coccidioidomycosis or histoplasmosis or *P. carinii*. Factors that may be helpful in identifying TB as a cause of illness include history of exposure to TB; characteristic radiographic findings, such as cavitation or apical infiltrates; presence of acid-fast bacilli (AFB) on sputum smear; and results of skin testing. The diagnosis of TB ultimately rests on the culture of *M. tuberculosis*, but culture may take several weeks.

Difficulty may arise in distinguishing disease due to *M. tuberculosis* from disease due to other mycobacterial species. A number of mycobacterial species other than *M. tuberculosis* have been identified. Many are ubiquitous in the environment and are usually contaminants when isolated, but some have been found to be human pathogens. *Mycobacterium avium* complex (MAC, also known as *Mycobacterium avium-intracellulare* [MAI]), *M. kansasii*, and other mycobacteria are rare causes of pulmonary disease; most other mycobacterial species are associated with skin, soft-tissue, and lymph node infections. AFB identified in sputum smears may represent colonization by nonpathogenic mycobacteria, but until they can be definitively identified as such by culture they should be considered to represent *M. tuberculosis* in a patient with a clinical picture consistent with TB.

MAC is the most common mycobacterial species isolated from persons with AIDS in the United States. Infection typically occurs as a systemic febrile illness in end-stage AIDS patients, rather than as a pulmonary infection in earlier stage AIDS patients, as with *M. tuberculosis*. A chest radiograph usually does not suggest mycobacterial disease, and pleuritis is uncommon. Acid-fast smears of stool and mycobacterial blood cultures are commonly positive, but acid-fast smears of sputum are often negative, suggesting that the gastrointestinal tract, rather than the lungs, is the portal of entry.

MAC infections in AIDS patients are often difficult to treat effectively, but they may respond to regimens containing clarithromycin or azithromycin, ethambutol, rifabutin, clofazimine, or ciprofloxacin (5). HIV-infected patients with suspected pulmonary mycobacterial disease should generally be given empiric therapy against *M. tuberculosis* initially. Therapy can be adjusted later if MAC or other nontuberculous mycobacteria are cultured.

EMERGENCY DEPARTMENT EVALUATION

The most important test in the initial evaluation of patients with suspected pulmonary TB is the chest radiograph. Findings strongly suggestive of pulmonary TB include nodular densities, with or without cavities that are commonly seen in the apical and posterior segments of the upper lobes or in the superior segments of the lower lobes (Fig. 144.1).

In disseminated TB, the chest radiograph often reveals a miliary pattern, but it may be normal in the early stages. TB may have many different radiographic appearances, ranging from lobar consolidation to a diffuse interstitial pattern. Patients with AIDS are especially likely to have TB without the typical radiographic pattern, and they are more likely to have lymphadenopathy on a chest x-ray (17). A diffuse interstitial pattern that is easily misdiagnosed as *P. carinii* pneumonia may be seen in patients with AIDS (Fig. 144.2).

If pulmonary TB is suspected, sputum samples should be obtained for AFB smear and culture. Collection of sputum can put health-care workers and other patients at risk for exposure to TB, and should be performed only in an isolation room adequately equipped with outside ventilation and filters or ultraviolet light. Emergency departments may consider having the patient step outside to provide a specimen if these facilities are not available. Ideally, three successive early-morning sputum samples should be obtained. In certain cases, they can be obtained on an outpatient basis.

A positive AFB smear supports a presumptive diagnosis of TB. A positive smear does not necessarily indicate infection with *M. tuberculosis*, however, because other mycobacteria (e.g., MAC) are also acid-fast. Patients with positive smears are potentially

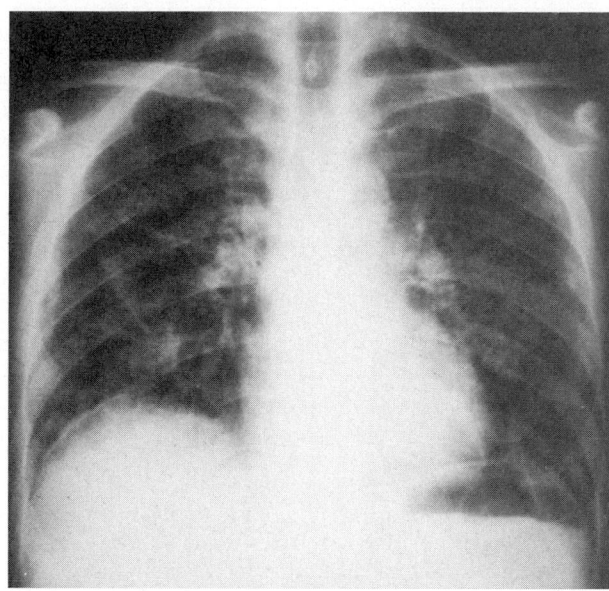

Figure 144.2. Chest radiograph of HIV-infected patient with tuberculosis, demonstrating hilar adenopathy and scattered interstitial infiltrates. This patient was initially misdiagnosed with *Pneumocystis carinii* pneumonia.

the most infectious, because they are usually coughing up large numbers of organisms. Because culture is more sensitive than AFB smear for the diagnosis of TB, the sample should be sent for culture even if the smear is negative.

AFB smear results are usually not available within the time frame of an emergency department visit. If there is a high likelihood of TB, the patient may be started on empiric therapy, with further AFB specimens obtained over the next couple of days. Empiric therapy will not significantly affect the diagnostic yield of specimens obtained over the next 1 to 2 days. Delays in diagnosis are a problem with current techniques, because culture usually takes 3 to 6 weeks, and susceptibility tests may take 8 weeks. Newer radiometric methods can provide results in as little as 10 to 15 days, but may not be available in many facilities. Nucleic acid amplification tests, such as polymerase chain reaction (PCR), can be used to rapidly verify *M. tuberculosis* (as opposed to other mycobacteria) in AFB smear–positive specimens (12).

Intradermal tuberculin skin testing is the standard method for identifying persons infected with *M. tuberculosis*. Tuberculin skin testing should be targeted at those persons who are at increased risk of recent latent TB infection or with conditions that increase the risk of developing active TB. Testing is discouraged for people at lower risk (14). The Mantoux test is performed by injecting 5 U (0.1 mL) of purified protein derivative (PPD) intradermally. The arm is then examined for 48 to 72 hours for induration at the site. Persons for whom TB skin testing is recommended are listed in Table 144.1, and interpretation of the test is summarized in Table 144.2.

A negative TB skin test does not rule out TB, because 60% of AIDS patients and up to 30% of those without HIV infection have a reaction of less than 5 mm even when they are infected. A skin test should nonetheless be performed in patients with AIDS, however, because it produces a positive reaction in up to 40% of those infected. False-positive reactions may be caused by cross-reaction with other mycobacteria, such as MAC.

A history of bacille Calmette-Guérin (BCG) vaccination generally does not alter the guidelines for interpretation of the skin test. BCG vaccination usually does not cause a reaction of more than 10 mm, and the extent of the reaction decreases with time. Because the vaccine is generally given only in areas with a high

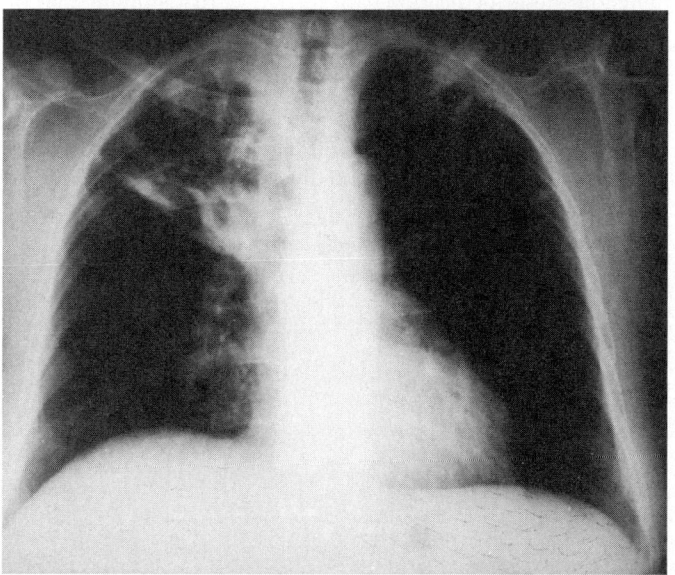

Figure 144.1. Chest radiograph demonstrating apical infiltrate with cavitation, typical of pulmonary tuberculosis.

TABLE 144.1. People in Whom PPD Skin Testing Is Indicated

People with signs, symptoms, or chest x-ray suggestive of active TB
Recent contacts of people known to have, or suspected of having, active TB
People with HIV infection
People with an abnormal chest x-ray compatible with past TB
People with other medical conditions that increase the risk of TB (e.g., intravenous drug use, diabetes, immunosuppressive therapy, renal failure, rapid weight loss)
Groups at high risk of recent infection with TB, such as immigrants from Asia, Africa, Latin America, and Oceania; medically underserved populations (e.g., homeless); personnel and residents in long-term care facilities and correctional institutions

TB, tuberculosis

incidence of TB, a reaction greater than or equal to 10 mm should still be considered positive in these patients (14).

The Centers for Disease Control and Prevention (CDC) recommend that facilities serving persons at high risk for HIV infection, TB infection, or both should provide screening for TB and encourage HIV testing. It is also recommended that TB case finding be part of the regular health care provided to all homeless people (8). Many persons at risk for TB and HIV come into contact with the health-care system only for episodic care in emergency departments.

Emergency department–based screening for TB could potentially identify many patients who require treatment (18). However, the cost and time commitment necessary for an effective TB screening program may preclude the development of such a program in many emergency departments. If a TB screening program cannot be established in the emergency department, then patients at risk for TB should be referred to local public health clinics for testing. It is essential that all persons with suspected active TB be reported to local public health authorities (6).

TABLE 144.2. Criteria for Interpretation of PPD Skin Tests as Positive

INDURATION = 5 MM

Recent contact with someone with active TB
Fibrotic changes on chest radiograph consistent with prior TB
HIV infection
Patients with organ transplants or other immunosuppression

INDURATION = 10 MM

Recent immigrants (<5 years) from an area with high TB prevalence
Intravenous drug users
Residents or employees of high-risk congregate settings (e.g., prison, nursing home, hospital, homeless shelter)
Mycobacteriology lab personnel
Persons with underlying disease that puts them at high risk for reactivation TB (e.g., diabetes, renal failure, malignancy, gastrectomy)
All children <4 years, as well as children and adolescents exposed to adults at high risk for TB

INDURATION = 15 MM

Persons with no risk factors for TB

(Adapted from Centers for Disease Control and Prevention. Targeted tuberculin testing and treatment of latent tuberculosis infection. *MMWR* 2000;49(No. RR-6):1–51.)

EMERGENCY DEPARTMENT MANAGEMENT

Treatment of Active Tuberculosis

Rapid initiation of an effective drug regimen is important to prevent the spread of TB. Presumptive therapy can begin in the emergency department on the basis of clinical grounds alone if the patient is at risk for TB and has signs, symptoms, and radiographic findings suggestive of TB. Specimens should still be sent for AFB smear, culture, and sensitivity for subsequent management. If cultures are negative or yield only nontuberculous mycobacteria, treatment can be stopped or adjusted accordingly. Considerations for hospital admission would include severity of illness, diagnostic uncertainty, and ability of the patient to avoid transmitting infection to others and to obtain and comply with outpatient management.

Active TB should always be treated with at least two drugs to which the organism is susceptible. Administration of a single drug can lead to the development of a bacterial population resistant to that drug. When two or more drugs are used simultaneously, each helps to prevent the emergence of TB resistant to the other. Because of concern about MDR-TB, the CDC recommends that initial therapy for TB include four drugs. The preferred initial regimen consists of daily INH, rifampin, PZA, and ethambutol (6). Doses of these drugs can be found in Table 144.3. If four drugs are used in the initial regimen, it is very likely that the organism will be sensitive to at least two of these drugs. The initial regimen is continued for 2 months, at which time the number of drugs and frequency of dosing can be reduced, depending in part on the results of susceptibility testing.

Immunocompetent patients usually cease to be infectious within 2 to 4 weeks of starting therapy, assuming the infecting organism is susceptible to the drugs being used and the patient is compliant. Treatment should be continued for at least 6 months in immunocompetent persons. Expert advice should be sought if a patient is suspected of having MDR-TB. Alternative regimens may be recommended for these patients, including drugs such as cycloserine, ethionamide, amikacin, or quinolones. Those who are at especially high risk for MDR-TB include anyone with HIV infection, those with known exposure to MDR-TB, and persons from a geographic area or demographic group with a high incidence of MDR-TB.

Because rifampin interacts with protease inhibitors and nonnucleoside reverse transcriptase inhibitors, HIV-infected patients on these medications are treated with regimens that do not contain rifampin (13). Rifabutin may be substituted in some cases, but is also contraindicated with some antiretroviral drugs.

TABLE 144.3. Daily Dosage Recommendation for the Initial Treatment of Tuberculosis

Drugs	Children <12	Adults
Isoniazid	10–15 mg/kg	5 mg/kg
	Max 300mg	Max 300mg
Rifampin	10–20 mg/kg	10 mg/kg
	Max 600 mg	Max 600 mg
Rifabutin	Unknown	5 mg/kg
		Max 300 mg
Pyrazinamide	15–30 mg/kg	15–30 mg/kg
	Max 2 g	Max 2 g
Ethambutol	15–20 mg/kg	15–20 mg/kg
	Max 1 g	Max 1600 mg

(Adapted from Centers for Disease Control and Prevention. Treatment of Tuberculosis, American Thoracic Society, CDC, and Infectious Diseases Society of America. *MMWR* 2003;52(No. RR-11):1–77.)

Expert consultation should be sought before initiating TB treatment for individuals taking antiretroviral drugs. HIV-infected patients who are unable to take rifampin or rifabutin may require 9 months of treatment.

Recommendations for treatment of extrapulmonary TB are generally the same as for pulmonary TB. However, longer courses of 9 to 12 months are usually recommended for TB meningitis, bone or joint TB, or children with miliary TB (6). Corticosteroids may be a useful adjunct for tuberculous meningitis or pericarditis.

Common side effects of these medications include hepatitis (INH, rifampin), peripheral neuropathy (INH), optic neuritis (ethambutol), and, rarely, purpura (rifampin). Adults should have baseline measurements of hepatic enzymes, bilirubin, serum creatinine or blood urea nitrogen, complete blood count, and platelet count. Serum uric acid should be measured if PZA is used, and a baseline examination of visual acuity should be obtained for patients to be treated with ethambutol. For this reason, unless resistance to other drugs is strongly suspected, ethambutol is not generally used for children younger than 6 years of age, in whom visual acuity cannot be assessed well.

Patients should be instructed to report any symptoms suggestive of hepatitis or thrombocytopenia. Pyridoxine (10 to 50 mg/d) may be given with INH to persons with conditions in which neuropathy is common, such as diabetes, alcoholism, or malnutrition. The rate of adverse reactions to antituberculous agents increases with age, and also appears to be higher in HIV-infected patients.

Management of Tuberculosis Exposure

Management of persons exposed to others with active TB involves several considerations: (1) the likelihood that the exposed person has been newly infected with *M. tuberculosis;* (2) the likelihood that the infecting strain is drug-resistant; and (3) the likelihood that the newly infected contact will develop active TB. Contacts who are not immunosuppressed and do not have a history of a positive PPD skin test should receive a tuberculin skin test and, if indicated by symptoms, a chest radiograph and sputum examination. Exposed persons who have a PPD skin test reaction equal to 5 mm should be considered newly infected and should be considered for preventive therapy once active TB has been ruled out.

Persons with a high-risk exposure and a negative PPD should have a follow-up skin test 12 weeks after the exposure has ended; if the PPD test is still negative at that time, no further evaluation is necessary. Because the risk of developing TB is higher for young children, preventive therapy may be considered for all children younger than 5 years of age who are close contacts of TB cases until repeat skin testing is done at 12 weeks after exposure.

Persons who are known to be HIV-infected or otherwise immunosuppressed and who are close contacts of patients with infectious TB should be carefully evaluated for evidence of TB. If there are no findings suggestive of active TB, preventive therapy with INH may be recommended, even if PPD skin testing is negative (14).

Management of Positive Tuberculosis Skin Tests

Persons with a positive TB skin test need to be evaluated for the presence of active TB with a chest radiograph. If the chest radiograph is abnormal or if symptoms suggest TB, an examination of sputum for AFB smear and culture is indicated. Those with no evidence of clinical disease should be referred for consideration of preventive therapy for TB. It is not necessary to initiate therapy urgently in this situation, but it is important that patients understand the importance of follow up to obtain preventive therapy. It has been shown in numerous studies that preventive therapy substantially reduces the risk of latent infection progressing to clinical disease. Immunocompetent persons who are not at risk for MDR-TB are generally treated with INH for 6 to 9 months (14). HIV-infected persons who are not at risk for MDR-TB should receive preventive therapy with INH for 9 months (13). Routine laboratory monitoring is not necessary for most patients receiving INH, but should be considered for those with HIV, pregnancy, liver disease, or regular alcohol use. A combination of rifampin plus PZA daily for 2 months had been recommended previously as an alternative, but is no longer recommended because of problems with liver toxicity (15).

The effectiveness of preventive therapy for people exposed to MDR-TB strains has not been prospectively studied, and guidelines for management of such patients are less clear. If the infecting strain of TB is known to be less than 100% resistant to INH, then INH should be included in the preventive regimen; rifampin should be included for those with less than 100% resistance to rifampin. Those with exposure to strains resistant to both INH and rifampin who are at increased risk for developing active disease may be treated with regimens of PZA plus ethambutol or PZA plus a fluoroquinolone (7).

Consultation with local infectious disease experts familiar with local patterns of resistance and current recommendations may be helpful in the management of such patients. Because the efficacy of drugs other than INH and rifampin for preventive therapy is unknown, persons on alternative therapies should have regular follow up.

Recommendations for TB therapy are likely to continue to change because of shifting patterns of infection and drug resistance. The most current recommendations can be found in *Morbidity and Mortality Weekly Report* and the publications of the American Thoracic Society.

Preventing the Spread of Tuberculosis

The basic principles for preventing the transmission of TB include early identification of persons with active TB, early initiation of AFB isolation precautions in persons with suspected TB, and initiation of effective therapy to render the patient noninfectious. Lapses in infection control measures have led to nosocomial transmission of MDR-TB between patients and from patients to healthcare workers (19).

The emergency department is potentially a high-risk area for the transmission of TB, because patients may be undiagnosed with TB when they present initially, and patients sometimes are crowded together for long periods of time, especially in busy inner-city emergency departments, which are likely to have a larger number of TB patients. There may be long delays in recognition and initiation of infection control measures for infectious TB patients in the emergency department, and HIV-infected patients appear to be even more likely to have delays in recognition, because they often have atypical presentations (20).

Emergency departments should have triage protocols to identify possible TB patients early. Those with possible TB should have an expedited chest radiograph, and can have a mask placed or wait outside while they are being evaluated for possible infectious TB. Note that HIV-infected patients with suspected pneumonia, such as due to *Pneumocystits carinii* or PCP, are at such increased risk of TB (and delayed recognition) that routine respiratory isolation is recommended.

Once a patient is suspected of having active TB, infection control measures should be initiated (2,9,10). These measures are aimed at isolating the source from other patients and reducing the microbial contamination of indoor air. Recommendations include the use of a private room for the source patient with negative pressure in relation to surrounding areas and a minimum of six air exchanges per hour. Air from the room should be exhausted directly to the outside. Use of ultraviolet lamps or high-efficiency particulate air filters to supplement ventilation may be considered.

Many emergency departments do not have the facilities to comply with these recommendations, and the costs associated with fitting a department with such facilities are substantial. If facilities that meet these standards are not available, it is important to at least designate an area for persons with possible TB that will keep them isolated from other patients and will minimize air exchange with other patient areas. Ordinary surgical masks may help reduce the amount of airborne droplets produced by patients who are coughing, but they are not truly effective for preventing the transmission of TB when worn either by TB patients or by those at risk for exposure. Masks used in the conventional manner are not designed to filter out particulates in the 1- to 5-micron range and can leak large amounts of air around the edges. The CDC recommends that health-care workers use masks capable of filtering out at least 95% of particles in the 1-micron range (commonly designated as N-95) for protection against TB. Individually fit-testing these masks may help ensure that they will provide adequate protection (11).

CRITICAL INTERVENTIONS

- Initiate infection control measures for patients suspected of TB
- Treat active TB with at least two drugs to which the organism is susceptible. Initial therapy usually consists of 4 drugs (INH, rifampin, PZA, and ethambutol) pending susceptibilities

DISPOSITION

Criteria for admission of patients with TB are similar to those for patients with other types of pneumonia. Patients who are not seriously ill and are not immunocompromised may safely be sent home with close follow up, but precautions must be taken to avoid the spread of TB to others. Any patient who is discharged home with possible TB must be reported to local public health authorities. It may be assumed that household contacts have already been exposed, and will need to be tested.

Patients should be instructed to avoid crowded, enclosed, public areas and to wear a mask for at least the first 2 weeks of therapy to reduce the amount of airborne droplets produced by coughing. Other factors, such as homelessness, degree of compliance with medications, follow up, and compliance with infection control measures should be considered when making decisions regarding admission. In the United States, laws vary among the states in regard to forced treatment and quarantine of patients who will not cooperate with therapy and are believed to be a public health hazard (16).

COMMON PITFALLS

✔ Failure to consider the possibility of TB in a patient presenting with nonspecific systemic complaints

✔ Risking the spread of TB in the emergency department by performing high-risk procedures such as sputum induction in infectious TB patients without proper isolation procedures
✔ Misdiagnosis of TB in AIDS patients as *P. carinii* or other infections
✔ Failure to refer patients at risk of TB for skin testing
✔ Failure to recognize and follow up patients whose cultures may become positive several weeks after an emergency department visit
✔ Failure to report persons with suspected TB to local public health authorities

References

1. American Thoracic Society. Diagnostic standards and classification of tuberculosis in adults and children. *Am J Respir Crit Care Med* 2000;161:1376–1395.
2. American Thoracic Society. Institutional control measures for tuberculosis in the era of multiple drug resistance. *Chest* 1995;108:1690–1710.
3. Bloom BR, Murray CJ. Tuberculosis: commentary on a reemergent killer. *Science* 1992;257:1055–1064.
4. Centers for Disease Control and Prevention. Trends in tuberculosis morbidity—United States, 1002-2002. *MMWR* 2003;52:217–222.
5. Center for Disease Control. Recommendations on prophylaxis and therapy for disseminated *Mycobacterium avium* complex for adults and adolescents infected with human immunodeficiency virus. *MMWR* 1993;42(RR-9):17–20.
6. Centers for Disease Control and Prevention. Treatment of Tuberculosis, American Thoracic Society, CDC, and Infectious Diseases Society of America. *MMWR* 2003;52(RR-11):1–77.
7. Center for Disease Control. Management of persons exposed to multidrug-resistant tuberculosis. *MMWR* 1992;41(RR11):61–71.
8. Center for Disease Control. Prevention and control of tuberculosis among homeless persons. Recommendations of the Advisory Council for the Elimination of Tuberculosis. *MMWR* 1992;41(RR5):13–23.
9. Centers for Disease Control and Prevention. Guidelines for environmental infection control in health-care facilities: recommendations of CDC and the Healthcare Infection Control Practices Advisory Committee (HICPAC). *MMWR* 2003;52(RR-10):1–44.
10. Centers for Disease Control and Prevention. Guidelines for preventing the transmission of *Mycobacterium tuberculosis* in health-care facilities, 1994. *MMWR* 1994;43(RR-13):1–132.
11. Centers for Disease Control and Prevention. Laboratory performance evaluation of N95 filtering facepiece respirators, 1996. *MMWR* 1998;47:1045–1049.
12. Centers for Disease Control and Prevention. Update: Nucleic acid amplification tests for tuberculosis. *MMWR* 2000;49:593–4.
13. Centers for Disease Control and Prevention. Prevention and treatment of tuberculosis among patients infected with HIV: principles of therapy and revised recommendations. *MMWR* 1998;47(RR-20):1–58.
14. Centers for Disease Control and Prevention. Targeted tuberculin testing and treatment of latent tuberculosis infection. *MMWR* 2000;49(RR-6):1–51.
15. Centers for Disease Control and Prevention. Update: adverse event data and revised American thoracic society/CDC recommendations against the use of rifampin and pyrazinamide for treatment of latent tuberculosis infection—United States, 2003. *MMWR* 2003;52:735–9.
16. Gostin LO. Controlling the resurgent tuberculosis epidemic—a 50-state survey of TB statutes and proposals for reform. *JAMA* 1993;269:255–261.
17. Havlir DV, Barnes PF. Tuberculosis in patients with human immunodeficiency virus infection. *N Engl J Med* 1999;340:367–373.
18. Kirsch TD, Chanmugam A, Keyl P, et al. Feasibility of an emergency department-based tuberculosis counseling and screening program. *Acad Emerg Med* 1999;6:224–231.
19. Menzies D, Fanning A, Yuan L, Fitzgerald M. Tuberculosis among health care workers. *N Engl J Med* 1995;332:92–98.
20. Moran GJ, Talan DA, Morgan MT, et al. Lack of recognition and infection control for tuberculosis patients admitted through the emergency department. *Ann Emerg Med* 1993;22:936.
21. Small PM, Fujiwara PI. Management of tuberculosis in the United States. *N Engl J Med* 2001;345:189–200.

Infectious Mononucleosis

David Anthony Jerrard

Infectious mononucleosis is clinically defined by the triad of fever, lymphadenopathy, and pharyngitis, combined with the development of heterophil antibodies and atypical lymphocytosis. It is caused by the Epstein-Barr virus (EBV), which is also strongly implicated in the etiology of nasopharyngeal cancer and Burkitt lymphoma. The causative organism for this disease remained unidentified until the 1960s. The virus is a member of the herpes virus family. It is a DNA virus that has the ability to become latent after an active infection. The most characteristic feature of the disease is its predilection for the young adult population, especially the 15- to 30-year age group. Early fall and spring are the two peak times of occurrence (5)

Epidemiologic studies have shown that the presence of antibody to EBV (indicating exposure) correlates strongly with immunity and that its absence is highly indicative of susceptibility (12). The age at which individuals develop the infection depends on socioeconomic factors as well as hygiene. Most children in developing countries have been exposed by the age of 3, whereas only 50% of those in economically advanced countries have antibodies by adolescence. Primary EBV infection during childhood is usually subclinical (12). By adulthood, most individuals are seropositive.

Epidemiologic and laboratory evidence indicates that transmission occurs through the oropharyngeal route. EBV may be found in throat washings many months after clinical symptoms have abated, and may even be cultured from 10% to 20% of completely asymptomatic individuals. It is likely to be found in nearly 100% of patients with acquired immunodeficiency syndrome (AIDS) (12). Most transmissions occur from asymptomatic individuals to previously uninfected members of the population.

When EBV is transmitted by saliva, the initial site of replication is in the oropharynx. Both B lymphocytes and oropharyngeal epithelial cells have specific surface receptors for EBV, and replication takes place within these cells. Both humoral and cellular components are important in the immune response to EBV infection. The cellular response, consisting of the elaboration of T lymphocytes having very similar characteristics to suppressor-cytotoxic T lymphocytes (12), is responsible for controlling B-cell proliferation.

CLINICAL PRESENTATION

The incubation period is 4 to 8 weeks. Humans are the only known reservoirs. Nonspecific symptoms such as malaise, anorexia, fatigue, and chills often herald the illness and are followed by the development of fever, pharyngitis, and lymphadenopathy. Most patients seek medical care because of sore throat, but headache and myalgia are often complaints as well. Abdominal pain is rare in the absence of splenic rupture.

Pharyngeal exudate is present about one-third of the time (12), and palatal petechiae may be observed. Anterior or posterior cervical lymphadenopathy is reported in about 90% of patients (10) and tends to be particularly impressive in these areas. Generalized adenopathy is often present; the nodes may be moderately tender or painless. Lymphadenopathy tends to be less prominent in patients older than the age of 40 (4).

Splenomegaly is noted in about 50% of patients, mostly in the second or third week of illness, and is usually not associated with pain. The spleen becomes infiltrated with large amounts of lymphoid cells with resultant thinning of the splenic capsule and trabeculae. The presence of pain should alert the clinician to the possibility of impending or actual splenic rupture, an uncommon but well-documented complication of the disease that may be life-threatening if not identified and treated promptly (1,2). Splenectomy is the most common treatment of choice. Splenic abscess has also been reported as a complication of infectious mononucleosis (8).

Tonsillitis may occur during any stage of the illness, although it is usually most pronounced during the first 2 weeks of the postprodromal period. Tonsils hypertrophied to the point of "kissing" in the midline are not at all unusual and do not, in themselves, mandate hospital admission. The distinction between severe pharyngitis and airway compromise is necessary for obvious reasons, but tonsillar hypertrophy only rarely causes airway compromise.

Complications of infectious mononucleosis are rare, but the clinician must be alert to recognize the complicatons. Autoimmune hemolytic anemia may appear within 1 to 2 months of initial symptoms; mild thrombocytopenia develops in approximately half of all cases. Both appear to be antibody mediated and are usually self-limited, lasting approximately 6 weeks. Glucocorticoids have been recommended for the treatment of both the thrombocytopenia and the hemolytic anemia, but there is little evidence to support their use (12).

A number of neurologic complications of infectious mononucleosis have been described. Cranial nerve palsies (especially Bell palsy) and various forms of encephalitis are the most common. Cerebellar dysfunction and episodes of Guillain-Barré syndrome have also been associated with infectious mononucleosis. Roughly 90% of patients with EBV-associated neurologic findings recover without sequelae (12).

About 90% of patients with infectious mononucleosis have transient elevation of hepatic enzymes, although significant hepatic dysfunction is exceedingly unusual. Roughly half of these patients have mild hepatic tenderness, but hepatomegaly is infrequent. Clinical jaundice may develop early in the illness, but resolution usually occurs within a few weeks. Subclinical illness that mimics mild viral hepatitis may in fact be due to infectious mononucleosis.

Although rare, airway obstruction secondary to extreme lymphoid hyperplasia of the tonsils is a potential complication. Airway compromise, as evidenced, for example, by stridor, requires active airway management.

DIFFERENTIAL DIAGNOSIS

The differential diagnosis of sore throat is lengthy (Table 145.1). Because several of the entities (e.g., foreign body, retropharyngeal abscess and hematoma, and, although less likely, adult epiglottitis) may be associated with airway compromise, it is vital to rule them out as possibilities. Compared with other causes of sore throat, infectious mononucleosis is likely to feature more prominent systemic complaints.

Generalized lymphadenopathy prompts consideration of other viral illness, AIDS, leukemia, lymphoma, or tuberculosis.

The differential diagnosis of splenomegaly is broad as well. Infectious endocarditis, abscess, and disseminated tuberculosis

TABLE 145.1. Differential Diagnosis of Sore Throat

Retropharyngeal abscess
Epiglottitis
Esophageal candidiasis
Peritonsillar abscess
Foreign body
Uvulitis
Pharyngitis (bacterial or viral)[a]
Laryngitis
Cervical adenopathy

[a]Includes infectious mononucleosis.

are all possible infectious etiologies of splenic enlargement. Infiltrative processes such as lymphoma and leukemia must also be included for consideration.

EMERGENCY DEPARTMENT EVALUATION

If there is suspicion of adult epiglottitis or retropharyngeal abscess or hematoma, a soft-tissue lateral radiograph of the neck should be performed. In any patient presenting with the complaint of sore throat, indications of airway compromise should be sought.

The diagnosis of infectious mononucleosis is based on clinical, hematologic, and serologic criteria. In a patient strongly suspected of having infectious mononucleosis, certain laboratory features may aid in making a firm diagnosis.

A relative and absolute lymphocytosis is seen in 39% to 75% of patients with infectious mononucleosis (7). The lymphocytosis is characterized by the presence of cells, roughly 10% of the total, that have atypical morphology. They are larger than mature lymphocytes and have large lobulated or indented nuclei and vacuolated or bluish cytoplasm. Lymphocytosis usually peaks in the second or third week of illness.

A significant number of patients with acute EBV infection, particularly those older than the age of 40 (4,7,11), do not fulfill the classic hematologic criteria for infectious mononucleosis, that is, lymphocytosis of at least 50%, with at least 10% atypical lymphocytes. Conversely, atypical lymphocytosis may be seen in other infections, such as toxoplasmosis, rubella, mumps, and hepatitis (13). Complicating matters further, mononucleosis-like syndromes may be associated with cytomegalovirus infection, toxoplasmosis, and hepatitis A and B, and sometimes cannot be distinguished clinically from infectious mononucleosis due to EBV.

Because so many of the symptoms of infectious mononucleosis are nonspecific, serologic evidence may be required to make the diagnosis. Heterophil antibodies (defined as antibodies that react with antigens not responsible for their production) are characteristically produced in infectious mononucleosis (3). The Monospot test is based on this tube dilution principle.

Heterophil agglutination is apparently almost never positive in persons of Japanese ancestry, for unknown reasons (13). False-positive results have been known to occur in leukemia, lymphoma, malaria, rubella, hepatitis, pancreatic cancer, systemic lupus erythematosus, and hepatic abscess (8,9,13). In addition, children younger than 4 years of age often fail to demonstrate heterophil antibody; likewise, the incidence of heterophil-negative infectious mononucleosis due to EBV increases with age (4). The false-positive rate for heterophil antibody in adults is roughly 2%, and the false-negative rate is 5% to 7%. Only 70% of patients tested in the first week of the illness have a positive test, but 85% to 90% are positive by the third week. One study reported that positive titers were associated with four physical findings: palatal petechiae, posterior auricular adenopathy, axillary adenopathy, and inguinal adenopathy (3).

More recently, latex agglutination tests have been developed for the detection of infectious mononucleosis–associated heterophil antibody (6).

Because many individuals are heterophil antibody negative during the first week of illness, it seems reasonable to omit this test in patients with an illness of recent onset, unless the physical examination raises a high suspicion for mononucleosis. Patients should be instructed to return for testing if symptoms persist beyond 7 days.

Individuals with infectious mononucleosis also produce specific antibody directed against EBV antigens. Even though the development of detectable heterophil antibodies may be delayed, EBV antibody tests are rarely necessary, because 90% of cases are heterophil positive, and false-positive heterophil results are rare; more practically, illness is usually mild and self-limited (6). Nevertheless, it should be noted that, as with heterophil antibodies, antibodies specific to EBV may sometimes not be detectable until several weeks after the onset of illness.

EMERGENCY DEPARTMENT MANAGEMENT

The treatment of infectious mononucleosis usually consists only of supportive care. There is no specific antiviral therapy. Fever and pharyngeal pain may be ameliorated by acetaminophen. Aspirin should probably be avoided because of the risk of increasing any bleeding tendency due to thrombocytopenia. Adequate rest should be advised, although this does not seem to expedite recovery. Ampicillin, via an unknown mechanism, causes a rash in roughly 90% of those with infectious mononucleosis. When treating presumed streptococcal tonsillitis in patients with infectious mononucleosis, therefore, erythromycin or penicillin should be prescribed instead. Because of the small but real risk of splenic rupture, contact sports should be avoided for 6 to 8 weeks after the onset of illness. Some authors recommend that college and intramural athletics be avoided for 6 months (10). Patients should be advised that feelings of malaise may linger, sometimes for months.

Severe pharyngitis may be treated with corticosteroids (prednisone, 40 to 60 mg/d, and tapered over 7 to 10 days). Impending airway obstruction or an inability to take oral medications may necessitate the use of dexamethasone. Symptoms of dysphagia and difficulty breathing are usually improved within 1 to 2 hours of administration of parenteral corticosteroids. As noted previously, active airway management is rarely necessary. Although corticosteroids do not decrease spleen size or reduce the likelihood of splenic rupture, some benefit may be obtained in decreasing neurologic, hematologic, and cardiac complications. Corticosteroid therapy is not generally recommended for uncomplicated infectious mononucleosis, however.

In patients presenting with abdominal pain, a computed tomography scan should be performed. Infectious mononucleosis may be the most common reason for splenic rupture (1). Splenic rupture is unlikely to occur in the first 2 weeks of the illness, however; the capsular and trabecular changes that are necessary to permit rupture to occur do not develop for 2 to 4 weeks.

CRITICAL INTERVENTIONS

- Perform a soft-tissue lateral radiograph of the neck for suspicion of adult epiglottitis, retropharyngeal abscess or hematoma
- Advise avoidance of contact sports for 2 to 6 months after the onset of illness due to risk of splenic rupture
- Treat severe pharyngitis with corticosteroids

DISPOSITION

Most patients with infectious mononucleosis do quite well without any intervention whatsoever and can be discharged from the emergency department with instructions to return should abdominal pain develop and breathing or swallowing become difficult.

Consultation with appropriate specialists is indicated for neurologic or hematologic complications.

Patients who are unable to maintain oral intake because of difficulty in swallowing should be admitted and begun on parenteral corticosteroids. This also holds true if airway compromise becomes a concern.

In the unlikely event of splenic rupture, a surgical consult is imperative. Should either computed tomographic scanning or surgical backup not be available, immediate transfer to a center that does have these resources is crucial.

COMMON PITFALLS

✔ The differential diagnosis of sore throat includes more than simple viral or bacterial pharyngitis. Other infections localized to the throat can have disastrous consequences if they go undetected. These include retropharyngeal abscess and epiglottitis

✔ Errors in management are usually the result of a failure to examine the patient thoroughly. This may result, for example, in a failure to diagnose splenic rupture (spontaneous is more common than posttraumatic), an uncommon but potentially dangerous complication

✔ Patients should be advised to seek medical attention promptly if they develop difficulty breathing or abdominal pain

✔ Ampicillin should be avoided because of the high likelihood that a rash will develop. The rash is morbilliform in nature. The rash from antibiotic use will develop 5 to 9 days after the antibiotic is started

References

1. Aldrete J. Spontaneous rupture of the spleen in patients with infectious mononucleosis. *Mayo Clin Proc* 1993;67:910.
2. Ali J. Spontaneous rupture of the spleen in patients with infectious mononucleosis. *Can J Surg* 1993;36:49.
3. Aronson M, Komaroff A, Puss T. Heterophil antibody in adults with sore throat. *Ann Intern Med* 1982;96:505.
4. Axelrod P, Finestone A. Infectious mononucleosis in older adults. *Am Fam Pract* 1990;42(6):1599.
5. Chatham M, Roberts K. Infectious mononucleosis in adolescents. *Pediatr Ann* 1991;20:208.
6. Dietrich W, Turner D, Vukich D. Use of the infectious disease laboratory in emergency medicine. *Emerg Med Clin North Am* 1991;9:263.
7. Fleisher G, Collins M, Fager S. Limitations of available tests for diagnosis of infectious mononucleosis. *J Clin Microbiol* 1983;17:619.
8. O'Dell K, Gordon R. Ruptured splenic abscess secondary to infectious mononucleosis. *Ann Emerg Med* 1992;21:1160.
9. Ridker P, Enders G, Lifton R. False positive mononucleosis screening test results associated with Klebsiella hepatic abscess. *Am J Clin Pathol* 1990;94:222.
10. Rutkow I. Rupture of the spleen in infectious mononucleosis. *Arch Surg* 1978;113:720.
11. Schmader K, Van der Horst C, Klotman M. Epstein-Barr virus and the elderly host. *Rev Infect Dis* 1989;2:64.
12. Schooley R. Epstein-Barr virus infections including infectious mononucleosis. In: Wilson J, Braunwald E, Isselbacher K, et al, eds. *Harrison's principles of internal medicine.* New York: McGraw-Hill, 1991:689.
13. Wallach J. Hematologic disease. In: Wallach J, ed. *Interpretation of diagnostic tests: a synopsis of laboratory medicine.* Boston: Little, Brown and Company, 1992:323.

CHAPTER 146
Influenza

Jonathan S. Olshaker

More people died in the 1918 influenza pandemic than in all of World War I (23). Today, influenza remains a major killer and causes more morbidity and mortality than the acquired immunodeficiency syndrome (AIDS). In nonpandemic years, 20,000 to 40,000 persons die of influenza-related illness in the United States alone; in pandemic years, deaths can exceed 100,000 (7). Influenza infections account for several billion dollars in healthcare expenditures each year (13).

Influenza is caused by large RNA viruses belonging to the myxovirus groups. Of the three immunologically distinct groups (A, B, and C), influenza A and B are encountered most frequently. Group A is responsible for the majority of the mortality and significant morbidity. It appears to cause more severe disease than type B, making secondary bacterial infection more likely, and is more common in older populations (23). Not surprisingly, the vast majority of deaths occur in elderly individuals and in those with chronic medical conditions, particularly chronic obstructive pulmonary disease (1).

CLINICAL PRESENTATION

Influenza is an extremely common respiratory illness, characterized by the abrupt onset of fever, sore throat, headache, myalgias, and nonproductive cough. The malaise is often much more extreme than that seen with most other common respiratory illnesses (4). Symptoms last from a few days to a week in most patients. More severe illness can result if there is pulmonary involvement due to primary viral or secondary bacterial pneumonia, which is the most common cause of death. This occurs almost exclusively in the elderly, in the immunosuppressed, and in patients with chronic cardiovascular or pulmonary disease.

DIFFERENTIAL DIAGNOSIS

The differential diagnosis of influenza includes the myriad respiratory and infectious diseases seen in the emergency department. The clinician's major task should be to recognize serious illness that requires specific antibiotic treatment or other aggressive interventions.

Prominent severe headache, meningeal signs, or changes in mental status make it mandatory to rule out meningitis. Sore throat, often seen with influenza, may be due to peritonsillar abscess, epiglottitis, or streptococcal pharyngitis. Myalgia may be due to bacteremia or sepsis, particularly in the elderly. A finding of hypotension or marked orthostasis mandates evaluation for sepsis or toxic shock syndrome, particularly if there is evidence of multiple organ system involvement. Cough or difficulty breathing may be due to bacterial or viral pneumonia, acute bronchospasm, or cardiac processes such as congestive heart failure or myocardial ischemia.

Unfortunately, the differentiation of viral from bacterial pneumonia in the patient with influenza is difficult. Antibiotics should be instituted early if there is any suspicion of a bacterial process.

Bioterrorism has brought anthrax front and center in recent years into the differential diagnosis of influenza-like illness. Although there is much overlap in symptoms, some clinical clues help distinguish the two. Nasal congestion and rhinorrhea are common with influenza-like illness and uncommon with anthrax. In the nonelderly adult, influenza-associated pneumonia is seen in less than 5%. Shortness of breath, which is common in anthrax, is seen in only a small percentage of influenza cases, unless pneumonia occurs. Also, all more recent cases of inhalation anthrax had abnormal chest radiographs on initial presentation.

Influenza may be difficult to differentiate from severe acute respiratory syndrome (SARS). Early to moderate symptoms of SARS can mimic influenza and should be considered in the individuals who have traveled within 10 days of onset of symptoms to an area with current or previously documented SARS, or who have close contact with a person known or suspected to have SARS. Likewise full blown SARS can have a very similar presentation to influenza associated pneumonia.

EMERGENCY DEPARTMENT EVALUATION

Initial management should focus on assessment of the airway, breathing, and circulation. Pulse oximetry is a simple, noninvasive test that may provide a quick indication of respiratory compromise. Physical examination should focus on the heart and lungs. A thorough examination of the skin should include a search for any cutaneous manifestations of infectious disease, such as purpura or petechiae.

Patients with significant cough, respiratory symptoms, or abnormalities on lung examination should have a chest radiograph. Lumbar puncture and urinalysis may be indicated if suggested by appropriate symptoms. A complete blood cell count, though nonspecific, may lend support to a diagnosis of superimposed bacterial infection. Tests to determine levels of electrolytes, blood urea nitrogen, creatinine, and blood glucose should be ordered in those patients with severe derangements of fluid balance or in those who have chronic medical problems or take medications, such as diuretics, that can affect electrolyte balance. Arterial blood gas analysis is appropriate when hypoxia or sepsis is suspected. Blood cultures should also be obtained if sepsis is a possibility.

Rapid ED influenza testing technology has become available more recently. The point-of-care tests are Zyme Tx Zstat (Zyme Tx, Inc., Oklahoma City, OK), and FLU OIA (Biostar, Inc., Boulder, CO) influenza tests. These tests have received heightened interest secondary to the bioterrorism scare with anthrax. At present, the true benefits of using these tests are unknown. Initial small studies have shown mixed results. In one study, the rate of positivity of the FLU OIA test was significantly lower than that of cell culture (2). In another study, the FLU OIA assay had a sensitivity of only 54% but a specificity of 97% (10). A study of 51 samples using the Zstat diagnostic assay for influenza A and B showed a sensitivity of 98% and specificity of 77% compared with culture (19). Recent small studies have shown awareness of a rapid diagnosis of influenza in pediatric emergency department patients has reduced the number of laboratory tests and radiographs, decreased antibiotic use, and increased antiviral use (3). It is hoped that larger studies in the near future will look at potential benefits in cost-effectiveness and in differentiating influenza from other diagnosis.

EMERGENCY DEPARTMENT MANAGEMENT

Initial treatment for patients with suspected influenza is directed at ensuring adequate oxygenation and hemodynamic stability. Patients with viral or bacterial pneumonia, particularly the elderly or those with chronic obstructive pulmonary disease, can present *in extremis* with an immediate need for endotracheal intubation and mechanical ventilation. Supplemental oxygen should be given to patients with significant respiratory symptoms or low pulse oximeter readings.

Patients who are tachycardic, hypotensive, or orthostatic should have a large-bore intravenous line placed and receive initial fluid resuscitation with normal saline. Care should be taken to avoid overhydration, particularly in the elderly or in those with a history of congestive heart failure. Standard bronchodilator therapy is indicated for any accompanying reactive airway disease.

If the patient has a coexisting pneumonia, antibiotics should be instituted in the emergency department, because it is, as a rule, difficult to differentiate viral pneumonia from bacterial pneumonia. Antibiotics should provide adequate coverage against *Haemophilus influenzae* and group B *Streptococcus*, as well as *Staphylococcus aureus*, which is a relatively common bacterial pathogen associated with influenza outbreaks (11).

Specific antiviral treatment until more recently has had limited usefulness. Rimantadine and amantadine previously were effective in reducing the severity and duration of illness in high-risk individuals who had not been vaccinated. These agents also potentially can reduce subsequent illness in nursing home residents exposed to an influenza outbreak (24,25). They do have significant limitations, however: rapid development of drug-resistant viral strains, lack of effects against influenza B, frequency of central nervous system and gastrointestinal side effects (particularly with amantadine), and unproven effects in reducing complications. If used, the normal adult dosage is 200 mg/d; 100mg/d is given to patients older than age 65.

The Food and Drug Administration (FDA) has approved a new class of antiviral drugs, neuraminidase inhibitors. Neuraminidase permits a virus to penetrate the surfaces of cells and is necessary for optimal release of virus from infected cells. Inhibitors now available are oseltamivir, given orally, and zanamivir, inhaled through the mouth at a high flow rate. These agents are approved for the treatment of influenza only in patients who have been symptomatic for fewer than 2 days. Initial studies showed only a 1- to 1.5-day decrease of symptoms, but subsequent research has supported further benefits and indications for these drugs. Both drugs have been shown to be effective in significantly reducing time to alleviation of symptoms, close contact prophylaxis, and reducing complications of high-risk individuals (12,14). Zanamivir was associated temporarily with termination of a nursing home outbreak that amantadine had failed to control (16).

The adult dose of oseltamivir for treatment of influenza is 75 mg twice daily for 5 days. The pediatric dose of oseltamivir is 30 mg twice daily for ≤15 kg, 45 mg twice daily for 15 to 23 kg, 60 mg twice daily for 23 to 40 kg and 75 mg twice daily for >40 kg. Treatment should begin within 2 days of onset of symptoms of influenza. The recommended oral dose of oseltamivir for prophylaxis of influenza in adults and adolescents 13 years and older following close contact with an infected individual is 75 mg once daily for at least 7 days. Therapy should begin within 2 days of exposure. Oseltamivir causes nausea and vomiting in about 10% of treated persons, although most continue taking the drug. When taken with food, the incidence of gastrointestinal side effects is reduced.

The dose of zanamivir for treatment of influenza in adult and pediatric patients ages 7 years and older is 2 inhalations (one 5 mg blister per inhalation for a total dose of 10 mg) twice daily (approximately 12 hours apart) for 5 days. Zanamivir should be used cautiously in patients with chronic respiratory disease because it can cause bronchospasm and reduction in airflow. A small percentage of patients have difficulty using the inhaler. Understanding proper use should be ensured.

Treatment recommendations for the neuraminidase inhibitors are as follows:

- All patients with high-risk factors (elderly, immunosuppressed, diabetics, adults and children with other chronic diseases)
- Patients with severe influenza
- Consider for other patients

Prophylaxis recommendations for the neuraminidase inhibitors are as follows:

- Give to high-risk patients who have not been vaccinated.
- Consider for immunosuppressed patients who have been vaccinated.
- Give to high-risk vaccinated patients who received vaccine in poor-match years.
- Give once daily × 6 weeks in season.
- Give × 14 days or until 7 days after onset of last case in nursing home outbreaks.

CRITICAL INTERVENTIONS

- Ensure adequate oxygenation
- Provide for staphylococcal coverage when treating pneumonia
- Initiate neuraminidase inhibitors for high-risk patients with influenza
- Administer influenza vaccine from late September through November to patients at risk for influenza complication and groups capable for influenza transmission

DISPOSITION

The majority of patients with influenza can be treated as outpatients. Close follow up should be ensured, and the patient should be given specific instructions to return immediately if symptoms progress.

There should be a low threshold for admission for elderly patients, the immunocompromised, and those with chronic pulmonary or cardiac disease. These patients should be admitted if there is any evidence of pneumonia, which can often progress rapidly in these individuals. Admission to an intensive care unit should be considered for patients who are hypoxic or show any signs of significant respiratory difficulty.

PREVENTION/VACCINATION

Influenza vaccines have been shown in a number of studies to be effective in preventing clinical disease (4,9). Each year, a different vaccine preparation is developed, using virus strains believed likely to appear in North America the following winter. As many as 90% of influenza cases can be prevented when there is a good match between vaccine and epidemic strains of the virus (6). Influenza vaccine has also been extremely effective in reducing morbidity and mortality (by up to 80%) in vaccinated individuals who nevertheless develop clinical disease, particularly the elderly and the immunocompromised (8). A number of studies have shown that vaccination reduces influenza-related hospitalizations and deaths in nursing home populations during epidemics (5,20). The World Health Organization says influenza vaccination may limit the number of false alarms for SARS. Adverse effects of the vaccine itself have been minimal and should not deter its use in the high-risk patient (17).

Despite the overwhelming evidence supporting the benefits and efficacy of influenza vaccines, many high-risk individuals go unvaccinated. Studies have shown poor vaccination rates in

TABLE 146.1. Influenza Vaccination Target Groups

GROUPS AT RISK FOR INFLUENZA COMPLICATIONS

Adults and children with chronic respiratory or cardiovascular disorders
Healthy persons 50 years of age or older
Immunocompromised persons

GROUPS CAPABLE OF INFLUENZA TRANSMISSION

Residents of nursing homes and chronic care facilities
Physicians
Nurses
Hospital personnel who have close contact with high-risk patients
Home health-care or nursing home care providers

both the elderly and younger persons with high-risk medical conditions such as asthma. Fewer than 50% of younger people with heart disease, lung disease and other chronic disorders are vaccinated (18). One study also showed that only 60% of pediatric emergency physicians received an influenza vaccine within the past year (15).

Emergency physicians can play a major role in educating patients and the general public about the need for vaccinations in high-risk groups. This should occur before the peak influenza season begins (6,13). Target groups for vaccination programs are listed in Table 146.1. Vaccinations should be offered between late September and early November, depending on when regional influenza activity is expected to begin. Many emergency departments offer the vaccine on-site. This approach has been shown to be both needed and feasible (22), even for most patients presenting with acute attacks of asthma requiring prednisone treatment (21).

Emergency physicians are also often in a position to recognize the outbreak of influenza in closed environments such as nursing homes.

COMMON PITFALLS

- ✔ Failure to realize that the elderly, the immunosuppressed, and those with chronic cardiac or pulmonary disease are at high risk for complications from influenza or acute worsening of their baseline chronic disease
- ✔ Failure to realize that *Staphylococcus aureus* has a significant role as a pneumonia pathogen during influenza outbreaks
- ✔ Failure to be on the alert for nursing home patients with influenza and to notify appropriate officials about potential outbreaks

References

1. Barker WH, Mullooly JP. Pneumonia and influenza deaths during epidemics: implications for prevention. *Arch Intern Med* 1982;142:85.
2. Boivin G. Hardy I, Kress A. Evaluation of a rapid optical immunoassay for influenza viruses (FLU OIA TEST) in comparison with cell culture and reverse transcription-PCR. *J Clin Microbiol* 2001;Feb:730–732.
3. Bonner AB, Monroe KW, Talley LI, et al. Impact of the rapid diagnosis of influenza on physician decision making and patient management in the pediatric emergency department: results of a randomized prospective controlled trial. *Pediatrics.* 2003;112:363–367.
4. Centers for Disease Control. Prevention and control of influenza. *MMWR* 1992;15:1.
5. Deguchi Y, Nishimera K. Efficacy of influenza vaccine in elderly persons in welfare nursing homes: reduction in risk of mortality and morbidity during an influenza A (H3V2) epidemic. *J Gerontol A Biol Sci Med Sci* 2001;56:M391–M394.
6. Douglas RG. Prophylaxis and treatment of influenza. *N Engl J Med* 1990;332:443.
7. Ghendon Y. Influenza—its impact and control. *World Health Stat Q* 1992;45:306.

8. Gross PA, Quinna GU, Rostein M. Association of influenza immunization with reduction in mortality in an elderly population: a prospective study. *Arch Intern Med* 1988;148:562.

9. Hermogenes AW, Gross PA. Influenza vaccine: a need for emphasis. *Semin Respir Infect* 1992;7:54.

10. Hindiyeh M, Gouldin C, Morgan H, et al. Evaluation of Biostar Flu-OIA assay for rapid detection of influenza A and B viruses in respiratory specimens. *J Clin Virol* 2000;17:19–26.

11. Jones A, MacFarlane J, Pugh S. Antibiotic therapy, clinical features and outcome of 36 adults presenting to hospital with proven influenza: do we follow guidelines? *Postgrad Med J* 1991;67:988.

12. Kaiser L, Wat C, Mills, T, et al. Impact of Oseltamivir treatment on influenza related lower respiratory tract complications and hospitalization. *Archives of Internal Medicine* 2003;163:1667–1672.

13. Kennedy MM. Influenza viral infections: presentation, prevention, and treatment. *Nurse Pract* 1998;23:17–28.

14. Lalezari J, Campion K, Keene O, et al. Zanamivir for the treatment of influenza A and B infection in high-risk patients. *Arch Intern Med* 2001;161:212–217

15. Lane NE, Paul RI, Bratcher DF, et al. Pediatric emergency physicians and communicable diseases: can we be trusted to take care of ourselves? *Pediatr Emerg Care* 1997;13:308–311.

16. Lee C, Loeb M, Phillips A, et al. Zanamivir use during transmission of amantadine resistant influenza A in a nursing home. *Infect Control Hosp Epidemiol* 2000;21:700–704

17. Margolis KL, Nichol KL, Poland GA, et al. Frequency of adverse reactions to influenza vaccine in the elderly. *JAMA* 1990;5:1139.

18. Prevention and control of influenza: recommendations of the Advisory Committee on Immunization Practices (ACIP). *MMWR Morb Mortal Wkly Rep* 2000;49(RR3):1–38.

19. Noyola PE, Paredes AJ, Clark B, Demmler GJ. Evaluation of a neuraminidase detection assay for the rapid detection of influenza A and B virus incidence in children. *Pediatr Dev Pathol* 2000;3:1627.

20. Ohmit SE, Arden NH, Monto AS. Effectiveness of inactivated influenza vaccine among nursing home residents during an influenza type A epidemic. *J Am Geriatr Soc* 1999;47:165–71.

21. Pak CL, Frank AL, Sullivan M, et al. Influenza vaccination of children during acute asthma exacerbation and concurrent prednisone therapy. *Pediatrics* 1996;98(2 Pt 1):196–200.

22. Slobodkin D, Zielske PG, Kithas J, et al. Demonstration of feasibility of emergency department immunization against influenza and pneumococcus. *Ann Emerg Med* 1998;32:537–543.

23. Small PA. Influenza: pathogenesis and host defense. *Hosp Pract* 1990;25:51.

24. Wintermeyer SM, Nahata MC. Rimantadine: a clinical perspective. *Ann Pharmacother* 1995;29:299–310.

25. Zimmerman RK, Ruben FL, Ahwesh ER. Influenza, influenza vaccine, and amantadine/rimantadine. *J Fam Pract* 1997;45:107–122.

decade (including early use of highly active antiretroviral therapy [HAART], and effective use of a broad range of prophylactic agents for opportunistic infections) the medical, social, and economic impact of this disease is enormous and continues to grow.

As of December, 2003 there were an estimated 790, 000 to 1.2 million persons living with HIV or AIDS in the United States (1). Despite widespread efforts to curtail the spread of disease, incident cases (number of new infections/year) have remained relatively stable with 36,000 to 54,0000 newly infected cases reported in 2003. The majority of AIDS cases occur in large metropolitan areas.

EPIDEMIOLOGY

HIV infection results in a broad spectrum of clinical conditions, ranging from an asymptomatic seropositive state to severe immunocompromise. The most recent Centers for Disease Control and Prevention (CDC) definition of AIDS published in 1993, is summarized in Table 147.1. The diagnosis of AIDS is made either by laboratory evidence of HIV infection and the presence of one or more "indicator" conditions, or laboratory evidence of severe immunosuppression (CD4 T-lymphocyte count of less than 200 cells/μL).

The majority of AIDS cases in the United States have occurred in men. Eighteen percent of cases are in women and less than 2% are in children. Between 1998 and 2002, nearly 90% of reported AIDS cases occurred in individuals 25 to 54 years of age. Nearly half of all people who acquire HIV in the United States initially become infected before they reach age 30, and most die before the age of 45. Minority groups are disproportionately affected, with at least 70% of AIDS cases in 2001 occurring in racial and ethnic minorities (4). Risk factors associated with an increased likelihood of acquiring HIV infection include homosexuality or bisexuality, intravenous drug use, heterosexual exposure to a partner at risk, blood transfusion before 1985, and vertical and horizontal maternal-to-neonatal transmission. Sexual partners of high-risk

CHAPTER 147
Human Immunodeficiency Virus Infection and Related Disorders

Richard E. Rothman, Samuel Yang, and Catherine A. Marco

Reports of Kaposi sarcoma (KS) and *Pneumocystis carinii* pneumonia (PCP) in previously healthy homosexual males appeared in the literature beginning in 1981. These are now recognized to represent the earliest cases of the disease known as the acquired immunodeficiency syndrome (AIDS), which has since escalated to become a global public health issue. Although significant therapeutic advances have been made over the past

TABLE 147.1. Indicator Conditions for Case Definition of AIDS

AIDS-Defining Illnesses*
CD4 cell count < 200/mm^3
Candidiasis, esophageal or pulmonary
Cervical cancer*
Coccidioidomycosis, extrapulmonary*
Cryptococcosis, extrapulmonary*
Cryptosporidiosis (with diarrhea for > 1 month)
Cytomegalovirus infection (of any organ system other than liver, spleen or lymph nodes)
Herpes simplex virus (mucocutaneous ulcer for > 1 mo, pneumonitis or esophagitis)
HIV-associated dementia (with functional impairment)
HIV wasting syndrome
Histoplasmosis, extrapulmonary*
Isosporiasis (with diarrhea for > 1 month)*
Kaposi sarcoma*
Lymphoma in patients < 60 yo (or > 60 yo*)
Mycobacterium tuberculosis (pulmonary or disseminated)*
Pneumocystis carinii pneumonia
Progressive multifocal leukoencephalopathy
Bacterial pneumonia (recurrent)*
Progressive multifocal leukoencephalopenia
Salmonella septicemia, recurrent*
Toxoplasmosis (of internal organ)

*Requires HIV-positive serology.
For a more comprehensive list, refer to the 1993 CDC Case Definition.

individuals are also at increased risk. A greater number of risk factors are associated with a higher likelihood of infection.

The pattern of infection among high-risk individuals is changing. Worldwide, heterosexual transmission is the most common route of transmission of HIV infection, and heterosexual transmission accounts for the largest proportionate increase in HIV infection. In the United States, new infections among the homosexual population have significantly decreased in many areas, although these downward trends have recently slowed. The proportion of AIDS cases in women has increased rapidly, with the male-to-female ratio in certain populations approaching 1:1. During the past several years, the greatest increase in reported AIDS cases has occurred among women, minority populations, and children. Because many of the populations at highest risk for disease are underinsured and have limited or no access to primary care, service emergency departments (EDs) are caring for increasing numbers of patients with HIV and AIDS.

PATHOPHYSIOLOGY AND TRANSMISSION

HIV is a cytopathic retrovirus that kills infected cells. In humans, HIV appears to selectively attack cells within the immune system (primarily CD4 T-lymphocytes), a characteristic that accounts for much of the immunodeficiency it produces in affected individuals. Following infection of host cells, the viral genes, which are encoded by a single-stranded RNA molecule, are reverse-transcribed into DNA (using the enzyme reverse transcriptase), and then permanently integrated into the host's genome. Once integrated, retroviral DNA may lay dormant, or may be actively transcribed and translated to produce virally encoded proteins and new HIV virions.

HIV protease converts viral protein precursors into functional enzymes required for virion infectivity. Antiretroviral therapy is directed at reducing levels of HIV RNA by interfering with the enzymes reverse transcriptase (nucleoside and nonnucleoside reverse transcriptase inhibitors) and HIV protease (protease inhibitors). Although the introduction of these agents has had a significant impact on disease progression, the emergence of mutant drug-resistant strains of HIV and the occurrence of drug toxicity have limited the ability to attain long-term and lasting inhibition of viral replication.

Proven modes of HIV transmission include via semen, vaginal secretions, blood or blood products, transplacental transmission *in utero*, and breast milk. There have been no documented cases of transmission by casual contact, although one report exists of possible salivary transmission (3). The HIV virion is extremely labile and can be easily neutralized by 50% ethanol, 0.3% hydrogen peroxide or a 1:10 solution of household bleach.

DIAGNOSIS OF HIV INFECTION

The standard procedure for diagnosing HIV in the United States is viral antibody detection by the enzyme-linked immunoassay technique (EIA), followed by a confirming Western blot on EIA-positive specimens. EIA detects binding of serum antibodies to HIV antigens; Western blot directly detects viral antigen based on their electrophoretic mobility. The sensitivity and specificity of the current tests are > 99.9%.

False-negative EIA tests occur primarily during acute disease before seroconversion. The vast majority of false-negative tests (> 98%) become positive by 6 months. Rates of false-negatives vary according to the prevalence of disease in the population, ranging from < 0.0001% in low prevalence populations, to 0.3% in high prevalence populations. False-positive tests are less common (< 0.004%) occurring among patients who have received transfusions containing HIV antibody or those with other cross-reactive antigens or antibodies (including antihepatitis A IgM, antihepatitis B core IgM, and antinuclear, antismooth muscle, antiparietal cell, and antimitochondrial antibodies). In children younger than 6 months of age, a positive test may be due to transplacentally acquired maternal antibodies and does not necessarily imply the presence of disease. False-positive results are most frequent in populations with a low seroprevalence for HIV.

Other less commonly used techniques for HIV testing include viral culture, p24 antigen assays, indirect immunofluorescence, monoclonal antibody detection, the production of reagent antigens by recombinant DNA techniques, and DNA amplification or polymerase chain reaction (PCR). These tests should generally only be used in patients with confusing serologic results requiring clarification. Emergency physicians should be familiar with the quantitative plasma HIV ribonucleic acid (RNA) assay, as it is used routinely for HIV staging and monitoring of response to retroviral therapy. Tests results are reported as copies per milliliter, with survival time directly correlated to viral burden. Emergency physicians may occasionally also consider using the quantitative RNA assay in cases where there is a high suspicion for acute HIV seroconversion, and diagnosis at the time of the ED visit is clinically important. CD4 lymphocyte count is routinely used to evaluate the clinical immunologic status of HIV-infected patients. When this test is available, and in cases in which stage of disease is unknown, the total lymphocyte count (TLC) can be used to approximate the CD4 count. A TLC of less than 1,000 cells/μL is highly predictive of a CD4 count of less than 200 cells/μL.

A variety of novel HIV tests have become available in the past few years, which will have increasing relevance to emergency physicians. The single use diagnostic system (SUDS) assay is a rapid HIV detection method that is analogous to an EIA screening tests, and can be performed in approximately 1 hour. This has generally been the most common method employed for management of occupational exposures to help guide decisions in the use of postexposure prophylaxis (PEP). Sensitivity is sufficient to report negative test results; positive test results should be described as 'reactive' to the patient and require confirmation with routine serology.

The most recent development in HIV testing is the release and FDA approval of the OraQuick Rapid HIV-1 Antibody Test (OraSure Technologies, Inc., Bethlehem, Pennsylvania), a simple, easy to use, point-of-care assay that can identify antibodies to HIV-1 in fingerstick or whole blood specimens. This test can be performed at the bedside with delivery of results in as little as 20 minutes (a similar saliva-based test is awaiting FDA approval). Sensitivity and specificity of OraQuick exceed 99%. Negative tests can be reported as negative; reactive tests require confirmatory followup testing with a Western Blot. The availability of this bedside point–of-care provides the first time opportunity to integrate HIV testing into routine medical care.

Although the traditional view has been that serologic testing of patients for HIV in the ED is not indicated (based on logistical difficulties associated with informed consent, counseling, and follow up for test results) the concept of ED testing for HIV is now being reexamined in light of new rapid testing methodologies and release of new guidelines by The Centers for Disease Control which include stream-lining the testing process (in appropriate venues) to meet the needs of specialty testing sites such as EDs (4). In support of this concept, a recent systematic review of the literature found objective evidence supporting the positive impact of routine HIV testing in appropriate high risk ED patients or populations. Primary beneficial outcomes included decreased transmission of disease in the community, delayed progression of disease (due to earlier initiation of therapy), reduced risk of opportunistic infections and decreased morbidity and mortality (5). Despite the potential promise of routine ED based HIV testing however, institutional issues (such as development of effective quality assurance and followup programs) must be addressed prior to implementation. For the time being, in cases where HIV is suspected, emergency physicians should provide urgent referral to primary care sites for testing, along with simple recommendations regarding risk reduction behavior.

Testing of patients for HIV in the ED to determine which patients require special infection control precautions is not recommended. Such practice has not been shown to alter rates of health care worker exposure to HIV-infected blood and detracts attention from other significant blood-borne infections.

DISEASE PROGRESSION

The spectrum of HIV-induced disease ranges from asymptomatic to acute retroviral infection, to a wide variety of opportunistic infections, malignancies, and other symptoms directly attributable to HIV infection. Several weeks after exposure to the virus, an acute "flulike" illness is reported to occur in 50% to 90% of patients. During this stage of infection, high-level HIV RNA viremia occurs, along with a precipitous decline in CD4 cell counts. Symptoms, including fever, sore throat, fatigue, myalgias, diarrhea and weight loss and typically last for 1 to 3 weeks, after which there is a significant reduction in HIV RNA levels and moderate increases in CD4 counts.

Although done infrequently in the ED, it is helpful to identify patients at this early stage, because it may be the optimal time to begin antiretroviral therapy. The best way to establish diagnosis during this acute stage is by quantitative plasma HIV RNA, because HIV antibody serology is usually negative until at least 4 weeks after infection. Median time from exposure to antibody detection has been estimated at 2.1 months, although delayed seroconversion of up to 11 months has been reported.

Disease progression varies among infected individuals. The average incubation time from initial infection to clinical AIDS is 10 to 12 years, although there are some patients who have remained free of AIDS-defining conditions for over 20 years (long-term nonprogressors). Laboratory variables that are most predictive of the stage of disease are CD4 cell counts and viral burden. Clinical characteristics that are predictive of clinically significant immunodeficiency include thrush, oral hairy leukoplakia, dermatomal varicella, and lymphadenopathy.

AIDS is defined by the appearance of any "indicator" condition (see Table 147.1) or a CD4 count of less than 200 cells/μL (6). During this stage, a variety of opportunistic infections and malignancies are common. Median survival time after CD4 cell count is less than 200 cells/μL is 3.7 years; median survival after an AIDS-defining complication is 1.3 years. In patients with CD4 cell counts less than 50 cells/μL, median survival is 12 to 18 months, with common life-threatening complications, including disseminated *Mycobacterium avium* complex (MAC) and disseminated cytomegalovirus (CMV). Immune reconstitution with highly active antiretroviral therapy (HAART) is indicated in patients with AIDS, and has been shown to delay onset to progression of opportunistic infections and death.

CLINICAL PRESENTATION AND EMERGENCY DEPARTMENT MANAGEMENT

It is reasonable to inquire about risk factors as part of the routine evaluation of all adult ED patients, especially in endemic areas, and particularly when patients present with atypical diseases or atypical presentations of common diseases. The infection rate may be surprisingly high, even in patients with presenting complaints not usually associated with HIV infection. Furthermore, inquiries about risk factors help in the medical evaluation, remind physicians of the potential for occupational exposure to blood-borne infections, and afford the opportunity to offer counseling and referral for testing to those who engage in high-risk behaviors.

Patients with HIV infection may present with any number of symptoms and diseases, ranging from complaints unrelated to HIV infection to life-threatening complications. Virtually any organ system may be involved. The following focuses on some of the more common presentations that may be encountered in the ED.

Constitutional Symptoms and Fever

Systemic symptoms such as fever, malaise, and weight loss are common among patients with HIV infection (7). For patients with newly acquired HIV, fever may occur in the course of primary infection, 8 to 12 weeks after exposure. When due to HIV infection alone, fever tends to occur in the afternoon or evening and is generally responsive to aspirin or acetaminophen. In patients with known HIV infection presenting with an acute febrile illness or a change in the patient's usual fever pattern, systemic infection and malignancy must be excluded. A thorough history and physical examination should be performed in an attempt to identify a site of infection and stage of disease.

Laboratory evaluation of fever may include blood cultures (aerobic, anaerobic, and fungal), blood tests for cryptococcal antigen and *Toxoplasma* and *Coccidioides* serologies, and chest radiography. Syphilis serology; viral hepatitis evaluation, purified protein derivative (PPD) with anergy panel; stool culture; stool examination for ova and parasites; urine culture for bacteria, fungus, and mycobacteria; and sputum smear and culture for fungus and mycobacteria may also be appropriate.

Two of the more common infectious etiologies of fever to consider in patients with advanced disease are disseminated MAC (*Mycobacterium avium* complex) and CMV (Cytomegalovirus) infection. MAC is the most common opportunistic bacterial infection in AIDS patients, causing disseminated disease in up to 50% of patients at some time during their illness. It is usually associated with severe weight loss, diarrhea, and constitutional symptoms such as fever, malaise, and anorexia. Infection occurs most often in patients with CD4 counts of < 100 cells/μL. The diagnosis may be made either with a Ziehl-Neelsen (acid-fast) stain of stool or other body fluids, or cultivation of the organism from blood. First line treatment is with azithromycin 600 mg qd with ethambutol 15 mg/kg/day; antimicrobial therapy reduces bacteremia and improves symptoms, but is not curative. Prophylaxis with azithromycin or clarithromycin for MAC is indicated in all patients with CD4 counts < 50 cells/μL.

CMV is the most common cause of opportunistic viral infection in HIV-positive patients. Disseminated disease usually involves the pulmonary or gastrointestinal system (esophagitis and colitis). Definitive diagnosis usually requires biopsy which demonstrates intranuclear inclusion bodies. Treatment is with foscarnet or ganciclovir; oral ganciclovir is used for prophylaxis.

A malignancy that frequently presents with fever is non-Hodgkin lymphoma. New central nervous system (CNS) symptoms, particularly a change in mental status in the presence of fever, should be evaluated with neuroimaging. Definitive diagnosis requires biopsy. Effective treatment regimens include combined radiotherapy and chemotherapy.

Intravenous drug users (IDUs) who present with fever have been shown to be at increased risk for infective endocarditis (IE). The current standard of care is to admit all febrile IDUs, because there are no reliable clinical or laboratory predictors of this disease (8). Inpatient evaluation for IE includes following blood culture results and findings on echocardiography. Recent studies suggest that a short ED-based evaluation for IE may be feasible, using echocardiography, culture, and new PCR-based technology as an alternative to blood culture (9,10). Currently, however, inpatient hospitalization is advised due to the significant morbidity and mortality of missed IE and the difficulties associated with outpatient follow up in this population.

Disposition of patients with fever depends on the patient's level of functioning and ability to maintain sufficient oral intake, the availability of timely medical follow up, and the physician's confidence that fever is due to a benign etiology that may be successfully managed on an outpatient basis. Admission criteria include inability to tolerate pos, toxic appearance, and neutropenia with fever.

Pulmonary Involvement

Pulmonary presentations are among the most frequent reasons for ED visits among patients with known HIV infection (7,11). More than 80% of AIDS patients develop pulmonary disease. Presenting complaints may include cough, hemoptysis, shortness of breath, and chest pain. The differential diagnosis includes viral, bacterial, mycobacterial, fungal, and protozoal pneumonias, as well as malignancies. The more common etiologies are shown in Table 147.2. Although differentiation of these entities in the ED may be difficult, appreciation of the epidemiology and the common findings associated with various pathogens can assist the emergency physician in arriving at a working diagnosis and instituting appropriate treatment and disposition decisions.

The physical examination itself is not likely to aid in establishing a diagnosis. CD4 counts are useful in assistance with determining the likely cause of a pulmonary disorder. Patients with CD4 counts > 500 cells/μL are most commonly infected with encapsulated bacteria or tuberculosis; for those with lower CD4 counts, *Pneumocystis pneumonia* (PCP), atypical mycobacteria, Kaposi sarcoma (KS), CMV, and lymphoma are seen with increasing frequency. Patients with fever and productive cough are likely to have a bacterial pneumonia, whereas a nonproductive cough is more likely to accompany PCP, CMV pneumonia, fungal infection, or neoplasm. Hemoptysis is most often associated with pneumococcal pneumonia and tuberculosis (TB). Fulminant respiratory failure is most likely to be caused by PCP or CMV.

Evaluation of HIV-infected patients who present with pulmonary complaints should generally include pulse oximetry and chest radiograph; hypoxia is more pronounced after exercise with PCP infection. Additional testing that may be helpful in certain situations includes a complete blood cell count, arterial blood gas analysis, serum lactate dehydrogenase, sputum culture, Gram stain, and special stains (Gomori, Giemsa, acid-fast). Obtaining blood cultures may cause delays in initiating antimicrobial therapy, and should be done in all patients that are being hospitalized.

Radiographic patterns are suggestive of certain specific disorders. A focal infiltrate often suggests bacterial pneumonia. A diffuse interstitial or perihilar granular appearance is associated with PCP or CMV. PCP is also suggested by an increased serum lactate dehydrogenase level and hypoxia more severe than expected from radiographic findings. Hilar adenopathy with diffuse pulmonary infiltrates suggests cryptococcosis, histoplasmosis, mycobacterial infection, or neoplasm. KS can present with cough, fever, and dyspnea; the chest radiograph may mimic that seen with PCP.

Pneumocystis Pneumonia

PCP is the most common opportunistic infection among AIDS patients. More than 80% of AIDS patients will acquire PCP at some time during their illness, and it is the initial opportunistic infection in 60% of cases. Widespread use of highly active antiretroviral treatment (HAART) has led to a recent decrease in incidence of PCP. PCP infections typically occur in HIV-infected adults with CD4 lymphocyte counts below 200/μL, although pediatric cases may be seen with higher CD4 counts. Disease is caused by the organism *Pneumocystis jiroveci* (formerly referred to as *Pneumocystis pneumonia*). Traditionally classified as a protozoan, its morphology more closely resembles a fungus.

Classic presenting symptoms of PCP are an insidious cough (typically nonproductive), dyspnea, and fatigue. A determined investigation of new or subtle symptoms may lead to an early diagnosis, which, in turn, may result in a better outcome. Typical chest radiographic findings are diffuse interstitial infiltrates. Atypical x-ray findings are more common in patients with CD4 counts less than 100 cells/μL, and negative chest x-rays have been reported in up to 20% of patients with PCP (12). Up to 10% of patients with PCP have been found to have pneumothoraces. In patients with PCP, arterial blood gas analysis may show hypoxemia and an increased alveolar–arterial oxygen gradient.

In the ED, a presumptive diagnosis of PCP is often made if there is hypoxia without any other explanation. Examination of induced sputum by indirect immunofluorescent staining using monoclonal antibodies has been shown to be a relatively easy and effective method of diagnosing PCP, although bronchoscopy (bronchoalveolar lavage, brush biopsy, transbronchial biopsy) is the mainstay of establishing the diagnosis. When PCP is suspected, treatment should be initiated without waiting to obtain a definitive diagnosis. Initial treatment is with 15 mg/kg/d of trimethoprim (TMP) and 75 mg/kg/d of sulfamethoxazole (SMZ), given either orally or intravenously in two to three daily divided doses for a total of 3 weeks (2 Bactrim DS every 8 hours). Alternative agents for those with adverse reactions to TMP/SMZ (which are typically rash, fever or neutropenia) include pentamidine isethionate, dapsone, clindamycin plus primaquine, atovaquone or trimetrexate. Systemic corticosteroid treatment is recommended for patients with a PaO$_2$ less than 70 mm Hg, or an alveolar–arterial gradient of more than 35 mm Hg. Prednisone should be administered in a dose of 80 mg for 5 days, with a 3 week taper. Prophylactic therapy for PCP (with Bactrim 1 DS po qd) is recommended to prevent reinfection, and in all patients with CD4 cell counts less than 200 cells/μL.

TABLE 147.2. Common Causes of Pulmonary Involvement in AIDS

INFECTION	Bacteria
	Streptococcus pneumoniae
Viral	*Haemophilus influenzae*
Cytomegalovirus	*Mycoplasma pneumonia*
Herpes simplex virus	*Legionella pneumonia*
Adenovirus	*Staphylococcus aureus*
Mycobacteria	*Pseudomonas aeruginosa*
M. tuberculosis	*Nocardia*
M. avium	
M. kansasii	**MALIGNANCY**
Fungi	
Histoplasma capsulatum	Lymphoma
Cryptococcus neoformans	Kaposi sarcoma
Coccidiodes	
Candida	**PNEUMONITIS**
Aspergillus fumigatus	
Blastomyces dermatitides	Lymphoid interstitial pneumonitis
Protozoa	
Pneumocystis carinii	
Toxoplasma gondii	

Tuberculosis

The incidence of *M. tuberculosis* in HIV-infected patients is increasing, particularly in socioeconomically disadvantaged groups, including the homeless, immigrant, and intravenous drug–using populations. The incidence of TB in the AIDS population is estimated to be 50 to 200 times that of the general population.(13). Increased incidence in the HIV population is thought to be due to a number of factors including increased rates of reactivation of latent infections, high rates of infection after exposure, increased at-risk groups, and rapid progression to clinically significant disease. Pulmonary TB may be the initial finding in HIV-infected patients, frequently occurring in patients with CD4 counts of 200 to 500 cells/μL.

Classic presenting symptoms of TB include cough (with hemoptysis), fever, night sweats, and weight loss. In patients with severe immunosuppression, clinical manifestations are increasingly atypical, and extrapulmonary findings may occur. Frequent sites of dissemination include peripheral lymph nodes, bone marrow, and the genitourinary system. Classic radiograph findings are upper lobe lesions with cavitation. Other associated findings include pleural effusions, mediastinal adenopathy and alveoloar opacities. In patients with CD4 counts < 200 cells/μL that have TB, atypical radiographic features or normal radiographs may be seen.(12).

In the ED, physicians should maintain a high index of suspicion for TB among HIV-infected patients with pulmonary symptoms. For any patient in whom the diagnosis is being considered, immediate isolation should be instituted because of the high rate of person-to-person transmission (14). Decisions for ongoing isolation and admission should be based on the results of chest x-ray and detailed historic and clinical information. Negative PPD tests are frequent among those infected. Attempts to diagnose TB by stain and culture of sputum may not be fruitful; bronchoscopy or biopsy of affected organs (e.g., lymph nodes, liver, and brain) may be required. AIDS patients with TB should receive four-drug initial empiric therapy with isoniazid, rifampin, pyrazinamide, and streptomycin for six months. Multidrug resistance TB is becoming an issue of increasing concern as well, and should be considered when making decisions about treatment regimens. This is best done in consultation with an infectious disease specialist. All HIV-infected patients with a positive PPD should receive isoniazid plus pyridoxine or rifampin plus pyrazinamide prophylaxis.

Bacterial Pneumonias

In HIV-infected patients, the most common pulmonary infections are nonopportunistic bacterial pneumonias, such as *Streptococcus pneumoniae*, *Mycobacterium pneumoniae*, and *Haemophilus influenzae*. In patients with severe immunosuppression, other pulmonary conditions to consider include opportunistic viral and fungal infections and malignancies. CMV is the most common viral pulmonary pathogen, occurs in late stage disease and has a radiograph appearance of alveolar infiltrates or ground glass opacities. The most common fungal pathogen is Cryptococcus neoformans, which also appears in late stage disease; radiograph findings are nonspecific and include consolidation and reticulonodular infiltrates. KS and lymphoma usually require biopsy for definitive diagnosis and should be treated with oncology consultation.

Disposition decisions for HIV-positive patients with pulmonary complaints are primarily dependent on respiratory status, oxygenation, and evidence of systemic toxicity. Recent pilot studies indicate that hospitalization decision guidelines derived in the nonimmunosuppressed population may not apply for this population (15). A staging system for predicting mortality from HIV-associated pneumonia found that clinical factors associated with increased mortality include presence of neurologic symptoms, RR ≥ 25 and creatinine > 1.2 (16).

Neurologic Involvement

CNS disease occurs in 90% of patients with AIDS, and 10% to 20% of AIDS patients initially present with CNS symptoms (7,17). Recent data show that the overall incidence of HIV-associated neurologic diseases and central nervous system (CNS) complications has decreased since the introduction of HAART, although this trend is expected to change as patients develop increased resistance of antiretroviral drugs (17).

A wide variety of neurologic symptoms are seen in patients with HIV, including altered mental status, coma, seizures, headache, and focal neurologic symptoms. Infection accounts for the vast majority of neurologic presentations and is often accompanied by fever. Noninfectious complications include HIV encephalopathy (AIDS dementia complex), lymphoma (primary and secondary), KS, intracerebral hemorrhage, subarachnoid hemorrhage, cerebral infarction, and cerebral edema.

A specific diagnosis may often be established with the aid of computed tomographic (CT) scanning, cerebrospinal fluid (CSF) studies, and, in some cases (e.g., lymphoma), biopsy. For patients with CD4 cell count > 200 cells/μL who present with fever and meningismus (in the absence of focal neurologic deficits) an immediate lumbar puncture (LP) should be performed. For those with focal deficits, or new seizures, neuroimaging should precede LP. Evaluation of patients with altered mental status or headache should proceed as in the non-HIV infected population with neuroimaging and LP reserved for those cases in which another cause is not clearly identified or with a clear indication for work up (i.e., worst headache of life) (18). For patients with CD4 cell counts of < 200 cells/μL, any of the above-described findings demand early neuroimaging followed by LP (19).

In general CT without contrast is considered adequate in the ED for initial evaluation. If the entire ED work up is unrevealing, and the patient has significant signs or symptoms, more advanced imaging should be pursued immediately, preferably in the inpatient setting. Specific CSF studies should include measurement of opening and closing pressures; cell count; glucose; protein; Gram stain; India ink stain; bacterial, viral, and fungal culture; and toxoplasmosis, cryptococcus, and coccidioidomycosis titers. Asking the laboratory to retain excess CSF for further testing, if necessary, is always prudent.

Toxoplasma gondii

Toxoplasma gondii is the most common cause of focal intracranial mass lesions in patients with HIV infection (incidence 3% to 4%). Typical manifestations include headache, confusion, and seizures. Focal deficits occur in up to 80% of cases. Serologic testing is not useful because antibody to *T. gondii* is prevalent in the general population. The presence of *T. gondii* in the CSF is helpful, although there is a high rate of false negatives. Diagnosis is usually made by the presence of multiple subcortical lesions on CT scan. In patients with suspicious lesions, or those with a high suspicion of clinical pathology but equivocal or negative noncontrast scans, contrast-enhanced head CT or MRI (even more sensitive) may be helpful. In these studies, toxoplasmosis appears as one or more ring-enhancing lesions associated with edema (Fig. 147.1).

Radiographic and clinical features of toxoplasmosis are similar to a wide variety of other CNS disorders (lymphomas, cerebral TB, fungi, CMV, KS and progressive multifocal leukoencephalopathy [PML]). Definitive diagnosis may require biopsy. Patients with suspected toxoplasmosis should be admitted and

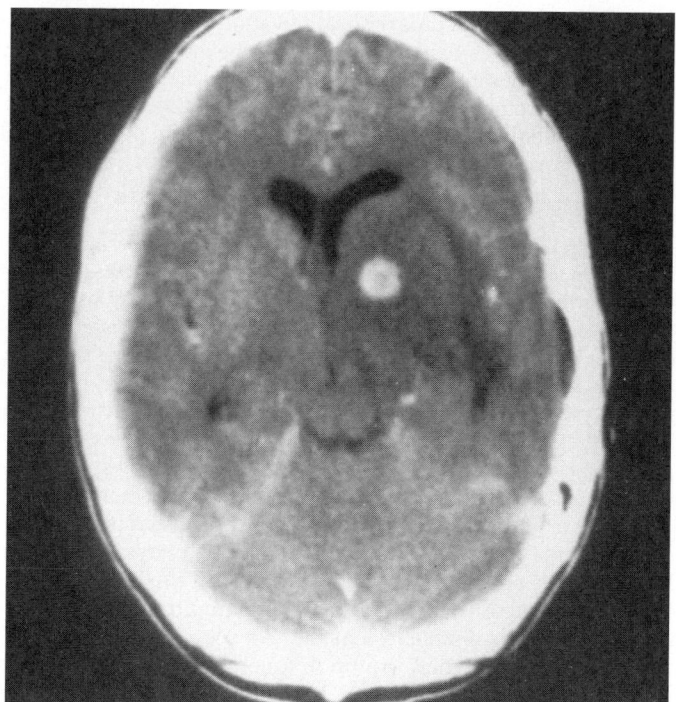

Figure 147.1.   Contrast-enhanced CT scan with typical ring-enhancing lesions of cerebral toxoplasmosis.

treated with sulfadiazine (4 to 8 g/d) and pyrimethamine (100 to 200 mg load, then 50 to 100 mg/d). Folinic acid should be added to decrease the incidence of pancytopenia. Short courses of high-dose corticosteroids may also be used, particularly in cases in which significant edema or mass effect is noted; seizure prophylaxis with phenytoin may be used in these cases as well. Presumptive treatment may be initiated before a definitive diagnosis is made. In cases in which the patient does not respond to therapy, alternative diagnoses should be considered. Chronic suppressive therapy is indicated after treatment to prevent relapse. Prophylaxis with Bactrim plus folinic acid is indicated for those with positive serology and CD4 cell counts < 100 cells/μl.

Cryptococcus neoformans occurs in up to 10% of AIDS patients and may cause either focal cerebral lesions or diffuse meningoencephalitis. Presenting symptoms are usually subtle (e.g., mild depression, headache, or dizziness without meningismus) but may be more dramatic (e.g., cranial nerve palsies and seizures). Mortality is up to 30%. Diagnosis of cryptococcus depends on identifying organisms in the CSF by cryptococcal antigen (nearly 100% sensitive and specific); other tests include India ink preparation (60% to 80% sensitive), fungal culture (95% to 100% sensitive) and serum cryptococcal antigen (95% sensitive). Treatment of cryptococcal meningitis is with intravenous amphotericin B (0.5 to 0.6 mg/kg/d), with or without 5-flucytosine, for 14 days. The initial course of therapy should be followed by 8 to 10 weeks of oral fluconazole. In patients with normal mental status, oral fluconazole, 400 mg/d orally, or itraconazole may be considered as alternative initial therapies. Because of the high relapse rate (about 50%), chronic suppressive therapy is often continued after successful treatment. Adverse effects of treatment for cryptococcal meningitis include marrow suppression (flucytosine) as well as fever and renal dysfunction (amphotericin).

Other infections, such as bacterial meningitis, TB meningitis, aseptic meningitis, brain abscess, CMV encephalitis, herpes simplex virus (HSV) encephalitis, aspergillosis, nocardial encephalitis, and neurosyphilis, may also be considered as causes of neu-

rologic symptoms. Noninfectious CNS processes include CNS lymphoma, cerebrovascular accidents, metabolic encephalopathy, and AIDS dementia complex (HIV encephalopathy).

CNS lymphoma is often made after patients with presumptive toxoplasmosis (based on CT findings) are unresponsive to therapy. These tumors originate from the B-cells, which express the Epstein Barr virus (EBV). PCR for EBV is helpful in the diagnostic work up but definitive diagnosis requires biopsy. Prognosis is poor with median survival of less than 1 month. Whole brain irradiation with steroid and chemotherapy may extend life expectancy to several months.

AIDS dementia or HIV encephalopathy is a common, progressive disorder characterized by impaired memory, lethargy, concentration difficulties, and other cognitive impairment. Physical findings may include frontal release signs, hyperactive deep tendon reflexes and other hallmarks of advanced AIDS (such as wasting, alopecia, generalized dermatitis and lymphadenopathy). It is important to recognize that AIDS dementia is a diagnosis of exclusion and is usually confirmed on the basis of neuropsychologic testing; thus even among patients with established HIV-related dementia, the acute appearance of signs or symptoms should prompt a work up to rule out other treatable CNS processes. CT scan in patients with HIV encephalopathy typically shows atrophy and diffuse deep matter hyperdensitivities; MRI shows patchy punctuate white matter lesions. HIV encephalopathy often responds to zidovudine therapy.

HIV-infected patients with new or changed CNS symptoms or signs should be considered for hospital admission, particularly if the ED evaluation is unrevealing. CT scan and lumbar puncture should usually be performed as part of the ED evaluation, although CSF culture and serologic results will not be available immediately. When CT and all CSF studies are unrevealing, magnetic resonance imaging may be helpful in identifying early CNS lesions.

Peripheral neuropathies are common in the HIV-infected population and may be caused by HSV, mononeuritis multiplex (possibly related to multifocal CMV), idiopathic sensory neuropathy, or drug reactions (specifically to dideoxyinosine and dideoxycytidine). In certain patients, symptomatic relief with pain-modifying agents such as amitriptyline or phenytoin may be helpful, although these agents should be used judiciously because of their potential for causing delirium in patients with concurrent HIV dementia. Ibuprofen may be used as first line therapy; narcotic analgesia should be reserved for more severe cases.

Gastrointestinal Involvement

About one-half of all AIDS patients have symptoms due to infection of the gastrointestinal tract at some time during the course of their illness. The most common symptoms are abdominal pain, bleeding, and diarrhea. Nonspecific GI-related symptoms are also common adverse effects of antiretroviral therapy, which may further complicate establishing the diagnosis. Treatment in the ED focuses on supportive care and obtaining appropriate studies for further investigation.

Oropharynx

Oral involvement is common, and may include a variety of etiologies, including infections, neoplasms, and autoimmune or idiopathic lesions. Oral lesions such as candidiasis and hairy leukoplakia are early indicators of disease progression.

Oral candidiasis is the most common oral manifestation of HIV infection and affects more than 80% of AIDS patients. *Candida albicans* typically involves the tongue and buccal mucosa. It can be distinguished from hairy leukoplakia by its characteristic whitish, lacy plaques, which are easily scraped away from an erythematous base. Microscopic examination of the material on potassium hydroxide smear can confirm the diagnosis in the ED. Oral and esophageal involvement with *Candida* is considered predictive of a progressive course of HIV infection. Most oral lesions can be managed symptomatically on an outpatient basis. Clotrimazole troches (10 mg, po, 5 times daily for 14 days) are the preferred treatment for oral candidiasis. Other treatment options include nystatin vaginal tablets and nystatin pastilles, both of which may be dissolved slowly in the mouth. Oral ketoconazole, fluconazole, or itraconazole may be considered for refractory cases.

Hairy leukoplakia, thought to be caused by the Epstein-Barr virus, results in a benign epithelial thickening and typically involves the lateral borders of the tongue. The tongue may appear to have hairlike projections. As it is often asymptomatic, therapy is not necessary, but when indicated, treatment may be initiated with acyclovir, foscarnet, gancyclovir, or Retin-A (although lesions often recur after cessation of therapy).

Painful oral and perioral ulcerations may be caused by herpes virus (HSV), which can be recognized by typical vesicular lesions and diagnosed in the ED by the identification of multinucleated giant cells in scrapings of the lesions. Oral HSV may be treated with oral acyclovir. Topical acyclovir is not effective. Aphthous ulcerations, also painful and recurrent, have an unknown etiology. These small, crateriform ulcers have a white to yellow membrane surrounded by an erythematous halo. Aphthous ulcers usually respond to topical steroids mixed with topical anesthetic, such as Orabase.

Oral KS may appear as nontender, well-circumscribed, slightly raised, violaceous lesions anywhere in the oropharynx. Definitive diagnosis and therapy should be carried out by a consultant.

Esophagus

Complaints of dysphagia or odynophagia are indicative of esophageal involvement. Candidal, HSV, and CMV infections may all cause painful esophagitis. The most cost-effective approach to evaluate patients with esophageal complaints is to initiate empiric therapy for presumptive candidiasis (which accounts for up to 70% of cases), with oral antifungal agents for 2 weeks before proceeding with endoscopy for patients who fail to improve (20). An air-contrast barium swallow may be obtained as part of the ED evaluation. An ulcerative pattern with plaques is characteristic of candidal esophagitis. HSV esophagitis typically produces easily seen punched-out ulcerations without associated heaped-up plaques. Endoscopy, fungal stains, viral cultures, and, occasionally, biopsy may be required to establish the definitive etiology.

Treatment for esophageal candidiasis should include either fluconazole (100 to 200 mg, PO, daily for 2 to 3 weeks) or ketoconazole (200 to 400 mg, PO, daily for 2 to 3 weeks). Relapses are common after cessation of treatment. Fluconazole has also been shown to be effective in prophylaxis against fungal infections with patients with a CD4 count of less than $100/mm^3$, although survival is unaffected by prophylactic therapy. Intravenous (IV) amphotericin B may be used for refractory cases, whereas disseminated candidiasis should be managed with IV amphotericin B and flucytosine.

Liver and Biliary Tract

Viral hepatitis occurs commonly among HIV-infected patients, and standard serologic testing and supportive care are indicated. Previous HBV infection may become reactivated following HIV infection, or acquired with increased prevalence following HIV infection. Several opportunistic organisms, including CMV, *M. avium*, *M. tuberculosis*, and *Histoplasma capsulatum*, can produce a hepatitis-like picture in patients with HIV infection. Most commonly, the patient presents with an elevation in the alkaline phosphatase level that is disproportionate to the levels of other liver enzymes. In HIV infected patients, hepatotoxicity may be seen as a result of side effects from a variety of medications, including indinavir. Acalculous cholecystitis may also occur in patients with HIV/AIDS as a result of infection with CMV or *Cryptosporidium*.

Anorectal Disease

Anorectal disease is common in AIDS patients, and careful examination is important in diagnosing such disorders. Proctitis is characterized by painful defecation, rectal discharge, and tenesmus. Common causative organisms include *Neisseria gonorrhoeae*, *Chlamydia trachomatis*, syphilis, and HSV. Proctocolitis presents with the same symptoms but is accompanied by diarrhea. Typical causative organisms include those just listed, plus bacterial agents such as *Shigella*, *Salmonella*, *Campylobacter*, and *Entamoeba histolytica*. Diagnostic evaluation in the ED should include anoscopy with evaluation of stool or pus (or both) by microscopic examination for leukocytes, ova and parasites, standard cultures as well as appropriate immunoassays or cultures for gonorrhea and chlamydial infections. HSV can be diagnosed by viral culture or by the identification of multinucleated giant cells on scrapings of anal lesions.

Diarrhea is extremely common among AIDS patients, and may vary in severity from a few loose stools per day to massive fluid loss with prostration, fever, chills, and weight loss. ED evaluation should be directed toward stabilization, hydration, and obtaining appropriate diagnostic studies.

The differential diagnosis of diarrhea in the HIV-positive population is broad. Common identified etiologies include parasites (*Cryptosporidium parvum*, *Enterocytozoon bieneusi*, *Isospora belli*, *Giardia lamblia*, *Entameba histolytica*, *Microsporidia*, *Cyclospora*, and others), bacteria (*Salmonella*, *Shigella*, *Campylobacter*, *Helicobacter pylori*, *Mycobacterium tuberculosis*, *Mycobacterium avium complex*, *Clostridium difficile*, and others), viruses (cytomegalovirus, herpes simplex, HIV, and others), and fungi (*Histoplasma capsulatum*, *cryptococcus neoformans*, *coccidioides imitis*, and others). Opportunistic infections are more commonly seen among patients with CD4 cell counts of less than 100 cells/mm^3. Significant gastrointestinal bleeding has been associated with many pathogens, particularly cytomegalovirus (CMV). *Salmonella* infection can be of particular concern in HIV-infected patients, often producing recurrent bacteremia and other significant clinical disease. Neoplastic GI involvement with KS or lymphoma may produce dysphagia, obstruction, intussusception, or diarrhea.

Two of the most common pathogens which result in a prolonged watery diarrhea in patients with HIV are *Cryptosporidium* and *Isospora belli* (21). Diagnosis may be sought using acid-fast staining of stool samples, or by monoclonal antibody, or enzyme-linked immunoabsorbent assays. Symptoms may be treated with diet modification or loperamide. *Cryptosporidium* infections may be treated with some success with paromomycin (500 to 750 mg, PO, 4 times daily for 2 to 4 weeks), or azithromycin (2,400 mg/day on day 1, followed by 1,200 mg/day for 4 weeks, followed by 600 mg/day). *Isospora* infections are often successfully treated with TMP-SMX (1 DS tablet, PO, 3 times daily for 10 days, followed by twice weekly therapy for 3 weeks). Pyrimethamine or metronidazole may be used as alternative therapy. HAART may also reduce duration and severity of symptomatology.

Initial studies should include microscopic examination of stool for leukocytes and of stool samples for bacterial culture, ova, and parasites (22). Often, no definitive diagnosis can be made in AIDS patients with diarrhea. In general, patients who can tolerate oral intake and are not orthostatic may be discharged from the ED, with outpatient follow up of test results. If bacterial infection is strongly suspected, empiric treatment with an antibiotic such as ciprofloxacin can be initiated. Patients who present with severe diarrhea may benefit from symptomatic therapy with agents such as attapulgite (Kaopectate), psyllium (Metamucil), and, if necessary, diphenoxylate hydrochloride with atropine (Lomotil).

Dermatologic Involvement

Skin disease may affect up to 90% of HIV-infected patients. Several cutaneous manifestations of AIDS are likely to be seen in the ED; neoplasms, cutaneous infection, and dermatitis are the most common. Viral infections may include HSV, herpes zoster, papillomavirus infection, and molluscum contagiosum.

The most common cutaneous neoplasm is KS, which has involved approximately 25% of known AIDS cases, occurring most often in homosexual men. KS typically presents as raised, irregular, nonblanching, brown-black or purple macules or nodules. Cutaneous KS is generally not associated with significant morbidity or mortality. Palliative therapy is indicated only for extensive, painful, or cosmetically disfiguring lesions. In addition to cutaneous involvement, KS may also involve the gastrointestinal tract, lungs, liver, spleen, and heart. Treatment may include cryotherapy, radiotherapy, infrared coagulation, sclerosing agents, intralesional vinblastine, or systemic chemotherapy (23).

Herpes simplex viruses are common in AIDS patients and can present as either a localized infection or systemic disease. Localized infections respond well to standard therapy with oral famciclovir (750 mg, PO, 3 times daily) or acyclovir (200 mg 5 times daily for 10 days). Intravenous therapy (5–10 mg/kg IV every 8 hours for 7–21 days) may be required in cases of disseminated infection or neurologic involvement. Suppressive therapy is effective.

Reactivation of varicella zoster virus is 17 times more likely to occur in patients with HIV than the general population. The clinical course is prolonged, and multidermatomal involvement is common. In patients with single dermatomal involvement who are not significantly immunosuppressed, outpatient treatment with acyclovir (800 mg PO five times a day), famciclovir (500 mg PO three times a day), or valcyclovir (1000 mg PO twice daily) for 7 days is usually sufficient. Patients with disseminated disease or ophthalmic zoster should be admitted to isolation beds for intravenous acyclovir.

Papillomavirus infection is manifested as warts, which may appear in various areas. Treatment may be initiated with topical salicylic acid, and referral to a dermatologist is generally indicated.

Molluscum contagiosum lesions are typically clusters of white umbilicated papules. Unless they are cosmetically significant, molluscum lesions are considered benign and treatment is not mandatory. If desired, referral to a dermatologist may be made for consideration of such therapy as cryosurgery or curettage.

Bacterial infections, such as staphylococcal infections (e.g., folliculitis, impetigo, cellulitis), are seen with increased frequency. Therapy involves standard antibiotic treatment, although the duration of treatment may need to be increased.

Intertriginous infections with either *Candida* or *Trichophyton* are common and may be diagnosed by microscopic examination of scrapings in potassium hydroxide. Treatment may include topical imidazole creams (e.g., clotrimazole, miconazole, or ketoconazole).

Scabies should be considered in all HIV-infected patients, particularly those with dermatitis with excoriations, or pruritus. The yield of microscopically evident mites is high. Preferred treatment is with 5% permethrin, single application. Sexual and household contacts should also be treated.

Other types of dermatitis are also commonly seen. Seborrheic dermatitis manifests as erythematous scaly eruptions typically involving the nasolabial folds, cheeks, and chest, and is treated with a topical corticosteroid preparation. Diffuse xerosis (dry skin) and pruritus are common among HIV-infected patients. Treatment with topical emollients, oatmeal baths, and oral antihistamines such as diphenhydramine or hydroxyzine may be of benefit.

Psychiatric Issues

HIV-infected patients may present with a variety of social and emotional issues, complicated by neuropsychiatric and cognitive components. Some of the common psychiatric conditions include depression, bipolar disease, psychosis, suicidal ideation, anxiety, addiction, and adjustment disorder. It is estimated that 60% of HIV-infected patients experience depression during their illness. Patients with depression tend to have lower CD4 counts, and they report more AIDS-related symptoms. All psychiatric symptoms should be evaluated with the goal of identifying treatable, reversible conditions, such as CNS or drug reactions (24). Many patients will benefit from initiation of pharmacologic therapy in conjunction with social intervention and support. Suicidal potential should be taken seriously, particularly in patients who have limited social support; management at an inpatient facility is often required.

Ophthalmologic Manifestations

Eye complaints are common among patients with AIDS. Although a wide range of ophthalmic disease can occur, recognition of two is critical for the emergency physician.

Cytomegalovirus (CMV) retinitis is the most serious ocular opportunistic infection and the leading cause of blindness in patients with AIDS, occurring in up to 30% of patients at some time during their illness. With advances in HAART, reduced incidences of CMV retinitis have been observed, but discontinuation of HAART may result in intraocular inflammation (25). Presenting complaints are variable and may include blurred vision, changes in visual acuity, floaters, flashes of light, photophobia, scotoma, eye redness, or pain (26). Fundoscopic examination typically shows fluffy white perivascular lesions with areas of hemorrhage. These findings may be easily confused with retinal cotton wool spots, a benign lesion with no prognostic significance seen in patients with AIDS (indicative of retinal microvasculopathy). Because of the risk of blindness associated with CMV retinitis, any patient in whom there is suspicion of CMV retinitis requires immediate ophthalmologic consultation. Patients with CMV require immediate treatment to prevent progression of disease. The treatment regimen consists of induction therapy with intravenous ganciclovir (5 mg/kg every 12 hours for 2 weeks), followed by 6 mg/kg/day maintenance therapy. Foscarnet may also be used at a dosage of 90 mg/kg every 12 hours. Intravitreal injection of fomivirsen or gancyclovir-containing intravitreal implants are other therapeutic options for patients unresponsive to traditional therapy (27,28).

Herpes zoster ophthalmicus is another common cause of ocular damage in patients with HIV. The typical presentation is pain or paresthesia in the distribution of cranial nerve V_1, followed by the emergence of the vesicular zoster skin rash. Complications include conjunctivitis, episcleritis, iritis, keratitis, secondary glaucoma, and, rarely, retinitis. As with CMV, early recognition and treatment can prevent morbidity. Immunocompetent patients can be treated with acyclovir on an outpatient basis in consultation with ophthalmology. Immunocompromised patients require admission for intravenous antibiotics.

available. Confidentiality should be rigorously protected while still ensuring that the appropriate information is provided to the exposed individuals. Finally, the identification of a seropositive patient should not affect the delivery of appropriate health care.

Patients may present to the ED seeking postexposure prophylaxis following a nonoccupational exposure. Because the CDC has not yet issued guidelines for nonoccupational PEP (citing the lack of data regarding efficacy of therapy in this population), decision regarding therapy must be considered on a case-by-case basis based on risk of the source, risk of the exposure, and risk for ongoing high-risk exposures. In house infectious disease consultation should be sought whenever possible; other invaluable resources for both occupational and nonoccupational exposure include a CDC 24-hour hotline (1-888-448-4911) as well as an on-line decision support tool at http//www.needlestick.mednet.ucla.edu.

CRITICAL INTERVENTIONS

- Make the presumptive diagnosis of PCP in patients with cough, dyspnea, fatigue and hypoxia without any other explanation
- Isolate HIV-infected patients with pulmonary symptoms until TB is excluded
- Perform a CT and LP to evaluate patients with CD4 cell counts of < 200 cell/μL who have an altered mental status or headache in which another cause is not clearly identified
- Admit patients with disseminated varicella zoster disease or ophthalmic zoster to isolation beds for intravenous acyclovir therapy

COMMON PITFALLS

✔ Failure to recognize undiagnosed infection. Because patients often may not volunteer information regarding HIV risk factors, this information must be actively sought whenever a patient with possible opportunistic infection or other symptoms suggestive of HIV infection (e.g., weight loss, fever) is being treated

✔ Failure to fully evaluate complaints of fever, headache, and shortness of breath in HIV-positive patients who appear well. Fever may indicate systemic infection; blood cultures should be obtained, even in patients who appear nontoxic. Chronic low-grade headache or headache different from a patient's usual pattern of headache may be suggestive of CNS infection or malignancy; a head CT and lumbar puncture are indicated in such patients. Subjective shortness of breath may be the only early sign of PCP

Acknowledgment

Thanks to the previous edition's chapter author Gabor D. Kelen.

References

1. Joint United Nations Programme on HIV/AIDS: AIDS epidemic update: 2003, available at *www.unaids.org.* Accessed December 11, 2003.
2. Centers for Disease Control and Prevention. Trends in the HIV and AIDS epidemic. CDC Web Site: *www.cdc.gov/nchspt/od/trends.htm, 2004.*
3. Centers for Disease Control and Prevention: Transmission of HIV possibly associated with exposure of mucous membrane to contaminated blood. *MMWR Morb Mort Wkly Rep* 1997;46:620.
4. Rothman RE. Current CDC Guidelines for HIV Counseling, Testing, and Referral: Critical Role of and a Call to Action for Emergency Department Physicians *Annals of Emergency Medicine* (in press).
5. Rothman RE, Ketlogetswe K, Dolan T, Kelen GD. Should emergency departments conduct routine HIV screening?: a systematic review *Academic Emergency Medicine,* 2003;10:278.
6. Centers for Disease Control and Prevention. 1993 revised classification system for HIV infection and expanded surveillance case definition for AIDS among adolescents and adults. *MMWR* 1993;41(RR-17):1.
7. Kelen GD, Johnson G, Digiovanna TA, et al. Profile of patients with human immunodeficiency virus infection presenting to an inner-city emergency department: preliminary report. *Ann Emerg Med* 1990;19:242.
8. Marantz PR, Linzer M, Feiner CJ, et al. Inability to predict diagnosis in febrile intravenous drug addicts. *Ann Intern Med* 1987;106:823.
9. Rothman RE, Mamjudar M, Kelen GD, et al. Detection of bacteremia in emergency department patients at risk for infective endocarditis using universal 16s rRNA primers in a decontaminated polymerase chain reaction assay. *J Infect Dis* 2002;186:1677.
10. Rothman RE, Londner M, Mehta, et al. Developing a 24-hour ED based diagnostic guidelines for "ruling out" endocarditis in intravenous drug users (IDUs). *Acad Emerg Med* 1999;6:453.
11. Kelen GD, Digiovanna T, Bisson K, et al. Human immunodeficiency virus infection in emergency department patients: epidemiology, clinical presentations and risk for health care workers: the Johns Hopkins experience. *JAMA* 1989;262:516.
12. Huang L, Stanell JD. AIDS and the lung. *Med Clin North Am* 1996;80:775.
13. Markowitz N, Hansen NI, Hopewell PC, et al. Incidence of tuberculosis in the United States among HIV-infected persons. *Ann Intern Med* 1997;126:123.
14. Moran GJ, McCabe F, Morgan TM, et al. Delayed recognition and infection control for tuberculosis in the emergency department. *Ann Emerg Med* 1995;26:290.
15. Khalil A, Ding M, Neuremberger et al. Community-acquired pneumonia (CAP) decision guidelines: Are the Pneuonia Patient Outcomes Research Team (PORT) guidelines a reliable tool for predicting mortality in the immunosuppressed population? *Acad Emerg Med* 2003;10:540.
16. Arozullah A, Parada J, Bennett CL, et al. A rapid staging system for predicting mortality from HIV-associated pneumonia. *Chest* 2003;123:1151.
17. Sacktor N. The epidemiology of human immunodeficiency virus-associated neurological disease in the era of highly active antiretroviral therapy. *J Neuro Virol* 21:1.
18. Rothman, RE, Keyl PM, McCarthur JC, et al. A decision guideline for emergency department utilization of noncontrast head CT in HIV-infected patients. *Acad Emerg Med* 1999;6:1010.
19. Graham CB, Wippold JF, Pilgram TK, et al. Screening CT determined by CD4 count in HIV-positive patients presenting with headache. *Amer J Neruorad* 2000;21:451.
20. Bonacini M. Medical management of benign oesophageal disease in patients with human immunodeficiency virus infection. *Dig Liver Dis* 2001;33:294.
21. Hunter PR, Nichols G. Epidemiology and clinical features of Cryptosporidium infections in immunocompromised patients. *Clin Microbiol Rev* 2002;15:145.
22. Oldfield EC III. Evaluation of chronic diarrhea in patients with human immunodeficiency virus infection. *Rev Gastroenterol Disord* 2002;2:176.
23. Nasti G, Errante D, Santarossa S, et al. A risk and benefit assessment of treatment for AIDS-related Kaposi's Sarcoma. *Drug Safety* 1999;20:403.
24. Treisman GJ, Angelino AF, Hutton HE. Psychiatric issues in the management of patients with HIV infection. *JAMA* 2001;286:1857.
25. Whitcup SM: Cytomegalovirus retinitis in the era of highly active antiretroviral therapy. *JAMA* 2000;283:653–658.
26. Wei LL, Park SS, Skiest DJ. Prevalence of visual symptoms among patients with newly diagnosed cytomegalovirus retinitis. *Retina* 2002;22:278.
27. Vitravene Study Group: Safety of intravitreous fomivirsen for treatment of cytomegalovirus retinitis in patients with AIDS. *Am J Ophthalmol* 2002;133:484.
28. Dhillon B, Kamal A, Leen C. Intravitreal sustained-release ganciclovir implantation to control cytomegalovirua retinitis in AIDS. *International J STD and AIDS.* 1998;9:227.
29. Ernst AA, Farley TA, Martin DH. Screening and empiric treatment for syphilis in an inner-city emergency department. *Acad Emerg Med* 1995;2:765.
30. Golden MR, Marra CM, Holmes KK. Update of syphilis: resurgence of an old problem. *JAMA* 2003;290:1510.
31. Mocroft A, Ledergerber B, Katlama et al. Decline in the AIDS and death rates in the EuroSIDA study: an observational study. *The Lancet* 2003;362:22.
32. Department of Health and Human Services, Panel on Clinical Practices for Treatment of HIV Infection: Guidelines for the use of antiretroviral agents in HIV-infected adults and adolescents. Available at: *www.hivatis.org.*
33. American College of Emergency Physicians: Code of Ethics for Emergency Physicians. Dallas, Texas, American College of Emergency Physicians, 1997.
34. Larkin GL. A code of conduct for academic emergency medicine. *Acad Emerg Med* 1999;6:45.
35. Kelen GD. Human immunodeficiency virus and the emergency department: risks and risk protection for health care providers. *Ann Emerg Med* 1990;19:242.
36. Kelen GD, Hansen KN, Green GB, et al. Determinants of emergency department procedure- and condition-specific universal (barrier) precaution requirements for optimal provider protection. *Ann Emerg Med* 1995;25:743.
37. Gerberding JL. Occupational exposure to HIV in health care settings. *N Engl J Med* 2002;343:826.
38. Cardo DM, Culver DH, Ciesielski CA, et al. A case-control study of HIV seroconversion in health-care workers after percutaneous exposure. Centers for Disease Control and Prevention Needlestick Surveillance Group. *N Engl J Med* 1997;337:1485.
39. Updated US Public Health Service guidelines for the management of occupational exposures to HBV, HCV and HIV and recommendations for postexposure prophyalixis. *MMWR Morb Mortal Wkly Rep* 50(RR-1):1, 2001.

CHAPTER 148
Toxic Shock Syndromes

Michelle J. Canham and Frederick M. Schiavone

STAPHYLOCOCCAL TOXIC SHOCK SYNDROME

Toxic shock syndrome (TSS), associated with *Staphylococcus aureus,* originally described in 1978 is recognized as a toxin-mediated, multi-system illness that occurs in primarily healthy people of any age group. The peak reported incidence, in 1980, was linked to the use of highly absorbant tampons. Due to federal regulations for tampons and public awareness, both the incidence and mortality from TSS have markedly declined. Currently, the number of cases of menstrual TSS is estimated to be about 1/100,000 and the case-fatality ratio is 1.8% (compared with 5.5% initially) (9,16).

Nonmenstrual cases of staphylococcal TSS have been found (17) and are associated with surgical procedures such as rhinoplasty, augmentation mammaplasty, liposuction, and burns. Cases have also been associated with influenza, sinusitis, tracheitis, intravenous drug use, human immunodeficiency virus (HIV) infection, cellulitis, gynecologic infections, and the postpartum period. Surveillance data for 1979 through 1996 recognized the decline in the incidence of TSS and the increase in the proportion of nonmenstrual cases (currently, at least 50% of cases) (7,9,16).

TSS is thought to be a superantigen-mediated disease. Superantigens are molecules that activate up to 20% of T cells at one time, resulting in massive cytokine production (20). These cytokines are responsible for capillary leak syndrome and account for many of the clinical signs of TSS (12). Toxic shock syndrome toxin-1 (TSST-1) was the initial exotoxin isolated from *S. aureus* isolates associated with TSS in 1981 (2,21). It has been isolated in over 90% of menstruation-associated cases (12). In contrast, TSST-1 has been detected in only 40% to 60% of the strains isolated in nonmenstrual TSS. Other toxins, such as staphylococcal enterotoxin B (SEB) and enterotoxins A (SEA) and C (SEC), are found in the remaining cases.

CLINICAL PRESENTATION AND DIFFERENTIAL DIAGNOSIS

The clinical manifestations of staphylococcal TSS are diverse based upon the action of the toxin(s). The patient often presents with an abrupt-onset of flu-like symptoms including fever, malaise, myalgias, and chills. The symptoms may progress over 2 to 3 days to a systemic shock–like syndrome. Some patients present with signs of hypovolemia due to diarrhea, generalized vasodilatation, or capillary leak. A major feature of TSS is the erythematous rash, resembling sunburn, which may be diffuse or patchy in distribution. Desquamation of the skin occurs in 7 to 14 days at the sites of the previous rash, with full-thickness peeling of the skin involving the palms, soles, and fingers.

Criteria for the diagnosis of staphylococcal TSS are provided in Table 148.1 (15). TSS can involve every organ system and can produce a wide constellation of symptoms. Patients

---

TABLE 148.1.   Criteria for Staphylococcal Toxic Shock Syndrome

1. Fever of 102°F (38.9°C)
2. Presence of diffuse macular erythroderma ("sunburn" appearance)
3. Desquamation 1 to 2 wk after onset of illness, particularly of the palms and soles
4. Hypotension, defined as a systolic blood pressure of 90 mm Hg for adults and less than the fifth percentile for children younger than 16 years; an orthostatic decrease in diastolic blood pressure of 15 mm Hg with a position change from lying to sitting; orthostatic syncope; or orthostatic dizziness
5. Involvement of three or more of the following organ systems:
   Gastrointestinal: history of vomiting or diarrhea at the onset of illness
   Muscular: elevated creatine phosphokinase level or severe myalgia
   Mucous membrane: nonpurulent conjunctivitis, oropharyngeal hyperemia, or vaginal hyperemia or discharge
   Renal: abnormal results or renal function tests or urinalysis
   Hepatic: elevated serum transaminase and bilirubin levels
   Hematologic: thrombocytopenia
   Central nervous system: disorientation or alteration in consciousness without focal neurologic signs and in the absence of hypotension or fever
   In addition, normal results of the following tests, if performed:
   Blood, throat, cerebrospinal fluid cultures (blood culture may be positive for *Staphylcoccus aureus*); antibody tests for Rocky Mountain spotted fever, ehrlichiosis, leptospirosis, and rubella

Toxic shock syndrome is "probable" when at least four of the five criteria are fulfilled.
Modified from American Academy of Pediatric. Staphylococcal toxic shock syndrome. In: Peter G, ed. *1997 Red book: report of the Committee on Infectious Diseases,* 24th ed. Elk Grove Village, IL: American Academy of Pediatrics, 1997:481.

---

often complain of severe myalgias or edema of the face and eyelids, with hyperemia of the pharynx, tongue, and vaginal mucosa. Gastrointestinal manifestations may include vomiting, diarrhea, abdominal pain, and hepatomegaly. There may be confusion, somnolence, lethargy, or agitation, without focal neurologic signs.

The differential diagnosis of TSS includes *streptococcal* toxic shock syndrome (discussion to follow), Kawasaki disease, staphylococcal scalded-skin syndrome, scarlet fever, Stevens-Johnson syndrome, Rocky Mountain spotted fever, ehrlichiosis, leptospirosis, meningococcemia, atypical measles, viral illness, anaphylaxis, heat stroke, gram-negative sepsis, and drug reactions.

EMERGENCY DEPARTMENT EVALUATION AND MANAGEMENT

The diagnosis of TSS is often made on clinical grounds. The disorder is toxin-mediated, therefore blood cultures are rarely positive (5%) (18). Laboratory examination may demonstrate a marked thrombocytopenia (platelets less than 100,000), elevated blood urea nitrogen and creatinine, and elevated liver function tests. The characteristic blanching macular or scarlatiniform rash often suggests the diagnosis.

Initial treatment consists of intravenous fluid replacement. Large volumes of crystalloid are often required to maintain normal perfusion. Hemodynamic monitoring and vasopressors are sometimes necessary. Tampons, nasal packs, or other foreign bodies must be removed. Surgical wounds or areas of infection need to be incised and drained.

Antibiotics may not affect the clinical course, however, may be beneficial if the patient is bacteremic or if there is a site of on-going infection. Antibiotic therapy reduces the likelihood of recurrent TSS in those that previously failed to develop an appropriate antibody response to staphylococcal toxins (1,5). Even in the absence of overt staphylococcal infection, most experts recommend a one to two week course of therapy with an antistaphylococcal agent such as clindamycin or dicloxacillin.

Adjunctive treatments for TSS have included intravenous immunoglobulin, steroids, and monoclonal antibodies. At present, these therapies have not demonstrated a clear benefit.

COMMON PITFALLS

✔ Failure to recognize TSS in young healthy patients with fever and an erythematous rash
✔ Failure to administer adequate fluid volumes to maintain tissue perfusion
✔ Failure to seek an occult source of staphylococcal colonization or infection

STREPTOCOCCAL TOXIC SHOCK SYNDROME

In the late 1980s, a disease similar to staphylococcal TSS, but caused by a strain of group A streptococci, was recognized (23). This illness, characterized by hypotension and multiorgan failure, was termed *streptococcal toxic shock syndrome* (STSS). The Centers for Disease Control and Prevention case definition of this syndrome is shown in Table 148.2 (4).

Cases of STSS are often associated with minor nonpenetrating trauma or soft-tissue infection (3,11). Viral infections, such as varicella (6) and influenza, are thought to provide a portal of entry in other cases, but, in many patients, no source of the organism can be identified. Bacterial toxins produced by group A streptococci (GAS), particularly streptococcal pyrogenic exotoxins (SPE), as well as host factors, are thought to play an important role in determining disease severity (24). Blood cultures are generally positive (60%). The young, the elderly, and the immunosuppressed are at greatest risk, but a large proportion of patients with STSS are young, healthy adults (10). Despite increased awareness, prevalence has remained approximately 3.5 cases per 100,000 people since the mid-1980s (13).

CLINICAL PRESENTATION AND EMERGENCY DEPARTMENT EVALUATION

A majority of patients have signs of a soft-tissue infection, such as localized swelling and erythema; of these, many progress to necrotizing fasciitis or myositis. The most common initial symptom is pain out of proportion to physical findings. The pain is usually severe and abrupt in onset, and occurs initially without associated tenderness. It may involve an extremity, the abdomen, the pelvis, or the chest. An ominous sign is the appearance of vesicles, which develop into violaceous or bluish bullae. These are an indication for emergent surgical exploration, both to establish the diagnosis of GAS infection and to debride nonviable tissue.

Half of patients have a normal blood pressure on admission but develop hypotension within a few hours of presentation. Many have other manifestations that include a flu-like syndrome of fever, malaise, myalgia, nausea, vomiting, and diarrhea. As with TSS, there might be multiorgan system involvement. Renal

---

TABLE 148.2.　Case Definition for the Streptococcal Toxic Shock Syndrome

1. Isolation of group A streptococci
   A. From a normally sterile site (e.g., blood, cerebrospinal fluid, peritoneal fluid, tissue biopsy, surgical wound)
   B. From a nonsterile site (e.g., throat, superficial skin lesion)
2. Clinical signs of severity
   A. Hypotension: systolic blood pressure 90 mm Hg in adults or less than fifth percentile for age in children, and
   B. Two or more of the following signs:
      Renal impairment: creatinine 2 mg/dL for adults or at least twice the upper limit of normal for age
      Coagulopathy: platelets less than 100,000/µL or disseminated intravascular coagulopathy
      Liver involvement: serum alanine aminotransferase (SGOT), aspartate aminotransferase (SGPT), or total bilirubin concentrations at least twice the upper limit or normal for age
      Adult respiratory distress syndrome
      A generalized erythematous macular rash that may desquamate
      Soft-tissue necrosis, including necrotizing fasciitis or myositis, or gangrene

An illness fulfilling criteria 1A and 2 (A and B) can be defined as a definite case.
An illness fulfilling criteria 1B and 2 (A and B) can be defined as a probable case if no other etiology for the illness is identified.
Modified from the Centers for Disease Control and Prevention. The Working Group on Severe Streptococcal Infection. Defining the group A streptococcal toxic shock syndrome: rationale and consensus definition. *JAMA* 1993;269:391.

---

dysfunction may be severe enough to require hemodialysis. Acute respiratory distress syndrome may require endotracheal intubation. In distinction to staphylococcal TSS, the diffuse scarlatina-like rash is uncommon in STSS (less than 10%). Despite prompt, aggressive medical and surgical management, the mortality rate of STSS is high, usually about 30% to 60% (23).

EMERGENCY DEPARTMENT MANAGEMENT

Early treatment with antibiotics is critical. Although *Streptococcus pyogenes* continues to be susceptible to beta-lactam antibiotics, including penicillin, several studies recommend treatment with both penicillin and clindamycin. Clindamycin suppresses the synthesis of bacterial toxins (8,22), thereby increasing survival rates. In addition to antibiotics, prompt and aggressive surgical exploration and debridement of suspected deep-seated *S. pyogenes* infections are mandatory. Areas of apparently minor, painful, erythematous swelling may represent the first sign of a serious group A streptococcus infection.

Massive quantities of intravenous fluids (up to 20 L/d) may be necessary. Vasopressors such as dopamine are frequently used, but outcome trials have not demonstrated their benefit. Cases of symmetrical gangrene of the digits have resulted with the use of vasopressors; however, it is difficult to determine whether this is due to pressors, infection, or both.

Case reports have described the successful use of intravenous gamma globulin infusions in a small number of patients with STSS (14). Anecdotal reports of hyperbaric oxygen have been used in a handful of patients (19), but it is unclear whether this treatment is useful.

COMMON PITFALLS

✔ Failure to consider the diagnosis of STSS early and to institute antibiotics promptly
✔ Failure to debride soft-tissue infections aggressively

CRITICAL INTERVENTIONS

- Administer aggressive intravenous fluid replacement to maintain perfusion
- Remove tampons, nasal packs, or other foreign bodies
- Incise and drain surgical wounds or areas of infection

References

1. Andrews, MM, Parent, EM, Barry, M, Parsonnet, J. Recurrent nonmenstrual toxic shock syndrome: clinical manifestations, diagnosis, and treatment. *Clin Infect Dis* 2001;32:1470.
2. Bergdoll, MS, Crass, BA, Reiser, RF, et al. A new staphylococcal enterotoxin, enterotoxin F, associated with toxic-shock-syndrome Staphylococcus aureus isolates. *Lancet* 1981;1:1017
3. Bisno AL. Streptococcal infections of skin and soft tissues. *N Engl J Med* 1996; 334:240.
4. Centers for Disease Control. The Working Group on Severe Streptococcal Infection. Defining the group A streptococcal toxic shock syndrome: rationale and consensus definition. *JAMA* 1993;269:391.
5. Davis, JP, Osterholm, MT, Helms, CM, et al. Tri-state toxic-shock syndrome study. II. Clinical and laboratory findings. *J Infect Dis* 1982;145:441.
6. Doctor A, Harper MB, Fleisher GR. Group A B-hemolytic streptococcal bacteremia: historical overview, changing incidence, and recent association with varicella. *Pediatrics* 1995;96
7. Gaventa, S, Reingold, AL, Hightower, AW, et al. Active surveillance for toxic shock syndrome in the United States, 1986. *Rev Infect Dis* 1989;11 Suppl 1:S28.
8. Gemmell, CG, Peterson, PK, Schmeling, D, et al. Potentiation of opsonization and phagocytosis of streptococcus pyogenes following growth in the presence of clindamycin. *J Clin Invest* 1981;67:1249.
9. Hajjeh, RA, Reingold, A, Weil, A, et al. Toxic shock syndrome in the United States: surveillance update, 1979 1996. *Emerg Infect Dis* 1999;5:807.
10. Hoge CW, Schwartz B, Talkington DF, et al. The changing epidemiology of invasive group A streptococcal infections and the emergence of toxic shock-like syndrome: a retrospective population-based study. *JAMA* 1993;269:384–389.
11. Kaul R, McGeer A, Low DE, et al. Population-based surveillance for group A streptococcal necrotizing fasciitis: clinical features, prognostic indicators, and microbiologic analysis of seventy-seven cases. *Am J Med* 1997;103:18–24.
12. Manders SM. Toxin-mediated streptococcal and staphylococcal disease. *Am Acad Dermatol* 1998;39:3.
13. O'Brien, KL, Beall, B, Barrett, NL, et al. Epidemiology of invasive group A streptococcus disease in the United States, 1995–1999. *Clin Infect Dis* 2002;35:268.
14. Perez CM, Kubak BM, Cryer HG, et al. Adjunctive treatment of streptococcal toxic shock syndrome using intravenous immunoglobulin: case report and review. *Am J Med* 1997;102:111–113.
15. Peter G, ed. *1997 Red book: report of the Committee on Infectious Diseases,* 24th ed. Elk Grove Village, IL: American Academy of Pediatrics, 1997:481.
16. Reduced incidence of menstrual toxic-shock syndrome: United States 1980–1990. *Morb Mortal Wkly Rep* 1990;39:421.
17. Reingold AL, et al. Nonmenstrual toxic shock syndrome: a review of 130 cases. *Ann Intern Med* 1982;96:871.
18. Reingold, AL, Dan, BB, Shands, KN, Broome, CV. Toxic-shock syndrome not associated with menstruation. A review of 54 cases. *Lancet* 1982;1:1.
19. Riseman JA. Hyperbaric oxygen therapy for necrotizing fasciitis reduces mortality and the need for debridements. *Surgery* 1990;108:847.
20. Schlievert, PM. Role of superantigens in human disease. *J Infect Dis* 1993;167:997.
21. Schlievert, PM, Shands, KN, Dan, BB, et al. Identification and characterization of an exotoxin from Staphylococcus aureus associated with toxic-shock syndrome. *J Infect Dis* 1981;143:509.
22. Stevens, DL, Maier, KA, Mitten, JE. Effect of antibiotics on toxin production and viability of Clostridium perfringens. *Antimicrob Agents Chemother* 1987;31:213.
23. Stevens DL, Tanner MH, Winship J, et al. Severe group A streptococcal infections associated with a toxic shock-like syndrome and scarlet fever toxin A. *N Engl J Med* 1989;321:1.
24. Stevens DL. Streptococcal toxic-shock syndromes: spectrum of diseases, pathogenesis, and new concepts in treatment. *EID* 1995;1:3

CHAPTER 149
Parasitic Disease

Keith T. Borg and Richard J. Ryan

Parasitic infestations are much more widespread than many realize. Parasites affect not only impoverished peoples in remote countries, but can also cause important health problems for rich and poor throughout the world, including the United States. Parasites are considered by many physicians to be the most undiagnosed infectious disease challenge in the United States today. Because of this, diagnosing parasitic infection in the emergency department can be challenging: the physician must be aware of the many potential manifestations of infestation by parasites, a large and varied group of organisms. Parasitic disease, however, can usually be diagnosed through methods available to most emergency physicians, and effective treatments are available that are generally minimally toxic to the human host (3,8). A history of foreign travel or habitation in an endemic area, including certain regions of the United States, should alert the clinician to the possibility of parasitic infection. As with many disease processes the key lies in considering parasitic infestation in the differential.

Symptoms may not manifest themselves until well after the traveler has returned home. In addition, over the last two decades, the proportion of the United States population born abroad has increased steadily, with newer immigrants typically coming from Latin America and Asia (18). The proper treatment of immigrants in the United States requires a familiarity with diseases common in the developing world, such as malaria, amebiasis, and neurocysticercosis. Given the constant change in the globalization of infectious disease, the clinician should always consult current references including the CDC website (www.cdc.gov/travel/). Parasitic infestation is a global problem. Here in the United States, the CDC cites food as the catalyst behind 80 percent of the pathogenic outbreaks.

Four major groups of organisms infest humans. *Protozoans* cause malaria, amebiasis, giardiasis, and many other diseases. Helminths or worms, including *nematodes* (roundworms), *cestodes* (tapeworms), and *trematodes* (flukes), are also responsible for a wide variety of human illnesses. A comprehensive review of parasitic diseases would encompass infections due to literally scores of organisms, so this chapter is limited to the parasitic diseases most common in emergency departments in the United States (Trichomoniasis is excluded). This chapter is divided into three discussions: systemic illnesses, predominantly gastrointestinal (GI) disease, and predominantly central nervous system (CNS) disease.

SYSTEMIC ILLNESS

CLINICAL PRESENTATION

Awareness about malaria and measures that travelers can take to avoid infective mosquito bites are more important than ever. Thus, fever in a patient with a history of recent travel or habitation in the tropics should suggest the diagnosis of malaria. Caused by four species of the protozoan *Plasmodium* (*P. vivax, P. ovale, P. falciparum,* and *P. malariae*), malaria is the most common parasitic disease in the world, accounting for an estimated 300 million cases and 1.5 to 2.7 million deaths annually. Although malaria is no longer considered endemic in the United States, increased immigration from and travel to countries where the disease is common has made malaria more frequent as a presenting complaint in emergency departments in this country (13). The number of cases of malaria acquired by international travel is growing due to the increased risk of malaria transmission where malaria control has faded and the spread of drug-resistant strains of malaria (21). Patients with malaria are frequently misdiagnosed on their initial presentation to the emergency department, thus increasing their risk for serious morbidity and mortality.

Classic symptoms of malaria include fever, chills, and rigors. These symptoms last 4 to 10 hours culminating in an episode of profuse diaphoresis followed by defervescence. This pattern may recur at 2- or 3-day intervals, depending on the species of *Plasmodium* involved. Other clinical signs and symptoms include general malaise, headache, and, occasionally, hypotension. Physical examination is not generally helpful. Splenomegaly and jaundice may be seen in established infections. Laboratory abnormalities include a mild anemia, neutropenia, thrombocytopenia, and increased prothrombin time. Clinical evidence of impaired hemostasis is rare.

The periodicity of the disease can be explained by examining the life cycle of the infecting organism. In the human, the life cycle of the parasite consists of two stages. The initial stage is known as the liver or exoerythrocytic stage. This is where the parasites multiply in hepatocytes and cause them to rupture. The second stage is known as the blood or erythrocytic stage and occurs when parasites are released into the bloodstream and invade the erythrocytes. This is the cause of clinical illness. *Plasmodium* species may be injected into the human circulation following the bite of the *Anopheles* mosquito, after sharing needles or receiving a blood transfusion, and by congenital transmission. Immature sporozoites migrate to the liver, beginning the exoerythrocytic phase, the duration of which is species-dependent. Ultimately, mature parasites (merozoites) are released into the circulation and invade red blood cells, beginning the erythrocytic phase. Replication within red cells is followed 48 to 72 hours later by red cell lysis and release of further merozoites into the circulation, which again invade erythrocytes and repeat the cycle. The fever corresponds to episodes of red cell lysis.

The classic pattern of periodic fever is not always seen, however, particularly early in the course of the illness. The variability of the clinical course also depends on the infecting species and the host's immune status. People living in endemic areas often have partial "immunity" that results in much less severe manifestations and symptoms. It is presumed to be an acquired immunity caused by frequent exposure to the infecting organism. Months after leaving an endemic area, these persons may experience relapses that resemble the acute form of the disease, probably caused by a loss of immunity and the release of exoerythrocytic parasites from the liver. *P. vivax* and *P. ovale* can persist for long periods in the exoerythrocytic state. Even patients who have received adequate antimalarial therapy may experience relapses associated with the release of exoerythrocytic organisms. Cases have been reported two months to four-and-a-half years after a traveler's return (21).

P. falciparum causes the most severe type of malaria and is responsible for most complications and deaths related to malaria (13). Falciparum malaria has two important features that account for differences in its presentation and in the severity of the disease it produces. First, this species causes widespread capillary obstruction, resulting in end-organ hypoxia and dysfunction, with severe complications that can include CNS dysfunction, hemolytic anemia, hypoglycemia, pulmonary edema, septicemia, renal failure, or splenic rupture. A second distinguishing feature of *P. falciparum* is that, unlike other malarial species that infect only the most mature red cells, it infects red cells of all ages, resulting in a greater degree of hemolysis and anemia and the potential for acute tubular necrosis. Finally, unlike *P. ovale and P. vivax*, cases of *P. falciparum* malaria in patients with late presentations are caused by blood-stage parasites that were drug resistant or had survived incomplete prophylaxis.

EMERGENCY DEPARTMENT EVALUATION

The diagnosis of malaria is a difficult one to make because of the disease's nonspecific clinical features—fever, chills, headache, and malaise. Because approximately 90% of travelers who contract malaria do not become ill until returning home, the diagnosis should be entertained for anyone presenting to the emergency department with a febrile illness and a history of travel or habitation in an endemic area (11). A high degree of suspicion is necessary for diagnosis by physicians who rarely encounter this disease. The most common incorrect diagnosis is a viral syndrome, but a history of recurrent fever generally distinguishes malaria from these disorders. Other disorders that cause fever and are endemic in foreign countries, such as viral hepatitis, dengue fever, typhoid fever, and amebiasis, should also be considered. Recent data suggest that a significant number of those presenting with malaria do so later than previously thought. Over 35% of malaria infested travelers in one study developed malaria more than 2 months after their return. This suggests that we may need to modify treatment to more aggressively treat the liver phase of the disease for effective prevention (21).

The standard way to make the diagnosis of malaria is through demonstration of intracellular forms of the parasite on a thin Giemsa-stained peripheral blood smear. If malaria is strongly suspected, negative blood films should be repeated every 12 hours for 2 days. Sometimes, it is necessary to use the thick-smear technique, which usually requires the expertise of a trained technician. Serologic tests may be helpful when there are very low levels of parasitemia, as in infection with *P. malariae* (10). New rapid testing by PCR and other methods are being developed and should aid in the rapid diagnosis of malarial infestations.

EMERGENCY DEPARTMENT MANAGEMENT

Management of malaria in the emergency department is guided by the severity of the infection. Assessment of airway patency and respiratory, circulatory, and neurologic status should be performed in a timely fashion. The emergency physician should be prepared to treat potential complications such as anemia, coagulopathies, pulmonary edema, azotemia, hypoglycemia, metabolic acidosis, and hypotensive shock (10).

Volume should be restored and fever controlled. Hypotension usually responds well to crystalloid infusion. Fever usually responds to standard cooling measures; for temperatures less than 104°F, oral antipyretics are likely to be effective. Acetaminophen is recommended rather than aspirin because of the common occurrence of thrombocytopenia. For patients with high-density parasitemia, altered mental status, pulmonary edema, or renal failure, exchange transfusion may be helpful (5).

Pharmacologic therapy of malaria is outlined in Table 149.1. Antimalaria pharmacotherapy and prophylaxis continue to pose difficult problems. Most antimalarial agents act on the parasites blood stage and therefore do not prevent late onset illness (21). Chloroquine remains the oral drug of choice for acute treatment of all infections except those due to chloroquine-resistant

TABLE 149.1. Treatment of Malaria

Indication	Drug	Adult Dosage	Pediatric Dosage
MALARIA			
Oral drug of choice:	Chloroquine phosphate	600 mg base (1 g), then 300 mg base (500 mg) 6 h later, then 300 mg base (500 mg)/d × at 24 and 48 hours	10 mg base/kg (max 600 mg base), then 5 mg base/kg 6 h later, then 5 mg base/kg/d × 2 d
Parenteral drug of choice	Quinidine gluconate	10 mg/kg loading dose (max 600 mg) in normal saline slowly over 1–2 h, followed by continuous infusion of 0.02 mg/kg/min until oral therapy can be started	Same as adult dose
	or Quinine dihydrochloride	20 mg/kg loading dose IV in 5% dextrose over 4 h, followed by 10 mg/kg over 2–4 h q8h (max 1800 mg/d) until oral therapy can be started	Same as adult dose
Alternative	Artemether	3.2 mg/kg IM, then 1.6 mg/kg a day	Same as adult dose
CHLOROQUINE-RESISTANT *P. FALCIPARUM* MALARIA			
Oral drugs of choice:	Quinine sulfate plus doxycycline *or* plus	650 mg q8h × 3 d–7 d 100 mg bid × 7 d	25 mg/kg/d in 3 doses × 3 d-7 d 2 mg/kg/d × 7 d (>8 yrs of age)
	pyrimethamine-sulfadoxine	3 tabs at once on last day of quinine	<1 yr – 1/4 tablet; 1–3 yrs – 1/2 tablet; 4–8 yrs – 1 tablet 9–14 yrs – 2 tablets
	or plus clindamycin	900 mg tid × 5 d	20–40 mg/kg/d in 3 doses × 5 d
Alternatives:	Mefloquine Halofantrine	750 mg followed in 12 hrs by 500 mg 500 mg q6h × 3 doses, repeat in 1 wk	25 mg/kg once (<45 kg) 8 mg/kg q6h × 3 doses (<40 kg); repeat in 1 wk
	Atovaquone	1000 mg qd × 3 d	11–20 kg: 250 mg 21–30 kg: 500 mg 31–40 kg: 750 mg
	plus proguanil	400 mg qd × 3 d	11–20 kg: 100 mg 21–30 kg: 200 mg 31–40 kg: 300 mg
	or plus doxycycline Artesunate plus mefloquine	100 mg bid × 3 d 4 mg/kg/d × 3 d 750 mg followed in 12 hrs by 500 mg	2 mg/kg/d × 3 d (>8 yrs of age)
CHLOROQUINE-RESISTANT *P. VIVAX* MALARIA			
Drug of choice	Quinine sulfate plus Doxycycline *or*	650 mg q8h × 3 d-7 d 100 mg bid × 7 d	25 mg/kg/d in 3 doses × 3 d-7 d 2 mg/kg/d × 7 d (>8 yrs of age)
	Mefloquine	750 mg followed in 12 hrs by 500 mg	15 mg/kg followed 8–12 hours later by 10 mg/kg
Alternatives	Halofantrine Chloroquine plus primaquine	500 mg q6 × 3 doses 25 mg base/kg in 3 doses over 48 hrs 2.5 mg base/kg in 3 doses over 48 hrs	8 mg/kg q6h × 3 doses
PREVENTION OF RELAPSES (*P. VIVAX* AND *P. OVALE* ONLY)			
Drug of choice:	Primaquine phosphate	15 mg base (26.3 mg)/d × 14 d or 45 mg base (79 mg)/wk × 8 wks	0.3 mg base/kg/d × 14 d

Adapted from Drugs for parasitic infections. Med Lett Drugs Ther April 2002 and the EMRA Antibiotic Guide 2004.

P. falciparum and *P. vivax*. For chloroquine-resistant *P. falciparum* infection or for severely ill patients with an unidentified malarial infection, quinine plus doxycycline or pyrimethamine and sulfadoxine or clindamycin is recommended.

In addition to acute therapy, patients infected with *P. vivax* or *P. ovale* require more prolonged treatment to prevent reactivation of exoerythrocyte forms. These patients should be treated with primaquine phosphate, 15 mg base/d for 14 days or 45 mg base/wk for 8 weeks. The pediatric dose is 0.3 mg base/kg/d for

14 days. Patients should be screened for G-6-PD deficiency before beginning primaquine therapy, and the drug is contraindicated during pregnancy (5).

To prevent fatal outcomes in cases of falciparum malaria, the following are required: improved health information and preventive measures for the 30 million travelers who visit regions where malaria is endemic, improved recognition of infection by physicians, and prompt initiation of effective therapy (11).

TABLE 149.2.   Treatment of Gastrointestinal Parasitic Infections

Infection	Drug	Adult Dosage	Pediatric Dosage
AMEBIASIS *(ENTAMOEBA HISTOLYTICAL)*			
Asymptomatic			
Drugs of choice:	Iodoquinol	650 mg tid × 20 d	30–40 mg/kg/d (max 2 g) in 3 doses × 20 d
	or Parmomycin	25–35 mg/kg/d in 3 doses × 7 d	25–35 mg/kg/d in 3 doses × 7 d
Alternative	Diloxanide furoate	500 mg tid × 10 d	20 mg/kg/d in 3 doses × 10 d
Mild to moderate intestinal disease			
Drugs of choice:	Metronidazole	500–750 mg tid × 10 d	35–50 mg/kg/doses × 10 d
	or Tinidazole	2 grams/d × 3d	50 mg/kg (max 2 g) qd c 3 d
Severe intestinal disease, hepatic abscess			
Drugs of choice:	Metronidazole	750 mg tid × 7–10 d	35–50 mg/kg/d in 3 doses × 10 d
	or Tinidazole	800 mg tid × 5 d	60 mg/kg (max 2 g) qd × 5 d
ASCARIASIS *(ASCARIS LUMBRICOIDES*, ROUNDWORM)			
Drugs of choice:	Albendazole	400 mg × 1 dose	400 mg × 1 dose
	or Mebendazole	100 mg bid × 3 d or 500 mg × 1 dose	100 mg bid × 3 d or 500 mg × 1 dose
	or Pyrantel pamoate	11 mg/kg × 1 dose (max 1 gram)	11 mg/kg × 1 dose (max 1 g)
***ENTEROBIUS VERMICULARIS* (PINWORM)**			
Drug of choice:	Pyrantel pamoate	11 mg/kg × 1 dose (max 1 g); repeat in 2 weeks	11 mg/kg × 1 dose (max 1 g); repeat in 2 weeks
	or Mebendazole	100 mg once; repeat in 2 weeks	100 mg once; repeat in 2 weeks
	or Albendazole	400 mg once; repeat in 2 weeks	400 mg once; repeat in 2 weeks
GIARDIASIS *(GIARDIA LAMBLIA)*			
Drug of choice:	Metronidazole	250 mg tid × 5 d	15 mg/kg/d in 3 doses × 5 d
Alternatives	Tinidazole	2 grams × 1 dose	50 mg/kg × 1 dose (max 2 g)
	Furazolidone	100 mg qid × 7–10 d	6 mg/kg/d in 4 doses × 7–10 d
	Paromomycin	25–35 mg/kg/d in 3 doses × 7 d	
HOOKWORM INFECTION *(ANCYLOSTOME DOUDENALE, NECATOR AMERICANUS)*			
Drugs of choice:	Albendazole	400 mg × 1 dose	400 mg × 1 dose
	or Mebendazole	100 mg bid × 3 d or 500 mg × 1 dose	100 mg bid × 3 d or 500 mg × 1 dose
	or Pyrantel pamoate	11 mg/kg (max 1 gram) × 3 d	11 mg/kg (max 1 g) × 3 d
STRONGYLOIDIASIS *(STRONGYLOIDES STERCORALIS)*			
Drug of choice:	Ivermectin	200 μg/kg/d × 1–2 d	200 μg/kg/d × 1–2 d
Alternative	Thiabendazole	50 mg/kg/d in 2 doses (max 3 g/d) × 2 d	50 mg/kg/d in 2 doses (max 3 g/d) × 2 d
TRICHURIASIS (TRICHURIS TRICHIURA, WHIPWORM)			
Drug of choice:	Mebendazole	100 mg bid × 3 d or 500 mg × 1 dose	100 mg bid × 3 d or 500 mg × 1 dose
Alternative	Albendazole	400 mg × 1 dose	400 mg × 1 dose

Adapted from Drugs for parasitic infections. Med Lett Drugs Ther April 2002 and the EMRA Antibiotic Guide 2004.

to symptomatic treatment, options for the treatment of neuro-cysticercosis include anticysticercal drugs, corticosteroids, CSF shunting, and surgical cyst removal (7). Most parasitic infections in the active phase with viable cysts are readily treated with safe and effective agents. Patients can commonly be treated as out-patients, with appropriate follow up.

If active neurocysticercosis is suspected, praziquantel (50 mg/kg/d in three divided doses for 15 days) or albendazole (400 mg two times a day for 8 to 30 days) should be initiated (5). Corticosteroids should be given for 2 to 3 days before and during drug therapy (5). Albendazole (400 mg two times a day for 28 days) has been used to treat echinococcal cysts. Surgical removal of cysts remains the most effective treatment (5,25). Patients who present with inactive disease (e.g., seizures secondary to parasitic calcifications) are not candidates for treatment with antihelminthic

agents. Seizures are treated no differently than seizures from other causes. Neurologic or neurosurgical consultation is appropriate for these patients.

CRITICAL INTERVENTIONS

- Diagnose malaria using a thin Giemsa-stained peripheral blood smear to demonstrate intracellular forms of the parasite. Repeat negative blood films every 12 hours for 2 days if diagnosis is strongly suspected
- Diagnose infestation with the pinworm *E. vermicularis* using clear cellulose tape placed against the perianal skin, lifted off, and then applied adhesive side down, to a glass slide and viewed under a microscope to identify the characteristic eggs

COMMON PITFALLS

✔ Failure to consider parasitic disease as a potential etiology for a variety of systemic, GI, CNS, and skin complaints. Parasitic disease should be considered in any patient presenting from an endemic area or with a travel history to an endemic area

✔ Failure to consider parasitic infestation in a traveler months after their return

✔ Failure to consult reference textbooks and current therapeutic guidelines concerning the appropriate diagnosis and treatment for these diseases

References

1. Avolio L, Avoltini V, Ceffa F, Bragheri R, et al. Perianal granuloma caused by *Enterobius vermicularis*: report of a new observation and review of the literature. *J Pediatr* 1998;132:1055.
2. Bainbridge CV, Klein GL, Neibart SI, Hassman H, Ellis K, Manring D, Goodyear R, Newman J, Micik S, Hoehler F, Walicke P. Comparative study of the clinical effectiveness of a pyrethrin-based pediculicide with combing versus a permethrin-based pediculocide with combing. *Clin Pediatr* 1998;37:17.
3. Beaver PC, Jung RC, Cupp EW. *Clinical parasitology.* Philadelphia: Lea & Febiger, 1984;240–245.
4. Burkhart CN, Arbogast J. Head lice therapy revisited. *Clin Pediatr* 1998;37:395.
5. Drugs for parasitic infections. *Med Lett Drugs Ther* April 2002.
6. Food-borne outbreak of cryptosporidiosis—Spokane, Washington, 1997. *JAMA* 1998;280:595.
7. Garg RK. Neurocysticercosis. *Postgrad Med J* 1998;74:321.
8. Becker BM, Cahill JD and Gibler WB. Parasites In: Marx JA, Hockberger RS and Walls RM, eds. *Emergency medicine—concepts and clinical practice.* St. Louis: Mosby, 2002.
9. Grencis RK, Cooper ES. Enterobius, trichuris, capillaria, and hookworm including *Ancylostoma caninum*. *Gastroenterol Clin North Am* 1996;25:579.
10. Jotte RS, Scott J. Malaria: review of features pertinent to the emergency physician. *J Emerg Med* 1993;11:729.
11. Kain KC, Keystone JS. Malaria in travelers: epidemiology, disease, and prevention. *Infect Dis Clin North Am* 1998;12:267.
12. Kramer MH, Sorhaqe FE, Goldstein ST, Dalley E, Wahlquist SP, Herwaldt BL. First reported outbreak in the United States of cryptosporidiosis associated with a recreational lake. *Clin Infect Dis* 1998;26:27–33.
13. Kyriacou DN, Spira AM, Talan DA, Mabey DC. Emergency department presentation and misdiagnosis of imported falciparum malaria. *Ann Emerg Med* 1996;27:696.
14. Lamont EB, Sayah A. An occult cause of persistent nausea and vomiting. *J Emerg Med* 1996;15:633.
15. Li E, Stanley SL. Protozoa: amebiasis. *Gastroenterol Clin North Am* 1996;25:471.
16. Nguyen V, Robert P. Treatment of head lice. *N Engl J Med* 1997;336:734.
17. Ortega YR, Adam RD. *Giardia:* overview and update. *Clin Infect Dis* 1998;25:545.
18. Shandera WX, Bollam P, Hashmey RH, Athey PA, Greenberg SB, White AC Jr. Hepatic amebiasis among patients in a public teaching hospital. *South Med J* 1998;91:829.
19. Villamazir E, Mizrahinn M. *Ascaris lumbricoides* infestation as a cause of intestinal obstruction in children: experience with 87 cases. *J Pediatr Surg* 1996;31:201.
20. Yamashita P, Kelsey J, Henderson SO. Subcutaneous cysticercosis. *J Emerg Med* 1997;16:583.
21. Schwartz E, Parise M, Kozarsky P, Cetron M. Delayed onset of malaria- implications for chemoprophylaxsis in travelers. *N Engl J Med* 2003;49:1510.
22. Korvek S, Villarin A. 2004 EMRA Antibiotic Guide, Irving Texas, 2003.
23. Willems TE, Miller LH. Two worlds of malaria. *NEJM,* 349;16:1496–1498.
24. DeMaeseneer J, Blokland I, Willems S, Vander Stichele R, Meersschaut F. Wet combing versus traditional scalp inspection to detect head lice in children. *BMJ* 321:1187–1188.
25. Garcia HH, Carleton CAW, Nash TE, Takayanagui O, White AC Jr, Boterc D, Rajshekar V, Tsang VCW, Schantz PM, Allan JC, Flisser A, Correa D, Sarti F, Friedland JS, Martinez SM, Gonzalez AE, Glman RH, Del Brutto OH., Current Consensus Guidelines for Treatment of Neurocysticerocosis. *Clin Microbio Reviews,* 2002;747–756.

CHAPTER 150
Blood and Body Fluid Exposures in the Health-Care Worker

Peter E. Sokolove

Despite the introduction of a safe and effective vaccine in 1982, hepatitis B (HBV) remains a serious occupational hazard among health-care workers. About 1.2 million Americans are chronically infected with HBV, forming a large pool of potential exposures to emergency care providers. In one study of paramedics and EMTs, about one in four remains unvaccinated against HBV (23). Seroprevalence studies indicate that health-care workers who have frequent contact with blood have a threefold to sixfold increase in seropositivity over that of the general population (15% to 30% vs. 5%) (8,25). It is also apparent that the more frequent the blood contact, the higher the rate of seroconversion. In studies of emergency medical personnel during the 1980s, emergency physicians exhibited a 12% to 16% seroprevalence rate (19,20), emergency medical services personnel a 16% to 25% rate (22,27,32), and emergency department nurses a 30% rate (16). While the incidence of hepatitis B infection in 2002 has declined by about two-thirds since 1990, unvaccinated health care workers remain at significant risk (7).

Although the acquired immunodeficiency syndrome (AIDS) accounts for a much smaller number of cases than does hepatitis B, it often causes more concern among health-care workers. When serving an emergency department patient population with a high prevalence of HIV, the cumulative career risk of occupational HIV infection has been estimated to be as high as 1.4% (33). Despite this estimate, as of December 2001, there were only 57 confirmed occupational human immunodeficiency virus (HIV) infections among health care workers in the United States, of which 7% occurred in an emergency department (17). Emergency physicians must be well versed in the management of HIV exposures, as both health-care workers and nonhealthcare workers visit the emergency department for exposure management (26).

Previously known as non-A non-B hepatitis, hepatitis C virus (HCV) is now the most common chronic blood-borne infection in the United States. About 3.9 million Americans are infected with this virus, with about 36,000 new infections each year. While the overall prevalence of HCV in health-care workers is similar to that of the general population (1% to 2%), emergency department personnel are at high risk of exposure (11). In one study from an urban emergency department, the prevalence of HCV infection among patients was 17%, many of whom had a history of intravenous drug use (4).

CLINICAL PRESENTATION

Health-care workers frequently present to the emergency department after exposure to material potentially infected with HBV, HCV, or HIV. First, the exposure must be assessed. Although blood is the single most important source of infection, other fluids may also transmit disease. Semen or vaginal secretions;

cerebrospinal, synovial, pleural, peritoneal, pericardial, or amniotic fluids and tissue are capable of transmitting HIV, HBV, and probably HCV. Unless blood is visible in them, feces, nasal secretions, sputum, sweat, and tears have not been identified as vehicles of transmission for HBV, HCV, or HIV infection. Transmission occurs most effectively through direct percutaneous exposure (e.g., needlestick); although far less likely, exposure through mucous membranes or open skin lesions can also result in HBV, HCV, and HIV transmission. Casual contact, airborne, and fecal–oral transmission have not been documented (9,11,18).

EMERGENCY DEPARTMENT EVALUATION

An initial evaluation should be made to assess the risk of disease transmission. Information about the injury should be gathered, including the infectious material, instrument procedure performed, depth of penetration, and volume of blood transferred. The source person should be evaluated for HIV and hepatitis risk factors, clinical signs of disease, previous HIV therapy, and viral load or CD4 count, if known.

The health-care worker should be evaluated for his or her medical history and immunization status for hepatitis B and tetanus. The source blood should be tested for hepatitis B surface antigen (HBsAg), HCV, and HIV antibodies. If the source is found to be positive for HBsAg, the source should also then be tested for hepatitis B e antigen (HBeAg). The health care worker should be tested for hepatitis B surface antibody (HBsAb), HCV, HIV, and pregnancy, as appropriate. Testing of sharp instruments is not recommended or reliable (13).

EMERGENCY DEPARTMENT MANAGEMENT

Hepatitis B Virus Exposure

Two types of products are available for the management of the exposed health-care worker. Hepatitis B immune globulin (HBIG), derived from plasma containing high titers of antibody to HBsAg, confers passive immunity. Side effects are minimal, and there is no evidence of HBV or HIV transmission with this product. For postexposure prophylaxis, the dose is 0.06 mL/kg intramuscularly. It should be administered within 72 hours of exposure (preferably within 24 hours), and is probably not useful beyond 7 days (8). The average wholesale cost (in 2003) was $684 per dose (28).

Hepatitis B vaccine is available for active immunization. It is a recombinant vaccine that is very safe, even in pregnancy. For postexposure prophylaxis of nonvaccinated individuals, 1 mL of vaccine is administered intramuscularly in the deltoid within 7 days of exposure and repeated at 1 month and 6 months (8). Because about 10% of adults will not initially achieve the recommended antibody titer following this series, antibody levels should be checked 4 to 6 weeks after the series is completed. Health-care workers who are smokers, obese, older than age 50, or immunocompromised are less likely to respond to the initial vaccination series (30,34)(4). Nonresponders should be given a second 3-dose series of vaccine and retested for antibody levels (13). For health care workers who achieve a level of at least 10 mIU/mL, the vaccine is essentially 100% effective in preventing subsequent HBV infection. The average wholesale price of HBV immunization is $180 per course (28).

Whether to administer HBIG, HBV vaccine, both, or neither is based on the HBsAg status of the source person and the vaccination status of the exposed health-care worker (Fig. 150.1) (13). A source person can transmit HBV if HBsAg is present, but the

degree of infectivity is best correlated with HBeAg positivity. The risk of developing clinical hepatitis after a percutaneous exposure to HBsAg-positive blood ranges from about 2% (HBeAg negative source) to as much as 40% (HBeAg positive source) (13). Overall, about 25% of those infected with HBV develop acute hepatitis, and 6% to 10% develop chronic infection (6). These patients are at increased risk of cirrhosis and hepatocellular carcinoma.

Hepatitis C Virus Exposure

There are currently no agents available for managing exposure of the health-care worker to HCV. (1,13). Immune globulin is not useful for postexposure prophylaxis of HCV (29) for a number of reasons. In contrast to HBsAb, HCV antibody is only a marker antibody, not a neutralizing antibody. Even if a neutralizing antibody did exist among the donor population, immune globulin is derived from plasma donors that are excluded from donation if they test positive for HCV. Finally, HCV mutates rapidly, and new variants may be unaffected by neutralizing antibodies.

There is currently no vaccine against HCV, as this virus demonstrates great genetic heterogeneity and a high mutation rate (14). Alpha-interferon, sometimes in combination with ribavirin, has been used successfully to treat patients with chronic hepatitis due to HCV (24). Early treatment of acute HCV infection with alpha-interferon can also prevent progression to chronic infection (21). Unfortunately, no clinical trials have been performed to support a role for such agents in postexposure prophylaxis (13). Given the lack of a vaccine against HCV or effective postexposure prophylaxis, the use of standard precautions and medical devices with safety features is crucial for preventing HCV exposures (2).

The average risk of acquiring HCV infection after percutaneous exposure is 1.8%, and ranges from 0% to 7% (13). This risk is similar to the risk of HBV transmission after percutaneous exposure to HBsAg-negative blood. Of those who acquire HCV infection, approximately 75% to 85% develop chronic infection, of whom 60% to 70% have liver enzyme elevations (10). About 10% to 20% of patients with chronic HCV infection, develop cirrhosis, and about 1% to 5% develop hepatocellular carcinoma (11).

Human Immunodeficiency Virus Exposure

Emergency department management of potential exposure to HIV materials consists of serologic testing of the exposed health-care worker and exposure source, counseling the health-care worker on the risk for infection, and consideration of postexposure prophylaxis. While the use of antiviral agents to prevent HIV seroconversion in exposed health-care workers was once considered highly controversial, an accumulation of evidence supports the use of certain drugs in many cases. The theoretical basis for postexposure prophylaxis is that there is a window of opportunity before HIV infection is established in the host. Antiviral agents may prevent or limit the replication of HIV in dendritic cells or regional lymph nodes, which appear to be the initial targets and route of spread of HIV (9).

Many animal studies have demonstrated that the use of postexposure antiviral agents can prevent or delay HIV infection (31). In human studies, when HIV-infected mothers were administered zidovudine (AZT) during pregnancy, perinatal transmission of HIV was decreased by 67% (15). While transmission during pregnancy is different from percutaneous exposure, these data clearly demonstrate that antiviral agents can be used to prevent blood-borne infection in an HIV-negative individual. The most compelling evidence of postexposure prophylaxis efficacy, however, was a multinational case-control study, performed by the CDC (5). In this study of health-care workers who had HIV exposures, mostly as a result of hollow-bore needlesticks, the risk for HIV infection was reduced by 81% if AZT was given following exposure. These data prompted the Public Health Service in 1998 to first recommend postexposure prophylaxis for health care workers exposed to HIV (9). These recommendations were updated and reaffirmed in 2001 (13).

AZT is a nucleoside reverse transcriptase inhibitor, and is administered in divided doses totaling 600 mg per day. Treatment should be continued for 4 weeks, but about one-third of health-care workers will discontinue therapy because of adverse symptoms. Short-term toxicity of AZT mostly consists of gastrointestinal (GI) discomfort and fatigue. Bone marrow suppression can be seen, but it is reversible and very rare in healthy individuals.

While AZT is the only drug with clinical data supporting its use for HIV postexposure prophylaxis in humans, multidrug regimens are often employed because of concerns about AZT-resistant strains of HIV, as well as a demonstrated synergistic effect of certain antiviral agents in the treatment of patients for AIDS. AZT resistance should be suspected if the source person is an HIV-positive patient who is not responding to AZT therapy.

However, AZT-resistant strains can be found in HIV-positive patients who have never taken AZT. In an occupational exposure study conducted at seven U.S. tertiary-care centers, the prevalence of antiviral drug resistance was 62% among source patients who had received HIV drug treatment and 17% among those who had not yet started HIV therapy (3).

Lamivudine (3TC) is another nucleoside reverse transcriptase inhibitor, and has been demonstrated to have synergistic antiviral activity when added to AZT to treat patients who have AIDS. The primary toxicity of 3TC is adverse GI symptoms, and pancreatitis is rare. 3TC is administered at a dose of 150 mg twice a day for 4 weeks. Because of the potential for increased efficacy without an increase in side effects, 3TC is usually added to the postexposure prophylaxis regimen whenever AZT is given (13).

Protease inhibitors should be considered for use as a third agent in the postexposure prophylaxis regimen for certain high-risk exposures. These agents inhibit HIV aspartyl protease and are very potent antiviral agents. Unlike the nucleoside agents, protease inhibitors do not require phosphorylation to become active, providing the theoretical benefit of having an active agent present in the bloodstream very rapidly following exposure.

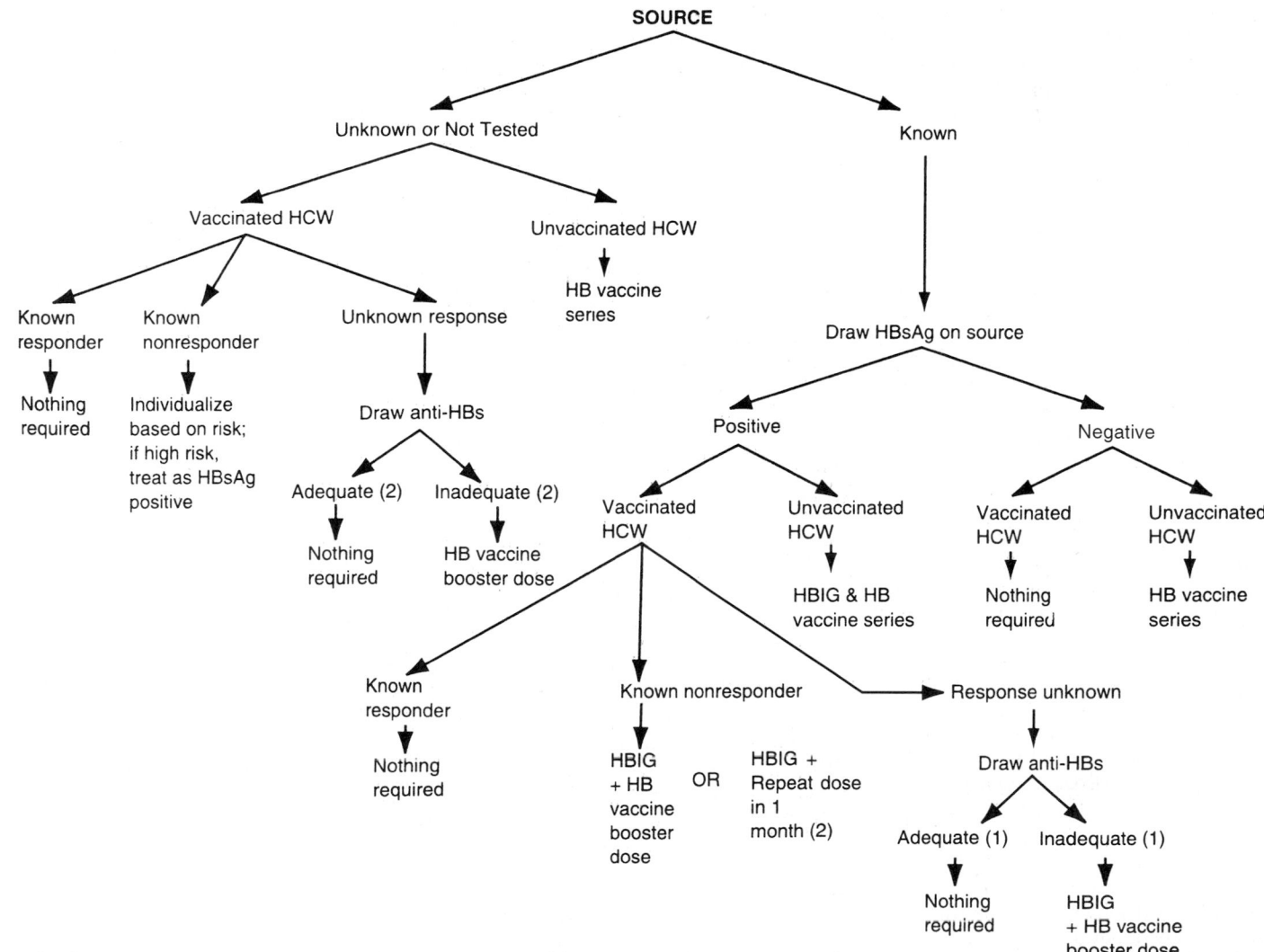

Figure 150.1. Hepatitis B exposure algorithm. *(1)* Adequate antibody greater than or equal to 10 mIU/mL. *(2)* Preferred for those who have failed to respond to a second 3-dose series of vaccine. (Adapted from CDC. Updated U.S. Public Health Service Guidelines for the Management of Occupational Exposures to HBV, HCV, and HIV and Recommendations for Postexposure Prophylaxis. *MMWR* 2001;50(RR-11):22.)

Indinavir or nelfinavir are generally the preferred protease inhibitors for postexposure prophylaxis because of their rapid bioavailability and the fact that patients are able to start treatment at full dose. Indinavir is administered at a dose of 800 mg three times a day for 4 weeks. Its major side effects are GI discomfort, hyperbilirubinemia (10%), and renal stones (4%). Patients should be instructed to drink at least 1.5 L of fluid each day to help prevent stones. Nelfinavir is administered at a dose of 750 mg three times a day for 4 weeks (9). This agent commonly results in diarrhea, so antimotility agents (e.g., loperamide) should be prescribed. All protease inhibitors may result in hyperglycemia. In rare cases, these agents may precipitate diabetic ketoacidosis, even in nondiabetic patients.

While AZT, 3TC and protease inhibitors are the agents most commonly used for HIV postexposure prophylaxis, there are a number of alternative agents available. The drug regimen chosen depends upon the exposure severity, the suspicion for antiviral resistance in the source, as well as the exposed patient's medical history. Expert consultation should be sought to assist with drug selection when source resistance is suspected.

When determining whether to initiate postexposure prophylaxis, as well as which agents to choose, the physician must consider a number of factors. The type of exposure helps determine the risk of seroconversion, and thus the potential benefit of postexposure prophylaxis. As of this writing, there have been no reported cases of HIV seroconversion when blood has come in contact with intact skin. If the skin integrity is compromised, or if mucous membranes are exposed, transmission is unlikely but can occur. The risk of transmission following a mucous membrane exposure to blood is about 0.1% (one in 1,000). The risk of transmission can be higher if a large volume of blood is involved or if prolonged contact occurs. The average risk for HIV transmission following percutaneous blood exposure is about 0.3% (one in 300) but depends on the severity of the exposure (9). Table 150.1 lists the risk factors for HIV transmission after percutaneous blood exposure, as reported in the previously described CDC case-control study (5).

The HIV status of the source person is also important when assessing the risk of transmission and choice of antiviral agents. If the source person is currently HIV-negative and has not had a recent retroviral-like illness (symptoms similar to those of acute mononucleosis), postexposure prophylaxis is not indicated. For HIV-positive source persons, the degree of infectivity is related to the patient's viral load. HIV-positive source patients can be categorized as either lower risk (class 1) or higher risk (class 2). Class 1 patients include those with asymptomatic HIV infection and a viral load of less than 1,500 RNA copies/mL. Class 2 patients include those with either symptomatic HIV, AIDS, acute seroconversion, or a viral load above 1,500 RNA copies/mL (13).

Based upon the severity of an exposure and the source HIV status (class 1 or 2), either a basic (2-drug) or an expanded (3-drug) regimen is recommended. For percutaneous exposures, an expanded regimen is usually used (Table 150.2). This most often consists of AZT, 3TC, and a protease inhibitor. The exception is for less severe percutaneous exposures (solid needle, superficial injury, *and* no blood visible on the device) from an HIV class 1 source. In such cases the basic regimen should be recommended (e.g., AZT and 3TC only) (13).

For skin and mucus membrane exposures, the PEP regimen chosen falls into three general categories (Table 150.3). For small volume exposures (few drops of blood) from an HIV class 1

TABLE 150.1. Risk Factors for HIV Transmission after Percutaneous Blood Exposure

Risk Factor	Odds Ratio	95% CI
Deep injury	15	6–41
Blood visible on device	6.2	2.2–21
Procedure with needle placed directly into artery or vein	4.3	1.7–12
Terminal AIDS in source patient	5.6	2–16
Postexposure zidovudine (AZT)	0.19	0.06–0.52

Adapted from Cardo DM, Culver DH, Ciesielski CA, et al. A case-control study of HIV seroconversion in health care workers after percutaneous exposure. N Engl J Med 1997;337:1487.

TABLE 150.2. Recommended HIV Postexposure Prophylaxis for Percutaneous Injuries

INFECTION STATUS OF SOURCE

Exposure Type	HIV-Positive Class 1*	HIV-Positive Class 2*
Less severe[¶]	Recommend basic 2-drug PEP	Recommend expanded 3-drug PEP
More severe[§§]	Recommend expanded 3-drug PEP	Recommend expanded 3-drug PEP

*HIV-Positive, Class 1—asymptomatic HIV infection or known low viral load (e.g., < 1,500 RNA copies/mL). HIV-Positive, Class 2—symptomatic HIV infection, AIDS, acute seroconversion, or known high viral load. If drug resistance is a concern, obtain expert consultation. Initiation of postexposure prophylaxis (PEP) should not be delayed pending expert consultation, and, because expert consultation alone cannot substitute for face-to-face counseling, resources should be available to provide immediate evaluation and follow up care for all exposures.

[¶]Less severe (e.g., solid needle and superficial injury).

[§§]More severe (e.g., large- bore hollow needle, deep puncture, visible blood on device, or needle used in patient's artery or vein).

Adapted from CDC. Updated U.S. Public Health Service Guidelines for the Management of Occupational Exposures to HBV, HCV, and HIV and recommendations for Postexposure Prophylaxis. MMWR 2001;50(RR-11):24.

TABLE 150.3. Recommended HIV Postexposure Prophylaxis for Mucous Membrane Exposures and Nonintact Skin Exposures

INFECTION STATUS OF SOURCE

Exposure Type	HIV-Positive Class 1[†]	HIV-Positive Class 2[†]
Small volume**	Consider basic 2-drug PEP[††]	Recommend basic 3-drug PEP
Large volume[¶¶]	Recommend basic 3-drug PEP	Recommend expanded 3-drug PEP

*For skin exposures, follow up is indicated only if there is evidence of compromised skin integrity (e.g., dermatitis, abrasion, or open wound).

[†]HIV-Positive, Class 1—asymptomatic HIV infection or known low viral load (e.g., < 1,500 RNA copies/mL). HIV-Positive, Class 2—symptomatic HIV infection, AIDS, acute seroconversion, or known high viral load. If drug resistance is a concern, obtain expert consultation. Initiation of postexposure prophylaxis (PEP) should not be delayed pending expert consultation, and, because expert consultation alone cannot substitute for face-to-face counseling, resources should be available to provide immediate evaluation and follow up care for all exposures.

**Small volume (i.e., a few drops).

[††]The designation, "consider PEP, " indicates that PEP is optional and should be based on an individualized decision between the exposed person and the treating clinician.

[¶¶]Large volume (i.e., major blood splash).

Adapted from CDC. Updated U.S. Public Health Service Guidelines for the Management of Occupational Exposures to HBV, HCV, and HIV and recommendations for Postexposure Prophylaxis. MMWR 2001;50(RR-11):25.

source, the basic regimen (two drugs) should be *considered*. If either the exposure is of large volume (major blood splash) or the source is HIV class 2, then the basic regimen should be *recommended*. In cases where there is both a large volume exposure and an HIV class 2 source, the expanded regimen (three drugs) should be recommended (13).

At times, emergency physicians need to make postexposure prophylaxis recommendations to patients who have sustained an exposure from either an unknown source (e.g., needle left on an open counter) or, more commonly, from a known source with unknown HIV status. In such circumstances the need for HIV postexposure prophylaxis should be decided on a case-by-case basis. In cases of an unknown source, postexposure prophylaxis is generally not recommended, but a two-drug regimen should be considered for exposures occurring in an HIV-likely setting (e.g., exposure to a discarded needle on an AIDS ward). For a source of unknown HIV status, rapid HIV testing can be used to quickly determine the need for postexposure prophylaxis (12). Postexposure prophylaxis can be withheld pending HIV test results, but only if a 1-hour rapid HIV test is available. Since this test is frequently not available, the decision to start postexposure prophylaxis should be made via discussion of risks and benefits with the exposed person, based upon the source person's likelihood of HIV infection. Postexposure prophylaxis can always be initiated and then stopped or modified once the source person's HIV status has been determined (13).

The timing of the initiation of postexposure prophylaxis is very important, as animal models have demonstrated an increased risk of infection with delays in AZT administration. It is best to initiate therapy promptly, preferably within 1 hour of exposure. Thus, potential HIV exposures should be treated as true emergencies. It is unclear how long following exposure treatment can be initiated and still be effective, but animal data suggest that some benefit may persist up to 36 hours (31).

Summary of Acute Management

Acute management includes thorough washing of the exposed area with soap and warm water or flushing of mucous membranes. As with all wounds, the need for tetanus toxoid administration should be considered. HBIG or hepatitis B vaccine or both should be administered as indicated (see Fig. 150.1). HIV postexposure prophylaxis should be recommended based on the exposure type and the source HIV status (see Tables 150.2 and 150.3). The health-care worker should be counseled regarding the risks of HBV, HCV, and HIV infection, as well as modifications of behavior (e.g., abstinence or condom use) to prevent secondary infection of others.

CRITICAL INTERVENTIONS

- Initiate therapy for post-HIV exposure within 1 hour
- Administer postexposure prophylaxis hepatitis B immune globulin within 72 hours of exposure (preferably within 24 hours) and hepatitis B vaccine within 7 days of exposure and repeated at 1 month and 6 months to unvaccinated health-care workers who are exposed to a HbsAg positive source

COMMON PITFALLS

✔ A common error in the management of health-care worker exposures is to provide either unnecessary or inadequate treatment. Unnecessary treatment usually results from an overestimation of the infectious potential of an exposure, such as providing three-drug antiretroviral therapy for a blood

splash onto intact skin. Undertreatment can occur if the treating physician is unaware of the benefit of postexposure prophylaxis, or if treatment for HIV exposure is delayed. These pitfalls can be avoided by applying a standardized protocol, such as the algorithms presented here. In uncertain or complex cases, consultation with an employee health service or an infectious disease specialist is advised

References

1. Alter MJ. Occupational exposure to hepatitis C virus: a dilemma. *Infect Control Hosp Epidemiol* 1994;15:742–744.
2. Alvarado-Ramy F, Beltrami EM, Short LJ, et al. A comprehensive approach to percutaneous injury prevention during phlebotomy: results of a multicenter study, 1993–1995. *Infect Control Hosp Epidemiol* 2003;24:97–104.
3. Beltrami EM, Cheingsong R, Heneine WM, et al. Antiretroviral drug resistance in human immunodeficiency virus-infected source patients for occupational exposures to healthcare workers. *Infect Control Hosp Epidemiol* 2003;24:724–730.
4. Brillman JC, Crandall CS, Florence CS, Jacobs JL. Prevalence and risk factors associated with hepatitis C in ED patients. *Am J Emerg Med* 2002;20(5):476–480.
5. Cardo DM, Culver DH, Ciesielski CA, et al. A case-control study of HIV seroconversion in health care workers after percutaneous exposure. Centers for Disease Control and Prevention Needlestick Surveillance Group. *N Engl J Med* 1997;337:1485–1490.
6. CDC. Guidelines for prevention of transmission of human immunodeficiency virus and hepatitis B virus to health-care and public-safety workers. *MMWR* 1989;38 Suppl 6:1–37.
7. CDC. Incidence of acute hepatitis B–United States, 1990–2002. *MMWR* 2004; 52:1252–1254.
8. CDC. Protection against viral hepatitis. Recommendations of the Immunization Practices Advisory Committee (ACIP). *MMWR* 1990;39(RR-2):1–26.
9. CDC. Public Health Service guidelines for the management of health-care worker exposures to HIV and recommendations for postexposure prophylaxis. Centers for Disease Control and Prevention. *MMWR* 1998;47(RR-7):1–33.
10. CDC. Recommendations for follow-up of health-care workers after occupational exposure to hepatitis C virus. *MMWR* 1997;46:603–606.
11. CDC. Recommendations for prevention and control of hepatitis C virus (HCV) infection and HCV-related chronic disease. Centers for Disease Control and Prevention. *MMWR* 1998;47(RR-19):1–39.
12. CDC. Revised guidelines for HIV counseling, testing, and referral. *MMWR* 2001;50(RR-19):1–57.
13. CDC. Updated U.S. Public Health Service Guidelines for the Management of Occupational Exposures to HBV, HCV, and HIV and Recommendations for Postexposure Prophylaxis. *MMWR* 2001;50(RR-11):1–52.
14. Colina R, Azambuja C, Uriarte R, Mogdasy C, Cristina J. Evidence of increasing diversification of hepatitis C viruses. *J Gen Virol* 1999;80 (Pt 6):1377–1382.
15. Connor EM, Sperling RS, Gelber R, et al. Reduction of maternal-infant transmission of human immunodeficiency virus type 1 with zidovudine treatment. Pediatric AIDS Clinical Trials Group Protocol 076 Study Group. *N Engl J Med* 1994;331:1173–1180.
16. Dienstag JL, Ryan DM. Occupational exposure to hepatitis B virus in hospital personnel: infection or immunization? *Am J Epidemiol* 1982;115(1):26–39.
17. Do AN, Ciesielski CA, Metler RP, et al. Occupationally acquired human immunodeficiency virus (HIV) infection: national case surveillance data during 20 years of the HIV epidemic in the United States. *Infect Control Hosp Epidemiol* 2003;24:86–96.
18. Gerberding JL. Management of occupational exposures to blood-borne viruses. *N Engl J Med* 1995;332:444–451.
19. Iserson KV, Criss E, Barrett S, et al. The prevalence of hepatitis B serological markers in emergency physicians. *Am J Emerg Med* 1984;2:394–398.
20. Iserson KV, Criss EA. Hepatitis B prevalence in emergency physicians. *Ann Emerg Med* 1985;14(2):119–122.
21. Jaeckel E, Cornberg M, Wedemeyer H, et al. Treatment of acute hepatitis C with interferon alfa-2b. *N Engl J Med* 2001;345:1452–1457.
22. Kunches LM, Craven DE, Werner BG, Jacobs LM. Hepatitis B exposure in emergency medical personnel. Prevalence of serologic markers and need for immunization. *Am J Med* 1983;75:269–272.
23. Lee DJ, Carrillo L, Fleming L. Epidemiology of hepatitis B vaccine acceptance among urban paramedics and emergency medical technicians. *Am J Infect Control* 1997;25:421–423.
24. McHutchison JG, Gordon SC, Schiff ER, et al. Interferon alfa-2b alone or in combination with ribavirin as initial treatment for chronic hepatitis C. Hepatitis Interventional Therapy Group. *N Engl J Med* 1998;339:1485–1492.
25. McQuillan GM, Townsend TR, Fields HA, et al. Seroepidemiology of hepatitis B virus infection in the United States. 1976 to 1980. *Am J Med* 1989;87:5S–10S.
26. Merchant RC, Becker BM, Mayer KH, Fuerch J, Schreck B. Emergency department blood or body fluid exposure evaluations and HIV postexposure prophylaxis usage. *Acad Emerg Med* 2003;10:1345–1353.
27. Pepe PE, Hollinger FB, Troisi CL, Heiberg D. Viral hepatitis risk in urban emergency medical services personnel. *Ann Emerg Med* 1986;15:454–457.
28. Red Book. 2003 ed. Montvale, NJ: Medical Economics Company; 2003.
29. Seeff LB, Zimmerman HJ, Wright EC, et al. A randomized, double blind controlled trial of the efficacy of immune serum globulin for the prevention of

post-transfusion hepatitis. A Veterans Administration cooperative study. *Gastroenterology* 1977;72:111–121.

30. Shaw FE, Jr., Guess HA, Roets JM, et al. Effect of anatomic injection site, age and smoking on the immune response to hepatitis B vaccination. *Vaccine* 1989; 7:425–430.

31. Shih CC, Kaneshima H, Rabin L, et al. Postexposure prophylaxis with zidovudine suppresses human immunodeficiency virus type 1 infection in SCID-hu mice in a time-dependent manner. *J Infect Dis* 1991;163:625–627.

32. Valenzuela TD, Hook EW, 3rd, Copass MK, Corey L. Occupational exposure to hepatitis B in paramedics. *Arch Intern Med* 1985;145:1976–1977.

33. Wears RL, Vukich DJ, Winton CN, et al. An analysis of emergency physicians' cumulative career risk of HIV infection. *Ann Emerg Med* 1991;20:749–753.

34. Wood RC, MacDonald KL, White KE, Hedberg CW, Hanson M, Osterholm MT. Risk factors for lack of detectable antibody following hepatitis B vaccination of Minnesota health care workers. *JAMA* 1993;270:2935–2939.

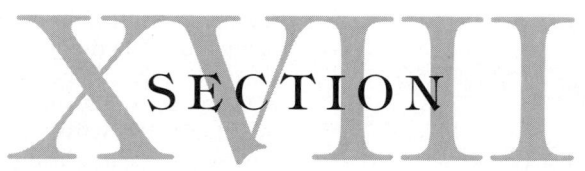

SECTION

XVIII

Section Editor: Jeffrey Schaider, MD

Hematologic/Oncologic Emergencies

CHAPTER 151
Bleeding Disorders

Kathleen C. Hubbell

Emergency physicians encounter bleeding on a daily basis: Bleeding lacerations, epistaxis, bruising, hematuria, gastrointestinal (GI) bleeding, and blunt and penetrating trauma are common complaints in the emergency department. Most of these patients have normal clotting function and are bleeding because of a local lesion. Their bleeding can be controlled by pressure, packing, suturing, or other local therapy aimed at the specific lesion, and bleeding does not recur if the lesion is properly treated.

On the other hand, a patient with a bleeding disorder may bleed spontaneously as well as after trauma, and treatment of the local lesion may not control the bleeding or prevent its recurrence. The disorder may be congenital or acquired, and may involve one or more components of the body's complex coagulation system.

PATHOPHYSIOLOGY

Hemostasis is normally maintained by the balanced functioning of four elements: the blood vessel wall, the platelets, the clotting factors (Table 151.1) and inhibitors, and the fibrinolytic system. Altered function of any of these components may lead to bleeding or thrombosis (4,16).

Normally, the *vascular endothelium* provides a barrier between the fluid blood and the adhesive proteins collagen, von Willebrand factor (vWF), and fibronectin, which are synthesized in the endothelial cells and secreted into the extracellular matrix. It also prevents coagulation through the action of thrombin inhibitors, such as thrombomodulin, that are bound to the endothelial cell membranes. When trauma, immune complexes, proteolytic enzymes, bacterial endotoxin, viruses, or other stimuli disrupt the endothelium, the adhesive molecules are exposed.

Platelets adhere to these proteins through their glycoprotein (GP) 1b/IX complexes. Adherence stimulates pseudopod formation and release of various substances involved in the coagulation process from the alpha and dense granules of the platelets. During the release, granule cell membranes merge with the platelet cell membranes, exposing other glycoproteins that serve as binding sites for coagulation factors. The release induces a change in the GP IIb/IIIa complexes that allows them to bind fibrinogen and link one platelet to another (aggregation). Products released from the injured endothelium and from the platelets, in addition to the presence of binding sites and cofactors for coagulation on the platelet membrane, encourage the initiation of the *clotting factor* cascade, which terminates in the formation of the fibrin clot.

The cascade has two initially separate pathways that join to form the common pathway (Fig. 151.1). The intrinsic pathway uses components normally found in plasma; the extrinsic pathway requires initial activation by tissue factor, previously known as thromboplastin. This classic version of the cascade has been supplemented by information from new studies, which shows additional interactions between the two pathways and a pre-

dominant role for the extrinsic pathway in the initiation of factor activation. The tissue factor (of the extrinsic pathway) released from the injured endothelial cells forms a complex with factor VII that activates not only factor X, as previously known, but also factor IX. Activated factor IX can then proceed through the last step of the intrinsic pathway to activate additional factor X, which, in turn, contributes to the formation of thrombin. Thrombin can activate factor XI, reinforcing the activation of the factors of the intrinsic pathway. As the extrinsic pathway initiates the cascade, an inhibitor called "tissue factor pathway inhibitor" is formed and prevents further activation of factors IX and X through the extrinsic arm of the cascade, leaving the intrinsic pathway as the main route to the activation of thrombin. These newly discovered coagulation mechanisms explain such previous observations as the lack of bleeding diathesis in patients with factor XII and prekallikrein deficiency, as contrasted to the severe disease seen in patients with low levels of factors VIII and IX. Several steps in the pathways require the presence of calcium and a platelet phospholipid surface. Platelets thus are necessary not only to fill the endothelial defect initially, but also to provide elements needed for the operation of the clotting cascade, which serves to localize thrombus generation to the area of endothelial injury (4,16).

Clotting *factor inhibitors*, such as antithrombin III (AT III), protein C, and tissue factor pathway inhibitor, provide a negative-feedback effect to limit the formation of clot.

The *fibrinolytic system* is activated by many of the same substances that activate the clotting cascade. Active plasmin cleaves fibrin to lyse the clot. Activation of plasminogen by substances found in the clot localizes fibrinolysis to the clot (4,16).

When all systems operate in a normal, balanced fashion, there is neither unchecked hemorrhage nor thrombosis in the vascular tree. However, when an inherited or acquired disorder produces an abnormality in one or more components of the system, bleeding may occur. The abnormality may be in the structure of the vascular tree; in the number of platelets; in the platelets' functional ability to adhere, aggregate, and release their dense-granule contents; in the activity of clotting factors; or in the activity of the fibrinolytic system. The emergency physician

---

TABLE 151.1. Concentration of Blood Clotting Factors Needed for Normal Hemostasis

Factor	Common Name	Concentration Required
I	Fibrinogen	100 mg/dL
II	Prothrombin	30%–40%
III	Tissue thromboplastin	—
IV	Calcium	—
V	Labile factor, proaccelerin	30%–40%
VII	Proconvertin	30%–40%
VIII	Antihemophilic globulin	30%–40%
IX	Christmas factor	30%–40%
X	Stuart–Prower factor	30%–40%
XI	Plasma thromboplastin antecedent	20%
XII	Hageman factor	None
XIII	Fibrin-stabilizing factor	1%
Prekallikrein	Fletcher factor	None
High-molecular-weight kininogen	Williams–Fitzgerald–Fleaujeac factor	None

Adapted from White GC, Marder VJ, Colman RW, et al. Approach to the bleeding patient. In: Colman RW, Hirsh J, Marder VJ, et al. (eds). Hemostasis and thrombosis, basic principles and clinical practice, 2nd ed. Philadelphia: JB Lippincott Co., 1987.

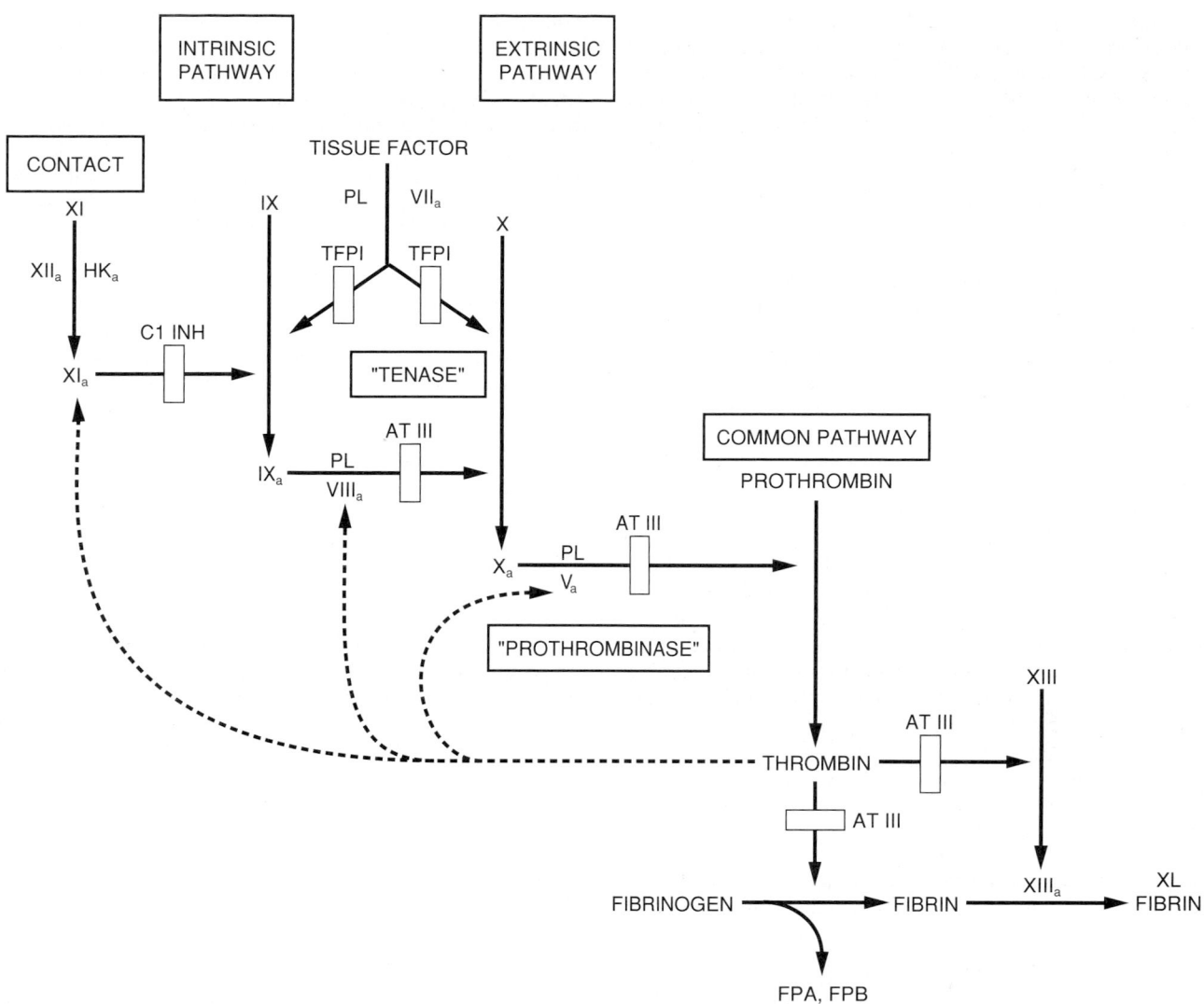

Figure 151.1. The clotting cascade. The central precipitating event is considered to involve tissue factor *(TF)*, which, under physiologic conditions, is not exposed to the blood. With vascular or endothelial cell injury, TF acts in concert with activated factor VIIa and phospholipid *(PL)* to convert factor IX to IXa and factor X to Xa. The "intrinsic pathway" includes "contact" activation of factor XI by the XIIa/activated high-molecular-weight kininogen *(HKa)* complex. Factor XIa also converts factor IX to IXa, and factor IXa, in turn, converts factor X to Xa, in concert with factors VIIIa and PL (the "tenase" complex). However factor Xa is formed, it is the active catalytic ingredient of the "prothrombinase" complex, which includes factor Va and PL and converts prothrombin to thrombin. Thrombin cleaves fibrinopeptides *(FPA, FPB)* from fibrinogen, allowing the resultant fibrin monomers to polymerize, and converts factor XIII to XIIA, which cross-links *(XL)* the fibrin clot. Thrombin accelerates the process *(interrupted lines)* by its potential to activate factors V and VIII, but continued proteolytic action also dampens the process by activating protein C, which degrades factors Va and VIIIa. Thrombin activation of factor XI to XIa is a proposed but not yet proven pathway. Natural plasma inhibitors retard clotting: C1-inhibitor *(C1 INH)* neutralizes factor XIIa, TF pathway inhibitor *(TFPI)* blocks factor VIIa/TF, and antithrombin III *(ATIII)* blocks factors IXa, Xa and thrombin. *Arrows,* active enzymes; *open rectangles,* sites of inhibitor action; *dashed lines,* feedback reactions.

must use information from the clinical and laboratory evaluation to identify the abnormal component and treat the patient correctly.

CLINICAL PRESENTATION

When taking the history in a bleeding patient, the physician should try to establish whether the bleeding is part of a systemic disorder and what the etiology of the disorder might be (i.e., congenital vs. acquired, vascular vs. platelet vs. coagulation factor disorder).

A *systemic* disorder is suggested by bleeding from multiple sites, either at the time of presentation or in the past; spontaneous bleeding from sites in the absence of trauma or a known lesion; or unusually severe bleeding (9). If a systemic disorder is suspected, further information regarding etiology is sought. Because of the large number of identified congenital bleeding disorders, the personal and family histories are closely scrutinized for clues to an inherited condition. Such patients often have had symptoms of bleeding since infancy (e.g., from the umbilical cord or after circumcision), have had unusual amounts of bleeding from previous trauma or surgery, and have a family history of bleeding.

Although these clues are helpful, mild forms of inherited bleeding disorders may be associated with significant bleeding only after severe trauma, and thus may not yet have caused any symptoms in the patient's life. The absence of a family history also does not rule out an "inherited" bleeding disorder: Up to 30% of cases of hemophilia A result from spontaneous mutation (9,22).

If the patient has a *family history of unusual bleeding*, the pattern of inheritance may help identify the disorder. Sex-linked recessive disorders, such as hemophilia A and B and the Wiskott-Aldrich platelet disorder, are seen in multiple generations of a family, primarily in males. Female carriers occasionally have clinically significant bleeding. Autosomal recessive conditions, such as deficiencies of factors II, V, VII, X, and XII, prekallikrein, and high-molecular-weight kininogen, are seen in both sexes and are manifested only in the proband's generation, because the parents are heterozygous and therefore asymptomatic. Autosomal dominant inheritance is seen in von Willebrand disease (vWD) and Osler-Weber-Rendu disease (hereditary telangiectasia); both sexes of multiple generations are affected (9).

Patients with *acquired bleeding disorders* are more likely to have an underlying illness that affects platelet number or function or clotting factor levels (e.g., hepatic or renal disorder, disseminated intravascular coagulation [DIC], cancer, or an immunologic process) (Table 151.2). The development of acquired inhibitors to individual clotting factors is rare in nonhemophiliac patients but is associated with severe, often fatal, bleeding (17). Factor VIII inhibitors are, by far, the most common. Patients are usually previously healthy individuals, often older, and often with a history of recent injury or surgery. Eighteen percent have an autoimmune disease; 5% note recent penicillin, sulfa, or other drug use. Some postpartum cases have been reported (17).

Acquired bleeding disorders are often linked to the use of medications that interfere with normal coagulation (e.g., coumadin, heparin, aspirin, and nonsteroidal antiinflammatory drugs [NSAIDs]) (9). Patients on these drugs who were involved in a fall or motor vehicle collision were almost five times more likely to die of a head injury than nonanticoagulated patients (15,23). The effects of aspirin on platelet function are irreversible, lasting the 7- to 10-day lifespan of the platelet (21); those of NSAIDs last about three to five drug half-lives, after which platelets again participate normally in clot formation. More than 100 drugs are associated with the development of thrombocytopenia. Heparin, quinidine, quinine, trimethoprim-sulfamethoxasole, and gold are some of the most common causes (Table 151.3) (8,9).

Hemorrhagic disease of the newborn due to inadequate vitamin K intake or absorption presents in the first days to weeks of life. Most cases can be prevented by prophylactic vitamin K administration in the newborn period (1).

Immune thrombocytopenic purpura (ITP) is seen both in children and adults who were previously healthy. In patients with this disorder, anti-platelet IgG antibodies coat the platelets leading to their rapid removal from circulation in the spleen. Most children with ITP are 2 to 6 years old and many have had a recent viral illness. Otherwise, the history and physical exam are lacking symptoms and signs such as fever, weight loss, anorexia, bone pain, adenopathy, masses, or hepatosplenomegaly that would suggest a more serious condition such as leukemia. Ten percent of children may have a palpable spleen tip, but massive splenomegaly is not seen. Generally the only exam abnormalities are signs of platelet-type bleeding such as petechiae, bruises, subconjunctival hemorrhage, and signs of mucosal bleeding such as epistaxis. Adult ITP is most common in patients between the ages of 18 and 40 years. The examination in both groups should emphasize detection of life-threatening bleeding, e.g., in the central nervous system, and of signs of other thrombocytopenic conditions such as DIC, TTP (thrombotic thrombocytopenic purpura), or leukemia (2).

TABLE 151.2. Acquired Hemostatic Defects Associated with Selected Underlying Clinical Conditions

Underlying Clinical Condition	Type of Hemostatic Defect	Cause
Liver disease	Factor deficiency	Decreased synthesis
	Fibrinolysis	Decreased clearance of activators
	Hypercoagulable state	Antithrombin III and protein C deficiency, decreased clearance of activated clotting factors
	Thrombocytopenia	Splenic sequestration
Renal disease	Thrombocytopenia	Decreased marrow production
	Platelet defect	Retained metabolites in the blood
Malabsorption	Multiple factor deficiency	Vitamin K malabsorption
Acute leukemia (especially promyelocytic)	Thrombocytopenia	Decreased megakaryocytopoiesis
	DIC	Increased cellular procoagulant activity
Myeloproliferative disease	Platelet defect	Abnormal thrombopoiesis
	Thrombocythemia/thrombocytopenia	Hyperplastic or replaced (fibrotic) marrow, splenic sequestration
Lymphoma/chronic lymphocytic leukemia	Decreased von Willebrand factor	Adsorption onto tumor, autoantibody
	Low factor VIII	Autoantibody
	Thrombocytopenia	Marrow replacement, splenic sequestration
Dysproteinemia	Thrombocytopenia	Decreased marrow production
	Prolonged thrombin time	Inhibition of fibrin monomer polymerization
Amyloidosis	Factor X deficiency	Adsorption by amyloid
	Capillary fragility	Amyloid vascular infiltration
Systemic lupus	Lupus inhibitor[a]	Antibody to acidic phospholipids
	Factor deficiency	Autoantibodies to coagulation proteins
	Thrombocytopenia/thrombocytopathia	Autoantibodies to platelet glycoproteins

[a] Although the lupus inhibitor produces prolongation of clotting assay results and may exist coincidentally in patients with thrombocytopenia or clotting factor deficiency that predisposes to bleeding, the lupus inhibitor itself is characterized by a thrombotic rather than a hemorrhagic tendency.

Adapted from White GC, Marder VJ, Colman RW, et al. Acquired disorders of hemostasis. In: Colman RW, Hirsh J, Marder VJ, et al., eds. Hemostasis and thrombosis, basic principles and clinical practice, 3rd ed. Philadelphia: JB Lippincott Co., 1994.

TABLE 151.3. Acquired Disorders of Hemostasis Associated with Drugs

PLATELET FUNCTION DEFECTS

Aspirin
Nonsteroidal antiinflammatory agents
Heparin
Dipyridamole
Theophylline
Penicillins
Cephalosporins
Tricyclic antidepressants
Phenothiazines
Clofibrate
Antihistamines
Ethanol
Dextrans

THROMBOCYTOPENIA

Immune Destruction
Heparin
Quinidine
Quinine
Gold
H$_2$ antagonists
Phenytoin
Antibiotics
Methyldopa
Decreased Production
Ethanol
Thiazides
Chemotherapeutic agents

COAGULATION FACTOR DEFICIENCIES

Coumadin
Penicillins
Cephalosporins

Further information as to the probable etiology of a bleeding disorder can be obtained by asking about the characteristics of the bleeding. Vascular and platelet abnormalities produce one pattern of bleeding, coagulation factor deficiencies another (1,9). Patients with vascular disorders, thrombocytopenia, platelet function disorders, and most types of von Willebrand disease complain of easy bruising, epistaxis, gingival bleeding, prolonged bleeding after dental extraction, hematuria, excessive menstrual flow, and GI bleeding. Bleeding may be either spontaneous or secondary to trauma. It may continue for hours, but, once stopped, does not recur.

Coagulation factor deficiencies, in contrast, typically cause deep intramuscular hematomas, retroperitoneal bleeding, or hemarthrosis. Thirty percent of neonates with hemophilia have profuse bleeding after circumcision; 1 to 5 percent have intracranial hemorrhage. Bleeding may not start until hours after trauma and may recur at a later time. This occurs because, although initial hemostasis is normal (due to properly functioning platelets), an adequate fibrin clot is not formed. Normal fibrinolysis then results in delayed bleeding (9).

Intracranial hemorrhage is the second most common cause of death in hemophiliacs, after AIDS, accounting for 33% of deaths (18). Only about half of hemophiliacs with intracranial hemorrhage have a history of recognized head trauma; even in patients with known trauma, neurologic manifestations may be delayed 1 to 6 days (5). Therefore, hemophiliacs with any neurologic symptom or sign should receive a computed tomography (CT) scan, even in the absence of trauma. The same approach should be followed in patients with signifi-

cant factor depletion due to an acquired disorder (e.g., coumadin therapy).

Several articles in the literature suggest that hemophiliac and anticoagulated patients with head trauma who have no history of loss of consciousness or posttraumatic amnesia, and who have a normal mental status and neurologic examination, may not need a CT scan of the head. These studies have shown either no CT abnormalities or no clinical findings of neurologic injury on follow up if CT is not done (6,12,24). However, these studies are retrospective and involve small numbers of patients. The physician should consider the patient's past as well as recent history, social circumstances, and the availability of followup care, and err on the side of obtaining a CT if there is even the slightest suspicion of intracranial injury or any problem with follow up.

Some bleeding disorders combine features of both platelet and clotting factor deficiencies. Examples include DIC, liver disease, and severe vWD. vWD results from a deficiency in the complex of two proteins, factor VIII and vWF, that circulate together in plasma. vWF promotes adhesion of platelets to the subendothelium of damaged vessels and induces platelets to bind fibrinogen, which facilitates the platelet interactions essential for formation of the hemostatic plug. Factor VIII plays its part in the clotting factor cascade in the activation of factor X. Most patients with vWD have bleeding typical of a platelet disorder, but those with severe disease display both mucosal and deep bleeding.

The physical examination is directed toward identifying all bleeding sites and recognizing signs of underlying illness. Jaundice, organomegaly, adenopathy, and abnormal masses are sought (9).

EMERGENCY DEPARTMENT EVALUATION

Laboratory Tests

When intelligently combined with a careful history and physical examination, a few basic laboratory tests are sufficient to screen for the existence of a bleeding disorder: the activated partial thromboplastin time (aPTT), the prothrombin time (PT), and a complete blood count (CBC) with platelet count. Other tests can pinpoint specific factor deficiencies or functional platelet disorders and can be ordered if indicated by the screening tests and clinical picture.

The aPTT detects abnormalities of the intrinsic and common pathways and is prolonged by deficiencies of high-molecular-weight kininogen; prekallikrein; factors XII, XI, IX, VIII, X, V, and II; and fibrinogen. The aPTT is also prolonged in the presence of antiphospholipid antibody (formerly termed the *lupus anticoagulant*) and by heparin, coumadin, and fibrin degradation products. The test is performed by exposing plasma to an activating surface such as kaolin and adding calcium and the necessary phospholipid (partial thromboplastin). The time required for clotting in this test is usually 25 to 40 seconds (9,16).

The PT reflects the activity of the factors of the extrinsic and common pathways. It is prolonged by deficiencies of factors VII, X, V, and II and fibrinogen; by coumadin; and by heparin in high concentrations. The test adds thromboplastin (a phospholipid-protein extract of lung, brain, or placental tissue) and calcium to the plasma. The time required for clotting is normally 10 to 14 seconds, shorter than the aPTT because the initial time-consuming steps of the intrinsic pathway have been bypassed with the direct activation of factor X by thromboplastin-activated factor VII. The PT is more affected by reduced levels of factors VII, V, and X than by decreases in factor II and fibrinogen (9,16).

When the PT is used to monitor coumadin therapy, the PT ratio (the ratio of the patient's PT to a control's PT) has been superseded by the international normalized ratio (INR): (9)

$$INR = (PT\ ratio)^{ISI}$$

The ISI is the international sensitivity index, which relates the thromboplastin's activity to that of a single batch of human brain thromboplastin, designated as the first international reference preparation by the World Health Organization in 1977. Using the ISI to standardize the PT ratio removes the variability in the determination of the PT caused by the use of thromboplastins manufactured from different organ sources and by different extraction techniques. The INR can be interpreted by the clinician as a reflection of the patient's degree of anticoagulation, whereas the PT ratio may reflect only the reactivity of the thromboplastin used to perform the test.

Recommended INR values for anticoagulant therapy monitoring are listed in Table 151.4 (13).

Patients with factor VIII and IX deficiencies (hemophilia A, B, and some forms of vWD) have a prolonged aPTT and a normal PT. Patients with a normal aPTT and a prolonged PT have a factor VII deficiency, because that is the only factor of the extrinsic pathway not involved in the common pathway. Isolated factor VII deficiency occurs as a rare congenital abnormality and is seen in the acquired form in mild liver disease and in the initial stages of oral anticoagulation or vitamin K deficiency. Although the aPTT, as well as the PT, are prolonged in the fully coumadinized patient, the PT is used for monitoring because of its simplicity. Both the PT and the aPTT are prolonged in moderate-to-severe liver disease, vitamin K deficiency, heparin and coumadin use, afibrinogenemia, and consumptive coagulopathies such as DIC (1,9,16).

Specific factor assays can be done to confirm the diagnosis suspected from the history or from abnormalities of the screening PT and aPTT and to provide exact activity levels. However, these assays are rarely available on an emergency basis, and emergency treatment must be initiated without the benefit of such tests.

The CBC is used to assess the degree of anemia produced by the bleeding. It also reveals abnormalities of the white blood cell count, which might suggest leukemia as the etiology of the more clinically obvious thrombocytopenia. Examination of the peripheral blood smear will detect platelet clumping which causes a falsely low platelet count as well as abnormalities of red and white blood cell number and morphology.

The platelet count is the first step in the evaluation of possible platelet disorders such as immune thrombocytopenic purpura (ITP) or thrombotic thrombocytopenic purpura (TTP). Patients with counts less than 100,000/μL are considered thrombocytopenic; if platelet function is normal, the bleeding time increases in direct proportion to the decrease of the count below 100,000/μL. Patients with platelet counts below 5,000 to 10,000/μL are at risk for spontaneous bleeding. Platelet counts above 50,000 to 60,000/μL are usually sufficient to control bleeding caused by trauma or local pathology. However, the platelet count should never be the only criterion considered when assessing a patient's risk of hemorrhage. The underlying condition leading to thrombocytopenia must be sought, and platelet function must also be considered (25).

No tests are available on an emergency basis that specifically screen for platelet function, as opposed to platelet number. A thorough history and physical examination, however, may suggest that the patient is at risk for a functional platelet disorder (e.g., alcohol or aspirin use). The bleeding time, a laboratory test that evaluates both platelet number and function is determined by measuring the time required for bleeding to stop after a standard incision 1 to 2 mm deep and 5 mm long is made on the patient's forearm while an inflated blood pressure cuff on the upper arm maintains venous pressure at 40 mm Hg. The normal bleeding time is 4 to 7 minutes. If the platelet count is normal, a prolonged bleeding time suggests a functional platelet disorder (9). A new lab device, the PFA-100, measures time to occlusion of an aperture in the machine by a platelet plug and is now thought to be a superior method for detecting many functional platelet disorders (1).

A few bleeding disorders produce no abnormalities in the available screening tests. Patients with vascular disorders, simple and senile purpura, factor XIII deficiency, and mild forms of other factor deficiencies (factor levels greater than 20% to 25% of normal) have normal aPTTs, PTs, and platelet counts (9,16).

EMERGENCY DEPARTMENT MANAGEMENT

Appropriate treatment of bleeding disorders depends on the physician's success in determining the most likely etiology of the bleeding.

The initial management of the bleeding patient includes airway control, if necessary, and adequate ventilation and oxygenation. If bleeding has led to hypovolemia, initiate crystalloid resuscitation and packed red blood cells as needed. Use local measures to control bleeding (e.g., pressure, packing, suturing, immobilization, gastric lavage). As these basic measures are instituted, information from the history, physical examination, and laboratory tests can be combined to assess the probability that a platelet, coagulation factor, or mixed disorder is present.

Platelet Disorders

If there is active bleeding unresponsive to local measures and typical of that caused by a platelet disorder and the platelet count is below 50,000/μL, initiate platelet transfusions (25). Active bleeding with a platelet count above 50,000/μL should prompt a search for another cause of bleeding, such as a functional platelet disorder or a coagulation factor deficiency. Controversy continues regarding the platelet count below which prophylactic transfusion to prevent spontaneous hemorrhage should be given. It is thought that platelets play an essential role in the maintenance of vascular endothelial integrity and that a minimum number are required to fulfill that function. Below this threshold, thinning and fenestration of the endothelium may lead to spontaneous bleeding. Studies suggest that 5,000 to 10,000 platelets/μL can maintain vascular integrity and that prophylactic transfusion should be given for values below that to prevent intracranial and other hemorrhage. However, factors such as fever, presence of an anatomic bleeding risk (e.g., a known GI lesion), rate of

---

TABLE 151.4. Recommended Values for Anticoagulant Therapy Monitoring

INR TARGET	ANTICOAGULANT INDICATION
2.0–3.0	Prophylaxis of venous thrombosis
	Treatment of venous thrombosis
	Treatment of pulmonary embolism
	Prevention of systemic embolism
	Tissue heart valves
	Acute myocardial infarction
	Valvular heart disease
	Atrial fibrillation
2.5–3.5	Mechanical prosthetic valves (high risk)

Adapted from Hirsh J, Dalen JE, Anderson DR, et al. Oral anticoagulants: mechanism of action, clinical effectiveness, and optimal therapeutic range. Chest 2001;119:8S–21S.

decrease of platelet count, presence of coexisting coagulation defects, and etiology of the thrombocytopenia affect the likelihood of bleeding and must be considered in the decision to transfuse. For these reasons, some experts recommend a higher level of 15,000/μL (25).

There are several benefits to decreasing unnecessary prophylactic platelet transfusions, including reduced cost and disease transmission. More importantly, avoidance of alloimmunization decreases the incidence of unresponsiveness to subsequent transfusions and may enhance the success of bone marrow transplantation, which may be a lifesaving procedure in some patients.

Patients who need prophylactic transfusion or who are actively bleeding because of thrombocytopenia should receive 10 bags of pooled random-donor platelets (RDPs) or a single-donor platelet (SDP) unit, which is equivalent to six to eight RDPs. One RDP unit raises the platelet count by 5,000 to 6,000/μL in healthy adults, and probably less in ill, bleeding patients and those with platelet-destructive or -consumptive disorders. A post-transfusion platelet count should be obtained to guide further transfusion (14,25).

Although immune destruction or consumption of transfused platelets may occur in patients with certain disorders, the temporary effect of the transfusion may be lifesaving in the actively bleeding patient; thus, platelets should be given while attempts are made to treat the underlying disorder. Two conditions are exceptions to this recommendation. In thrombotic thrombocytopenia purpura and in heparin-induced thrombocytopenia, platelet transfusions are considered to be harmful, because they can lead to increased microangiopathic thrombosis (25).

In ITP the initial treatment depends on the age of the patient (2). In both adults and children, life-threatening bleeding is treated with platelet transfusions as described above. Such patients also receive high-dose steroids and intravenous immune globulin (IVIg) at a dose of 1 gram per kilogram body weight per day for 2 to 3 days. In the absence of immediately life-threatening bleeding, however, management is tailored to the expected disease course, which is acute and self-limited in 85% to 90% of children but chronic in most adults.

In children with ITP the management plan should be coordinated with the patient's pediatrician or hematologist. Most patients without bleeding are treated as outpatients. Bone marrow aspiration is rarely done if history, exam, CBC, and peripheral smear provide no suspicion of another diagnosis. When steroid treatment is planned, some will first perform bone marrow aspiration to rule out the possibility of leukemia, since a course of steroids may produce a temporary remission of the leukemia. The need for treatment in nonbleeding children with ITP is controversial. The goal of treatment is to prevent intracranial bleeding which occurs in 0.2% to 1% of children, usually within the first month of disease. It has not been shown that any treatment prevents intracranial hemorrhage. Since most children recover completely without treatment and without complications, many hematologists recommend an expectant management strategy. Others prefer to decrease the duration of thrombocytopenia by treating, especially if the patient's medical history or lifestyle suggest an increased risk for head trauma or if antiplatelet drugs have been taken. IVIg and IV anti-D globulin have both been shown to produce a rapid, significant elevation in the platelet count. Side effects are few, but these are expensive preparations. Oral steroids in conventional or high doses are also effective, but side effects such as weight gain, hyperglycemia, osteopenia, and behavioral changes can occur even with brief courses of therapy.

Half of adults with ITP present with platelet counts less than 10,000 per cubic millimeter and thus merit immediate treatment. Diagnostic bone marrow aspiration is recommended for adults greater than 40 to 60 years of age and for those with any other exam or blood count abnormalities. The same agents, IVIg and steroids, are used in adults, but the response to treatment is dramatically different from that seen in children. Although 50% to 85% of patients respond to the initial course of steroids, only 5% to 30% sustain an adequate platelet count. Adults usually receive steroids as the initial treatment, either at conventional doses of 1 to 1.5 mg per kilogram of prednisone per day or at extremely high doses of 40 mg per day of dexamethasone (2,3). Those that do not respond are given IVIg or IV anti-D immune globulin. Possible intervention for those who do not respond or who suffer relapse includes splenectomy, danazol, dapsone, and immunosuppressive drugs.

Hemostatic defects in uremia are multifactorial, but are primarily related to defects in platelet function. Only in the severely nephrotic patient should significant coagulation factor deficiencies be suspected. Platelet counts are somewhat decreased, but rarely below 100,000/μL. The functional platelet defect is due to toxic-retained metabolites, which can quickly reduce the effectiveness of newly transfused platelets. Dialysis at least partially reverses this toxic effect but may not be immediately available for the bleeding patient. Two pharmacologic adjuncts can help (14). DDAVP can shorten the bleeding time within 2 hours in uremia. The effect lasts only 12 hours and decreases with repeated doses. The mechanism of action is not known. Conjugated estrogens decrease the bleeding time within 6 hours, and a 5-day course will maintain the effect for 2 weeks. Along with the administration of platelets, these should be considered primary therapy of bleeding in the uremic patient. If they fail, cryoprecipitate can be given. Its efficacy is controversial, and its mechanism of action unclear.

Maintaining a hematocrit greater than 25% also appears to decrease bleeding time in uremia. It has been proposed that an adequate number of red cells distribute the platelets closer to vessel walls, where they can fulfill their function (14).

Coagulation Disorders

If the clinical evaluation suggests a congenital single-factor deficiency (e.g., hemophilia A or B), the location of the bleeding determines the therapeutic approach. Bleeding into the central nervous system (CNS), neck, sublingual, or retroperitoneal spaces, and GI tract is immediately life-threatening. All hemophiliacs with suspected bleeding in these high-risk sites should receive immediate factor replacement therapy to achieve a factor level of 100% of normal. One unit of factor VIII per kilogram of body weight will raise the patient's level by 2%, so 50 U/kg should be given. One unit of factor IX per kilogram raises the level by only 1%, so patients with hemophilia B require 100 U/kg in life-threatening situations (18). This should be initiated without waiting for the results of the aPTT, factor levels, or head CT or other scans. The half-life of factor VIII is 8 to 12 hours, so maintenance therapy should be infused 2 to 3 times per day or given as a continuous infusion. Factor IX maintenance therapy is given every 18 to 24 hours. Factor administration should be continued for 14 days if bleeding is located in the CNS, neck, or retroperitoneum (18,20). Admission for observation should be strongly considered in those patients with injury or suspected bleeding in the high-risk sites.

Minor bleeding in the soft tissues, muscles, oral cavity, urinary tract, and limited hemarthrosis can be treated with 20 to 40 U/kg (10,18,20). Patients with massive hemarthrosis and bleeding into large joints such as the hip and shoulder should receive at least three doses of 50 U/kg. The presence of limb hematomas should prompt a thorough search for signs of compartment syndrome. If suspected, 50 U/kg of factor should be administered and a surgical consultation placed. However, most patients are observed 6 to 8 hours after the infusion to observe for spontaneous resolution (10). Rest, ice, and compression, as well as crutches and limited weight bearing, should be prescribed after joint and limb bleeds, followed by physical therapy. The addition of antifibrinolytic therapy (tranexamic acid mouthwash and oral epsilon-aminocaproic acid) to combat the effects of saliva in cases of bleeding from oral mucosa, gums, anterior tongue, and dental extraction sites may hasten effective coagulation when used with factor infusion.

Recognition of the role of pooled plasma products in the transmission of hepatitis, the human immunodeficiency virus (HIV), and other viral diseases to a majority of severe hemophiliacs spurred the development of the safer and more highly purified products available today. The emergency physician should be knowledgeable about selecting the appropriate product for each patient. No HIV, hepatitis B, or hepatitis C seroconversion has been reported in previously unexposed hemophiliacs since 1987. However, there have been outbreaks of thermoresistant and nonlipid-enveloped hepatitis A and parvovirus B19 infection associated with virucidally treated factor VIII preparations (22).

Another problem associated with pooled plasma factor concentrates is the large amount of nonfactor VIII plasma proteins included in the preparations. Repeated exposure to these contaminants has been associated with significant and progressive alterations in immune function (e.g., lowering of CD4 counts and development of anergy) in HIV-infected hemophiliacs. A purification method called "immunoaffinity," that uses monoclonal antibodies against factor VIII or vWF to separate the factor from the other proteins, produces an extremely pure product that should be used in the HIV-positive hemophiliac (20,22).

Recombinant factor VIII (produced in hamsters) has been shown to have full hemostatic function and a normal half-life in humans. Although there was concern initially that the recombinant factor would be more likely to induce the production of inhibitors than plasma-derived factor, these effects have been no greater than with any other factor VIII preparation (22). Recombinant factor VIII products are usually more expensive than the other products.

Recombinant factor IX is now available for treatment of hemophilia B and is made without the use of any human or animal protein. This product eliminates the risk of viral infection and of thrombosis posed by older products.

The choice of appropriate factor VIII product for each hemophilic patient is one that should be made in concert with the patient's hematologist, if possible. All currently marketed factor VIII products are considered safe from the standpoint of HIV and hepatitis B and C transmission. High-purity products are those from which nonfactor VIII protein contaminants have been removed. Intermediate-purity products contain plasma protein, but not viral contaminants. Recombinant factor products cost 2 to 3 times more than plasma-derived products and are sometimes in short supply because of limited manufacturing capacity. They are prescribed most often for newly diagnosed hemophiliacs and in those in whom no blood-borne infections have developed.

Gene therapy for hemophilia is now under study in humans. Trials involve injection of virus vectors that have been modified to contain the DNA for factor VIII, or the implantation of cells that contain the DNA. Small, transient elevations of factor VIII have been found in these patients (22).

Another approach to the treatment of non-life-threatening bleeding in patients with mild or moderate hemophilia A or with type I vWD is the use of DDAVP. The intravenous dose is 0.3 μg/kg, and the intranasal dose is 1 spray in children and 1 spray in each nostril in adults. A two- to threefold increase in factor VIII and vWF is seen, peaking about 30 to 60 minutes after the dose (20).

Patients with types II and III vWD who have abnormal or absent vWF do not benefit from DDAVP, which simply stimulates factor release from the endothelial cells. A factor VIII preparation that also contains significant vWF, such as Humate P, must be used for these individuals (20).

Antibodies against factor VIII, termed *inhibitors,* develop in 15% to 20% of hemophiliacs (18), usually early in life and after relatively few factor VIII transfusions. These inhibitors render the patient unresponsive in varying degrees to factor VIII given to treat bleeding episodes. In patients with low inhibitor titers, regular or high doses of factor VIII usually continue to be effective. Another approach is administration of activated prothrombin complex concentrates (aPCCs) (Autoplex T, FEIBA VH), which "bypass" factor VIII and are effective in controlling 50% to 60% of bleeding episodes, as compared to the 85% to 90% success rate when using factor VIII products in patients without inhibitors (22). However, repeated use is associated with thrombotic complications, and factor levels cannot be monitored to assess therapy (20). Most recently, recombinant factor VIIa has become available and has been shown to be safe and effective in patients with inhibitors, achieving a control rate of 80%. It is given as an IV bolus at a dose of 90 to 120 micrograms/kg every 2 hours for at least 2 to 4 doses. It works by activating factor X which then plays its role in the common pathway of the clotting cascade (11,22). The cost is $1 per microgram. Thus this expensive product is often reserved for patients with inhibitors who have life-threatening bleeding or are undergoing major surgery.

Inhibitors also occur *de novo* in nonhemophiliac patients, those directed against factor VIII being the most common. Treatment of life-threatening bleeding is similar to that described previously, which uses high doses of human factor VIII, porcine factor VIII, aPCCs, and recombinant factor VII. To arrest synthesis of the inhibitor, steroids and immunosuppressants, such as azathioprine or cyclophosphamide, are given. Spontaneous remission is thought to be fairly common (17).

Patients with complex conditions such as liver disease or DIC usually have deficiencies of multiple coagulation factors and, often, of platelets as well. If laboratory tests confirm these abnormalities and the patient is actively bleeding, fresh-frozen plasma and platelets are given to replace the needed components.

When heparin or coumadin is implicated as a cause of bleeding, knowledge of the mechanisms by which it anticoagulates the blood helps the physician to treat the bleeding logically. Heparin acts immediately on administration by accelerating 1,000-fold the reaction by which thrombin combines with the plasma protease inhibitor antithrombin III (AT III). The complex is inactive, and the AT III–bound thrombin cannot activate fibrinogen. Heparin is not consumed in the reaction and is available for further activity. Fortunately, the half-life of heparin is short, about 1 hour at usual doses and longer at higher doses. Therefore, when bleeding occurs in the heparinized patient, discontinuation of the drug leads to a rapid fall in the plasma heparin concentration. For severe bleeding, it may be necessary to administer protamine sulfate, a specific heparin antidote that combines with heparin to form a stable complex with no anticoagulant activity. One milligram of protamine neutralizes 100 U of heparin. The physician should estimate the amount of heparin remaining in the plasma and give the protamine at a rate no faster than 50 mg over 10 minutes (21).

The mechanism of action of coumadin is quite different. It interferes with the carboxylation of the vitamin K–dependent clotting factors II, VII, IX, and X in the liver. Factor synthesis is decreased 30% to 50%, and biologic activity is decreased to 10% to 40% of normal because of inadequate carboxylation. The onset of anticoagulant activity is delayed 8 to 12 hours because it depends on the gradual decrease in factor levels that is a consequence of the decreased rate of their synthesis, although their normal rate of degradation is unchanged. Factor VII has the shortest half-life (about 6 hours), and some anticoagulant effect is noted as factor

VII levels drop. However, the longest-lived of the four factors, factor II, has a half-life of 60 hours, so that 2 to 3 days are required before the full anticoagulant effect of coumadin can be expected (21).

The effects of coumadin cannot be reversed rapidly by discontinuing it, because time is required for synthesis of the factors. If severe hemorrhage occurs in a patient on coumadin, fresh-frozen plasma must be given to provide the needed coagulation factors immediately.

Because of the large volume and, possibly, repeated doses of fresh-frozen plasma needed to reverse an intensely anticoagulated patient, some authors recommend the use of aPCCs, which specifically contain the vitamin K–dependent coagulation factors (14). There is a small risk of thrombosis associated with the use of this product because of the presence of activated factors. The risk is greatest in patients with liver disease or previous thrombotic events. Vitamin K_1, 5 to 10 mg by slow intravenous injection, should also be given to promote factor synthesis in patients with severe or life-threatening bleeding. In patients with elevated INR greater than 5 but no significant bleeding, vitamin K_1 1 to 5 mg orally will safely correct the INR (19). One should always maintain an awareness of the risk of thrombotic complications occurring as a result of the reversal of anticoagulation, and careful judgment should be exercised (7).

Because so many bleeding disorders are associated with underlying diseases, attention should always be directed to the potential associated condition while immediate lifesaving transfusions of blood components are provided.

CRITICAL INTERVENTIONS

- Initiate platelet transfusion if there is active bleeding unresponsive to local measures and typical of that caused by a platelet disorder and the platelet count is below 50,000/μL
- Replace factor to achieve a factor level of 100% of normal for hemophiliacs with suspected bleeding in high-risk sites. Give 50 U/kg of factor VIII or 100 U/kg of factor IX depending on which factor deficiency exists

DISPOSITION

An acutely bleeding patient should be transferred to another facility only if a service unavailable at the initial hospital can be provided at the second facility. For example, a child with a head injury and hemophilia would benefit from transfer to a hospital where neurosurgical services are available, despite the risk of transport. The ABCs must always be attended to and the hematologic parameters normalized as much as possible by transfusion of the appropriate components before transfer.

COMMON PITFALLS

✔ Bleeding is a common occurrence in the emergency department, and most patients have no bleeding disorder. In most cases, the history and a physical examination directed toward the identification of a congenital or acquired bleeding disorder constitute adequate screening

✔ Delayed bleeding is characteristic of coagulation factor deficiencies. Because the initial stage of hemostasis is normal, these patients may appear to have their bleeding well controlled in the emergency department and may be discharged, only to experience life-threatening hemorrhage a few hours later. Factor transfusion should be given immediately in the emergency department to patients with potential bleeding in high-risk sites such as the CNS, neck, and retroperitoneal space without waiting for results of coagulation or imaging studies. Admission for observation should be strongly considered in these patients

✔ The emergency physician must use judgment in deciding whether to perform invasive procedures in patients with bleeding disorders. When possible, such procedures should be delayed until appropriate treatment has normalized clotting parameters

References

1. Allen GA, Glader B. Approach to the bleeding child. *Pediatr Clin N Am* 2002;49:1239–56.
2. Cines DB, Blanchette VS. Immune thrombocytopenic purpura. *N Engl J Med* 2002;346:995–1008.
3. Cheng Y, Wong RSM, Soo YOY, et al. Initial treatment of immune thrombocytopenic purpura with high-dose dexamethasone. *N Eng J Med* 2003;349:831–836.
4. Colman RW, Clowes AW, George JN, Hirsh J, Marder VJ. Overview of hemostasis. In: Colman RW, Hirsh J, Marder VJ, Clowes AW, George JN, eds. *Hemostasis and thrombosis: basic principles and clinical practice,* 4th ed. Philadelphia: Lippincott Williams & Wilkins, 2001:3–16.
5. DeBehnke DJ, Angelos MG. Intracranial hemorrhage and hemophilia: case report and management guidelines. *J Emerg Med* 1985;8:423–427.
6. Dietrich AM, James CD, King DR, Ginn-Pease ME, Cecalupo AJ. Head trauma in children with congenital coagulation disorders. *J Pediatr Surg* 1994;29:28–32.
7. Ferrera PC, Bartfield JM. Outcomes of anticoagulated trauma patients. *Am J Emerg Med* 1999;17:154–156.
8. George JN, Raskob GE, Shah SR, et al. Drug-induced thrombocytopenia. A systematic review of published case reports. *Ann Intern Med* 1998;129:886–890.
9. Greaves M, Preston FE. Approach to the bleeding patient. In: Colman RW, Hirsh J, Marder VJ, Clowes AW, George JN, eds. *Hemostasis and thrombosis: basic principles and clinical practice,* 4th ed. Philadelphia: Lippincott Williams & Wilkins, 2001:783–793.
10. Hampers LC, Manco-Johnson M. Emergency department management of musculoskeletal injuries in children with inherited bleeding disorders. *Clin Ped Emerg Med* 2002;3:138–144.
11. Hedner U. Recombinant factor VIIa (NovoSeven®) as a hemostatic agent. *Disease-A-Month* 2003;49:39–48.
12. Hennes H, Losek JD, Sty JR, Gill JC. Computerized tomography in hemophiliacs with head trauma. *Pediatr Emerg Care* 1987;3:147–149.
13. Hirsh J, Dalen JE, Anderson DR, et al. Oral anticoagulants: mechanism of action, clinical effectiveness, and optimal therapeutic range. *Chest* 2001;119:8S–21S.
14. Humphries JE. Transfusion therapy in acquired coagulopathies. *Hematol Oncol Clin North Am* 1994;8:1181–1201.
15. Karni A. Traumatic head injury in the anticoagulated elderly patient: a lethal combination. *Am Surg* 2001;67:1098–1100.
16. Kottke-Marchant K. Laboratory diagnosis of hemorrhagic and thrombotic disorders. *Hematol Oncol Clin North Am* 1994;8:809–853.
17. Kunkel LA. Acquired circulating anticoagulants. *Hematol Oncol Clin North Am* 1992;6:1341–1357.
18. Lozier JN, Kessler CM. Clinical aspects and therapy of hemophilia. In: Hoffman R, Benz EJ, Shattil SJ, Furie B, Cohen HJ, Silberstein LE, McGlave P, eds. *Hematology: basic principles and practice,* 3rd ed. Philadelphia: Churchill Livingstone, Inc., 2000:1883–1904.
19. Lubetsky A, Yonath H, Olchovsky D, et al. Comparison of oral vs. intravenous phytonadione (vitamin K_1) in patients with excessive anticoagulation. *Arch Intern Med* 2003;163:2469–2473.
20. Lusher JM. Transfusion therapy in congenital coagulopathies. *Hematol Oncol Clin North Am* 1994;8:1167–1780.
21. Majerus PW, Tollefsen DM. Anticoagulant, thrombolytic, and antiplatelet drugs. In: Hardman JG, Limbird LE, eds. *Goodman and Gilman's the pharmacological basis of therapeutics,* 10th ed. New York: McGraw-Hill, 2001:1519–1538.
22. Mannucci PM, Tuddenham EGD. The hemophilias – from royal genes to gene therapy. *N Engl J Med* 2001;344:1773–1779.
23. Mina AA, Knipfer JF, Park DY, et al. Intracranial complications of preinjury anticoagulation in trauma patients with head injury. *J Trauma* 2002;53:668–672.
24. Morgan LM, Kissoon N, deVebber BL. Experience with the hemophiliac child in a pediatric emergency department. *J Emerg Med* 1993;11:519–524.
25. Rintels PB, Kenney RM, Crowley JP. Therapeutic support of the patient with thrombocytopenia. *Hematol Oncol Clin North Am* 1994;8:1131–1157.

CHAPTER 152
Antithrombotic Therapy and Its Complications

John Bailitz

The antithrombotics have multiple life-saving indications and life-threatening complications within emergency medicine. In acute coronary syndromes, venous thromboembolism and acute ischemic stroke, the antithrombotics save lives. Unfortunately, patients may develop life-threatening iatrogenic complications in the emergency department (ED). Furthermore, patients may present to the ED with subtle, but life-threatening complications related to outpatient use. Emergency physicians must understand the basic mechanisms, indications, and complications of antithrombotic therapy. This chapter provides a practical review of the current antithrombotics including the antiplatelet, anticoagulant and fibrinolytic agents.

ANTIPLATELET AGENTS

Aspirin

Originally discovered by Hoffman in the late 1800s, aspirin today remains the most effective, safest, and least expensive of all antithrombotic drugs (1). At doses as low as 75 mg, aspirin irreversibly blocks platelet synthesis of thromboxaneA2, a potent inducer of platelet aggregation and vasoconstriction. Conversely, aspirin only partially blocks endothelial cell synthesis of prostacyclin, a potent inhibitor of platelet aggregation and vasodilatation. This irreversible inhibition of platelet thromboxane and comparatively insignificant inhibition of prostacyclin results in the predominant antithrombotic effects of low doses of aspirin (31).

Aspirin is commonly prescribed for the prevention and management of cerebrovascular and coronary artery disease, as well as the prevention of stroke in low-risk patients with atrial fibrillation or with contraindications to anticoagulant therapy. Other indications include the treatment of pain, rheumatic fever, preeclampsia, and Kawasaki Syndrome. The recommended dose in acute coronary syndromes (ACS) is 162 mg (31). Nonenteric-coated aspirin is rapidly absorbed in the stomach and inhibits platelet function within 1 hour versus 3 to 4 hours for enteric coated. Antithrombotic effects last the 10-day life span of the individual platelet with 50% replacement of the platelet pool within 5 days (31). Given the significant benefit in ACS, occult gastrointestinal (GI) bleeding requires close monitoring, but is not an absolute contraindication to aspirin therapy.

ADP Inhibitors

The thienopyridines, ticlodipine and clopidogrel, selectively inhibit ADP induced platelet aggregation. Delayed onsets, and significant side effects such as thrombotic thrombocytopenic purpura (TTP) and neutropenia, have limited the use of ticlodipine. The CAPRIE (Clopidogrel vs Aspirin in Patients at Risk of Ischemic Events) trial demonstrated a lower incidence of new ischemic stroke, new myocardial infarction (MI), or vascular death with plavix compared to aspirin therapy. Patients given plavix had a 9.8% incidence of adverse outcome versus 10.6% for patients given aspirin with an overall risk reduction of 8.7% (5). The CURE Trial (Cloperidogrel in Unstable Angina to Prevent Recurrent Ischemic Events) demonstrated a lower incidence of CV death, MI, or stroke with plavix in addition to standard therapy versus standard therapy alone. Patients given plavix had a 9.3% incidence of adverse outcome versus 11.4% for patients given placebo with an overall risk reduction of 20% in the clopidogrel group.

Current FDA indications for clopidogrel include unstable angina, non Q wave MI, ACS with aspirin intolerance, and reduction of secondary atherosclerotic events in patients with recent MI, recent stroke or peripheral vascular disease. Plavix is commonly prescribed after stent placement (35). The recommended dose in ACS is 300 mg PO on day one followed by 75 mg PO QD. Contraindications include previous hypersensitivity reaction, active peptic ulcer disease, and intracerebral hemorrhage.

Glycoprotein IIb/IIIa Receptor Inhibitors

Studies of the rare bleeding disorder, Glanzmann thromboasthenia, led to the discovery of the glycoprotein IIb/IIIa receptor. Fibrinogen binding to the IIb/IIIa receptor is the "final common pathway" of platelet activation and aggregation. If the IIb/IIIa receptor is nonfunctional, thrombus will not form. Several glycoprotein IIb/IIIa receptor inhibitors (GPI) have been developed within three broad categories; abciximab (ReoPro) is a monoclonal antibody, eptifibatide (Integrilin) is a synthetic peptide and tirofiban (Aggrastat) a nonsynthetic peptide. GPI's have been extensively studied and proven to be beneficial in patients with unstable angina or non-Q wave MI undergoing percutaneous coronary interventions (32). Use in low-risk patients with unstable angina who are not undergoing PCI is not recommended (21). However, in high-risk patients where PCI is not possible, GPI's, specifically eptifibatide or tirofiban, may be considered in consultation with the admitting cardiologist (32). The recommended dosage of abciximab is a 0.25 mg/kg IV bolus before percutaneous coronary interventions (PCI), followed by continuous infusion of 0.125 μg/kg/min (to a maximum of 10 μg/min) for 12 hours. Eptifibatide is administered as a 180 μg/kg IV bolus followed by a continuous infusion of 2.0 μg/kg/min until 18 to 24 hours after PCI. The dose of eptifibatide should be lowered in patients with renal insufficiency. Tirofiban is administered at an initial rate of 0.4 μg/kg/min for 30 minutes and then continued at 0.1 μg/kg/min. Contraindications are similar to fibrinolytic therapy.

ANTICOAGULANTS

Heparin

Heparin, derived from the latin "hepar" meaning liver, was first discovered by McLean in 1916 from a liver extract. By inducing a conformational change in Antithrombin III, heparin produces a very rapid inhibitor of thrombin (13). This complex inactivates several enzymes of the coagulation cascade's intrinsic system including IXa, XIa, and XIIa and highly sensitive enzymes of the common pathway Xa and IIa (Thrombin). Heparin also inhibits platelet function and binds to endothelial cells contributing to hemorrhagic complications. Heparin is unable to inhibit clot-bound thrombin since the heparin-binding site of thrombin is not accessible when bound to a fibrin clot (40). In contrast to fibrinolytics, heparin has no effect on clot already present but prevents new clot formation and existing clot propagation.

For immediate anticoagulant effect in the ED, an IV bolus is necessary in order to saturate heparin's multiple nonspecific binding sites followed by continuous IV infusion. The IV route is preferred in acute thrombosis due to variable bioavailablity with SC administration. An 80 IU/kg bolus followed by continuous infusion of 18 IU/kg/hr of UFH provides anticoagulation more rapidly and prevents recurrent thromboembolic events more effectively compared to fixed dose nomograms. In patients with ACS receiving fibrinolytic or GPI therapy, a lower dose, 60 IU/kg bolus followed by a continuous infusion of 12 IU/kg/hr of heparin is equally effective and safer compared to higher-dose nomograms (14).

The anticoagulant response to heparin varies among patients necessitating dose adjustments based on the activated partial thromboplastin time (APTT), the standard PTT reagent with additional chemical activators that increase the sensitivity to heparin. The *in vivo* validity of this measure has been called into question, and no relationship exists between APTT and therapeutic efficacy in ACS (13). Other methods such as factor Xa and heparin levels have been studied, but the APTT remains the most common method to indirectly measure the anticoagulant effects of heparin. The continuous IV dose is adjusted based on the APTT measured 6 hours after the bolus with a typical therapeutic range 1.5 to 2.5 times the normal APTT.

IV heparin is indicated in the ED for acute deep venous thrombosis (DVT), pulmonary embolism (PE), atrial fibrillation (AF), and acute coronary syndromes (ACS). In hospitalized patients, IV heparin is used for patients undergoing cardiac bypass, vascular surgery, coronary angioplasty, and select patients with DIC (13). In contrast to coumadin, both heparin and LMWH are safe to use in pregnancy since neither crosses the placenta.

Low Molecular Weight Heparins

In the 1970s, work to improve heparin's anticoagulant effect while minimizing hemorrhagic side effects led to the depolymerization of heparin into fragments approximately one third the size producing the low molecular weight heparins (LMWHs). Interaction with thrombin is the major difference in mechanism between heparin and LMWHs. To inactivate thrombin, both ATIII and a long-chained heparin molecule must bind to thrombin forming a tertiary complex. In contrast, to inactivate factor Xa, only antithrombin III needs to bind factor Xa catalyzed by heparin molecules of any length. Most unfractionated heparin molecules have the required 18 saccharide units needed to form a tertiary complex with ATIII and thrombin compared with only 25% of LMWH molecules resulting in significantly less thrombin inhibition with LMWH (13). This results in an anti-Xa to antithrombin inhibition ratio of 1:1 for heparin and 4:1 for LMWHs.

Additionally, LMWH has less of an effect on platelet function and vascular permeability, theoretically reducing hemorrhagic complications. Clinical effects of these differences are summarized in Table 152.1.

The depolymerization of unfractionated heparin into LMWHs reduces the negative charge of unfractionated heparin producing less nonspecific binding (17). This results in improved bioavailablity, prolonged half-life, predictable clearance, and predictable antithrombotic response based on bodyweight dosing. LMWH undergo slow consistent renal elimination resulting in a two to fourfold longer half-life versus heparin (13). LMWH may be dosed once or twice daily without the need for laboratory monitoring except in the patient with renal failure or morbid obesity. Anti-Xa levels are measured at 4 hours after SC injection with morbid obesity or chronic renal failure with therapeutic range of 0.6 to 1.0 IU/mL for twice daily dosing. The reduction in the need for routine laboratory monitoring and theoretical potential for fewer complications makes LMWH more cost effective than heparin. Despite the higher cost per does of LMWH, evidence for overall cost savings has been demonstrated in studies of DVT and ACS management, as well as improved quality of life assessments in patients treated at home for DVT (17). Contraindications to heparin and LMWH include hypersensitivity to heparin, thrombocytopenia, coagulopathies, and the presence of or potential for uncontrolled active bleeding.

Multiple studies have recently compared LMWH to heparin in the management of ACS, DVT, and pulmonary embolism. Enoxaparin has been found to result in fewer recurrent cardiac events, with equal rates of hemorrhagic complications, at considerable cost savings when compared to heparin following fibrinolytic therapy for acute myocardial infarction (AMI) (4). Enoxaparin is also recommended over heparin in unstable angina and Non-Q wave MI patients not undergoing coronary artery bypass grafting in the next 24 hours (32). Recent work has found enoxaparin to be as safe as heparin in patients undergoing percutaneous coronary intervention (28). Outpatient enoxaparin has been shown to be safe, efficacious, and cost effective when compared with inpatient heparin in the management of DVT (41). Multiple studies have demonstrated comparable safety and efficacy in the management of PE. "Off label" uses of LMWHs include long-term management of hypercoagulable states, ulcerative colitis exacerbations, cerebral sinus thrombosis, anticoagulation for hemodialysis, acute ischemic stroke and outpatient management of upper extremity DVT (17).

The FDA has approved several LMWHs each with unique pharmokinetic profiles resulting from different depolymerization techniques that prevent easy interchangeable use. Current FDA indications include acute management of DVT with or

---

TABLE 152.1. Clinically Significant Differences of Heparin and LMWH

Characteristic	Heparin	LMWH	Clinical Advantage
Nonspecific protein binding	High	Minimal	Improved consistency,
Dose response	Poor	Predictable	safety, and decreased
Bioavailablity	30%	> 90%	need for laboratory monitoring with LMWH
Platelet binding	More	Less	Theoretically decreased
Inhibition of platelet function	More	Less	bleeding complications
Vascular permeability	Increased	No effect	and HIT syndrome with LMWH
Half-life	30–150 min	12–24 hr	Lack of therapeutic "Off
Protamine reversal	Good, predictable	Poor	Switch" and poor reversibility with LMWH

LMWH, low molecular weight heparin.

without PE with enoxaparin or tinzaparin, outpatient DVT with enoxaparin, postsurgical DVT prophylaxis with enoxaparin or dalteparin, and unstable angina and non-Q wave myocardial infarction (NQWMI) with enoxaparin or dalteparin (17). Recently, lovenox has been proven to be more effective than tinzaparin in the conservative management of NQWMI (25). Emergency physicians need to know which LMWHs on formulary at their institution, specific approved indications, dosing, and sensitivity to protamine reversal.

Coumadin

In 1941, Link isolated dicoumarol from moldy sweet clover that was later developed and marketed as a rat poison by the Wisconsin Alumni Research Foundation (WARFarin) (1). Coumadin, the brand name of sodium warfarin, is the most commonly prescribed oral anticoagulant. Coumadin inhibits regeneration of the Vitamin K cofactor required for hepatic carboxylation of factors II, VII, IX, X and the anticoagulant proteins C and S. The coagulation cascade's extrinsic system and common pathway is thereby blocked. The relatively short half-life of the anticoagulant Protein C (6–8 hours) compared to the four coagulation factors (6–60 hours) results in an iatrogenic hypercoaguable state for 24 to 36 hours necessitating anticoagulation with heparin or LMWH prior to beginning therapy with coumadin (15). In addition to this hypercoaguable state, physicians must be aware of the dissociation of laboratory response and the clinical response to coumadin. Reduction in factor VII (half-life 6 hours) results in an increased INR within 24 to 36 hours. However, a reduction in thrombin levels (half-life 60 hours) and hence a reduction in significant clot formation does not occur until the fifth day of coumadin therapy necessitating continued effective anticoagulation with IV heparin or LMWH therapy during the initial 5 days of management of acute thrombosis (13).

Coumadin therapy is typically begun with a maintenance dose of 5 mg that results in an INR of 2.0 in 4 to 5 days in the majority of patients. Less than 5 mg is typically used in the elderly, those with poor nutrition, liver disease or patients at high risk for bleeding. Loading doses of 10 mg may result in increased bleeding complications due to a dramatic reduction in factor VII and increased hypercoaguable complications due to increased sensitivity of factor C to a 10-mg dose without increased sensitivity of thrombin (2). Coumadin is completely absorbed from the GI tract achieving peak levels within 4 hours with a mean effective half-life of 40 hours. Adjustments in coumadin dosing are made based on the International normalization ratio (INR), a standardized measurement of prothrombin time (PT) that corrects for differing laboratory reagents. The typical therapeutic range is 2.0 to 3.0 for most indications with the exception of mechanical valves and antiphospholipid syndromes requiring a higher INR of 2.5 to 3.5. Frequent monitoring is necessary to determine the ideal dose in each patient since many factors such as age, use of other drugs, diet, comorbidities, and even race may affect patient response. Table 152.2 provides a brief listing of factors that may increase or decrease the response to coumadin.

Coumadin is most commonly indicated for the management of venous thromboembolism and prevention of embolism with prosthetic heart valves or atrial fibrillation. Coumadin is pregnancy class X since the drug crosses the placenta and may causes multiple birth defects and spontaneous abortions. Contraindications include any condition in which the risk of hemorrhage or adverse reaction outweighs the clinical benefit including prior hypersensitivity, skin reactions, recent surgeries, active or potential gastrointestinal, intracerebral or genitourinary bleeding, and fall risk.

TABLE 152.2.   Factors That May Increase or Decrease INR/PT Response to Coumadin

Increase	Decrease
Medications	**Medications**
— Multiple antibiotics including azithromyocin, penicillins, cephalosporins and flouroquinolones, tertacyclines, flagyl	— Carbamazepine, haloperidol
	— Naficillin, dicloxacillin, prednisone, ranitidine
— NSAIDs including ibuprofen, indomethacin, celecoxib, naproxen, acetaminophen and aspirin	**Alternative Medicine**
	— St. John's Wort
— Cardiovascular drugs including amiodarone, propranolol, streptokinase, TPA	**Diet Changes**
	— Excess dietary vitamin K
— Prednisone, cimetidine	**Patient Factors**
— Influenza virus vaccine	— Edema, hereditary coumadin resistance, hyperlipidemia, hypothyroidism
Alternative Medicine	
— Ginko biloba, garlic	
Diet	
— Dietary deficiency or malabsorbtion of Vitamin K	
— Altered intestinal flora by antibiotics	
Patient Factors	
— Cancer, collagen vascular disease, congestive heart failure, diarrhea, hyperthyroidism, steatorrhea, advanced, age, liver disease, fever	

INR, international normalized ratio; NSAID, nonsteroidal antiinflammatory drug; PT, prothrombin time.

Direct Thrombin Inhibitors

Leeches were first used in the middle ages to rid the body "black humors." Derived from a salivary extract of the leech hirudo medicinalis, hirudin tightly binds to and inactivates thrombin. Leeches became endangered species in the 1970s ending medical research until the advent of recombinant technology and r-hirudin or lepirudin. Other direct thrombin inhibitors include bivalirudin, argatroban, efegatran, and inogatran (29). Hirudin has several advantages over heparin including the ability to inhibit clot-bound thrombin, lack of inactivation by activated platelets, and lack of a required cofactor (29,40). The APTT may be used to monitor therapy with a range of 2 to 3 times prolongation from median. Warfarin titration may be difficult due to prolongation of the PT. Half-life is 40 minutes IV, 3 hours SQ, and is prolonged up to 2 days in renal failure. Hirudin is FDA approved for the treatment of thrombotic complications of the heparin induced thrombocytopenia (HIT) syndrome and has been used for anticoagulation in patients with antithrombin III deficiency. Recent work demonstrates that hirudin may be more effective than heparin in DVT prophylaxis, as well as unstable angina and non-ST segment elevation myocardial infarction (NSTEMI) (40).

Fibrinolytics

Streptokinase was the first fibrinolytic agent to be discovered by Tillett and Garner in 1932. The use of fibrinolytics for reperfusion in acute MI was first reported in 1958 (29). Today's many different agents have one common mechanism: the conversion of plasminogen to plasmin which then degrades fibrin and hence thrombus. First-generation, less-fibrin specific agents included streptokinase, anistreplase, and urokinase. Second-generation, more fibrin-specific agents include recombinant tissue plasminogen activator (alteplase) and several mutants of tissue plasminogen activator including reteplase (r-PA) and tenecteplase (TNK-tPA).

Streptokinase (SK) is a purified preparation of a bacterial protein of group C β-hemolytic streptococci. Streptokinase binds to plasminogen, forming an activator complex that activates both fibrin-bound plasminogen and free circulating plasminogen producing localized thrombus breakdown and a generalized "systemic lytic state." This systemic fibrinolytic state persists for 3 to 4 hours despite a short half-life of 23 minutes. For acute ST segment elevation MI (STEMI), the dose is typically 1,500,000 IU over 60 minutes. Anistreplase is a modified streptokinase molecule with a longer half-life (100 min) allowing for single-bolus dosing. For STEMI, the dose is 30 units over 2 to 5 minutes. IV or SQ heparin therapy is typically delayed four hours after SK and anistreplase to reduce bleeding complications. Urokinase (UK) is a plasminogen activator produced by the human kidney. When compared to SK, UK directly activates plasminogen and is less antigenic. UK has been used to treat occlusive peripheral vascular disease but availability has been limited by production difficulties (29).

Vascular endothelial cells produce tissue plasminogen activator. Alteplase is a commercially produced recombinant TPA molecule. Alteplase has several advantages compared to SK including increased fibrin specificity resulting in less systemic fibrinolysis, a lower rate of allergic reactions, and an ability to lyse more highly linked fibrin clots theoretically resulting in increased effectiveness in patients with prolonged symptoms (29). Recommended dose of rt-PA (alteplase) for STEMI is 100 mg IV administered "front loaded," beginning with a bolus of 15 mg followed by 50 mg over 30 minutes and the remaining 35 mg over the next hour. Reteplase is a deletion mutation of TPA with less fibrin specificity but a longer serum half-life of 18 minutes versus 5 minutes for rt-TPA allowing for bolus administration. No antigenicity has been reported with reteplase. Although early trials demonstrated improved reperfusion rates, mortality, clinical outcomes, and complications have been similar to SK (3). Dose in STEMI is two 10-unit bolus injections, each administered over 2 minutes, 30 minutes apart. Tenecteplase (TNK) is a triple substitution variant mutant of TPA with improved fibrin specificity and a longer half-life again allowing bolus administration. A weight-based bolus, not exceeding 50 mg, is administered over 5 seconds. Mortality benefits have not been demonstrated, but a significant reduction in bleeding with TNK compared to TPA was demonstrated in the one study (29). A 60 unit/kg heparin bolus followed by 12 units/kg/hour infusion is recommended as an immediate adjunctive therapy to the TPA-derived agents.

Fibrinolytics clearly reduce mortality and improve vessel patency in AMI (29). A meta-analysis of nine clinical trials of fibrinolytics demonstrated an 18% reduction in mortality at 35 days (10). Indications for fibrinolytic therapy in acute MI include history consistent with AMI, less than 12 hours since symptom onset, ST elevation greater than 1.0 mm in 2 leads or new onset left bundle branch block. Absolute contraindications include prior hemorrhagic stroke, CVA within previous year, intracranial neoplasm or AVM, active noncompressible bleeding other than menses, and suspected aortic dissection or pericarditis. Relative contraindications include severe uncontrolled hypertension greater than 180/110, elevated INR, CVA greater than 1 year prior, pregnancy, bleeding diathesis, acute peptic ulcer or other internal bleeding within 4 weeks, recent trauma within 4 weeks, and noncompressible vascular puncture site (24). Patients with a history suggestive of AMI with ST depression, T wave changes or normal EKGs may actually be harmed by fibrinolytic therapy, an exception being the patient with ST segment depression in V1-V4 consistent with a posterior wall MI. Increased bleeding complications occur in patients over 75 requiring a careful discussion of risks and benefits with elderly patients and their family. SK and subcutaneous heparin therapy may be preferred in the elderly to reduce bleeding complications when a cath lab is not available (24).

Second-generation agents are recommended over first-generation agents. The GUSTO-1 Global Use of Streptokinase and t-PA for Occluded coronary arteries trial demonstrated slightly reduced mortality at 30 days and 1 year with accelerated t-PA versus streptokinase (11). None of the second-generation agents has demonstrated clear clinical superiority. The GUSTO III Trial comparing alteplase and reteplase found no significant differences between the two agents (12). In patients with prolonged symptoms, alteplase may be more effective due to its theoretical ability to lyse more highly linked fibrin clots.

Although the in vitro advantages of newer fibrinolytics have yet to result in improved clinical outcomes, bolus therapy has distinct advantages including faster door to drug times, easier prehospital administration, and fewer medication errors (29). Choice of agent is not as important as speed with a goal of a door to drug time less then 30 minutes or door to stent of 90 minutes. Multiple recent studies suggest the benefits of percutaneous coronary intervention over fibrinolytic therapy especially in cardiogenic shock. (8). However, when such facilities are not immediately available, fibrinolytics remain the best option.

The clinical role of fibrinolytics in venous thromboembolism is less well defined. In DVT, fibrinolytics have been shown to decrease pain, swelling, valve damage and the incidence of postphlebetic syndrome. Catheter infusion has not been proven to be more effective than systemic therapy (15). Risks and benefits of fibrinolytic therapy for DVT must be carefully considered until further data exists. Fibrinolytic therapy for PE results in a more rapid improvement in lung scan and hemodynamic stability the heparin alone. However, there is an associated 2.2% incidence of fatal intracranial hemorrhage with alteplase use compared to a 2% mortality with PE treated with standard heparin and coumadin therapy alone (15). Due to this high rate of complications, and low overall mortality with standard treatment, fibrinolytics are currently recommended only for massive hemodynamically unstable PE without contraindications to therapy (15). However, more recent work demonstrates a reduction in clinical deterioration with similar death rates in patients with submassive PE treated with alteplase versus placebo (18). Currently approved agents include streptokinase, urokinase, and alteplase.

The National Institute of Neurological Disorders and Stroke (27) rt-PA Stroke Study Group in 1995 published the still controversial landmark study of fibrinolytic therapy in acute ischemic stroke. Treatment with alteplase resulted in a 30% greater likelihood of minimal or no disability at three months and one year in patient meeting strict inclusion criteria (19,27,39). Despite the fact that patient treated with alteplase were ten times more likely to experience ICH within the first 10 days, there was no significant difference in mortality at 3 months or one year. Patients and family members must be educated and included in decision making. Several trials demonstrated unacceptably high rates of ICH when the strict NINDS criteria were not followed (37). Emergency physicians must work with other departments including pharmacy, neurology, neurosurgery, and critical care to establish up-to-date, safe and effective evidence-based institutional practice policies.

CLINICAL PRESENTATION

Patients with complications related to antithrombotic therapy may present to the ED in many different ways. Presentations may be occult, or dramatic, reported by the patient, or detected only during a meticulous history, physical examination, and work up. Regardless of the presentation, a high index of suspicion is necessary to rule out life threats in the patient on antithrombotic therapy.

GI bleeding is the major complication of aspirin therapy. Patients on outpatient antiplatelet agents such as aspirin or plavix may present with occult or massive GI bleeds. Although risk of bleeding is dose dependent, bleeding may occur even with low-dose therapy. In one large multicenter study, enteric-coated aspirin did not offer any benefit (16).

The majority of patients presenting to the ED on outpatient anticoagulant therapy are taking coumadin. Up to 15% of patients will suffer bleeding complications each year, 4.9% major bleeding complications, and up to 0.8% fatal, most commonly intracerbral hemorrhage (23). The risk of bleeding is directly related to the INR, increasing dramatically above 4.0, and is inversely related to the amount of time spent in the therapeutic range. Risk factors for bleeding include age greater than 75, past GI bleeding, hypertension, cerebrovascular disease, severe heart disease, renal insufficiency, alcoholism, known malignancy and occult GI and genitourinary malignancies (22). Recent changes in drug doses, diet, and addition or discontinuation of other drugs may interact with coumadin as described in Table 152.2.

Several types of skin lesions may result from anticoagulation therapy. The classic lesions of coumadin skin necrosis begin on the third to eighth day of therapy resulting from capillary thrombosis in subcutaneous fat. Commonly associated with protein C deficiency, skin necrosis may also occur with protein S deficiency and in patients with normal levels. Unique skin lesions may occur with heparin and less commonly LMWH. A urticarial rash secondary to local histamine release is becoming less common due to improved heparin purification techniques. LMWHs are well purified and preservative free, rarely causing this urticarial rash. Well-circumcised plaques may occur at injection sites up to 20 days later, typically in obese or pregnant women. Heparin skin necrosis may occur within 1 day but typically at 1 week after starting therapy. The lesions start as an erythematous plaque before becoming hemorrhagic, necrotic, and often puritic and painful. Biopsy often reveals antibodies and thrombocytopenia may occur as part of the heparin-induced thrombocytopenia syndrome (17). Skin necrosis with LMWH typically occurs in patients with prior heparin exposure, often without thrombocytopenia, and with less thrombotic complications. In contrast, heparin-induced skin lesions typically occurs in patients without prior exposure, and is more often accompanied by thrombocytopenia and thrombotic complications.

Within the ED, patients treated with antithrombotic medications require constant reevaluation. Minor bleeding such as bleeding from puncture sites, or life-threatening gastrointestinal or intracerebral hemorrhage must be detected and treated early to minimize further harm. For IV heparin, the risk of bleeding is less than 6% depending on indication (22). Bleeding risk with heparin is directly related to dose and patient response as indirectly measured by the APTT. Dose adjustments based on every 6 hour APTT have been the traditional method of reducing hemorrhagic complications but bleeding can occur even within the therapeutic range (22). Risk factors for bleeding complications include recent surgery or trauma, renal failure, aspirin use, GPI's, fibrinolytics, and age greater than 70. Although the theoretical risk of bleeding is less with LMWH than heparin, more recent studies have failed to demonstrate a significant difference. Furthermore, LMWH have been associated with more bleeding complications after subcutaneous administration when compared with subcutaneous heparin as well as unusual bleeding episodes such as intrahepatic and psoas hematoma (17).

ED patients started on GPI or direct thrombin inhibitors may develop bleeding from vascular puncture sites, GI bleeding, or ICH, especially when treated with fibrinolytic therapy. Lower heparin dose reduces the risk of bleeding with GPI's and fibrinolytics. Rates of life-threatening bleeding and intracranial bleeding for GPI's and direct thrombin inhibitors are low compared to fibrinolytics in ACS. Patients started on fibrinolytic therapy in the ED may develop transient hypotension, mild to severe allergic reactions, and mild to life-threatening bleeding complications. In the absence of contraindications, risk factors for fibrinolytic associated bleeding include older age, female sex, lower body weight, and hypertension.

EMERGENCY DEPARTMENT EVALUATION

Many chief complaints are complicated by anticoagulation. The emergency department physician should question the patient and family about the reason for anticoagulation, any recent dose changes, compliance with, recent INR testing, other prescriptions, over the counter and alternative medicines. Discussions with primary care physicians often help fill in historical blanks. The ED physician should also question the family about subtle changes in mental status, recent "minor falls," or bleeding. Pay close attention to vital signs for evidence of early hemorrhagic shock or intracerebral hemorrhage (ICH). Hypertension may be secondary to Cushing response in ICH. Remember that other concomitant medicines often mask important changes in vital signs. Examine carefully for pallor, contusions, abrasions, ecchymosis, and other skin lesions. Perform a rectal exam with any suspicion of bleeding and in any patient beginning anticoagulation in the ED.

In patients with complaints related to antithrombotic therapy, check hemoglobin, platelets, PTT, INR and other tests as indicated. Patients with bleeding related to aspirin therapy may have normal platelet levels but functional deficits. Bleeding time and aspirin levels may be helpful, but are often difficult to obtain and unnecessary with a thorough history. Untold noncompliance, medication changes, diet factors, and concurrent illness may affect the adequacy of anticoagulation necessitating laboratory screening.

GPI therapy may have mild or dramatic effects on platelet levels. Mild thrombocytopenia occurs in 5% of patients that are treated. Lower dose heparin also reduces thrombocytopenia with abciximab. Severe thrombocytopenia (< 50,000) occurs in 2% of patients receiving abciximab versus 1% of eptifibatide and tirofiban. Acute profound thrombocytopenia (< 20,000) occurs within 24 hours of administration of abciximab in 0.7% of patients but is much more rare eptifibatide and tirofiban. Platelet counts must be checked daily in patients receiving GPI to detect this rare but life-threatening complication (36).

Similarly, heparin and LMWH may have mild or dramatic affects on platelets. An early nonimmune-mediated transient thrombocytopenia occurs in 25% of patients resolving in the majority within 3 days despite ongoing treatment. Heparin-induced thrombocytopenia (HIT) develops in up to 3% of patients typically presenting 5 days after initial heparin exposure but earlier in patients with prior exposure. The clinicopathologic syndrome is characterized by HIT antibody formation accompanied by a fall in the platelet count of greater than 50% or skin lesions at injection sites. A hypercoagulable state may result in producing both venous and arterial thrombosis as well as DIC. The HIT antigen is platelet factor IV conformationally modified by interaction with medium chain heparin molecules. This accounts for the lower incidence of HIT with low molecular weight, shorter chained heparins (17).

In patients presenting to the ED with new thrombosis, an evaluation for hypercoagulable states should be considered. The common primary hypercoagulable states include antithrombin deficiency, protein C and S deficiency, activated protein C resistance (Factor V Leiden mutation), the prothrombin gene mutation and hyperhomocystinemia. Patients with arterial thrombosis should generally only be tested for hyperhomocystinemia. Decreased levels of antithrombin, protein C and S may result from acute thrombosis necessitating repeat confirmatory levels two weeks after finishing oral therapy for acute thrombosis or testing of family members. Secondary hypercoagulable states include malignancy, postoperative, posttrauma, postpartum, oral contraceptive use, myeloproliferative disorders, and antiphospholipid antibody syndromes (38).

A low threshold for imaging of patients on antithrombotic therapy is required to detect occult, but life-threatening bleeding. Even with minor mechanisms of blunt head trauma without loss of consciousness or blunt abdominal trauma without significant tenderness, head and abdominal CT scans are recommended to diagnose occult life-threatening bleeding in patients on daily coumadin therapy (9,26). With 100% sensitivity at 3 hours, CT may detect ICH presenting with only mild symptoms of headache and nausea, before the classic gradual progression of symptoms to focal deficits and coma (33).

For patients started on fibrinolytic therapy in the ED, repeat physical examinations are essential to the detection of bleeding. The majority of bleeding will occur at vascular puncture sites. Check labs every 6 hours for 24 hours after therapy to detect occult blood loss. A fall in hemoglobin without an obvious source of blood loss necessitates a more diligent search. Repeat rectal exams and CT scan of the abdomen and pelvis may be necessary. Any change in mental status requires discontinuing therapy, and an immediate head CT.

EMERGENCY DEPARTMENT MANAGEMENT

Patients with gastrointestinal bleeding related to outpatient antiplatelet agents such as aspirin and plavix require standard treatment including large bore IV access, volume replacement and packed red blood cell replacement as indicated, proton pump inhibitor therapy, and specialty consultation for endoscopy. Despite normal levels, a functional platelet deficiency exists, requiring platelet transfusion of 5 to 10 units of random donor platelets to raise platelet levels by 50,000. A summary of the management of bleeding complications from antithrombotic therapy is presented in Table 152.3.

Rapid reversal of GPI blockade may be necessary in patients who need emergent CABG or develop massive bleeding due to a previously occult bleeding disorder. Abciximab is a long-acting receptor blocker with 50% receptor blockade and platelet inhibition at 24 hours. Fortunately, the plasma half-life of the drug is only 15 to 30 minutes. Discontinuation of infusion and platelet transfusion are effective in reversing Abciximab. Eptifibatide and tirofiban are competitive dose-dependent receptor blockers with return of normal hemostasis only after 4 hours. Reversal of these two agents requires discontinuation of the drug and time for clearance. With renal failure, hemodialysis may be necessary. Platelet transfusion is of little use since the high number of drug molecules will easily saturate new glycoprotein receptors on transfused platelets. Treatment of GPI thrombocytopenia includes discontinuation of the GPI and heparin and platelet transfusion (36).

Careful consideration must be given to the appropriate management of the anticoagulated patient even without bleeding. A subtherapeutic INR requires anticoagulation with heparin or LMWH while the coumadin dose is increased. For the 50 year old with a mechanical valve who "ran out of coumadin a week ago" and now has an INR of 1, simply restarting coumadin may result in an iatrogenic hypercoagulable state and breakthrough

thromboembolism. A supra-therapeutic INR may require little more than holding the next dose. Specific management depends on the degree of elevation, presence of bleeding and the reason for anticoagulation. Methods to lower the INR include withholding or lowering the next dose, vitamin K1 (Phytonadione), and replacement products such as fresh frozen plasma (FFP) and prothrombin concentrate complex (PCC). The American College of Chest Physicians evidence-based guidelines for the asymptomatic patients with an elevated INR are summarized in Table 152.3. Major bleeding has not been clearly defined in the literature but for practical purposes may be considered to be any life-threatening bleeding or bleeding requiring transfusion.

Vitamin K1 is not without risk. Anaphylaxis may occur at any dose when given IV and IM. Subcutaneous absorption is unpredictable. Intramuscular administration may result in hematoma formation. Complete correction of the INR may result in breakthrough thromboembolism. High-dose vitamin K1 risks prolonged warfarin resistance and may precipitate thromboembolism for up to 1 week. Of the three routes, oral administration is considered the safest and most predictable with effects beginning in 6 to 10 hours. Recent work demonstrates that one milligram of oral vitamin K1 more rapidly lowers an elevated INR between 4 to 10 in an asymptomatic patient than 1 milligram subcutaneously without an increased risk of thromboembolism (7). IV infusion over 10 minutes is recommended for life-threatening active bleeding with effects beginning in 1 to 2 hours. Vitamin K1 is not effective in advanced liver failure when coagulation factors are no longer synthesized. In the anticoagulated patient with bleeding, several factors must be considered. What is the severity of this bleeding episode? Why is the patient on anticoagulation and what is the risk of reversal? What other modalities such as endoscopy and proton pump inhibitors may be efficacious? In the setting of controlled bleeding, maintain the INR at the lower level of therapeutic efficacy, 1.5 to 2.0 for atrial fibrillation and 2.0 to 2.5 with a mechanical heart valve. The treatment of life-threatening bleeding related to coumadin requires holding the next dose and administering vitamin K1 10 mg by slow IV infusion along with factor replacement with fresh frozen plasma (FFP) or prothrombin complex concentrate (PCC). Traditionally 3 to 4 units of FFP (1L) are given to control continued bleeding in the short term without excessive risk of thromboembolism but patient response is variable and may not correlate with correction of the INR (23).

Prothrombin concentrate complex (PCC) provides a more rapid reversal of coumadin-associated coagulopathy than FFP (23). First used to treat hemophilia B, PCC is a fractionation product of FFP containing equal amounts of factors II, VII, IX, and X. Long shelf life and easy reconstitution into a highly concentrated volume (500–1000 units/20 cc versus 1 L of FFP per dose) allowing for rapid and quick reversal without volume overload. Exact dosing with either FFP or PCC remains empiric. Dosing of PCC in coumadin coagulopathy has been extrapolated from studies of life-threatening bleeding in severe hemophilia B. For patients with an INR of 2.0 to 3.9, administer 25 units/kg, 4.0 to 5.9, 35 units/kg, and > 6.0, 50 units/kg. In contrast to FFP, thrombosis has been reported with PCC (23). Virus transmission has been reported with both products but inactivation procedures are possible with PCC. The risk of thrombosis must be balanced against the more rapid, although institution dependent, availability when considering treatment options. Emergency physicians must be familiar with availability of PCC at their institution.

The trauma patient on daily coumadin therapy with evidence of active bleeding requires aggressive evaluation and management including reversal of anticoagulation, early replacement of blood loss, and aggressive surgical management. Indications for

TABLE 152.3.   Management of Bleeding Complications Related to Antithrombotic Therapy

ASPIRIN OR PLAVIX

Major*	Transfuse 5–10 U of random donor platelets to raise platelet levels by 50,000

GLYCOPROTEIN IIB/IIIA INHIBITORS

Major or Reversal for CABG	Abciximab: Discontinue all antithrombotics. Infuse 5–10 U of random donor platelets to raise platelet levels by 50,000 Eptifibatide and Tirofiban: Discontinue all antithrombotics. Platelets ineffective

HEPARIN

Minor Bleeding	Hold Heparin Close observation and serial APTT
Major Bleeding	Hold Heparin Protamine 1 mg per 100 mg of heparin in last 4 hrs

LMWH

Major Bleeding	Protamine 1 mg/mg of enoxaparin, 1 mg/100 U dalteparin, or 1 mg/ 100 U ardeparin Repeat protamine dosing often needed at 0.5mg/mg of enoxaparin, 1 mg/100 U of dalteparin, or 1 mg/100 U ardeparin

COUMADIN

INR < 5 without bleeding	Lower or omit next dose Recheck INR in 24 hrs
INR 5–9 without bleeding	Omit next one or two doses Recheck INR in 24 hrs Resume therapy at lower dose once INR is at therapeutic level If at increased risk for bleeding, then administer Vitamin K 1–2.5 mg PO
INR > 9 without bleeding	Hold Coumadin Vitamin K 3–5 mg PO Recheck INR in 24 hrs Resume therapy at lower dose once INR is at therapeutic level
INR > 20 with minor bleeding OR Life threatening bleeding	Hold Coumadin Vitamin K 10 mg by slow IV infusion FFP 3–4 U OR PCC If INR of 2.0–3.9, then administer 25 U/kg, 4.0–5.9 then 35 U/kg, and > 6.0 then 50 U/kg

DIRECT THROMBIN INHIBITORS

Major	Discontinuing therapy. No antidote is available, half-life is short. Replace coagulation factors with 2–4 U of FFP.

FIBRINOLYTICS

Major bleeding	Start with 10 U of cryoprecipitate and 2 U of fresh frozen plasma. Persistent bleeding or ICH: Above with 5–10 U of platelets and aminocaproic acid: loading dose of 5 g or 0.1 g/kg over 30–60 min followed by continuous infusion of 0.5 to 1.0 g/h.

*Major Complications = Life-threatening, ICH, or requiring blood transfusion.
PCC, Prothrombin concentrate complex.

the rapid reversal of anticoagulant therapy include CNS bleeding, active bleeding, need for surgery and vascular compromise from expanding hematomas (30). Suggested treatment includes 4 to 6 units of FFP given to rapidly reverse anticoagulation with careful monitoring for volume overload (9).

Management of heparin-associated bleeding begins with stopping therapy with a remaining half-life of 30 to 150 minutes for doses of 25 to 400 units/kg. With life-threatening bleeding, protamine may be used to reverse heparin anticoagulation in a dose of 1 mg per 100 units of heparin administered in the previous 4 hours. As with vitamin K, protamine is not a benign

drug. Hypotension, bradycardia, flushing and fatal anaphylactic reactions have been reported. Dose is limited to 50 mg and must be given slowly over 10 minutes. As the duration from last treatment with heparin increases, heparin activity decreases, requiring less protamine for reversal. Although reversal is rapid, the half-life of protamine is shorter than heparin, necessitating repeat dosing if rebound bleeding occurs. In contrast to heparin, LMWHs cannot be turned off after subcutaneous administration. The long half-life and lack of a therapeutic off switch must be weighed against the benefits when deciding on LMWHs versus heparin. The dose of protamine is compound specific: 1 mg/mg of enoxaparin, 1 mg/100 U dalteparin, or 100 U ardeparin. Repeat dosing is often needed at 0.5 mg/mg of enoxaparin, 1 mg/100 U of dalteparin, or 100 U ardeparin. To date, only a few case reports of neutralization of LMWH have been published with relatively poor efficacy in comparison to heparin neutralization (17).

Management of HIT syndrome and coumadin skin necrosis includes discontinuing all heparin or coumadin products and administration of a rapid-acting anticoagulant such as danaparoid, a mixture of anticoagulant glycosaminoglycans with predominant antifactor Xa activity, or a direct thrombin inhibitor such as lepirudin or argatroban.

Management of complications of direct thrombin inhibitor therapy is straightforward. Allergic reactions, most commonly bronchospasm, have been reported in up to 10% of patients and are treated with standard therapies. Minimizing vascular punctures may help to minimize bleeding from other sites. Treatment of bleeding begins with discontinuing therapy. No antidote is available but the half-life is short. With persistent bleeding, replace coagulation factors with fresh frozen plasma (FFP).

The best way to reduce complications from fibrinolytic therapy is to carefully review indications and contraindications before administration. Each institution should create separate "clot box" for acute myocardial infarction, acute ischemic stroke and massive PE, containing an easy to follow pathway of indications, contraindications, patient consents, consultants to notify, adjunctive medications, and treatment of complications. Avoid unnecessary procedures and blood draws. Nasal intubation and nasogastric tubes may precipitate massive epistaxis. Arterial lines are rarely essential for ED management. If central access is absolutely required, femoral vein cannulation is preferred since manual pressure of a missed jugular or a subclavian site and a chest tube for an iatrogenic pneumothorax are unnecessarily challenging. Transthoracic is preferred over transvenous pacing if required in arterial cannulation support.

The majority of fibrinolytic bleeding will occur from puncture sites requiring only direct point pressure to the wound without discontinuing fibrinolytic therapy. Management of life-threatening gastrointestinal bleeding requires aggressive volume replacement with crystalloid and packed red blood cells as indicated, reversal of fibrinolytic therapy, and adjunctive measures including proton pump inhibitors and endoscopy. Management of ICH requires cryoprecipitate, FFP, platelets, an antifibrinolytic agent and neurosurgical evaluation.

Most life-threatening hemorrhage related to fibrinolytic therapy will respond to the administration of 10 units of cryoprecipitate and 2 units of fresh frozen plasma (34). With persistent bleeding or ICH, administer 5 to 10 units of platelets and an antifibrinolytic agent such as aminocaproic acid with a loading dose of 4 to 5g or 0.1 g/kg over 30 to 60 minutes followed by continuous infusion of 0.5 to 1.0 g/h until bleeding is controlled. Tranexamic acid has also been recommended but has a longer half-life preventing titration and balance of thrombosis and thrombolysis. Be careful to avoid antifibrinolytics in the patient with DIC. Detailed use of fibrinogen levels and bleeding times has been described, but may not be practical in the acutely hemorrhaging patient. Baseline and repeat CBC, PT/PTT fibrinogen levels, and d-dimers are indicated during continued management. Reverse heparin with protamine as previously directed.

With either streptokinase or anistreplase, allergic reactions may occur typically with mild symptoms of chills, fever, and rigors but in severe forms may include anaphylaxis. Treat with standard therapy including antihistamines, epinephrine, steroids, and airway management. Although controversial, repeat dosing or readministration within 1 year is not recommended (29). Hypotensive episodes secondary to bradykinin generation respond well to decreasing rate of infusion, vasopressors and IV fluids.

CRITICAL INTERVENTIONS

- Inquire about recent changes in drug doses, diet, and addition or discontinuation of other drugs that may interact with coumadin when evaluating INR response to coumadin dosage
- Maintain a low threshold for imaging the head or abdomen in patients with minor trauma on antithrombotic therapy to detect occult, but life-threatening bleeding
- Administer reversal agents for major bleeding complications associated with antithrombotic therapy (Table 152.3)

DISPOSITION

Most patients who present with or develop complications related to antithrombotic therapy require hospitalization for their primary disease. The patient with complications related to outpatient antiplatelet therapy with aspirin or plavix often need hospitalization for monitoring and replacement of blood loss, and consultation with a gastroenterologist for endoscopy. The patient who develops bleeding complications while on GPI therapy requires hospitalization for continued ACS treatment, monitoring and replacement of blood loss, and cardiology consultation. The patient on GPI therapy who develops major bleeding complications from a missed central venous or arterial line may require vascular surgery for control of bleeding.

The subtherapeutic patient on coumadin often requires adequate anticoagulation with inpatient heparin or LMWH to prevent a paradoxical hypercoagulable state and breakthrough thromboembolism. Outpatient lovenox therapy followed by increased coumadin, with close follow up prevents unnecessary hospitalization. The asymptomatic patient with a supratherapeutic INR need not be an automatic admission for "coagulopathy." Although the rate of serious bleeding increase with an INR of greater than 4, the overall rate remains low. The indication for anticoagulation, reason for supra-therapeutic level, underlying comorbidities, overall risk of bleeding, fall risk, social situation, reliability, and availability of follow up must all be considered. Holding a dose, discharge to home, and repeating an INR in the next day is appropriate for a 50-year-old patient with a mechanical valve who presents with a sprained ankle and is found to have an incidental INR of 6.0 after a recent dose increase. In contrast, the "wobbly " 80-year-old with a recurrent UTI and an INR of 12.0 after an outpatient course of antibiotics needs inpatient observation. Arrange appropriate follow up with primary care physicians. HIT syndrome and skin lesions require admission for anticoagulation with alternative agents in consultation with a hematologist.

Anticoagulated patients with active bleeding require hospitalization for complete or partial reversal of anticoagulation, definitive control of bleeding, replacement of significant blood loss, and management of potential thromboembolism. Specialty consultation and critical care monitoring is often necessary. GI or GU bleeding after starting anticoagulation requires aggressive evaluation for malignancy. Up to 25% of these patients will have an otherwise occult malignancy detected during evaluation for anticoagulant related bleeding (20).

For the asymptomatic anticoagulated patient with minor trauma, therapeutic INR, stable hemoglobin, normal imaging studies, and reliable caretakers, discharge with close follow up is appropriate. The symptomatic anticoagulated trauma patient with evidence of active bleeding requires aggressive management including reversal of anticoagulation, blood replacement, early surgical consultation for operative intervention, and hospitalization. These patients often require transport to a level one-trauma center after initial stabilization for definitive care.

Patients treated with fibrinolytic therapy obviously require admission to an intensive care unit for treatment of the primary disease, close observation and treatment of complications, and cardiology, neurology, and/or neurosurgery consultation.

COMMON PITFALLS

✔ Not asking about anticoagulation; indication for, changes in dose, timing and result of last INR, compliance, bleeding or skin lesions, comorbidities, new medicines, changes in diet, and changes in mental status or back pain

✔ Inappropriate use of vitamin K and protamine. Both have serious potential complications. High-dose IV vitamin K results in coumadin resistance for up to 1 week. FFP or PCC is often the most effective, easily monitored, and adjustable short-term therapy

✔ The safest place for an asymptomatic supra-therapeutic patient may be at home "resting on their couch." Decide on admission versus close follow up on a case-by-case basis in consultation with the patient's primary physician

✔ The patient with a mechanical valve who ran out of coumadin a week ago with an INR of 1.0 cannot be simply sent home with a "little extra" coumadin. Adequate anticoagulation with heparin or lovenox is necessary prior to and after restarting coumadin for 5 days

✔ Failing to work together with cardiology, neurology, neurosurgery, critical care, and pharmacy to create up-to-date indication-specific "clot boxes" containing detailed pathways with indications, contraindications, easy to understand patient consents, consultant notification phone numbers, exact dosing of fibrinolytics, adjunctive agents, and reversal agents

References

1. Abu-Hajir M. The Pharmacology of Antithrombotic and Antiplatelet agents. *Anesth Clin N Am* 1999;17:749–786.
2. Ansell J, Hirsh J, Dalen J, et al. Managing oral anticoagulant therapy. *Chest* 2001;119(1 Suppl):22S–38S.
3. Armstrong PW, Collen D, Antman E. Fibrinolysis for acute myocardial infarction: the future is here and now. *Circulation* 2003;107:2533–2537.
4. Baird S, Menown I, McBride S, et al. Randomized comparison of enoxaparin with unfractionated heparin following fibrinolytic therapy for acute myocardial infarction. *Ann Emerg Med* 2003;41:588.
5. Bhatt DL, Hirsch AT, Ringleb PA, et al. Reduction in the need for hospitalization for recurrent ischemic events and bleeding with clopidogrel instead of aspirin. CAPRIE Trial. *American Heart Journal* 2000;140:67–73.
6. Clopidogrel in Unstable Angina to Prevent Recurrent Events Trial Investigators. Effects of clopidogrel in addition to aspirin in patients with acute coronary syndromes without ST-segment elevation. *N Engl J Med* 2001;345:494–502.
7. Crowther MA, Douketis JD, Schnurr T, et al. Oral vitamin K lowers the international normalized ratio more rapidly than subcutaneous vitamin K in the treatment of warfarin-associated coagulopathy. A randomized, controlled trial. *Ann Int Med* 2002;137:251–254.
8. Dalby M, Bouzamondo A, Lechat P. Montalescot G. Transfer for primary angioplasty versus immediate thrombolysis in acute myocardial infarction: a meta-analysis. *Circulation* 2003;108:1809–1814.
9. Ferrera P, Bartfield J. Brief Reports: Outcomes of Anticoagulated Trauma Patients. *Amer J Emerg Med* 1999;154–163.
10. Fibrinolytic Therapy Trialists' (FTT) Collaborative Group. Indications for fibrinolytic therapy in suspected acute myocardial infarction: Collaborative overview of early mortality and major morbidity results from all randomized trials of more than 1000 patients. *Lancet* 1994;343:311–322.
11. GUSTO Angiographic Investigators. The effects of tissue plasminogen activator, streptokinase, or both on coronary-artery patency, ventricular function, and survival after acute myocardial infarction. *N Engl J Med* 1993;329:1615–1622.
12. GUSTO-III Investigators. An international, multicenter, randomized comparison of reteplase with alteplase for acute myocardial infarction. *N Engl J Med* 1997;337:1118–1123.
13. Hirsh J, Warkentin TE, Shaughnessy SG, et al. Heparin and LMW Heparin, Mechanisms of Action, Pharmacokinetic, Dosing, Monitoring Efficacy and Safety. *Chest* 2001;1119(Suppl 1):64S–94S.
14. Hochman JS, Wali AU, Gavrila D, et al. A new regimen for heparin use in acute coronary syndromes. *Am Heart J* 1999;138:313–318.
15. Hyers TM, Agnelli G, Hull RD, et al. Antithrombotic therapy for venous thromboembolic disease. *Chest* 2001;119(1 Suppl):176S–193S.
16. Kelly JP, Kaufman DW, Jurgelon JM, et al. Risk of aspirin-associated major upper-gastrointestinal bleeding with enteric-coated or buffered product. *Lancet* 1996;348:1413–1416.
17. Kleinschmidt K, Charles R. Pharmacology of low molecular weight heparins. *Emerg Med Clin North Am* 2001;19:1025–1049.
18. Konstantides S, et al. Heparin plus alteplase compared with heparin alone in patients with submassive PE. *N Eng J Med* 2002;347:1143–1150.
19. Kwiatkocoumadinki TG, Libman RB, Frankel M, et al. Effects of tissue plasminogen activator for acute ischemic stroke at one year. *N Engl J Med* 1999;340:1781–1787.
20. Landefeld CS, Rosenblatt MW, Goldman L. Bleeding in outpatients treated with warfarin: relation to the prothrombin time and important remedial lesions. *Am J Med* 1989;87:153–159.
21. Lang ES. Evidence based medicine. Use of platelet glycoprotein IIb/IIIa inhibitors in patients with unstable angina and non-ST-segment elevation MI. *Ann Emerg Med* 2002;40:518–520.
22. Levine MN, Raskob G, Landefeld S, et al. Hemorrhagic Complications of Anticoagulant Treatment. *Chest* 2001;119(1 Suppl):108S–121S.
23. Makris M, Watson HG. The management of coumarin-induced over-anticoagulation. *Br J Haematol* 2001;114:271–280.
24. McPherson JA. Reperfusion therapy for acute myocardial infarction. *Emerg Med Clin North Am* 2001;19:433–449.
25. Michalis LK, et al. Enoxaparin versus tinzaparin in non-ST-segment elevation in ACS: The EVET trial. *Am Heart J* 2003;146:304–310.
26. Mina A, Bair H, Howells G, Bendick P. Complications of preinjury warfarin use in the trauma patient. *J Trauma* 2003;54:842–847.
27. The National Institute of Neurological Disorders and Stroke rt-PA Stroke Study Group. Tissue plasminogen activator for acute ischemic stroke. *N Engl J Med* 1995;333:1581–1587.
28. Niemann JT. Percutaneous coronary intervention after subcutaneous enoxaparin pretreatment in patients with unstable angina pectoris. *Ann Emerg Med* 2002;39;209.
29. Ohman EM, Harrington RA, Cannon CP, et al. Intravenous thrombolysis in acute myocardial infarction. *Chest* 2001;119(1 Suppl):253S–277S.
30. O'Mara K, Mavichak V. Trauma and oral anticoagulants. *Ann Emerg Med* 1983;12:700–703.
31. Patrono C. Platelet-active drugs: the relationships among dose, effectiveness, and side effects. *Chest* 2001;119(1 Suppl):39S–63S.
32. Pollack C. 2002 update to the ACC/AHA guidelines for the management of patients with unstable angina and non-ST-segment elevation myocardial infarction: Implications for emergency department practice. *Ann Emerg Med* 2003;41:355–369.
33. Panagos PD, Jauch EC, Broderick JP. Intracerebral hemorrhage. *Emerg Med Clin North Am* 2002;20:631–655.
34. Sane DC, Califf RM, Topol EJ, et al. Bleeding during thrombolytic therapy for acute myocardial infarction: Mechanisms and Management. *Ann Int Med* 1989;111:1010–1020.
35. Steinhubl S. What is the role for improved long-term antiplatelet therapy after percutaneous coronary intervention? *Am Heart J* 2003;145:971–978.
36. Tcheng JE. Clinical challenges of platelet glycoprotein IIb/IIIa receptor inhibitor therapy: bleeding, reversal, thrombocytopenia, and retreatment. *Am Heart J* 2000;139(2 Pt 2):S38–S45.
37. Thurman RJ. Acute ischemic stroke: emergent evaluation and management. *Emerg Med Clin North Am* 2002;20:609–630.
38. Van Cott EM, Laposata M. Coagulation Disorders and Treatment Strategies: Laboratory Evaluation of Hypercaoguable States. *Hem Onc Clin N Amer* 1998;12:1141–1166.
39. Wardlaw JM, Zoppo G, Yamaguchi T, et al. Thrombolysis for acute ischaemic stroke. Cochrane Stroke Group. *Cochrane Database of Systematic Review* 2003.
40. Weitz JI. New anticoagulant drugs. *Chest* 2001;119(1 Suppl):95S–107S.
41. Yusen RD, et al. Outpatient treatment of acute venous thromboembolic disease. *Clin Chest Med* 2003;24:49–61.

Disseminated Intravascular Coagulation, Thrombotic Thrombocytopenic Purpura, and Hemolytic–Uremic Syndrome

Kathleen C. Hubbell

A number of disease processes lead to thrombus formation in the microvascular circulation with resultant consumption of clotting components and, ultimately, organ dysfunction. The underlying pathologies of these conditions differ, but the clinical presentation of multisystem involvement with hemorrhage and thrombosis may be very similar. Careful history, physical examination, and laboratory analysis enables the emergency physician to differentiate these conditions and begin appropriate treatment and referral.

Disseminated intravascular coagulation (DIC), thrombotic thrombocytopenic purpura (TTP), and hemolytic-uremic syndrome (HUS) are characterized by thrombocytopenia, microangiopathic hemolytic anemia, varying degrees of coagulation factor depletion, and multisystem involvement. Red cells are damaged as they encounter microthrombi in the small vessels, forming the schistocytes seen on the peripheral blood smear and causing laboratory evidence of hemolysis such as anemia, increased indirect bilirubin, decreased haptoglobin, and increased reticulocyte count.

The unique pathophysiology, laboratory findings, and treatments of each condition are discussed in the following sections.

DISSEMINATED INTRAVASCULAR COAGULATION

DIC is a condition of deranged and unbalanced activity of the clot-forming and clot-dissolving systems that normally function to maintain unimpeded blood flow through the body. DIC occurs only in conjunction with a variety of well-recognized conditions that have in common the release of procoagulant substances into the circulation. These conditions include sepsis; malignancy; trauma, including burns, crush injuries, and head injuries; obstetric conditions, such as abruptio placenta and retained fetus; and intravascular hemolysis, as with transfusion reactions (3,16) (Tables 153.1 and 153.2).

The procoagulant substances released activate the coagulation cascade through the tissue factor pathway, leading to the formation of thrombin. Thrombin plays its normal pivotal role in coagulation, cleaving fibrinogen to form fibrin, activating factor XI of the intrinsic pathway, and activating platelets. Thrombin is also involved in the body's normal method of terminating the clotting process, by inhibiting coagulation through a number of mechanisms. As the procoagulant substances are continuously released into the circulation as part of the patient's illness, they drive the coagulation cascade and the coactive inhibitory mechanisms, yielding both fibrin clots throughout the vascular system and large amounts of inactivated factors. Levels of antithrombin III, the most important inhibitor of thrombin, are reduced by consumption and decreased synthesis. The fibrin mesh of the clots traps platelets as they flow past. An eventual depletion of factors, inhibitors, and platelets occurs, causing hemorrhage.

Further contributing to this clotting disorder is activation of the fibrinolytic system. Plasmin attacks fibrinogen and fibrin, producing fibrin degradation products (FDPs). FDPs interfere with the polymerization of fibrin, which is necessary to create functional clots, and they cause a severe functional platelet defect, which exacerbates the quantitative platelet disorder.

In most patients, fibrinolysis does not keep pace with the intravascular coagulation, due to an increase in plasminogen-activator inhibitor type 1, the major regulating enzyme of the fibrinolytic system. Consequently, the microvasculature fills with occlusive thrombi. The resultant tissue ischemia and necrosis manifest as severe organ dysfunction, which is the usual cause of death in DIC. Although bleeding can be dramatic and many physicians think of DIC as a hemorrhagic disorder, it is essential to realize that it is a thrombohemorrhagic condition. Interventions to arrest the clotting process must be a part of the therapy (3,5,24).

The procoagulant substances that initiate the thrombohemorrhagic processes vary according to the underlying illness with which the DIC is associated. In sepsis, bacterial endotoxin and cytokines induce the production and surface expression of tissue factor by circulating monocytes and endothelial cells (5,11,24). Many tumor cells also make tissue factor in large amounts. Severe trauma, intravascular hemolysis, and obstetric conditions such as abruptio placenta all release large quantities of tissue factor into the general circulation from damaged cells.

CLINICAL PRESENTATION AND DIFFERENTIAL DIAGNOSIS

DIC occurs in an acute, fulminant form and in a low-grade, chronic form. The acute form usually is associated with sepsis, trauma, transfusion reactions, and acute obstetric events. The incidence of DIC in severe sepsis is 18% and in septic shock, 38% (24). Bleeding in these clinical settings should cause suspicion of DIC. Bleeding may occur from surgical or traumatic wounds despite local treatment and from venipuncture and arterial puncture sites. Petechiae, purpura, hemorrhagic bullae, and subcutaneous hematomas can be seen. Gastrointestinal, urinary tract,

TABLE 153.1. Frequency of Conditions Associated with DIC

Condition	% of Total
Infection	26–29
Malignancy	18–24
Surgery	18–20
Liver disease	8–10
Obstetric	4–6
Trauma	2–5
Other	18–23

TABLE 153.2.   Conditions Associated with DIC

INFECTIONS	MALIGNANCIES	SURGERY, TRAUMA
Bacterial	**Carcinomas**	Extracorporeal circulation
Gram-negative sepsis	Lung	Extensive surgery
Neisseria meningitidis	Colon	Severe burns
Neisseria gonorrhoeae	Stomach	Head trauma
Klebsiella	Pancreas	Trauma with shock, acidosis
Serratia	Breast	
Proteus mirabilis	Gallbladder	**OBSTETRIC**
Pseudomonas aeruginosa	Esophagus	
Escherichia coli	Kidney	Abruptio placenta
Salmonella	Melanoma	Amniotic fluid embolism
Gram-positive sepsis	Prostate	Saline or septic abortion
Streptococcus pneumoniae		Missed abortion
Staphylococcus aureus	**Leukemias**	Eclampsia
Staphylococcus albus	Acute promyelocytic	
Legionnaires' disease	Acute myelocytic	**MISCELLANEOUS**
Bacteroides	Chronic myelocytic	
Haemophilus meningitis	Eosinophilic	Collagen vascular diseases
Typhoid fever	Hairy cell	Major transfusion reactions
Shigella		Snake bites
Clostridium welchii	**Other**	Heat stroke
	Pheochromocytoma	Cardiac arrest
Mycoplasmal	Neuroblastoma	Conditions of anoxia, acidosis
Mycoplasma pneumonia	Sarcomas	Giant hemangiomas
	Histiocytosis X	Aortic aneurysms
Rickettsial	Polycythemia vera	Intra-aortic balloon-assist devices
Rocky Mountain spotted fever		Peritoneovenous shunt devices
		Pleurovenous shunt devices
Viral		
Varicella, disseminated		
Measles pneumonia		
Dengue fever		
Herpes simplex		
Influenza		
Yellow fever		
Rubella, congenital		
Chlamydial		
Psittacosis		
Fungal		
Aspergillosis		
Candidiasis		
Histoplasmosis		
Mycobacterial		
Tuberculosis		
Protozoal		
Malaria (*P. falciparum*)		

and pulmonary bleeding are common. Typical patients with DIC bleed from at least three sites. They are often febrile and hypotensive. Signs of thromboses may be more subtle and manifest as abnormal mental status, dyspnea, abdominal pain, deteriorating renal function, acral cyanosis, and gangrene (3,4).

Patients with the chronic form of DIC usually have malignancy, liver disease, collagen vascular disease, or an obstetric condition such as retained fetus. Bleeding is rarely severe; instead, thrombotic disorders such as thrombophlebitis, pulmonary embolism, and nonbacterial thrombotic endocarditis predominate. Diagnosis of a thrombotic event, followed by recognition of typical laboratory abnormalities of DIC, may lead to the diagnosis of an occult malignancy (16).

EMERGENCY DEPARTMENT EVALUATION

An appropriate clinical setting with a typical physical examination is highly suggestive of DIC and should spur the physician to seek laboratory evidence of the diagnosis. To support a diagnosis of DIC, results should show abnormalities in four areas: (1) depletion of coagulation factors; (2) depletion of coagulation inhibitors; (3) activation of the fibrinolytic system; and (4) evidence of end-organ damage (3,4). The tests that are most sensitive and specific for detecting abnormalities in these areas may not be available on an emergency basis. Those that are available may not be sensitive or specific and must be used with an understanding of their limitations.

Examination of the peripheral blood smear will show schistocytes in 50% of patients with fulminant DIC (3). Thrombocytopenia is usually evident on the smear, and large platelet forms (young platelets) are commonly seen because of increased platelet turnover.

Readily available laboratory tests that confirm depletion of coagulation factors include the PT and PTT and the fibrinogen level (3,4). The PT and PTT are prolonged in only about 50% of cases of DIC, because activated factors and degradation products may interfere with these tests. Therefore, normal PT or PTT values do not rule out DIC. The fibrinogen level is less than 150 mg/dL in only 70% of cases, probably because it is an acute-phase reactant and its baseline level can be increased in acute illness. Other, more reliable tests exist but are not generally available in the emergency department.

The consumption of coagulation inhibitors can be measured directly by checking the antithrombin III (AT III) level, which is decreased in 89% of patients with DIC, but will rarely be available to the emergency physician.

Activation of the fibrinolytic system is best demonstrated by elevation of the D-dimer level, which is seen in 93% of patients with DIC and has an 80% specificity (3,5). D-dimer is produced by the action of plasmin on cross-linked fibrin. FDPs, which are increased in 75% to 100% of patients with DIC, are not as specific for DIC as the D-dimer level.

Laboratory test results reflecting end-organ damage are increased lactic dehydrogenase (LDH) and serum creatinine levels, and arterial blood gases showing acidosis and hypoxia. Other useful tests are hemoglobin and platelet count, urinalysis, pregnancy test, and imaging studies as guided by history and examination to search for the inciting illness. Platelet counts range from 20,000 to 100,000/μL, averaging about 60,000/μL (3).

Thus, of the laboratory analyses available to the emergency physician for the diagnosis of DIC, the most sensitive is D-dimer. The PT, PTT, fibrinogen, and FDP should be ordered, but may be normal in patients with early DIC and may be abnormal in other clinical conditions. Prothrombin fragment 1+2, antithrombin III, and fibrinopeptide A levels may not be available on an emergency basis, but, with D-dimer, are the most reliable tests for DIC (3). Similarly, in cases of mild or chronic low-grade DIC, the PT, PTT, fibrinogen level, and platelet count may all be normal, because the bone marrow and liver can increase the synthesis and release of the clotting components. FDPs and D-dimer are elevated, however, and the peripheral smear is abnormal.

Appropriate coagulation studies should be drawn early in patients with sepsis, trauma, and other conditions with high risk for DIC. Laboratory abnormalities are usually present before severe hemorrhage occurs.

EMERGENCY DEPARTMENT MANAGEMENT

Treatment of DIC is an area lacking consensus and clarity. The heterogenicity of underlying causes has made it difficult to perform prospective clinical trials with results applicable to the individual patient. Treatment must be individualized and based on a current understanding of the pathologic basis of the condition underlying the DIC. An expanding choice of agents is becoming available as knowledge of hemostasis grows.

There is one area of universal agreement in DIC treatment. The underlying illness must be aggressively attacked with surgery, antibiotics, chemotherapy, or other appropriate therapy so as to stop the continuous release of the procoagulant factor and persistent activation of the coagulation cascade (3,4,5,11). For example, in abruptio placenta, DIC terminates immediately upon evacuation of the uterus. Correction of hypovolemia, hypotension, acidosis, and hypoxia should also begin in the emergency department, and disease-specific interventions should be initiated promptly whenever possible.

If the patient is bleeding, transfusion with packed red blood cells and platelets to correct anemia and thrombocytopenia is indicated. A platelet count less than 50,000/μL should prompt transfusion in the bleeding patient, and the additional contribution of functional platelet disorders to the bleeding tendency should be remembered (5). Although some clinicians fear "fueling the fire" of coagulation by giving fresh-frozen plasma (FFP) or cryoprecipitate to patients with DIC, this event has not been shown to occur in most cases, especially if concurrent therapy

to arrest the consumption of coagulation factors is under way (4,5). Six units of cryoprecipitate will raise fibrinogen by about 50 mg/dL. A level of at least 100 mg/dL is desired.

Other specific treatments for DIC are generally initiated after admission. A number of agents, including heparin, AT III, antifibrinolytics, protein C, hirudin, tissue factor pathway inhibitor (TFPI), thrombomodulin, and tissue plasminogen activator (TPA), have been investigated (11). Several are associated with improvement in coagulation abnormalities, lung function, and duration of symptoms and show promise to decrease mortality when used in appropriately selected conditions in concert with aggressive supportive care.

Heparin must be used selectively in DIC. It is more useful in chronic than acute DIC. Some recommend it in conditions such as purpura fulminans, in which devastating thrombi are obvious. Many specifically recommend against its use in fulminant acute DIC, in cases in which potential central nervous system (CNS) bleeding is of concern (e.g., head trauma), in cases of fulminant liver failure, and in obstetric catastrophes other than retained fetus (4,5,11).

AT III appears promising in acute DIC. It has been shown to decrease duration of symptoms, improve coagulation parameters, improve oxygenation, and decrease intensive care unit (ICU) and ventilator days and the need for dialysis in patients with sepsis and trauma. It also has been associated with a trend toward decreased mortality. Most agree that it should be given in doses that achieve very high serum levels, 125% to 150% of normal (4,5,11,16).

Fibrinolytic inhibitors such as epsilon amino caproic acid (EACA) or tranexamic acid are usually contraindicated in DIC because the thrombotic aspects of the condition are those most associated with morbidity. However, in certain conditions, such as acute promyelocytic leukemia, fibrinolysis is the predominant pathology and improvement is seen with fibrinolytic inhibitor therapy (4,6,11).

DISPOSITION

The primary role of the emergency physician in the management of DIC is to be aware of its association with severe illness and injury, to perform the appropriate physical examination and laboratory screening tests to identify its presence, and to initiate immediate stabilization of airway, breathing, and circulation. The importance of immediate specialty consultation once DIC is suspected cannot be overemphasized, owing to the importance of treating the underlying cause. Antibiotics, correction of hypotension and hypoxia, and replacement blood component therapy (as well as preparation of the patient for surgery, if needed) should be initiated in the emergency department.

The prognosis in patients with DIC is poor. The appearance of DIC signifies severe illness or injury and extensive tissue damage. In trauma patients, mortality rises from 14% in those without DIC to 59% in those with it. Mortality quadruples from 10% to 40% in meningococcal sepsis in children when DIC supervenes (13).

Patients with acute DIC are very ill and should not be transferred from an institution that has facilities to care for them. However, because treatment of the underlying condition is so essential to the termination of the coagulation abnormalities, transfer should be arranged after initial stabilization if the hospital does not offer the required surgical, obstetric, or intensive care services. If transfer is anticipated, the emergency physician must ensure adequate airway, breathing, and circulation and should initiate appropriate blood component replacement. Other modalities, such as antibiotic therapy, should also be started prior to transfer, preferably after consultation with the accepting physician.

COMMON PITFALLS

✔ Failing to consider DIC in the appropriate clinical setting. Because of its association with severe illness or injury and its effect on mortality, signs of DIC should be sought in all patients at risk. The identification of such signs should prompt the physician to order the appropriate laboratory tests to confirm the diagnosis

✔ Allowing the bleeding associated with DIC to distract the physician from the search for and treatment of the underlying causative illness. Any therapeutic plan that fails to include measures directed against the underlying cause is likely to be unsuccessful

THROMBOTIC THROMBOCYTOPENIC PURPURA AND HEMOLYTIC–UREMIC SYNDROME

TTP and adult HUS appear to be clinically similar disorders that each present with some of the elements of the classic pentad of microangiopathic hemolytic anemia, thrombocytopenia, neurologic abnormalities, fever, and renal dysfunction. In TTP, neurologic abnormalities predominate, and renal dysfunction is seen less often; the opposite is characteristic of HUS. These syndromes occur twice as often in women and peak in the fourth and fifth decades of life (15). In the United States, mortality data from the years 1968 through 1991 seem to suggest that the incidence of TTP is increasing (21).

There is an epidemiologically distinct form of HUS seen in children 6 months to 4 years of age, with an equal distribution between the sexes. This childhood illness is often preceded by diarrheal illness caused by infection with cytotoxin-producing strains of *Escherichia coli* and *Shigella* that damage the renal vascular endothelium. About 90% of cases of pediatric HUS are associated with *E. coli* enterocolitis (2).

Most cases of TTP occur in previously healthy patients. A rare familial form usually manifests during infancy or childhood and recurs at regular intervals. Acquired idiopathic TTP is most often a single episode seen in older children and adults, although up to one-third of patients may experience recurrence. TTP is also seen in association with the use of drugs such as ticlopidine, clopidogrel, cyclosporine, mitomycin, quinine, and combinations of chemotherapeutic agents. It also occurs concurrently with other conditions, such as pregnancy; autoimmune diseases; cancer; and bacterial and viral infections, including HIV and HTLV-1 (1,12,15,19).

The pathophysiology of familial and idiopathic TTP (and perhaps the other forms) involves the formation of occlusive small vessel thrombi made up of platelets held together by unusually large von Willebrand factor (ULvWF) multimers with little or no fibrin. These large multimers are produced by and released from endothelial cells. In healthy people, they are immediately cleaved into the smaller vWF molecules normally found in the circulation by a metalloprotease enzyme referred to as ADAMTS-13. This enzyme is synthesized in the liver and has a binding site on endothelial cells. During an episode of TTP, ADAMTS-13 activity is undetectable in the plasma, probably due to the action of IgG inhibitory antibodies. The ULvWF multimers are not cleaved and their large size and configuration induce active adhesion and aggregation of platelets, leading to thrombus formation. Fibrin is not detected in these clots and there is no depletion of clotting factors. Smaller sized, cleaved vWF molecules do not bind platelets under conditions of normal blood flow. Patients with familial TTP do not have inhibitors. Instead, genetic mutations interfere with the synthesis or activity of the metalloprotease enzyme (8,14). IgG inhibitors have been detected in some patients with clopidogrel-associated TTP (1).

In HUS, the Shiga toxin released from the causative *E. coli* and *Shigella* strains is transported by neutrophils to target organs such as the brain and kidney whose cells have globotriaosylceramide receptors. The toxin activates platelets and induces the secretion of ULvWF from the endothelial cells. However, unlike patients with TTP, those with HUS have normal metalloprotease activity and microthrombi in HUS contain fibrin and platelets with little or no vWF (8,14,23). Only smaller, not ultra-large, vWF fragments are found in the plasma of HUS patients (23). A prothrombotic state with biochemical evidence of thrombin generation and inhibition of fibrinolysis has been detected as early as the fourth day of diarrheal illness in children who go on to develop HUS (6). As HUS becomes clinically obvious, levels of molecular markers for these processes increase further.

Thus it is clear that despite some clinical similarity, the pathophysiologies of TTP and HUS are distinct. Plasma exchange, a therapy which removes inhibitory antibodies and provides active metalloprotease enzyme is usually curative in TTP, but ineffective in HUS. A laboratory test for the metalloprotease may provide a diagnostic tool for differentiating these two syndromes in the future.

CLINICAL PRESENTATION AND DIFFERENTIAL DIAGNOSIS

Although the pentad of symptoms and laboratory findings is considered classic in these diseases, it is important to realize that only about 40% of patients manifest all 5 criteria. In those with a diagnosis of TTP, 50% to 70% have neurologic dysfunction and 50% to 75% have renal involvement. Less than 15% have severe renal dysfunction with creatinine greater than 5 mg/dL (12,15). Only about one-third of HUS patients have neurologic dysfunction. Fever has been reported in 60% to 100% of patients (20).

The most frequent initial neurologic abnormality is altered mental status, which may be manifested by subtle personality change, lethargy, agitation, or confusion. Seizures, hemiplegia, aphasia, paresthesias, and visual disturbances occur in somewhat less than half of patients and more often in the later stages of the disease. Visual symptoms may be caused by thromboses in the CNS or in the retinal vessels.

Although 20% of patients may complain of gross hematuria, renal dysfunction is usually discovered only on laboratory studies. Bleeding (e.g., epistaxis, hematuria, gastrointestinal or vaginal hemorrhage) is seen in about 30% to 40% at initial presentation. Abdominal pain, usually without an identifiable source, may be part of the presentation in 30% to 40%.

This type of multisystem symptomatology requires the emergency physician to entertain a broad differential diagnosis that includes DIC, CNS infection, collagen vascular disease, bacterial endocarditis, and malignant hypertension, among others. History and physical examination directed to the identification of salient characteristics of each condition may narrow the differential. Laboratory studies can be very helpful in confirming the diagnosis of TTP or HUS, as the laboratory abnormalities of the pentad are more consistently present than the clinical symptoms.

EMERGENCY DEPARTMENT EVALUATION

Laboratory studies directed toward the etiology of fever, bleeding, and neurologic and renal abnormalities should be ordered. Complete blood count, platelet count, PT, PTT, fibrinogen, fibrin degradation products, D-dimer, and examination of the peripheral blood smear often suggest the diagnosis. All patients with TTP-HUS are anemic; 90% have hemoglobin less than 10 g/dL, and 40% have less than 6 g/dL. The peripheral smear reveals schistocytes and a decreased number of platelets; 50% of patients have a platelet count less than 20,000/μL. The PT and PTT are normal in 90%, and fibrinogen is less than 100 mg/dL in only 5% of TTP-HUS patients. In DIC, by contrast, tests reflective of coagulation factor consumption are usually abnormal (15).

The LDH, blood urea nitrogen (BUN), creatinine, electrolytes, blood cultures, and computed tomography (CT) scan of the head can provide further important diagnostic information. Lumbar puncture should be considered, but severe thrombocytopenia may lead the clinician to defer this procedure. Serum LDH is uniformly and greatly elevated in TTP patients; median levels are often six times normal. This is a much larger elevation than is seen in other hemolytic anemias, suggesting tissue sources in addition to red blood cell lysis. LDH measurements show LDH5 from liver and skeletal muscle to be the isoenzyme most elevated (7). It has been suggested that because LDH is greatly elevated in most cases and decreases rapidly in response to therapy, it should be considered a sensitive marker of TTP (20). The combination of a greatly elevated LDH, microangiopathic hemolytic anemia, and thrombocytopenia is often considered sufficient to make a diagnosis of TTP, even in the absence of fever and renal or neurologic abnormalities.

Abnormalities of BUN and creatinine are universal in patients in whom HUS is diagnosed, and are seen in 40% to 50% of patients with TTP.

EMERGENCY DEPARTMENT MANAGEMENT

As always, airway, breathing, and circulation should receive primary attention. In febrile patients in whom infection is suspected, antibiotic therapy should be initiated after obtaining appropriate cultures in the emergency department. When the diagnosis of TTP-HUS is suspected on clinical and laboratory grounds, a hematologist should be consulted. The emergency physician should be aware that despite significant thrombocytopenia and clinical bleeding, platelet transfusions are contraindicated in TTP (15). Several case reports note clinical deterioration following platelet administration, and it is assumed that more thrombi are formed in the tissues when additional platelets are supplied. Platelet transfusions are sometimes given as a stopgap measure in patients with intracranial bleeding demonstrated on CT.

The mainstay of current therapy for TTP is plasma exchange which removes metalloprotease inhibitors and ULvWF and provides active ADAMTS-13 (12,17). An infusion of approximately 10 U of FFP per 24-hour period should be started, and arrangements made for plasmapheresis if there is not prompt improvement. An exchange of one plasma volume per day is recommended initially, with an increase or decrease according to the patient's response. Seriously ill patients with coma, cardiac failure, or renal dysfunction should have plasmapheresis as soon as possible (15). In familial TTP, plasma infusion to replace functionally defective metalloprotease is adequate therapy because there are no inhibitor antibodies to remove through plasmapheresis. In the future, purified metalloprotease may be available, replacing plasma infusion for patients with familial TTP. The gene sequence for ADAMTS-13 has been determined, holding promise of gene therapy in familial TTP (14).

The benefits of plasma exchange using FFP are clear. In a study comparing plasma exchange with plasma infusion, 47% of those receiving exchange had an increased platelet count after the first treatment cycle, compared with 26% of those receiving infusion. The death rate was four times greater in the infusion group (17). Another study noted an 81% reduction in the risk of

development of end-stage renal disease in patients who received plasma exchange, compared with those who did not (10). Red cell transfusions are rarely needed, but should be considered if the patient is symptomatic from severe anemia.

Prednisone in doses of 1 mg/kg/d or greater is often given on the basis of historic precedent. Thirty of 100 patients were noted to have complete resolution of symptoms and laboratory abnormalities after receiving prednisone only, without plasma therapy. Inhibitors of platelet function, such as aspirin, dipyridamole, sulfinpyrazone, and prostacyclin, are often given, despite conflicting reports of their efficacy (15).

PEDIATRIC HEMOLYTIC–UREMIC SYNDROME

E. coli O157:H7 is now recognized as the leading cause of HUS in the United States, Canada, and Europe (2), although cases associated with HIV infection, chemotherapeutic agents, and radiation therapy continue to be reported.

E. coli O157:H7 is transmitted by contaminated food and water. In the United States, the largest outbreak was associated with undercooked, contaminated hamburger meat. More recently, there have been outbreaks related to unpasteurized apple juice, lettuce, and alfalfa sprouts in the United States and to radish sprouts in Japan. Well water contaminated with run-off from cattle pastures led to infection of more than 100 people in New York in 1999. Person-to-person spread is also reported in institutions, childcare centers, and within families (2).

Five percent to 15% of children with *E. coli* O157:H7 infection develop HUS with microangiopathic hemolytic anemia, thrombocytopenia, and renal dysfunction. HUS is usually evident 5 to 13 days after onset of the diarrheal illness. Most laboratory abnormalities resolve within 2 weeks. Twenty-five percent of patients will have severe HUS with more than 7 days of anuria, more than 14 days of oliguria, or stroke. Five to 9% die, usually from thrombotic CNS involvement, which occurs in about 30% of pediatric HUS cases. Thirty-five percent to 50% of survivors have chronic kidney damage; 3% have end-stage disease (2,9).

The role of antibiotics in the development or prevention of HUS remains unclear due to the lack of appropriate studies (18,25). An orally administered Shiga toxin–binding resin is under study but, so far, has shown no efficacy in preventing HUS (22).

The general management of pediatric diarrhea-associated HUS is supportive, with careful management of fluids, electrolytes, and blood pressure, and dialysis when needed. Plasma exchange is generally reserved for those more severe cases that resemble TTP with CNS involvement (2,14).

CRITICAL INTERVENTIONS

- For DIC treat the underlying illness aggressively with surgery, antibiotics, chemotherapy, or other appropriate therapy so as to stop the continuous release of the procoagulant factor and persistent activation of the coagulation cascade
- In suspected DIC, order a D-dimer because it is the most sensitive rapidly available laboratory test, since PT, PTT, fibrinogen, and FDP may be normal in patients with early DIC
- Avoid platelet transfusions in TTP-HUS except as a stopgap measure in patients with intracranial bleeding demonstrated on CT since administration of platelets is associated with deterioration in TTP-HUS
- In TTP initiate plasma exchange with FFP and arrange for plasmapheresis

DISPOSITION

Patients with TTP-HUS require high levels of nursing care and blood bank support, and should be admitted to an ICU. If plasmapheresis is not available, transfer to another institution should be arranged while plasma infusion therapy is begun.

Response to plasma therapy generally follows a predictable pattern in TTP. Neurologic abnormalities are the first to resolve, usually within 3 days. LDH levels normalize in about 5 days, and platelet counts in 10 days. Renal function is the last to normalize, typically requiring about 2 weeks to return to baseline. It usually takes about nine plasmapheresis treatments to produce sustained improvement (20).

Other treatments that may be used by the admitting physician, if there is rapid deterioration or no response to plasmapheresis, include immunosuppressive agents such as vincristine and splenectomy (15,20). In one series of 44 patients, about 30% underwent splenectomy.

Relapse is fairly common in TTP. Most relapses (84%) occur within the first month after diagnosis, and 97% within 2 months. A small percentage of relapses occur years after the initial episode.

Since the advent of plasma therapy, overall survival in patients with TTP has been about 90% (14). Recovery from neurologic, hematologic, and renal abnormalities is usually complete.

COMMON PITFALLS

✔ Only about a third of patients have all five criteria of the classic diagnostic pentad of TTP-HUS at the time of presentation. The clinical components of the syndrome are variable in their appearance, and may be subtle or absent

✔ The multisystem abnormalities seen in cases of TTP-HUS suggest a wide variety of possible diagnoses. Despite its rarity, TTP-HUS should always be considered in patients with neurologic, renal, or hemostatic abnormalities

✔ No specific laboratory abnormality is diagnostic of TTP-HUS. However, the combination of microangiopathic hemolytic anemia, thrombocytopenia, an extremely high LDH, and normal PT and PTT is characteristic of the syndrome and distinguishes it from DIC

References

1. Bennett CL, Connors JM, Carwile JM, et al. Thrombotic thrombocytopenic purpura associated with clopidogrel. *N Engl J Med* 2000;342:1773–1777.
2. Besser RE, Griffin PM, Slutsker L. *Escherichia coli* O157:H7 gastroenteritis and the hemolytic uremic syndrome: an emerging infectious disease. *Annu Rev Med* 1999;50:355–367.
3. Bick RL. Disseminated intravascular coagulation: current concepts of etiology, pathophysiology, diagnosis, and treatment. *Hemato/Oncol Clin North Am* 2003;17:149–176.
4. Bick RL. Disseminated intravascular coagulation. In: Rakel RE, Bope ET, eds. *Conn's Current Therapy,* 55th ed. Elsevier, 2003;449–453.
5. Carey MJ, Rodgers GM. Disseminated intravascular coagulation: clinical and laboratory aspects. *Am J Hematol* 1998;59:65–73.
6. Chandler WL, Jelacic S, Boster DR, et al. Prothrombotic coagulation abnormalities preceding the hemolytic-uremic syndrome. *N Engl J Med* 2002;346:23–32.
7. Cohen JA, Brecher ME, Bandarenko N. Cellular source of serum lactate dehydrogenase elevation in patients with thrombotic thrombocytopenic purpura. *J Clin Apheresis* 1998;13:16–19.
8. Furlan M, Robles R, Galbusera M, et al. Von Willebrand factor-cleaving protease in thrombotic thrombocytopenic purpura and the hemolytic-uremic syndrome. *N Engl J Med* 1998;339:1578–1584.
9. Garg AX, Suri RS, Barrowman N, et al. Long-term renal prognosis of diarrhea-associated hemolytic-uremic syndrome. *JAMA* 2003;290:1360–1370.
10. Hollenbeck M, Kutkuhn B, Aul C, et al. Haemolytic-uraemic syndrome and thrombotic-thrombocytopenic purpura in adults: clinical findings and prognostic factors for death and end-stage renal disease. *Nephrol Dial Transplant* 1998;13:76–81.
11. Levi M, ten Cate H. Disseminated intravascular coagulation. *N Engl J Med* 1999; 341:586–592.
12. Martinez FA, Pereira A, Ordinas A. Thrombotic thrombocytopenic purpura and hemolytic uremic syndrome (TTP/HUS). Description of a series of 35 patients. *Med Clin (Barc)* 1997;109:49–52.
13. Mertens R, Peschgens T, Granzen B, et al. Diagnosis and stage-related treatment of disseminated intravascular coagulation in meningococcal infections. *Klin Paediatr* 1999;211:65–69.
14. Moake JL. Thrombotic microangiopathies. *N Engl J Med* 2002;347:589–600.
15. Moake JL, Eisenstaedt RS. Thrombotic thrombocytopenic purpura and the hemolytic uremic syndrome. In: Colman RW, Hirsh J, Marder VJ, et al., eds. *Hemostasis and thrombosis: basic principles and clinical practice,* 3rd ed. Philadelphia: JB Lippincott Co, 1994;1064–1075.
16. Penner JA. Disseminated intravascular coagulation in patients with multiple organ failure of non-septic origin. *Semin Thromb Hemost* 1998;24:45–52.
17. Rock GA, Shumak KH, Buskard NA, et al. Comparison of plasma exchange with plasma infusion in the treatment of thrombotic thrombocytopenic purpura. Canadian apheresis study group. *N Engl J Med* 1991;325:393–397.
18. Safdar N, Said A, Gangnon RE, Maki DG. Risk of hemolytic uremic syndrome after antibiotic treatment of *Escherichia coli* O157:H7 enteritis: a meta-analysis. *JAMA* 2002;288:996–1001.
19. Sutor GC, Schmidt RE, Albrecht H. Thrombotic microangiopathies and HIV infection: report of two typical cases, features of HUS and TTP, and review of the literature. *Infection* 1999;27:12–15.
20. Thompson CE, Damon LE, Ries CA, Linker CA. Thrombotic microangiopathies in the 1980s: clinical features, response to treatment, and the impact of the human immunodeficiency virus epidemic. *Blood* 1992;80:1890–1895.
21. Török TJ, Holman RC, Chorba TL. Increasing mortality from thrombotic thrombocytopenic purpura in the United States—analysis of national mortality data, 1968–1991. *Am J Hematol* 1995;50:84–90.
22. Trachtman H, Cnaan A, Christen E, et al. Effect of an oral Shiga toxin-binding agent on diarrhea-associated hemolytic uremic syndrome in children. *JAMA* 2003;290:1337–1344.
23. Tsai HM, Chandler WL, Sarode R, et al. Von Willebrand factor and von Willebrand factor-cleaving metalloprotease activity in *Escherichia coli* O157:H7-associated hemolytic uremic syndrome. *Pediatric Research* 2001;49:653–659.
24. Vervloet MG, Thijs LG, Hack CE. Derangements of coagulation and fibrinolysis in critically ill patients with sepsis and septic shock. *Semin Thromb Hemost* 1998;24:33–44.
25. Wong CS, Jelacic S, Habeeb RL, Watkins SL, Tarr PI. The risk of the hemolytic-uremic syndrome after antibiotic treatment of *Escherichia coli* O157:H7 infections. *N Engl J Med* 2000;342:1930–1936.

CHAPTER 154
Sickle Cell Disease

Donald M. Yealy and Michele L. Dorfsman

Sickle cell disease is a hereditary disorder of hemoglobin structure and function. Hemoglobin S (for "sickle") differs from the normal hemoglobin A in that valine is substituted for glutamic acid in position 6 of the globin beta chain. Both hemoglobin A and C function similarly in the oxygenated state, but deoxygenated hemoglobin S tends to polymerize and gelate, leading to red cell sickling. Erythrocytes with less total hemoglobin or less hemoglobin S are more resistant to sickling, as are younger and small cells.

Individuals who are homozygous for the sickle cell gene (SS) are said to have **sickle cell disease**. Their erythrocytes contain at least 90% hemoglobin S. Patients who are heterozygous for the sickle cell gene (SA) are said to have **sickle cell trait**. Their erythrocytes contain both hemoglobin A (50–60%) and hemoglobin S (30%–40%). **Common sickle variants** include **SC disease** (in which patients are heterozygous for both hemoglobin S and hemoglobin C) and **sickle-thalassemia**. These variants display lower red blood cell (RBC) levels of hemoglobin S and are associated with less morbidity than sickle cell disease.

An estimated 8% to 10% of black Americans carry the sickle cell gene and about 1 in 400 to 600 manifests sickle cell disease. The sickle variant diseases are less common and are regarded as less severe disorders compared to homozygous disease (19,20). Most patients with sickle trait or variants have a normal life span and rare crises, although an increased risk for sudden death during exertion exists.

The anemia of sickle cell disease is due to both chronic and acute hemolysis. The red cell membranes are damaged with repeated episodes of sickling, leading to increased fluid and electrolyte permeability and fragility. RBCs have an average life-span of about 10 to 20 days in SS disease, compared to 120 days in normal subjects. During an acute painful event (also called 'pain crisis'), the involved red cells undergo sickling. Initially this is a reversible process, but after repeated episodes the RBCs become irreversibly sickled and are destroyed. The microvascular circulation is slowed or obstructed because of the sickling, the increased viscosity, and the increased endothelial adherence of RBCs. Local tissue ischemia and acidosis leads to further sickling, and organ damage results because of tissue ischemia and infarction.

The clinical severity of sickle cell disease is variable. Some patients follow a mild clinical course with infrequent pain events or crises, but others are more severely affected. An increased frequency of painful crises, particularly chest crises (see later), is associated with a shorter life expectancy (19,20). Most homozygous patients develop painful events before the age of 1 year, and by 5 years nearly all sickle cell disease patients have experienced a pain event. Neonates and infants are often spared from crisis symptoms because of the protective effects of fetal hemoglobin (hemoglobin F), which persists in significant amounts during the first 6 to 12 months of life. Those patients with sickle trait may develop painful crises when stressed or at higher elevations.

Infection is a leading cause of mortality in patients with sickle cell disease. The life expectancy of these patients is increasing because of aggressive medical therapy, particularly treatment of infection. Currently, most sickle cell patients survive into middle adulthood (19,20). Sickle trait, SC, and sickle-thalassemia patients all have near normal life expectancies and suffer far fewer symptoms.

CLINICAL PRESENTATION AND DIFFERENTIAL DIAGNOSIS

Painful vasoocclusive events are the most common presenting problem for sickle cell patients in the emergency department. Although a proximate instigator is not always discovered, many triggers have been identified, including infection, systemic acidosis, dehydration, hypoxia, cold exposure, pregnancy, and physical or emotional stress. Identifying one or more of these factors helps guide therapy and may prevent sequelae. Episodes of painful sickle events commonly last 48 hours to several days.

Bony pain is very common during acute vasoocclusive crises. In young children, pain and swelling often occur in the metacarpal and metatarsal areas, where older children and adults usually complain of back and proximal extremity pain. When evaluating a patient with suspected bony vasoocclusive pain, other causes, such as trauma or infection, must be considered. The association between sickle cell anemia and *Salmonella* osteomyelitis is well described, yet *Staphylococci* remain the most common pathogen causing osteomyelitis. Repeated episodes of bony ischemia can lead to aseptic necrosis, particularly in the femoral head (14) and carpal navicular areas, causing persistent pain frequently mistaken for acute vasoocclusion.

Abdominal pain, nausea, and vomiting are common with episodes of vasoocclusion. Local ischemia is thought to be the cause of these symptoms. However, a careful evaluation to rule out other causes of abdominal pain is mandatory in these patients. Because of the persistent hemolysis, sickle cell patients develop calcium bilirubinate gallstones and symptomatic cholelithiasis. In addition, other causes of acute abdominal pain, including pancreatitis, appendicitis, renal colic, and peptic ulcer disease should be considered before concluding that a vasoocclusive event is the sole cause. The presence of active bowel sounds and a lack of high fever or signs of peritonitis favor a nonsurgical etiology. The risk of infectious hepatitis is higher in sickle cell patients because of previous transfusion therapy and an increased incidence of drug abuse. Jaundice does not necessarily indicate liver disease, since it is commonly due to chronic hemolysis.

The pregnant sickle cell patient with abdominal pain poses a diagnostic and therapeutic challenge. Identifying appendicitis or cholecystitis is more difficult because of the anatomic changes associated with pregnancy. Pre-term labor, placental ischemia and abruption, and spontaneous abortion are also more common in sickle cell patients than the general population.

Low-grade fever during a vasoocclusive episode is not uncommon. If the temperature exceeds 38°C, an infectious source should be sought. Viruses probably account for most infections, but because of functional asplenia these patients are at risk for bacteremia, especially with encapsulated organisms such as *Streptococcus pneumoniae* and *Hemophilus influenza*. The functional asplenia of sickle disease is due to auto-infarction of the spleen, which is usually completed by school age in those with homozygous disease. Patients with sickle trait or sickle cell variants generally have normal splenic function and immunity.

The clinical entity known as the acute chest syndrome (ACS) is a leading cause of death in patients with sickle cell disease. Patients with ACS present similarly to those with pneumonia. They have fever, chest pain, cough, and hypoxia, and have new infiltrates on chest x-ray. Although the exact cause is unknown, ACS is thought to be caused by many mechanisms, from infection and fat embolism from infarcted bone, to pulmonary microvascular sludging and infarction. The most common infectious etiologic agents of ACS are *Chlamydia pneumoniae, Mycoplasma pneumoniae,* and respiratory syncytial virus (29).

Chest pain is very common in vasoocclusive events (1,15, 19–21). Sickle cell patients have a higher frequency of hypercoagulable diseases and thrombotic events, including pulmonary embolism and infarction. Thus, pleuritic pain can be due to vasoocclusion (red cell microocclusion) with or without pulmonary infarction (platelet and coagulation protein-based clot) or due to infectious etiology. Low-grade fever, hypoxemia, and leukocytosis are common in vasoocclusive events, pulmonary embolism and pneumonia. The radiographic diagnosis of an infiltrate is difficult because chronic interstitial changes are present in many patients and some new opacities represent atelectasis or infarction. A productive cough, high fever, elevated total and immature neutrophil count, or Gram stain evidence of infection supports the diagnosis of pneumonia. The best clinical indicator of infarction is the absence of these infectious clues and the presence of occlusive symptoms in another area. *Streptococcus pneumoniae* and *Hemophilus influenza* are the most frequent causes of bacterial pneumonia in sickle cell patients (21). It is also important to remember that in adults, chest pain can result from myocardial ischemia.

Focal or generalized neurologic signs and symptoms (including seizures) can follow vasoocclusion in the cerebral circulation, with both small and large vessels affected. Acute retinal ischemia with visual loss and "floaters" from vitreous hemorrhages secondary to vessel disruption are also reported in sickle cell patients.

Priapism is a manifestation of local sequestration and vasoocclusion and may present in all age groups. It often responds to vigorous medical therapy, including hydration, analgesia, local ice packs, or exchange transfusions. In refractory cases, surgical decompression is indicated. Testicular or ovarian ischemia can also result from vasoocclusion, presenting with pain in the affected area. Another complication of vasoocclusion is rhabdomyolysis, which requires aggressive fluid therapy to diminish the risk of acute renal failure.

Most sickle cell and many sickle trait or variant patients are at increased risk for dehydration because of a renal concentrating defect. Chronic renal failure (from repeated infarction and papillary necrosis) is common in sickle disease and may be associated with hypertension.

Besides painful vasoocclusive events, the patient with sickle cell disease is subject to other less common episodic hematologic crises. These are categorized as sequestration, hemolytic, megaloblastic, or aplastic crises. In **sequestration crisis**, acute anemia, hypotension, and even shock occur because of sequestration of RBCs in the spleen. This often follows a viral illness and usually occurs in younger children with SS disease before auto-infarction, or in older patients with sickle cell variants. **Hemolytic crisis** can occur during a fulminant vasoocclusive episode when large numbers of irreversibly sickled cells are lost. Severe anemia with increased reticulocytosis and jaundice is found. Marrow failure, resulting from either **megaloblastic crisis** (often from folate deficiency) or **aplastic crisis,** presents with a falling hematocrit and deficient reticulocytosis.

In addition to the organ ischemia induced by RBC sickling, sickle cell disease patients frequently have enhanced coagulation, leading to arterial and venous thrombotic events. This is due to a variety of procoagulant syndromes seen more often in these patients, including Protein C and S deficiency and circulating antiphospholipid antibodies (31).

EMERGENCY DEPARTMENT EVALUATION

The rapid evaluation and treatment of the sickle cell patient with acute pain is a formidable challenge. Vasoocclusive crises are common and may mask other serious pathology, while other types of sickle crises are less frequent and easily overlooked.

The diagnosis of uncomplicated vasoocclusive event is one of exclusion but common; a dangerous error is to attribute all pain in sickle cell patients to this cause. The initial investigation should seek evidence of an acute infection or other precipitating events. Chest pain can result from acute chest syndrome, pneumonia, pulmonary embolism, pulmonary infarction, or myocardial ischemia; abdominal pain may reflect a surgical emergency. By the third decade of life, many sickle cell patients have undergone cholecystectomy and appendectomy, either because of demonstrable pathology or because abdominal pain during a previous vasoocclusive crisis suggested an acute abdominal emergency. This eases the task of evaluating later episodes of acute abdominal pain by eliminating certain possibilities.

A focused history and examination are the cornerstones of the evaluation of sickle cell patients. Knowledge of the frequency and severity of past pain events and complications, the medication history, and baseline laboratory values are helpful in tailoring the initial evaluation and treatment of patients with acute pain. Especially ominous are any new neurologic signs or symptoms, which may require magnetic resonance imaging (MRI), computed tomography (CT) scanning, transcranial ultrasound, or (rarely) lumbar puncture.

Based primarily on dogma, a complete blood and reticulocyte count (CBC and RC) are commonly ordered in sickle cell patients presenting for ED care. These can help screen for marrow failure (from sickle disease or hydroxyurea therapy), sequestration crisis, or infection. In a clinically uncomplicated vasoocclusive pain event that is similar to previous episodes in patients not treated with hydroxyurea, these tests add little to the clinical management. In other patients, especially those with suspected infection or nonocclusive crisis, the CBC and RC should be obtained.

When interpreting a blood count, a few points must be kept in mind. Most sickle cell patients have a persistent mild leukocytosis and a moderate anemia (hematocrit of 20%–30%, although lower values are seen in some individuals). The total leukocyte count should be adjusted for nucleated RBCs to avoid factitious elevation. Because of ongoing hemolysis and anemia, the reticulocyte count is elevated (usually to 8% or greater) compared to normal subjects. An abrupt drop in the hematocrit suggests a sequestration or hemolytic crisis, while an abnormally low reticulocyte count suggests marrow failure. The erythrocyte sedimentation rate (ESR) is low in most patients with SS disease and is not helpful unless it is extremely elevated (12).

The urine should be screened for evidence of infection or infarction, especially in patients with pelvic or back pain. If symptoms of urinary tract infection are present with pyuria or bacteriuria, a urine culture should be obtained to help guide followup therapy.

Some authors believe that all sickle cell patients with acute pain deserve routine chest radiography to screen for occult infection (21), but data validating this routine practice in low-risk patients is lacking. Clearly, fever, chills, or any pulmonary symptoms or signs suggesting a new abnormality mandate chest radiography, since the difference between acute chest syndrome and pneumonia can be difficult to assess from clinical history and examination alone (15,21). Because of the risk of bacteremia and sepsis, blood cultures should be obtained when there is evidence of pneumonia or pyelonephritis, or when high fever or leukocytosis occurs without an apparent source.

Other tests may have a role, depending on the clinical presentation. An electrocardiogram (ECG) is indicated with chest pain or other symptoms suggestive of myocardial ischemia. Serum electrolytes, blood urea nitrogen (BUN), and creatinine determinations are sometimes helpful to assess hydration and renal function, but are not mandatory in clinically uncomplicated mild to moderate crises. In cases of unexplained abdominal pain, a serum amylase, liver enzymes, abdominal x-rays, gallbladder ultrasound, or computed tomography (CT) scan may be indicated (26). Helical CT or radionuclide tests of the chest can help detect pulmonary embolism in patients where pneumonia or vasoocclusion do not explain the findings. A d-dimer is not usually helpful in these cases due to false-positive results.

In previously undiagnosed cases, a sickle prep and hemoglobin electrophoresis will confirm the diagnosis. Although quantifying fetal hemoglobin levels may aid in assessing long-term prognosis, electrophoresis for this or other reasons is not helpful in the acute management of painful crisis. In those patients with stroke, myocardial ischemia, pulmonary embolism, or other arterial/venous thrombotic findings, a hypercoagulable work up, beginning with prothrombin and partial thromboplastin time tests may help, though these are not needed in other sickle crises.

An assessment of oxygen saturation is important, especially if any pulmonary or chest symptoms or abnormal physical exam findings exist. The pulse oximeter is minimally affected by sickle cell disease (18) and can be used in the absence of other acquired hemoglobin abnormalities; reserving arterial blood analysis for those with a suspected acid-base abnormality, inadequate oximetry signal or severe hypoxemia (as a confirmatory test).

EMERGENCY DEPARTMENT MANAGEMENT

In unstable patients, airway stabilization and circulatory assistance are the primary immediate concern. Otherwise, routine emergency department management can proceed after starting an appropriate diagnostic work up. Treatment is usually supportive, since definitive treatment of crisis based on the underlying pathophysiology is still lacking. Often the best treatment is rehydration and analgesia, with oral regimens preferred whenever possible (1,5,30).

The choice of fluids is controversial; those with orthostasis or hypotension should receive isotonic saline initially. However, in the absence of significant volume depletion, hypotonic fluids have theoretical benefits. Experimentally induced hyponatremia decreases the mean corpuscular hemoglobin concentration and interferes with gelation of hemoglobin S. In one trial, desmopressin (DDAVP) combined with a diuretic and a low-sodium diet induced hyponatremia and decreased the frequency and duration of painful events (24). In spite of these investigations, there are no clinical data to support routine parenteral hypotonic solutions in vasoocclusive crises. Outside of the United States, oral regimens are often used successfully. Irrespective of the fluid chosen, the physician must pay attention to the total volume administered to avoid iatrogenic pulmonary edema (12).

Traditionally, all sickle cell patients received supplemental oxygen during painful crises. Although oxygen reverses some sickling *in vitro*, it has never been shown to affect the incidence, duration, or severity of clinical vasoocclusive events. Oxygen can depress erythropoietin levels and reticulocytosis, potentially interfering with a natural compensatory response and paradoxically increasing the number of irreversibly sickled cells (4). Currently, there are no clinical data supporting or refuting the routine use of oxygen, although pragmatism suggests that those with clinically important hypoxemia are most likely to benefit. The latter threshold has not been defined rigorously, though oxygen saturation of <85% or a drop of >5% from known baseline is often used to initiate therapy.

Achieving adequate pain control in vasoocclusive events is challenging (13). By late adolescence, many patients with sickle disease require opioid analgesics to gain relief. Complicating the management of these patients are physician and nursing fears of drug abuse and secondary gain. Subjectively reported pain is generally the only tool available to measure discomfort; it is not possible to reliably identify "feigned" pain on clinical grounds. Optimal treatment of vasoocclusive pain is based on multifaceted, inexpensive regimens that offer the best chance of timely relief with a minimum of complications. Additionally, the patient must be educated to actively participate in the process of pain relief rather than reinforcing a passive "lie there and we'll take care of it" approach. This means a frank discussion about the goals of therapy (pain relief, albeit not always immediate pain extinction, without harm) and the need for nonpharmacologic adjuncts including counseling and behavior modification. The goals of pain management in sickle cell disease and metastatic cancer are analogous, since both are terminal diseases (3). Analgesia must be titrated to need rather than to arbitrary ceiling doses, using regimens that rapidly achieve and sustain effective levels of therapeutic agents.

Oral analgesics are the mainstays for most patients with mild to moderate pain, with parenteral regimens reserved for those who cannot tolerate oral agents or are in severe pain. Aside from young children, most patients presenting for care in the United States receive opioids in addition to hydration and ac-

etaminophen. Since the pain of vasoocclusion is incited by ischemia, the analgesic effects of NSAIDs are less prominent than in other syndromes where prostaglandin excess is the major biochemical trigger (e.g., inflammatory or postoperative pain) (33). Additionally, the risk of renal failure may be higher than in non-sickle cell patients due to the renal arterial ischemia frequently present (10); given this, NSAIDs are best avoided in these patients.

Hydrocodone, oxycodone, morphine, and hydromorphone are good choices of an opioid for those with refractory or more intense pain who can tolerate oral therapy. Other agents that have been found to be useful in the management of other chronic pain syndromes (e.g., antidepressants or phenothiazines) have been suggested for sickle cell pain, but their effectiveness is not supported by controlled trials.

For those who require parenteral therapy, there is no ideal opioid. The key is choosing an adequate dose and dosing regimen based on individual patient response; the ceiling dose is whatever relieves pain or causes side effects. Intravenous regimens (either by repeated injections, continuous infusion, or patient-controlled administration) offer ease of titration, rapid analgesia, and less risk of side effects (7). Intramuscular injections should be reserved for selected cases when oral therapy is impractical and venous access unobtainable.

Meperidine is commonly used for sickle cell-related pain events but has some disadvantages, primarily related to its short duration of action and the accumulation of toxic metabolites, which can cause seizures. Morphine is inexpensive, but it is short-acting and frequently causes nausea, requiring the use of antiemetic agents. In patients who are not on outpatient opioid therapy, a mixed or partial opioid agonist (e.g., butorphanol, pentazocine, nalbuphine, or buprenorphine) offers analgesia with less euphoria and a ceiling on respiratory depression. For others, a longer-acting opioid agonist (e.g., hydromorphone) may be an ideal choice.

A minority of sickle cell patients are deliberate opioid abusers. This has led some centers to initiate "contracts" with their patients in an effort to limit abuse while ensuring prompt and humane treatment when a painful crisis occurs. Often, the patient agrees in writing to take oral opioids only for severe pain and to contact a designated physician or emergency department during a crisis. The patient also agrees to not seek alternate opioid sources. This provides adequate care while limiting the total amount of opioid prescribed over a specified period.

For documented or suspected bacterial infections, a broad-spectrum antibiotic should be administered early while awaiting culture results. Sickle cell patients should take folic acid supplements daily to avoid megaloblastic crisis.

Transfusion therapy is indicated in selected sickle syndromes. In patients with priapism or aplastic, sequestration, or hemolytic crisis, exchange transfusion is preferable to simple transfusion since it avoids the risk of iron overload and is generally more effective. With CNS vasoocclusion, exchange transfusion can reverse some neurologic symptoms and lower the incidence of recurrence (9). Prophylactic transfusion is best reserved for patients requiring immediate surgery and those in impending or active labor. Anemia alone is not an indication for emergency transfusion in the absence of signs or symptoms of deficient oxygen delivery to the heart or brain.

Several new approaches to the treatment of SS disease are currently under evaluation. Hydroxyurea (HU) disrupts RBC endothelial adhesion, enhances Hemoglobin F production, promotes the formation of hemoglobin S polymers, may mediate nitric oxide release (see below) and can diminish the frequency and severity of crises (8,23,27). The long-term safety of this treatment is still not completely defined, with marrow failure a limiting side effect, as well as the drug having potential mutagenic and carcinogenic properties. It may also cause nausea, vomiting, and skin rashes. A recent long-term observational followup study of adult patients documented that patients taking HU actually decreased mortality (28). Other methods to alter hemoglobin production, through gene manipulation, a combination of HU and recombinant erythropoietin, or a combination of HU and L-Arginine therapy show promise in reducing clinical vasoocclusive crisis frequency (16,23). Bone marrow transplant remains the only curative therapy for sickle cell to date.

High dose corticosteroids (dexamethasone 0.3 mg/kg every 12 hours for 3 doses) may augment inpatient analgesic regimens in children and adolescents with sickle crisis, especially the acute chest syndrome (2,6). The mechanism and true effect of this therapy are debated, and the lack of data confirming utility in the initial treatment in acute sickle crisis makes routine use of corticosteroids speculative currently.

Purified poloxamer 188 is a nonionic surfactant with antithrombotic properties. It is thought to improve microvascular blood flow and reduce whole blood viscosity, diminish erythrocyte aggregation, and limit erythrocyte adhesion to the vascular endothelium. It is administered as an intravenous infusion, and under investigational use has shown some promise, especially in patients receiving concomitant HU. It is an investigational agent currently to try to shorten the duration of acute vasoocclusive events (17).

Inhaled nitric oxide has been shown to increase the oxygen affinity of Hemoglobin S in humans both *in vivo* and *in vitro*. Therapeutic inhalation is thought to exert direct effect on the pulmonary vasculature to increase oxygenation through diminished shunting and reduce pulmonary hypertension (22). Clinical experience is limited, and its long-term efficacy and toxicity are unknown. It has been found to provide pain relief, especially with chest syndromes, together with standard therapies but remains investigational.

CRITICAL INTERVENTIONS

- Seek evidence of an acute infection or other precipitating events for patients with vasoocclusive events
- Rehydrate patients with sickle cell crisis using oral regimens rather than parenteral fluids if possible
- Initiate broad-spectrum antibiotic for documented or suspected bacterial infections

DISPOSITION

Patients with uncomplicated painful crises who are adequately hydrated and obtain sufficient pain relief in the emergency department can be discharged with close follow up. There is no absolute rule to determine how long an "adequate" analgesia and hydration trial in the ED should be, since individual patients, physicians, and local resources vary. If pain relief is obtained in uncomplicated vasoocclusive events, oral analgesics should be prescribed for 3 to 5 days to treat milder recurrence, a common phenomenon. Each patient should be encouraged to obtain further care from the same institution or a single physician (or group) to ensure continuity.

The inability to control pain is the most common indication for admission in adults. Patients with proven or suspected sequestration, aplastic, or hemolytic crisis require admission. The presence of any new neurologic sign or symptom, priapism, or an acute abdomen also mandates hospitalization.

In general, the presence of an invasive bacterial infection mandates admission, since it is largely through the aggressive treatment of infections that the life expectancy for SS patients has been increased. Two groups of patients may be discharged home with treatment if close outpatient follow up within 24 hours can be arranged–adults with a minor pharyngeal or respiratory tract infection; and nontoxic appearing children (age 6 months to 12 years) with fever less than 40°C; no clinical evidence of pneumonia or pyelonephritis, and a leukocyte count between 5,000 and 30,000 (32). In the latter group, blood cultures should be obtained to screen for bacteremia, and ceftriaxone (50 mg/kg IM) or a similar oral regimen should be given before discharge. Besides these specific instances, admission is indicated for patients with fever, unexplained leukocytosis (especially with immature forms), or uncertain compliance with followup schedules.

Since continuity of care is especially important in sickle cell disease, the patient's primary physician should be contacted during the emergency department visit. Consultation with the internal medicine or hematology service is advisable for routine admissions, with other subspecialist consultation obtained as needed.

Finally, patients should be counseled to avoid any sympathomimetic drugs (including over the counter decongestants and illicit cocaine) and alcohol (which may suppress a stressed marrow). Pneumococcal and influenza vaccines can be offered or made available in follow up, along with potential long-term oral penicillin prophylaxis for those with frequent bacterial infections.

COMMON PITFALLS

✔ Do not assume that abdominal pain is due to a vasoocclusive event without considering other causes, especially surgical pathology

✔ It is easy to overdiagnose pneumonia in sickle cell patients, but underdiagnosis can be fatal. Since an acute infiltrate often represents an infarct rather than infection, other signs and symptoms of pneumonia should be sought. It is prudent to err on the side of caution and begin antibiotic therapy if uncertainty exists

✔ Some complications of sickle disease are mistaken for "crisis" pain (e.g., osteomyelitis, aseptic necrosis of bone)

✔ Although transfusions are ordered too frequently and unnecessarily, exchange transfusion therapy is often not started early enough in the setting of neurologic changes or priapism

✔ Do not undertreat pain, but do not seek 'zero' pain in all. The goal is not necessarily complete relief, but rather, a clear path toward relief to be completed as either an inpatient or outpatient. Nontraditional destinations, like observation units or other outpatient centers, can add to the disposition options when no complications exist. Make the patient an active part of the analgesic plan, not a passive recipient

✔ Abuse concerns are common in patients with sickle cell pain events who access the ED, though often not possible to validate. Give those with pain 'the benefit of the doubt' while being prudent with the total number of doses (if being prescribed as an outpatient). In those with frequent visits, developing a clear plan to be used by all ED providers and having the patient enter into a written treatment contract with their primary care providers can ease concerns

✔ Educate sickle cell patients about avoiding triggers, maintaining hydration, and early, self-titrated analgesia to limit the need for recurrent ED visits

Acknowledgment

We would like to thank the previous edition's chapter author Larry D. Weiss.

References

1. Athanasou NA, Hatton C, McGee JO, et al. Vascular occlusion and infarction in sickle cell crisis and the sickle chest syndrome. *J Clin Pathol* 1985;38:659.
2. Bernini JC, Rogers ZR, Sandler ES, et al. Beneficial effect of intravenous dexamethasone in children with mild to moderate severe acute chest syndrome complicating sickle cell disease. *Blood* 1998;92:3082.
3. Brookoff D, Polomano R. Treating sickle cell pain like cancer pain. *Ann Int Med* 1992;116:364.
4. Embury SH, Garcia JF, Mohandas N, et al. Effects of oxygen inhalation on endogenous erythropoietin kinetics, erythropoiesis, and properties of blood cells in sickle cell anemia. *New Eng J Med* 1984;311:291.
5. Friedman EW, Webber AB, Osborn HH, et al. Oral analgesia for treatment of painful crisis in sickle cell anemia. *Ann Emerg Med* 1986;15:787.
6. Griffin TC, McIntire D, Buchanan GR. High-dose intravenous methylprednisolone therapy for pain in children and adolescents with sickle cell disease. *New Engl J Med* 1994;330:733.
7. Gonzalez ER, Bahal N, Hansen LA, et al. Intermittent injection vs. patient-controlled analgesia for sickle cell crisis pain. Comparison of patients in the emergency department. *Arch Intern Med* 1991;151:1373.
8. Halsey C, Roberts IA. The role of hydroxyurea in sickle cell disease. *Br J Haematol* 2003;120:177.
9. Haruda F, Friedman JH, Ganti SR, et al. Rapid resolution of organic mental syndrome in sickle cell anemia in response to exchange transfusion. *Neurology* 1981;31:1015.
10. Hardwick WE, Givens TG, Monroe KW, et al. Effect of ketorolac in pediatric sickle vaso-occlusive pain crisis. *Pediatric Emerg Care* 1999;15:179.
11. Haynes J, Allison RC. Pulmonary edema: Complication in the management of sickle cell pain crisis. *Amer J Med* 1986;80:833.
12. Lawrence C, Fabry ME. Erythrocyte sedimentation rate during steady state and painful crisis in sickle cell anemia. *Amer J Med* 1986;81:801.
13. Maxwell K, Streetly A, Bevan D. Experiences of hospital care and treatment seeking for pain from sickle cell disease: A qualitative study. *BMJ* 1999;318:1585.
14. Milner PF, Kraus AP, Sebes JI, et al. Sickle cell disease as a cause of osteonecrosis of the femoral head. *N Engl J Med* 1991;325:1476.
15. Morris C, Vichinsky E, Styles L. Clinician assessment for acute chest syndrome in febrile patients with sickle cell disease: Is it accurate enough? *Ann Emerg Med* 1999;34:64.
16. Morris CR, et al. Hydroxyurea and arginine therapy: Impact on nitric oxide production in sickle cell disease. *J Pediatr Hematol Oncol* 2003;25:629.
17. Orringer EP, et al. Purified poloxamer 188 for treatment of acute vaso-occlusive crisis of sickle cell disease. *JAMA* 2001;286:2099.
18. Ortiz FO, Aldrich TK, Nagel RL, Benjamin LJ. Accuracy of pulse oximetry in sickle cell disease. *Am J Respir Crit Care Med* 1999;159:447.
19. Platt OS, Brambilla DJ, Rosse WF, et al. Mortality in sickle cell disease. Life expectancy and risk factors for early death. *New Engl J Med* 1994;330:1639.
20. Platt OS, Thorington BD, Brambilla DJ, et al. Pain in sickle cell disease. Rates and risk factors. *N Engl J Med* 1991;325:11.
21. Pollack CV, Jorden RC, Kolb JC. Usefulness of empiric chest radiography and urinalysis testing in adults with acute sickle cell pain crisis. *Ann Emerg Med* 1991;20:1210.
22. Reiter CD, Gladwin, MT. An emerging role for nitric oxide in sickle cell disease vascular homeostasis and therapy. *Curr Opin Hematol* 2003;10:99.
23. Rodgers GP, Dover GJ, Uyesaka N, et al. Augmentation by erythropoietin of the fetal-hemoglobin response to hydroxyurea in sickle cell disease. *N Engl J Med* 1993;328:73.
24. Rosa RM, Bierer BE, Thomas R, et al. A study of induced hyponatremia in the prevention and treatment of sickle cell crisis. *New Engl J Med* 1980;303:1138.
25. Schaller S, Kaplan BS. Acute nonoliguric renal failure in children associated with nonsteriodal antiinflammatory agents. *Pediatr Emerg Care* 1998;14:416.
26. Serafini AN, Spolianski G, Skafianakis GN, et al. Diagnostic studies in patients with sickle cell anemia and acute abdominal pain. *Arch Intern Med* 1987;147:1061.
27. Steinberg MH. Management of sickle cell disease. *N Engl J Med* 1999;340:1021.
28. Steinberg MH, et al. Effect of hydroxyurea on mortality and morbidity in adult sickle cell anemia. *JAMA* 2003;289:1645.
29. Vichinsky EP, et al. Causes and outcomes of the acute chest syndrome in sickle cell disease. *N Engl J Med* 2000;342:1855.
30. Ware MA, Hambleton I, Ochaya I, Serjeant GR. Day-care management of sickle cell painful crisis in Jamaica: A model applicable elsewhere? *Br J Haematol* 1999;104:93.
31. Westerman MP, Green D, Gilman-Sachs A, et al. Antiphospholipid antibodies, protein C and S, and coagulation changes in sickle cell disease. *J Lab Clin Med* 1999;134:352.
32. Williams JA, Flynn PM, Harris S, et al. A randomized study of outpatient treatment with ceftriaxone for selected febrile children with sickle cell disease. *N Engl J Med* 1993;329:472.
33. Wright SW, Norris RL, Mitchell TR. Ketorolac for sickle cell vaso-occlusive crisis pain in the emergency department: Lack of a narcotic sparing effect. *Ann Emerg Med* 1992;21:925.

CHAPTER 155
Anemia

Louis S. Binder and George S. Kim

Anemia is defined as a decrease in the number of circulating red blood cells, with a concomitant decrease in the capacity of the blood to carry oxygen to tissues. Anemia is a manifestation of disease rather than a diagnostic entity in and of itself.

Anemia can be classified into disorders of decreased red cell production, disorders of increased red cell destruction, and anemia resulting from blood loss (10,15). Each of these diagnostic groups has its own clinical presentation and differential diagnosis (Table 155.1) and, in general, requires its own approach to emergency department evaluation and management.

Anemia of any cause may present acutely or chronically, and the aggressiveness of intervention and management depends on the acuteness of onset and on the severity of the clinical presentation. For example, anemia secondary to acute gastrointestinal blood loss may require vigorous fluid resuscitation, transfusion therapy, and intensive care management; anemia secondary to chronic occult gastrointestinal bleeding leads to a well-compensated iron deficiency anemia that can be evaluated and treated on an outpatient basis (16).

Defective red blood cell production may be caused by interruption in the availability or synthesis of any of the three moieties of the hemoglobin molecule: iron, heme, and globin. Hence, anemia may result from iron deficiency, from toxins or enzymatic deficits that interfere with heme synthesis, or from genetic defects in globin synthesis. Disorders and deficiencies that affect the proliferation of erythroid stem cells in the bone marrow may also result in anemia from decreased red cell production (12,18).

Red cell destruction may result from either intrinsic or extrinsic causes. Intrinsic abnormalities of hemoglobin, enzymes, or red cell membranes may result in hemolytic anemia (18). Extrinsic destruction may be due to immunologic, mechanical, or environmental causes, or to hypersequestration (hypersplenism) (10,15,18).

Blood loss resulting in anemia may be acute or chronic and may originate from intraperitoneal, retroperitoneal, pelvic, pleural, gynecologic, or gastrointestinal sources (15).

CLINICAL PRESENTATION

Patients with anemia secondary to acute blood loss present with hypovolemia. A source of blood loss may be readily identifiable on clinical evaluation; menstrual blood loss and losses from the gastrointestinal tract are the most common sources for occult bleeding if the locus is unclear (8). A history of underlying disease (e.g., cirrhosis, bleeding diathesis, malignancy, or infection) or of medication use (e.g., use of salicylates, nonsteroidal antiinflammatory drugs, or anticoagulants) may be useful in guiding initial evaluation and management. Hypovolemia may be relatively well tolerated in the young patient without underlying disease, but can be a significant stress to elderly or chronically ill individuals whose compensatory mechanisms may be overwhelmed and whose tissue perfusion may be marginal at baseline (1,13).

TABLE 155.1. Differential Diagnosis of Anemia (9)

ANEMIA SECONDARY TO BLOOD LOSS (ACUTE OR CHRONIC)

Intraperitoneal
Retroperitoneal
Pelvic
Urinary tract
Gastrointestinal tract
Gynecologic (vaginal bleeding, placenta previa, abruption)
Epistaxis
Hemoptysis
External bleeding
Drug-related (coumadin, heparin)
Traumatic

ANEMIA SECONDARY TO DECREASED RBC PRODUCTION
(Insidious-Onset, Decreased Reticulocyte Count)

Hypochromic/Microcytic
Iron deficiency
Thalassemia
Sideroblastic (including lead)
Chronic disease (infection, chronic inflammation, neoplasm,
    diabetes, liver failure, uremia, thyroid disease)

Macrocytic
Hypothyroidism
Folic acid deficiency
Chemotherapy, radiotherapy, immunosuppressive therapy
Liver disease
Vitamin B_{12} deficiency
Scurvy

Normocytic
Primary bone marrow disorder (aplastic anemia, myeloid metaplasia,
    myelofibrosis, myelophthistic anemia)
Secondary bone marrow disease (endocrinopathy, uremia, chronic
    inflammation, liver disease, ethanol ingestion)

ANEMIA SECONDARY TO INCREASED RBC DESTRUCTION
(Increased Reticulocyte Count, Free Hemoglobin, RBC Fragmentation)

Intrinsic
Enzyme defect (G6PD, pyruvate kinase)
Membrane abnormality (spherocytosis, elliptocytosis, spur cell,
    paroxysmal nocturnal hemoglobinuria)
Hemoglobin abnormality (hemoglobinopathy, thalassemia)

Extrinsic
Immunologic (alloantibody, autoantibody, cold agglutinins, e.g.,
    mononucleosis)
Neoplastic (especially leukemia, lymphoma)
Collagen vascular (lupus, rheumatoid arthritis, periarteritis nodosa)
Infections (mycoplasma, syphilis, malaria, bartonella, viral)
Other (thyroid disease, ulcerative colitis)
Mechanical (microangiopathic hemolytic anemia, prosthetic valve)
Abnormal sequestration (hypersplenism)
Environmental (drugs, toxins, hyperthermia, drowning)

Patients with anemia secondary to chronic blood loss or to decreased red cell production often present with progressive fatigue, malaise, and a "washed-out" feeling. Dizziness, dyspnea on exertion, decreased exercise tolerance, or exacerbation of congestive heart failure may also be prominent symptoms. Gastrointestinal symptoms such as anorexia or nausea may reflect compensatory hypoperfusion of the splanchnic bed. Patients with asymptomatic underlying atherosclerotic vascular disease may present with angina pectoris, claudication, syncope, or focal neurologic deficits when decreased oxygen-carrying capacity is superimposed on local ischemia from vascular lesions. Other important historic information includes ethnicity and family history (predisposition to certain hemoglobinopathies and pernicious anemia), drug use, dietary history, use of ethanol, recent hospitalization (anemia of chronic disease is common in hospitalized patients), and history of underlying disease (renal, hepatic, thyroid, collagen vascular, or neoplastic disease; previous anemia; or recurrent jaundice) (1,3,4,7,8,10,11, 15,17).

Pallor of the skin or mucous membranes is the cardinal sign of anemia, although it may be difficult to ascertain in some patients. Jaundice is suggestive of a hemolytic process. Tachycardia with a wide pulse pressure and hyperdynamic precordium (reflecting increased cardiac output) and a systolic ejection murmur may be present (10,14).

Petechia and purpura may indicate a concomitant thrombocytopenia. Signs of chronic disease (rheumatologic, endocrine, hepatic, or neoplastic disease) manifest as lymphadenopathy, rash, thyromegaly, myxedema, or the stigmata of liver failure (1,6,14). Hepatosplenomegaly may suggest underlying disease or extramedullary hematopoiesis (15).

Other signs may suggest specific causes of anemia. Vitamin B_{12} deficiency affects exfoliating cell populations and demyelination of the dorsal columns, resulting in atrophy and tenderness of mucous membranes (particularly glossitis) and stocking–glove anesthesia of the distal lower extremities with impaired position and vibratory sense (11,12).

The symptoms, signs, and laboratory findings of anemia may be the initial presenting manifestations of pancytopenia (10). The etiology of pancytopenia is multifactorial. Pancytopenia is most commonly idiopathic (50%), but may result from chemical and physical agents, autoimmunity, or vitamin B_{12} or folic acid deficiency. Pancytopenia may follow viral illness, including upper respiratory infection, hepatitis, Epstein-Barr infection, and human immunodeficiency virus infection (4,10). It may also be associated with hypersplenism, myelodysplasia, bone marrow failure, or marrow replacement (15). Clinically, pancytopenia may present as a viral illness, preceding the symptomatic presentation of anemia over several weeks, or as an insidious presentation of anemia with clinical evidence of thrombocytopenia (petechia, purpura, or mucous membrane bleeding) (10).

Patients with anemia secondary to acute hemolysis are likely to present with signs and symptoms similar to those seen with mild chronic anemia. In more severe presentations, there may be jaundice and dark urine. Fever, prostration, abdominal and back pain, and hemoglobinuria suggest acute intravascular hemolysis, similar to that associated with transfusion reaction (10,18). A family history of anemia suggests an intrinsic cause of hemolysis, whereas exposure to drugs or toxins suggests an extrinsic cause (10,15). Immunologic destruction of red blood cells may be due to autoantibodies (18). Mechanical destruction is seen in some patients with prosthetic heart valves (15). Disseminated intravascular coagulation leading to microangiopathic hemolytic anemia is suggested by diffuse bleeding (14). A finding of hepatosplenomegaly may suggest either sequestration or an autoimmune process (10,15).

DIFFERENTIAL DIAGNOSIS

A complete differential diagnosis is presented in Table 155.1.

EMERGENCY DEPARTMENT EVALUATION

After anemia is identified by a complete blood count or hematocrit determination in the emergency department, further laboratory evaluation includes the measurement of red blood cell indices and reticulocyte count. Examination of a peripheral smear may show heterogeneity of cells, evidence of hemolysis, basophilic stippling, ringed sideroblasts, or hypersegmented leukocytes (10,15). Additional diagnostic tests are normally neither necessary nor available in the emergency department. However, serum iron, total iron-binding capacity (TIBC), and serum ferritin determinations should be considered in hypochromic, microcytic anemia; folate and vitamin B_{12} levels, liver function tests, and thyroid function tests in macrocytic anemia; and direct and indirect Coombs' tests, fractionated serum bilirubin count, and plasma and urine tests for free hemoglobin in hemolytic anemia (1,4,10,15,18). Inpatient evaluation may include further laboratory evaluation for specific disease and a bone marrow biopsy for evaluation of any unexplained anemia or pancytopenia (1,7,10,12,15).

Potential diagnostic errors of importance include the following:

1. Not suspecting acute blood loss and impending hypovolemic shock with any unexplained normocytic normochromic anemia
2. Confusing anemia with other entities that also cause constitutional symptoms (e.g., uremia, collagen vascular disease, fluid and electrolyte imbalance, infections, drug effects)
3. Confusing iron deficiency anemia, which presents with low iron, increased TIBC, and low ferritin, with anemia of chronic disease, which presents with low iron, low TIBC, and normal ferritin associated with a chronic disease or recent hospitalization (1,10,15)
4. Confusing hemolytic anemia with other entities that also cause acute jaundice (particularly acute hepatitis)
5. Overlooking pancytopenia by focusing on a clinical picture of anemia and low hemoglobin, while neglecting findings of leukopenia and thrombocytopenia

EMERGENCY DEPARTMENT MANAGEMENT

The need for rapid intervention in both prehospital and emergency department patients is limited to identifying and treating hypovolemic shock. For certain anemic patients, treatment is best begun in the emergency department without waiting for definitive outpatient evaluation. Anemia of pregnancy is treated with prenatal vitamins (one daily) and iron replacement (ferrous sulfate 325 mg three times per day), and hypochromic microcytic anemia associated with an identified source of blood loss (presumed to be due to iron deficiency anemia) is treated similarly, with iron replacement therapy (1,5,16). These patients should be reevaluated after 4 to 6 weeks to assess the adequacy of the therapeutic response (1,16). A reticulocyte count may be checked after a few days of therapy if more immediate confirmation of a therapeutic response is desired (9).

In megaloblastic anemia presumed to be due to folic acid or vitamin B_{12} deficiency, treatment may be initiated with 1 mg/d of oral folic acid or with 100 μg/d of cobalamin parenterally for 1 week, after specimens for serum vitamin B_{12} and folic acid levels are drawn and follow up is arranged (1,4,9,11,12). In mild or asymptomatic anemia of chronic disease, therapy is generally directed to control the underlying disease (15). For severe or symptomatic anemia, however, consultation and, usually, hospital admission are advisable.

In many cases of newly identified anemia, drug therapy and other interventions including the use of erythropoietin have been shown to be beneficial but are frequently not indicated in the emergency department setting, and patients are referred to a consultant for further evaluation and management (3,4,7,8,16).

CRITICAL INTERVENTIONS

- For hypochromic, microcytic anemia, order serum iron, total iron-binding capacity (TIBC), and serum ferritin
- For macrocytic anemia, order folate and vitamin B_{12} levels, liver function tests, and thyroid function tests
- For hemolytic anemia, order direct and indirect Coombs' tests, fractionated serum bilirubin count, and plasma and urine tests for free hemoglobin

DISPOSITION

Consultation or referral for follow up, in most cases, is to the patient's primary care physician. Most anemic patients have iron deficiency anemia, vitamin B_{12} or folic acid deficiency anemia, or anemia of pregnancy; these cases can be treated and followed up on an outpatient basis.

Urgent consultation and hospital admission should be sought for the following indications (1,9,15):

1. Hypovolemia or ongoing bleeding
2. Need for urgent transfusion, generally because of a hemoglobin level less than 9 g/dL in a bleeding or symptomatic patient (2)
3. Severe symptoms (e.g., chest pain, dyspnea, syncope) that impair the patient's ability to function at home
4. Pancytopenia requiring diagnostic evaluation (4,10)
5. Anticipated need for extensive diagnostic or therapeutic intervention

Unless active bleeding is present or the patient is hemodynamically unstable, there is usually no contraindication to routine transfer for specialized evaluation.

COMMON PITFALLS

✔ Failure to suspect and identify bleeding and hypovolemia
✔ Failure to appreciate the possibility of anemia from the clinical presentation, and, hence, not ordering a hemoglobin or hematocrit determination. This is especially likely in hemolytic anemia or when chest pain, dyspnea, dizziness, or claudication is the presenting complaint
✔ Failure to ensure referral or appropriate follow up for evaluation of therapeutic response or the need for additional diagnostic testing

References

1. Balducci L. Epidemiology of anemia in the elderly: information on the diagnostic evaluation. *J Am Geriatr Soc* 2003;51:2–9.
2. Bratton S, Annich G. Packed red blood cell transfusions for critically ill pediatric patients: When and for what conditions? *J Pediatr* 2003;142:95–97.
3. Cella D, Dobrez D, Glaspy J. Control of cancer related anemia with erythropoietic agents: a review of evidence for improved quality of life and clinical outcomes. *Ann Oncol* 2003;14:511–519.
4. Claster S. Biology of anemia, differential diagnosis, and treatment options in human immunodeficiency virus infection. *J Infect Dis* 2002;185:105–109.
5. Cogswell M, Parvanta I, Ickes L, et al. Iron supplementation during pregnancy, anemia, and birth weight: a randomized controlled trial. *Am J Clin Nutr* 2003;78:773–781.
6. Ershler W. Biological Interactions of Aging and Anemia: A Focus on Cytokines. *J Am Geriatr Soc* 2003;51:18–21.
7. Furuland H, Linde T, Ahlmen J, et al. A randomized controlled trial of hemoglobin normalization with epoetin alfa in pre-dialysis and dialysis patients. *Nephrology Dialysis Transplantation* 2003;18:353–361.
8. Groopman J, Itri L. Chemotherapy-Induced Anemia in Adults: Incidence and Treatment. *Journal of the National Cancer Institute* 1999;91:1616–1634.
9. Hamilton GC, Braen GR. Anemia and white blood cell disorders. In: Rosen P, Barkin RM, Braen GR, et al., eds. *Emergency medicine: concepts and clinical practice*, 5th ed. St. Louis: Mosby, 2002:1665.

10. Hermiston M, Mentzer W. A Practical Approach to the Evaluation of the Anemic Child. *Pediatr Clin North Am* 2002;49:877–891.
11. Lane L, Rojas-Fernandez C. Treatment of Vitamin B$_{12}$-deficiency anemia: oral versus parenteral therapy. *Ann Pharmacotherapy* 2002;36:1268–1272.
12. Oh R, Brown D. Vitamin B$_{12}$ Deficiency. *Am Fam Phys* 2003;67:979–986.
13. Robinson B. Cost of Anemia in the Elderly. *J Am Geriatr Soc* 2003;51:14–17.
14. Sadowitz P, Amanullah S, Souid A. Hematologic emergencies in the pediatric emergency room. *Emerg Med Clin North Am* 2002;20:177–198.
15. Schnall S, Berliner N, Duffy T, et al. Approach to the Adult and Child with Anemia. In: Hoffman R, Banz J, Shattil S, et al, eds. *Hematology: basic principles and practice*, 3rd ed. Orlando: Churchill Livingstone, 2000:368.
16. Sifakis S. Anemia in Pregnancy. *Ann New York Acad Sci* 2000;900:125–136.
17. Turner R, Anglin P, Burkes R, et al. Epoietin Alfa in Cancer Patients: Evidence-Based Guidelines. *J Pain & Symptom Management* 2001;22:954–965.
18. Trivedi D, Bussel J. Immunohematologic disorders. *J Allerg and Clin Immunol* 2003;111:669–676.

CHAPTER 156
Transfusion Reactions and Complications

Gregory W. Hendey

Each year approximately 29 million units of blood components are transfused to patients in the United States (1). The incidence of transfusion reactions is estimated to be only 1%, and the majority of reactions are simple febrile or minor allergic reactions (17). The exceptionally low rate of serious transfusion reactions is mainly due to strict adherence to blood-banking techniques, careful transfusion practices, and extensive testing of donated units.

Life-threatening reactions occur rarely, but it is critical that physicians recognize them quickly and respond appropriately in order to avert a disastrous outcome. Transfusion reactions may be divided by severity and time of onset (Table 156.1).

CLINICAL PRESENTATION

Acute, Severe Reactions

Acute Hemolysis

One of the most serious (and most preventable) blood transfusion reactions is acute hemolysis caused by incompatibility between recipient and donor ABO blood groups. The incidence is between one in 250,000 and one in 1 million PRBC units transfused (7). The resulting IgM–antigen complex fixes complement, leading to rapid intravascular hemolysis, with massive release of hemoglobin, acute renal failure, disseminated intravascular coagulopathy (DIC), and cardiovascular collapse.

The most common cause is simple clerical error—the wrong unit is given to the wrong patient. For that reason, painstaking efforts must be taken to double-check every step in the identification process prior to a transfusion.

The clinical signs of an acute hemolytic reaction are usually not subtle in patients that are awake but may be difficult to recognize quickly in unconscious, intubated patients. In an acute reaction, patients experience a rapid onset of fever, chills, back pain, vomiting, tachycardia, and hypotension.

Anaphylaxis

Anaphylaxis is, fortunately, rare during a blood transfusion, but when it does occur, it is most often in IgA-deficient individuals who react to the IgA present in the transfused unit. The incidence has been estimated to be between one in 20,000 and one in 150,000 transfusions (15,17). Unfortunately, these reactions cannot be reliably predicted, even by testing for the presence of IgA antibody in the patient's serum (15).

The onset is generally within the first minutes of transfusion and may present as sudden flushing, pruritus, laryngospasm, bronchospasm, and hypotension.

Sepsis

Another potentially fatal transfusion reaction occurs when a contaminated blood product is transfused. This is a rare event with PRBC transfusions, with reported bacteremia in approximately one per 5 million units transfused (11). The risk is higher, however, in platelet transfusions (approximately one in 100,000 units) because they are stored at room temperature to maintain platelet activity (3,7,11). Single-donor apheresis platelet units carry a slightly lower risk for bacterial contamination than do random-donor pooled platelets, as do fresher units with less storage time (3,7,11). Many bacteria have been implicated in platelet transfusions, including *Staphylococcus aureus* and gram negatives, and the mortality has been reported at 26% (7,11). The most common agent in PRBC units is *Yersinia enterocolitica*, which grows well under refrigerated conditions (3,7).

When the contaminated unit is transfused, it may produce the acute onset of a sepsis syndrome, with fever, chills, and hypotension. A septic reaction, especially when caused by a

---

TABLE 156.1. Blood Transfusion Reactions and Complications

ACUTE, SEVERE REACTIONS

Acute hemolysis
Anaphylaxis
Septic
Transfusion-related acute lung injury
Congestive heart failure

ACUTE, MINOR REACTIONS

Simple febrile
Allergic

DELAYED REACTIONS

Delayed hemolysis
Graft-versus-host disease
Hepatitis
HIV
CMV
Other infections: Epstein-Barr virus, Cytomegalovirus, Syphilis, Trypanosomiasis, Babesiosis, Malaria, Toxoplasmosis, Brucellosis, West Nile Virus

MASSIVE TRANSFUSION

Coagulopathy
Hypothermia
Hypocalcemia (Citrate toxicity)
Hyperkalemia
Lactic acidosis

gram-negative organism, could easily be confused with the early stages of hemolytic or anaphylactic reactions in the early stages.

Transfusion-Related Acute Lung Injury

Transfusion-related acute lung injury (TRALI) is a noncardiogenic pulmonary edema occurring unpredictably in one in 5,000 to one in 10,000 units of PRBC transfused (7,17). Antileukocyte antibodies in the donor unit reacting with the patient's white blood cells (WBCs) probably cause TRALI. This reaction leads to increased pulmonary capillary permeability and produces an adult respiratory distress syndrome (ARDS) during or just following transfusion. It should be differentiated from acute congestive heart failure (CHF) by the patient's history and the typical chest x-ray finding of diffuse interstitial edema without cardiomegaly.

Congestive Heart Failure

The cardiovascular systems of most patients can easily accommodate the rapid change in intravascular volume that a blood transfusion provides. Elderly patients, however, and those with preexisting cardiomyopathy or diastolic dysfunction may have difficulty handling an acute change in volume and preload, and the result is pulmonary edema. Acute, progressive dyspnea and rales may develop over minutes or hours, during or soon after a blood transfusion.

Acute, Minor Reactions

Simple Febrile Reaction

This is the most common transfusion reaction, with an incidence of 1%. It is thought to be due to antileukocyte and antiplatelet antibodies, or to transfused pyrogenic cytokines that accumulate in stored blood as leukocytes break down. It is characterized as an isolated fever during transfusion, without the more serious signs and symptoms of vomiting, back pain, hypotension, or evidence of hemolysis.

Allergic Reaction

Minor allergic reactions occur largely in response to transfused plasma proteins. The incidence is estimated to be 0.1%, but it may be underreported (17). The reaction is more common with platelet or plasma transfusions, but PRBC units also carry some residual plasma. The patient develops urticaria or flushing and pruritus, without any dyspnea or hypotension.

Delayed Reactions

Adverse transfusion reactions may occur days to months after the transfusion. These include delayed hemolysis, graft-versus-host disease (GVHD), and a number of infections. Many infectious diseases may be transmitted by blood transfusion, including the human immunodeficiency virus (HIV), hepatitis, syphilis, malaria, cytomegalovirus (CMV), Epstein-Barr virus (EBV), trypanosomiasis, toxoplasmosis, babesiosis, brucellosis, and West Nile virus (1,3,6). The most clinically significant in the United States are hepatitis, HIV, and CMV.

Delayed Hemolysis

Delayed hemolysis is unusual, but may occur 5 to 7 days posttransfusion. The incidence is between one in 1,000 and one in 2,500 units transfused (3,6). It is most commonly caused by reactivation of antibodies to the minor RBC antigen systems such as Rh, Kell, Kidd, and Duffy. It presents in a less severe and dramatic way than the acute hemolytic reaction, though progression to renal failure is still a concern. In contrast to acute hemolysis, there is usually less free hemoglobin circulating at any given time, and thus the renal insult tends to be less severe (17). Low-grade hemolysis and progressively worsening anemia are the most common clinical findings of this reaction.

Graft-Versus-Host Disease

GVHD occurs when lymphocytes from a donated unit of blood attack an immunocompromised host who is unable to combat the foreign cells, or when lymphocytes from an immunologically similar donor are not recognized as foreign by the host. Signs and symptoms may include fever, rash, nausea, and vomiting, as well as elevation of transaminases and pancytopenia. This is a particular danger in neonates and bone marrow transplant recipients.

Hepatitis

Transfusion-associated hepatitis was a major problem in the 1970s and 1980s. It has been estimated that during the early 1970s, transfusion-associated hepatitis occurred in up to 33% of transfusions (12). Since then, aggressive screening of donors and the development of specific assays for hepatitis B (HBsAg and anti-HBc) and C (anti-HCV and nucleic acid amplification) have greatly reduced the risk.

Donahue reported a decrease in the risk of posttransfusion hepatitis C from approximately one in 200 during 1985 to one in 3,300 in 1991, after hepatitis C testing became available (2). With further advances in testing, the current estimated risk of transfusion-transmitted hepatitis B is one in 137,000, and that of hepatitis C is one in 1,000,000 (1). Although hepatitis C testing has successfully eliminated the majority of non-A, non-B hepatitis, the small risk of non-A, non-B, non-C hepatitis remains.

Human Immunodeficiency Virus

Although it is now exceedingly rare, the transfusion complication that has received the most public attention is HIV infection. It has been estimated that the risk of HIV transmission in some metropolitan areas was as high as one in 100 units transfused in 1983, before HIV testing was available to blood banks in March of 1985 (7). Now, thanks to aggressive pre-donation screening along with testing for HIV-1 and HIV-2 antibody, p24 antigen testing, and nucleic acid amplification testing (NAT) technology for HIV, the current risk is estimated to be one in 1.9 million units of blood (1). NAT technology allows for the detection of viral genetic materials prior to the antibody response, but its cost-effectiveness has recently been challenged (10).

The use of concentrated pooled plasma products resulted in a majority of hemophiliacs in the 1980s contracting the acquired immunodeficiency syndrome or hepatitis. Highly purified, lyophilized factor VIII concentrate and recombinant products have eliminated these tragic complications of therapy.

Cytomegalovirus

Although CMV is generally not a significant pathogen in immunocompetent individuals, the immunosuppressed, especially premature neonates, HIV patients, and bone marrow and organ transplant recipients, are especially susceptible to CMV infection transmitted by blood transfusion. The risk may be greatly reduced through the use of blood collected from CMV-negative donors, or by using leukocyte-reduced or frozen–deglycerolized units of blood (2).

Massive Transfusion

Several alterations are present in stored blood that are insignificant in small transfusions but may become clinically relevant in the setting of massive transfusion. *Massive transfusion* is usually defined as transfusion of the equivalent of one blood volume, or 10 to 12 units of PRBC, within 24 hours. Although this situation is unusual in the ED, it may be encountered in the setting of major trauma or gastrointestinal (GI) bleeding when definitive care is delayed for whatever reason.

Hyperkalemia and lactic acidosis may result from the transfusion of multiple units of older stored blood, but the effects tend to be relatively mild and transient. Hypocalcemia due to citrate toxicity was a significant clinical issue in the past when it was common to transfuse whole blood units. However, in the era of component therapy, whole blood is rarely (if ever) available or indicated, and PRBC units contain far less citrate. Transfusing large amounts of cold blood may also cause hypothermia, which in turn may worsen coagulopathy. Blood warmers lessen this problem, but they also slow the rate of transfusion, which is problematic in the hypotensive, hemorrhaging patient. Methods of mixing PRBC units with heated crystalloids, making the transfusion both faster and warmer, have been described (4,9).

The coagulopathy associated with massive transfusion is multifactorial and difficult to predict. Dilutional effects play a part, since the multiple units of PRBC transfused contain only negligible amounts of clotting factors and platelets. Coagulation times may rise beyond 1.5 times control, and clinically relevant bleeding occurs in some patients. Trauma patients who receive more than 10 units in 24 hours are more likely to develop serious coagulopathy in the presence of hypothermia, acidosis, or hypotension (5). Although platelet counts fall during massive transfusion, the decrease is much less than would be predicted from dilution alone (14). This is thought to be due to an "auto-transfusion" effect, or release of stored platelets into the circulation from the spleen or bone marrow. Platelet counts usually remain above 50,000 until 20 units of PRBC are transfused, but coagulation times exceed 1.5 times control in patients receiving more than 12 units (13).

DIFFERENTIAL DIAGNOSIS

The patient who develops any adverse symptoms early in a blood transfusion must be carefully evaluated for the possibility of one of the acute, severe reactions. However, many patients who receive emergent transfusions have underlying disease that may have symptoms in common with transfusion reactions. For example, when trauma patients or those with GI bleeding become hypotensive during a transfusion, the hypotension may represent either increasing hemorrhage or an acute, severe transfusion reaction. Sepsis and some drug overdoses (i.e. salicylates) may also present with symptoms that are similar to those of a transfusion reaction. Hypotensive reactions to platelet transfusions have also been reported. These are not thought to be allergic in origin but may initially lead the clinician to suspect anaphylaxis. These reactions appear to be uncommon and resolve quickly with cessation of the platelet transfusion (8). Patients with fever may have infectious causes unrelated to the blood transfusion, and those with allergic symptoms may be reacting to an allergen other than a blood product.

Although many of the signs and symptoms of transfusion reactions are nonspecific and can be confused with many disease processes, most transfusion reactions occur during or soon after a transfusion. The temporal relationship is less clear with the delayed reactions. A delayed hemolytic reaction must be differentiated from other causes of jaundice and anemia, but the indirect hyperbilirubinemia should cue the physician that hemolysis has occurred. A new diagnosis of hepatitis or other transmissible diseases may be traceable to the blood supply, but may also have occurred independently.

EMERGENCY DEPARTMENT EVALUATION

In the patient with an acute reaction, the clinician must rapidly decide whether the signs and symptoms are consistent with one of the severe reactions or one of the more benign febrile or allergic reactions (Fig. 156.1). Differentiation may sometimes be done clinically by evaluating the constellation of findings, without extensive testing. One may also employ quick, simple testing, such as observing the serum (after centrifugation of a blood sample) or the urine for pink discoloration during a hemolytic reaction.

The evaluation should also involve immediate reporting to the laboratory and sending blood samples for testing. Based on the clinical setting, the laboratory will often confirm the ABO types of the patient and donor unit, perform a direct Coombs' test, and search for evidence of hemolysis (an elevated indirect bilirubin, decreased haptoglobin, schistocytes on a peripheral smear, or hemoglobinuria). Testing may also include Gram staining and cultures, especially after platelet transfusions, if bacterial contamination is suggested.

The transfusion should be stopped during this evaluation in case the patient is in the early stages of a severe reaction. In some cases of minor reactions, especially allergic ones, the clinician may choose to treat the symptoms and restart the transfusion after determining that a severe reaction is not present, although this procedure is controversial. One should quickly involve the laboratory and transfusion service for consultation when a reaction occurs. Most institutions have policies or guidelines to help the clinician in evaluating and reporting transfusion reactions.

EMERGENCY DEPARTMENT MANAGEMENT

Treatment, of course, depends on which type of reaction has occurred (Fig. 156.1). The first step is always to stop the transfusion and carefully evaluate the patient to determine whether a transfusion reaction is occurring and, if so, which type.

The treatment of *acute hemolysis* is largely supportive, with special attention to maintaining renal perfusion. In hemodynamically unstable patients, early use of invasive monitoring is warranted, along with vasopressors and forced diuresis with crystalloids and loop diuretics (e.g., furosemide). Dopamine may be added—in "renal" doses (2 to 3 μg/kg/min)—for its potential benefit in increasing renal blood flow. Other treatments, such as steroids, mannitol, or heparin for DIC, are more controversial.

Anaphylaxis should be treated with epinephrine, steroids, diphenhydramine, and IV fluids. Patients with a history of serious allergic reactions to blood products may be given washed RBCs or frozen–deglycerolized RBCs in an effort to prevent allergic reactions. IgA-deficient donors are often available when the transfusion can be planned in advance.

Sepsis from bacterial contamination requires aggressive supportive care, including IV fluids, vasopressors, and broad-spectrum antibiotics. Antibiotic coverage for a contaminated platelet transfusion should include an antistaphylococcal agent as well as a third-generation cephalosporin. Coverage for a contaminated PRBC transfusion must include a third-generation cephalosporin or quinolone to cover *Yersinia*.

TRALI and *CHF* are treated with ventilatory support, as well as nitrates and diuresis for CHF. Transfusions must be done carefully in elderly patients and in those with a history of CHF or renal failure. It may be sufficient to transfuse each unit slowly (over 3 to 4 hours) and allow a period of time between subsequent units transfused, usually in the inpatient setting. Administration of a loop diuretic (e.g., furosemide) between units may also be helpful. In high-risk patients, invasive monitoring of right or left

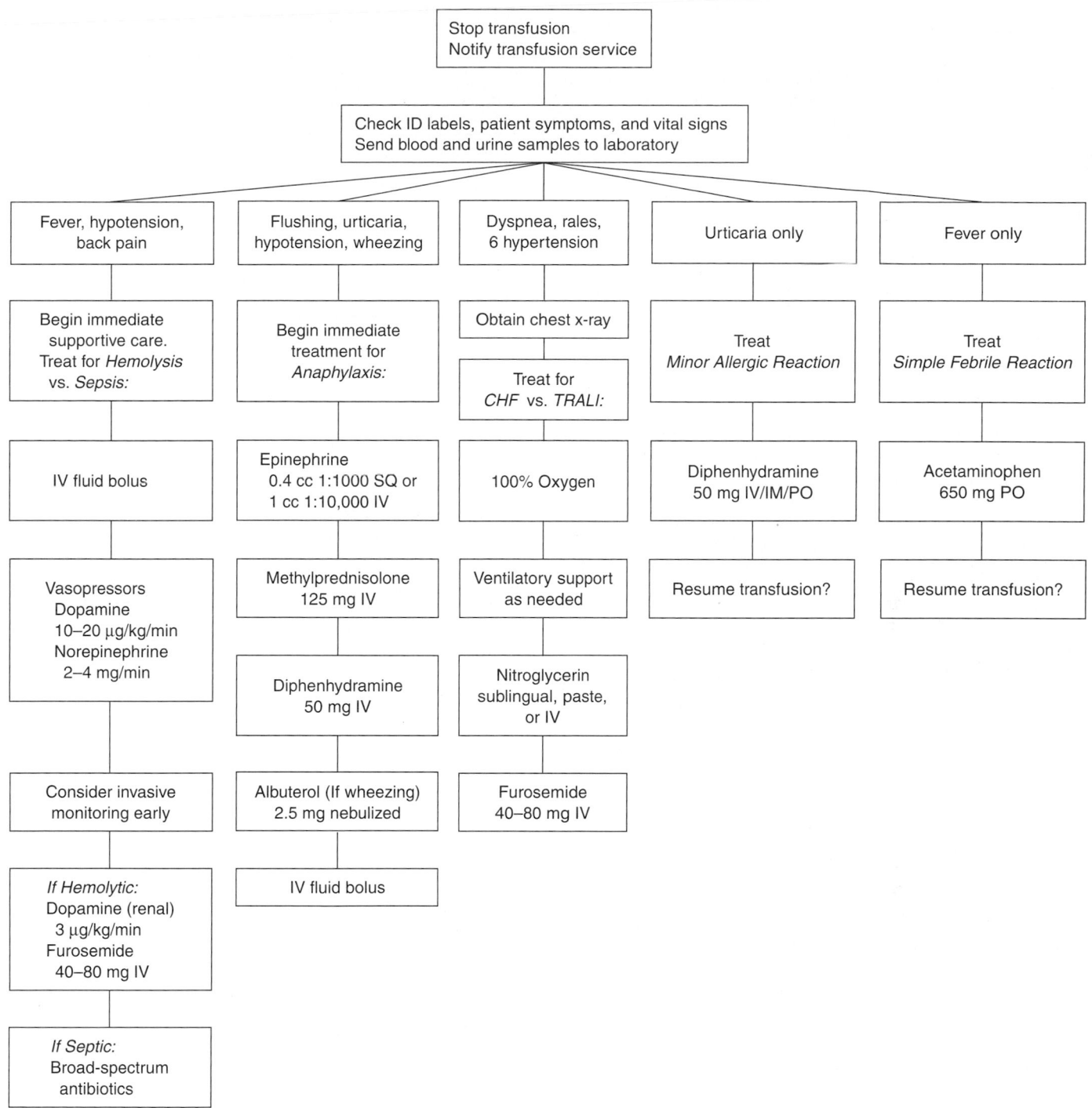

Figure 156.1. Clinical algorithm for suspected transfusion reaction. Many hospitals have developed policies and guidelines for actions to be taken in case of a transfusion reaction. Physicians should be informed regarding local hospital policy. TRALI = transfusion-related acute lung injury.

ventricular filling pressures in the ICU may be necessary, and transfusions may be accomplished during dialysis for renal failure patients.

Simple febrile and *allergic* reactions are treated with acetaminophen and diphenhydramine, respectively, but must be differentiated from the more dangerous transfusion reactions. Patients who receive frequent transfusions or who have a history of minor reactions may be given leukocyte-reduced units to reduce the risk of a febrile reaction, or pretreatment with diphenhydramine to reduce allergic symptoms. There is controversy about whether the transfusion may be carefully resumed after clinical observation and appropriate laboratory testing have ruled out a more serious reaction.

For graft-versus-host disease (GVHD), there is no specific treatment beyond supportive care, but some preventive measures exist. Irradiation of PRBC and platelet units suppresses white blood cells that may be transfused along with the desired component, and may prevent GVHD in high-risk immunocompromised patients.

Problems associated with *massive transfusion* should generally be treated as they arise. Hyperkalemia, hypocalcemia, and hypothermia should be treated if clinically significant.

TABLE 156.2. Medication Dosages for Transfusion Reactions

Fever and Hypotension

IV Fluid bolus	NS or LR, 1–2L
Dopamine	10–20 U/kg/min IV infusion

Anaphylaxis

IV Fluid bolus	NS or LR, 1–2L
Epinephrine	1:1,000 0.4 cc SQ
Methylprednisolone	125 mg IV
Diphenhydramine	50 mg IV
Albuterol	5 mg nebulized (if bronchospasm)

CHF

Nitroglycerin	0.4 mg SL, or
	1"paste, or
	20–40 U min IV infusion
Furosemide	40–80 mg IV

Coagulopathy is difficult to predict, making the routine prophylactic transfusion of platelets and clotting factors problematic. However, increased vigilance and a low threshold for treating coagulopathy and bleeding complications are recommended when patients are transfused beyond 10 units of PRBC. Administer FFP after massive transfusion when there are other complicating factors, such as hypothermia, acidosis, or hypotension because individuals with these conditions are at greater risk for developing significant coagulopathy (5).

CRITICAL INTERVENTIONS

- Stop transfusion
- Send samples from patient and transfusion unit to lab

See Table 156.2 for medication dosages for transfusion reactions.

DISPOSITION

Most patients receiving blood transfusions in the emergency department are ultimately admitted to the hospital, whether or not they have a transfusion reaction. However, acute, severe reactions usually necessitate ICU admission, regardless of the patient's original disposition. Simple febrile or allergic reactions do not necessarily require a change in the patient's treatment plan.

COMMON PITFALLS

✔ Failure to carefully identify patients when drawing pretransfusion blood samples, and to carefully match identities of blood components, their paperwork, and the recipient. This is the most frequent cause of fatal hemolytic reactions

✔ Failure to adequately evaluate a patient who develops symptoms during a blood transfusion. The large majority of reactions are simple febrile or allergic reactions, but the few dangerous reactions must be discovered and treated immediately

✔ Failure to recognize a severe reaction in an intubated patient. Because the patient cannot complain of symptoms, it is more difficult to differentiate a transfusion reaction from underlying disease. An acute, severe reaction may initially appear as isolated hypotension, fever, or hematuria

✔ Rapidly transfusing an elderly patient who is inadequately observed. Congestive failure can be avoided by slow, intermittent transfusion and diuresis

References

1. American Association of Blood Banks. (http://www.aabb.org)
2. Donahue J, Munoz A, Ness P, et al. The declining risk of post-transfusion hepatitis C virus infection. *N Engl J Med* 1992;327:369–373.
3. Chamberland M, Khabbaz R. Emerging issues in blood safety. *Infect Dis Clin North Am* 1998;12:217–229.
4. Cohn S, Stack G. In vitro comparison of heated saline-blood admixture with a heat exchanger for rapid warming of red blood cells. *J Trauma* 1993;35:688–690.
5. Cosgriff M, Moore M, Sauaia M, et al. Predicting life-threatening coagulopathy in the massively transfused trauma patient: hypothermia and acidoses revisited. *J Trauma* 1997;42:857–862.
6. Dobroszycki J, Herwaldt B, Boctor F, et al. A cluster of transfusion-associated babesiosis cases traced to a single asymptomatic donor. *JAMA* 1999;281:927–930.
7. Goodnough L, Brecher M, Kanter M, et al. Transfusion medicine. First of two parts. Blood transfusion. *N Engl J Med* 1999;340:438–447.
8. Hume H, Popovsky M, Benson K, et al. Hypotensive reactions: a previously uncharacterized complication of platelet transfusion? *Transfusion* 1996;36:904–909.
9. Iserson K, Knauf M, Anhalt D. Rapid admixture blood warming: technical advances. *Crit Care Med* 1990;18:1138–1141.
10. Jackson B, Busch M, Stramer S, AuBuchon J. The Cost-effectiveness of NAT for HIV, HCV, and HBV in Whole-blood Donations. *Transfusion* 2003;43:721–729.
11. Kuehnert M, Roth V, Haley N, et al. Transfusion-transmitted Bacterial Infection in the United States, 1998 through 2000. *Transfusion* 2001;41:1493–1499.
12. Labadie L. Transfusion therapy in the emergency department. *Emerg Med Clin North Am* 1993;11:379–406.
13. Leslie S, Toy P. Laboratory hemostatic abnormalities in massively transfused patients given red blood cells and crystalloid. *Am J Clin Pathol* 1991;96:770–773.
14. Reed R, Ciavarella D, Heimbach D, et al. Prophylactic platelet administration during massive transfusion. *Ann Surg* 1986;203:40–47.
15. Sandler S, Mallory D, Malamut D, et al. IgA Anaphylactic transfusion reactions. *Transfus Med Rev* 1995;9:1–8.
16. Schreiber G, Busch M, Kleinman S, et al. The risk of transfusion-transmitted viral infections. The Retrovirus Epidemiology Donor Study. *N Engl J Med* 1996;334:1685–1690.
17. Sloop G, Friedberg R. Complications of blood transfusion. How to recognize and respond to noninfectious reactions. *Postgrad Med* 1995;98:159–162.

CHAPTER 157
The Cancer Patient in the Emergency Department

Austen Chai

The emergency physician often makes or suspects a diagnosis of cancer and provides the initial care before turning to a specialist for a more definitive care. More commonly, the emergency physician faces patients with a known history of cancer that present to the emergency department with a recurrence of the disease in remission, significant progression of the underlying disease, or the complications of therapy for the cancer. In any case, the emergency physician is left with a difficult task of managing a wide range of complicated emergencies that pose significant challenges. This task has been made more difficult by the advent of earlier detection and improved therapies that have resulted in longer patient survival and the increasing frequency of catastrophic emergencies that present with subtle complaints and findings. As such, cancer patients deserve special attention for even minor problems. For example, mild radicular back pain may be the first sign of impending spinal cord compression in a patient with a history lung or prostate cancer. Likewise, a patient with a malignant pericardial effusion that has progressed nearly to a point of frank tamponade may only complain of vague dyspnea or malaise. Thus, a heightened sense of suspicion is needed when treating a patient with a suspected or known history of cancer.

SHORTNESS OF BREATH

Airway Obstruction

Most cases of upper airway obstruction involve advanced cases of cancers of the larynx or the hypopharynx, neck and mediastinum. These patients often present with a history of gradual worsening dyspnea over the course of weeks to months. There is often associated increasing hoarseness and dysphagia.

Initial assessment may include soft tissue x-ray of the neck and chest x-ray, which are rarely diagnostic. Computed tomography (CT) with contrast of the neck and chest with three-dimensional airway reconstruction is more helpful. Direct laryngoscopy assesses the size of the airway lumen. Typically, the tumors acutely cause airway compromise when exacerbated by infection, hemorrhage, or excessive secretions leading to critical obstruction at the time of presentation. In such situations, one must be prepared to establish an emergent surgical airway. Early involvement of an ear, nose, and throat (ENT) surgeon is recommended as the local anatomy of the airway can be greatly distorted. This is particularly true if the patient has been treated previously with radiotherapy. Initial interventions include oxygen, heliox when available, administration of steroids, racemic epinephrine and antibiotics. Further therapy may involve surgery, radiation, and chemotherapy.

Tumors can also cause dyspnea by impinging directly on the trachea. Most commonly, carcinoma of the lung, esophagus and the thyroid and lymphoma grow and impinge on the trachea. Tracheal obstruction is also a complication of edema secondary to radiation therapy or due to tracheomalacia following prolonged intubation. Tracheostomy is often necessary in these patients as endotracheal intubation is unlikely to be successful as the obstruction may be below the cricoid membrane.

Bronchial obstruction is usually the result of primary lung carcinoma. Rarely endobronchial metastasis from other primaries as breast, colon, and renal carcinoma can also cause significant bronchial obstruction with wide spread endobronchial metastasis. Typically there must be greater than 75% obstruction before a patient becomes symptomatic. The patient may present with dyspnea on exertion, cough, hemoptysis, wheezing and rhonchi.

When patients present with dyspnea, fever and sputum production, pneumonia should be suspected. Patients with obstructing lesions are more prone to pneumonia. This is particularly true of immune-compromised patients.

Additionally, shortness of breath can be the result of agents such as bleomycin, cyclophosphamide, and radiation therapy to the chest causing granulomatous and fibrotic changes in the lung tissue, leading to restrictive lung disease.

Malignant Pleural Effusion

Malignant pleural effusion is caused most commonly by lymphoma, lung, breast or ovarian cancer. It is estimated that up to 30% of cancer patients develop malignant pleural effusion.

Patients typically present with dyspnea on exertion or when supine and may complain of a dry cough. Examination typically reveals decreased breath sounds on the affected side, dullness to percussion and occasionally a pleural friction rub. Rarely,

pleural effusion can be due to congestive heart failure resulting from cardiomyopathies caused by certain chemotherapeutic treatments.

Chest x-ray confirms the diagnosis. Approximately 300cc of fluid is needed to see the effusion on an upright chest x-ray. The amount needed for detection on a decubitus film is 100cc. Therapy includes supplemental oxygen if the patient is hypoxemic. Thoracentesis should be performed for both diagnosis and to provide therapeutic relief. The pleural fluid obtained should be sent for cytology, gram stain, culture, cell count, protein and LDH determinations. If infection is suspected, antibiotics should be started after a sample is obtained. For recurrent effusions, an oncologist should be consulted for more definitive therapeutic modalities such as sclerosis, pleurectomy, or chemotherapy.

Pericardial Effusion

Pericardial effusion occurs most commonly in patients with lung and breast cancer, but virtually any tumor can involve the pericardium. Patients complain of shortness of breath. Pericardial effusions leading to tamponade are usually the result of long-standing processes that may evolve into critical problems over the course of a few hours. The severity of tamponade is related to the rapidity with which fluid accumulates, because the pericardium can usually stretch a great deal to accommodate a slow growing effusion. If the pericardium is thickened by fibrosis, as is often the case in patients that have received radiation therapy to the mediastinum, a small effusion can cause significant compression due to the constricting pericardium. In such cases, chest radiograph may show a small heart and cardiac tamponade can be confirmed by the use of a bedside echocardiogram.

Nonconstricting pericardial effusion usually does not cause specific symptoms. However, as the pericardium distends and compression worsens, patients develop dyspnea, chest pain relieved by leaning forward, cyanosis, dysphagia, hoarseness, epigastric discomfort, or hiccups. Initially the patient may present like a patient with congestive heart failure. On physical examination, the patient is typically anxious and diaphoretic with decreased systolic and pulse pressure. Lungs are usually clear, the neck veins distended and the heart sounds distant. An increased pulsus paradoxus and inspiratory swelling of the neck veins may be noted. If the effusion is long standing, patients may also have peripheral edema, hepatojugular reflux, hepatomegaly and even ascites, further giving the impression that the patient may have congestive heart failure.

Chest x-ray shows cardiomegaly or a globular cardiac silhouette. The most common electrocardiogram (ECG) finding is sinus tachycardia and low voltage QRS complexes or occasionally global ST elevation. Electrical alternans is pathognomonic of significant pericardial effusion, but is commonly missed as it can disappear as compression worsens. Definitive diagnosis can be made by echocardiography. A temporizing treatment is the deliverance of vigorous intravenous fluids to maintain filling pressure in patients that may be fluid depleted. This often provides the time to get the patient to surgery for a pericardial stripping procedure. Emergent pericardiocentesis should be performed in case of shock, cyanosis, and decreased level of consciousness.

Pulmonary Embolism

Cancer patients are at an increased risk for thrombosis especially due to their underlying hypercoagulable state that predisposes them to thromboembolism. Development of venous thromboembolism is particularly common in patients with brain tumors with an incidence of about 25%. As such, pulmonary embolism (see Chapter 38) must always be considered as a potential cause of dyspnea in cancer patients. Even in cases of brain metastasis, because of the greater danger and urgency with pulmonary embolism, patients are generally treated with anticoagulation. Another available option is the placement of an inferior vena cava filter (IVC). Studies have shown increasing complications with IVC filters and advantage over anticoagulation should be established before its placement.

Superior Vena Cava Syndrome

In superior vena cava syndrome, the insidious obstruction of blood flow to the superior vena cava results in elevation of venous pressure to the lower airway, arms, neck, face and the brain. This leads to edema of the lower airway and results in hoarseness, dysphagia, chest fullness and headache. Physical findings include venous distension of the neck, facial redness, and swelling. The patient's symptoms are usually exacerbated by positional change such as bending forward, stooping, or lying down. As the venous pressure rises, intracranial pressure also elevates and may lead to syncope.

Malignancy is the most common etiology and these patients will have evidence of a mass on chest radiograph, usually in the right hilum. Other causes of superior vena cava syndrome include mediastinal fibrosis, thyroid mass, tuberculosis, or thrombosis around indwelling venous catheters and rarely renal cell carcinoma whose tumor may have extended up the vena cava. Furosemide and steroids may reduce venous pressure and provide some time before radiation therapy can be initiated. Emergent radiation therapy is indicated when there is compromised cardiac function, significant upper airway edema leading to respiratory dysfunction, or cerebral dysfunction secondary to brain edema.

HEADACHES, SEIZURES AND ALTERED SENSORIUM

Brain Metastasis

Lung, breast, melanoma, colon and rectal cancers are the most common tumors that spread to the brain. Forty to 50% of patients with brain metastasis complain of headache. The headache is typically worse on awakening and improves during the course of the day. Since 80% of the metastasis is located in the cerebrum, patients may additionally present with a history of progressive lethargy, memory loss, cognitive dysfunction, aphasia, paresis, or sensory disturbance. Cerebellar metastasis, which account for less than 10% of metastasis, usually cause dysmetria or gait disturbance. Papilledema is seen in less than 10% of the patients. A new seizure may be the first presenting complaint for about 15% of the patients with brain metastasis. Patients found to have brain metastasis without known primary should have the lung as the focus of evaluation since 60% of such patients will have lung primary or metastasis.

CT scan, ideally with contrast or magnetic resonance imaging of the brain identifies brain metastasis. Corticosteroids reduce headache and improve function in 60% to 75% of patients with brain metastasis. Dexamethasone 10 mg intravenous (IV) loading dose followed by 4 mg four times a day should be promptly started for patients with brain metastasis. Dexamethasone is the drug of choice because of its high central nervous system penetration. When there are physical or radiographic signs of increased intracranial pressure, the head of the patient should be elevated to at least 30 degrees, fluid restriction instituted, an intravenous bolus of 0.75 mg to 1 gram/kg of mannitol administered followed by 0.25 to 0.5 g/kg every 3-5 hours and consideration given to radiation therapy. Diuretics may be given

and hyperventilation is an effective short-term measure to reduce intracranial pressure. When a patient has had a seizure, anticonvulsant therapy should be begun. The decision to give anticonvulsants to patients with brain metastasis that have not had a seizure should be left to the oncologist. Additionally, all patients with brain metastasis will have a potential to have a seizure in the future and they should be warned against driving or operating machinery.

Meningitis

When patients with a predisposing cancer present with headache, lethargy, or other vague central nervous system (CNS) symptoms, meningitis including carcinomatous meningitis should be considered (see Chapter 138). After obtaining a CT scan to ascertain that there are no brain masses, a spinal tap should be performed. An opening pressure greater than 160 mm H_2O, cerebrospinal fluid (CSF) leukocytosis, increased CSF protein concentration and decreased CSF glucose concentration should raise suspicions about the presence of meningitis. An additional tube of CSF should be obtained for malignant cells evaluation.

Cancer patients with impaired cellular immunity like patients with leukemia, lymphoma or recent steroid can also have meningitis caused by cryptococcus neoformans or Listeria monocytogenes. Treat Listeria with ampicillin as the organism is resistant to third generation cephalosporins. In patients with other bacterial infections such as sinusitis, otitis, or dental abscesses are at risk for contiguous CNS infections including brain abscess.

METABOLIC DISTURBANCES

Hypercalcemia

Hypercalcemia is relatively common in patients with cancer, occurring in about 10% to 20% of cases (see Chapter 167). The most common cancers associated with hypercalcemia include breast, lung and prostate cancers with bony metastasis, multiple myeloma, renal cell carcinoma and lymphomas. The mechanism for development of hypercalcemia includes matrix destruction by the cancer (multiple myeloma, bony metastasis from breast, lung and prostate); the secretion of parathormone-like hormone by certain lung cancers; and the secretion of osteoclastic-activating factor by certain lymphomas and leukemias.

Mildly elevated levels of serum calcium are usually symptom free but with increasing levels, patients may present with nausea and vomiting, constipation, hypertension, gradual increase in lethargy and depressed mental status. Generally, serum levels of calcium greater than 13 mg/dL require treatment. Elevated levels of ionized calcium causes neuromuscular dysfunction and ECG changes and should be interpreted in conjunction with serum albumin, phosphorus and serum pH levels.

The majority of patients with hypercalcemia will respond to intravenous saline infusion. Careful evaluation of the patient's cardiac and renal function should be done, especially in patients with multiple myeloma who may already have compromised renal function or patients with a history of cardiomyopathy or congestive heart failure, so as not to iatrogenically overload the patient with fluid. In such patients, loop diuretics such as furosemide can be added along with intravenous fluids. Initial IV fluid load of 1 to 2 liters with 80 mg of furosemide is sufficient. Potassium as well as magnesium should be replenished. For severe hypercalcemia, dialysis may be needed. Additional initial treatments can include glucocorticoids, pamidronate, mithramycin and calcitonin.

Hyponatremia

Hyponatremia in cancer patients is due to secretion of inappropriate antidiuretic hormone or syndrome of inappropriate antidiuretic hormone (SIADH) from an ectopic source (see Chapter 165). It most commonly occurs with lung (especially small cell), pancreatic, and ovarian cancer, lymphoma, thymoma, and brain tumors. SIADH causes hyponatremia by interfering with urinary dilution and thus preventing the excretion of ingested water. The definitive treatment is the removal of the ectopic source. However, the initial treatment is fluid restriction. Patients with hyponatremia will not have symptoms unless there is an acute drop in the sodium level or if the level falls below 120 meq/dl. Symptoms of precipitous sodium loss include muscle twitching, seizures and coma.

Treat actively seizing patients due to hyponatremia with hypertonic 3% saline solution. It should be administered at 25 to 100 cc per hour until the seizure stops. Additionally, furosemide can be given to reduce fluid volume in the body. In cases of chronic hyponatremia, correction of sodium should be done as slowly as possible at rates no faster than 10 to 12 meq/dL per day. Use of hypertonic and isotonic solutions to rapidly increase the serum sodium levels in patients that have had long standing hyponatremia are known to cause osmotic demyelination, also known as, central pontine myelinolysis (CPM).

Hypernatremia

Most causes of hypernatremia in cancer patients are due to reduced water intake or caused by excessive fluid loss due to treatment of cancer. Generally, in cases of acute hypernatremia, sodium correction can be achieved rapidly without problems, but if the patient is chronically hypernatremic, correction should be gradual, especially in children. Additionally, monitor patients with cardiac histories for fluid overload and administer furosemide to reduce sodium along with excess fluid.

Tumor Lysis Syndrome

Tumor lysis syndrome is a metabolic complication after treatment of neoplastic disorders. Findings include acute renal failure due to urate nephropathy, hyperphosphatemia, hypocalcemia, hyperuricemia and hyperkalemia. This syndrome is most commonly associated with lymphoma, acute lymphocytic leukemia, myelogenous leukemia and other tumors with high rate of tumor cell turnovers in patients that have received combination chemotherapy.

Diagnosis should be suspected in patients with a large tumor burden who develop acute renal failure in the presence of marked hyperuricemia greater than 15 mg/dL and hyperphosphatemia greater than 8 mg/dL. The incidence of significant tumor lysis syndrome has been significantly reduced due to pretreatment with allopurinol prior to chemotherapy or radiation plus fluid loading. Treatment includes IV hydration, diuretics and allopurinol. Hemodialysis should be used in those patients in whom diuresis cannot be induced and volume overload is a concern.

MUSCULOSKELETAL PAIN

Spinal Cord Compression

Any vertebral pain in patients with a history of cancer should alert the emergency physician of the possibility of spinal cord compression. The incidence of spinal cord compression in cancer patients is estimated at 5% to 10% of all cancer patients. Metastatic tumor from any primary site can produce cord compression but the most common are metastasis from prostate cancer, breast cancer, lung cancer, renal cell carcinoma, non-Hodgkin's lymphoma and multiple myeloma. Approximately 20% of cord compressions are the first manifestations of malignancy with 60% of the cases occurring in the thoracic spine, 30% in the lumbosacral spine, and 10% in the cervical spine.

Pain is the initial symptom of spinal cord syndrome in 80% to 95% of patients at the time of diagnosis. On average pain precedes other neurologic symptoms by 7 weeks. Pain upon recumbency should raise a higher suspicion. Over time, the pain may develop a radicular quality. Abrupt worsening of pain may herald a pathologic compression fracture. Motor findings are present in 60% to 85% of patients at the time of presentation. Typically there is increasing weakness until there is gait disturbance and paralysis. Patients frequently complain of ascending numbness and paresthesias. Bladder and bowel dysfunction due to cord compression is generally a late finding that occurs in one-half of patients.

Plain radiographs are inadequate to define the lesion. MR imaging is the imaging modality of choice to evaluate the patient's thecal sac and epidural space. Treatment includes pain control, avoidance of complications, and attempts to preserve or improve neurologic function. Corticosteroid and opiate analgesic should be used for pain management. Administer a bolus of 10 mg of dexamethasone followed by 4 mg every 6 hours for patients with neurologic findings. Radiation therapy is the definitive treatment of choice for most patients. Depending on the type of tumor involved, debulking surgery followed by radiation may improve patient outcome. Thus prompt neurosurgical consultation should be obtained when spinal cord compression is suspected.

Bony Metastasis

Sudden onset of pain, commonly in the extremities and pelvis may be due to pathologic fractures in cancer patients, in particular those with prostate, breast, or lung cancer or multiple myeloma. Recent bone scans may be negative in cancers that form purely lytic lesions (myeloma and some prostate cancers). Plain radiographs establish the diagnosis and emergent orthopaedic consultation is required for followup care.

Pain Control

Pain is a common feature in many cancer patients. Opiates should be administered for severe pain. Respiratory depression from additional narcotic doses does not occur in patients who continue to have severe pain after the initial dose.

COMPLICATIONS OF CANCER THERAPY

Neutropenia with Fever

Fever in a neutropenic patient is a medical emergency. Fever is defined as a temperature > 38 degrees C (100.4 degrees F). There are situations where neutropenic patients may not develop a fever yet may still have a serious infection. This may be the case with the elderly, those receiving corticosteroids, patients that are hypothermic and or hypotensive. With such patients if there is deterioration, investigate and treat as a serious infection.

Neutropenia is defined as absolute neutrophil count (ANC) < 500 cells/μL or < 1000 cells/μL with a predicted nadir of < 500 cells/μL. The ANC is the total number of white blood cell (WBC) count multiplied by the percentage of neutrophils plus bands. As the total number of neutrophils decreases, the incidence of occult infection increases with the highest incidence of infection in those with ANC < 100 cell/μL. When a cancer patient receives chemotherapy or radiation or when tumor invasion occurs, there is a breakdown of normal skin and mucosal barriers leading to bacteremia, which can overwhelm a depressed immune system. Approximately 80% of the infections arise from the patient's endogenous flora. Historically, infections due to gram negative bacilli, particularly P. aeruginosa, were the most common but with the use of indwelling catheters, there has been an increase in gram-positive infections.

Patients should have a very thorough history and examination with careful attention to the skin, indwelling catheters, and perianal areas. However, digital rectal examination and rectal temperature measurements are not recommended until broad spectrum antibiotics have been administered. Laboratory evaluation includes a CBC, electrolytes, urinalysis, BUN, Cr, urine culture, CXR and at least two sets of blood cultures including a sample from any indwelling catheters.

Treatment includes initial empiric antibiotic therapy. A dual antibiotic regimen includes an extended spectrum beta-lactam (piperacillin or ceftazime) plus an aminoglycoside. Monotherapy is also frequently used and may include ceftazidime, meropenem or cefepime. Vancomycin should be added for patients with catheter site infection, methicillin resistant *staphylococcus aureus* infection, hypotensive patients or when recent quinolone prophylaxis was applied. Colony stimulating factors should only be added to critically ill patients with pneumonia, hypotension, or organ dysfunction.

Chemotherapy-induced Vomiting and Dehydration

From the cancer patient's point of view, one of the most feared side effects of cancer treatment is nausea and vomiting. Promethazine (Phenergan) or Prochlorperazine (Compazine) are indicated for mild to moderate nausea and vomiting. For more severe cases, serotonin receptor antagonists such as ondansetron (Zofran) are indicated. High dose metoclopramide (Reglan) can also be employed. Additionally, the administration of dexamethasone in conjunction with metoclopramide or serotonin receptor antagonist has been shown to significantly reduce nausea and emesis. For those that are receiving the highest emetogenic chemotherapeutic agents, Neurokinin 1 receptor antagonists may be used in conjunction with serotonin receptor antagonists and dexamethasone.

HEMATOLOGIC MALIGNANCIES

Acute Leukemia

Increased production of malignant cells in the bone marrow result in the reduction of normal red blood cells, neutrophils, and platelets. Thus, leukemic patients generally present with symptoms related to complications of pancytopenia, and have increased risk of infections, anemia and bleeding. Patients generally complain of weakness and fatigue and on physical examination may reveal gingival bleeding, petechiae, ecchymoses, epistaxis, or menorrhagia, and less commonly lymphadenopathy, splenomegaly, or sternal tenderness. Provisional diagnosis is dependent upon complete blood count and the evaluation of peripheral blood smear showing blast cells constituting more than 5% of the circulating white cells. Definitive diagnosis is made with appropriate evaluation of the bone marrow.

Infection

The most common complication of leukemia seen in the emergency department is infection. When fever is present in a leukemic patient, an infection site must be immediately and vigorously sought and the patient treated empirically with broad spectrum antibiotics. Since most patients with leukemia tend to have qualitative defects of the circulating neutrophils, febrile patients should be presumed to be septic. Monotherapy using a broad spectrum antipseudomal antibiotic (ceftazidime, meropenem, or cefipime) or dual therapy using an extended spectrum beta lactam (piperacillin or ceftazidme) and an aminoglycoside may be administered.

Hemorrhage

Bleeding occurs due to thrombocytopenia. Thrombocytopenic patients may develop petechiae and ecchymoses but typically will not suffer fatal hemorrhagic complications without first developing extensive mucous membrane bleeding such as epistaxis, bleeding gums, hematuria, GI bleed, and bleeding from catheter or surgical sites. The threshold of 10,000/μL can be used to transfuse patients with no signs of bleeding or just petechiae and ecchymoses. More aggressive therapy is indicated for active bleeding or other risk factors such as fever, coagulation abnormalities, hyperleukocytosis or minor surgery. In such patients, the threshold should be increased to at least 20,000/μL. A prophylactic transfusion of 50,000/μL in the absence of any coagulation abnormalities is indicated in patients about to have a major invasive procedure. Lumbar puncture in children is safe at a platelet count > 10,000/μL.

The goal of transfusion is to prevent bleeding and to raise the platelet count to about 50,000/μL. One unit of platelet usually raises the total platelet count by about 5000 μL. Patients that have had repeated transfusions in the past may require HLA-matched platelets. Leukoagglutinin reaction, a common complication of transfusion, manifested by fever, rigors, body aches, or shortness of breath can be prevented or treated by use of acetaminophen and diphenhydramine prior to transfusion and the use of leukapor filter.

Disseminated intravascular coagulation (DIC) is a less common cause of bleeding. DIC prolongs both the prothrombin and partial thromboplastin time with decreased levels of fibrinogen and increased concentration of fibrinogen degradation products. See Chapter 153, Disseminated Intravascular Coagulation, Thrombotic Thrombocytopenic Purpura, and Hemolytic-Uremic Syndrome.

Hyperleukocytotic Syndrome

Hyperleukocytosis and leukostasis occur in acute leukemias as the total white blood cell count exceeds 50,000 to 100,000/μL and blood flow in the microcirculation becomes impeded by the more rigid blast cells. There is local hypoxemia by the high metabolic activity of the leukemic cells with resultant endothelial damage and hemorrhage. In patients with chronic myelogenous leukemia, a cell count greater than 250,000/μL is needed for leukostasis to occur. With chronic lymphocytic leukemia, the problems related to leukostasis do not develop until the cell count exceeds 1 million/μL.

Patients with hyperleukocytotic syndromes can be treated with emergent leukapheresis. If this modality is not available in a timely fashion, cytotoxic drugs can be used to reduce the peripheral white blood cell count. Cytotoxic therapy, however, carries the risk of "tumor lysis syndrome," manifested by the rapid onset of hyperuricemia, hyperphosphatemia, hyperkalemia, and lactic acidosis. A commonly used cytotoxic agent that is easy to administer is hydroxyurea, an oral medication given in doses of 500 to 2,000 mg four times per day. Patients with hyperleukocytosis who will be treated with hydroxyurea should be given allopurinol at least 3 to 6 hours before the first dose; the serum electrolytes and blood counts must also be monitored closely. Tumor lysis syndrome is also associated with rapidly growing lymphomas.

Hyperviscosity Syndrome

Hyperviscosity Syndrome is seen in approximately half of the patients with macroglobulinemia and in about 2% of the patients with multiple myeloma. The normal range of relative serum viscosity is 1.4 to 1.8. As values exceed 4, symptoms such as epistaxis, purpura, GI bleeding, visual impairment, and neurologic deficits begin to appear. For symptomatic patients, emergent plasmapheresis is needed.

Polycythemia

Overproduction of erythrocytes or platelets may also precipitate medical emergencies. A hemoglobin level greater than 17 g/dL or a hematocrit greater than 55% in women or 60% in men may signal polycythemia vera, an uncontrolled clonal overproduction of erythrocytes. Other conditions that should be considered in patients presenting with a high hematocrit include volume depletion, hypoxia, and polycythemia due to cigarette smoking or exposure to high altitudes. Patients with polycythemia vera are usually middle-aged and generally have a normal arterial oxygen saturation (greater than 92%) and splenomegaly. They often have leukocytosis (> 12,000 white blood cells/mL) as well as thrombocytosis (> 400,000 platelets/mL).

Emergencies due to polycythemia are related to hypervolemia and hyperviscosity. Patients may present with headache, vertigo, angina pectoris, or claudication. Other clinical features include generalized pruritus, especially after a shower or bath and erythromyalgia (burning in the feet or hands with erythema). Thirty percent of patients with polycythemia vera suffer thrombotic episodes, and stroke is a common complication and cause of death. Elevated hematocrit findings can also interfere with platelet function; thus, some patients with uncontrolled polycythemia suffer hemorrhagic complications, most commonly in the gastrointestinal tract. Many patients with polycythemia also have thrombocythemia (platelet counts greater than 600,000/mL), a finding that is also associated with abnormal bleeding.

Polycythemic patients with signs or symptoms of hyperviscosity or thrombotic complications should have their blood volume and hemoglobin concentration reduced to normal as quickly as possible.

Even without symptoms, a hemoglobin level of 18 g/dL or a hematocrit reading of 60% or higher is also an indication for emergent phlebotomy or cytapheresis. Patients who are otherwise healthy can usually tolerate a rapid phlebotomy of 500 mL, although more gradual treatment may be required in the elderly or in those with known coronary artery disease. With the attainment of a normal hematocrit, the platelet defect that gives rise to thrombosis and bleeding is eventually corrected, but this can take weeks to occur. Elective surgery and dental procedures in polycythemic patients should thus be delayed until the red cell mass and platelet count have been normalized for at least 2 months. Polycythemic patients in need of emergency surgery require emergent phlebotomy or cytapheresis.

Administer low-dose aspirin if not contraindicated. Antihistamines are indicated for pruritus. Other chemotherapeutic agents may be used with the guidance of a hematologist.

Thrombocytosis

Primary thrombocytosis, also known as essential thrombocytosis, is a subgroup of chronic myeloproliferative disorders that describes a chronic thrombocythemic state that is not due to infection, inflammation or other causes of reactive thrombocytosis or other myeloproliferative disorders. Platelet count > 600,000/μL is seen and typically will not be symptomatic or require treatment until the count is > 1,000,000/μL. High-risk patients are those with a count > 1.5 million/μL and age > 60.

Clinically, 25% to 50% of the patients will have splenomegaly and many will have vasomotor symptoms or thrombohemorrhagic complications. Vasomotor manifestations include headache, lightheadedness, syncope, chest pain, acral paresthesia, visual disturbance or erythromyalgia. Despite the high platelet count, patients may present with varying degrees of bleeding. Thrombotic events include strokes, transient digital ischemia. Treatment includes the use of low-dose aspirin up to 325 mg. Other chemotherapeutic agents as hydroxyurea and anagrelide may be used with the guidance of a hematologist.

CRITICAL INTERVENTIONS

- Administer broad spectrum antibiotics in patients with neutropenia and fever after obtaining the appropriate cultures
- Administer adequate analgesia for patients with severe, chronic pain
- Arrange emergent radiation therapy for patients who present with spinal cord compression

COMMON PITFALLS

✔ Failing to recognize functional neutropenia, especially in cancer patients receiving chemotherapy
✔ Failing to adequately treat pain and vomiting in patients receiving therapy
✔ Failing to seek out treatable causes of mental status changes or personality changes in cancer patients
✔ Failing to recognize that back pain in a cancer patient should alert the clinician of the possibility of cord compression
✔ Failing to adequately resuscitate patients who have significant therapeutic options and are not known to have a well-documented advanced refractory disease

Acknowledgments

Thanks to the previous edition's chapter author Daniel Brookoff.

References

1. Abner A. Approach to the patient who presents with superior vena cava obstruction. *Chest* 1993;103:394.
2. Carroll MF, et al. A practical approach to hypercalcemia. *Am Fam Physician* 2003;67:1959–1966.
3. Elting LS, et al. Outcomes of bacteremia in patients with cancer and neutropenia: Observations from two decades of epidemiological and clinical trials. *Clin Infect Dis* 1997;25:247.
4. Feusner J, et al. Role of intravenous allopurinol in the management of acute tumor lysis syndrome. *Semin Oncol* 2001;28:13.
5. Fiocco M, et al. The management of malignant pleural and pericardial effusions. *Hematology Oncol Clin North Am* 1997;11:253.
6. Flombaum, CD. Metabolic emergencies in the cancer patient. *Semin Oncol* 2000;27:322.
7. Giles FJ, et al. Leukapheresis reduces early mortality in patients with acute myeloid leukemia with high white cell counts but does not improve long-term survival. *Leuk Lymphoma* 2001;42:67.
8. Glantz MJ, et al. Practice parameter: Anticonvulsant prophylaxis in patients with newly diagnosed brain tumors: Report of the Quality Standards Subcommittee of the American Academy of Neurology. *Neurology* 2000;54:1886.
9. Gralla RJ, et al. Recommendations for the use of antiemetics: Evidence-based, clinical practice guidelines. *J Clin Oncol* 1999;17:2971.

10. Harrison CN. Current trends in essential thrombocythaemia. *Br J Haematol* 2002;117:796.

11. Hughes WT, et al. 2002 Guidelines for the use of antimicrobial agents in neutropenic patients with cancer. *Clin Infect Dis* 2002;34:730.

12. Husband DJ. Malignant spinal cord compression: Prospective study of delays in referral and treatment. *BMJ* 1998;317:318.

13. Laham RJ, et al. Pericardial effusion in patients with cancer: outcome with contemporary management strategies. *Heart* 1996;75:67.

14. Loblaw DA, Laperriere NJ. Emergency treatment of malignant extradural spinal cord compression: An evidence-based guideline. *J Clin Oncol* 1998; 16:1613.

15. Mermel LA, et al. IDSA guidelines for the management of intravascular catheter-related infections-I. *Clin Infect Dis* 2001;32:1249.

16. Mndy GR, et al. Hypercalcemia of malignancy. *Am J Med* 1997;103:134–145.

17. Ozer H, et al. 2000 update of recommendations for the use of hematopoietic colony-stimulating factors: Evidence-based, clinical practice guidelines. *J Clin Oncol* 2000;18:3558.

18. Patchell, R. Brain metastases. *Handbook of Neurology* 1997;25:135.

19. Roberts JR, et al. Multimodality treatment of malignant superior vena caval syndrome. *Chest* 1999;116:835.

20. Rose BD, et al. *Clinical Physiology of Acid-Base and Electrolyte Disorders*, 5th ed, McGraw-Hill, New York, 2001, pp. 707–711.

21. Rowell NP, et al. Steroids, radiotherapy, chemotherapy and stents for superior vena caval obstruction in carcinoma of the bronchus: a systematic review. *Clin Oncol* 2002;14:338.

22. Schiff D, et al. Neuroimaging and treatment implication of patients with multiple epidural spinal metastases. *Cancer* 1998;83:1593.

23. Schiffer CA, et al. Platelet transfusion for patients with cancer: Guidelines of the American Society of Clinical Oncology. *J Clin Oncol* 2001;19:1519.

24. Tefferi A, et al. A Clinical update in polycythemia vera and essential thrombocythemia. *Am J Med* 2000;109:141.

25. Rowell NP, et al. Steroids, radiotherapy, chemotherapy and stents for superior vena caval obstruction carcinoma of the bronchus: a systematic review. *Clin Oncol* 2002;14:338.

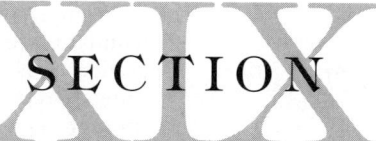

Section Editor: Jeffrey Schaider, MD

Endocrine and Metabolic Emergencies

CHAPTER 158
Acid–Base Disturbances

Robert Shesser and Tina Rosenbaum

Severe acid–base abnormalities lead to diffuse cellular dysfunction and represent important sequelae of a wide variety of serious illnesses. The immediate treatment of a serious acid–base disturbance is simply accomplished, but precise analysis of the patient's acid–base status will often provide a critical clue for the identification of the disturbance's underlying etiology. A thorough understanding of the principles of acid–base pathophysiology permits the physician to expand the diagnostic considerations and may help to identify a previously unsuspected pathology.

BASIC PHYSIOLOGY

The hydrogen ion concentration or its negative logarithm (pH) is a fundamental measure of the character of all solutions. A neutral pH of 7.0 indicates that the numbers of H^+ and OH^- ions resulting from the dissociation of water ($H_2O \rightarrow H^+ + OH^-$) are equal. At body temperature, this equilibrium is pushed further right, resulting in a greater concentration of both free hydrogen and hydroxyl ions with a more acidic pH of 6.8.

Intracellular pH varies among different tissues; brain pH is 7.0, erythrocyte pH is 7.19, and liver has a pH of 7.27 (26). The pH of normal blood is 7.4. Extracellular fluids such as blood are more alkaline than intracellular fluid (higher ratio of OH^-/H^+) due to the greater transmembrane permeability of H^+ compared to OH^-. Cellular enzyme systems function optimally over a narrow range of hydrogen ion concentrations, and prolonged, significant deviations of hydrogen ion concentration from normal are not well tolerated (26). Nevertheless, the body maintains a stable internal milieu most of the time, so that deviations from the norm invariably point to disturbances (26).

Three homeostatic systems help to maintain pH close to baseline after the addition of acid or alkali to the body:

1. *Nonvolatile, soluble buffer systems* provide an immediate response by either releasing or capturing hydrogen ion. In the extracellular compartment, which includes red blood cell contents, hemoglobin represents the largest single contribution to buffering capacity with lesser contributions from plasma proteins and inorganic compounds such as phosphates and sulfates. These extracellular buffers, although responsible for most of the immediate response, account for only one-third of the body's total buffering capacity and intracellular tissue proteins are responsible for the remaining two-thirds.
2. *Respiratory response* leads to changes in ventilation causing either retention or excretion of carbon dioxide which in turn changes the hydrogen ion concentration mediated through the carbonic acid system: $\Delta pCO_2 + H_2O^- \leftrightarrow H_2CO_3 \leftrightarrow H^+ + HCO_3^-$
3. *Renal mechanisms* mediate a slower response to changes in the total body hydrogen ion load by causing net excretion or generation of hydrogen ions through the urine.

From a clinical perspective, the carbonic acid system and ventilatory response is the body's single most important buffer system. This is because changes in respiratory rate permit the rapid excretion (or retention) of large quantities of hydrogen ions through changes in the PCO_2, which in turn affects the serum bicarbonate and pH. Ventilatory change is rapid and open-ended, resulting in greater buffering capacity than the soluble systems. In addition, the carbonic acid system's components are easily measured. Although inferences concerning systemic acid–base balance can be made by analyzing any buffer system, ease of measurement makes the carbonic acid system the most attractive for clinical use. In fact, common clinical terminology relies exclusively on the carbonic acid system's components to define a patient's acid–base status.

PATHOPHYSIOLOGY

Pathologic processes perturb the body's acid–base equilibrium in two fundamental ways: either through an increase or decrease the body's soluble hydrogen ion activity (a metabolic disturbance) or through an increase or decrease ventilation (a respiratory disturbance). The disruption of acid–base equilibrium by a single disease process is termed a *primary disturbance*. This disruption initiates a series of compensatory responses that tend to return the pH toward normal. A compensatory response to a primary disturbance rarely returns the pH to the normal range and never overshoots the normal range.

The body responds to a primary metabolic disturbance by adjusting the respiratory rate and, thus, the PCO_2 (*respiratory compensation*). It responds to a primary respiratory disturbance by increasing or decreasing renal hydrogen ion excretion (*metabolic compensation*) (Table 158.1).

A disease process causing a single primary acid–base abnormality is termed a *simple acid–base disturbance*. A *mixed acid–base disturbance* occurs when two or more primary acid–base abnormalities occur simultaneously, possibly as a result of more than one disease process.

Although the degree and rapidity of compensatory responses to simple acid–base disturbances vary from patient to patient, empiric data have defined a range of the expected compensatory response for each type of simple disturbance. Table 158.2 lists the anticipated compensatory responses for the different types of primary, simple acid–base disturbances (17). Patients with metabolic or respiratory profiles falling outside the predicted compensation range for a simple acid–base disturbance should be suspected of having a mixed disorder.

Tables 158.3 and 158.4 list the causes of the simple or mixed acid–base disturbances most common in the emergency department patient. The emergency physician must be able to differentiate simple and mixed acid–base abnormalities and to identify and treat the underlying disease processes operative in a given patient.

EMERGENCY DEPARTMENT EVALUATION AND MANAGEMENT

Acid–base disturbances should be suspected when a patient appears critically ill, has an abnormal respiratory rate, abnormal mental status, or complains of vomiting or diarrhea. Arterial blood gas and serum electrolyte determinations provide enough data for the initial metabolic assessment. Blood gas determination on a venous sample can often suffice for measuring the pH and pCO_2.

TABLE 158.1. Primary Disturbances and Compensatory Responses in Terms of Changes in Carbonic Acid Constituents

	Usual pH	Hydrogen Ion Concentration	Serum Bicarbonate (Measured as Total CO_2 Content)	P_{CO_2}
Metabolic acidosis	< 7.38	Primary increase	Immediate decrease	Rapid compensatory decrease
Metabolic alkalosis	> 7.42	Primary decrease	Immediate increase	Variable compensatory increase
Acute respiratory acidosis	< 7.38	Secondary increase	Immediate small compensatory increase	Primary increase
Chronic respiratory acidosis	< 7.38	Secondary increase	Slow larger compensatory increase	Primary increase
Acute respiratory alkalosis	> 7.42	Secondary decrease	Immediate small compensatory decrease	Primary decrease
Chronic respiratory alkalosis	7.40–7.42	Secondary decrease	Slow larger compensatory decrease	Primary decrease

A history and physical examination is mandatory before considering the acid–base status, as the physician should attempt to interpret these abnormalities only after formulating a set of preliminary hypotheses about the disease processes most likely present in the patient. To identify acid–base abnormalities accurately, the physician should then ask three questions:

1. Does the patient have an acidemia or an alkalemia? *Acidemia* is defined as a pH less than 7.38, and *alkalemia* as a pH greater than 7.42. An *acidosis* is any process that causes acid to accumulate; an *alkalosis* is a process that causes hydrogen ion depletion. If the patient is acidemic, at least one of the processes present must be an acidosis.

2. Is the primary disturbance respiratory or metabolic? Look at the serum bicarbonate and arterial P_{CO_2}. Patients with a simple metabolic acidosis have both a low bicarbonate resulting from the combination of this buffer with exogenous hydrogen ion and a low P_{CO_2} resulting from increased respiratory compensation. Similarly, patients with a primary simple respiratory disturbance have an abnormal P_{CO_2} with changes in serum bicarbonate resulting from renal compensation (Table 158.5).

3. Is the acid–base disturbance simple or mixed? In order to identify a mixed disturbance, the physician must employ a series of formulas that quantify the expected compensatory response to a simple acid–base disturbance. When the appropriate formula (see Table 158.2) is applied, a significant deviation from the parameters expected for the compensatory response, to a simple disturbance, indicates the presence of a mixed disorder. These formulae were developed in populations that were in steady state for 12 to 24 hours (17). Accordingly, the emergency physician should avoid their rigid application in situations where the clinical situation is rapidly changing.

Simple Metabolic Acidosis

This is the most common acid–base disturbance in hospitalized patients and is often present in emergency department patients (7). The diagnosis of the underlying cause is aided by determining the *anion gap,* defined as serum sodium (chloride + CO_2 content). This gap is a misnomer because it reflects the difference between the cations and anions that are not measured by commonly used clinical laboratory assays. As the electric neutrality of the plasma is always maintained, there are actually equal numbers of cations and anions. The gap is simply a phenomena of commonly available assays. The normal range for the anion gap is 5 to 12 ± 3 mEq/L (20,24,25).

A normal anion gap in a patient with a simple metabolic acidosis indicates the presence of excess hydrochloric acid; an anion gap greater than 14 mEq/L may indicate an excess of organic acids. Table 158.3 classifies the causes of metabolic acidosis according to the presence or absence of an abnormal anion gap (8). The emergency physician is likely to evaluate many patients with an increased anion gap. When using the anion gap diagnostically, several factors must be kept in mind:

1. A moderate increase in the anion gap (12 to 20 mEq/L) is noted in many situations in which a metabolic acidosis is not present. These include dehydration, alkalosis, spurious laboratory values, and treatment with citrate, lactate, or certain antibiotics.
2. An anion gap greater than 25 mEq/L is seen only with lactic acidosis, ketoacidosis, and the toxin-associated acidoses (10).
3. Common sense indicates that in a high anion gap metabolic acidosis, the degree to which the anion gap exceeds normal limits should be matched by an equal decrease in the serum bicarbonate level. This does not occur for several reasons. Nonbicarbonate intracellular buffers accept hydrogen ions, blunting the decrease in serum bicarbonate. The longer the duration of acidosis, the greater the contribution from intracellular buffers (25). The unmeasured anions associated with different acidoses have different volumes of distribution.

TABLE 158.2. Formulas Describing Expected Compensatory Response to Primary Acid–Base Disturbances

Simple Metabolic Acidosis
Predicted decreased P_{CO_2} mm Hg = 1.2 × $\Delta(HCO_3^-)$ mEq/L
Predicted P_{CO_2} mm Hg = 1.5(HCO_3-) mEq/L + 8 ± 2
Anticipated P_{CO_2} approximates last two digits of arterial pH

Simple Metabolic Alkalosis
Predicated increased ΔP_{CO_2} mm Hg = 0.67 × $\Delta(HCO_3^-)$ mEq/L

Simple Acute Respiratory Acidosis
Predicted decreased ΔpH units = 0.8 × ΔP_{CO_2} mm Hg
Predicted increased $\Delta(HCO_3^-)$ mEq/L = 0.1 × ΔP_{CO_2} mm Hg

Simple Chronic Respiratory Acidosis
Predicted decreased ΔpH units = 0.3 × ΔP_{CO_2} mm Hg
Predicted increased $\Delta(HCO_3^-)$ mEq/L = 0.35 × ΔP_{CO_2} mm Hg

Simple Acute Respiratory Alkalosis
Predicted increased ΔpH units = 0.8 × ΔP_{CO_2} mm Hg
Predicted decreased $\Delta(HCO_3^-)$ mEq/L = 0.2 × ΔP_{CO_2} mm Hg

Simple Chronic Respiratory Alkalosis
Predicted increased ΔpH units = 0.17 × ΔP_{CO_2} mm Hg
Predicted decreased $\Delta(HCO_3^-)$ mEq/L = 0.5 × ΔP_{CO_2} mm Hg

TABLE 158.3. Causes of Simple Acid–Base Disturbances

SIMPLE METABOLIC ACIDOSIS

Elevated Anion Gap (MUDPILES)
Methanol
Uremia/Renal failure
Diabetic ketoacidosis/Alcoholic ketoacidosis/Starvation
Paraldehyde/Propylene glycol
Iron/INH
Lactic acidosis
Ethylene Glycol
Salicylates

Normal Anion Gap (FUSED CRASH)
Fistulas
Uretoenteric conduits
Saline
Endocrine (hyperparathyroidism)
Diarrhea
Carbonic anhydrase inhibitor therapy
Renal tubular acidosis
Arginine/Lysine/Chloride (e.g., TPN)
Spironolactone
Hydronephrosis

SIMPLE METABOLIC ALKALOSIS

Vomiting/gastric suctioning
Volume depletion
Diuretic therapy
Corticosteroid therapy

SIMPLE RESPIRATORY ACIDOSIS

CNS lesion
Sedative therapy/overdose
Neuropathies
Myopathies
Chest wall abnormalities
    Trauma
    Kyphosis
Pleural disease
Obstructive airway disease

SIMPLE RESPIRATORY ALKALOSIS

Anxiety
Progesterone therapy/increased exogenous progesterone
Sympathomimetic therapy
Fever
Hyperthyroidism
Hypoxia
Liver disease

The greater the exogenous anion's ability to diffuse intracellularly, the lower the drop in the serum bicarbonate and the lower the anion gap. Also, acidemia itself decreases the anion gap by decreasing the negative charge on serum proteins that makes a major contribution to the normal anion gap (25). Finally, exogenous anions that are rapidly cleared from the plasma will result in a lower anion gap for a given degree of academia (6).

Several conditions may lower the anion gap. These include hypoalbuminemia, which decreases the anion gap by 3 mEq/L for every 1-g/L decrease in the serum albumin, hypercalcemia, lithium intoxication, paraproteinemia secondary to multiple myeloma, and hypertriglyceridemia, which can spuriously elevate the serum chloride determination (12). Organic acidoses in these patients may thus result in a smaller anion gap than otherwise predicted (25).

TABLE 158.4. Mixed Acid–Base Disturbances

METABOLIC ACIDOSIS-RESPIRATORY ALKALOSIS

Salicylate ingestion
Liver disease
Sepsis
Pulmonary embolism or pulmonary edema with hypotension
Pulmonary-renal syndrome

METABOLIC ACIDOSIS-RESPIRATORY ACIDOSIS

Cardiopulmonary arrest
Pulmonary edema
Drug overdose

METABOLIC ALKALOSIS-RESPIRATORY ALKALOSIS

Critical illness
Pregnancy
Mechanical ventilation-induced chronic hypercapnea

METABOLIC ALKALOSIS-RESPIRATORY ACIDOSIS

Chronic hypercapnea with:
    Diuretic overuse
    Dehydration
    Hypokalemia

METABOLIC ACIDOSIS-METABOLIC ALKALOSIS

Diarrhea/vomiting
Organic acidosis/vomiting
Metabolic acidosis with excessive bicarbonate administration

The serum potassium level must be closely monitored in patients with suspected metabolic acidosis (1). The emergency physician should perform a rapid assessment of the serum potassium level (by seeking electrocardiographic evidence of hyperkalemia) in patients with suspected acidosis. In general, the serum potassium level increases as the patient becomes more acidemic. This increase may result from the interaction of the excess hydrogen ion with intracellular buffer systems (18). There is no reliable formula by which to estimate the expected change in serum potassium arising from a given change in pH and inorganic acidoses (hydrochloric acid, toxins) tend to increase the serum potassium more than organic (keto and lactic) acidoses (1).

Persistent acidemia (pH <7.2) can lead to decreased cardiac output, cardiac dysrhythmias secondary to increased sympathetic discharge and decreased ventricular fibrillation threshold, decreased renal and hepatic blood flow, inhibition of anaerobic glycolysis, decreased hepatic lactic uptake, increased protein breakdown, and hyperkalemia (32). Treatment of the underlying disorder in both lactic and ketoacidosis can lead to rapid replenishment of bicarbonate stores (see below) but inorganic acidoses such as diarrhea-induced lactic acidosis may require exogenous treatment.

TABLE 158.5. Respiratory vs. Metabolic Acidosis/Alkalosis

	pH	PCO$_2$	HCO$_3$
Metabolic acidosis	Decrease	Decrease	Decrease
Metabolic alkalosis	Increase	Increase	Increase
Respiratory acidosis	Decrease	Increase	Increase
Respiratory alkalosis	Increase	Decrease	Decrease

In these instances, treatment with intravenous bicarbonate at a dose that will restore the serum bicarbonate levels to 8 to 10 mmol/liter should be considered. Since the volume of distribution is about 50% of body weight, the following formula will determine the dose in mmoles of bicarbonate: weight (kg) $\times$ 0.5 $\times \Delta$ HCO$_3^-$(mmol/L). Given the risks of overshoot alkalosis and volume overload, the clinician should be extraordinarily conservative in estimating dosage. In addition, bicarbonate should be administered as an infusion and not as a bolus (32).

Simple Metabolic Alkalosis

Metabolic alkalosis is a common condition that should be suspected in a patient with a very high value for the total serum CO$_2$ content. Most metabolic alkaloses are initiated by the combination of volume, potassium, and chloride depletion. Patients with mild metabolic alkalosis generally require both normal saline and a potassium chloride administration to correct the acid–base disturbance.

The compensatory responses to metabolic alkalosis are weak. The ventilatory response (requiring hypoventilation to increase the Pco$_2$) is limited by systemic defenses against hypoxia, and the kidney cannot alkalize the urine if the patient is hypokalemic or significantly volume-depleted (21). Metabolic alkalosis, therefore, tends to be self-perpetuating if untreated (17).

Patients with a pH >7.6 from metabolic alkalosis are at risk for cardiovascular and cerebrovascular ischemia, and hypoventilation. They require rapid reduction of the serum bicarbonate below 40 mmol/l. The most common causes of this condition are chloride-responsive and include loss of gastric acid and loop diuretics (33). Severe metabolic alkalosis often leads to a decrease in bicarbonate's space of distribution (contraction alkalosis) resulting in high extracellular bicarbonate levels in the presence of massive peripheral edema and total body chloride depletion.

Primary Respiratory Disturbances

Primary respiratory abnormalities are classified as acute or chronic according to their duration. Because the renal compensatory process becomes effective only with the passage of time (48 to 72 hours), patients with primary acute respiratory disturbances have a larger ΔpH for any given ΔpCO$_2$ than a patient with a chronic respiratory disturbance. Chronic respiratory alkalosis is alone among the primary acid–base disturbances where the compensatory mechanism can return the pH into the normal range (2).

The immediate treatment of a severe, primary respiratory disturbance involves a mechanical airway intervention, such as increasing ventilation for respiratory acidosis or decreasing the minute ventilation for respiratory alkalosis. Longer-term treatment involves identifying and treating its underlying cause. The physician must avoid a treatment that suddenly normalizes the Pco$_2$ in a patient with chronic respiratory disturbance. In instances where renal compensatory mechanisms have corrected the pH, rapid normalization of the respiratory parameters risks a dangerous overshooting of pH until the kidneys adapt to the new respiratory situation.

Patients with respiratory acidosis require the most emergent intervention, because the Pco$_2$ can rise quickly to cause both a life-threatening acidosis and serious encephalopathy (CO$_2$ narcosis) (7). An arterial blood gas determination is mandatory for patients with abnormal mental status, especially if they manifest any clinical evidence of ventilatory dysfunction.

Acute respiratory alkalosis is the most common acid–base disorder in emergency practice, being present in fever, pregnancy, and high altitude living. Although most cases of this acid–base abnormality do not require treatment, it should lead to a search for a specific underlying cause.

Mixed Acid–Base Disturbances

When a mixed disorder is present, the patient may be acidemic or alkalemic, or may have a normal pH. Any two primary acid–base disturbances other than acute respiratory acidosis and acute respiratory alkalosis can coexist. As mentioned above, clinical context must be established before performing an analysis to determine the presence of a mixed disturbance.

Metabolic acidosis with respiratory acidosis or alkalosis is diagnosed when the Pco$_2$ deviates significantly from that predicted (see Table 158.2) in a simple metabolic acidosis. Combined metabolic acidosis and respiratory acidosis is seen in situations such as cardiac arrest or the postictal state, in which ventilation is inadequate for the degree of metabolic acidosis. Combined metabolic acidosis and respiratory alkalosis is commonly noted in salicylate poisoning, in which salicylate induces metabolic acidosis and also directly stimulates ventilation in excess of the ventilatory drive induced by the acidosis.

One should be cautious in diagnosing mixed disturbances for patients with a rapidly changing clinical status, because the formulae for the expected response to simple metabolic acidosis were derived from Pco$_2$ levels in patients who had achieved a steady state. Thus, there is an increased chance of overdiagnosing a mixed disorder in many acutely ill patients (17).

The combination of *metabolic acidosis and metabolic alkalosis* often manifests with a relatively normal pH and an anion gap elevation significantly exceeding the decrease in total CO$_2$ content (19). A common setting for this mixed disturbance is the patient with alcoholic ketoacidosis who has been vomiting. If combined metabolic acidosis and metabolic alkalosis occurs in a patient with a normal anion gap acidosis, however, there is no anion gap elevation to serve as a marker for the disturbance.

An example would be a patient with severe diarrhea (metabolic acidosis caused by loss of sodium bicarbonate in the stool) associated with vomiting (metabolic alkalosis caused by loss of gastric hydrochloric acid). Unless this disturbance is suspected because of the clinical setting, the presence of a mixed acid–base abnormality becomes evident only after one of the deficits is corrected. In the vomiting and diarrhea example, rapid volume correction with normal saline but without concomitant bicarbonate replacement might unmask the normal anion gap acidosis, with the serum bicarbonate decreasing as volume is restored.

CONTROVERSIES IN MANAGEMENT

Diabetic Ketoacidosis

Insulin administration, rehydration, and close monitoring and replacement of potassium are the mainstays of emergent therapy of diabetic ketoacidosis (DKA). Although bicarbonate has traditionally been recommended for patients with DKA whose pH is below 7.1, even patients with a pH between 6.9 and 7.1 do not benefit from receiving bicarbonate (30). Judicious administration of bicarbonate may be useful in patients with severe acidosis and cardiovascular compromise (16) and in patients with a pH below 6.9 (14). Authors (30) have even questioned regarding the necessity of bicarbonate therapy in DKA patients with a pH below 6.9, but there is not yet universal agreement on withholding bicarbonate in this circumstance.

Adverse effects of excessive bicarbonate administration in DKA include tissue hypoxia from bicarbonate's leftward shifting of the oxyhemoglobin dissociation curve; augmentation of hepatic ketogenesis; hypertonicity and sodium overload; hypokalemia; and late alkalemia, when bicarbonate is regenerated from ketoacids (9). Some patients have deteriorated after aggressive bicarbonate treatment from either a "paradoxical" central nervous system acidosis (11) (bicarbonate does not cross the blood–brain barrier) or cerebral edema from activation of a membrane Na^+–H^+ exchanger by the organic acidosis (29).

Lactic Acidosis

This common acidosis occurs with a pH below 7.35 and a serum lactate level >5 mmol/L and is often divided into type A (low tissue oxygen delivery) and type B (hyperlacticemia in the absence of tissue hypoxia) (13). Common causes of lactic acidosis are listed in Table 158.6. Most patients with lactic acidosis have some degree of tissue hypoxia leading to overproduction (e.g., hypoperfusion, cyanide poisoning, etc.) or underutilization (e.g., liver disease) of tissue-generated lactate.

The treatment of patients with lactic acidosis should focus on improvement of tissue oxygenation and identification and treatment of its underlying cause. There remains no evidence or basis for recommending bicarbonate treatment of severe lactic acidosis, and no basis for a suggestion that peripheral bicarbonate administration could worsen intracellular pH in lactic acidosis (34). However, a slow bicarbonate infusion of 1 to 2 mEq/kg should be considered as a temporizing measure in the presence of severe lactic acidemia (pH <7.0), while its underlying cause is being addressed.

Emergency physicians should be aware of cases of potentially life-threatening lactic acidosis in HIV patients taking nucleoside-analog reverse transcriptase inhibitors, particularly stavudine (35). Recent analysis also questions the association of metformin to lactic acidosis, but emergency providers should be aware of case reports describing this association in patients with renal failure and chronic hypoxia (36).

Cardiac Arrest

A common emergency department setting in which the use of bicarbonate is considered is cardiac arrest. These patients would be expected to manifest a combined metabolic and respiratory acidosis, although the actual acid–base status varies depending on the cause and duration of the cardiac arrest. Neither animal nor human data have demonstrated the effectiveness of bicarbonate in increasing survival after cardiac arrest, and there have been reports of severe hyperosmolality, alkalosis, hypernatremia, and even pediatric intracerebral hemorrhage from injudicious bicarbonate administration (3,4,22,23).

TABLE 158.6.   Common Causes of Lactic Acidosis

Hypotension
Sepsis
Methanol, ethylene glycol
Metformin, nitroprusside, Beta-agonist, Reverse transcriptase
  inhibitors
Diabetes mellitus
Alcoholism
Congenital
Thiamine deficiency
Short bowel syndrome
Hematologic malignancies

The 2001 American Heart Association *Advanced Cardiac Life Support* guidelines (5) unequivocally support the use of bicarbonate in cardiac arrest associated with hyperkalemia, in tricyclic overdose, salicylate ingestion, and in patients with preexisting bicarbonate-responsive metabolic acidosis. Bicarbonate therapy may also be considered during prolonged cardiopulmonary resuscitation in which the patient has been adequately ventilated but is not responding to standard resuscitative measures. When bicarbonate is used, the initial dose should be 1 mEq/kg, with subsequent doses and timing determined by the arterial pH.

Toxin-Induced Acidosis

Methanol and ethylene glycol are two low-molecular-weight alcohols that can produce severe metabolic acidosis when ingested. If treatment begins promptly, recovery can be excellent despite severe acidemia. Parenteral sodium bicarbonate is an effective interim treatment. In contrast with other high anion gap acidoses, the organic anions generated in these poisonings cannot be converted back to bicarbonate by the liver.

The physician should administer 1 mEq/kg of bicarbonate if the pH is below 7.20 and gauge the quantity and frequency of further doses by the response. Additional treatment includes administration of ethanol or 4-methylpyrazole (fomepizole, Antizol) to delay the formation of toxic intermediates, and hemodialysis for removal of the alcohol and its toxic metabolites. Note that in these ingestions, the elevation in anion gap and osmolar gap may not be present simultaneously. Initially patients present with elevated osmolar gaps, and then the anion gap increases as the osmolar gap decreases (15).

Salicylate ingestion produces a characteristic picture of metabolic acidosis-respiratory alkalosis. Unless the serum is highly alkaline, judicious administration of sodium bicarbonate to alkalinize the urine, while keeping the blood pH less than 7.50, will trap the salicylate ion in the renal tubules. With the addition of forced diuresis, urinary alkalinization will enhance excretion of the ingested salicylate.

Use of Alternative Alkalinizing Agents

A number of alternatives to bicarbonate for the treatment of metabolic acidosis have been investigated. These include Carbicarb (a mixture of sodium bicarbonate and sodium carbonate that generates less carbon dioxide during the buffering process), and THAM, a commercially available solution of tromethamine that buffers both metabolic and respiratory acids. Neither of these bicarbonate alternatives is currently recommended for emergency department use (2).

CRITICAL INTERVENTIONS

- Monitor the serum potassium level and cardiac rhythm in patients with suspected nonorganic metabolic acidosis
- Avoid therapy that suddenly normalizes the Pco_2 in a patient with chronic respiratory disturbance as this may lead to a dangerous overshooting of normal pH
- One should be cautious in diagnosing mixed disturbances in patients with a rapidly changing clinical status, because the formulas for the expected response were developed in patients who had achieved a steady state

COMMON PITFALLS

✔ Emergency physicians must be proficient in differentiating simple from mixed acid–base disturbances. They should search for and aggressively treat any underlying causes of significant disturbances. The limitations of the standard formulas that assist in the categorization of acid–base disturbances must be understood

✔ There is significant controversy about the indications for and appropriate doses of sodium bicarbonate in several common emergency conditions. Bicarbonate should be used in hyperkalemia, toxin-induced metabolic acidosis, or severe DKA, and can be used for alkalization after appropriate overdoses. In selected cases of suspected lactic acidosis, bicarbonate can be given cautiously and with close monitoring. Bicarbonate should be avoided in hypoxic lactic acidosis. In metabolic acidosis of unknown cause, bicarbonate should not be withheld if there is cardiovascular compromise and a pH below 7.0

References

1. Adrogue HJ, Ledeier ED, Suki WW, et al. Determinants of plasma potassium levels in DKA. *Medicine* 1986;65:165.
2. Adrogue HJ, Madias NE. Management of life-threatening acid–base disorders. *N Engl J Med* 1998;338:26–33.
3. Bishop RL, Weisfelt ML. Sodium bicarbonate administration during cardiac arrest. *JAMA* 1976;235:506.
4. Chazan JA, Stenson R, Kurland GS. The acidosis of cardiac arrest. *N Engl J Med* 1968;278:360.
5. Cummins Richard O, ed. *Advanced cardiac life support: provider manual.* Dallas: American Heart Association, 2001:83.
6. DiNubile MJ. The increment in the anion gap: overextension of a concept? *Lancet* 1988;2:951.
7. Dulfano MJ, Ishikawa S. Hypercapnia: mental changes and extrapulmonary complications. *Ann Intern Med* 1963;63:829.
8. Elkington JR. Clinical disorders of acid–base regulation. *Med Clin North Am* 1966;50:1325.
9. Fleckman AM. Diabetic ketoacidosis. *Endocrinol Metabol Clin North Am* 1993; 22:181.
10. Gabow PA, Kaehny WD, Fennessey PV, et al. Diagnostic importance of an increased serum anion gap. *N Engl J Med* 1980;303:854.
11. Hale PJ, Crase J, Nattras M. Metabolic effects of bicarbonate in the treatment of DKA. *BMJ* 1984;289:1035.
12. Jurado RL, Del Rio C, Nassar G, et al. Low Anion Gap. *South Med J* 1998;91:624.
13. Mizack B. Controversies in lactic acidosis. *JAMA* 1987;258:497.
14. Morris LR, Murphy MB, Kitabchi AZ. Bicarbonate therapy in severe DKA. *Ann Intern Med* 1986;105:836.
15. Mycyk MB, Aks SE. A visual schematic for clarifying the temporal relationship between the anion and osmol gaps in toxic alcohol poisoning. *Am J Emerg Med* 2003;21:333–335.
16. Narins RG, Cohen JJ. Bicarbonate therapy for organic acidosis: the care for its continued use. *Ann Intern Med* 1987;106:615.
17. Narins RG, Emmett M. Simple and mixed acid–base disorders: a practical approach. *Medicine* 1980;59:161.
18. Oster JR, Perex GO, Vaamonde CA. Relationship between blood pH, potassium, and phosphorus during acute metabolic acidosis. *Am J Physiol* 1978;135:F345.
19. Paulson WD. Anion gap—bicarbonate relation in DKA. *Am J Med* 1986;81:995.
20. Paulson WD, Roberts WL, Lurie AA, et al. Wide variation in serum anion gap measurements by chemistry analyzers. *Am J Clin Path* 1998;110:735–742.
21. Pierce NF, Fedson DS, Brighton KL, et al. The ventilatory response to acute acid–base deficit in humans. *Ann Intern Med* 1970;72:633.
22. Redding JS, Pearson JW. Resuscitation from ventricular fibrillation. *JAMA* 1968; 203:93.
23. Redding JS, Pearson JW. Metabolic acidosis: a factor in cardiac resuscitation. *South Med J* 1967;601:926.
24. Roberts WL, Johnson RD. The serum anion gap. Has the reference interval really fallen? *Arch Path Lab Med* 1997;121:568–572.
25. Salem MM, Mujais SK. Gaps in the anion gap. *Arch Intern Med* 1992;152:1625.
26. Schlichtig R, Grogono AW, Severinghaus JW. Current status of acid–base quantitation in physiology and medicine. *Anesth Clin North Am* 1998;16:211–233.
27. Stacpoole PW. Lactic acidosis: the case against bicarbonate therapy. *Ann Intern Med* 1986;105:276.
28. Stacpoole PW. Lactic acidosis. *Endocrinol Metab Clin North Am* 1993;22:221.
29. Van der Meulen JA, Klip A, Grinsten S. Possible mechanism for cerebral edema in DKA. *Lancet* 1987;2:306.
30. Viallon A, Zeni F, Lafond P, et al. Does bicarbonate improve the management of severe diabetic ketoacidosis? *Crit Care Med* 1999;27:2690–2693.
31. Simon N, Ramaut C, Getti R, Abderrahim N. Can venous blood gas replace arterial blood gas in emergency patients? *Acad Emerg Med* 2003;10:563.
32. Adrogue HJ, Madias NE. Management of Life-Threatening Acid–Base Disorders: First of Two Parts. *New Engl J Med* 1998;338:26–34.
33. Adrogue HJ, Madias NE. Management of Life-Threatening Acid–Base Disorders: Second of Two Parts. *New Engl J Med* 1998;338:107–111.
34. Levraut J, Giunti C, Ciebiera JP, et al. Initial effect of sodium bicarbonate on intracellular pH depends on the extracellular nonbicarbonate buffering capacity. *Crit Care Med* 2001;29:1033–1039.
35. Falco V, Crespo M, Ribera E. Lactic acidosis related to nucleoside therapy in HIV-infected patients. *Expert Opinion on Pharmacotherapy* 2003;4:1321–1329.
36. Salpeter S, Greyber E, Pasternak G, Salpeter E. *Risk of fatal and nonfatal lactic acidosis with metformin use in type 2 diabetes mellitus (Cochrane Review).* In: The Cochrane Library, Issue 4, 2003 Chichester, UK: John Wiley & Sons, Ltd.

CHAPTER 159
Diabetes Mellitus

Scott R. Votey and Anne L. Peters

Diabetes mellitus currently affects over 18 million Americans, and this number is likely to reach 20 million by the year 2010. It is a disproportionately expensive disease; patients with diabetes accounted for 6.2% of the United States population, yet were responsible for 18.5% of all health care expenditures in 2002. This chapter focuses on the emergency department (ED) evaluation and treatment of the acute and chronic complications of diabetes other than those directly associated with hypoglycemia and severe metabolic disturbances.

Diabetes is a chronic disease that requires long-term medical attention to limit the development of its devastating complications and to manage them when they do occur. Approximately 90% of diabetics have type 2 (or ketosis-resistant) diabetes (T2DM), and the remainder has type 1 (ketosis-prone) diabetes (T1DM). Although the frequency of the acute and chronic complications of diabetes differs between the two types of patient, both groups are at risk for the microvascular, macrovascular, and neuropathic complications of diabetes.

Microvascular complications of diabetes include retinopathy and nephropathy. Macrovascular complications are peripheral vascular, cerebrovascular, and coronary artery disease. Hypertension eventually occurs in approximately 50% of patients with diabetes. Chronic, poorly controlled hyperglycemia, in addition to the metabolic consequences associated with glycosuria, can lead to impaired immune function and delayed wound healing. The development of complications is related to the duration of diabetes and the degree of glycemic control.

EMERGENCY DEPARTMENT EVALUATION

A diabetes-related history is important in assessing any patient with diabetes who presents to an ED. The first fact to be determined is which type of diabetes the patient has (Table 159.1). Type 1 diabetes mellitus (T1DM) generally occurs in younger, lean patients and is characterized by an autoimmune process that leads to the marked inability of the pancreas to secrete insulin. The distinguishing characteristic of a patient with T1DM is that if insulin is withdrawn, ketosis, and eventually ketoacidosis, develops. These patients are therefore insulin-dependent (i.e., insulin is life-sustaining), because they produce no endogenous insulin. Although the onset of T1DM often occurs in childhood, 30% of patients with new onset T1DM are greater than 30 years of age. In adults T1DM seems to have a slower course to total islet-cell failure than it does in children, and is called latent autoimmune diabetes of adulthood (LADA) (26).

TABLE 159.1.   Metabolic and Clinical Characteristics of the Two Major Types of Diabetes Mellitus

Characteristic	Type 1 Diabetes (DM1)	Type 2 Diabetes (DM2)
Synonyms	Juvenile-onset diabetes, IDDM	NIDDM
Age of onset	Usually <30 yr; sometimes in older adults	Usually >40 yr; sometimes in younger persons, even children
Genetic predisposition	Moderate (requires environmental factor[s] for expression); only 50% of identical twins develop DM1 if one sibling affected	Strong; 80%–100% of identical twins develop DM2 if one sibling is affected. More common among Native Americans, Hispanic, African Americans.
Precipitating factors	Viral/toxic/other trigger precipitating autoimmune response	Obesity, age
Findings at diagnosis	80% ICA-positive at diagnosis	Most patients had asymptomatic diabetes for 4–7 yr prior to "diagnosis"
Endogenous insulin levels	Very low to none	Present
Insulin resistance	Only present when blood glucose levels high	Almost always present
Response to prolonged fast	Hyperglycemia, ketoacidosis	Normal blood glucose levels
Response to stress, withdrawl of insulin	Ketoacidosis	Hyperglycemia without ketosis
Response to diet alone	Negligible	Always present to some degree
Response to sulfonylurea agents	Absent	Present

IDDM, insulin-dependent diabetes mellitus; NIDDM, non-insulin-dependent diabetes mellitus; ICA, islet cell antibody.

Type 2 diabetes mellitus (T2DM) typically occurs in older (>40 years of age) patients who have a family history of diabetes. However, T2DM is occurring in younger and younger individuals. Children as young as 2 years old have been diagnosed with T2DM, and increasingly teenagers of Hispanic, Native American, and African American descent are developing prediabetes (abnormal glucose tolerance) and diabetes (19). Patients who develop T2DM have a genetic predisposition to do so and develop insulin resistance along with insufficient pancreatic β-cell secretion of insulin. Most patients (90%) who develop T2DM are obese, and obesity itself is associated with insulin resistance, which further worsens the diabetic state. Because patients with T2DM retain the ability to secrete some endogenous insulin, those who take insulin rarely develop diabetic ketoacidosis (DKA) when insulin is stopped. Therefore, they are considered insulin-requiring, not insulin-dependent. Moreover, patients with T2DM often do not require treatment with oral antidiabetic medication or insulin if they lose weight or do not over eat.

Differentiating between the two types of diabetes based on age has become less reliable. Almost always a lean child with no family history of diabetes who presents in DKA will have T1DM. However, an overweight child from a high risk group who has a family history of T2DM may present in DKA yet ultimately have T2DM, and be treatable with diet or oral medications. Defining the type of diabetes can, therefore, be challenging, but a good clinical history often allows the distinction to be made. A strong family history of T2DM, obesity, and Hispanic, African-American, or Native-American heritage all make the diagnosis of type 2 diabetes more likely, regardless of age. The presence of anti-GAD antibodies confirms the diagnosis of T1DM, and the presence of an elevated or even normal C-peptide level in patients who have been treated with insulin for several years confirms a diagnosis of T2DM. The presence of measurable C-peptide levels at the time of diagnosis is not usually helpful since C-peptide levels can be elevated or absent in both new onset type 1 and type 2 diabetes depending on the level of hyperglycemia and other clinical circumstances. Although neither of these tests is likely to be available on a stat basis in the ED, an understanding of their results may be useful to emergency physicians. The duration of the diagnosis of diabetes is important also, because the chronic complications of diabetes are related to the length of time the patient has had the disease. Patients with T2DM have often had diabetes for 5 to 7 years before the diagnosis is made, and can present with the complications of diabetes at the time of diagnosis (15).

Patients should be asked if they self-monitor their blood glucose levels, what their usual blood glucose levels are, and what the recent values have been. Patients should be asked about the types and doses of their diabetes medications. A sense of patients' level of knowledge about managing their diabetes is useful, as is a sense of their degree of compliance with diet and medications. The date and value of the most recent A1C level determination is a useful indicator of both the quality of glycemic control and the patients' monitoring of their disease.

Symptoms of hypoglycemia and hyperglycemia (polyuria, polydipsia, nocturia, weight loss) should be elicited, with their time course and severity.

Although complications are often diagnosed by physical examination or by laboratory testing, the presence of known complications of diabetes should also be assessed in the patient history. Specifically, a history of retinopathy, nephropathy, vasculopathy (hypertension and coronary, peripheral, and cerebrovascular disease), neuropathy, or diabetic foot complications (ulcers and amputations) should be sought.

A diabetes-focused physical examination includes the following components: vital signs, funduscopic examination, limited vascular and neurologic examinations, and a foot assessment. Other organ systems should be examined as indicated by the patient's clinical situation.

Vital signs are useful for several reasons. Obviously, it is important to note whether the patient has hypertension or hypotension. Orthostatic vital signs may be useful in assessing volume status, as well as in suggesting the presence of an autonomic neuropathy. If the respiratory rate and pattern suggest Kussmaul respiration, DKA must be immediately considered and appropriate tests ordered.

The funduscopic examination should include a careful view of the retina, including both the optic disc and the macula. If hemorrhages or exudates are seen, the patient should be seen by an ophthalmologist as soon as possible, because nonophthalmologists tend to underestimate the severity of retinopathy, especially if the pupils have not been dilated.

The dorsalis pedis and posterior tibialis pulses should be palpated and their presence or absence noted. This is particularly important among patients with foot infection, because poor lower extremity blood flow can delay healing and increase the risk of amputation.

Documenting lower extremity sensory neuropathy is useful among patients who present with foot ulcers, because decreased sensation limits the patient's ability to protect the feet and ankles. If peripheral neuropathy is found, the patient should be made aware that foot care (including daily foot examinations) is very important for the prevention of foot ulcers and possible subsequent lower extremity amputation.

Diabetes Medications

In addition to sulfonylurea agents and insulin, a variety of new drugs have become available for the treatment of T2DM (16). These drugs allow for the use of combination oral therapy, often with improvement in glycemic control. The sulfonylurea agents (e.g., glyburide and glipizide) and meglitinides (e.g., repaglinide and nateglinide) increase insulin secretion and are considered long- and short-acting insulin secretatogues, respectively. Their most common serious adverse reaction is hypoglycemia. The biguanides (e.g., metformin) primarily decrease hepatic glucose production and may also slightly lower insulin resistance. These drugs commonly cause gastrointestinal symptoms such as nausea, abdominal cramping, and diarrhea (20). Rarely, they can cause severe lactic acidosis, especially among patients with renal insufficiency and congestive heart failure. The α-glucosidase inhibitors (e.g., acarbose and miglitol) decrease intestinal absorption of carbohydrate, often producing flatulence and, rarely, causing small bowel obstruction. The newest class of drugs are the thiazolidinediones (troglitazone, rosiglitazone, and pioglitazone) which act as insulin sensitizers. Troglitazone was withdrawn from the market due to cases of severe hepatotoxicity. Rosiglitazone and pioglitazone both require measurement of liver function tests every other month for the first year of use, but despite widespread use, have not proven to be particularly hepatotoxic. Both increase plasma volume and can cause fluid retention. The most common side effect is mild to moderate pedal edema. Congestive heart failure (CHF) rarely occurs in patients who are at risk. The thiazolidinediones have been found to be well tolerated in New York Heart Association (NYHA) Class I and II congestive heart failure (CHF), but should be avoided in patients with more advance congestive heart failure (23).

Abnormalities Caused by Hyperglycemia

Acute hyperglycemia, even when not associated with DKA or the hyperglycemic hyperosmolar syndrome (HHS) is harmful for a number of reasons. If the blood glucose level exceeds the renal threshold for glucose (greater than 240 mg/dL in a healthy person, but diminished with advancing age, renal insufficiency, and pregnancy), an osmotic diuresis ensues, with loss of glucose, electrolytes, and water. Hyperglycemia impairs leukocyte function through a variety of mechanisms. Patients with diabetes have an increased rate of wound infection (4), and hyperglycemia may also independently impair wound healing.

Chronic hyperglycemia is associated with an increased risk for the development of the microvascular and neuropathic complications of diabetes, as elegantly demonstrated in the Diabetes Control and Complications Trial (DCCT) for T1DM (9) and the United Kingdom Prospective Diabetes Study (UKPDS) for T2DM (32). In the DCCT, intensive therapy designed to maintain normal blood glucose levels greatly reduced the development and progression of retinopathy, microalbuminuria, proteinuria, and neuropathy as assessed over a 7-year period. Intensive therapy

was not associated with increased mortality or major macrovascular events and did not decrease the quality of life, although it did increase the likelihood of severe hypoglycemic episodes (8). In the UKPDS, aggressive treatment of blood glucose levels and hypertension was shown to decrease the risk of microvascular complications in patients with T2DM.

Among patients with known diabetes that is poorly controlled, there is no absolute level of blood glucose elevation that necessitates admission to the hospital or the administration of insulin. Admission is appropriate for the following:

1. *Diabetic ketoacidosis* (see Chapter 160). Plasma glucose >250 mg/dl (>13.9 mmol/l) with 1) arterial pH <7.30 and serum bicarbonate level <15 mEq/l and 2) moderate ketonuria or ketonemia. DKA can occur in patients with normal blood glucose levels, particularly if they are vomiting frequently. Therefore, any blood sugar level in the setting of ketoacidosis can be indicative of DKA, even though an elevated blood sugar level is most common.
2. *Hyperglycemic hyperosmolar syndrome* (see Chapter 161). Impaired mental status and elevated plasma osmolality in a patient with hyperglycemia. This usually includes severe hyperglycemia (e.g., plasma glucose >600 mg/dl [> 33.3 mmol/l]) and elevated serum osmolality (e.g., >320 mOsm/kg [>320 mmol/kg]).
3. *Hypoglycemia* (see Chapter 162).
4. *Severely symptomatic patient.* Patients with T1DM who cannot tolerate oral fluids require hospitalization. Likewise, if the patient is severely symptomatic or the precipitating cause of hyperglycemia cannot be adequately treated in the emergency department, the patient needs to be admitted.

Generally, lowering the blood glucose level in the emergency department does not correct the underlying cause of hyperglycemia and has no long-term impact on the patient's blood glucose levels. Therefore, a plan must be formulated as to how the patient's blood glucose level will be lowered and how it will subsequently be monitored. The adequacy of follow up is an extremely important consideration. Whether to give insulin in the emergency department is of lesser consequence and can be decided on an individual basis.

EMERGENCY DEPARTMENT MANAGEMENT

New-Onset Diabetes

Most patients with diabetes have T2DM, and most of those are asymptomatic at diagnosis. The initial treatment for patients with newly discovered, asymptomatic diabetes is a trial of diet therapy. Therefore, if an asymptomatic patient is noted incidentally to have an elevated blood glucose level in the emergency department, this can be followed up by the patient's outpatient physician. Patients who have mild-to-moderate symptoms of poorly controlled diabetes but have not previously been diagnosed can usually be treated on an outpatient basis, often with the initiation of low-dose oral antidiabetic agent therapy.

Controversy exists over the management of markedly symptomatic patients with newly discovered T2DM and blood glucose levels over 400 mg/dL. If close follow up can be arranged, these patients can be started on maximal doses of a sulfonylurea agent and treated as outpatients. Generally, the patient feels better within 1 to 2 days, and, within a week, the blood glucose levels are markedly lower (25). These patients can often have their sulfonylurea agent dose tapered as they comply with diet therapy, and, in some cases, diabetes can subsequently be controlled by diet alone. However, patients who cannot drink adequate amounts of fluid, who have serious coexisting medical conditions (e.g., myocardial infarction [MI] or systemic infection), or who do not have reliable follow up should generally be hospitalized for initiation of therapy.

Patients with new-onset T1DM need to be started on lifelong insulin therapy. Many present in DKA. An occasional patient with new-onset T1DM who presents with mild manifestations and is judged to be very compliant can be started on insulin as an outpatient. T1DM patients begun on insulin as outpatients require basic education on insulin administration and close follow up. At follow up, patients should receive thorough education concerning the use of insulin; the signs, symptoms, and treatment of hypoglycemia; and self-monitoring of blood glucose levels.

Management of Hyperglycemia during Medical Illness and Surgery

Serious medical illness and surgery produce a state of increased insulin resistance and relative insulin deficiency. Hyperglycemia can occur, even in nondiabetic patients, because of stress-induced insulin resistance plus the administration of dextrose-containing intravenous fluids. Increases of glucagon, catecholamines, cortisol, and growth hormone antagonize the effects of insulin, and insulin secretion is itself inhibited by the β-adrenergic effect of increased catecholamine levels. The counterregulatory hormones also directly increase hepatic gluconeogenesis.

To maintain normal blood glucose levels, treatment regimens must be modified to compensate for both the decreased caloric intake and increased physiologic stress. Near-normal blood glucose levels should be maintained in medical and surgical patients with diabetes for four basic reasons:

1. To prevent the development of ketosis in patients with T1DM
2. To prevent electrolyte abnormalities and volume depletion secondary to osmotic diuresis
3. To prevent the development of impaired leukocyte function that occurs when blood glucose levels are elevated
4. To prevent the impaired wound healing that occurs when blood glucose levels are elevated

A variety of approaches have been described for the management of patients with diabetes who undergo surgery (17, 22) or are otherwise unable to maintain oral caloric intake. Patients with T1DM must have insulin and carbohydrate given at all times to prevent the development of ketosis. For seriously ill patients and those undergoing general anesthesia, the optimal regimen involves continuous intravenous infusions of dextrose and insulin. This technique requires that the blood glucose level be measured with a glucose meter every hour, and that the insulin and dextrose infusion rates be adjusted accordingly to prevent hypoglycemia or persistent hyperglycemia (17).

Frequent blood glucose monitoring is not always possible for every patient, and patients with less serious illness or those undergoing minor surgery may do just as well with subcutaneously injected insulin. In patients going to surgery who have not received a dose of intermediate-acting insulin that day, an injection of half of the patient's total daily dose as neutral protamine Hagedorn (NPH) insulin or 80% of the dose as glargine (Lantus) insulin before surgery is often effective. At the same time, an intravenous infusion containing 5% dextrose should be started at a rate of 125 mL/h. Blood glucose levels should be checked every 2 hours during surgery, and small doses of regular or rapid-acting insulin (lispro [Humalog] or aspart [Novolog]) insulin given if values are greater than 250 mg/dL.

The same principles of providing a constant source of insulin and carbohydrate apply to patients with T1DM who are not going to surgery but who must remain NPO due to other medical reasons. One approach is to give sliding-scale regular or rapid-acting insulin every 4 hours, the dose based on the patient's blood glucose level. To avoid hypoglycemia, the regular insulin should not be given more frequently than every 3 to 4 hours, because the previous dose will peak in 2 to 4 hours and last up to 6 hours. Rapid-acting insulin can be given every 3 hours.

Patients with T2DM who are on insulin can follow similar guidelines. However, because patients with T2DM secrete some endogenous insulin and do not develop ketosis, they can often be managed for brief periods without either insulin or dextrose. However, if the blood glucose is less than 80 mg/dL, or more than 250 mg/dL, appropriate treatment is required.

Patients who have been taking sulfonylurea agents or other oral antidiabetic agents should have their blood glucose levels monitored when oral intake is not allowed and intravenous dextrose with or without insulin should be given to keep blood glucose levels between 100 and 250 mg/dL. Metformin should not be given to hospitalized patients until it is clear that their renal function is stable. In general, for the initially hospitalized patients, oral antidiabetic medication should be held and then restarted once the patient is less acutely ill.

The presence of cardiovascular disease and renal dysfunction increases surgical morbidity and mortality in patients with and without diabetes. The emergency physician caring for the diabetic patient who requires emergent surgery must notify the surgeon and the anesthesiologist of the patient's condition, obtain medical consultation when appropriate, and promptly initiate a thorough medical evaluation so as not to delay surgery.

Infections

Infections cause considerable morbidity and mortality among patients with diabetes. Infections may precipitate metabolic derangements, and, conversely, the metabolic derangements of diabetes may facilitate infection. Depending on the population studied, infections have been identified as the precipitant in 26% to 77% of cases of DKA (2). A few infections, such as malignant otitis externa, rhinocerebral mucormycosis, and emphysematous pyelonephritis, occur almost exclusively in patients with diabetes. Certain infections, such as staphylococcal sepsis, occur more frequently and result in greater mortality among patients with diabetes, while others, such as pneumococcal pneumonia, affect diabetic patients no differently than the general population (18).

Although diabetes can compromise all aspects of host defenses against infection, all diabetic patients are nevertheless not equally susceptible to infection. Impairments in humoral immunity and polymorphonuclear leukocyte and lymphocyte function are exacerbated by hyperglycemia and acidemia but are substantially, if not entirely, reversed by normalization of pH and blood glucose levels (7). Although the exact level above which impaired leukocyte function occurs has not been well defined, in vitro evidence suggests that glucose levels above 250 mg/dL impair leukocyte function (3).

Patients with long-standing diabetes also tend to develop microvascular and macrovascular disease, with resulting poor tissue perfusion and an increased risk of infection. The ability of skin to act as a barrier to infection may also be compromised when the diminished sensation of diabetic neuropathy results in unnoticed injury.

Ear, Nose, and Throat Infections

Two head and neck infections that are associated with high morbidity and mortality, malignant otitis externa and rhinocerebral mucormycosis, are seen almost exclusively in diabetic patients.

Malignant or necrotizing otitis externa principally occurs in diabetic patients older than 35 years of age and is almost always caused by *Pseudomonas aeruginosa*. The infection starts in the external auditory canal and spreads to the adjacent soft tissue, cartilage, and bone. Patients typically present with severe ear pain and otorrhea; and although they often have a preexisting otitis externa, the progression to invasive disease is usually rapid. Examination of the auditory canal may reveal granulation tissue, but spread of infection to the pinna, the preauricular tissue, and the mastoid often makes the diagnosis apparent. Involvement of cranial nerves, particularly the facial nerve, is common; when there is extension to the meninges, the outcome is often fatal. Computed tomography (CT) is useful to define the extent of disease.

Prompt surgical consultation is mandatory for malignant otitis externa, because surgical debridement is often an essential part of therapy. Intravenous antipseudomonal antibiotic therapy should be started at once in patients with invasive disease. Diabetic patients with severe otitis externa but no evidence of invasive disease can be treated with an otic antibiotic drop and oral ciprofloxacin, but they require close follow up.

Mucormycosis is the name given collectively to the infections caused by various ubiquitous molds. Invasive disease occurs in poorly controlled diabetic patients, especially in conjunction with DKA. In these patients, the organism colonizes the nose and paranasal sinuses, spreading into adjacent tissues by invading blood vessels and causing soft-tissue necrosis and bony erosion. Patients usually present with periorbital or perinasal pain and various degrees of swelling and induration. There may be a bloody nasal discharge. Involvement of the orbits, with lid swelling, proptosis, and diplopia, is common. The nasal turbinates may appear dusky red or frankly necrotic. The appearance of black necrotic tissue is an important visual clue. As the illness progresses, there is invasion of the cranial vault through the cribriform plate, which may result in cerebral abscess, cavernous sinus thrombosis, or internal carotid artery thrombosis. Wet smears of the necrotic tissue often reveal broad hyphae and distinguish mucormycosis from a severe facial cellulitis.

CT helps to delineate the extent of disease. Treatment consists of control of the predisposing hyperglycemia and acidemia, intravenous amphotericin B, and immediate surgical debridement. Until the diagnosis is confirmed, treatment with antistaphylococcal antibiotics is appropriate.

Urinary Tract Infection

Patients with diabetes have an increased risk for cystitis and, more importantly, for serious upper urinary tract infection (27). Intrarenal bacterial infection should be considered in the differential diagnosis of any patient with diabetes who presents with flank or abdominal pain.

The treatment of cystitis is essentially the same as in nondiabetic patients, although individuals with a neurogenic bladder due to diabetic neuropathy may not empty the bladder well and may require urologic referral. Sulfonamide antibiotics can cause hypoglycemia among patients taking sulfonylurea agents by displacing the sulfonylurea agents from their binding sites and increasing their hypoglycemic effect.

The principles of treatment of pyelonephritis do not differ for diabetic patients, but a lower threshold for hospital admission is appropriate for at least two reasons. First, pyelonephritis makes control of diabetes more difficult by causing insulin resistance; in addition, nausea may limit the patient's ability to maintain normal hydration. The ensuing hyperglycemia further compromises the immune response. Second, diabetic patients are more susceptible to the complications of pyelonephritis, including renal abscess, emphysematous pyelonephritis, renal papillary necrosis, and gram-negative sepsis.

Emphysematous pyelonephritis can occur in patients with diabetes (30). This is an uncommon necrotizing infection of the kidney caused by *Escherichia coli, Klebsiella pneumoniae,* or other organisms capable of fermenting glucose to carbon dioxide. The presentation is usually similar to that of uncomplicated pyelonephritis. The diagnosis is established by identifying renal gas on plain radiography, ultrasonography, or noncontrast helical CT urography, and surgical intervention is indicated once the diagnosis is made.

Skin and Soft-Tissue Infection

Sensory neuropathy, atherosclerotic vascular disease, and hyperglycemia all predispose diabetic patients to skin and soft-tissue infections. These can affect any skin surface but most commonly involve the feet. Even the smallest wound can be complicated by cellulitis, lymphangitis, and, more ominously, staphylococcal sepsis. Minor wound infections and cellulitis are typically caused by *Staphylococcus aureus* or hemolytic streptococci and can be treated with a penicillinase-resistant synthetic penicillin or a first-generation cephalosporin.

Outpatient treatment of minor infections is appropriate if the patient is reliable, performs self-monitoring of blood glucose levels (and urine ketones for T1DM patients), and has close follow-up available. Wounds and, in particular, cutaneous ulcers can also be complicated by necrotizing infections of the skin, subcutaneous tissues, fascia, or muscle. These infections are typically polymicrobial, involving group A streptococci, enterococci, *S. aureus,* Enterobacteriaceae, and various anaerobes. Radiographs should be taken of any spreading soft-tissue infection in a diabetic patient to look for the soft-tissue gas that characterizes these infections. Surgical debridement is necessary for necrotizing infections. Gram stains and surface cultures are not helpful; antibiotic coverage should reflect the range of potential pathogens.

Osteomyelitis

Contiguous spread of a polymicrobial infection from skin ulcer to adjacent bone is common in diabetic patients. In one study, osteomyelitis was found underlying 68% of diabetic foot ulcers, and physical examination and plain radiographs each failed to make the diagnosis in one half of patients (24). Use of MR imaging is also effective, if it is available. Often physical examination and plain films are the only diagnostic modalities available in the emergency department, and the diagnosis is suspected but cannot be established. If osteomyelitis is apparent by radiograph or physical examination (e.g., if wounds are deep enough to expose tendons or bone), the patient should be admitted for intravenous administration of antibiotics. If osteomyelitis is suspected but admission is not necessitated by the soft-tissue infection or metabolic disturbances, the patient can be discharged to have an outpatient work up.

Other Infections

Although cholecystitis is probably no more common in patients with diabetes than in the general population, severe fulminating infection, especially with gas-forming organisms, is. The early clinical manifestations of emphysematous cholecystitis are indistinguishable from those of usual cholecystitis. The diagnosis can be made by finding gas in the gallbladder lumen, wall, or surrounding tissues. Even with immediate surgery, mortality is high. Clostridial species are found in over 50% of cases.

Diabetic patients have a greater incidence of staphylococcal and Klebsiella pneumonia than do persons without diabetes. Diabetes is also a risk factor for reactivation of tuberculosis. Cryptococcal infections and coccidioidomycoses are more virulent in diabetic patients.

Ophthalmologic Abnormalities

Diabetes is the leading cause of blindness in the United States; therefore, visual complaints by diabetic patients should be taken very seriously (11). Diabetes can affect the lens, the vitreous, and the retina, causing visual symptoms that may prompt the patient to come to the emergency department. Visual blurring may develop acutely as the lens changes shape with marked changes in blood glucose concentrations. This effect, which is caused by osmotic fluxes of water into and out of the lens as the blood glucose concentration varies, usually occurs as hyperglycemia increases, but it may also be seen when high blood glucose levels are lowered rapidly. In either case, recovery to baseline visual acuity can take up to a month, and some patients are almost completely unable to read small print or do close-up work during this period.

Rarely, patients with T1DM who are in extremely poor control (e.g., those with frequent episodes of DKA) can acutely develop a "snowflake" (or "metabolic") cataract. Named for their snowflake or flocculent appearance, these cataracts can progress rapidly and create total opacification of the lens within a few days. Surgery is often required to restore vision. Patients with diabetes also tend to develop senile cataracts at a younger age than do persons without diabetes, although not in relation to the degree of glycemic control.

Some degree of diabetic retinopathy can be expected to develop in more than 90% of patients with T1DM and in 40% to 60% of patients with T2DM who have had the disease for 15 years or more. Patients with T2DM may already have diabetic retinopathy at the time their diabetes is diagnosed (l5). There are five stages in the progression of diabetic retinopathy:

1. Dilation of the retinal venules and formation of retinal capillary microaneurysms
2. Increased vascular permeability
3. Vascular occlusion and retinal ischemia
4. Proliferation of new blood vessels on the surface of the retina
5. Hemorrhage and contraction of the fibrovascular proliferation and the vitreous

Patients with T2DM do not develop proliferative retinopathy as often as those with T1DM.

The first two stages of diabetic retinopathy are known as "background" or nonproliferative retinopathy. Initially, there is dilatation of the retinal venules, followed by the appearance of microaneurysms, which appear as tiny red dots on the retina and cause no visual impairment. However, as the microaneurysms or retinal capillaries become more permeable, hard exudates appear, reflecting the leakage of plasma. These are sharply defined yellow deposits composed mostly of lipid material. Rupture of intraretinal capillaries results in hemorrhage. If these ruptures occur deep in the retina, they appear as "dot blot" hemorrhages that can be difficult to distinguish from microaneurysms. If a more superficial capillary ruptures, a flame-shaped hemorrhage appears. Hard exudates are often found in partial or complete rings (circinate pattern), which usually include multiple microaneurysms. These rings usually mark an area of edematous retina.

Many patients with macular edema are unaware of its presence. No change in visual acuity may be noted by the patient, unless the center of the macula is involved. Macular edema can cause visual loss, however, so it is extremely important to refer patients with suspected macular edema to an ophthalmologist for evaluation and possible laser therapy. Laser therapy is very effective in decreasing macular edema and preserving vision, but it is less effective in restoring vision once it is lost.

Preproliferative and proliferative diabetic retinopathy are the next stages in the progression of the disease. Cotton-wool spots can be seen in preproliferative retinopathy. These represent reti-nal microinfarcts due to capillary occlusion and are off-white to gray patches with poorly defined margins.

Proliferative retinopathy is characterized by neovascularization, the development of networks of fragile new vessels that are often seen on the optic disc or along the main vascular arcades. The vessels undergo cycles of proliferation and regression. During proliferation, fibrous adhesions develop between the vessels and the vitreous. Subsequent contraction of the adhesions can result in traction on the retina and retinal detachment. Contraction also tears the fragile new vessels, which hemorrhage into the vitreous.

Often, the first hemorrhage is small and is noted by the patient as a fleeting, dark area, or "floater," in the field of vision. Because subsequent hemorrhages can be larger and more serious, the patient should be referred immediately to an ophthalmologist for possible laser therapy. Patients with retinal hemorrhage should be advised to limit their activity and keep their head upright (even while sleeping), so that the blood settles to the inferior portion of the retina, thus obscuring less central vision.

Patients with active proliferative diabetic retinopathy are at increased risk for retinal hemorrhage if they receive thrombolytic therapy, so this is a relative contraindication to the use of thrombolytic agents.

Diabetic Nephropathy

Nephropathy occurs eventually in 20% to 30% of patients with diabetes (1). All patients with diabetes should be considered to have the potential for renal impairment unless proven otherwise. Thus, extreme care should be exercised when using any nephrotoxic agent in a patient with diabetes. The use of contrast media can precipitate acute renal failure in patients with underlying diabetic nephropathy, and, although most recover within 10 days, some develop irreversible renal failure. Patients with diabetes who must undergo contrast medium–enhanced studies should be well hydrated before, during, and after the procedure and should have careful monitoring of renal function (21). A better solution is to get equivalent clinical information by using an alternative study that does not require contrast medium administration (e.g., ultrasonography or noncontrast helical CT urography).

Potentially nephrotoxic drugs should be avoided whenever possible. Renally excreted or potentially nephrotoxic drugs should be given at reduced dosage as appropriate to the patient's serum creatinine level or creatinine clearance.

Because chronic blood pressure elevation contributes to the decline in renal function, it is extremely important that patients with diabetes who are found to be hypertensive be referred for chronic blood pressure management. If antihypertensive therapy is to be started in the emergency department, an angiotensin-converting enzyme (ACE) inhibitor or angiotensin receptor blocker (ARB) is a good choice (6,33) because these agents have been found to reduce the rate of decline in renal function, independent of their effect on blood pressure. They also decrease proteinuria among patients with diabetic nephropathy. It should be kept in mind, however, that ACE inhibitors and ARBs tend to increase the serum potassium level and should thus be used with caution in patients with renal insufficiency or somewhat elevated serum potassium levels. Data is emerging as to the benefits of combining both ACE inhibitors and ARB agents for enhanced benefit (28).

Diabetic Neuropathy

Diabetic neuropathy is common. Distal symmetric sensorimotor polyneuropathy (in a "glove and stocking" distribution) is the most frequent pattern (29). In addition to the pain often experienced in its early stages, this type of neuropathy eventually leads to loss of sensation. The combination of decreased sensation and peripheral arterial insufficiency often leads to foot ulceration and eventual amputation.

A variety of acute-onset neuropathies occur in diabetic patients, including acute cranial mononeuropathies, mononeuropathy multiplex, focal lesions of the lumbosacral plexus, and radiculopathies. Among cranial neuropathies, third oculomotor nerve palsy is the most common, followed by sixth (abducens) and fourth (trochlear) nerve palsies. All can present with diplopia and eye pain. In diabetic third-nerve palsy, the pupil is usually spared, whereas in third-nerve palsy due to intracranial aneurysm or tumor, the pupil is affected in 80% to 90% of cases. It is important to consider nondiabetic causes for cranial nerve palsies, because 42% have been found to be due to causes other than diabetes. Evaluation should therefore include either nonenhanced and contrast medium–enhanced CT or magnetic resonance imaging of the optic nerve. Neurologic consultation is generally recommended. Acute cranial nerve mononeuropathies usually resolve within 2 to 9 months. These neuropathies are thought to be caused by acute thrombosis of the blood vessels supplying the nervous system structure involved.

Autonomic dysfunction can involve any part of the sympathetic or parasympathetic chains and produces myriad manifestations. Patients likely to seek care in the emergency department include those with diabetic gastroparesis and vomiting, those with severe diarrhea, and those with bladder dysfunction and urinary retention. Symptoms tend to wax and wane over time. Treatment is only symptomatic. Patients with gastroparesis may benefit from the use of metoclopramide, or erythromycin. Alleviating the functional abnormalities associated with the autonomic neuropathy is often difficult and frustrating for both doctor and patient. The patient's primary physician, and often an appropriate subspecialist, should be involved in devising a long-term treatment plan.

The Diabetic Foot

Fifty percent to 70% of all nontraumatic lower extremity amputations occur in diabetic patients (12). At one clinic, however, the rate of amputation was halved after the institution of a program that ensured that patients removed their shoes for a foot examination at every clinic visit. Although foot care is a lifelong challenge for the diabetic patient, the emergency physician can play an important role in this process. This is most obvious in the case of the acutely injured or infected limb, but extends to the recognition of feet at risk and appropriate referral for podiatric care.

The insensate, poorly perfused foot is at risk for ulcers from pressure necrosis or inflammation from repeated skin stress and unnoticed minor trauma. Either can evolve into cellulitis, osteomyelitis, or nonclostridial gangrene and end in amputation.

Wounds, infections, or ulcers of the feet demand particular attention in the diabetic patient. In addition to appropriate use of antibiotics, it is mandatory to avoid further trauma to the healing foot through use of crutches, a wheel chair, or bed rest. If bone or tendon is visible, osteomyelitis is present, and hospitalization for intravenous antibiotics is often necessary. Many patients need a vascular evaluation in conjunction with local treatment of the foot ulcer, because, in some cases, a revascularization procedure may be required to provide adequate blood flow for wound healing. For patients who may be discharged, every attempt should be made to ensure frequent follow up or, if necessary, home nursing visits. If such follow up is not available, hospitalization may be necessary for initial treatment. Followup care by a podiatrist or an orthopaedist with experience in the care of a diabetic foot is optimal.

Because curing ulcers and foot infections are so difficult, it is better to prevent them. The emergency physician can facilitate this by briefly inspecting the feet of each patient with diabetes and educating the patient about the need for proper foot care and maintenance of near normal blood sugar levels (5). Patients with distal sensory neuropathy to pinprick or light touch, decreased peripheral pulses, moderate-to-severe onychomycosis, or impending skin breakdown deserve referral to a podiatrist for foot care.

Macrovascular Complications

Macrovascular disease is the leading cause of death in patients with diabetes. It is responsible for approximately 75% of deaths in patients with diabetes, compared with approximately 35% of deaths in the general population. The presence of diabetes causes a twofold increase in myocardial ischemia (MI) in males and a fourfold increase in females that is in addition to the other known risk factors. The risk of stroke is doubled, and the risk of developing peripheral vascular disease is increased fourfold. Although the disease process itself is the same as in patients without diabetes, atherosclerosis develops earlier and follows a more malignant course among patients with diabetes. Patients with T1DM are predisposed to develop coronary artery disease at a younger age than are patients without diabetes; it is not rare for patients in their 30s and 40s to die of ischemic heart disease. Hypertension is twice as common among patients with T2DM, which also increases the risk of atherosclerosis. In fact, it has been shown that patients with T2DM who have never had an MI have the same risk of having an MI as nondiabetic patients who have had a prior MI (14). Patients with diabetes must therefore have their hypertension and lipid abnormalities treated aggressively to lessen their risk of developing atherosclerotic vascular disease (13).

Patients with diabetes have been said to have an increased incidence of silent ischemia. However, silent ischemia is common in many patients with coronary artery disease, and the apparent higher incidence among patients with diabetes may simply be related to the fact that they are more likely to have coronary artery disease to begin with (10). Nevertheless, it is prudent to order an electrocardiogram on patients with diabetes who have a serious illness or who present with generalized weakness, malaise, or other nonspecific symptoms that are not generally expected to be due to myocardial ischemia. Because of their high risk profile, most patients with type 2 diabetes should be taking a daily aspirin (81 mg to start), an HMG-CoA-reductase inhibitor (statin) and an ACE-inhibitor or an ARB agent. Aggressive global risk reduction, reinforced by all health care providers, is needed to lower the morbidity and mortality associated with diabetes.

CRITICAL INTERVENTIONS

- Maintain the blood glucose levels of patients with wounds or active infections below 250 mg/dL to enhance healing
- Provide adequate hydration to patients with mild diabetic nephropathy before contrast material is given to avoid precipitating acute renal failure

COMMON PITFALLS

✔ Failure to provide patients who have T1DM with a continuous source of insulin and glucose when they are unable to receive oral intake

The absence of detectable ketonuria or ketonemia in DKA is a theoretical concern, which may confound the treating physician. Despite consistent increase in blood ketoacid levels, the relative ratio of AcAc and BHBA is dynamic and varies from patient to patient depending upon the patient's redox state. Because the nitroprusside test for qualitative ketones in serum and urine detects AcAc but not BHBA, patients with a high BHBA/AcAc ratio may appear nonketonuric and the diagnosis may be missed. However, the potential for a false negative urine dipstick may be overestimated; a negative urine dip test has been demonstrated to reliably exclude DKA in hyperglycemic patients with any symptoms of illness (19). A blood sample sent for detection of BHBA as well as serum AcAc might be the best solution if the diagnosis of DKA is not readily apparent.

EMERGENCY DEPARTMENT MANAGEMENT

Once the diagnosis is established, treatment requires correction of hypovolemia, reversal of ketoacid production, enhancement of glucose and ketoacid metabolism, replacement of electrolytes and treatment of precipitating causes. Normalization of the metabolic state should occur gradually to avoid complications such as volume overload, hypoglycemia, hypokalemia and cerebral edema (21). Volume replacement should begin as soon as hypovolemia is recognized. Fluid deficits in DKA average 5 L (24); normal saline effectively restores intravascular volume while avoiding a rapid fall in extracellular osmolality. The initial rate of infusion should be rapid, with the first liter given in the first hour of treatment (1). An infusion rate of 500 mL/h for the first 4 hours followed by 250 mL/h for the next 4 hours has been shown to be effective in patients without extreme volume deficit (1). Smaller volumes of bicarbonate-free solutions tend to lessen the dilutional effect on existing bicarbonate and avoids excessive washout of ketone bodies; if retained, ketone bodies are eventually metabolized to bicarbonate in the presence of insulin. Ultimately, the initial infusion rate is dictated by the patient's hemodynamic stability and response to therapy as reflected by the urine output.

Volume replacement lowers serum glucose and ketone levels and helps to correct metabolic acidosis and electrolyte abnormalities. Insulin must be given for ketogenesis to be reversed, for ketone bodies to be metabolized to bicarbonate, and for glucose to be utilized as a substrate for cellular energy production. Treatment is commonly begun with a bolus dose of regular insulin, 0.15 units/kg IV. Although this practice appears safe, evidence for its necessity is lacking. A subsequent continuous infusion of 0.1 units/kg/h lowers serum glucose concentrations reliably and predictably, and is considered safer and more efficacious than high dose or intermittent bolus therapy (15,23). Intramuscular and subcutaneous injections are not recommended in volume-depleted patients (8,17).

The osmotic diuresis associated with hyperglycemia produces clinically significant deficits in total body potassium, sodium, phosphate and bicarbonate. Acidosis, insulin deficiency and hyperosmolality all shift potassium and phosphate extracellularly, often masking total body deficits (2). Regardless of the initial serum potassium, all patients in DKA will require replacement. Elevated potassium on presentation is common; supplementation should take place when the serum potassium decreases below 5. Patients with normal or low potassium should receive replacement as soon as urine output is confirmed. The administration of fluids and insulin and correction of acidosis causes intracellular shifts of potassium, leaving patients with low total body potassium vulnerable to cardiac dysrhythmias and respiratory arrest. An infusion rate of 10 to 30 mEq/h will correct typical deficits within 24 hours.

Hyperphosphatemia is commonly seen, although total body stores are depressed. With appropriate restoration of volume and administration of insulin, phosphate levels fall, reaching a nadir 24 to 48 hours after initiation of therapy. Phosphate administration can be associated with undesirable side effects such as hypocalcemia. In addition, phosphate replacement has not been shown to affect the outcome of patients with DKA (7). Phosphate supplementation should be reserved for patients with severe hypophosphatemia and it is not routinely indicated in the initial management of DKA.

Sodium deficits are corrected with normal saline infusion. The use of bicarbonate to correct base deficit is controversial. Although systemic acidosis has deleterious effects on cellular function throughout the body, patients in DKA maintain a higher central nervous system pH through a poorly understood buffering mechanism (20). The administration of bicarbonate increases systemic levels of CO_2, which diffuses freely across the blood-brain barrier and combines with water to form carbonic acid. Because bicarbonate crosses the blood-brain barrier much less readily than does CO_2, cerebrospinal fluid (CSF) acidosis ensues.

Other cellular membranes exhibit this differential permeability to CO_2 and bicarbonate as well, suggesting that bicarbonate administration may cause a paradoxical intracellular and CSF acidosis. In addition, it has been shown that administration of bicarbonate confers no therapeutic benefit in patients with a presenting pH of 6.9 or greater, and may actually increase ketone-body formation or delay the metabolism of ketoacids to bicarbonate (9,13,20).

Other potential hazards of bicarbonate therapy include tissue hypoxia through shifting of the oxyhemoglobin dissociation curve, hypokalemia, and rebound alkalosis. Overall, it appears that bicarbonate administration, although it may transiently increase serum pH, does not improve clinical outcome and may be deleterious in the patient with DKA. Adjunctive bicarbonate therapy should be considered only for those patients presenting with a pH less than 6.9, in order to prevent complications of decreased cardiac contractility, cardiac dysrhythmias and peripheral vasodilatation commonly associated with severe academia.

Initially, the patient's blood glucose should be monitored at least every 1 to 2 hours during treatment. Serum electrolytes should also be monitored closely to ensure that metabolic derangements are being corrected. A fall in blood glucose of 75 to 100 mg/dL/h is a reasonable goal and insulin infusions should be adjusted accordingly. The serum potassium level generally reaches a minimum 1 to 4 hours after the initiation of therapy. Although obtaining an initial pH through ABG is an accepted practice, recent trails have demonstrated that ABG results rarely influence physician's decisions regarding diagnosis, treatment, or disposition in suspected DKA patients (4). In addition, since venous pH correlates well with arterial values, arterial sampling may be avoided altogether in this patient population (4).

Ketone monitoring is not helpful and may demonstrate a paradoxical increase in quantitative ketones despite clinical improvement, as BHBA is oxidized to AcAc in the presence of insulin (19). Cardiac monitoring is indicated for patients who present with hemodynamic instability or hypokalemia. Urinary output should be monitored; fluid resuscitation should be adjusted to maintain a urine output of at least 30 cc/hr. A diligent search for underlying precipitating causes should be undertaken.

Insulin therapy must be continued for ketonemia and academia to be corrected. To avoid hypoglycemia and to reduce osmotic gradients between blood and brain, 5% dextrose should be added to the intravenous infusion when the blood glucose level reaches 250 mg/dL (2); the insulin infusion is also reduced by half at this point.

Complications of therapy for DKA include hypoglycemia, hypokalemia, hypophosphatemia, fluid overload and cerebral edema. Careful electrolyte and fluid monitoring and the use of 5% dextrose, as indicated, substantially reduce the risk of treatment complications. Vascular thrombosis, rhabdomyolysis and disseminated intravascular coagulation are rare but often are fatal complications of DKA (3).

CRITICAL INTERVENTIONS

- Aggressive volume infusion (at least 2 liters in the first 4 hours)
- Maintain low-dose insulin infusion until anion gap is normal
- Begin potassium replenishment when serum potassium is ≤ 5
- Administer dextrose when serum glucose reaches 250 mg/dL

DISPOSITION

Proper management of DKA may require close observation and alteration of the therapeutic plan as fluids and electrolytes are replenished; complications tend to occur early and rapidly with potentially severe consequences. Most patients with DKA will be admitted to an intensive care setting. Intermediate-level specialty units with monitoring capability and low patient-to-nurse ratios have also been used safely; these telemetry units provide a cost-effective alternative for patients not requiring cardiorespiratory support.

In very mild cases, patients may be treated in the emergency department and released. At a minimum, these patients should have a mild presentation that responds rapidly to therapy, no precipitating illness requiring hospitalization, normal vital signs, pH and anion gap, blood glucose less than 300 mg/dL, and bicarbonate level greater than 15 mEq/L. Moreover, the patient should be tolerating oral fluids well, have appropriate family support, should be compliant and reliable, and finally, should have follow up scheduled with their family physician within 24 hours.

If needed, transfer to another facility should occur after vital signs have been stabilized and volume resuscitation is well underway. Continuous cardiac monitoring by personnel capable of providing advanced cardiac life support should be provided. The transferring physician should provide a detailed flow sheet of fluid and electrolyte therapy in addition to the usually transfer documentation.

COMMON PITFALLS

✔ Failure to administer dextrose to diabetic patients presenting in coma

✔ Failure to diagnose DKA in patients who are euglycemic, have a negative nitroprusside test or do not present with a high anion-gap acidosis
✔ Failure to monitor glucose frequently and add dextrose to the infusion when the blood glucose level reaches 250 mg/dL
✔ Failure to search diligently for precipitating causes

Acknowledgment

Thanks to the previous edition's chapter author Michael D. Rush.

References

1. Adrogue HJ, Barrero J, Eknoyan G. Salutary effects of modest fluid replacement in the treatment of adults with DKA. *JAMA* 1989;262:2108–2113.
2. Alberti KGMM, Hockaday TDR. Diabetic coma: A reappraisal after 5 years. *Clin Endocrinol Metab* 1977;6:421–455.
3. Basu A, Close CF, Jenkins D, et al. Persisting mortality in DKA. *Diabet Med* 1993;10:282–284.
4. Ma OJ, Rush MD, Godfrey MM, Gaddis G. Arterial blood gas results rarely influence emergency physician management of patients with suspected diabetic ketoacidosis. *Acad Emerg Med* 2003;10:836–841.
5. ADA Position Statement. Hyperglycemic crisis in patients with diabetes mellitus. *Diabetes Care* 2002;25:100–108.
6. Faich GA, Fishbein HA, Ellis SE. The epidemiology of diabetic acidosis: A population-based study. *Am J Epidemiol* 1983;117:551–558.
7. Fisher JN, Kitabchi AE. A randomized study of phosphate therapy in the treatment of diabetic ketoacidosis. *J Clin Endocrinol Metab* 1983;57:177–180.
8. Fisher JN, Shahshahani MN, Kitabchi AE. Diabetic ketoacidosis: Low dose insulin therapy by various routes. *N Engl J Med* 1977;297:238–241.
9. Gamba G, Oseguera J, Castrejon M, et al. Bicarbonate therapy in severe diabetic ketoacidosis. A double blind, randomized, placebo-controlled trial. *Rev Invest Clin* 1991;43:234–238.
10. Gamblin GT, Ashburn RW, Kemp DG, et al. DKA presenting with a normal anion gap. *Am J Med* 1986;80:758–760.
11. Guerin JM, Meyer FP, Sergrestaa JM. Hypothermia in diabetic ketoacidosis. *Diabetes Care* 1987;10:801–802.
12. Goldman JM, Chiriboga M. DKA with alkalemia. *J Emerg Med* 1989;7:369–372.
13. Hale PJ, Crase J, Nattrass M. Metabolic effects of bicarbonate in the treatment of diabetic ketoacidosis. *BMJ* 1984;289:1035–1038.
14. Kaminska ES, Pourmotabbed G. Spurious laboratory values in DKA and hyperlipidemia. *Am J Emerg Med* 1993;11:77–80.
15. Kitabchi AE, Umpierrez GE, Kreisberg RA, et al. Management of hyperglycemic crisis in patients with diabetes. *Diabetes Care* 2001;24:131–153.
16. Knight AH, Williams DN, Ellis G, et al. Significance of hyperamylasemia and abdominal pain in DKA. *BJM* 1973;3:128–131.
17. Luzi L, Barret EJ, Groop LC, et al. Metabolic effects of low-dose insulin therapy on glucose metabolism in diabetic ketoacidosis. *Diabetes* 1988;37:1470–1477.
18. Malone ML, Klos SE, Glennis VM, Goodwin JS. Frequent hypoglycemic episodes in the treatment of patients with DKA. *Arch Intern Med* 1992;152:2472–2477.
19. Schwab TM, Hendey GW, Soliz TC. Screening for ketonemia in patients with diabetes. *Ann Emerg Med* 1999;34:342–346.
20. Morris LR, Murphy MB, Kitabchi AE. Bicarbonate therapy in severe DKA. *Ann Intern Med* 1986;105:836–840.
21. Munro JF, Campbell IW, McCuish AC, et al. Euglycemic diabetic ketoacidosis. *BJM* 1973;2:578–580.
22. Okuda Y, Adrogue HJ, Field JB, et al. Counterproductive effects of sodium bicarbonate in diabetic ketoacidosis. *J Clin Endocrinol Metab* 1996;81:314–320.
23. Page MM, Alberti KGMM, Greenwood R, et al. Treatment of diabetic coma with continuous low-dose infusion of insulin. *BMJ* 1974;2:687–689.
24. Waldhausl W, Kleinberger G, Korn A, et al. Severe hyperglycemia: Effects of rehydration on endocrine derangements and blood glucose concentration. *Diabetes* 1979;28:577–584.
25. Westphal SA. The occurrence of diabetic ketoacidosis in non-insulin dependent diabetes and newly-diagnosed diabetic adults. *Am J Med* 1996;101:19–24.

CHAPTER 161
Hyperosmolar Hyperglycemic State

Michael E. Chansky and Renee L. Riggs

Hyperosmolar hyperglycemic state (HHS) is a syndrome of profound dehydration that develops insidiously as a consequence of prolonged osmotic diuresis. HHS is defined by the following laboratory values: serum glucose level of greater than 600 mg/dL, a plasma osmolarity greater than 320 mOsm/L, and absence of ketoacidosis (1,14,15). However, it must be remembered there is a wide spectrum of hyperglycemic illness with variations in laboratory findings. Commonly referred to as *hyperosmolar hyperglycemic nonketotic coma* in the past, this appears to be somewhat of a misnomer, as some degree of ketosis is often present. Coma is reported to occur in approximately 10% of patients with HHS and carries an increased mortality rate (3,14). HHS should be treated as a medical emergency, as it is associated with a high mortality rate often secondary to severe underlying illness (1,12,14).

CLINICAL PRESENTATION

The typical patient who develops HHS is elderly, with a dependence on others for care and often with some degree of underlying renal insufficiency and undiagnosed type II diabetes (5,14,15). The average age of the HHS patient is between 55 and 70 (12,15), but HHS has also been reported in the pediatric population (6,10). There is no history of diabetes mellitus in one-third of patients who develop HHS, although on recovery most previously undiagnosed patients will prove to have mild type II diabetes (15). HHS accounts for less than 1% of all diabetes-related admissions (1). The reason for lack of ketonemia is not known. Theories include glucagon resistance and presence of enough portal vein insulin to inhibit hepatic production of ketones. A common risk factor for patients who develop HHS is lack of access to or inability to request fluids, for example nursing home residents and infants (1).

Patients with HHS often have severe concurrent illnesses, which may precipitate HHS (3). Infection is the most common precipitating event (1,5,12,15), and identified in 40% to 60% of patients with HHS. Pneumonia is the most common infectious source identified (40% to 60%) (15), followed by urinary tract infection (5% to 16%) (15), and sepsis (14). Chronic renal insufficiency, myocardial infarction, pancreatitis, gastrointestinal bleeding, cerebrovascular accident, severe burns, pulmonary embolism, subdural hematoma, and heat stroke have also been identified as precipitants (2). Other etiologies reported are hypothermia, intestinal obstruction, and peritoneal dialysis (14). Many drugs have also been implicated in the development of HHS: thiazide diuretics, corticosteroids, phenytoin, propranolol, chlorthalidone, furosemide, ethacrynic acid, diazoxide, cimetidine, chlorpromazine, *l*-asparaginase, immunosuppressive agents, loxapine, and total parenteral nutrition (14). Noncompliance with diabetic medications may also be a factor in the development of HHS (14).

HHS has a reputation for being under recognized prior to presentation. The mortality rate of 20% to 60% is likely due to delay in presentation, failure to treat aggressively, and the high incidence of serious underlying disease (3,9,14). Poor prognostic indicators are hypothermia (1), hypotension, or coma on presentation (1,3).

Many patients who develop HHS experience polyuria and polydipsia for days or weeks before coming to medical attention (5). Insidious dehydration progresses until mental status is altered. The most common reason patients are brought to medical attention is diminished or complete lack of responsiveness (3). This delay explains the increased severity of dehydration, as compared to patients with diabetic ketoacidosis (DKA). On average, patients diagnosed with DKA present within 3 days of symptom onset, whereas patients with HHS typically present after an average of 12 (3,9). Ketoacidosis causes symptoms of nausea, vomiting, and dyspnea, which bring patients to medical attention earlier.

The severity of dehydration is dependent on multiple factors, including underlying illnesses. Standard signs of dehydration such as poor skin turgor and dry mucous membranes may not be evident. Laboratory values may not correctly reflect the degree of dehydration (3). Urine output is often maintained by the glucose-mediated osmotic diuresis, which may lead one to underestimate the degree of dehydration.

The degree of altered mental status does correspond with the degree and rate of development of hyperosmolarity. Many neurological symptoms have been described, including seizures, hemiparesis, confusion, and coma (14). Other neurological findings reported include: bilateral or unilateral major motor hyperreflexia or hyporeflexia, aphasia, muscle fasciculations, central hyperthermia, hemianopsia, nystagmus, visual hallucinations, visual loss, acute quadriplegia, dysphagia, and urinary retention.

DIFFERENTIAL DIAGNOSIS

The differential diagnosis of altered mental status and decreased level of consciousness is extensive and focuses primarily on metabolic or structural etiologies. The metabolic etiologies would include, but certainly are not limited to: hypoglycemia, hypo- and hyperthermia, myxedema, intoxication/ingestion, carbon monoxide, acidosis, hepatic failure, and uremia. Structural causes include intracranial hemorrhage, acute ischemic stroke with edema, central nervous system infections, and trauma. The simplest, yet crucial test, appropriate for all patients with altered mental status, is fingerstick blood glucose measurement. This quickly confirms the diagnosis of hypo- or hyperglycemia.

The differential diagnosis of HHS includes DKA, alcoholic ketoacidosis (AKA), and lactic acidosis. Patients with DKA often demonstrate Kussmaul respirations, and an acetone odor may be detected on their breath. Also, DKA patients frequently present with nausea, vomiting, and abdominal pain. An anion-gap metabolic acidosis, ketosis, and mild to marked hyperglycemia are diagnostic. AKA characteristically presents in a known alcoholic with recent abstinence secondary to abdominal pain and vomiting. Marked ketosis, anion gap metabolic acidosis, and mild hyperglycemia (<200 mg/dL) support the diagnosis of AKA. The acidosis responds to D_5NS and appropriate supportive care. Lactic acidosis is often suspected when patients are gravely ill and display signs of shock.

HHS must be included in the differential diagnosis when an elderly patient presents to the emergency department with coma, change in mental status, or dehydration. Delay in diagnosis and therapy is partly responsible for the high mortality rate. It is imperative for the physician to have a high level of suspicion for HHS in any patient who presents with hyperglycemia and alteration of mental status or shock.

EMERGENCY DEPARTMENT EVALUATION

The initial approach to an acutely ill elderly patient includes the "ABCs," a rapid bedside determination of serum glucose and venous or arterial blood gas (13), an electrocardiogram (ECG), and bedside urine dipstick for glucose and ketones. Fluid resuscitation begins immediately with normal saline. Additional laboratory evaluation for a patient suspected of having HHS should include determination of serum electrolytes, blood urea nitrogen (BUN), creatinine, and serum osmolarity, a complete blood cell count, and urinalysis. It is important to identify the precipitating event and to identify any underlying illnesses. A chest radiograph, blood and urine cultures, serum lipase, liver profile, coagulation studies, and, in some cases, cardiac enzymes should be considered.

Typically the serum blood glucose concentration in HHS is greater than 600 mg/dL and may well exceed 2,000 mg/dL (8). Caution must be exercised in the interpretation of rapid finger-stick readings when the blood glucose concentration is either very high or very low, as the accuracy of the meters declines with increasingly abnormal values. In addition, most bedside or home glucose monitors will not read glucose values over 600 mg/dL and will only give a text statement, such as "High." Therefore, any significantly abnormal value must be confirmed by a serum glucose measured by the laboratory.

Serum sodium and potassium concentrations may be low, normal, or high, and the values may not reflect total body losses. If the initial serum sodium concentration is normal or elevated, significant water loss can be assumed to have occurred. Hyperglycemia tends to artificially lower measured serum sodium concentration. Standard teaching of adding 1.6 mEq to the reported sodium concentration for every 100 mg of glucose over 100 mg/dL is accurate only for glucose concentrations under 400 mg/dL (11). A factor of 2.4 mEq/L appears to be more accurate for glucose levels over 400 mg/dL (11). Potassium depletion secondary to ongoing osmotic diuresis is the rule, and profound deficits are usually encountered. Initial hypokalemia reflects profound total body potassium depletion.

All patients with HHS are initially azotemic due to both pre-renal and renal causes. The BUN to creatinine ratio may exceed 30:1. In one series the average initial BUN and creatinine values were 87 mg/dL and 5.5 mg/dL, respectively. After treatment, the average values had fallen to 24 mg/dL and 2.0 mg/dL, respectively (3).

The serum osmolarity can be calculated using the traditional formula:

$$\text{Osmolarity (mOsm/kg water)} = 2 \text{ (serum Na)} + \text{(blood glucose)}/18 + \text{(BUN)}/2.8.$$

Although the measured and calculated osmolarity values follow similar trends, there is not always a reliable correspondence between the values. The calculated osmolarity is by definition greater than 320 mOsm/kg in patients with HHS.

Because urea is freely permeable across cell membranes, it does not create an osmotic gradient between intracellular and extracellular spaces. The effective osmolarity should be calculated by excluding the BUN value from the equation, because azotemia may mask actual hypotonicity of the extracellular fluid. If a patient presents with hyperglycemia and a normal or low effective plasma osmolarity, it is potentially dangerous to administer hy-

potonic fluids or insulin, because lowering the tonicity of the extracellular fluid too rapidly may lead to cerebral edema.

About half the patients with HHS have a mild metabolic acidosis, with an anion gap about twice normal (3). Various explanations of the acidosis are offered: accumulation of lactic acid or β-hydroxybutyric acid (not measured by routine urine tests) or renal insufficiency with accumulation of fixed acid metabolites.

The complete blood cell count may show an elevated white blood cell (WBC) count suggestive of a serious underlying infection. Because of profound dehydration, hemoconcentration can be expected to elevate the hemoglobin and hematocrit, so a patient with an initially normal hematocrit should be suspected of being anemic. Urinalysis may show only modest glycosuria, and ketonuria need not be absent to make the diagnosis of HHS.

EMERGENCY DEPARTMENT MANAGEMENT

When the diagnosis of HHS is being entertained, the patient should be in a monitored bed with i.v. access and an adequate airway ensured. The priority of specific therapy is fluids, potassium and/or insulin, and phosphate (Fig. 161.1). Fluid resuscitation should be initiated prior to receiving electrolyte results. The main goal of treatment is to replace fluid loss (14). Adult patients have profound fluid deficits which average 9 L (1,14) and require aggressive initial fluid resuscitation with 2 L of 0.9% normal saline (1,7,14,15). The choice of fluids thereafter remains somewhat controversial. A reasonable plan is to use 0.45% normal saline infusion, replacing half of the total fluid deficit the first 12 hours at a rate of approximately 200 to 500 mL per hour and the remaining deficit over the following 12 hours (14,15). Normal saline is always the fluid of choice if the patient displays signs of shock or hypoperfusion. Intravenous fluid resuscitation alone decreases the serum blood glucose level by 25 to 50 mg/dL per hour on average (15).

Initial serum potassium concentration determines utilization of insulin and/or potassium. Intravenous regular insulin infusion of 0.1 units/kg/h should be initiated in patients who have a K^+ greater than 3.3 mEq/L, have received at least 1 L of normal saline, and have adequate urine output (5,14,15). A one-time i.v. bolus of regular insulin, 0.15 units/kg, is optional. In the rare patient with an initial K^+ of <3.3 mEq/L, hold insulin and give 10 to 15 mEq KCl per hour i.v. until K^+ is documented to be over 3.3 mEq/L (1). Remember to monitor patients closely, including hourly glucose and potassium measurements. When the glucose level has reached 250 mg/dL, dextrose is added to the i.v. fluids (1,3,14,15). The glucose level should be maintained between 250 and 300 mg/dL until hyperosmolarity resolves and mental status is at baseline (1,5).

Initial potassium concentration may not reliably predict total body potassium stores because of profound total body potassium deficits. Fluids and insulin rapidly decrease serum potassium concentration, and severe hypokalemia may develop during therapy. If the initial serum K^+ is greater then 3.3 but less than 5.0 mEq/L, give 20 to 30 mEq K^+ in each L of i.v. fluid. If serum K^+ is greater than 5.0 mEq/L, continue with fluid resuscitation and insulin therapy until serum K^+ falls below 5.0 mEq/L. Initial hypokalemia (<3.3 mEq/L) mandates potassium therapy *prior to* insulin, as outlined above.

Fluid and insulin therapy will decrease serum phosphate concentration, necessitating careful monitoring. Severe hypophosphatemia, <1.0 mg/dL, can lead to skeletal muscle weakness, respiratory depression, decreased oxygen delivery to the tissues, and rhabdomyolysis. If necessary, 20 to 30 mEq/L of potassium phosphate can be added to replacement fluid, or, if possible, oral phosphate replacement initiated.

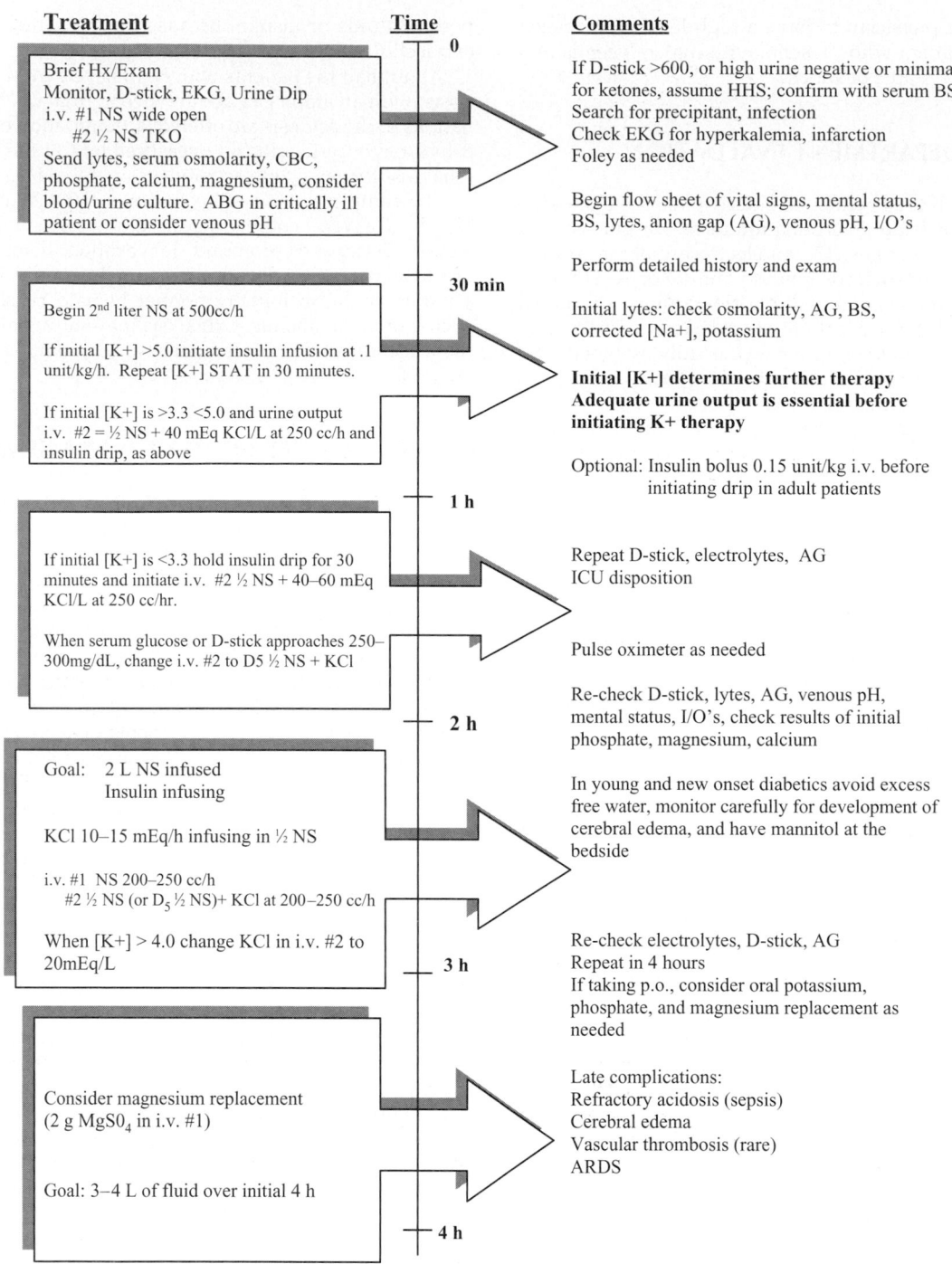

Figure 161.1.   Timeline for the typical adult patient with suspected HHS. (Modified from: Chansky ME, Lubkin CL. Diabetic ketoacidosis. In: Tintinalli J, et al., eds. *Emergency Medicine, A Comprehensive Study Guide.* 6th ed. New York: McGraw-Hill, 2004:1290, with permission.)

The use of sodium bicarbonate is not recommended in the specific treatment of DKA or HHS (4,15).

If seizures develop in patients diagnosed with HHS, the commonly used anticonvulsants are usually ineffective (14). Phenytoin, which inhibits the release of endogenous insulin, may further exacerbate seizures in the setting of HHS and, therefore, should be avoided (14). Seizures carry a grave prognosis.

If bacterial infection is strongly suspected or the WBC count is >25,000/mm^3 appropriate antibiotics should be started promptly, even if the source has not yet been identified (15). It is appropriate to have a low threshold for initiating broad spectrum antibiotics in the emergency department.

Critically ill patients often board in emergency departments until an ICU bed becomes available. Complications that may occur during therapy include venous or arterial thrombosis, pancreatitis, acute respiratory distress syndrome, secondary pneumonia, and disseminated intravascular coagulopathy.

Fatal cases of cerebral edema have been rarely reported with HHS (1). Pediatric patients with HHS may be at higher risk, as in DKA. Rapid deterioration of level of consciousness coupled with seizures, incontinence, bradycardia, and respiratory arrest are seen and worsen as herniation occurs. Etiology of cerebral edema is most likely multifactorial and may be related to generation of intracellular idiogenic osmoles during the hyperosmolar state. Therapy with insulin promotes glucose to move intracellularly prior to the dissipation of intracellular osmoles, promoting cerebral edema. A change in neurologic condition during therapy of HHS, particularly in children, should prompt therapy with i.v. mannitol (1 g/kg). The clinician must consider more aggressive therapy, including intubation and hyperventilation prior to confirmatory CT scan.

CRITICAL INTERVENTIONS

- Obtain adequate i.v. access and place patient on cardiac monitor
- Initiate intravascular support with aggressive infusion of normal saline
- Ensure adequate urine output prior to initiating potassium replacement
- Replace potassium prior to starting insulin therapy if initial potassium is <3.3 mEq/L
- Perform hourly monitoring of blood glucose and electrolytes

DISPOSITION

With the high mortality rate and severity of underlying medical illness, patients diagnosed with HHS require admission to an intensive care setting. Because of the need for immediate and closely monitored treatment for at least 24 hours, it is usually preferable to avoid transfer to another facility until after the fluid deficits and hyperosmolarity have been corrected and treatment for any serious underlying illness has been maintained.

COMMON PITFALLS

✔ Failure to obtain initial fingerstick blood sugar on all at-risk patients
✔ Failure to initially replace fluid and potassium deficit before starting insulin therapy
✔ Failure to identify and address the precipitating event

Acknowledgments

The authors gratefully acknowledge the contribution of Dana Pope, M.D. and Leslie Zun, M.D., who wrote the previous version of this chapter, and Susan E. Kirk, M.D. and Cary L. Lubkin, M.D. for their thoughtful editorial comments.

References

1. American Diabetes Association. Hyperglycemic crisis in patients with diabetes mellitus. *Diabetes Care* 2002;25:S100–S108.
2. Arieff AI, Carroll HJ. Cerebral edema and depression of sensorium in nonketotic hyperosmolar coma. *Diabetes* 1974;23:525–531.
3. Arieff AI, Carroll HJ. Nonketotic hyperosmolar coma with hyperglycemia: clinical features, pathophysiology, renal function, acid-base balance, plasma-cerebrospinal fluid equilibria and the effects of therapy in 37 cases. *Medicine* 1972;51:73–94.
4. Boord JB, Graber AL, Christman JW, et al. Practical management of diabetes in critically ill patients. *Am J Respir Crit Care Med* 2001;164:1763–1767.
5. Chiasson JL, Aris-Jilwan N, Belanger R, et al. Diagnosis and treatment of diabetic ketoacidosis and the hyperglycemic hyperosmolar state. *Can Med Assoc J* 2003;168:859–866.
6. Ellis EN. Concepts of fluid therapy in diabetic ketoacidosis and hyperosmolar hyperglycemic nonketotic coma. *Pediatr Clin North Am* 1990;37:313–321.
7. Feig PU, McCurdy DK. The hypertonic state. *N Engl J Med* 1977;297:1444–1454.
8. Filbin MR, Brown DF, Nadel ES. Hyperglycemic hyperosmolar nonketotic coma. *J Emerg Med* 2001;20:285–290.
9. Gerich JE, Martin MM, Recant L. Clinical and metabolic characteristics of hyperosmolar nonketotic coma. *Diabetes* 1971;20:228–238.
10. Gottschalk ME, Ros SP, Zeller WP. The emergency management of hyperglycemic-hyperosmolar nonketotic coma in the pediatric patient. *Pediatr Emerg Care* 1996;12:48–51.
11. Hillier TA, Abbott RD, Barrett EJ. Hyponatremia: evaluating the correction factor for hyperglycemia. *Am J Med* 1999;106:399.
12. Kitabchi AE, Murphy MB. Diabetic ketoacidosis and hyperosmolar hyperglycemic nonketotic coma. *Med Clin North Am* 1988;72:1545–1563.
13. Ma OJ, Rush MD, Godfrey MM, et al. Arterial blood gas results rarely influence emergency physician management of patients with suspected diabetic ketoacidosis. *Acad Emerg Med* 2003;10:836–841.
14. Trence DL, Hirsch IB. Hyperglycemic crisis in diabetes mellitus type 2. *Endocrinol Metab Clin North Am* 2001;30:817–831.
15. Umpierrez GE, Khajavi M, Kitabchi AE. Review: diabetic ketoacidosis and hyperglycemic hyperosmolar nonketotic syndrome. *Am J Med Sci* 1996;311:225–233.

CHAPTER 162
Hypoglycemia

Scott R. Votey and Anne L. Peters

Hypoglycemia is defined as a plasma glucose value less than 50 mg/dL, accompanied by signs and symptoms of adrenergic excess (sweating, nervousness, tachycardia, shakiness) or alterations in mental status, or both, that are relieved by the administration of carbohydrate. The glucose concentration at which clinical hypoglycemia occurs varies. Completely healthy women may have glucose levels less than 45 mg/dL during a fast without symptoms of hypoglycemia. Conversely, adrenergic symptoms of "hypoglycemia" may occur in patients without low blood glucose levels. Therefore, the diagnosis of hypoglycemia must be based on the presence of both biochemical hypoglycemia and concomitant hypoglycemic symptoms.

Although there are many causes of hypoglycemia, the vast majority of episodes encountered in the emergency department (ED) occur as complications of the treatment of diabetes with insulin or an oral antidiabetic agent. Hypoglycemia is an important and growing concern for the approximately 17 million individuals with diabetes in the United States. The publication of the Diabetes Treatment and Control Trial (DCCT) (6) in 1993 and the United Kingdom Prospective Diabetes Study (UKPDS) (17) in 1998 has proven that tight control of blood glucose delays the development and progression of complications in patients with both type 1 and type 2 diabetes. From these studies has come a greater emphasis on maintaining euglycemia.

Unfortunately, tight control also increases the frequency of hypoglycemia, especially in patients treated with insulin (7). Although mild episodes of hypoglycemia (defined as episodes recognized and treated by the patient) are not harmful and should not dissuade patients from adequately treating their diabetes, recurrent severe episodes (involving altered mentation and requiring assistance to treat) may be associated with progressive cognitive decline (12). Goals for emergency physicians in the management of hypoglycemia are: (1) recognition of each episode of hypoglycemia, (2) prompt and adequate treatment, (3) identification of the cause of the episode, (4) identification of the need for hospital admission to prevent recurrent episodes, and (5) establishment of a plan to prevent future episodes.

A balance between glucose utilization and production maintains normal blood glucose levels. In health, preprandial blood glucose levels are usually 70 to 100 mg/dL, with a small postprandial rise peaking 1 hour after eating and returning to baseline within 4 hours. The major glucose-requiring tissues are the brain and red blood cells. Muscle, fat, and a variety of other tissues take up glucose but are also capable of utilizing other fuels. The brain, with its absolute requirement for glucose, is what drives the need to maintain adequate blood levels of glucose. During fasting, glucose production occurs through hepatic glycogenolysis (breakdown of glycogen) and gluconeogenesis (biosynthesis of glucose from nonglucose substrates). Insulin levels are high in the postprandial period and fall with fasting.

Glucoreceptors in the hypothalamus sense low blood glucose levels and cause the secretion of counterregulatory hormones. Glucagon is the primary counterregulatory hormone in nondiabetic patients. Patients with type 1 diabetes lose their glucagon response to hypoglycemia within the first 5 years of disease.

The onset of action of glucagon is rapid, and it acts by enhancing glycogenolysis and gluconeogenesis. If glucagon is not present, epinephrine serves as the major counterregulatory hormone. It also has a rapid onset of action and acts by inhibiting glucose utilization by muscle, increasing gluconeogenesis, and inhibiting insulin secretion. Cortisol and growth hormone are secreted as part of normal hypoglycemic counterregulation, but their release is delayed and they do not contribute to the acute recovery from hypoglycemia.

CLINICAL PRESENTATION

The signs and symptoms of hypoglycemia fall into two categories: adrenergic (those caused by increased activity of the sympathetic autonomic nervous system) and neuroglycopenic (those caused by depressed activity of the central nervous system [CNS]) (Table 162.1). Although there is much individual variation, the adrenergic symptoms of hypoglycemia typically start at approximately 60 mg/dL, and evidence of neuroglycopenia occurs at approximately 50 mg/dL. Symptoms vary from person to person but, within an individual, remain fairly constant from episode to episode.

Not all patients experience the adrenergic symptoms of hypoglycemia (10). Autonomic neuropathy, which occurs in more than 25% of patients with long-standing (more than 10 years) type 1 diabetes, can diminish adrenergic symptoms (4). Patients who are chronically hypoglycemic, particularly patients with tightly controlled type 1 diabetes, accommodate to hypoglycemia and may not have adrenergic symptoms until the blood glucose is less than 50 mg/dL and neuroglycopenic symptoms develop. This phenomenon, termed *hypoglycemia-associated autonomic failure*, is the combined result of a downregulation of the adrenergic response to hypoglycemia, due to intensive insulin therapy or recent hypoglycemia, and autonomic dysfunction (3).

Patients who lack adrenergic symptoms often fail to recognize impending hypoglycemia and are at increased risk for severe neuroglycopenia.

Because the CNS is almost entirely glucose-dependent for function, hypoglycemia manifests neurologically within minutes. Measurable cognitive deficits commonly begin at blood glucose levels less than 50 mg/dL, but some patients remain awake and alert at much lower levels (13). Patients may fail to perceive their cognitive dysfunction and deny having any CNS symptoms. The blood glucose at which seizures occur varies, but a seizure at a glucose greater than 40 mg/dL should prompt investigation for an alternative cause. Focal neurologic deficits, including hemiparesis, are the presenting symptoms in a small percentage of patients (19).

Long-term cognitive deterioration is a function of the severity, duration, and number of hypoglycemic episodes (12). Mild episodes consisting only of adrenergic symptoms do not result in CNS injury. Severe episodes, particularly those resulting in loss of consciousness or seizures, are damaging. Time to recovery and completeness of recovery depend on the severity and duration of hypoglycemia. Elderly patients and those with a history of prior CNS injury, such as a stroke, appear to be at higher risk for a prolonged or incomplete recovery.

DIFFERENTIAL DIAGNOSIS

Although chronic treatment of diabetes with insulin or a sulfonylurea agent is the root cause of the vast majority of hypoglycemic episodes encountered in the ED, there is invariably an acute precipitant perturbing the patient's usual glucose homeostasis. The key to preventing future hypoglycemic episodes is the identification of the precipitant of the current episode. A good history is the principal tool in achieving this goal and will identify the precipitant in approximately 50% of cases. Common precipitants can be grouped according to their physiologic mechanisms (Table 162.2). Inadequate glucose availability is the most commonly identified cause of hypoglycemia, followed by

TABLE 162.2.   Precipitants of Hypoglycemia in Patients with Diabetes

INADEQUATE GLUCOSE AVAILABILITY

Decreased caloric consumption: missed or delayed meal, fasting
Decreased hepatic gluconeogenesis: suppression by alcohol, hepatic failure
Insufficient counter-regulatory hormones: glucagon, epinephrine, cortisol

INCREASED CALORIC UTILIZATION

Exercise
Illness and injury

MEDICATIONS—INCREASED INSULIN EFFECT

Accidental overdose: poor vision, misunderstanding, change in syringe size, change in insulin concentration, pharmacy error
Intentional overdose

DIMINISHED EXCRETION OR METABOLISM

Renal insufficiency: insulin and sulfonylurea agents undergo renal excretion
Hepatic failure: sulfonylurea agents undergo hepatic metabolism

TABLE 162.1.   Signs and Symptoms of Hypoglycemia

Adrenergic	Neuroglycopenia
Weakness	Headache
Tremor	Mental dullness
Sweating and warmth	Confusion
Tachycardia and palpitations	Amnesia
Nervousness	Incoordination
Irritability	Visual disturbances
Tingling of face and fingers	Seizures
Hunger	Coma
Nausea	Focal neurologic deficits

increased caloric utilization, medication error, and diminished excretion of antidiabetic medication.

Patients who take oral sulfonylurea agents can have prolonged periods of hypoglycemia (sometimes lasting up to a week) because of the long elimination half-life of many of these agents; this phenomenon occurs particularly in elderly patients and those with renal insufficiency or hepatic failure (11,16). The possibility of declining renal function should be assessed in any patient who develops recurrent unexplained episodes of hypoglycemia while taking these agents. These individuals often require admission to the hospital, continuous intravenous administration of dextrose, and frequent blood glucose monitoring until blood glucose levels stabilize. In addition, ingestions of even small doses of sulfonylurea agents may produce severe hypoglycemia in young nondiabetic children, and any sulfonylurea ingestion in these patients should be taken seriously (15).

Repaglinide (Prandin) and nateglinide (Starlix) are short-acting insulin secretagogues which increase insulin secretion and may cause hypoglycemia. The hypoglycemia associated with these agents is of shorter duration than the hypoglycemia associated with the sulfonylurea agents, nevertheless, repaglinide and nateglinide can cause severe symptoms (e.g., seizure) if given after, instead of before, a meal (8). On the other hand, metformin (Glucophage), the α-glucosidase inhibitors (acarbose [Precose], miglitol [Glyset]), and the thiazolidinediones (rosiglitazone [Avandia], and pioglitazone [Actos]) do not increase insulin secretion and rarely cause hypoglycemia when used alone. In combination with insulin or a sulfonylurea, however, these drugs may exacerbate an episode of hypoglycemia.

Due to frequent miscommunication among patients, pharmacists, and medical care providers about the currently available types of insulin, it is necessary to be familiar with these products (Table 162.3). Patients often confuse the type of insulin with the brand name, referring to their insulin as "Humulin" for instance, when they mean the "Lilly brand of human NPH insulin." If patients have their insulin vials with them, it helps to look at them. If not, and they cannot name the insulins they take, it is helpful to remember that all the rapid- and short-acting insulins are clear, as is glargine insulin (Lantus). NPH insulin as well as mixtures that contain NPH insulin are cloudy. Ultralente insulin is also cloudy. Most of the types of insulin, except for glargine insulin, come in insulin pens.

Some patients, particularly the elderly, are not aware that they are being treated for diabetes. Therefore, it is helpful to review all medications the patient is currently taking when investigating the cause of an unexplained episode of hypoglycemia. Surreptitious use of medication is a consideration in healthy-appearing patients with unexplained hypoglycemia, especially if it is severe or recurrent.

Aside from insulin and sulfonylurea agents, a number of other drugs can precipitate hypoglycemia, either at therapeutic doses or in overdose (Table 162.4). Patients taking β-blockers are at increased risk for severe hypoglycemia both because of a blunted counterregulatory response and diminished adrenergic symptoms when hypoglycemia does develop. Salicylate overdoses occasionally precipitate hypoglycemia, particularly in children.

Many serious illnesses may result in hypoglycemia; the most common are renal failure, hepatic failure, malnutrition (including anorexia nervosa), and sepsis (9). Others include severe right heart failure and malignancy. The etiology is often multifactorial. Adrenal insufficiency itself rarely causes symptomatic hypoglycemia, but it may be a contributing factor during times of physiologic stress. Cortisol is necessary for gluconeogenesis, and, without it, glucose levels (especially fasting levels) fall (see Chapter 164, "Adrenal and Pituitary Disorders").

Ethanol ingestion can precipitate hypoglycemia in patients with or without diabetes by suppressing gluconeogenesis, usually in association with inadequate intake of food. This phenomenon occurs most commonly in children, malnourished chronic alcoholics, binge drinkers, and diabetics who neglect to eat adequately when consuming alcohol.

Insulinomas are a rare cause of hypoglycemia. Patients with these tumors have recurrent episodes of hypoglycemia, typically presenting with neuroglycopenic rather than adrenergic symptoms; insulinomas often go undiagnosed for years. Weight gain from eating large amounts of food to self-treat the hypoglycemia

---

TABLE 162.3. Time Course of Action of Insulins (times are approximate, insulins may act differently in different individuals)

Type	Onset (h)	Peak (h)	Duration (h)	Mixability
Rapid Acting				
• Lispro (Humalog)	0.25–0.50	1.0–2.0	3.0–5.0	Good
• Aspart (Novolog)	0.25–0.50	1.0–2.0	3.0–5.0	Good
Short Acting				
• Regular	0.50–1.0	2.0–4.0	6.0–8.0	Good
Intermediate Acting				
• NPH	1.0–3.0	4.0–12.0	18.0–24.0	Good
Long Acting				
• Glargine (Lantus)	2–4	None	~24	Never mix
• Ultralente	4–8	8–12 (variable)	18–36	Avoid mixing
• Determir (Levamir)	2–4	None	~20	Fair
Mixtures				
• 70/30 (Two mixtures are marketed: 70% NPH + 30% regular, and 70% NPH + 30% Aspart)	Actions based on components of the mixture			
• 75/25 (75% NPH + 25% Lispro)				
• 50/50 Varies (50% X and 50% Y)				

TABLE 162.4. Selected Causes of Hypoglycemia

FASTING

Healthy-Appearing Individuals
Drugs
    Exogenous insulin
    Oral hypoglycemic agents—sulfonylurea agents, repaglinide and
      nateglinide
    Beta-adrenergic blocking agents
    Salicylates
    Disopyramide
    Quinine
    Pentamidine
Others
    Ethanol and other alcohols
    Insulinomas and non β cell tumors
    Inherited disorders of metabolism

Ill-Appearing Individuals
Hepatic failure: depleted glycogen stores and impaired
    gluconeogenesis
Renal failure
Adrenal insufficiency
Sepsis
Shock
Malnutrition, including anorexia nervosa
Congestive heart failure, especially severe right heart failure
Pregnancy

FED (REACTIVE)

Impaired glucose tolerance
Alimentary
Idiopathic reactive

is common. Non–β-cell tumors, including mesenchymal tumors, hepatocellular carcinomas, adrenal carcinomas, and others, can also produce hypoglycemia.

Newborns, especially premature infants, are at risk for hypoglycemia during times of physiologic stress due to small glycogen stores and limited hepatic gluconeogenesis. In addition, several inborn errors of metabolism can cause hypoglycemia in children. These include glucose-6-phosphatase deficiency, galactosemia, hereditary fructose intolerance, and carnitine deficiency. Inborn errors of metabolism usually present in the first year of life. Infants experiencing unexplained hypoglycemia should be hospitalized and evaluated for these disorders.

Although hypoglycemia occurs most commonly in the fasting state, there are several causes of fed, or reactive, hypoglycemia. Alimentary hypoglycemia occurs in patients who have undergone gastrointestinal surgery, most commonly gastrectomy. Patients have symptoms of hypoglycemia 30 to 120 minutes after eating. The hypoglycemia is thought to occur because of a more rapid emptying of food into the duodenum, leading to both an accelerated absorption of glucose and an exaggerated insulin response.

Some patients with "mild" diabetes, including patients treated with diet alone and those with risk factors for type 2 diabetes but who have not yet been diagnosed as having diabetes, experience postprandial hypoglycemia. The insulin response to food is initially delayed; the enhanced insulin secretion that follows produces postprandial hypoglycemia.

Idiopathic reactive hypoglycemia is a rare disorder that is substantially overdiagnosed, particularly in young women. In general, patients with this diagnosis have adrenergic symptoms on fasting or postprandially but are rarely documented to have a glucose less than 50 mg/dL.

EMERGENCY DEPARTMENT EVALUATION

In the ED, the biochemical diagnosis of hypoglycemia is usually made by using a bedside glucose meter. A blood glucose level should be checked immediately on any patient presenting with adrenergic or neuroglycopenic symptoms, including behavioral abnormalities, decreased level of consciousness, and acute focal deficits. An immediate check should be done on patients with syncope and trauma patients in whom hypoglycemia as a precipitant may be overlooked.

Most glucose meters are now calibrated to give results that are consistent with plasma glucose levels, but plasma glucose levels measured in the laboratory are still considered the most accurate determination of the blood glucose level. In addition, arterial blood has a glucose level 5% to 10% higher than that of venous blood. Test strips and meters are highly sensitive for the diagnosis of hypoglycemia but may give falsely *high* readings in the setting of severe anemia and acetaminophen overdose (2,14). Test strip accuracy also deteriorates with prolonged storage, so strips should not be used beyond their printed expiration date.

Laboratory confirmation of hypoglycemia diagnosed by bedside testing is usually not necessary, however, unless results are ambiguous. Laboratory glucose levels measured by the glucose oxidase method (and presumably test strips and meters, which also rely on this reaction) may be falsely low in the setting of high levels of ascorbic acid, levodopa, tolbutamide, and bilirubin (14).

When the patient has recovered adequately, a focused history should be taken, investigating the cause of the episode, including the timing and doses of medications, food eaten, and activity. For diabetic patients, the history should include an assessment of diabetic control, whether home glucose monitoring is performed, usual values, and the frequency and severity of hypoglycemic episodes. The presence of comorbidities, including renal insufficiency and liver disease, should be ascertained.

Additional laboratory testing, including measurements of the serum creatinine or hepatic transaminases, is necessary only if the history fails to reveal the cause of the episode and contributory comorbidities are suspected.

Hypoglycemia has been associated with silent and symptomatic myocardial ischemia and infarction in diabetic patients both with and without known coronary artery disease (5). The possibility that an episode of hypoglycemia has induced myocardial ischemia should be considered in all diabetic patients at risk for coronary artery disease.

Nondiabetic patients who are suspected of having hypoglycemia, but for whom the diagnosis was not established in the ED, can be referred for an outpatient diagnostic workup.

EMERGENCY DEPARTMENT MANAGEMENT

Hypoglycemia should be considered in every patient with an altered sensorium or any acute neurologic deficit. Ideally, a fingerstick blood glucose level should be obtained to confirm the diagnosis before treatment with glucose is initiated, but glucose should be given empirically if the level cannot be obtained immediately. Although animal studies and retrospective human studies have found a correlation between hyperglycemia and poor neurologic outcome among patients with stroke and severe brain injury, there is no evidence that the doses of glucose given to correct hypoglycemia are harmful. Only 15 to 20 g of carbohydrate is generally required to restore euglycemia, although, occasionally, more is required. Glucose can be administered orally or intravenously, depending on the patient's level of consciousness.

The initial treatment for a confused or comatose adult with hypoglycemia is a 50-mL bolus of 50% glucose intravenously. Less concentrated glucose solutions are recommended for children (25%) and neonates (10%) due to concerns about hyperosmolality. The mean increase in the serum glucose level following this bolus is 150 mg/dL, but it varies greatly and is not predictable (1). The bolus should be followed by the continuous infusion of 5% or 10% glucose at a rate sufficient to keep the glucose level over 100 mg/dL until the patient is capable of eating. If there is any reason to suspect thiamine deficiency, thiamine 100 mg intravenously should be given concomitantly with glucose to avoid precipitating Wernicke-Korsakoff syndrome.

Patients who are alert enough to eat may be treated with glucose tablets or gel, orange juice, hard candy, or any form of concentrated sugar. If a patient is taking an α-glucosidase inhibitor (acarbose or miglitol), absorption of oral carbohydrate may be inhibited. These patients must be treated with dextrose (which is in glucose tablets) as opposed to sucrose (which is in table sugar). They can also be effectively treated with milk, because the drug does not inhibit lactase.

Adults with hypoglycemia who are unable to eat and in whom intravenous access cannot be secured can be given glucagon 1 mg intramuscularly (18). Children should receive 0.5 mg. Available data have shown glucagon to be safe and effective in restoring euglycemia, with neurologic recovery occurring generally within 10 minutes.

Adrenergic symptoms respond to glucose therapy within minutes. The time to recovery of neuroglycopenic symptoms is more variable, ranging from minutes to (in rare cases) days (13). A patient failing to show clear signs of neurologic recovery within 10 minutes should have the glucose level rechecked to verify that euglycemia has been restored, because an additional bolus of glucose is occasionally needed. Alternative etiologies should be considered if there are no signs of neurologic recovery within 30 minutes.

To prevent recurrence, a meal or snack should be given after treatment. The simple carbohydrate given to raise the blood glucose level quickly does not produce a sustained elevation of blood glucose (50 mL of D50 and an 8-oz glass of orange juice contain only about 100 calories each), so a more complete meal, containing protein, fat, and complex carbohydrate, should be given to produce a more sustained rise in blood glucose levels. If hypoglycemia is due to administration of a long-acting insulin or an oral hypoglycemic drug, low glucose levels will typically last for an extended time. It is important to continue treatment and close observation to prevent relapse.

Long-term therapy depends on the cause of the hypoglycemia. If the hypoglycemia is secondary to a disorder such as hepatic failure or adrenal insufficiency, treatment of the underlying disorder is necessary to prevent recurrent hypoglycemia.

Dietary therapy is the treatment of choice for reactive and alimentary hypoglycemia. Patients should avoid sugars and eat frequent small snacks that contain a mixture of carbohydrate, fat, and protein. Restricting carbohydrate intake to 40% of total calories also may help.

In insulin-treated patients who become hypoglycemic, whether the usual insulin dose should be adjusted depends on the severity of the reaction. If the reaction is minor (easily detected and treated by the patient) and there is an explanation for the reaction (e.g., a missed meal or increased exercise), no insulin dose adjustment is indicated. However, if the reaction is more severe or is unexplained, or if there is a pattern of hypoglycemia occurring at the same time each day, the insulin dose should be decreased. Close monitoring of blood glucose levels is necessary to prevent hypoglycemia or hyperglycemia when the insulin dose has been changed.

Recurrent hypoglycemia acutely downregulates the adrenergic response to additional episodes of hypoglycemia. A moderately severe episode of hypoglycemia on day 1 will induce

hypoglycemia unawareness on day 2, resulting in a more severe episode on the second day. Therefore, on the day following a moderate-to-severe hypoglycemic episode, the insulin dose should be reduced by 25%.

TABLE 162.5.   Discharge Criteria Following a Symptomatic Hypoglycemic Episode

Brief episode
Fully neurologic recovery
Able to eat
No major co-morbidities that require hospital admission
Cause of the episode found and addressed
Treatment plan to prevent future episodes understood by the patient
Hypoglycemia accidental
Relapse unlikely—no long-acting insulin or oral agent, nor prolonged excretion or metabolism
Ability to do home glucose monitoring*
Responsible person to be with the patient*
Follow-up arranged*

*Imperative for severe episodes requiring assistance for recovery

CRITICAL INTERVENTIONS

- Administer glucose based on patients' symptoms rather than waiting for laboratory confirmation of hypoglycemia
- Feed patients in the ED following a response to intravenous glucose
- Administer glucagon to any hypoglycemic patient with neuroglycopenic symptoms who is unable to take oral glucose and in whom intravenous access has failed
- Admit patients with hypoglycemia secondary to long-acting oral hypoglycemic agents (sulfonylureas) or long-acting insulin preparations

DISPOSITION

Most patients seen in the ED for hypoglycemia meet discharge criteria (Table 162.5). Hospital admission is indicated for patients failing to meet these criteria. Hypoglycemic patients with type 2 diabetes require hospitalization more frequently due to the need for monitoring in patients with sulfonylurea-induced hypoglycemia, poor general condition, and a higher rate of concomitant disease requiring treatment (11).

Patients who are discharged should receive specific instructions on how best to avoid recurrent episodes (most commonly by increasing caloric intake or decreasing the insulin dose), should be instructed to perform self-monitoring of blood glucose, and should carry some form of oral glucose at all times. Family members of patients who have experienced a severe episode requiring assistance should be instructed in how to recognize and treat hypoglycemia, including use of a glucagon emergency kit.

COMMON PITFALLS

- ✔ Failure to consider hypoglycemia in all patients with acute neurologic or psychiatric symptoms, regardless of any history of diabetes
- ✔ Failure to consider hypoglycemia in any physiologically stressed infant

✔ Failure to follow a bolus of intravenous glucose with a continuous glucose infusion in patients who remain unable to eat

✔ Prematurely discharging a patient whose episode of hypoglycemia is due to a long-acting insulin or a sulfonylurea agent

✔ Failure to consider intentional overdose as the cause of hypoglycemia

✔ Failure to consider that hypoglycemia may have induced clinically significant myocardial ischemia

✔ Failure to reinforce the need for self-monitoring of blood glucose and, in particular, failure to discuss the need for monitoring blood glucose levels prior to driving

References

1. Adler PM. Serum glucose changes after administration of 50% dextrose solution: pre- and in-hospital calculations. *Am J Emerg Med* 1986;4:504.
2. Cartier LJ, Leclerc P, Pouilet M, et al. Toxic levels of acetaminophen produce a major positive interference on Glucose Elite and Accu-Chek Advantage glucose meters. *Clin Chem* 1998;44:893.
3. Cryer PE, Davis SN, Shamoon H. Hypoglycemia in diabetes. *Diabetes Care* 2003;26:1902.
4. Davidson MB. *Diabetes mellitus, diagnosis and treatment.* 3rd ed. New York: Churchill Livingston, 1991.
5. Desouza C, Salazar H, Cheong B, et al. Association of hypoglycemia and cardiac ischemia: a study based on continuous monitoring. *Diabetes Care* 2003;26:1485.
6. Diabetes Control and Complications Trial Research Group. The effect of intensive treatment of diabetes on the development and progression of long-term complications in insulin-dependent diabetes mellitus. *N Engl J Med* 1993;329:977.
7. The Diabetes Control and Complications Trial Research Group. Hypoglycemia in the Diabetes Control and Complications Trial. *Diabetes* 1997;46:271.
8. Flood TM. Serious hypoglycemia associated with misuse of repaglinide. *Endo Pract* 1999;5:137.
9. Fischer KF, Lees JA, Newman JH. Hypoglycemia in hospitalized patients. *N Engl J Med* 1986;315:1245.
10. Heller SR, MacDonald IA, et al. Influence of sympathomimetic nervous system on hypoglycemia warning symptoms. *Lancet* 1987;2:359.
11. Holstein A, Plaschke A, Egberts EH. Incidence and costs of severe hypoglycemia. *Diabetes Care* 2002;25:2109.
12. Langan SJ, Deary IJ, Hepburn DA, et al. Cumulative cognitive impairment following recurrent severe hypoglycemia in adult patients with insulin treated diabetes mellitus. *Diabetologia* 1991;34:337.
13. Malouf R, Brust JCM. Hypoglycemia: causes, neurologic manifestations, and outcome. *Ann Neurol* 1985;17:421.
14. Pointer JE. Glucose analysis: indications for ordering and alternatives to the laboratory. *Ann Emerg Med* 1986;15:372.
15. Quadrani DA, Spiller HA, Widder P. Five year retrospective evaluation of sulfonylurea ingestion in children. *J Toxicol Clin Toxicol* 1996;34:267.
16. Shorr RI, Ray WA, Daugherty JR, et al. Incidence and risk factors for serious hypoglycemia in older persons using insulin or sulfonylureas. *Arch Intern Med* 1997;157:1681.
17. UK prospective Diabetes Study (UKPDS) Group. Intensive blood-glucose control with sulphonylureas or insulin compared with conventional treatment and risk of complications in patients with type 2 diabetes (UKPDS 33). *Lancet* 1998;352:839.
18. Vukmir RB, Paris PM, Yealy DM. Glucagon: prehospital therapy for hypoglycemia. *Ann Emerg Med* 1991;20:375.
19. Wattoo MA, Liu HH. Alternating transient dense hemiplegia due to episodes of hypoglycemia. *West J Med* 1999;170:170.

CHAPTER 163
Thyroid Emergencies

Scott C. Sherman

NORMAL PHYSIOLOGY

The thyroid gland begins to appear 1 month after conception as a thickening of the epithelium at the base of the pharyngeal floor. As development ensues, the gland undergoes caudal displacement into the neck, leaving in its track the thyroglossal duct, which normally dissolves by the second month of conception. If the thyroglossal duct does not close, a cyst, most commonly found in the midline between the hyoid bone and thyroid cartilage, can form.

The thyroid gland is composed of two major cell types. Follicular cells are the source of production of the thyroid hormones, while parafollicular cells secrete the calcium-lowering hormone, calcitonin. Production of the thyroid hormones, thyroxine (T_4) and triiodothyronine (T_3) starts with the active transport of iodide (I^-) into the follicular lumen. There it is oxidized to iodine (I_2) by a peroxidase enzyme. Organification occurs when thyroglobulin, synthesized within the follicular cell, is bound to one or two iodine molecules. The resultant iodinated thyroglobulins—monoiodotyrosine (MIT) and diiodotyrosine (DIT)—are then coupled to produce T_4 and T_3.

The storage capacity of the thyroid gland for T_4 and T_3 is tremendous, and normal turnover occurs at a rate of 1% per day. The normal human thyroid has storage capacity of T_4 for approximately 50 days (14). The administration of antithyroid agents that halt the synthesis of de novo thyroid hormone production will not impact the serum T_4 concentration for up to 2 weeks.

Regulation of thyroid hormone secretion occurs via the negative feedback loop of the hypothalamic–pituitary axis. Thyrotropin-releasing hormone (TRH) is produced by the hypothalamus and stimulates the release of thyroxine-stimulating hormone (TSH) from the anterior pituitary. TSH promotes production and release of T_4 and T_3, which in turn negatively impact further production of TSH.

Further regulation of thyroid hormone secretion occurs via iodine. The relationship between iodine and the thyroid gland is dependent upon the dose of iodine, rate of administration, presence of underlying thyroid dysfunction, and previous iodine status. Iodine is not only necessary for proper production of thyroid hormone, but, depending on the clinical scenario, iodine administration can also cause both hyper- and hypothyroidism.

Administration of excess iodine in the normal thyroid gland results in decreased production of T_4 and T_3, the so-called Wolff-Chaikoff effect, and decreased release of preformed thyroid hormone. The normal thyroid autoregulates the production of T_4 and T_3 based on the concentration of iodine within the gland. When the thyroid is saturated with iodine, there is a decrease in production and release of thyroid hormone. The end result is the rapid lowering of the serum T_4 concentration. Susceptibility to the Wolf-Chaikoff effect is further increased in two clinically important situations: (1) the hyperthyroid state, where follicular iodide uptake is already elevated and (2) after propylthiouracil (PTU) therapy blocks conversion of iodide to iodine. It is this effect that makes iodine administration beneficial in thyroid storm.

Eventually, after continued iodine administration, the thyroid gland escapes the acute Wolff-Chaikoff effect and the production and release of hormone returns to normal. Iodine-induced hypothyroidism occurs in some patients due to a failure to escape the Wolff-Chaikoff effect. In this scenario, continued suppression of thyroid hormone production results in clinical hypothyroidism. The mechanism is not completely understood, but susceptible individuals include those with Hashimoto's disease, Graves' disease after radioiodine ablation, and patients with cystic fibrosis.

Iodine-induced hyperthyroidism, the jodbasedow effect, occurs most commonly in areas of endemic iodine deficiency. The sudden administration of large quantities of iodine present in drugs, contrast media, or foods can cause hyperthyroidism in patients possessing an autonomously functioning thyroid, most commonly multinodular goiter. Less commonly, iodine-induced hyperthyroidism occurs in patients with previously normal thyroid function and in areas of iodine sufficiency or excess. Patients previously treated for Graves' disease are prone to developing iodine-induced hyperthyroidism.

Upon release from the thyroid, T_4 and T_3 are bound in the serum by thyroxine-binding globulins (TBG) with less than 1% of the hormone circulating in the unbound state. Binding to TBG is in a steady state, and while some medications and disease states change the amount of TBG, the amount of T_4 and T_3 in the free, unbound state remains relatively constant. T_3 is bound with less affinity and therefore undergoes a greater peripheral turnover—60% per day versus 10% for T_4. T_3 is more potent than T_4 by a factor of three to four. Conversion of T_4 to T_3 takes place in peripheral tissues, thereby maximizing hormone function.

Thyroid hormone acts to stimulate the production of cellular proteins, which promote the functions of the body's organ systems. The net result is an increase in bone growth, central nervous system activity, basal metabolic rate, and oxygen consumption. Metabolic effects include increased absorption of glucose from the intestine, increased glycogenolysis, gluconeogenesis, and lipolysis—producing an overall catabolic effect. Cardiovascular function is stimulated and an increased heart rate and stroke volume is observed, while the gastrointestinal system increases intestinal transit time. The respiratory system is likewise affected by an increase in ventilatory rate and an increase in the ventilatory response to hypoxia and hypercapnia.

THYROID FUNCTION TESTS

The wider availability of the measurement of free, unbound thyroid hormones has made interpreting the tests simpler. A free thyroid hormone measurement allows the clinician to make an accurate determination of the patient's physiologic thyroid state with less concern for the medications and illnesses that affect thyroid binding globulin capacity.

Rarely, medications will alter the measurement of unbound thyroid hormone without altering the physiologic thyroid state. Examples include phenytoin, carbamazepine, phenobarbital, fenclofenac, and corticosteroids, which can all decrease the measurement of free T_4, while maintaining the euthyroid state. Conversely, heparin, β-blockers, phenylbutazone, and aspirin can all result in increased measurements of free T_4, in patients who are clinically euthyroid. Another medication, amiodarone, causes almost universal alterations in thyroid function tests during administration but is different in that it can cause both clinical hypothyroidism and thyrotoxicosis. Thyroid function abnormalities during amiodarone administration are due to inhibition of 5-deiodinase activity. This enzyme is responsible for the peripheral conversion of T_4. The resultant thyroid function abnormalities include an elevated free T_4, decreased free T_3, and elevated TSH (may also be normal or low).

The American Thyroid Association has recommended initial screening of thyroid function with a TSH level and a free-T_4 level (13). The TSH and free T_4 level will reliably distinguish the euthyroid state from thyrotoxicosis and hypothyroidism. A normal TSH and free T_4 level make thyroid disease highly unlikely. A low TSH and high free T_4 confirm the diagnosis of thyrotoxicosis, while a high TSH and a low free T_4 accurately diagnosis primary hypothyroidism. Other variations of these tests are listed in Table 163.1.

TABLE 163.1. Interpretation of Thyroid Function Tests*

TSH	Free T_4	Disease State
Normal	Normal	None
Normal	Low	Euthyroid hypothyroxemia; severe nonthyroidal illness
Normal	High	Euthyroid hyperthyroxemia
Low	Normal	Subclinical hyperthyroidism; T_3 toxicosis (rare)
Low	Low	Central hypothyroidism; euthyroid sick syndrome
Low	High	Thyrotoxicosis
High	Normal	Subclinical hypothyroidism
High	Low	Primary hypothyroidism
High	High	TSH-mediated hyperthyroidism

*Adapted from (22)

THYROTOXICOSIS

Clinical Presentation

Thyrotoxicosis refers to all disorders in which the patient has increased circulating thyroid hormone concentrations. Hyperthyroidism is a disease state in which the thyroid gland is responsible for thyrotoxicosis due to overproduction of thyroid hormone. Hyperthyroidism is a common disorder and affects 2% of woman and 0.2% of men (8). The most common signs and symptoms of thyrotoxicosis are listed in Table 163.2 and include heat intolerance, excessive sweating, myalgias, and palpitations. Weight loss may be present despite increased appetite.

TABLE 163.2. Signs and Symptoms of Thyrotoxicosis

General
- Excessive sweating
- Flushing
- Heat intolerance
- Weight loss
- Gynecomastia
- Irritability
- Dyspnea

Cardiovascular
- Palpitations
- Tachycardia
- Atrial fibrillation
- Systolic hypertension
- Congestive heart failure

Head/Neck
- Ophthalmopathy (Graves')
- Goiter

Gastrointestinal
- Abdominal pain
- Anorexia or increased appetite
- Diarrhea

Neurologic
- Nervousness
- Hyperreflexia
- Tremor

Muscular
- Muscle weakness
- Myalgias, myopathies
- Periodic paralysis (rare)

Dermatologic
- Hair loss
- Velvety skin
- Palmar erythema

Neurological symptoms include nervousness and tremor. If altered mental status is present, the clinician should be considering thyroid storm, not thyrotoxicosis.

The most common cause of hyperthyroidism, accounting for 80% of cases, is *Graves' disease*. Graves' disease is 10 times more frequent in women than men and usually occurs by the fourth decade. The etiology of Graves' disease is an antibody—thyroid-stimulating immunoglobulin (TSI)—that mimics the action of TSH by binding to and activating the TSH receptor.

Extrathyroidal manifestations of Graves' disease include infiltrative ophthalmopathy and dermopathy. Ophthalmologic disease is evident clinically in 50% of patients and on CT scan in almost all patients. This condition occurs via a similar autoimmune mechanism, with the end result being increased orbital connective tissue and edema of the extraocular muscles. The increased tissue mass causes proptosis and paresis of extraocular muscle function and may be accompanied by diplopia. The skin manifestations of Graves' disease range from thickened patches of skin, most commonly in the pretibial area, to massive lymphocytic infiltration of the entire leg. Almost all patients with the dermopathy will also have eye disease (5).

The second most common cause of thyrotoxicosis is *toxic multinodular goiter* (TMG), which encompasses 5% to 15% of the remaining cases. In this condition, at least two autonomously functioning thyroid nodules produce excess thyroid hormone. The exact etiology is not known. Not all multinodular goiters are thyrotoxic, but in patients 55 years and older, TMG is the most common cause of thyrotoxicosis, accounting for over 40% of cases. Like Graves' disease, it is also more common in women.

Thyroiditis comes in three common forms—subacute, Hashimoto's, and postpartum. In subacute thyroiditis, symptoms of thyrotoxicosis usually follow an upper respiratory infection. The thyroid is generally very tender, and systemic symptoms include fatigue, fever, and myalgias. Pain may radiate to the jaw or ear. The thyrotoxicosis of Hashimoto's thyroiditis (silent thyroiditis) is usually transient if it occurs at all. Symptoms last 2 to 3 months and then resolve spontaneously with many patients passing into a hypothyroid period. Postpartum thyroiditis is a transient hyperthyroid state that occurs 6 weeks to 6 months postpartum and is purported to occur in 5% to 10% of all women (5).

Elderly may not present with the typical signs and symptoms of thyrotoxicosis but often present with apathetic hyperthyroidism. Apathetic hyperthyroidism is due to an attenuated end-organ responsiveness and occurs in up to 10% of elderly patients. In these patients, cardiac manifestations and depressed mental status are more often present. One study reported cognitive impairment in 52% of elderly patients (15). A goiter is much less common in the elderly patient and is absent in 50% of patients over age 70. Anorexia and atrial fibrillation are much more common, occurring in 32% and 35% of patients, respectively. Rarely, apathetic hyperthyroidism can occur in young patients (25).

Medications, dietary supplements, or radiographic contrast agents with a high concentration of iodine can induce thyrotoxicosis. Amiodarone is an iodine-rich drug that with standard doses can contribute a 50- to 100-fold increase in the optimal daily iodine intake. The clinical presentation of amiodarone-induced thyrotoxicosis (AIT) is subtler because the anti-adrenergic actions of amiodarone obscure the typical signs and symptoms of thyrotoxicosis. The overall incidence of AIT is 2% in the United States but higher in countries with lower dietary iodine intake. A longer duration of therapy increases the risk of developing AIT (16). In addition, radiographic contrast agents possess large quantities of organic iodine—30 to 50 g per study or approximately 200 to 300 times the recommended daily allowance.

Other causes of thyrotoxicosis include factitious thyrotoxicosis, toxic adenoma, metastatic follicular thyroid carcinoma, struma ovarii (ectopic thyroid tissue), and a pituitary adenoma secreting TSH. Trophoblastic tumors (choriocarcinoma, hydatidiform mole, and embryonal carcinoma of the testes) and hyperemesis gravidarum can induce thyrotoxicosis by elaboration of an altered hCG molecule that can activate the TSH receptor.

Differential Diagnosis

Thyrotoxicosis may be confused with pheochromocytoma or sympathomimetic ingestion as they share many of the same hyperadrenergic effects. In elderly patients, cognitive impairment such as dementia and delirium must be differentiated from apathetic hyperthyroidism. Thyrotoxicosis must be distinguished from other causes of congestive heart failure. Psychiatric conditions such as psychosis and depression should be considered, but are generally considered a diagnosis of exclusion. Finally, if gastrointestinal symptoms predominate, gastroenteritis or hepatitis must be considered.

Emergency Department Evaluation

Most patients with thyrotoxicosis will have either a history consistent with the condition or a goiter on physical examination (Fig. 163.1). Diagnosis in the elderly requires a higher index of suspicion. Evaluation consists of obtaining free T_4 and TSH levels.

Graves' disease can be diagnosed based on clinical or laboratory findings. Laboratory findings include an elevated free T_4, low TSH, and the presence of TSI antibodies. In general, use of TSI antibody measurement is reserved for situations in which the diagnosis is in question. Rarely, thyrotoxicosis will manifest with an elevated free T_3 and normal free T_4, termed T_3 *toxicosis*. This condition seems to be more common in elderly patients and should be suspected in patients with the signs and symptoms of thyrotoxicosis, a normal free T_4, and a suppressed TSH.

The electrocardiogram (ECG) will almost universally yield tachycardia, most commonly sinus. Atrial fibrillation is present in 9% to 22% of patients with thyrotoxicosis. Conversely, in studies of patients with atrial fibrillation, <1% will be due to thyrotoxicosis. Rarely, heart block and ventricular dysrhythmias are seen.

Computed tomography (CT) with iodinated contrast should be avoided in patients with thyrotoxicosis for two important

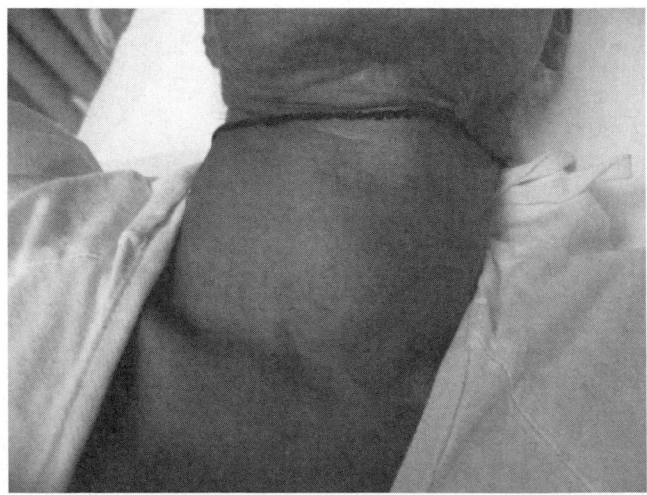

Figure 163.1.   Goiter.

reasons. First, thyroid storm has been precipitated in patients with untreated or poorly controlled thyrotoxicosis receiving iodine-containing contrast agents as early as 5 hours following the radiographic study. This complication is thought to be rare but, nonetheless, worth avoiding. Second, iodinated contrast diminishes the effectiveness of nuclear thyroid imaging used for both diagnostic and treatment purposes. This effect persists for several weeks after an iodine load.

Emergency Department Management

Management of uncomplicated thyrotoxicosis consists of administration of a thionamide. Thionamides work by inhibiting the synthesis of thyroid hormone. In the United States, the two most widely available thionamides are methimazole (Tapazole) and propylthiouracil (PTU). Many endocrinologists favor methimazole for uncomplicated thyrotoxicosis because PTU has a shorter half-life and it can decrease the effectiveness of radioactive iodine therapy. Methimazole is started at 15 mg twice a day with maintenance doses of 5 to 10 mg per day. PTU is initiated at a dose of 100 to 150 mg every 8 hours and can be reduced to 50 mg two to three times a day once the euthyroid state is reached. Up to 40% of patients receiving thionamides will undergo remission after 6 to 18 months of therapy. Serious complications of thionamides include cholestatic jaundice, thrombocytopenia, lupus-like syndrome, and hepatitis. Agranulocytosis is seen in 1 of 400 patients taking thionamides (5).

β-blocker therapy is adjuvant treatment in patients with moderate to severe thyrotoxicosis. The most commonly prescribed β-blocker is propranolol because it blocks the hyperadrenergic state as well as the peripheral conversion of T_4. β-blockers are a mainstay of therapy, but care should be taken when administered to elderly patients, especially those with congestive heart failure. In addition, case reports have also recommended propranolol for treatment of thyrotoxic periodic paralysis (7,19).

Definitive treatment is with radioactive therapy (RAI) or thyroidectomy. In some, especially younger patients, the endocrinologist may elect to administer RAI prior to antithyroid therapy. The desired end result is a euthyroid state, but continued hyperthyroidism (10%) and, more commonly, hypothyroidism (20% initially and increasing 3% to 5% per year) can occur. Finally, thyroidectomy is rarely employed and is reserved for patients with allergy to thionamides, pregnancy, compressive symptomatology, or personal choice. Adverse outcomes include recurrent laryngeal nerve damage and permanent hypoparathyroidism (5).

Management of subacute thyroiditis differs in that the condition is usually self-limited. Nonsteroidal medications or prednisone 40 to 60 mg per day for 1 week with reduction over the following 3 weeks is usually sufficient to treat the pain. β-blockers are provided for symptomatic relief (5).

Graves' disease complicates pregnancy in 1 of 500 women. Left untreated, it is associated with miscarriage, premature labor, low birthweight, and eclampsia. Radioactive iodine is contraindicated in the pregnant patient and surgery is considered a measure of last resort. Antithyroid medications are appropriate, however, with PTU at the lowest therapeutic dose being the drug of choice in the U.S. Complications include neonatal hypothyroidism. Antithyroid drugs are considered safe in nursing mothers.

Disposition

The majority of patients with uncomplicated thyrotoxicosis can be discharged with referral to an endocrinologist and the initiation of therapy from the emergency department. Admit elderly patients with concomitant congestive heart failure or cognitive dysfunction. Patients with thyroid storm (see below) should be admitted to an intensive care unit.

Common Pitfalls

✔ Not recognizing thyrotoxicosis in an elderly patient with apathetic hyperthyroidism
✔ Administration of iodine contrast to a thyrotoxic patient without recognizing the risk of developing thyroid storm

THYROID STORM

Clinical Presentation

Thyroid storm and thyrotoxic crisis are synonymous and represent the extreme manifestation of thyrotoxicosis. Differentiating uncomplicated thyrotoxicosis from thyroid storm may be difficult. Classically, the clinical presentation of thyroid storm consists of a triad of hyperthermia (temperatures as high as 106°F), exaggerated tachycardia, and extreme central nervous system dysfunction. However, all three of these symptoms may not be present and the patient may still be considered to have thyroid storm. Burch and Wartofsky developed a diagnostic criteria (Table 163.3) as an aid to the clinician in distinguishing uncomplicated thyrotoxicosis from impending thyroid storm and thyroid storm (2).

Another important aspect of thyroid storm is recognition and treatment of a precipitating event. Surgery was historically described as the most common precipitating event, but today surgery is relatively uncommon as a precipitating event and other illnesses constitute a greater proportion of causes. Reported precipitating events are listed in Table 163.4. With advances in CT and its greater application, the number of patients receiving iodinated contrast will increase and extra attention should be paid to screening patients for goiter and thyroid dysfunction before infusion. In 25% to 44% of cases of thyroid storm, a precipitating illness cannot be identified.

Differential Diagnosis

Other entities that may present similarly to thyroid storm include sepsis, adrenal insufficiency, bacterial meningitis, encephalitis, serotonin syndrome, neuroleptic malignant syndrome, and sympathomimetic ingestions (i.e., cocaine). Rhabdomyolysis with renal failure has been reported in thyroid storm.

Emergency Department Evaluation

Because thyroid storm occurs in patients with untreated or partially treated thyrotoxicosis, evaluation consists initially of recognition of thyrotoxicosis. This can be based on a combination of past medical history, a thorough review of the patient's historical features, and a finding on examination such as a goiter or eye findings consistent with Graves' disease. Thyroid storm occurs most commonly in patients with Graves' disease but may also occur in patients with toxic multinodular goiter. A low TSH and elevated free T_4 further confirm the diagnosis of thyrotoxicosis but are not useful in distinguishing thyroid storm from thyrotoxicosis. A free T_3 level should be obtained in the extreme case that the level of free T_4 remains within the normal range. Use of Burch and Wartofsky's diagnostic criteria (Table 163.4) will increase recognition and treatment of thyroid storm.

The next important step in evaluation is recognizing and treating a precipitating event. Infection is potentially the most

TABLE 163.3.   Diagnostic Criteria for Thyroid Storm

Thermoregulatory Dysfunction
Temperature (°F)

99–99.9	5
100–100.9	10
101–101.9	15
102–102.9	20
103–103.9	25
≥104.0	30

Central Nervous System Effects

Absent	0
Mild	10
Agitation	
Moderate	20
Delirium	
Psychosis	
Extreme lethargy	
Severe	30
Seizure	
Coma	

Gastrointestinal–Hepatic Dysfunction

Absent	0
Moderate	10
Diarrhea	
Nausea/vomiting	
Abdominal pain	
Severe	20
Unexplained jaundice	

Cardiovascular Dysfunction
Tachycardia

99–109	5
110–119	10
120–129	15
130–139	20
≥140	25
Congestive heart failure	
Absent	0
Mild	5
Pedal edema	
Moderate	10
Bibasilar rales	
Severe	15
Pulmonary edema	
Atrial fibrillation	
Absent	0
Present	10
Precipitant history	
Negative	0
Positive	10

In patients with severe thyrotoxicosis, points are assigned to the highest weighted description applicable in each category and scores totaled. When it is not possible to distinguish the effects of an intercurrent illness from those of the severe thyrotoxicosis per se, points are awarded such as to favor the diagnosis of storm and hence empiric therapy. A score of 45 or greater is highly suggestive of thyroid storm; a score of 25–44 is suggestive of impending storm, and a score below 25 is unlikely to represent thyroid storm.
From Burch HB, Wartofsky L. Life-threatening thyrotoxicosis: thyroid storm. Endocrinol Metab Clin North Am 1993;22:263–277, with permission.

treatable precipitating event, and, therefore, a chest radiograph, urinalysis, and blood and urine cultures should be obtained.

Emergency Department Management

Therapy consists of correcting the thyrotoxicosis, treating the precipitating event, and normalizing decompensated organ systems. Management of thyroid storm is summarized in Table 163.5.

Correcting the thyrotoxicosis begins with administration of a thionamide. In thyroid storm, PTU is the drug of choice because, unlike methimazole, it functions to decrease hormone synthe-

sis and reduces the peripheral conversion of T_4. It can be given rectally or via a nasogastric tube if necessary.

Inorganic iodine (Lugol's solution or SSKI) is used 1 hour after the administration of PTU to block the release of preformed thyroid hormone. Large doses of iodine will also reduce the organification of thyroglobulin. The delay in initiating this therapy is necessary to ensure that further substrate cannot be used for thyroid hormone production. In patients with an anaphylactic reaction to iodine, lithium carbonate can be administered at a dose of 300 mg every 6 hours. Another alternative is the radiocontrast agent, ipodate (Oragrafin). Ipodate inhibits peripheral

TABLE 163.4.   Precipitants of Thyroid Storm

Infection
Surgery/trauma
Vigorous palpation of the thyroid gland
Thyroid hormone ingestion
Cerebrovascular accident
Congestive heart failure
Pulmonary embolism
Diabetic ketoacidosis
Parturition
Toxemia of pregnancy
Emotional stress
Iodinated contrast dyes
Pseudoephedrine
Amiodarone

TABLE 163.5.   Treatment of Thyroid Storm

(1) **Propylthiouracil (PTU) 600–1000 mg PO/PR then 200–250mg every 4 hours**
(2) **Inorganic Iodine (1 hour after PTU)**
  Lugol's solution 8 drops PO/PR every 6 hours *or*
  Saturated solution of potassium iodide (SSKI) 5 drops PO/PR every 6 hours
(3) **Corticosteroids**
  Dexamethasone 2 mg i.v. every 6 hours *or*
  Hydrocortisone 300 mg i.v. then 100 mg every 8 hours
(4) **β-blocker (If NO CHF)**
  Esmolol 250–500 μg/kg i.v. bolus then 50–100 μg/kg/min infusion *or*
  Propanolol 60–80 mg PO every 4 hours *or*
  Propanolol 0.5–1 mg i.v. every 1 hour (infuse slowly)
(5) **Supportive care**
  Acetaminophen, cooling blankets, intravenous fluids
(6) **Treat the precipitating event**

T_4 conversion in addition to blocking thyroid hormone release. The dose of ipodate is 0.5 to 3 g per day (24).

Corticosteroids function to decrease peripheral conversion of T_4 and inhibit release of hormone from the thyroid gland. They have been shown to improve survival in patients with thyroid storm. The beneficial effects are also due to their ability to treat a relative adrenal insufficiency that often occurs concomitantly with thyroid storm.

β-blockers are considered a cornerstone of therapy for thyroid storm. Typical contraindications apply, including asthma, bronchospasm, and congestive heart failure. Special attention should be given to congestive heart failure, as this is a common presentation of thyroid storm, especially in older patients. Propranolol has been the agent of choice because it inhibits adrenergic overactivity and blocks conversion of T_4. It can be administered orally or intravenously. Disadvantages include its long half-life (2.3 hours) and depression of cardiac output. One study found that in patients with uncomplicated thyrotoxicosis, a dose of 2 mg of propranolol caused a reduction in cardiac output by 13%. In patients with thyrotoxic cardiac failure given the same 2 mg dose, cardiac output fell by 30% (10).

An alternative agent is esmolol, which has the advantage of a short duration of action and a half-life of only 9 minutes. Esmolol also has beta-1 selectivity and, therefore, is less of a concern in patients with bronchospasm (1). Esmolol does not possess the same membrane-stabilizing properties as propranolol and therefore has no activity inhibiting peripheral conversion of T_4. In patients with contraindications to β-blockers, diltiazem has been used successfully to ameliorate thyrotoxic symptoms, but its benefits are unproven yet in thyroid storm. Guanethidine (1 to 2 mg/kg/day) or reserpine (2.5 to 5 mg every 4 to 6 hours) can also be considered but are no longer agents of choice.

Congestive heart failure and atrial dysrhythmias, both common to thyroid storm, are treated in the usual fashion. Oxygen, diuresis, and digoxin are all appropriate. Further supportive care consists of attempts to lower temperature with cooling blankets and acetaminophen. Intravenous fluids are administered as needed, but care should be taken in the setting of heart failure.

Identification and treatment of a precipitating event will improve survival. Special attention should be given to a search for an underlying infection. If no focus can be identified, and no other obvious precipitant is readily apparent, administration of broad-spectrum antibiotic coverage is warranted in the emergency department until the results of cultures can be obtained (24).

CRITICAL INTERVENTIONS

- In an ill patient with a history of thyrotoxicosis or a goiter, suspect and treat thyroid storm early
- In the treatment of thyroid storm, administer PTU 1 hour before inorganic iodine
- Administration of a beta-blocker. Consider the short-acting agent esmolol in unstable patients or patients with signs of congestive heart failure

Disposition

All patients with thyroid storm or impending thyroid storm should be admitted to an intensive care setting with appropriate consultation from endocrinology.

Common Pitfalls

✔ Diagnosing and treating thyroid storm without considering, searching for, and treating the precipitating event

✔ Failure to consider thyroid storm in a patient with a history of hyperthyroidism and treating the precipitating illness only
✔ Inducing cardiogenic shock by overly aggressive attempts to lower heart rate with long-acting β-blockers in the emergency department

HYPOTHYROIDISM

Clinical Presentation

Hypothyroidism is second only to diabetes mellitus as the most common endocrine disorder in the United States. The incidence is 0.5% of the U.S. population and increases to 2% to 3% in the elderly. Women are much more commonly affected than men. The condition is due to a primary process within the thyroid in 95% of patients. Secondary hypothyroidism is due to dysfunction of the hypothalamic–pituitary axis and is much less common.

Hypothyroidism can manifest in all of the body's organ systems. Signs and symptoms are listed in Table 163.6. Deep tendon reflexes may exhibit a characteristic delayed-relaxation phase. Hypothyroidism affects the cardiovascular system by reducing stroke volume and heart rate. Peripheral vascular resistance is increased and blood volume is reduced. The decrease in cutaneous circulation is responsible for coolness and pallor of the skin. The respiratory system can be compromised by pleural effusion. In severe hypothyroidism, depression of hypoxic and hypercapnic ventilatory drives may cause alveolar hypoventilation and CO_2 retention.

Constipation is present in over half of patients. Weight gain despite reduced appetite is seen in many patients. Fatigue and lethargy are almost universally present with nervousness occurring in less than half of patients. Other neurologic manifestations include memory deficits with dementia in elderly patients. Depression is not uncommon.

A list of the causes of hypothyroidism is in Table 163.7. Autoimmune thyroiditis (Hashimoto's) is the most common cause of hypothyroidism followed closely by radioiodine therapy given to treat hyperthyroidism. Lithium causes overt hypothyroidism in 5% to 15% of patients being administered the drug, with one-third of patients developing subclinical hypothyroidism. Goiter develops in 37% of patients taking lithium.

The mechanism of amiodarone-induced hypothyroidism appears to be related to an inability to escape from the acute Wolff-Chaikoff effect after an iodine load. Amiodarone causes clinical hypothyroidism more frequently in susceptible patients with previous damage by Hashimoto's thyroiditis. The overall incidence of amiodarone-induced hypothyroidism is approximately 5% to 15%. Treatment does not necessitate withdrawal of

---

TABLE 163.6. Signs and Symptoms of Hypothyroidism

	% of cases		% of cases
Weakness	99	Weight gain	59
Dry, coarse skin	97	Hair loss	57
Lethargy	91	Dyspnea	55
Slowed speech	91	Peripheral edema	55
Cold sensation	89	Hoarseness	52
Coarseness of hair	76	Anorexia	45
Pallor of skin	67	Nervousness	35
Memory impairment	66	Menorrhagia	32
Constipation	61	Palpitations	31

Data from Means JH. The thyroid and its diseases. 2nd ed. Philadelphia: JB Lippincott, 1948:233.

TABLE 163.7. Causes of Hypothyroidism

Autoimmune thyroiditis (Hashimoto's)
Radioablation with ^{131}I for hyperthyroidism
Thyroidectomy
Infiltrative process
  Neoplasia
  Sarcoidosis
  Tuberculosis
  PCP
Medications
  Lithium
  Amiodarone
  Iodine
  Iodinated contrast
  Sulfonamides
  Thionamides
  Iodine deficiency
Secondary hypothyroidism
  Sheehan's syndrome
  Pituitary tumors

amiodarone, but thyroid hormone replacement should be instituted (16).

Differential Diagnosis

Hypothyroidism should be considered in patients with symptoms of congestive heart failure, liver failure, carpal tunnel syndrome, rheumatologic symptoms, depression, dementia, and psychosis.

Emergency Department Evaluation

Evaluation should consist of liberal screening of patients with the signs and symptoms of hypothyroidism (Table 163.6). An elevated TSH and a low free T$_4$ level confirm the diagnosis. Further laboratory studies may reveal low serum glucose or sodium levels. Anemia may be present and is either microcytic or macrocytic. Up to 40% of hypothyroid patients will have elevations in creatine kinase levels, while approximately one-third will have elevations in liver enzymes. The ECG may reveal sinus bradycardia, prolongation of the PR interval, low amplitude QRS complex, and flattening or inversion of T waves. An enlarged heart on chest radiograph may be due to pericardial effusion or cardiomegaly. Pericardial effusion is rarely significant enough to cause cardiac tamponade. Pleural effusions may also be evident on CXR.

Emergency Department Management

Levothyroxine preparations (Synthroid, Unithroid, Levothroid, Levoxyl, and generic) for thyroid hormone replacement appear to be equivalent (3). In otherwise healthy adults, replacement therapy is initiated at 50 to 75 μg per day and increased slowly until symptoms resolve and the TSH level normalizes. Correction of TSH levels trails the initiation of therapy or adjustments in dosing by up to 4 to 8 weeks. Adequately treated patients will have normalization of the serum free T$_4$ level. In elderly patients with increased risk of cardiovascular compromise, starting doses are lower (25 to 50 μg per day). The dose should be raised during pregnancy and should also be monitored and possibly increased after the addition of many commonly prescribed medications, including amiodarone, lithium, coumadin, phenobarbital, carbamazepine, ferrous sulfate, furosemide, and salicylates. Due to the long half-life of thyroxine, patients unable to take thyroxine for several days need not take any additional doses (9).

Disposition

Admission is rarely indicated in uncomplicated hypothyroidism. Patients with cardiovascular compromise secondary to a large pericardial effusion or hypoxia due to a pleural effusion should be admitted. The majority of patients are managed on an outpatient basis.

Common Pitfalls

✔ Failure to consider hypothyroidism in elderly patients with cognitive deficits or patients with an unexplained pleural effusion or anemia
✔ Failure to consider the effect of many commonly prescribed drugs and pregnancy on thyroid function
✔ Expecting the rapid return of the TSH level in a patient recently started on hormone replacement for hypothyroidism

MYXEDEMA COMA

Clinical Presentation

Myxedema coma represents an exaggerated form of thyroid disease associated with a precipitating event. The name is misleading, however, because patients may not present with either myxedema, a dry nonpitting edema due to the accumulation of mucopolysaccharides, or coma. This form of decompensated hypothyroidism occurs most commonly in the elderly and during the winter months when adaptive mechanisms are most stressed. Precipitating events are listed in Table 163.8. All patients will have signs and symptoms of hypothyroidism prior to developing myxedema coma.

The principal clinical features of myxedema coma are hypothermia and altered mental status. Temperature is usually less than 95.9°F but may be as low as 80°F. A normal temperature is seen in up to 20% of patients. Mental status changes range from unconsciousness to slowed verbal responses and mentation. Delirium with hallucinations, the so-called myxedema madness, is an uncommon manifestation. The respiratory rate is usually reduced due to a diminished ventilatory drive, and CO_2 narcosis can result. The combination of reduced cardiac contractility, bradycardia, and reduced intravascular volume may result in hypotension, which is present in up to 50% of cases.

Differential Diagnosis

The differential diagnosis of myxedema coma includes adrenal insufficiency, sepsis, meningitis, cold exposure, stroke, SIADH (syndrome of inappropriate secretion of antidiuretic hormone),

TABLE 163.8. Precipitants of Myxedema Coma

Infection
Trauma, burns
Cerebral vascular accident
Congestive heart disease
Gastrointestinal bleeding
Lung disease/CO_2 retention
Hypothermia
Hypoglycemia
Untreated hypothyroidism
Discontinuation of thyroid replacement
Medications
• Drug overdose
• Diuretics, amiodarone, β-blockers
• Sedatives, lithium, phenytoin

and seizure disorder. Myxedema may superficially resemble congestive heart failure, liver failure, renal failure, and nephrotic syndrome.

Emergency Department Evaluation

The large majority of patients with myxedema coma will carry a concurrent diagnosis of hypothyroidism. Therefore, a history of hypothyroidism, treatment for Graves' disease, or discontinuation of thyroid replacement therapy is helpful, if elicited. Physical examination may reveal a scar on the anterior aspect of the neck. If the history is not obtainable due to an altered mental status and the physical examination does not give clues to the diagnosis of hypothyroidism, an elevated TSH and low free T_4 level, if it can be obtained on an emergent basis, is confirmatory of the diagnosis of hypothyroidism.

A search for precipitants of myxedema coma should include a thorough review of the patient's medications. An aggressive search for an infectious source should be sought. Laboratory testing in addition to a TSH and free T_4 should include electrolytes, white blood cell (WBC) count, urinalysis, and cortisol level. A chest radiograph will identify infiltrates and effusions. An ECG will most likely reveal sinus bradycardia, but transient third degree heart block has been reported. Other ECG abnormalities including low voltage QRS complexes are similar to hypothyroidism. Any ischemic abnormalities on the ECG should initiate consideration for an acute coronary syndrome.

Emergency Department Management

The treatment of myxedema coma is based on two principles: replacing thyroid hormone and identifying the precipitant event. Thyroid hormone replacement occurs with the administration of i.v. levothyroxine. Bacterial infection is the most common precipitant and should be presumed to be present until proven otherwise. Consequently, a low threshold for the administration of empiric antibiotics should be maintained (18).

Table 163.9 summarizes treatment of myxedema coma. There is some debate regarding the best method of thyroid hormone replacement, but most authors agree that i.v. levothyroxine (T_4) is the most appropriate therapy. Intravenous T_3 is more biologically active but has a major drawback in that it has the potential to precipitate dysrhythmias and sudden death. A dose of 500 μg i.v. is enough to restore the free T_4 concentration to 50% of the normal euthyroid pool. Intravenous levothyroxine is safe and effective and is recommended in all patients with presumed myxedema coma. If levothyroxine is administered to a patient with sick euthyroid (low TSH, low free T_4) mistakenly, the likelihood it will produce any detectable adverse effect is small (18).

Peripheral vasoconstriction and low intravascular blood volumes present in myxedema coma make rapid re-warming potentially hazardous. Re-warming should take place with blankets and elevated ambient room temperatures because electric heating blankets and other active forms of re-warming may cause hypotension due to peripheral vasodilation in a patient with an already low intravascular volume.

TABLE 163.9. Treatment of Myxedema Coma

(1) Levothyroxine 200–500 μg i.v. followed by 75–100 i.v./PO μg per day
(2) Intravenous fluids, pressors, and mechanical ventilation as needed
(3) Passive rewarming
(4) Hydrocortisone 100 mg i.v. or dexamethasone 6 mg i.v.
(5) Treat any precipitants with special attention to a potential infectious etiology

---

Fluid overload and congestive heart failure can result from overzealous use of i.v. fluids and pressors, so these agents should be instituted as needed only. Dopamine is preferable to other vasopressors because it maintains coronary perfusion, but patients may be refractory because of decreased beta-receptor responsiveness. Pressors should be used only as a last resort (11).

Hypoglycemia and hyponatremia should be sought and treated promptly. Hypoglycemia may result from concomitant adrenal insufficiency. Therapy with dextrose and stress dose steroids is indicated. Dexamethasone is preferred if the patient may undergo a cosyntropin stimulation test, as this steroid will not alter the results. Hyponatremia should be treated if the level is <120 mEq/L, however, hyponatremia usually resolves with levothyroxine therapy alone. Hypertonic saline is indicated in the presence of active seizures. A sodium level greater than 120 mEq/L usually resolves with levothyroxine therapy.

CRITICAL INTERVENTIONS

- Intravenous levothyroxine should be administered in an ill hypothyroid patient with possible myxedema coma
- Judicious use of i.v. fluids should be administered before i.v. pressor agents
- Passive re-warming should be instituted in myxedema patients because active re-warming may precipitate hypotension

Disposition

Patients with myxedema coma should be admitted to an intensive care unit. The diagnosis carries a mortality of 30% to 60%. Factors that increase mortality include advanced age, core temperature less than 93°F, bradycardia less than 44 beats per minute, hypotension, and concomitant sepsis or myocardial infarction (11).

Common Pitfalls

✔ Failure to consider the diagnosis of myxedema coma in a patient with altered mental status and a history of hypothyroidism
✔ Use of active re-warming that may precipitate hypotension
✔ Failure to search for and treat precipitating events, especially infectious causes

THYROID NODULES

The prevalence of a thyroid nodule is estimated to be about 5% in the general population and up to 50% in ultrasound and autopsy studies. In general, patient reassurance is indicated in the emergency department, as the prevalence of thyroid cancer in patients with a thyroid nodule ranges from 4% to 6%. Some factors that increase the likelihood of a malignancy include a history of radiation therapy, male, female of reproductive age, or a nodule that has poorly defined borders, is irregular, firm, and fixed to the underlying tissue.

A thyroid nodule (Fig. 163.2a) can be confused with other neck masses if a careful physical examination is not performed. Thyroglossal duct cysts are more common in children but are also seen in adults. They are found in the midline of the anterior neck but superior to the thyroid cartilage. Thyroglossal duct cysts have an average size of 2.5 cm and usually are smaller than 4 cm. If they become larger, they may be confused with a goiter (Fig. 163.2b). A branchial cleft cyst (Fig. 163.2c) is located laterally along the anterior border of the lower sternocleidomastoid muscle. These cysts are more common in children and may

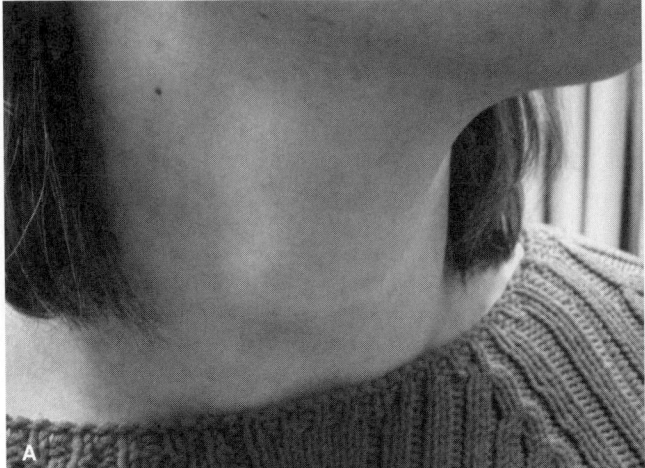

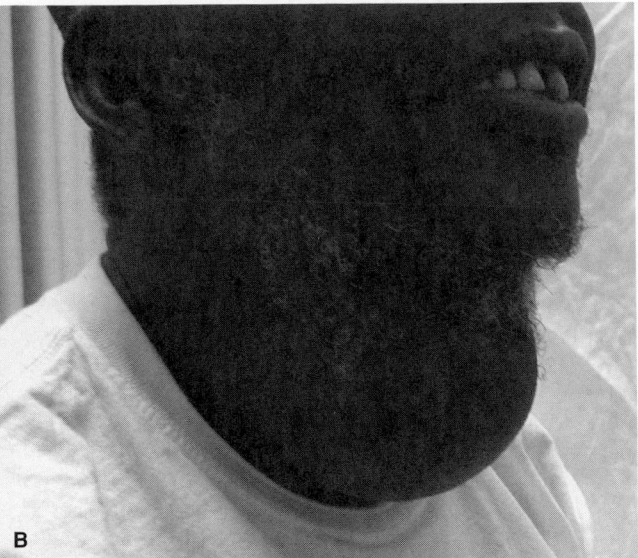

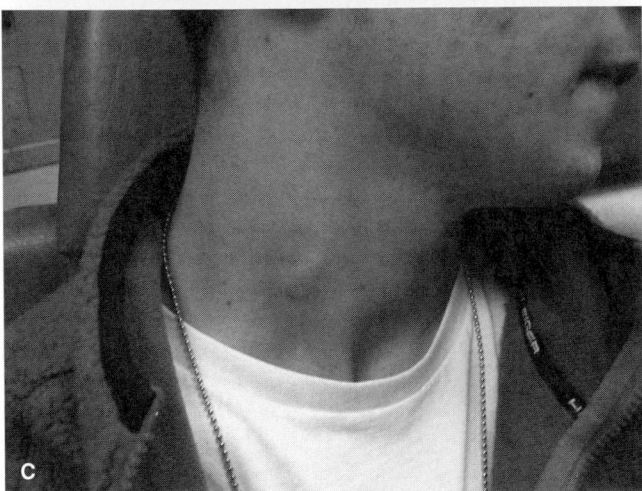

Figure 163.2.   (A) Thyroid nodule. (B) A large thyroglossal duct cyst. (C) Branchial cleft cyst.

present to the emergency department when they become infected. Other considerations include reactive lymphadenopathy, lymphoma, and Hodgkin's disease.

An asymptomatic thyroid nodule should be referred for an evaluation by an endocrinologist. Work-up should commence with a TSH level. A normal TSH level is followed up by a fine needle biopsy of the nodule to determine if the nodule is malignant or benign. In the instance of a low TSH level, the patient should undergo a radiolabeled ^{123}I thyroid scan, and all "cold" nodules should undergo biopsy. "Hot" nodules in thyrotoxic patients are treated with surgery or radioactive iodine ablation (23).

MECHANICAL ISSUES

The thyroid gland can be problematic to the patient and clinician beyond its inherent endocrine function. Mechanical issues caused by an enlarged thyroid or ectopic thyroid tissue (substernal and lingual) can have a significant impact on the airway and blood vessels in and around the neck.

A goiter can compress, displace, and on rare occasions infiltrate the airway (4). Upper airway obstruction demonstrated by pulmonary function tests is present in one-third of patients with a goiter, but it is difficult to determine by physical examination which enlarged thyroids will cause upper airway obstruction (8). The most common symptoms of obstruction include dyspnea, orthopnea, dysphagia, choking sensation, and a fullness or pressure in the neck. However, not all patients with airway obstruction by pulmonary function testing and radiographs will

be symptomatic, and, in turn, many without documented airway obstruction will have symptoms of obstruction due to their goiter. Other causes of the thyroid gland precipitating airway obstruction include trauma, thyroid malignancy, or following radioactive iodine treatment (21). Other less common manifestations are acute respiratory distress and superior vena cava syndrome.

Studies have shown that orotracheal intubation has a good success rate, but in large goiters, some orotracheal intubations may be difficult. McHenry and Piotrowski reported uncomplicated intubation in 91 patients undergoing thyroidectomy due to Graves' disease, toxic multinodular goiter, adenoma, or carcinoma. (17). In another study, 11 of 13 patients with airway compromise secondary to goiter were successfully orotracheally intubated, with the other 2 requiring a bougie to successfully place the endotracheal tube (6). In the event that an enlarged thyroid causes subglottic narrowing, smaller endotracheal tubes should be available when the endotracheal tube will not advance despite passing through the vocal cords. A large goiter will also make attempts at cricothyroidotomy more difficult. Alternative methods, including awake fiberoptic intubation and laryngeal mask airways should be considered.

A final cause of airway obstruction occurs in the setting of a lingual thyroid. In this condition, reported to occur in 1 in 200,000 people, there is a failure of the normal embryological descent of the gland such that it remains situated at the base of the tongue. This condition is more problematic in childhood, but obstruction can also occur in adults. Any enlargement will obstruct the airway and attempts at endotracheal intubation in this situation will be difficult due to poor visualization of the glottis. An awake fiberoptic intubation or a surgical airway may be necessary (12).

Additionally, central venous access in the internal jugular vein of the neck should be avoided in patients with an enlarged thyroid. Distorted vascular anatomy will make blind insertion using external landmarks difficult, and every effort to find an alternative means of gaining i.v. access should be sought (20).

Common Pitfalls

✔ Confusing orthopnea due to goiter with congestive heart failure
✔ Attempting central line placement in the internal jugular vein in a patient with an enlarged thyroid
✔ Failure to recognize an enlarged thyroid or ectopic thyroid tissue as a cause of airway compromise or superior vena cava syndrome

References

1. Brunette DD, Rothong C. Emergency department management of thyrotoxic crisis with esmolol. *Am J Emerg Med* 1991;9:232–233.
2. Burch HB, Wartofsky L. Life-threatening thyrotoxicosis: thyroid storm. *Endocrinol Metab Clin North Am* 1993;22:263–277.
3. Dong BJ, Hauck WW, Gambertoglio JG, et al. Bioequivalence of generic and brand name levothyroxine products in the treatment of hypothyroidism. *JAMA* 1997;277:1205–1213.
4. Dossing H, Jorgensen KE, Oster-Jorgensen E, et al. Recurrent pregnancy-related upper airway obstruction caused by intratracheal ectopic thyroid tissue. *Thyroid* 1999;9:955–958.
5. Fisher JN. Management of thyrotoxicosis. *South Med J* 2002;95:493–505.
6. Gauger PG, Guinea AI, Reeve TS, et al. The spectrum of emergency admissions for thyroidectomy. *Am J Emerg Med* 1999;17:591–593.
7. Gittoes NJL, Franklyn JA. Hyperthyroidism: current treatment guidelines. *Drugs* 1998;55:543–553.
8. Gittoes NJL, Miller MR, Daykin J, et al. Upper airway obstruction in 153 patients presenting with thyroid enlargement. *BMJ* 1996;312:484.
9. Guha B, Krishnaswamy G, Peiris A. The diagnosis and management of hypothyroidism. *South Med J* 2002;95:475–480.
10. Ikram H. Haemodynamic effects of beta-adrenergic blockade in hyperthyroid patients with and without heart failure. *BMJ* 1977;1:1505–1507.
11. Jordan RM. Myxedema coma: pathophysiology, therapy, and factors affecting prognosis. *Medl Clin North Am* 1995;79:185–194.
12. Koch CA, Picken C, Clement SC, et al. Ectopic lingual thyroid: an otolaryngologic emergency beyond childhood. *Thyroid* 2000;10:511–514.
13. Ladenson PW, Singer PA, Ain KB, et al. American Thyroid Association Guidelines for the Detection of Thyroid Dysfunction. *Arch Intern Med* 2000;160:1573–1575.
14. Larson PR, Davies TF, Hay ID. The thyroid gland. In: Wilson JD, Foster DW, Kroneberg HM, et al, eds. *Williams Textbook of Endocrinology.* 9th ed. Philadelphia: WB Saunders Company, 1998;389–515.
15. Martin FI, Deam DR. Hyperthyroidism in elderly hospitalized patients. Clinical features and treatment outcomes. *Med J Aust* 1996;164:200–203.
16. Martino E, Bartalena L, Bogazzi F, et al. The effects of amiodarone on the thyroid. *Endocr Rev* 2001;22:240–254.
17. McHenry CR, Piotrowski JJ. Thyroidectomy in patients with marked thyroid enlargement: airway management, morbidity, and outcome. *Am Surg* 1994;60:586–591.
18. Nicholoff JT, LoPresti JS. Myxedema coma: a form of decompensated hypothyroidism. *Endocrinol Metab Clin North Am* 1993;22:279–290.
19. Shayne P, Hart A. Thyrotoxic periodic paralysis terminated with intravenous propranolol. *Ann Emerg Med* 1994;24:736–740.
20. Silva FS. Neck haematoma and airway obstruction in a patient with goitre: complication of internal jugular vein cannulation. *Acta Anaesthesiol Scand* 2003;47:626–629.
21. Smallridge RC. Metabolic and anatomic thyroid emergencies: a review. *Crit Care Med* 1992;20:276–291.
22. Supit EJ, Peiris AN. Interpretation of laboratory thyroid function tests for the primary care physician. *South Med J* 2002;95:481–485.
23. Supit E, Peiris AN. Cost-effective management of thyroid nodules and nodular thyroid goiters. *South Med J* 2002;95:514–519.
24. Tietgens ST, Leinung MC. Thyroid storm. *Med Clin North Am* 1995;79:169–184.
25. Trivalle C, Doucet J, Chassagne P. Differences in the signs and symptoms of hyperthyroidism in older and younger patients. *J Am Geriatr Soc* 1996;44:50–53.

CHAPTER 164
Adrenal and Pituitary Disorders

Christine A. Kletti and Clare T. Sercombe

ADRENAL INSUFFICIENCY

Adrenal insufficiency refers to a failure of the adrenal cortex to produce adequate quantities of cortisol, aldosterone, or both. The disorder can be primary adrenal insufficiency, due to adrenal tissue loss, or can be secondary to adrenal insufficiency, due to inadequate adrenocorticotropic hormone (ACTH) production by the pituitary gland.

Primary adrenal insufficiency, or Addison's disease, is an uncommon disorder, affecting approximately 100 persons per 1,000,000. In the United States, autoimmune disease is the most common cause of primary adrenal insufficiency after the newborn period (17). Autoimmune adrenalitis is believed to account for over 70% of all cases. Over 90% of the gland must be destroyed before symptoms become apparent. This disorder is more common in women, with a peak onset at about 30 years old. It is sometimes associated with other autoimmune diseases, such as early ovarian failure, hyperthyroidism and hypothyroidism, insulin-dependent diabetes, hypoparathyroidism, vitiligo, and pernicious anemia. Table 164.1 summarizes the various causes of primary adrenal failure.

In an otherwise healthy person, acute primary adrenal failure is exceedingly rare. Most primary adrenal insufficiency results from disease processes that slowly progress. However, patients with unrecognized asymptomatic adrenal insufficiency can present in acute life-threatening crisis when experiencing physiologic stress.

The most common cause of *secondary* adrenal insufficiency is suppression of the hypothalamic–pituitary–adrenal (HPA) axis by exogenous glucocorticoids. The likelihood of such

TABLE 164.1.   Causes of Primary Adrenal Failure

Autoimmune disease
Metastatic cancer
  Lung
  Breast
  Leukemia
Infection
Tuberculosis
Viral (CMV, HIV/AIDS)
Bacterial (meningococcemia)
Fungal (histoplasmosis, coccidiomycosis)
Infiltrative diseases
  Sarcoidosis
  Amyloidosis
  Hemochromatosis
Hemorrhage
  Anticoagulant therapy
  Abdominal trauma
Congenital adrenal hyperplasia
Adrenalectomy
Adrenal infarction
  Overwhelming sepsis (Waterhouse-Friderichsen syndrome)

suppression is based on the dose of glucocorticoids and the duration of treatment. Suppression is unlikely with doses equivalent to <5mg/day of prednisone and duration of less than 2 weeks (9,14). Depending on the dose and duration of therapy, it may require several months to 1 year after withdrawal of glucocorticoids before the HPA axis again functions normally. Other drugs that have been noted to suppress adrenal cortisol synthesis include etomidate, ketoconazole, fluconazole, aminoglutethimide, methyrapone, and suramin (1,16).

Secondary adrenal insufficiency is otherwise caused by disorders that destroy or compromise pituitary or hypothalamic integrity, such as pituitary or parasellar tumors (prolactinoma, acromegaly, meningioma, craniopharyngioma), hypothalamic tumors, head trauma, infarction, infiltrative or inflammatory processes, and hemorrhage. With the exceptions of trauma, infarction, and hemorrhage, pituitary and hypothalamic disease tends to result in gradual rather than sudden loss of function. Aldosterone secretion is usually normal in secondary adrenal insufficiency.

Adrenal insufficiency is seen in patients with human immunodeficiency virus (HIV) at a rate higher than the general population. Patients with HIV can have both primary and secondary adrenal insufficiency. The diagnosis is often not made because the vague symptoms are attributed to the patient's medications or to the virus itself. One study found that 25% of asymptomatic patients with early HIV infection had insufficient adrenal reserve. It appears that many factors contribute to adrenal insufficiency in this population, including HIV itself, opportunistic infections, malignancy, and medications often used by HIV-infected patients. CMV is the opportunistic infection most frequently associated with adrenalitis (5).

Clinical Presentation

The historical hallmarks of adrenal insufficiency include weakness, fatigue, anorexia, nausea and vomiting, abdominal pain, diarrhea, dizziness, musculoskeletal pain, and weight loss. Commonly, the presenting complaint is related to the gastrointestinal tract. The manner in which adrenal insufficiency presents clinically is determined by how rapidly it develops.

Acute adrenal insufficiency, or Addisonian crisis, is a medical emergency that requires rapid intervention. It usually occurs in an individual with underlying chronic adrenal insufficiency or with adrenal suppression due to chronic steroid use who experiences an acute stress, such as severe infection, sepsis, alcohol withdrawal, trauma, surgery, or myocardial infarction. Thus, it is important that the physician try to identify a concurrent illness that could have precipitated the acute episode. Physical examination of a patient in Addisonian crisis often reveals mental status changes, tachycardia, and hypotension. The patient may be hypothermic or have fever, particularly if infection is triggering the crisis.

The classic physical finding in chronic primary adrenal failure is hyperpigmentation, which is present in 98% of patients and is described as a "suntan that doesn't fade." These patients have pigmentation of skin creases or folds that are not exposed to the sun; the nails, buccal mucosa, and gingiva may also be hyperpigmented. Other findings that may suggest chronic adrenal insufficiency include vitiligo, premature graying, and calcification of the ear lobes. Personality changes, irritability, and restlessness can also be noted.

Patients with secondary adrenal insufficiency may have additional symptoms and signs related to hypothalamic or pituitary disease, such as loss of sexual performance and libido, menstrual disturbances, headache, visual disturbances, galactorrhea, features of acromegaly, or evidence of head trauma. Hyperpigmentation is rare, because circulating levels of ACTH and related peptides are low. Loss of ACTH is often accompanied by loss of thyroid-stimulating hormone (TSH) secretion, so signs of hypothyroidism may be present.

Laboratory findings consistent with adrenal insufficiency include hyponatremia, hyperkalemia, hypercalcemia, and hypoglycemia. Hyponatremia is the most classic laboratory abnormality and the one found in about 90% of cases (10). Complications that result from hyponatremia and hyperkalemia should be considered but are not commonly encountered. The blood cell count may show lymphocytosis or eosinophilia. The urine sodium value is inappropriately high for a state of hypoperfusion. In secondary adrenal failure, the potassium level is usually normal because aldosterone secretion has not been impaired.

Differential Diagnosis

Acute adrenal failure may present as hypovolemic shock, hypoglycemia, or both. The diagnosis should be pursued in any patient with a history of chronic glucocorticoid use. The differential diagnosis of acute adrenal crisis includes other causes of cardiovascular collapse and shock: myocardial infarction, heart failure, hypovolemia, sepsis, pulmonary embolism, and so forth. The diagnosis should be considered in all patients with dehydration, hypotension, orthostasis, or obtundation. Hyperpigmentation and typical laboratory abnormalities also suggest adrenal insufficiency.

Chronic adrenal insufficiency is difficult to diagnose because the symptoms may develop over months to years. It is often confused with a "flu-like" illness because many of the complaints are nonspecific: fatigue, weakness, abdominal discomfort, poor appetite, and musculoskeletal complaints. The examination is often unremarkable. Laboratory evaluation may not be particularly revealing in all cases, especially with secondary insufficiency.

Emergency Department Evaluation and Management

After attention has been given to the ABCs, a thorough history and physical examination should be performed, noting altered mental status, fever, tachycardia, hypotension or orthostatic changes, abdominal discomfort, cutaneous and oral hyperpigmentation, or vitiligo.

In general, hypotension and hypoglycemia pose the greatest threat to the patient presenting with acute adrenal failure. The first step of treatment is to reverse shock. Normal saline and vasopressors are administered as needed. Central venous lines for hemodynamic monitoring may be necessary, and cardiac monitoring should always be instituted. Laboratory studies are ordered as necessary, including electrolytes, glucose, creatinine, baseline plasma ACTH, and serum cortisol. Because plasma ACTH is extremely labile, the blood sample must be placed on ice before being transported to the laboratory. The results of these tests can often take days to become available, so if adrenal insufficiency is suspected, treatment should be initiated promptly, particularly because the condition can progress rapidly to circulatory collapse and death. If no apparent cause for cardiovascular collapse is apparent, blood cultures, urine culture, and chest radiography should be performed to seek evidence of occult infection.

If hypoglycemia is noted, it should be reversed. In severe cases, it may be necessary to treat the hyperkalemia immediately. The total body potassium level is often low, however, and the serum potassium value can be expected to decrease after glucocorticoids are administered. Symptomatic hyponatremia should also be treated. The next step is to administer glucocorticoids. Dexamethasone, 6 to 8 mg i.v., is recommended because it will not interfere with the ACTH (cosyntropin) Stimulation Test, which may be used later to try to establish the diagnosis

TABLE 164.2.   Treatment of Acute Adrenocortical
Insufficiency (Adrenal Crisis)

1. Obtain adequate IV access. Consider central access to assist
   hemodynamic monitoring.
2. Normal saline boluses to correct hypovolemia. Monitor carefully
   for signs of fluid overload.
3. Obtain glucose level and replace accordingly.
4. Send additional laboratory studies including electrolytes,
   creatinine, and baseline cortisol and ACTH levels.
5. Hydrocortisone 100 mg i.v. (Use dexamethasone 6–8 mg i.v. if
   ACTH stimulation test to be performed later for diagnostic
   purposes.)
6. General supportive measures as indicated.
7. Further evaluation to determine potential cause of crisis (ECG,
   chest x-ray, blood and urine cultures).

(Table 164.2). If the cause of adrenal insufficiency is pituitary failure, treatment with levothyroxine is also indicated. Desmopressin may also be necessary if diabetes insipidus is present.

Patients with known chronic adrenal insufficiency require three to four times their normal glucocorticoid replacement dose during illness and stress. Patients with illnesses severe enough to require hospitalization may need an even higher dose. Those receiving exogenous steroids as therapy for other illnesses must be given adequate doses during surgery, illness, or stress.

The hallmark of adrenal insufficiency is loss of adrenal reserve. The diagnosis cannot always be made on the basis of a single cortisol level, which may be in the normal range. A low baseline cortisol level, especially in the presence of physiologic stressors, however, suggests adrenal failure: primary adrenal insufficiency if the ACTH level is high and secondary adrenal insufficiency if both cortisol and ACTH levels are low.

Although not necessary in the emergency department, more definitive evaluation of adrenocortical function may be performed with the short ACTH (cosyntropin) Stimulation Test. Immediately after a baseline serum cortisol and plasma ACTH level are drawn, ACTH 0.25 mg is administered i.v. or i.m., and a serum cortisol value is obtained 60 minutes later. A cortisol level of <500nm/L defines a positive test (4). If prednisone or hydrocortisone has been administered, it will interfere with this test; however, dexamethasone does not interfere with the assay and, furthermore, has no acute effect on the response of the adrenal gland to ACTH.

After the short ACTH test, glucocorticoid replacement is continued with hydrocortisone (100 to 200 mg i.v. bolus, then 20 to 25 mg/hour as a continuous infusion). Alternatively, one may give 100 to 200 mg of hydrocortisone every 6 hours as an i.v. infusion over 30 minutes. Fluids and vasopressors are administered as needed. The clinical picture of shock should improve within 6 to 12 hours. When the acute adrenal crisis resolves, the infusion can be replaced with an oral regimen of hydrocortisone. Most patients do well with 15 to 25 mg/day divided into a morning and afternoon dose. Three to four times this dose is needed for patients under continuing stress. Replacement of mineralocorticoid, if necessary, is accomplished with fludrocortisone acetate (Florinef), 0.05 to 0.2 mg daily (14).

Disposition

After treatment for shock and glucocorticoid deficiency is begun in the emergency department, all patients with *acute* adrenal insufficiency should be admitted to an intensive care unit. Subspecialty consultation should be requested. The short ACTH test may be performed at this time. Endocrine consultation should be obtained in situations when *chronic* adrenal insufficiency is suspected.

Common Pitfalls

✔ Because adrenal insufficiency is uncommon and the symptoms are often nonspecific, the emergency physician may fail to consider the diagnosis
✔ Patients may be potassium-depleted even when the serum potassium concentration is high. The serum potassium value may drop substantially with glucocorticoid replacement and must be monitored closely during treatment
✔ Patients with pituitary failure may not show evidence of diabetes insipidus until after deficiencies of glucocorticoids and thyroid hormone have been corrected
✔ Patients receiving exogenous steroid therapy should always have the dose increased (to two to four times the usual replacement regimen) when there is concurrent illness or stress
✔ The clinician should not fail to institute appropriate fluid resuscitation and steroid replacement while performing the ACTH stimulation test

CUSHING'S SYNDROME

Cushing's syndrome, also known as hypercortisolism, occurs whenever there is symptomatic glucocorticoid excess, regardless of the cause of that excess. The syndrome as originally described by Harvey Cushing in 1932 includes truncal obesity, hypertension, proximal muscle weakness, and striae. The most common cause of Cushing's syndrome is prolonged exogenous steroid administration.

Cushing's disease refers to the situation in which this syndrome is specifically due to excessive ACTH secretion from the pituitary; this accounts for 60% to 80% of individuals with naturally occurring Cushing's syndrome (3). Cushing's disease typically occurs in women between 20 and 40 years of age, is of gradual onset and slowly progressive, and produces only mild symptoms. Most of these patients have pituitary microadenomas; macroadenomas can develop, however, and may present as headaches or visual changes due to pressure on the optic chiasm.

Cushing's syndrome can also be caused by an ectopic ACTH-secreting tumor (e.g., small-cell carcinoma, pancreatic cancer, bronchial carcinoid, or carcinoma of the thymus). The peak incidence is in men between the ages of 40 and 60; the typical course is very rapid, and the tumor is usually advanced when discovered.

Adrenal neoplasms are another cause of Cushing's syndrome, comprising about 20% of cases. Typically, these tumors produce signs and symptoms of glucocorticoid excess but not of androgen excess; they are usually unilateral, and approximately 50% are malignant (10). Adrenal carcinoma has a rapid onset and rapid progression, with hypokalemia and abdominal pain as common symptoms. Benign adrenal tumors have a slow, progressive course.

Clinical Presentation

The clinical manifestations of Cushing's syndrome can vary widely. Obesity and hypertension are common findings. Depending on the source, 75% to 80% of patients have deposition of fat in the face, described as "moon facies," and around the neck and shoulders, classically known as a "buffalo hump." Other fat accumulation occurs within the mesentery, producing truncal obesity. There also may be atrophy of the skin, which, in combination with rapid weight gain, causes many patients to develop striae. The face can appear red and flushed. Patients also complain of fatigue and weakness; a proximal myopathy can be detected in about 60% of patients (3).

Osteoporosis develops from mobilization of calcium, resulting in vertebral compression and pathologic fractures. Glucose

medical treatment. Dialysis is required for some individuals. If renal consultation and dialysis are not available at the treating institution, transfer to a facility with those capabilities should be initiated.

COMMON PITFALLS

✔ Failure to consider rhabdomyolysis in patients with alcoholism, unconsciousness, prolonged immobilization, seizures, hyperthermia, or infection

✔ Failure to pharmacologically control agitation, seizures, or abnormal posturing in patients who are at risk for rhabdomyolysis

✔ Failure to evaluate for compartment syndrome

✔ Failure to realize that the diagnosis of rhabdomyolysis cannot be ruled out on the basis of the serum or urine myoglobin alone

✔ Failure to provide adequate hydration and to prevent or treat acidosis in patients with rhabdomyolysis

References

1. Anonymous. Haff disease associated with eating buffalo fish—United States, 1997. *MMWR* 1998;47:1091–1093.
2. Bedry R, Baudrimont I, Deffieux G, et al. Wild-mushroom intoxication as a cause of rhabdomyolysis. *N Engl J Med* 2001;345:798–802.
3. Better OS, Stein JH. Early management of shock and prophylaxis of acute renal failure in traumatic rhabdomyolysis. *N Engl J Med* 1990;322:825–829.
4. Brody SL, Wrenn KO, Wilber MM, et al. Predicting the severity of cocaine-associated rhabdomyolysis. *Ann Emerg Med* 1990;19:1137–1143.
5. Callaway CW, Clark RF. Hyperthermia in psychostimulant overdose. *Ann Emerg Med* 1994;24:68–74.
6. Curry SC, Chang D, Connor D. Drug- and toxin-induced rhabdomyolysis. *Ann Emerg Med* 1989;18:1068–1084.
7. Counselman FL, McLaughlin EW, Kardon EM, et al. Creatine phosphokinase elevation in patients presenting to the emergency department with cocaine-related complaints. *Am J Emerg Med* 1997;15:221–223.
8. Gabow PA, Kaehny WD, Kelleher SP. The spectrum of rhabdomyolysis. *Medicine* 1982;61:141–152.
9. Homsi E, Barreiro MF, Orlando JM. Prophylaxis of acute renal failure in patients with rhabdomyolysis. *Ren Fail* 1997;19:283–288.
10. Kimmick G, Owen J. Rhabdomyolysis and hemolysis associated with sickle cell trait and glucose-6-phosphate dehydrogenase deficiency. *South Med J* 1996;89:1097–1098.
11. Knottenbelt JD. Traumatic rhabdomyolysis from severe beating—experience of volume diuresis in 200 patients. *J Trauma* 1994;37:214–219.
12. Laios ID, Clark R, Wult B. Myoglobin clearance as an early indicator for rhabdomyolysis-induced acute renal failure. *Ann Clin Lab Sci* 1995;25:179–184.
13. Lofberg M, Jankala H, Paetau A, et al. Metabolic causes of recurrent rhabdomyolysis. *Acta Neurol Scand* 1998;98:268–275.
14. Oda J, Tanaka H, Yoshioka T, et al. Analysis of 372 patients with crush syndrome caused by the Hanshin-Awaji earthquake. *J Trauma* 1997;42:470–475.
15. Poels PJ, Gabreels FJ. Rhabdomyolysis: a review of the literature. *Clin Neurol Neurosurg* 1993;95:175–192.
16. Richards JR, Johnson EB, Stark RW, et al. Methamphetamine abuse and rhabdomyolysis in the ED: a 5-year study. *Am J Emerg Med* 1999;17:681–685.
17. Richards JR. Rhabdomyolysis and drugs of abuse. *J Emerg Med* 2000;19:51–56.
18. Shimazu T, Yushioka T, Nakata Y, et al. Fluid resuscitation and systemic complications in crush syndrome: 14 Hanshin-Awaji earthquake patients. *J Trauma* 1997;42:641–646.
19. Sinert R, Kohl L, Rainone T, et al. Exercise-induced rhabdomyolysis. *Ann Emerg Med* 1994;23:1301–1306.
20. Singh U, Scheld WM. Infectious etiologies of rhabdomyolysis: three cases and a review. *Clin Infect Dis* 1996;22:642–649.
21. Slater MS, Mullins RJ. Rhabdomyolysis and myoglobinuric renal failure in trauma and surgical patients: a review. *J Am Coll Surg* 1998;186:693–716.
22. Thompson PD, Clarkson P, Karas RH. Statin-associated myopathy. *JAMA* 2003;289:1681–1690.
23. Vanholder R, Sever MS, Erek E, et al. Rhabdomyolysis. *J Am Soc Nephrol* 2000;11:1553–1561.
24. Ward MM. Factors predictive of acute renal failure in rhabdomyolysis. *Arch Intern Med* 1988;148:1553–1557.
25. Welch RD, Todd K, Krause GS. Incidence of cocaine-associated rhabdomyolysis. *Ann Emerg Med* 1991;20:155–157.

Trauma

PART

I

General Considerations

CHAPTER 169
General Principles of Trauma

Eric L. Legome and Peter Rosen

Accidental trauma is the leading cause of death in the United States in the 1- to 44-year-old age group and the fourth leading cause overall (41). Injuries cost the United States an estimated $117 billion dollars in medical expenditures each year. This represents approximately 10% of total medical spending; similar in magnitude to the medical costs associated with other leading public health concerns such as obesity and smoking. The true economic burden of injuries is much greater. These estimates do not include the lost productivity, nonmedical expenditures, insurance costs, property damage, litigation, decreased quality of life, and long-term noninjury health consequences (e.g., mental health care costs) (9). In addition, the personal and social cost due to premature loss of life or livelihood is immeasurable.

Optimal care of the trauma patient begins in the prehospital setting, continues throughout the emergency department course, and extends into the intensive care and rehabilitation phases. All of these parts must work in concert in order to provide for the best outcome. Although not always feasible, the best outcome for the multiple trauma patient occurs when they are initially treated at, or expeditiously transferred to, a regional trauma center with expertise in and dedication to all facets of trauma care (12,15,39).

In addition to treatment of the individual patient, it is imperative that resources and manpower be allocated to the prevention of trauma, an often underappreciated but highly important aspect of trauma care. Even minor changes in traffic safety, alcohol and drug use, and gun safety have a tremendous potential to decrease trauma morbidity (46,52).

CLINICAL PRESENTATION

Prehospital

The appropriate care of the major trauma patient begins in the prehospital setting. Currently, after extrication and immobilization, rapid transport to a trauma center is the one prehospital trauma intervention that has proven useful. Many prehospital interventions such as MAST for hypotensive patients have not been found to be helpful, and even interventions such as rapid sequence intubation (RSI) in the head-injured patient, once thought invaluable, have become controversial. The use of intravenous fluids has likewise become controversial, with timing, amount, and end point a current focus of contention. Current EMS policies and treatments are undergoing scrutiny, and, in the future, which interventions are useful will be better understood (17,38,50,51).

There are many reasons for rapid transport to a trauma center. While many community hospitals have physicians with excellent skills in managing trauma patients, major trauma centers evaluate a significantly higher number of major trauma patients and must maintain their skills. In addition, they generally have appropriate ancillary staffing, up-to-date technology, readily available consultants, rapid operating room (OR) capability, intensive care unit (ICU) capability, and rehabilitative care to restore a patient to full health. Some areas do not have an available trauma center; for example, there are no major level 1 trauma centers in such rural states as Idaho or Montana (55). In these areas, it may be prudent to go directly to a center with an available surgeon or computed tomography (CT) capability, even if it means bypassing a closer hospital. Often a local hospital will have to stabilize a patient prior to transfer to a convenient trauma center. It is therefore wise to have the transfer agreements and routes as well as the mechanics of evacuation worked out well in advance of the individual patient's need. These decisions are often community-specific and based on an understanding of local resources, demographics, and transport times.

Emergency Department

On arrival at the ED, patients assessed as having a major mechanism of injury or having a potentially serious injury should be triaged immediately to a suitable treatment area capable of major resuscitation. Human nature is such that, once a patient has been labeled "not serious," it is difficult to change the label and achieve appropriate care for the patient. Patients can always be downgraded to a less acute ED area after it is clear that they are not seriously injured. Appropriate personnel should accompany the patient to the resuscitation room to ensure that adequate life-support measures are being accomplished en route. Details regarding the mechanism of injury may offer important clues in predicting potential injuries (Table 169.1). While mechanism must always be taken seriously and is a proper place to begin triage, a significant mechanism may not lead to major injury while a trivial mechanism may cause severe morbidity. The most specific way to prognosticate major injury and need for extensive care is by physiologic parameters. Unfortunately,

TABLE 169.1.   Important Details about Mechanism of Injury

BLUNT TRAUMA

Motor Vehicle Collision

1. Estimated speed of both vehicles on impact
2. Orientation of the vehicles (e.g., head-on, broadside)
3. Location of the patient in the vehicle
4. Trajectory and extent of damage to patient's vehicle
5. Amount of intrusion into the vehicle
6. Was there an explosion or fire?
7. Was the patient restrained?
8. Were airbags deployed?
9. Was the windshield intact?
10. Was the steering wheel intact?
11. Was there an initial loss of consciousness at the scene?
12. Were any alcohol or drugs recovered from the patient or car?
13. How long did it take to extricate the patient?
14. What is the ambient temperature (potential for hypothermia)?
15. Was any person killed in the crash?

Fall

1. Estimated height
2. Possible reason for fall (e.g., electrocution; explosion; medical cause of syncope such as a dysrhythmia)
3. Was there an initial loss of consciousness at the scene?
4. Were any alcohol or drugs recovered from the patient or scene?
5. How long was the patient down?
6. What is the ambient temperature (potential for hypothermia)?

PENETRATING TRAUMA

Stab Wound

1. Description of the weapon (e.g., length, width)

Gunshot Wound

1. Description of the weapon (including caliber)

---

sensitivity may suffer if these are looked at alone, so mechanism of injury should alert the triage nurse or physician to the possibility of underlying injury. It is far better to overtriage and not miss an injury than to undertriage and have a catastrophic outcome from underappreciation of possible pathology (21,33).

Triage must take into account the immediate threat to life and limb as well as patient discomfort and anxiety. The means to appropriate evaluation is a rapid but adequate history and physical examination. In many hospitals, an emergency nurse fulfills the triage function. Larger centers may use a highly trained and experienced trauma nurse or a triage physician.

Major trauma is best evaluated by a dedicated trauma team. The team must have a captain. The training and experience of this person may vary and should be appropriate to the specific hospital. Usually, the captain is initially an emergency physician (EP). In some settings, an EP may be the only physician physically present in the ED (and, for that matter, in the hospital). Ideally, surgical support personnel are available within 10 to 30 minutes.

In trauma centers, surgical support is immediately available within the hospital. In this system, the EP may assume the role of trauma captain for the initial assessment and resuscitation. When the attending trauma surgeon arrives, a defined transition of leadership should occur. The team concept must be maintained at all times.

If the responsibility for the major orchestration is formally handed over to the attending trauma surgeon, it does not relieve the EP of responsibility for the patient. The EP should stay and assist until the patient physically leaves for the OR, ICU, or special diagnostic study. Exceptions of course are made if there

are other critical patients who demand the attention of the EP. When the EP has to leave the patient, the departure should always be made in coordination with the team and the team leader. The team may summon subspecialty consultations, as needed, for stabilization, but there must be a single person in charge of the orchestration of total patient needs. Too often, resuscitation becomes chaotic, with multiple subspecialists tunneled into the concerns of their own specialty. The trauma surgeon or EP must stay in command of the overall care.

Nurses who care for trauma patients should have the requisite special knowledge and skills. In large urban centers, there is usually an abundance of physicians to perform resuscitative procedures, but in the rural ED, the trauma nurse may require technical skills ordinarily reserved for physicians. Prehospital personnel who do not need to immediately return to the field may be requested to remain in the ED so that their technical skills can be utilized.

The area of the radiology department designated for emergency patients should be located adjacent to the ED. Portable or built-in x-ray equipment in the trauma resuscitation room is also necessary for proper care of the seriously injured patient. As radiology has become essential to the management of trauma, the radiologist must be considered a member of the trauma team and should be available for consultation at all hours. The radiologist should be integrated into the trauma team and should participate in planning the protocols and guidelines that guide the resuscitation. Protocols and guidelines should be available regarding expectations of all ancillary staff. A coordinated, knowledgeable response from the blood bank, laboratory, respiratory therapy, and radiology department is vital to an effective trauma system. Social workers, clergy, and lay support should be included in the team framework.

The OR must be immediately accessible to the ED for operative resuscitation of critically injured patients. Some centers have emphasized this relation by having an OR as part of the ED or by reserving a single OR for trauma use.

EMERGENCY DEPARTMENT MANAGEMENT

Prior to Arrival

When notice is given by EMS that a patient is en route, the ED should consider potential needs to speed treatment. For example, if there is significant loss of blood at the scene or the patient is hypotensive from presumed hemorrhage, the team may want to have blood immediately available. This may also apply to medications for intubation or pain control. The trauma team should dress in a manner to insure universal precautions. All patients should be presumed to be potentially infectious from bloodborne or body-fluid-borne diseases such as hepatitis B or human immunodeficiency virus (HIV) infection and should be treated accordingly until risk can be fully assessed. Universal precautions apply to blood and to other body fluids containing visible blood, along with cerebrospinal fluid (CSF), synovial fluid, pleural fluid, peritoneal fluid, pericardial fluid, amniotic fluid, semen, and vaginal secretions. In the trauma setting, universal precautions consists of gloves, gowns, masks, and protective eyewear (35).

Primary Survey

The approach to the multiple trauma patient begins with a rapid initial examination; this takes no more than 1 minute and is done in concert with vital signs assessment. On arrival the patient must be immediately undressed. Care should be taken to avoid hypothermia by placing warm blankets on the patient after the initial assessment is performed.

The physician should immediately ascertain the patency of the airway. Can the patient speak clearly or control secretions? Is there a foreign body or relaxed tongue obstructing the airway? The neck is examined for direct trauma, carotid pulsation, tracheal position, and character of neck veins. The physician should observe the chest for sucking wounds or paradoxical motion; palpate for bony crepitus or subcutaneous air, and auscultate for breath sounds. While the lack of breath sounds and subcutaneous air signify a pneumothorax, an inability to appreciate either does not rule them out. Severe dyspnea, hypoxia, or tachypnea in the presence of penetrating chest trauma should lead to the presumption of an underlying hemo- or pneumothorax.

The extremities should be palpated; if they are cool, moist, or pale, shock must be presumed. Patients with penetrating trauma, in the absence of contraindications, should be rolled on their side to ensure that there are no wounds on the back, buttocks, or in the axillae. In the field, it may be impossible to auscultate the blood pressure because of extraneous noise, but in the ED, an attempt to auscultate both the systolic and diastolic pressures must be made. Locating a palpable pulse provides information about the perfusion pressure.

When intravenous lines are placed, blood is drawn for typing and other tests. If possible, the prehospital providers may draw blood, but not every hospital laboratory accepts field blood samples. While it may be more efficient to use a large, 50-mL syringe and simultaneously draw all needed blood samples, as well as measure arterial blood gas from the femoral artery, this may also increase the possibility of needle sticks if the blood is transferred. It is the trauma captain's responsibility to ensure that blood is obtained in a timely manner.

The cervical spine should be immobilized until it is cleared of injury by radiographic or clinical criteria. Oxygenation of the tissues is of primary importance, and clearing the airway is the initial step in delivery. In the unconscious patient, the physician can use a finger to sweep vomitus, blood, teeth, bone, or other debris from the oral cavity. A chin lift or jaw thrust will usually relieve upper airway obstruction. The neck should not be extended if a concern exists for cervical spine injury. A suction apparatus may be used to clear the upper airway. The patient with facial injuries, but no neck injuries, may be turned onto a side or sat up leaning forward to allow rapid clearing of the airway. A patient may also be turned on the backboard or while maintaining spinal immobilization (log rolling) if the condition of the cervical spine is unknown.

An oral airway may be placed in the trauma victim to allow for oxygenation, but only in cases where the patient is unconscious and a plan to rapidly intubate has been made. In some cases of severe maxillofacial trauma or direct tracheal injury, cricothyrotomy is indicated. The need for intubation and active airway management is a clinical decision and should never be withheld pending a blood gas. Once the airway is patent, breath sounds should be rechecked.

If the patient is not breathing spontaneously or adequately, ventilation must be controlled. Initial control may be by bag-valve-mask ventilation with high-flow oxygen. Once the patient is oxygenated and hypercapnia has been corrected, intubation is less hazardous, but undertaking bag-valve-mask ventilation must always be weighed against the risk of distending an already full stomach.

Major trauma victims often need active airway management, even if they are breathing spontaneously. Patients may have injuries that can distort their airways (e.g., a gunshot wound to the neck). It is always prudent to intubate these patients early in their course before the anatomy becomes distorted and intubation is impossible to perform. It will also be much harder, if not disastrous, to attempt a surgical airway when the neck is filled with a massive hematoma. In addition to airway protection and maintenance of anatomical function, other reasons to intubate exist in the major trauma patient. Intubation will decrease the metabolic work of breathing in the seriously injured patient and allow for multiple tests and transport in patients with serious injuries or altered mental status. In addition, in some cases airway management is indicated due to the expectation that the injuries are so severe that the patient will eventually need intubation, either in the ICU or OR. Patients with severe or suspected head injury with a Glasgow Coma Score (GCS) <8 or a declining mental status benefit from intubation. It protects the airway, prevents hypoxia and allows for controlled breathing. Finally, because few trauma patients have an empty stomach at the time of injury, intubation can help lower the risk of vomiting and aspiration of the vomitus.

Oral intubation using an RSI has been very successful and has virtually eliminated the need for cricothyrotomy (2). The preferred approach to intubation in the patient with a possible cervical spine injury is to keep the neck immobilized by in-line stabilization to prevent hyperflexion, hyperextension, or hyperdistraction and perform RSI. While a second pair of hands other than those of the intubator provides in-line stabilization of the head and neck, it is necessary to open the anterior portion of the cervical collar. It is almost never possible to intubate orally with the anterior collar closed.

While RSI has largely replaced cricothyrotomy, optimal management of some patients with midface injuries and severe oral trauma is by placement of a surgical airway. A surgical airway is also necessary if there is extensive damage to the patient's larynx or if there is complete tracheal separation. In the latter instance, the trachea may not separate because the cervical fascia holds it together. Before making an incision in the neck of a patient with this suspected injury (as seen in motorcyclists who have run into a chain or wire strung across their paths), it is prudent to grasp the distal stump of the trachea with a towel clip. Then, when the incision is made, the distal stump will not retract into the anterior mediastinum, where it cannot be reached without splitting the sternum. The need for active airway management is the most critical question in the patient with multiple trauma; universally accepted criteria for mandatory intubation, however, have never been established. Table 169.2 lists criteria that serve as guidelines

---

TABLE 169.2.   Criteria for Airway Management

MANDATORY

Massive facial injuries
Head injury with Glasgow Coma Scale <8
Penetrating injury to the cranial vault
Missile penetrating injury to the neck
Blunt injury to the neck, with expanding hematoma, painful phonation, or alteration of the voice
Bilateral missile penetrating injuries of the thorax
Multisystem trauma with persistent shock

RELATIVE INDICATIONS

Upper airway obstruction from any cause
Any patient with injuries impairing ventilation
Flail chest with increasing respiratory rate or deteriorating blood gases
Bilateral pneumothorax
Expanding hemothorax that recurs or does not respond to thoracostomy
Any patient developing severe hypovolemic shock or with extensive burns, or pulmonary or facial or neck burns

for this decision. Nasal intubation, while occasionally necessary, should be avoided. While still occasionally performed in some prehospital systems, in the ED the optimal approach to the airway is via the oral route.

After evaluation and management of the airway, breathing and circulation must be assessed. In the severely injured patient, dysfunction of either one or both may contribute to a shock state. *Shock* is defined as inadequate perfusion of the tissues. Cool, pale, moist skin indicates shock. Other indicators include a low systolic blood pressure coupled with tachycardia, low urine output, and altered mental status. The major etiology of shock in the acutely traumatized patient is hemorrhagic, usually from bleeding into the peritoneal or retroperitoneal cavity or from blunt or penetrating extremity injuries. Less common but still important etiologies that need to be rapidly treated or ruled out are tension hemo- and pneumothorax. Other less common etiologies include neurogenic (spinal) shock, pericardial tamponade, and cardiac contusion.

Noting the character of the neck veins of the trauma patient is invaluable in identifying the cause of shock. If the neck veins are collapsed, hypovolemia must be presumed. If they are distended, then cardiogenic shock, tension pneumothorax, or pericardial tamponade must be excluded. However, the neck veins may not be distended if the patient is concomitantly hypovolemic. *Most trauma patients in shock are hypovolemic.* The major causes of pulmonary dysfunction in the trauma patient are hemo- and pneumothorax. The patient may also hypoventilate due to multiple rib fractures or underlying pulmonary contusions.

Tension pneumothorax causes shock by increasing intrathoracic pressure, shifting the mediastinum, and compressing the great veins, thereby preventing venous return. The diagnosis is probable in a trauma patient in shock who has distended neck veins and an increased resistance to bagging. An ipsilateral decrease in breath sounds may be noted, as well as a contralateral tracheal shift. Unfortunately, these physical findings are often not present in the acute trauma situation, and the only clues to the presence of this correctable cause of patient collapse may be a sudden rise in pulse, a drop in blood pressure, and an increased resistance to ventilation (6). If tension pneumothorax is suspected in the field, it should be immediately decompressed with a large-bore over-the-needle catheter in the fifth intercostal space in the window between the pectoralis major and the latissimus dorsi muscles. This location is easier to find than the second intercostal space, in the mid-clavicular line. It overcomes the problem of a highly muscular patient in whom the catheter won't be long enough to reach the pleural cavity, and avoids injury to the internal mammary artery that may not be lying below the sternum. Treatment of a suspected tension pneumothorax should not be delayed to obtain radiographic confirmation. The patient may arrest while the film is being obtained. The physician should needle decompress the chest or perform thoracostomy by inserting a large-bore chest tube in the fifth intercostal space, midaxillary line, to evacuate any blood or air.

If shock is not due to pulmonary compromise, circulation must be rapidly assessed. Vascular access is critical. There is no single answer to which method of intravenous access is the best. Each patient must be evaluated individually, and the risk–benefit ratio of the chosen routes weighed. In general, it is best to insert a minimum of two large-bore (14–16 gauge) peripheral lines, adding more as necessary. Sometimes, this scenario is impossible to achieve, however, and it is necessary to proceed immediately to a central line or peripheral cutdown to gain access.

If veins are collapsed or sclerosed, cutdowns, either in the antecubital or saphenous veins, can be rapidly placed. A femoral line may be placed rapidly for access, although it must be balanced with consideration for complications such as deep venous thrombosis or hematoma (40). A central venous catheter may be helpful in monitoring central volume, in addition to delivering fluid and blood. Central line placement utilizing an ultrasound probe has become a much safer procedure, and will not only give access with a large bore catheter, but allow successful central venous pressure monitoring (26,47). In the child under age 3, infusion through an intraosseous needle may be the only available route. Most traumatized adults can tolerate generous fluid infusions because they are usually young and previously in good health. If there is any question about underlying cardiac disease, it is wise to control the amount of intravenous fluids. An initial dose of 20 mL/kg is always safe. If the patient still shows signs of significant volume deficit after administration of 50 mL/kg or 2 L of crystalloid, type-specific or O-negative blood should be started. In the patient who has an injury that obviously will produce a major volume deficit (e.g., shotgun blast with marked tissue destruction and loss), blood should be given immediately. When massive transfusions are necessary, one must remember the need for additional platelets and other clotting factors. Blood should be warmed whenever possible.

In children, fluids should be given as aliquots rather than infused wide open. An aliquot of 20 mL/kg is safe as an initial bolus. This dose can be repeated once and then halved, at a dose of 10 mL/kg. At this time, blood is started at 10 mL/kg.

In all cases, the amount of fluids given depends on continued losses, which should be minimized as much as possible. While intraabdominal bleeding may require definitive surgical or angiographic intervention, interventions in the ED such as proper splinting, bandaging, and avoidance of probing large soft-tissue wounds will maximize hemorrhage control. The degree to which long-bone and pelvic fractures bleed is not generally appreciated; it is far more effective to administer blood when these injuries are recognized than to wait until the patient is in shock. Direct pressure should be applied to control external hemorrhage. Blind probing and clamping deep within a wound may cause further injury to vessels and nerves. A soft-tissue injury, especially to the scalp, may result in large amounts of bleeding. The best treatment of hypovolemia is to locate the source of bleeding and stop the blood loss. Hemostasis can be rapidly obtained in a scalp laceration either by the use of Raney clips (the neurosurgical skin clips that can be quickly applied to the scalp laceration edges) or by placement of a 2-0 nylon running locked stitch.

Both the end point and the aggressive use of fluid resuscitation are controversial. Due to concerns, based mostly on animal studies, that aggressive fluid resuscitation to normotension may lead to increased mortality, a less assertive response to hypovolemia has been advocated. This mortality is due to factors such as increased bleeding due to increased arterial and venous pressure, dilution of clotting factors, clot disruption, and decrease in blood viscosity. Multiple animal studies have upheld this idea of "hypotensive resuscitation." In clinical practice, however, it is unclear if this is beneficial. Only two significant studies have been performed in human beings, one with penetrating and one with a combination of penetrating and blunt trauma patients (5,20). Although one study found a benefit to not actively resuscitating, there have been many concerns about the methodology and validity of the study (29). In addition, patients with severe head injury have a worsened outcome with hypotension, making this approach unlikely to be helpful in this group of patients. At the moment, the standard practice is to resuscitate the patient actively. However, many clinicians and academic centers believe strongly in the concept of less aggressive resuscitation. This approach should be considered while awaiting more definitive research in this area.

Cardiac causes of shock must not be overlooked. Pericardial tamponade is rare with survivable closed-chest injuries; another source of the shock should probably be sought. It must always be considered with penetrating injuries, even if the entrance wound appears anatomically remote. The physiologic response to tamponade is to compensate for the fall in cardiac output by raising the pulse rate. The classic physical findings in this disorder may also be absent in the acute situation. Thus, one may not see distended neck veins if the patient is profoundly hypovolemic. Furthermore, heart sounds may be difficult to appreciate in the ED. If the patient still has vital signs, a pericardiocentesis can be performed. If, on the other hand, the patient has lost vital signs or has suddenly become bradycardic (an ominous sign in a patient with this potential pathology), an immediate thoracotomy should be performed.

Myocardial contusion, most commonly from blunt trauma, may cause dysrhythmias, often within the first hour after injury. An electrocardiogram (ECG) should be obtained in patients with significant anterior blunt chest trauma. Continuous cardiac monitoring is indicated. Myocardial infarction may occur as a result of the stress associated with blood loss and catecholamine release, or it may have preceded the traumatic injury. Coronary arterial air embolization rarely occurs with penetrating neck and chest trauma or serious rib fractures after intubation and positive-pressure ventilation. Air passes from the airway into the pulmonary veins and embolizes to the arterial circulation, often involving the cerebral and coronary arteries. If air embolization is suspected, the patient should be immediately turned to the left lateral decubitus position (i.e., right side up); fluid infusion should be increased, and immediate thoracotomy with bypass arranged. It may be possible to salvage some of these patients with immediate femorofemoral bypass while preparing the OR.

The presence of spinal cord trauma with loss of sympathetic vascular tone can be assessed by rectal examination and examination of peripheral reflexes.

If the patient has a cardiac arrest from hypovolemia or pericardial tamponade, immediate emergency thoracotomy is indicated. While there are no absolute guidelines on when to perform this procedure, thoracotomy offers the only chance for salvage. In general, thoracotomy in the presence of penetrating injury and a patient who arrests in the ED or just prior to arrival offers the best prognosis. Maximal benefits are obtained in the presence of low velocity penetrating injury to the chest, particularly the heart. Blunt trauma arrests in general have an extremely poor prognosis, especially with a prehospital arrest or multiple concomitant injuries (8). It is probably of little benefit to perform a thoracotomy unless the surgical expertise and institutional resources to render definitive care are readily available.

Operative intervention is part of the resuscitation of the unstable trauma victim. In the patient unable to be resuscitated from shock without an obvious source of blood loss, immediate exploration is indicated. A chest radiograph helps determine whether the chest or the abdomen is the site of initial exploration.

The priorities of definitive management are still vigorously debated, and it is often necessary to perform invasive procedures without the luxury of confirming diagnostic studies. In general, one should attempt to approach the pathology that poses the most immediate threat to the patient's life—usually in the abdomen.

Secondary Survey

In the patient who stabilizes during resuscitation, the next priority is a complete head-to-toe examination, which includes performing repeat maxillofacial, cardiopulmonary, abdominal, neurologic, and orthopedic examinations. In addition to the examination, a history about the timing and mechanism of the injury should be obtained as well as the past medical history, medications the patient is taking, and allergies.

If the patient is unconscious, determining the level of brainstem function and the presence of a herniation syndrome is paramount. Most trauma victims die of central nervous system–related injuries. A rectal examination may reveal displacement of the prostate, or gross blood, and provide for neurologic assessment of the anal sphincter tone and sensation. The absence of tone or sensation may indicate a spinal cord injury in a patient previously assessed to have only head injury.

It is necessary to immobilize the spinal column until its status can be ascertained, but it is not necessary to spend long periods of time trying to clear the cervical or other spinal column before dealing with more life-threatening injuries. The patient can be maintained on a backboard with a hard collar while more immediate life threats are determined.

Open fractures should be gently irrigated (realizing that this procedure will not substitute for more effective and complete irrigation and debridement under anesthesia) and splinted to prevent further injury and reduce pain and bleeding. Open fractures should be covered with clean dressings, and intravenous antibiotics administered, to provide antistaphyloccal coverage. Definitive care may have to be delayed while surgical treatment of more serious, life-threatening injuries occurs.

Laboratory and Diagnostic Studies

After completion of the physical examination, the ABCs have been addressed, and external hemorrhage control and splinting have been performed, laboratory and radiologic studies are performed. Laboratory analysis of the trauma patient is generally more extensive than necessary. Routine laboratory studies on pre-operative patients are not useful or cost-effective when a complete history and physical is performed. However, due to the limitations in obtaining this information in the multiple trauma patient, an extensive array of tests is often completed, usually without obtaining beneficial information. While testing based on clinical parameters has been shown to be cost-effective without compromising care, most trauma centers use some type of protocol in order to standardize and speed the laboratory evaluation of patients (14,28). The patient who is fully awake, alert, who has sustained minimal trauma and has no distracting injuries may require no testing. Rational laboratory analysis of most patients with moderate trauma can probably be limited to a complete blood count, basic electrolytes, blood type and screen, and urinalysis. The multiple trauma patient or one about to undergo urgent operative management may require more thorough testing. Women of childbearing age should have a pregnancy test performed.

The sequencing of radiologic studies should be prioritized in the same manner as the other components of the resuscitation. While cervical spine imaging is essential in the patient who cannot be clinically cleared, the film may be delayed and the patient kept in a collar and immobilized while addressing more pressing issues. In victims of blunt trauma, chest and pelvic films should be obtained next and, if necessary, extremity films obtained thereafter. The chest radiograph should be taken as soon as possible in the patient with penetrating injury. Obviously, empiric treatment of a presumed pneumo- or hemothorax should take priority if the patient is unstable. There is recent work to strongly suggest that though clinical evaluation of the pelvis without radiographic study is accurate to exclude fracture, it is still wise to routinely obtain a study on the patient with any component of altered mental status or significant distracting injury (23,24,34).

One of the most important decisions in the management of the multiple trauma patient is when and how to obtain an objective evaluation of the abdomen. With a major mechanism of injury, no matter how well a patient looks, it is wise to assess the abdomen for occult hemorrhage. The physical examination of the abdomen is extremely unreliable when there are multiple injuries, competing pain from skeletal trauma, or altered mental status form head injury, shock, or substance abuse (27,48). In the presence of any of these factors, objective evaluation must be obtained. Finally, in any patient who demonstrates vital sign instability without obvious source, it is prudent to evaluate the abdomen for hemorrhage.

Objective evaluation of the abdomen is generally performed by one of three common methods, diagnostic peritoneal lavage (DPL), CT scan, or ultrasound (US). In some instances, these methods are combined to increase diagnostic specificity or speed.

DPL is highly accurate, and is one of the few tests in medicine that has reliable significance when negative. However, it has largely been supplanted by CT scan and US, both noninvasive tests. DPL is still recommended in the unstable patient with an unclear US result or in the stable patient with a significant concern for a hollow viscous or mesenteric injury, either by examination or after an equivocal CT scan. DPL also plays a major role when CT scan and US are unavailable. If there is no institutional access to US or CT, DPL may provide information that will avoid a transfer to another institution or mandate a laparotomy prior to transfer. While CT can accurately identify the intraperitoneal pathology causing the hemorrhage in an unstable patient, the CT gantry is an unsafe place to manage an unstable patient.

The accuracy of DPL in evaluating intraabdominal hemorrhage ranges between 92% and 98%. The specificity for a therapeutic laparotomy is somewhat less and it should be interpreted in light of the overall clinical picture. That is, a positive DPL in a hemodynamically stable patient should not automatically lead to laparotomy. It is estimated that up to 30% of grossly positive lavages lead to nontherapeutic laparotomies (22). With advances in nonoperative management of solid organ injuries, this number is probably even higher. The other limitation of DPL is that it is insensitive for retroperitoneal injuries.

The only absolute contraindication for DPL is the need for emergency laparotomy. Ultrasonography can also be performed at the bedside, which is occurring with greater frequency in many institutions. The focused assessment with sonography for trauma (FAST), a four-view, directed US examination, is able to reliably find fluid within the abdomen, as well as within the pericardial sac. It is felt to be accurate with significant intraabdominal hemorrhage, and since it s noninvasive, it is replacing the DPL. FAST is performed on the supine patient with the examiner positioned on the right side. Four locations are scanned: (1) the right upper quadrant (RUQ), (2) the left upper quadrant (LUQ), (3) the suprapubic region, and (4) the pericardium. The examiner looks for unclotted blood, a black or anechoic finding on the ultrasound's screen. It is reliable, especially with enough bleeding to cause hemodynamic instability, but may need to be performed more than once if the patient is seen very soon after the trauma when there has not been enough time to produce visible bleeding. The level of accuracy is independent of whether an EP, surgeon, radiologist, or US technician performs the study; they all have comparable results. As with DPL, the US shows fluid in the abdomen, but not its source or the magnitude of injury. This is the major limitation of using DPL as the sole diagnostic test, especially in the stable patient (13,27). Another advantage of US is that the heart can be assessed for pericardial effusion. More recent studies have also shown the bedside ultrasound has good diagnostic accuracy for long bone fractures and pneumothorax (11,31).

While the main use for US is in blunt abdominal trauma, a positive FAST in a penetrating trauma patient has an extremely high positive predictive value for an operative lesion. A negative test cannot rule one out (53).

CT is a diagnostic test that offers both quantitative and qualitative information. It is the gold standard for evaluation of the abdomen in the hemodynamically stable blunt trauma patient. It also is used to evaluate penetrating trauma, although in limited circumstances. With the advent of the very rapid spiral or helical CT scanner, and now the multidetector CT, the test is performed rapidly with excellent sensitivity and specificity. The newer generation scanners also allow for reformations of areas of concern for pathology, including the spine and aorta (43,18). The major limitation of abdominal CT scan is the decreased sensitivity for bowel, mesenteric, and pancreatic injury (1,30). A major advantage of abdominal CT is that a normal CT in trauma has an extremely high negative predictive value for operative intraabdominal pathology (36,37). That is, a normal CT should provide clinicians with a very high probability that they are not missing an operative lesion. Of course, technology and those who interpret its data are not infallible. If the clinical examination still suggests the possibility of injuries not revealed on CT, the patient should undergo further testing or observation.

Additional evaluation depends of specific concerns. Gross hematuria is significant and should prompt evaluation of the genitourinary (GU) tract. Microscopic hematuria is poorly sensitive and specific for significant GU injury, and in the absence of a pelvic fracture or unexplained hypotension after blunt trauma, does not mandate workup (19). Penetrating trauma with any hematuria should be followed by a formal evaluation of the GU tract. Gross penile bleeding should be evaluated by retrograde urethrography before passage of a Foley catheter.

The advent of the multidetector CT has changed the trauma evaluation in many centers. The increased speed and accuracy and the ability to obtain reformations of information rapidly obtained have led to significantly increased usage of CT. Many modern EDs have a scanner either in or immediately adjacent to the ED. Even though the radiology suite is close by, unstable patients should not be sent there, except under rare circumstances. However, the speed of the newest scanners along with their proximity to the ED has allowed for safer use in patients who previously would not have been scanned due to borderline blood pressure or concern over absolute stability. One approach that some trauma centers are now using is to perform a CT from head to pelvis. This may actually be cost effective since the extra time is measured in minutes, there is no increased use of film if the images are stored on a picture archival retrieval system (PACS), and scans of the bones can be included, obviating the need for plain films. Reformations allow for the ability to image the aorta and have essentially replaced aortography in the diagnosis of aortic injury.

Interventional angiography is becoming increasingly important in the management of trauma patients. Angiography is the definitive modality in controlling hemorrhage from major pelvic fractures. In patients with ongoing hemorrhage from major pelvic trauma, angiography with embolization has been shown to be more effective and definitive than external fixation devices or operative packing (16,44). For stable patients with intraperitoneal injuries, if an actively bleeding spleen, liver, or kidney is visualized, a dedicated angiography team may be able to embolize the lesion and avoid laparotomy. While effective, angiography still remains resource-intensive and is not readily available at many centers (18,56).

Angiography may also be used to diagnose arterial injuries in the neck or extremities. Doppler US may reveal flow impairment in the carotid or vertebral vessels after a whiplash trauma to the neck. Arteriography is then used to define the injury. Some centers utilize magnetic resonance angiography in the stable patient. Another place for angiography is in the patient with a penetrating wound near a large vascular structure with massive tissue damage or evidence of distal pulse deficits. If the patient is unstable, however, it is more prudent to take the patient to the OR, obtain vascular control, and perform the angiography intraoperatively.

Transesophageal echocardiography is also very accurate for the diagnosis of aortic transection and has the added advantage that it can be performed at the bedside or in the OR and requires no contrast material.

Unfortunately, not all of these modalities are available 24 hours a day, especially in rural institutions, and the patient will need to be transferred to an appropriate institution to obtain the diagnostic information.

While the management priorities in patients with head, chest, and abdominal injuries still present a challenge, spiral CT scan has made the job of the trauma surgeon and EP much easier because of the availability and speed of this technique. In general, the critical ordering should be to diagnose and treat injuries to the abdomen, head, and then chest (aorta), in that order. However, the specific patient and clinical judgment may alter this approach. The initial priority is to assess for intraperitoneal bleeding. US or DPL that shows blood in the abdomen does not reveal the specific organ injured or the amount of damage, and the patient may also have evidence of intracranial injury. A head CT requires transfer to the radiology suite, but the speed of the procedure may enable a quick assessment of the head en route to the OR for laparotomy. It also adds little time to the assessment to take cuts of the chest and abdomen. If intraperitoneal bleeding is present in the unstable patient, then management of pelvic fractures or aortic injury must be delayed until after laparotomy.

Finally, it is imperative to recognize that the trauma patient needs prompt definitive care. Time wasted in the field, the ED, or the radiology suite may increase mortality. Sometimes, the trauma surgeon must proceed to the OR with a paucity of diagnostic information rather than have the patient continue to hemorrhage.

Trauma in Children

Many important anatomic differences must be kept in mind when caring for injured children. Children under age 6 months are obligate nose breathers, so nasal obstruction in these infants may have serious consequences. The infant's oral cavity is small, and the tongue is relatively larger than the adult's. The larynx is located more cephalad in the infant, and the vocal cords are more distensible. Moreover, the vocal cords are anterior and inferior to their usual location in the adult. If these differences are not appreciated, an endotracheal tube may become lodged in the anterior commissure or may be passed into the esophagus.

Since the trachea is short, right mainstem bronchial intubation or perforation can easily occur. The infant has a large occiput, so the neck is already flexed and the head is slightly extended, even in the "neutral" position. Oral intubation is easier than nasal intubation in infants and young children, and cricothyrotomy is virtually impossible in children under age 8. Needle jet insufflation by way of the cricothyroid membrane may be an appropriate temporizing technique if there is no upper airway obstruction.

The normal systolic blood pressure of a young child should be approximately 80 mm Hg plus twice the age in years; the diastolic pressure should be about two-thirds of the systolic pressure.

The high ratio of body surface area to body mass in young children greatly affects their ability to regulate core temperature. Their lack of substantial subcutaneous tissue and the presence of thin skin contribute to increased evaporative heat loss and caloric expenditure. The resulting hypothermia leads to catecholamine secretion and shivering, resulting in a metabolic acidosis. The young child who is hypothermic may be refractory to therapy for shock. Therefore, the child's temperature should be maintained at 37°C by overhead heaters.

A child's chest wall is very compliant and allows energy to transfer to the intrathoracic structures, frequently without any evidence of injury to the ribs. The result is a higher frequency of pulmonary contusion and intrapulmonary hemorrhage than in adults. Injury to the great vessels is infrequent, however.

Almost all infants and young children who are stressed and crying swallow a large amount of air, and it is particularly important to decompress the stomach by inserting a small nasogastric tube. The tenseness of the abdominal wall often decreases as the gastric distention is relieved. Deep palpation should be avoided at the onset of the examination, as the child will voluntarily guard against subsequent abdominal compression. When performing a diagnostic peritoneal lavage, a fluid volume of 10 to 15 mL/kg of warmed normal saline should be infused.

Blood loss associated with long-bone and pelvic fractures is proportionately greater in children than in adults.

Head injuries are more common in children than in adults. However, long episodes of unconsciousness in children do not necessarily correlate with a poorer prognosis. Conversely, children may sustain a significant concussion without an observed loss of consciousness. Children are also prone to have apneic episodes at the time of injury.

Trauma in Pregnancy

The pregnant mother who sustains trauma has special constraints, not only because there are two lives at risk, but because the physiology of pregnancy makes the management of the mother more complicated. Death due to trauma is the leading cause of mortality in the pregnant female. Most injuries are secondary to motor vehicle collisions; however, pregnant women also sustain a disproportionate amount of domestic violence. In general the blunt trauma mortality rates are similar to those for nonpregnant women. Unique concerns of pregnancy include placental abruption, premature rupture of membranes, and fetomaternal hemorrhage.

In the first trimester, blunt trauma to the infant is less concerning because the fetus is protected by the amniotic fluid. In the second trimester, placental abruption becomes a concern, and in the third trimester, even minor trauma may lead to abruption and fetal demise in as many as 5% of patients. Major trauma has been reported to result in abruption with an incidence that ranges from 44% to 66%. These patients require fetal monitoring, and it is prudent to have early obstetric consultation while the mother is being evaluated. The best protection for the fetus results from optimal care of the mother. Radiologic studies should never be withheld if they are indicated in the mother, and are of lesser concern past the first trimester. Although the hematocrit decreases during pregnancy, the mother's plasma volume will increase, which may give the appearance of stability when the mother is actually losing volume rapidly. The blood pressure is normally low in the second and third trimesters, and this should not be overcorrected from a fear of volume depletion. In the late third trimester, the mother may need to be resuscitated in the left lateral decubitus position, or with manual displacement of the gravid uterus to avoid hypotension from pressure on the vena cava.

After evaluation of the mother, cardiotocographic monitoring should be instituted on patients in the second or third trimester of pregnancy, even without any evidence of significant injury. This is the best way to assess for placental abruption and is the best predictor of adverse outcomes. Usually 4 hours is sufficient with minor trauma; after major trauma, or, if patients have uterine contractions, vaginal bleeding, or abnormal fetal heart tracings, then 24 hours of monitoring is required.

DISPOSITION

The stable trauma patient may spend a number of hours between the ED and the radiology department during the completion of diagnostic tests. During this time, the patient must be monitored to ensure that deterioration does not occur or that a quick transfer to the OR has not become necessary.

The patient remains the responsibility of the ED until he or she is admitted. Once admitted, overall ED care of the patient may depend on institutional policies and resources; but regardless, the EP should assist in care of any patient who remains in the ED. Even if the trauma team monitors the patient in the radiology department, when the patient returns to the ED, it again becomes the EP's responsibility to become involved in the care of the patient, unless preexisting protocols are in place and the trauma service has the proper manpower to observe the patient.

After careful evaluation and a period of observation, many patients can be discharged from the ED. However, any patient who has had a significant mechanism of injury is likely to develop areas of pain and may have occult injuries not identified in the ED. It is therefore prudent, although not mandatory, to provide a period of observation and care in the hospital.

Transfer of the patient to another institution depends on multiple factors. If the patient is unstable, the only rationale for transfer is to achieve a level of care higher than what is available at the original treating facility. It may be necessary to care for life-threatening injury (e.g., removal or salvage of a torn spleen) and then transfer the patient for more sophisticated neurosurgical, orthopedic, or thoracic management.

TRAUMA SCORING SYSTEMS

Trauma scores are an imperfect but commonly used tool in trauma systems. Prehospital providers, EPs, and inpatient trauma services use these scores for planning purposes and as a quality assurance screen to monitor system performance. Regional trauma planners use these scoring systems to compare institutions and assess resource needs and as a tool for performing research on the effects of different interventions.

Economic and geographical constraints have dictated that many trauma patients cannot be cared for in a trauma center. Therefore, a system has been developed to enable the accurate triage of seriously injured trauma patients. Unfortunately, it is extremely difficult to devise a system based on inpatient data that is accurate in the prehospital setting for triaging patients. Prehospital triage protocols are complicated by factors such as drugs, alcohol, and competing injuries, and many serious injuries are often hidden until there is a catastrophic decompensation. For example, most of the trauma scores utilize the Glasgow Coma Score (GCS) as part of their scoring estimation. Although the GCS is often applied in the field, it was not intended to be used until after all alcohol has been metabolized. Since at least half of all major trauma involves patients who are intoxicated, the GCS is not likely to represent solely brain injury. It is also difficult to calculate the GCS in the intubated and paralyzed patient. Even mechanism of injury, which provides useful clues to the seriousness of the forces involved, is inaccurate because the recipients of those forces sustain such variable degrees of injury. Newer data suggests that physiologic criteria and altered mental status are the best predictors of the need for major interventions; however, these criteria are bound to miss serious occult injuries which may not present until later in the ED or hospital course (25,33,42). Even at the trauma center, the initial recognition of injury severity is often difficult, and the variations of response to what appears to be minor trauma can lead to disaster. An example of this is admission of a trauma patient to a neurosurgical or orthopedic service without recognition of an underlying splenic injury (54).

The optimal scoring system should be easy to apply to patients, have validity and good interrater reliability. It must have easily measured and understandable criteria and should not be so complex that it is difficult to calculate or understand the out-come measurements. Most scoring systems are based on mechanism of injury, physiologic criteria, anatomic injury sites, or some combination thereof.

In the prehospital system, scores may be used to monitor quality assurance and to assist in deciding if a patient requires a major trauma center. They may also aid trauma centers in formulating their needs and levels of response prior to patient arrival. In the ED, scores may be chosen to assess the need for a trauma team response, the need for prophylactic intubation, the likelihood of occult injury, or the need for ICU admission.

Physiologic Scores

These are employed in prehospital decision making, to evaluate the appropriateness and efficacy of injury treatment, and to prognosticate outcome.

Revised Trauma Score

The original Trauma Score evaluated respiratory rate, respiratory expansion, systolic blood pressure, capillary refill, and GCS. Due to variability in assessing several of the components, a revised score was developed in 1989, using data from the Washington Hospital Trauma Center and the Major Trauma Outcome Study. The Revised Trauma Score (RTS) was broken into three components: GCS, systolic blood pressure, and respiratory rate. Numbers were assigned to each parameter, with a higher number representing improved function. An RTS less than 12 identified 97.2% of all fatally injured patients. As this score is based entirely on physiologic variables, there is a risk of inappropriate decision making when patients are scored early after injury. While the RTS is a commonly used score, several factors contribute to decreasing its specificity. This score is partially driven by the GCS score. As mentioned above, the GCS is skewed by alcohol and drugs, but it is also skewed by how quickly the patient is evaluated after the head trauma. For example, many patients who are ultimately deemed minor head injuries would actually have a low GCS if examined immediately after being struck on the head.

Anatomic Scores

Injury Severity Score

The Injury Severity Score (ISS) was developed as an extension of the Abbreviated Injury Scale (AIS) (46), one of the original scoring systems. The AIS grade was developed by dividing the body into six regions (the thorax, abdomen and visceral pelvis, head and neck, face, bony pelvis and extremities, and external structures) and utilizing the site with the worst injury from each region when calculating the overall score. The original ISS was devised by summing the squares of the highest AIS grade in each of the three most severely injured areas. This modified scale was shown to correlate with fatality from trauma. Death from trauma begins to rise significantly when the ISS is above 15. Unfortunately, both the AIS and the ISS can be calculated accurately only after the full extent of the patient's injuries is known. The ISS is now commonly used as a quality assurance tool, but it has no role in decision making either in the ED or in the prehospital setting.

Other Scoring Systems

Trauma and Injury Severity Score

While the ISS accounts for patients' injuries, prediction of mortality should take into account factors that affect likelihood of survival. The Trauma and Injury Severity Score (TRISS) methodology incorporates the patient's age and ISS into a score that predicts the chance of survival. Patients with outcomes different from those predicted by the formula may be candidates for quality assurance review. TRISSs are heavily weighted toward head injury. The W statistics, derived by comparison of a hospital's results to those from the Major Outcome Trauma Study, portray the number of excess survivors per 100 patients (7).

ASCOT

A severity characterization of trauma system (ASCOT) was developed based on analysis of the shortcomings of TRISS seen in the Major Trauma Outcome Study. In addition to the revised trauma score variables, ASCOT adds scoring assignments for injury to three body regions (brain/spinal cord, thorax/neck, and abdomen/major vessel). In comparison, ASCOT seems to perform better than TRISS for adults with blunt trauma. Both TRISS and ASCOT appear adequate for pediatric patients (5).

Prehospital Index

Another widely used trauma score is the Prehospital Index (PHI) (32). The PHI was developed using 313 trauma patients, who were considered to have major trauma if they died within 72 hours of injury or required surgical intervention within 24 hours. Originally, this trauma score utilized only physiologic parameters. The authors realized, however, that the addition of a measure of anatomic injury (penetrating injuries of the abdomen or chest) would improve the accuracy of the score. The PHI was validated in a multicenter study of 3,581 patients. In the validation study; the PHI had a positive predictive value of 52.1% and a negative predictive value of 99.4% (32).

Clinical Judgment

After reviewing the available scores and methodologies for triaging trauma patients, the practicing physician may wish to consider the role of clinical judgment. One study noted that the inclusion of advanced EMT injury perception, in addition to standard out-of-hospital triage criteria, improved accuracy of field trauma triage (49). In a large study evaluating the ability of urban EMTs to assess trauma, none of the scores were found to perform better than EMT judgment. The physician considering the use of these scores will need to consider the setting in which the scores will be used. Most urban EMTs have the ability to recognize major trauma patients (3,49).

New trauma-scoring systems continue to be devised. Until there is an agreement over a gold standard against which these scores can be measured, there is likely to be disagreement over the optimal scoring system. Hospital trauma services continue to use both the RTS and the ISS because of their usefulness in assessing quality assurance through the TRISS methodology.

Depending on the purpose for which they are being used, EDs have a number of scoring systems available for their use. The RTS may be used to monitor changes in a patient's condition during the course of the patient's initial resuscitation. Clearly, the use of mechanism of injury to activate the trauma team will lead to an overutilization of that resource, but a degree of overtriage is accepted in the effort to include all potentially injured trauma patients. EMS systems commonly use the PHI or the RTS. The Baxt Trauma Triage Rule (TTR) is also used in some systems because it has been demonstrated to be valid and easy to use. It uses several common variables, (systolic BP <85mm Hg, GCS motor score <5, or penetrating injury to the trunk, head or neck) to define major trauma victims who should be taken to the nearest trauma center. While the Baxt rule is easy to use, it's principle advantage is as a teaching tool for paramedics and physicians who do not have extensive experience and need help to identify potentially serious injuries (45).

COMMON PITFALLS

- ✔ Failure to appreciate the severity of the mechanism of injury
- ✔ Ascribing positive physical findings to a benign cause
- ✔ Failure to anticipate patient needs prior to arrival
- ✔ Failure to have a visible trauma captain throughout the resuscitation
- ✔ Failure to use a well thought out, systematic approach to the patient
- ✔ Chaotic and inefficient resuscitation because of poor use of team members or because too many physicians are trying to give orders
- ✔ Focusing on subspecialty needs at the expense of real or potential life threats
- ✔ Overemphasizing diagnostic tests in an unstable patient

Acknowledgments

Thanks to previous edition chapter authors Charles L. Emerman and Thomas E. Collins.

References

1. Akhrass R, Yaffe MB, Brandt CP, et al. Pancreatic trauma: a ten-year multi-institutional experience. *Am Surg* 1997;63:598–604.
2. Bair AE, Filbin MR, Kulkarni RG, et al. The failed intubation attempt in the emergency department: analysis of prevalence, rescue techniques, and personnel. *J Emerg Med* 2002;23:131–140.
3. Baker SP, O'Neill B, Haddon W, Jr., et al. The injury severity score: a method for describing patients with multiple injuries and evaluating emergency care. *J Trauma* 1974;14:187–196.
4. Baker SP, O'Neill B. The injury severity score: an update. *J Trauma* 1976;16:882–885.
5. Bickell WH, Wall MJ, Jr., Pepe PE, et al. Immediate versus delayed fluid resuscitation for hypotensive patients with penetrating torso injuries. *N Engl J Med* 1994;331:1105–1109.
6. Bokhari F, Brakenridge S, Nagy K, et al. Prospective evaluation of the sensitivity of physical examination in chest trauma. *J Trauma* 2002;53:1135–1138.
7. Boyd CR, Tolson MA, Copes WS. Evaluating trauma care: the TRISS method. Trauma Score and the Injury Severity Score. *J Trauma* 1987;27:370.
8. Branney SW, Moore EE, Feldhaus KM, et al. Critical analysis of two decades of experience with postinjury emergency department thoracotomy in a regional trauma center. *J Trauma* 1998;45:87–94.
9. CDC. Medical expenditures attributable to injuries in the United States, 2000. *MMWR* 2004;53:1–4.
10. Champion HR, Sacco WJ, Copes WS, et al. A revision of the Trauma Score. *J Trauma* 1989;29:623–629.
11. Chan SS. Emergency bedside ultrasound to detect pneumothorax. *Acad Emerg Med* 2003;10:91–94.
12. Chiara O, Cimbanassi S. Organized trauma care: does volume matter and do trauma centers save lives? *Curr Opin Crit Care* 2003;9:510–514.
13. Chiu WC, Cushing BM, Rodriguez A, et al. Abdominal injuries without hemoperitoneum: a potential limitation of focused abdominal sonography for trauma (FAST). *J Trauma* 1997;42:617.
14. Chu UB, Clevenger FW, Imami ER, et al. The impact of selective laboratory evaluation on utilization of laboratory resources and patient care in a level-I trauma center. *Am J Surg* 1996;172:558–562.
15. Clancy TV, Gary Maxwell J, Covington DL, et al. A statewide analysis of level I and II trauma centers for patients with major injuries. *J Trauma* 2001;51:346–351.
16. Cook RE, Keating JF, Gillespie I. The role of angiography in the management of haemorrhage from major fractures of the pelvis. *J Bone Joint Surg Br* 2002;84:178.
17. Davis DP, Hoyt DB, Ochs M, et al. The effect of paramedic rapid sequence intubation on outcome in patients with severe traumatic brain injury. *J Trauma* 2003;54:444–453.
18. Demetriades D, Velmahos G. Technology-driven triage of abdominal trauma: the emerging era of nonoperative management. *Annu Rev Med* 2003;54:1–15.
19. Dreitlein DA, Suner S, Basler J. Genitourinary trauma. *Emerg Med Clin North Am* 2001;19:569–590.
20. Dutton RP, Mackenzie CF, Scalea TM. Hypotensive resuscitation during active hemorrhage: impact on in-hospital mortality. *J Trauma* 2002;52:1141–1146.
21. Esposito TJ, Offner PJ, Jurkovich GJ, et al. Do prehospital trauma center triage criteria identify major trauma victims?. *Arch Surg* 1995;130:171–176.
22. Fryer JP, Graham TL, Fong HM, et al. Diagnostic peritoneal lavage as an indicator for therapeutic surgery. *Can J Surg* 1991;34:471–476.
23. Gonzalez RP, Fried PQ, Bukhalo M. The utility of clinical examination in screening for pelvic fractures in blunt trauma. *J Am Coll Surg* 2002;194:121–125.
24. Heath FR, Blum F, Rockwell S. Physical examination as a screening test for pelvic fractures in blunt trauma patients. *W V Med J* 1997;93:267–269.

25. Henry MC, Alicandro JM, Hollander JE, et al. Evaluation of American College of Surgeons trauma triage criteria in a suburban and rural setting. *Am J Emerg Med* 1996;14:124–129.
26. Hind D, Calvert N, McWilliams R, et al. Ultrasonic locating devices for central venous cannulation: meta-analysis. *BMJ* 2003;327:361.
27. Hoff WS, Holevar M, Nagy KK, et al. Practice management guidelines for the evaluation of blunt abdominal trauma: the East practice management guidelines work group. *J Trauma* 2002;53:602–615.
28. Jacobs IA, Kelly K, Valenziano C, et al. Cost savings associated with changes in routine laboratory tests ordered for victims of trauma. *Am Surg* 2000;66:579–584.
29. Jacobs LM. Timing of fluid resuscitation in trauma. *N Engl J Med* 1994;331:1153–1154.
30. Killeen KL, Shanmuganathan K, Poletti PA, et al. Helical computed tomography of bowel and mesenteric injuries. *J Trauma* 2001;51:26–36.
31. Kirkpatrick AW, Brown R, Diebel LN, et al. Rapid diagnosis of an ulnar fracture with portable hand-held ultrasound. *Mil Med* 2003;168:312–313.
32. Koehler JJ, Malafa SA, Hillesland J, et al. A multicenter validation of the prehospital index. *Ann Emerg Med* 1987;16:380–385.
33. Kohn MA, Hammel JM, Bretz SW, et al. Trauma team activation criteria as predictors of patient disposition from the emergency department. *Acad Emerg Med* 2004;11:1–9.
34. Krantz BE, Bell RM. Clinical examination in screening for pelvic fractures in blunt trauma. *J Am Coll Surg* 2002;195:740.
35. Leads from the MMWR. Update: universal precautions for prevention of transmission of human immunodeficiency virus, hepatitis B virus, and other bloodborne pathogens in health-care settings. *JAMA* 1988;260:462.
36. Livingston DH, Lavery RF, Passannante MR, et al. Admission or observation is not necessary after a negative abdominal computed tomographic scan in patients with suspected blunt abdominal trauma: results of a prospective, multi-institutional trial. *J Trauma* 1998;44:273–280.
37. Livingston DH, Lavery RF, Passannante MR, et al. Emergency department discharge of patients with a negative cranial computed tomography scan after minimal head injury. *Ann Surg* 2000;232:126–132.
38. Mackersie RC, Christensen JM, Lewis FR. The prehospital use of external counterpressure: does MAST make a difference? *J Trauma* 1984;24:882–888.
39. Mann NC, Mullins RJ, MacKenzie EJ, et al. Systematic review of published evidence regarding trauma system effectiveness. *J Trauma* 1999;47:S25–S33.
40. Mian NZ, Bayly R, Schreck DM, et al. Incidence of deep venous thrombosis associated with femoral venous catheterization. *Acad Emerg Med* 1997;4:1118–1121.
41. National Center for Health Statistics (NCHS) Vital Statistics System. 10 Leading Causes of Death, United States All Races, Both Sexes, Office of Statistics and Programming, National Center for Injury Prevention and Control, CDC, 2001
42. Norwood SH, McAuley CE, Berne JD, et al. A prehospital glasgow coma scale score < or = 14 accurately predicts the need for full trauma team activation and patient hospitalization after motor vehicle collisions. *J Trauma* 2002;53:503–507.
43. Novelline RA, Rhea JT, Bell T. Helical CT of abdominal trauma. *Radiol Clin North Am* 1999;37:591–612.
44. O'Neill PA, Riina J, Sclafani S, et al. Angiographic findings in pelvic fractures. *Clin Orthop:* 1996;60–67.
45. Roth R.Prehospital care: trauma scoring systems and trauma triage. In: Ferrera PC CS, Marx JA, Verdile VP, et al, eds. *Trauma Management An Emergency Medicine Approach.* St. Louis: Mosby, 2001.
46. Sampalis JS, Denis R, Frechette P, et al. Direct transport to tertiary trauma centers versus transfer from lower level facilities: impact on mortality and morbidity among patients with major trauma. *J Trauma* 1997;43:288–295.
47. Scalea TM, Sinert R, Duncan AO, et al. Percutaneous central venous access for resuscitation in trauma. *Acad Emerg Med* 1994;1:525–531.
48. Schurink GW, Bode PJ, van Luijt PA, et al. The value of physical examination in the diagnosis of patients with blunt abdominal trauma: a retrospective study. *Injury* 1997;28:261–265.
49. Simmons E, Hedges JR, Irwin L, et al. Paramedic injury severity perception can aid trauma triage. *Ann Emerg Med* 1995;26:461–468.
50. Spaite DW, Tse DJ, Valenzuela TD, et al. The impact of injury severity and prehospital procedures on scene time in victims of major trauma. *Ann Emerg Med* 1991;20:1299–1305.
51. Spivak M. Trauma care in EMS: where are we? A look at the nature, origins, controversies and future of prehospital trauma services. *Emerg Med Serv* 1999;28:29–34, 37–42.
52. Stewart RM, Myers JG, Dent DL, et al. Seven hundred fifty-three consecutive deaths in a level I trauma center: the argument for injury prevention. *J Trauma* 2003;54:66–70.
53. Udobi KF, Rodriguez A, Chiu WC, et al. Role of ultrasonography in penetrating abdominal trauma: a prospective clinical study. *J Trauma* 2001;50:475–479.
54. Van Natta T, Morris J Jr. Injury scoring and trauma outcomes. In: Moore GE, Mattox KL, Feliciano DV (ed.) *Trauma.* 4th edition. McGraw-Hill, 2000.
55. Verified Trauma Sites, American College of Surgeons Website www.facs.org, 2004.
56. Willmann JK, Roos JE, Platz A, et al. Multidetector CT: detection of active hemorrhage in patients with blunt abdominal trauma. *AJR Am J Roentgenol* 2002;179:437–444.

CHAPTER 170
Trauma Airway Management

Kevin R. Ward

Expert management of the airway is the single most important skill that must be acquired and maintained by the emergency physician (EP). Many victims of trauma will benefit from early control of the airway to ensure adequate oxygenation and ventilation and to protect against aspiration. This chapter discusses the unique aspects of airway management in patients with multisystem trauma.

CLINICAL PRESENTATION

Airway management in the trauma patient is problematic for many reasons. The five most immediate concerns are listed in Table 170.1. The EP should assume the presence of cervical spine (c-spine) injury in most blunt trauma victims. Due to an altered mental status, hemodynamic instability, and difficulty in obtaining adequate c-spine radiographs rapidly, cervical spine injury cannot be excluded in most patients requiring emergent intubation. The methods for assessing the difficulty of intubation (i.e., MOAN and LEMONS) that are discussed in Chapter 1 (Airway Management) are helpful, but most methods used to predict the difficulty of intubation require either a cooperative patient or the ability to fully extend the neck. The inability to optimally position the airway can be problematic in obtaining an adequate laryngeal view during intubation. Coexisting facial and penetrating neck trauma add to this problem. Therefore, the ability to predict the difficulty of intubation in the setting of trauma is limited.

Hypovolemia complicates airway management because the drugs given to facilitate airway management can cause secondary hemodynamic deterioration. All major trauma patients should be assumed to have occult hypovolemia or compensated shock. Only after the patient has lost 30% to 40% of his or her blood volume does shock uniformly manifest itself. This is especially true for the pediatric and geriatric populations.

Due to the unpredictability of the timing of traumatic injuries, all trauma patients should be presumed to have a full stomach. Furthermore, patients may be nauseated or vomiting due to pain or head injury. Patients who are immobilized in a cervical collar and on a long board are not able to fully protect their airways. All of these conditions place trauma patients at risk for aspiration.

TABLE 170.1. Factors Complicating Trauma Airway Management

1. Inability to optimally position the airway for intubation due to the possibility of C-spine injury
2. Presence of hypovolemic shock or occult hypovolemia
3. Presence of full stomach and risk of aspiration
4. Possibility of concomitant head injury
5. Known or unknown preexisting disease states

Concomitant head injury also alters the approach to airway management in the trauma patient. Adequate cerebral perfusion pressure should be maintained and intracranial pressure (ICP) may need to be controlled. Drugs or alcohol, which may cause altered mental status and combative behavior, further complicate the determination of the presence of closed head injury and the need for emergent airway management.

In addition, laryngoscopy and intubation result in circulatory responses that can cause bradycardia, tachycardia, hypertension, increased ICP, and disturbances in cerebral blood flow. All of the factors mentioned must be considered when managing the airway of a trauma patient.

EMERGENCY DEPARTMENT MANAGEMENT

Indications for Airway Management in the Trauma Patient

Trauma patients require airway management for a variety of reasons. The inability of the patient to adequately oxygenate and ventilate and the need for airway protection are the most common reasons for deciding to perform endotracheal intubation (ETI). These issues are not separate but combined in many cases, especially in the victim with multisystem trauma. The inability to adequately oxygenate and ventilate may be due to many causes, including severe chest injury, severe hemorrhage, traumatic brain injury, and airway obstruction. The inability of a patient to protect the airway may be due to depressed mental status from traumatic brain injury or severe alcohol intoxication or upper airway trauma. Lastly, many situations arise in which early active airway management is warranted because of the complexity of the workup to exclude serious injuries and because of the anticipated future course of the patient. Examples include penetrating neck trauma prior to taking the patient to surgery, inhalation injury prior to evidence of stridor, and taking patients out of the ED for diagnostic testing, such as computed tomography and angiography. Occasionally, patients at risk for severe injury who are combative and resistant to chemical restraint may require short term ETI to expedite their diagnostic evaluation to exclude serious injury. The increasing number of elderly trauma patients with potentially severe injuries may also lower the clinician's threshold for early intubation for various reasons ranging from preexisting active diseases such as COPD to the need for systemic analgesia and sedation for fracture reduction of long bones.

Techniques of Airway Management

Orotracheal intubation (OTI), blind nasotracheal intubation (NTI), and surgical cricothyrotomy are the major choices for definitive airway management in the trauma patient. Regardless of technique, proper preparation is essential. The use of the mnemonic SOAPME is helpful to ensure readiness (Table 170.2).

Orotracheal Intubation and Rapid Sequence Induction

OTI may be performed in several ways, ranging from having the patient totally awake to performing it in conjunction with rapid sequence induction (RSI). OTI with RSI has become the procedure of choice in managing the trauma airway. It is also being used in the prehospital setting (26). Although different pharmacologic agents may be chosen, the major components of this technique remain the same: preoxygenation, administration of agents that cause loss of consciousness, administration of paralytics, and administration of postintubation analgesia and sedation.

TABLE 170.2.   Preparation for Airway Management: Mnemonic

S: Suction should be readily available with Yankauer or tonsil tip apparatus.

O: High-flow oxygen (15 L/min) with appropriate methods of delivery such as bag-valve mask device and nonrebreathing masks should be available.

A: Airway supplies should be present in various sizes. These include naso- and ororpharyngeal airways, endotracheal tubes with stylets and 10-mL syringes, and functioning straight- and curved blade laryngoscopes. Airway adjuncts should be available for difficult airways. Adequate assistance to keep the airway positioned and to provide cricoid pressure is essential.

P: Pharmacology in the form of induction, sedative, analgesic and neuromuscular blocking agents, as well as local anesthetics should be available for immediate administration.

ME: Monitoring equipment such as ECG, pulse oximetry, end-tidal CO_2 monitoring, and stethoscopes should be applied and in working condition.

Preoxygenation is performed to prevent hypoxemia during the intubation process. It is achieved either actively, such as with use of a bag-valve mask (BVM), or by letting the patient with spontaneous respiration (and adequate minute ventilation) inhale 100% oxygen. Active preoxygenation should be avoided, if possible, to reduce the risk of gastric insufflation. However, some argue that a brief attempt should be made to assist the patient with a BVM to ensure the patient can be adequately ventilated prior to inducing paralysis. Optimal application of a BVM in the trauma patient may require two people (one to make the seal with the mask and one to squeeze the bag). Preoxygenation should begin in all trauma patients by placement of a nonrebreathing oxygen mask upon arrival.

Application of cricoid pressure (Sellick maneuver) is essential during RSI, or any other active ventilation technique, to prevent gastric insufflation. This maneuver is applied until the endotracheal tube cuff is inflated and tube position is confirmed. Unless lung or chest trauma exists, it should be possible to significantly denitrogenate the lungs within 30 seconds if the patient receiving 100% oxygen can take four maximally deep breaths or if the equivalent can be delivered actively with a BVM (9). This will provide the patient a reservoir of oxygen lasting up to five minutes before desaturation of hemoglobin occurs. Difficulty in providing maximal preoxygenation may occur in patients with chest trauma producing decreased chest wall compliance, pulmonary contusions, hemothoraces or pneumothoraces, or those with bronchospasm (from smoke inhalation or preexisting reactive airway disease). In cases where pneumothorax is strongly suspected, consideration should be given to delaying intubation and mechanical ventilation until after performance of tube or needle thoracostomy. Artificial ventilation may rapidly turn a simple pneumothorax into a tension pneumothorax with one or two ventilations.

Paralysis is performed during RSI for a number of reasons. It reduces the chance of regurgitation and aspiration by eliminating the gagging and coughing response to the stimulus of laryngoscopy. Paralysis also totally relaxes the upper airway musculature to allow the physician an optimal view of the larynx. It also prevents spontaneous movements by the patient with cervical spine injury that might produce spinal cord injury during the peri-intubation period.

Because of the challenge in predicting the degree of difficulty in intubating the trauma patient who has facial and neck injuries, inhalation injuries, or potential c-spine injuries, care must be taken in using paralytic agents if there is likely to be a problem in providing other forms of artificial ventilation. Rescue airway adjuncts, as well as cricothyrotomy equipment, must be immediately available at all times during RSI. In cases in which a difficult airway is anticipated, RSI may be modified to provide adequate sedation, sometimes in conjunction with topical or intravenous anesthesia, but the paralysis component is deleted. This combination may be the best alternative since it will partially blunt the physiologic response to laryngoscopy and intubation. Paralytics may then be given immediately after endotracheal tube position is confirmed. Despite the attractiveness of this approach in theory, it may still be difficult to obtain optimal views of the glottis during laryngoscopy (5).

Placement of a nasogastric tube prior to intubation can be extremely problematic, depending on the patient's level of consciousness. Although gastric emptying prior to RSI would appear to offer advantages, many patients in distress will not tolerate its placement. This sometimes results in dangerous movement of the c-spine as well as gagging and vomiting that may lead to aspiration or deleterious changes in cerebral hemodynamics.

Blind Nasotracheal Intubation

NTI has long been advocated as the method of choice for intubating patients with suspected c-spine injury and patients in whom sedation is contraindicated. It requires a patient who is spontaneously breathing and in whom the operator can recognize inspiration and expiration. Patients with significant midface trauma have not been considered candidates for NTI, although clinical studies demonstrate its safety in patients with demonstrated cribriform plate fractures (19).

NTI has several drawbacks. Because optimal performance requires proper preparation of the nasal mucosa, it can be time-consuming and can take several minutes to complete. NTI often requires multiple attempts. Even after mucosal preparation, significant epistaxis may occur, placing the patient at risk for aspiration and possibly making subsequent OTI more difficult. NTI may cause intense cardiovascular stimulation and may result in increased ICP in those at risk for head injury or movement of the c-spine in those at risk for cord injuries.

During NTI, oxygen should be administered by high-flow delivery throughout the procedure to prevent desaturation. The larger naris should be chosen. The nasal mucosa should be prepared using a topical anesthetic and vasoconstrictive agent (e.g., 4% lidocaine and 1% phenylephrine) if possible. Adequate sedation may decrease the incidence of the previously discussed side effects. Attention should be paid to maintaining c-spine immobilization if indicated, as well as to the application of cricoid pressure. Special endotracheal tubes have been designed in which the tip of the tube can be manipulated by a proximal trigger, thus enhancing the success of blind placement in the trachea.

Surgical Airway Management

Cricothyrotomy equipment should be immediately available for any patient undergoing RSI. Even with the development of percutaneous kits, experience remains essential. The major indication for cricothyrotomy is failure of other methods of intubation (OTI or NTI) and when BVM then fails to provide adequate oxygenation. Many of these situations involve patients with significant facial trauma and upper airway hemorrhage who require airway protection. Patients with anterior neck trauma (penetrating and blunt) deserve special consideration since they have a relative contraindication to cricothyrotomy. In the case of tracheal trauma, even the small incision used for the technique may convert a partial cricotracheal separation into a complete one. In addition, the release of the neck hematoma may cause significant bleeding, making the procedure extremely difficult. There will always be a small percentage of patients whose oral anatomy or body habitus makes OTI or NTI impossible and limits the feasibility of using airway adjuncts for more than a very limited amount of time. Perhaps the biggest mistake regarding the use of cricothyrotomy is its timing; it is frequently used too late in the course of management when the patient is already severely hypoxemic.

Special Maneuvers and Intubation Adjuncts

Displacement of the thyroid cartilage backward against the cervical vertebrae, upward or as superiorly as possible, and laterally to the right (BURP maneuver) has been described and found to significantly improve the view of the glottis during laryngoscopy (Fig. 170.1) (35). It is finding widespread acceptance as an aid in management of the difficult airway. The mechanism by which BURP improves visibility may lie in the ability to move the glottis back into the line of vision since laryngoscopy itself tends to push the tongue and possibly the larynx towards the left. The use of BURP in the setting of potential c-spine injury in which

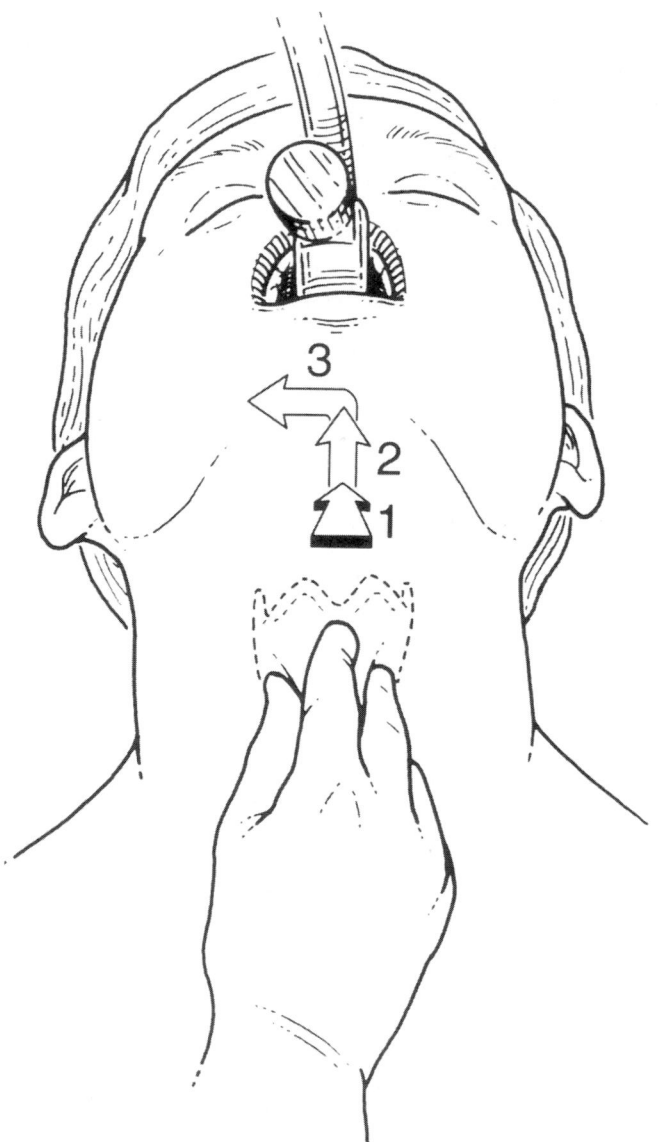

Figure 170.1. Diagram of application of the BURP maneuver to improve the glottic view during laryngoscopy. The thyroid cartilage is moved backward against the cervical vertebrae, upward or as superiorly as possible, and laterally to the right. See text for further explanation.

in-line immobilization of the neck is necessary has not been studied. It is therefore unknown if the laryngeal view in this setting is significantly improved. It is also unknown how displacement of the thyroid cartilage might effect an unstable c-spine injury. However, its use in patients without suspected c-spine injuries would seem to be advantageous and without contraindications. It should be remembered that BURP does not replace the need for cricoid pressure in any patient undergoing intubation.

Several airway adjuncts either aid in the intubation process or are designed to temporarily substitute for intubation if it cannot be performed (3,20). See Chapter 2, Airway Procedures, for a complete discussion of these methods. Several intubation adjuncts such as the lighted stylet and gum elastic bougie allow blind placement of an endotracheal tube without manipulation of the cervical spine (6,18). Different laryngoscopes and laryngoscopic blades have been marketed in an attempt to help improve the glottic view, especially during difficult intubations in which minimum or no movement of the c-spine is desired. These include the Bullard and McCoy laryngoscope and the Belscope blade (7,8,37). The Bullard laryngoscope is rigid and uses fiberoptic technology to obtain an indirect view of the larynx. The McCoy laryngoscope has a blade with a hinged tip allowing elevation of the epiglottis from a fulcrum deep within the pharynx. The Belscope blade is specially angulated with a detachable prism allowing indirect visualization of the larynx. The Bullard laryngoscope and Belscope blade take more time to use and master. A large ED experience has not been reported with any of these devices.

Pharmacologic Agents

Pharmacologic agents are chosen to accomplish several goals, including topical anesthesia, sedation, analgesia, amnesia, and paralysis. Judicious use of these agents may facilitate rapid intubation while avoiding such complications as increased ICP and regurgitation. Selecting the wrong agent can cause life-threatening complications such as prolonged paralysis with inability to ventilate, or cardiovascular collapse. Unfortunately, there are no agents that are rapid-acting, of short duration, and totally void of complications in all situations.

Local Anesthetics

Lidocaine is an amide that can be used topically, locally, or intravenously to aid in airway management. Maximum doses are 3 to 4 mg/kg. When applied topically in a 4% solution, lidocaine may be used with topical vasoconstrictors to aid in NTI. Nebulization of a 4% solution to a spontaneously breathing patient can produce complete topical anesthesia of the oro- and nasopharynx and the vocal cords in 5 to 7 minutes (4). Although somewhat controversial, when given intravenously in a dose of 1.5 to 2.0 mg/kg 2 to 3 minutes before intubation, lidocaine may attenuate much of the hemodynamic and cough reflex-mediated rise in ICP and appears to be comparable to the use of a β-blocker (14,29).

Induction Agents

Sedatives and hypnotics, as well as potent opioid analgesics, can be used as pharmacologic adjuncts to achieve states ranging from light sedation to loss of consciousness. There is a risk/benefit ratio for each of these agents in the trauma setting. Although adverse effects on respiration can be countered in most instances with artificial ventilation, there is no simple maneuver to counteract the cardiac dysfunction that may be produced by these agents in the trauma victim. The choice of agent should be based on the following factors: (1) the agent's reliability of induction at a given dose; (2) the need to maintain spontaneous respiration; (3) the patient's level of consciousness and risk of head injury; (4) the patient's hemodynamic or suspected hemodynamic status; and (5) the patient's preexisting physiologic state.

The barbiturates thiopental and methohexital are very short-acting sedative and hypnotic agents that provide no analgesia. Their onset of action is within 1 minute; their duration of action is between 5 and 10 minutes (30). The benefits of these agents are their induction reliability and rapidity of onset. The major disadvantage is that they can result in myocardial and respiratory depression (30). Although this is not a major factor in the normal host, their use may cause sudden and profound hypotension in the presence of preexisting myocardial dysfunction or hypovolemia. Even in "normal" subjects this may result in mild-to-moderate decreases in blood pressure and increases in heart rate. Thiopental doses ranging from 3 to 5 mg/kg in the setting of normal hemodynamics, and 0.5 to 1.0 mg/kg in the unstable patient, have been recommended for induction (30).

Barbiturates can reduce ICP by reducing cerebral blood flow in a dose-dependent fashion. Concomitant matched reductions in the cerebral metabolic rate must also occur to prevent cerebral ischemia. Whether matched reductions occur after a single bolus or lower titrated doses in the injured area of brain is unclear. Although barbiturates may be safely used in victims of isolated head trauma in whom preexisting disease states are known, their widespread use in trauma patients in whom volume status and past history is unknown may be risky.

Propofol is a substituted isoprophylphenol that is highly lipophilic and capable of producing profound sedation hypnosis and amnesia, but it has no analgesic properties (33). Its major unique characteristic is its rapid metabolic clearance and redistribution, which is approximately 10 times faster than thiopental. Clinical recovery is extremely rapid (4 to 8 minutes) with little residual sedation even after prolonged administration. A large experience with the use of propofol as an induction agent in the initial resuscitation of the critically ill or injured patient is lacking. Its major drawbacks are those of respiratory and cardiovascular depression, even in healthy normovolemic individuals (33). Extreme caution must therefore be exercised if propofol is used in the undifferentiated trauma patient. Favorable cerebral hemodynamics can be produced similar to that of the barbiturates if decreases in mean arterial pressure (MAP) can be minimized. Again it is unclear if this extends to injured brain areas after single dose use. Since trauma patients remain intubated for prolonged time periods for resuscitation and diagnostic purposes, the advantages of propofol's rapid redistribution is limited in this setting. If used, slowly administered doses ranging from 1.5 to 2.5 mg/kg are recommended. Its main use may be as a postintubation sedative once significant hemorrhage has been ruled out or volume resuscitation has taken place.

Etomidate is a nonbarbiturate, nonnarcotic sedative-hypnotic induction agent with no analgesic properties (33). In doses of 0.2 to 0.3 mg/kg, induction is reliably produced in less than 1 minute, and the duration of action is between 4 and 6 minutes. This drug has several properties that make it attractive for use in the multisystem trauma victim. When given in single induction boluses it evokes minimal changes in heart rate and cardiac output compared with equipotent doses of thiopental (33). This may be particularly advantageous in patients with hypotension or compensated shock, as well as in those with preexisting myocardial dysfunction. Etomidate also causes significantly less respiratory depression than barbiturate agents, although when given rapidly transient apnea may occur (33). Etomidate may in fact stimulate ventilation independent of action on the medullary respiratory centers. For this reason it may be advantageous when maintenance of respiration is desirable, such as during sedation with NTI or modified RSI. Similar to the barbiturates, etomidate can reduce ICP by causing a dose-dependent reduction in cerebral blood flow and cerebral metabolic rate. Whether consistent improvements in cerebral hemodynamics are obtained after a single induction bolus of etomidate remains to be determined.

Etomidate occasionally causes side effects, but none should contraindicate its use as a single injection in the trauma patient. Side effects include transient burning on injection, transient myoclonus after administration, and transient suppression of endogenous cortisol production. The occasional temporary suppression of cortisol production has not been shown to affect outcome and should not limit the use of etomidate in the ED (21,33).

Ketamine is a phencyclidine derivative that produces dissociative anesthesia. It is the only agent that possesses sedative, hypnotic, analgesic, and amnestic properties (33). It provides the most cardiovascular and respiratory support of any agent. Although it is a direct myocardial depressant, heart rate and blood pressure are usually maintained or increased because of centrally mediated sympathetic stimulation. Central sympathetic stimulation also results in transient bronchodilation. Unless given rapidly, apnea does not occur. The major advantage of ketamine lies in the setting of the hypovolemic patient, especially when the heart is directly involved, such as in pericardial tamponade (33). Its onset of action is within 1 minute when given intravenously (1 to 2 mg/kg), and its duration of action ranges from 5 to 15 minutes. It may also be given intramuscularly (4 mg/kg), with the onset of action delayed by several minutes. This is advantageous when rapid control of the patient without venous access is needed.

The disadvantages of ketamine are few. It may result in worsening hypotension if given to patients who are either sympathetically depleted or those who have severe coronary artery disease and may not tolerate increased myocardial oxygen demand. However, administration of any induction agent in this setting is hazardous. Use in hypertensive patients with suspected traumatic aortic injuries may also be problematic. Because it is a phencyclidine derivative, ketamine can cause an emergence delirium. While this is a concern during conscious sedation, it should never prohibit its use as an intubation adjunct in a critically ill trauma patient. Intubated trauma patients are usually kept sedated and paralyzed for many hours after their initial presentation, and emergence delirium at that time is rare (33). Continued sedation with benzodiazepines virtually eliminates its occurrence.

An additional concern with the use of ketamine is its potential to affect ICP due to its ability to increase cerebral blood flow by 30% to 60% (33). Even though the cerebral metabolic rate is increased with ketamine, cerebral blood flow is probably sufficient to meet demand. Evidence is accumulating that this increase in cerebral blood flow does not increase ICP (16,17). In fact, there is evidence that ketamine is neuroprotective in the setting of head trauma because it is an NDMA receptor antagonist (27). Despite this, there is still reluctance to use ketamine in the presence of potential head injury. Its use may still be warranted in the setting of head injury when induction is needed in a hypotensive patient. Any reduction in MAP has more potential to worsen cerebral ischemia than will a transient rise in ICP. In addition, ketamine is useful for awake oral intubations in patients with penetrating neck trauma.

Benzodiazepines (diazepam and midazolam) have been used alone, and in combination with opioids, as induction agents. They provide good anxiolysis and amnesia, but large doses are usually needed to produce predictable states of induction equivalent to those of the agents discussed above (31). No analgesia is provided. Midazolam is currently the most commonly used benzodiazepine for airway management. It is two to four times as potent as diazepam. An induction dose of midazolam (0.3 mg/kg) takes effect within 1 to 2 minutes and has a duration of action of between 30 and 60 minutes. Even at doses of 0.3 mg/kg, induction is not always predictable. This dose can be

accompanied by side effects such as severe respiratory depression (even more than equivalent doses of thiopental). Significant decreases in MAP and cardiac contractility can also occur, especially in patients with hypovolemia or heart disease (1). All of these effects are more pronounced when opioids are given simultaneously. Subinduction doses (0.03 to 0.05 mg/kg) of midazolam are not commonly associated with these complications and can serve as valuable adjuncts in providing continued sedation for patients after intubation.

The newer synthetic opioid agonists (fentanyl family), which include fentanyl, sufentanil, and alfentanil, are 100, 500 to 1000, and 20 times more potent than morphine, respectively (34). They are fast-acting, having an onset of action of less than 1 minute, and their duration of action is between 15 and 60 minutes. Fentanyl has gained widespread popularity in emergency medicine as a fast-acting analgesic used in conscious sedation, and it is also commonly used as an induction agent in emergency medicine. Depending on the existing state of consciousness and the presence of drugs such as alcohol, the dose necessary to produce unconsciousness can range from 2 to 20 μg/kg or more. The effect of fentanyl on ventilation varies, but doses above 2 μg/kg result in a high incidence of respiratory depression in "normal" subjects (2). This incidence is even higher when used together with other agents. Fentanyl results in little or no histamine release, and its cardiovascular effects in the normal host are minimal. At higher doses, however, small but potentially significant decreases in blood pressure may occur (34). Fentanyl is used as a preinduction adjunct for intubation of the head-injured patient because of its ability to attenuate the hemodynamic response to intubation. However, when given in sufficient doses to achieve this (at least 2 to 3 μg/kg, 2 to 3 minutes before laryngoscopy), increases in ICP may occur which may negate any advantage to its use in the setting of traumatic brain injury (28). This has been studied in intubated patients with severe head trauma undergoing ICP monitoring in an ICU. This increase in ICP has also been shown with sufentanil and alfentanil administration. Decreases in MAP were also noted to occur after administration of fentanyl at these doses. Coupled with the potential for producing premature hypoventilation and apnea, this makes the routine use of these agents as induction or preinduction agents in the setting of multisystem trauma controversial. The other role for fentanyl in trauma airway management is to provide postintubation sedation and analgesia to attenuate the hyperdynamic responses from pain and intubation and for patient comfort.

Despite the most careful use, any induction agent may result in sudden and profound hypotension not responsive to simple fluid boluses. In cases of head injury, hypotension, even if transient, can result in prolonged cerebral hypoperfusion even after blood pressure and oxygen delivery are restored to normal levels (22). For this reason, it is advisable to have an agent such as phenylephrine immediately available for administration in bolus form (50 to 200 μg) to help immediately restore MAP until the offending induction agent is sufficiently redistributed or metabolized. Phenylephrine is a synthetic noncatecholamine that stimulates principally alpha-1 adrenergic receptors by a direct effect. Its onset is very rapid and its effect is relatively short-lived when given in bolus form.

Neuromuscular Blocking Agents

The use of neuromuscular blocking agents (NMBAs) to facilitate intubation has become widespread in emergency airway management. These agents are classified as *depolarizing* and *nondepolarizing*.

The only *depolarizing* NMBA in use in the United States is succinylcholine. Succinylcholine (1.0 to 2.0 mg/kg) is the agent of choice during emergent RSI. No agent has a faster onset

(<1 minute) or is of shorter duration (4 to 6 minutes). The disadvantages of succinylcholine are relatively minor and should never prohibit its use in the acutely injured patient. These include fasciculations, hyperkalemia, and transient rises in intragastric, intraocular, and intracranial pressure (32). Succinylcholine-induced hyperkalemia in burns and crush injuries does not occur in the acute setting. If fasciculations and elevated intraocular, intragastric, and intracranial pressure are major concerns, administration of a defasciculating dose of a nondepolarizing agent (i.e., vecuronium 0.01 mg/kg) 2 to 3 minutes before succinylcholine administration may help prevent these occurrences (32). If a defasciculating dose of a nondepolarizing agent is used, the dose of succinylcholine should be increased to 1.5 to 2.0 mg/kg to maintain its rapidity of onset. Although difficult to predict, a few patients may develop vagally mediated bradycardia, histamine-induced hypotension, and malignant hyperthermia with succinylcholine administration. Succinylcholine can also be given intramuscularly (4 mg/kg), but its onset is delayed by 2 to 4 minutes.

There are several *nondepolarizing* NMBAs in current use; vecuronium and rocuronium are the major agents used in trauma airway management. The advantages of these agents are that they are longer-acting, cause no fasciculations, and cause no reported increase in intraocular, intragastric, or intracranial pressure. They also have little effect on the cardiovascular system (12,32). The major disadvantage of vecuronium is that it may take up to 2 to 3 minutes to take full effect. Time to onset can be reduced with the priming principle, in which an initial smaller subparalyzing dose is given 1 to 2 minutes before the paralyzing dose (32). This would appear to have no advantage in managing an emergent trauma airway, where time is the issue. Priming and defasciculating doses of nondepolarizing agents may produce significant respiratory impairment in elderly patients, so meticulous care of the airway is necessary (15). Large doses of vecuronium (0.25 mg/kg), used as an initial bolus, can achieve paralysis within 90 seconds but may last as long as 90 minutes. The standard dose of vecuronium for paralysis is 0.1 mg/kg. This results in complete paralysis within 2 to 3 minutes, with a duration of action of 30 to 40 minutes. The onset of action of rocuronium (0.6 mg/kg) is similar to that of succinylcholine, although its duration of action is similar to that of vecuronium (25 to 40 minutes) (32). The other major disadvantage to the use of the nondepolarizing NMBAs is that their duration of action is long, creating significant problems if intubation attempts are unsuccessful. Nondepolarizing agents can be reversed to some extent by drugs that block cholinesterases, such as neostigmine, edrophonium, and pyridostigmine. Their routine use is not advised because of potential cardiovascular complications.

Since the peak onset of both succinylcholine and rocuronium approaches 1 minute, and the onset of action of induction agents such as etomidate, thiopental, and ketamine essentially is less than 1 minute, it may be advantageous to administer the paralytic first followed by the induction agent (timing principle) (25). Because clinical weakness will occur at about 30 seconds with both agents, administration of an induction agent such as etomidate 10 to 20 seconds after administration of either succinylcholine or rocuronium will produce adequate intubating conditions approximately 1 minute after paralytic administration. For patients who are not being actively oxygenated with a BVM prior to RSI this helps to both guard against premature apnea and hypoventilation (thus preserving the functional residual capacity of oxygen) while ensuring adequate induction at the time of laryngoscopy. Patients intubated with the timing principle do not demonstrate restlessness prior to loss of consciousness and do not report any dissatisfaction postoperatively (25).

Special Considerations

Cervical Spine Injury

In most urgent situations a detailed neurologic examination cannot be performed before the need to intubate. Even in the face of normal radiographs, the patient would need to be able to fully cooperate with a physical exam to exclude c-spine injury. The blunt trauma or penetrating neck trauma patient requiring intubation after trauma is unlikely to be able to meet this criterion. The role of c-spine radiography before intubation is, therefore, controversial. Lateral c-spine radiography can miss up to 20% to 30% of c-spine injuries. It is estimated that a small but significant percentage (1.2%) of all blunt trauma victims will have an occult c-spine injury, assuming a 6% total incidence of injury and a 20% miss rate on lateral c-spine radiography (36). If time permits, a lateral c-spine radiograph that reveals an unstable injury may cause the operator to choose a particular intubation technique. However, it is imperative to remember that a negative radiograph does not exclude injury. Recent studies have indicated that certain patients traditionally intubated with c-spine precautions may not require such precautions, including victims of penetrating head trauma (13).

OTI utilizing RSI is now the procedure of choice in achieving definitive airway control in patients with suspected c-spine injury (23). Since positioning the airway in this setting is limited, use of a straight laryngoscope blade may be preferable to a curved blade since it will lift the epiglottis directly. Removal of the front of the cervical collar while maintaining in-line immobilization (not traction) significantly improves the view of the larynx during intubation (11). When manual immobilization is being performed, an intact c-collar offers no additional advantage. Regardless of approach, airway management in the setting of potential c-spine injury is optimally performed with at least three people: one is the intubator, one provides in-line immobilization of the c-spine, and one applies cricoid pressure. Rational use of airway adjuncts such as special laryngoscopes, the gum elastic bougie, and the LMA may be indicated based on the experience of the operator.

Penetrating Neck Trauma

In cases of penetrating neck trauma with possible altered upper airway anatomy or signs of airway obstruction, OTI with RSI is still the procedure of choice in many circumstances (24). Administration of paralytics may be strategically deleted if proper sedation and upper airway anesthesia is provided. Use of induction agents with less effect on ventilation (etomidate and ketamine), along with i.v. or nebulized lidocaine, will aid in reduction of gagging and further hemorrhage and anatomical distortion of the neck. Ketamine, without paralysis, is an alternative as it preserves respiratory drive. This may be essential for intubating patients who have anatomical distortion due to an expanding hematoma that makes intubation very difficult. Patients with anterior neck trauma have a relative contraindication to cricothyrotomy.

Head Injury

The pathophysiology of traumatic brain injury is complex and involves a combination of mechanical and biochemical events initiated by the trauma itself, followed by secondary injury in the form of ischemia. The most preventable forms of secondary brain injury are systemic hypoxemia and hypotension. Traditional approaches to the head trauma victim who required intubation assumed that the brain had lost some degree of its ability to autoregulate its blood flow. The MAP minus the ICP determines cerebral perfusion pressure and hence cerebral blood flow in this setting. Emphasis has been placed on blocking the rise in ICP during intubation with the use of agents such as barbiturates. However, maintaining the MAP is also critical since cerebral blood flow will be directly related to it. Because ICP is not known at the time of initial resuscitation, a mean systemic arterial pressure between 80 and 100 mm Hg should be maintained. Although an attempt to block the rise in ICP during intubation is of theoretical benefit, it has never been demonstrated to affect outcome. Attempts to manage ICP during intubation must be carefully balanced with the drug's effect on blood pressure, since lowering mean arterial blood pressure may lower cerebral blood flow and cause secondary ischemic brain injury (22). No airway drug affects ICP more than patient struggling or the pain of procedures performed during the initial examination and resuscitation. Because most head injuries occur in association with multisystem trauma, a more reasonable approach would be to administer agents that cause a predictable loss of consciousness, cause no increase in ICP, and maximize the chance to maintain MAP. Use of paralytic agents and adjuncts such as lidocaine prevents the largest and most harmful increases in ICP caused by gagging and coughing during laryngoscopy. Administration of fentanyl should also be considered, in order to decrease the hemodynamic effects of intubation such as tachycardia and hypertension, which may increase ICP by exaggerated increases in cerebral blood volume. However, in the multisystem trauma patient with potential traumatic brain injury care should be taken to avoid hypotension, since this will result in a decrease in cerebral perfusion pressure. This is of particular concern in elderly patients with limited cardiac reserve. Cerebral hemodynamics are probably best managed immediately after intubation with limited hyperventilation and continued paralysis along with concomitant sedation and analgesia guided by heart rate and blood pressure. A similar logic should be used in patients with spinal cord injuries to maintain spinal perfusion pressure (10).

Facial Trauma

Patients with facial injuries represent an airway management challenge, especially when there is severe upper airway hemorrhage. The airway management technique of choice depends on several factors, including the patient's level of consciousness, level of oxygenation, amount of upper airway hemorrhage, and risk of other injuries such as c-spine injury. The availability of one or more large-volume suctioning devices is critical if upper airway hemorrhaging is present. OTI with RSI is still the best first choice in the majority of cases. Airway adjuncts should be readily available. If orotracheal intubation is unsuccessful, placement of the esophageal tracheal combitube or laryngeal mask airway can reverse hypoxemia and temporarily protect the airway while cricothyrotomy is performed. Fiberoptic laryngoscopy is of limited use, as blood and other secretions make it difficult to view the glottis. Although previously considered a contraindication, patients with midface trauma, including those with cribriform plate fractures, can be safely intubated using properly performed NTI.

Suggested Approaches

The final decision on airway management depends primarily on the urgency of the situation and how comfortable the physician feels with a particular approach. The most immediate mortality and morbidity are usually due to hypoxemia and hypotension that are not quickly reversed. In most urgent situations, OTI with RSI using cervical stabilization is the best approach. This is followed with sedation and analgesics as tolerated.

Although each patient is unique, several assumptions should be made to prevent iatrogenic harm when a patient needs

---

TABLE 170.3.   Major Presentations of Trauma Patients

1. Blunt trauma with suspected head, maxillofacial, neck, and multisystem injury involvement at risk for hypovolemic shock
2. Isolated blunt or penetrating head or neck trauma requiring c-spine control but not at risk for hypovolemia
3. Penetrating injury below the head and neck not at risk for c-spine and head injury but at risk for hypovolemia.

---

aggressive airway control. In trauma victims with possible thoracic and abdominal injury, the physician should assume that the patient has occult hypovolemia, even if no signs of shock are present. In victims of blunt trauma or penetrating head injuries, the EP should assume that there has been intracranial injury, with loss of cerebral blood flow autoregulation. In victims of blunt multisystem trauma, the physician should assume that there has been a c-spine injury. Based on these assumptions, trauma patients are grouped into three categories based on the possibility of head and neck injuries and hypovolemia. This grouping is helpful in choosing the approach to airway management (Table 170.3). With these groups in mind, the following goals should be achieved during the preparation period and during intubation:

1. The patient should not experience further decreases in MAP secondary to administration of medications or maneuvers.
2. The patient should not develop premature apnea or hypoventilation.
3. The patient should not develop large increases in ICP.

Tables 170.4 and 170.5 demonstrate intubation sequences that will meet the needs of the majority of severely injured patients, while resulting in few complications.

After intubation, most patients benefit from continued sedation and analgesia. Small and frequent doses of midazolam (1 to 3 mg) and fentanyl (50 to 100 μg) are appropriate and do not have major associated side effects. Longer acting agents such as lorazepam and morphine may also be used. Once large cavitary bleeding has been ruled out, easily titrated agents such as propofol should be considered as continuous infusions.

TABLE 170.4.   Example of RSI Protocol for Trauma Patients with Suspected Hypovolemia and Head and Neck Injuries

1. Prepare and preoxygenate passively or actively with BVM. Use Sellick maneuver if using BVM. Manually immobilize c-spine but remove front of c-collar.
2. Lidocaine 1.5–2.0 mg/kg i.v., consider fentanyl 2–3 μg/kg (2–3 minutes prior to laryngoscopy).
3. Sellick maneuver; consider defasciculating dose of nondepolarizing agent if using succinylcholine in step 4 (vecuronuim 0.01 mg/kg). Give at least 2 minutes prior to succinylcholine administration. May be given simultaneously with lidocaine.*
4. Succinylcholine 1.5–2.0 mg/kg i.v.
5. Etomidate 0.2–0.3 mg/kg i.v. (reduce to 0.1–0.2 mg/kg if hypotensive) 10–20 seconds after paralytic administration.
6. Intubate trachea, inflate cuff, confirm placement with auscultation and end-tidal CO_2. After placement is confirmed, release cricoid pressure.
7. Continue paralysis with nondepolarizing agent if desired. Provide appropriate sedation and analgesic as allowed.

*If using rocuronium, step 3 may be deleted (with exception of Sellick maneuver). Rocuronium administered in place of succinylcholine in step 4 at dose of 0.6 mg/kg followed by induction agent (step 5) 10–20 seconds later.

TABLE 170.5.   Example of RSI Protocol for Patient at Risk for Shock but Not Head or Neck Injuries

1. Prepare and preoxygenate passively or actively if required. Apply Sellick maneuver if using BVM. Optimally position airway.
2. Ensure Sellick maneuver and give succinylcholine (1–2 mg/kg) or rocuronium (0.6 mg/kg) i.v.
3. 10–20 seconds later administer etomidate 0.2–0.3 mg/kg (0.1–0.2 mg/kg if hypotensive) or ketamine 1–2 mg/kg (0.5–1.0 mg/kg if hypotensive).
4. Intubate trachea, inflate cuff, confirm placement with auscultation and end-tidal CO_2. Release Sellick maneuver after placement confirmed.
5. Continue paralysis if desired along with appropriate sedation and analgesia.

Continued or newly initiated paralysis simultaneous with provision of analgesia and sedation may be required to optimize resuscitation and diagnostic workup. Especially in the head-injured patient, continued paralysis and sedation will prevent the patient from fighting and bucking the ventilator during the ensuing resuscitation. Early removal of patients from backboards, proper splinting of fractures, and application of local anesthetics to wounds will significantly decrease patient discomfort.

COMMON PITFALLS

✔ Failure to consider occult hypovolemia, shock and preexisting disease states when choosing induction agents
✔ Failure to provide cricoid pressure during intubation until proper endotracheal tube placement is confirmed
✔ Failure to maintain meticulous stabilization of the C-spine during intubation in patients with suspected c-spine injuries
✔ Failure to have airway rescue adjuncts available for difficult airway situations
✔ Failure to provide adequate ongoing post-intubation sedation and analgesia

References

1. Adams P, Gelman S, Reves JG, et al. Midazolam pharmacodynamics and pharmacokinetics during acute hypovolemia. *Anesthesiology* 1985;63:140–146.
2. Bailey PL, Pace NL, Ashburn MA, et al. Frequent hypoxemia and apnea after sedation with midazolam and fentanyl. *Anesthesiology* 1990;73:826–830.
3. Blostein PA, Koestner AJ, Hoak S. Failed rapid sequence intubation in trauma patients: esophageal tracheal combitube is a useful adjunct. *J Trauma* 1998;44:534–537.
4. Bourke DL, Katz J, Tonneson A. Nebulized anesthesia for awake endotracheal intubation. *Anesthesiology* 1985;63:690–692.
5. Bozeman WP Young S. Etomidate as a sole agent for endotracheal intubation in the prehospital air medical setting. *Air Med J* 2002;21:32–35; discussion 35–37.
6. Davis L, Cook-Sather SD, Schreiner MS. Lighted stylet tracheal intubation: a review. *Anesth Analg* 2000;90:745–756.
7. Gabbott DA. Laryngoscopy using the McCoy laryngoscope after application of a cervical collar. *Anaesthesia* 1996;51:812–814.
8. Gajraj NM, Chason DP, Shearer VE. Cervical spine movement during orotracheal intubation: comparison of the Belscope and Macintosh blades. *Anaesthesia* 1994;49:772–774.
9. Gold MI, Duarte I, Muravchick S. Arterial oxygenation in conscious patients after 5 minutes and after 30 seconds of oxygen breathing. *Anesth Analg* 1981;60:313–315.
10. Hadley MN. Blood pressure management after acute spinal cord injury. *Neurosurgery* 2002;50:S58–62.
11. Heath KJ. The effect of laryngoscopy of different cervical spine immobilisation techniques. *Anaesthesia* 1994;49:843–845.
12. Hunter JM. New neuromuscular blocking drugs. *N Engl J Med* 1995;332:1691–1699.
13. Kaups KL, Davis JW. Patients with gunshot wounds to the head do not require cervical spine immobilization and evaluation. *J Trauma* 1998;44:865–867.
14. Levitt MA, Dresden GM. The efficacy of esmolol versus lidocaine to attenuate the hemodynamic response to intubation in isolated head trauma patients. *Acad Emerg Med* 2001;8:19–24.
15. Mahajan RP, Hennessy N, Aitkenhead AR. Effect of priming dose of vecuronium on lung function in elderly patients. *Anesth Analg* 1993;77:1198–1202.
16. Mayberg TS, Lam AM, Matta BF, et al. Ketamine does not increase cerebral blood flow velocity or intracranial pressure during isoflurane/nitrous oxide anesthesia in patients undergoing craniotomy. *Anesth Analg* 1995;81:84–89.
17. Nimkoff L, Quinn C, Silver P, et al. The effects of intravenous anesthetics on intracranial pressure and cerebral perfusion pressure in two feline models of brain edema. *J Crit Care* 1997;12:132–136.
18. Nolan JP, Wilson ME. Orotracheal intubation in patients with potential cervical spine injuries. An indication for the gum elastic bougie. *Anaesthesia* 1993;48:630–633.
19. Rosen CL, Wolfe RE, Chew SE, et al. Blind nasotracheal intubation in the presence of facial trauma. *J Emerg Med* 1997;15:141–145.
20. Rosenblatt WH, Murphy M. The intubating laryngeal mask: use of a new ventilating-intubating device in the emergency department. *Ann Emerg Med* 1999;33:234–238.
21. Schenarts CL, Burton JH, Riker RR. Adrenocortical dysfunction following etomidate induction in emergency department patients. *Acad Emerg Med* 2001;8:1–7.
22. Schmoker JD, Zhuang J, Shackford SR. Hemorrhagic hypotension after brain injury causes an early and sustained reduction in cerebral oxygen delivery despite normalization of systemic oxygen delivery. *J Trauma* 1992;32:714–720; discussion 721–712.
23. Shatney CH, Brunner RD, Nguyen TQ. The safety of orotracheal intubation in patients with unstable cervical spine fracture or high spinal cord injury. *Am J Surg* 1995;170:676–679; discussion 679–680.
24. Shearer VE, Giesecke AH. Airway management for patients with penetrating neck trauma: a retrospective study. *Anesth Analg* 1993;77:1135–1138.
25. Sieber TJ, Zbinden AM, Curatolo M, et al. Tracheal intubation with rocuronium using the "timing principle". *Anesth Analg* 1998;86:1137–1140.
26. Sloane C, Vilke GM, Chan TC, et al. Rapid sequence intubation in the field versus hospital in trauma patients. *J Emerg Med* 2000;19:259–264.
27. Smith DH, Okiyama K, Gennarelli TA, et al. Magnesium and ketamine attenuate cognitive dysfunction following experimental brain injury. *Neurosci Lett* 1993;157:211–214.
28. Sperry RJ, Bailey PL, Reichman MV, et al. Fentanyl and sufentanil increase intracranial pressure in head trauma patients. *Anesthesiology* 1992;77:416–420.
29. Splinter WM, Cervenko F. Haemodynamic responses to laryngoscopy and tracheal intubation in geriatric patients: effects of fentanyl, lidocaine and thiopentone. *Can J Anaesth* 1989;36:370–376.
30. Stoelting RK. Barbiturates. In: Stoelting RK, ed. *Pharmacology and anesthesiology in anesthetic practice.* 2nd ed. Philadelphia: J.B. Lippincott, 1991:102.
31. Stoelting RK. Benzodiazepines. In: Stoelting RK, ed. *Pharmacology and anesthesiology in anesthetic practice.* 2nd ed. Philadelphia: J.B. Lippincott, 1991:118.
32. Stoelting RK. Neuromuscular blocking drugs. In: Stoelting RK, ed. *Pharmacology and anesthesiology in anesthetic practice.* 2nd ed. Philadelphia: J.B. Lippincott, 1991:172.
33. Stoelting RK. Nonbarbiturate induction agents. In: Stoelting RK, ed. *Pharmacology and anesthesiology in anesthetic practice.* 2nd ed. Philadelphia: J.B. Lippincott, 1991:134.
34. Stoelting RK. Opioid agonist and antagonist. In: Stoelting RK, ed. *Pharmacology and anesthesiology in anesthetic practice.* 2nd ed. Philadelphia: J.B. Lippincott, 1991:70.
35. Takahata O, Kubota M, Mamiya K, et al. The efficacy of the "BURP" maneuver during a difficult laryngoscopy. *Anesth Analg* 1997;84:419–421.
36. Walls RM. Airway management in the blunt trauma patient: how important is the cervical spine? *Can J Surg* 1992;35:27–30.
37. Watts AD, Gelb AW, Bach DB, et al. Comparison of the Bullard and Macintosh laryngoscopes for endotracheal intubation of patients with a potential cervical spine injury. *Anesthesiology* 1997;87:1335–1342.

Traumatic Shock

Christopher B. Colwell

Shock refers to inadequate tissue perfusion, which may be manifested clinically by hemodynamic disturbances and organ dysfunction. At the cellular level, shock results from the insufficient delivery of required metabolic substrates, principally oxygen, to sustain aerobic metabolism. In the setting of trauma, shock is most often related to loss of circulating blood volume due to hemorrhage, although inadequate oxygenation, mechanical vascular obstruction, neurologic dysfunction, and cardiac dysfunction may be either primary or contributing factors (4,7).

Shock is a common and potentially treatable cause of death in injured patients. Traumatic shock usually results from one or more of the following conditions: hemorrhage from solid-organ injury, major vascular injury, pelvic fracture or multiple long-bone fractures; tension pneumothorax; hemothorax; pericardial tamponade; pulmonary contusion or hemorrhage; myocardial contusion and dysfunction; or neurologic injury that adversely affects ventilation or hemodynamics.

The pathophysiology of traumatic shock is largely related to an imbalance in oxygen supply and demand. In the early phase of acute trauma, this imbalance is often due to hypoperfusion, although low arterial blood oxygen saturation may be a significant contributing factor. Aggressive resuscitation with fluids having low or no oxygen-carrying capacity in the setting of severe and ongoing hemorrhage may lead to a critically low hemoglobin concentration that further contributes to tissue oxygen debt.

Acute blood loss elicits compensatory hemodynamic changes that serve to maintain vital organ perfusion. These changes include increased heart rate and vasoconstriction primarily in the peripheral circulation and splanchnic vascular beds. The term *compensated shock* generally indicates varying degrees of tachycardia and peripheral vasoconstriction that maintain adequate vital organ perfusion. Arterial blood pressure in compensated shock states may be moderately low or within the normal range. The term *uncompensated shock* generally indicates significant hypotension with inadequate vital organ perfusion.

Vasoconstriction in response to hemorrhage and hypovolemia is a protective response that preserves perfusion to the vital organs at the expense of peripheral and abdominal organ perfusion. In the hypoperfused tissues, however, oxygen demand exceeds oxygen delivery, and the numerous cellular processes that depend on oxidative metabolism and adenosine triphosphate (ATP) begin to fail. Acidosis results when aerobic metabolism slows as protons are not being used up as quickly to synthesize ATP from ADP (adenosine diphosphate). If the pathologic processes are not stabilized or corrected, cellular dysfunction and organ failure can result.

There are four general pathophysiologic types of shock: (1) hemorrhagic or hypovolemic, (2) cardiogenic, (3) neurogenic or vasogenic, and (4) septic (4). *Hemorrhagic* or *hypovolemic shock* involves the loss of circulating intravascular volume caused by blood loss internally, externally, or both. *Cardiogenic shock* indicates a process that prevents the normal pumping of the heart and can be caused by pericardial tamponade that prevents normal ventricular filling, tension pneumothorax with vena caval compression and reduction in venous return to the heart, or direct cardiac damage with loss of contractile force (myocardial contusion).

Neurogenic or *vasogenic shock* may result from spinal cord injury with loss of peripheral vascular resistance. Major spinal cord injury results in acute vasodilatation but generally does not cause impaired tissue perfusion unless other injuries are present. These injuries result in a loss of sympathetic tone and are therefore accompanied by bradycardia (spinal shock). *Septic shock* refers to the hyperdynamic responses (elevated cardiac output, tachycardia, and low systemic vascular resistance), followed by decreased cardiac output, increased systemic vascular resistance, and organ function deterioration associated with the metabolic demands and toxic mediators accompanying infection.

If the acute stress of the traumatic shock state is sufficiently severe or prolonged, organ dysfunction may subsequently develop, including acute tubular necrosis (ATN), adult respiratory distress syndrome (ARDS), systemic inflammatory distress syndrome (SIRS), and multiple organ failure (MOF). These entities can develop within a few hours to several days after the acute injury.

CLINICAL PRESENTATION

Initial findings in a patient with traumatic shock may include tachycardia, hypotension, signs of poor peripheral perfusion, and alteration in mental status. In response to a loss of circulating volume, the heart rate will increase to sustain normal cardiac output. Continued blood loss will eventually result in a decrease in blood pressure. Peripheral vasoconstriction and central venoconstriction shunt blood centrally and result in a narrowed pulse pressure. Clinically, decreases in peripheral perfusion manifest as cool, pale, clammy extremities, with prolongation of capillary refill.

The skin may become mottled in appearance, but cyanosis is not a common finding. The narrowed pulse pressure can make the pulse quality weak or thready. Alterations in mental status caused by hypoperfusion may be subtle initially and can be difficult to distinguish from associated head injury or intoxication. Therefore, altered mental status on presentation or a subsequent decline in mental status, especially in patients with no evidence of head trauma, should raise concern of systemic hypoperfusion and impending circulatory collapse.

Shock may exist even in the setting of "normal" vital signs. Young, healthy patients with substantial blood loss may maintain a blood pressure within the normal range by compensatory vasoconstriction and increases in heart rate. Heart rate can even occasionally be in the upper normal range. In such patients, signs of peripheral hypoperfusion and subtle changes in mental status may be the only warning signs preceding rapid hemodynamic decompensation. Elderly patients may not develop a tachycardic response to blood loss because of preexisting medical conditions or medications. A bradycardic response to abdominal trauma that may be vagally mediated has been described (22). Conversely, hypotension and tachycardia may be exacerbated in a pregnant trauma patient for a given degree of blood loss due to compression of the inferior vena cava by the gravid uterus, resulting in decreased venous return (14).

Decline in urine output due to renal hypoperfusion and renal fluid reabsorption is an important manifestation of shock physiology. Monitoring urine output may be useful in the emergency department (ED); later, it is a critical parameter for the trauma surgeon and intensivist. Therefore, a urinary catheter should be placed in patients who exhibit evidence of shock, and the bladder should be drained to begin urine output monitoring and check for hematuria.

DIFFERENTIAL DIAGNOSIS

The most common cause of traumatic shock is hemorrhage-induced hypovolemia. Several pathologic entities must be considered, however, as either potential contributors or primary causes of shock. These include cardiac tamponade, tension pneumothorax, pulmonary contusion or hemorrhage affecting oxygenation, myocardial contusion with dysfunction, myocardial infarction associated with trauma, autonomic dysfunction or spinal cord shock, and effects of toxicologic or pharmacologic agents. Other entities to consider include pneumothorax, hemothorax, flail chest, air or fat embolism, and diaphragmatic rupture extensive enough to effect oxygen saturation and hemodynamic status.

Pericardial tamponade is classically described as exhibiting Beck's triad of hypotension, distended neck veins, and muffled heart sounds. A pulsus paradoxus of greater than 10 mm Hg may also be seen. All of these markers may not be present or detected at the same time. In a hypovolemic patient, the neck veins may be flat. Muffled heart sounds may be difficult to distinguish in a busy trauma resuscitation room, and detection of a pulsus paradoxus is not reliable. Pericardial tamponade should be considered whenever there is penetrating chest trauma, there are rib fractures near the heart or when there has been significant blunt trauma to the chest. The immediate availability of ultrasonography (US) or echocardiography offers the best potential for rapid and accurate diagnosis.

A large pneumothorax or hemothorax can usually be detected by diminished breath sounds, although auscultation can be unreliable. Confirmation with a chest radiograph is usually prudent if the patient is stable. A tension pneumothorax may also result in deviation of the trachea away from the affected side, cardiac displacement, and hypotension related to inferior vena caval compression that limits venous return to the heart. However, tracheal deviation and cardiac displacement are late findings and may be difficult to detect by physical examination. Animal studies have suggested that hypoxemia may be an earlier sign of a tension pneumothorax than hypotension (3). If a patient is hypotensive and has clinical evidence of a pneumothorax, placement of a chest tube or needle thoracostomy before diagnostic imaging is appropriate.

Myocardial contusion resulting in significant contractile dysfunction is a difficult diagnosis to make in the ED unless echocardiography is immediately available. Myocardial contusion should be suspected when blunt trauma involves the sternum and anterior left chest, particularly if ventricular ectopy, dysrhythmias, or electrocardiographic demonstration of ST segment elevations (especially in the anterior precordial leads) are present. Evidence of cardiogenic shock (hypotension, tachycardia, elevated central venous pressure) should alert the physician to the possible presence of a myocardial contusion or pericardial tamponade.

Spinal cord trauma with neurogenic shock may present with hypotension due to loss of peripheral vascular resistance. In addition, due to the loss of the sympathetic tone, these patients will not have the usual tachycardic response to hypotension, but will demonstrate bradycardia instead. In this setting, presence of neurologic deficits and lack of signs of peripheral vasoconstriction should arouse suspicion for this entity. Such patients generally have warm extremities and good urine output. Volume status must be carefully monitored, because excess fluid administration in patients with spinal shock may be detrimental.

Signs of shock in a trauma patient may not be a direct consequence of the injury. For example, a myocardial infarction in a patient may cause a motor vehicle collision, or the physiologic stress associated with trauma may cause a myocardial ischemic event in a patient with coronary artery disease. A history, examination, or electrocardiographic findings consistent with myocardial infarction should arouse suspicion of combined medical and surgical processes. Another rare medical cause of hypotension in a trauma patient is anaphylaxis that may have preceded the trauma. Pharmacologic agents such as β-adrenergic blockers and recreational agents such as ethanol and cocaine may significantly affect the clinical picture in the setting of acute trauma.

EMERGENCY DEPARTMENT EVALUATION

According to the Advanced Trauma Life Support (ATLS) guidelines, the initial step in managing shock in the injured patient is to recognize its presence. Effective management of the acute trauma victim exhibiting signs of shock requires that initial assessment and treatment begin simultaneously (1). Assessment of airway patency, adequacy of ventilation (respiratory excursion and lung auscultation), hemodynamic status (pulse rate, central and peripheral pulse quality, blood pressure), and evidence of controllable hemorrhage should be immediately linked with interventions to (1) secure the airway while protecting the cervical spine, (2) enhance oxygenation, (3) provide ventilatory assistance, (4) limit further hemorrhage, (5) gain intravenous access, (6) initiate volume replacement, and (7) obtain blood for laboratory and blood bank testing (Fig. 171.1).

After the primary assessment and initiation of treatment, a thorough secondary assessment should be initiated to identify potential injuries to the head, neck, chest, abdomen, pelvis, back, extremities, and neurologic system. Hypothermia can markedly depress hemodynamics and should be aggressively treated. Acute trauma is a highly dynamic disease process that requires frequent and careful reassessment of ventilation and hemodynamic status and physical examination to optimally adjust therapeutic interventions and identify evolving pathologic processes.

Initial laboratory studies in patients with major trauma should include (1) complete blood count (CBC); (2) arterial blood gases (base deficit); (3) electrolytes; (4) coagulation studies; (5) type and crossmatch for 4 to 8 units of packed red blood cells (PRBC); and (6) toxicologic studies (Table 171.1). Urine should be obtained and checked for blood. Lactate and ketone levels may be useful when there is metabolic acidosis, although some studies suggest admission base deficit may be of better prognostic value than serum lactate (18).

Initial radiographs should include the lateral view cervical spine, chest, and pelvis. The initial chest radiograph will identify pneumothorax, hemothorax, and pulmonary contusion, and the initial pelvic radiograph will identify major pelvic fractures as the cause of hypotension. Completion of the cervical spine series when appropriate and other radiographs should be performed after the patient has been stabilized and it has been determined that immediate surgery is not required. Spine plain radiographs are indicated in any patient with suspected spinal fractures or spinal shock, followed by computed tomography (CT) or magnetic resonance imaging.

Ultrasound (US) has become part of the initial evaluation of the trauma patient. During the initial resuscitation, the *focused assessment with sonography for trauma* or FAST exam should be performed to obtain views of the heart and abdomen to assess for pericardial effusion and intraperitoneal bleeding. Serial US exams can be performed to increase the sensitivity for detecting intraperitoneal bleeding. In addition, recent studies document its use for detecting hemothorax and pneumothorax. An alternative means of detecting intraperitoneal bleeding is diagnostic peritoneal lavage (DPL). The unstable trauma patient should

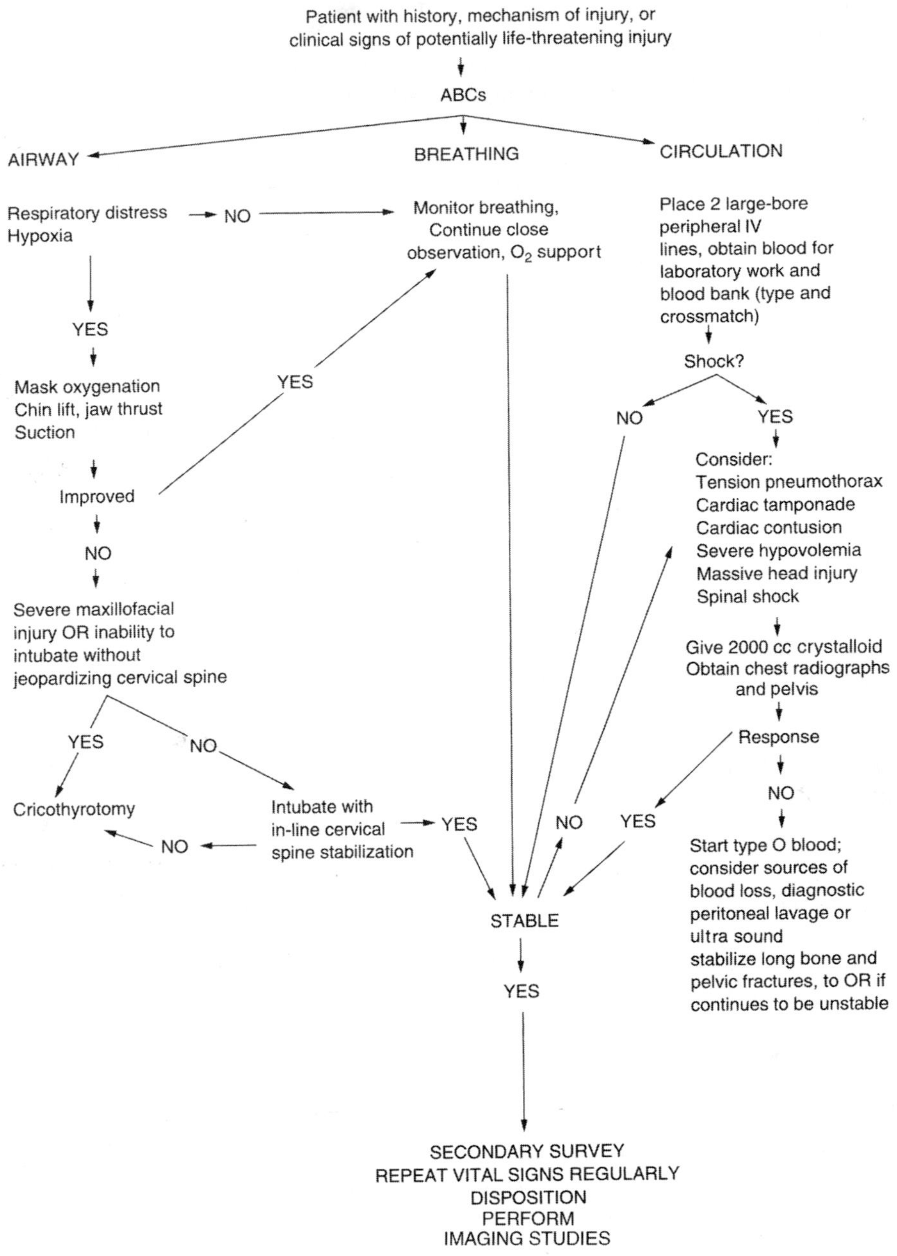

Patient with history, mechanism of injury, or
clinical signs of potentially life-threatening injury

↓

ABCs

↓

AIRWAY ← → BREATHING → CIRCULATION

Respiratory distress → NO → Monitor breathing,   Place 2 large-bore
Hypoxia   Continue close   peripheral IV
                               observation, O₂ support lines, obtain blood for
↓   laboratory work and
                                                       blood bank (type and
YES   crossmatch)
↓   ↓
Mask oxygenation   YES   Shock?
Chin lift, jaw thrust
Suction   NO ← → YES
↓   ↓
Improved   Consider:
↓   Tension pneumothorax
NO   Cardiac tamponade
↓   Cardiac contusion
Severe maxillofacial   Severe hypovolemia
injury OR inability to   Massive head injury
intubate without   Spinal shock
jeopardizing cervical spine   ↓
                                                       Give 2000 cc crystalloid
YES   NO   Obtain chest radiographs
                                                       and pelvis
Cricothyrotomy   Intubate with → YES   ↓
                 in-line cervical   NO   YES   Response
     NO ←   spine stabilization   ↓
                                                       NO
                                                       ↓
                              STABLE   Start type O blood;
                                ↓   consider sources of
                              YES   blood loss, diagnostic
                                                       peritoneal lavage or
                                                       ultra sound
                                                       stabilize long bone and
                                                       pelvic fractures, to OR if
                                                       continues to be unstable

SECONDARY SURVEY
REPEAT VITAL SIGNS REGULARLY
DISPOSITION
PERFORM
IMAGING STUDIES

Figure 171.1.   Treatment algorithm for traumatic shock.

TABLE 171.1.   Initial Laboratory and Radiographic Studies in Major Trauma

LABORATORY

Complete blood count
Arterial blood gases
Electrolytes (including BUN, creatinine, glucose)
Coagulation studies (PT, PTT)
Type and crossmatch for 4–8 units of blood
Toxicologic studies (as indicated)
Urinalysis

RADIOGRAPHS

Chest x-ray, portable AP
Cross-table lateral cervical spine
Pelvis x-ray, AP view

undergo DPL when US is not available or if the US results are equivocal.

Monitoring of heart rate, respiratory rate, blood pressure, temperature, is pulse oximetry are important. Placement of arterial pressure catheters and central venous pressure lines should be considered in patients who do not rapidly stabilize or are suspected of having cardiogenic or neurogenic shock components. Placement of a nasogastric or orogastric tube for decompression reduces the chances of aspiration and may improve ventilation if the stomach is distended with air. A urinary drainage catheter should be placed after a search for potential urethral injury has been performed.

Urethral injury should be suspected in patients with pelvic fractures in the area of the symphysis pubis, anterior lacerations on rectal or vaginal examination, or abnormal position of the prostate gland. As noted, urine output becomes an important indicator of the adequacy of organ perfusion. Quantitative end-tidal carbon dioxide (ETCO₂) monitoring, if available, is useful in intubated patients. $ETCO_2$ can help avoid hypoventilation, prevent excessive therapeutic hyperventilation, and detect decreases in cardiac output. Sequential assessment of hemoglobin/hematocrit and arterial blood gases during therapy for traumatic shock may be useful. These should be interpreted together in terms of oxygen-carrying capacity and blood oxygen content. For example, an O_2 saturation of 90% with a hematocrit of 35% may be more favorable than an O_2 saturation of 100% with a hematocrit of 20% in terms of actual tissue oxygen delivery. In the trauma patient, the presence of metabolic acidosis in the early phase of resuscitation indicates poor tissue perfusion and should be considered an indicator of inadequate volume resuscitation or ongoing hemorrhage.

Constant reassessment of ventilation and oxygenation, hemodynamic response to volume replacement therapy, and physical examination findings is crucial to detect clinical deterioration, adjust therapy, and identify previously missed injuries. Trauma resuscitations involve multiple individuals performing numerous tasks. During the process of resuscitation, tubes and catheters can become dislodged or disconnected, pneumothoraces can develop or enlarge, external or internal injuries may bleed again as blood pressure increases, pulmonary congestion may develop in response to volume therapy, core temperature may drop substantially in an exposed patient receiving large amounts of intravenous fluids, or the previously unremarkable abdomen may become distended or rigid. These are examples of significant changes that can occur rapidly during the trauma resuscitation. Careful and constant attention with frequent reassessment is crucial to ensure optimal outcome.

EMERGENCY DEPARTMENT MANAGEMENT

Walter Cannon wrote in 1923 "since acidosis in shock indicates a deficient delivery of oxygen to active tissues, the rational move is not to treat the effect, but the cause, that is, to provide a better supply of oxygen by early and permanent improvement of the circulation." This remains prudent management today. Initial treatment in traumatic shock occurs concurrently with initial evaluation and is focused on restoring adequate oxygen delivery. Oxygen should be administered to all major trauma patients, regardless of presenting pulse oximetry readings. Insertion of oral or nasal airways, assisted ventilation, endotracheal intubation, hemorrhage control, and vascular access are all essential components of the initial trauma resuscitation. Early control of the airway in the patient with traumatic shock may be lifesaving and should take priority over all other interventions.

Gaining intravenous access rapidly is essential to begin volume replacement and support the hemodynamics of the patient in traumatic shock. The antecubital fossa is an excellent site to initiate intravenous access. Large-bore catheters (14- or 16-gauge) and high-flow intravenous tubing should be used to maximize delivery rate of fluids. At least two intravenous sites should be secured. If adequate intravenous access cannot be established within a few minutes, percutaneous femoral venous access, ankle venous cutdown, greater saphenous venous cutdown at the proximal thigh, or subclavian/jugular venous access should be considered.

Fluid therapy in trauma is an area of on-going controversy (13). Intravascular volume replacement to compensate for blood loss and restore tissue perfusion has been accepted standard therapy for many years. The historical justification for aggressive intravenous fluid resuscitation was to maintain organ perfusion and improve survival. This was, however, based on models of *controlled* hemorrhage. Recent studies suggest that aggressive fluid resuscitation in patients with *uncontrolled* or ongoing hemorrhage (prior to operative control) may increase blood loss and mortality. Research has questioned which intervention should take priority, reversal of hypovolemia or control of hemorrhage, when both cannot be achieved simultaneously. Restoring blood volume before active hemorrhage is controlled may result in increased blood loss due to clot disruption, hemodilution, and loss of clotting factors. Some studies have criticized aggressive fluid administration as being ineffective (5,16). Other studies suggest that limited volume replacement, termed *hypotensive resuscitation*, that maintains minimally adequate organ perfusion may result in improved outcome (19). A clinical trial of patients with penetrating torso trauma documented higher survival rates in patients who underwent delayed fluid resuscitation at the time of operative intervention instead of immediate fluid resuscitation starting in the field (5). It is important to remember that most clinical trials evaluating fluid administration have involved penetrating trauma victims. Whether the same principles can be applied to blunt trauma victims is not clear. In fact, this approach may be detrimental to blunt trauma patients with traumatic brain injury (TBI), since hypotension increases mortality in these patients (24). A clear end point of fluid therapy in terms of an optimal blood pressure to have as a goal has not been defined (20). Based on the current literature, it appears reasonable to have a goal of a systolic blood pressure of approximately 90 to 100 mm Hg in penetrating trauma and somewhat higher, 110 to 120 mm Hg, for blunt trauma patients, particularly in those with suspected TBI.

The optimal fluid for volume replacement has also been the subject of considerable debate. Crystalloid solutions, such as normal saline or lactated Ringer's solution, have long been considered the standard. Hypertonic saline has been extensively studied, and has shown a benefit in clinical trials (12,23), although it has not become an accepted standard for resuscitation in clinical trauma care. Replacing a significant percentage of the patient's blood volume with fluids that have not been warmed ("room temperature" is significantly cooler than body temperature) can render a patient hypothermic very quickly. Fluids may be warmed ahead of time or administered through a fluid warmer. In an average-sized adult showing signs of shock, infusion of 2 L of crystalloid and immediate reassessment of hemodynamics is a reasonable course of action (see Chapter 209, "General Approach to Pediatric Trauma," for pediatric resuscitation). The point in volume resuscitation at which blood transfusion is initiated has not been well defined. Factors that influence the decision to start blood transfusion include severity of shock, initial response to crystalloid, initial hemoglobin/hematocrit, and general health of the patient. In general, if hemodynamics do not improve after administration of 2 to 3 L of crystalloid (or about 40 to 50 mL/kg) given rapidly, further volume replacement with blood should be considered. Certain patients may also require transfusion based on their initial injuries. For instance, those with major pelvic trauma should be transfused upon arrival to the ED, prior to the development of hemodynamic instability.

The value of colloids in the treatment of traumatic shock is uncertain. Colloids, such as albumin, hetastarch, and dextran, can effectively increase intravascular volume and maintain plasma oncotic pressure at more normal levels compared with crystalloids. However, substantial data demonstrate that crystalloid and colloids are equally effective in resuscitation from hemorrhagic shock (17,21). Furthermore, some evidence suggests that colloids may have deleterious effects in patients with hemorrhagic shock. Therefore, until well-designed clinical trials are performed showing the benefit of colloids, crystalloids should remain the fluid of choice for the resuscitation of trauma patients in hemorrhagic shock (15).

Red blood cell substitutes consisting of hemoglobin that has been modified by polymerization and biochemical alteration have been extensively studied recently in both animal and human trials. Studies have suggested these red blood cell substitutes, with their ability to carry oxygen, may be superior to the current, more conventional methods of resuscitation from hemorrhagic shock (9). A trial is currently underway studying the effect of a red blood cell substitute in the resuscitation of human trauma victims in the prehospital setting.

Typed and cross-matched PRBC are the best choice for blood transfusion, although this usually takes an hour to obtain. If the need for transfusion does not permit the time required for cross-matching, however, type-specific blood is an appropriate alternative (this usually takes 20 to 30 minutes). If traumatic shock is severe and immediate transfusion is critical, type O Rh-positive blood for males and type O Rh-negative for girls and women of childbearing age should be used until type-specific or typed and cross-matched blood is available. Type O negative blood should be immediately available in the trauma room.

If several units of blood are required to manage profound hypovolemia or ongoing hemorrhage, fresh-frozen plasma (FFP) and platelets may be needed to stabilize the coagulation system and limit further "nonmechanical" hemorrhage. In otherwise healthy individuals, FFP is rarely required until blood transfusion approaches 6 units. Empiric administration of FFP and platelets is not indicated (8). Coagulation studies and platelet counts should be used to help guide such decisions.

Pneumothorax or hemothorax should be managed by the placement of a large chest tube (32F or 36F) in the lateral chest with the tubes oriented toward the apicoposterior chest wall. If a tension pneumothorax is suspected and the patient is hypotensive, needle thoracostomy using a long, large-gauge angiocatheter or needle inserted at the second intercostal space in the midclavicular line or the fifth intercostal space in the midaxillary line is an appropriate measure until a chest tube can be inserted.

If pericardial tamponade is suspected and the patient is hypotensive and worsening despite volume resuscitation, pericardiocentesis is indicated. A pericardiocentesis needle is inserted in the left subxiphoid area and directed 45 degrees toward the left shoulder or sternal notch while suction is maintained on an attached syringe. If possible, the needle should be hooked to an electrocardiographic lead to show evidence of needle contact with the myocardium. Blood in the pericardium often forms clots, thus precluding the value of pericardiocentesis. If the patient is profoundly hypotensive or has lost discernible blood pressure for only a few minutes, an emergency left lateral thoracotomy should be considered to open the pericardium. Patients who have not shown signs of life after sustaining blunt trauma are poor candidates for ED thoracotomy (2).

Traumatic shock due to hemorrhage is most often caused by intraabdominal injury. The clinical presentation and response to initial therapy dictate the subsequent assessment of the abdomen. Hemodynamically unstable patients with physical examination or US evidence of abdominal injury should undergo exploratory laparotomy. Patients with suspected abdominal trauma who have exhibited transient hemodynamic instability should undergo a FAST exam, which will reliably identify free intraabdominal fluid, provided that the person performing the examination is adequately proficient (6,10). If US is not available, then DPL is an alternative method of detecting intraperitoneal hemorrhage. Hemodynamically stable patients with potential abdominal trauma are candidates for abdominal CT scanning.

The role of a pneumatic antishock garment (PASG) or military antishock trousers (MAST) is much more limited than once thought (11). One potential indication for the use of these devices is in the patient with pelvic fractures. The MAST trousers provide fracture stability and pelvic compression that limits further blood loss until the patient is surgically stabilized. Simply tying a sheet firmly around the pelvis may provide equal benefit, but this has not been adequately studied.

A quick maneuver to treat the hypotensive pregnant trauma patient is to place the patient in the left lateral decubitus position or tilt the backboard up 15 degrees on the right in order to move the gravid uterus off of the inferior vena cava. This will improve venous return and may result in normotension.

In general, vasopressors and inotropic agents are not used in the ED management of traumatic shock. In cases of neurogenic or vasogenic shock (e.g., spinal cord injury) in which peripheral vasodilatation causes or contributes to hemodynamic instability, vasopressors such as dopamine, phenylephrine, or norepinephrine may be useful after fluid resuscitation. From the ED perspective, shock rarely, if ever, results from isolated head trauma. In cases of myocardial infarction associated with trauma or significant myocardial contusion, inotropic support with dobutamine, for example, may be appropriate.

CRITICAL INTERVENTIONS

- When possible, recognize and treat shock aggressively before hypotension develops. Remember that shock may exist in a patient with "normal" vital signs
- Wrap potentially unstable pelvic fractures with a sheet prior to transfer or extended diagnostic testing
- When possible, place the hypotensive pregnant trauma patient in the left lateral decubitus position to release possible compression of the inferior vena cava
- Search for other causes of hypotension in the head injured trauma patient. Isolated head trauma rarely causes hypotension

DISPOSITION

Definitive management of the patient with traumatic shock often requires emergency surgery. Consultation with a surgeon should be initiated as soon as possible in all victims of significant trauma who might require operative or critical care interventions. If information from prehospital care providers indicates potentially serious injury, the surgeon (or trauma team) should be notified before the patient arrives in the ED. If transfer to another hospital is required, early mobilization of resources (ambulance, staff, or air medical transport service) should be initiated concurrently with assessment and stabilization.

The criteria for transfer to a trauma center include lack of an experienced trauma surgeon, lack of adequate critical care or support services, and lack of adequate resources to manage a patient's injuries. The use of scoring systems such as the Trauma Score (TS), Revised Trauma Score (RTS), and the Glasgow Coma Scale (GCS) for triage may be useful in identifying patients with severe injury. Patients with a TS less than 12, an RTS of 8 or less, or a GCS less than 10 generally have serious injuries and should be managed within an organized trauma system. The emergency physician must determine which interventions and diagnostic studies are essential before transfer. These decisions are affected by mode of transport, distance to the trauma center, and the capabilities of the referring hospital. For example, delaying transfer to obtain a head and abdominal CT scan or plain radiographs is of no benefit if there is no neurosurgeon, general surgeon, or orthopedist available or if no immediate intervention will take place at the referring hospital. On the other hand, if a head CT scan is indicated and can be obtained while waiting for the ambulance or helicopter to arrive (and will not cause a delay in transfer), it is optimal to proceed with the study.

COMMON PITFALLS

- ✔ Failure to recognize the severity of trauma or that the state of shock exists; normal vital signs can be misleading
- ✔ Failure to realize that altered mental status is a sign of shock, particularly when there is no evidence of head trauma
- ✔ Failure to carefully monitor and perform repeated exams to detect changes in clinical status and to respond with appropriate interventions. An initial favorable response to volume replacement should not lull the emergency physician into being less vigilant in trauma management. Adequate resuscitation can temporarily mask ongoing significant hemorrhage
- ✔ Delaying surgical consultation or transfer to a trauma center
- ✔ Missing subtle injuries, especially in patients with severe multiple trauma

Acknowledgments

Thanks to previous edition chapter authors James Manning and Samir M. Fakhry.

References

1. American College of Surgeons Committee on Trauma. *Advanced trauma life support: providers' manual.* Chicago: American College of Surgeons, 1997.
2. Baker CC, Thomas AN, Trunkey DD. The role of emergency room thoracotomy in trauma. *J Trauma* 1980;20:848–855.
3. Barton ED, Rhee P, Hutton KC, et al. The pathophysiology of tension pneumothorax in ventilated swine. *J Emerg Med* 1997;15(2):147.
4. Baue AE. Physiology of shock and injury. In: Gelder ER, ed. *Shock and resuscitation.* New York: McGraw-Hill, 1993.
5. Bickell WH, Wall MJJ, Pepe PE, et al. Immediate versus delayed fluid resuscitation for hypotensive patients with penetrating torso injuries. *N Engl J Med* 1995;332:681.
6. Block EFJ. Diagnostic modalities in acute trauma. *New Horiz* 1999;7:10.
7. Britt LD, Weireter LJ, Riblet JL, et al. Priorities in the management of profound shock. *Surg Clin North Am* 1996;76:645.
8. Fakhry SM, Sheldon GF. Blood transfusion and disorders of surgical bleeding. In: Sabiston DC, Lyerly HK, eds. *Textbook of surgery: the biological basis of modern surgical practice.* Philadelphia: WB Saunders, 1997:118.
9. Gould SA, Moore EE, Hoyt DB, et al. The life sustaining capacity of human polymerized hemoglobin when red cells might be unavailable. *J Am Coll Surg* 2002;195(4):445–452.
10. Ma OJ, Mateer JR, Ogata M, et al. Prospective analysis of a rapid trauma ultrasound examination performed by emergency physicians. *J Trauma* 1995;38:879.
11. Mattox KL, Bickell WH, Pepe PE, et al. Prospective randomized evaluation of antishock MAST in posttraumatic hypotension. *J Trauma* 1986;26:779.
12. Mattox KL, Maningas PA, Moore EE, et al. Prehospital hypertonic saline/dextran infusion for post-traumatic hypotension: the U.S.A. Multicenter Trial. *Ann Surg* 1991;213:482–491.
13. Mattox KL, Brundage SI, Hirshberg A. Initial resuscitation. *New Horiz* 1999;7:1.
14. Pearlman MD, Tintinalli JE, Lorenz RP. Blunt trauma during pregnancy. *N Engl J Med* 1990;323:1609.
15. Rizoli SB. Crystalloids and colloids in trauma resuscitation: a brief overview of the current debate. *J Trauma* 2003;54:S82–S88.
16. Roberts I, Evans P, Bunn F, et al. Is the normalisation of blood pressure in bleeding trauma patients harmful? *Lancet* 2001;357:385–387.
17. Shierhout G, Roberts I. Fluid resuscitation with colloid or crystalloid solutions in critically ill patients: a systematic review of randomised trials. *BMJ* 1998;316:961.
18. Siegal JH, Rivkind AI, Dalal S, et al. Early physiologic predictors of injury severity and death in blunt multiple tauma. *Arch Surg* 1990;125:498–508.
19. Stern SA, Dronen SC, Birrer P, et al. The effect of blood pressure on hemorrhage volume and survival in a near-fatal hemorrhage model incorporating a vascular injury. *Ann Emerg Med* 1993;22:155.
20. Tisherman SA. Trauma fluid resuscitation in 2010. *J Trauma* 2003;54:S231–S234.
21. Velanovich V. Crystalloid versus colloid fluid resuscitation: a meta-analysis of mortality. *Surgery* 1989;105:65.
22. Vayer JS, Henderson JV, Bellamy RF, et al. Absence of a tachycardic response to shock in penetrating intraperitoneal injury. *Ann Emerg Med* 1988;17:227.
23. Wade CE, Grady JJ, Kramer GC. Efficacy of hypertonic saline dextran fluid resuscitation for patients with hypotension from penetrating trauma. *J Trauma* 2003;54:S144.
24. Winchell RJ, Simons RK, Hoyt DB. Transient systolic hypotension. A serious problem in the management of head injury. *Arch Surg* 1996;131(5):533.

CHAPTER 172
Wound Management

Judd E. Hollander and Adam J. Singer

Nearly 11 million patients with traumatic wounds are treated annually in emergency departments (EDs) in the United States (26). The ultimate goals are to restore the physical integrity and function of the injured tissue in a cosmetically pleasing manner and to reduce the risk of infection. Treatment of these wounds involves a series of decisions that determine the methods of evaluation, wound preparation, wound closure, and postoperative care most likely to help attain these goals.

CLINICAL PRESENTATION

Lacerations occur predominantly in young adults; the majority of patients with lacerations are males (18). Most wounds are located on either the head or neck (50%) or the upper extremity (35%), usually involving the fingers or hands. The most common mechanism of injury is application of a blunt force, such as bumping the head against a coffee table. Such contact crushes the skin against an underlying bone, causing the skin to split. Other causes of injury include sharp instruments, glass, and wooden objects (18). While mammalian bites continue to receive much attention, they are a relatively infrequent cause of puncture wounds and lacerations (18).

EMERGENCY DEPARTMENT EVALUATION

Evaluation of the patient with a traumatic wound begins with an expeditious, comprehensive assessment of the patient. This assessment can be divided into primary and secondary surveys, following Advanced Trauma Life Support Algorithms (see Chapter 169). Unless the wound compromises the ABCs, formal wound evaluation and management occurs during the secondary survey and management phase of the trauma evaluation.

Proper wound management begins with a thorough patient history. Particular emphasis should be placed on the various factors that can have adverse effects on wound healing. Host factors such as the extremes of age, diabetes mellitus, chronic renal failure, obesity, malnutrition, and the use of immunosuppressive medications such as steroids and chemotherapeutic agents all increase the risk of wound infection and can impair wound healing. Wound healing can also be impaired in the presence of inherited and acquired connective-tissue disorders such as Ehlers-Danlos syndrome, Marfan syndrome, osteogenesis imperfecta, and protein and vitamin C deficiencies. The tendency of patients to form keloids should be ascertained since the development of keloids can result in a scar with less than acceptable cosmesis. Black and Asian populations are more prone to keloid formation (39).

Identification of the mechanism of injury is essential to help ascertain the presence of potential wound contaminants and foreign bodies that might result in chronic infection and delayed healing (39). Failure to diagnose foreign bodies in wounds is the fifth leading cause of litigation against emergency physicians. Missed tendon and nerve injuries and failure to prevent infection are other common wound-related causes of litigation. Associated symptoms should be sought as part of the history. In patients with scalp lacerations, a history of loss of consciousness and any neurologic complaints should be obtained. In patients with hand injuries, a history of neurologic deficits should be obtained in order to help predict the presence of tendon or nerve injury.

A careful history can also predict the likelihood of foreign bodies. Organic and inorganic components of soil can potentiate infection. Wounds contaminated by these fractions will become infected with lower doses of bacterial inoculum. The major inorganic particles that potentiate infection are the clay fractions, which reside in heaviest concentration in the subsoil rather than in the topsoil. Injuries that occur in swamps or excavations are at high risk of being contaminated by these fractions. Other soil contaminants, such as sand grains, are relatively innocuous. The black dirt on the surface of highways appears to have minimal chemical reactivity.

Knowledge of the types of forces applied at the time of injury also helps predict the likelihood of infection. Thus, crush injuries that tend to cause greater devitalization of tissue are more susceptible to infection than are wounds resulting from the more commonly seen shearing forces (8). Impact injuries with low energy levels may not result in division of the skin; they can, however, disrupt vessels and produce an ecchymosis.

The presence of allergies to local anesthetics, latex, and antibiotics should be determined. The tetanus status of all patients should be assessed, and patients should receive immunization in accordance with current Centers for Disease Control and Prevention recommendations (Table 172.1). Before inspecting the wound, the emergency physician should question the patient regarding the time and mechanism of injury. The amount of time elapsed since the accident may influence treatment decisions.

Adequate wound examination should always be conducted under optimal lighting conditions in a field where bleeding has been controlled. Cursory examination under poor lighting conditions or when the depths of the wound are obscured by blood may result in underdetection of embedded foreign bodies and damage to important structures such as tendons, nerves, and arteries. One way to minimize the possibility of missing an injury to a vital structure is to start the wound examination with a careful neurovascular assessment of pulses, motor function, and sensation distal to the laceration. Finger tourniquets or a blood pressure cuff may then be used to obtain a bloodless field, but they should not be used for more than 30 to 60 minutes.

The anatomic location of the injury helps to predict the likelihood of infection. Moist areas of the body, such as the axillae, perineum, toe webs, and intertriginous areas, harbor millions of bacteria per square centimeter. Lacerations of the oral cavity are usually heavily contaminated with facultative species and obligate anaerobes. Wounds with human or animal fecal contaminants run a high risk of infection despite therapeutic intervention.

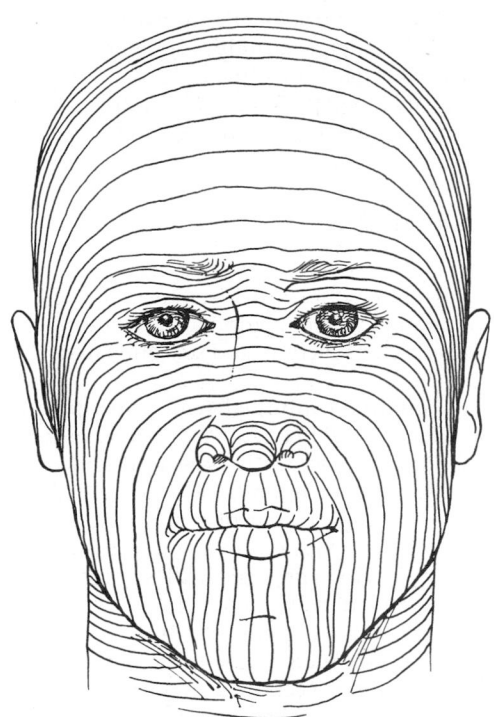

Figure 172.1. Langer's lines of least skin tension. Lacerations parallel to these lines will have less evident scarring.

Anatomic variation in regional blood flow also plays a role in determining the likelihood of infection. Wounds located on highly vascular areas, such as the face and scalp, are less likely to be infected than are wounds located in less vascular areas, such as the extremities (18). Lacerations of the scalp and face have a very low infection rate regardless of the intensity of cleansing (19).

Wound location also contributes to the cosmetic appearance of the scar by affecting static and dynamic skin tensions (Fig. 172.1). Lacerations over joints are subject to large, dynamic skin tensions and will have a wider scar than will similar lacerations subject to less tension. Wounds that run perpendicular to the lines of minimal skin tension will also be prone to the development of wider and more visible scars.

EMERGENCY DEPARTMENT MANAGEMENT

Aseptic Technique

The use of sterile gloves makes common sense, despite the lack of clinical evidence supporting their use (36,49). While more costly, use of powder-free gloves may reduce the risk of foreign-body reaction or infection that can theoretically occur from the introduction of talc particles into the wound. While the practice of universal precautions is recommended in all patients, double-gloving is recommended when caring for patients who can transmit serious infections to the health-care provider. Patients who harbor the human immunodeficiency virus or hepatitis are among those for whom the health-care provider may wish to take extra precautions, such as double-gloving.

Latex Allergy

Concerns have been raised about the safety of latex. Absorption of water-soluble proteins through intact mucosa or the surgical wound is believed to elicit an immunoglobulin-E (IgE)–mediated anaphylactic response in sensitive individuals. Severe reactions have resulted in fatalities. Populations that

TABLE 172.1. Recommendations for Tetanus Prophylaxis

	Clean Minor Wounds		All Other Wounds*	
History of tetanus immunization	Td	TIG	Td	TIG
<3 or uncertain doses	Yes	No	Yes	Yes
≥3 doses				
Last dose within 5 years	No	No	No	No
Last dose within 5–10 years	No	No	Yes	No
Last dose >10 years ago	Yes	No	Yes	No

*For example, contaminated wounds, puncture wounds, avulsions, burns, crush injuries.

Td, tetanus–diphtheria toxoid; TIG, tetanus immune globulin.

From Singer AJ, Hollander JE, Quinn JV. Evaluation and management of traumatic lacerations. *N Engl J Med* 1997;337:1142.

appear to be at increased risk for allergic reactions to latex include patients who have undergone multiple operations, patients with atopic disease, children with spina bifida, and medical personnel with frequent latex exposures (28). Careful screening should identify patients who may be at increased risk for latex hypersensitivity.

Wound Examination

Wound examination should always be conducted under optimal lighting conditions and with bleeding in the field controlled. Wound examination should begin with a neurovascular assessment of pulses, motor function, and sensation distal to the laceration.

Bleeding should be controlled with direct pressure. When possible, skin flaps should be returned to their original position prior to application of pressure, to prevent vascular compromise of the injured area. When lacerations continue to bleed despite reasonable pressure, placement of a sphygmomanometer cuff proximal to the injury, with inflation to a pressure greater than the patient's systolic blood pressure, will help contain bleeding to allow proper examination. Palpation of the bones adjacent to the injured site may detect tenderness, a defect, or instability consistent with an underlying injury. Use of radiography should be liberal to detect fractures. Detection of an open fracture will dictate a change from usual management. Carefully evaluate wounds occurring adjacent to a joint for joint violation. This condition requires meticulous cleaning and possibly debridement, usually in the operating room.

Amputated parts should be cared for as outlined in the chapters on hand injuries and replantation emergencies (Chapters 191 and 198). Digits should be covered with a protective saline-soaked dressing, placed within a waterproof bag, and then placed in a container of ice for preservation and consideration of future reattachment.

Complicated injuries involving most open fractures, joint penetration, flexor tendon injuries, nerve injuries, or arterial injuries are usually treated in the operating room. In most other cases, wound repair will occur in the ED.

The ultimate appearance and function of a scar can be predicted by the static and dynamic skin tensions on the surrounding skin (see Fig. 172.1). The most aesthetically pleasing scar occurs when the long axis of the scar is parallel to the direction of maximal skin tension, because the static skin tensions continually pull on the wound edges even after wound closure. The ultimate width of the scar is proportional to the magnitude of the static skin tensions.

Dynamic skin tensions may have considerable impact on the magnitude and extent of scar formation. These changing tensions are caused by a combination of forces that are associated with joint movement or mimetic muscle contraction. The clinical significance of dynamic tensions is particularly apparent in skin of changing dimensions in which elasticity is needed for normal function. In general, a linear scar intersecting the transverse axis of a joint or running perpendicular to the wrinkle lines can result in a serious contracture because the scar does not stretch or recoil like uninjured tissue. The patient should be warned that an unattractive scar may result. An appreciation of the effects of various dynamic tensions can be used to determine the need for absorbable sutures in addition to the nonabsorbable skin closure.

Wound Anesthesia

Most lacerations will require some form of anesthesia prior to wound closure. The administration of anesthesia prior to wound cleansing will enable more vigorous wound cleansing and possibly surgical debridement. All visibly contaminated wounds and wounds that will require anesthesia for closure should receive anesthesia prior to cleansing so that adequate mechanical removal of bacteria, soil, and other debris can be more readily accomplished.

Local Infiltration

The most common form of anesthesia for traumatic injuries is local infiltration. Unfortunately, local anesthesia is painful. In order to reduce the pain associated with local infiltration, several strategies can be employed. The addition of sodium bicarbonate to lidocaine (pK_a, 7.9) in a 1:9 ratio increases the ratio of uncharged to charged ions and results in more rapid diffusion of anesthetic agent into nerve endings. It reduces the pain associated with local infiltration without altering the ability of host defenses to prevent infection (3). The use of warm anesthetic solutions, small needles, slow rates of infiltration, injection through the wound edges in noncontaminated wounds, and pretreatment with topical 4% tetracaine or LET (lidocaine, adrenaline, and tetracaine) are additional strategies that can be used to decrease the pain of infiltration (5,20,22).

For injection of local anesthesia, use a 27- to 30-gauge needle attached to a 10-mL syringe. The needle should be passed into the wound edge rather than the intact skin because subdermal (wound edge) injections are less painful. Full anesthesia to pinprick is present 5 to 6 minutes after subdermal injection. The local anesthetic agent should be instilled slowly to decrease the pain that accompanies tissue infiltration (22). The needle should be passed through the dermal tissue initially; then the anesthetic agent can be injected as the needle is slowly withdrawn. This technique minimizes distention and pain by providing a potential space for the anesthetic solution. Aspiration of the syringe before injection is recommended to prevent inadvertent intravascular injection.

The two major classes of local anesthetics are the esters and amides (Table 172.2). Because the amides cause less sensitivity and allergic reactions than the esters, lidocaine and bupivacaine are most commonly used for local anesthesia. Because the duration of local anesthesia induced by bupivacaine is nearly four times longer than that of lidocaine, bupivacaine (0.25%) should be used when longer durations of anesthesia are desirable (Table 172.3).

Many patients with "allergies" to lidocaine are really allergic to methylparaben, the preservative used in multidose vials. One alternative for this situation is to use single dose lidocaine (cardiac lidocaine), which does not contain a preservative. Another option is to use an anesthetic agent unrelated to the "caines," such as diphenhydramine or benzyl alcohol.

Vasoconstrictors such as epinephrine can be used as adjuncts to the local anesthetic agents. They will reduce bleeding and oozing within the laceration, which will make exploration and closure easier to accomplish. Clinical studies have not found that the vasoconstriction associated with epinephrine use results in differences in infection rates. The use of vasoconstrictors is generally discouraged in areas with end-organ blood supply, such as the fingers and toes.

TABLE 172.2. Classification of Local Anesthetics

Amides	Esters
Lidocaine	Procaine
Bupivacaine	Cocaine
Etidocaine	Tetracaine
Mepivacaine	Benzocaine
	Chloroprocaine

TABLE 172.3. Properties of Commonly Used Local Anesthetics

Agent	Trade Name	Local Anesthetic Class	Concentration	Maximal Safe Dose	Onset	Duration
Procaine	Novocaine	Ester	0.5%–1.0%	7 mg/kg	2–5 min	15–45 min
With epinephrine				9 mg/kg		30–90 min
Lidocaine	Xylocaine	Amide	0.5%–2.0%	4.5 mg/kg	2–5 min	1–2 h
With epinephrine				7 mg/kg		2–4 h
Bupivacaine	Marcaine	Amide	0.125%–0.25%	2 mg/kg	2–5 min	4–8 h
With epinephrine				3 mg/kg		8–16 h

Regional Anesthesia

When the nerve supply to a wound is easily accessible, a regional nerve block is a valuable alternative to local anesthesia. The use of regional nerve blocks will prevent distortion of the wound edges, facilitating approximation and increasing the likelihood of an excellent cosmetic result. Additionally, a regional nerve block is more useful than local anesthesia in areas with abundant sensory nerve supplies, such as the fingers, palms, and soles. Regional nerve blocks can be accomplished by only one or two needle passages through skin proximal to the injury site. Often these areas have a considerably higher threshold of pain. Regional nerve blocks of the supraorbital, infraorbital, and mental nerves are useful for facial lacerations; however, they are more painful and less reliable than local infiltration (47). Median, radial, and ulnar nerve blocks may be useful for lacerations of the hand. Digital or metacarpal nerve blocks can be used for finger lacerations. Regional nerve blocks can also be used for lacerations of the feet. Field blocks can be considered for more proximal extremity injuries.

A 27- or 25-gauge needle is preferred to a 30-gauge needle for a regional nerve block, because either one is more resistant to deflection during passage through tissue. The duration of sensory analgesia can be significantly prolonged when epinephrine (1%) is added to the anesthetic solution. When the needle puncture site is the mucous membrane, anesthetizing the mucous membrane with a topical anesthetic agent makes the introduction of the needle painless.

Topical Anesthesia

Topical anesthesia eliminates needle use and the risk of inadvertent needle sticks while allowing the application of painless anesthesia. Various combinations of lidocaine (1% to 4%), adrenaline (1 : 1,000 to 1 : 2,000), and tetracaine (0.5% to 2.0%) (14,15) are as effective as EMLA cream (eutectic mixture of local anesthetics) (41). Application of LET at triage also reduces the length of stay in the ED. EMLA has a slower onset of action and is more expensive than LET; therefore it is not recommended for use in the ED.

Preparation of Skin

Removal of the hair surrounding a laceration may facilitate meticulous wound closure. Because many bacteria normally reside in hair follicles, shaving the hair prior to repair may increase wound infection rates (37). Reduced damage to hair follicles may be achieved by using hair clippers instead of a razor. Removal of the eyebrow hair should be avoided because it does not always grow back. Additionally, the presence of hair serves as a guide to approximation of wound edges during laceration repair.

The skin surrounding the wound should either be cleansed with normal saline or disinfected with an iodophor (such as Betadine) or chlorhexadine; avoid contacting the wound itself with disinfectant. Although these agents can reduce the bacterial concentration on intact skin, they appear to damage wound defenses, making the wound more susceptible to development of infection. Consequently, any contact of these agents with the wound should be avoided. Also take care to avoid antiseptic contact with the eyes.

Debridement

Appropriate debridement is an important factor in the management of contaminated wounds (17). Retained devitalized soft tissue, fat, muscle, and skin can damage wound defenses and increase the likelihood of infection through the promotion of bacterial growth and the inhibition of phagocytosis. Identification of the exact limit of devitalized tissue in wounds may be difficult. Evaluation of the color, consistency, contraction, and circulation is useful.

In some anatomic sites, such as the trunk, debridement is best accomplished by complete excision of the skin and deep tissues. Heavily contaminated wounds with serpiginous defects in these regions can be converted to clean wounds by more generous tissue excision. When a heavily contaminated wound contains specialized tissues, such as the nerves or tendons that perform important physical functions, complete excision often is not feasible. In such instances, mechanical wound cleansing followed by excision of all fragments of tissue that are not clearly viable is indicated.

The benefits of debridement must be weighed against the consequences of excision of the tissue. Debridement of skin and underlying tissue leaves a significant soft-tissue defect that makes reapproximation more difficult. The increased static skin tensions produced may result in a wider scar. In some cases, debridement may be best performed in the operating room, where sterile conditions, lighting, and assistants may offer an advantage.

Assessment for Foreign Bodies

On occasion, wound imaging for detection of foreign bodies may be necessary. Most foreign bodies commonly found in wounds are more dense than the surrounding tissue and are readily apparent on plain radiographs. Metal, bone, teeth, pencil graphite, certain plastics, glass, gravel, sand, some fish bones, some wood, and some types of aluminum are visible on plain radiographs. Almost all glass fragments 2 mm or larger are visible on radiographs (12). If the wound was caused by metal or glass and no foreign body is found on wound exploration or on plain films, it is unlikely that a foreign body exists. Some objects will not be identifiable with plain radiography. Computed tomography (CT) and magnetic resonance imaging (MRI) are useful for identifying and locating objects that have densities similar to soft tissue. Sonography may also be useful, particularly for wooden foreign bodies.

Cleansing the Wound

The two basic methods of wound cleansing are hydraulic forces (irrigation) and direct contact (scrubbing).

Irrigation

Some debate exists over both the optimal method of irrigation and the preferred solution. The efficacy of wound irrigation can be correlated with the pressure at which the irrigant is delivered to the wound (13). In an experimental model involving a contaminated animal wound, high-pressure (>7 psi) irrigation was more effective than low-pressure (<7 psi) irrigation in reducing both bacterial wound counts and wound infection rates (46). High-pressure irrigation successfully cleans wounds of small particulate matter, such as bacteria and soil. Such cleansing has reduced the infection rate of experimentally contaminated wounds. In contrast, low-pressure syringe irrigation, even with large volumes of fluid, demonstrates negligible capability for removing small particles (bacteria), but removes large particulate matter, such as detached devitalized tissue.

Wound impact pressures of more than 8 psi (high pressure) can be easily obtained using a 30- to 60-mL syringe and a 19-gauge needle (46) or Zerowet splash shield (29). However, it must be noted that sustained high-pressure irrigation can result in tissue damage. As a result, at very high pressures, infection rates may actually increase (13). Thus, the optimal irrigation pressure lies somewhere in between.

For individual wounds, the benefits of high-pressure irrigation should be weighed against the potential risks. Thus, for noncontaminated wounds in highly vascularized areas containing loose areolar tissue, such as the eyelid, high pressures should be avoided. In fact, high-pressure irrigation has not been found to offer any advantages for cleansing clean, noncontaminated facial lacerations (19). Conversely, high-pressure irrigation is clearly indicated for contaminated wounds of the lower extremity. Very high pressure irrigation (Pulsivac) is not recommended for use in the ED but may be used for extraordinarily difficult to cleanse wounds in the operative setting.

The choice of irrigation solution is relatively straightforward. Normal saline is the most cost-effective and readily available choice. It has compared favorably with more expensive, less easily available alternatives (11). Because of their tissue toxicity, detergents, hydrogen peroxide, and concentrated forms of povidone–iodine should not be used to irrigate wounds (13). A recent study of pediatric lacerations found that irrigation of wounds with tap water resulted in comparable infection rates versus irrigation with sterile saline (48). Irrigation volume should be individualized based on patient characteristics and such wound characteristics as location and etiology. Use of a device designed to reduce splatter will minimize the health-care provider's risk of exposure to potentially infectious materials.

Scrubbing

Direct scrubbing of the wound with a sterile surgical brush helps remove both bacteria and particulate matter, which potentiate the risk of wound infection. However, scrubbing also contributes to the tissue damage and reduces the ability of the wound to resist infection. The magnitude of the damage to the local tissue resistance is correlated with the porosity of the sponge. Sponges with a low porosity (45 pores per inch [ppi]) are more abrasive and exert more damage to the wound than do sponges with a higher porosity (90 ppi). The addition of a nontoxic surfactant to a sponge minimizes the tissue damage the sponge inflicts while maintaining the bacterial removal efficiency of mechanical cleansing. Because the use of high-porosity sponges and surfac-

tant adds to the cost of wound care, their use is probably justified only for highly contaminated wounds.

Use of Drains

The potential benefits of the use of surgical drains in a clinical setting must be weighed against its harmful effects. Drains evacuate potentially harmful collections of pus and blood from wounds. When no definite localized fluid exists, drains must be considered prophylactic, and its potentially harmful effects become more important. Drains act as retrograde conduits through which skin contaminants gain entrance into the wound. Placement of both Silastic and Penrose drains within experimental wounds exposed to subinfective inoculations of bacteria greatly enhanced the rate of infection compared with that observed in undrained controls (24).

The general use of drains is not indicated in the management of most wounds in the ED.

Open Wound Management

After wound cleansing, the physical integrity and function of the injured tissue must be restored. The technique of wound closure largely depends on whether the wound has lost tissue and the risk of wound infection. With *primary closure* the wound is immediately closed. Primary closure results in a reduction in healing time in comparison with other closure methods. It also may reduce the bleeding and discomfort often associated with open wounds. *Secondary wound closure*, in which the wound is left open and allowed to close on its own, is particularly well suited for highly contaminated or infected wounds. While this method may reduce the risk of infection, it is relatively slow and uncomfortable. *Delayed primary* (or *tertiary*) *closure* combines the advantages of both primary and secondary closure. The wound is left open for a period of 3 to 5 days, after which it may be closed if no infection supervenes. For wounds with associated significant tissue loss, grafts or flaps are often required to close the defect. These procedures are usually performed in the operating room. They are relatively infrequent occurrences in the ED.

The timing of laceration closure is critical. Most wounds should be closed primarily in order to reduce patient discomfort and speed healing. While there is a direct relationship between the time interval from injury to laceration closure and the risk of subsequent infection, the length of this "golden period" is highly variable (39). A study of forearm lacerations found that closure within 4 hours had a lower infection rate than later closure (30). A large series of pediatric patients (2,834 patients) with lacerations did not find a difference in infection rate for lacerations closed within or greater than 6 hours from the time of injury (2). Facial lacerations healed well regardless of the time to closure. In contrast, trunk and extremity lacerations exhibited lower rates of healing if they were closed more than 19 hours from the time of injury (63% to 75%) as compared to earlier (75% to 91%) (4).

On the basis of these data, it seems appropriate to consider each laceration separately, taking the time from injury until presentation into account, along with laceration location, degree of contamination, risk of infection, and importance of cosmetic appearance, before deciding whether to perform primary wound closure. For example, a 19-hour-old laceration on the face of a healthy 5-year-old child may be closed primarily, while a deep laceration from a puncture in the dirty foot of a diabetic patient will be at very high risk of infection and should not be closed primarily. Thus, the timing during which wound closure is deemed safe must be individualized (39). Wounds that are not closed primarily due to a high risk of infection should be considered

TABLE 172.4. Advantages and Disadvantages of the Common Wound-Closure Techniques

	Advantages	Disadvantages
Suture	Time-honored Meticulous closure Greatest tensile strength Lowest dehiscence rate	Requires removal Requires anesthesia Greatest tissue reactivity Highest cost Slowest application
Staples	Rapid application Low tissue reactivity Low cost Low risk of needlestick	Less meticulous closure May interfere with some older generation imaging techniques (CT, MRI)
Tissue adhesives	Rapid application Patient comfort Resistant to bacterial growth No need for removal Low cost No risk of needlestick	Lower tensile strength than sutures Dehiscence over high-tension areas (joints) Not useful on hands Cannot bathe or swim
Surgical tapes	Least reactive Lowest infection rates Rapid application Patient comfort Low cost No risk of needlestick	Frequently falls off Lower tensile strength than sutures Highest rate of dehiscence Requires use of toxic adjuncts Cannot be used in areas of hair Cannot get wet

for delayed primary closure after 3 to 5 days, when the risk of infection decreases.

Wound Closure

Careful handling of tissues and judicious use of electrocautery are necessary in order to reduce further trauma that may lead to poor cosmetic outcome (42). The ideal wound-closure technique should allow a meticulous closure, be accomplished rapidly with ease, be painless, pose a low risk to the health-care provider, be inexpensive, result in minimal scarring, and involve a low infection rate. The optimal wound-closure technique varies with the clinical situation. Sutures are the most commonly employed wound-closure technique. Tissue adhesives can be used in up to one-third of ED laceration repairs. Staples and surgical tapes can be used in selected situations. The advantages and disadvantages of various wound-closure techniques are summarized in Table 172.4.

Sutures

The choice of suture technique should be determined by the configuration and biomechanical properties of the wound, in combination with an assessment of its risk of infection. Percutaneous sutures pass through the epidermal and dermal layers of the skin. They are used alone for low-tension lacerations and in combination with dermal (subcuticular) sutures for higher tension lacerations. The dermal suture reapproximates the divided edges of the dermis without penetrating the epidermis. Often, dermal and percutaneous sutures are used together.

Most often, percutaneous sutures are performed with nonabsorbable sutures (Table 172.5), such as nylon and polypropylene. Both nylon and polypropylene retain most of their tensile strength for more than 60 days and are relatively nonreactive (39). Removal of nonabsorbable sutures is required. Percutaneous sutures of either monofilament nylon or polypropylene exert the least damage to the wound defenses. Polybutester suture has greater elasticity than other sutures, allowing the suture to return to its original length once tension is removed. Polybutester sutures are useful when sutures are subject to wound edema and

may be expected to stretch. Nylon, polypropylene, and silk resist extension under low forces, thereby lacerating encircled tissue and creating unsightly marks on the skin.

Nonabsorbable sutures made from natural fibers potentiate infection more than synthetic nonabsorbable sutures, correlating with the reaction of tissue to these sutures in clean wounds. The use of silk and cotton should be avoided in wounds that have significant bacterial contamination. The incidence of infection in contaminated tissue containing monofilament sutures is lower than in those containing multifilament sutures. Although use of absorbable sutures is generally reserved for dermal closures, more rapidly absorbing forms can be used to close skin in children and avoid the discomfort and inconvenience of suture removal.

Dermal closures are generally accomplished with absorbable sutures (Table 172.6). They increase the duration of time the wound retains 50% of its tensile strength from 1 week to as much as 8 weeks. Chromic gut lasts for up to 2 weeks, but it is associated with increased tissue reactivity. Polyglactin (Vicryl) and polyglycolic acid (Dexon) maintain tensile strength for 20 to 28 days and have less tissue reactivity. Some synthetic absorbable sutures, such as polydioxanone (PDS) and polyglyconate (Maxon), retain their tensile strength for as long as 2 months. They are particularly useful in areas with high static and dynamic tensions. These sutures should be used only in the deeper areas, because they can become extruded after long periods of time.

The use of dermal sutures relieves skin tension, decreases dead space and hematoma formation, and, theoretically, should improve cosmetic outcome. Research in experimental animal

TABLE 172.5. Characteristics of Nonabsorbable Sutures

Suture	Knot Security	Tensile Strength	Tissue Reactivity	Workability
Nylon (Ethilon)	Good	Good	Minimal	Good
Polypropylene (Prolene)	Least	Best	Least	Fair
Silk	Best	Least	Most	Best

TABLE 172.6.   Characteristics of Absorbable Sutures

Suture	Knot Security	Tensile Strength	Wound Security (50% Tensile Strength)	Tissue Reactivity
Surgical gut	Poor	Fair	5–7 d	Most
Chromic gut	Fair	Fair	10–14 d	Most
Polyglactin (Vicryl)	Good	Good	30 d	Minimal
Polyglycolic acid (Dexon)	Best	Good	30 d	Minimal
Polydioxanone (PDS)	Fair	Best	45–60 d	Least
Polyglyconate (Maxon)	Fair	Best	45–60 d	Least

models has found that deep sutures increase the risk of infection in highly contaminated wounds, but they do not do so in clean, noncontaminated lacerations (1,27). Sutures placed through adipose tissue do not reduce tension, and they increase the infection rate. Deep sutures should not be placed in adipose tissue and should not be used in contaminated wounds (10). No studies of traumatic lacerations have demonstrated any benefit to the use of deep sutures. Many practitioners prefer to use deep sutures in gaping lacerations and in cosmetically important lacerations despite a lack of evidence. Deep sutures should not be used in the hand as they may inadvertently cause damage to important structures such as nerves and tendons.

Undermining the wound margin decreases the forces required for wound closure. Theoretically, it should limit the width of the ultimate scar. However, this benefit must be weighed against its potential damage to the skin blood supply, which may limit the patient's defenses, increasing the likelihood of infection. Consequently, undermining should be reserved for clean, noncontaminated wounds subjected to strong static and dynamic tensions.

The magnitude of the suture's damage to the local tissue defenses is related to the quantity of the suture within the wound. As a result, the narrowest diameter suture (5/0 or 6/0) that is strong enough to resist disruption of the skin should be used (Table 172.7). Approximation of the midportion of the laceration first, with subsequent bisection of the remaining portion, will enable the use of least amount of suture. Interrupted dermal sutures placed in each quadrant of the wound subjected to strong static and dynamic skin tensions provide sufficient strength to permit early suture removal.

Tissue Adhesives

The only tissue adhesives that are strong enough to close wounds are the cyanoacrylate polymers. Shorter alkyl chain molecules (methyl, ethyl) are more reactive and have greater histotoxicity and weaker tissue binding than longer alkyl chain cyanoacrylates. The *n*-butyl-cyanoacrylates are less toxic than shorter chain cyanoacrylates and maintain a stronger bond. 2-Octylcyanoacrylate (Dermabond) is even more stable, has greater flexibility, and maintains a stronger bond. It has a breaking strength three to four times greater than the butylcyanoacrylates, and degrades much more slowly. It is considered nontoxic. Dermabond also has the advantage of forming a microbial barrier to further wound contamination.

Observational studies of children with small scalp, face, or limb lacerations treated with Histoacryl Blue (Braun, Germany), a butyl-2-cyanoacrylate, found low infection rates (less than 2%) and low dehiscence rates (0.6% to 1.8%). Histoacryl Blue results in similar long-term cosmetic outcomes to 5-0 or 6-0 sutures when used for repair of small facial lacerations (32).

Several clinical studies have compared the use of 2-octylcyanoacrylate to 5-0 and 6-0 sutures. Quinn et al. (33) found the long-term cosmetic outcomes to be equivalent. The use of 2-octylcyanoacrylate was faster and less painful than the use of sutures. The largest study to date enrolled 818 patients from a variety of office-based and ED sites (43). Patients were randomized to receive skin closure with either 5-0 or 6-0 sutures or 2-octylcyanoacrylate. Of the 818 patients enrolled, 333 had subcuticular or subcutaneous sutures placed prior to laceration closure. Comparing the group of patients who received 2-octylcyanoacrylate with the group of patients who received skin closure with sutures, the 3-month cosmetic outcomes, short-term infection rates, and wound dehiscence rates were all similar. The time to wound closure was reduced by more than 50% in the group treated with 2-octylcyanoacrylate. Likewise, subgroup analysis of patients from both adult and pediatric EDs found equivalent 3-month cosmetic outcomes (6,40).

Although *in vitro* and *in vivo* studies have found that cyanoacrylate tissue adhesives possess Gram-positive antimicrobial properties, it is imperative that clinicians adhere to standard wound preparation and wound cleansing procedures. When tissue adhesives have been used without anesthesia, and wound cleansing is not performed in a thorough manner, an increased rate of wound infection has been observed.

The application of tissue adhesives is rapid and relatively painless. Adhesives also have the advantage that they do not require later removal, as do sutures. They will usually slough off in 7 to 10 days as the keratinized layer of epithelium sloughs. They should be used only topically. Tissue adhesives should not be placed within the wound or between wound margins. Octylcyanoacrylate tissue adhesives provide greater three-dimensional tensile strength than do butylcyanoacrylates. Both polymers are needleless alternatives to sutures for the closure of most facial lacerations, providing an excellent cosmetic appearance, comparable to that provided by sutures.

2-Octylcyanoacrylate is packaged in a sterile, single-use ampule and is colored with violet dye. After the inner glass portion of the ampule is manually crushed, the polymerization process begins. The adhesive should be painted on top of the skin as

TABLE 172.7.   Suture Selection Based on Anatomic Location

Location	Suture Size*
Face	6-0 or 7-0
Oral Mucosa	4-0 or 5-0
Scalp	5-0
Chest	3-0 or 4-0
Back	3-0 or 4-0
Forearm	4-0 or 5-0
Fingers	4-0 or 5-0
Hand	4-0 or 5-0
Lower extremity	4-0 or 5-0
Foot	4-0 or 5-0

*Larger suture sizes may need to be used for wounds with higher tension.

the laceration edges are manually approximated. If lacerations cannot be manually approximated and the skin edges cannot be held together without tension, the use of tissue adhesives is inappropriate. 2-Octylcyanoacrylate is available as a low or high viscosity formulation. When low viscosity 2-octylcyanoacrylate is painted on the laceration, the clinician should apply at least three coats to provide adequate strength to the wound closure. With the high viscosity formulation, only two layers are required. The high viscosity formulation is nearly four times less likely to result in inadvertent runoff (44). The physician should take care to avoid applying too much tissue adhesive, because polymerization is associated with an exothermic reaction (heat release). Increased rates and amounts of polymerization may be associated with the perception of increased heat sensation by the patient.

2-Octylcyanoacrylates can be used in locations that could otherwise be closed with 5-0 or 6-0 nonabsorbable sutures. 2-Octylcyanoacrylates should be used in higher-tension areas only if subcutaneous or subcuticular absorbable sutures are placed to relieve tension on the skin. They should not be used over high-tension areas or areas involved in repetitive movement, such as joints. When tissue adhesive application leads to a suboptimal wound closure, antibiotic ointment, petroleum jelly, or bathing can be used to accelerate removal. Acetone can be used when more rapid removal is necessary.

The butylcyanoacrylates possess less tensile strength than 5-0 sutures and only approximately two-thirds the tensile strength of the octylcyanoacrylates (45). Studies have found that for the repair of very small facial lacerations, the butylcyanoacrylates are equivalent to 5-0 and 6-0 sutures or octylcyanoacrylates (31). In general, the butylcyanoacrylates are more brittle and friable than octylcyanoacrylates and do not allow the same degree of movement and flexibility of the skin.

Staples

Staples can be applied more rapidly than sutures. Staples are associated with a lower rate of foreign-body reaction and a lower infection rate (34). In general, staples are considered particularly useful for scalp, trunk, and extremity wounds (39). They can also be used when time is limited, such as in situations of mass casualties or multiple trauma (39). On the other hand, they do not allow as meticulous a skin closure as sutures, and their use is limited when cosmetic appearance is of utmost importance. They are slightly more painful to remove than sutures. In experimental animal models, staples have shown lower rates of bacterial growth and lower infection rates than sutures (21), although these effects appear to have limited clinical significance.

Adhesive Tapes

The ideal adhesive tape should be strong enough, even when wet, to withstand the forces disrupting the wound, sufficiently adherent to the skin and able to maintain approximation of the wound edges (35). Although a secure bond to skin is necessary for wound security, it also appears to be beneficial for the tape to stretch slightly under constant stress. This ability to elongate under moderate loads reduces the shear forces on the underlying edematous skin, thereby preventing blister formation. The tape construction should provide an environment on the skin surface that is resistant to bacterial growth.

The ease with which wounds can be closed by tape varies according to the anatomic and biomechanical properties of the wound site. Linear wounds in skin subjected to minimal static and dynamic tensions are easily approximated by tape. The relatively lax skin of the face and abdomen is amenable to wound closure by tape. With tape closures, patients are spared the discomfort of suture removal and the development of suture puncture scars. An additional benefit of this technique is that patients need not be subjected to the painful injection of the local anesthetic agent required for suturing.

Surgical tapes are intrinsically less reactive than staples (21). However, adhesive tapes require the use of adhesive adjuncts (e.g., tincture of benzoin), which are tissue-toxic and increase local induration and wound infection rates. Adhesive adjuncts are toxic to wounds, and care should be taken that they do not enter the wound. Although the various surgical tapes have different degrees of adhesion, porosity, breaking strength, and elasticity (35), tapes alone will not maintain wound integrity in areas subject to tension (39). They are seldom recommended for primary wound closure in the ED but are often used after suture removal to decrease tension on the wound until they fall off. The outcome of highly select, small, short, linear, low tension facial lacerations that are closed with surgical tape is comparable to closure with a tissue adhesive (25).

Complex Issues in Wound Care

Bite Wounds

An estimated 1 to 2 million animal bites are treated each year in the United States. The most frequent complication from bites is infection. Dog bites have an infection rate of 1.4% to 30%, cat bites 15.6% to 50%, and human bites 9% to 18% (7). Most bite wounds are minor. Local wound care always begins with a thorough evaluation of the injury. The location, number, type, and depth of wound are noted. The wound is also assessed for signs of infection. Bite wounds are frequently puncture wounds. Meticulous examination is of utmost importance, since they are notoriously deceptive and may be more extensive than they initially appear to be. The physician should evaluate all bite wounds for injuries to deep structures such as tendons, joint capsules, blood vessels, nerves, and bone. Local or regional anesthetic should be used to facilitate wound exploration, and a proximal tourniquet may be used when necessary to create a bloodless field. If bony involvement or foreign body is suspected, a plain radiograph should be obtained. Meticulous cleansing, irrigation, and debridement are the essential components of all bite wound care. Irrigation of puncture wounds is controversial. Their small openings do not allow the irrigant solution to drain out appropriately. This may result in infiltration of the tissue. Surgical debridement may be necessary to remove compromised or necrotic tissue that may contain embedded organisms, soil, and clots that cannot be removed by irrigation alone.

Primary closure should not be performed for any human or cat bites. Primary closure of dog bite wounds is controversial. Recent studies support primary closure of selected dog bite wounds (7). In one study, 145 head and neck dog bite wounds underwent primary closure without the use of antibiotics and the wound infection rate was only 1.4% (16). Dog bite wounds to the head and neck that are >1.5 cm in length can be closed primarily with sutures. Small bite wounds (<1.5 cm) behave like puncture wounds and should be left open to allow for drainage. Patients with bite wounds that require reconstructive surgery should be immediately referred to the appropriate specialist. Hand wounds should be managed without immediate primary closure. However, for cosmetic reasons, facial wounds should be repaired. Other bite lacerations can be closed using delayed primary closure techniques. All injured extremities should be immobilized and elevated. Bites are tetanus-prone wounds, and the recommendations of the Advisory Committee on Immunization Practices (ACIP) for immunoprophylaxis should be followed. Domestic and wild animal bite victims should be assessed for the need for rabies postexposure immunoprophylaxis (see Chapter 350, "Mammalian Bites and Associated Infections").

Puncture Wounds

The feet are the most common site for puncture wounds. There are many different views on the management of plantar puncture wounds (7,23). Some physicians prefer expectant therapy, reacting to complications as they develop. Others pursue invasive exploration for and removal of foreign bodies with subsequent antibiotics in the hopes of preventing unusual but devastating infections that can develop.

Infections of plantar wounds can often have serious consequences and lead to disability or amputation. Osteomyelitis, osteochondritis, and septic arthritis are the worst of the complications. *Staphylococcus aureus* and *Pseudomonas aeruginosa* are the most common isolates from plantar puncture wound infections. *Pseudomonas* infections are associated with puncture wounds through tennis shoes.

Exploration of plantar puncture wounds for foreign bodies is technically difficult. Foreign bodies that penetrate the plantar fascia are almost impossible to locate through a narrow puncture wound. Irrigation of deep puncture wounds may not be beneficial because the irrigant does not completely drain out of the wound. Some authors recommend enlarging the puncture wound to allow for deeper irrigation and exploration, especially if bone or joint involvement is suspected. Others believe that removing a block of tissue down to the subcutaneous layer allows adequate visualization of accessible foreign bodies and removal of most of the contaminated tissue. And still others simply trim jagged epidermal skin edges. Simple probing and blind grasping have unknown false-negative rates and may force foreign bodies deeper into the wound. If a wound infection is present, the risk of foreign body is very high, and imaging or exploration is mandated.

Another controversy involves the use of prophylactic antibiotics for this type of injury. Many experts do not recommend the use of antibiotics for new plantar puncture wounds. They argue that antibiotics will not compensate for inadequate initial wound care, they are ineffective in wounds with retained foreign bodies, they may contribute to a Gram-negative infection, and wound infections that do not have a retained foreign body respond quickly to initiation of antibiotics. Due to the difficulty of cleaning and exploring plantar puncture wounds, physicians should reevaluate these wounds for infection within 2 to 3 days of initial presentation. If infection develops, they should be aggressively explored for a foreign body.

Facial Lacerations

Due to their cosmetic significance and proximity to important structures, several points concerning the repair of facial lacerations are noteworthy. Due to their rich vascular supply, facial lacerations have a relatively low rate of infection. The risks of high-pressure irrigation (edema making it more difficulty to perfectly approximate wound edges) should be weighed against the benefits (cleansing), and individual decisions regarding use of wound irrigation should be made accordingly. For example, an upper eyelid laceration resulting from a blunt impact with the corner of a table requires minimal irrigation, while a contused cheek laceration resulting from a fall onto a rough and dirty surface requires larger volume irrigation.

Whether nongaping facial lacerations routinely require deep sutures is a subject of ongoing debate. Gaping (>5 to 10 mm in width) lacerations as well as those in which underlying muscle are involved should be repaired in multiple layers. Meticulous wound approximation should follow important anatomical landmarks such as the forehead or nasolabial creases, the eyebrow, and the vermillion border. When these structures are

within a laceration, initial placement of key sutures aligning the landmarks is crucial. Eyebrows should never be removed since they may not grow back.

With lip lacerations it is important to exclude any underlying dental injuries. If a fractured tooth is not found, careful exploration of the lip wound should be performed to rule out an embedded tooth fragment. Through and through lacerations of the lips should be closed in three layers. The first layer should be placed within the oral labial mucosa using a 4-0 or 5-0 absorbable suture. The laceration should then be recleansed now that it is sealed off from the oral flora. The second layer should be placed in the muscle using a 5-0 absorbable suture and the third layer should be placed in the skin using a 6-0 nonabsorbable suture. The first suture in the skin should be placed at the vermillion border. Patients should be advised to eat a soft diet and carefully rinse out their mouth after each meal. Prophylactic use of oral antibiotics for lacerations of the oral mucosa is recommended.

With ear lacerations it is important to identify any underlying injuries to the cartilage. A field block performed at the base of the ear is helpful with extensive ear injuries. With simple lacerations primary repair of the overlying skin, ensuring complete coverage of the cartilage, suffices using nonabsorbable 6-0 sutures. Large or gaping lacerations of the cartilage may be closed with a 6-0 monofilament nonabsorbable suture. Any hematoma beneath the skin needs to be evacuated and a compressive dressing should be placed to ensure adequate contact between the skin and the cartilage. Due to its relative avascularity, necrosis of the cartilage with subsequent formation of a "cauliflower" ear may result if the cartilage is deprived of its vascular supply. With exposure of cartilage, prophylactic oral antibiotic coverage for staphylococcus and pseudomonas is recommended.

With eyelid lacerations it is crucial to exclude any injury to the lacrimal duct or the tarsal plate. These lacerations, as well as those involving the lid margins and inner surface, should be repaired by a specialist. The presence of ptosis should always prompt referral. See Chapter 176, "Eye Trauma."

Post Repair Wound Care

Post repair wound care should optimize healing. It must be tailored to both the type of wound and method of wound closure. Sutured or stapled lacerations should be covered with a protective nonadherent dressing for 24 to 48 hours until enough epithelization takes place to protect the wound from gross contamination. Maintenance of a moist wound environment increases the rate of reepithelization. Additionally, pressure dressings minimize the accumulation of the intercellular fluid dead space. When possible, the site of injury should be elevated above the patient's heart to limit the accumulation of fluid in the wound interstitial spaces. The wound with little edema heals more rapidly than one with marked edema.

Topical antibiotic ointments may help reduce infection rates and prevent scab formation (12). Patients whose lacerations are closed with tissue adhesives should not have topical ointments applied. They will loosen the adhesive and result in dehiscence.

Prophylactic antibiotic administration should not be used as a regular adjunct to wound care. Several studies and a metaanalysis have found no benefit to prophylactic antibiotics for routine laceration repair (9). Use of antibiotics should be individualized on the basis of the degree of bacterial contamination, the presence of infection-potentiating factors (e.g., soil), the mechanism of injury, and presence or absence of host predisposition to infection. In general, decontamination is far more important than antibiotics. Antibiotics should be used in most human, dog, and cat bites; intraoral lacerations; open fractures; and exposed joints or tendons (39). Additionally, patients with soft-tissue lacerations who are prone to the development of infective endocarditis,

TABLE 172.8. Optimal Time from Placement of Sutures until Suture Removal

Location	No. of Days
Face	3–5
Oral Mucosa	3–5
Scalp	7
Chest	8–10
Back	10–14
Forearm	10–14
Fingers	8–10
Hand	8–10
Lower extremity	8–12
Foot	10–12

patients with prosthetic joints and other permanent "hardware," and patients with lymphedema should receive antimicrobial therapy. Intravenous antibiotics can be given prior to wound care in patients at high risk for systemic complications of infected soft-tissue injuries.

Sutured or stapled wounds should be kept clean and gently cleansed after 24 to 48 hours. Patients with tissue adhesives may shower, but they should avoid bathing and swimming; prolonged moisture will loosen the adhesive bond. Gentle blotting should be used to dry the area, as wiping could result in dehiscence. Elevation of the injured area decreases edema formation. Splinting may prove helpful in areas subject to high tension (e.g., in lacerations across joints). Patients should be instructed to observe the wound for erythema, warmth, swelling, and drainage, as these findings may indicate infection. Use of standardized wound-care instructions improves patient compliance and understanding.

Sutures or staples in most locations should be removed after approximately 7 days (Table 172.8). Facial sutures should be removed sooner (within 3 to 5 days) to avoid the formation of unsightly sinus tracts. Sutures subject to high tension (e.g., in joints, hands) should be left in for 10 to 14 days. When tissue adhesives are used, take care to avoid picking or scrubbing the area or exposure of it to water for more than brief periods until the previously noted times. When tissue adhesives remain on the skin for prolonged periods, antibiotic ointment, petroleum jelly, or bathing can accelerate removal. Acetone can be used when more rapid removal is required. Patients should be told when and with whom to follow up for suture removal or wound examination.

Abraded skin may develop permanent hyperpigmentation after exposure to the sun (38). Consequently, abraded skin should be protected with a sun-blocking agent for at least 6 to 12 months after injury.

Prevention of Tetanus

Two-thirds of the recent tetanus cases in the United States have followed lacerations, puncture wounds, and crush injuries. For every wounded patient, information about the mechanism of injury, the characteristics of the wound and its age, previous active immunization status, history of a neurologic or severe hypersensitivity reaction after a previous immunization treatment, and plans for follow-up should be recorded in a permanent medical record.

Proper immunization plays the most important role in tetanus prophylaxis. Recommendations on tetanus prophylaxis are based on the condition of the wound and the patient's immunization history. A summary guide to tetanus prophylaxis of the wounded patient, as recommended by the CDC, is outlined in Table 172.1. As noted, passive immunization with tetanus immunoglobulin (TIG) is indicated only under specific conditions.

The only contraindication to tetanus and diphtheria toxoids is a history of neurologic or severe hypersensitivity reaction after a previous dose. Local side effects do not preclude repeated use. Local reactions, generally erythema and induration with or without tenderness, are common after the administration of vaccines containing diphtheria, tetanus, and pertussis antigens. These reactions are usually self-limited and require no therapy. If a systemic reaction is suspected to represent allergic hypersensitivity, immunization should be postponed until appropriate skin testing is undertaken. If the use of a tetanus toxoid is contraindicated, passive immunization against tetanus should be considered in a tetanus-prone wound. In those patients who have not completed a primary tetanus immunization series, appropriate follow-up should include referral to a physician who can complete active immunization.

CRITICAL INTERVENTIONS

- Obtain a tetanus immunization history and administer tetanus toxoid if it has not been given within the past 10 years (5 years if the wound is tetanus-prone)
- Perform and document a neurovascular assessment distal to the laceration
- Perform and document a careful wound exploration to exclude foreign bodies and tendon lacerations

DISPOSITION

The appropriate surgical specialist should be consulted for patients with open fractures of long bones, nerve or vascular injuries, flexor tendon disruptions, repair of specialized structures such as the parotid or lacrimal duct, replacement of skin loss by a flap or graft, or extensive debridement.

Few patients with lacerations will require admission to the hospital. Even those patients requiring surgical intervention can often be discharged with appropriate follow-up arrangements. Often, definitive repair can be accomplished via same-day surgery.

If the initial receiving hospital does not have the appropriate emergency or surgical specialist, transfer is necessary. The patient should be transferred in the most expeditious manner possible.

COMMON PITFALLS

✔ Failure to detect sensory, motor, and vascular complications or injuries to specialized tissues
✔ Failure to detect and remove foreign bodies
✔ Using vasoconstrictors in anesthetic agents in areas with terminal end-arteriole blood supply
✔ Removing hair with a razor since it may increase the infection rate
✔ Using antiseptic agents such that there is contact between the agent and the wound
✔ Using drain placement as a replacement for meticulous hemostasis; drains should be reserved for removal of harmful collections of fluid
✔ Using tissue adhesives without appropriate cleansing and exploration
✔ Using tissue adhesives in high-tension wounds or over joints
✔ Failure to understand the different indications for using butyl- and cyanoacrylate tissue adhesives

References

1. Austin PE, Dunn KA, Eily-Cofield K, Brown CK, Wooden WA, Bradfield JF. Subcuticular sutures and the rate of inflammation in noncontaminated wounds. *Ann Emerg Med* 1995;25:328–330.
2. Baker MD, Lanuti M. The management and outcome of lacerations in urban children. *Ann Emerg Med* 1990;19:1001–1005.
3. Bartfield JM, Gennis P, Barbera J, Breuer B, Gallagher EJ. Buffered versus plain lidocaine as a local anesthetic for simple laceration repair. *Ann Emerg Med* 1990;19;1387–1389.
4. Berk WA, Osbourne DD, Taylor DD. Evaluation of the "golden period" for wound repair: 204 cases from a third world emergency department. *Ann Emerg Med* 1988;17:496–500.
5. Brogan GX, Giarrusso E, Hollander JE, Cassara G, Maranga MC, Mode Jr. HC. Comparison of plain, warmed, and buffered lidocaine for anesthesia of traumatic wounds. *Ann Emerg Med* 1995;26:121–125.
6. Bruns TB, Robinson BS, Smith RJ, Kile DL, Davis TP, Sullivan JV. A new tissue adhesive for laceration repair in children. *J Pediatr* 1998;132:1067–1070.
7. Capellan O, Hollander JE. Management of lacerations in the emergency department. In: Peth HA, ed. *High Risk Presentations. Emergency Medicine Clinics of North America.* Philadelphia: WB Saunders, 2003;21:205–231.
8. Cardany CR, Rodeheaver G, Thacker J, Edgerton MT, Edlich RF. The crush injury: a high risk wound. *JACEP* 1976;5(12):965–970.
9. Cummings P, Del Beccaro MA. Antibiotics to prevent infection of simple wounds: a meta-analysis of randomized studies. *Am J Emerg Med* 1995;13(4):396–400.
10. deHoll D, Rodeheaver G, Edgerton MT, Edlich, RF. Potentiation of infection by suture closure of dead space. *Am J Surg* 1974;127:716.
11. Dire DJ, Welsh AP. A comparison of wound irrigation solutions used in the emergency department. *Ann Emerg Med* 1990;19:704–708.
12. Dire DJ, Coppola M, Dwyer DA, Lorette JJ, Karr JL. A prospective evaluation of topical antibiotics for preventing infections in uncomplicated soft-tissue wounds repaired in the ED. *Acad Emerg Med* 1995;2:4–10.
13. Edlich RF, Rodeheaver GT, Morgan RF, Berman DE, Thacker JG. Principles of emergency wound management. *Ann Emerg Med* 1988;17:1284–1302.
14. Ernst AA, Marvez-Valls E, Mall G, et al. 1% Lidocaine versus 0.5% diphenhydramine for local anesthesia in minor laceration repair. *Ann Emerg Med* 1994;23:1328–1332.
15. Ernst AA, Marvez-Valls E, Nick TG, et al. LAT versus TAC for topical anesthesia in face and scalp lacerations. *Am J Emerg Med* 1995;13:151–154.
16. Guy RJ, Zook EG. Successful treatment of acute head and neck dog bite wounds without antibiotics. *Ann Plastic Surg* 1986;17:45–48.
17. Haury B, Rodeheaver G, Vensko J, Edgerton MT, Edlich RF. Debridement: an essential component of traumatic wound care. *Am J Surg* 1978;135:238–242.
18. Hollander JE, Singer AJ, Valentine S, Henry MC. Wound registry: development and validation. *Ann Emerg Med* 1995;25:675–685.
19. Hollander JE, Richman PB, Werblud M, Miller T, Huggler J, Singer AJ. Irrigation in facial and scalp lacerations: does it alter outcome? *Ann Emerg Med* 1998;31:73–77.
20. Hollander JE, Singer AJ. State of the art laceration management. *Ann Emerg Med* 1999;34:356–367.
21. Johnson A, Rodeheaver GT, Durand LS, Edgerton MT, Edlich RF. Automatic disposable stapling devices for wound closure. *Ann Emerg Med* 1981;10:631–635.
22. Krause RS, Moscatti R, Filice M, Lerner EB, Hughes D. The effect of injection speed on the pain of lidocaine infiltration. *Acad Emerg Med* 1997;4:1032–1035.
23. Lammers R. Plantar puncture wounds. In: Singer AJ, Hollander JE, eds. *Lacerations and Acute Wounds. An Evidenced-Based Guide.* Philadelphia: FA Davis, 2003;157–160.
24. Magee C, Rodeheaver GT, Golden GT, et al. Potentiation of wound infection by surgical drains. *Am J Surg* 1976;131:547.
25. Mattick A, Clegg G, Beattie T, et al. A randomised, controlled trial comparing a tissue adhesive (2-octylcyanoacrylate) with adhesive strips (Steristrips) for paediatric laceration repair. *Emerg Med J* 2002;19:405–4057.
26. McCaig LF, Burt CW. National Hospital Ambulatory Medical Care Survey: 2001 emergency department summary. Advance data from vital health statistics; no 335. Hyattsville, Maryland: National Center for Health Statistics, 2003.
27. Mehta PH, Dunn KA, Bradfield JF, Austin PE. Contaminated wounds: infection rates with subcutaneous sutures. *Ann Emerg Med* 1996;27:43–48.
28. Merguerian PA, Klein RB, Graven MA, Rozychi AA. Intraoperative anaphylactic reaction due to latex hypersensitivity. *Urology* 1991;308:301.
29. Mittra ES, Singer AJ, Bluestein D, et al. Simulated wound irrigation impact pressures. *Israeli J Emerg Med* 2003;3:9–16.
30. Morgan WJ, Hutchison D, Johnson HM. The delayed treatment of wounds of the hand and forearm under antibiotic cover. *Br J Surg* 1980;67:140–141.
31. Osmond MH, Quinn JV, Sutcliffe T, et al. A randomized, clinical trial comparing butylcyanoacrylate with octylcyanoacrylate in the management of selected pediatric facial lacerations. *Acad Emerg Med* 1999;6:171–177.
32. Quinn JV, Drzewiecki A, Li MM, Stiell IG, Elmslic TJ, Wood WE. A randomized, controlled trial comparing a tissue adhesive with suturing in the repair of pediatric facial lacerations. *Ann Emerg Med* 1993;22:1130–1135.
33. Quinn JV, Wells GA, Sutcliffe T, Jarmuske M, May J, Stiell I, Johns P. Tissue adhesive vs. suture wound repair at one year: randomized clinical trial correlating early, three-month, and one-year cosmetic outcome. *Ann Emerg Med* 1998;32:645–649.
34. Ritchie AJ, Rocke LG. Staples versus sutures in the closure of scalp wounds: a prospective, double-blind, randomized trial. *Injury* 1989;20:217–218.
35. Rodeheaver GT, Halverson JM, Edlich RF. Mechanical performance of wound closure tapes. *Ann Emerg Med* 1983;12:203–207.
36. Ruthman JC, Hendricksen D, Miller RF, Quigg DL. Effect of cap and mask on infection rates. *Illinois Med J* 1984;165:397–399.
37. Seropian R, Reynolds BM. Wound infections after preoperative depilation versus razor preparation. *Am J Surg* 1971;121:251–254.
38. Ship AG, Weiss PR. Pigmentation after dermabrasion: an avoidable complication. *Plast Reconstr Surg* 1985;75:528.
39. Singer AJ, Hollander JE, Quinn JV. Evaluation and management of traumatic lacerations. *N Engl J Med* 1997;337:1142–1148.
40. Singer AJ, Hollander JE, Valentine SM, Turque TW, McCuskey CF, Quinn JV. Prospective randomized controlled trial of tissue adhesive (2-octylcyanoacrylate) vs standard wound closure techniques for laceration repair. *Acad Emerg Med* 1998;5:94–99.
41. Singer AJ, Stark MJ. LET vs. EMLA for pretreating lacerations—a randomized trial. *Acad Emerg Med* 2001;8:223–230.
42. Singer AJ, Quinn JV, Thode HC Jr., et al. Determinants of poor outcome after laceration and surgical incision repair. *Plast Reconstr Surg* 2002;110:429–435.
43. Singer AJ, Quinn JV, Hollander JE, et al. Closure of lacerations and incisions with Octylcyanoacrylate: A multi-center randomized clinical trial. *Surgery* 2002;131:270–276.
44. Singer AJ, Giordano P, Fitch JL, et al. Evaluation of a new high viscosity octylcyanoacrylate tissue adhesive for laceration repair. A randomized control trial. *Acad Emerg Med* 2003;10:1134–1137.
45. Singer AJ, Zimmerman T, Rooney J, et al. Comparison of wound bursting strength and surface characteristics of FDA approved tissue adhesive for skin closure. *J Adhesion SciTech*, 2003:in press.
46. Stevenson TR, Thacker JG, Rodeheaver GT, Bacchetta C, Edgerton MT, Edlich RF. Cleansing the traumatic wound by high pressure syringe irrigation. *JACEP* 1976;5:17–21.
47. Tarsia V, Singer AJ. Comparison of regional and local anesthesia for facial lacerations. *Acad Emerg Med* 2002;9:449.
48. Valente JH, Forti RJ, Freundlich LF, et al. Wound irrigation: tap water or saline? *Acad Emerg Med* 2001;8:539.
49. Whorl GJ. Repairing skin lacerations: does sterile technique matter? *Can Fam Physician* 1987;33:1185–1187.

PART II

Specific Injuries

CHAPTER 173
Head Injuries

Pierre Borczuk and Stephen H. Thomas

Data from the National Institute of Neurologic Disorders and Stroke estimate that there are 2,000,000 cases of traumatic brain injury (TBI) in the United States per year, with approximately 500,000 patients requiring hospitalization. There are many more patients who do not seek any medical attention after mild head trauma. A review of U.S. mortality data reveals that head injury is responsible for 26% of trauma-related deaths. TBI deaths are bimodal, with a peak in the 15- to 24-year-old age group due to motor vehicle collisions and a second peak due mostly to falls in the 75-year-old and older group (19). The economic impact of head injury in the U.S. is estimated to exceed $25 billion annually (19).

Primary brain injury refers to the irreversible damage that occurs at the time of the head injury. The nature of crucial interventions in the emergency department (ED) depends on the severity of the head injury. In patients with moderate TBI (Glasgow Coma Scale [GCS] score of 9 to 12) (Table 173.1) and severe TBI (GCS less than or equal to 8), the goal is to adequately resuscitate the patient to halt any further central nervous system (CNS) damage, referred to as secondary brain injury. This includes treatment and prevention of hypotension, hypoxia, seizures, herniation, and possible CNS infections. Primary brain injury prevention refers to the public health initiatives, such as automobile seat belt laws or motorcycle helmet laws, that can decrease the incidence of serious head injury. In patients with mild head trauma (GCS 13 to 15), the initial challenge is to identify which patients harbor a significant intracranial lesion that may lead to neurologic deterioration and require neurosurgical intervention (2).

CLINICAL PRESENTATION

The clinical presentation of patients with head trauma has been arbitrarily divided into mild, moderate, and severe categories based on the GCS. Over 80% of patients seen by emergency physicians will have a GCS of 13 to 15. Alcohol and other drugs are the most common causes of a loss in points on the GCS for verbal response. Patients may complain of headache, nausea, or vomiting; have a history of loss of consciousness or amnesia; or have external signs of head trauma. The possibility of a coexisting cervical spine injury should be considered, and the patient should be placed in cervical spine precautions until injury has been ruled out. In addition, the patient with an altered sensorium from TBI may require radiologic imaging and observation to determine whether there is coexisting intraabdominal injury. Concurrent medical conditions may need prompt identification and treatment.

Seizures increase the metabolic requirements of the brain and produce hypoxia and hypercarbia, which promote secondary brain injury. Transtentorial herniation from a laterally based intracranial hematoma causes downward pressure on the uncus, which in turn causes compression of the ipsilateral third cranial nerve, and therefore produces pupillary dilation on the same side as the hematoma (Fig. 173.1). Central herniation from brain lesions in deeper structures will present with obtundation and hydrocephalus. Subfalcine herniation involves midline shift of the cingulate gyrus. This may entrap the anterior cerebral artery, causing contralateral leg weakness.

Skull fractures span a continuum from linear, nondisplaced and nonpalpable to depressed cranial defects that may be open and extruding brain matter. Fractures involving the lateral

---

TABLE 173.1.   Glasgow Coma Scale

EYE OPENING

Opens Spontaneously	4
Opens Eyes to Verbal Command	3
Opens Eyes to Pain	2
Does Not Open Eyes	1

VERBAL RESPONSE

Alert and Oriented	5
Converses But Disoriented	4
Speaking But Nonsensical	3
Moans or Makes Unintelligible Sounds	2
No Response	1

MOTOR RESPONSE

Follows Commands	6
Localizes Pain	5
Movement or Withdrawal to Pain	4
Abnormal Flexion (Decorticate)	3
Abnormal Extension (Decerebate)	2
No Response	1
	3–15

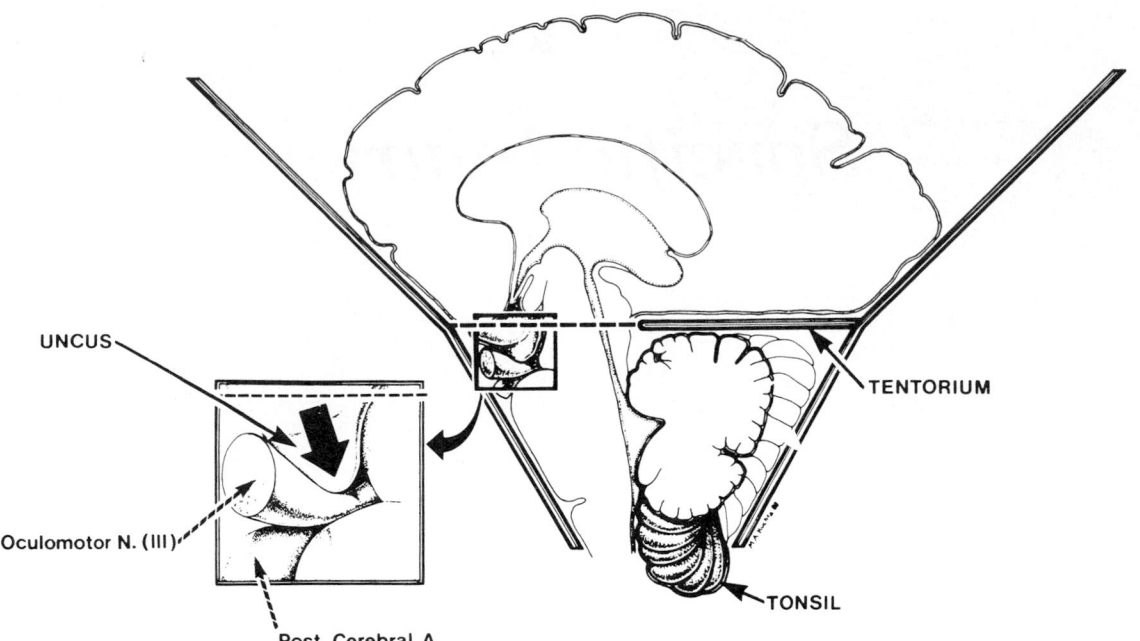

Figure 173.1. The intracranial cavity depicted as a funnel and subdivided by the tentorium into the supratentorial and the infratentorial compartments. Note herniation of the ipsilateral uncus with compression of the adjacent third cranial nerve and the posterior cerebral artery. Note also cerebellar tonsillar herniation with compression against the medulla.

aspects of the skull may involve the middle meningeal artery groove. Since this vessel is associated with epidural hematomas, computed tomography (CT) investigation is warranted. Basilar skull fractures may present as periorbital ecchymosis ("raccoon eyes"), retroauricular ecchymosis (*Battle's sign*), hemotympanum, or a cerebrospinal fluid (CSF) leak from the ears or nose. Open fractures, especially ones that are depressed, and CSF leaks place the patient at risk for infection.

Epidural hematomas (EDHs) usually result from a blow to the head that fractures the skull immediately adjacent to the middle meningeal artery (Fig. 173.2). The arterial pressure is able to dissect the dura away from the inner skull table. This occurs less commonly in elderly patients, as the dura is more closely attached to the periosteum. The classic history of a blow to the head, loss of consciousness, a lucid interval, and subsequent deterioration is seen in less than 30% of patients. EDH is an operative emergency. Prompt neurosurgical intervention is important, as operative patients who exhibit intact neurologic examinations have a mortality of close to zero. Mortality in unconscious operative patients is approximately 20% (16). EDHs can also involve middle meningeal veins, diploic veins and venous sinuses; these lower pressure collections are more commonly seen in the pediatric population, are not associated with skull fractures, and can develop over longer periods of time.

Subdural hematomas (SDH) are more common than EDHs, and they can be present in as many as 70% of patients with moderate and severe head trauma. Individuals with brain atrophy (i.e., elderly and chronic alcoholic patients) are more susceptible to damage to bridging veins in the increased subdural space produced by rotational or acceleration–deceleration mechanisms. Subdural hematomas are characterized by the time it takes for patients to become symptomatic after injury (Fig. 173.3). Acute SDH appears as a crescent-shaped, hyperdense (whiter than brain tissue) mass on CT scan. As the time to presentation increases, the SDH becomes less dense and can appear isodense when compared with brain tissue. Chronic SDHs are hypodense and become symptomatic more than 2 weeks after injury. In elderly

patients, there may be no history of trauma, and patients may present with a more subtle change in cognition and mental status (Fig. 173.4). SDHs exhibit a higher mortality than do EDHs; this can approach 70%. Patients with signs of neurologic dysfunction usually require clot evacuation.

Cerebral contusions are the most common lesions seen on cranial CT scans in patients with mild head trauma. They are found in frontal, temporal, and occipital regions and are frequently seen

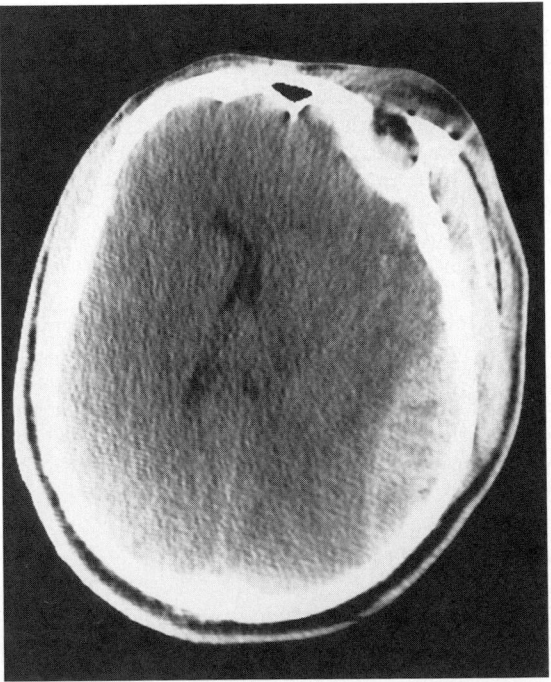

Figure 173.2. A case of EDH. Note the classic biconvex, hyperdense lesion on the CT scan. This patient underwent urgent clot evacuation in the ED.

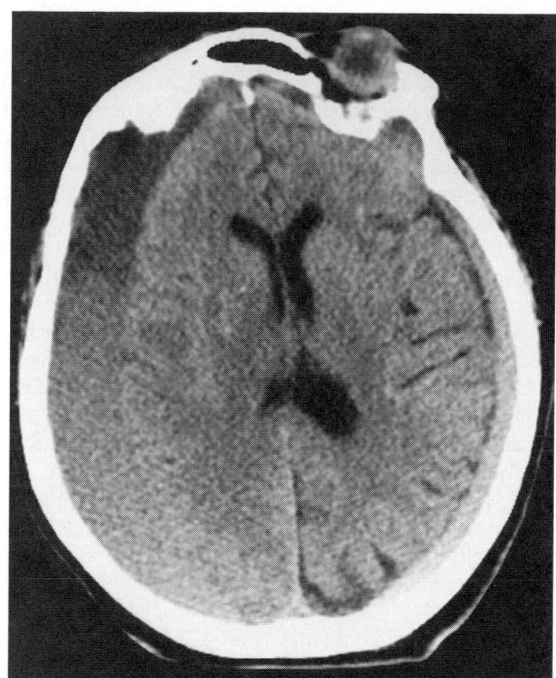

Figure 173.3.   An elderly woman with change of mental status after a fall. Note the bilateral, subacute SDHs, with varying densities and layering.

on the inferior surfaces of these lobes (because the skull base has a rough interior). Contusions can vary from punctate (millimeters in size) to several centimeters in size collections of blood, necrotic brain tissue, and edema. Complications include worsening edema and rebleeding from injured vessels. Patients may exhibit focal neurologic deficits if contusions occur in the sensorimotor strip.

Traumatic subarachnoid hemorrhages (SAH), while causing headache and nausea, are otherwise inconsequential and have

an excellent prognosis. However, one must be certain that the patient's head trauma is not secondary to a ruptured CNS aneurysm causing the traumatic head injury and SAH seen on CT. Blood near the circle of Willis is of concern for an aneurysmal bleed.

Diffuse axonal injury (DAI) is used to describe a clinical syndrome in which the patient is in a coma, but no culprit lesion is discovered on CT scan. Deceleration and rotational mechanisms of injury cause shear forces that can disrupt axons in the white matter of the brain and brainstem. Patients with milder forms of DAI may be in coma for several hours, while more severe cases can suffer from cerebral edema, herniation, or persistent coma states. Magnetic resonance imaging (MRI) may be used to detect abnormalities in patients with DAI but is usually not performed in the ED.

Concussion is very common and ranks third highest in incidence among all neurologic diseases, behind migraine headache and herpes zoster. Symptoms include headache, nausea, blurry vision, unsteadiness, vertigo, sleep disturbance, emotional lability, and difficulty with concentration. Concussions are usually associated with a period of altered consciousness, that can include amnesia. A certain number of patients remain symptomatic after trauma. These patients usually undergo CT scanning. If the CT does not show any traumatic lesions, then the patient is diagnosed with a *postconcussive syndrome*. The duration of symptoms noted after a head injury is related to the patient's age and the length of posttraumatic amnesia and can last from days to years after the initial trauma.

Penetrating head trauma most commonly results from firearm injuries. The projectile may traverse the skull or may ricochet intracranially, making anatomic prediction of injury clinically difficult. The overall mortality of patients who arrive in the ED with penetrating head trauma is greater than 60%. Cranial CT will demonstrate bleeding, skull fragments, bullet fragments, and intracranial air (pneumocephalus) (Fig. 173.5). Impaled objects should be left in place in the ED and removed in the operating room.

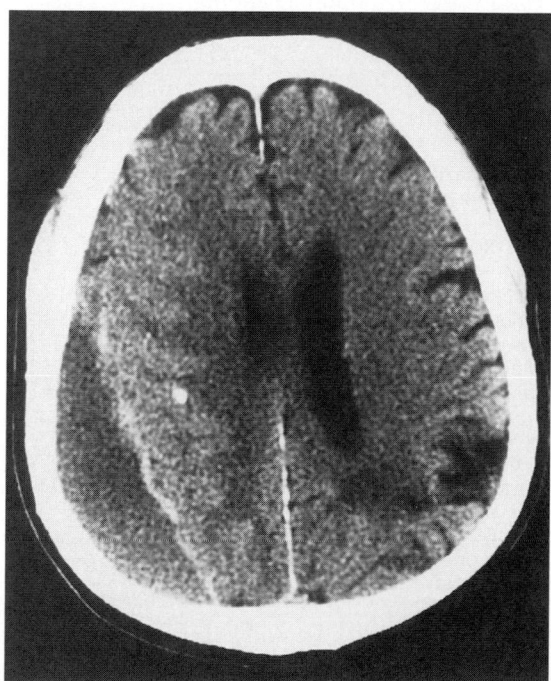

Figure 173.4.   A male presents 3 weeks after a fall, with increased sleepiness and change in personality. Cranial CT scan demonstrates a chronic SDH.

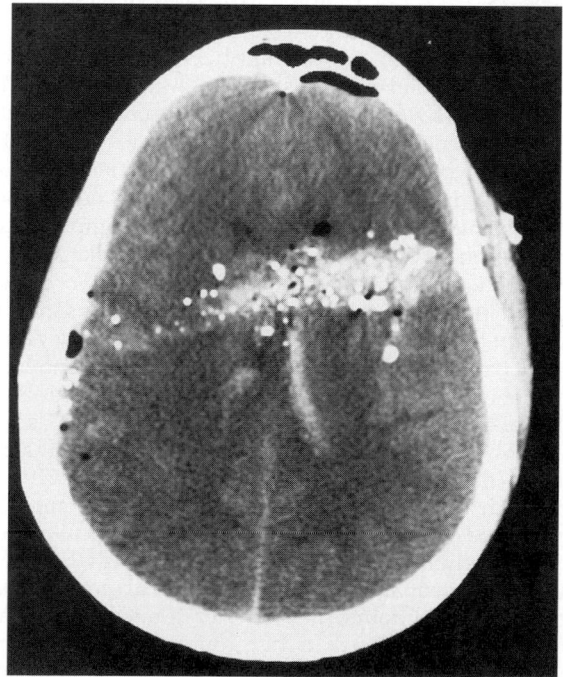

Figure 173.5.   A self-inflicted wound from a handgun. CT scan reveals injury to the bilateral hemispheres and intracranial fragments of bone, bullet, and air.

DIFFERENTIAL DIAGNOSIS

The dramatic presentation of the trauma patient should not detract the physician from considering other medical conditions that could have contributed to the trauma or that may be causing a change in mental status. Myocardial infarction, dysrhythmia, a cerebrovascular event, or a seizure may have been the primary insult that precipitated the head trauma. Causes of hypotension, including infection and sepsis, and gastrointestinal bleeding should also be considered. Secondary factors should especially be considered in patients involved in single automobile collisions or falls. The etiology of an altered sensorium in a patient with TBI may also be multifactorial. One should consider metabolic causes, including hypo- and hyperthermia and hypo- and hyperglycemia. Drugs, both legal and illicit, may also play a role in the patient with a change in mental status, with alcohol the most common ingestion noted. Frequently, a complete and reliable history cannot be obtained, and proper management by the clinician requires maintenance of a broad differential diagnosis and systematic exclusion of medical conditions through testing.

EMERGENCY DEPARTMENT EVALUATION

The general goal in the management of patients with head trauma is to minimize further brain injury from secondary insults such as hypotension, hypoxia, herniation, seizures, and infection (7). Prehospital information such as mechanism of injury, vehicle speed, airbag deployment, height of a fall, loss of consciousness, posttraumatic seizures, or alterations in neurologic function since the accident will determine the need for urgent neuroimaging and for neurosurgical consultation. Other important historical components include a history of cardiac disease or stroke, diabetes mellitus, as well as conditions that suggest the patient may be coagulopathic (cirrhosis, hemophilia, or, more commonly, warfarin use).

The crucial initial intervention is based on the patient's general appearance and vital signs. All resuscitations begin with the ABCs. Both hypotension (systolic blood pressure less than 90) and hypoxia (PaO₂ less than 60) have been shown to be independent predictors of poor outcome. Hypotension has been associated with a doubling of mortality, even when controlled for trauma to extracranial organ systems (6). As many as one-fourth of patients with severe brain injury are hypoxic and hypotensive. The emergency physician needs to be aggressive at volume-resuscitating hypotensive head injury patients, without the fear that excess fluids will lead to brain swelling and herniation.

After the initial ABCs, the clinician should complete the primary and secondary surveys, with a focus on pupillary size, symmetry, and motor function. Intervention is necessary if there is evidence of increased intracranial pressure (ICP) or signs of herniation, or if the patient demonstrates seizure activity. After stabilization, patients with severe head injury should undergo CT.

In patients with *mild head injury*, ED evaluation focuses on the selection of those patients who need urgent cranial CT scans, as well as the evaluation of any other medical conditions that might have led to the trauma. The prevalence of a positive CT scan in patients with a GCS of 13 to 15 is in the 7% to 18% range, while the prevalence of lesions that require a neurosurgical procedure is approximately 1% (19). A subgroup of patients who "talk and deteriorate" present to the ED with GCS verbal scores of 4 and 5. However, within 24 hours, they deteriorate and will have a total GCS less than or equal to 8. In this group, mortality is high, and the survivors tend to be severely disabled. The most common CT finding is an SDH, which causes a greater than 10-mm midline shift (Fig. 173.4) (12).

Many investigators have tried to elucidate risk factors that identify which of these apparently low-risk patients harbor sig-

nificant intracranial pathology. Some clinicians use the presence of loss of consciousness or amnesia as a marker to screen patients for urgent cranial CT scan (2,8,14,20). The alcoholic patient who experiences head trauma is a frequent visitor to the ED. A strategy of serial observation until sobriety is achieved is a common one, although, as previously stated, once the patient has undergone deterioration, the outcome is significantly worse. There have been two prospective studies aimed at defining which ED patients with mild head trauma and loss of consciousness or amnesia require a cranial CT scan. Both studies involved the development of a set of decision rules to order a CT scan based on maximizing sensitivity for finding acute intracranial pathology. In these studies, the rules or algorithms were then validated on another large patient group. The Charity hospital group (9) included pediatric patients and developed a seven-variable decision rule that included age >60, trauma above the clavicles, headache, vomiting, intoxication, short-term memory deficits and seizure. Ordering a CT scan based on the presence of any of these criteria yields a sensitivity of 100% (95% CI 95–100) and a specificity of 25% (95% CI 22–28). The Canadian Head CT (21) rule has a sensitivity of 98.4% (95% CI 96–99) and a specificity of 49.6% (95% CI 48–51) using the presence of any one of the following as an indication for CT scan: age ≥65, signs of a basilar skull fracture, GCS <15 2 hours post injury, vomiting ≥2 episodes, suspected open or depressed skull fracture, amnesia before impact >30 minutes, and a dangerous mechanism of injury. One can conclude that elderly patients compose a high-risk subgroup for acute intracranial pathology. In the mild head trauma patient, the moderate risk factors listed in Table 173.2 may prompt the physician to order a cranial CT scan.

Skull films should not be used to rule out intracranial injury, as they can have a false-negative rate as high as 80% (13). Skull fractures, however, should raise the suspicion for further

---

TABLE 173.2.   Categorizations for Imaging Head Trauma Patients

LOW-RISK GROUP

Asymptomatic
Headaches
Dizziness
Scalp hematoma, laceration, contusion
Adequate home observation

MODERATE-RISK GROUP

History of altered consciousness
History of progressive headache
Alcohol or drug intoxication
Unreliable or inadequate history of injury
Age <2 years and >60 years (unless trivial injury)
Posttraumatic seizure
Vomiting
Posttraumatic amnesia
Multiple trauma
Serious facial injury
Signs of basilar skull penetration or depressed fracture
Possible skull penetration or depressed fracture
Suspected physical child abuse

HIGH-RISK GROUP

Depressed level of consciousness not clearly caused by *alcohol or drug use* or other causes
Focal neurologic signs
Decreasing level of consciousness
Penetrating skull injury or palpable depressed fracture

intracranial injury; the range of associated injury is between 7% and 50%, depending on the study reviewed (13).

MRI scans are generally more difficult to obtain and take longer to perform than cranial CT scans. They are useful in those instances when posterior fossa injuries or nonhemorrhagic injuries, especially diffuse axonal injury, are suspected. However, cranial CT scans are much better than MRI scans for the detection of skull fractures and hemorrhage (17).

EMERGENCY DEPARTMENT MANAGEMENT

The prehospital phase begins with secondary injury prevention. Airway management, intravenous access, and fluid resuscitation, as well as spinal immobilization, should be initiated by paramedics. Determination of a scene GCS, detection and treatment of hypoglycemia, control of seizures, and "coma cocktail" administration should also begin in the prehospital phase. Prehospital personnel are frequently the sole source of information from scene witnesses regarding trauma mechanism or details regarding loss of consciousness.

ED management begins with the primary survey and the ABCs. Managing the airway includes use of rapid-sequence techniques (22). (See Chapter 170, "Trauma Airway Management.") Patients with an initial GCS less than or equal to 8 or a decreasing level of consciousness are unable to protect their airway and require intubation. As laryngeal stimulation can reflexively increase ICP, blood pressure, and heart rate, the emergency physician should utilize drugs that blunt those increases (e.g., fentanyl and lidocaine) prior to intubation. The FIO_2 should be set at 100%. A patient should not be hyperventilated unless signs of herniation exist. Shock should be treated aggressively with crystalloids and blood. Patients should undergo frequent hemodynamic monitoring, cardiac monitoring, and pulse oximetry. Initial blood analysis, depending on both the degree of head injury and coexistent injury, may include complete blood count, rapid glucose determination, blood urea nitrogen and creatinine, type and screen or cross, a coagulation profile, and a serum ethanol level. Urine screening for drugs of abuse may also be appropriate.

If the patient exhibits signs of intracranial hypertension, several therapeutic options are available (6). Hyperventilation can decrease cerebral blood flow and decrease intracranial hypertension, as cerebral arteries constrict when there is a decrease in hydrogen ions in the CSF. A PCO_2 of 30 is the hyperventilation target. Because of regional imbalances in cerebral perfusion and loss of autoregulation in the early postinjury period, hyperventilation can worsen an ischemic insult. A growing body of evidence indicates that prophylactic hyperventilation in patients with TBI has been shown to be detrimental at 3 and 6 months postinjury (15). Sedation, mannitol, and ICP bolt placement with direct drainage of CSF (if possible) demonstrate a lower risk-to-benefit ratio than hyperventilation (5).

Osmotic diuresis is another modality used to reduce ICP (4,5). Recommended doses of mannitol range from 0.25 to 1.0 g/kg. The duration of action of mannitol ranges from 90 minutes to more than 6 hours. Repeated mannitol use may allow it to concentrate within brain tissue, causing a reverse effect and a worsening of ICP. This occurs in patients with TBI due to disruption of the blood–brain barrier. To avoid accumulation of mannitol within brain tissue, it should be administered as boluses to treat signs of herniation rather than as a continuous infusion. Like hyperventilation, mannitol should be used only in patients who exhibit signs of increased ICP. The patient's fluid status should be carefully monitored to avoid osmotic dehydration. When given as a rapid bolus, mannitol serves as a small-volume resuscitation fluid and will expand intravascular volume and cause an increase in cerebral blood flow (4).

While steroids can decrease edema in patients with intracerebral malignancies, they have no utility in head injury; this finding is supported by prospective randomized trials (3). Active seizures are treated with either diazepam (0.1 mg/kg up to 5-mg bolus i.v. every 5 minutes) or lorazepam (0.05 mg/kg up to 2-mg bolus every 5 minutes), followed by i.v. phenytoin (13- to 18-mg/kg load). Seizure prophylaxis with phenytoin is also commonly used to prevent secondary injury in patients with EDH, SDH, SAH, cortical contusions, depressed skull fractures, severe head injury (GCS ≤8), and penetrating head wounds.

Once the patient's vital signs and neurologic function have been stabilized, the emergency physician should complete the primary and secondary surveys. Patients with severe or moderate head injuries require urgent cranial CT scanning. Any patient with a suspicion of significant intracranial injury requires prompt neurosurgical consultation. Severely compromised patients may go from the CT scanner directly to the operating room for hematoma evacuation. Emergency burr holes may be indicated in the patient who rapidly deteriorates despite the use of conventional ICP-lowering treatments. Neurologic intensive care management of patients with severe intracranial injury is based on the optimization of cerebral perfusion pressure (CPP). Indications for ICP monitoring are severe head injury (GCS 3–8) and a CT scan that reveals hematomas, contusions, edema, or hydrocephalus. ICP and mean arterial blood pressure (MAP) are directly measured. Then, using the relationship CPP = ICP—MAP, CPP should be maintained at a minimum of 60 mm Hg (4).

Basilar skull fractures commonly involve the temporal bone, can cause bleeding in the middle ear and disruption of the auditory bones, and may cause permanent hearing loss. These patients will need ENT consultation. Mastoid air cells can also be affected, and dural tears can present an opportunity for upper respiratory organisms to cause meningitis. However, the incidence of meningitis is small (.7% to 5%) and there is no data to suggest that antibiotic prophylaxis is effective (18).

Linear skull fractures are generally clinically nonsignificant and can be managed on an outpatient basis. However, if the fracture spans a vascular structure, such as the middle meningeal artery groove, or a venous or dural channel, then the patient should be admitted for observation.

Patients with cerebral contusions and nonoperative SDHs are generally admitted for observation with serial examinations, seizure prophylaxis, and follow-up imaging. Patients who have sustained a concussion who are young and have not had a loss of consciousness may have symptoms for days to weeks. Patients who are 55 years old and older who exhibit prolonged posttraumatic amnesia may require months to clear, if they ever have a full recovery. Treatment options include analgesics, antiemetics, cyclic antidepressants, as well as psychotherapy and neurorehabilitation (1).

CRITICAL INTERVENTIONS

- Manage the airway and volume; resuscitate patients with severe head injury to ensure SBP >90 mm Hg and PaO_2 >60 mm Hg
- Protect the cervical spine in patients with head trauma, until radiologic or clinical clearance
- Perform a careful physical examination and prompt CT scanning to identify intracranial mass lesions before the patient suffers a clinical deterioration
- Hyperventilate and administer mannitol only in cases of transtentorial herniation or progressive neurologic deterioration
- Use clinical guidelines, including loss of consciousness, age, and signs of a basilar skull fracture to determine who should undergo cranial CT, in patients with mild head trauma

DISPOSITION

Patients who have documented intracranial pathology and depressed neurologic function (GCS ≤8) should be managed in a facility with immediately available neurosurgical capability and an intensive care unit that can monitor ICP and CPP. This may require safe and expeditious transfer from facilities that lack these capabilities.

A negative cranial CT scan in patients with mild head trauma is useful in deciding who can be safely discharged home, even if a home observer is not available (11). A patient with mild head trauma, in whom a cranial CT scan was not obtained, who has a lack of risk factors for significant injury (e.g., minor mechanism, no loss of consciousness or amnesia) may be discharged home as long as the patient and a competent observer can understand and execute post head injury discharge instructions. This requires the observer to assess the patient every 2 to 3 hours for changes in consciousness, focal neurologic deficits, worsening pain, or persistent vomiting and be able to use a telephone in case help is needed. Medications that cause an alteration in mental status or bleeding should not be used during this observation period of 12 to 24 hours. Patients with mild head injury, for whom a CT scan cannot be obtained, should be transferred to an institution with CT capability.

Protocols have been designed to help manage the patient with a sports-related head injury (10). These management recommendations incorporate the concept and risk of the second impact (reports of severe neurologic sequelae after multiple minor concussions). Concussions are graded on the basis of duration of confusion (15 minutes is the threshold) or loss of consciousness (even if only for seconds). Depending on the number and grade of concussion, the physician may recommend that the athlete remain inactive for a day, a week, or the entire season.

COMMON PITFALLS

✔ Not adequately fluid-resuscitating the hypotensive head-injured patient for fear of worsening brain injury by increasing the risk for swelling

✔ Failure to consider other conditions that contribute to changes in mental status, including stroke, hypoglycemia, or drugs and toxins (including alcohol), that may be present in the head-injured patient

✔ Failure to limit the use of hyperventilation and mannitol to patients with signs of intracranial hypertension

✔ Failure to remember that patients with mild head trauma may have an intracranial injury that can cause neurologic deterioration

✔ Failure to remember that patients 60 years and older with mild head trauma are in a higher risk group for intracranial pathology

References

1. Alexander MP. Mild traumatic brain injury: pathophysiology, natural history, and clinical management. *Neurology* 1995;45:1253.
2. Borczuk P. Predictors of intracranial injury in patients with mild head trauma. *Ann Emerg Med* 1995;25:731.
3. Braakman R, Schouten HJ, Blaaw-van Dishoeck M, et al. Megadose steroids in severe head injury: results of a prospective double blind clinical trial. *J Neurosurg* 1983;58:326.
4. Brain Trauma Foundation. *Management and prognosis of severe traumatic brain injury.* www.braintrauma.org. 2000.
5. Bullock R, Chestnut RM, Clifton G, et al. *Guidelines for the management of severe head injury.* New York: Brain Trauma Foundation, 1996.
6. Chesnut R. Guideline for the management of severe head injury: what we know and what we think we know. *J Trauma* 1997;42(5)[Suppl]:19S.
7. Chesnut RM, Marshall LF, Klauber MR, et al. The role of secondary brain injury in determining outcome from severe head injury. *J Trauma* 1993;34:216.
8. Cheung DS, Kharasch M. Evaluation of the patient with closed head trauma: an evidence based approach. *Emerg Clin North Am* 1999;17(1):9–23.
9. Haydel M. Micelle J.; Preston et al. J.; Indications for computed tomography in patients with minor head injury. *N Engl J Med* 2000;343:100.
10. Kelly J, Rosenberg JH. Diagnosis and management of concussion in sports. *Neurology* 1997;48:575.
11. Livingston DH, Loder PA, Koziol J, et al. The use of CT scanning to triage patients requiring admission following minimal head injury. *J Trauma* 1991;31:343.
12. Marshall LF, Toole BM, Bowers SA. The National Coma Data Bank. Part II. Patients who talk and deteriorate. Implications for treatment. *J Neurosurg* 1983;59:285.
13. Masters SJ. Evaluation of head trauma: efficacy of skull films. *Am J Radiol* 1980;135:539.
14. Miller EC, Derlet RW, Kinser D. Minor head trauma: is computerized tomography always necessary? *Ann Emerg Med* 1996;27:290.
15. Muizelaar JP, Marmarou A, Ward JD, et al. Adverse effects of prolonged hyperventilation in patients with severe head injury: a randomized clinical trial. *J Neurosurg* 1991;75:731.
16. Narayan RK. Closed head injury. In: Rengachary SS, Wilkens RH, eds. *Principles of neurosurgery.* London: Wolfe Publishing, 1994.
17. Orrison WW, Gentry LR, Stimac GK, et al. Blinded comparison of cranial CT and MR in closed head injury evaluation. *Am J Neuroradiol* 1994;15:351.
18. Rathore MH. Do prophylactic antibiotics prevent meningitis after basilar skull fracture? *Pediatr Infect Dis J* 1991;10:87–88.
19. Sosin DM, Sacks JJ, Smith SM. Head injury–associated deaths in the United States from 1979-1986. *JAMA* 1989;262:2251.
20. Stein SC, Ross SE. Minor head injury: a proposed strategy for emergency management. *Ann Emerg Med* 1993;22:1193–1196.
21. Stiell IG, et al. The Canadian CT head rule for patients with minor head injury. *Lancet* 2001;357:1391.
22. Walls RM. Rapid sequence intubation in head trauma. *Ann Emerg Med* 1993;22:1008.

CHAPTER 174
Maxillofacial Injuries

Jayne MacLaughlin and Stephen Colucciello

Over the past decades, the rise in maxillofacial injuries has paralleled the increase in motor vehicle collisions and to a lesser extent, interpersonal violence. The wide variety of traumatic mechanisms and the complexity of the facial structures produce disparate injuries. The most frequently fractured facial bones include the nasal bones, zygoma, maxilla, and mandible, while orbital, ethmoidal, and frontal bone injuries are less common (5,12,31).

CLINICAL PRESENTATION

The presentation of maxillofacial trauma depends largely on the mechanism of injury. Patients who sustain significant blunt trauma (e.g., motor vehicle collision) often suffer multiple injuries and their initial evaluation and stabilization should follow a standard trauma protocol. Neglecting potentially serious chest, abdominal, or pelvic injuries in the multiple trauma patient with distracting facial deformity is a dangerous error. Facial injuries may also be the presenting complaint of a more serious condition—intimate partner violence. In particular, women with facial fractures should be asked whether they are the victim of partner violence; especially if the supposed mechanism of injury is "fall down stairs" or "ran into door."

Victims of penetrating maxillofacial trauma are less likely to have serious injuries to distant organ systems but may experience injury to the globe, brain, or neck. Nearly a third may require urgent airway control, either intubation or cricothyrotomy (17,21). The emergency physician must be particularly attuned to central nervous system (CNS) injury, which occurs in about 20% of victims of penetrating facial trauma (5,6,10,25,29). Loss of vision is another significant concern. Careful examination of the globe and periorbital area may reveal important clues to ocular or periorbital injury, such as decreased visual acuity, visual field cuts, eye pain, limitation of extraocular movements, subconjunctival hemorrhage, lid laceration, diplopia, or infraorbital anesthesia.

Maxillofacial injury becomes a treatment priority when the airway is compromised and less commonly when brisk bleeding occurs. Airway problems result from dislodged teeth, oral hemorrhage, or injury to the soft tissues surrounding the airway. In addition to these immediate risks, delayed edema and hematoma formation may compromise the airway 24 to 48 hours after trauma (24). While this delayed risk of airway compromise has prompted some authors to recommend intubating patients who present with significant intraoral blood or moderate-size hematomas in the neck or face, definitive support in the literature is lacking (6).

The significant vascularity of facial structures may result in substantial blood loss with maxillofacial trauma, occasionally producing hypotension and, rarely, exsanguination. However, the tamponade effect of facial musculature combined with the relative accessibility for direct pressure makes life-threatening hemorrhage in adults unlikely (30).

DIFFERENTIAL DIAGNOSIS

The dramatic appearance of some patients with facial trauma may distract the examining physician from more serious injuries. Once the airway is assured and brisk facial bleeding controlled, other life-threats must be quickly and systematically excluded. Only after life-threatening injuries have been excluded should the emergency physician attempt to specifically address bony and soft-tissue facial injuries.

Head injury is the most common associated injury. This link suggests a low threshold for head computed tomography (CT) in patients with blunt or penetrating maxillofacial injuries who have altered mental status, neurologic deficit, and perhaps a worrisome mechanism of injury (6,31). The converse is also true. In one study, 10% of comatose blunt trauma victims had significant unsuspected facial bone fractures that were diagnosed by routine facial CT (26).

Recent studies cast doubt on the classical association of maxillofacial trauma with cervical spine (c-spine) fracture (6,31). Use of the Nexus or Canadian Cervical Spine Rules provides evidence-based guidelines for cervical radiography (4,13). See Chapter 179, "Cervical Spine Fractures."

EMERGENCY DEPARTMENT EVALUATION

Aside from airway concerns, maxillofacial injuries are seldom life-threatening. However, other organ system injuries occur frequently and carry significant morbidity and potential mortality (5,6,9,12,21,31). After resuscitation and significant injuries to other organ systems are addressed, the emergency physician should perform a thorough and directed examination of the face. Performing an optimal physical examination may be challenged by anatomic complexity, swelling, lacerations, pain, and altered level of consciousness. A systematic approach can help surmount these challenges.

The emergency physician should begin with inspection and evaluate the patient from several perspectives (include looking down from above—"bird's eye view"—and up from below—"worm's eye view") to reveal subtle facial asymmetries. Loss of contours, edema, ecchymosis, and hemorrhage are clues to soft-tissue and underlying bony injuries (Fig. 174.1). Facial elongation in the frontal plane can occur with high-grade Le Fort fractures (11,18). Ecchymoses around the eyes (raccoon eyes) and over the mastoid areas (Battle's sign) are associated with basilar skull fractures. Raccoon eyes, however, are nonspecific and may be

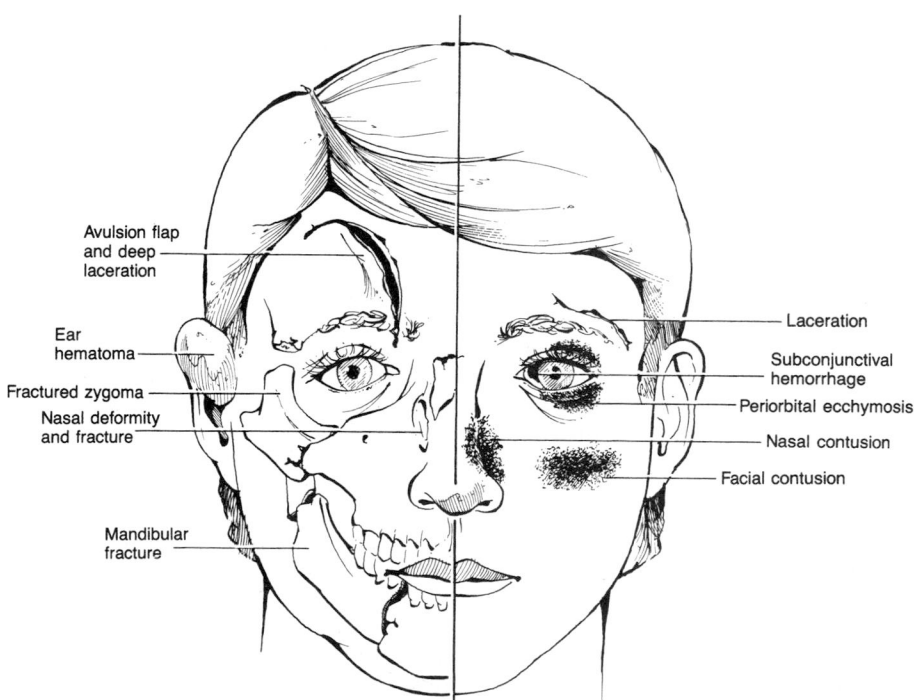

Figure 174.1. Superficial facial injuries provide important visual clues to underlying soft-tissue and bony injuries.

information on the symphysis and body of the mandible, and the lateral oblique view that adds delineation of the mandibular rami.

Open mandibular fractures usually require intravenous antibiotic coverage of oral pathogens. Penicillin G (2 to 4 million units i.v.) is the drug of choice, with clindamycin (600 to 900 mg i.v.) and first-generation cephalosporins serving as alternatives (11). Most closed mandibular fractures can be treated on an outpatient basis with open reduction and internal fixation 3 to 5 days post-injury to allow for swelling to decrease. A Barton's bandage (ace bandage wrapped around the head and jaw) may aid in patient comfort while awaiting definitive treatment. Also, patients will need to eat a soft or liquid diet. The specific treatment plan should be formulated with the appropriate consultant.

Mandibular Dislocations

The temporomandibular joint (TMJ) is also subject to dislocation; this may occur during yawning, singing, or other movements that involve opening the mouth very widely. Dislocation can also occur during seizures or after trauma, and it is often recurrent.

With mandibular dislocation, often the history is difficult to obtain because the patient has difficulty speaking. During inspection, asymmetry of the jaw is a clue to the diagnosis. A unilateral dislocation will often cause deviation of the mandible away from the affected side. A bilateral dislocation of both condyles will give the patient an underbite appearance (bottom teeth more anterior than upper teeth). The teeth will not occlude normally. Often there is significant masseter muscle spasm that can make reduction difficult.

Mandibular dislocations can be reduced by the emergency physician, sometimes requiring benzodiazepines or local anesthetic to relax the masseter or pterygoid muscles. Occasionally, conscious sedation may be required. There are two simple reduction techniques that are often used. In the first technique, the clinician faces the patient with thumbs wrapped in gauze. The physician's thumbs are then placed under the posterior molars or on the mandibular ridge and the inferior surface of the mandible is grasped placing downward pressure on the molars. This will free the condyles and allow them to be pushed forward into place (28). In the second technique, the clinician stands behind the patient with thumbs on the posterior molars and fingers grasping the mandible anteriorly. Pressure is exerted downward and forward until the joint snaps into place (18).

Rarely, neither of the above techniques will work and reduction under general anesthesia may be required. Once reduction is accomplished, the patient's jaw should be wrapped in a Barton's bandage and the patient should be instructed to avoid opening the mouth widely to prevent repeat dislocation. While some physicians obtain x-rays to confirm the relocation of the condyles and to exclude any fractures that occurred during reduction, others do not find this necessary (11,28).

Soft-Tissue Injuries

Almost all patients with facial fractures have associated cutaneous injuries. These do not need to be closed in the patient who will undergo surgical evaluation in the ED, as the opening may be used for examination or repair. Rapid suture ("whip stitching") is appropriate to achieve hemostasis in some cases, as the sutures can be easily removed by the consultant. Laceration repair is discussed in Chapter 172. In addition to lacerations, oral, ocular, salivary, lacrimal, otologic or neurologic injuries may be associated with maxillofacial trauma (Fig. 174.10).

Any dental appliances present should be removed to prevent their aspiration from compromising the airway. These appliances

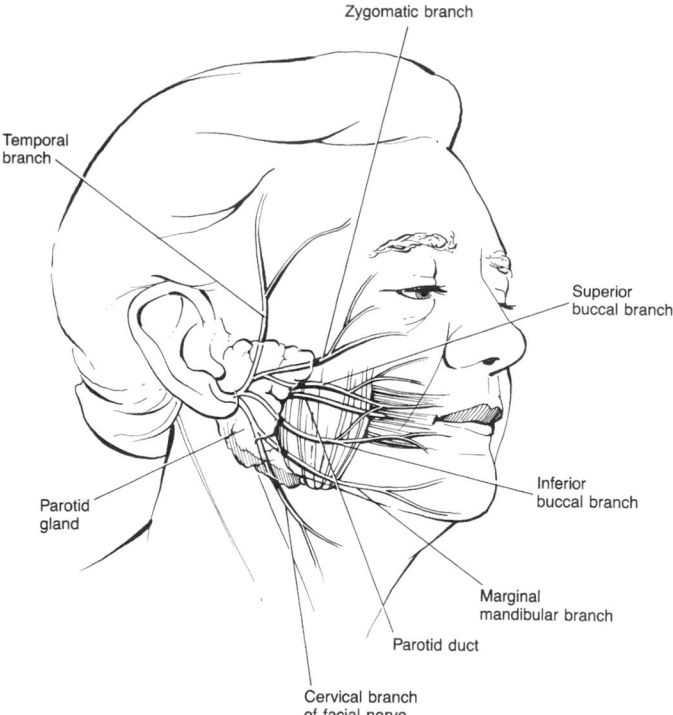

Figure 174.10.   Important soft-tissue structures of the face.

should be saved as they are expensive and may provide important guides to pretraumatic oral alignment.

The significant incidence of ocular injuries associated with various facial fractures necessitates meticulous ophthalmologic evaluation in all patients sustaining maxillofacial trauma. Injuries to the lacrimal system, with associated findings such as epiphora, may be present in patients with midface fractures. Lacrimal disruption is rare in blunt trauma, even in patients with significant craniofacial injury (27). These injuries are discussed in Chapter 176, "Eye Trauma."

Clear or pink fluid leakage from the cheek suggests parotid gland laceration or Stensen's duct damage. Glandular laceration does not require repair, as commonly occurring salivary fistulas resolve spontaneously in less than a month. Stensen's duct may be repaired by suturing the ends together over a stent; this is most appropriately performed by a surgical consultant.

Tympanic membrane rupture can occur when there is significant force applied to the condyles that fractures the temporal bone. They generally heal spontaneously but referral may be necessary in those with large disruptions.

Pediatric Considerations

Fracture patterns and management of fractures differ in children because of the immature facial anatomy and the future growth and development of the maxillofacial structures. There are two major points to consider with facial trauma in children. First, children have a larger head to body mass ratio. Thus, the prominence of the calvarium takes more of the impact in blunt trauma "protecting" the remainder of the face from injury. This accounts for the higher incidence of frontal bone injuries and associated head injuries in children. Up to 60 percent of children with facial fractures have associated intracranial injury (9). Second, because sinuses in children are rudimentary and poorly pneumatized, this further decreases the likelihood of pediatric midface fractures. Once the sinuses are formed, they weaken the bones of the face and predispose older children and adolescents to Le Fort fractures.

There are two fractures that impact future facial development; mandibular condyle fractures and fractures to the nasal septum (16). Condylar fractures can result in growth disturbances, deformity, and ankylosis secondary to damage to the growth centers. Overall, mandibular fractures account for 75% to 90% of facial fractures in children. Displaced nasal injuries can also affect future development of the naso-maxillary buttress. It is important to discuss possible complications with the child's family and refer these children to a surgeon shortly after injury. The initial assessment of pediatric maxillofacial injuries is similar to the adult, but there are some important differences. Because children are more prone to tracheomalacia and subglottic stenosis, cricothyrotomy should be avoided in children less than age 12 (11). If orotracheal intubation is not feasible, laryngeal mask airway (LMA) or transtracheal jet ventilation are useful until a formal tracheostomy can be performed.

Although adults rarely have hemodynamically significant bleeding from facial trauma, children can develop shock from facial blood loss. Bleeding in children is controlled in the same fashion as adults, with direct pressure as a first-line treatment.

Although plain films can be used as initial screening tools, they are not particularly useful in children. Children have a higher proportion of cancellous to cortical bone, making fracture lines difficult to delineate on plain films (16). Facial CT scanning is preferred for evaluation of facial fractures in children.

In addition to the fact that pediatric facial fractures can lead to significant deformity and cosmetic problems, fractures in children heal faster than in adults. Thus it is important that all facial fractures in children be referred for early follow-up. It is preferable that follow-up be within 1 to 3 days, because, within a week, callous formation can complicate reduction (11).

CRITICAL INTERVENTIONS

- Secure the airway in patients with evidence of progressive swelling or airway obstruction using rapid sequence orotracheal intubation
- Have equipment for "back-up" cricothyrotomy readily available when managing the airway of a patient with significant maxillofacial trauma
- Perform CT as the initial radiologic study in patients with a high probability of fracture of the periorbital bones, midface, or frontal sinus. Plain radiographs should be reserved for patients with a low likelihood of fracture
- Perform cranial CT scanning in patients with significant facial fractures to rule out intracranial injury
- Obtain urgent neurosurgical consultation for patients with posterior table fractures of the frontal sinus
- Obtain urgent ophthalmologic consultation for patients with orbital fractures who have paralysis of extraocular motions, ptosis, and periorbital anesthesia (superior orbital fissure syndrome)
- Administer intravenous antibiotics (penicillin or clindamycin) to patients with open facial fractures

DISPOSITION

In the vast majority of patients with maxillofacial trauma, the emergency physician can perform the initial resuscitation and stabilization without the need for consultation with maxillofacial specialists. The role of emergent surgical consultation in patients with airway compromise or refractory facial hemorrhage has been discussed.

Involvement of the appropriate surgical specialist is now recommended at an earlier time than had been standard in the past. Delays in treatment have been shown to result in suboptimal outcome in some facial injuries (7,22,25).

Patients with CSF leak must be evaluated by a neurosurgeon in addition to a facial specialist. Some neurosurgeons initiate prophylactic antibiotics for CSF oto- or rhinorrhea, and this decision is best left to the consultant. However, the literature shows no clear benefit to this practice (32).

The surgical therapy of maxillofacial trauma is a rapidly evolving field. Patients with significant injuries should be transferred to referral centers if local consultants lack expertise in treating the injury in question. Before transfer, the patient who requires definitive care of maxillofacial injuries must be evaluated for life- or limb-threatening injuries. Even in the setting of isolated maxillofacial trauma, the potential for airway deterioration may be present, and pretransfer stabilization in these instances may include intubation. The potential for airway compromise, as well as the high frequency of significant associated injuries, dictates a high level of training for personnel involved in the prehospital or interhospital transport of the patient with significant maxillofacial trauma.

COMMON PITFALLS

✔ Failure to manage the airway aggressively with intubation or cricothyrotomy when indicated. Waiting for swelling or hemorrhage will convert an elective procedure into an emergent one

✔ Failure to consider the presence of subtle injuries. Particular attention should be paid to the neurologic and ophthalmologic examinations

✔ Ordering c-spine radiographs on all patients with facial fractures. Evidence-based guidelines such as the Nexus or Canadian C-spine rules should be followed (4,13)

✔ Failure to realize that frontal bone injuries are associated with intracranial injury

Acknowledgments

The authors wish to thank previous edition chapter authors Suzanne Moore Shepherd, Iris M. Reyes, and Barry Steinberg for their contributions.

References

1. Ardekian L, Rosen D, Klein Y, et al. Life-threatening complications and irreversible damage following maxillofacial trauma. *Injury* 1998;29(4):253.
2. Assael LA. Clinical aspects of imaging in maxillofacial trauma. *Radiol Clin North Am* 1993;31:209.
3. Azevedo AB, Trent R, Ellis A. Population-based analysis of 10,766 hospitalizations for mandibular fractures in California, 1991 to 1993. *J Trauma* 1998;45:1084.
4. Bandiera G, Stiell IG, Wells GA, et al. Canadian C-Spine and CT Head Study Group. The Canadian C-spine rule performs better than unstructured physician judgment. *Ann Emerg Med* 2003:42(3):395.
5. Cook HE, Rowe M. A retrospective study of 356 midfacial fractures occurring in 225 patients. *J Oral Maxillofac Surg* 1990;48:574.
6. Dolin J, Scalea T, Mannor L, et al. The management of gunshot wounds to the face. *J Trauma* 1992;33:508.
7. Ellis E. Sequencing treatment for naso-orbito-ethmoid fractures. *J Oral Maxillofac Surg* 1993;51:543.
8. Ellis E, Scott K. Oral-facial emergencies: assessment of patients with facial fractures. *Emerg Med Clin North Am* 2000;18(3).
9. Gentry LR. Facial trauma and associated brain damage. *Radiol Clin North Am* 1984;27:435.
10. Greene D, Raven R, Carvalho G, et al. Epidemiology of facial injury in blunt assault: determinants of incidence and outcome in 802 patients. *Arch Otolaryngol Head Neck Surg* 1997;123:923.
11. Hasan N, Colucciello S. Maxillofacial trauma. In: Tintinalli J, et al: *Emergency Medicine: A Comprehensive Study Guide.* New York: McGraw-Hill, 2000.
12. Haug RH, Prather J, Indresano AT. An epidemiologic survey of facial fractures and concomitant injuries. *J Oral Maxillofac Surg* 1990;48:926.

optic nerve may be injured along its course by direct or indirect mechanisms.

Symptoms are often lacking, or they are nonspecific. They include blurred vision, curtain of darkness, flashes of light, floaters, pain, and red eye. Important signs are blurring of fundus detail, decreased acuity, and RAPD. Anatomic findings are not necessarily apparent on direct funduscopy performed in the emergency department, even with dilatation. They are best identified by an ophthalmologist using dilated indirect funduscopy. Emergency department ultrasonography may be helpful in identifying posterior segment injuries at the bedside.

Retrobulbar Hematoma

Retrobulbar hematoma (*orbital compartment syndrome*) is a very rare condition. It is associated with intraoperative retrobulbar injections and occurs postoperatively. It is less often associated with trauma (Fig. 176.10). Signs and symptoms include severe eye pain, nausea, vomiting, decreasing vision, diplopia, RAPD, decreased ocular motility, hemorrhagic chemosis, proptosis, and resistance to retropulsion of the globe. The retina can withstand total ischemia for only about 90 minutes before damage may be permanent, so rapid treatment without any delays is required. Initiating conservative management (head elevation, ice packs, acetazolamide, mannitol, timolol) while preparations are underway (including consultation) is appropriate, as long as the definitive treatment is not delayed. The definitive treatment is to decompress the eye by lateral canthotomy and cantholysis in order to maximize the chance of preserving vision. After local injection of an anesthetic agent, the lateral canthus is crushed with a small hemostat to reduce bleeding, then incised with scissors 1 cm into the tissue, taking care to avoid injury to the globe. The inferior arm of the lateral canthal tendon is cut to release the globe (Fig. 176.11). An ophthalmologist must be consulted as soon as this condition is suspected.

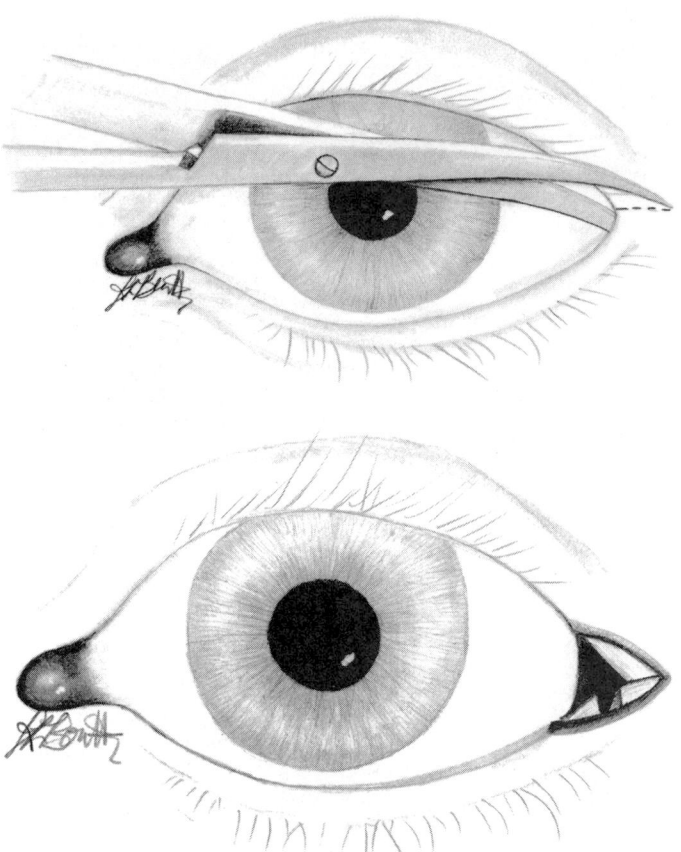

Figure 176.11.   Lateral canthotomy and cantholysis. The inferior arm of the lateral canthal tendon has been incised to release to globe. (Adapted from Cullom RD Jr, Chang B, eds. *The Wills eye manual.* Philadelphia: Lippincott–Raven Publishers, 1994.)

COMPLICATIONS OF EYE TRAUMA

Eye trauma (25% of cases) and eye surgery (62% cases) predispose to *endophthalmitis*. It develops in 8% to 13% of patients with eye trauma when there is a retained FB. The percentage rises to 26% if the FB is organic material from a rural setting. The onset is sudden and begins from hours to 2 months after the injury. *Bacillus cereus* infection has been reported to develop within 24 hours, streptococci within 2 days, and *Staphylococcus epidermidis* within 4 days (16). Treatment of endophthalmitis is intravitreal injection of vancomycin and amikacin by an ophthalmologist. Delay in treatment of even a few hours, particularly with *Bacillus* species, can lead to the loss of an eye. The symptoms are blurred vision, fever, a red eye, and severe pain. The signs are anterior chamber reaction, markedly decreased acuity, cells, and opacities in the vitreous, conjunctival hyperemia, corneal ring abscess, decreased red reflex, hypopyon, increased IOP, and proptosis. There is a noted association between *B. cereus* infections, metallic intraocular FBs, and injuries related to soil. Early diagnosis is imperative for the best outcome. Therefore, endophthalmitis should be considered in any patient presenting with a history of previous eye trauma.

Sympathetic ophthalmia is an immune-mediated inflammatory condition that occurs in the uninjured eye days to years after severe trauma to the opposite eye. After a penetrating or rupturing injury, antigens in the injured eye are exposed and an immune response is mounted against the uninjured eye. The incidence is 0.2% after penetrating eye trauma and 0.01% after routine eye surgery. Sixty-five percent of cases begin between 2 and 8 weeks after the insult and 90% within 1 year (range of 5 days to decades). The signs and symptoms in the sympathetic eye begin as a mild anterior uveitis, which progresses over time to anterior and posterior uveitis. In about 5% of the cases, only the posterior uveitis occurs (blurred vision, floaters, pain, photophobia,

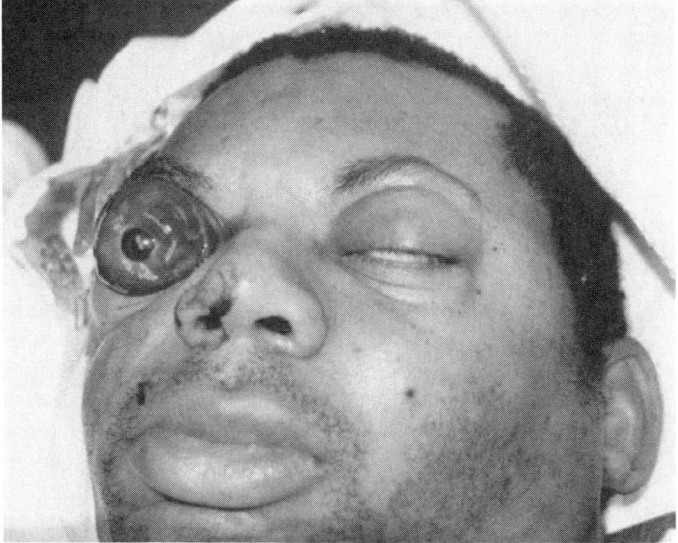

Figure 176.10.   Retrobulbar hemorrhage demonstrating dramatic proptosis and subconjunctival hemorrhage after a fist strike in a man on warfarin.

with or without redness). The condition of the injured eye may worsen at the same time. Enucleation of a severely traumatized eye, with no hope for useful vision, appears to eliminate the risk of sympathetic ophthalmia.

CRITICAL INTERVENTIONS

- Assess the patient for nonocular injuries; always assess the ABC's first
- Document the best-corrected visual acuity. Failure to improve with pinhole suggests a posterior segment injury
- In patients with chemical burns, continue eye irrigation in the ED until pH is normal and the injury has been assessed
- Obtain a history of contact lens use (corneal ulcer) or striking metal on metal (globe perforation) in patients with suspected corneal abrasion
- Protect the eye when globe penetration is suspected; confirm with Seidel's test
- Perform a lateral canthotomy or obtain immediate ophthalmology consultation in patients with retrobulbar hematoma

DISPOSITION

Disposition of patients with ophthalmologic trauma is arranged on a case-by-case basis. Immediate consultation in the emergency department or transfer to an appropriate center when an ophthalmologist is not available should take place for patients with globe penetration (or suspicion thereof), complex eyelid lacerations, penetrating foreign bodies, orbital fracture with entrapment, ocular burns, anterior chamber injuries, hypopyon, hyphema (>25% of anterior chamber, associated with increased IOP or blood disorders), globe luxation, orbital compartment syndrome and traumatic endophthalmitis. All but the most trivial of ocular injuries should be discussed with an ophthalmologist and appropriate outpatient follow up and care arranged; even apparent trivial injuries may harbor significant occult injury.

COMMON PITFALLS

✔ Failure to test visual acuity
✔ Using Nitrazine paper (measures pH only up to 7.4) to assess alkaline injuries
✔ Inadequate visualization of the eye on exam; use a slit lamp for best magnification
✔ Failure to evert the upper lid to diagnose foreign body

Acknowledgments

The authors recognize the many contributions by William H. Shoff and Suzanne Moore Shepherd to this chapter through the previous edition of the textbook.

References

1. Blaivas M, Theodoro D, Sierzenski PR. A study of bedside ocular ultrasonography in the emergency department. *Acad Emerg Med* 2003;9:791.
2. Bryden FM, Pyott AA, Bailey M, et al. Real time ultrasound in the assessment of intraocular foreign bodies. *Eye* 1990;4:727–731.
3. Catone GA, Morrissette MP, Carlson ER. A retrospective study of untreated blow-out fractures. *J Oral Maxillofac Surg* 1988;46:1033.
4. Crikelair GF et al. A critical look at the "blowout" fracture. *Plast Reconstr Surg* 1972;49:374.
5. Emmanuella J, et al. Predictors of blinding or serious eye injury in blunt trauma. *J Trauma* 1992;33:19.
6. Flynn CA, D Amico F, Smith G. Should we patch corneal abrasions? A meta-analysis. *J Fam Pract* 47(4):264,1999.
7. Gossman MD, Roberts DM, Rarr CC. Ophthalmic aspects of orbital injury. *Clin Plast Surg* 1992;19:71.
8. Harlan JB, Pieramici DJ. Evaluation of patients with ocular trauma. *Ophthalmol Clin North Am* 2002;15(2).
9. *Impact protection and polycarbonate lenses.* Schamburg, IL: Prevent Blindness America, 1995.
10. Kylstra JA, Lamkin JC, Runyan DK. Clinical predictors of scleral rupture after blunt ocular trauma. *Am J Ophthalmol* 1993;115:530.
11. Lubeck D. Penetrating ocular injuries. *Emerg Med Clin North Am* 1988;6:127.
12. Martin XD. Normal intraocular pressure in man. *Ophthalmologica* 1992;205:57.
13. McCaig LF, Burt CW. National Hospital Ambulatory Medical Care Survey: 2001 Emergency Department Summary. Advance Data from Vital and Health Statistics; No. 335.
14. O'Hare TH. Blow-out fractures: a review. *J Emerg Med* 1991;9:253.
15. Rothova A et al. Clinical features of acute anterior uveitis. *Am J Ophthalmol* 1987;103:137.
16. Shemmer GB, Driebe WT Jr. Posttraumatic *Bacillus cereus* endophthalmitis. *Arch Ophthalmol* 1987;105:342.
17. Talbot ME. A simple test to diagnose iritis. *Br Med J* 1987;295;812.
18. Tso MM, LaPiana RG. The human fovea after sungazing. *Trans Am Acad Ophthalmol Otolaryngol* 1975;79:788.
19. Vachon CA, Warner DO, Bacon DR. Succinylcholine and the open globe. Tracing the teaching. *Anesthesiology* 2003;99(1):220–223.
20. Walton W. Management of traumatic hyphema. *Surv Ophthalmol* 2002;47(4):297.

CHAPTER 177
Blunt Neck Trauma

Edward Ullman

The majority of blunt neck trauma occurs in conjunction with other significant injuries to the head, cervical spine, and face (13). The most common reported injury is the "padded dash syndrome." This occurs when the unrestrained driver decelerates against the steering wheel or dashboard. There have been case reports of isolated neck trauma due to a "clothesline" mechanism in motorcycle, jet ski, snowmobile, and ATV users (18). Other etiologies include blunt impact secondary to a punch, kick, or strike by a baseball bat or other object.

CLINICAL PRESENTATION

There is a wide range of presentations in patients with blunt neck trauma; patients may be asymptomatic, have minimal symptoms, or present in extremis. Therefore, it is crucial to recognize that a lack of obvious soft tissue trauma does not rule out a significant injury (21,4).

Airway injuries can present with hoarseness, stridor, subcutaneous emphysema, hemoptysis, or respiratory distress (17). Laryngotracheal injuries include vocal cord damage or disruption, dislocation of the arytenoid cartilage, tracheal transection, and fractures of the thyroid or cricoid cartilage or hyoid bone (Fig. 177.1) (15). Patients with any alteration in voice should be assumed to have a laryngeal injury. However, a normal voice does not rule out this injury. Development of a soft tissue hematoma or edema can externally compress the airway and cause respiratory compromise. Therefore, continuous airway reassessment is required in patients with blunt neck trauma. Palpation of the thyroid and cricoid cartilages will reveal tenderness and crepitus as an indication of injury, especially in men, since these landmarks

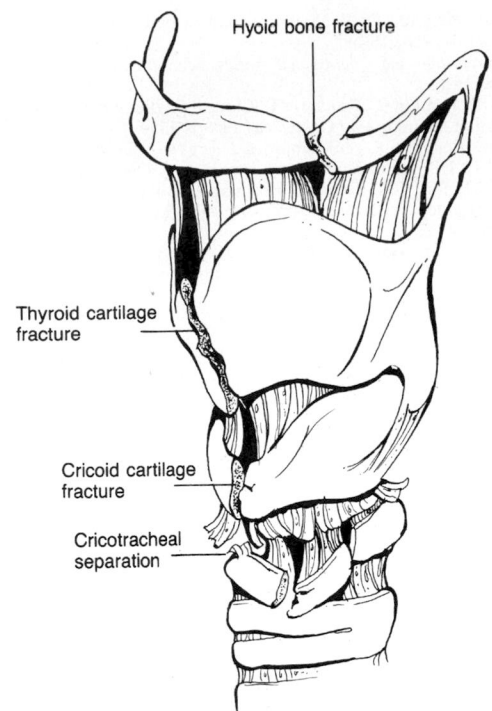

Figure 177.1.   Types of laryngeal injuries: hyoid bone fracture; thyroid cartilage fracture; cricoid cartilage fracture; cricotracheal separation.

are prominent. If there is loss of definition or deviation of these structures, the likelihood of underlying injury is high.

Blunt vascular injuries to the carotid or vertebral arteries are often diagnosed after admission (10). The incidence of vascular injury in blunt trauma patients is 0.08% to 1.00% (4). The majority of these injuries occur at the carotid bifurcation or higher and involve multiple vessels (19). Carotid injuries include intimal tears, hematoma, thrombosis, and pseudo-aneurysms. Injuries that cause hyperextension and rotation can stretch the carotid artery and compromise the vessel. Acute flexion injuries may crush the carotid artery between the mandible and the cervical spine leading to thrombosis or intimal damage. An intraoral blow to the soft palate can cause carotid thrombosis, especially in the pediatric population. This usually occurs when a child has an object in his or her mouth and falls, forcing the object into the soft palate. Carotid injuries can present with isolated ipsilateral cerebral findings which include: contralateral hemiplegia, sensory loss, and aphasia (17). The presence of a bruit can indicate partial disruption of the carotid by either intimal dissection or thrombus formation. Patients may also present with Horner's syndrome (ipsilateral miosis, ptosis, and anhidrosis) due to disruption of the thoracic sympathetic chain that encircles the carotid artery. Vertebral artery involvement can be difficult to diagnose. Often these patients complain of vague symptoms such as dizziness, visual disturbances, nausea, and vertigo. Furthermore, since the vertebral artery connects to the basilar artery, an embolic event from trauma could affect either the ipsilateral or contralateral posterior circulation. This can leave the patient with a variety of neurologic deficits, without an apparent vascular source (6).

DIFFERENTIAL DIAGNOSIS

The existence of other associated injuries and the lack of external neck findings make vascular injuries difficult to diagnose. Neurologic deficits are often delayed; only 10% of those with

vascular injury have initial findings. The diagnosis should be suspected in patients with neurologic deficits not explained by head computed tomography (CT) and in hemiparetic patients without alteration in mental status. In a series of 66 patients, 34% of those with neck vascular injuries had incongruent neurologic findings (4). The emergency physician should consider this diagnosis in patients with basilar skull fractures and marked external cervical trauma, since associated vascular injuries are often present. The diagnosis should also be considered in patients with anterior neck soft tissue injury such as abrasions, edema, or hematoma.

There are only 10 reported cases of isolated gastrointestinal injury in blunt neck trauma (3). The majority of these injuries occur in conjunction with laryngotracheal injury. Gastrointestinal injury should be considered in patients with pain on swallowing or subcutaneous emphysema; the latter group have a higher incidence of airway compromise.

EMERGENCY DEPARTMENT EVALUATION

Because of the difficulty in diagnosing vascular, airway, and gastrointestinal injury in blunt neck trauma, a systematic evaluation is critical. Table 177.1 lists factors which should raise the suspicion of a vascular injury.

In the patient with acute findings (Table 177.1), four vessel angiography is recommended regardless of the zone of injury (4,10). In the asymptomatic patient or those who have sustained a low-risk event (minor trauma without evidence of acute findings), color-flow Doppler ultrasonography may identify arterial dissection. It has been shown to have sensitivities as high as 92% to 100% in detecting *penetrating* injuries. For *blunt* neck trauma, there are retrospective reports of sensitivities as high as 92%; however, no study has looked prospectively at the effectiveness of ultrasound (US) versus the gold standard, angiography (10). Furthermore, since the majority of carotid artery injury occurs near the bifurcation, where US visualization is less reliable, this modality is limited. Given the "miss rate" for US detecting carotid injury is reported to be as high as 8% in the literature, when evaluated retrospectively (9), it is difficult to recommend US as a sole diagnostic modality in the high-risk patient. Initial research has shown that helical computed tomography angiography (CTA) is able to diagnose vascular injury and to decrease the time to diagnosis (16). However, Miller et al. showed a low sensitivity and specificity (47% and 59%, respectively); this raises doubt about the effectiveness of this modality (12). Magnetic resonance angiography (MRA) has a reported sensitivity as high as 95% (19). However, difficulty in obtaining this modality in an acute trauma setting limits its usefulness in the emergency department.

Evaluation of the airway is crucial in patients with blunt neck trauma. Fiberoptic visualization of the endolarynx allows for identification of function and pathology. Plain films have limited value but may indicate evidence of subglottic narrowing of the air column, prevertebral soft tissue swelling, fractured calcified larynx, or the presence of subcutaneous air. CT can

TABLE 177.1.   Signs and Symptoms of Vascular Injury

Decreased level of consciousness
Hemiparesis without CT-scan evidence of pathology
Neck hematoma
Horner's syndrome
Carotid bruit
Vomiting and dizziness

TABLE 177.2.	Signs and Symptoms of Gastrointestinal Injury

Pain on swallowing
Subcutaneous air
Bloody saliva

identify cartilage disruption and define anatomical relationships (7). Some authors feel that CT should be performed regardless of the fiberoptic findings if the suspicion for injury is high (11).

Although isolated esophageal injuries after blunt trauma are rare, those patients with signs of gastrointestinal injury (Table 177.2) require additional examination. Gastrograffin swallow is often the initial study of choice because it causes less pleural irritation if extravasation occurs. Barium provides a more sensitive study, but has an increased risk of pulmonary complications. Recently, several studies have shown endoscopy as an adequate modality to evaluate for perforation (20).

EMERGENCY DEPARTMENT MANAGEMENT

Blunt trauma can create difficult airway situations. As delays in presentation are common, any evidence of respiratory compromise requires prompt action. Evidence of air hunger, stridor, or sonorous respirations should be addressed immediately. The emergency physician should prepare all airway management equipment upon recognition of possible airway compromise. If time permits, anesthesiology or otolaryngology should be alerted due to the potential for a difficult airway. The current literature indicates that orotracheal intubation is the first-line airway management technique for all blunt neck trauma patients requiring airway control (15). Surgical or needle cricothyrotomy is contraindicated in the presence of bruising, hematoma over the cricothyroid membrane, or suspected laryngotracheal injury. In these cases, emergency tracheotomy is recommended to avoid the risk of converting a partial to a complete cricotracheal disruption. The development of subcutaneous emphysema and a large air leak after intubation and initiation of positive-pressure ventilation indicates a tracheal injury distal to the cuff of the endotracheal tube. This situation requires immediate tracheotomy, and in some cases median sternotomy, to regain control of the distal tracheal segment. Nasotracheal intubation is relatively contraindicated given the high rate of failure and the possibility of worsening an already difficult airway by extending the laryngeal injury.

In patients with marked laryngeal injuries, bleeding and edema can obscure landmarks. In those with complete laryngeal transection, use of neuromuscular blockade can make endotracheal intubation nearly impossible. Upon muscular paralysis, the muscles which provide internal stabilization become relaxed; this may result in the endotracheal tube creating a false lumen in the soft tissues of the neck (8). Given this concern, oral-awake intubation is an alternative to rapid sequence intubation, especially in the presence of an anterior neck hematoma. Due to the increased incidence of cervical injury in blunt neck trauma patients, careful in-line stabilization should be performed with any airway management technique.

Fiberoptic laryngoscopy has replaced direct laryngoscopy as the standard method of evaluating upper airway injuries. It is useful in assessing airway patency, vocal cord mobility, and the presence of endolaryngeal lacerations or hematoma without causing movement of the cervical spine. Fiberoptic bronchoscopy permits additional visualization of the subglottic airway and may be used to facilitate endotracheal intubation.

There is an increased incidence of pneumothorax, hemothorax, and pulmonary contusion in patients with blunt neck trauma. Tension pneumothorax is a clinical diagnosis; the combination of hypotension, unilateral decreased breath sounds, and respiratory distress is an indication for needle decompression and tube thoracostomy. This may be difficult to evaluate in the patient with altered neck anatomy; however, the emergency physician should have a low threshold for decompressing the chest.

It is rare for patients with blunt neck trauma to have life-threatening hemorrhage. However, concern for expanding neck hematoma should always be addressed. This requires aggressive, early airway management, as well as ENT or general surgery consultation. In the case of suspected gastrointestinal injury, broad-spectrum antibiotics with anaerobic coverage should be administered.

As the majority of vascular injuries result in luminal narrowing and thrombosis, anticoagulation is the recommended therapy; it results in improved neurologic outcomes in patients with blunt neck trauma (14). Since the majority of blunt cervical vascular injuries are high in the internal carotid artery, surgical repair is difficult. Furthermore, in one study the majority of injuries were "long dissections" not amenable to surgery (12). There is growing evidence that endovascular repair of pseudoaneurysms produces favorable results. This may prove to be a rational approach in patients with cervical vascular injuries (2).

CRITICAL INTERVENTIONS

- Perform early orotracheal intubation in blunt neck trauma patients with evidence of airway compromise
- Perform four vessel angiography in patients who are at high risk for vascular injuries
- In patients with suspected blunt laryngeal injury, order a neck CT to elucidate the injury pattern
- Administer broad-spectrum antibiotics to patients with esophageal injuries to prevent abscess formation

DISPOSITION

Patients with evidence of blunt neck trauma that involves the airway or vascular or gastrointestinal systems should be admitted or carefully observed. For these patients, early consultation with ENT or general surgery should be obtained. If the patient is asymptomatic and has a negative work-up, discharge is recommended. Comprehensive instructions are critical for patient education in discharged patients. Symptomatic patients should be admitted or transferred to a trauma center where an ENT surgeon and general surgeon are available. It is critical to secure the airway in those symptomatic patients who are transferred, given the potential for respiratory compromise.

COMMON PITFALLS

✔ Failure to secure the airway early and failure to prepare for a difficult airway that may require specialty intervention
✔ Failure to recognize potential vascular injury in the patient with neurologic deficits and a normal head CT
✔ Failure to recognize that vascular injuries frequently have a delayed presentation

Acknowledgments

Thanks to previous edition chapter authors Gerard R. Cox and Brigitte M. Baumann.

References

1. Bent JP, Silver JR, Porubsky ES. Acute laryngeal trauma: a review of 77 patients. *Otolaryngol Head Neck Surg* 1994;109:441–449.
2. Coldwell DM, Novak Z, Ryan RK, et al. Treatment of posttraumatic internal carotid arterial pseudoaneurysms with endovascular stents. *J Trauma* 2000;48: 470–472.
3. Duchynski R. Neck injury. In: Ferrera PC, Colucciello SA, Marx JA, et al., eds. *Trauma Management*. St. Louis: Mosby, 2001:218–231.
4. Fabian TC, Patton JH, Croce MA, et al. Blunt carotid injury. Importance of early diagnosis and anticoagulation therapy. *Ann Surg* 1996;223(5):513–522.
5. Furhman GM, Stieg FH, Buerk CA. Blunt laryngeal trauma: classification and management protocol. *J Trauma* 1990;30:87–92.
6. Jacobs I, Niknejad G, Kelly K, et al. Hypopharyngeal perforation after blunt neck trauma: case report and review of the literature. *J Trauma* 1999;46(5):957–958.
7. Jordan R.Blunt neck trauma. In: Rosen P, Barkin R, Danzl DF, et al., eds. *Emergency Medicine*. 4th ed. St. Louis: Mosby; 1998:505–514.
8. Kasantikul V, Ouellet JV, Smith TA. Head and neck injuries in fatal motorcycle collisions as determined by detailed autopsy. *Traffic Inj Prev* 2003;4(3):255–262.
9. Kraus RR, Bergstein JM, DeBoard JR. Diagnosis, treatment, and outcomes of blunt carotid arterial injuries. *Am J Surg* 1999;178(3):190–193.
10. Kumar SR, Weaver FA, Yellin AE. Cervical vascular injuries. *Surg Clin North Am* 2001;81(6):1331–1344.
11. Mace S. Blunt laryngotracheal trauma. *Ann Emerg Med* 1986;(15):836–842.
12. Miller PR, Fabian TC, Bee TK, et al. Blunt cerebrovascular injuries: diagnosis and treatment. *J Trauma* 2001;51(2):279–286.
13. Miller PR, Fabian TC, Croce MA, et al. Prospective screening for blunt cerebrovascular injuries: analysis and of diagnostic modalities and outcomes. *Ann Surg* 2002;236(3):386–393.
14. Pretre R et al. Blunt carotid artery injury: difficult therapeutic approaches for an under-recognized entity. *Surgery* 1994;115:375–381.
15. Reese GP, Shatney CH. Blunt injury of the cervical trachea, a review of 51 patients. *South Med J* 1988;81;1542–1548.
16. Rogers FB, Baker EE, Osler TM, et al. Computer tomographic angiography as a screening modality for blunt cervical arterial injuries: preliminary results. *J Trauma* 1999;46:380–385.
17. Sanzone AG, Torres H, Doundoulakis SH. Blunt trauma to the carotid arteries. *Am J Emerg Med* 1995;13:327–330.
18. Schaefer SD. The acute management of external laryngeal trauma: a 27 year experience. *Arch Otolaryngol Head Neck Surg* 1992;118:598–604.
19. Schaider J, Bailitz J. Neck trauma. *Emerg Med Pract* 2003;5:1–28.
20. Srinivasan R, Haywood T, Horowitz B, et al. Role of flexible endoscopy in the evaluation of possible esophageal trauma after penetrating injuries. *Am J Gastroenterol* 2000;95:1725–1729.
21. Watridge CB, Muhlbauer MS, Lowery RD. Traumatic carotid artery dissection: diagnosis and treatment. *J Neurosurg* 1989;71:854–857.

CHAPTER 178
Penetrating Neck Trauma

Andrew L. Knaut and John L. Kendall

Penetrating wounds of the neck present a therapeutic and diagnostic challenge to the emergency physician. Mortality among patients who suffer penetrating neck injuries in the civilian population approaches 6%. Fatality rates escalate dramatically, however, if injury involves such vital structures as the esophagus (19%) or the major vessels (67%) (3,8). Successful management of a penetrating neck wound demands an understanding of the regional anatomy and those structures vulnerable to injury, familiarity with the options for proper airway management, and appreciation of the evolving concepts in the diagnosis and treat-

ment of significant injuries. Even the most benign-appearing wound may belie serious pathology, and extreme vigilance is essential to avert catastrophic airway, vascular, neurologic, and gastrointestinal complications.

A number of anatomic factors predispose structures within the neck to serious injury in the setting of penetrating trauma. Vital components of the respiratory, vascular, neurologic, and gastrointestinal systems course through the neck. Dense musculature and the structural integrity of the cervical spine afford some protection to these structures posteriorly, but the lack of similar shielding anteriorly exposes them to significant injury. Moreover, the majority of the vital structures of the neck are contained within dense, tightly confined fascial compartments, rendering them vulnerable to distortion and compression when bleeding occurs within the deep tissues (Fig. 178.1). For these reasons, penetrating wounds to the neck are best approached conceptually with regard to the site of external penetration, the depth of the wound, and the potential pathway of injury within the deeper compartments.

Most sources concur in dividing the external neck anatomically into *posterior* and *anterior* triangles. The *posterior triangle* connotes an area bordered by the posterior aspect of the sternocleidomastoid muscle anteriorly, the anterior edge of the trapezius muscle posteriorly, and the clavicle inferiorly (Fig. 178.2). The defining sides of the *anterior triangle* consist of the mandible superiorly, the anatomic midline anteriorly, and the anterior aspect of the sternocleidomastoid posteriorly. The anterior triangle is further subdivided into three zones, with penetrating injury to each zone and its underlying structures carrying distinct and important implications for diagnostic evaluation and clinical management (Fig. 178.3).

Zone I defines the region between the clavicles and the inferior rim of the cricoid cartilage. Vital structures susceptible to injury after penetrating trauma to zone I include the proximal common carotid, vertebral, and subclavian arteries, the thoracic outlet, the apex of the lung, the trachea, the esophagus, the thoracic duct, and the thyroid. Mortality rates for penetrating wounds to zone I are the highest of the three zones because of the inherent inability to achieve rapid proximal control of vascular injuries and the overall difficulty in gaining exposure to injuries within the thoracic cavity (15).

Zone II spans the distance from the superior edge of the cricoid to the angle of the mandible. Injuries to zone II threaten the carotid and vertebral arteries, the jugular veins, the vagus and recurrent laryngeal nerves, the cervical spinal cord, the trachea and larynx, and the esophagus. As the most exposed anatomic region of the neck, zone II injuries are the most common penetrating wounds in most series (5,10,21).

Zone III extends superiorly from the angle of the mandible to the base of the skull. Vulnerable structures in this region include the distal carotid and vertebral arteries, the salivary and parotid glands, the pharynx, the spinal cord, and cranial nerves IX, X, XI, and XII. As with zone I, management of zone III wounds may be problematic because of the difficulty in gaining surgical access to injured structures and control of bleeding vessels.

Within the anterior neck, the superficial fascia lies immediately beneath the skin and envelopes the platysma, a thin sheet of muscle that extends upward from the upper thorax over the clavicles to cover the entirety of the anterior triangle as well as the anteroinferior portion of the posterior triangle. As it extends cephalad, the platysma crosses the mandible to merge with the musculature of the face. This superficial structure is an important landmark in gauging the potential severity of a wound—violation of the platysma by a penetrating mechanism signifies injury to vital underlying structures until proven otherwise. Beneath the platysma, the investing, pretracheal, and prevertebral layers of the deep cervical fascia divide the deep, tightly-packed

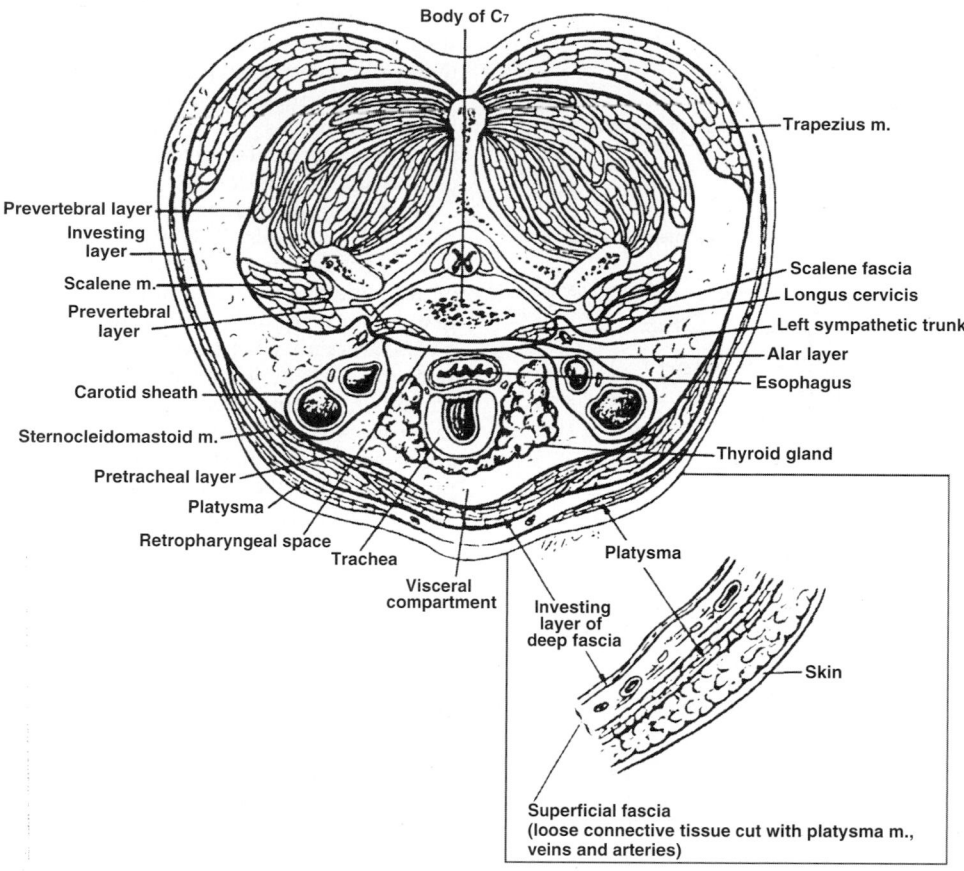

Figure 178.1.   Cross-sectional anatomy of the neck. (From Gray SW, Skandalakis JE, McClusky DA. *Atlas of surgical anatomy.* Baltimore: Williams & Wilkins, 1985, with permission.)

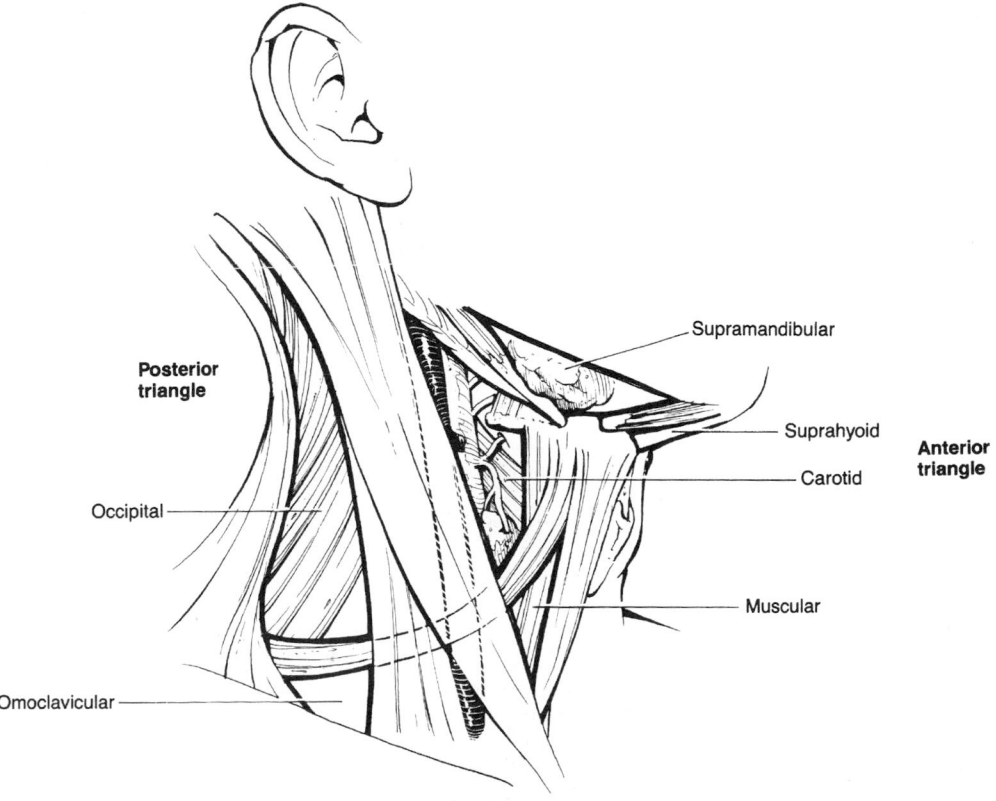

Figure 178.2.   Anatomy of the neck: anterior and posterior triangles.

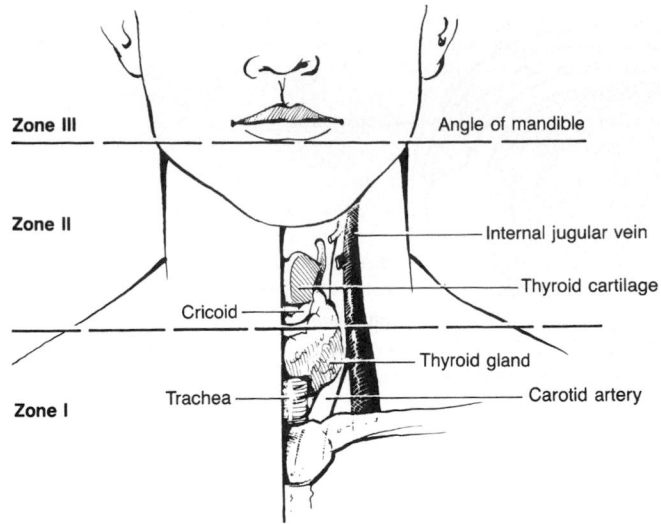

Figure 178.3.   Anatomy of the neck: zones I, II, and III.

compartments of the neck and the anatomic structures contained within.

CLINICAL PRESENTATION

Penetrating neck trauma is usually the result of a violent attack. This is reflected in the fact that the majority of victims are young adult males, and that most victims have ingested alcohol or other abusive substances immediately prior to the trauma (6,10,21). Other mechanisms of injury include unintentional impalements and bites from animals such as dogs. In most societies, stabbings outnumber gunshot and other wounds as the most common cause of penetrating neck trauma. In the United States, however, gunshot wounds account for an increasing proportion of injuries, particularly among the pediatric and young adult population (16,21).

Low-energy penetrations occur through such injuries as stabbings with knives or other cutting instruments, impalements, or wounds inflicted by air guns, low-caliber handguns, or shotguns at long range. High-energy mechanisms include discharges from rifles and shotguns at close range as well as shrapnel from explosive devices.

Stab wounds to the neck are typically unilateral and more frequently involve the left side because of the higher likelihood of right hand dominance in a facing attacker. As the most exposed portion of the anterior neck, zone II is the area injured most frequently, accounting for 50% to 80% of stab wounds to the

neck in most series (5,21). Information relating to an assault, such as the size of the instrument and the angle of the attack, may yield some insight into the potential depth and tract of a wound. Nevertheless, the external appearance of a stab injury to the neck correlates poorly with its underlying severity, and even the most superficial-appearing injury should be approached as potentially life threatening.

Because of the higher kinetic energy imparted to the tissues by an offending missile, a large percentage of gunshot wounds to the neck results in clinically significant injury. In one series of 312 patients with penetrating neck wounds that violated the platysma, 45% of those with gunshot wounds suffered injury to a vital structure, whereas only 23% of those who presented with stab wounds experienced significant pathology (5). As with stab wounds, the depth and pathway of injury of a gunshot wound to the neck can be difficult to predict based upon its external appearance, particularly when it is secondary to a low-velocity projectile. When the wound traverses the anatomic midline of the neck, however, the likelihood of significant injury doubles (9,14).

DIFFERENTIAL DIAGNOSIS

Penetrating trauma to the neck demands consideration of potential injury to vital respiratory, vascular, neurologic, and gastrointestinal structures (Table 178.1). This differential diagnosis should guide the clinician through an initial evaluation that is rapid yet thorough. Moreover, subtle signs of significant injury may not be appreciable initially and can evolve rapidly. Frequent reevaluation of the patient for developing clinical signs and symptoms is therefore essential to avoiding a disastrous outcome.

Respiratory Injuries

Structures of the respiratory tract that are vulnerable to penetrating neck wounds include the oropharynx, larynx, trachea, and lung apices. Assessment for airway and respiratory compromise takes the highest priority during the initial and subsequent evaluations, and obvious signs of injury include dyspnea, cyanosis, and stridor. Air bubbling at the wound site, subcutaneous emphysema, pneumomediastinum, hemoptysis, voice change, tenderness over the larynx, and unilaterally diminished breath sounds are other important indications of respiratory injury.

Vascular Injuries

Vascular injuries are present in approximately one fourth of patients and are the leading cause of mortality in the setting of penetrating neck trauma (10). Death results most often from

---

TABLE 178.1.   Signs and Symptoms of Specific System Injuries

Vascular	Aerodigestive	Neurologic
Hematoma	Respiratory distress	Altered sensorium
Persistent hemorrhage	Stridor	Hemiplegia/quadriplegia
Neurologic deficit	Cyanosis	Respiratory paralysis
Pulse deficit	Hemoptysis	Brown-Sèquard syndrome
Horner's syndrome (carotid injury)	Tracheal deviation	Extremity paresis or sensory loss
Hypovolemic shock	Subcutaneous emphysema	Horner's syndrome (stellate ganglion)
Vascular bruit or thrill	Pneumothorax	Hoarseness (recurrent laryngeal nerve)
Altered sensorium	Sucking wound	Cranial nerve deficit (VII, XI, and XII)
Harsh, machinery-like pre-cordial murmur (venous air embolism)	Dysphonia, aphonia, hoarseness	
	Dysphagia	
	Odynophagia	

exsanguination secondary to arterial injury, venous injury, or both. Unequivocal signs of a major vascular insult include shock either with or without active hemorrhage, an expanding or pulsatile hematoma, carotid bruit or thrill, absent radial or ulnar pulses, hemiplegia consistent with hemispheric stroke, and airway compromise or obstruction. More subtle indications of vascular injury include diminished pulses in the temporal or facial arteries, decreased breath sounds as a consequence of hemothorax, bleeding within the oropharynx, and signs of venous air embolism such as hemodynamic collapse unresponsive to standard resuscitative measures or the presence of a loud, machinery-like murmur over the precordium. See Chapter 54, "Venous Gas Embolism."

Gastrointestinal Injuries

When present, violation of the pharynx and esophagus is frequently unrecognized during the initial evaluation of the patient with a penetrating neck injury, and yet the consequences of such an injury can be devastating. Extravasation of saliva, gastric acid, digestive enzymes, and bacteria through a penetrating wound can ignite an aggressive necrotizing inflammatory reaction within the neck and mediastinum. Mortality and morbidity increase sharply when there is a delay in diagnosis and treatment in this setting (3). Pertinent signs and symptoms include dysphagia, odynophagia, hematemesis, and air within the soft tissues as manifested by subcutaneous emphysema or radiographic free air within the retropharyngeal space or mediastinum.

Nervous System Injuries

A number of neurologic injuries can manifest as distinct clinical syndromes after penetrating neck trauma. Gunshot wounds and, occasionally, stabbings that enter the spinal canal from a posterior orientation can partially or completely transect the spinal cord. Complete transection of the cord above the level of C5 is fatal due to paralysis of the diaphragm. Transection at a lower point will cause paraplegia and loss of upper extremity function according to the level of injury. Hemisection of the spinal cord, or the Brown-Séquard syndrome, yields ipsilateral hemiplegia and loss of tactile and proprioceptive sensation and contralateral loss of pain and temperature sensation. Injury to the cervical sympathetic ganglia can present with the ipsilateral ptosis and myosis of Horner's syndrome. Damage to the recurrent laryngeal nerve as it courses in the groove between the trachea and the esophagus impairs vocal cord movement, resulting in dysphonia or hoarseness. Cranial nerve transection may result in ipsilateral drooping of the corner of the mouth (CN VII), inability to shrug the shoulders (CN XI), or tongue deviation (CN XII). Injury to a nerve root as it travels from the vertebral foramen to the brachial plexus causes sensory and motor deficits in the corresponding upper extremity.

Cervical Spine Considerations

There is controversy as to whether cervical spine immobilization should be routine practice for victims of gunshot wounds to the neck. While such injury is unlikely to result from a stab wound, high-energy projectiles such as bullets can destabilize the cervical spine. The reported incidence of cervical spine injury as a result of gunshot wound ranges from 2.7% to 22% (7,22). A majority of victims of gunshot wounds to the cervical spine suffer neurologic deficit either from direct injury to the spinal cord by a transecting bullet or as a consequence of the concussive force imparted to the cord by a projectile passing in close proximity (7,22). Victims of gunshot wounds to the neck who do not manifest a neurologic deficit, on the other hand, are very unlikely to have an unstable cervical spine. At present, only one such case report exists in the literature (1). Moreover, a retrospective review by Arishita et al. of 472 cases of penetrating neck injury during the Vietnam conflict identified only four (1.4%) of 296 casualties who survived long enough to receive first aid with cervical spinal column injuries that might have benefited from neck stabilization (2). Among the civilian population, one retrospective review of 28 patients with low-velocity gunshot wounds to the cervical spine failed to identify any cases of spinal instability as the result of penetrating injury (18).

At the same time, the small potential benefit of routine cervical spine immobilization for penetrating wounds to the neck must be weighed against its dangers. Stabilization devices deprive the clinician of direct visualization and easy palpation of the neck, thus increasing the likelihood that signs of life-threatening complications of injury might be missed. In reviewing 44 cases of penetrating neck wounds in Israel, Barkana et al. identified 8 instances in which significant clinical signs were identified only after patient transport and the removal of a stabilization apparatus in the emergency department (4). Moreover, cervical spine immobilization may make visualizing vocal cords more difficult, further complicating an already challenging intubation. Thus, routine cervical spine immobilization after penetrating neck trauma in the absence of a focal neurologic deficit is not supported by the existing literature and is not recommended.

EMERGENCY DEPARTMENT EVALUATION

Attention to airway patency and protection is the central focus of the initial evaluation of any patient with penetrating neck trauma. Vigilance for signs of actual or impending airway compromise begins with the initial patient contact in the prehospital setting and must continue throughout the victim's emergency department evaluation.

While several acceptable options for establishing definitive airway control in this clinical setting exist, each possesses inherent challenges and the risk of failure or complication. The emergency physician must therefore be familiar with and capable of quickly implementing an array of airway management techniques when confronted with the victim of a penetrating neck wound. At the same time, rapid and thorough assessment of the patient's circulatory status, the need for emergent operative intervention, and the potential for injury to the major structures of the neck is essential.

In the prehospital setting all patients with penetrating neck trauma should be considered to have a life-threatening injury. If circumstances allow, prehospital personnel can gather pertinent information such as the circumstances related to the trauma, the character and size of the weapon responsible for the injury, the position of an attacker relative to the patient, and an estimation of the amount of blood lost at the scene.

Immediate airway management in the field is indicated for any patient with acute respiratory distress, stridor, or cardiopulmonary arrest. If transport to an appropriate trauma center will be rapid, attempts at intubation may otherwise be deferred until arrival in the emergency department. High-flow oxygen should be provided, but ventilation via bag-valve mask should be avoided because of its potential to force air through a tracheolaryngeal wound and into the surrounding tissues, distorting neck anatomy and further compromising the airway. Orotracheal intubation is preferred for establishing airway control because it allows for passage of an endotracheal tube under direct visualization. It may prove difficult, however, because of hemorrhage or distortion of normal airway anatomy by an expanding hematoma, air within the surrounding tissues, or direct injury to the larynx or trachea. Blind nasotracheal intubation (BNTI) has traditionally been avoided in patients with penetrating neck trauma because of the theorized potential to worsen any existing tracheolaryngeal injury, complete an airway obstruction through misplacement, or induce gagging and coughing that might aggravate existing respiratory or vascular injuries. A recent review of 45 patients with penetrating neck wounds managed with BNTI in the prehospital setting, however, revealed a 90% success rate for the technique and no identifiable complications as the result of any attempts (26). Cricothyrotomy may be warranted in the presence of massive facial trauma, complete airway obstruction not relieved by standard repositioning maneuvers, or failed endotracheal intubation attempts. Cricothyrotomy should be avoided when hematoma is present across the anterior neck. Rarely, direct insertion of an endotracheal tube through an open tracheal wound may be necessary. As the airway is secured, breathing assessment should include inspection, palpation, and auscultation of the chest for signs of tension pneumothorax, pneumothorax, or hemothorax, particularly when injury to zone I is present. Direct pressure should be applied to sites of hemorrhage, and at least one large-bore i.v. catheter should be placed at a site contralateral to any potential vascular injury.

Upon arrival to the emergency department, the primary survey must be quickly and thoroughly repeated. Indications for emergent airway stabilization not accomplished in the prehospital setting include acute respiratory distress or persistent stridor, copious blood or secretions threatening the airway, extensive subcutaneous emphysema, visible expanding hematoma or tracheal shift, and altered mental status. When such frank signs of airway compromise are absent, however, the emergency physician must remain vigilant for subtle indications of airway compromise such as voice change or odynophagia. Early airway management is warranted, as deterioration can be rapid and catastrophic.

A number of options exist for appropriate airway management after penetrating neck trauma. Intubation over a fiberoptic bronchoscope in the awake patient may allow for effective visualization of the vocal cords and passage of an endotracheal tube despite the presence of airway distortion or excessive blood and secretions. It may also identify specific laryngotracheal injuries. Its disadvantages include the need for specialized equipment and expertise and, like BNTI, the potential to induce gagging and coughing. Orotracheal intubation with an induction agent such as ketamine (2 mg/kg i.v.) but without induced paralysis may be preferable in some instances when preservation of the patient's respiratory drive is needed, as may occur, for example, when associated facial trauma renders bag-valve mask ventilation impossible.

In most emergency departments, rapid sequence intubation (RSI) using a neuromuscular paralytic agent is the primary modality of airway management after penetrating neck trauma. In two series of patients with penetrating neck injuries intubated in the emergency department, the rate of success for RSI was 100% (19,26). Some authors recommend using caution with RSI in this setting, however, arguing that a decrease in muscle tone following paralysis holds the potential to worsen airway distortion and thus invite airway disaster. In one series of 20 patients requiring airway management in the emergency department and ultimately diagnosed with laryngotracheal injury after penetrating neck trauma, RSI was successful among only 77% of those with gunshot wounds and 80% of those with stab wounds (24). Appropriate caution and, more importantly, preparation for an alternative means of airway management in the event of failure are therefore essential before attempting RSI after penetrating neck trauma.

The establishment of a surgical airway is the most commonly used rescue technique for airway management after failed RSI among patients with penetrating neck injuries (11,24). Cricothy-

roidotomy should be performed with a vertical incision to allow for extension of the incision if the cricothyroid membrane is not easily identified initially. Significant hematoma overlying the cricothyroid membrane is a contraindication to cricothyroidotomy because of the potential to convert a partial cricotracheal separation into a complete disruption. Emergent tracheostomy is warranted in this setting.

Assessment of circulatory status, direct pressure to active bleeding sites, and appropriate volume resuscitation must occur in tandem with proper airway evaluation and management. If direct pressure fails to control hemorrhage, insertion and inflation of a Foley catheter balloon within the wound may tamponade bleeding.

When the patient is stable, the wound itself should be inspected *but never probed* to determine if it has violated the platysma. Wounds that do not penetrate the platysma may be irrigated and closed. Otherwise, a thorough secondary assessment for the signs and symptoms of significant vascular, respiratory, neurologic, and gastrointestinal injury described above should proceed in order to determine further appropriate evaluation and management in the emergency department.

EMERGENCY DEPARTMENT MANAGEMENT

Historically, surgeons advocated mandatory operative exploration of all penetrating neck wounds because of the high mortality and morbidity associated with delays to diagnosis and treatment observed during the First World War. For much of the twentieth century, this practice was extended to wounds suffered by the civilian populace as well. However, the rate of negative neck explorations conducted under this recommendation approached 90% (10). As effective adjunctive diagnostic modalities have emerged, selective operative management for victims of penetrating neck trauma based on clinical assessment and supplementary diagnostic imaging has become standard.

Thorough clinical examination is essential to differentiating those patients in need of operative intervention from those who may be observed and further evaluated without immediate surgery. Exsanguinating hemorrhage, shock unresponsive to volume resuscitation, rapidly expanding neck hematoma, evolving signs of stroke, or obvious air bubbling from a wound are indications to transfer the patient to the operating room immediately.

Those patients who do not present with signs mandating immediate surgery may be divided into two groups: those who are asymptomatic and those with findings or symptoms suggestive of vascular, neurologic, or aerodigestive injury. Persistent bleeding, evolving hematoma, dysphonia, hemoptysis, subcutaneous crepitance, hematemesis, hemoptysis, and peripheral pulse or neurologic deficits are some of the manifestations of penetrating neck injury that define the latter group (Table 178.1).

The specific zone of injury determines the approach to further evaluation and management for patients in either group (Fig. 178.4). Patients with *zone I* injury who do not proceed emergently to surgery should undergo further diagnostic evaluation regardless of whether or not they manifest any of the vascular, neurologic, or aerodigestive symptoms described above. Asymptomatic patients may harbor occult injury to the structures of the lower neck and upper thorax that may not become apparent until catastrophic decompensation occurs. Stable but symptomatic patients should likewise receive further diagnostic study to identify the specific nature and sites of any vascular or aerodigestive injury in order to facilitate planning for proper operative approach.

Asymptomatic patients with injuries to *zone II* may be safely observed without further intervention. Those who present with

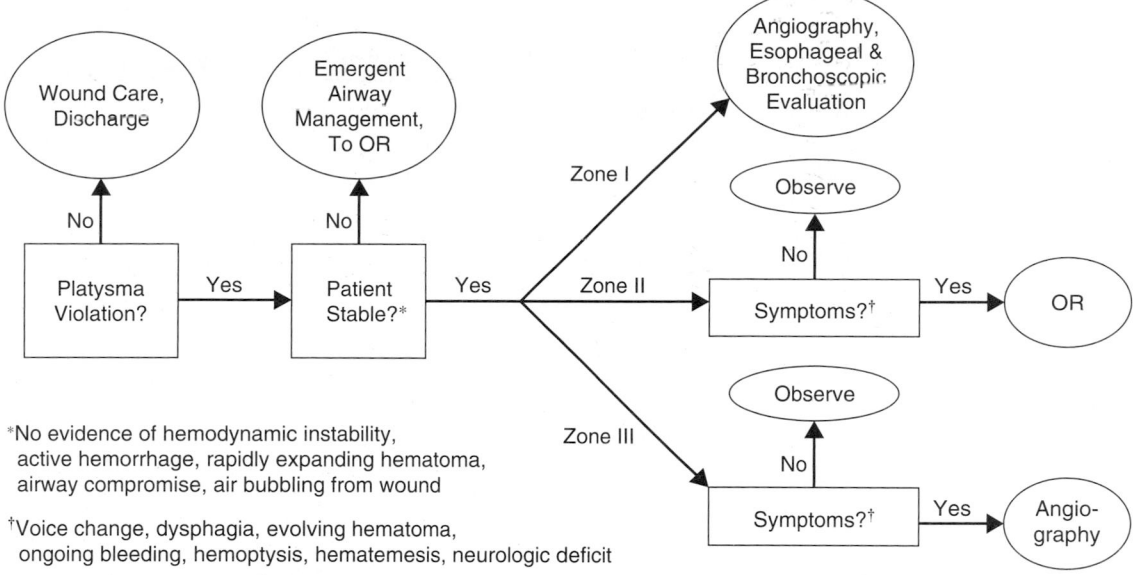

*No evidence of hemodynamic instability,
active hemorrhage, rapidly expanding hematoma,
airway compromise, air bubbling from wound

†Voice change, dysphagia, evolving hematoma,
ongoing bleeding, hemoptysis, hematemesis, neurologic deficit

Figure 178.4.   The emergency department management of penetrating neck trauma.

or develop persistent bleeding, evolving hematoma, hemoptysis or hematemesis, voice change, difficulty swallowing, or neurologic deficit should undergo expeditious surgical exploration.

Asymptomatic victims of zone III injury may be likewise observed, whereas those who are stable but manifest signs of vascular or neurologic injury should receive further diagnostic imaging to assist in determining the optimal method of surgical repair. The safety and cost-effectiveness of this and similar algorithms have been prospectively validated by several large series (5,10,17,21).

Several diagnostic modalities may assist in the nonoperative definition of vascular, respiratory, and digestive tract injuries resulting from penetrating neck trauma. Because of its high sensitivity and specificity, arteriography is the gold standard for diagnosing vascular injuries and may also allow for selective embolization of identified vascular lesions resulting from zone III injuries. Its disadvantages include high cost, limited availability in some institutions, and potential for iatrogenic vascular and anaphylactic complications. Duplex sonography can identify such vascular lesions as dissection, occlusion, and pseudoaneurysm with a reported sensitivity and specificity that approximate those of angiography and may be an acceptable alternative to more invasive vascular imaging (10). Its drawbacks include a limited ability to visualize the internal carotid artery above the angle of the mandible or major vascular structures directly under the clavicle. Helical CT angiography demonstrated a 93% positive predictive value and a 100% negative predictive value for significant vascular injury among 145 patients in one prospective study (20). Its advantages include its speed and noninvasive nature. It may be less definitive in the inferior portion of zone I, however, because of streak artifact from the shoulder and the parallel course of the subclavian vessels within axial imaging planes.

All patients with signs or symptoms suggestive of aerodigestive injury should receive standard radiographs of the chest and neck looking for evidence of air in the soft tissues or pneumothorax. Plain radiographs may demonstrate subcutaneous emphysema not appreciated by clinical exam. Moreover, while it may be difficult to distinguish air from an esophageal or tracheobronchial injury from air tracking through a penetrating wound, any positive finding should prompt strong consideration of and further evaluation for these often occult and potentially fatal injuries (24). Suspected tracheolaryngeal injuries are best evaluated by formal laryngoscopy and bronchoscopy.

Esophageal injuries are often occult, and delays in their diagnosis and management are associated with significantly increased morbidity (3). Contrast esophagography and fiber-optic esophagoscopy are the mainstays of diagnosis. Esophagography is reported to yield false negative rates of between 10% and 43%, prompting most authors to recommend proceeding to flexible endoscopy for those patients with a negative screening esophagram, because the sensitivity of the two modalities in combination approaches 100% (23,24,25). Helical CT may assist in identifying potential injuries based on 3-dimensional reconstruction of injury pathways after penetrating neck trauma. Each modality may yield false negative results, however, and persistent clinical vigilance for evolving signs and symptoms of esophageal violation is warranted (12,13,23).

CRITICAL INTERVENTIONS

- Perform early airway management for patients with acute respiratory distress, stridor, copious blood or secretions, extensive subcutaneous emphysema, expanding hematoma, tracheal shift, or altered mental status
- Apply direct pressure to active bleeding sites
- If direct pressure fails to control hemorrhage, insert and inflate a Foley catheter balloon within the wound to tamponade bleeding
- Evaluate patients with zone I injuries for vascular, esophageal, and airway injuries

DISPOSITION

Patients with wounds that do not violate the platysma should receive standard wound care, after which they may be discharged safely. All patients with injuries deep to the platysma must receive emergent surgical consultation and should undergo systematic evaluation as described above. Even the most benign-appearing wound that violates the platysma in an asymptomatic patient must be observed for 12 to 24 hours; hospital admission or transfer to an appropriate trauma center for such patients is therefore appropriate.

COMMON PITFALLS

✔ Failure to appreciate the potential severity of a small or "trivial" penetrating neck wound

✔ Failure to appreciate subtle signs and symptoms of impending airway compromise

✔ Delaying definitive airway management until airway distortion or patient respiratory compromise have rendered intubation exponentially more problematic

✔ Failure to anticipate difficulties in airway management and implement effective alternative strategies

✔ Failure to complete a thorough physical exam to detect subtle vascular, aerodigestive, and neurologic injuries

Acknowledgments

Thanks to previous edition chapter authors Gerard R. Cox and Brigitte M. Baumann.

References

1. Apfelbaum JD, Cantrill SV, Waldman N. Unstable cervical spine without spinal cord injury in penetrating neck trauma. *Am J Emerg Med* 2000;18:55–57.
2. Arishita GI, Vayer JS, Bellamy RF. Cervical spine immobilization of penetrating neck wounds in a hostile environment. *J Trauma* 1989;29:332–337.
3. Asensio JA, Chahwan S, Forno W, et al. Penetrating esophageal injuries: multicenter study of the American Association for the Surgery of Trauma. *J Trauma* 2001;50:289–296.
4. Barkana Y, Stein M, Scope A, et al. Prehospital stabilization of the cervical spine for penetrating injuries of the neck—is it necessary? *Injury* 2000;31:305–309.
5. Biffle WL, Moore EE, Rehse DH, et al. Selective management of penetrating neck trauma based on cervical level of injury. *Am J Surg* 1997;174:678–682.
6. Bumpous JM, Whitt PD, Ganzel TM, et al. Penetrating injuries of the visceral compartment of the neck. *Am J Otolaryngol* 2000;21:190–194.
7. Carducci B, Lowe RA, Dalsey W. Penetrating neck truama: consensus and controversies. *Annals Emerg Med* 1985;15:208–215.
8. Demetriades D, Skalkides J, Costas S, et al. Carotid artery injuries: experience with 124 cases. *J Trauma* 1989;29:91–94.
9. Demetriades D, Theodorous D, Cornwell E, et al. Transcervical gunshot injuries: mandatory operation is no necessary. *J Trauma* 1996;40:758–760.
10. Demetriades D, Theodorou D, Cornwell E, et al. Evaluation of penetrating injuries of the neck: prospective study of 223 patients. *World J Surg* 1997;21:41–48.
11. Desjardins G, Varon AJ. Airway management for penetrating neck injuries: the Miami experience. *Resuscitation* 2001;48:71–75.
12. Gonzalez RP, Falimirski M, Holevar MR, et al. Penetrating zone II neck injury: does dynamic computed tomographic scan contribute to the diagnostic sensitivity of physical examination for surgically significant injury? A prospective blinded study. *J Trauma* 2003;54:61–65.
13. Gracias VH, Reilly PM, Philpott J, et al. Computed tomography in the evaluation of penetrating neck trauma. *Arch Surg* 2001;136:1231–1235.
14. Hirshberg A, Wall MJ, Johnston RH, et al. Transcervical gunshot injuries. *Am J Surg* 1994;167:309–312.
15. Kendall JL, Anglin D, Demetriades D. Penetrating neck trauma. *Emerg Med Clin North Am* 1998;16:85–105.
16. Kim MK, Buckman R, Szeremeta W. Penetrating neck trauma in children: an urban hospital's experience. *Otolaryngol Head Neck Surg* 2000;123:439–443.
17. Klyachkin ML, Rohmiller M, Charash WE, et al. Penetrating injuries of the neck: selective management evolving. *Am Surg* 1997;63:189–194.
18. Kupcha PC, An HS, Cotler JM. Gunshot wounds to the cervical spine. *Spine* 1990;15:1058–1063.
19. Mandavia DP, Qualls S, Rokos I. Emergency airway management in penetrating neck injury. *Ann Emerg Med* 2000;35:221–225.
20. Mnera F, Soto JA, Palacio DM, et al. Penetrating neck injuries: helical CT angiography for initial evaluation. *Radiology* 2002;224:366–372.
21. Nason RW, Assuras GN, Gray PR, et al. Penetrating neck injuries: analysis of experience from a Canadian trauma centre. *Canadian J Surg* 2001;44:122–126.
22. Ordog GJ, Albin D, Wasserberger J, et al. 110 bullet wounds to the neck. *J Trauma* 1985;25:238–246.
23. Srinivasan R, Haywood T, Horwitz B, et al. Role of flexible endoscopy in the evaluation of possible esophageal trauma after penetrating neck injuries. *Am J Gastroenterol* 2000;95:1725–1729.
24. Vassiliu P, Baker J, Henderson S, et al. Aerodigestive injuries of the neck. *Am Surg* 2001;67:75–79.
25. Weigelt JA, Thal ER, Snyder WH, et al. Diagnosis of penetrating cervical esophageal injuries. *Am J Surg* 1987;154:619–622.
26. Weitzel N, Kendall JL, Pons P. Blind nasotracheal intubation in patients with penetrating neck trauma. *J Trauma* 2004;56:1097–1101.

CHAPTER 179
Cervical Spine Fractures

William R. Mower, Jerome R. Hoffman, and Swaminatha V. Mahadevan

Each year United States emergency physicians evaluate nearly one million patients for cervical spine injury. Two percent to 3% of these patients actually have spine injuries, including nearly 11,000 who suffer catastrophic injury and permanent paralysis. Lifetime medical care exceeds $1 million per injury victim, while the cost of annual nationwide care for these patients exceeds $2 billion (14). Medical costs reflect only a portion of the burden produced by catastrophic cervical spine injuries. Affected patients also encounter severe limitations on activity and mobility, loss of income, productivity, and independence, and increased rates of medical illness, depression, and suicide (3,8,14).

CLINICAL PRESENTATION

Cervical spine injury (CSI) most frequently occurs following blunt trauma and is often accompanied by other significant injuries, particularly head injuries. CSI may be severe and life-threatening and may require immediate attention (14). Conversely, unstable CSI can present with subtle clinical findings. While truly occult injury rarely if ever occurs, patients may be unaware of a serious neck injury if they are intoxicated, have another painful injury that distracts their attention, or if they have an altered level of alertness that impairs their ability to appreciate the spine injury (6). While cervical spine injury should be suspected in the setting of new-onset neurologic impairment, a normal neurologic examination does not preclude serious and potentially unstable spine injury (6).

Classification Based On Mechanism

Injuries to the cervical spine tend to reflect the vector forces acting on the spine at the time of injury. Specific injury patterns tend to result from specific forces, while the extent and severity of injury are determined by duration of loading and final magnitude of the applied force. An understanding of injury biomechanics allows clinicians to focus on identifying specific families of injury and reduces the need for exhaustive evaluation for unrelated injuries (5,22).

The specific injuries associated with a given force reflect both compressive and tensile stresses generated by the force. In general, compressive forces produce failure (fracture) in osseous elements, while distractive or tensile forces can result in failure of either ligament or bone, depending on the strength of the involved bone and the rate of loading (ligamentous failure is more likely at high rates of loading) (22). For example, forced flexion generates compressive stress along the anterior spine and posterior tensile or distractive stresses. The anterior compression can produce mechanical failure of the vertebral body resulting in wedge compression and flexion teardrop fractures, while the posterior tensile forces can cause stretching and tearing of the posterior ligament complex, as seen in anterior subluxation, or failure across the spinous process, as found in clay shoveler's fractures. Severe flexion forces may destroy the entire posterior ligament complex and obliterate all middle and anterior support, and produce bilateral interfacetal dislocation (5).

Hyperextension and lateral flexion also produce forced curvature of the spine, generating compressive stresses along the concave side of the curvature and tensile stresses along the convexity. Alternatively, pure vertical compression generates only compressive stresses, while some combined actions (rotation coupled with hyperflexion or hyperextension) produce relatively complex force distributions. Each of these mechanisms generates specific stress patterns and is associated with a particular family of injuries (5,22).

It is not possible to classify all CSI in terms of specific applied forces. Injuries involving the occipital articulation and atlantoaxial complex, such as occipito-atlantal and atlanto-axial dissociations, as well as fractures of the dens, appear to have multiple etiologies (5,22). These injuries indicate the application of significant forces capable of producing other spine injuries and should prompt a careful search for additional lesions.

Classification Based On Stability

Functionally, the spine is considered stable if it is able to support physiologic loads without developing displacement or structural changes that cause irritation of the spinal cord or nerve roots, or incapacitating deformity or pain (22). While this definition is relatively straightforward, determining the stability following

specific spine injuries can be extremely difficult. Consequently, general principles have been developed to aid in assessing stability (22).

The two-column concept of the spine is particularly useful in understanding pathophysiology and assessing stability of injuries to the lower cervical spine (base of the second cervical vertebra through first thoracic vertebra) produced by predominantly flexion or extension. This construct divides the spine into anterior and posterior columns based on anatomic elements. The anterior column consists of the posterior longitudinal ligament and all anatomic elements anterior to it, including the vertebral body, annulus fibrosus, intertransverse ligaments, and anterior longitudinal ligament. The posterior column consists of all elements posterior to the posterior longitudinal ligament, including the facet and capsular ligaments, the lamina and ligamentum flavum, and the spinous process and interspinous and supraspinous ligaments (Fig. 179.1) (22). Biomechanical studies demonstrate that clinical stability is preserved if all of the elements from one column and any single element from the other column remain intact (i.e., all of the anterior elements plus one posterior element, or all of the posterior elements plus one anterior element) (16,21).

The two-column concept is not useful in assessing stability for injuries involving the occipital articulation and atlanto-axial complex, and it is of limited utility in assessing injuries associated with lateral flexion (5,22). With a very limited number of

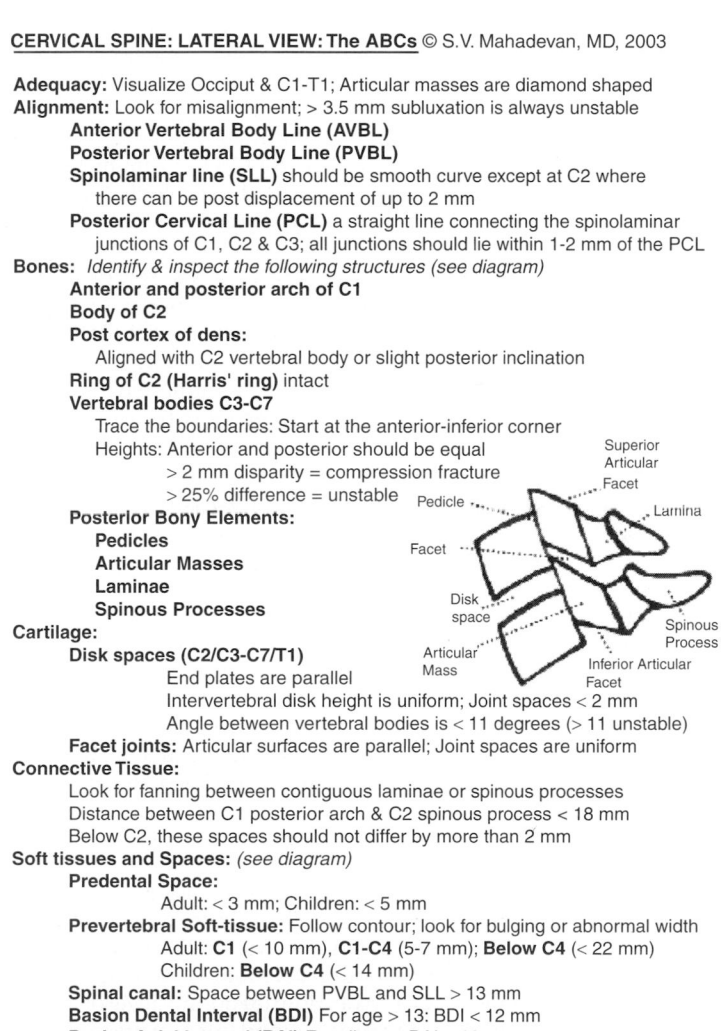

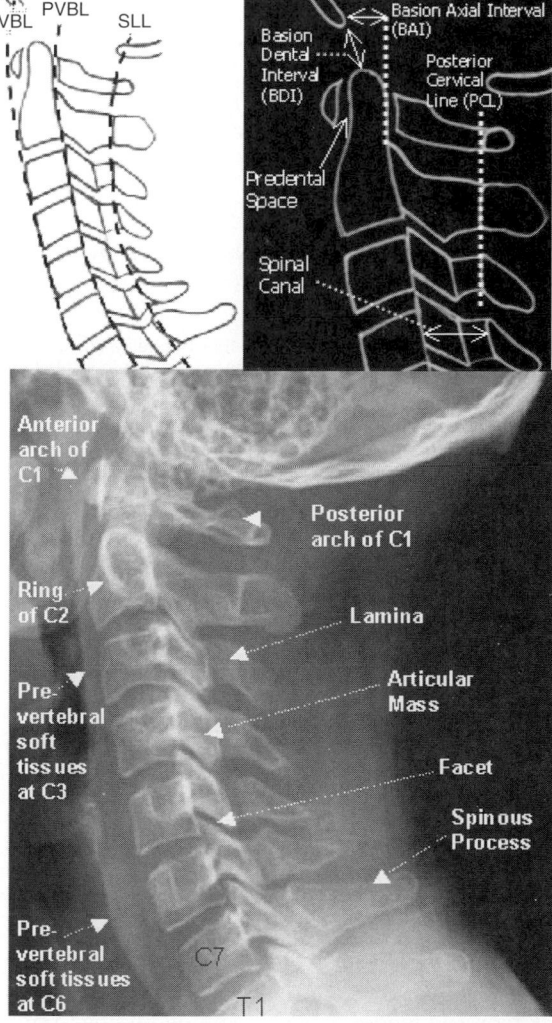

CERVICAL SPINE: LATERAL VIEW: The ABCs © S.V. Mahadevan, MD, 2003

Adequacy: Visualize Occiput & C1-T1; Articular masses are diamond shaped
Alignment: Look for misalignment; > 3.5 mm subluxation is always unstable
  Anterior Vertebral Body Line (AVBL)
  Posterior Vertebral Body Line (PVBL)
  Spinolaminar line (SLL) should be smooth curve except at C2 where
    there can be post displacement of up to 2 mm
  Posterior Cervical Line (PCL) a straight line connecting the spinolaminar
    junctions of C1, C2 & C3; all junctions should lie within 1-2 mm of the PCL
Bones: *Identify & inspect the following structures (see diagram)*
  Anterior and posterior arch of C1
  Body of C2
  Post cortex of dens:
    Aligned with C2 vertebral body or slight posterior inclination
  Ring of C2 (Harris' ring) intact
  Vertebral bodies C3-C7
    Trace the boundaries: Start at the anterior-inferior corner
    Heights: Anterior and posterior should be equal
      > 2 mm disparity = compression fracture
      > 25% difference = unstable
  Posterior Bony Elements:
    Pedicles
    Articular Masses
    Laminae
    Spinous Processes
Cartilage:
  Disk spaces (C2/C3-C7/T1)
    End plates are parallel
    Intervertebral disk height is uniform; Joint spaces < 2 mm
    Angle between vertebral bodies is < 11 degrees (> 11 unstable)
  Facet joints: Articular surfaces are parallel; Joint spaces are uniform
Connective Tissue:
  Look for fanning between contiguous laminae or spinous processes
  Distance between C1 posterior arch & C2 spinous process < 18 mm
  Below C2, these spaces should not differ by more than 2 mm
Soft tissues and Spaces: *(see diagram)*
  Predental Space:
    Adult: < 3 mm; Children: < 5 mm
  Prevertebral Soft-tissue: Follow contour; look for bulging or abnormal width
    Adult: **C1** (< 10 mm), **C1-C4** (5-7 mm); **Below C4** (< 22 mm)
    Children: **Below C4** (< 14 mm)
  Spinal canal: Space between PVBL and SLL > 13 mm
  Basion Dental Interval (BDI) For age > 13: BDI < 12 mm
  Basion Axial Interval (BAI) For all ages BAI < 12 mm

Figure 179.1.   Cervical spine lateral view: the ABCs.

TABLE 179.1. Injury Mechanism and Clinical Stability of Common Isolated Cervical Spine Injuries

Forced flexion
  Spinous process fracture (Clay shoveler's fracture) (S)
  Anterior subluxation (D)
  Wedge compression fracture (D)
  Bilateral interfacetal dislocation (U)
  Flexion teardrop fracture (U)
Extension
  Avulsion of anterior arch of the atlas (S)
  Fracture of posterior arch of atlas (S)
  Laminar fracture (S)
  Traumatic spondylolisthesis (Hangman's fracture)
    Nondisplaced—type I (S)
    Displaced—types II and III (U)
  Extension teardrop fracture (U)
  Hyperextension dislocation (U)
  Hyperextension fracture dislocation (U)
Vertical compression
  Jefferson burst fracture (U)
  Vertebral body burst fractures (U)
Hyperflexion and rotation
  Unilateral interfacetal dislocation (S*)
  Unilateral interfacetal fracture dislocation (U)
Hyperextension and rotation
  Pillar fracture (S)
  Unilateral pedicolaminar fracture-separation (S)
  Bilateral pedicolaminar fracture-dislocation (U)
Lateral flexion
  Unilateral occipital condyle fracture (U)
  Unilateral fracture of the C1 lateral mass (U)
  Uncinate process fracture (U)
  Transverse process fracture (U)
Injuries due to multiple or poorly understood mechanisms
  Torticollis (atlantoaxial rotatory displacement or fixation) (S)
  Dens fractures
    Type I (S)
    Type II or high (U)
    Type III or low (U)
  Os odontoideum (U)
  Occipitoatlantal subluxation or dislocation (U)
  Occipitoatlantal dissociation (U)
  Atlantoaxial rotatory dissociation (subluxation or dislocation) (U)
  Atlantoaxial dissociation (U)
  Occipital condyle fractures (U)

(S) = Stable injury, (D) = Initially stable, but delayed instability possible, (U) = Unstable or potentially unstable injury; consider consultation with experienced spine specialist. See text for definitions.
*May occasionally be associated with spinal cord or nerve root injury.
Modified from Harris JH Jr, Mirvis SE. The radiology of acute cervical spine trauma. 3rd ed. Baltimore: Williams & Wilkins, 1996, with permission.

exceptions (fractures to the posterior arch of the atlas, small avulsion fractures of the anterior arch, and type I dens fractures), consultation with an experienced spine specialist is recommended to determine the stability of these injuries.

Table 179.1 summarizes the injury mechanism and clinical stability associated with common cervical spine injuries. This table presents a conservative interpretation of clinical stability in that many of the injuries described as unstable may actually have stable variants, but the detailed considerations required for a definitive assessment are beyond the scope of this text. Consultation with an experienced spine specialist is recommended in cases of uncertainty. Table 179.2 describes the specific injuries that characterize common cervical spine fractures.

DIFFERENTIAL DIAGNOSIS

Neck pain and tenderness are common findings among trauma patients, but significant cervical spine injury is rare. Most patients have minor strains and contusions that require no specific therapy. As such, it is not necessary to identify specific soft tissue injuries in most cases but rather to exclude serious injuries that could result in permanent dysfunction or catastrophic disability.

Injury to the spine and spinal cord should be suspected in any trauma patient presenting with a new-onset neurologic deficit. At the same time, it is important to recognize that these same deficits can be due to a variety of other etiologies outside the cervical spine, such as vascular injury, intracranial injury, lower spine injury, or injury to one or more peripheral nerves (5,6). Respiratory distress in blunt trauma patients may also be due to a variety of causes, including upper CSI. The neck contains a remarkable number of vital structures, including the spinal cord, carotid and basilar arteries, jugular veins, the trachea, and the esophagus. All are susceptible to injury and may produce pain indistinguishable from that produced by cervical spine injury. It is important to note that trauma patients frequently have multiple injuries and identifying a specific injury does not preclude the presence of other injuries. Spine injuries in particular provide evidence of significant axial forces and should prompt clinicians to evaluate affected patients for secondary cervical spine injuries, as well as injuries to other axial elements, including the lower spine.

EMERGENCY DEPARTMENT EVALUATION

Once the ABCs have been addressed, patients should undergo a meticulous examination to detect other injuries and ascertain baseline function. Patients should be assessed for mental status changes that may limit the reliability of clinical evaluations. Careful attention should be placed on assessing the face and calvarium. Many of the force vectors that cause cervical spine injuries originate in the head and meticulous evaluation may disclose such injuries as well as provide information relating to potential spine injuries. The neck and spine should be examined to detect areas of pain and swelling. A detailed neurologic examination is essential and should include an assessment of reflexes and pathologic findings associated with spine injury (bulbocarvernosus reflex, priapism, decreased rectal tone). Sensory innervation follows dermatomal distributions and is particularly helpful in localizing lesions in patients with cord injuries (Table 179.3). Similarly, deficits in motor function are associated with specific nerve root levels and may also prove informative in determining injury levels (Table 179.3). Any patient with suspected spine injury should also undergo a careful evaluation of the remaining axial anatomy.

Because cervical spine injuries can be permanent and devastating, all trauma patients should be evaluated for potential cervical spine injuries. Radiographic imaging provides the definitive means of assessment, but is unnecessary in many cases. Clinical assessments based on decision guides such as the NEXUS low-risk criteria (Table 179.4) (6) and Canadian c-spine rule (Fig. 179.2) (19) allow clinicians to identify patients who are at very low risk of cervical spine injury and who can be safely spared the expense and radiation exposure associated with imaging. While these instruments reliably detect injury (high sensitivity) and preclude injury in patients deemed "low risk" (high negative predictive value), they exhibit poor positive predictive value, and the majority of "non-low-risk" patients do not have cervical spine injuries.

The NEXUS criteria are based on five historical and physical examination findings. Patients are at low risk and may safely be spared radiographic imaging provided they exhibit all of the following criteria: (1) no posterior midline cervical spine tenderness; (2) no evidence of intoxication; (3) normal level of alertness; (4) no focal neurologic impairment; and (5) no distracting painful injuries. The criteria are subject to interpretation by individual physicians. Although they are not precisely defined, each criterion is further clarified as follows (15).

TABLE 179.2. Pathophysiologic Lesions Associated with Common Cervical Spine Injuries

Injury	Pathophysiology
Occipitoatlantal dislocation	Separation or disruption of the craniovertebral junction.
Burst fracture of the atlas (Jefferson burst fracture)	Fracture of the anterior and posterior arches of the atlas (C1) that may be accompanied by disruption of the transverse atlantal ligament. Unilateral and bilateral variants exist.
Dens fractures (Odontoid fractures)	Fractures of the axis (C2) involving the dens. Subclassification is based on fracture location with respect to the dens and has important implications for stability and treatment.
Type I	Fracture of the superolateral odontoid process.
Type II	Fracture at the base of the dens.
Type III	Fracture of the axis body caudal to the junction with the dens.
Traumatic spondylolisthesis (Hangman's fracture)	Bilateral fractures of the pars interarticularis of the axis (C2). Subclassification is based on displacement of the posterior ring of the axis and disruption of the C2–C3 disk space and reflects important mechanistic and therapeutic implications.
Type I	Minimal (hairline) displacement of fracture fragments with preservation of the disk space.
Type II	Displacement between anterior and posterior fragments with abnormal disk space.
Type III	Displacement between anterior and posterior fragments with bilateral interfacetal dislocation of C2 and C3.
Vertebral body burst fractures	Compressive fracture of the vertebral body, producing circumferential dispersion of bone fragments.
Flexion teardrop fracture	Fracture of the anteroinferior corner of the vertebral body, with associated disruption of the anterior and posterior longitudinal ligaments and intervertebral disk.
Extension teardrop fracture	Avulsion fracture of the anteroinferior corner of the vertebral body of the axis (C2).
Wedge compression fracture	Impaction and angulation of the superior endplate and anterior cortical margin of the vertebral body. Frequently accompanied by injuries to the posterior ligament complex.
Bilateral interfacetal dislocation	Disruption of the posterior ligament complex, posterior longitudinal ligament, and intervertebral disk, with bilateral anterior dislocation of the articular masses.
Unilateral interfacetal dislocation	Unilateral rotation and dislocation of the articular mass (perched or locked facet). Usually accompanied by disruption of the articular capsule and posterior ligament complex but may also involve disruption of the contralateral articular capsule.
Hyperextension dislocation	Disruption of both anterior and posterior longitudinal ligaments, and disruption or detachment of the intervertebral disk. Frequently reduces spontaneously with no apparent osseous abnormality. Diagnosis may depend on the detection of soft tissue abnormalities.
Anterior subluxation (Hyperflexion sprain)	Disruption of the posterior ligament complex and posterior longitudinal ligament. Frequently involves injury to the posterior disk elements. The remainder of the disk and anterior longitudinal ligament remain intact.
Spinous process fracture (Clay shoveler's fracture)	Avulsion fracture of the spinous process of the lower vertebrae.

- Midline posterior bony cervical spine tenderness is present if the patient complains of pain on palpation of the posterior midline neck from the nuchal ridge to the prominence of the first thoracic vertebra, or if the patient has pain with direct palpation of any cervical spinous process.
- Patients should be considered intoxicated if they have either of the following: (a) a recent history by the patient or an observer of intoxication or intoxicating ingestion; or (b) evidence of intoxication on physical examination such as odor of alcohol, slurred speech, ataxia, dysmetria or other cerebellar findings, or any behavior consistent with intoxication. Patients may also be considered to be intoxicated if tests of bodily secretions are positive for drugs (including but not limited to alcohol) that affect level of alertness.
- An altered level of alertness can include any of the following: (a) Glasgow Coma Scale score of 14 or less; (b) disorientation to person, place, time, or events; (c) inability to remember 3 objects at 5 minutes; (d) delayed or inappropriate response to external stimuli; or, (e) other evidence of cognitive impairment or altered alertness.
- Any focal neurologic complaint (by history) or finding (on motor or sensory examination).
- No precise definition for distracting painful injury is possible. It includes any condition thought by the clinician to be producing pain sufficient to distract the patient from a second (neck) injury. Examples may include, but are not limited to: (a) any long bone fracture; (b) a visceral injury requiring surgical consultation; (c) a large laceration, degloving injury, or crush injury; (d) large burns; or (e) any other injury producing acute functional impairment. Physicians may also classify any injury as distracting if it is thought to have the potential to impair the patient's ability to appreciate other injuries.

Radiographic imaging, if indicated, should be individualized according to the patient's clinical presentation and potential for cervical spine injury. A three-view series of plain radiographs (lateral, anterior-posterior and odontoid) currently provides the minimal acceptable standard for radiographically evaluating most blunt trauma patients (5). Such imaging is highly sensitive in detecting the presence of cervical spine injury but frequently fails to reveal the specific form of injury (13). Many centers employ oblique views to increase sensitivity and improve detection of specific injuries involving the lateral and posterior spine elements, although the benefit is only marginal.

Plain radiography requires correct exposure and positioning; injury cannot be reliably excluded if images are incomplete or inadequate. Abnormal radiographs should also cause concern, even though no specific injury is evident. Misalignment of spine elements and changes in soft tissue contours may indicate the

TABLE 179.3. Sensory and Motor Examination

Spinal Cord Level	Sensory Distribution	Functional Ability
C4	Neck	Spontaneous breathing
C5	Shoulder and arm	Shrug shoulders
C6	Thumb	Elbow flexion
C7	Third digit	Elbow extension
C8	Fifth digit	Flexion of fingers

TABLE 179.4.   NEXUS Low-Risk Criteria*

Patients are at low risk and may safely be spared radiographic imaging provided they exhibit all of the following criteria:

1) No posterior midline cervical spine tenderness
2) No evidence of intoxication
3) Normal level of alertness
4) No focal neurologic impairment
5) No distracting painful injuries

See text for explanation.

*Copyright © 2000. Reproduced with permission.

presence of serious injuries. The interpretation of plain radiographs can be difficult and requires comprehensive knowledge of the subtle findings that may indicate significant injury, as well as a detailed understanding of the normal variants that may simulate injury patterns (5). The inexpert interpretation of inadequate cervical spine radiographs is a recipe for disaster. Figures 179.1, 179.3, and 179.4 present a detailed and systematic approach to reviewing and interpreting screening radiographs.

Despite the limitations associated with plain radiography, it remains the most effective means of excluding significant CSI in most patients. Such imaging is particularly useful in patients deemed to have relatively low risk of injury (5,10,13).

Computed tomography (CT) provides the most definitive means of evaluating the bony cervical spine and is generally indicated in the initial evaluation of patients with high risk of cervical spine injury (major multiple trauma patients, those with significant intracranial injury or evidence of neurologic injury) (2) and in cases where plain radiographs are either abnormal or inadequate (5). CT has also been advocated as a means of excluding fractures in patients who have normal plain radiographs but exhibit unexplained persistent neck pain. CT imaging is highly sensitive in detecting bony injury but may miss fractures of the dens, as well as injuries in the plane of the scanner such as dislocations and subluxations, particularly if imaging is completed using early generation scanners (23). The cross-table lateral

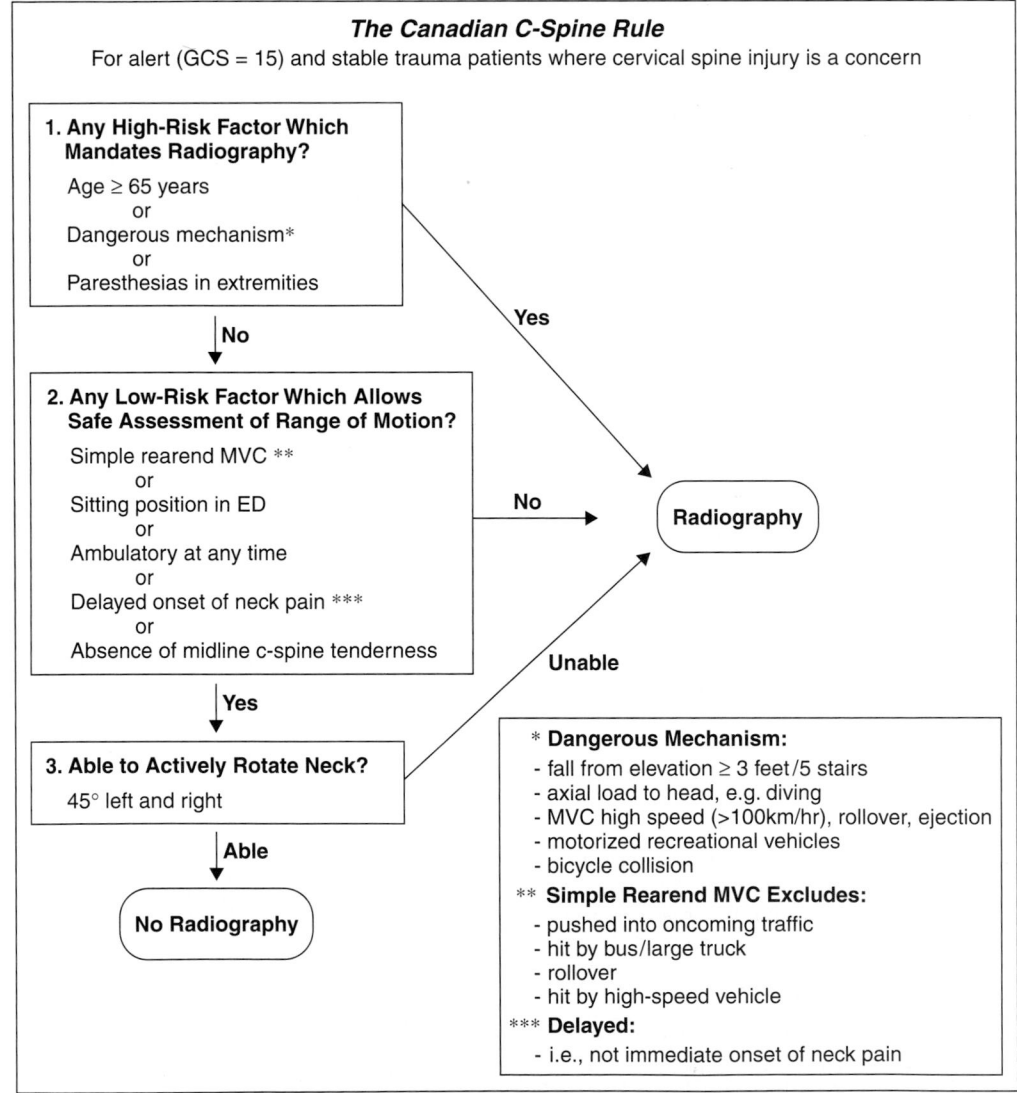

Figure 179.2.   Canadian C-spine rule. Patients are excluded from low-risk classification if they: **(1)** are younger than 16 years; **(2)** have a Glasgow Coma Scale (GCS) score lower than 15; **(3)** have grossly abnormal vital signs; **(4)** were injured more than 48 hours previously; **(5)** have penetrating trauma; **(6)** present with acute paralysis; **(7)** have known vertebral disease (ankylosing spondylitis, rheumatoid arthritis, spinal stenosis, or previous cervical surgery), as determined by the examining physician; **(8)** are returning for reassessment of the same injury; or **(9)** are pregnant (19).

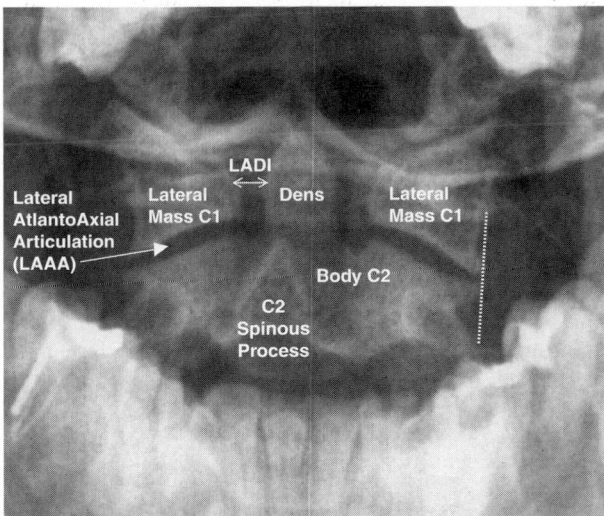

CERVICAL SPINE: OPEN MOUTH: The ABCs © S.V. Mahadevan, MD, 2003
Adequacy: The dens and lateral masses (C1 and C2) are visible
including the entire **Lateral AtlantoAxial Articulation (LAAA)**
Rotation is minimized: Dens and C2 spinous process are in the midline
Alignment: Lateral margins of the articular surfaces of C1-C2 are aligned
About 1-2 mm symmetric overriding is allowable
medially or laterally
Bones: *Identify & inspect the following structures (see diagram above)*
Lateral masses of C1
Body and spinous process of C2
Peg and base of the dens
Cartilage: The **Lateral AtlantoAxial Articulation (LAAA)** of C1-C2 form
parallel joint surfaces
Spaces: Lateral AtlantoDental Intervals (LADI) are similar
but not necessarily equal

Figure 179.3.   Cervical spine open mouth view: the ABCs.

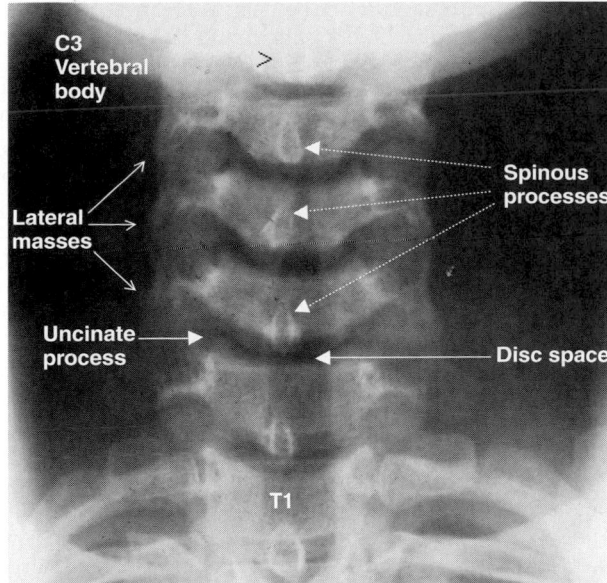

CERVICAL SPINE: AP : The ABCs © S.V. Mahadevan, MD, 2003
Adequacy: No tilt or rotation
The vertebral bodies of C3-T1 are visible
Alignment: The spinous processes are aligned in the midline
The articular masses form a smooth, undulating and
continous lateral margin
Bones: *Identify & inspect the following structures (diagram above)*
Vertebral bodies: Are rectangular and of uniform height & width
Uncinate processes
Lateral masses
Spinous processes
Cartilage: Disk spaces are of uniform height
Articular surfaces are parallel
Spaces: Spinous processes are equidistant

Figure 179.4.   Cervical spine anteroposterior view: the ABCs.

radiograph provides a reliable means for detecting these potentially missed injuries, and, consequently, still plays an important role in the initial evaluation of blunt trauma patients undergoing radiographic imaging (5).

Radiography, whether plain film or CT, must be of high quality, with complete visualization of the spine and soft tissues from the base of the skull to the top of the first thoracic vertebra. High technical quality is essential, with proper film exposure, proper patient positioning, removal of foreign bodies and avoidance of motion artifact (5).

Magnetic resonance imaging (MRI) offers an effective and discriminating means for assessing the soft tissues of the cervical spine. Bony injuries are frequently missed on MRI, hence it is not an adequate substitute for CT or plain film imaging. MRI is most useful in assessing injuries to the cord, intervertebral disks, and paracervical tissues, including supporting ligaments. Use of this modality should be limited to patients with post-traumatic myelopathy or radiculopathy, patients with pain disproportionate to their physical and radiographic findings, those with plain radiographs demonstrating occipito-atlantal subluxation, and to assess the acuity of anterior subluxations. MRI and MR angiography may also be valuable in assessing the vertebral arteries, particularly in patients who have pedicolaminar fracture separations (5).

Flexion-extension radiographs have been advocated in the acute evaluation of suspected anterior subluxation when plain films are nondiagnostic. However, this type of imaging is known to miss acute anterior subluxations, presumably because of reflex cervical spasm, and has not been shown to enhance the early detection of this initially stable injury (18,20). Consequently, the value of flexion-extension imaging is questionable in the emer-

gency setting and may provide false security to patients with missed injuries. A better approach to the diagnosis and management of patients with suspected anterior subluxation is to employ MRI to evaluate patients with typical radiographic findings or those with neurologic symptoms such as radiculopathy. The remaining patients appear to be best evaluated by delayed flexion-extension imaging once their spasm has resolved (12,18).

Motion fluoroscopy has been used to assess spine stability in select patients, particularly those who cannot cooperate with flexion-extension imaging. Use of this modality, particularly passive fluoroscopy, is controversial because of its potential to produce permanent cord injury. Currently, there are no emergent indications for the use of this imaging (11).

EMERGENCY DEPARTMENT MANAGEMENT

The primary goal of the emergent treatment of spine injury is to prevent further injury and disability. While cervical spine injury can be devastating, initial management must focus on ensuring other vital functions, including adequate airway, breathing and circulation. Trauma patients should always be presumed to have an unstable spine injury until proven otherwise, and their entire spine should be protected until an appropriate evaluation can be completed.

Special care must be exercised in managing patients who require mechanical ventilation. While all methods of securing an adequate airway, including surgical approaches, can produce movement of the cervical spine, it should not result in neurologic deterioration if performed appropriately, and of course ventilatory support should not be delayed because of concerns related to spine injury. Inadequate ventilation not only places other organ systems at risk but also increases the potential for ischemic and hypoxic injury to the spine.

The airway should be secured using familiar techniques that are least likely to require repeated attempts. Most patients can be orotracheally intubated, while those with extensive neck and facial injuries may require a surgical airway. Adequate preparation and equipment are essential, as is careful technique. An assistant who can help stabilize the spine and ensure anatomic alignment may prove particularly helpful (7). Axial traction may produce harmful distractive forces and is contraindicated (1).

Protecting the spine from additional mechanical injury is essential. Cervical spine "precautions" should be used to maintain an anatomically neutral position. Immobilization may include the use of various collars, backboards, and supplemental devices such as braces and sandbags. However, the use of these devises should be directed towards the primary goal of maintaining appropriate spine alignment. Ill-fitting collars and poor patient positioning may actually produce further injury, despite the fact that the spine is immobilized. Backboards and cervical collars can be removed as soon as the spine has been cleared in patients who are uninjured, or as soon as alternative measures have been initiated to provide support for patients with spine injuries.

Specific treatments for spinal cord injuries are currently limited. Meticulous supportive care, including optimization of ventilatory and circulatory support, is essential and plays a substantial role in the preservation of neurologic function. Injury to the spinal cord may produce loss of sympathetic and vasomotor tone and subsequent spinal shock. Intravenous crystalloids should be administered as initial treatment, and patients should be carefully assessed for other sources of hypotension, particularly other traumatic injuries. Vasopressors may be required to attain adequate perfusion pressures, but these agents should be used carefully, with an appreciation of their ability to temporarily mask the hypovolemia produced by coexisting injuries. Spinal shock may also be complicated by bradycardia, which may require specific pharmacologic treatment if accompanied by hypotension.

Corticosteroids and GM-1 gangliosides have been advocated in the treatment of acute cord injuries, but there is insufficient evidence to support the use of either agent. They are recommended as options in the treatment of spinal cord injuries but have no demonstrated benefit. Treatment with methylprednisolone in particular appears to be more likely to produce harmful side effects as opposed to clinical benefit (17).

CRITICAL INTERVENTIONS

- Suspect cervical spine injury in all trauma patients. While cervical spine injury frequently occurs in the setting of multisystem trauma, presentation can be subtle. Geriatric patients are particularly at risk of injury following relatively minor trauma such as ground-level falls (9)
- Support the airway, ensure ventilation, and treat other life-threatening injuries. Assume cervical spine injuries are present in all blunt trauma patients until they are sufficiently stable to permit a thorough evaluation
- Maintain normal cervical anatomy (cervical immobilization). Provide physical support for the spine to prevent further injury
- Perform an adequate diagnostic evaluation. Obtain radiographic imaging in any cases in which injury cannot reliably be excluded on the basis of clinical evaluation. Obtain adequate radiographic imaging and ensure that the images are interpreted by clinicians familiar with the subtle radiographic findings associated with many cervical spine injuries

DISPOSITION

Patients who have minor spine injuries, including those with cervical strains and isolated stable fractures that do not require further intervention, may be discharged with analgesia and instructions to avoid uncomfortable or painful activities. Soft cervical collars are frequently dispensed to these patients but have little proven benefit (4).

An experienced spine specialist should be involved in the care of all patients with evidence of neurologic injury, those with clinically unstable or potentially unstable spine injuries, those with fractures that are displaced or otherwise interfere with normal function, and any patient in whom injury status is uncertain. Rigorous protection from additional injury is indicated in all cases involving unstable fractures and those with neurologic injury. Consultation with a spine specialist should be initiated as soon as the patient's condition permits.

COMMON PITFALLS

- ✔ Failure to suspect injury, particularly in patients without localized tenderness or neurologic deficits, and among intoxicated patients, those with altered levels of alertness, and those with other painful or distracting injuries
- ✔ Performing an inadequate physical examination. Clinical clearance is impossible in patients who cannot cooperate with a detailed exam (intoxicated patients and those with altered mentation or other painful distracting injuries). Detailed and complete neurologic examination is essential with careful attention to dermatomal function and pathologic reflexes
- ✔ Performing inadequate radiographic evaluation. Radiographs must be of high technical quality with complete visualization of the spine from the base of the skull to the cervicothoracic junction. Films must be free of foreign bodies and motion artifacts. Radiographs must be reviewed carefully, with appreciation for the subtle soft tissue and alignment abnormalities that may indicate serious cervical spine injury

References

1. Bivins HG, Ford S, Bezmalinovic Z, et al. The effect of axial traction during orotracheal intubation of the trauma patient with an unstable cervical spine. *Ann Emerg Med* 1988;17:25–29.
2. Blackmore CC, Emerson SS, Mann FA, et al. Cervical spine imaging in patients with trauma: determination of fracture risk to optimize use. *Radiology* 1999;211:759–765.
3. Elliot TR, Frank RG. Depression following spinal cord injury. *Arch Phys Med Rehabil* 1996;77:816–823.
4. Gennis P, Miller L, Gallagher EJ, et al. The effect of soft cervical collars on persistent neck pain in patients with whiplash injury. *Acad Emerg Med* 1996;3:568–573.
5. Harris JH Jr, Mirvis SE. *The Radiology of Acute Cervical Spine Trauma.* 3rd ed. Baltimore: Williams & Wilkins, 1996.
6. Hoffman JR, Mower WR, Wolfson AB, et al. Validity of a set of clinical criteria to rule out injury to the cervical spine in patients with blunt trauma. *N Engl J Med* 2000;343:94–99.
7. Holley J, Jordan R. Airway management in patients with unstable cervical spine fractures. *Ann Emerg Med* 1989;18:1237–1239.
8. Johnson RL, Gerhart KA, McCray J, et al. Secondary conditions following spinal cord injury in a population-based study. *Spinal Cord* 1998;36:45–50.
9. Lomoschitz FM, Blackmore CC, Mirza SK, et al. Cervical spine injuries in patients 65 years old and older: epidemiologic analysis regarding the effects of age and injury mechanism on distribution, type, and stability of injuries. *Am J Roentgenol* 2002;178:573–577.
10. Mirvis SE, Diaconis JN, Chirico PA, et al. Protocol driven radiographic evaluation of suspected cervical spine injury: efficacy study. *Radiology* 1989;170:831–836.
11. Mirvis SE. Fluoroscopically guided passive flexion-extension views of the cervical spine in the obtunded blunt trauma patient: a commentary. *Emergency Radiology* 2001;8:3–5.
12. Mower WR, Clements CM, Hoffman JR. Anterior subluxations of the cervical spine. *Emergency Radiology* 2001;8:194–199.
13. Mower WR, Hoffman JR, NEXUS Group, et al. Use of plain radiography to screen for cervical spine injuries. *Ann Emerg Med* 2001;38:1–7.

anterior to the nucleus pulposus and the anter[ior]
ligament. If the distraction forces are great enoug[h]
[mid]dle and posterior columns may be disrupted.

Chance fractures are usually seen in victims [of]
airplane accidents who are wearing lap seat bel[ts] [Examina]tion may reveal ecchymosis of the lower abdo[men]
[tender]ness at the fracture site, but the absence of the[se]
preclude the diagnosis. Although neurologic de[ficits occur in less]
than 5%, Chance fractures are commonly asso[ciated with]
abdominal injuries, such as intestinal perforati[on]
and contusions.

Chance fractures are best seen on a lateral r[adiograph which]
demonstrates a horizontal disruption throug[h the spinous pro]cess, laminae, transverse process, pedicles, a[nd vertebral]
body (8). The height of the vertebral body is i[ncreased and the]
distance between the spinous processes above [and below the in]jury may appear to be widened (Fig. 180.3). [The AP film may]
demonstrate an increased interspinous distan[ce as well as]
the transverse processes. Routine axial CT sca[ns may fre]quently miss these fractures, since the image [is parallel to]
the level of the injury. Thus, sagittal reconstru[ction]
is recommended if a Chance fracture is suspe[cted.]

Burst Fractures

Burst fractures comprise 14% of all TLS injuri[es and are due to a]
compressive force causing a fracture of the e[ndplate and]
the nucleus pulposus on the vertebral body, a[nd the fragments]
being retropulsed into the spinal canal. Bur[st fractures]
without posterior element injuries occur in [...]
and those with posterior element involveme[nt are more likely]
for neurologic deficits (11).

Burst fractures are most commonly asso[ciated with]
motor vehicle collisions. All burst fracture[s are consid]ered unstable, since standard radiography [...]

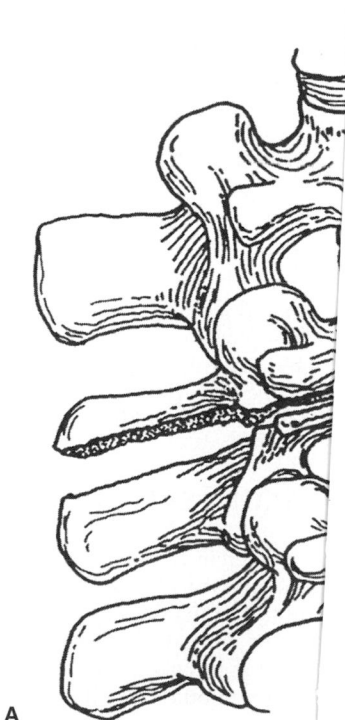

A

Figure 180.3. A Chance fracture [...]
(From Fractures, dislocations, and [...]
Emergency orthopaedics: the spine [...]

14. National Spinal Cord Injury Statistical Center (NSCISC). *Spinal Cord Injury: Facts and Figures at a Glance.* Birmingham, AL: National Spinal Cord Injury Statistical Center, 2003.
15. Panacek EA, Mower WR, NEXUS Group, et al. Test performance of the individual NEXUS low-risk clinical screening criteria for cervical spine injury. *Ann Emerg Med* 2001;38:22–25.
16. Panjabi MM, White AA, Johnson RM. Cervical spine mechanics as a function of transection of components. *J Biomech* 1975;8:327–336.
17. Pharmacological therapy after acute cervical spinal cord injury. *Neurosurgery* 2002;50(3 Suppl):S63–72.
18. Pollack CV Jr, Hendey GW, Martin DR, et al. NEXUS Group. Use of Flexon-extension radiographs of the cervical spine in blunt trauma. *Ann Emerg Med* 2001;38:8–11.
19. Stiell IG, Clement CM, McKnight RD, et al. The Canadian C-spine rule versus the NEXUS low-risk criteria in patients with trauma. *N Engl J Med* 2003;25;349:2510–2518.
20. Vandemark RM. Radiology of the cervical spine in trauma patients: practice pitfalls and recommendations for improving efficacy and communication. *Am J Roentgenol* 1990;155:465–472.
21. White AA, Johnson RM, Panjabi MM, et al. Biomechanical analysis of clinical stability in the cervical spine. *Clin Orthop* 1975;109:85–96.
22. White AA, Panjabi MM. *Clinical biomechanics of the spine.* 2nd ed. Philadelphia: J. B. Lippincott Company, 1990.
23. Woodring JH, Lee C. The role and limitations of computed tomographic scanning in the evaluation of cervical trauma. *J Trauma* 1992;33:698–708.

CHAPTER 180
Thoracolumbar Spine Fractures

Amy Kaji and Robert S. Hockberger

Thoracolumbar spine (TLS) injuries are relatively uncommon in the United States; however, of all blunt trauma patients presenting to the emergency department (ED), the rate of TLS injury is as high as 6.3% in those who undergo TLS radiographs (12). Predominantly afflicting productive young adults, 55% percent of spinal cord injuries (SCI) occur among those 16 to 30 years of age. There is a 4:1 male predominance, and the total annual cost to society from medical expenses and lost productivity is estimated to be $5 billion. Statistics from the National Spinal Cord Injury Database (NSCID) reveal that motor vehicle-related accidents account for 38.5% of all spinal injuries, while the second largest contributor is intentional acts of violence (24.5%), followed by falls (21.8%), and sports-related injuries (7.2%) (18).

The human spine consists of 33 bony vertebrae: 7 cervical, 12 thoracic, 5 lumbar, 5 sacral, and 4 coccygeal. Due to its highly exposed location above the torso and its inherent flexibility, the cervical spine is the most commonly injured part of the spinal column (see Chapter 179, "Cervical Spine Fractures"). In contrast, the thoracic spine is rigidly fixed. The thoracic ribs articulate with the respective transverse processes and sternum, and a great amount of force is necessary to damage the thoracic spine. The second most commonly injured region is the thoracolumbar junction. The transition zone from thoracic to lumbar vertebrae is vulnerable to injury because of the juxtaposition of a rigidly fixed thoracic spine against a flexible lumbar spine. The spinal column also changes from a kyphotic curve to a lordotic curve at this level, and, of all TLS injuries, 90% of the fractures occur in

the region between T11 and L4. Since the spinal canal is relatively wide at this level, thoracolumbar junction injuries rarely result in complete cord lesions and more commonly result in incomplete cord lesions (17).

CLINICAL PRESENTATION

Classification

White and Panjabi first described the concept of spinal instability, which they defined as the inability of the spine to maintain the anatomical relationships between vertebrae necessary to prevent neurologic injury or compromise (21). Since then, numerous classification schemes for TLS injuries have been reported. Utilizing results from a retrospective review of over 400 TLS injuries, Denis delineated a means to assess stability of vertebral fractures in which he divided the spinal column into three columns: anterior, middle, and posterior. The anterior column includes the anterior longitudinal ligament, the annulus fibrosus, and the anterior half of the vertebral body; the middle column comprises the posterior longitudinal ligament, the posterior annulus fibrosus, and the posterior half of the vertebral body; while the posterior column includes the supraspinous and interspinous ligaments, as well as the facet joint capsule (8) (Fig. 180.1). According to this scheme, the stability of the spine is based upon the integrity of two of the three spinal columns. More specifically, Denis stipulated that the stability of the middle column determined the

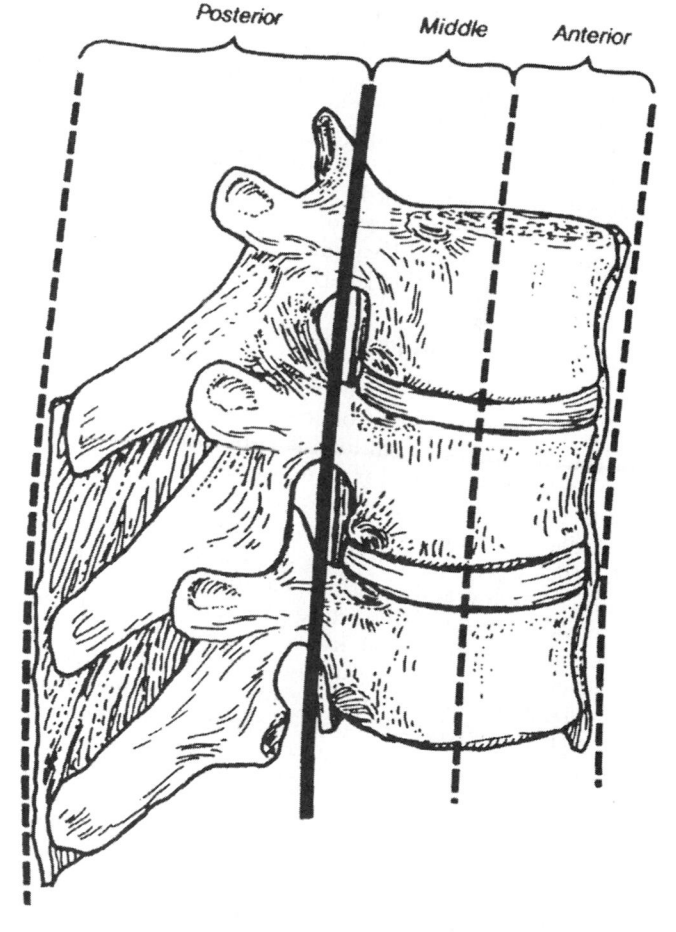

Figure 180.1. The three-column concept used to classify thoracic and lumbar spine fractures. (From Fractures, dislocations, and major ligamentous injuries. In: Galli RL, Spaite DW, Simon RR, eds. *Emergency orthopaedics: the spine.* Appleton and Lange, 1989 with permission.)

TABLE 180.1. Thoracolumbar Spine Injury Classi…

Major Fracture/Dislocation	Minor Fra…
Wedge compression fracture: isolated anterior column fracture	*Transverse proc…*
Chance fractures: horizontal vertebral avulsion injury with center of rotation anterior to vertebral body	*Spinous proces…*
Stable burst fractures: anterior and middle column compression failure with posterior column intact	*Pars interarticu…*
Unstable burst fractures: compressive failure of anterior and middle columns with disruption of the posterior column	
Flexion-distraction injuries: compressive failure of anterior column with tensile failure of the posterior column	
Translational injuries: disruption of the spinal canal in the transverse plane, usually due to a shear mechanism	

integrity of the spine, and he used his three col…
distinguish major and minor TLS fractures.

McAfee subsequently classified TLS injuries :
ent patterns: wedge compression fractures, Ch
stable and unstable burst fractures, flexion-distr
and translational injuries. All of these fractures
or more of three mechanisms of injury: axial cor
distraction, and translation (8). In McAfee's clas
and unstable burst fractures are distinguished
the integrity of the posterior ligament comple;
nation of Denis' division of major and minor f
and McAfee's fracture-dislocation scheme is c
accepted and utilized (Table 180.1).

Wedge Compression Fractures

Wedge compression fractures account for 50%
fractures and usually result from compressive
terior column after an axial load is applied i
wedge fractures are defined as demonstrating l
pression, and there is generally no neurologic
the middle column remains intact. Simple w
stable, since pure flexion injuries do not dis
ligament complex, and an additional rotatio
sary to cause an unstable fracture pattern. H
severe compression (>50%), kyphosis greate
multilevel compression fractures, or a rotatic
the injury, then the posterior ligamentous
and progress to involve the middle column,
instability (21).

Wedge compression fractures generally re
tor vehicle collisions, and occasionally gene
seizures. Bilateral calcaneal fractures should
physician to the possibility of a TLS fractu
pression from a vertical plunge (11). Associa
mon, and fractures frequently coexist at o
is important to image patients greater tha
complain of back pain, even after apparentl
the incidence of osteoporotic compression
this age group. In conscious patients who
tracting injury, there is invariably pain or t

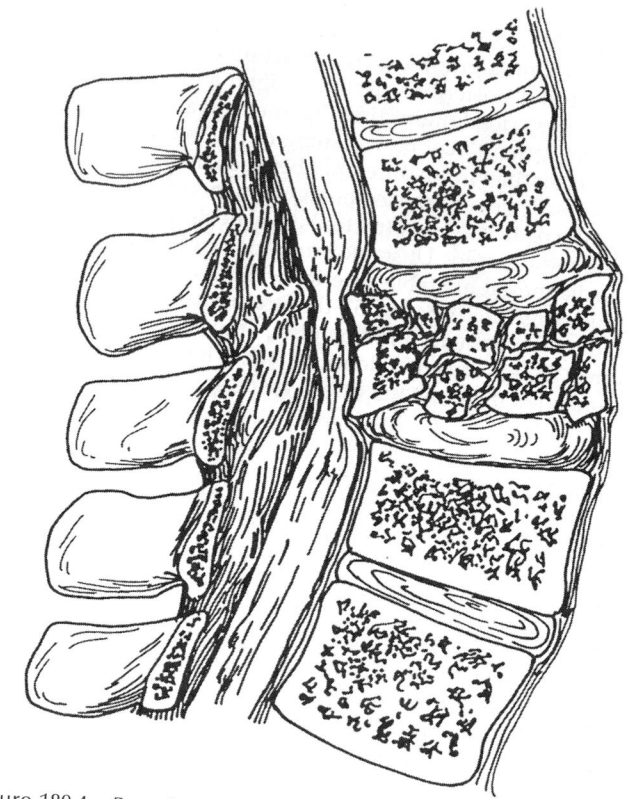

Figure 180.4. Burst fracture without posterior element disruption. Note retropulsion of bone fragments posteriorly into the spinal canal with cord injury. (From Fractures, dislocations, and major ligamentous injuries. In: Galli RL, Spaite DW, Simon RR, eds. *Emergency orthopaedics: the spine.* Appleton and Lange, 1989 with permission.)

translational component, displacement is unusual. As with Chance fractures, flexion-distraction injuries are frequently missed on routine axial CT scans since the disruption is oriented in the horizontal plane. Thus, it is important to obtain sagittal reconstructions of CT images if a flexion-distraction injury is suspected.

Translational Injuries

Translational injuries result in failure of all three columns from massive direct trauma to the back. This mechanism results in several injury patterns, including the "slice" fracture, rotational fracture-dislocations, shear injuries, and pure dislocations.

The classic mechanism that creates flexion-rotation forces on the thoracolumbar spine, often resulting in a "slice" fracture, is a fall ending in the "tuck and roll" landing. The majority of these injuries occur at the level of the thoracolumbar junction (T10 to L2), and examination usually reveals tenderness at the fracture site. There may be significant kyphosis and a widening of the spinous processes at the level of the dislocation (11). Those with shear fractures in the lumbar region may present with large contusions in the lumbosacral area due to direct trauma. Patients with a complete vertebral dislocation usually have sustained massive trauma, and their exam will invariably demonstrate neurologic deficits.

Among patients who are rendered paraplegic from TLS trauma, the majority have sustained a fracture-dislocation injury. In fact, 60% to 80% of these injuries result in permanent neurologic deficits, and most patients also sustain serious trauma to other organ systems (11). Shear fractures and pure dislocations

also result in severe neurologic sequelae, with complete paraplegia occurring in nearly all patients.

With plain radiographs, the classic "slice" fracture is best seen on the lateral view and appears as the superior segment being anteriorly subluxed on the inferior segment with a slice through the upper portion of the vertebral body below it. The spinous processes will appear widened due to posterior ligament rupture. If there is also a rotational component, the alignment of the spinous processes will be distorted (11). Pure dislocations are generally not subtle and appear as a complete displacement of the superior vertebrae on the one below it. CT scan is very helpful in evaluating these injuries, since it demonstrates and objectively quantifies the extent of spinal canal compromise and cord impingement.

Minor Spinal Fracture Patterns

Minor spinal fracture patterns account for 14% of all TLS injuries and include isolated transverse process fractures, spinous process fractures, facet or laminar fractures, bipedicular fractures, and fractures of the pars interarticularis.

Most minor spinal fractures occur in the lumbar region and are usually caused by direct blows, but sudden contraction of the psoas muscles may also result in avulsion of the transverse processes. While transverse process fractures are considered to be stable, it is important to realize that in high velocity trauma, transverse process fractures frequently do not occur in isolation. In one retrospective analysis of 28 patients who initially appeared to have isolated transverse process fractures by plain radiographs, 3 patients were subsequently found to have compression and burst fractures by CT scan (14). Additionally, high thoracic fractures may be associated with injury to the brachial plexus, and lumbar and sacral fractures may result in injury to the lumbosacral plexus. In order to ensure the appropriate diagnosis and management of SCI, CT should be considered when transverse process fractures are seen on plain radiographs.

DIFFERENTIAL DIAGNOSIS

The differential diagnosis in any patient who presents with back pain after trauma includes vertebral fractures, SCI, epidural hematoma, paraspinous hematoma, "lumbar strains" and "sprains," *spinal cord injury without radiographic abnormality* (SCIWORA), major aortic disruptions (intimal tear or rupture of a pre-existing aneurysm), retroperitoneal hematoma, intraabdominal injury, and simple contusions. However, in patients on corticosteroids, those with metastatic cancer to the spine, or in the elderly who are at risk for compression fractures related to osteoporosis, the absence of a history of trauma should not dissuade the physician from considering a diagnosis of a TLS fracture. Additionally, the most difficult diagnostic task for the emergency physician may be to correctly classify each of the fracture patterns and to assess spinal stability.

EMERGENCY DEPARTMENT EVALUATION

TLS injuries should be suspected in victims of motor vehicle collisions, falls, sport-related injuries who complain of mid to lower back pain, and in all trauma victims with a suggestive mechanism of injury who cannot be clinically assessed because of an altered mental status or other associated painful injuries (16). To assess for TLS injury, the spine should be palpated for evidence of deformity, tenderness, and muscle spasm. Palpation of the spine may reveal an interspinous gap, which may indicate posterior ligamentous disruption. The back should also be visually inspected for contusions, lacerations, and abrasions. Next, the neurologic status of the patient should be determined and carefully documented to establish a baseline. The neurologic exam should include a quantitative evaluation of motor function, and sensory testing must include an evaluation of the sacral dermatomes and an examination of anal sphincter tone. Dorsal and ventral cord function should also be assessed, and serial exams should be performed whenever deficits are found in order to identify patients exhibiting progressive neurologic dysfunction.

Although there has been much work done with regard to the clinical clearance of the cervical spine, there has been relatively little research into establishing guidelines for diagnosing and imaging TLS fractures. In the latest edition (sixth) of the Advanced Trauma Life Support (ATLS) manual, the authors state, "any patient with an altered level of consciousness or cognitive dysfunction, GCS <15, multi-system injuries, or a palpable gap or tenderness in the thoracolumbar area requires spinal protection until AP and lateral spine x-rays are obtained to exclude any injury... Anteroposterior films of the thoracic and lumbar areas are standard"(1).

A summary of the current literature reveals that TLS imaging is indicated for those who have sustained a high-energy mechanism of injury (a fall greater than 10 feet, high-speed motor vehicle collisions, etc.) PLUS any of the following: (1) back pain or midline back tenderness; (2) abnormal neurologic signs; (3) any other spine fracture; (4) GCS <15; (5) major distracting injury; or (6) alcohol or drug intoxication (2,10,13,19,20).

The advantages of CT over plain radiography include superior fracture-detection rates, spinal canal evaluation, paravertebral soft-tissue assessment, and reduced manipulation of the patient. As noted above in the section on wedge compression and burst fractures, CT scan is recommended for all patients in whom spinal instability is in question, as plain radiographs do not adequately evaluate the posterior vertebral body cortex. Unclear fractures or displacements on standard radiographs should be further evaluated by a CT scan.

Magnetic resonance imaging (MRI), with its superior resolution and definition of the spinal canal, multi-planar capabilities, and lack of ionizing radiation, has become the optimal imaging modality in the general evaluation of spinal disease. The primary advantage of MRI is its ability to directly image nonosseous structures, including ligamentous injuries, and intramedullary and extramedullary spinal abnormalities. However, plain films and CT are superior to MRI in evaluating osseous anatomy and fractures, particularly posterior-element fractures. MRI is also not universally available, and there are numerous contraindications to its use, such as the presence of a pacemaker, cerebral aneurysm clips, and metallic foreign bodies. Although there are no clear evidence-based indications for MRI after spinal injury, MRI should be considered in patients with neurologic signs and symptoms and those with intractable pain that cannot be accounted for by osseous disruption on plain radiographs and CT.

EMERGENCY DEPARTMENT MANAGEMENT

The patient who has sustained TLS trauma has typically been subjected to high-energy forces, and initial resuscitation efforts should focus on the evaluation and treatment of life-threatening injuries. However, it is important to assure that resuscitative maneuvers do not compromise neurologic function. Patients should remain immobilized on a spine board with a rigid cervical collar until neurologic and radiographic evaluation can be performed.

Hypotension in a trauma victim may be due to SCI causing neurogenic hypotension, but this should be a diagnosis of exclusion. Other causes of hypotension, such as hemorrhagic shock, cardiac tamponade, and tension pneumothorax must first be excluded. Neurogenic hypotension results in vasodilation and bradycardia, and mild cases (generally seen with TLS injuries) most often respond to fluid resuscitation but occasionally require vasopressor support.

Neurosurgical consultation, if available, should be obtained promptly when neurologic deficits are present or when spinal instability is suspected. TLS fractures are rarely treated as an operative emergency, however, unless there is evidence of progressive neurologic dysfunction, or in the presence of a significant epidural hematoma with cord or cauda equina compression.

Pharmacologic agents, such as glucocorticoids, naloxone, thyrotropin-releasing hormone, insulin-like growth factor, dimethyl sulfoxide, calcium channel blockers, tirilazad mesylate, and GM-1 gangliosides have been found to improve neurologic outcome in experimentally induced SCI (5). However, of these, only methylprednisolone is currently routinely used, and its use remains highly controversial.

The National Acute Spinal Cord Injury Study (NASCIS) Group has published several studies showing that the administration of high-dose methylprednisolone improves neurologic outcome after blunt SCI, if it is administered within 8 hours (5). However, other studies have reported that patients treated with methylprednisolone had higher rates of respiratory and gastrointestinal complications than the placebo-treated patients, and the NASCIS studies have been criticized for methodologic flaws (15). The administration of steroids also resulted in a worse outcome when started after 8 hours. Recent guidelines published jointly by the American Association of Neurological Surgeons and the Congress of Neurological Surgeons state that "treatment with methylprednisolone... is recommended... only with the knowledge that the evidence suggesting harmful side effects is more consistent than any suggestion of clinical benefit" (3). In contrast, a Cochrane Database Systematic Review article concludes that "high dose methylprednisolone steroid therapy is the only pharmacological therapy shown to have efficacy in a Phase Three randomized trial when it can be administered within 8 hours of injury" (6). Given this conflicting evidence, high-dose steroids should only be administered with neurosurgical consultation, and only if the patient presents within 8 hours post-injury.

Intestinal ileus is common following TLS injury, and a nasogastric tube may be required to prevent gastric dilation. Urinary bladder atony, due to autonomic dysfunction, is also common. Thus, placement of a Foley catheter will help prevent bladder distension and monitor fluid balance. Since gastrointestinal bleeding from stress ulcers occurs in up to 20% of spinal trauma patients, ulcer prophylaxis is indicated. Denervated skin is especially susceptible to pressure necrosis, so the spinal immobilization backboard should be removed, or pressure points padded, as soon as possible. Frequent patient repositioning should be instituted if the patient is insensate and immobilized. Prophylaxis against deep venous thrombosis should also be provided.

CRITICAL INTERVENTIONS

- Address the ABCs
- Provide spinal immobilization until an unstable fracture is excluded
- Perform a thorough baseline neurologic exam followed by serial exams
- Order and interpret appropriate radiographs, CT scans, and MRI scans
- Obtain prompt neurosurgical consultation if there is evidence of spinal instability or neurologic deficits
- Provide adequate analgesia
- Institute nasogastric suction if an ileus is present
- Order Foley catheter drainage to help with fluid management

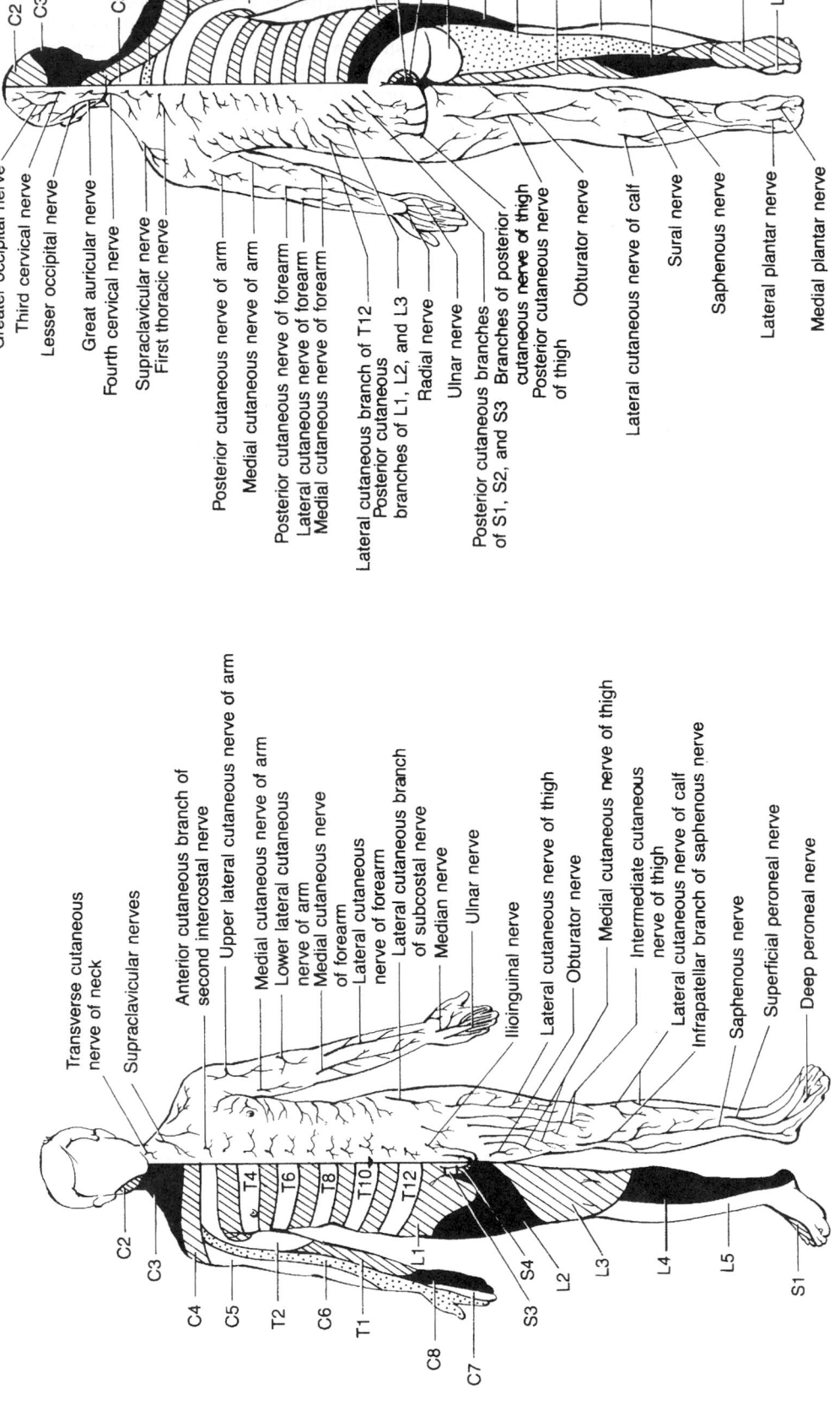

Figure 181.1.   Sensory dermatomal segments. (*Left*) Anterior view. (*Right*) Posterior view.

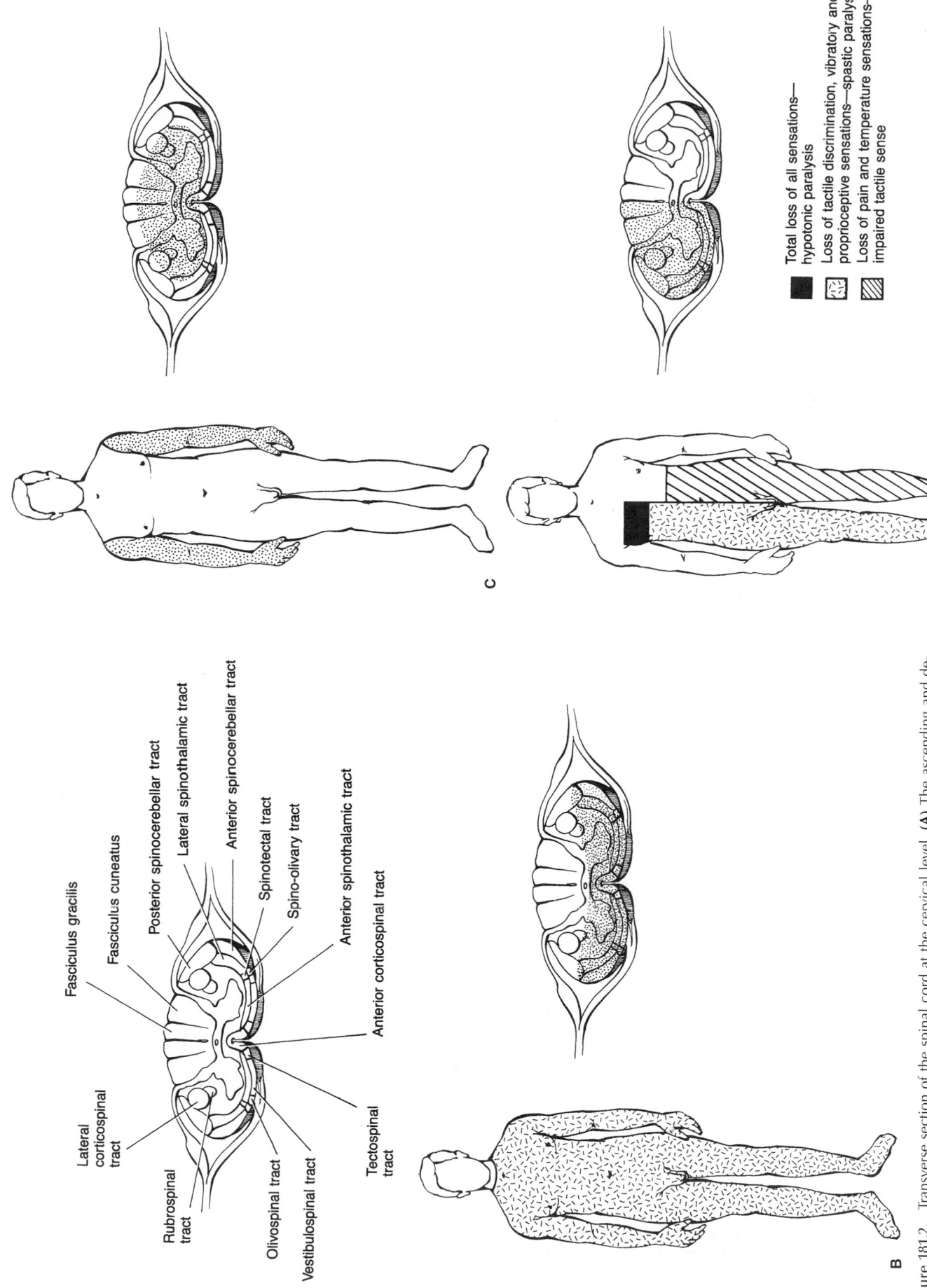

Lateral
corticospinal
tract

Fasciculus gracilis

Fasciculus cuneatus

Posterior spinocerebellar tract

Lateral spinothalamic tract

Anterior spinocerebellar tract

Spinotectal tract

Spino-olivary tract

Anterior spinothalamic tract

Anterior corticospinal tract

Rubrospinal tract

Olivospinal tract

Vestibulospinal tract

Tectospinal tract

A

B

C

D

■ Total loss of all sensations—hypotonic paralysis

▨ Loss of tactile discrimination, vibratory and proprioceptive sensations—spastic paralysis

▧ Loss of pain and temperature sensations—impaired tactile sense

Figure 181.2. Transverse section of the spinal cord at the cervical level. (A) The ascending and descending tracts. (B) Tracts that may be damaged in the anterior spinal artery syndrome. (C) Tracts that may be damaged in the central cord syndrome. (D) Involved tracts and the superimposed areas of deficit from an injury at T4, resulting in the Brown-Séquard syndrome.

The *anterior spinal cord syndrome* (see Fig. 181.2B) is the result of either direct blunt injury to the cord itself or compression of the anterior spinal artery by disc, bone, or hematoma, causing ischemic damage to the anterior cord. The patient presents with a loss of motor and pain sensation bilaterally below the level of the lesion, but posterior column function is preserved. Posterior column function is tested with a tuning fork for vibratory sensation or by plantarflexing and dorsiflexing the great toe to assess for gross proprioception. After CT, the patient should have an urgent attempt at reduction and reestablishment of the normal diameter of the spinal canal. This is typically performed by the neurosurgeon using Gardner-Wells tongs applying in-line traction guided by serial x-rays and serial neurologic examinations after each incremental addition of weight. Endpoints are successful reduction, any sign of distraction which can cause additional cord injury, or the neurosurgeon's acceptable maximum weight limits for the level of the injury. Computed tomography (CT) myelography or magnetic resonance imaging (MRI) should follow to assess for possible soft tissue masses, such as an extruded disc or hematoma that may continue to exert extrinsic pressure on the spinal cord or anterior spinal artery. If found, these should be relieved by laminectomy. Unfortunately, the prognosis for recovery after this injury is poor.

The acute *central cord syndrome* (see Fig. 181.2C) usually afflicts patients with a narrowed spinal canal. This may be due to degenerative spine disease causing bony ridges and thickened ligaments in the spinal canal, a congenital stenotic canal, or acute fracture and disc herniation. Degenerative spine disease is more common in the elderly but also may be present in younger patients. The mechanism of injury is usually hyperextension. The hallmark of this lesion is greater damage to the central portion of the cord than to the periphery. This leads to a variable sensory loss and bladder dysfunction but a predictable motor loss, with motor function of the upper extremities below the level of the lesion more impaired than that of the lower extremities. This is because the motor fibers in the lateral corticospinal tract lie in a lamellar fashion; cervical segments are most medial, and thoracic, lumbar, and sacral motor fibers are progressively more lateral. The diagnosis is confirmed by MRI. Management of this injury is usually nonoperative though surgical decompression is recommended if the cord is compressed and particularly if the compression is focal and anterior (5). There is a relatively good prognosis for recovery of at least partial neurologic function. Three-fourths of these patients are walking at 1 year; however, there is usually much less recovery of hand function.

The *Brown-Séquard syndrome* (Fig. 181.2D) is a hemicord injury that presents with a crossed sensory and motor deficit. Motor function is lost ipsilateral to the cord lesion, but sensory function is preserved on the ipsilateral side. Sensory function is lost on the contralateral side, where motor function is preserved. The crossed lesion is explained by the decussation of motor fibers in the medulla and the decussation of sensory fibers about two segments above the segment at which their sensory root enters the spinal cord. Causes include penetrating injuries, tumor, and disc disease. The prognosis is poor with penetrating injuries.

DIFFERENTIAL DIAGNOSIS

Determination of a cord injury is straightforward in the patient with acute quadri- or paraplegia. It becomes more difficult in patients with partial cord syndromes, particularly in those with acute central cord syndrome. This is due to both the patchy nature of the sensory loss and preservation of at least some motor function in the lower extremities. Evaluation for cord injury is also difficult in the unconscious patient. Most patients who present to the emergency department with complaints of neck or back pain or tenderness are found to have muscular strains or ligamentous sprains and no associated cord injury. The clinician should not be fooled by the absence of a fracture. A third-degree ligamentous sprain can render the spinal column unstable, allowing motion between vertebral bodies and subsequent cord or spinal root injury. In addition, children, as well as adults, may have *spinal cord injury without radiographic abnormality* (SCIWORA). It is recommended that these patients have an MRI and external immobilization until spinal stability is confirmed by flexion-extension views or MRI; in addition, they should avoid high risk activities for up to 6 months (4). See Chapter 211, "Evaluation of the Cervical Spine."

EMERGENCY DEPARTMENT EVALUATION

The principles of evaluation are the same for all significantly injured patients. Initial attention should be paid to airway, breathing, circulation, disability, exposure, and environment (the ABCDEs), with simultaneous resuscitation involving high-flow oxygen, two large-bore intravenous lines, a Foley catheter, and serial vital sign determinations. Early in their course, patients often have an atonic bladder. A Foley catheter is used to monitor urine output during the resuscitation and to prevent damaging distention of the bladder. Early in the hospitalization, the Foley catheter is removed and replaced by intermittent catheterization to decrease the chance of developing an ascending urinary tract infection.

In the critically injured patient, the primary survey should be followed by x-rays (lateral cervical spine, chest, and pelvis films), ultrasound of the pericardium and abdomen, and the secondary survey. In many centers, the use of emergent CT of the cervical spine obviates the need for the lateral cervical spine x-ray. During the secondary survey, a careful neurologic examination must be performed. This examination is carefully recorded so that an ascending lesion or deterioration in function can be identified by serial examinations. Motor function for all muscle groups is tested and recorded on a 0 to 5 scale (0, no voluntary muscle contraction; 1 flicker or trace of muscle contraction; 2, muscle activity apparent but cannot overcome gravity; 3, can overcome gravity but not active resistance; 4, active motion against mild to strong but reduced resistance from normal; 5, full normal active motion against resistance). The level of sensory loss is plotted to identify the level on which to concentrate with radiographic imaging. This level can be marked on the body in ink to identify any changes. Gross proprioception or vibratory function is measured to examine posterior column function. Deep tendon reflexes, anogenital reflexes (bulbocavernosus, anal wink), and perianal sensation are elicited to identify spinal shock or sacral sparing. Serial vital sign determinations should be obtained. One common diagnostic error is performing an inadequate neurologic examination and specifically failing to examine for posterior column function (gross proprioception, vibratory sensation). A second error is failing to examine for sacral sparing, which is needed to differentiate a partial cord lesion from a physiologically complete injury. Serial neurologic examinations are performed to identify any important change in functional status, which would have a profound influence on the management of the patient by the neurosurgeon or orthopaedic surgeon. Deterioration of function despite vertebral alignment implies the need for a CT myelogram or MRI to check for the presence of an extrinsic soft tissue mass compressing the cord, which might be surgically correctable. No specific laboratory studies aid in this evaluation.

After the history and physical examination have identified the level of the lesion, plain films help characterize the lesion. For a complete discussion of x-rays and fracture management see Chapter 179, "Cervical Spine Fractures" and Chapter 180, "Thoracolumbar Spine Fractures."

EMERGENCY DEPARTMENT MANAGEMENT

In the patient with a spinal cord injury, the immediate focus should be on identifying and managing life-threatening injuries, while avoiding secondary injury. The patient should be immobilized without applying traction until after films carefully define the lesion. Traction that causes distraction on the cord or roots may cause severe, possibly irreparable neurologic damage. The first priority is to ensure that the patient survives, by attending to the ABCDEs. The second priority is to prevent secondary injury through unnecessary motion, hypoxia, hypotension, or infection.

The physician must not allow, or cause, the patient to have unnecessary motion of the unstable spinal column. However, at times, such motion may be necessary to preserve the patient's life, such as in the patient with an obstructed airway who needs immediate management when initial maneuvers have proven unsuccessful. In-line immobilization with Sellick's maneuver should be used, allowing only as much motion as is needed to successfully control the airway. The physician should prepare to logroll and suction if the patient regurgitates, while keeping the patient's spinal column as straight as possible. Although x-ray studies show that logrolling is associated with some motion of the thoracolumbar spinal column (21), it must be done to prevent aspiration and obstruction in the patient who regurgitates without a protected airway.

The spinal cord and column should be protected with a long board and semirigid collar while attending to the ABCDEs of the primary survey and resuscitation. The semirigid collar can be removed in a supine, immobilized patient, as needed, to examine the neck. When this examination is complete, the collar is replaced. It should otherwise be left on until clinical evaluation or the full series of cervical films shows the spine to be stable.

The NEXUS study provides a reliable decision instrument to help the physician decide if the patient needs cervical x-rays after blunt trauma (15). The 5 NEXUS criteria are as follows: no posterior midline cervical tenderness; no focal neurologic deficit; the patient must be alert; the patient must not be intoxicated; and no distracting painful injury. If the patient meets all 5 exclusion criteria then the physician can reliably continue the evaluation without performing cervical spine x-rays. When the patient has none of these indications for cervical x-rays the physician may remove the collar and gradually have the patient move the neck to assess for pain with range of motion. An untoward amount of pain with motion should lead to replacing the collar and obtaining films. No similar national multicenter study has defined exclusion criteria for thoracic and lumbar spine x-rays, but many physicians apply these cervical criteria to the rest of the spinal evaluation.

Typically as the last step in the exposure phase the patient is removed from the long board and logrolled to examine the back. The backboard is then removed but the semirigid collar is left in place. Further movement of the patient is accomplished using spinal precautions to move the patient as a unit, using sliding boards, logrolling, or multiple-person horizontal lifts. The long board is an important tool in immobilizing and protecting the spinal cord, but it also causes serious complications such as aspiration, impaired ventilation, and decubitus ulcers (1). For these reasons the patient should be removed from the long board as soon as is practical and other spinal precautions put in place.

The patient must be protected against unnecessary movement until the history, physical examination, and, if indicated, radiologic studies are complete that show that the spinal column is stable. The physician should not be fooled into thinking films are unnecessary by the fact that the patient was walking after the injury. If such a patient presents, the 5 NEXUS discriminating factors listed above should be used to determine if the patient needs x-rays.

The phrenic nerve, providing motor innervation to the diaphragm, arises from the C3 through C5 segments of the spinal cord. An otherwise healthy patient can maintain adequate long-term ventilation with diaphragmatic breathing alone. However, if a traumatic lesion affects C3 through C5, or if the level of the lesion ascends, as sometimes happens, the patient will become ventilator-dependent. In addition the patient may need intubation and ventilation early on, despite preserved diaphragmatic breathing, if there are additional injuries that combine with the cord injury to make oxygenation or ventilation inadequate.

The ultimate outcome of any spinal cord injury is determined by a combination of the initial mechanical injury and a cascade of secondary injuries. Timely reduction of the displaced column is vital to achieve decompression of the spinal cord. Timely reduction has been associated with recovery from otherwise devastating spinal cord injury (13). The secondary vascular and biochemical injuries are the subject of numerous animal and human studies for their mechanism of injury and treatment. Various monotherapy and combination therapy protocols attempt to interrupt this cascade of injury at various points in its course.

Unfortunately, the one therapy (methylprednisolone) shown in prospective case-controlled human research to positively impact this cascade of destruction is the subject of great controversy. The National Acute Spinal Cord Injury Studies (NASCIS) demonstrated a statistically significant though modest improvement in neurologic outcome without causing a statistically significant increase in wound complications or gastrointestinal bleeds (9,10). There are several criticisms of the NASCIS studies. The primary benefits analysis was negative and only the post hoc subgroup analysis showed a modest improvement in outcome that was of questionable clinical significance. The study has also been criticized for using questionable statistical tests (17). The American Association of Neurological Surgeons recommends following the NASCIS protocol but only with the knowledge that the evidence suggesting harmful effects to other body systems is more consistent than any suggestion of clinical benefit (3). Others have argued that high-dose methylprednisolone used according to the NASCIS protocol is a class II (randomized clinical trial with methodological flaws, prospective controlled trial) modestly efficacious treatment, with a favorable risk-benefit ratio, no known better alternative, and therefore a recommended therapy (14). Bracken argues that it is a safe and modestly effective therapy but that research is needed to identify other treatments that may be used alone or in combination to achieve an even better result (12).

Decisions about whether or not to use methylprednisolone are based on consultation with a neurosurgeon and institutional protocols. If the emergency physician chooses to follow the NASCIS protocols, then for blunt cord injury in adults within 8 hours of spinal cord injury, high doses of methylprednisolone are given (9-11). The dose is 30 mg/kg as a bolus, followed by a continuous drip of 5.4 mg/kg/h for the subsequent 23 hours. High-dose methylprednisolone is not indicated after penetrating spinal cord injury (19). It has not been adequately studied in children less than 13 years old, or in patients with cauda equina or spinal root injury.

CRITICAL INTERVENTIONS

- Perform in-line immobilization with Sellick's maneuver for airway interventions
- When using high-dose methylprednisolone for blunt injury in adults, start the bolus and continuous drip as soon as possible, but not after 8 hours
- In the hypotensive patient with suspected spinal neurogenic shock, after completing a negative search for occult hemorrhage, use volume resuscitation and then pressors if needed to raise blood pressure initially above 90 systolic
- Remove the patient from the backboard, while maintaining spinal precautions, as soon as practical to avoid decubitus ulcerations and limit the risk of aspiration that results from being immobilized supine

DISPOSITION

The emergency physician must decide if a spinal column or cord injury exists. Next, the physician must decide whether the column is stable. Consultation should be obtained once cord or spinal nerve root injury is identified by physical examination or radiologic studies. The timing of consultation is urgent; it should be obtained while the patient is in the emergency department. It should be requested after attention is focused on the primary survey and initial resuscitation.

Patients are admitted if there is a cord injury or unstable column injury, for pain control, or for an anticipated complication such as the association of ileus with a thoracolumbar compression fracture. Patients with cord or unstable column injuries are admitted to the intensive care unit; circle beds, rotating frames, or serial inflating devices are used to protect from pressure sores.

Patients discharged home should be instructed to return immediately for a recheck if there is any sign of worsening, such as the development of numbness, weakness, hyperesthesia, paresthesias, cauda equina syndrome with urinary retention, fecal incontinence, or saddle hypoesthesia. Paresthesias are a sign of potential instability.

The patient should be transferred to a specialized trauma facility if the trauma team cannot meet all the special requirements for extensive rehabilitation and specialized care of the cord-injured patient. Deteriorating or unstable internal injuries are best managed before transfer. Transport personnel should be, at a minimum, advanced life support-certified to ensure the continuous administration of intravenous methylprednisolone. For the emergent transfer, the patient should remain immobilized on a spinal board with a semirigid collar.

COMMON PITFALLS

- Failure to ensure survival by attending to the ABCDEs and initial resuscitation
- Applying cervical spine traction instead of immobilization. The patient is at the highest potential risk for traction injury during prehospital placement on a spinal board or during intubation (8,16,20) when in-line immobilization and Sellick's maneuver, not traction, should be used
- Blaming hypotension on spinal neurogenic shock without completing the search for occult injury
- Failure to identify other injuries in the anesthetic or hypoesthetic patient. Since the patient cannot feel pain or tenderness below the lesion, common historical and physical examination findings will be absent. The patient requires a very thorough examination, and areas with significant bruises should be imaged
- Misreading x-rays or accepting inadequate films and failure to identify an unstable spinal segment
- Failure to place a Foley catheter in a cord-injured patient to prevent acute bladder distention
- Failure to perform an adequate neurologic examination, and failure to identify changes in the neurologic status. These changes may lead to CT myelography or MRI and possible decompressive surgery
- Failure to record an accurate baseline motor, sensory, posterior column, and rectal tone examination as well as repeat examinations

References

1. Anonymous. Cervical spine immobilization before admission to the hospital. *Neurosurgery* 2002;50(3):S7–S17.
2. Anonymous. Blood pressure management after acute spinal cord injury. *Neurosurgery* 2002;50(3):S58–S62.
3. Anonymous. Pharmacological therapy after acute cervical spinal cord injury. *Neurosurgery* 2002;50(3):S63–S72.
4. Anonymous. Spinal cord injury without radiographic abnormality. *Neurosurgery* 2002;50(3):S100–S104.
5. Anonymous. Management of acute central cervical spinal cord injuries. *Neurosurgery* 2002;50(3):S166–S172.
6. Atkinson PP, Atkinson JLD. Spinal shock. *Mayo Clin Proc* 1996;71:384–389.
7. Bicknell JM, Kirsch WM, Seigel R, et al. Atlantoaxial dislocation in rheumatic fever. *J Neurosurgery* 1987;66:286.
8. Bivins HG, Ford S, Bezmalinovic Z, et al. The effect of axial traction during orotracheal intubation of the trauma victim with an unstable cervical spine. *Ann Emerg Med* 1988;17(1):25.
9. Bracken MB, Shepard MJ, Collins WF, et al. A randomized, controlled trial of methylprednisolone or naloxone in the treatment of acute spinal-cord injury. *N Engl J Med* 1990;322:1405.
10. Bracken MB, Shepard MJ, Collins WF, et al. Methylprednisolone or naloxone treatment after acute spinal cord injury: 1-year follow-up data (results of the Second National Acute Spinal Cord Injury Study). *J Neurosurg* 1992;76:23.
11. Bracken MB, Shepard MJ, Holford TR, et al. Administration of methylprednisolone for 24 or 48 hours or tirilazad mesylate for 48 hours in the treatment of acute spinal cord injury. Results of the Third National Acute Spinal Cord Injury Randomized Controlled Trial. National Acute Spinal Cord Injury Study. *JAMA* 1997;277(20):1597–1604.
12. Bracken MB. Methylprednisolone and acute spinal cord injury—an update of the randomized evidence. *Spine* 2001;26(24S):S47–S54.
13. Brunette DD, Rockswold GL. Neurologic recovery following rapid spinal realignment for complete cervical spinal cord injury. *J Trauma* 1987;27:445–447.
14. Fehling MG. Editorial: recommendations regarding the use of methylprednisolone in acute spinal cord injury—making sense out of the controversy. *Spine* 2001;26(24S):S56–S57.
15. Hoffman JR, Mower WR, Wolfson AB, et al for the National Emergency X-Radiography Utilization Study Group. Validity of a set of clinical criteria to rule out injury to the cervical spine in patients with blunt trauma. *N Engl J Med* 2000;343(2):94–99.
16. Holley J, Jorden R. Airway management in patients with unstable cervical spine fractures. *Ann Emerg Med* 1989;18:1237.
17. Hurlbert RJ. The role of steroids in acute spinal cord injury. *Spine* 2001;26(24S):S39–S46.
18. Lali HS, Sekhon MB, Fehlings MG. Epidemiology, demographics, and pathophysiology of acute spinal cord injury, *Spine* 2001;26(24S):S2–S12.
19. Levy ML, Gans W, Wijesinghe HS, et al. Use of methylprednisolone as an adjunct in the management of patients with penetrating spinal cord injury: outcome analysis. *Neurosurgery* 1996;39(6):1141–1149.
20. Majernick TG, Bieniek R, Hughes HG. Cervical spine movement during orotracheal intubation. *Ann Emerg Med* 1986;15:417.
21. McGuire RA, Neville S, Green BA, et al. Spinal instability and the logrolling maneuver. *J Trauma* 1987;27:525.
22. Panjabi MM, White AA. Basic biomechanics of the spine. *Neurosurgery* 1980;7(1):76.
23. Trafton PG. Spinal cord injuries. *Surg Clin North Am* 1982;62(1):61.
24. Trafton PG, Boyd CA. Computed tomography of thoracic and lumbar spine injuries. *J Trauma* 1984;24:506.

CHAPTER 182
Blunt Chest Trauma

Vincent J. Markovchick

Blunt chest trauma (BCT) is a very common emergency department (ED) presentation. It can range from the most minor chest wall contusion to catastrophic and fatal intrathoracic injury such as a rupture of the thoracic aorta or myocardium. BCT is involved in nearly one-third of acute admissions to trauma centers and accounts for about 25% of all trauma related deaths in the United States (23). Most of these injuries are the result of blunt force trauma secondary to motor vehicle collisions, ejections from motorcycles, falls, or interpersonal violence. BCT is often associated with multiple system trauma including injury to the abdomen, head, spine and extremities. In contradistinction to penetrating injuries, BCT usually occurs when a large force is applied over a relatively larger area. Injury kinetics include acceleration and deceleration forces as well as transmittal of blunt force injury to internal structures. Blunt force chest trauma, when it involves multiple trauma, must be evaluated in the context of other injuries and, at times, more imminent life threats.

CLINICAL PRESENTATION

Chest Wall Injuries

Chest wall contusions and rib fractures account for the majority of blunt chest wall trauma. Fractures typically occur at the site of the impact or the posterior angle where the rib is structurally the weakest. Fractures are more common in adults than children because of the relative inelasticity of the mature thorax. Elderly patients have a higher morbidity and mortality associated with rib fractures than younger patients (4). Although the 4th through the 9th ribs are most commonly involved, fractures of ribs 9 through 11 deserve special concern as there is an increased incidence of associated splenic or liver injuries. Multiple rib fractures or the presence of a flail chest wall segment is often associated with intrathoracic injury, usually a pulmonary contusion. Rib fractures in young children should raise the suspicion for child abuse.

Clinical findings typically include pleuritic pain, tachypnea, splinting and point tenderness intensified by deep breathing or coughing. Bony crepitus may be palpable. The presence of subcutaneous emphysema over the ribs in an intact chest wall makes the diagnosis of a pneumothorax. Compression over the rib anteriorly or posteriorly produces referred pain to the fracture site; if there is no fracture present there should not be referred pain to the localized area of tenderness.

Sternal Fractures

Sternal fractures usually result from high-energy forces to the mid-anterior chest wall. This most commonly occurs from motor vehicle collisions in which the chest strikes the steering wheel, dashboard or shoulder belt at high velocity. This may result in a sternal fracture or costochondral separation, and in rare instances, an anterior flail chest when the sternum is disarticulated from the ribs. Though usually nondisplaced, sternal fractures

may be 100% subluxed. In either case, there is a low likelihood of associated cardiac trauma (4). Nonetheless, the major concern when presented with a patient with chest wall contusion or rib or sternal fractures is injury to underlying intrathoracic or mediastinal structures such as the pulmonary parenchyma, bronchi, heart or great vessels.

Flail Chest

Flail chest occurs when three or more ribs are fractured in two or more places. In a patient who is breathing spontaneously, the increased negative intrathoracic pressure with inspiratory effort results in a paradoxical movement of the chest wall (the flail segment moves in during inspiration and out during expiration). There is usually no significant ventilatory compromise caused by the flail segment per se. In these patients, respiratory compromise is related to the degree of pulmonary contusion, which almost inevitably occurs with blunt force trauma significant enough to cause a flail chest. All patients experience significant pain secondary to the respiratory movement of multiple rib fracture fragments. Patients with flail chest will also have tenderness, crepitus, and paradoxical movement of the chest wall. In some patients who are splinting or in those on positive pressure ventilation, the flail segment may not be readily apparent. Palpation of the chest can help detect the injury.

Pulmonary and Pleural Injuries

Blunt force trauma may result in pneumothorax, hemothorax or hemopneumothorax, usually secondary to a rib fracture penetrating the visceral pleura and lung parenchyma. Hemothorax usually results from disruption of an intercostal artery (see Chapter 183, "Penetrating Chest Trauma").

Pulmonary Contusion

The most common injury to the pulmonary parenchyma in blunt chest trauma is pulmonary contusion. This results from blunt force trauma to the pulmonary parenchyma causing an alveolar-capillary membrane permeable pulmonary edema. Depending upon the extent, this results in minimal to life-threatening symptoms. Leakage of fluid into the alveoli results in localized pulmonary edema. This results in areas of the lung that are perfused but not ventilated (i.e., a ventilation perfusion mismatch), resulting in hypoxia, hypercarbia and acidosis. Pulmonary contusion is a common sequela of blunt chest trauma in children because of the elasticity of the chest wall resulting in forces being transmitted to the pulmonary parenchyma rather than being dissipated by fracturing the ribs.

A patient with a pulmonary contusion usually presents with dyspnea and tachypnea. There may be tenderness or obvious ecchymosis and deformity over the injured chest wall. Large pulmonary contusions are associated with tachycardia, hypotension, cyanosis and low oxygen saturation. Patients with multiple rib fractures or flail segments of the chest wall are more likely to have associated pulmonary contusion.

Tracheal and Bronchial Injuries

Tracheal and bronchial injuries must be considered in any patient with a history of significant BCT such as a severe, sudden deceleration of any kind or a direct blow to the chest. The majority of these injuries occur within 2 cm of the carina or at the origin of the lobar bronchi (21,43). Occasionally minimal symptoms may occur, even with severe tracheal or bronchial injury. Dyspnea, hoarseness, aphonia and hemoptysis may occur.

Subcutaneous mediastinal emphysema is likely to be present. This injury should be considered if there is a persistent air leak from a chest tube (with all the holes inside the thorax) and difficulty in fully reexpanding the lung.

Blunt Cardiac Injuries

Blunt cardiac injury is a spectrum of injuries which ranges from myocardial concussion to myocardial contusion, to myocardial infarction and myocardial rupture. Since there is no gold standard to make the diagnosis, their true incidence is unknown. By virtue of its location in the chest, the heart is susceptible to injury from compression of the chest wall and upper abdomen and from deceleration forces. The right ventricle is most commonly injured due to its relatively vulnerable position immediately behind the sternum.

Some patients will sustain a *myocardial concussion* (commotio cordis), which is a ventricular dysrhythmia or asystole secondary to a direct blow to the myocardium. If the dysrhythmia or asystole does not spontaneously reverse and the patient cannot be resuscitated, a postmortem will not reveal any cardiac pathology. *Myocardial concussion* is the most common cause of sudden death in young athletes (22,33,45). The remainder who survive after having sustained blunt cardiac injury usually have little or no long-term sequelae from their blunt cardiac injury. *Myocardial contusion* is characterized by localized edema and hemorrhage into cardiac muscle. This trauma may involve segments of the cardiac conduction system most commonly the right bundle branches. *Traumatic myocardial infarction* is rare but can occur from disruption of the coronary artery intima and subsequent thrombosis. The most severe form of blunt cardiac injury is *cardiac rupture*; which is a rare injury. These patients will present with hypotension or in extremis and usually have a right atrial or ventricular injury.

Physical findings in blunt cardiac injury may be nonspecific. Chest pain from either chest wall trauma or ischemia may be present. Seventy to eighty percent of patients with blunt cardiac injury have external signs of chest trauma including contusions, abrasions, palpable crepitus and flail segments (13). The presence of a fractured sternum, once thought to be a marker for blunt cardiac injury, has not been shown to reliably correlate with the presence of a blunt cardiac injury (2,34). The most common vital sign abnormality is persistent sinus tachycardia after other causes have been treated. Hypotension is a serious sign and should raise the possibility of acute pericardial tamponade, myocardial rupture or rupture of an internal cardiac structure such as a chordae tendineae or valve. Cyanosis of the upper torso, head and neck may be present in some patients with cardiac rupture.

Great Vessel Injuries

Great vessel injuries in the mediastinum are most commonly caused by rapid and sudden deceleration in the setting of motor vehicle collisions (16,25). Most often, these injuries involve the aorta, but can involve the brachiocephalic artery and inferior vena cava (37,46). Up to 15% of automobile fatalities are due to traumatic disruption of the aorta. Eighty percent of patients with aortic injuries die in the field (31). Those patients who present to the ED with a contained traumatic aorta tear usually have a several hour window during which the diagnosis must be made and definitive treatment instituted; otherwise mortality is high. Patients with rupture of the vena cava have a poorer outcome because of continued ongoing significant blood loss and difficulty in controlling the bleeding and repairing the defect at surgery (29).

Disruption of the great vessels usually results from high-speed motor vehicle collisions, falls from a height or ejection from motorcycles or other vehicles. The classic mechanism associated with an MVC is a head-on collision, although the injury can occur after side impacts or rear impacts. Several mechanisms have been postulated to explain these injuries. First and foremost, rapid horizontal deceleration produces shearing forces at the aortic isthmus just distal to the origin of the left subclavian artery. Ninety percent of traumatic aortic tears originate at this site (3,6). Anatomically, this can be explained by the fact that the descending aorta is tethered by the ligamentum arteriosum and the intercostal arteries. The ascending aorta is relatively mobile, and, during deceleration, continues to move forward while the descending aorta is held in place, resulting in shearing forces that cause a rent in the aorta (Fig. 182.1). In seat-belted motor vehicle victims, descending thoracic tears are more common, while ascending aortic disruption is seen more often in unrestrained drivers, those who are ejected or fall from a height and experience vertical deceleration forces (16). Although the aorta may withstand intraluminal pressures of up to 350 mm Hg, this pressure may be surpassed in high-speed MVCs producing a burst or "water-hammer" effect directly compressing the aorta and propagating a pressure wave which can also lead to aortic injury (14,32). Another proposed mechanism is the "osseous pinch" model in which the aorta is pinched between the sternum and the vertebral column resulting in shearing forces that cause injury to the aorta (11).

The tear of the aorta is usually a circumferential transverse laceration that disrupts the physical integrity of the intima and muscularis layers of the aorta. If the tear is complete, involving all three layers, this results in death due to immediate exsanguination. In survivors, the adventitia remains intact and blood is contained by a false aneurysm formed by the adventitia and surrounding mediastinal structures. If this injury is unrecognized, there is a significant risk of a free rupture and sudden death in the hours to days following this injury (32).

In the setting of blunt trauma, aortic injury may be obscured by concomitant, significant injuries to the head, spine, abdomen, pelvis and extremities. This injury should be suspected whenever there have been major acceleration-deceleration forces

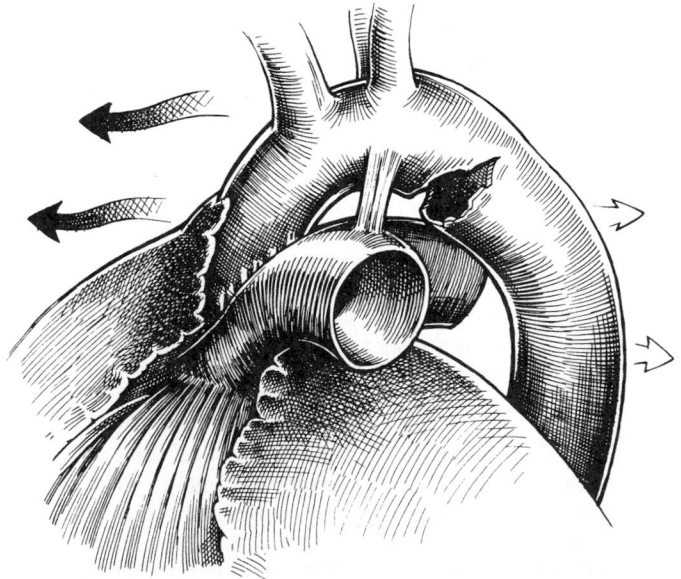

Figure 182.1. Rapid decelerative injury causing a tear in the thoracic aorta. The ascending (anterior) aorta tends to continue moving forward, while the more fixed descending aorta is held stationary. The rupture occurs just distal to the ligamentum arteriosum at the level of the isthmus.

involving the chest. This occurs when the body is moving forward at a high speed and the chest wall strikes a blunt object, such as a dashboard. This should be considered in significant ejection mechanisms, falls from heights greater than ten feet, and motor vehicle collisions with speeds greater than 30 mph and a lack of proper vehicle restraints.

The symptoms and signs of traumatic great vessel disruption are often absent or missed due to coexisting painful injuries. The most frequently recorded complaints are chest pain, dyspnea and back pain. Other symptoms include dysphagia, hoarseness and ischemic pain of the extremities.

Physical examination may reveal ecchymosis, abrasion, or tenderness of the anterior chest wall consistent with the impact of this area on a steering wheel. Thirty-one percent of patients with an aortic disruption present with the *pseudocoarctation syndrome* (15). In these cases, upper extremity hypertension is present with decreased or absent femoral pulses, due to compression of the aortic lumen by surrounding periaortic hematoma. Reflex stretching of the cardiac sympathetic fibers at the aortic isthmus may account for the observation that 72% of patients with aortic rupture manifest a relative hypertension (average blood pressure 152/98) (15). A harsh systolic murmur over the precordium or interscapular area (thought to be due to turbulent flow across the area of transection) has been reported to be present in 26% of cases (42). The presence of great vessel injury cannot be confirmed or ruled out on the basis of physical examination. In confirmed cases of traumatic aortic injury, one-third to one-half of the patients have no external evidence of chest injury on initial presentation to the ED (40). Furthermore, many patients have associated CNS, abdominal, or bony injuries that may distract the physician from considering injury to the great vessels. Thus, the treating physician must consider this diagnosis in any patient with blunt chest trauma and a concerning mechanism.

Diaphragmatic Injuries

Blunt traumatic diaphragmatic injury results from a violent blunt force compression trauma to the lower chest and upper abdomen. Sixty percent to 90% of traumatic rupture of the diaphragm from blunt trauma occurs on the left side since the liver is protective on the right (28,43). Blunt trauma typically produces diaphragmatic defects of greater than 10 centimeters on average and has a higher mortality rate than penetrating injury to the diaphragm because of the higher incidence of serious associated injuries to abdominal and chest structures.

Signs and symptoms of diaphragmatic rupture are highly variable depending upon the size of the defect, the mechanism, the abdominal viscous that herniates through the defect and the degree of cardiopulmonary compromise. Common symptoms include cough, dyspnea, nonspecific chest or abdominal pain radiating to the shoulder and the perception of peristalsis in the chest. Signs include an immobile left hemithorax, decreased breath sounds, and tympany or borborygmi in the left chest. Significant herniation of abdominal viscera into the thoracic cavity usually results in severe respiratory distress and may be clinically confused with a tension pneumothorax (19). A tension viscero-thorax (gastro-thorax) occurs when the resulting increase in intrapleural pressure causes shift of the mediastinum and hemodynamic collapse. Therefore, great care should be taken when performing a thoracostomy to verify a free pleural space before inserting the chest tube.

Esophageal Injuries

Esophageal injuries secondary to blunt trauma are rare occurrences. However, they have been reported from sharp blows or when force is applied to the upper abdomen in which air and gastric contents are violently forced into the esophagus causing a perforation in the distal esophagus similar to that which occurs secondary to retching and vomiting (i.e., Boerhaave syndrome). The perforation typically occurs in the left side of the distal esophagus, the area physiologically weakened due to the paucity of circular muscular fibers. Although falls and motor vehicle accidents account for most injuries by this mechanism, there have been reported cases of perforation caused by attempts at the Heimlich maneuver (26). Finally, chest wall compressions during cardiopulmonary resuscitation may cause injury to the esophagus (24). Injuries to the esophagus can also occur with compression of the esophagus against the spine, producing longitudinal tears in the upper thoracic esophagus. These lesions are sometimes accompanied by a laceration in the membranous (i.e., posterior) portion of the trachea, resulting in a traumatic tracheoesophageal fistulas. Injuries to the esophagus can also occur from barotrauma, since the esophagus is a hollow, air-containing organ. An example of this is forceful insufflation of the esophagus from inhalation of aerosol cans, air compressors or inflation devices (47). This has been reported in children from the biting of inner tubes and eruption of bottled carbonated beverages into the esophagus (10). Perforations of the esophagus can result from alkali ingestion, foreign bodies, and iatrogenic misplaced tubes or endoscopes.

Signs and symptoms of esophageal injury are pain, subcutaneous emphysema (especially in the neck or supraclavicular fossa), unexplained tachycardia, dyspnea, dysphagia, odynophagia, cyanosis, pneumomediastinum, pneumothorax, pleural effusion, and hematemesis.

Traumatic Asphyxia

Traumatic asphyxia occurs when the thorax is squeezed between two objects for a prolonged period of time. This results in compression of the vena cava with resultant prolonged increased venous pressure to the neck and head. This prolonged squeeze and compromised venous return results in intense cyanosis of the upper chest, neck and face as well as petechiae and subconjunctional hemorrhage. Some patients may have retinal hemorrhage and loss of consciousness due to cerebral hypoxia. Sometimes there are associated chest wall and pulmonary parenchymal injuries such as pulmonary contusion and hemopneumothorax.

DIFFERENTIAL DIAGNOSIS

The differential diagnosis for chest wall injuries includes rib fractures, flail chest, sternal fracture, costochondral separation and chest wall contusion.

After blunt trauma, the differential diagnosis for pulmonary and pleural injuries includes pulmonary contusion, pneumothorax, hemothorax, hemopneumothorax, lung parenchymal injury, tension pneumothorax and acute pericardial tamponade. Tension pneumothorax must be differentiated from acute pericardial tamponade since both cause tachycardia hypotension and an elevated CVP. In patients with tension pneumothorax breath sounds are absent or markedly diminished and pericardial ultrasound is normal.

The differential diagnosis for tracheal and bronchial injuries includes other traumatic causes of pneumomediastinum, such as a ruptured esophagus or an iatrogenic perforation of the esophagus, posterior pharynx or pyriform sinus during attempts at endotracheal intubation.

In patients with blunt cardiac injury rupture of the valves or cordae tendinea may result in acute cardiac failure. In rare instances, blunt cardiac injury may cause acute pericardial tamponade. This can be differentiated from tension pneumothorax by the presence of a pericardial effusion on ultrasound.

The majority of patients who suffer from blunt thoracic aortic injury have coexisting serious injuries. These include fractures of the sternum and ribs, hemothorax, pneumothorax, hemopneumothorax, tracheobronchial disruption, diaphragmatic rupture, esophageal perforation, acute pericardial tamponade and blunt trauma to the myocardium.

Traumatic rupture of the diaphragm can be confused with a pneumothorax or a tension pneumothorax when abdominal viscera have herniated into the thoracic cavity resulting in respiratory distress and diminished or absent breath sounds, usually on the left side.

EMERGENCY DEPARTMENT EVALUATION

Chest Wall Injuries

The diagnosis of rib fracture should be made on clinical grounds because up to 50% of these injuries are missed on the initial chest radiographs; 10% do not visualize radiographically for 1 to 2 weeks after the injury regardless of the views taken. Chest radiographs are not indicated in isolated, localized chest wall trauma when there are no physical findings and no respiratory distress manifested by tachypnea or decreased oxygen saturations. A chest radiograph is valuable, however, when looking for complications of rib fractures such as hemothorax, pneumothorax, pulmonary contusion, atelectasis and pneumonia. Oxygen saturation should also be measured in these patients. Since elderly patients have a greater morbidity and mortality from complications of rib fractures, there should be a lower threshold for evaluating these patients with a chest x-ray (4,17).

Consideration should be given to observation, performance of the FAST exam or abdominal computed tomography (CT) when multiple ribs are fractured overlying the liver or spleen and the patient exhibits any abdominal upper quadrant pain or tenderness. Pain referred to either shoulder may indicate the presence of either hemothorax or pneumothorax or subdiaphragmatic hemorrhage from injury to the spleen or liver. Patients who present several days after their initial trauma with increasing pain, dyspnea or fever following chest wall trauma should have a chest x-ray to ascertain if there are any late complications such as atelectasis or pneumonia.

Flail Chest

Patients with evidence of a flail chest on physical examination should be evaluated with oxygen saturation monitoring and a radiograph of the chest to detect the presence of underlying pulmonary contusion, pneumothorax or hemothorax. Parenteral analgesics or regional nerve blocks are necessary for adequate analgesia. Most of these patients will require contrast-enhanced helical CT scans of the chest to evaluate the severity and extent of underlying pulmonary contusions and to determine if there is any injury to the great vessels.

Pulmonary and Pleural Injuries

During the initial resuscitation of the patient with blunt chest trauma, clinical signs of tension pneumothorax or massive hemothorax (decreased breath sounds or subcutaneous emphysema in association with hypotension, tachycardia and respiratory distress) mandate initial placement of a chest tube prior to obtaining chest radiography. Ideally, tension pneumothorax should be a clinical diagnosis and should not be captured on a chest x-ray. If the patient is hemodynamically stable, then a portable chest radiograph is the initial study of choice; this will demonstrate hemothorax, pneumothorax, and pneumomediastinum.

Pulmonary Contusion

The radiographic evidence for pulmonary contusion may not be evident initially on the chest x-ray since these injuries tend to get worse over the ensuing 6 to 12 hours following blunt force trauma, and the radiographic findings usually lag behind the clinical findings. A contrast enhanced helical CT scan of the chest will detect the presence of pulmonary contusions before they become visible on standard chest radiographs. CT scans may be used to measure the extent of the pulmonary contusion and to determine the prognosis (7,28). All patients should be placed on O_2 and have continuous O_2 saturation monitoring. If the O_2 saturation is low, an arterial blood gas can be obtained to calculate an alveolar-arterial gradient and followed serially to determine subsequent therapy.

Tracheal and Bronchial Injuries

This injury should be suspected when there is a persistent air leak despite the proper placement of a tube thoracostomy on the involved side. All patients should have a chest x-ray to rule out associated pneumothorax and to confirm that all the holes on the chest tube are within the thoracic cavity, since a hole outside of the thorax will result in a persistent air leak and inability to reexpand the lung. Consideration should also be given to diagnostic studies which rule out the presence of an esophageal disruption (discussed later in this chapter). In addition, surgical consultation should be obtained so bronchoscopy can be performed for definitive diagnosis.

Blunt Cardiac Injuries

All patients in whom this injury is suspected should have their cardiac rhythm and oxygen saturation continuously monitored. An electrocardiogram should be obtained to ascertain the presence of any dysrhythmia, bundle-branch block or new changes on the electrocardiogram (ECG). An initial ED ultrasound of the pericardium to detect the presence of pericardial effusion and to ascertain, if possible, the quality of cardial wall motion should be performed. New murmurs or acute congestive failure after chest trauma should raise the suspicion of a ruptured intraventricular septum, valve leaflet or chordae tendineae. Traumatic ventricular septal rupture presents with a pansystolic murmur heard over the entire precordium, especially at the left sternal border. This may not be appreciated, however, until the patient has been resuscitated to a euvolemic state. In patients exhibiting hemodynamic instability and clinical signs of cardiac failure, a formal echocardiogram should be obtained to look for the presence of pericardial tamponade, valvular or cordae tendinea disruption and to ascertain cardiac output.

Unfortunately, there is no gold standard to make the diagnosis of myocardial contusion. Chest radiographs are not helpful in diagnosing cardiac trauma per se, but may be helpful in identifying other thoracic injuries. Although nondiagnostic, multiple ECG abnormalities have been described which range from persistent sinus tachycardia to ST and T wave changes and bundle-branch blocks (the most common being right bundle branch block). If ECG abnormalities are present or if there is persistent chest pain, the patient should be admitted for 24 to 48 hours of continuous cardiac monitoring. Recently it has been reported that cardiac enzymes and troponin-I and T determinations may be helpful in making the diagnosis and in the stratification of those at risk for life-threatening conditions (9,38,41). If the troponin is not elevated at 4 to 6 hours post injury and the ECG is normal, the patient may be discharged from the ED. There is little or no role for radionuclide imaging studies in diagnosing this entity.

Great Vessel Injuries

In patients with a major traumatic mechanism, a chest x-ray is a helpful screening tool in detecting, not only great vessel, but also other associated thoracic abnormalities. There are multiple radiographic features of great vessel injury (Fig. 182.2). Despite the many radiographic signs of traumatic aortic injury that have been described, no single radiographic criterion is diagnostic or can rule out this entity (Table 182.1). If any of these are present, then further diagnostic studies are indicated. The most sensitive finding in patients with aortic injury is a wide mediastinum (>6 cm upright and >8 cm supine anteroposterior view) (20). However, only 10% of patients with a wide mediastinum will end up having an aortic injury; other causes include sternal, rib, or spine fractures and the supine technique (5,18,35,49). Sitting the patient up after the cervical spine has been cleared will decrease the incidence of a wide mediastinum. Even in the presence of a completely normal upright chest x-ray, if there is a significant mechanism, it is reasonable to consider further diagnostic studies. In 7% to 28% of cases of aortic injury, the chest radiograph will be normal (16).

TABLE 182.1.   Radiographic Features of Great Vessel Injury

Widening of the superior mediastinum at the level of the aortic knob on an upright radiograph
Mediastinal width–chest width ratio of more than 0.25
Deviation of the trachea or endotracheal tube to the right
Deviation of the nasogastric tube (representing the esophagus) to the right
Narrowing of the carinal angle
Depression of the left mainstem bronchus
Irregularity of the aortic knob contour
Left apical cap
Opacification of a clear space between the aorta and pulmonary artery ("aortic pulmonary window")
Widening of the left or right paraspinous stripe
Hemothorax, sternal, or rib fractures

Dynamic CT scanning of the chest with contrast has become the procedure of choice when the diagnosis of mediastinal great vessel injury is considered, with reported sensitivity and specificity of 96% to 100% and 98% to 100%, respectively. An added benefit to CT is the detection of other pulmonary processes, such as pulmonary contusions or small pneumothoraces not visible on the initial chest x-ray (3,30,44). Furthermore, CT is noninvasive and can be completed in a short period of time. Dynamic contrast enhanced CT of the chest should be performed in those patients who have any findings on chest x-ray associated with

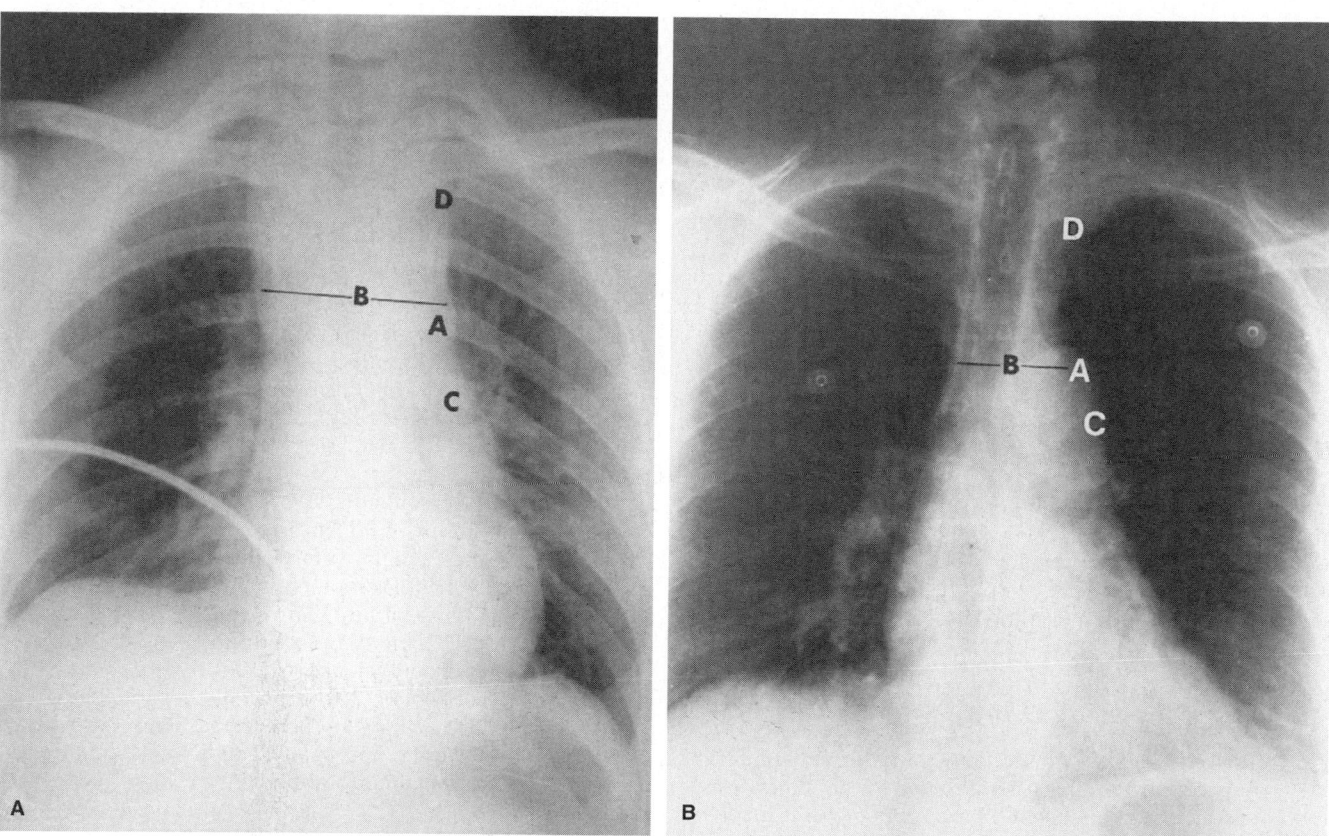

Figure 182.2.   Upright posteroanterior chest radiographs of a 20-year-old man involved as a driver in a head-on motor vehicle collision **(A)** compared with that of a normal person **(B).** The first radiograph has several abnormalities suggestive of a great vessel disruption. **(A)** Loss of detail of aortic knob with blurring of the aortic outline. **(B)** Widened mediastinum (mediastinal width–chest width ratio greater than 0.28). **(C)** Opacification of the clear space between the aorta and pulmonary artery (aortopulmonary window). **(D)** Obliteration of the medial aspect of the left upper field. The aortogram revealed rupture of the aortic arch. (Radiographs courtesy of the Department of Radiology, St. Luke's Hospital, Milwaukee, Wisconsin.)

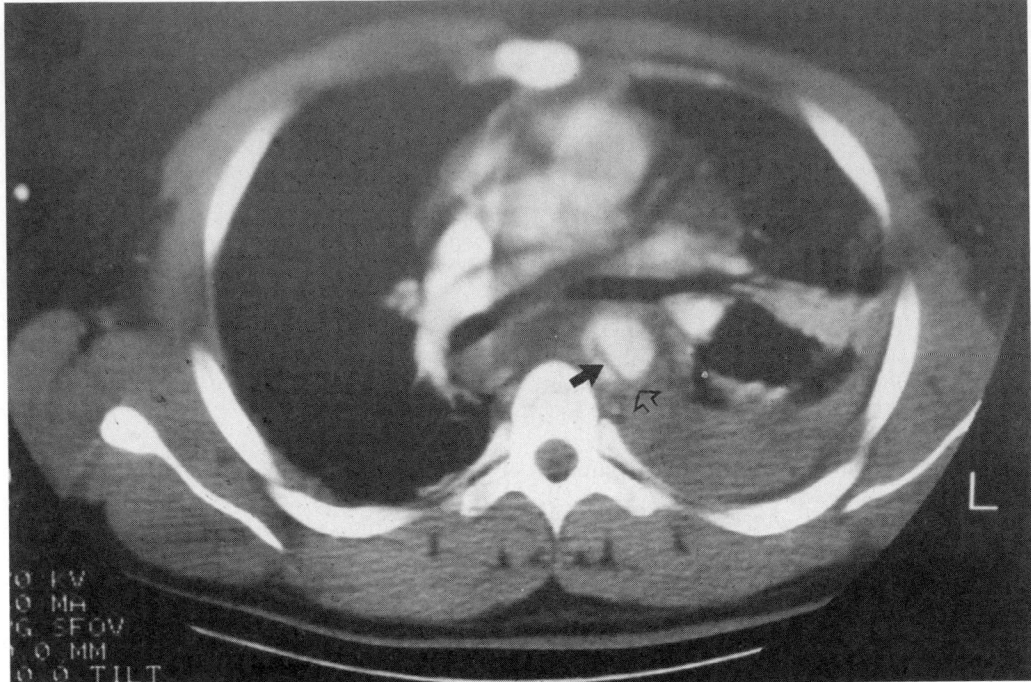

Figure 182.3.   Dynamic chest computed tomography reveals an intimal flap (*solid arrow*) and surrounding periaortic hematoma (*open arrow*). This patient underwent successful operative repair of a traumatic disruption located at the "classic" site (ligamentum arteriosum).

traumatic aortic injury, are hemodynamically stable and have sustained significant acceleration/deceleration blunt force chest trauma such as high speed motor vehicle collisions or falls from a significant height. Positive criteria for the diagnosis of great vessel injury include periaortic hematoma, an irregular aortic contour, change in caliber of the aorta, and intraluminal irregularity (intimal flap) (Fig. 182.3) (1).

Transesophageal echocardiography (TEE) is reported to have a sensitivity and specificity comparable to helical CT in the diagnosis of blunt aortic injury (44,48). In contrast to CT, it can be performed at the bedside in an unstable patient. However, in contrast to helical chest CT, its availability is limited in most EDs. It may be performed in an ICU setting or the operating room to diagnose aortic injury in unstable patients and those with other life-threatening injuries. This technique is contraindicated in patients with esophageal injury or unstable cervical spine injuries.

Aortography is still the gold standard for making the diagnosis of traumatic aortic injury, but it is now only used in a small number of cases with equivocal findings on helical CT and when planning the surgery in some selected cases. This is the definitive study for determining whether or not the periaortic hemorrhage is secondary to disruption of minor vessels in the mediastinum or is due to a traumatic aortic injury.

Diaphragmatic Injuries

An immediate chest x-ray should be obtained when blunt traumatic rupture of the diaphragm is suspected by the clinical examination (i.e., decreased or absent breath sounds on the involved side, bowel sounds audible in the chest, severe respiratory distress) and the patient has sustained major blunt force trauma to the lower chest or upper abdomen. In most instances of blunt traumatic rupture, the left hemidiaphragm is not visualized on the radiograph and stomach or bowel is often visualized in the left hemithorax. The evaluation of suspected penetrating trauma to the diaphragm is much more difficult since many of these pa-

tients exhibit little or no clinical findings. Small diaphragmatic tears may not be obvious on initial chest x-ray but may be diagnosed with contrast enhanced abdominal CT.

Esophageal Injuries

The presence of particulate matter in chest tube drainage as well as the presence of supraclavicular subcutaneous emphysema should lead the physician to consider esophageal perforation. This diagnosis has a very high morbidity and mortality if not recognized early and treated aggressively. When this diagnosis is suspected, it is imperative to move rapidly to a definitive diagnostic study to rule out this entity. The choice of the initial diagnostic procedure is somewhat controversial and is dependent upon the suspected injury. Some authors advocate esophagography, and others esophagoscopy. *Contrast esophagraphy* has the disadvantage of potentially introducing contrast material into the mediastinum or peritoneum. Therefore, this study should first be performed with a water-soluble contrast material (i.e., Gastrografin), which has a much lower risk of mediastinitis or peritonitis than does barium. However, care should be taken in patients at risk for aspiration, as the entry of water-soluble contrast into the tracheobronchial tree can lead to pulmonary edema. If this study is negative, it can be followed by *esophagoscopy*, since Gastrografin will not obscure the lining of the esophagus. Ultimately, a barium esophagram may be needed to detect the presence of very small perforations.

Traumatic Asphyxia

Since these patients can sustain rib fractures and pulmonary contusions, one should consider chest CTs to evaluate these injuries. Also, any patient with a neurologic deficit should have a CT of the head.

EMERGENCY DEPARTMENT MANAGEMENT

Chest Wall Injuries

Chest wall contusions and rib fractures with no underlying pulmonary parenchymal injury should be managed with adequate analgesics as well as careful aftercare instructions encouraging the patient to cough and deep breathe every hour while awake in order to prevent the complications of atelectasis and subsequent pneumonia. Patients may be discharged with a spirometer to aid them in following these instructions. Consideration can be given to regional nerve blocks for multiple rib fractures, but these may only give significant pain relief for up to 12 hours.

Flail Chest

Pain can be controlled with administration of narcotics, regional nerve blocks, or in severe cases, epidural anesthesia. Intubation should be considered if there is respiratory distress or ventilatory failure as manifested by a P_aO_2 of less than 60 mm Hg on a nonrebreather bag reservoir mask at sea level or low oxygen saturation. In elderly patients with flail chest, the physician should have a lower threshold for intubation, as their cardiac and pulmonary reserves are limited.

Sternal Fractures

Patients with suspected sternal fractures should have a standard PA and lateral chest x-ray. The lateral chest x-ray is the best view to determine if a fracture is present. Because of the anatomical location of the injury, all patients with sternal fractures should be on a cardiac monitor and have an ECG.

Pulmonary and Pleural Injuries

Tension pneumothorax, pneumothorax, and hemothorax should be treated emergently with tube thoracostomy (see Chapter 184). Patients with clinical evidence of tension pneumothorax should undergo immediate needle chest decompression with a 14- or 16-gauge needle or tube thoracostomy with a 28- to 36-French tube for adults or a 16 to 24-French tube for children before chest x-rays are obtained. Small (less than 15%) simple pneumothoraces, such as those visualized on CT only (occult pneumothorax), can often be observed and treated without thoracostomy. Patients with occult pneumothorax who will undergo transfer in an ambulance or helicopter or positive pressure ventilation are at risk for development of a larger pneumothorax (or tension pneumothorax), and should undergo tube thoracostomy.

Patients with pulmonary contusions should be placed on continuous, high-flow oxygen via a nonrebreather bag reservoir mask, and their oxygen saturation continuously monitored. Excessive crystalloid administration should be avoided since it may exacerbate the pulmonary edema. Those who exhibit falling oxygen saturations or hypercarbia should be considered for rapid sequence intubation (RSI) and positive pressure ventilation. Independent lung ventilation with low tidal volume and PEEP has been reported to be efficacious in the treatment of unilateral pulmonary contusions (8). Until the pulmonary contusion resolves, this treatment will mechanically force fluid out of the effected alveoli, enabling better ventilation and improving ventilation-perfusion mismatch.

Patients with an initial thoracostomy tube output of greater than 20cc/Kg or an ongoing blood loss of greater than 7cc/Kg/hr are candidates for operative thoracotomy.

Tracheal and Bronchial Injuries

In a patient who clinically has a major airway disruption or problems with maintaining adequate oxygen saturation, endotracheal intubation should be performed. In some instances, selective intubation of the nontraumatized mainstem bronchus is indicated. All tracheobronchial lacerations and disruptions require a surgical consultation, further diagnostic studies (bronchoscopy) and definitive management.

Blunt Cardiac Injuries

All patients should be on oxygen and monitored for dysrhythmias, which should be treated with the proper antidysrhythmic agent. A patient in shock may benefit from pulmonary artery pressure monitoring in order to optimize fluid resuscitation. Care must be taken not to fluid overload patients with myocardial contusion as their compromised cardiac output may lead to pulmonary edema. Patients who remain hemodynamically compromised after adequate volume resuscitation may benefit from pressor support with dobutamine. Acute pericardial tamponade should be treated as outlined in Chapter 183, "Penetrating Chest Trauma." These patients have cardiac rupture and require operative thoracotomy. Unstable patients with this injury require pericardiocentesis or ED thoracotomy if they are in extremis. Patients with abnormalities detected on echocardiography such as chordae tendinea or valvular disruption should be referred to a cardiac surgeon for definitive repair of these lesions. In those rare instances where blunt cardiac trauma results in myocardial infarction from intimal disruption and thrombosis of the coronary artery, these patients should undergo emergency angioplasty since the use of thrombolytics is contraindicated. The last option for refractory cardiogenic shock is placement of an intraaortic balloon pump. The prognosis for patients with blunt cardiac trauma is most closely correlated with the severity and number of other associated injuries as most patients who have an isolated myocardial contusion do well.

Great Vessel Injuries

In patients in whom a traumatic aortic injury is strongly suspected or proven via dynamic CT scan of the chest, blood pressure should be controlled via the use of a beta-blocker and antihypertensive agent (usually nitroprusside). Beta-blocking agents are usually started first; because it is easily titratable, esmolol is ideal for this purpose. The objective of lowering blood pressure is to decrease the shearing jet effect of the elevated pulse pressure, thus decreasing the possibility of free rupture. Using nitroprusside without a beta-blocking agent may result in a reflex tachycardia and increased intraluminal pressure. The systolic blood pressure should be maintained between 100 to 120 mm Hg, and all patients must be emergently referred for definitive surgical management. Many patients with aortic injury will have associated life-threatening injuries that require management before operative repair of the aorta. Management of intraperitoneal injuries, intracranial hematomas, and sometimes unstable pelvic trauma or other orthopaedic injuries will take priority over aortic repair.

Diaphragmatic Injuries

A nasogastric tube should be placed and tube thoracostomy performed in patients with traumatic diaphragmatic rupture. Emergent surgical consultation for operative repair of the diaphragm should be obtained. Some of these patients may require RSI intubation, sedation and mechanical ventilation if there is significant respiratory compromise.

Esophageal Injuries

Once the presence of an esophageal injury is confirmed by a contrast study of the esophagus or by esophagoscopy, surgical consultation for definitive surgical repair and drainage should be obtained to minimize the subsequent morbidity and mortality of this lesion. Intravenous antibiotics should be administered preoperatively.

Emergency Department Thoracotomy

For those patients with blunt trauma who sustain cardiac arrest prior to arrival in the ED, an ED thoracotomy is a futile procedure. Those patients who arrest after arrival in the ED and undergo ED thoracotomy have a 1.4% survival rate. Patients with isolated cardiac or pulmonary injuries have the best chance of survival after ED thoracotomy (36).

CRITICAL INTERVENTIONS

- Perform tube thoracostomy immediately for patients with clinical signs of tension pneumothorax or massive hemothorax (decreased breath sounds or subcutaneous emphysema in association with hypotension, tachycardia and absent breath sounds)
- Obtain an electrocardiogram in patients with external evidence of chest trauma or sternal fractures
- Obtain an echocardiogram in unstable patients with clinical signs of cardiac failure to detect pericardial tamponade and valvular or chordae tendinea disruption
- Administer beta-blocking agents then nitroprusside to control blood pressure in patients in whom a traumatic aortic injury is strongly suspected or proven via CT scan

---

DISPOSITION

Patients with contused ribs and isolated rib fractures may be discharged from the ED. They should be instructed to return if they develop any increasing shortness of breath, fever, chills, cough or other new symptoms. Patients with multiple rib fractures should be admitted for continued monitoring and observation, and in some selected circumstances, consideration of epidural anesthesia for pain. In particular, elderly patients with multiple rib fractures should be admitted for pain control and appropriate management to prevent pulmonary complications.

All patients with flail chest should be admitted to the hospital and carefully monitored via continuous oxygen saturation for an evolving pulmonary contusion, which almost always accompanies this injury. In addition, these patients have significant pain and usually require parenteral analgesics and consideration of regional or epidural nerve blocks.

Patients with fractures of the sternum sometimes need admission for analgesics because of associated injuries to the bony thorax and intrathoracic cavity. If the fracture is displaced, surgical reduction is needed. However, patients with isolated nondisplaced sternal fractures may be discharged after appropriate measures have been taken to rule out the presence of underlying cardiac or pulmonary contusion (ECG and chest x-ray). Even though there is a low incidence of proven associated cardiac injury, appropriate measures should be taken to rule out a myocardial injury if there is any abnormality on the ECG, including persistent sinus tachycardia, when all other causes have been treated or ruled out.

Patients with pneumothorax, hemothorax, hemopneumothorax and, of course, tension pneumothorax must be admitted to the appropriate inpatient surgical service for continued observation and treatment. Most patients with a pneumothorax and hemothorax only require a tube thoracostomy and do not require subsequent thoracotomy. However, in those patients in whom active, continued bleeding occurs or a persistent air leak is present, additional studies and surgery may be necessary.

All patients with a suspected or proven pulmonary contusion should be admitted to the hospital for continued monitoring and treatment since most pulmonary contusions will gradually worsen over the first 24 hours.

Patients with tracheal and bronchial injuries must be admitted and often require surgical repair if they do not spontaneously resolve.

Patients who have sustained blunt anterior chest trauma, have no associated injury necessitating admission and have a normal EKG may be discharged from the ED. Because the prognosis of patients with blunt cardiac injury is related to the magnitude of the initial trauma, the preexisting condition of the heart, the size and location of the cardiac injury and the patient's other traumatic injuries, patients who have coronary artery disease, significant dysrhythmias or any new abnormality on an EKG should be admitted for continuous monitoring for 12 to 24 hours. Patients with operable blunt trauma to the heart, such as myocardial and valve rupture or acute pericardial tamponade, need early and aggressive cardiac surgical treatment.

Traumatic disruption of the great vessels is a surgical emergency, and as soon as the diagnosis is suspected or confirmed, trauma or vascular surgery consultation should be obtained. After other more immediate life threats have been treated, these lesions should receive definitive surgical repair.

All patients with diaphragmatic injuries must be admitted to a trauma surgeon for definitive repair of the tear in the diaphragm as well as associated intraabdominal and intrathoracic injuries that often accompany these injuries.

All patients with confirmed esophageal perforation require admission and immediate surgical consultation. Nearly all patients with esophageal perforation require surgical intervention. Rarely, a patient with a very small lesion and a localized infection may be successfully managed with antibiotics alone. However, most require mediastinal drainage with esophageal repair and temporary esophageal exclusion (creation of a cervical esophagostomy and distal esophageal ligature). A few patients require esophagectomy with subsequent reconstruction using the stomach and colon. Surgical management is then supplemented by hyperalimentation or tube feedings by way of operatively placed jejunostomy tube and continuation of antibiotic therapy. Patients should be transferred to an appropriate surgeon and facility if resources for this definitive management are not available.

Those patients who have sustained traumatic asphyxia but have no evidence of significant chest wall, intrathoracic, or neurologic injury may be discharged home. Those with associated intrathoracic or neurologic injury should be admitted for continued observation and treatment.

Patients who must be transferred to another trauma facility for definitive treatment or critical care management should undergo a chest x-ray prior to transfer. Tube thoracostomy should be performed prior to transfer in patients with pneumothorax, hemothorax, or those with an occult pneumothorax detected only by CT. Patients with significant chest wall trauma or flail chest, especially the elderly, should be intubated prior to transfer. Any blunt chest trauma patient with suspected aortic injury should be transferred to a trauma center.

COMMON PITFALLS

✔ Failure to appreciate a serious deceleration mechanism of injury

✔ Failure to recognize the potential morbidity of rib fractures in the elderly

✔ Delaying transfer of a patient to an appropriate level trauma center for definitive management of aortic injury

✔ Failure to consider esophageal perforation in any patient with mediastinal emphysema

✔ Insertion of a chest tube into an abdominal viscous in patients with a ruptured diaphragm

✔ Overzealous fluid administration in patients with pulmonary and myocardial contusions

✔ Failure to provide adequate analgesia and pulmonary care to patients with rib fractures, leading to the development of atelectasis and pneumonia

Acknowledgments

The author wishes to thank Drs. Joanne Edney, Brian Tiffany, Robert Jordan, Daniel Gabbay, Patrick Reilly, Lee Shockley, C. Keith Stone, and Ron Koury who authored the chapters relevant to blunt chest trauma in the previous edition.

References

1. Agee CK, Metzler MH, et al. Computed tomographic evaluation to exclude traumatic aortic disruption. *J Trauma* 1992;33:876.
2. Bar I, Friedman T, Rudis E, et al. Isolated sternal fractures: A benign condition. *Isr Med Assoc J* 2003;5:105–106.
3. BenMenachem Y. Rupture of the thoracic aorta by broadside impacts in road traffic and other collisions: further angiographic observations and preliminary autopsy findings. *J Trauma* 1993;35:363.
4. Bulge EM, Arenson MA, Mock CN, et al. Rib fractures in the elderly. *J Trauma* 2000;48:1040–1046.
5. Burney RE, Gundry SR, et al. Chest roentgenograms in diagnosis of traumatic rupture of the aorta. *Chest* 1984;84:605.
6. Cernaianu AC, Cilley JH Jr, et al. Determinants of outcome in lesions of the thoracic aorta in patients with multiorgan system trauma. *Chest* 1992;101:331.
7. Christin F, Meyer N, Launoy A, et al. Lung contusion: Relevance of initial injured pulmonary volume measurement by CT. *Ann Fr Anesth Reanim* 2003;22:408–413.
8. Cinnella G, Dambrosio M, Brienza N, et al. Independent lung ventilation in patients with unilateral pulmonary contusion: Monitoring with compliance and ETCO2. *Intensive Care Med* 2001;27:1860–1867.
9. Collins JN, Cole FJ, Weireter LJ, et al. The usefulness of serum troponin levels in evaluating cardiac injury. *Am Surg* 2001;67:821–825.
10. Conlan AA, Wessels A, Hammond CA, et al. Pharyngoesophageal barotrauma in children: a report of six cases. *J Thorac Cardiovasc Surg* 1984;88:452.
11. Crass JR, Cohen AM, Motta AO, Tomashefski JF Jr, Wiesen EJ. A proposed new mechanism of traumatic aortic rupture: the osseous pinch. *Radiology* 1990;176:645–649.
12. Dowd MD, Krug S. Pediatric blunt cardiac injury: epidemiology, clinical features, and diagnosis. Pediatric emergency medicine collaborative research committee: working group on blunt cardiac injury. *J Trauma* 1996;40:61.
13. Dyer DS, Moore EE, Ilke DN, et al. Thoracic aortic injury: How predictive is mechanism and is chest CT a reliable screening tool? A prospective study of 1561 patients. *J Trauma* 2000;48:673–682.
14. Feczko JD, Lynch L, et al. An autopsy case review of 142 nonpenetrating (blunt) injuries of the aorta. *J Trauma* 1992;33:846.
15. Fox S. Pierce WS, Waldhausen JA. Acute hypertension: its significance in traumatic aortic rupture. *J Thorac Cardiovasc Surg* 1979;77:622.
16. Frick E, Cipolle MD, Pasquale MD, et al. Outcome of blunt thoracic aortic injury in a level I trauma center: an 8-year review. *J Trauma* 1997;43:844–851.
17. Holcomb JB, McMulllin NR, Kozar AA, et al. Morbidity from rib fractures increase after age 45. *J Am Coll Surg* 2003;196:549–555.
18. Hunt MD, Schwab FJ.Chest trauma. In: Rosen P, Doris PE, et al, eds. *Diagnostic radiology in emergency medicine.* St. Louis: Mosby–Year Book, 1992.
19. Kanowitz A, Marx JA. Delayed traumatic diaphragmatic hernia simulating acute tension pneumothorax. *J Emerg Med* 1989;7:619.
20. Kirshner R, Seltzer S, D'Orsi C, De Weese JA. Upper rib fractures and mediastinal widening: indications for aortography. *Ann Thorac Surg* 1983;35:450–454.
21. Kiser AC, O'Brien SM, Detterbeck FC. Blunt tracheobronchial injuries: Treatment and outcomes. *Ann Thorac Surg* 2001;71:2059–2065.
22. Lateef F. Commotio cordis: An under appreciated cause of sudden death in athletes. *Sports Med* 2000;30:301–308.
23. Maenza RL, Seaberg D, D'Amico F. A meta-analysis of blunt cardiac trauma: ending myocardial confusion. *Am J Emerg Med* 1996;14:237.
24. McGrath RB. Gastroesophageal lacerations: a fatal complication of closed chest cardiopulmonary resuscitation. *Chest* 1983;83:570.
25. McGwin G Jr, Reiff DA, Moran SG, et al. Incidence and characteristics of motor vehicle collision-related blunt thoracic aortic injury according to age. *J Trauma* 2002;52:859–865.
26. Merriedith M, Liebowitz R. Rupture of the esophagus caused by the Heimlich maneuver. *Ann Emerg Med* 1986;15:106.
27. Mihos P, Potaris K, Gakidis J, et al. Traumatic rupture of the diaphragm: Experience with 65 cases. *Injury* 2003;34:169–172.
28. Mizushima Y, Hiraide A, Shimazu T, et al. Changes in contused lung volume and oxygenation in patients with pulmonary parenchymal injury after blunt chest trauma. *Am J Emerg Med* 2000;18:385–389.
29. Ochsner JL, Crawford ED, DeBakey ME. Injuries of the vena cava caused by external trauma. *Surgery* 1961;49:397.
30. Parker MS, Matheson TL, Rao AV, et al. Making the transition: The role of helical CYT in the evaluation of potentially acute traumatic aortic injury. *AJR Am J Roentgenol* 2001;176:1267–1272.
31. Parmley LF, Mattingly TW, Manion WC, et al. Nonpenetrating traumatic injury of the aorta. *Circulation* 1958;17:1086.
32. Patel NH, Stephens KE, Mirvis SE, et al. Imaging of acute thoracic aortic injury due to blunt trauma: a review. *Radiology* 1998;209:335–348.
33. Perron AD, Brady WJ, Erling BF. Commotio cordis: An under-appreciated cause of sudden death in young patient: Assessment and management in the emergency department. *Am J Emerg Med* 2001;19:406–409.
34. Potaris K, Gakidis J, Mihos P, et al. Management of sternal fractures: 239 cases. *Asian Cardiovasc Thorac Ann* 2002;10:145–149.
35. Raptopoulos V, Sheiman RG, et al. Traumatic aortic tear: screening with chest CT. *Radiology* 1992;182:667.
36. Rhee PM et al: Survival after emergency department thoracotomy: review of published data from the past 25 years. *J Am Coll Surg* 2000;190:288.
37. Rosengart MR, Smith DR, Melton SM, et al. Prognostic factors in patients with inferior vena cava injuries. *Am Surg* 1999;65:849–856.
38. Salim A, Velharnos GC, Jindal A, et al. Clinically significant blunt cardiac trauma: Role of serum troponin level combined with electrocardiographic findings. *J Trauma* 2001;50:237–243.
39. Simpson J, Lobo DN, Shah AB, et al. Traumatic diaphragmatic rupture: Associated injuries and outcome. *Ann R Coll Surg Engl* 2000;82:97–100.
40. Sturm JT et al: Significance of symptoms and signs in patients with traumatic aortic rupture, *Ann Emerg Med* 1984;13:876.
41. Sybrandy KC, Cramer MJ, Burgersdijk C. Diagnosing cardiac contusion: Old wisdom and new insights. *Heart* 2003;89:485–489.
42. Symbas PN, et al. Traumatic rupture of the aorta. *Ann Surg* 1973;178:6.
43. Tintinalli JE, Gabaor D, Saphcynski JS, eds. *Emergency medicine: a comprehensive study guide.* 5th Ed. New York: McGraw-Hill 2000:1675–1699.
44. Vignon P, Boncoeur MP, Francois B, et al. Comparison of multilane transthoracic echocardiography and contrast enhanced helical CT in the diagnosis of blunt traumatic cardiovascular injury. *Anesthesiology* 2001;94:615–622.
45. Wang JN, Tsai YC, Chen SL, et al. Dangerous impact—Commotio cordis. *Cardiology* 2000;93:124–126.
46. Weiman DS, McCoy DW, Haan CK, et al. Blunt injuries of the brachiocephalic artery. *Am Surg* 1998;64:383–387.
47. Weissbert D, Kaufman M. Compressed air injury to the esophagus. *J Trauma* 1991;31:150.
48. Wintermark M, Wicky S, Schnyder P. Imaging of acute traumatic injury of the thoracic aorta. *Eur Radiol* 2002;12:431–442.
49. Woodring JH, King JG. Determination of normal transverse mediastinal width and mediastinal-width to chest-width (M/C) ratio in control subjects: implications for subjects with aortic or brachiocephalic arterial injury. *J Trauma* 1989;29:1268.

In the setting of a gunshot wound to the heart, loss of an extremity pulse or focal neurologic deficits should raise the question of arterial embolization of the bullet, pellet, or fragment. New murmurs or acute congestive heart failure after chest trauma should raise the suspicion of intraventricular septum, valve leaflet, or chordae tendineae injuries. Ventricular septal lacerations present with a pansystolic murmur auscultated over the entire precordium, especially at the left lower sternal border. This may not be appreciated, however, until the patient has been resuscitated to euvolemia.

Penetrating chest trauma can also result in injury to abdominal structures. During expiration, diaphragmatic excursion can extend as high as the nipple line anteriorly and the inferior border of the scapula posteriorly. Wounds below this level have the potential for injuring abdominal organs. Further, bullet and other missiles can enter the chest, traverse the diaphragm, and injure abdominal organs. Similarly, stab wounds from long-bladed weapons can also traverse the diaphragm and injure abdominal organs.

EMERGENCY DEPARTMENT EVALUATION

Physical Examination

The initial physical examination of the chest in patients with penetrating trauma should focus on signs of pneumothorax or hemothorax and include an assessment for breath sounds and palpation for subcutaneous air. If there are signs of pneumothorax or hemothorax, then a tube thoracostomy is placed. In a stable patient the next part of the physical examination should focus on searching for all of the wounds. This is accomplished by having the patient sit up or by rolling the patient and carefully inspecting areas where wounds are initially missed such as the buttocks, back, and axillae.

Physical examination alone is insufficient to rule out pneumothorax or hemothorax in penetrating chest trauma patients (10). Furthermore, as many as 31% of patients with penetrating diaphragm injuries have no abdominal tenderness and 40% have normal chest radiographs (32). Probing chest wounds with a finger or cotton-tip applicator does not add to the evaluation of the penetrating trauma patient. There is no diagnostic benefit to performing this technique and it may actually cause bleeding or pneumothorax. In addition, the examining physician may be blamed for causing a pneumothorax that is noted subsequently.

Wounds directly over the precordium and epigastrium (the "cardiac box") are more likely to involve cardiac injury than those in more posterior or lateral locations. The most common vital sign abnormality in penetrating cardiac trauma is sinus tachycardia. Bradycardia or pulseless electrical activity (PEA) is often a preterminal sign. Hypotension is a serious sign and should raise the possibility of cardiac tamponade, massive hemothorax from the cardiac wound, other noncardiac trauma with hypovolemia, or valvular injury. Measuring the central venous pressure (CVP) early in the course of resuscitation will help differentiate tamponade (CVP greater than 15 to 20 cm H_2O) from hypovolemia (CVP less than 5 cm H_2O) in the patient with systemic hypotension. However, the CVP may not be elevated in the severely hypovolemic patient in tamponade until a reasonable circulating volume has been restored.

In penetrating trauma to the great vessels, physical findings are not insidious. Usually, there is overt bleeding from a visible wound, a massive hemothorax, or continuous bleeding from a thoracostomy tube. In the proper context, an absent or diminished pulse in the arm represents subclavian artery injury, while the presence of a murmur or bruit suggests an aneurysm or arteriovenous fistula.

Chest Radiography

The single most helpful diagnostic study in the evaluation of penetrating chest trauma is the chest radiograph. Ideally, a high quality, posterior-anterior, upright view should be obtained with a similar high quality lateral view. In the case of a suspected small pneumothorax, an expiratory view may demonstrate the extrapleural air better than the inspiratory view. Portable, supine, anterior-posterior chest radiographs offer a great deal of information, should be immediately available, and do not require altering the patient's position. However, 20% to 35% of pneumothoraces may be missed on these initial radiographs. A three-hour repeat chest x-ray appears to be as effective as a six-hour x-ray in identifying delayed pneumo- and hemothoraces in patients with blunt or penetrating chest trauma (23). One helpful finding suggestive of pneumothorax on the supine view is the *deep sulcus sign*-a deep costophrenic angle. A minimum of 200 to 300 ml of blood must be present in the pleura in order for it to be detected on standard chest radiographs.

A pathognomonic but rare chest x-ray finding for bronchial rupture is the fallen lung sign; the lung is displaced ("fallen") away from the hilum, laterally and posteriorly (36).

Chest radiographs are not very helpful in diagnosing penetrating cardiac trauma *per se,* but they are useful in identifying other thoracic injuries associated with penetrating cardiac injuries. The radiograph may demonstrate a hemothorax, pneumothorax, pneumopericardium, or the offending missile(s). The blurry image of a bullet overlying the cardiac silhouette should raise the question of an intracardiac location and "movement artifact" on the film.

Chest radiograph findings that suggest great vessel injuries include large hemothorax, foreign bodies (i.e., bullets) near the great vessels, out of focus foreign bodies overlying the heart, a confusing trajectory (indicating a migrating intravascular bullet), and a "missing" bullet (suggesting distal arterial embolization).

Central Venous Pressure Monitoring

In patients with penetrating cardiac trauma, a rise in central venous pressure may be one of the first signs of accumulating pericardial fluid, even prior to the onset of hypotension. It is prudent to measure central venous pressure (CVP) early in the course of a patient with penetrating chest trauma in whom a cardiac injury is possible, and to monitor the pressure frequently. If, however, the diagnosis of pericardial blood has been made (by ultrasound, for example), CVP offers little additional information and attempts at placing a central line may delay definitive repair of the injury.

Computed Tomography

As noted previously, up to 35% of pneumothoraces and small hemothoraces may not be visible on standard chest radiographs, only to be found on chest CT. The clinical significance of these "occult" pneumothoraces is a subject of debate and is discussed in the management section.

CT has been used to aid in the evaluation of tracheobronchial injuries but, so far, has not replaced bronchoscopy as the diagnostic procedure of choice. CT scanning is not a primary diagnostic study for thoracic esophageal perforation, but it can reveal nonspecific findings suggestive of perforation, such as air in soft tissues or abscess cavities. CT scanning can also be helpful in detecting postoperative leaks and abscess formation (22).

Chest CT has a low sensitivity in the diagnosis of diaphragm injuries because the imaging plane is parallel to the dome of the diaphragm, and the dome is not well visualized (27). Chest CT is a useful test for diagnosing hemopericardium in stable patients with penetrating chest trauma (34). It has a sensitivity approaching 100% when compared to subxyphoid pericardial window. However, its greatest utility is in hemodynamically stable patients in whom bedside echocardiography is not available or is inadequate.

Echocardiography and Abdominal Ultrasonography

Echocardiography has several advantages in the evaluation of patients with penetrating cardiac injuries. A noninvasive test that can be performed at the bedside, it can quickly give information about pericardial fluid collections, valve injuries, and septal lacerations. Bedside two-dimensional echocardiography is the most expedient and accurate diagnostic test for pericardial fluid, with a sensitivity and specificity of 97% to 100% and 90% to 97%, respectively, compared to a subxyphoid pericardiotomy standard in the absence of hemothorax (21,29,42). The presence of a hemothorax makes the study more difficult to interpret and lowers its sensitivity to only 56% (29). As little as 20 to 50 ml of pericardial blood can be detected by M-mode echocardiography.

Echocardiography is indicated in the evaluation of the patient at risk for a penetrating cardiac injury who exhibits signs of hemodynamic instability (persistent tachycardia, hypotension, elevated pulsus paradoxus, elevated CVP, new heart murmurs, or significant dysrhythmias) (42). However, echocardiography with the advantages of being noninvasive, at the bedside, and repeatable is becoming an important tool in the stable patient who may have sustained an occult cardiac injury. Bedside echocardiography performed by emergency physicians significantly reduces the time to diagnosis, mortality, and neurologic impairment of patients with penetrating cardiac injuries (38).

Ultrasound has also been used as a rapid, bedside technique to detect hemothorax and pneumothorax. Compared to a portable chest radiograph, ultrasound has a sensitivity of 92% to 97.5% and a specificity of 99.7% to 100% for detecting hemothorax (12,44). The technique can be hampered, however, by subcutaneous air.

If available, *focused assessment with sonography for trauma* (FAST) may help in the diagnosis of penetrating chest injuries which violate the peritoneum as well. FAST is particularly indicated in patients with stab wounds below the nipple line (4th intercostal space) anteriorly or the inferior tip of the scapula posteriorly. These guidelines are based on the excursion of the diaphragm during ventilation. FAST is also indicated in gunshot wound trauma to the chest in which the bullet trajectory indicates a potential for peritoneal violation. A FAST exam that demonstrates hemoperitoneum is helpful in making diagnostic and treatment decisions but a negative FAST does not rule out abdominal injury. One of the limitations of the FAST exam in penetrating trauma is that it will miss small amounts of intraperitoneal hemorrhage (<250cc) that may result from injuries to the bowel or diaphragm.

Diagnostic Peritoneal Lavage

Diagnostic peritoneal lavage (DPL) is indicated for patients with penetrating chest trauma in whom there is a potential for transdiaphragmatic violation. In general, this includes patients with stab wounds below the nipple line (4th intercostal space) anteriorly or the inferior tip of the scapula posteriorly. These guidelines are based on the excursion of the diaphragm during ventilation. DPL has a 25% false-negative rate in the detection of isolated diaphragmatic injury using the criteria of 100,000 RBCs/mm³.

Some authors advocate lowering the RBC count considered positive to 5000 RBCs/mm³ when evaluating injuries at high risk for diaphragmatic injury (i.e., lower chest or upper abdominal penetrating wounds), however, even at this level, DPL will miss some injuries (3,19,30) (see Chapter 185, "Penetrating Abdominal Trauma").

Laparoscopy and Thoracoscopy

Although not performed in the emergency department, laparoscopy and thoracoscopy may offer the best diagnostic accuracy for diaphragm injuries, short of exploratory laparotomy or thoracotomy (28). In many centers, it is replacing DPL for the evaluation of potential diaphragm injuries. Since the incidence of diaphragmatic injuries is high in patients with penetrating left thoracoabdominal trauma (26%) and clinical and radiographic findings are unreliable in making the diagnosis (false-negative rates of 31% and 40% respectively), laparoscopy is indicated for evaluation of these injuries in patients who have no other indication for laparotomy but who are at risk because of the location of their wounds (33). In addition, some diaphragm injuries can be repaired via the laparoscope. Although less frequently employed, video-assisted thoracoscopy (VATS) is as accurate as laparoscopy in detecting diaphragm injuries.

Pericardiocentesis

Because of an unacceptable incidence of false positives and false negatives, pericardiocentesis is not a reliable technique for diagnosing cardiac tamponade.

Aortography

Aortography remains the gold standard for depicting the extent and location of penetrating thoracic vascular injury (17). With a complication rate of less than 1% for the percutaneous transfemoral approach, aortography has been consistently shown in the literature to have a sensitivity approaching 100% and a specificity of nearly 98%. This is largely because it is the only imaging modality that allows complete evaluation of the thoracic aorta from the aortic root to the diaphragmatic hiatus as well as the brachiocephalic arteries and their branches.

Esophagography

In stable patients with transmediastinal penetrating injuries, esophagography should be performed prior to aortography because of the greater likelihood of esophageal injury in this setting (17). Contrast esophagraphy has the disadvantage of potentially introducing contrast material into the mediastinum or the tracheobronchial tree. For this reason, the study should first be performed with a water-soluble contrast material that has a much lower risk of mediastinitis or pneumonitis than barium does. Water-soluble contrast studies, however, can miss up to 15% of small esophageal leaks subsequently seen with a barium study (45). Therefore, a negative water-soluble contrast study should be followed by a barium study, which provides better detection of small perforations.

Esophagoscopy

Both flexible and rigid esophagoscopy have been used in evaluating esophageal injuries, with sensitivities of 90% to 100% (20). Because esophagoscopy may detect esophageal perforations missed by contrast studies, it should be considered in high risk patients even in the setting of negative esophagography.

Bronchoscopy

Bronchoscopy is useful in the evaluation of tracheobronchial injuries. Indications for bronchoscopy include large pneumomediastinum, refractory pneumothorax, large air leak, persistent atelectasis, and marked subcutaneous emphysema.

Diagnostic Approach to Cardiac Injury

A diagnostic and treatment algorithm for penetrating cardiac injury has been proposed (46) (Fig. 183.1). This algorithm relies heavily on access to reliable diagnostic ultrasound; its utility is severely limited if ultrasound is not readily available.

The diagnostic approach to a suspected penetrating cardiac injury is dictated by the patient's stability. A patient in extremis is a candidate for a resuscitative thoracotomy without further diagnostic tests. In a patient who is hemodynamically compromised,

bedside echocardiography may yield an expedited diagnosis. If echocardiography is unavailable or technically inadequate, subxyphoid pericardial window is indicated. It is minimally invasive and allows direct inspection of the heart. It is typically done in the operating room with preparation for open thoracotomy if the window identifies pericardial blood. In the hemodynamically stable patient with a potential for a penetrating cardiac injury, a helical chest CT scan or serial physical exams combined with serial echocardiographs and serial determinations of the central venous pressure are reasonable approaches.

Diagnostic Approach to Diaphragmatic Injury

A diagnostic and treatment algorithm for penetrating diaphragmatic injury during the acute phase (immediately postinjury) has been proposed (4) (Fig. 183.2). This algorithm is based on chest

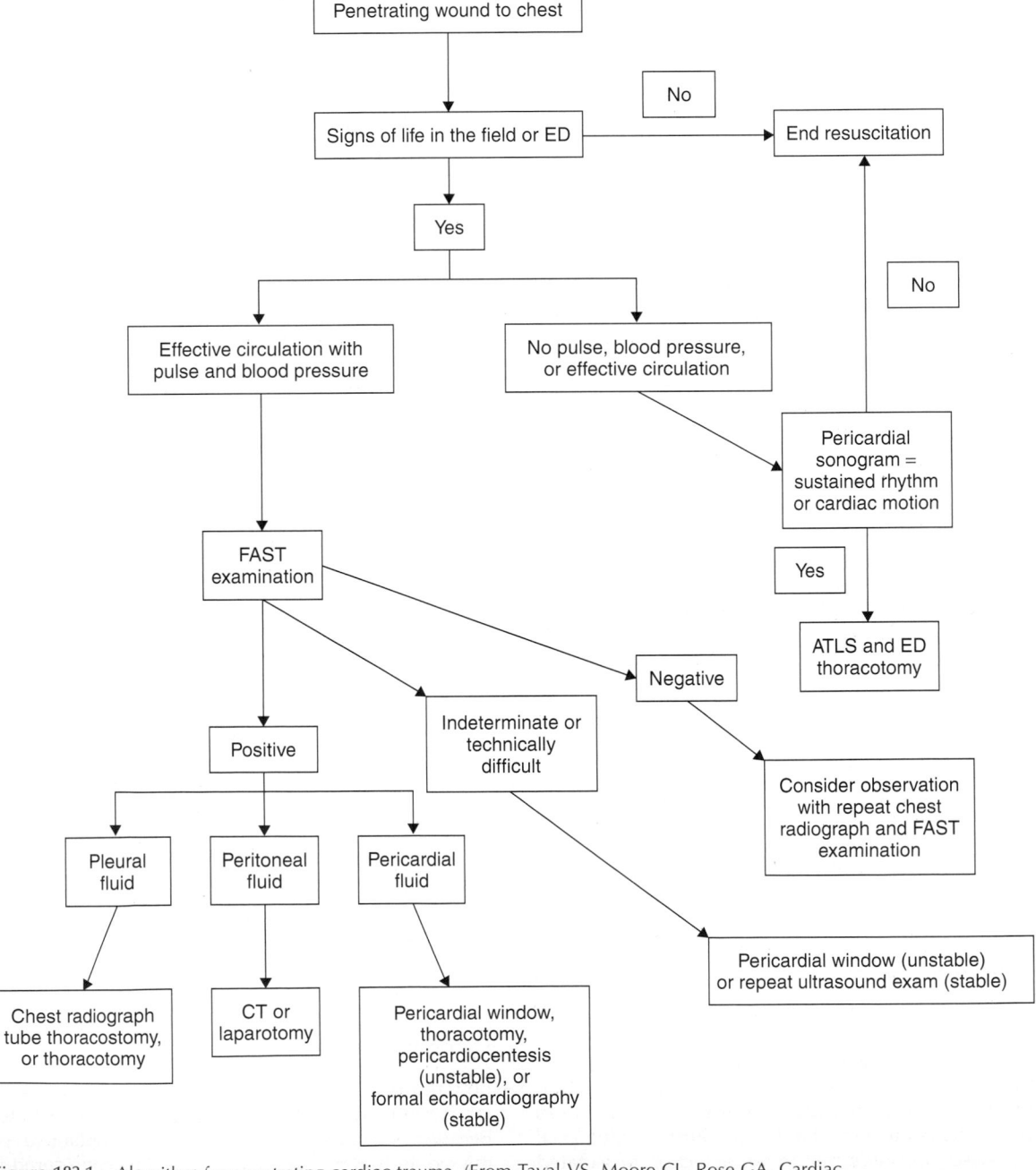

Figure 183.1.   Algorithm for penetrating cardiac trauma. (From Tayal VS, Moore CL, Rose GA. Cardiac. In: Ma OJ, Mateer JR (eds). *Emergency ultrasound,* New York, McGraw-Hill, 2003, p. 93, Fig. 5.1, with permission.)

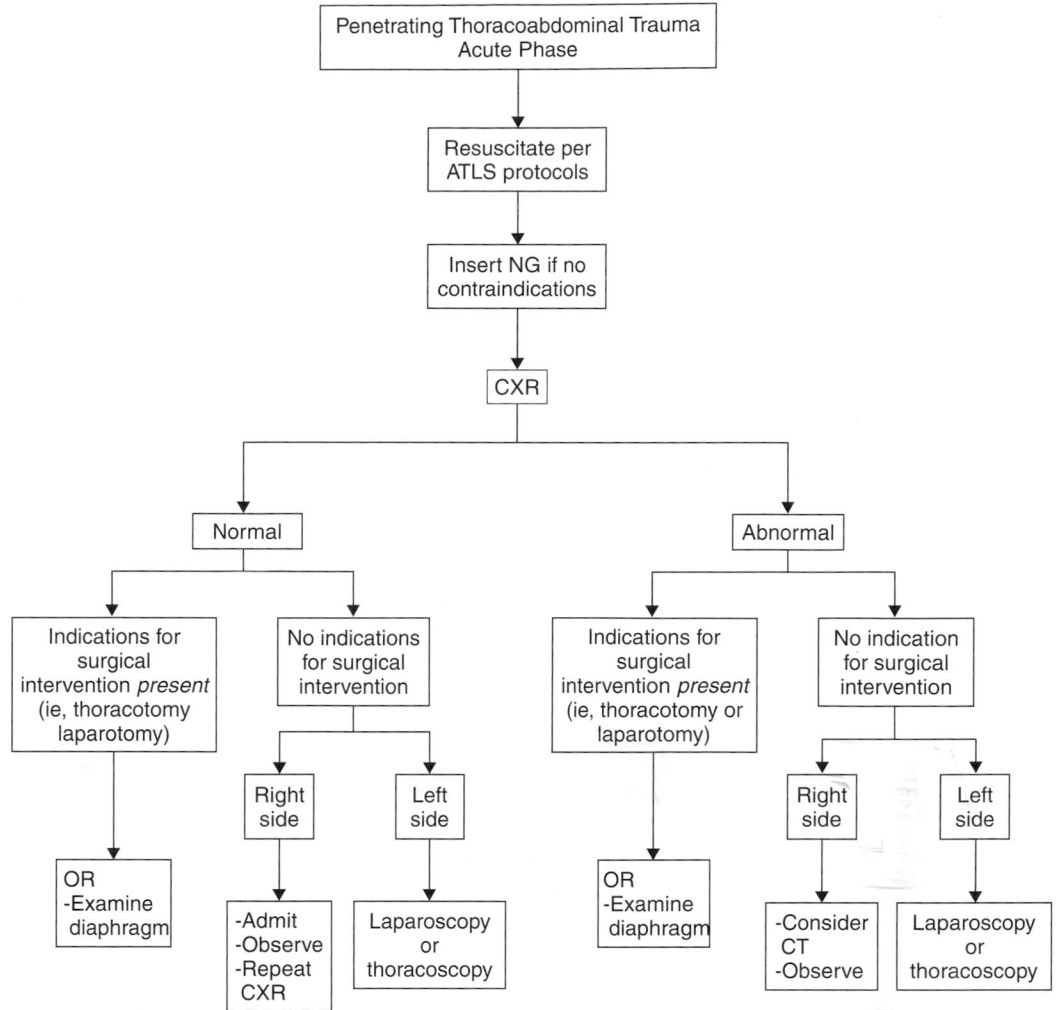

NG, nasogastric tube; OR, operating room.

Figure 183.2.   Algorithm for penetrating thoracoabdominal trauma. (From Asensio JA, Petrone P, Demetriades D. Injury to the diaphragm. In: Moore EE, Feliciano DV, Mattox KL (eds): *Trauma*, 5th ed, McGraw-Hill, New York, 2004, p. 629, Fig. 30.14, with permission.)

radiography findings. Of note, this algorithm favors thoracoscopy and laparotomy and does not rely on the diagnostic peritoneal lavage. It should be considered as one way of approaching this challenging diagnosis. A similar algorithm for the work up of diaphragm injury during the chronic phase (delayed presentation) suggests greater latitude in the diagnostic options (5) (Fig. 183.3).

EMERGENCY DEPARTMENT MANAGEMENT

There are several conditions that require treatment immediately after the primary survey in patients with penetrating chest trauma. These include respiratory failure, tension pneumothorax, cardiac tamponade, massive hemothorax, and open pneumothorax.

Intubation

Indications for intubation and ventilatory support in patients with penetrating chest trauma include: (1) hypoxia, tachypnea, bradypnea, apnea; (2) impaired ventilation in spite of an open airway; (3) shock; (4) multiple injuries; (5) coma; and (6) large hemopneumothorax. Other factors that may prompt the emergency physician to intubate early include preexisting pulmonary disease, a requirement for multiple transfusions, and elderly pa-

tients. In most cases, a standard rapid sequence intubation (RSI) technique is adequate.

Chest Decompression

A tension pneumothorax should be relieved immediately. The decompression should not be delayed while waiting for confirmatory radiographs. One of the most expeditious methods for relieving the tension involves placing a 12- or 14- gauge angiocatheter (catheter-over-needle) into the pleural space through the chest wall in either the 2nd intercostal space in the mid-clavicular line anteriorly or 4th or 5th intercostal space at the anterior axillary line. If a tension pneumothorax was present and the catheter enters the pleura, a rush of high-pressure air should be noted. Placing a catheter in this manner is merely temporizing; the patient requires a tube thoracostomy.

Tube Thoracostomy

Tube thoracostomy is the only invasive procedure that is required in approximately 85% of chest trauma patients. It is the definitive emergency department treatment for traumatic pneumothorax. A small (less than 15%) pneumothorax or an occult pneumothorax that is only identified on CT in a patient who will not undergo general anesthesia or receive positive-pressure ventilation may

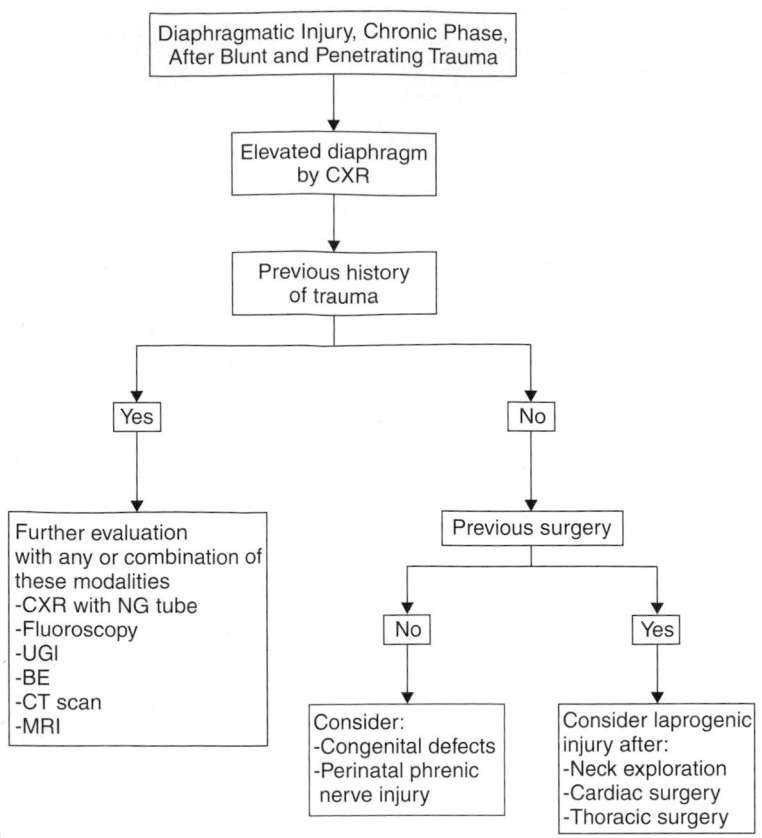

Figure 183.3. Algorithm for diaphragmatic injury, chronic phase, after blunt and penetrating trauma. (From Asensio JA, Petrone P, Demetriades D. Injury to the diaphragm. In Moore EE, Feliciano DV, Mattox KL (eds). *Trauma*, 5th ed, McGraw-Hill, New York, 2004, p. 631, Fig. 30.16, with permission.)

NG, nasogastric tube; UGI, upper gastrointestinal series; BE, barium enema.

be managed with observation while the pleural air collection spontaneously resorbs. If observation is selected, the physician must be prepared to immediately place a thoracostomy tube in the event of clinical deterioration. The preferred site of insertion for a chest tube is in the 4th or 5th intercostal space at the midaxillary line for two reasons: this location is usually safely above the diaphragm and it is the area of the chest wall where the musculature is the thinnest. The tube should be placed through a fresh incision made for this purpose; it should not be placed through a gunshot wound or stab wound hole because of an increased risk of infectious complications. If the chest tube is being placed for a pneumothorax alone (with minimal blood expected), a 20- or 22-French tube is adequate. There is a growing interest and experience in the use of "skinny" catheters or "pig-tail" catheters instead of conventional chest tubes for the drainage of simple pneumothoraces. These techniques appear to be safe and effective.

Great care must be exercised in placing chest tubes because as many as 26% are malpositioned (6). Further, the complication rate for tube thoracostomy is as high as 25%, including failure to drain the hemothorax or pneumothorax, posttube removal complications, empyema, improper placement with subsequent injuries to the lung or vessels (18). Prophylactic antibiotics reduce intrathoracic infection rates in patients sustaining isolated penetrating chest injuries requiring tube thoracostomy (the number needed to treat is six). The most appropriate regimen appears to be a 24-hour course of a first-generation cephalosporin (15).

Chest tubes are placed in the treatment of hemothorax for three reasons: to re-expand the lung and allow for proper ventilation, to stop intrathoracic bleeding by expanding the lung against the inner chest wall to tamponade bleeding vessels, and to monitor for ongoing blood loss. In the majority of cases, this is all that is necessary. However, an initial output of greater than 1.5 liters of blood, ongoing blood loss of greater than 250 ml/hr, or the

failure to drain a significant hemothorax (clotted or "caked" hemothorax) are indications for operative thoracotomy. Uncontaminated blood obtained from the intrapleural space with a cell-saver device can be reinfused into the hypovolemic trauma patient. A hemothorax may not be adequately drained with a small chest tube or catheter (as used for a simple pneumothorax). Many experts recommend thoracostomy tubes as large as 38- or 40-French for hemothoraces in adults.

Chest Wall Seal

An open pneumothorax in a spontaneously breathing patient should be sealed with an occlusive dressing, taped into place on three of the four sides. The reason to leave one side untaped is to have the dressing act as a one-way valve and allow an egress of air from the chest. If the patient deteriorates (and tension pneumothorax is suspected) or if the patient is subjected to positive pressure ventilation, the dressing should be removed immediately.

Pericardiocentesis

Pericardiocentesis is a temporizing procedure to reduce intrapericardial pressure as a prelude to thoracotomy. An indwelling pericardial catheter can be placed in the pericardial sac via a subxyphoid approach to allow for repeated aspirations while preparations are made for an expeditious thoracotomy. It is best to perform pericardiocentesis under ultrasound guidance, if available.

Resuscitative Thoracotomy

Resuscitative thoracotomy is a heroic procedure that can be lifesaving. There has been a good deal of research into determining a

TABLE 183.1. Predictors of Outcome and Rationale for
Selective Application of Emergency Department
Thoracotomy in Trauma

Parameter	SURVIVORS' NEUROLOGIC STATUS		
	Patients	Intact	Invalid
No SOL scene	177	1	2
No SOL ED			
Blunt	150	0	1
No cardiac activity	139	1	0
Penetrating	166	4	3
SBP <70 after aortic occlusion	180	0	0

ED, emergency department; SOL, signs of life; SBP, systolic blood
pressure

*From Cogbill TH, Moore EE, Millikan JS, et al. Rationale for selective
application of Emergency Department thoracotomy in trauma.* J Trauma
1983;23(6):453–460, with permission.

selective approach for thoracotomy, providing it only for patients who have a reasonable chance of survival. The best candidates for the procedure are victims of penetrating chest trauma from stab wounds who have vital signs in the prehospital setting and in the emergency department initially, who then lose their vital signs and receive a prompt resuscitative thoracotomy. In such patients, up to 37.5% survive neurologically intact (11). Even in patients suffering penetrating chest trauma caused by gunshot

wounds who have no vital signs in the field, there have been neurologically intact survivors after resuscitative thoracotomy, given rapid transportation and intervention (11). The key predictors of survival are the mechanism of injury, the location of the primary injury, and presence or absence of signs of life (SOL) at various times prior to thoracotomy (40).

The probability of neurologically intact survival following a resuscitative thoracotomy is correlated with the mechanism of injury (penetrating or blunt), the presence or absence of electrical cardiac activity, and signs of life (8) (Table 183.1). A decision algorithm for the selective use of resuscitative thoracotomy should take these factors into account in determining potential candidates with a chance of neurologic survival (9) (Fig. 183.4).

Several life sustaining procedures can be performed during the resuscitative thoracotomy. These include internal (open chest) CPR, which produces a greater cardiac output and coronary perfusion pressure than closed chest CPR. By performing a pericardiotomy as part of the procedure, pericardial tamponade is decompressed and the heart can be inspected for wounds and for filling. Wounds to the heart, great vessels, and lungs may be controlled directly, thereby limiting blood loss, tamponade, and air embolism. The majority of heart wounds can be controlled with digital pressure. Definitive repair can then be attempted in the emergency department or in the operating room. Several techniques for repair have been described including repair with pledgeted sutures (to keep the suture material from pulling out through the cardiac muscle fibers) and repair with skin staples.

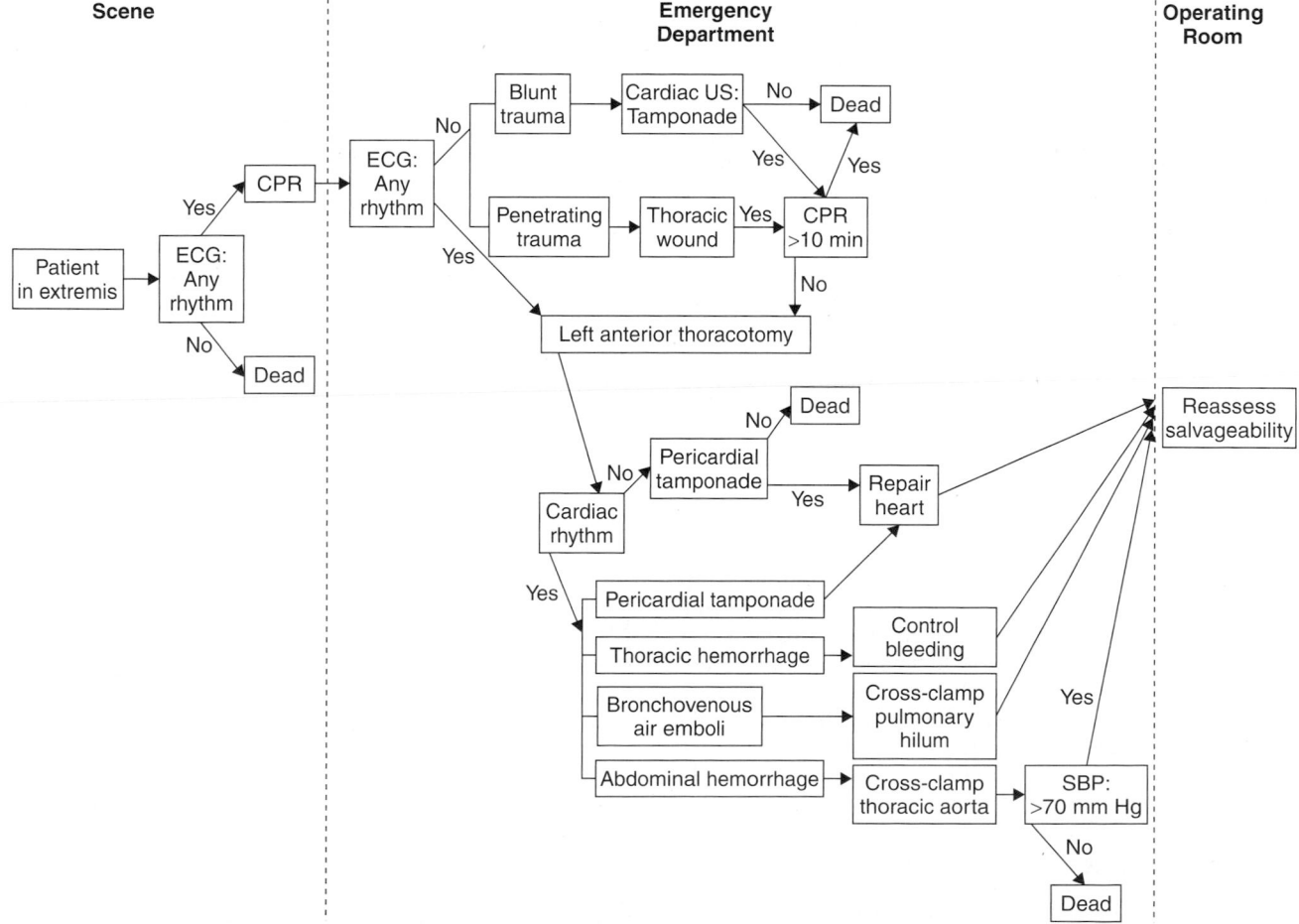

Figure 183.4. Decision algorithm for the selective use of resuscitative thoracotomy in the emergency department. (From Biffl WL, Moore EE, Johnson JJ. Emergency Department Thoracotomy. In: Moore EE, Feliciano DV, Mattox KL (eds). *Trauma*, 5th ed, McGraw-Hill, New York, 2004, p. 249, Fig. 14.7, with permission.)

A Foley catheter can be used to control a heart wound. Wounds amenable to this technique are small stab wounds and small gunshot wounds that are not close to a coronary artery or the inflow or outflow tracks of the cardiac chamber (to avoid interrupting cardiac output or coronary circulation when the Foley balloon is inflated). The tip of the Foley is placed into the chamber of the heart through the wound. A clamp is applied to the drainage tube end of the Foley and the balloon is inflated with saline. The physician can then apply traction to the Foley to create a seal between the balloon and the inner wall of the heart. With the Foley in place, a purse-string suture is placed around the wound. In a coordinated movement, the Foley balloon is deflated, the Foley catheter is removed, and the purse-string suture is tightened and tied.

The aorta can be cross-clamped, limiting distal hemorrhage and increasing afterload. Similarly, the hilum of an injured lung can be clamped reducing hemorrhage and the risk of air embolism. Intracardiac resuscitation drugs can be administered. There is probably no advantage and greater risk to delivering resuscitation drugs in this manner over a central venous catheter. However, the intracardiac route is preferred over a peripheral IV site in the setting of traumatic cardiac arrest. Lastly, the heart can be cardioverted or defibrillated directly during the thoracotomy.

The decision to provide a resuscitative thoracotomy for selected trauma patients implies an institutional commitment of trained personnel, facilities, and resources. Without that commitment, even the best candidate for the procedure will not benefit.

Cardiac Injuries

Cardiac wounds in patients with a degree of hemodynamic stability are best managed in the operating room. In patients with suspected tamponade, pericardiocentesis may buy some time by stabilizing the patient before surgery. However, false-negative taps can be misleading; they occur because pericardial blood is often clotted. Thus, pericardiocentesis is better as a therapeutic rather than a diagnostic tool. Surgical therapy should not be delayed with repeated attempts at pericardiocentesis.

External CPR in the victim of arrest from cardiac trauma is likely to be ineffective. Patients with penetrating trauma to the chest that have a rapidly deteriorating clinical course, uncontrolled hemorrhage, or cardiac arrest may benefit from a resuscitative thoracotomy in the emergency department. Since only 10% of penetrating cardiac trauma patients require extracorporeal bypass, it is typically not necessary to transfer cardiac trauma patients away from otherwise equipped trauma centers (14).

Diaphragmatic Injuries

The definitive treatment of diaphragmatic injuries is repair in the operating room. However, tension gastrothorax is an immediately life-threatening emergency that should be addressed in the proper sequence. Chest tube placement can have a paradoxical effect by decompressing the chest and allowing more of the abdominal contents to herniate through the rent in the diaphragm. In order to avoid that complication, these patients are typically intubated first. After intubation, a nasogastric or orogastric tube is placed and connected to suction to decompress the stomach. Then tube thoracostomy is performed.

Great Vessel Injuries

As with cardiac wounds, patients with suspected great vessel injuries and a degree of hemodynamic stability are best managed in the operating room. Large bore lower extremity intravenous lines are indicated when major injuries to the major thoracic venous branches are suspected. There are great controversies surrounding volume resuscitation in patients with an uncontrolled major vascular injury. Some experts believe that a degree of hypotension may be protective by compensatorily serving to reduce bleeding (7). Aggressive fluid resuscitation may be counterproductive until the hemorrhaging vessel can be controlled. Patients with penetrating trauma to the chest that have a rapidly deteriorating clinical course, uncontrolled hemorrhage, or cardiac arrest may benefit from a resuscitative thoracotomy in the emergency department and control of a great vessel hemorrhage prior to definitive repair in the operating room.

Tracheobronchial Injuries

Small penetrating wounds to the tracheobronchial tree may be treated effectively with endotracheal intubation and tube thoracostomy. Larger injuries require operative repair.

Esophageal Injuries

The decision to repair an esophageal perforation is a surgical one based on adequate diagnostic studies. The initiation of antibiotic therapy is indicated early. The antibiotic regimen chosen should be broad in spectrum and should include anaerobic coverage.

Venous Air Embolism

The treatment of venous air embolism involves prohibiting the accumulation of additional air in the venous tree, removal of a portion of the air that is present, and reducing the effects of the air that cannot be removed. Prohibiting the accumulation of additional air in the venous tree may involve cross-clamping the hilum of an injured lung to control bronchovenous communication and maintaining perfusion pressures (49). In addition, patients with suspected venous air embolism should be promptly treated with 100% oxygen in order to facilitate nitrogen washout. Removal of a portion of the air that is present in the vascular system may involve the use of the Trendelenberg position in an attempt to trap the venous bubbles in the apex of the right ventricle followed by aggressive aspiration of the frothy venous blood via a large central venous catheter. Such patients may also benefit from hyperbaric oxygen therapy (HBO), however, facilities for HBO in a multiplace chamber in which the patient's trauma can be assessed and treated by a team working in the hyperbaric environment may not be readily available. Cardiopulmonary bypass has been used with anecdotal success in treating patients with venous air embolism (39). The use of steroids and antiplatelet drugs for the treatment of traumatic venous air embolism has not been proven.

CRITICAL INTERVENTIONS

- Completely undress the patient and examine the entire body (including the back, buttocks, and axilla) to search for other injuries. Even minor-appearing exterior wounds (such as from an ice pick) can cause serious cardiac wounds
- Perform tube thoracostomy on any patient with clinical evidence of pneumothorax without waiting for confirmatory radiographs
- Perform tube thoracostomy in a patient with a small pneumothorax who will undergo positive-pressure ventilation or transfer in an aircraft
- Perform an emergency department thoracotomy on any patient with a chest stab wound who loses vital signs enroute to the ED or in the ED

DISPOSITION

Discharge after a limited observation period (6 hours) is safe and cost-effective in asymptomatic patients with stab wounds to the chest in whom serial inspiratory and expiratory chest x-rays are negative (13). Patients presenting with asymptomatic isolated stab wounds of the chest should undergo observation and repeat chest x-rays after six to eight hours. Patients with persistently negative chest x-rays and absence of symptoms may be discharged with outpatient follow up after 2 days. Patients with small but nonprogressive pneumothoraces should be observed for 48 hours (37). Although a very rare patient with a small pneumothorax may be discharged with a drainage device (such as a pigtail catheter or Heimlich valve) after a period of observation in the ED, the vast majority should be admitted. All patients with penetrating chest trauma resulting in hemothorax should be admitted.

All patients with penetrating chest trauma resulting in tracheobronchial injuries should be admitted. Many of them will require diagnostic studies and operative intervention. All patients with penetrating chest trauma resulting in diaphragm injuries should be admitted. Nearly all require operative intervention.

Patients with penetrating chest trauma resulting in heart or great vessel injuries require operative intervention. However, cardiopulmonary bypass is rarely necessary (47).

Patients with confirmed esophageal perforation require admission. Suspicion of the injury is sufficient for admission for further evaluation because there may be as much as a twofold increase in mortality when the diagnosis is delayed beyond 24 hours. Nearly all patients with thoracic esophageal perforation require operative intervention.

COMMON PITFALLS

✔ Delaying early intubation or tube thoracostomy
✔ Attempting to probe chest wounds
✔ Waiting for radiographic confirmation of tension pneumothorax before performing tube thoracostomy in patients with unilateral diminished breath sounds and shock
✔ Failure to place a tube thoracostomy after performing needle decompression
✔ Failure to insert a finger to ensure that the tube will not be placed through the lung, diaphragm, liver, or spleen when inserting a chest tube
✔ Failure to consider that all patients with penetrating trauma below the scapula tips posteriorly or nipple level anteriorly are at high risk for diaphragmatic perforation
✔ Failure to follow a negative water-soluble contrast study with the more sensitive barium swallow, when evaluating for an esophageal injury. When the suspicion for esophageal injury is high, esophagoscopy should be performed if contrast studies are negative

Acknowledgments

Some material is based on the previous edition's chapters written by C. Keith Stone, Ron Forrest Koury, Daniel S. Gabbay, Patrick M. Reilly, Vincent J. Markovchick, Joanne Edney, Brian Tiffany, and Robert C. Jorden.

References

1. Adegboye VO, Ladipo JK, Adebo OA, Brimmo AI. Diaphragmatic injuries. *Afr J Med Med Sci.* 2002;31:149–153.
2. Adegboye VO, Ladipo JK, Brimmo IA, Adebo AO. Penetrating chest injuries in civilian practice. *Afr J Med Med Sci.* 2001;30:327–331.
3. Aitken RJ, Immelman EJ. Traumatic diaphragmatic hernias—pitfalls in the barium meal. *Injury* 1986;17:224–225.
4. Asensio JA, Petrone P, Demetriades D. Injury to the diaphragm. In: Moore EE, Feliciano DV, Mattox KL (eds): *Trauma,* 5th ed, McGraw-Hill, New York, 2004:629.
5. Asensio JA, Petrone P, Demetriades D. Injury to the diaphragm. In: Moore EE, Feliciano DV, Mattox KL (eds): *Trauma,* 5th ed, McGraw-Hill, New York, 2004: 631.
6. Baldt M, Bankier A, Germann P, et al. Complications after emergency tube thoracostomy: Assessment with CT. *Radiology.* 1995;195:539–543.
7. Bickell WH, Wall MJ, Pepe PE, et al. Immediate versus delayed fluid resuscitation for hypotensive patients with penetrating torso injuries. *N Engl J Med* 1994;331:1105–1109.
8. Biffl WL, Moore EE, Johnson JJ. Emergency department thoracotomy. In: Moore EE, Feliciano DV, Mattox KL (eds): *Trauma,* 5th ed, McGraw-Hill, New York, 2004: 248.
9. Biffl WL, Moore EE, Johnson JJ. Emergency department thoracotomy. In: Moore EE, Feliciano DV, Mattox KL (eds): *Trauma,* 5th ed, McGraw-Hill, New York, 2004: 249.
10. Bokhari F, Brakenridge S, Nagy K, Roberts R, Smith R, Joseph K, An G, Wiley D, Barrett J. Prospective evaluation of the sensitivity of physical examination in chest trauma. *J Trauma* 2002;53:1135–1138.
11. Branney SW, Moore EE, Feldhaus KM, et al. Critical analysis of two decades of experience with postinjury resuscitative thoracotomy in a regional trauma center. *J Trauma* 1998;45:87–94.
12. Brooks A, Davies B, Smethhurst M, Connolly J. Emergency ultrasound in the acute assessment of haemothorax. *Emerg Med J* 2004;21:44–46.
13. Brown PF 3rd, Larsen CP, Symbas PN. Management of the asymptomatic patient with a stab wound to the chest. *South Med J* 1991;84:591–593.
14. Buchman TG, Phillips J, Menker JB. Recognition, resuscitation and management of patients with penetrating cardiac injuries. *Surg Gynecol Obstet* 1992;174: 205–210.
15. Butler J. Antibiotics in patients with isolated chest trauma requiring chest drains. *J Accid Emerg Med* 2002;19:553.
16. Campbell NC, Thomson SR, Muckart DJ, et al. Review of 1198 cases of penetrating cardiac trauma. *Br J Surg* 1997;84:1737–1740.
17. Demetriades D. Penetrating injuries to thoracic great vessels. *J Card Surg* 1997;12:173–180.
18. Deneuville M. Morbidity of percutaneous tube thoracostomy in trauma patients. *Eur J Cardiothorac Surg.* 2002;22:673–678.
19. Gurney J, Harrison WL, Anderson JC. Omental fat stimulating pleural fluid in traumatic diaphragmatic hernia: CT characteristics. *J Comput Assist Tomogr* 1985;9:1112.
20. Horwitz B, Krevsky B, Buckman RF Jr, Fisher RS, Dabezies MA. Endoscopic evaluation of penetrating esophageal injuries. *Am J Gastroenterol.* 1993;88:1249–1253.
21. Jimenez E, Martin M, Krukenkamp I, Barrett J. Subxiphoid pericardiotomy versus echocardiography: a prospective evaluation of the diagnosis of occult penetrating cardiac injury. *Surgery.* 1990;108:676–679, 680.
22. Jones WG 2nd, Ginsberg RJ. Esophageal perforation: a continuing challenge. *Ann Thorac Surg* 1992;53:534–543.
23. Kiev J, Kerstein MD. Role of three hour roentgenogram of the chest in penetrating and nonpenetrating injuries of the chest. *Surg Gynecol Obstet.* 1992;175:249–253.
24. Kim HH, Shin YR. Blunt traumatic rupture of the diaphragm. *J Ultrasound Med* 1997;16:593–598.
25. Kiss SS, Toth P, Kollar S, Nabradi Z, Boni J. Five-year study on the injury of the great thoracic vessels after penetrating chest injury. *Acta Chir Hung* 1999;38:75–78.
26. Mattox KL, Feliciano DV, Burch J, et al. Five thousand seven hundred sixty cardiovascular injuries in 4459 patients. Epidemiologic evolution 1958 to 1987. *Ann Surg* 1989;209:698–705; discussion 706–7.
27. McHugh K, Ogilvie BC, Brunton FJ. Delayed presentation of traumatic diaphragmatic hernia. *Clin Radiol.* 1991;43:246–250.
28. McQuay N Jr, Britt LD. Laparoscopy in the evaluation of penetrating thoracoabdominal trauma. *Am Surg.* 2003;69:788–791.
29. Meyer DM, Jessen ME, Grayburn PA. Use of echocardiography to detect occult cardiac injury after penetrating thoracic trauma: a prospective study. *J Trauma* 1995;39:902–909.
30. Moore JB, Moore EE, Thompson JS. Abdominal injuries associated with penetrating lower chest trauma. *Am J Surg.* 1980;140:724–730.
31. Morgan AS, Flancbaum L, Esposito T, Cox EF. Blunt injury to the diaphragm: an analysis of 44 patients. *Trauma.* 1986;26:565–568.
32. Murray JA, Demetriades D, Arsensio JA, et al. Occult injuries to the diaphragm: Prospective evaluation of laparoscopy in penetrating injuries to the lower left chest. *JACS* 1998;187:626–630.
33. Murray JA, Demetriades D, Cornwell EE, et al. Penetrating left thoracoabdominal trauma: The incidence and clinical presentation of diaphragm injuries. *J Trauma* 1997;43:824.
34. Nagy KK, Gilkey SH, Roberts RR, Fildes JJ, Barrett J. Computed Tomography Screens Stable Patients at Risk for Penetrating Cardiac Injury. *Acad Emerg Med* 1996;3:1024–1027.
35. Nesbitt JC, Sawyers JL. Surgical management of esophageal perforations. *Am Surg.* 1987;53:183–191.
36. Oh, KS, Fleischner FG, Wyman SM. Characteristic pulmonary finding in traumatic complete transection of a main-stem bronchus. *Radiology* 1969;92:371–372.

37. Ordog GJ, Wasserberger J, Balasubramanium S, Shoemaker W. Asymptomatic stab wounds of the chest. *J Trauma*. 1994;36:680–684.

38. Plummer D, Brunette D, Asinger R, Ruiz E. Emergency department echocardiography improves outcome in penetrating cardiac injury. *Ann Emerg Med* 1992;21:709–712.

39. Rawlins R, Momin A, Platts D, El Gamel A. Traumatic cardiogenic shock due to massive air embolism. A possible role for cardiopulmonary bypass. *Eur J Cardiothorac Surg* 2002;22:845–846.

40. Rhee PM, Acosta J, Bridgeman A, et al. Survival after emergency department thoracotomy: review of published data from the past 25 years. *J Am Coll Surg* 2000;190:288–298.

41. Rodriguez-Morales G, Rodriguez A, Shatney CH. Acute rupture of the diaphragm in blunt trauma: analysis of 60 patients. *J Trauma* 1986;26:438–444.

42. Rozycki GS, Feliciano DV, Ochsner MG, et al. The role of ultrasound in patients with possible penetrating cardiac wounds: a prospective multicenter study. *J Trauma* 1999;46:543–551.

43. Shatz DV, de la Pedraja J, Erbella J, Hameed M, Vail SJ. Efficacy of follow-up evaluation in penetrating thoracic injuries: 3-vs. 6-hour radiographs of the chest. *J Emerg Med* 2001;20:281–284.

44. Sisley AC, Rozycki GS, Ballard RB, et al. Rapid detection of traumatic effusion using surgeon-performed ultrasonography. *J Trauma* 1998;44:291–297.

45. Tanomkiat W, Galassi W. Barium sulfate as contrast medium for evaluation of postoperative anastomotic leaks. *Acta Radiol* 2000;41:482–485.

46. Tayal VS, Moore CL, Rose GA, et al. (eds). Emergency Ultrasound, New York, McGraw-Hill, 2003:93.

47. Wall MJ, Mattox KL, Chen C, Baldwin JC. Acute management of complex cardiac injuries. *J Trauma* 1997;42:905–912.

48. White RK, Morris DM. Diagnosis and management of esophageal perforations. *Am Surg* 1992;58:112–119.

49. Yee ES, Verrier ED, Thomas AN. Management of air embolism in blunt and penetrating thoracic trauma. *J Thorac Cardiovasc Surg* 1983;85:661–668.

CHAPTER 184
Blunt Abdominal Trauma

Eric L. Legome and William Goldberg

Blunt abdominal trauma (BAT) accounts for a minority of all traumatic deaths, but represents an important source of morbidity. The variety of clinical presentations, limitations of the physical examination, and the absence of consistent clinical markers make patients with blunt abdominal trauma a particularly challenging population. Death due to abdominal injury may be prevented by early recognition of intraabdominal hemorrhage. After initial resuscitation, one of the primary objectives of the emergency physician is to decide which patients require early surgical intervention and obtain timely surgical consultation. Although injuries to solid organs are most frequently involved after BAT, the clinician must also search for the more subtle injuries to the bowel, mesentery, and pancreas. The history and physical examination continue to be essential components of the evaluation; the addition of the *focused assessment with sonography for trauma* (FAST) and abdominal computed tomography (CT) scanning has significantly enhanced the emergency physician's diagnostic ability and therapeutic approach.

CLINICAL PRESENTATION

The signs and symptoms of blunt abdominal trauma are highly variable and the assessment is often complicated by the presence of multiple other injuries. While historical factors and physical findings may offer insight into the likelihood of intraabdominal injury, neither are highly sensitive or specific (66,70). The initial assessment may be unreliable due to altered sensorium from head injury, medications, substance abuse, multisystem trauma, distracting injuries, spinal cord injuries, or shock.

Although hypotension in the field or on arrival increases the likelihood of severe bleeding, vital signs may be normal upon presentation to the ED. Injuries that produce minimal bleeding, such as bowel or diaphragm perforation, and those isolated to the retroperitoneum, typically result in a paucity of physical findings.

DIFFERENTIAL DIAGNOSIS

The differential diagnosis of injury in blunt abdominal trauma includes both intraabdominal and extraabdominal etiologies. The most common intraabdominal concerns are the solid organ injuries (i.e., the spleen or liver). Next are the hollow viscous structures, or the small and large bowel. These comprise only about 5% to 10% of intraabdominal injuries. The gallbladder, pancreas or vascular structures may also be injured, although these injuries are infrequent and found in combination with hollow or solid viscous injuries. Occasionally there is an isolated injury to the bowel mesentery.

In addition to these intraabdominal injuries, there may be extraabdominal findings that mimic intraabdominal injury. These include muscle strains, contusions or rectus sheath hematomas. Muscle injuries tend to cause pain mainly over the involved muscular area, do not lead to hemodynamic instability, and the pain may intensify when palpation is performed on the contracted muscle. However, the ability of these findings to exclude an intraabdominal injury has never been proven useful.

EMERGENCY DEPARTMENT EVALUATION

The assessment of the blunt trauma patient must be performed within the context of the patient's hemodynamic status and potential for life- or limb-threatening injuries. The ABCs of resuscitation are rapidly performed on arrival, and the patient should be fully unclothed. The secondary survey, including the abdominal examination, should proceed only after the primary survey is complete. In general, the more critically injured the patient, the faster the emergency physician must determine the need for laparotomy, blood transfusion or angiography and obtain early surgical consultation.

History

A brief initial history is obtained upon arrival. One common approach is the AMPLE format (allergies, medications, past medical history, last meal, and events surrounding the injury). In addition, the patient should be questioned about pain in the abdomen or other areas. Obtaining the history also allows the EP to judge the mental status of the patient.

In addition to the patient, valuable sources of information are the prehospital care providers and witnesses or passengers who may arrive with the patient. After a description of the mechanism and events of the injury, most paramedic reports indicate mental status changes, vital signs, evaluation of the ABCs, interventions, and significant complaints. Certain historical factors, such as prehospital vital signs and mechanism of injury, have classically been associated with a greater chance of serious injury. Recent reports however, have shown mechanism alone to be poorly predictive of the need for operative intervention or advanced therapeutic maneuvers (2,24,27,35,42,48). A history of prehospital hypotension, significant fluid resuscitation or declining mental status must be taken very seriously (27,59).

Physical Examination

Despite the necessity of a well-directed physical examination, the EP must be aware of its limitations. The physical examination is not sensitive enough to diagnose all patients with operative intraabdominal injuries, nor is it specific enough to rule in an injury, even in patients with guarding and rigidity. The literature has cited a wide variability in the physical examination. For example, one study found the examination to be 65% accurate in the setting of BAT, while another trauma center reported abdominal examination alone as adequate in 35% of patients (36,52,64,66,70). While not well stratified in the literature, the physical examination alone is probably adequate in the minimally injured patient with a normal mental status and benign physical findings without significant extraabdominal injuries.

To perform the physical examination, the patient should be completely undressed and life threats addressed first. Concomitant evaluation and therapeutic interventions of the airway, breathing and circulation are first priority. The abdominal examination should begin with inspection for abrasions or ecchymosis. Ecchymosis over the lower abdomen in a lapbelt distribution is suspicious for hollow viscus injury and vertebral fractures (11,76). Although Cullen's sign (ecchymosis around the umbilicus) and Turner's sign (ecchymosis of the flanks) are associated with retroperitoneal bleeding, they are highly insensitive and often take hours to manifest. Auscultation for bowel sounds has not been formally studied, but probably has no utility in the initial examination.

Palpation of the abdomen begins with examination of the lower chest. Lower rib fractures, especially with high-energy trauma, are associated with a significant rate of associated intraabdominal injury. The abdomen should be carefully palpated, paying particular attention to the right and left upper quadrants. The finding of Kehr's sign (pain in the shoulder unrelated to shoulder tenderness or range of motion) indicates the presence of blood irritating the diaphragm and is often secondary to splenic or liver injury (52,61,66,70).

Pelvic stability is assessed by applying distraction and compression forces over the iliac crest and over the symphysis pubis. Care should be taken not to use excessive force to avoid disrupting an unstable fracture and increasing bleeding. Patients with pelvic fractures have a significant incidence of intraabdominal injury, ranging from over 30% to greater than 50% in those with severe or unstable fractures (20,65).

Rectal examination is rarely useful in seriously injured patients with pelvic fractures or concern for gastrointestinal disruption. It may demonstrate a high-riding or boggy prostate in patients with urethral disruption. Gross blood on rectal examination may indicate gastrointestinal rupture and mandates surgical consultation. Stool evaluation for occult blood has not been shown to be predictive of traumatic injury (62). The external genitalia should be inspected for blood at the meatus, scrotal hematoma, or urethral outlet bleeding, which may signify a bladder or urethral injury. The patient should then be log-rolled with palpation of the lumbar and thoracic area. Lumbar fractures, particularly those in conjunction with the seatbelt sign, are markers of hollow viscus injury.

Plain Radiographs

The plain abdominal radiograph has no utility in the evaluation of blunt abdominal trauma. Although it has been used in the past, it rarely contributed to operative decision-making. It is not reliable in diagnosing intraabdominal pathology, and therapeutic interventions should not be made on the basis of the results. A chest radiograph should be performed to assist in evaluating the aorta, lungs and rib cage. It may show evidence of a ruptured diaphragm in anywhere from 20% to 80% of patients with this injury (12,30,38,72). Pelvic films should be obtained based on the reliability of the examination and on physical findings. The current evidence shows that in the stable and alert blunt trauma patient without distracting injuries, a normal clinical examination can rule out a clinically important pelvic fracture (23,31,33,43).

Laboratory Tests

Laboratory analysis of most trauma patients is generally more extensive than necessary. It rarely offers insight into diagnosing an occult injury. While laboratory testing based on clinical parameters is cost-effective without compromising care, most trauma centers use some type of protocol in order to standardize and speed the laboratory evaluation of patients (14,39). The patient who is fully awake, alert, has sustained minimal trauma and has no distracting injury may require no testing. Rational laboratory analysis in most patients with blunt abdominal trauma can be limited to a complete blood count, basic electrolytes, blood type and screen and urinalysis. Women of child-bearing age should have a pregnancy test performed.

The hematocrit level is influenced by many factors, including the rate of blood loss, dilutional effects of intravenous fluids, fluid shifts from the interstitium to the intravascular space, and preinjury level. While an initial low hemoglobin < 8 gm/dl may be useful to prognosticate major injury and outcome (41), the main value is as a baseline blood count. Leukocytosis may be present, but is a nonspecific finding. Baseline chemistries provide information regarding blood glucose, creatinine and evidence of acidosis. Gross hematuria is significant and should prompt evaluation of the genitourinary tract. Microscopic hematuria is poorly sensitive or specific for significant genitourinary (GU) injury, and in the absence of a pelvic fracture or unexplained hypotension, does not mandate workup (22).

Other studies to consider, mostly for the severely injured patient or elderly patient, include liver function studies, coagulation profiles, arterial blood gas, and alcohol and drug screening. Liver function enzymes that are significantly elevated to two to three time normal may represent hepatic injury, although it is unclear how much they add to objective radiologic testing based on mechanism and physical examination (68,74). Coagulation studies are useful in anti-coagulated patients, those with a history or stigmata of liver disease, pregnant patients, or with the possibility of disseminated intravascular coagulation due to shock.

Analysis of the arterial blood gas, specifically for the base deficit, may provide diagnostic and prognostic information in the major trauma patient. Those patients with deficits less than −6 (i.e., −7 or greater) have an increased risk of intraabdominal hemorrhage. Serial base deficits or serial lactates indicate trends in patient status. Monitoring the deficit for improvement or normalization helps discern whether ongoing resuscitation is effective. The failure to normalize a base deficit by several hours predicted a significantly greater morbidity and mortality in one study (17,18).

Serum amylase and lipase are insensitive and nonspecific for pancreatic injury. One study showed that 53% of blunt abdominal trauma patients had at least one elevation during an initial or subsequent measurement, yet less than 2% had a pancreatic injury. Other studies have confirmed the lack of utility of a screening amylase or lipase in the blunt trauma patient (10,57).

Ethanol levels and drug screens may provide additional information about the reliability of the physical examination.

Diagnostic Peritoneal Lavage

Diagnostic peritoneal lavage (DPL), introduced in 1965 by Root et al, is a rapid and accurate test for determining the existence of intraperitoneal blood. Although it is invasive, DPL has a low (< 1%) complication rate of bleeding, perforation or infection. (5,19,29). Once part of the standard evaluation of blunt abdominal trauma patient, it has been replaced by CT scan in the stable patient. In the hemodynamically unstable patient, ultrasound has replaced DPL in many trauma centers. DPL is still recommended in the unstable patient with an unclear ultrasound result or in the stable patient with a significant concern for a hollow viscous or mesenteric injury, either by examination or after an equivocal CT scan. DPL also plays a major role when CT scan and ultrasound are unavailable (36).

The two main techniques are open and closed. The *closed* technique is faster and is not associated with a significant increase in complication rate. The *open* technique relies on direct visualization and incision of the peritoneum, while the closed technique is performed using the Seldinger technique after skin incision. While generally performed in the infraumbilical area, a supraumbilical approach should be performed in patients with pelvic fractures, previous surgical scars, and in the pregnant patient (16,19,37,44). In some cases, a *semi-open* technique may be performed. With this technique, the skin, and sometimes the fascia, is incised and the catheter (placed over a trocar) is inserted blindly into the peritoneal cavity. Most centers perform the open or closed technique. The sensitivity and specificity of DPL for intraabdominal blood are both in the 95% to 99% range, with accuracy ranging between 92% and 98%. The specificity of DPL for predicting the need for a therapeutic laparotomy is somewhat lower and it should be interpreted in light of the overall clinical picture. A positive DPL in a hemodynamically stable patient should not automatically lead to laparotomy. It had previously been estimated that up to 30% of grossly positive lavages lead to nontherapeutic laparotomies (29). With the advances in nonoperative management of solid organ injuries, this number is probably even higher. The lavage is insensitive for retroperitoneal injuries involving the duodenum or parts of the colon, is not specific for site and extent of injury and may diagnose injuries that do not require operative intervention. The only absolute contraindication for DPL is the need for emergency laparotomy.

Criteria for a positive test after blunt trauma include an initial aspirate of more than 10 mL of blood (grossly positive lavage) or greater than 100,000 RBC/mm^3 in the lavage fluid. Patients with a grossly positive lavage (initial aspiration of 10 mL of blood) who are unstable should undergo immediate laparotomy. If less than 10 mL is aspirated, then this amount of blood should be added back into the peritoneal cavity and counted toward the final lavage fluid red blood cell determination. Those patients with RBC counts between 25,000 and 100,000 RBC/mm^3 should undergo CT scan. Patients with counts greater than 100,000 RBC/mm^3 should be seriously considered for CT scanning if they remain hemodynamically stable. Other lavage criteria based on the leukocytes count and amylase are less sensitive and more controversial and should be interpreted in light of the clinical exam. Gross bile or fecal material should be considered a positive lavage.

Computed Tomography

Computed tomography (CT) scan of the abdomen and pelvis has become the best method for radiographic evaluation of the hemodynamically stable patient. Initially, generalized adoption of this modality over DPL was slow as it was more costly, time consuming and in an often remote location from ED. Newer generation scanners, commonly found within or adjacent to the ED, have made it a quicker, cheaper and safer test to obtain. Improvements in technology have led to less artifact, lower radiation and higher accuracy. Due to limitations in the physical examination of the trauma patient, almost all except the minimally injured patient will require some sort of diagnostic test or prolonged observation. The CT offers the ability to perform, in a relatively rapid fashion, a quantitative and qualitative diagnostic test (8,36,60,63).

Abdominal CT after blunt trauma is indicated in patients with an unreliable physical examination. This includes patients with altered sensorium, spinal cord trauma, distracting injuries, or when general anesthesia is planned for another injury. CT also evaluates for suspected retroperitoneal, small bowel, renal or pancreatic injury. It also provides excellent visualization of pelvic fractures. Helical CT scanners may also reveal pneumothorax or hemothorax and fractures missed on initial plain radiograph. The newest generation CT scanner, the multidetector CT (MDCT), allows for greatly enhanced image reconstructions with thinner slices, higher spatial resolution and increased speed. Artifacts caused by motion, respiration and pulsations are significantly decreased.

Multidetector CT images more anatomic area as the IV contrast material goes through the body, resulting in better detail of structures. Thus, because of the greater anatomic coverage during optimal IV contrast material opacification, vascular structures and parenchymal organs are imaged more effectively and the ability to construct 3D reformations is greatly enhanced (26,73,78). For example, instead of visualizing a lumbar fracture and then returning to perform dedicated views, the MDCT allows for small slice accurate reformations with the original data. This clinically translates into less time, less radiation and possibly fewer films. An approach some trauma centers are now using is to perform a CT from head to pelvis. While seemingly cost prohibitive, it may actually be less expensive given that the extra time to perform the scan takes minutes, there is no increased use of film when images are stored on a picture archival retrieval system (PACS), and scans of the bones can be included, obviating the need for plain films.

An ongoing controversy regarding abdominal CT is the need for oral contrast medium to opacify the bowel. Although the major disadvantages (the delay to scan and possibility of aspiration) are very small, it remains unclear exactly how much it contributes to care. It can assist in diagnosing bowel and pancreatic injury, although the incidence of injury to these structures is low. Extravasated contrast is a pathognomonic finding; however, it has a low sensitivity. Contrast improves the ability to see bowel wall thickening, although most patients with this finding alone do not need intervention. Several retrospective reviews and case series have led to mixed conclusions and it remains an institutional judgment at this point (15,25,58,77). Given its limited assistance, if oral contrast is administered, CT should not be delayed while waiting for passage of the contrast material, unless there is a strong suspicion for bowel or pancreatic injury and the patient is stable.

Aside from the limitation of having to move an unstable patient out of the trauma room in order to perform the CT, the other major limitation of abdominal CT scan is the decreased sensitivity for bowel, mesenteric and pancreatic injury. Hollow viscous injury has historically been one of the most elusive diagnoses to make by CT in trauma. It is found in approximately 1% to 5% of patients with significant blunt abdominal trauma and may be higher with certain mechanisms such as a seat belt injury. Well described findings of bowel injury on CT help determine the need for surgical intervention versus observation. Air, extravasated contrast, active mesenteric bleeding or bowel injury with mesenteric hematoma are indications for surgical intervention. Unfortunately, these are relatively insensitive and rare findings. The significance of isolated free intraperitoneal fluid is much more controversial; several studies have found a high likelihood of bowel or mesenteric injury and others document a low likelihood (9,46). Findings such as mesenteric infiltration or hematoma or bowel thickening are often seen in patients with less serious lesions; these patients may be safely observed. In the past reported sensitivities for diagnosing bowel injury with CT were as low as 41%. Helical CT has been noted to have improved accuracy, with sensitivities above 90%, however, the actual numbers of injuries are small in the published studies. The newer scanners have improved resolution and should provide better diagnostic acumen (25,26,40,61).

Pancreatic injury remains a difficult diagnosis. As discussed earlier, elevations of amylase or lipase are neither sensitive nor specific for detecting this injury. While the incidence of pancreatic injury in BAT patients is less than 1%, and the need for operative intervention is even lower, CT is only 50% to 78% sensitive and tends to underestimate the extent and magnitude of the injuries. These patients, however, often undergo exploration for other concomitant injuries (3,4).

Diaphragmatic injuries, while relatively rare, remain diagnostic dilemmas. Studies of helical CT in diaphragmatic injury have found it better in the acute phase and with visceral herniation. Pathognomonic signs for this injury include the "collar sign"—a waistlike constriction of the abdominal viscera, intrathoracic herniation of abdominal contents, and discontinuity of the diaphragm. In one small study of helical CT these signs were highly specific, with a moderately high sensitivity; CT detected approximately 80% of left sided and 50% of right-sided herniations. The newer scanners have improved sensitivity and specificity, with values reaching 84% and 77%, respectively, using coronal and sagittal reconstructions. Familiarity and greater use of the MDCT should improve the ability to make this diagnosis in the acute phase (32,38,45,60,72).

CT remains the diagnostic test of choice in the stable patient. It is also being used with increasing frequency in the patient who is moderately stable (i.e., the patient who is able to maintain their vital signs, although they may be fluctuating, or the patient with ongoing hemorrhage who can be adequately resuscitated) in whom nonoperative management is still a possibility. A multi-institutional prospective study of 2,774 patients with suspected BAT found that a negative CT scan has a negative predictive value of 99.63%. This has tremendous implications for cost savings. A patient without other significant injuries, pain or social concerns with a normal abdominal CT can be safely discharged. The chance of a missed significant abdominal injury is extremely low (47).

Ultrasound

Focused assessment with sonography for trauma (FAST) is a directed assessment of the abdomen and pericardium with the goal of detecting hemoperitoneum or pericardium. The FAST exam is performed on the supine patient with the examiner positioned on the patient's right side. Four locations are scanned: (1) the right upper quadrant (RUQ), (2) the left upper quadrant (LUQ), (3) the suprapubic region, and (4) the pericardium. The examiner looks for unclotted blood, which appears black or anechoic on the ultrasound screen. The RUQ view is generally the initial

view since it is the easiest to obtain. This view detects blood in Morison's pouch, a dependent space between the kidney and liver. Although this location has the greatest yield, the addition of all abdominal views has been found to significantly increase the sensitivity by up to 40%. The LUQ is examined next, specifically looking for blood in the splenorenal space. Either view of the upper quadrants may also reveal a hemothorax or pneumothorax. Trendelenburg positioning may improve the sensitivity of either of these views. The suprapubic view evaluates the cul-de-sac between the rectum and bladder (the pouch of Douglas) and the heart and pericardium are examined by a subxiphoid view. The suprapubic view should be performed before the Foley catheter is placed, since the full bladder acts as an acoustic window and enhances visualization of peritoneal fluid (34,49,50,67).

The FAST exam has become a standard part of the EP and trauma surgeon's evaluation of the blunt trauma patient. Initially used over 20 years ago in Europe, it has gained tremendous popularity and widespread acceptance in the United States over the last 12 years. In many centers it is considered the first line diagnostic study to identify or exclude significant hemoperitoneum. Clear benefits of ultrasound are that it is rapid, noninvasive, inexpensive, repeatable and relatively portable. The test can be performed in conjunction with resuscitation, usually takes less than 5 minutes and has a relatively steep learning curve. Its sensitivity and specificity ranges from 81% to 98% and 94% to 98% respectively. The sensitivity and specificity vary somewhat depending on the amount of free fluid present and the expertise of the examiner (51,54,55,75). While ultrasound is moderately sensitive for as little as 100 to 200 ml of fluid, sensitivities increase to over 90% with volumes of fluid close to 700 ml. In other words, ultrasound is highly sensitive in patients with enough blood loss to cause hemodynamic instability. The sensitivity of the FAST exam also increases when serial exams are performed, separated by 30 minutes. Accuracy has been reported to range between 96% and 98% (7,36). The level of accuracy is independent of whether an emergency physician, surgeon, radiologist, or ultrasound technician performs the study; they all have comparable results. While there is controversy over the exact number of studies and instructional time needed for proficiency, current studies appear to support that several hours of instruction and roughly twenty hands on studies lead to excellent accuracy in defining hemoperitoneum (1,28,53,56,69,71).

In the United States, FAST has largely supplanted the diagnostic peritoneal lavage, especially in unstable patients, and has been used as a diagnostic adjunct in the stable patient in conjunction with physical exam or, more commonly, CT scan. Compared to diagnostic peritoneal lavage, ultrasound allows for a quicker, safer and noninvasive test without interference with other resuscitative procedures. Unlike DPL, it does not require extra time or modification for the pregnant patient or patients with pelvic fractures, previous surgery or coagulopathy.

Most centers use some variation of the algorithm from Denver published in 1997 (6). The initial test in all BAT patients is the ultrasound. If the patient is unstable and the FAST is positive, immediate laparotomy is performed. In the unstable patient, if the FAST is negative or equivocal and intraabdominal injury is a concern, a DPL is performed. A CT scan follows a positive ultrasound in a stable patient. A negative ultrasound is followed by a subsequent CT scan or serial ultrasounds, physical examination and hematocrit six hours later. A concerning change in physical examination, ultrasound findings or significant drop in hematocrit is followed by either a CT scan or laparotomy. Branney et al., along with others, have shown this to be a cost effective approach in decreasing CT usage. This has to be balanced however, with the increased use of ED or hospital resources since these patients may require an increased length of stay (6).

While ultrasound clearly is valuable in the unstable patient, it has some disadvantages compared to CT scan in the stable patient. Although highly sensitive for large amounts of hemoperitoneum, it is less so with small amounts, and it is not reliable at providing a qualitative assessment of a solid organ injury. The sensitivity of ultrasound for identifying solid organ injury is approximately 30% when performed by sonographers trained for limited bedside ultrasound. It also does not provide information about bowel or pancreatic injury or evaluate the retroperitoneum (7,13,26). Patients at significant risk for intraperitoneal injury such as those with abdominal abrasions, lower rib fractures, multiple traumatic injuries, pelvic or long bone fractures or inability to be clinically followed may be poor candidates for ultrasound as the only modality for evaluation. At a minimum, these patients should not be evaluated using a single exam at a single point in their course.

Overall, ultrasound provides a very useful initial test in blunt abdominal trauma. While it can potentially predict the need for surgical repair based on the amount of fluid observed, its main utility has been in the unstable patient as a replacement for diagnostic peritoneal lavage. As it does not reliably grade or even diagnose solid organ injury, it is most valuable as an adjunct to CT in the stable patient. In most centers, given the increasing availability of CT and the high negative predictive value, a negative or equivocal ultrasound is often followed by abdominal CT scanning. However, from the beginning of the resuscitation, ultrasound alerts the team to the presence of intraperitoneal injury within seconds to minutes and can be used to rapidly triage patients to the operating room or radiology suite. In addition, due to its portability and accessibility, ultrasound can be repeated in the trauma room several times to detect hemoperitoneum when the hemodynamic status of the patient changes.

Angiography

Interventional angiography is becoming increasingly important and is being used more frequently in the treatment of blunt abdominal trauma patients. As the technology of CT improves, active hemorrhage is increasingly identified faster and more accurately. If an actively bleeding spleen, liver, or kidney is visualized and the patient is clinically stable, a dedicated angiography team may be able to intervene to rapidly embolize the lesion and avoid laparotomy. While effective, the technique is resource intensive and is not fully implemented at many centers (21,78).

EMERGENCY DEPARTMENT MANAGEMENT

In Level I trauma centers, prehospital criteria such as vital signs, level of consciousness, and mechanism of injury will alert a trauma team before arrival of the patient. In most hospitals, however, the emergency physician is solely responsible for initial trauma management. The seriously injured patient with blunt abdominal trauma should undergo standard ATLS resuscitation. First, the airway should be addressed while maintaining cervical spine immobilization. High-flow oxygen should be administered by nonrebreather mask, oxygenation should be assessed by pulse oximeter, and the patient should be placed on a cardiac monitor. Vascular access is obtained using two large-bore (14-gauge or 16-gauge) intravenous catheters connected to normal saline or lactated Ringer. The neurologic status is evaluated by assessing the pupils and using the *AVPU* method (Alert, responds to Voice, responds to Pain, Unconscious) or the Glasgow Coma Scale. The patient should be fully undressed and then covered with blankets to prevent the development of hypothermia. By this point, the emergency physician should classify the victim of blunt abdominal trauma as stable or unstable.

Unstable Patients

In the hypotensive or tachycardic patient large-bore intravenous lines should be inserted and the patient should receive crystalloid infusion. A nasogastric or orogastric tube should be inserted as well as a Foley catheter, after ensuring that there is no urethral injury. If crystalloid resuscitation does not restore hemodynamic stability, blood products should be administered early. The choice of initial blood product (type O blood versus type-specific blood or fully crossed-matched blood) depends on the degree of instability. Patients with hemodynamic instability in whom an abdominal injury is clearly the source, such as an injury with a traumatic bowel wall hernia and abdominal wall ecchymosis, should be taken directly to the operating room. For unstable patients, particularly those with multisystem trauma, in whom intraabdominal injury is a possibility, options include DPL or the FAST examination. Special consideration should be given to the unstable patient with significant pelvic fractures (Fig. 184.1).

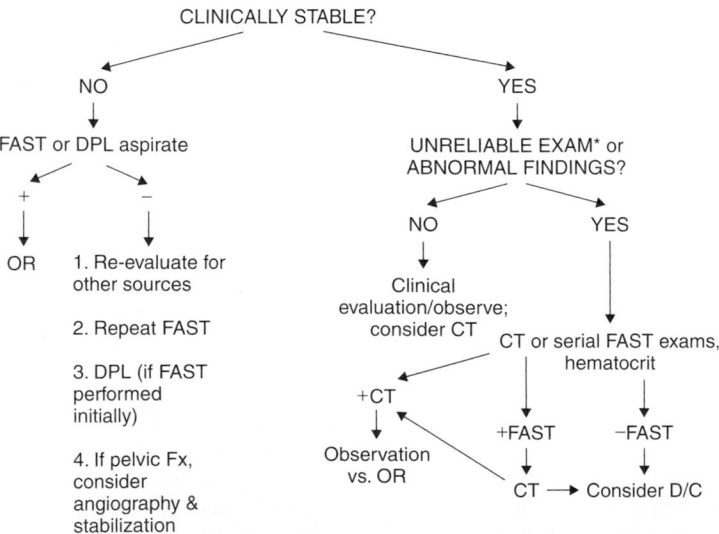

*Change in mental status, multisystem trauma, distracting injury, intoxication

Figure 184.1. Blunt abdominal trauma algorithm.

The speed and sensitivity of the FAST examination for diagnosing intraabdominal hemorrhage make it the best means of initially evaluating the unstable blunt abdominal trauma patient. A positive test in this setting mandates laparotomy. Management options in the unstable patient with a negative examination include DPL, a repeat FAST examination or laparotomy.

For unstable patients in whom a FAST examination is not available, the peritoneal aspirate component of the DPL remains a useful tool. An initial aspirate of more than 10 mL of blood is an indication for surgery. Despite the improved speed of the current generation of scanners, CT does not have a role in the persistently unstable victim of blunt abdominal trauma.

While the ranking of priorities in patients with head, chest, and abdominal injuries is still very difficult, there are some advantages from the modern spiral or multidetector CT scan speed. The speed of the newer CT scan may allow a few quick cuts of the head and chest to screen for obvious pathology. The time of the scan is now often measured in seconds to minutes. This may enable a quick assessment of the head en route to the operating room for laparotomy. In general, the critical ordering is to manage injuries to the abdomen first, and then the head, and then aorta; but, obviously, decisions must be colored by the actual pathologies present.

Stable Patients

For the hemodynamically stable patient with blunt abdominal trauma, the approach to management is guided by several factors. Victims of blunt abdominal trauma who are awake and alert, with a reliable, benign abdominal examination, can be followed clinically with serial examinations in the emergency department or hospital. For stable patients with positive abdominal findings, an unreliable examination, significant distracting injuries, or possible retroperitoneal injury, abdominal CT is the diagnostic test of choice. Occasionally, some patients with a significant mechanism of injury may undergo CT or a period of observation, in spite of negative clinical findings.

Although an initial FAST examination should be performed, a subsequent CT is indicated in most patients. Some centers, however, follow patients with serial ultrasounds, physical examinations and hematocrits. CT can often help determine whether underlying injury can be managed nonoperatively. CT in patients with a negative FAST examination may identify significant injuries that have not resulted in intraabdominal bleeding such as bowel injury. In addition, it will detect injuries in the retroperitoneum, pelvis, spine, and lower chest.

CRITICAL INTERVENTIONS

- Address the basic ABCs of resuscitation prior to examination of the abdomen
- In stable patients with significant pain, tenderness or an unreliable examination, perform a CT scan, serial examinations and ultrasounds
- In unstable patients perform an ultrasound or DPL to evaluate for intraabdominal injury
- Obtain surgical consultation early in hemodynamically unstable patients or those with intraabdominal pathology by examination, DPL, ultrasound or CT scan

DISPOSITION

For stable patients who require evaluation by CT, disposition can be made based on a combination of physical findings and CT findings. The sensitivity of CT scanning has been evaluated in several recent studies (6,21). These studies indicate that patients

with a normal CT scan and a brief period of observation in the ED can be safely discharged from ED. Patients who are awake and alert, with a reliable, benign abdominal examination, who are not candidates for CT, can be followed clinically with serial abdominal examinations in the ED over a 4- to 6-hour period.

Operative delay is the primary cause of preventable deaths in patients with blunt abdominal trauma. At a very early stage, the emergency physician should evaluate the services available at his or her institution and determine whether a patient is a candidate for transfer. It is imperative that a patient is initially resuscitated prior to transfer with careful attention paid to the airway and hemodynamic status. In consultation with the receiving institution, a decision is made to have a patient transferred on the basis of the primary and secondary surveys alone. Multiple diagnostic studies at the transferring hospital will only delay care and therefore only essential tests should be ordered. Two large-bore intravenous lines, a Foley catheter, and a nasogastric or orogastric tube should be placed in most patients. A chest x-ray should be obtained and chest tubes placed for hemothorax or pneumothorax.

COMMON PITFALLS

✔ Failure to obtain early surgical consultation in the unstable patient
✔ Attributing hypotension to extraabdominal causes, such as chest trauma, spinal shock, or external blood loss
✔ Failure to evaluate the abdomen in the patient with an unreliable examination. All patients who have multiple injuries, altered mental status or a distracting injury should be considered to have an unreliable examination
✔ Performing an abdominal CT scan in the hemodynamically unstable patient
✔ Relying on a negative ultrasound to rule out inraperitoneal injury
✔ Delaying transfer while performing unnecessary studies

Acknowledgments

Thanks to Kevin M. Curtis and Vicente H. Gracias who contributed to this chapter in a previous edition.

References

1. American College of Emergency Physicians. ACEP emergency ultrasound guidelines-2001. *Ann Emerg Med* 2001;38:470.
2. American College of Emergency Physicians: Clinical policy for the initial approach to patients presenting with acute blunt trauma. *Ann Emerg Med* 1998;31:422.
3. Akhrass R, Kim K, Brandt C: Computed tomography: an unreliable indicator of pancreatic trauma. *Am Surg* 1996;62:647.
4. Akhrass R, Yaffe MB, Brandt CP, et al: Pancreatic trauma: a ten-year multi-institutional experience. *Am Surg* 1997;63:598.
5. Bilge A, Sahin M: Diagnostic peritoneal lavage in blunt abdominal trauma. *Eur J Surg* 1991;157:449.
6. Branney SW, Moore EE, Cantrill SV, et al: Ultrasound based key clinical pathway reduces the use of hospital resources for the evaluation of blunt abdominal trauma. *J Trauma* 1997;42:1086.
7. Branney SW, Wolfe RE, Moore EE, et al: Quantitative sensitivity of ultrasound in detecting free intraperitoneal fluid. *J Trauma* 1995;39:375.
8. Brasel KJ, Borgstrom DC, Kolewe KA, et al: Abdominal computed tomography scan as a screening tool in blunt trauma. *Surgery* 1996;120:780.
9. Brasel KJ, Olson CJ, Stafford RE, et al: Incidence and significance of free fluid on abdominal computed tomographic scan in blunt trauma. *J Trauma* 1998;44:889.
10. Buechter KJ, Arnold M, Steele B, et al: The use of serum amylase and lipase in evaluating and managing blunt abdominal trauma. *Am Surg* 1990;56:204.
11. Chandler CF, Lane JS, Waxman KS: Seatbelt sign following blunt trauma is associated with increased incidence of abdominal injury. *Am Surg* 1997;63:885.
12. Chen JC, Wilson SE: Diaphragmatic injuries: recognition and management in sixty-two patients. *Am Surg* 1991;57:810.
13. Chiu WC, Cushing BM, Rodriguez A, et al: Abdominal injuries without hemoperitoneum: a potential limitation of focused abdominal sonography for trauma (FAST). *J Trauma* 1997;42:617.

cluster in a 9-inch diameter (if a normal choke barrel is used), whereas at 20 yards (25% loss in velocity), pellets will spread out over an 18-inch diameter, markedly decreasing lethality. SGWs are categorized based on distance and pattern of injury. Type I wounds are greater than 7 yards from the victim and only penetrate deep fascia and subcutaneous tissue. Type II wounds occur at a distance of 3 to 7 yards, have a pellet spread of 10 cm to 25 cm, and create deeper wounds, frequently into the thoracic or abdominal cavities. Finally, type III wounds (less than 3 yards distance) create massive destruction of tissue and organs due to their close range. Debris is also forced into these wounds and there is substantial morbidity associated with them (12).

DIFFERENTIAL DIAGNOSIS

While there may be an obvious penetrating abdominal injury, other wounds to the head, neck, and extremities must also be sought. Unstable vital signs usually result from intracavitary hemorrhage, but tension pneumothorax and pericardial tamponade may also be responsible. Rapid physical examination, chest x-ray, and ultrasound are invaluable in delineating hemoperitoneum, hemothorax, tension pneumothorax, cardiac tamponade, or some combination of these potential contributors to hypotension.

EMERGENCY DEPARTMENT EVALUATION

All patients with suspected trauma must be completely undressed and scrupulously examined. In penetrating trauma in particular, the scalp, axilla, and perineum easily hide narrow but deep and dangerous wounds. The examiner should not be swayed by prehospital or patient testimony or by the identification of a single site of penetration.

The principal tenet in the evaluation and management of penetrating abdominal trauma is to discern the presence of organ injury that requires immediate laparotomy. For patients without clinical mandates for laparotomy, a careful evaluation for indications of peritoneal violation and the need for operative management may proceed. Finally, any equivocal findings of peritoneal violation require further observation, adjuvant testing, or both. Standard practices of resuscitation and stabilization prevail.

EMERGENCY DEPARTMENT MANAGEMENT

The earliest notification possible should be made to the on-call trauma surgeon, trauma team, and operating room personnel. Information gleaned from prehospital communication alone can be a sufficient prompt to alert consultants.

Stab Wounds

Peritoneal violation occurs in 50% to 70% of anterior abdominal SWs; laparotomy is required in approximately half of these cases. Therefore, only one-fourth to one-third of patients who sustain SWs to the anterior abdomen ultimately requires operative intervention. Selective management is widely accepted, but use depends on the type of injury, hemodynamic stability of the patient and standard of care within the hospital and community. Three sequential questions form the basis for an algorithm for patients with stab wounds to the abdomen (Fig. 185.1).

1. Are There Indications for Immediate Laparotomy?

There are six clinical indicators that suggest a high likelihood of intraperitoneal injury requiring laparotomy after anterior abdominal SW. If one of these is present then immediate surgical consultation and operative management should ensue.

Unstable vital signs: Any patient with unstable vital signs has a potential major solid visceral or vascular injury and requires immediate surgical consultation (11). Other causes of hemodynamic instability must be considered as causal or contributory, such as tension pneumothorax and tension hemopericardium.

Evisceration: In patients with evisceration of any abdominal contents, approximately two thirds have coincident intraperitoneal injury that requires laparotomy (15). Many surgeons adopt these odds and simply proceed to laparotomy. Others reduce the omentum or small bowel and proceed with other diagnostic studies.

Peritoneal signs: Peritoneal signs on physical examination, although neither sensitive nor specific, may indicate peritoneal injury and the need for exploratory laparotomy (11).

Diaphragmatic injury: Diaphragmatic injuries due to SW are often small and thus difficult to impossible to discern using routine chest x-ray and PE. These may lead to significant morbidity or mortality due to herniation of abdominal contents into the chest, often months to decades following the original insult. Very conservative centers conduct mandatory laparotomy or thoracotomy for SW's to the left low chest or upper abdomen to avoid missing diaphragmatic tears. The chance of herniation of bowel or mesentery through SW's of the right hemidiaphragm is mitigated by the presence of the liver, so that diagnostic tests are not considered necessary. Other centers use DL or DPL to evaluate for diaphragmatic injury instead of mandatory laparotomy (9,17,19).

Gastrointestinal (GI) hemorrhage: Evidence of upper GI hemorrhage after SW suggests hollow visceral injury, particularly to the stomach or duodenum, and the need for operative intervention.

Implement in situ: Dogma states that implements in situ require removal in the operative setting so potential hemorrhage may be rapidly controlled. There are exceptions to this maxim. Patients with severe comorbid illness or pregnant women may sustain greater harm from general anesthesia. In rare instances in other patients, it is necessary to remove the implement in order to provide adequate prehospital or ED resuscitation.

2. Is There Evidence of Peritoneal Violation?

If there is no clinical mandate for immediate laparotomy, then the next step is to assess the wound tract to determine presence of peritoneal penetration. Several diagnostic studies can be used in this process as described below.

Plain radiographs: The presence of free air on an upright chest or left lateral decubitus radiograph establishes that the stabbing implement penetrated the peritoneal cavity and drew air in with it. It does not, however, establish that a hollow viscous injury has necessarily occurred. Due to poor positive and negative predictive value, an upright chest radiograph is not routinely warranted.

Local wound exploration: LWE can be performed safely on the anterior abdomen, flank or back. A negative LWE establishes that the end of an SW tract is anterior to the rectus fascia. Such patients can be discharged from the emergency department after appropriate wound care (14,18). An indeterminate local wound exploration must be considered positive. Patients who have multiple wounds or who pose technical obstacles, such as being massively obese, may not be candidates for this procedure.

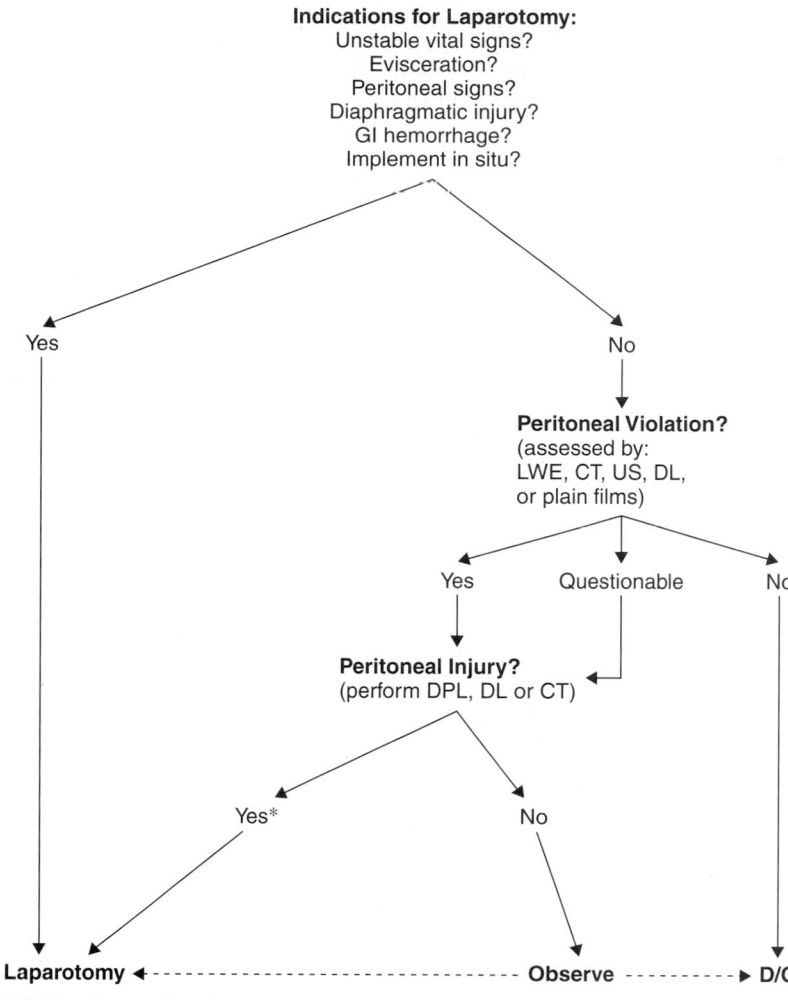

Figure 185.1. Algorithm for emergency department management of abdominal stab wounds.
*Selective Nonoperative Management is used in some centers in conjunction with CT or DPL.

LWE, local wound exploration; DL, diagnostic laparoscopy.

CT scan: CT scans for SWs of the abdomen can exclude peritoneal violation, sometimes predict the need for laparotomy, and facilitate nonoperative management of certain injuries (most commonly hepatic wounds) (6). However, CT lacks sensitivity for injuries to the small bowel, pancreas and diaphragm. In addition, CT's exquisite sensitivity for diagnosing intraperitoneal free air may lead to unnecessary operation.

Ultrasound: This can be helpful in evaluating the intraperitoneal, pleural and pericardial spaces in wounds that may have violated the mediastinum or diaphragm. A positive *focused assessment with sonography for trauma* (FAST) exam is helpful; laparotomy or thoracotomy is indicated, depending on whether free intraperitoneal or intrapericardial hemorrhage is discovered. However, a negative FAST exam does not rule out injury, particularly to hollow viscera and the diaphragm, as these tend to bleed minimally (3,22).

Diagnostic laparoscopy: This can be used to evaluate the depth of a wound tract and while it compares favorably with LWE, it is far more invasive and can only be performed by a surgeon trained in its use. DL is more useful for inspecting the diaphragm in left low chest and upper abdominal wounds. Additionally, it may allow immediate repair of diaphragmatic and certain organ injuries, often decreasing the cost and length of stay of patients who otherwise would have had an exploratory laparotomy (17,19).

If the wound tract is determined to be superficial, that is, it does not penetrate the peritoneum, then the patient may be safely discharged after wound care. There is no credible data that address specifically the question of whether to primarily close SW's. A slash-type wound that can be readily explored and irrigated can generally be closed. Puncture-type wounds, on the other hand, are generally left open. Prophylactic antibiotics are not indicated.

3. Is There Evidence of Peritoneal Injury?

If peritoneal violation is present or if there are equivocal findings of peritoneal violation, further diagnostic evaluation with DPL, CT, or DL is indicated in order to determine whether injury requiring operative intervention is present.

Diagnostic peritoneal lavage: DPL, although invasive, is a rapid, reliable indicator of intraabdominal injury and need for operative management (9,14,21). It is also effective in determining hollow viscous or diaphragmatic injury. The presence of 10cc of gross blood or lavage fluid with 100,000 RBC/HPF indicates the presence of visceral injury with a sensitivity of greater than 90%. A count of 20,000–100,000 RBCs/HPF should be considered indeterminate and the patient observed for at least 12 to 24 hours. When low chest wounds are present, the RBC criterion needs to be lowered to 5,000 to 10,000 RBCs/HPF to discern potential isolated diaphragmatic injury (12). False-positive peritoneal aspiration results may be caused by drainage of free blood from the torso muscle and subcutaneous tissue at the SW site into the peritoneal cavity.

CT scan: The CT is an integral diagnostic procedure following blunt trauma, as it is excellent for detecting solid visceral injury and hemoperitoneum. Its role in hemodynamically stable patients with penetrating abdominal trauma is expanding, and can facilitate nonoperative management of selected injuries (most notably hepatic lacerations) (1,6,8,20). However, it remains insensitive for small diaphragmatic tears and has moderate sensitivity for isolated hollow viscous trauma. Triple contrast CT (intravenous, oral, and rectal) is generally reserved for low abdominal, flank and back wounds in order to detect colorectal injury.

Diagnostic laparoscopy: DL has been used for direct inspection of the diaphragm, detection of peritoneal violation and evaluation of solid viscera. However it remains inadequate in identifying hollow viscus and retroperitoneal injury (17,19). In centers experienced with DL, it is usually undertaken for low chest, upper flank and upper back penetration on the left side where diaphragmatic penetration is far more vulnerable to future herniation of abdominal contents into the chest.

If peritoneal injury is discovered, then most centers proceed to laparotomy. However, several recent studies have shown good outcomes utilizing *selective nonoperative management* (SNOM) of hemodynamically stable patients with SWs to the abdomen who undergo serial clinical evaluations over 12 to 24 hours. Others advocate this approach in conjunction with diagnostic modalities such as CT or DPL. Although safely employed in selected trauma centers, SNOM requires meticulous, ongoing observation, which may be impractical on a hectic trauma service (4,7).

Stab Wounds to the Flank and Back

The chance of retroperitoneal injury is significantly greater after a SW to the flank and back than after one to the anterior abdomen. Yet, the risk of intraperitoneal organ injury ranges from 15% to 40% after SWs to these sites. Local wound exploration can be very difficult to perform in these areas because of the lack of a definite fascial plane of demarcation with the peritoneal cavity. CT scans in hemodynamically stable patients with flank and back wounds may be used to safely triage patients to operative versus nonoperative management (1). In addition, CT scan will assess for renal injuries. A triple contrast CT is recommended to assess for colorectal perforation, should the wound tract appear to have entered that region. DPL can discern the presence of intraperitoneal and diaphragmatic injury and may be used in conjunction with CT (4).

Stab Wounds in Proximity to the Diaphragm

Because missed injuries to the diaphragm may eventually cause substantial morbidity and mortality, certain centers promote mandatory exploration to inspect the diaphragm when it is considered at risk, based on the wound entry site alone. Although exploratory laparotomy is the most sensitive technique of injury determination, it incurs an unacceptably high unnecessary laparotomy rate. Thus, laparoscopy, thoracoscopy, and DPL are more commonly employed to aid in diagnosing an injury. When DPL is utilized, the RBC criterion should be lowered to 5 to 10,000 RBCs/HPF in order to raise the sensitivity of the procedure for identifying a structure that ordinarily bleeds little when injured.

Gunshot Wounds

In most institutions, the knowledge or strong suspicion of peritoneal violation is enough to prompt laparotomy. In contrast to SWs, older studies showed that cavity entry and multiple-organ injury was the rule in GSWs, with a mortality that was ten times greater. However, selected recent studies show that GSW to the anterior abdomen incur peritoneal violation and resultant intraabdominal organ injury in 30% to 74% of patients, rather than the almost 90% reported in older papers citing mostly military experience (25). As for SW's, an algorithm for patients with abdominal gunshot wounds can be predicated on 3 sequential questions (Fig. 185.2).

1. Are There Indications for Immediate Laparotomy?

As with abdominal stab wounds, GSWs to the abdomen have accepted criteria for immediate surgical consultation and operation. If any of the following are found, surgical consultation and operative intervention should generally proceed. If none of these is present, then the physician should continue to the next step in the algorithm.

Unstable vital signs: Any victim of a GSW with unstable vital signs requires immediate surgical consultation as injury to a major vessel or solid organ is presumed. If the GSW is to the abdomen, there are relatively few cases that are managed outside the operating theater. Associated hemopneumothorax or hemopericardium may contribute to the clinical situation, and requires management in the ED or operating room.

Peritoneal signs: As with SW, there is a well-documented lack of specificity of peritoneal signs with GSW, but patients with initial diffuse abdominal tenderness after GSW to the abdomen may require surgical exploration (25).

Gastrointestinal hemorrhage: As is true for patients with SWs, gastrointestinal bleeding in association with a GSW to the abdomen, flank, or back mandates surgical exploration for potential intestinal injury.

Evisceration: Because of the greater energy transference and cavitation that occurs with GSWs to the abdomen (compared with SW), evisceration warrants surgical exploration.

2. Is There Evidence of Peritoneal Penetration by the Missile?

The following methods can determine if the missile has penetrated the peritoneum. In some centers, evidence of peritoneal penetration is enough to prompt laparotomy.

Plain films: If performed in two planes, radiographs can help determine the trajectory of the missile. However, this is generally unhelpful in those injuries that are through and through. Ricochet off the ribs and pelvic girdle or multiple missiles make the interpretation of plain films much more difficult.

Local wound exploration: This is less useful for GSWs than SWs because there is more tissue destruction and difficulty in visualizing the entire tract. It is best used for low-velocity missiles with superficial wounds.

Ultrasound: As with stab wounds, US can be reliably used to detect the presence of hemoperitoneum and pericardial fluid in patients with GSWs to the abdomen. However, a negative FAST does not rule out the presence of intraabdominal injury, particularly to hollow viscera and the diaphragm (3,22).

Diagnostic laparoscopy: DL may help identify the presence of peritoneal violation and the need for conversion to celiotomy, but it is inadequate to evaluate for hollow viscous injury. Laparoscopy is also useful for identifying diaphragmatic injury. DL is an invasive procedure that when used incorrectly can increase risk and cost to the patient. Its role in the evaluation of patients with abdominal GSWs is still evolving (17).

High-velocity GSWs impose tremendous energies and can cause serious intraperitoneal damage despite an extraperitoneal course. If no peritoneal violation is determined, these patients should be observed for 12 to 24 hours unless their injury was of low velocity with a superficial missile path. These patients may be discharged home after wound care and clear instructions for return. GSWs are not typically closed. If peritoneal penetration

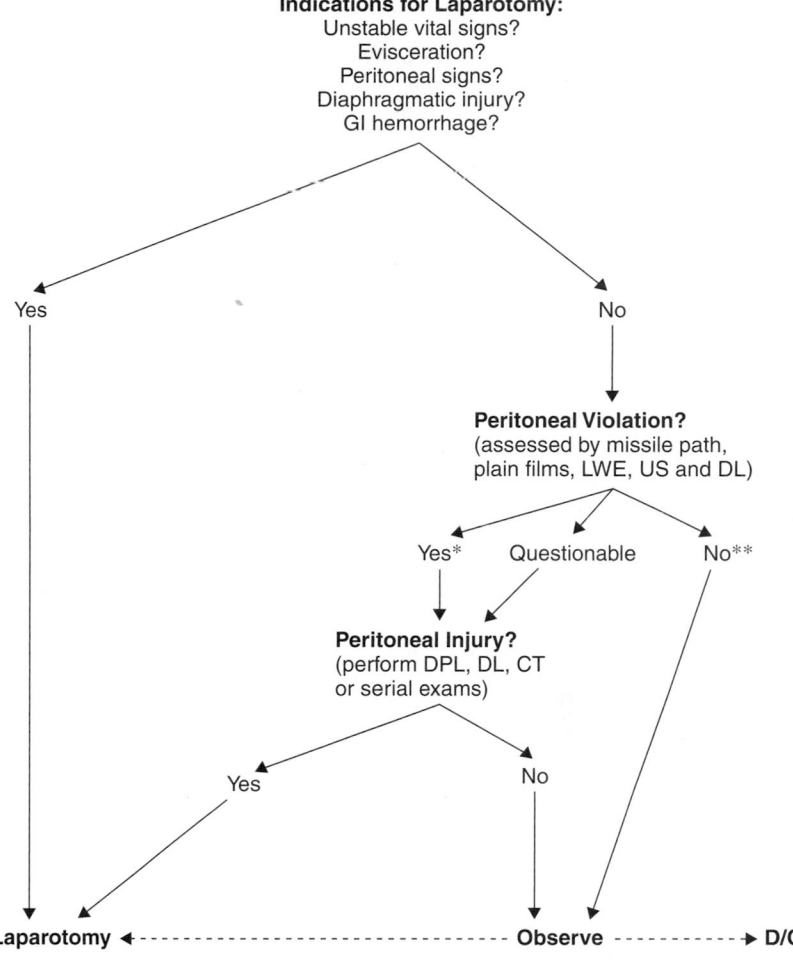

Figure 185.2. Algorithm for emergency department management of abdominal gunshot wounds.
*Most centers proceed to laparotomy if peritoneal entry is suspected.
**Patients with low velocity superficial injuries may be discharged; unknown depth or high-velocity injuries require further testing and observation.

is discovered or if it is suspected, then most centers proceed with laparotomy. However, some trauma centers advocate a selective nonoperative management approach in a setting that employs the opportunity for close serial physical examinations and additional diagnostic testing, such as DPL, CT, and DL (24,25). This next step in the algorithm should be reserved for stable patients without clinical indications for laparotomy.

3. Is There Evidence of Peritoneal Injury?

In those centers not proceeding to laparotomy when peritoneal violation is found or strongly indicated, several diagnostic techniques have been utilized to include or exclude peritoneal injury following GSWs to the abdomen. Of these, DPL and CT have received the most attention, with a smaller number of studies evaluating DL.

Diagnostic peritoneal lavage: The use of DPL to determine peritoneal injury after GSW has been shown to have a sensitivity of 87.5% to 99% with a specificity of 95% to 98% (5,13). DPL, with a RBC threshold lowered to 5,000 RBC/hpf, coupled with clinical examination can help guide the need for laparotomy (10).

CT scan: In patients with torso injuries, CT has been used in an attempt to determine peritoneal violation and avoid nontherapeutic invasive procedures, including laparotomy (8). A more common use for CT is to provide information and assist in the management of select hemodynamically stable patients with penetrating trauma to the abdomen, flank, or pelvis (6).

Diagnostic laparoscopy: DL is best used in those patients with tangential GSW to the abdomen who do not have a clear indication for laparotomy or in those with GSW to the left low chest without indication for thoracotomy or laparotomy (17).

CRITICAL INTERVENTIONS

- Completely undress and carefully examine all patients with suspected penetrating trauma to the abdomen
- Obtain early surgical consultation for patients with penetrating abdominal trauma
- Perform local wound exploration as the initial screening test in stable patients with anterior abdominal stab wounds to determine the potential for peritoneal penetration
- For patients with left low chest or upper abdominal stab wounds, perform a work up for diaphragmatic injury (laparoscopy, thoracoscopy, or DPL)

DISPOSITION

In most centers, patients who undergo a negative DPL, CT, or DL should be held for 12 to 24 hours to ensure absence of injury resulting from the original mechanism or the diagnostic procedure. However, one recent retrospective study of 107 patients with penetrating abdominal trauma who were managed with selective ED work up (LWE, CT, serial examinations) and discharged to home from the ED, showed no significant adverse outcomes (7).

Ideally, all patients with a SW or a GSW to the torso are triaged from the point of injury directly to a Level I or Level II trauma center. When this does not occur, transfer to such a center at the earliest opportunity is recommended. Only life-saving maneuvers such as endotracheal intubation, tube thoracostomy, pericardial aspiration, and fluid resuscitation are indicated before initiating transfer.

COMMON PITFALLS

✔ Failure to recognize a stab wound or gunshot wound

✔ Minimizing the injury. Always assume that peritoneal injury is present

✔ Delaying transport to the operating suite for patients with indications for laparotomy

✔ Blind probing with digits or instruments into wound tracts, as this is inaccurate and hazardous

✔ Relying on a negative physical examination or abdominal ultrasound to rule out injury after penetrating abdominal trauma

✔ Failure to observe and admit the penetrating abdominal trauma patient for repeated examinations after a negative DPL or CT

✔ Failure to obtain early consultation with a trauma surgeon

✔ Failure to properly monitor and observe a trauma patient with abdominal wounds while in the radiology suite undergoing CT scan

Acknowledgments

The authors gratefully acknowledge the contributions of Vicente H. Gracias and Kevin M. Curtis, who wrote the previous version of this chapter.

References

1. Albrecht RM, Vigil A, Schermer CR, Demarest III GB, Davis VH, Fry DE. Stab wounds to the back/flank in hemodynamically stable patients: evaluation using triple contrast computed tomography. *American Surgeon* 1999;65:683–687.
2. Bailey H, ed. *Surgery of modern warfare*. 3rd edition, vol. 2. Baltimore: Williams & Wilkins, 1944.
3. Boulanger BR, Kearney PA, Tsuei BM, Ochoa JB. The routine use of sonography in penetrating torso injury is beneficial. *J Trauma-Injury Infection & Critical Care* 2001;51:320–325.
4. Boyle EM, Maier RV, Salazar JD, et al. Diagnosis of injuries after stab wounds to the back and flank. *J Trauma-Injury Infection & Critical Care* 1997;42:260–265.
5. Brakenridge SC, Nagy KK, Joseph KT, et al. Detection of intra-abdominal injury using diagnostic peritoneal lavage after shotgun wound to the abdomen. *J Trauma-Injury Infection & Critical Care* 2003;54:329–331.
6. Chiu WC, Shanmuganathan D, Mirvis SE, Mirvis SE, Scalea TM. Determining the need for laparotomy in penetrating torso trauma: A prospective study using triple-contrast enhanced abdominopelvic computed tomography. *J Trauma-Injury Infection & Critical Care* 2001;51:860–869.
7. Conrad MF, Patton JH, Parikshak M, Kralovich KA. Selective management of penetrating truncal injuries: is emergency department discharge a reasonable goal? *American Surgeon* 2003;69:266–272.
8. Ginzburg E, Carrillo CH, Kopelman T, et al. The role of computed tomography in selective management of gunshot wounds to the abdomen and flank. *J Trauma-Injury Infection & Critical Care* 1998;45:1005–1009.
9. Gonzalez RP, Turk B, Falimirski ME, Holevar MR. Abdominal stab wounds: diagnostic peritoneal lavage criteria for emergency room discharge. *J Trauma-Injury Infection & Critical Care* 2001;51:939–943.
10. Kelemen JJ, Martin RR, Obney JA, Jenkins D, Kissinger DP. Evaluation of diagnostic peritoneal lavage in stable patients with gunshot wounds to the abdomen. *Archives of Surgery* 1997;132:909–913.
11. Leppaniemi AK, Voutilainen PE, Haapiainen RK. Indications for early mandatory laparotomy in abdominal stab wounds. *British Journal of Surgery* 1999;86:76–80.
12. Marx JA. Abdominal trauma. In: Marx JA, ed. Rosen's *Emergency Medicine: Concepts and Clinical Practice* 5th ed. St. Louis: Mosby, 2002;415–436.
13. Nagy KK, Krosner SM, Joseph KT, et al. A method of determining peritoneal penetration in gunshot wounds to the abdomen. *J Trauma-Injury Infection & Critical Care* 1997;43:242–245.
14. Nagy KK, Roberts RR, Joseph KT, et al. Experience with over 2500 diagnostic peritoneal lavages. *Injury* 2000;31:479–482.
15. Nagy K, Roberts R, Joseph K, An G, Barrett J. Evisceration after abdominal stab wounds: is laparotomy required? *J Trauma-Injury Infection & Critical Care.* 1999;47:622–632.
16. Otis GA.The medical and surgical history of the war of the rebellion, part 2, vol II. In: *Surgical history.* Washington, DC: U.S. Government Printing Office, 1877.
17. Poole GV, Thomae KR, and Hauser CJ. Laparoscopy in trauma. *Surgical Clinics of North America* 1996;76:547–556.
18. Rosenthal RE, Smith J, Walls RM, et al. Stab wounds to the abdomen: failure of blunt probing to predict peritoneal penetration. *Ann Emerg Med* 1987;16:172.
19. Simon RJ, Rabin J, Kuhls D. Impact of increase use of laparoscopy on negative laparotomy rates after penetrating trauma. *J Trauma-Injury Infection & Critical Care* 2002;53:297–302.
20. Soto JA, Morales C, Munera F, Sanabria A, Guevara JM, Suarez T. Penetrating stab wounds to the abdomen: use of serial US and contrast-enhanced CT in stable patients. *Radiology.* 2001;220:365–371.
21. Sriussadaporn S, Pak-art R, Pattaratiwanon M, et al. Clinical uses of diagnostic peritoneal lavage in stab wounds of the anterior abdomen: a prospective study. *European Journal of Surgery* 2002;168:490–493.
22. Udobi KF, Rodriguez A, Chiu WC, Scalea TM. Role of ultrasonography in penetrating abdominal trauma: a prospective clinical study. *J Trauma-Injury Infection & Critical Care* 2001;50:475–479.
23. Van Brussel M and Van Hee R. Abdominal stab wounds: a five-year patient review. *European Journal of Emergency Medicine* 2001;8:83–88.
24. Velmahos GC, Demetriades DF, Foianini E, et al. A selective approach to the management of gunshot wounds to the back. *American Journal of Surgery* 1997;174:342–346.
25. Velmahos GC, Demetriades, D, Toutouzas KG, et al. Selective nonoperative management in 1,856 patients with abdominal gunshot wounds: should routine laparotomy still be the standard of care? *Ann of Surgery.* 2001;234:395–403.

CHAPTER 186
Genitourinary Trauma

Carrie D. Tibbles

The genitourinary (GU) system is involved in approximately 10% of acutely injured patients (22). The presentation of genitourinary trauma may be occult, and is often overshadowed by more dramatic and immediate life-threatening injuries. However if these injuries are not identified and properly treated, the patient may experience delayed complications and significant long-term morbidity. Clues to suggest the possibility of GU trauma lie in the mechanism of injury, a constellation of associated injuries, and physical examination findings identified during the secondary survey. For diagnosis and management, genitourinary trauma is generally divided into upper tract injuries (kidney and ureter), and lower tract injuries, (bladder, urethra, and external genitalia). The evaluation of the urologic system is unique in that it should occur in a retrograde fashion, (i.e., a urethral injury is ruled out before assessment of the bladder and upper tract). A systematic approach and thorough understanding of the available diagnostic modalities are necessary for the emergency physician to effectively manage these injuries.

CLINICAL PRESENTATION

Upper Tract Injury

The kidneys and ureters lie securely in the retroperitoneum, beneath the lower ribs and musculature of the back. Therefore, injuries to the upper urinary tract typically occur in the setting of high-energy, multisystem trauma. Blunt force to the back, flank, or abdomen; falls from height; or, less commonly, rapid deceleration may result in injuries to the kidneys or ureters (13). Upper tract injuries may occur in isolation. However, more commonly, trauma that results in renal injuries produces associated bony, vascular, and visceral injuries that directly contribute to the observed morbidity and mortality (9). Penetrating injury, which accounts for 6% to 11% of renal injuries, is suggested by transaxial wounds or wounds in anatomic proximity to the kidneys and ureter. The majority of blunt trauma patients with upper tract injuries present with hematuria, but renal pedicle injury and penetrating injuries to the ureter may not cause hematuria. A vascular pedicle injury may present as refractory hypotension following severe blunt trauma; this injury usually results from a deceleration mechanism.

The American Association for the Surgery of Trauma has established a classification system for renal injuries based on the anatomic location and severity (16) (Table 186.1) (Fig. 186.1). Grade I and Grade II injuries consist of contusions and lacerations confined to the cortex respectively and are considered minor injuries. Eighty five percent of renal injuries are classified as minor injuries. Grade III injuries are deeper lacerations that extend into the corticomedullary junction. A laceration into the collecting system or lacerations involving segmental arteries are Grade IV injuries. The most severe injuries are classified as Grade V and include a shattered kidney, thrombosis of the main renal artery, or avulsion of the renal hilum.

Lower Tract Injuries

Blunt trauma to the lower urinary tract (bladder and urethra) is usually associated with pelvic rami fractures and symphyseal diastasis. *Anterior urethral injuries* (penile and bulbous urethra, below the urogenital diaphragm) are associated with self-instrumentation, falls, and straddle injuries. *Posterior urethral injuries* (membranous and prostatic urethra, above the urogenital diaphragm) commonly accompany pelvic fractures (Fig. 186.2). As the urinary continence mechanism and autonomic innervation responsible for erection are contained in the

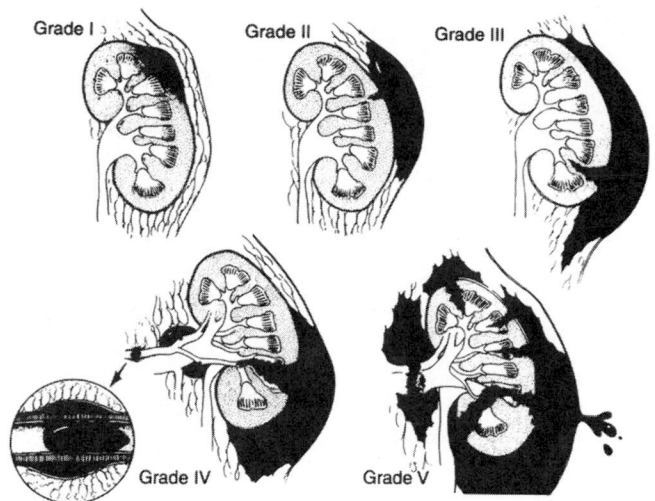

Figure 186.1. Grading system of renal injuries. (From: Santucci RA, McAninch JW, Safir M, et al. Validation of the American Association for the Surgery of Trauma Organ Injury Severity Scale for the Kidney. *J Trauma* 2001;50:195, with permission.)

posterior urethra, posterior urethral injuries may result in permanent incontinence and erectile dysfunction. Signs of anterior urethral injury depend on the integrity of Buck fascia. If this fascial layer is torn, blood and urine may pass into the penis, scrotum, and abdominal wall. Clinical signs of urethral injury are blood at the urethral meatus, high-riding prostate, scrotal or perineal hematoma, and difficulty voiding. However, these signs can be absent in patients with urethral injury.

There are two types of bladder ruptures after blunt trauma: extraperitoneal and intraperitoneal. Extraperitoneal bladder injuries are most commonly associated with pelvic fractures and bladder laceration by bony fragments. There is leakage of urine into the perivesicular space. Intraperitoneal bladder injuries result from compressive forces in the presence of a full bladder, and rupture occurs at the dome of the bladder through the peritoneum into the abdominal cavity. The presence of a pelvic fracture and gross hematuria is virtually diagnostic of bladder rupture. Ninely eight percent of patients with bladder rupture will have gross hematuria. Other signs of bladder injury are suprapubic or lower abdominal pain and tenderness, inability to void, and blood at the urethral meatus.

As with penetrating trauma to the upper GU tract, penetrating injuries to the lower tract are suggested by location of wounds. Any penetration of the lower abdominal wall in the region of the pelvis raises the possibility of urinary tract injury. Given the variability of the projectile tract, any gunshot wound in the region should include consideration of GU tract injury.

External Genitalia Trauma

Testicular injuries are often the result of a fall or direct trauma. They include lacerations, contusions, dislocations, or fractures. Symptoms include pain, nausea, lightheadedness, and acute urinary retention. A swollen, tender testicle or a hematoma may be seen on physical examination. Penile injuries range from small lacerations and contusions to complete amputations. The incidence of penetrating trauma to the external genitalia resulting from gunshot wounds and stabbing has been increasing (4). Penile fracture, which involves rupture of the tunica albuginea, most commonly occurs during overzealous vaginal intercourse, although several other mechanisms have been reported (21). Any constricting object placed around the penis can result in marked edema and eventual incarceration and necrosis distal to the

---

TABLE 186.1.   Grading System for Renal Injuries*

MINOR INJURIES

Grade I: Contusions and contained subcapsular hematomas
Grade II: Nonexpanding perirenal hematomas and cortical
    lacerations

MAJOR INJURIES

Grade III: Parenchymal lacerations into the corticomedullary
    junction and thrombosis of a segmental artery without an
    associated parenchymal laceration
Grade IV: Renal lacerations involving segmental renal vessels,
    lacerations violating the collecting system, and contained
    injuries to the renal vessels
Grade V: Avulsion of the renal hilum, thrombosis of the main renal
    artery, shattered kidney

*American Association for the Surgery of Trauma Grading System

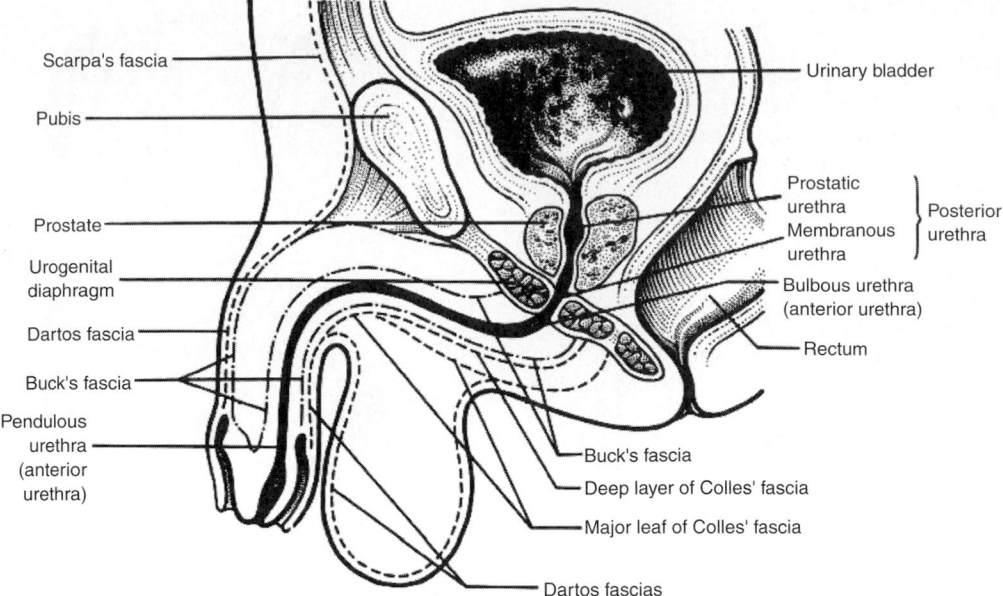

Figure 186.2.   Normal anatomy of the male urethra. (From Schneider RE *Genitourinary System*. In Marx JA, Hockberger RS, and Walls RM eds. Rosen's emergency medicine concepts and clinical practice 5th ed. St. Louis: Mosby;2002:438, with permission.)

constriction. Entrapment of the penis in a zipper occurs most often in uncircumcised young boys.

Vaginal injuries are frequently complications of pelvic fractures, but may also be seen following sexual assault or other penetrating injuries. The majority of patients present with vaginal bleeding. A careful vaginal exam is required in any female patients suspected of having a pelvic fracture. According to a recent series, up to one-third of patients with vaginal trauma unrelated to childbirth, will have concurrent urethral injuries (8).

EMERGENCY DEPARTMENT EVALUATION

Upper Tract Injury

The emergency department (ED) evaluation of a multitrauma patient begins with the standard Advanced Trauma Life Support assessment and resuscitation. In this manner, immediately life-threatening injuries are identified and treated. In the unstable patient requiring emergency laparatomy for other reasons, gross hematuria and signs of a pelvic fracture should be noted during the secondary survey. Definitive evaluation of the GU tract can be performed once the patient has been stabilized. In the stable patient, the emergency physician must determine the necessity of further evaluation and diagnostic imaging.

The first task is to identify those patients at risk for significant renal injuries. Mee et al. published the influential article establishing criteria for the evaluation of blunt renal trauma. Their 10-year prospective study of 1,007 consecutive blunt trauma patients established markers associated with increased risk of major renal lacerations. Gross hematuria, microscopic hematuria (greater than 5 red blood cells [RBC]/HPF) with shock either in the prehospital setting or in the ED, or, less commonly, a history of significant deceleration, were associated with renal injuries. The authors concluded that if radiographic evaluation were limited to those patients, no significant renal injuries would be missed (14). These guidelines have been supported by subsequent studies and have become the criteria defining the population of patients who require further radiographic evaluation (7,9,10). It

should be noted, however, that this approach is based on the assumption that patients with microscopic hematuria in the absence of hemodynamic instability or high-energy mechanism are likely to have minor injuries (i.e., renal contusions) that would be managed by simple observation.

Traditionally it has been recommended that children with any degree of traumatic hematuria undergo renal imaging. Children are more prone to renal injuries than adults because the pediatric kidney is proportionally larger and has less protection from surrounding tissues. However, recent studies have challenged this recommendation. Santucci et al. reviewed 720 pediatric blunt trauma patients and found that the adult criteria would not have missed any significant injuries in this population. He concluded that the decision to image pediatric patients utilizing the adult criteria is appropriate (23).

Most authors advocate radiologic imaging in the setting of penetrating trauma to evaluate for upper urinary tract injuries, as a substantial percentage of patients may have significant injury in the absence of hematuria (1,15). Table 186.2 lists the indications for radiologic evaluation in patients at risk for renal injuries.

Urine dipstick analysis for blood is reliable as a screening test for traumatic hematuria. Daum and associates demonstrated urine dipstick analysis to be 100% sensitive and 58% specific for identifying patients with greater than 5 RBC/HPF by spun urine microscopy (5). Other authors and subsequent studies have confirmed these findings.

Computed tomography (CT) scan has largely supplanted intravenous pyelography (IVP) as the preferred diagnostic

---

TABLE 186.2.   Indications for Radiologic Evaluation of Suspected Renal Injury

Penetrating trauma
Blunt trauma with gross hematuria
Blunt trauma with microscopic hematuria and hemodynamic instability (hypotension or tachycardia)
High-energy deceleration mechanism or suspected associated intra-abdominal injuries

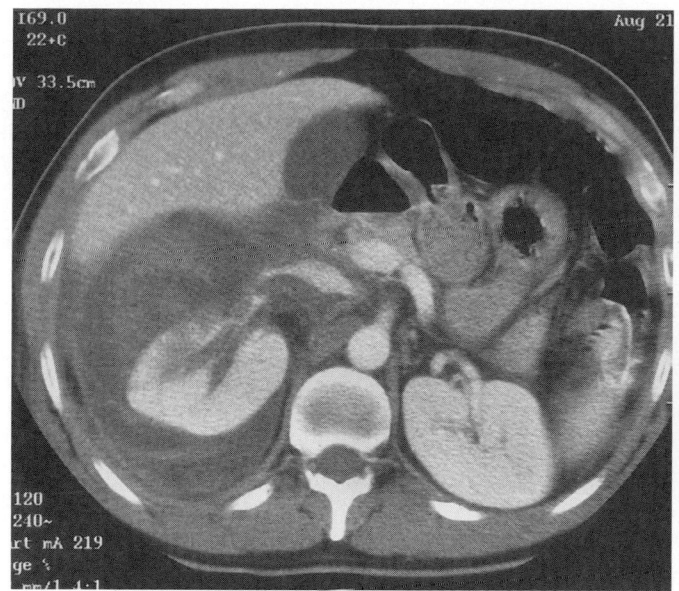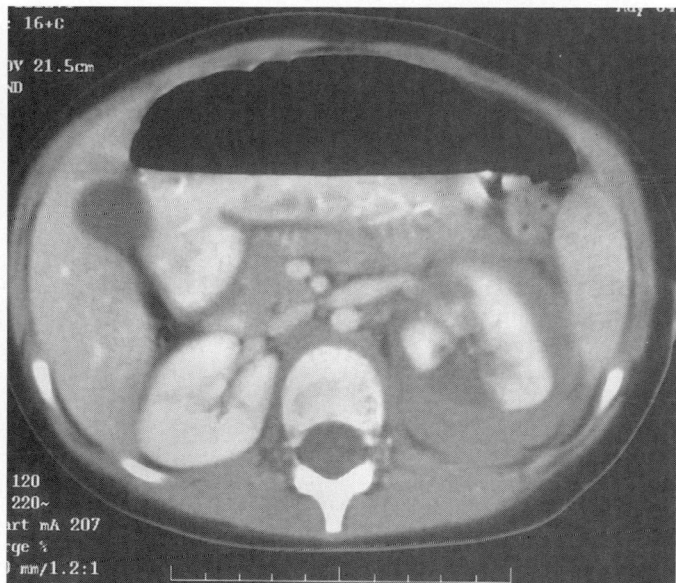

Figure 186.3. **(A,B)** Renal lacerations with perirenal hematoma.

modality for evaluating the hemodynamically stable patient with blunt or penetrating trauma. CT clearly defines parenchymal lacerations, hematomas, and the presence of urinary extravasation and may identify renal vascular injuries (Fig. 186.3). Furthermore, the findings of IVP, when abnormal, are frequently nonspecific and require CT scan to better define the extent of the renal injury (9,10,13). Finally, patients at risk for blunt or penetrating injuries to the upper GU tract usually have sustained a high-energy mechanism and have associated bony, visceral, and vascular injuries. CT scan is required to adequately assess these associated injuries, as well as the GU injury.

The most significant findings on CT scan are either a nonfunctional renal unit or extravasation of urine. Nonfunction suggests extensive trauma to the kidney, pedicle injury, or severely shattered kidney. Extravasation of contrast material implies trauma involving the capsule, parenchyma, and collecting system. Other findings are less reliable and require additional evaluation and staging (1).

In rare circumstances, after penetrating trauma, IVP still has a distinct role in the evaluation of the patient requiring resuscitation or immediate operative intervention who is not stable enough to have an abdominal CT scan. It may be performed in the operating room. A bolus of contrast media is injected intravenously (2 mL/kg to a maximum of 100 mL). An anterior–posterior (AP) abdominal radiograph is then obtained 5 minutes after contrast bolus. In this setting, IVP may confirm the presence of bilateral kidneys, and may suggest the extent of the injury (17).

Arteriography has a very limited role in the evaluation of renal injuries, and is reserved for stable patients requiring further clarification of pedicle injuries. Arteriography may demonstrate intimal tears and complete or partial disruption of the renal vasculature. CT findings requiring further evaluation by arteriography include large perirenal hematomas, major renal fractures, or segmental areas of nonenhancement. Penetrating trauma with renal laceration or retroperitoneal hematoma requires arteriography (or surgical exploration) because of the high risk of associated renal vascular injury. Small hematomas may not require further evaluation. The major limitation of arteriography is the time it takes to perform the test; delays may result in worsening renal ischemia and loss of the kidney. Nonenhance-

ment of the kidney on CT scan is diagnostic of renal artery thrombosis and is sufficient indication for surgery without additional studies.

The role of magnetic resonance imaging (MRI) and ultrasound remains limited. Several studies have suggested that the performance of MRI approximates that of CT scan. The additional time and expense required limit its clinical application (11). Ultrasound has performed poorly in the evaluation of patients with suspected injuries to the upper GU tract (20).

Ureteral injury remains a diagnostic dilemma. A third of ureteral injuries are not identified on initial evaluation. Hematuria is an unreliable indicator for the detection of isolated ureteral injuries (3). If a ureteral injury is suspected, a contrast enhanced helical CT with delayed images or IVP with delayed films should be obtained. Extravasation of contrast visualized on the delayed images may be the only sign of ureteral injury (Fig. 186.4). Retrograde pyelography may be used if the initial studies are inconclusive.

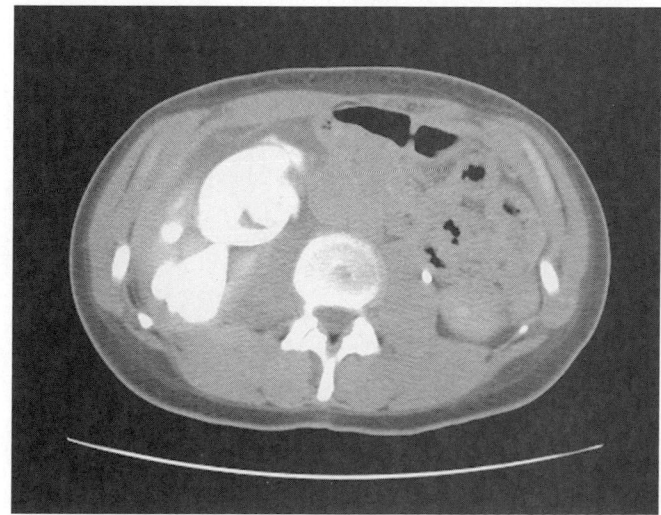

Figure 186.4.   Delayed CT image demonstrating extravasation of contrast diagnostic of ureteral disruption following blunt trauma.

Lower Tract Injury

Genitourinary injuries should be evaluated in a retrograde fashion. Once the potential for injury has been identified based on mechanism of injury, physical findings (i.e., scrotal hematoma, blood at the urethral meatus, or a high-riding prostate), or radiographic evidence of associated high-risk injuries (i.e., pelvic fracture), the urethra should be evaluated first. The presence of urethral injury should be ruled out prior to Foley catheter placement, since catheter placement may potentially convert a partial urethral tear to a complete urethral disruption. A retrograde urethrogram is the diagnostic modality for evaluating the urethra.

A retrograde urethrogram is performed with the patient supine to avoid movement of the patient; oblique views, advocated by some authors, add little and risk disrupting a retroperitoneal hematoma. An initial KUB is obtained for comparison. A Foley catheter is then passed approximately 1 to 2 cm to the fossa navicularis, and the balloon is inflated with 1 to 2 mL of saline. Alternatively a 60-cc Toomey syringe with a Christmas tree or Cooke adapter may be gently inserted until snug. Lateral traction is applied to the penis and 60 mL of water-soluble contrast material is injected over 30 to 60 seconds. The radiograph is exposed as the last 10 mL of contrast material is injected (22). Extravasation of contrast material or failure of contrast material to reach the bladder is diagnostic of urethral injury, mandates urologic consultation, and precludes the passage of a urethral catheter by the emergency physician (Fig. 186.5).

If a team member places a urinary catheter prior to adequate evaluation for urethral injury, *it should not be removed.* It is not necessary to remove the catheter to perform a retrograde urethrogram. Instead, the presence or absence of urethral injury should be documented by passing a small feeding tube beside the catheter and performing a modified retrograde urethrogram (22).

The integrity of the bladder is evaluated with either a retrograde cystogram or computed tomography with retrograde contrast (CT cystogram). A diagnostic work up for bladder injury is indicated for patients with gross hematuria, inability to void, or a pelvic ring fracture in association with microscopic hematuria. After exclusion of urethral injury and placement of catheter, a retrograde cystography is performed by first obtaining a scout KUB for comparison. Then, radiocontrast dye is instilled by gravity through the catheter to a total volume of 400 mL. The Foley catheter is clamped and a full-bladder AP radiograph is performed. If bladder contraction occurs prior to administration of 400 mL, the physician should wait a few minutes and then reintroduce the contrast material to the volume that stimulated contraction previously. An additional 50 mL is gently administered, the catheter is clamped, and a full-bladder AP radiograph is performed (22). Post-void radiographs are performed after allowing the bladder to empty. In the presence of intraperitoneal rupture, contrast material will extravasate, outlining intraperitoneal structures. In the presence of extraperitoneal rupture, contrast material will extravasate at the pubic symphysis or pelvic outlet (Fig. 186.6). A "tear drop" appearance of the bladder is seen when a pelvic hematoma compresses the bladder from the side. Spilling of contrast externally may produce false-positive findings or obscure the findings. Multiple studies have demonstrated false-negative cystography, particularly in penetrating trauma, due to insufficient contrast material (less than 400 cc). Inadequate distention of the bladder may allow a tenuous seal of a penetrating wound, and fail to demonstrate extravasation of contrast (2,22).

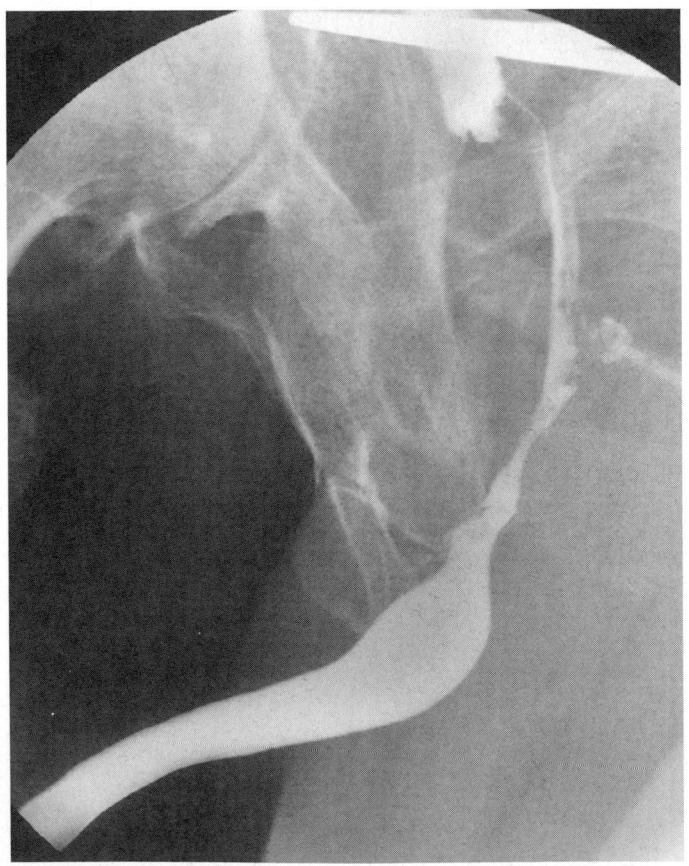

Figure 186.5. Retrograde urethrogram with partial tear of membranous urethra.

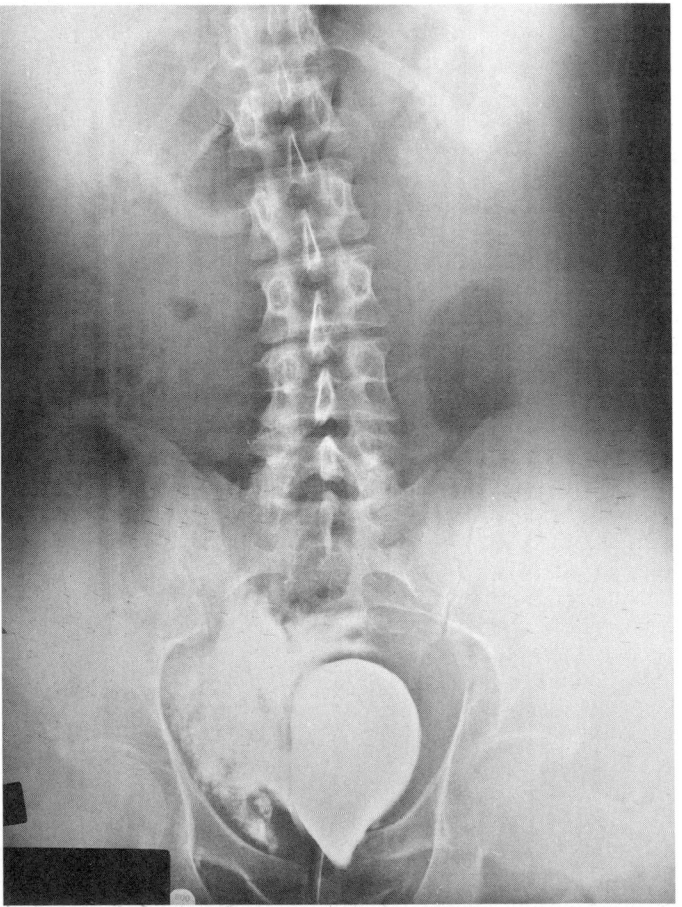

Figure 186.6. Cystogram with extraperitoneal bladder rupture.

A routine CT of the abdomen and pelvis is not sensitive for bladder rupture. However, a CT scan with retrograde contrast (CT cystography) has accuracy comparable to plain film cystography. CT cystography is performed in the same manner as retrograde cystography, with retrograde instillation of 400 mL of dye into the bladder in order to cause bladder distension. In a review of 316 blunt trauma patients with 44 cases of bladder rupture, Deck and colleagues reported a sensitivity of 95% and a specificity of 100% for the detection of bladder rupture with CT cystography and recommended it as the test of choice for patients with other clinical indications for a CT scan of the abdomen and pelvis (6).

External Genitalia Injury

Clinical examination of the scrotum after blunt trauma is often difficult because of severe pain and swelling. If there is a clinical suspicion of a testicular injury, a testicular ultrasound should be performed (19). Since the sensitivity of ultrasound for testicular injury is at best 90%, if the ultrasound is negative and there are clinical findings suggestive of injury, then a urologist should be consulted; operative exploration may be indicated. Any patient with significant external genitalia trauma with hematuria, urinary retention, or pain with urination should have a retrograde urethrogram to evaluate for a urethral tear.

EMERGENCY DEPARTMENT MANAGEMENT

Upper Tract Injury

The principles of care for the patient with multi-system trauma apply to the patient with trauma to the upper GU tract. Airway management, if necessary and hemodynamic stabilization with crystalloid and blood products are the initial priorities. Once immediately life-threatening injuries are addressed, evaluation of the GU tract and associated injuries can occur as outlined in the previous section.

A recent review of over 2,500 trauma patients demonstrated a very strong correlation between AAST renal injury grade and the subsequent need for surgical intervention (24). It is generally accepted that patients with minor renal injuries (grades I and II) may be managed nonoperatively, and patients with Grade V injuries require early surgical intervention. There is disagreement concerning other major injuries (grades III and IV). Several authors have reported series of selective nonoperative management of major renal injuries (9,12,13). In general, the majority of blunt renal trauma may be successfully managed nonoperatively. Delayed interventions may be necessary in a small subset of patients managed nonoperatively. Those most likely to require delayed intervention include patients with extravasation of urine, or devitalized renal segments on initial CT scan. Recent advances in percutaneous and endourologic techniques have decreased the morbidity of these complications (2).

There is a lower threshold for operative exploration and intervention after penetrating trauma. Most penetrating injuries are explored and repaired. Ureteral injuries are repaired surgically and stented or repaired in a staged fashion (1).

Lower Tract Injuries

If a urethral disruption is identified, urologic consultation should be obtained and a suprapubic cystostomy should be performed to allow drainage of the bladder. This may be performed in the resuscitation bay if the patient is stable. If the patient is unstable and requires operative intervention for associated injuries, it can be performed in the operating room. If a catheter was placed prior to identifying the injury, it should be left in place. Occasionally, a catheter may be placed through a partial urethral tear. Once the partial disruption is identified, however, any gentle and limited attempts at urethral catheterization should be done by a urologist.

The acute management of bladder rupture is bladder drainage via Foley catheter. Patients with intraperitoneal bladder rupture undergo primary surgical repair. Those patients with extraperitoneal bladder rupture are typically managed nonoperatively, with simple urinary drainage by Foley catheter or cystostomy. However, if the patient is undergoing exploratory laparotomy for another indication, some authors advocate primary repair at that time (2).

External Genitalia Injury

Diagnosis of testicular rupture or dislocation should prompt urgent urologic consultation, as surgical repair within 72 hours dramatically improves the salvage rate.

There have been several reported cases of microvascular reimplantation following amputation of the penis. Successful repair depends on the condition of the severed part and the ischemia time. In the prehospital and emergency setting, the amputated penis should be preserved in a manner similar to that for other amputated parts. Prompt urologic and microvascular consultation is imperative for successful reimplantation (26). Penetrating trauma to the external genitalia mandates early surgical exploration and conservative debridement; this is followed by primary repair in most cases (4). Some authors have also advocated operative repair of penile fractures, proposing that it decreases the incidence of erectile deformity and may speed recovery. There is, however, no accepted standard of treatment (21). For patients with penile zipper entrapment, Nolan and associates described the successful atraumatic removal by cutting the median bar of the zipper with bone cutters. The upper and lower shields of the zipper device separate, releasing the skin with minimal injury (14). Penile incarceration may be managed by the string technique, similar to that described for removal of rings from fingers (25).

CRITICAL INTERVENTIONS

- Address immediately life-threatening injuries first. If the patient is hemodynamically unstable, evaluation of the genitourinary system can be performed after operative intervention for other injuries (i.e., intraperitoneal injuries)
- Rule out a urethral injury by clinical exam, and retrograde urethrogram if necessary, before placement of a Foley catheter
- Obtain an urgent urology consultation if testicular disruption is diagnosed
- Perform a vaginal exam in all female patients with pelvic fractures

DISPOSITION

The majority of patients with blunt renal injuries will require admission to the hospital. Select patients with microscopic hematuria in the absence of any hemodynamic instability, and no associated injuries, may be discharged with a follow up repeat urinalysis in 1 week to ensure resolution. All patients with penetrating renal or ureteral trauma require admission or transfer to a facility capable of providing definitive diagnostic and therapeutic care. Disposition following trauma to the external genitalia depends on the complexity and severity of the injury as well as any associated injuries. Many of these patients will require a urology consultation in the ED or close outpatient urology follow up.

COMMON PITFALLS

✔ Failure to consider upper tract injury in the absence of hematuria. Patients with renal pedicle injury resulting from a deceleration mechanism or ureteral injury resulting from penetrating trauma may not have hematuria

✔ Delaying an urgent laparotomy to perform further diagnostic imaging of the genitourinary tract

✔ Ruling out significant injury following penetrating trauma to the flank based on a suboptimal local wound exploration. If the wound is in anatomic proximity to the GU tract, the patient requires further diagnostic evaluation

✔ Attempting to rule out bladder injury with routine abdominal CT without adequate distension of the bladder (i.e., instillation of 400 mL of contrast dye)

Acknowledgments

Thanks to the previous edition's chapter authors B. Tilman Jolly and Scott D. Weir.

References

1. Baniel J, Schein M. The management of penetrating trauma to the urinary tract. *J Am Coll Surg* 1994;178:417.
2. Bodner DR, Selzman AA, Spirnak JP. Evaluation and treatment of bladder rupture. *Semin Urol* 1995;13:62.
3. Campbell EW, Filderman PS, Jacobs SC. Ureteral injury due to blunt and penetrating trauma. *Urology* 1992;40:216.
4. Cline KJ, Mata JA, Venable DD, et al. Penetrating trauma to the male external genitalia. *J Trauma* 1998;44:492.
5. Daum GS, Krolikowski FJ, Reuter KL, et al. Dipstick evaluation of hematuria in abdominal trauma. *Am J Clin Pathol* 1988;89:538.
6. Deck AJ, Shaves S, Talner L, et al. Computed tomography cystography for the diagnosis of traumatic bladder rupture. *J Urol* 2000;164:43.
7. Eastham JA, Wilson TG, Ahlering TE. Radiographic assessment of blunt renal trauma. *J Trauma* 1991;31:1527.
8. Goldman HB, Idom CB, Dmochowski RR. Traumatic Injuries of the Female External Genitalia and their Association with Urological Injuries. *J Urol* 1998;159:956.
9. Goff CD, Colin GR. Management of renal trauma at a rural, level 1 trauma center. *Am Surg* 1998;64:226.
10. Herschorn S, Radomski SB, Shoskes DA, et al. Evaluation and treatment of blunt renal trauma. *J Urol* 1991;146:274.
11. Leppaniemi A, Lamminen A, Tervahartiala P, et al. Comparison of high-field magnetic resonance imaging with computed tomography in the evaluation of blunt renal trauma. *J Trauma* 1995;38:420.
12. Mansi MK, Alkhudair WK. Conservative management with percutaneous intervention of major blunt renal injuries. *Am J Emerg Med* 1997;15:633.
13. Matthews LA, Smith EM, Spirnak JP. Nonoperative treatment of major blunt renal lacerations with urinary extravasation. *J Urol* 1997;157:2056.
14. Mee SL, McAninch JW, Robinson AL, et al. Radiographic assessment of renal trauma: a 10-year prospective study of patient selection. *J Urol* 1989;141:1095.
15. Miller KS, McAninch JW. Radiographic assessment of renal trauma: our 15 year experience. *J Urol* 1995;154:352.
16. Moore EE, Shockford SR, Pachter HL, et al. Organ injury scaling: spleen, liver and kidney. *J Trauma* 1989;29:1664.
17. Morey AF. McAninch JW, Tiller BK, Duckett CP, Carroll PR. Single Shot Intraoperative Excretory Urography for the Immediate Evaluation of Renal Trauma. *J Urol* 1999;161:1088.
18. Nolan JF, Stillwell TJ, Sands JP Jr. Acute management of the zipper-entrapped penis. *J Emerg Med* 1990;8:305.
19. Pantil MG, Onora VC. The value of ultrasound in the evaluation of patients with blunt scrotal trauma. *Injury* 1994;25:177.
20. Perry MJ, Porte ME, Urwin GH. Limitations of ultrasound evaluation in closed renal trauma. *J R Coll Surg Edinb* 1997;42:420.
21. Ruckle HC, Hadley HR, Lui PD. Fracture of penis: diagnosis and management. *Urology* 1992;40:33.
22. Schneider RE. Genitourinary trauma. *Emerg Med Clin North Am* 1993;11:137.
23. Santucci RA, Langernburg SE, Zachareas MJ. Traumatic Hematuria in Children can be Evaluated as in Adults. *J Urol* 2004;171:822.
24. Santucci RA, McAninch JW, Safir M, et al. Validation of the American Association for the Surgery of Trauma Organ Injury Severity Scale for the Kidney. *J Trauma* 2001;50:195.
25. Vahasarja VJ, Hellstrom PA, Serlo W, et al. Treatment of penile incarceration by the string method: two case reports. *J Urol* 1993;149:372.
26. Wells MD, Boyd JB, Bulbul MA Penile Replantation. *Ann Plast Surg* 1991;26:577.

CHAPTER 187
Peripheral Vascular Injuries

Peter T. Pons

Prompt recognition and management of peripheral vascular injuries are crucial to limb salvage and preservation of function. Penetrating trauma accounts for approximately 85% of vascular injuries in the United States; blunt trauma and iatrogenic causes are responsible for the rest. Until the advent and widespread use of antibiotics, these wounds were treated by ligation or amputation. Once infection could be controlled, the previously developed methods of primary vessel repair were applied and are now the mainstay of management.

Vascular injury may result from direct or indirect trauma. Direct injury may produce partial or complete transection, contusion, laceration, or arteriovenous fistula. Indirect injury may cause spasm, external compression, mural contusion, thrombosis, or aneurysm formation. The vessels most often involved are the brachial and axillary arteries in the upper extremity and the femoral and popliteal arteries in the lower extremity.

Vascular damage should be suspected in penetrating trauma when the penetrating object has traversed the path of a vessel or is in proximity to one. Blunt vascular injury may be more subtle in presentation. Stretching, tearing, or shearing forces may damage a vessel, yet leave little external evidence. The classic example is dislocation of the knee, with associated popliteal artery injury. Often there are few visual clues indicating vascular injury. Failure to recognize this complication frequently leads to amputation of the leg, which can be prevented by appropriate evaluation. The emergency physician must obtain a careful, complete history and be aware of the mechanics that produce vascular injury, even if there are minimal or absent physical findings that suggest vessel damage.

CLINICAL PRESENTATION

The most obvious visible sign of arterial injury is profuse, spurting red blood. Venous laceration may be manifested by a continuous flow of dark blood, which also may be profuse. Significant blood loss may produce shock. However, many vascular injuries, either blunt or penetrating in origin, appear relatively innocuous at first glance. Penetrating wounds of an extremity can present with a small entrance site that harbors significant underlying vascular damage. Blunt injury may be quite misleading because of minimal obvious external signs. The vessel wound, either arterial or venous, may produce a significant soft tissue hematoma. Occasionally, a pulsatile mass is felt or a rapidly expanding hematoma is noted.

The absence of a palpable pulse distal to the site of injury in a normotensive patient is pathognomonic of vessel injury. However, the presence of a pulse does not exclude a significant wound. Collateral circulation or transmitted pressure waves through a small clot or intimal flap can produce a distal pulse, misleading the physician. A patient in shock must have repeated examinations of the peripheral pulse to assess vascular status, as the physical findings may change once the patient is resuscitated.

The presence of a palpable thrill or bruit suggests an arteriovenous fistula.

Classic signs of arterial compromise of an extremity have been described as "the five P's": pallor, pulselessness, pain, paresthesias, and paralysis. Additional findings may include tenseness of the extremity, coolness to touch, and delayed capillary refill (greater than 3 seconds). Unfortunately, some of these signs require a patient who can relate these complaints, and many multiply injured patients cannot. In addition, concomitant neurologic injury of the extremity may present with similar findings. Careful examination is necessary to differentiate the paresthesias of vascular insufficiency from those of neurologic injury. As many as 70% of upper and 30% of lower extremity vascular injuries have associated nerve damage, of which 40% to 45% result in permanent deficit.

Doppler examination of distal blood flow can assist in the evaluation of patients with swelling, hematoma, displaced fractures, or obesity. Pulse deficits and limb comparisons can be performed with greater sensitivity using the Doppler device.

Finally, the structural integrity of the skeletal system must be evaluated. About 18% of patients with peripheral vascular injuries have an associated fracture.

A growing body of literature documents the importance and value of the physical examination, including Doppler blood pressure index, in determining the presence or absence of a peripheral vascular injury (6,7,13).

EMERGENCY DEPARTMENT EVALUATION

The first step in the evaluation of a patient with suspected peripheral vascular injury is the assessment of the physical examination and the determination of whether or not the so-called "hard" signs of vascular injury are present (Fig. 187.1). These include pulsatile hemorrhage, expanding or pulsatile hematoma, bruits or thrills, or a combination of the findings of the "five Ps." Immediate surgery is indicated if the peripheral pulse is absent, obvious "hard" signs of major vessel injury are present, or the location of the injury is apparent from physical examination. In these cases, operative intervention should not be delayed for other diagnostic studies or radiographic imaging, unless the location of the vessel injury cannot be determined clinically (10).

Further diagnostic evaluation is warranted for patients with so-called "soft" signs of peripheral vascular injury. These include patients with diminished (but present) pulses, large hematomas that are not expanding or pulsatile, peripheral nerve injury, and delayed capillary refill.

Measurement and comparison of systolic blood pressure using a Doppler (Doppler pressure index or DPI) is extremely helpful in evaluating for the potential arterial injury (14). Doppler blood pressure at the ankle or wrist of the injured extremity is compared to the Doppler blood pressure at the brachial artery of an uninjured arm. If the ratio of the blood pressures (injured extremity over uninjured extremity) is less than 0.9, vascular injury is suggested (14,19) and arteriography is indicated.

The mainstay of evaluation and diagnosis has been contrast arteriography. Angiography has been used in patients with so-called "soft signs" of vascular injury and in those with wound trajectories in proximity to a major vessel but without obvious signs of damage. Arteriography is 97% to 99% sensitive in detecting arterial injury.

Digital subtraction angiography has also been used with significant success to evaluate vascular injuries. This study may be performed by either intravenous or intraarterial injection. This technique appears to be more sensitive in detecting extravasation of contrast material, whereas conventional arteriography is better for subtle findings, such as intimal disruption. Digital subtraction studies require a cooperative patient who can remain still, as it is very sensitive to motion artifact.

Studies have focused on the need for angiography in patients without obvious physical signs (including Doppler pressure index) of vessel injury, "soft signs" of injury, and in those with "proximity" wounds (2,3,5–8,14,17,20,25). Several studies have shown that surgically important lesions in these patients are rare and that most of these patients do not need surgery. Instead of angiography, serial physical examination with Doppler measurement of blood pressures in the injured extremity compared with an uninjured extremity (5–8,13–15), and in some cases evaluation with color-flow duplex Doppler ultrasonography (2,3,9,17,20) have been advocated as the primary methods of evaluation in this select group of patients. Color-flow duplex Doppler ultrasonography interprets the sound of blood flow and shows it as red and blue colors based on the speed and direction of the flow relative to the ultrasound probe. This sonographic technique will

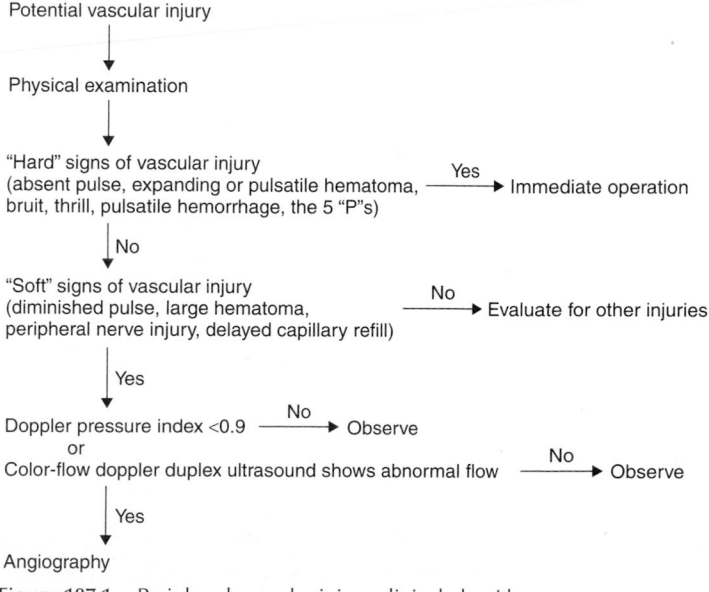

Figure 187.1. Peripheral vascular injury clinical algorithm.

easily demonstrate absence of arterial flow but is less valuable for more subtle injuries such as intimal flaps or pseudoaneurysms which may not interrupt blood flow in the damaged vessel (2). Lastly, preliminary work utilizing spiral computed tomographic angiography and magnetic resonance angiography has demonstrated that both imaging modalities can be used to diagnose vascular injury, however the clinical application and utility of both remain limited (11,12,16,21,22,35).

Shotgun wounds to an extremity have a much higher incidence of vascular injury due to the nature of the weapon (i.e., multiple missiles and multiple trajectories) (5,20). Therefore, angiography is indicated in these patients unless the physical examination, including DPI, suggests that the potential for vascular injury is remote. If angiography is not performed, a period of observation is warranted.

Special mention must be made of knee dislocation and the potential for associated popliteal artery injury. Traditional teaching has been that all patients presenting with a knee dislocation must undergo arteriography to rule out popliteal artery injury as there is a high rate of amputation if the injury is missed. Recent work indicates that physical examination, including DPI, can be used to reliably determine which patients should undergo immediate angiographic study and which patients can be observed (18,23).

Each institution should determine in advance how it plans to evaluate patients with potential peripheral vascular trauma by having protocols in place agreed upon by the emergency medicine and surgery departments.

EMERGENCY DEPARTMENT MANAGEMENT

Prehospital and emergency department (ED) management priorities include control of hemorrhage, fluid resuscitation, and assessment and management of other life threats (15).

Hemorrhage should be controlled by direct pressure over the bleeding site. Blind clamping of bleeding vessels deep in a wound is to be condemned, as adjacent structures such as nerves and tendons may be crushed in the attempt to stop hemorrhage (5). If a bleeding vessel can be identified and isolated, it may be clamped using a noncrushing vascular clamp. Recent work in animals suggests that hemostatic agents may be of benefit in controlling exsanguinating hemorrhage secondary to proximal vascular injury such as femoral artery or vein injury in the groin (1). This may be particularly important in the prehospital setting. Fluid restoration is accomplished by initiating one or more intravenous lines (as the trauma mechanism and vital signs dictate) and infusing crystalloid. After bleeding is controlled and resuscitation started, a careful examination for other life-threatening injuries is performed. As with all trauma patients, a patent airway and adequate ventilation must be ensured while circulation is being addressed. Vascular injuries are treated after other potential life-threats have been assessed and managed.

Angulated fractures associated with pulse deficits should be anatomically repositioned and splinted. This may restore perfusion to an ischemic extremity.

Blood for type and crossmatch should be sent to the laboratory, and appropriate preparations made for transfusion if blood loss or anticipated surgical needs indicate. Unless indications for immediate surgery are present, complete evaluation for possible vascular injury should follow.

Tetanus immunization status should be ascertained and the patient immunized, if necessary. Prophylactic antibiotics are indicated when operative repair or vascular grafts are to be undertaken, and if there is an open fracture. Anticoagulants should generally not be given until surgical consultation has been obtained, the absence of other major injuries has been determined, and the patient is ready to undergo arterial repair.

CRITICAL INTERVENTIONS

- Control hemorrhage by using direct pressure over the bleeding site
- Resuscitate with crystalloid infusion and blood when indicated
- After bleeding is controlled, perform a general examination for other life-threatening injuries
- Measure the Doppler pressure index in all patients with penetrating extremity trauma
- Reduce angulated fractures associated with pulse deficits immediately

DISPOSITION

Surgical consultation must be obtained as early as possible, as the amount of time elapsed from injury until operative repair is a crucial determinant of successful repair and decreased morbidity in the ischemic extremity. Endovascular embolization may be an option for treatment of nonessential vessels in select situations. Observation for a period of 12 to 24 hours is appropriate for patients without obvious signs of vessel injury and normal Doppler pressure index. In fact, one study suggests that asymptomatic patients with a DPI ≥ 1.0 may be safely discharged from the ED (4). If surgical intervention or arteriography is unavailable in the primary receiving institution, the patient should be transferred as soon as possible, after appropriate stabilizing procedures have been performed, to a facility capable of providing the necessary therapy.

COMMON PITFALLS

✔ Failure to realize that vascular injuries may be subtle in origin and misleading on physical examination
✔ Failure to appreciate injury mechanics or vessel proximity to a penetrating wound
✔ Failure to recognize that delays in diagnosis of vascular compromise may lead to permanent deficit or loss of the limb
✔ Blind clamping of bleeding vessels deep in a wound

References

1. Alam HB, Uy GB, Miller D, et al. Comparative analysis of hemostatic agents in a swine model of lethal groin injury. *J Trauma* 2003;54:1077–1082.
2. Bergstein JM, Blair JF, Edwards J, et al. Pitfalls in the use of color-flow duplex ultrasound for screening of suspected arterial injuries in penetrated extremities. *J Trauma* 1992;33:395–402.
3. Bynoe RP, Miles WS, Bell RM, et al. Noninvasive diagnosis of vascular trauma by duplex ultrasonography. *J Vasc Surg* 1991;14:346–352.
4. Conrad MF, Patton JH Jr, Parikshak M, et al. Evaluation of vascular injury in penetrating extremity trauma: Angiographers stay home. *Amer Surg* 2002;68:269–274.
5. Dennis JW, Frykberg ER, Crump JM, et al. New perspectives on the management of penetrating trauma in proximity to major limb arteries. *J Vasc Surg* 1990;11:84–93.
6. Dennis JW, Frykberg ER, Veldenz HC, et al. Validation of nonoperative management of occult vascular injuries and accuracy of physical examination alone in penetrating extremity trauma: 5- to 10-year follow-up. *J Trauma* 1998;44:243–253.
7. Francis H, Thal ER, Weigelt JA, et al. Vascular proximity: is it a valid indication for arteriography in asymptomatic patients? *J Trauma* 1991;31:512–514.
8. Frykberg ER, Dennis JW, Bishop K, et al. The reliability of physical examination in the evaluation of penetrating extremity trauma for vascular injury: results at 1 year. *J Trauma* 1991;31:502–511.
9. Gagne PJ, Cone JB, McFarland D, et al. Proximity penetrating extremity trauma: the role of duplex ultrasound in the detection of occult venous injuries. *J Trauma* 1995;39:1157–1163.
10. Gonzalez RP, Falimirski ME. The utility of physical examination in proximity penetrating extremity trauma. *Amer Surg* 1999;65:784–789.
11. Grainger ML, Wilson CH, Augustine SJ, et al. Radiologic Case Study. Traumatic Dislocation of the knee. *Orthopaedics* 2003;26:351–354.
12. James CA. Magnetic resonance angiography in trauma. *Clin Neurosci* 1997;4:137–145.

13. Johansen K, Lynch K, Paun M, et al. Non-invasive vascular tests reliably exclude occult arterial trauma in injured extremities. *J Trauma* 1991;31:515–522.
14. Lynch K, Johansen K. Can Doppler pressure measurement replace "exclusion" arteriography in the diagnosis of occult extremity arterial trauma? *Ann Surg* 1991;214:737–741.
15. Modrall JG, Weaver FA, Yellin AE. Diagnosis and management of penetrating vascular trauma and the injured extremity. *Emerg Med Clin North Am* 1998;16:129–144.
16. Nunez D Jr, Rivas L, McKenney K, et al. Helical CT of traumatic arterial injuries. *Am J Roentgenol* 1998;179:1621–1626.
17. Ordog GJ, Balasubramanium S, Wasserberger J, et al. Extremity gunshot wounds. Part 1: identification and treatment of patients at high risk of vascular injury. *J Trauma* 1994;36:358–368.
18. Pretre R, Bruschweiler I, Rossier J, et al. Lower limb trauma with injury to the popliteal vessels. *J Trauma* 1996;40:595–601.
19. Schwartz MR, Weaver FA, Bauer M, et al. Refining the indications for arteriography in penetrating extremity trauma: a prospective analysis. *J Vasc Surg* 1993;17:116–124.
20. Schwartz M, Weaver F, Yellin A, et al. The utility of color-flow Doppler examination in penetrating extremity arterial trauma. *Am Surg* 1993;59:375–378.
21. Soto JA, Munera F, Cardoso N, et al. Diagnostic performance of helical CT angiography in trauma to large arteries of the extremities. *J Comput Assist Tomogr* 1999;23:188–196.
22. Soto JA, Munera F, Morales C, et al. Focal arterial injuries of the proximal extremities: Helical CT arteriography as the initial method of diagnosis. *Radiology* 2001;218:188–194.
23. Treiman GS, Yellin AE, Weavver FA, et al. Examination of the patient with knee dislocation: The case for selective arteriography. *Arch Surg* 1992;127:1056–1062.
24. Weaver FA, Yellin AE, Bauer M, et al. Is arterial proximity a valid indication for arteriography in penetrating extremity trauma? *Arch Surg* 1990;125:1256–1260.
25. Yaquinto JJ, Harms SE, Siemers PT, et al. Arterial injury from penetrating trauma: Evaluation with single acquisition fat-suppressed MR imaging. *Am J Roentgenol* 1992;158:631–633.

Orthopaedic Trauma

CHAPTER 188

Approach to Musculoskeletal Injuries

Andrew D. Perron

Musculoskeletal injury has been cited as the second most common reason for emergency department (ED) visits in the United States (9). Additionally, missed fracture has been cited as a common reason for medical malpractice lawsuits against emergency physicians (5). A coherent and systematic approach to the assessment and management of patients with orthopaedic injuries and other musculoskeletal complaints is essential. Musculoskeletal injuries range from mild (tendinosis, sprains, strains, and contusions) to potentially life- and limb-threatening trauma (pelvis fracture, femur fracture, knee dislocation). Most of the time, acute trauma is responsible for the presenting complaints; and usually the primary impairment is an inability to move a part of the body due to pain or discomfort. The mechanisms of trauma include sports injuries, assaults, motor vehicle crashes, falls in the home, and industrial catastrophes. When acute trauma is absent, overuse syndromes or repetitive movements are often the culprit.

The immediate tasks of the emergency physician evaluating a patient with a musculoskeletal complaint include:

- Accurately determining those injuries that need only symptomatic care and distinguishing them from ones that require more complex, timely specialist intervention.
- Differentiating injuries that can be handled solely by an emergency physician (the vast majority of musculoskeletal injuries) from those that require emergent consultation or timely referral to an orthopaedic surgeon (e.g., open fractures, compartment syndrome, growth plate injuries, and flexor tendon injuries).
- Formulating a logical, cost-effective algorithm for the diagnosis and management of each patient.
- Aggressively managing the pain associated with these injuries early and effectively, recognizing, for example, that "a mere contusion" can be the source of exquisite pain.

- Recognizing that care for many musculoskeletal injuries is not complete when emergency care has been delivered. Successful management of the patient is only complete when appropriate follow-up has been arranged, as a large percentage of acute musculoskeletal injuries require reevaluation and ongoing care (e.g., physical therapy and rehabilitation) for optimal recovery.

CLINICAL PRESENTATION

Sprains

A sprain is a ligamentous injury. Ligaments link bone to bone. Damage to the fibers of the ligament range from microscopic damage to complete disruption. A sprain can result from an abnormal (nonbiomechanical) force vector applied to a joint, an excessive force applied along a normal vector, or a combination of the two mechanisms. The phrase "just a sprain" is probably best relegated to the past; it is possible to sustain a sprain that is significantly more severe than an analogous fracture. For example, a complete lateral ankle ligament rupture and a transverse avulsion fracture of the distal fibula cause the same pattern of instability. However, because bone regenerates without scarring, the outcome for the latter injury is usually much better. The grading of sprains is based on the severity of the damage, recognizing that with an acute injury, there may be too much pain and spasm to accurately determine the grade of the sprain:

(1) *Grade I sprain:* A grade I sprain (in older terminology, "first-degree") represents microscopic tears of the ligament, which lead to localized hemorrhage and inflammation as the healing process evolves. Active range of motion is usually preserved but painful. Abnormal movement of the joint stabilized by the sprained ligament is not elicited by stress maneuvers, but these maneuvers may produce focal pain and the area overlying the sprained ligament is tender to palpation.

(2) *Grade II sprain:* In a grade II sprain ("second-degree") or partial tear, the overall architecture of the ligament is preserved, with the majority of fibers still in continuity, but some of them have been completely ruptured. Hemorrhage is more extensive and swelling is pronounced. Loss of function secondary to decreased and painful range of motion is the hallmark. When the joint that the ligament stabilizes is stressed, there may be some gapping of the joint or abnormal motion. However, frank instability does not occur and a clearly defined end point is reached.

(3) *Grade III sprain:* A grade III sprain ("third-degree") denotes a complete tear of the ligament and is synonymous with a complete rupture. Hemorrhage is more extensive and healing

involves the formation of scar tissue in the area between the fragments of the ligament. Stressing the joint reveals greater gapping than in the case of a grade II sprain, and frank instability without a well-defined end point may be elicited. This frank instability can be summed up by the examiner's thought, "I should stop stressing this joint, as it isn't going to resist my efforts." This is tempered by the knowledge that with acute injury, the physical examination may be severely limited due to acute pain and muscular spasm.

Common ligament sprains seen in the ED include lateral ankle sprains, injuries to the anterior cruciate and collateral ligaments of the knee, and ligamentous injuries of the shoulder, associated with either glenohumeral dislocations or acromioclavicular separations.

The clinical signs of a sprain typically include point tenderness to palpation, swelling, painful or decreased range of motion, and ecchymosis. A complete sprain, with no fibers in continuity, may be completely pain-free when stressed. Often, athletes will continue to play after a grade III sprain of the medial collateral ligament of the knee, but it is rare that they continue activities after a grade II sprain. In fact, pain may be inversely proportional to the severity of the injury. A grade I sprain is extremely painful when stressed, as there are many intact but damaged and inflamed fibers that will be stretched, triggering the discharge of pain fibers as the ligament is loaded with force. With a grade III sprain, the same maneuver does not cause any stretching of the ligament, as it cannot be loaded by force and the only pain fibers triggered by the stress maneuver will lie in surrounding soft tissue. Bone can be injured at the same time as a ligament is damaged. For example, grade III sprains of the medial, deltoid ligament of the ankle are often accompanied by fibula fractures. Bony evidence of sprains on x-ray includes small avulsion fractures at the point of insertion of the ligament into the bone, impaction injuries, and simple joint-space widening.

Strains

Tendons connect muscles to bone. A strain is an injury to this musculotendinous unit, which can range from mild "pulled muscles" to complete tendon ruptures. The mechanisms of injury are twofold: (1) stretching a muscle beyond its normal range of motion by forced extension ("overstretching injury") and (2) tearing of muscle or tendon fibers by a violent, uncontrolled contraction or repetitive, prolonged contractions, often in attempted compensation for an unexpected change in direction of movement, unanticipated variations in terrain, or a sudden force applied to the antagonist muscle group (an "overexertion injury").

Strains are graded from first-degree to third-degree, reflecting the severity of damage:

- In a first-degree strain, microscopic damage occurs to the musculotendinous unit, with associated localized hemorrhage, inflammation, and tenderness to palpation. Active range of motion is often unrestricted, but pain can be elicited by resisted contraction or forced extension of the muscle group.
- A second-degree strain involves more severe damage, with rupture of some fibers of the muscle or tendon. Hemorrhage is usually visible, swelling more severe, and range of motion limited by pain.
- In a third-degree strain, the muscle or tendon is completely ruptured. The rupture can occur in the muscle belly, at the musculotendinous junction, within the tendon itself, or at the point of insertion of the tendon into bone.

Common strains seen in the ED include those to the quadriceps, hamstring, and rotator cuff muscles; "groin pulls"; and Achilles tendon ruptures.

The clinical signs of a strain include pain, ecchymosis, edema, and decreased or painful range of motion. With complete disruption of the muscle or tendon, a palpable defect is often present. Physical examination should include inspection of the injured area, observation of active and passive range of motion, palpation of the affected area, and provocative maneuvers (either resisted contraction or passive stretching) to elicit the location and extent of injury. In addition, with certain suspected injuries, specific tests should be performed. For example, if an Achilles' tendon rupture is suspected, then a Thompson test is performed. While the patient lies prone with his or her foot and ankle hanging off the end of the stretcher, the examiner squeezes the calf on the affected side and observes whether the foot plantar flexes in response to the calf being squeezed. The presence of plantar flexion indicates an Achilles' tendon that is at least partially intact.

Contusions

A contusion is a bruise caused by a direct blow to a body part. Contusions can occur to bone, with significant pain from periosteal bruising and bone edema, or, more commonly, to soft tissue, especially fat and muscle. In these crush injuries, the degree of injury is proportional to the force of the blow and the surface area of impact. Tissue damage occurs as the energy transmitted by the impact dissipates into or is absorbed by surrounding structures.

The diagnosis of contusion is one of exclusion, with fracture, sprain, and strain being the most important diagnoses that must be ruled out. Common contusions seen in the ED include bruised quadriceps muscles, rib cage contusions, contusions of the ulnar aspect of the forearm in "defensive maneuvers" during an assault, and direct blows to the anterior tibia.

Either the blow itself or the body's reaction to it causes signs and symptoms that prompt the patient to seek emergency care. Typically, they include pain, swelling, ecchymosis, and decreased range of motion of the affected part.

Usually, the entities that are ruled out (e.g., fracture, sprain, and strain) are potentially more serious than the diagnosis of contusion itself. However, the clinician must remember that contusions can lead to serious complications, including severe pain, rhabdomyolysis, compartment syndrome, and *myositis ossificans.*

Severe pain: One of the most common reasons that patients seek reevaluation in an emergency room is inadequate analgesia following a soft-tissue injury. Initial attention to adequate analgesia ensures patient comfort and decreases the need for reevaluation. A number of studies have confirmed that physicians notoriously under-treat painful conditions. This is particularly true in both the pediatric and geriatric patient populations.

Rhabdomyolysis: Severe muscle breakdown can occur after strenuous exercise without an acute, isolated injury or after a significant contusion to a muscle body. Rhabdomyolysis results from the destruction of myocyte cell membrane integrity. The subsequent release of intracellular contents, including potassium, myoglobin, uric acid, phosphate, and the enzyme creatine kinase, into the bloodstream can result in a number of systemic complications, including metabolic abnormalities and acute renal failure. The emergency physician must assess the extent of tissue involvement, the degree of tissue destruction, and the potential for systemic complications. If rhabdomyolysis is suspected, urinalysis should be performed to look for evidence of myoglobinuria (dipstick positive for blood without microscopic evidence of erythrocytes), and the serum creatine kinase level should be checked (see Chapter 168, "Rhabdomyolysis" for details.)

Compartment syndrome: Compartment syndrome occurs when pressure within soft tissues in a fixed body compartment increases to the point at which it compromises venous blood flow and limits capillary perfusion. This leads to muscle ischemia and necrosis. Most commonly associated with long-bone fractures, it can occur in the setting of severe contusion, crush injury, or excessive exertion and must be considered in any patient with pain out of proportion to physical findings or with swelling causing obvious tautness in a nonexpansible compartment, such as the anterior tibial compartment. When this diagnosis is considered, it must be objectively ruled out by manometry (see Chapter 199 for details.)

Myositis ossificans: Severe hemorrhage into a muscle can initiate a cascade of "healing," which can lead to the formation of ectopic bone within the muscle. A large number of these cases have occurred in athletes treated with early, aggressive nonsteroidal antiinflammatory drugs (NSAIDs), heat, massage, and physical therapy in the hope of facilitating early return to athletic competition. This is of concern to the emergency physician for a number of reasons. If severe quadriceps tear and resultant hemorrhage and ecchymosis are suspected, the initial management should include ice, a brief period (24 hours) of immobilization in a stretched position (knee flexed to 120 degrees for severe quadriceps contusion), and acetaminophen, instead of NSAIDs, for pain control. This regimen limits the ongoing bleeding and inflammation in the area. These patients must be referred for appropriate long-term followup care. In addition, a patient's complaint of decreased range of motion, ongoing pain, and a mass or firmness in soft tissue weeks to months after sustaining a contusion should suggest the possibility of *myositis ossificans*. A soft-tissue x-ray is the best way to evaluate for heterotopic bony formation. If heterotopic bone is present, the patient should be referred to an orthopaedic surgeon for close followup care and potential resection of the bone when it has matured (usually at 9 to 12 months).

Fractures

Most fractures require urgent medical attention. Without appropriate emergency care, many will not heal properly or healing will be accompanied by unnecessary complications. A *fracture* is defined as a partial or complete break in a bone. Bone is unique in that it is the only tissue in the human body, other than the liver, that heals by regeneration, not by scarring (1,8,10). For regeneration to occur, however, the bone must be immobilized to allow uninterrupted formation of new bone. Ensuring appropriate immobilization is one of the fundamental tasks of the emergency physician when dealing with musculoskeletal problems.

The process of new bone formation begins with hematoma bridging the realigned fracture fragments. Hematopoietic cells in the hematoma secrete growth factors, which stimulate the formation of granulation tissue at the fracture ends, resulting in slow resorption of the hematoma. Over the next several weeks, a primary callus is formed, beginning as a soft callus and progressing to a hard callus. The final phase of healing is remodeling, during which the bone reassumes its original architecture as it is exposed to the normal stresses of weight bearing and movement (1,10).

Fractures also require immediate attention for several other reasons. Virtually all fractures are painful. The vast majority of fractures result from high-energy trauma (relative to sprains, strains, and contusions) and, because of force vectors, are accompanied by well-known associated injuries (e.g., 15% of calcaneal fractures sustained in a fall from height have associated lumbar vertebral fractures). In addition, many fractures place the patient at risk for specific complications (e.g., compartment syndrome in long-bone fractures, blood loss in pelvic fractures, avascular necrosis in scaphoid fractures of the hand).

A working knowledge of the nomenclature of fractures is essential to the successful management of fractures in the ED, and to ensure clear communication with radiologists and consulting orthopaedic surgeons. Adequate description of a fracture includes the bone(s) involved, whether it is open or closed, the location and direction of the fracture within the bone, the number of fragments, the alignment of the fracture fragments, the displacement of the fragments, and notation of associated complications (e.g. compartment syndrome, neurologic or vascular deficits).

The description of the injury should include the side of the body, the specific bone, and the location within the bone. By convention, long bones are divided into proximal, middle, and distal thirds and these divisions are used to describe the fracture location. Alternatively, long bone injuries can be described as diaphyseal (shaft), metaphyseal (flared ends), or epiphyseal (rounded ends). If the fracture lies at the junction of any two thirds of the bone, it should be described as such. Fractures in children deserve special mention. In this group, fractures occur frequently through the physis (growth plate), and can disrupt future bone growth if not recognized and adequately treated. These injuries are described with the Salter-Harris classification system (Fig. 188.1).

Closed Versus Open Fractures

The old terminology of simple (closed) and compound (open) fractures should be abandoned. In a closed fracture, the skin and soft tissue overlying the fracture have not been violated. Therefore, no communication exists between the outside environment and the fracture fragments. Any break in the skin overlying a fracture must be considered an open fracture until proven

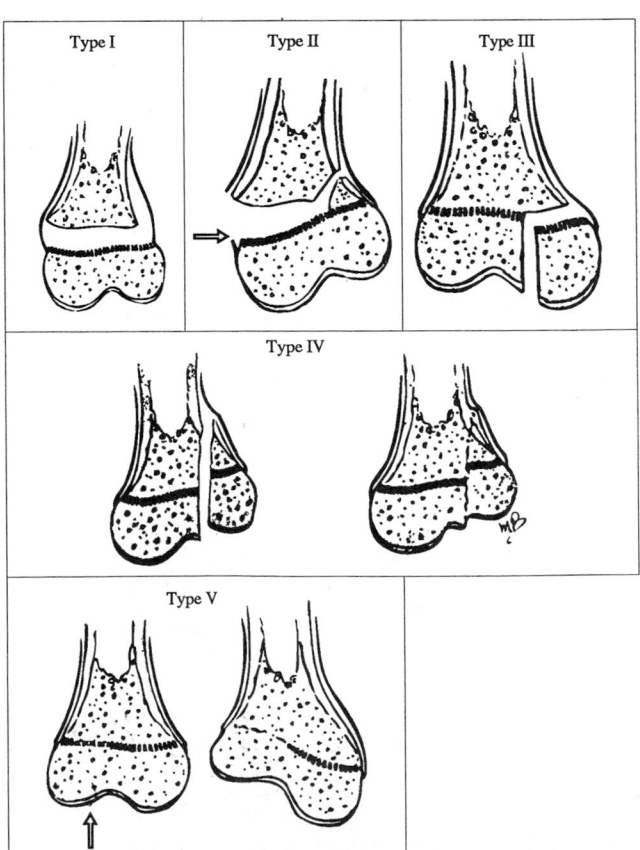

Figure 188.1. Salter-Harris fracture classification. (From Rang M. The growth plate and its diseases. In: Rockwood CA Jr, Wilkins KE, King RE, eds. *Fractures in children,* 3rd edition. Philadelphia: Lippincott-Raven Publishers, 1991:128, with permission.)

otherwise. It is frequently difficult to tell whether there has been actual communication between the bone and the environment or whether the patient has simply sustained an abrasion to the skin overlying the fracture.

Open fractures are traditionally classified into three types based on the size of the wound and the amount of soft-tissue injury. Type I wounds are less than 1 cm long, the energy dissipated by the mechanism of injury is low, and there is minimal soft-tissue trauma. Type II wounds are less than 10 cm long, the mechanism of injury has dissipated a low or moderate amount of energy, and there is moderate soft-tissue trauma but no gross contamination of the wound, major crush injury, or soft-tissue defects or flaps. Type III wounds are greater than 10 cm long. These include high-velocity gunshot wounds, close-range shotgun wounds, open fractures with major vascular injuries, fractures more than 8 hours old, or open fractures sustained in environments where exposure to fecal contents is a concern (e.g., open pelvic fractures with perineal exposure), or extensive soft-tissue or periosteal stripping of bone, or evidence of gross contamination or significant crush injury (2).

Open fractures are orthopaedic emergencies. These injuries require immediate control of hemorrhage which can frequently be accomplished with appropriate splinting. Additionally, open fractures may require emergent reduction if neurovascular compromise exists. Principles of care include irrigation, early administration of sufficient analgesia and appropriate antibiotics, tetanus prophylaxis, and emergent consultation with orthopaedic surgery for definitive irrigation, debridement, reduction, and fracture repair in the operating room. Appropriate early intervention is the best way to prevent future complications, as the incidence of infection following open fracture is directly proportional to the time from injury to definitive irrigation and debridement.

Direction and Description of Fractures

The *direction* of a fracture refers to the configuration of the fracture—the way the fracture disrupts the bone. By convention this descriptive modifier communicates the direction of the fracture in relation to the long axis of the involved bone (Fig. 188.2). A *transverse* fracture disrupts the bone perpendicular to its long axis; an *oblique* fracture lies at an angle to the long axis of the bone; a *spiral* fracture results from a rotational force and spirals around the center of the long axis of the bone.

Additional terms are used to describe the configuration of a fracture. A *comminuted* fracture has three or more fragments. *Segmental* refers to the presence of two or more fractures in a bone, creating at least one segment of bone that is not connected to either end of the bone. An *avulsion fracture* occurs when a piece of bone is pulled off at the site of insertion of a tendon or ligament. Avulsion fractures are usually the result of traction injuries. Their presence indicates potential instability at the joint, which is caused by the loss of stabilization normally provided by the avulsed ligament or tendon. An *impacted* fracture occurs when the fractured surfaces of the bone are forced into each other, foreshortening the bone. On computed tomography (CT) scan, impacted fractures are often comminuted with numerous small fragments wedging across the main fracture line. *Compression* refers to a fracture in which the trabeculae of the bone are compressed, decreasing the overall volume of the affected part of the bone.

Fracture Alignment

A fracture is also described in terms of its alignment—the relationship of the fracture fragments to each other. The fracture may be *displaced*, *angulated*, or *rotated*.

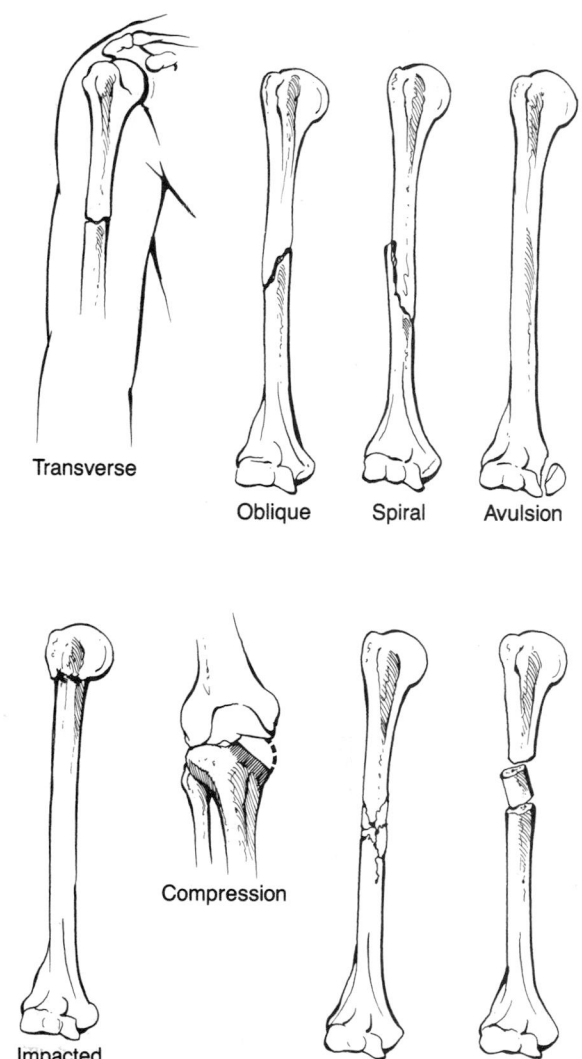

Figure 188.2.   Fracture configuration.

A fracture is *displaced* if the fragments are offset in a transverse or longitudinal plane. The position of the distal fragment in relation to the proximal fragment is described. The distal fragment may be displaced in an anterior, posterior, medial, lateral, radial, ulnar, proximal, or distal direction. The amount of displacement is commonly measured in terms of the width of the fractured shaft, using fractions of the width in the description.

A fracture is *angulated* if there is a deviation from the normal relationship of the bony fragments along the longitudinal axis of the bone (Fig. 188.3). The direction of angulation may be described in two ways. It may be described in terms of the direction of the apex of the angle formed at the fracture site by the two main fracture fragments. The apex may point in an anterior, posterior, lateral, or medial direction. The direction of the apex may also be described by other adjectives, including ulnar, radial, dorsal, or volar, depending on the involved bones. A second way to describe the angulation of the fracture is in terms of the relation of the distal fragment to the proximal fragment. If the distal fragment is angled away from the midline of the body, there is *valgus* angulation (the fracture is in valgus). If the distal fragment angles toward the midline, there is *varus* angulation to the distal fragment (the fracture is in *varus*).

Rotation refers to twisting of the distal fragment in relation to the proximal fragment around the center of the long axis of the fractured bone. When viewed along the long axis of the bone from the most distal point on the bone, if the distal fracture

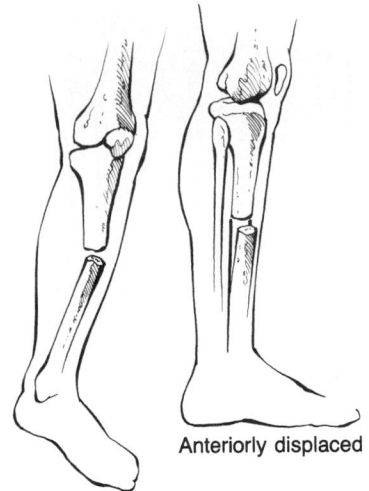

Anteriorly displaced

Anteriorly angulated

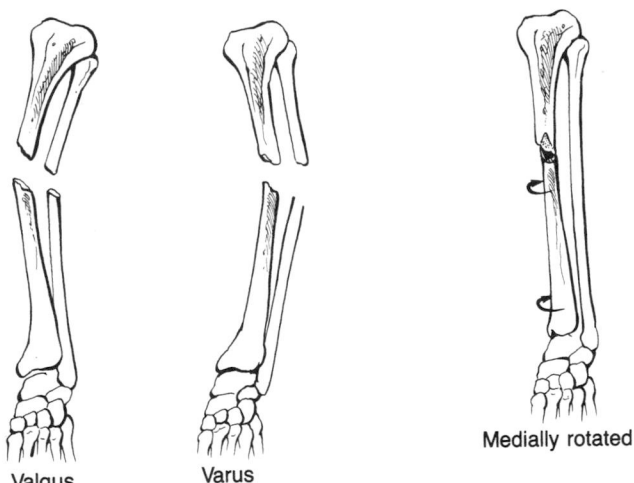

Valgus   Varus   Medially rotated

Figure 188.3.   Fracture alignment.

TABLE 188.1. Complication of Fractures and Dislocations	
Vascular injuries	Ischemic necrosis
Nerve injuries	Delayed union
Compartment syndrome	Nonunion
Infection	Malunion
Shock	Joint stiffness
Cast-induced injuries	Posttraumatic arthritis
DVT	Reflex sympathetic dystrophy
Fat embolism	

DVT, deep vein thrombosis.

fragment has rotated toward the midline in relation to the proximal fragment, it is *medially rotated*; if it has rotated away from the midline, it is *laterally rotated*.

Other Descriptive Modifiers

An *incomplete* fracture involves only one cortex of the bone; a *complete* fracture disrupts both cortices. A *pathologic* fracture occurs in an area of abnormal bone, weakened by disease or prior trauma, and is often the result of apparently trivial trauma or a biomechanically routine force applied along a natural vector. Pathologic fractures occur at sites of old fractures, through primary osteosarcomas, at sites of tumor metastases, near cysts, and in bone weakened by Paget disease, rickets, osteomalacia, tuberculosis, osteomyelitis, chronic steroid therapy, obesity, anorexia, and many other disease processes. A *stress* fracture is the result of the bony cortex becoming fatigued by repeated low-level loading rather than disrupted by one acute episode of trauma. The repeated stress to the cortex causes bone resorption and may result in overt fracture if adequate healing is not allowed. Clinically, patients have pain with activity and tenderness to palpation over the affected bone. Eating disorders and amenorrhea predispose to stress fractures in female athletes. Stress fractures are most

common in the proximal tibia but have also been described in the spine, pelvis, femur, ribs, tarsal navicular, and metatarsals bones, among other sites.

Complications of Fractures

No assessment and description of a fracture is complete without a thorough assessment for, and identification of, possible associated complications (Table 188.1). Well-recognized complications of fractures are suggested by the site of the fracture and the mechanism of injury.

Blood Loss and Shock. Bone has a generous blood supply, and fractures can disrupt the blood vessels, causing localized bleeding. If this bleeding results in the loss of a significant percentage of the patient's blood volume, hypovolemic shock can result. Rarely, exsanguination occurs. An isolated long-bone fracture is rarely the cause of shock, with a unilateral tibia and fibula fracture typically resulting in loss of approximately 500 mL of blood. Certain femur fractures can result in 3 or 4 units of blood loss into the thigh with subsequent development of shock. Hemorrhagic shock can occur with pelvic fractures, in which typical blood loss is between 1,500 and 3,000 mL (1). If a bleeding disorder such as hemophilia A, thrombocytopenia, or marked anemia is present, a fracture that typically results in modest blood loss may be the source of life-threatening hemorrhage. This is also true in patients on anticoagulation therapy. In these patients, isolated long-bone fractures may require administration of vitamin K, fresh-frozen plasma, and transfusion of packed red blood cells.

Vascular Injuries. Vascular injuries occur most commonly in open fractures, widely displaced fractures, or fracture-dislocations, and at sites where the vessels lie close to the bone or are held in a relatively fixed position. Vulnerable sites include the popliteal artery at the knee, which may be injured in supracondylar fractures of the distal femur or in fracture–dislocations of the knee; the axillary artery at the shoulder, injured in fractures of the proximal humerus and humeral head; and the brachial artery at the elbow, which is at risk in supracondylar fractures of the distal humerus (Fig. 188.4). Even at the most vulnerable sites, these injuries are rare, but if they are not diagnosed in a timely fashion, the consequences can be devastating.

The classic signs of vascular injury are the "Five P's": pain, pallor, pulselessness (or diminished pulse), paresthesia, and paralysis. The Five P's are present only in a complete injury to the vessel. A partial injury can have subtle clinical signs and symptoms or be completely asymptomatic. In addition, collateral circulation may maintain distal flow around a vascular injury. Vascular compromise may also be delayed, as in the case of an initial vascular intimal injury leading to progressive thrombosis. Therefore, the location of the fracture and the mechanism of injury determine the need to assess for a potential vascular injury in the asymptomatic patient. Initial evaluation should involve assessment of pulses, evaluation with a Doppler stethoscope if palpable

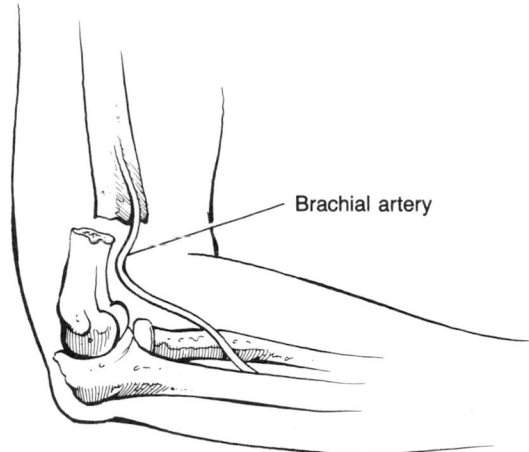

Figure 188.4.   Fracture-associated vascular injury.

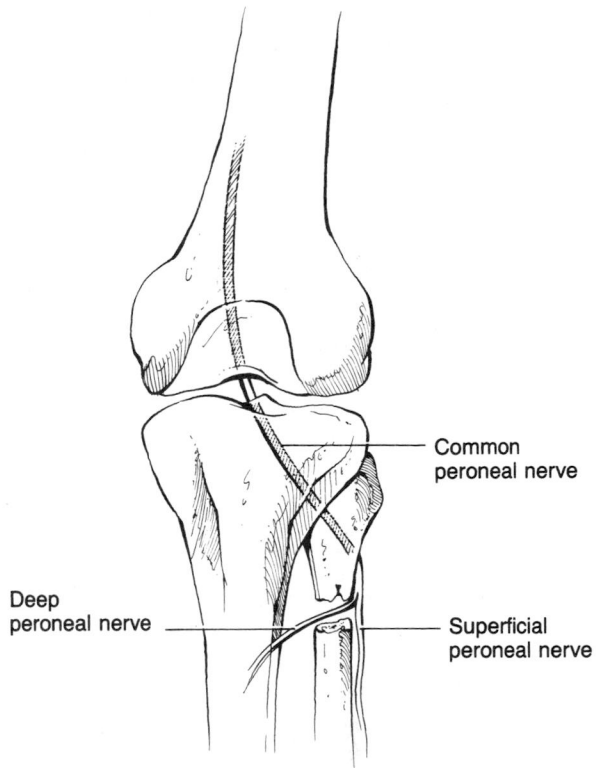

Figure 188.5.   Peroneal injury associated with a knee fracture.

pulses are diminished or absent, observation of the color of the distal extremity, and assessment of capillary refill. If vascular injury is suspected, further evaluation with angiogram, color-flow Doppler ultrasound, magnetic resonance angiography (MRA), or surgical exploration is usually warranted. Complications of fracture-associated vascular injuries include *in situ* thrombosis, false aneurysms, true aneurysms, compartment syndrome, arteriovenous fistulas, and distal limb ischemia with mechanical dysfunction.

Nerve Injuries. Nerves are more frequently injured than vessels in association with fractures. They can be damaged by blunt trauma, along the trajectory of penetrating trauma causing an associated fracture, or by the fracture fragments themselves. Nerves are at increased risk of injury when they are superficial to the skin, lie close to the bone, or span the joint, making them susceptible to stretch injury.

The most frequently injured nerves in association with specific fractures include the axillary and musculocutaneous nerves in shoulder fracture–dislocations; the radial nerve in fractures of the distal third of the humerus; the radial, median, and ulnar nerves in supracondylar elbow fractures; the median nerve in fracture-dislocations about the wrist; the peroneal and tibial nerves in knee fracture-dislocations; and the peroneal nerve in fractures of the fibular head or proximal fibula (Fig. 188.5).

Nerve injuries are classified based on the amount of damage to the nerve according to Seddon staging system:

- *Neuropraxia:* The least severe injury, neuropraxia involves a contusion to the nerve, with minor injury to the myelin sheath. Sensory loss and transient paralysis may occur, but spontaneous and complete recovery occurs over a period of several days to weeks (occasionally, a few months).
- *Axonotmesis:* In axonotmesis, more severe crush injury to the nerve occurs with axonal breakdown followed by distal Wallerian degeneration. The epineurium and the continuity of Schwann tubes are maintained. Prolonged paresthesias and muscle weakness are the clinical hallmarks. Recovery can be complete but takes months to years. The axon has to regenerate proximally to distally; and for functional conduction to occur, the myelin sheath must be fully repaired. Recovery is often incomplete.
- *Neurotmesis:* The most severe form of nerve damage is neurotmesis-disruption of the axon, epineurium, and Schwann cell sheath (complete severance of the nerve). When complete disruption occurs, all functions controlled by the injured nerve are interrupted.

The emergency evaluation of a nerve injury should involve assessment of motor strength, deep tendon reflexes, light touch, and two-point discrimination. Formal testing can be performed using electromyogram (EMG); however, this is not necessary in the ED.

Compartment Syndrome. Compartment syndrome (fully discussed in Chapter 199) should be suspected in long-bone fractures and fractures associated with significant vascular injuries or pronounced swelling, especially when the patient has pain out of proportion to physical examination findings or paresthesias. Manometry should be performed if compartment syndrome is suspected, as the clinical signs are variable and may be delayed. Compartment syndrome is a surgical emergency and requires prompt decompression to prevent or minimize the associated morbidity.

Infection. Infections occur primarily in open fractures, especially in those in which there is a delay in treatment. Infection can also occur with extensive hematoma or after open reduction internal fixation repair. It may also occur without a fracture in cases of osteomyelitis, septic arthritis, and abscesses eroding to bone. Septic arthritis should be suspected in the patient with monoarticular arthritis and ruled out in those who present with a swollen, erythematous, hot joint. If the diagnosis is in question, aspiration for crystal analysis, Gram stain, cell count, and culture should be performed. Most orthopaedic surgeons recommend aggressive arthroscopic lavage to prevent destruction of the joint space by bacteria and inflammatory-mediated damage.

Casts and Splints. Immobilization devices have the potential to cause postinjury problems. They may become too tight as swelling increases during the first 24 to 48 hours postinjury and cause pain and impair circulation. Pressure sores may occur on the skin in areas where a cast or external fixation device exerts localized excessive pressure (e.g., over the heel in a patient with a bimalleolar fracture). Immediate steps should be taken to correct the problem. A cast that is too tight can be split lengthwise; the underlying padding can then be cut and the cast spread open. A cast that is pressing on a particular site can have a window cut out. The window may be replaced more loosely with plaster or covered with soft dressing. An ill-fitting splint can be trimmed. The clinician should take great care in the selection of the appropriate splint (type and material), its placement (to make sure that it adequately immobilizes the intended joint), and perform a postsplinting examination to ensure neurovascular integrity.

Fat Emboli Syndrome. Single or multiple long-bone fractures in the young and hip fractures in the elderly predispose to fat emboli. Twenty percent of patients with pelvic or long-bone fractures have detectable fat droplets in their blood. However, the clinical significance of this is not clear, as the vast majority of these patients remain asymptomatic. Fat emboli syndrome is the most common form of nonthrombotic embolism and has a characteristic clinical course. Its etiology is unclear, but three main hypotheses have been postulated: (1) After fat droplets enter the bloodstream, the liberation of free fatty acids from marrow fat by circulating lipase causes a toxic vasculitis and capillary leak syndrome; (2) it is the end result of extensive platelet–fibrin thrombosis; and (3) it results from direct obstruction of distal vascular lumen by fat emboli. After the injury, the patient often remains asymptomatic for 12 to 36 hours before suddenly and unexpectedly developing a life-threatening syndrome that is characterized by rapid cardiopulmonary and neurologic deterioration. Patients develop agitation, hallucinations, delirium, coma, hypoxia, dyspnea, tachypnea, tachycardia, and a petechial rash. If this deterioration is not quickly reversed, refractory hypotension, anemia, thrombocytopenia, disseminated intravascular coagulopathy (DIC), and adult respiratory distress syndrome (ARDS) often ensue, with an associated high morbidity and mortality.

Ischemic or Avascular Necrosis. Ischemic or avascular necrosis is characterized by bone death that occurs following the interruption of blood supply to bone. Avascular necrosis (AVN) is most frequently associated with carpal scaphoid fractures, lunate dislocations, hip dislocations, femoral neck fractures, and complex fractures of the talus. The time required for an injury to result in AVN is extremely variable and its location and patient specific.

Delayed Complications. Other complications of fractures may occur some time after the initial injury. Many fractures require reduction of the displaced fracture fragments in the ED or the operating room. The goal in reduction is always to reestablish anatomic position; eliminate displacement, angulation, and other forms of malalignment; and immobilize the broken bone in the reestablished anatomic position to promote healing. Sometimes, this ideal condition is not achieved and the systematic progression from hematoma to callus formation to bony union is delayed or interrupted. *Delayed unions* are fractures that take longer than usual to heal; *malunions* are fractures that heal in a faulty position; *nonunions* occur when the process of fracture healing stops before the fracture is united.

Joint stiffness, *posttraumatic arthritis*, and *complex regional pain syndrome* (CRPS) – *type I* (formerly known as reflex sympathetic dystrophy or RSD) may also occur as delayed complications of extremity trauma. Any intraarticular fracture of a weight-bearing joint predisposes the patient to early degenerative changes. The patient may present to the ED years after a fracture, complaining of *perceived* sudden onset of joint pain and decreased range of motion. Radiographs typically demonstrate extensive *osteoarthritis.*

CRPS is a three-stage, posttraumatic syndrome of unclear etiology, the development of which has no known correlation to the severity of the initial injury (14). The first, or early, stage, characterized by continuous burning and aching in the posttraumatic extremity, is exacerbated by weight bearing and by movement. After a variable period of time, the middle, or dystrophic, stage

ensues, characterized by the development of shiny, cool skin over the affected extremity and a progressively decreased range of motion. In the final, or atrophic, stage, the skin atrophies, the muscles waste, and flexion contractures develop.

In 1992, Gibbons and Wilson, in the *Clinical Journal of Pain*, developed an RSD score, which was proposed as a strict system for the clinical diagnosis of RSD. The scoring system consists of nine criteria and has more than academic interest. Early diagnosis improves outcome, interrupting the progression from burning to dystrophy to atrophy. The nine criteria are (1) allodynia—the phenomenon whereby pain is increased by stimuli that activate the involved nerve, such as a breeze blowing on the area, temperature changes, or emotional outbursts [hyperpathia]; (2) burning pain; (3) edema; (4) change in color or hair growth in the affected area; (5) change in sweating; (6) change in temperature; (7) demineralization of bone in the involved limb, as documented in radiographs; (8) quantitative measurements of vasomotor disturbances; and (9) a triple-phase bone scan consistent with RSD. A score of five points qualifies as a clinical diagnosis of RSD; one point is given for each positive criterion, zero points for each negative criterion, and one-half point for each equivocal criterion. Application of heat or cold, exercises, early sympathetic blockade, or sympathectomy to the affected limb can halt the progression to atrophy. A minority of patients have been helped by a short course of high-dose prednisone (a 3-week taper) in conjunction with heat, cold, and exercise therapy (4).

Subluxations and Dislocations

Acute or chronic ligamentous laxity or tearing can result in subluxation or dislocation of a joint. Chronic ligamentous laxity is usually the result of an overuse syndrome, in which repetitive microtrauma leads to an attenuation of the static restraints of the joint. Acute ligamentous tears are the result of excessive or abnormal forces applied to the joint. The classic example is subluxation or dislocation of the glenohumeral joint. *Subluxation* occurs when one bone becomes partially disarticulated from the other bone that forms the joint. The articular surfaces forming the joint remain partially intact. *Dislocation* occurs when the bones are completely disarticulated and no parts of their articular surfaces are in contact. Dislocations can occur in isolation or with an associated fracture (Fig. 188.6). Often, the fracture is anatomic evidence of the direction of the pathologic force vector resulting in the dislocation. For example, 90% to 95% of shoulder dislocations occur anteriorly, disrupting the continuity of the anterior capsule and the labrum. Sometimes, these structures resist the forces producing dislocation to the point that a fracture occurs, avulsing a piece of bone from the anterior glenoid rim, known as a bony Bankart lesion.

The nomenclature of subluxations and dislocations is straightforward. Most subluxations and dislocations occur at a joint formed by two bones, and the subluxation or dislocation is named after the affected joint (e.g., posterior dislocation of the distal interphalangeal (DIP) joint of the fourth finger of the right hand). If a joint is formed by three bones, and the two major bones are disarticulated, the subluxation or dislocation is named after the joint involved (e.g., posterior dislocation of the knee). If the joint is formed by three bones, and the minor bone is subluxed or dislocated, the abnormality is named after the minor bone (e.g., lateral dislocation of the patella). As for fractures, direction is assigned referential to the distal segment.

Specific subluxations and dislocations are frequently seen in the ED and should be skillfully and efficiently reduced, with restoration of anatomic position, by the emergency physician. These include anterior and posterior dislocations of the shoulder joint; anterior and posterior dislocations of the sternoclavicular joint; posterior dislocations of the elbow joint; posterior

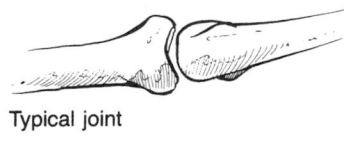

Typical joint

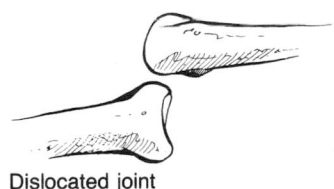

Dislocated joint

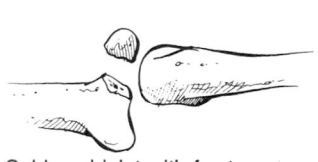

Subluxed joint with fracture

Figure 188.6.　Joint subluxation and dislocation.

dislocations of the proximal interphalangeal (PIP) and DIP joints, often with accompanying avulsion fractures; posterior dislocations of the hip joint; posterior dislocations of the knee joint; lateral dislocations of the patella; and fracture–dislocations of the ankle.

The hallmarks of subluxations and dislocations are pain, deformity, and decreased range of motion. Certain dislocations are associated with specific complications, and these must be ruled out in the evaluation and treatment of the injury. For example, the aorta and trachea are at risk in posterior dislocations of the sternoclavicular joint, and injury to them can lead to rapid respiratory compromise or intrathoracic hemorrhage. The axillary nerve and, less commonly, the musculocutaneous nerve are at risk in anterior shoulder dislocations. Their function must be clearly assessed prior to any attempted reduction and then reassessed after the reduction is complete. The popliteal artery can be stretched, torn, or completely disrupted in a posterior dislocation of the knee. Many experts recommend angiogram followed by close observation for patients with knee dislocation. Radiographs should be obtained prior to attempts at reduction and after the reduction has been achieved in order to document the position of the bones, restoration of anatomic position, and the presence of associated fractures.

Techniques for the reduction of specific joints are discussed in the chapters dedicated to those joints, but certain principles hold true for all subluxations and dislocations. The length of time between injury and relocation corresponds proportionally to the severity of spasm and swelling that will occur and the difficulty involved in reducing the joint. Adequate pain control and sedation facilitate smooth reduction; excess force applied during the reduction can result in fractures, nerve damage, and vascular injury. The technique used to reduce the dislocation should initially replicate the mechanism of injury to release the dislocated bone from the anatomic structure that is keeping it dislocated. In certain dislocations, the incidence of delayed complications is directly proportional to the time from injury to relocation. For example, avascular necrosis of the femoral head occurs in 10% to 20% of hip dislocations. The rate is directly proportional to the total time from injury to successful reduction. Similarly, myositis ossificans is a well-recognized complication of posterior dislocation of the elbow. The incidence of myositis ossificans is directly related to three variables: the number of attempts at reduction, the length of time from injury to successful reduction, and whether the joint is adequately immobilized after reduction.

Tendinosis

Tendinosis is a subset of strain since it is an injury to the musculotendinous unit, but it is more appropriately considered a separate entity. Tendinosis was felt to represent inflammation to the musculotendinous unit, and was hence termed *"tendinitis."* Recent work has indicated that a more correct term is *tendinosis*, as there is no significant inflammatory response by the body in these conditions (7). Instead, there is a degeneration of the collagen portion of the tendon in the absence of inflammatory cells. Tendinosis differs from strain in that the pathologic changes are *isolated* to the tendon and *involve the insertion of the tendon into the bone,* which occurs via a transitional, calcified fibrocartilage known as Sharpey's fibers. Tendinopathy can result from chronic use or from one acute episode of overuse. In acute tendinopathy, the tendon is irritated and an acute response occurs. Microscopically, there is loss of collagen continuity with an associated increase in ground substance, vascularity, and cellularity. The cellularity results from the presence of fibroblasts and myofibroblasts, not inflammatory cells. If this cycle is not interrupted, permanent changes in the architecture of Sharpey's fibers and atrophy of the tendon fibers occur.

Common tendons involved in acute or chronic tendinosis presenting to the ED include patellar, quadriceps, rotator cuff, and the Achilles' tendons.

Clinically, tendinosis presents with pain during active range of motion, loss of function, point tenderness over the affected tendon near its insertion into bone, and, often, localized edema and erythema. Forced contraction of the affected muscle against resistance elicits pain, which is exacerbated by pressure over the point of insertion. Pain can also be elicited by forced extension of the tendon, stretching the inflamed fibers.

Calcific tendinitis is an entirely different entity, representing a truly inflammatory response by the body. It is usually associated with chronic inflammation and consists of calcium deposition within the body of the tendon. It is often an indication of tendinous degeneration altering the macrostructure of the tendon. Calcific tendinitis has a characteristic radiographic appearance, revealing the calcium depositions within the tendon. For example, a band of calcification can be seen passing over the bicipital groove in calcific biceps tendinitis at the shoulder.

Muscle Spasms

Muscle spasms are a poorly understood phenomenon in which a voluntary muscle undergoes sustained involuntary contraction, leading to depletion of stored glycogen, localized build-up of lactic acid, and severe pain. The causes of muscle spasm are not known, but hypotheses include localized alterations in blood flow, regional or systemic electrolyte imbalances (especially sodium and calcium; less often, potassium), and postural abnormalities that place a bone in a nonanatomically neutral position, causing attached musculature to fire continuously. For example, overdevelopment of the muscles on one side of the body in a racquet-sports athlete can cause latissimus dorsi spasm, as the proprioceptors present in the latissimus sense that the arm is out of the neutral position and cause repetitive muscle contraction in attempted compensation.

Muscle spasms typically seen in the ED include spasms of the gastrocnemius, levator scapulae, trapezii, rhomboids, and latissimus dorsi. Rectus abdominus muscle spasm can mimic an acute abdomen.

Treatment may be frustrating for both the patient and the clinician, as complete relief is difficult to achieve. The treatments are not perfect, and many are controversial. Treatment options includes freezing the muscle belly with fluoroethane spray, followed by passive, gentle, forced range of motion to "break the spasm;" massage; treatment with muscle relaxants, including diazepam and other benzodiazepines; pain control with acetaminophen, NSAIDs, or opioid analgesics. Recent research indicates that treatment with muscle relaxants for these conditions may not be as good as basic analgesia (13).

EMERGENCY DEPARTMENT EVALUATION

The ED evaluation of any injured patient begins with the basic ABCs- airway, breathing, and circulation. If the patient is reliable, not intoxicated, and has an isolated injury, and the mechanism of injury does not suggest other possible injuries, then evaluation and treatment are limited to the injured joint along with the joints immediately proximal and distal to the injury. The contralateral side of the injured joint or limb should be examined for comparison of range of motion, anatomy, and laxity.

In patients with multiple injuries, head trauma, amnesia, intoxication, or medical illnesses resulting in their musculoskeletal injury (e.g., a distal radial fracture after syncope), a complete physical evaluation is mandatory and should follow basic trauma guidelines. This should begin with a primary survey and assessment of the ABCs; evaluation of neurologic disability and Glasgow Coma Scale; then continue with complete exposure of the patient and a search for any accompanying injuries. Once this is complete, the emergency physician should systematically evaluate the underlying medical problem that could have produced the trauma; if a problem is identified, it should be addressed before moving on to the next step in the systematic evaluation. For example, the motorcyclist thrown from the cycle, who presents with an open fracture of the tibia and fibula and flail chest, needs breathing stabilized before the leg is further evaluated. In extremity wounds, hemorrhage can often be rapidly but temporarily controlled with a direct-pressure dressing, ensuring continued circulatory stability until the source of bleeding can be systematically evaluated. After the primary survey, each joint should be palpated and ranged systematically, and the integrity of long bones assessed by inspection, palpation, and range of motion.

As alluded to previously, certain extremity injuries are true orthopaedic emergencies, meriting expeditious evaluation and management. These include vascular injuries, compartment syndromes, open fractures and dislocations, and certain dislocated joints (Table 188.2). They should be addressed immediately after the ABCs have been evaluated, stabilized, and recorded on a trauma flow sheet. If vascular compromise is suspected, immediate consultation with an orthopaedic or vascular surgeon is advised. When vascular insufficiency is caused by stretching of the vessel across the site of a dislocation or displaced fracture, reduction of the fracture or dislocation may correct the problem.

Pulses should be documented after the reduction. If an injury to the vessel itself is suspected, arteriography, color-Doppler ultrasound, magnetic resonance angiography, or surgical exploration may be indicated. Color-Doppler ultrasound evaluation, followed by close observation with serial neurovascular examinations, is a relatively newer option, and is still being validated as a modality. These decisions should be left to the consulting surgeon. Blood flow to an ischemic extremity should, ideally, be reestablished within 6 to 8 hours to prevent permanent injuries, including ischemia and necrosis.

Similarly, if compartment syndrome is suspected, it should be ruled out by manometry. This is usually accomplished through emergent consultation with an orthopaedic surgeon. If compartment pressures are elevated, emergent fasciotomy is mandatory.

After all life- and limb-threatening injuries have been addressed, attention can be directed toward the identification of individual injuries—fractures, dislocations, sprains, strains, tendinitis, and spasm. This evaluation begins with a *thorough history* to ascertain the mechanism of injury, timing of the injury, previous injury to the limb, handedness where applicable, and medical problems potentially contributory to current disability. The history should include questions about associated symptoms of pain, paresthesia, weakness, signs of pallor or deformity.

Inspection follows. On physical examination, the emergency physician should note the appearance of the injury, looking for deformity, swelling, erythema, ecchymosis, and exposed bone. Other physical findings include the presence of grease spots at puncture wounds, purulent fluid drainage from the wound, abrasions, or lacerations over the injured area.

Palpation follows. The emergency physician should palpate for deformity, local or diffuse tenderness, edema, calor, and induration. Palpation should include a careful assessment of neurovascular integrity. Patients with vascular compromise will have dusky or mottled skin, diminished distal pulses, and delayed capillary refill. Sensation to light touch may be decreased, and hypesthesia often occurs over an area of acute injury. Active range of motion should be tested. In the majority of acute injuries, the patient is not enthusiastic about actively ranging the joint and passive range of motion and provocative maneuvers are of limited utility due to pain.

Radiographs are the cornerstone of further evaluation and management of most musculoskeletal complaints. Many fractures can be diagnosed clinically. However, in the vast majority of cases, the diagnosis should be supported radiographically. Radiographs frequently determine the need for operative reduction, the length of time the fracture needs to be immobilized, and potential complications during the rehabilitation process. Criteria for obtaining radiographs of specific injuries are formalized but constantly evolving, and are beyond the scope of this chapter. They are addressed in the chapters on injuries to specific joints. The goals of objective criteria for obtaining radiographs include reduction in unnecessary imaging, increased efficiency of patient flow in the ED, decreased exposure to radiation, and containment of health-care costs. For example, the Ottawa Ankle Rules are objective criteria for obtaining an ankle series after an ankle injury. They state that ankle films are required in patients over 18 years old if pain in the malleolar area is accompanied by inability to bear weight (defined as walking four steps) immediately after the injury and in the ED, or by bony tenderness over the posterior aspect of the distal 6 cm of the medial or lateral malleolus. Strict implementation of the Ottawa Ankle Rules has been shown to reduce the number of ankle films ordered by 28%, increase ED efficiency, and decrease ED costs without increasing the percentage of missed fractures (12).

When the decision is made to obtain roentgenograms, the correct views must be obtained, they need to be of sufficient quality

---

TABLE 188.2. Orthopaedic Emergencies

Vascular injuries
Compartment syndrome
Open fractures
Open joints
Dislocated hip
Dislocated joint with vascular compromise or threat to skin integrity

to competently evaluate for fracture, and they need to be read thoroughly, in a systematic fashion. Poor-quality films should not be accepted. Many fractures have been missed because of technically inadequate films. In addition, thorough examination of the soft tissue and every bone in the x-ray is essential to avoid missing subtle findings that may indicate fracture or dislocation. For example, the fat pad sign on an elbow x-ray may be the sole indication of a radial head fracture.

Other pitfalls in interpretation include the following:

- A nutrient foramen, housing a nutrient artery, may be misinterpreted as a fracture. A nutrient foramen will appear less radiolucent than a fracture (very smooth-edged) and will angle obliquely from the edge of the bone through the cortex, and then terminate without involving the cortex on the other side of the marrow.
- Sesamoid bones or accessory ossicles may be confused with fractures. These anatomic variants usually have smooth edges and are well corticated, and no defect in the adjacent bone will be noted. In some instances, a comparison view of the unaffected side can help clarify the structure in question. For example, the patient with pain over the patella following a dashboard injury, who is found to have a two-part patella on x-ray, may have bipartite patella, which is confirmed by its presence on an x-ray of the unaffected knee.
- Fat and clothing folds, casts, or splints may be misinterpreted as fractures; and jewelry or body piercings may be misinterpreted as foreign bodies.

Every x-ray series should include a minimum of two views that are *shot at right angles to each other*. If the plane of the fracture is at 90 degrees (perpendicular) to the plane of the x-ray beam, the fracture may not be evident on that view but would be readily visible on an x-ray taken in a plane parallel to the plane of the fracture line.

Fractures in the shaft of long bones are often accompanied by additional fractures in that bone proximal or distal to the main fracture site or by dislocations at the joints at either end of the bone. Therefore, all long-bone shaft fractures require imaging of the entire length of the bone, including adequate views of its joints. For example, a midshaft femur fracture requires x-rays of the entire shaft, a two-plane knee series, and a two-plane hip series.

Fractures to paired long bones, such as the radius and ulna or the tibia and fibula, present with different associated fractures: A fracture to one bone is sometimes accompanied by a distant fracture to the other bone in the pair. For example, medial malleolar ankle fractures resulting from a lateral twisting mechanism sometimes have an associated proximal fibular or fibular head fracture or dislocation. The mechanism of injury explains this association: The twisting force that breaks the medial malleolus is transmitted up the shafts of the tibia and fibula and is dissipated at the weakest point, the proximal fibula, resulting in either fracture or dislocation. Thus, more complex ankle fractures require imaging of the entire shafts of the fibula and tibia and a two-way series of the knee. Certain forearm fractures are commonly associated with a fracture–dislocation of the other bone of the forearm, such as a radial shaft fracture and distal radioulnar joint dislocation, known as a Galeazzi fracture (Fig. 188.7).

Additional views are sometimes helpful. A dedicated scaphoid view can aid in the detection of a subtle scaphoid fracture. An axial view of the calcaneus can reveal a fracture missed on standard ankle and foot series. Many posterior dislocations of the shoulder are not evident, except on an axillary view of the glenohumeral joint, clearly depicting the relationship between the humeral head and the glenoid fossa. In certain instances, comparison views to the patient's other side are helpful. For ex-

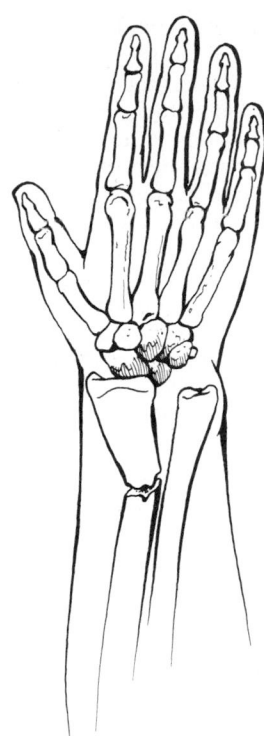

Figure 188.7. Galeazzi fracture dislocation.

ample, in distal clavicle osteolysis, characterized by pain and osteolysis of the distal clavicle, bilateral clavicle views help confirm the diagnosis when a larger separation is seen at the affected acromioclavicular joint compared with the unaffected side. Distal clavicle osteolysis occurs in power lifters and in contact athletes suffering significant blunt trauma to the point (acromion) of the shoulder.

Adequate films, correctly interpreted, are not 100% sensitive for fractures. Growth plate injuries (aka Salter-Harris injuries) may appear entirely normal on plain radiographs. The diagnosis may not become evident until there has been new bone deposition or resorption at the site of injury. Similarly, nondisplaced, hairline fractures often become visible, or radiolucent, only on radiographs 7 to 10 days after injury, as bone resorption widens the fracture line, hematoma develops, and new bone formation proceeds. If there is potential morbidity associated with a missed fracture on plain x-rays, a clinically fractured bone should be treated as a fracture, or more sophisticated imaging studies should be obtained. A patient with a story and examination consistent with a femoral neck fracture, which has normal plain radiographs and remains nonweight bearing in the ED, should be treated as having a nondisplaced hip fracture. Assessment of a patient's ability to ambulate is essential prior to discharge, and the inability to ambulate can further confirm the presence of an occult lower extremity fracture. These patients should be kept nonweight bearing and magnetic resonance imaging should be performed to demonstrate the fracture; a bone scan may also be diagnostic.

Similarly, tenderness in the snuff box (the space on the radial side of the wrist between the extensor pollicis longus tendon and the paired extensor pollicis brevis and adductor pollicis longus tendons) following a *fall on an outstretched hand* (FOOSH) needs to be treated as a scaphoid fracture, *even if the radiographs are normal*. If the radiographs show no fracture, immobilization in a thumb spica with followup examination and repeat radiographs in 10 days is mandatory (11).

EMERGENCY DEPARTMENT MANAGEMENT

In general, the initial management of musculoskeletal injuries includes immobilization of the affected extremity and administration of pain medication. Once a fracture or dislocation is identified, reduction should be performed as needed; this is determined by the location of the injury and the amount of distraction or angulation. The management of specific injuries is discussed in subsequent chapters.

The initial management of open fractures and joints should be directed toward reducing the chances of infection. Gross particulate debris in the wound should be removed. Exposed bone *should not be replaced in the wound,* because this may further introduce contamination. A sterile dressing should be applied. The extremity is splinted to prevent further tissue and neurovascular injury. Intravenous antibiotic therapy, usually with a first- or second-generation cephalosporin, is instituted (if not contraindicated by drug allergies), and tetanus prophylaxis (sometimes including tetanus immune globulin) given when indicated. A macrolide antibiotic or trimethoprim–sulfamethoxazole is a good choice for the penicillin-allergic patient. An aminoglycoside such as gentamycin is frequently added to the cephalosporin when there is heavy contamination of the wound. After these initial management steps have been taken, orthopaedic consultation should be obtained. Most open fractures and dislocations require formal debridement in the operating room, which should be performed within 8 hours of the injury. The incidence of infection is directly proportional to the length of time from injury until irrigation and formal debridement occurs.

Certain dislocations require expeditious reduction. Dislocated hips are at risk for development of ischemic necrosis, and dislocated elbows are at risk for development of Volkmann ischemic contracture (compartment syndrome, decreased blood flow, necrosis, and contracture following a dislocation). Avascular necrosis of the hip is thought to be caused by damage to the vessels supplying the femoral head. In general, these vessels are not completely torn in the dislocation; rather, they are stretched and blood flow through them is compromised. Therefore, the incidence of avascular necrosis is directly related to the length of time from injury to adequate relocation of the hip. Similar principles apply to the development of Volkmann ischemic contracture following elbow dislocation. Therefore, reduction should be accomplished as soon as is feasible.

CRITICAL INTERVENTIONS

> - Once the patient has stabilized, palpate every bone and put every joint through a range of motion to search for occult injury
> - Relocate or re-align any fractures or dislocations that result in neurovascular compromise in an attempt to alleviate the neurovascular deficit as expeditiously as possible
> - Splint fractures as quickly as is possible in order to minimize pain, prevent injury to adjacent structures, and reduce blood loss associated with these injuries
> - Perform manometry and obtain early consultation for patients with suspected compartment syndrome
> - Administer intravenous antibiotics (first- or second-generation cephalosporin and gentamycin) early for patients with open fractures

DISPOSITION

Emergency department care is not complete when the diagnosis is made. Appropriate immobilization should be instituted, and instructions for immediate care and follow up given. These should be tailored to the specific injury but, in general, involve rest, ice, and elevation. These simple, cost-effective steps are often overlooked in the rush to discharge patients from the ED and can, in some cases, affect more than the patient's comfort. For example, the simple application of ice to a lateral ankle sprain during the first 24 hours after injury has been shown to decrease time to return of full function by 50% (6).

Depending on the injury, the patient may be instructed to remain nonweight bearing or keep the injured joint immobilized. In other cases, activity as tolerated is appropriate and may speed recovery (e.g., low-back strain). Pain control must be achieved in the ED, and the pain medications given for the outpatient setting should be commensurate with the injury. For example, the patient who requires morphine in the ED for a rib cage contusion is mismanaged if he or she is discharged with instructions to take acetaminophen as needed for pain. Adequate postinjury pain control improves outcome and decreases repeat visits to the ED.

Patients should be instructed to return to the ED if they experience any signs or symptoms of neurovascular compromise, excessive pain, coldness, erythema, fevers, chills, cough, pleuritic chest pain, or a cast or splint that feels too tight or causes pain. Appropriate follow up depends on the nature and extent of the injury and can range from a visit to the patient's primary care doctor in 2 weeks, to orthopaedic referral in 10 days' time, to being seen by a hand surgeon in the next few days for operative repair of a flexor tendon laceration.

COMMON PITFALLS

- ✔ Ordering the wrong x-ray because of an inadequate physical examination
- ✔ Not recognizing all injuries because the physician's attention is focused on one specific injury. For example, the patient who falls off a ladder and presents with a grade II lateral ankle sprain may have a calcaneal fracture from the initial impact
- ✔ Relying on poor-quality x-rays or on a single view without obtaining an additional view at 90 degrees to the initial one
- ✔ For patients with long-bone fractures, failure to include the length of the bone, the joint above, and the joint below in adequately exposed radiographs
- ✔ Failure to rule out infection or similar condition (olecranon bursitis) in a patient presenting with a swollen joint. It may be a mistake to assume that the swollen joint in the patient with a history of gouty arthritis is another flare of gout if the presentation is atypical or there are other concerning signs
- ✔ Failure to realize that drops of blood or small abrasions on the skin in the area of a fracture are signs of an open fracture
- ✔ Not checking or documenting a complete neurovascular examination on initial presentation and after reduction of a fracture or dislocation
- ✔ Not obtaining radiographs prior to and after reducing a fracture or dislocation to rule out accompanying avulsion fractures from the dislocation or from the reduction procedure. X-rays should not be obtained only when the delay caused by waiting for the x-ray could contribute to morbidity
- ✔ Attributing pain to the fracture itself, rather than thoroughly investigating other potential sources of pain, such as a cast problem, neurovascular compromise, or compartment syndrome
- ✔ Not evaluating a patient for compartment syndrome with manometry after considering the diagnosis
- ✔ Not pursuing additional studies when the plain radiographs are normal in patients with a suspected fracture, especially if they are unable to bear weight

Acknowledgments

Thanks to the previous edition's chapter authors David F. Gaieski and Joseph Bernstein.

References

1. Swiontkowski MF. The multiply-injured patient with musculoskeletal injuries. In: Bucholtz RW, Heckman JD. (eds). *Rockwood & Green's Fractures in Adults.* 5th ed. Philadelphia: Lippincott Williams & Wilkins, 2001:47–84.
2. DeLong WG Jr., Born CT, Wei SY, Petrik ME, et al. Aggressive treatment of 119 open fracture wounds. *J Trauma-Injury Infect & Critical Care* 1999;46(6):1049–1054.
3. Freedman KB. The adequacy of medical school education in musculoskeletal medicine. *J Bone & Joint Surg (American Vol)* 1998;80(10):1421–1427.
4. Gibbons JJ, Wilson PR. RSD score: a criteria for the diagnosis of reflex sympathetic dystrophy and causalgia. *Clin J Pain* 1992;8:260.
5. Henry GL, George JE. Specific high-risk clinical presentations. In: Henry GL, Sullivan DJ, (eds). *Emergency medicine risk management.* Dallas: American College of Emergency Physicians, 1997:475–494.
6. Hocutt JE, Jaffe R, Rylander R, et al. Cryotherapy in ankle sprains. *Am J Sports Med* 1982;10:316.
7. Khan KM, Cook JL, Bonnar F, et al. Histopathology of common tendinopathies: update and implications for clinical management. *Sports Med* 1999;27:393–408.
8. Marder RA, Chapman MW. Principles of management of fractures in sports. *Clin Sports Med* 1990;9:1.
9. McCaig LF, Burt CW. National hospital ambulatory medical care survey: 2001 emergency department summary. *Advance Data* 2003;335:1–36.
10. McKibbin B. The biology of fracture healing in long bones. *J Bone Joint Surg* 1978;60:150.
11. Perron AD, Brady WJ, Keats TE, Hersh RE. Orthopaedic Pitfalls in the Emergency Department: Scaphoid Fracture. *Am J Emerg Med*, 2001;19:310–316.
12. Stiell IG, Greenberg GH, McKnight RD, et al. Decision rules for the use of radiography in acute ankle injuries: refinement and prospective validation. *JAMA* 1993;269:1127.
13. Turturro MA, Frater CR, D'Amico FJ. Cyclobenzaprene with ibuprophen vs. ibuprophen alone in acute myofascial strain: a randomized double-blind clinical trial. *Ann Emerg Med* 2003;41:818–826.
14. Wasner G, Schattschneider J, Binder A, et al. Complex regional pain syndrome-diagnosis, mechanisms, CNS involvement and therapy. *Spinal Cord* 2003;41:61–75.

CHAPTER 189

Shoulder Injuries

Jeffrey Schaider and Robert R. Simon

The shoulder joint is composed of three bones and three joints. The bones are the humeral head, clavicle, and scapula; the joints are the sternoclavicular (SC), acromioclavicular (AC), and glenohumeral. Figures 189.1 and 189.2 demonstrate the essential osseous and ligamentous anatomy of the shoulder, respectively. The rotator cuff surrounds the glenohumeral joint and is composed of the teres minor, infraspinatus, and supraspinatus muscles attaching to the greater tuberosity of the humerus, and the subscapularis muscle attaching to the lesser tuberosity of the humerus. Superficial to these muscles is the deltoid muscle.

The glenohumeral joint and scapulothoracic articulation function as a unit in abducting the humerus. The ratio of scapular to glenohumeral movement is 1:2; therefore, for every 30 degrees of abduction of the arm, the scapula moves 10 degrees and the glenohumeral joint moves 20 degrees. If the glenohumeral joint is completely immobilized, the scapulothoracic articulation can provide 65 degrees of abduction.

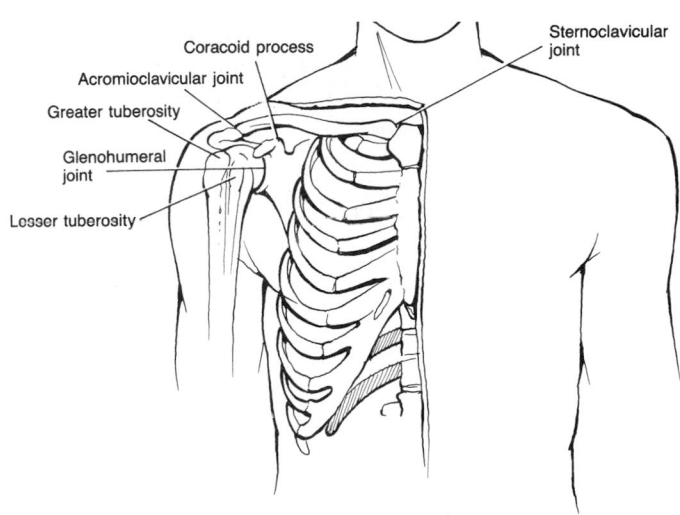

Figure 189.1.   The essential anatomy of the shoulder. (Adapted from Simon RR, Koenigsknecht SJ. *Emergency orthopaedics.* Norwalk, CT: Appleton & Lange, 1994.)

EMERGENCY DEPARTMENT EVALUATION

The clavicle is anchored to the scapula by the AC and coracoclavicular ligaments. The SC and costoclavicular ligaments anchor the clavicle medially. The SC joint is palpable immediately lateral to the suprasternal notch. The AC joint is palpated by pushing in a medial direction against the distal end of the clavicle as it protrudes above the flattened acromion process.

The greater tuberosity of the humerus lies laterally to the acromion process, and can easily be palpated by following the acromion process to its lateral edge and then sliding the fingers inferiorly. The bicipital groove, which contains the biceps tendon, is located anterior and medial to the greater tuberosity and is bordered laterally by the greater tuberosity and medially by the lesser tuberosity. External rotation places the groove in a more exposed position for palpation, and permits the examiner to palpate the greater tuberosity first, then the bicipital groove, and finally the lesser tuberosity by moving from a lateral to a medial position. The articular surface of the proximal humerus articulates with the glenoid, forming the glenohumeral joint. Because the articular surface ends at the *anatomic* neck, fractures located proximal to the anatomic neck are considered articular surface fractures. The *surgical* neck is the narrow portion of the proximal humerus distal to the anatomic neck, just below the greater and lesser tuberosities (Fig. 189.3).

The examiner must consider injury to proximate structures. The subclavian vessels and the brachial plexus lie in close proximity to the clavicle; so displaced clavicular fractures can be associated with injuries to these structures, but this is rare. The brachial plexus, axillary nerve, and axillary artery lie in close proximity to the proximal humerus, and injuries to these structures frequently accompany proximal humerus fractures.

The scapula covers ribs 2 through 7 posteriorly. It is covered with thick muscles over its entire body and spine. The scapula is connected to the axial skeleton solely by the AC joint. The examiner should test function of the associated muscles and range of motion of this joint.

Routine clavicular radiographs include an anteroposterior (AP) view of the upper thorax to define the structures. Occasionally, an AP view with the tube directed 45 degrees cephalad (apical lordotic) is needed to detect medial-third fractures. At times, cone-down views, upper rib radiographs, and tomograms may be necessary to delineate fractures adequately.

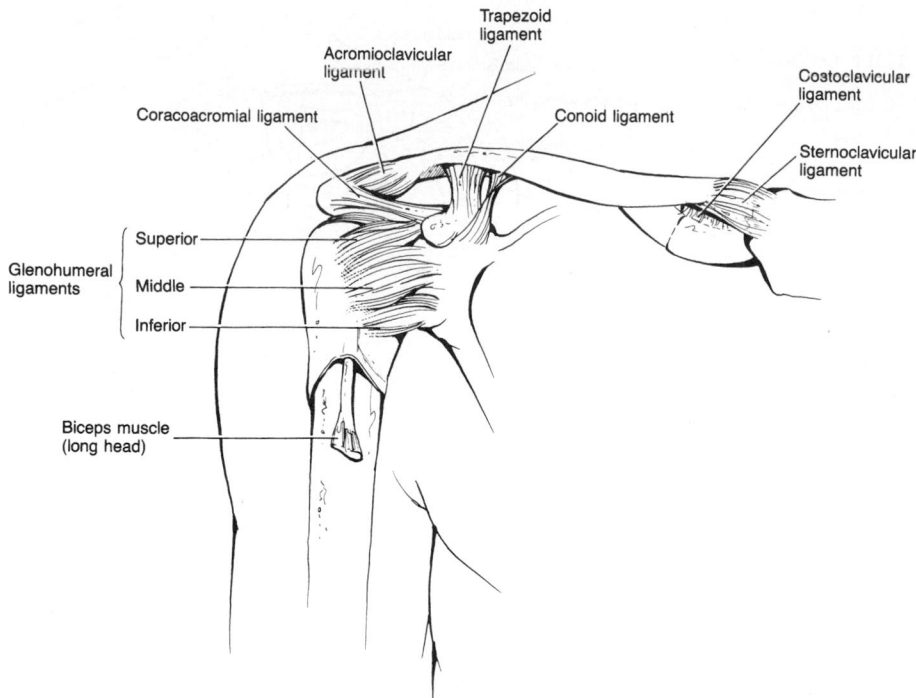

Figure 189.2. The ligaments around the shoulder.

Four views of the shoulder are optimal to evaluate the proximal humerus and glenoid joint for fractures and dislocations. The trauma series recommended by Neer (25) includes an AP view of the shoulder in addition to a transscapular projection commonly known as the Y view. The transscapular view is obtained by placing the radiographic film along the lateral side of the humerus, with the beam projected along the length of the scapula. This view is helpful in identifying shoulder dislocations. In addition to the two-view trauma series, an AP internal rotation view of the humerus and an axillary view permit full evaluation of the shoulder and proximal humerus, including the articular surface.

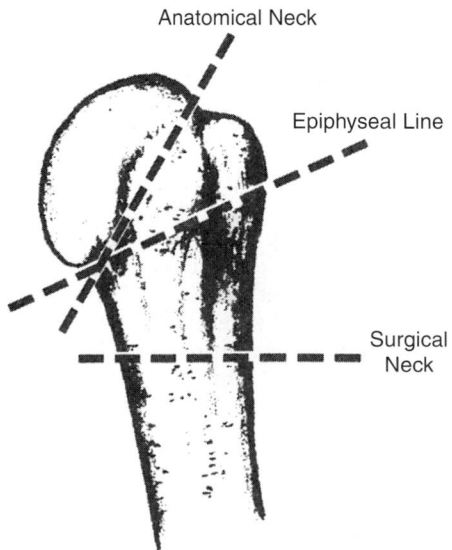

Figure 189.3. Anatomy of the proximal humerus. (From Aldred B. Proximal and Midshaft Humeral Injuries. In: Hart RG, Rittenberry TJ, Uehara DT (eds): *Handbook of orthopaedic emergencies.* Philadelphia, Lippincott-Raven, 1999, with permission.)

EMERGENCY DEPARTMENT MANAGAMENT

Clavicular Fractures

Clavicular fractures are the most common childhood fracture. They are often encountered in newborns secondary to birth trauma. Clavicular fractures account for 5% of all fractures seen for all age groups. Two mechanisms are commonly responsible: (1) force applied directly to the clavicle and (2) force applied to the outer end of the clavicle, which can push the shoulder inward toward the chest, causing a shearing force and fracture of the clavicle (29). Most patients have swelling and tenderness over the fracture site. Middle-third clavicular fractures usually result in a downward and inward slump of the involved shoulder due to loss of support.

Eighty percent of all clavicular fractures occur in the middle third. Nondisplaced middle-third fractures in adults have an intact periosteum. These require a sling for support and ice to reduce swelling. Figure-of-eight splints can be used for reduction and maintenance of position for displaced middle-third clavicular fractures in adults and children; however, they show no benefit over a simple sling. There are a number of studies that demonstrate no benefit whatsoever in either pain control or fracture reduction by using a figure-of-eight instead of a simple sling (17). Complications of middle-third clavicular fractures include malunion; excess callus formation, resulting in cosmetic defect; and neurovascular compromise. Rarely, nonunion occurs in fractures treated with open reduction and internal fixation.

Fifteen percent of clavicular fractures occur in the distal third. Nondisplaced fractures of the distal clavicle are splinted by the surrounding intact ligaments and muscles. They are usually treated symptomatically with ice, analgesics, a sling, and early motion. Fractures of the distal clavicle which are Type II fractures (displacement of the distal clavicle) may require surgical intervention because of rupture of the coracoclavicular ligament (1,17). There is a relatively high risk of nonunion in these displaced fractures (1). Complications include delayed union of displaced fractures treated conservatively, and degenerative arthritis with intraarticular involvement.

Medial-third fractures represent only 5% of all clavicular fractures. Considerable force is required to fracture the medial clavicle, so associated injuries, such as vascular injuries, should be sought. Management includes ice, analgesics, and a sling for support. Displaced fractures require orthopaedic referral for reduction. Degenerative arthritis frequently accompanies these fractures.

Proximal Humerus Fractures

Proximal humeral fractures account for 5% of all fractures. They are most common in the elderly (36). Anatomically, proximal humeral fractures include all humeral fractures proximal to the surgical neck. Two mechanisms of injury commonly produce proximal humeral fractures: (1) a direct blow on the lateral aspect of the arm and (2) a fall on an outstretched arm. Patients present with pain and swelling over the upper arm and shoulder. Most commonly, the arm is held adducted. Patients who present with the arm abducted have a much higher incidence of neurovascular injury.

Using the Neer classification system for proximal humerus fractures, the proximal humerus is divided into four segments: greater tuberosity, lesser tuberosity, anatomic neck, and surgical neck (25,26). This classification system has both prognostic and therapeutic implications, and depends on the relation of the bone segments involved and their displacement. The Neer system divides the fractures into one-part, two-part, three-part, and four-part fractures, depending on the displacement and angulation of the fracture (Fig. 189.4).

If all the proximal humeral fragments are nondisplaced and without angulation (less than 45 degrees), the injury is classified as a one-part fracture. The humeral fragments are held in place by the periosteum, rotator cuff, and joint capsule. Examples of one-part fractures are a surgical neck fracture with less than 45 degrees of angulation, a nondisplaced anatomic neck fracture, and a nondisplaced greater tuberosity fracture. Therapy for one-part fractures requires immobilization in a sling and swathe and orthopaedic referral within 4 to 5 days. Circumduction exercises should begin as soon as tolerated, and should be followed by passive exercise of the elbow and shoulder at 2 to 3 weeks. Shoulder motion exercises can usually be started within 3 to 4 weeks.

Two-part fractures have either a fragment with more than 1 cm of displacement or one with over 45 degrees of angulation to the intact proximal humerus. Surgical neck fractures with over 45 degrees of angulation, and displaced anatomic neck fractures, require immobilization with a sling and swathe and emergent orthopaedic referral for reduction. There remains significant controversy regarding the treatment of two-part fractures. Some authors feel that conservative therapy should be the primary modality while others feel that anatomic reduction is essential to prevention of avascular necrosis and, thus, advocate surgical intervention (2,37,38). Anatomic neck fractures have a high incidence of avascular necrosis.

The insertions of the supraspinatus, infraspinatus, and teres minor on the greater tuberosity complicate fractures in this region. Displaced greater tuberosity fractures (two-part fractures) are always associated with a tear of the rotator cuff. Greater tuberosity fractures are also seen in about 15% of all anterior shoulder dislocations (12,33). Therapy for displaced greater tuberosity fractures depends on the patient's age. Young patients require internal fixation or excision of the fragment, with repair of the torn rotator cuff. Older patients are usually not candidates for surgical repair and require ice, immobilization with a sling and swathe, and early orthopaedic referral. Complications of greater tuberosity fractures include impingement on the long head of the biceps, resulting in chronic tenosynovitis and eventually tendon rupture; nonunion; and myositis ossificans.

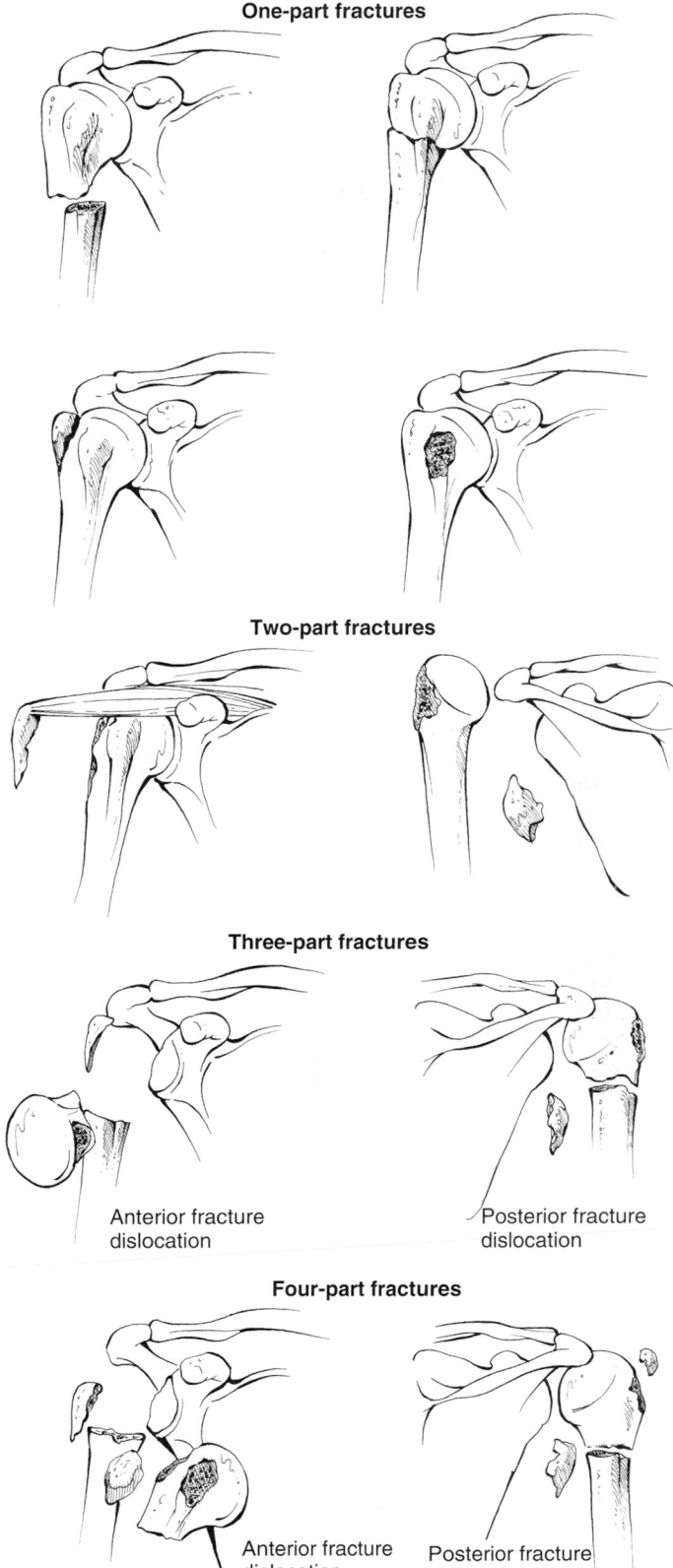

One-part fractures

Two-part fractures

Three-part fractures

Anterior fracture dislocation

Posterior fracture dislocation

Four-part fractures

Anterior fracture dislocation

Posterior fracture dislocation

Figure 189.4.   Examples of one-, two-, three-, and four-part fractures as described by Neer.

Lesser tuberosity fractures commonly occur in conjunction with posterior shoulder dislocations, due to intense contraction of the subscapularis muscle, which inserts on the lesser tuberosity. Management of these fractures includes sling and swathe immobilization. Most orthopaedic surgeons recommend 3 to 5 days of immobilization, followed by gradually increasing range-of-motion exercises. Some orthopedists prefer surgical fixation, so early consultation is advised.

Combination fractures (Neer three- and four-part fractures) result from severe forces. Three-part fractures involve two fragments that are individually displaced from the proximal humerus. Four-part fractures involve three fragments individually displaced from the remaining proximal humerus. Combined proximal humeral fractures are associated with shoulder dislocations, rotator cuff injuries, and neurovascular compromise. Therapy includes sling immobilization and emergent orthopaedic referral. These complex injuries usually require admission. Most authors feel that three and four-part fractures require surgical intervention and four-part fractures may require a prosthesis (2,14,19,23,24,32,37,38). However, some authors feel that even with these fractures conservative therapy should be considered, especially in the elderly (10,39). Virtually all combined fractures require surgical repair. Many four-part fractures require the insertion of a prosthesis, as a high incidence of avascular necrosis of the humeral head occurs secondary to compromised blood supply.

Articular surface fractures, also referred to as impression fractures, often result from direct trauma to the lateral arm. Fractures that involve less than 20% of the joint surface can be treated with sling and swathe immobilization in external rotation and early referral. Fractures involving more than 20% of the joint surface require surgical repair, and possibly prosthesis insertion. Complications of these fractures include joint stiffness, arthritis, and avascular necrosis with severely comminuted fractures.

Scapular Fractures

Scapular fractures represent only 1% of all fractures and 5% of fractures involving the shoulder (15). Many fracture patterns are associated with scapular fractures.

Because a great deal of force is usually required to fracture the body or spine of the scapula, these fractures are often associated with other more serious injuries. Typically, there is little displacement, due to the support of the investing muscles and periosteum. Treatment includes sling and swathe immobilization, early limited exercise, and orthopaedic referral.

Acromion fractures result from a direct downward blow to the shoulder. Due to the large amount of force required to produce these fractures, they are often accompanied by associated injuries, including brachial plexus injuries, rotator cuff tears, and superior shoulder dislocations. Nondisplaced fractures may be treated with sling immobilization in conjunction with an elastic circular dressing that pushes the elbow up and the lateral clavicle down. Displaced fractures require internal fixation.

Glenoid rim fractures are associated with two mechanisms of injury. A direct blow may result in a stellate fracture. An upward force, secondary to a fall on the flexed elbow, may cause a displaced glenoid rim fracture. Therapy for fractures with small fragments consists of sling immobilization, ice, and analgesia. Large or widely displaced fragments and stellate fractures require surgical fixation.

Coracoid process fractures may occur from a direct blow to the superior part of the shoulder, or from violent contraction of one of the inserting muscles, causing an avulsion fracture. The patient presents with tenderness to palpation over the coracoid process. Radiographs should include an axillary lateral view for delineation of any displacement of the fragment. Coracoid fractures are usually treated symptomatically with a sling, ice, and analgesics.

Anterior Shoulder Dislocation

Anterior shoulder dislocation is one of the most common dislocations, accounting for half of all dislocations presenting to the emergency department. This injury occurs when a blow to an abducted, externally rotated arm disrupts the anterior capsule and the glenohumeral ligaments (12). There are three types of anterior dislocations: subclavicular, subcoracoid, and subglenoid.

The patient presents with the arm held to the side. The acromion is prominent, and there is loss of the normal rounded contour of the shoulder. There is a gap beneath the acromion because of displacement of the greater tuberosity anteriorly and inferiorly. Axillary nerve injury is the most common associated neurologic injury in anterior shoulder dislocations, occurring in about 12% of cases. Nerve injury is assessed by testing pinprick sensation over the lateral aspect of the deltoid. A defect in the posterior lateral portion of the humeral head is often seen on radiographs. This impaction fracture of the humeral head is known as the Hill-Sachs deformity. The physician should determine the position of the humeral head in order to ascertain if there are associated injuries. The typical position is subcoracoid. If, however, the humeral head is in a subglenoid or subclavicular position, the patient either has a greater tuberosity fracture or a rotator cuff tear.

Adequate analgesia and muscle relaxation improves patient comfort and the success rate of reduction. Some have used intraarticular lidocaine with good results. There are numerous reduction techniques.

External Rotation Technique. The external rotation technique (Hennepin technique) requires little manipulation and permits the shoulder muscles to reduce the dislocation with minimal analgesia. The patient is seated upright or at 45 degrees. One of the physician's hands supports the elbow, and the other hand slowly externally rotates the patient's arm (Fig. 189.5). The arm is externally rotated to 90 degrees. The rotation must be performed gradually, and the patient must remain relaxed. After reaching 90 degrees, the shoulder may have reduced spontaneously. If not, the arm is slowly elevated, and the humeral head is lifted into the socket if it does not spontaneously reduce on elevation. Each of the aforementioned techniques requires little or no sedation or anesthesia and can be successfully performed within a few minutes (13).

Scapular Manipulation Technique. The patient lies prone on the table, with the affected arm hanging off the table and suspended with about 5 to 10 lbs of weight, similar to the Stimson technique (discussion follows). The physician pushes the tip of the scapula medially and the superior aspect of the scapula laterally (22). This technique may be performed on an upright patient, with an assistant grasping the patient's arm and applying mild traction while the physician rotates the scapula in a similar fashion. For patients are immobilized in the supine position due to multiple trauma; the scapular manipulation technique involves placing the affected extremity in adduction and 90-degree flexion at both the shoulder and elbow joints. Steady, gentle, upward traction is applied on the arm while the inferior tip of the scapula is gently manipulated with a force directed medially (11).

Stimson Technique. The patient is placed in the prone position, with the arms dependent over a pillow or folded sheet and hanging over the side of the stretcher. A strap is added to the wrist and weights are applied (10 to 15 lbs) over 20 to 30 minutes (26,36). If unsuccessful, the examiner may rotate the humerus gently, externally and then internally with mild force, which usually reduces the dislocations.

Traction and Countertraction. With the patient lying in the supine position, an assistant applies countertraction with a folded sheet around the upper chest while the examiner applies

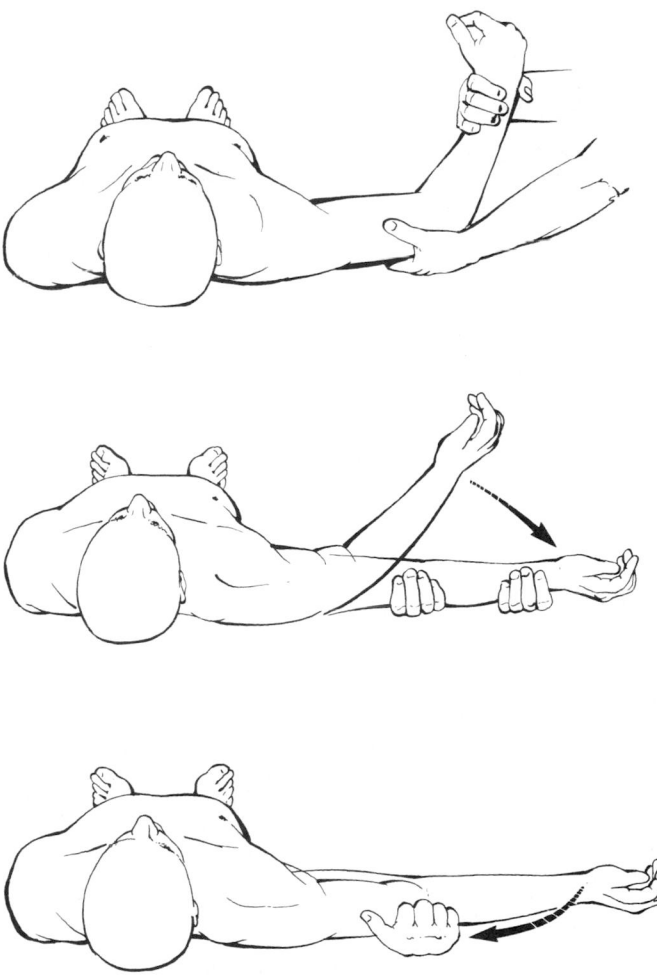

Figure 189.5. Hennepin technique for anterior shoulder dislocation reduction. (Adapted from Simon RR, Koenigsknecht SJ. *Emergency orthopaedics.* Norwalk, CT: Appleton & Lange, 1994.)

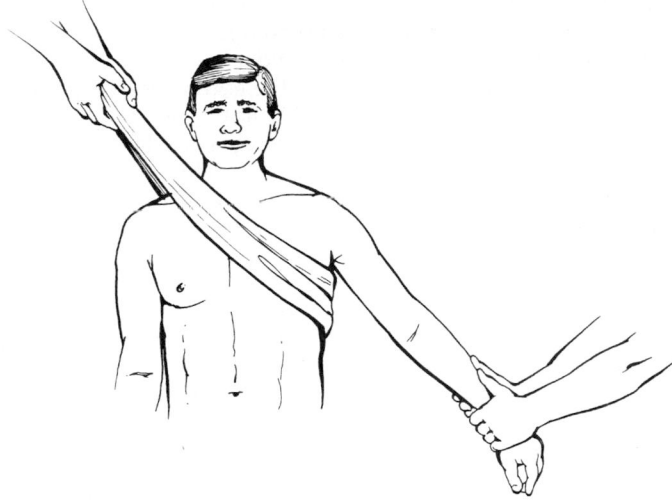

Figure 189.6. Traction–countertraction technique for reducing anterior shoulder dislocations. (Adapted from Simon RR, Koenigsknecht SJ. *Emergency orthopaedics.* Norwalk, CT: Appleton & Lange, 1994.)

traction to the arm (Fig. 189.6). Additional lateral traction may be added with a second sheet applied to the proximal portion of the humerus, with lateral force applied to this area. To prevent avulsion injuries (16) when using this maneuver, the patient must have good muscle relaxation. Alternatively, traction can be applied with the patient seated in an upright position of a chair. The patient sits as straight as possible. Traction is provided by a 3-ft loop of 4-in.-wide cast stockinette placed around the proximal forearm of the involved extremity, with the elbow flexed at 90 degrees. Countertraction is provided by the chair. An assistant maintains the patient upright by standing adjacent to the unaffected shoulder and clasping his or her hands around the chest in the axilla of the affected side. The physician places a foot in the stockinette loop to provide firm downward traction (9).

The external rotation and scapular manipulation techniques should be attempted first as they have no associated complications. If these are unsuccessful then the traction-countertraction or Stimson techniques should be attempted. If the dislocation cannot be reduced by these methods, general anesthesia should be considered and reduction attempted in the operating room. Irreducible dislocations are usually due to soft-tissue interposition. For patients less than 30 years old, after reduction the shoulder is immobilized for 3 weeks, followed by gentle active range-of-motion exercises. The patient should avoid abduction and external rotation for an additional 3 weeks. For patients over

age 30, the shoulder is immobilized for 1 week, followed by active range-of-motion exercises, avoiding abduction and external rotation (35). Patients should follow up with an orthopedist within one week. There is now controversy regarding whether the patient should be placed in a simple sling or whether nonoperative therapy should include a pillow supporting the arm or device whereby some external rotation is allowed (24). Most authors continue to feel that the optimal therapy would be a sling and swathe followed by circumduction exercises (6). The shoulder may be kept immobilized for circumduction exercises. The older the patient, the earlier the mobilization should be instituted to avoid stiffness. Exercises forcing internal rotation of the arm strengthen the subscapularis muscle, helping to prevent recurrent anterior shoulder dislocations.

Complications of anterior shoulder dislocations include tears of the rotator cuff, avulsion of the greater tuberosity, axillary nerve injury, and fracture of the humeral head. Operative repair is indicated in patients who have sustained more than three dislocations.

Postreduction radiographs are not necessary if the reduction was performed smoothly and postreduction physical examination shows no suspicion of unsuccessful reduction (16).

Posterior Shoulder Dislocation

Posterior dislocations are less common than anterior dislocations and are the most frequently missed major dislocation. There are three types of posterior dislocations: subacromial, subglenoid, and subspinous. Almost all dislocations are the subacromial type. The mechanisms involved in this injury include violent internal rotational force occurring during a fall on the forward-flexed, internally rotated arm; and internal rotational force following a generalized tonic–clonic seizure.

On physical examination, the arm is held in adduction and internal rotation, with abduction severely limited. External rotation of the shoulder is blocked. The blocking of external rotation is one of the critical features that help to determine that there is, in fact, a posterior dislocation of the shoulder. Whenever a patient has had a grand mal seizure, the physician should always check for external rotation in both shoulders. If external rotation is blocked, then a posterior shoulder dislocation should be considered. This is one of the most commonly missed injuries, and one of the common mechanisms is a seizure. There is a prominence in the posterior aspect of the shoulder, accompanied by a flattening of the normal anterior shoulder contour.

Radiographically, there is loss of the normal elliptic pattern produced by overlap of the humeral head and the posterior glenoid rim. The greater tuberosity is internally rotated. Isolated fractures of the lesser tuberosity are associated with posterior shoulder dislocations.

Posterior shoulder dislocations may be reduced using the Stimson method, or other techniques that push the posteriorly displaced humeral head forward. If there is severe pain or muscle spasm, general anesthesia may be necessary to reduce the dislocation. Surgical intervention is needed for major displacement of the lesser tuberosity that cannot be reduced on reduction of the dislocation. Reduction of a posterior shoulder dislocation either by closed or open techniques is the optimal treatment of these injuries (6,28). Neurovascular compromise is uncommon.

Inferior Shoulder Dislocation (Luxatio Erecta)

Inferior dislocations of the shoulder are uncommon, and occur due to hyperabduction. These injuries are always associated with detachment of the rotator cuff.

On physical examination, the patient is in severe pain and holds the arm at 180 degrees of elevation. The humeral head can be palpated along the lateral chest wall. Compression of the axillary artery and brachial plexus may occur as the humeral head tears through the inferior capsule. Vascular injury is more common with inferior dislocations than with any other form of shoulder dislocation (22). Associated fractures of the acromion, inferior glenoid rim, and greater tuberosity may occur (21).

To reduce the dislocation, the physician applies traction in the longitudinal axis of the humerus while an assistant applies countertraction with a folded sheet wrapped around the supraclavicular region. With traction maintained, the arm is rotated inferiorly in an arc toward a position of complete adduction. After reduction, the shoulder is immobilized for 2 to 4 weeks.

Occasionally, general anesthesia may be required to reduce the dislocation and repair the torn rotator cuff.

Acromioclavicular Joint Injury

The AC joint functions to elevate and abduct the arm. Stability is provided by two ligaments—the AC and the coracoclavicular. Most injuries of the AC joint are caused by a direct force applied to the point of the shoulder.

The diagnosis of an AC joint injury is made by examining the patient in the upright position and looking for a deformity at the tip of the shoulder. This deformity represents a prominence of the distal clavicle, created by a tear of the AC ligament, and possibly the coracoclavicular ligament. Coracoclavicular ligament injury may involve the conoid ligament, the trapezoid ligament, or both. Patients will also have tenderness at the AC joint.

For suspected AC joint injury, stress views taken in the AP position with 5 to 10 lbs of weight should be obtained only when one cannot clinically demonstrate the classical features of third-degree injury. Hand-held weights temper the actual degree of separation, so weights should be suspended from the arm or wrist for full effect.

The therapy for AC joint injuries depends on the degree of AC and coracoclavicular ligament injury. The traditional three-part *Aliman classification* of AC joint injuries has been expanded to a six-part classification system.

Type I injuries are a simple sprain of the AC ligament and involve an incomplete tear of that structure. The patient complains of pain and has tenderness over the AC joint. Swelling is minimal and no subluxation is present. Radiographs are negative, even with stress views. Therapy includes rest, ice, and a sling, with early range of motion.

Type II injuries involve disruption of the AC ligament, with sprain of the coracoclavicular ligament (Fig. 189.7). There is a partial subluxation of the distal end of the clavicle from the acromion. The patient experiences tenderness to mild palpation, and moderate swelling is present. Routine radiographs are usually normal, although subluxation with stress views is noted. The

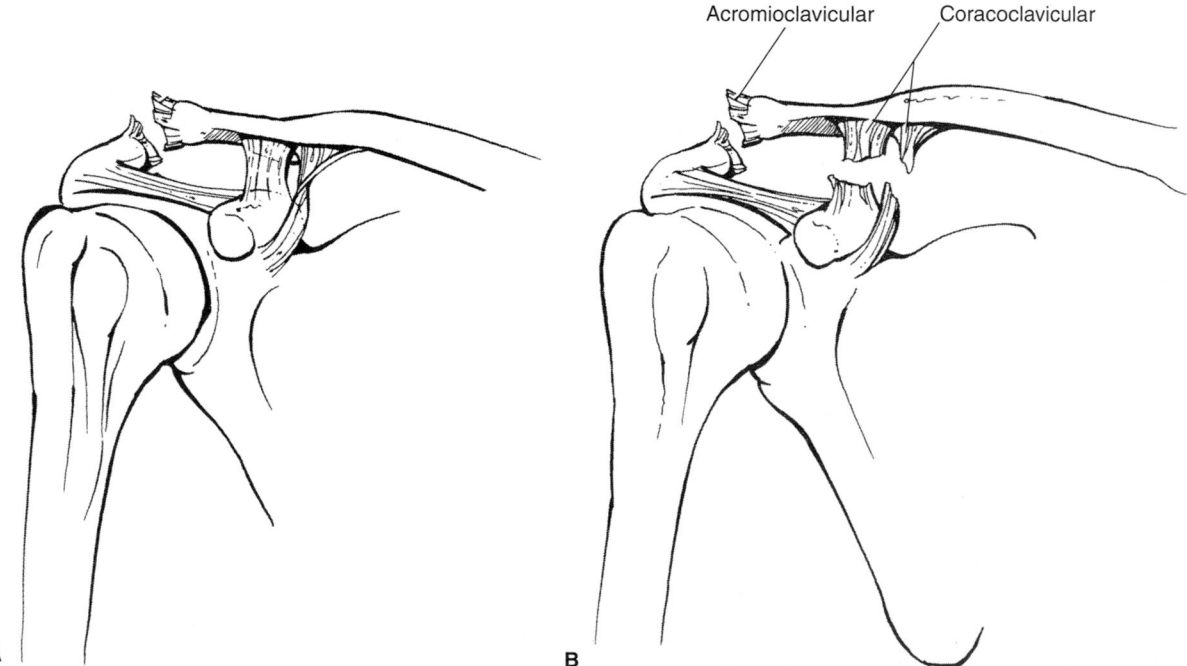

Figure 189.7. Acromioclavicular subluxation and dislocation. **(A)** A grade II sprain with tear of the acromioclavicular ligament. **(B)** A grade III sprain with tear of both the acromioclavicular and coracoclavicular ligaments.

pathognomonic radiographic finding is a separation of the distal clavicle by no more than half its diameter from the acromion on stress films. Separation of the clavicle by more than half its diameter indicates a type III injury. Type II injuries are treated conservatively with ice, rest, and immobilization in a sling. Additional measures for reducing the clavicle and holding it in place with a brace-strap (Kenny-Howard sling) may be used, but clavicular support has not been shown to produce superior improvement in long-term function over that produced by a sling (7).

Type III injuries result in complete dislocation at the AC joint, with upward displacement of the clavicle and disruption of both the AC and coracoclavicular ligaments (Fig. 189.7). Controversy exists regarding therapy. In the past, type III injuries were treated surgically in young patients. With the advent of arthroscopic surgery, Type III injuries are often treated arthroscopically (27). However, there remains significant controversy regarding conservative versus operative management of these patients in all age groups. Thus, patients with these injuries should be referred to an orthopedist within one week (4,18,27). However, conservative treatment similar to type II therapy has been shown to produce results as good as those after surgical intervention (25,30). Immobilization in the Kenny-Howard sling should be used for 3 weeks. Type III injuries require orthopaedic referral. In *type IV* injuries, the clavicle is displaced posteriorly into or through the trapezius muscle.

Type V injuries are severe injuries that involve disruption of all ligaments above the joint. The clavicle is displaced far cephalad toward the base of the neck.

In *type VI* injuries, the clavicle is dislocated inferiorly, with the lateral end displaced under the acromion or the coracoid process. Type VI injuries are associated with clavicle fractures, rib fractures, or brachial plexus injuries.

Types IV, V, and VI injuries require surgical intervention.

Sternoclavicular Joint Injuries

The SC joint is stabilized by the SC ligament and the costoclavicular ligament. The most common mechanism of injury to this joint is a force that thrusts the shoulder forward.

First-degree SC joint injury is a sprain of the SC joint and involves incomplete tears of the SC and costoclavicular ligaments. The patient experiences minimal swelling and has tenderness at the joint. Therapy includes ice, analgesics, and a sling for 3 to 4 days.

Second-degree SC joint injury involves subluxation of the clavicle from its manubrial attachment. Complete rupture of the SC ligament and partial rupture of the costoclavicular ligament occur. There is pain on abduction of the arm, and swelling is noted over the joint. Treatment includes 6 weeks of immobilization with a figure-of-eight clavicle strap and a sling to hold the clavicle in its normal position. This immobilization permits ligamentous healing (40).

Third-degree SC joint injury involves complete rupture of the SC and costoclavicular ligaments, permitting the clavicle to dislocate from its manubrial attachment. Anterior dislocations are much more common, but posterior dislocations result in much more serious injuries. Patients experience severe pain, increased by any motion of the shoulder. Posterior dislocations may constitute a true orthopaedic emergency since respiratory embarrassment may occur secondary to tracheal compression or a pneumothorax, or venous congestion may occur secondary to compression of vessels in the neck. These associated injuries necessitate emergency reduction of the SC joint dislocation by the physician in the emergency department.

Reduction is accomplished by placing a folded sheet between the shoulders, with the patient supine, which serves to separate the clavicle from the manubrium. The arm is abducted and trac-

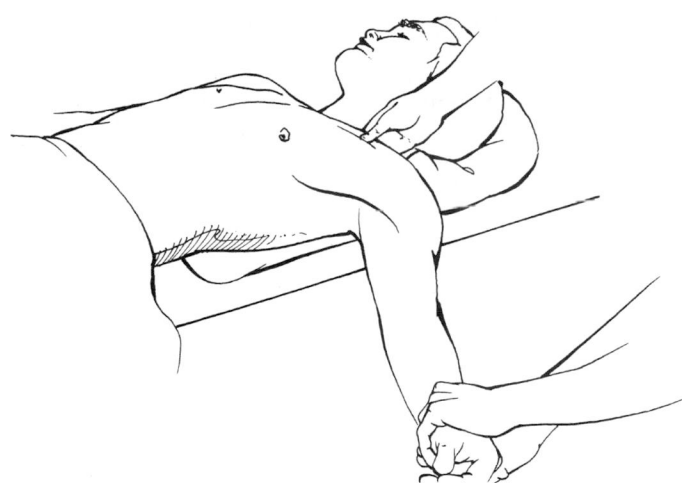

Figure 189.8. Reduction of a displaced sternoclavicular joint injury. The arm is abducted and traction is applied. With traction maintained, an assistant pushes the clavicle back into its normal position for anterior dislocations (*not shown*). With posterior dislocations, the clavicle is pulled back into its normal position. In difficult cases, the clavicle can be grasped with a towel clip. (Adapted from Simon RR, Koenigsknecht SJ. *Emergency orthopaedics.* Norwalk, CT: Appleton & Lange, 1994.)

tion is applied. For anterior dislocation, while traction is maintained, the clavicle is pushed in place (Fig. 189.8). For posterior dislocations, using the same maneuver, the clavicle should be grasped near its medial border with a towel clip (following the instillation of local anesthesia) and pulled out of its posterior position. Unstable sternoclavicular joint dislocations may require surgical intervention (1). General anesthesia may be required to relocate a posterior dislocation of the SC joint.

Complications of an anterior SC dislocation are cosmetic, with chronic swelling around the joint. Although some authors have stated that up to 25% (3) of posterior dislocations are associated with complications, including pneumothorax, laceration of the superior vena cava, occlusion of the subclavian artery or vein, and rupture or compression of the trachea, this may overestimate the incidence.

Rotator Cuff Injury

Tears of the rotator cuff are more common in the elderly because of degenerative changes that occur with advancing age. In young patients, a tear requires much more trauma. The mechanism of injury is a sudden forceful elevation of the arm against resistance in an attempt to cushion a fall, heavy lifting, or a direct impact to the shoulder. The most common area of disruption of the cuff is at its anterior superior portion, at the attachment of the supraspinatus muscle. At this point, the tendon is worn down by the compressive forces between the humeral head and the coracoacromial arch.

Patients complain of pain, aggravated by activity that radiates to the anterior aspect of the arm. Abduction and external rotation of the arm are painful and weak. Tenderness is present over the insertion at the greater tuberosity.

The *drop arm test* is positive in patients with significant tears. This is performed by horizontally elevating the arm to the 90-degree position and asking the patient to continue to hold the arm in this position. Slight pressure on the distal forearm will cause the patient to drop the arm suddenly. In addition, the patient cannot bring the arm from the abducted position to the side in a slow fashion, but drops it precipitously.

Thirty percent or more of the tendon must be ruptured to produce a significant reduction of strength. The extent of the tear is directly related to the limitation of shoulder abduction (8). Arthrography may be used to detect the location and extent of the tear.

Emergency treatment includes ice, immobilization, and orthopaedic referral within 4 to 5 days. Conservative therapy results in a good outcome in only 50% of patients. Arthroscopic treatment can be performed in a number of rotator cuff tears, particularly in the young. Anterior tears have been shown to have the best outcome with arthroscopic repair (17,20). Patients with large posterior rotator cuff tears are poor candidates for arthroscopy. In the young, early surgical repair is indicated for complete tears of the rotator cuff (3). In the elderly patient who has a more sedentary life, repair may not be indicated.

CRITICAL INTERVENTIONS

- In patients with scapular fractures, evaluate for other associated thoracic injuries with careful physical examination, radiographs, and further testing when indicated
- In patients who have had a grand mal seizure, check for external rotation in both shoulders to evaluate for posterior shoulder dislocation
- Use the towel clip method to reduce posterior sternoclavicular dislocations as they are associated with respiratory distress due to tracheal compression or pneumothorax and they can cause vascular compression

COMMON PITFALLS

✔ Failure to obtain a transscapular radiographic view (Y view) when assessing the shoulder for dislocation
✔ Forgetting that lesser tuberosity fractures are often associated with posterior shoulder dislocations
✔ Failure to search for other injuries in patients with scapular fractures

References

1. Anderson K. Evaluation and treatment of distal clavicle fractures. *Clin Sports Med* 2003;22:319–26.
2. Bathis H. Surgical treatment of proximal humeral fractures. Is the T-plate still adequate osteosynthesis procedure? *Zentralbl Chi* 2001;12:211–216.
3. Bicos J, Nicholson G. Treatment and results of sternoclavicular joint injuries. *Clin Sports Med* 2003;22:359–370.
4. Bradley J, Elkousy H. Decision making: operative versus nonoperative treatment of acromioclavicular joint injuries.
5. Burkhart SS. Arthroscopic treatment of massive rotator cuff tear. *Clin Orthop* 1991;267:45.
6. Burra G, Andrews J. Acute shoulder and elbow dislocations in the athlete. *Orthop Clin North Am* 2002;33:479–495.
7. Clarke HD. Acromioclavicular joint injuries. *Orthop Clin North Am* 2000;31:177–187.
8. Cofield RF. Current concepts review: rotator cuff disease of the shoulder. *J Bone Joint Surg Br* 1981;63B:198.
9. Craig DW, Gill EA, Noyes ME, et al. Anterior shoulder dislocation, a simple and rapid method for reduction. *Am J Sports Med* 1995;23:369–371.
10. De la Hoz Marin J. Surgical treatment of three-part proximal humeral fractures. *Acta Orthop Belg* 2001;67:226–232.
11. Doyle WL, Ragar. Use of the scapular manipulation method to reduce an anterior shoulder dislocation in the supine position. *Ann Emerg Med* 1996;27:92–94.
12. Flatlow EL, Cuomo F, Maday MG, et al. Open reduction and internal fixation of two-part displaced fractures of the greater tuberosity of the proximal part of the humerus. *J Bone Joint Surg Am* 1991;73:1213.
13. Graeme KA, Jackimczyk KC. The extremities and spine. *Emerg Med Clin North Am* 1997;15:365–379.
14. Hessman MH. Osteosynthesis techniques in proximal humeral fractures. *Chirurg* 2001;72:1235–1245.
15. Herscovici D, Fiennes AG, Allgower M, et al. The floating shoulder: ipsilateral clavicle and scapular neck fractures. *J Bone Joint Surg Br* 1992;74:362.
16. Kaufman ML, Leung J. Evaluation of the patient with extremity trauma: an evidence based approach. *Emerg Med Clin North Am* 1999;17:77–95.
17. Kao FC. Treatment of distal clavicle fracture using Kirschner wires and tension band wires. *J Trauma* 2001;51:522–525.
18. Kwon Y, Iannotti J. Operative treatment of acromioclavicular joint injuries and results. *Clin Sports Med* 2003;22(2):291–300.
19. Lill H. Conservative treatment of dislocated proximal humeral fracture. *Zentralbl Chir* 2001;126:205–210.
20. Lyons AK, Tomlinson JE. Clinical diagnosis of tears of the rotator cuff. *J Bone Joint Surg Br* 1992;74B:414.
21. Mallon WJ, Bassett FH, Goldner RD. Luxatio erecta: the inferior glenohumeral dislocation. *J Orthop Trauma* 1990;4:19.
22. McNamara RM. Reduction of anterior shoulder dislocation by scapular manipulation. *Ann Emerg Med* 1993;21:1140.
23. Misra A. Complex proximal humeral fractures in adults—a systematic review of management. *Injury* 2001;32:363–372.
24. Murrell GA. Treatment of shoulder dislocation: is a sling appropriate? *Med J Aust* 2003;179:370–371.
25. Neer CS II. Displaced proximal humeral fractures. Part I: classification and evaluation. *J Bone Joint Surg* 1970;52:1077.
26. Neer CS II. Fractures about the shoulder: a classification. *J Bone Joint Surg* 1970;52:1081.
27. Nuber G, Bowen M. Arthroscopic treatment of acromioclavicular joint injuries and results. *Clin Sports Med Apr* 2003;22:301–317.
28. Ogawa K. Posterior shoulder dislocation associated with fracture of the humeral anatomic neck: treatment guidelines and long-term outcome. *J Trauma* 1999;46:318–323.
29. Post M. Current concepts in the treatment of fractures of the clavicle. *Clin Orthop* 1989;245:89.
30. Press J, Zuckerman JD, Gallagher M, et al. Treatment of grade III acromioclavicular separations, operative versus nonoperative management. *Bull Hosp Jt Dis* 1997;56:77–83.
31. Riebel GD, McCabe JB. Anterior shoulder dislocation: a review of reduction techniques. *Am J Emerg Med* 1991;9:180.
32. Robinson CM. Primary hemiarthroplasty for treatment of proximal humeral fractures. *J Bone Joint Surg Am* 2003;85-A):1215–1223.
33. Rockwood CA, Green DP, (eds). *Fractures.* Philadelphia: JB Lippincott Co, 1991.
34. Serin E. Two-prong splint in treatment of proximal humeral fracture. *Arch Orthop Trauma Surg* 1999;119:368–370.
35. Simon RR, Koenigsknecht SJ. Emergency orthopaedics. Norwalk, CT: Appleton & Lange, 1994.
36. Stimson BB. *A manual of fractures and dislocations,* 2nd ed. Philadelphia: Lea & Febiger, 1947.
37. Szyszkowitz R. Fractures of the proximal humerus. *Unfallchirurg.* 1999;102:422–428.
38. Takeuchi R. Minimally invasive fixation for unstable two-part proximal humeral fractures: surgical techniques and clinical results using j-nails. *J Orthop Trauma* 2002;16:403–408.
39. Tingart M. The displaced proximal humeral fracture: is there evidence for therapeutic concepts? *Chirurg* 2001;72:1284–1291.
40. Yeh GL. Conservative management of sternoclavicular injuries. *Orthop Clin North Am* 2000;31:189–203.

CHAPTER 190
Elbow Injuries

Andrew D. Perron

The elbow is a synovial hinge joint consisting of three articulations between the distal humerus, radius, and ulna. The humerus widens distally to form the lateral and medial condyles. The capitellum is a spheroidal cartilaginous structure of the lateral condyle that articulates with the radial head, permitting pronation and supination. The trochlea is a spoon-shaped cartilaginous projection of the medial condyle that articulates with the deep trochlear notch of the ulna, permitting flexion and extension at the elbow. The articulating surfaces of the head of the radius and ulna are held together by the annular ligament. The anterior capsule combined with the radial and ulnar collateral ligaments provide stability at the elbow joint.

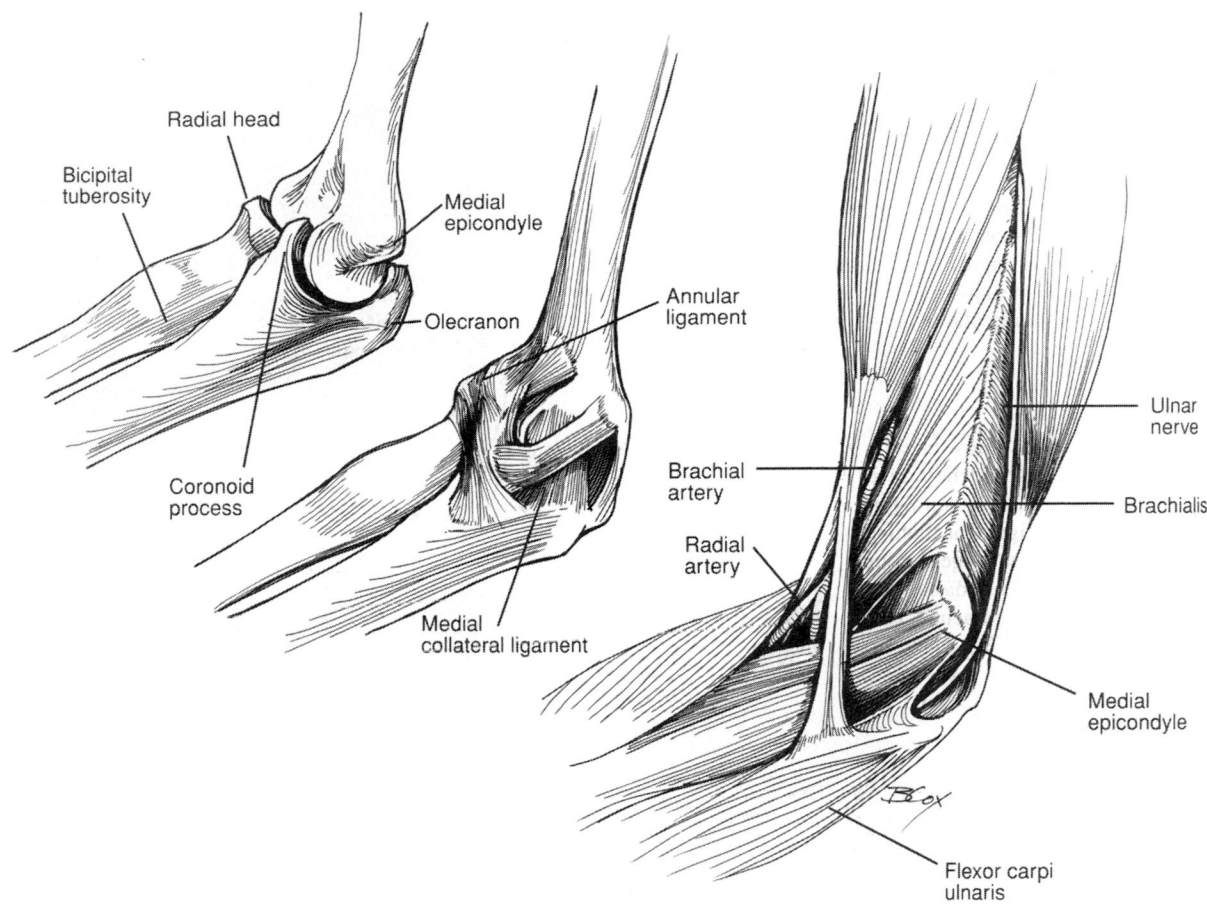

Figure 190.1. Elbow anatomy. (From McCue FC III, Sweeney T, and Urch S. The elbow, wrist, and hand. In: Perrin DH (Ed): *The injured athlete,* 3rd edition. Philadelphia: Lippincott-Raven, 1999, with permission.)

The wrist flexor and pronator muscles originate from the medial epicondyle. The wrist extensor and supinator muscles attach to the lateral epicondyle. The brachial artery is palpable medial to the biceps tendon in the antecubital space. The median nerve traverses deep in the antecubital fossa medial to the brachial artery. The ulnar nerve courses posteriorly in the cubital tunnel between the medial epicondyle and olecranon process. The radial nerve passes between the heads of the triceps in the posterior humerus and may be injured in humeral shaft fractures.

There are several bursal structures in the elbow. The superficial olecranon bursa lies beneath the skin over the olecranon process and is particularly vulnerable to traumatic and infectious processes. Figure 190.1 illustrates the anatomy of the elbow.

EMERGENCY DEPARTMENT EVALUATION

The assessment of elbow injuries should include a detailed history of the mechanism of injury. The most common complaints are pain, restriction of movement, and swelling. A description of the location and duration of pain, aggravating factors, and presence of paresthesias or loss of movement is important. Elbow pain may also be referred from injuries to the shoulder, forearm, or wrist. Injuries to the elbow may refer pain to the wrist. Identification of one injury should not preclude the search for other injuries. An occupational history may provide a clue to the diagnosis in patients presenting with chronic pain.

Inspection of the involved extremity for swelling, open wounds, deformities, effusions, and discoloration is the first step in the physical examination of the patient with elbow pain. The involved joint should not be extensively manipulated until radiographs have been obtained to exclude fracture and dislocation. The shoulder, forearm, wrist, and hand should also be carefully examined. Laceration over the medial epicondyle should raise suspicion of an ulnar nerve injury. Any abnormality noted in the involved extremity should be compared with the contralateral extremity.

An effusion is best palpated over the soft-tissue area lateral to the radial head. The bony prominences of the medial and lateral condyles, olecranon, and radial head should be palpated for tenderness. The radial head is best palpated with the thumb of one hand while pronating and supinating the forearm with the examiner's other hand. With the elbow flexed to 90 degrees, the medial and lateral condyles and the olecranon should form a triangle. In an elbow dislocation, this triangle is disrupted with displacement of the olecranon. A posterior dislocation or extension-type fracture is suggested by a prominent olecranon. Loss of the olecranon prominence suggests an anterior dislocation or supracondylar fracture. The triangular relationship is maintained in supracondylar fracture. Each of the muscle groups should be tested against resistance and the muscle belly palpated during contraction.

Careful neurovascular examination is of critical importance. Brachial, radial, and ulnar pulses should be palpated and capillary refill assessed. The brachioradialis, biceps, and triceps reflexes should be elicited. The radial nerve is best tested by evaluating wrist and finger extension. Wristdrop results from radial nerve injury. Flexion of the wrist and digits and pronation of the forearm are the functions of the median nerve. Inability to flex and abduct the thumb is diagnostic of median nerve injury. Loss of strength of the interossei muscles and adduction of the thumb suggests ulnar nerve injury. The sensory component of the radial nerve innervates the dorsum of the hand and is best tested in the web space between the thumb and index finger. Median nerve sensation is tested over the palmar aspect of the thumb and the digits to the radial one-half of the ring finger; at the volar tip of the index finger there is no overlap from the radial or median nerves. The ulnar nerve is tested at the volar tip of the fifth digit. The neurovascular examination of the extremity should be repeated after manipulation and at regular intervals since edema from a fracture may result in neurovascular compromise.

The radiographic examination of the elbow should consist of a minimum of two views at right angles to each other (anteroposterior and lateral). Radiographs are most commonly misread because a true lateral view of the elbow is not obtained. In one university emergency department setting, the incidence of missed elbow fractures was 12% (2). Oblique views may be obtained to provide additional information. Specialized views, such as the radial head–capitellum view, are indicated when a suspicion for particular injury exists.

On the lateral radiograph, a line parallel to the anterior border of the humerus should intersect the anterior portion of the middle third of the capitellum (Fig. 190. 2) (11). If this intersection is displaced, usually anterior to the capitellum, a supracondylar fracture should be suspected.

The radiocapitellar line extends from the center of the radius and should intersect the middle third of the capitellum on the lateral view (11). Disruption of this line suggests radial head dislocation or fracture and is most useful in evaluating subtle fractures in children.

Fat pad signs are helpful in diagnosing occult fractures within the joint capsule. The *anterior fat pad* is a combination of fat in the coronoid and radial fossa. This radiolucent fat overlaps and normally appears as a triangular area over the distal humerus on a lateral radiograph of the elbow. The *posterior fat pad* is located in the olecranon fossa and is normally hidden by the overlying humeral condyles on a lateral radiograph.

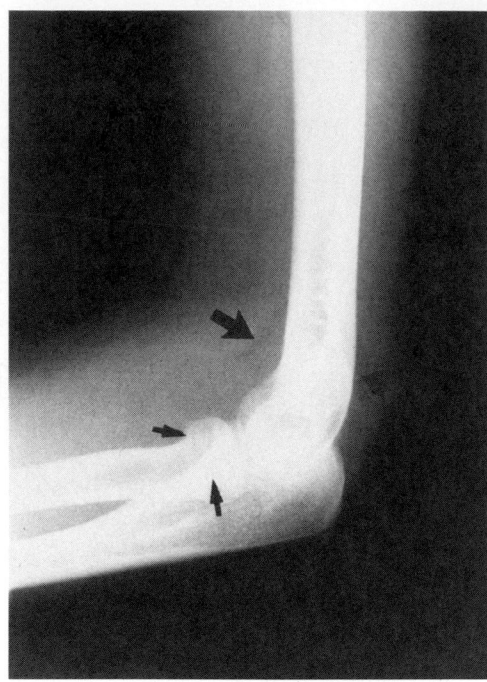

Figure 190.3.   Anterior and posterior fat pad signs are indicated by the *large arrows. Small arrows* indicate the radial head fracture that produced the effusion displacing the fat pads.

When an effusion is present, it distends the joint capsule and displaces the fat pads (Fig. 190.3). The *anterior fat pad* displaces anteriorly and superiorly and appears as a "ship's sail." The *posterior fat pad* becomes visible on radiography and is highly indicative of intraarticular disease. In the setting of elbow trauma, a visible posterior fat pad or a prominent anterior fat pad in the absence of visible fracture should mandate a search for occult fracture, most commonly of the radial head.

Positive fat pad signs can also be present with any intraarticular disease process and thus are not strictly pathognomonic for fracture. Fat pad signs may be seen with arthritis, gout, pseudogout, infection, neoplasia, or other disease process causing an intraarticular fluid collection (8). A fat pad sign may not be present with severe injury causing disruption of the joint capsule.

While not usually necessary in the ED evaluation of these patients, computed tomography (CT) scanning may be useful in delineating complex fractures in adults. Magnetic resonance imaging has become the procedure of choice for evaluating soft tissues, cartilaginous surfaces, joint space, and trabecular bone (6).

EMERGENCY DEPARTMENT MANAGEMENT

Supracondylar Fractures

Supracondylar fractures occur in the distal humerus proximal to the epicondyles and are most commonly seen in children. In adults, because of their stronger bones, elbow dislocations from ligamentous disruption are more common. These fractures most commonly result from a fall on the outstretched hand with the elbow in extension.

Twenty-five percent of supracondylar fractures are nondisplaced. Treatment of a nondisplaced fracture is a posterior splint from axilla to palm, with the elbow flexed to 90 degrees. These patients should be urgently referred to an orthopaedic surgeon for follow up within 24 to 48 hours. The patient and parents should be carefully counseled regarding warning signs of compartment

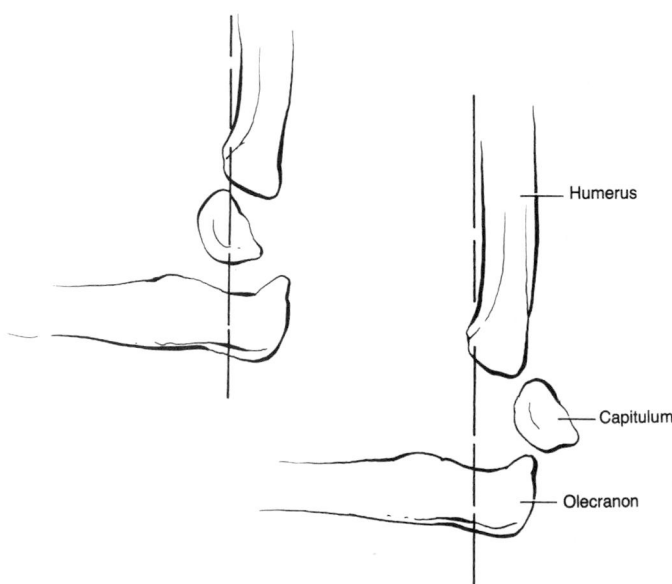

Figure 190.2.   Anterior humeral line. The anterior humeral line is a line drawn on the lateral radiograph along the anterior surface of the humerus through the elbow. Normally this line transects the middle of the capitellum (**left**). With an extension fracture of the supracondylar region, this line will either transect the anterior third of the capitellum or pass entirely anterior to it (**right**). (Adapted, with permission, from Simon RR, Koenigsknecht SJ. *Emergency orthopaedics: the extremities,* 2nd ed. Norwalk, CT: Appleton & Lange, 1987.)

syndrome. A child with elbow tenderness and swelling should be splinted, even without a demonstrable radiographic fracture, because of the possibility of occult fracture (16).

In displaced fractures, the distal fragment is usually displaced posteriorly (extension injury), and an abnormal anterior humeral line will be visualized on the lateral radiograph. Anterior displacement of the distal fragment (flexion injury) occurs less frequently and is caused by a direct blow to the posterior aspect of the flexed elbow.

Assessment of neurovascular function is essential, especially with extension injuries, because occult injury to the brachial artery may occur. A strong pulse does not completely rule out arterial injury, and a vascular study should be performed if injury is clinically suspected. Closed reduction of displaced fractures should be attempted as soon as possible if neurovascular compromise is present.

Displaced fractures require internal fixation or percutaneous pinning if good alignment is not maintained with closed reduction. Patients with displaced fractures should be admitted because of the risk of delayed swelling and neurovascular compromise, including compartment syndrome, and the potential for Volkmann ischemic contracture. Flexion fractures may also require internal fixation and should be splinted in extension. Range-of-motion exercises after internal fixation are encouraged and will generally be started within 1 to 2 weeks.

A common complication of supracondylar fracture is an abnormal carrying angle. The normal carrying angle is 10 degrees to 15 degrees of valgus. Measurement of Baumann's angle, formed by a line perpendicular to the humeral shaft and a line through the lateral humeral condyle, is predictive of an acceptable carrying angle (15). This angle normally measures about 75 degrees. A discrepancy of greater than 5 degrees to 10 degrees, compared with the uninjured extremity, is an unacceptable reduction, as it may impair useful function of the arm (Fig. 190.4).

Intercondylar Fractures

Intercondylar fractures usually occur in older patients as a result of direct trauma to the flexed elbow. They usually occur in "T" and "Y" configurations, and treatment is based on the amount of displacement of the humeral condyles from each other and from the proximal humerus. Neurovascular complications are uncommon and these fractures rarely require manipulation by the emergency physician.

Nondisplaced fractures are treated in a posterior splint for 3 weeks, and then active range of motion is begun. Displaced fractures are treated with internal fixation and early range of motion beginning after 1 week. Severely comminuted fractures may be treated with olecranon traction for 3 to 4 weeks if operative repair is not possible.

Humeral Condyle Fractures

Isolated humeral condyle fractures are caused by a fall on the outstretched hand, by direct trauma, or by avulsion of bone from the pull of the flexor or extensor muscles from the medial and lateral condyles, respectively. Lateral condyle fractures are more common than medial fractures and frequently involve the joint surface.

Nondisplaced lateral condyle fractures are immobilized in a posterior splint, with the elbow flexed to 90 degrees and the forearm in supination with the wrist extended. The forearm should be in pronation and the wrist flexed for medial condyle fractures. Active range of motion is begun as early as 2 to 3 weeks after injury. Operative fixation is required for displaced fractures, owing to instability caused by the pull of the forearm muscles.

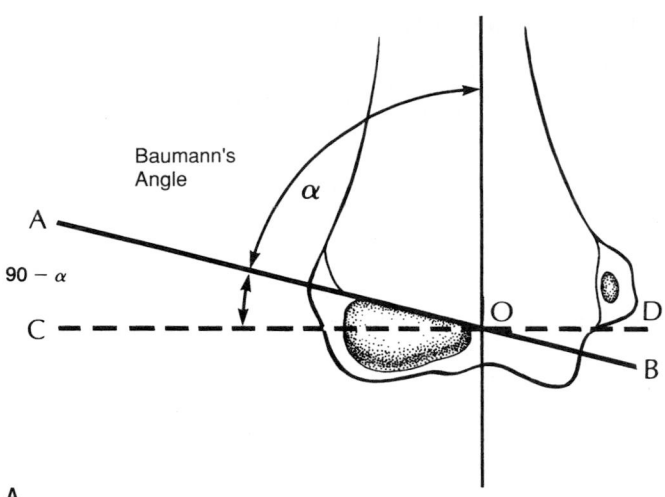

A

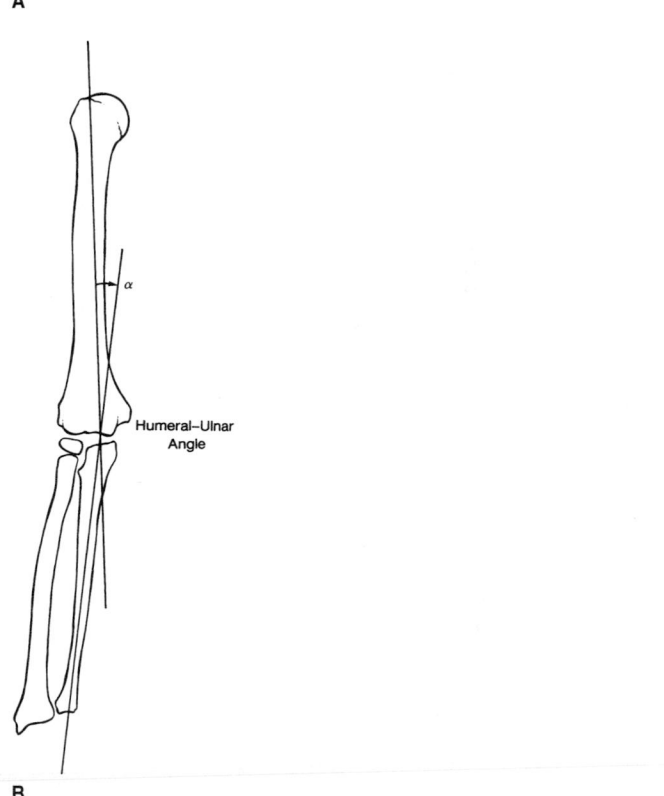

B

Figure 190.4. **(A)** Line drawing of Baumann's angle **(B)** Line drawing of humeral-ulnar angle. (From O'Brien WR, Eilert RE, Chang FM, et al. The metaphyseal-diaphyseal angle as a guide to treating supracondylar fractures of the humerus in children. Unpublished data; with permission.)

All of these patients should be treated in consultation with an orthopaedic surgeon.

Epicondyle Fractures

Epicondyle fractures in adults are usually caused by a direct blow. The medial epicondyle is involved more commonly than is the lateral epicondyle, and ulnar nerve function should be evaluated, as it is in close proximity to the epicondyle at the elbow.

Nondisplaced fractures may be treated with immobilization and early range of motion. If displacement of more than 10 mm is present, then surgical fixation may be required. Intraarticular fragments may impede joint mobility and are difficult to visualize radiographically. Entrapment of the ulnar nerve is a possible complication.

Articular Surface Fractures

Fractures of the capitellum and trochlea usually occur as a result of a posterior elbow dislocation. Isolated fractures are rare, and joint stability is maintained because the condyles remain intact, but motion may be impeded.

Nondisplaced fractures with normal anatomic alignment can be treated with immobilization for 2 to 3 weeks. Displaced small fragments may be excised, whereas larger fragments require internal fixation with early range of motion. Common complications of capitellar fractures include restriction of motion and, rarely, nonunion and avascular necrosis.

Olecranon Fractures

Olecranon fractures are usually intraarticular and may result from a direct blow or an avulsion injury from the pull of the triceps muscle (Fig. 190.5). On examination, the patient is unable to extend the elbow against resistance. Because of its proximity, the ulnar nerve may be injured, and its function should be assessed.

Treatment of these injuries varies with the amount of displacement and usually requires orthopaedic consultation. Nondisplaced fractures may be splinted with the elbow in a semiflexed position and with early range of motion begun in 2 to 3 weeks. Complete healing generally occurs in 6 to 8 weeks. If greater than 2 mm of displacement is present, then operative intervention is usually indicated. Treatment options include tension band wiring, olecranon screws, or plates (5). Range-of-motion exercises may be started in 1 week. Management of severely comminuted fractures is controversial and may require removal of the loose fragments.

Radial Head Fractures

Radial head fractures are the most common elbow injuries in adults. They usually occur as a result of a fall on the outstretched hand, which drives the radial head into the capitellum. On examination, patients have tenderness to palpation over the radial head and pain with pronation and supination of the forearm.

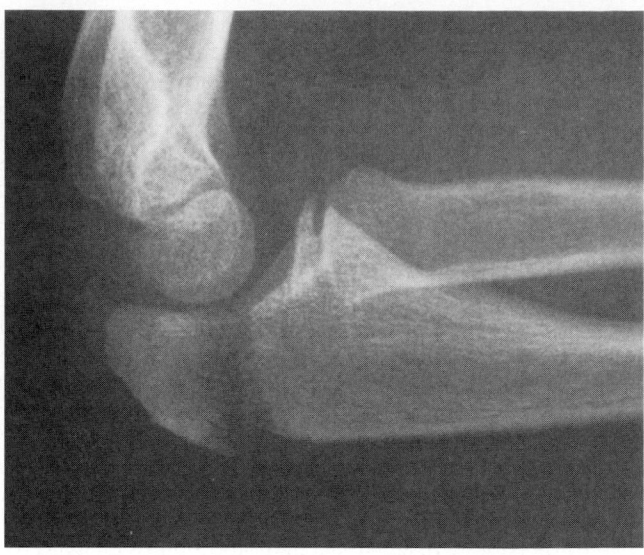

Figure 190.5.   Olecranon fracture. (From Chambers H, Jose Fernando DLG, O'Brien E, et al. Fractures of the radius and ulna. In: Rockwood CA, Wilkins KE, Beaty JH [eds]: *Fractures in children*, 4th edition. Philadelphia, Lippincott Raven, 1996. Fig 9.217 C p.633, with permission.)

Fractures are classified as nondisplaced, displaced, or comminuted. Nondisplaced fractures may be difficult to visualize on standard radiographs. Any disruption of the normally smooth, concave cortical contour of the radial head suggests fracture. A positive fat pad sign on a lateral radiograph without evidence of fracture should raise suspicion for an occult radial head fracture. This fracture may be better visualized radiographically with a radial head–capitellar view.

Nondisplaced fractures are treated with a posterior splint or sling, followed by early range of motion after a few days. Aspiration of the hemarthrosis in the emergency department may provide pain relief and expedite mobilization. Minimally displaced fractures may be treated in a similar manner. Fractures displaced more than 3 mm or involving more than one-third of the joint surface will likely be treated with operative fixation (Fig. 190.6).

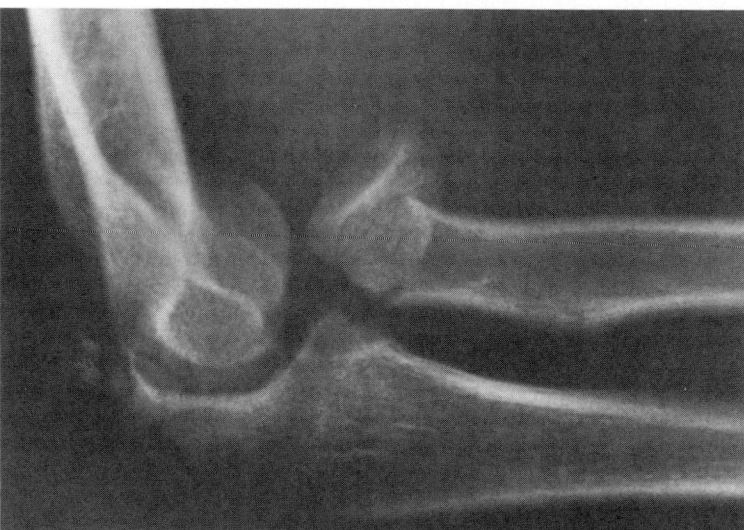
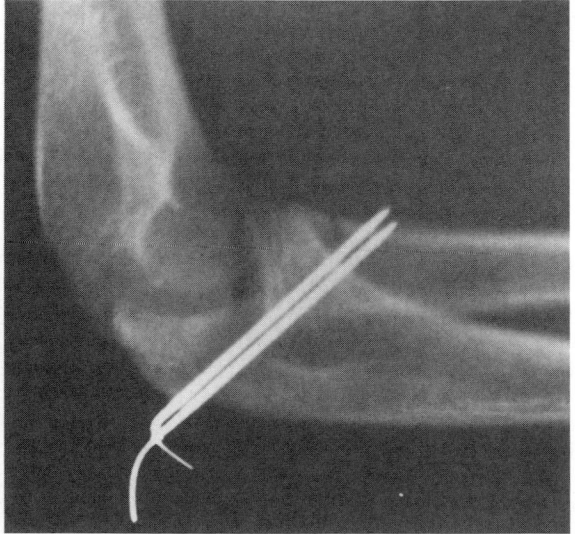

Figure 190.6.   Displaced radial head fracture. (From Wilkins KE [ed]: *Operative management of upper extremity fractures in children.* American Academy of Orthopaedic Surgeons Monograph Series, p. 57. Rosemont, Ill., AAOS, 1994.)

These patients should begin early range of motion postoperatively.

Comminuted fractures may be treated with a sling and early range of motion in 1 to 2 weeks. Joint aspiration and injection of a local anesthetic can aid in assessing joint mobility. The treatment of severely comminuted and displaced fractures is controversial and may include excision of fragments or complete radial head excision, with or without prosthetic implants.

Any patient with a radial head fracture should also be examined for wrist tenderness. The Essex-Lopresti lesion, a radial head fracture with disruption of the distal radioulnar joint ligaments and forearm interosseous membrane, must be recognized early since internal fixation produces the best results (1).

Aspiration of the radiohumeral joint is indicated to relieve pain, promote early range of motion and assess joint mobility with radial head fractures. This can be performed in the acute setting to the great relief of the patient. Elbow joint aspiration is also indicated to diagnose a septic joint. The aspiration should be performed over the lateral elbow in the center of the triangle that connects the radial head, lateral epicondyle, and olecranon process (Fig. 190.7) (13). No neurovascular structures are located in this area, and the joint capsule is present beneath the skin and the thin anconeus muscle. Under sterile technique, the skin over this area is anesthetized with a local anesthetic. An 18-gauge needle on a 10- to 20-mL syringe is directed into the center of the triangle and perpendicular to the skin. Aspiration of up to 5 mL of blood from the joint and injection of 1 to 2 mL of a long-acting anesthetic provide relief of pain and allow assessment of joint mobility.

Nursemaid's Elbow

Subluxation of the radial head is most commonly seen in children 1 to 3 years of age, but has been described even into the early teen years. The mechanism of injury is a sudden longitudinal pull of the forearm, causing fibers of the annular ligament to become stuck between the capitellum and the radial head. The child is unwilling to move the arm, and the elbow is held in slight flexion with pronation of the forearm.

When a child presents with the characteristic history for radial head subluxation, radiographs are not necessary. However,

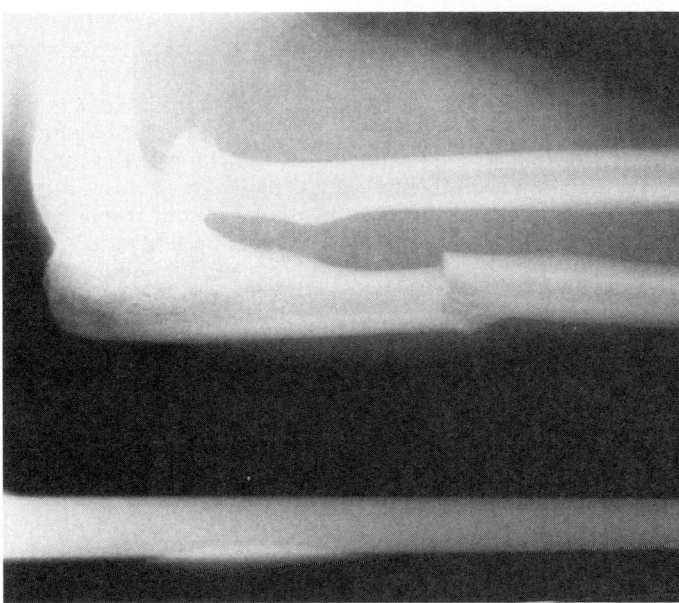

Figure 190.8. Monteggia fracture. The first component is fracture of the proximal one-third of the ulna; the second component is dislocation of the radial head.

the presence of swelling or deformity, or the child's refusal to resume normal use of the arm after reduction, is an indication for a radiograph.

Treatment usually consists of supination and flexion of the forearm in one continuous motion. The examiner's thumb can be used to apply pressure over the radial head. If unsuccessful with this reduction maneuver, supination with extension is also described as an option. With successful reduction of a nursemaid's elbow, the child will resume using the arm normally within several minutes, and no further treatment is necessary.

Monteggia Fracture

Fracture of the proximal one-third of the ulna with dislocation of the radial head is a Monteggia fracture (Fig. 190.8). Based on the position of the radial head, there are four types of Monteggia fractures. The radial head dislocates anteriorly in 60% of cases, with posterolateral, lateral, and posterior dislocations being less common. The mechanism of injury involves direct trauma, forced hyperpronation, or hyperextension. The most commonly associated injury is paralysis of the radial nerve. The usual treatment is open reduction with internal fixation. Any patient found to have an ulnar fracture should be carefully examined for elbow pain or limitation of range of motion. The radio-capitellar line should be closely examined on the lateral elbow radiograph to assure a normal relationship (10).

Elbow Dislocation

Dislocation of the elbow accounts for 20% of all dislocations and is described by the direction in which the forearm is displaced in relationship to the distal humerus. Posterior and posterolateral dislocations account for 90% of all elbow dislocations. Dislocation may also occur between the radius and ulna. Posterior dislocations are caused by a fall on an extended and abducted arm. Patients present with significant swelling, tenderness, and deformity, with the elbow held in flexion and prominence of the olecranon. Anterior dislocation is the result of a blow to the

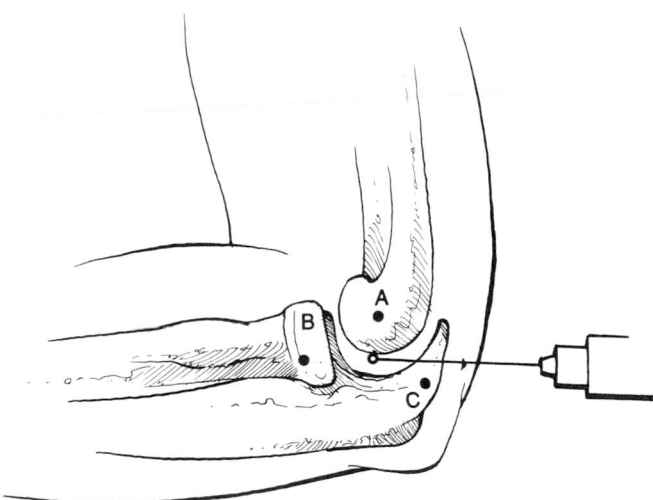

Figure 190.7. Elbow aspiration. The safest place to aspirate the elbow is in the center of a triangle produced by connecting **(A)** the lateral epicondyle of the humerus, **(B)** the radial head, and **(C)** the olecranon. (Adapted, with permission, from Simon RR, Koenigsknecht SJ. *Emergency orthopaedics: the extremities,* 2nd ed. Norwalk, CT: Appleton & Lange, 1987.)

olecranon while the elbow is held in extension with the forearm supinated and is associated with loss of the olecranon prominence.

Radiographs should be obtained before reduction to exclude associated fractures, which occur in up to 60% of patients with elbow dislocation. Supracondylar fractures in the younger patient and avulsion fractures of the medial epicondyle are the most common. A complete neurovascular examination must be performed on presentation. Neuropraxia is present in 20% of patients, most commonly involving the ulnar and median nerves. As with most nerve injuries associated with dislocations and fractures, these deficits are usually transient (9). Brachial artery injury is most commonly associated with open dislocations and those with concomitant fractures. The incidence of vascular injury is greater with anterior dislocations.

Analgesia and muscle relaxation are required for closed reduction. Posterior, medial, and lateral dislocations are reduced using the same technique. With the patient lying supine, the area of the wrist and forearm is grasped and traction is applied along the long axis of the forearm. An assistant provides countertraction to the upper arm. Any medial or lateral displacement is corrected. While forearm traction is continued, the elbow is flexed and a palpable clunk should be felt as the elbow is reduced. Downward pressure over the proximal forearm may aid in disengaging the coronoid from the olecranon fossa (Fig. 190.9). After reduction, the neurovascular examination should be repeated and postreduction films obtained. The elbow should be flexed to 90 degrees as long as good pulses are maintained and then immobilized in a posterior splint. Patients should be assessed serially following reduction for vascular injury to the brachial artery. Any concern for vascular compromise

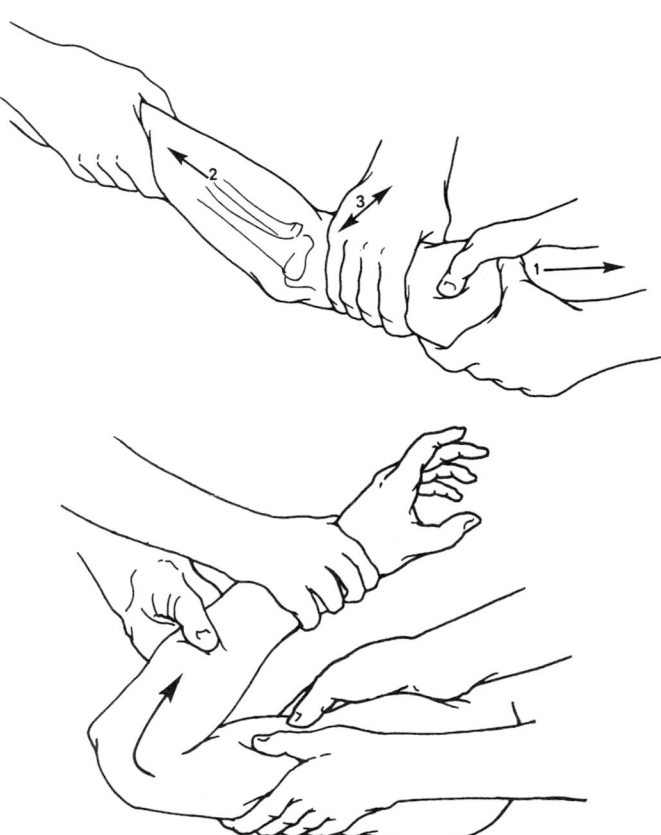

Figure 190.9. Technique for reduction of posterior dislocation of the elbow.

should prompt consultation with an orthopaedic surgeon. All patients should follow up with an orthopaedic surgeon within 1 week to begin early range-of-motion exercises and help prevent contractures.

Indications for open reduction include an associated fracture, open dislocation, neurovascular injury, or inability to accomplish a closed reduction. Long-term complications include stiffness, contractures, neurovascular injury, heterotropic bone formation, and ankylosis. Recurrent elbow dislocations are rare.

Epicondylitis

Tennis elbow, or *lateral epicondylitis*, is an "overuse syndrome" characterized by inflammation at the radiohumeral joint or the lateral epicondyle. It is believed to represent a failure of the extensor carpi radialis brevis attachment to bone in this region (12). It is most commonly seen in athletes or adults with occupations requiring repeated rotary motion, as in twisting or grasping (e.g., tennis players, pipefitters, and carpenters) (3). The gradual onset of a dull ache appears over the lateral epicondyle and radiates into the forearm. Dorsiflexion of the wrist and supination of the forearm against resistance with the elbow extended will reproduce the pain. Radiographs should be obtained to exclude an associated fracture. In chronic conditions, calcification may be seen over the lateral epicondyle.

The mainstay of treatment is avoidance of the offending activity and immobilization. A posterior splint is applied with the elbow flexed 90 degrees, the forearm supinated, and the wrist slightly dorsiflexed. Moist heat, nonsteroidal antiinflammatory agents, and physical therapy may be helpful. Local infiltration of the affected area with 1 to 2 mL of a corticosteroid and anesthetic mixture will give dramatic relief. All patients should have an orthopaedic or sports medicine referral.

Medial epicondylitis, or *"golfer's elbow,"* is similar to tennis elbow and involves the common flexor origin at the medial epicondyle of the humerus. It is seen in golfers but occurs more frequently in people who routinely perform household chores, manual labor, and other tasks involving repetitive movements. Maximal tenderness is localized over the medial aspect of the elbow and medial epicondyle. Treatment is similar to that for lateral epicondylitis, and routine orthopaedic follow-up (in 7 to 10 days) should be arranged.

Olecranon Bursitis

Olecranon bursitis is inflammation of the bursa overlying the olecranon process at the proximal aspect of the ulna. The bursa functions to provide a mechanism for the skin to glide freely over the olecranon process, preventing tissue tears. Inflammation of the bursa can be caused by a variety of mechanisms, including acute trauma; chronic friction (due to overuse, aka "draftsman's bursitis"); crystal deposition (e.g., gout, pseudogout); local infection; and systemic diseases such as rheumatoid arthritis, scleroderma, uremia, and oxalosis. Regardless of the etiology, patients usually present with focal swelling and pain exacerbated by pressure over the posterior aspect of the elbow. Flexion of the elbow may be slightly restricted, due to tightening of the skin over the inflamed bursa. Regardless of etiology, the area may be warm and tender, so this is not a reliable determinant of infectious versus other etiologies. Repetitive trauma can result in a chronic inflammatory process and a thickened, rubbery, and usually painless bursa.

Aspiration of the bursa is essential for both diagnostic and therapeutic purposes if infection is suspected. The aspirated fluid should be analyzed for crystals, gram stain, cell count and cultures. The cell count should be interpreted in light of the clinical picture and other synovial fluid results, as there is considerable overlap between expected counts in noninflammatory, inflammatory, and infectious conditions. Cell counts greater than 50,000 to 100,000 WBC per mm^3 and cell counts with PMN predominance are strongly suspicious for infectious etiologies. However, cell counts can be as low as 5,000 WBC per mm^3 in cases of early infection. In these situations, the gram stain and culture become critical in the evaluation of the fluid results. The bursa is aspirated utilizing an 18-guage needle from a posterior-lateral approach so that the ulnar nerve is not inadvertently injured. Care should be taken to avoid, if possible, aspiration of the bursa through an area of superficial cellulitis, to avoid seeding of a noninfected bursa. Patients suspected of having septic bursitis should be treated with antibiotics while awaiting culture results. *Staphylococcus aureus* is the most commonly identified organism in septic olecranon bursitis, and high resistance to penicillin has been reported (4). Antistaphylococcal coverage should be provided. Besides antibiotics in cases of suspected infectious bursitis, other measures that can be utilized include analgesia (NSAID and narcotic), moist heat, and splinting for comfort. Occasionally, cases of septic bursitis will require serial aspiration (every 1-3 days) to resolve. Rarely, in cases that progress despite drainage and antibiotics, open incision and drainage will be required by an orthopaedic or general surgeon.

In simple non-infectious olecranon bursitis, drainage of the bursa should be considered with subsequent compression dressing, NSAIDs, and protective measures to prevent recurrence. Symptoms may be recurrent, and serial drainage may be required. In refractory cases, bursal excision by a surgeon may be performed.

Rupture of the Distal Biceps or Triceps Tendon

Distal rupture of the biceps tendon may be the result of degenerative changes or sudden, forceful flexion of the elbow against resistance. Patients present with a history of a painful snap at the elbow. Flexion of the elbow and supination of the forearm are weakened. On flexion, the belly of the biceps retracts, producing a bulbous swelling in the upper arm. The treatment is surgical if significant motor weakness is present, and should occur within 2 weeks postinjury (14).

Avulsion of the triceps tendon should be considered in patients with pain, swelling, and weakness with arm extension. A defect is often palpable just proximal to the olecranon. Associated injuries include radial head and neck fractures and wrist fractures. The diagnosis is confirmed radiographically when a bony avulsion is seen on the lateral view of the elbow. Orthopaedic consultation in the ED or within 24 to 48 hours should be assured, and early surgical treatment is usually recommended.

Osteochondritis Dissecans

Osteochondritis dissecans is a process of avascular necrosis of the subchondral bone and the overlying articular cartilage, and is most common in males and adolescents. There is usually a history of trauma or sports-related activities. Patients may complain of the gradual onset of dull, aching pain; limited extension; intermittent swelling; and catching, locking, or clicking of the affected elbow (7). The capitellum is the most common site of involvement, and joint effusion may be present. Treatment consists of immobilization with a sling or cast, avoidance of all throwing activities, and nonsteroidal antiinflammatory agents. Loose bodies within the joint may restrict movement of the elbow and should be surgically removed. Prognosis is usually good.

CRITICAL INTERVENTIONS

- Assess the radial head for dislocation in patients with a fracture of the proximal ulna. Monteggia fractures require internal fixation, whereas isolated ulna fractures are treated with immobilization
- In patients with radial head fractures examine the wrist for the Essex-Lopresti lesion. These patients require internal fixation, whereas radial head fractures are usually treated conservatively
- Obtain radiographs before reducing an elbow dislocation to exclude associated fractures, except with nursemaid's elbow. Postreduction films should always be obtained
- Measure the anterior humeral line to aid in diagnosing supracondylar fractures in children. Splint the arm if a significant mechanism of injury or swelling exists, and refer for orthopaedic consultation

DISPOSITION

Disposition of patients with elbow injuries is important, as deformity or loss of motion at the elbow can affect proper function of the forearm, wrist, and hand. Clearly, any patient with an open fracture or neurovascular compromise following elbow injury needs urgent ED consultation. Compartment syndrome, due to the location of the brachial artery, and neurologic entrapment may occur following injuries to this region. All pediatric supracondylar fractures are concerning for complications and future disability, and orthopaedic consultation in the ED may be necessary. Occasionally patients in this group with nondisplaced supracondylar fractures can be splinted and discharged, but only if urgent orthopaedic follow up is assured (24–48 hours), and the patient and parents are fully cognizant of warning signs that would require return to the ED. Most nondisplaced elbow fractures in adults seen in the ED will require urgent orthopaedic follow up (24–48 hours), but this decision should be made in phone consultation with the orthopedist who will be seeing them subsequently.

COMMON PITFALLS

- ✔ Failure to diagnose an occult radial head fracture. This injury should be suspected when a positive fat pad sign is present on radiography without demonstrable fracture. Oblique views of the radial head may demonstrate the fracture
- ✔ Making the assumption that a negative radiograph rules out elbow injury. Injuries to cartilaginous and ligamentous structures, as well as soft tissues, may be present. Splinting of the elbow and orthopaedic referral should be considered when a significant mechanism of injury is present
- ✔ Failure to diagnose neurovascular injury. A careful neurovascular examination should be documented, in addition to interval reexamination
- ✔ Failure to diagnose avulsion of the biceps muscle from the bicipital tuberosity of the radius. The patient will still be able to flex the elbow with the brachialis muscle

Acknowledgments

Thanks to the previous edition's chapter authors Jefferson D. Bracey and Alok Saxena.

References

1. Edwards GS, Jupiter JB. Radial head fractures with acute distal radioulnar dislocation: Essex-Lopresti revisited. *Clin Orthop Rel Res* 1988;234:61.

2. Freed HA, Shields NN. Most frequently overlooked radiographically apparent fractures in a teaching hospital emergency department. *Ann Emerg Med* 1984;13:900.

3. Gellman H. Tennis elbow (lateral epicondylitis). *Orthop Clin North Am* 1992;23:75.

4. Ho G, Tice AD, Kaplan SR. Septic bursitis in the prepatellar and olecranon bursae: an analysis of 25 cases. *Ann Intern Med* 1978;89:21.

5. Horne JG, Tanzer TL. Olecranon fractures: a review of 100 cases. *J Trauma* 1981;21:469.

6. Miller TT. Imaging of elbow disorders. *Orthop Clin North Am* 1999;30:21.

7. Mitsunaga MM, Adishian DA, Bianco AJ. Osteochondritis dissecans of the capitellum. *J Trauma* 1981;22:53.

8. Murphy WA, Siegel MJ. Elbow fat pads with new signs and extended differential diagnosis. *Radiology* 1977;124:659.

9. Nelson AJ, Izzi JA, et al. Traumatic nerve injuries about the elbow. *Orthop Clin North Am* 1999;30:91.

10. Perron AD, Brady WJ, Keats TE, Hersch, RE. Orthopaedic pitfalls in the emergency department: galeazzi and monteggia fracture-dislocation. *Am J Emerg Med* 2001;19:225–228.

11. Pitt MJ, Speer DP. Imaging of the elbow with an emphasis on trauma. *Radiol Clin North Am* 1990;28:295.

12. Putnam MD, Cohen M. Painful conditions around the elbow. *Orthop Clin North Am* 1999;30:109.

13. Quigley TB. Aspiration of the elbow joint in the treatment of fractures of the head of the radius. *N Engl J Med* 1949;240:915.

14. Strauch RJ. Biceps and triceps injuries of the elbow. *Orthop Clin North Am* 1999;30:95.

15. Worlock P. Supracondylar fractures of the humerus: assessment of cubitus varus by the Baumann angle. *J Bone Joint Surg Br* 1986;68:755.

16. Wu MJ, Perron AD, Miller MD, Powell SM, Brady WJ. Orthopaedic pitfalls in the emergency department: pediatric supracondylar humerus fractures. *Am J Emerg Med* 2002;20:544–550.

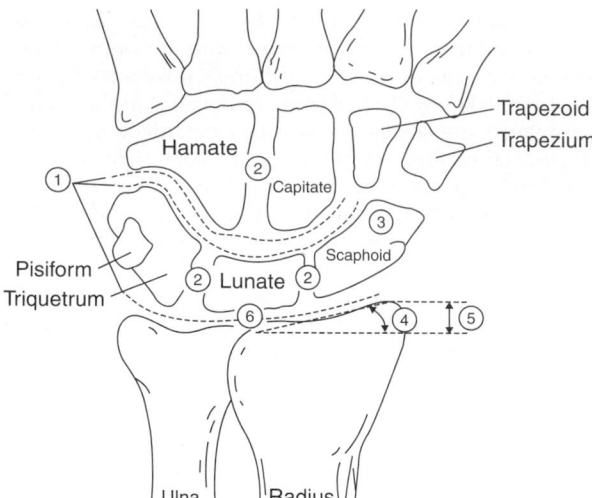

Figure 191.1. Key elements on a normal posteroanterior view. (1) The carpal bones are arranged in two rows forming three smooth arcs. (2) The carpal bones are separated by a uniform 1- to 2-mm space. (3) The scaphoid is elongated. (4) The radius has an ulnar inclination of 13 to 30 degrees. (5) The radial styloid projects 8 to 18 mm, with an average of 13 mm. (6) Half the lunate articulates with the radius, with equal length over the ulna (neutral ulnar variance). (From Uehara DT, Wolanyk D, Escarza RH. *Wrist injuries* in *emergency medicine:* a comprehensive study guide, Tintinalli JE, Kelen GD, Stapczynski JS, (eds). 6th ed., New York: McGraw Hill, 2004, with permission).

CHAPTER 191

Wrist and Forearm Injuries

Joel Kravitz and Carl R. Chudnofsky

Anatomically, the wrist is the area from the distal ulna and radius to the carpometacarpal joints, and the bones of the wrist form complex articulations at both the proximal and distal borders mentioned above. A thorough understanding of the various injuries to the wrist is essential to the emergency physician for numerous reasons; wrist injuries are common, often difficult to diagnose, and they may result in decreased use of the associated hand if left undiscovered and untreated. Outcome depends on accurate assessment of the injury, appropriate initial management, and prompt recognition of those injuries that require immediate specialty consultation or outpatient referral.

The 8 carpal bones of the wrist are arranged in two rows (Fig. 191.1), which form three concentric arches on a posteroanterior (PA) radiograph (Fig. 191.2). The proximal row (radial to ulnar) consists of the scaphoid, lunate, triquetrum, and pisiform. The distal row (radial to ulnar) comprises the trapezium, trapezoid, capitate, and hamate, which has a hook-like process that forms a fibroosseous tunnel through which the ulnar artery and nerve travel (called *Guyon's canal*). The distal row is generally more stable, and moves as a unit with the metacarpals. The proximal row is less stable by virtue of its increased mobility with respect to wrist motion. This is particularly true of the

scaphoid bone, which acts as a link between the two carpal rows. This stabilizing function means that most forces applied to the wrist are eventually applied to the scaphoid, explaining why this bone is the most commonly injured or fractured of all the carpal bones. With the exception of the pisiform (which is in actuality a sesamoid bone in the tendon of the flexor carpi ulnaris), none of the carpal bones have any muscular attachments. Hence, the carpal bones move passively as a function of hand position, and wrist motion is produced by midcarpal and radiocarpal joint movement.

The carpal bones are further stabilized by three ligamentous bands, two volar and one dorsal, and by numerous interosseous ligaments. The volar ligaments are the strongest, forming two concentric arches extending from the radial styloid to the distal ulna. The distal ligamentous complex arches across the proximal capitate while the proximal band crosses and stabilizes the lunate. The *space of Poirier*, which overlies the junction of the lunate and capitate bones, lies between these two bands creating a weak spot that accounts for the injury patterns seen with lunate and perilunate dislocations. Also, both volar ligamentous bands have their attachment on the radial styloid, making a fracture in this area potentially unstable.

The *flexor retinaculum* is a dense band of fibrous tissue that attaches to the hook of the hamate and pisiform bone on the ulnar aspect and the trapezium and scaphoid radially. This structure forms the roof of the *"carpal tunnel,"* through which the tendons of the flexor digitorum superficialis, flexor digitorum profundus, and flexor pollicis longus pass, as well as the median nerve.

The *forearm* consists of the radius and ulna, and is the origin of most of the muscles of the hand. The distal radius is the only forearm bone that directly articulates with the carpal bones, specifically the lunate and scaphoid. The distal radius has three articular surfaces: the *distal radioulnar joint (DRUJ)*, the *radiocarpal joint*, and the *triangular fibrocartilage complex (TFCC)*. The TFCC is the main stabilizer of the radioulnar joint, and is further supported by volar and dorsal radioulnar ligaments. The TFCC also stabilizes the lunate and triquetrum as they abut on the distal ulna.

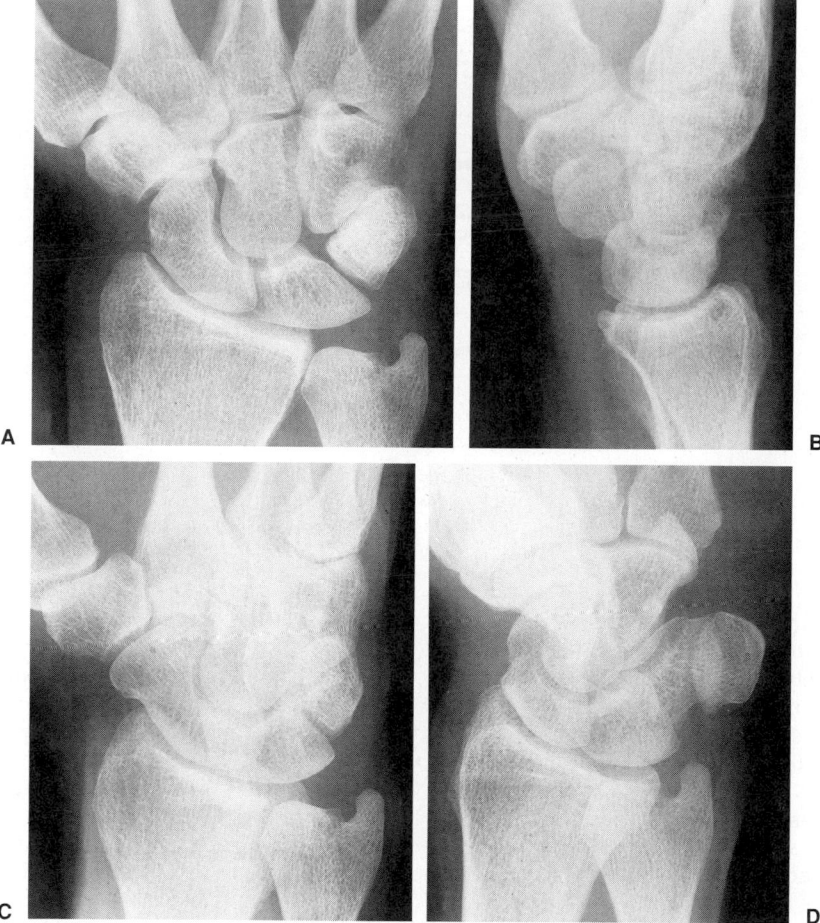

Figure 191.2.   Normal adult wrist in (a) Frontal view. (b) Lateral view, and both oblique projections (c&d). (From Harris JH Jr, Harris WH. *The radiology of emergency medicine*, 4th ed. Philadelphia: Lippincott Williams & Wilkins, 2000, p. 372, with permission).

In contrast to the outward bowing radius, the ulna is relatively straight and fixed. The concave notch on the ulnar aspect of the radius permits rotation of the radius around the curved ulnar head during pronation and supination. A fibrous interosseous membrane joins these bones along their entire length. Injury to either bone often results in a fracture of the other or causes a dislocation of either the distal or proximal joints (see Galeazzi and Monteggia fracture–dislocations below).

The median, radial, and ulnar nerves course through the wrist and provide sensory and motor innervation to the hand (see Chapter 192, "Hand Injuries"). The *ulnar nerve* innervates the flexor carpi ulnaris and the ulnar portion of the flexor digitorum profundus; it then travels through Guyon canal to innervate all the remaining intrinsic muscles of the hand. The *radial nerve* innervates those muscles of the forearm that provide extension of the wrist and digits and extension and abduction of the thumb.

The arterial supply to the hand is provided by the radial and ulnar arteries, which arise from the brachial artery in the antecubital fossa. The radial artery passes through the anatomic snuff box and terminates as the *deep palmar arch*. The ulnar artery passes into the hand through the Guyon canal superficial to the flexor retinaculum to form the *superficial palmar arch* (see Chapter 192 Hand Injuries).

CLINICAL PRESENTATION

Patients with a wrist or forearm injury will complain of pain, swelling, and limited range of motion in the wrist or forearm. However, the presentation will vary, depending on the na-

ture and severity of the injury. Fractures of the distal radius or ulna may be confused with, or accompanied by, a carpal injury. Chronic wrist conditions such as carpal tunnel syndrome often present with wrist pain, though there is commonly a more protracted history of pain with repetitive motions. These conditions generally present in a more indolent fashion, and often have a waxing and waning pattern to the symptoms.

The carpal bones in children are primarily cartilaginous; as such, carpal injuries are rare. Children are more likely to injure the weakest part of the wrist complex—the immature radial metaphysis or its epiphyseal growth plate. In contrast, the elderly more commonly injure the distal radius because of increased osteoporosis.

EMERGENCY DEPARTMENT EVALUATION

Evaluation of wrist and forearm injuries should never precede the initial resuscitation or a proper assessment of the patient to detect other significant injuries or control hemorrhage.

A focused, but thorough history is essential in the evaluation and treatment of the injured wrist and forearm. Important historic information includes hand dominance, occupation and avocations (e.g., musician, sculptor, mechanic), prior hand injuries and preinjury hand function, past medical history (e.g., diabetes mellitus, immunosuppression) including previous tetanus immunization, time of injury, and mechanism and circumstances of injury (e.g., position of the hand at the time of injury, contaminated environment, chemical exposures, potential for foreign bodies). Mechanism of injury is particularly important, as

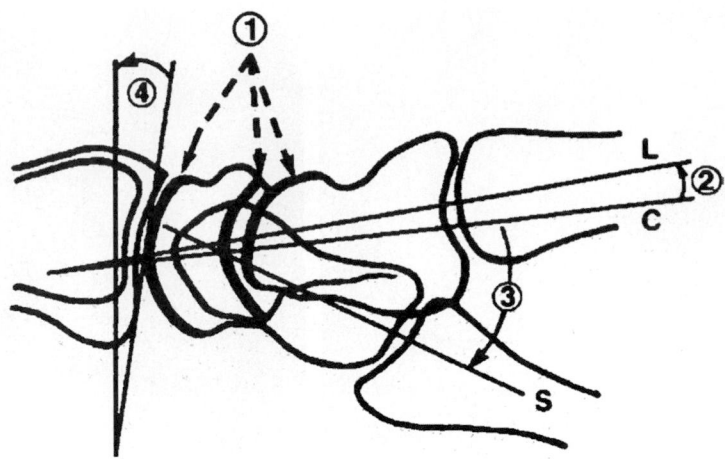

Figure 191.3.   Lateral radiograph. (1) Three C's sign, (2) capitolunate angle <20 degrees, (3) scapholunate angle of 30 to 60 degrees, and (4) volar tilt of the radius of 10 to 15 degrees. (From *Handbook of orthopaedic emergencies.* Hart RG, Lippincott-Raven, 1999, Figure 2, p. 204.)

the precise position of the hand and wrist during the injury can guide investigation and treatment. For example, a fall onto the thenar eminence is more likely to cause a scaphoid injury, while impact on the hypothenar eminence is more likely to cause a triquetral injury.

Correlation of surface anatomy and clinical complaints to underlying structures is the key to an accurate diagnosis of wrist injuries. The volar wrist crease marks the location of the proximal carpal row. The *anatomic snuff box* (ASB) is perhaps the best-known and most useful anatomic landmark of the wrist. The scaphoid lies on the floor of this triangle, which is formed by the radial styloid at its base, the extensor pollicis brevis tendon radially and the abductor pollicis longus tendon at the ulnar aspect. Moving in an ulnar direction from the radial styloid, a small bony prominence of the radius known as *Lister's tubercle* can be palpated on the dorsal surface. The *scapholunate joint* lies immediately distal to this prominence. The *capitolunate joint* lies immediately ulnar to the scapholunate joint. The capitate can also be found on the dorsum of the wrist; with the hand in the neutral position, a small depression can be palpated midway between the base of the 3rd metacarpal and Lister tubercle. The proximal capitate can be felt distal to this depression. Upon flexion of the wrist, the depression disappears and the lunate can be palpated.

The ulnar styloid is the largest bony prominence on the ulnar aspect of the wrist—the triquetrum and TFCC are located distally. The pisiform is palpable at the base of the hypothenar muscles just distal to the wrist crease. The hook of the hamate may be palpated in the soft tissue of the palm, 1 cm distal and radial to this point.

Wrist and forearm injuries may be complicated by damage to peripheral nerves and arteries. Hence, testing neurovascular function is imperative following a wrist or forearm injury. This is best performed in the hand, and is described in detail in Chapter 192. *Allen's test*, which is used to test the patency of the radial and ulnar arteries and the palmar arches, is performed at the level of the wrist. The test is performed by having the patient clench the fist to exsanguinate the hand while the examiner occludes the radial and ulnar arteries. Once the hand is blanched, pressure over one of the arteries is released. Normal hand color should return in 3 to 5 seconds. The test is then repeated, releasing the other artery.

Radiographs of the wrist and forearm should be obtained in all but the most trivial of injuries. Standard views of the wrist include posteroanterior (PA), lateral, and oblique views

(Fig. 191.2). These are adequate in most cases, but additional views can be requested as clinically indicated. On an adequately positioned PA view, the distal radius and ulna should not overlap, and the 3rd metacarpal axis should be in line with that of the radius. The radial styloid should project between 9 and 15 mm beyond the DRUJ and should create an ulnar inclination of 15 to 30 degrees. A normal PA radiograph should also demonstrate three arcs outlining the carpal bones. The proximal and distal surfaces of the scaphoid, lunate and triquetrum make up the two proximal arcs, while the distal third is outlined by the proximal surfaces of the capitate and hamate in the midcarpal area. Disruption of any of these arcs is abnormal. The carpal bones are all separated from each other by a space of no more than 2 mm; increased intercarpal spaces imply ligamentous disruption and potential wrist instability.

The lateral projection should be examined closely for the normal volar tilt of the radius (which should be 10–15°), as well as the normal linear alignment of the radius, lunate, and capitate (Fig. 191.3). The lunate appears as a "cup in a saucer" articulating with the distal radius. The radius, lunate and capitate should all line up on a lateral view, and their articular surfaces should make three neatly overlapping 'C's; this provides a simple assessment of carpal dislocation. The axes of the lunate and capitate should almost overlap; an angle of 10 to 20 degrees is considered normal. The scaphoid and lunate axes should form an angle of 30 to 60 degrees (the scapholunate angle). Oblique radiographs project the pisiform and triquetrum away from other carpal bones making identification of fractures to these bones easier. Oblique views may also help delineate other carpal bone fractures seen on PA and lateral radiographs.

Additional radiographic views may be requested as clinically indicated. A *scaphoid view* is a cone-down view of the scaphoid in ulnar deviation, resulting in the scaphoid being viewed lengthwise, which can assist in detecting subtle fractures. A *carpal tunnel view* is helpful in assessing the hook of the hamate. Clenched fist views force the capitate into the proximal carpal row and will force the proximal bones apart in the event of ligamentous disruption.

EMERGENCY DEPARTMENT MANAGEMENT

Emergency department management of wrist and forearm injuries includes ice application and elevation of the extremity to reduce swelling. Analgesics are recommended as needed

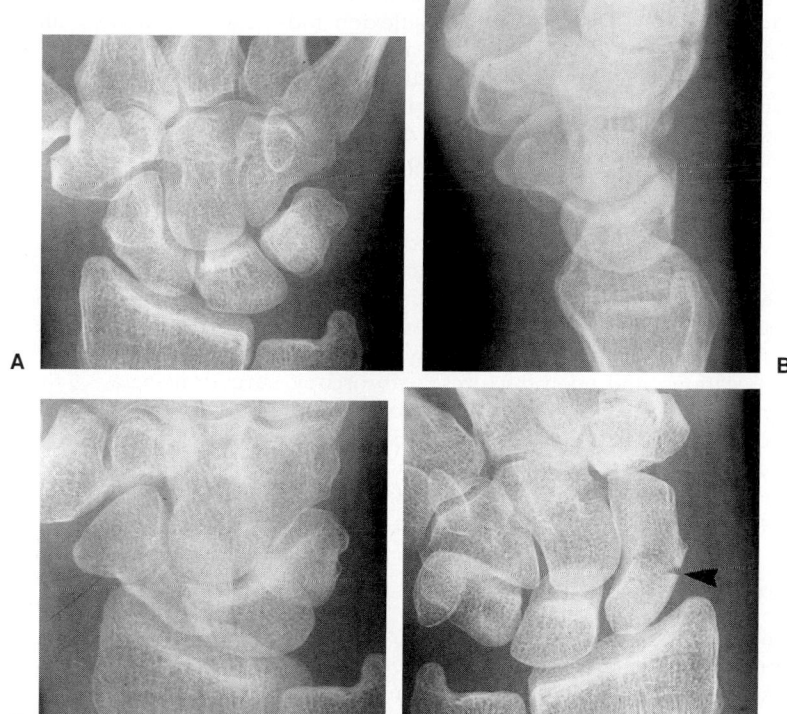

Figure 191.4. Scaphoid view of the wrist demonstrating a minimally displaced fracture of the waist of the scaphoid not seen in the frontal **(A)**, lateral **(B)**, or oblique **(C)** projections but clearly evident on the navicular view **(D).** (From Harris: *The radiology of emergency medicine*, 4th ed. Philadelphia: Lippincott Williams & Wilkins, 2000, p. 401, with permission.)

to control pain. Intravenous antibiotics are indicated for open fractures and dislocations and for severely contaminated or infected wounds. Tetanus immunization status should be assessed and updated appropriately (see Chapter 172, "Wound Management"). Open wounds should be covered with sterile, moist gauze pending radiographs, surgical consultation, or wound closure. In addition, suspected fractures should be temporarily immobilized with an appropriate splint while awaiting radiographs, reduction, or surgical consultation. This is best accomplished with the wrist neutral or in slight extension (e.g., 10–25 degrees), the metacarpophalangeal joints in 60 degrees of flexion, and the proximal and distal interphalangeal joints in 15 and 10 degrees of flexion, respectively. This position is generally safe and comfortable pending complete evaluation.

Carpal Injuries

Most carpal injuries are caused by a *fall on an outstretched hand* (i.e., *FOOSH* injury), resulting in forced dorsiflexion of the wrist, or by a direct blow to the wrist. Carpal fractures account for 7% to 10% of all hand and wrist injuries and are among the most frequently missed fractures in the emergency department (6,7). The scaphoid is fractured most commonly (60% to 70% of carpal fractures), followed by the triquetrum, lunate, trapezium, pisiform, hamate, capitate, and trapezoid (27). Carpal dislocations are less common but are associated with severe sequelae if not diagnosed and treated appropriately.

Scaphoid Fractures

The unique position of the scaphoid among the carpal bones explains its status as the most commonly fractured carpal bone. The scaphoid acts as a stabilizer for both the proximal and distal carpal rows. Therefore, any force applied to the carpal bones will at least in part be transmitted to the scaphoid. This fact, coupled with its location proximal to the thumb metacarpal makes the scaphoid a frequently injured bone. The injury is most commonly caused by a FOOSH mechanism with the main impact on the

thenar eminence. Patients usually complain of pain to the radial wrist, particularly with pressure or movement.

Tenderness on palpation of the anatomic snuff box is a common feature. Examining the wrist in ulnar deviation brings the scaphoid up from the floor of the ASB, making it easier to assess. Scaphoid loading, where the examiner gently grasps the thumb and applies axial pressure onto the scaphoid, is believed by some to be a more sensitive test for scaphoid fractures. Resisting pronation or supination due to radial wrist pain is another diagnostic clue.

Most scaphoid fractures (70%) occur at the waist of the bone (Fig. 191.4), and as many as 10% of scaphoid fractures are not evident on the initial x-ray. Approximately 12% to 15% of scaphoid fractures have other associated injuries, such as fractures of the radius or adjacent carpal bones (2,12).

The blood supply to the scaphoid enters the bone distally via small branches off the radial artery. Scaphoid fractures thus have an associated risk of avascular necrosis (3%), nonunion (5%–10%) and pseudoarthrosis (2,7). For this reason, patients with suspicion of a scaphoid fracture (i.e., those with snuff box tenderness) have historically had their injuries immobilized and reevaluated in 10 to 14 days. Another option to consider is to have the patient return for a bone scan in 72 to 96 hours; a negative scan at this time rules out a fracture. Recently, magnetic resonance imaging (MRI) has recently been shown to be an excellent modality to rule out the presence of a scaphoid fracture in the acute setting (4), and has been shown to be as cost-effective as immobilization and reevaluation in 10 to 14 days (9).

One small study (20) demonstrated 100% sensitivity for initial detection of scaphoid fractures using six radiographic views (PA, lateral, extreme ulnar deviation, radial deviation, 25-degree pronation and supination views), while another demonstrated a specificity of 98% in detecting occult scaphoid fractures using high-resolution sonography (15). However, the number of patients in both studies was small, and larger corroborating studies are needed before these techniques can be used to definitively rule out a scaphoid fracture. Until then, patients with clinical signs of a scaphoid fracture, despite negative radiographs, should be placed in a thumb spica splint and referred for follow up in 10 to 14 days (slight dorsiflexion and radial deviation compresses the fracture fragments and may improve healing).

Patients with nondisplaced fractures may be treated initially with immobilization in a thumb spica splint (with the forearm and wrist positioned as described above) and timely follow up with a hand surgeon. Immobilization of the elbow, using a long-arm versus a short-arm thumb spica splint, is controversial and evidence exists to support both practices; therefore, discussion with the on-call specialist is advised.

As many as 95% of nondisplaced fractures will heal with simple immobilization (2). Immediate consultation should be obtained for unstable fractures, fractures with displacement of 1 mm or more, those associated with other wrist fractures or dislocations, and open fractures. Arthroscopic surgery using a screw to adjoin the fragments is a promising alternative to open reduction and internal fixation (ORIF), allowing earlier use of the hand. Prognosis is dependent on the location of the fracture and the presence of any displacement; oblique and proximal pole fractures are associated with a worse prognosis.

Triquetrum Fractures

The majority of triquetral fractures are dorsal avulsion fractures due to a FOOSH or they occur when pronation or supination of the hand is suddenly resisted, causing the hamate or ulnar styloid to forcefully impact the triquetrum. Fracture of the triquetral body, in contrast, is generally due to direct trauma and is often associated with other carpal injuries (e.g., carpal dislocations). Patients complain of pain to the dorsum of the wrist, and are maximally tender just distal to the ulnar styloid. Triquetrum fractures are best seen on lateral or oblique radiographs of the wrist, where the fractured fragment appears as a small piece of bone dorsal to the triquetrum.

Triquetrum fractures generally heal well with proper immobilization but may be complicated by damage to the deep branch of the ulnar nerve, with subsequent motor impairment. These fractures are rarely displaced, and avascular necrosis is not known to occur. Emergency department management involves immobilizing the wrist in a short-arm volar splint in neutral position and close surgical follow up. Unstable fractures and those with concomitant carpal dislocations should be referred for immediate evaluation by a hand surgeon.

Lunate Fractures

Isolated lunate fractures are relatively rare, accounting for only about 3% of traumatic wrist injuries. More commonly, lunate fractures occur in association with other wrist injuries. Given the anatomical location of the lunate in the space of Poirier (a weak spot between the proximal and distal volar ligamentous bands), the application of large forces to the lunate is more likely to produce a perilunate or lunate dislocation than a fracture. Patients will complain of tenderness in the middle of the wrist, and axial loading of the 3rd metacarpal causes pain. Examination reveals tenderness over the lunate, which is palpable just distal to Lister tubercle.

Like the scaphoid, the blood supply to the lunate enters distally giving these injuries a high incidence of avascular necrosis (known as *Kienbock's disease*), nonunion, and subsequent carpal instability. Patients with Kienbock disease present with pain localized in the area of the lunate, stiffness, occasional swelling, and marked loss of grip strength; a history of significant wrist trauma is often lacking. In some cases, patients present with a *carpal tunnel syndrome*. It is believed that people with a shorter ulna are more likely to develop Kienbock disease, as their ulna provides less support to the lunate. The diagnosis is usually con-

firmed by plain radiographs that demonstrate sclerosis, collapse, and, ultimately, fragmentation of the lunate. However, radiographs may be normal early in the course of the disease. This is also true of acute lunate fractures, which also may not be evident on initial radiographs. Therefore, patients suspected of having an acute lunate fracture or those with Kienbock's disease should be immobilized in a long-arm thumb spica splint and referred to a hand specialist.

Trapezium Fractures

The trapezium lies proximal to the thumb metacarpal, and fractures are often due to a direct blow to the thumb or forced dorsiflexion. There is tenderness at the anatomic snuff box and thenar eminence, and painful thumb movement is noted on examination. Decreased thumb pinch strength secondary to pain is another diagnostic clue. These fractures are often intraarticular and can extend distally, where they are analogous to a *Bennett* or *Rolando* fracture of the thumb metacarpal (see Chapter 192, "Hand Injuries"). Treatment consists of immobilization in a thumb spica splint and elevation. Surgical consultation should be arranged within 7 to 10 days for possible open reduction and internal fixation (ORIF) if displaced.

Hamate Fractures

The classic history described by patients with this rare fracture is sudden pain to the ulnar wrist when a swinging motion (i.e., golf club, bat) has been interrupted. Pain is maximal over the hamate, which is located 1 cm distal to the pisiform. The hook is fractured much more frequently than the body of the hamate, and suspicion must be high, as hook fractures are best demonstrated on a carpal tunnel view. As the hook of the hamate forms one of the borders of Guyon's canal, special attention must be paid to ensure the integrity of the ulnar nerve and artery. Treatment consists of a short arm cast or splint and follow up with a hand surgeon within 1 week.

Other Carpal Fractures

Fractures of the pisiform, capitate and trapezoid are extremely rare. The capitate is rarely fractured in isolation; usually the scaphoid is fractured first, followed by the capitate and then the lunate (creating a so-called *arc fracture*). Capitate fractures, although rare, bear mention for two reasons; the capitate has a distal blood supply, placing it at risk for avascular necrosis, and a fracture of the capitate is often missed due to the more obvious surrounding bony and ligamentous injuries that accompany it. Treatment consists of immobilization in a short arm thumb spica with the wrist in slight dorsiflexion and the thumb immobilized to the IP joint, and consultation with a hand specialist prior to discharge. ORIF is often necessary due to the concomitant injuries, or if attempts at closed reduction are unsuccessful. The timing of surgery is best left to the discretion of the hand surgeon, but consultation should take place while the patient is in the ED.

Scapholunate Dissociation

Scapholunate dissociation is a subtle injury often misdiagnosed as a simple wrist sprain. The mechanism of injury is forced dorsiflexion (i.e., FOOSH) with impact on the thenar eminence, resulting in a torn scapholunate ligament. Patients usually present with pain, swelling, and a clicking sensation in the wrist. Tenderness on examination is maximal on the dorsal wrist just distal and radial to Lister tubercle. The diagnosis is confirmed radiographically. A gap of greater than 3 mm between the scaphoid and the lunate on a PA view of the wrist is diagnostic (Fig. 191.5), and is

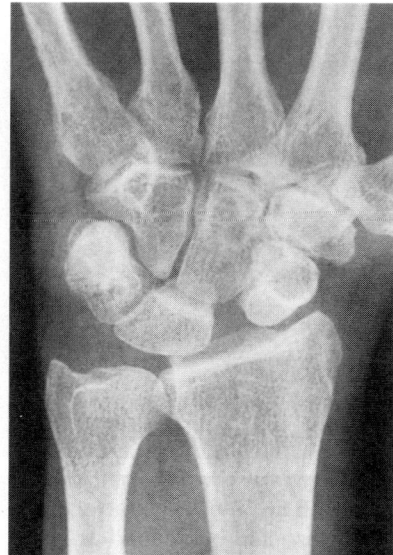

Figure 191.5.   Terry Thomas sign (increased space between the scaphoid and the lunate) indicating scapholunate dissociation. (From Greenspan A. *Orthopaedic radiology*, 3rd ed. Philadelphia: Lippincott, Williams and Wilkins, 2000:182, with permission.)

called the '*Terry Thomas sign*' (named for a British comedian with a gap between his front teeth). The PA view may also demonstrate a '*signet ring*' sign, which occurs because the scaphoid has rotated toward the x-ray beam exposing its rounded cortical end, giving it the appearance of a signet ring. A clenched fist view may be helpful for more subtle presentations, and will usually demonstrate rotatory subluxation of the scaphoid (e.g., a radio-scaphoid angle greater than 60 degrees). Emergency department management includes immobilization in a volar splint with the wrist neutral, and specialty referral within a week. Although some controversy exists regarding optimal treatment, most hand surgeons favor open reduction and repair of the scapholunate ligament.

Triquetrolunate Dissociation

This rare injury is the ulnar counterpart to scapholunate dissociation. The mechanism is usually a FOOSH with impact on the hypothenar eminence. The triquetrum may have a palpable click on examination. When the triquetrolunate ligament is disrupted, the triquetrum is no longer able to counterbalance the flexion torque of the scaphoid. The lunate tilts in the volar direction,

and the capitate tilts in the dorsal direction as a consequence of the lunate's movement. PA radiographs reveal widening of the triquetrolunate space. Treatment consists of an ulnar gutter or short-arm volar splint and referral to a hand surgeon, who will often place the patient in a cast for 8 weeks.

Lunate and Perilunate Dislocations

Lunate and perilunate dislocations can be viewed as similar injuries, and represent the final disruptions that occur with extreme progressive dorsiflexion of the wrist. The forces initially cause a tear in the scapholunate and triquetrolunate ligaments widening the space of Poirier, the weakest spot in the volar arcades. At this point, one of two events occurs. Either the capitate is displaced dorsal to the lunate, producing a *perilunate* dislocation, or the capitate 'pushes back' on the lunate, forcing it through the space of Poirier and into the palm, creating a *lunate* dislocation. As more force is applied, any or all of the carpal bones surrounding the lunate may fracture. The *arc fracture* occurs when the radial styloid, scaphoid, capitate and triquetrum (in various combinations) fracture in a semicircular arc around the lunate.

Lunate and perilunate dislocations are best seen on the lateral radiographic view (Fig. 191.6). An imaginary straight line should be drawn through the distal radius, lunate, and capitate. If this line does not pass through the centers of the lunate or capitate, a lunate or perilunate dislocation should be suspected, respectively. In a *perilunate* dislocation, the lateral radiograph demonstrates disarticulation of the capitolunate joint, with the capitate dorsally displaced and the lunate remaining in normal alignment with the distal radius (Fig. 191.7). With a *lunate* dislocation, the capitate has a near linear alignment with the radius, but the lunate is volarly rotated and displaced giving it the appearance of a "spilled teacup." Another clue to a lunate dislocation may be seen on the PA view, where the rotated lunate takes on a triangular shape known as the 'piece of pie' sign (Fig. 191.8).

Emergency department management of a lunate or perilunate dislocation includes immobilizing the wrist in the neutral position in a volar splint and consultation with a hand surgeon for immediate reduction. Some surgeons believe that if reduction is not accomplished and maintained early, open reduction and internal fixation (ORIF) with repair of the damaged ligaments is required.

Distal Radial Fractures

Distal radial fractures are the most common wrist fractures seen in adults. These injuries are produced by either a direct blow or FOOSH in forced pronation. Factors that affect the type and

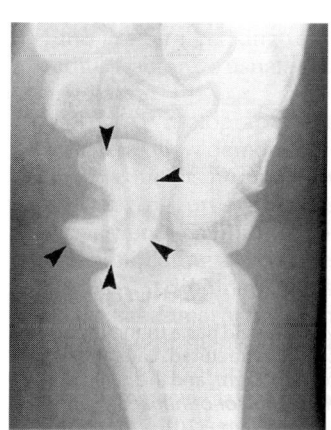
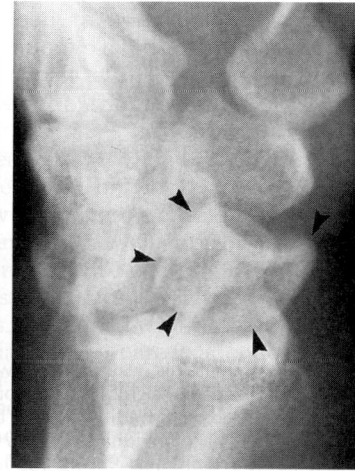

Figure 191.6.   Lunate (a) and perilunate (b) dislocations seen in the lateral views. (From Harris JH Jr, Harris WH. *The radiology of emergency medicine*, 4th ed. Philadelphia: Lippincott Williams & Wilkins, 2000), pp. 397 and 398, with permission.)

A   B

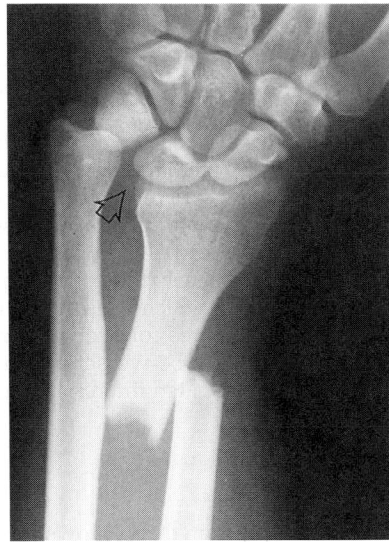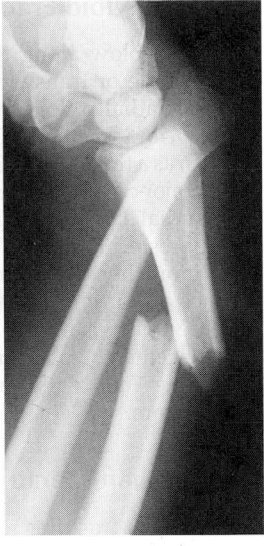

Figure 191.12. Severely displaced Galeazzi fracture–dislocation in frontal (**A**) and lateral (**B**) projections. The distal radioulnar dislocation (*open arrow*) is secondary to the marked shortening of the radius caused by the severe ulnar displacement and dorsal angulation of the distal radial fragment. (From Harris JH Jr, Harris WH. *The Radiology of Emergency Medicine*, 4th ed. Philadelphia: Lippincott–Raven, 2000, p. 390, with permission.)

the Monteggia fracture–dislocation. This is usually a diaphyseal fracture in the proximal one-third of the ulna, with an associated anterior dislocation of the radial head. Occasionally, posterolateral or anterolateral radial head dislocation or a metaphyseal ulnar fracture may occur. Clinically, the forearm may appear angulated and shortened. The ulnar fracture is clearly noted. Although less obvious than the ulnar findings, there is usually pain and swelling at the elbow, and the radial head may be palpated in a posterior or anterior location. On plain radiography, the apex of the ulnar fracture points toward the radial head dislocation, and the radial head may not point toward the capitellum on all views. In adults, these are treated with open reduction and internal fixation (ORIF) of the ulna and closed reduction of the radial head dislocation. In children, adequate reduction may be achieved by closed reduction of both bones. In either case, Monteggia fracture–dislocations require specialty evaluation in the ED. Complications include re-dislocation, infection, paralysis of the posterior interosseous nerve, and nonunion.

Ligamentous Injuries

Radioulnar joint disruption is usually seen with fractures of both bones of the forearm, or intra-articular or distal radial shaft fractures. Because attention is usually given to the more obvious fracture, DRUJ disruption is missed in almost half the cases (4,6). The diagnosis is often not made until chronic pain and decreased wrist mobility are noted. Localized tenderness is present over the wrist and distal radius. Weak grip and decreased pronation and supination are noted; subtle prominence of the ulnar head may also be seen. The more commonly seen dorsal dislocation is usually produced by falls on a hyperpronated wrist, while volar dislocation is produced by forced hypersupination. Dorsal or volar displacement of the ulna can be seen on lateral films. AP radiography demonstrates narrowing of the distal radioulnar joint, which may be subtle. Emergency department management includes cold application, elevation, and immobilization (in supination to reduce dorsal ulnar dislocation; in pronation to reduce volar ulnar dislocation). These injuries have a high recurrence rate and may require surgical repair, hence consultation within 5 to 7 days is recommended.

Soft Tissue Lacerations

All wrist and forearm lacerations, regardless of the depth, must be carefully explored, because injury to significant underlying structures can occur with even very small surface wounds. In addition, exploration should be carried out through a full range of motion, otherwise injury to underlying structures, particularly tendons, may be missed. Simple lacerations are cleaned, irrigated, and repaired in the same fashion as in other areas of the body (see Chapter 172, "Wound Management"). As with hand wounds, deep sutures should be avoided when repairing wrist

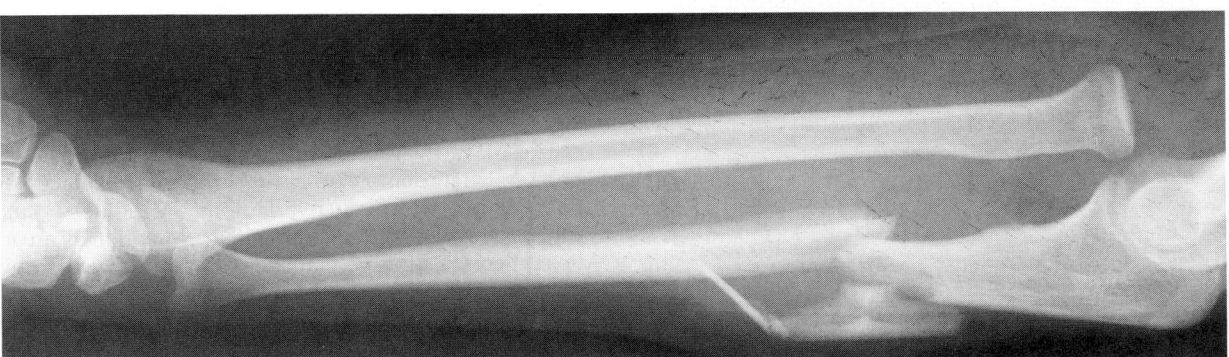

Figure 191.13. In this variation of the Bado I Monteggia injury, the fracture site is comminuted and the volar angulation less than usual. The volar dislocation of the radial head and the ulnar fracture make this a Bado I fracture–dislocation. (From Harris JH Jr, Harris WH. *The Radiology of Emergency Medicine*, 4th ed. Philadelphia: Lippincott–Raven, 2000, p. 365, with permission.)

lacerations. After repair, lacerations over areas of motion and areas of dynamic skin tension should be splinted until the skin edges are well adherent. In addition, lacerations that cross the flexor surface of joints may create a flexion contracture as they heal. Performing a Z-plasty, which creates a transverse scar, can prevent this. Antibiotics are generally not required for simple wrist or forearm lacerations in otherwise healthy patients.

Tendon Lacerations

Tendon injuries can be seen with wrist lacerations. A detailed examination and careful wound exploration are essential for detecting these injuries. Partial tendon tears may have entirely normal function passively, but pain occurs with active motion. In this case, only meticulous wound exploration will prevent the possible complications associated with a missed partial tendon laceration (i.e., adhesions, delayed rupture, triggering, bow-stringing). Once identified, management of a tendon laceration depends on the type of tendon injured, the cross-sectional area of tendon involved, and the location of the laceration. Consultation with an appropriate surgeon is recommended for most tendon lacerations.

Multiple tendon lacerations or those with underlying fractures will require repair in the operating suite. In addition, all tendon lacerations at the level of the wrist and distal forearm will require operating room repair, because proximal extension of the wound is often needed to search for retracted tendons. The repair does not have to be performed at the time of injury, but should be accomplished within 72 hours whenever possible.

Patients whose tendon lacerations are not repaired at the time of ED presentation should be seen by the hand specialist within 24 hours to arrange definitive repair. Prior to discharge, the wound should be thoroughly cleaned and irrigated and the skin edges approximated. The wrist and hand should be immobilized in a well-padded splint and the patient should be encouraged to elevate the extremity. Many emergency physicians will also administer an intravenous dose of an antistaphylococcal antibiotic (e.g., cephazolin), followed by a short course of an oral antibiotic with similar coverage. However, there is no evidence that this practice improves outcome.

Patients who undergo tendon repair in the ED should be referred to a hand specialist within 48 hours for a wound check. In addition, this will allow the surgeon to arrange timely physical therapy when needed.

Nerve Injuries

The emergency physician should be proficient in the diagnosis of hand and wrist injuries complicated by nerve injury, because outcome is improved with early diagnosis. It is imperative that a careful examination of the hand and wrist is performed before the instillation of any local anesthetics. If suspicion of a peripheral nerve injury exists, anesthetics should be withheld until consultation with the hand surgeon. Nerve repair requires microsurgical techniques and can be performed down to the level of the digital nerve proximal to the DIP flexor crease. Reapproximated peripheral nerves will regenerate at a rate of 1 to 4 mm per day. When nerve injuries occur in fresh, clean, well-perfused tissue, most surgeons prefer immediate repair. However, when necessary, repair can be delayed for 2 weeks to 3 months.

Arterial Injuries

Arterial injuries may complicate either blunt or penetrating trauma and are frequently associated with nerve injuries due to their close proximity to peripheral nerves. In some cases these injuries are obvious (i.e., a history or observation of pulsating hemorrhage). However, in others, the diagnosis requires a thorough physical examination (e.g., capillary refill, Allen test) and careful wound exploration. Even complete arterial lacerations may spasm and the bleeding will have stopped by the time the patient is evaluated.

Management of arterial injuries depends on the structures involved, and the extent and location of the injury. Because the hand has a dual blood supply, ischemia is uncommon with a single artery injury. Consequently, isolated injury to the radial or ulnar artery without distal ischemia or sensory impairment is often managed by simple ligation. In contrast, arterial injuries with distal ischemia or associated nerve injury usually require surgical repair. If a severed digital artery is not repaired, both the proximal and distal ends should be ligated to avoid rebleeding. Consultation with a specialist is strongly recommended prior to repair or discharge.

Carpal Tunnel Syndrome

The carpal tunnel is formed by the proximal carpal row and is overlaid by the flexor retinaculum, which acts as a sling for the extrinsic wrist flexors and also houses the median nerve. This common chronic wrist condition is often seen in people who perform repetitive wrist movement (e.g. typists, jackhammers), but is also seen in conjunction with numerous systemic illnesses (rheumatoid arthritis, diabetes mellitus, collagen vascular diseases) and pregnancy.

Compression of the median nerve produces paresthesias and pain in the distribution of the median nerve in the hand (i.e. the palmar surface of digits 1-3 and the radial half of the 4th digit). These are frequently reported to be worse at night and after strenuous exercise or repeated activity. Examination may reveal atrophy of the thenar eminence (although this is a late finding) and weakness of finger and wrist flexion and thumb pincer function. A positive *Phalen's test* (paresthesias produced or worsened by holding the wrist in palmar flexion for one minute) has a sensitivity of 76% and specificity of 80% for carpal tunnel syndrome (CTS) (16,25). *Tinel's sign* (paresthesias produced or worsened by tapping on the flexor retinaculum) has a sensitivity and specificity of only 64% and 55%, respectively (16,25). The diagnosis is usually clinical, although nerve conduction studies (EMGs) are often obtained as confirmation.

Treatment is generally conservative, consisting of NSAIDs and wrist splinting for 3 to 4 weeks. The splinting should be continuous at first, with eventual nightly use only. Preventive measures (such as wrist guards for keyboards) should also be undertaken if possible. 'Intra-tunnel' steroid injections may provide relief comparable with surgical release; however, the duration of this relief has been questioned. Surgical release of the carpal tunnel is reserved for refractory cases. Patients diagnosed in the emergency department should be referred to a hand specialist for evaluation and follow up.

CRITICAL INTERVENTIONS

- For patients with clinical signs of a scaphoid fracture, despite negative radiographs, immobilize the wrist in a thumb spica splint and refer them for follow up in 10 to 14 days
- Arrange timely (i.e., within 1 week) follow up for complex distal radial fractures in order to minimize long-term complications
- Carefully explore all wounds for partially torn or retracted tendons or severed arteries
- Obtain hand surgery consultation for repair of tendon lacerations at the level of the wrist

DISPOSITION

The disposition of patients with a wrist or forearm injury depends on the nature and severity of the injury. Institutional and regional protocols may influence the indications and timing of consultation as well as the specialty background of surgical consultants (e.g., orthopaedic surgeon, plastic surgeon, hand surgeon). However, certain injuries (discussed above) require immediate specialty evaluation and treatment; consultation in these cases should occur in the emergency department before the patient is discharged.

For discharged patients, elevation of the extremity and the intermittent use of ice for the initial 24 to 48 hours should be stressed. Instructions regarding signs of infection, the timing of return visits for complications, wound checks, and suture removal are mandatory. Patients with injuries that are splinted should receive instructions regarding splint care, as well as signs or symptoms that should prompt an immediate return to the emergency department. Appropriate and timely followup arrangements should be provided for all patients treated in the emergency department.

COMMON PITFALLS

✔ Failure to splint or immobilize a wrist injury in spite of negative radiographs when clinical suspicion of a fracture is high (e.g., scaphoid fracture)

✔ Misdiagnosing a scapholunate or triquetrolunate dissociation as a wrist sprain and not providing adequate immobilization and follow up

✔ Failure to appreciate radiographic evidence of a lunate or perilunate dislocation and obtain immediate consultation

✔ Failure to achieve proper restoration of volar tilt during reduction of a Colles fracture

✔ Failure to assess for carpal instability with Barton and Hutchison fractures

✔ Failure to recognize the associated dislocations that occur with Galeazzi and Monteggia fractures

✔ Failure to recognize potential DRUJ disruption

✔ Failure to perform a thorough neurologic evaluation prior to the administration of anesthesia

Acknowledgments

Thanks to the previous edition's chapter authors Suzanne Moore Shepherd, Jeffrey Desmond, and William H. Shoff.

References

1. Annamalai G, Raby N. Scaphoid and pronator fat stripes are unreliable soft tissue signs in the detection of radiographically occult fractures. *Clin Rad* 2003;58:798.
2. Amadio PC. Scaphoid fractures. *Orthop Clin North Am* 1992;23:7.
3. Blasier RD. White R. Intravenous regional anesthesia for management of children's extremity fractures in the emergency department. *Ped Emer Care* 1996;12:404.
4. Brydie A, Raby N. Early MRI in the management of clinical scaphoid fracture. *Br J Rad* 2003;76:296.
5. Chin HW, Visotsky J. Ligamentous wrist injuries. *Emerg Med Clin North Am* 1993;11:717.
6. Chin HW, Visotsky J. Wrist fractures. *Emerg Med Clin North Am* 1993;11:703.
7. Cooney WP, Linsceid RL, Robyns JH. Fractures and dislocations of the wrist. In: Rockwood CA, Green DP, Bucholz RW (eds.). *Fractures in adults*, 4th ed., Philadelphia: Lippincott-Raven, 1996.
8. Deminci S, Kutluhan S, Kayuncougla HR, et al. Comparison of open carpal tunnel release and local steroid treatment. *Rheum Intl* 2002;22:33.
9. Dorsay TA, Major NM, Helms CA. Cost-effectiveness of immediate MR imaging versus traditional follow-up for revealing radiographically occult scaphoid fractures *AJR* 2001;177:1257.
10. Farrell RG, Swanson SL, Walter JR. Safe and effective IV regional anesthesia for use in the emergency department. *Ann Emer Med* 1985;14:288.
11. Feuerstein M, Burrell LM, Miller VI, et al. Clinical management of carpal tunnel syndrome: a 12-year review of outcome. *Am J Ind Med* 1999;35:232.
12. Green DP. Carpal dislocations and instabilities. In: Green DP (ed.). *Operative hand surgery*, 3rd ed., New York: Churchill Livingstone, 1993.
13. Griggs SM, Weiss AC. Bony injuries of the wrist, forearm and elbow. *Clin Sports Med* 1996;15:373.
14. Harris JHJ, Harris WH, Novelline RA. *The radiology of emergency medicine*, 4th ed. Baltimore: Williams & Wilkins, 1993.
15. Herneth AM, Siegmeth A, Bader, TR, et al. Scaphoid fractures: evaluation with high-spatial-resolution US initial results. *Radiology* 2001;220:231–235.
16. Kanaan N, Sawaya RA. Carpal tunnel syndrome: modern diagnostic and management techniques. *Br J Gen Prac* 2001;51:311.
17. Kirk M, Orlinsky M, Goldberg R, et al. The validity and reliability of the navicular fat stripe as a screening test for detection of navicular fractures. *Ann Emerg Med* 1990;19:1371.
18. Lacey JD, Hodge JC. Pisiform and hamulus fractures: easily missed wrist fractures diagnosed on a reverse oblique radiograph. *J Emerg Med* 1998;16:445.
19. Larsen CF, Lauristen J. Epidemiology of acute wrist trauma. *Int J Epid* 1993;22:911.
20. Mehta M, Brautigan MW. Fracture of the carpal navicular: efficacy of clinical findings and improved diagnosis with six-view radiography. *Ann Emerg Med* 1990;19:255.
21. Murphy DG, Eisenhauer MA. Utility of a bone scan in the diagnosis of clinical scaphoid fracture. *J Emerg Med* 1994;12:709.
22. Propp DA, Chin HW. Forearm and wrist radiology. *J Emerg Med* 1989;7:393.
23. Roberts JR. Intravenous regional anesthesia. In: Roberts JR, Hedges JR, et al (eds). *Clinical procedures in emergency medicine*, 4th ed. Philadelphia: WB Saunders and Co, 2004.
24. Sloan EP. Nerve injuries in the hand. *Emerg Med Clin North Am* 1993;11:651.
25. Sternbach G. The carpal tunnel syndrome. *J Emer Med* 1999;17:519.
26. Watson HK, Weinzweig J. Physical examination of the wrist. *Hand Clinics* 1997;13:17.
27. Uehara DT, Wolanyk D, Escarza RH. Wrist Injuries. In: Tintinalli JE, Kelen GD, Stapczynski JS (eds). *Emergency medicine: a comprehensive study guide*, 6th ed., New York: McGraw-Hill Companies, Inc., 2004.

CHAPTER 192

Hand Injuries

Kenneth Jackimczyk, Suzanne Moore Shepherd, and Paul Blackburn

Hand injuries are a common problem in the emergency department, accounting for 5% to 20% of emergency department visits (2,6,15). Emergency physicians must be skilled in the evaluation and management of hand injuries since outcome depends on accurate assessment of the injury, appropriate initial management, and prompt recognition of those injuries that require immediate specialty consultation or outpatient referral.

An understanding of the anatomy and terminology of the hand is crucial for the evaluation and treatment of hand injuries. The surfaces of the hand and digits are referred to as dorsal, palmar (or volar), ulnar, and radial. The palmar surface is divided into the thenar (overlying the thumb metacarpal), hypothenar (overlying the little finger metacarpal), and midpalm areas. The digits are named thumb, index, middle (or long), ring, and little fingers. Each digit has a metacarpophalangeal (MCP) joint and interphalangeal (IP) joints. The thumb has one IP joint, while the fingers have both a proximal interphalangeal (PIP) joint and a distal interphalangeal (DIP) joint (Fig. 192.1). Finger motion is described as extension, hyperextension (i.e., greater than 180° at the MCP or IP joints), flexion, and abduction and adduction (as related to the midline of the long finger). In addition, the thumb can perform opposition to touch the pads of all the fingers. There

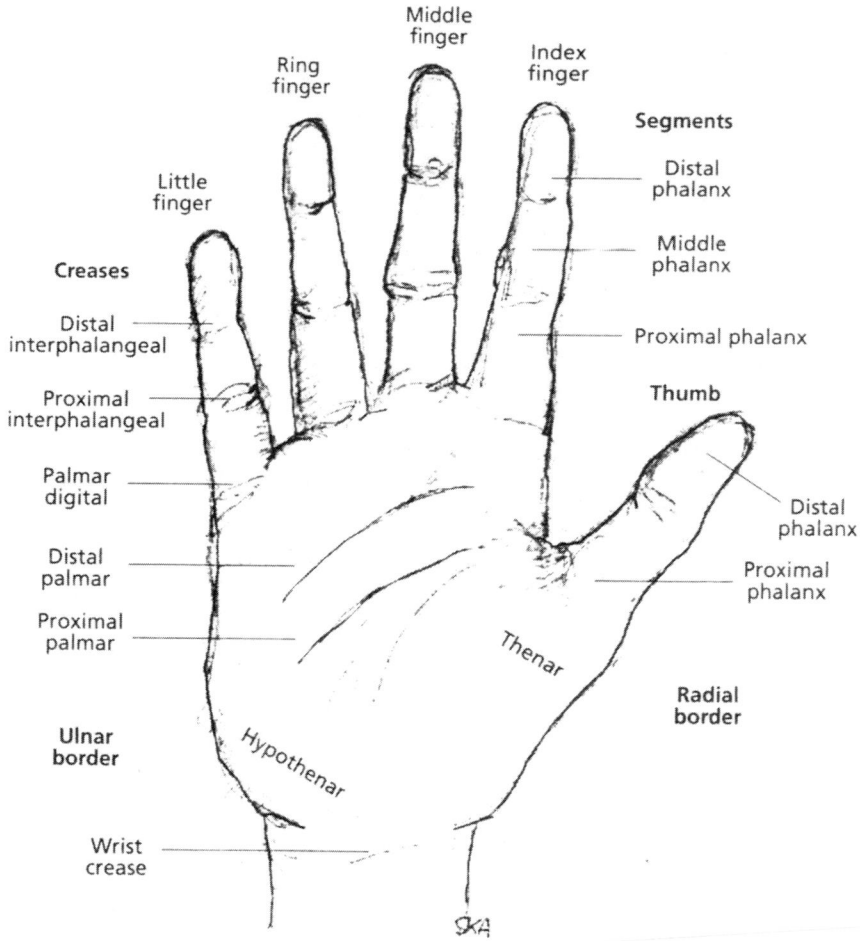

Figure 192.1.   Palmar (volar) surface anatomy.

are 19 separate bones of the hand, including 5 metacarpals and 14 phalanges.

Muscles that control hand motions are divided into flexors and extensors, each of which may be intrinsic or extrinsic to the hand. The intrinsic muscles (thenar and hypothenar muscles, adductor pollicus, lumbricals, and interossei) have their origins and insertions within the hand. The thenar muscles and adductor pollicis are tested by flexing, adducting and abducting the thumb. The four lumbricals originate from the flexor digitorum profundus tendons and insert on the radial aspect of the extensor expansion of the extensor digitorum. The four dorsal and three palmar interossei originate from the lateral metacarpals and insert on the base of the proximal phalanxes and extensor expansion (Fig. 192.2). Motor function of the lumbricals and interossei are tested by placing the hand on a flat surface and moving each finger from side to side. The hypothenar muscles are tested by adducting the little finger.

The extrinsic muscles have their origins in the forearm and exert their effect on hand motion by means of tendinous insertions in the hand. The extensor tendons pass under the extensor retinaculum at the wrist and affect extension of the fingers by their dorsal attachments on the metacarpals and phalanges. Because there are many interconnections (junctura tendineae) between the extensors, care must be taken in evaluating suspected extensor tendon injuries, since normal movement may be preserved via these interconnecting bands.

The nine extrinsic finger flexors enter the hand via the carpal tunnel. The flexor pollicis longus inserts on the distal phalanx of the thumb and is tested by flexing the thumb against resistance. The other four fingers each have two flexors. The flexor digitorum superficialis (FDS) attaches to the base of the middle phalanx and provides flexion at the wrist, MCP and PIP joints. The flexor digitorum profundus (FDP) attaches at the base of the distal phalanx and provides flexion at the wrist, MCP, PIP and DIP joints. The FDP tendon of each finger is tested individually by flexing the DIP joint against resistance with the PIP and MCP joints held in extension. The FDS tendons are tested by flexing the PIP joint of each finger against resistance with the other fingers held in extension. It is important to test both FDS and FDP function in each finger individually in order to avoid missing an isolated injury.

The median, radial, and ulnar nerves provide sensory and motor innervation to the hand. The sensory innervation of the hand is detailed in Figure 192.3. The median nerve supplies motor function to the extrinsic flexors of the hand (only the radial

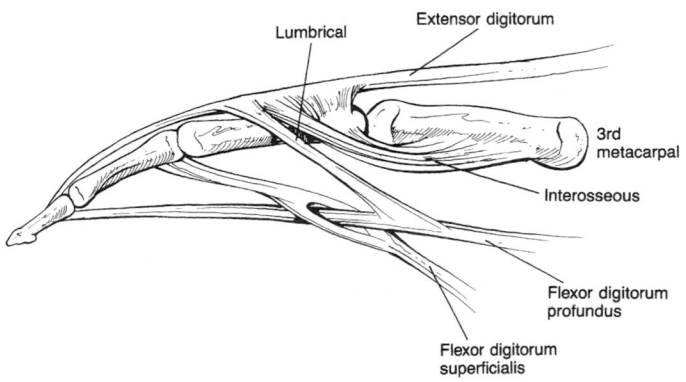

Figure 192.2.   Musculotendinous anatomy of the finger.

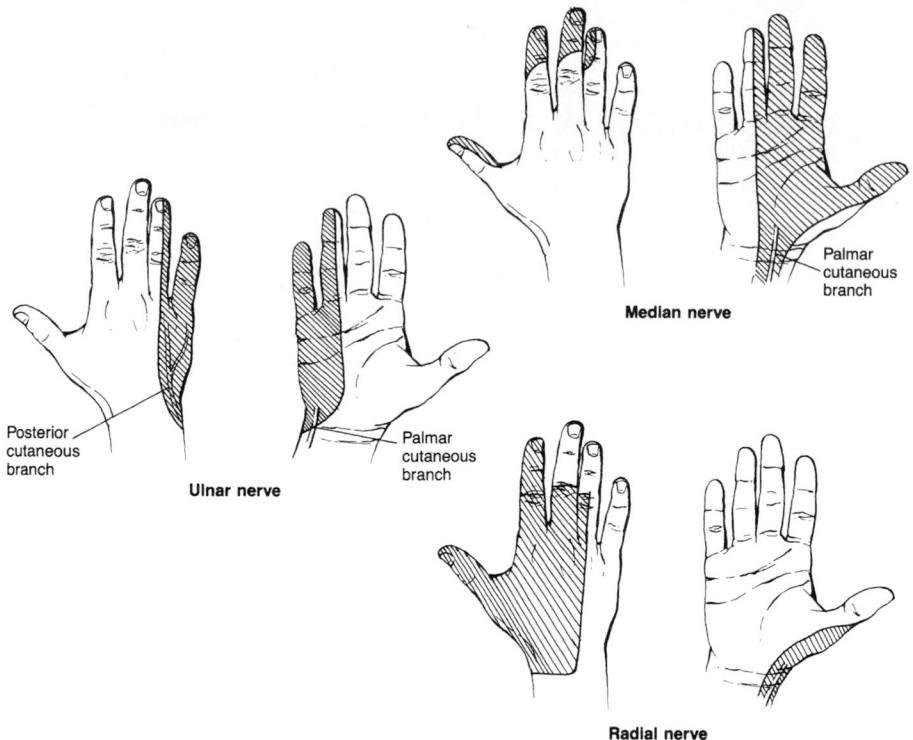

Figure 192.3. Sensory innervation of the hand.

portion of the flexor digitorum profundus), the intrinsic thenar muscles (abductor pollicis brevis, a portion of the flexor pollicis brevis, and the opponens pollicis), and first and second lumbricals. The ulnar nerve innervates the flexor carpi ulnaris and the ulnar portion of the flexor digitorum profundus; it then travels distally to innervate all the remaining intrinsic muscles of the hand. The radial nerve innervates those muscles of the forearm that provide extension of the wrist and digits and extension and abduction of the thumb. The radial nerve does not innervate any of the intrinsic hand muscles.

The arterial supply to the hand is provided by the radial and ulnar arteries. Extensive collateralization occurs between the two vessels. The radial artery passes through the anatomic snuffbox and terminates as the deep palmar arch. The ulnar artery passes into the hand through Guyon's canal superficial to the flexor retinaculum to form the superficial palmar arch. A deep branch of the ulnar artery anastomoses with the deep palmar arch, and a superficial branch of the radial artery anastomoses with the superficial palmar arch. The four common digital arteries arise from the superficial palmar arch and then divide to form the proper digital arteries.

The thick palmar skin is adherent to the underlying palmar aponeurosis by numerous fibrous bands. The palmar aponeurosis forms the triangular, thick, deep fascia of the palm. It is attached to the distal flexor retinaculum, where it receives the insertion of the palmaris longus tendon and spreads distally to the base of the four fingers. In contrast to that of the palm, the dorsal skin of the hand is thin and supple, with little underlying adipose or fibrous tissue. For this reason, edema from hand injuries is often more pronounced on the dorsal surface.

An appreciation of fingertip and nail bed anatomy is essential when evaluating distal finger injuries. The soft tissue of the fingertip is segmented by several fibrous septae, which provide stability to the finger pad (Fig. 192.4). The nail plate emerges from the proximal nail fold and is bordered on each side by the lateral nail folds. The nail grows from the germinal matrix and is tightly adherent to the nail bed (sterile matrix).

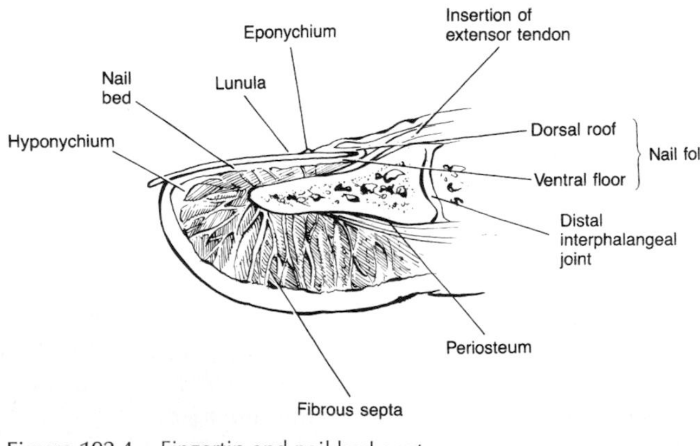

Figure 192.4. Fingertip and nail bed anatomy.

CLINICAL PRESENTATION

Patients with acute blunt or penetrating hand injuries present with varying degrees of pain, swelling, and loss of function. Deformity may or may not be present or may be obscured by associated swelling. In contrast, injuries resulting from repetitive motions or systemic or bone diseases usually present more insidiously, with chronic waxing and waning symptoms (See Chapter 102, "Painful Syndromes of the Hand and Wrist" and Chapter 103, "Bursitis and Tendinopathy").

Patients with metacarpal injuries generally present with pain, swelling, deformity, and limitation of movement after a direct blow to the hand, a crush injury, a missile injury, or striking an object with a closed fist. The location of maximal tenderness and the presence of crepitus and deformity will help localize the area

nerve block is accomplished by injecting 5 to 7 mL of local anesthetic 1 cm proximal to the distal wrist flexion crease just radial and deep to the flexor carpi ulnaris tendon. The ulnar artery at this level lies in close proximity to the ulnar nerve, so aspiration before injection is important to avoid intravascular injection of the anesthetic. The dorsal sensory branch of the ulnar nerve is blocked by subcutaneous infiltration of anesthetic just distal to the ulnar styloid. A radial nerve block is performed by subcutaneous infiltration of 5 mL of anesthetic agent just distal to the radial styloid. If paresthesias are elicited during insertion of the needle, it should be withdrawn before injection, because direct injection into the nerve may cause neuritis. A hematoma block is performed by injecting a local anesthetic into the hematoma surrounding a fracture. A 27- to 30-gauge needle is inserted over the fracture site. When blood is aspirated into the syringe, indicating correct needle placement, 5 to 10 mL of anesthetic is injected. Ten to 15 minutes are often required before complete anesthesia is obtained with regional and hematoma nerve blocks.

Metacarpal Injuries

Diagnosis and correction of rotational malalignment (Fig. 192.5) is particularly important with metacarpal injuries. Nondisplaced metacarpal fractures are managed by immobilization in an ulnar gutter splint (metacarpals 4 and 5), radial gutter splint (metacarpals 2 and 3), or thumb spica splint (metacarpal 1) and by prompt referral. It is imperative that malalignment, especially rotational malalignment, is excluded by radiographs and careful physical examination (Fig. 192.5). The wrist should be splinted in 20 degrees of extension, the MCP joints at 90 degrees flexion, and IP joints in extension. This is the functional position of the hand which relaxes all of the intrinsic muscles of the hand. All open fractures, unstable fractures, multiple metacarpal fractures, and fractures that cannot be reduced by closed technique require surgical consultation for open reduction and internal fixation.

Metacarpal Neck Fractures

Most commonly seen in the fifth metacarpal (i.e., boxer fracture), neck fractures are usually the result of striking an object with a closed fist. Metacarpal neck fractures are easily reduced, but reduction is often difficult to maintain due to comminution of the volar cortex. Because metacarpals 2 and 3 are relatively fixed and immobile, reduction of these fractures must be nearly anatomic. Any volar angulation will project the metacarpal head into the palm and impair grip strength. Greater angulation is acceptable in metacarpals 4 and 5 because they have greater mobility and can move dorsally without impairment of grip strength. Most hand surgeons will allow up to 40 degrees of angulation in fractures of the fifth metacarpal neck and 30 degrees of angulation in fractures of the fourth metacarpal neck. In contrast, as little as 10 degrees of angulation is unacceptable for metacarpals 2 and 3.

Reduction of a metacarpal neck fracture is accomplished by taking advantage of the fact that the MCP joint collateral ligaments are taut in flexion and the proximal phalanx can be used as a lever to manipulate the distal fracture fragment. Reduction techniques are the same regardless of which metacarpal is fractured. However, surgical consultation is recommended before reduction of metacarpals 2 and 3, because some surgeons prefer operative fixation. After adequate anesthesia has been obtained, the MCP and PIP joints are flexed to 90 degrees and pressure is applied to the PIP joint in a dorsal direction to force the metacarpal head into its normal position. Stabilizing volar pressure should be applied with the physician's other thumb just proximal to the fracture site (Fig. 192.6). If reduction is difficult, longitudinal distraction may be needed to disimpact the fracture before successful reduction can be accomplished.

of injury. In patients with a metacarpal head fracture, axial compression of the extended digit causes severe discomfort, whereas in patients with a metacarpal base fracture, flexion, or extension of the wrist or longitudinal compression exacerbates the pain. Metacarpal fractures are classified according to the bone that is injured and the fracture site. Fractures of metacarpals 2 through 5 are classified together and divided into head, neck, shaft, and base fractures. First metacarpal fractures are classified separately as extraarticular base and shaft fractures and intraarticular base fractures.

Patients with phalangeal injuries present with varying degrees of pain, swelling, and tenderness; limited or complete loss of function; and deformity of the involved digit.

Hand lacerations range from clean, superficial wounds to severely contaminated crush injuries or amputations. Associated tendon injuries may cause a partial or complete loss of motor function, and injury to surrounding nerves, may result in loss of both motor and sensory function. Due to their close proximity, digital nerve and flexor tendon injuries frequently occur together.

Patients with fingertip injuries may present with a minor laceration or a severe injury with significant tissue loss or destruction. There may be considerable discomfort, particularly with crush injuries and amputations. Bleeding is usually not severe unless there is associated injury to a digital artery.

DIFFERENTIAL DIAGNOSIS

Metacarpal injuries include fractures, dislocations, or combinations of the two. Carpal–metacarpal dislocations may be confused with proximal metacarpal injuries, while proximal phalangeal injuries and MCP joint dislocations must be included in the differential diagnosis of distal metacarpal injuries. If an injury is associated with an open wound, the possibility of infection of the underlying structures should be considered (see Chapter 104, "Hand Infections").

The differential diagnosis of acute phalangeal injuries includes fractures, fracture–dislocations, and ligamentous injuries. Associated metacarpal injuries must always be excluded, especially in the presence of a proximal phalanx injury.

The diagnostic challenge of hand lacerations lies in the detection of underlying injuries that may threaten function of the hand. Tendon lacerations and injury to bones, joints, nerves, and arteries must be excluded by examination, radiography, and direct exploration of the wound. In older wounds, the patient must be evaluated for the possibility of a developing deep space infection. Wounds that do not heal or have persistent pain with movement should be evaluated for an occult foreign body.

EMERGENCY DEPARTMENT EVALUATION

Initial emergency department evaluation should focus on the need for resuscitation, followed by a general assessment of the patient to detect other significant injuries. Direct pressure should be used to control bleeding from hand wounds. In the rare instances when direct pressure is not sufficient, careful and intermittent use of a tourniquet (i.e., proximal blood pressure cuff) will usually gain control of the bleeding and allow adequate visualization of the wound. Blind clamping of bleeding vessels should be avoided because adjacent nerves and tendons may be injured.

A focused history is essential in the evaluation and treatment of the injured hand. Important historical information includes the patient's age, dominant hand, occupation, prior hand injuries, previous tetanus immunization and past medical history.

Details of the traumatic event should be obtained including time and mechanism of the injury, position of the hand during the accident and treatment administered before arrival.

A detailed systematic examination of the hand is important for accurate diagnosis of hand injuries. All dressings should be removed to completely expose the hand. Rings should be removed from all fingers because swelling may create a tourniquet effect. The location and type of wounds, skin loss, ecchymosis, pallor, swelling, and resting attitude of the digits should be noted. The normal resting cascade of the fingers reveals progressive flexion of the digits from the index to the little finger, which is generally symmetric.

Alterations in the normal stance may indicate an underlying tendon injury. For example, a flexor tendon injury may appear as an extended digit because of unopposed extensor tone, while an extensor tendon injury may reveal a flexion deformity. The hand should also be observed during passive flexion and extension of the wrist. With wrist extension, the fingers naturally assume a flexed posture, and with wrist flexion, the fingers will passively extend (13). This may be particularly helpful in evaluating children or patients who are uncooperative because of intoxication or pain.

The hand should be carefully palpated to identify areas of tenderness, bony step-off, and crepitus. In patients with phalangeal or metacarpal fractures the presence of rotational malalignment must be sought. Rotational deformity may be diagnosed by having the patient make a fist. Normally, all of the fingers point to the same spot on the scaphoid (Fig. 192.5). Scissoring of the digits and loss of the usual parallel relationship of the fingernails are additional signs of rotational deformity.

Nerve integrity is assessed by testing both sensory and motor function. Sensation should always be evaluated and documented before the administration of any anesthetic agent. Digital nerve sensory function is best assessed by two-point tactile discrimination. This test may be easily performed with a paper clip bent into a U shape. The volar lateral aspects of the digits are lightly stroked in a longitudinal direction with the two points. Normal discrimination is 2 to 5 mm at the fingertips and 7–12 mm at the base of the palm but may vary among individuals (4,19). Comparison with the opposite hand may be helpful. Motor function of the median nerve is tested by opposing the thumb against resistance (touching the thumb to the little finger) and palmar abducting the thumb against resistance (elevating the thumb of the pronated hand lying on a flat surface). Radial nerve function is checked by extending the wrist and fingers. Ulnar function is tested by spreading the fingers apart against resistance.

In young children or uncooperative patients, it can be difficult to accurately perform two-point tactile discrimination. In these circumstances, nerve integrity can be assessed by testing for the presence of sympathetically mediated skin wrinkling and skin sweating. Soaking the hand in warm water for 30 minutes should cause wrinkling of the normally innervated skin. Skin sweating can be assessed by stroking the digit with a smooth object (e.g., the barrel of a pen). Less resistance (due to loss of sweating) should be noted over the denervated area. Alternatively, the hand can be painted with povidone–iodine solution, allowed to dry completely, and then placed in a sterile glove. Normal digital sweating will moisten the povidone–iodine and cause the talc in the glove to turn black.

Vascular integrity of the hand is evaluated by looking for cyanosis or pallor, noting skin temperature, assessing capillary refill, and by palpating the ulnar and radial arteries at the wrist (13). The Allen test is utilized to evaluate the patency of the radial and ulnar arteries and the palmar arches. The test is performed by having the patient clench the fist to exsanguinate the hand while the examiner occludes the radial and ulnar arteries. When the hand is blanched, pressure over one of the arteries is released. Normal hand color should return in 3 to 5 seconds. The test

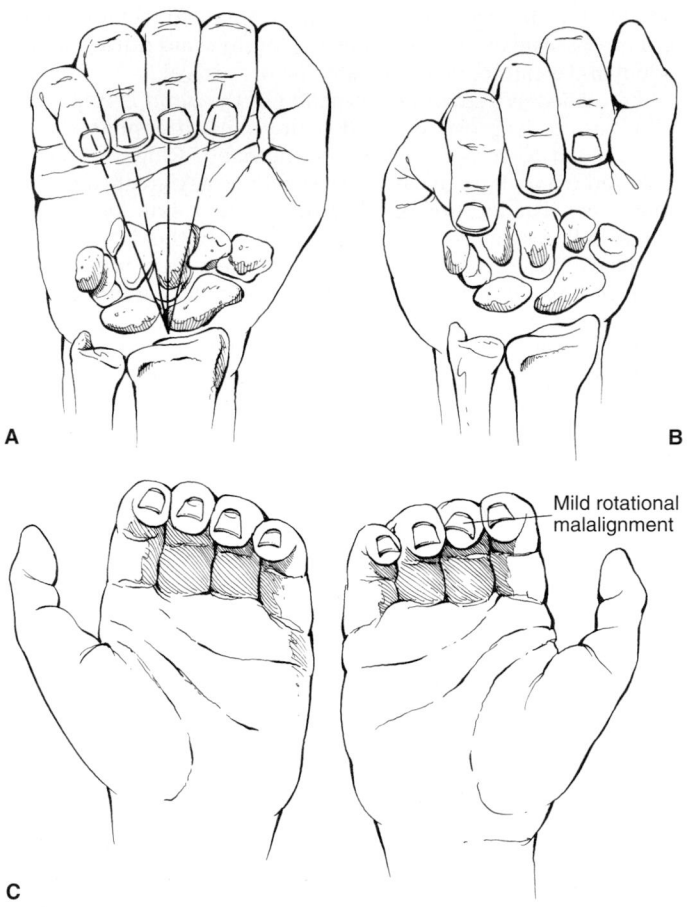

Figure 192.5.   Clinical signs of rotational malalignment. (A) Normally, all fingers point to the same spot on the scaphoid when making a fist. (B) With rotational malalignment, the affected finger does not point to the scaphoid. (C) Loss of the usual parallel relationship of the finger nails with rotational malalignment. (Redrawn from Simon RR, Koenigsknecht SJ. *Emergency Orthopaedics: The Extremities,* 3rd ed. Norwalk, CT: Appleton & Lange, 1995:64.)

is then repeated releasing the other artery. A digital Allen test performed in a similar fashion has also been described (13).

Testing for musculotendinous integrity of both the extrinsic and intrinsic hand muscles is another important aspect of the hand examination. When evaluating finger lacerations, the digit should be moved through a full range of motion against light resistance, because a tendon laceration may be proximal or distal to the skin wound, depending on the position of the hand when the injury occurred. Partial tendon lacerations may have full function and are easily missed. If there is any concern about the possibility of a foreign body or injury to a deep structure, the wound should be evaluated under bright lighting with a dry field. A bloodless field is obtained by first emptying the veins by elevating the extremity and then inflating a proximally placed blood pressure cuff above systolic pressure. The blood pressure cuff may be left in place for up to 20 minutes while the wound is explored. A dry field can be obtained in individual digits by placing a sterile glove on the injured hand, cutting off the tip of the glove on the injured finger, and rolling the end of the cut glove proximally to simultaneously exsanguinate and tourniquet the finger.

Radiographs of the hand should be obtained whenever the mechanism might result in bony disruption, joint instability, or a retained foreign body. Standard views of the hand and fingers include posteroanterior (PA), lateral, and external oblique views. If a thumb injury is suspected, PA and lateral views of

apex of the fracture and dorsal pressure on the flexed MCP joint. It is essential that any rotational deformity be corrected. If reduction is successful, the hand is splinted as described earlier and the patient is referred for follow up in 3 to 5 days. If a transverse fracture cannot be reduced, or if an oblique, spiral, or comminuted fracture is present, consultation with a hand surgeon for operative repair is indicated.

Metacarpal Base Fractures

Fractures of the base of the metacarpals are generally stable, but even slight rotational deformity will be greatly amplified at the fingertip (5). Nondisplaced fractures without rotational deformity may be treated by immobilization in a gutter or volar splint and by surgical referral. Displaced or intraarticular base fractures require hand surgery consultation for open reduction and internal fixation.

First Metacarpal Fractures

First metacarpal fractures are uncommon fractures and are usually the result of a direct injury to the thumb. These fractures most often occur at or near the base and may be either extraarticular or intraarticular. Extraarticular fractures are more common and are usually transverse or, less often, oblique. Because of the mobility of the first metacarpal, as much as 20 to 30 degrees of angulation may be present without loss of mobility or function. Transverse fractures with less than 30 degrees of angulation are treated with immobilization in a short-arm thumb spica splint and prompt follow up. A transverse fracture with greater than 30 degrees of angulation requires reduction, which involves manipulation of the fracture, using the thumb for distraction. After reduction, the thumb is splinted as described earlier, and the patient is referred for follow up. Oblique fractures are often unstable and frequently require percutaneous pinning for adequate immobilization. Therefore, consultation is advised before manipulation or discharge.

There are two types of intraarticular fractures: the Bennett fracture and the Rolando fracture. A *Bennett fracture* is a two part intraarticular fracture of the metacarpal base. Because of the pull of the abductor pollicis longus, the metacarpal base is subluxed or dislocated proximally and radially. A *Rolando fracture* is a comminuted, usually T- or Y-shaped intraarticular fracture of the base of the first metacarpal. Both fractures result from an axial blow to the metacarpal, commonly sustained by striking an object with a closed fist. Emergency department management includes immobilization in a thumb spica splint and expeditious follow up with a hand surgeon. Definitive therapy for a Bennett fracture frequently requires pinning for a stable anatomic reduction. A Rolando fracture often requires open reduction and has a poor prognosis, even with optimal management (4,5).

Metacarpal Dislocations

Dislocations involving the metacarpals are either carpometacarpal (CMC) or metacarpophalangeal (MCP). CMC dislocations are uncommon, require a significant force and are usually caused by a crush injury, a direct longitudinal blow along the metacarpals or a levering dorsiflexion force. These dislocations are generally dorsal and often associated with metacarpal or carpal fractures and significant soft-tissue trauma. The presence of a displaced proximal metacarpal fracture should prompt a careful search for an associated CMC dislocation. The lateral view is the most helpful standard view for diagnosing CMC dislocations. However, overlapping densities on standard wrist radiographs may make the detection of CMC dislocations difficult so special views (e.g., anteroposterior [AP] in supination, 30-degree radial, and ulnar obliques) may be needed to detect

CMC dislocations. Emergency department care is supportive pending hand surgery consultation. CMC dislocations are easily reduced, but operative fixation (i.e., Kirschner pinning) is usually required to maintain reduction. Complications of CMC dislocations are ulnar and median nerve injuries, extensor tendon injuries, and circulatory compromise.

MCP dislocations usually occur dorsally and are generally well visualized on standard radiographs of the hand. Dorsal MCP dislocations are classified as simple (reducible) or complex (irreducible). Simple dorsal dislocations are the most common and can usually be reduced in the emergency department. With complex dorsal dislocations, the volar plate is interposed between the metacarpal head and the proximal phalanx, trapping the metacarpal head between the flexor tendons and the lumbricals; these are irreducible by closed techniques (Fig. 192.7). On examination, complex dislocations often appear less deformed than simple dislocations and are associated with puckering of the palmar skin overlying the metacarpal head. Radiographically, the presence of a sesamoid bone within the MCP joint space is pathognomonic of a complex dislocation (5). Simple dorsal dislocations are reduced by slight flexion of the wrist to relax the extrinsic flexors, followed by gentle hyperextension of the MCP joint and firm pressure on the dorsal aspect of the proximal phalanx. Longitudinal traction and extreme hyperextension should be avoided because this may entrap the volar plate, converting a simple dislocation into a complex one. After reduction, the hand is immobilized, with the wrist in 20 degrees of extension, the MCP joint in 60 degrees of flexion, the PIP joint in 20 degrees of flexion, and the DIP joint in 15 degrees of flexion. One attempt at reduction of a possible complex dislocation may be warranted, but multiple attempts should be avoided. These patients require open reduction and repair of the volar plate injury.

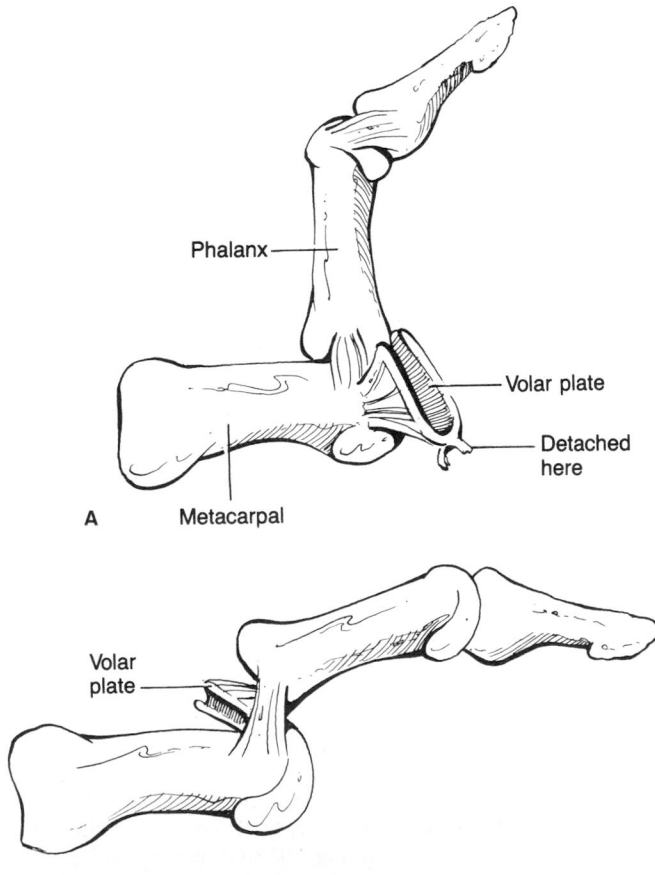

Figure 192.7.   Dorsal dislocation of the MCP joint. (A) Simple dorsal dislocation. (B) Complex dorsal dislocation; note entrapment of the volar plate.

Collateral MCP ligament injuries occur infrequently and are often missed acutely. The presence of an avulsion fracture from the metacarpal head or corner fracture of the base of the proximal phalanx suggests an MCP collateral ligament injury. Consultation with a hand surgeon is recommended for patients with a collateral ligament injury, because some surgeons prefer operative reduction and repair of these injuries (5). Emergency department care involves immobilization in a gutter splint, with the MCP in at least 50 degrees of flexion, and appropriate referral.

Ulnar Collateral Ligament Injury (Gamekeeper's Thumb)

Initially described as a chronic laxity of the thumb MCP joint ulnar collateral ligament in Scottish gamekeepers (a result of the technique by which they killed wounded rabbits), the term *gamekeeper's thumb* has come to include all injuries to the thumb ulnar collateral ligament. Today, acute rupture of the ulnar collateral ligament caused by sudden abduction of the thumb is much more common and is most often due to falls while skiing, earning the eponym *skier's thumb*.

Plain radiographs may be normal or may reveal an avulsion fracture from the base of the proximal phalanx. If plain radiographs do not reveal a fracture, stressing the ligament may help determine if a complete tear has occurred. The joint should be stressed both in extension and in 30 degrees of flexion to reduce the stabilizing effect of the volar plate. A difference of greater than 10 degrees between the injured and uninjured thumb is considered indicative of a ligamentous tear. Unless the joint is grossly unstable, local anesthesia may be needed for reliable stress testing (5).

Emergency department management includes immobilization in a thumb spica splint and early referral to a hand surgeon. A frequent complication of ulnar collateral ligament rupture is chronic laxity of the MCP joint due to interposition of the adductor aponeurosis between the ends of the torn ligament, referred to as a Stener lesion (5,7,11). Because of this, many surgeons prefer routine operative repair of the ulnar collateral ligament tears. The presence of a fracture involving greater than 25% of the articular surface or of a displaced avulsion fracture is also an indication for open repair (5).

Phalangeal Injuries

Phalangeal injuries can result in significant functional disability if not recognized and treated appropriately. Injuries to the fingers are usually a result of direct trauma to the digit. As with all hand injuries, a detailed history and physical examination are essential. The presence of rotational deformity must be carefully sought (Fig. 192.5) and corrected, particularly with proximal phalangeal fractures. Radiographs are indicated in most injuries.

Treatment of closed phalangeal injuries depends on the nature of the injury (discussion follows). Open phalangeal fractures, with the exceptions of distal amputations and distal phalanx fractures, are managed in a fashion similar to that for other open fractures.

Proximal and Middle Phalangeal Fractures

Stable, nondisplaced middle and proximal phalangeal fractures without angulation or rotational deformity can be managed with dynamic splinting (i.e., "buddy taping") to an adjacent normal digit. An absorbent material should be placed between the digits for padding and to prevent maceration of the skin. The patient should bend the fingers normally and use the hand as comfort allows. Radiographs are obtained in 7 and 14 days to assess angu-

lation and healing. Unstable fractures of the proximal and middle phalanges (e.g., oblique, condylar, displaced, or angulated transverse fractures) and displaced intraarticular fractures generally require operative reduction or fixation. Emergency department management of these fractures includes immobilization in a gutter splint and surgical consultation.

Avulsion fractures off the dorsal aspect of the base of the middle phalanx are of special concern. If not recognized and treated appropriately, these fractures can result in a *boutonniere deformity* (i.e., fixed flexion of the PIP joint and fixed hyperextension of the DIP joint). This deformity is caused by avulsion of the central slip of the extensor tendon, with loss of extensor function at the PIP joint and unopposed force from the flexor digitorum superficialis (Fig. 192.2). With time, the lateral bands of the extensor expansion sublux laterally and volarly, will become PIP joint flexors and DIP joint extensors. Contractures make this a fixed deformity. These fractures should be immobilized in a volar splint with the PIP joint in extension, and promptly referred to a hand surgeon for evaluation. Avulsion fractures from the volar aspect of the base of the middle phalanx may be indicative of a volar plate injury. These injuries should be immobilized in a volar splint in 15 degrees of flexion, followed by appropriate referral.

Distal Phalanx Fractures

Distal phalanx fractures are divided into intra- and extraarticular fractures. Extraarticular fractures usually result from a direct blow to the distal phalanx. These injuries are often associated with injury to the fingernail or nail bed. Nondisplaced extraarticular fractures are managed with elevation, oral analgesics and placement in a protective splint for 3 to 4 weeks. A U-shaped splint can be constructed using commercially available aluminum and foam splints. Displaced extraarticular fractures are reduced by applying dorsal traction to the distal fragment. If reduction is successful, the digit is immobilized in a volar splint and the patient is referred to a hand surgeon. Otherwise, hand surgery consultation should be obtained in the ED.

Intraarticular fractures often involve the dorsal surface of the joint and may result in loss of extension of the DIP, commonly referred to as a *mallet finger*. This injury is frequently caused by a ball striking the tip of an extended finger. This results in forced flexion of the distal phalanx with the finger in taut extension, causing rupture of the extensor tendon or an intraarticular avulsion fracture of the dorsal aspect of the distal phalanx with loss of extensor function. Patients typically present with tenderness and swelling over the dorsal aspect of the DIP joint and loss of extension at the DIP joint.

Emergency department management includes immobilization using a padded dorsal aluminum splint with the DIP joint in extension. If the fracture involves less than 25% of the articular surface, immobilization is maintained for 6 weeks to coapt the tendon or fracture segments. If the fracture involves more than 25% of the articular surface, the patient should be referred for surgical fixation. Untreated mallet finger may result in a swan neck deformity characterized by hyperextension of the PIP joint and flexion at the DIP joint (9). Open distal phalanx fractures are treated by copious irrigation and wound closure, ensuring complete soft-tissue coverage of exposed bone. If the nail bed has been injured it must be repaired. Prophylactic antibiotics are generally administered.

Proximal Interphalangeal Joint Dislocations

Dislocation of the PIP joint is the most common dislocation of the hand. Dorsal dislocations result from hyperextension forces, such as those that occur when the outstretched finger is struck by a ball. Dorsal PIP dislocations are accompanied by partial or complete rupture of the volar plate or collateral ligaments. Volar dislocations occur less often but are associated with complete rupture of the volar plate and collateral ligaments, as well as the central slip of the extensor mechanism. Patients usually present with pain, swelling, and deformity of the PIP joint. Rarely, severe swelling will mask an otherwise obvious deformity. The presence of pain and a locking sensation with flexion suggests a volar plate injury. Radiographs are diagnostic for acute dislocations, but small avulsions of the volar plate may not be visible or are seen only on the lateral post-reduction view. Most dorsal dislocations are easily reduced, but the volar plate may become interposed in the joint space, preventing reduction by closed techniques. If this occurs, open reduction is required. For closed reduction, a digital nerve block provides adequate anesthesia. The distal portion of the digit is firmly grasped and slightly hyperextended. Then, with gentle traction parallel to the middle phalanx, the base of the middle phalanx is pressed back into position and the PIP joint is flexed. The PIP joint should be immobilized using a volar splint, in 15 to 20 degrees of flexion for 2 to 5 weeks.

Some authors recommend dynamic splinting (buddy taping) for 3 to 6 weeks if the collateral ligaments are stable and there is no evidence of a fracture (5,21). If there is instability after reduction, the patient should be immobilized in a gutter splint and expeditiously referred to a hand surgeon. Volar PIP dislocations can be problematic. They can be reduced by traction with both the MCP and PIP joints flexed; but consultation with a hand surgeon before reduction is recommended, since some surgeons prefer to treat these dislocations operatively to prevent a boutonniere deformity. Joint stiffness is a common complication after both volar and dorsal dislocations.

Distal Interphalangeal Joint Dislocations

Dislocations of the DIP joint are relatively uncommon injuries. They are almost exclusively dorsal and often associated with an open wound. DIP joint dislocations can usually be reduced with digital block anesthesia and simple traction. After reduction, the DIP joint should be immobilized in extension using a dorsal splint and the patient referred to a hand surgeon in 3 to 7 days.

Hand Lacerations

The objectives of emergency department care of hand lacerations are to preserve function, prevent infection, minimize scar formation, and provide the optimal wound environment for rapid healing. Simple lacerations (clean, less than 6 hours old, and not involving tendons, joints, or neurovascular structures) are managed in the same manner as lacerations elsewhere (see Chapter 172, "Wound Management"). However, in many areas of the hand, vital structures are extremely superficial, and injuries to these structures are not always readily apparent. Therefore, great care must be taken in the evaluation of hand lacerations to identify associated injuries, particularly injuries to tendons, nerves, or arteries.

Evaluation of a hand laceration begins with a pertinent history and meticulous examination. Adequate exploration of the wound requires a clean, bloodless, well-illuminated field and adequate anesthesia. A proximal blood pressure cuff (for hand wounds) or finger tourniquet (for digit wounds) provides optimal visualization of the wound. Blind clamping of bleeding vessels may injure adjacent nerves or tendons and should be avoided. Anesthesia may be obtained by direct infiltration of a local anesthetic or regional nerve block but should not be attempted until a sensory examination has been performed. When a complex injury requiring hand surgery consultation is apparent from the initial evaluation, the instillation of local anesthetic should await examination by the consultant. Pain control can be provided with systemic analgesics. Radiographs are indicated in cases in which the mechanism of injury could produce a fracture, dislocation, joint capsule injury, or retained foreign body.

All hand lacerations, regardless of the depth, must be carefully explored, since injury to significant underlying structures can occur with even small surface wounds. Exploration should be carried out through a full range of motion, otherwise injury to underlying structures, particularly tendon lacerations, may be missed. Simple lacerations are cleaned, irrigated, and repaired in the same fashion as in other areas of the body. Deep sutures should be avoided. After repair, lacerations over areas of motion should be splinted until the skin edges are well adherent. Antibiotics are generally not required for simple hand lacerations in otherwise healthy patients.

Clenched-Fist Injuries (Fight Bites)

Lacerations over the MCP joints are often a result of striking an object (e.g., an opponent's teeth during an altercation) with a clenched fist and may be associated with extensor tendon injury, joint capsule violation, or metacarpal neck fracture. Because of the devastating consequences of inadequate treatment (e.g., wound infection, septic arthritis), any laceration over the MCP joints must be approached with suspicion and assumed to be a human bite wound until proven otherwise. Human bites are particularly prone to infection, usually with *Staphylococcus aureus* and *Streptococcus* or anaerobes such as *Eikenella corrodens* (4). Patients with an uncomplicated wound (i.e., no tendon or joint capsule damage) who present within 24 hours with uninfected wounds may be treated with copious irrigation, immobilization and follow up within 24 hours. Prophylactic antibiotics are given. Options for outpatient antibiotics include amoxicillin-clavulanic acid 500/125 mg tid, cephalexin 500 mg qid plus penicillin 500 mg qid or dicloxicillin 500 mg qid plus penicillin 500 mg qid. All other patients with clenched fist injuries are copiously irrigated and splinted in the emergency department and admitted for possible debridement in the operating room by a hand surgeon. Admitted patients receive parental antibiotics. Inpatient antibiotic choices include ampicillin-sulbactam 1.5 gm IV q 6 hours, cefoxitin 2 gm q 8 hours or ticarcillin-clavulanic acid 3.1 gm q 6 hours.

Tendon Lacerations

Tendon injuries are frequently associated with hand lacerations. A detailed examination and careful wound exploration are essential for detecting these injuries since a partially cut tendon may demonstrate normal function. Once identified, management of a tendon laceration depends on the type of tendon injured, the cross-sectional area of tendon involved, and the location of the laceration.

Because of their complex structure, deep location, and high complication rate after injury all suspected flexor tendon lacerations require consultation and repair by a hand surgeon. In circumstances in which a hand surgeon is not immediately available, the wound can be copiously irrigated and the skin closed primarily without tendon repair. The hand is then immobilized in a volar splint, with the wrist in 20 degrees of flexion, the MCP joint in 60 degrees of flexion, and the IP joints in 15 degrees of flexion; and the patient is referred to a hand surgeon for delayed repair within 10 days. Broad-spectrum antibiotic coverage is generally recommended for tendon lacerations.

In contrast to flexor tendons, extensor tendons are anatomically less complex, have a more superficial location, and are associated with fewer complications after repair. As a result, emergency department repair of many simple extensor tendon lacerations is an accepted practice. Tendon lacerations at or distal to the DIP joint (open mallet finger) and lacerations over the metacarpals, middle phalanges, and proximal phalanges (not involving the PIP joint) are amenable to emergency department repair. Lacerations over the PIP joint may involve the lateral bands or the central slip of the extensor mechanism, which, if not repaired meticulously and followed closely, can result in a boutonniere deformity. Therefore patients with extensor tendon injuries over the PIP joint should be referred to a hand surgeon for repair. Partial extensor tendon lacerations involving greater than 20% of the cross-sectional area of the tendon should also be repaired.

Because increased attention is now being given to rehabilitation after extensor tendon repairs, particularly dynamic splinting and early mobilization, timely hand surgery referral should be arranged for all patients undergoing tendon repair in the emergency department.

Technique of Laceration Repair

Wound preparation of a hand injury is similar to that for injuries to other areas of the body (see Chapter 172, "Wound Management"). However, the entire hand should be sterilely prepped and draped so that the laceration and all digits can be manipulated during exploration. Exploration of the wound should be performed under good lighting with a bloodless field. As always, copious irrigation with normal saline is essential. Extension of the wound may be necessary to visualize the tendon laceration or locate the proximal tendon slip. Extending incisions should start from one corner of the wound and generally follow the course of the involved tendon, avoiding obvious veins. Scar contractures are less problematic on the dorsum of the hand than on the palm. Once the involved tendon is identified, a holding stitch can be placed through the proximal tendon for traction during repair. The tendon can then be repaired with 4-0 or 5-0 nonabsorbable sutures using simple, interrupted sutures or a horizontal mattress suture with the knot "buried" between the ends of the tendon. Sutures should be placed 5 to 10 mm from the cut edge of the tendon to avoid the suture tearing through the end of the tendon.

The hand or digit should be splinted in a position with the extensor mechanism relaxed. Tendon repairs at the DIP joint can be treated with a mallet finger splint, leaving the PIP joint mobile. Injuries at or proximal to the PIP joint should be splinted with the wrist in 30 degrees of extension, the MCP joint in 10 to 20 degrees of flexion, and the IP joints in slight flexion. Splinting may be required for up to 6 weeks, although some surgeons prefer to allow early protected motion.

Nerve Injuries

The emergency physician should be proficient in the diagnosis of hand injuries complicated by nerve injury, because outcome is improved with early diagnosis. It is imperative that a careful examination of the hand is performed before the instillation of any local anesthetics. If suspicion of a peripheral nerve injury exists, anesthetics should be withheld until consultation with the hand surgeon. Nerve repair requires microsurgical techniques and can be performed down to the level of the digital nerve proximal to the DIP flexor crease (19). When nerve injuries occur in fresh, clean, well-perfused tissue, most surgeons prefer immediate repair. However, when necessary, repair can be delayed for 2 weeks to 3 months (19).

Arterial Injuries

The hand has a dual blood supply with abundant collateral flow via the palmar arches, and ischemic injuries to the hand are rare. Arterial lacerations may spasm and stop bleeding by the time the patient is evaluated, so careful wound exploration is important. Arterial injuries with distal ischemia or associated nerve injury usually require surgical repair. However, isolated injuries to the radial or ulnar artery without distal ischemia or sensory impairment are often managed by simple ligation.

Fingertip Lacerations, Avulsions, and Amputations

Fingertip injuries are classified according to the extent and level of injury. Simple lacerations and small avulsion injuries are easily managed by the emergency physician. However, injuries that involve significant tissue loss or bony exposure should be referred to a hand surgeon for repair. Partial or complete amputations should also be managed by a hand surgeon (see Chapter 198, "Replantation").

Evaluation should include a focused history and careful hand examination. Standard radiographs of the injured hand should also be performed.

Crush injuries, amputations, and avulsion injuries in which there is significant soft-tissue or bone loss or bone exposure require evaluation and repair by a hand surgeon. These injuries frequently necessitate split- or full-thickness skin grafts or the use of skin flaps for adequate coverage. Pending consultation, emergency department care includes administration of a parenteral antistaphylcoccal antibiotic, appropriate analgesia, wound cleansing, and elevation. Avulsion injuries with minimal soft-tissue loss (wound area less than 10 mm^2) and no bone loss or exposure may be allowed to heal by secondary intention, with excellent cosmetic and functional results. This is particularly true in children, who have excellent regenerative capacity. The technique consists of debriding all dead and devitalized tissue, followed by copious irrigation. The digit is then bandaged with a nonadherent dressing (e.g., Xeroform) and gauze and splinted for comfort and protection. The patient then performs daily dressing changes. Complications include cold intolerance, hypersensitivity in the area of the scar, and a volar curving of the nail at the amputation site.

Subungual Hematoma

A subungual hematoma is a collection of blood under the nail plate. It commonly occurs after a direct blow to the fingertip and may be associated with a nail bed laceration or distal phalanx fracture.

Patients frequently complain of severe throbbing pain. A variable amount of blood will be visible beneath the nail plate and appears as a blue or black discoloration. There may also be associated injury to the nail bed and surrounding nail folds.

When distal phalanx pain and swelling is not related to a recent identifiable traumatic event, the possibility of an infection such as a felon or paronychia should be considered (see Chapter 104, "Hand Infections").

One study suggests that all subungual hematomas, regardless of size or the presence of a distal phalanx fracture may be treated by simple nail trephination as long as the nail plate and surrounding nail folds are intact (17). Others recommend trephination for hematomas that occupy greater than 25% of the nail (4). The use of a battery-operated microcautery device is an effective, and painless method to drain a subungual hematoma. Use of a needle or drill is also effective but can be painful and often requires the use of a digital block. Heated paper clips have been commonly used but may introduce carbon particles into the nail bed. After trephination, the digit should be dressed with absorbent gauze and if a distal phalanx fracture is present, it should be splinted. If there is significant disruption of the nail plate or surrounding nail folds, the nail plate should be removed and proper alignment of the nail bed assured through careful wound repair.

Nail Bed Lacerations

Nail bed lacerations include simple lacerations, stellate lacerations, crush injuries, and avulsions. Failure to properly repair these lacerations can result in a split nail deformity, irregular nail surface, or failure of the nail to adhere to the nail bed. These deformities are significant from both a cosmetic and a functional standpoint.

Presentation varies from innocuous-appearing injuries to those with severe deformity and tissue loss. There is usually throbbing pain, swelling, and tenderness. The nail plate may be intact, broken, partially avulsed, or completely torn away. Bleeding is usually not significant, but if a digital artery is injured, it can be profuse.

Management depends on the type and severity of the injury. Crush and avulsion injuries often require a grafting procedure and are best repaired by a hand surgeon. However, management of simple and stellate lacerations may be performed in the emergency department under digital block anesthesia and tourniquet hemostasis using a 1-in. sterile Penrose drain placed securely around the proximal portion of the finger. The broken nail can be removed with a small hemostat or iris scissors by gently opening and closing the instrument beneath the distal free edge of the nail until the nail plate is loose. The distal end of the nail is then grasped with a Kelly clamp and gently removed. The lacerations should be explored carefully for foreign bodies and then irrigated copiously. Debridement of the wound margins should be avoided, because removal of even small amounts of tissue can lead to enhanced scar formation. Simple lacerations should be closed with interrupted 6-0 absorbable sutures. The use of loop magnification may aid in accurate approximation of the wound edges. The sutures should be tied with only three to four knots so that they do not interfere with nail replacement. Stellate lacerations are repaired in a similar manner, keeping in mind that accurate approximation of each arm of a stellate laceration is essential for normal nail growth.

After repair, the involved nail (if available) should be used as a protective covering for the injured nail bed. The nail should be inspected for debris or foreign matter and rinsed in normal saline before replacement. No tissue should be removed from the undersurface of the nail, because replacing the nail in its normal position often replaces avulsed tissue as well. This tissue acts as a free graft that reduces nail bed scarring. A hole should be placed in the center of the nail to permit blood drainage. The proximal end of the nail is inserted under the eponychium until the nail is in its normal position on the nail bed. A 5-0 monofilament nylon suture placed through the fingertip and the distal free border of the nail secures the nail plate. The suture is cut in 2 to 3 weeks, allowing growth of the new nail to push out the old one. If the nail is missing or damaged, various materials such as metal foil, adaptic or Xeroform can be used to cover the injured nail bed. It is important to insert foil or other material into the proximal nail fold between the eponychium and the nail so that adhesions do not impair normal nail regrowth. An absorbent gauze dressing and application of a splint for comfort and protection are important adjunctive measures.

High-Pressure Injection Injuries

A high-pressure injection injury of the hand may at first appear innocuous, but clinical sequelae are devastating if the initial recognition or management is inadequate or delayed. Three types of industrial equipment (grease guns, spray guns, and diesel injectors) account for most injection injuries (18). Injection often occurs as the operator uses a finger to wipe the plugged nozzle. At the time of the injury, the patient may feel temporary stinging or no pain at all, which, unfortunately, may result in delay in seeking treatment (18).

Several factors determine the type and degree of high-pressure injection injury (14). The *type of material* is the most important element in determining the subsequent morbidity. Paint and paint thinner create the greatest tissue inflammatory response and result in a high rate of amputation. Conversely, grease gun injuries do not create much inflammation. The *amount of material* injected determines tissue distention, compression, and mechanical distortion of blood flow.

The clinical appearance is determined by the time elapsed between injury and presentation. At the time of high-pressure injection, the patient may feel a stinging sensation at the site of penetration. The examiner may note a small puncture wound, which may or may not have a droplet of the injected material at the site.

Within several hours, increased discoloration and swelling occur, accompanied by pain severe enough to be unrelieved by narcotics. This may appear similar to an infectious process, but conservative therapy will almost certainly lead to the need for amputation of the affected part (18).

If the injury is not treated aggressively with operative debridement a poor functional and cosmetic outcome will result.

Taking a thorough history and performing a complete physical examination greatly limits the differential diagnosis. If a wound is noted, the patient should be assumed to have a high-pressure injection injury.

Patients usually present to the emergency department in significant pain within hours of the injury. The affected area should be meticulously inspected to find the site of injection. The amount and location of swelling, tendon function, and joint range of motion are evaluated. Plain films of the involved extremity are useful in determining the extent of the dispersed material and may help guide the extent of surgical debridement. Material can be dispersed at a considerable distance from the site of penetration. Therefore, imaging to the elbow is mandatory (18).

Emergency department treatment must be rapid and definitive if a catastrophic outcome is to be avoided. The time from injury to proper treatment is the prime determinant of prognosis (16). Emergency department care includes elevation of the extremity, administration of broad-spectrum antibiotics, tetanus prophylaxis, and preparation for surgery. Pain control is provided through opiates or proximal extremity nerve blocks. Digital nerve blocks are absolutely contraindicated because of the additional fluid volume and tissue and vascular compression added to the already compromised digit (14,18,20). Warm soaks also are contraindicated since they increase blood flow to the compromised extremity and cause increased tissue compression. Immediate surgical consultation is mandatory.

CRITICAL INTERVENTIONS

- Perform a systematic examination including a careful neurovascular assessment in all patients with hand injuries and document the results
- Carefully explore all wounds for tendon lacerations and foreign bodies using a tourniquet to obtain a bloodless field and document the results
- For patients with a *fight bite*, copiously irrigate and splint in the ED, obtain hand surgery consultation, and admit for intravenous antibiotics and possible operative debridement
- For most injuries, splint the hand with the wrist in 20 degrees of extension, the MCP joint in 60 degrees of flexion, and the IP joints in 15 degrees of flexion

DISPOSITION

Most patients with metacarpal injuries can be discharged from the emergency department with appropriate immobilization and instructions. Those patients with open fractures, irreducible fractures or dislocations, or circulatory compromise should be evaluated by a hand surgeon in the emergency department. Patients with stable fractures, anatomically reduced dislocations, and ligamentous injuries can be discharged with early follow up, because operative repair or fixation can be performed 3 to 5 days after the injury.

Patients with stable, anatomically reduced phalangeal injuries can be discharged from the emergency department with appropriate follow up. Patients with open fractures or nonreducible or unstable fractures or dislocations require consultation with a hand surgeon.

Patients with simple hand or extensor tendon lacerations repaired in the emergency department can be discharged. Reevaluation in 36 to 48 hours for signs of wound infection is advisable for all but minor lacerations. Surgical referral should be made for any complex injury. Discharge instructions should include strict hand elevation, intermittent application of ice for the first 24 hours, and splint precautions. Patients should receive written instructions on specific signs or symptoms which should prompt a return to the emergency department.

Patients with simple fingertip lacerations and minor avulsion injuries may be discharged from the emergency department. A followup visit at 48 hours to check for infection is advised. Patients with more significant injuries require surgical consultation.

Patients with a subungual hematoma may be discharged from the emergency department. If a fracture was detected on radiographs, the digit should be immobilized as described previously under distal phalanx fractures. All patients should be informed about the possibility of nail loss or deformity. Patients with a significantly avulsed nail matrix should be referred to a hand surgeon. Follow up in 48 hours is recommended for patients with a distal phalanx fracture and those with nail bed lacerations that required nail removal and suturing. Antibiotics are unnecessary in immunocompetent patients with clean, fresh wounds. For high-risk patients (e.g., immunosuppressed, delayed care, contaminated wound), many practitioners still recommend prophylactic use of an antibiotic, such as cephalexin or dicloxacillin, for 3 days.

The patient with a high-pressure injection injury should receive immediate surgical consultation, with expectation of wide debridement and copious irrigation of all involved areas.

Discharge instructions for all patients with hand injuries should include elevation of the extremity and the use of ice for the initial 24 to 48 hours. Instructions regarding signs of infection, the timing of return visits for complications, wound checks, and suture removal are mandatory. Patients with injuries that are splinted should also receive instructions regarding splint care and problems that should prompt an immediate return to the emergency department. Appropriate and timely followup arrangements should be provided for all patients treated in the emergency department.

COMMON PITFALLS

✔ Failure to provide adequate analgesia and sedation for patients requiring fracture or joint reduction

✔ Failure to appreciate and correct rotational deformity in metacarpal and phalangeal fractures
✔ Failure to appreciate CMC dislocation on standard hand films due to overlapping densities
✔ Failure to appreciate the extent of a PIP joint injury, which may lead to a Boutonniere deformity
✔ Failure to appreciate the extent of a DIP injury, which may lead to a Swan-neck deformity
✔ Failure to recognize a partial tendon laceration due to inadequate wound exploration
✔ Failure to identify a foreign body in a wound as a result of inadequate exploration or omission of a radiograph
✔ Failure to appreciate the significance of a high-pressure injection injury. The patient may have felt only a transient stinging sensation, and the entrance wound may be minuscule or absent

Acknowledgments

Thanks to the previous edition's chapter authors Carl R. Chudnofsky, William H. Shoff, and Paul Blackburn.

References

1. Bowman SH, Simon RR. Metacarpal and phalangeal fractures. *Emerg Med Clin North Am* 1993;11:671.
2. Clark DP, Scott RN, Anderson IW. Hand problems in an accident and emergency department. *J Hand Surg [Br]* 1985;10:297.
3. Harris JHJ, Harris WH. *The radiology of emergency medicine*, 4th ed. Philadelphia: Lippincott Williams & Wilkins, 2000:655.
4. Harrison BP, Hilliard MW. Emergency department evaluation and treatment of hand injuries. *Emerg Med Clin North Am* 1999;17:793.
5. Henry M. Fractures and dislocations in the hand. In: Bucholz RA, Heckman JD. eds. *Rockwood and Green's fractures in adults*, 5th ed. Philadelphia: Lippincott Williams & Wilkins, 2001:441.
6. Jarvik JG, Dalinka MK, Kneeland JB. Hand injuries in adults. *Semin Roentgenol* 1991;26:282.
7. Kahler DM, McCue F. Metacarpophalangeal and proximal interphalangeal joint injuries of the hand, including the thumb. *Clin Sports Med* 1992;11:57.
8. Lammers RL. Soft tissue foreign bodies. *Ann Emerg Med* 1988;17:1336.
9. Lee SJ, Montgomery K. Athletic hand injuries. *Ortho Clin North Am* 2002;33:547.
10. Mason ML, Queen FB. Grease gun injuries to the hand. *Q Bull Northwest Med School* 1941;15:122.
11. Mastey RD, Weiss AC, Akelman E. Primary care of hand and wrist athletic injuries. *Clin in Sports Med* 1997;16:705.
12. Melone CJ, Isani A. Anesthesia for hand injuries. *Emerg Med Clin North Am* 1985;3:235.
13. Overton DT, Uehara DT. Evaluation of the injured hand. *Emerg Med Clin North Am* 1993;11:585.
14. Proust AF. Special injuries of the hand. *Emerg Med Clin North Am* 1993;11:767.
15. Redmon HA. Acute hand injuries: emergency room management. *J Fla Med Assoc* 1989;76:633.
16. Schnall SB, Mirzayan R. High-pressure injection injuries to the hand. *Hand Clin* 1999;15:245.
17. Seaberg DC, Angelos WJ, Paris PM. Treatment of subungual hematomas with nail trephination: a prospective study. *Am J Emerg Med* 1991;9:209.
18. Sirio CA, Smith JS, Graham WP. High-pressure injection injuries of the hand. *Am Surg* 1989;55:714.
19. Sloan EP. Nerve injuries in the hand. *Emerg Med Clin North Am* 1993;11:651.
20. Stark HH, Ashworth CR, Boyle JH. Paint-gun injuries of the hand. *J Bone Joint Surg Am* 1967;49:637.
21. Street JM. Radiographs of phalangeal fractures: importance of the internally rotated oblique projection for diagnosis. *AJR* 1993;160:575.
22. Stern PJ. Fractures of the metacarpals and phalanges. In: Green DP, Hotchkiss RN, Pederson WC (eds.). *Green's operative hand surgery*, 4th ed. New York: Churchill Livingstone, 1999:711.

CHAPTER 193
Pelvic Fractures

Michael A. Gibbs and Carrie D. Tibbles

Pelvic fractures are a common and often life-threatening consequence of major trauma. A pelvic fracture suggests a significant force of injury, mandating a careful evaluation for multi-system involvement. Many of these patients are hemodynamically unstable and require aggressive volume resuscitation. Pelvic fractures are frequently complicated by injuries to the genitourinary tract, pelvic vessels, and abdominal viscera, and are also associated with chest and central nervous system injuries. Early resuscitation, stabilization of the pelvis, diagnosis of associated injuries, and appropriate specialty consultation are the priorities in the emergency department (ED) management of these complex injuries.

Motor vehicle crashes and auto-pedestrian trauma are responsible for 60% to 70% of pelvic fractures. Falls from a height account for 10% to 20%, and the balance is made up of athletic and direct crush injuries (9,16). After traumatic brain injury and blunt aortic disruption, pelvic fractures are the third most common cause of death after motor vehicle collisions. The overall mortality associated with pelvic trauma can be as high as 20%, with disproportionate lethality in the elderly (1,19).

CLINICAL PRESENTATION

An understanding of both the anatomy of the pelvis and the mechanism of injury is necessary to manage patients with significant pelvic trauma. It is useful to visualize the pelvis as a ring with anterior and posterior components (Fig. 193.1). The posterior pelvic ring, which is critical for stability, is strengthened by several ligaments: the anterior and posterior sacroiliac ligaments, sacrospinous ligament, and sacrotuberous ligament (Figs. 193.2A,B). Disruption of this powerful ligamentous complex is a marker of tremendous energy transfer. In addition, major blood vessels traversing the posterior pelvic ring are directly vulnerable when fractures occur here. Anteriorly the pubic symphysis acts as a strut. Disruption of the symphysis alone does not lead to instability, provided that the posterior ligamentous structures remain intact.

Several different pelvic fracture classification systems have been developed. The most widely used is based on the direction of force causing the injury (5,31). Three force vectors are described: *lateral compression, anteroposterior (AP) compression,* and *vertical shear.* "Complex patterns" describe injuries that are the result of more than one force vector. Each of these vectors breaks or dislocates the pelvic ring in a predictable pattern, and is associated with varying degrees of mechanical instability. In addition, each injury type has a different impact on pelvic volume. The associated blood loss can be predicted by the stability of the fracture and this effect on pelvic volume. Fractures that destabilize the pelvis and those that result in an increase in pelvic volume are associated with pelvic and retroperitoneal hemorrhage. Conversely, mechanically stable fractures and those that decrease pelvic volume or leave it unchanged are less likely to precipitate life-threatening bleeding. The objective of this classification scheme is to assess for pelvic stability using imaging studies (AP plain film, computed tomography) available during the early phase of resuscitation. Using this approach the emergency physician can identify patients at risk for hemorrhage and hemodynamic deterioration, predict associated injuries, formulate a comprehensive diagnostic plan, and communicate effectively with consultants.

Lateral Compression

Lateral compression fractures account for almost 50% of pelvic fractures. The force is delivered to the pelvis from the side. Lateral compression fractures are common after a "T-bone" motor vehicle collision or when a pedestrian is struck from the side. The affected hemipelvis is crushed *inward* (Fig. 193.3). Stability is usually maintained, and pelvic volume is *reduced.* For this reason lateral compression injuries are typically not associated with major pelvic hemorrhage, and morbidity is secondary to coincident blunt force trauma to the head and torso, rather than the pelvic fracture itself.

One type of fracture that results from lateral compression is the "stove-in," or *pelvic wing fracture* that was first described by Duverney in 1751 (Fig. 193.4). It may produce an unstable fragment off the iliac crest, but the load-bearing stability of the pelvic ring is not jeopardized.

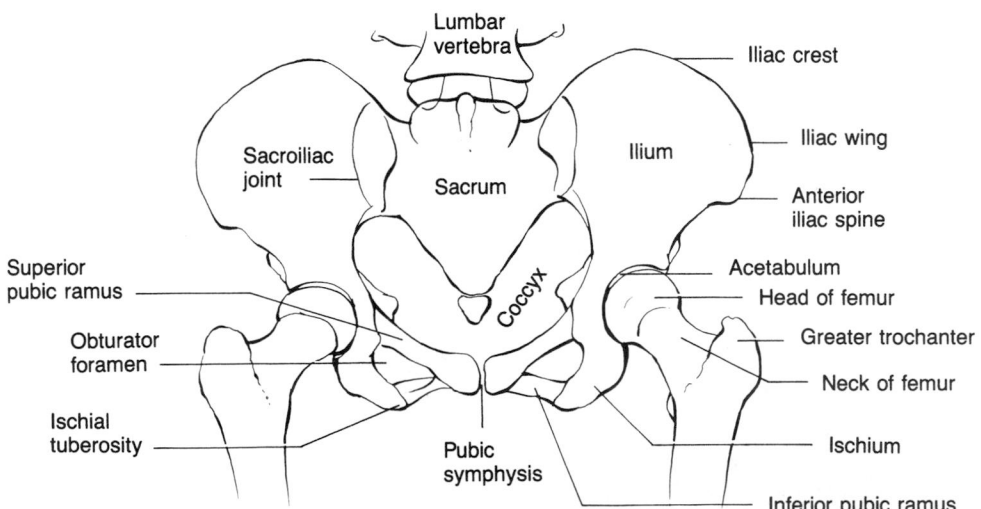

Figure 193.1.   The pelvis.

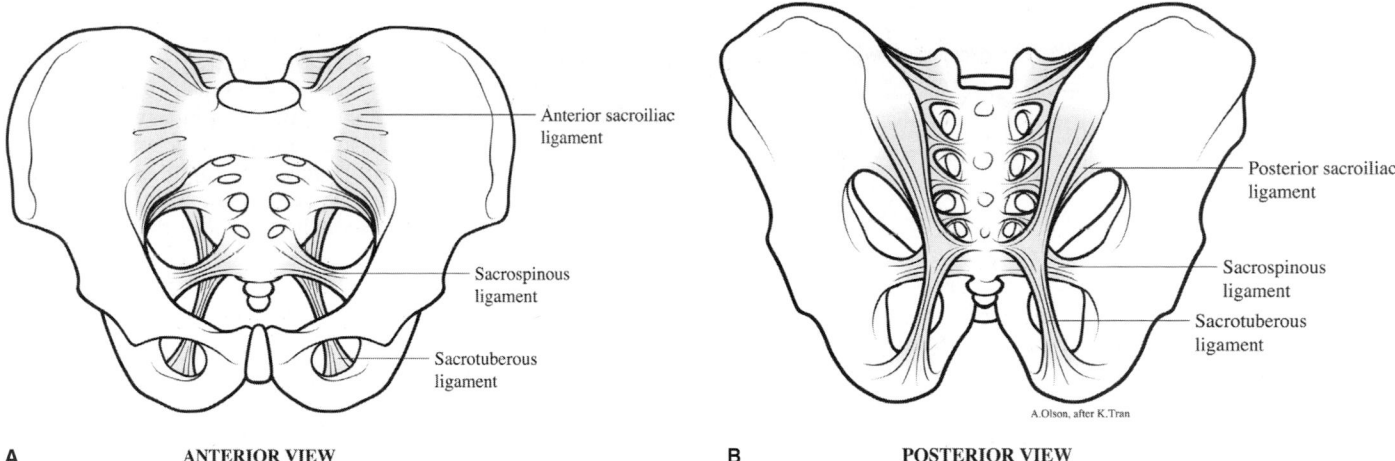

A   **ANTERIOR VIEW**   **B**   **POSTERIOR VIEW**

Figure 193.2.   Ligamentous support of the bony pelvis, **(A)** anterior, and **(B)** posterior views. The posterior pelvic ring is stabilized by several strong ligaments. Disruption in this region implies major energy transfer and the potential for significant multisystem injury.

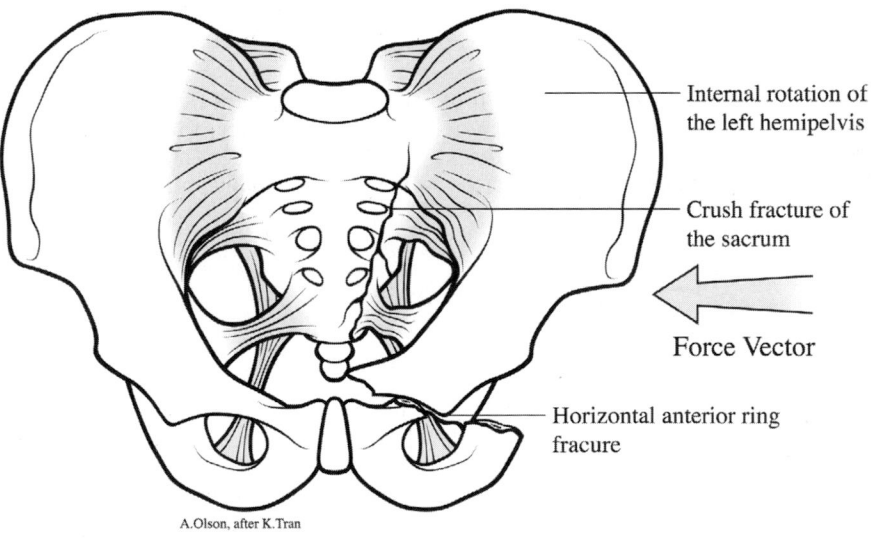

Figure 193.3.   Lateral compression injury. The causative force vector is delivered from the side, crushing the affected hemipelvis inward. Lateral compression injuries typically reduce pelvic volume. Instability is variable.

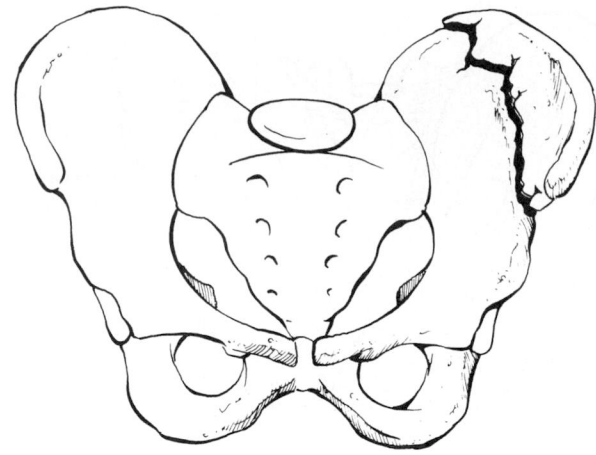

Figure 193.4.   Duverney fracture. Pelvic wing or "stove-in" fracture.

Anteroposterior Compression

Nearly one third of pelvic fractures are anteroposterior compression injuries. Anteroposterior compression fractures are seen following head-on motor vehicle crashes, or when a pedestrian is struck head-on by an oncoming vehicle. Forces may also be delivered in a posterioranterior direction. Both iliac wings are forced *outwards* (Fig. 193.5). AP compression injuries are unstable, and pelvic volume is *increased*. For these reasons, AP compression injuries are often associated with brisk pelvic and retroperitoneal hemorrhage. Coincident injuries of the thorax and abdomen are the rule.

Vertical Shear Fractures

Vertical shear injuries occur when a vertically oriented force is delivered to the pelvis via the extended femurs. These rare injuries are usually the result of a fall from a height or follow a head-on motor vehicle collision in which the occupant has the leg fully extended. Alternatively, vertical shear injuries can result from a downward force delivered to the pelvis via the spine, as may occur when a heavy object falls on the back or shoulders. Because one hemipelvis is driven up (or down) compared to the other (Fig. 193.6), these injuries produce major instability and pelvic volume is increased. The hemodynamic consequences are similar to those associated with AP compression injuries.

The Malgaigne fracture, first described in 1859, is characterized by anterior disruption of the pubic symphysis or 2 to 4 pubic rami fractures and ipsilateral sacroiliac joint disruption. Because of involvement of the posterior arch, these injuries can be complicated by significant neurologic and vascular injury. These patients are often hypotensive and the mortality rate approaches 20%.

Straddle Injuries

A straddle injury is an unstable injury characterized by bilateral double pubic rami fractures. Classically, this fracture is caused by falling while straddling a solid object between the legs. However, both lateral and anteroposterior compressive forces can cause straddle injuries as well. The lower genitourinary tract is particularly susceptible to injury by this mechanism. These are usually closed fractures. Patients will have perineal tenderness, ecchymosis, and gross hematuria; males may be unable to void. The incidence of hemorrhage and bowel injury is high.

Avulsion Fractures

These are among the most trivial of pelvic fractures and are often sustained by athletes who stress muscular or ligamentous insertions onto the bony pelvis (Fig. 193.7). Avulsions of the anterior superior iliac spine generally occur in adolescent hurdlers and long jumpers and reflect forceful contraction of the sartorius muscle or abdominal musculature transmitted to the iliac epiphysis. Less commonly, the anterior inferior iliac spine may be avulsed by intense contraction of the straight head of the rectus femoris muscle; this injury may occur in athletes playing sports that involve kicking (e.g., soccer and rugby). Avulsion fractures of the ischial tuberosity are even less common. This injury usually results from strenuous stretching of the pelvic ring, as in hurdling or pole vaulting. Patients with avulsion fractures generally present with a characteristic history and local tenderness. In isolated trauma, there are usually no associated complaints or injuries. These are stable fractures because the integrity of the pelvic ring remains intact.

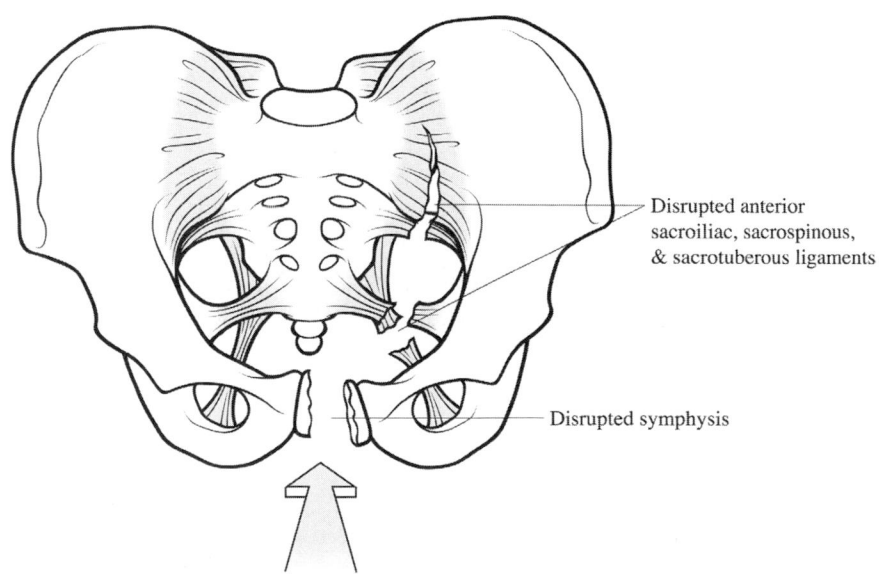

Disrupted anterior sacroiliac, sacrospinous, & sacrotuberous ligaments

Disrupted symphysis

Force Vector

Figure 193.5.   AP compression injury. The causative force vector is delivered from the front (or back), causing the pelvic ring to 'open like a book.' These injuries are mechanically unstable, and associated with increases in pelvic volume.

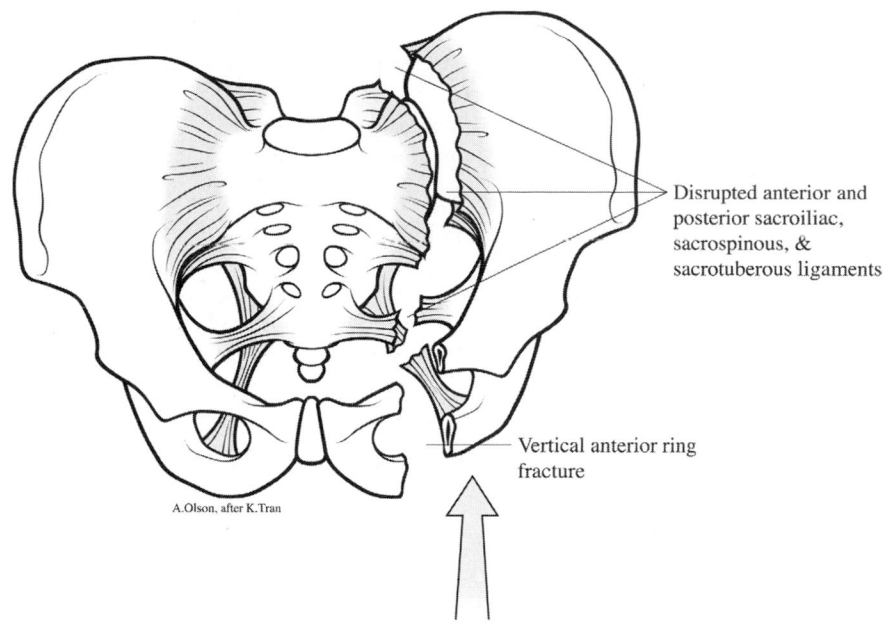

Disrupted anterior and posterior sacroiliac, sacrospinous, & sacrotuberous ligaments

Vertical anterior ring fracture

A.Olson, after K.Tran

Force Vector

Figure 193.6. Vertical shear injury. The causative force is transmitted up the ipsilateral femur, driving the affected hemipelvis upwards. Vertical shear injuries are extremely unstable and associated with increases in pelvic volume.

Other Types of Pelvic Fractures

Patients who *fall from a standing height* frequently present with pelvic pain localized to the bony prominences. Areas such as the iliac spine, ischial tuberosities, superior pubic rami, and coccyx are particularly susceptible to direct trauma. These fractures are stable injuries and are particularly common in elderly osteopenic patients. Presentation involves localized pain, swelling, and ecchymosis. There are usually no associated injuries.

Sacral fractures are defined by the orientation of the fracture line and occur in transverse upper, transverse lower, and vertical planes. Upper sacral fractures are frequently difficult to recognize both radiographically and clinically, often presenting only as buttock and perianal pain. These fractures may injure sacral nerve roots, resulting in decreased anal sphincter tone and loss of perineal sensation. Lower sacral fractures are equally painful but are rarely complicated by neurologic injury. A careful physical exam to exclude rectal tears is important. Vertical sacral fractures occur as a result of vertical shear injury.

Associated Injuries

Significant force is required to disrupt the pelvic ring. Consequently, associated injuries, both to adjacent viscera as well as organs distant to the pelvis, are common following major pelvic trauma. In one series of 348 patients with pelvic fractures, only 32 patients (9%) had injury isolated to the pelvic ring (33). Fox et al reviewed over one thousand pelvic fractures and found associated neurologic injury in 27% of patients, thoracic injury in 26%, and abdominal injury in 14% (14). Specific injuries can be anticipated based on the mechanism of injury and the fracture type.

Thoracic aortic injury is associated with pelvic fractures and dislocations. Patients with AP compression fractures are particularly vulnerable. Aortic injuries are eight times more frequent in patients with AP compression fractures as compared to the total blunt trauma population (9).

Approximately one-fourth of pelvic fractures are complicated by injuries to the urethra and/or bladder (30). Additionally, over 95% of patients with an injury to the posterior urethra and 70% to 95% of patients with a bladder injury following blunt trauma have a pelvic fracture (6). Bladder injury is usually the result of perforation by fracture fragments, and is especially likely in patients with symphyseal diastasis and with multiple pubic rami fractures. The posterior urethra is also prone to injury following anterior pelvic fractures because it is firmly attached to the pubis by the puboprostatic ligament.

Injuries to the vagina are a rare but important complication of pelvic trauma (27). While seldom life-threatening, these injuries can be associated with severe morbidity if they are not recognized and managed appropriately. Vaginal and rectal lacerations tend to coexist, and the presence of one should prompt a search for the other. Pelvic fractures associated with vaginal and/or rectal lacerations are considered open and should be treated accordingly.

Upper sacral fractures, vertical shear fractures, fractures of the sciatic notch, and sacroiliac joint injuries are frequently complicated by injuries to the lumbosacral plexus. The overall incidence of neurologic injury in patients with pelvic fractures is reported to be 10% to 21% (34) and is as high as 50% in fractures with posterior disruption. Such patients may present with distal motor weakness (impaired dorsiflexion or plantar flexion of the great

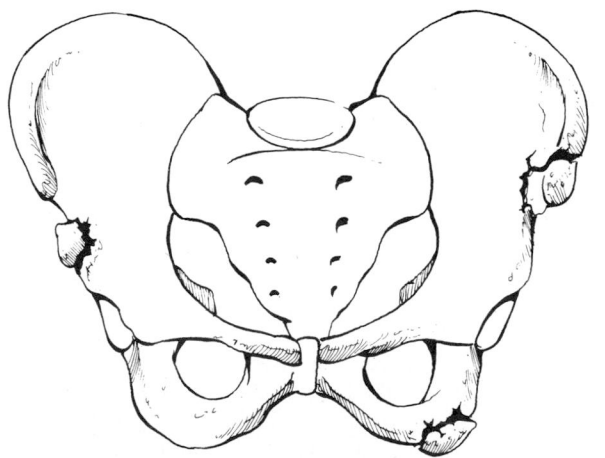

Figure 193.7. Fractures due to stress on muscular or ligamentous insertions onto the bony pelvis.

toe), numbness on the dorsal and lateral aspect of the foot, a diminished Achilles tendon reflex, or evidence of cauda equina syndrome, including perianal anesthesia and loss of sphincter tone.

Open pelvic fractures are defined as a fracture with direct communication with a vaginal, rectal, or skin wound. These fractures are invariably associated with severe injuries of the pelvic viscera. Early mortality is attributed to severe blood loss or associated chest or intracranial injuries, and historically may be as high as 30% to 50% (4). Following the initial resuscitation phase, heavy contamination of perineal wounds resulting from damage of the rectum and genitourinary tract increases the risk of delayed complications, including abscess formation, sepsis, and multiorgan failure.

EMERGENCY DEPARTMENT EVALUATION

Physical Examination

During the initial resuscitation of the severely injured trauma patient, the priorities are to rapidly identify immediately life-threatening injuries and to begin hemodynamic stabilization. In the patient with a pelvic fracture, hypotension is an ominous sign and a search for the cause should be rapidly initiated. Following these critical first steps, the physician can perform a systematic examination of the pelvis.

The objectives of the examination of the pelvis are to estimate the likelihood of a pelvic fracture and to identify any complications and associated injuries. The physician should systematically inspect and palpate the front and back of the pelvis noting any abrasions, contusions, lacerations, tenderness, or crepitance. In a patient that is awake, inability to actively flex the hip is predictive of a pelvic fracture, with a sensitivity of 90% and a specificity of 95% (18). While the identification of an unstable pelvic ring is important, overzealous 'rocking' of the disrupted pelvis may cause additional retroperitoneal bleeding. Instead, it is preferable to apply gentle steady downward and lateral pressure on the iliac wings to detect or exclude tenderness. If tenderness is present appropriate imaging should follow. In the obtunded blunt trauma patient imaging should be performed.

Signs of urethral injury include blood at the urethral meatus, penile or scrotal hematoma and an abnormal prostate examination. Patients with these findings should have a urethrogram *before* insertion of a Foley catheter to avoid worsening of an incomplete urethral tear. Female patients should have a careful bimanual and speculum examination. Perineal lacerations may have associated intravaginal mucosal tears. Bleeding is the hallmark of vaginal trauma, although it may not be immediately apparent because of muscle spasm. Vaginal injury should also be suspected if hematuria is present or it is difficult to pass a Foley catheter. While it is important to evaluate associated gynecologic and urologic complications following pelvic trauma, these injuries are not immediately life-threatening. Urgent laparotomy or angiography should not be delayed by the evaluation of the genitourinary system in the unstable patient.

The lumbosacral plexus is prone to injury in pelvic fractures and a neurologic examination of the lower extremity should be performed, with particular attention to the L5 and S1 nerve roots. In the patient that is awake, motor function of the L5 nerve root is tested by assessing dorsiflexion of the great toe against resistance, and the S1 nerve root is tested by having the patient plantar flex the great toe. L5 supplies sensation to the dorsum of the foot and S1 to the lateral aspect of the foot. The Achilles tendon reflex, perianal sensation and sphincter tone should also be assessed.

Diagnostic Imaging

During the early resuscitation of the blunt trauma patient, the identification of a pelvic fracture on x-ray has important implications for management. It is a marker for serious multisystem injury, reflecting a major force vector at the time of injury. It provides clues to the likelihood of pelvic soft tissue and vascular injuries and rapidly identifies a potential source of blood loss in the hypotensive patient. Finally, it may alter the method or sequence of further diagnostic testing, helping the clinician formulate a management plan.

Traditionally, routine pelvic radiography has been recommended in all patients following blunt trauma. While an effective strategy to exclude injury, this results in a large number of negative radiographs. The severely injured blunt trauma patient who is either hemodynamically unstable, obtunded, or who has clinical evidence of abdominopelvic injury requires pelvic imaging. For the rest of the less severely injured patients, there is a growing body of literature suggesting that a thorough physical examination can be used to identify the patient at low risk for pelvic fracture who can be managed safely without radiography. In a study of 717 blunt trauma patients, no pelvic fractures were diagnosed in 125 patients who were hemodynamically stable, alert, and without pelvic pain or tenderness, gross hematuria, or the presence of a femur fracture (24). Yugeeros et al prospectively studied 608 blunt trauma patients and demonstrated a negative predictive value of 99% for a normal physical examination (37). In another series, only 3 of 810 (0.4%) alert, asymptomatic blunt trauma patients had pelvic fractures. Each of these injuries was minor and did not affect the clinical course (36). In a recent prospective trial of 2,176 alert blunt trauma patients, Gonzalez et al demonstrated that the physical examination was 93% sensitive for detecting pelvic fractures and 100% sensitive for detecting those requiring operative repair (15). These data support a selective approach to pelvic radiography.

Once the decision to image the pelvis is made, this typically proceeds with either plain-film radiographs, computed tomography (CT), or both. This decision should be influenced by the patient's clinical stability, anticipated treatment priorities, and practice setting. As a general rule, the unstable blunt trauma patient being prepared for urgent transfer should have imaging restricted to a single AP view of the pelvis. Resuscitation should not be delayed or interrupted to obtain additional plain films or CT, especially when there is an indication for immediate laparotomy or pelvic angiography. Additional images are justifiable in stable patients and in those for whom computed tomography is already planned.

Plain Radiographs

A single AP radiograph will identify the large majority of pelvic fractures and provides sufficient information to guide early management. The film should visualize the iliac crests, each hip joint, the fifth lumbar vertebrae and the proximal portion of each femur. Important landmarks include the pubic symphysis, superior and inferior rami, anterior-superior, and anterior-inferior iliac spines, sacroiliac joints, sacral ala, sacral foramen, and L5 transverse processes. The AP radiograph provides specific clues that will help identify the various injury patterns and fractures described in the previous section.

Inlet and outlet views are helpful for identifying certain sacral fractures and SI joint disruption. To obtain the inlet view the x-ray beam is directed from the head to the midpelvis at an angle of 35 to 40 degrees. The resultant projection is perpendicular to the pelvic brim and demonstrates a view of the entire pelvic rim, and is useful for demonstrating anterior and posterior displacement.

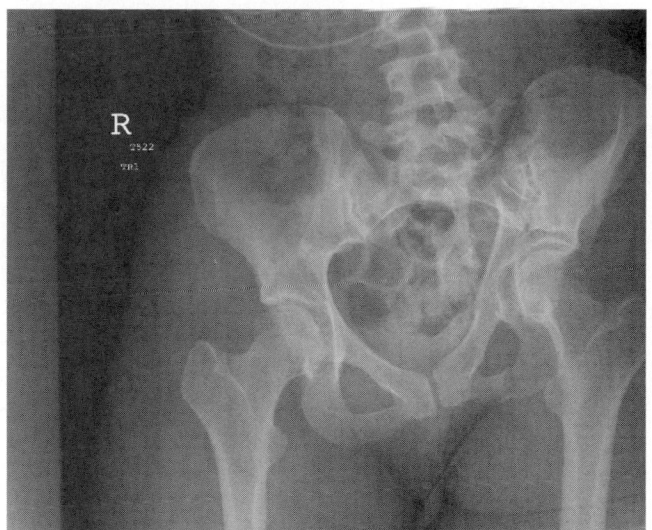

Figure 193.8. AP plain film of a severe lateral compression injury. The left hemipelvis is crushed inwards.

The outlet view is obtained with the beam perpendicular to the sacrum, directed cephalad from the foot to the symphysis at an angle of 30 to 40 degrees. This view demonstrates sacral fractures and sacroiliac joint disruption.

Lateral Compression Fracture

Compressive forces directed laterally to the pelvis cause inward movement of the ipsilateral hemipelvis, hinging on the sacroiliac joint (Figs. 193.8 and 193.9). Essential radiographic features of lateral compression fractures include *horizontal* pubic rami fractures. These fractures are visible 80% of time on the AP view, and this feature alone is highly suggestive of lateral compression injury. Crush fractures of the sacrum are seen in 88% of cases. This may only be visible as a disruption of the arcuate lines. The combination of a crush fracture of the sacrum and a horizontal pubic ramus fracture is diagnostic for a lateral compression injury. Fractures of the acetabulum or hip dislocations can also

be seen. Sacroiliac joint diastasis in combination with any of the other findings also suggests a lateral compression injury.

AP Compression Fracture

An anterior compressive force causes rupture of the symphyseal ligament and diastasis of the anterior pelvic ring. The posterior ligaments will tolerate up to 2.5 cm of symphyseal diastasis. Progressive widening of the symphysis beyond this point results in disruption of the anterior sacroiliac and sacrospinous ligaments, and is commonly referred to as an *"open book"* pelvic fracture. Severe trauma will disrupt the posterior sacroiliac ligaments as well (Figs. 193.10 and 193.11). In these circumstances, the sacroiliac joint is widely displaced on x-ray.

Radiographs of anterior compression injuries will demonstrate vertically oriented pubic rami fractures, symphyseal diastasis, or both, and a variable degree of sacroiliac joint disruption. An acetabular fracture is seen in up to one-half of patients.

Vertical Shear Fractures

Vertical shear fractures are associated with disruption of both the anterior and posterior ring. These mechanically unstable injuries result from a severe vertical force delivered over one or both sides of the pelvis lateral to the midline. Asymmetry of the hip joints in the vertical plane is a useful clue to vertical migration of one hemipelvis relative to the other (Fig. 193.12). The outlet view is used to evaluate the extent of superior displacement of the fracture fragments. Radiographs of a vertical shear fracture demonstrate severe posterior disruption; this appears as either complete sacroiliac joint disruption, a vertical sacral

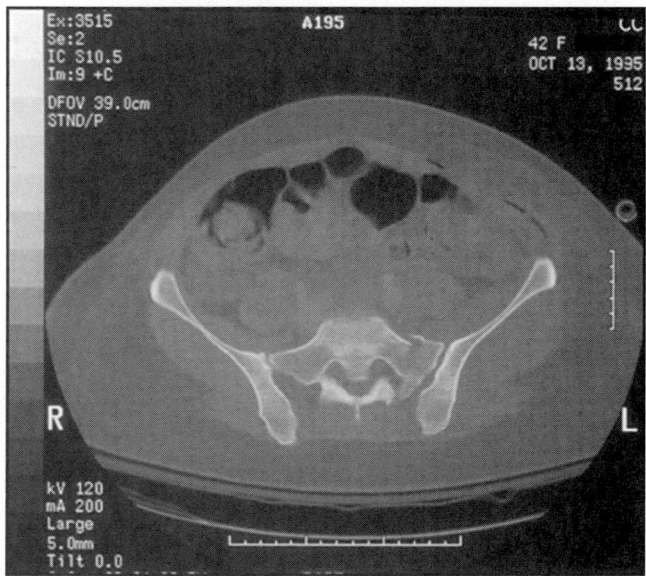

Figure 193.9. CT scan of a left lateral compression injury with a crush fracture of the affected sacrum.

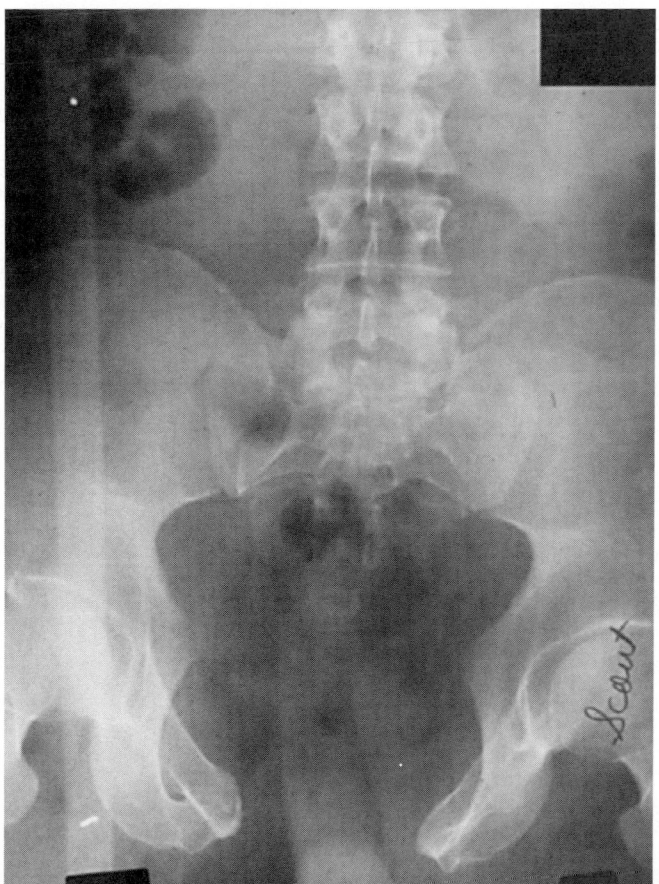

Figure 193.10. AP plain film of a severe AP compression injury with symphysis diastasis and left posterior sacroiliac joint disruption.

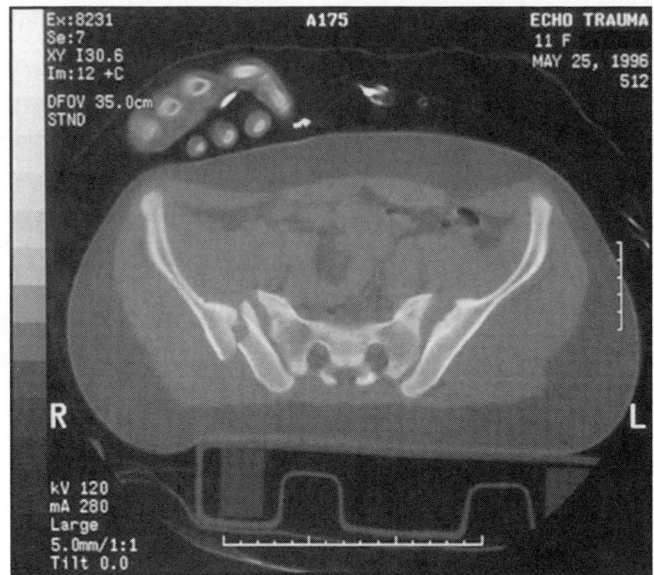

Figure 193.11. CT scan of an AP compression injury with major disruption of the posterior pelvic ring.

fracture, or a medial iliac wing fracture, with associated symphyseal disruption or pubic rami fractures.

Acetabular Fractures

A significant number of patients with pelvic ring injuries also have acetabular fractures. Acetabular fractures can be easily missed on the AP film. Judet oblique views can be used to supplement the AP radiograph if an acetabular fracture is suspected (21). CT images are preferred, however, as they provide superior fracture definition and give important preoperative information to the orthopedist.

Computed Tomography

The use of computed tomography has revolutionized the assessment of injured patients, and pelvic trauma is no exception. When compared to plain films, CT has a higher sensitivity for the detection of fracture in both adults and children. Other

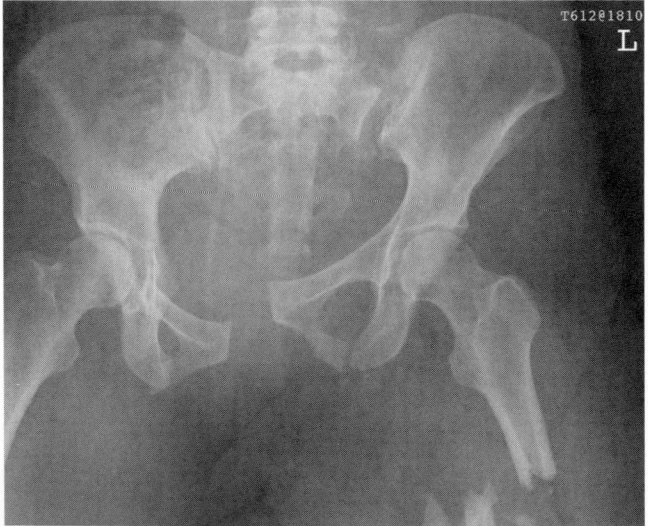

Figure 193.12. AP plain film of vertical shear injury with symphysis diastasis and upward-migration of the left hemipelvis.

advantages include a more accurate assessment of pelvic instability, the ability to provide reconstructed three-dimensional images, and visualization of adjacent pelvic and abdominal viscera. In addition, contrast extravasation seen on abdominopelvic CT accurately predicts the need for therapeutic angiography (32). Computed tomography plays an important role in planning operative management of pelvic fractures and is performed in most patients with significant or unstable pelvic fractures identified by plain radiographs.

EMERGENCY DEPARTMENT MANAGEMENT

During the initial resuscitation of the patient with significant pelvic injury, the physician should *anticipate* hypotension and initiate early aggressive resuscitation. Adequate intravenous access and careful monitoring are crucial. A blood sample should be sent for a crossmatch for type-specific blood. Hemoglobin, serum lactate (26) and the base deficit (10) are also used to guide resuscitation. The critically ill patient requires vigorous resuscitation with warmed crystalloid and early transfusion, as well as precautions to prevent hypothermia.

Pelvic Stabilization

Vascular injuries and substantial blood loss often complicate displaced pelvic fractures. Mechanically unstable injuries and those that increase pelvic volume create a potential space for ongoing hemorrhage. Pelvic stabilization can tamponade venous bleeding and reduce pelvic volume, as well as stabilize displaced fracture segments. This can be accomplished by several simple measures in the ED. Wrapping a sheet tightly around the pelvis will close the pelvic ring to some degree. The use of a pneumatic antishock garment (PASG) is especially well-suited for the prehospital setting and may be applied before interfacility transport (7). This device should be considered a temporizing measure, as prolonged use of the PASG has been reported to cause lower extremity compartment syndrome (3). Several vacuum-splints that envelope the patient and compress the pelvis are also available, although controlled trials using these devices are limited.

The role of external fixation in the ED remains controversial. Proponents argue that external fixation reduces transfusion requirements (13) and improves survival (35). Opponents point out that the application of an external fixator expends valuable time, requires expertise not usually available, and offers little advantage over the less invasive techniques described above. When transfer to a regional trauma center is imminent, time should not be wasted waiting for an orthopaedic surgeon to apply a fixator. Instead, a temporary device should be applied and transport should proceed without delay. In the setting of a tertiary trauma center, the use of external fixation can be individualized.

Therapeutic Angiography

In the blunt trauma patient with pelvic trauma, venous bleeding accounts for the majority of bleeding in the pelvis. Pelvic stabilization will slow the venous bleeding in most cases. Conversely, injury to pelvic arteries results in brisk hemorrhage which is not controlled by pelvic stabilization alone. Arterial injury is found in up to 20% of patients with AP compression and vertical shear injuries, but is uncommon in lateral compression injury (29). The most commonly injured vessels include the superior gluteal, internal pudendal, obturator, and lateral sacral arteries (23). In the presence of arterial injury, vascular embolization is effective in 86% to 100% of cases and improves outcome (2,17). Early mobilization of the angiography team is essential, as the time to embolization impacts survival.

Management Priorities in the Unstable Patient

During the initial assessment of the unstable patient with pelvic trauma, it is essential to quickly identify the predominant site of hemorrhage. Immediate angiography and pelvic stabilization is indicated if pelvic bleeding poses the primary life-threat. An exploratory laparotomy should be performed first, however, if there is evidence of intraabdominal hemorrhage. Two important steps can help the emergency physician make the right decision: (1) the rapid detection or exclusion of hemoperitoneum, and (2) classification of the pelvic fracture as 'stable' or 'unstable.'

In the unstable blunt trauma patient, the presence of hemoperitoneum points to the abdomen as the primary source of hemorrhage. This determination can be made within minutes at the bedside using either diagnostic peritoneal lavage (DPL) or ultrasound (US). DPL is used in this situation to detect significant abdominal hemorrhage, not the mere presence of blood in the abdomen. Therefore, the DPL *aspirate* should be used to guide decision-making as the results of the DPL cell count can be misleading in patients with pelvic fractures, and the results are slow to return (20). The aspiration of 10 cc of gross blood is indicative of life-threatening abdominal hemorrhage. In patients with pelvic fractures, the open supraumbilical technique is preferred and has higher specificity (8). Bedside ultrasound is an alternative to DPL. In experienced hands, US has a high sensitivity for hemoperitoneum and can be performed within minutes during the secondary survey (11,25). It should be recognized that US cannot discern blood from other sources of fluid, and that uroperitoneum resulting from bladder rupture may precipitate a false-positive study (22).

Pelvic fracture patterns can also be used to predict the most important source of bleeding in the unstable patient. Eastridge et al recently described the injury patterns in 231 hypotensive patients with pelvic trauma. In persistently hypotensive patients with 'stable' fractures (i.e., lateral compression and AP compression injuries with minor displacement), abdominal hemorrhage was the culprit in 85% of cases. Conversely, in patients with 'unstable' fracture patterns (i.e., lateral compression and AP compression injuries with major displacement and all vertical shear injuries), hemorrhage was predominantly from a pelvic source, and pelvic angiography was positive in 59% of cases (12).

CRITICAL INTERVENTIONS

- Aggressively resuscitate with crystalloid and early blood transfusion
- Rapidly detect or exclude hemoperitoneum at the bedside using DPL or ultrasonography
- Evaluate for associated visceral injuries (torso, genitourinary, and neurologic)
- Immobilize fractures that open the pelvic ring using a wrapped sheet or PASG
- Initiate timely transfer to a Level I Trauma Center

DISPOSITION

Patients with complex pelvic fractures require the resources of a Level I trauma center. Rapid transport to a hospital capable of handling such injuries is essential, as these patients may deteriorate quickly. Preparation of the pelvic fracture patient for interfacility transport includes appropriate clinical stabilization, temporary pelvic stabilization, and communication with the accepting physician.

A small minority of patients with pelvic fractures can be discharged from the ED and managed as outpatients. The mechanism of injury, the age and social supports of the patient should be factored into this decision. An example of this might be an isolated pubic ramus fracture in an otherwise healthy person. Consultating with an orthopaedic surgeon, careful discharge instructions, close outpatient follow up are essential.

COMMON PITFALLS

✔ Failure to recognize that pelvic trauma can be a cause of life-threatening hemorrhage
✔ Failure to order an anteroposterior pelvic radiograph in all unconscious blunt trauma patients
✔ Failure to diagnose associated intraperitoneal, retroperitoneal, and neurovascular injuries
✔ Delaying transfer to a Level 1 Trauma Center

Acknowledgments

Thanks to the previous edition's chapter authors Paula S. Wadbrook and Charles V. Pollack, Jr.

References

1. Adams JE, Davis GG, Alexander CB, et al. Pelvic trauma in rapidly fatal motor vehicle accidents. *J Orthopaedic Trauma* 2003;17:406.
2. Agolini SF, Shah K, Jaffe J. Arterial embolization is a rapid and effective technique for controlling pelvic fracture hemorrhage. *J Trauma* 1997;43:395.
3. Aprahamian C, Gessert G, Bandyk DF, et al. MAST-associated compartment syndrome (MACS): A review. *J Trauma* 1989;29:549.
4. Birolini D, Steinman E, Utiyama EM, et al. Open pelvicoperineal trauma. *J Trauma* 1990;30:492.
5. Bucholz RW. Pathomechanics of pelvic ring disruptions. *Adv Orthop Surg* 1987;10:167.
6. Cass AS, Ireland GW. Bladder trauma associated with pelvic fractures in severely injured patients. *J Trauma* 1973;13:205.
7. Clarke G, Mardel S. Use of MAST to control massive bleeding from pelvic injuries. *Injury* 1993;24:628.
8. Cochran W, Sobat WS. Open versus closed diagnostic peritoneal lavage: A multiphasic prospective randomized comparison. *Ann Surg* 1984;200:24.
9. Dalal SA, Burgess AR. Pelvic fracture in multiple trauma: Classification by mechanism is key to pattern of organ injury, resuscitative requirements, and outcome. *J Trauma* 1988;29:981.
10. Davis JW, Mackersie RC, Holbrook TL, et al. Base deficit as an indicator of significant abdominal injury. *Ann Emerg Med* 1991;20:842.
11. Dolich MO. 2,576 ultrasounds for blunt abdominal trauma. *J Trauma* 2001; 50:108.
12. Eastridge BJ, Starr A, Minei JP, et al. The importance of fracture pattern in guiding therapeutic decision-making in patients with hemorrhagic shock and pelvic ring disruptions. *J Trauma* 2002;53:446.
13. Edwards CC, Meier PJ, Browner BD, et al. Results treating 50 unstable pelvic injuries using primary external fixation. *Orthop Trans* 1985;9:434.
14. Fox MA, Mangiante EC, Fabian TC, et al. Pelvic fractures: An analysis of factors affecting pre-hospital triage and patient outcome. *South Med J* 1990;83:785.
15. Gonzalez RP, Fried PQ, Bukhalo. PQ, The utility of clinical examination in screening for pelvic fractures in blunt trauma. *J Am Coll Surg* 2002;194:121.
16. Gustavo Parreira J, Coimbra R, Rasslan S, et al. The role of associated injuries on outcome of blunt trauma patients sustaining pelvic fractures. *Injury* 2000;31:677.
17. Hagiwara A, Minakawa K, Fukushima H, et al. Predictors of death in patients with life-threatening hemorrhage after successful transcatheter arterial embolization *J Trauma* 55:696–703, 2003.
18. Ham SJ, van Walsum AD, Vierhout PA. Predictive value of the hip flexion test for fractures of the pelvis. *Injury* 1996;27:543.
19. Henry SM, Pollak AN, Jones AL, et al. Pelvic fracture in geriatric patients: a distinct clinical entity. *J Trauma* 2002;53:15.
20. Hubbard SG, Bivins BA, Sachatello CR, et al. Diagnostic errors with peritoneal lavage in patients with pelvic fractures. *Arch Surg* 1979;114:844.
21. Hunter JC, Brandser EA, Tran KA. Pelvic and acetabular trauma. *Radiol Clin North Am* 1997;35:559.
22. Jones AE, Mason P, Tayal VT, et al. Uroperitoneum presenting as a positive FAST in a patient with bladder rupture. *Am J Emerg Med* 2003;25:373.
23. Kam J, Jackson H, Ben-Menachem Y. Vascular injuries associated with blunt pelvic trauma. *Radiol Clin North Am* 1981;19:171.
24. Koury HI, Peschiera JL, Welling RE. Selective use of pelvic roentgenograms in blunt trauma patients. *J Trauma* 1993;34:236.
25. Ma OJ. Operative versus nonoperative management of blunt abdominal trauma: Role of ultrasound-measured intraperitoneal fluid levels. *Am J Emerg Med* 2001;19:284.
26. Mizock BA, Falk JL. Lactic acidosis in critical illness. *Crit Care Med* 1992;20:80.
27. Niemi TA, Norton. Vaginal injuries in patients with pelvic fractures. *J Trauma* 1985;25:547.

28. Ochsner MG Jr., Hoffman AP, DiPasquale D, et al. Associated aortic rupture–pelvic fracture: An alert for orthopaedic and general surgeons. *J Trauma* 1993;33:429.

29. O'Neill PA, Riina J, Sclafani S, et al. Angiographic findings in pelvic fractures. *Clin Orthop* 1996;329:60.

30. Palmer JK, Benson GS, Corriere JN. Diagnosis and initial management of urologic injuries associated with 200 consecutive pelvic fractures. *J Urol* 1983;30:712.

31. Pennal GF, Tile M, Waddel JP, et al. Pelvic disruption: assessment and classification. *Clin Orthop Rel Res* 1980;151:12.

32. Pereira SJ, O'Brien DP, Luchette FA, et al. Dynamic helical computed tomography scan accurately detects hemorrhage in patients with pelvic fracture. *Surgery* 2000;1128:678.

33. Poole GV, Ward EF. Causes of mortality in patients with pelvic fractures. *Orthopaedics* 1994;17:691.

34. Reilly MC, Zinar DM, Matta JM. Neurologic injuries in pelvic ring fractures. *Clin Orthop* 1996;329:28.

35. Riemer BL, Butterfied SL, Diamond DL, et al. Acute mortality associated with injuries of the pelvic ring: The role of early patient mobilization and external fixation. *J Trauma* 1993;35:671.

36. Salvino CK, Esposito TJ, Smith D, et al. Routine pelvic X-ray in awake blunt trauma patients: A sensible policy? *J Trauma* 1992;33:413.

37. Yugueros P, Sarimiento JM, Garcia AF, et al. Unnecessary use of pelvic X-ray in blunt trauma. *J Trauma* 1995;39:722.

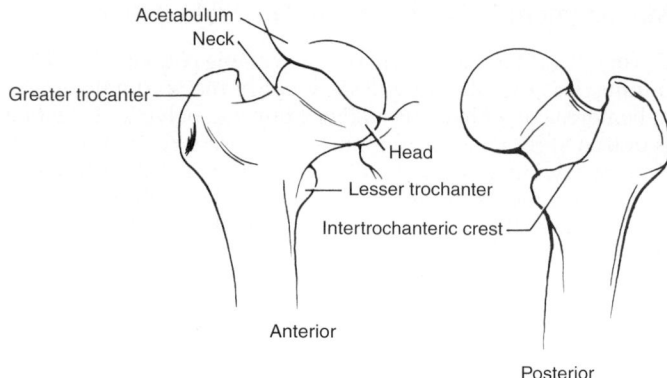

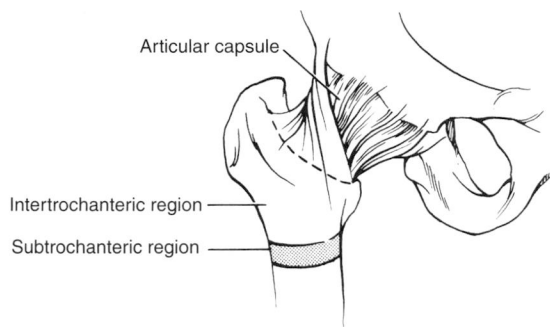

Figure 194.1. Anatomy of the hip. (**Top**) Anterior and posterior views of the femur. (**Bottom**) Division of the proximal femur.

CHAPTER 194
Hip and Femur Injuries

Norberto Adame, Jr., and Timothy Seay

Injuries to the hip are a major cause of morbidity and mortality, and the associated morbidity is becoming more important as the population ages. For the elderly, as many as 37% of hip fractures result in death within 1 year, and half of these deaths are thought to be directly due to the fracture (9). Causes of hip fractures are primarily pathologic (from osteopenia) and due to falls (primarily a disease of the elderly), whereas motor vehicle crashes account for the majority of dislocations (primarily a disease of the young). The frequency of traumatic hip dislocations and proximal fracture–dislocations of the femur has declined with the use of seatbelts. Although this decline is encouraging, early recognition of hip dislocations and proximal femur fractures will minimize the likelihood of developing avascular necrosis of the femoral head. In traumatic hip dislocations, the incidence of associated osteoarthritis is 26% (2,10,13). For avascular necrosis, the incidence ranges from 8% to 30%, depending on the degree of displacement (10). The incidence of these complications can be minimized by prompt diagnosis, evaluation, and definitive treatment in the emergency department (ED).

Anatomically, the hip is an articulation between the femoral head and the acetabulum, joined together by the ligamentum teres and the capsular ligament of the hip joint. It is a very stable articulation, requiring violent injury to dislocate. Primary sources of blood flow for the femoral head are the retinacular branches of the circumflex femoral artery. These enter the femur in the region of the femoral neck, and fractures proximal to their entry can result in disruption of blood flow and cause avascular necrosis of the femoral head. The other source of blood for the femoral head comes from the artery of the ligamentum teres. Often, this artery is absent or vestigial, and its loss is rarely of clinical significance.

In addition to the capsule, the hip joint is reinforced by the hip abductor muscles (gluteus medius and minimus, obturator, gamelli, and piriformis) attached to the greater trochanter and the hip flexor (iliopsoas), which is attached to the lesser trochanter (Fig. 194.1).

EMERGENCY DEPARTMENT EVALUATION

The initial radiographic studies in patients with suspected hip and femur injuries are the anteroposterior (AP) and lateral views. When analyzing the AP view of the hip, there are two important radiographic lines that help identify femur fractures and *slipped capital femoral epiphysis* (SCFE): the Klein and Shenton lines. The *Klein line* is a line drawn along the superior aspect of the femoral neck that projects through the superior portion of the femoral head (Fig. 194.2). The Klein line will project superior to a subtle fracture of the femoral head. More importantly, the Klein line will project superior to the epiphysis of a subtle case of SCFE. The *Shenton line* is a gentle arc seen on the AP view of the hip radiograph that overlies the inferior aspect of the femoral neck and extends to the curvature of the obturator foramen, along the inferior aspect of the pubic bone (Fig. 194.3). The Shenton line will have a step off or discontinuity in subtle cases of femoral neck and head fractures. It may also appear disrupted in the radiograph of a normal hip if it is not a true AP view.

EMERGENCY DEPARTMENT MANAGEMENT

Posterior Hip Dislocations

Posterior hip dislocations are the most common type of dislocation and result from force applied to a flexed knee and hip. When the knee hits the dashboard during a motor vehicle crash,

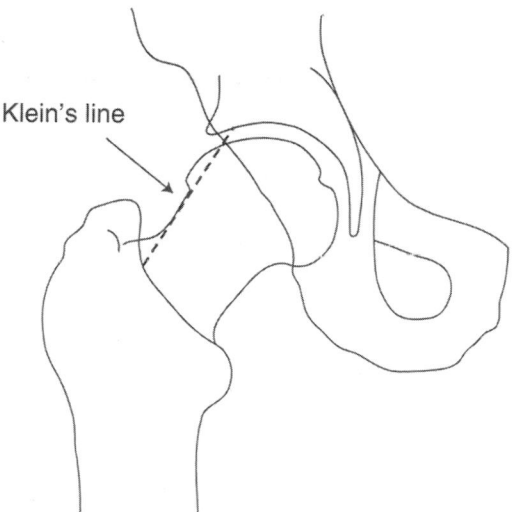

Figure 194.2. Klein's line. (From Gruber JE, Gibbs MA, Ferrara PC, et al. *Trauma management an emergency medicine approach.* St. Louis: Mosby, 2001:398 (Figure 26-3) with permission).

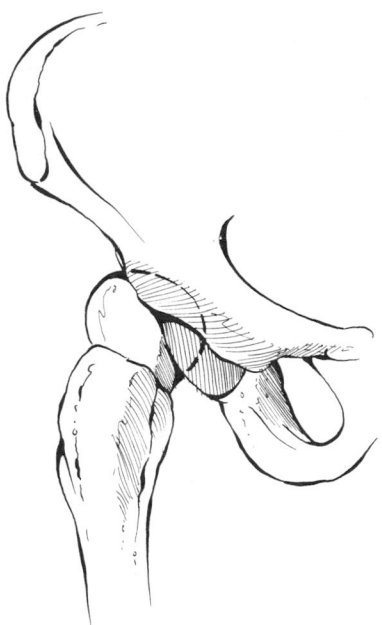

Figure 194.4. Posterior dislocation of the hip.

the hip is forcefully adducted and flexed while it is simultaneously pushed posteriorly. This is prevented by the use of a lap belt.

In posterior hip dislocations, the limb is flexed, adducted, and internally rotated, with limb shortening. If the patient is thin, the femoral head can often be palpated in the buttocks region (Figs. 194.4 and 194.5). Examination of the leg should ensure vascular function (rarely compromised) and include neurologic evaluation for possible sciatic nerve injury. The sciatic nerve lies posterior to the femoral head, separated from it by the capsule and by the obturator and gamelli muscles. Up to 50% have an associated acetabular or femoral head fracture (discussion follows).

Posterior dislocations optimally need reduction within 6 hours to minimize the risk for avascular necrosis (6,12). This should be attempted in the ED (Fig. 194.6). Adequate analgesia and muscle relaxation must be obtained by using a short-acting

narcotic (e.g., fentanyl) and a short-acting benzodiazepine (e.g., midazolam) with proper conscious sedation monitoring. The more recent short-acting anesthetics used for procedural sedation in the emergency department are etomidate and propofol. Both have a very fast onset and short recovery time. Etomidate is administered in doses of .1 to .3 mg/kg intravenously. One of the most common side effects is myoclonus which can be generalized thus making the reduction procedure difficult. Propofol has a rapid onset time of 30 to 60 seconds and patients recover in 5 to 15 minutes. Propofol is administered as an initial bolus of 1 mg/kg then titrated in doses of .5 mg/kg as needed. It has very good antiemetic qualities that help in the recovery phase (1,5). Further analgesia can be accomplished with a short-acting opiate such as fentanyl. The dose of fentanyl for procedure sedation is recommended at 1 to 2 µg/kg.

After the patient is adequately sedated, an assistant should apply pressure to the iliac crests, stabilizing the pelvis from lifting off the bed. While straddling the patient, the physician applies traction in line with the deformity and gently begins to flex the hip to 90 degrees. The hip is then rotated internally and externally with continued longitudinal traction. Successful reduction is often felt by a dull click. After reduction, the extremity should be placed in extension and neurovascular function of the extremity frequently reassessed. Postreduction radiographs should be obtained. General anesthesia is occasionally necessary if procedural sedation in the emergency department is unsuccessful. Orthopaedic consultation should be obtained for all patients with dislocations, and patients should be admitted to the hospital.

Anterior Hip Dislocations

Anterior hip dislocations occur most commonly from a direct blow to the abducted hip. A distally applied force causes the femoral head to tear through the anterior capsule. Anterior dislocations may be classified as *obturator, iliac,* and *pubic* (Fig. 194.7). *Obturator-type* hip dislocations occur when the hip is abducted and in flexion. The *pubic* and *iliac* types occur most commonly when the hip is abducted and in extension.

Careful neurovascular examination is mandatory, owing to the risk of arterial damage and venous thrombosis (11). *Anterior obturator* dislocations present as abduction, external rotation, and

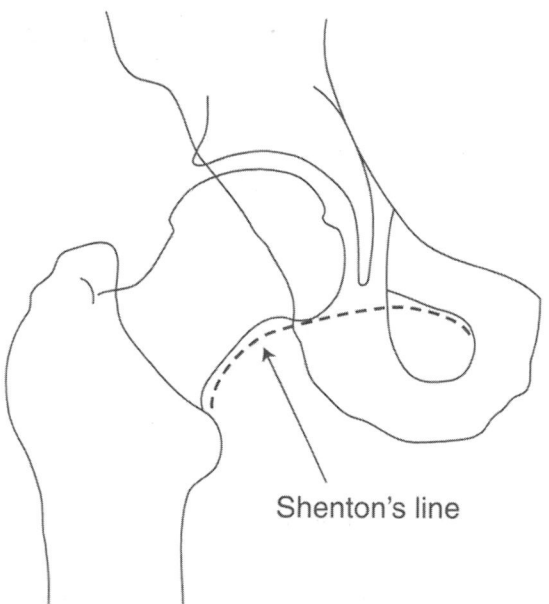

Figure 194.3. Shenton's line. (From Gruber JE, Gibbs MA, Ferrera PC, et al. *Trauma management an emergency medicine approach.* St. Louis: Mosby, 2001: 398 (Figure 26-2) with permission.)

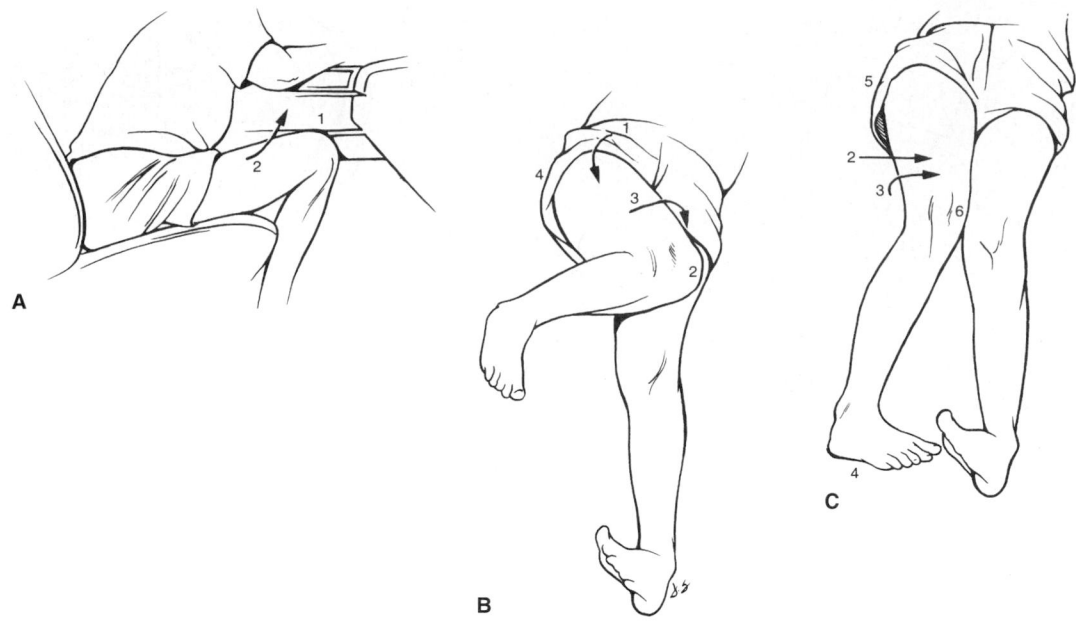

Figure 194.5. Posterior dislocation of the hip. **(A)** Mechanism of injury. The knee *(1)* strikes the dashboard. The thigh *(2)* is forced into flexion and adduction, and the femoral head is driven backward out of the acetabulum. **(B)** Ischial dislocation. The hip *(1)* is flexed. The hip is markedly adducted so that the knee *(2)* of the affected limb lies on the opposite thigh. The limb *(3)* is in extreme internal rotation. The greater trochanter and buttock *(4)* on the affected side are unusually prominent. **(C)** Iliac dislocation. As in **(B)**, the hip is flexed and is adducted *(2)*. It is internally rotated *(3)*. The affected extremity *(4)* appears shortened. The greater trochanter and buttock *(5)* on the affected side are unusually prominent. The knee *(6)* of the affected extremity rests on the opposite thigh.

flexion of the involved extremity. *Anterior iliac* and *pubic* dislocations present as slight abduction, external rotation, and extension of the involved extremity (Fig. 194.8).

Anterior dislocations are best treated with closed reduction with the patient under general anesthesia if reduction is unsuccessful in the ED using common procedural sedation techniques (discussed in the previous section). Emergent orthopaedic consultation for early reduction is extremely important because of associated vascular injuries. This will minimize major sequelae, such as avascular necrosis of the femoral head. These patients should undergo frequent neurovascular checks of the affected limb.

Hip Fractures

Fractures of the hip are one of the common injuries seen in the ED, especially among elderly patients. It is estimated that 5% to 10% of those reaching their 80s will have a femoral neck fracture. The increasing elderly population could double the number of hip fractures seen over the next 20 years. A third of those over age 65 who live at home and half of institutionalized individuals are estimated to fall yearly. Morbidity in this age group is staggering, with a third dying within 1 year (9). Thirty percent of those who were independently ambulatory prefracture require permanent postinjury crutches or a walker, and 7% of them become permanently bedridden (3). For the emergency physician, the diagnosis becomes the important step, as, almost invariably, these patients are repaired intraoperatively with an Austin-Moore–type femoral head prosthesis. The emergency physician should determine prior level of function, including the degree of independent ambulation, mental status, and any associated illnesses, as they are important factors in the ED and in the definitive management of these patients.

The term *hip fracture* refers to a fracture of the femur proximal to the subtrochanteric region. Hip fractures are broadly classified into six anatomic groups: femoral head and neck fractures, intertrochanteric fractures, subtrochanteric fractures, and isolated fractures of greater or lesser trochanters. Pertinent anatomy is shown in Figure 194.1.

Femoral Head Fractures

Isolated fractures of the femoral head are relatively uncommon. These fractures usually occur in conjunction with dislocations of the femoral head (unlike most other types of hip fractures). Three-fourths are due to motor vehicle crashes, generally in younger patients. As with dislocations of the hip, acetabular fracture may also be seen.

Femoral head fractures may not be visualized on routine radiographs; additional studies, such as tomography, radionuclide scans, CT, or MRI may be required. Persistent pain in the absence of radiographic findings should prompt further investigation. In one report, one in seven changes in the femoral head noted after trauma, which were typically thought to be due to avascular necrosis, were actually due to impaction of the femoral head (4).

These fractures may be subdivided into two types: single fragment (*type I*) and comminuted (*type II*). The site of fracture and the accompanying complications are also related to the type of dislocation associated with the fracture (8). Posterior dislocations are more likely to result in fracture of the inferior aspect of the femoral head and may have concomitant sciatic nerve injury. Anterior dislocations tend to result in fracture of the anterior femoral head and may have associated vascular injury.

Precise and early reduction is important to maximize range of motion and subsequent function and to minimize complications such as avascular necrosis or degenerative joint disease. Unfortunately, complications occur regardless of proper intervention and result in the need for prosthetic replacement. Urgent orthopaedic consultation is mandatory.

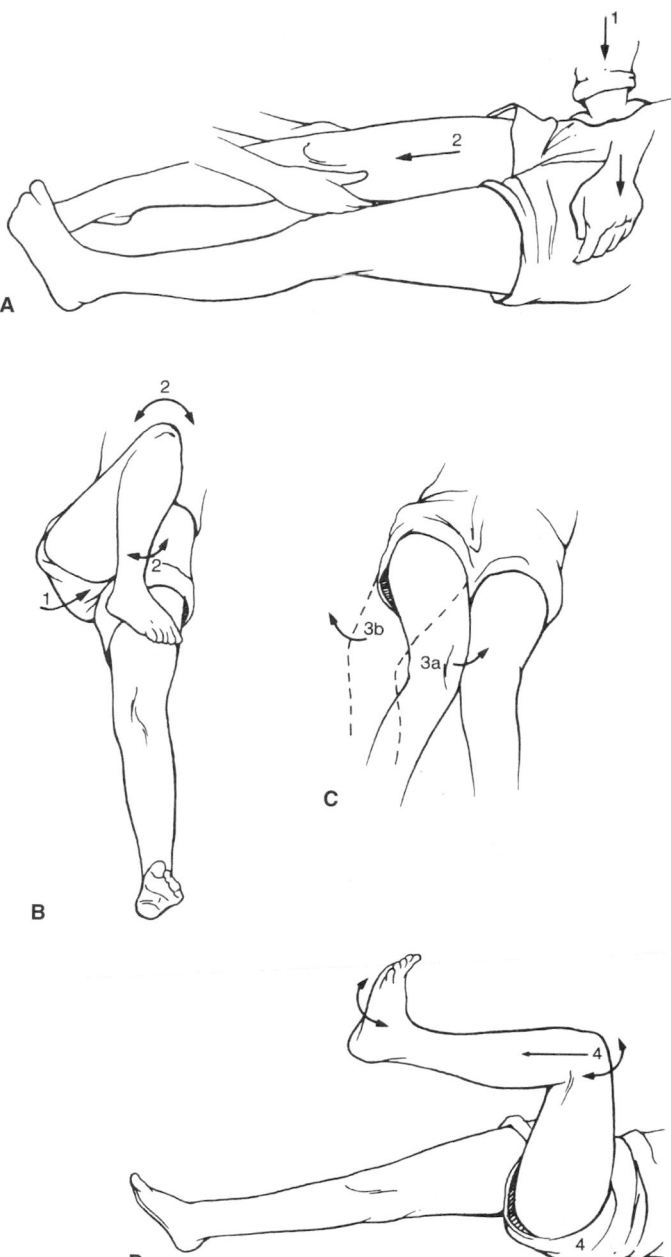

Figure 194.6. Posterior dislocation of the hip: method of manipulative reduction. **(A)** The assistant holds downward pressure *(1)* on the anterior–superior iliac spine. With the knee flexed *(2)*, the operator pulls on the limb in the line of deformity. **(B)** The assistant slowly brings the thigh *(1)* to 90 degrees of flexion. The assistant gently rotates the thigh internally and externally and rocks the thigh *(2)* backward and forward to disengage the head from the external rotator muscles and the posterior capsule. **(C)** The assistant relocates the femoral head by further internal rotation and extension of the thigh *(3a)*, or external rotation and extension of the thigh *(3b)*. **(D)** The assistant pushes firmly on the trochanter to direct the femoral head into the acetabulum while the limb is rotated and extended *(4)*. Forceful rotation should be avoided, because it can fracture the femoral neck. If the reduction is not accomplished with two adequate attempts, open reduction is indicated.

Femoral Neck Fractures (Transcervical or Intracapsular Fractures)

These fractures occur below the femoral head and above the greater trochanter and are much more common than femoral head fractures. They are located within the joint capsule and include subcapital fractures (which occur through the fused epi-

physeal plate). In the elderly, these fractures are pathologic, occurring with little or no trauma. In younger patients they are usually the result of violent, unrestrained motor vehicle trauma. Osteoporosis is a major risk factor, making the injury four times more common in women than in men. Indeed, the fracture may sometimes occur due to angular or torsional forces placed on the neck before a fall (2).

Classifications of these fractures have been based on both patient and fracture characteristics. The system proposed by Garden is one of the most commonly used (Table 194.1). In *type I,* there is impaction or incomplete fracture. *Type II* is a complete transcervical fracture with displacement. *Type III* is a complete fracture with partial displacement of the distal fragment, and *type IV* is a fracture with total displacement or comminution. Ambulation does not imply absence of a fracture, because patients with *type I* and *II* fractures commonly walk after these injuries. Patients with *type III* and *IV* fractures are unable to ambulate and usually present with a shortened, externally rotated extremity and an abducted hip.

Stress fractures represent a unique type of femoral neck fracture. They most commonly occur in young, athletic individuals, but also occur in those with pathologic bone, such as in rheumatoid arthritis, renal osteodystrophy, and chronic steroid use. They may be bilateral and are usually the result of repetitive abnormal stress on normal bone or repetitive normal stress on abnormal bone. The pain is often gradual in its onset. Ambulation is common, and patients complain of pain with weight bearing. The usual signs of fracture are missing, both clinically and radiographically. Bone scan and MRI is indicated in any high-risk individual who cannot bear weight. Treatment centers on the degree of injury and the state of the underlying bone; the range is from resting the affected hip to prosthetic hip replacement.

Type I fractures may be managed nonoperatively, but patient compliance is mandatory, and the likelihood of complications make operative management the preferred modality (pinning, most commonly). *Types II, III,* and *IV* fractures require open reduction and internal fixation (compression screw and plate or Austin-Moore–type femoral head prosthesis). Early and precise anatomic reduction, within 12 hours, reduces the risk of avascular necrosis. Prompt recognition and orthopaedic consultation in the ED may help minimize avascular necrosis and the other sequelae associated with these types of fracture.

Avascular necrosis of the femoral head is a common early complication of fracture of the femoral neck. It is identified on x-ray films as an increase in density in the region of the femoral head, thought to be new bone deposition onto necrotic spicules.

Intertrochanteric Fractures

These are the most common types of hip fractures. They are usually extracapsular, and the vast majority are due to falls in the elderly. These are considered pathologic fractures; the most common reason for the pathologic fracture is osteoporosis. Other causes include cancer or metastatic disease and less commonly, Paget disease. DeLee (2) found these to be four times as common as femoral neck fractures. X-ray findings usually show comminution, with only 20% composed of two pieces, 65% composed of three or four fragments, and 15% highly comminuted (10).

Emergency diagnosis is usually straightforward. Any movement causes extreme pain, and the hip may be tender to palpation. The affected leg is shortened and externally rotated, and weight bearing is not possible. The diagnosis is usually confirmed radiographically with a single anteroposterior (AP) view of the hip. A lateral or groin view may be necessary to evaluate the degree of comminution.

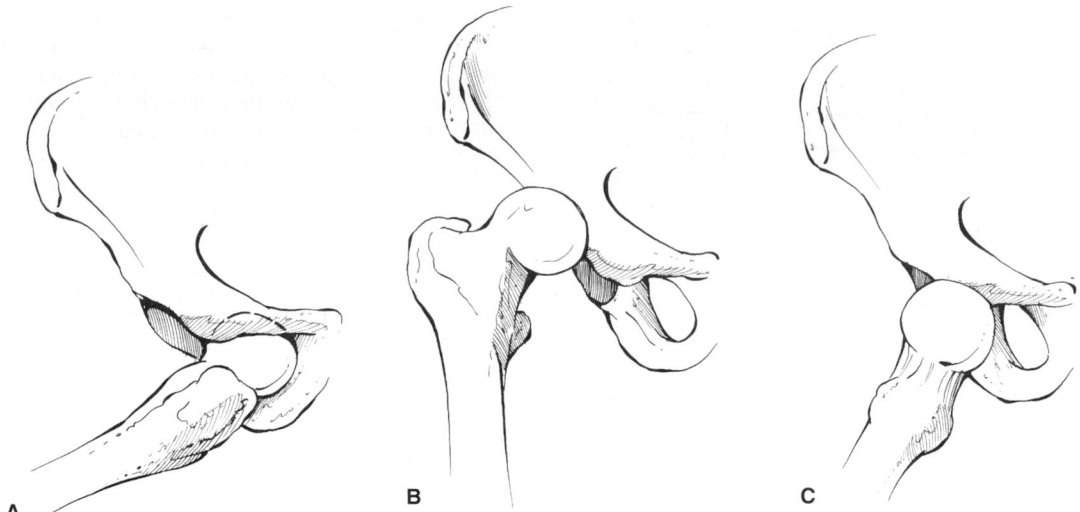

Figure 194.7.   Anterior hip dislocations. **(A)** Anterior obturator hip dislocation. **(B)** Anterior iliac hip dislocation. **(C)** Anterior pubic hip dislocation.

The intertrochanteric fracture is extraarticular, but transarticular forces clearly play a major role in its occurrence. The fracture typically extends in a relatively straight line between the greater and lesser trochanters (Fig. 194.9). A variety of classifications are used to describe these fractures, and there is no universal agreement. The Boyd and Griffin classification uses four categories (Fig. 194.9). *Type I* is nondisplaced. *Type II* fracture lines parallel those in type I, but there is displacement. *Types III* and *IV* fracture lines run nearly perpendicular to types I and II. *Type III* is nondisplaced, whereas *type IV* is displaced. Another system uses stability and comminution as criteria. When obtaining orthopaedic consultation, precise anatomic description may be more useful than a specific classification type.

Initial management consists of immobilization with sandbags or Buck traction (2 to 4 kg). This helps to decrease blood loss until definitive therapy can be performed. Intravenous volume replacement, with crystalloid or blood, may be necessary, because patients can lose 1 to 2 L of blood with these fractures. Many of these patients have concomitant chronic medical problems. These should be addressed (including the cause of the fall) and will help to establish whether the patient is an operative candidate. Laboratory evaluation should include the standard preoperative laboratory assessment, as well as other analysis necessary to ascertain the cause of the fall. This may include neurologic and cardiovascular evaluations.

Operative repair has historically been considered safer than conservative therapy. This is due to the morbidity and mortality associated with extended immobilization. As a result, the treatment of choice is surgical. Surgical reduction and fixation should be considered urgent rather than emergent, and all patients should have a thorough preoperative evaluation. Selected fractures may be managed by splinting, traction, or spica immobilization, as determined by the consulting orthopedist and the patient's underlying medical condition. Complications are common after these injuries and reflect the frail status of most of these patients; about a third of these patients will die within 1 year of injury. Avascular necrosis is an uncommon complication.

Greater Trochanteric Fractures

These injuries are quite uncommon. They occur as a result of direct trauma (generally in adults, including the elderly). Greater trochanteric fractures also occur secondary to avulsion of the apophysis as a result of forceful muscular contraction in those with preepiphyseal plate fusion (ages 7 to 17). When caused by direct trauma, they are rarely displaced and can be difficult to see on routine radiographic views. Radiographic imaging frequently requires comparison views.

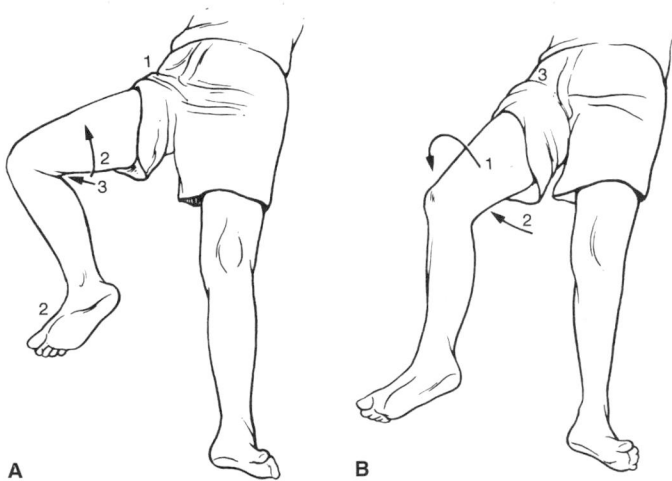

Figure 194.8.   Anterior dislocations of the hip. **(A)** Obturator dislocation. The hip *(1)* is slightly flexed. The limb *(2)* is externally rotated. The thigh *(3)* is abducted. **(B)** Pubic dislocation. The extremity *(1)* is in severe external rotation (90° degrees). The extremity *(2)* is abducted only slightly (15 to 20° degrees), and it is slightly flexed. The femoral head *(3)* can readily be palpated in the inguinal region.

TABLE 194.1.   Garden Classification of Femoral Neck Fractures

Type	Definition
Type I	Impaction or incomplete fracture
Type II	Complete transcervical fracture with displacement
Type III	Complete fracture with partial displacement of the distal fragment
Type IV	Fracture with total displacement or comminution

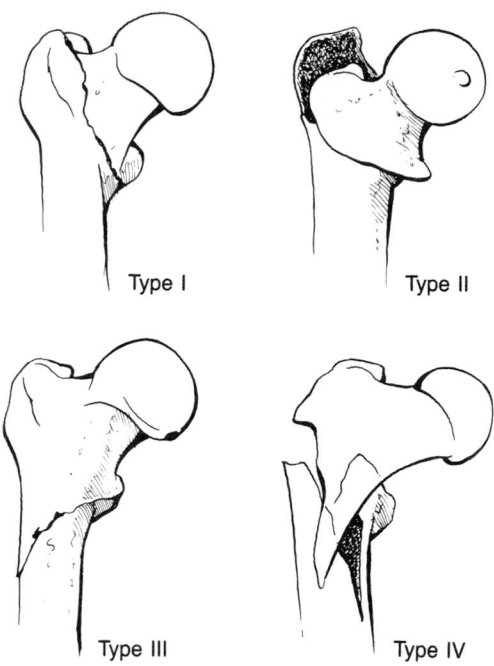

Figure 194.9.   Boyd and Griffin classification of intertrochanteric fractures. (Adapted from Rockwood CA Jr, Green DP, Bucholz RW. *Rockwood and Green's fractures in adults,* 3rd ed. Philadelphia: Lippincott Co., 1991.)

Tenderness to palpation is usually present over the greater trochanter. Patients are usually ambulatory, and frequently with a limp. The fracture in adults, due to a direct blow, is usually comminuted without significant displacement. The epiphyseal avulsion type of injury is usually displaced but not comminuted.

Management varies from adduction splint and bed rest, to open reduction and internal fixation (ORIF). In most instances, the prognosis is good, regardless of the method used. DeLee (2) recommends ORIF for greater than 1-cm displacement of either a large isolated fragment for the direct trauma (adult) type or the entire apophysis in the epiphyseal avulsion (youth) type.

Lesser Trochanteric Fractures

Lesser trochanteric fractures usually occur in the young; 85% occur before age 20 (2). They usually occur from forceful contraction of the iliopsoas muscle during strenuous activities. The lesser trochanter can be displaced up to 1 cm. This type of injury in an adult mandates a search for pathologic bone.

Patients will have pain and tenderness in the femoral triangle. They will be unable to lift the affected extremity when in the sitting position if there is complete avulsion (*Ludloff sign*). Radiographic imaging frequently requires comparison views.

Treatment is usually bed rest, unless there is significant displacement. Some orthopedists favor nonoperative management, regardless of the degree of separation, because the outcome is uniformly good (2).

Subtrochanteric Fractures

Subtrochanteric fractures are defined as fractures occurring between the lesser trochanter and a point 5 cm (or 2 in.) distally. They account for 10% of hip fractures and are associated with more severe trauma, or they occur in pathologic bone (such as severe osteoporosis, Paget disease or cancer metastasis).

Clinical presentation is similar to that of intertrochanteric fractures. The forces of the muscles extending across this region frequently result in abduction, flexion, and external rota-

tion. Young patients with these fractures are subject to violent forces; associated injuries are common. Blood loss can be substantial in fractures of the midshaft femur, and these fractures fall into this subset. Subtrochanteric fractures may occur in combination with other hip fractures. Classification is varied and complex. Accepted anatomic description is best used when describing these fractures.

Treatment involves immobilization, analgesia, volume replacement (if indicated), and timely orthopaedic intervention. Associated neurovascular injury to the profunda femoris artery, ascending and descending branches of the lateral circumflex femoral arteries, and the lateral femoral cutaneous nerve and branches of the femoral nerve should be suspected. They occur with severe displacement and angulation of the proximal femur. The presence of a tense, swollen upper thigh should be evaluated with angiography or Doppler for an acute vascular injury. Prompt vascular surgery consultation should be obtained, if indicated. Operative reduction and fixation (usually some type of intramedullary nail) is used based on specific patient and fracture characteristics.

Acetabular Fractures

Acetabular fractures should be considered in patients with either type of femoral head dislocation and, more commonly, in patients with pelvic fractures. The force of injury applied to the femur from impact onto the dashboard is transmitted to the acetabulum.

There are four types of acetabular fractures. The *posterior lip* fracture is the most common and is associated with posterior hip dislocations. The *transverse acetabulum* fracture is best seen on AP view as it crosses the acetabulum. The third is the anterior fracture, which disrupts the arcuate or iliopubic line. The fourth is the *ilioischial* (or *posterior*) fracture. In the *ilioischial or posterior* type of fracture, the entire posterior column (the bone extending from the ilium to the ischium) becomes separated from the pelvis. An occult acetabular fracture should be suspected when the patient gives a history of a recent fall, but the pelvic radiograph is normal. Always consider the use of oblique views to diagnose these fractures, as the first films generally do not visualize the injury. It is frequently necessary to consider CT scan, MRI, and bone scan to diagnose these injuries.

Acetabular fractures are managed in consultation with an orthopaedic surgeon. ED management involves immobilization, analgesia, volume replacement (if necessary), and identification of associated injuries.

Slipped Capital Femoral Epiphysis

Slipped capital femoral epiphysis (SCFE) is the most common hip abnormality in adolescents who present to an orthopedist, and if untreated, can result in profound lifelong morbidity due to avascular necrosis. The diagnosis is frequently missed in the ED. SCFE is a Salter-Harris type 1 fracture of the femoral capital epiphysis in which the head of the femur slips to a varying degree, posteriorly and inferiorly. It occurs in boys twice as often as in girls; affected boys can be as young as 10 years old. SCFE prior to age ten mandates a metabolic workup for endocrine disorders, although the ED treatment remains the same. Most affected children are obese, suggesting a primary mechanical problem. However, the disease is multifactorial and may have a genetic component. About half of SCFE's present bilaterally, and surgical repair is usually bilateral because of the high association of SCFE in the contralateral hip within 18 months. Because of referred pain from the hip, a common presentation is with knee pain, often with an associated history of injury, but a normal knee exam and radiograph.

The most common presentation is that of a limping obese 12-year-old male, complaining of pain in the hip. In this setting, SCFE must be aggressively sought. The hip is externally rotated and there is an antalgic gait. However, the diagnosis should also be considered in a thin adolescent girl (average age of 13.5) with knee or groin pain. There is progressive hip flexion and external rotation as the condition becomes chronic. The physician should carefully document an acute, chronic, or acute-on-chronic presentation and whether the limp has been episodic. Bilateral hip radiographs are mandatory. The projection of the Klein line over the head of the femur should be noted; if SCFE is present the line will not project through the femur head.

All patients with SCFE should be nonweight bearing and all need operative percutaneous fixation of the femoral head, usually without reduction unless there is significant displacement. Fixation should be performed within a few days; if nonweight bearing before surgery cannot be assured, admission is necessary. The most common complication of SCFE is avascular necrosis, which is thought to be caused by the shearing and movement at the epiphysis, primarily at the time of injury, but also possibly at the time of attempted reduction. Avascular necrosis ultimately requires hip replacement. Chondrolysis, another potential complication, is usually associated with violation of the hip capsule during fixation, but this is rare with current single screw percutaneous fixation methods. However, chondrolysis occurs in about 5% of SCFE cases with or without fixation (13).

CRITICAL INTERVENTIONS

- Evaluate patients with hip dislocations for associated acetabular, femur, and knee injuries (especially ligamentous); computed tomography (CT) or magnetic resonance imaging (MRI) may be necessary
- Perform early closed reduction of hip dislocations (less than 6 hours is ideal); this lowers the risk of avascular necrosis and posttraumatic osteoarthritis
- Perform a CT, MRI, or other diagnostic tests in patients with persistent hip pain in the absence of radiographic findings in order to identify an occult hip fracture

DISPOSITION

Orthopaedic consultation is recommended for all hip dislocations and fractures. Hip dislocations require careful observation with frequent neurovascular checks. Unstable anterior dislocations may require traction to maintain reduction. Young healthy patients with nondisplaced femoral neck fractures are typically managed with nonweight bearing and crutches. Occasionally they will require surgical fixation. Both elderly and young patients with intertrochanteric and subtrochanteric fractures require surgical fixation. Hospital admission for all elderly patients with acute hip fractures is recommended. They generally require evaluation and consultation for preoperative medical clearance, as well as frequent neurovascular checks of the affected limb.

COMMON PITFALLS

✔ Failure to consider SCFE in adolescent patients with knee or hip pain
✔ Failure to realize that persistent pain after reduction of a dislocated hip may indicate entrapment of neurologic or vascular structures within the joint
✔ Failure to evaluate an elderly patient with a history of a recent fall and a complaint of knee pain for hip fracture
✔ Failure to evaluate young, athletic adults with pain in the femoral triangle for lesser trochanteric fracture
✔ Failure to realize that hip pain and inability to walk, even in the absence of trauma, may be due to hip fracture
✔ Failure to look for acetabular fractures in patients with hip dislocations and inferior pubic rami fractures

References

1. Bassett KE, Anderson JL, Pribble CG, Guenther E. Propofol for Procedural Sedation in Children in the Emergency Department. *Ann Emer Med* 2003:42:773–782.
2. DeLee JC. Fractures and dislocations of the hip. In: Rockwood CA Jr, Green DP, Bucholz RW. *Rockwood and Green's fractures in adults*, 3rd ed. Philadelphia: JB Lippincott Co, 1991:1481.
3. Finsen V, Borset M, Rossvoll I. Mobility, survival and nursing-home requirements after hip fracture. *Ann Chir Gynaecol* 1995;84:291–294.
4. Gruen GS, Mears DC, Tauxe WN. Distinguishing avascular necrosis from segmental impaction of the femoral head following an acetabular fracture: preliminary report. *J Orthop Trauma* 1980;2:5.
5. Guenther E, Pribble CG, Junkins EP Jr, et al. Propofol sedation by emergency physicians for elective pediatric outpatient procedures. *Ann Emer Med* 2003;42:783–791.
6. Jasulka RA, Fischer G, Fenzl G. Dislocation and fracture-dislocation of the hip. *J Bone Joint Surg Br* 1991;73:459–465.
7. Loder, RT. Slipped capital femoral epiphysis. *American Family Physician* 1998;57:2135–42, 2148–2150.
8. Meislin RJ, Zuckermann JD. Case report: bilateral posterior hip dislocations with femoral head fractures. *J Orthop Trauma* 1989;3:358.
9. Parker MJ, Anad JK. What is the true mortality of hip fractures? *Publ Health* 1991;105:443–446.
10. Rogers LF. The radiology of skeletal trauma, 2nd ed. New York: Churchill Livingstone, 1992.
11. Simon RR, Koenigsknecht SJ. Emergency orthopaedics—the extremities, 3rd ed. Norwalk CT: Appleton & Lange, 1995.
12. Vecsei V, Schwendenwein E, Berger G. Hip dislocation without bone injuries. *Orthopade* 1997;26:317–326.
13. Yang RS, Tsuang YH, Hang YS, et al. Traumatic dislocations of the hip. *Clin Orthop Rel Res* 1991;265:218.

CHAPTER 195
Knee Injuries

John E. Gough and Luis E. Rodriguez

The knee is a synovial hinge joint with a complex architecture of bone, ligament, muscle, and cartilage (Fig. 195.1). The three bones that make up the knee are the distal femur, patella, and proximal tibia. The femoral condyles articulate with the proximal tibia (tibial plateau) to form the weight-bearing portion of the knee joint. The femoral condyles also articulate with the posterior portion of the patella in the trochlear groove. The patellofemoral articulation does not function in weight bearing. However, the patella provides protection to the femur, as well as improved stability and strength of the extensor mechanism. The proximal fibula is not part of the knee joint proper, although it does serve as the site of attachment of the lateral collateral ligament (LCL).

The bony structures of the knee offer the joint little stability; the knee relies on fibrinous soft-tissue components for stability and proper function. Stability of the medial aspect of the knee is provided mainly by the medial collateral ligament (MCL). The MCL has a superficial and deep layer. The superficial portion originates from the medial femoral epicondyle and inserts on

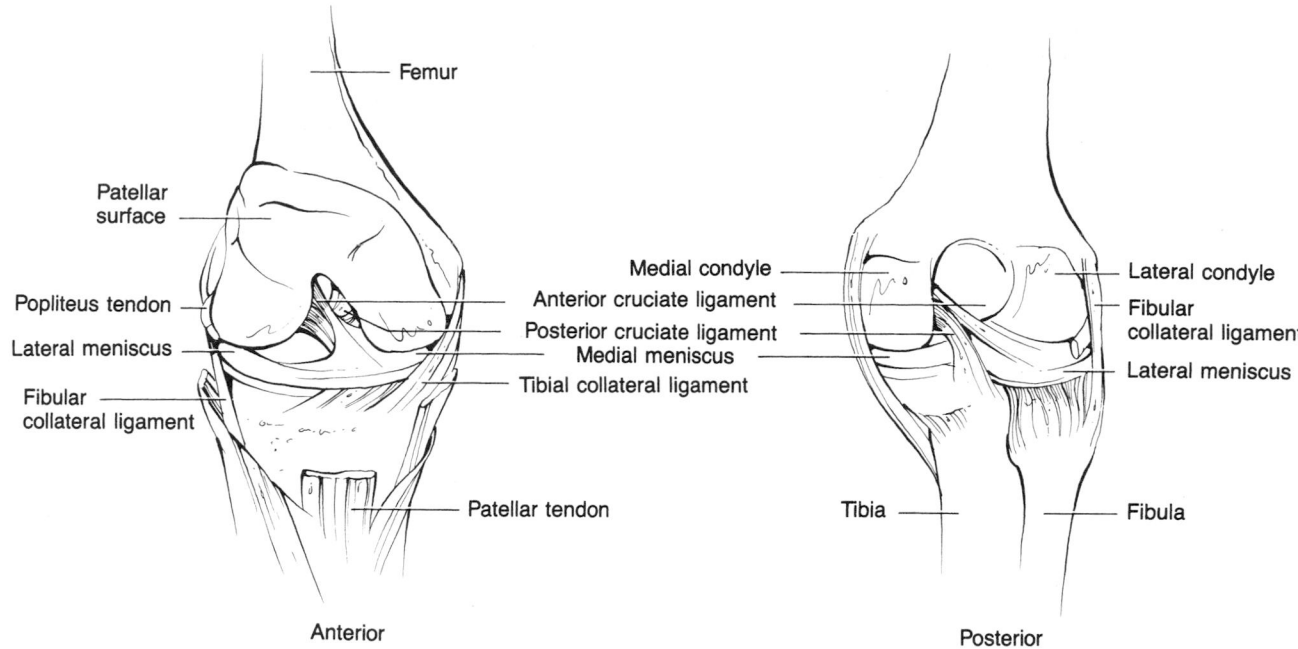

Figure 195.1.   Anatomy of the knee.

the medial aspect of the tibia just distal to the tibiofemoral joint and provides most of the resistance to valgus forces. The deep portion of the MCL helps to stabilize the medial meniscus. The LCL protects the knee from varus stresses and originates from the lateral femoral epicondyle.

The cruciate ligaments are located within the intercondylar notch. The anterior cruciate ligament (ACL) originates from the posterior aspect of the lateral femoral epicondyle and inserts into the anterior tibia at the tibial spine. The posterior cruciate ligament (PCL) arises from the medial femoral condyle, crosses behind the ACL, and inserts on the posterior tibial spine. The ACL prevents anterior displacement of the tibia relative to the femur; the PCL helps to prevent posterior displacement. Both cruciate ligaments also play a minor role in resisting varus and valgus rotation within the knee.

The menisci are cartilage positioned on the articulating surface of the tibia. They provide a contact surface between the tibia and femur and distribute and dissipate forces within the knee. The menisci also aid in stabilizing the knee by preventing abnormal motion of the tibia and femur. They have only peripheral vasculature, which is of clinical importance in the healing process following injury.

The muscles involved with normal knee function can be divided into extensors and flexors. Extension is primarily provided by the quadriceps muscles, composed of the vastus medialis, vastus intermedius, vastus lateralis, and rectus femoris. The tendons of these muscles combine to form the quadriceps tendon, which inserts into the superior patella and the medial and lateral retinaculum of the joint capsule. The tendon then becomes the patellar tendon, which connects the inferior portion of the patella to the tibial tubercle.

The hamstring muscles of the posterior thigh are the primary flexors of the knee. The four muscles of the hamstring are the semimembranosus, semitendinosus, and the two heads of the biceps femoris. The biceps femoris attaches to the proximal fibula. The semitendinosus and semimembranosus form the medial aspect of the hamstrings and insert into the tibia and medial joint capsule of the knee.

The major vascular structures around the knee pass posteriorly and are of extreme clinical importance. The popliteal artery

is fixed proximally at the hiatus of the adductor magnus and distally at the tendinous arch of the soleus muscle. This tethering makes it susceptible to injury by traction forces, as seen with dislocations. The popliteal artery is also at risk of disruption by fractures or penetrating wounds. The collateral circulation is generally poor, so significant damage to the popliteal artery places the viability of the lower limb in jeopardy.

Proximal to the knee, the sciatic nerve separates into the tibial and peroneal nerves. The tibial nerve passes posteriorly and is therefore susceptible to the same mechanisms of injury as the popliteal artery. The peroneal nerve courses superficially around the lateral aspect of the knee to the proximal fibula. Because of its superficial location, the peroneal nerve may be injured in trauma involving less significant forces than those needed to affect the deeper tibial nerve.

EMERGENCY DEPARTMENT EVALUATION

The history is extremely helpful in directing the evaluation of a knee injury. The chief complaint, mechanism of injury, and the nature and duration of symptoms help to differentiate acute trauma from chronic problems or reinjury.

The mechanism of injury is a key piece of the history. The force, direction, and placement of traumatic stresses, as well as the position of the knee at the time of injury, should be identified. Associated complaints, such as locking of the joint, effusions (and how quickly the fluid accumulated), popping sensations, and ability to ambulate, should be elicited. Any associated injuries, particularly to the hip and ankle, should be evaluated.

The physical examination begins with inspection of the knee and entire limb for obvious deformity, ecchymosis, erythema, edema, or cutaneous lesions. The presence of scars should be noted, as they may indicate previous trauma or surgery. Careful palpation will identify tenderness, crepitus, abnormal skin temperature, or the presence of an effusion.

At this point, if a fracture is suspected, appropriate radiologic studies should be obtained before performing extensive manipulation of the knee. Several clinical decision rules for the use of radiographs in the acutely injured knee have recently been

TABLE 195.1. Decision Rules for the Use of Radiographs in the Acutely Injured Knee

Pittsburgh	Ottawa
Mechanism of injury (blunt trauma, falls)	Age (>55)
	Tenderness at fibula head
Age (<12, >55)	Isolated tenderness of the patella
Inability to walk (4 weight bearing steps)	Inability to flex to 90 degrees
	Inability to transfer weight for 4 steps (either immediately following injury or in the ED)

developed; the most common being the Ottawa and Pittsburgh Rules (7,13) (Table 195.1). Prospective validation has shown the sensitivity of the rules to be 100% in both pediatric and adult patients. These studies suggest a potential x-ray reduction of up to 49% (2,4).

If radiographs are not indicated or are negative, the assessment of potential injuries should continue. The physician should perform a systematic examination of the soft tissues, as well as determination of weight bearing and gait. When possible, the unaffected knee should be examined for comparison. Often, it is useful to examine the uninjured joint first to assess normal variability for the patient. Discrepancies between the patient's joints are more important than absolute laxity. Examining the uninjured knee also permits the physician to demonstrate the maneuvers that will be performed, allaying the patient's fears and improving cooperation.

The presence of excessive tenderness or joint effusions may make the examination difficult. Effusions and tensing of the musculature secondary to pain may give the impression of more joint stability than is actually present. Therefore, although it is important to evaluate the patient acutely, it is often necessary to immobilize the injured knee in the emergency department (ED) and arrange for a followup examination within 5 to 7 days.

Specific Tests for Soft-Tissue Injuries

During each of the following tests, the patient should be as relaxed as possible. The physician should explain the examination to the patient and compare the findings with those of the uninjured knee. If the patient cannot cooperate because of pain, appropriate analgesia or sedation may be necessary. In certain cases, it may be necessary to have the orthopedist perform these tests with the patient under general anesthesia.

Collateral Ligaments

The knee is examined in both full extension and at 30 degrees of flexion (Fig. 195.2). The tibia and femur should be stabilized with the examiner's hands while applying varus and valgus stresses to the knee, testing the stability of the LCL and MCL, respectively (8). With a *first-degree* sprain, there is no laxity at either extension or flexion. A *second-degree* sprain demonstrates some laxity in flexion (with a solid end-point) but no laxity in extension. With a *third-degree* sprain, there is some laxity in extension and significant laxity in flexion, without a solid end-point. Marked opening of the joint in both flexion and extension indicates the possibility of a cruciate ligament disruption in addition to the collateral ligament injury.

Cruciate Ligaments

The *Lachman test* is the best way to evaluate the ACL (12). The patient should be in the supine position, the tibia and femur are stabilized with the examiner's hands and the knee is flexed to 20 to 30 degrees. The tibia is then pulled anteriorly. Excessive anterior displacement of the tibia relative to the femur and a lack of a distinct end-point indicate an ACL rupture (12).

Although not as sensitive as the Lachman test, the *anterior drawer test* may also be utilized to evaluate the ACL. The knee is flexed to 90 degrees with the foot flat on the stretcher in a neutral position and stabilized (Fig. 195.2). Anterior force is placed on the tibia. Significant displacement of the tibia anteriorly (compared with the unaffected knee) suggests ACL rupture (8). This test can also be performed with the foot in 15 degrees of external rotation (*Slocum test*) and 15 degrees of internal rotation.

Another test for ACL injury is the *pivot shift*, which has a good positive predictive value (12). With the knee in full extension, the leg is lifted by the distal tibia. With an ACL rupture, the tibia is subluxed anteriorly in this position. Then the examiner applies a mild valgus force while the knee is carefully flexed to 20 to 40 degrees. At this point, the tibia jumps into a reduced position. Pain may hinder the performance of this test in the acutely injured knee (8).

The *posterior drawer test*, the reverse of the anterior drawer, is the most accurate physical examination test used to evaluate PCL injuries (3). The knee is flexed to 90 degrees and the foot is secured in a neutral position. Then the examiner applies posterior force to the tibia. If the tibia moves posterior to the femoral condyles, the test is positive, representing PCL injury (8).

An alternative test for PCL injury is the *posterior sag*. The examiner holds the knee in 90 degrees of flexion with the thigh supported by a pillow and the foot secured. In this position, the tibia will displace posteriorly, or sag, if the PCL is ruptured (3).

Meniscus

The *McMurray test* is used to identify meniscal injury. The examiner holds the knee in one hand and the lower leg or foot in the other. Then the examiner applies internal and external rotation to the lower leg while flexing and extending the knee (8) (Fig. 195.2). The knee should be palpated for catching or clicking sensations. A medial meniscal tear should be suspected if clicking occurs as the leg is extended and externally rotated after being completely flexed. Clicking with internal rotation during extension is used to help identify a lateral meniscal injury. While a positive test does not guarantee a meniscal injury, it does suggest an intraarticular injury warranting further evaluation. Joint line tenderness is very suspicious for potential injury to the lateral meniscus; however, it is not as sensitive with medial meniscus injuries (5).

Another test used to identify meniscal injury is the *Apley test*. The patient is in the prone position and the knee is flexed to 90 degrees. The examiner applies upward force to the tibia while it is rotated and the knee is extended (8) (Fig. 195.2). Pain and clicking in the joint suggest a meniscal injury.

Patellar Subluxation

The *apprehension sign* is seen with patellar subluxation. The knee is in extension and the examiner attempts to displace the patella laterally. With patellar subluxations, this manipulation is painful, and the patient, who is typically anxious and apprehensive about this maneuver, will contract the quadriceps (8).

Extensor Mechanism

The extensor mechanism includes the quadriceps muscle, quadriceps tendon, patella, patellar tendon and retinacula. Disruption of any of these may lead to the inability to extend the leg. Other causes include meniscal rupture (with "bucket-handle" tears), ACL injuries, synovitis, and intraarticular tumors (11). The patient should be evaluated for an injury to the extensor

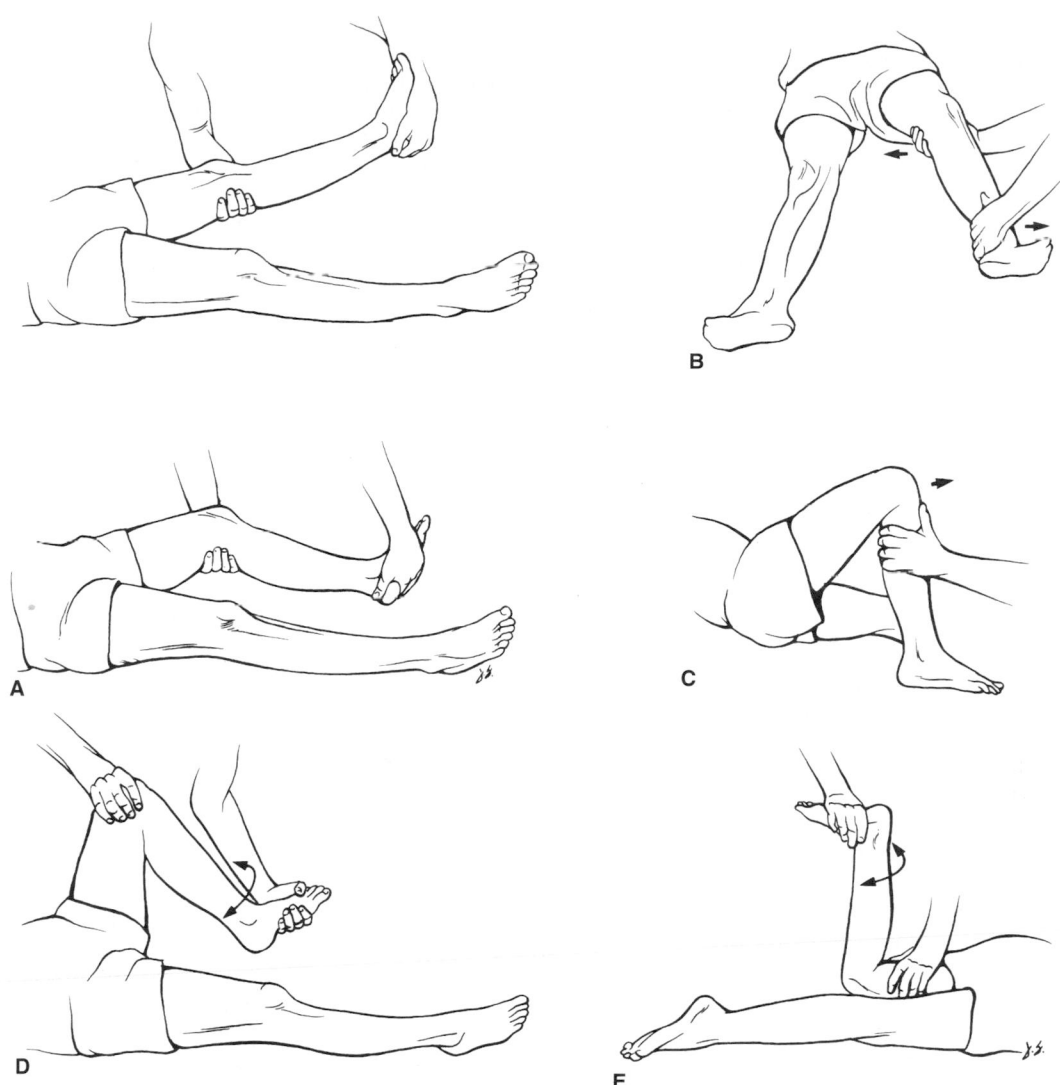

Figure 195.2.   Examination of the knee. **(A)** Valgus stress at 0-degree and 30-degree flexion, as viewed from the side. **(B)** Valgus stress at 0-degree flexion, as viewed from above. **(C)** Anterior drawer test. **(D)** McMurray test. **(E)** Apley test.

mechanism by having him or her extend the leg. The patient should be instructed to lift the leg off the bed. Limited or loss of ability to extend is indicative of an injury to the extensor mechanism.

Diagnostic Tests

Plain radiographs are indicated in many knee injuries. Standard anteroposterior and lateral views should be supplemented with *sunrise* (skyline) and *tunnel* views to evaluate the patellofemoral joint and intercondylar notch, respectively. Plain films help diagnose fractures, effusions, dislocations, foreign bodies, and calcified loose bodies. Fluid–fluid levels seen on plain radiographs have traditionally been thought to represent lipohemarthrosis (fat floating on synovial fluid) and are thought to be an indication of an occult fracture. While not all fluid–fluid interfaces seen on plain films represent lipohemarthrosis, the presence of such a finding warrants further evaluation utilizing tomography, computed tomography (CT) scanning, or magnetic resonance imaging (MRI). Although not as common as other modalities, recently sonography has been utilized to evaluate acute knee injuries (6,10).

Plain radiographs give little information about soft-tissue structures, but stress views and arthrography may be used to evaluate soft-tissue injuries. More recently, MRI scanning has become the test of choice for evaluating the soft tissues of the knee. Although MRI is more expensive than plain films, it has many advantages over plain radiography. MRI involves no ionizing radiation and clearly defines soft-tissue structures. It can also identify subtle injuries, such as bone contusions and occult fractures that are not seen on plain films.

Angiography, utilized to evaluate the presence of vascular injury, is indicated in the presence of any penetrating trauma in proximity to vascular structures. Furthermore, it is frequently indicated in the presence of a knee dislocation to rule out an occult injury to the popliteal artery.

Arthrocentesis and joint fluid analysis can be helpful in determining the etiology of a knee effusion. It may be difficult to differentiate hemarthrosis from an infective or inflammatory effusion clinically, particularly if the history is difficult to obtain. An analysis of the joint fluid may be helpful in making a diagnosis. An acute hemarthrosis may suggest an ACL tear, and the presence of lipid droplets in a bloody effusion may signify an occult fracture. The presence of white blood cells may indicate inflammatory or infectious processes. White blood cell counts in the range of 20,000 to 60,000 WBCs/mm^3 are associated with inflammatory processes, and higher counts (greater than 100,000 WBCs/mm^3) usually represent infection (see Chapter 107, "Monarticular Arthritis").

Further studies, such as Gram stain, cultures, crystal analysis, and glucose and protein determinations, are generally performed and provide clues to the etiology of the effusion. Some authors advocate arthrocentesis of acute hemarthrosis for pain relief; others, however, note that after evacuation of an acute hemarthrosis, it may quickly reaccumulate. Therefore, it may be preferable to use arthrocentesis in a diagnostic rather than a therapeutic role.

For patients with deep lacerations of the knee, it is important to ensure that the wound does not extend into the joint. Methylene blue should be injected into the joint and the wound should be inspected for extravasation.

EMERGENCY DEPARTMENT MANAGEMENT

Distal Femur Fractures

The distal femur is the lower third of the bone. Fractures in this area are typically described relative to the femoral condyles and are separated into *supracondylar* or *intercondylar* (Fig. 195.3). Distal femur fractures account for 4% to 7% of all femur fractures (31% if hip fractures are excluded). They are most often associated with high-energy trauma (e.g., knee to dashboard in high-speed motor vehicle crashes [MVCs]), but they may occur with less violent forces, particularly in the elderly.

The physical examination typically demonstrates a tender, edematous knee and distal femur. Obvious deformity may be present, and crepitus may accompany movement. If a fracture is suspected, the knee should be immobilized and radiographs obtained. Although neurovascular injuries are uncommon, the proximity of the femoral artery and peroneal nerves to the bone requires that the neurovascular status of the extremity be evaluated and documented. Differential diagnoses include patellar

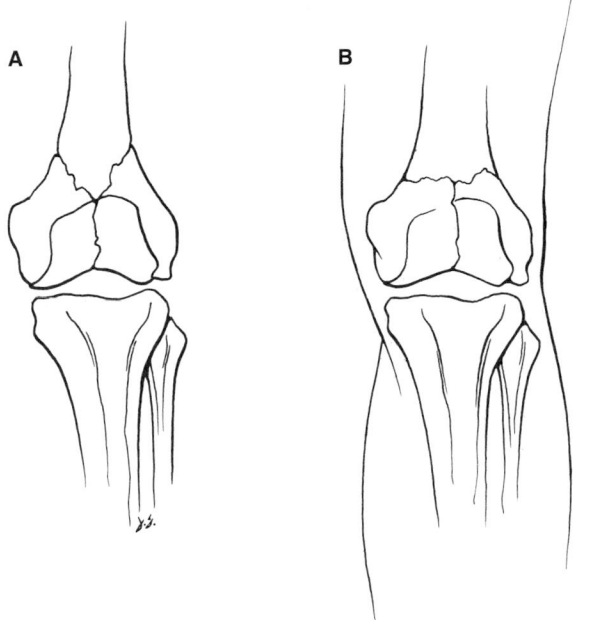

Figure 195.3. Distal femur fractures. **(A)** Y-shaped intercondylar. **(B)** T-shaped intercondylar.

fractures, knee dislocations, and soft-tissue injuries with resulting effusions. Associated injuries, such as hip fractures and dislocations, acetabular fractures, knee dislocations, and proximal tibial fractures, should be suspected and evaluated.

Standard diagnostic tests include anteroposterior and lateral radiographs. Oblique views and tomography help evaluate intracondylar and intraarticular injuries. If vascular trauma is suspected, arteriography should be performed.

Initial management includes immobilization, pain management, and evaluation of concomitant injuries. Early orthopaedic consultation is indicated for definitive care (skeletal traction or surgical repair).

Proximal Tibia Fractures

Tibial plateau fractures occur as a result of varus–valgus forces, from axial loads, or both. Fractures of the tibial plateau may cause a major impairment in the stability and function of the knee joint. The lateral portion of the tibial plateau is most commonly involved (approximately 80% of cases).

Clinical findings vary with the severity and type of fracture. There may be gross or only minimal deformity. The knee is usually swollen and tender. The potential for neurovascular injuries is much higher in proximal tibial fracture than in distal femoral fracture. The physician should maintain a high level of suspicion for such injuries and carefully evaluate the neurovascular status. The potential for the development of a compartment syndrome is also significant. Paresthesias and paralysis from compartment syndromes may be mistaken for a primary nerve injury. Injuries to the menisci, as well as to the collateral and cruciate ligaments, should be suspected. Deep venous thrombosis (DVT) is another common complication seen with tibial plateau fracture.

Diagnostic tests include plain radiographs, tomography, and CT scans. Plain radiographs will identify most tibial plateau fractures and therefore remain the initial test that is used. However, it is important to obtain oblique as well as the standard anteroposterior and lateral views to better evaluate the articular surface. CT scanning has advantages over plain radiography in that it is more sensitive for detecting subtle nondisplaced fractures as well as being able to identify occult lesions. With severely comminuted fractures, CT scanning can quantify the extent of the articular surface involved and the amount of displacement or depression of the fracture line. This information will be helpful to the orthopedist in planning operative repair. While not commonly obtained in the ED, bone scans and MRI may also be used to identify subtle findings (e.g., stress fractures). If a vascular injury is suspected, an arteriogram should be obtained. Doppler studies and venograms may be indicated to exclude DVT. If compartment syndrome is clinically suspected, compartment pressures should be measured.

In addition to the standard management of immobilization and evaluation of other injuries, orthopaedic consultation is indicated. Simple fractures may be treated with immobilization, and depressed fractures require surgical reduction.

Tibial Spine Fractures

Fractures of the tibial spines generally represent avulsion injuries caused by trauma to the cruciate ligaments. Tibial spine fractures are more common in children, as their ligaments are stronger than their bones. The anterior spine is most commonly affected.

Clinical examination generally reveals a swollen, tender knee. Because there is a high correlation with ACL injuries, hemarthrosis is common. The most common diagnostic test needed is a plain radiograph. Fractures are usually seen on plain films, but

MRI scanning or arthroscopy may be needed to identify associated injuries.

Management involves immobilization and orthopaedic referral within a week. Some fractures may be treated nonsurgically, but if significant displacement is present, surgical intervention may be necessary.

Tibial Tuberosity Fractures

A fracture of the tibial tuberosity represents an avulsion injury caused by the patellar tendon. This uncommon fracture occurs with either strong flexion or extension of the knee against resistance. It most commonly occurs before closure of the epiphysis.

Examination reveals tenderness and possible deformity at the site of injury. As this is an extraarticular injury, joint effusion is rare. The differential diagnosis must include Osgood-Schlatter disease in adolescents. *Osgood-Schlatter disease* is a traction injury to the apophysis of the tibial tuberosity. Although most common in boys ages 10 to 13, it may be seen in girls, usually ages 8 to 13. It is thought that repetitive trauma to the epiphysis results in incomplete separation of parts of the cartilaginous and chondroosseous portions of the tibial tuberosity. Diagnosis is based on the history and physical examination. The tubercle is painful, tender, and usually enlarged. Pain is exacerbated by extension of the knee, particularly against resistance.

The diagnosis of a tibial tuberosity fracture is generally made on plain radiographs. If Osgood-Schlatter disease is suspected, plain radiographs may be difficult to interpret, as fragments of the tuberosity may be a normal variant.

Tibial tuberosity fractures may require open reduction but are usually treated with immobilization. Osgood-Schlatter disease is treated with rest, sometimes plaster cast immobilization, and, rarely, surgical excision of loose ossicles to relieve symptoms.

Patellar Fractures

Patellar fractures may result from direct or indirect forces. Direct forces, as seen with falls and MVCs, are most common. Less common are fractures resulting from severe tension placed on the patella by strong contraction of the quadriceps; the usual result is a transverse fracture, which may disrupt the extensor mechanism.

Examination generally reveals pain and tenderness over the patella, inability to walk, and, commonly, a joint effusion. If the fracture is significantly displaced, a defect may be palpable. Diagnosis is generally made with plain radiographs. Tomograms and CT scans may identify an occult fracture. A bipartite patella may be confused with a fracture. Often, the margins of a bipartite patella are rounded, but in the setting of acute trauma, it may be difficult to differentiate from an acute fracture.

Therapy is based on the type of fracture, degree of separation, and condition of the extensor mechanism. Orthopaedic referral is indicated. Simple nondisplaced fractures are treated with immobilization. The patient should receive an outpatient orthopaedic referral within a week for cast placement for approximately 4 to 6 weeks. Fractures that disrupt the extensor mechanism, typically displaced transverse or severely comminuted fractures, will require open reduction and internal fixation for optimal results. As with all fractures about the knee, posttraumatic arthritis is a significant complication.

Tibiofemoral Joint Dislocation (Knee Dislocation)

Knee dislocations are orthopaedic emergencies and require immediate attention. Dislocation of the tibiofemoral joint is rare. It is generally associated with high-energy trauma but may be

seen with low-energy forces (e.g., stepping in a hole, jumping on a trampoline). The dislocation is described as anterior, posterior, medial, lateral, or rotary based on the position of the tibia relative to the femur. For a dislocation to occur, significant trauma to the surrounding soft tissue is generally seen, including the collateral ligaments, cruciate ligaments, menisci, joint capsule, and neurovascular structures (14).

Physical examination may be difficult, and some dislocations spontaneously reduce before the patient arrives at the ED. The patient may describe a history of abnormal position of the joint before reduction. Tenderness, swelling, joint effusion, and deformity may be present. Because of a high incidence of peroneal nerve and popliteal artery injury, specific attention should be devoted to this aspect of the physical examination. The absence of distal pulses highly correlates with significant vascular injury; the presence of pulses, however, does not eliminate the possibility of vascular damage (1,9). Considering the common high-force mechanisms of injury and the potential for vascular damage, compartment syndrome is a significant potential complication.

Diagnosis is based on history, physical examination, and plain radiographs, and CT scanning may also be useful. MRI scanning will identify intraarticular injuries, but it is not commonly used in the acute setting.

For years, arteriography has been used in evaluating knee dislocations. If there are hard signs of vascular injury (absent pulses, expanding hematoma, hemorrhage, ischemia or bruit) the patient requires an arteriogram. Those without hard signs or a negative clinical examination are more of a diagnostic dilemma. They may be admitted for serial examinations. Some authors have advocated the selective use of arteriography. These authors argue that although some patients with intact normal pulses may demonstrate arteriographic evidence of injuries, such as intimal tears, these lesions rarely need surgical intervention (1,9). Traditionally it was taught that arteriography is indicated in all patients because of the devastating complications of missed injuries that can lead to limb ischemia and amputation.

Emergency management involves rapid reduction of the dislocation, especially if vascular compromise is evident. It can be accomplished by longitudinal traction (Fig. 195.4). If the clinical status permits, intravenous sedation and analgesia may facilitate the reduction. The limb's neurovascular status must be reassessed periodically, particularly after manipulation. If the patient is stable, appropriate diagnostic tests and orthopaedic and vascular surgery consultations should be quickly obtained.

Patellar Dislocation

The patella may be completely dislocated or subluxed from the intercondylar groove as a result of a direct blow or by hyperflexion of the knee joint. The patella almost always displaces laterally, and this injury is common in adolescent girls. The patient often reports previous episodes in which subluxations were spontaneously reduced.

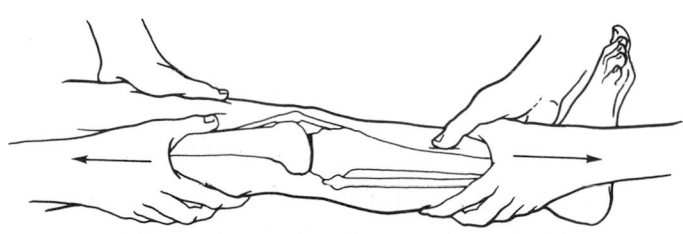

Figure 195.4. Technique for reduction of knee dislocation.

The physical examination generally reveals an inability to extend the knee and an obvious deformity. A joint effusion is commonly present, and the subluxed patella may often reduce spontaneously. The apprehension sign may suggest this injury. Plain radiographs help confirm the diagnosis if it is not apparent on clinical examination. If the patella has spontaneously reduced, plain films will confirm proper placement and identify any bony injury. If subluxations are recurrent, plain films may assist in the evaluation of the anatomy of the patellofemoral joint and help direct further treatment.

Emergency management of subluxations involves acute reduction. It is usually performed by applying medial force to the patella while the knee is being extended. Appropriate sedation and analgesia are often necessary. Once reduced, the knee is immobilized and the patient treated with elevation, ice, and crutches. Complete dislocations often require surgical repair to decrease the incidence of recurrence or subluxation.

Collateral Ligamentous Injuries

The collateral ligaments protect the knee from varus and valgus stresses. The MCL is the most commonly injured ligamentous structure in the knee. It is typically injured in sporting events when a direct valgus force is applied to the knee while the foot is relatively stationary. The LCL can also be injured, but injury to it is less likely to occur during athletic events. LCL injuries are more commonly seen after falls and MVCs. MCL and LCL tears are associated with cruciate ligament injuries, with the LCL injury less likely to occur as an isolated event.

The patient generally presents with tenderness along the distribution of the ligament. There is often a history of "popping" and abnormal bending of the knee. The physical examination should include the previously listed diagnostic tests, with varus and valgus forces applied to the knee at extension and 30 degrees of flexion (8). The presence of an associated effusion may complicate the examination, warranting a few days of elevation and immobilization prior to reexamination.

Treatment is based on the severity of the injury. First- and second-degree sprains are treated with immobilization, ice, and crutches. Followup examination by an orthopedist is required to reevaluate the patient's progress and the need for further intervention (e.g., arthroscopy, surgical repair).

Cruciate Ligamentous Injuries

Injuries to the cruciate ligaments are common with low-velocity trauma (e.g., football, basketball) as well as with high-energy forces. The patient usually reports a direct anterior or posterior blow to the knee. The cruciates can also be injured by rotational forces, usually in association with other soft-tissue trauma (e.g., collateral ligaments, menisci). The ACL is weaker than the PCL and is more commonly injured.

The patient often presents with a swollen, tender knee. Seventy percent of patients presenting with an acute, traumatic hemarthrosis have a tear of the ACL. Because the cruciate ligaments are located deep in the articular surface and are associated with a high incidence of joint effusions, clinical diagnosis is often difficult.

Tests for ACL injuries include the Lachman, anterior drawer, and pivot shift tests. The Lachman test is the most sensitive. PCL stability is evaluated by the posterior drawer and posterior sag tests. Plain radiographs are of little value. MRI scanning is the best imaging test to evaluate the cruciate ligaments.

Arthroscopy is used for both diagnosis and treatment. Definitive treatment is based on factors such as the patient's age, level of activity, and the severity of the injury. Initially, immobilization and orthopaedic consultation are necessary.

Meniscal Tears

Meniscal injuries generally occur with a twisting force applied to the knee. The twisting may result from relatively minor forces, such as those produced when rising from a squatting position. Patients frequently complain of hearing a "snap" or "pop," which is common but not specific to meniscal injuries. Often, the patient reports locking of the knee, usually a result of a "bucket handle" tear of the meniscus, with a free central portion of the cartilage becoming lodged in the intercondylar notch. The medial meniscus is most commonly affected.

The patient usually presents with a joint effusion. Unlike the hemarthrosis seen with an ACL rupture, the effusion accumulates much more slowly, generally over 12 to 24 hours. Pain is usually localized to the side of the knee where the tear is located. A decrease in the range of motion is often noted and may be related to the effusion or a loose body. Diagnostic tests include the McMurray and Apley tests. MRI scanning is very helpful in defining the anatomy of the meniscus and in pinpointing injuries.

Arthroscopy is generally reserved for treatment, as the accuracy of the MRI is well documented. Initial treatment consists of immobilization, analgesia, and outpatient orthopaedic referral within 1 week. Definitive treatment is based on clinical evaluation. If symptoms persist, meniscectomy is generally performed arthroscopically.

Tendon Injuries

The extensor mechanism includes the quadriceps tendon, the patella, and the patellar tendon. Injuries to these structures, or avulsion of the tibial tubercle, can disrupt the extensor mechanism. Disruption may result from high-energy or penetrating trauma, but is also seen with low-energy forces. Tendon ruptures associated with low-energy trauma commonly occur when the tendons are weakened (e.g., by gout, arthritis, infection, metabolic diseases, tenosynovitis, previous trauma). If the tendon is already weakened, rupture may occur with forceful contraction of the quadriceps.

Generally, the patellar tendon is least likely to rupture. The quadriceps tendon is more commonly ruptured, and this is usually seen in elderly patients. The quadriceps tendon usually ruptures just proximal to the patella. The patellar tendon frequently ruptures at the insertion into the patella.

The physical examination generally reveals a swollen, tender knee, and a palpable deficit may be present. Tenderness is usually identified at the site of injury. To evaluate the tendons properly, the patient's ability to extend the knee fully against resistance must be tested. The diagnosis is usually suspected clinically. Partial injuries may be difficult, if not impossible to detect in the ED. X-ray findings may include a high-riding patella (patella alta) with a patellar tendon rupture, or low-riding patella (patella baja) with quadriceps tendon rupture. CT or MRI may be needed but can be performed on an outpatient basis.

A complete rupture requires surgical repair. Incomplete ruptures usually will heal in 6 to 8 weeks with immobilization. They necessitate outpatient orthopaedic referral within 5 to 7 days for further evaluation and definitive management.

Bursitis

Local inflammation and subsequent bursitis may be a complication of knee trauma. The bursae of the knee are illustrated in Fig. 195.5.

The physical examination often reveals a swollen, tender knee with a localized effusion that is warm to the touch. Other causes of knee swelling (hemarthrosis, infection) should be considered

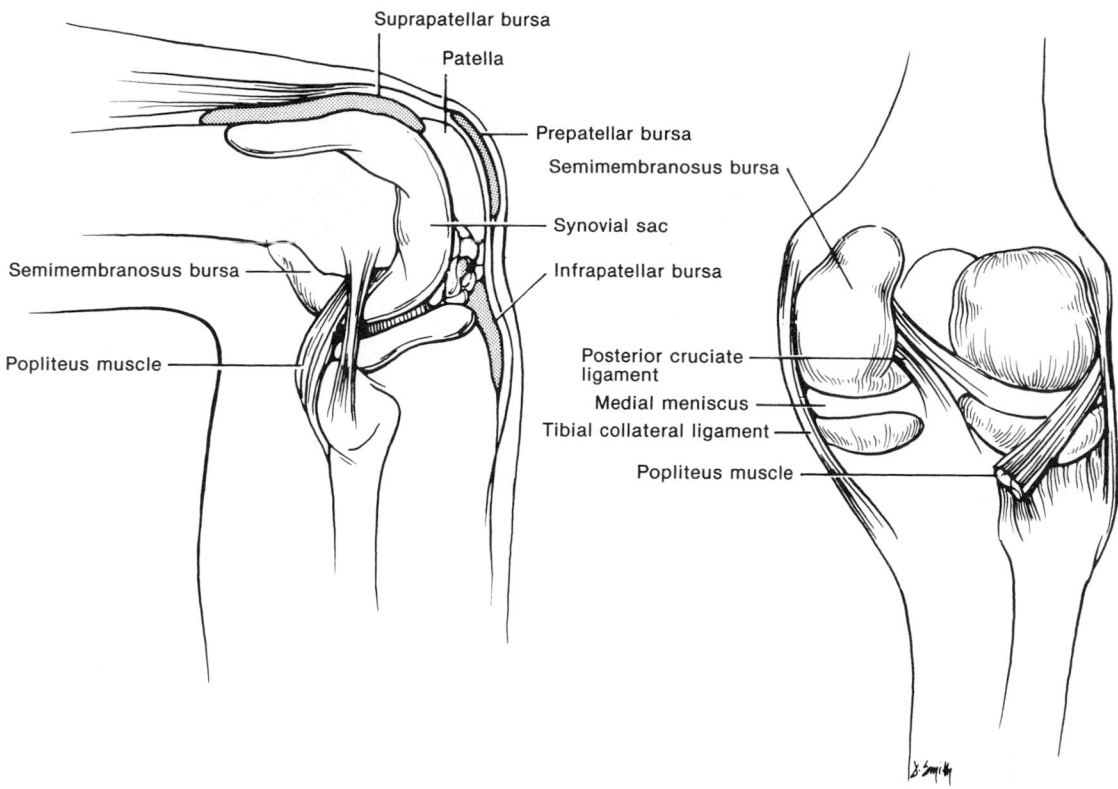

Figure 195.5. Bursae of the knee.

and evaluated. Arthrocentesis and joint fluid analysis are performed if an effusion is present.

If bursitis is suspected, rest, ice, and nonsteroidal antiinflammatory medications are prescribed. The patient is referred to an orthopedist for follow up.

CRITICAL INTERVENTIONS

- Rapidly reduce knee dislocations utilizing longitudinal traction after intravenous sedation and analgesia, especially when vascular compromise is present
- Perform arteriography in patients with knee dislocations if there are hard signs of vascular injury (absent pulses, expanding hematoma, hemorrhage, ischemia or bruit)

DISPOSITION

Many of the knee injuries described may be evaluated in the ED and safely referred for orthopaedic follow up as an outpatient. The physician should ensure that the patient is properly immobilized, has appropriate analgesia, has instructions on specific restrictions (weight-bearing, crutches), and is provided with an orthopaedic referral. Follow-up appointments should generally take place within 1 week. Common injuries that may be handled in this manner include tibial spine fractures, suspected ligament or tendon injuries, nondisplaced patella fractures, tibial tuberosity fractures, and reduced patellar subluxations.

More severe injuries will mandate hospital admission. Significantly displaced fractures, open fractures, fractures with associated vascular or nerve damage, and injuries with the potential to develop compartment syndrome should all be admitted for further evaluation and treatment. Injuries which typically will fall into this category include distal femur fractures, tibial

plateau fractures, patella fractures (with disruption of the extensor mechanism), significant ligamentous injuries, and knee dislocations.

COMMON PITFALLS

✔ Performing an examination while the patient is sitting in a wheelchair
✔ Failure to examine the hip carefully. Knee pain is often referred from the hip, and knee trauma may precipitate hip injuries
✔ Performing a soft-tissue examination in the face of joint effusion and muscle guarding. A period of immobilization and reexamination is indicated after the effusion resolves
✔ Mistaking bipartite patella for a patellar fracture
✔ Failure to examine the knee in full extension against resistance, when evaluating the extensor mechanism
✔ Failure to diagnose a proximal fibula fracture or dislocation resulting from an ankle injury
✔ Failure to consider Osgood-Schlatter disease in an adolescent with knee pain

Acknowledgment

Thanks to the previous edition's chapter author Nicholas H. Benson.

References

1. Barnes CJ, Pietrobon R, Higgins LD. Does the pulse examination in patients with traumatic knee dislocation predict a surgical arterial injury? A meta-analysis. *J Trauma* 2002;53:1109–1114.
2. Bulloch B, Neto G, Plint A, et al. Validation of the Ottawa knee rules in children: A multicenter study. *Ann Emerg Med* 2003;42:48–55.
3. Cosgarea AJ, Jay PR. Posterior cruciate ligament injuries: Evaluation and management. *J Amer Acad Orthoped Surg* 2001;9:297–307.
4. Emparanza JI, Aginaga JR. Validation of the Ottawa knee rules. *Ann Emerg Med* 2001;38:364–368.

5. Eren OT. The accuracy of joint line tenderness by physical examination in the diagnosis of meniscal tears. *Arthroscopy: J Arthroscopic Rel Surg* 2003;19:850–854.

6. Fuchs S, Chylarecki C. Sonographic evaluation of ACL rupture signs compared to arthroscopic findings in acutely injured knees *Ultrasound in Med & Biol* 2002;28:149–154.

7. Jackson JL, O'Malley PG, Kroneke K. Evaluation of acute knee pain in primary care. *Ann Intern Med* 2003;139:575–588.

8. Malanga GA, Andrus S, Nadler SF, McLean J. Physical examination of the knee: A review of the original test description and scientific validity of common orthopaedic tests. *Arch Phys Med Rehabil* 2003;84:592–603.

9. Miranda FE, Dennis JW, Veldnez HC, et al. Confirmation of the safety and accuracy of physical examination in the evaluation of knee dislocation for injury of the popliteal artery: A prospective study. *J Trauma* 2002;52:247–251.

10. Miller TT. Sonography of injury of the posterior cruciate ligament of the knee. *Skeletal Radiol* 2002;31:149–154.

11. Sarimo J, Rantanen J, Heikkila J, Orava S, Acute traumatic extension deficit of the knee. *Scand J Med Sci Sports* 2003;13:155–158.

12. Scholten RJ, Opstelten W, van der Plas CG, Bijl D, et al. Accuracy of physical diagnostic tests for assessing ruptures of the anterior cruciate ligament: A meta-analysis. *J Fam Prac* 2003;52:689–694.

13. Tandeter HB, Shvartzman P. Acute knee injuries: use of decision rules for selective radiograph ordering. *Am Fam Physician* 1999;60:2599–2608.

14. Twaddle BC, Bidwell TA, Chapman JR. Knee dislocations: Where are the lesions? *J Ortho Trauma* 2003;17:198–202.

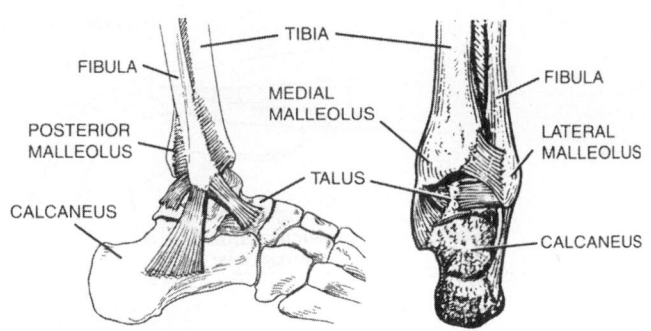

Figure 196.1. The ankle. (From Ankel F. The Ankle. In: Hart RG, Rittenberry TJ, Uehara DT (eds). *Handbook of orthopaedic emergencies.* Philadelphia: Lippincott Raven, 1999, with permission.)

CHAPTER 196
Ankle and Foot Injuries

Kaushal Shah

Ankle injuries are among the most common sports-related and extremity injuries presenting to the emergency department (ED) (1,12,14). Although the vast majority are benign injuries, there are instances when immediate action and emergent consultation are necessary.

The ankle and foot are relatively simple structures. The ankle is formed by: (1) the tibia which forms the medial malleolus, posterior malleolus and the plafond (ceiling); (2) the fibula which forms the lateral malleolus; and (3) the talus (Fig. 196.1). The ankle is held together by (1) the medial ligaments (collectively termed deltoid ligament); (2) the lateral ligaments (anterior talofibular ligament [ATFL], calcaneofibular ligament [CFL] and posterior talofibular ligament [PTFL]) and (3) the syndesmosis between the distal tibia and fibula (Fig. 196.2). The foot has 3 general parts: the hindfoot (calcaneus and talus), the midfoot (navicular, cuboid and cuneiforms) and the forefoot (metatarsals and phalanges) (Fig. 196.3).

CLINICAL PRESENTATION

Ankle sprains comprise 75% of ankle injuries with approximately 90% due to inversion of the ankle resulting in sprain of the lateral ligaments, most commonly the ATFL (1). Significant injuries from an eversion mechanism are far less common because the broad deltoid ligament is strong and resistant to tears. Key historical factors include the ability to ambulate and a history of previous injuries.

Ankle fractures can present after a significant traumatic mechanism or after a simple ankle inversion or eversion twisting injury. Most common "red flags" suggestive of a fracture rather than a sprain are inability to bear weight or significant swelling or tenderness. The ankle should be considered a closed ring with the tibia, fibula and talus as the main parts held together by ligaments. A break in two or more places results in instability.

EMERGENCY DEPARTMENT MANAGEMENT

Ankle Ligamentous Injuries

The clinical findings associated with ankle sprains range from mild pain and swelling to severe pain with edema and ecchymosis. Neurovascular status (palpable posterior tibial and dorsalis pedis pulses, rapid capillary refill, and distal sensation) should be checked. However, it is extremely unlikely that the neurovascular status will be compromised in a sprain without gross deformity. Palpation of the medial and lateral malleoli and the base of the 5th metatarsal for focal tenderness is critical to evaluate for associated fracture. The Ottawa Ankle and Foot Rules have been demonstrated to be useful in determining which patients do not need radiographic evaluation for an ankle injury; the sensitivities range from 97% to 100% (Table 196.1) (4,5,10). In the pediatric population, the Ottawa Ankle Rules have been shown to be 100% sensitive for predicting significant ankle and midfoot fractures in one study of 670 children 2 to 16 years of age (8). If x-rays are obtained, the physician should inspect the AP view for talar shift and malleolar fractures, the mortise view for widening of the tibial-talar joint, and the lateral view for posterior malleolar fracture and general alignment.

Provocative tests for ankle stability are necessary to determine the grade of injury. The *anterior drawer test* assesses the integrity of the ATFL (Fig. 196.4). The test is positive if greater subluxation is noted on the injured ankle than the opposite one. The *talar tilt test* can be used to assess the lateral and medial ligaments (Fig. 196.5). If there is significant subluxation with inversion, tears of the ATFL or CFL should be suspected. Significant subluxation with eversion raises suspicion for a tear of the deltoid ligament. Integrity of the tibiofibular syndesmosis can be

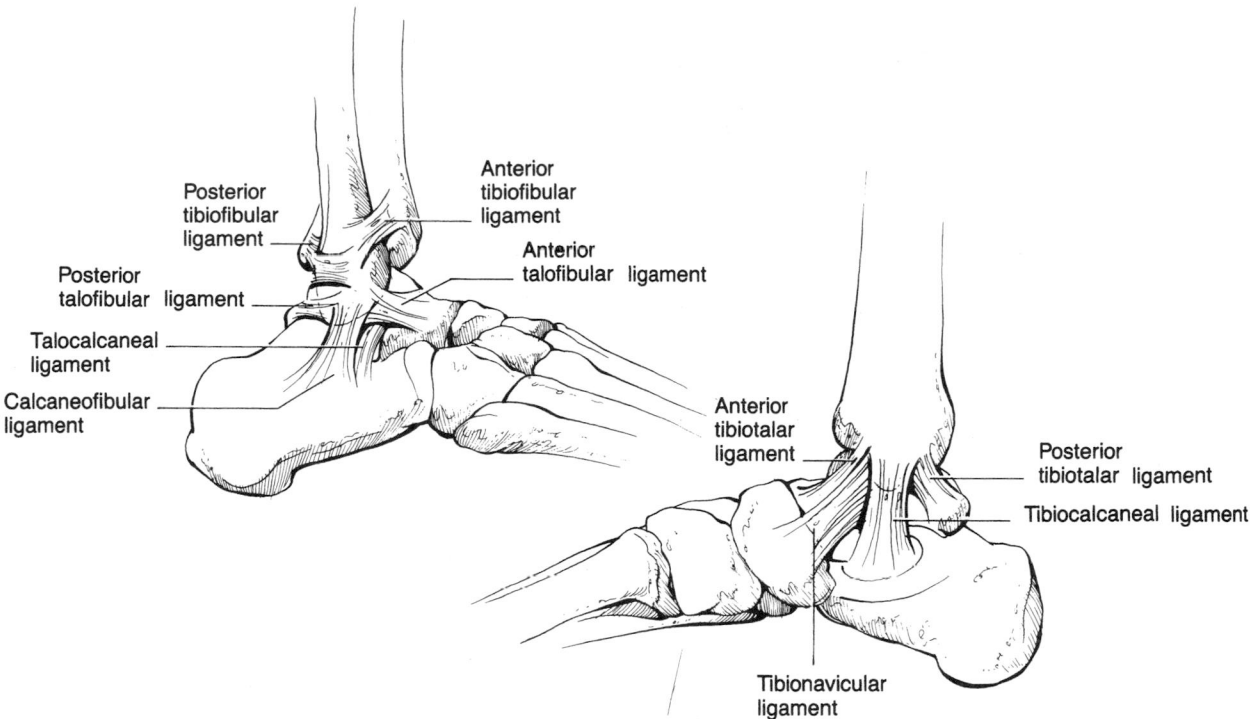

Figure 196.2.   The ankle ligaments: (**A**) lateral view; (**B**) medial view.

tested via the *squeeze test* which involves squeezing the proximal tibia and fibula together. If pain is elicited, the test is positive (Fig. 196.6).

Acutely, ibuprofen 10 mg/kg (not to exceed 800 mg) PO or acetaminophen 15 mg/kg (not to exceed 1000 mg) PO should be administered for pain. Toradol 30 to 60 mg IM or IV, in an adult, is also effective. General management guidelines follow the "*RICE*" mnemonic: *r*est ankle and avoid re-injury which may entail use of crutches; *i*ce the ankle for 20 minutes 3 to 4 times per day for the first day to reduce swelling; *c*ompress with an elastic ACE wrap or ankle brace to reduce swelling and pain; *e*levate the extremity as often as possible to reduce swelling. Table 196.2 describes the management based on the grade of the injury. If serious ligamentous injury is suspected, resulting in joint laxity (i.e., Grade II and higher sprains), more rigid splinting methods should be considered. An air stirrup splint is moderately effective in preventing inversion and eversion of the ankle and is appropriate for Grade I and II ankle sprains. For Grade III injuries, a short leg posterior rigid splint (e.g., plaster) that runs from mid-calf to the toes should be used to further immobilize the ankle in order to prevent worsening of the injury and promote healing.

All patients with ankle sprains can be discharged home but should have appropriate follow up within 1 week. Although pain, swelling and the ability to ambulate should improve with time, occult fractures and high-grade sprains may require further orthopaedic or sports medicine care. Other indications for orthopaedic referral include: (1) a "pop" that is heard or felt, (2) a history of several previous injuries, (3) medial ankle tenderness, (4) a positive squeeze test or other stress test, and (5) Grade II and higher sprains in children with open growth plates (11). In children, less force is required to sustain a Salter-Harris I fracture than is required to tear a ligament. Thus, any patient who is suspected of having a significant ankle sprain and no clear fracture on x-ray should be splinted and referred to an orthopaedic surgeon for followup.

Ankle Fractures

There are several types of ankle fractures that should be considered in the differential diagnosis. A *lateral malleolus* fracture is the most common type of ankle fracture.

Isolated *medial malleolus* fractures are less common because the injury requires more force than a lateral malleolus fracture. Therefore, other associated fractures and joint instability should be suspected. Patients with *bi-* or *tri-malleolar fractures* present with significant pain, swelling and ecchymosis. Associated dislocations are common. Orthopaedic consultation is necessary. A *plafond fracture* is a fracture through the articular surface of the distal tibia resulting from the talus striking the distal tibia in the dorsiflexed position with high energy (Fig. 196.7). A *pilon fracture is a* comminuted fracture of the distal tibia and fibula that results from an axial compression force to the tibial plafond (Fig. 196.8). The *Maisonneuve fracture* is an oblique fracture of the proximal fibula associated with a medial malleolus fracture or deltoid ligament tear. It can easily be missed if the proximal fibula is not routinely palpated in patients with ankle twisting injuries.

As with ankle sprains, neurovascular status should be checked immediately. The history and physical exam is identical to that of ankle sprains. If there is gross deformity, a dislocation should be considered and should be reduced emergently if there is neurovascular compromise. Lacerations and wounds should be examined closely to ensure that an open fracture is not present.

Suspected ankle fractures require x-rays in three views. The two most common classification systems for ankle fractures are the *Lauge-Hansen* and *Danis-Weber*. The Danis-Weber Classification system is simpler and is based on the location of the fibular fracture (Fig. 196.9). A fibular avulsion fracture below the tibiotalar joint line is called a *Weber type A* fracture. If the fibular fracture is in the joint line, it is a *Weber type B* fracture. Fractures above the joint line disrupting the syndesmosis ligament are termed *Weber type C* fractures.

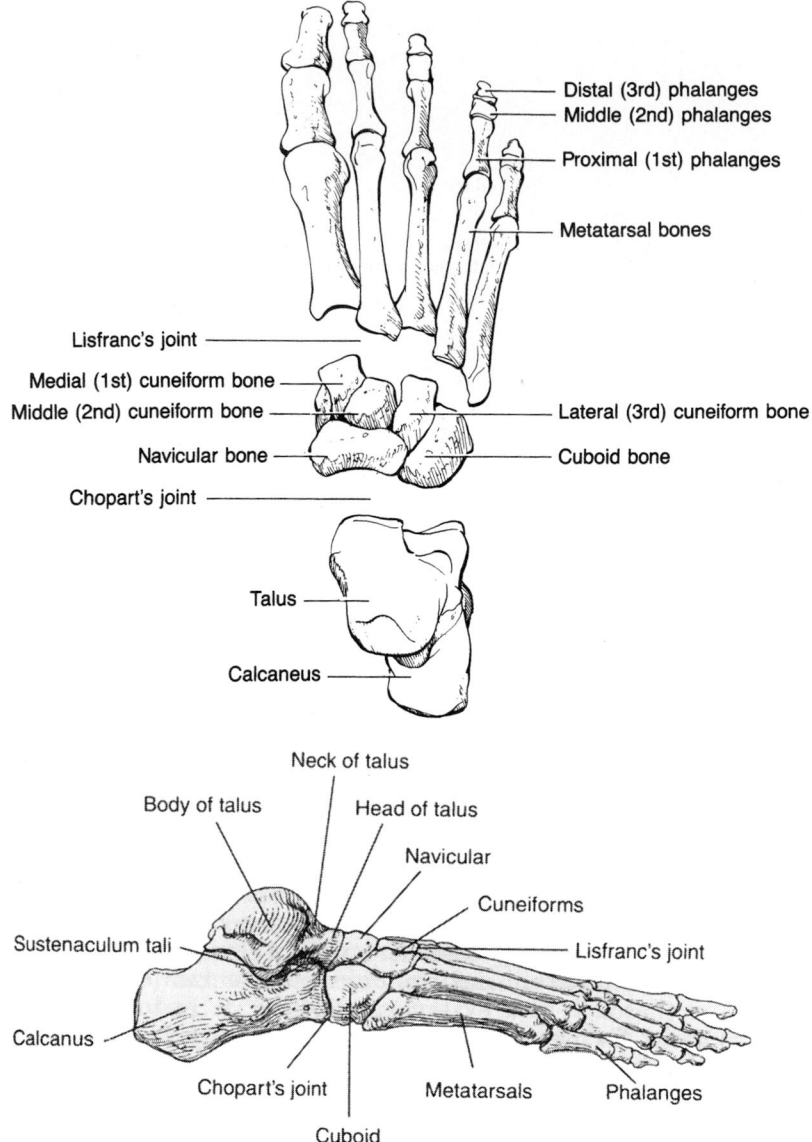

Figure 196.3.   Bones of the Foot. (Bottom from Ankel F. The Foot. In: Hart RG, Rittenberry TJ, Uehara DT (eds). *Handbook of orthopaedic emergencies.* Philadelphia: Lippincott Raven, 1999, with permission.)

Patients should receive adequate analgesia. Intravenous (IV), intramuscular (IM), and subcutaneous (SQ) injections are preferred (rather than oral administration) until it is certain the patient will not require an operative procedure. Isolated lateral or medial malleolar fractures without instability can be safely discharged home without orthopaedic consultation in the ED. The emergency physician should first place the ankle in a posterior splint, provide crutches for nonweight bearing, provide adequate analgesia and ensure close orthopaedic follow up. All other ankle fractures require orthopaedic consultation in the ED.

Isolated fractures of the distal tibia and fibula should be immobilized in a short leg posterior splint. A *sugar tong* splint (U-splint) can also be used; it wraps along both the medial and lateral sides of the leg with the base of the "U" under the foot (similar to an air stirrup) and is more effective in stabilizing the medial and lateral ligaments. Patients with severe injuries to the ankle, such as bi- and trimalleolar fractures, should be placed in both a posterior splint and a sugar tong splint

TABLE 196.1.   Ottawa Criteria for Ankle Radiographs

An ankle radiographic series is required in patients aged 18–55 only if there is any malleolar pain and any of the following findings:
1. Bone tenderness at the posterior edge or tip of the medial malleolus
2. Bone tenderness at the posterior edge or tip of the lateral malleolus
3. Inability to bear weight for four steps both immediately and in the emergency department

(From Ankel F. The Ankle. In: Hart RG, Rittenberry TJ and Uehara DT (eds). *Handbook of Orthopaedic Emergencies.* Philadelphia: Lippincott-Raven Publishers, 1999, with permission.)

TABLE 196.2. Classification of Ankle Sprains

Severity	Symptoms	Signs	Examination	Treatment
Grade I	Mild pain and swelling, able to bear weight	Slight edema	Negative anterior drawer and talar tilt	RICE* and referral to primary care physician in 1 week
Grade II	Moderate pain and swelling, difficulty bearing weight	Moderate edema and ecchymosis	Positive anterior drawer (4–14 mm) and talar tilt test (5–15 degrees)	Rigid splint and referral to orthopaedist in a week
Grade III	Severe pain and swelling, inability to bear weight	Severe edema and ecchymosis	Positive anterior (>15 mm) and tilt test (>15 degrees)	Rigid splint and referral to orthopaedist within a week

*Rest, ice, compressive dressing, and elevation.
(From Ankel F. The Ankle. In: Hart RG, Rittenberry TJ and Uehara DT (eds). *Handbook of orthopaedic emergencies.* Philadelphia: Lippincott–Raven Publishers, 1999, with permission.)

("AO" splint). This provides immobilization similar to that of casting.

Ankle Dislocations

In order for the talus to dislocate from the distal tibia, multiple ligaments are torn and there are often associated malleolar fractures. Significant force is required and there is always gross deformity and inability to bear weight.

The emergency physician should perform immediate reduction if there is neurovascular compromise or significant skin tenting with concern for conversion into an open fracture-dislocation. In cases of uncomplicated dislocations, x-ray evaluation should precede reduction.

Reduction of the ankle requires conscious sedation and 2 assistants. For posterior dislocations, the first assistant flexes the knee to 45 degrees and applies counter-traction over the calf while the second assistant pushes down on the front of the lower leg. The physician applies traction to the heel and forefoot after first plantar flexing the foot and then lifting the heel (Fig. 196.10). For anterior dislocations, the first assistant flexes the knee to

45 degrees and applies counter-traction over the calf while the second assistant lifts up on the lower leg. The physician should dorsiflex the foot initially to disengage the talus and then push downward on the foot (Fig. 196.11). For lateral dislocations, the physician applies longitudinal and medial traction while an assistant applies counter-traction.

Orthopaedic consultation is necessary for all fracture-dislocations of the ankle. If a patient needs to be transferred, the emergency physician should reduce the ankle and place the ankle in a short leg posterior splint (with or without a sugar tong splint). Prior to transfer, IV antibiotics should be administered if the dislocation is open. Cefazolin 1 to 2 gm IV in adults is usually adequate but patients with contaminated wounds should also receive gentamicin 2 mg/kg IV.

Achilles Tendon Rupture

The classic presentation is a middle-aged man complaining of ankle pain and inability to bear weight after hearing a "pop" while playing sports. Risk factors for rupture include steroid injections and tendonitis. The Achilles tendon usually ruptures at the narrowest segment approximately 5 cm above its attachment to the calcaneus.

Occasionally an obvious defect in the Achilles tendon can be palpated. However, the most useful signs of this injury are weakness of plantar flexion and a positive *Thompson test* (the foot does not plantar flex when the calf is squeezed). The test is performed with the patient prone and the knee flexed to 90 degrees.

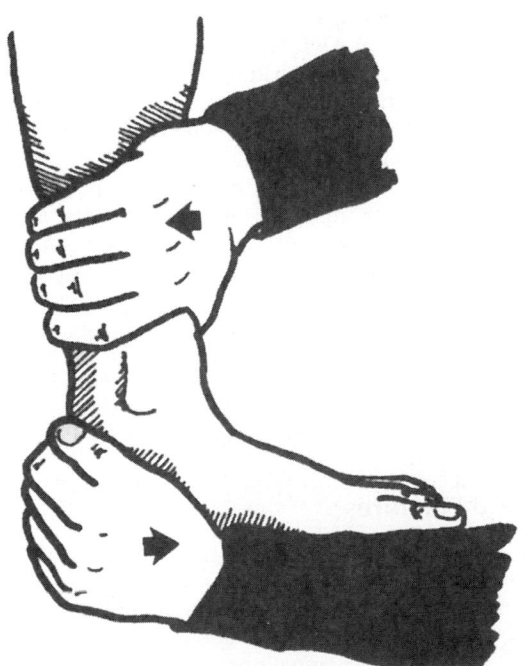

Figure 196.4. The anterior drawer test. (From Ankel F. The Ankle. In: Hart RG, Rittenberry TJ, Uehara DT (eds). *Handbook of orthopaedic emergencies.* Philadelphia: Lippincott Raven, 1999, with permission.)

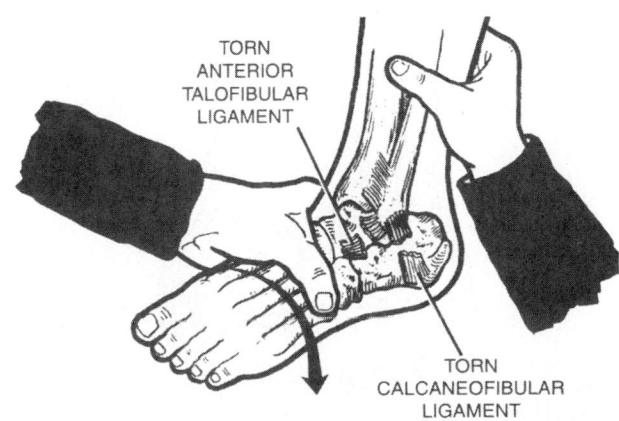

TORN ANTERIOR TALOFIBULAR LIGAMENT

TORN CALCANEOFIBULAR LIGAMENT

Figure 196.5. The talar tilt test. (From Ankel F. The Ankle. In: Hart RG, Rittenberry TJ, Uehara DT (eds). *Handbook of orthopaedic emergencies.* Philadelphia: Lippincott Raven, 1999, with permission.)

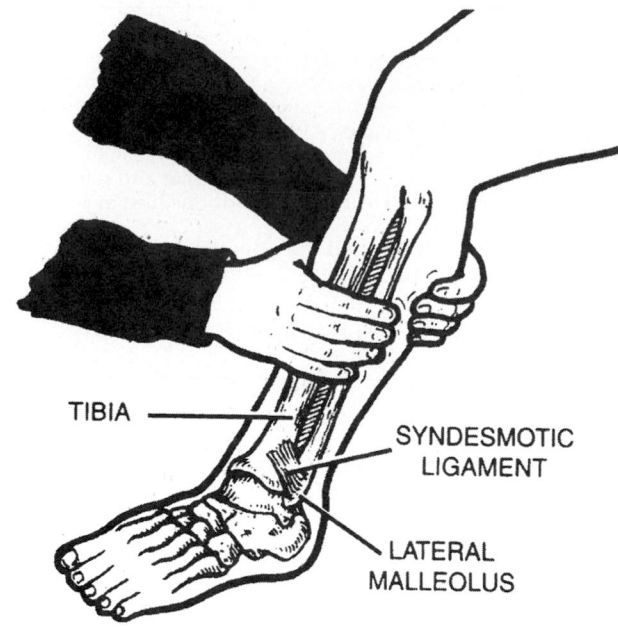

Figure 196.6.   The squeeze test. (From Ankel F. The Ankle. In: Hart RG, Rittenberry TJ, Uehara DT (eds). *Handbook of orthopaedic emergencies.* Philadelphia: Lippincott Raven, 1999, with permission.)

Orthopaedic consultation should be obtained since early surgical repair results in better outcomes (2). It is also appropriate to place a posterior splint with the foot in plantar flexion and refer to an orthopedist within 48 to 72 hours.

Peroneal Tendon Subluxation

These patients present very similar to those with a simple ankle sprain. However, the mechanism is different. The injury is caused by dorsiflexion and eversion of the ankle resulting in contraction of the peroneal muscle and disruption of the peroneal retinaculum. Because the peroneal tendon subluxes out of its groove along the posterior lateral malleolus, the ankle is swollen, tender and ecchymotic around the lateral malleolus.

Although x-rays are negative for bony disruptions, these patients should be placed in a sugar tong splint with extra lateral

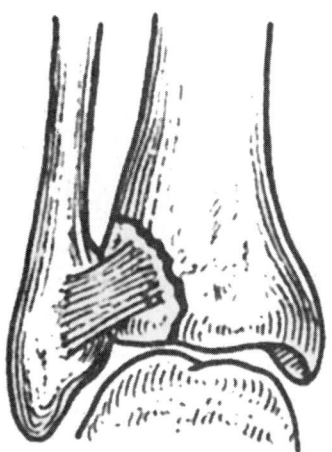

Figure 196.7.   Plafond fracture. (From Ankel F. The Ankle. In: Hart RG, Rittenberry TJ, Uehara DT (eds). *Handbook of orthopaedic emergencies.* Philadelphia: Lippincott Raven, 1999, with permission.)

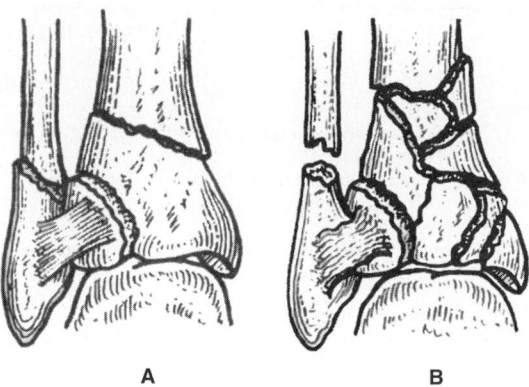

Figure 196.8.   Pilon fracture. (From Ankel F. The Ankle. In: Hart RG, Rittenberry TJ, Uehara DT (eds). *Handbook of orthopaedic emergencies.* Philadelphia: Lippincott Raven, 1999, with permission.)

malleolar padding. Patients should be referred to an orthopedist within a week for casting and should remain nonweight bearing for 4 to 6 weeks. Occasionally, surgery is recommended for athletes, those who fail nonoperative management and those with chronic subluxations (13).

Lisfranc Fracture-Dislocation

The Lisfranc joint is the joint between the midfoot and forefoot (metatarsals and phalanges). Direct trauma or hyperdorsiflexion of the Lisfranc joint (e.g., motor vehicle accident) can result in a Lisfranc fracture-dislocation defined as a fracture at the base of the 2nd metatarsal or 2nd cuneiform with dislocation of the lateral 4 metatarsals. The occurrence is rare but results in significant morbidity when there is a delay in treatment. This particular fracture has a high misdiagnosis rate of approximately 20%.

The foot is usually very swollen and tender. Plantar ecchymosis has been described as a relatively common finding in patients with Lisfranc fracture-dislocations (9).

When examining an AP foot x-ray, the physician should look for a fracture at the base of the 2nd metatarsal and assess alignment of the cuneiform bones with the metatarsals. The space between the bases of the 1st and 2nd metatarsal bones is widened, especially on the oblique view (Fig. 196.12).

Lisfranc fracture-dislocations require orthopaedic consultation in the ED. These injuries require open reduction and internal fixation to improve outcome and reduce complications. If an orthopaedic consultant is not immediately available, the physician should provide analgesia and place the patient in a short leg posterior splint, preferably with a sugar tong splint. The patient should be nonweight bearing. Orthopaedic follow up should occur within 24 to 48 hours, and the timing of definitive treatment and the degree of reduction are critical to the outcome.

Calcaneal Fractures

A vertical compression force, such as jumping or falling from a height and landing directly on the feet is the most common etiology of calcaneal fractures. They occur more commonly in men who are 30 to 50 years old. Patients complain of heel pain and have difficulty bearing weight.

Three radiographic views (AP, lateral, and axial) of the heel should be obtained. Fractures are often not clearly visible due to a predominantly compressive force. A helpful measurement

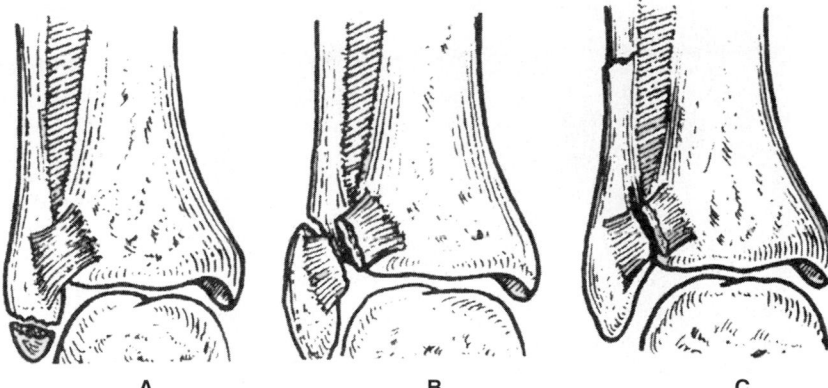

Figure 196.9. The Weber classification. (From Ankel F. The Ankle. In: Hart RG, Rittenberry TJ, Uehara DT (eds). *Handbook of orthopaedic emergencies.* Philadelphia: Lippincott Raven, 1999, with permission.)

to make the diagnosis is determination of *Boehler's angle* on the lateral view (Fig. 196.13). A normal angle is 20 to 40 degrees and an angle less than 20 degrees indicates a calcaneal fracture.

Due to the mechanism and force required, a thorough trauma evaluation is important. Calcaneal fractures are specifically associated with lumbar spine injuries in 10% of patients.

Patients with calcaneal fractures require emergent orthopaedic evaluation. Operative verses nonoperative management is controversial. However, both are associated with a high incidence of chronic pain and loss of joint mobility and function. If orthopaedic consultation is not immediately available and the patient has no associated injuries warranting admission, the physician should provide analgesia and place the patient in a short leg posterior splint. The patient should be nonweight bearing. Orthopaedic follow up should occur within 24 to 48 hours.

Talus Fractures

A high-impact mechanism is required to fracture the talus. A hyperdorsiflexion injury from a motor vehicle collision or fall from a height is necessary to compress the talus between the tibia and calcaneus. Osteochondral fractures of the talar dome (also termed *"osteochondritis dessicans"*) occur after an inversion mechanism. Patients usually present with chronic pain after the diagnosis is missed on the initial visit because physical findings are nonspecific and plain radiographs may be normal.

Unlike talar dome fractures, fractures through the body and neck are usually visible on plain radiographs. It is particularly important to evaluate for the commonly associated *subtalar dislocation*. In addition, the *os trigonum* (accessory bone) can occasionally be mistaken for a posterior process fracture. Suspected talar dome fractures require bone scan, CT or MRI for further evaluation and classification.

Talus fractures require evaluation and continued care by an orthopaedic surgeon because the bone has a tenuous blood supply and, as a result, there is a high rate of avascular necrosis. Most talar fractures require short-leg casting for 6 to 8 weeks but some require open reduction and internal fixation. Patients should be nonweight bearing. Disposition is based on recommendations by the orthopedist. Patients can be referred for an outpatient CT or MRI for suspected talar dome fractures.

Subtalar Dislocation

A subtalar dislocation involves the talocalcaneal and talonavicular joints (without disruption of the tibiotalar joint). This injury results from a significant torsional force usually causing a medial or lateral dislocation. There is usually an obvious deformity of the foot, but swelling can occasionally mask the deformity.

As with any dislocation, assessing the neurovascular status is important. Although uncommon, compromised neurovascular status is an indication for immediate reduction. Plain films of the foot are diagnostic; the AP view is most likely to reveal the subtalar dislocation.

Subtalar dislocations require urgent closed reduction either under conscious sedation or general anesthesia. Reduction is preformed by flexing the knee and applying longitudinal traction on the foot with initial reproduction of the injury followed

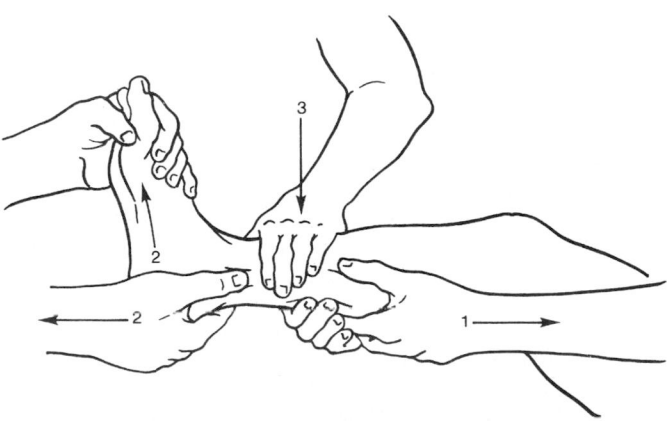

Figure 196.10. Technique of reduction of posterior dislocation of the ankle.

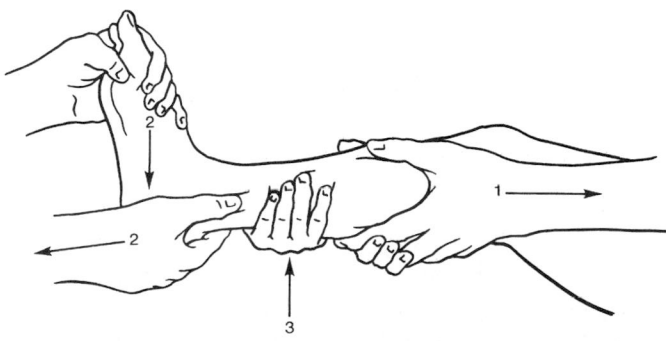

Figure 196.11. Technique of reduction of anterior dislocation of the ankle.

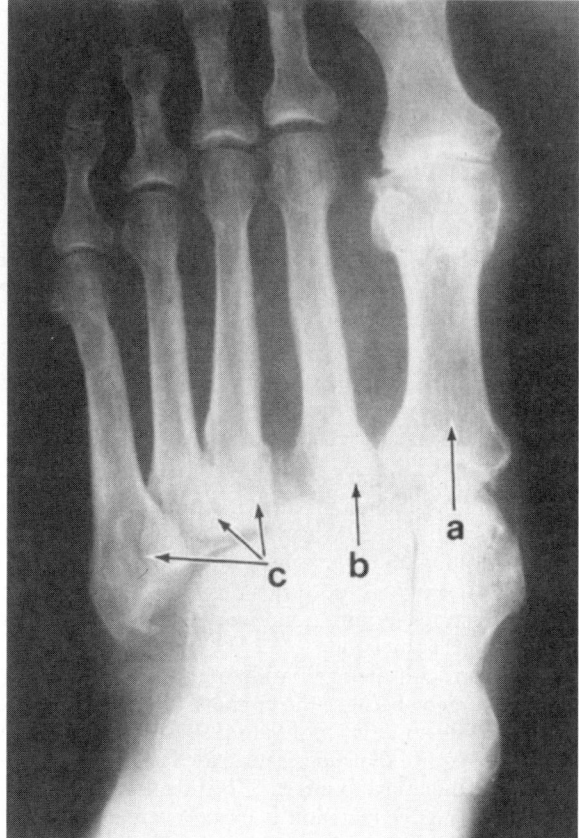

Figure 196.12. Radiograph of a Lisfranc dislocation: (**A**) first metatarsal; (**B**) second metatarsal; (**C**) third, fourth, and fifth metatarsals, which have been discolated laterally.

by reversal of the deformity. If closed reduction in the ED is unsuccessful, orthopaedic consultation is essential. Successfully reduced subtalar dislocations should be immobilized with a short leg posterior splint and sugar tongs (U-splint). After reduction, if orthopaedic consultation is not available in the ED, follow up should occur within 24 to 48 hours.

Midfoot Fractures

Fractures of the midfoot (cuboid, navicular and cuneiforms) are rare and usually occur from direct, blunt trauma. Isolated bone fractures are the exception and most injuries involve a combina-

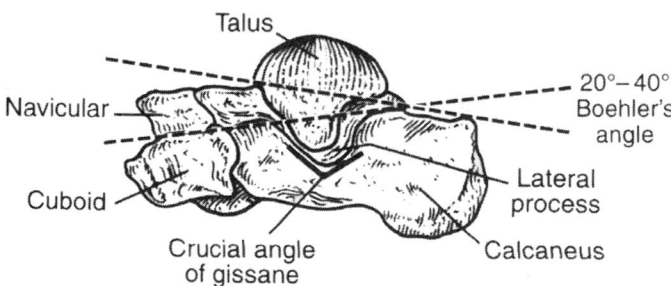

Figure 196.13. Boehler's angle. (From Ankel F. The Ankle. In: Hart RG, Rittenberry TJ, Uehara DT (eds). *Handbook of orthopaedic emergencies.* Philadelphia: Lippincott Raven, 1999, with permission.)

tion of fractures. There is usually focal tenderness and swelling over the fractured bones.

Midfoot fractures are usually visible on plain radiographs. Nondisplaced fractures can be immobilized with a posterior splint and patients can be discharged with prompt orthopaedic follow up for evaluation and a short leg cast (for 6–8 weeks). Patients should be nonweight bearing; ice and elevation should be used in the first 24 hours to keep swelling to a minimum.

Fifth Metatarsal Fractures

Fractures of the 5th metatarsal usually result from an ankle inversion mechanism. The *Jones* fractures and *Pseudo-Jones* (also termed *"Dancer's"*) fractures present with pain over the base of the 5th metatarsal. A *Jones fracture* is a transverse fracture at the proximal diaphysis of the 5th metatarsal. A *pseudo-Jones* or *Dancer's fracture* is an avulsion fracture by the peroneus brevis tendon (resulting from plantar flexion and inversion of the foot) that occurs at the very proximal end of the 5th metatarsal.

Palpation of the 5th metatarsal is essential in any patient with an ankle twisting injury to determine the need for foot films; ankle films are not adequate to make the diagnosis of Jones or pseudo-Jones fractures.

Jones fractures have a high incidence of delayed healing or nonunion. Orthopaedic evaluation in the ED is recommended. If immediate consultation is not available, the foot should be immobilized with a posterior splint with or without a sugar tong splint and the patient should have an orthopaedic referral in 24 to 48 hours. Athletes are usually treated operatively and nonathletes are treated with a walking cast for 4 to 6 weeks.

Pseudo-Jones fractures are stable and can be treated with a hard-sole shoe or a *Jones dressing* with weight-bearing as tolerated. A *Jones dressing* is a bulky dressing used for injuries that require moderate immobilization when swelling is expected. The dressing consists of multiple layers: a thick layer of Webril (cotton roll), followed by an ACE wrap (elastic bandage), then another layer of Webril and another layer of ACE wrap.

Forefoot Injuries

The most common metatarsal and phalangeal fractures result from direct trauma and present with swelling, tenderness and ecchymosis. Dislocations of the metatarsophalangeal (MP) and interphalangeal (IP) joints are caused by dorsiflexion and compression of the phalanges. In addition to swelling and tenderness, there is usually visible deformity.

More subtle stress fractures can occur to the 2nd and 3rd metatarsal bones. During push-off the maximum load is placed on the forefoot. As a result, these bones are prone to stress fractures. Patients usually have a history of increased walking, jogging, or marching activity and they complain of poorly localized pain in the foot with minimal swelling.

The neurovascular status of the foot should be documented, especially the presence of the dorsalis pedis pulse. Dislocations with neurovascular compromise should be reduced immediately; otherwise it is prudent to assess the plain films for fractures before manipulation.

Plain films are adequate to evaluate for dislocations and fractures incurred by direct trauma. However, initial radiographs will often not reveal stress fractures. Stress fractures are usually apparent 2 to 3 weeks later as callus formation or periosteal reaction, but they can also be detected earlier by bone scan.

In patients with MP joint dislocations the phalanx is usually dorsally displaced. Reduction is performed by hyperextension, followed by longitudinal traction and dorsal pressure. Patients can be discharged with a dorsal toe splint, crutches and orthopaedic follow up. IP joint dislocations can occur in a dorsal or volar direction. The reduction technique is similar for both types. Patients can be discharged after the injured toe is buddy taped to the adjacent toe. Patients should follow up with an orthopedist in a week because of the possibility of unstable dislocations.

Nondisplaced fractures should be placed in a short-leg splint and follow up should be arranged. Displaced fractures require reduction by an orthopedist. Stress fractures or suspected stress fractures require close orthopaedic follow up and discontinuation of any pain-producing activity.

Turf Toe

Turf toe is a sprain of the metatarsophalangeal joint of the great toe that results from pushing off of a hyperdorsiflexed toe. The toe is tender and swollen. An x-ray should be obtained to rule out fracture. Like most sprains, the treatment is joint rest with a hard-soled shoe limiting dorsiflexion, ice and analgesia, and ibuprofen or acetaminophen for pain. Orthopaedic consultation is only necessary for patients with persistent pain beyond 1 to 2 weeks.

Plantar Fasciitis

Patients with plantar fasciitis complain of pain in the arch and heel of the foot that is worse in the morning or when climbing stairs. There is usually a history of overuse (hill running or sprinting) or poor arch support. Evaluation reveals tenderness over the plantar fascia and reproduction of the pain with dorsiflexion of the toes. If there is focal tenderness or a stress fracture is suspected, plain films of the foot are indicated. Treatment involves rest, ice, analgesia and, splinting for comfort. Follow up with an orthopedist, sports medicine specialist or physical therapist is recommended. These patients may require evaluation for an orthotic device or exercise program.

Puncture Wounds

Plantar puncture wounds have the potential for serious complications (e.g., soft tissue infection and osteomyelitis). Wounds should be inspected, cleansed, irrigated and explored, especially if a foreign body is suspected. Deep probing, extensive coring or debridement of vital tissue does not improve outcome. Radiographic studies are warranted if the history suggests a foreign body and exploration is inconclusive. Tennis shoes have been implicated in pseudomonal infections, but most soft tissue infections are due to *streptococcus* and *staphylococcus* species. Most cases of osteomyelitis are due to *pseudomonas* (3,6,7). The use of prophylactic antibiotic for puncture wounds to the foot is controversial. Given the risk of complications such as osteomyelitis, its use should be considered. If the decision is made to use antibiotics, a first generation cephalosporin should be given. For clean, superficial wounds with no concern for retained foreign body, local wound care is sufficient treatment. A wound check in 48 hours is recommended for contaminated wounds and those with possible retained foreign bodies.

Patients presenting with infection after a puncture wound should be treated with broad-spectrum antibiotics and the physician should search for a foreign body via exploration, radiographs, or CT scan. Surgical consultation may be needed.

CRITICAL INTERVENTIONS

- In a patient with neurovascular compromise and a visibly deformed extremity, reduce the fracture emergently to restore sensation and blood flow
- Obtain radiographic confirmation in patients with dislocated joints without neurovascular compromise, and then reduce the joint
- In patients with open fractures administer antibiotics and obtain emergent orthopaedic consultation for wash-out and admission
- Provide appropriate followup care for all patients with ankle and foot injuries

DISPOSITION

Most patients with ankle or foot injuries should have close follow up in the event that symptoms do not improve and further investigation and treatment are required. Exceptions are minor ankle sprains and turf toe. Patients who are sent home in a posterior short leg or sugar tong splint should have orthopaedic follow up within 24 to 72 hours for reassessment and definitive immobilization with a cast.

Orthopaedic consultation should be obtained in the ED for the following fractures and dislocations: bi- or tri-malleolar fractures; calcaneal, talar or Jones fractures; Lisfanc fracture/dislocation; ankle and subtalar dislocations. If orthopaedic consultation is not immediately available, appropriate reduction or splinting should be performed and arrangements should be made for orthopaedic evaluation within 24 to 48 hours. Open fractures require immediate orthopaedic consultation.

COMMON PITFALLS

✔ Failure to palpate the base of the 5th metatarsal to evaluate for a Jones fracture
✔ Failure to squeeze the proximal tibia-fibula area to evaluate for a Maisonneuve fracture in patients with presumed ankle sprains
✔ Applying the Ottawa Ankle Rules to patients over 55 years old
✔ Failure to recognize a Lisfranc fracture
✔ Treating a Jones fracture as a pseudo-Jones fracture
✔ Treating grade I and II ankle sprains with prolonged immobilization rather than early mobilization and exercise

Acknowledgments

Thanks to Daniel R. Martin and Wenzel Tirheimer upon whose previous edition chapter some of this material was based.

References

1. Balduini FC, Vegso JJ, Torg JS, Torg E. Management and rehabilitation of ligamentous injuries to the ankle. *Sports Med* 1987;4:364–380.
2. Cetti R, Christensen SE, Ejsted R, Jensen NM, Jorgensen U. Operative versus nonoperative treatment of Achilles tendon rupture. A prospective randomized study and review of the literature. *Am J Sports Med* 1993;21:791–799.
3. Jacobs RF, McCarthy RE, Elser JM. Pseudomonas osteochondritis complicating puncture wounds of the foot in children: a 10-year evaluation. *J Infect Dis* 1989;160:657–661;1989.
4. Leddy JJ, Smolinski RJ, Lawrence J, Snyder JL, Priore RL. Prospective evaluation of the Ottawa Ankle Rules in a university sports medicine center. With a modification to increase specificity for identifying malleolar fractures. *Am J Sports Med* 1998;26.158–65.
5. Markert RJ, Walley ME, Guttman TG, Mehta RA. Pooled analysis of the Ottawa ankle rules used on adults in the ED. *Am J Emerg Med* 1998;16:564–567.

6. Niall DM, Murphy PG, Fogarty EE, Dowling FE, Moore DP. Puncture wound related pseudomonas infections of the foot in children. *Ir J Med Sci* 1997;166:98–101.

7. Pennycook A, Makower R, O'Donnell AM. Puncture wounds of the foot: can infective complications be avoided? *J R Soc Med* 1994;87:581–583.

8. Plint AC, Bulloch B, Osmond MH, et al. Validation of the Ottawa Ankle Rules in children with ankle injuries. *Acad Emerg Med* 1999;6:1005–1009.

9. Ross G, Cronin R, Hauzenblas J, Juliano P. Plantar ecchymosis sign: a clinical aid to diagnosis of occult Lisfranc tarsometatarsal injuries. *J Orthop Trauma* 1996;10:119–122.

10. Stiell IG, Greenberg GH, McKnight RD, et al. Decision rules for the use of radiography in acute ankle injuries. Refinement and prospective validation. *JAMA* 1993;269:1127–1132.

11. Swain RA, Holt WS, Jr. Ankle injuries. Tips from sports medicine physicians. *Postgrad Med* 1993;93:91–92, 97–100.

12. Title CI, Katchis SD. Traumatic foot and ankle injuries in the athlete. *Orthop Clin North Am* 2002;33:587–598.

13. Trevino S, Baumhauer JF. Tendon injuries of the foot and ankle. *Clin Sports Med* 1992;11:727–739.

14. Wedmore IS, Charette J. Emergency department evaluation and treatment of ankle and foot injuries. *Emerg Med Clin North Am* 2000;18:85–113.

PART IV

Special Considerations

CHAPTER 197
Burns

Luis H. Haro, Steve Miller, and Wyatt W. Decker

The incidence of burn injuries in the United States has declined from 2 million burns annually in the 1960s to an estimated 1.25 million annual burn injuries as of the most recently reported data from 1991 to 1993 (6). In the early 1990s burn injuries resulted in 700,000 annual emergency department visits but only 45,000 burn patients were hospitalized (1). The majority of burn patients are treated as outpatients. Thus, emergency physicians must be skilled in the evaluation and management of acute burns.

Seventy-six percent of burn or fire deaths in 2002 resulted from residential fires (7). Many of these deaths were actually related to smoke inhalation. Children less than 5 years of age and adults greater than 65 years of age have higher mortality rates (9). Burns remain the third leading cause of unintentional death in children, surpassed only by motor vehicle collisions and drownings (7). Approximately 70% of pediatric burns are scalds from hot liquids associated with cooking or bathing (whereas flame burns occur more typically in working age adults), and nearly 20% of these burns involve neglect or abuse, particularly water immersion. The remaining 30% of pediatric burns are due to flame burns, contact burns, chemical burns, high-voltage electrical burns, or tar injuries (16).

CLINICAL PRESENTATION

The severity of thermal trauma is most closely related to the depth and extent of injury, but may also be related to inhalation injury, circumferential burns or specific locations of the burn injury, such as hands, feet, major joints, face, or genitalia (2). Other factors that contribute to the severity of the injury include the causative factors, age of the patient, toxic exposures, concomitant traumatic injuries, and comorbidities. The depth of injury depends on the source type, the source temperature, and the length of exposure. A scald injury usually results in partial-thickness burns, while a flame injury typically results in full-thickness burns. Infants, young children, and the elderly have a thinner dermal layer of skin, which gives them a greater propensity for deep burns. Certain causative agents, such as grease, chem-

icals, and electricity, have the potential to cause a deeper, more severe injury because of their higher temperature, greater heat-transferring ability, sustained effect, and internal effect. The systemic response to burn injuries is driven by the loss of the skin's barrier functions, the release of vasoactive mediators from the wound, and from the subsequent infections that are commonly encountered (16).

Depth of burn trauma refers to the level of destruction of the epidermis and the dermis (Fig. 197.1). Superficial burns (first-degree), such as those from sunlight or very short flash, involve the superficial epidermal layers. They are erythematous, painful, do not have blisters, are sensate, and heal without scars. These burns are not included in calculations of total body surface area (TBSA).

Second-degree burns are divided into *superficial* and *deep partial-thickness* burns. *Superficial partial-thickness* burns, from scalds or short flashes, involve the full epidermis and cause varying levels of destruction in the dermis, but spare important structures and leave epidermal appendages in the dermis. They generally heal without scarring in 3 weeks as epidermal cells migrate from the remaining appendages. They are erythematous, blistered, weeping, and painful. *Deep partial-thickness* burns are usually caused by flames, oil, or grease. They involve deeper areas of the dermis, with fewer remaining dermal structures and epidermal appendages. Such burns may have areas that are waxy and dry in addition to blisters, and they can be difficult to distinguish from *full-thickness* burns. *Deep partial-thickness* burns usually scar when they heal, and may require skin grafting for an optimal functional result.

Full-thickness burns can be caused by flames, scalds, and chemical and electrical contact. They destroy dermal structures (third-degree) or underlying tendons, muscle, and bone (fourth-degree). The skin appears dry and leathery, with a pale-to-brown color, is inelastic, and had thrombosed vessels. The patient will not have pain on palpation. These injuries will not heal spontaneously unless the injury is very small, and these wounds will scar with contracture.

Differentiating between *deep partial-thickness* and *full-thickness* burns may be difficult in the emergency department. Despite various advances in technology, serial examinations by an experienced clinician are the standard to accurately determine the depth of a burn (2). Pain is related to the depth of injury but is not reliable for determining the depth of injured dermis, since pain receptors may not function in the acute phase of injury.

DIFFERENTIAL DIAGNOSIS

Burn injuries to the skin do not occur in isolation. The emergency physician must consider associated injuries. Internal

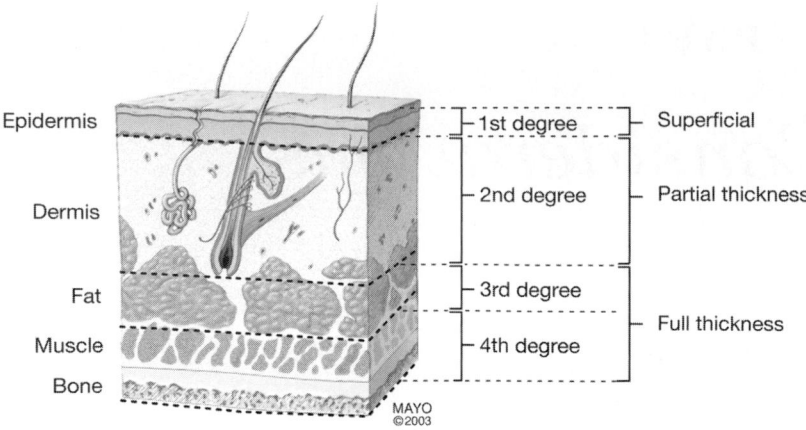

Epidermis

Dermis

Fat

Muscle

Bone

1st degree — Superficial

2nd degree — Partial thickness

3rd degree

4th degree — Full thickness

MAYO
©2003

Figure 197.1.   Cross-section of skin demonstrating various depths of burn.

injuries may be sustained as burn victims attempt to escape the fire. Furthermore, they may have been thrown during an explosion. Patients with inhalation injuries often require immediate airway management. In patients with CNS or cardiopulmonary depression, carbon monoxide poisoning and cyanide toxicity should be considered, particularly in industrial settings.

Although burn-injured patients usually present with a straightforward history, this is not the rule. Such presentations may be the result of self-inflicted injury or nonaccidental injury. Children with unreported hot liquid ingestion or steam inhalation have been misdiagnosed as having croup, laryngomalacia, and tracheobronchitis (18). Several dermatologic conditions such as toxic epidermal necrolysis, Stevens-Johnson Syndrome, staphylococcal scalded skin syndrome, and purpura fulminans may present with bullae and skin sloughing much like burn patients. These patients are often referred to burn centers for definitive management of the large wounds (16).

Since up to 20% of pediatric burns are a result of abuse or neglect, the emergency physician must consider the possibility of abuse when evaluating burn injured children. Intentional burn injuries are suggested by a history inconsistent with injuries or the child's developmental stage, conflicting histories from caregivers and child, a delay in seeking treatment, and a history of previous injury. Immersion injuries are common intentional burns and key physical examination findings include uniformity of burn depth, absence of splash marks, sharply defined circumferential wound margins, flexor surface sparing, and stocking glove patterns. Suspected abuse must be reported and the child may need to be admitted for further evaluation and protection (16).

Another consideration in children is that household cleaners often cause chemical burns. Ingestion should also be suspected in any young child with a chemical burn. The burn should be copiously irrigated with warm water or normal saline for 20 minutes after removal of the child's clothing. Then the extent and depth of the burn can be assessed and treated. See Chapter 307, "Corrosives and Chemical Burns."

EMERGENCY DEPARTMENT EVALUATION

All burn-injured patients should be evaluated first as a trauma patient using a systematic approach following the Advanced Trauma Life Support (ATLS) guidelines. Adhering to an organized approach improves physician response and patient outcomes (2).

Airway evaluation in the burn patient primarily centers on the presence of inhalation injury. A history of closed space exposure to hot gases, steam, or products of combustion support inhalation injury as do physical exam findings of carbonaceous

sputum, singed facial hairs, tachypnea, stridor, wheezing, cough, dysphonia, loss of consciousness, and altered mental status. Although elevated carboxyhemoglobin or cyanide levels also raise suspicion of inhalation injury (2), reliance on lab tests or radiographs cannot be utilized to determine the need for intubation. Patients with suspected inhalation injury may require prophylactic intubation as progressive airway edema may preclude successful intubation once the patient is in respiratory distress. (See Chapter 316, "Smoke Inhalation.")

All burn patients should receive 100% humidified oxygen via nonrebreather mask during the evaluation of their respiratory status. Inhalation injury, comorbidities, as well as circumferential burns of the neck and chest may lead to respiratory compromise and require intubation. Serial chest x-rays are of value, but the emergency department chest x-ray is often normal. Arterial blood gas (ABG) measurement of carboxyhemoglobin should be obtained on patients with headache, syncope, nausea, or altered mental status. Although of limited utility in the emergency department, other tests to evaluate for inhalation injury include $P_{A}O_2/F_{IO_2}$ ratio and xenon and technetium scanning. Bronchoscopy is considered the "gold standard" when diagnosing inhalation injury. These tests guide ventilatory management and decision-making regarding transferring patients to specialized burn centers although clinical impression suffices for the majority of situations in the ED (2).

Evaluation of the circulatory system is often difficult in the severely burned patient. Level of consciousness may be altered due to inhaled toxins, blood loss from coexisting trauma, or "burn shock." Burn shock refers to hypovolemic shock caused by increased blood flow to the wound, capillary leak, decreased cardiac output, and "third spacing" (2) (extracellular and extravascular fluid shifts). Blood pressure measurement and peripheral pulses may be difficult to obtain and unreliable secondary to pain and catecholamine response. Capillary refill and skin color may also be difficult to assess in severely burned patients (3). Circulation distal to circumferential burns should repeatedly be evaluated. Emergent escharotomy is indicated if distal perfusion remains poor despite adequate intravenous volume resuscitation.

The neurologic status of the patient should be quickly determined. Any alteration of mental status should prompt immediate reevaluation of the patient's oxygenation, ventilation, and perfusion. Concern for CNS trauma warrants head CT scanning (3,16).

The patient should be completely undressed to facilitate a thorough examination and halt ongoing injury. Usually the burning process has ceased prior to the emergency department evaluation, but certain fabrics can ignite and melt into residues that continue to burn the patient. Chemicals or other substances may be embedded in the clothing as well. Any substance should be

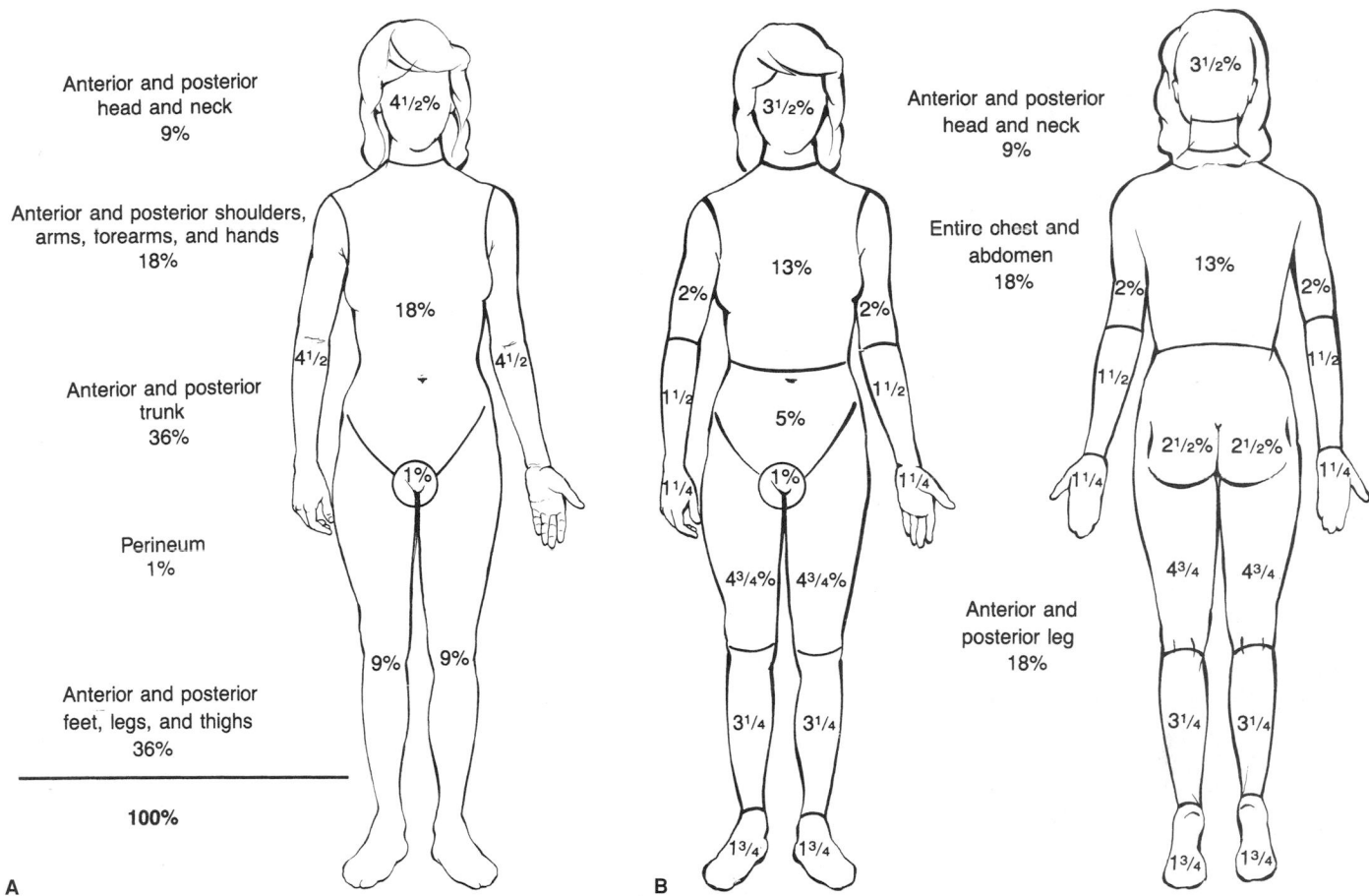

Figure 197.2. Methods to evaluate the percentage of body surface area burned. **(A)** Rule of nines **(B)** Lund and Browder chart.

safely removed and the involved skin surface copiously irrigated with water (3).

The secondary survey includes a systematic head-to-toe thorough examination. Key components of the history should now be obtained. These include documentation of the mechanism and time of injury, closed-space exposure, substances consumed by flames, and prehospital interventions.

After the initial stabilization of the burn patient, the physician should determine the extent of the burn injury by calculating the percentage of *total body surface area* (TBSA) that is burned. The TBSA burn should be subdivided into *partial-thickness and full-thickness* percentages as this will facilitate further patient management and categorization of the injury severity. There are various methods for calculating the TBSA of burn injury. Classically, the "rule of nines" has been used in adult patients (Fig. 197.2). The head, each arm, and each half of each leg approximates 9% TBSA. The torso is assigned 18% each for the anterior and posterior aspects. The genitals are 1% TBSA. The "rule of nines" is not applicable in the pediatric population as the head compromises a larger TBSA (18%) and the legs a smaller TBSA (14%). This evaluation is a good rough estimate but can lead to overestimation and inappropriate patient transfer to burn centers. Lund and Browder charts are more accurate in all age groups and should be used after the initial resuscitation is complete. A modified Lund and Browder chart is used for infants and children (Fig. 197.3). Another method is to use the patient's hand to estimate the TBSA. The palmar surface of the hand (excluding fingers) represents approximately 0.5% TBSA (2).

Further radiographic evaluation including x-rays and CT scans should be performed based on the mechanism of injury (16). In addition to arterial blood gas determination, baseline hematocrit, electrolytes, and glucose, a pregnancy test should be obtained in females of childbearing age. Cardiac monitoring may be necessary for burns associated with electrical injuries (3,16) (see Chapter 357, "Electrical Injuries"). Human studies in critically ill patients have demonstrated that blood lactate (BL) levels are highly accurate as a guide to the efficacy of resuscitation. Persistently elevated BL has also been shown to distinguish survivors from nonsurvivors (10).

EMERGENCY DEPARTMENT MANAGEMENT

The ED management of burn patients is focused on four main aspects of care: (1) airway management, (2) fluid resuscitation, (3) pain control, and (4) appropriate management of associated injuries.

As with all emergency patients, the physician should consider the ABCs as part of the initial assessment. All clothing should be removed as soon as possible. If there has been associated trauma, the neck should be immobilized until a cervical spine injury has been ruled out. Until a good history about the circumstances of the injuries is obtained, significantly burned patients should be given humidified 100% oxygen by a nonrebreathing mask.

Airway Management

In severely burned patients, an expeditious decision must be made regarding potential airway damage. Intubation should be performed *before* the airway is lost. Intubation must be performed immediately in unconscious patients with a history of prolonged smoke or fire exposure in a confined space and in those with a

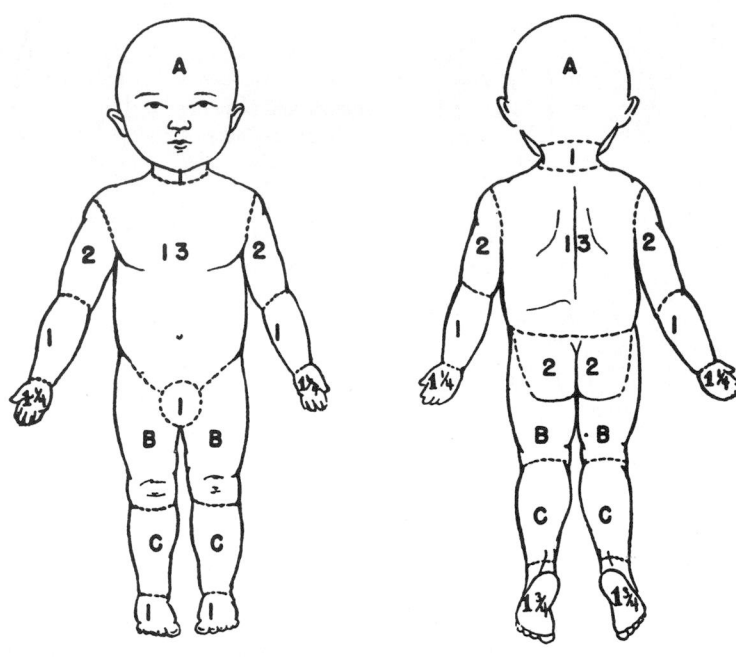

RELATIVE PERCENTAGES OF AREAS AFFECTED BY GROWTH

Area	Age 0	1	5
A = ½ of Head	9½	8½	6½
B = ½ of One Thigh	2¾	3¼	4
C = ½ of One Leg	2½	2½	2¾

% BURN BY AREAS

Probable 3rd° Burn { Head_____ Neck_____ Body_____ Up. Arm_____ Forearm_____ Hands_____
Genitals_____ Buttocks_____ Thighs_____ Legs_____ Feet_____

Total Burn { Head_____ Neck_____ Body_____ Up. Arm_____ Forearm_____ Hands_____
Genitals_____ Buttocks_____ Thighs_____ Legs_____ Feet_____

Sum of All Areas_____ Probably 3rd°_____ Total Burn_____

Figure 197.3. Modified Lund and Browder chart for estimation of body surface area burn involvement in infants and children.

high suspicion for airway edema (stridor, increasing respiratory distress, hypoxia despite 100% oxygen, and poor peak flow). Airway management should be performed using rapid-sequence orotracheal intubation technique. Succinylcholine can be safely administered within 12 to 24 hours of a burn injury. Succinylcholine should be avoided in patients 24 to 48 hours following a thermal injury and for at least one year after the burned skin has healed (15). The rise in serum potassium that normally follows succinylcholine administration is markedly exaggerated in these victims. Apparent proliferation of extra-junctional receptors to these agents occurs. As a result cells depolarize distant to the neuromuscular junction and subsequently, the release of potassium occurs. Potassium levels as high as 13 mEq/L, resulting in ventricular tachycardia, fibrillation, and cardiac arrest, have been reported. The magnitude of the hyperkalemic response does not appear to closely correlate with the magnitude of the burn. A marked hyperkalemic response has been noted following a burn of only 8% TBSA. Whereas susceptibility to hyperkalemia may persist for only several weeks to months, an altered response to nondepolarizing relaxants has been reported in one patient as long as 463 days after the thermal injury.

Many patients require positive end-expiratory pressure (PEEP) to keep the distal airways open; PEEP should begin at 5 cm H_2O. Bronchodilators may be effective if secretions or particulate inhalation leads to bronchospasm.

In the more stable patient, whose clinical examination is suggestive of the potential for airway damage (singed nasal hair, carbonaceous deposits in the pharynx and sputum), immediate nasolaryngoscopy or bronchoscopy is warranted. If unavailable, the emergency physician should have a low threshold for intubation.

Fluid Resuscitation

The critical concept in burn shock is that massive fluid shifts can occur even though total body water remains unchanged. Therefore each resuscitation formula whether it includes colloids, proteins, or crystalloid alone, should be effective in the resuscitation of the burn patient in the immediate postburn period. This assumes that close attention is paid to the individual's clinical response to therapy and that fluid replacement therapy is modified according to this response. Although it is critical to adequately resuscitate the burn patient, over resuscitation is deleterious since it produces an exaggerated edema response. The volume of fluid necessary to resuscitate burn patients depends on the severity of injury, physiological status, age, and associated injuries (13). Two large-bore intravenous lines should be placed through unburned skin if possible. The patient should be placed on a monitor, and a urinary catheter should be placed to monitor output. The amount of fluid needed to treat the burn shock should be calculated keeping in mind the additional fluid loss from other sources, i.e., trauma and inhalation injury.

In adults, crystalloid remains the intravenous fluid of choice for the first 24 hours. Calculation of fluid requirements should be based on the time of the burn, *not* the time the patient arrives in the emergency department. The quantity of crystalloid needed is in part dependent upon the parameters used to monitor resuscitation. If a urinary output of 0.5 cc × kg of body weight × hour is considered to indicate adequate perfusion, approximately 3 cc × kg × % burn will be needed in the first 24 hours. If a urine output of 1 cc × kg of body weight × hour is the target, then of course more edema will occur. Most institutions managing burns of greater than 15% TBSA use the Parkland formula

(4 mL/kg of lactated Ringer's (LR) solution × percentage TBSA burn) as an estimate of the total fluid required during the first 24 hours. One-half is given during the first 8 hours, and the remainder during the next 16 hours. In most instances, this formula will provide the ideal urine output of 0.5–1cc-kg of body weight-hour. However, several other things need to be considered before adapting a formula for all.

The modified Brooke formula recommends beginning burn shock resuscitation at 2 cc/kg/% burn in the first 24 hours. Their proponents argue that this results in less edema. However, more effort is placed into adjusting the rate according to urine output, which is a real challenge in a busy ED. Patients with special fluid management problems such as heart failure, renal insufficiency, or those on dialysis may benefit from this formula.

Several authors recommend the use of hypertonic saline solutions based on studies demonstrating less edema and less fluid requirements. However, prospective randomized studies were not able to demonstrate significant advantages. Experienced burn centers and authorities in burn care recommend the use of modified hypertonic saline (LR + 50 mEq of NaHCO$_3$) for the first 8 hours using the Parkland Formula in patients with massive burns (> 40% TBSA), pediatric patients, and those with associated inhalation injury (2).

Plasma proteins are extremely important in the circulation since they generate the inward oncotic force that counteracts the outward capillary hydrostatic force. The optimal amount of protein or time to infuse remains undefined. Fresh frozen plasma (0.5 to 1 cc/kg/% burn) administered during the first 24 hours, beginning at 8 to 10 hours postburn will result in the development of less edema and will result in more optimal maintenance of hemodynamic stability in certain patients. This treatment is beneficial in older patients, patients with burns and concomitant inhalation injury, and patients with burns in excess of 50% TBSA (17). In most cases, this treatment is left to the burn surgeon, since most patients will be out of the ED within 8 hours from their burn time.

Dextran is rarely used in the emergency department. It is expensive, not readily available, carries the risk of allergic reactions and interferes with blood typing. Most importantly, it has not been demonstrated to be of any clinical benefit in the first phase of the resuscitation.

The burned child continues to represent a special challenge, since resuscitation therapy must be more precise than for an adult with a similar burn. Children require more fluid for burn shock resuscitation than adults with similar thermal injury; fluid requirements for children average 5.8 cc/kg/% burn (2). In addition, children commonly require intravenous resuscitation for even relatively small burns (10%–20% TBSA). The use of hypertonic saline and albumin has become standard therapy in children and is better accepted than in adults. There are two major schools of thought with regard to fluid resuscitation in pediatrics (Table 197.1) (17). Both formulas are relatively easy to use, and both appear to result in similar outcomes. Urine output should be maintained between 0.5 and 1.0 ml/kg/h in children less than 30 kg.

The presence of inhalation injury increases fluid requirements for resuscitation from burn shock after thermal injury. Several authors have documented that patients with inhalation injury require crystalloid at a rate of 5.7 cc/kg/% burn (2). Fluid resuscitation utilizing a calculation of 6 cc/kg/% burn (over the first 24 hours) should work well in the ED. The first half should be given in the first 8 hrs and the rest in the next 16 hrs.

Pain Management

Pain can be severe, particularly in patients with partial-thickness burns. Full-thickness burns tend to be painless because nerve endings have been destroyed. All pain medication should be given *intravenously* in small, frequent aliquots, titrated to pain relief; otherwise, the vasodilatory effect of the narcotics may cause hypotension. Morphine remains the narcotic of choice; doses of 0.1 mg/kg in the young patient and 0.05 mg/kg in the elderly are usually well tolerated. Fentanyl in doses of 50 to 100 mcg IV over 1 to 3 minutes is also a safe option. However, because of its shorter duration (45–90 minutes) and potential for hypotension with rapid administration this medication should be used as an alternative for patients intolerant to morphine. If the patient is extremely anxious, and is not hypoxic or hypotensive, small doses of intravenous lorazepam may be used. In stable patients with severe pain that require procedures, such as hand escharotomies, major debridement or fracture reductions, moderate or deep sedation is warranted.

Management of Associated Injuries

The standard treatment for burn patients with concomitant carbon monoxide exposure is to administer 100% oxygen for 6 to 12 hours. Hyperbaric oxygen therapy should be considered for those with documented serious exposure to carbon monoxide (carboxyhemoglobin level >25% with depressed mental status). Patients must be hemodynamically stable and not requiring ongoing burn resuscitation (see Chapter 306, "Carbon Monoxide").

Cyanide is another product of incomplete combustion that may be inhaled by house fire victims. Recently the contribution of cyanide toxicity in acute smoke inhalation syndrome has been debated (5). Cyanide-related fatalities are rare and tend to be associated with high carboxyhemoglobin levels. Furthermore laboratory confirmation of cyanide poisoning is always a retrospective event. The diagnosis must be considered and treatment administered long before laboratory definitive tests are available. Burn victims with inhalational exposures do not require specific antidotal therapy if significant recovery has occurred before reaching medical attention. Many patients have survived cyanide poisoning with supportive care alone. Patients who exhibit persistent acidosis despite adequate fluid resuscitation, normal carbon monoxide levels, and the absence of other major injuries, should be treated for cyanide toxicity with the Taylor Cyanide Antidote Kit (4,9). See Chapter 308, "Cyanide" and Chapter 316, "Smoke Inhalation" for further discussion.

TABLE 197.1. Formulas for Estimating Pediatric Resuscitation Needs

	Calculation	Time	Fluid and Mixture
Cincinnati Shriners Burns Hospital (modified Parkland)	4 ml × kg × % TBSA burn + 1500 cc × m^2 BSA	½ total volume over 1st 8 hours ¼ total volume over 8 hours ¼ total volume over 8 hours	Lactated Ringer's + 50 mg NaHCO$_3$ Lactated Ringer's Lactated Ringer's + 12.5 g albumin
Galveston Shriners Burns Hospital*	5000 ml/m^2 BSA burn + 2000 ml/m^2 BSA	½ volume over 1st 8 hrs ½ over the next 16 hrs	Ringers Lactate + 12.5 g albumin

* The Galveston resuscitation solution is prepared by mixing 50 ml of 25% human serum albumin (12.5 g) with 950 ml of LR.

Hypothermia can contribute to coagulopathy, and result in decreased circulation to the wound and extension of a partial-thickness burn. Thus, hypothermia should be prevented during resuscitation. Patients who have sustained a burn greater than 25% TBSA should have a nasogastric tube placed since they may develop an ileus secondary to splanchnic vasoconstriction. The emergency physician should update tetanus prophylaxis for all burn patients, as needed.

Full-thickness burns create a leathery coagulum of necrotic tissues known as the eschar. If the full-thickness burn is circumferential in an extremity, the inflexible eschar and progressive edema beneath the eschar can lead to increased compartment pressures that impede venous return initially and arterial inflow ultimately. If this circumferential burn involves the chest and upper abdomen, the restriction of chest expansion and diaphragm excursion can result in respiratory compromise. If the patient is in severe respiratory distress and has sustained circumferential burns to the chest, an immediate escharotomy may be necessary. If a surgeon is not available or is delayed, emergent escharotomy may be necessary to preserve a limb or a life in the case of thoracic circumferential burns. Incision should be made in the anterior axillary line connected by a third incision in the form of an inverted V (Fig. 197.4). An incision through the burn eschar to the underlying subcutaneous fat can be accomplished by using a scalpel or electrocautery. Because the eschar and underlying tissue are insensate, analgesia is not required, but sedation should be considered. Bleeding should be minimal and can be treated effectively with gentle pressure.

Escharotomy is indicated in limbs with distal cyanosis, decreased capillary refill, decreased pulses, or progressive neurologic change. Serial Doppler flow measurements of vessels distal to the burn are useful in deciding whether an escharotomy is adequate. Incisions should be made on the radial and ulnar borders of the arm and forearm and along the midaxial lines of the digits. Incisions are made on the medial and lateral borders of the lower extremities including involved joints, with care to avoid superficial blood vessels and nerves (Fig. 197.4) (17).

Wound Care

Patients with major wounds that require admission to a burn unit should have sterile dressings or sterile sheets placed over their wounds to decrease exposure to in-hospital multiresistant organisms. If the patient's burns are such that hospitalization is not necessary, they should be irrigated with sterile saline and cleaned with mild soap. For very superficial, small burns, nonadherent dressings with or without antibiotic ointment should be used.

The most commonly used topical therapy is silver sulfadiazine (SSD), which is a nontoxic, broad-spectrum antibiotic. SSD has several disadvantages. Patients experience a 5% to 7% incidence of allergic reaction. It should not be used in pregnant patients or nursing mothers and should not be used on the face because of staining. SSD should not be used in patients who will be transferred to a burn center, since it makes wound assessment significantly more difficult. Each time the dressing is changed the old SSD should be completely washed off (8). The efficacy of SSD has been controversial for many years. Published reports show that other methods of outpatient topical treatment might be superior. DuoDerm is a flexible sterile dressing that has an outer layer of polyurethane foam and an inner adhesive layer of a hydrocolloid polyurethane complex. DuoDerm-dressed wounds have been shown to heal faster, have better appearance, and require fewer and less elaborate dressing changes than SSD, and it is less expensive (15). Other synthetic occlusive dressings (Biobrane, OpSite, and Inerpan) have been compared with silver sulfadiazine. Patients in whom these dressings were used had a decrease in the frequency of dressing changes, better compliance,

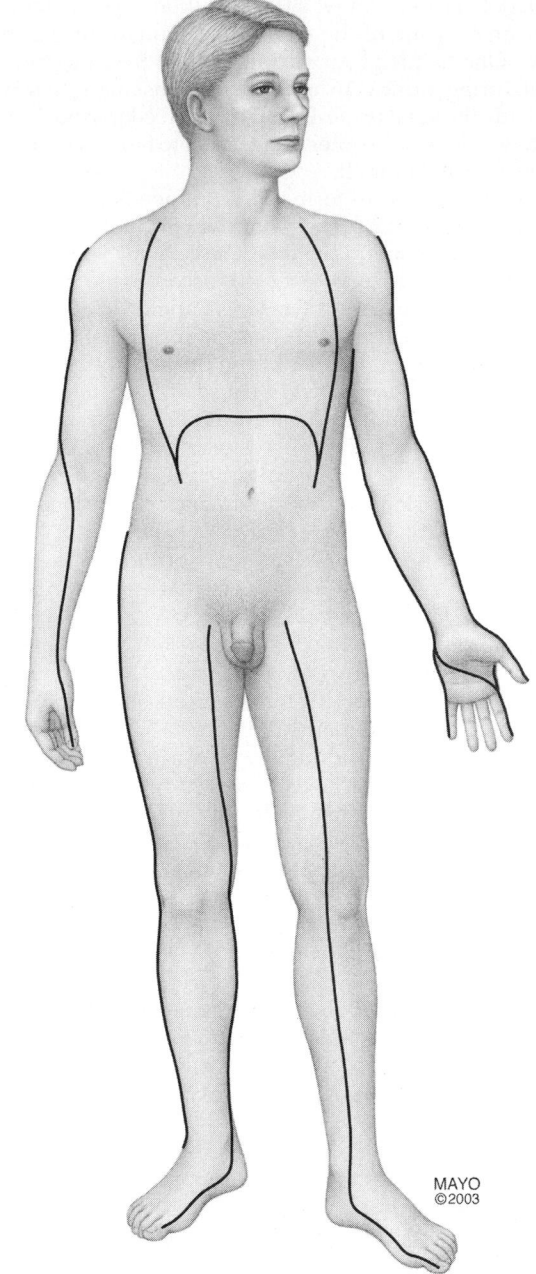

Figure 197.4.   Escharotomy sites.

and marginally faster healing at lower cost. However, none of the dressings were found to produce superior healing (8).

When choosing a dressing many things need to be considered. SSD has been a traditional therapy in burn wound care, mostly because it is readily available in most emergency departments. Regardless of what is used, the outer covering should be absorbent gauze and stockinette, which is changed twice daily while the burn weeps, and once daily thereafter. Necrotic skin should be sharply debrided, and broken bullae should be unroofed and debrided, especially over joints. Controversy exists about the management of small intact bullae. Some authorities believe that the intact bullae provide protection for the new skin. Others believe that the fluid contains toxic products of the inflammatory reaction and recommend debridement of bullae larger than 2 cm, or sterile aspiration of the fluid (14).

Burns to the hand represent a particular challenge. Separate dressings should be used for each finger and the hand should be immobilized in the position of function (wrist extension, metaphalangeal flexion, interphalangeal extension), which

TABLE 197.2. Criteria for Transfer of a Burn Patient
to a Burn Center (2)

Second-degree burns greater than 10% total body surface area
(TBSA)
Third-degree burns
Burns that involve the face, hands, feet, genitalia, perineum, and
major joints
Chemical burns
Electrical burns including lightning injuries
Any burn with concomitant trauma in which the burn injuries pose
the greatest risk to the patient
Inhalation injury
Patients with preexisting medical disorders that could complicate
management, prolong recovery, or affect mortality
Hospitals without qualified personnel or equipment for the care of
the critically burned children.

is opposite of the position assumed by the burned hand. The
extremity should be elevated and joints must be exercised, particularly in the case of burns that cross joints.

If a deep partial-thickness or full-thickness burn heals untreated, new collagen is formed randomly resulting in piling
up of excessive tissue and hypertrophic scar formation. Two
approaches exist for the management of deep partial- and full-
thickness burns-early excision and grafting versus delayed grafting after the eschar separates. The former approach appears to be
the most accepted one at the present time. Finally, patients should
be cautioned that burned skin is sun-sensitive for up to a year
(13), skin should be protected by using SP25 sunblock agents.

CRITICAL INTERVENTIONS

- Completely undress the burn patient to facilitate a thorough
  examination and halt ongoing injury
- Manage the airway immediately in unconscious patients and
  in those with suspected inhalation injury (stridor, increasing
  respiratory distress, hypoxia despite 100% oxygen, and poor
  peak flow)
- Administer 100% oxygen by face mask to patients with suspected carbon monoxide exposure
- Calculate the amount of fluid needed to treat the burn shock,
  keeping in mind the additional fluid loss from other sources,
  i.e., trauma and inhalation injury
- Administer pain medication intravenously in small, frequent
  aliquots, titrated to pain relief
- As soon as the patient is stabilized, initiate transfer to a burn
  center when indicated

DISPOSITION

Burns should be rechecked in 24 to 48 hours. Some emergency
departments manage their own followup burn care for *superficial* partial-thickness burns. Patients with small *deep* partial-
thickness or full-thickness burns should be referred to a plastic
surgeon or other burn-care specialist in 2 to 4 days for consideration of skin grafting and physical therapy. Hospitalization
should be considered, even for minor burns, for patients who
are immunocompromised, the very young and the elderly, and
those with poor home situations or possible abuse. Published
criteria for admission or transfer to a burn center are outlined in
Table 197.2.

COMMON PITFALLS

✔ Waiting too long to intubate a patient with a compromised
  airway

✔ Failure to detect child abuse in suspected immersion burns
✔ Failure to diagnose compartment syndrome, especially in the
  hand
✔ Failure to calculate fluid requirements from the time of the
  burn
✔ Overestimating or underestimating the size of the burn

Acknowledgments

*Thanks for the contributions of Donna A. Caniuno, Marc Dwoning
(Pediatric Chapter) and Janet Talbot-Stern to this chapter.*

References

1. American Burn Association. Burn Incidence and Treatment in the US: 2000 Fact
   Sheet. Available at http://www.ameriburn.org. [2003 Oct 16].
2. American Burn Association. Practice Guidelines for Burn *Care J Burn Care Rehabilitation.* April 2001, (Supplement).
3. American College of Surgeons Committee on Trauma. Advanced trauma life
   support for doctors. Chicago: *American College of Surgeons,* 1997.
4. Berlin CM. The treatment of cyanide poisoning in children. *Pediatrics*
   1970;46:793–796.
5. Barillo DJ, Goode R, Esch V. Cyanide poisoning in victims of fire: analysis of
   364 cases and review of the literature. *J Burn Care Rehabil* 1994;15:46–57.
6. Brigham P, McLoughlin E. Burn incidence and medical care use in the United
   States: estimates, trends, and data sources. *J Burn Care Rehabil* 1996;17:95.
7. Centers for Disease Control and Prevention. Web-based Injury Statistics Query
   and Reporting System (WISQARS) [Online]. (2003). National Center for Injury Prevention and Control, Centers for Disease Control and Prevention (pro-
   ducer). Available from: URL: www.cdc.gov/ncipc/wisqars. [2003 Oct 16].
8. Clayton MC, Solem LD. No ice, no butter: advice on management of burns for
   primary care physicians. *Postgrad Med* 1995;97:151.
9. Deaths resulting From residential fires and prevalence of smoke alarms-United
   States, 1991–1995. *MMWR* 1998;47:803–806.
10. Jeng JC. Serum lactate, not base deficit, rapidly predicts survival after major
    burns. *Burns* 2002;28:161–166.
11. Jones J, McMullen MJ, Dougherty J. Toxic smoke inhalation: Cyanide poisoning
    in fire victims. *Am J Emerg Med* 1987;5:318–321.
12. Osguthorpe JD. Head and neck burns: evaluation and current management.
    Arch Otolaryngol Head Neck Surg 1991;117.
13. Peate WF. Outpatient management of burns. *Am Fam Physician* 1992;45:1321.
14. Robson MC, Burns BR, Smith DJ. Acute management of the burned patient.
    Plast Reconstr Surg 1992;89:6.
15. Schwinn DA, Steven LS. *Basic principles of pharmacology related to anesthesia.* In:
    Miller: Anesthesia, 5th ed., New York: Churchill Livingstone, Inc. 2000.
16. Sheridan RL. The seriously burned child: resuscitation through reintegration.
    Curr Probl Pediatr 1998;28:105–127, 139–167.
17. Warden Glenn. Fluid Resuscitation and early management. In: Hernon D. *Total
    Burn Care.* 2nd ed. Philadelphia: W.B Saunders – Hartcourt publishers 2002.
18. Whitelock-Jones L, Bass DH, Millar AJ, Rode H. Inhalation burns in children.
    Pediatric Surgery International 1999;15:50–55.
19. Wyatt D, McGowan DN, Najarian MP. Comparison of hydrocolloid dressing
    and silver sulfadiazine cream in the outpatient management of second degree
    burns. *J Trauma* 1990;30:857–865.

CHAPTER 198
Replantation

James L. Larson

CLINICAL PRESENTATION

Advances in microsurgery have enabled surgeons to perform
viable replantation procedures on virtually any part of the body.
Viability, however, is only one consideration when evaluating
for replantation. The most important factor is the ultimate function of the replantation. Decisions by the emergency physician

in the first few minutes can significantly impact the viability and function of the replantation.

The majority of replantations involve digits injured in industrial accidents (4). Cutting machines, press machines and belts are the leaders in producing amputations. A significant cause of injury and amputations in children are bicycle chain-rings and spokes, including those on stationary exercise bikes (5).

DIFFERENTIAL DIAGNOSIS

An amputated part is a completely severed part of the body, and replantation is the reattachment of an amputated part. An incomplete amputation is partially attached but has loss of arterial circulation. The repair of an incomplete amputation is a revascularization. Revascularization is more successful than replantation because the venous outflow system is often intact.

EMERGENCY DEPARTMENT EVALUATION

Identification and treatment of life-threatening injuries takes precedence over the evaluation for potential replantation. A systematic approach to patients with traumatic injuries is necessary to avoid distraction from amputations (Chapter 169). Serious undetected concomitant injuries have been found in patients after transfer to a tertiary care facility for replantation (7).

Indications and Contraindications for Replantation

The evaluation of a patient with an amputation or near-amputation should be expeditious. The key considerations are identifying the injuries and potential for replantation. Amputations that are considered for replantation are listed in Table 198.1. The decision to proceed with replantation is based on potential viability and long-term function. A working knowledge of factors that impact on the decision will facilitate patient care and case discussion with the surgeon.

The mechanism of the amputation and resulting condition of the anatomic structures are most significant. Guillotine-like "sharp" amputations are most amenable to surgical repair in

---

TABLE 198.1. Replantation Candidates

UPPER EXTREMITY (8)

Indications:
Any part in a child
Thumb
Multiple digits
Palm
Wrist
Forearm
Elbow and above (sharp mechanism of injury)
Finger distal to flexor digitorum superficialis insertion

Contraindications:
Single digits proximal to flexor digitorum superficialis insertion
Crushed or mangled parts
Multiple level amputations

OTHER REPLANTATION CANDIDATES:

Lower extremity amputation (sharp mechanism of injury)
Ear
Scalp
Lip
Nose
Penis

---

contrast to crush and avulsion mechanisms. Injuries at one level are easier to replant than multiple insults along an extremity.

There are several potential contraindications to replantation. Multiply injured patients that require surgery or prolonged resuscitation for traumatic injuries are not candidates for a prolonged replantation procedure. Patients with complex medical problems that affect vascular integrity, immune function, and healing may be poor candidates for replantation. Patients without sufficient mental capacity or judgment to comply with postoperative rehabilitation are not likely to have success with replantation (8). Ultimately the decision to proceed with replantation is made by the consulting surgeon. All potential replantation candidates, even with relative contraindications, should be discussed with a replantation surgeon.

Replantation surgeons have less stringent criteria for attempting replantation in children. Children are slightly less likely to have success with viability of a replantation, due in part to the small size of their vessels; however, they have better functional results. As an example, fingertip amputations distal to the lunula of the fingernail can be sewn on as a composite graft with greater success in children (2).

Replantation Sites

The digits of the hand are the most frequent site of replantations. Replantation of the thumb is considered even when function of the replanted thumb is potentially limited. Even a nonfunctioning thumb is important due to its role in opposition. Single finger replantation proximal to the insertion of the flexor digitorum superficialis (mid portion of middle phalanx) is not performed because of poor functional outcomes. These patients have almost no return of flexion. In contrast, replantation of amputations at the level of the distal interphalangeal joint usually results in a good functional outcome. Multiple finger amputations are usually considered for replantation. Replantation of hand and wrist amputations results in more function than a prosthesis and therefore are considered for replantation. Replantation of forearm, elbow, and proximal arm injuries are more successful after a sharp mechanism in young healthy patients.

Replantation of lower extremity amputations is less common. Injuries to the lower extremity often result from a crushing mechanism and the large muscle mass of the lower extremity is less tolerant of ischemia (8). Children and younger adults with noncrushing injuries are the best candidates for repair. Other amputations in which replantation should be considered include ears, lips, nose, scalp, and penis.

EMERGENCY DEPARTMENT MANAGEMENT

The priorities in management of an amputation are decreasing the ongoing ischemia in the amputated part and expediting the time to the operating room for definitive repair. Hemorrhage is a frequent complication in amputations. Direct pressure is the preferred method to control bleeding. Tourniquets may be used to control hemorrhage temporarily and for evaluation of the wound but should not be used as the primary means of hemostasis. Prolonged use of a tourniquet can produce more loss of function. Blind clamping or ligation should not be performed to avoid damage to vessels and nerves that may be needed for the definitive repair.

Care of the amputated part can prolong its viability and improve the success of the surgical repair. All tissues that are available should be kept, even smaller portions of skin can be used for wound coverage. The amputated part should be cleaned with normal saline solution to remove gross contaminants; alcohol, iodine, formaldehyde or other "cleaning" solutions should not be used (9). The amputated part should be wrapped in saline moistened gauze and placed in a sealed plastic bag or container. The sealed bag or container with the amputated part is then placed in a water and ice bath. To avoid freezing the tissue, the amputated part should not be placed directly on ice and "dry" ice should not be used. An amputated limb can survive 6 hours of warm ischemia and 12 hours of cold ischemia. Amputated digits can tolerate ischemia for longer periods of time (6). Incomplete amputations should be splinted to minimize further trauma and maintain vascular integrity. Radiographs of the involved extremity and amputated part should be obtained only if it does not delay transfer.

Tetanus prophylaxis (0.5 ml tetanus toxoid) should be administered to patients who are more than five years from their last booster. Tetanus immune globulin should be given to those who have not been primarily immunized. Patients with open fractures or contaminated wounds should receive a first generation cephalosporin and an aminoglycoside as prophylactic antibiotics (3).

CRITICAL INTERVENTIONS

- Contact replantation surgeon early
- Control hemorrhage with direct pressure
- Wrap the amputated part in saline gauze
- Place the amputated part in a waterproof container and place the container in an ice and water bath
- Administer tetanus and antibiotics

DISPOSITION

Early communication with a replantation surgeon is critical because replantation is a time-sensitive process. Having protocols in place that identify specialists and medical centers capable of performing replantations is important to expedite definitive care. One group has used internet transmission of photographs and radiographs to evaluate potential replantation candidates prior to transfer (1). To avoid disappointment, the patient and family should not be told that a replantation will occur, but that a replantation surgeon will evaluate them for possible replantation.

COMMON PITFALLS

- ✔ Failure to recognize concomitant serious injury
- ✔ Failure to notify replantation surgeon early
- ✔ Indiscriminant use of clamps or prolonged tourniquets to control hemorrhage
- ✔ Failure to properly cool the amputated part

Acknowledgment

Thanks to the previous edition's chapter author Iris M. Reyes.

References

1. Buntic RF, Siko PP, Ruebeck GM. Using the internet for rapid exchange of photographs and x ray images to evaluate potential extremity replantation candidates. *J Trauma* 1997;342–344.
2. Cheng GL, Pan DD, Yang ZX, et al. Digital replantation in children. *Ann Plast Surg* 1985;15:325–331.
3. Gosselin RA, Roberts I, Gillespie WJ. Antibiotics for preventing infection in open limb fractures (Cochrane Review). In: *The Cochrane Library*, Issue 1, 2004. Chichester, UK: John Wiley & Sons, Ltd.
4. Kim WK, Lim JH, Han SK. Fingertip replantations: Clinical evaluation of 135 digits. *Plast Reconstr Surg* 1996;470–476.
5. Lehrer MS, Bozentka DJ, Partington MT, et al. Pediatric hand injuries due to exercise bicycles. *J Trauma* 1997:100–102.
6. Morgan RF, Reisman NR, Curtis RM. Preservation of upper extremity devascularizations and amputations for replantation. *Am Surg* 1982:481.
7. Partington MT, Lineaweaver WC, O'Hara M, et al. Unrecognized injuries in patients referred for emergency microsurgery. *J Trauma* 1993;34:238–241.
8. Pederson WC. Replantation. *Plast Reconstr Surg* 2001:823–841.
9. Schlenker JK, Koulis CP. Amputations and replantations. *Emerg Med Clin* 1993:739–753.

CHAPTER 199
Acute Compartment Syndrome

John A. Siefert

Acute compartment syndrome is the presence of pathologically elevated intramuscular pressures (IMP) within confined osseofascial compartments resulting in tissue ischemia, infarction and subsequent contractures (5). This clinical entity was named for Dr. Richard Von Volkmann. In 1881, he described this pathologic condition of muscle ischemia, paralysis, and subsequent contracture in a child with a supracondylar fracture (11). Although known by many names including *Volkmann ischemic contracture* it is now termed *compartment syndrome* (11). The osseofascial compartments are delineated by bony and fascial tissue planes, have limited pressure elasticity, and contain various muscles, nerves and blood vessels. Elevated pressure in these spaces, beyond normal physiologic ranges, compromises capillary blood flow and produces unique clinical signs and symptoms. Delays in treatment result in myonecrosis, permanent nerve damage, and muscle contracture. Compartment syndrome is relatively rare; the incidence in patients with tibial shaft fractures is reported to range from 3% to 10% (12). The most frequently involved compartments are the lower leg and forearm (11). Table 199.1 lists the common locations of compartment syndromes.

A number of pathologic mechanisms have been proposed to explain the development of a compartment syndrome and complication of Volkmann ischemic contracture. These include arteriolar vasoconstriction or spasm, critical closure pressures for affected vessels, and microvascular capillary occlusions by various hematologic components. Ultimately, interruption of the capillary blood flow delivering the tissues' metabolic needs results in ischemia, loss of function and finally infarction. Normal tissue pressure is 0 to 8 mm Hg. Direct capillary pressures have been measured at 20 to 33 mm Hg (4). Capillary blood flow depends on the pressure differences between the arterial and venous sides. As tissue pressure increases the blood flow across the capillary bed decreases. The *arteriovenous gradient theory* has been proposed by a number of investigators to explain experimental and clinical findings, and it is the most widely accepted theory. It states that increases in tissue pressure reduce the local arteriovenous gradient and blood flow to the point where the metabolic demands of the tissues are not met. Then functional abnormalities and compartment acute syndrome occur (11). Two mechanisms result in elevated compartment pressures: either an extrinsic force constricts the compartment (e.g., a cast) or there is

TABLE 199.1. Common Locations of Compartment Syndromes

Upper Limb Compartments	Lower Limb Compartments	Miscellaneous Compartments
ARM	**BUTTOCK**	**PELVIC**
• Deltoid	• Gluteal	• Iliacus
• Biceps		
	THIGH	
FOREARM		
	• Quadriceps	
• Dorsal		
• Volar	**LEG**	
HAND	• Anterior	
	• Lateral	
• Interosseous	• Superficial posterior	
	• Deep posterior	

(Modified From Matsen FA. *Compartmental syndromes*. New York: Grune & Stratton, 1980.)

an increase in the size of the compartment due to edema or hemorrhage.

Studies have shown that reductions in blood flow and blood oxygenation occur at tissue pressures above 20 mm Hg (8,13). Cellular metabolic derangements are closely associated with the difference between mean arterial blood pressure and compartment pressure. This difference is known as the *delta P*. In one study, the lowest delta P that was compatible with a normal metabolic state was 30 mm Hg in normal muscle and 40 mm Hg in traumatized muscle (7). The length of time that tissue can tolerate elevated pressures is less clear; some authors use a 6-hour limit (15). Other factors should also be considered when assessing the effect of increased tissue pressure on an osseofascial compartment. Externally applied pressures (i.e., casting) tends to produce less compartment pressure elevations when compared to similar levels of internally developed pressures (i.e., edema or hemorrhage) (17). Postischemic swelling and edema can increase muscle weight by 30% (6). Reperfusion injury leads to the release of vasoactive factors resulting in fluid extravasation and elevated pressures. Concurrent hypotension, hypoxia, and associated premorbid conditions such as peripheral vascular disease adversely affect the ability of ischemic tissue to tolerate even mildly elevated tissue pressures.

CLINICAL PRESENTATION

Pain out of proportion to exam is the key clinical finding in acute compartment syndrome. The pain is often described as deep, aching, and poorly localized and does not respond to immobilization or analgesic medications. Increasing analgesic requirements may be the only clue to a developing compartment syndrome. Passive stretching of involved muscles produces intense pain. Weakness or paresis of muscle function is a late finding. Distal hypesthesias or paresthesias are noted in the distributions of nerves transiting through the compartment. Two-point discrimination and light-touch should be assessed and are considered more sensitive than pinprick sensation. Tenseness of externally palpable compartments is the earliest and most objective finding though tenseness of certain compartments, such as the deep posterior compartment of the lower leg and the iliacus compartment, are very difficult to assess. Findings of compartment syndrome are often present within 2 hours of injury but may first occur up to 6 days later (11). Progressive worsening over time is

expected and helps to distinguish compartment syndrome from those injuries with primary nerve and muscle damage.

Griffith's mnemonic, the *5 P's* (Pain, Pallor, Pulselessness, Paresthesias, and Paresis), is used for this clinical entity. However, pulses are most often maintained and the skin does not typically develop pallor (5). These signs are useful to assess an extremity at risk for compartment syndrome, but more accurately reflect the late findings of acute arterial obstruction or insufficiency. The reliance on the clinical exam makes it difficult to assess patients with altered sensorium, acute intoxication, spinal cord injuries, overlying extensive burns, and children. Obtunded patients are often at risk for compartment syndrome by compression, entrapment or unknown mechanisms of trauma. Overdose-related compartment syndromes tend to affect the lower extremities (12). Critically ill pediatric and adult patients may experience iatrogenic causes of compartment syndrome produced by intravenous infiltrations, transfusions under pressure or tourniquet malfunction. Table 199.2 lists common etiologies of compartment syndrome. Compartment syndrome may develop in more than one compartment simultaneously as reported in one case of thrombolytic therapy for cocaine induced myocardial infarction (16). Severely burned patients lose most, if not all, clinical signs of compartment syndrome. In these complex cases a lower threshold for use of invasive monitoring may be necessary.

The clinical findings for specific anatomic compartments are summarized in Table 199.3. Figure 199.1 illustrates the anatomy for the two most common sites. Overall the three most common causes of an acute compartment syndrome are fractures, crush injury and reperfusion of an ischemic limb. The lower extremity and forearm have relatively "tight" compartments and are the most common sites for compartment syndrome. In the pediatric population, fractures are the most common cause, specifically supracondylar fractures. Despite apparent loss of compartment

TABLE 199.2. Common Etiologies of Compartment Syndromes Seen in Emergency Medicine

INCREASED COMPARTMENT CONTENT

Infiltrated infusion
Bleeding
• Vascular injury
• Coagulation defect
Increased capillary permeability
• Reperfusion after ischemia
• Trauma
• Fracture
• Contusion
• Intensive use of muscles
• Exercise
• Seizures
• Eclampsia
• Tetany
• Burns
• Cold
• Snakebite
Increased capillary pressure
• Venous obstruction
Diminished serum osmolarity
• Nephrotic syndrome

EXTERNALLY APPLIED PRESSURE

• Casts, dressings, splints, pneumatic garment
• Lying on limb

(From Matsen FA. *Compartmental syndromes*. New York: Grune & Stratton, 1980, with permission.)

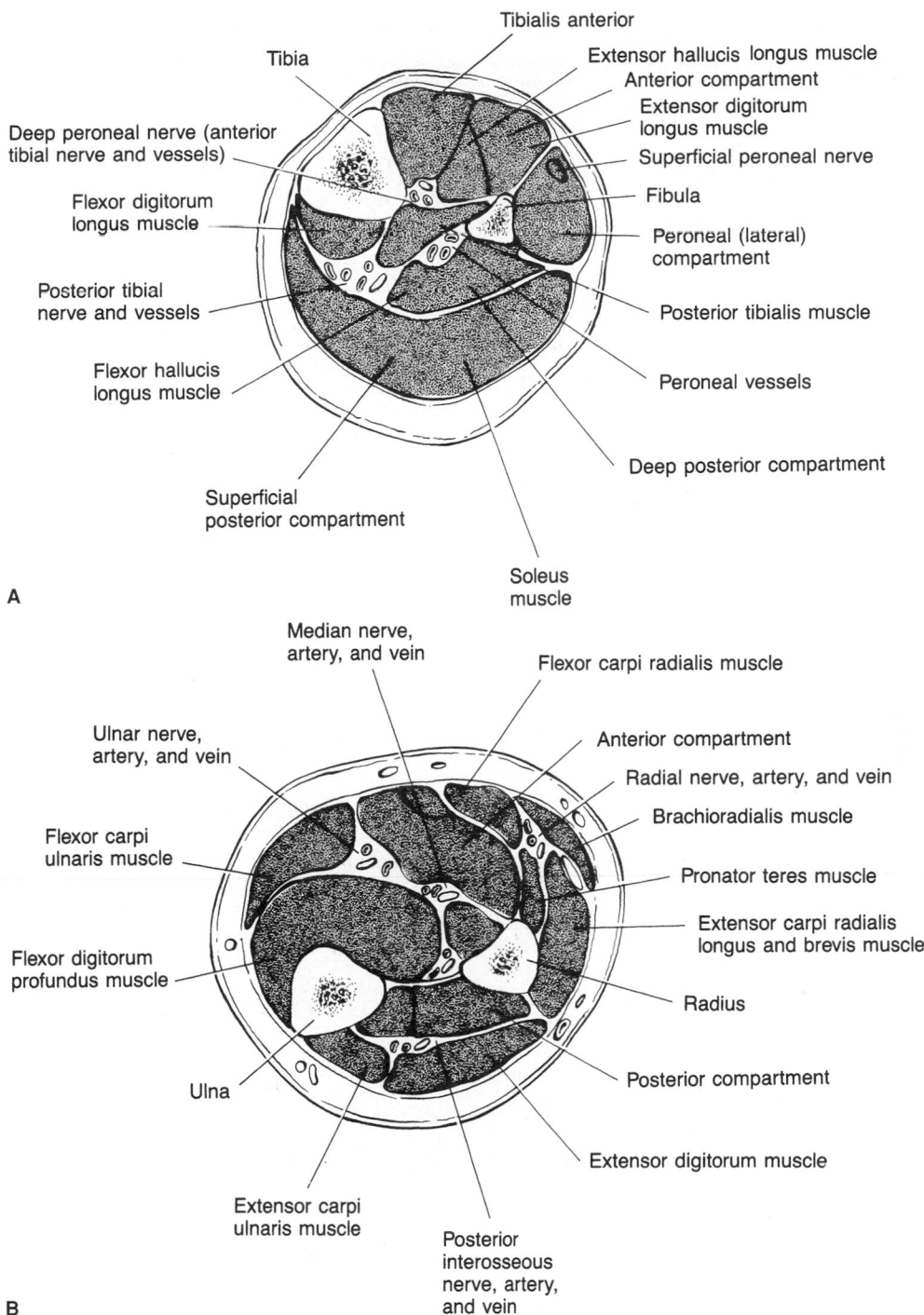

Figure 199.1.   Compartments of the leg (**A**) and forearm (**B**).

integrity open fractures can still develop this syndrome. Common fracture etiologies for compartment syndrome include tibial plateau, supracondylar and forearm fractures (12).

Differential diagnostic considerations include deep vein thrombosis, necrotizing fasciitis, arterial embolus or insufficiency, gas gangrene, and myositis.

EMERGENCY DEPARTMENT EVALUATION

Laboratory and radiologic studies do not assist in the diagnosis of compartment syndrome but may help in assessing for other etiologies and secondary complications such as rhabdomyolysis.

The best diagnostic test for compartment syndrome is measurement of elevated intracompartmental pressures. This is especially important in those patients who are unreliable because of age or altered sensorium. These direct tissue measurements can also be used to provide ongoing monitoring in patients who are at high risk for development of a compartment syndrome, as in the case of a crush injury. Various pressure measurement techniques are used such as the needle-manometer, the wick catheter, the slit catheter and the portable Stryker hand-held monitor. All devices provide acceptable accuracy though the least expensive, and self-assembled needle-manometer is the least accurate and least reproducible (11). Most compartments are superficial, but access to deeper ones such as the gluteal and deep posterior

TABLE 199.3. Compartment Syndromes and Associated Physical Signs

Compartment	Painful Passive Movement	Location of Tenseness	Muscles Weakened	Sensory Loss
FOREARM				
Dorsal	Thumb and finger flexion	Dorsal forearm	Thumb and finger extensors	—
	Thumb and finger extension	Volar forearm	Thumb and finger flexors	Ulnar and median nerves
HAND				
Interosseous	Adduction, abduction of metacarpophalangeal joints	Dorsum of hand between metacarpals	Interosseous	—
LEG				
Anterior	Toe flexion	Anterior aspect of leg	Toe extensors and tibialis anterior	Deep peroneal nerve
Lateral	Foot inversion	Lateral aspect of leg over fibula	Peroneal muscles	Superficial and deep peroneal nerves
Superficial posterior	Foot dorsiflexion	Calf	Soleus and gastrocnemius	—
Deep posterior	Toe extension	Distal medial leg between Achilles tendon and tibia	Toe flexors and tibialis posterior	Posterior tibial nerve
PELVIC				
Iliacus	Hip extension	Not palpable	Iliacus, psoas major and psoas minor	Femoral nerve

(Modified from Matsen FA. Compartmental syndromes. *Clin Orthop* 1975;113:8.)

compartments may require a spinal needle. Once the compartment pressure has been obtained there is ongoing debate over which pressures warrant a fasciotomy. Various investigators have suggested absolute pressures ranging from 30 to 45 mm Hg. Other investigators choose pressures anywhere from 10 to 40 mm Hg below the diastolic blood pressure (11,14,18). These pressure measurements must be assessed in the context of hypotension, anemia, hypoxia or other factors that would increase the tissue sensitivity for ischemia at less elevated pressures. Noninvasive measures of a compartment can provide indirect assessment of tissues status, although they are not widely used. These include the use of laser Doppler, magnetic resonance imaging, and P-NMR. Nerve conduction studies and arteriography are used primarily to distinguish primary nerve and arterial injuries and not to diagnose compartment syndrome.

EMERGENCY DEPARTMENT MANAGEMENT

The key to management of patients with compartment syndrome is to consider the diagnosis early. Surgical fasciotomy is the definitive treatment and surgical consultation must be initiated early. Surgical decompression should ideally be performed less than 6 hours after the onset of symptoms (15). Supportive care is aimed at resuscitation and stabilization of the patient and preparation for appropriate operative intervention.

In patients with fractures who are in casts, bivalving and spreading of the cast may be necessary and can produce an almost 65% reduction in applied external pressures while maintaining alignment (2). Elevation of an extremity at risk can produce a 0.8 mm Hg drop in arterial pressure for each centimeter of leg elevation (9). Placing the affected extremity in a neutral position is important to prevent ongoing injury and swelling. The emergency physician should address aggravating factors specific to the extremity involved such as MAST suits or pneumatic splints as well systemic factors such as hypotension, anemia and hypoxia.

CRITICAL INTERVENTIONS

- Immobilize the involved extremity in the least restrictive dressing with minimal elevation
- Initiate surgical consultation early
- Measure intracompartmental pressures

DISPOSITION

Patients with suspected compartment syndrome should be admitted for observation and repeated clinical examinations. This should be done after surgical or orthopaedic consultation is obtained. Patients with multiple trauma may require intensive care unit admission for management of other associated injuries.

COMMON PITFALLS

✔ Failure to recognize early signs and symptoms of compartment syndrome
✔ Attributing the signs and symptoms of compartment syndrome to other types of injury
✔ Failure to do a thorough extremity and neurologic examination, especially in those patients who are intoxicated or unreliable

Acknowledgment

Thanks to the previous edition's chapter author Steven C. Larson.

References

1. Davey JR, Rorabeck CH, Fowler PJ. The tibialis posterior muscle compartment. *Am J Sports Med* 1984;12:391–397.
2. Garfin SR, Mubarak SJ, Evans K, et al. Quantification of intracompartmental pressures and volume under plaster casts. *J Bone Joint Surg* 1981;63:449–453.
3. Hargens AR, Botte MJ, Swanson MR, et al. Effects of local compression on peroneal nerve function in humans. *J Orthop Res* 1993;11:818–827.
4. Hargens AR, Mubarak SJ, Owen CA, et al. Interstitial fluid pressure in muscle and compartment syndrome in man. *Microvasc Res* 1977;14:1–10.

5. Hargens AR, Mubarak SJ. Current concepts in the pathophysiology evaluation and diagnosis of compartment syndrome. *Hand Clinics* 1998;14:371.
6. Harman JW. The significance of local vascular phenomena in the production of ischemic necrosis in skeletal muscle. *Am J Pathol* 1948;24:625–642.
7. Heppenstall RB, Sapega AA, Scott R, et al. The compartment syndrome: An experimental and clinical study of muscular energy metabolism using phosphorus nuclear magnetic resonance spectroscopy. *Clin Orthop* 1988;226:138.
8. Matsen FA, Krugmire RB, King RV. Increased tissue pressure and its effect on muscle oxygenation in level and elevated human limbs. Nicholas Andry Award. *Clin Orthop Relat Res* 1979;144:311–320.
9. Matsen FA, Wyss CR, Krugmire RB, et al. The effects of limb elevation and dependency on local arteriovenous gradient in normal human limbs with particular reference to limbs with increased tissue pressure. *Clin Orthop Relat Res* 1980;150.
10. Matsen FA. Compartmental syndromes. *Clin Orthop* 1975;113:8.
11. Matsen FA. *Compartmental syndromes*. New York: Grune & Stratton, 1980.
12. Mubarak SJ, Hargens AR. *Compartment Syndromes and Volkmann's Contracture*. Philadelphia: W.B. Saunders Company, 1981;85.
13. Rorabeck CH, MacNab I. The pathophysiology of the anterior tibial compartment syndrome. *Clin Orthop Relat Res* 1975;113:52–57.
14. Rorabeck CH, Castle GSP, Hardie R, et al. Compartmental pressure measurements: an experimental investigation using the slit catheter. *J Trauma* 1981;21:446
15. Simon RR, Koenigknecht SJ. Complications. In: *Emergency orthopaedics: the extremities*, 2nd ed. Norwalk, CT: Appleton & Lange, 1987.
16. Thomas WO, Harris CN, D'Amore TF, et al. Bilateral forearm and hand compartment syndrome following thrombolysis for acute myocardial infarction: A case report. *J Emerg Med* 1994;12:467–472.
17. Whitesides TE, Harada H, Morimoto K. Compartment syndromes and the role of fasciotomy, its parameters and techniques, in Instructional Course Lectures. The American Academy of Orthopaedic Surgeons, Vol. 26. St. Louis, Mosby, 1979;179.
18. Whitesides TE, Haney TC, Morimoto K, et al. Tissue pressure measurements as a determinant for the need for fasciotomy. *Clin Orthop* 1975;113:43.

CHAPTER 200
Ballistics and Blast Injuries

Leon D. Sanchez

BALLISTICS

Ballistics is the science of the motion of a projectile. *Wound ballistics* refers to the motion of the projectile through tissue. The majority of projectiles that cause significant injury in the United States population are in the form of firearm injuries. In 2001 there were 20,308 homicides in the United States of which 11,348 were due to firearms (19). These injuries can be classified as violence-related, accidental or self inflicted (23).

Firearms include two basic types: rifled firearms and shotguns. A rifled firearm (pistol and rifle) has spiral grooves in its barrel. When the cartridge is fired, the burning of the powder generates gas in a contained space. The pressure generated by the gas propels the bullet forward. The bullet accelerates while inside the barrel and reaches its maximum speed upon exit (muzzle velocity). Bullets are rotated around their long axes by the rifling of the barrel, which gives them sufficient gyroscopic stability to maintain the point-forward position while traveling through air. Without gyroscopic stabilization, bullets would preferentially travel in the more stable *base forward* orientation where the greater mass of the bullet is. Bullets fired from a properly designed rifle barrel *yaw* no more than a few degrees during flight. The yaw angle is the angle between the long axis of the bullet and the line of flight. This angle is greatest as the bullet exits the barrel and is reduced as the gyroscopic spin stabilizes the bullet's flight through the air. Once a bullet enters a denser medium the gyroscopic spin is insufficient to stabilize the bullet. As the bullet enters tissue it will begin to tumble and deform. Depending on the makeup of the bullet and the properties of the tissue through which it travels it may expand, fragment or remain in one piece (6,8,22).

The majority of bullets in use today are at least partially jacketed. The jacket is a layer of hard metal that surrounds what is typically a lead core. Without a jacket, lead bullets fired at speeds of greater than 600 m/s would have some of the lead stripped by the rifling of the barrel (6). Jacketing allows bullets to reach greater muzzle velocities. Military bullets are fully jacketed (24).

While military bullets are fully jacketed, civilian bullets usually have the lead core exposed at the tip (soft point). The tip is often further modified into different varieties of hollow point bullets. The exposure of lead at the tip will cause the softer lead to deform much more than a fully jacketed bullet upon entry into tissue. Hollow point bullets are designed to expand and deform as they penetrate tissue. A soft point or hollow point bullet will deform earlier in its travel through tissue than a comparable fully jacketed projectile. Therefore, the injury patterns will be different, although the claims that soft or hollow point bullets cause more tissue destruction are not consistently borne out.

Shotguns differ from rifles and pistols in that they have a smooth barrel that discharges hot gases, wad, and either multiple projectiles or a single projectile (rifled slug). Shot charges contain multiple projectiles that spread out from the muzzle in a conelike pattern. The distance from the muzzle of the shotgun to the point of impact of the projectiles is a key determinant of the magnitude of injury. At short range (less than 6 m), the shot charge containing multiple projectiles results predominantly in a single-hole wound (diameter of less than or equal to 6 cm) that communicates with a deep underlying wound with massive tissue destruction. At this short range, soft-tissue impact deforms the individual pellets, increasing their original cross section with a concomitant increase in tissue crush or hole size. The multiple pellets result in severe disruption between the multiple wound channels. A gradual decrease in the amount of pellet deformation and tissue destruction occurs as the distance of the impact range increases. When the impact range exceeds 7 m, the multiple projectiles result in numerous discrete wounds that are not associated with underlying massive tissue destruction (6).

Shotguns also can discharge rifled slugs that are designed for killing larger animals. The muzzle velocity of rifled slugs (487 m/s) is approximately half that of nonexpanding, fully jacketed rifle projectiles. The rifled slug does not hold the point orientation that it has as it is propelled from the muzzle of the gun, but drifts toward a sideways orientation as it moves toward the target. The rifled slugs experience a 25% decrease in velocity as the impact range increases from 5 to 45 m. At short range (less than or equal to 45 m), the slug deforms on striking the tissue, thereby enhancing the size of the permanent and temporary cavities.

Tissue is injured by a bullet by two mechanisms: tissue crush and tissue stretch. These two mechanisms correspond to the permanent and temporary cavities created by passage of the projectile (8,9). As the bullet travels through tissue it will crush tissue that is directly in its path; this is the primary method of injury from gunshot wounds. The most important determinant of injury is the properties of the tissue that the bullet crushes. The tissue that is crushed corresponds to the permanent cavity formed by the bullet. Passage of the projectile at a high rate of speed also displaces other tissue away from the path of the projectile. As the tissue stretches away from the path of the projectile a temporary cavity that exists for a brief time (measured in milliseconds) is formed. By definition no tissue is present in the temporary cavity. The stretch of tissue away from the temporary cavity can injure tissue to different degrees; the resistance of tissue to stretch depends on tissue elasticity. The same stretch that causes moderate contusion and functional changes in relatively elastic muscle, skin, lung, and bowel wall can cause catastrophic disruption of the inelastic liver, heart, and brain. Muscle, skin, and lung are flexible and elastic, having the physical characteristics of good energy absorbers. While temporary cavitation stretches these tissues, their elastic properties allow them to maintain their structure and function. For example, muscle, when disrupted, will have an area of devitalized nonfunctioning tissue surrounding the permanent cavity; but tissue farther away which was stretched by the temporary cavity is still structurally sound and maintains its contractile function. In comparison, the inelastic liver is fractured and rendered nonviable to a much greater degree by the temporary cavity (24). The brain is a special case of inelastic tissue. Not only is brain tissue very sensitive to structural disruption but this is magnified by the fact that the brain is encased in a solid container (the skull) which prevents tissue displacement. As a bullet penetrates the skull temporary cavitation will increase pressure within the skull and this pressure will be relieved either through the entrance or exit wound.

The size of the temporary cavity depends on the energy of the projectile, the surface area the projectile presents to the tissue as it moves through it, and the mass of tissue displaced. As the bullet tumbles through tissue from the point-forward orientation to the final base-forward orientation it will present its greatest surface area at 90 degrees of rotation. It is at this point where maximal tissue displacement will occur and the size of the temporary cavity is greatest.

These permanent and temporary cavities are the sole wounding mechanisms of missiles. The sonic shock wave generated by supersonic missiles does not cause either tissue displacement or detectable damage. Projectile fragmentation can greatly enhance the effects of the temporary cavity by providing points of weakness on which the stretching effects of cavitation are focused, rather than being absorbed evenly by the tissue mass.

CLINICAL PRESENTATION

Patients who are awake should be asked how many shots they heard and any other information they have relating to the event such as their distance from the weapon and the type of weapon utilized.

The physical examination should focus on the detection of penetrating or perforating injuries. A careful examination of the patient including the back, under the hair, axillae and gluteal folds will help identify injuries. The identification of an initial wound should not negate the need for a complete survey of the patient to avoid missing other injuries. Attempts to differentiate entrance from exit wounds are at best educated guessses. It is best to simply note the size and location of wounds as accurately as possible rather than attempting to designate individual wounds as entrance or exit wounds.

EMERGENCY DEPARTMENT EVALUATION

Initial evaluation is similar to that of any multiple trauma victim. This includes an assessment of the ABCs, followed by the secondary survey and ongoing monitoring of vital signs and pulse oximetry. Radiographs of the areas the bullet is thought to have

traversed are indicated to identify the position of the projectiles. Laboratory studies should be ordered if clinically indicated. The evaluation and management of injuries should follow the algorithms presented in previous chapters. See Chapters 178, "Penetrating Neck Trauma," 183, "Penetrating Chest Trauma," 185, "Penetrating Abdominal Trauma," and 187, "Peripheral Vascular Injuries."

Gunshot wounds must be reported to the appropriate authorities, and the medical record and patient property become evidence. If a patient's clothing is cut, care should be taken to avoid cutting through bullet holes. Location of all wounds identified should be listed in the medical record with comments on the presence of any powder residue observed surrounding the wound. If a bullet is recovered and must be marked to preserve the chain of evidence, it should be marked at the nose or base and not the side, as marking the side will interfere with the evaluation of rifling patterns (6).

EMERGENCY DEPARTMENT MANAGEMENT

The management should proceed as it would for any other victim of multiple trauma in both the prehospital setting and the emergency department (ED). For prehospital personnel, it is important that the scene be secured and declared safe before approaching the victims. Treatment of gunshot wounds is best conducted in consultation with a trauma surgeon. If resources are unavailable the decision to transfer the patient should be made early.

Wounds that may have crossed the mediastinum require a thorough evaluation even in stable patients. Evaluation of the aorta, heart, pericardium, and esophagus is indicated. Patients that present with unstable vital signs or become unstable during evaluation should receive bilateral chest tubes. Bedside ultrasound should be used to identify the presence of pericardial tamponade; pericardiocentesis and ED thoractomy may be necessary. Surgical exploration is often indicated in these patients (22). See Chapter 183, "Penetrating Chest Trauma."

Patients with gunshot wounds to the abdomen, even with stable vital signs, require an exploratory laparotomy. Stable patients with back or flank wounds can be evaluated by CT and observation but these patients may also benefit from surgical exploration. This decision must be made in conjunction with the trauma surgeon. See Chapter 185, "Penetrating Abdominal Trauma."

Injuries of the extremities require evaluation of the distal neurovascular status. A bullet does not need to transect a vessel to cause injury. The development of compartment syndrome as swelling of the injured area develops should be considered. If arterial injury is suspected angiography is indicated. Fractures from a gunshot wound should be treated as open fractures and early antibiotics should be administered. Debridement of devitalized soft tissue is often necessary (22).

Gunshot wounds to the head are often nonsurvivable. For patients that arrive at the hospital alive, consultation with a neurosurgeon is indicated. Injuries to the spine can occur even when the bullet does not actually pass through the vertebral canal, as temporary cavitation can damage the cord without the presence of crushed tissue. Use of steroids is not indicated for penetrating cord injuries. Presence of a CNS injury should not delay the assessment for thoracoabdominal injuries, which can be rapidly fatal.

BLAST INJURY

Blast injury is a general term used to describe the harmful effects produced by the sudden change in environmental pressure originating from an explosion. In the United States, blast injuries usually result from civilian industrial accidents (12) and occasionally from intentional bombing. Injuries produced by explosions can be divided into four categories. *Primary blast injuries* are caused by the sudden change in environmental pressure as the explosion-produced shock wave passes by. *Secondary blast injuries* result from the victim being struck by flying debris. *Tertiary blast injuries* are sustained when the victim is hurled against a stationary object. Both secondary and tertiary blast injuries are due to the accelerative force imparted to loose objects, (debris or the human body) by the shock wave. Although the duration of an explosion-produced shock wave is brief, the accelerative force is significant. For a 70-kg adult, a shock wave with a peak overpressure of 15 pounds per square inch (psi) produces an instantaneous acceleration of 450 ft per second squared or about 14 *g*. *Miscellaneous blast injuries* include exposure to dust, chemicals, direct thermal burns, and burns from blast-ignited fires.

There are four energy sources for explosions.

1. *Mechanical* (hydraulic): This is due to sudden structural failure of a pressurized container.
2. *Electrical:* As an electrical arc passes through the air, intense heat is generated that produces a sudden increase in pressure.
3. *Nuclear:* Intense heat is generated by the process of fission or fusion.
4. *Chemical*
   a. Diffuse reactants: Flammable gases or particulate matter are mixed with air.
   b. Condensed reactants: These are liquid or solid, and can be either low-order (e.g., black powder) or high-order (e.g., TNT) explosives.

Chemical explosions are the most common cause of accidental or intentional blast injuries. Once ignited, a solid or liquid explosive undergoes a chemical decomposition into a gas. The space previously occupied by the explosive is now filled with gas under high pressure and temperature. This pressure is transmitted through the surrounding medium and propagates outward as a shock wave at speeds of 6 to 8 km/s. As measured at a position away from the explosion, the passing shock wave produces a rapid increase in environmental pressure to a peak above the ambient pressure (the peak overpressure), followed by a slow decline of pressure back to baseline. The peak overpressure can be very intense but brief, especially close to an explosion; at a distance of 10.2 m (33 ft), from 0.364 kg (0.8 lb) of TNT, the peak overpressure is about 45 kPa (6.5 psi), with a duration of about 2 ms (7).

As the shock wave expands, the overpressure decreases, the duration lengthens, and the velocity of propagation diminishes. For free field air blast, the peak pressure of the shock wave falls off as the inverse of the distance from the explosion to the third power. For a bomb to produce twice the damage, it must be eight times as large. In denser media, such as water, explosions produce shock waves that have a much higher peak overpressure and a shorter duration, and propagate at a faster velocity than comparable explosions in air. In addition, the overpressure is lower just below the surface than at greater depths. Parts of the body submerged to a greater depth sustain more damage than body parts submerged just below the surface or those that are above the surface.

If the explosion is contained within a closed space, reflections of the shock wave lead to greater overpressure, longer duration, and an increased incidence of primary blast injuries and death (16).

Primary blast injuries are unique to this form of trauma. As the shock wave passes through biologic tissue, the injury is greatest at the interface between tissues of different densities, such as the lungs (which contain both blood and air), the tympanic membrane (which separates two air-filled cavities), and the bowel (which contains a slurry of solid and gas) (18). The potential for primary blast injuries correlates with both the height and duration of the peak overpressure. The likelihood of primary blast injury can be illustrated for a specific clinical outcome (e.g., threshold for lung damage or 50% lethality [LD50]) by pressure-duration graphs. By the late 1960s, the Lovelace Foundation of Albuquerque, New Mexico, had assembled enough animal data to make an estimate of human tolerance to shock waves using pressure-duration graphs (14). The most vulnerable organ to primary blast injury is the tympanic membrane, followed by the lungs (18).

The most common primary blast injury is a linear tear in the inferior portion of the tympanic membrane (10). Depending on the orientation of the external auditory canal in relation to the source of the shock wave, tympanic membranes may rupture at pressures as low as 2 to 5 psi. Explosions also commonly produce damage to the cochlea, which results in sensorineural hearing loss and tinnitus (6).

In the lungs, primary blast injury produces a diffuse lung contusion; damage to the alveolar parenchyma leads to edema and hemorrhage into the interstitial and interalveolar spaces (18). The threshold for lung damage is about 15 psi of peak overpressure, and moderate-to-severe lung damage can be seen with 50 psi (7). Lacerations of the delicate parenchyma may occur in many locations, rupturing alveolar walls, tearing visceral pleura, and creating fissures between the alveolar spaces and the pulmonary veins. The latter allows air to enter into the pulmonary venous system, which can then travel to the left side of the heart and enter the systemic circulation. Systemic air emboli are the likely cause of sudden death, abnormal neurologic findings, and myocardial ischemia seen in some victims in the immediate post blast period.

Primary blast injury to the bowel requires even higher peak overpressures. Such injuries are relatively rare in air explosions, but are more common in water explosions, where the victim is completely or partially submerged. The most common injuries are serosal tears, subserosal and intramural hemorrhages, as well as bowel perforations, usually involving the ileocecal region (18).

CLINICAL PRESENTATION

Casualty analysis of terrorist bombing incidents documents that secondary, tertiary, and miscellaneous injuries account for the vast majority of injuries in victims (13,16,17). The following principles are important to remember.

1. Terrorist explosions often occur within a populated and confined space, producing a large number of casualties.
2. The most common type of injury from terrorist bombs is superficial soft-tissue damage to exposed areas of the body from flying debris. The nonaerodynamic shape of most debris fragments means that they have marked air resistance and limited range for causing serious injury.
3. Serious injuries from terrorist bombings are usually major soft-tissue damage, flash burns, fractures, and eye injuries. Most of these victims are within 10 to 15 m of the source of the explosion.
4. While flash burns commonly injure exposed skin, the temperature content of gas is low and the duration of exposure is brief so that skin underlying clothing and the upper respiratory tract are rarely burned. However, burns and smoke from blast-ignited fires can be more damaging.

5. Other than tympanic membrane rupture, primary blast injuries are uncommon and account for less than 10% of the victims in open-air explosions but up to 38% in closed-space (e.g., bus) explosions (13,16).

A triad of hypotension, bradycardia, and apnea has been observed in experimental animals exposed to moderate thoracic blast injury (11). The first two responses—hypotension and bradycardia—have been observed in human victims immediately after the explosion.

The clinical presentation of patients with primary blast injuries is usually related to damage to the ears, lungs, brain, and bowel. The most common respiratory symptoms are dyspnea, chest pain, and hemoptysis. Physical examination will disclose rales, rhonchi, and, occasionally, the presence of a pneumothorax or pneumomediastinum. Frothy, blood-tinged sputum is seen in severe cases. Radiographic progression of pulmonary injury can occur during the first 48 hours after the explosion and corresponds to the clinical development of respiratory failure.

Tympanic membrane rupture usually presents with decreased hearing, occasionally accompanied by bleeding into the external auditory canal. Perforations are usually small and located in the inferior portion of the membrane (10,15). The degree of associated conductive hearing loss is related to the size of the perforation. Sensorineural hearing loss can occur from damage to the sensory structures in the cochlear basal membrane (20).

Concussion with amnesia is common in blast-injured victims. Focal neurologic findings usually result from cerebral air emboli. If the victim was exposed to underwater blast, concussion of the spinal cord may present as lower extremity weakness, paralysis, or paresthesias lasting from seconds to minutes.

Bowel injuries are more common in victims exposed to underwater explosions, compared with those exposed to air blasts. Clinical symptoms and signs include abdominal pain, tenderness, nausea, vomiting, and an urge to defecate.

Systemic air emboli may be difficult to detect, and the diagnosis depends on clinical suspicion. Definitive diagnosis of systemic air emboli can be made if air emboli are visualized in retinal vessels or on computed tomography of the brain. Air emboli usually develop immediately or very soon after the explosion. However, the presentation may be delayed in patients with pulmonary blast injury until positive-pressure ventilation is initiated; and subsequent cardiac arrest or hemodynamic collapse occur.

DIFFERENTIAL DIAGNOSIS

The key to diagnosis is to obtain a history of injury associated with an explosion. Finding a tympanic perforation may be a clue to potential blast injuries, but the absence of tympanic membrane perforation does not exclude potential blast injury. Nonexplosive blast injury to the ear can occur from a blow that seals the external auditory meatus and causes a sudden increase in air pressure (4). Tympanic membrane perforations and conductive hearing loss are common. Such perforations almost always heal with improvement in the conductive hearing loss.

EMERGENCY DEPARTMENT EVALUATION

The initial evaluation is similar to that of any multiple trauma victim, and begins with the ABCs, followed by the secondary survey and ongoing monitoring, including vital signs, electrocardiographic monitoring, and pulse oximetry. The focus of the examination is the detection of primary blast injury, which may be obscured by secondary and tertiary injury. After the primary and secondary assessments, further examination is directed toward identifying emergent life-threatening arterial emboli. A chest radiograph is indicated because of pulmonary susceptibility to primary blast injury. Radiographic injuries seen with primary blast injury include pneumothorax, pneumomediastinum, hemothorax, subcutaneous emphysema, pulmonary interstitial emphysema, interstitial infiltrates, and alveolar edema.

Laboratory studies should be ordered if clinically indicated, but routine arterial blood gas analysis is particularly useful. In blast-injured patients, the arterial blood gas may be the first sign of lung damage, preceding radiographic changes.

All patients exposed to blast explosions should be observed to exclude delayed manifestations of primary blast injuries. For patients with only soft-tissue injuries, the observation period can be as short as the time it takes for evaluation of such injuries in the emergency department or treatment center.

EMERGENCY DEPARTMENT MANAGEMENT

Evaluation, resuscitation, and ongoing management should proceed as it would for any other victim of multiple trauma in both the prehospital setting and the emergency department. For prehospital personnel, it is important that the scene be secured and declared safe before approaching the victims. Accurate triage is an important determinant of survival for critically injured casualties from terrorist bombings and industrial accidents. High-flow oxygen should be administered, because injury to the lungs may not be initially recognized and hypoxemia may develop insidiously. Because excessive fluid accumulation may occur in damaged lungs, fluid resuscitation should be carefully monitored to avoid exacerbation of pulmonary insufficiency.

For victims with systemic air emboli, hyperbaric oxygen therapy is the treatment of choice. It can be dramatically effective for cerebral air emboli, even up to 12 hours after the acute event. Although unproven, the Trendelenburg position is sometimes advocated to reduce embolization to the brain. However, experimental models and anecdotal reports find no clear benefit to this position, as compared with the standard supine position for assessment and treatment of the trauma patient.

Primary blast lung injury requires careful management (2). For trauma patients with respiratory failure, the standard approach is endotracheal intubation and positive-pressure ventilation. However, positive-pressure ventilation in patients with blast-injured lungs may produce or exacerbate pneumothorax, increase the alveolar-to-pulmonary vein pressure gradient, and potentiate systemic air embolization. The immediate use of mechanical ventilation during the first 2 hours in a dog model of blast-injured lungs resulted in an increased rate of air embolism and mortality. In addition, general anesthesia is poorly tolerated in patients with primary blast injury during the first 24 to 48 hours; therefore, regional or spinal anesthesia should be used, if possible. Intravenous fluid management should be carefully monitored, and pulmonary artery and arterial catheters may be required to manage fluids appropriately. For patients with severe pulmonary blast injuries, a regimen of volume-controlled, synchronized, intermittent, mandatory ventilation with small tidal volumes and permissive hypercapnia ($PaCO_2$ 57 mm Hg) appears beneficial (21).

Abdominal blast injury is managed just like that of any other blunt-force trauma to the abdomen. Lacerations, abrasions, fractures, and burns resulting from secondary and tertiary blast injury can be managed the same as trauma caused by other mechanisms. Fragments generated by small explosions (e.g., from a hand grenade) tend to produce wounds with little damage and can usually be managed without extensive wound exploration and fragment removal (5). However, high-velocity fragment wounds (e.g., from a terrorist bomb incident) should have as many fragments excised as possible and the wound left open for delayed primary closure.

Tympanic membrane perforation has a high rate of spontaneous healing, especially if it is small and marginal in location (15). For large and central perforations, immediate paper patching has been advocated (15). If a perforation (large or small) does not heal after 10 months, tympanoplasty should be performed. In general, the external auditory canal should be kept clean and dry; there is no need for routine irrigation or use of topical solutions. One potential long-term sequela to bear in mind is the development of cholesteatoma. The ruptured tympanic membrane can distribute small pieces of keratinizing squamous epithelium throughout the middle ear and mastoid sinuses, viable fragments of which may grow into a mass of keratinous debris known as a cholesteatoma. Cholesteatoma may lead to varying degrees of sensorineural or conductive hearing loss and may erode into surrounding structures.

DISPOSITION

Blast injuries that result in multiple trauma require consultation with the hospital trauma service or referral and transfer to the regional trauma center. If systemic air embolism is suspected, urgent consultation with a hyperbaric specialist is required for definitive therapy. Patients with signs of blunt-force trauma and those with tympanic membrane rupture should be observed for occult injuries during the first 24 hours. Outpatient management is acceptable for patients who were a distance from the blast origin and received relatively minor lacerations, abrasions, fractures, or burns (17).

Patients with serious blast injuries should be transferred to a regional trauma center. Those with suspected systemic air embolism may require transfer to a hyperbaric therapy facility. If air transport is used, pressurized aircraft or flights at low altitude are important to prevent further exacerbation of air emboli or pneumothoraces from barometric changes during flight.

CRITICAL INTERVENTIONS

> - Carefully examine the back, scalp, axillae, and gluteal folds for wounds in patients with penetrating trauma
> - In blast victims, examine for ruptured tympanic membrane since this is an indicator of the potential for primary blast injuries to the lungs
> - Obtain trauma surgery consultation early in the management of patients with gunshot wounds and blast injuries

COMMON PITFALLS

✔ Delaying the evaluation for thoracoabdominal injuries in stable patients with gunshot wounds
✔ Delaying the transfer of gunshot victims to another facility
✔ Failure to appreciate that accurate triage at the scene is an important determinant of survival for critically injured victims of explosions
✔ Failure to recognize symptoms suggestive of cerebral emboli or myocardial ischemia resulting from systemic air embolism in blast victims
✔ Failure to appreciate that positive-pressure ventilation poses a significant risk of worsening pneumothorax or producing systemic air embolization in blast victims

Acknowledgments

Thanks to the previous edition's chapter authors J. Stephan Stapczynski, Judd E. Hollander, and Adam Singer.

References

1. Aboutanos MB, Baker SP. Wartime civilian injuries: epidemiology and intervention strategies. *J Trauma* 1997;43:719.
2. Argyros GJ. Management of primary blast injury. *Toxicology* 1997;121:105.
3. Barach E, Tomlanovich M, Nowack R. Ballistics: A pathophysiologic examination of the wounding mechanisms of firearms, Part I. *J Trauma* 1986;26:225–235. Part II. *J Trauma* 1986;26:374–383.
4. Berger G, Finkelstein Y, Avraham S, et al. Patterns of hearing loss in nonexplosive blast injury of the ear. *J Laryngol Otol* 1997;111:1137.
5. Coupland RM. Hand grenade injuries among civilians. *JAMA* 1993;270:624.
6. Di Maio V. *Gunshot wounds.* CRC Press LLC, 1999:1–62.
7. Elsayed NM. Toxicology of blast overpressure. *Toxicology* 1997;121:1.
8. Fackler ML. Ballistic Injury. *Ann Emerg Med* 1986;15:1451–1455.
9. Fackler ML. Wound ballistics: A review of common misconceptions. *JAMA* 1980;259:2730.
10. Garth RJ. Blast injury of the ear: an overview and guide to management. *Injury* 1995;26:363.
11. Guy RJ, Kirkman E, Watkins PE, et al. Physiologic responses to primary blast. *J Trauma* 1998;45:983.
12. Karmy-Jones R, Kissinger D, Golocovsky M, et al. Bomb-related injuries. *Milit Med* 1994;159:536.
13. Katz E, Ofek B, Adler J, et al. Primary blast injury after a bomb explosion in a civilian bus. *Ann Surg* 1989;209:484.
14. Kokinakis W, Rudolph RR. An assessment of the current state-of-the-art of incapacitation by air blast. *Acta Chir Scand* 1982;508[Suppl]:135.
15. Kronenberg J, Ben-Shoshan J, Wolf M. Perforated tympanic membrane after blast injury. *Am J Otol* 1993;14:92.
16. Leibovici D, Gofrit ON, Stein M, et al. Blast injuries: bus versus open-air bombings—a comparative study of injuries in survivors of open-air versus confined-space explosions. *J Trauma* 1996;41:1030.
17. Mallonne S, Shariat S, Stennies G, et al. Physical injuries and fatalities resulting from the Oklahoma City bombing. *JAMA* 1996;276:382.
18. Mayorga MA. The pathology of primary blast overpressure injury. *Toxicology* 1997;121:17.
19. NCHS. Vital statistics mortality data, underlying cause of death detail, 2001. US Department of Health and Human Services, Public Health Service, CDC, 2001.
20. Patterson JH, Hamerik RP. Blast overpressure induced structural and functional changes in the auditory system. *Toxicology* 1997;121:29.
21. Sorkine P, Szold O, Kluger Y, et al. Permissive hypercapnia ventilation in patients with severe pulmonary blast injury. *J Trauma* 1998;45:35.
22. Swan KG. Missile injuries: Wound ballistics and principles of management. *Milit Med* 1987;152:29–34.
23. WRISS. Weapon related injury update October 1999. Massachusetts Department of Public Health, Bureau of Health Statistics, Research and Evaluation, 1999:1–4.
24. Zajychuck R (ed). *Textbook of military medicine* Part I, Volume 5. Conventional Warfare: ballistics, blast and burn injuries. TMM Publications, 1989:83–220.

CHAPTER 201
Hanging and Strangulation Injuries

Leon D. Sanchez and Richard Wolfe

Strangulation occurs when pressure is applied to the neck. This common traumatic injury accounts for 2.5% of deaths worldwide. Men are 3 to 5 times more likely to be victims than women, and those injured are most often between the ages of 21 to 40 years (17). Causes of death from strangulation have been attributed to asphyxia, arterial occlusion, spinal cord injuries, and cardiac arrest due to pressure on the vasoactive centers of the great vessels. The specific role played by each of these causes as well as the types of injuries depend on the method used to apply pressure, the force, and the duration of the strangulation. To better manage this injury, it is helpful to subdivide strangulation by the methods used to apply the pressure: hanging, garroting, or throttling.

Hanging occurs when the ligature pressure is applied by the weight of the individual's body as part of a judicial, homicidal, suicidal or accidental event. Although judicial hangings are rarely performed today, hanging is the third most common form of suicide after firearms and ingestions. Men attempt hanging 3 times more often than women do. Newly jailed prisoners are at particular risk. Complete hanging refers to the body being suspended and incomplete hanging describes situations where the body exerts pressure but is not suspended. Accidental hangings are most commonly incomplete. Children and individuals who practice autoerotic asphyxiation are the most common victims of accidental hanging (17).

Garroting or ligature strangulation involves pressure being applied to the neck by a ligature just like in hanging. The difference is that the force used to exert this pressure is something other than the individual's body weight. Throttling can be considered a type of garroting where the ligature is the assailant's hands which exert the pressure directly.

CLINICAL PRESENTATION

Hanging or strangulation may result in injury to vascular structures in the neck. Venous obstruction results from forces applied to the jugular system (10,11). This leads to vascular congestion and cerebral hypoxia. As a result of the hypoxia, the neck musculature is thought to relax leading to further compression which can lead to arterial and airway occlusion (10). Injury to the arteries is caused by hyperextension and rotation of the head. The carotid artery can be stretched over the transverse process of C2 or compressed by direct pressure over the transverse process of C6 (10,12). This results in an intimal tear (3,12). Vertebral artery flow is not affected by direct pressure except at the extremes of rotation and lateral flexion (10).

Neurologic injury after hanging results from a combination of hypoxia and ischemia. Autonomic stimulation from pressure on the carotid bodies or vagal sheath can lead to cardiac arrest (11,14). Hypoxia secondary to upper airway obstruction plays a role in the development of neurologic injury or death but is thought to be second in importance to ischemia. Ischemic injury is caused by venous vascular congestion and arterial compression, both of which result in decreased cerebral flow (2,4,11,21). Increased intracranial pressure secondary to cerebral edema is common in patients with altered mental status (6,14). Nevertheless, delayed neurologic sequellae are rare (4,11), and even patients who present with a low Glasgow coma scale (GCS) often recover fully (21).

Injury to the laryngotracheal apparatus may be caused by compression or traction of the involved structures. Manifestations of these injuries may be evident at presentation or may have a delayed course (18). Most airway injuries by themselves are not life-threatening (11). In one study which looked at 112 deaths and 59 survivors of strangulation, only one case required emergent operative management. None of the deaths could be attributed to airway injury (13). Fractures of the hyoid bone and thyroid cartilage are seen with some regularity while cricoid fractures are less common (13,16). The incidence of these fractures increases with greater age of the patient probably due to calcification of the structures (16). Throttling victims have a much higher incidence of fractures compared to hanging victims. The

incidence of thyroid and hyoid fractures in hanging victims is in the 10 to 15% range; cricoid fractures are rare. Throttling victims have an incidence of fractures in the 30% to 40% range (11,13,16). Even with the higher rates of injury in throttling victims, injuries to the laryngotracheal apparatus are rarely life-threatening. Asphyxia from upper airway obstruction due to the ligature itself is also rare, although pressure from the ligature can displace the tongue upwards and obstruct the airway (15,21).

In the late 19th and early 20th centuries, British postmortem studies of judicial hanging demonstrated that a minimum drop force (patient weight multiplied by the length of the drop) was needed to cause a cervical spine fracture. The required drop height varies depending on factors such as the weight of the subject, the neck musculature and the strength of the bone itself. Although generally a drop height greater than the patient's height is required to cause a spinal fracture, in rare circumstances shorter drop heights can produce these injuries. The minimum reported drop height is 3 feet (1,21). The most common spinal injury with long drops is disjointing of the second from the third cervical vertebra and bilateral fractures of the second cervical vertebra, the classic Hangman's fracture. The position of the knot is important. In typical hangings, the knot is placed under the occiput and has the greatest ability to cause arterial occlusion rather than a spinal fracture. A Hangman's fracture will most likely occur when the knot is placed under the chin to ensure hyperextension, yet one study reported routine occurrence with the knot in the suboccipital position (1). Despite drops from body height and knot placement under the chin, even "proper" judicial hangings do not always cause cervical spine fractures (9,16). In complete suicidal and accidental hangings, most victims have negligible drop distances and few if any cervical spine fractures occur (2,5,20,21).

Pulmonary complications from strangulation injury include pulmonary edema, aspiration pneumonia and adult respiratory distress syndrome. Aspiration pneumonia following vomiting in patients with a depressed mental status is reported in case series of strangulation victims (6,11,21). Pulmonary edema is thought to be caused by inspiratory efforts against an occluded upper airway (19). The adult respiratory distress syndrome (ARDS) in strangulation victims is secondary to the perfusion of the brain with hypoxic blood (7). Brain hypoxia leads to autonomically mediated vasoconstriction of the pulmonary venules, leading to ARDS (7,15). This mechanism may also play a role in the formation of pulmonary edema.

The clinical presentation of a patient with a strangulation injury can vary from being normal to a full cardiac arrest, and from an alert mental status to deep coma. The presenting mental status and GCS is related to the duration of hanging. The GCS is a poor predictor of the patient's final outcome and patients presenting with very low scores have a strong likelihood of surviving the injury with a normal mental status. Ligature marks are often present but may be absent (21). Subconjunctival, gingival and oral petechial hemorrhages may be observed. These are thought to be caused by vascular congestion (13). Patients may also present with hoarseness or voice change (14), both of which may represent injury to the laryngotracheal apparatus. Subcutaneous emphysema can also be present (13). Occasionally, patients will present with frank stridor. Tachypnea can be an early sign of aspiration pneumonia or pulmonary edema (14,19).

Mental status changes may be secondary to brain anoxia, preexisting mental illness or posttraumatic response to the event (14,21). In many of these patients the evaluation may be more difficult due to the presence of alcohol or other substances (14). One study found that 70% of hanging patients had concomitant drug or alcohol ingestion (20). Throttling victims often present after a domestic abuse incident and frequently will not volunteer the fact that they were throttled, unless specifically asked (8).

EMERGENCY DEPARTMENT EVALUATION

After immediate life-threats have been addressed, a more extensive history and physical should be performed. The presence of alcohol and other substances in these patients is common and may complicate the exam. In alert patients attention should be paid to the evaluation of the laryngotracheal apparatus and to the pulmonary status. The presence of hoarseness, difficulty swallowing or other complaints that raise suspicion for laryngotracheal injury should prompt a more extensive work up. Cervical spine films are of little benefit for the evaluation of cervical spine injuries as these are extremely rare. However, they may reveal soft tissue swelling or a hyoid bone fracture. Evidence of laryngeal edema should be followed by prompt ear nose and throat (ENT) consultation. Computed tomography (CT) of the neck can be very helpful in delineating any injury to the laryngeal skeleton. Early control of the airway should be considered in these patients.

Pulmonary complications are the leading cause of death in patients that survive to hospital admission. Pulse oximetry and chest radiographs should be routinely performed in these patients. Pulmonary edema and ARDS may present early or there may be a delay of several hours. Aspiration pneumonia is also common and more likely in those patients with an initial depression of their mental status.

Vascular injuries that are clinically significant are essentially restricted to the arterial tree. Although extremely rare, clinical signs of arterial dissection should prompt further work up. The most common signs which should raise suspicion for dissection are neurologic abnormalities consistent with a transient ischemic attack or cerebrovascular accident, Horner syndrome, amaurosis fugax, unexplained nausea or vomiting and vertigo. Headache and neck pain are also common presenting complaints, although they are not very specific.

The gold standard for this evaluation is four-vessel angiography. Magnetic resonance angiography (MRA) and CT angiography are reasonable alternatives if angiography is unavailable or if they are available faster than angiography, as they may help delineate injury and expedite the work up. However, these "techniques" may miss injuries. A negative MRI or CT does not completely rule out the diagnosis. Doppler ultrasonography is not useful for the evaluation of the vertebral arteries but can provide useful information about the carotid arteries. However, the sensitivity of duplex ultrasound is not high enough to completely rule out carotid injury. In patients with a high suspicion for arterial injury four-vessel angiography remains the test of choice and if unavailable, transfer of the patient to another institution should be considered.

EMERGENCY DEPARTMENT MANAGEMENT

The initial presentation of the patient may dictate early management of the airway due to respiratory distress or poor neurologic status. Cervical spine injury is extraordinarily rare in strangulation victims and excessive cervical spine precautions need not be taken. Airway injuries severe enough to interfere with airway management are uncommon and intubation using rapid sequence intubation is recommended. When possible, intracranial pressure (ICP) blunting techniques should be used during the intubation. Positive end expiratory pressure should be instituted early as these patients are at high risk for the development of pulmonary edema and ARDS.

Once the life-threats have been addressed, special attention should be paid to psychosocial issues. Throttling and ligature strangulation victims are often victims of domestic abuse. It may not be safe for these patients to be discharged even in the absence of medically important injuries. In the adult population, hanging victims are predominantly victims of suicide attempts. Ingestion of toxic substances in these patients is common and should be ruled out. These patients should be separated from their property and placed under direct observation to avoid further attempts at harming themselves. Psychiatric consultation is indicated.

CRITICAL INTERVENTIONS

- Ensure a patent airway. Monitor the respiratory status closely and manage the airway if needed
- Obtain early ENT consultation for suspected laryngotracheal injuries
- Consider the possibility of increased ICP in patients with a depressed sensorium
- If there is any evidence of increased ICP, obtain neurosurgical consultation and initiate measures to decrease ICP
- Consider toxic ingestions
- Address the psychiatric or social issues that are at the root of the strangulation once immediate life-threats have been managed

DISPOSITION

Due to the presence of delayed neurologic and pulmonary complications in strangling victims, admission for at least a 24-hour period is recommended. Otolaryngology and neurosurgical consultation should be considered when warranted. Psychiatric consultation as well as social work involvement may be necessary.

COMMON PITFALLS

- ✔ Failure to consider early airway management
- ✔ Failure to diagnose vascular dissections
- ✔ Failure to involve ENT and neurosurgery when needed
- ✔ Failure to consider interpersonal violence
- ✔ Failure to consider toxic ingestions
- ✔ Failure to involve psychiatry
- ✔ Early discharge of the patient

Acknowledgments

Thanks to the previous edition's chapter authors Yevgeniy Gincherman and Edward T. Dickinson.

References

1. Anonymous. Hanging from a historical and physiological point of view. *Med Times Gazette* 1871;10:669–671.
2. Aufderheide TP, Aprahamian C, Mateer JR, et al. Emergency airway management in hanging victims. *Ann Emerg Med* 1994;24:879.
3. Berne JD, Norwood SH, McAuley CE, et al. The high morbidity of blunt cerebrovascular injury in an unscreened population: more evidence of the need for mandatory screening protocols. *J Am Coll Surg* 2001;192:314.
4. Dooling EC, Richardson EP. Delayed encephalopathy after strangling. *Arch Neurol* 1976;33:196.
5. Elfawal MA, Awad OA. Deaths from hanging in the Eastern Province of Saudi Arabia. *Med Sci Law* 1994;34:307.
6. Feldman KW, Simms RJ. Strangulation in childhood: epidemiology and clinical course. *Pediatrics* 1980;65:1079.
7. Fischman CM, Goldstein MS, Gardner LB. Suicidal hanging: An association with adult respiratory distress syndrome. *Chest* 1977;71:225.
8. Funk M, Schuppel J. Strangulation injuries. *WMJ* 2003;102:41.
9. Hammond GM. On the proper method of executing the sentence of death by hanging. *Med Rec* 1882;22:426–428.
10. Iserson KV. Strangulation: A review of ligature, manual, and postural neck compression injuries. *Ann Emerg Med* 1984;13:179.

11. Kaki A, Crosby ET, Lui ACP. Airway and respiratory management following non lethal hanging. *Can J Anaesth* 1997;44:445.
12. Kumar SR, Weaver FA, Yellin AE. Cervical Vascular Injuries: carotid and jugular venous injuries. *Surg Clin North Am* 2001;81:1331.
13. Line WS, Stanley RB, Choi JH. Strangulation: a full spectrum of blunt neck trauma. *Ann Otol Rhino Laryngol* 1985;94:543.
14. McClane GE, Strack GB, Hawley D. A review of 300 attempted Strangulation cases Part II: Clinical evaluation of the surviving victim. *J Emerg Med* 2001;21:311.
15. McHugh TP, Stout M. Near hanging injury. *Ann Emerg Med* 1983;12:774.
16. Morild I. Fractures of neck structures in suicidal hanging. *Med Sci Law* 1996;36:80.
17. National Safety Council: *Injury facts*, Itasca, Ill, 1999, The Council.
18. Noto R. Les traumatisms laryngo-tracheaux au cours des pendaisons. *Ann Anesth Franc* 1976;17:751.
19. Oswalt CE, Gates GA, Fritz MG, et al. Pulmonary Edema as a complication of acute airway obstruction. *JAMA* 1977;238:1833.
20. Penney DJ, Stewart AH, Parr MJ. Prognostic outcome indicators following hanging injuries. *Resuscitation* 2002;54:27.
21. Vande Krol L, Wolfe R. The emergency department management of near hanging victims. *J Emerg Med* 1994;12:285.

CHAPTER 202
Trauma in Pregnancy

Susan B. Promes and Charles J. Gerardo

TABLE 202.1.   Changes in Maternal Physiology During Pregnancy

Body Water Metabolism	↑ total body water
Cardiovascular System	↑ cardiac output
	↑ pulse to 80–95 bpm
	↓ BP in second trimester
	↓ central venous pressure
	left axis deviation on electrocardiogram
	↓ venous return when patient supine
Respiratory System	↑ respiratory rare
	↑ tidal volume
	↑ minute ventilation
	↓ functional residual capacity
	+ respiratory alkalosis
	↑ oxygen consumption
Hematologic System	↑ blood volume producing a dilutional anemia
	↑ white blood cell count
	↓ platelet count
	↑ erythrocyte sedimentation rate
	↑ fibrinogen, factors VII, VIII, IX and X
	↑ risk thromboembolic disease
Urinary System	↓ motility in collecting system
	↑ glomelular filtration rate
	↓ BUN and creatinine levels
	↑ glucose excretion
Gastrointestial System	↓ motility
	↓ tone in lower esophageal sphincter
	↑ dilation of hemorrhoidal veins
	↑ risk of gallstone formation
	↑ spider angiomas & palmar erythema
	↓ albumin & total protein levels
	↑ serum alkaline phosphatase
Mosculoskeletal System	↓ total calcium levels
	↑ ligamentous laxity
Endocrine System	↑ aldosterone & cortisol levels
	↑ peripheral resistance to insulin
Central Nervous System	↓ coordination in late gestation
	↑ emotional lability

Adapted from Gordon MC. Maternal Physiology in Pregnancy. In: Gabbe SG, Niebly JR, Simpson JL, eds. *Obstetrics: Normal and Problem Pregnancies*. New York: Churchill Livingstone, 2002;63–91.

Significant trauma affects approximately 8% of pregnant women (1). In fact, trauma is the leading cause of maternal death during pregnancy (5). The pregnant trauma patient presents unique challenges to the emergency department (ED) team caring for her. Not only is the physician caring for two patients, but both of the patients have their own unique needs. The emergency medicine mantra in the setting of the pregnant trauma patient is to resuscitate the mother first. The well being of the unborn fetus is dependent upon the homodynamic stability of the mother.

It is imperative that the physician caring for the gravid woman be aware of the physiologic changes that occur during pregnancy and the impact these changes may have on the resuscitation of the pregnant woman and her unborn fetus (Table 202.1). This knowledge is critical to the evaluation and treatment of the pregnant trauma patient and the unborn child.

Pregnancy is a high-flow, low-resistance state of cardiovascular homeostasis. Heart rate increases until the end of the second trimester, when it plateaus at 10 to 15 beats above baseline. Systolic and, to a greater degree, diastolic blood pressures decrease 5 to 15 mm Hg during the first and second trimesters, returning to prepregnancy baseline levels during the third trimester. Cardiac output increases 40% by the end of the first trimester and persists at this level, causing a systolic flow murmur in 90% of pregnant women. By the third trimester, there is increased vascular congestion in the pelvis and a 50% decrease in the velocity of venous flow in the lower limbs associated with a 10 mm Hg increase in venous pressure (2). These changes predispose the gravida to deep vein thromboses, as well as increased bleeding with lower extremity trauma.

The diaphragm is gradually pushed up 3 to 4 cm, causing the QRS axis on the electrocardiogram to shift an average of 15 degrees to the left. Other pregnancy-related electrocardio-graphic changes include Q waves in leads III and aVF and flattened or inverted T waves in lead III.

Elevation of the diaphragm causes a 25% decrease in functional residual capacity, resulting in decreased maternal oxygen reserve. Pulmonary function is further compromised by increased oxygen consumption. Starting in the first trimester, stimulation of the medullary respiratory center by progesterone gradually increases minute ventilation by up to 50% (a result of increased tidal volume). This is accompanied by a 10 mm Hg increase in Po_2, a 10 mm Hg decrease in Pco_2, and a compensatory decrease in bicarbonate to about 19.5 mEq/L, producing a net slight respiratory alkalosis.

Progesterone also causes smooth muscle relaxation in the gastrointestinal tract, which leads to decreased motility and decreased gastroesophageal sphincter competence, producing a greater risk of aspiration. Urologic changes begin at the end of the first trimester. The bladder becomes hyperemic and rises out of the pelvis, and the ureters dilate and become laterally displaced. After the third month, the uterus is no longer protected by the pelvis. Uterine blood flow increases tenfold by term. The uterine vascular bed has no autoregulatory capability and is completely dependent on maternal blood pressure for perfusion.

Several hematologic changes accompany pregnancy. A 50% increase in blood volume, accompanied by only a 20% to 30% increase in red blood cell mass, results in a 3% to 6% drop in hematocrit. The white blood cell count increases to 12,000 to

18,000/μL by the second trimester and may increase to 25,000/μL with stress. The prothrombin and partial thromboplastin times are somewhat shortened. Coagulation factors rise gradually and, by the third trimester, exceed fibrinolytic activity.

The fetus has a higher hemoglobin concentration than the mother, and fetal hemoglobin has a greater affinity for oxygen. As a result, fetal oxygen consumption does not decrease until oxygen delivery decreases by 50% (15). This allows the fetus to tolerate brief periods of maternal hypoxia and hypoperfusion. Furthermore, late in pregnancy, the fetus is capable of the mammalian diving reflex by which blood can be redistributed to the heart and brain (15).

CLINICAL PRESENTATION

Critically ill pregnant trauma patients may present with normal vital signs due to the physiologic changes that occur in pregnancy; this should not give the emergency physician a false sense of security. Pregnant women have increased blood volume as they near term so blood loss must be excessive before hypotension occurs. Abdominal pain in the pregnant trauma patient may be due to common intraabdominal injuries associated with blunt trauma. However, other causes of life-threatening problems include uterine rupture, placental abruption, and premature labor.

After penetrating trauma, the emergency physician can expect slightly different injuries due to the change in maternal anatomy with increasing gestational age. The diaphragm and intraabdominal contents are displaced upwards by the enlarging uterus and hence the injury patterns will vary. For example, someone with a stab wound to the left upper quadrant is at increased risk for intestinal injury since the uterus displaces the intestinal contents superiorly.

Whether the pregnant patient is involved in blunt or penetrating trauma, the fetus in addition to the mother is at risk for injury. Even minor maternal injuries can lead to placental abruption, uterine rupture, fetal-maternal hemorrhage and premature birth. The physician should look for signs of occult injury that can be manifested by uterine irritability, vaginal bleeding and fetal tachycardia.

DIFFERENTIAL DIAGNOSIS

The emergency physician caring for the pregnant trauma patient should first consider the typical injury patterns that are associated with a given mechanism of injury. The pregnant trauma patient is not immune to common traumatic injuries. While the emergency physician is evaluating the pregnant patient for common injuries, the physician should also consider the unique role the gravid uterus plays in the traumatic event. As the uterus enlarges during pregnancy, changes in intraabdominal anatomy alter the injury pattern. For example, the diaphragm moves cephalad into the thoracic cavity. Subsequently, in a pregnant patient who sustains a penetrating injury to the chest, the physician should have a greater suspicion for a diaphragmatic injury. Additionally, the large gravid uterus displaces the intraabdominal contents making bowel injuries less common and injury to the uterus more common in blunt trauma. A few important injuries associated with pregnancy include placental abruption, uterine rupture, maternal-fetal hemorrhage and premature labor. The greater the severity of maternal trauma, the more likely a significant fetal insult will occur. Pearlman, et al reported a fetal loss rate of 41% with life-threatening maternal injuries while the fetal loss rate was 1.6% with non-life-threatening injuries (17).

Seizures in trauma patients are generally associated with head injuries. However, in the gravid trauma patient, the emergency physician must also consider *eclampsia* as the etiology of the seizure and subsequent trauma.

EMERGENCY DEPARTMENT EVALUATION

Since the survival of the fetus is dependent upon maternal resuscitation, the evaluation of the pregnant trauma patient should proceed in a step-wise fashion. Advanced Trauma Life Support principles should be followed as in the nonpregnant trauma patient. However, during the primary and secondary trauma surveys, the emergency physician must apply a detailed understanding of the physiologic changes that occur in the pregnant state in order to detect potentially life-threatening conditions. The airway must be managed aggressively. All pregnant trauma patients should be placed on oxygen, since oxygen consumption is increased with pregnancy and it is important to avoid fetal hypoxia. When evaluating the circulatory status, the physician should remember that the second trimester pregnant patient without significant injuries may have an elevated heart rate and lower blood pressure. Conversely, she may also have significant life-threatening hemorrhage without alteration in vital signs due to the physiologic increase in cardiac output and intravascular volume.

Once the primary survey is completed a complete history should be obtained including last menstrual period, estimated date of delivery, previous pregnancy history and any problems associated with the pregnancy.

The fetus is evaluated during the secondary survey. The fundal height should be assessed, recognizing that a fundal height at or above the level of the umbilicus may indicate a potentially viable fetus. The distance between the symphysis pubis and the uterine fundus measured in centimeters approximates gestational age in weeks (Fig. 202.1). The threshold for fetal viability is 23 to 24 weeks depending on the resources available at the facility to care for the neonate (4). The presence of fetal heart tones should be documented. In patients 20 weeks or greater, gestation and cardiotocographic monitoring should be obtained as soon as possible. This gives the physician information regarding fetal-maternal well-being. A normal fetal heart rate is between 120 and 160 bpm. Fetal tachycardia, fetal bradycardia, contractions, loss of beat–to-beat variability, late or prolonged decelerations after contractions, may be signs of fetal distress heralding such pathologic states as placental abruption or occult maternal shock. If the patient has vaginal bleeding, then a vaginal speculum examination should be performed to identify the source of bleeding. Aside from evaluation of the pregnancy itself, a speculum exam may reveal signs of genitourinary trauma such as lacerations from pelvic fractures or penetrating trauma.

Upon completion of the primary and secondary surveys the clinician should tailor further diagnostic studies to the individual patient. Diagnostic tests and therapy should be directed primarily at the care of the mother and should not be delayed because of the pregnancy. As signs of shock may be late, a more aggressive work up is appropriate in pregnancy. The hematologic changes of pregnancy must be considered when evaluating any laboratory results. Pregnant women have a "dilutional anemia" due to their increased blood volume (Table 202.2). They also have an elevated white blood cell count and sedimentation rate. Fibrinogen levels are increased, as are coagulation factors. All pregnant trauma patients should have blood type determination since all Rh-negative women require Rho (D) immune globulin (RhoGAM). The recommended dose for all Rh-negative gravidas is 300 micrograms regardless of gestational age. A Kleihauer-Betke test is indicated only for those Rh-negative women at risk for massive isoimmunization (greater than 16 weeks estimated gestational age [EGA] with significant trauma). The

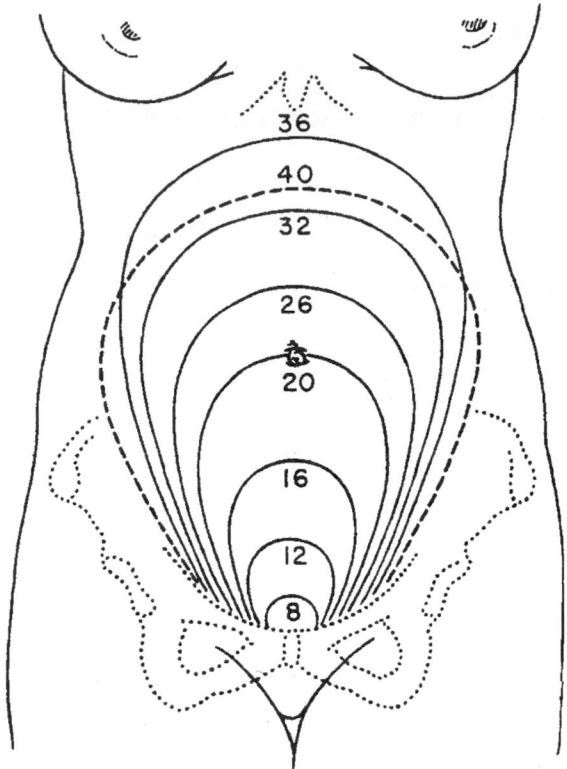

Figure 202.1. The height of the uterine fundus at different gestational dates.

Kleinhauer-Betke test uses a citric acid elution technique on maternal blood to stain the fetal cells present in the maternal blood sample. This test quantifies the degree of fetal-maternal hemorrhage allowing the clinician to adjust the dose of RhoGAM to treat the Rh-negative gravida.

Ultrasound is another diagnostic modality, which may be used in pregnancy (13). The ultrasound examination can be used to evaluate for a traumatic pericardial effusion and tamponade or to demonstrate free fluid in the abdomen. Additionally, it may help determine fetal age, position, and amniotic fluid volume. However, its limitations must be recognized. Ultrasound may easily miss placental abruption; the reported sensitivity is 2% to 20% (14). This diagnosis is made by signs of maternal compromise or fetal distress on cardiotocographic monitoring.

Since fetal outcome is dependent upon maternal condition and resuscitation, radiographic studies should not be withheld in

TABLE 202.2. Hemoglobin Values in Pregnancy

Weeks' Gestation	Mean Hemoglobin (g/dL)	Fifth Percentile Hemoglobin (g/dL)
12	12.2	11.0
16	11.8	10.6
20	11.6	10.5
24	11.6	10.5
28	11.8	10.7
32	12.1	11.0
36	12.5	11.4
40	12.9	11.9

Adapted from U.S. Department of Health and Human Services: *MMWR* 189;38:400–404.

TABLE 202.3. Estimated Radiation Dose to Fetus Per Radiograph

Cervical spine	< 1 mrad
Chest	1–3 mrad
Abdomen	200–500 mrad
Pelvis	200–500 mrad
Lumbar spine	600–1,000 mrad
Hip/femur	100–450 mrad
CT head/chest with shielding	< 1,000 mrad
CT abdomen	3,000 mrad
CT pelvis	3,000–9,000 mrad

order to prevent fetal radiation exposure. However, knowledge of the underlying principles of fetal radiation exposure must be understood by the practitioner in order to address patient concerns and guide evaluation (Table 202.3). In the first 10 days of pregnancy, the response to significant radiation exposure is an all-or-none response. From 10 days to 10 weeks the fetus is at greatest risk for radiation related malformation. After 20 weeks the fetus does not appear to be at increased risk of malformation (8). Fortunately, exposure to less than 5 to 10 rads does not increase the baseline risk. Most shielded plain film radiographs and head or chest CT scans are well below this level. An abdominal CT scan may deliver 3 to 9 rads of radiation to the fetus. In patients less than 20 weeks pregnant the emergency physician may consider shielding the uterus and scanning only the upper abdomen to rule out solid organ injury. The patient must also be followed clinically for signs of increasing abdominal pain, worsening anemia, fetal distress, or maternal hemodynamic changes.

Diagnostic peritoneal lavage (DPL) may be performed in pregnancy using the supraumbilical technique. As with ultrasound, DPL cannot be used to evaluate the retroperitoneum. Exploratory laparotomy may be necessary during pregnancy, especially in patients with penetrating trauma to the upper abdomen. Previously, surgical exploration was recommended for all pregnant patients with penetrating trauma. However, based on case series some authors advocate nonoperative management with observation for penetrating wounds directly to the uterus (7,9). The determination of whether or not to perform a cesarean section at the time of exploration is based on evidence of fetal-maternal compromise detected on cardiotocographic monitoring.

EMERGENCY DEPARTMENT MANAGEMENT

As with all trauma patients, the initial management of the pregnant trauma patient occurs simultaneously with the ED evaluation. Emphasis is placed on maternal resuscitation in order to maximize both maternal and fetal outcomes. Special care should be taken if the patient requires intubation. The pregnant patient is at increased risk of aspiration secondary to delayed gastric emptying and decreased lower esophageal sphincter tone. Gravidas have decreased oxygen reserves and may desaturate rapidly after paralysis (12). Due to the patient's lack of reserve, they may require early intubation in order to maximize oxygenation and ventilation. If the patient requires a chest tube in later pregnancy, it should be placed one to two rib spaces higher as the diaphragm will be elevated. This along with palpation of the diaphragm with a finger during thoracostomy placement will prevent inadvertent intraabdominal placement of the tube.

After the 20th week of pregnancy the trauma patient is at risk for the *supine hypotensive syndrome*. This is caused by uterine compression of the inferior vena cava leading to decreased venous return to the heart. There is a subsequent decrease in preload and in cardiac output. All pregnant trauma patients of 20 weeks or greater gestation that are supine should be placed in the left lateral decubitus position. This is accomplished by tilting the backboard so the uterus is not compressing the inferior vena cava and compromising venous return to the heart. The gravida should be aggressively resuscitated early since gravid patients may not develop overt signs of hypovolemia until they are in the late stages of shock. Changes in uterine blood flow, which can lead to fetal distress, occur before maternal vital signs change. Crystalloid fluid replacement should be started, and blood administered as necessary. Vasopressor support should be avoided. These medications significantly decrease uterine blood flow and do not address the likely underlying pathology of hemorrhage. Hemodynamic instability secondary to dysrhythmias that are amenable to defibrillation or cardioversion should be treated as such without concern for fetal injury.

In addition to the basic trauma management principles discussed above, there are unique situations that the emergency physician must consider in the gravid patient. Pelvic fractures may be particularly dangerous during pregnancy. They may lead to increased blood loss from dilated pelvic veins. They also may lead to direct fetal injury, resulting in a high incidence of fetal morbidity and mortality. Medical Anti-shock Trousers (MAST) have no role in the management of the gravid trauma patient.

Uterine injury is uncommon in the first trimester as the pelvis protects the small gravid uterus. However, later in pregnancy minor uterine injury, such as contusion, is relatively common. This usually presents with uterine contractions, 90% of which will resolve spontaneously. Rarely blunt abdominal trauma may lead to uterine rupture that can present with catastrophic blood loss causing peritonitis and fetal demise (16,17). This may be diagnosed on physical examination by palpating a flattened uterus or fetal parts free in the abdominal cavity. Ultrasound can also be used to identify a traumatic uterine rupture.

Placental abruption is defined as a premature separation of the placenta from the uterine wall, and is common with blunt abdominal trauma and can cause fetal distress. It occurs in 1% to 3% of pregnant women with minor trauma and in 40% to 50% of pregnant women with major life-threatening trauma (6,17). Abruption may present with vaginal bleeding, abdominal pain and tenderness, uterine contractions or fetal distress. However, it may be occult with no vaginal bleeding in up to 20% of cases. Moreover, it may be missed on ultrasound examination. The gold standard for the evaluation of placental abruption is cardiotocographic monitoring to detect uterine irritability and fetal distress. A cesarean section may be necessary to save the fetus in severe cases of placental abruption.

Amniotic fluid embolism can occur with trauma and placental abruption. In the setting of an amniotic fluid embolism, debris and amniotic fluid become lodged in the maternal respiratory system causing sudden dyspnea, hypoxia and hypotension. These patients are also at risk for developing disseminated intravascular coagulation. Treatment of amniotic fluid embolism patients is supportive, but unfortunately, mortality is high.

Fetal outcomes in pregnant patients with *burns* are directly related to the extent of the burn and the gestational age of the fetus. Less than a 20% total body surface area burn usually does not lead to pregnancy complications, but extensive burns may lead to fetal demise or premature labor (18). Conversely, maternal outcomes in the setting of burns are not affected by pregnancy. The patient should also be assessed for carbon monoxide exposure. There is increased binding of carbon monoxide by fetal hemoglobin, resulting in increased carbon monoxide exposure to the fetus. Any symptomatic patient or patient with carboxyhemoglobin level greater than 15% should be placed on 100%

oxygen by mask and should be considered for hyperbaric oxygen therapy (11).

If the pregnant trauma patient arrests, the clinician should consider a perimortem cesarean section if there is a potentially viable fetus with signs of life. As time is critical to the survival of the fetus, the procedure should begin early and be performed by the most experienced physician available. Delivery within five minutes of maternal arrest leads to a higher fetal survival rate with good neurologic outcomes. This rapidly declines to 5% survival with neurologic sequelae at 15 minutes (10). A midline vertical incision using a #10 blade scalpel should be made from the epigastrium to the pubic symphysis. Ideally, the clinician should make one incision that goes from the skin down to the uterus. The uterine incision is performed vertically from the fundus to the reflection of the bladder. The placenta is incised if necessary. The child is delivered and the cord clamped and cut. Neonatal resuscitation should be aggressive and begin immediately. This procedure may actually improve the maternal hemodynamics by increasing venous return.

CRITICAL INTERVENTIONS

- Adequately resuscitate the mother in order to resuscitate the fetus
- Identify and treat early shock prior to development of abnormal vital signs
- Position the patient in a 15-degree tilt to prevent the *supine hypotensive syndrome*
- Admit all pregnant trauma patients with a potentially viable fetus for cardiotocographic monitoring for at least 4 hours
- Administer RhoGam 300 µg intramuscularly (IM) to Rh-negative trauma patients

DISPOSITION

Appropriate consultation is necessary for the best management of the pregnant trauma patient. Trauma surgery, obstetric and gynecological care as well as the care of a neonatalogist may be necessary for the multidisciplinary care of the pregnant trauma patient. The necessary consulting services are determined by the patient's injuries and the estimated gestational age of the fetus. It is best to be proactive and obtain consultation early rather than delaying necessary care.

The disposition for a pregnant trauma patient is the same as for a nonpregnant trauma patient. The only exception is that all patients carrying a potentially viable fetus should undergo at least 4 hours of cardiotocographic monitoring. This includes gravid trauma patients with little or no evidence of maternal injury. If monitoring detects an abnormality (vaginal bleeding, abdominal pain, contractions and/or fetal heart rate abnormalities) during this 4-hour evaluation period, it should be acted upon or the monitoring period should be extended to 24 to 48 hours (4). Although the fetus is not viable until 23 weeks, at the earliest, with a 10% survival at 5 years, some recommend monitoring for anyone over 20 weeks pregnant (4). This recommendation is based on the fact that some obstetricians will attempt tocolysis if there is evidence of premature labor in this group.

Prior to disposition, injury prevention issues must be addressed. The possibility of interpersonal violence or intentional injury cannot be overstated. Data suggests that there is a rise in the rate of domestic violence as the pregnancy progresses. The healthcare provider should also discuss appropriate seatbelt use prior to discharge. The lap belt should be worn low over the iliac crest and the shoulder restraint should cross above the uterus. As always, the emergency physician must remember tetanus prophylaxis. Standard guidelines for tetanus prophylaxis should be followed. No adjustments are needed in pregnant women.

COMMON PITFALLS

✔ Inadequate early maternal resuscitation
✔ Failure to perform cardiotocographic monitoring
✔ Failure to perform necessary radiographs
✔ Failure to treat fetal-maternal hemorrhage in Rh-negative trauma patients
✔ Delaying performing a perimortem cesarean section during maternal cardiopulmonary arrest

Acknowledgments

Thanks to the previous edition's chapter authors Andy Jagoda and Stu G. Kessler.

References

1. Ali J, Yeo A, Gana TJ, et al. Predictors of fetal mortality in pregnant trauma patients. *J Trauma* 1997;42:782.
2. Barron WM. The pregnant surgical patient: medical evaluation and management. *Ann Intern Med* 1984;101:683.
3. Connolly AM, Katz VL, Bash KL, et al. Trauma and pregnancy. *Am J Perinatol* 1997;14:331–336.
4. Doyle LW. Outcome at 5 years of age of children 23–27 weeks gestation: Refining the prognosis. *Pediatrics* 2001;108:134–141.
5. Fildes J, Reed L, Jones, et al. Trauma: The leading cause of maternal death. *J Trauma* 1992;32:643–645.
6. Fleming AD. Abruptio placentae. *Crit Care Clin* 1991;7:865–875.
7. Franger AL, Buchsbaum HJ, Peaceman AM. Abdominal gunshot wounds in pregnancy. *Am J Obstet Gynecol* 1989;160:1124–1128.
8. Goldman SM, Wagner LK. Radiologic management of blunt abdominal trauma in pregnancy. *American Journal of Radiology* 1996;166:763–767.
9. Grubb DK. Nonsurgical management of penetrating uterine trauma in pregnancy: A case report. *Am J Obstet Gynecol* 1992;166:583–584.
10. Katz VL, Dotters DJ, Droegemueller W. Perimortem cesarean delivery. *Obstet Gynecol* 1986;68:571.
11. Koren G, Shavrav T, Pastuszak A, et al. A multicenter, prospective study of fetal outcome following accidental carbon monoxide poisoning in pregnancy. *Reprod Toxicol* 1991;5:397.
12. Lewin SB, Cheek TG, Deutschman CS. Airway management in the obstetrical patient. *Critical Care Clinics* 2000;16:505–513.
13. Ma OJ, Mateer JR, DeBehnke DJ. Use of ultrasonography for the evaluation of pregnant trauma patients. *J of Trauma: Injury, Infection and Critical Care* 1996;40:665–668.
14. Nyberg DA, Cyr DR, Mack LA, et al. Sonographic spectrum of placental abruption. *AJR* 1987;148:161–164.
15. Pearlman MD, Tintinalli JE, Lorenz RP. Blunt trauma during pregnancy. *N Engl J Med* 1992;323:1609.
16. Pearlman MD, Tintinalli JE, Lorenz RP. A prospective controlled study of outcome after trauma during pregnancy. *Am J Obstet Gynecol* 1990;162:1502–1510.
17. Pearlman MD, Tintinalli JE. Evaluation and treatment of the gravida and fetus following trauma during pregnancy. *Obstet Gynecol Clin North Am* 1991;18:371.
18. Rayburn W, et al. Major burns during pregnancy: effects on fetal well-being. *Obstet Gynecol* 1984;63:392–395.

CHAPTER 203
Trauma in the Elderly

Shahram Lotfipour and Federico E. Vaca

In the United States, the elderly population (those 65 years and older) has continued to experience a rapid growth rate, accounting for more than 15% of the nation's inhabitants (35 million) in the 2000 census, and is projected to represent 20% of the population by 2030 (27). In this age group, both unintentional and intentional injuries are common reasons for emergency department (ED) visits (13).

In 2002 the Center for Disease Control and Prevention (CDC) noted that *unintentional injury* was the leading cause of nonfatal injury among the elderly (30). Falls accounted for the majority of these (6,30). Motor vehicle collisions (MVC) were a close second; the elderly have a higher fatality rate per mile driven than any other age group except drivers under the age of 25 (26). The fatality rate for drivers 85 years and older is 9 times higher than the rate for drivers age 25 to 69 years (26).

Intentional injury was the 15th leading cause of nonfatal injury among the elderly in 2002 (30). During the same year, over five thousand deaths were due to suicide, accounting for 85% of elderly intentional injury deaths (30). White males account for 90% of all elderly suicide attempts and the ratio of men to women who successfully commit suicide is 4 to 1. Predominant methods of elderly suicide are through the use of firearms, suffocation, and poisoning (30). For homicide deaths (nearly 14% of the annual elderly intentional injury deaths), firearms are also the most common mechanism of injury (30).

CLINICAL PRESENTATION

When assessing elderly trauma patients, the physician should pay special attention to the physiologic changes and limited reserves in this patient population, which contribute to increased morbidity and mortality.

Pathophysiology

Cardiovascular

With aging, as the heart and pericardium stiffen, resting cardiac output and stroke volume begin to fall (4,7,9). Although the resting heart rate often does not change, fibrosis of the conduction system and the loss of specialized conduction cells impede the heart's ability to increase its rate when necessary (3). Also, aging is often accompanied by the development of atherosclerotic coronary disease. The combination of fixed coronary artery lesions, decreased cardiac compliance, increased wall tension, and the inability to increase the heart rate limits myocardial oxygen delivery. Because cardiac output often needs to increase after injury or blood loss, these patients are at risk for developing myocardial ischemia. Ischemia, in turn, may further impair cardiac output.

Many elderly patients are on prescription medications that tend to limit the heart's ability to respond to stress (i.e., beta blockers, calcium channel blockers, clonidine). Afterload-reducing agents and diuretics may limit preload, thereby decreasing blood pressure under stress.

The changes in the vascular system are similar to those in the heart. Loss of compliance tends to make vessels more easily injured by shearing forces, producing vascular rupture, occlusion from intimal disruption, or aneurysm formation (4,23).

Pulmonary

As the lungs age, they undergo numerous changes. The same loss of elasticity that impedes the cardiovascular system tends to occur in the lung. As the lungs stiffen, forced vital capacity and maximal expiratory flow are reduced. Residual volume rises and vital capacity decreases as the total lung capacity does not change. These alterations, combined with a decrease in lung surface area due to emphysematous changes, contribute to a decrease in ventilation (25). As perfusion does not change, ventilation–perfusion mismatch occur, characterized by a fall in Po_2.

Loss of elasticity also occurs in the muscle and connective tissue of the chest wall. Combined with osteoporosis of the ribs and the pulmonary parenchymal changes, this condition makes the elderly more prone to rib fractures and pulmonary contusion, which may occur even with seemingly minor forces.

Renal

With aging, the kidneys lose structure and function due to a loss of glomeruli and nephrons. Creatinine clearance decreases (15). Diminution of renal function is characterized by an inability to concentrate urine, as the kidneys cannot retain free water.

Serum creatinine and urine output, two of the clinical tools often used to estimate renal function, are not reliable in the elderly. The loss of concentrating ability means that patients may continue to produce seemingly adequate amounts of dilute urine, even in the face of significant hypovolemia. Patients with an impaired myocardium may also not make adequate amounts of urine in response to a fluid challenge, making urine output an unreliable indicator of intravascular volume.

Osteoporosis

Osteoporosis is present to some degree in almost every elderly patient; this makes bones much more susceptible to fractures. Osteoporosis accounts for an estimated 1.5 million fractures in the United States every year (17,29). The most common osteoporotic fractures in the elderly are vertebral compression fractures and fractures of the wrist, hip, pelvis, and skull.

A seemingly straightforward fracture may carry substantial morbidity and mortality in the elderly patient. Fractures often require operative fixation, subjecting the elderly patient to myriad postoperative complications. Nonoperative therapy puts the patient at risk for skin breakdown, pulmonary embolus, and pneumonia.

Central Nervous System

The central nervous system undergoes substantial changes with aging. The brain progressively loses volume, and the dura becomes more tightly adherent to the skull, limiting the occurrence of epidural hematoma. The loss of volume stretches the parasagittal bridging veins, making them prone to rupture. Therefore, in this age group, subdural hematomas are more common. The increased space around the brain can also hold a remarkable amount of blood before the hematoma produces clinical signs. Neurotrauma is second only to shock as a predictor of death in the traumatized elderly patient (14).

Mechanisms of Injury

Motor vehicle collisions, falls, and burns account for over 80% of the cases of accidental injury in the elderly.

Falls

Falls remain the leading cause of injury in the elderly (5,30). Whether they occur as a result of a mechanical (environmental) or medical-related event, the injuries suffered may initially appear to be benign, yet significant injuries (head injury, intraabdominal and thoracic injury, spine or extremity fractures and lacerations) are frequent (24). Falls in the elderly are more likely to be a symptom of underlying pathology, and are associated with greater morbidity and mortality (8). In the elderly, the initial clinical presentation may appear to be mild, such as a complaint of a nondescript headache, fleeting or intermittent mental status changes, or a subtle new gait change.

Motor Vehicle Collisions

National crash statistics have shown that older drivers are actually more careful while driving than younger drivers are. Older drivers tend to use self-modification of driving habits for the sake of safety (i.e., driving at slower speeds, driving shorter distances, and avoidance of driving at night and in adverse weather conditions) (16). However, even though there may be fewer crashes in this age group, the consequences are more severe. The physiologic changes associated with aging translate into increased fragility. These changes are apparent after age 60 (11). Factors that play a role in older driver motor vehicle crashes (MVCs) include slower reaction times, sensory or cognitive deficits, distractions, medications, and medical conditions. Impaired driving due to drugs and alcohol has also been shown to be a significant contributor to collisions.

The prehospital personnel may uncover important clues to the cause of the crash (i.e., hypoglycemic or seizure event) as well as the mechanism of injury. This information will help in the evaluation of the elderly trauma patient and can help guide the use of diagnostic studies.

Injuries that are particularly common and devastating in older drivers include head, thoracic aorta, rib fractures, pelvic and extremity bony fractures, and solid organ injuries. Preexisting comorbid conditions and limited physiologic reserve place the elderly trauma victim at an increased mortality risk (28).

Intentional Injuries

Depression continues to be the most prevalent mental illness that leads to suicidal ideation, gestures and attempts in the elderly. Suicide risk factors in the elderly include previous attempts, psychiatric problems, history of alcohol or drug abuse, living alone, chronic or terminal illness and male gender (24). Strong social ties have been shown to have a significantly favorable influence on decreasing the risk of suicide among older adults (2). Although suicide is attempted most often in the young female age groups, those with the greatest rate of success are elderly male patients (2). The increased mortality found in elderly suicide victims is attributed to decreased physical resilience of the population, concomitant medical problems, increased determination and often greater physical isolation of these patients from society (2). Elderly patients contemplating suicide give fewer warning signs to family and caretakers, apply more deadly resolve, and have better planning (2). Therefore it is important to incorporate screening and intervention methods into the emergency care of these patients.

Elder neglect is an important cause of intentional injuries in the elderly. It is estimated that up to 85% of cases remain unreported (10). Factors contributing to abuse and neglect include socio-demographic factors such as family stressors, financial strains, decreasing importance of traditional age roles, increasing life-expectancy, and prolongation of life in patients with chronic illnesses (10). Because caretakers and the elderly patient may minimize the symptoms, these potentially deadly cases are difficult to recognize. Some of the warning signs for elder abuse and neglect include delays in seeking medical attention, inconsistent history between caregiver and patient, unexplained injuries (fractures or bruising), discrepancy between history and physical examination findings and diagnostic testing, severe malnutrition and poor personal hygiene (10).

Common Patterns of Injury

Elderly trauma victims exhibit a greater extent of injury for a given amount of energy (12). The majority of injuries in the elderly are musculoskeletal.

Spinal Injuries

Chronic bony changes and stiffening of the spine place the elderly at increased risk for spinal injuries. The spinal cord can be damaged by bony spur impingement into the spinal canal caused by minor force. In addition, elderly patients are at risk for cord contusions or the central cord syndrome that results from a hyperextension mechanism. These patients will have weakness affecting the upper extremities and will have negative plain cervical radiographs.

Fractures

Pathologic conditions associated with fractures include Paget disease, metabolic derangements, malignancy, infection, marrow dysplasia, and osteomalacia. Due to trabecular bone thinning and weakening in the elderly, fractures involving the proximal humerus, tibia, pubic rami, vertebral bodies and hip are more common. Distal radius and proximal humerus fractures frequently result from falls onto an outstretched hand. Hip fractures are one of the most common fractures seen in the elderly and commonly involve the femoral neck or greater trochanter. Intertrochanteric fractures, when displaced, leave the affected leg shortened and externally rotated. Pelvic rami fractures are common after a fall from a standing position. Fractures of the tibial plateau are more common after an auto versus pedestrian mechanism, due to lateral bending forces and angulation of the leg. A misstep while walking and routine lifting or bending in patients with underlying osteoporosis can result in vertebral body compression fractures in the elderly. These are frequently asymptomatic, found incidentally on x-ray examination and have no neurologic deficits. The typical wedge-shaped deformity is seen on x-ray (5).

Head Trauma

Head injury is second only to shock as a cause of trauma-related deaths in the elderly. Although epidural hematomas are relatively rare, subdural hematomas are more common due to the stretching of the bridging veins associated with cerebral atrophy. Additionally, many elderly patients are at increased risk for bleeding due to age-related clotting deficiencies or use of anticoagulants.

Chest and Abdominal Trauma

The elderly are at increased risk for rib fractures, hemothorax and pneumothorax. In addition, due to the risk of occult intraperitoneal injuries, liberal use of CT is recommended especially in head-injured or intoxicated patients with chest and abdominal trauma, or those with an altered mental status (5).

DIFFERENTIAL DIAGNOSIS

Patients with falls that present as a result of a medical cause should be carefully evaluated for their musculoskeletal injuries as well as for concomitant life-threats such as cerebral vascular accidents, transient ischemic attacks, myocardial infarctions, and malignant cardiac dysrhythmias. A subgroup of elderly patients will present without a clear history or mechanism of injury; such patients frequently reside in assisted living conditions and may have concurrent psychiatric or neurologic conditions (e.g., Alzheimer dementia). Communication with primary caregivers may help determine the cause of the fall. Involvement of a social worker or adult protective services is necessary if there is a suspicion of elder neglect or abuse.

EMERGENCY DEPARTMENT EVALUATION

The initial evaluation of the elderly trauma patient is similar to that of the younger injured patient. The American College of Surgeons' Advanced Trauma Life Support (ATLS) protocols are used for guidance in the management of the multisystem elderly trauma patient with some additional considerations. Particular attention should be paid to the adequacy of ventilation, oxygenation and to preventing aspiration. Elderly patients have limited pulmonary reserve due to preexisting comorbid conditions. In addition, significant cardiovascular disease is common. Medication history, especially the use of anticoagulants and beta-blockers, is important in the initial evaluation of the trauma patient. Cardiac monitoring, pulse oximetry, and rapid glucose assessment are essential. Testing should be directed at identifying metabolic derangements or a precipitating cardiac event (CBC, electrolytes, CPK, serum lactate and arterial blood gas), 12-lead ECG, and a CT of the head as clinically indicated. Admission for serial ECGs, cardiac enzymes and cardiac monitoring are necessary if a cardiac etiology is suspected or cannot be ruled out. When evaluating patients with dementia, the possibility of elder neglect and abuse should be considered (1).

Elderly patients require careful neurologic evaluation. Patients on coumadin or with an altered mental status should have a head CT performed even after minor head trauma. The physician should also have a lower threshold for evaluating the cervical spine after blunt trauma. Special attention should be paid to the integrity of the ring of C2 on the lateral view and to the odontoid and lateral masses of C1 on the open mouth view. It may be necessary to obtain CT scans of the spine after equivocal plain films or in patients with persistent pain or neurologic deficits (5,12). Due to the inability of demented patients to provide an accurate history and their often unreliable physical examinations, these patients may also require further evaluation beyond plain radiographs (e.g., CT or MRI).

Patients who have persistent hip pain with ambulation or weight-bearing or who are unable to ambulate should undergo further evaluation to rule out occult fractures either with CT or MRI, if the plain radiographs are normal.

EMERGENCY DEPARTMENT MANAGEMENT

The initial management of the elderly trauma patient begins with an assessment for shock. The approach should be aggressive and may commonly require invasive monitoring. Routine blood pressure monitoring should be supplemented by invasive hemodynamic monitoring such as central venous pressure (CVP),

TABLE 203.1. High-Risk Geriatric Patients
Auto versus pedestrian mechanism
Initial systolic blood pressure < 130 mm Hg
Acidosis (pH < 7.35)
Multiple long-bone fractures
Head injury

central venous oximetry (ScvO$_2$), noninvasive cardiac output, and pulmonary artery catheterization (9). Rivers et al found that early goal-directed therapy resulted in improved outcomes in elderly patients with septic shock (18). Although this study is not specific to trauma patients, the outcome of critically ill patients who progress to multiorgan failure has been shown to be dependent on the care provided in the emergency department (18).

Certain elderly patients are at high risk for significant morbidity and mortality after trauma (Table 203.1). Although these patients may be relatively normotensive in the ED, the combination of soft-tissue injury, long-bone fractures, and head injuries produces tissue oxygen deficits that are difficult to compensate for. If the oxygen delivery deficits are not met early on, the oxygen debt worsens, resulting in early death from heart failure or late death from multiorgan failure (22). Failing to recognize this oxygen debt is one of the main reasons for the high mortality rate in the traumatized elderly patient. Invasive hemodynamic monitoring can be extremely helpful in guiding resuscitation in these patients (20). Early aggressive trauma care (i.e., fluid resuscitation, transfusion, and invasive hemodynamic monitoring) increases survival in the elderly (21). A normotensive elderly patient in the high-risk group should not be assumed to be stable. Although skeletal surveys are necessary to complete the trauma evaluation, they almost never affect the immediate management and take much longer than planned. The same is true for studies such as precautionary head CT scans or the evaluation of microscopic hematuria. These are of lower priority than invasive monitoring and should be deferred until the patient's cardiovascular status has been optimized. Other important considerations include preventing and treating hypothermia, monitoring urine output, and having a lower threshold for intubation. Early ventilatory support should be considered for patients with multiple rib fractures, pulmonary contusions, or any evidence of impending respiratory compromise.

Factors that predict a poor outcome in elderly trauma patients include: (1) Glascow coma scale of less than 8, (2) age greater than 75 years, (3) severe head injury, (4) the presence of shock on admission, and (5) the development of sepsis during the admission for the traumatic event.

CRITICAL INTERVENTIONS

- Measure lactate levels and perform invasive hemodynamic monitoring and central venous oximetry (ScvO$_2$) for elderly patients after moderate or major mechanism trauma
- Consider elder abuse and neglect; identify abusive situations and report them to the appropriate authorities

DISPOSITION

Because the presence of serious occult injury with subsequent clinical deterioration is a well recognized threat in the elderly, most patients should be admitted for observation, unless the mechanism is very minor. The mechanism of injury, past medical history, and extent of the current injuries should be considered when making disposition decisions. Patients with multiple comorbid conditions, limited capacity to follow through with important discharge instructions, or poor social support at home should be admitted. Patients with seemingly minor injuries, such as multiple rib fractures, require admission for observation and pain control, as they are at risk for complications. Appropriate social work consultation and home safety evaluations should be arranged prior to discharge.

COMMON PITFALLS

- ✔ Assuming that a patient with normal vital signs is "stable"
- ✔ Failure to consider that a change in mental status may be the only indication of an intracranial bleed in an elderly trauma patient
- ✔ Failure to recognize abuse and neglect as the cause of the injuries
- ✔ Failure to recognize occult fractures
- ✔ Failure to admit elderly trauma patients to the hospital, at least for a period of observation

Acknowledgments

The authors wish to acknowledge the contributions of Vanaja Menon for editorial assistance, Ian Nipomnick for the literature review, and Suzanne Moore Shepherd and William H. Shoff, who wrote the previous version of this chapter.

References

1. Appleton W. Elder abuse–diagnose, treat, cure. *Ann Emerg Med* 1988;17:1104–1105.
2. Conwell Y, Duberstein PR, et al. Risk factors for suicide in later life. *Society of Biological Psychiatry* 2002;52:193–204.
3. Darr KC, Bassett DR, Morgan BJ, Thomas DP. Effects of age and training status on heart rate recovery after peak exercise. *Am J Physiol* 1988;254:H340–H343.
4. Davies M. Pathology of the aging heart. In: Brocklehurst HM Fillit, et al. *Textbook of geriatric medicine and gerontology.* Edinburgh, Chruchill Livingstone: 1992:181.
5. Evans R. Trauma and Falls. *Emergency care of the elder person.* Sanders AB (ed). St. Louis: Beverly Cracom Publishing 1996:153–170.
6. Francis RM. Falls and fractures. *Age and Ageing* 2001;30:25–28.
7. Gibson TC, Klainer LM. The prevalence of congestive heart failure in two rural communities. *J Chronic Dis* 1996;19:141.
8. Haentjens P, Autier P, Collins J, et al. Colles fracture, spine fracture, and subsequent risk of hip fracture in men and women. A meta-analysis. *J Bone Joint Surg Am* 2003;85:1936–1943.
9. Lakatta EG. Determinants of cardiovascular performance: modification due to aging. *J Chronic Dis* 1983;36:15–30.
10. Levine JM. Elderly neglect and abuse: A primer for primary care physicians. *Geriatrics* 2003;58:37–44.
11. Li G, Braver E, et al. Fragility versus excessive crash involvement as determination of high death rates per vehicle-mile of travel among older drivers. *Accident Analysis and Prevention* 2003;35:227–235.
12. Lowe DK, Trunkey DD. Response to trauma in the elderly: introduction and general considerations. In: Bosker G, Schwartz FR, Jones JS, Sequeira M (eds). *geriatric emergency medicine* St Louis: Mosby 1990:393–397.
13. National Hospital Ambulatory Medical Care Survey: 2001 Emergency department summary. *Advance Data: From Vital and Health Statistics,* U.S. Department of Health and Human Services 2003:1–34.
14. Osler T, Baack B, et al. Trauma in the elderly. *Am J Surg* 1988;156:537.
15. Papper S. The effects of age in reducing renal function. *Geriatrics* 1973;28:83.
16. Preusser D, Williams A, et al. Fatal crash risk for older drivers at intersections. *Accident analysis and prevention,* 1998;30(2):151–159.
17. Riggs BL, Melton LJ 3rd. Involutional osteoporosis. *N Engl J Med* 1986;26;314:1676–1686.
18. Rivers E, Nguyen B, et al. Early goal-directed therapy in the treatment of severe sepsis and septic shock. *The New England Journal of Medicine* 2002;345:1368–1377.

19. Rivers E, Nguyen H, et al. Critical care and emergency medicine. *Curr Opin Crit Care* 2002;8:600–606.

20. Scalea TM, Holman M, Fuortes M, et al. Central venous blood oxygen saturation: an early, accurate measurement of volume during hemorrhage. *J Trauma* 1988;28:725–732.

21. Scalea TM, et al. Geriatric trauma. In: Feliciano DV, Mattox KL, et al. (eds). *Trauma*. Nowalk, CT: Appleton & Lange, in press.

22. Scalea TM, Simon HM, Duncan AO, et al. Geriatric blunt multiple trauma: improved survival with early invasive monitoring. *J Trauma* 1990;30:129–134.

23. Schlag G, Heinz R, et al. Cardiopulmonary response of the elderly to traumatic and septic shock. *Perspectives in shock research.* Vienna, Ludwig Boltzman Institute for Experimental Traumatology: 1988:223.

24. Tiscott JAC, Edmonton AB, et al. Evidence-based care of the elderly health-guide. *Geriatrics Today* 2003;6:36–42.

25. Tockman M. Aging of the respiratory system. In: WR Hazzard, JP Blass, et al (eds). *Principles of geriatric medicine and gerontology.* New York, McGraw-Hill 1994:555.

26. Traffic Safety Facts 2002: Older Population, U.S. Department of Transportation, National Highway Traffic Safety Administration, 2003.

27. US Census Bureau: Age Data, U.S. Department of Commerce, 2000.

28. Victorino GP, Chong TJ, Pal JD. Trauma in the elderly patient. *Arch Surg* 2003;138:1093–1098.

29. Washington DC, National Academy Press, 1990.

30. Web-based Injury Statistics Query and Reporting System, Centers for Disease Control: National Center for Injury Prevention and Control, 2002.

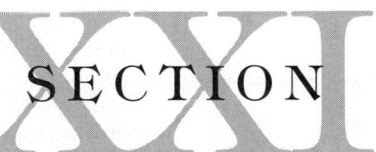

SECTION XXI

Section Editors: Phyllis L. Hendry and
Ghazala Q. Sharieff

Pediatrics

CHAPTER 204
General Approach to the Pediatric Emergency Patient

Robert A. Wiebe

Approximately 30% of the 91 million emergency department (ED) visits annually in the United States are for the care of infants and children in crisis (8). Although true medical emergencies in Pediatrics are relatively rare, they must be recognized in a timely fashion and treated in a manner that addresses the special needs of children and families in an ED setting. When providing care to pediatric patients, there are always two "patients": the child and the caretaker. Because emergencies are uncommon, it is not unusual that the most important aspect of treatment is to address the fears and concerns of the caretaker. Parental perceptions of urgency, if not addressed, can result in dissatisfaction. Always consider the family unit, treat the family, and be aware of caretaker attitudes and perceptions that need to be managed as a part of overall emergency care.

Every ED must be prepared to care for patients of all ages. Most children in the United States are seen in community hospitals, and it is imperative that these hospitals have available equipment and supplies necessary to stabilize critically ill and injured children (1). Hospitals that do not have in-patient definitive-care resources for children should have triage and transfer agreements and protocols. This will enable rapid access to definitive care for the critically ill and injured children (6).

PEDIATRIC TRIAGE

Increasing use of the ED as the healthcare *safety net* has resulted in ED overcrowding and longer wait times. Access to primary care for infants and children is a problem in most communities. Triage provides the first point of service for the ED and allows the categorization of patients sorted by acuity. The process of triage depends on the acuity level and age of the patient and differentiates patients into meaningful groups based on expected resource needs. An effective triage system will improve efficiency and effectiveness of care and decrease the risk of negative outcomes (9).

The Canadian Pediatric Triage and Acuity Scale (CPTAS) serves as an outstanding basic template for categorizing pediatric emergency patients (3). Five levels of triage categories are described. Pediatric triage categories clearly must be age-specific because serious or critical problems are often more difficult to recognize in younger infants.

Patients who are considered to be critical and cannot wait for care are categorized as *Level I*. Immediate recognition of level I patients is the most important aspect of the triage process. The pediatric assessment triangle (PAT) is a useful tool to quickly identify even the smallest infant who is in critical need of emergency care (5). Figure 204.1 demonstrates the 3 limbs of the PAT that can be used as a rapid and simple tool to identify infants and children in need of stabilization. Before touching the patient, a quick 15- to 20-second period of observation to look and listen

can provide important cues for early identification of shock, respiratory failure, and other critical problems needing emergency attention. The infant/child's appearance, work of breathing, and circulation to the skin can be quickly assessed from across the room and together can provide a quick assessment of the child's oxygenation, ventilation, perfusion, and the functional status of the brain.

The appearance limb of the PAT is actually a mental status examination. It not only assesses brain function but also helps to determine adequacy of circulation, ventilation, and oxygenation. Is the child irritable or lethargic? How does she respond to her environment? Does she console when rocked or cuddled? Does she interact appropriately with her environment and caregiver? Is her look/gaze age appropriate? The vacant, "nobody-home stare" must be recognized as altered mental status in infants. Is the character of the cry weak, high-pitched, cephalic, muffled or atypical in any way? Often the caretaker can describe a change in the character of the cry when it is not noticeable to the healthcare provider.

Work of breathing in infants and young children can best be assessed before touching the patient. Listen carefully for both inspiratory and expiratory sounds. Is there wheezing, stridor, or grunting? Once a child is agitated and crying, it is very difficult to differentiate important sounds related to respiratory distress from either upper or lower airway obstruction. Are there intercostal, subcostal, or supraclavicular retractions? Is there nasal flaring or head bobbing? What is the preferred position of the patient? Are they sitting up, leaning forward or in a tripod position in an attempt to make best use of accessory muscles and maintain a patent airway?

Assessment of circulation to the skin can be assessed by observing for pallor, cyanosis, or mottling. The first objective indicator of compensated shock is a combination of tachycardia and pallor. The pale infant or young child should be considered in shock until proven otherwise. As circulation to the skin becomes further compromised, patches of erythema or cyanosis interspersed with pallor (mottling) will appear. Mottling should not be confused with cutis marmorata or the vascular instability often seen in a young infant when placed in a cool ambient environment.

Figure 204.2 provides an algorithm for sorting the five levels of triage acuity. This model is adapted from the CPTAS (3), and the Emergency Severity Index of Eitel and Wuerz (7). The PAT when used as an observation tool can be expected to identify *all Level I* triage category patients and many *Level II* patients as well. Triage *Level II* patients include any conditions that are a potential threat to life, limb, or function. The time-frame to assessment and stabilizing care should be less than 15 minutes. Included in the emergent category are any physiologically unstable children with altered consciousness, moderate respiratory

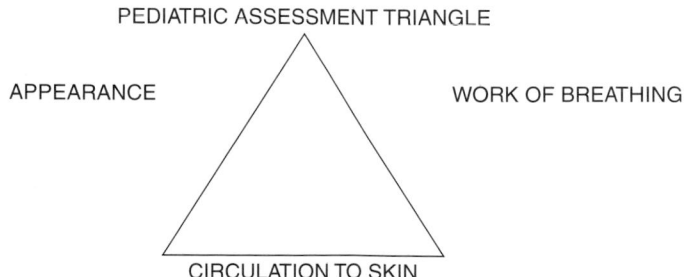

Figure 204.1.   Pediatric assessment triangle. (From Dieckmann RA. Pediatric Assessment. In: Gausche-Hill M, Fuch S, Yamamoto L, eds. APLS: *The Pediatric Emergency Medicine Resource.* Boston: Jones and Bartlett, 2004.)

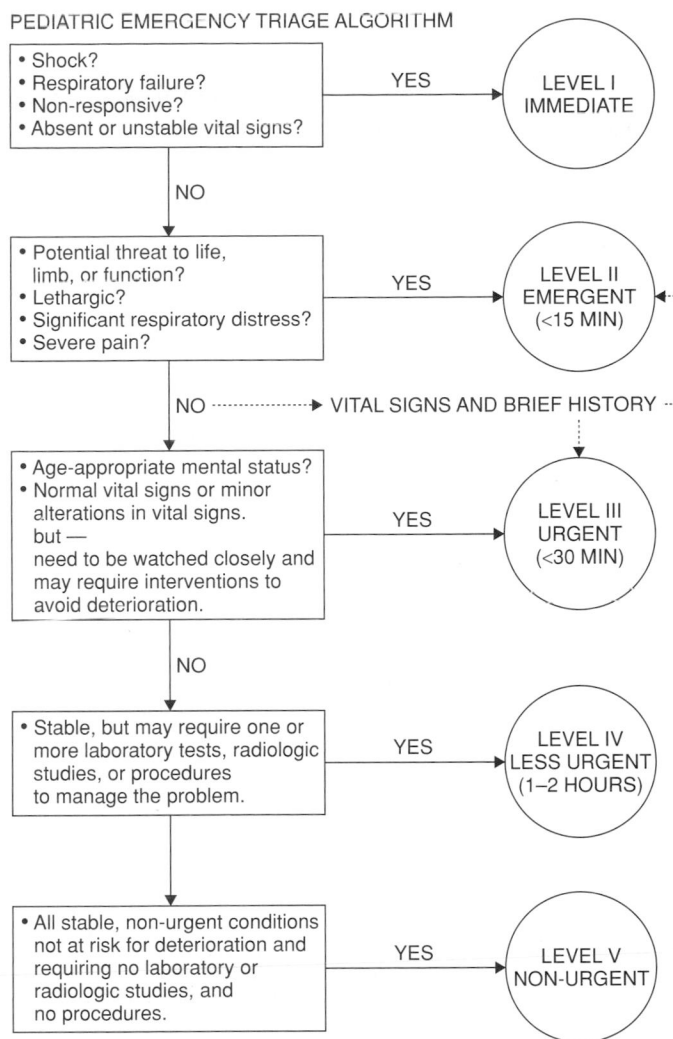

PEDIATRIC EMERGENCY TRIAGE ALGORITHM

Figure 204.2. Pediatric emergency triage algorithm. (Modified from the Canadian Association of Emergency Physicians. Canadian paediatric triage and acuity scale: implementation guidelines for emergency departments. *Canad J Emerg Med* 2001;13, www.caep.ca; and Gilboy N, Tanabe P, Travers D, Eitel D, Wuerz R. The emergency severity index implementation handbook. Des Plaines, IL: Emergency Nurses Association 2003.) (ESI Conceptual v3 by Eitel D, and Wuerz R with permission.)

distress, significant dehydration, or any child who requires medical intervention in order to avoid further deterioration of the patient's condition. The patient triaged as *Level III* is one who is alert, has age-appropriate mental status, and normal or only minor alterations in vital signs.

Age-related risk differences may determine whether a patient is *Level II, III, or IV* by triage. For example, a neonate with fever must be considered Level II until further detailed assessment can be performed. A febrile infant from 1 to 3 months of age may be considered *Level III* because they would need to be watched closely and may require interventions to avoid deterioration. Older children who are alert and stable but have fever may be considered *Level IV* or *Level V* depending on the need for further laboratory tests, radiologic studies, or procedures necessary to manage the problem.

A *Level IV* patient is stable but may require a procedure or ancillary resource in order to manage the problem. *Level V* patients are nonurgent conditions that require no laboratory studies or procedures for definitive care. *Level V* patients may be triaged to definitive care resources outside the hospital when appropriate.

Table 204.1 from the CPTAS (3), provides examples of problems in each triage category by organ system.

PEDIATRIC VITAL SIGNS

Normal vital signs for infants and children are age-dependent. Table 204.2 provides guidelines for normal respiratory and heart rates for age (4). In early and compensated shock, the first sign will always be an increased heart rate. However, heart rate is a very nonspecific finding and is also increased with fear, anxiety, and fever. The heart rate must be compared with pulse quality and mental status in order to determine the significance of either an abnormally fast or slow rate. The most common cause of a slow heart rate is respiratory compromise and hypoxemia. The quality of pulses can be an extremely important physical exam tool to monitor during stabilization and resuscitation of seriously ill or injured children. A central and peripheral pulse should be compared simultaneously. The femoral and dorsalis pedis, or the brachial and radial pulses palpated at the same time can give the healthcare provider an objective measure of pulse quality when assessing a child in compensated shock.

Blood pressure measurements are often difficult to obtain when infants and young children are agitated and crying. Cuff size, when improperly measured, can cause incorrect readings. In order to obtain an accurate blood pressure, the cuff width should be at least 2/3 the length of the upper arm of the child. Time should not be wasted during resuscitation and stabilization with attempts to obtain an accurate blood pressure. If the child is alert, crying and responding to his environment, blood pressure measurements can wait until stabilizing interventions are complete. The lower limit for blood pressure (5th percentile) by age can easily be determined from the formula: *Systolic blood pressure = 70 + (2 times age in years).*

Capillary refill should always be less than two–three seconds when an infant or child is in a neutral-thermal environment. Delays up to four to five seconds can occur in a cool ambient environment. When an infant compensates for hypovolemia or hemorrhage, early skin signs not only include pallor and decreased peripheral pulses, but also cool distal skin temperature. The *reverse thermometer sign* can be useful during resuscitation. An infant who is cool peripherally to the mid-region of the arm will warm distally as resuscitation occurs.

Respiratory rate is also very age dependent. Table 204.2 includes guidelines for normal respiratory rates by age. Although rates above 60/minute can periodically be normal for short periods of time in an infant, any rate above 60/minute must be considered abnormal until proven otherwise. Slow respiratory rates must alert the healthcare provider to consider respiratory failure. The respiratory rate must always be interpreted in conjunction with heart rate and mental status when determining whether ventilatory efforts are adequate or insufficient.

An age-appropriate pain scale should be used to objectively measure pain whenever significant pain is a complaint. Although the perception of pain is very subjective, intense pain should always be an issue of concern to the healthcare provider (see Chapter 269, "Pediatric Sedation and Pain Management," for pain scales).

ASSESSMENT BY DEVELOPMENTAL AGE

A basic understanding of how developmental age affects child behavior is necessary in order to get the most out of assessment techniques. Knowledge of language development and the sequence of behavioral milestones can be quite helpful in determining the optimal approach to the assessment of an infant

TABLE 204.1.   Canadian Pediatric Triage and Acuity Scale

LEVEL I TRIAGE CATEGORY

Respiratory	Airway compromise
	Severe respiratory distress, inadequate breathing
	Critical asthma
	Chest trauma with respiratory distress
Neurological	Major head injury
	Unconscious or unresponsive
	Active seizure state
Cardiovascular	Cardiac arrest
	Shock or hypotension
	Exsanguinating hemorrhage
Musculoskeletal	Major trauma
	Traumatic amputation – extremity
	Major cold injury – hypothermia
Skin	Burn, > 25% body surface area (BSA) or airway involvement
Gastrointestinal	Difficulty swallowing, with airway or respiratory compromise
	Abdominal trauma – penetrating or blunt – signs or symptoms of shock
Gynecologic	Vaginal bleeding, patient with abnormal vital signs
Hematologic/ Immunologic	Anaphylaxis
Endocrine	Diabetic – altered consciousness
Behavior	Unresponsive
Infection	Septic shock
Child Abuse	Unstable situation or conflict

LEVEL II TRIAGE CATEGORY

Respiratory	Marked stridor
	Moderate respiratory distress
	Severe asthma
	Foreign body aspiration with respiratory distress
	Inhalation of toxic substances
Neurologic	Moderate head injury with altered mental state
	Altered consciousness
	Shunt dysfunction – patient appears ill
	Sudden onset of confusion, weakness, severe headache
Cardiovascular	Significant tachycardia
	Bradycardia
	Severe dehydration
	Uncontrolled major hemorrhage
Musculoskeletal	Traumatic amputation – digit
	Fracture, open or with neurovascular impairment
	Back pain with neurologic deficit
	Avulsed permanent tooth
Skin	Burn, >10% BSA or face, hand or foot involvement
	Burn, chemical or electrical
	Purpuric rash
Gastrointestinal	Acute bleeding, vomitus or rectal
	Abdominal pain with vomiting, diarrhea, or abdominal vital signs
Genitourinary	Severe testicular pain
	Urine retention > 24 hours
	Paraphimosis, priapism
Gynecologic	Possible ectopic pregnancy with normal vital signs
	Severe vaginal bleeding
Eye/ear/nose/throat	Chemical substance in eye
	Burn, penetration, of eye
	Orbital infection
	Impaled object or amputation of ear
	Uncontrolled epistaxis/post T & A bleeding
	Sore throat with drooling, stridor, or difficulty swallowing

	Hoarseness, sudden onset with history of trauma to larynx
Hematologic/ Immunologic	Bleeding disorder
	Fever – neutropenia/sickle cell disease
Endocrine	Diabetic – ketoacidosis/hypoglycemia
Psychiatry	Toxic overdose
	High risk of harm to self or others
	Violent behavior
Behavior	Lethargic child
	Infant > 7 days old
Infection	Any infant or child with toxic appearance
	Infant > 3 months, temperature > 36° or > 38 C°
Child Abuse	History of ongoing risk
Pain	Severe pain 810/10

LEVEL III TRIAGE CATEGORY

Respiratory	Stridor
	Mild respiratory distress
	Moderate asthma
	Foreign body aspiration, cough present, with no distress
	Constant cough, appears distressed
Neurological	Minor head injury, GCS 3/4 15
	History of altered consciousness
	Headache
	Possible shunt obstruction with no distress
	Seizure prior to emergency visit, not actively seizing
Cardiovascular	Tachycardia
	Signs of dehydration
	Uncontrolled minor hemorrhage
Musculoskeletal	Probable fracture with no neurovascular deficit
	Tight cast with possible neurovascular impairment
	Joint pain with fever
	Dental trauma
Skin	Burn, partial thickness and > 10% BSA
	Burn, full thickness > 5% BSA
	Localized cold injury
	Cellulitis – patient appears ill, or is febrile
	Complex lacerations
Gastrointestinal	Persistent or bilious vomiting
	Vomiting or diarrhea > 2 years
	Possible appendicitis
Genitourinary	Moderate testicular pain or swelling
	Inguinal bulge with pain
	Urinary retention > 8 hours
Gynecologic	Vaginal bleeding with normal vital signs
Eye/ear/nose/throat	Foreign body in nose causing pain or possible risk or aspiration
	Epistaxis, controlled/history of post T & A bleeding
	Puncture wound of soft palate
	Tonsil pustules with difficulty swallowing
	Hearing problem – acute onset
	History of postoperative bleeding – tonsillectomy or adenoidectomy
	Foreign body in ear
	Periorbital swelling with fever
	Sudden vision change
Hematologic/ Immunologic	Sickle cell crisis
	Moderate allergic reaction
Endocrine	Diabetic – Hyperglycemia
Psychiatry	Ingestion requiring observation
	Moderate risk of harm to self or others
	Disruptive or distressed

(continued)

TABLE 204.1.   *Continued*

Behavior	Inconsolable infant	Eye/ear/nose/throat	Corneal foreign body or abrasion
	Infant not feeding		Crusting, matting, discharge from eye
Infection	Infant 3–36 months, temperature		Ear drainage
	> 38.5 °C		Earache
Child Abuse	Physical assault	Hematologic/	Local allergic reaction
	Sexual assault > 48 hours	Immunologic	
Pain	Moderate pain 47/10	Psychiatry	Low risk of harm to self or others
			Depression

LEVEL IV TRIAGE CATEGORY

Respiratory	Mild asthma
	Possible foreign body aspiration with no history of distress
	Minor chest injury with no respiratory distress
Neurological	Minor head injury – no vomiting or altered consciousness, GCS = 15
	Chronic or repeating headache with no acute distress
Cardiovascular	Chest pain with normal vital signs
Musculoskeletal	Possible extremity fracture, green-stick or buckle
	Sprain or strain
	Extremity swelling
Skin	Minor cold injury – no discoloration – minimal pain
	Localized cellulitis
	Minor burn
Gastrointestinal	Constipation; not eating; cramps
	Abdominal pain with vomiting or diarrhea > 2 years old
Genitourinary	Scrotal trauma
	Possible urinary infection

Behavior	Irritable consolable infant
	Atypical behavior
Infection	Child > 36 months with temperature > 38.5°C, non toxic appearance
Child Abuse	Signs or history of family violence
Pain	Mild pain 13/10

LEVEL V TRIAGE CATEGORY

Skin	Superficial burn
	Minor lacerations, abrasions, contusions
	Localized rash
	Minor bite
Gastrointestinal	Vomiting or diarrhea, no pain or dehydration, normal vital signs
Eye/ear/nose/throat	Sore throat, laryngitis, minor mouth sores
	Nasal congestion, allergy or upper respiratory infection
	Conjunctivitis
Psychiatry	Chronic symptoms with no acute changes
Pain	Minor pain

(Reprinted from the Canadian Association of Emergency Physicians. Canadian paediatric triage and acuity scale: implementation guidelines for emergency departments. Canad J Emerg Med 2001; 13(4) Suppl: www.caep.ca. with permission.)

or young child. Table 204.3 summarizes age-related pediatric differences in language development, behavioral activities, and motor/physiologic milestones. Abdominal breathing, a sign of respiratory distress in older infants and children, is a normal physiologic process that reflects increased reliance on the diaphragm for ventilation in the infant. Seesaw movement of the chest and abdomen, however, is abnormal and suggests increased work of breathing. Acrocyanosis and marbled skin (cutaneous marmorata) reflects only vascular instability with poor peripheral vasomotor control. This is normal in the first two months of life. Approximately twenty hours per day in early infancy is spent sleeping. The infant's expression of need is by crying and is generally a sign of hunger or discomfort.

Infants from 2 to 6 months of age begin appropriate interaction with their environment such as smiling with pleasure and recognition of familiar faces. Babbling sounds emerge as the beginning of language development and motor activities begin to mature. When performing assessments on infants under 6 months of age, emphasis should be on the most important and least traumatic aspects of the examination first. Keeping hands and instruments warm and using distractions and a quiet soothing voice can assist in gaining cooperation and facilitating the examination process. The majority of the exam should be done in the caretaker's arms whenever possible. It is important to be aware of the increased risk of heat loss from a high surface area to weight ratio and try to maintain a neutral-thermal environment during the examination process.

Examination of the 6-month to 1-year-old infant can be a challenge, especially if they have had previous negative experiences with a healthcare provider. Always anticipate and expect separation anxiety and perform as much of the examination on the caregiver's lap as possible. It is often helpful to get at or below eye level of the infant during the examination. Toys and distracting sounds can be used to keep the infant from losing control. The *toe-to-head* approach to examining the infant should always concentrate on the least traumatic aspects of examination first. The ears and mouth should be examined last.

The early toddler years are manifested by increasing mobility and curiosity about everything. There is absolutely no fear of danger and the risk of needless and predictable-preventable injury events increases dramatically as mobility progresses. "The terrible two's" begins at approximately eighteen months of age with "no" being the most widely used word in the toddler's progressing vocabulary. Whenever examining a toddler, obtain as much information through observation before laying on hands or a stethoscope. Magical games often help with difficult portions of an examination. As the caretaker palpates the abdomen

---

TABLE 204.2.   Normal Vital Signs for Age

Age	Respiratory Rate (Breaths/Min)	Heart Rate (Beats/Min)
>1 Y	30–60	100–160
1–2	24–40	90–150
2–5	22–34	80–140
6–12	18–30	70–120
>12	12–16	60–100

(Adapted from: Dieckman R, Brownstein D, Gausche-Hill M, eds. Pediatric education for prehospital professionals. Sudbury, MA: Jones and Bartlett Publishers, American Academy of Pediatrics; 2000: 43–45.)

TABLE 204.3. Age-Related Pediatric Differences

Age	Language	Behavioral	Motot/physiologic
Birth	• Express needs and discomfort by crying	• No/limited eye contact • No social smile • No recognition of caretaker	• Acrocyanosis • Abdominal breathing • Irregular head control
2 Months	• Vowel sounds with pleasure • Babbles • Laughs aloud	• Social smile • Recognizes caretaker	• Tracks light • Grasps objects • Rolls over • Sits with support

6 Months	• Repetitive vowel sounds
	• Repetitive consonant sounds
		• Stranger anxiety
		• Oral exploration
		• Imitative behavior
		• Independent activities
			• Sits alone
			• Increasing mobility
			  Creeps
			  Crawls
			  Stands

12 Months	• Variable and progressive language capabilities • Jargon speech • Speaks in 2–3 word phrases	• Increasing curiosity • No fear of danger • Strong opinions • Egocentrism • Problem solve by trial and error	• Walks alone • Stiff running • Climbs stairs
2 Years	• Comprehension greater than expression • Speaks in short sentences • Rapidly progressing language development	• Development of acceptable social patterns • Toilet training • Nightmares; fears of separation, bodily injury	• Refinement of both fine and gross motor skills
4 Years	• Good verbal skills	• Cooperative during exam • Gain in independence • Ability to reason with adults • Fear of pain, procedures	• Specialized motor skills emerge (games) • Common respiratory infections as immune system matures • Lymphoid tissue response causes variable "benign" adenopathy, and tonsil adenoid hypertrophy.
Adolescence	• Expressive and comprehensive language skills mature	• Peer pressures replace parent control. • Abstract thinking • Rational thought/analysis • Risk-taking	• Very mobile

he can "guess what the toddler had for breakfast earlier." Reassurance and praise goes a long way and any painful procedure should be explained in very simple terms.

In the early school age, young children begin to understand cause and affect relationships and learn to reason with adults. Their increasing independence outside the home becomes evident. This newfound independence will often crumble during stressful situations. It is not unusual for a 4-year-old to express plans for complete cooperation during a painful procedure, but when the procedure begins they may lose control and become combative. Information given to a young child can often be misinterpreted and create unwarranted fear and anxiety. It is important to speak directly to the child, and obtain information from the child, supplementing that information by parental report. Praise and compliments go a long way. The examiner should do their best to avoid ridicule if the young child loses control. It is best to anticipate questions and address fears with simple and clear explanations during the examination. Always respect the patient's modesty. When there are options in performing a procedure, allow the child limited control. For example, one cannot negotiate the need for a blood draw, but they can negotiate whether the procedure is performed in the left arm or the right arm.

In many ways adolescent behavior is similar to the toddler. They are very mobile, risk taking and often have no fear of danger. They may not anticipate consequences, and fail to use common sense before performing risk-taking activities. Peer pressure becomes very important. During a history and physical examination, adolescents should be separated from parents and information should be obtained from the patient, not the caretaker. Privacy and confidentiality must be respected. Explanations

of procedures and examination findings must be simple and concrete.

The child with special healthcare needs or developmental delays can be a challenge. The patient's caretaker must be able to provide assistance in establishing a normal baseline functional level. The caretaker of special needs children will usually be a valuable source of critical information. Parents of children with chronic conditions and high-tech gear are usually quite aware of important signs and symptoms that may alert the healthcare worker of impending problems. Listen to the caretaker. Always maintain a low threshold for seeking subspecialty consultation when in doubt about the signs and symptoms of special needs children.

EMERGENCY DEPARTMENT PREPARATION FOR CHILDREN

The ED must have resources necessary for the stabilization of critically ill or injured children and when necessary, written transfer agreements for further definitive care. A joint policy statement by the American College of Emergency Physicians and the American Academy of Pediatrics, *Care of Children in the Emergency Department: Guidelines for Preparation* provides a handy road map for a pediatric emergency-ready ED (1). Because most children who require emergency care are not brought to a hospital with comprehensive pediatric services, EDs must be prepared to care for children (2). All hospitals that serve as pediatric receiving facilities for emergency care, no matter what their size, pediatric volume, or available inpatient services must be prepared to stabilize pediatric emergencies.

A physician and nursing coordinator with special interests and knowledge in pediatrics should take responsibility for pediatric care. In very rural communities where there is a lack of resources, there may be shared professional responsibilities with a definitive care facility. The coordinator's roles are to oversee pediatric quality improvement processes, development of policies and procedures, review of medications and supplies, and serve as liaison for in-hospital and community committees addressing pediatric emergency care issues. The ED configuration should be child-friendly and safe. It is understood that not every hospital can afford the luxury of having separate pediatric and adult emergency departments. It is relatively simple, however, to have a child-friendly area in a community ED that is separated for children and decorated to meet the needs of the pediatric patient. Whenever possible, a separate waiting area should also be considered.

Acknowledgment

Thanks to the previous edition's chapter author John P. Santamaria.

References

1. American Academy of Pediatrics, Committee on Pediatric Emergency Medicine; American College of Emergency Physicians, Pediatric Committee: Care of children in the emergency department: guidelines for preparedness. *Ann Emerg Med* 2001;37:423–427 and *Pediatrics* 2001;107: 777–781.
2. Athey J, Dean JM, Ball J, Wiebe RA, Melise-d'Hospital I. Ability of hospitals to care for pediatric emergency patients. *Pediatr Emerg Care* 2001;17(3):170–174.
3. Canadian Association of Emergency Physicians. Canadian Paediatric Triage and Acuity Scale: Implementation Guidelines for Emergency Departments. *Canad J Emerg Med* 2001;13(4)Suppl: www.caep.ca. (Revised July 11, 2003).
4. Gausche-Hill M, Brownstein D, Dieckmann R, eds. *Pediatric education for prehospital professionals.* Boston: Jones and Bartlett, 2000:43,45.
5. Gausche-Hill M, Fuchs S, Yamamoto L, eds. APLS: *The pediatric emergency medicine resource.* Boston: Jones and Bartlett, 2004:20–50.
6. Gausch-Hill M, Wiebe RA. Guidelines for preparedness of emergency departments that care for children. *Ann Emerg Med* 2001;37:389–391 and *Pediatrics* 2001;107:773–774.
7. Gilboy N, Tanable P, Travers D, Eitel D, Wuerz R. *The Emergency Severity Index Implementation Handbook.* DesPlaines, IL: Emergency Nurses Association 2003.
8. Weiss HB, Mathers LJ, Farjuoh SN, et al.Child and adolescent emergency department datebook. Pittsburgh: Center for Violence and Injury Control, Allegheny University of the Health Sciences, 1997.
9. Wiebe RA, Rosen LM. Triage in the emergency department. *Emerg Med Clin North Am* 1991;9:491–505.

CHAPTER 205
Newborn Resuscitation

Rodney B. Boychuk

Approximately 5% to 10% of all newborns require resuscitation following birth to establish spontaneous respirations (8). However, all newborns delivered in or transported to the emergency department (ED) must be considered a true emergency as nearly 40% require some form of resuscitation (9). Although the majority of these infants will respond to simple maneuvers such as drying, suctioning, oxygen, and stimulation (S.O.S) more invasive resuscitation efforts may be required. The key to successful neonatal resuscitation in the ED is to equip and train all personnel in the aspects of neonatal resuscitation. At every delivery, there should be at least 1 person whose primary responsibility is the baby, and who is capable of performing a complete resuscitation, including endotracheal intubation and medication administration (8).

Pathophysiology

The goal of newborn resuscitation is to facilitate the transition from fetal to extrauterine life. Prior to delivery, fetal lungs are fluid-filled, gas exchange occurs through the placenta, and intra- and extra-cardiac circulation shunts blood through the foramen ovale and ductus arteriosus, largely bypassing the left side of the heart and lungs. After clamping the umbilical cord and the newborn's first breath, physiologic changes must occur to allow survival in the extrauterine environment. Establishment of adequate ventilation is essential for extrauterine survival.

During the first initial respirations, fetal lung fluid is displaced, functional residual capacity is established, and pulmonary vascular resistance decreases. Clamping of the umbilical cord leads to increased systemic vascular resistance, resulting in closure of the foramen ovale and ductus arteriosus. The combination of these events leads to increase in pulmonary blood flow and the establishment of normal extrauterine circulation. This normally smooth transition can be precluded by antepartum or postpartum events that cause asphyxia (9). It is not possible to predict every asphyxiated newborn; however, certain prenatal factors should alert the ED to the possibility of a problem (Table 205.1).

TABLE 205.1. Significant Maternal History

1. Prematurity: Most require intubation.
2. Multiple gestations: Multiple resuscitation set-ups; more personnel required.
3. Meconium: Suction at perineum/trachea (if nonvigorous) before stimulation.
4. Maternal drug (opiate) abuse: Avoid naloxone; it may precipitate seizures.
5. Maternal opiate administration: Consider naloxone for respiratory depression if the mother has received narcotics within 4 hours of delivery;
6. "Maternal" bleeding: May require fluid or O-negative blood resuscitation.

The principles of asphyxia and newborn resuscitation are as follows:

1. All newborn infants have some degree of respiratory acidosis and hypoxia at birth.
2. The asphyxiated newborn has more profound respiratory acidosis and hypoxia and, in addition, develops metabolic acidosis when respiratory efforts are ineffective. The pH falls at a rate of approximately 0.2 pH unit/min, whereas carbon dioxide rises at a rate of about 10 mm Hg/min. Oxygen content of the blood decreases to a level near 0 mm Hg within 2.5 minutes of asphyxia.
3. The type and degree of resuscitation necessary depends on when resuscitation is started in relation to the onset of asphyxia. Deprivation of oxygen leads to progressive bradycardia, decreased neuromuscular tone, and finally, primary apnea (8,9). Free-flow oxygen and stimulation will induce spontaneous respirations in most newborns at this stage. If asphyxia continues, however, irregular gasping respirations occur with profound bradycardia, hypotension, and flaccidity until the infant takes his or her last gasp and enters into secondary apnea. Once secondary apnea occurs, death is imminent unless resuscitation with assisted ventilation and oxygen is initiated. From a practical standpoint, it is difficult to distinguish primary apnea; therefore, all apneic newborns assumed to be in secondary apnea must be treated with ventilatory assistance.
4. The most important and effective action is ventilating oxygen into the lungs. Therefore one essential component of an asphyxiated neonatal resuscitation is 100% oxygen. Oxygen is a very potent chemical stimulant of the respiratory center in the brain, resulting in increased ventilatory drive. Oxygen also decreases pulmonary vascular resistance, resulting in

increased pulmonary blood flow and, therefore, increased oxygen and carbon dioxide exchange in the lungs. Once oxygenated blood reaches the bradycardic hypoxic heart, heart rate, myocardial contractility, cardiac output, and tissue perfusion increase. Therefore, free-flow oxygen should be used if indicated initially at 5 liters per minute flow (to avoid heat loss). Recently 21% (room air) oxygen resuscitations. have been studied. Until further evidence supports this practice, be liberal with oxygen.

5. Distention of the alveoli stimulates stretch and other pulmonary receptors, which are connected to and result in excitation of the respiratory center. Ventilation alone, therefore, has a beneficial effect; thus, the principle (if not contraindicated) of "do not hesitate—ventilate" should be followed quickly even if oxygen is NOT available.

6. Resuscitation of the asphyxiated newborn, therefore, should include correction of the three above-mentioned components, namely, ventilation for treatment of respiratory acidosis, 100% oxygen for correction of hypoxia, and, if indicated, sodium bicarbonate for correction of documented severe metabolic acidosis (usually prolonged resuscitation).

7. Neonates may not respond to standard resuscitation measures for a variety of reasons and reevaluation is a key step. The causes of resuscitation failure or deterioration must be sought and corrective action begun (Table 205.2).

8. Cooling results in increased oxygen consumption, increased metabolic rate with utilization of glucose and glycogen, increased lactic acid production, and increased acidosis (both respiratory and metabolic); therefore, the infant must be kept warm (4). Hypothermia and hypoglycemia are common occurrences in neonates requiring resuscitation and must be treated if present. Preventing hyperthermia is also important (10).

Practical Aspects of Resuscitation

Every ED delivery should be considered an emergency until proven otherwise. The worst scenario must be anticipated. Following notification of an impending (or completed) "incoming" delivery, the ED resuscitation "team" sets in motion the following practical aspects: (1) preparation, (2) assessment, and (3) management. Preparation must occur well in advance of the delivery. The resuscitation of a severely depressed and asphyxiated newborn requires at least two people, and ideally three: the resuscitation team. A trained physician, nurse, and respiratory therapist make-up an ideal trio to perform the two basic principles of resuscitation: (Fig. 205.1) (1) SOS (suction, oxygen, and stimulation) and (2) don't hesitate—ventilate, (i.e., if not breathing, start positive pressure ventilation (PPV). Assignments must be made quickly and personnel must adhere to their assigned duties.

Preparation

Table 205.3 outlines equipment that should be maintained in every ED and readily accessible at all times. This equipment is useless, however, unless personnel in the ED are familiar with its location and operation. It is advisable, therefore, that all EDs are equipped with an easily accessible neonatal resuscitation tray that includes not only emergency resuscitation equipment, but also medication dose and algorithm charts specific for neonates. It is essential that all ED personnel familiarize themselves with the resuscitation tray, and that daily checks be made to ensure presence and proper function of all types of equipment noted. In addition, a radiant warmer should be kept on at all times, and personnel skilled in newborn resuscitation must be immediately available.

TABLE 205.2.   Special Situations Resulting in Nonresponse to Resuscitation

TECHNICAL PROBLEMS

- Equipment failure
- Inadequate airway/ventilation
- Inadequate mask-face seal
- Inadequate pressure
- Inadequate oxygen
- Obstruction (mucus/meconium)
- ETT in esophagus
- ETT down too far

UNRECOGNIZED PULMONARY PROBLEMS

- Pneumothorax
- Diaphragmatic hernia
- Intrauterine pneumonia/sepsis
- Hypoplastic lungs
- Pleural effusion(s)

SEVERE METABOLIC PROBLEMS

- Hypoglycemia
- Acidosis
- Hypothermia

OTHER PROBLEMS

- Extreme prematurity
- Central nervous system
  injury
  narcosis
- Congenital anomalies
  upper airway
  lower airway
  pulmonary
  cardiac
  neurologic

SEVERE ANEMIA, HYPOVOLEMIA

Assessment

Assessment, the second and most important aspect of resuscitation, is the physician's responsibility when a full "team" is present. If this is not the case, then the most skilled nurse or respiratory therapist must perform this role. From the instant of birth until resuscitation is complete, this individual evaluates the infant dynamically, assessing the degree of asphyxia, the initial resuscitation measures necessary, the response to resuscitation, and further resuscitation measures required. This dynamic assessment begins immediately after the baby's exit from the vagina, even before the cord is clamped, with evaluation of the neonate's respiratory effort, heart rate, and then color. The compromised neonate may exhibit cyanosis, bradycardia, depressed respiratory drive, and poor muscle tone, and low blood pressure.

Although the Apgar score is determined by five factors, respiratory effort, heart rate, and color are most relevant to the resuscitation (Table 205.4). First, respiratory effort, then, heart rate and, finally, color are dynamically monitored throughout the resuscitation on a second-by-second basis. Because the Apgar score is assigned at 1 and 5 minutes after delivery, it should not be used as a guide to resuscitation. Improvement in HR, respiratory effort, and eventually color should serve as the guides to successive steps of resuscitation immediately after delivery. If the 5-minute

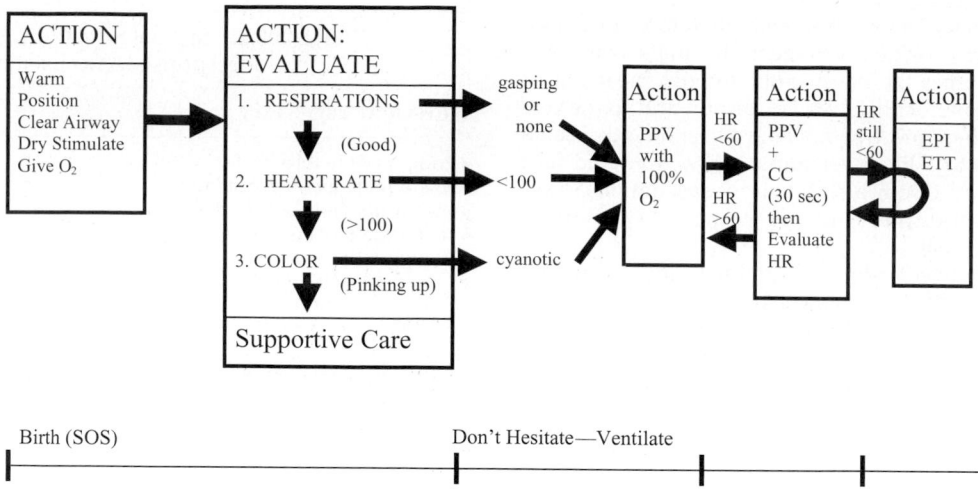

PPV = positive pressure ventilation   CC = chest compressions   EPI = epinephrine   HR = heart rate
ETT = endotracheal tube
*see text for initial management of nonvigorous meconium birth.   Adapted and modified in part from reference 8.

Figure 205.1.   Neonatal Resuscitation Algorithm (excluding nonvigorous meconium birth): Action vs. Time (sec).

score is less than 7, continue to document additional scores every 5 minutes for up to 20 minutes. It should be emphasized that several interventions occur simultaneously and not in isolated, consecutive steps.

Initial Resuscitation

The initial steps of newborn resuscitation are: position, clear airway (including tracheal suctioning if necessary), dry, remove linen, reposition, give oxygen as necessary, then simultaneously evaluate the infant's respiratory effort, HR, and color (8). These steps must be done quickly, so that more advanced resuscitation efforts can be performed if required. After delivery the umbili-

cal cord is clamped and cut, and the newborn is placed under a radiant warmer. The infant is positioned supine, or lying on its side with the head in a neutral or slightly extended position. This will facilitate optimal opening of the airway. Suctioning of the mouth, then the nose can be accomplished with a bulb syringe or mechanical suction device. If mechanical suction is used, do not suction for a prolonged period, deeply or vigorously, as vagally mediated apnea and bradycardia will occur (6). Unless meconium is present, the newborn is thoroughly dried with warm blankets to prevent heat loss and stimulate spontaneous respirations. Wet blankets should be removed immediately. Reposition if needed, and give oxygen as necessary. Stimulation is provided by rubbing the back or flicking the soles of the feet. Following this process again simultaneously evaluate respiratory effort, HR, and color. Spontaneous respiratory effort is adequate if the infant is able to maintain HR greater than 100 beats/min and becomes pink. Following delivery, most infants respond to initial resuscitation by crying, the heart rate immediately rising, and gradually becoming pink. Some infants, however, require additional brief stimulation and 100% free-flow oxygen. Free-flow oxygen is required during initial resuscitation if the neonate is breathing but cyanotic, or if an apneic neonate begins to breathe during initial resuscitation.

Infants who remain apneic throughout the initial steps or who have gasping respirations require PPV with bag-mask ventilation (BVM), with 100% oxygen. It is important NOT to delay PPV by prolonging free flow oxygen and stimulation! If the neonate remains apneic provide PPV (don't hesitate—ventilate!). Ventilate for about 30 seconds, then reassess. Once the

---

TABLE 205.3.   Practical Aspects of Resuscitation: Preparation of Equipment

1. Overhead radiant warmer: on and working. Warm blankets, caps.
2. Suction: on and working; catheters (sizes 8F, 12F, 14F) immediately available; blue bulb suction open and ready.
3. Oxygen supply: on and working.
4. Laryngoscope and number 0 and 1 straight blades: batteries fresh, bulb secure, light a bright "white" intensity when turned on.
5. Endotracheal intubation tubes: sizes 2–4 mm ready.
6. Pressure-monitored anesthesia bagging apparatus: set up and ready. Face masks in premature and newborn sizes. Resuscitation Bags: 250 ml for premature, 450 ml for term infant.
7. Nurse: ready to start the timer and monitor the infant's heart rate.
8. Physician: ready to evaluate, suction, laryngoscope, ventilate, intubate, and carry out further procedures.
9. Respiratory therapist: ready to administer oxygen, suction, and assist with ventilation and intubation.
10. Other equipment: meconium aspirators, umbilical catheters (3.5F and 5F), syringes, three way stopcock, catheterization trays, chest tube trays, and drugs-epinephrine, volume expanders, naloxone, glucose, saline flush-immediately available or drawn up.

TABLE 205.4.   Apgar Score

Sign	0	1	2
Heart rate	Absent	Slow (<100)	>100
Respirations	Absent	Slow, irregular	Good; crying
Muscle tone	Limp	Some flexion	Active motion
Reflex irritability	No response	Grimace	Vigorous
Color	Blue, pale	Acrocyanosis	Pink

respiratory effort has been evaluated and appropriately managed, HR can be assessed. HR is determined by palpating the base of the umbilical cord. If a pulse is not palpable, auscultate the central left chest with a stethoscope. In the uncompromised infant, the HR should remain greater than 100 beats/min. HR less than 100 needs to be closely monitored and PPV initiated (or continued). If the HR remains less than 60, further intervention with chest compressions, medications, and appropriate diagnostic evaluation is indicated.

The color of a healthy newborn will become and remain pink without supplemental oxygen. Acrocyanosis, or peripheral cyanosis, is not an unusual finding at birth. It is thought to occur secondary to cold stress and initially sluggish circulation, not to hypoxemia (2). True cyanosis, or central cyanosis (hypoxemia) is determined by examining central structures particularly the mucous membranes. Infants with central cyanosis, regardless of HR and respiratory effort, require supplemental oxygen and may require BVM and endotracheal intubation, depending on the etiology of the hypoxemia.

The Distressed Newborn

Following the initial assessment and resuscitation, the newborn will generally follow one of two paths. Either the newborn is vigorous and requires minimal or no further intervention other than close observation and postresuscitative care, or the newborn is distressed, mandating further resuscitative efforts. One situation that precludes normal resuscitation is that of the infant born with meconium in the amniotic fluid.

Meconium staining of the amniotic fluid generally implies fetal distress. It is found in approximately 12% of all deliveries, predominantly in small for gestational age (SGA) and postterm-stressed newborns (15). The clinical concern is to avoid meconium aspiration, with the resultant complications of meconium aspiration syndrome (hypoxemia, acidosis, and pulmonary hypertension) (7).

Clearing meconium from the airway begins at the mother's perineum after delivery of the head, but before delivery of the shoulders, at which time a bulb syringe (12) or 12F or 14F suction catheter is used to suction the mouth, pharynx, and nose (3). After the body delivers, the appropriate management of the airway depends not only on the presence of meconium but also the neonates' level of activity (i.e., vigorous vs. nonvigorous.) A vigorous newborn is defined as one who has strong respiratory effort, a heart rate greater than 100 per minute and good muscle tone (16). In the vigorous infant with meconium, simply repeat what was done on the perineum. However, if the meconium-stained newborn is nonvigorous with depressed respirations, depressed muscle tone, and/or a heart rate less than 100 beats per minute, direct suctioning of the trachea is indicated, before many respirations have occurred. In this scenario the trachea is then intubated and meconium suctioned from the lower airway (16). Repeat intubation and suctioning can be performed until meconium is no longer recovered, provided the infant's HR remains above 60 beats/min. Suction negative pressure (vacuum) should not exceed 100 mm Hg when the suction tubing is clamped. Following tracheal suctioning, the infant should be resuscitated like other infants.

Advanced Resuscitation

Distressed newborns may require ongoing resuscitation (Fig. 205.2). Following the initial evaluation, any infant who has apnea, gasping respirations, HR less than 100, or persistent central cyanosis requires BVM (using the E-C technique: E = resuscitators fingers 3, 4, and 5 pulling the chin up into the mask (into a sniffing position); C = fingers 1 and 2 holding the mask

onto the face) with 100% oxygen at 40 to 60 breaths per minute. Initial BVM "breaths" may require >30 cm H_2O pressure to establish adequate lung volumes, but all subsequent breaths should be delivered at the lowest possible pressure. Good chest rise should be observed; if not, reposition the infant's head and attempt ventilation again. It is important to ensure a good seal between the mask and the infant's face, and if necessary, use the two-person technique. Placement of an 8F orogastric tube, to prevent gastric distension, will be necessary if prolonged BVM is required. After 30 seconds of PPV, the HR should be reevaluated. If oxygen is not available, initiate PPV with room air, and if nothing is immediately available, mouth (resuscitator) to mouth and nose (neonate), with appropriate precautions, may be utilized. The HR is an internal monitor of ventilation adequacy, and will rise immediately if ventilation is adequate. Once the HR is greater than 100, observe for spontaneous, effective respirations and discontinue PPV once they occur. If the HR remains <100, continue PPV and reassess the HR in 2 to 3 minutes. If the HR is less than 60 after the initial 30 seconds of PPV, or if, at any time, the HR is absent, chest compressions should accompany PPV with 100% oxygen (2). After 30 seconds of chest compressions and ventilation, stop long enough to determine the heart rate (palpable umbilicus). Continue ventilation if pulse is palpable. If pulse is not palpable, check the heart rate by auscultating the chest. Then continue resuscitation based on heart rate, ventilatory effort and color.

Chest Compressions

The best technique for neonatal chest compression utilizes both thumbs placed on the lower third of the infant's sternum, with the resuscitator's hands encircling the neonate's torso with the fingers supporting the spine. Pressure is applied to the lower third of the sternum. The sternum should be depressed one third of the total diameter of the chest, accompanied by PPV at a rate of 1 ventilation for every 3 compressions, delivering 120 events per minute (90 chest compressions + 30 ventilations) (8). Chest compressions should be smooth, with the thumbs not leaving the infant's sternum between compressions and sufficiently deep to generate a palpable pulse. Care should be taken to avoid applying pressure to the xiphoid process, as this may injure abdominal organs. Compressions may be discontinued when the neonates spontaneous HR exceeds 60 beats/min.

Endotracheal Intubation

Endotracheal intubation is necessary whenever BVM is ineffective or prolonged, when tracheal suctioning for meconium is required, if endotracheal medication administration is desired, or when chest compressions are performed. It is also indicated when a congenital diaphragmatic hernia is suspected, (to avoid gastric distension) or after birth of an extremely low birth weight premature. Equipment size for intubation can be selected based on the infant's estimated weight and gestational age (Table 205.5). In general, premature newborns require a

TABLE 205.5. Equipment Size Based on Estimated Age and Weight

Age (wk)	Weight (kg)	ETT (mm)	Insertion Depth (cm)	Blade
<28	<1	2.5	7	0
28–34	1–2	3.0	8	0
35–38	2–3	3.5	9	0–1
>38	>3	3.5–4.0	10	1

2.5-mm endotracheal tube (ETT), while term newborns need a 3.0- to 3.5-mm ETT. A laryngoscope with a straight (Miller) blade is preferred (size 0 to premature, size 1 to term infants) to visualize the newborn's glottis and vocal cords. If a stylet is used, care must be taken to prevent the tip from protruding beyond the end of the ETT and injuring the airway. After intubation, proper ETT placement should be determined by careful physical examination capnography or end tidal CO_2 monitoring (exhaled CO_2 detection) (1), and chest radiograph. Lack of chest rise, asymmetry of chest movement, and the lack of rise of HR and/or color are signs of inappropriate ETT placement (8). The laryngeal mask airway (LMA) may be an effective alternate when used by appropriately trained providers.

Medications

Medications are rarely indicated during a newborn resuscitation and are reserved for specific situations (2,13). Epinephrine is recommended for asystole or bradycardia (HR less than 60) if no response to PPV with 100% oxygen and chest compressions for a minimum of 30 seconds. Volume expansion with 10 mL/kg of crystalloid (normal saline, lactated Ringer) or colloid (0 negative blood for large volume blood loss) is indicated when acute blood loss is suspected and signs of hypovolemia are present (pallor, poor perfusion, weak pulse). Volume is given by slow intravenous push, usually over 5 to 10 minutes. Naloxone is useful when there is severe respiratory depression and a history of maternal narcotic administration within 4 hours of delivery (recommended dose 0.1 mg/kg IV, ETT or if good perfusion IM). Naloxone should not delay other resuscitation efforts, such as airway management, and should never be used if chronic maternal narcotic drug use is suspected, as it can precipitate withdrawal signs in the newborn. Sodium bicarbonate (4.2%) is only indicated during a prolonged arrest that does not respond to other therapy after adequate ventilation is established and metabolic acidosis is documented. Two to four ml/kg of Glucose (DIOW) should be administered for documented hypoglycemia (less than 30 mg/dL in preterm, less than 40 mg/dL in term infants). The usual dose is 2 to 4 ml/kg intravenously (IV). A dopamine infusion should be considered when signs of shock continue despite volume expansion (5-20 micrograms/kg/minute IV continuous). High-dose epinephrine is not recommended in neonatal resuscitations (Table 205.6).

The administration of medications can occur via several routes. In general, the quickest route to give epinephrine or naloxone is down the ETT. Medications given down an ETT

should be 2 to 3 times the intravenous dose, flushed with 1 to 2 mL of normal saline and followed by BVM (11).

Vascular Access

When intravenous access cannot be established and vascular access is needed, the umbilical vein is the most accessible site. Using sterile technique, a tie is placed around the base of the umbilical stump to control bleeding, and a scalpel is used to cut the cord 0.5 to 1.0 cm above the skin. The umbilical vein (always at the 12:00 o'clock position towards the head) is easily distinguished from the two smaller arteries, which are usually constricted. Flush a sterile 3.5F (premature) or 5.0F (term) umbilical venous catheter with normal saline and attach it to a three-way stopcock. The catheter is advanced into the umbilical vein just below the skin level until good blood return is obtained (usually of 2 to 4 cm). Wedged hepatic positions are recognized by subsequent failure of free blood return after introduction. If this occurs, the catheter should be withdrawn to a position where blood can be easily aspirated. Secure the umbilical venous catheter to the skin with tape (Fig. 205.2). When other means of vascular access are not available, the intraosseous route may be attempted; however, its use is not common (5).

Special Situations Resulting in "Nonresponsive" Resuscitations

If the neonate is not responding, other causes of asphyxia must be considered and sought. Generally, the etiology falls into 1 or more of 5 major categories: (1) technical problems, (2) unrecognized pulmonary problems, (3) severe metabolic problems, (4) congenital anomalies of the organ systems involved, and (5) severe anemia (Table 205.2).

By far, technical problems are the most common, and of these, inadequate ventilation either because of not opening the airway, poor seal of the mask to the face or malposition of the ETT are the most frequent. The ETT may be in the esophagus instead of the trachea, or it may have been advanced too far, the tip being in the right main stem bronchus. First, check the tube position by relaryngoscoping or reintubating the neonate. If the infant is correctly intubated, chest expansion should be seen with ventilation and good air entry heard bilaterally. No air entry should be heard in the stomach. Hearing good air entry on the right side and no or poor air entry on the left side suggests that the ET tube is down the right main stem bronchus. If this occurs, the ET tube should be pulled back until good air

---

TABLE 205.6.   Medications

Medication	Concentration	Dose	Route
Epinephrine	1:10,000	0.1–0.3 mL/kg	i.v., ETT*
Volume expanders	Normal saline Ringer's lactate O⁻ blood, 5% albumin	10 mL/kg	i.v.
Naloxone	1.0 mg/mL	0.1 mL/kg	i.v., ETT i.m., SQ
Sodium bicarbonate	4.2% solution (0.5 mEq/mL)	2–4 mL/kg	i.v. (1–2 mEq/kg)
Glucose	$D_{10}W$	2–4 mL/kg	i.v.
Dopamine	$\dfrac{\text{wt (kg)} \times 6 \times \mu g/kg/min}{mL/h} = $ mg in 100 mL fluid For example, if kg × 6 × 5, then 1 mL/h = 5 μg/kg/min Continuous i.v. infusion at 5–20 μg/kg/min		

*ETT = endotracheal tube

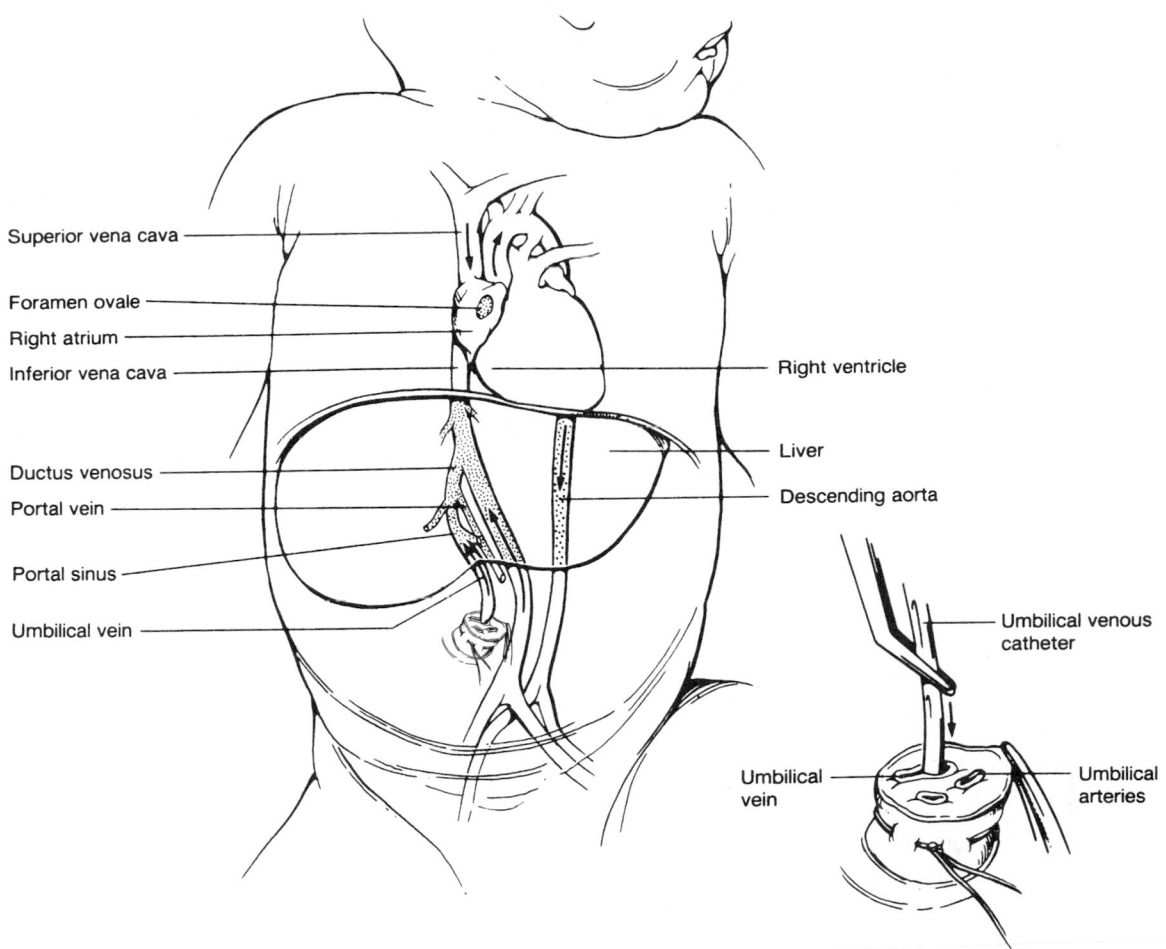

Figure 205.2. Insertion of the umbilical venous catheter.

entry is heard on both sides. Another possible cause of poor left-sided air entry is a pneumothorax on the left side, although this may occur on either side. PPV with esophageal intubation may result in "apparent" air entry when auscultating the lungs; however, the chest will not move and air will be heard entering the stomach. Therefore, one should auscultate both lungs (in the axilla) and the epigastric area for initial ET tube position confirmation.

Other technical problems include an inadequate flow, pressure, oxygen concentration, or a "malfunctioning" ventilation system. When there is inadequate response, always use, 100% oxygen with enough flow and adequate pressure to ventilate the neonate. Excessive pressures are harmful, yet adequate pressure must be administered for ventilation to occur. Always use enough pressure to move the chest.

The second category of failures in resuscitation is unrecognized pulmonary problems. Although these must be suspected clinically, they are ultimately confirmed radiologically. Problems such as pneumothorax, diaphragmatic hernia, hypoplastic lungs, intrauterine pneumonia/sepsis and other severe restrictive lung problems may result in an "unresuscitatible" infant. Once the condition is recognized, further emergency treatment is indicated.

Those born with hypovolemia or severe anemia may not have a history suggesting anemia and frequently are unrecognized, not responding to appropriate resuscitation techniques. Other failures in resuscitation may be secondary to metabolic problems. The most common problems include severe metabolic acidosis, hypoglycemia, and hypothermia. All will interfere with resus-

citative efforts and, therefore, must be prevented, appropriately recognized, and treated.

Those born with congenital or acquired conditions involving the lungs, airway, heart, central nervous system, neuromuscular system, or hematopoietic system may not respond to resuscitation. Radiographic and other evaluations are frequently required for the diagnosis to be made.

Two other important groups of neonates requiring resuscitation include the premature newborn and multiple births.

Specific Conditions Requiring Resuscitation

Pneumothorax

Pneumothorax is not uncommon in the newborn who receives aggressive resuscitation. Symptomatic pneumothoraces are relieved with needle decompression at the second intercostal space, midclavicular line, or the anterior axillary line at the level of the nipples. Chest tube placement usually is needed after stabilization.

Congenital Diaphragmatic Hernia

Infants with a diaphragmatic hernia present in respiratory distress and persistent cyanosis immediately after birth, often with a scaphoid abdomen and displaced cardiac impulse. Ventilation by BVM should be avoided, because it increases gastric distension and further compromises lung expansion. Infants must be immediately endotracheally intubated with a nasograstic (NG) tube passed for gastric decompression.

Congenital Heart Disease

Infants who remain cyanotic despite adequate resuscitation efforts may have cyanotic congenital heart disease or persistent fetal circulation. Referral to a pediatric cardiologist for echocardiography is required. Prostaglandin E_1 may be necessary to maintain patency of the ductus arteriosus.

Pneumonia/Sepsis

Prolonged rupture of the membranes may result in chorioamnionites, with the newborn presenting with respiratory distress and signs of pneumonia/sepsis. Common bacterial causes include group B *Streptococcus*, *Escherichia coli*, and *Listeria monocytogenes*. After appropriate cultures and stabilization, treatment with ampicillin and cefotaxime is indicated.

Multiple Births

Additional equipment and personnel will be required to manage multiple births. Resuscitation is frequently required secondary to mechanical complications of delivery and compromised cord blood flow. Twin B, in particular, is at risk of birth asphyxia.

Prematurity

Premature newborns are prone to respiratory distress secondary to immature lungs and surfactant deficiency. Most will require intubation. They are also at increased risk for hypoglycemia, heat loss, and intraventricular hemorrhage during resuscitation (6). Expeditious transfer to a neonatal intensive care unit (NICU) is mandatory.

Maternofetal Hemorrhage/Acute Blood Loss

Vaginal bleeding may be a sign of placenta previa or abruptio placenta with acute fetal blood loss. Transplacental fetal to maternal blood transfusion may also occur. These infants are at increased risk for severe anemia/hypovolemia and if unrecognized may be unresuscitatible. Usually during the resuscitation the neonate will become pale white rather than pink, with poor tissue perfusion. This situation requires volume expansion/blood. Immediate O-negative blood transfusion may be life-saving.

Postresuscitative Care and Disposition

Early consultation (including the physical presence) of a neonatologist or pediatrician is ideal in order to assist with resuscitation and determine the level of postresuscitative care needed. Depending on the etiology of and the degree of resuscitation required, the neonate will now require 1 of 3 levels of care: routine (standard observation), supportive (frequent evaluation) or ongoing care (continuing evaluation and monitoring in a nursery environment). If transfer is required, it is best accomplished by a tertiary care facility that has a neonatal transport team.

Following stabilization of the newborn, special care should be taken to maintain temperature, avoid and treat hypoglycemia, and monitor respiratory rate and effort, oxygen saturation, administered oxygen concentration, HR, blood pressure, and muscle tone/activity. Infants remaining in the ED for any prolonged time should have labs sent, including CBC, arterial blood gas (ABG), and glucose and calcium level. A chest x-ray to assess ETT placement and rule out occult pathology is recommended. If needed, the neonate can be ventilated at a rate of 40 to 60 breaths per minute with end tidal CO_2 and pulse oximeter monitoring until the ABG results are obtained. Maintenance intravenous fluids can be started with $D_{10}W$ at 80 cc/kg/d, as electrolytes are generally not required in the first 24 hours of life. Lorazepam 0.1 mg/kg (or equivalent) is effective to sedate the intubated newborn if needed. In addition, treatment of possible infection, seizures, or hypotension (with volume expanders or pressors), and documentation of resuscitation are indicated. The parents must be informed of the newborn's condition and must be allowed to see and touch the baby, with their questions answered as frankly and honestly as possible.

CRITICAL INTERVENTIONS

- Advance and immediate neonatal resuscitation preparation plans or policies including equipment, medications, contact information (NICU, transport team, labor and delivery, etc), mock resuscitations and staff education
- Obtain critical history elements as soon as possible (multiple births, prematurity, meconium, bleeding or maternal drug use)
- Reassess heart rate, color and respirations after each intervention
- Remember the resuscitation basics, S.O.S. (suction, oxygen, and stimulation), and don't hesitate—ventilate.

COMMON PITFALLS

✔ Failure to have specific neonatal resuscitation equipment set up and readily accessible, including a radiant warmer
✔ Lack of an individual with skills required to perform a complete newborn resuscitation
✔ Failure to recognize the "high risk" mother/fetus
✔ Failure to initiate basic resuscitation techniques, including giving free-flow oxygen as necessary
✔ Failure to recognize the neonate with secondary apnea, therefore delaying the initiation of PPV
✔ Failure to adequately clear meconium from the hypopharynx and trachea before stimulating the neonate in the nonvigorous neonate
✔ Failure to consider "other causes" in a nonresponsive neonate (Table 205.2)

SUMMARY

For most newborns, the asphyxial stress of birth is mild and brief and there is no need for sophisticated intervention. When the stress is excessive or the neonate's ability to compensate is decreased, resuscitation is necessary. The ABCs (Airway–clear and position; breathing–stimulate to breathe; circulation–assess HR and color; drugs) of resuscitation (8), adequately describe the essential steps; however, to simplify neonatal resuscitation remember the acronym SOS—suction, oxygen, and stimulation. Even infants with moderate depression (occasional respiratory effort) will generally respond to brief suctioning of the airway, 100% free flow oxygen, and stimulation. If SOS is ineffective, PPV must be administered without hesitation. Resuscitation of the newborn is not a simple procedure, but rather a dynamic process involving continuous evaluation, action, and reassessment before, during, and after the actual resuscitation.

Acknowledgment

The author gratefully acknowledges the contribution of Brian P. Gilligan, who wrote the previous edition of this chapter.

References

1. Aziz HF, Martin JB, Moore JJ. The pediatric disposable end-tidal carbon dioxide detector role in endotracheal intubation in newborns. *J Perinatol* 1999;19:110–113.
2. Burchfield DJ. Medication use in neonatal resuscitation. *Clin Perinatol* 1999; 26:683–691.
3. Carson BS, Losey RW, Bowes WA Jr, Simmons MA. Combined obstetric and pediatric approach to prevent meconium aspiration syndrome. *Am J Obstet Gynecol* 1976;126:712–715.
4. Dahm LS, James LS. Newborn temperature and calculated heat loss in the delivery room. *Pediatrics* 1972;49:504–513.

5. Ellemunter H, Simma B, Trawoger R, Maurer H. Intraosseous lines in preterm and full term neonates. *Arch Dis Child Fetal Neonatal Ed* 1999;80:F74–F75.

6. Estol PC, Piriz H, Basalo S, Simini F, Grela C. Oro-naso-pharyngeal suction at birth: effects on respiratory adaption of normal term vaginally born infants. *J Perinatal Med* 1992;20:297–305.

7. Greenough A. Meconium aspiration syndrome: prevention and treatment. *Early Hum Dev* 1995;41:183–192.

8. International Guidelines for Neonatal Resuscitation: An Excerpt From the Guidelines 2000 for Cardiopulmonary Resuscitation and Emergency Cardiovascular Care: International Consensus on Science. *Circulation* 2000;102:I–343–I–357.

9. Khan N, Luten R. Neonatal resuscitation. *Emerg Med Clin North Am* 1994;12:239–256.

10. Lieberman E, Lang J, Richardson DK, et al. Intrapartum maternal fever and neonatal outcome. *Pediatrics* 2000;105:8–13.

11. Lindemann R. Resuscitation of the newborn: endotracheal administration of epinephrine. *Acta Paediatr Scand* 1984;73:210–212.

12. Locus P, Yeomans E, Crosby U. Efficacy of Bulb versus DeLee suction at deliveries complicated by meconium stained amniotic fluid [see comments]. *Am J Perinatol* 1990;7:87–91.

13. Perlman JM, Risser R. Cardiopulmonary resuscitation in the delivery room: associated clinical events. *Arch Pediatr Adolesc Med* 1995;149:20–25.

14. Slywka B, Whitelaw C, Goldsmith L. Comparison of the two finger vs. the two thumb compression. *Acad Emerg Med* 1998;5:398 (Abstract).

15. Wiswell TE, Tuggle JM, Turner BS. Meconium aspiration syndrome: have we made a difference? [see comments] *Pediatrics* 1990;85:715–721.

16. Wiswell TE. Meconium in the Delivery Room Trial Group: delivery room management of the apparently vigorous meconium-stained neonate: results of the multi-center collaborative trial. *Pediatrics* 200;105:1–7.

CHAPTER 206
Pediatric Resuscitation

John A. Brennan and Neil Schamban

Resuscitation of an infant or child can be one of the most challenging and anxiety-producing experiences any physician will encounter in the emergency department (ED). The ability to recognize and treat life-threatening conditions requires prior preparation, experience, a substantial knowledge base, adequate airway and vascular access skills, and appropriate use of all resources.

Throughout this chapter, fundamental differences, similarities, and intragroup differences related to size and age are highlighted as they affect resuscitation. Management goals of pediatric resuscitation are to correct hypoxemia and ventilation abnormalities, correct metabolic abnormalities (e.g., acidemia), and improve coronary, renal, and cerebral perfusion. A successful outcome depends on adequate alveolar oxygenation and carbon dioxide exchange, maintaining vascular perfusion, and correcting the underlying cause of the cardiopulmonary arrest.

The events just before, during, and after a pediatric resuscitation are all critical components to the successful resuscitation of an infant or child. The physician must be able to treat the family, as well as the patient, during and after the resuscitation. He or she must help the parents have some sense of understanding and control as their child is taken to a pediatric intensive care unit or help the parents begin the grieving process if the resuscitation efforts have been unsuccessful.

Annually there are 12.7 to 19.7 (17) pediatric arrests in the United States per every 100,000 children (5). Approximately half of the arrests are in children less than 1 year old (17). The survival rate of a child with cardiopulmonary arrest is between 0% and 13%. The most common initial rhythm is asystole.

Because most EDs have very few "true" pediatric emergencies, preparedness and education are crucial aspects of pediatric resuscitation (8). Less than 5% to 7% of pediatric ED visits are considered critical, and in less than 1% is cardiac or respiratory resuscitation required.

The pathophysiology of cardiopulmonary arrest and shock in children differs from that of adults in many aspects. Most pediatric cardiopulmonary arrests are caused by progressive deterioration in respiration or circulation due to medical or less commonly traumatic illness. Children have remarkable physiologic compensatory mechanisms which tend to obscure common signs of shock that are readily recognizable in adults. For this reason, recognition of pediatric cardiopulmonary decompensation can be problematic, as significant intracellular hypoxemia and acidosis that decrease the cardiovascular system's ability to respond to medications and defibrillation can occur without early detection.

CLINICAL PRESENTATION

In the vast majority of cases, respiratory failure precedes overt cardiopulmonary arrest in children. This is in stark contrast to adults where primary cardiac disease is the root of most arrests. The causes of respiratory arrest can be divided into two categories. First, there is upper airway pathology, which includes anatomic abnormalities, infectious disease, inflammatory reactions, and foreign bodies. The second category is lower airway pathology, which includes interstitial disease, alveolar disease, and bronchus or bronchiole disease.

Shock (inadequate cellular energy supply) is the next most common pathway predisposing the child to cardiopulmonary arrest. Shock has many different etiologies, the most common of which is hypovolemia, either from dehydration or bleeding. Distributive shock is secondary to anaphylaxis, spinal cord injuries, or sepsis. Cardiogenic shock is secondary to an arrhythmia or mechanical abnormality, whether structural or infectious (i.e., myocarditis). Obstructive shock, secondary to cardiac tamponade or tension pneumothorax, and dissociative shock, secondary to hemoglobin abnormalities (carbon monoxide poisoning or methemoglobinemia), complete the list.

Thus, a rapid assessment of cardiopulmonary stability is of paramount importance. An assessment tool (known as the Pediatric Assessment Triangle [10]) allows rapid evaluation of the child's appearance, breathing, and circulation status. This assessment correlates with a child's state of oxygenation and perfusion and can be completed in 15 to 30 seconds of initial presentation.

Specifically, the parameters involved include the rapid assessment of the child's airway, breathing, and cardiac status; general appearance (10), skin color, and capillary refill; and a general neurologic assessment of the child that includes the child's mental status and best verbal, motor, and eye responses.

EMERGENCY DEPARTMENT MANAGEMENT

Cardiopulmonary Resuscitation Overview

Single-rescuer cardiopulmonary resuscitation (CPR) should activate EMS after 1 minute of rescue breathing and compressions if the patient is less than 8 years old (more likely respiratory than cardiac) (7). Infants and children should have a compression rate of 100 per minute and 20 ventilations per minute (5:1). The resuscitator's hand should be on the lower half of the sternum and a depth of one-third to one-half the depth of the chest. Foreign-body maneuvers include back blows and chest thrusts for infants and the Heimlich maneuver for children. There are many investigational alternative methods for CPR, but none has been shown to have better outcomes than those described in the American Heart Association (AHA) guidelines for CPR.

Airway

The foundation of all pediatric resuscitative attempts is appropriate airway management. Because the airway in childhood changes with age, the clinician must be aware of variables such as anatomic location, caliber, and length. Further consideration must be given to variability in head circumference (occipital prominence), as well as the relative size of the tongue and mandible size as compared to the head (7).

As the child grows, the larynx descends from a relatively superior and anterior position in infancy to the adult location. This change is complete by about age 10 years (range, 8 to 12 years). The narrowest portion of the extrathoracic airway in a child younger than 8 years is the cricoid ring, while in older children and adults it is the glottic opening. This anatomic difference is the reason why uncuffed endotracheal tubes are generally in children younger than 8 years of age. Head size, equal to or larger than chest circumference in the neonate, grows to adult proportions by adolescence.

Given these anatomic differences, positioning of the infant requires careful attention to the tendency of the prominent occiput to cause neck flexion and resultant airway occlusion. Mild extension of the head (nontraumatic arrest) to achieve the "sniffing" position will provide airway patency in the child with adequate mandibular muscle tone. Overextension may cause airway obstruction by compressing the compliant trachea.

The large tongue may still occlude the airway, even with proper head–neck position. When hypotonia occurs, the mandible will no longer be maintained in a stable open position by the child, so the tongue will fall against the posterior pharyngeal wall, obstructing the airway. Appropriate maneuvers, such as a chin lift or jaw thrust, will move this block of tissue anteriorly and will open the airway. Airway devices, such as nasopharyngeal tubes for conscious children or oropharyngeal airways in unconscious patients, may be helpful once the airway has been opened manually. When the airway cannot be maintained using these maneuvers, or when other indications exist, an endotracheal tube (ETT) may need to be placed.

There are many physiologic and anatomic differences between adult and pediatric airways. The physician taking care of children must also be prepared to treat patients with less common but still prevalent congenital malformations such as webs, tracheolaryngeal malacia, hemangiomas, cranial facial disorders, subglottic stenosis, and extrinsic and intrinsic foreign bodies. Resuscitation and airway management in these children present special challenges to even the most experienced caregiver.

Physiologic differences between adults and children include a higher metabolic and oxygen consumption of children (which causes them to become hypoxic sooner), the smaller functional reserve capacity of children, their exaggerated vagal responses, and the higher airway resistance of children. For the practitioner the importance of these physiologic differences is that there is even a smaller window of opportunity from recognition of respiratory or cardiorespiratory arrest to age-appropriate management when compared with adults.

In general if the child has inadequate oxygenation or ventilation unresponsive to basic airway treatment, intubation is indicated. Preparations for this procedure should be started while the child is being properly positioned and oxygenated. A bag-valve-mask device with supplemental oxygen and oxygen reservoir can provide a 90% inspired concentration of oxygen, and the child can be ventilated until intubation preparations are complete.

Endotracheal intubation offers the following advantages:

- It affords significant airway protection against aspiration
- It provides a conduit for suctioning of secretions and debris
- It permits alveolar ventilation which can correct respiratory acidosis without compromising chest compressions
- It permits 100% oxygen instillation to the trachea with the possibility of applying positive end-expiratory pressure

Full preparation includes an adequate large-bore suction device for clearing the oral and hypopharynx, a range of ETT sizes, smaller suction catheters for the ETT following insertion, and a laryngoscope with the proper size and shape of blade.

In general, a straight blade is preferable in children 4 years of age and younger. The curved blade should be used for older children. The epiglottis is floppy in younger children and its position along with the larynx are more cephalad and anterior. These anatomic and physiologic differences in the pediatric airway compared with the adult airway make a straight blade preferable for the initial intubation attempt. The straight blade can hook the epiglottis directly and be placed in proper position easier than the curved blade. The curved blade must be placed in the vallecula for ideal use, whereas the straight blade is placed posterior to the epiglottis and does not require strict anatomic matching to the curvature of the tongue. The child's anterior and superior anatomy may preclude visualization of the entire anteroposterior dimensions of the glottic opening, even with sufficient help, lighting, positioning, and preparation. In fact, the clinician may be able to visualize only the posterior one-third of that opening.

A rapidly available supply of endotracheal tubes in a wide range of sizes is needed to accommodate the size- and age-related differences of childhood. In most instances, ETTs without cuffs should be used in children younger than 7 or 8 years of age because the cricoid ring is small enough to produce an air seal. Controversy exists regarding the use of tubes with cuffs in children younger than 8 when a child has ingested a poison, because gastric lavage may potentially lead to aspiration. Theoretically, a cuff could provide better airway protection than an uncuffed tube. As with any cuffed ETT, cuff pressure must be monitored and maintained at 20 cm H_2O or less to minimize the risk of mucosal ischemia and necrosis. This complication can also be avoided by using an uncuffed tube small enough to allow a minimal leak audible on positive-pressure ventilation.

The appropriate-sized ETT can be found by using a table of approximate sizes. These tables, however, require an accurate age or weight estimation for access of appropriately sized equipment. Length has been shown to be the most accurate predictor of correct ETT size in children (13). The Broselow pediatric resuscitation tape (a length-based resuscitation tape) provides accurate equipment selection as well as resuscitation drug doses with a single length measurement. Two additional tubes should be available, one-half size smaller and one-half size larger. The child's small finger can serve as an approximation of his or her tracheal diameter, and an infant's length corresponds to the ETT size.

Because ETTs for children are short and easily dislodged from the trachea, one must be wary of tube movement and carefully secure the tube in position. Holding the tube and the corner of the mouth together until the tube is taped or otherwise held in position usually maintains this security. Once the ETT has passed between the vocal cords, proper position must be determined by auscultating the lung fields in both axillas. An endotracheal vapor cloud may be seen, and apparent breath sounds may be heard, even with esophageal intubation. The latter is especially common in small infants. The *sine qua non* of proper ETT placement is a patient whose vital signs improve, whose chest rises, and whose tissue perfusion improves and who exhibits end tidal carbon-dioxide exhalation. If the patient does not improve or if doubt exists, tube position may be checked by direct visualization using a laryngoscope. Alternate airway methods and personnel must be available for the difficult airway that cannot be ventilated or intubated.

Breathing

Once the airway is secured, attention should focus on breathing. The physiologic goals of oxygenation and ventilation require patency of airway and alveoli, normal alveolar capillary membranes, and matching of perfusion with ventilation. Patients with patent airways who require ventilatory support with bag-valve-mask devices must have the proper "bagging" technique employed to avoid complications.

Proper bag-valve-mask use demands a good mask–face seal with an appropriately sized mask and the use of a bag that allows the provider to supply the necessary tidal volume. The mask must fit over the nose and mouth without compressing the eyes (compression of the eyes may lead to vagal-induced bradycardia) and without extending beyond the chin. A properly sized mask minimizes artificial airway dead space. A self-inflating bag is most commonly used. Overventilation may lead to unilateral or bilateral pneumothoraces; underventilation will lead to carbon dioxide retention and respiratory acidosis.

Whether using a mask or ETT, the clinician should provide a tidal volume that causes the chest to rise. A pop-off valve, if present, allows for a preset maximum inspiratory pressure. Additional tidal volume can be delivered at higher pressures by holding a finger on the valve while delivering the breath with the self-expanding bag. Ideally, an in-line manometer should be used to monitor peak inspiratory pressure.

Resting tidal volume in children and adults is 5 to 7 mL/kg, while ventilatory supported tidal volume may be 10 to 15 mL/kg. Rather than calculating a value, attention should be paid to lung and chest wall compliance while bagging and the volume should be varied according to chest rise. Resuscitation bags for premature neonates should have a 250-mL capacity; 500-mL bags should be used for term newborns, infants, and small children. Adolescents require 750-mL bags.

Circulation

Adequacy of circulation is a clinical determination based on physical examination. The primary indication for assisting circulation with chest compressions is pulselessness. In neonates, chest compressions are also indicated when the heart rate remains below 60 beats/min, despite effective maneuvers to oxygenate and ventilate the patient, or when the heart rate is between 60 and 80 beats/min and not increasing.

Access to the vascular space of infants and small children is required when there is an immediate need to restore circulating blood volume or to infuse medications that can be given by no other route. The most common cause of cardiopulmonary failure in children older than 1 year of age is trauma; most of these children are large enough to allow for rapid intravenous cannulation. Nontraumatic arrests in children younger than 1 year old are most often secondary to respiratory failure. Consequently, appropriate airway management may preclude full arrest, and if cardiac arrest does ensue, the endotracheal cannula provides a route for administration of certain necessary medications.

The most common sites for intravenous cannulation are dorsal hand veins, superficial veins on the dorsum of the foot, antecubital veins of the forearm, superficial scalp veins, the external jugular veins, and the femoral vein in the inguinal canal. Once the airway is patent and maintained, any one or more of these sites

may be used. Standard cleansing and cannulation techniques should be used.

Both the external jugular vein and the femoral vein may provide passage to the central venous circulation through guidewire and long-line insertion. These procedures should not be first-line attempts; rather, short, reasonably large-bore cannulas should be placed first. When the patient is stable, these lines can be replaced under more controlled conditions.

An alternate site for access to the vascular space is the bone marrow. Infusion of blood, fluids, and medications into the circulation using the bone marrow has been done for over 50 years (11). Intraosseous (IO) cannulation can be accomplished using either the distal femur (proximal to the physis) or the proximal tibia (distal to the physis).

The bone marrow can be used to facilitate infusion of all resuscitation drugs and for volume resuscitation with fluids or blood (2). These sites are used in the patient in full cardiopulmonary arrest who needs intravenous medications when intravenous access is not obtainable within 90 to 120 seconds.

Disposable IO infusion needles are available in various sizes for infants and children and can be used in all age groups. Standard aseptic technique should be used. The IO needle can be removed once one or more intravenous catheters have been placed and are stabilized.

For most resuscitation medications, the intravenous doses are well recognized and standardized. For optimum action, these drugs should be given as close as possible to the heart. In the absence of specific pediatric recommendations, accepted intravenous dosage schedules should be used. Drugs given through the ETT should be delivered deep into the bronchial system for optimum mucosal absorption via a feeding tube (two to three times the dosage for lidocaine, atropine, and naloxone, and ten times the intravenous epinephrine dose). Drugs given through the bone marrow have dosages identical to the intravenous dosage and should be followed with a 2- to 5-mL saline flush to aid delivery to the central circulation. Some authorities also recommend a 2- to 5-mL saline flush after bolus intravenous medication administration.

Equipment selection, medication, and defibrillation dosing errors can be minimized by using standardized charts, forms, tables, and the Broselow pediatric resuscitation tape (Table 206.1). All information should be displayed in large type in an easy-to-read format and should be prominently located for reference during critical situations. The AHA publishes resuscitation algorithms and drug dosages in the *Handbook of Emergency Cardiovascular Care for Healthcare Providers and* pocket cards (Fig. 206.1). In 2001, the American College of Emergency Physicians and the American Academy of Pediatrics published joint policy statements regarding the care if children in the ED and guidelines for preparedness including equipment, medications, and staffing suggestions.

Resuscitation Medications

All of the drugs used during adult CPR can be used for children. For the most part, they function through the same molecular mechanisms. Thus, alpha- and beta-adrenergic receptors must be stimulated by exogenous agonists, as must the dopaminergic receptors. However, children may have fewer available receptors because of underlying maximal endogenous stimulation or incomplete development. The concerns after restoration of cardiovascular function include prolonged tachycardia and potential hypertension.

Oxygen, the mainstay of any resuscitation attempt, is the most important "drug" used during pediatric resuscitation. It has no contraindications, and airway management must be the first therapeutic modality instituted.

TABLE 206.1.   Length-Based Equipment Chart

Item	Length (cm)						
	54–70 (4–7 kg)	70–85 (8–11 kg)	85–95 (12–14 kg)	95–107 (14–17 kg)	107–124 (18–23 kg)	124–138 (24–30 kg)	138–155 (>30 kg)
ET tube size (mm)	3.5	4.0	4.5	5.0	5.5	6.0	6.5
Lip-tip length (mm)	10.5	12.0	13.5	15.0	16.5	18.0	19.5
Laryngoscope	1 straight	1 straight	2 straight	2 straight or curved	2 straight or curved	2–3 straight or curved	3 straight or curved
Suction catheter	8F	8F–10F	10F	10F	10F	10F	12F
Stylet	6F	6F	6F	6F	14F	14F	14F
Oral airway	Infant/small child	Small child	Child	Child	Child/small adult	Child/adult	Medium adult
Bag-valve-mask	Infant	Child	Child	Child	Child	Child/adult	Adult
Oxygen mask	Newborn	Pediatric	Pediatric	Pediatric	Pediatric	Adult	Adult
Vascular access catheter/butterfly	22–24/23–25, intraosseous	20–22/23–25, intraosseous	18–22/21–23, intraosseous	18–22/21–23, intraosseous	18–20/21–23	18–22/21–22	16–20/18–21
Nasogastric tube	5F–8F	8F–10F	10F	10F–12F	12F–14F	14F–18F	18F
Urinary catheter	5F–8F	8F–10F	10F	10F–12F	10F–12F	12F	12F
Chest tube	12F–12F	16F–20F	20F–24F	20F–24F	24F–32F	28F–32F	32F–40F
Blood pressure cuff	Newborn/infant	infant/child	Child	Child	Child	Child/adult	Adult

Directions
1. Measure patient length with centimeter tape.
2. Using measured length in centimeters, access appropriate equipment column.
Alternatively, this same information can be accessed from a single measurement directly from a Broselow tape.
Modified from Luten RC, Wears RL, Broselwo J, et al. Length-based endotracheal tube sizing for pediatric resuscitation. *Ann Emerg Med* 1995;21:900–904.

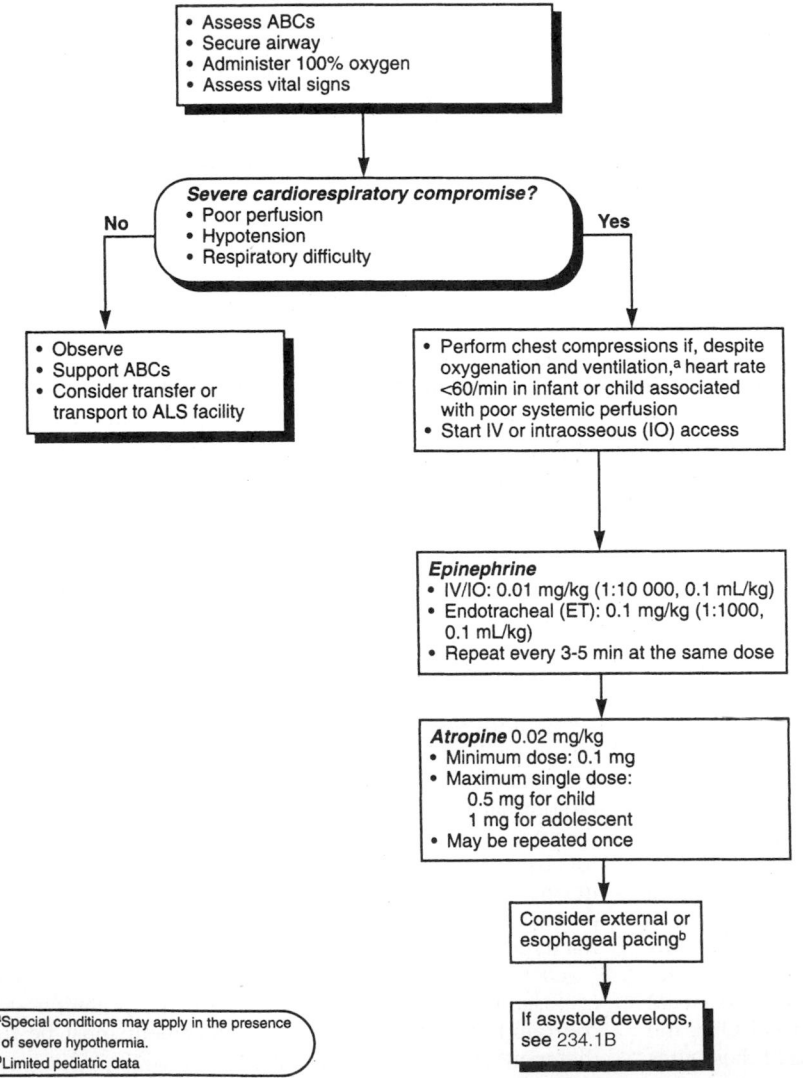

Figure 206.1. Treatment algorithms for pediatric advanced life support. (A) Bradycardia algorithm. *(Continued)*

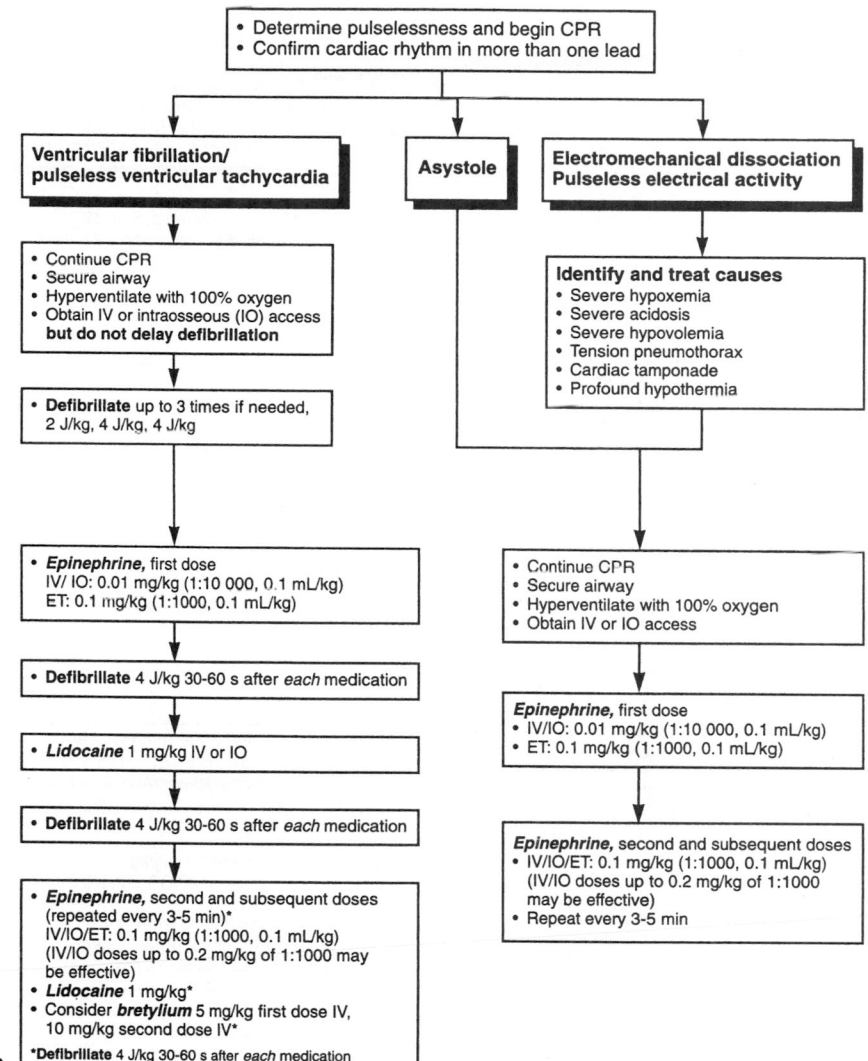

Figure 206.1. *(Continued)* **(B)** Asystole and pulseless arrest algorithm.

Fluids such as normal saline or Ringer lactate should be used in the hypotensive infant or child. The initial fluid bolus is 20 cc/kg, which may be repeated up to three times, depending on the clinical condition. Packed red blood cells are dosed at 10 cc/kg.

Epinephrine, with both alpha- and beta-receptor action, is a potent medication to help reverse cardiac collapse, treat lethal arrhythmias, treat symptomatic bradyarrhythmias, and treat hypotension not related to hypovolemia. The cardiac beta-receptor action may improve output when heart rate is slow. Thus, epinephrine is often used in neonates and young infants to accelerate heart rate.

The alpha-adrenergic receptor activity that predominates in the doses used for cardiopulmonary arrest has many effects. It increases coronary and cerebral perfusion pressures; increases intravascular resistance of the skin, muscles, and splanchnic vessels; prevents arterial collapse of intrathoracic arteries; increases heart rate, myocardial contractility, and cardiac automaticity; and increases myocardial oxygen demand. All neonatal dosages are 0.01 mg/kg. Higher doses are not used because of the increased incidence of intracranial bleeding in this age group.

The initial intravenous/IO dose of epinephrine for patients outside the neonatal range in pulseless arrest is 0.01 mg/kg (0.1 mL/kg) of the 1:10,000 solution. All endotracheal doses (2) are 0.1 mg (0.1 mL/kg) of the 1:1,000 solution for pulseless arrest. Note that intravenous epinephrine and endotracheal epinephrine doses have the same amount of milliliters; only the concentration of the drug changes. These doses may be administered every 3 to 5 minutes during arrest. There is no evidence-based literature to support the use of high-dose epinephrine. High-dose epinephrine may increase return of spontaneous circulation (ROSC) but it does not improve survival to hospital discharge (6,9). In addition to increasing myocardial oxygen demand, epinephrine postresuscitation may cause prolonged hypertension and tachycardia after ROSC. Therefore, although high dose epinephrine may be used for subsequent intravenous doses, it is not routinely recommended. For bradycardia, epinephrine may be given intravenously or IO at 0.01 mg/kg of the 1:10,000 solution, or 0.1 mg/kg of the 1:1,000 solution per ETT.

Atropine is a parasympatholytic drug used in cardiorespiratory arrest. It accelerates sinus and atrial pacemakers, reduces cardiac vagal tone, and increases atrioventricular conduction. Atropine increases heart rate and therefore improves cardiac output. In children, an improvement in cardiac output generally relies much more on heart rate than on an increase in stroke volume. Atropine is indicated for symptomatic bradycardia after oxygenation–ventilation and epinephrine have been given. It also attenuates vagolytic effects of infants and children during intubation.

The recommended dose of atropine is 0.02 mg/kg, with a minimum dose of 0.1 mg and a maximum single dose for a child of 0.5 mg and for an adolescent of 1.0 mg. The initial dose may

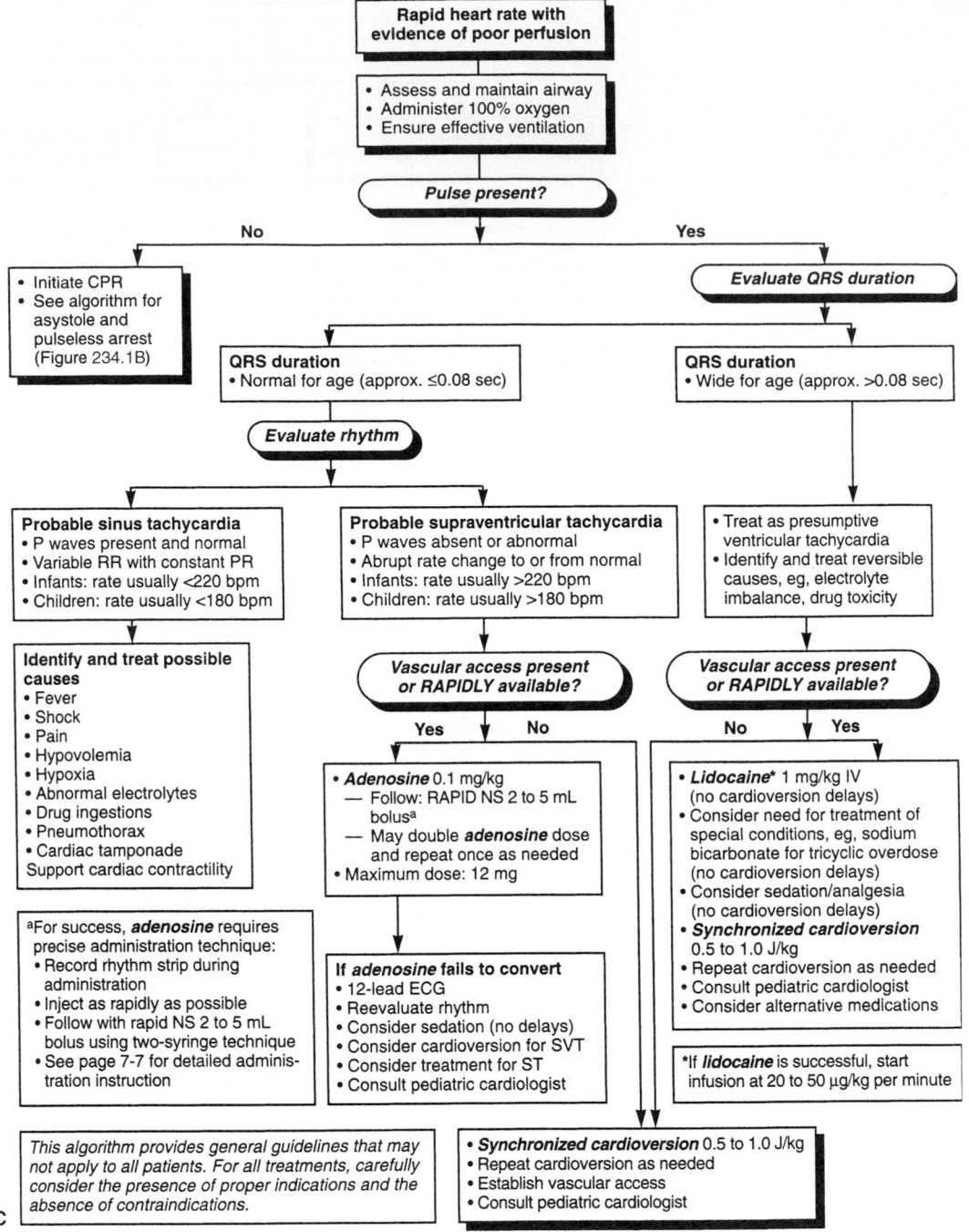

Figure 206.1. *(Continued)* **(C)** Tachycardia with poor perfusion algorithm. (From American Heart Association. *Textbook of pediatric advanced life support.* Dallas: American Heart Association, 2002, with permission.)

be repeated once. The total of the two doses should not exceed 1.0 mg for the child or 2.0 mg for the adolescent. The endotracheal dosage of atropine is unknown but is generally given at higher than the intravenous dose (2 to 3 times the intravenous dose). Side effects of atropine include paradoxical bradycardia and tachycardia, and increased myocardial oxygen demand.

Glucose is a medication uncommonly used during adult cardiorespiratory arrest. In infants and small children, the small reserve of endogenous glucose in the form of hepatic glycogen is readily exhausted during stress. Rapid bedside glucose testing, with easily usable equipment that provides accurate results, is mandatory in any location that resuscitation of a child may occur. Serum glucose and its anaerobic end product lactate can be monitored during the resuscitation process. If needed, glucose can be given intravenously or intraosseously in a dose of 2 to 4 mL/kg of 25% dextrose in water. Because dextrose concentrations over 12.5% may cause loss of integrity of small peripheral veins, it should be given in as large a vein as possible. The 10% solution should be used in neonates.

Naloxone is a narcotic antagonist and is used for potential narcotic overdose. The dosage is 0.1 mg/kg up to 20 kg, and 2 mg for anyone over 20 kg. There are no adverse side effects, but it does have a short half-life. It needs to be monitored, especially if the child has taken a long-acting narcotic.

Recommended indications for *calcium* are calcium-channel blocker toxicity, hypocalcemia, hyperkalemia, and hypermagnesemia. If given, calcium chloride should be used in a dose of 20 mg/kg (0.2 mL/kg). The recommended calcium solution is calcium chloride. Magnesium in a dose of 25 to 50 mg/kg (maximum 2 grams) may be used for hypomagnesemia or torsades de pointes.

Respiratory and lactic acidosis are secondary to hypoventilation and hypoperfusion. Correction of acidemia is primarily by ventilation–oxygenation and restoration of circulation. *Sodium bicarbonate* is indicated for acidemia after a prolonged arrest when adequate ventilation–oxygen and cardiac compressions are being performed. During CPR, sodium bicarbonate should be given intravenously or intraosseously. The dose of sodium bicarbonate is 1 mEq/kg of the 8.4% solution. In the neonate, the dose is the same, but the solution should be 4.2%. The 8.4% solution can be converted to 4.2% by diluting it 1:1 with sterile water (not sterile saline). Side effects include hypernatremia, hyperosmolarity, alkalemia, and paradoxical cerebrospinal fluid and intracellular acidosis.

Dopamine is used to enhance urine output and treat hypotension not related to hypovolemia. Renal dosages are 2 to 5 µg/kg/min; beta-adrenergic effects, 2 to 10 µg/kg/min; and alpha-adrenergic effects, 15 to 20 µg/kg/min.

Lidocaine is used in ventricular tachycardia (VT) and ventricular fibrillation (VF) or symptomatic ventricular arrhythmias. The initial dosage is a 1-mg/kg bolus, followed by a 20- to 50-µg/kg/min drip.

Amiodarone may be used for ventricular tachycardia without a pulse and ventricular fibrillation and should be administered as a 5 mg/kg bolus. It can also be used for ventricular tachycardia with a pulse and supraventricular tachycardia and is administered as 5 mg/kg for 20 to 60 minutes.

Procainamide may also be used for ventricular tachycardia with a pulse. The dose is 15 mg/kg given for 30 to 60 minutes. Amiodarone and procainamide should not be routinely administered together.

Electrical Treatment of Rhythm Disturbances

Electrical dysfunction of cardiac muscle in childhood is most often secondary to respiratory failure and/or congenital heart disease. The most common rhythm disturbance after asystole is sinus bradycardia. It will respond to adequate ventilation and oxygenation, if provided early enough, and rarely requires medication. Sinus tachycardia is also seen and may present as the earliest sign of impending cardiopulmonary arrest. Both of these rhythms must be interpreted in light of possible causes, and the underlying cause should be treated. The ventricular dysrhythmias in pediatrics are more difficult to treat, because children have a prolonged compensatory stage and therefore are much more acidotic and hypoxic than an adult who has a sudden collapse secondary to a ventricular dysrhythmia. Electricity is the immediate treatment for pulseless VT or VF.

Electrical conversion energy levels for supraventricular tachycardia are 0.25 to 1.0 J/kg, while delivered energy for VF or pulseless VT starts at 2 J/kg. Figure 206.1 illustrates current treatment algorithms for potentially lethal dysrhythmias.

When electricity is being used to convert an unstable rhythm, appropriate-sized paddles must be placed in an appropriate position. The recommended paddle size for small children (less than 10 kg) is 4.5 cm in diameter, and up to 8 cm in diameter in larger children and adolescents. If only large paddles are available, they should be placed in the anteroposterior position. Regardless of position, a proper conducting medium must be used with full paddle contact on the chest wall.

Automatic external defibrillators are being used more commonly and may be effective in children as young as 1 year of age (15). Their use is not recommended in infants due to the potential for myocardial damage.

Paying attention to the underlying ionic, metabolic, or mechanical causes of the unstable rhythm in a child is the mainstay of therapy. The child should be assessed for hypothermia or hyperthermia, hypoglycemia or hyperglycemia, and alterations in oxygen, potassium, calcium, sodium, and magnesium. Acid–base alterations must be corrected. Mechanical causes of pulseless electrical activity (PEA), such as hypovolemia due to dehydration, cardiac tamponade, tension pneumothorax, and ETT obstruction or misplacement should be rapidly addressed.

Implementing Resuscitation Principles

Successful resuscitation requires applying the principles of resuscitation, practicing psychomotor skills, and using proper equipment and drugs. One barrier to optimal results can be the difficulties caused by variations in the size of pediatric patients: It is not uncommon for valuable resuscitation time to be lost calculating drug doses or selecting appropriately sized equipment. This is compounded by the provider's anxiety and the potential for error inherent in this process (12). In adults, this problem is virtually nonexistent, because size variations and, therefore, drug and equipment needs do not change significantly from one patient to another. See Table 206.2 for a list of recommended ED equipment and supplies (3,8).

A system based on length has been introduced. The Broselow pediatric resuscitation tape relates the patient's length to his or her weight and, therefore, to the appropriate drug dosage and also to appropriate equipment sizes. The tape provides immediate access to the correct drug dosage, as well as equipment selection, based on a single measurement. It is not enough to have the knowledge and the skills to resuscitate; any barriers to implementation of that knowledge must also be eliminated. Appropriate personnel, training, equipment and medications, and preparedness are the keys to a successful resuscitation. ED nursing and physician staff should be trained in Pediatric Advanced Life Support and aware of national pediatric emergency resource materials and policies. (3,7,10).

Postresuscitation Stabilization

Avoiding secondary injury and frequent assessment of the ABCs, neurologic status, urine output, fluid administration, monitors, laboratory results, and vital signs are mandatory for successful postresuscitation stabilization. Sedation and pain management must also be appropriately addressed and monitored. Family members and friends must be continuously updated on the status of the patient.

Outcome Predictors

Respiratory arrests without cardiac arrests have a much higher survival rate. Patients in whom return of spontaneous circulation has occurred with less than 5 minutes of CPR and with fewer than two doses of epinephrine (vs. multiple doses) have a better chance of survival. Those patients who arrested because of VF and are treated rapidly have better outcomes than all other causes of cardiopulmonary arrest. Patients who arrest secondary to sepsis have the lowest rate of survival. Those patients who arrest and have a family member begin CPR have higher survival rates than patients who do not get immediate CPR (16).

Family Presence in Pediatric Resuscitation

Parent surveys have indicated that most parents find being at their child's bedside during a code helps them begin the grieving

TABLE 206.2. Guidelines for Minimum Equipment and Supplies for Care of Pediatric Patients in Emergency Departments

MONITORING

Cardiorespiratory monitor with strip recorder
Defibrillator (0- to 400-J capability) with pediatric and adult paddles (4.5 cm and 8.0 cm)
Pediatric and adult monitor electrodes
Pulse oximeter with sensor sizes for newborn through adult
Thermometer/rectal probe[a]
Sphygmomanometer
Doppler blood pressure device
Blood pressure cuffs (neonatal, infant, child, adult, and thigh sizes)
Method to monitor endotracheal tube and placement[b]

VASCULAR ACCESS

Butterfly needles (19- to 25-gauge)
Catheter-over-needle devices (14- to 24-gauge)
Infusion device[c]
Tubing for the above
Intraosseous needles (16- and 18-gauge)[d]
Arm boards (infant, child, and adult sizes)
Intravenous fluid/blood warmers
Umbilical vein catheters (sizes 3.5F and 5F)[e]
Seldinger technique vascular access kit (with pediatric sizes 3F, 4F, 5F catheters)

AIRWAY MANAGEMENT

Clear oxygen masks (preterm, infant, child, and adult sizes)
Nonrebreather masks (infant, child, and adult sizes)
Oral airways (sizes 00–5)
Nasopharyngeal airways (12F–30F)
Bag-valve-mask resuscitator, self-inflating (450- and 1,000-mL sizes)
Nasal cannulae (infant, child, and adult sizes)
Endotracheal tubes: uncuffed (sizes 2.5 to 8.5) and cuffed (sizes 5.5 to 9.0)
Stylets (pediatric and adult)
Laryngoscope handle (pediatric and adult)
Laryngoscope blades, curved (sizes 2 and 3) and straight (sizes 0 to 3)
Magill forceps (pediatric and adult)
Nasogastric tubes (sizes 6F–14F)
Suction catheters: flexible (sizes 5F–16F) and Yankauer suction tip
Chest tubes (sizes 8F–40F)
Tracheotomy tubes (sizes 00 to 6)[f]

[a] Suitable for hypothermic and hyperthermic measurements with temperature capability from 25°C to 44°C.
[b] May be satisfied by a disposable $ETCO_2$ detector, bulb, or feeding tube methods for endotracheal tube placement.
[c] To regulate rate and volume.
[d] May be satisfied by standard bone marrow aspiration needles, 13- or 15-gauge.
[e] Available within the hospital.
[f] Ensure availability of pediatric sizes within the hospital.
(From the Committee on Pediatric Equipment and Supplies for Emergency Departments, National Emergency Medical Service for Children Resource Alliance. Guidelines for pediatric equipment and supplies for emergency departments. Ann Emerg Med 1998;31:56.)

process if the resuscitation is unsuccessful. Prewritten protocols and a healthcare professional who can be with the family and answer questions as the code proceeds are a must for successful implementation (1). These healthcare providers can help explain procedures and recognize potential problems parents may encounter during the resuscitative effort.

Terminating an Unsuccessful Cardiopulmonary Arrest and Informing the Parents

Patients in cardiopulmonary arrests continuing longer than 30 minutes, unless they are hypothermic, have very little chance of survival. Informing the parents of a child's death is a skill in which very few physicians have any formal training. Most training focuses on interactions with the dying patient, not the bereaved family. Some general guidelines include telling both parents together, knowing the name of the deceased, telling the parents their child has *died* (not that their child is *dead*), looking professional, preparing the patient before the family enters the room, having counselors available, having a private grieving room, and making sure the staff has an adequate debriefing (12). (See Chapter 270, "Dealing with Death for Catastrophic Illness in children.")

PEDIATRIC RESUSCITATION PEARLS AND CRITICAL INTERVENTIONS

Preparation and competent personnel are mandatory to adequately resuscitate children. Team approaches, with clear identification of individual roles, helps to prevent confusion and potential chaos during a pediatric code. Resuscitation rooms in the ED, which are designed to facilitate pediatric resuscitations, help lower the stress of a very stressful situation. They have the appropriate equipment, medications, and room to facilitate the resuscitative efforts. Carts, which are color coded by length, have helped decrease medication errors during these resuscitative efforts.

Neonatal patients are usually not given atropine for bradycardia. The second dose of epinephrine for neonates in VF or pulseless VT is not increased as it is with all other VF and pulseless VT arrests. If the neonatal patient requires sodium bicarbonate, it is given at half strength. The umbilical vein is an excellent vascular access site in neonates. Suction pressure should not exceed 100 mm Hg in neonates and should not last greater than 2 to 3 seconds in any pediatric patient.

All medications given by intravenous, IO, or ETT routes should be followed by a small normal saline bolus. All children in cardiopulmonary arrest should have their glucose immediately checked. A bedside warmer should be used during all pediatric resuscitations. Pediatric patients should be kept in a slight Trendelenburg position during resuscitation efforts, to help prevent aspiration. Airway equipment and alternative airway equipment must be checked every shift to make sure it is always in working condition. The most important medication for any pediatric patient is oxygen.

Appropriate airway management and ventilation of an arrested child can be the difference between a successful and an unsuccessful resuscitation. The rhythm strip should be carefully examined in any pediatric arrest. Cardiopulmonary arrest secondary to sepsis has a very high mortality rate. Always consider child abuse or neglect if there are any inconsistencies in the caregivers' history or the physician's physical examination. Finally, be prepared to help a family begin their grieving process if the resuscitative efforts are unsuccessful.

COMMON PITFALLS

✔ Failure to have an organized system for stocking appropriate pediatric equipment and supplies
✔ Failure to perform routine mock codes and assessments of pediatric preparedness in the ED
✔ Failure to understand anatomic and physiologic differences between pediatric and adult airway management
✔ Failure to provide advance preparation and staff education for emergency neonatal resuscitation, equipment and medications.

Acknowledgment

Thanks to the previous edition's chapter author Neena Gupta.

References

1. Adams S, Whitlock M, Baskett PJF, et al. Should relatives be allowed to watch resuscitation? *BMJ* 1994;308:1687.
2. American Academy of Pediatrics: Committee on Drugs. Alternative routes of drug administration: advantages and disadvantages (subject review). *Pediatrics* 1997;100:143.
3. American College of Emergency Physicians and American Academy of Pediatrics. Care of children in the emergency department: guidelines for preparedness. *Ann Emerg Med* 2001;37:423–427.
4. American College of Emergency Physicians and American Academy of Pediatrics. APLS: The pediatric emergency resource, 4th ed. Jones and Bartlett, 2003.
5. Appleton GO, Cummins RO, Larson MP, et al. CPR and the single rescuer: at what ages should you "call first" rather than "call fast?" *Ann Emerg Med* 1995;25:492.
6. Carpenter TC, Stenmark KR. High-dose epinephrine is not superior to standard-dose epinephrine in pediatric in-hospital cardiopulmonary arrest. *Pediatrics* 1997;99:403.
7. Pediatric airway management. In: Chameides L, Hazinski MF (eds). *Textbook of pediatric advanced life support*. Dallas: American Heart Association, 2002.
8. Committee on Pediatric Equipment and Supplies for the Emergency Department, National Emergency Medical Service for Children Resource Alliance. Guidelines for pediatric equipment and supplies for emergency departments. *Ann Emerg Med* 1998;31:54–57.
9. Dieckmann RA, Vardis R. High-dose epinephrine in pediatric out-of-hospital cardiopulmonary arrest. *Pediatrics* 1995;95:901.
10. Gausche M (ed). The pediatric emergency medicine course: instructor manual, 3rd ed. Dallas: American College of Emergency Physicians and Elk Grove Village, IL: American Academy of Pediatrics, 1998.
11. Hodge D. Intraosseous infusions: a review. *Pediatr Emerg Care* 1985;1:215.
12. Knazik S, Gausche-Hill M, Dietrich A, et al. The death of a child in the emergency department. *Ann Emerg Med* 2003;42:519–529.
13. Luten RC, Wears RL, Broselow J, et al. Length-based endotracheal tube sizing for pediatric resuscitation. *Ann Emerg Med* 1992;21:900.
14. Oakley P. Inaccuracy and delay in decision making in pediatric resuscitation and a proposed reference chart to reduce errors. *BMJ* 1988;297:817.
15. Samson R, Berg R, Bingham R. Use of external defibrillators for children: an update-an advisory statement from the pediatric advanced life support task force, international liaison committee on resuscitation. *Pediatrics* 2003;112:163–168.
16. Sirbaugh PE, Pepe PE, Shook JE, et al. A prospective population-based study of the demographics, epidemiology, management, and outcome of out-of-hospital pediatric cardiopulmonary arrest. *Ann Emerg Med* 1993;33:174.
17. Young KD, Seidel JS. Pediatric cardiopulmonary resuscitation: a collective review. *Ann Emerg Med* 1999;33:195.

CHAPTER 207
Rapid-Sequence Induction

Robert C. Luten and Stephen Andy Godwin

All patients requiring emergent intubation must be assumed to have a full stomach, as they are at risk for aspiration, and intubation must be done with all precautions taken to prevent this complication. Also, manipulating the airway can cause hemodynamic changes, including increases in intracranial pressure (ICP), which, in the head-injured patient, may lead to further central nervous system insult. Using rapid-sequence induction (RSI) with the aid of potent induction agents, muscle relaxants, and cricoid pressure to prevent passive regurgitation, patients can be quickly rendered fully unconscious, facilitating intubation and preventing the side effects of airway manipulation, es-

pecially iatrogenic ICP increases. The exposure time to the risk of aspiration can also be reduced. RSI helps facilitate endotracheal intubation in the combative or seizing patient, or in other patients in whom inadequate muscle relaxation prevents endotracheal intubation (3,4,5,10,12,15,16).

The procedure of RSI in children varies little from the adult procedure. Tables 207.1 and 207.2 respectively outline some of the key physiologic and anatomic differences which must be accommodated when managing the child's airway (8). Additionally, because children vary so much in size, logistical issues are introduced which must be also be addressed. These issues mainly relate to performance of calculations, many times under the stress of an acute crisis. Examples of the variables are presented in Table 207.3. The solution to reducing these logistical problems is the use of reference/resuscitation aids that precalculate or select these variables according to different sizes (7).

The decision to employ the technique of RSI for emergent intubation should be based on a structured assessment of patient stability and the perceived difficulty of obtaining successful endotracheal intubation with the standard oral laryngoscopic technique. Figure 207.1 demonstrates the Universal Emergency Airway Algorithm adapted from the *National Emergency Airway Management Course* (14). Defined plans or algorithms for crash, difficult, and failed airways must be part of the armamentarium of any practitioner who utilizes RSI, and patients must be selected accordingly.

Details of this process are beyond the scope of this chapter, but are discussed in "Airway Management" (adult), Chapter 1. Proper implementations of these principles are critical to ensuring a safe and efficient RSI process.

The steps of RSI are:

- 1. Preparation
- 2. Preoxygenation
- 3. Premedication
- 4. Induction and paralysis
- 5. Cricoid pressure
- 6. Intubation

Figure 207.2 presents a timed flowchart of the procedure. Tables 207.4 to 207.7 outline the medications used in the scheme.

PREPARATION

Without adequate preparation, no amount of skill or expertise can ensure successful intubation. Lack of preparation also increases the likelihood of complications. *Advance preparation* includes equipment, medications, and team function, education, and orientation. *Immediate preparation* includes selecting appropriate equipment, selecting and preparing appropriate medications, and assigning team roles.

Advance Preparation

Table 207.8 lists the equipment needed to perform RSI in children. Most pediatric equipment is age- or size-appropriate. Because the child's age and weight are usually not known in emergencies, using a length-based measurement such as the Broselow pediatric emergency tape allows for correct selection of equipment and drug dosages.

Adequate training for team participants is critical. Physicians must be skilled in advanced airway management and RSI, and nursing personnel also need practice with the mechanics of the procedure (e.g., cricoid pressure and the logistics of medication preparation). The Advanced Pediatric Life Support and Pediatric Advanced Life Support courses include chapters and skill stations on RSI, and there are now several national advanced airway

TABLE 207.1.   Anatomic Differences Between Adults and Children

Anatomy	Clinical Significance
Large intraoral tongue occupying relatively large portion of the oral cavity	High anterior airway position of the glottic opening compared with that in adults
High tracheal opening: C-1 in infancy versus C-3 to C-4 at age 7, C-4 to C-5 in the adult	Straight blade preferred over curved to push distensible anatomy out of the way to visualize the larynx
Large occiput that may cause flexion of the airway, large tongue that easily collapses against the posterior pharynx	Sniffing position is preferred. The larger occiput actually elevates the head into the sniffing position in most infants and children. A towel may be required under shoulders to elevate torso relative to head in small infants
Cricoid ring is the narrowest portion of the trachea as compared with the vocal cords in the adult	Uncuffed tubes provide adequate seal as they fit snugly at the level of the cricoid ring. Correct tube size essential because variable expansion cuffed tubes not used
Consistent anatomic variations with age with fewer abnormal variations related to body habitus, arthritis, chronic disease	< 2 years, high anterior 2 to 8, transition > 8, small adult
Large tonsils and adenoids may bleed. More acute angle between epiglottis and laryngeal opening results in nasotracheal intubation attempt failures.	Blind nasotracheal intubation not indicated in children. Nasotracheal intubation failure
Small cricothyroid membrane	Needle cricothyrotomy difficult, surgical cricothyrotomy impossible in infants and small children

(Adapted from Luten, R, Approach to the pediatric airway. In: The Manual of Emergency Airway Management, 2nd ed. Walls R, Murphy M, Luten R, Schneider R (eds). Lippincott Williams & Wilkins, Philadelphia. p. 218 , Box 19–1, 2004, with permission.)

courses available for training (1,14). Mock codes and practice sessions help prepare the team and ensure that resources are available.

Immediate Preparation

Early, prehospital length measurement permits timely equipment selection and drug dosage preparation. Team roles (e.g., leader, cricoid pressure designee) are immediately assigned, and the timing of the procedure is monitored by the team leader.

PREOXYGENATION

During RSI, the patient sustains a variable period of complete apnea. To prevent hypoxia by extending the time of adequately saturated blood, the patient must be preoxygenated. The purpose of preoxygenation is to produce nitrogen washout by having the patient breathe 100% oxygen, creating an oxygen reservoir.

In the patient who is spontaneously breathing, 2 to 5 minutes of 100% oxygen delivery by a nonrebreather mask should allow 2 to 4 minutes of apnea without hypoxia. In the apneic

or inadequately ventilated patient, preoxygenation with a bag-valve-mask for 1 to 2 minutes should produce the same result. Cricoid pressure is applied during bag-valve-mask ventilation to prevent gastric insufflation.

PREMEDICATION

Certain medications used as adjuncts to RSI are given before the muscle relaxant (Table 207.4). *Lidocaine* 1.5 mg/kg is of benefit in lowering ICP. *Atropine* 0.02 mg/kg pf dries secretions and prevents reflex vagal tone and bradycardia due to airway manipulation and succinylcholine administration. Atropine is recommended for all children younger than 5 years or 20 kg, and any child receiving succinylcholine as the muscle relaxant. An alternative is to give atropine as a premedication to all children, regardless of age or paralyzing agent used. It is a relatively benign drug and can help maintain heart rate—and therefore perfusion—in the face of potential hypoxia- or drug-induced bradycardia and also eliminates another decision, reducing the complexity of an already complex process.

If succinylcholine is used as a muscle relaxant, a pretreatment dose of a nondepolarizing agent is given to prevent muscle fasciculations and ICP elevations secondary to the succinylcholine. For children less than 5 years old or 20 kg (less muscle mass than older children and adolescents), this additional step seems unnecessary. The reality is that this recommendation is only theoretical as there are no studies documenting the effectiveness of the nondepolarizing agent in children as there are in adults. For

---

TABLE 207.2.   Physiologic Differences

Physiologic difference	Significance
Basal O_2 consumption is twice for equivalent adult values (> 6mL/kg/min).	Shortened period of protection from hypoxia adult preoxygenation time as compared with adults. Infants and small children often require BMV while maintaining cricoid pressure to avoid hypoxia.
Proportionally small FRC as compared with adults.	

(Adapted from Luten, R. Approach to the pediatric airway. In: The manual of emergency airway management, 2nd ed. Walls R, Murphy M, Luten R, Schneider R (eds). Lippincott Williams & Wilkins, Philadelphia. p. 219, Box 19–2, 2004, with permission.)

TABLE 207.3.   Sources of Logistical Issues Particular to Pediatric Airway Management

1. Weight estimation
2. Equipment selection
3. Recall/referencing doses
4. Calculation of doses
5. Calculation of drug volumes
6. Calculation of fluid volumes
7. Calculation of ventilatory volumes

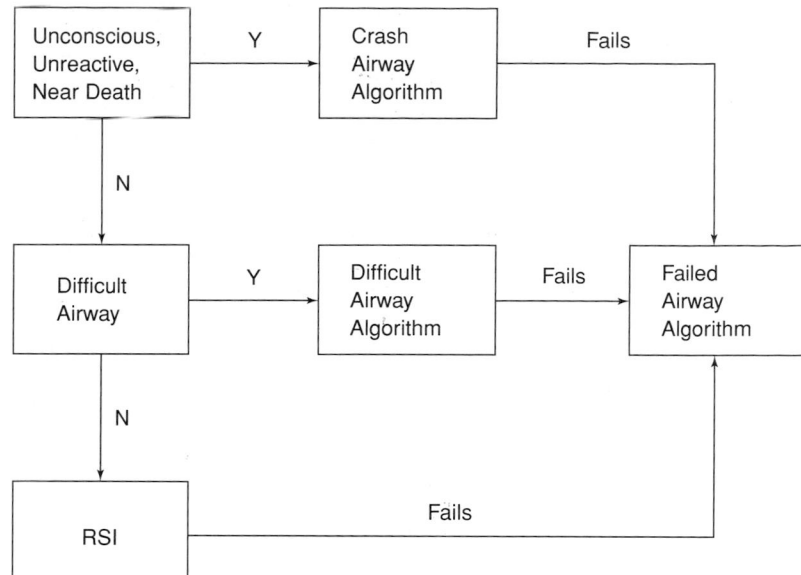

Figure 207.1.   The Universal Emergency Airway Algorithm, adapted from the *National emergency airway management course.*

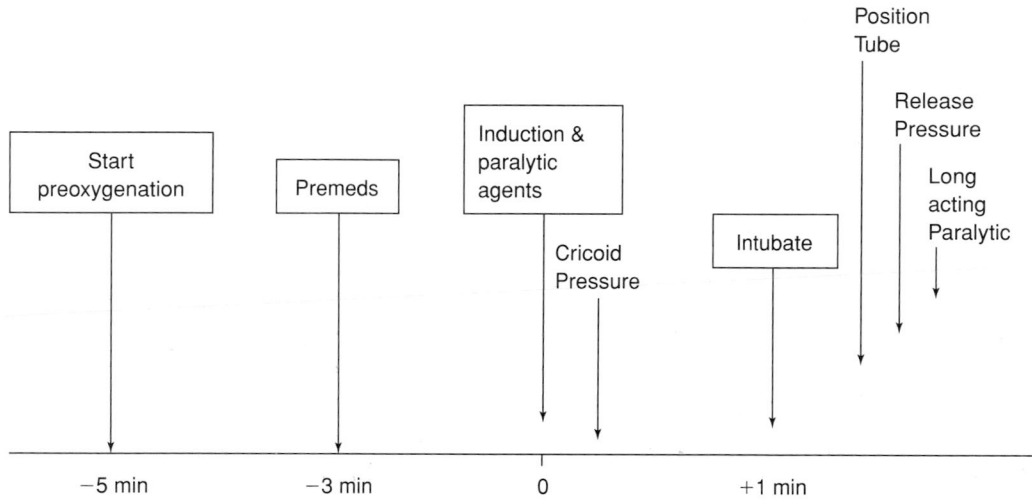

Figure 207.2.   Rapid-sequence induction. This chart reflects details of timed activity of the procedure in the stable patient. All time intervals may be abbreviated by the clinician, if deemed necessary, because of less than optimal or deteriorating clinical status.

TABLE 207.4.   Common Premedications in Rapid-Sequence Induction

Drug	Dose (i.v.)	Action
Lidocaine	1.5 mg/kg	Lowers ICP
Atropine	0.02 mg/kg	Prevents bradycardia associated with airway manipulation and succinylcholine
Pancuronium/ vecuronium (defasciculating dose)	0.02 mg/kg	Prevents fasciculations and ICP elevations from succinylcholine in patients >5 years of age
Fentanyl (optional)	1–3 μg/kg	Attenuates sympathetic discharge and resultant elevations in ICP. Use with caution. May cause respiratory depression or blunt compensatory sympathetic tone

TABLE 207.5.   Common Agents for Induction of Unconsciousness in RSI

Drug	Dose (i.v.)	Onset	Duration
Thiopental	3–5 mg/kg	10–30 s	10–30 min
Ketamine	1–2 mg/kg	1–2 min	15–30 min
Midazolam	0.2 mg/kg (maximum 5 mg)	1–2 min	30–60 min
Etomidate	0.2–0.4 mg/kg	1 min	30–60 min
Propofol	1.0–2.0 mg/kg	30–60 s	10–15 min

TABLE 207.6.   Medications Required
for Rapid-Sequence Induction

PREMEDICATIONS

Atropine
Lidocaine
Defasciculating agent

SEDATION

Ketamine
Thiopental
Midazolam
Propofol
Etomidate

MUSCLE RELAXANTS

Succinylcholine
Vecuronium
Pancuronium
Rocuronium

TABLE 207.8.   Equipment Required
for Rapid-Sequence Induction

Oxygen source
Bag-valve masks
Face masks (100% nonrebreather)
Oral airways
Laryngoscope handles
Laryngoscope blades
Suction system
Endotracheal tubes
Stylet
Cardiac monitor
Pulse oximeter
Cricothyroidotomy supplies
End-tidal CO_2 detector

the sake of simplicity it appears reasonable to reserve defasciculation premedications for adults and adolescents. All premedications may be given 3 minutes prior to the administration of the induction and paralytic agent.

SEDATION/INDUCTION

The choice of induction agent depends on two variables: clinical condition and perfusion status. Advantages and disadvantages of the commonly used sedatives are listed in Tables 207.5 and 207.6 gives examples of the use of thiopental, midazolam, and ketamine, based on the child's perfusion status and clinical condition (9). Other agents frequently used include propofol, etomidate, and diazepam, and all have advantages and disadvantages (2,4).

Of the agents mentioned, etomidate is an agent that can be used in almost any clinical situation, and it has one of the best cardiovascular profiles. It is the agent of choice in RSI for many emergency department (ED) physicians.

CRICOID PRESSURE: THE SELLICK MANEUVER

The Sellick maneuver consists of digital cricoid pressure to occlude the esophagus and prevent passive regurgitation. The anatomic structure of the cricoid cartilage—a complete

ring—prevents collapse of the airway while occluding the esophagus. If the patient vomits, cricoid pressure is immediately released to avoid esophageal rupture. Pressure is initiated as soon as the patient becomes sedated and is not released until the position of the endotracheal tube is verified. Cricoid pressure is always applied when using a bag-valve-mask to ventilate an apneic patient.

PARALYSIS

Paralytic agents are used to provide total muscle relaxation for optimal intubating conditions. There are two categories of muscle relaxants: the depolarizing agents (succinylcholine is the principal agent) and nondepolarizing agents (e.g., vecuronium, pancuronium, atracurium, and the newer, shorter-acting agent rocuronium). See Table 207.7. The ideal agent acts quickly, thereby reducing the time to intubation. It should have a short duration of action, because if the patient cannot be intubated, he or she will require bag-valve-mask ventilation until the paralysis wears off. The agent should have minimal side effects (4,6,11).

The ideal drug for RSI is succinylcholine. Although it has many side effects, in the acute situation, they are rarely of practical concern. Pretreatment with a defasciculating dose of a nondepolarizing agent prevents rises in ICP. As noted, this is necessary only in adolescents and adults. Atropine pretreatment prevents the bradycardia associated with succinylcholine; such bradycardia is especially common if a second dose of succinylcholine is needed to achieve or prolong paralysis.

Nondepolarizing agents such as vecuronium or rocuronium can also be used as the paralyzing agent and require no pretreatment with defasciculating doses (13). However, the time to intubation is prolonged with the nondepolarizing agents. They also

TABLE 207.7.   Common Agents for Muscle Relaxation in RSI

Drug	Dose (i.v.)	Onset	Duration
Succinylcholine	1.0–1.5 mg/kg (>10kg)	30–60 s	4–10 min
	1.5–2.0 mg/kg (<10kg)		
Vecuronium	0.2–0.25 mg/kg (RSI)	60–90 s	90 min
	0.1 mg/kg (standard dose)	2–3 min	25–40 min
	0.01 mg/kg (defasciculating dose)		
Pancuronium	0.1 mg/kg	2–5 min	45–90 min
	0.01 mg/kg (defasciculating dose)		
Rocuronium	1.0–1.2 mg/kg	30–60 s	25–60 min

have a longer duration of action (11). Newer nondepolarizing agents, such as rocuronium, offer the advantage of short onset of action without the potential side effects of succinylcholine or the need for a defasciculating dose for the older child.

INTUBATION

The intubation procedure during RSI is no different from the procedure in other situations. Patience is needed to await complete paralysis (approximately 45 seconds). A stylet is recommended for better control of the endotracheal tube. Tube position should be verified by auscultating the chest and colorimetric CO_2 detection before releasing cricoid pressure. After succinylcholine administration, a nondepolarizing agent should be given to continue paralysis.

Table 207.7 summarizes the medications used in the pediatric patient undergoing RSI. The scheme is one approach only and can be modified using alternative induction agents and paralytics if preferred.

CRITICAL INTERVENTIONS

- Have a system in place for RSI that includes all participants (i.e., medical specialists and nursing personnel) and addresses medications, equipment, failed airway, education and mock training exercises
- Select premedications, sedative and paralytic agents on an individual patient basis taking history, age and physiologic status into consideration

COMMON PITFALLS

✔ Lack of preparation of equipment and drugs before initiating the procedure
✔ Failing to preoxygenate
✔ Using bag-valve-mask ventilation in the spontaneously breathing patient
✔ Failing to perform the Sellick maneuver; failing to relax cricoid pressure if active regurgitation occurs
✔ Attempting intubation before muscle relaxation
✔ Failing to secure the endotracheal tube adequately after intubation
✔ Failing to preceed succinylcholine with atropine for *all* pediatric patients
✔ Confusing a defasciculating dose with a paralyzing dose of a nondepolarizing agent before using succinylcholine
✔ Failing to follow succinylcholine with a nondepolarizing agent in patients requiring prolonged mechanical ventilation
✔ Failing to verify endotracheal tube position both clinically and with an end-tidal CO_2 detector

Acknowledgment

Thanks to the previous edition's chapter author Phyllis Hendry.

References

1. American College of Emergency Physicians, American Academy of Pediatrics. *APLS: the pediatric emergency medicine resource.* Jones and Bartlett Publishers. 2004:153–180.
2. Bergen JM, Smith DC. A review of etomidate for rapid sequence intubation in the emergency department. *J Emerg Med* 1997;15:221.
3. Berry FA, Yemen TA. Pediatric airway in health and disease. *Pediatr Clin North Am* 1994;41:153.
4. Gerardi MJ, Sacchetti AD, Cantor RM, et al. Rapid sequence intubation of the pediatric patient. *Ann Emerg Med* 1996;28:55.
5. Gnauck K, Lungo JB, Scalzo A, et al. Emergency intubation of the pediatric medical patient: use of anesthetic agents in the emergency department. *Ann Emerg Med* 1994;23:1242.
6. Gronert BJ, Brandom BW. Neuromuscular blocking drugs in infants and children. *Pediatr Clin North Am* 1994;41:73.
7. Luten, R, Wears R, Broselow J, Croskerry P, Joseph M, Frush K. Managing the Unique size related issues of pediatric resuscitation: Reducing Cognitive load with resuscitation aids. *Acad Emerg Med* 2002;9:840–847.
8. Luten R. Approach to the Pediatric Airway. In: Walls R, Murphy M, Luten R, Schneider R (eds.), The manual of emergency airway management, second edition. Lippincott Williams & Wilkins, Philadelphia, 2004:212–250.
9. L'Hommedieu CS, Arens JJ. The use of ketamine for the emergency intubation of patients with status asthmaticus. *Ann Emerg Med* 1987;16:568.
10. Nakayama DK, Gardner MJ, Rowe MI. Emergency endotracheal intubation in pediatric trauma. *Ann Surg* 1990;211:218.
11. Nugent SK, Lavarvuso R, Rogers MC. Pharmacology and use of muscle relaxants in infants and children. *J Pediatr* 1979;94:481.
12. Perkin R, Van Stralen D, Mellick LB. Managing pediatric airway emergencies: anatomic considerations, alternative airway and ventilation techniques, and current treatment options. *Pediatr Emerg Med Rep* 1996;1:1–12.
13. Tullock WC, Diana P, Cook DR, Wilks DH, et al. Neuromuscular and cardiovascular effects of high-dose vecuronium. *Anesth Analg* 1990;70:86.
14. Walls RM, Luten RC, Murphy et al. *National Emergency Airway Management Course manual,* 3rd ed. Wellesley, MA: Airway Management Education Center, 1999.
15. Walls RM. Rapid sequence intubation in head trauma. *Ann Emerg Med* 1993;22:1008.
16. Yamamoto LG, Yim GK, Britten AG. Rapid sequence anesthesia induction for emergency intubation. *Pediatr Emerg Care* 1990;6:200.

CHAPTER 208
Shock and Vascular Access

Tonia J. Brousseau

Shock is a complex syndrome resulting from insufficient substrate and oxygen delivery to meet tissue metabolic demands. Untreated, it leads to metabolic acidosis, organ dysfunction, and death. Although shock may be a result of many etiologies, the end result is inadequate cardiac output (CO) to maintain effective tissue perfusion. In children the most common causes of shock are hypovolemia and sepsis. When compared to adults with septic shock the pediatric mortality rate is 9% versus 28% in adults (1). As a result, prompt recognition, diagnosis, and treatment prior to irreversible organ failure can substantially reduce morbidity and mortality.

PATHOPHYSIOLOGY

Maintaining CO and systemic vascular resistance are the primary mechanisms by which children compensate for shock. In the late phases of shock children lose their ability to maintain CO and SVR. Once CO is decreased there is a higher mortality rate (18). Understanding the factors that affect CO in children will help to direct therapy that may be life-saving.

Heart rate (HR) has the largest effect on CO. The child's ability to increase HR to maintain CO is preserved until late in shock. Therefore, bradycardia in children is a late and ominous finding as the patient is no longer able to compensate for the physiologic state. In addition a fast HR as in supraventricular tachycardia (SVT) may be the underlying cause of shock.

The second factor that affects CO is stroke volume (SV). SV is determined by preload, afterload, and cardiac compliance. Because most shock states in children have a relative hypovolemia, improving preload with volume resuscitation is the initial intervention. Children are usually able to maintain afterload (systemic vascular resistance), but when shock is unresponsive to fluid therapy, then inotropic and vasopressor agents are used to improve both afterload and contractility.

By maintaining CO there is also improvement of oxygen delivery which is a major determinant of oxygen consumption in children (5). The other factors include hemoglobin concentration, oxygen saturation, and dissolved oxygen in serum. Initial management remains volume replacement and providing 100% oxygen. In states of severe anemia or hemorrhage, replacement of blood products may be necessary.

CLINICAL PRESENTATION

The early diagnosis of shock requires a high index of suspicion based on an understanding of conditions that predispose children to shock. The diagnosis is made by a thorough physical examination that focuses on all physiologic systems. Septic shock can be recognized by the clinical triad of hypo-or hyperthermia, altered mental status, and peripheral vasodilatation with either warm or cool extremities.

Although shock affects all organ systems, the observable clinical features include:

Skin and Extremities: In general, shock is manifested by cool, mottled extremities with a decrease in peripheral pulses and prolongation of capillary refill. In septic shock there is an early and a late clinical presentation. These two phases of shock are apparent in the examination of the skin and extremities. The clinical picture is dependent on when the patient presents to the emergency department (ED). In early or "warm" shock the patient may have warm, flushed extremities with intact and bounding pulses. In addition, the pulse pressure may be widened. Recognition of warm shock and early volume replacement can significantly improve outcome (4,19). As warm/early shock progresses it is referred to as cold or late shock. In order to maintain vital organ perfusion, circulation to the skin and extremities will be diverted. The skin and mucous membranes may be cool, with pallor, cyanosis, and mottling. Capillary refill at the nail beds will be greater than 2 seconds, and peripheral pulses at the wrist and ankles may be weak or absent. Poor muscle tone reflects decreased muscle perfusion.

The presence of rashes that are consistent with classical meningococcemia, viral, or rickettsial infections may give some insight to a possible etiology. Petechial and purpuric rashes should always prompt a thorough evaluation even when the patient looks well (6).

Cardiopulmonary: Tachypnea and tachycardia may be the only cardiopulmonary signs in early, compensated shock, as increases in HR compensate for decreased SV, and hyperpnea compensates for metabolic acidosis. Auscultation of the chest is often normal unless the source of the shock is pulmonary edema, pneumonia, supraventricular tachycardia, pneumothorax, cardiac tamponade, or undiagnosed congenital heart disease. Findings in children with congestive heart failure include tachycardia, tachypnea, and hepatomegaly. Edema and jugular venous distention are not reliable findings in children.

Neurologic: Fluctuating mental status is a hallmark of poor cerebral perfusion, beginning with agitation, combativeness, lethargy, and progressing to unresponsiveness. This is a late finding in the progression of shock and requires immediate intervention. In infants without meningitis the anterior fontanelle may be sunken which is reflective of the relative hypovolemia.

Renal: As organ perfusion diminishes, so does glomerular filtration rate. The first compensation for decreased perfusion is urinary concentration, followed by decreased-to-absent urine output. This decrease will not be readily apparent by examination but may be elicited by history or bladder catheterization.

Hematologic: Coagulation abnormalities may be apparent by bleeding from the patient's orifices, petechiae or purpura, or prolonged bleeding from sites where intravascular access has been attempted. Evaluation should include a complete blood count with platelets, prothrombin time (PT), and partial thromboplastin time (PTT). Any abnormalities should be corrected with replacement of platelets and/or fresh frozen plasma (FFP).

DIFFERENTIAL DIAGNOSIS

Although there are many classifications of shock (Table 208.1), it is important to recognize that precise identification may be arduous and requires prolonged laboratory examination. Time

---

TABLE 208.1.   Etiologic Classification of Shock States

HYPOVOLEMIC SHOCK

Hemorrhage
  Internal
  External
Serum/plasma loss
  Burn
  Third-spacing (i.e., nephrosis, bowel ischemia)
  Septic
  Diabetes insipidus and mellitus
  Gastrointestinal loss
Drugs (i.e., diuretics, laxatives)

CARDIOGENIC SHOCK

Myocardial
  Ischemia
  Infectious/septic
  Toxic/drugs (i.e., hypocalcemia, beta blockers, etc.)
Dysrhythmia
Congenital
  Usually ductus arteriosus-dependent lesion (i.e., coarctation,
    hypoplastic left heart, critical aortic stenosis)

DISTRIBUTIVE SHOCK

Anaphylactic
Neurogenic
  Increased intracranial pressure
  Spinal cord injury
Septic

OBSTRUCTIVE SHOCK

Pneumothorax
Pericardial tamponade
Dissecting aortic aneurysm

METABOLIC/TOXIC SHOCK

Heat
CO, cyanide
Endocrine
  Thyroid
  Adrenal
  Parathyroid

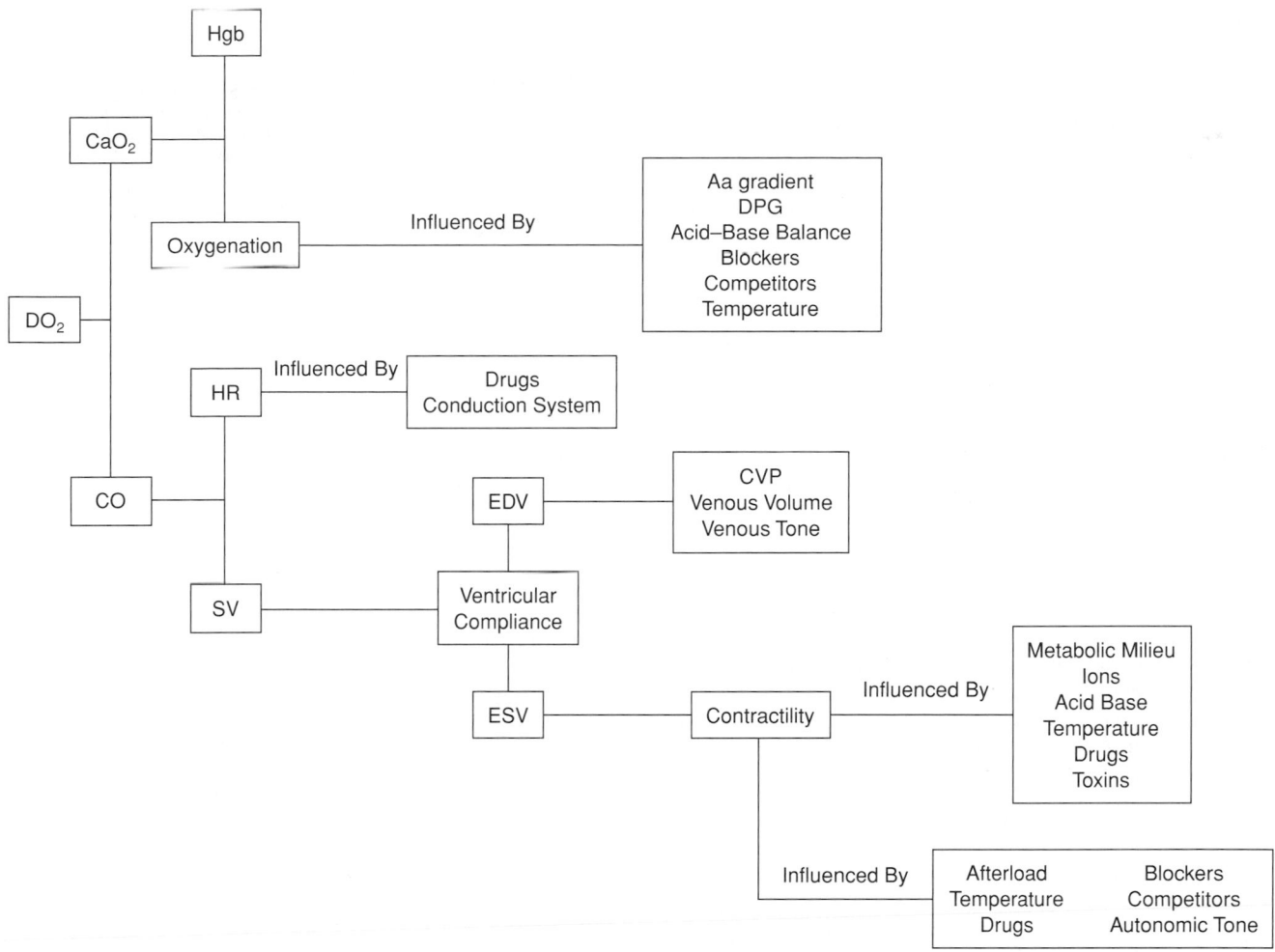

Figure 208.1. Factors affecting oxygen delivery.

is critical, and treatment cannot wait for precise classification. Lacking immediate physical signs that indicate precise etiology, the history and, occasionally, the laboratory findings may help to differentiate the causes of shock. Physiologically, with the exception of some forms of cardiogenic shock, absolute or relative hypovolemia is usually present, causing decreased preload and decreased SV. With the exception of pericardial tamponade, the size of the cardiac shadow on chest radiogram reflects the intracardiac volume and can be used as a determinate of the need for volume replacement (Fig. 208.1).

EMERGENCY DEPARTMENT EVALUATION

The initial systematic assessment of a sick child or infant is the same regardless of the etiology. The initial survey will give you an idea of the general condition and need for aggressive interventions. When a child is awake and alert there is time for a more thorough evaluation and history before intervening however, a child with mental status changes and/or hemodynamic instability always requires immediate management.

Airway patency is assessed and, in the absence of cervical instability, can be corrected by positioning or provision of an artificial airway. Assessment of breathing may be difficult. Hypoventilation in the face of shock signals central nervous system dysfunction and requires immediate attention. Hypoxia also requires immediate attention. Hyperventilation may be compensatory for metabolic acidosis instead of a primary pulmonary or cardiac etiology.

Circulation is evaluated by inspection of the skin for signs of vasoconstriction such as pallor, mottling, cool extremities, and prolonged capillary. Palpation of the peripheral pulse correlates better with tissue blood flow than does the blood pressure, which may be preserved by intense vasoconstriction until just prior to cardiac arrest. Hypotension and bradycardia require immediate intervention.

Once the initial survey is completed and resuscitation airway, breathing, and circulation (ABC's) are instituted, a secondary survey may be undertaken to investigate the etiology and extent of the shock state. There should be a complete physical examination, with emphasis placed on the primary shock organs, including the neurologic, pulmonary, and cardiac systems and a careful abdominal examination. A complete blood count, serum electrolytes, blood glucose, blood urea nitrogen, creatinine, and acid–base determination are usually necessary. The patient's history guides the remainder of the laboratory examination and may include a reticulocyte count, PT, PTT, serum protein and albumin, liver or cardiac enzymes, drug screens, and cultures. Arrhythmias require sequential electrocardiograms, and when congenital heart disease is considered, a pediatric echocardiogram is helpful if immediately available.

A plain film of the chest has both diagnostic and therapeutic significance. In addition to revealing heart or lung disease, including pneumothorax, the size of the heart can be used as an indicator of volume status. The size of the cardiac silhouette on serial x-rays may be used to guide the degree of volume replacement.

EMERGENCY DEPARTMENT MANAGEMENT

All children in shock should be maintained at physiologic temperatures and provided with sufficient oxygen to maintain oxygen saturation above 92% by pulse oximetry. Heart rate and rhythm should be continuously monitored, and blood pressure, temperature, fluid intake, and fluid output must be assessed frequently. A calm and reassuring manner may reduce pain and anxiety, thus decreasing wasted oxygen consumption without resorting to the use of analgesics or sedatives that might impede physiologic compensation.

Endotracheal intubation is indicated for any patient with a compromised or unstable airway. Provision of positive-pressure ventilation is indicated for respiratory arrest, persistent apnea, hypoventilation, presumed intracranial hypertension, and acute hypercapnea, or when deep anesthesia is required for definitive therapeutic interventions. When absolute indications are lacking, mechanical ventilation should be postponed until adequate preload is established, because positive-pressure ventilation may impede right heart return. When the etiology of the shock is clearly discernible (i.e., anaphylaxis, chest trauma, known hypoparathyroidism, known steroid dependency) and definitive treatment is quickly available, early attempts should then be made for primary correction (i.e., removal of antigen, insertion of chest tube, correction of profound hypocalcemia, administration of steroids). In most cases, however, a general approach to the treatment of shock is required.

Intravascular access (IV) access remains an anxiety provoking and challenging skill to master in the pediatric population. In an acute setting, intravenous access is needed for the delivery of resuscitation medications, antibiotics, volume expanders, correction of electrolyte abnormalities, and blood sampling for diagnostic tests. Selection of site and mechanism for vascular access is primarily dependent on the clinical situation. The stable patient may allow for more time and attempts at peripheral access, whereas the unstable patient requires immediate rapid access that is most commonly obtained via an intraosseous (IO) line. The neonate has the unique option of umbilical venous (UV) cannulation.

In all situations, the area should be properly immobilized and sterilized prior to any attempts. After successful access is obtained, the area should be adequately secured to prevent dislodging the line. Vascular access sites in children include:

Peripheral IV Lines

This is a safe and appropriate procedure in the stable, nonemergent patient. The large peripheral veins including the antecubital and saphenous are good options at all ages. A small 20- to 24-gauge catheter may be necessary. The scalp vein cannulation has a high rate of complications and is not recommended for use in resuscitation. In the unstable patient, peripheral access is satisfactory if it can be obtained rapidly.

IO Access

The IO route is probably the most useful and versatile of the emergency nonperipheral vascular access sites and should be considered in patients of all ages when emergent access is crucial and attempts at peripheral vascular sites are unsuccessful. Any drug or fluid that can be administered intravenously can be infused through the IO route with the exception of sodium

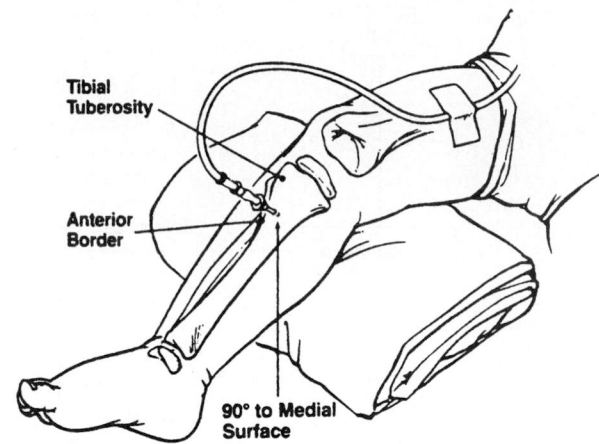

Figure 208.2.   Intraosseus cannulation technique. (From American Heart Association. *Textbook of pediatric advanced life support.* Dallas: American Heart Association, 1997, with permission.)

bicarbonate (7,9,22). The IO route also provides a means for rapid and effective volume resuscitation using crystalloids, colloids, or blood products (8). Bone marrow can also be a source of laboratory studies for diagnostic as well as therapeutic interventions (11). The preferred site at all ages for IO infusion is the flat, anteromedial surface of the proximal tibia, 1 cm inferior to and 1 cm medial to the tibial tubercle (Fig. 208.2), but alternatives include the distal femur, the medial malleoli, distal humerus and the anterior-superior iliac crests. Older children and adults may also have attempts in the distal tibia and the distal radius and ulna. In addition, a sternal IO system is available for use in adults (13). There are several styles of commercially available IO infusion needles, and Jamshidi-type bone marrow aspiration needles can be used. The skin over the anterior tibia or alternative site should be sterilized. Starting 1 to 3 cm below the tibial tuberosity (to avoid damaging the growth plate), the needle is directed at a 90-degree angle to the medial surface of the tibia. Several signs help to confirm that the needle is in the marrow cavity: sudden decrease in resistance as the needle passes through the cortex; the needle stands upright without support; when a syringe is attached to the needle, bone marrow may be aspirated (if you are unable to aspirate marrow, attempt to infuse flush fluid); fluid infuses freely without signs of subcutaneous infiltration.

Complications of IO infusions are rare but include osteomyelitis, compartment syndrome, tibial fracture, and skin necrosis (20).

Central Venous Access

The central venous catheter is a commonly used invasive tool in the monitoring and management of critically ill children. Indications in emergent situations include inability to establish peripheral venous or IO access, or for monitoring in the hemodynamically unstable patient. Because complications occur more frequently in children than adults, attempts should be done by the person who is most skilled at central venous access in children.

Percutaneous central venous catheter kits are available in various sizes. A 3.0F or 4.0F catheter should be used in infants younger than 1 year, while 4.0 to 5.5F catheters can be used in children 1 to 12 years of age. Catheters may be inserted percutaneously into the subclavian, femoral, or internal and external jugular veins using the Seldinger technique (21).

The femoral vein is the easiest and safest central vein to cannulate in emergencies because of its anatomic landmarks and large size. It can be accessed without interfering with resuscitation (15). The leg is slightly externally rotated and the area is sterilized and draped. The femoral vein is located medial to the femoral artery, which can be palpated as a guide. During cardiopulmonary resuscitation (CPR) there may be palpable pulsations in either the artery or vein. The area below the inguinal ligament, medial to the femoral artery is infiltrated with 1% lidocaine. In children the introducer needle is directed at a 30- to 40-degree angle to the skin starting about 1 cm below the inguinal ligament and aiming toward the contralateral shoulder or umbilicus. Once complete, the catheter should be sutured in place and a radiograph is performed to confirm proper position. Internal jugular and subclavian venous approaches also can be performed by experienced personnel, but these procedures carry the additional risks of pneumothorax and hemothorax.

Vascular Cutdown

Surgical venous cutdown has decreased in popularity since the resurgence of the IO technique, but remains useful in emergency situations when attempts at peripheral, IO, and central access have failed or cannot be performed. This mechanism is time consuming even in skilled hands and has a higher rate of complications when compared with alternative routes. The long saphenous vein that courses anterior to the medial malleolus at the ankle is the preferred site for cutdown. The lower extremity is immobilized, with the foot turned laterally, exposing the saphenous vein anterior to the medial malleolus. A sterile field is prepared, and 1% lidocaine is injected subcutaneously over the vein and a tourniquet should be placed proximal to this site. An incision perpendicular to the vein is made, and the vein is gently isolated by blunt dissection with a curved hemostat. Two silk sutures are looped around the vein; the distal one may be used to ligate the vein. With tension applied to the proximal suture loop, a venotomy is made with a no. 11 blade inserted into the lateral wall of the vessel and drawn upward. This avoids complete transection of the vessel. Finally, the cannula is inserted into the vein, advanced, and secured in place by tying a proximal suture loop. The tourniquet is then removed and the wound is then closed with simple nylon sutures and dressed.

Umbilical Vascular Access

In neonates, the umbilical vessels may be directly accessed during the first several days of life, directly or by intraumbilical cutdown. The umbilical vein (UV) may be used for blood sampling, fluid or drug infusion, and monitoring blood pressure and central venous pressure. Normally, two UAs and one UV exist. At skin level, the UV is usually in the 12 o'clock position and has a thinner wall and wider lumen than does the UA. The umbilicus is scrubbed with a bactericidal solution and draped, and a silk suture is looped around the base of the umbilicus stump. The distal end of the stump is cut off, and the vessels are occluded to prevent blood loss. A 3.5F to 5.0F catheter is flushed with saline and inserted into the lumen of the desired vessel. Advancement of a UV catheter should be just to the point where good blood return is obtained. This will be approximately 1 to 4 cm deep. Plain radiographs should be taken to confirm placement. Complications of umbilical catheters include hemorrhage, infection, air embolism, and perforation of a blood vessel.

Arterial Access

Arterial cannulation for continuous blood pressure and arterial blood gas monitoring may be necessary in critically ill infants and children. Sites available for arterial access include the radial, axillary, femoral, posterior tibial, and dorsalis pedis arteries, but the most commonly used sites are the radial and femoral arteries. The hand is secured on an arm board with dorsiflexion of the wrist to 45 degrees. The area should be sterilized and the fingertips should be left exposed when the hand is taped down so that any peripheral ischemic changes can be observed. Palpate the artery for maximal pulsation and introduce a 20- to 24-gauge cannula at a 30-degree angle. Blood is aspirated to confirm the intraarterial position of the cannula. This can also be accomplished with a Seldinger technique. A similar technique is used to cannulate other arteries. The most common complications of arterial catheterization include minor skin lesions, localized hematoma, arterial bleeding, and arterial thrombosis with distal ischemia. The catheter should be removed immediately if any evidence of tissue ischemia develops.

Volume Expansion

Volume resuscitation is the mainstay of all forms of shock therapy and is oriented toward restoring intravascular volume relative to the vascular space and optimizing ventricular preload. Even in shock due to myocardial failure, judiciously optimizing left ventricular preload (using aliquots of 5 cc/kg of 0.9% saline) can improve stroke volume. Initially, the resuscitation fluids of choice are either normal saline (0.9% NaCl) or lactated Ringer solution. Except for shock due to myocardial failure, aliquots of 20 mL/kg are given rapidly over 2 to 10 minutes and may require from 40 to 60 cc/Kg to 200 cc/Kg in the first hour of resuscitation (4). The end-point of volume resuscitation is clinical improvement in perfusion as assessed by a decrease in HR and compensatory hyperventilation, an increase in blood pressure, capillary refill, muscle tone and strength of peripheral pulses, improvement in affect and skin color, and improvement of urine output to >1 cc/Kg/hr. If no improvement is seen after 40 to 60 cc/Kg of resuscitation fluid has been given, consider ongoing fluid losses, alternative causes of shock, adrenal insufficiency, intestinal ischemia, pericardial effusion, or pneumothorax. When central venous access is obtainable, determination of central venous pressure may be useful in guiding further volume therapy. Early determination of serum glucose, electrolytes, calcium, acid–base status, and hemoglobin concentration will help to guide the choice of solutions for definitive therapy.

Cardiotonic Infusions

The lack of unusual fluid losses by history, preexisting heart disease, hepatomegaly, rales, cardiomegaly, and failure to improve perfusion with provision of adequate oxygenation, ventilation,

TABLE 208.2.   Pharmacologic Treatment of Pediatric Shock

Medication	Dose
Dopamine	2–20 mcg/Kg/min IV
Epinephrine	0.1–1 mcg/Kg/min IV
Norepinephrine	0.1–2 mcg/Kg/min IV
Dobutamine	2–20 mcg/Kg/min IV
Hydrocortisone	25–50 mg IV

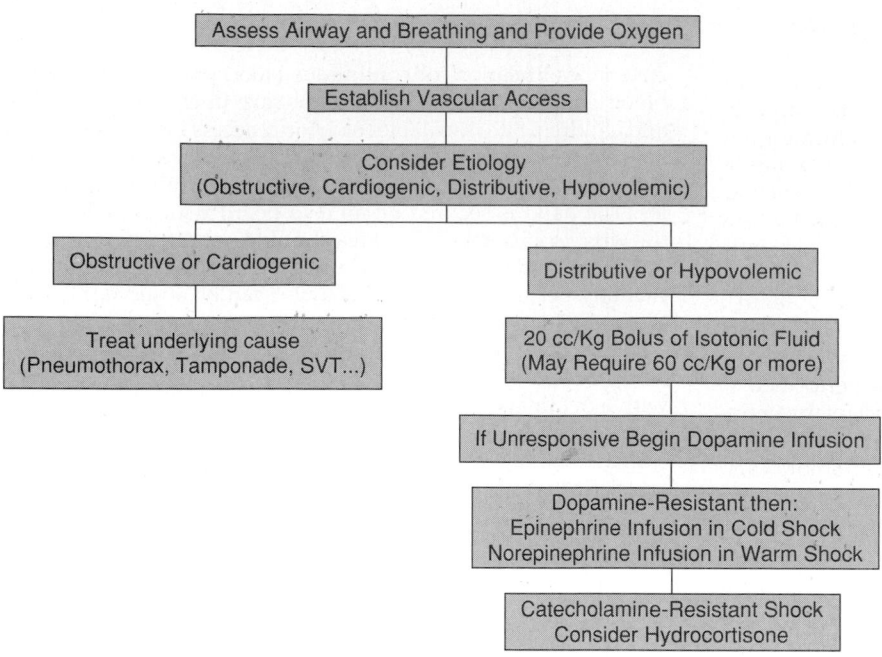

Figure 208.3. Algorithm for management of shock.

HR, and volume expansion should suggest a cardiogenic or distributive component to the patient's shock state. Cardiotonic and vasoactive drug infusions can further improve cardiac output and tissue perfusion by inotropy, chronotropy, or altering blood flow distribution. Prior to the administration of cardiotonic–vasoactive drugs, the goals of therapy and the criteria for monitoring the end-point must be established. Although a variety of agents are available, only a few drugs are appropriate for the acute resuscitation period in pediatric patients. Dopamine is the first line in the pharmacologic therapy of shock. It is important to recognize that dopamine resistant shock is common in children and if there is no response to dopamine, then norepinephrine should be considered in warm shock and epinephrine in cold shock (3,14,15). Dobutamine may also used for inotropic support, but also has the difficulty of resistance in children (16) (Table 208.2).

Metabolic Support

Blood glucose should be evaluated initially and periodically during the resuscitation and promptly replaced if hypoglycemia is present (12). Calcium should be measured and replaced if hypocalcemia is present. In addition, the patient who remains unresponsive despite conventional therapies may have adrenal suppression and may benefit from hydrocortisone replacement (10). See Figure 208.3 for a management algorithm of shock.

The child's outcome is dependent on both the expeditious reversal of the shock state and the definitive treatment of the underlying cause. Administration of antibiotics, antihistamines, hormones, antidotes or surgical intervention may preclude the need for prolonged cardiotonic treatment.

DISPOSITION

Specific subspecialty referral is dependent on the etiology of the child's shock. In all cases, these children will require admission to an inpatient facility with the trained staff and facilities to care for a critically ill child. The child in shock should be transported by appropriate transport personnel that have pediatric experience and necessary equipment and medications.

CRITICAL INTERVENTIONS

- Shock that is unresponsive to volume resuscitation and cardiotonic administration requires a broadened differential diagnosis that should include adrenal crisis, hypoglycemia, and hypocalcemia, as well as obstructive shock and abdominal crisis
- When a child is in shock and peripheral IV access cannot be rapidly obtained, an IO should be placed
- Children may be dopamine resistant and norepinephrine or epinephrine should be considered as alternatives

COMMON PITFALLS

✔ Failure to recognize pediatric shock, either due to the child's ability to maintain blood pressure by increasing HR and systemic resistance or due to early hyperdynamic septic shock where perfusion is maintained. To avoid this, the physician must have a high index of suspicion and perform a complete physical examination, with emphasis on the shock organs

✔ Do not assume that all "shocky" children are septic when the true diagnosis may be a neurologic or cardiologic problem or an abdominal vascular crisis (i.e., volvulus or intussusception)

✔ Failure to rapidly administer the appropriate amount of volume expansion. Children have a higher blood volume relative to weight than do adults, and thus may require substantial volumes of resuscitation fluid

Acknowledgments

Thanks to previous edition's chapter authors Lucian K. DeNicola, James H. McCrory, and Talaat A. Abdelmoneim.

References

1. Angus DC, Linde Zwirble WT, Liddicker J, et al. Epidemiology of severe sepsis in the United States: Analysis of incidence, outcome, and associated costs of care. *Crit Care Med* 2001;29:1303–1310.
2. Berg RA. Emergency infusion of catecholamines into bone marrow. *Am J Dis Child* 1984;138:810–811.
3. Bollaert PE, Bauer P, Audibert G, et al. Effects of epinephrine on hemodynamics and oxygen metabolism in dopamine-resistant septic shock. *Chest* 1990;98:949–953.

4. Carcillo JA, Davis AL, Zaritsky A. Role of early fluid resuscitation in pediatric septic shock. *JAMA* 1991;266:1242–1245.

5. Carcillo JA, Pollack MM, Ruttiman UE, et al. Sequential physiologic interactions in cardiogenic and septic shock. *Crit Care Med* 1989;17:12–16.

6. DiGuilio GA. Fever and petechiae: No time for a rash decision. *Clin Pediatr Emerg Med* 2000;1:132–137.

7. Ellemunter H, Simma B, Trawoger R, Maurer H. Intraosseous lines in preterm and full term neonates. *Arch Dis Child Fetal Neonatology Ed* 1999;80:F74–F75.

8. Fiser DH. Intraosseous infusion. *N Engl J Med* 1990;322:1579–1581.

9. Glaeser PW, Hellmich TR, Szewczuga D, Losek JD, Smith DS. Five-year experience in prehospital intraosseous infusions in children and adults. *Ann Emerg Med* 1993;22:1119–1124.

10. Hatherhill M, Tibby SM, Hilliard T, et al. Adrenal Insufficiency in septic shock. *Arch Dis Child* 1999;80:51–55.

11. Johnson L, Kissoon N, Fiallos M, Abdelmoneim T, et al. Use of intraosseous blood to assess blood chemistries and hemaglobin during cardiopulmonary resuscitation with drug infusions. *Crit Care Med* 1999;27:1147–1152.

12. Losek JD. Hypoglycemia and the ABC's (sugar) of pediatric resuscitation. *Ann Emerg Med* 2000;35:43–46.

13. Macnab A, Christenson J, Findlay J, et al. A new system for sternal intraosseous infusion in adults. *Prehosp Emerg Care* 2000;4:173–177.

14. Meadows D, Edwards JD, Wilkins RG, et al. Reversal of intractable septic shock with norepinephrine therapy. *Crit Care Med* 1988;16:663–666.

15. Padbury JF, Agata Y, Baylen BG, et al. Pharmacokinetics of dopamine in critically ill newborn infants. *J Pediatr* 1990;117:472–476.

16. Perkins RM, Levin DL, Webb R, et al. Dobutamine: A hemodynamic evaluation in children with septic shock. *J Pediatr* 1982;100:977–983.

17. Pollack MM, Fields AI, Ruttimann UE, et al. Sequential cardiopulmonary variables of infants and children in septic shock. *Crit Care Med* 1984;12:554–559.

18. Pollack MM, Fields AI, Ruttimann UE. Distributions of cardiopulmonary variables in pediatric survivors and nonsurvivors of septic shock. *Crit Care Med* 1985;13:454–459.

19. Rivers E, nguyen B, Havstad S, et al. Early goal directed therapy in the treatment of severe sepsis and septic shock. *N Engl J Med* 2001;345:1368–1377.

20. Rosovsky M, Fitzpatrick M, Goldfarb CR, et al. Bilateral osteomyelitis due to intraosseous infusion: case report and review of the English-language literature. *Pediatr Radiol* 1994;24:72–73.

21. Strauss RH. Pediatric vascular access. In Fuhrman BP, Zimmerman JJ, eds. *Pediatric Critical Care.* St Louis; Mosby, 1998:126–139.

22. Waisman M, Waisman D. Bone marrow infusion in adults. *J Trauma* 1997;42:288–293.

PART II

Pediatric Trauma

CHAPTER 209

General Approach to Pediatric Trauma

Rick C. Place and Thom A. Mayer

Over 17,000 children under the age of 20 die of unintended injuries each year; this is more than any other cause of pediatric mortality. Nonfatal and minor trauma is even more prevalent, accounting for over 10 million emergency department (ED) visits in the United States every year (17). The majority of ill and injured children are initially cared for in community EDs. While commonalities exist, the significant differences between adult and pediatric trauma victims preclude complete extrapolation of adult skills and algorithms to pediatric trauma patients. A protocol-oriented approach to the care of the child with multiple trauma, accentuating differences between adults and children, is presented in this chapter.

Most important to the care of the pediatric multiple trauma victim is preparation of the entire ED and surgical backup teams to care for pediatric patients with acute injuries. There is a small margin for error in caring for severely injured children and therefore clinicians must be familiar with the appropriate elements in the evaluation and resuscitation, including normal baseline physiologic parameters in children. As with many other low frequency, high-risk conditions, appropriate preparation can result in a well-organized resuscitation with excellent outcomes. Guidelines for ED preparedness for the care of pediatric patients have been published (1).

Causes of pediatric injury largely depend on the age and developmental characteristics of children. Major causes of nonfatal injuries in young children (less than age 5) include falls, drowning, burns, motor vehicle crashes, and child abuse. In addition, suffocation and drowning are major causes of fatalities. School-age children suffer similar events but are more likely to be victims of automobile crashes, while in the adolescent years the vast majority of injuries are attributed to falls, motor-vehicle crashes (with or without the influence of drugs and alcohol), homicides (firearms), and in urban areas, gunshot wounds (many of which are self-inflicted) predominate (17).

ANATOMIC AND PHYSIOLOGIC DIFFERENCES

It is important to review pertinent anatomic and physiologic differences between adults and children as well as variations in evaluation and management (13,18). These differences dictate age-specific differences in the epidemiology, pathophysiology, and approach to pediatric traumatic injuries. In many respects, such as the airway and cervical spine, the child will physically transition into a more adult physiology at approximately 8 years of age. This review will focus primarily on the pediatric patient under this age.

Published charts and tables can be placed on the wall of the resuscitation area that provides typical age-specific weights allowing for appropriately sized tube and drug calculations. Better still, the Broselow resuscitation tape can be used to measure the child's length; from this measurement, the child is placed in a color zone that provides estimated fluid and drug dosages, as well as resuscitative equipment (11,12). The advantage of the Broselow resuscitation tape is that predicted weights are extremely accurate for infants and young children and color-coding the child eliminates cumbersome, time-consuming, and error-prone calculations (11).

The extent and severity of head injury is the primary determinant of outcome in the pediatric trauma victim (23). The increased relative weight of the child's head and the more prominent occiput partly explains this excess vulnerability, the head acting as the leading edge of impact in much the same way as the head of a hammer tossed across a room. The prominence of the occiput also affects positioning of the airway in the course of the resuscitation. The child's cranial sutures are open at birth and gradually fuse by 12 to 18 months of age; bulging of the fontanels may indicate increased intracranial pressure. The infant brain also differs from its mature counterpart and may experience more diffuse injury and be more vulnerable to secondary injury (15). On the other hand, children with head injuries of similar degrees of severity and with similar global injury scores fare better in terms of both morbidity and mortality compared with adults (23).

The shorter neck and increased subcutaneous tissue make evaluating the neck veins and midline position of the trachea considerably more difficult in respiratory emergencies. The larynx is more cephalad and anterior position in children. The glottic opening is at the level of C1 in infancy, C3–4 by age 7 and C4-5 in adults (14). This high, anterior position causes difficulties in cord visualization in children up to the age of 8, when the airway assumes more adult characteristics, making intubation more challenging (14). Until the age of 8, the narrowest portion of the pediatric airway is not glottic, but rather subglottic, at the level of the cricoid cartilage. Furthermore, the comparative narrowness and laxity of the subglottic mucosa means that traumatic or toxic edema is more poorly tolerated.

Cervical spine fractures are less common in children than in adults (18). Nonetheless, fractures and/or cervical cord injuries do occur, and the type and pattern of these injuries differ as well. The baby's head comprises 25% of its entire weight, compared with 10% in an adult; this results in a higher fulcrum about which flexion and extension occurs (C2–C3 in infants vs. C5–C6 in adults). The weaker neck muscles and relatively greater weight of the head leads to a proportionately increased number of devastating high cervical spine injuries; up to 50% of spinal injuries in children under the age of 3 years occur at the C1 and C2 levels (18). Unfortunately, the cervical spine of infants and young children is less ossified, making fracture of the spine difficult to recognize radiographically. Moreover, physiologic anterior pseudosubluxation between C2 and C3, a widened predental space, and incomplete ossification at the base of the dens can make interpretation of pediatric cervical radiographs problematic. Ligamentous laxity, relatively horizontal facet joints, and wedge-shaped vertebral bodies allow serious cord injury in the absence of bony fracture. The pediatric spinal column does not take on adult characteristic until around the age of 8. These factors all combine to permit a condition aptly named spinal cord injury without radiographic abnormality (SCIWORA). Severe SCIWORA is found almost exclusively in children under the age of 8 and is a devastating injury with a poor prognosis for significant recovery (18) (see Chapter 211, "Evaluation of the Cervical Spine").

The pediatric abdominal wall is thin and less muscular and therefore is less effective at preventing internal force transmission. The result is a significant risk of internal injury in the absence of external findings. In particular, the bladder, well protected by the overlying pubic bone in adults, is an abdominal structure in young children and is far more prone to injury from blunt trauma. A high index of suspicion for intrathoracic and intraabdominal injury should be maintained with a low threshold for imaging studies.

Infants are "belly" breathers, meaning they require full diaphragmatic excursion to produce normal respirations. Horizontal diaphragmatic insertion provides less mechanical advantage and they are less able to recruit the intercostal muscles to assist in respiration than are adults. Also, a child's diaphragm is much more compliant and gastric distention frequently results in pulmonary compromise by pushing the diaphragm upward.

Children accommodate bony growth through the epiphyseal growth plate, radiographically lucent until their mid to late teens. In younger children, ligamentous structures are actually stronger than the growth plate junction, and compared with adults, children are more likely to experience a fracture than a sprain. Unfortunately, a Salter I epiphyseal fracture (a linear fracture only through the growth plate), like a sprain, is radiographically invisible, making differentiation of the two conditions problematic. It is therefore wise to maintain a low threshold for splinting extremity injuries with an equivocal exam.

THE PRIMARY AND SECONDARY SURVEYS

The fundamental primary survey—secondary survey format initially described by the American College of Surgeons Committee on Trauma in the *Advanced Trauma Life Support* (ATLS) course remains the most effective and efficient manner of evaluating the injured child (2). The primary survey is the focused initial assessment of the patient's airway, ventilation, circulation, and overall level of consciousness. It is a physiologic survey that assesses any acute and immediate threat to the child's life. The primary survey resuscitative phase is brief but gives the emergency physician an accurate baseline assessment of the child's overall physiologic status. The more extensive systematic secondary survey identifies less acute life-threatening and nonlife-threatening injuries. Life-sustaining therapies should be guided by findings on the initial assessment while injury treatment therapies are guided by findings elicited on the secondary survey. By using a protocol approach to patient assessment, the emergency physician can be assured that potential threats to life and limb are identified in sequential yet complete fashion. The essential tenets of the survey are the same but one must remember critical differences between adults and children in: recognition of cervical spine injuries; provision of an airway and use of appropriate ventilation techniques; recognition of circulatory stability and shock; provision of vascular access; management of pediatric head injury; maintenance of core body temperature.

Severe pediatric trauma, in its initial phases, is a disease of the airway. Victims are far more likely to suffer problems with adequate ventilation than circulatory failure. As with other critically ill children, the focus should initially lie there. However, most pediatric victims with multisystem trauma have suffered a concurrent traumatic brain injury (TBI) and prevention of secondary injury following TBI is dependent on adequate oxygenation and ventilation as well as hemodynamic parameters (4). For that reason, close attention needs to be paid to circulatory status in pediatric multisystem injuries.

AIRWAY

The highest priority in caring for either adult or pediatric patients with multiple traumatic injuries is ensuring and/or providing a patent airway with adequate ventilation and oxygenation while protecting the cervical spine. However, significant differences in the pediatric airway may require a modified approach different from that for an adult (Table 209.1).

Although cervical spine injuries are less common in children than in adults, it is equally important to protect the cervical spine throughout all airway manipulations. A high index of suspicion must be maintained in caring for children who are at high risk for cervical spine injury (e.g., unrestrained infants in motor vehicle crashes, children struck by automobiles, or children suffering a fall from a significant height). In these children, due to the significant risk of SCIWORA, even if the initial lateral cervical spine radiograph is normal, cervical spine integrity must be preserved.

As in adults, the mechanism of protecting the cervical spine in children is in-line cervical immobilization. With a struggling child, one rescuer holds the cervical position while maintaining the airway, while another ensures that the distal portions of the body are also immobilized until more permanent means of cervical spine immobilization can be obtained. All emergency medical services providers should have rigid pediatric cervical spine collars available. Inappropriate sizing may cause excessive

---

TABLE 209.1. Anatomic Differences in the Pediatric Airway[†]

Proportionately larger tongue
Large floppy epiglottis
Anterior and cephalad glottic opening
Narrowest portion of trachea is subglottic
Tiny cricothyroid membrane

[†]These differences especially apply to children under the age of 2. The pediatric airway then assumes a transitional state until around the age of 8 where it more closely resembles the adult airway (10).

distraction, hyperextension, or flexion of the neck that might worsen high cervical injuries or cause airway compromise. If the appropriate collar is not available, the head of the supine child should be braced in a neutral position with blocks or rolled towels and tape. A flattened towel may need to be placed under the shoulders to prevent natural flexion of the infant neck due to the large occiput. However, without a high-risk mechanism, rigid insistence on immobilizing the alert, struggling child with no obvious injury should not be done at the risk of injuring the child further.

Concurrently with stabilization of the cervical spine, the airway should be evaluated. The most frequent and critical error is failure to position the airway properly. A relaxed-head position in infants and young children results in excess flexion of the neck and airway occlusion. In addition, in severely injured children, the tongue and other muscular tissue attached to the mandible often falls posteriorly, obstructing the airway. To ensure that the airway is patent, the child is placed in the "sniffing position" (with the neck slightly extended or rotated at the atlantooccipital junction and the head slightly raised above the neck) (Fig. 209.1). In practical terms, this position can be obtained by placing a flattened towel under the shoulders of younger children. While the head tilt-chin lift maneuver ensures that the mandibular block of tissue does not fall posteriorly and obstruct the airway, it should be avoided in cases of possible cervical spine injury in favor of the jaw thrust (8). Unless the airway is appropriately positioned as described here, it may be difficult to provide appro-

priate oxygenation or ventilation, even with an intact airway and in the presence of otherwise proper bag-mask-ventilation (BMV) technique.

Once the airway has been appropriately positioned, a rapid assessment should be made for airway patency and adequacy of ventilation. If airway obstruction exists, and repositioning is unsuccessful, manual clearing or suction with a rigid tonsillar suction catheter should be performed. Up to about age 4 to 6 months, children are obligate nasal breathers, so nasal obstruction must be quickly and effectively relieved to allow spontaneous ventilation. In addition, the respiratory effort, adequacy of air excursion, and the presence or absence of cyanosis should be assured. Because children have small tidal volumes, chest wall rise may be subtle. Normal respiratory and heart rates should be posted or easily accessible in the trauma care area (see Chapter 204, "General Approach to the Pediatric Emergency Patient" Table 204.2).

Oropharyngeal and Nasopharyngeal Airways

In unconscious adult patients, oral or nasal airways are sometimes used to assist in ensuring airway patency. However, such airways are less commonly used in children. In the semiconscious child, oral or nasal airways can produce vomiting or laryngospasm, or even worse airway obstruction if sized incorrectly. Also, the posterior pharynx of a child consists of highly vascular adenoidal tissue, which is easily traumatized by the insertion of a nasal tube, and the resultant bleeding may then interfere with more definitive efforts to secure the airway. Rarely, an oral airway may be useful in the unconscious child when the tongue continues to prevent adequate BMV despite optimal airway positioning. Likewise, a nasal airway may assist in ventilating the child with unusual head and neck anatomy due to syndromic or congenital anatomic abnormalities, such as the Pierre-Robin sequence, or in children with excessive adenoidal or tonsillar tissue.

Bag-and-Mask Ventilation

In pediatric multiple trauma patients with a compromised airway, there is a natural tendency to rush toward endotracheal (ET) intubation even in the face of suboptimal intubating conditions, such as in the prehospital setting. This is a common but potentially fatal mistake. Almost all children can be initially ventilated adequately by BMV, assuming the clinician remembers several factors. First, BMV in children is much easier than in adults because of the child's smaller size and more compliant physiology; it is much easier to generate appropriate tidal volumes and airway pressures. As discussed above, proper airway positioning is the key to effective BMV. Second, providing an adequate seal by face-mask is usually easier in children. The appropriately sized mask can be selected by choosing one that easily fits from the bridge of the nose to the chin. In small children or infants, the thumb and index finger can be placed on the mask and the remaining three fingers underneath the angle and length of the mandible (EC clamp) (8). The latter three fingers firmly pull the jaw into the mask while the thumb and index fingers maintain a tight seal *without pushing* the mask into the face. The adequacy of assisted ventilation should be assessed by ensuring that there is equal and full bilateral chest wall rise.

One of the most frequent criticisms of BMV versus ET intubation is the inability to protect the airway from aspiration. Overly aggressive BMV may result in significant gastric distention, ventilatory compromise, and subsequent aspiration. However, judicious application of cricoid pressure by another person helps to reduce the possibility of aspiration. This maneuver consists of placing pressure on the cricoid cartilage and occluding

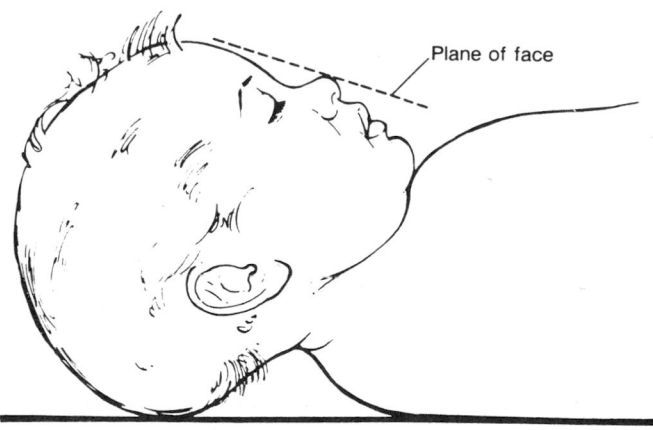

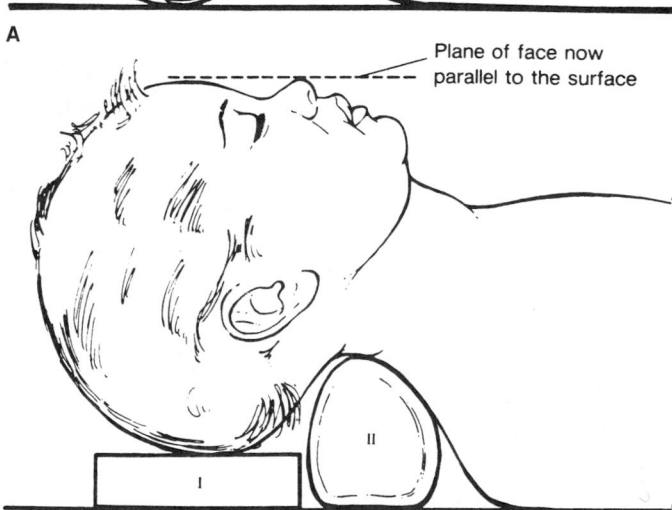

Figure 209.1.   **(A)** Airway at high risk for occlusion. Flexion of the neck on the thorax is caused by a prominent occiput. **(B)** Sniffing position, which gives maximum possibility for a patent airway.

the esophagus against the spinal column, thereby preventing regurgitation by preventing gastric distention.

Early placement of a nasogastric tube should be considered if BMV is likely to be prolonged. This will prevent further gastric insufflation and distention and reduce the chances for subsequent aspiration. It will also allow for more effective ventilation by preventing upward pressure on the diaphragm.

The tendency to overly ventilate the young child in an emergency situation, both in terms of rate and depth, should be resisted. In addition to potential barotrauma, an excessive tidal volume may overwhelm the benefit of cricoid pressure, causing gastric distension, upward pressure on the diaphragm, impaired diaphragmatic excursion, emesis and aspiration. Furthermore, hyperventilation may be detrimental to the child with TBI, inducing cerebral vasoconstriction, worsening focal or global ischemia. Inadvertently hyperventilating the child may be controlled by consciously saying, "squeeze, release, release" and squeezing only to the point of visible chest rise (21).

Endotracheal Intubation

A length-based system can be used to select the appropriately sized ET tube and intubation equipment (2). A curved laryngoscope blade that is adequately lodged in the vallecula may not allow adequate visualization of the vocal cords because the pediatric larynx is more anterior, more cephalad, and may be obscured by a large, floppy epiglottis. A straight (Miller) blade allows better visualization in children by directly compressing the large tongue and epiglottis out of the orolaryngeal line of site. An uncuffed tube is generally used in children less than age 8, since the narrow subglottic region provides a snug seal, serving as a natural cuff. If a cuffed tube is used, care should be taken to inflate the cuff only to the point of preventing air leak; a high-pressure cuff easily produces mucosal necrosis.

Airway positioning is critical during pediatric ET intubation. The child is placed in the sniffing position, and the Sellick maneuver is used to prevent vomiting and aspiration. Pulse oximetry readings should be followed closely to monitor oxygenation. Infants and young children have a basal oxygen consumption approximately twice that of adults and a proportionately smaller functional residual capacity from which to sustain saturation (14). Pre-oxygenating children with 100% oxygen prior to intubation attempts is an essential feature of pediatric intubation, except in rare situations in which "crash intubation" is necessary to secure the airway.

Once the tube has been placed within the trachea, the best way to ensure proper position is by the use of CO_2 colorimetry. Chest auscultation may be deceiving and inaccurate since the chest transmits sound very easily in children, especially in infants. It is not uncommon for the rescuer to hear relatively clear breath sounds in both axillae, even though the tube is either in the esophagus or right main bronchus. The short trachea also makes mainstem intubation more likely; a rule of thumb for depth of placement is that tube length in centimeters at the lips should be three times the size of the endotracheal tube (14,21).

Rapid sequence induction (RSI) is the standard for intubating critically injured trauma patients. Most patients will have an uncleared cervical spine and will require intubation before adequate radiographs and definitive examination. Appropriate measures must be taken to stabilize the cervical spine, and a neurologic examination must be done before RSI. Ideally, the RSI technique in a trauma patient requires one person to stabilize the cervical spine, one to hold cricoid pressure, and a third to intubate and supervise the airway (see Chapters 206–207).

In those exceedingly rare instances in which severe orofacial or direct laryngeal injury is present precluding ET intubation,

needle cricothyrotomy should be performed. Although surgical cricothyrotomy has been performed successfully in numerous adult series, surgical cricothyrotomy is essentially contraindicated in children under the age of 8 to 10 years and needle cricothyrotomy would be the only alternative (14,21). Because the child can almost always be ventilated by bag-mask techniques, even with severe laryngeal injury, needle cricothyrotomy should be a procedure of last resort.

CIRCULATION

Once the airway has been secured and adequate ventilation and oxygenation is provided, attention is turned to the patient's circulation. The major goals are to assess overall circulatory status, including pulse and perfusion, while obtaining reliable venous access with the fewest possible complications, and controlling any internal or external hemorrhage. Assessing and treating the circulatory system corresponds closely to an accurate assessment of the presence and degree of shock in the pediatric patient.

The initial assessment of the overall circulatory status of pediatric multiple trauma patients involves determining the patient's heart rate and perfusion. Although tachycardia is a normal response to hypovolemia in both adult and pediatric patients, reliance on the tachycardic response is much more profound in children than in adults. In infants, stroke volume is essentially fixed and maintaining cardiac output becomes much more dependent on heart rate (8). Charts with age-specific norms should be available and easily visible in the resuscitation room. (Chapter 204, "General Approach to the Pediatric Emergency Patient," Table 204.2) In general, any heart rate over 140 to 150 in a child over 1 year of age mandates close attention.

Looking for a low blood pressure is less useful for identification of shock than in adults. Children tend to remain in compensated shock much longer than adults and are more likely to maintain a normal blood pressure in the face of significant blood loss. The formula 70 + (2 times age in years) = systolic blood pressure for children over the age of one is a good marker to gauge the lower limit of blood pressure. Any children below this should be considered hypotensive and in decompensated shock until proven otherwise (8). It should be emphasized that a normal blood pressure in a child does not exclude shock. Hypotension is a late finding (see Chapter 208, "Shock and Vascular Access in Children").

Assessing the child's overall tissue perfusion lies at the heart of the recognition and early diagnosis of shock. Basic measures of peripheral perfusion include assessment of capillary refill and pallor of the mucous membranes. However, capillary refill time is easily affected by the ambient temperature and may be an unreliable indicator of shock. Likewise, pallor is generally only seen with profound blood loss. Indicators of central perfusion are specific measures of total peripheral resistance and include diastolic blood pressure and pulse pressure, maintenance of central nervous system (CNS) perfusion, and measures of renal blood flow (urine output). Level of consciousness is generally an excellent clue to central perfusion in young children; however, because concurrent TBI is common in children with serious multisystem trauma, and measuring urine output requires at least 30 to 60 minutes to ensure accuracy—blood pressure, the quality of central and peripheral pulses, and tachycardia may be the only initially reliable indicators. Even then, normal vital signs do not exclude the possibility of compensated shock (6).

Clues to the presence of an early shock state may be subtle and difficult to appreciate in children and a high index of suspicion should be maintained. The earliest finding of shock in pediatric patients is tachycardia. It should be remembered that children often move from a state of compensated to decompensated shock abruptly; once clear, unequivocal signs of shock are visible, the rate of deterioration may be dramatic and even irreversible if not immediately corrected. A rapid infusion of 20 ml/kg of a crystalloid solution (normal saline or lactated Ringer solution) is given over 0 to 20 minutes as the situation warrants. This bolus may be given by intravenous push with a 60cc syringe in extreme circumstances until blood becomes available. Once two crystalloid boluses have been given, if the child remains hypotensive, they likely will require an immediate transfusion. A single "unit" equivalent in pediatric patients is generally considered to be 10cc/kg of warmed packed red blood cells. Inadequate volume resuscitation is one of the leading causes of preventable mortality in pediatric trauma victims (8). Strict attention is paid to preinfusion and postinfusion parameters to assess the patient's response to fluid therapy. Other causes of hypotension should be sought out simultaneously: tension pneumothorax, pericardial tamponade, and neurogenic shock.

Venous Access

Rapid, efficient venous access is one of the most challenging problems facing the emergency physician responsible for caring for pediatric multiple trauma victims. Alternatives include peripheral venous catheters, intraosseous infusion, peripheral venous cutdown, and percutaneous central venous access. One should select the route that is the most rapid and yet involves the fewest possible complications for the child as guided by the urgency of the situation.

In most cases, the pediatric patient will be well served by the initial placement of one or two peripheral venous catheters whenever possible. In a truly emergent situation, if this is not successful within 90 seconds, an intraosseous (IO) line should be placed immediately in the proximal tibia or distal femur (see Chapter 208, "Shock and Vascular Access in Children"). If IO placement is unsuccessful, one must decide whether to pursue central venous cannulation (generally via the femoral vein) or peripheral venous cutdown.

HEAD INJURY

Because the primary survey is a resuscitative survey of the critically injured patient, assessment of the extent of head injury is secondary to maintaining a patent airway with adequate ventilation and ensuring adequate central and peripheral perfusion. Clearly, providing the "ABCs" is critical to the survival of head-injured children.

During the primary survey, the goal is simply to assess the *general* level of injury, and the best way to assess overall CNS injury is the patient's level of consciousness. At this stage, the AVPU mnemonic is preferred over the Glasgow coma scale (GCS) until there is time for a more in-depth evaluation:

A: **A**lert
V: Responsive to **V**erbal stimuli
P: Responsive to **P**ainful stimuli
U: **U**nresponsive

By using this brief, simple assessment the emergency physician can gain a sense of whether significant CNS injury is present. In general, a patient who responds only to painful stimuli or does not respond at all should be presumed to have a major head injury. In addition to assessing the overall level of consciousness, the examiner should quickly check for the size and reactivity of the pupils and the presence of any posturing or lateralizing findings. Failure to briefly check peripheral neuromuscular function in all four extremities before rapid sequence intubation may re-

sult in delayed recognition of critical spinal or CNS lesions. A more detailed neurologic examination may be performed in the secondary survey.

When significant brain injury is noted, secondary injury and outcome are closely related to a stable respiratory and hemodynamic status. The brain of the young child and infant differ from that of the adult. The higher water content, incomplete myelinization, and biomechanical vulnerability to impact and shearing injuries make the young child more likely to suffer diffuse brain injury. Outcome may be as dependent on meticulous management of the injured child's cardiopulmonary status as the primary brain trauma itself. Hypoxia and hypercarbia from inadequate ventilation increase cerebral blood flow and worsen cerebral edema in TBI, while hyperventilation may cause significant reactive vasoconstriction, and has little role in the treatment of pediatric TBI except in the setting of impending herniation (9,15). On the other hand, even a transiently low blood pressure lowers cerebral blood flow and worsens ischemic injury. Cerebral hypoperfusion is common in the first 24 hours and is associated with a poor outcome (4) (see Chapter 210, "Head Trauma").

SECONDARY SURVEY

After an overall survey of the patient's respiratory, circulatory, and neurologic status, the patient is fully undressed for an adequate secondary survey. Although it is important to ensure that the child is undressed rapidly and completely, infants and small children are especially vulnerable to hypothermia and may require warming lights or blankets to maintain their body temperature. Young children have a greater body surface area for weight and are much more vulnerable to heat loss. While mild hypothermia may be beneficial in TBI, study results are mixed and this is not the standard of practice at this time (4,15). While temperature is the forgotten vital sign in a critical resuscitation and it should be followed closely.

Trauma is a dynamic process and because the condition of pediatric patients may deteriorate rapidly and because they often present with subtle signs and symptoms, the elements of the primary survey must continually be reassessed over the course of the patient's initial ED resuscitation. The examiner must keep updated on the status of the airway, breathing, circulation, response to shock therapy, neurologic disability, and core body temperature.

Early in the secondary survey, a focused history is taken from the patient, the family, or the paramedics who brought the patient to the ED. This may be done concurrently with the physical examination by another clinician. The history should include all events leading up to the accident, the mechanism/biomechanics of the injury, initial status, and clinical course during transportation. The AMPLE mnemonic provides a quick outline of vital information (2):

A: Allergies
M: Medications
P: Past medical history
L: Last meal eaten before injury
E: Events preceding the injury

The secondary survey is usually performed in a head-to-toe fashion, which allows for an easily followed approach that adheres to protocol. Although head injury is the most common cause of death in pediatric multiple trauma victims, one must not neglect closer *reassessment* of the cardiorespiratory system during the secondary survey. Providing oxygenation and ventilation, as well as central perfusion, addresses the earliest threats to life and meticulous attention to vitals is necessary for optimal outcomes in traumatic brain injury. Finding a striking and severe injury during the evaluation should not cause the physician to pause in the evaluation, except to treat life-threatening injuries. Multiple system injuries are common in pediatric patients, and a detailed, systematic evaluation of each body system is necessary.

Head and Neck

The secondary survey should begin with an in-depth evaluation of the child's head and neck. Any signs of obvious trauma are noted. Bleeding is stemmed with firm, direct pressure. Mucous membranes are examined for color and hydration status. The eyes are examined for pupil size and reactivity, the presence of hyphema, and easily overlooked foreign bodies (e.g., glass fragments). The bones and soft tissues of the midface are palpated for evidence of fracture or instability. Raccoon eyes or the postauricular Battle sign indicates a likely basilar skull fracture. The tympanic membranes should be examined for perforation or hemotympanum. The patient's upper airway, including the nasopharynx and oropharynx, is examined for blood or tooth fragments. Blood or clear fluid (CSF) from the nares should be noted. In children younger than age 2, one should carefully examine the fontanels as they may reveal important information regarding intracranial pressure. Tracheal deviation and distended neck veins may be a sign of tension pneumothorax or cardiac tamponade and are both more difficult to determine in children because of their inherent anatomic differences. Examination of the occiput in the supine, collared child is easily forgotten.

Evaluation for cervical spine injury should include detailed information regarding the mechanism of injury. Unrestrained victims of high-speed motor vehicle crashes, automobile–pedestrian collisions, and falls from greater than 10 to 15 ft are all at higher risk of cervical spine injury. Muscular spasm seems to be less common or more difficult to assess in young children. Since children with spinal cord injury may have no radiographic abnormality, therefore when focal splinting is present, the neck should remain immobilized, even if the cross-table lateral cervical spine film is normal. Early immobilization is also good clinical practice if there is a truly high-risk mechanism and the child is not verbal (see Chapter 211).

Chest

Examination of both the chest and the abdomen should follow the "look, listen, and feel" rule. One of the most neglected aspects of the chest examination in children is simply looking at the patient's spontaneous respirations and chest wall movement. Impaired respiratory excursion may be due to chest wall contusion and splinting, rib fracture, or tension pneumothorax. Because the chest wall in children is much more compliant, it is not uncommon for forces applied to the external thorax to be transmitted internally to underlying structures without any external or radiographic manifestations of chest wall damage. While rib fractures are seen less frequently in children, underlying pulmonary contusion is much more common (9). When multiple rib fractures are present, they are highly correlated with the presence of other intrathoracic injuries. Other findings statistically correlated with intrathoracic injury include hypotension, elevated respiratory rate, low GCS, femur fracture, and abnormal findings on chest auscultation (9).

Breath sounds are easily transmitted across the child's small, resilient chest, so the presence of normal lung sounds is less reassuring in children than in adults. Nonetheless, the chest should still be carefully auscultated; when present, abnormal breath sounds have a high predictive value of thoracic injury (9). Parenchymal crackles or diminished breath sounds may indicate the presence of hemothorax, pneumothorax, or early pulmonary contusion. Infants are at potentially increased risk of tension pneumothorax because of a pliable, easily compressed mediastinum. Hemothorax may also be found in children and should be managed with appropriately sized chest tubes and judicious surgical intervention based on weight specific bleeding criteria as noted in Chapter 212. While many traumatic intrathoracic injuries are rare in children, such as blunt aortic, esophageal, tracheal-bronchial, and diaphragmatic injuries, they have been reported and children should be evaluated and worked up in the same fashion as their adult counterparts (6). Clearly these injuries will be seen in critically ill children who have sustained massive multisystem trauma and will be found in varying combinations.

Abdomen and Pelvis

Examination of the abdomen in children is begun by carefully looking for evidence of abrasions, ecchymosis, splinting, or distention. The seat belt sign is a marker for possible intestinal perforation or a Chance fracture of the lumbar spine. Both injuries are difficult to identify and require a high index of suspicion. Children who are inappropriately restrained with a seat belt that rides high across the lower abdomen, rather than the pelvis, are most at risk for these injuries. As booster seats become more widespread, the incidence of these injuries should decline.

The most helpful aspect of the pediatric abdominal examination is palpation (10). Verbal children should be asked where they hurt, and the examination is then begun away from that site. The child should be reassured or distracted as much as possible, and the examination should be performed gently while closely observing the child's face and reaction. Young children are frequently frightened and verbal responses to questions regarding either the presence or absence of pain should be interpreted cautiously. Spontaneous complaints of pain should be taken very seriously. Repeat examination of the abdomen may be necessary for accurate assessment and may reveal significant findings missed on the initial exam.

Stable children with blunt abdominal injury are evaluated with abdominal/pelvic CT scanning the same as their adult counterparts. Many clinicians have a low threshold for imaging young children, as they are considered relatively unreliable historians, or as with adults, if they have an altered level of consciousness (10). Patients with microscopic hematuria (>50 RBC/hpf) should also undergo imaging to detect renal injury (see Chapters 228, "Hematuria," and 212, "Chest and Abdominal Trauma"). The two most common intraabdominal injuries are blunt hepatic and splenic lacerations and the vast majority of these may be managed nonoperatively with close observation and judicious blood transfusion (6,10). Pancreatic and duodenal injuries, e.g., hematoma and perforation, should be sought out in children who suffer bicycle handle bar injuries, a relatively unique form of childhood trauma.

For the child who is unstable or who has retroperitoneal vascular disruption, penetrating intraperitoneal abdominal wounds, or documented perforation of a hollow viscous, a trip to the operating room is indicated. However, some children will have a negative work up and mild to moderate persistent abdominal discomfort without a clear indication for surgical intervention. Due to the low sensitivity of physical examination and diagnostic testing for bowel injury, these children should at the very least receive surgical consultation and probably warrant hospital admission for observation.

After the abdomen is examined, the bony pelvis and the perineum are inspected. The entire bony pelvis is palpated and compressed for tenderness or instability. While hemodynamically significant pelvic fractures are less common in children, like rib fractures, they are indicative of high-impact forces and other injuries should be looked for. The hips are gently flexed as this may detect more subtle pelvic fractures. Examination of the urethral meatus for blood, evidence of scrotal hematoma or swelling should be noted, and a rectal examination performed in children with demonstrated or suspected pelvic injury or direct trauma to the groin.

Peripheral Musculoskeletal Evaluation

The examiner should carefully palpate the entire bony skeleton for tenderness or swelling. All bony areas are examined visually for deformity, abrasion, contusion, or hematoma. Significant bleeding should be controlled with pressure dressings, avoiding tourniquets or blind clamping with hemostats. Close attention should be paid to distal perfusion in limbs with obvious deformities or fractures, identifying potential arterial disruption.

Any splinting or asymmetric activity of the extremities should be noted, particularly in preverbal children, as this may be a subtle sign of injury. In otherwise normal-appearing extremities, range-of-motion maneuvers may identify undetected injuries. Finally, the child should be logrolled while holding in-line cervical stabilization for inspection and palpation of the back. The examiner should evaluate and document the pulse and neuromotor status of each extremity.

Neurologic Examination

In completing the secondary survey, a more detailed neurologic examination is done. Close attention to the history and mechanism of injury is critical in assessing the likelihood of a neurologic injury. The pupils are examined for size, symmetry, and reactivity. Focal abnormalities are indicative of underlying CNS injury and remind the physician of the urgency of radiologic evaluation and neurosurgical consultation.

The integrity of the spinal cord should be assessed. Asymmetries in motor activity or strength, proximal and distal, should be noted, particularly in the absence of obvious extremity injury. Assessing only grip strength and plantar flexion, allow the risk of missing a central cord syndrome. Absent or asymmetric reflexes and rectal tone may be informative in the unresponsive child.

By far the most critical aspect in the evaluation of the head-injured patient is the overall level of consciousness. The Glasgow coma scale (GCS) is the most widely applied and demonstrably reliable method of describing this. The GCS assesses patient alertness with regard to eye opening, verbal, and motor responses to stimulus. This scale has been extensively evaluated and found to correlate extremely well with outcome (15). In preverbal children, a modified GCS is sometimes used (see Chapter 210). Patients with a GCS score of 12 or less are considered to have a potentially serious head injury and neurosurgical consultation is obtained after ensuring adequate ventilation, oxygenation, and perfusion. As in adults, a GCS score of 8 is considered an indication for ET intubation and possibly monitoring of intracranial pressure (8,15). The primary goal of treatment for severe TBI is the prevention of secondary insults. The marked increase in morbidity and mortality experienced by children with TBI who have even minor additional extracranial injuries underscores the importance of critical management techniques of multisystem trauma (23).

Laboratory Studies and Radiologic Evaluation

A complete set of trauma laboratory studies should be ordered on any patient in shock with an altered level of consciousness or evidence of multisystem injury. Studies include bedside glucose testing, complete blood count; electrolyte panel with creatinine; microscopic urinalysis; coagulation panel, and type and

screen or type and cross-match with the knowledge that the total blood volume of a young child is 70cc/kg (3). An arterial blood gas should not be neglected in intubated patients. The interpretation of these labs may differ in children; for instance, while imaging the renal system in adults may depend on the presence of gross hematuria, finding microscopic hematuria on urinalysis is a well-recognized indication in children (10). In teenagers, alcohol or other intoxicants may contribute to an altered level of consciousness, so appropriate toxicologic studies are indicated. The need for additional laboratory studies should be guided by the patient's physical findings and clinical course. With severe, multiple trauma victims, coagulopathy and acidosis may become life-threatening and should be sought after and aggressively treated.

Radiography has an important role in the management of the pediatric trauma victim. Vital signs and the physical examination are the clinician's first resource in caring for all injured pediatric patients; radiographic studies should simply confirm or verify suspicions and should be ordered in a focused and thoughtful manner. In evaluating the pediatric multiple trauma victim, chest, pelvis, and cervical spine radiographs have the highest priority, while extremity films are less time-dependent. A lower threshold should be maintained to obtain these films in younger children because of the inability to use symptom-driven criteria and the greater possibility of internal injuries in the absence of visible external manifestations.

Additional radiographic studies, such as computed tomography of the head, chest, and abdomen, and vascular contrast studies, should be guided by the patient's physical findings, mechanism of injury, clinical course, and the availability of such resources. It should be noted that while focused abdominal sonography for trauma (FAST) is an effective method of identifying serious intraabdominal injury in adults, its use in children has been found to be less sensitive. A FAST exam may be useful to identify serious intraabdominal injury in the unstable multiple trauma child, however, it should not be relied upon to exclude such injuries and is currently inferior to CT scanning as a diagnostic modality (20). A more extensive treatment of chest and abdominal trauma may be found in Chapter 212.

DISPOSITION AND DEFINITIVE CARE

Whether the pediatric multiple trauma victim is resuscitated in a general hospital ED or a pediatric trauma center, the best available resources for the child's care should be implemented at the earliest possible time. Immediate surgical consultation is required for any pediatric multiple trauma victim with either single-system or multisystem injury or in whom there is sustained alteration of the level of consciousness. Although an increasing number of pediatric multiple trauma victims are being managed without surgery, this in no way implies that the evaluation and care of such patients be handled without bedside surgical input. Indeed, the decision whether to operate is ultimately a surgical decision.

Indications for Admission and Transfer to a Pediatric Center

Any child with a significant head injury and major cardiovascular instability should be admitted to the pediatric intensive care unit. A pediatric trauma score was devised to assist pediatric surgeons and emergency physicians in calculating injury severity in the prehospital setting. This trauma score is helpful in deciding which patients should be transported to a pediatric trauma center and also which patients warrant hospital

TABLE 209.2.   Checklist for Sudden Deterioration

AIRWAY

Adequate airway position?
Adequate tidal volume?
Adequate rate?
Pneumothorax?
Tension pneumothorax?

ENDOTRACHEAL TUBE

Dislodged?
Plugged?
Right main stem bronchus?

INTRAVENOUS ACCESS

Functional?
Adequate size?
Medications infusing?

UNRECOGNIZED BLEEDING

Pelvis
Chest
Abdomen
Thighs
Retroperitoneum

UNRECOGNIZED INJURIES

CRITICAL INTERVENTIONS

- Complete the primary survey before starting the secondary assessment
- Have the proper equipment available including an endotracheal tube that is one size smaller and one size larger than predicted
- Reassess using the "ABCs" whenever a patient decompensates or has a change in status
- Try to perform a brief neurologic examination prior to performing rapid sequence intubation
- Do not wait for a C-spine radiograph in order to intubate the patient

COMMON PITFALLS

✔ Failure to recognize that trauma is a dynamic process and that failure to continuously reevaluate the multiple trauma patient may lead to a poor outcome

✔ Lack of advance preparation and organization of equipment, medications, resources, and personnel will result in a chaotic resuscitation with the potential for poor outcomes

✔ Inexperience and/or discomfort with children may be distracting to an otherwise competent physician and lead to a disorganized approach, missing frequently subtle but important details in preverbal and uncooperative children

---

admission (19) (Table 209.2). Overnight observation should be considered for any child with significant head injury who has not completely returned to baseline or has sustained multiple trauma with a negative work up for significant, life-threatening injury. This continued observation of the child allows a clear delineation of the extent and severity of injuries and possible identification of injuries missed on the initial evaluation, such as small bowel perforation.

The decision to transfer a pediatric multiple trauma patient to a higher level of care depends largely on the patient's stability, identified injuries, and on the availability of resources at the closest pediatric trauma center versus the resources of the referring institution. In some cases, severe intraabdominal bleeding may require immediate operative intervention to obtain appropriate hemostasis and preclude immediate transfer. However, such cases represent a small minority of pediatric trauma cases. For that reason, it is important to consult with the appropriate pediatric trauma centers within each EDs geographic area to ensure that the initial resuscitation reflects the standards of the nearby center. As much as possible, the initial resuscitative and management approach in the ED should reflect standards similar to those of the tertiary pediatric critical care center to which the patient may be transferred. The overall outcome of the pediatric patient depends less on how long it takes the child to reach the pediatric critical care center than it does on ensuring that the regional center's expertise is applied as early as possible at the referring hospital (16).

Currently, there are two forms of recognition as a designated pediatric trauma center: one is individual state designation and the other is an external verification process through the American College of Surgeons. Transfer and management of pediatric trauma at dedicated trauma centers with pediatric expertise have been shown to significantly improve outcome, particularly in children with severe internal or CNS injuries (5). This improvement in outcome seems to be concentrated in critically ill, yet salvageable trauma victims (5,16).

References

1. American Academy of Pediatrics, Committee on Pediatric Emergency Medicine and American College of Emergency Physicians, Pediatric Committee. Care of children in the emergency department: guidelines for preparedness. *Ann Emerg Med* 2001;37:423–427.
2. American College of Surgeons Committee on Trauma. *Advance Trauma Life Support*. 6th ed. Chicago: 1997.
3. Barkin AZ, ed. *Emergency Pediatrics: a Guide to Ambulatory Care*. 6th ed. St. Louis: Mosby, Inc., 1999.
4. Bayri H, Kochanek PM, Clark RSB. Traumatic brain injury in infants and children: mechanisms of secondary damage and treatment in the intensive care unit. *Crit Care Clin* 2003;19:529–549.
5. Cooper A, Barlow B, Di Scala C, et al. Efficacy of pediatric trauma care: results of a population-based study. *J Ped Surg* 1993;28:299–305.
6. Garcia VF, Brown RL. Pediatric trauma beyond the brain. *Crit Care Clin* 2003; 19:552–561.
7. Gausche M, Lewis RJ, Stratton SJ, et al. Effect of out-of-hospital pediatric endotracheal intubation on survival and neurological outcome: a controlled clinical trial. *JAMA* 2000;283:783–790.
8. Hazinski MF, ed. *PALS Provider Manual*. Dallas: American Heart Association, 2002.
9. Holmes JF, Sokolove PE, Brant WE, Kuppermann N. A clinical decision rule for identifying children with thoracic injuries after blunt torso trauma. *Ann Emerg Med* 2002;39:492–499.
10. Holmes JF, Sokolove PE, Brant WE, et al. Identification of children with intraabdominal injuries after blunt trauma. *Ann Emerg Med* 2002;39:500–509.
11. Lubitz DS, Seidel JS, Chameides L, et al. A rapid method for estimating weight and resuscitation drug dosages from length in the pediatric age group. *Ann Emerg Med* 1988;17:576.
12. Luten RC, Wears RL, Broselow J, et al. Length-based endotracheal tube sizing for pediatric resuscitation. *Ann Emerg Med* 1990;19:476.
13. Luten RC. Pediatric Airway Techniques. In: Walls RM, ed. *Manual of emergency airway management*. Philadelphia: Lippincott Williams & Wilkins, 2000;105–111.
14. Luten RC. The pediatric patient. In: Walls RM, ed. *Manual of emergency airway management*. Philadelphia: Lippincott Williams & Wilkins, 2000;143–152.
15. Mazzola CA, Adelson PD. Critical care management of head trauma in children. *Crit Care Med* 2002;30:S393–S401.
16. Nakayama DK, Copes WS, Sacco W. Differences in trauma care among pediatric and nonpediatric trauma centers. *J Ped Surg* 27;1992:427–431.
17. National Center for Injury Prevention and Control. Available at: http://www.cdc.gov/ncipc/wisqars/. Accessed Nov 19, 2003.
18. Proctor MR. Spinal Cord Injury. *Crit Care Med* 2002;30:S489–S499.
19. Ramenofsky ML, Ramenofsky MB, Jurkovich IJ, et al. The predictive validity of the Pediatric Trauma Score. *J Trauma* 1988;4:1038.
20. Rothrock SG, Green SM, Morgan R. Abdominal trauma in infants and children: Prompt identification and early management of serious and life-threatening injuries. Part 1: injury patterns and initial assessment. *Ped Emerg Care* 2000;16: 106–112.

21. Santamaria JP. Office-based emergencies. In: APLS: *The pediatric emergency medicine resource*. 4th ed. Sudbury: Jones and Bartlett Publishers, 2003:269–321.
22. Skippen P, Seear M, Poskitt K, et al. Effect of hyperventilation on regional cerebral blood flow in head-injured children. *Crit Care Med* 1997;25:1402–1409.
23. Tepas III JJ, DiScala C, Ramenofsky ML, Barlow B. Mortality and head injury: the pediatric perspective. *J Ped Surg* 1990;25:92–96.

CHAPTER 210
Head Trauma

Dee Hodge III and Kimberly S. Quayle

Trauma is the leading cause of death in children older than 1 year in the United States; 75% or more of these deaths are associated with significant central nervous system (CNS) injury (25). Approximately 150,000 to 300,000 children are hospitalized each year as a result of head injury (3,15). Falls are the leading cause of head injuries in children, especially in those younger than 5 years of age.

Motor-vehicle collisions with bicyclists and pedestrians become more significant in school-age children, while motor-vehicle occupant injuries, assaults, and sports injuries are more common in the adolescent age group. Motor-vehicle collisions are the leading cause of severe and fatal head injuries for all pediatric age groups, except for infants, for whom nonaccidental trauma is the most common cause of serious injury (1,32).

HEAD INJURY CLASSIFICATION

Anatomy

Figure 210.1 shows the cross-sectional anatomy of the head and associated CNS injuries (26). The types of injury can be grouped by location.

Injuries to the scalp are the most common complication of head injury. These injuries include swelling, contusions, and lacerations. Causes of swelling of the scalp must be differentiated. Subgaleal hematomas are common in children. In neonates, subgaleal hematomas present with diffuse swelling that does not transilluminate. This presentation differs from that of the cephalohematoma, which is focal swelling. Porencephalic or leptomeningeal cysts also present as focal swelling, but these have increased transillumination.

The presence of skull fractures means that significant force has been applied to the cranium, but the presence of fractures does not guarantee intracranial hemorrhage. Likewise, intracranial hemorrhage is seen in the absence of skull fracture. Seventy-five percent of skull fractures are linear fractures. Basilar skull fractures involve the frontal, ethmoid, sphenoid, temporal, and occipital bones. Signs of basilar skull fracture include "raccoon eyes," the Battle sign, cerebrospinal fluid (CSF) otorrhea or rhinorrhea, and hematotympanum. Compound fractures, those with laceration of the scalp, carry a risk of complicating infection of the CNS.

Depressed skull fractures are seen when force is applied over a small surface area. A depressed fracture greater than a few mil-

limeters needs surgical elevation. Diastatic fractures are unique to children and are seen in the first 4 years of life. These fractures represent separation of the sutures. "Growing" fractures are caused by the formation of porencephalic or leptomeningeal cysts in the site of linear or diastatic fractures. These cysts occur during the first 6 months after injury and are most often seen in children younger than 3 years of age.

Traumatic intracranial hemorrhage includes subdural, epidural, and subarachnoid hemorrhages. Subdural hemorrhages occur 5 to 10 times as often as epidural hemorrhages. There is a relatively slow onset of symptoms because these are usually venous in origin. Signs and symptoms of the hemorrhage are secondary to increased intracranial pressure. In infants, these hemorrhages may present with seizures. Although rare in children, the mortality rate of 10% to 20% associated with epidural hematomas makes their early recognition essential. The usual presentation is one of rapid and focal neurologic deterioration. The classic triad is of concussion with an intervening lucent phase, followed by deterioration. These hemorrhages usually represent a tear in the middle meningeal artery. In the child, hemorrhages from the meningeal and diploic veins are also seen. Although these hemorrhages are always associated with fractures in adults, this association is observed in only 50% of the pediatric patients. Subarachnoid hemorrhages are a common computed tomographic (CT) finding in severe pediatric head trauma.

Penetrating head injuries are less common in children. Puncture wounds are seen with lawn darts, other missile-type projectiles, and dog-bite wounds in young children. These injuries are often associated with lacerations of the brain.

Contusions and lacerations of the cerebral cortex are often adjacent to sites of significant focal impact or at locations that predispose the brain to accelerative forces. Coup injuries represent contusions directly beneath the site of impact, while contrecoup injury occurs against the skull surface opposite the site of impact. The signs are often focal and are associated with local swelling on a CT scan. These injuries are not necessarily the cause of unconsciousness.

Concussions are a functional injury. While there is no universally accepted definition, concussions are characterized by deficits in one or more of the following: cognition, mental status, memory, attention, and coordination (21). Associated symptoms include anorexia, vomiting, pallor, or abnormal behavior lasting up to several hours. There are several grading systems used to classify the severity of concussion. The grading system of the American Academy of Neurology is shown in Table 210.1 (2,5,21). Alternative presentations in infants and younger children include lethargy, irritability, and vomiting not associated with loss of consciousness. These symptoms usually subside within 48 hours. Headache, impaired memory and concentration may last up to 6 months (i.e., post concussive syndrome). A second impact syndrome may occur when a second head injury is sustained before symptoms of the first concussion have fully cleared (9).

Pathophysiology

The types of injuries can also be classified as primary and secondary. Primary injuries occur at the time of impact and cannot be prevented. These include fractures, concussions, contusions, lacerations, and neuronal or vascular injury on impact. Secondary injuries occur after the initial impact and include cerebral hyperemia, vascular autoregulatory dysfunction, cerebral edema, hemorrhagic lesions, and seizures. These CNS reactive lesions are either preventable or may be minimized by good medical management. If untreated, these lesions lead to mechanical distortion, ischemia, and hypoxic injury.

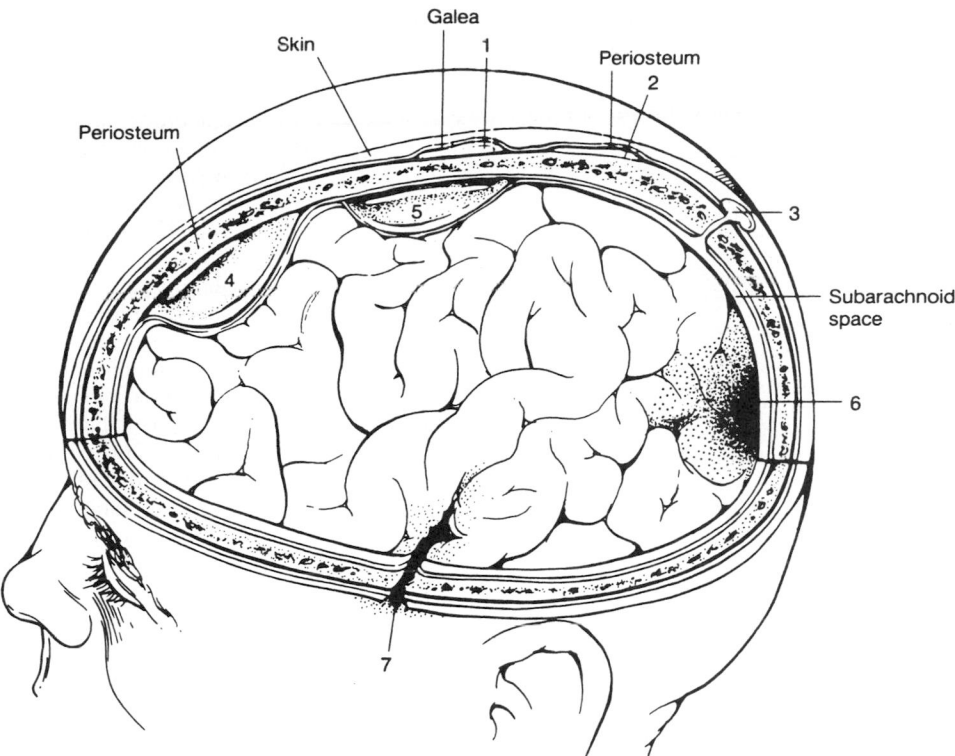

Figure 210.1. Cross-sectional anatomy of the head and associated central nervous system injuries. *1,* Subgaleal hematoma; *2,* cephalohematoma; *3,* porencephalic cyst; *4,* epidural hematoma; *5,* subdural hematoma; *6,* cerebral contusion; *7,* cerebral laceration. (Modified from Rosman NP, Oppenheimer EY, O'Conner JF. Emergency management of pediatric head injuries. *Emerg Med Clin North Am* 1983;1:141 with permission.)

Cerebral edema and increased intracranial pressure account for a large degree of the morbidity in the pediatric head trauma patient. Injury occurs because the volume of the cranium is fixed. The relationship is expressed by the following formula:

$$\text{Volume CSF} + \text{volume blood} + \text{volume brain} + \text{volume other} = \text{constant.}$$

An increase in the volume of one means a reduction in the size of the others. A buffering capacity is important in the early stages of increasing pressure. With an increase in brain volume or a mass lesion, CSF is displaced, followed by a decrease in blood flow. Once the intracranial volume increases beyond the buffering capacity, the intracranial pressure increases and the brain subsequently herniates (12).

Differences in the growth and maturation of head structures account for the different injuries seen in children and adults. The prevalence of head trauma in children is due partly because the young child's proportionally larger head size and weight give a higher center of gravity. The cranial vault is more pliable and less dense in young infants. The open fontanelle and sutures in the younger child, along with the larger subarachnoid space and cisterns, offer a greater extracellular space. This allows better tol-

erance of expanding mass lesions, up to a point. The dura mater's tight adherence to the skull accounts for the lower incidence of mass hemorrhages in children (less than 30%, compared with 40% to 50% in adults) and the variable and occasional subacute presentation of epidural hemorrhage. Because myelination continues for the first 6 months of life, subcortical white matter tears are often present in this age group, as opposed to the contusions and hemorrhages seen in toddlers. Finally, cerebral edema and increased intracranial pressure as a result of severe head injury occur in 80% of pediatric cases, as opposed to 40% to 50% of the cases in adults (1,16,23).

EMERGENCY DEPARTMENT EVALUATION

As with most emergencies, evaluation, assessment, and management is a multifaceted, ongoing process until the patient is stabilized and appropriate disposition is made. Although the classic systematic approach of history, physical examination, radiographic evaluation, and management are presented here, these often occur simultaneously.

The history is often obtained from an adult caretaker who may or may not have been present at the time of injury. One must elicit and document details of the accident, including height of fall and type of surface struck, and include history of loss of consciousness, memory loss, disorientation, and visual disturbance. A brief seizure at the time of impact may be part of the history but may have no diagnostic or prognostic significance, in contrast to seizures that occur after injury. Vomiting is another useful symptom, especially when it is protracted or occurs more than 6 hours after injury.

The physical examination should not be limited to the head; significant physical findings may be found elsewhere. The initial respiratory rate and pattern are noted, and pulse and blood pressure are measured. The examiner should quickly evaluate the level of consciousness using the mnemonic AVPU (*a*lert, responds to *v*oice, responds to *p*ainful stimuli, *u*nconscious). The

TABLE 210.1. Grading System for Severity of Concussion

Grade 1	Grade 2	Grade 3
Transient confusion	Transient confusion	Any LOC
No LOC	No LOC	
Symptoms or mental status change (MSE) resolve < 15 min	Symptoms or MSE last ≥ 15 min	

LOC = Loss of consciousness
(Adapted from American Academy of Neurology. Practice parameter: The management of concussion in sports. Neurology 1997;48:581–585.)

TABLE 210.2.   Glasgow Coma Scale Modified
for the Preverbal Child

EYE OPENING

Spontaneous	4
To voice	3
To pain	2
None	1

VERBAL RESPONSE

Coos, babbles	5
Irritable cries	4
Cries to pain	3
Moans to pain	2
None	1

MOTOR RESPONSE

Spontaneous movements	6
Withdraws to touch	5
Withdraws to pain	4
Abnormal flexion	3
Extensor response	2
None	1
E + V + M = 3 to 15	

From Raimondi AJ, Hirschauer J. Head injury in the infant and toddler.
Childs Brain *1984;11:12.*

Glasgow coma scale, a fast, objective, and reproducible scoring system, evaluates the best eye opening, verbal, and motor response of the patient and has been modified for the preverbal child (Table 210.2) (18). Ocular signs, including pupil size and response and extraocular movement, should be checked, and an early funduscopic examination, looking for retinal hemorrhages and papilledema, should be done. The head is examined for signs of trauma, including scalp lacerations and abrasions, hematomas, hematotympanum, the Battle sign, raccoon eyes, and CSF leaks from the ears or nose. A complete neurologic examination should be part of the secondary survey. This should also include a search for signs of injury at other sites (23).

Recommendations for imaging remain somewhat controversial; however, most experts do not advocate routine skull radiographs in the evaluation of head-injured children. Although the risk for intracranial injury is increased with the presence of a skull fracture, as many as 50% of intracranial injuries occur without skull fractures (8,14,17,22). Head CT has become the imaging modality of choice for the evaluation of possible intracranial injury, including epidural and subdural hematomas, and parenchymal contusions and edema. The head CT can also delineate facial, orbital, and sinus injuries, as well as linear and depressed skull fractures.

Clinical features, such as altered level of consciousness, focal neurologic deficits, palpable skull depressions, seizures, and signs of a basilar skull fracture, indicate children at higher risk for intracranial injuries (8,18,22). These children should undergo head CT imaging. Recently published data indicated that symptoms of headache and vomiting were also predictive of traumatic brain injury, and should also prompt a head CT scan (20). In 1999, the American Academy of Pediatrics published a practice parameter for management of children with minor closed head injury (6). The parameter recommended no imaging studies for children with minor head injury and no loss of consciousness, and a choice of no imaging with close observation or head CT scans for children with minor injury and a brief loss of consciousness. Head CT imaging should be considered in symptomatic children

who are neurologically normal; however, careful observation by a reliable caretaker may be another option.

The presentation of intracranial injury in infants may be very subtle, often occurring without symptoms (11,13,22). Unlike older children, the great majority of intracranial injuries in infants occur in association with a skull fracture. Moreover, most skull fractures in infants are associated with scalp hematomas or contusions (1,29). In asymptomatic infants with scalp hematomas, skull radiographs may serve as a screen for serious head injury. If a skull fracture is present, these infants should undergo head CT imaging. Any symptomatic infant should undergo head CT imaging. In 2001, Schutzman and colleagues published a detailed guideline for management of head-injured children younger than 2 years (28). Infants with depressed mental status, focal neurologic findings, signs of depressed or basilar skull fracture, seizure, irritability, an acute skull fracture, bulging fontanelle, excessive or persistent vomiting, and loss of consciousness longer than one minute were considered high risk for intracranial injury and should undergo head CT scan (28). Infants with other symptoms or a high energy mechanism should also be considered for head CT scan (28).

EMERGENCY DEPARTMENT MANAGEMENT

Major Head Trauma

Patients with major head trauma are at the highest risk for intracranial injury. They may have findings of depressed level of consciousness, focal neurologic signs, decreasing level of consciousness, penetrating injury or palpable depressed skull fracture, or a combination of these problems.

Airway and cervical spine control are critical in these patients. Airway patency is assessed and any obstructions are removed. Once the airway has been opened, ventilatory effort is assessed and assisted with bag-valve-mask ventilation in an attempt to keep the PaO_2 above 100 mm Hg. Good cerebral oxygenation is necessary for the prevention of secondary injury. Cricoid pressure is useful to avoid regurgitation and aspiration. A secure airway must be maintained. Endotracheal intubation should be considered in children with a Glasgow coma scale score less than 8; rapid-sequence intubation is the method of choice in this situation. An appropriate sedative and amnestic agent (diazepam, midazolam, thiopental, or etomidate) should be administered. Etomidate is preferred in the hypotensive patient. (See Chapter 207, "Rapid-Sequence Induction in Children.")

Circulation is maintained within normal physiologic limits. Shock may be explained by large scalp lacerations in older children or epidural hemorrhage in infants, but, more commonly, the source of blood loss is elsewhere. Shock is treated with crystalloid boluses. Once normal blood pressure is established, fluids are given at one-half to two-thirds of the maintenance rates.

The goal of treatment of increased intracranial pressure is to prevent displacement (herniation) of the brain. Elevating the patient's head to 30 degrees promotes venous drainage. Controlled hyperventilation reduces cerebral blood flow by reducing arteriolar diameter. Some studies have promoted the use of moderate hyperventilation. $PaCO_2$ is maintained in the 30 mm Hg range (19,30). Diuretic therapy is used in an attempt to shift water from the brain into the vascular compartment, but these agents should be used with caution in the hypovolemic patient. Intravenous mannitol at 0.25 g/kg is generally recommended. Intracranial pressure increases initially after mannitol administration as a result of an increase in cerebral blood flow secondary to expansion of the vascular volume and increased cardiac output. Intravenous furosemide (Lasix) 0.5 to 1.0 mg/kg is useful in cases of diffuse cerebral edema.

Patients with major head trauma require emergency CT scanning as soon as they are stable enough to tolerate the procedure. Neurosurgical consultation should be obtained as soon as possible (12).

Minor Head Trauma

Children with altered mental status, focal neurologic deficit, signs of a basilar skull fracture, palpable skull depression, or seizure should undergo head CT imaging. Neurologically normal children who have a history of vomiting, headache, or loss of consciousness should be considered for head CT imaging as well. Careful observation of these children at home by a reliable caretaker may be an alternative strategy. Children with progressive or persistent symptoms should return for reevaluation and head CT imaging. Children who have a normal head CT scan after minor head injury will very rarely develop delayed intracranial sequelae (7). They can be safely discharged home for further observation. Neurologically normal children without symptoms may also be discharged home without imaging studies.

Skull radiographs are often included in the Kempe series as part of the evaluation of nonaccidental trauma and for asymptomatic infants with scalp hematomas or contusions in which abuse is suspected. Asymptomatic infants with skull fractures should have head CT imaging to exclude intracranial injury. Infants younger than 12 months who develop symptoms following head trauma should also undergo head CT imaging.

CRITICAL INTERVENTIONS

- Prompt airway management in the patient with a GCS of less than 8
- Neuroimaging should be performed in infants less than 12 months of age who are symptomatic and also in infants with skull fractures
- Appropriate removal from competitive sports after a concussion. Athletes with grade 1 concussion and no previous concussion can return to play. Individuals with grade 2 injury may return after 1 week and grade 3 after 2 weeks to a month
- Mild hyperventilation (no less than a PCO_2 of 30 mm hg) in patients with severe head injury

DISPOSITION

Neurosurgical consultation should be sought for patients with major head trauma, including those with abnormal head CT scans, altered mental status, focal neurologic deficit, penetrating injury, or depressed skull fracture. A patient with major head trauma should be stabilized and transported to a facility with a pediatric intensive care unit. The patient should be transported by personnel experienced in caring for critically ill and injured children. Vital signs and neurologic status must be followed closely. The patient's head should be elevated at 30 degrees, and adequate ventilation should be maintained in intubated patients. An intravenous infusion of dextrose 5% in an isotonic solution should be given at one-half to two-thirds of maintenance rates.

Children with minor head trauma should be hospitalized for intracranial injuries identified on the head CT and for persistent neurologic abnormality despite a normal head CT. Children with suspected child abuse and children without a reliable caretaker should also be admitted for observation. Discharge instructions for home observation following head trauma should include in-

dications to return for persistent vomiting, weakness, worsening headache, pupillary asymmetry, lethargy, or difficulty with gait or balance. Symptomatic children and children with isolated skull fractures should be seen by their physician 24 hours after discharge from the ED. In general, athletes with Grade 1 concussion and no previous concussion can return to play. Individuals with Grade 2 injury may return after 1 week and Grade 3 after 2 weeks to a month (Table 210.1) (2). Return to sport should be delayed until neuropsychologic and possible neuroimaging has been performed if one or two previous concussions. Preliminary data suggests that younger athletes have a longer recovery period from concussion. A referral to a primary care provider for systematic evaluation before return to competition is warranted (9,31).

COMMON PITFALLS

✔ Failure to recognize the protean manifestations of head injury in children. Open fontanelles and sutures in the younger child, along with larger subarachnoid space and cisterns, create a greater extracellular space thereby allowing better tolerance of expanding mass lesions up to a critical point

✔ Failure to take an adequate history, to perform a complete examination, and recognize signs of retinal hemorrhage and increased intracranial pressure. This can lead to a delay in diagnosis and treatment

✔ Failure to suspect child abuse, especially shaken-impact syndrome

✔ Failure to consider other causes of altered mental status, such as CNS infections, metabolic disorders such as hypoglycemia, and toxins, when there are no obvious signs of trauma

References

1. Adelson PD, Kochanek PM. Head injury in children. *J Child Neurol* 1998;13:2–15.
2. American Academy of Neurology. Practice parameter: The management of concussion in sports. *Neurology* 1997;48:581–585.
3. Bruce DA. Head injuries in the pediatric population. *Curr Probl Pediatr* 1990;20:61–107.
4. Cantu RC, Voy R. Second Impact Syndrome–A Risk in Any Contact Sport. *Phys Sportsmed* 1995;23:27–34.
5. Collins MW, Lovell MR, Mckeag DB. Current Issues in Managing Sports-Related Concussion. *JAMA* 1999;282:2283–2285.
6. Committee on Quality Improvement, American Academy of Pediatrics. The management of minor closed head injury in children. *Pediatrics* 1999;104:1407–1415.
7. Davis RL, Hughes M, Gubler KD, et al. The use of cranial CT scans in the triage of pediatric patients with mild head injury. *Pediatrics* 1995;95:345–349.
8. Dietrich AM, Bowman MJ, Ginn-Pease ME, et al. Pediatric head injuries: can clinical factors reliably predict an abnormality on computed tomography? *Ann Emerg Med* 1993;22:1535–1540.
9. Field M, Collins MW, Lovell MR, Maroon J. Does Age Play a Role in Recovery from Sports-Related Concussion? A Comparison of High School and Collegiate Athletes. *J Pediatr* 2003;142:546–553.
10. Greenes DS, Schutzman SA. Infants with isolated skull fractures: What are their clinical characteristics, and do they require hospitalization? *Ann Emerg Med* 1997;30:253–259.
11. Greenes DS, Schutzman SA. Occult intracranial injury in infants. *Ann Emerg Med* 1998;32:680–686.
12. Griffith JE, Brasfield JC. Increased intracranial pressure. *Pediatr Rev* 1981;2:269.
13. Gruskin KD, Schutzman SA. Head trauma in children younger than 2 years. Are there predictors for complications? *Arch Pediatr Adolesc Med* 1999;153:15–20.
14. Hahn YS, McLone DG. Risk factors in the outcome of children with minor head injury. *Pediatr Neurosurg* 1993;19:135–142.
15. Kraus JF, Rock A, Hemyari P. Brain injuries among infants, children, adolescents, and young adults. *Am J Dis Child* 1990;144:684–691.
16. Lillehei KO, Hoff JT. Advances in the management of closed head injury. *Ann Emerg Med* 1985;14:789–795.
17. Lloyd DA, Carty H, Patterson M, et al. Predictive value of skull radiography for intracranial injury in children with blunt head injury. *Lancet* 1997;349:821–824.
18. Masters SJ, McClean PM, Arcarese JS, et al. Skull x-ray examinations after head trauma. Recommendations by a multidisciplinary panel and validation study. *N Engl J Med* 1987;316:84–91.

19. Muizelaar JP, Marmarou A, Ward JD, et al. Adverse effects of prolonged hyperventilation in patients with severe head injury: a randomized clinical trial. *J Neurosurg* 1991;75:731–739.

20. Palchak MJ, Holmes JF, Vance CW, et al. A decision rule for identifying children at low risk for brain injuries after blunt head trauma. *Ann Emerg Med* 2003;42:492–505.

21. Poirier MP, Wadsworth MR. CME Review Article. Sports-Related Concussions. *Ped Emerg Care* 2000;16:278–283.

22. Quayle KS, Jaffe DM, Kupperman N, et al. Diagnostic testing for acute head injury in children: when are head computed tomography and skull radiographs indicated? *Pediatrics* 1997;99:1–8.

23. Raimondi AJ, Hirschauer J. Head injury in the infant and toddler. *Childs Brain* 1984;11:12–35.

24. Rekate HL. Head injuries: management of primary injuries and prevention of secondary damage. *Childs Nervous System* 2001;17:632–634.

25. Rivara FP. Pediatric injury control in 1999: where do we go from here? *Pediatrics* 1999;103:883–888.

26. Rosman NP, Oppenheimer EY, O'Conner JF. Emergency management of pediatric head injuries. *Emerg Med Clin North Am* 1983;1:141–174.

27. Schunk JE, Rodgerson JD, Woodward GA. The utility of head computed tomographic scanning in pediatric patients with normal neurologic examination in the emergency department. *Pediatr Emerg Care* 1996;12:160–165.

28. Schutzman SA, Barnes P, Duhaime AC, et al. Evaluation and management of children younger than two years old with apparently minor head trauma: proposed guidelines. *Pediatrics* 2001;107:983–993.

29. Shane SA, Fuchs SM. Skull fractures in infants and predictors of associated intracranial injury. *Pediatr Emerg Care* 1997;13:198–203.

30. Stringer WA, Hasso AN, Thompson JR, et al. Hyperventilation induced cerebral ischemia in patients with acute brain lesions: demonstration by xenon-enhanced CT. *Am J Neurosurg Res* 1993;14:475–484.

31. Wojtys EM, Hovda D, Landry G, Boland A, Lovell M, et al. Current concepts: concussions in sports. *Am J Sports Med* 1999;27:676–687.

32. Zuckerman GB, Conway EE. Accidental head injury. *Pediatr Ann* 1997;26:621–632.

CHAPTER 211
Evaluation of the Cervical Spine

Jeffrey R. Avner

Evaluation of a child for a cervical spine injury is a diagnostic challenge because, unlike the adult cervical spine, the developing pediatric cervical spine has unfused synchondroses, incomplete ossification centers, and epiphyseal growth plates. Due to dynamic changes that occur with bone and ligament development in the pediatric cervical spine, distribution patterns of fractures and dislocations within the cervical spine itself differ from the distribution of injuries in the adult spine. Furthermore, a significant percentage of pediatric spinal cord injuries occur in the absence of radiographically identifiable fractures and dislocations.

DEVELOPMENTAL ANATOMY

The first cervical vertebra (atlas) develops from three primary ossification centers: the body and two neural arches (Fig. 211.1). The neural arches ossify *in utero* and fuse posteriorly at approximately the third year of life. The body of C1 is not ossified at birth and does not become visible until approximately 1 year of age. The synchondroses between the body and neural arches

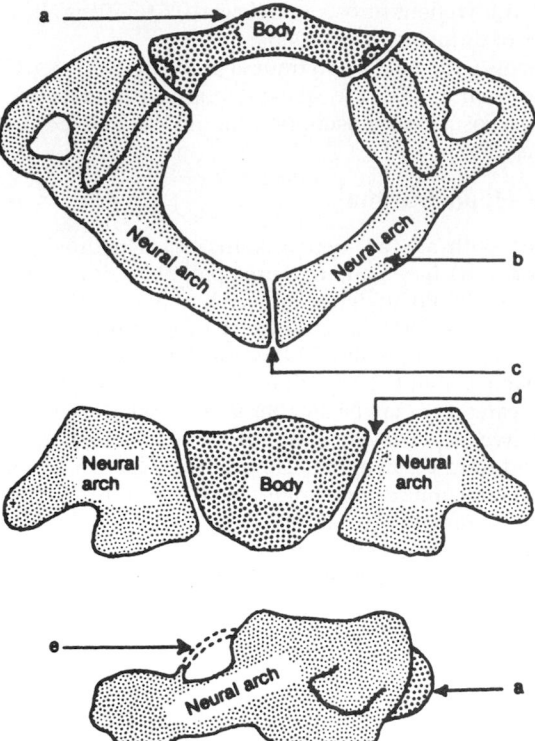

Figure 211.1.   The first cervical vertebra (atlas). **(a)** Body: ossification center becomes visible during first year of life. **(b)** Neural arches: ossification center appears *in utero* at approximately the seventh fetal week. **(c)** Synchondrosis of spinal process: fuses at approximately the third year of life. **(d)** Synchondrosis about the body (neurocentral synchondrosis: fuses at approximately the seventh year of life). **(e)** Ligament surrounding the superior vertebral notch: may ossify later in life. (From Fielding JW. Cervical spine injuries in children. In: The Cervical Spine Research Society, (eds). *The cervical spine.* Philadelphia: JB Lippincott Co, 1983,pp.268–281, with permission.)

(neurocentral synchondroses) fuse at approximately the seventh year of life (9).

The second cervical vertebra (axis) is the most difficult to interpret radiographically because of its four primary ossification centers: the odontoid, body, and two neural arches (Fig. 211.2). All four ossification centers are visible at birth. A secondary ossification center appears at the apex of the odontoid (summit ossification center) at approximately 3 to 6 years and fuses with the odontoid by the twelfth year of life. The synchondroses of the posterior neural arches fuse at approximately the third year. The synchondrosis between the odontoid–body of C2 and the neural arches fuses at approximately the third to sixth year. Before fusion, these synchondroses may be confused with fracture lines. The fusion line of the synchondrosis between the odontoid and the body of C2 commonly remains visible until age 11, and one-third of individuals have a visible fusion line throughout life.

In the remaining C3 to C7 cervical vertebrae, there are three major ossification centers—the body and two neural arches—all of which are visible at birth (Fig. 211.3). The posterior synchondroses of the neural arches fuse at approximately the third year of life. The neurocentral synchondroses fuse at approximately the third to sixth year of life. Secondary ossification centers appear at puberty along the superior and inferior aspects of the cervical bodies (superior and inferior epiphyseal rings) and at the tips of the spinous processes. Before fusion, these ossification centers may be mistaken for chip fractures of the cervical bodies and clay shoveler's fractures of the spinous processes, respectively. These

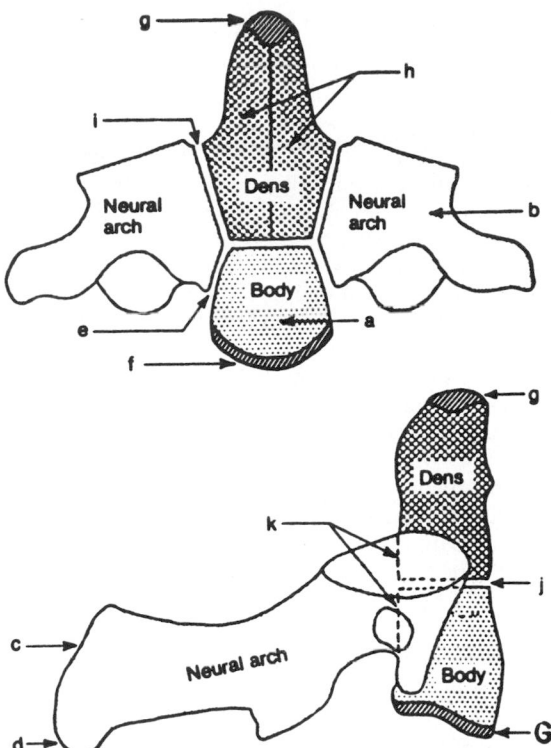

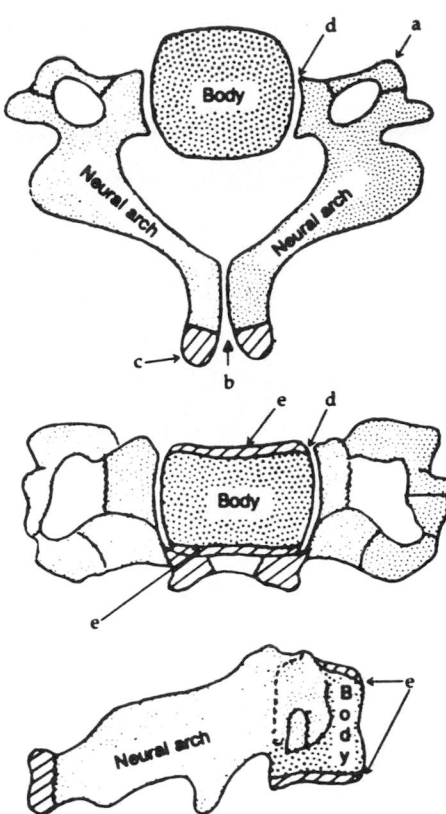

Figure 211.2. The second cervical vertebra (axis). **(a)** Body: ossification center appears by the fifth fetal month. **(b)** Neural arches: appear by the seventh fetal month. **(c)** Synchondrosis of spinous process: fuses by the third to sixth year of life. **(d, e)** Neurocentral synchondrosis: fuses by the third to sixth year. **(f, G)** Inferior epiphyseal ring: appears at puberty and fuses to body at approximately 25 years of life. **(g)** Summit ossification center for odontoid: appears at approximately the third to the sixth year and fuses with the odontoid by the twelfth year of life. **(h)** Odontoid: develops from two ossification centers that fuse by the seventh fetal month. **(i)** Synchondrosis between the odontoid and body: fuses at approximately the third to sixth year of life. (From Fielding JW. Cervical spine injuries in children. In: The Cervical Spine Research Society, eds. *The cervical spine.* Philadelphia: JB Lippincott Co, 1983:268–281, with permission.)

Figure 211.3. Typical cervical vertebrae (C3-C7). **(a)** Anterior portion of transverse process: may develop from a separate ossification center that fuses by the sixth year. **(b)** Synchondrosis between the spinous processes: fuse by third year. **(c)** Secondary centers for bifid spinous processes: appear at puberty and fuse by 25 years of life. **(d)** Neurocentral synchondrosis: fuses at approximately third to sixth year of life. **(e)** Superior and inferior epiphyseal rings: appear at puberty and fuse with body by 25 years of life. (From Fielding JW. Cervical spine injuries in children. In: The Cervical Spine Research Society, eds. *The cervical spine.* Philadelphia: JB Lippincott Co, 1983:268–281, with permission.)

secondary ossification centers fuse with the main body by age 25 years. Table 211.1 summarizes the major radiographic changes seen in the development of the pediatric cervical spine.

NORMAL VARIANTS AND CONGENITAL ANOMALIES

The development of the cervical vertebrae during childhood results in a range of normal anatomic and radiologic variants (Fig. 211.4). In particular, the weak support provided by relatively immature axial muscles, elastic interspinous ligaments and flat interfacet joints create laxity of the vertebrae. In addition, during the ossification process of the immature cervical bodies, an appearance of anterior wedging is produced. Thus, there is more mobility of the vertebral structures in a child compared to an adult whose vertebral alignment is relatively fixed. Due to this ligamentous laxity, absent lordosis is a frequent finding on the lateral radiograph in the pediatric cervical spine, while in adults, this finding may signify ligamentous injury. In one study, lordosis was absent in 14% of 160 healthy children aged 16 years and younger (6).

The extreme laxity of ligaments can also exaggerate the vertebral override (pseudosubluxation) of adjacent vertebrae in 46% of children younger than 8 years old (6). This finding is most pronounced at the level of C2 to C3 (see Fig. 211.4). To

TABLE 211.1. Radiographic Development of the Pediatric Cervical Spine

Age	Developmental Change
6 mo.	Body of C1 not visible; all synchondroses open
1 yr.	Body of C1 visible
3 yr.	Synchondroses of posteriorly located spinous processes fuse
3–6 yr.	Neurocentral syncondroses fuse; synchondrosis between odontoid and body of C2 fuses; summit ossification center appears at superior aspect of odontoid; anterior wedging of vertebral bodies resolves
8 yr.	Pseudosubluxation and widening of predental space resolve; spine assumes a more lordotic appearance
Puberty	Secondary ossification centers appear at the tips of the spinous processes; superior and inferior epiphyseal rings appear; summit ossification center of odontoid fuses
25 yr.	Secondary ossification centers at tips of spinous processes fuse; superior and inferior epiphyseal rings fuse to the main body

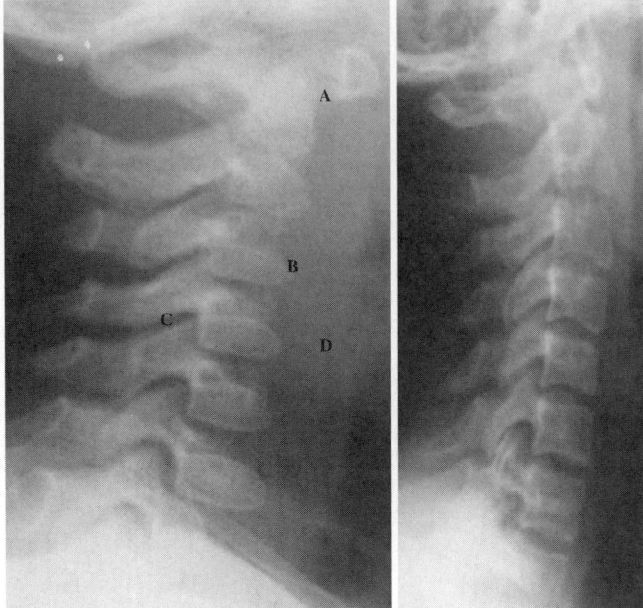

Figure 211.4.   Comparison of a normal lateral cervical spine x-ray of a child (left) and adult (right). Normal anatomic differences notable in the pediatric spinal x-ray include: nonpathologic, widened predental space of 4.5 mm **(A)**, anterior wedging of the vertebral bodies **(B)**, flat interfacet joints **(C)**, increased soft-tissue space anterior to the cervical spine **(D)** and an anterior pseudosubluxation of C2 on C3. (Reprinted from Loren G. Yamamoto, http://www2.hawaii.edu/medicine/pediatrics/pemxray/v5c02.html, with permission.)

distinguish pseudosubluxation from true subluxation, Swischuk (24) has developed the concept of the posterior cervical line (Fig. 211.5). This line is drawn by connecting the anterior aspects of the spinous processes of C1 and C3. If the anterior aspect of the spinous process of C2 misses this line by 2 mm or more (1.5 mm is borderline), this finding is suggestive of a true subluxation or a hangman's fracture of the neural arches of C2. This posterior cervical line can be applied only in children demonstrating subluxation or pseudosubluxation of C2 on C3. If no subluxation or pseudosubluxation exists, the anterior aspect of the spinous pro-

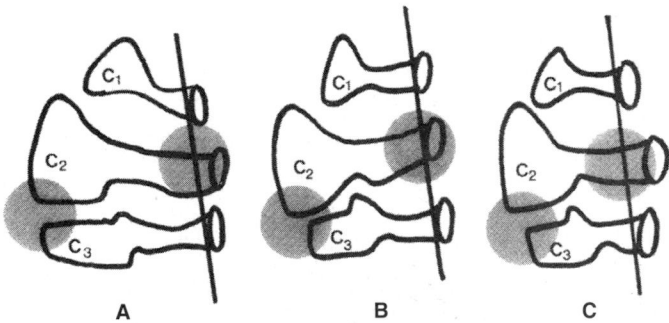

Figure 211.5.   The posterior cervical line (PCL) is drawn by connecting the anterior aspect of the spinous processes of C1 and C3. The concept of the PCL can be applied only if subluxation or pseudosubluxation is present. **(A)** Pseudosubluxation is absent: The anterior aspect of the spinous process of C2 will commonly miss the PCL by 2 mm—*Normal or Abnormal* (PCL cannot be applied). **(B)** Pseudosubluxation is present: The anterior aspect of the spinous process of C2 lies on the PCL—*Normal.* **(C)** Subluxation is present: The anterior aspect of the spinous process of C2 misses the PCL by 2 mm. This finding is suggestive of a hangman's fracture of the neural arches of C2—*Abnormal.* (From Fesmire FM, Luten RC. The pediatric cervical spine: developmental anatomy and clinical aspects. *J Emerg Med* 1989;7:133–142, with permission.)

cess of C2 commonly misses the posterior cervical line by more than 2 mm.

In adults, widening of the predental space (greater than 2.5–3 mm) frequently signifies a rupture of the transverse ligament or subluxation of C1 on C2. However, in children younger than 8 years old, distances of 3 to 4 mm are common and normal; even distances up to 5 mm may be seen in nonpathologic instances (6), although they should be considered abnormal, however, until proven otherwise.

Widening of the prevertebral soft tissue due to hemorrhage and edema is an important adult radiographic finding. In children, suggested norms have included soft-tissue space less than 7 mm anterior to C2 or less than three-fourths of the adjacent vertebral body's width (1). The younger the child, the more unreliable these norms, because dramatic increases in soft-tissue density occur during expiration or when the neck is held in mild flexion.

Excluding major congenital malformations, os odontoideum and ossiculum terminale are two congenital malformations that occasionally occur. Os odontoideum is a failure of the odontoid to fuse with the body of C2. The odontoid is separated from the body of C2 by a thin layer of hyaline cartilage, and fairly insignificant trauma can result in odontoid subluxation, resulting in death or quadriplegia. Os odontoideum can also occur secondarily from the failure of an odontoid fracture to heal. Ossiculum terminale is a failure of the apical segment of the odontoid (summit ossification center) to fuse with the main body of the odontoid. This is generally a benign condition, but one case of this anomaly has led to progressive atlantoaxial dislocation, resulting in quadriplegia and death (22).

CLINICAL PRESENTATION

Cervical spine injury occurs in only 2% to 3% of all patients with significant blunt trauma who have radiologic studies performed (23). Furthermore, of all cervical spinal injuries, only 2% to 4% occur in children younger than 16 years old, and only approximately 1% of all pediatric cervical spine radiographs reveal an abnormality (10,13,25).

The incidence of cervical spine fractures and dislocations increases with age. Radiographically apparent cervical spine injury, excluding birth trauma, is virtually nonexistent in children younger than 16 months of age (1,2,8,10,12,25). The cause of cervical spine fractures and dislocations is broad and the epidemiology of injury may reflect regional differences. In general, motor vehicle accidents and falls account for the majority injuries in children younger than 8 years old while sports injuries are more common in the older child (2,8,15,20). Pediatric cervical injuries related to the use of front-passenger airbags have been increasingly described in the literature. Airbag deployment has produced a pattern of cervical injuries in older children traveling in front seats and crush injury to the skull of infants in rear-facing safety seats (18). Currently, the National Highway Traffic Safety Administration recommends placing infants in rear-facing child safety seats in the back seat until about 1 year old, in forward-facing child safety seats until about 4 years old and in belt-positioning booster seats until they are at least 8 years old (19). Children under 12 should ride seat-belted in a rear seat at all times.

Types of pediatric cervical spine injuries can be divided into those of the upper cervical spine (C1 to C3) and those of the lower cervical spine (C4 to C7). Injuries most commonly seen in the upper cervical spine are fracture or synchondral separation of the odontoid with atlantoaxial dislocation, and hangman's fracture of the neural arches of C2. Abnormalities most frequently encountered in the lower cervical spine are anterior subluxation or dislocation, compression fractures, teardrop fractures, and spinous process fractures. The distribution of the level of cervical spine injury varies with age, reflecting the effect of the relatively large head of the child, coupled with the laxity of ligaments and nearly horizontal facet joints. This combination results in high torques and shear forces being applied to the C1 to C3 regions. Thus, younger children tend to have higher cervical spine injuries (1,2,8,10,12,20). Children younger than 8 years old have more upper cervical spine fractures and dislocations, whereas children older than 12 years have a distribution of injuries resembling that of adults, with more low cervical lesions. Children aged 8 to 12 years are in a transition state between the two. The incidence of neurologic deficit with cervical spine fractures and dislocations also increases with age, with neurologic deficit occurring in 20% of children younger than 8 years of age and in approximately 40% of children aged 8 to 16 years (1,10,12).

In addition to vertebral injuries seen on plain x-rays, the pediatric patient may also suffer Spinal Cord Injury WithOut Radiographic Abnormality (SCIWORA), a term defined before widespread use of MRI. In the child, the flexibility and elasticity of the vertebral column are more than that of the spinal cord. Thus, a distraction injury may cause cord traction or ischemia without anatomic defects. The pathophysiology of SCIWORA is thought to result from a combination of a diverse multitude of mechanisms, all resulting in a disruption of microvascular blood supply. Mechanisms proposed include spinal cord traction, spinal cord concussion from transmission of externally applied energy, hyperextension with inward bulging of the interlaminar ligaments, reversible disc prolapse, flexion compression of the cord, and vertebral artery spasm.

There is a large range in the reported incidence of SCIWORA although 2 large recent studies found an incidence of 18% to 38% of all pediatric spinal injuries (4,16). Because of the age-related anatomic differences, it is not surprising that SCIWORA injuries usually occur in younger children (mean age between 9 and 11 years) and involve the upper cervical spine in up to 80% of cases (4,16). Interestingly, in one series (4), sports-related activities were associated with 54% of cases of SCIWORA and involved older children and adolescence. Most cases of SCIWORA present with some type of neurologic symptoms, most commonly parasethesias, and have partial cord syndromes (4,16). However, delayed onset of neurologic deficit and complete cord transection can occur.

EMERGENCY DEPARTMENT EVALUATION AND MANAGEMENT

All children with potential cervical spine injury should have their necks immobilized. Prehospital cervical spine immobilization is best accomplished using a rigid plastic cervical collar and a backboard, combined with tape, sandbags, or a commercially available head-immobilization device (14). However, neutral position is difficult to achieve and may be present in as little as 11% to 20% of children who were immobilized on presentation to the ED (7,16). The disproportionate head size of young children causes cervical flexion to occur in children younger than 7 years old when they are immobilized on a standard flat backboard (11). This flexion can be prevented either by placing padding underneath the back to raise the level of the thoracic spine or by using a spinal backboard with a recess for the occiput. The cervical spine is properly positioned when a line drawn through the external auditory meatus and the anterior aspect of the shoulder is parallel to the backboard. When an alert child vigorously resists attempts at immobilization, the injury may worsen. As a general rule, children rarely ingest central nervous system depressants

such as ethanol and, if alert, will not move a significantly injured portion of the body. Thus, it is acceptable to not immobilize the cervical spine of a young alert child with no obvious injuries who is vigorously resisting all attempts. It should also be noted that there are no randomized controlled trials of cervical spine immobilization in trauma patients (17). Furthermore, improper spinal immobilization may cause neurologic injury, airway obstruction, pain, and increased intracranial pressure. Therefore, extreme care must be used when immobilizing a trauma patient.

All children who arrive at the ED with a new neurologic deficit consistent with a spinal cord injury and a history of trauma or suspected trauma should undergo treatment with high-dose methylprednisolone as soon as possible (3). Recommended dosing consists of a loading dose of 30 mg/kg over 15 minutes, followed by a maintenance infusion of 5.4 mg/kg/h for either 24 hours (if initiated less than 3 hours after injury) or 48 hours (if initiated 3 to 8 hours after injury). Due to the existence of SCIWORA, work up should not delay the initiation of high-dose methylprednisolone in patients with spinal cord injury.

The management of the threatened airway in a child can be an urgent dilemma. Ventilation can frequently be accomplished with a chin lift alone (which elevates the tongue off the hypopharynx) or in combination with bag-valve-mask ventilation. Oral intubation, which is preferred in younger children, is best performed using manual in-line stabilization *without* traction to maintain cervical immobilization. Manual traction may aggravate a distracting injury. Young children require little, if any, extension to visualize the glottis. Nasotracheal intubation should be attempted only in older children with spontaneous respirations.

Although the incidence of cervical spine injury is small, the consequence of severe neurologic disability from an unrecognized injury has raised concern about the overuse of radiography in this setting. In fact, there are many reasons for a missed cervical spine injury including altered mental status, distracting injury, inadequate examination, SCIWORA, not obtaining x-rays and not seeking medical care (21). Still, investigators have sought to develop clinical algorithms to identify children at high risk for cervical spine injury who need radiographic studies while at the same time avoiding unnecessary x-rays in low-risk children. Jaffe and coworkers (15) retrospectively analyzed 206 children with suspected cervical spine injury and found that the clinical criteria of any one of the following—history of direct neck trauma; neck pain; neck tenderness; limitation of mobility; abnormality in flexion, strength, or sensation; or decreased mental status—had a sensitivity of 98% and a specificity of 54% for detecting cervical spine injuries. Recently, a prospective, multicenter study by the National Emergency X-Radiography Utilization Study (NEXUS) group (25) applied the following set of 5 predictors for low risk of cervical spine injury: no midline cervical tenderness, no focal neurologic deficit, normal alertness, absence of intoxication and no painful distracting injury. Thirty (0.98%) of the 3,065 patients who were younger than 18 years old, had a cervical spine injury. These clinical criteria correctly identified all cervical spine injury victims (sensitivity of 100%) and correctly designated 603 patients as low risk for cervical spine injury (negative predictive value of 100%). However, the positive predictive value was only 1.2%. Furthermore, there were only a small number of infants and toddlers, thus limiting the applicability of the criteria in this age group.

In light of the existing data, a conservative approach to clearing the cervical spine with clinical criteria in children seems reasonable. If a child is brought to the ED with the neck immobilized but no history of direct neck trauma, and is awake, alert, cooperative with no distracting injury, no complaint of neck pain and no neurologic deficit (or history of transient paralysis), the cervical collar can be removed for further neck examination. The child should try to maintain his neck in neutral position (with help from a clinician if necessary) while the neck is inspected and the spine palpated. If there is no neck tenderness, allow gentle active range of motion of the neck. Children with a spinal injury will often limit their neck motion secondary to pain in order to protect the area of injury; therefore, never passively extend or flex the child's neck. If there is neck tenderness or limitation of movement due to pain, the cervical collar should be replaced and appropriate radiographic examination performed. Otherwise, immobilization can be removed and the cervical spine cleared clinically.

Radiographic examination begins with a lateral cervical spine x ray with the collar in place. However, this single view may miss 5% to 20% of injuries (2,15). Therefore, the standard 3-view series (lateral, anteroposterior and odontoid x-rays) should be obtained, recognizing that the open-mouth odontoid view is frequently impossible to obtain in young children. Due to the potential of SCIWORAs developing despite normal radiographs, all children with potential spinal injury should be questioned specifically concerning transient paresthesias at the time of the injury. Such children should be assumed to have a spinal injury until a neurosurgical consultation establishes otherwise. The diagnosis of SCIWORA should be a diagnosis of exclusion and should not be made until occult bony, ligamentous, or disc injuries are ruled out by fluoroscopically guided flexion and extension radiographs, computed tomography scanning, magnetic resonance imaging, or myelography.

CRITICAL INTERVENTIONS

- Use a properly fitted hard cervical collar to maintain the neck in neutral position
- If emergent airway management is needed, continue in-line immobilization without traction to avoid creating or exacerbating neurologic injury
- Obtain radiologic examination beginning with a lateral neck x-ray if the child has any of the following symptoms: cervical tenderness or pain, focal neurologic deficit, altered consciousness, intoxication or painful distracting injury
- If there is limitation of neck movement, persistent cervical pain or neurologic symptoms even in the face of unremarkable 3-view cervical spine x-rays, maintain immobilization and proceed with additional radiographic studies (e.g., CT or MRI) and neurosurgical consultation
- Begin intravenous methylprednisolone therapy if there are new neurologic deficits consistent with a spinal cord injury

DISPOSITION

All children suspected of having a cervical spine injury on the basis of clinical findings and/or radiographic studies should have neurosurgical consultation to help assess the severity of injury, need for further radiographic studies and disposition. Pending further studies concerning the nature of cervical spine fractures and dislocations, as well as the nature of SCIWORA, it seems prudent to conservatively admit to the hospital all children with suspected cervical spine injury. Adolescents with clinically insignificant vertebral injury (e.g., type 1 odontoid fracture, spinous process fracture) and a normal neurologic examination may be considered for outpatient management. Any child with a potentially unstable vertebral fracture or with a spinal column injury without cord damage should be admitted to an in-patient unit for observation. All children with proven spinal cord injury should be admitted to the Pediatric Intensive Care Unit.

COMMON PITFALLS

✔ Physicians may confuse open synchondrosis and secondary ossification centers with fractures

✔ Physicians may not realize that absent lordosis, anterior wedging of cervical bodies, pseudosubluxation of C2 on C3, increased prevertebral soft-tissue density, and widening of the predental space can be normal

✔ A normal radiograph does not rule out cervical spinal cord injury in the pediatric age group, because spinal cord injuries frequently occur in the absence of radiographically detectable injuries. All children with suspected neck injury should be questioned specifically for transient paresthesias at the time of the injury, because approximately one-half of all patients with delayed onset of SCIWORA have this finding

✔ A young alert child with no obvious injuries who is vigorously resisting all attempts at immobilization should not be forced into a restraining device as secondary injury may occur

Acknowledgments

Thanks to the previous edition's chapter authors David M. Cosentino and Francis M. Fesmire.

References

1. Apple JS, Kirks DR, Merten DF, et al. Cervical spine fractures and dislocations in children. *Pediatr Radiol* 1987;17:45–49.
2. Baker C, Kadish H, Schunk JE. Evaluation of pediatric cervical spine injuries. *Am J Emerg Med* 1999;17:230–234.
3. Bracken MB, Shepard MJ, Holford TR, et al. Administration of methylprednisolone for 24 or 48 hours or tirilazad mesylate for 48 hours in the treatment of acute spinal cord injury. Results of the Third National Acute Spinal Cord Injury Randomized Controlled Trial. National Acute Spinal Cord Injury Study. *JAMA.* 1997;277:1597–1604.
4. Brown RL, Brunn MA, Garcia VF. Cervical spine injuries in children: A review of 103 patients treated consecutively at a level 1 pediatric trauma center. *J Pediatr Surg* 2001;36:1107–1114.
5. Burke D. Spinal cord trauma in children. *Paraplegia* 1971;9:1–14.
6. Cattell HS, Filtzer DK. Pseudosubluxation and other normal variations in the cervical spine in children. *J Bone Joint Surg* 1965;47A:1295–1309.
7. Curran C, Dietrich AM, Bowman MJ, Ginn-Pease ME, King DR, Kosnik E. Pediatric cervical-spine immobilization: achieving neutral position? *J Trauma* 1995;39:729–732.
8. Dietrich AM, Ginn-Pease ME, Bartkowski HM, et al. Pediatric cervical spine fractures: predominately subtle presentation. *J Pediatr Surg* 1991;26:995–999.
9. Fesmire FM, Luten RC. The pediatric cervical spine: developmental anatomy and clinical aspects. *J Emerg Med* 1989;7:133–142.
10. Henrys P, Lyne ED, Lifton C, et al. Clinical review of cervical spine injuries in children. *Clin Orthop* 1977;129:172–176.
11. Herzenberg JE, Hensinger RN, Dedrick DK, et al. Emergency transport and positioning of young children who have an injury of the cervical spine: the standard backboard may be hazardous. *J Bone Joint Surg Am* 1989;71:15–22.
12. Hill SA, Miller CA, Kosnik EJ, et al. Pediatric neck injuries: a clinical study. *J Neurosurg* 1984;60:700–706.
13. Hoffman JR, Mower WR, Wolfson AB, Todd KH, Zucker MI, for the National Emergency X-Radiography Utilization Study Group Validity of a set of clinical criteria to rule out injury to the cervical spine in patients with blunt trauma. *N Engl J Med* 2000;343:94–99.
14. Huerta C, Griffith R, Joyce SM. Cervical spine stabilization in pediatric patients: evaluation of current techniques. *Ann Emerg Med* 1987;16:1121–1126.
15. Jaffe DM, Binns H, Radowski NA, et al. Developing a clinical algorithm for early management of cervical spine injury in child trauma victims. *Ann Emerg Med* 1987;16:270–276.
16. Kokoska ER, Keller MS, Rallo MC, Weber TR. Characteristics of pediatric cervical spine injuries. *J Pediatr Surg* 2001;36:100–105.
17. Kwan I, Bunn F, Roberts I. Spinal immobilisation for trauma patients. *Cochrane Database Syst Rev* 2001;CD002803.
18. Marshall KW, Koch BL, Egelhoff JC. Air bag-related deaths and serious injuries in children: injury patterns and imaging findings. *Am J Neuroradiol* 1998; 19:1599–1607.
19. National Highway Traffic Safety Association. Child passenger safety. 2003; URL: http://www.nhtsa.dot.gov/CPS.
20. Nitecki S, Moir CR. Predictive factors of the outcome of traumatic cervical spine fracture in children. *J Pediatr Surg* 1994;29:1409–1411.
21. Orenstein JB, Klein BL, Ochsenschlager DW. Delayed diagnosis of pediatric cervical spine injury. *Pediatrics* 1992;89(6 Pt 2):1185–1188.

22. Sherk H, Nicholson J. Rotary atlanto-axial dislocation associated with os-siculum terminale and mongolism. *J Bone Joint Surg Am* 1969;51A:957–964.
23. Spinal Cord Injury Statistics. Birmingham, AL: National Spinal Cord Injury Association Resource Center, 1999.
24. Swischuk LE. *Emergency imaging of the acutely ill or injured child*, 4th ed. Baltimore: Williams & Wilkins, 2000.
25. Viccellio P, Simon H, Pressman BD, et al. A prospective multicenter study of cervical spine injury in children. *Pediatrics* 2001;108(2). URL: http://www.pediatrics.org/cgi/content/full/108/2/e20.

CHAPTER 212
Chest and Abdominal Trauma

Christine E. Koerner and Brent R. King

EPIDEMIOLOGY

Injuries to the chest and abdomen are not uncommon among infants, children, and adolescents (2,6,10,11,13,14,21,23). Young children have pliable rib cages and poorly developed abdominal musculature and these features place them at risk for thoracic and abdominal injuries (2,3,10,21,23). As is the case for adult patients, blunt trauma causes most injuries and blunt abdominal trauma is more common than blunt chest trauma (3,10,21,23). Most injuries are caused by motor vehicle and automobile versus pedestrian accidents (3,6,10,14,21,23). Penetrating injuries are exceedingly rare in infants and young children (3,23) but are more common among older children and adolescents (3,6,13).

CLINICAL PRESENTATION

Children who have sustained blunt thoracic and abdominal trauma may have clinical findings on a spectrum from little or no evidence of serious injury to obvious life-threatening injuries. In most cases, however, patients can be divided into two broad categories, those with evidence of physiologic compromise and those with no evidence of physiologic compromise (3,5,6,10,13,16,19,21). This distinction is important because those patients in the former category will require resuscitation prior to or concurrent with their diagnostic evaluation while those in the latter group require diagnostic evaluation only (1,3,5,6,10,12,13). It is important, however, to recognize that patients can move up and down the spectrum of illness during their ED evaluation and frequent reassessment is mandatory to insure that significant clinical deteriorations have not been missed (2,3,6,21).

Attention to the physical examination can be helpful in predicting thoracic and abdominal injury. For instance, predictors of thoracic injury in children include tachypnea, abnormal thoracic and chest auscultation findings, low systolic blood pressure, and the presence of a femur fracture (3,15,20). However, there may be no evidence of thoracic injury secondary to rib cage pliability in young children (3,13,15). Patients who have incurred abdomi-

nal trauma may have evidence of external injury such as bruises, tenderness, and distention (3,14,21). Like thoracic injury, abdominal injury may not always be apparent. This is typically the case for children with altered sensorium, neurologic impairment, or painful distracting injuries (21,24,25).

DIFFERENTIAL DIAGNOSIS

Given that most of the vital organs are located in the thorax and abdomen, trauma, whether blunt or penetrating, can and often does injure more than one organ (3,6,10,11,13,17,19,21,24). This fact makes the differential diagnosis necessarily broad. However, in many cases the patient's clinical presentation allows the practitioner to focus on a few key diagnoses (2,10,19,21,23,25). For example, the child with blunt chest trauma who has primarily respiratory symptoms is likely to have sustained a pneumothorax or a pulmonary contusion (2,3,12,13,15). The same child with both respiratory and hemodynamic compromise may have sustained a hemothorax or a tension pneumothorax (3,5,6,13). Likewise, the child who presents with hypotension after a blunt abdominal injury has, in all probability, an injury of the liver or spleen (3,10). It is also important to recognize injury patterns that suggest the diagnosis of "Seat Belt syndrome" (see specific injury section below) (3,9,23). And, although uncommon, abdominal and chest trauma secondary to child abuse (8,11,23) should always be suspected in cases where the history is inconsistent with the mechanism of injury (3).

While it is appropriate to use initial clinical findings to narrow the differential diagnosis and focus the patient's evaluation, care must be taken not to prematurely exclude certain diagnoses (2,6, 3,21). In many cases the early symptoms of injury may be subtle and the practitioner is well advised to perform a thorough initial assessment followed by frequent reassessments (2,3,6,13,14,17,21).

EMERGENCY DEPARTMENT EVALUATION

Early ED evaluation follows a pathway familiar to most (3,10,21,23,24). The evaluation begins with an assessment of the airway followed, if necessary, by definitive airway management. The second step is the evaluation of the adequacy and effectiveness of respiratory efforts. The patient with hypoxemia should receive supplemental oxygen while respiratory failure should be treated with mechanical ventilation. Significant injuries to the chest may be identified or at least suspected based upon the initial or secondary physical examination. The examining physician should be alert for crackles, diminished breath sounds, crepitus over the chest wall, and external marks indicating either significant blunt or penetrating trauma. An initial chest radiograph (3,11,15,21,25) is often a useful adjunct to the physical examination as it can identify subtle pneumothoraces, pulmonary contusions, and rib fractures as well as abnormalities in the cardiac and aortic silhouettes, which can signify cardiac or aortic injury (3,10,11,13,15,16,19,25).

Once the patient is assured of a stable airway and adequate respirations, attention is directed to the evaluation of the circulatory system (3,10). Victims of blunt trauma with hemodynamic compromise are evaluated differently from those without physiologic abnormalities (1,3,5,6,10,13,19,21,24). While patients with hemodynamic compromise and those without physiologic abnormalities undergo an initial physical examination intended to identify areas of tenderness, guarding, and signs of peritoneal indication, patients in the former group require urgent resuscitation. They should also have an evaluation aimed at identifying intraabdominal pathology as soon as possible (3,10,19,21).

Currently, the preferred examination is the Focused Abdominal Sonogram in Trauma (FAST examination). The FAST examination is an ultrasound scan performed at the bedside, often during the resuscitation phase of care. The FAST examination is intended to identify fluid (assumed, in the trauma patient to be blood) in the peritoneal cavity. A minimum of four sonographic views are used. The right and left upper quadrant scans are used to identify fluid in Morison's pouch and the spleno-renal recess. A suprapubic view is used to find fluid collected behind the bladder. Finally, the subxiphoid view helps to exclude nonabdominal causes of hypotension by evaluating the heart and the pericardium. If the FAST examination reveals intraabdominal fluid in an unstable child, surgery is usually indicated (10,21,23). If the FAST examination is unavailable or is negative in a patient with hemodynamic compromise who has no other source for his/her symptoms, then a diagnostic peritoneal lavage should be strongly considered (3,23). However, neither DPL nor FAST can identify the exact source of bleeding, and the decision for surgical intervention in the unstable patient should not be dependent on these studies (3,10,23). Likewise, immediate surgical intervention to control bleeding in an unstable patient should not be delayed to obtain chest and pelvic radiographs (3).

Further evaluation of the hemodynamically unstable patient should include laboratory values for hemoglobin, and blood type and cross-match (10,23), amylase for diagnosing pancreatic and small bowel injury, and transaminase levels as markers for hepatic injury (10,21). In females of childbearing age, a blood or urine specimen should be sent for pregnancy test. In all patients urine should also be sent for urinalysis and drug screen if indicated (3).

The child with blunt abdominal trauma who is hemodynamically normal may be evaluated somewhat less aggressively. In recent years, contrast-enhanced computed tomography (CT) has become the study of choice in the evaluation of victims of blunt trauma with abnormal abdominal examinations and those whose examinations are unreliable based upon the presence of distracting injuries, poorly developed verbal skills, or altered sensorium (10,21,25). An alternative in such patients is observation and serial examination (21).

Baseline laboratory values in the hemodynamically stable patient should include hemoglobin, amylase, urinalysis, and type and screen (23). Pregnancy tests should be performed in females of childbearing age (3). Plain films of the lateral cervical spine, chest, and pelvis should be considered (3,10,25).

Penetrating abdominal or thoracic trauma injuries always necessitate evaluation by a surgeon (3,13,19). It is important to note that thoracic gunshot wounds and any penetrating injury below the nipples anteriorly and the scapula posteriorly, may also involve the diaphragm and the abdominal cavity (3,6,19,23). Hemodynamically stable patients with penetrating trauma and suspected thoracoabdominal injury should receive an upright chest roentgenogram to exclude an associated hemo-or pneumothorax, and to document the presence of peritoneal air (3). Using clips to mark all entrance and exit wounds, the stable patient with a gunshot wound should also undergo a supine abdominal roentgenogram to assist in identification of the missile track and the presence of retroperitoneal air (3). However, the hypotensive unstable child with penetrating abdominal trauma requires prompt operative treatment, and there should be no screening radiographs in the ED if a surgeon is available (3). Likewise, if the patient is hemodynamically stable with penetrating injury and has microscopic or gross hematuria then further evaluation for urologic injury should be done (1). However, in children who require immediate laparotomy, an intraoperative one-shot IVP is useful in identifying renal injuries (1,3,24).

EMERGENCY DEPARTMENT MANAGEMENT

All patients with thoracic or abdominal injury should undergo resuscitation according to established guidelines (3,10,23,24). Prompt consultation of a surgeon is indicated if intrathoracic or intraabdominal injury is suspected (24). After a functional airway is established, one should assess breathing. Patients may have respiratory distress because of pneumothorax, hemothorax and hemopneumothorax (3,13). A chest roentgenogram may be helpful in establishing the diagnosis in these patients and placement of a tube thoracostomy is necessary. If there is a continued air leak or blood loss the patient should have a thoracotomy in the operating room (3,13). Flail chest is rare in young children because the pliability of their chest wall makes for infrequent disruption; however, when present it is almost always associated with underlying pulmonary contusion and an initial chest roentgenogram should be obtained (2). These patients require admission to the intensive care unit for monitoring and observation (2). Chest roentgenograms can also be helpful in identifying rupture of the thoracic aorta. A widened mediastinum may be visualized on chest radiograph with abnormal contour of the aortic knob, presence of a pleural or apical cap, and tracheal deviation (3,13,16). On physical examination, the patient with rupture of the thoracic aorta may have paraplegia as a result of poor spinal cord perfusion that may be confused initially with a spinal cord injury (6,13,16). A high index of suspicion for traumatic aortic rupture is needed to make the diagnosis. To confirm the diagnosis in stable patients the contrast-enhanced aortogram has been the "gold" standard. However, many centers currently rely upon CT, instead. Aortic injury identified by either technique is an indication for urgent consultation with a thoracic or vascular surgeon (16). However, if the patient is unstable, consultation should occur early and the surgical team should dictate further evaluation (3).

Patients with hemodynamic instability should receive a 20-ml/kg bolus of normal saline or Ringer's lactate administered rapidly via intravenous or intraosseous access (3,10,24). While blood is obtained for hemoglobin and hematocrit, and type and cross-match (3,24), nasogastric tubes (NGT) and urinary drainage catheters (Foley) may be placed (21,24). An NGT should not be placed if there is visible blood or cerebrospinal fluid in the nose, significant facial injury, or a basilar skull fracture (3). Foley catheters should be avoided when blood is seen at the urethral meatus, there is a perineal or scrotal hematoma, or there is a high-riding prostate (1,3,21).

If a child remains hemodynamically unstable after 40 ml/kg of crystalloid fluid, then 10 to 20 ml/kg or more of blood should be transfused, and the source of bleeding identified (3,10,24). After intrathoracic or CNS causes for the hemodynamic instability are excluded, abdominal sources of bleeding should be sought. DPL or FAST is performed to determine the presence of intraperitoneal blood, and if positive necessitates a laparotomy (3,10). Other indications for surgical exploration in the hemodynamically unstable child include abnormal vital signs; transfusion needs exceeding 40 ml/kg, peritoneal signs, abdominal distension, hypovolemia, and base deficit (23,24,25). It is important to note that abdominal distention secondary to aerophagia can mimic an acute abdomen, and insertion of a nasogastric tube can decompress the stomach (10,21). Intravenous antibiotics, analgesics and tetanus should be administered as indicated (3).

In contrast, management of patients who present with abdominal trauma but are hemodynamically stable depends on the injuries identified and investigations planned (23). Children who are hemodynamically stable with suspected abdominal injury should have a hemoglobin, amylase, urinalysis, blood type and screen. Females of childbearing age should undergo a pregnancy test (3,23). Other laboratory values and radiographic studies are performed for specific indications (3,23). Although an

IV heplock may be administered, nasogastric tubes and Foley catheters are not routinely placed.

CT is the diagnostic study of choice for evaluating stable patients with suspected blunt abdominal trauma as most blunt solid-organ (liver, kidney, spleen, and pancreas) injury in children can be successfully managed nonoperatively (10,21,23,25). Observation should be done in hospitals equipped and staffed to care for children with these injuries (3,21,23). Therefore, once the patient's workup is complete, he or she should be admitted to the hospital or transferred to a facility capable of monitoring him/her and of managing his/her injuries. In most cases, a surgeon should be involved in the patient's care (3,21,23). Patients should receive serial abdominal examination and hemoglobin levels (3,10,24). Children with hemoglobin that remains > 7 gm% can be treated conservatively without blood transfusion (21,23). Indications for surgical exploration based on CT imaging are evidence of bowel injury, renovascular injury, bladder rupture, ureteral transection, pancreatic injury, and contrast extravasations (1,3,7,9,10).

Children with penetrating wounds of the thorax or abdomen require surgical consultation, as children are more likely to require surgical intervention for these injuries than adults (3,13). Initial management of patients with thoracic injury follows the standard guidelines previously discussed with stabilization of the airway followed by fluid resuscitation, and chest wound care. An experienced surgeon should evaluate all superficial stab and gunshot wounds to determine the extent of the injury (3). Patients with deeper wounds or those that have penetrated the thoracic cavity will need further interventions such as a chest roentgenogram, hemoglobin and hematocrit, and type and cross match. Most penetrating thoracic injuries result in a pneumothorax or hemothorax that requires a tube thoracostomy (3,13). Some patients with penetrating chest injuries may have large chest wall defects that result in an open pneumothorax with a "sucking" chest wound (3,13). In these patients, air passes through the chest wall defect, rather than the tracheal lumen, causing impairment of ventilation (3,13). Temporizing treatment consists of application of sterile gauze dressing to occlude the open wound taped on three sides. This will act as a flutter type valve so that when the child inspires, the dressing is sucked tightly to the chest wall and when the child exhales trapped air is permitted to escape from the untaped side of the dressing. Ultimate therapy includes surgical repair of the chest wall defect with tube thoracostomy (3,13).

Patients with penetrating injuries near the mediastinum who are hemodynamically unstable should be suspected of having haemopericardium and tamponade (4). The classic findings of Beck triad (venous pressure elevation, decline in arterial pressure, and muffled heart tones) (3,19) may not be evident. In the unstable patient with suspected tamponade rapid evacuation of pericardial blood is indicated for patients not responding to treatment for hemorrhagic shock. A pericardiocentesis may be life-saving and result in rapid hemodynamic improvement if tamponade exists. If immediately available, bedside ultrasound can be used to identify the presence of a tamponade and as a guide for drainage (3). In the stable patient an ultrasound or echocardiogram may, likewise be helpful in determining if the patient has fluid in the periocardial sac (3). If the child has a cardiopulmonary arrest after a penetrating thoracic injury then immediate resuscitative thoracostomy is indicated (3). Similar to the situation in adults, the outcome for this procedure is likely to be poor even if vital signs are present. Thoracotomy should only be undertaken when a surgeon can be available in a timely fashion to provide definitive management (4).

Penetrating wounds of the abdomen and associated hypotension, peritonitis, evisceration or ongoing hemorrhage require operative intervention (1,3,19,23,25). Pneumoperitoneum, unexplained fever, or leukocytoses are additional indications for laparotomy (19,23). Children with abdominal gunshot wounds require mandatory surgical exploration (3,19,23,24,25), and hemodynamically unstable children with stab wounds also require surgery (19,23,25). However, children with anterior stab wounds who are asymptomatic may be managed expectantly by pediatric and trauma surgeons (3,23,24), and stable children with posterior penetrating stab wounds to the flank should receive a CT with triple contrast (24).

SPECIFIC INJURIES

Rib Fractures

Rib fractures in young children are infrequent (2,3,6,13,21), and when present are a marker of severe injury (3,11). In infants and young children, rib fractures may be an indication of child abuse (6,11,13). The diagnosis of rib fracture is usually made by chest roentgenogram, and the presence of multiple rib fractures suggests significant injury and is associated with a greater risk of death and disability (6,13). These patients should be admitted for observation to exclude associated injuries such as pneumothorax, or hemothorax (6,13). The management of this injury is largely supportive and is primarily centered upon pain control (6,11).

Pulmonary Injury

Pulmonary contusion is a prevalent injury that is caused by a direct bruise of the lung resulting in hemorrhage, interstitial edema, alveolar collapse and consolidation (2,6,15). Although evidence of chest wall injury may be absent, suspicion of a pulmonary contusion should be raised by the history of the mechanism of injury and the presence of hypoxemia or rib fractures (2,3,6). Initially, the pulmonary contusion may not be visualized on the initial chest roentgenogram but may appear on subsequent films, usually within 6 hours of the injury. Its radiographic appearance is that of an opacified lung segment (2,13). If a patient has unexplained respiratory distress after blunt trauma, CT might be helpful as it is somewhat more sensitive for the presence of a pulmonary contusion (2,6). Any patient with a significant pulmonary contusion should be admitted to the ICU for monitoring (3,13). Management of patients with pulmonary contusion includes oxygen, cardiopulmonary monitoring, appropriate ventilatory equipment, fluid restriction, and pain control (3,6). Progressive respiratory distress is a worrisome sign and the physician should be prepared to provide ventilatory support, if needed.

A *pneumothorax* is an abnormal accumulation of air in the pleural space that causes collapse of the affected lung (3,6,12,13). Patients with pneumothoraces have variable presentations, from subtle findings to the more classic description of respiratory distress, decreased breath sounds and hyperesonance to percussion of the affected side (12,13). Although a chest roentgenogram aids in the diagnosis in stable patients (3,6), sometimes pneumothoraces are missed. It is in these cases that chest CT may be helpful in establishing the diagnosis (6). Once a pneumothorax is identified the goal of therapy should be to reexpand the involved lung and return respiratory function to normal (3,12). Patients who are asymptomatic and have small pneumothoraces may be managed conservatively with observation if they will not be undergoing anesthesia or receiving positive pressure. In most cases these patients receive 100% oxygen by nonrebreather mask until their lung is reexpanded (3,12). However, symptomatic patients require definitive treatment for a pneumothorax that consists of tube thoracostomy placement in the fourth or fifth intercostal space at the anterior to midaxillary line with underwater seal drainage (3,12). A length-based device such as the Broselow Resuscitation Tape™ can be used to determine chest tube size in small children. A chest roentgenogram should be obtained after insertion of the chest tube to confirm placement (3). In some cases, an intermediate step is possible. Rather than a formal chest tube, these patients can have a Heimlich valve placed. The Heimlich valve is a one-way valve that allows air to escape the chest cavity but does not permit air to enter. Using this device, a spontaneously breathing or ventilated patient can be effectively treated without thoracostomy drainage.

A *tension pneumothorax* is life-threatening and occurs when air is trapped under pressure in the pleural space causing collapse of the affected lung, shift of the mediastinum, dramatically elevated intrathoracic pressure and decreased venous return (3,6,13). The diagnosis can and should be made clinically without radiographic confirmation in patients with respiratory distress, unilateral absent breath sounds and tracheal deviation (3,5,6,13). In order to decompress the tension pneumothorax a 14-gauge angiocatheter should be inserted into the affected side at the second intercostal space, midclavicular line. A rush of air and improvement of the patient's respiratory status confirms the diagnosis. This should be followed immediately by tube thoracostomy placement in the fifth intercostal space, between the anterior and midaxillary line with underwater seal drainage (3). At the completion of the procedure, a chest roentgenogram is indicated to verify lung expansion (13).

A *hemothorax* may result from injury to any of the intrathoracic vessels or the lung parenchyma (6). Each hemithorax can hold approximately 40% of a child's blood (6,13), and as a result hypotension or shock may develop. Patients with hemothoraces usually have decreased breath sounds on the affected side and trachea deviation towards the opposite side. The diagnosis of a hemothorax is confirmed by aspiration of blood (13), and treatment requires insertion of a tube thoracostomy to monitor the rate and volume of blood loss. Most patients can be managed nonoperatively; however, surgical intervention is indicated for hemorrhage through the tube greater than 100 mL/h or more than 20% of the child's blood volume (13). Shock and hypotension are treated with crystalloids and blood. In many cases, blood shed through the thoracostomy tube can be collected and retransfused to the patient. Antibiotic prophylaxis is controversial in the management of chest injury, and is used more often in care of patients penetrating trauma (6).

Airway injury to the tracheobronchial tree is rare in children and potentially fatal (3,6,20). Patients with tracheobronchial injury may present with hemoptysis, subcutaneous emphysema, or tension pneumothorax (3,6,20). A tracheobronchial injury must be suspected any time a well placed tube thoracostomy continues to demonstrate a significant air leak or is unable to reexpand the lung (3,6). Bronchoscopy is required for definitive diagnosis (3,6,20), and endotracheal intubation of the opposite main stem bronchus may be necessary to improve oxygenation (3). Identification of the injury necessitates prompt surgical repair (6), although some lesser injuries may be treated nonoperatively (6). However, all patients with tracheobronchial tree injury should be admitted to a surgical ICU (20).

Mediastinal Injuries

Aortic injuries are rare in children (6,16). Patients with aortic injuries may have retrosternal pain, hoarseness, dysphagia, and paraplegia (13). The diagnosis of aortic injury should be suspected if the chest roentgenogram shows mediastinal widening and abnormal contour of the aortic knob. However, these chest film findings are sensitive but nonspecific and the gold standard for diagnosis of aortic injury is arch aortography although CT is often substituted (6,13,16). The recommended treatment for aortic injuries is emergency surgical repair (6,13,16), but delayed operation has evolved with early institution of beta-blockers (6).

Blunt cardiac injury (BCI) can cause impairment of the myocardium or any cardiac valve (4). *Myocardial contusion* is the most common BCI (4,13), and patients with myocardial contusion may present with dysrhythmias, unexplained hypotension, or elevation of cardiac specific enzymes (3,4,6,13). Serum cardiac treponin 1(cTn1) levels can establish the diagnosis (4,6) Two-dimensional echocardiography is essential for inspection of valves, the pericardial space, and wall motion (3,4,13). The treatment in children with serious myocardial contusion should follow the same guidelines as acute myocardial infarction in adults (6,13). It is important to note that symptoms of myocardial contusion may not be observed for 24 hours after injury (3,13). In most cases injuries are not serious and management is usually supportive including continuous monitoring for rhythm disturbance and hypotension (3,6,13).

Commotio cordis is a syndrome of blunt chest impact producing cardiac arrest in the absence of cardiovascular disease. Typically it is seen in athletes who receive a blow to the chest, resulting in a rhythm disturbance, rapid cardiovascular collapse, and in most cases sudden death (6,13,18).

Esophageal injuries are rare, but can occur after penetrating injury or a severe blow to the upper abdomen (3,6,13). Patients with esophageal injury may have fever, chest or epigastric pain with unexplained mediastinal air or pleural effusion (6,13). Both water-soluble contrast esophagram and rigid esophagoscopy are necessary for assessment (3,6,13). Treatment can include broad-spectrum antibiotics, intravenous fluid resuscitation, drainage of the pleural space and mediastinum with surgical repair (3,6).

Diaphragm

Diaphragmatic injuries caused by blunt or penetrating thoracoabdominal trauma are rare in children (6,17,24), and there is no "gold standard" for early diagnosis. Chest roentgenograms in patients with diaphragmatic injury may show an irregular contour of the hemidiaphragm, but this finding is present in less than 50% of patients (3,17). Diagnostic tools such as ultrasound (17) and CT scan are not always accurate (6,17,24), and the diagnosis may be missed initially (10). Surgical repair remains the standard of care for these patients (17).

Spleen and Liver

The spleen and liver are the most commonly injured abdominal organs in children (10,24). A history of left-sided trauma and physical findings of left upper quadrant tenderness, left shoulder pain (Kerh sign) and anemia may accompany splenic injury but in some cases physical findings are initially subtle (10,24). Stable children with hepatic injuries usually complain of right upper quadrant pain and/or right shoulder pain. Additionally, elevated transaminases are often noted (10,21,24). Liver injuries in children are generally more severe than splenic injuries and are associated with a higher morbidity and mortality.

The CT can accurately identify and grade both splenic and hepatic injury (10,21,22,23,24), and a surgeon can manage many of these injuries nonoperatively if the patient remains hemodynamically stable, and requires less than 40 ml/kg of blood (one-half blood volume) in the first 24 hours (3,10,21). It is important to note that liver injuries have a tendency to rebleed and some authors suggest that a lower transfusion cutoff of ≥ 30 ml/kg in the first 24 hours is a more accurate indicator for the need for surgery (24).

Intestinal Perforation

Intestinal perforations are atypical in children unless associated with "Seat Belt syndrome" (see below) (10,14). The diagnosis is often not made until peritonitis occurs (14,24), and surgical intervention is always required (14). If there is no clear mechanism of injury for the intestinal perforation then child abuse should be suspected (10,14).

Kidney, Bladder, Urethra

Renal injuries are commonly seen in children following blunt abdominal trauma, and the majority of these can be managed nonoperatively (1,3). Hemodynamically stable children with gross hematuria, microscopic hematuria ($\geq$ 50 RBCs/HPF), or rapid–deceleration injury should be evaluated with CT (1,3,21, 23,25). Stable patients with isolated microscopic hematuria (< 50 RBCs/HPF) and suspected renal contusions may be observed without initial radiographic imaging, but should be followed with serial urinalyses and bed rest (1).

Children with gross hematuria should also be evaluated for lower tract injury. Bladder perforation can be diagnosed with cystography or CT and usually requires surgical repair (1,3,21,23). Urethral injury in boys should be suspected with pelvic fracture, blood at the meatus, scrotal hematoma, a high-riding prostate, and inability to void or pass a Foley catheter. A retrograde urethrogram must be performed in these patients to evaluate the urethra and guide surgical repair (1,3,21,23). CT is also being utilized to diagnose urethral injuries because it can detect urinomas and visualize the entire retroperitoneal space (1).

Pancreas

Pancreatic injuries are uncommon (7). Serum amylase levels, lipase levels, and abdominal CT can be useful in making this diagnosis, although the CT scan may not be accurate in determining the location and type of injury (7,10,24,25). Patients with distal transection of the pancreas require operative management (10,24), and patients with pancreatic contusions but no major ductal injury can be managed nonoperatively (10,24). Those patients with major ductal injury may be treated initially with nonoperative treatment, or by endoscopic retrograde cholangiopancreatography (ERCP) with stent placement (7,10,23).

Pelvis

Pelvic fractures are uncommon in children (22), and they are more likely to be present in patients with multiple injury and high injury severity scores (10,22). Contrary to adult findings, pelvic fractures in children usually do not cause massive bleeding, and only a small number of patients have associated genitourinary tract injuries (10). The pelvic roentgenogram is used routinely to establish the diagnosis (3,10,22), although in most cases the physical examination alone is reliable (10,22). In children the majority of pelvic fractures are stable ring fractures (22), and treatment tends to be nonoperative with most being treated with bed rest (22).

Seat Belt Syndrome

Also called the "Lap Belt Complex," the seat belt syndrome consists of characteristic patterns of bruising, and intraabdominal and lumbar spine injuries that result from compression, burst, or shearing, which are associated with restraint in lap seat belts. Children who are prematurely graduated to seat belts are at risk for this injury (9,14). The "seat belt sign" (contusion) may be found on the abdomen and hips (9,10), and small bowel perforations may be present even when the abdominal CT scan is negative (3,9,10,23,25). Therefore, patients with the "seat belt sign" should be admitted for serial abdominal examinations (9,10,24).

Lumbosacral injuries, i.e., compression and Chance fractures, may also occur with the "seat belt sign" and small bowel perforations. Chance fractures are caused by hyperflexion over the fulcrum of the seatbelt (3,9,10,14), which results in bony and ligamentous injuries (9). Plain radiographs are the diagnostic study of choice (10), and treatment includes hyperextension in cast or brace for bony injuries and spinal fusion for ligamentous injuries (9). Such injuries should be considered in children with other signs of the "Seat Belt Syndrome."

CRITICAL INTERVENTIONS

PHYSIOLOGICALLY UNSTABLE PATIENT WITH CHEST OR ABDOMINAL TRAUMA	PHYSIOLOGICALLY STABLE PATIENT WITH CHEST OR ABDOMINAL TRAUMA
Airway 100% Oxygen; evaluate the necessity for an ET tube or needle thoracostomy	**Airway** 100% Oxygen initially
Fluids 20 ml/kg NS or Ringer lactate via bolus Repeat bolus 1 or 2 times if needed Transfuse 10–20 ml/kg of blood for $\downarrow$ BP If vital signs are unstable, repeat the blood transfusion and proceed to laparotomy	**Fluids** IV heplock
Laboratory Studies, Tube Placement Hb, hct, type and cross, nasogastric tube, foley catheter, pregnancy test in child bearing females	**Laboratory Studies, Tube Placement** Hb, hct, amylase, urinalysis, type and screen, pregnancy test in child bearing females
Diagnostic Studies FAST or DPL to check for intraabdominal bleeding	**Diagnostic Studies** Chest radiograph to rule out chest injury; CT scan of the abdomen for blunt abdominal trauma
Needle thoracostomy and chest tube Tension pneumothorax	**Chest tube** Pneumothorax
Laparotomy Stab wounds and gun shot wounds	**Laparotomy** GI perforation, bladder rupture, pelvic fractures
Disposition Operating Room or the ICU	**Disposition** Admit the majority of thoracic injuries; solid organ injuries; abdominal pain; and a small subset of anterior stab wounds in asymptomatic patients

Hb, hemoglobin; hct, hematocrit.

DISPOSITION

Role of the Consultant

The patient's clinical assessment, the injury severity, and diagnostic results must be considered (3,6,13) when deciding on the necessity of surgical consultation. However, a surgeon familiar with pediatric trauma should be contacted as early as possible if intrathoracic or intraabdominal injury is suspected (1,3,6,17,19,21,23,24,25). All children with penetrating injury should be evaluated by a surgeon because of the likelihood of exploratory surgery (3,19,24).

Additionally, other specialists may also be needed for consultation. For instance, if a heart injury is suspected; consultation with an echocardiographer or cardiologist may be necessary to aid in imaging (3,4,6,13). Likewise, once the diagnosis of urologic injury is made the urologist should be consulted for a definitive plan of therapy (1).

Indications for Admission

The majority of children with thoracic and abdominal trauma should be admitted to the hospital for observation. The determination of which hospital unit is most appropriate for the care of these children depends on the severity of the injury and the type of monitoring required (24). For example, most children with thoracic injury are admitted to the ICU for observation, serial examination and management (2,11,13,20). All patients with penetrating chest trauma even without air or fluid accumulation within the chest should be admitted for observation (19). Patients with hemothorax require admission for serial examinations of the chest and monitoring of ongoing blood loss through the chest tube (3,6,13). In addition, all patients with traumatic pneumothorax require surgical consultation and admission (6). However, if there are no other significant injuries present then admission to general pediatric unit is adequate.

When considering disposition of patients with abdominal trauma one should keep in mind that there are no laboratory tests that reliably diagnose solid or visceral injury. Intestinal injuries can be especially difficult to diagnose (25). Therefore, all children with persistent abdominal tenderness on examination, a "seat belt sign" (9), laboratory abnormalities or radiologic evidence of intraabdominal organ injury must be admitted for monitoring (21). The majority of children who require an abdominal CT should also be admitted for observation, and most require surgical consultation (10). Patients with a major solid organ injury should be admitted to an area capable of providing intensive monitoring or transferred to an appropriate facility. Since at least some of these patients will ultimately require surgery; surgeons should be involved in their care (3). Children with suspected solid organ injury based on laboratory abnormalities alone may be admitted to the general ward for observation. A small group of children with minimal abdominal pain and a history of abdominal trauma may be discharged home if they appear well, and if no significant injuries have been detected after a complete ED evaluation. In most cases, these patients should be observed in the ED for a few hours, and be reexamined. After discharge they should have follow up with their primary care physician.

Transfer Considerations

All patients admitted for observation of thoracic and abdominal injuries should be managed in concert with pediatric or trauma surgical specialists (3,19,24). If a patient with thoracic or abdominal injuries arrives at a hospital not equipped to care for children or the type of injury the patient has then the patient should be rapidly stabilized and transferred to a regional pediatric or general trauma center (3,19,23,24). All patients with a pediatric trauma score of ≤ 8 (Table 209.2), or a revised trauma score < 12 should be transferred to a designated trauma facility (24). Similarly, children with multiple rib fractures at risk for splenic and liver injury may require transfer to a specialized center (13), as these injuries should be managed by surgeons familiar with nonoperative solid organ injury in facilities equipped to handle sequelae promptly (3,23).

COMMON PITFALLS

- ✔ Failure to recognize that chest injury may occur in young children without physical evidence
- ✔ Failure to recognize that gastric distension may compromise oxygenation and ventilation
- ✔ Failure to suspect diaphragm injury with any penetrating trauma to the chest or abdomen
- ✔ Verifying radiographic confirmation of a tension pneumothorax prior to tube thoracostomy
- ✔ Inability to promptly recognize hemodynamic instability in children
- ✔ Failure to administer adequate crystalloid and blood products for significant blood loss
- ✔ Missing rupture of the small bowel in "Seat Belt Syndrome"
- ✔ Failure to recognize evidence of child abuse
- ✔ Failure to recognize aerophagia as a cause of abdominal distention in children
- ✔ Failure to repeatedly reevaluate an injured child while he/she is in the ED

Acknowledgments

Thanks to the previous edition's chapter authors Khaled Mutabagani and Donna A. Caniano.

References

1. Ahn JH, Morey AF, McAnich, JW. Workup and management of traumatic hematuria. *Emerg Med Clin North Am* 1998;16:145–164.
2. Allen GS, Cox CS. Pulmonary Contusion in children: diagnosis and management. *South Med J* 1998;91:1099–1106.
3. American College of Surgeons. In: *Advanced Trauma Life Support (ATLS) for doctors student course manual*. 6th ed. Chicago: American College of Surgeons, 1997.
4. Baum VC. Cardiac trauma in children. *Pediatr Anaesth* 2002;12:110–117.
5. Baumann MH, Sahn SA. Tension pneumothorax: diagnostic and therapeutic pitfalls. *Crit Care Med* 1993;21:177–179.
6. Bliss D, Silen M. Pediatric thoracic trauma. *Crit Care Med* 2002;30:S409–S415.
7. Canty TG, Weinman D. Management of major pancreatic duct injuries in children. *J Trauma* 2001;50:1001–1007.
8. DiGiacomo JC, Frankel H, Haskell RM, Rotondo MF, Schwab W. Unsuspected child abuse revealed by delayed presentation of periportal tracking and myoglobinuria. *J Trauma* 2000;49:348–350.
9. Durbin DR, Arbogast KB, Moll EK. Seat belt syndrome in children: a case report and review of the literature. *Pediatr Emerg Care* 2001;17:474–477.
10. Gaines BA, Ford HR. Abdominal and pelvic trauma in children. *Crit Care Med* 2002;30:S416–S423.
11. Garcia VF, Gotschall CS, Eichelberger MR, Bowman LM. Rib fractures in children: a marker of severity. *J Trauma* 1990;30:695–700.
12. Genc A, Özcan C, Erdener A, Mutaf O. Management of pneumothorax in children. *J Cardiovasc Surg* 1998;39:849–851.
13. Grisoni ER, Volsko TA. Thoracic injuries in children. *Respir Care Clin N Am* 2001;7:25–38.
14. Holland A, Cass DT, Glasson MJ, Pitkin J. Small bowel injuries in children. *J Paediatr. Child Health* 2000;36:265–269.
15. Holmes JF, Sokolove PE, Brant WE, Kuppermann N. A clinical decision rule for identifying children with thoracic injuries after blunt torso trauma. *Ann of Emerg Med* 2002;39:492–499.
16. Hormuth D, Cefali D, Rouse T, et al. Traumatic disruption of the thoracic aorta in children. *Arch Surg* 1999;134:759–763.
17. Karnak İ, Senocak ME, Büyükpamukcu TC. Diaphragmatic injuries in children. *Surg Today* 2001;31:5–11.
18. Lateef F. Commotio cordis an underappreciated cause of sudden death in athletes. *Sports Med* 2000;30:301–308.
19. Murray JA, Berne J, Asencio JA. Penetrating thoracoabdominal trauma. *Emerg Med Clin North Am* 1998;16:107–128.
20. Ozdulger A, Guven C, Gulhan SE, et al. A review of 24 patients with bronchial ruptures: is delay in diagnosis more common in children? *Eur J of Cardio-thoracic Surg* 2003;23:379–383.
21. Rance CH, Singh SJ, Kimble R. Blunt abdominal trauma in children. *J Paediatr Child Health* 2000;36:2–6.
22. Rees MJ, Aickin R, Kolbe A, Teele RL. The screening pelvic radiograph in pediatric trauma. *Pediatr Radiol* 2001;31:497–500.
23. Rothrock SG, Green SM, Morgan R. Abdominal trauma in infants and children: prompt identification and early management of serious and life-threatening injuries. Part I: Injury patterns and initial assessment. *Pediatr Emerg Care* 2000;16:106–115.

24. Rothrock SG, Green SM, Morgan R. Abdominal trauma in infants and children: prompt identification and early management of serious and life-threatening injuries. Part II: Specific injuries and ED management. *Pediatr Emerg Care* 2000;16:189–195.
25. Vane DW. Imaging of the injured child: important questions answered quickly and correctly. *Surg Clin North Am* 2002;82:315–323.

CHAPTER 213
Fractures and Sports Injuries

Christopher S. Kennedy and Robert D. Yniguez

Fractures account for up to 10% to 15% of emergency department (ED) visits of children, owing to their high activity level, youthful fearlessness, poor judgment, and underdeveloped motor coordination. High-energy trauma has become more significant, although the incidence may decrease with stricter child passenger seat laws and enforcement. Over the past decade as participation in organized youth sports programs has increased, so has the spectrum of injuries that are sustained by children.

Because their bones are actively growing, children have a distinct bony architecture different from that of adults, and active growth may make different growth areas more susceptible at different stages. Actively growing bones are described by three areas: the epiphysis, metaphysis, and diaphysis.

Generally, children's bones are more porous, more pliable, and overall have less strength than those of adults. Likewise, because ligamentous attachments are stronger than their bony attachments, fractures (e.g., avulsions) are more common than sprains, strains, or dislocations. Children's fractures have a high rate of healing and potential for deformity correction through remodeling. Pediatric fracture healing is complicated by problems such as plastic deformation, growth arrest, and progressive angulation.

A thorough examination is necessary, not only of the fracture site, but also to rule out any associated or occult injury. This can be challenging with a frightened, uncooperative patient who is in pain, and with concerned parents hovering nearby. After taking a history and performing a detailed physical examination, further diagnostic studies, usually plain radiographs, are obtained. Laboratory evaluation has minimal utility in most fracture decision-making. If an isolated extremity injury is the presumptive diagnosis, adequate pain control should be strongly considered and may be started before plain films are performed. Occasionally, pelvic fractures and multiple long-bone fractures may cause enough blood loss to result in hemodynamic compromise. Barring suspicion of these injuries, hemodynamic instability merits a careful examination to seek others sources of blood loss.

Treatment is based on the complete diagnosis and should include pain control. Options include definitive treatment by the emergency physician, splinting and referral, or immediate consultation with orthopaedic or other specialists.

DESCRIPTION OF FRACTURES

Proper use of fracture nomenclature can do much to elevate the status of the emergency physician in the eyes of the consultant. Simplicity is the key, avoiding unfamiliar eponyms and references to bony landmarks.

The description should begin by naming the injured bone. In the hand, use of the terms *thumb, index finger, long finger, ring finger,* and *small finger* is preferable to numeric description, due to confusion as to whether the thumb is counted or if the count starts medially or laterally.

Fractures are classified by where they are on the bone. Shaft fractures are diaphyseal. The flare is the metaphysis. The radiolucent growth plate is the physis, and the epiphysis is the secondary ossification center. "Proximal" or "distal" is the best way to distinguish one end of the bone from the other.

Displacement is relative to the width of the shaft. Nondisplaced fractures show only a hairline fracture. Displacement of only 5% to 10% of the shaft width is termed *minimally displaced.* Further displacement is described by percentage.

Angulation is described separately from displacement, by both degrees of angulation and direction, with the apex as the reference direction. For example, the common Colles' fracture is volar angulation, even though the hand is deformed in a dorsal direction.

Various fracture configurations are described below (Fig. 213.1). Growth plate injuries are classified by the Salter-Harris scheme (Fig. 213.2), with the risk of growth problems increasing with grade. Salter III and IV are further complicated by the potential for intraarticular displacement. Salter V fractures are often diagnosed only in retrospect.

It is important to describe any associated injuries, particularly the nature of the injury (i.e., open or closed) and the child's neurovascular status, as these can alter crucial treatment decisions.

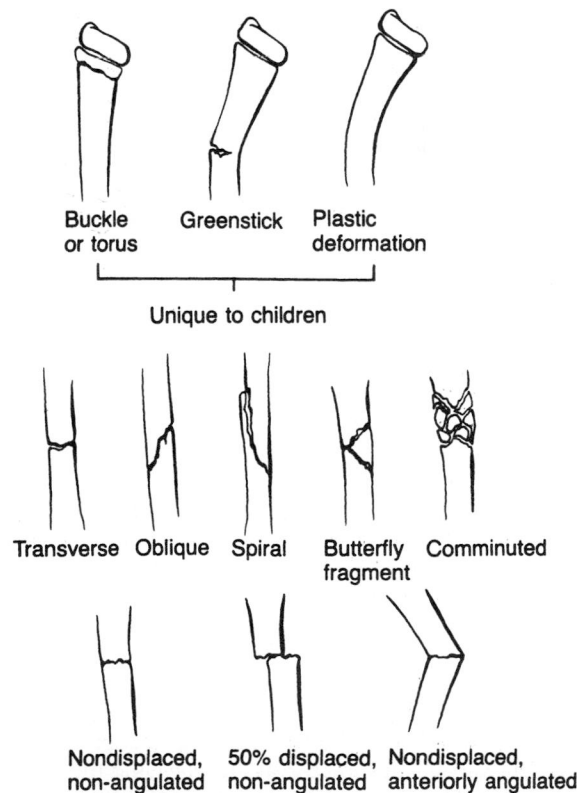

Figure 213.1. Descriptive terminology for pediatric fractures.

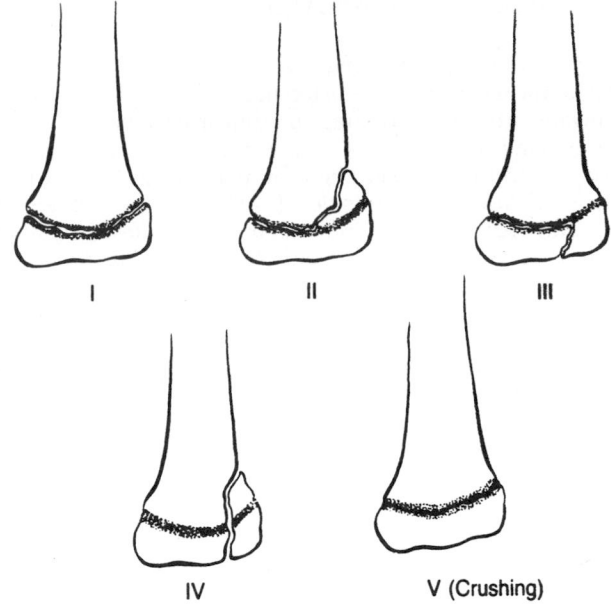

Figure 213.2. Salter-Harris nomenclature of representative fractures involving the growth plate in children.

EMERGENCY DEPARTMENT EVALUATION

Accurate, complete diagnosis is of paramount importance. Common fracture patterns and associations are easily recognized if the treating physician is familiar with them. Management, based on some knowledge of the natural history, is usually straightforward if the diagnosis is correct and complete. An incorrect or delayed diagnosis can result in complications. Although the rapid healing of children's fractures is generally beneficial, it can decrease the time-frame in which interventions are possible, usually to about a week.

History

While it may be tempting to take a quick history, believing that the x-rays will show everything, it is very important to establish the circumstances and mechanism of injury. The time spent obtaining the history also allows the physician time to establish rapport with the parent and to calm and gain the trust of the child.

When the nature of the injury seems implausible, child abuse must be considered. If high-energy trauma was involved, occult intraabdominal or intracranial injury must be sought. If the cause of the fracture is a mystery to the child, the physician must consider the possibility of seizures, leading to a fall.

The mechanism of injury provides clues as well. The common fall on an outstretched arm can produce wrist, forearm, or elbow fractures, or a combination of these. Falls from a height may result in calcaneus fractures associated with lumbar spine fractures. A dashboard injury can fracture the patella and can cause a hip fracture or dislocation.

Physical Examination

It is difficult to overemphasize the importance of the physical examination. The uninjured extremities and the spine are examined first; the physician should reassure the child that he or she will not cause pain unexpectedly. This may reveal occult injuries while the child is most cooperative and least upset.

When examining the injured extremity, the examiner should start at the end farthest from the painful area. Careful and thorough palpation of the entire limb is important. Any significantly tender areas should be x-rayed. When possible, joints should be taken through a range of motion to assess for possible dislocation, particularly in the older child. This is most important for the shoulder, elbow (including pronation and supination), and hip. The joints should be palpated as well; radial head and proximal fibula fractures are frequently missed.

The skin should be thoroughly assessed, including the part hidden by splints applied as first aid. A laceration over a joint requires exploration to rule out an arthrotomy, a condition requiring urgent management. A break in the skin associated with a fracture is usually an open fracture, particularly if it has a continuous, slow oozing of dark blood, characteristically associated with fat droplets. This requires emergent intervention as well.

Neurologic and vascular examinations must not be omitted. Frequently, the child will cooperate with at least a sensory examination for light touch. More encouragement may be rewarded with a limited motor examination. A wiggle is better than nothing.

Compartment syndrome must not be overlooked. It is most common in the forearm and lower leg as a result of either fracture or crushing injuries, leading to bleeding and swelling within inelastic fascial compartments. Elevated pressures lead to ischemia at the capillary level and, untreated, can threaten the entire limb from muscle and nerve necrosis. The hallmarks are pain out of proportion to the degree of injury, and extreme pain with passive range of motion of the fingers or toes. Paresthesias, pulselessness, and pallor are all late manifestations. A compartment syndrome is a true orthopaedic emergency, and early consultation with an orthopedist is warranted. Definitive diagnosis should be in concert with an orthopedist to measure compartment pressure. Emergent fasciotomy is required to preserve limb function.

Unfortunately, a fracture during childhood may be a manifestation of child abuse in up to 5% to 18% of cases. Suspicion for child abuse should be high when an infant (less than 1 year old) has a fracture, there are inconsistencies between the history and the fracture type or developmental abilities of the child, there are multiple fractures in different stages of healing, or there are multiple, complex or depressed fractures. Certain fracture types are associated with child abuse. Especially noteworthy is a spiral fracture of the femur or tibia in a nonambulating child, spiral fracture of the humerus, avulsion of the clavicle or acromion process, posterior rib, scapular, sternal, or metaphyseal chip fracture. Any suspicious finding constitutes grounds for reporting to local social service officials and consultation with the nearest center providing comprehensive care for the abused child.

Radiographic Evaluation

Obtaining high-quality radiographs is almost as important as the physical examination. Performing an inadequate examination and accepting poor radiographs can mean missing a fracture. Long bone fractures should be splinted before taking x-rays. Unstable joint injuries also may be splinted, although this sometimes obscures crucial detail.

X-rays should be made at 90 degrees (orthogonal) to each other. With diaphyseal fractures, radiographs should be taken of the joint above and below, particularly if there is any tenderness or if the physical examination is limited. The wrist and elbow cannot be adequately evaluated with regular forearm films. Foregoing additional radiographs and missing an associated fracture is, obviously, a false economy.

Comparison views can be helpful, but should not be routine. Start with an oblique view then move on to comparison films if necessary. An anteroposterior view of the pelvis, with a lateral view of the affected hip, should be routinely ordered, rather than an anteroposterior and lateral view of the hip. Elbows can be difficult to evaluate without a contralateral control, even for the subspecialist. Comparison views are also frequently indicated for ankle fractures or shoulder injuries. Oblique x-rays can aid in diagnosis as well, particularly in the knee, ankle, and elbow.

Some injuries have a high rate of missed associated fractures. Cervical spine and pelvic radiographs should be part of the protocol for high-energy trauma. Chest x-rays should be evaluated for bony injuries. A calcaneus fracture due to a fall should prompt lumbar spine films. Suspected child abuse should be routinely pursued with a skeletal survey, especially with a preverbal or developmentally delayed child.

Poor-quality films must not be accepted. The child may be uncomfortable and the radiologic technician may shy away from getting high-quality films, but the duty of diagnosis ultimately rests with the physician, who should insist on films with good anteroposterior views and a true lateral. Excessive obliquity easily obscures subtle fractures. Administering pain medications prior to obtaining radiographs may help by reducing the patient's discomfort and allowing more adequate positioning.

Additional imaging techniques are sometimes helpful. Stress views are commonly used to evaluate acromioclavicular joint injuries and occult knee-joint growth plate or ligament injuries. Computed tomography (CT) scanning is frequently used for spine injuries. More intensive techniques, such as arthrography, arteriography, bone scanning, and magnetic resonance imaging are of great benefit when indicated, but are typically considered to be the domain of the consultant.

EMERGENCY DEPARTMENT MANAGEMENT

The treatment options are for the ED practitioner to treat the fracture definitively, to splint and provide temporary treatment with later referral to a specialist, or to seek immediate consultation.

Some simple fractures with low risk of problems and uniformly good outcomes may be cared for completely in the ED. Factors in this decision include the physician's degree of confidence in fracture management, ease of providing followup care, and acceptance by the parents of the treatment plan.

Temporary splinting with later referral is more common. Common indications are nondisplaced or minimally displaced fractures and fractures with a low risk of short-term complications such as neurovascular compromise or compartment syndrome.

Immediate consultation should be sought for all open fractures, arthrotomies, moderately displaced fractures and unreduced dislocations. Open fractures should be regarded as orthopaedic emergencies. They should be treated with prophylactic intravenous antibiotics (e.g., broad-spectrum cephalosporins), tetanus prophylaxis, and orthopaedic consultation. Neurovascular injury and compartment syndrome require emergent surgical intervention. Consultation is also indicated when there is a high index of suspicion but adequate evaluation has failed to establish a diagnosis. Triage of displaced fractures that require reduction depends on the relationship between the emergency physician and the orthopedist. Many orthopedists prefer to see the child initially and perform the reduction in the ED, where there is appropriate equipment and support personnel.

Immobilization

Immobilization decreases the discomfort in the injured limb. It also can maintain the fracture in a reduced position and prevent further injury by jagged fracture fragments.

Choices for immobilization are varied. Splints are the most popular, and plaster of Paris is best, owing to its ease of molding, although prepadded, fiberglass splint material is being used in many areas. A good plaster splint requires adequate padding, with particular attention to bony prominences. The splint should hold the joint above and below the fracture. Too long is better than too short. Fifteen layers of plaster is the standard. It should be applied and overwrapped while wet for a good mold. Movement while hardening greatly weakens the splint. Commercial splints are much less desirable due to the difficulty of proper fitting and the resulting poor immobilization. Inflatable splints may exert external pressure on already traumatized tissue.

Casts are less commonly used by emergency physicians due to problems associated with swelling inside a rigid cast. This difficulty may be alleviated to some degree by splitting the cast. Ice and elevation are critically important in managing swelling in all fractures. Proper cast application requires skill and practice to achieve the proper balance between being tight enough to maintain the immobilization and loose enough to avoid problems with swelling. Overall, a splint is more easily applied and is superior to a poorly fitting cast. Neurovascular status distal to the affected limb should be evaluated and documented both before and after splinting.

If the child is being transferred or referred for later treatment, the fracture fragments must not be left in a position that tents the skin. Skin necrosis can result in conversion to an open fracture in only a few hours.

Operative Treatment

A detailed discussion is beyond the scope of this chapter. Operative intervention is usually indicated for fractures with a high degree of instability. A nontype I supracondylar fracture will likely require reduction with pinning. Open fractures require thorough cleaning and removal of contaminated, necrotic tissue to reduce the risk of infection. Other high-risk fractures include those with the potential for neurovascular compromise secondary to displacement, intraarticular fracture or severe growth plate injury. Internal fixation is also used to make overall management easier in head-injured and multiply injured children.

Complications

Neurovascular injury and compartment syndrome, discussed previously, may result in loss of function or even loss of the limb. Angular deformity is common, but many deformities remodel if sufficient growth remains and the deformity is in the plane of joint motion. A general rule is that remodeling will be adequate if the child's deformed bone fits within the outline of the adult bone. No remodeling is to be expected in rotational deformity, nor in displaced Salter III and IV fractures.

The child's growth potential can lead to problems with physeal fractures. Partial or complete growth arrest leads to progressive angular malalignment or limb-length discrepancy, respectively, and requires surgery for correction, often with compromised results.

Discharge Instructions

The parents should be taught routine care of the cast or splint, the importance of frequent neurovascular checks, and that adequate pain medication should be provided. The importance of ice and elevation must be stressed. The parents must understand the need for followup care and the risk of complications if this is neglected.

Treatment of Specific Fractures

Shoulder

The clavicle is the most commonly fractured bone in childhood, specifically the middle third in about 80% of cases. Usually resulting from falls or direct blows, the majority can be managed without orthopaedic referral. Clavicular fractures in children less than 2 years of age should raise concern for intentional injury. Fractures of the clavicle can be treated with an arm sling for children less than 12 years and should be worn for at least 2 weeks. Children older than 12 years may require use of a figure-of-eight strap and a sling for at least 4 weeks to allow for adequate healing. Range of motion exercises, limited activity, and intermittent follow up is needed once the sling is removed. Fractures of the humerus usually involve the metaphysis and are Salter Harris type I or II. Nongrowth plate involved fractures heal remarkably well without reduction in children less than 11 years and can remodel with up to 20 degrees of angulation and 2 cm of shortening. Proximal humeral fractures are typically managed with the use of a sling. Range of motion exercises commence after a brief period of immobilization, but sling use is continued for at least 2 weeks. Older children will require immediate orthopaedic intervention with anatomic reduction.

Elbow

Pediatric elbow fractures have high rates of complications, even in the hands of experts. In order to confirm the diagnosis, a true lateral film of the elbow is required. A true lateral will show a figure of eight or hour glass appearance at the distal humerus. Radiographic evidence of a torus fracture may be subtle, and a nondisplaced fracture may be difficult to diagnose. Secondary ossification centers may be confused with fractures if one is not familiar with the ages of their appearances and closures. Radiographs must be carefully inspected for the presence of abnormal fat pads, anterior or posterior to the distal humerus. Also important is the alignment of the radial head with the capitellum. To evaluate this alignment, a line drawn through the central axis of the radius should pass through the center of the capitellum. The anterior humeral line also aids in evaluation for fracture. A line is drawn down the anterior aspect of the humerus and it should pass though the anterior aspect of the capitellum or just in front of it. Comparison views of the unaffected extremity may prove helpful if the diagnosis is not clear. Isolated abnormalities in the fat pads should be considered signs of occult fracture; immobilization and prompt follow up should be arranged in consultation with an orthopedist. In general, any displaced distal humerus fracture requires pinning. Supracondylar fractures have an extremely high risk for neurovascular injury and compartment syndrome and potential for significant complications if not managed properly. Late deformity results from less-than-anatomic reduction. Medial epicondyle fractures in younger children have a high association with elbow dislocation. Minimally displaced radial head fractures are usually treated with early motion.

Forearm

Forearm fractures are common fractures in childhood. Good results are the norm, even with growth plate injury. It is important to view the wrist and elbow when a forearm fracture is present. A Monteggia fracture (radial head dislocation with a proximal ulna fracture) can be missed if attention is focused on the forearm fracture and radial head alignment is overlooked. Isolated distal ulna torus fractures usually have an associated distal radius physeal fracture. True buckle fractures require only 3 to 4 weeks of immobilization, initially with a sugar tong splint followed by a short arm cast. Fractures with angulation or displacement should be promptly referred to an orthopedist for possible reduction. The majority of reductions can be performed nonoperatively by an orthopedist via deep sedation.

Hand/Wrist

Children's hand fractures, unless the injury is severe, are generally free of the stiffness problems that plague adults. Phalangeal fractures involving the growth plate or through the joint should be followed up by an orthopedist, but can be splinted in the ED. Before splinting, each phalangeal injury should be examined for the presence of rotational or malrotation deformity, which may be missed if the digit is examined only in extension. To examine for rotational deformity, the fingers should be flexed to make sure all fingers point in the same direction. Overlapping of the digits occurs if rotational deformity is present and reduction is needed. A nailbed injury with the nail pulled out proximally and overlying the eponychial fold is generally associated with a Salter fracture of the distal phalanx. This is an easily overlooked open fracture. Nailbed injuries require precise repair. Carpal bone fractures can be difficult to assess in an anxious child. One must not overlook these fractures with the most common being the scaphoid and lunate. These will need splinting and orthopaedic follow up. If a scaphoid injury is suspected (i.e., tenderness at anatomic snuffbox) but not seen on radiograph, a thumb spica splint with radiographic follow up in 2 weeks is necessary.

Hip

Hip fractures in children are not very common but carry a high potential for serious injury if not dealt with appropriately. Usually a high-energy event precedes these types of fractures, such as a motor vehicle crash or fall from significant height. Once the patient is medically and hemodynamically stable, patient care is coordinated with the orthopedist. Apophyseal avulsion should be suspected when hip pain is present after sudden onset of pain during an activity and the patient's flexion and range of motion of the hip do not elicit pain. Radiographs will rule out fracture to the hip but may show the avulsed bony fragment. Treatment includes pain management and rest with a gradual return to previous activities. Fractures of the proximal femur will warrant reduction with fixation by the orthopedist. A slipped capital femoral epiphysis is easily missed. The child usually presents with no or minimal trauma, groin aching, or simply medial thigh and knee pain. Hallmarks on physical examination are mandatory abduction and external rotation when the hip is brought into flexion. Delay in diagnosis is associated with progressive slipping. Radiographic findings can be subtle, especially in early cases; therefore, good lateral radiographs are required.

Knee

Knee pain can be referred from the hip. Strong consideration should be given to the routine use of anteroposterior pelvic and lateral hip x-rays when evaluating knee pain. Ligament injuries are less common in children's knees than are occult growth plate injuries. The most common injury involving the distal femoral physis follow by the proximal tibia. Stress views can establish the diagnosis only if the child is relaxed and cooperative. After proper reduction (closed or open) by the orthopedist, a long-leg cast is applied with the duration of 6 to 8 weeks. A dislocated patella may be reduced simply by bringing the knee into extension.

Leg

Fractures of the femur and tibia will require urgent orthopaedic referral. The decision for use of traction, spica cast placement, external fixation, or internal fixation will be individualized to the patient according to age and other factors by the orthopedist.

If the tibia or fibula fracture are nondisplaced then the patient can be placed in a long-leg cast with nonweight bearing and given orthopaedic follow up in 1 week. Tibia fractures may be a cause of compartment syndrome. If a patient has increasing pain after simple measures of elevation and pain medications then compartment syndrome should be suspected. The term *toddler fracture* refers to an oblique nondisplaced fracture of the distal tibia, usually occurring in children under 4 years of age. These children may present to the ED with complaints of a limp and a history of a minor accident or no witnessed event. The physical findings may be subtle. Pain with gentle twisting of the leg may be the only localizing physical finding. Because they may poorly localize, complete radiographs of both lower extremities are needed. Immobilization in a posterior long-leg splint usually provides relief of symptoms, and at least telephone consultation with a pediatric orthopedist is advisable.

Ankle

Young children rarely sustain "sprains" and therefore this diagnosis should be used with caution. Salter-Harris type I and II can usually be managed conservatively with possible closed reduction followed by short leg splint immobilization for 3 to 4 weeks. Salter-Harris types III, IV, and V will likely require operative intervention some time during their management. Pain over the distal fibula physis with a normal radiograph in a child should be managed as a Salter-Harris type I fracture. The fracture pattern varies with age. An example of this age variation is the distal tibia fracture called a "Tillaux fracture," which is unique to adolescents. As skeletal maturity is achieved and growth plates are beginning to close, the medial distal tibial epiphysis closes prior to the lateral. This creates a fulcrum through which a Salter-Harris III fracture may occur, just lateral to the point of fusion. Due to growth plate involvement and a potential need for open fixation, a prompt orthopaedic consultation is indicated. Intraarticular injury is common. CT scans are useful in evaluating complex fracture patterns and comparison views may help in difficult cases.

Foot

Lawn mower injuries are a common cause of open fractures including 60,000 U.S. emergency ED visits in 1998 with 20% of cases involving children. (1) Severe contamination and degree of injury may require operative debridement. Athletes are subject to metatarsal stress fractures, particularly in adolescence. Fractures at the very base of the fifth metatarsal require only minimal treatment, but proximal metaphyseal fractures outside the articular area (Jones fractures) need cast immobilization and a period of nonweightbearing. Jones fracture requires close orthopaedic follow up due the high incidence of nonunion. Malalignment at the base of the metatarsals, particularly the second, suggests a Lisfranc dislocation, which has a high risk of associated complications.

Sports Injuries

Over the past decade, larger numbers of children began participating in organized youth sports programs. This has led to an increase in sports-related injuries. Common among these injuries, other than various acute fractures, are overuse injuries, avulsion fractures, stress fractures, and ligamentous injuries. The following are specific examples.

Peripheral Nerve Injuries: The Stinger

A "stinger" is a peripheral nerve injury that involves an upper limb unilaterally. This nerve injury is most commonly caused by a compressive overload of the head and neck, such as tackling in football. The athlete experiences a burning pain in the affected limb over the C5 to C6 dermatome, which may last from seconds to 60 minutes, and there may be associated weakness. More than single-limb involvement should raise concern for possible cervical spine injury. The athlete should be immobilized on the field and transported to the ED. Most athletes transported to the ED with cervical immobilization for a tackling injury require cervical spine radiographs before removing the cervical collar. Cervical spine fracture is a rare diagnosis. Most patients should be advised in the ED to discontinue play until cleared by a follow up visit with their primary care, sports medicine, or orthopaedic specialist, and some will require aggressive physical therapy.

Overuse Injuries

Stress Fractures. Stress fractures are becoming more common in children. Risk factors include a "high-volume" or repetitive activity and improper training or overtraining. The most common sites of injury in children are the tibia, fibula, and the pars interarticularis segment of the vertebra (i.e., spondylolysis). Each of these stress fractures may cause localized tenderness; most require more than plain films, and so are not usually diagnosed in the ED. One exception may be spondylolysis, the most common cause of back pain in a child to yield an anatomic diagnosis. The thin segment of bone between facet joints is subject to high forces, especially with marked lordosis, or heavy lifting. Most commonly seen in the early teen years, the frequency may reach 20% of those athletes competing in wrestling, gymnastics, or weight lifting. While pain will be exacerbated by straight-leg raising, radiation of pain into the legs is rare. Plain film radiography may reveal the diagnosis and is best visualized on oblique views. The most frequent location is at L5, followed by L4. Management is conservative, and the athlete should be discouraged from sports participation if activity is painful. Outpatient follow up with a bone scan may be needed.

Little League Elbow. Little League elbow is an overuse injury seen in young pitchers. The usual presentation is elbow pain, history of intense throwing and a subtle flexion contracture, most commonly caused by valgus strain during the acceleration phase of throwing. Plain films of the elbow may be normal or difficult to assess due to the immature physis and secondary ossification centers. Treatment should include ice, NSAIDs, physical therapy, and rest from play until clearance by a qualified physician. No immobilization is needed.

Iliac Crest Apophysitis. Iliac crest apophysitis is an overuse injury commonly seen in runners and hockey, soccer, or football players. The main symptom is pain over the affected iliac crest that is worsened with running. Plain radiographs are normal. Treatment is conservative.

Patellofemoral Stress Syndrome. Patellofemoral stress syndrome is the most common complaint in young female athletes. The common presentation is of aching knees, with pain increased by jumping or climbing. Physical findings usually include pain on compression of the patellar region; joint effusion and swelling are rare. Plain films are normal and treatment includes relative rest and physical therapy.

Sever Disease. Sever disease, or calcaneal apophysitis, is a common complaint of adolescent boys. The chief complaint is pain in the heel that is worsened by running. No swelling or deformity is noted on physical examination; only tenderness is noted at the posterior heel at the Achilles tendon insertion site. Radiographs are not helpful and treatment includes rest, NSAIDs, and Achilles tendon stretching exercises. The disease is usually self-limited.

Osgood-Schlatter disease. This disease is seen in adolescents who usually participate in jumping sports such as basketball.

There is a repetitive stress to the apophysis of the tibial tuberosity, a secondary ossification center. The athlete will complain of pain at the site of the distal patellar ligament. Physical examination may reveal swelling of the proximal tibia and tenderness with palpation over the distal tibial tubercle. Fragmentation of the tibial tubercle may be seen on radiography. Treatment is conservative with rest and NSAIDs (see Chapter 282).

Avulsion Fractures

Avulsion fractures may occur at virtually any muscular insertion point. Two noteworthy examples in children include avulsions about the pelvis and avulsions about the tibial spine or intercondylar eminence. Avulsion fractures of the hip may occur at a muscular attachment typically pulled off during strong, active resistance. Pain is localized but may be significant with weight bearing. Often, the diagnosis can be made by plain film radiographs, and treatment is conservative, with partial or no weight bearing for 2 or more weeks.

Intercondylar eminence or tibial spine fracture occurs from anterior cruciate ligament injury caused by either noncontact or collision trauma. Typically, this happens with abrupt decelerating or direction changes, with or without an audible "pop." Gross swelling about the knee joint is a prominent physical finding, as is intense pain. Plain film radiographs may reveal the fragment as nondisplaced (type I), minimally displaced (type II), or with rotation or significant displacement (type III). This injury should prompt consultation with an orthopedist, and treatment may include drainage of the associated effusion or open reduction and pinning.

CRITICAL INTERVENTIONS

- If a scaphoid injury is suspected (i.e., tenderness at anatomic snuffbox) but not seen on radiograph, a thumb spica splint should be applied
- Obtain radiographs of a joint above and a joint below the fractured area

COMMON PITFALLS

✔ Children rarely sustain sprains. When in doubt immobilize and instruct on proper follow up
✔ Child abuse should be considered when there are inconsistencies between the history of injury, developmental stage, and the fracture type
✔ Children with fractures need adequate outpatient pain control

Acknowledgment

The authors gratefully acknowledge the contribution of John Churchill, who wrote a previous version of this chapter.

References

1. Anderson SJ. Lower extremity injuries in youth sports. *Pediatr Clin N Am* 2002;49:627–641.
2. Cramer KE. Orthopaedic aspects of child abuse. *Pediatr Clin North Am* 1996;43:1035–1051.
3. Green NE, Swiontkowski MF, eds. *Skeletal trauma in children*. Philadelphia: WB Saunders, 1994.
4. Gomez JE. Upper extremity injuries in youth sports. *Pediatr Clin N Am* 2002;49:593–626.
5. Kay RM, Matthys GA. Pediatric ankle fractures: evaluation and treatment. *J Am Acad Orthop Surg* 2001;9:268–278.
6. Luckstead EF, Patel DR. Catastrophic pediatric sports injuries. *Pediatr Clin N Am* 2002;49:581–591.
7. Marsh JS, Daigneault JP. Ankle injuries in the pediatric population. *Curr Opin Pediatr* 2000;12:52–60.
8. Outerbridge AR, Micheli LJ. Overuse injuries in the young athlete. *Sport Med Clin North Am* 1995;14:503–516.
9. Perron AD, Miller MD, Brady WJ. Orthopaedic pitfalls in the ED: pediatric growth plate injuries. *Am J Emerg Med* 2002;20:50–54.
10. Rockwood CA, Wilkins KE, Beaty JH, eds. *Fractures in children*, 4th ed. Philadelphia: JB Lippincott Co, 1996.

Selected Readings

Centers for Disease Control and Prevention (2003, November 18). National Hospital Ambulatory Medical Care Survey. Retrieved February 18, 2004, from http://www.cdc.gov/nchs/about/major/ahcd/injurytable.htm.
England SP, Sundberg S. Management of common pediatric fractures. *Pediatr Clin North Am* 1996;43:991–1012.
Hogan KA, Gross RH. Overuse injuries in pediatric athletes. *Orthop Clin N Am* 2003;34:405–415.

PART III

Chief Complaints

CHAPTER 214
Abdominal Pain

Loren G. Yamamoto

Abdominal pain is a common complaint in children presenting to emergency departments (EDs). The differential diagnosis of abdominal pain is extensive. Clinical presentations vary based on the age of the child and underlying disease. The emergency physician must be able to identify the patients with serious causes, which vary among different age groups (Table 214.1).

CLINICAL PRESENTATION

The most common condition of infancy, presenting with apparent abdominal pain, is colic (8). The predominant symptom is prolonged, continuous crying. The infant may have mild abdominal distention, and may pull the knees up against the abdomen, giving the caregiver the impression that the infant is experiencing abdominal pain. The infant may be inconsolable, although rocking, swinging, or a car ride may calm the baby. The pattern of the pain is predictable, coming on suddenly in the late afternoon or evening. The physical examination, except for the infant's crying, is often unremarkable. Management options are limited to encouraging breast feeding or a trial of a protein hydrolysate formula such as Nutramigen, Pregestimil or Alimentum. It is prudent for breast-feeding mothers to avoid stimulants and spicy foods. It may be difficult to confidently rule out a more serious condition. A period of prolonged observation in the ED may be useful to be more confident of a benign diagnosis. However, laboratory or imaging studies may be required if a serious diagnosis cannot be excluded.

Vomiting in neonates is abnormal and suggests an obstruction or a potentially serious infection (i.e., gastroenteritis is unlikely). Vomiting due to gastroenteritis in older infants and children can be common, but abdominal distention or bilious vomiting suggests a more serious abdominal disorder. Vomiting in conjunction with observational evidence of abdominal pain (often based on parental observation) should be considered to be potentially serious since gastroenteritis more commonly results in vomiting without abdominal pain. The presence of nasal congestion, coughing, fever, or diarrhea, may be present in viral infections, but these findings do not rule out acute surgical conditions since young children are frequently enduring viral infections that do not afford them immunity against acute surgical conditions. Nonsurgical causes of bilious vomiting include sepsis, urinary tract infection, and inborn errors of metabolism. Surgical causes include intussusception, appendicitis, and malrotation complicated by midgut volvulus.

Intussusception can be defined as a telescoping of a proximal section of bowel (the lead point is called the intussusceptum) into a more distal segment (called the intussuscipiens). This results in a bowel obstruction with ischemia of the involved bowel. The typical age group is under 24 months of age, but it occurs with lesser frequency in older children. It typically has a dramatic, acute onset usually associated with vomiting. The key differentiating point here is that there is noticeable pain (manifested by crying and/or curling up) which appears to come in cycles every 3 to 20 minutes, with the child relatively normal or drowsy between attacks. The classic triad for intussusception includes colicky abdominal pain, emesis, and currant jelly stool (poorly defined, but most agree that this refers to bloody, mucous-like stool) that is typically a late finding. This can be misleading since any presenting form of blood in the stool (dysentery, maroon stool, etc.) may be due to intussusception (24). Additionally, younger infants may present with profound lethargy (presumably from an intussusception-induced endogenous opioid

---

TABLE 214.1. Differential Diagnosis of Abdominal Pain in Children

Infants	Toddlers	School-Aged	Teenager
Colic	Acute gastroenteritis	Idiopathic	Appendicitis
Intussusception	Urinary tract infection	Appendicitis	Pelvic Inflammatory Disease
Malrotation	Constipation	Acute gastroenteritis	Peptic ulcer disease
Volvulus	Referred pain	Constipation	Ectopic pregnancy
Hirschsprung disease	Appendicitis	Urinary tract infection	Mittelschmerz
Necrotizing enterocolitis		Peptic ulcer disease	
Incarcerated hernia			

secretion [16]) without vomiting or abdominal pain. A right-sided abdominal mass (classically sausage shaped) is often palpable with deep, careful palpation when the child is relaxed or drowsy to minimize abdominal muscle tone. Intussusception usually starts in the cecum, with the ileum intussuscepting into the ascending colon. Most clinical and radiographic investigations should focus on the right side (10,20,25).

Malrotation complicated by midgut volvulus is a surgical emergency. The term malrotation focusses attention on its embryology which is less important than its resulting clinical abnormality of mesentery fixation. In normal bowel anatomy, the mesentery attaches in a broad fan-like attachment to the entire posterior abdominal wall. However, in a malrotation, the mesentery (and all the vessels perfusing the bowel) attach to a single point on the abdominal wall forming a stalk (called "guts on a stalk") (10,12,18), which can twist on itself, resulting in a catastrophic midgut volvulus (as opposed to a sigmoid volvulus). Necrosis of the entire small bowel develops rapidly, occurring in 1 to 2 hours. These infants often present with an acute onset of pain followed, by distention and bilious emesis. Most patients with a malrotation will present with an acute midgut volvulus during infancy, but an occult malrotation could present at any age subsequently, with an acute midgut volvulus. In some patients with a malrotation, they may experience an early volvulus that spontaneously reduces. They may have intermittent symptoms to suggest an "intermittent volvulus." An upper GI series (a lower GI study may miss some malrotation cases) is the best test to identify an occult malrotation if intermittent volvulus is suspected (10,12,18).

Appendicitis in the infant will present as peritonitis in over 90% of cases (13). Irritability, crying, refusal of feeding, and vomiting, in conjunction with fever, distention, and shallow, grunting respirations, constitute the clinical presentation. In advanced cases, the infant may present in shock. The physical examination may reveal an indurated and erythematous abdominal wall in these delayed presentations. Older children can present with more classic symptoms of appendicitis, such as low-grade fevers, anorexia, and periumbilical pain that localizes to the right lower quadrant. On physical examination, McBurney point tenderness and peritonitis may be noted. Appendicitis is the most common of the serious abdominal surgical emergency conditions, and it frequently presents in an atypical fashion making appendicitis possible in anyone with abdominal pain. The diagnosis of appendicitis must be made in a timely manner. This urgency is highlighted by the increased risk of appendiceal perforation with time, as the majority of cases will perforate within 48 hours of symptom onset (2). Since it is often difficult to confirm the diagnosis of appendicitis (especially early in its course) it is often necessary to employ an advanced imaging study such as a CT scan or ultrasound for confirmation (10,15,23).

Meckel diverticulum is a special diverticulum located in the jejunum or ileum. It has several distinct clinical consequences. It contains gastric mucosa, so it may secrete acid and cause a bleeding ulcer, presenting with painless rectal bleeding. Meckel diverticulum is a tubular pouch, therefore, it may become inflamed similar to the appendix resulting in Meckel diverticulitis, which will be clinically similar to acute appendicitis, but the pain may be in an atypical location. The Meckel diverticulum may occasionally ulcerate and perforate which may present as a bowel perforation without the preceding diverticulitis symptoms. A Meckel diverticulum may be attached to the abdominal wall (near the umbilicus) and form a stalk-like connection, around which a volvulus can occur. It may also form a lead point for an intussusception (often ileo-ileal intussusception). Meckel diverticulum presents with a diverse set of serious acute surgical conditions. Many textbooks describe Meckel diverticulum following the rule of 2's: 2% of the population are born with a Meckel. only 2% of those with a Meckel manifest clinical prob-

lems, usually located 2 feet proximal to the terminal ileum and the diverticulum is usually 2 inches long, and symptoms commonly manifest at age 2 years (10,19,21).

Hirschsprung disease (congenital aganglionosis of the distal colon), will usually present subacutely or insidiously with constipation, episodes of crampy, recurrent abdominal pain and/or poor weight gain. They may present acutely with peritonitis, acute abdominal pain or bowel obstruction. The diagnosis is made on rectal biopsy or by a barium enema demonstrating of a "transition zone" between the dilated proximal colon (normal ganglionic colon) and the nondilated (abnormal aganglionic) distal colon. Patients who have had a surgical resection of the distal aganglionic colon are at risk for "enterocolitis," a condition of severe gastroenteritis functionally resulting in a bowel obstruction, requiring hospitalization for IV fluid and rectal dilatation.

Gastroesophageal reflux may present with only a vague suggestion of abdominal or esophageal pain but a perplexing array of symptoms. They include failure to thrive, respiratory disturbances (obstructive apnea, stridor, pneumonia, bronchospasm), or neurobehavioral aberrations (seizure-like episodes) (11). Peptic ulcer disease (PUD) is uncommon in infants, but should be considered in adolescents. It is difficult to diagnose in the ED and if suspected, such patients should be referred to a gastroenterologist.

Recurrent abdominal pain is the most common somatic complaint of school-age children and is usually psychophysiologic in origin (9). Subjective pain with associated pallor, sweaty palms, and anxiety may be present during examination. The child is more likely to be female (2:1), with periumbilical or epigastric pain that lasts less than 3 hours and does not awaken the child from sleep.

Recurrent abdominal pain associated with fever, diarrhea, and growth or sexual maturational arrest may indicate the presence of inflammatory bowel disease.

Cholecystitis may occur as right upper quadrant pain and is uncommon in the younger child unless associated with a chronic hemolytic anemia (sickle cell disease, thalassemia, spherocytosis) or Kawasaki disease (1). As the teen years approach, cholelithiasis and cholecystitis become more common. They are often associated with female gender, obesity, pregnancy, and previous ileal surgery.

Abdominal pain following trauma may be the chief and only complaint with blunt abdominal contusion. Signs of hemodynamic instability suggest spleen or liver injury. Peritoneal signs suggest a hollow viscus injury or free peritoneal blood. Delayed presentation with recurrent emesis may indicate a mural duodenal hematoma. Handlebar injuries may result in traumatic pancreatitis.

A postpubertal female presenting with abdominal pain should be carefully examined for evidence of reproductive tract sources, such as ectopic pregnancy, pelvic inflammatory disease (PID), tuboovarian abscess, and corpus luteal cyst. Secondary sexual maturity characteristics (Tanner stage) suggesting puberty in a female who has not had her first menstrual period (pre-menarche) suggests the possibility of an imperforate hymen and hematocolpos (6).

The presentation of abdominal pain and fever in the child with immunodeficiency, nephrotic syndrome, or ascites suggests primary peritonitis.

Sexual abuse may also manifest itself as a vague abdominal complaint in some children. A high degree of suspicion is therefore required by the emergency physician to include this diagnosis as part of the differential that must be thoroughly investigated. Once sexual abuse is suspected, prompt involvement by the appropriate local and state authorities is required.

The most common cause of pediatric abdominal pain presenting to an ED is abdominal cramps due to stool that is not moving forward with normal peristalsis. As stool moves distally through the colon, it may fail to move forward, e.g., at the splenic flexure. If normal peristalsis fails to move this forward, the colon contracts more forcefully, resulting in severe crampy abdominal pain. This pain will suddenly remit, once the stool moves forward and normal peristalsis resumes. This is facilitated with an enema which helps to establish the diagnosis. This is sometimes called "constipation," but this term is not accurate since "constipation" is poorly defined and more often refers to not stooling every day, painful defecation, difficulty with defecation, and/or hard stools.

DIFFERENTIAL DIAGNOSIS

Abdominal pain in children may indicate a primary abdominal process or a condition far removed. Evaluation by the emergency physician should establish first whether there is a surgical emergency (ischemia, obstruction, or peritonitis). Ischemic pain is often of sudden onset and associated with torsion or volvulus. Obstruction is most commonly associated with the mnemonic "double-AIM" (A-A-I-I-M-M): appendicitis, adhesions, incarcerated inguinal hernia, intussusception, malrotation/midgut volvulus, Meckel diverticulum. If the evaluation suggests peritonitis, the most frequent etiology is appendicitis, but other acute surgical conditions are possible as well. Nonbowel conditions such as pyelonephritis or sickle cell disease must also be considered.

EMERGENCY DEPARTMENT EVALUATION AND MANAGEMENT

A detailed history is useful, but it can be misleading as well. Many patients with appendicitis have nontypical histories. Characterizing the quality and assessing the severity of pain is difficult and unreliable in young children. Some children with appendicitis are fairly stoic, ambulatory and complaining of only mild abdominal pain.

The emergency physician should approach the physical examination in a friendly manner, with younger children remaining in the parent's lap or while being carried. For young children, parents can be asked to bounce the child gently while carrying them or while sitting on their lap to look for facial signs suggesting discomfort with this (peritoneal signs). Since most children are comforted by this, paradoxical crying or signs of discomfort may suggest peritonitis. If the parent is carrying the child, an examiner can palpate the abdomen from behind the child, by bringing his/her hands around the child's abdomen. Close inspection for distention, asymmetry, or abdominal wall erythema is followed by auscultation with a warm stethoscope. Palpation in the supine position, should then proceed with a soft, warm hand on the abdomen, palpating very slowly for tenderness or masses, initially in the area of the abdomen away from the suspected pathology. The groin and genitals should always be examined for inguinal hernias, scrotal/testicular abnormalities, or vaginal abnormalities. A rectal examination should be performed only if there is a specific indication (e.g., checking for stool impaction or for occult blood) (3,5,7,14). A pelvic examination may be indicated in sexually active or pubertal females.

Very ill-appearing patients will require resuscitation (ABCs), IV fluids, and other indicated treatments. A rapid surgical consultation should be obtained if the patient is at risk for bowel infarction. A consultation with a radiologist is likely to be helpful as well.

In some instances, a specific set of signs and symptoms may lead to a particular diagnosis. For example, painless rectal bleeding suggests a Meckel diverticulum or vomiting, bloody stools and intermittent crampy abdominal pain suggest intussusception. Imaging studies are very helpful in leading to a diagnosis. There should be a low threshold for ordering an advanced imaging study if this will benefit the patient by leading to the early diagnosis of a serious condition.

A "Meckel scan" (nuclear medicine scintigraphy) can be done to identify a Meckel diverticulum. The radioisotope is taken up by gastric mucosa, so it will typically image the stomach, but if a Meckel diverticulum is present, the scan will identify the stomach plus an ectopic source of acid secreting gastric mucosa. Barium enema and upper GI series will often fail to identify the Meckel diverticulum.

Plain abdominal radiographs can identify a bowel obstruction in most instances. Criteria for identifying a bowel obstruction in children are different from that of adults (4). Plain film radiographic signs of intussusception include the target sign, crescent sign, absence of the subhepatic angle, and a bowel obstruction (10,20,25). Appendicitis may present with an ileus or an appendicolith (22). Pneumonia is a common cause of abdominal pain and it is frequently missed because the lung portion of the abdominal films is at the upper margin of the film and is not carefully reviewed (17).

CT scan and ultrasound are emerging as the best advanced imaging studies to identify most serious abdominal conditions. Published ultrasonography study results are often from ultrasound specialty centers that are not necessarily applicable to general radiologists. CT scans are more diagnostic, but they are more difficult to do. The choice between these two depends on the expertise of the radiologists and availability of the equipment at a particular hospital. CT scans which include the abdomen and pelvis are capable of diagnosing appendicitis, intussusception, some Meckel cases, midgut volvulus, hematocolpos, ovarian cysts, colitis, neoplasms, pancreatitis, genitourinary obstruction, cholecystitis, and many other conditions (10,15,23).

If intussusception is suspected, this can be confirmed by ultrasound or contrast enema. An ultrasound should be avoided if the interpreting radiologist cannot confidently rule out intussusception by ultrasound. If the ultrasound identifies an intussusception, then a contrast enema must still be done. Contrast enemas can be done with air, barium, or water-soluble contrast under fluoroscopy. Some radiologists have published literature regarding their experience with saline enemas done under ultrasound visualization. Although air contrast has some advantages, the type of contrast should be chosen by the radiologist performing the procedure based on their personal expertise (10,23).

Laboratory tests are not helpful in most instances. Pregnancy testing is useful in ruling out pregnancy. A CBC is often ordered, but it is of limited diagnostic value. The commonly ordered electrolytes/glucose/renal function panel is useful to detect electrolyte abnormalities, metabolic acidosis, hypoglycemia, and hyperglycemia (e.g., diabetic ketoacidosis). A lipase (better than an amylase) can diagnose the occasional patient with pancreatitis. Liver enzymes can diagnose the presence of hepatitis. Urinalysis can identify pyuria which can mislead the clinician to diagnose the patient with a urinary tract infection. However, appendicitis can cause pyuria as well, due to inflammation surrounding the ureter.

Unless there is a specific diagnosis that is suspected, an approach that is commonly used is to obtain an abdominal series. If this confirms a specific diagnosis, then further management proceeds toward that diagnosis. If the abdominal films demonstrate a large amount of stool, an enema is given as a test to determine if stool movement will result in the resolution of the abdominal pain. If the pain resolves completely, then a benign diagnosis is most likely and the patient can be discharged home. If any pain remains (even if it has improved) and the diagnosis is still in question, then a CT scan of the abdomen/pelvis is ordered to look for evidence of appendicitis or other serious intraabdominal conditions. However, this algorithm is greatly simplified and other approaches may be indicated as well.

DISPOSITION

Role of the Consultant

For seriously ill patients with a surgical abdomen, a surgeon should be consulted immediately in conjunction with resuscitation measures. In the past, surgeons would be consulted for cases of diagnostic uncertainty. However, the availability of abdominal CT scans and other advanced imaging modalities, has changed this, such that the imaging studies are generally ordered first and the surgeon is contacted only if a surgical condition is confirmed or if the diagnosis is still uncertain, despite the advanced imaging studies that are done. This is not true for all hospitals since this depends on the availability of surgeons and advanced imaging studies (23).

Indications for Admission

Advanced imaging studies should permit the diagnosis to be made in the ED with clear indications for hospitalization in most instances. In unclear cases, patients should be admitted for observation until the suspected abdominal emergency can be excluded. Parental exhaustion or the inability to deal with a fussy child is a legitimate reason to hospitalize a child.

Transfer Considerations

Surgical emergencies in infants require a surgeon with specific expertise. If one is not available, the patient may need to be transferred to a pediatric facility.

Discharge Home

Low-risk cases can be discharged home without an advanced imaging study. It may be useful to present the option of doing an advanced imaging study to the family. If they are reliable and reasonable, and they decline the study, this greatly limits liability. Regardless of the diagnostic impression at discharge, it may be beneficial to discharge the patient with a standardized set of instructions. Such an "Abdominal pain sheet" should state that the diagnosis is never totally certain and abdominal pain causes can be difficult to determine. Signs and symptoms of serious causes of abdominal pain requiring an immediate return to the ED (such as appendicitis, intussusception, bowel obstruction, GI bleeding, etc.) should be listed on this sheet. Parents should be encouraged to monitor the child for these symptoms and to call the ED or return to the ED if these symptoms occur.

COMMON PITFALLS

✔ Intussusception is easily missed. Abdominal pain or blood in the stool should raise suspicion

✔ Bloody diarrhea is often due to bacterial dysentery such as shigella. However, intussusception is a possible cause

✔ Currant jelly stools occur in the minority of cases. Any type of blood in the stool may be due to intussusception

✔ Appendicitis is fairly common and approximately half of these cases present with atypical features

✔ It is preferable to be conservative with children in whom the diagnosis is unclear. An advanced imaging study can be em-

ployed to obtain greater certainty. In patients with a high clinical probability of appendicitis with a negative abdominal CT scan or ultrasound, it may be preferable to hospitalize them for continued observation since CT and ultrasound are not perfectly accurate

CLINICAL TIPS

- For all patients who present with vomiting, ask parents about the presence of abdominal pain.
- Plain film showing signs of intussusception are subtle. Review the sample radiographs in the online references to familiarize yourself with these findings (20,24).
- A pediatric bowel obstruction has a different appearance than an adult bowel obstruction. Most pediatric bowel obstructions are due to serious intestinal conditions requiring immediate intervention (4).
- For patients at a low risk of intussusception, document that the patient does not exhibit a crampy abdominal pain pattern on observation.
- Have the patient cough, and then jump up and down. For infants and young children, have the parents bounce the child and observe them for discomfort.
- Examine small children and infants from the back while the parent is carrying them.
- Vomiting in younger infants (especially neonates) should be worrisome and not routinely assumed to be gastroenteritis.

Acknowledgments

The author gratefully acknowledges the contributions of Lowell Clark, Javier I. Escobar II, and Steven A. Godwin, who wrote previous versions of this chapter.

References

1. Bailey PV, et al. Changing spectrum of cholelithiasis and cholecystitis in infants and children. *Am J Surg* 1990;158:585.
2. Braveman P, Schaff VM, Egerter S, et al. Insurance related differences in the risk of ruptured appendix. *N Engl J Med* 1994;331:444–449.
3. Brewster GS, et al. Medical myth: A digital rectal examination should be performed on all individuals with possible appendicitis. *West J Med* 2000;173:207.
4. Chan Nishina CC, Tim Sing PML. Test your skill in distinguishing obstruction from ileus. In: Yamamoto LG, Inaba AS, DiMauro R (eds). *Radiology Cases in Pediatric Emergency Medicine*, 1995, volume 3, case 18. Available online at: www.hawaii.edu/medicine/pediatrics/pemxray/v3c18.html.
5. Dickson AP, et al. Rectal examination and acute appendicitis. *Arch Dis Child* 1985;60:666.
6. Halm B. Right lower quadrant pain in a 13-year old female. In: Yamamoto LG, Inaba AS, DiMauro R (eds). *Radiology Cases In Pediatric Emergency Medicine*, 1996, Volume 4, Case 8. Available online at: www.hawaii.edu/medicine/pediatrics/pemxray/v4c08.html.
7. Jesudason EC, et al. Rectal examination in paediatric surgical practice. *Br J Surg* 1999;86:376.
8. Miller A, Barr R. Infantile colic: Is it a gut issue? *Pediatr Clin North Am* 1991;38:1407.
9. Oberlander T, Rappaport L. Recurrent abdominal pain during childhood. *Pediatr Rev* 1993;14:313.
10. Okada P, Hicks B. Non-traumatic surgical emergencies. In: Gausche Hill M, Fuchs S, Yamamoto L, (eds). *APLS: The Emergency Medicine Resource*, 4th edition. Sudbury, MA: Jones & Barlett, 2004:360–409.
11. Orenstein SR. Gastroesophageal reflux. *Pediatr Rev* 1992;13:174.
12. Rosen LM, Yamamoto LG. Abdominal pain and vomiting in a 7-year old. In: Yamamoto LG, Inaba AS, DiMauro R (eds). Radiology Cases in Pediatric Emergency Medicine, 1995, volume 2, case 8. Available online at: www.hawaii.edu/medicine/pediatrics/pemxray/v2c08.html.
13. Rothrock SG, Skeock G, et al. Clinical features of misdiagnosed appendicitis in children. *Ann Emerg Med* 1991;20:45.
14. Scholer SJ, et al. Use of the Rectal examination on children with acute abdominal pain. *Clin Pediatr* 1998;37:311.
15. Sivit CJ, Applegate KE, Stallion A, et al. Imaging evaluation of suspected appendicitis in a pediatric population: effectiveness of sonography versus CT. *Am J Roentgenol* 2000;175:977–998.
16. Tenebien M, Wiseman NE. Early coma in intussusception: endogenous opioid induced? *Pediatr Emerg Care* 1987;3:22–23.

17. Yamamoto LG. Abdominal pain with a negative abdominal examination. In: Yamamoto LG, Inaba AS, DiMauro R (eds). *Radiology Cases In Pediatric Emergency Medicine*, 1994, Volume 1, Case 3. Available online at: www.hawaii.edu/medicine/pediatrics/pemxray/v1c03.html.

18. Yamamoto LG. Bilious Vomiting in a 3-month old. In: Yamamoto LG, Inaba AS, DiMauro R (eds). *Radiology Cases In Pediatric Emergency Medicine*, 1995, volume 3, case 17. Available online at: www.hawaii.edu/medicine/pediatrics/pemxray/v3c17.html.

19. Yamamoto LG. Bowel obstruction with intra-intestinal sand (A case of a bowel obstruction and midgut volvulus due to a Meckel's diverticulum). In: Yamamoto LG, Inaba AS, DiMauro R (eds). *Radiology Cases In Pediatric Emergency Medicine*, 1996, Volume 5, Case 19. Available online at: www.hawaii.edu/medicine/pediatrics/pemxray/v5c19.html.

20. Yamamoto LG. Find the intussusception target and crescent signs. In: Yamamoto LG, Inaba AS, DiMauro R (eds). *Radiology Cases in Pediatric Emergency Medicine*, 2003, volume 7, case 18. Available online at: www.hawaii.edu/medicine/pediatrics/pemxray/v7c18.html.

21. Yamamoto LG. Periumbilical abdominal pain (Meckel's diverticulitis case). In: Yamamoto LG, Inaba AS, DiMauro R (eds). *Radiology Cases in Pediatric Emergency Medicine*, 1996, volume 4, Case 9. Available online at: www.hawaii.edu/medicine/pediatrics/pemxray/v4c09.html.

22. Yamamoto LG, Goto CS. Appendicoliths. In: Yamamoto LG, Inaba AS, DiMauro R (eds). *Radiology Cases in Pediatric Emergency Medicine*, 1999, volume 6, case 18. Available online at: www.hawaii.edu/medicine/pediatrics/pemxray/v6c18.html.

23. Yamamoto LG, Isaacman DJ, Knapp JF. Emergency medicine. In: Metzl K (ed). AAP *Pediatric Update*, 2002, volume 22, number 11.

24. Yamamoto LG, Morita SY, Boychuk RB, et al. Stool appearance in intussusception: assessing the value of the term "currant jelly." *Am J Emerg Med* 1997;15293–298.

25. Young LL, Yamamoto LG. The stomach flu?—The target, crescent, and absent liver edge signs. In: Yamamoto LG, Inaba AS, DiMauro R (eds). *Radiology Cases In Pediatric Emergency Medicine*, 1994, volume 1, case 2. Available online at: www.hawaii.edu/medicine/pediatrics/pemxray/v1c02.html.

CHAPTER 215
Altered Mental Status

S. Margaret Paik and Mark A. Hostetler

Consciousness is a state of awareness of one's self and the surrounding environment, and is a product of arousal. *Altered mental status* (AMS) is a generic term for any change in the level of consciousness. Terms such as *lethargy, obtundation, delirium, stupor, and coma* are often used interchangeably, but are not synonymous. They can be thought of as occurring along a continuum with lethargy indicating the least amount of dysfunction, and coma the most (Table 215.1). In order for coma to occur, there must be *bilateral* cerebral dysfunction, injury to the ascending reticular activating system (ARAS), or both. The (ARAS) activates the cerebral cortex, resulting in wakefulness, attention, and a normal level of consciousness. It is located within the brainstem, and acts via connections within the caudal medulla, upper pons, and rostral midbrain.

Encephalopathy describes a state of global brain dysfunction with at least two of the following symptoms: altered level of consciousness, altered behavior or cognition, and/or seizures. Encephalopathic states can be acute or chronic, progressive or static. Acute mental status changes associated with cerebrospinal fluid pleocytosis are most often seen in individuals with acute *encephalitis*.

Structural abnormalities, as seen with trauma or tumors, can lead to compression of the ARAS and produce focal deficits.

TABLE 215.1.   Terms Used to Describe Altered Mental Status

Term	Description
Lethargy	Difficulty maintaining a state of wakefulness but arouses to vocal stimuli
Obtundation	Blunted state of alertness when responding to stimulation other than pain
Delirium	Decompensation in mental status characterized by one or more of the following: disorientation, trepidation, misinterpretation of sensory stimuli, or hallucinations
Stupor	Responsive only to painful stimuli, usually that is forceful and continuous
Coma	Unresponsive to painful stimuli

Supratentorial lesions of sufficient size to cause compression of underlying structures can cause shifting of the intracranial contents and herniation.

In uncal herniation, an expanding lesion in the temporal fossa or temporal lobe displaces the uncus and hippocampal gyrus towards the midline and the edge of the tentorium. The initial complaint may be of headache that then progresses toward AMS. A unilateral dilated pupil is most often noted on the ipsilateral side of the lesion. Further expansion of the lesion will result in progression of symptoms including decerebrate posturing and transtentorial or central herniation.

Central or transtentorial herniation occurs as a consequence of downward herniation of the hemispheres and the basal nuclei. This is usually due to increased intracranial pressure that affects both cerebral hemispheres evenly. There is caudal displacement of the thalamus and hypothalamus through the foramen magnum and into the posterior fossa. Compression of the brainstem results in abnormal posturing, abnormal breathing patterns and pupillary changes that can range from small and reactive to mid-position and fixed. In cingulate herniation, expansion of a lesion results in lateral shifting of the cingulate gyrus under the falx cerebri, subsequent compression of the adjacent blood vessels, particularly the ipsilateral anterior cerebral artery, and associated ischemia.

Subtentorial lesions cause coma by either destroying the ARAS or via external compression of the brainstem and the ARAS, as with cerebellar tonsillar herniation. Expansion of a subtentorial lesion can also cause reverse transtentorial herniation by pushing the brainstem in a cephalad direction. Sudden and abrupt onset of coma coupled with a rapidly deteriorating clinical course suggests an acute subtentorial lesion.

In pediatric patients the majority of cases of coma are due to nonstructural causes (infection, toxic ingestion, metabolic abnormalities), and result in bilateral cerebral hemisphere dysfunction with global but symmetric deficits. Generally, confusion, stupor, and obtundation are seen initially, and precede any motor deficits. Pupillary responses remain preserved, but the respiratory rate and pattern may be altered.

DIFFERENTIAL DIAGNOSIS

Several different schemas have been used in the evaluation of a patient with AMS. The "AEIOU-TIPS" coma mnemonic (Table 215.2) is often used for adult patients with AMS. Although clinically useful as a starting point, several diagnoses specific to the pediatric patient need to be highlighted on the list. Most notable of these are infection, intussusception, inborn errors of metabolism, child abuse, and the markedly higher rate of accidental ingestions. The causes of AMS specific to children will be discussed in this chapter.

TABLE 215.2. Pediatric Altered Mental Status:
The "AEIOU–TIPS" Mnemonic

A
Alcohol
Abuse (nonaccidental trauma)
E
Encephalopathy (infectious, metabolic, toxic, Reye)
Electrolyte abnormalities (hypoglycemia, hypo-, hypernatremia,
   hypocalcemia)
Endocrinopathy (diabetic ketoacidosis, congenital adrenal
   hyperplasia)
I
Infection (meningitis, encephalitis, sepsis)
Intussusception
Inborn errors of metabolism (fatty acid oxidation disorder, urea
   cycle defect)
O
Opiates
U
Uremia
T
Trauma (intracranial hemorrhage)
Tumor
Toxins (lead)
I
Insulin
P
Poisonings (see Table 214.3)
Psychogenic (pseudoseizure, conversion disorder)
S
Seizure (neonatal, atypical, complex)
Shock
Shunt malfunction (increased ICP, infection)

Abuse

Physical abuse is the primary cause of serious head injury in infants. Findings consistent with the diagnosis of "shaken-baby syndrome" or "shaken-impact syndrome" include subdural hematoma, subarachnoid hemorrhage, retinal hemorrhage, and fractures in the ribs and metaphyseal region of the long bone. Discrepancies between the history and findings from the more detailed physical examination should alert the physician to the possibility of child physical abuse. Children may present with AMS and a paucity of external physical findings on the initial evaluation. Retinal hemorrhages seen on the fundoscopic examination are suspicious for child physical abuse. Previously, it was postulated that retinal hemorrhages could be a result of vigorous resuscitative efforts, but recent studies do not support this. Evidence of papilledema is suggestive of increased intracranial pressure and should alert the physician to the possibility of child physical abuse. Children may present with AMS and no external evidence of trauma.

Encephalopathy

Reye syndrome is a progressive encephalopathy, occurring either during or following a viral illness. The syndrome occurs more often with the concurrent use of salicylates. Initially the child will have unrelenting vomiting which can be followed by lethargy and then coma. Laboratory studies demonstrate elevated liver function tests and serum ammonia. Fatty infiltration of the liver is seen on biopsy specimens. The decreased usage of salicylates in children has been temporally associated with a marked decrease in the incidence of Reye Syndrome. In addition, there have been concurrent improvements in the recognition and diagnosis of fatty acid oxidation disorders, particularly medium-chain acyl-CoA dehydrogenase deficiency (MCAD), which many believe mimic most of the symptoms commonly associated with Reye Syndrome.

Intussusception

Intussusception occurs most often in children between the ages of 3 and 12 months with a male to female ratio of 4:1. Although patients typically present with complaints of abdominal pain and vomiting, up to 10% of infants will present solely with a depressed level of consciousness. It is postulated that endogenous opioids are released from the bowel wall. The commonly taught "classic triad" of colicky abdominal pain, vomiting and currant jelly stools is seen infrequently (less than 25% in some reports).

Inborn Errors of Metabolism

Inborn errors of metabolism should be considered in a young infant with a history of vomiting, poor feeding, failure to thrive and AMS. Although commonly thought of as only occurring in the neonatal period, these conditions can also present later in childhood. Seizures can also be a presenting symptom, especially in the neonatal period. Inborn errors of metabolism can be divided into 2 large groups, those associated with metabolic acidosis and those associated with hyperammonemia. The initial presentation can be triggered by a mild viral illness. Even though the diagnosis is unlikely to be made in the emergency department (ED), additional laboratory studies such as serum pyruvate, lactate and ammonia can be helpful. Early identification and treatment of these children can prevent long-term neurologic damage.

Toxins

AMS due to lead encephalopathy is still seen in children, especially those living in older buildings or those who live near construction sites. Lead encephalopathy can present with a prodrome of vomiting, abdominal pain and fatigue. Ingestion of paint chips or dust coating the surface of objects commonly put into a child's mouth, can cause a rapid and acute rise in the serum lead level resulting in AMS. Specific symptoms include seizures, cranial nerve palsy, lethargy and coma.

Poisonings

Accidental ingestions are a major reason for visits to the ED. Ingested substances associated with AMS are listed in Table 215.3. Many substances can cause altered mental status in small amounts, and more than a handful can be truly toxic or deadly. All exposures should be reported to the regional poison control center; they are the only national organization currently tracking all poisonous and injurious plants, and their input is invaluable.

Seizures

Neonatal seizure patterns vary greatly from older infants and children. Generalized tonic-clonic seizures are generally not seen in neonates. This is because the neural pathways of neonates are incompletely myelinated and incapable of propagation along an entire pathway long enough to cause a true tonic-clonic seizure. In addition, many newborns thought to be having generalized tonic-clonic movements are actually exhibiting jittery behavior. Patterns more typical of seizure in neonates include apnea with tonic stiffening of the body, focal clonic movement of one limb or one side, myoclonic jerking, tonic deviation of the eyes to one side or upward, or patterned stereotypical behavior such as paroxysmal laughing (see Chapter 231, "Seizures").

TABLE 215.3.   Substances Associated with Altered Mental Status

Alcohols
Anticholinergics
Amphetamines
Anticonvulsants
Barbiturates
Carbon monoxide
Clonidine
Cocaine
Cyclic antidepressants
Gamma hydroxybutyrate (GHB)
Heavy metals
Insulin
   Lithium
   Lysergic acid diethylamide (LSD)
   Narcotics
   Nonsteroidal anti-inflammatory drugs
Nicotine
Organophosphates
Phencyclidine (PCP)
Theophylline

TABLE 215.4.   Pediatric Glasgow Coma Score and Glasgow Coma Score (GCS)

Best Response	Score	Pediatric GCS	GCS
Eye	1	No eye opening	No eye opening
	2	Eye opening to pain	Eye opening to pain
	3	Eye opening to speech	Eye opening to verbal command
	4	Eyes open spontaneously	Eyes open spontaneously
Verbal	1	No verbal response	No vocal response
	2	Inconsolable, agitated	Incomprehensible sounds
	3	Persistent crying or screaming	Inappropriate words
	4	Cries, but consolable	Confused conversation
	5	Smiles, interactive	Orientated
Motor	1	No motor response	No motor response
	2	Extension to pain	Extension to pain
	3	Flexion to pain	Flexion to pain
	4	Withdraws from pain	Withdraws from pain
	5	Localizing pain	Localizing pain
	6	Obeys commands	Obeys commands

EMERGENCY DEPARTMENT EVALUATION

The initial evaluation of a child with AMS begins with attention to the *ABCs*: ensuring the protection and patency of the airway, adequacy of breathing and maintenance of a normal circulatory status. Following the ABCs, there are a variety of important clues that can and should be sought during the initial history and physical examination. An effort should be made toward obtaining at least an "AMPLE" history: allergies, medications, past medical history, last meal, and events of recent occurrence. Of particular note these would include any possible ingestions or exposures, vomiting, trauma, fever, or unusual behavior. It is extremely important to obtain an accurate timeline regarding the progression of symptoms and alteration in mental status.

If the child is an infant with an open anterior fontanelle, it can be palpated as an approximation of intracranial pressure and hydration. It is helpful to try and smell the clothes and breath of the patient in order to determine if there may have been any ingestions or exposures. The child should be completely undressed, viewed, rolled and palpated from head to toe, and from front to back to evaluate for any signs of trauma. The abdomen should be palpated for any evidence of hepatosplenomegaly, mass or tenderness. The skin should be examined for any signs of rashes, and the extremities for tone and capillary refill.

Assessment of the child's level of consciousness can be determined by using either the AVPU (Alert; responds to Verbal Stimuli; responds to Painful stimuli; Unresponsive) or the Glasgow coma scale (GCS). Since its introduction in 1976, the GCS has been used extensively in adult patients both with and without traumatic injuries. A modified scoring system has been developed for use in nonverbal pediatric patients (Table 215.4). In general a score of 13 or higher is associated with mild brain injury, a score between 9 and 12 denotes moderate injury and a score of 8 or less signifies severe brain injury.

Abnormal respiratory patterns can also be very helpful as they imply either a metabolic insult or a structural lesion. In *Cheyne-Stokes respiration*, regular periods of hyperpnea alternate with apneic periods, with the hyperpneic period lasting longer than the apneic phase. There is usually a lesion deep inside both cerebral hemispheres or within the diencephalon. It is seen in bilateral cerebral infarction, metabolic and hypertensive encephalopathy. *Central neurogenic hyperventilation* is marked by persistent rapid respirations in spite of normal oxygenation and hypocarbia and indicates midbrain dysfunction.

Abnormal pupillary responses can help to localize the level of the lesion, and the regions in the brain that affect level of consciousness and pupillary response to light are in close proximity to each other. Small but reactive pupils imply either a metabolic or diencephalic lesion. A fixed, dilated pupil can be seen with expanding supratentorial lesions involving the uncus and the ipsilateral third nerve. Pupils that are unresponsive to light and remain midsized imply a midbrain lesion whereas pupils totally unresponsive to light and widely dilated imply brainstem pathology.

Induced eye movements that are useful in the evaluation of a comatose patient are the oculocephalic, or Doll eye reflex, and the oculovestibular responses, or caloric testing responses. A positive, normal response to the Doll eye reflex is the conjugate deviation of the eyes opposite to the direction in which the head is turned. When testing the oculovestibular reflex in an unconscious individual with an intact brainstem, the fast component is absent with the eyes moving toward the side irrigated with cold water and then remaining tonically deviated for one minute or longer. The response to the Doll eye reflex and caloric testing are initially brisk for most causes of metabolic coma, but will become more difficult to elicit as the coma state deepens.

There are three basic types of reflex posturing that may be seen in response to pain. Decorticate posturing (arm flexion and lower leg extension) occurs when there is injury to the cerebral hemispheres (diencephalons) with intact brainstem function. Decerebrate posturing (internal rotation and extension of the arms with lower leg extension) occurs with damage to the midbrain and pons at the level of the brainstem (brainstem dysfunction and therefore worse prognosis). Flaccid posturing (no response), is seen with compression of the medulla and signifies a grave prognosis.

EMERGENCY DEPARTMENT MANAGEMENT

The initial management of a patient begins with stabilization and control of the *ABCs*. An immediate bedside glucose determination should be obtained. Intravenous access should be obtained and initial laboratory studies including a complete blood count, electrolytes (including calcium, magnesium, and phosphorus) and a serum ammonia level should be obtained. A urinalysis and cultures of the blood and urine should be obtained if there is any concern for infection. A blood gas, either venous or arterial, should also be sent to evaluate blood pH and acid-base balance. The child should have continuous cardiopulmonary and oximetry monitoring. An EKG is recommended in cases of dysrhythmia and selected poisonings. A trial dose of naloxone (0.1 mg/kg) should be administered, particularly if the pupils are miotic.

Signs and symptoms of herniation or increased intracranial pressure warrant immediate intubation and mild hyperventilation to reduce the PCO_2 to 30 to 35 mm Hg. Addition of IV mannitol (0.5 gm/kg) may be helpful but careful monitoring of the child's intravascular status and avoidance of hypotension is mandatory. Children with focal deficits, evidence of herniation, increased intracranial pressure and those with suspected head injury require imaging with a head CT. Lumbar puncture is indicated in patients suspected of having meningitis.

Further management and treatment options are based on the history, signs, symptoms, and physical examination findings. Therapeutic options include administration of broad spectrum antibiotics for patients with suspected infection, antidote therapy for suspected poisonings, antiepileptic medications for seizures, and correction of any fluid, electrolyte or acid-base abnormalities. In addition, young children, due to their proportional body surface area, can have or develop hypothermia when exposed to the ambient temperatures; active attention is therefore required toward maintaining normal temperatures, particularly in unclothed young infants undergoing resuscitation in a cold ED. External or overhead warming devices are strongly recommended to prevent hypothermia.

CRITICAL INTERVENTIONS

- Assess, stabilize, and maintain *airway, breathing, and circulation*, maintaining cervical immobilization if indicated
- Obtain IV access, administer high flow oxygen, and place on monitor
- Determine rapid bedside glucose and administer trial dose of naloxone
- Administer antibiotics if infection suspected
- Evaluate for evidence of ingestion, signs of increased intracranial pressure, or nonaccidental trauma

DISPOSITION

Final disposition is dependent on the suspected diagnosis and condition of the child. Generally, a child with AMS will warrant further inpatient evaluation in an intensive care unit. Until transfer of care is complete, continual reevaluation, reassessment and modification of therapy is essential.

COMMON PITFALLS

- Failure to adequately assess, and aggressively manage, the ABCs
- Failure to obtain a rapid bedside glucose
- Failure to consider an electrolyte disturbance as a cause for altered mental status in an infant (hyponatremia, hypernatremia, hypocalcemia)
- Failure to consider an inborn error of metabolism as a cause for altered mental status in an infant (fatty acid oxidation disorder, hyperammonemia)
- Failure to consider diagnoses that may present as AMS in children: seizures without tonic–clonic activity (atypical or subtle seizures), intussusception, accidental ingestions, and child physical abuse (nonaccidental trauma)
- Failure to reassess and modify therapy as needed

Acknowledgments

Thanks to the previous edition's chapter author Lindsey Alan Johnson.

References

1. American Academy of Pediatrics. Altered levels of consciousness. In: *APLS: the Pediatric Emergency Medicine Course*, 3rd ed. Elk Grove Village, IL: American Academy of Pediatrics/American College of Emergency Physicians, 1998; 159–166.
2. Birkhahn R, Fiorini M, Gaeta TJ. Painless intussusception and altered mental status. *Am J Emerg Med* 1999;17:345–347.
3. Fenichel GM. *Clinical Pediatric Neurology.* 4th ed. Philadelphia: WB Saunders, 2001.
4. Hostetler M. An 18-month-old child with previously undiagnosed fatty acid oxidation disorder. *Hospital Physician* 2003;39:36–45.
5. King D, Avner JR. Altered Mental Status. *CPEM* 2003;4:171–178.
6. Marcin JP, Pollack MM. Triage scoring systems, severity of illness measures, and mortality prediction models in pediatric trauma. *Crit Care Med* 2002;30:S457–S467.
7. Parvizi J, Damasio A. Consciousness and the brainstem. *Cognition* 2001;79:135–160.
8. Piomelli S. Childhood lead poisoning. *Pediatr Clin North Am* 2002;49:1285–1304.
9. Plum F, Posner JB. *The Diagnosis of Stupor and Coma,* 3rd ed. Philadelphia: Oxford University Press, 1980.
10. Yager JY, Johnston B, Seshia SS. Coma scales in pediatric practice. *Am J D Child* 1990;144:1088–1091.
11. Zenel J, Goldstein B. Child abuse in the pediatric intensive care unit. *Crit Care Med* 2002;30:S515–S523.

CHAPTER 216
Apnea and Apparent Life-Threatening Events (ALTE)

Ghazala Q. Sharieff

Apnea is one of the many different types of breathing problems presented to the emergency department, and is seen predominantly in the neonate and young infant. In 1987, the Consensus Statement of the National Institutes of Health Consensus Development Conference on Infantile Apnea and Home Monitoring was published in an effort to serve as a guide for future research (2). The definitions published in the consensus statement will be used in this chapter (Table 216.1). The focus of this chapter is on the evaluation, differential diagnosis, and management of the neonate and young infant with apnea and briefly mentions other causes of apnea in older children.

EPIDEMIOLOGY

ALTEs have been reported to occur in up to 3% of all children (1). The mortality of patients with apnea in infancy varies in the literature from 2% to 6%. Infants presenting with apnea during sleep may have up to 10% mortality, with the risk of death

TABLE 216.1.   Definitions of Apnea

Apnea—Cessation of respiratory airflow. The respiratory pause may be central or diaphragmatic (i.e., no respiratory effort), obstructive (usually due to upper airway obstruction), or mixed. Short (<15 s) central apnea can be normal at all ages.

Pathologic Apnea—A respiratory pause is abnormal if it is prolonged (>20 s) or associated with cyanosis; abrupt, marked pallor or hypotonia; or bradycardia.

Periodic Breathing—A breathing pattern in which there are three or more respiratory pauses of greater than 3 seconds' duration with less than 20 seconds of respiration between pauses. Periodic breathing can be normal.

Apnea of Prematurity—Periodic breathing with pathologic apnea in a premature infant. Apnea of prematurity usually ceases by 37 weeks' gestation (menstrual dating) but occasionally persists for several weeks past term.

Apparent Life-Threatening Event (ALTE)—An episode that is frightening to the observer and that is characterized by some combination of apnea (central or occasionally obstructive), color change (usually cyanotic or pallid but occasionally erythematous or plethoric), marked change in muscle tone (usually marked limpness), choking, or gagging. In some cases, the observer fears the infant has died.

Apnea of Infancy—An unexplained episode of cessation of breathing for 20 seconds or longer, or a shorter respiratory pause associated with bradycardia, cyanosis, pallor, or marked hypotonia. The term *apnea of infancy* generally refers to infants who are greater than 37 weeks' gestational age at onset of pathologic apnea. Apnea of infancy should be reserved for those infants for whom no specific cause of an ALTE can be identified. In other words, these are infants whose ALTEs were idiopathic and believed to be related to apnea.

From Consensus Statement. National Institute of Health Consensus Development Conference on Infantile Apnea and Home Monitoring. *Pediatrics* 1987;79:293.

tripling with two or more recurrences. In over 50% of ALTEs, no definitive cause can be found (1).

Sudden infant death syndrome (SIDS) occurs in about two per 1,000 live births in the United States. SIDS has been defined as "the sudden death of an infant less than 1 year of age that remains unexplained after a thorough case investigation, including performance of a complete autopsy, examination of the death scene and review of clinical history" (13). The National Institute of Child Health and Development Cooperative Epidemiological Study of SIDS found that only 2% to 4% of cases had a hospital record of apnea of prematurity, and less than 7% had a history of an acute life-threatening event (ALTE). Prone sleeping has been found to be a significant risk factor for SIDS. Even with the implementation of infant supine sleeping campaigns, SIDS still occurs twice as often in African-Americans as in Caucasians (6).

PATHOPHYSIOLOGY

In general, apnea is the final common pathway of many pathophysiologic processes, especially in the neonate and young infant. Respiratory function is a complex, precise system regulated in the pons and medulla, which receive afferent stimuli from numerous receptors. These vary from chemoreceptors to stretch receptors found in the bronchioalveolar tree. The efferent impulses from respiratory centers are mainly found in the vagus, phrenic, and intercostal nerves. The neonate has more nerve endings and smooth muscle surrounding the walls of small airways and a thinner pulmonary arterial wall, contributing to the decreased vascular resistance.

These changes, coupled with the immaturity of all the systems, may translate into sudden changes in both pulmonary vascular and distal airway resistance, causing ventilatory-perfusion

disturbances, with possible intrapulmonary shunting and hypoxemia. Also, gastroesophageal reflux has been associated with central, obstructive, or mixed apnea due to reflex hypoxemic episodes.

CLINICAL PRESENTATION

There is no typical clinical setting or presentation of a child with apnea. Most children are brought to the emergency department in stable condition by the parents, who say the child "stopped breathing." The child may present, however, in cardiopulmonary arrest or in respiratory distress with an unstable airway (Fig. 216.1). It is important to determine the child's position, activity, and exact sequence of events before and during the apneic episode (9). The child may have a spontaneous inspiratory effort or require stimulation after an apneic episode. The child may also experience a change in color, usually cyanosis, but the color may vary from pallid to erythematous. Associated changes in muscle tone can be seen before or during the apneic event. This change in tone may vary from arching or extension of the extremities to marked hypotonia and limpness (12). An understanding of the specific event sequence may help guide the diagnosis; for instance, arching with apnea after feeding, with or without formula in the oronasal passages, can be seen in gastroesophageal reflux (5).

In general, there are two clinical types of apnea: obstructive and central. An absence of respiratory airflow with effort in respiration and chest wall movement suggests obstructive apnea. The absence of respiratory effort, chest wall movement, and respiratory airflow is consistent with central apnea.

The parents are usually extremely frightened by what they have seen, and frequently believe that their child is dying. In most cases, parents administer some form of cardiopulmonary resuscitation (CPR) or stimulation. A thorough history is vital in order to determine whether the CPR was actually clinically indicated.

DIFFERENTIAL DIAGNOSIS

The differential diagnoses of apnea in neonates, infants, and older children are shown in Tables 216.1 through 216.4. Davies et al. (3) found that the most common discharge diagnoses in patients admitted with an ALTE were: gastroesophageal reflux (26%), seizures (9%), pertussis (9%), urinary tract infection (5%). In a septic child, there may be associated hypothermia or hyperthermia, thready pulses, prolonged capillary refill, or mottled skin. Apnea may be the only manifestation of a seizure, or a seizure may be precipitated by a hypoxic event. In the toddler and young child, foreign-body ingestion and poisoning should also be considered.

The clinician must differentiate between a breath-holding spell and an ALTE: A breath-holding spell is an involuntary event that occurs during an awakened state in a healthy toddler or young child during expiration. The most common type is the cyanotic or classic spell, which begins with crying, usually after a known precipitating event. The child then stops breathing in end expiration, with resultant cyanosis and loss of consciousness. The spell usually resolves spontaneously, with resumption of breathing and gradual recovery to the patient's baseline state. There may be associated body jerks and urinary incontinence (5). The clinical sequence and definition of a breath-holding spell does not apply to spells occurring during sleep. The pallid breath-holding spell involves a sudden painful incident, with resultant vagally mediated bradycardia or asystole. The patient turns pale and limp and may experience tonic-clonic seizure activity, but then ultimately resumes normal behavior.

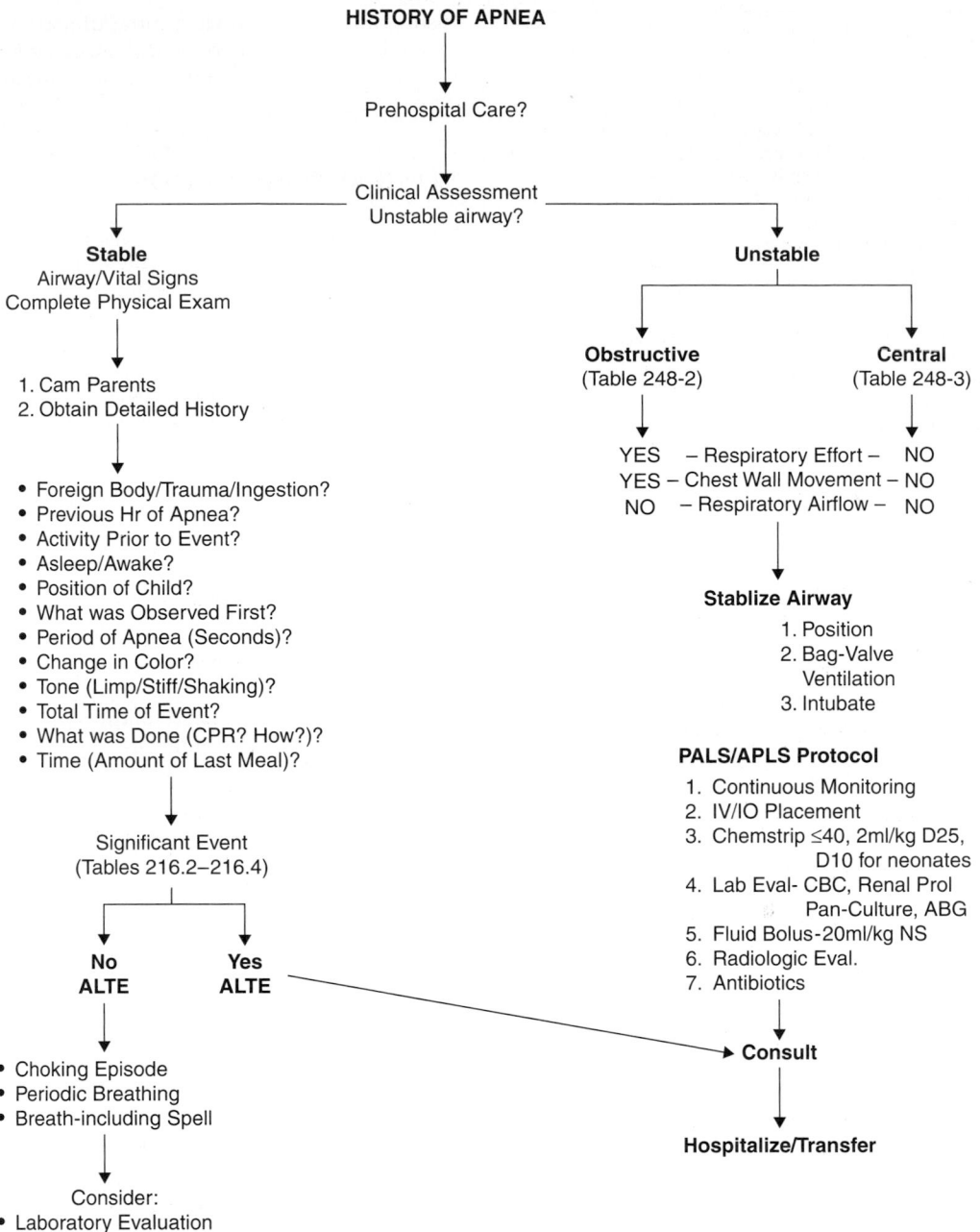

Figure 216.1. Algorithm for emergency department management and evaluation of apnea in an infant/young child.

Child abuse has been detected in 2.3% of patients presenting with an ALTE (10). Therefore, child abuse should be considered especially if retinal hemorrhages or signs of increased intracranial pressure are present. Cyanotic congenital heart disease usually presents in the first few weeks of life. The cause of the cyanosis is the right-to-left shunt, and it can vary in degree, depending on the pulmonary blood flow (i.e., the lower the pulmonary blood flow, the greater the degree of cyanosis). These children tend to have difficulty feeding, with associated diaphoresis and poor weight gain. The administration of 100% oxygen can clinically differentiate pulmonary from cardiac causes of cyanosis. The oxygen saturation measurement and PaO_2 increase when the cyanosis is secondary to a pulmonary cause, and typically fail to increase in the cardiac patient.

Many infants with known apnea who are on home monitors are brought to the emergency department for "frequent alarms." False alarms account for greater than 90% of monitor alarm events (7) and typically are due to shallow breathing or loose lead placement (11). A thorough history usually helps to differentiate between a true apneic event and a false alarm. However, if there is any doubt, the child should be admitted for further evaluation.

EMERGENCY DEPARTMENT EVALUATION AND MANAGEMENT

Most infants who present to the emergency department with a history of apnea are in stable condition and have a normal physical examination. The clinician must ensure a stable airway, because positioning (i.e., excessive neck flexion or extension) may predispose to upper airway obstruction, especially in patients with anatomic anomalies. A thorough physical

TABLE 216.2. Differential Diagnosis of Obstructive Apnea

Neonate/Infant	Both	Toddler/Young Child
STRIDOR		
Vascular ring	Vocal cord paralysis Foreign body Croup/epiglottitis	
PREMATURITY		
	Positional Laryngomalacia Tracheomlacia	Laryngeal web Tracheostomy plug Subglottic stenosis Bronchopulmonary dysplasia
ABNORMAL AIRWAY		

Choanal atresia/
  stenosis
Tracheoesophageal
  fistula
	Craniofacial
	  abnormalities
		Large tonsils/
		  adenoids

OTHER		

	Gastroesophageal
	  reflux
	Hemangioma/
	  lymphangioma
	Pharyngeal/
	  retropharyngeal
	  mass	

examination, correlating the vital signs with chest wall movements, respiratory effort, and airflow, helps to differentiate between obstructive and central apnea. All patients presenting with apnea should be placed on a pulse oximeter and cardiac monitor, and an intravenous line should be placed.

The questions in Figure 216.1 can be used to determine high-risk groups, such as those that meet the criteria for an ALTE, patients with previous events, occurrence during sleep, and events requiring either vigorous stimulation or any form of CPR (8). In addition, these questions may help to differentiate between events that appear similar.

After taking a methodical history and performing a complete physical examination, the physician should be able to conclude whether the child has had an ALTE and whether the apneic

TABLE 216.3. Differential Diagnosis of Central Apnea

Neonate/Infant	Both	Toddler/Young Child
CENTRAL NERVOUS SYSTEM		

CNS immaturity
Aberrant thermo
  regulation
	Seizures
	Brainstem tumor
	Chiari type 1
	  malformation
	Increased intracranial
	  pressure
	Vascular malformation/
	  hemorrhage
	Congenital central
	  hypoventilation
	  syndrome
		Apneustic breathing
		(achondroplasia)

TABLE 216.4. Other Causes of Apnea

Neonate/Infant	Neonate/Infant and Toddler/Young Child
CARDIOVASCULAR	
	Shock Dysrhythmias Congenital heart disease Prolonged QT syndrome
INFECTIOUS DISEASES	
Infant botulism Respiratory syncytial Virus	Sepsis Pertussis Meningitis Encephalitis Pneumonia
MISCELLANEOUS	
	Anemia Trauma Poisoning Neuromuscular disorders Munchausen syndrome by proxy Metabolic disorders

event was obstructive, central, or mixed (see Tables 216.2 through 216.4). If there is a significant event consistent with ALTE, a consultant should be notified for further inpatient evaluation and management.

If the patient has an unstable airway, positioning, oxygen, and bag-valve ventilation may be the only necessary immediate support to stabilize the child. If there is no improvement, endotracheal intubation is necessary to secure the airway. Continuous monitoring and intravenous access are also indicated.

A common error is failing to obtain an immediate bedside glucose level; hypoglycemia, commonly seen in sepsis, can be treated with 2 to 4 mL/kg of D_{25} solution intravenously or intraosseously. Neonates should be treated with 3 to 10 mL/kg of D_{10} solution (starting with 2 cc/kg), because higher glucose concentrations can cause sclerosis. The laboratory evaluation consists of a complete blood count, renal profile, pan-cultures, and possible pertussis and respiratory syncytial virus studies. Testing for respiratory syncytial virus should be performed in infants who were premature and in patients with congenital heart disease; this virus is associated with an increased risk of apnea in these populations (7).

A lumbar puncture should be strongly considered in patients less than 2 months of age, regardless of whether they are febrile, to rule out meningitis/encephalitis. Pertussis and chlamydia cultures should be obtained if these diseases are clinically suspected. The radiographic evaluation consists of a chest radiograph and, if upper airway obstruction is suspected, anteroposterior and lateral soft-tissue radiographs of the neck. Occasionally patients with apnea take caffeine or aminophylline; therefore, a theophylline level should be checked, with a therapeutic range of 8 to 12 µg/mL (9).

An electrocardiogram should be obtained to rule out arrhythmias and prolonged QT syndrome. In addition, obtain a CT scan of the head or cranial ultrasound in patients with an altered level of consciousness, abnormal muscle tone, focal neurologic findings, or retinal hemorrhages. Further inpatient evaluation may include an electroencephalogram, swallowing studies, esophageal pH probe, and polysomnography (1).

CRITICAL INTERVENTIONS

- Obtain bedside glucose
- Check electrocardiograph for dysrhythmias and prolonged QT syndrome
- Perform a full septic work up especially in infants less than 2 months of age
- Consider pertussis and respiratory syncytial virus studies
- Perform neuroimaging in patients with altered mental status or abnormal neurologic findings

DISPOSITION

Any child who meets the criteria for an ALTE, despite a normal work up and physical examination, should have the appropriate consultation and be admitted for further evaluation, observation, and parental education. The stable child can be admitted to a general pediatric ward with an apnea-bradycardia monitor to help determine the frequency and length of the apneic episodes and any associated bradydysrhythmias. Children who required any type of resuscitative measures in the prehospital course or in the ED should be monitored in a pediatric step-down or pediatric intensive care unit, depending on the severity of the event.

Indications for transfer depend on whether the facility has a pediatric intensive care unit or is capable of the necessary work up. The transfer should ideally be conducted by personnel trained in pediatric advanced life support.

COMMON PITFALLS

✔ Failing to believe the caretaker about the event, particularly when the child is happy and alert or if the parents are young
✔ Failing to obtain an immediate bedside glucose level. It should be repeated within 5 minutes after giving the dextrose bolus. Sepsis can present with respiratory instability, and hypoglycemia must be treated
✔ Failing to hospitalize all patients with apparent life-threatening events

Acknowledgment

The author gratefully acknowledges the contribution of Manuel Carmona Jr., who wrote the previous version of this chapter.

References

1. Brooks JG. Apparent life-threatening events. *Pediatr Rev* 1996;17:257.
2. Consensus Statement. National Institutes of Health Consensus Development Conference on Infantile Apnea and Home Monitoring. *Pediatrics* 1987;79:292.
3. Davies F, Gupta R. Apparent life threatening events in infants presenting to an emergency department. *Emerg Med J* 2002;19:11–16.
4. Evans OB. Breath-holding spells. *Pediatr Ann* 1998;26:410.
5. Halstead LA. Role of gastroesophageal reflux in pediatric upper airway disorders. *Otolaryngol Head Neck Surg* 1999;120:208.
6. Hauck F, Moore C, Herman S et al. The contribution of prone sleeping position to the racial disparity in sudden infant death syndrome: The Chicago Infant Mortality Study. *Pediatrics* 2002;110:772–780.
7. Kneyber MC, Brandenburg AH, de Groot R, et al. Risk factors for respiratory syncytial virus associated apnoea. *Eur J Pediatr* 1998;157:331.
8. Palfrey S. Overcoming ALTE phobia: a rational approach to "spells" in infants. *Contemp Pediatr* 1999;16:132.
9. Palfrey S. When and how to manage infants who have "spells." Part 2. *Contemp Pediatr* 1999;16:79.
10. Pitetti R, Maffei F, Chang K et al. Prevalence of retinal hemorrhages and child abuse in children who present with an apparent life-threatening event. *Pediatrics* 2002;110:557–562.
11. Rosenbaum RA, Levine BJ, Sweeney TA. Another false alarm? Apnea monitor activation in a neonatal intensive care unit graduate. *J Emerg Med* 1997;15:855.
12. Steinschneider A, Richmond C, Ramaswamy V, et al. Clinical characteristics of an apparent life-threatening event (ALTE) and the subsequent occurrence of prolonged apnea or prolonged bradycardia. *Clin Pediatr* 1998;37:223.
13. Willinger M, James LS, Catz C. Defining the sudden infant death syndrome (SIDS): deliberation of an expert panel convened by the National Institute of Child Health and Human Development. *Pediatr Pathol* 1991;11:677–684.

CHAPTER 217
Ataxia

Peter S. Auerbach and Erin E. Endom

Ataxia is an uncommon reason for a child to present to the emergency department (ED), but can be a highly distressing symptom when it occurs. Acute ataxia is usually due to a benign and self-limited process, with an excellent prognosis for full recovery in a previously healthy child. The emergency physician must have an awareness of the rare but life-threatening causes of ataxia, so that potentially serious diagnoses are not overlooked.

As a general term, ataxia refers to any disturbance in the coordination of movement and can result from dysfunction at virtually any level of the nervous system. Ataxia is most commonly of cerebellar origin, however, and thus the majority of cases can be referred to as *cerebellar ataxia*. The other major aspects of the nervous system involved in motor coordination are the sensory, motor and vestibular systems, and problems with any of these pathways may manifest as ataxia. In addition, any general metabolic disturbance of the central nervous system (CNS), such as hypoglycemia or drug or toxin exposures, can result in ataxia, usually by affecting the cerebellum which is particularly sensitive to metabolic derangements.

Cerebellar ataxia usually manifests as a wide-based, staggering gait, abnormal gross motor movements (dysmetria), or swaying of the trunk or head while at rest (titubation). In contrast, *sensory ataxia* is associated with a cautious, steppage gait (exaggerated elevation of the feet, which are then brought down suddenly in a flopping manner), an abnormal Romberg sign (loss of balance with the eyes closed), problems with fine motor movements, and loss of position and vibration sense. *Vestibular ataxia* presents with vertigo, nausea and nystagmus, while *motor ataxia* (sometimes also called *pseudoataxia*) results from muscle weakness and may be associated with loss of reflexes and tone.

For evaluation purposes ataxia can be classified by temporal course into acute, episodic or recurrent, and chronic causes. Acute ataxia, which can be defined as a new-onset ataxia present for less than 72 hours in a previously healthy child, is of primary concern to the emergency physician and will therefore be the focus of the majority of this chapter. Episodic and chronic ataxias are usually associated with other CNS abnormalities and genetic or metabolic disorders. Acute ataxia is generally due to benign, self-limited processes which require no treatment in children once serious problems (e.g., posterior fossa tumors, brainstem encephalitis) have been ruled out.

CLINICAL PRESENTATION

Most previously well children with acute ataxia will be brought to the ED for an unsteady gait or refusal to walk. Other less common complaints include difficulty in reaching for toys, abnormal eye movements, or a change in speech. As the two most common causes of acute ataxia are postinfectious cerebellitis (also referred to as acute cerebellar ataxia or ACA) and drug ingestions, features which might clearly indicate one of these two etiologies should be sought. These include a history of recent viral-type illness (fever, upper respiratory or gastrointestinal symptoms), vaccination (e.g., varicella), or medication, drug or toxin exposures. In contrast, features indicating a more serious cause of ataxia, such as encephalitis or a mass lesion, include a change in behavior or personality, significant headache or vomiting, and double vision. Other important aspects to be sought in the history include recent head injury or seizures, a loss of developmental milestones, and a family history of neurologic disorders.

Physical assessment should likewise be focused towards eliminating the possibility of a life-threatening cause of ataxia. This includes looking for focal neurologic deficits and signs of elevated intracranial pressure (ICP) such as papilledema or a bulging fontanelle, which may indicate a mass lesion; signs of head or neck trauma; and signs of CNS infections (fever, meningismus, altered mental status). Children with postinfectious cerebellitis should have a normal mental status and general physical examination, including vital signs, with the exception of ataxia. Clues to a toxicologic cause of ataxia should also be sought on physical examination, such as evidence of a specific toxidrome (e.g., anticholinergics) and an altered level of consciousness.

Detailed neurologic examination may be difficult in a young child. In addition to the general categories of mental status, cranial nerves, motor function and tone, reflexes, and sensation (depending on age), coordination testing should focus on careful observation of gait, truncal position and stability, the ability to reach for toys and manipulate objects, and eye movements. Assessment of speech is important in older children, specifically to detect the scanning type of dysarthria which can occur with cerebellar dysfunction (characterized by abnormal variation in volume and separation of syllables).

Through a combination of careful history and physical examination, the emergency physician should be able to narrow the differential diagnosis of ataxia and eliminate the possibility of most potentially serious etiologies. This will allow for a focused approach toward laboratory testing and further diagnostic evaluation.

DIFFERENTIAL DIAGNOSIS

Although many different entities can potentially cause ataxia, it is important to recognize that acute ataxia in a previously healthy child is almost always due to a very limited number of etiologies which are listed in Table 217.1. In fact, over 60% of children with acute ataxia have either postinfectious cerebellitis or drug ingestion (6). For comparison, Table 217.2 lists a number of

---

TABLE 217.1.   Common Causes of Acute Ataxia in Children

- Postinfectious cerebellitis (acute cerebellar ataxia)
- Drug ingestion
- Guillain-Barré syndrome

TABLE 217.2.   Life-Threatening Causes of Acute Ataxia in Children

- Hypoglycemia
- Drug overdose
- Encephalitis/meningitis
- Intracranial mass lesion
- Hydrocephalus
- Intracranial bleed
- Vertebrobasilar dissection
- Stroke
- Vasculitis
- Paraneoplastic syndrome (e.g., *opsoclonus-myoclonus syndrome* from neuroblastoma)

---

rare but serious causes of acute ataxia that should not be missed in the ED. These conditions almost never present with isolated ataxia.

Postinfectious cerebellitis accounts for over one-third of acute ataxia cases and is thought to result from cerebellar demyelination following an antecedent illness, either as an autoimmune phenomenon or from direct infection (6). It is seen most commonly in children younger than 6 years old and has most often been linked to varicella infection (1). It has also been reported in association with Epstein-Barr virus, enterovirus, herpes viruses, influenza A and B, hepatitis A, general viral upper respiratory infections, and a long list of other viral and bacterial infections, as well as following routine childhood vaccinations including varicella (10). The symptoms of postinfectious cerebellitis generally appear suddenly within 1 to 3 weeks after an illness, should be maximal at onset, and include dramatic truncal ataxia and gait instability. Most children recover completely without treatment within three months (3). Postinfectious cerebellitis is not associated with fever, seizures, altered mental status, or focal neurologic deficits and the presence of any of these factors make the diagnosis highly unlikely (6).

Drug ingestion and toxin exposure should always be considered early in the differential diagnosis, as this etiology is a close second to postinfectious cerebellitis as a cause of acute ataxia. Children less than 6 years old often present with ataxia due to ingestion of anticonvulsants (e.g., phenytoin, phenobarbital, carbamazepine, valproic acid), antihistamines, benzodiazepines, dextromethorphan, or alcohol. Older children often present after recreational drug and/or alcohol use. In both age groups the ataxia is usually accompanied by mental status changes, which should be a clue to the ingestion. Since drug ingestions are such a common cause of ataxia in children, and the history may not always be readily forthcoming, a high index of suspicion must be maintained and a toxicologic screen should almost always be ordered.

Guillain-Barré syndrome, which is an acute ascending inflammatory demyelinating polyneuropathy, presents with a sensory ataxia in up to 15% of pediatric cases (4). Because this syndrome affects the peripheral nerves and spreads from distal to proximal, the extremities will be affected much more than the trunk. Like postinfectious cerebellitis, Guillain-Barré syndrome is usually a postinfectious autoimmune phenomenon, and the key to the diagnosis lies in the finding of a sensory ataxia in the extremities in combination with areflexia (or hyporeflexia early in the course of the disease). The Miller-Fisher variant of this syndrome is characterized by the triad of ataxia, areflexia and ophthalmoplegia, with other cranial nerve abnormalities commonly found as well (8). Unlike postinfectious cerebellitis, Guillain-Barré syndrome requires hospitalization and may progress to respiratory failure in severe cases. Treatment options include intravenous immunoglobulin (IVIG) and plasmapheresis, although most patients recover completely without treatment (2). Other less common postinfectious neurologic syndromes also present with ataxia, such as acute disseminated encephalomyelitis (ADEM) and transverse myelitis, and are treated in a similar way (7).

The most worrisome cause of acute (or apparently acute) ataxia is an intracranial mass lesion. Over half of all childhood brain tumors are located in the brainstem and cerebellum, and often produce ataxia either through direct effects of the mass or via the development of hydrocephalus. Usually a history of gradually progressive ataxia can be elicited, along with other symptoms such as headache, visual changes, vomiting, and personality change. The physical examination may reveal signs of elevated intracranial pressure (ICP), such as papilledema, or focal neurologic deficits. The most common primary posterior fossa tumors in childhood include medulloblastoma, ependymoma, cerebellar astrocytoma and brainstem glioma. Metastatic lesions can affect the cerebellum as well.

Other serious causes of acute ataxia include head injury, resulting in intracranial hemorrhage with mass effect, cerebellar contusion or postconcussive ataxia, and neck trauma, which can cause vertebrobasilar dissection leading to cerebellar and brainstem ischemia or infarction. Cerebellar strokes, although rare in children, can result from bleeding disorders, arteriovenous malformations or CNS vasculitis (as in Kawasaki disease). CNS infections such as viral encephalitis often affect the cerebellum and brainstem preferentially and may present with ataxia as a prominent symptom. Finally, occult distant malignancies can present with ataxia in association with opsoclonus (rapid, chaotic eye movements) and myoclonus (rapid, chaotic contractions of individual muscles or muscle groups). This so-called *opsoclonus-myoclonus syndrome* occurs most commonly in children between the ages of 6 months and 3 years and is thought to result from a paraneoplastic autoimmune phenomenon primarily affecting the cerebellum. It is associated with neuroblastoma in over 50% of cases and should prompt admission for further evaluation including chest and abdominal computed tomography (CT) (9).

Less serious causes of ataxia include childhood migraine variants, epilepsy, postconcussive syndrome, conversion disorder, and labyrinthitis. Migraine variants may explain most forms of episodic or recurrent ataxia in children and can present with cerebellar ataxia, as in basilar migraine, or vestibular ataxia, as in benign paroxysmal vertigo (BPV). Basilar migraine most commonly affects adolescents while BPV affects infants and preschool children. In both cases a family history of migraine can almost always be elicited (5). Epilepsy will rarely manifest primarily as ataxia, usually in association with some degree of alteration in consciousness (complex partial seizures). More commonly, patients with known epilepsy are ataxic as a side-effect of their seizure medications. Postconcussive syndrome is a diagnosis of exclusion following head trauma and normal brain imaging. Conversion disorder should also be considered a diagnosis of exclusion but can usually be identified by characteristic features (e.g., complex lurching movements which require a high degree of coordination; absence of a wide-based stance; variability in physical findings, especially when the patient is unaware of being observed) in combination with an otherwise normal neurologic exam. Labyrinthitis is associated with the acute onset of severe vertigo and is typically worsened with head movements.

Causes of chronic ataxia are less of a concern in the ED, as they are usually known to the family and ataxia is rarely the reason for presentation. Examples of this include a long list of genetic and metabolic disorders with ataxia as but one component. A number of congenital malformations are associated with chronic ataxia as well, such as cerebellar aplasias and Chiari malformations. Most of these entities are associated with other significant neurologic and developmental abnormalities in addition to ataxia.

EMERGENCY DEPARTMENT EVALUATION

With the understanding that most cases of acute ataxia in otherwise healthy children are due to either postinfectious cerebellitis or drug ingestion, the primary goal of the ED evaluation is to eliminate the possibility of a more serious etiology. The first and most important step is a thorough history and physical examination, which together can help eliminate most life-threatening disease processes. If there are no concerning features in the history, and the physical examination is normal except for cerebellar ataxia, the only laboratory test which has been shown to be of significant yield is a comprehensive toxicology screen. This is often positive even when an ingestion is unsuspected by history. A "drugs of abuse" screen alone is less useful as it will miss the majority of ingestions in younger children. "Routine" laboratory studies, such as electrolytes and a complete blood count, are extremely low-yield in the evaluation of acute ataxia in the absence of underlying medical issues (6). Children taking antiepileptic drugs, as well as those with family members taking such medications, should have levels checked.

Lumbar puncture should be considered in all but the mildest cases of acute ataxia and those with a known etiology (e.g., drug ingestion by history and verified by toxicologic screening). This is particularly true of patients with altered mental status and/or fever. Cerebrospinal fluid (CSF) analysis is often normal in postinfectious cerebellitis, though there may be mild pleocytosis and protein elevation in up to 50% of cases (3). A significantly elevated cell count in the CSF suggests encephalitis or meningitis, and an elevated protein in combination with a normal cell count (cytoalbuminologic dissociation) is supportive of Guillain-Barré syndrome.

A CT or magnetic resonance image (MRI) of the brain should be performed whenever a mass lesion, hydrocephalus, elevated ICP or trauma is suspected. Although CT is more readily available than MRI from the ED, it is of limited value in visualizing the posterior fossa and brainstem. If a mass lesion is strongly suspected, an MRI must be obtained despite a normal CT, though not necessarily on an emergent basis. In addition to posterior fossa tumors, brain MRI may show other abnormalities missed by CT, such as areas of increased signal intensity or focal demyelination from encephalitis or postinfectious encephalopathy.

Electroencephalography (EEG) may be helpful if epilepsy or a migraine-variant is suspected by history as the cause of ataxia, although consultation with a neurologist should be considered at this point.

EMERGENCY DEPARTMENT MANAGEMENT

The management of acute ataxia is focused on the treatment of identifiable causes such as hypoglycemia, encephalitis/meningitis, elevated ICP and drug overdoses. Most children with postinfectious cerebellitis recover completely within 3 months of symptom onset and there is no specific treatment (3). Children with drug ingestions are managed according to the specific drug(s) involved, but a social services and/or Children's Protective Services (CPS) referral should be considered in many cases depending upon the specific details surrounding the ingestion.

Guillain-Barré and other postinfectious neurologic syndromes (e.g., ADEM) may require emergent airway management if severe, and require admission even if mild. Early consultation with a neurologist is appropriate. Other causes of ataxia, such as tumors and CNS infection, are treated according to the specific etiology and also require admission.

DISPOSITION

Children who are mildly symptomatic, appear well, and have a history and physical examination consistent with postinfectious cerebellitis may require no further ED evaluation. These patients are candidates for discharge home as long as close outpatient follow-up can be assured. If discharge is planned, parents should be counseled on injury prevention as children with postinfectious cerebellitis will be at increased risk of injury until recovery is complete. Children in whom this diagnosis is in doubt should have further testing done to rule out other diagnostic possibilities (e.g., toxicologic screen, brain imaging, lumbar puncture) as indicated by the history and physical examination. If a brain MRI is considered, it can often be done on an outpatient basis.

Most other causes of acute ataxia require admission for specific treatment or further diagnostic evaluation, including consultation with appropriate specialty services (e.g., neurosurgery for a posterior fossa tumor or acute hydrocephalus; neurology and infectious disease for suspected encephalitis). In the case of minor ingestions which would normally not require admission, discharge from the ED should be considered only after the home environment and social situation are judged to be safe.

CRITICAL INTERVENTIONS

- Rule out life-threatening etiologies of ataxia
- Reassure parents of the benign and self-limited nature of most causes of acute ataxia in childhood

COMMON PITFALLS

✔ Failure to obtain a thorough history and perform a careful neurologic examination prior to ordering extensive laboratory tests

✔ Failure to obtain a comprehensive toxicologic screen even in the absence of a history of ingestion

✔ Discharge home when the diagnosis is in doubt or when prompt outpatient follow up cannot be assured

✔ Failure to counsel on injury prevention prior to discharge

References

1. Adams C, Diadori P, Schoenroth L, Fritzler M. Autoantibodies in childhood post-varicella acute cerebellar ataxia. *Can J Neurol Sci* 2000;27:316–320.
2. Asbury AK. New concepts of Guillain-Barré syndrome. *J Child Neurol* 2000;15:183–191.
3. Connolly AM, Dodson WE, Prensky AL, Rust RS. Course and outcome of acute cerebellar ataxia. *Ann Neurol* 1994;35:673–679.
4. Delanoe C, Sebire G, Landrieu P, Huault G, Metral S. Acute inflammatory demyelinating polyradiculopathy in children: clinical and electrodiagnostic studies. *Ann Neurol* 1998;44:350–356.
5. Fenichel GM. Ataxia, In: *Clinical Pediatric Neurology*, 4th ed. Philadelphia: WB Saunders, 2001:223–242.
6. Gieron-Korthals MA, Westberry KR, Emmanuel PJ. Acute childhood ataxia: 10-year experience. *J Child Neurol* 1994;9:381–384.
7. Hynson JL, Kornberg AJ, Coleman LT, et al. Clinical and neuroradiologic features of acute disseminated encephalomyelitis in children. *Neurology* 2001;56:1308–1312.
8. Mori M, Kuwabara S, Fukutake T, Yuki N, Hattori T. Clinical features and prognosis of Miller Fisher syndrome. *Neurology* 2001;56:1104–1106.
9. Schor NF. Nervous system dysfunction in children with paraneoplastic syndromes. *J Child Neurol* 1992;7:253–258.
10. Sunaga Y, Hikima A, Ostuka T, Morikawa A. Acute cerebellar ataxia with abnormal MRI lesions after varicella vaccination. *Pediatr Neurol* 1995;13:340–342.

CHAPTER 218
Chest Pain

Steven M. Selbst

Children frequently present to the emergency department (ED) with the complaint of chest pain. One study found that 6 out of 1,000 children who presented to an urban pediatric emergency department or walk-in clinic complained of chest pain (13). Chest pain occurs equally in boys and girls, and is found in children of all ages and races. The mean age of children with this complaint is 12 years (13).

Unlike adult patients with chest pain, most studies have shown that children with chest pain rarely have serious organic pathology (1,13,15,22). Infrequently, a child with chest pain will present with significant distress and require immediate resuscitation in the ED. Even though most patients are not in extremis, chest pain should be taken seriously because underlying heart disease or other serious pathology can sometimes exist.

Certainly many patients and their families often associate their chest pain with heart disease and they are understandably frightened by media reports of sudden death in young athletes. Although serious, fatal heart disease is extremely rare in the pediatric population, the symptom of chest pain often disturbs the child's daily routine. About one-third of children with this complaint are awakened from sleep by the pain, while one-third misses school because of the pain (13). In general, a thorough history and careful physical examination can be used to guide the emergency physician as to when to order laboratory studies, and when to refer a child with chest pain to a specialist for further evaluation.

DIFFERENTIAL DIAGNOSIS OF PEDIATRIC CHEST PAIN

Age is a factor in the etiology of pediatric chest pain. Young children are more likely to have a cardiorespiratory cause for their pain, such as cough, asthma, pneumonia, or heart disease, while adolescents are more likely to have pain associated with stress or a psychogenic disturbance (13). Because there are occasional children with serious pathology related to chest pain, the ED physician must carefully contemplate an extensive differential diagnosis when evaluating a child with chest pain (Tables 218.1 and 218.2).

Cardiac Disease

Cardiac disease that was previously undiagnosed is a rare cause of chest pain in children, but should be considered. One study showed that less than 5% of children with chest pain had previously unrecognized heart disease as the etiology for the pain (13). Myocardial infarction can result from anomalous coronary arteries, and there may be no warning of this underlying condition. However, some children will have a pansystolic, continuous or mitral regurgitation murmur or gallop rhythm that suggests myocardial dysfunction. In many cases, exercise induces the chest pain because coronary blood flow is limited. Myocardial ischemia or infarction should be considered in any child who has pain with exertion. Syncope may also be an associated complaint in these patients (4,11,20).

TABLE 218.1. Cardiac Disorders Leading to Chest
Pain in Children

Coronary artery disease-ischemia/infarction
  Anomalous coronary arteries
  Kawasaki disease (coronary arteritis)
  Diabetes mellitus (long standing)
Arrhythmia
  Supraventricular tachycardia
  Ventricular tachycardia
Structural abnormalities of the heart
  Hypertrophic cardiomyopathy
  Severe pulmonic stenosis
  Aortic valve stenosis
Infection
  Pericarditis
  Myocarditis

Some children may have a history of a disease that results in a higher likelihood of angina or infarction. For instance, children who have long standing diabetes mellitus may have coronary artery disease, and may develop chest pain or myocardial infarction. Furthermore, those with a past history of Kawasaki disease are at risk because they may have coronary artery aneurysms that can produce problems long after the original illness. Likewise, those with chronic anemia are at risk for eventual cardiac pathology. Angina pectoris has been reported in a young child with sickle cell disease whose chronic anemia led to hypoxemia during exercise (15). Furthermore, teenagers who abuse cocaine are at risk for ischemia and myocardial infarction. Cocaine causes tachycardia, increased oxygen demand, vasoconstriction and hypertension as well as chest pain (7).

Moreover, some children may have an arrhythmia that causes symptoms such as palpitations, or an abnormal cardiac exam. Supraventricular tachycardia is the most common of these arrhythmias in childhood, but premature ventricular tachycardia, can also lead to brief, sharp chest pain (5).

Some children with structural abnormalities of the heart may develop ischemia and chest pain. One structural abnormality

TABLE 218.2. Noncardiac Causes of Pediatric Chest Pain

Musculoskeletal disorders
  Chest wall strain
  Direct trauma/contusion
  Rib fracture
  Costochondritis
Respiratory disorders
  Severe cough
  Asthma
  Pneumonia
  Pneumothorax/pneumomediastinum
  Pulmonary embolism
Psychological disorders
  Stress related pain
Gastrointestinal disorders
  Reflux esophagitis
  Pill induced esophagitis
  Esophageal foreign body
Miscellaneous disorders
  Sickle cell crises
  Abdominal aortic aneurysm (Marfan syndrome)
  Pleural effusion (collagen vascular disease)
  Shingles
  Pleurodynia (coxsackievirus)
  Breast tenderness (pregnancy, physiologic)
Idiopathic

that deserves mention is hypertrophic obstructive cardiomyopathy. This disorder has an autosomal dominant pattern of inheritance, so there is often a family history of this condition. Children with this disorder have a murmur that may be heard when the patient is standing or performing a Valsalva maneuver. The electrocardiogram (ECG) may reveal left ventricular hypertrophy and may show ST segment depression and T wave inversion. The risk for ischemic chest pain increases when a child with this condition exercises (7,15,20).

Most other structural disorders of the heart rarely cause chest pain. However, severe pulmonic stenosis with associated cyanosis, coarctation of the aorta and aortic valve stenosis can lead to ischemia (4,5,6). The pain in these conditions may be described as squeezing, choking, or as a pressure sensation in the sternal area. Children with aortic valve stenosis often have a harsh ejection murmur that is heard best at the upper right sternal border, radiating to the carotid arteries. These conditions are almost always diagnosed before the child presents with pain, and the associated murmurs are found on physical examination. Finally, mitral valve prolapse (MVP) may cause chest pain by papillary muscle or left ventricular endocardial ischemia. With this disorder, a midsystolic click and late systolic murmur are found in many cases. However, one study showed that MVP is no more common in children with chest pain than in the general population (13).

Cardiac infections should also be considered in children with chest pain. Patients with pericarditis may present with sharp stabbing midsternal chest pain that improves when the patient sits up and leans forward. The child with this infection is usually febrile, in respiratory distress, and has a friction rub, distant heart sounds, neck vein distention and pulsus paradoxus (7,15). Myocarditis is a more common infection and can sometimes present more subtly. The condition is often misdiagnosed because the signs and symptoms mimic other conditions. Children with myocarditis have chest pain for several days albeit mild and not disruptive (15,16). After a few days of fever and other systemic symptoms such as vomiting and lightheadedness, the patient may develop chest pain with exertion and shortness of breath. Examination may reveal muffled heart sounds, low-grade fever, a gallop rhythm, or tachycardia that is out of proportion to the degree of fever present. The patient also may have orthostatic changes in pulse or blood pressure (pulse increase >30 beats/min, blood pressure decrease by >20 mm hg when moving from supine to standing position). This is often misinterpreted as volume depletion since the child with this infection may not be taking oral fluids well and may indeed have mild dehydration. However, cardiogenic causes such as myocarditis should be suspected when orthostatic changes do not improve with fluid resuscitation. A chest x-ray will usually show cardiomegaly, in both myocarditis and pericarditis infections and the electrocardiogram will be abnormal prompting a further evaluation, such as an echocardiogram (15).

Musculoskeletal Pain

Musculoskeletal pain is one of the most common diagnoses in children with chest discomfort (13,15,22). Active children frequently strain chest wall muscles while wrestling, carrying heavy books, or exercising. Some children will suffer direct trauma to the chest, resulting in a mild contusion of the chest wall or, with more significant force, a rib fracture, hemothorax or pneumothorax. In most such cases, there is a straightforward history of trauma, and the diagnosis is clear. Generally, a careful physical examination will reveal chest tenderness or bruising, or pain with movement of the torso or upper extremities.

Costochondritis is a related musculoskeletal disorder that is common in children. This disorder is characterized by mild to moderate anterior chest wall pain that may radiate to the chest, back or abdomen. Exercise or an upper respiratory infection may precede pain. The pain may be bilateral, and it is generally sharp and exaggerated by physical activity or breathing. Eliciting tenderness over the costochondral junctions with palpation makes the diagnosis. Such pain may persist for several months (15).

Respiratory Conditions

Respiratory conditions frequently lead to chest pain. For instance, children with severe, persistent cough or asthma may complain of chest pain due to overuse of chest wall muscles. The diagnosis is made by the history and the findings of rales, wheezes, tachypnea, or decreased breath sounds. Some children who complain of chest pain with exercise may be found to have exercise-induced asthma, which can be determined quite readily with a treadmill test (21). In addition, some patients may develop a spontaneous pneumothorax or pneumomediastinum and complain of pain associated with respiratory distress. Children at high risk for these conditions are those with asthma, cystic fibrosis, and Marfan syndrome (17). However, previously healthy children may rupture an unrecognized subpleural bleb with minimal precipitating factors, such as coughing or straining. Patients with pneumothoraces present with respiratory distress, possibly decreased breath sounds on the affected side (if the pneumothorax is significant), and possibly palpable subcutaneous air (15,17). In addition, adolescents who snort cocaine are at risk for similar barotrauma and may complain of severe, sudden chest pain with associated anxiety, hypertension, and tachycardia (19).

Chest pain associated with fever should prompt concern about an acute infection such as pneumonia (13). Most of these children have a history of a cough and may be tachypneic on examination. A pleural effusion that develops from a systemic disease such as lupus erythematosis may also cause chest pain. Pleural effusion may cause pain that is worsened by deep inspiration. Although radiographs are helpful in confirming the presence of effusion, auscultation of decreased breath sounds should raise suspicion about this condition.

Finally, pulmonary embolism is extremely rare in pediatric patients, but may be considered in the adolescent girl with dyspnea, fever, pleuritic pain, cough and hemoptysis. The likelihood of this diagnosis is increased if she is using birth control pills, or has recently had an abortion. Young males with recent leg trauma are also at some risk for pulmonary embolism (2).

Psychogenic Disturbances

Psychogenic disturbances can precipitate chest pain in both boys and girls at equal rates. Stress-related pain accounts for about 10% of children with chest pain who present to the ED (13). Often the anxiety and stress that results in somatic complaints are not apparent as not all of these children will present with hyperventilation, or an anxious appearance. A careful history is essential. If the child has had a recent major stressful event such as separation from friends, death or divorce in the family, or school failure that correlates temporally with the onset of the chest pain, it is reasonable to conclude that the symptoms are related to the underlying stress (12,15). However, it is still imperative to rule out more serious pathology.

Gastrointestinal Disorders

Gastrointestinal disorders such as reflux esophagitis, often cause chest pain in young children and adolescents. The pain is classically described as burning, substernal in location, and worsened by reclining or eating spicy foods. The diagnosis can be made clinically, or with a therapeutic trial of antacids. Manometric studies to confirm the diagnosis are rarely needed (15).

Some young children will complain of acute chest pain following the ingestion of a coin or other foreign body that lodges in the esophagus. These children are occasionally in significant pain and may have drooling or dysphagia if the coin is trapped in the upper esophagus. In general, the child or parent can give a clear history that the foreign body was recently ingested and a simple radiograph can confirm the diagnosis.

Likewise, some adolescent patients may present to the ED with pill-induced esophagitis. Teenagers who take pill medications, especially tetracycline or doxycycline, can develop esophagitis particularly when the patient takes the medication with minimal water and then lies down (10). Prior history of esophageal dysmotility or stricture will make the pain more likely. However, many normal teenagers also report this pain. Due to the pH of the drug, doxycycline produces an acidic solution or gel as it dissolves and thus it is caustic when it remains in the esophagus. Symptoms may be noted several days after beginning the medication, but frequently pain occurs after taking the first dose. Physical examination will likely be unremarkable. The diagnosis is made by taking a careful history. These medications are often taken by adolescents for treatment of acne, and since they are used chronically the teen may fail to reveal that they take the medication unless asked specifically (10).

Miscellaneous

Miscellaneous causes of chest pain include pain related to underlying diseases. For instance, a child with sickle cell disease may have a vasoocclusive crisis, which localizes to the chest or produces acute chest syndrome (9). Marfan syndrome may result in chest pain and fatal dissection of an abdominal aortic aneurysm. Herpes zoster infection, or shingles, may produce severe chest pain that precedes the classic vesicular rash by several days or occurs simultaneously. Likewise, coxsackievirus may rarely lead to pleurodynia with paroxysms of sharp pain in the chest or abdomen ("devil's grip"). Teenagers or pre-teens may complain of chest pain when there is breast tenderness from physiologic changes of puberty or from early changes of pregnancy. A child with a thoracic tumor (Hodgkin disease or nonHodgkin lymphoma) may present with chest pain but undoubtedly would have other signs and symptoms of disease as well (7,15).

One should also consider the precordial catch syndrome (Texidor Twinge or "Stitch in the Side") as an explanation for unilateral chest pain that lasts a few seconds or minutes, and is associated with bending or a slouched posture. It is believed the pain arises from the parietal pleura or from pressure on an intercostal nerve, but the etiology is unclear. Sitting upright and taking shallow breaths or one deep breath relieves the pain. The pain may recur often or remain absent for months (7,15).

Slipping rib syndrome is a rare "sprain disorder" caused by trauma to the costal cartilages of the 8th, 9th, and 10th ribs, which do not attach to the sternum. Children with slipping rib syndrome complain of pain under the ribs or in the upper abdominal quadrants (8). They also hear a clicking or popping sound when they lift objects, flex the trunk, or even with walking. It is believed the pain is caused by one of the ribs hooking under the rib above and irritating the intercostal nerves. The pain can be duplicated and the syndrome confirmed by performing the "hooking maneuver" whereby the affected rib margin is grasped and then pulled anteriorly. Surgery is thought to be the only definitive management, though most patients are treated satisfactorily with nonopioid analgesics (8).

Unfortunately, in 20% to 45% of cases of pediatric chest pain, no diagnosis can be determined with certainty. The child's pain is labeled as *idiopathic* in many of these cases (13,22).

EMERGENCY DEPARTMENT EVALUATION

History

A complete history will reveal the etiology of chest pain in most cases. Family history may be helpful because disorders like hypertrophic obstructive cardiomyopathy are familial. Patients with hypertrophic cardiomyopathy may relate a family history of sudden death (5,7). Past medical history may reveal asthma that places the patient at risk for more serious causes for pain. Previous heart disease or conditions like diabetes mellitus (hyperlipidemia) or Kawasaki disease may increase the risk for cardiac pathology. The emergency physician should determine if the pain is frequent, severe, or interrupts the child's daily activity. Children who wake from sleep because of the pain are more likely to have an organic etiology, athough not necessarily serious (13). The emergency physician should then ask about the location and description of the pain. This is not always helpful because young children are vague in their descriptions. However, burning pain in the sternal area suggests esophagitis, and sharp stabbing pain that is relieved by sitting up and leaning forward, suggests pericarditis in a febrile child. The onset of pain should also be determined, as children with acute onset are again more likely to have an organic etiology (13). Those with chronic pain who have gone for extended periods without a diagnosis are much more likely to have an idiopathic or psychogenic etiology (13).

A history of trauma, rough play, or choking on a foreign body may be quite relevant. Also chest pain that occurs with exercise should be taken seriously, as this may relate to cardiac disease, or more commonly, exercise-induced asthma. Associated complaints should be assessed since chest pain that is associated with syncope or palpitations is more significant and may also relate to cardiac disease. Similarly, associated fever would make an infectious process such as pneumonia or myocarditis more of a concern. Likewise, the emergency physician may determine that the pain is part of an underlying systemic disorder such as a collagen vascular disease if joint pain, rash, or fever has been present. The physician should inquire about possible stressful conditions at home or school, and the diagnosis of psychogenic pain should not be just a diagnosis of exclusion. Finally, in some cases of adolescents with chest pain, it may be appropriate to ask about substance abuse (cocaine, in particular), or use of birth control pills. It is also wise to ask about prescribed and over the counter medications, considering the possibility of pill-induced esophagitis (1,10). Table 218.3 summarizes the history that is important in a child with chest pain.

Physical Examination

A careful physical examination is likely to point to the cause of pain. Vital signs have first priority. A quick general assessment should differentiate the child in severe distress who needs immediate treatment for life-threatening conditions such as a tension pneumothorax. Hyperventilation should be distinguished from respiratory distress by the absence of cyanosis or nasal flaring. Signs of chronic disease (pallor, poor growth) should be noted as these may suggest that chest pain is one symptom of a more complex problem like a tumor, or collagen vascular disease. Furthermore, consider the possibility that the child could have Marfan syndrome if the patient is tall and thin with upper extremity span that exceeds his or her height.

The skin should be examined for rashes or other skin lesions. Bruises on parts distant from the chest may indicate unrecognized trauma to the chest. The abdomen deserves careful evaluation, because it may be a source of pain that is referred to the chest. In the course of the examination, the emergency physician should note any signs of anxiety that could indicate the presence of emotional stress.

A complete chest examination is essential. This is likely to reveal rales, wheezes, or decreased breath sounds if there is pulmonary pathology. Murmurs, rubs, muffled heart sounds, or arrhythmias may be noted if there is cardiac pathology (4,5). A murmur that intensifies with Valsalva and the standing position is the hallmark of hypertrophic cardiomyopathy. The chest wall should be evaluated for signs of trauma, tenderness (suggesting musculoskeletal pain) or subcutaneous air (suggesting a pneumothorax or pneumomediastinum) (15,17).

Laboratory Evaluation

If the history and the physical examination do not lead to a specific diagnosis for the chest pain, it is unlikely that laboratory tests will be helpful. Laboratory studies usually confirm previously known disorders or abnormal findings that are suspected clinically. In general, chest radiographs and electrocardiograms should not be routinely ordered unless indicated by the history and/or physical examination (13,15,18). See Table 218.4.

If the history reveals pain that is acute in onset (within the past 2 or 3 days) or is otherwise concerning for pulmonary problems or cardiac disease, a chest x-ray and/or electrocardiogram are indicated. If there is pain with exertion, one should be

---

TABLE 218.3. History Questions for Children with Chest Pain

When did the pain begin?
How severe is the pain?
How often does the pain occur?
How long does the pain last?
What is the pain like?
What seems to bring on the pain?
Are there associated symptoms?
What is the child's past medical history?
Is there a family history of heart disease or chest pain or sudden death?
What treatments for the pain have been tried?
What is the patient or guardian concerned about?

TABLE 218.4. Indications for Laboratory Studies in Children with Chest Pain

WORRISOME HISTORY

Acute onset of pain
Pain on exertion
History of heart disease
Serious associated medical problems (diabetes mellitus, asthma, Marfan syndrome, Kawasaki disease, anemia, lupus erythematosus)
Use of drugs (cocaine, oral contraceptives)
Associated complaints (syncope, dizziness, palpitations)
Significant trauma
Foreign body ingestion/aspiration
Fever

ABNORMAL PHYSICAL EXAMINATION

Respiratory distress
Palpation of subcutaneous air
Decreased breath sounds
Cardiac findings (murmurs, rubs, arrhythmias)
Fever
Trauma

particularly concerned about cardiac disease or asthma and obtain an ECG and chest x-ray (13,15,18).

Certainly if the physical exam is abnormal, laboratory studies are justified. A chest x-ray can be quite helpful if the patient has fever, respiratory distress, decreased or abnormal breath sounds. Fever with chest pain is highly correlated with pneumonia. Pericarditis or myocarditis should also be considered in the febrile child with chest pain. The chest film may lead to these diagnoses if cardiomegaly is found. Moreover, an abnormal cardiac exam, including unexplained tachycardia, arrhythmia, murmur, rub, or click, warrants an electrocardiogram.

Laboratory studies are probably not necessary in the child with chronic pain, a normal physical examination, and no history to indicate cardiac or pulmonary disease. The family should be reassured that the child is unlikely to have a serious etiology for the pain and studies will be unhelpful. If this strategy is not successful, then noninvasive studies should be considered to alleviate the family's anxiety. Likewise, it is not necessary to obtain an echocardiogram on all children with ill-defined chest pain to look for mitral valve prolapse (13).

Blood counts and sedimentation rates are of limited value unless the physician suspects sickle cell disease, collagen vascular disease, infection, or malignancy. A drug screen for cocaine may be indicated in the older child with acute pain that is associated with anxiety, tachycardia, hypertension or shortness of breath. Cardiac enzymes are rarely of value unless there are specific concerns from the history or examination.

EMERGENCY DEPARTMENT MANAGEMENT

When a specific etiology for the pain is found, such as pneumonia or asthma, it can be specifically treated. In most cases of musculoskeletal, psychogenic or idiopathic pain the child will respond to reassurance, acetaminophen or nonsteroidal antiinflammatory analgesics, and rest. Heat and relaxation techniques may also be useful to manage pain. If esophagitis is suspected, a trial of antacids may be beneficial. When pill-induced esophagitis is suspected, some physicians prefer to perform endoscopic evaluation to document esophageal ulcers (midesophageal ulcers are most common, as the tablets are most likely to lodge in that region). Others prefer to omit endoscopy, discontinue the offending medication and treat with sucralfate. This approach is both diagnostic and therapeutic (10). The emergency physician can provide appropriate counseling to patients with chest pain related to minor stress and anxiety. Appropriate reassurance is very helpful in most cases of pediatric chest pain with a benign etiology.

CRITICAL INTERVENTIONS

- Assess the child's vital signs and the general appearance of the patient to determine if immediate treatment is needed
- Determine if the chest pain is due to thoracic trauma
- Assess the child's degree of pain and the impact of pain on the child's life
- Determine if chest pain is part of a chronic underlying condition
- Consider serious associated conditions such as asthma, lupus, sickle cell disease, Marfan syndrome
- Consider serious organic pathology if the child has fever or pain induced by exercise
- Consider laboratory studies if the history is concerning or the physical examination is abnormal. Avoid expensive, invasive laboratory studies with chronic pain and normal physical examination if there is evidence of benign history

DISPOSITION

The child in severe distress or with abnormal vital signs should be admitted to the hospital for monitoring, further diagnostic studies and extended treatment. Patients who have pain with exertion should be referred for exercise stress tests, or pulmonary function tests. Those with suspected esophageal foreign body should be referred to a specialist for removal of the foreign object. Likewise, referral to a mental health specialist should be considered if the patient has a serious emotional problem that cannot be managed by the ED staff. The child with known or suspected heart disease may be best served by a visit to the cardiologist, even if the pain proves to be unrelated. Children with chest pain associated with exercise, syncope, dizziness or palpitations should also be referred for further evaluation, and perhaps a Holter monitor and or echocardiogram to look for an arrhythmia or structural heart disease (3,5,7,15,22).

In all cases, appropriate follow up should be arranged since many children with ill-defined chest pain have persistent symptoms for many months. While serious organic pathology is unlikely to be found in the future, some patients are kept from participating in their usual activities because of the pain, and some manifest significant psycho-emotional problems or exercise-induced asthma that was not recognized at the initial ED visit (14).

COMMON PITFALLS

- ✔ Immediately ruling out serious pathology in the child with chest pain before observation and follow up evaluation
- ✔ Assuming that pediatric chest pain is either cardiac or musculoskeletal
- ✔ Failure to consider pneumonia or viral myocarditis in patients with a fever and chest pain
- ✔ Failure to recognize that pain associated with exertion, syncope, and dizziness is suspicious for cardiac disease
- ✔ Failure to consider stress or emotional upset as the cause of pain, if an important life event is temporally correlated
- ✔ Failure to consider esophageal foreign body (coin ingestion) in a young toddler with acute onset of chest pain

References

1. Anzai AK, Merkin TE. Adolescent chest pain. *Am Fam Phys* 1996,535:1682–1690.
2. Bernstein D, Coupey S, Schonberg SK. Pulmonary embolism in adolescents. *Am J Dis Child* 1986;140:667–671.
3. Brumund MR, Strong WB. Murmurs, fainting, chest pain: Time for a cardiology referral? *Contem Ped* 2002;19:155–166.
4. Graneto JW, Turnbull TL, Marciniak SA. An unusual cause of chest pain in an adolescent presenting to the emergency department. *Ped Emerg Care* 1997;13:33–36.
5. Gutgesell HP, Barst RJ, Humes RA, et al. Common cardiovascular problems in the young Part I. Murmurs, chest pain, syncope and irregular rhythms. *Am Fam Phys* 1997;567:1825–1830.
6. Hallagan LF, Dawson PA, Eljaiek LF. Pediatric chest pain: case report of a malignant cause. *Amer Journ Emerg Med* 1992;10:43–45.
7. Kocis KC. Chest pain in pediatrics. *Ped Clin NA* 1999;46:189–203.
8. Mooney DP, Shorter NA. Slipping rib syndrome in childhood. *Journ Ped Surg* 1997;32:1081–1082.
9. Morris C, Vichinsky E, Styels L. Clinical assessment for acute chest syndrome in febrile patients with sickle cell disease: is it accurate? *Ann Emerg Med* 1999;34:64.
10. Palmer KM, Selbst SM, Shaffer S, Proujansky R. Pediatric chest pain induced by tetracyline ingestion. *Ped Emerg Care* 1999;15:200–201.
11. Perry RF, Garlisi AP, Allison EJ, Hamrick CW, McConnell ME. Acute myocardial infarction in a 16 year old boy with no predisposing risk factors. *Ped Emerg Care* 1997;13:413–416.
12. Porter SC, Fein JA, Ginsburg KR. Depression screening in adolescents with somatic complaints presenting to the emergency department. *Ann Emerg Med* 1997;291:141–145.

13. Selbst SM, Ruddy RM, Clark BJ, Henretig FM, Santulli T. Pediatric chest pain: a prospective study. *Pediatr* 1988;82:319–323.
14. Selbst SM, Ruddy R, Clark BJ. Chest pain in children: follow-up of patients previously reported. *Clin Pediatr* 1990;29:374–377.
15. Selbst SM. Chest pain in children. *Ped in Rev* 1997;18:169–173.
16. Shetty AK. A child with chest pain. *Clin Pediatr* 1998;37:317–320.
17. Stack AM, Caputo GL. Pneumomediastinum in childhood asthma. *Ped Emerg Care* 1996;122:98–101.
18. Swenson JM, Fischer DR, Miller SA. Are chest radiographs and electrocardiograms still valuable in evaluating new pediatric patients with heart murmurs and or chest pain? *Pediatr* 1997;991:1–3.
19. Uva JL. Spontaneous pneumothoraces, pneumomediastinum, and pneumoperitoneum: consequences of smoking crack cocaine. *Ped Emerg Care* 1997;13:24–26.
20. Washington RL. Most sudden deaths in adolescent athletes caused by cardiac conditions. *Ped Ann* 2003;32:751–756.
21. Weins L, Sabath R, Ewing L, et al. Chest pain in otherwise healthy children and adolescents is frequently caused by exercise-induced asthma. *Pediatr* 1992;90:350–353.
22. Zavarus-Angelidou KA, Weinhouse E, Nelson DB. Review of 180 episodes of chest pain in 134 children. *Ped Emerg Care* 1992;8:189–193.

CHAPTER 219
Constipation

Elisa Alter Zenni

Although there are relatively few situations in which disorders of bowel control are truly emergent, concerns about constipation frequently result in emergency room visits. The emergency physician should be able to discern abnormal situations as well as advise concerned parents about the developmental process of bowel control, including normal stooling patterns and normal makeup of stool.

There is a wide variation in "normal" stool patterns. The normal newborn passes a meconium stool in the first 48 hours of life and then passes a mean of four stools per day during the first week, with a range of zero to 12 (7). Meconium stools are sticky, greenish-black, and odorless. Transitional stools, which are passed within 3 to 5 days, are thinner, greenish-brown, and commonly mixed with milk curds if the newborn is bottle-fed. The stools of breast-fed infants are pale yellow, occasionally slightly green, and are homogeneously mushy. Breast-fed newborns often pass a small stool after each feeding, which may be as frequent as eight to 15 times daily, although an occasional infant may not have a bowel movement for 7 to 10 days (9). In contrast, bottle-fed infants tend to have firm, formed, yellow, putty-like stools 1 to 4 times daily. Many infants strain, grunt, and turn red in the face during bowel movements, and parents often erroneously interpret this behavior as signaling constipation. When infants are 3 to 4 months of age stool frequency decreases, with the occasional bottle-fed infant passing only one stool every other day. For children beyond infancy, the normal frequency ranges from passing 1 stool every other day to passing 3 daily. Most children develop the adult pattern of having a mean of 1.2 stools per day by age 4 years (7).

During the first year of life, defecation is a reflex act (5). Maturational voluntary control of the external anal sphincter occurs in the second year, and bowel continence then becomes physiologically possible. Between the ages of 2 and 3 years, most American parents begin to toilet train their children, although the techniques and timing vary between cultural and socioeconomic groups. An important pathophysiologic concept relative to bowel control is that of stool retention (9). Stool retention usually occurs in boy toddlers, with the common starting point being simple constipation, which leads to painful passage of stool. Parents may describe their children as spending long periods of time straining and trying to have a bowel movement, when, in reality, the children are trying not to have a bowel movement. The association of pain with defecation leads to the cycle of pain, retention to avoid painful defecation, increasing fecal mass and further retention to avoid pain. Anal fissures are common and may start the process because of their associated pain or may exacerbate the problem by causing pain with the passage of each large stool. The rectum and sigmoid become dilated, the anal canal shortened, and the normal stretch-defecation reflexes blunted. Eventually, the fecal mass may become impacted, and unformed liquid stool leaks around the impaction, resulting in soiled pants. The process becomes established and may continue into the child's school years, at which time, hectic schedules and unsuitable school toilet facilities tend to worsen the situation. Because such fecal soilage occurs beyond the normal training period, the child's emotional or psychological constitution is invariably questioned. If emotional problems are found, they are as likely to be the result of this form of encopresis as the cause. There is also an association between stool retention and recurrent urinary tract infections, enuresis, and urinary incontinence (3).

A single definition of *constipation* has not been agreed upon in the pediatric population. Although many parents focus on the length of time between bowel movements, any determination of *normal* should encompass stool consistency and the ease with which the stool is passed. A child who defecates twice daily but painfully passes only small and dry pellets is constipated, whereas a child who produces a large, soft stool every other day is probably normal. It is simplest to define *constipation* as the difficult passage of large or hard stools, irrespective of frequency. The epidemiology and clinical scenarios commonly associated with constipation vary with age (7). In infants and toddlers, constipation occurs equally in boys and girls. In older, prepubertal children, constipation is more common in boys, with a male-to-female ratio of 3:1. This ratio reverses during adolescence, with constipation being 3 times more common in postpubertal girls.

CLINICAL PRESENTATION

A newborn infant discharged before 48 hours of age will occasionally present to the emergency department (ED) with a history of constipation, progressive abdominal distention, and vomiting, which may become bilious. In relation to constipation, this may be caused by imperforate anus, anal stenosis, meconium plug syndrome, meconium ileus, or Hirschsprung disease.

Constipation in the older infant or child is far less likely to be a serious or life-threatening process, yet is a source of great anxiety and frustration for some parents. Onset of constipation is commonly related to changes in diet, especially from breast milk to prepared formula or baby foods. Inadequate fluid intake is a common predisposing factor, as is any illness that may produce dehydration and inactivity. Constipation may arise with overly zealous efforts at toilet training. The school-aged child may present with constipation simply from reluctance to use the school bathroom.

The child with rectal retention and encopresis has fecal soiling of the underpants and may paradoxically complain of diarrhea. A lower abdominal mass may be found by palpation, and a shortened anal canal with huge fecal impaction may be found on rectal examination. Older children may present with abdominal pain, on occasion mimicking an acute abdomen.

DIFFERENTIAL DIAGNOSIS

Although there are many primary pediatric diseases with constipation as a symptom, most constipation does not suggest serious underlying disease. Anatomic malformations and congenital intestinal disorders are more likely to present in infancy than at a later age, but nonorganic causes of constipation predominate at all ages (7). The more common serious causes of constipation in the newborn are imperforate anus, anal stenosis, meconium plug syndrome, meconium ileus, Hirschsprung disease, volvulus, hypothyroidism, and any of the numerous causes of newborn bowel obstruction. Imperforate anus is easily diagnosed by inspection, which reveals no anal opening. In anal stenosis, the anus appears small, with a central black dot of meconium. In meconium plug syndrome or meconium ileus, there is scanty or no meconium and progressive signs of intestinal obstruction. Meconium plug syndrome is strongly related to Hirschsprung disease. Gentle digital examination produces passage of a dry, hard plug of meconium. Hirschsprung disease is suggested by an empty rectal vault and a long, sleevelike anal canal around the examining finger. It may be complicated by enterocolitis with paradoxical diarrhea, abdominal distention, and shock. In meconium ileus, there is delayed or no passage of meconium, with progressive intestinal obstruction and, often, serious complications (e.g., volvulus or perforation). Meconium ileus is strongly associated with cystic fibrosis; however, the respiratory symptoms of cystic fibrosis are usually absent in the newborn, and the clinical picture is dominated by the bowel obstruction. In an infant presenting with constipation, inadequate fluid intake should always be considered.

When the infant is beyond the immediate newborn period, constipation tends to be less emergent in nature, with most cases having either an idiopathic or dietary cause (8). The more common identifiable causes of constipation include excessive cow's milk intake, lack of dietary roughage, anal fissure, cerebral palsy, anterior displacement of the anus, and dehydration. Less common causes include Hirschsprung disease, drug intake (e.g., phenytoin, methylphenidate, imipramine, codeine), spinal cord lesions, chronic intestinal pseudoobstruction, infant botulism, prune-belly syndrome, presacral teratoma and other tumors, hypocalcemia, hypercalcemia, and hypothyroidism.

Hirschsprung disease is considered whenever there is significant constipation in the pediatric patient. It is caused by the congenital absence of submucosal and myenteric ganglion cells in a segment or all of the colon. It is more common in boys and is occasionally associated with Down syndrome. The cardinal sign is failure to pass meconium within the first 48 hours of life, followed by ongoing constipation and small-diameter (ribbonlike) stools in infants. Hirschsprung disease is the cause of 20% to 25% of neonatal intestinal obstruction. Necrotizing enterocolitis (toxic megacolon) is a complication that may develop in infants. Newborns who are not diagnosed may present later in childhood with chronic constipation, abdominal distention, and, often, failure to thrive.

A rectal examination of a child should be performed gently and deliberately. The physical examination may reveal well-formed fecal masses suprapubically or in either lower quadrant. Pertinent findings may include an anteriorly displaced anus (anal ectopy), a tight and stenotic anus (anal stenosis), anal fissure, or a sleevelike anal canal with empty ampulla (Hirschsprung disease). The signs of hypothyroidism (coarse facial features, umbilical hernia, macroglossia) should raise suspicion of that diagnosis.

EMERGENCY DEPARTMENT EVALUATION AND MANAGEMENT

The Constipation Subcommittee of the Clinical Guidelines Committee was formed by the North American Society for Pediatric Gastroenterology and Nutrition to develop a clinical practice guideline for the evaluation and management of constipation (1). Their recommendations are summarized below. Evaluation of the constipated patient should include a careful history and physical examination, which often provide the diagnosis without requiring further studies in the ED. Information regarding the time after birth of the first bowel movement, length of time the condition has been present, frequency of bowel movements, consistency and size of stools, presence of pain and blood, and toilet use habits (if applicable) should be obtained. Dietary habits, medications, and associated fever, abdominal distention, anorexia, vomiting, and weight loss or poor weight gain, should be assessed. A thorough physical examination should be done, including abdominal palpation for masses, especially fecal masses in the left lower quadrant; inspection of the perineum and perianal area for fissure, anterior displacement, or stenosis; and inspection of the sacrum for signs of myelodysplasia. Gentle rectal examination with a well-lubricated little finger should be attempted but not forced on an unwilling child, assessing perianal sensation, anal tone, size of the rectum, presence of an anal wink, and amount and consistency of stool within the rectum. It is recommended that a test for occult blood in the stool be performed in all infants with constipation, as well as in any child who also has abdominal pain, failure to thrive, intermittent diarrhea, or a family history of colon cancer or colonic polyps. If the history is chronic, a urine culture should be taken to avoid missing the occult urinary tract infection. Exhaustive laboratory and radiographic investigation is not appropriate in the ED, although occasionally a plain abdominal radiograph is helpful in confirming the diagnosis when the history and/or physical examination are confusing or inconclusive.

The first step in management of constipation is education of the child and family and "demystification" of constipation (10). If fecal impaction is present, disimpaction is necessary. This can be accomplished by using oral medications, rectal medications, or a combination of the two. All approaches have been determined to be effective in uncontrolled clinical trails (11), and the individual approach should be discussed with the child and family. Oral disimpaction can be achieved with mineral oil 1 to 4 mL/kg/dose once or twice a day (contraindicated in infants and in children at risk for aspiration), milk of magnesia 1 to 3 mL/kg/dose once or twice per day, lactulose 1 to 2 mL/kg/dose once or twice per day, or with medications containing polyethylene glycol (PEG), sorbitol, senna, or bisacodyl (6,11). MiraLax is a new electrolyte-free PEG solution that is tasteless and can be mixed with any clear liquid beverage (2). It is prepared by dissolving 1 capful (17g) of powder in 8 ounces of liquid (0.07 g/ml), and giving the child 0.7 to 0.9 g/kg or 10 to 14 mL of this solution per kilogram of body weight per day in 2 divided doses.

Maintenance therapy of constipation, best managed by a primary care clinician, consists of dietary changes, behavioral modification and laxatives (1). Dietary management includes increasing fluid intake, adding bulk to the diet, and adding fruits such as prunes or plums to the diet. Maltsupex (barley malt extract) or Karo syrup can be safely recommended for infants in a dosage of 1 to 2 teaspoons 2 to 4 times daily, added to formula, juice, or food. Behavioral modification for the older child includes regular toilet sitting, stool diaries and reward systems. Medications are often useful as part of maintenance therapy. Cathartics, suppositories (other than small glycerin suppositories), and, especially, enemas should generally be avoided in infants. Hypertonic phosphate enemas have been associated with severe, acute hypocalcemia and cardiac arrest in infants (10). Tap water enemas have been associated with acute hyponatremia, seizures, and death (12). In the older infant and toddler, milk of magnesia, mineral oil or lactulose can be used. Docusate (Colace) 5 to 10 mg/kg/d or senna extract (Senokot) 5 to 10 mL daily can be safely used in older children.

If an anal fissure is discovered, management includes frequent, gentle, thorough cleansing of the anus and liberal lubrication with petroleum jelly. A stool softener must be used, and a topical anesthetic ointment such as dibucaine may be necessary (4). Aggressive care of the simple fissure is necessary to prevent the pain-retention cycle from becoming established.

CRITICAL INTERVENTIONS

- Avoid cathartics, most suppositories, and enemas in infants
- Laxatives and cathartics can be used in older children
- Aggressively treat anal fissures

DISPOSITION

Role of the Consultant

Consultation for simple constipation is unnecessary. Infants with suspected Hirschsprung disease or bowel obstruction should be expeditiously referred to a pediatrician or pediatric surgeon, and prompt response to the ED should be expected, because such conditions may constitute a surgical emergency. Older children with chronic constipation with or without encopresis should be referred to a pediatrician for long-term management. Older children with suspected Hirschsprung disease should be referred to a pediatric gastroenterologist or pediatric surgeon.

Indications for Admission

The following are indications for admission: failure to pass meconium, bowel obstruction, and toxic megacolon complicating Hirschsprung disease. Occasionally, the need for complicated disimpaction and initiation of a therapeutic regimen for chronic constipation with encopresis may require admission, but this is quite rare in the current era of cost containment and emphasis on ambulatory care.

Transfer Considerations

Bowel obstruction or toxic megacolon in the newborn requires specific pediatric expertise on an emergent basis, and transfer to a pediatric facility may be necessary. Before transfer, venous access should be secure, gastric suction and decompression begun, and antibiotics considered. Hypothermia should be vigorously avoided.

COMMON PITFALLS

✔ The newborn or young infant who presents with constipation should be carefully evaluated, so that Hirschsprung disease with subsequent necrotizing enterocolitis is considered in the differential diagnosis and not missed
✔ Enemas, especially hypertonic phosphate enemas, should be avoided in infants

References

1. Baker SS, Liptak GS, Colletti RB, et al. Constipation in infants and children: evaluation and treatment. A medical position statement of the North American Society for Pediatric Gastroenterology and Nutrition. *J Pediatr Gastroenterol Nutr* 1999;29:612–626.
2. Bishop WP. Miracle Laxative? *J Pediatri Gastroenterol Nutr* 2001;32:514–515.
3. Dohil R, Roberts E, Jones KV, et al. Constipation and reversible urinary tract abnormalities. *Arch Dis Child* 1994;70:56.
4. Felt B, Wise CG, et al. Guideline for the management of pediatric idiopathic constipation and soiling. *Arch Pediatr Adolesc Med* 1999;153:380.
5. Green M. *Constipation in pediatric diagnosis.* Philadelphia: WB Saunders, 1986: 234.
6. Ingebo KB, Heyman MB. Polyethylene glyco-electrolyte solution for intestinal clearance in children with refractory encopresis: A safe and effective therapeutic program. *AJDC AM J Dis Child* 1988;142:340–342.
7. Lewis LG, Rudolph CD. Practical approach to defecation disorders in children. *Pediatr Ann* 1997;26:260.
8. Loening-Baucke V. Chronic constipation in children. *Gastroenterology* 1993; 105:1557.
9. Rappaport L, Levine M. The prevention of constipation and encopresis: a developmental model and approach. *Pediatr Clin North Am* 1986;33:859.
10. Reedy J, Zwiren J. Enema-induced hypocalcemia and hyperphosphatemia leading to cardiac arrest during induction of anesthesia in an outpatient surgery center. *Anesthesiology* 1983;59:578.
11. Tolia V, Lin CH, Elitsur Y. A prospective randomized study with mineral oil and oral lavage solution for treatment of faecal impaction in children. *Aliment Pharmacol Ther* 1993;7:523–529.
12. Ziskind A, Gellis SS. Water intoxication following tap water enemas. *Am J Dis Child* 1958;96:699.

CHAPTER 220
Crying, Fussy Infant

Naghma S. Khan

Crying is one of the most important forms of communication between infants and their caretakers (2). Few studies exist on normal infant crying patterns during the first year of life, but they tend to agree that crying follows a circadian rhythm (8). Crying is generally considered to signal an unmet need or distress, and as such, evokes significant apprehension in both the parents and healthcare providers. In addition, persistent infant crying can contribute to family stress and has been shown to play a role in child abuse (3). Parental temperament and experience greatly determine the crying limit at which medical help is sought. An emergency department (ED) encounter is likely to be precipitated by prolonged, inconsolable, and recurrent episodes of crying that are usually two or three times longer than normal controls (8), or if a single act of crying is abnormally high-pitched or associated with an appearance of pain or anxiety. This behavior provokes anxiety in both parents and physicians. Emergency physicians must be able to distinguish between the more prevalent "normal crying" and colic and the more serious acute illnesses, some of which may be life-threatening and require immediate intervention.

CLINICAL PRESENTATION

Parents tend to seek assistance from healthcare providers when they cannot identify the cause of their infant's crying or cannot console the infant, or when crying continues for longer than usual. Most commonly, the presentation is in the late evening or the middle of the night. A febrile infant with extreme irritability and fussiness does not pose as much of a diagnostic dilemma as does an afebrile child with the same symptoms (12).

DIFFERENTIAL DIAGNOSIS

It is important to differentiate recurrent benign crying syndromes such as colic from the single episode of excessive crying that may be a symptom of some life-threatening pathologic process (13). Therefore, it is essential that a thorough head-to-toe exam be performed when a child presents with excessive crying.

The presence of fever with acute-onset, high-pitched, inconsolable crying may suggest meningitis or infection, although fever is not always present in young infants with serious bacterial infection. Occult urinary tract infections may present as recurrent crying possibly related to episodes of urination or as a single episode of excessive crying possibly secondary to bladder irritation. Urinary tract infections should be ruled out in all patients without another obvious cause for excessive crying.

Excessive, persistent crying (>3 hours) is a well-documented side-effect of the diphtheria-pertussis-tetanus (DPT) vaccination and is probably related to an extremely painful local reaction at the site of inoculation (1).

With the use of disposable diapers, an open diaper pin is seldom a cause for excessive crying, but this should be ruled out in infants wearing cloth diapers.

A strangulated digit, penis, or clitoris, usually with an encircling hair or a sock fiber, and insect bites, especially brown recluse spider bites, may go unrecognized by parents, as may burns, particularly scald burns on the buccal mucosa or tongue (most common caused when milk bottles are heated in the microwave oven).

Unlike older patients, infants with corneal abrasions do not present with easily recognizable signs and symptoms like foreign body sensation, photophobia, and tearing. Instead, crying may be the only presenting complaint. Complete resolution of irritability with use of short-acting anesthetics in the eye confirms the diagnosis (4). It is difficult to visualize the tympanic membrane in infants, especially neonates. The ear canal is narrow and the tympanic membrane is in a horizontal rather then vertical alignment. Assistance may be required to immobilize the infant so that the examiner can visualize the red, bulging, immobile ear drum diagnostic of acute suppurative otitis media.

Effortless tachypnea associated with irritability should suggest metabolic acidosis or salicylate poisoning. Supraventricular tachycardia may present with irritability as the sole manifestation.

Head trauma, fractures, and other signs of child abuse and neglect should be sought carefully, lest these potentially life-threatening entities be missed.

A high degree of suspicion is needed to rule out intussusception, anal fissures, testicular torsion, and incarcerated hernias.

Cocaine exposure (including passive inhalation) and drug withdrawal should be considered as part of the differential diagnosis.

Finally, "infantile colic" is arbitrarily defined by the rule of threes: an otherwise healthy, thriving infant crying for more than 3 hours a day, more than 3 days in a week, for more than 3 weeks (9). The typical colic episode is described as paroxysmal crying that develops into a piercing scream, with legs drawn up, abdominal distention, and passage of flatus. The infant appears to be in severe abdominal pain (6,9). Normal infant crying peaks in the afternoon and evening hours from 1 to 3 months of age and is reported to last a mean of 2.0 to 2.5 hours a day. Cow's milk allergy, infant temperament, overstimulation and gastroesophageal reflux have been implicated in the cause of "colic," while others regard it as the extreme end of normal crying (5,11). It is obvious from the foregoing that the cause of infantile colic is unknown, but we do know that it subsides spontaneously by 3 to 4 months of age.

Table 220.1 lists conditions associated with abrupt onset of inconsolable crying in young infants.

EMERGENCY DEPARTMENT EVALUATION

A methodical approach to the evaluation of the crying infant yields the most information with the least morbidity to the parents and the infant. The importance of a careful history, documenting the onset, frequency, duration, and associated events (vaccinations, particularly pertussis) cannot be overemphasized. A thorough physical examination of a completely undressed infant (including the diaper) yields vital information in nearly 54% of patients (7), circumventing the need for invasive procedures. The initial history and physical examination must focus on ruling out potentially life-threatening causes of crying, such as meningitis, shaken-baby syndrome and other forms of child abuse, acute abdominal catastrophes (e.g., intussusception), incarcerated hernias, metabolic disorders, and intoxications; the less critical causes are collectively more common. A review of the vital signs is essential to rule out cardiac dysrhythmias and respiratory problems. A catheterized or suprapubic urine specimen should be obtained in all infants when the cause is not obvious.

Fluorescein staining and ultraviolet light eye examination is essential to rule out corneal abrasions. Eversion of the eyelids may be needed to visualize a foreign body in the eye. A fundoscopic examination should be attempted; if visualization is difficult and the index of suspicion is high for shaken-baby syndrome, this examination should be repeated after dilating the pupils. A careful otoscopic examination may show an unsuspected otitis media.

The head should be examined for any signs of trauma and for a bulging fontanel. The extremities and joints (especially the hips) should be carefully palpated and maneuvered to rule out fractures, osteomyelitis, and septic joint.

An abdominal examination is difficult to perform in a crying infant. It is important to examine the abdomen and chest and listen to the heart before attempting any invasive or painful procedures; if possible, this should be done while the infant is in the mother's lap and sucking on a bottle or pacifier. Flexing the legs at the hip may help relax the abdominal muscles enough to allow a good abdominal examination. Before attempting a rectal examination, the physician should check the anal area for signs of trauma or anal fissures.

If a careful history and physical examination do not reveal or suggest a cause for crying, further studies are indicated. Skeletal roentgenography and cranial computed tomography scanning are indicated in suspected child abuse. If an abnormal cardiac rhythm is auscultated, initial cardiac monitoring and a subsequent 12-lead electrocardiogram may reveal the diagnosis. Suspected gastrointestinal problems should be confirmed with appropriate studies, such as a barium enema, ultrasound, CT or upper GI. A sepsis work up is indicated if there is any suspicion of an infectious etiology. An elevated anion gap or abnormal urinalysis and electrolyte levels may point toward an inborn error of metabolism or endocrinopathy.

EMERGENCY DEPARTMENT MANAGEMENT

Most infants have a completely normal examination and workup. If the history and physical examination are compatible, a diagnosis of colic should be entertained. Parents who present to the emergency department with a crying infant usually do not readily accept the diagnosis and the inability to treat the cause with medications. Multiple studies have shown the danger of

TABLE 220.1. Causes of Excessive Crying in Afebrile Infants

HEAD AND NECK

Head
Head trauma (intracranial hemorrhage,
 shaken-baby syndrome)
Meningitis
Encephalitis
Pseudotumor cerebri

Eye
Corneal abrasions
Ocular foreign body

Ear
Otitis media

Throat
Oral mucosal burns
Teething
Herpangina
Herpes stomatitis
Foreign body in oropharynx
Oral thrush

CHEST

Cardiac
Supraventricular tachycardia
Congestive heart failure
Coarctation of the aorta
Anomalous left coronary artery

Respiratory
Pneumonia
Rib fractures

ABDOMEN

Intussusception, volvulus
Appendicitis
Gastroenteritis
Constipation
Gastroesophageal reflux

GENITOURINARY

Urinary tract infection
Incarcerated hernia
Strangulated penis, clitoris (hair tourniquet
 syndrome)
Torsion testis

EXTREMITIES

Fractures
Strangulated digit (hair tourniquet syndrome)
Osteomyelitis
Septic arthritis
Open pin in diaper
Pain at vaccination site (especially after DPT)
Insect bites (brown recluse)

METABOLIC

Inborn errors of metabolism
Metabolic acidosis
Aspirin overdose

MISCELLANEOUS

Colic
Night terrors
Overstimulation
Maternal depression
Environmental deprivation (starvation,
 neglect)
Idiopathic

---

using alcohol-based preparations and Dramamine–Donnatal combinations (10). About 4% of infants may benefit from changing to a protein hydrolysate formula due to cow's milk allergy (5). It is important to empathize with the parents and to take time to counsel them on methods to console the child early; possible intervention techniques include rocking slowly in a quiet room, warm compresses to the abdomen, feeding, frequent burping, and diaper changing.

Other etiologies of crying should be managed as outlined in the appropriate chapters of this book.

CRITICAL INTERVENTIONS

- Search thoroughly for the cause of crying and do not assume that colic is the diagnosis
- Perform fluorescein staining in order to check for a corneal abrasion. Similarly, retinal hemorrhages may not be noted on a cursory ophthalmoscopic examination in a crying, uncooperative patient unless the pupils are dilated

DISPOSITION

All children who present to the ED with crying need appropriate follow up to ensure an adequate weight gain and no progression of symptoms, especially if the diagnosis is "colic." Consultation with subspecialists and admission are determined by the diagnosis.

COMMON PITFALLS

✔ A hurried and superficial history and physical examination on this group of infants will lead to misdiagnosis and inadequate care. On the other hand, doing complete sepsis work ups in all infants with crying would subject a large population of colicky infants to unnecessary tests with extremely low yield. A rational approach is to tailor the work up based on a reliable history and physical examination

✔ Careful attention should be paid to the vital signs, lest the physician miss the presence of fever, tachypnea, and supraventricular tachycardia

✔ Listen to the parents. Do not underestimate their distress and ability to determine the degree of illness in their infant

✔ Avoid terms and diagnoses such as "difficult infant" (8)

✔ If neglect can be safely ruled out, reassure the parents about their parenting skills

Acknowledgment

Thanks to the previous edition's chapter author Agoritsa G. Baka.

References

1. Blumberg DA, Lewis K, Mink CM, et al. Severe reactions associated with DPT vaccine: detailed study of children with seizures, hypotonic-hyporesponsive episodes, high fevers, and persistent crying. *Pediatrics* 1993;91:1158.
2. Brazelton TB. Crying in infancy. *Pediatrics* 1962;29:579.
3. Frodi A. When empathy fails: aversive infant crying and child abuse. In: BM Lester, CFK Boukydis, eds. *Infant crying: theoretical and research perspectives.* New York: Plenum Publishing, 1985.

4. Harkness MJ. Corneal abrasion in infancy as a cause of inconsolable crying. *Pediatr Emerg Care* 1989;5:242.
5. Lucassen PLBJ, Assendelft WJJ, et al. Effectiveness of treatments for infantile colic: systematic review. *BMJ* 1998;316:1563–1569.
6. Miller AR, Barr RG. Infantile colic: is it a gut issue? *Pediatr Clin North Am* 1991;38:1407.
7. Poole SR. The infant with acute, unexplained, excessive crying. *Pediatrics* 1991;88:448.
8. St. James SR. Roberts I, Halil T. Infant crying patterns in the first year: normal community and clinical findings. *J Child Psychol Psychiatry* 1991;32:951.
9. Wessell MA, Cobb SC, Jackson EB, et al. Paroxysmal fussing in infancy sometimes called "colic." *Pediatrics* 1954;14:421.
10. Williams J, Watkin-Jones R. Dicyclomine: worrying symptoms associated with its use in some small babies. *BMJ* 1984;288:901.
11. Sutphen JL. Is it colic or is it gastroesophageal reflux? *J Pediatr Gastroenterol Nutr* 2001;110–1.
12. Ruiz-Contreras J, Urquia L, Bastero R. Persistent crying as predominant manifestation of sepsis in infants and newborns. *Pediatr Emerg Care.* 1999;113–115.
13. Trocinski DR, Pearigen PD. The crying infant. *Emerg Med Clin North Am* 1998;895–910.

CHAPTER 221
Dehydration

Todd Wylie

Dehydration in pediatric patients is commonly encountered. Approximately 200,000 children less than 5 years of age are hospitalized annually in the United States for acute gastroenteritis (5). Worldwide, 1.5 to 2.5 million children under the age of 5 years die every year from diarrheal disease (10). Although usually nonfatal in developed nations, dehydration does account for significant morbidity in the pediatric population.

Diagnosis and management of dehydration in pediatric patients requires a basic understanding of fluid and electrolyte balance. Total body water varies with age, ranging from approximately 75% in the term newborn to 65% in a 1-year-old, and decreasing to 55% to 60% in adolescents and adults (7,9). Total body water is distributed between the extracellular and intracellular fluid compartments. Distribution of total body water between the two fluid compartments is age dependent, with the extracellular fluid comprising slightly greater than half the total body water in a newborn and decreasing to about one-third the total body water in adults. The extracellular fluid compartment includes the intravascular plasma and extravascular interstitial fluid. The majority of effective solutes in the extracellular fluid are Na and Cl. The intracellular fluid compartment comprises less than half the total body water in a newborn, but makes up two-thirds of the total body water in adults. Potassium is the primary intracellular solute. Although infants have a greater percentage of total body water than adults, this does not provide extra protection from dehydration. Pediatric patients, and in particular infants, have larger surface area to body weight ratios, greater resting metabolic rates, and a higher rate of fluid turnover. In fact, fluid turnover in infants is roughly double that seen in adults (11). The increased rate of fluid turnover makes infants susceptible to dehydration stemming from excessive losses or lack of fluid intake.

Multiple organ systems and a variety of mechanisms are involved in maintaining electrolyte and fluid balance. Volume status, including the intravascular and intracellular compartments, is inextricably linked to amount and concentration of solute. Sodium is the primary extracellular solute, and therefore the focus of mechanisms aimed at maintaining osmolality, and subsequently, volume status. Antidiuretic hormone, aldosterone, the renin-angiotensin system and the kidneys all act in concert to maintain sodium concentration and volume status.

Isonatremic dehydration is the most common form of dehydration encountered. In isonatremic dehydration there is a proportional loss of both water and electrolytes, as occurs in children with short bouts of diarrhea. Children may also present with hyponatremic dehydration (Table 221.1). Hyponatremia is generally thought of in terms of hypovolemia, euvolemia, and hypervolemia. Causes of hypovolemic hyponatremia include viral gastroenteritis, renal losses (proximal renal tubular acidosis, diuretic use, salt-wasting nephropathy), and cystic fibrosis patients exposed to high environmental temperatures. Euvolemic hyponatremia is most commonly secondary to SIADH. Hypervolemic hyponatremia occurs in conditions in which water is retained in greater proportion than sodium, such as congestive heart failure, cirrhosis, and renal failure. Hypernatremic dehydration results from a greater loss of water relative to sodium. Diarrhea in conjunction with persistent fever and decreased oral intake may produce hypernatremic dehydration. Other causes of hypernatremia include diabetes insipidus, excessive exogenous sodium (i.e., sodium bicarbonate, hypertonic saline, improperly diluted infant formula), and inability to regulate fluid intake.

Decreased intake through fasting and vomiting, increased losses through diarrhea, or an increase in insensible losses secondary to fever or respiratory distress can easily leave an infant deficient in total body water. For this reason, any infant who presents with fever, vomiting, diarrhea, or respiratory distress, regardless of etiology, must be assessed for potential dehydration.

EMERGENCY DEPARTMENT EVALUATION

History

An accurate history is important to evaluate the etiology and severity of dehydration. Multiple factors and disease states contribute to dehydration in pediatric patients, but the source of dehydration is simplified by focusing on factors that decrease fluid intake, increase fluid losses, or cause translocation of fluids (e.g., burns, ascites). Decreased fluid intake may be secondary to pharyngitis, stomatitis, vomiting, respiratory distress, or an inability to obtain fluids due to physical limitations (particularly in infants). Sources of increased fluid losses include gastrointestinal losses, insensible losses, and renal losses. Conditions that may increase insensible losses include fever, increased respiratory rate, and environmental conditions. These conditions have a more significant effect on infants and small children than adults. Fever in an infant can increase insensible water losses by approximately 0.42 ml/kg/degree Celsius for each degree above 37°C (6). Increased renal losses may result from hyperglycemia, diabetic ketoacidosis, congenital adrenal hyperplasia, proximal

TABLE 221.1.   Type of Dehydration Based on Serum Sodium Concentration

Dehydration Type	Serum Sodium Concentration
Hyponatremic	< 130 mEq/L
Isonatremic	130–145 mEq/L
Hypernatremic	> 145 mEq/L

renal tubular acidosis, diuretic use, and diabetes insipidus. Increased gastrointestinal losses in the form of diarrhea and vomiting are probably the most common source of dehydration in pediatric patients. Fulminant diarrhea can rapidly progress to cause dehydration, particularly when associated with vomiting, fever, and decreased intake. The potential for dehydration in this situation is inversely proportional to the child's age. Total body water and the percentage of daily fluid turnover are highest in infants less than 6 months old. In these infants, fulminant rotaviral gastroenteritis, shigellosis, or salmonellosis can cause dehydration in minutes to hours. Therefore, even if the infant does not appear clinically dehydrated at the time of examination, continued close observation is necessary to prevent progression.

Other pertinent historical items include recent body weight, and urinary output. The preillness body weight should be compared with the current weight if possible. This information, along with physical examination findings, allows an estimate of the percent dehydration. Frequency and amount of urine output should be clarified. The physician must obtain an accurate history of the volume and composition of oral intake; the frequency, consistency, and volume of diarrhea; the presence or absence of fever and vomiting; recent body weight; and frequency of urination.

Physical Evaluation

The diagnosis of dehydration is based on clinical criteria, not on laboratory values (8,12,16). The degree of dehydration is best determined by measurement of acute weight loss. Since an accurate preillness weight is not often known in the acute setting, clinical assessment is used to estimate fluid deficits. Signs and symptoms used for clinically assessing the degree of dehydration are listed in Table 221.2. The degree of dehydration is generally expressed as a percentage of the preillness body weight. Body fluid deficits of 3% to 5%, 6% to 9%, and ≥10% correspond to "mild," "moderate," and "severe" dehydration respectively for infants and small children (1). In teenagers and adults, mild, moderate, and severe dehydration correspond to approximately 3%, 5% to 6%, and 7% to 9% fluid deficit (14). The reliability of clinical parameters for evaluation of dehydration has been evaluated by Gorelick et al (8). In this study it was found that the median number of clinical findings in children with mild dehydration was 1, in those with moderate dehydration it was 5, and in severe dehydration the median number of clinical findings was 8 (8). Four specific findings were found to be independently associated with dehydration, including: general appearance, capillary refill >2 seconds, dry mucous membranes, and reduced tears (8).

In hypernatremic dehydration, redistribution of fluid out of the intracellular compartment into the extracellular compartment masks the signs of dehydration, even in the face of significant weight loss. The skin consistency is doughy. In hyponatremic dehydration, the intravascular volume is severely compromised as fluid translocates into the intracellular compartment to maintain osmotic equilibrium. Infants with hyponatremic dehydration may exhibit signs of shock in the face of minimal weight loss.

Before initiating fluid therapy, it is important to feel the liver to assess its size. Cardiogenic shock, although rare, may be misdiagnosed as hypovolemic shock. The patient must be reevaluated after every bolus, because it is easy to overshoot and cause congestive cardiac failure with only a few hundred milliliters of extra fluid.

The diagnosis of dehydration does not require the use of laboratory values; these are only confirmatory in nature. Treatment should never be delayed while awaiting the results of laboratory tests. If the degree of dehydration is estimated to be less than 5%, and there is an obvious etiology, measurement of electrolytes is not necessary. With moderate or severe dehydration, laboratory studies should be obtained to evaluate for electrolyte abnormalities and acidosis. Elevation of the urea nitrogen (BUN) may be present, but usually only occurs when the glomerular filtration rate is significantly reduced (14). The serum bicarbonate is usually decreased with dehydration (12,13,17). One study demonstrated that a serum bicarbonate concentration <17 mEq/L was 77% sensitive for predicting moderate dehydration, and 94% sensitive for predicting severe dehydration (17). A low serum bicarbonate (less than or equal to 13 mEq/L) appears to correlate with more severe dehydration and an inability to tolerate oral fluids (13,17). The hematocrit may be elevated due to hemoconcentration. The urine-specific gravity may be elevated, but can be altered by other medical conditions (e.g., SIADH, pyelonephritis). In addition, the concentrating ability of the kidneys is reduced in neonates and young infants, with renal blood flow and glomerular filtration not reaching adult values until approximately 1 year of age (2).

EMERGENCY DEPARTMENT MANAGEMENT

In severe dehydration and shock, the immediate goal is to rapidly expand the intravascular volume with intravenous fluids. In the presence of decompensated shock, if intravenous access is not rapidly obtainable, intraosseous access is a reasonable alternative (18). Once access is obtained, successive fluid boluses of 20 ml/kg of an isotonic solution (lactated Ringer or normal saline) are given until clinical improvement is noted. It is

TABLE 221.2. Clinical Assessment of Hydration Status and Percentage Dehydration

Extent of Dehydration	Mild (3%–5%)	Moderate (6%–9%)	Severe (≥10%)
Eyes	Normal	Sunken	Markedly sunken
Skin turgor	Normal	Decreased	Tenting
Heart rate	Normal	Slightly increased	Significantly increased
Blood pressure	Normal	Normal to orthostatic	Shock
Mental status	Normal	Normal to listless	Depressed/lethargic
Thirst	Slight increase	Moderate increase	Marked increase
Mucous membranes	Normal	Dry	Parched
Tears	Normal	Decreased	Absent
Anterior fontanelle	Normal	Sunken	Markedly sunken
Skin/Capillary refill	Normal	Delayed capillary refill	Cool/mottled/delayed refill
Urine output	Minimally decreased	Decreased	Anuric

reasonable to administer up to 60 cc/kg of isotonic solution in the initial fluid resuscitation phase. Subsequent boluses may be given as needed with reevaluation after each bolus. Close attention to cardiopulmonary status must be maintained to avoid iatrogenic pulmonary edema. This is particularly true for children with underlying pulmonary or cardiac conditions. If the child is not in shock but is clinically dehydrated, the 20-mL/kg fluid bolus may be given more slowly (i.e., over a period of 30 minutes to 1 hour). Blood should be drawn for laboratory studies, which should include electrolyte levels and a bedside serum glucose screening to rule out hypoglycemia.

Subsequent management consists of calculating the deficit of fluids and evaluating the acid-base and electrolyte disturbances, but this kind of management is not necessarily the responsibility of the emergency physician. In the consolidation phase, the total volume of fluid needed is determined by calculating deficit fluids, maintenance fluids, and ongoing losses.

To Calculate Fluid Deficits:

1. If the normal baseline weight of the patient is known, the fluid deficit (in liters) is easily calculated with the formula:

   Fluid deficit (liters) = normal wt (kg) − present wt (kg)

   Since the normal weight often is not known, the deficit is based on the estimated percent dehydration of the patient.
2. Determine the present weight. The normal weight can then be calculated using: Normal wt = present wt × (100/[100 − % dehydration])
3. Calculate the free water deficit. The fluid deficit in liters = normal wt (kg) − present wt (kg)
4. Calculate the sodium and potassium deficits. First determine whether the dehydration is hypotonic, isotonic, or hypertonic, based on the criteria in Table 221.1.
5. Calculate the rate of deficit replacement. For isotonic dehydration, half of the deficit is replaced in the first 8 hours, and the second half is replaced over the next 16 hours. This should be given in addition to (and in conjunction with) the maintenance fluids required for the 24-hour period.

To Calculate Maintenance Fluids:

1. Free water needs for a 24-hour period are 100 ml/kg/24 hrs for the first 10 kg of body weight; 50 ml/kg/24 hrs for the second 10 kg; and 20 ml/kg/24 hrs for every kg of body weight >20 kg. Alternatively, to calculate per hour, needs are 4 ml/kg/hr for the first 10 kg; 2 ml/kg/hr for the next 10 kg; and 1 ml/kg/hr for every kg >20 kg. For example, maintenance fluids for a 25 kg child will be (1,000 ml + 500 ml + 100 ml)/24 hrs = 65 ml/hr.
2. Sodium requirements are 2 to 3 mEq/kg/d.
3. Potassium requirements are 1 to 2 mEq/kg/d.

An alternate method is to replace the remaining deficit over the first 8 hours with $D_5 0.45 NS$ + 20 mEq/L of K^+ (14). Then, the 24 hours worth of maintenance fluid are given over the next 16 hours. Since 24 hours worth of maintenance fluid is given over 16 hours, the rate of fluid administration is 1.5 times the usual hourly maintenance rate (14).

To accommodate for ongoing losses, fluid losses from vomiting and diarrhea can be replaced milliliter for milliliter with normal saline every 4 to 6 hours, unless the losses are severe; if so, more frequent replacement may be required. Usually, however, once parenteral fluids are initiated, these losses diminish rapidly to an insignificant level and do not need to be taken into consideration.

Patients with hyponatremic dehydration may present with nausea, vomiting, seizures and coma. These symptoms typically resolve when the serum sodium is increased above 125 meq/L.

The amount of 3% saline needed for the correction can be calculated by subtracting the current serum sodium level from the desired level and then multiplying by 0.6 and the patient's weight in kilograms. Three percent saline contains 0.5 mEq NaCl/ml and therefore, the desired increase in mEq/L must be multiplied by a factor of 2 to obtain the milliliters of 3% NaCl needed. An alternative acceptable approach in patients with hyponatremic seizures is to administer 4-5cc/kg of 3% saline as a bolus over 10 minutes in order to terminate the seizure.

It is very important to note that hypertonic dehydration is not approached in the same manner. Rapid fluid administration in the setting of hypertonic dehydration can result in fluid shifts with catastrophic repercussions, including cerebral edema and intracranial bleeding. For hypertonic dehydration, fluids should be given over an extended period of time. The rate of decline in serum sodium should not exceed 10 mEq/L/24 hours. Rehydration is distributed over the number of days necessary to decrease the serum sodium to 150 mEq/L, by decreasing no more than 10 mEq/L/24 hours.

Oral Rehydration

Intravenous rehydration is not necessary in all cases of dehydration. Multiple sources support oral rehydration in children with mild and even moderate dehydration secondary to acute gastroenteritis (1,3,4,9,10). This is accomplished by giving small frequent amounts of an appropriate oral rehydration solution over 3 to 4 hours. The goal is to provide 50 ml/kg over 3 to 4 hours in mildly dehydrated children, and 100 ml/kg over 4 hours in moderately dehydrated children (1,3,9). Therapy is initiated with 5 ml (1 teaspoon) every 1 to 2 minutes (1). Frozen rehydration solutions are sometimes successful in patients that initially refuse oral fluids, or have difficulty tolerating oral fluids (15). Juices and sodas are not appropriate for oral rehydration therapy. Pedialyte is a maintenance fluid and is not adequate replacement therapy for losses secondary to vomiting and diarrhea. Rehydralyte and the WHO (World Health Organization) oral rehydration formulation are more appropriate replacement fluids (see Table 221.3). Clear liquids should not be continued for longer than 24 hours, and if losses continue, the patient should return for evaluation. Refusal of oral fluids or failure to tolerate oral fluids should prompt initiation of intravenous hydration. Children who do not improve with oral rehydration, or have any signs of severe dehydration, require intravenous rehydration.

DISPOSITION

In many centers, the clinical diagnosis of dehydration mandates intravenous therapy and, therefore, admission. This is the more classical and accepted management, but some centers advocate intravenous rehydration for selected infants in the ED over a period of 3 to 4 hours; the physician then determines the need for admission. Infants with severe dehydration by clinical criteria,

TABLE 221.3.   Contents of Commercial Oral Hydration Solutions

Solution	Na (mEq/L)	K (mEq/L)	Cl (mEq/L)	Base (mEq/L)	Carbohydrate (g/L)
Pedialyte	45	20	35	30	25
Infalyte	50	25	45	30	30
Rehydralyte	75	20	65	30	25
WHO solution	90	20	80	30	20

acidosis, ongoing losses, electrolyte abnormalities, intolerance to oral fluids, or social needs should be admitted.

CRITICAL INTERVENTIONS

- Obtain a bedside glucose measurement in patients with altered mental status or signs of dehydration
- Use isotonic solutions for bolus intravenous therapy. Never use glucose-containing or hypotonic fluids for bolus therapy
- Reevaluate the patient after every intravenous bolus of fluids is completed before giving another bolus
- Aggressively treat severely dehydrated patients with adequate volumes of intravenous isotonic fluids
- In the setting of hypernatremia, reduce the serum sodium concentration slowly

COMMON PITFALLS

✔ Failing to appreciate the acuity of the ongoing process
✔ Failing to recognize and treat shock secondary to dehydration. This includes failing to give boluses of 20 ml/kg until end-organ perfusion is improved, or the use of nonisotonic fluids to accomplish this task
✔ Failing to monitor ongoing therapy, which may result in over-hydration or underhydration
✔ Failing to address associated abnormalities of electrolyte and acid-base balance
✔ Failing to address the underlying cause of dehydration (e.g., pyloric stenosis, diabetic ketoacidosis, child abuse or neglect)
✔ Misdiagnosing cardiogenic shock as hypovolemic shock

Acknowledgment

The author would like to thank Naghma S. Khan for her work on the previous version of this chapter.

References

1. American Academy of Pediatrics, Provisional Committee on Quality Improvement, Subcommittee on Acute Gastroenteritis. Practice Parameter: The Management of Acute Gastroenteritis in Young Children. *Pediatrics* 1996;97:424–435.
2. Arant BS Jr. Developmental patterns of renal functional maturation compared in the human neonate. *J Pediatr* 1978;92:705.
3. Armon K, Stephenson T, MacFaul R, Eccleston P, Werneke U. An evidence and consensus based guideline for acute diarrhea management. *Arch Dis Child* 2001;8:132–142.
4. Atherly-John YC, Cunningham SJ, Crain EF. A Randomized Trial of Oral vs. Intravenous Rehydration in a Pediatric Emergency Department. *Arch Pediatr Adolesc Med* 2002;156:1240–1243.
5. Cicirello HG, Glass RI. Current concepts of the epidemiology of diarrheal diseases. *Semin Pediatr Infect Dis* 1994;5:162–167.
6. D'Angio Fann B. Fluid and Electrolyte Balance in the Pediatric Patient. *Journal of Intravenous Nursing* 1998;21:153–159.
7. De Bruin WJ, Greenwald BM, Notterman DA. Fluid Resuscitation in Pediatrics. *Critical Care Clinics* 1992;8:423–438.
8. Gorelick MH, Shaw KN, Murphy KO. Validity and reliability of clinical signs in the diagnosis of dehydration in children. *Pediatrics* 1997;99:E6.
9. Jospe N, Forbes G. Fluids and Electrolytes–Clinical Aspects. *Pediatrics in Review* 1996;17:395–403.
10. King CK, Glass R, Bresee JS, Duggan C. Centers for Disease Control and Prevention. Managing acute gastroenteritis among children: oral rehydration, maintenance, and nutritional therapy. *MMWR Recomm Rep* 2003;21:1–16.
11. Kooh SW, Metcoff J. Physiologic considerations in fluid and electrolyte therapy with particular reference to diarrheal dehydration in children. *J Pediatr* 1963;62:107.
12. Narchi H. Serum bicarbonate and dehydration severity in gastroenteritis. *Arch Dis Child* 1998;78:70–71.
13. Reid SR, Bonadio WA. Outpatient rapid intravenous rehydration to correct dehydration and resolve vomiting in children with acute gastroenteritis. *Ann Emerg Med* 1996;28:318–323.
14. Roberts KB. Fluid and Electrolytes: Parenteral Fluid Therapy. *Pediatrics in Review* 2001;22:380–387.
15. Santucci KA, Anderson AC, Lewander WJ, Linakis JG. Frozen oral hydration as an alternative to conventional enteral fluids. *Arch Pediatr Adolesc Med* 1998;152:142–146.
16. Teach SJ, Yates EW, Feld LG. Laboratory predictors of fluid deficit in acutely dehydrated children. *Clin Pediatr* 1997;36:395–400.
17. Vega RM, Avner JR. A prospective study of the usefulness of clinical and laboratory parameters for predicting percentage of dehydration in children. *Pediatr Emerg Care* 1997;13:179–182.
18. Zaritsky AL, Nadkarni VM, Hickey RW, Schexnayder SM, Berg RA, eds. American Heart Association: PALS Provider Manual, 2002:155.

CHAPTER 222
Diarrhea

James E. Colletti

Diarrheal illness continues to be a significant cause of pediatric morbidity and mortality. In the United States, approximately 220,000 children less than 5 years of age are hospitalized annually for acute gastroenteritis, which accounts for more than 925,000 inpatient hospital days and an annual 3.7 million acute care visits (2). Dehydration secondary to diarrhea is responsible for 300 to 500 pediatric deaths per year. The incidence of diarrhea in children less than 3 years of age is estimated to be 1.3 to 2.5 episodes per child per year, with higher rates in children enrolled in daycare (11).

The pathophysiologic insult most often leading to diarrhea is infectious. Enteroinvasive pathogens cause osmotic diarrhea by invading and destroying enterocytes of the villous tip, resulting in failure of water and electrolyte absorption and damage to the brush border disaccharidase enzymes. Unabsorbed carbohydrates are fermented to organic acids, which impart an acid reaction to the stool (pH less than 5.5), and undigested carbohydrates may appear as reducing substances. In addition, the organic acids increase the osmotic load and result in increased water loss into the stool. Invasion of the mucosa by bacterial pathogens may produce a leukocytic reaction in the stool, demonstrable by staining with methylene blue. In contrast, enterotoxigenic pathogens generally result in secretory diarrhea, in which enterotoxins affect cAMP and cGMP pumps. Secretion of chloride and sodium followed by water and potassium, results in large-volume diarrhea, usually without acid reaction or reducing substances.

CLINICAL PRESENTATION

The most common presenting etiology of children with diarrhea is infectious gastroenteritis, with viral agents accounting for 75% of cases. Acute diarrhea typically lasts less than 2 weeks, and the history is one of a distinct change in stool frequency, volume, and color. The stools may be less well formed and yellowish, loose and green, or watery and voluminous. The presence of bloody, mucoid stools increases the possibility of a bacterial cause. Vomiting is common, especially with viral disorders. However, bilious vomiting requires close attention and raises the possibility of intestinal obstruction. Intussusception may complicate an otherwise mild gastroenteritis. Low-grade fever is common, but fever in excess of 40°C suggests a bacterial etiology.

TABLE 222.1.   Signs and Symptoms of Dehydration

Clinical Findings	Mild (≤ 5%)	Moderate (6–9)	Severe (≥ 10)
Mental status	Alert	Irritable	Lethargic
Tears	Present	Decreased	Absent
Mucous membranes	Moist	Dry	Very dry
Urine output	Normal	Oliguric	Anuric
Systolic blood pressure	Normal	Normal	Decreased
Heart rate	Normal	Normal-rapid	Rapid
Fontanelle	Normal	Flat	Sunken
Eyes	Normal	Sunken	Glassy
Capillary refill	< 2 s	2–3 s	> 3 s

Important history to obtain from the caretaker includes antibiotic use, recent travel, or other exposures, such as daycare, pets, or unsanitary water supply. The patient's prior weight, duration of illness, and associated signs and symptoms, such as fever, abdominal pain, vomiting, rash, seizures, and activity level can aid in determining the degree and severity of dehydration. A vital component of the history is the type of oral intake given to the child. The use of hyperosmolar fluids, such as carbonated soft drinks, apple juice, or excess sodium due to improper formula preparation, can result in hypernatremia, while hypotonic fluid replacement can result in hyponatremia.

Of foremost clinical importance on presentation is the presence of signs of dehydration. Infants may become critically dehydrated over a period of only a few hours and may present with sepsis. The signs and symptoms of progressive dehydration are listed in Table 222.1. As the vascular space contracts, the extremities become cool with decreased distal pulses, and alterations in mental status occur. Gorelick et al (9) discovered that the findings of 3 or fewer of the clinical signs of dehydration correlated with a 5% fluid deficit, three to five signs correlated with 5% to 9% dehydration, and more than 6 signs, with a fluid deficit of 10% or greater.

A recent review found parental report to accurately predict degree of dehydration as well as clinically significant acidosis (18). A parental report of a normal tearing state was associated with a reduced likelihood of significant dehydration and acidosis. However, parental reporting of a sunken fontanelle and decreased tears were associated with an increased likelihood of hospital admission (18).

Rotavirus is the most important cause of severe diarrhea in childhood in both developed and developing countries (27). Rotaviral gastroenteritis accounts for 30% to 60% of acute diarrheal disease, with a peak incidence in children between the ages of 4 and 23 months (17). However, up to 25% of severe cases occur in patients over 2 years of age. Rotavirus is responsible for at least 50% of the hospitalizations for gastroenteritis during the peak season of October to May (6). Transmission occurs by the fecal-oral route and by person-to-person distribution. The illness presents with fever and vomiting prior to the onset of diarrhea; bloody stools are uncommon. The patient may have concomitant respiratory disease. A recent investigation by Staat et al, found that rotavirus detection was highest when the constellation of diarrhea, vomiting, and fever occurred simultaneously (27).

Norwalk virus is responsible for up to 40% of diarrheal illness in older children. Transmission is via airborne droplets, person-to-person contact, contaminated food, and contaminated water. The incubation period is 12 to 48 hours, with symptoms consisting of nonbloody diarrhea, vomiting, fever, headache, myalgias, and abdominal cramping. Other viruses associated with enteritis include adenovirus, astrovirus, calicivirus and torovirus (25).

Campylobacter species are the leading cause of bacterial diarrhea in the United States. The organism's reservoirs are newborn puppies, chicken, and turkey, with person-to-person transmittal. The incubation period is 2 to 5 days, with symptoms consisting of fever, abdominal pain, bloody stools, vomiting, myalgias, and headache.

The *Salmonella enteritidis* are transmitted by the fecal-oral route, and have an incubation period ranging from 6 to 72 hours. The minimum infective dose is 10 million organisms. The highest attack rate involves those less than 1 year of age. Complications such as pneumonia, bacteremia, septic arthritis, osteomyelitis, meningitis, endocarditis, and urinary tract infections may be seen. *Salmonella typhi* presents with fever, headache, myalgias, organomegaly, and rose spots. Infection with this agent causes a prolonged gastroenteritis.

Shigella species are extremely virulent in that the minimum infective dose is only 100 organisms, with an incubation period of 1 to 5 days. Typical presenting symptoms include fever, malaise, febrile seizures, and tenesmus, with possible resultant rectal prolapse.

Yersinia presents with fever, vomiting, headache, and pharyngitis and may mimic appendicitis, with severe right lower quadrant pain. Erythema multiforme and a reactive arthritis may also be present.

Diarrhea associated with *Escherichia coli* 0157:H7 may result in hemolytic-uremic syndrome (4). The organism has a bovine reservoir and is transmitted by undercooked meat, contaminated water, unpasteurized milk, or person-to-person contact. The illness usually begins as nonbloody diarrhea and may progress to grossly bloody stools. Severe abdominal pain is common, at times mimicking an acute surgical condition. In the case of hemolytic uremic syndrome, after the gastroenteritic phase of the disease seems to have resolved, the patient may develop irritability, pallor, and oliguria. Laboratory examination then reveals anemia with schistocytes and helmet cells, thrombocytopenia, and azotemia. Peritoneal or renal dialysis may be required for acute renal failure.

Profuse sudden-onset diarrhea, especially when associated with vomiting and abdominal cramps but no fever, raises the possibility of bacterial toxin food contamination, such as that caused by *Staphylococcus aureus* or *Clostridium perfringens*. Such illnesses tend to be explosive in onset but brief in duration. Acute-onset diarrhea associated with cranial nerve weaknesses suggests botulism.

Noninfectious diarrhea is less likely to be accompanied by fever or lead to dehydration. Food intolerance, such as to sorbitol in candy and gum, hyperosmolar juices (pineapple), or even simply overfeeding may precipitate a brief bout of diarrhea. Allergic diarrhea such as with infant formulas presents, sometimes explosively, soon after exposure to the offending food and may be part of a larger picture of anaphylaxis. Breast milk colitis, caused by sensitivity to maternally ingested proteins, occurs in breast-fed infants and presents as bloody diarrhea with negative microbial studies in an otherwise thriving infant.

A key observation in the child with chronic diarrhea is the presence of failure to thrive, as determined by anthropometric measurements. Such children often lose calories in the stool by malabsorption and do not grow normally. Usually, the malabsorption is accompanied by bulky, malodorous stools that may be oily on close inspection. Disorders with such a presentation include chronic giardiasis, cystic fibrosis, pancreatic diseases, celiac disease, and immunodeficiency disorders, including acquired immunodeficiency syndrome.

The presence of chronic diarrhea without failure to thrive suggests irritable bowel syndrome. These children tend to have frequent, large, occasionally explosive stools early in the day but otherwise appear well. Questioning often reveals a history

TABLE 222.2. Common Causes of Acute Diarrheal Illness

BACTERIAL	PARASITIC
Campylobacter	*Giardia lamblia*
Salmonella	*Cryptosporidium*
Shigella	*Entamoeba histolytica*
Yersinia	
Escherichia coli	**OTHER**
Clostridium perfringens	
Clostridium botulinum	Medication-induced
Clostridium difficile	Parenteral: otitis media, upper respiratory
Cholera	infection, urinary tract infection
Staphylococcus aureus	Food intolerance
Aeromonas	Psychogenic: anxiety
	Necrotizing enterocolitis
VIRAL	Cystic fibrosis
	Adrenal insufficiency
Rotavirus	Organophosphates
Norwalk virus	Heavy metals (iron)
Adenovirus	Hirschsprung disease
Calicivirus	Intussusception
Astrovirus	
Torovirus	

of colic as an infant and a family history of irritable bowel syndrome.

Acquired disaccharide intolerance is common and presents with flatulence, bloating, cramps, and watery diarrhea. The history often reveals a preceding bowel insult, most commonly infectious. Disaccharide intolerance may also complicate cystic fibrosis, celiac disease, or postoperative states.

In children, especially infants, diarrhea may accompany almost any acute or chronic illness, especially if antibiotics are given. Although fulminant pseudomembranous enterocolitis is uncommon, milder antibiotic-associated diarrhea is often seen. The most frequent drugs that can result in pseudomembranous colitis are clindamycin, third-generation cephalosporins, and anticancer drugs.

DIFFERENTIAL DIAGNOSIS

The differential diagnosis of diarrheal illness is broad. Diarrhea may accompany almost any pediatric illness at any given point in its course. The differential diagnosis may be categorized as acute or chronic. There may be important diagnostic clues based on the child's age, character of the stool, associated symptoms, and effect on the child's general health.

The most common causes of acute diarrheal disease are listed in Table 222.2. Some causes of chronic diarrhea are listed in Table 222.3 (29). The presence or absence of blood, leukocytes, reducing substances, an acid reaction, or fat in the stool can be helpful in the differential diagnosis. Blood and white cells suggest bacterial gastroenteritis or inflammatory bowel disease. Reducing substances and an acid pH suggest disaccharide intolerance. Fat on Sudan stain suggests malabsorption, most commonly cystic fibrosis, celiac disease, or chronic giardiasis.

EMERGENCY DEPARTMENT EVALUATION AND MANAGEMENT

The goals of diarrhea management include prevention of dehydration by early fluid administration, treatment of dehydration with an oral rehydration solution (ORS), continued feeding during the diarrhea, selective use of antibiotics and avoidance of antidiarrheal medications (8,20).

A thorough history should determine acute or chronic status. Preliminary studies that may be indicated for chronic diarrhea include a stool examination for blood, parasites, culture, Sudan fat stain, and alpha-1-antitrypsin. If there is significant failure to thrive or dehydration, the child should be hospitalized. Otherwise, the patient should be referred to a pediatrician for further evaluation.

If the diarrhea is acute, the primary concern is the existence of dehydration, acidosis, electrolyte disturbances, shock, or, associated sepsis. The physical examination determines dehydration according to the signs previously described. If dehydration is not present, laboratory studies may be unnecessary. However, the presence of significant dehydration calls for the measurement of electrolytes, blood urea nitrogen, and glucose (12). In particular, a serum bicarbonate level may prove useful in the evaluation of dehydration as well as a need for prolonged intravenous (IV) therapy. A serum bicarbonate concentration of less than 17 mEq/L when utilized along with clinical parameters increases the sensitivity of detecting moderate to severe dehydration (30,32). Furthermore, a bicarbonate value of 13 mEq/L or less is associated with a need for prolonged IV fluid replacement (18,21).

TABLE 222.3. Causes of Chronic Diarrhea

Postinfectious disaccharide intolerance
Irritable bowel syndrome
Milk or soy protein intolerance
Food allergy
Urinary tract infection
Giardiasis
Maternal deprivation syndrome
Cystic fibrosis
Celiac disease
Immunodeficiency disorders
Short bowel syndrome (postoperative)
Inflammatory bowel disease
Tumors (neuroblastoma, carcinoid)
Stagnant loop syndrome
Acrodermatitis enteropathica
Adrenal insufficiency or hyperthyroidism
Chronic constipation with overflow diarrhea

TABLE 222.4. Contents of Commercial Oral Rehydration Solutions

Solution	Na (mEq/L)	K (mEq/L)	Other (mEq/L)	Cl (mEq/L)	Base (mEq/L)	Carbohydrate (g/L)
Pedialyte	45	20		35	30	25
Rehydralyte	75	20		65	30	25
Infalyte	50	25		45	34	30
Resol	50	20	8	50	34	20
WHO solution	90	20		80	30	20

Other than a guaiac test or culture, stool studies such as fecal leukocytes, Rotazyme, pH, reducing substances, and ova and parasites are usually not helpful in the emergency setting. A complete blood count may aid in diagnosis, as patients with *Shigella* typically have a white blood cell count less than 10,000 with a marked left shift. If the ratio of bands to total polymorphonuclear leukocytes (PMNs) is greater than 0.10, a bacterial etiology such as *Shigella, Salmonella,* or *Campylobacter* should be suspected.

Dehydration exceeding 5% to 10% or significant electrolyte disturbances are considerations for admission, with rehydration beginning in the emergency department. In children who are mildly to moderately dehydrated and refusing oral intake, a nasogastric tube can be placed to initiate replacement therapy. An option for the moderately dehydrated child is rapid nasogastric hydration or rapid intravenous hydration. A recent investigation examining rapid nasogastric hydration and rapid intravenous hydration found them to be safe, efficacious and cost-effective alternatives to standard therapy for moderately dehydrated children (16). When rapid nasogastric hydration was compared to rapid intravenous hydration, no significant difference was discovered. In this trial, rapid nasogastric hydration was achieved by administering a continuous infusion of 50 mL/kg of Pedialyte over 3 hours and rapid intravenous hydration was performed by a continuous infusion of 50 mL/kg of normal saline over 3 hours (16).

In severely dehydrated children, intravenous fluids should be initiated. Normal saline boluses of 20 cc/kg should be initiated, with repeat boluses, as needed, to restore intravascular volume. It is common to administer 60 to 80 cc/kg in the initial phase of fluid resuscitation. To avoid iatrogenic pulmonary edema, close monitoring of the pulmonary status is important in children with underlying cardiac or pulmonary conditions,. Once intravascular volume has been restored, dextrose-containing maintenance fluid should be initiated, avoiding potassium replacement until the patient is spontaneously voiding and is known to have normal renal function.

In mild dehydration and in selected cases of moderate dehydration, outpatient oral rehydration therapy (ORT) should begin with a commercially available ORS (13,14). ORT is an inexpensive, effective therapy for dehydration that is currently underutilized in the United States (7). When compared to IV therapy in mildly to moderately dehydrated children, ORT was as effective as IV therapy. Furthermore ORT was found to be associated with higher parental satisfaction as well as decreases in both length of stay and staff time (2,7,20).

Homemade solutions and electrolyte-glucose beverages for athletes should be avoided; in the former, serious errors may be made in preparation, and the latter contain too little sodium, too much sugar, and almost no potassium. Moreover, the use of carbonated beverages, apple juice, and jello water should be discouraged as they consist of high concentrations of carbohydrates and low concentrations of required electrolytes. The high osmotic load of these fluids results in an increase in stool output and their low sodium content may contribute to hyponatremia (5,24). Each liter of a commercial ORS contains about 45 to 75 mEq sodium, 20 to 25 mEq potassium, 2% glucose, and a mixture of chloride and base as anions (Table 222.4). This ratio of electrolytes and glucose promotes the coupled mucosal transport of sodium and glucose, with water absorption following.

If oral rehydration is chosen, it is best started during an extended period of monitored therapy in the ED, and it may be implemented in any child who can drink and is not in shock. Even in the child presenting with emesis accompanying diarrhea the efficacy of ORT has been established. In these children, ORT should be administered in small frequent quantities (5 ml q 1–2 minutes) (5,24). A safe program for infants with less than 5% dehydration is listed in Table 222.5. After successful oral rehydration, a prompt return to age-appropriate diet is indicated. It should be stressed to parents that the objective is to "feed through" the diarrhea, and that loose stools will persist for a few days but should decrease in volume and frequency (28). Continued feeding is safe and may reduce the duration and volume of diarrhea (24). In general, smaller but more frequent feedings should be given so that the total daily intake approaches normal (8).

Subsequent diet depends on the child's dietary status before the illness. If formula was the primary nutrition, a return to half-strength formula for 12 to 24 hours, followed by full-strength formula, is advised. If there is impressive return of diarrhea following refeeding of a standard cow's milk-based formula (Enfamil or Similac), a lactose-free formula (Lactofree, ProSobee, or Isomil) may be tried, again gradually advancing through half- to full-strength formulas. Continued diarrhea on these

TABLE 222.5. Emergency Department Management of Acute Diarrhea with Mild Dehydration

- Estimate daily fluid requirements and degree of dehydration.
- Maintenance: 100 mL/kg for first 10 kg body weight, 50 mL/kg for each additional kg over 11–20 kg, and 20 mL/kg for each kg over 20 kg.
- Deficit requirement for 5% dehydration is 50 mL/kg.
- While patient is being monitored in the ED, give 50 mL/kg ORS over 4 h. ORS is best tolerated as small, frequent volumes rather than larger boluses. If vomiting occurs, give the solution 1–2 teaspoons every 5–10 min.
- Replace ongoing losses with 10 mL/kg ORS for each diarrheal stool.
- If stable and retaining fluids, the child may be discharged after deficit fluid is replaced, with phone contact 4–6 h later.
- The remainder of calculated fluids (deficit plus maintenance) should be given at home as maintenance ORS, such as Pedialyte, Infalyte, or Resol. Any fluid intake desired by the child beyond calculated should be provided as water or dilute juice.
- Infants should be offered breast milk or half-strength formula in increasing amounts. Older infants and children should be offered rice cereal, rice, potatoes, toast, bananas, and noodles, and rapidly advanced to full caloric intake.

TABLE 222.6. Indications for Admission
Dehydration greater than 5%
Significant electrolyte disturbances
Suspected sepsis
Intractable vomiting
Bilious vomiting
Complicated chronic diarrhea with failure to thrive
Poor social situation
Parental noncompliance or inability to follow prescribed therapy
Suspected deprivation or neglect
Neonate with dehydration

preparations may require an elemental formula such as Alimentum or Pregestimil. For older children on a mixed diet, a bland diet of rice or rice cereal, bananas, potatoes, noodles, crackers, and toast should be offered in increasing quantities and then advanced to a balanced intake over 24 to 48 hours. Although lactose in milk may cause an osmotic diarrhea, fermented milk products such as yogurt are generally well tolerated. The breastfed infant with diarrhea generally has a milder illness for which evaluation and reassurance alone may suffice. If significant dehydration exists, oral rehydration should proceed using the previously mentioned guidelines with no or minimal interruption of breast-feeding. Indications for hospital admission are listed in Table 222.6.

Most episodes of diarrhea do not require antimicrobial therapy. Bloody diarrhea with PMNs probably represents a bacterial cause, and antibiotic therapy may be considered if *Escherichia Coli O157:H7* and *Salmonella* have been excluded. The association of antibiotic therapy in children with Escherichia coli 0157:H7 and the development of hemolytic uremic syndrome (HUS) is controversial. It is currently unknown whether empiric antibiotic therapy increases the risk of HUS (15). A few investigations have determined an increased risk of HUS with empiric antibiotic therapy (26,31). In contrast others have reported a protective effect or lack of association (10,19,23). Therefore, the physician contemplating empiric antibiotic therapy for bloody diarrhea should give careful consideration to the possibility of *E. Coli O157:H7* infection and the potential for increased HUS risk with empiric antibiotics. Antibiotics should be avoided in *Salmonella* gastroenteritis, because they prolong the carrier state. Exceptions include certain populations prone to *Salmonella* bacteremia, such as infants less than 3 months old and patients with immunodeficiency or hemoglobinopathies (1). These high-risk patients should be admitted and given intravenous antibiotics.

In cases where *Escherichia Coli* 0157:H7 and Salmonella have been excluded, antibiotic selection should be made and adjusted based on stool culture and sensitivity results. For *Shigella*, the episode may be treated with trimethoprim-sulfamethoxazole (TMP/SMX) (TMP 8 mg/kg/d divided b.i.d.) or erythromycin (40 mg/kg/d q.i.d.) for 5 to 7 days. *Campylobacter* enteritis has been shown to be resistant to TMP/SMX, and should be treated with erythromycin for 5 to 7 days. If *Giardia is* demonstrated by stool testing, furazolidone (6 mg/kg/d divided q.i.d. for 7 days) or metronidazole (15 mg/kg/d divided t.i.d. for 7 days) is indicated. If C. *difficile* cytotoxin is found in the stool, oral vancomycin (50 mg/kg/d divided q.i.d. for 7 days) or metronidazole is usually effective.

The American Academy of Pediatrics does not recommend the use of antiemetic, antisecretory, or antiperistaltic drugs (20). The use of narcotic-based agents are specifically contraindicated in bacterial gastroenteritis, because they may induce bowel stasis and promote more aggressive bacterial invasion.

Parents should be instructed on hygienic precautions for diaper handling and good hand-washing practices. Strict hand-washing techniques have been demonstrated to reduce the incidence of acute infectious diarrhea in daycare facilities (3,22). The child should be excluded from the daycare center if there is diarrhea not contained by diaper or toilet use, if stools contain mucus or blood, or if there is associated fever.

CRITICAL INTERVENTIONS

- Recognition and correction of dehydration, acidosis, electrolyte disturbances, hypoglycemia, shock, or associated sepsis
- Prompt return to an age-appropriate diet once rehydration is achieved
- Selective utilization of antibiotics
- Avoidance of antisecretory or antiperistaltic medications
- Instruct parents on hygienic precautions

DISPOSITION

If more than 5% dehydration is present, a pediatrician should be consulted for probable admission, with rehydration efforts beginning in the ED. With chronic diarrhea, consultation with a pediatrician or pediatric gastroenterologist is in order. Diarrhea may paradoxically complicate surgical conditions (e.g., Hirschsprung disease), in which case, a pediatric surgeon should be consulted.

Indications for hospitalization are listed in Table 222.6. Sepsis and serious illness in infants less than 1 month old may be clinically subtle or occult. Even mild dehydration in young infants deserves careful consideration for admission.

Simple diarrhea with dehydration requires only judicious oral or intravenous rehydration and rarely requires transfer unless there are no inpatient pediatric services. Complicated cases of dehydration (e.g., hypernatremic) or those of chronic duration usually require specific pediatric expertise.

COMMON PITFALLS

- ✔ The young infant with diarrhea may initially appear well but develop serious dehydration over a short period
- ✔ Because of renal immaturity, infants less than 3 months of age may continue to produce urine even when dehydrated
- ✔ Not relying on the caregiver's history of decreased or absent urine output, lethargy, or inability to tolerate fluids may lead to inappropriate management and disposition
- ✔ Underestimating the degree of hypovolemia and missing the subtle signs of shock
- ✔ Antidiarrheal agents should be avoided. The narcotic-based antidiarrheals may cause apnea in infants or predispose to systemic invasion of certain bacterial pathogens

Acknowledgments

The authors gratefully acknowledge the contributions of Lowell Clark and Ghazala Sharieff, who wrote the previous versions of this chapter.

References

1. American Academy of Pediatrics: Salmonella infections. *In:* Pickering LK (ed). 2003 Red Book: Report of the Committee on Infectious Diseases, 26th edition. Elk Grove Village: American Academy of Pediatrics, 2003:541–547.
2. Atherly-John YC, Cunningham SJ, Crain EF. A randomized trial of oral vs intravenous rehydration in a pediatric emergency department. *Arch Pediatr Adolesc Med* 2002;156:1240–1243.
3. Black RE, Dykes AC, Anderson KE, et al. Handwashing to prevent diarrhea in day-care centers. *Am J Epidemiol* 1981;113:445–451.

4. Bolton FJ, Aird H. Verocytotoxin producing *Escherichia Coli* 0157: public health and microbiological significance. *Br J Biomed Sci* 1998;55:127–135.
5. Burkhart DM. Management of acute gastroenteritis in children. *Am Fam Physician* 1999;60:2555–2566.
6. Committee on Infectious Diseases, American Academy of Pediatrics. Prevention of rotavirus disease: guidelines for use of rotavirus vaccine. *Pediatrics* 1998;1484–1489.
7. Conners GP, Barker WH, Mushlin AI, Goepp JGK. Oral versus intravenous: rehydration preferences of pediatric emergency medicine fellowship directors. *Pediatr Emerg Care* 2000;16:335–338.
8. Gastanaduy AS, Begue RE. Acute gastroenteritis. *Clin Pediatr* 1999;38:1–12.
9. Gorelick MH, Shaw KN, Murphy K. Validity and reliability of clinical significance in the diagnosis of dehydration in children. *Pediatrics* 1997;99:5.
10. Ikeda K, Ida O, Kimoto K, et al. Effect of early fosfomycin treatment on prevention of hemolytic uremic syndrome accompanying *Escherichia coli* O157:H7 infection. *Clin Nephrol* 1999;52:357–362.
11. Kilgore PR, Holman RC, Clark MJ, et al. Trends of diarrheal disease associated mortality in US Children, 1968–1991. *JAMA* 1995;27:1143–1148.
12. Liebelt EL. Clinical and laboratory evaluation and management of children with vomiting, diarrhea, and dehydration. *Curr Opin Pediatr* 1998;10:461–469.
13. Lifschitz CH. Treatment of acute diarrhea in children. *Curr Opin Pediatr* 1997;9:498–501.
14. Merrick N, Davidson B, Fox S. treatment of acute gastroenteritis: too much and too little care. *Clin Pediatr* 1996;35:429–435.
15. Molbak K, Mead PS, Griffin PM. Risk of hemolytic uremic syndrome after antibiotic treatment of *Escherichia coli* O157:H7 enteritis: a meta-analysis. [Abstract]. *J of Pediatri* 2003;142:353–354.
16. Nager AL, Wang VJ. Comparison of nasogastric and intravenous methods of rehydration in pediatric patients with acute dehydration. *Pediatrics* 2002;109:566–572.
17. Parashar UD, Holman RC, Bresee JS, et al. Epidemiology of diarrheal disease among children enrolled in four West Coast health maintenance organizations. Vaccine Safety Datalink Team. *Pediatr Infect Dis J* 1998;17:605–611.
18. Porter SC, Fleisher GR, Kohane IS, Mandl KD. The value of parental report for diagnosis and management of dehydration in the emergency department. *Ann Emerg Med* 2003;41:196–205.
19. Proulx F, Turgeon JP, Delage G, Lafleur L, Chicoine L. Randomized, controlled trial of antibiotic therapy for *Escherichia coli* O157:H7 enteritis. *J Pediatr* 1992;121:299–303.
20. Provisional Committee on Quality Improvement, Subcommittee on Acute Gastroenteritis, American Academy of Pediatrics Practice parameter. The management of acute gastroenteritis in young children. *Pediatrics* 1996;97:424.
21. Reid SR, Bonadio WA. Outpatient rapid intravenous rehydration to correct dehydration and resolve vomiting in children with acute gastroenteritis. *Ann Emerg Med* 1996;28:318–323.
22. Roberts L, Jorm L, Patel M, et al. Effect of infection control measures on the frequency of diarrheal episodes in child care: a randomized, controlled trial. *Pediatrics* 2000;105:743.
23. Safdar N, Said A, Gangnon RE, Maki DG. Risk of hemolytic uremic syndrome after antibiotic treatment of *Escherichia coli* O157:H7 enteritis. A Meta-analysis. *JAMA* 2002;288:996–1001.
24. Santosham M. Oral rehydration therapy: reverse transfer of technology. *Arch Pediatr Adolesc Med* 2002;156:1177–1179.
25. Sherman PM, Petric M, Cohen M. Infectious gastroenterocolitides in children. An update on emerging pathogens. *Pediatr Clin North Am* 1996;43:391–405.
26. Slutsker L, Ries AA, Maloney K, et al. A nationwide case-control study of *Escherichia coli* O157:H7 infection in the united states. *J Infect Dis* 1998;177:962–966.
27. Staat MA, Azimi PH, Berke T, et al. Clinical presentations of rotavirus infection among hospitalized children. *Pediatr Infect Dis J* 2002;21:221–227.
28. Sullivan PB. Nutritional management of acute diarrhea. *Nutrition* 1998;14:758–762.
29. Vanderhoof JA. Chronic diarrhea. *Pediatr Rev* 1998;19:418–422.
30. Vega RM, Avner JR. A prospective study of the usefulness of clinical and laboratory parameters for predicting percentage of dehydration in children. *Pediatr Emerg Care* 1997;13:179–182.
31. Wong CS, Jelacic S, Habeeb RL, Watkins SL, Tarr PI. The risk of the hemolytic-uremic syndrome after antibiotic treatment of *Escherichia coli* O157:H7 infections. *N Engl J Med* 2000;342:1930–1936.
32. Yilmaz K, Karabocuoglu M, Citak A, Uzel N. Evaluation of laboratory tests in dehydrated children with acute gastroenteritis. *J Paediatr Child Health* 2002;38:226–228.

CHAPTER 223
Failure to Thrive

Robert E. Sapien

Failure to thrive is a constellation of symptoms and is not in itself a diagnosis (16). The concept of failure to thrive is commonly used in the pediatric literature but lacks a clear definition (12). Failure to thrive is frequently defined as a failure to gain weight (weight less than the third percentile for age, or weight for height below the fifth percentile); however, the definition should be more global and should include any decrease of growth velocity leading to a decline of 2 major percentiles, using the National Center for Health Statistics growth charts. The term failure to thrive is used less and less by some experts; terms such as undernutrition or malnutrition are preferred (4). Measurements of weight, height, and head circumference are necessary to define and classify growth failure. Failure to thrive has been reported as the seventh most common reason for hospitalization in Children's Hospitals (11). It is common in inner-city emergency departments (EDs), with rates from 15% to 30% reported (5).

DIAGNOSIS

Except for familial short stature and constitutional growth delay, the etiology of failure to thrive is malnutrition. Failure to thrive can be arbitrarily classified into three groups (Table 223.1). The most common form is secondary to caloric insufficiency. This can be due to inadequate caloric intake, caloric wasting, increase caloric needs, or abnormal regulation. Decreased caloric intake most commonly is caused by psychosocial impairment in the child's environment such as poverty, behavioral feeding difficulties, neglect, or child abuse. The child presents with a markedly decreased weight compared with height and head circumference. Social history and environmental circumstances are important keys in this assessment. Less commonly, caloric intake can be impaired by diseases causing regurgitation (e.g., severe gastroesophageal reflux, pyloric stenosis, rumination syndrome),

TABLE 223.1.   Classification of Failure to Thrive

GROUP I

Most common type. Normal head circumference; weight reduced out of proportion to height. In most cases of failure to thrive, malnutrition is present as a result of either deficient caloric intake or malabsorption.

GROUP II

Normal or enlarged head circumference for age; weight only moderately reduced, usually in proportion to height; structural dystrophies, constitutional dwarfism, endocrinopathies.

GROUP III

Subnormal head circumference; weight reduced in proportion to height; primary CNS deficit; intrauterine growth retardation.

(From Kempe CH, Silver HK, O'Brien D, eds. Current pediatric diagnosis and treatment, 6th ed. Los Altos, CA: Lange, 1980:624.)

mechanical problems (e.g., sucking/swallowing abnormalities, neurologic disease, perinatal asphyxia), or malabsorption (e.g., cystic fibrosis, lactase deficiency, renal tubular acidosis). A history of chronic disease may explain the malnutrition.

The second group of children presents with weight and height equally affected. The head circumference is normal or enlarged. Most of these patients have a metabolic disorder (e.g., hypothyroidism, growth hormone deficiency, galactosemia, renal tubular acidosis).

The third group consists of children whose weight, height, and head circumference are all reduced. This category includes patients with genetic disorders (e.g., Turner syndrome, structural dystrophies) or congenital problems (e.g., fetal alcohol syndrome, small for gestational age).

Often a child does not clearly fit into any one particular group, making the differential diagnosis of growth deficiency difficult. Even after hospitalization and a thorough evaluation, 24% of patients will not have a definite etiology for their failure to thrive (10). Similarly, another study reports that of children hospitalized with failure to thrive, 32% have a psychosocial etiology (social or environmental), 20% have either gastroesophageal reflux or chronic diarrhea, and 15% have some "other" etiology. In 33% of the children, however, the etiology is undetermined (1).

The major challenge for the emergency physician is to recognize growth deficiency. This is more difficult to do when caretakers use the ED as their primary care center. When a child is brought to the ED with an acute illness, it is common for both parents and physicians to fail to recognize the insidious and potentially more serious problem of growth failure. Weight measurement should be part of the initial evaluation of any child seen in the ED, and it should be routinely charted on a growth chart. When the diagnosis of failure to thrive is suspected, a thorough history, physical examination, and growth pattern evaluation must be done.

EMERGENCY DEPARTMENT MANAGEMENT

The emergency physician's responsibility is to recognize the condition, not to determine its cause. Environmental factors are the leading cause of failure to thrive, principally maternal deprivation. If child abuse or neglect is suspected, proper referral to child protective services should be made. Laboratory tests are of limited value in most cases of failure to thrive, but they can help diagnose serious conditions that require immediate attention. Tests commonly performed in the ED are a complete blood count with differential, a urinalysis with culture, and routine chemistries. More specific tests should be individualized, such as thyroid function tests and human immunodeficiency virus.

CRITICAL INTERVENTIONS

- Recognition of malnutrition
- Recognition of possible abuse or neglect
- Limited laboratory tests
- Indications for admission include:
  - Abuse/neglect
  - Medical instability
  - Severe undernourishment
  - Laboratory abnormalities leading to medical instability

DISPOSITION

Traditionally, patients with failure to thrive were admitted and evaluated in the hospital, but outpatient treatment has been advocated (6,7). When failure to thrive is mild, with no obvious organic cause, outpatient management is encouraged if private physician follow up is possible (3). Ensuring the child has a medical home is imperative. A multidisciplinary team approach, involving a social worker, psychiatrist, and nutritionist, is more likely to be successful than the private doctor alone in both inpatient and outpatient treatment. A recent randomized, controlled trial showed that the use of a health visitor significantly improved the growth rate of children, compared with conventional management (14). Inpatient evaluation and treatment are reserved for cases in which outpatient management has failed. In addition, severe cases of failure to thrive in which there is severe malnutrition or laboratory abnormalities leading to medical instability (15) (e.g. hyponatremia, anemia, etc.), the presence of an organic etiology, young age, or concerns that the child is at risk for abuse should prompt inpatient management (2). In all cases of failure to thrive, communication between the emergency physician and the primary physician helps in decisionmaking.

COMMON PITFALLS

- ✔ Failing to recognize failure to thrive by addressing only the acute illness of presentation
- ✔ Failing to look for signs and symptoms of neglect
- ✔ Failing to screen for serious disease
- ✔ Failing to provide adequate follow up

Acknowledgments

Thanks to the previous edition's chapter authors Marc Linares and Bruce J. Quinn.

References

1. Berwick DM, Levy JC, Kleinerman R. Failure to thrive: diagnostic yield of hospitalization. *Arch Dis Child* 1982;57:347–351.
2. Bithoney W, Dubowitz H, Egan H. Failure to thrive/growth deficiency. *Pediatr Rev* 1992;13:453.
3. Bithoney W, McJunkin J, Michalek J, et al. Prospective evaluation of weight gain in both nonorganic and organic failure-to-thrive children: an outpatient trial of a multidisciplinary team intervention strategy. *J Dev Behav Pediatr* 1989;10:27.
4. Cahagan S, Holmes R. A stepwise approach to evaluation of undernutrition and failure to thrive. *Pediatr Clin North Am* 1998;1:169–187.
5. Frank D, Zeisel S. Failure to thrive. *Pediatr Clin North Am* 1988;35:1187.
6. Kirkland R. Failure to thrive. In: Oski F, DeAngelis C, Feigin R, et al., eds. *Principles and practice of pediatrics*. Philadelphia: JB Lippincott Co, 1990:969.
7. Schmitt B, Mauro R. Nonorganic failure to thrive: an outpatient approach. *Child Abuse Negl* 1989;13:235.
8. Schwartz ID. Failure to thrive: an old nemesis in a new millennium. *Pediatr Rev* 2000;21:257–264.
9. Shah MD. Failure to thrive in children. *J Clin Gastroenterol* 2002;35:371–374.
10. Sills R. Failure to thrive—the role of clinical and laboratory evaluation. *Am J Dis Child* 1978;132:967.
11. Srivastava R, Homer CJ. Length of stay for common pediatric conditions: teaching versus nonteaching hospitals. *Pediatrics* 2003;112:278–281.
12. Wilcox W, Nieburg P, Miller D. Failure to thrive: a continuing problem of definition. *Clin Pediatr* 1989;28:391.
13. Wright CM. Identification and management of failure to thrive a community perspective. *Arch Dis Child* 2000;82:5–9.
14. Wright CM, Callum J, Birks E, et al. Effect of community based management in failure to thrive: randomized controlled trial. *BMJ* 1998;317:571–574.
15. Yetman RJ, Coody DK. Failure to thrive: a clinical guideline. *J Pediatr Health Care* 1997;11:134–137.
16. Zenel, JA. Failure to thrive: a general pediatrician's perspective. *Pediatr Rev* 1997;18:371–378.

CHAPTER 224
Fever of Acute Onset

Maureen D. McCollough and David A. Talan

Fever is present in 25% of infants and children brought to the emergency department (ED), either as the sole complaint or in conjunction with other symptoms. Fever produces tremendous parental anxiety, often reinforced by healthcare personnel. Fever, in and of itself, is usually not harmful, but it may be an early sign of an emergency condition, such as meningitis or other bacterial infections (26).

The ED evaluation of fever focuses first on identifying life-threatening sepsis syndromes. A source of infection is also sought through a careful history and physical examination. The extent of laboratory testing (to confirm a suspected focus of infection or evaluate the likelihood of occult infection) and the decision to initiate empirical antimicrobial therapy depends on several variables. The patient's age, degree of fever, illness severity, and presence or the absence of a clinically suspected source of infection are most important in determining the need for further diagnostic testing. Other factors that must be considered include the patient's history of vaccinations and underlying medical conditions, the examiner's skill, the child's course during a period of observation, laboratory resources, and availability of follow up.

Both the likelihood and consequences of serious infections are increased in febrile children with immunocompromising diseases, such as sickle cell anemia and leukemia.

Signs of serious illness, such as meningitis, can be subtle. When the examiner's experience is limited, greater laboratory evaluation may be justified. For example, most experts recommend a lumbar puncture for febrile infants less than 1 month old. The ability to determine signs of meningitis in older infants depends on the physician's experience in interpreting infant behavior and clinical examination findings.

Assessing behavior in young children can be difficult, even for experienced examiners. Observation of trends in behavior over time, including alertness, consolability, social interactions, and feeding, is perhaps the most sensitive means to discern the presence or absence of a serious infection in a child with an initially equivocal presentation. Expectant antibiotic therapy for young children with fever without source and presumed occult bacteremia may be justified when a hospital's laboratory requires 48 hours to identify and report on a positive blood culture. But in a hospital that uses radioisotope techniques to identify positive cultures in 12 hours, the justification for empiric antibiotic therapy is less.

AVAILABILITY OF FOLLOW UP

When follow up is uncertain, extensive evaluation and cautious disposition are justified. For example, a 3-year-old nontoxic, toilet-trained girl with reliable follow up might be discharged to return with a voided urine specimen for urinalysis and culture in 12 hours. But if follow up is uncertain, it might be appropriate to catheterize the child during the ED visit. Children at risk for unreliable follow up include those with parents who are young, who have no access to transportation, or who believe their child is not ill (30).

DEFINITION, MEASUREMENT, AND INTERPRETATION OF FEVER

Traditionally, a rectal temperature (for neonates and young children) or oral temperature (older children and adolescents) at or above 38°C (100.4°F) has been defined as fever. Note that temperature varies diurnally 0.5°C or 1.0°F, and a temperature of 37.0°C (98.6°F) in the early morning hours (e.g., 4 a.m.) may represent a low-grade fever (24,36). Rectal temperatures are generally about 0.3°C or 0.5°F higher and less variable than oral temperatures (16). Bundling of a nonfebrile child should not cause a fever when the temperature is taken rectally (20). Axillary temperatures have been shown to be unreliable (27). Although previously not advocated, tympanic thermometers, when used after proper training, may be more reliable than previously thought (34).

Recent antipyretic use could interfere with fever identification, although, typically, fever is not eliminated and the antipyretic effect dissipates approximately 2 hours after the last dose (37). It should be noted that the degree of fever response to antipyretic therapy bears no relation to the likelihood of bacterial infection, and thus is irrelevant in clinical decisionmaking (5,11). Elevated body temperature is not generally harmful unless the temperature rises above approximately 106.5°F (26).

INITIAL EVALUATION

All children who are evaluated for fever should receive a thorough physical examination. The initial examination should start with an evaluation of the child's ABCs. Signs of respiratory distress, hypoperfusion, or shock should be treated immediately. The child's mental status and interaction with the environment are especially important to evaluate. A happy and playful infant with a fever of 40.0°C is less concerning than a lethargic child with no eye contact with a fever of 38.5°C. Febrile children should be undressed to look for skin infections and rashes, including petechiae (e.g., meningococcemia) and vesicles (e.g., *coxsackie* or *varicella* virus infection). Walking an ambulating child will help evaluate for occult joint infections. Table 224.1 lists other key symptoms and signs that should be pursued as part of the emergency evaluation of febrile infants and children.

DIFFERENTIAL DIAGNOSIS AND EMERGENCY DEPARTMENT MANAGEMENT BY AGE

Tables 224.2 and 224.3 list noninfectious and infectious causes of fever, respectively, along with the clinical features that should trigger their consideration. Table 224.4 presents an approach to the evaluation of the acutely febrile infant or child. This protocol assumes the absence of underlying chronic medical conditions and the presence of a skilled examiner and laboratory, as well as reliable follow up. A few of the more common fever syndromes by age and clinical findings are discussed below.

Fever in the Neonate (0 to 28 Days)

Neonates, once infected with a bacterial process in one area, such as the urinary tract, are at risk for seeding of the bacteria into other areas, such as the meninges. Because bacterial sepsis and meningitis can have such subtle presentations in this age group (e.g., change in sleep or feeding pattern, diarrhea, jaundice), a complete septic work up, including lumbar puncture, and hospital admission are generally recommended (13,28). In most circumstances, neonates should be treated with intravenous antibiotics until the culture results are known. Ampicillin (200 mg/kg/d) and cefotaxime (150 mg/kg/d) are recommended as

TABLE 224.1.   Key Historic and Physical Findings Relevant to the Evaluation of the Acutely Febrile Infant or Child

HISTORY

Behavior: activity level, consolability, irritability when moved (may be sign of meningitis), lethargy
Hydration status: fluid intake, urine output
Respiratory symptoms: cough, difficulty breathing
Gastrointestinal symptoms: vomiting, diarrhea (with blood), travel
Renal symptoms: abdominal pain, dysuria, frequency, urgency, hematuria
Other: focal pain (e.g., limp, sore throat, earache, abdominal pain, rash)
Medical history: immunization status, chronic medical conditions, ill contacts

PHYSICAL EXAMINATION

General appearance: activity, eye contact, muscle tone, color, consolability
Hydration status: mucous membranes, fontanelle, capillary refill, skin color, mottling
Respiratory: respiratory rate, grunting, nasal flaring, rales, bronchial breath sounds (may be only finding in child with pneumonia), retractions
HEENT: adenopathy, meningismus (may not be present in meningitic infants < 1 yr old), pharyngitis, otitis media (bulging, decreased mobility; redness as the only sign is insufficient to diagnose otitis)
Cardiovascular: heart rate, murmur
Abdomen: tenderness, guarding, organomegaly, CVA* tenderness
Skin: rash (including viral, Kawasaki disease, measles, Coxsackie virus, scarlet fever, roseola, Henoch-Schönlein purpura, varicella), petechiae
Musculoskeletal: bone or joint tenderness, swelling, erythema, ability to ambulate

*CVA = costovertebral angle.

TABLE 224.2.   Noninfectious Causes of Acute Fever in Infancy and Childhood

ENVIRONMENTAL

Overbundling (may raise skin temperature but not rectal temperature[17])
Heat stroke

COLLAGEN-VASCULAR

Rheumatic fever (prolonged fever, recent sore throat, rash, arthralgia)
Juvenile rheumatoid arthritis (prolonged fever, rash, arthritis)

POISONING

Atropine or other anticholinergics (dry mucous membranes, flushed)
Salicylates (tinnitus, hyperventilation)
Amphetamines (pupillary dilation, agitation, tremor, hypertension, tachycardia, hyperreflexia)
Antidepressants

OTHER

Kawasaki disease (prolonged fever, conjunctivitis, rash, adenopathy, erythematous mucous membranes)
Drug reaction
Prolonged seizures
Hemolysis

TABLE 224.3.   Common Infectious Processes Causing Fever in Children*

CNS

Meningitis
Encephalitis

HEENT

Pharyngitis/tonsillitis
Gingivostomatitis
Common cold/influenza
Sinusitis
Parotitis (viral or suppurative)
Tonsillar/pharyngeal abscess (uncommon)
Peritonsillar cellulitis/abscess (uncommon)

RESPIRATORY

Pneumonia
Croup
Epiglottitis (uncommon)
Bronchliolitis
Bronchitis

CARDIOVASCULAR

Myocarditis (uncommon)
Endocarditis (uncommon)

GI

Acute gastroenteritis
Appendicitis

GU

Urinary tract infection
Acute salpingitis (fever generally not the primary symptom)
Epididymitis (fever generally not the primary symptom)

CELLULITIS/SUPPURATIVE ADENITIS

Periorbital cellulitis
Facial cellulitis
Cervical adenitis
Inguinal adenitis

MUSCULOSKELETAL

Osteomyelitis
Septic arthritis

SYSTEMIC

Bacterial sepsis/bacteremia
Viremia
Rocky Mountain spotted fever
Toxic shock syndrome

*Boldface indicates common emergency conditions.

---

initial empirical therapy (and continued therapy for confirmed meningitis), with gentamicin (7.5 mg/kg/d, or 5 mg/kg/d if less than 1 week postterm age) later substituted for cefotaxime if the cerebrospinal fluid (CSF) is negative. These combinations will provide adequate coverage for the most common bacterial pathogens in this age group, including group B *Streptococcus*, *Listeria monocytogenes*, and *Escherichia coli*. Studies have shown that implementing a standard febrile young infant protocol in the emergency department (ED) can decrease

TABLE 224.4. Evaluating the Acutely Febrile Child[a]

Age	
<28 d[b,c]	Septic work up,[d] empirical antimicrobials, supportive care and monitoring, and hospital admission
1–3 mo[b]	Septic work up[d]
	Ill appearing infants or those with positive septic work up or not meeting Rochester criteria (see Table 249.5) should receive empirical antimicrobials, supportive care and monitoring, and hospital admission.
	If nontoxic with a negative septic work up (i.e., meeting Rochester criteria), discharge home with close follow up with or without intramuscular antibiotics[d]
3–36 mo	Ill-appearing infants and young children should receive empirical antimicrobials, supportive care and monitoring, and hospital admission.
	If non-toxic-appearing, temperature > 39.0°C to 39.5°C,[e] and no source on examination[f]:
	UA and UC for girls < 2 to 3 years old and for uncircumcised boys < 6 to 12 months old
	Chest x-ray if signs of lower respiratory tract disease
	Additional laboratory work up and management considerations in this age group are dependent on general appearance and change over time or specific physical findings, such as meningismus or bulging fontanelle (e.g., lumbar puncture), painful swollen joint (e.g., arthrocentesis), and petechial rash (e.g., possible meningococcemia requiring parenteral antimicrobials and hospital admission).
	If no infectious source is identified, various approaches include discharging home, with close follow up; blood cultures and empirical antimicrobial therapy for all febrile children, or for those with peripheral WBC >15,000/µL or ANC >10,000/µL, or for those with special risk (i.e., temperature > 40.0°C to 41.0°C, lack of complete HIB vaccination, sickle cell disease, unreliable follow up).
>36 mo	History and physical examination are usually reliable to identify presence of serious (e.g., meningitis or septic shock) or localized infection, and will dictate the extent of laboratory work up and management. UA and UC should be considered for girls if no source found on examination, or if vomiting, abdominal pain, or tenderness exists.

[a]Simplified approach to evaluation of fever; many variables must be taken into account, including prematurity, past medical conditions, ability to follow up.
[b]Fever defined as 38.0°C in this age group.
[c]Age is defined as postterm age; body weight and past medical conditions should be considered when determining category for workup.
[d]CBC, blood culture, urinalysis (UA), urine culture (UC), stool for WBCs and culture if diarrhea, chest x-ray if symptoms or signs of lower respiratory infection are present. Lumbar puncture and CSF analysis recommended < 1 month of age; 1 to 3 months of age optional if no signs of CNS infection, but recommended if antimicrobials are to be prescribed.
[e]The risk of bacterial infection as a cause for the fever increases with the level of the fever.
[f]Otitis media, upper respiratory infections and gastroenteritis are not necessarily considered reliable sources of fever, such that other diagnoses can be excluded.

the time to antibiotic therapy for these at-risk infants (31). Studies suggest that some febrile, well-appearing neonates with negative initial septic work ups can be successfully managed with admission and observation without empiric antibiotic treatment, or even discharged (4). However, currently, this is not considered a standard approach.

Fever in the Young Infant (1 to 3 Months)

Infants 1 to 3 months of age also may have subtle manifestations of serious infection, and, until just a few years ago, febrile infants as old as 12 weeks were routinely admitted to the hospital after a complete septic work up. Several studies now support the use of specific guidelines in order to stratify the risk of serious bacterial infection in children 1 to 3 months of age. The Rochester criteria (Table 224.5) are a well-validated set of clinical and laboratory criteria that, if met, place a young infant at low risk for a bacterial infection, such that he or she can be managed as an outpatient (9,10). Based on these criteria, the estimated risk of bacteremia and meningitis is 1.1% and 0.5%, respectively. For children meeting the Rochester criteria, urine and blood cultures are recommended, and routine lumbar puncture and empirical antimicrobials are considered to be optional (3,15). If an empiric antibiotic is to be used, intra-

muscular ceftriaxone (50 mg/kg) is recommended. Because of difficulty in clinically evaluating meningitis in this age group, and the concern for undiagnosed partially treated meningitis, it is recommended that lumbar puncture be performed if antimicrobials are to be administered. Discharged infants should be followed up in 24 hours. Standard management is to administer a second dose of ceftriaxone until the cultures are finalized as negative.

TABLE 224.5. The Rochester Criteria for Evaluating Young Infants

Previously healthy, nontoxic-appearing[a] term infant
No previous antimicrobial use
No focal infection on examination
WBC count 5,000–15,000/µL
Band count > 1,500/µL
Stool WBC count ≤ 5 WBC/HPF when diarrhea present
≤ 10 WBCs/HPF in spun urine

[a]Includes activity, alertness, color, strength of cry, consolability, irritability, eye contact, social responsiveness, and respiratory effort

Fever in Infants and Children Older Than 3 Months by Clinical Findings

In children older than 3 months of age, signs such as mentation and behavior are more reliably present when serious bacterial infections are present. Young infants with meningitis may have a bulging fontanel, and infants older than 12 to 18 months usually have meningeal signs. Careful, repeated assessments of the patients' general appearance, especially just before discharge from the ED, are the key to reasonably excluding meningitis in children 3 to 36 months of age. If the febrile child becomes lethargic or is persistently irritable or inconsolable, then a lumbar puncture is recommended, regardless of other physical findings or laboratory parameters. Children with cancer, sickle cell anemia, or other immunocompromised conditions should be more carefully evaluated for the source of their fever (e.g., white blood cell count, chest radiograph, urinalysis, and blood cultures), and are more likely to need empiric antibiotics and hospital admission.

Fever and Headache

Febrile children with significant headache as the only other chief complaint should be considered to have meningitis until proven otherwise. Fever itself may cause a headache and so a trial of an antipyretic is warranted. Meningeal signs such as stiff neck, Kernig or Brudzinski signs are not consistently found in children less than 12 to 18 months old with meningitis. Analgesia with either EMLA topical cream (prilocaine and lidocaine) or injectable lidocaine prior to a lumbar puncture is encouraged. Laboratory evaluation should include cell count, glucose, protein, gram stain and culture. A well appearing child diagnosed with viral meningitis that has reliable follow up may be discharged home.

Fever and Rash

Vesicles or ulcers isolated to the oropharynx are possibly herpes simplex or Coxsackie virus. If vesicles are also present on the hands or feet, then hand-foot-mouth disease is likely. Diffuse vesicular lesions on an erythematous base suggest the presence of varicella.

A febrile, ill-appearing child with an acute onset of a petechial or purpuric rash should be considered to be meningococcemic until proven otherwise.

Petechiae may develop on the face or neck area due to severe coughing or vomiting. It is recommended that any child with fever and petechiae not thought to be due to vomiting or coughing should undergo a complete septic work up. If the child remains well-appearing after a period of observation, no new petechiae have developed, and the child has a negative septic work up, then it may be possible to discharge the child with close follow up (25). Henoch-Schönlein purpura (HSP), a multisystem vasculitis, is suggested by subacute onset of a petechial or purpuric rash of the lower extremities, associated with painful swollen joints and abdominal pain in a slightly older child. As opposed to meningococcemia, these children rarely appear acutely ill. If HSP is suspected, stool for occult blood and urine for hematuria should be evaluated.

The pink maculopapular rash of roseola infantum will develop after a high fever has defervesced in an otherwise well-appearing infant. The maculopapular rash of measles will usually be associated with an ill-appearing young child with fever, cough, coryza, conjunctivitis, and Koplik spots in the mouth. Kawasaki disease is uncommon but has the potential for serious morbidity. Kawasaki disease usually presents in a young child with a several-day history of high fever that progresses to a macular–papular diffuse rash, conjunctivitis, erythematous or fissured lips, strawberry tongue, cervical lymphadenopathy, and edema or desquamation of hands or feet. Children with Kawasaki disease are at risk for developing aneurysms of the coronary arteries. The treatment includes high-dose aspirin, immunoglobulin therapy, and serial echocardiograms.

Fever and a Red Tympanic Membrane

Acute otitis media remains one of the most common discharge diagnoses for young children with fever. Because an erythematous tympanic membrane can result from the fever alone or from crying, this finding alone is not sufficient to diagnose acute otitis media. A bulging membrane or immobility during insufflation is necessary for this diagnosis to be reasonably considered.

Fever and Pharyngitis

Group A beta-hemolytic *Streptococcus* remains a concern as a cause of pharyngitis and fever in children generally older than 5 years of age. This infection is often associated with prominent gastrointestinal symptoms in children. Scarlet fever is likely when a fine, "sandpapery," raised maculopapular rash is also present. A rapid streptococcal antigen test is a relatively specific aid to diagnosis. If it is negative, however, a throat culture is necessary to exclude this diagnosis. Adolescents with exudative pharyngitis accompanied by prominent cervical adenopathy and splenomegaly may have mononucleosis; atypical lymphocytes on a blood smear or a Monospot test help to confirm this diagnosis.

Fever and Cough, Wheezing, or Tachypnea

Upper respiratory symptoms associated with fever in the winter and early spring are often due to respiratory syncytial virus (RSV) bronchiolitis and can range in severity from mild cough and wheezing to severe respiratory distress with tachypnea, retractions, grunting, and nasal flaring. The chest x-ray typically shows hyperinflation with peribronchial cuffing. A nasal wash for rapid RSV antigen testing can quickly be obtained. If the child clinically appears to have bronchiolitis and the RSV antigen test is positive, the yield from blood cultures and urine cultures looking for other sources of fever is low (2,35).

Pneumonia in pre–school-age children is most often due to viral infection; *Mycoplasma* pneumonia is more common in older children and adolescents. Toxic-appearing, febrile children of any age may have pneumonia due to pyogenic bacteria such as *Streptococcus pneumoniae*. The signs of pneumonia in young children that are indications to consider a chest radiograph include tachypnea, retractions, nasal flaring, grunting, abnormal auscultatory findings, and a pulse oximeter reading of less than 92% (14).

Fever and Vomiting, Diarrhea, or Abdominal Pain

Fever presenting with vomiting, diarrhea, or abdominal pain has a variety of causes, depending on the child's age. Acute gastroenteritis is a very common cause of fever with vomiting or diarrhea in young children and can have a viral or bacterial etiology. The most common cause of gastroenteritis in young children is *Rotavirus*. The vomiting frequently precedes the diarrhea by 24 hours. Rehydration is the cornerstone in treating the vomiting and diarrhea. If oral rehydration appears as an option, encourage the parents to try small amounts of fluids (e.g., 5 cc or 1 teaspoon every 2 to 3 minutes for young children). The child's diet should be advanced to a regular diet as soon as possible.

Bacterial causes of enteritis include *Shigella, Salmonella, Campylobacter,* and enterotoxic *E. coli.* Laboratory evaluation of children with fever, hematochezia, and abdominal pain may include a stool culture. A persistently symptomatic child found to have a bacterial pathogen as the cause of the diarrhea, with the exception of *Salmonella,* should be treated with the appropriate antimicrobial. Antibiotic treatment of *Salmonella* causes an increased duration of stool carriage and is recommended only for infants less than 3 months of age, patients with immunosuppressive illness, and toxic patients. The fluoroquinolones are relatively contraindicated in young children due to concern for arthropathy found in animal toxicity studies, which, however, has not been observed in human pediatric experience.

Appendicitis also remains a serious cause of fever and abdominal pain in young children. Young children have higher perforation rates compared with older children, due in part to the difficulty in making the diagnosis. Children with appendicitis are often discharged home with diagnoses of gastroenteritis or urinary tract infection (UTI) before the final diagnosis of appendicitis is made. The omentum in young children is less capable of walling off focal areas of infection, such as appendicitis. Peritonitis with diffuse abdominal tenderness is therefore more common. Ultrasound and computed tomography (CT) scan are two modalities that are now used more commonly to diagnose appendicitis in young children.

Streptococcal pharyngitis in older children may present with fever, abdominal pain, and associated dysphagia. Lower lobe pneumonia can sometimes present with abdominal pain and fever. Adolescent girls with fever and abdominal pain should be questioned regarding sexual activity and possibly evaluated for pelvic inflammatory disease. UTIs are also a common cause in girls with fever and abdominal pain. In young children, UTIs may present with fever and vomiting, often without abdominal pain. UTI should be considered in febrile girls less than 2 years old and in uncircumcised boys less than 1 year old.

Fever and vomiting without diarrhea can be a sign of a neurologic process. Meningitis, particularly bacterial meningitis, is the most serious cause. Children with a central nervous system (CNS) ventricular shunt should be evaluated for the possibility of obstruction and meningitis. This evaluation may include a head CT scan and lumbar puncture or shunt tap for CSF evaluation. Finally, acute otitis media can also present with fever and diarrhea in young children.

Fever and Swollen Joint or Limp

Febrile children who are nonambulatory, walk with a limp, or have local joint symptoms should be evaluated for a joint infection. Toxic synovitis, a benign condition related to coincident viral infection, must be differentiated from septic arthritis, which can rapidly be destructive. Joint effusions should be aspirated and analyzed for cell counts, Gram stain, and culture. If the hip joint is suspected, ultrasound appears to be a reliable test to evaluate the presence of an effusion, and can then be used to guide joint aspiration. The absence of a hip effusion makes the likelihood of septic arthritis of the hip infection low. However this does not completely exclude this infection or osteomyelitis, and therefore patients should still be carefully followed. Sexually active adolescents may have arthritis or tenosynovitis due to disseminated gonococcal infection.

Fever without Source in Young Children (3 to 36 Months)

After a thorough physical examination, often no identifiable infection source for the fever is found in infants and children younger than 36 months of age. The presence of some clinical diagnoses can reasonably explain fever, including Coxsackie pharyngitis (and hand-foot-mouth disease) and chickenpox. The presence of acute otitis media does not necessarily exclude other diagnoses as the cause of fever.

Fever may be the only indication of a UTI in a young child. Up to 7% of febrile young children without a source found on physical examination have a UTI as a cause of their fever (33). In one study, up to 4% of young febrile children less than 2 years old, with either acute otitis media or gastroenteritis as a source for the fever, also had a UTI (32). A urinalysis and culture are recommended as part of the work up of girls less than 2 years old and of uncircumcised boys less than 12 months old. Urinalysis is insufficiently accurate to be used alone to evaluate the presence of UTI in young children (21). Therefore, a urine culture should be sent in addition to the urinalysis. Enhanced urinalysis, defined as either a positive Gram stain or presence of pyuria by hemocytometer has been shown to improve the capabilities of the urinalysis (21). Bag urine specimens are also more likely to produce contaminant flora, compared with catheterized specimens. Pneumonia is rarely present without signs of disease (see previous discussion) (17).

When no source is found on physical examination, and pneumonia and UTI have been ruled out by either physical examination or laboratory tests, the potential for occult bacteremia should be considered. The evaluation and management of children with possible occult bacteremia has changed dramatically in the last 10 to 15 years. Previous studies showed that 3% to 5% of children with no focus of infection and with temperatures above 39.5°C were bacteremic with *S. pneumoniae* (85%), *Haemophilus influenzae* (10%), or *Neisseria meningitides* (3%) (7). Previously, 5% to 10% of children treated as outpatients without antibiotics who had *H. influenzae* bacteremia would have seeded other areas, causing other serious bacterial infections, such as meningitis or septic arthritis (7). Due to *H. influenzae* type b vaccine (Hib) which was introduced in 1988, this virulent bacteria is now almost nonexistent as a cause of occult bacteremia. Large studies from the mid1990s showed that the overall bacteremia rate had declined to 1% to 2% with *S. pneumoniae* accounting for over 90% of cases (1,22).

The risk of meningitis resulting from pneumococcal bacteremia is also much lower than that occurring after *H. influenzae* bacteremia (1% to 3%) (1,29).

Although occult pneumococcal bacteremia ultimately spontaneously resolves in the vast majority of children, previous studies showed that both oral and parenteral antimicrobial agents may reduce the risk of focal bacterial infections and possible meningitis in children with occult bacteremia. Approaches to the management of fever without a source have included: (1) blood cultures and empiric antimicrobials for all nontoxic children 3 to 36 months of age with fever without source; (2) for only those at high risk (e.g., temperature greater than 41.0°C, under- or nonimmunized children, or a combination of temperature greater than 39.0°C and total white blood cell count greater than 15,000/mm³ or absolute neutrophil count [ANC] greater than 10,000/μL); and (3) close follow up without testing or treatment (6,19). If empiric antibiotics are to be utilized, intramuscular ceftriaxone (50 mg/kg) is appropriate, especially for the child who is not fully immunized. For other children, oral amoxicillin (60 to 90 mg/kg/d) is a reasonable alternative.

In 2000, the *Streptococcus pneumoniae* vaccine (Prevnar) was added to children's primary immunization schedule here in the United States. This new protein conjugate vaccine appears to be 80% to 100% effective in preventing invasive disease by *Streptococcus pneumoniae* (11). Currently there are no data regarding the overall bacteremia rate in the post*pneumooccal,* post*haemophilus influenzae* era. There is evidence however that the overall rate of invasive pneumococcal disease including bacteremia is decreasing (23). If the overall bacteremia rate drops below 1%, the management options using empiric testing and treatment may no longer be cost-effective. For a child who has received even 2 doses of the pneumococcal vaccine, the risk of occult pneumococcal bacteremia and the sequelae of bacterial meningitis is so low, that the use of white blood cell count criteria, blood cultures, and empiric antibiotics does not appear to be warranted (6).

Clearly, the management of young febrile children without a defined source for that fever is rapidly changing. The development of new or resistant strains of bacteria must continue to be monitored through multicenter surveillance studies.

EMERGENCY DEPARTMENT DISPOSITION AND INSTRUCTIONS TO PARENTS

Fever control with acetaminophen (15 mg/kg every 4 to 6 hours) or ibuprofen (10 mg/kg every 4 to 6 hours); cool, clear liquids; and light dressing are advised. Sponging may be used but is of questionable value. Body temperature is determined by the temperature regulatory center in the hypothalamus. Acetaminophen resets the regulatory center, but sponging has no effect on it and a minimal effect on lowering the temperature for any significant period of time. Sponging usually results in an irritated and agitated child (18).

Although experimental evidence suggests that fever may be adaptive and stimulate the immune system, fever reduction has not proven to be deleterious, and does lead to increased patient comfort and decreased metabolic demands and fluid loss. Therefore, fever control is recommended.

The second component of discharge instructions consists of the indications for urgent return for reevaluation (Table 224.6). The most important indications for urgent reevaluation are lethargy and persistent irritability. Even with continued fever, if the child's behavior and disposition improve, urgent reevaluation is not necessary. A child less than 3 months old or a child

---

TABLE 224.6. Indications for Reevaluation[a]

AGE OR TREATMENT

Any child less than 3 mo old
Any child given antibiotics for fever without a source

BEHAVIOR

Persistent lethargy or irritability

HYDRATION STATUS

Signs of dehydration (decreased urine output, decreased tears)

RESPIRATORY

Worsening cough
Difficulty breathing

GASTROINTESTINAL

Persistent vomiting
Bilious vomiting
Worsening diarrhea

OTHER

New rash
Pain

[a]Telephone contact my be sufficient in some cases.

---

given empiric antibiotics should generally be followed up in 12 to 24 hours by a primary care physician or clinic. That follow up may consist of a telephone call to the caretaker or, if there is reason for additional concern, a repeat examination.

CRITICAL INTERVENTIONS

- Perform a complete evaluation for the source of the fever including lumbar puncture and antibiotics for febrile infants less than 1 month of age
- Perform a complete evaluation for the source of the fever in febrile infants 1 to 3 months of age; if empiric antibiotics are to be prescribed, then a lumbar puncture should be done prior to their administration
- A selected evaluation for well-appearing febrile infants and children over 3 months of age can be performed
- Avoidance of blood cultures and empiric antibiotics in previously healthy nontoxic appearing infants and children with fever and no source who have received a complete immunization series including the *Haemophilus influenzae* and *Streptococccus pneumoniae* vaccines
- Perform aggressive resuscitation, evaluation for the source of the fever, and antibiotic treatment for ill-appearing or immuno-compromised febrile infants and children

COMMON PITFALLS

✔ Do not forget to consider noninfectious disease processes as a cause for the fever
✔ Remember to account for an infant's age in determining the extent of the fever evaluation
✔ Do not forget to carefully evaluate and document the child's general appearance
✔ Remember to undress all febrile children; petechiae may be an early indication of meningococcal disease
✔ Do not over rely on acute-phase reactants such as the white blood cell count or ANC

Acknowledgments

Thanks to the previous edition's chapter authors R. Kemp Crockett and Elizabeth Rincon.

References

1. Alpern ER, Alessandrini EA, Bell LM et al. Occult bacteremia from a pediatric emergency department: current prevalence, time to detection, and outcome. *Pediatrics* 2000;106:505–511.
2. Antonow JA, Hansen K, McKinstry CA, et al. Sepsis evaluations in hospitalized infants with bronchiolitis. *Pediatr Infect Dis J* 1998;17:231–236.
3. Baker MD, Bell LM, Avner JR. Outpatient management without antibiotics of fever in selected infants. *N Engl J Med* 1993;329:1437–1441.
4. Baker MD, et al. The applicability of an established outpatient management protocol for febrile 0–1 month old infants. SAEM 1997 Annual Meeting. *Acad Emerg Med* 1997;427(abst258).
5. Baker MD, Fosarelli PD, Carpenter RO. Childhood fever: correlation of diagnosis with temperature response to acetaminophen. *Pediatrics* 1987;80:315–318.
6. Baraff LJ. Editorial: Clinical policy for children younger than three years presenting to the emergency department with fever. *Ann Emerg Med* 2003;42:546–549.
7. Baraff LJ, Bass JW, Fleisher GR, et al. Practice guideline for the management of infants and children 0 to 36 months of age with fever without a source. Agency for Health Care Policy and Research. *Ann Emerg Med* 1993;22:1198–1210.
8. Baraff LJ. Management of fever without source in infants and children. *Ann Emerg Med* 2000;36:602–613.
9. Baskin MN, Fleisher GR, O'Rourke EJ. Outpatient management of febrile infants 28 to 90 days of age with intramuscular ceftriaxone. *Am J Dis Child* 1988;142:391(Abstract).
10. Baskin MN, O'Rourke EJ, Fleisher GR. Outpatient treatment of febrile infants 28 to 89 days of age with intramuscular administration of ceftriaxone. *J Pediatr* 1992;120:22–27.
11. Berkowitz CD, Schiff D, Black JL, et al. Effect of acetaminophen on clinical assessment of febrile infants. *Am J Dis Child* 1988;142:393(Abstract).

12. Black S, Shinefield H, Ray P, et al. Efficacy of heptavalent conjugate pneumococcal vaccine in 37,000 infants and children: results of the Northern California Kaiser Permanente Efficacy Trial (abst LB-9). 1998 Interscience Conference on Antimicrobial Agents and Chemotherapy, San Diego, California, September 1998.

13. Bonadio WA. Incidence of serious infections in afebrile neonates with a history of fever. *Pediatr Infect Dis J* 1987;6:911–914.

14. Bramson RT, Meyer TL, Silbiger ML, et al. The futility of the chest radiograph in the febrile infant without respiratory symptoms. *Pediatrics* 1993;92:524–526.

15. Brik R, Hamissah R, Shehada N, et al. Evaluation of febrile infants under 3 months of age: is routine lumbar puncture warranted?. *Isr J Med Sci* 1997;33:93–97.

16. Chamberlain JM, Grandner J, Rubinoff JL. Comparison of a tympanic thermometer to rectal and oral thermometers in a pediatric emergency department. *Clin Pediatr* 1991;30[Suppl 4]:24–29; discussion, 34–35.

17. Crain EF, Bulas D, Bijur PE, et al. Is a chest radiograph necessary in the evaluation of every febrile infant less than 8 weeks of age?. *Pediatrics* 1991;88:821–824.

18. Friedman AD, Barton LL. Efficacy of sponging vs acetaminophen for reduction of fever. Sponging Study Group. *Pediatr Emerg Care* 1990;6:6–7.

19. Green SM, Rothrock SG. Evaluation styles for well-appearing febrile children: are you a "risk-minimizer" or a "test-minimizer"?. *Ann Emerg Med* 1999;33:311–214.

20. Grover G, Berkowitz CD, Lewis RJ, et al. The effects of bundling on infant temperature. *Pediatrics* 1994;94:669–673.

21. Hoberman A, Wald ER, Penchansky L, et al. Enhanced urinalysis as a screening test for urinary tract infection. *Pediatrics* 1993;91:1196–1199.

22. Lee GM, Harper MB. Risk of bacteremia for febrile young children in the post-*Haemophilus influenzae* type b. *Arch Peds Adol Med* 1998;152:624–628.

23. Ling Lin P, Michaels MG, Janosky J, et al. Incidence of invasive Pneumococcal disease in children 3–36 months of age at a tertiary care pediatric 2 years after licensure of the Pneumococcal conjugate vaccine. *Pediatrics* 2003;111:896–899.

24. Mackowiak PA, Wasserman SS, Levine MM. A critical appraisal of 98.6 degrees F, the upper limit of the normal body temperature, and other legacies of Carl Reinhold August Wunderlich. *JAMA* 1992;268:1578–1580.

25. Mandl KD, Stack AM, Fleisher GR. Incidence of bacteremia in infants and children with fever and petechiae. *J Pediatr* 1997;131:398–404.

26. May A, Bauchner H. Fever phobia: the pediatrician's contribution. *Pediatrics* 1992;90:851–854.

27. Morley CJ, Hewson PH, Thornton AJ. Axillary and rectal temperature measurements in infants. *Arch Dis Child* 1992;67:122–125.

28. Roberts KB, Borzy MS. Fever in the first eight weeks of life. *Johns Hopkins Med J* 1977;141:9–13.

29. Rothrock SG, Harper MB, Green SM, et al. Do oral antibiotics prevent meningitis and serious bacterial infections in children with *Streptococcus pneumoniae* occult bacteremia? A meta-analysis. *Pediatrics* 1997;99:438–444.

30. Scarfone RJ. Compliance with scheduled visits to a pediatric emergency department. *Acad Emerg Med* 1994;1:(Abstract 41).

31. Sharieff GQ, Hoecker C, Silva PD. Effects of a pediatric emergency department febrile infant protocol on time to antibiotic therapy *J Emerg Med* 2001;21:1–6.

32. Shaw K, Gorelick M, McGowan K, et al. Prevalence of urinary tract infections in febrile young children in the emergency department. *Pediatrics* 1998;102:E16.

33. Shaw K. Predicting urinary tract infections in febrile young children in the emergency department. SAEM 1997 Annual Meeting. *Acad Emerg Med* 1997;427(Abstraact 257).

34. Terndrup TE, Rajk J. Impact of operator technique and device on infrared emission detection tympanic thermometry. *J Emerg Med* 1992;10:683–687.

35. Titus MO, Wright SW. Prevalence of serious bacterial infections in febrile infants with respiratory syncytial virus infections. *Pediatrics* 2003;112:282–284.

36. van der Bogert. *J Pediatr* 1937;10:795.

37. Vauzelle-Kervroedan F, d'Athis P, Pariente-Khayat A, et al. Equivalent antipyretic activity of ibuprofen and paracetamol in febrile children. *J Pediatr* 1997;131:683–687.

CHAPTER 225
Gastrointestinal Bleeding

Michael Gayle and Niranjan Kissoon

Gastrointestinal (GI) bleeding is uncommon in relatively healthy children. In fact, published data of the incidence of GI bleeding in children is limited to the pediatric intensive care population (2). The causes of gastrointestinal bleeding vary with the child's age. Moreover, the site of bleeding and character of the blood is important in diagnosis and therapy, and can often be determined by the presenting symptoms. For instance, hematemesis is the vomiting of blood and implies a source proximal to the ligament of Treitz. Vomited blood may have the appearance of coffee grounds or may be bright red, implying ongoing bleeding. Blood from the upper GI tract or proximal small bowel, when passed per rectum, is typically black or tarry, is sticky, has a characteristic aroma, and is called *melena*. Bright red blood per rectum or maroon stools (hematochezia) implies a more distal GI source. Upper GI bleeding, however, may present as gross blood rectally (hematochezia), if blood loss is considerable and transit time is short.

GI bleeding is an alarming problem in children with many causes common to children and adults. However, there are lesions such as necrotizing enterocolitis or allergic colitis, that are unique to children (6). Tables 225.1 and 225.2 outline the causes of GI bleeding in children and illustrate the wide, age-related differential diagnosis.

CLINICAL PRESENTATION

Bleeding from anal fissures or bleeding from the upper GI tract are the most common reasons children with GI bleeding visit the emergency department (ED). Life-threatening hemorrhage is a rare presentation to the ED. Under these circumstances children may present in hypovolemic shock. The GI tract as the source of bleeding is the obvious source although more commonly, GI bleeding in the child presents as anemia from chronic upper GI bleeding (typically microcytic) or occult bleeding in the stool (e.g., cow's milk protein sensitivity) (7). However, with the more frequent use of NSAIDs, such as ibuprofen, naproxen and ketorolac in children, there may be an increase in the cases of gastric ulcerations and erosions (11).

Acute bleeding can be classified as occult, overt, or massive. Massive bleeding (e.g., variceal bleeding) is the most dramatic presentation and is usually accompanied by compromised cardiac output or tissue oxygenation.

DIFFERENTIAL DIAGNOSIS

Determination of the exact diagnosis in a child with GI bleeding is usually unnecessary in the ED, because most patients are stable and the differential diagnosis is large (see Tables 225.1 and 225.2). A thorough history and clinical examination can usually lead to the diagnosis. For the emergency physician, it is most important to determine whether the source of bleeding is in the upper or the lower GI tract. The easiest method is to atraumatically insert

TABLE 225.1.   Differential Diagnosis of Lower GI Bleeding

Newborn (0–1 mo)	Preschool (2–5 yrs)
Anal fissure	Anal fissure
Local trauma	Polyps
Swallowed maternal blood	Infectious colitis
Upper GI bleeding	Meckel diverticulum
Necrotizing enterocolitis	Hemolytic–uremic syndrome
Malrotation with volvulus	Henoch-Schönlein purpura
Infectious colitis	Inflammatory bowel disease
Hirschsprung disease	Intussusception
Allergic colitis	Pseudomembranous colitis
Coagulopathy	Lymphonodular hyperplasia
Infant (1 month–2 yrs)	**School Age (>5 yrs)**
Anal fissure	Anal fissure
Hirschsprung disease	Polyps
Allergic colitis	Infectious colitis
Intussusception	Hemorrhoids
Infectious colitis	Inflammatory bowel disease
Meckel diverticulum	Pseudomembranous colitis
Intestinal duplication	Lymphonodular hyperplasia
Lymphonodular hyperplasia	Hemolytic–uremic syndrome
Pseudomembranous colitis	
Polyps	

a small, soft, nasogastric tube and perform a gastric lavage with tap water or normal saline at room temperature. Normal Saline at room temperature (not chilled or "iced) should be used as the lavage fluid to avoid central hypothermia, especially in the infant or young child who are more prone to heat loss (20). If blood is not evident on lavage, it is unlikely that the bleeding is above the ligament of Treitz (i.e., bleeding from the nose, esophagus, and stomach).

Measuring the ratio of blood urea nitrogen to creatinine (BUN/Cr), as described by Felber and colleagues (5), may also provide supportive evidence of upper GI bleeding. A ratio exceeding 30 suggests bleeding from the upper GI tract; less than 30 might be consistent with either an upper or a lower GI bleeding site. This ratio also provides a useful means of assessing the amount of blood loss and predicting when a significant bleed has ceased (15).

The performance of radiologic and nuclear medicine imaging studies are rarely necessary in the ED. Plain x-ray film is useful if a foreign body, bowel perforation or bowel obstruction is suspected. Ultrasonography is useful when intussusception, liver disease, portal hypertension or vascular anomalies, are suspected (16).

TABLE 225.2.   Differential Diagnosis of Upper GI Bleeding

Newborn (0–1 mo)	Preschool (2–5 yr)
Idiopathic	Esophagitis
Swallowed maternal blood	Gastritis
Esophagitis	Peptic ulcer
Gastritis	Varices (esophageal, gastric)
Stress ulcer	Mallory-Weiss tear
Vitamin K deficiency	Foreign body
Bleeding disorders	Bleeding disorders
Vascular anomalies	Vascular anomalies
Infant (1 mo–2 yr)	**School Age (>5 Years)**
Esophagitis	Esophagitis
Gastritis	Gastritis
Stress ulcer	Peptic ulcer
Mallory-Weiss tear	Varices (esophageal, gastric)
Vascular anomalies	Mallory-Weiss tear
Foreign body	Inflammatory bowel disease
Duplication	

Newborn (0 to 1 Month)

Most causes of bleeding in neonates are never identified, as most bleeding usually stops between 24 and 48 hours of life. Significant upper GI bleeding may result from stress ulcers or hemorrhagic gastritis in the neonate with sepsis, an intracranial lesion, or other major illness. Hematemesis in the neonate may also result from hemorrhagic disease of the newborn (vitamin K deficiency) or congenital bleeding disorders such as hemophilia. The swallowing of a mixture of amniotic fluid and maternal blood is a frequent cause of hematemesis but may also present as dark red rectal bleeding. Swallowed maternal blood (adult hemoglobin) can be easily differentiated from upper GI bleeding in the fetus (fetal hemoglobin) by adding sodium hydroxide to a blood sample. This test is known as the Apt-Downey test. Fetal hemoglobin resists alkaline degradation and remains pink while adult hemoglobin gives a brownish color (18).

Anal fissure and local trauma are the most common causes of rectal bleeding in the first month of life. However, both necrotizing enterocolitis and enterocolitis due to Hirschsprung disease may present with occult or overt rectal bleeding. Necrotizing enterocolitis is more common in the preterm infant but may also be seen in the stressed term infant. Bilious vomiting, abdominal distention, and rectal bleeding are the most common clinical features and may also be due to surgical emergencies such as midgut volvulus. A finding of air in the bowel wall (pneumatosis intestinalis) on an abdominal radiograph is pathognomonic for necrotizing enterocolitis.

Infant (1 Month to 2 Years)

Upper GI bleeding is frequently caused by esophagitis, gastritis, or stress ulcers. However, congenital malformations such as duodenal web, although more likely to present in the newborn period, can present after 1 month of life.

Lower GI bleeding is most commonly due to anal fissure, but other anorectal lesions, such as juvenile polyps, should also be considered (4). Intussusception, which classically presents with currant jelly stools, is most common in infants 7 to 12 months old. Infectious colitis is usually secondary to species of *Salmonella* and *Shigella* and to *Campylobacter jejuni, Yersinia enterocolitica,* and both enterohemorrhagic and enteroinvasive *Escherichia coli.* Other organisms that should be considered include *Aeromonas hydrophila* and *Entamoeba histolytica.* With the increasing number of children with the acquired immunodeficiency syndrome, cases of GI bleeding due to opportunistic infections such as cytomegalovirus will be seen with increased frequency (25).

Preschool (2 to 5 Years)

Varices in both the upper and the lower GI tracts can lead to massive, life-threatening hemorrhage in this age group. Two-thirds of patients with portal hypertension sustain bleeds before 5 years of age, and 85% do so by age 10 years. On physical examination, other signs of portal hypertension or liver disease, such as splenomegaly, hepatomegaly, and dilated abdominal veins are present (1). Foreign-body ingestion, although uncommon, should also be considered as a cause of upper GI bleeding.

Anal fissure and juvenile polyps are the most frequent causes of lower GI bleeding. These polyps are usually solitary and nonmalignant and can usually be felt on rectal examination. Massive GI bleeding from Meckel diverticulum is sometimes seen in preschool children. Infectious enterocolitis from infectious agents similar to those described for the infant may also present with bloody stools. Multisystem diseases such as hemolytic–uremic syndrome and Henoch-Schönlein purpura are less common causes of bloody stools.

School Age (Over 5 Years)

Esophagitis, gastritis, and peptic ulcer disease account for most cases of upper GI bleeding. Erosions of the gastric mucosa may occur acutely after any major stressful situation, such as trauma, shock, burns, or sepsis. Peptic ulcer disease may be either primary or secondary to other conditions, such as medications used in patients with cystic fibrosis (e.g., corticosteroids and non-steroidal antiinflammatory agents).

Anal fissure and juvenile polyps account for most cases of lower GI bleeding. Intestinal lymphonodular hyperplasia of childhood has a peak incidence between 6 and 10 years; inflammatory bowel diseases (e.g., Crohn's disease and ulcerative colitis) have a peak incidence in children over 5 years (9). With the increased prevalence of cocaine use, drug intoxication should be considered in cases of unexplained shock and hemorrhagic diarrhea in this age group (17).

EMERGENCY DEPARTMENT EVALUATION

If the patient presents with signs and symptoms of cardiovascular compromise, immediate attention to restoring intravascular volume is necessary. Usually, however, the evaluation can be done in a leisurely manner, beginning with a thorough history and physical examination.

Under these circumstances, the emergency physician's initial step is to determine the site and magnitude of bleeding and whether it is ongoing.

Important elements of the history and physical examination are outlined in Table 225.3. A nasogastric tube should be inserted and fluid aspirated, unless a distal source is obvious. A positive aspirate for blood almost certainly indicates that the site of bleeding is proximal to the ligament of Treitz. However, a negative aspirate does not exclude an upper GI bleeding site beyond the pylorus.

In most cases, the cause of bleeding is evident, but sometimes, before beginning an expensive and possibly invasive work up, it may be necessary to confirm that the patient is actually passing blood. Many foods and medications (e.g., tomato or cranberry juice, flavored gelatin, Kool-Aid, red licorice, ampicillin,

rifampin, iron, and bismuth preparations [Pepto-Bismol]) can give stools a bloody appearance or test positive for blood (20). In most hospitals, guaiac benzidine or benzidine derivative test pads (Hemoccult or Hematest) are used to detect blood. These tests use a hydrogen peroxide developer and are based on the peroxidase activity of hemoglobin and its derivatives. In the presence of hydrogen peroxide, these substances catalytically oxidize substrates such as guaiac or benzidine. The oxidation produces a color change in the substrate, indicating a positive test. However, false-negative results can be obtained if the patient has ingested large doses of ascorbic acid or if intestinal bacteria have degraded the hemoglobin to porphyrin. False-positive results can be seen if the patient has eaten rare red meat or peroxidase-containing fruits and vegetables such as broccoli, radishes, cauliflower, cantaloupe, or turnips. A new test, HemoQuant®, appears to be more sensitive (8).

Laboratory studies (Table 225.4) should include a complete blood count with platelet and reticulocyte counts and a coagulation profile. An elevated eosinophil count signifies milk allergy or parasitic infestation. If bleeding is severe, blood should also be sent for a cross-match. The BUN/Cr ratio is useful in localizing the source of bleeding to the upper GI tract and may provide an estimate of the severity of blood loss from the upper GI tract. An elevated BUN level is more likely to be associated with an upper than a lower GI bleed (15). Hepatic and renal function tests (to assess liver function and to obtain the BUN/Cr index) should be obtained. If an infective cause is likely, stool should be examined promptly for fecal leukocytes, aerobic, and anaerobic cultures, and microscopy for ova and parasites (19).

Plain radiography and sonography are noninvasive and minimally distressing for a child and may give definitive information, such as a classic appearance of multiple short fluid levels in the abdomen in a neonate with volvulus, or the appearance of an intraluminal mass on sonography, in a case of intussusception.

If the source of bleeding is not obvious after these investigations, more detailed testing, including endoscopy and complex radiographic procedures, is necessary. However, most of these will not be conducted as part of the ED work up. In children with a positive nasogastric aspirate, endoscopy within the first 24 hours can determine the source of upper GI bleeding in 90% of cases. Fiberoptic endoscopy in children has shown that the most common causes of bleeding are gastritis, esophagitis, duodenal ulcers, and esophageal varices (10). Endoscopy is especially recommended in children with a history of esophageal varices, because the source of bleeding may be from other lesions. Upper GI barium studies are less accurate than endoscopy and may interfere with subsequent endoscopic examination.

Both endoscopy and barium studies may fail to determine the source of bleeding in patients with massive bleeding (greater than 0.5 mL/min, making endoscopic examination impossible). In these patients, arteriographic examination of the superior and mesenteric arteries and the celiac axis may reveal some common causes of bleeding, as well as some unusual causes, such

---

TABLE 225.3.   History and Physical Examination
for GI Bleeding

HISTORY

Bleeding (duration, quantity, color, rectal vs. oral)
Associated pain
Vomiting/diarrhea
Medication history
(e.g., aspirin, alcohol)
Illicit drugs (e.g., cocaine)
Systemic diseases
Family history
Social history

PHYSICAL EXAMINATION

Vital signs
Site of bleeding (nose, mouth, outside GI tract)
Acuity or chronicity
Anthropometric data
Cutaneous signs (e.g., spider nevi)
Abdominal tenderness/mass
Hepatomegaly
Splenomegaly
Anorectal examination

TABLE 225.4.   Laboratory Studies

Blood count: CBC with reticulocyte count
Coagulation profile: platelet count, prothrombin time, partial
   thromboplastin time, fibrinogen
Hepatic profile: bilirubin, SGPT, SGOT
Renal profile: BUN/Cr
Blood bank: type and crossmatch
Stools: leukocytes, aerobic and anaerobic stool cultures,
   microscopy for ova and parasites

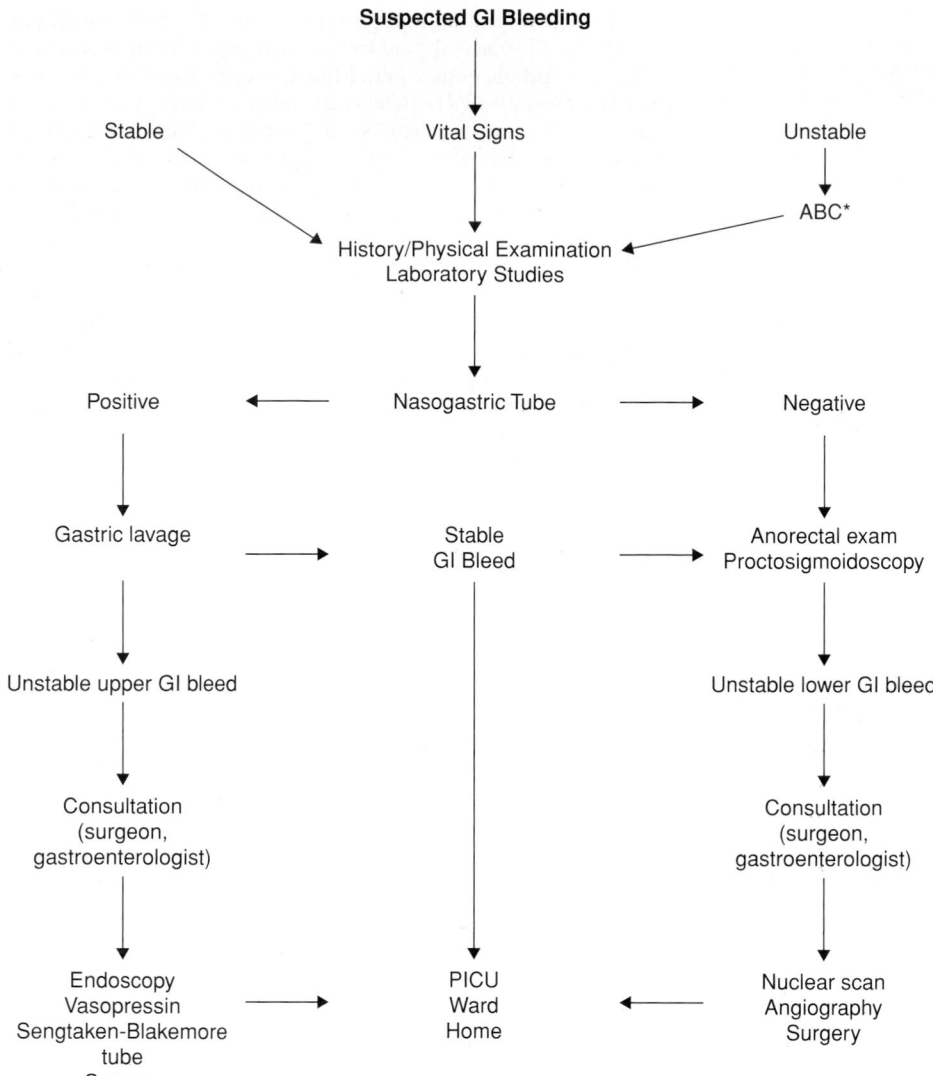

Suspected GI Bleeding

Figure 225.1. Flow diagram of suggested management of GI bleeding in the emergency department. ABCs (*) include attention to respiratory status (may include endotracheal intubation) and cardiovascular support (including vascular access, crystalloid and blood infusions).

as hepatic artery aneurysms, traumatic hematobilia, or malformations (e.g., arteriovenous lesions and hemangiomas). Nuclear medicine scans have fewer complications and are preferred by some clinicians (13).

If the nasogastric aspirate does not contain blood, a rectal examination and proctosigmoidoscopy can identify the source of rectal bleeding in 80% of cases. Additional studies are needed to identify the other 20%. Dark blood mixed with stool, in the absence of abdominal pain or diarrhea, may indicate Meckel diverticulum, intestinal duplication, or right-sided colonic polyps. A bleeding Meckel diverticulum is the cause in 80% of cases and can often be diagnosed by a nuclear medicine scan. Colonoscopy and, ultimately, an air-contrast barium enema should be performed if the scan is inconclusive.

CRITICAL INTERVENTIONS

- Assessment of cardiorespiratory status—determine if shock or respiratory distress is present and resuscitate appropriately
- If the patient has a massive GI bleed, start 2 large bore IVs. Send blood for type and cross-match, and coagulation factors
- Quick history and physical examination—determine source of bleeding
- Pass an NG tube and perform gastric lavage if the source is not obvious or is suspected to be from the upper GI tract
- Check stools to see if blood is present

EMERGENCY DEPARTMENT MANAGEMENT

Management depends on the child's clinical status and the severity and site of bleeding (Fig. 225.1).

Assessment of Cardiovascular Status

Initial management is based on the child's condition, including factors such as age, source, rate, and amount of bleeding, and associated medical illnesses. Assessment of cardiopulmonary status and prompt attention to any derangements should be a priority. Oxygen administration and venous access, followed by fluid boluses of crystalloids (20 mL/kg lactated Ringer or normal saline), are mandatory, particularly if the patient has signs of volume compromise (anxiety, tachycardia, weak pulses, delayed capillary refill, hypotension, tachypnea). Additional fluid boluses are given as indicated by frequent reevaluations. A nasogastric tube is then placed in the stomach, and lavage with tap water or saline should be started.

Occult Bleeding

In the stable child with occult bleeding, management is geared toward making the diagnosis and excluding more serious conditions. Investigations are dictated by the history and physical examination, but most tests, including cultures, radiologic and nuclear medicine scans, and endoscopy, can be performed on an outpatient basis. The cause of occult upper GI bleeding in children is often not from the GI tract. Although anal fissures account for most cases of occult blood in stools, the physician should always consider the possibility of a less benign cause (e.g., necrotizing enterocolitis or intussusception in the ill-looking neonate or infant). Occult bleeding may also presage other serious events, such as Meckel diverticulum.

Overt Bleeding

Administration of crystalloids (normal saline or Ringer lactate) to restore intravascular volume is the management priority. Blood is sent for urgent type and cross-match, or O-negative blood is made immediately available. The child who has lost 10% to 20% of his or her blood volume does not necessarily require blood replacement, provided that the bleeding has stopped. If, after 20% of the blood volume has been replaced by crystalloid and the child still has orthostatic hypotension, blood should be given. The child's age and physical condition may also dictate the need for blood; for example, children with heart and chronic lung disease may require earlier transfusion. Platelets, fresh-frozen plasma, or vitamin K (1 mg per year of age, up to 10 mg) is given as necessary to correct an identified coagulopathy. In the neonate suspected of vitamin K deficiency, vitamin K (1 mg) is given intramuscularly. Antacid therapy, H_2 blockers, and sucralfate have proven to be efficacious in minimizing or preventing bleeding in patients with stress or peptic ulcer from trauma, shock, or sepsis, if gastric pH levels are kept above 4. H_2 blockers are best given intravenously by continuous infusion. Ranitidine is the recommended agent at an intravenous dosage of 1.5 to 6 mg/kg/d, depending on the patients age (3).

Massive Bleeding

Aggressive fluid resuscitation and administration of blood components is the usual management, however, in some cases, endotracheal intubation, to secure the airway and decrease the work of breathing, is needed in a patient with low cardiac output. Endotracheal intubation allows adequate sedation without the risk of hypoventilation or aspiration, and also facilitates endoscopy. Continuous monitoring of vital signs, urine output with a urinary catheter, and oxygen saturation with pulse oximetry is essential. Central venous catheter placement, although not mandatory, may be helpful in monitoring the vascular volume status.

Management of the child with massive variceal bleeding from portal hypertension may include intravenous vasopressin (0.1 to 0.4 U/min), variceal injection, or ligation using endoscopy (1). Recently, the use of intravenous somatostatin has been shown to control variceal bleeding in approximately 80% of patients. A loading dose of 1 to 2 µg/kg is administered intravenously over 2 to 5 minutes, followed by a continuous infusion of 1 to 2 µg/kg/hour (3).

Massive bleeding can also occur in children with Meckel diverticulum; these patients also require aggressive resuscitation initially. Following cardiovascular stabilization, the site of bleeding can be confirmed by a nuclear medicine scan or by arteriography.

If massive bleeding precludes stabilization, immediate laparotomy may be required.

DISPOSITION

Conditions that require urgent surgical evaluation include volvulus, vascular malformations, and necrotizing enterocolitis in the neonate. Some cases of GI bleeding from stress ulcers,

variceal bleeding, or intussusception may also require urgent surgical evaluation. The emergency physician should always be in direct communication with specialists who will assume inpatient care of the child. Consultation with a pediatric gastroenterologist, pediatric surgeon, and/or pediatric intensivist may be necessary early in management. Panendoscopy to establish a specific diagnosis and to assess the rapidity of bleeding, the risk of rebleeding, and, possibly, the administration of definitive therapy may be required.

During interhospital transfer, the child with GI bleeding is prone to compromise of the cardiorespiratory system. Oxygenation and vascular access with the administration of crystalloid are priorities if there is evidence of vascular compromise. Continuous monitoring to ensure an adequate airway and stable vital signs is mandatory. Although personnel skilled in advanced pediatric life support should accompany the child, attention to stabilization before transport should minimize the need for interventions during transport.

COMMON PITFALLS

- ✔ Assuming the colored material is blood. Many foods and medicines can give secretions or stools a bloody appearance
- ✔ Failing to perform an Apt test on a neonate's stool to rule out swallowed maternal blood
- ✔ Using the wrong-sized nasogastric tube. Smaller bore tubes may be adequate for assessing bleeding, but not for removing clots
- ✔ If the nasogastric aspirate does not sample duodenal contents, or if bleeding is intermittent, a false-negative aspirate may result
- ✔ A carelessly placed nasogastric tube may yield a false-positive aspirate and cause distress to the patient. Iodine, supplemental iron, and ingestion of red meat may cause false-positive results
- ✔ A normal hemoglobin level does not exclude significant, rapid GI bleeding
- ✔ A normal or increased blood pressure in children does not exclude hypovolemia
- ✔ Performing a barium study before endoscopy
- ✔ Not considering sexual abuse as a cause of anal fissures
- ✔ Failing to consider nonorganic causes (e.g., Munchausen syndrome by proxy) of GI bleeding

References

1. Alvarez F. Long-term treatment of bleeding caused by portal hypertension in children. *J Pediatr* 1997;131:798.
2. Chaibou M, Tucci M, Dugas MA, et al. Clinically significant upper gastrointestinal bleeding acquired in a pediatric intensive care unit: a prospective study. *Pediatrics* 1998;102:933.
3. Barnard JA Gastrointestinal polyps and polyposis syndromes in children. *Curr Opin Pediatr* 2002;14:576.
4. Erdman SH, Barnard JA Gastrointestinal polyps and polyposis syndromes in children. *Curr Opin Pediatr* 2002;14:576.
5. Felber S, Rosenthal P, Henton D. The BUN/Creatinine ratio in localizing GI bleeding in pediatric patients. *J Pediatr Gastroenterol Nutr* 1988;7:685.
6. Fox VL. Gastrointestinal bleeding in infancy and childhood. *Gastroenterol Clin North Am* 2000;29:37.
7. Fuchs G, Dewier M, Hutchinson S, et al. GI blood loss in older infants: impact of cow milk vs. formula. *J Pediatr Gastroenterol Nutr* 1993;16:4.
8. Gopalswamy N, Stelling HP, Markert RJ, et al. A comparative study of eight fecal occult blood tests and HemoQuant in patients in whom colonoscopy is indicated. *Arch Fam Med* 1994;12:1043.
9. Grand RJ, Ramakrishna J, Calenda KA. Inflammatory bowel disease in the pediatric patient. *Gastroenterol Clin North Am* 1995;24:613.
10. Kay MH, Wyllie R. Alcohol isn't for kids: endoscopic hemostasis of bleeding peptic ulcers in pediatric patients. *J Pediatr* 1998;133:802.
11. LiVoti G, Acierno C, Tulone V, et al. Relationship between upper gastrointestinal bleeding and nonsteroidal anti-inflammatory drugs in children. *Pediatr Surg Int* 1997;12:264.

12. McRury JM, Barry RC. A modified Apt test: a new look at an old test. *Pediatr Emerg Care* 1994;10:189.

13. O'Hara SM. Pediatric gastrointestinal nuclear imaging. *Radiol Clin North Am* 1996;34:845.

14. Pearl RH, Irish MS, Caty MG, et al. The approach to common abdominal diagnoses in infants and children. Part II. *Pediatr Clin North Am* 1998;45: 1287.

15. Peters JM. Management of Gastrointestinal bleeding in children. *Curr Treat Options Gastroenterol* 2002;5:399.

16. Racadio JM, Agha AK, Johnson ND, et al. Imaging and radiological interventional techniques for gastrointestinal bleeding in children. *Semin Pediatr Surg* 1999;8:181.

17. Riggs D, Weibley RE. Acute hemorrhagic diarrhea and cardiovascular collapse in a young child owing to environmentally acquired cocaine. *Pediatr Emerg Care* 1991;7:154.

18. Rogers BM. Gastrointestinal Hemorrhage *Pediatr Rev* 1999;20:171.

19. Sarda AK, Cannan R. Massive lower GI hemorrhage due to ascariasis. *Am J Gastroenterol* 1992;87:1233.

20. Squires RH. Gastrointestinal Bleeding. *Pediatr Rev* 1999;20:95.

21. Stringer, RH. McClean. RH. Treatment of oesophageal varices. *Arch Dis Child* 1997;77:476.

22. Teach SJ, Fleisher GR. Rectal bleeding in the pediatric emergency department. *Ann Emerg Med* 1994;32:1252.

23. Thompson EC, Brown MF, Bowen EC, et al. Causes of gastrointestinal hemorrhage in neonates and children. *South Med J* 1996;89:370.

24. Treem WR. Gastrointestinal bleeding in children. *Gastrointest Endosc Clin N Am* 1994;4:75.

25. Ukarapol N, Chartapisak W, Lertprasertsuk N, et al. Cytomegalovirus-associated manifestations involving the digestive tract in children with human immunodeficiency virus infection. *J Pediatr Gastroenterol Nutr* 2002;35:669.

CHAPTER 226
Headache

Laurie J. Burton and Harold K. Simon

Headaches are a common complaint among children presenting to the emergency department (ED), and are often associated with other systemic signs and symptoms that can help to determine their etiology. Headaches can be acute or chronic, recurrent or of new onset, and often vary in how they progress or resolve. The child's description of the duration, specific location and intensity is often difficult to elicit and make classification and treatment a challenge for the physician in the ED.

While often a diagnostic and management problem for physicians, headaches in children are equally frustrating and concerning for families. Families confronted with a child who complains of headache are often concerned with severe, life-threatening possibilities such as meningitis or intracranial lesions. For this reason, many families bring their children to an emergency center for evaluation. In addition, for those with chronic headaches, lack of symptomatic relief is a major precipitating factor for bringing a child for evaluation.

Even though most children with acute or chronic headaches do not have life-threatening etiologies or intracranial lesions, these must be of foremost concern for the ED physician and must be ruled out by a careful and detailed history and physical examination (3,4,6). An in-depth knowledge of the various presentations and causes of headache is therefore paramount for the ED physician.

Most children presenting to the ED are found to have headaches related to viral illnesses, sinusitis, stress, or migraines. Serious neurologic conditions are found in less than 7% of cases,

many of these being viral meningitis (2). Even so, one cannot be lulled into thinking that all children with the complaint of headache have relatively benign, nonlife-threatening concerns.

CLINICAL PRESENTATION

Headache is often a chief complaint, but it is more often part of a series of concerns. The complaint can be acute or chronic, intermittent or persistent, localized or focal, and mild to extremely intense. The severity of the presentation is related to the general appearance of the child, historic, and physical findings, as well as associated signs and symptoms. Most commonly, the concern of headache is associated with viral or self-limited illnesses. Emotional problems and new types of stress (school or home) should be identified.

Certain historical and physical findings raise the suspicion for significant medical conditions. These include historical findings of sudden onset of headache, visual disturbances, weight loss, morning vomiting, neck pain, significant changes in behavior, and persistent and unremitting headache. Chronic progressive headaches, or headaches that are increasing in frequency or severity over time, have a significant association with intracranial pathology. Physical findings on presentation that would point toward more worrisome conditions include ill appearance of the child, change in mental status, focality on neurologic examination, papilledema, retinal hemorrhages, cranial bruits, nuchal rigidity, fever with petechiae or purpura, café-au-lait spots, hypertension, or signs of nonaccidental trauma.

The two most commonly seen primary headache disorders in the pediatric population are migraine and tension headaches. It may be difficult to distinguish the two types in some pediatric patients, but it is important to do so, because the treatments are somewhat different. Children with migraine headaches usually have a positive family history. Migraines are often bilateral in children, as opposed to the unilateral presentation commonly seen in adults. The pain is often throbbing or pulsatile located in the regions of the eye, forehead, and temple. The headache may last anywhere from less than an hour up to 72 hours. It is often associated with nausea and vomiting, and it may be preceded by an aura. Light, noise, and movement usually aggravate the pain. A history of motion sickness can often be elicited in children with migraine headaches. Tension headaches, on the other hand, are usually bandlike and nonpulsatile in quality; lack the nausea, vomiting, photophobia, and phonophobia components; and do not have an aura (1,8). Environmental triggers, anxiety, and depression are often associated with tension headaches.

DIFFERENTIAL DIAGNOSIS

The differential diagnosis of pediatric headache is outlined in Figure 226.1.

EMERGENCY DEPARTMENT EVALUATION

A complete history often points the clinician toward the correct diagnosis and helps identify concerns for an underlying serious neurologic condition, including central nervous system (CNS) infection or structural pathology. All patients seen in the ED with a complaint of headache must have a complete set of vital signs, including measurement of temperature and blood pressure. A complete physical examination is useful diagnostically, and there are several highlights to mention.

The best assessment of CNS "well-being," or perfusion and oxygenation, is the level of consciousness. In the HEENT exam, any signs of trauma, minor infections such as pharyngitis, otitis

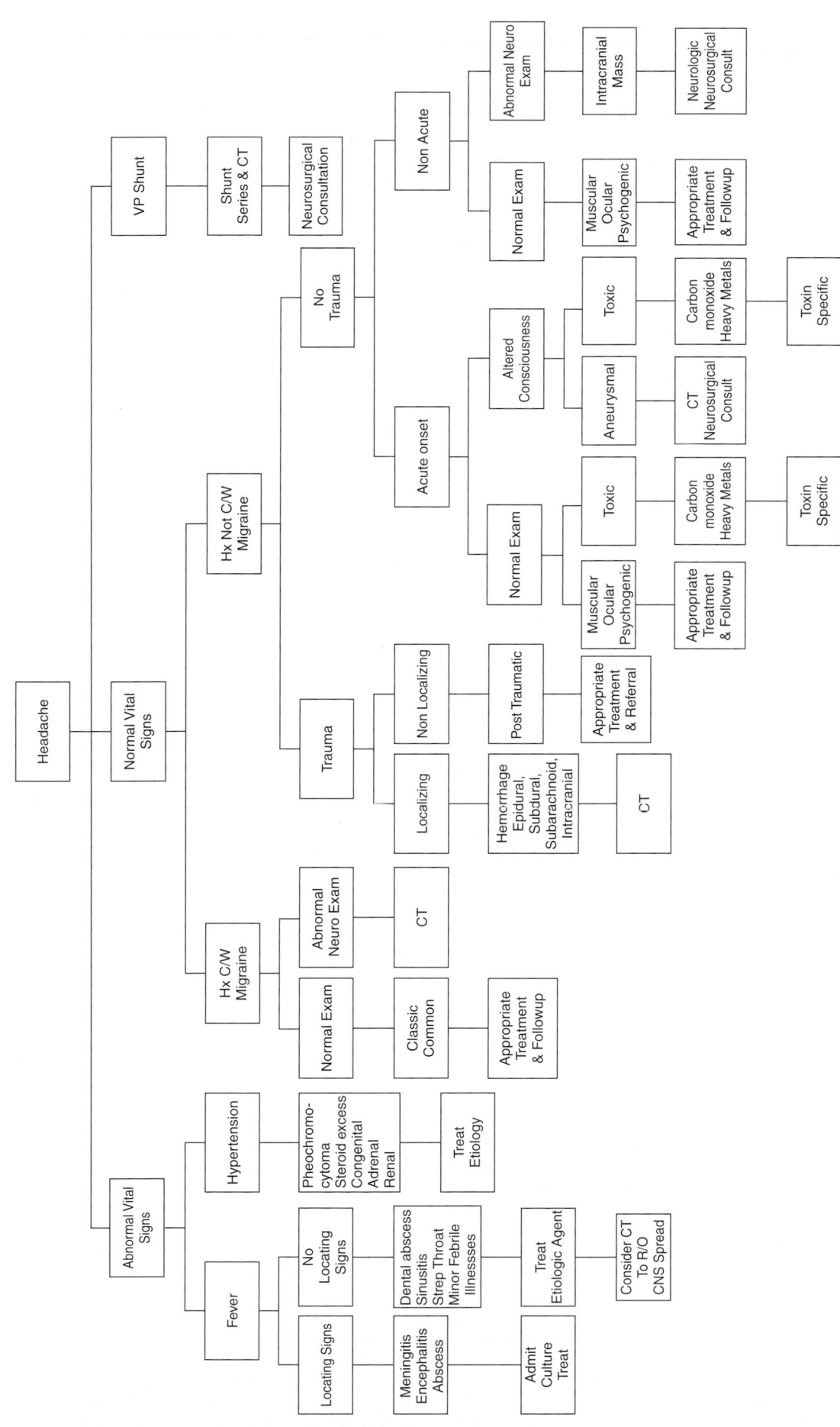

Figure 226.1. Differential diagnosis of headache in the pediatric patient.

media, or sinus tenderness could be diagnostic. Given that the frontal sinuses become pneumatized between the ages of 6 to 10 years, there is potential for frontal sinus infection in children aged 6 and older. The patient with frontal sinusitis may have tenderness in the forehead above the inner canthus of the eye. The teeth and gums should be checked carefully for signs of caries or abscesses.

Auscultation for a cranial bruit, a very rare finding, can be attempted. The neck should be examined carefully for signs of meningismus, especially for Brudzinski and Kernig signs. In the infant, the fontanelle should be checked for bulging, indicative of increased intracranial pressure from such causes as CNS infection or structural pathology. Fundoscopy should be attempted on every patient with headache. Although papilledema may not be present early in the patient with increased intracranial pressure, the presence of venous pulsations would effectively rule it out. Retinal hemorrhages are indicative of child abuse until proven otherwise. Performing a neurologic examination is fundamental in the evaluation of patients with headache.

Laboratory evaluation is clinically guided and may include a rapid streptococcal throat screen or culture, sinus radiographs or sinus CT, lumbar puncture, toxicology assays in patients with altered consciousness or carbon monoxide exposure, and pregnancy testing. Radiographic evidence of sinusitis on plain films includes air-fluid levels, mucosal thickening of greater than 4 to 5 mm, or complete opacification. Indications for lumbar puncture include any patient with fever and meningismus, bulging fontanelle, or suspicion of subarachnoid hemorrhage.

In the child who has abnormal neurologic findings, controversy exists over whether to perform a lumbar puncture prior to or after a computed tomography (CT) scan. A CT scan confirms there are no signs of increased intracranial pressure that could precipitate herniation. If a lumbar puncture is undertaken prior to CT scan, the risk can best be minimized with the use of a small-bore needle. Obtaining an opening pressure is critical if there is suspicion of intracranial hypertension.

Indications for a CT scan of the head include abnormal neurologic findings without a clear etiology. More specific indications include recurrent morning headaches, persistent emesis without clear etiology, paroxysmal onset of excruciating headache, or head trauma with severe headache. The clinician should have a low threshold for obtaining a head CT scan in the following types of pediatric patients: the infant with persistent irritability of unclear etiology, the child under 5 years of age with severe headache, the sickle cell or bleeding diathesis patient with headache, and the ventriculoperitoneal (VP) shunt patient with headache. For the patient with a VP shunt and headache, a shunt series should also be obtained to ensure there is no shunt disconnection or migration. Lastly, the pediatric patient with sinus tenderness and severe persistent headache could have contiguous CNS spread from the sinuses best diagnosed by CT of head and sinuses.

In the patient with a migraine headache associated with neurologic deficits, or a "complicated migraine," CNS imaging is recommended to confirm the diagnosis. The preferred imaging test, if available, is magnetic resonance imaging with and without gadolinium. Otherwise, a head CT without contrast will suffice.

EMERGENCY DEPARTMENT MANAGEMENT

Treatment of the patient with headache should be based on the presumptive diagnosis. Most tension headaches or headaches due to minor illnesses can be treated successfully in the pediatric population simply with analgesics such as ibuprofen (in patients over 6 months of age) and acetaminophen. Migraines deserve special mention. Currently, there are no specific practice guidelines for migraine headaches in the pediatric population. Several classes of drugs are used to treat the acute migraine, including various analgesics, vasoconstrictors, serotonin agonists and antiemetic sedatives. If the patient suffers from chronic migraines, the best approach might be to ask what medications have successfully aborted attacks in the past. Milder migraine pain often responds to acetaminophen, ibuprofen, a quiet dark room, and rest. With more moderate pain, ketorolac can be given parenterally in lieu of ibuprofen, at a dosage of 1 mg/kg (maximum 30 mg IV, 60 mg IM.)

Management of a child over 12 years of age is similar to that of an adult, and a serotonin agonist such as sumatriptan can be given intranasally or orally at a dose of 25 mg or subcutaneously at a dose of 6 mg (1). When using these agents, it is important to made a correct diagnosis of migraine, because the serotonin agonists do not work well in patients with tension or other types of headache. Care should be taken not to mix the serotonin agonists with the ergotamines, because side effects can be potentiated. Neither the serotonin agonists nor the ergotamines should be used to treat complicated migraines. Ergotamines are often chosen to treat the most severe migraine attacks. They are contraindicated in the pregnant patient. A frequently used ergotamine in the intractable migraine patient aged is dihydroergotamine (DHE) at a dose of 0.5 mg IV or 1 mg subcutaneously in children >10 years of age (1,4,7). Opioids should be avoided in patients with recurrent headache disorders to avoid dependency (4).

Regarding the younger child, analgesics such as acetaminophen and ibuprofen are first-line therapy. In a vomiting child, acetaminophen can be given rectally at a dose of 30 mg/kg (1). Anecdotally, sumatriptan has been shown to be effective even in children as young as 4 years of age. Dosages of sumatriptan in the young child are 1 mg/kg, maximum 50 mg orally; 0.6 mg/kg, maximum 6 mg subcutaneously; or 5 to 10 mg intranasally (1,7). Another option in the younger child with more severe migraine pain is to induce sleep. Antiemetic-sedatives are employed for this purpose, such as promethazine (Phenergan) 1 mg/kg per dose PO, PR, IM or IV, maximum 25 mg. This approach is especially useful if the patient is nauseated or vomiting (4).

Of late, overuse of analgesics of any class has been recognized as a cause of headache. These "analgesic abuse headaches" have been well described in adults but are being more widely recognized as occurring in children of all ages. There should be a high index of suspicion especially if the child is regularly receiving analgesia more than three days a week. Limiting the analgesic use provides the headache relief (4,5,7).

DISPOSITION

There are several scenarios involving the pediatric patient with headache wherein consultation is indicated. Neurosurgical consultation should be sought for any patient with CNS hemorrhage or midline shift. If the etiology of the bleed is from trauma and no neurosurgical support is available at the site of care, stabilization and transfer should be expedited. Consultation with a neurologist should be considered for a patient with focal neurologic findings or unexplained altered mental status, as well as for patients with papilledema, severe migraine unresponsive to medical management, and head CT showing mass lesion that is not felt to be a CNS bleed. Complicated migraines also warrant consultation with a neurologist. Such migraines, by definition, are associated with abnormal neurologic findings. Examples include migraine with hemiplegia, ataxia, transient blindness or visual field defect, acute confusional state, Alice-in-Wonderland syndrome (visual hallucinations wherein objects appear distorted in size), and olfactory or gustatory hallucinations. Toxicology consultation with the local poison center should be considered in high-risk populations, such as the adolescent with altered mental status.

Indications for hospital admission include pain control that cannot be maintained in an outpatient setting, altered mental status or focal neurologic findings, suspected increased intracranial pressure, possible bacterial meningitis or encephalitis, severe headache after head trauma, complicated frontal sinusitis, or any CNS pathology.

Patients discharged from the ED should be encouraged to seek medical attention if the headache worsens, changes, or persists for more than 2 to 3 days. They should also be encouraged to see their primary care provider to ensure proper follow up and to avoid delays in diagnosis of inapparent or undeclared structural lesions. The patient and family should be encouraged to keep a headache diary (time of onset, activity, symptoms, medications, etc) to present to the primary care provider or neurologist.

CRITICAL INTERVENTIONS

- All children with headache should have a screening blood pressure. The normal value for the systolic blood pressure in children can be approximated by the formula 2 x patient's age (in years) + 90 mm Hg. Diastolic blood pressure is approximately two-thirds of that value
- In the setting of head trauma, do not forget about the possibility of occult neck injury
- Always perform an opening pressure on the patient with headache who is undergoing a lumbar puncture. Many pediatric lumbar puncture kits do not come with manometers. One should be secured in advance, ideally before the first drop of cerebrospinal fluid is obtained
- Have a low threshold for obtaining a head CT in children with frontal sinusitis and severe, persistent headache. Frontal sinusitis spreading to CNS involvement is not uncommon, particularly in the adolescent population
- Perform a full physical examination including a neurologic examination. Always palpate the anterior fontanelle in infants less than 1 year of age. It may be "full," especially if the infant is crying, but it should not bulge over the dimensions of the scalp. Life-threatening causes of a bulging fontanelle include not only CNS infection, but also CNS hemorrhage or edema, possibly from abuse. In the ambulatory child, the presence of up-going toes is indicative of CNS pathology, whereas the preambulatory child has a Babinski reflex normally

COMMON PITFALLS

✔ Assuming that a child is just sleepy because it is either naptime or late at night. Subtle signs of altered mental status can be easy to miss during the overnight hours. In this scenario, one should have a lower threshold to obtain ancillary testing such as head CT and toxicology screening

✔ Meningismus can be a sign not only of CNS infection, but also of occult cervical spine injury or subarachnoid hemorrhage, the latter seen in the pediatric patient almost exclusively in the perinatal period

✔ Failure to perform a head CT with contrast in a patient presenting more than 7 days posttrauma. CT scanning of the head without contrast beyond this period may miss an intracranial bleed, because the breakdown of blood often causes it to be isodense with surrounding tissue. The use of contrast may be warranted

✔ Failure to recognize that recurrent headaches awakening a child from sleep, occurring upon morning awakening, or associated with head tilt are well known signs of a mass lesion, especially in the young child

References

1. Annequin D, Tourniaire B, Massiou H. Migraine and headache in childhood and adolescence. *Pediatr Clin North Am* 2000;47:617–631.
2. Burton L, Quinn B, Pratt-Chaney J, Pourani M. Headache etiology in the pediatric emergency department. *Pediatr Emerg Care* 1997;13:1–4.
3. Cruz MN, Schor J, Simon HK. The emergency department headaches conundrum. *Pediatr Emerg Care* 1997;13:437–440.
4. Forsyth R, Farrell K. Headache in childhood. *Pediatr Rev* 1999;20:39–45.
5. Guidetti V, Galli F. Recent development in paediatric headache. *Curr Opin Neurol* 2001;14:335–340.
6. Lewis DW, Ashwal S, Dahl G, et al. Practice parameter: evaluation of children and adolescents with recurrent headaches: report of the Quality Standards Subcommittee of the American Academy of Neurology and the Practice Committee of the Child Neurology Society. *Neurology* 2002;59:490–498.
7. Linder SL, Winner P. Pediatric headache. *Med Clin North Am* 2001;85:1037–1053.
8. Pakalnis A. New avenues in treatment of paediatric migraine: a review of the literature. *Fam Pract* 2001;18:101–106.

CHAPTER 227
Heart Murmurs

Annalise Sorrentino and Steven Baldwin

The discovery of a heart murmur or other abnormal auscultatory finding during assessment of a pediatric patient in the emergency department (ED) is often anxiety provoking for the patient, family, and clinician because of fear of finding a serious underlying cardiovascular problem. Such findings are usually nonspecific and their definitive evaluation is not usually part of the repertoire of emergency physicians. There is no universally applicable algorithm that allows the ED clinician to sort out the numerous potential issues and conditions. Referral of all heart murmur patients to a specialist is costly, further escalates patient/caretaker anxiety, and has a low yield of significant findings. On the other hand insightful recognition of characteristics that make significant cardiovascular issues more likely can make a difference in outcomes.

This chapter will address abnormal auscultation findings in pediatric patients that may arise during patient assessment in the ED. Referral to a more expansive or condition-specific resource may be needed for particular cases. Involvement of a pediatric cardiologist may be needed for patients with equivocal or definite risk for significant cardiac disease.

CLINICAL PRESENTATION

Most commonly, a heart murmur will be detected on a child as an incidental finding. The ED physician should be aware of factors that may increase the chances of a murmur indicating potential underlying cardiac pathology. These factors include:

1. Other significant symptoms (i.e., chest pain, syncope, shortness of breath, failure to thrive, cyanosis)
2. Positive family history for sudden death or Marfan syndrome
3. Loud/harsh sounding murmur
4. Underlying congenital syndrome (i.e., Down syndrome)
5. Active precordium

6. Decreased pulses, especially femoral
7. Abnormal S2
8. Clicks
9. Murmur that becomes louder with standing
10. Hepatosplenomegaly (3)

EMERGENCY DEPARTMENT EVALUATION

There are essentially two phases to applying cardiac auscultation clinically. The first phase is to perform the physical examination. The second phase is combining the physical exam with the history to detect potential pathology. Studies have shown that auscultatory skills in pediatric residents have room for improvement (2). For physicians who do not evaluate children on a regular basis, this can be even more challenging.

Before beginning the examination the clinician should try to restrict the amount of ambient noise as much as possible. Trying to establish rapport with young patients will often help improve patient cooperation and reduce the problem of crying during the examination. Allowing the patient to be held by their caretaker is often of benefit as is distraction. A pacifier or nursing may help quiet crying infants. It is better to perform auscultation prior to performing other more noxious portions of the patient examination.

Most heart sounds in infants and children can be adequately heard with an adult stethoscope, although a pediatric-sized stethoscope may be of some benefit when evaluating a small child.

It is helpful to perform a screening survey of the precordium with the stethoscope. The examiner then needs to rigorously listen to the heart in each of the cardinal positions (right upper sternal border (RUSB), left upper sternal border (LUSB), left lower sternal border (LLSB), and the apex in turn for several cardiac cycles (see Figure 227.1 for diagram of auscultation positions). S1 and S2 should be clearly defined. Distinguishing S1 and S2 can often be facilitated by palpating a central pulse simultaneously with auscultation. Once S1 and S2 are clearly defined the examiner should focus on the interval between S1 and S2 (systole) exclusively and identify whether or not there are any murmurs (or other sounds) heard during this interval. The same process of exclusively listening should then be applied to the interval between S2 and S1 (diastole). Again any murmurs or other sounds should be carefully noted and characterized. The clinician should likewise identify S1, S2, extra sounds between S1 and S2, and

extra sounds between S2 and S1 at each of the cardinal positions on the chest. Next determine the point of maximal loudness and points of radiation of the extra sounds between S1 and S2 and between S2 and S1. This can be done by moving the stethoscope back and forth between the areas where the sounds are heard. In addition, specifically listening over the carotids, subclavian areas, and the back may identify some radiation patterns.

By correlating the timing of the noise with the cardiac cycle one can generate a preliminary differential diagnosis of the sounds heard. This can be further refined by correlating the anatomical position where the noise is best heard and the radiation pattern. See Tables 227.1 and 227.2 for differential diagnoses of systolic and diastolic murmurs, respectively.

In classifying pediatric heart murmurs, certain characteristics are important to note. They include intensity, timing, location, transmission, and quality. Intensity is typically graded on a scale of 1 to 6:

Grade I	Barely audible
Grade II	Soft, but easily audible
Grade III	Louder; heard in a noisy child
Grade IV	Louder; + thrill
Grade V	Audible with edge of stethoscope on chest wall
Grade VI	Audible with stethoscope off chest wall

This can be a very subjective finding, and is also affected by certain physiologic states commonly seen in children, such as fever or anxiety (1).

If there is concern for a pathologic murmur, further testing may be indicated. If hypoxia is demonstrated during oximetry monitoring, then a trial of oxygen with note of response is typically documented. Chest radiographs are usually obtained, and may be of assistance in evaluating heart size and shape, as well as pulmonary vasculature. Some "classic" chest x-ray findings of congenital heart disease include:

1. Transposition of the great arteries = "egg on a string" with ↑ pulmonary markings
2. Tetralogy of Fallot = "boot shaped" with ↓ pulmonary markings
3. Total anomalous pulmonary venous circulation = normal heart with ↓ pulmonary markings
4. Ebstein anomaly (tricuspid regurgitation) = cardiomegaly with ↓ pulmonary markings (6)

Electrocardiograms are often done, although studies have shown that they are unlikely to change the clinical diagnosis made by auscultation. If clinical suspicion is high for cardiac pathology, an echocardiogram should be performed (5).

DIFFERENTIAL DIAGNOSIS

Heart murmurs and other abnormal auscultatory findings related to the cardiovascular system are believed to be related to abnormal vibrations induced in cardiac structures, vessel walls, or blood. The underlying cause of the vibrations that lead to the abnormal sound(s) can be induced by abnormal anatomic and/or physiologic conditions. The anatomic and/or physiologic pathology can be primary or secondary to other conditions. Many specific conditions can therefore result in associated abnormal cardiovascular auscultatory findings. (See Table 227.3 for pathophysiologic themes that can cause or affect heart murmurs and related auscultatory findings.)

Innocent Murmurs

More than 80% of children have what are known as innocent, or functional, murmurs (1). They usually begin around age 3 years.

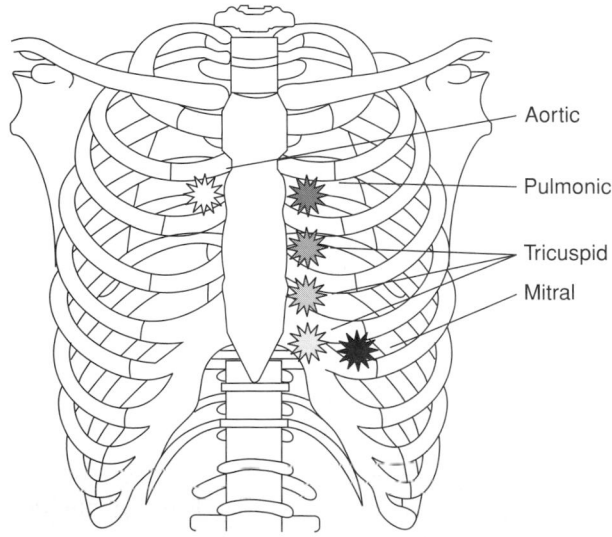

Aortic

Pulmonic

Tricuspid

Mitral

Figure 227.1. Auscultation positions.

TABLE 227.1.   Differential Diagnosis of Systolic Murmurs

Condition	Type/Physical Findings	Location
Pulmonary valve stenosis	Ejection ± thrill	LUSB
Atrial septal defect	Ejection Fixed, split S2	LUSB
Pulmonary flow murmur	Ejection Transmission to back	LUSB/Back
Pulmonary artery stenosis	Ejection Transmission to back	LUSB/Back
Aortic stenosis	Ejection ± thrill	LUSB
Tetralogy of Fallot	Ejection Cyanosis	LUSB
Coarctation of the aorta	Ejection Weak femoral pulses	LUSB
Patent ductus arteriosus	Continuous Bounding pulses	LUSB/ Infraclavicular
Total anomalous pulmonary venous circulation	Ejection Cyanosis	LUSB
Aortic valve stenosis	Ejection Transmission to neck	RUSB/ Neck
Ventricular septal defect	Regurgitant May be holosystolic	LLSB
Vibratory murmur	Ejection	LLSB
Idiopathic hypertrophic subaortic stenosis	Ejection	LLSB
Tricuspid regurgitation	Regurgitant cyanosis	LLSB
Mitral regurgitation	Regurgitant Transmission to left axilla	Apex/Left axilla
Mitral valve prolapse	Click Thoracic skeletal abnormalities	Apex

LUSB, left upper sternal border; RUSB, right upper sternal border.

All functional murmurs are heightened in high output states such as fever. Innocent murmurs are associated with a normal electrocardiogram (ECG) and chest x-ray. The challenge comes in deciding which murmurs are innocent, and which need referral to the cardiologist. Referral is recommended for the following: cyanosis, diastolic murmur, Grade 3 or greater systolic murmur, abnormal ECG, abnormal heart size or pulmonary markings on CXR, and abnormal pulses or heart sounds.

TABLE 227.2.   Differential Diagnosis of Diastolic Murmurs

Condition	Type/Physical Findings	Location
Aortic regurgitation	Early diastolic Transmission to apex Bounding pulses	LUSB
Pulmonary regurgitation	Early diastolic	LUSB
Mitral stenosis	Middiastolic "rumble"	Apex
Tricuspid stenosis	Middiastolic	LLSB

TABLE 227.3.   Pathophysiologic Factors Affecting Auscultation

Underlying Pathology	Examples
Primary anatomic defects	Congenital heart disease Vascular abnormalities
Secondary anatomic defects	Acquired cardiac or vascular disease due to: Illness Injury Surgery
Primary physiologic defects	Cardiomyopathy
Secondary physiologic defects	Anemia Hypertension Surgical devices Fever

TABLE 227.4. "Normal" Murmurs in Infants and Children

Murmur	Characteristics
Still's	Vibratory, musical quality at LLSB to apex: louder in supine position; disappears with Valsalva
Pulmonary flow	Raspy quality at ULSB; normal S2; not heard in back
Venous hum	Loudest in seated position; disappears when supine; continuous (systolic-diastolic)
Carotid bruits	Short ejection murmurs over one or both clavicles to carotids
"Physiologic" PPS	Short ejection murmur with quality of breath sounds; heard in axillae and back; age <6 months

LLSB, lower left sternal border; PPS, peripheral pulmonic stenosis; S2, second heart sound; ULSB, upper left sternal border.

Two types of innocent murmurs are vibratory murmurs (i.e., Still murmurs) and pulmonary flow murmurs. Vibratory murmurs are typically detected in children greater than 2 years of age. They are midsystolic, ejection type murmurs, most audible along the midleft sternal border, or between the LLSB and the apex. They are best heard with the bell of the stethoscope, with the patient in the supine position. The murmur may disappear with a Valsalva maneuver. Occasionally, these murmurs may be confused with a VSD, but a VSD is usually accompanied by a thrill, and is regurgitant in character.

Pulmonary flow murmurs are seen in infancy, and then again in adolescence. They are best heard at the LUSB, and are midsystolic, ejection-type murmurs. In infants, it usually disappears by the age of 3 to 6 months. Characteristically, they radiate to the axillae and back.

Another type of innocent murmur is a venous hum. Classically, venous hums are heard in children 3 to 6 years of age. This sound is produced by turbulent flow through the jugular veins. This is a continuous murmur best heard in the infra- and supraclavicular areas. These are only heard when the patient is upright, and can be extinguished by placing the patient in the supine position, or by rotating the head. A venous hum can sometimes be confused with the murmur of a patent ductus arteriosus (PDA), but can be distinguished by performing the above measures. See Table 227.4 for a summary of innocent murmurs.

Systolic Murmurs

Most pediatric heart murmurs occur between S1 and S2, making them systolic in nature. Murmurs that occur during systole result from events related to ventricular contraction and consequent blood movement. Because blood flow through a ventricular septal defect begins almost simultaneously with the onset of ventricular contraction and ceases essentially simultaneously with the end of systole, these murmurs tend to be holosystolic (S1 may even be unidentifiable). Systolic murmurs due to valvular abnormalities are usually heard sometime after systole begins and end sometime before systole ends. This is because the blood flow across the valve takes a moment to escalate as systole begins and slows as systole is ending. As a result these types of murmurs tend to be midsystolic and crescendo-decrescendo in character.

Systolic murmurs are further classified into one of two groups: ejection or regurgitant, depending on the onset of the murmur in relation to S1. Ejection type murmurs are typically caused by a stenotic valve, and are usually crescendo-decrescendo. There is a brief interval between S1 and the beginning of the murmur, which, in less severe cases, will end prior to S2. Any systolic murmur that is not regurgitant can be classified as an ejection-type murmur.

A systolic murmur caused by a regurgitant valve begins at the same time as S1, and often times will continue through to S2. These murmurs are only seen with ventricular septal defect (VSD), mitral regurgitation (MR), and tricuspid regurgitation (TR).

Once a systolic murmur is classified as either ejection-type or regurgitant, it is important to note where the murmur is best heard. This can help to differentiate between otherwise very similar sounding murmurs. Usually, this is documented as either left upper sternal LUSB, LLSB, RUSB, or apical. See Table 227.1 for murmurs typically heard at each of these locations. Transmission of the murmur is also very helpful in determining the etiology. Murmurs that transmit to the back are often pulmonary valve or artery in nature, while those transmitted to the neck are typically aortic in origin (4).

Diastolic Murmurs

Diastolic murmurs are less common than systolic murmurs, and are heard between S2 and S1 (4). Murmurs that occur during diastole result from blood flow problems that arise either due to problems with atrial to ventricular flow or problems with backflow from either of the great arteries. They are divided into 3 categories: early diastolic, middiastolic, and presystolic.

Early diastolic murmurs start immediately after S2 and are caused by a regurgitant aortic or pulmonary valve. Aortic regurgitation (AR) is heard best with the diaphragm of the stethoscope, and radiates to the apex. Bounding distal pulses may be present. These murmurs are typically heard with congenital bicuspid aortic valve, rheumatic heart disease, subaortic stenosis, and postoperative aortic stenosis (AS) (s/p valvotomy).

Pulmonary regurgitation (PR) is also heard early in diastole, and radiates along the left sternal border. This murmur is heard with postoperative Tetralogy of Fallot (surgically induced), pulmonary hypertension, postoperative pulmonary stenosis (PS), and congenital malformation of the pulmonary valve.

Middiastolic murmurs start with an S3 and are heard either in early or middiastole. They are best heard with the bell of the stethoscope. These murmurs are originated by stenosis of the mitral or tricuspid valves. Mitral middiastolic murmurs are best heard at the apex and often referred to as an "apical rumble." These are often caused by mitral stenosis (MS), or possibly a VSD or patent ductus arteriosus (PDA) causing relative MS. Tricuspid middiastolic murmurs are best heard along the LLSB. These are most often associated with an atrial septal defect (ASD), or total anomalous pulmonary venous return (TAPVR), as these conditions cause relative tricuspid stenosis (TS).

Presystolic murmurs result from active atrial contraction propelling blood into the ventricle, as opposed to the passive filling of the ventricle from a pressure gradient. These occur late in diastole, or just prior to systole, and are due to true MS or TS.

Continuous Murmurs

Continuous heart murmurs begin in systole and continue throughout diastole. They are caused by arteriovenous or aortopulmonary connections (PDA, arteriovenous fistula, surgical shunt), venous flow disturbance (hums), and arterial flow disturbance (coarctation of the aorta, pulmonary artery stenosis). Murmurs associated with a PDA are best heard over the LUSB, and are crescendo-decrescendo in nature. Pulmonary artery stenosis may be heard over the anterior chest and also radiating to the sides and back.

Anatomic Localization/Radiation Patterns

The area of the chest where a murmur is heard can help suggest the underlying lesion. Beware that anatomic correlation is not always accurate or reliable but it is still worthwhile. Systolic murmurs tend to be heard best over the forward moving blood that is causing the noise. Hence aortic valve stenosis problems are usually heard best superior to the aortic valve (RUSB) and pulmonic valve stenosis problems are usually heard best superior to the pulmonic valve (LUSB). Aortic valve lesions also will tend to create murmurs that radiate to the carotids. In contrast, ventricular septal defect murmurs are usually heard loudest at the mid or lower sternal border and tend to radiate in the direction of the cross-septal jet. Patent ductus arteriosus murmurs tend to localize to the left sternal border/subclavian area and radiate to the back or scapula in the direction of the patent ductus arteriosus jet (from the posterior wall of the aorta to the anterior wall of the pulmonary artery). Diastolic murmurs tend to be heard best behind the flowing blood that is causing the murmur. Mitral murmurs tend to be heard over the apex/left lateral chest wall and tricuspid murmurs tend to be heard at the lower sternal border.

Some children have pulmonary to systemic shunts done as a palliative measure for congenital heart defects. These shunts can be of several types. Some connect the pulmonary artery to a subclavian artery (usually right side). Others connect the pulmonary artery to the aorta. Children with these types of shunts should have a murmur. If such a child has a known history of such a shunt or a suggestive surgical scar on the chest the examiner should carefully auscultate the entire chest to ascertain whether or not a shunt murmur is present. If the child has new or progressive cardiac and/or pulmonary symptoms and no shunt murmur can be heard then a clotted/nonfunctioning shunt should be considered as a possible problem and a cardiologist should probably be contacted emergently to evaluate the shunt more definitively with ultrasound or other means.

EMERGENCY DEPARTMENT MANAGEMENT

Findings on cardiac auscultation must be placed into context with a physical examination that focuses on the cardiovascular and pulmonary systems. Key components include examination of skin perfusion and color, pulses with respect to intensity and regularity, liver and spleen size, presence or absence of edema, respiratory rate, lung sounds, fingertips (looking for clubbing), and precordial palpation (for heaves and thrills). By synthesizing such findings the clinician can usually get an impression of whether or not there is a pathophysiologic syndrome present and possibly some sense of an underlying anatomic correlate. For example signs of peripheral edema, hepatosplenomegaly, and systemic venous congestion would suggest right heart failure syndrome. Signs of cyanosis suggest a right-to-left shunt syndrome. An example of anatomic correlation would be coarctation of the aorta suggested by left heart failure syndrome with decreased pulse amplitude in the lower extremities.

For the patient that has significant pathology associated with a murmur, treatment should be targeted toward treating the underlying condition or symptoms. Attempts should be made to maintain adequate airway, breathing, and circulation. Once those are achieved, further therapy should be initiated as needed by each particular patient. This may include fluid resuscitation, diuretics, antihypertensives, or vasoactive pressors. Often these decisions are made with the assistance of a pediatric cardiologist.

Electronic stethoscopes are becoming available and include recording of heart sounds with download recording features in real or slowed time. The sound file can be converted to a phonocardiogram very quickly after it is downloaded to a computer. This may facilitate interpretation of auscultation findings and telemedicine opportunities. The phonocardiogram tracing or actual sound recording file can be attached to the medical record to allow more effective communication among the team caring for the patient.

Patients with known or suspected valvar heart disease, prosthetic cardiovascular grafts or patches, or other indications should receive appropriate antibiotics for perioperative prophylaxis against subacute bacterial endocarditis whenever a procedure that poses this risk is performed.

CRITICAL INTERVENTIONS

- Take a good history. Find out if there is a known heart murmur or history of cardiac surgery. The absence of a pulmonary to systemic shunt murmur in a child known to have such a shunt is worrisome. Children who become dehydrated may clot off their grafts or shunts. This can cause significant circulatory problems and lead to cardiovascular collapse if not recognized
- Determine if the patient has significant pulmonary or cardiovascular symptoms and clinical findings that mandate a chest x-ray or ECG to facilitate diagnosis and followup
- Determine if the patient has a physiologic stressor that could cause a secondary auscultatory finding. This is commonly seen in anemia states

DISPOSITION

The vast majority of pediatric patients evaluated in the ED with a heart murmur will not need cardiology referral. Children that require referral or immediate hospitalization are the ones that reveal other concerning symptoms in addition to the heart murmur.

Many times, reassurance for the family is the only therapy needed. If there is any doubt that a murmur is innocent, however, referral to a pediatric cardiologist is warranted. If this is the case, communication with the family as well as the child's primary physician is essential. Parents should know what symptoms to monitor for, and when to return to the ED. Often times, school-age children are given activity restrictions until follow up can be arranged.

COMMON PITFALLS

✔ Assuming all heart murmurs are innocent in children
✔ Failing to recognize that innocent murmurs are accentuated by high output states such as anemia and fever
✔ Alarming parents and patients when a murmur is heard during ED evaluation before completing a full history and exam
✔ Failing to provide SBE when indicated

Acknowledgment

Thanks to the previous edition's chapter author Edward J. Bayne.

References

1. Feit, LR. The heart of the matter: Evaluating murmurs in children. *Contemporary Pediatrics* 1997;14:97–122.
2. Gaskin, PR, et al. Clinical Auscultation Skills in Pediatric Residents. *Pediatrics* 2000;105:1184–1187.
3. McConnell, ME, et al. Heart Murmurs in Pediatric Patients: When do you refer? *American Family Physician* 1999;60:558–565.
4. Park MK. Physical Examination. In: *Pediatric Cardiology for Practitioners*, 3rd ed. St. Louis: Mosby, 1996:22–33.
5. Smythe, JF, et al. Initial evaluation of heart murmurs: are laboratory tests necessary? *Pediatrics* 1990;86:497–500.
6. Welch J. Pediatric Heart Sounds and Murmurs. http://gucfm.georgetown.edu. Cited: October 2003.

CHAPTER 228
Hematuria

Lina Abujamra and Madeline Matar Joseph

Hematuria is the presence of blood in the urine, which usually alarms the patient, the parents, and the physician. It can be macroscopic (visible to the naked eye) or microscopic. Microscopic hematuria represents one of the most frequently encountered genitourinary abnormalities in children, occurring in 0.5% to 6.0% of school-age children undergoing routine screening (23). Currently, the American Academy of Pediatrics recommends performance of a screening urinalysis at school entry (ages 4 to 5 years) and one time during adolescence. The prevalence of hematuria is 0.5% for boys and 1.0% for girls, with an annual new case incidence of 0.4% for both sexes. In the absence of gross hematuria, the primary tool for hematuria screening is a urine dipstick. Blood +1 and greater is considered positive. The dipsticks used for detection of blood in the urine are very sensitive in detecting red blood cells (RBCs) as well as minute amounts of free hemoglobin and myoglobin. All positive dipstick screens should be confirmed by a microscopic examination of the urine to confirm the presence of RBCs and exclude false positive and negative dipstick results. Causes of false-positive dipstick reactions include myoglobinuria (rhabdomyolysis); hemoglobinuria (seen in conditions causing hemolysis); oxidizing contaminants, such as bacterial peroxidases from a urinary tract infection (UTI); delay in reading the dipstick; and interfering compounds, such as beets or aniline dyes. A false-negative dipstick result can occur in urine with high specific gravity and in urine containing large amounts of a reducing agent, such as ascorbic acid.

The definition of *hematuria* is somewhat arbitrary. The presence of five to ten erythrocytes by high power field (HPF), in a-centrifuged urine, is considered significant by a number of authors (24). Hematuria can originate from any part of the urinary tract. Localizing the source of the bleeding to the kidney or the lower urinary tract can facilitate the work up and assist the emergency physician in developing the most efficient diagnostic plan. A good approach is to classify the origin of hematuria anatomically from the glomeruli, renal tubules–interstitium, or urinary tract. In children, the cause is more often glomerular in origin. Glomerulonephritis is usually accompanied by proteinuria and RBC casts in the urine. The nonglomerular causes of hematuria can be further subdivided into renal parenchymal disease and extrarenal disease (Table 228.1) (24).

CLINICAL PRESENTATION

Once the presence of hematuria is confirmed by microscopic urinalysis, further information regarding the presentation will help guide the investigation. Children with glomerular bleeding will present with cola-colored urine, red cell casts (pathognomonic), renal insufficiency, and proteinuria, whereas lower tract bleeding colors the urine red or pink. Passing blood clots in the urine usually points to the bladder or urethra as the source of bleeding (23). A recent upper respiratory tract infection is often seen with immunoglobulin-A (IgA) nephropathy (Berger disease). Poststreptococcal glomerulonephritis is generally preceded with sore

TABLE 228.1.   Causes of Hematuria

GLOMERULAR

Primary Glomerulonephritis
Poststreptococcal glomerulonephritis
IgA nephropathy (Berger disease)
Membranoproliferative glomerulonephritis
Focal glomerulosclerosis
Secondary Glomerulonephritis
Systemic lupus erythematosus
Henoch-Schönlein purpura
Hemolytic-uremic syndrome
Familial
Alport syndrome
Thin basement membrane disease

EXTRARENAL

Tumors: Wilms', tuberous sclerosis
Other
Drugs and toxins
Trauma and exercise
Coagulopathy
Dehydration
Other: menstruation, masturbation, fever

NONGLOMERULAR

Renal Parenchymal
Anatomic: hydronephrosis
Ureteropelvic junction obstruction
Polycystic kidney disease
Vascular Malformation
Renal vein thrombosis
Arteriovenous fistula
Sickle cell disease
Metabolic
Hypercalciuria
Hyperuricosuria
Infectious
Urinary tract infection, pyelonephritis
Tuberculosis
Foreign Body to Urethra or Bladder

throat or impetiginous lesions 7 to 21 days earlier. Dysuria, frequency, or abdominal pain suggests a UTI.

A history of recent trauma, strenuous exercise, menstruation, or bladder catheterization may account for transient hematuria and exclude the need for further work up. An adolescent's history should include certain habits, such as masturbation, excessive bicycle riding, or urethral foreign-body insertions. A recent or earlier history of renal colic or passage of a stone in the urine, as well as a family history of hypercalciuria and renal stones should be elicited, because hypercalciuria is one of the most common causes of hematuria in children.

Certain medical conditions are commonly associated with hematuria. Children with hemoglobinopathies (sickle cell trait) and coagulopathies should be carefully evaluated. The use of drugs such as furosemide for congenital heart disease can lead to hypercalciuria and, subsequently, hematuria. Antibiotics and over-the-counter medications may cause interstitial nephritis. Chemotherapy and radiation for malignancies can explain isolated hematuria in children. In the neonatal period, hematuria can be caused by thrombosis of the renal vein or artery after use of umbilical catheters. A history of tuberculosis exposure is important to identify children with genitourinary tuberculosis, which is a rare but reported cause of hematuria (3).

A family history can be extremely critical in elucidating the cause of hematuria in the presenting child. Alport syndrome is frequently seen in family members with hearing deficits and renal failure. Other diseases that carry a genetic origin include systemic lupus erythematosus (SLE), sickle cell anemia, hemophilia, and other coagulation factor deficiencies. Nephrolithiasis and IgA nephropathy also have a familial association. The thin basement membrane of the glomerulus is a common cause of benign familial hematuria in children. Family members may not be aware that they have microscopic hematuria and should be screened with a microscopic urinalysis.

The physical examination of the patient with hematuria is not specific, but several elements deserve attention. An accurate blood pressure is essential, because the presence of elevated blood pressure should alert the emergency physician to the possibility of a more severe underlying condition. The height and weight of the child should be plotted carefully to detect failure to thrive associated with long-standing acidosis or chronic renal insufficiency. A funduscopic examination of the retina, looking for evidence of long-standing hypertension or lenticonus as seen in Alport syndrome, should be performed. Periorbital edema is frequently the first site of edema in children. The chest should be examined for signs of fluid overload. Costovertebral angle tenderness may indicate a UTI. Recent trauma can be detected by findings of flank bruises and pain. Examining the abdomen for masses is critical for the identification of malignancies (Wilms' tumor), polycystic kidneys or hydronephrosis. Ascites suggests nephrosis. The examination of the skin can give evidence of pallor or rashes. This may be significant in diseases such as hemoglobinopathies, leukemia, HSP (Henoch-Schönlein purpura; petechial or purpuric lesions on the lower extremities), and SLE (malar rash). The genital examination should be included to identify abuse or trauma, discharge, and meatal stenosis, all of which can cause hematuria.

DIFFERENTIAL DIAGNOSIS

The causes of hematuria are numerous (20). A careful history and physical examination are essential in guiding the investigation for the correct etiology. It is important to first determine the site of bleeding in the presenting child. In infants, blood on the diaper can originate from the vagina or rectum and be confused with hematuria. In the menstruating girl, vaginal bleeding can be confused with urinary blood (obtain a catheterized urine specimen). The "red diaper syndrome" in infants has two causes: One is a group of healthy infants whose soiled diapers develop a red color after 24 to 36 hours, which is attributed to *Serratia marcescens;* the second is due to urate crystals. The former is rarely seen, due to the popularity of disposable diapers.

The differential diagnosis for childhood hematuria can be remembered by using the alphabetic sequence A through I (14):

*A*natomy/vascular (renal cysts, arteriovenous malformations, obstruction with hydronephrosis)
*B*oulders (renal stones, hypercalciuria and hyperuricosuria)
*C*ancer (Wilms' tumor or adenocarcinoma and infiltration of the kidney by leukemia or solid tumors)
*D*rugs (over-the-counter or illicit drugs, methicillin, cyclophosphamide, anticoagulants)
*E*xercise-induced hematuria
*F*oreign body, familial (Alport) or factitious
*G*lomerulonephritis
*H*ematology (hemoglobinopathy, coagulopathy)
*I*nfection (cystitis caused by adenovirus, tuberculosis, schistosomiasis in patients with recent travel to the Middle East or Africa)

EMERGENCY DEPARTMENT EVALUATION

The diagnosis of hematuria requires an organized and systematic approach. Figure 228.1 suggests an approach to the emergency department evaluation. If the history and physical examination fail to disclose the diagnosis of hematuria, a stepwise laboratory evaluation is necessary. Hematuria can be categorized into three types: gross hematuria, microscopic hematuria without abnormal findings, and microscopic hematuria with abnormal findings (17). Gross hematuria and the presence of blood on a urine dipstick must be followed up with a microscopic analysis of the urine to confirm the presence of RBCs. The absence of RBCs in the urine with a positive dipstick reaction suggests hemoglobinuria or myoglobinuria. The child with gross hematuria and a history of abdominal trauma should have renal imaging (computed tomography) for the diagnosis and grading of renal injuries. It is important to note that gross hematuria is not the only presentation for renal injuries of significant grade. In fact significant injuries may present with microscopic hematuria, as well as with normal urine analysis findings. Therefore, the decision of renal imaging for the diagnosis and grading of these injuries should not be based on urine analysis alone in isolation from clinical status, and mechanism of injury (15).

In addition, a high index of suspicion must be maintained regarding pathologic lesions of the urinary tract when a patient presents with gross hematuria with a minimal force blunt abdominal trauma. The diagnostic and therapeutic approach to blunt renal trauma should be modified in these cases (1,4). Some authors recommend that a CT scan study of the abdomen and pelvis should be performed in patients with 50 or greater red blood cells on urinalysis, hypotension at the time of ED presentation, or if there is a serious mechanism of injury such as high speed motor vehicle accident deceleration injuries). In a recent study, Perez-Brayfield et al found that patients with ureteropelvic junction avulsion without hematuria underwent diagnostic imaging based on the mechanisms of injury and number of associated injuries (18). If blood is noted at the urethral meatus, a retrograde urethrogram must be done prior to catheterization to verify urethral integrity.

The presence of dysuria and urinary frequency or the presence of systemic signs (fever, vomiting, diarrhea, and abdominal pain) should suggest the possibility of a urinary tract infection, and a urine culture must be sent. The urine culture is especially important in the child with white blood cells on microscopic urinalysis because UTIs are the most common cause of macroscopic hematuria and a third of UTIs are associated with hematuria (24). If the culture is negative for bacterial growth and the signs and symptoms are strongly suggestive of cystitis, a possible cause is adenovirus, which is well known to cause hemorrhagic cystitis. Another common cause is chemical cystitis due to bubble bath.

The child with gross hematuria and severe episodic flank or abdominal pain must be evaluated for urolithiasis (13). In this case, the initial work up consists of radiologic imaging and testing the urine for calcium excretion. If the kidney-ureter-bladder (KUB) is negative for stones, a renal sonogram or abdominal and pelvic spiral computed tomography (CT) scan should be obtained. A urologic consultation is appropriate if a stone is detected. Gross hematuria and the presence of proteinuria suggest glomerulonephritis. Proteinuria should not exceed 2+ if the only source of protein is from the blood. Pertinent laboratory evaluation includes a complete blood count (hemolytic–uremic syndrome), throat culture, streptozyme panel, serum C3 and C4 concentrations (acute post streptococcal glomerulonephritis), and serum creatinine and potassium concentrations (looking for renal insufficiency). The complement C3 level is low in

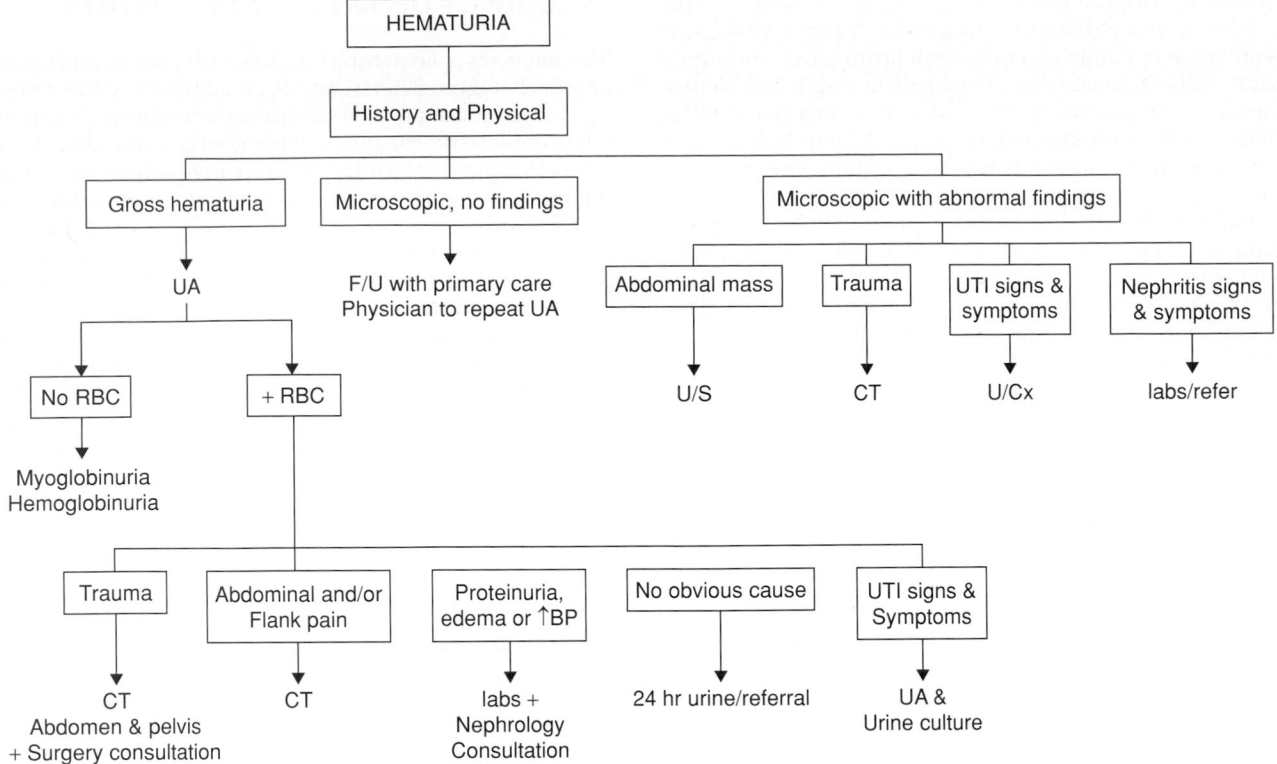

Figure 228.1.   Approach to the diagnosis of hematuria in children.

acute poststreptococcal glomerulonephritis, membranoproliferative glomerulonephritis, and SLE.

The presence of RBC casts on microscopic urinalysis is also significant. RBC morphology by phase contrast microscopy can be helpful in localization of hematuria. Dysmorphic cells indicate glomerular bleeding. However, this is thought to be a costly test, offering little additional information to the evaluation of microscopic hematuria in children and of limited use in the ED (23).

Less common causes of gross hematuria include hypercalciuria, nephrocalcinosis, sickle cell trait, and glomerular basement membrane defects (Alport syndrome and benign familial hematuria). Diagnosis begins with a urine Cr/Ca ratio or a 24-hour urinary calcium excretion, serum creatinine, and renal sonography. Consultation with a pediatric nephrologist is recommended.

It is important for the emergency physician to address pain management in the uncomfortable child. Ketorolac provides comparable analgesia to morphine, meperidine, or acetaminophen in children undergoing myringotomy, hernia repair, tonsillectomy, or other surgery associated with mild to moderate pain (12). Contrary to the adult literature demonstrating the efficacy of ketorolac in the pain management of renal colic, to date, there has been no study evaluating the analgesic effects of ketorolac in renal colic in the pediatric population.

The second category of hematuria includes the child presenting with asymptomatic microscopic hematuria without proteinuria. Persistent hematuria is defined as the presence of hematuria in at least 2 to 3 urine analyses obtained during a 2- to 3-week period (5,14,17). Persistent hematuria warrants further evaluation. For the emergency physician, a careful review of the history and physical examination is mandatory. Laboratory investigation can be tailored to the need of the child. Such an evaluation can include a spot urinary Ca/Cr ratio or parental urinalysis to look for hypercalciuria and benign familial hematuria (19). A ratio of 0.2 or greater is typically considered hypercalciuria (16). There have been reports of recurrent abdominal and flank pain

in children with idiopathic hypercalciuria (IH) (21). In addition, some recent studies proposed that noncalculous IH as an important contributing factor to recurrent UTI in children (22).

In African-American children, hemoglobin electrophoresis should be considered. A renal sonogram and checking renal function have a low diagnostic yield in the emergency department (ED) evaluation (8). The emergency physician can help arrange follow up with a pediatric nephrologist at a later time.

Finally, there are children with microscopic hematuria and the presence of abnormal physical examination findings (edema, pain, hypertension), or the presence of proteinuria. This group of patients can have a wide range of diagnostic possibilities (6,10). The presence of proteinuria on urinalysis suggests glomerulonephritis. A child may show evidence of edema or hypertension on physical examination. The ED evaluation should include measurements of serum BUN and creatinine, electrolytes, C3 and C4 levels, an ASO titer, an albumin level, and a complete blood count. The presence of proteinuria, edema, and hypoalbuminemia suggest nephrotic syndrome. Consultation with a pediatric nephrologist is recommended.

Less common causes of hematuria in children exist and can be pursued in the ED based on the level of suspicion raised by the history and physical examination. Such causes include coagulation abnormalities and some anatomic and vascular problems (24). Most of the conditions requiring advanced work up (Table 228.2) should be referred to a pediatric nephrologist or urologist.

There is rarely a reason for performing cystoscopy or retrograde urography in the emergency department. The renal ultrasound is capable of detecting gross lesions as effectively as can intravenous urography, and has replaced the latter as the diagnostic study of choice. The renal ultrasound can rule out polycystic kidney disease, Wilms tumor, renal stones, and obstruction as possible causes of hematuria. Children thought to need further diagnostic imaging should be referred to a pediatric urologist.

TABLE 228.2. Evaluation of the Child with Hematuria

INITIAL EVALUATION OF CHILD WITH HEMATURIA

History
Physical examination
Family history
Initial laboratory evaluation
Urinalysis with microscopy, protein measurement
Red blood cell morphology
Urine culture
Calcium—creatinine ratio
Sickle cell screen, if applicable
Complete blood count, creatinine and blood urea nitrogen levels
Urine of first-degree relatives
Renal ultrasound

ADVANCED EVALUATION OF CHILD WITH HEMATURIA

Complement level
Membranoproliferative glomerulonephritis
SLE, postinfectious glomerulonephritis
Antistreptolysin-O and anti-DNAase B
Acute poststreptococcal glomerulonephritis
Antinuclear antibody
SLE
Audiogram
Alport syndrome
Anti-glomerular basement membrane antibodies
Antineutrophil cytoplasmic antibodies
Active crescenteric glomerulonephritis
Tuberculosis testing
Renal biopsy

EMERGENCY DEPARTMENT MANAGEMENT

The patient with hematuria should be managed according to the etiology of the disease condition. Asymptomatic hematuria does not need acute management in the emergency department. An exception to this rule includes evaluation for UTIs. Younger infants and dehydrated or ill-appearing patients with UTI warrant hospitalization and intravenous antibiotics. Some authors recommended treating UTI even in the very young children 1 to 24 months with oral cefixime for 14 days (11). Older patients may be treated orally.

Children with suspected hypercalciuria should increase water intake to attempt to decrease the concentration of calcium in the urine. A low-calcium diet and hydrochlorothiazide therapy have been shown to decrease urinary calcium excretion; a short course can result in the disappearance of microscopic hematuria. Parekh et al recommended that thiazide diuretic should only be used with intractable hematuria associated with hypercalciuria, a markedly increased urine calcium-to-creatinine ratio and family history of urolithiasis (16). A child with a suspected renal calculus should have a urologic consultation in the ED.

When there are no indications for immediate medical intervention, the parents can be reassured that a life-threatening condition does not exist and that most cases of isolated hematuria do not require treatment (2).

CRITICAL INTERVENTIONS

- A urine culture should be sent regardless of the results of the urine analysis in the presence of signs and symptoms of urinary tract infection
- The decision for renal imaging in blunt trauma for the diagnosis and treatment of renal injuries should not be based on urine analysis alone. Clinical status, history, and mechanism of injury should also be considered

DISPOSITION

Referral to a pediatric nephrologist should occur if the child has gross hematuria, a coexistent significant proteinuria, hypertension, abnormal kidney function tests, persistent hypocomplementemia, or findings suggesting a systemic disease; or if there is a family history of glomerulonephritis, nerve deafness, chronic renal failure, end-stage renal disease, or familial hematuria. If parental anxiety is high, referral to a pediatric nephrologist may help alleviate compounding fears and serve as additional reassurance to the family that dangerous and treatable conditions have been ruled out by the primary physician. Parents are often concerned that their child is losing large amounts of blood due to the color of the urine and they should be reassured and reminded that as little as 1 ml of blood in 1 L of urine can make the urine red (17).

Rarely does a patient with hematuria need to be hospitalized. Patients with newly diagnosed renal disease should be admitted with pediatric nephrologist consultation. A toxic-appearing child with a UTI is admitted for intravenous antibiotics. Inadequate outpatient pain management may lead to hospitalization.

Follow-up urinalysis should be arranged every 2 to 4 months for at least a one-year period for patients with persistent hematuria without any other abnormalities (such as hypertension, proteinuria, or RBC casts). This is usually done by the primary care or subspecialty physicians. Blood pressure and a dipstick test for proteinuria should also be checked periodically. If proteinuria or gross hematuria develops during this followup period, the patient should be referred to a nephrologist.

It is important to remember that the most common causes of microscopic hematuria without casts or proteinuria are benign and untreatable. The prognosis for these children is very good. A poor prognosis is associated with proteinuria at presentation, persistent hematuria, and hypertension.

COMMON PITFALLS

✔ Failure to perform a urine dipstick and urinalysis to confirm the presence of blood in the "red urine" can lead to unnecessary performance of numerous laboratory tests
✔ Failure to obtain relevant information in the history (recent pharyngitis, trauma, or a family history of renal stones) can make the determination of the cause of hematuria more cumbersome
✔ Most children with microscopic hematuria have an excellent prognosis. Failure to detect proteinuria, hypertension, and the subtle signs of fluid overload can be detrimental to the prognosis of such patients

References

1. Ahmed Z, Lee J. Asymptomatic urinary abnormalities. *Med Clin North Am* 1997;81:641–651.
2. Benbassat J, Gergawi M, et al. Variability in management of symptomless microhaematuria in schoolchildren. *Postgrad Med J* 1998;74:161–164.
3. Chattopadhyay A, Bhatnagar V, et al. Genitourinary tuberculosis in pediatric surgical practice. *J Pediatr Surg* 1997;32:1283–1286.
4. Chopra P, St-Vil D, Yazbeck S. Blunt renal trauma-blessing in disguise? *J Pediatr Surg* 2002;37:779–782.
5. Cilento BG, Stock JA, Kaplan GW. Hematuria in children. *Urol Clin North Am* 1995;22:43–54.
6. Diven SC, Travis LB. A practical primary care approach to hematuria in children. *Pediatr Nephrol* 2000;14:65–72.
7. Feld LG, Waz WR, et al. Hematuria. *Pediatr Clin North Am* 1997;44:1191–1209.
8. Feld LG, Waz WR, Perez LM, et al. Hematuria: an integrated medical and surgical approach. *Pediatr Clin North Am* 1997;44:1191–1210.
9. Feld LG, Meyers KE, Kaplan BS, et al. Limited evaluation of microscopic hematuria in pediatrics. *Pediatrics* 1998;102:E42.
10. Fitzwater DS, Wyatt RJ. Hematuria. *Pediatr Rev* 1994;15:102–108.

11. Hoberman A, Wald ER, et al. Oral versus initial intravenous therapy for urinary tract infections in young febrile children. *Pediatrics* 1999;104:79–86.
12. Gillis JC, Brogden RN. Ketorolac. A reappraisal of its pharmacodynamic and pharmacokinetic properties and therapeutic use in pain management. *Drugs* 1997;53:139–188.
13. Levy FL, Kemp RD, et al. Macroscopic hematuria secondary to hypercalciuria and hyperuricosuria. *Am J Kidney Dis* 1994;24:515–518.
14. Neiberger RE. The ABC's of evaluating children with hematuria. *Am Fam Physician* 1994;49:623–628.
15. Nguyen MM, Das S. Pediatric renal trauma. *Urology* 2002;59:762–766.
16. Parekh DJ, Pope CJ IV, Adams MC, Brock JW III. the association of an increases urinary calcium-to-creatinine ratio, and asymptomatic gross and microscopic hematuria in children. *J Urol* 2002;167:274.
17. Patel HP, Bissler JJ. Hematuria in children. *Pediatr Clin North Am* 2001;48:1519–1537.
18. Perez-Brayfield MR, Gatti JM, Smith EA, et al. Blunt traumatic hematuria in children. Is a simplified algorithm justified? *J Urol* 2002;167:2543–2546.
19. Perrone HC, Stapleton FB, et al. Hematuria due to hyperuricosuria in children: 36-month follow-up. *Clin Nephrol* 1997;48:288–291.
20. Roy S. Hematuria. *Pediatrics Annals* 1996;25:284–287.
21. Vachvanichsanong P, Malagon M, Moore ES. Recurrent abdominal and flank pain in children with idiopathic hypercalciuria. *Acta Paediat* 2001;90:643–648.
22. Vachvanichsanong P, Malagon M, Moore ES. Urinary tract infection in children associated with idiopathic hypercalciuria. *Scand J Urol Nephrol* 2001;35:112–116.
23. Ward JF, Kaplan GW, et al. Refined microscopic urinalysis for red blood cell morphology in the evaluation of asymptomatic microscopic hematuria in pediatric population. *J Urol* 1998;160:1492–1495.
24. Yadin O. Hematuria in children. *Pediatr Ann* 1994;23:474–485.

CHAPTER 229
Limp

Jonathan I. Singer

Locomotion is accomplished by a graceful succession from a stance phase to a swing phase. The stance phase is initiated by the heel striking the ground and terminates with toeing-off. The swing phase begins with flexion of the knee and hip, followed by extension of the knee, and ends with dorsiflexion of the foot, which permits heel contact. Altered locomotion and gait disturbance are generic terms for any deviation from this rhythmic movement (1). Paralysis implies loss or impairment of neuromuscular mechanisms. Pseudoparalysis is a physiologically intact neuromuscular apparatus but with a refusal to walk or an inability to support weight (12,20). A child who limps has faulted cadence of the swing and stance phase. When pain is the cause of acute loss of rhythm, the gait is described as antalgic (18).

Lesions of the central nervous system, spine, peripheral nervous system, intraabdominal contents, hip, knee, ankle joints, feet, or any of the weight-bearing long bones can lead to distinct patterns of altered locomotion. By organizing the characteristic history, demonstrating the accompanying physical findings, and adjunctive laboratory features the emergency physician may establish the affected organ system (18,22).

CLINICAL PRESENTATION

Take the history in a setting comfortable for both the parent and the child. The physician should attempt to remain as inconspicuous as possible, and the historian should be encouraged to distract the child's attention from the physician. The physician should inquire about the length of time the child has been symptomatic. With gait disturbance, symptoms may be acute, constant, of a brief duration, or insidious with inconstant manifestations.

Are there temporal relationships or patterns related to physical activity? Ask the parent what part of the body appears to be the source of the child's problem. Determine whether there is pain associated with the gait disturbance. Attempt to identify the site, if pain is present. Focus on posture during sleep and rest, avoidance of a particular position, and discomfort with handling a specific body part.

Seek the history of an acute traumatic event, such as a fall, a twisting injury, a direct blow, or penetration by a foreign body. Inquire about the presence of fever, which may accompany an inflammatory or infectious problem. Is there exposure to contagion? Is there an antecedent infectious process? Is the child currently being treated with antibiotics for an intercurrent infection? The review of symptoms should emphasize cutaneous lesions such as a scarlatiniform erythroderma, erythema marginatum, erythema migrans, erythema nodosum, urticaria, or purpura. Make inquiry regarding weight loss, morning stiffness, decreased motor strength and agility, a change in bladder or bowel control, altered mental status, headache, rhinorrhea, cough, anorexia, nausea, vomiting, and abdominal pain. Exclude exposures to animals, ticks, and potential intoxicants, such as heavy metals, insecticides, alcohol, or various medications, such as hydantoin, isoniazid, antimetabolites, and steroids.

Determine whether there have been recent intramuscular injections, including immunizations. Is there a history of previous joint disease, prior lumbar puncture, known anatomic spinal canal defects or underlying disease state, such as endocrinopathy, sickle hemoglobinopathy, diabetes mellitus, or immunocompromised state? Is there a family history of inflammatory bowel or joint disease? Is there any suggestion of physical abuse, sexual assault, or psychosocial disturbances that would predispose to a conversion reaction? Has there been acquisition of any new footwear? (6,19).

In the preschool-aged child, first carry out the physical examination with the child on a parent's lap. Begin with inspection. Observe the position of the patient at rest, and look at the child's passive movements. Focus on the skin, looking for evidence of hemorrhagic diathesis, occult trauma, and penetrating wounds. Look for soft-tissue swelling and skin changes that suggest pyoderma, varicella, cellulitis, or a deeper plane infection. Look for asymmetry of gluteal, thigh, and popliteal creases. Determine whether there is effusion or distension of the joint capsules of the hip, knee, or ankle.

Only after inspection should the physician palpate for localized induration, warmth, or tenderness over the bones, particularly metaphyseal regions of long bones. Gently examine the joints for motion, avoiding the probable area of pathology until last. Handle the limb systematically and delicately, providing anxiolytic, distracting speech. Determine the degree of restriction of flexion, extension, abduction, and rotation. Palpate the spine in the midline, looking for paraspinal muscle spasm or scoliosis. Determine whether there is any sensory disturbance, asymmetry of deep tendon reflexes, loss of motor strength, cranial nerve abnormalities, or nuchal rigidity. Finally, examine the feet and footwear for embedded foreign objects.

Transfer the patient onto an examining table. Readdress positive physical findings. With the patient recumbent, look for abdominal guarding or palpable mass in the iliac fossa. Perform a pelvic rock. With a rectal examination, exclude a mass in the pelvic floor. Perform a Valsalva maneuver, heel strike, and straight leg raise (11,18). Remove the patient from the examining table, and place him or her on the floor in a sitting position. Observe the method chosen to achieve the erect position. If the child refuses to arise, stand the child on the floor at a distance from the parent. Determine whether the child refuses to bear weight on one of the limbs or simply walks with an antalgic gait.

DIFFERENTIAL DIAGNOSIS

A wide variety of problems have a presenting complaint of limp. The ones most common in the emergency department are listed in Table 229.1. Because of their frequency, overt or occult trauma and infectious diseases should be part of the differential diagnosis for any child with an acute gait disturbance (7,19).

Trauma to the lower extremities is the principal cause of gait disturbance, especially in early childhood (1). In children less than 5 years old, multiple obstacles may impede this diagnosis. A fracture of the tibia or fibula should be considered the probable diagnosis in an afebrile child less than 5 years old who suddenly refuses to walk or place any weight on a single lower extremity. The absence of direct trauma should not rule out the diagnosis, because these fractures may occur as the result of trivial, indirect injury associated with the child's daily activity (21).

Older children may limp from stress fractures of the femoral head, tibial tubercle, and tibial or fibular shaft. They also may limp from avulsion of the ischial apophysis, lesser trochanter, or navicular tuberosity, or from lacerations and compression of cartilage plates, fracture of the epiphyseal ossification centers, shaft fractures, and infractions at various levels of the long-bone metaphyses. These traumatic lesions may present singly or in various combinations. They may appear acutely or insidiously, caused by repeated injury during sports. Trauma and repeated stress may be important factors in the genesis of slipped capital femoral epiphysis, transient synovitis, and Legg-Calvé-Perthes disease, three of the most common hip afflictions associated with antalgic gait (10).

Among the nontraumatic conditions that can cause altered locomotion, potentially serious infectious diseases predominate (16). A history of an antecedent infectious process with or without fever in the preceding 2 weeks should heighten concern for a serious infectious disease in the child with a gait disturbance. Similarly, current treatment with antibiotics for a recognized infection, especially of the skin or respiratory tract, in a child with gait disturbance should raise suspicion for a more serious infection.

The most common infectious conditions associated with gait disturbance are focal cellulitis of the lower extremity, unifocal pyarthrosis of a weight-bearing joint, and osteomyelitis of the femoral or tibial metaphyses. On clinical grounds alone, it may be difficult to differentiate these three conditions. The final

---

TABLE 229.1. Principal Causes for
Altered Childhood Locomotion

Overt and occult trauma
Cellulitis
Osteomyelitis
Pyarthrosis
Sickle cell, vasoocclusive crisis
Drug intoxication
Transient synovitis
Legg-Perthes disease
Appendicitis
Juvenile rheumatoid arthritis

(Modified and reproduced with permission from Singer J. The cause of gait disturbance in 425 pediatric patients. In: Ludwig S, Fleisher G, eds. Pediatric emergency care, vol 1. Baltimore: Wiliams & Wilkins, 1985:7.)

---

diagnosis rests with isolation of an offending organism from skin and soft tissues, synovial fluid, or subperiosteal space (18).

Patients with sickle hemoglobinopathy may present acutely with a gait disturbance from dactylitis, stasis of blood in tendons and periarticular and synovial tissues, bone infarction, osteomyelitis of the long bones, and avascular necrosis of a femoral head (19).

Dose-dependent toxic reactions from alcohol or diphenylhydantoin and prolonged exposure to heavy metals, insecticides, and toluene-containing compounds may produce clumsiness, incoordination, and unsteady gait with overt ataxia or inability to walk. This diagnosis depends on the medication history and potential exposure to toxins (19).

In acute synovitis, there is a transient, unilateral inflammatory reaction in the hip. There may be antecedent minor trauma or recent upper respiratory tract symptoms, possibly associated with low-grade fever. An affected child presents with either acute or progressive discomfort in the hip, anteromedial thigh, or ipsilateral knee, eventually leading to an antalgic gait. Clinically, this condition is indistinguishable from Legg-Calvé-Perthes disease. In both cases, children do not appear systemically ill. They will choose a position with the thigh flexed, abducted, and externally rotated. They guard the hip during examination and have pain with internal rotation of the hip and, to a lesser extent, with hip extension (10).

Patients with uncomplicated appendicitis, or a perforated or abscessed appendix, exhibit a gait disturbance manifested by a cautious, slow gait, often accompanied by flexion of the trunk. An outright right-sided limp is seen occasionally. The gait resembles that seen with cervicitis or any pelvic inflammatory disease (16).

The clinical manifestations of juvenile rheumatoid arthritis are so varied that it may be difficult to recognize this disease when first encountering a patient. The mode of onset varies considerably, from involvement of a single joint with no constitutional reactions, to a more widespread polyarthritis of varying severity, to a generalized systemic onset with extraarticular manifestations (19).

Major Emergency Entities

An early presumptive diagnosis for the cause of gait disturbance must be established for a few conditions (Table 229.2). Failing to consider these conditions at the initial encounter may lead to deformity, functional disability, or death (14,17).

Pain associated with osteomyelitis of the long bones is primarily located over the affected metaphysis. Direct pressure over the affected metaphysis produces extreme discomfort. Swelling is limited to the immediate metaphyseal area initially, but it can spread rapidly to involve an entire extremity or adjacent periarticular tissue. Joints adjacent to the infected metaphysis may have some limitation of motion caused by voluntary guarding or sympathetic effusion. If the joints are handled gently, slowly, and persistently, motion is not as restricted as in septic arthritis, and full range may be possible. Neck pain, back pain, and refusal to walk may signal the presence of osteomyelitis of the spine. Fever associated with back, buttock, or hip pain with gait disturbance may be the initial expression of osteomyelitis of the pelvis (19,23).

Patients with pyarthrosis are readily diagnosed because of the protective posturing imposed by joint capsule distention. When there is hip involvement, children assume a position of comfort, with the thigh on the affected side in moderate flexion, abduction, and external rotation. Children place the affected limb on the ground in the same position as when it is supine, and often hold the foot in plantar flexion (13). If the knee or ankle is involved, it is erythematous, warm, swollen, and painful to

TABLE 229.2. Disease States Associated with Limp That Require Prompt Recognition

Osteomyelitis
Long bone, spine, pelvis
Pyarthrosis
Hip, knee, ankle
Sacroiliac infection
Psoas abscess
Deep-plane infection
Epidural abscess
Intramedullary abscess of the spinal cord
Slipped capital femoral epiphysis
Cord tumor
Guillain-Barré syndrome
Tick paralysis
Meningitis
Encephalitis
Cerebral abscess
Appendicitis

(Modified and reproduced with permission from Singer J. Evaluation of acute and insidious gait disturbance in children less than 5 years of age. In: Barness LA, et al., eds. Advances in pdiatrics, vol. 26. Chicago: Year Book, 1979.)

palpate, with limited range of motion. Minimal active motion, extreme muscle spasm, and pain with passive movement are distinguishing features of pyarthrosis in weight-bearing regions (19).

Suppuration may be limited to the sacroiliac joint and causes gait disturbance in rare cases. Patients have pain in the buttocks and lower back that radiates to the hip, lateral thigh, lower leg, or abdomen. They may hold a single hip guarded, abducted, and externally rotated, but flexion, abduction, external rotation, and hip extension are permitted. Another differentiating feature is pain caused by direct compression of the sacroiliac joint or pain in the sacroiliac joint during rectal examination or from compression of the ileal wings. Often, the straight leg-raising test is positive (4).

Hip, groin, abdomen, lower back, buttock, or upper thigh pain associated with fever and limping may occur with a psoas abscess. Like patients with septic arthritis of the hip, those with psoas abscess may assume the position of hip flexion, abduction, and external rotation. Hip extension and internal rotation that stretches the iliopsoas muscle may cause increased pain. Rotation of the fully flexed hip is typically pain-free. When they attempt to walk, patients keep the affected extremity advanced in relation to the unaffected side, with the trunk deviated toward the affected side, the pelvis tilted down, and the knee and hip flexed slightly. Several findings may differentiate psoas abscess from septic arthritis or osteomyelitis: the presence of abdominal guarding with tenderness in both lower quadrants, or a palpable mass in the iliac fossa or pelvic floor that may be detectable by rectal examination. Patients also may have bulging of the flank with or without cutaneous edema, scoliosis, immobility of the spine with spasm of the paravertebral muscles, or decreased excursions of the diaphragm (5).

Deep-plane infection refers to suppuration that extends to the depth of fascia or muscle (8). In necrotizing fasciitis, fat and fascia are destroyed. Muscle is typically uninvolved, and skin, on occasion, may be spared (2). In bacterial myositis, the striated muscle is involved, and there may be localized abscess formation within the muscle (pyomyositis) (3).

Clinical features of fasciitis and myositis overlap. Neither is common in immunologically intact children. Predisposing conditions including diabetes mellitus, chronic cardiac or pulmonary disease, collagen vascular disease, varicella complicated by pyoderma, and antecedent blunt trauma. There is a predilec-

tion for involvement of the lower extremities, especially the groin and thigh. Symptoms are often insidious, starting with poorly localized extremity pain that impairs gait. Fever may be absent or only of low grade. Pain that is out of proportion to the degree of physical findings may be the only clue to the correct diagnosis at the initial encounter (2).

With varicella, a violaceous hue about a cluster of pox lesions may be the clue to deep-plane infection. In those without varicella, rapidly developing skin changes suggest the diagnosis. These include a localized soft-tissue swelling, erythema, and either darker discoloration of the skin (pyomyositis) or bullae formation, and spontaneous sloughing (necrotizing fasciitis). If misdiagnosed at the time there is painful gait without skin changes, children may return in extremis within 24 to 48 hours in septic shock (2,3).

Hip pain and limp may be the presenting complaints with epidural abscess, but most patients seek medical attention because of abdominal pain or unremitting back pain. At the onset, most patients exhibit fever, headache, malaise, and aching midline back pain. Patients may have tenderness on palpation of the spinous processes at the level of the subjective back pain. Neck stiffness is present in more than one-third of patients, and when altered sensorium is an accompanying feature, the disease may mimic meningitis. Overt cord involvement may be heralded by weakness of voluntary muscles and bowel and bladder sphincters, or by sensory abnormalities, most often characterized as ascending anesthesia (15).

Intramedullary abscess of the spinal cord results from either a hematogenous spread from a distant infection or a direct spread of infection from the skin to the cord. The major predisposing factor to cord abscess is anatomical abnormality such as dermal sinus or meningocele. The defect may not be appreciated until the child develops the abscess. Presentation is typically insidious with low grade fever and prolonged back pain made worse when lying flat. Examination demonstrates increased pain at the site of infection with movement and exacerbation with neck flexion, straight leg raising or Valsalva maneuvers. Delayed recognition of the disease process can lead to paralysis (17).

Deep groin pain and hip, distal medial thigh, or knee pain may be of sudden onset or progressive over weeks as result of acute or chronic slipped capital femoral epiphysis. Classically, pain is vague, dull at rest, and exacerbated by ambulation. Children seek comfort by externally rotating the leg when walking. They limp, and there is often a truncal shift with ambulation to accommodate hip abductor weakness. Examination demonstrates a partially flexed, irritable hip maintained in external rotation. Maximal hip flexion is restricted, and complete internal rotation is not possible. Delay in recognition of an acute slip may result in further displacement or may increase the risk for avascular necrosis (6,11).

A diagnosis of cord tumor must be considered in any child with a gait disturbance who also has a recent history of altered bowel pattern or an insidious onset of motor weakness of the lower extremities, subjective sensory disturbance (including leg and neck pain), or back pain that is usually progressive. The back pain associated with a cord tumor is classically increased in the supine position and increased in intensity by the Valsalva maneuver. Physical examination may reveal weakness of the lower extremities, paraspinal or hamstring muscle spasm, nuchal rigidity, scoliosis, back stiffness, spine tenderness, relaxed sphincter tone, and absence of fever. Even when cord tumors present precipitously, the absence of systemic manifestations helps to discriminate them from acute epidural abscess (9,19).

Alterations in gait seen with Guillain-Barré syndrome can be secondary to subjective complaints of foot or leg pain, impairment of position sense, or profound leg weakness with loss of voluntary movement. The clinical hallmark of Guillain-Barré syndrome is rapidly progressive, relatively symmetric motor impairment. The motor deficit may range from isolated lower limb weakness to total paralysis of the muscles of all four extremities and the trunk. Mild sensory symptoms or signs strongly support the diagnosis. Severe sensory dysfunction with pain as a dominant expression is a clinical variant. Such patients may experience bilateral pain in the large proximal muscles, including the lower back, buttocks, and anterior and posterior aspects of the thighs. Such sensory disturbances can precede the onset of clinically demonstrable weakness (19).

The prognosis for full functional recovery from tick paralysis depends on establishment of the diagnosis. After a brief period with nonspecific symptoms, patients experience a progressive weakness of the lower extremities, usually without pain or paresthesias. The weakness or attendant ataxia can lead to inability to walk, and the patient may seek medical attention before the development of a generalized flaccid paresis (19).

Children may be reluctant to assume an upright position or to walk because of cephalalgia, myalgia, electrolyte imbalance, compromised circulatory status, and altered sensorium from encephalitis or meningitis. The cardinal symptoms of cerebral abscess include severe and intractable headache, altered sensorium, vomiting, fever, and neurologic abnormalities that include seizure, paresthesias, incoordination, unsteady gait, or hemiparesis (19). Early recognition of these intracranial infections can prevent significant morbidity and mortality.

EMERGENCY DEPARTMENT EVALUATION

Among the benign and potentially life- or limb-threatening causes of gait disturbance, several have a classic profile. By recognizing the characteristic history and subsequently demonstrating the accompanying physical findings, the physician may establish a diagnosis. Where the pathogenesis is clear, no diagnostic investigation is an option. When the provisional diagnosis is elusive, ancillary tests from phlebotomy or imaging may be helpful.

A complete blood count may facilitate the diagnosis of systemic infection, hemoglobinopathy, or blood dyscrasia. The erythrocyte sedimentation rate (ESR) correctly identifies over 75% of all patients with limb pain who have an inflammatory or infectious disease. About 70% of patients with an ESR of more than 30 mm/h have arthralgia or arthritis of infectious or inflammatory origin (11). Those with an ESR of 40 mm/h or more have bacterial infections as the cause of their refusal to walk.

When the area of pain has been localized, radiographs limited to the area of interest have proven diagnostic efficacy. Plain radiographs may aid in the diagnosis of periostitides, osteochondroses, benign and malignant tumors, mechanical disturbances, metabolic derangements, and infectious diseases. Films that appear negative should never hinder therapeutic strategies. Several noteworthy conditions that present with gait disturbance, such as tibial fracture in the toddler, septic hip in the child over 1 year old, osteomyelitis of the long bone or pelvis, sacroiliac joint infection, and intervertebral disk infection, may be associated with normal radiographs. Radiographs are often insensitive and unreliable, especially in the early course of these disorders (1,11,14).

Ultrasonography may be helpful in the investigation of hip irritability. Sonography may demonstrate intraarticular effusion when plain films are normal.

Radionuclide scans rarely establish an unexpected diagnosis, but they do provide important positive and negative information central to inpatient management. A positive technetium scan reflects any condition that results in increased bone formation or blood flow. A negative technetium scan does not rule out an infectious process and should be followed by a gallium scan.

Gallium accumulates in leukocytes independent of blood supply. A positive gallium scan supports a provisional diagnosis of infection, and negative technetium and gallium scans refute it. The diagnostic accuracy of these procedures is augmented only when both scans are performed sequentially.

Computed tomography (CT) scanning is useful for the study of tumors and inflammatory and infectious problems of the musculoskeletal system in children. Magnetic resonance imaging (MRI) is superior to both plain films and CT scans for soft-tissue detail. MRI may be the most sensitive means of establishing an early diagnosis of Legg-Calvé-Perthes disease, differentiating bone infarction from osteomyelitis in the sickle cell patient and benign from malignant bone tumors. MRI may be useful in certain anatomic regions that are difficult to evaluate with plain films (e.g., region of the sacroiliac joint, vertebral bodies, and intervertebral disks) (13). All of these imaging modalities, however, are of limited assistance to the emergency physician, who must make a prompt diagnosis (17,19,22).

EMERGENCY DEPARTMENT MANAGEMENT

The intensity of the emergency department (ED) management of patients with gait disturbances rests with the physiologic derangement at the time of presentation. Rarely, a patient with limp, pseudoparalysis, or paresis requires establishment of an airway or ventilatory support. Cardiovascular instability, which can occur with a few of the infectious diseases (notably deep-plane infection, meningitis, and appendiceal abscess), requires fluid resuscitation. Neurologic deficits may be rapidly progressive in a few conditions associated with gait disturbance. Continuous monitoring of neurologic status is warranted for patients suspected of having Guillain-Barré syndrome, poliomyelitis, acute transverse myelitis, tick paralysis, brain abscess, meningitis, and cerebral vascular accident. A few conditions associated with gait disturbance require specific ED treatment to forestall functional disability. Various therapeutic modalities include splinting of fractures, antibiotic administration, arthrocentesis to reduce intraarticular pressure, and removal of a tick to definitively treat tick paralysis.

CRITICAL INTERVENTIONS

- Infectious diseases must be considered as a prime cause of altered locomotion in the young
- Uncommon infectious diagnoses must be entertained early in the evaluation of febrile children with gait disturbance

DISPOSITION

When presented with a child who has a gait disturbance, the physician has a major responsibility to distinguish between those children who require ED intervention and immediate hospitalization and those who have self-limited conditions. The following features, when present, may be helpful in characterizing patients who require greater scrutiny. Be more cautious when the gait disturbance is more likely to be from illness rather than from injury. In nontraumatic states, have a heightened awareness for adverse outcome when a gait disturbance is associated with a rapid progression of signs and symptoms or when there is an indolent illness with sudden change.

Admission is warranted for children with gait disturbance in certain circumstances. Admit all patients who appear to have a serious bacterial infection. History and physical examination are more likely to uncover serious bacterial infection than are ancillary laboratory investigations (14,23). Maintain a high index of suspicion for serious bacterial diseases in those patients who have recently been febrile or are currently being treated with antibiotics for benign intercurrent illness.

Certain clinical findings suggest that serious bacterial illness is present. They include fever, even if of low grade; nuchal rigidity; limitation of joint motion; lower limb direct metaphyseal pain; compression tenderness over a spinal process; pain in the sacroiliac joint, with pelvic rock; and back pain enhanced with Valsalva movement, heel strike, or straight leg raising. Additional features that suggest serious bacterial infection include pain that is disproportionate to physical findings or neurologic abnormalities. In the context of a likely infectious disease, do not be dissuaded by a normal white blood cell count or normal ESR. Conversely, do not admit a child who has no historic or clinical findings to suggest serious bacterial infection when there is an isolated finding of leukocytosis or elevated sedimentation rate.

Admission is warranted for all patients with neurologic abnormalities, such as altered consciousness, cranial nerve involvement, subjective or objective sensory disturbance, ataxia, alteration of sphincter tone, urinary retention, altered deep tendon reflexes, or loss of voluntary movement. Admit patients with gait disturbance who might have been physically abused.

COMMON PITFALLS

✔ Think of trauma when there is an abrupt onset of gait disturbance without prodromal events in a previously healthy child

✔ Deemphasize the history of trauma, even if witnessed, when there is an antecedent or current infectious process; this scenario suggests serious bacterial infection

✔ Fever, leukocytosis, and elevated ESR may not uniformly accompany infectious diseases associated with gait disturbance

References

1. Barkin RM, Barkin SZ, Barkin AZ. The limping child. *J Emerg Med* 2000;18:331–9.
2. Barton LL, Jeck DT, Vaidya VU. Necrotizing fasciitis in children: report of two cases and review of the literature. *Arch Pediatr Adolesc Med* 1996;150:105–108.
3. Boyle MF, Singer J. Necrotizing myositis and toxic strep syndrome in a pediatric patient. *J Emerg Med* 1992;10:577–579.
4. Carlson SA, Jones JS. Pyogenic sacroiliitis. *Am J Emerg Med* 1994;12:639–641.
5. Chern CH, Hu SC, Kao WF, et al. Psoas abscess: making an early diagnosis in the ED. *Am J Emerg Med* 1997;15:83–88.
6. Clark MC, Iwiniski HJ. The limping child: meeting the challenge of an accurate assessment and diagnosis. *Pediatr Emerg Med Rep* 1997;2:123–133.
7. Felter RA, Venglarcik J, Winograd S. Bone and Joint infections in children: diagnosis and treatment. *Pediatr Emerg Med Rep* 1999;3:221–227.
8. Halsey NA, Abramson JS, Chesney PG, et al. Severe invasive group A streptococcal infections: a subject review. *Pediatrics* 1998;101:136–140.
9. Hardasmalani MD, Naim FA, Kroning D, Bithoney WG. Emergency department presentations of a rare tumor–extraosseous cervical paraspinal Ewing's sarcoma. *J Emerg Med* 2003;24:271–275.
10. Koop S, Quanbeck D. Three common causes of childhood hip pain. *Pediatr Clin North Am* 1996;43:1053–1066.
11. Lawrence LL. The limping child. *Emerg Med Clin North Am* 1998;16:911–929.
12. McLario DJ, Burton LJ, Bruce RW, Whipple TJ, Simon HK. Pseudoparalysis of the lower extremity in an infant. *Pediatr Emerg Care* 1998;14:277–279.
13. Myers MT, Thompson GH. Imaging the child with a limp. *Pediatr Clin North Am* 1997;44:637–658.
14. Rosenbloom JS, Barton LL, Rekate HL. Abdominal and leg pain in a twenty-three-month-old child. *Pediatr Infect Dis J* 1998;17:441–442, 443–445.
15. Schneider P, Givens TG. Spinal subdural abscess in a pediatric patient: a case report and review of the literature. *Pediatr Emerg Care* 1998;14:22–23.
16. Sharieff GQ, Lee DM, Anshus JS. A rare case of salmonella-mediated sacroiliitis, adjacent subperiosteal abscess, and myositis. *Pediatr Emerg Care* 2003;19:252–254.
17. Simon JK, Lazareff JA, Diament MJ, Kennedy WA. Intramedullary abscess of the spinal cord in children: a case report and review of the literature. *Pediatr Infect Dis J* 2003;22:186–192.
18. Singer J. Altered locomotion: an approach to the assessment of the child with a limp. In: Barkin RM, (ed). *The emergently ill child.* Rockville, MD, Aspen, 1987:260–268.
19. Singer J. Evaluation of acute and insidious gait disturbance in children less than five years of age. *Adv Pediatr Chicago Year Book* 1979;26:209–273.
20. Singer J. Neonatal psoas pyomyositis simulating pyarthrosis of the hip. *Pediatr Emerg Care* 1993;9:87–89.
21. Singer J, Towbin R. Occult fractures in the production of gait disturbance in childhood. *Pediatrics* 1979;64:192–196.
22. Singer JI. The cause of gait disturbance in 425 pediatric patients. *Pediatr Emerg Care* 1985;1:7–10.
23. Zvulunov A, Gal N, Segev Z. Acute hematogenous osteomyelitis of the pelvis in childhood: Diagnostic clues and pitfalls. *Pediatr Emerg Care* 2003;19:29–31.

CHAPTER 230
Respiratory Distress

Richard Cantor and Bruce Quinn

Respiratory distress represents a compensatory state in response to impaired oxygen delivery to the tissues, with or without decreased carbon dioxide elimination. When the child's capacity for compensation is overwhelmed, respiratory failure occurs.

The respiratory tract can be divided into two anatomic categories: the lungs, or gas-exchange portion; and the "respiratory pump," consisting of the nervous system, respiratory muscles, and thorax (13). Pathology involving any of these areas can potentially present with signs and symptoms of respiratory distress. Depending on the etiology of the respiratory compromise and the time until presentation to the emergency department (ED), these signs and symptoms may be subtle.

A number of differences exist between the pediatric and the adult patient that place the child at greater risk for respiratory compromise. Infants and young children have a subglottic airway that is smaller and has less cartilaginous support, making it easier for obstruction to occur secondary to edema, secretions, constriction, or compression (4). The smaller the airway, the greater the resistance for a given decrease in luminal diameter. Dynamic collapse of a partially obstructed airway, as can be seen in croup during inspiration, is a direct consequence of the high compliance of the pediatric airway (4). Children less than 1 to 2 years of age may not have the anatomic pathways or "collateral ventilation" that allows aeration distal to an obstructed airway, thereby increasing the risk of atelectasis and ventilation–perfusion mismatching (13). Due to the increased chest wall compliance of the pediatric patients, diaphragmatic efforts may be wasted distorting the rib cage rather than expanding the lungs (13). The younger the child, the greater the pliability of the chest wall; placing the neonate at greatest risk for fatigue, respiratory failure, and cardiopulmonary arrest.

In addition to anatomic differences, the higher metabolic rate in children, compared with that in adults, places them at a further disadvantage by increasing their oxygen demand. With the onset of hypoventilation, hypoxemia and acidosis will occur more rapidly in the child (4).

CLINICAL PRESENTATION

The presentation of a child in respiratory distress varies, depending on a number of factors, including the specific etiology, duration of illness, age, underlying medical conditions, and

TABLE 230.1. Indicators of Actual or Possible Respiratory Compromise

Visual	Audible
Chest retractions	Cough
Abnormal behavior	Stridor
Altered mental status	Wheezing
Tachypnea/bradypnea	Grunting
Shallow/deep respirations	Abnormal voice or cry
Nasal flaring	
Head bobbing	
"See-saw" respirations	
Cyanosis	

interventions prior to arrival in the ED. Any degree of respiratory compromise must be rapidly recognized and appropriate therapy instituted, in order to avoid potential deterioration to respiratory failure and cardiopulmonary arrest.

Signs of respiratory distress can be separated into two categories: visual and audible (Table 230.1). Initially, simply looking at a child and listening, avoiding prolonged eye contact and use of a stethoscope, can provide a great deal of information with minimal, if any, anxiety being produced in the patient.

Visual inspection begins with the child's behavior. Normal behavior in a child does not rule out underlying pathology, but it does inform the clinician that the child is comfortable and in no need of urgent intervention. However, a quiet, serious child, who prefers sitting upright in a sniffing position, is a cause for concern and requires immediate assessment. Behavioral changes such as restlessness or irritability can be subtle clues of hypoxemia. Any alteration in mental status can represent either generalized central nervous system (CNS) disease or hypercarbia, with or without hypoxemia.

The presence of either tachypnea or bradypnea is taken as evidence of respiratory compromise. It is important, therefore, to be aware of the normal range of respiratory rates in the pediatric population. Hooker et al (15) found normal respiratory rates to be higher than in previously published studies with a wide range of "normal." In addition, fever, pain, and anxiety increase the respiratory rate in the absence of pulmonary disease. In Hooker's study, patients younger than 1 year of age had a mean respiratory rate of 39 $\pm$ 11 with a minimum of 22 breaths per minute to a maximum of 65 (15). Patients 2 to 3 years of age had a mean rate of 28 $\pm$ 4, with rates at 8 years of age falling into the adult range (20 $\pm$ 4) (15).

Rather than an absolute respiratory rate, a better marker of respiratory distress may be a change in the respiratory rate for a particular child, as well as an assessment of the depth of respirations. Shallow respirations are often seen in diseases associated with lower airway obstruction, while deep respirations are often representative of central compensatory mechanisms in response to underlying metabolic acidosis (23). The presence of chest retractions indicates respiratory distress. They begin subcostally with mild disease, and progress upward as the disease process worsens (36). Nasal flaring can be a subtle sign that is more commonly present in the infant and younger child, and is usually associated with lower tract disease. Head bobbing with each breath and "see-saw" or "rocky" respirations, in which the chest pulls in while the abdomen thrusts out, are signs of severe distress; the latter is an inefficient means of ventilation that can quickly lead to respiratory failure (4). Cyanosis is not apparent until at least 5 g of desaturated hemoglobin per deciliter of capillary blood is present; this usually correlates with a PO_2 below 40 and an arterial oxyhemoglobin saturation of 85% or less (5,21). Because anemic patients can be acyanotic and profoundly

hypoxic, cyanosis should not be considered a reliable or early indicator of hypoxemia (4).

Certain indicators of respiratory distress can be heard without the use of a stethoscope. Persistent, forceful, nonproductive coughing may indicate a foreign body lodged in the upper airway, with the potential for complete obstruction. Stridor is a harsh, crowing sound, occurring during inspiration (30) and commonly seen in the pediatric population. It signifies upper airway pathology being produced by rapid, turbulent air flow through a narrowed area (36). Wheezing represents expiratory obstruction of the lower airways (23). If heard without chest auscultation, it clearly indicates serious disease and the need for urgent intervention. Grunting, an end-expiratory sound is produced by glottic closure during exhalation in an attempt to provide physiologic positive end-expiratory pressure (PEEP) (23). When detected, it indicates a disease process causing alveolar and/or interstitial fluid (23). An abnormal voice or cry, particularly if muffled in quality, should alert the clinician to possible upper airway disease and the need for prompt, nonthreatening evaluation.

In the absence of visual and audible signs of respiratory distress, the likelihood of an infant or child having serious respiratory pathology requiring emergent intervention is small.

DIFFERENTIAL DIAGNOSIS

Determining the precise etiology of respiratory distress in the pediatric patient can be challenging; the differential diagnosis is substantial (Table 230.2). The clinician needs to recognize the signs and symptoms of respiratory distress in a child and determine the degree of severity. In moderate-to-severe degrees of distress, a rapid assessment of the likely etiology is necessary so that proper therapy can be initiated.

The presence of stridor indicates some form of upper airway obstruction and, when associated with fever, one should suspect an infectious etiology. Croup classically presents between 6 months and 3 years of age, with a history of a low-grade fever

TABLE 230.2. Etiologies of Respiratory Distress

INFECTIOUS	TRAUMA/MECHANICAL
Respiratory Tract	Hemothorax
Upper	Pneumothorax
Croup	Pulmonary contusion
Epiglottitis	Flail chest
URI	Spinal cord injury
Bacterial tracheitis	Intracranial hemorrhage
Peritonsillar abscess	Abdominal distension
Retropharyngeal abscess	
Lower	**ENVIRONMENTAL**
Pneumonia	
Bronchiolitis	Foreign body
	Smoke inhalation
Central Nervous System	Near drowning
Meningitis	Ingestions
Encephalitis	
Brain abscess	**OTHER**
HYPERACTIVE AIRWAY	Seizures
	Cardiac failure
Asthma	Cystic fibrosis
Anaphylaxis	Metabolic acidosis
	Vocal cord dysfunction
	Congenital anomalies
	Hypocalcemia

and upper respiratory infection (URI) symptoms for a few days, followed by the gradual onset of a barking cough, hoarseness, and stridor, with or without chest retractions.

In any child thought to have croup, the diagnosis of epiglottitis must be considered and ruled out. Although the incidence of epiglottitis has declined dramatically since the introduction of the *Haemophilus influenzae* type b conjugate vaccine (14,37), the physician must remain vigilant for this potentially life-threatening disease. Epiglottitis usually occurs between 3 and 8 years of age, although it can be seen as early as 6 months and as late as adulthood (35). Sudden onset of high fever is often the earliest manifestation (5). Losek et al (22) reported that among children with epiglottitis, 95% of those aged 2 years and older had a history of sore throat, and that 92% of all children had a change in voice or cry. At physical examination, the most common signs of epiglottitis were found to be stridor (88%), retractions (81%), and temperature 38°C or higher (85%); drooling (66%) and a preference for sitting (58%) were less common (22). The time course from first clinical sign to respiratory failure can be rapid, usually occurring within 12 hours (5).

In distinguishing between epiglottitis and croup in a child presenting with fever, stridor, and retractions, the importance of the history cannot be overemphasized. Drooling in the absence of spontaneous cough is the most specific indicator of acute epiglottitis (25). It is important to note, though, that cough can be seen in epiglottitis, and that its presence in no way eliminates it from the differential diagnosis (5,22).

Not infrequently, a URI alone will cause signs of mild-to-moderate respiratory distress in the very young infant. Simply suctioning the nares, using several drops of normal saline and a bulb syringe, is usually all that is required.

Other, less common etiologies to consider in a child with fever and stridor include bacterial tracheitis and peritonsillar or retropharyngeal abscesses. Patients with bacterial tracheitis typically have the initial symptoms of croup with progressive development of high fever, toxicity, and purulent tracheal secretions, resulting in airway compromise (5). Peritonsillar abscesses are most common in older adolescents and young adults in their early 20s (12). There is sudden elevation of temperature, toxicity, and unilateral throat pain following an earlier tonsillitis (5). The patient complains of trismus and has drooling, difficulty speaking, and a muffled voice (8). Examination may reveal bilateral tonsillar hypertrophy, or unilateral tonsillar enlargement with uvular deviation contralaterally (8). Unlike peritonsillar abscesses, retropharyngeal abscesses usually present in young children, from infancy to 3 years of age (5). The clinical picture is similar to that seen with epiglottitis, but with a less sudden onset (8). If the child is stable, radiographs of the soft tissues of the neck (either plain films or CT scanning) should be ordered.

Infectious etiologies of the lower respiratory tract that may cause respiratory distress include bronchiolitis and pneumonia. Bronchiolitis presents as any wheezing-associated illness in the first year of life that is preceded by a URI (41). Differentiation from acute attacks of asthma, often triggered by viral infections, may be difficult.

In those patients presenting in respiratory distress not clearly associated with infection, the history and physical examination should quickly solve the mystery. Most commonly, a diagnosis of reactive airway disease will be made. An important etiology to include in the differential diagnosis is anaphylaxis, a multisystem syndrome involving the cutaneous, respiratory, cardiovascular, and gastrointestinal systems; involvement of two or more systems is required for the diagnosis (7). Both the upper and lower airways can be involved, leading to hoarseness, stridor, wheezing, and cough. Early diagnosis and distinction of anaphylaxis from more benign conditions is essential, as these patients can progress rapidly to anaphylactic shock (7).

Environmental causes of respiratory distress, such as smoke inhalation and near drowning, will usually be evident from the history. Others, particularly foreign-body aspirations, may be difficult to determine. An infant or young child found in the midst of peanuts or similar sized objects, who subsequently develops a persistent cough with stridor, should obviously be evaluated for foreign-body aspiration. Often, however, the history of a foreign-body aspiration is less apparent, with the parents reporting only that their previously well child suddenly "began coughing out of the blue." Stridor or wheezing not responsive to appropriate therapy requires further evaluation, beginning with lateral and anteroposterior x-rays of the neck and chest, preferably during both inspiration and expiration.

Etiologies of respiratory distress associated with trauma should be evident from clinical examination. Tension pneumothorax and hemothorax need to be rapidly diagnosed and treated. Respiratory depression in the trauma patient without obvious respiratory tract pathology should raise the possibility of injury to the CNS.

Other important causes of respiratory compromise in the child include seizures, congestive heart failure, cystic fibrosis, and metabolic acidosis due to sepsis, diabetic ketoacidosis, renal disease, and certain ingestions (e.g., salicylate, methanol). Neuromuscular diseases, including Guillain-Barré, botulism, and myasthenia gravis, also need to be considered. Vocal cord dysfunction, believed to represent a conversion disorder, results in either inspiratory or expiratory stridor that may be confused with wheezing (38). Congenital anomalies should be considered in infants less than 6 months old who present with stridor; such anomalies include vascular rings, laryngeal webs, vocal cord paralysis, and laryngomalacia (21). Hypocalcemia, in addition to having neurologic, cardiovascular, and psychiatric manifestations, can also result in apnea, laryngeal spasm, bronchospasm, or biphasic respiratory noises and needs to be included in the differential diagnosis of any patient with respiratory distress (1).

EMERGENCY DEPARTMENT EVALUATION

The goals of the ED evaluation are to reach a diagnosis quickly, with minimal stress on the patient, and to promptly begin appropriate therapy and monitoring. Assessing the degree of respiratory distress is important, but mild distress must not be underestimated, as some diseases or conditions can progress rapidly (e.g., epiglottitis). The initial evaluation begins when the physician enters the room, noting any visual and audible indicators of actual or possible respiratory compromise. The child in respiratory distress must be approached in a gentle, reassuring manner and allowed to find the most comfortable position, whether it be on the examining table or on a parent's lap. In the child who is alert and behaving normally, the evaluation can proceed with the history and physical examination. However, any child who has an altered mental status, or one who is irritable or restless, with other signs of distress, needs to have an immediate assessment of airway, breathing pattern, and circulatory status, the ABCs of resuscitation. Further assessment or therapeutic intervention follows this initial evaluation.

Important historic points include underlying medical problems (e.g., asthma, cystic fibrosis, or seizure disorder), the onset and type of current symptoms, and the possibility of a foreign-body aspiration or ingestion or poisoning. If epiglottitis is suspected, forced visualization of the pharynx should be avoided in the ED (35). Although such attempts by Mauro and colleagues (25) in six patients did not lead to complications, forced visualization may result in a vasovagal response, causing cardiopulmonary collapse, respiratory obstruction, and death (9). We recommend the traditional approach of taking the child with suspected epiglottitis to the operating room for direct visualization of the airway in the presence of personnel skilled in establishing the airway.

After the history and physical examination, the etiology of the respiratory distress is usually clear. Noninvasive monitoring can be used to help with clinical assessment. Pulse oximetry provides a continuous, generally valid measure of the arterial hemoglobin oxygenation status and arterial pulse. Obtaining blood gas measurements stress an already distressed child, and should therefore generally be avoided early in the evaluation.

Sometimes, the diagnosis may not be obvious from the history and examination, and further evaluation may be needed. In situations in which aspiration of a foreign body is suspected, lateral and anteroposterior neck and/or chest x-rays should be obtained; if normal, either an assisted expiratory film, bilateral decubitus x-rays, or fluoroscopy should be done (3). If the distinction between croup and epiglottitis is not obvious, and the child is stable and only mildly ill, a lateral neck radiograph with close monitoring has been traditionally viewed as appropriate. However, Ragosta and colleagues (32) found lateral neck films to be of limited value in the initial evaluation of suspected epiglottitis and recommend against their use.

Repeated evaluations at regular intervals, as well as noninvasive monitoring, are essential in any child presenting to the ED in respiratory distress. Once the diagnosis is determined and appropriate therapy instituted, the response to therapy must be constantly reassessed. Often, the best way to determine whether an adult or older child is improving is simply to ask, "Are you feeling better?" In the nonverbal or frightened child, however, the response to therapy must be assessed by using changes in clinical parameters. Repeated examinations, although difficult in busy ED, can be lifesaving for the child in respiratory distress.

EMERGENCY DEPARTMENT MANAGEMENT

The importance of a gentle, nonthreatening approach cannot be overemphasized. Interventions of any sort are usually poorly tolerated by young children and, at least temporarily, may result in a worsening of their condition. The benefit of any intervention must always be weighed against its potential for adversely affecting the child.

Management of the child in respiratory distress generally involves two goals: keeping the patient as calm and comfortable as possible, and providing appropriate therapy. Therapy begins with humidified oxygen. Infants and some children often do not tolerate masks well, and depending on their oxygen requirement, may best be served with blow-by oxygen administered by the parent. In addition to the physical examination, pulse oximetry is useful in determining oxygenation status. Normal pulse oximetry readings have been reported as 91.5% to 100% in infants 6 months and younger who are awake (26), and 96% to 100% (median, 99.5%) in children 2 to 16 years of age who are asleep (29). If the anxiety produced by the administration of oxygen to children in mild distress worsens their condition, then the oxygen is clearly doing more harm than good and should be avoided. However, the anxiety elicited by the administration of oxygen is usually transient. An attempt at oxygen delivery should be made for all children in respiratory distress, except, perhaps, for the rare patient with chronic obstructive pulmonary disease (COPD). For severely distressed or cyanotic patients, 100% humidified oxygen must be provided quickly, irrespective of their acceptance.

The next step in management is to provide disease-specific therapy. Common diagnoses that respond to specific medical therapy include croup, asthma, and bronchiolitis. Children presenting with croup and stridor at rest can be provided a trial of humidified air. However, a beneficial effect of mist therapy on the upper airway edema found with croup has not been established (11,24,27). Steroids, given orally, parenterally, or via nebulizer, have been shown to be effective in the management of croup (6,11,24). A single oral dose of dexamethasone (0.15 mg/kg) significantly reduced the need for follow up in children discharged from an ED with mild croup; 16.7% of the placebo group required additional medical care versus 0% of the steroid group (10). In patients with moderately severe croup, parenteral dexamethasone and, to a lesser extent, nebulized budesonide were shown to provide clinical improvement; both significantly reduced hospital admissions (16). For severe croup, nebulized epinephrine can rapidly relieve distress, but its effect lasts only 1 to 3 hours (34). Either racemic epinephrine or L-epinephrine can be used, the latter having been shown to be as safe and effective as the more commonly prescribed racemic form (40). Although nebulized epinephrine's activity is short lived, studies indicate that when it is used with steroids (e.g., dexamethasone, 0.15–0.6 mg/kg, intramuscularly or orally), patients can be safely discharged home after 2 to 4 hours if clinically well (e.g., without retractions and stridor at rest) (17,19,20,31,34). Caution should be used when employing nebulized epinephrine if epiglottitis is suspected, as it may precipitate airway obstruction (18).

The mainstays of therapy for acute asthma are inhaled beta-adrenergic bronchodilators and corticosteroids, either orally or parenterally (39). Anticholinergic agents, widely recognized as important therapy for chronic asthma and COPD, have been shown to be effective for asthma exacerbations as well (2). Combining a nebulized anticholinergic agent with a beta-adrenergic agent appears to provide better bronchodilation than either drug alone (28). Although the effectiveness of inhaled bronchodilators in the management of bronchiolitis is controversial, an initial trial of inhaled beta-adrenergic agents is recommended (39,41). In addition, Reijonen and colleagues (33) found nebulized racemic epinephrine to be safe and useful.

CRITICAL INTERVENTIONS

- Keep the patient in their position of comfort for as long as possible
- Consider a foreign body in the patient who presents with paroxysmal cough or new onset wheezing
- Give steroids when administering epinephrine for croup

DISPOSITION

The disposition of the child in moderate-to-severe distress depends on the hospital's capacity to accommodate the patient's needs. Often, an inpatient pediatric floor or a pediatric intensive care unit (PICU) is required.

For the stable child in moderate distress, admission to an inpatient pediatric floor is appropriate. When there is a concern that the patient may deteriorate due to the particular disease process (e.g., anaphylaxis) or medical history (e.g., an asthmatic previously requiring intubation), admission to a PICU should be considered. If necessary, transfer to the nearest hospital having a PICU should be arranged in accordance with federal guidelines. The transfer should be done by personnel skilled in airway management (i.e., an advanced cardiac life-support unit or the pediatric transfer team of the receiving hospital). Ground transport is adequate for the stable child in only moderate distress.

Any child in severe distress should be admitted to a PICU. If transfer is necessary, consideration should be given to intubating and stabilizing the airway before departure, rather than risk deterioration and the need for a potentially difficult intubation en route. Transfer by ground units with personnel skilled in airway management is adequate for most patients in severe distress. However, the need for ground versus air transport must always be individualized.

COMMON PITFALLS

✔ Taking a blood pressure before giving therapy to the well-perfused patient

✔ Starting an intravenous line not needed for initial therapy (23)

✔ Forcing oxygen on the child in mild distress who will not tolerate it

✔ Obtaining blood for blood gas analysis in a severely distressed patient before providing therapy

✔ Doing a detailed history and physical examination before intervening in the severely distressed child (23)

✔ Misinterpreting decompensation for improvement

✔ During pulse oximetry monitoring, determining a sleeping infant to be hypoxic without further evaluating him or her in an awakened state

Acknowledgments

The authors would like to thank Marc Linares for his assistance with the previous version of this chapter.

References

1. Abrunzo TJ. An infant fatality associated with inspiratory and expiratory wheezing: another wheeze that wasn't asthma. *Pediatr Emerg Care* 1995;11:48.
2. Beakes DE. The use of anticholinergics in asthma. *J Asthma* 1997;34:357.
3. Brownstein DR. Foreign bodies of the gastrointestinal tract and airway. In: Barkin RM, (ed). *Pediatric emergency medicine concepts and clinical practice*, 2nd ed. St. Louis: Mosby-Year Book, 1997:371.
4. Chameides L, Hazinski MF, (eds). *Pediatric advanced life support*. Dallas: American Heart Association, American Academy of Pediatrics, 1997.
5. Davis HW, Gartner JC, Galvis AG, et al. Acute upper airway obstruction: croup and epiglottitis. *Pediatr Clin North Am* 1981;28:859.
6. Donaldson D, Poleski D, Knipple E, et al. Intramuscular versus oral dexamethasone for the treatment of moderate-to-severe croup: a randomized, double-blind trial. *Acad Emerg Med* 2003;10:16–21.
7. Edwards KH, Johnston C. Allergic and immunologic disorders In: Barkin RM, (ed). *Pediatric emergency medicine concepts and clinical practice*, 2nd ed. St. Louis: Mosby-Year Book, 1997:619.
8. Fleisher GR. Infectious disease emergencies. In: Fleischer GR, Ludwig S, (eds). *Textbook of pediatric emergency medicine*, 3rd ed. Baltimore: William & Wilkins, 1993:613.
9. Fulginiti VA. Acute supraglottitis (epiglottitis): to look or not? *Am J Dis Child* 1988;142:597.
10. Geelhoed GC, Turner J, MacDonald WBG. Efficacy of a small single dose of oral dexamethasone for outpatient croup: a double blind placebo controlled clinical trial. *BMJ* 1996;313:140.
11. Geelhoed GC. Croup. *Pediatr Pulmonol* 1997;23:370.
12. Hammerschlag PE, Hammerschlag MR. Peritonsillar, retropharyngeal, and parapharyngeal abscesses. In: Feigin RD, Cherry JD, (eds). *Textbook of pediatric infectious diseases*, vol. 1, 4th ed. Philadelphia: WB Saunders, 1998:164.
13. Helfaer MA, Nichols DG, Rogers MC. Developmental physiology of the respiratory system. In: Rogers MC, (ed). *Textbook of pediatric intensive care*, 3rd ed. Baltimore: Williams & Wilkins, 1996:98.
14. Hickerson SL, Kirby RS, Wheeler JG, et al. Epiglottis: a 9-year case review. *South Med J* 1996;89:487.
15. Hooker EA, Danzl DF, Brueggmeyer M, et al. Respiratory rates in pediatric emergency patients. *J Emerg Med* 1992;10:407.
16. Jonson DW, Jacobson S, Edney PC, et al. A comparison of nebulized budesonide, intramuscular dexamethasone, and placebo for moderately severe croup. *N Engl J Med* 1998;339:498.
17. Kelly PB, Simon JE. Racemic epinephrine use in croup and disposition. *Am J Emerg Med* 1992;10:181.
18. Kissoon N, Mitchel I. Adverse effects of racemic epinephrine in epiglottitis. *Pediatr Emerg Care* 1985;1:143.
19. Kunkel NC, Baker MD. Use of racemic epinephrine, dexamethasone, and mist in the outpatient management of croup. *Pediatr Emerg Care* 1996;12:156.
20. Ledwith CA, Shea LM, Mauro RD. Safety and efficacy of nebulized racemic epinephrine in conjunction with oral dexamethasone and mist in the outpatient treatment of croup. *Ann Emerg Med* 1995;25:331.
21. Letourneau MA, Schuh S, Gausche M. Respiratory disorders. In: Barkin RM, (ed). *Pediatric emergency medicine concepts and clinical practice*, 2nd ed. St. Louis: Mosby-Year Book, 1997:1056.
22. Losek JD, Dewitz-Zink BA, Melzer-Lange M, et al. Epiglottitis: comparison of signs and symptoms in children less than 2 years old and older. *Ann Emerg Med* 1990;19:55–58.
23. Luten R. Respiratory distress. In: Harwood-Nuss A, Linden C, Shepherd S, et al., (eds). *The clinical practice of emergency medicine*. Philadelphia: JB Lippincott Co, 1991:681.
24. MacDonald WBG, Geelhoed GC. Management of childhood croup. *Thorax* 1997;52:757.
25. Mauro RD, Poole SR, Lockhart CH. Differentiation of epiglottitis from laryngotracheitis in the child with stridor. *Am J Dis Child* 1988;142:679.
26. Mok JYQ, McLaughlin J, Pintar M, et al. Transcutaneous monitoring of oxygenation: what is normal? *J Pediatr* 1986;108:365.
27. Neto G, Kentab B, Klassen T, et al. A Randomized Controlled Trial of Mist in the Acute Treatment of Moderate Croup. *Academic Emergency Medicine* 2002;9:873–879.
28. Nichols DG. Emergency management of status asthmaticus in children. *Pediatr Ann* 1996;25:394.
29. Poets CF, Stebbens VA, Samuels MP, et al. Oxygen saturation and breathing patterns in children. *Pediatrics* 1993;92:686.
30. Poole SR, Mauro RD, Fan LL, et al. The child with simultaneous stridor and wheezing. *Pediatr Emerg Care* 1990;6:33.
31. Prendergast M, Jones JS, Hartman D. Racemic epinephrine in the treatment of laryngotracheitis: can we identify children for outpatient therapy? *Am J Emerg Med* 1994;12:613.
32. Ragosta KG, Orr R, Detweiler MJ. Revisiting epiglottis: a protocol—the value of lateral neck radiographs. *J Am Osteopath Assoc* 1997;97:227.
33. Reijonen T, Korppi M, Pitkäkangas S, et al. The clinical efficacy of nebulized racemic epinephrine and albuterol in acute bronchiolitis. *Arch Pediatr Adolesc Med* 1995;149:686.
34. Rizos JD, DiGravio BE, Sehl MJ, et al. The disposition of children with croup treated with racemic epinephrine and dexamethasone in the emergency department. *J Emerg Med* 1998;16:535.
35. Ruddy RM. Respiratory distress in a child in the office. *Pediatr Emerg Care* 1990;6:314.
36. Saipe C. Respiratory emergencies in children. *Pediatr Ann* 1990;19:637.
37. Schroeder LL, Knapp JF. Recognition and emergency management of infectious causes of upper airway obstruction in children. *Semin Respir Infect* 1995;10:21.
38. Snyder HS, Weiss E. Hysterical stridor: a benign cause of upper airway obstruction. *Ann Emerg Med* 1989;18:1991.
39. Stempel DA, Redding G. Management of acute asthma. *Pediatr Clin North Am* 1992;39:1311.
40. Waisman Y, Klein BL, Boenning DA, et al. Prospective randomized double-blind study comparing L-epinephrine and racemic epinephrine aerosols in the treatment of laryngotracheitis (croup). *Pediatrics* 1992;89:302.
41. Welliver JR, Welliver RC. Bronchiolitis. *Pediatr Rev* 1993;14:134.

CHAPTER 231
Seizures

Craig R. Warden and Christopher S. Kennedy

A seizure in a child can be a dramatic event, provoking fear and panic in parents and caregivers. The majority of parents will bring their child to the emergency department (ED) for evaluation, even if the child has seemed to fully recover. The initial step in this process requires determining whether the seizure has stopped and whether the child has returned to his or her prior neurologic baseline. If the child is continuing to have seizure activity on arrival to the ED, managing the ABCs and stopping the seizure are the first priorities.

A seizure is a series of excessive, abnormal electrical discharges from cerebral neurons that produce transient involuntary alterations in functioning, including consciousness, motor activity, behavior, and/or autonomic regulation. Affecting 4% to 6% of children by age 16, seizures are the most common childhood neurologic disorder. The incidence is highest in newborns with a decreasing frequency as children get older (12).

During seizure activity, consumption of oxygen and glucose is increased in cerebral tissues. Early physiologic changes include hypertension, hyperglycemia, and hypoxemia. With subsequent or prolonged seizure activity, progressive lactic acidosis, rhabdomyolysis, hyperkalemia, hyperthermia, and hypoglycemia may develop, leading to possible permanent neurologic damage.

Most childhood seizures are brief, isolated and have a good outcome. However, in some children, seizures are prolonged and recurrent. *Status epilepticus*, defined as recurrent or continuous seizure activity that lasts longer than 30 minutes without recovery of baseline mental functioning, is one of the most common neurologic emergencies encountered in children. As seizure cessation and prevention of complications are time dependent, the ED physician should be familiar with all aspects of seizure management. These aspects include initial stabilization, primary investigation of cause, acute management, and disposition.

CLINICAL PRESENTATION

The single most important clinical finding when a child presents with a seizure is whether there is ongoing seizure activity. Seizures are classified as either generalized or partial. Generalized seizures may be convulsive or nonconvulsive and may manifest with an altered level of consciousness and with or without bilateral motor activity. Partial seizures may be simple, without affecting consciousness; or complex, with impaired mental status. In the ED, ongoing seizures may manifest with a wide array of clinical presentations, from tonic, clonic, tonic–clonic, or myoclonic activity; or by clouding of, or loss of, consciousness; eye deviations; repetitive, stereotyped movements; or by isolated behavioral changes, such as continuous crying or bicycling movements seen in infants. Whether the child responds to a caregiver's presence or voice can also be a useful clinical clue.

If the seizure has already stopped, additional related clinical findings include presence of a postictal phase, loss of bowel and/or bladder control, or focal neurologic deficit. A hemiparesis or other focal neurologic deficit (without signs of increased intracranial pressure, ICP), also called a Todd's paralysis, is an important localizing sign and suggests that the seizure had a focal component. If the focal deficit is new and persists, a structural cause for the seizure should be sought. Fever is the most common cause of seizures in childhood; discussion of febrile seizures follows in a subsequent section. Clinical signs of neurologic disease or remote neurologic events that predispose a child to seizures include skin findings associated with neurocutaneous disorders (such as ash leaf spots or adenoma sebaceum, suggesting tuberous sclerosis; café-au-lait spots, suggesting neurofibromatosis; or port-wine staining of the face, suggesting Sturge-Weber syndrome), microcephaly, dysmorphic features, spasticity, hemiplegia, or quadriplegia. Stroke, increased ICP, or meningitis may be associated with acute clinical findings such as hemiparesis, papilledema and bulging fontanelle, or stiff neck. Unexplained superficial bruising should raise the suspicion of a bleeding disorder or child abuse. Eclampsia should be considered in the potentially pregnant patient.

DIFFERENTIAL DIAGNOSIS

A seizure is not a diagnosis but a clinical symptom of an underlying disease or process with many potential causes, which vary with age (Table 231.1). Other entities that may be confused with seizures include underlying neurologic disease, such as spasticity, and acute dystonic reactions, neither of which has an associated loss of consciousness. A detailed history of the seizure event from a witness is the single most important feature for accurate diagnosis. It is important to determine whether the child has actually had a seizure, because many childhood conditions can easily be mistaken for a seizure. These disorders can be classified by one of three presentations: sudden loss of consciousness, paroxysmal movements, or sudden change in behavior.

Disorders with sudden loss of consciousness include breath-holding spells, syncope, cardiac dysrhythmias, and complicated migraines, and each is differentiated from a seizure because a postictal state is rare. Breath-holding spells occur in two forms,

TABLE 231.1. Acute Causes of Seizures by Age

NEONATAL

Congenital CNS abnormalities
Hypoxic-ischemic CNS insult
Intracranial hemorrhage
Intrauterine drug exposure/drug withdrawal
Metabolic disorders (e.g., hypoglycemia, hyponatremia, hypernatremia, hypomagnesemia, hyperphosphatemia, hypocalcemia)
Inborn errors of metabolism
Hypertension
Infections/sepsis
Epilepsy (e.g., infantile spasms)
Pyridoxine deficiency
Benign familial neonatal seizures/benign idiopathic neonatal seizures ("fifth day fits")

EARLY CHILDHOOD

Past birth-related injury
Febrile seizures (6 mo to 6 yr)
Meningitis/encephalitis
Metabolic disorders
Neurocutaneous syndromes
Cerebral degenerative disorders
Tumors
Head trauma (shaking or direct injury)
Epilepsy (± medication noncompliance)

CHILDREN AND ADOLESCENTS

Head trauma
Meningitis/encephalitis
Epilepsy (medication noncompliance)
Cerebral degenerative disorders
Tumors
Idiopathic

ANY AGE GROUP

Ventriculoperitoneal shunt malfunction or infection
Toxins
  Pesticides, phenothiazines, phencyclidine
  Lidocaine, lindane, lithium
  Alcohol, amphetamines, antihistamines, antidepressants, anticholinergics
  Salicylates
  Theophylline
  Insulin, isoniazid, Inderal
  Camphor, caffeine, carbon monoxide, cocaine

cyanotic and pallid, usually in children between 6 months and 5 years of age. Cyanotic spells begin with vigorous crying, followed by apnea, cyanosis, and, occasionally, myoclonus. Pallid spells begin with a painful or fear-producing stimulus, followed by pallor and loss of consciousness. Vasovagal syncope, the most common cause of syncope in childhood, may be preceded by light-headedness and dizziness, followed by loss of consciousness. The loss of consciousness is brief, and recovery is rapid and may be occasionally accompanied by a brief generalized seizure. Syncopal events from cardiac dysrhythmias are usually associated with a positive family history; they are characterized by a brief loss of consciousness, with myoclonic movements, and rapid recovery. Electrocardiographic or Holter monitoring as an outpatient may be needed for confirmation. With complicated migraines, loss of consciousness may be associated with or preceded by blurred vision, blindness, dizziness, or loss of postural tone.

Disorders with paroxysmal movements include tics, shuddering attacks, benign sleep myoclonus, and pseudoseizures. These are differentiated from seizures because a loss of consciousness is rare. Tics are brief, stereotyped, nonrhythmic movements that may be precipitated by stress; usually, some voluntary control is exhibited. Shuddering attacks are characterized by rapid tremors of the entire body, which may occur up to 100 times a day. They are usually inherited, are self-limited, may be precipitated by stress, and may require an electroencephalogram (EEG) (which is normal) to convince the family that they are not seizures. Benign sleep myoclonus usually presents in infancy with benign, self-limited, sudden, jerky movements of one or more extremity. Although more common when the child is falling asleep, they may occur throughout sleep. Pseudoseizures may be difficult to distinguish from seizures in the ED and may require video EEG monitoring for diagnosis. They present with paroxysmal movements, lack of coordination, and moaning or talking during the episode, and can even be seen in patients with an underlying seizure disorder.

Disorders with sudden behavioral changes include night terrors. These are differentiated from seizures by their characteristic findings. Night terrors, a form of parasomnia, occurs in preschoolers, with sudden awakening from sleep with fits of crying, sweating, and rapid breathing, and there may be associated stereotyped movements.

EMERGENCY DEPARTMENT EVALUATION

The history and physical examination are the most useful tools in ED evaluation. History should focus on a detailed description of the seizure including seizure duration, type of seizure (focal or generalized), associated loss of consciousness, presence of incontinence or cyanosis, length of postical period, any postical neurologic abnormalities, and for patients with known seizure disorders whether the current seizure is different or the frequency has increased. Further history taking should focus on potential causes: trauma, infection, recent immunization, presence of a CSF shunt, or intoxication, and a history of seizures, anticonvulsant use and compliance or use of the ketogenic diet. An important component of the history is to differentiate true seizures from mimics. The history should include any prehospital observations and treatment by either caretakers or emergency medical service (EMS) providers. This may include the use of rectal diazepam by caretakers or other benzodiazepines by EMS providers that may explain a prolonged postical phase.

The physical examination should focus on signs of trauma (including retinal hemorrhages), increased ICP, focal neurologic abnormalities, and meningeal irritation. In addition, one should assess hepatosplenomegaly for possible metabolic or glycogen

storage diseases and the skin for café-au-lait spots (neurofibromatosis), vitiliginous lesions (tuberous sclerosis) and port-wine stains (Sturge-Weber syndrome).

Laboratory testing should be guided by the history and examination. A rapid bedside glucose should be done on all seizure patients. Serum electrolytes, calcium, magnesium, ammonia, complete blood count, and a urine toxicology screen may be indicated depending on the clinical scenario. These tests have been shown in several studies to have a low yield in patients without identifiable risk factors compared to a well-done history and physical examination (12,17). Hyponatremia has been most associated with age less than one month, hypothermia (temperature < 36.5°C) and active seizures in the ED (8).

A lumbar puncture is not indicated for the typical child with a seizure without any other clinical indications of meningitis (4,9,14). An LP should be considered in all neonates with a seizure with a low threshold to perform one in young infants who are difficult to evaluate for meningitis and may not be febrile. Magnetic resonance imaging has become the imaging modality of choice for new-onset seizure in children when imaging is indicated, but is usually not required on an emergent basis. Brain imaging studies for the ED patient at most institutions consist of a cranial computed tomography (CT) scan. Indications for CT in the ED include a focal deficit on neurologic examination, signs of increased ICP, an infant less than 6 to 12 months old without another cause of the seizure, patients with ventriculoperitoneal shunts, status epilepticus, any immunocompromising states, exposure to area endemic for cysticercosis, suspected cerebrovascular disease, hypercoagulable states (including sickle cell disease), and suspected head trauma (16,23). In general, a well-appearing child over 6 to 12 months of age with a first-time unprovoked seizure does not need emergent neuroimaging. EEG monitoring is rarely used emergently, except for refractory status or if a diagnosis of nonconvulsive status is considered (EEG may be the only way to accurately diagnose this disorder) (3).

EMERGENCY DEPARTMENT MANAGEMENT

Seizure activity upon arrival in the ED should be considered status epilepticus until further history can be obtained, and the main priorities should be resuscitation of the child and stopping the seizure. A brief history should focus on finding an acute cause of the seizure, such as trauma, infection, or intoxication, and history of seizures and anticonvulsant use. A rapid physical examination should search for signs of trauma, increased ICP, and meningeal irritation. If meningitis is a concern, appropriate antibiotics should be given expeditiously.

CRITICAL INTERVENTIONS

- The following protocol is suggested to manage status epilepticus (7,10,11,13,15,18,20)

At 0 to 5 minutes
- Maintain airway, give oxygen, support ventilation, and consider cervical spine immobilization for trauma patients
- Obtain IV access, check bedside glucose, and send blood samples for electrolytes, CBC, glucose, and anticonvulsant levels, as appropriate
- Monitor vital signs, pulse oximetry, and ECG
- Administer first dose of benzodiazepine (see Table 231.2) IV. If delay in obtaining IV access, administer midazolam or lorazepam IM or diazepam PR
- Consider intravenous glucose 2 mL/kg of D_{25} (Use D10 solution in newborns) for documented hypoglycemia only and pyridoxine (50–100 mg IV) for neonates (or for isoniazid overdose)

At 5 to 15 minutes, if seizure continues
- Administer second dose of benzodiazepine (see Table 231.2)
- Start loading dose of phenytoin or fosphenytoin, consider phenobarbital for neonates (see Table 231.2)
- Search for reversible causes of seizures: trauma, toxins, shunt malfunction, and electrolyte abnormalities and initiate appropriate management
- Continue monitoring of VS including pulse oximetry and now core temperature for hyperthermia

At 15 to 30 minutes, if seizure continues
- Start loading dose of phenobarbital (see Table 231.2)
- Reevaluate airway and strongly consider need for intubation
- Consider initiating contact with referral PICU and transferring patient if necessary
- Continue search for reversible causes of seizure and initiate appropriate management
- Check electrolyte results; consider need for intravenous hypertonic saline for symptomtic hyponatremia

At > 30 minutes, if seizure continues
- Consider additional phenobarbital
- Consider consultation with pediatric neurologist. Discuss need for continuous EEG monitoring
- Consider need for continuous pentobarbital, midazolam, or propofol infusions. Consider general anesthesia in consultation with an anesthesiologist (rarely required)
- Intubate now if not previously done
- Consider central venous access for multiple infusions and CVP monitoring. Consider continuous arterial pressure monitoring

At beyond 60 minutes, if seizure continues
- Begin alternative continuous infusion regimen with pentobarbital, midazolam or propofol or general anesthesia while awaiting transfer or admission to PICU

Brief Overview of Pharmacotherapy

First-line drugs for the management of status include benzodiazepines, fosphenytoin or phenytoin, and phenobarbital (discussed above). Benzodiazepines are the current drugs of choice for initial management of all seizures. Lorazepam may be pre-ferred due to its long half-life. Benzodiazepines cause respiratory depression and, in higher doses, may cause hypotension. Diazepam may be given rectally via a short 8 French feeding tube or a needleless 1-mL Tb syringe. Midazolam or lorazepam may be given IM if intravenous access is not available. Recently developed Diastat®, a viscous solution for rectal administration, is available in prefilled, rectal-tipped syringes in a variety of doses for use especially at home. One strategy for the patient with a known seizure disorder who has a breakthrough seizure is to administer a dose of a benzodiazepine such as lorazepam to stop a seizure or prevent its recurrence while checking the patient's antiepileptic drug (AED) level and/or loading that AED or another long-acting AED.

Fosphenytoin or phenytoin is utilized if a seizure continues after benzodiazepine use. Fosphenytoin, a newly developed prodrug of phenytoin, is often preferred for use in children because it causes fewer side effects such as hypotension with IV infusion and tissue necrosis with accidental infiltration. Fosphenytoin can also be given intramuscularly if vascular access has not been established.

Phenobarbital is considered by many to be the drug of choice for neonatal seizures and for complex febrile seizures that are unresponsive to benzodiazepines. Noteworthy is the increased risk of respiratory depression when phenobarbital is given concomitantly with benzodiazepines, more likely with diazepam than lorazepam (6).

DISPOSITION

Children with first-time seizures can be followed as outpatients if they appear well, the parents are comfortable with outpatient management, and follow up can be assured. These children frequently do not require maintenance anticonvulsant therapy, but the decision to start therapy, and which agent to use, should be done in consultation with a pediatric neurologist and the primary care physician (12). Hospital admission is reserved for children with a prolonged seizure or status epilepticus, even if successfully treated in the ED. Children requiring intubation and ventilatory support or those with prolonged refractory status

TABLE 231.2.   Medications Used in the ED for Seizures and Status Epilepticus

Use	Drug	Route/Dosage	Adverse Effects
First-line agents	Midazolam	IV: 0.1 mg/kg IM: 0.2 mg/kg	Loss of airway control, hypoventilation Hypotension: rare
	Diazepam	IV: 0.2–0.3 mg/kg PR: 0.5 mg/kg	Loss of airway control, hypoventilation Hypotension: rare PR: erratic absorption IM: sterile abscess
	Lorazepam	IV: 0.1 mg/kg IM: 0.2 mg/kg	IM: erratic absorption, accumulation of drug with multiple doses
Second-line	Phenytoin	IV: 20 mg/kg over 30–45 minutes	Hypotension & arrhythmias with rapid infusion
	Fosphenytoin	IV: 20 mg PE/kg over 15–20 minutes IM: same, several sites needed	Expensive
Third-line	Phenobarbital	IV: 20 mg/kg over 30 minutes	Loss of airway control, hypoventilation, hypotension, prolonged obtundation
Fourth-line	Pentobarbital	IV: 5–15 mg/kg slow bolus then 1–3 mg/kg/hr	Loss of airway control, hypoventilation, hypotension, prolonged obtundation
	Midazolam	IV: 0.1–0.2 mg/kg slow bolus then 0.06–0.12 mg/kg/hr (1–2 µg/kg/min) titrate by 0.06 mg/kg/hr (1 µg/kg/min) every 10 mins as needed	Loss of airway control, hypoventilation, hypotension, prolonged obtundation
	Valproic acid	IV: 10 mg/kg over 20 mins	Hepatoxicity

PE, phenytoin equivalents; IV, intravenous; IM, intramuscular; PR, per rectum.

should be transported to a tertiary care facility with a PICU and pediatric subspecialists.

SPECIAL CONSIDERATIONS: FEBRILE SEIZURES

Febrile convulsions are the most common form of seizures in childhood, occurring in 2% to 5% of children. Generally, febrile seizures are defined by a seizure in association with a febrile illness, without central nervous system infection, previous afebrile seizures, known brain disorder or electrolyte imbalance. They usually occur between the ages of 6 months and 5 years; peak incidence is approximately 18 months of age. Febrile seizures are classified as simple or complex. A febrile seizure is complex if it is focal, lasts longer than 15 minutes, or multiple (more than one seizure during the febrile illness). The majority of febrile seizures are simple febrile seizures that are brief, isolated, and generalized. Although the pathophysiology of febrile seizures remains unclear, it appears that the absolute peak temperature plays a key role. Mortality is extremely rare, and there are no differences in cognitive abilities after a febrile seizure, even when prolonged (1,2,24).

To diagnose a febrile seizure, meningitis, encephalitis, electrolyte imbalances, and other acute neurologic disease must be ruled out. Most of these can be eliminated by a careful history or physical examination. In 1996, the American Academy of Pediatrics issued guidelines for the evaluation of children with simple febrile seizures who are between the ages of 6 months and 5 years (1). According to these guidelines, a lumbar puncture should strongly be considered in all infants less than 12 months of age, should be carefully considered in all children between 12 and 18 months, and should not be considered necessary in well-appearing children over 18 months, without symptoms of meningitis. Neuroimaging of any kind is not routinely required, and additional routine laboratory studies are of limited value. Patients with febrile seizures have the same risk of serious bacterial illness including meningitis as matched febrile patients without seizures (5,22). If the child arrives in the ED in apparent status from a febrile seizure, it should be treated as such. Benzodiazepines are the drugs of choice, but the most studied agent is diazepam, as discussed above.

Other than evaluation and treatment of the underlying cause of the fever, the majority of cases will require only reassurance and education of parents about febrile seizures. Anticonvulsant prophylaxis is not routinely recommended.

SPECIAL CONSIDERATIONS: NEONATAL SEIZURES

Neonatal seizures are often clinically subtle and may present as apnea, subtle eye deviations, abnormal chewing movements, and abnormal extremity movement such as "bicycling" (21). Associated autonomic changes seen with older infants and children may not be seen. Occasionally, an excessively "jittery" baby may be thought to be having seizures but these movements can be suppressed with gentle restraint. Most neonatal seizures are provoked by an underlying insult and a vigorous evaluation for an etiology is necessary. The most common etiology accounting for 50% to 65% of neonatal seizures is hypoxic-ischemic encephalopathy from a perinatal anoxic insult. An intracranial hemorrhage accounts for another 15% of neonatal seizures and an additional 10% is due to inborn errors of metabolism, sepsis, metabolic disorders, and toxins (19). Pyridoxine deficiency is an autosomal recessive disorder that is a rare cause of neonatal seizures but will not readily respond to the usual treatment of status epilepticus and is eminently treatable with supplemental pyridoxine and needs to be thought of early in the evaluation.

There are two benign neonatal seizure disorders which are diagnoses of exclusions: *benign familial neonatal convulsions* which present in the first three days of life with a strong family history of epilepsy or neonatal seizures and *benign idiopathic neonatal convulsions* ("fifth day fits") which present on the fifth day of life but may continue until the 15th day of life.

Neonatal seizures mandate an aggressive work up for the underlying etiology and will always include an imaging study; the modality depends on presentation (MRI, cranial ultrasound, or CT). Similarly, an aggressive laboratory work up is usually indicated. Laboratory work up will include electrolytes (including magnesium, calcium, and phosphate), bedside glucose determination, and toxicology studies when indicated. If an inborn error of metabolism is suspected, blood for amino acids, lactate, pyruvate, and ammonia and urine for organic acids are indicated. Sepsis is always high on the differential in any sick neonate and the work up generally includes a complete blood count with differential, blood culture, urine for analysis and culture, and CSF including consideration for testing for herpes simplex.

The management of neonatal seizures is initially the same as for older infants and children with attention to the ABCs and terminating the seizure with a parenteral dose of a benzodiazepine. Most neonates with a seizure will be loaded with a long-acting anticonvulsant. In this age group, phenobarbital is usually preferred over phenytoin due to the latter's myocardial depressant effect and unpredictable hepatic metabolism (19). Pyridoxine therapy should be considered early if seizures are refractory to first-line agents. Electrolyte and glucose abnormalities should be aggressively sought and treated with appropriate agents. Most neonates with seizures are initially treated with antibiotics for potential sepsis with ampicillin and either an aminoglycoside such as gentamicin or a third-generation cephalosporin such as cefotaxime. In patients with a suspicion for herpes, acyclovir should be initiated pending results of confirmatory tests. All neonates having had a seizure are admitted to an appropriate monitored bed.

COMMON PITFALLS

✔ Failure to address airway, breathing, and circulation as the first priority in status epilepticus management
✔ Failure to expeditiously treat ongoing status epilepticus with loading doses of anticonvulsants in addition to benzodiazepines
✔ Failure to recognize and treat the underlying disease causing the seizure
✔ Failure to consider child abuse in young children
✔ Failure to diagnose meningitis in infants with a febrile seizure

References

1. American Academy of Pediatrics. Provisional Committee on Quality Improvement, Subcommittee on Febrile Seizures. Practice parameter: the neurodiagnostic evaluation of the child with a first simple febrile seizure. *Pediatrics* 1996;97:769–772; discussion 773–765.
2. American Academy of Pediatrics. Committee on Quality Improvement, Subcommittee on Febrile Seizures. Practice parameter: long-term treatment of the child with simple febrile seizures. *Pediatrics* 1999;103:1307–1309.
3. Alehan FK, Morton LD, Pellock JM. Utility of electroencephalography in the pediatric emergency department. *J Child Neurol* 2001;16:484–487.
4. Al-Eissa YA. Lumbar puncture in the clinical evaluation of children with seizures associated with fever. *Pediatr Emerg Care* 1995;11:347–350.
5. Chamberlain JM, Gorman RL. Occult bacteremia in children with simple febrile seizures. *Am J Dis Child* 1988;142:1073–1076.
6. Chiulli DA, Terndrup TE, Kanter RK. The influence of diazepam or lorazepam on the frequency of endotracheal intubation in childhood status epilepticus. *J Emerg Med* 1991;9:13–17.

7. Crawford TO, Mitchell WG, Snodgrass SR. Lorazepam in childhood status epilepticus and serial seizures: effectiveness and tachyphylaxis. *Neurology* 1987;37:190–195.

8. Farrar HC, Chande VT, Fitzpatrick DF, Shema SJ. Hyponatremia as the cause of seizures in infants: a retrospective analysis of incidence, severity, and clinical predictors. *Ann Emerg Med* 1995;26:42–48.

9. Green SM, Rothrock SG, Clem KJ, Zurcher RF, Mellick L. Can seizures be the sole manifestation of meningitis in febrile children? *Pediatrics* 1993;92:527–534.

10. Haafiz A, Kissoon N. Status epilepticus: current concepts. *Pediatr Emerg Care* 1999;15:119–129.

11. Hanhan UA, Fiallos MR, Orlowski JP. Status epilepticus. *Pediatr Clin North Am* 2001;48:683–694.

12. Hirtz D, Berg A, Bettis D, et al. Practice parameter: treatment of the child with a first unprovoked seizure: Report of the Quality Standards Subcommittee of the American Academy of Neurology and the Practice Committee of the Child Neurology Society. *Neurology* 28 2003;60:166–175.

13. Holmes GL, Riviello JJ, Jr. Midazolam and pentobarbital for refractory status epilepticus. *Pediatr Neurol* 1999;20:259–264.

14. Joffe A, McCormick M, DeAngelis C. Which children with febrile seizures need lumbar puncture? A decision analysis approach. *Am J Dis Child* 1983;37:1153–1156.

15. Lowenstein DH, Alldredge BK. Status epilepticus. *N Engl J Med* 1998;338:970–976.

16. Maytal J, Krauss JM, Novak G, Nagelberg J, Patel M. The role of brain computed tomography in evaluating children with new onset of seizures in the emergency department. *Epilepsia* 2000;41:950–954.

17. Nypaver MM, Reynolds SL, Tanz RR, Davis AT. Emergency department laboratory evaluation of children with seizures: dogma or dilemma? *Pediatr Emerg Care* 1992;8:13–16.

18. Pellock JM. Use of midazolam for refractory status epilepticus in pediatric patients. *J Child Neurol* 1998;13:581–587.

19. Rennie JM, Boylan GB. Neonatal seizures and their treatment. *Curr Opin Neurol* 2003;16:177–181.

20. Rivera R, Segnini M, Baltodano A, Perez V. Midazolam in the treatment of status epilepticus in children. *Crit Care Med* 1993;21:991–994.

21. Scher MS. Controversies regarding neonatal seizure recognition. *Epileptic Disord* 2002;4:139–158.

22. Trainor JL, Hampers LC, Krug SE, Listernick R. Children with first-time simple febrile seizures are at low risk of serious bacterial illness. *Acad Emerg Med* 2001;8(8):781–787.

23. Warden CR, Brownstein DR, Del Beccaro MA. Predictors of abnormal findings of computed tomography of the head in pediatric patients presenting with seizures. *Ann Emerg Med* 1997;29:518–523.

24. Warden CR, Zibulewsky J, Mace S, Gold C, Gausche-Hill M. Evaluation and management of febrile seizures in the out-of-hospital and emergency department settings. *Ann Emerg Med* 2003;41:215–222.

CHAPTER 232
Syncope

Sharon E. Mace

Syncope is the sudden transient loss of consciousness accompanied by an inability to maintain postural tone with spontaneous resolution. Syncope is a common complaint in patients of all ages, accounting for 3% of (ED) visits (2) and 1% to 6% of adult hospital admissions (5,6,8). In children and adolescents, syncope accounts for 2% of pediatric ED visits (10) and 1% of pediatric hospital admissions (11). In the pediatric population, syncope occurs more often in females than males, and most often in adolescents with the highest incidence in the fifteen to nineteen-year old age group (4). From 15% to 50% of all adolescents will have had at least one syncopal episode (3,9,11,12). Syncope is less common in children ≤ 5 years of age in whom primary cardiac dysrhythmias, seizures, and breath holding spells are the main considerations. Although the general categories of

disorders that can result in syncope are similar in adults and children; the specific causes and the evaluation may differ between adults and children/infants (Table 232.1). In addition, there are a few causes of syncope that are unique to the pediatric population.

TABLE 232.1. Causes of Syncope in the Pediatric Patient

- **Vasodepressor (vasovagal, neurocardiogenic, neurally mediated, reflex)**
  - Triggers: pain, fear, prolonged standing, heat exposure
  - Situational syncope: posttussive, micturition, defecation, deglutition
  - Carotid sinus sensitivity
  - Autonomic insufficiency
- **Cardiovascular**
  1. *Dysrhythmias: congenital or acquired*
     - Bradyarrhythmias: sinus node disease, atrioventricular block (Stokes Adams syndrome)
     - Tachyarrhythmias: long QT syndromes, Wolf-Parkinson White syndrome, ventricular tachycardia, supraventricular tachycardia, torsades de pointes, ventricular fibrillation, arrhythmogenic right ventricular dysplasia
     - Postoperative congenital heart disease patients, certain congenital heart defects (tetralogy of Fallot, Ebstein anomaly, others) are especially high risk for dysrhythmias and sudden death.
     - Pacemaker malfunction, AICD malfunction
  2. *Outflow Obstruction*
     - Hypertrophic obstructive cardiomyopathy, pericarditis with tamponade, severe aortic stenosis, pulmonary hypertension, prosthetic valve dysfunction, pulmonary emboli, some cyanotic congenital heart disease defects, severe coarctation, severe mitral stenosis, Eisenmenger syndrome, right ventricular dysplasia, cardiac tumor mass (atrial myxoma)
  3. *Myocardial Disease*
     - Cardiomyopathy, myocarditis, coronary artery abnormalities (congenital: anomalous coronary artery, or acquired: Kawasaki disease), rheumatologic/immunologic/vasculitis disorders: amyloidosis, sarcoidosis, others
  4. *Vascular*
     - Aortic dissection, connective tissue disorders: Marfan disease, Ehlers Danlos syndrome
     - Subclavian steal
     - Thoracic outlet syndrome
- **Orthostatic (Postural)**
  - Decreased intravascular volume: vomiting, diarrhea, diuretics, hemorrhage, or relative hypovolemia: sepsis, extended bedrest
- **Neurologic**
  - Subarachnoid hemorrhage
  - Transient ischemic attack
  - Peripheral neuropathies
  - Autonomic neuropathies
    - Primary: Shy-drager syndrome, Parkinson disease
    - Secondary: Diabetes mellitus, amyloidosis
- **Metabolic/Endocrine**
  - Hypoglycemia
- **Respiratory/Pulmonary**
  - Pulmonary Emboli (see also cardiac)
  - Cough (posttussive)
  - Hyperventilation
  - Breath-holding
  - Hypoxia
    - Pulmonary disease or respiratory failure causing hypoxia
    - Carbon monoxide poisoning, other toxins
    - Severe anemia
- **Drugs**
  - Poisons, toxins
  - Substance abuse: alcohol, opiates
  - Prescription drugs: antidepressants (tricyclics, phenothiazines) antihypertensives (alpha and beta blockers, hydralazine, ACE inhibitors, ganglionic blockers), vasodilators (calcium channel blockers, nitrates)
- **Psychiatric**
  - Hysteria

PATHOPHYSIOLOGY

The pathophysiology of syncope involves dysfunction of the reticular activating system in the brainstem, or both cerebral hemispheres, generally from an acute decrease in cerebral blood flow. The decreased cerebral blood flow is most often a result of systemic hypotension but can occur from cerebral vasoconstriction or regional hypoperfusion of the CNS. Reduced cardiac output causes decreased cerebral perfusion with impaired delivery of substrate (e.g., oxygen and glucose) to the brain. Less commonly, cardiac output and blood flow to the brain are adequate but there is deficient substrate as with hypoglycemia, carbon monoxide poisoning, severe anemia, or asphyxia.

CLINICAL PRESENTATION

Vasovagal syncope, also known as neurocardiogenic, neurally mediated, vasodepressor, and reflex syncope; is the most common cause of pediatric syncope and is responsible for at least half of all cases of pediatric syncope (10,11). Typical examples are: the individual who passes out at the sight of blood or while experiencing pain, anger, or fear; or while standing erect for a prolonged time in a warm environment (as in the military, a parade, or a religious service).

The classic explanation of vasovagal syncope has been a vagally mediated reflex causing bradycardia, and a decreased peripheral vascular resistance with venous pooling in the periphery resulting in hypotension. The decreased venous return leads to a relatively empty ventricle. Strong myocardial contractions against an empty ventricle stimulates the vagal reflex causing bradycardia, and sympathetic withdrawal results in decreased peripheral vascular resistance and a drop in arterial blood pressure. However, the occurrence of "vasovagal" syncope in heart transplant patients indicates that other mechanisms must be occurring. Possibilities include: neurohumoral-mediated sympathoinhibition, impaired responses in the peripheral vessels (affecting peripheral vascular resistance), and abnormal central CNS control mechanisms or a combination of such factors.

Cardiovascular causes of syncope can be categorized into several groups: dysrhythmias, obstruction to flow, myocardial dysfunction, and vascular. The common pathophysiology is a decrease in cardiac output resulting in decreased cerebral perfusion causing syncope. Cardiac syncope occurs when cardiac output (CO) is decreased from inadequate stroke volume (SV) or an abnormal heart rate (HR) leading to inadequate filling of the ventricles where $CO = SV \times HR$.

Although dysrhythmias are a less frequent cause of syncope in pediatric patients than adults, this possibility should be in the differential because of the association with sudden death. Patients with heart disease, whether congenital or acquired, are at high risk for dysrhythmias and sudden cardiac death. Congenital heart disease is the number one cause of dysrhythmias resulting in syncope in pediatric patients. Most sudden cardiac deaths associated with arrhythmias occur in pediatric patients who are status postcorrective cardiac surgery, especially repair of tetralogy of Fallot, or a baffle (Mustard or Senning procedure) for transposition of the great vessels. Estimates of the incidence of sudden cardiac death with congenital heart disease are: tetralogy of Fallot = 2.5% to 10%, Eisenmenger syndrome = 10% to 47%, and Ebstein anomaly = 2/5% to 20% (1). Other cardiac disorders associated with dysrhythmias include: Ebstein anomaly, arrhythmogenic right ventricular dysplasia, and cardiac tumors.

In patients with a structurally "normal" heart, syncope and sudden death can occur with: the Wolff-Parkinson White syndrome (WPW), long QT syndrome, ventricular tachycardia, complete heart block, and the Brugada syndrome.

The diagnostic hallmark of WPW is a short PR interval and a delta wave. Supraventricular tachycardia results from reentrant conduction down the atrioventricular node and up the accessory pathway (Kent bundle). Rapid conduction over the Kent bundle can proceed to ventricular fibrillation and sudden death. An electrophysiologic study with radio frequency ablation is the recommended treatment.

The long QT syndrome is due to a disorder of ventricular depolarization resulting in a prolongation of the refractory period. This can cause torsades de pointes with the potential to degenerate into ventricular fibrillation and sudden death. The long QT syndrome is characterized by QT interval prolongation. There are several forms of the long QT syndrome. The congenital types of long QT syndrome include the Romano-Ward syndrome, and the Jervell and Lange-Nielsen syndrome. The Romano-Ward syndrome has an autosomal dominant inheritance, while the Jervell and Lange-Nielson syndrome has an autosomal recessive inheritance and deafness. Acquired prolongation of the QT interval can be due to: electrolyte abnormalities (hypocalcemia, hypokalemia), drugs/overdose, and increased intracranial pressure. Medications associated with prolongation of the QT interval include: psychotropics (tricyclic antidepressants, phenothiazines), antihistamines, and promotility drugs (such as cisapride) especially in combination with other medications (for example, erythromycin and ketoconazole).

Bradyarrhythmias, which can cause syncope and sudden death, include complete heart block and sick sinus syndrome. Atrioventricular block may be congenital or acquired. Acquired causes are most commonly after cardiac surgery but rheumatologic diseases, infections, and neuromuscular diseases (e.g., Lyme disease, acute rheumatic fever, endocarditis, diphtheria, myotonic dystrophy, certain forms of muscular dystrophy, and Kearns-Sayre disease) are other etiologies for complete heart block. Congenital heart block can occur as an isolated condition or with structural heart disease especially defects of the atrioventricular septum, L-transposition of the great vessels, or ventricular inversion. Infants born to mothers with systemic lupus erythematosis may have complete heart block due to transplacental antibodies cross-reacting with fetal cardiac tissue.

Sinus node dysfunction most commonly occurs in patients who have undergone cardiac surgery especially atrial surgery. These patients are also at risk for atrial arrhythmias (e.g., atrial flutter and atrial fibrillation). The combination of atrial flutter/fibrillation with a rapid ventricular response plus sinus node dysfunction can lead to syncope from hemodynamic compromise and is a harbinger for dysrhythmias and sudden death.

Ventricular tachycardia/fibrillation leading to syncope and sudden death can occur in patients with myocardial disease (such as myocarditis, cardiomyopathy and myocardial ischemia) and with ventricular damage or scarring post cardiac surgery (even years after surgical repair).

The second category of cardiac syncope involves obstruction to blood flow. The classic example is hypertrophic obstructive cardiomyopathy (HOCM), which is the most common cause of sudden death in young athletes. Aortic stenosis with outflow obstruction may cause syncope, anginal chest pain, and dyspnea on exertion. Severe coarctation of the aorta or severe mitral valvular disease can also present with syncope. Similarly, patients with primary pulmonary hypertension or severe pulmonic stenosis may develop syncope. Sudden death in Eisenmenger syndrome is probably due to a drop in blood flow from a sudden increase in pulmonary vascular resistance. Tumors such as an atrial myxoma causing decreased cardiac output are a rare cause of cardiac syncope.

Myocardial disease is the third category of cardiac syncope and includes cardiomyopathies, myocarditis, myocardial ischemia (congenital from anomalous coronary arteries or acquired as in Kawasaki disease) and diseases infiltrating/destroying the myocardium such as amyloidosis or Chagas disease.

Vascular causes of syncope include: aortic dissection, subclavian steal, and thoracic outlet syndrome. Other uncommon causes of cardiac syncope include pericarditis leading to tamponade and aortic dissection.

Respiratory diseases ranging from status asthmaticus, severe pneumonia, or any cause of respiratory failure resulting in hypoxemia can cause syncope from decreased oxygen delivery to the brain. Posttussive or cough syncope, occurring after severe coughing, is due to the decreased venous return (and thus, decreased cardiac output), caused by the Valsalva maneuver. Cough syncope is a type of vasodepressor syncope. Pulmonary emboli exerts its effect by obstruction to blood flow.

Other respiratory/pulmonary causes of syncope include breath-holding spells, which are unique to pediatrics, and hyperventilation. Hyperventilation syncope generally occurs when there is an emotional upset or pain or anxiety, and is often associated with light-headedness, tachypnea, dyspnea, chest pain, and paresthesias. The pathophysiology is thought to be from decreased oxygen/glucose delivery to the brain caused by vasoconstriction of the cerebral arteries from the hypocapnia caused by hyperventilation.

Breath holding spells are common, occurring in about 4.6% of children (7). Breath holding spells usually begin between 6 to 18 months of age (with a range from the first week of life to 3 years) and end by 6 years of age in most (90%) of children. There are two types of breath holding spells: cyanotic and pallid. Cyanotic spells are more common. Both spells are due to transient cerebral anoxia.

Typically, the cyanotic breath holding spell is precipitated by the child/infant crying after being angered. The vigorous crying results in transient cerebral ischemia caused by: (1) cerebral arterial vasoconstriction from hypocapnia, (2) hypoxemia from apnea, and (3) decreased cardiac output from a prolonged Valsalva effect. The pallid breath holding spell generally occurs after a painful or anxiety-producing incident such as a minor fall. The transient cerebral ischemia occurring with the pallid breath-holding spell is due to an exaggerated vagal response to pain causing prolonged asystole or bradycardia. Breath-holding spells are a benign entity with no sequelae although they are commonly misdiagnosed as seizures.

Neurologic syncope can occur as a result of cerebral hypoperfusion from cerebral vasoconstriction (as with hyperventilation syncope) or from focal hypoperfusion of CNS structures. Cerebrovascular disease (generally in adults) could cause syncope but usually there are other neurologic signs and symptoms. Other causes of syncope from focal hypoperfusion of CNS structures include: subarachnoid hemorrhage, vasculitis (affecting cerebral vessels), CNS tumors, CNS trauma, and basilar artery migraine.

Psychiatric "disorders" are in the differential diagnosis of syncope. "Hysterical syncope" usually occurs before an audience, with no injuries occurring to the patient, and often is accompanied by dramatic moaning/gestures and attention seeking behavior with secondary gain.

DIFFERENTIAL DIAGNOSIS

Seizures are often mistaken for a syncopal event and vice versa. Brief tonic clonic movements may occur with vasodepressor syncope. Akinetic seizures may present like a syncopal episode. The history may help distinguish between syncope and a seizure. The following suggest a seizure not syncope: focal neurologic signs,

bowel/bladder incontinence, prolonged loss of consciousness or confusion, tongue biting, and a prodromal aura. With a syncopal episode, the period of unconsciousness is brief (only seconds), and has a rapid recovery to a normal mental status.

EMERGENCY DEPARTMENT EVALUATION AND MANAGEMENT

The history and physical examination are the key indicators in the evaluation of the pediatric patient with syncope. After ruling out mimickers of pediatric syncope, such as seizures and breath-holding spells, the first consideration is to determine whether the etiology of the syncope is benign or potentially life threatening. With near syncope or presyncope, the syncopal symptoms resolve before loss of consciousness occurs. The evaluation of the near syncope patient is similar to that of the syncope patient.

The history and physical examination should guide the choice of laboratory and ancillary tests. If the history is pathognomonic, for example: vasodepressor syncope (e.g., teenager who passed out while getting a routine immunization) or an infant with a breath-holding spell, further testing may not be necessary. If the history suggests orthostatic syncope due to dehydration from vomiting or diarrhea then checking the electrolytes and providing intravenous fluids may be all that is needed.

The physical examination can provide clues to the diagnosis. Cardiac findings (such as a murmur, loud S2, the presence of a click or S3 or S4) suggests cardiac syncope. The presence of neurologic symptoms and signs may indicate CNS disease or a seizure. Simple cost effective tests such as orthostatic vital signs or hemoccult of the stool can suggest orthostatic syncope or gastrointestinal bleeding. A pregnancy test should be considered in female syncopal adolescents since bleeding during pregnancy as with ectopic pregnancy can cause syncope. Diabetics with hypoglycemic symptoms can present with syncope and thus a serum glucose or accucheck might be useful in a diabetic. When pallor is present or bleeding is suspected, a hematocrit is appropriate.

If cardiac syncope is being considered, an ECG and chest roentgenogram are indicated. An electrocardiogram is a simple, noninvasive, inexpensive test that should be considered in any syncopal patient regardless of age, although the yield may be low. Additional studies for cardiovascular syncope such as an echocardiogram, Holter monitoring, and referral to a pediatric cardiologist or hospital admission may be warranted.

If autonomic syncope is being considered, then referral for tilt testing may be appropriate. Routine CT scans are usually not helpful, but a head CT scan may be indicated if neurologic signs/symptoms are present or seizures are a likely diagnosis. A chest CT scan or ventilation perfusion scan can be done if pulmonary emoboli is a consideration.

CRITICAL INTERVENTIONS

- Obtain a clear history of the events prior to, during, and immediately after the syncopal event
- Perform an accucheck on patients with altered level of consciousness
- Perform a thorough physical examination (particularly cardiac and neurologic) in addition to orthostatic vital signs
- Obtain an EKG on patients with possible cardiac syncope to check for long QT syndrome, WPW syndrome and other causes of cardiac syncope
- Consider all patients with a history of cardiac disease (congenital or acquired, especially those status post cardiac surgery) to have a potentially life-threatening dysrhythmia as a cause of their syncope until proven otherwise

DISPOSITION

Generally, testing, referrals, and the decision for admission are guided by the findings on the history and physical examination. Most causes of syncope are benign but some are life-threatening (Table 232.1). Syncope may be a warning sign for sudden death. Thus, patients with cardiac syncope require referral and probably admission. Patients experiencing vasopressor syncope or breath-holding spells may be discharged home without additional testing, after the history and physical examination. Patients with orthostatic syncope from dehydration can usually be treated with intravenous fluids in the emergency department then discharged home, while other patients such as those with a neuropathy may need referral for further outpatient evaluation.

COMMON PITFALLS

✔ Failure to differentiate syncope from seizures and breath-holding spells
✔ Failure to recognize potentially life-threatening causes of syncope such as cardiac syncope
✔ Failure to identify the high risk patient (such as the patient who has congenital heart disease and/or has a history of cardiac surgery) and make a referral and/or admit to the hospital
✔ Failure to perform a pregnancy test on sexually active adolescent females

References

1. Berger S, Dhala A, Friedberg DZ. Sudden cardiac death in infants, children, and adolescents. *Pediatr Clin N Amer* 1999;46:221–234.
2. Day SC, Cook EF, Funkestein H, et al. Evaluation and outcome of emergency room patients with transient loss of consciousness. *Am J Med* 1982;73:15–23.
3. Dermksian G, Lamb LE. Syncope in a population of healthy young adults. *JAMA* 1958;168:1200–1207.
4. Driscoll DJ, Jacobsen SJ, Porter CJ, et al. Syncope in children and adolescents: a population based study of incidence and outcome. *Circ* 1996;94:1–54.
5. Gendelman HE, Linzer M, Gabelman M, et al. Syncope in a general hospital patient population. *NY State J Med* 1983;83:1161–1165.
6. Kapoor WN, Karpf M, Wieand S, et al. A prospective evaluation and follow-up of patients with syncope. *N Engl J Med* 1983;309:197–204.
7. Lombroso CT, Lerman P. Breathholding spells (cyanotic and pallid infantile syncope). *Pediatrics* 1967;39:563–581.
8. Martin GJ, Adams SL, Maritno HG, et al. Prospective evaluation of syncope. *Ann Emerg Med* 1984;13:499–504.
9. Murdoch BD. Loss of consciousness in healthy South African men. *S Afr Med* 1980;57:771–774.
10. Owens TR. Sudden cardiac death: is your patient at risk? *J Resp Dis* 1998;19:384–396.
11. Pratt JL, Fleisher GR. Syncope in children and adolescents. *Pediatr Emerg Care* 1989;5:80–82.
12. Williams RL, Allen BD. Loss of consciousness: incidence, causes and electroencephalographic findings. *Aerospace Med* 1962;33:545–551.

Selected Readings

American College of Emergency Physicians. Clinical policy: critical issues in the evaluation and management of patients presenting with syncope. *Ann Emerg Med* 2001;37:771–776.
Brignole M, Alboni P, Benditt D, et al. Guidelines on management of syncope. *Eur Heart J* 2001;22:1256–1306.
Driscoll D, Jacobsen S, Porter C, et al. Syncope in children and adolescents. *J Am Coll Cardiol*, 1997;29:1039–1045.
Kilic A, Ozmer S, Turanli G, et al. Dysrhythmia as a cause of syncope in children without neurological or cardiac morphological abnormalities. *Pediatr International* 2002;44:358–362.
Klitzner TS. Sudden cardiac death in children. *Circulation* 1990;82:629–632.
Linzer M, Yang EH, Estes M, et al. Clinical efficacy assessment project of American College of Physicians. Clinical guideline: Diagnosing syncope – part 2: unexplained syncope. *Ann Intern Med* 1997;126:989–996.
Linzer M, Yang EH, Estes M, et al. Clinical efficacy assessment project of American College of Physicians. Clinical guideline: Diagnosing syncope, Part 1: Value of history, physical examination, and electrocardiography. *Ann Intern Med* 1997;126:989–99.
Martin GJ, Adams SL, Martin HG, et al. Prospective evaluation of syncope. *Ann Emerg Med* 1984;13:499–504.
Martin TP, Hanusa BH, Kapoor W. Risk stratification of patients with syncope. *Ann Emerg Med* 1997;29:459–466.
McHarg ML, Shinnar S, Rascoff H, et al. Syncope in childhood. *Pediatr Cardiol* 1997;18:367–371.
Ozme S, Alshan D, Valaz K, et al. Causes of syncope in children: a prospective study. *Int J Cardiol* 1993;40:111–114.
Quinn JV, Stiell IG, Sellers KA, et al. The San Francisco syncope rule to predict patients with serious outcomes. (Abstract). *Acad Emerg Med* 2002;9:358.
Sarasin FP, Louis-Simonet M, Carballo D, et al. Prospective evaluation of patients with syncope: a population-based study. *Am J Med* 2001;111:177–184.
Soteriades ES, Evans JC, Larson MG, et al. Incidence and prognosis of syncope. *N Engl J Med* 2002;347:878–933.

CHAPTER 233
Vomiting

Ronald A. Furnival

Vomiting is the coordinated action of the pharyngeal, esophageal, stomach, and diaphragmatic musculature to expel gastric contents, directed by the medullary vomiting center. This center receives input from the chemoreceptor trigger zone in the floor of the fourth ventricle, and from higher cortical centers that receive and process external stimuli. While vomiting may provide a survival advantage by expelling ingested toxins, it more frequently occurs with disorders from a variety of organ systems (12).

The infant or child with vomiting commonly presents to the emergency department (ED) for diagnosis and treatment. For most pediatric patients, vomiting is associated with a relatively minor self-limited condition, for a few it may be a manifestation of serious surgical or medical illness. In the ED, the first priority must be to determine whether an emergent surgical or medical condition exists, and whether clinical stabilization is immediately required. If no evidence of serious illness is identified, the next priority becomes recognizing and initiating therapy for the less urgent clinical conditions associated with vomiting.

CLINICAL PRESENTATION

The ED history and physical examination initially should identify and address any evidence of systemic illness or toxicity. Persistent vomiting with severe dehydration or metabolic abnormalities may require treatment prior to establishing a definitive diagnosis. Because pediatric vomiting may be a nonspecific symptom associated with severe systemic illness (i.e., meningitis, sepsis, respiratory distress, drug overdose, closed head injury, etc.) the ED evaluation must consider or "rule out" these possible etiologies for each child, based upon the initial history and physical examination.

For the vomiting child, the initial history should define whether the emesis is bilious or nonbilious. Bilious vomiting generally indicates a mechanical or functional bowel obstruction below the ampulla of Vater, with presence of pancreatic secretions in the bowel. Nonbilious emesis implies either a more proximal obstruction in the duodenum, or a functional disorder with no mechanical bowel obstruction (12). Yellow bile-stained emesis may occur with persistent vomiting and no bowel obstruction, possibly from temporary reversal of gastric peristalsis. Fecal material in the emesis indicates a colonic obstruction, with severe obstipation, Hirschsprüng disease, or other large bowel disorders. Although recent studies have found that only 10% to 38% of infants and children presenting to the ED with bilious (either yellow or green) vomiting have a surgical emergency, every child must be assumed to have a bowel obstruction until proven otherwise (5,22).

History of the duration of vomiting, the number of episodes each day, and any additional gastrointestinal symptoms should be defined next, including abdominal pain, distention, anorexia, diarrhea, constipation, and blood in the emesis or stools. The history should also note presence of systemic, (fever, weight loss, nutritional status, hydration status) neurologic, (headache, neck pain or stiffness, coordination or behavioral changes) genitourinary, (dysuria, hematuria, urine output, vaginal discharge or bleeding) respiratory, (cough, evidence of distress) and head and neck (otalgia, sore throat, dysphagia, nasal drainage) symptoms to further direct care and diagnostic evaluation. A past history of similar severe episodes of vomiting may lead to the diagnosis of a recurring condition, such as cyclic vomiting, an inborn error of metabolism, or malrotation with an intermittent volvulus.

The physical examination should initially seek evidence of systemic toxicity, including severe dehydration, cardiovascular insufficiency, or altered mental status. In a recent prospective pediatric study, the combination of 4 objective physical findings (dry mucous membranes, absent tears, abnormally lethargic or restless appearance, prolonged capillary refill) was found to be quite accurate for the clinical diagnosis of dehydration, with 2 of 4 findings present at 5% dehydration, and 3 or more present with more severe states of dehydration (6). On abdominal examination, auscultation for bowel sounds prior to palpation may reveal diminished activity with an ileus from surgical or medical illness, or increased activity (borborygmi) with a partial bowel obstruction or diarrheal disorder. Next, palpation for abdominal tenderness, distention, mass, or enlargement of the liver or spleen may be diagnostic. Gentle one-or two-finger percussion, rather than the less accurate gross abdominal wall movement with the compression-rebound technique, may demonstrate peritoneal findings from surgical conditions such as appendicitis. Finally, a thorough general evaluation for nonabdominal conditions associated with vomiting, including the head and neck, pulmonary, genitourinary, and neurologic examination may identify the etiology, and direct or obviate further diagnostic work up.

DIFFERENTIAL DIAGNOSIS

While viral gastroenteritis is one of the most common causes of vomiting for infants and children of all ages, the differential diagnosis for vomiting generally varies according to age at presentation. Table 233.1 lists the life-threatening causes of vomiting.

For the infant from birth to 2 months of age, the most common condition associated with vomiting is gastroesophageal reflux, often resulting from overfeeding, and occurring within 30 to 60 minutes of a feeding in an otherwise healthy appearing infant. Occult gastroesophageal reflux may present as positional fussiness, persistent cough and congestion, or truncal arching (Sandifer syndrome) that may mimic tonic seizure activity. Reflux precautions, with small frequent feedings and subsequent upright positioning for 30 minutes, will effectively treat the majority of infants, but persistent reflux may require medical therapy. Pyloric stenosis is the most common surgical condition to differentiate from gastroesophageal reflux. Most affected infants will present at 3 to 4 weeks of age, with a history of 1 to 2 weeks of progressive forceful "projectile" nonbilious vomiting, and weight loss from severe dehydration with more advanced disease. While palpation of the hypertrophied pylorus or 'olive' is diagnostic in over half of all cases, an ultrasound or upper gastrointestinal (UGI) series may be required for

TABLE 233.1. Life-Threatening Causes of Vomiting

NEWBORN (BIRTH TO 2 WK)

Anatomic anomalies–esophageal stenosis/atresia, intestinal obstructions (T.49.1.E), especially malrotation and volvulus, Hirschsprung disease
Other GI causes(necrotizing enterocolitis, peritonitis)
Neurologic—kernicterus, mass lesions, hydrocephalus
Renal—obstructive anomalies, uremia
Infectious—sepsis, meningitis
Metabolism—inborn errors, especially congenital adrenal hyperplasia

OLDER INFANT (2 WK TO 12 MO)

Gastroesophageal reflux, severe
Esophageal disorders
Rumination
Intestinal obstruction (T.49.1, II.E), especially pyloric stenosis, intussusception, incarcerated hernia
Other GI causes, especially gastroenteritis (with dehydration)
Neurologic—mass lesions, hydrocephalus
Renal—obstruction, uremia
Infectious—sepsis, meningitis, pertussis
Metabolic—inborn errors
Drugs—aspirin, theophylline, digoxin

OLDER CHILD (> 12 MO)

GI obstruction, especially intussusception (T.49.1, III.A)
Other GI causes, especially appendicitis, peptic ulcer disease
Neurologic—mass lesions
Renal—uremia
Infectious—meningitis
Metabolic—diabetic ketoacidosis, Reye syndrome, adrenal insufficiency
Toxins, drugs—aspirin, ipecac, theophylline, digoxin, iron, lead

OLDER CHILD AND ADOLESCENT

Gastroenteritis
Appendicitis/peritonitis; pancreatitis
Reflex vomiting due to stimuli from GU tract; pyelonephritis; calculi
Labyrinthine disorders (e.g., motion sickness)
Metabolic disorders
Intracranial lesions
Migraine
Drugs and alcohol
Pregnancy
Ulcers
Functional or self-induced

CAUSES COMMON TO ALL AGE GROUPS

Head trauma
Intracranial infections or space-occupying lesions
Drug overdose
Chemotherapeutic agents and radiation
Intestinal obstruction
Food poisoning

Henntig FM, Vomiting. In: Fleisher G, Ludwig S eds. *Textbook of pediatric emergency medicine.* Baltimore: Williams & Wilkins, 1988:331.

diagnosis in younger infants. ED treatment includes prompt evaluation for electrolyte disturbances (the classic presentation with hypochloremic metabolic alkalosis has become increasingly rare) and intravenous (IV) fluid rehydration, with appropriate surgical referral for suspected cases (1,4).

Other emergent surgical causes of vomiting in the first 2 months of life include congenital gastrointestinal anomalies, (intestinal stenosis or duplications, duodenal or antral webs, annular pancreas, etc.) incarcerated inguinal hernia, malrotation with volvulus, and Hirschsprüng disease. Most upper gastrointestinal congenital anomalies will present within the first few days of life, and are infrequently seen in the ED setting. An inguinal hernia may be noted on examination of the diaper area, with presence of an inguinal, scrotal, or labial mass. Steady and gentle pressure at the external inguinal ring and on the mass will successfully reduce the majority of hernias, and occasional patients may require sedation and surgical consultation if the initial ED attempt is unsuccessful. The young infant presenting to the ED with bilious emesis (even one episode) must be assumed to have gastrointestinal malrotation with volvulus until proven otherwise. Eighty-five percent of patients with volvulus present in the first year, and most (60%) within the first month of life. The abdominal physical examination may be normal in 50% to 75% of cases but diminished bowel sounds, distention, a palpable mass, or tenderness may be noted in 10% to 25% of infants with volvulus (16,17). Hypovolemic shock at presentation from prolonged intestinal ischemia is uncommon, but must be considered in the moribund infant. Immediate evaluation with an UGI series (a contrast enema may miss the diagnosis in up to 20% of patients) is a must for all suspected cases, with emergent surgical consultation and laparotomy for any symptomatic patient with an identified malrotation (3,21). Hirschsprüng disease, or aganglionosis, is a fairly common cause of intestinal obstruction in the newborn, infant, or young child, with an incidence of 1 in 5000 live births; more than 80% of cases are diagnosed within the first year of life. A congenital absence of ganglion cells in the colonic submucosa results in uncoordinated intestinal contractions and the clinical presentation of chronic constipation, abdominal distention, and vomiting in affected infants. Abdominal radiographs may demonstrate dilated proximal bowel loops with air-fluid levels; a contrast enema may be diagnostic for more than 80% of cases. ED treatment consists of IV fluid resuscitation, nasogastric (NG) decompression, broad-spectrum antibiotics (with anaerobic coverage) and surgical consultation for biopsy and corrective surgery (10,11).

Many medical conditions, in addition to gastroesophageal reflux, may cause vomiting in the young infant. Infections such as generalized sepsis, meningitis, encephalitis, hepatitis, pharyngitis, stomatitis, or otitis media may present with vomiting as an initial symptom. Gastroenteritis, with vomiting, diarrhea, and fever is common year-round, with seasonal peaks during summer and winter viral outbreaks. Urinary tract infections are the most common bacterial source for a fever in the infant with a normal physical examination, and may appear as vomiting without diarrhea (24). Intracranial pathology, from occult closed head injury, abuse, hydrocephalus, or hemorrhage may present with neurologic findings and associated vomiting. Respiratory distress from pertussis, pneumonia, asthma, bronchiolitis, or aspiration in the developmentally-impaired patient, may also be noticed only after the infant has been vomiting. Finally, metabolic conditions such as inborn errors of metabolism, renal tubular acidosis, or congenital adrenal hyperplasia may show up as vomiting with a severe metabolic acidosis, hyperkalemia in combination with hyponatremia, or other laboratory abnormalities (13).

While a number of the conditions outlined above may also affect the older infant or child, gastroesophageal reflux, congenital anomalies, and inborn metabolic disorders become less likely with increasing age. Two of the most common surgical disorders to consider for the older infant or child with vomiting are appendicitis and intussusception. While only 10% of appendicitis occur in children under 10 years of age, and only 1% in infants less than two years, it continues to be the most frequent indication for emergent pediatric surgery. The "classic" findings of right lower quadrant abdominal pain, vomiting, and fever are uncommon in younger patients, who may have an atypical history of diarrhea or respiratory distress, evidence of generalized sepsis, and atypical laboratory findings at presentation (7,8,14).

Because of the often nonspecific nature of such symptoms, and perhaps a more rapid progression to perforation, appendicitis in the child less than 4 years of age is often associated with an 80% perforation rate at the time of diagnosis, and a significant mortality risk among younger infants (7,8). Older children are more likely to have the 'classic' presentation of appendicitis. Presence of at least 2 of 4 clinical findings (vomiting, abdominal tenderness, right lower quadrant pain, guarding) was noted in 97% of children with appendicitis, but fewer than 25% of nonappendicitis patients in one recent study (20). Contrast pelvic CT scan has been quite accurate for the diagnosis of pediatric appendicitis, and probably has the greatest utility for the child with an atypical presentation (15,18,19). Intussusception, from a spontaneous invagination of the intestine upon itself, compromises the vascular supply to the inner segment or intussusceptum. Approximately 95% of intussusception is ileo-colic, beginning at the ileocecal valve, the remaining 5% are ileo-ileal, or occur within the colon or sigmoid. Sixty-five percent of intussusception occurs in infants under one year of age, most frequently (45%) between 5 and 9 months of age. The typical infant presents with the sudden onset of intermittent severe abdominal pain and vomiting, and may appear well between episodes. Bilious vomiting, lethargy, passage of bloody mucus or "currant-jelly" stool, peritonitis, or evidence of cardiovascular compromise are late findings indicating more pronounced intestinal ischemia. The abdominal examination may identify a palpable mass, but is usually normal, often with only a positive stool guaiac test to confirm the clinical suspicion for intussusception; abdominal radiographs are generally normal to nonspecific. Air- or barium-contrast enema is diagnostic for nearly 100% of cases, and allows therapeutic reduction of the intussusception, although recent studies have also successfully used ultrasound as both a screen for suspected cases, and as a guide for the air-enema reduction (9,26).

A number of medical conditions may cause vomiting in the older infant or child. Metabolic disorders often present with vomiting, including new onset insulin-dependent diabetes, diabetic ketoacidosis, and renal or adrenal insufficiency. Henoch-Schönlein purpura, with characteristic purpuric lesions concentrated on the lower extremities in an otherwise nontoxic child, may cause abdominal pain and vomiting, and is associated with an increased risk for intussusception. An accidental drug ingestion in the exploring toddler, or an intentional overdose in the adolescent may present with vomiting among a variety of other toxin-specific findings. Pancreatitis, cholecystitis, inflammatory bowel disease, and nephrolithiasis, while more often seen in older patients, may present in the school-age child (23,25). Migraine headaches, cyclic vomiting, and some seizure variants may also cause recurrent vomiting episodes. With the U.S. average for onset of menstruation at approximately 12 years of age, pregnancy, ovarian pathology, and pelvic inflammatory disease must also be considered in the differential for the vomiting adolescent (2).

EMERGENCY DEPARTMENT EVALUATION AND MANAGEMENT

The initial ED therapy for the vomiting infant or child should focus on identifying and addressing evidence of systemic toxicity. IV access should be established, with fluid administration of 20 ml/kg boluses of isotonic normal saline or lactated Ringer solution, and with repeat boluses as needed. An NG tube for decompression should be placed in all patients with an ileus or bowel obstruction, and for gastric lavage in infants or children with significant upper gastrointestinal bleeding. Initial diagnostic laboratory studies, ideally obtained with placement of the IV catheter, should include serum electrolytes, glucose, and renal function tests with clinical evidence of dehydration. Additional tests may also be indicated, including a complete blood count (CBC) with a type and cross-match for surgical patients, liver function tests, amylase, and lipase for undiagnosed medical conditions, and a urinalysis and urine culture for the febrile patient with vomiting but no diarrhea.

After initial stabilization, diagnostic imaging studies may be necessary to identify the cause of vomiting. A chest x-ray should be considered for the vomiting patient with respiratory symptoms, and may lead to the diagnosis of pneumonia or other pulmonary conditions. If the infant or child is suspected of having a bowel obstruction, ileus, mass, or evidence of peritonitis, 'flat and upright' abdominal x-rays may confirm the diagnosis and direct further care. For the young infant with bilious vomiting, the initial test of choice is the UGI series, which is more sensitive for the diagnosis of malrotation than contrast enema studies. The air- or barium-contrast enema may be both diagnostic and therapeutic for the older infant or toddler with a suspected intussusception. Barium-contrast enema may also diagnose Hirschsprüng disease in the infant with chronic constipation, demonstrating a funnel-shaped 'transition zone' at the border between the normal and abnormal bowel segments. While ultrasound is quite sensitive for the recognition of pyloric stenosis, with a number of reports advocating its use for this indication, a number of studies have found the UGI series to be a more cost-effective initial study, since the infant with a negative ultrasound may then require a follow-up UGI series for diagnosis. Ultrasound is effective for the diagnosis of intussusception, uretero-pelvic obstruction, and gynecologic disorders as causes of vomiting in the pediatric patient. Appendicitis may be documented by ultrasound or pelvic computed tomography (CT) scan, but most pediatric studies note better diagnostic accuracy with CT scan. CT scan is also the test of choice for evaluation of abdominal masses, nephrolithiasis, abdominal trauma, and intracranial pathology as causes of vomiting.

CRITICAL INTERVENTIONS

- Address clinical instability prior to efforts at definitive diagnosis
- Check a bedside serum glucose and blood gas for the infant or child with altered mental status, or other evidence of systemic toxicity
- Give initial IV fluid boluses with nonDextrose-containing isotonic solutions, and add Dextrose as needed for documented hypoglycemia
- Give stress-dose corticosteroids (hydrocortisone 50–100 mg IV bolus) to the ill-appearing steroid-dependent patient as soon as possible
- Presence of bilious vomiting or evidence of peritonitis must be considered due to an emergent surgical condition until proven otherwise

---

DISPOSITION

For the vomiting infant or child with a self-limited condition and no evidence of dehydration or systemic illness, outpatient oral rehydration is appropriate, with defined discharge instructions and a clear followup plan. Oral rehydration can also be effective for the patient with mild to moderate illness. IV fluid rehydration should be utilized for the vomiting patient with an inability to tolerate oral fluids, with demonstrated electrolyte abnormalities, or with more severe illness. While two 20 ml/kg IV fluid boluses may improve most mildy- to moderately-dehydrated patients enough for safe discharge home, those with persistent vomiting, with significant serum electrolyte or glucose abnormalities, or with a more complex diagnosis may benefit from

continued inpatient rehydration and observation. The infant or child with evidence of bowel obstruction or peritonitis requires an emergent surgical referral and hospitalization.

COMMON PITFALLS

- ✔ Forgetting to assess for hypoglycemia in a vomiting infant or child. A rapid glucose test should be checked with the first blood draw
- ✔ Giving IV fluid boluses with Dextrose-containing solutions that may result in hyperglycemia and hyperosmolarity
- ✔ Failing to aggressively evaluate and treat the young infant with bilious emesis, even if physical examination and laboratory studies appear normal. You do not want to miss the diagnosis of malrotation

Acknowledgment

Thanks to the previous edition's chapter author Anthony P. Pohlgeers.

References

1. Barksdale EM. Pyloric stenosis. In: Ziegler MM, Azizkhan RG, Weber TR, (eds). *Operative Pediatric Surgery.* New York: McGraw-Hill Companies, 2003:583–588.
2. Chumlea WC, Schubert CM, Roche AF, et al. Age at menarche and racial comparisons in U.S. girls. *Pediatrics* 2003;111:110–113.
3. Clark LA, Oldham KT.Malrotation. In: Ashcraft KW, (ed). *Pediatric Surgery,* 3rd ed. Philadelphia: W. B. Saunders Co, 2000:425–434.
4. Dillon PW, Cilley RE. Lesions of the stomach. In: Ashcraft KW, (ed). *Pediatric Surgery.* Philadelphia, PA: W. B. Saunders Company; 2000:391–405.
5. Godbole P, Stringer MD. Bilious vomiting in the newborn: how often is it pathologic? *J Pediatr Surg* 2002;37:909–911.
6. Gorelick MH, Shaw KN, Murphy KO. Validity and reliability of clinical signs in the diagnosis of dehydration in children. *Pediatrics* 1997;99:E6.
7. Graham JM, Pokorny WJ, Harberg FJ. Acute appendicitis in preschool age children. *Am J Surg* 1980;139:247–250.
8. Grosfeld JL, Weinberger M, Clatworthy HW. Acute appendicitis in the first two years of life. *J Pediatr Surg* 1973;8:285–293.
9. Harrington L, Connolly B, Hu X, et al. Ultrasonographic and clinical predictors of intussusception. *J Pediatr* 1998;132:836–839.
10. Hirschsprüng's Disease. In: O'Neill JA, Grosfield JL, Fonkalsrud EW, et al. (eds). *Principles of Pediatric Surgery, 2nd ed.* St. Louis: Mosby, 2003:573–586.
11. Holschneider A, Ure BM. Hirschsprüng's Disease. In: Ashcraft KW, (ed). *Pediatric Surgery.* 3rd ed. Philadelphia: W. B. Saunders Co, 2000:453–472.
12. Murray KF, Christie DL. Vomiting. *Pediatr Rev* 1998;19:337–341.
13. Nadel FM, Weinzimer SA. The case of the missing "olive." *Pediatr Ann* 2000;29:119–122.
14. Nelson DS, Bateman B, Bolte RG. Appendiceal perforation in children diagnosed in a pediatric emergency department. *Pediatr Emerg Care* 2000;16:233–237.
15. Pena BM, Taylor GA, Lund DP, Mandl KD. Effect of computed tomography on patient management and costs in children with suspected appendicitis. *Pediatrics* 1999;104:440–446.
16. Pickhardt PJ, Bhalla S. Intestinal malrotation in adolescents and adults: spectrum of clinical and imaging features. *AJR Am J Roentgenol* 2002;179:1429–1435.
17. Powell DM, Otherson HB, Smith CD. Malrotation of the intestines in children: The effect of age on presentation and therapy. *J Pediatr Surg* 1989;24:777–780.
18. Rao PM, Rhea JT, Novelline RA, et al. Effect of computed tomography of the appendix on treatment of patients and use of hospital resources [see comments]. *N Engl J Med* 1998;338:141–146.
19. Rao PM, Rhea JT, Rattner DW, Venus LG, Novelline RA. Introduction of appendiceal CT: impact on negative appendectomy and appendiceal perforation rates. *Ann Surg* 1999;229:344–349.
20. Reynolds SL, Jaffe DM. Diagnosing abdominal pain in a pediatric emergency department. *Pediatr Emerg Care* 1992;8:126–128.
21. Rotational Anomalies and Volvulus. In: O'Neill JA, Grosfield JL, Fonkalsrud EW, et al, (eds). *Principles of Pediatric Surgery,* 2nd ed. St. Louis: Mosby, 2003:477–483.
22. Sadow KB, Atabaki SM, Johns CM, Chamberlain JM, Teach SJ. Bilious emesis in the pediatric emergency department: etiology and outcome. *Clin Pediatr* 2002;41:475–479.
23. Santos-Victoriano M, Brouhard BH, Cunningham RJ, 3rd. Renal stone disease in children. *Clin Pediatr* 1998;37:583–599.
24. Shaw KN, Gorelick M, McGowan KL, Yakscoe NM, Schwartz JS. Prevalence of urinary tract infection in febrile young children in the emergency department. *Pediatrics* 1998;102:e16.
25. Takiff H, Fonkalsrud EW. Gallbladder disease in childhood. *Am J Dis Child* 1984;138:565–568.
26. Zheng JY, Frush DP, Guo JZ. Review of pneumatic reduction of intussusception: evolution not revolution. *J Pediatr Surg* 1994;29:93–97.

PART IV

Specific Diseases

CHAPTER 234
Abuse: Sexual

J. M. Whitworth

Until recent years, sexual abuse in children was considered an uncommon problem. It is now clear that sexual abuse or sexual molestation affects at least one in four girls and one in seven boys before age 18 (7). The short- and long-term physical and psychological effects of sexual abuse depend on many factors, including the severity of the abuse, the length of time of involvement, the relationship of the abuser to the child, and the sensitivity of intervening professionals and family members after the problem has come to light.

The needs of sexually abused children differ from the needs of sexually assaulted adults. Although children are sometimes raped, the usual case is characterized by a long-term process perpetrated by an older person who is well known to the child, and results in totally different evidentiary, evaluation, and treatment approaches. The "child sexual abuse accommodation syndrome" describes characteristics seen in these children and points out the challenges in approaching child victimization, as compared with adults. Children are gradually entrapped in a secret arrangement with a trusted adult or adolescent and feel helpless. They accommodate to the abuse and often display delayed and conflicting disclosure, followed by retraction of the allegation (25). A specially trained professional interviewer is needed to begin addressing these specific issues often seen in children.

The emergency department (ED) response to sexual abuse of children must address the child's medical needs and must be equally considerate of his or her psychological needs. The ED visit can serve as the first step in a therapeutic process. The forensic examination is a small part of a multidisciplinary effort to evaluate and protect the child; the examiner must have the time, effort, and skill to minimize the traumatic aspects of the encounter. If such a commitment cannot be ensured, the ED should consider referring cases to another facility for evaluation.

CLINICAL PRESENTATION

A few child sexual abuse cases present to the ED as a medical emergency, usually with a history of genital bleeding or clinical suggestions of acute abdominal trauma or peritoneal irritation.

In these cases, matters of evidence collection, forensic evaluation, and reporting are secondary to the need for immediate intervention to stabilize the child's condition. Resuscitation takes precedence.

More typically, patients present in one of two ways. First, the child may present with a chief complaint of sexual abuse by personal report or because of a caretaker's suspicion. Second, the child may present with a seemingly unrelated chief complaint and the examiner suspects sexual abuse because of findings in the history or physical examination.

The approach to these presentations may be different, but the examiner's immediate reaction should always be the same. After an assessment to determine whether there are immediate medical needs, a team of professionals must become involved to obtain a detailed interview, to recommend and perform necessary interventions, and to ensure the child's safety. Psychosocial assessment and treatment plans must be addressed early in case development. This requires the involvement of the local child protection agency, law enforcement, and, ideally, a multidisciplinary child protection team in the community (2,3).

Whenever sexual abuse is suspected, the health-care professional must make a report to child protective services or to a law enforcement agency in the community (23). Local and state laws determine the physician's responsibility for reporting.

EMERGENCY DEPARTMENT EVALUATION

History

In the sexually abused child, the medical history is separate from the detailed interview. The medical history focuses on the information necessary to make a diagnosis, determine assessment needs, determine public health issues, and plan treatment. Taking a medical history should not be seen as an opportunity to do a detailed interview, unless there is no other resource available in the community.

The exact history and source of the information should be clearly recorded in the chart. If possible, the history should come from the child to ensure greatest reliability. It should be taken in the least threatening environment possible; adequate time must be taken to develop rapport with the child. Generally, the child should be interviewed alone. The examiner must spend enough time with the child to ascertain his or her names for body parts and bodily functions. If the child volunteers specific information, it is recorded as direct quotes. Information gathered from others is considered hearsay. Questions must be presented in a format that does not lead the child; if a question can be answered "yes" or "no," it is probably leading. If the child says nothing, this fact should be recorded in the chart, documenting that the child was asked to give information about the case.

The history should also include an assessment of evidence for other kinds of abuse, family violence, and any other significant medical problems.

The decision as to the type and extent of medical intervention should be made by a health-care professional. It should not be based on the supposed needs of the legal system or a child protection agency. This medical responsibility for protecting the child cannot be abrogated to others who may not understand the potential trauma of a forensic examination in a child.

Physical Examination

Before the examination, the child should be told what to expect, and he or she should receive constant reassurance during the procedure.

The examination of the genitalia of a sexually abused child should always be done in the context of a complete standard pediatric physical examination. This approach is necessary to ensure that other significant problems are documented and addressed, and it is also necessary to reassure the child that he or she has been completely examined by a health professional and is intact. Abused children generally perceive themselves as "damaged goods."

Abnormal findings should never be reported in the child's presence. Likewise, assurances by the physician that the child is not at fault and is believed are remembered by the child long after the minor trauma of the examination has faded. The physician should approach the child in a warm, friendly, age-appropriate manner and should not engage in extensive play or subterfuge to accomplish the examination, because playing games and subterfuges are often approaches used by an abuser.

If the child will not or cannot cooperate, the examination can be done at another time or in another place. With adequate preparation and patience, examination under anesthesia or with sedation is rarely necessary.

In a busy emergency department, an examination for sexual abuse of a child may have unanticipated negative effects. Other patients and the procedures performed on them may frighten the child. The examination should be done in a quiet environment. A support figure—never the suspected abuser—should be present and should be selected by the child. Blood samples, if necessary, can be obtained shortly after the examination.

The examination of the genitalia of a prepubertal child is primarily a process of description and observation based on the knowledge of normal structures and deviations from normal. A child's genitalia differ in appearance from adult structures, so review of a standard pediatric gynecology reference is essential (24).

Proper positioning of the child for a genital examination varies depending on the child's age, comfort, and degree of cooperation. An adequate examination can be performed with a small child on the mother's lap. Preferable positions, from the examiner's viewpoint, are the knee–chest and frog-leg positions. In the frog-leg position, direct inspection while grasping the labia majora and pulling toward the examiner allows adequate visualization of all structures germane to the examination. In the knee–chest position, structures can usually be visualized directly without pressure or traction on the labia, but this position is often difficult to accomplish because it makes the child feel more vulnerable.

There are significant differences in the appearance of normal anatomic structures in different positions, as well as with different degrees of relaxation in the same child. For this reason, only findings that clearly indicate scarring from trauma, con-

sistent changes in reflex response, or active infection should be considered definitive.

Invasion with a speculum or digit is seldom necessary or helpful, except in much older children or children who are sexually active. Cultures or specimen collection should be done with the smallest swab available. Inspection of the labia and introitus should include attention to evidence of old or new lacerations or abrasions.

Hymenal configuration should be noted and may be described as annular, crescentic, cribriform, septate, or imperforate (13). Congenital absence of the hymen does not occur (15). Thickness of the membrane should be described, along with any scarring located, and recorded as related to the face of a clock. In the past, the lateral hymenal diameter was considered extremely important in making the diagnosis of sexual abuse or molestation, but currently, this measurement seems less important than evidence of chronic scarring or acute injury.

If the vaginal canal can be visualized, a description of general appearance, rugous folds, and any scars may be important.

Abnormalities in the prepubertal child fall into several categories (1,6,13,14,18–21):

1. Findings diagnostic of sexual abuse
   a. Presence of sperm or semen in a prepubertal child
   b. Presence of a sexually transmitted disease with no reasonable possibility of nonsexual transmission (i.e., gonorrhea, syphilis, HIV, chlamydia (before puberty))
   c. Witnessed or photographically documented sexual abuse with or without physical findings
2. Findings diagnostic of penetration and consistent with a history of sexual abuse
   a. Healed or fresh vaginal tear
   b. Healed or fresh hymenal tear
   c. Missing section(s) of hymen in the posterior half
   d. Fresh or healed rectal tears
3. Findings diagnostic of genital trauma (insult) and consistent with a history of sexual abuse
   a. Microlacerations of the posterior fourchette
   b. Abrasions of the fossa navicularis or perihymenal tissues
   c. Bruises of genital tissues
   d. Presence of other sexually transmitted diseases (a disease not exclusively sexually transmitted, such as chlamydia or herpes)
   e. Rectal fissures
4. Findings that neither support nor negate an allegation of sexual abuse
   a. Redness or irritation of the genital area
   b. Agglutination of the labia minora
   c. Variations in the vascular pattern seen without attendant scars
   d. Enlargement of the hymenal opening
   e. Attenuated hymen without scarring
   f. Vaginitis (other than sexually transmitted diseases)

In cases of documented sexual abuse, definite physical findings are present in a very small numbers of cases; this is also true in many cases of known penetration (22). Most recent research strongly suggests that the only definitive finding for healed hymeneal trauma in sexually abused children is a scar that indicates complete transaction (27). The physical examination, therefore, can never be used to negate an allegation of sexual abuse.

Findings should be recorded, for future reference, on a standard anatomic chart. Color photography is strongly recommended but is not always readily available in the ED.

When reaching a conclusion, external pressures always suggest that a definitive "yes" or "no" answer is necessary. This is not always possible, and the examiner should not be tempted to make definitive statements if the history and physical examination are not definitive. The physician may conclude that the examination is diagnostic of sexual abuse, consistent with sexual abuse, or neither confirms nor negates a history of sexual abuse. The examiner will probably be asked to support his or her conclusions at a later date.

Laboratory Evaluation

Useful forensic evidence in small children is almost never found beyond a few hours after an assault (26). Evidence of sperm or semen is more often found on clothes or bedclothes. In older children, if forensic evidence collection is needed, an evidence collection packet must be sought from local law enforcement sources, and the physician must be knowledgeable about the use of the kit before doing the examination. Thorough training in maintaining the chain of evidence and evidence collection techniques is mandatory and varies from jurisdiction to jurisdiction. Training is available from adult sexual assault centers or from police departments.

Sexual abuse victims must always be assessed for sexually transmitted diseases, but the extent of the search is a matter of clinical judgment. Cultures for *Neisseria gonorrhoeae* should be obtained from the vagina, rectum, and throat, assuming a reasonable history or finding that suggests potential transmission. Cultures for *Chlamydia trachomatis* are useful if facilities are available. The use of screening or presumptive tests for chlamydia or gonorrhea is not recommended (12).

Wet mounts are done with anogenital discharges, and dark-field examinations are done on genital ulcers. Viral cultures for herpes simplex are indicated with vesicular lesions, and routine bacteriologic cultures should be done in all patients with a demonstrable discharge. The utility of cultures for herpes and human papillomavirus in determining sexual transmission is limited. Routine serologic tests for syphilis should not be done unless there are clinical indications.

Human immunodeficiency virus transmission can occur with sexual abuse but is uncommon. Routine testing is not recommended but should be available for any patient with high-risk exposure, or on request (9). There are compelling clinical reasons for testing only in a setting where adequate preparation and follow up with counseling services are provided.

EMERGENCY DEPARTMENT MANAGEMENT

The first priority is to alleviate any urgent or life-threatening medical needs. Subsequent treatment should be responsive to time-sensitive evidence collection and the treatment of sexually transmitted diseases. Presumptive treatment is never advisable; treatment should be undertaken only after definitive culture evidence exists or when there are life-threatening infectious disease issues.

In selecting treatment choices, the physician should always seek a history of drug sensitivity and should be familiar with the expected sensitivity of organisms in the community. Treatment recommendations are shown in Table 234.1 (5,8,10).

CRITICAL INTERVENTIONS

- Proper positioning of the child is imperative in order to identify genital abnormalities
- The use of a speculum or digit is rarely needed in young children
- Never report abnormal findings in the presence of the child
- Do not use leading questions while obtaining a history

TABLE 234.1. Treatment Recommendations for Children Who Have Contracted a Sexually Transmitted Disease through Sexual Abuse

Agent	Drug	Dosage
Neisseria gonorrhoeae	Ceftriaxone	125 mg i.m. or
	Azithromycin	2 g PO if ≥45 kg, otherwise 20 mg/kg
Herpes genitalis	Acyclovir	400 mg PO t.i.d. for 7–10 d
Chlamydia trachomatis	Erythromycin Ethylsuccinate or Azithromycin	50 mg/kg/d for 10 d 1 g PO if ≥45 kg
Treponema pallidum	Benzathine (Penicillin G)	50,000 U/kg i.m. (max, 2.4 million units)
Trichomonas vaginalis	Metronidazole	15 mg/kg/d divided as a single dose t.i.d. for 7 d, or 40 mg/kg (max, 2 g)

COMMON PITFALLS

✔ The examiner should not become confused when a child recants a history of sexual abuse. This phenomenon is common and often results from fear, parental coaching, the observed response of authority figures, or the realization that intervention may result in jail for a family member or family separation. Recantation is so common that it does not necessarily interfere with prosecution or with therapy for the patient. Documentation of the ED visit assumes greater importance in these cases

✔ Believing that the absence of physical findings means that sexual abuse did not occur or that a case cannot be prosecuted. This is contrary to current knowledge and experience with sexually abused children and can actually lead to further victimization. Because a child's disclosure of sexual abuse is generally accurate, and because serious sexual abuse can occur without physical findings, the history is the critical piece of evidence. The absence of physical findings does not hinder the ability to obtain a conviction (9,16,22)

✔ Failure of the examiner to record all data. This is important because he or she may need to recall the information in detail months or years later in a courtroom. Meticulous attention to detail in the examination and in the recording of the history and examination findings is essential to minimize this problem

References

1. Adams JA, Harper K, Knudsen S. A proposed system for the classification of anogenital findings in children with suspected sexual abuse. *Adolesc Pediatr Gynecol* 1992;5:73.
2. American Academy of Pediatrics Committee on Child Abuse and Neglect. Guidelines for the evaluation of sexual abuse of children. *Pediatrics* 1991;87:254.
3. AMA guidelines for the evaluation of child sexual abuse. Chicago: American Medical Association, 1992.
4. Atabaki S, Paradise JE. The medical evaluation of the sexually abused child: lessons from a decade of research. *Pediatrics* 1999;104:178.
5. Barone MA, ed. The Harriet Lane handbook, 14th ed. St. Louis: Mosby–Year Book, 1996.
6. Berenson A, Heger A, Hayes J, et al. Appearance of the hymen in prepubertal girls. *Pediatrics* 1992;89:387.
7. Berkowitz CD. Child sexual abuse. *Pediatr Rev* 1992;13:443.
8. Committee on Infectious Diseases, American Academy of Pediatrics. Report of the Committee on Infectious Diseases (red book), 24th ed. Elk Grove Village: IL: American Academy of Pediatrics, 1997.2003.
9. DeJong A, Rose M. Legal proof of child sexual abuse in the absence of physical evidence. *Pediatrics* 1991;88:506.

10. Gellert G, Durfee M, Berkowitz C, et al. Situational and sociodemographic characteristics of children infected with HIV from pediatric sexual abuse. *Pediatrics* 1993;91:39.
11. Hammerschlag M. Sexually transmitted diseases in sexually abused children. *Adv Pediatr Infect Dis* 1988;3:1.
12. Hammerschlag MR, Rettig PJ, Shields ME. False-positive results with the use of chlamydial antigen detection tests in the evaluation of suspected sexual abuse in children. *Pediatr Infect Dis J* 1988;7:11.
13. Heger A, Emans S, Muram D. Evaluation of the sexually abused child. New York: Oxford University Press, 1993/2000.
14. Hobbs C, Wynne J. Sexual abuse of English boys and girls: the importance of anal examination. *Child Abuse Negl* 1989;13:195.
15. Jenny C, Kuhns MLD, Arakawa F. Hymens in newborn female infants. *Pediatrics* 1987;80:399.
16. Jones D, McGraw J. Reliable and fictitious accounts of sexual abuse to children. *J Interpers Viol* 1987;2:27.
17. Kini N, Brady WJ, Lazoritz S. Evaluating child sexual abuse in the emergency department: clinical and behavioral indicators. *Acad Emerg Med* 1996;3:966.
18. McCann J, Voris J. Perianal injuries resulting from sexual abuse: a longitudinal study. *Pediatrics* 1993;91:390.
19. McCann J, Voris J, Simon M. Genital injuries resulting from sexual abuse: a longitudinal study. *Pediatrics* 1992;89:307.
20. McCann J, Voris J, Simon M, Wells R. Perianal findings in prepubertal children selected for nonabuse: a descriptive study. *Child Abuse Negl* 1989;13:179.
21. McCann J, Wells R, Simon M, Voris J. Genital findings in prepubescent girls selected for nonabuse: a descriptive study. *Pediatrics* 1990;86:428.
22. Muram D. Child sexual abuse: relationship between sexual acts and genital findings. *Child Abuse Negl* 1989;13:211x.
23. Ricci LR. Child sexual abuse: the emergency department response. *Ann Emerg Med* 1986;7:711.
24. San Philippo JS. Pediatric and adolescent gynecology. Philadelphia: WB Saunders, 1994.
25. Summit R. The child sexual abuse accommodation syndrome. *Child Abuse Negl* 1983;7:177.
26. Christian C, Lavelle J, DeJong A, et al. Forensic evidence findings in prepubertal victims of sexual assault. *Pediatrics* 2000;106:100–104.
27. Hegar A, Ticson L, Guerra L, et al. Appearance of the genitalia in girls selected for non-abuse: review of hymeneal morphology and non-specific findings. *J of Adol and Ped Gynecol* 2002;15:27–35.

CHAPTER 235
Abuse and Neglect: Physical

J. M. Whitworth

An awareness of child abuse and neglect is of particular importance in the emergency department (ED) setting. Any visit by a child may afford the health-care professional an opportunity to protect a child from further harm. The visit may also provide a rare window into a family that may desperately need intervention and supportive services.

Approximately 3 million cases of child maltreatment were reported in the United States in the year 2000 with 879,000 confirmed cases and 1,200 substantiated deaths. Most deaths occur in children less than age 3 years old. For each case reported there are one to two cases that go unrecognized (14,15). Because many of these children receive only episodic medical care or care at a time of medical crisis, the ED or acute care clinic plays a special role in identification and reporting of child abuse and neglect. Although the physician is legally required to report suspected child abuse and is protected from liability for making a report in all states, the more important responsibility of the physician

is to protect the child from further harm, and, therefore, cause an investigation to be done by the appropriate agency (2). More detailed information as to state reporting requirements and procedures should be sought from local law enforcement or child protection agencies.

PHYSICAL ABUSE

Physical abuse occurs in all cultural, ethnic, socioeconomic, and racial groups. There are some geographic and regional differences in the prevalence of given types of abuse, but not in overall incidence. The incidence of abuse in a socioeconomic subgroup is most closely related to the presence of significant stresses in that population (i.e., joblessness, homelessness, drug and alcohol abuse). In any parent dyad, the parent with caretaking responsibilities is more likely to abuse a child. Abusive parents are usually not psychotic and generally respond to their children in a pattern similar to that experienced in their own childhood. They often have unrealistic expectations of their children, with limited knowledge of developmental norms, and are unable to cope with the failure of the child to meet expectations. Triggering behaviors in the child, such as excessive crying or colic, are frequently seen.

EMERGENCY DEPARTMENT EVALUATION

Presentation

The history from an abused child or an abusive parent remains the most important evaluative tool for the physician. The veracity of a child's history must be assumed until there is good reason to assume otherwise. If children lie, they usually do so to hide the abuse rather than to bring it to light. The history from an abusive parent usually reflects a significant delay in seeking medical attention, and if a primary physician exists, parents have usually not sought his or her advice. There is almost always a history disparate from the severity or type of injury. If repeated questions are used to elicit the history, there is usually considerable variation in detail. Injury may be attributed to a sibling or to someone not present to verify the occurrences.

Caregiver histories often are clearly insufficient to explain the injuries, such as a history of a fall from the sofa in the presence of a subdural hematoma with cerebral edema. Parents often simply cannot relate any explanation for the injuries sustained. A brief interview of witnesses to trauma can often quickly obviate a need for investigation of a case.

Physical Assessment

The initial physical assessment of the child may show findings that are strong indicators that further evaluation for abuse is necessary:

1. Bruises in unusual locations or where an accidental etiology is implausible due to the age or developmental status of the child (e.g., nonambulatory infant with multiple bruises)
2. Bruises that have a characteristic pattern, suggesting an object used to inflict the injury (e.g., hand print, belt mark)
3. Second degree burns without bullae that show a characteristic pattern (e.g., the sole plate of an iron)
4. Second degree burns with bullae and no evidence of splash marks and an unusually sharp line of demarcation (e.g., glove or stocking burns of an extremity)
5. Burns limited to the perineum

6. Swelling of any part of the body out of proportion to the severity of described injury (e.g., may indicate underlying fracture)
7. Unexplained or implausibly explained sudden changes in neurologic status
8. Retinal hemorrhages
9. Failure to thrive without a history suggestive of chronic or debilitating disease

The physical finding most commonly present in abused children is a bruise. Bruises are also the most commonly found accidental injury in children. Accidental bruises are located in areas most frequently exposed to injury in play or other normal childhood activities. These areas include the elbows, knees, and skin over the anterior tibia. The occasional bruise in less usual locations is of little concern and generally occurs over a bony prominence. The only commonly occurring lesion that may be mistaken for a bruise is the Mongolian spot. Mongolian spots are most common in darker skinned infants and are characteristically shiny and blue-black and may be limited to the back.

Bruises that occur in clusters and in unusual locations, such as on the abdomen, the back, or buttocks, and that show unusual severity or varying stages of resolution should cause concern, because they are rarely accidental. Resolution of bruises takes place in a sequence related to the severity and location of the injury. While there are findings that indicate an acute injury, such as swelling and tenderness, the color of a bruise cannot be used to date the injury accurately. A bruise has usually resolved after about 2 to 4 weeks (13). Photographic documentation of these findings may become critically important to those pursuing the investigation of abuse, and this must be anticipated in completing the medical record.

Children who have been injured in falls from a height often present challenges in assessment for abuse versus an accidental cause. Although there have been poorly designed papers in the literature that would suggest otherwise, a significant head injury requires a fall from a distance of 4 feet or higher. Falls from a bed or sofa never result in serious injury beyond an uncomplicated fracture or bruise (4).

Laboratory Evaluation

Laboratory evaluation in suspected physical abuse cases should include bleeding and clotting studies when bruises are present and when there is any suggestion of easy bruisability. At a minimum, these studies should include a prothrombin time, partial thromboplastin time, and platelet count. In addition, a photographic record of any finding is always preferable to a written or schematic description alone. Radiographic studies are indicated when evidence of trauma is noted and in children for which abuse is identified by some other means. These studies should include the chest, skull, and long bones in addition to the area of suspected injury. Films should be reviewed for fractures as well as evidence of osteopenia, increased trabeculation, and presence of excessive numbers of wormian bones in the skull. These findings, along with an appropriate family history, might suggest the presence of osteogenesis imperfecta. If fractures are seen, they should be related to the history of the type of injury. For example, spiral fractures occur in response to a torsional force, and chip fractures of the metaphysis occur with traction of the extremity or with a shearing force across the end of the bone. Metaphyseal chip fractures are rarely accidental (9).

In addition, it is often necessary to estimate the age of fractures in comparison to the history. Fractures of differing ages without good evidence of multiple accidental trauma are virtually diagnostic of physical abuse. Healing of a fracture takes place in a predictable sequence. Periosteal new bone is formed as early as 4 to 10 days after the fracture, and soft callus formation may be seen as early as 10 to 14 days. Hard callus formation may occur as early as 14 days, and remodeling may begin by 3 months after the acute fracture (10).

Computed axial tomography of the head is indicated in those children with retinal hemorrhages or evidence of acute neurologic deterioration. The presence of intracranial hemorrhage with or without skull fracture and in the absence of a history of major trauma is diagnostic of child abuse until proven otherwise (7). Magnetic resonance imaging is a useful tool in identifying small areas of bleeding and to more carefully determine areas of bleeding that have occurred at different times (1). The use of bone scans is usually not indicated, except under special circumstances in which abuse is clearly a likely possibility and in which fractures may be suspected that are not yet visible on routine films.

With abdominal trauma, one might expect to see evidence of acute anemia associated with intraabdominal bleeding or an elevated amylase with trauma to the pancreas. Hematuria is not an uncommon occurrence with paddling or spanking, in which one or more blows has strayed cephalad.

ASSOCIATED SYNDROMES

Shaken-Baby Syndrome (Acceleration–Deceleration Injury) and Shaken-Impact Syndrome

Shaken infants rarely present with a history of shaking. The most common presentation is that of respiratory difficulty, apnea, or unexplained seizures. The basic insult is the presence of intracranial bleeding, which may be characterized as subdural, epidural, interhemispheric, or intraparenchymal. Symptoms are usually a result of increased intracranial pressure. Retinal hemorrhages are the single most common physical finding and, outside the newborn period, provide presumptive evidence of intracranial trauma. Although retinal hemorrhages may be seen with other head trauma, they should be considered the hallmark of the shaken-baby syndrome until another plausible explanation is found. The hemorrhages seen are usually superficial and diffuse, as compared with the deeper flame-type hemorrhages seen in hypertension. Trauma-related retinal hemorrhages are much more common in the periphery of the retina. The diagnosis is made by a careful history after documentation of intracranial bleeding by computed tomography or magnetic resonance imaging. The mechanism of injury was once believed to be totally due to rotational and shear forces created by the to-and-fro motion of the head in shaking, hence the term "Shaken Baby." Later studies suggest that similar lesions can be caused by significant increased venous pressure transmitted from squeezing of the chest as part of shaking or in any type of injury in which significant increases in intraabdominal or intrathoracic pressure are sustained (7). The latest studies suggest that impact of the head is necessary to produce the full clinical picture and that repetitive acceleration–deceleration forces are important (5). Because impact with even a soft surface can cause diffuse axonal injury, the concept of "shaken-impact syndrome" developed. Diffuse axonal injury is suspected to be the primary mechanism of neuronal injury after abuse (6).

As might be expected, other skeletal injuries can be seen with shaking. The child is commonly held by the thorax or the extremities with enough force to cause fractures at those sites. The combination of intracranial bleeding, as described here and metaphyseal chip fractures of the distal tibias is sometimes indicative of the child being held by the feet and cracked like a whip. The clinical outcome in this syndrome is dismal, in that approximately 65% of children will die or have significant neurologic sequelae as a result. Milder forms of this syndrome undoubtedly exist with milder neurologic sequelae but are yet to be carefully documented. This syndrome is frequently missed or misdiagnosed in the clinical setting, and missing the diagnosis can have disastrous results. In a recently published study reporting 173 cases presenting to emergency departments, 31.2% were misdiagnosed at initial presentation, 27.8% were abused again before an accurate diagnosis was made, and 2 were killed before an accurate diagnosis was made (8).

Failure to Thrive

Failure to thrive is often categorized as organic and nonorganic, although there are often some elements of both types in most individual cases. The child presents with the weight being greater than two standard deviations below the mean expected for age, and there may be associated growth failure as well. In most cases of organic failure to thrive, a strong suggestion of the underlying etiology will be evident from the history or physical examination. Suggestions of a nonorganic etiology may be evident in observing the interactions between the mother and child. The mother and child often show little interaction, and nonnurturing behavior is evident on the part of the mother. The child often shows little eye contact and is generally withdrawn from the environment (3). Most commonly, nonorganic failure to thrive requires a period of observation in a hospital setting for accurate diagnosis, (see Chapter 223, "Failure to Thrive").

Munchausen Syndrome by Proxy

This unusual type of child abuse occurs when a caretaker describes or produces factitious illness in a child as a response to their own psychiatric pathology. This is a diagnosis of which the emergency physician should be aware of but it is not a diagnosis to be made in the emergency department. This diagnosis requires intense record review and, usually, inpatient evaluation (11).

EMERGENCY DEPARTMENT MANAGEMENT

After a decision to report has been made, the next dilemma is to decide whether to tell the parents about the report. Under most circumstances, the physician should calmly inform the parents that a report is being made because he or she is required to do so by state law and therefore has no choice in the matter. It is generally good to relieve some of the mystery of what will happen after the report is made by informing the parents about the steps in the investigation process. The circumstance when it is better not to inform the parents is one in which the physician feels the parents are likely to flee with the child and further endanger the child's health and welfare.

Meticulous attention to the chart is essential in all abuse cases. The examiner is often called on to recall the encounter with the patient and parents in great detail months or years later. The use of direct quotes from the child is helpful in avoiding questions of hearsay information. The use of detailed body charts to delineate injuries and findings, including careful measurements, is important. Even better is the inclusion of photographs of findings as part of the medical record.

The emergency department physician should be aware of community agencies that provide investigative and intervention services to abusive families and abused children, so that he or she has immediate access to information and consultation on individual cases. If the services of a multidisciplinary team are available, participation in the activities of the team is often very valuable in receiving feedback as to case outcome and progress.

CRITICAL INTERVENTIONS

- Meticulous attention to documentation of physical findings is imperative
- The provider must recognize history components that are inconsistent with the developmental stage of the child
- In patients with bruising, obtain a prothrombin time, a partial prothrombin time and a platelet count
- Report all suspicious cases to appropriate law enforcement and state child agencies

COMMON PITFALL

✔ The most common pitfall in the diagnosis of child abuse is the failure of the physician to seriously consider this etiology in the differential diagnosis of trauma to children. The presence of documented findings of trauma with an implausible history should provide more than adequate impetus for further evaluation and careful documentation

References

1. Alexander RC, Schor DP, Smith WL. Magnetic resonance imaging of intracranial injuries from child abuse. *J Pediatr* 1986;109:975.
2. American Medical Association. *Guidelines for the management of physical abuse of children*. Chicago: American Medical Association, 1992.
3. Bithoney WG, Dubowitz H, Egan H. Failure to thrive/growth deficiency. *Pediatr Rev* 1992;13:453.
4. Chadwick D, Chin S, Salerno C, et al. Deaths from falls in children: how far is fatal? *J Trauma* 1993;31:1353.
5. Duhaime AC, Alario AJ, Lewander WJ, et al. Head injury in very young children: injury types and ophthalmologic findings in 100 hospitalized patients younger than 2 years of age. *Pediatrics* 1992;90:179.
6. Duhaime AC, Christian CW, Rorke LB, et al. Nonaccidental head injury in infants- the "Shaken-Baby syndrome." *N Eng J Med* 1998;338:1822–1828.
7. Dykes LJ. The whiplash shaken infant syndrome: what has been learned? *Child Abuse Negl* 1986;10:211.
8. Jenny C, Hymel K, Ritzen A, et al. Analysis of missed cases of abusive head trauma. *JAMA* 1999;281:621.
9. Leventhal JM, Thomas SA, Rosenfield NS, et al. Fractures in young children: distinguishing child abuse from unintentional injuries. *Am J Dis Child* 1993; 147:87.
10. O'Conner JF, Cohen J. Dating fractures. In: Kleinman PK, ed. *Diagnostic imaging of child abuse*. Baltimore: Williams & Wilkins, 1987.
11. Rosenberg DA. Web of deceit: a literature review of Munchausen syndrome by proxy. *Child Abuse Negl* 1987;11:547.
12. Schimdt BD. The child with nonaccidental trauma. In: Helfer ME, ed. *The battered child*. 3rd ed. Chicago: University of Chicago Press, 1983.
13. Schwartz A, Ricci L. How accurately can bruises be aged in abused children? *Pediatrics* 1996;97:254.
14. U.S. Department of Health and Human Services Releases 2000 Child Abuse Report Data. AHA Legislative Activities. American Human association. http://www.americanhumane.org/actnoww/2000abuse.data.htm
15. U.S. Department of Health and Human Services, Administration on Children, Youth and Families. Child Maltreatment 1999. Washington, DC: U.S. Government Printing Office, 2001.

CHAPTER 236
Appendicitis

Maureen D. McCollough

Appendicitis is the most common surgical emergency in childhood, with an estimated 80,000 children affected annually (2). Despite the decline in mortality since the introduction of antibiotics, morbidity has remained unchanged over the past 40 years, due primarily to perforation because of delays in diagnosis. Perforation rates are higher in children, occurring in 50% to 70% of preschoolers with appendicitis, versus 10% to 20% in an adult population (12,16). This highlights the importance of early diagnosis and treatment in the prevention of significant morbidity.

Obstruction of the appendiceal lumen, caused most commonly by a fecalith (calcified fecal material), is the primary cause of appendicitis. Other less common causes of obstruction include inflamed lymphoid tissue; vegetable and fruit seeds; intestinal worms (especially Ascaridae); bacterial infection with *Yersinia*, *Salmonella*, or *Shigella;* and, rarely, retained barium from previous radiographic studies, or anomalies of mucus-secreting glands, as in cystic fibrosis (15,22).

Luminal obstruction of the appendix causes distention and increased intraluminal pressure, resulting in obstruction of the blood supply. Bacterial invasion occurs, and, ultimately, the ischemic appendix becomes gangrenous and perforates. Bacteriologic cultures of perforated appendices have revealed polymicrobial organisms, including *Escherichia coli, Bacteroides fragilis*, and enteric streptococci (10).

The progression from appendiceal obstruction to perforation is more rapid in children. What starts as vague abdominal complaints can quickly progress to ileus, nausea, vomiting, fever, tachycardia, localized pain, and, finally, peritonitis. The inability of omentum in young children to wall-off localized infections contributes to the development of diffuse peritonitis. Therefore, appendicitis must be recognized early and proper management instituted without delay (16).

CLINICAL PRESENTATION

The symptoms of acute appendicitis correlate with the pathophysiology of the disease. Obstruction and distention of the appendix stimulates stretch receptors, relaying pain through visceral nerve fibers to the tenth thoracic ganglion, resulting in the perception of periumbilical pain. Bacterial invasion and inflammation then lead to fever, nausea, or vomiting in up to 80% of children. As the inflammation extends to surrounding tissues, localized pain depends on the location of the appendix. Up to one-third of appendices are located in areas other than the usual intraperitoneal location. This results in up to 30% of children with appendicitis having localized pain in areas other than the right lower quadrant. A retrocecal location of the appendix may cause back or flank pain, a pelvic appendix may cause suprapubic pain, and a retroileal location may cause referred pain to the testicle.

If appendicitis is allowed to progress without surgical intervention, appendiceal rupture will occur. The diagnosis of perforation is easier to make. The child is usually ill appearing, toxic, and dehydrated. Particularly in younger children, the in-

completely developed greater omentum is incapable of walling off the inflammatory process. Therefore, the abdominal pain is more diffuse and may decrease in intensity just after perforation, becoming much more severe as peritonitis develops.

Examining a young child with abdominal pain is often fraught with difficulty. Because young children are often frightened of doctors and "white coats," observing the child from the doorway or across the room can be revealing. A young child who is ambulating easily around the room, interested in his or her surroundings, is less concerning than a child who is ill appearing and lying very quietly. A slight limp in the child's gait, hesitation to climb onto the examination table, and inability to stretch the right leg may suggest appendicitis even before the full evaluation. The child usually prefers to lie still in the supine position with the thighs, particularly the right, drawn up, because any motion increases pain. Vital signs are essentially normal, but a child with simple appendicitis may show a mild temperature elevation. Tachycardia may be present if the child is dehydrated, febrile, or in pain.

Examination of the abdomen for bowel sounds and tenderness can often frighten young children. Distraction of the young child, using a hand puppet or other toy, may help achieve a better examination. Bowel sounds are usually normal in early appendicitis. Advanced inflammation, perforation, or both, usually result in an ileus and a quiet abdomen.

Abdominal palpation should start away from the painful area. Muscular resistance to palpation of the abdomen parallels the severity of the inflammatory process. Early in the disease process, resistance, if present, consists of voluntary guarding. With the progression of peritoneal irritation, muscle spasm increases and becomes involuntary. The classic physical finding is point tenderness at McBurney point (3 to 5 cm from the anterior–superior iliac spine on a straight line drawn from that process to the umbilicus) (22).

Physical signs usually associated with acute appendicitis are as follows (28):

1. Rovsing sign. This may be found if local peritoneal inflammation is present. By testing for tenderness in the left lower quadrant, referred tenderness can be elicited in the right lower quadrant.
2. Psoas sign. The child lies on the left side, stretches the psoas muscle by slowly extending the right thigh. Alternatively, the child lies supine and flexes the right hip against a hand placed just above the knee. Pain elicited by either maneuver can indicate an irritating focus in proximity to the psoas muscle.
3. Obturator sign. A positive obturator sign occurs when passive internal rotation of the flexed thigh with the patient supine produces right-sided abdominal pain. This sign indicates irritation around the obturator internus muscle.

A positive psoas or obturator sign suggests retrocecal or retrocolic inflammation. Although these signs (Rovsing, psoas, and obturator) are often quoted as associated with appendicitis, there have been few studies published evaluating the accuracy of the clinical examination for appendicitis (28). A metaanalysis regarding the clinical signs most likely to identify patients (both children and adults) at increased likelihood for appendicitis was published. The clinical signs with the highest positive likelihood ratios were right lower quadrant pain, rigidity, and migration of initial periumbilical pain to the right lower quadrant. Clinical signs with the highest negative likelihood ratios for ruling out appendicitis were absence of right lower quadrant pain and presence of similar previous pain (28). The diagnostic value of the rectal examination in children is limited; rectal tenderness is present in 50% of all children with or without appendicitis (3).

DIFFERENTIAL DIAGNOSIS

The differential diagnosis in children depends on three major factors: the anatomic location of the inflamed appendix, the stage of the process (simple or ruptured), and the age and sex of the patient. The five main groups of differential diagnoses are as follows (15,21,22,26):

1. Intestinal diseases: mesenteric adenitis, viral and bacterial enteritis, Meckel diverticulitis, intussusception, enteric duplication
2. Uterine or tuboovarian pathology: ovarian or testicular torsion, acute epididymitis, pelvic inflammatory disease, ectopic pregnancy, endometriosis, mittelschmerz
3. Urinary tract pathology: acute pyelonephritis, cystitis, renal stones
4. Respiratory and systemic diseases: basal pneumonia, Henoch-Schönlein purpura, sickle cell crisis, diabetic ketoacidosis
5. Trauma: accidental or nonaccidental injury

Acute Mesenteric Lymphadenitis

Mesenteric adenitis is most often confused with acute appendicitis in children. A careful history almost invariably reveals the presence of upper respiratory symptoms in these patients. Laboratory procedures are usually of limited value in differentiation, although a relative lymphocytosis may suggest mesenteric adenitis or a generalized viral syndrome. The abdominal pain is usually more diffuse and less severe, and generalized lymphadenopathy may be noted on physical examination.

Pelvic Inflammatory Disease

A history of vaginal discharge in a sexually active adolescent can often be elicited. Interviewing adolescents alone, without parental presence, may offer a more revealing and true history regarding sexual activity. Pain is most often bilateral and lower in location. Physical examination reveals Chandelier sign (pain with motion of the cervix).

Acute Gastroenteritis

Acute gastroenteritis usually can be differentiated from appendicitis. Often, there is a history of other ill contacts. These patients have nausea, vomiting, watery diarrhea, and intermittent, crampy abdominal pain. Often, the vomiting precedes the diarrhea by 24 hours. Localizing signs on the abdominal examination are usually absent.

Meckel's Diverticulitis

Preoperative differentiation is unnecessary, because the signs and symptoms of Meckel diverticulitis are similar to those of acute appendicitis, and surgical treatment is indicated for both.

Intussusception

Differentiating between intussusception and acute appendicitis is important and relatively straightforward. Appendicitis is rare in children younger than 2 years of age, whereas nearly all intussusceptions occur in children younger than age 2 years. Intussusception typically occurs suddenly in an otherwise healthy infant. The infant "doubles up" with apparent colicky pain, but is usually without pain between attacks. A bloody mucoid stool is usually passed several hours after the onset of pain. Physical examination may reveal a sausage-shaped mass in the right lower quadrant. Occasionally, infants with intussusception present with altered mental status. Treatment of intussusception is reduction by barium or air enema (see Chapter 251, "Intussusception").

Henoch-Schönlein Purpura

Henoch-Schönlein purpura, a diffuse vasculitis, classically presents with joint pain and swelling and purpura. Abdominal pain may also be a prominent symptom. Rectal examination should be performed for occult blood. Urinalysis to evaluate for hematuria due to nephritis should also be performed.

Mittelschmerz

These patients are at the midpoint of their menstrual cycle. The pain of Mittelschmerz is usually sudden in nature and may be localized to one side of the lower abdomen, or diffuse in nature.

Ovarian or Testicular Torsion

A number of nonspecific symptoms may exist, including anorexia, nausea, and vomiting. The correct diagnosis can be made by always including the genitalia in the physical examination, which usually reveals the subtle findings of asymmetry in gonadal size or position. A normal examination of the ovarian or testicular size or position does not completely rule out the diagnosis of torsion, however.

Urinary Tract Infection

Bacteria or white blood cells may be present in the urine specimen of approximately 17% of children with acute appendicitis (1). This occurs if the appendix lies near the ureter or bladder. With the exception of an elevated specific gravity due to dehydration, the urinalysis is normal in more than 80% of children with acute appendicitis.

EMERGENCY DEPARTMENT EVALUATION

The most important steps in making a correct diagnosis of appendicitis are eliciting a complete history and performing a complete physical examination, including examining the external genitalia in boys and performing an internal pelvic examination in adolescent girls. However, because the sensitivity of the clinical examination has been reported to be as low as 63%, other modalities have been utilized to improve diagnostic capabilities (7).

Indicated laboratory studies include a complete blood count with differential and urinalysis. Moderate leukocytosis (10,000 to 18,000 white blood cells/mL) with a predominance of polymorphonuclear cells is classically seen but does not necessarily correlate with the severity of the disease (5,29). A left shift in the differential may precede a total leukocytosis in children. It must be noted that a normal white blood cell count does not rule out the diagnosis of appendicitis.

Abdominal radiographs are not particularly helpful, as the presence of a fecalith is shown in only 10% to 20% of children with appendicitis (15). Nonspecific findings on plain abdominal films include isolated distended loops of bowel in the right lower quadrant and obliteration of the psoas shadow. Because lesions that irritate nerves at the T10 to T12 level may simulate the referred pain distribution of appendicitis, a chest film may be required to rule out right lower lobe pneumonia, especially if signs or symptoms of lower respiratory tract disease exist.

Other noninvasive imaging studies, such as ultrasonography or computed tomography (CT), may help make the diagnosis and have gained popularity. Ultrasound in children has been shown to have a sensitivity and specificity of 90% and 97%, respectively, with an overall accuracy of 96% (13). The classic finding of appendicitis, when viewed by ultrasound, is a thickened, noncompressible, nonperistaltic appendix. Ultrasonography in adolescent girls is especially useful to differentiate appendicitis from tuboovarian disease (e.g., a tuboovarian abscess or ovarian cyst). A normal appendix should be visualized to rule out the diagnosis of appendicitis (13,19,23). CT scan of the abdomen, with rectal contrast, has been shown to have sensitivity and specificity of 94% and negative predictive value of 97% (7). CT also has been shown to reduce the number of inpatient prediagnosis observation days, operations, and negative laparotomies (4,6,9,27). CT scanning is best utilized in the pediatric patient with atypical history or examination for appendicitis when the clinical suspicion is high enough to warrant further testing (25).

It has been shown that 20% to 40% of children with acute appendicitis are given the wrong diagnosis on the first visit to a physician (8,16,20). The most common erroneous preoperative diagnoses, in descending order of frequency, are acute mesenteric lymphadenitis, no organic pathologic condition, acute pelvic inflammatory disease, ovarian cyst, Mittelschmerz, and acute gastroenteritis. These account for more than 75% of all missed diagnoses. A thorough history and physical examination should result in a higher degree of accuracy (21). There is a higher incidence of perforation in younger children and in children with a history of prolonged symptoms. Symptoms suggestive of perforation are as follows (26):

- Duration of symptoms more than 36 hours
- Temperature greater than 102°F
- White blood cell count of more than 15,000/mL
- Physical findings of peritonitis

The surgical consultant should be contacted as soon as the diagnosis of acute appendicitis is entertained, to avoid the complication of late diagnosis and perforation. Perforated appendicitis has a mortality rate of 5% and a morbidity rate of up to 46% in some series, compared with a mortality rate of 0.1% for nonperforated appendicitis (6,14,21).

EMERGENCY DEPARTMENT MANAGEMENT

Appendicitis is a surgical emergency. All children thought to have an abdominal surgical emergency should be seen by a surgeon as soon as possible. The initial emergency department management of simple and perforated appendicitis is essentially the same. Once the diagnosis is made, the child must be fluid-resuscitated intravenously and kept NPO. In a child who has been vomiting, obtaining serum electrolyte levels should be considered while intravenous fluid therapy is begun. Those children who have clinical signs or symptoms of dehydration should receive 0.9 NaCl or Ringer lactate boluses at 20 mL/kg to maintain urine output at 1 to 2 mL/kg/h. Once the child is considered fluid-resuscitated, dextrose 5% in 0.45 or 0.225 normal saline and 20 mEq/L KCl at 1.5 times maintenance should be given, as long as the child is not oliguric. If the patient has eaten or vomited within a few hours of the operation, insertion of a nasogastric tube to empty the stomach may be requested by the surgeon. If the child is febrile, an acetaminophen suppository may be given.

The use of routine antibiotic coverage in children with uncomplicated appendicitis continues to be debated. It appears that short-term perioperative antibiotic prophylaxis in children with acute nonperforated appendicitis may decrease the rate of postoperative infectious complications (24). Absolute indications for extended therapy and a broader spectrum of antibiotic coverage are systemic signs of toxicity, sepsis, suspected perforation, and the presence of underlying conditions that predispose the patient to complications of bacteremia (i.e., infants younger than 6 months of age and children with congenital or acquired cardiac anomalies, sickle cell disease, diabetes mellitus, chronic renal failure, or other states of immune suppression) (21). One commonly used regimen includes ampicillin (100 mg/kg/24 h in four doses), gentamicin (5 mg/kg/24 h in three doses), and clindamycin (40 mg/kg/24 h in four doses). This particular regimen ensures coverage of aminoglycoside-resistant enterococci, gram-negative bacilli, and anaerobes, respectively (6,18). Other antibiotic combinations or single-drug therapy can be used as long as the same microbial coverage is obtained in the setting of acute noncomplicated disease.

CRITICAL INTERVENTIONS

- Maintain a high index of suspicion in children with abdominal pain. A retrocecal location of the appendix may cause back or flank pain, a pelvic appendix may cause suprapubic pain, and a retroileal location may cause referred pain to the testicle
- Administer 0.9 NaCl or Ringer lactate boluses at 20 ml/kg in children with clinical signs or symptoms of dehydration to maintain urine output at 1 to 2 ml/kg/h
- Obtain a surgical consult as soon as possible in order to avoid the complications of late diagnosis and perforation

DISPOSITION

All children with appendicitis should be admitted to the hospital for surgical exploration. In certain cases of appendiceal abscess, a surgeon may opt for admission to the hospital for intravenous antibiotics or percutaneous drainage, with an interval appendectomy several weeks later (17).

If there is doubt about the correct diagnosis, but the suspicion for appendicitis is still high, the child should be admitted to the hospital for serial physical examinations. If the suspicion is low but still a consideration, the child may be discharged with clear instructions to return in 6 to 8 hours for a reexamination of the abdomen. If there is any doubt about the ability of the child to return for a revisit, the child should be admitted to the hospital for serial physical examinations.

The child may require transfer to another facility if appropriate surgical staff is unavailable at the initial hospital. This should be done expediently after resuscitation has been started.

COMMON PITFALLS

✔ Immediate diagnosis of acute appendicitis in children is essential. Rapid progression of disease in this age group necessitates early suspicion, diagnosis, and operation if perforation is to be avoided. Late diagnosis results in significantly higher morbidity and mortality
✔ The evaluating physician must be thorough in obtaining the history and performing the physical examination. In some cases, children or adolescents have been admitted to the hospital for observation with a diagnosis of "rule out appendicitis," when the actual, unrecognized diagnosis was testicular torsion or pelvic inflammatory disease, which could have been recognized if a complete physical examination had been performed

Acknowledgment

The author gratefully acknowledges the contribution of Bonnie Beaver, who wrote the first version of this chapter.

References

1. Arnbjornsson E. Bacteriuria in appendicitis. *Am J Surg* 1988;155:356.
2. Ballantine TVN. Appendicitis. *Surg Clin North Am* 1981;6:117.
3. Bower RJ, Bell MJ, Ternberg JL, et al. Controversial aspects of appendicitis management in children. *Arch Surg* 1981;116:885.
4. Christopher FL, Lane MJ, Ward JA, et al. Unenhanced helicial CT scanning of the abdomen and pelvis changes disposition of patients presenting to the emergency department with possible acute appendicitis. *J Emerg Med* 2002;23:1–7.
5. Coleman C, Thompson JE Jr, Bennon RS, et al. White blood cell count is a poor predictor of severity of disease in the diagnosis of appendicitis. *Am Surg* 1998;64:983.
6. Douville C, Birinyi L, Stevenson RJ. Complicated appendicitis in children. *Hosp Physician* 1986;22:33.
7. Garcia Pena BM, Mandl KD, Kraus SJ, et al. Ultrasonography and limited computed tomography in the diagnosis and management of appendicitis in children. *JAMA* 1999;282:1041.
8. Garcia Pena BM, Taylor GA, Lund DP. Effect of computed tomography on patient management and costs in children with suspected appendicitis. *Pediatrics* 1999;104:440.
9. Garcia-Pena BM, Taylor GA, Fishman SJ, et al. Effect of an imaging protocol on clinical outcomes among pediatric patients with appendicitis. *Pediatrics* 2002;110:1088–1093.
10. Gilbert SR, Emmens RW, Putnam TC. Appendicitis in children. *Surg Gynecol Obstet* 1985;161:261.
11. Gilchrist BF, Lobe TE, Schropp KP, et al. Is there a role for laparoscopic appendectomy in pediatric surgery? *J Pediatr Surg* 1992;27:209.
12. Graham JJ, Pokorny WJ, Harberg FJ, et al. Acute appendicitis in preschool age children. *Am J Surg* 1980;139:247.
13. Hahn HB, Hoepner FU, Kalle T, et al. Sonography of acute appendicitis in children: 7 years experience. *Pediatr Radiol* 1998;28:147.
14. Karp MP, Caldarola VA, Cooney DR, et al. The avoidable excesses in the management of perforated appendicitis in children. *J Pediatr Surg* 1986;21:506.
15. Kottmeier PK. Appendicitis. In: Welch KJ, Randolph JG, Ravitch MM, et al, eds. *Pediatric surgery,* 3rd ed. Chicago: Year Book, 1986:989.
16. Linz DN, Hrabovsky EE, Franceschi D, et al. Does the current health care environment contribute to increased morbidity and mortality of acute appendicitis in children? *J Pediatr Surg* 1993;28:321.
17. Mazziotti MV, Marley EF, Winthrop AL, et al. Histopathologic analysis of interval appendectomy specimens: support for the role of interval appendectomy. *J Pediatr Surg* 1997;32:806.
18. Neilson IR, Laberge JM, Nguyen LT, et al. Appendicitis in children: current therapeutic recommendations. *J Pediatr Surg* 1990;25:1113.
19. Rubin SZ, Martin DJ. Ultrasonography in the management of possible appendicitis in childhood. *J Pediatr Surg* 1990;25:737.
20. Savrin RA, Clatworthy HW. Appendiceal rupture: a continuing diagnostic problem. *Pediatrics* 1979;63:37.
21. Scherer LR. Acute appendicitis. In: Cameron JL, ed. *Current surgical therapy,* 4th ed. St. Louis: Mosby–Year Book, 1992:217.
22. Schwartz SI. Appendix. In: Schwartz SI, ed. *Principles of surgery,* 6th ed. New York: The McGraw-Hill Companies, 1994:1307.
23. Siegel MJ, Carel C, Surratt S. Ultrasonography of acute abdominal pain in children. *JAMA* 1991;266:1987.
24. Soderquist-Elinder C, Hirsch K, Bergdahl S, et al. Prophylactic antibiotics in uncomplicated appendicitis during childhood—a prospective randomised study. *Eur J Pediatr Surg* 1995;5:282.
25. Stephen AE, Segev DL, Ryan DP. The diagnosis of acute appendicitis in a pediatric population: to CT or not to CT. *J Ped Surg* 2003;38:367–371.
26. Stone HH, Sanders SC, Martin JD. Perforated appendicitis in children. *Surgery* 1971;69:673.
27. Torbati SS, Gus DA. Impact of helical computed tomography on the outcomes of emergency department patients with suspected appendicitis. *Acad Emerg Med* 2003;10:823–829.
28. Wagner JM, McKinney WP, Carpenter JL. Does this patient have appendicitis? *JAMA* 1996;276:1589.
29. Williams R, Mackway-Jones K. White cell count and diagnosing appendicitis in children. *Emerg Med J* 2002;19:428–429.

Asthma

Jeffrey F. Linzer

Almost 4.2 million children had an acute asthma attack in 2001 (2). The number of asthma-related emergency department (ED) visits for children were almost twice that for adults (16) (104 vs. 54 per 10,000 population). African-American children continue to have the highest exacerbation rate versus white or Latino children (7.7% vs. 5.4% vs. 4.0%) (2).

Asthma can simply be defined as recurrent reversible bronchospasm due to a trigger (Table 237.1). There are underlying inflammatory and neural mechanisms that make the airways more sensitive to the triggers and result in bronchial hyperresponsiveness. A number of preformed and generated mediators cause the airway epithelium to become fragile and denuded and the epithelial subbasement membranes to thicken. Also, mucus production and consistency increase, and endothelial leakage results in mucosal edema (3). Mediator-induced abnormalities in the parasympathetic and nonadrenergic noncholinergic nervous systems may also lead to increased bronchial hyperresponsiveness.

CLINICAL PRESENTATION

Acute asthma exacerbations vary in severity and duration. An asthma attack can be divided into two phases: early and late asthmatic responses. The early asthmatic response (EAR) occurs soon after trigger exposure, producing bronchospasm, and usually lasts 1 to 2 hours. About 50% of patients go on to develop a late asthmatic response (LAR), with reoccurrence of bronchospasm about 4 hours after the initial trigger exposure. The LAR episode usually lasts 12 to 24 hours but may persist up to several days in some children.

Clinical events such as symptoms, spirometry, and ventilation–perfusion measurements poorly correlate with each other (14). Spirometry tends to reflect the degree of bronchoconstriction in large and medium airways. Ventilation–perfusion mismatch is more related to obstructive changes in the peripheral airways. Patients who are admitted to a hospital tend to have more severe airway obstruction (6).

Classically, with an acute asthma attack, the child presents with wheezing and respiratory distress. Bronchospasm, however, can also present as cough, chest pain, shortness of breath, and fatigue with exertion which can make the diagnosis and appropriate management more difficult. Acute asthma attacks can be divided into mild, moderate, severe, and impending respiratory failure (17) (Table 237.2).

With a mild attack, the child usually has been symptomatic for a short period of time and may still be in the EAR. There may be some increase in the respiratory rate, with a tight, hacking cough or end-expiratory wheezing. There is good air exchange, with minimal breathlessness and no accessory muscle use. Room air oxygen saturation (SaO_2) is greater than 95%, and peak expiratory flow rate (PEFR) or forced expiratory volume in one second (FEV_1) greater than 80% predicted or personal best.

In a more moderate attack, symptoms may have been ongoing for several hours to days, indicating LAR. There is an increase

TABLE 237.1.   Triggers of Asthma Symptoms in Various Age Groups

	Infancy	Early Childhood	Late Childhood	Adolescence
Viral infections	++++	+++	±	+++
Exercise	+	++	+++	+++
Irritants	+	++	+++	+++
Foods	++	+	()	()
Indoor inhalants	±	+++	+++	+++
Pollens	()	++	+++	++
Emotions	()	+	+	+

Adapted from Pearlman DS, Lemanske RF Jr. Asthma (bronchial asthma): principals of diagnosis and treatment. In: Bierman CW, Pearlman DS, Shapiro GG, et al., eds. *Allergy, asthma and immunology from infancy to adulthood*. Philadelphia: WB Saunders, 1996:492.

TABLE 237.2.   Classification of Severity of Asthma Exacerbation

	Mild	Moderate	Severe	Respiratory Arrest Imminent
SYMPTOMS				
Breathlessness	While walking	While talking (infant softer, shorter cry; difficulty feeding)	While at rest (infant stops feedings)	
	Can lie down	Prefers sitting	Sits upright	
Talks in	Sentences	Phrases	Words	
Alertness	May be agitated	Usually agitated	Usually agitated	Drowsy or confused
SIGNS				
Respiratory rate	Increased	Increased	Often > 30/min	

Guide to normal rates of breathing in awake children:

Age	Normal rate
< 2 mo	< 60/min
2–12 mo	< 50/min
1–5 yr	< 40/min
6–8 yr	< 30/min

	Mild	Moderate	Severe	Respiratory Arrest Imminent
Use of accessory muscles; suprasternal retractions	Usually not	Commonly	Usually	Paradoxical thoracoabdominal movement
Wheeze	Moderate, often only end expiratory	Loud; throughout exhalation	Usually loud; throughout inhalation and exhalation	Absence of wheeze
Pulse/minute	< 100	100–120	> 120	Bradycardia

Guide to normal pulse rates in children:

Age	Normal rate
2–12 mo	< 160/min
1–2 yr	< 120/min
2–8 yr	< 110/min

	Mild	Moderate	Severe	Respiratory Arrest Imminent
Pulsus paradoxus	Absent (< 10 mm Hg)	May be present (10–25 mm Hg)	Often present (20–40 mm Hg)	Absence suggest respiratory muscle fatigue

FUNCTIONAL ASSESSMENT

	Mild	Moderate	Severe	
PEF % predicted or % personal best	> 80%	Approx. 50%–80% or response lasts < 2 h	< 50% prdicted or personal best	
PaO_2 (on air)	Normal (test not usually necessary)	> 60 mm Hg (test not usually necessary)	< 60 mm Hg: possible cyanosis	
and/or PCO_2	< 42 mm Hg (test not usually necessary)	< 42 mm Hg (test not usually necessary)	≥ 42 mm Hg; possible respiratory failure	
SaO_2% (on air) at sea level	> 95% (test not usually necessary)	91%–95%	< 91%	

Hypercapnia (hypoventilation) develops more readily in young children than in adults and adolescents.

Adapted from National Heart, Lung, and Blood Institute, National Institutes of Health. *Expert panel report 2: guidelines for the diagnosis and management of asthma*. NIH Publication No. 97-4051, Bethesda, MD, 1997.

in the work of breathing, with tachypnea and accessory muscle use. Expiratory wheezing may be audible on entering the examination room, and inspiratory–expiratory wheezing may be present. The child may become breathless while talking and be somewhat agitated. An infant may have a less vigorous but more irritable cry and pull away from an offered bottle. Oxygen saturation will be in the low normal range, and PEFR/FEV$_1$ will be less than 80% predicted or personal best.

Severe attacks are similar to moderate exacerbations in their time of onset and duration. There is marked respiratory distress, work of breathing, and tachypnea. Accessory muscle use is associated with intercostal and tracheosternal retractions and nasal flaring. Breath sounds can range from inspiratory–expiratory wheezing to a somewhat quiet chest. The child will be breathless at rest. Neurologically, the child may range from anxious and agitated to somnolent and difficult to arouse. Infants will range from very agitated to unusually quiet and will refuse to take a bottle. Hypoxia is present, and the PaCO$_2$ may rise above 40 mm Hg. PEFR/FEV$_1$ will be less than 50% predicted or personal best.

While type I respiratory failure (hypoxia without CO$_2$ retention) can develop with a moderate-to-severe asthma attack, type II failure (hypoxia with CO$_2$ retention) develops as the child becomes fatigued from the increased work of breathing. Respiratory efforts are labored to the point of paradoxical respiratory movement. The chest may be quiet because of the inability to move any air. The level of consciousness will be depressed. Bradycardia may develop because of hypoxia. Oxygenation may remain significantly low (SaO$_2$ less than 92% and PaO$_2$ less than 60 mm Hg) despite adequate supplementation (greater than or equal to 40% O$_2$).

It is important to remember that a child may present with symptoms from any and all of the mentioned categories, and symptoms thus do not always lend themselves to easy classification.

DIFFERENTIAL DIAGNOSIS

The clinician's careful history and physical examination can help locate from which part of the respiratory tract the symptoms originate. It is important to note that the term reactive airways disease refers to a group of conditions that affect the lower airways. The diagnosis "reactive airway disease" defaults to "asthma" under the International Classification of Disease 9th Revision, Clinical Modification. Generally, the diagnosis of asthma can be made after documentation of three or more episodes of bronchodilator responsive bronchospasm (30).

Cough or rattling chest sounds that could mimic asthma are most commonly heard with upper airway pathology. These sounds can occur in children with an upper respiratory infection and in older children and adolescents with allergic rhinitis and sinusitis. These conditions also can contribute to an asthma exacerbation. Similar sounds can be produced in infants with choanal atresia and in children with hypertrophy of the tonsils or adenoids. The examiner should especially be aware of the potential of foreign bodies in toddlers and young children.

Middle-airway pathology can not only cause cough, but also result in wheezing and chest sensations that a young or preverbal child may indicate to be chest pain. Stridor, which is an inspiratory sound, should not be confused with wheezing. Examples of conditions that produce stridor include croup, epiglottitis, and pharyngeal foreign bodies. Fortunately, epiglottitis in the post-*Haemophilus influenzae b* vaccination era has become rare in children although group A streptococcus may produce a similar picture. Unfortunately, laryngotracheobronchitis ("wheezy croup") and tracheal foreign bodies can also produce wheezing.

In infants, anatomic conditions that can cause cough and wheeze include laryngomalacia, tracheomalacia, tracheoe-

sophageal fistula, and hemangiomas. Laryngeal webs, vascular rings, and slings are seen in older infants and toddlers. Vocal cord dysfunction is rare and usually seen in older children and adolescents. In all of these conditions, there is minimal, if any, improvement in symptoms with asthma therapy.

The lower airway causes of asthma-like symptoms are more difficult to differentiate from asthma. Cystic fibrosis can present with symptoms that initially respond well to asthma therapy. Children with cystic fibrosis can go on to develop digital clubbing, which is rarely seen with asthma. Now less common due to surfactant therapy, bronchopulmonary dysplasia can occur in ex-premature infants who required prolonged ventilatory support. Chronic aspiration and gastroesophageal reflux, which can exacerbate underlying asthma, can produce cough and wheezing on their own. Inhalation of chemical and toxic substances and foreign bodies must also be considered.

Bronchiolitis, both RSV and non-RSV variants, is a common cause of wheezing in children under 2 years of age, although viral infections can trigger wheezing in any age group. This disease occasionally will respond to asthma treatment. Bronchitis should be considered an adult or adolescent disease. Chlamydia trachomatis (infants under 3 months), pertussis (especially in infants under 6 months of age), pneumonia, and chronic Chlamydia pneumoniae in asthmatics can present like or worsen asthma.

Rare lower airway conditions to consider include complications of congenital cardiac conditions, alpha$_1$-antitrypsin deficiency, pulmonary hemosiderosis, and pulmonary eosinophilia (Löffler syndrome).

EMERGENCY DEPARTMENT EVALUATION

Determination of the severity of the attack is based on a rapid initial assessment that includes a brief history, directed physical examination, and baseline SaO$_2$ measurement, which should be done in a calm and reassuring manner. PEFR or FEV$_1$ should be obtained in all children 6 years of age and older (Fig. 237.1).

The presentation and duration of symptoms and response to any therapy prior to arrival in the ED help determine whether the child is in LAR. Identifying contributing factors (e.g., fever, choking) assists in determining the need for ancillary tests or other therapy. Assessment of the risk of severity of an acute exacerbation includes:

The number and timing of similar episodes,

1) Prior ED visits and hospitalizations (including intensive care unit admissions),
2) Prior need for aggressive interventions including bilevel positive airway pressure (bipap), continuous positive airway pressure (cpap), heliox and/or intubation, and
3) Medication history (including last use of systemic steroids).

The physical examination should rapidly determine the child's work of breathing by evaluating the degree of breathlessness, use of accessory muscles and nasal flaring, and listening to breathing sounds. A great deal of information can easily be gleaned simply by removing or opening the child's top and watching the breathing effort. Neurologic status is reflected by the degree of irritability and interaction with the examiner and caretaker. Measurement of PEFR or FEV$_1$ allows objective monitoring of lung function. It should be expressed as a percentage of a predicted value based on height, age, and sex from any of several available tables. A better comparison is the child's own personal best value that was obtained during a symptom-free period.

Routine radiographs are not needed for the straightforward asthma attack that improves with ED treatment. Plain chest films should be considered if there is a fever or suspicion of

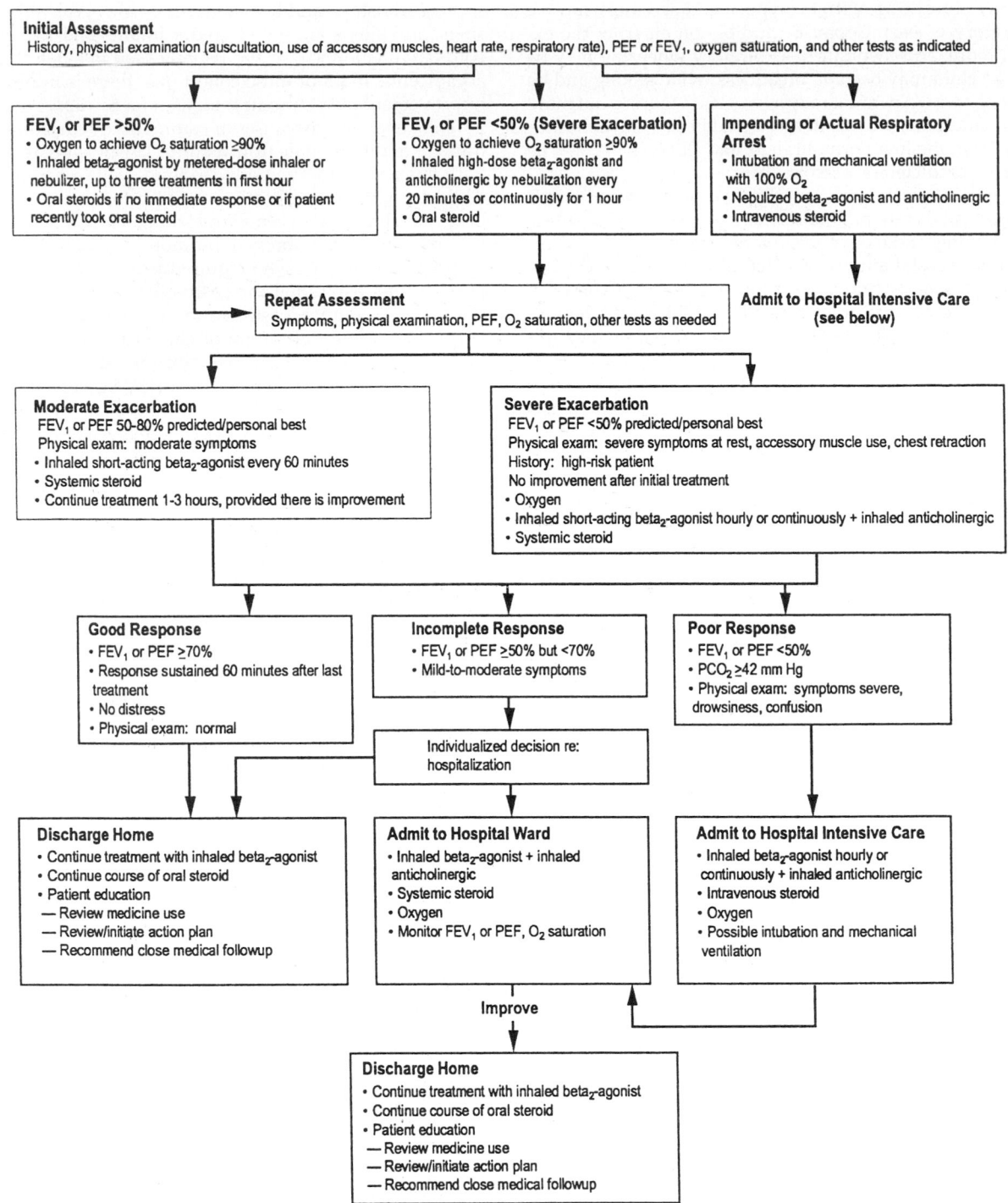

Initial Assessment
History, physical examination (auscultation, use of accessory muscles, heart rate, respiratory rate), PEF or FEV_1, oxygen saturation, and other tests as indicated

FEV_1 or PEF >50%
• Oxygen to achieve O_2 saturation ≥90%
• Inhaled beta$_2$-agonist by metered-dose inhaler or nebulizer, up to three treatments in first hour
• Oral steroids if no immediate response or if patient recently took oral steroid

FEV_1 or PEF <50% (Severe Exacerbation)
• Oxygen to achieve O_2 saturation ≥90%
• Inhaled high-dose beta$_2$-agonist and anticholinergic by nebulization every 20 minutes or continuously for 1 hour
• Oral steroid

Impending or Actual Respiratory Arrest
• Intubation and mechanical ventilation with 100% O_2
• Nebulized beta$_2$-agonist and anticholinergic
• Intravenous steroid

Repeat Assessment
Symptoms, physical examination, PEF, O_2 saturation, other tests as needed

Admit to Hospital Intensive Care (see below)

Moderate Exacerbation
FEV_1 or PEF 50-80% predicted/personal best
Physical exam: moderate symptoms
• Inhaled short-acting beta$_2$-agonist every 60 minutes
• Systemic steroid
• Continue treatment 1-3 hours, provided there is improvement

Severe Exacerbation
FEV_1 or PEF <50% predicted/personal best
Physical exam: severe symptoms at rest, accessory muscle use, chest retraction
History: high-risk patient
No improvement after initial treatment
• Oxygen
• Inhaled short-acting beta$_2$-agonist hourly or continuously + inhaled anticholinergic
• Systemic steroid

Good Response
• FEV_1 or PEF ≥70%
• Response sustained 60 minutes after last treatment
• No distress
• Physical exam: normal

Incomplete Response
• FEV_1 or PEF ≥50% but <70%
• Mild-to-moderate symptoms

Poor Response
• FEV_1 or PEF <50%
• PCO_2 ≥42 mm Hg
• Physical exam: symptoms severe, drowsiness, confusion

Individualized decision re: hospitalization

Discharge Home
• Continue treatment with inhaled beta$_2$-agonist
• Continue course of oral steroid
• Patient education
— Review medicine use
— Review/initiate action plan
— Recommend close medical followup

Admit to Hospital Ward
• Inhaled beta$_2$-agonist + inhaled anticholinergic
• Systemic steroid
• Oxygen
• Monitor FEV_1 or PEF, O_2 saturation

Admit to Hospital Intensive Care
• Inhaled beta$_2$-agonist hourly or continuously + inhaled anticholinergic
• Intravenous steroid
• Oxygen
• Possible intubation and mechanical ventilation

Improve

Discharge Home
• Continue treatment with inhaled beta$_2$-agonist
• Continue course of oral steroid
• Patient education
— Review medicine use
— Review/initiate action plan
— Recommend close medical followup

Figure 237.1.   NHLBI ED/Hospital Care management algorithm. (Modified from National Heart, Lung, and Blood Insititute, National Institutes of Health. *Expert panel report 2: guidelines for the diagnosis and management of asthma.* NIH Publication No. 97-4051, Bethesda, MD, 1997:112.)

pneumothorax or pneumomediastinum. Care should be taken not to "over read" the x-ray. Hilar prominence and patchy atelectasis are common findings and sometimes misinterpreted as pneumonic infiltrates. Inspiratory–expiratory (or left and right lateral decubitus in infants and toddlers) chest views showing unilateral hyperinflation are useful in evaluation for possible inhaled foreign bodies. Portable chest films are appropriate for any child who has a worsening of symptoms in the ED or is in impending respiratory failure. Children with chronic reoccurring exacerbations may benefit from radiographic determination for the presence of sinusitis (plain sinus films or limited sinus CT). An untreated or undertreated sinusitis may be the cause of recur-

rences. Upper airway radiographs should be obtained if middle airway pathology is suspected.

The use of pulse oximetry and noninvasive end-tidal CO_2 monitors has diminished the need for arterial and capillary blood gases. Blood gases are indicated for patients who have persistent hypoxia on greater than 40% O_2, elevated end-tidal CO_2 trends, or impending respiratory failure. Routine complete blood counts or electrolyte determinations generally do not provide useful information in uncomplicated asthma attacks. A serum level should be obtained for all patients taking theophylline.

Clinical asthma scores (CAS) are an additional method of monitoring the child's progress in the ED. Many CAS have been developed over the years and are variations and improvements of the Wood-Downes-Lecks respiratory failure score (33). An ED can develop and validate a simple scoring system based on the current National Heart, Lung, and Blood Institute (NHLBI) guidelines.

EMERGENCY DEPARTMENT MANAGEMENT

Beta-Agonists

Inhaled, intermediate-acting beta-agonists (albuterol, levalbuterol (R-albuterol), bitolterol, pirbuterol) are the mainstay of acute asthma therapy (18). The inhaled medications are preferred because they have been shown to be more effective and have fewer side effects than their oral or parenteral counterparts (1,15,22). Children respond better to aggressive high-dose albuterol therapy than do adults. There is a significant relationship between albuterol dosing and improvement in pulmonary function (19). Higher and more frequent administration also leads to greater bronchodilatation (29).

The initial dosage of albuterol or bitolterol is 0.15 mg/kg (2.5 mg minimum) by oxygen-powered nebulizer. This dose may be repeated at 20-minute intervals during the first hour, as indicated by the patient's response. Subsequent doses at 0.15 to 0.3 mg/kg (10 mg maximum) may be given every 1 to 4 hours, depending on the child's response. Children with moderate-to-severe exacerbations may benefit from continuously nebulized albuterol (20). The dosage is 0.5 mg/kg/h (7.5-mg minimum) or the equivalent of three intermittent treatments over 1 hour. This may be repeated in severe attacks or impending respiratory failure. The levalbuterol dose is one-half that of albuterol (0.075 mg/kg, 1.25-mg minimum).

A metered-dose inhaler (MDI) with spacer has been shown to be equivalent to nebulized albuterol in mild-to-moderate exacerbations (12). Four to eight puffs (each puff taken at 30- to 60-second intervals) of albuterol, pirbuterol, or biosterol are taken every 20 minutes, as needed, in the first hour. The dose may then be repeated every 1 to 4 hours, as needed, while the patient is in the ED. Though part of the NLHBI Expert Panel recommendations, bitolterol (both nebulized and MDI) and pirbuterol have not been studied in acute pediatric asthma and are considered not as potent as albuterol on a milligram per milligram basis.

Subcutaneous injections of epinephrine or terbutaline have no advantage over the inhaled beta-agonists. Their use should be limited to those patients with very poor air exchange. The dose for terbutaline (1 mg/mL) and epinephrine (1:1000 solution) is the same: 0.01 mL/kg (0.1 mL minimum, 0.3 mL maximum). This may be repeated at 15- to 20-minute intervals to a maximum of three doses.

There is no intravenous beta-agonist approved in the United States. The injectable preparation of terbutaline has been used for children with impending respiratory failure (8). A loading dose of 10 µg/kg is given over 10 minutes, followed by a maintenance infusion of 0.4 µg/kg/min. The dose is titrated in increments of 0.2 µg/kg/min until desired respiratory effects are achieved or unacceptable tachycardia occurs. The usual effective dose is 3 to 6 µg/kg/min. The most common side effects of beta-agonists, tremors and tachycardia, are dose related.

Ipratropium

Ipratropium bromide is a quaternary ammonium derivative of atropine. This greatly diminishes its systemic absorption and side effects. By itself, ipratropium has a relatively long onset but a prolonged duration of action when compared with the beta-agonists. Its anticholinergic activity does provide an additional mechanism of bronchodilation. When given with albuterol, there appears to be greater improvement in pulmonary function than when the same medications are given individually (23). This appears to be especially true for children with moderate-to-severe attacks (28). Also, because cough is more a large-airway (rich in cholinergic innervation) function, this medication may be of benefit when there is a significant cough component.

The dose for ipratropium is 0.25 mg for infants and 0.5 mg for older children and adolescents. It may be repeated at 20-minute intervals during the first hour and is mixed in the same nebulizer with the albuterol. Repeated doses are given every 2 to 4 hours. Add 0.5 to 1.0 mg to any continuous albuterol treatment.

Corticosteroids

Systemic corticosteroids are important in controlling LAR. They also decrease the relapse rate during the first week after an asthma exacerbation. Oral and parenteral forms appear equally effective. The onset of antiinflammatory activity is approximately 4 to 8 hours (27); however, corticosteroids appear to upregulate the beta-receptors in about 1 hour (5). Some recent studies have shown benefit to using inhaled steroids acutely as well.

Oral prednisone, prednisolone, or methylprednisolone, 1 to 2 mg/kg (60 mg maximum), should be given within the first hour of ED arrival to children with moderate-to-severe attacks. If the child is unable to tolerate oral medications, then 1 to 2 mg/kg (120 mg maximum) of methylprednisolone intravenously, or 0.15 to 0.6 mg/kg (30 mg maximum) of dexamethasone intramuscularly, may be given. There may be no benefit in using corticosteroids in children with EAR. The oral and intravenous doses may be repeated every 6 hours, up to 48 hours. Because of its prolonged half-life, the higher dose of intramuscular dexamethasone will provide 2 to 3 days of systemic corticosteroid coverage.

Oxygen

Any child with significant respiratory distress will benefit from oxygen, even with a normal SaO2. Low-flow oxygen (1 to 2 L/m) by nasal cannula is usually sufficient. Warm, humidified oxygen is preferable because dry oxygen can irritate the respiratory tree. High-flow oxygen should be administered via a nonrebreather mask whenever the child is hypoxic.

Alternative Therapies for Refractory Asthma

Treatment of acute refractory asthma, either an exacerbation not responding to standard therapy or impending respiratory failure continues to be limited. Medications such as ketamine, magnesium and heliox as well as modalities such as BiPAP have been investigated. The use of these and other medications and therapies are controversial and still subject to more detailed study.

Ketamine is a dissociative anesthetic that improves pulmonary compliance and decreases airway resistance in moderate to severe bronchospasm (26). Its mechanism of action is unclear but is thought to result from a combination of drug-induced increases in circulating catecholamines, direct smooth muscle relaxation, and inhibition of vagal outflow (32). Children but not adults tend to tolerate doses needed to obtain bronchodilation (9,11). Ketamine at a loading dose of 1 mg/kg (over 15 minutes) with a maintenance drip of 0.5–0.75 mg/kg/h have shown some promise in decreasing the severity of a severe attack and need for intubation (21). Side effects including emergence reactions or hypertension can be treated with a benzodiazapine and/or discontinuance of the drip.

Magnesium appears to be a smooth muscle relaxant (31). While its role as a primary drug in acute asthma has come into question (25), studies have shown benefits in children with

Take These Long-Term-Control Medicines Each Day (include an anti-inflammatory)

GREEN ZONE: Doing Well

- No cough, wheeze, chest tightness, or shortness of breath during the day or night
- Can do usual activities

And, if a peak flow meter is used,
Peak flow: more than _____
(80% or more of my best peak flow)

My best peak flow is: _____

Before exercise ☐ _____ ☐ 2 or ☐ 4 puffs 5 to 60 minutes before exercise

FIRST ⬆

YELLOW ZONE: Asthma Is Getting Worse

- Cough, wheeze, chest tightness, or shortness of breath, or
- Waking at night due to asthma, or
- Can do some, but not all, usual activities

-Or-

Peak flow: _____ to _____
(50% - 80% of my best peak flow)

Add: Quick-Relief Medicine – and keep taking your GREEN ZONE medicine

☐ _____ ☐ 2 or ☐ 4 puffs, every 20 minutes for up to 1 hour
(short-acting beta₂-agonist)   ☐ Nebulizer, once

SECOND ⬆ If your symptoms (and peak flow, if used) *return to GREEN ZONE after 1 hour of above treatment:*

☐ Take the quick-relief medicine every 4 hours for 1 to 2 days.
☐ Double the dose of your inhaled steroid for _____ (7-10) days.

-Or-

If your symptoms (and peak flow, if used) *do not return to GREEN ZONE after 1 hour of above treatment:*

☐ Take: _____ ☐ 2 or ☐ 4 puffs or ☐ Nebulizer
(short-acting beta₂-agonist)

☐ Add: _____ _____ mg. per day For _____ (3-10) days
(oral steroid)

☐ Call the doctor ☐ before/ ☐ within _____ hours after taking the oral steroid.

RED ZONE: Medical Alert!

- Very short of breath, or
- Quick-relief medicines have not helped, or
- Cannot do usual activities, or
- Symptoms are same or get worse after 24 hours in Yellow Zone

-Or-

Peak flow: less than _____
(50% of my best peak flow)

Take this medicine:

☐ _____ ☐ 4 or ☐ 6 puffs or ☐ Nebulizer
(short-acting beta₂-agonist)

☐ _____ _____ mg.
(oral steroid)

Then call your doctor NOW.   Go to the hospital or call for an ambulance if:
- You are still in the red zone after 15 minutes AND
- You have not reached your doctor.

DANGER SIGNS

- Trouble walking and talking due to shortness of breath
- Lips or fingernails are blue

⬆ ■ Take ☐ 4 or ☐ 6 puffs of your quick-relief medicine *AND*
■ Go to the hospital or call for an ambulance (_____) *NOW!*

Figure 237.2.   NHLBI ED/Hospital Care asthma action plan form. (Modified from National Heart, Lung, and Blood Institute, National Institutes of Health, *Practical guide for the diagnosis and management of asthma.* NIH Publication No. 97-4053, Bethesda, MD, 1997:45.)

severe exacerbations (4). A dose of 25 to 40 mg/kg of magnesium sulfate (2 grams. maximum) given over 20 minutes may be useful for children not responding to conventional therapy.

The use of a helium-oxygen mixture (heliox) remains very controversial. Studies have shown that heliox may improve the deposition of bronchodilator particles in the lungs (10), but positive clinical outcomes have been elusive (24). One study in children showed a reduction in pulsus paradoxus and aversion of respiratory failure with an 80/20 mixture (13). Heliox may best work when given to severe asthmatics within the first hour of ED care primarily as the driver for bronchodilator delivery. It should be discontinued if there is no positive clinical response or after 8 hours of administration, whichever comes first.

BiPAP has been shown to be of benefit in children with moderate hypoxia as an alternative to intubation (7). Theophylline is no longer considered first-line therapy for an acute asthma attack.

Antibiotics

There is no benefit to the routine use of antibiotics in the management of an acute asthma attack. They should be used when findings are consistent with pneumonia or other clinical bacterial infection. Therapy is directed to the most likely organism (see Chapter 261, "Pneumonia").

CRITICAL INTERVENTIONS

- Asthma is a diagnosis of exclusion in the first year of life and uncommon during the second year. Don't fall into the trap of treating this group of patients without considering other reasons for the respiratory symptoms (foreign body, anatomic variants, bronchiolitis)
- Asthma is an inflammatory disease. Viral infections are an important trigger. There is no need to routinely use antibiotics unless there is clearly a bacterial focus of infection
- Corticosteroids are like any other medication with appropriate and inappropriate uses. Not every child who comes to the ED with an asthma attack needs corticosteroids
- Use the diagnosis of "asthma if the child has findings consistent with asthma. The diagnosis "reactive airway disease" will code to "asthma" and bronchitis is generally not considered a pediatric entity. If the child has not been diagnosed with asthma, then use symptom- and complaint-based terminology (e.g., wheezing, shortness of breath, respiratory distress)

DISPOSITION

Patient disposition depends on the severity of the attack, response to treatment, and contributing risk factors. It is important that the patient be reassessed after initial therapy and observed for an appropriate period of time for relapse while in the ED.

A child who has had a mild attack, required no more than one or two albuterol treatments, and whose PEFR or FEV1 was not less than 70% may be sent home after a short (30-minute) observation period. All other patients should be observed for at least 1 hour for signs of relapse. Patients with an incomplete or poor response to therapy should be considered for admission. The decision to watch a patient in an observation unit or an inpatient ward is dependent on local policy and capabilities. Children presenting in impending or actual respiratory failure or who have deteriorated in the ED should be admitted to a pediatric intensive care unit.

Discharged children should be sent home with inhaled beta-agonists (albuterol, levalbuterol, pirbuterol, biosterol) if they do not already have the medication. Normal oxygen saturation and a respiratory assessment should be documented at time of discharge. An MDI and appropriate spacer (with or without a mask)

can be used in children as young as 1 month of age. Older children and adolescents can use an MDI with autoactuator or dry powder inhaler otherwise all patients should have a spacer for their MDI. The initial MDI dose is two to six puffs (each separated by 1 minute) every 6 to 8 hours for the first 24 to 48 hours following ED treatment. For patients with a home nebulizer, the dose is 2.5 to 5 mg of albuterol (1.25–2.5 mg of levalbuterol) per treatment. Additional medication may be used every 3 to 4 hours, as needed for rescue therapy. A good rule of thumb is to use this intensive course of beta-agonist for as long as the patient is taking corticosteroids (up to 5 days).

Children respond well to short courses ("bursts") of corticosteroids and generally do not need to be "weaned" from the systemic steroid effects. The dose of prednisone, prednisolone, or methylprednisolone is 1 to 2 mg/kg (60 mg maximum) in one or two divided doses. The length of treatment is a 3- to 7-day course, depending on patient's severity and rapidity of response. Use a tapering dose if the child has taken systemic corticosteroids in the previous 30 to 60 days, has had three bursts in the past 6 months, or four bursts in the past 12 months. The taper should be over 7 to 14 days. Because of the potential risk of disseminated disease and death, the risks of using systemic (not inhaled) steroids in children with active varicella must be carefully weighed against the benefits. Use of appropriate antivirals should be considered. In some cases, it is appropriate to start preventative therapy with inhaled corticosteroids on discharge from the ED.

Children should be sent home with an asthma plan that details what treatment the patient received and how they should manage continuing problems at home. Children 6 years old and older should be sent home with a PEFR meter. The PEFR is done two to four times a day, and the results used to trigger part of the action plan (Fig. 237.2).

All children who have an ED visit for asthma exacerbation should be referred back to their primary care physician or specialist for follow up. At a minimum, the parent should make phone contact within 24 hours of discharge to advise the physician of the child's progress.

COMMON PITFALLS

✔ Failure to provide early, aggressive treatment can lead to unnecessarily prolonged ED care or hospitalization. Children tolerate relatively higher, more frequent doses of inhaled bronchodilator then adults

✔ Do not assume that all children who wheeze have asthma, the conditions are not synonymous. Be alert to other possible etiologies such as foreign body aspiration or laryngotracheobronchitis

✔ Do not assume just because a child is not wheezing there is no asthma attack. Asthma can present as cough (cough variant asthma), chest pain, shortness of breath, and fatigue with exertion

✔ Failure to educate parents and children about potential triggers and how to avoid them. Smoking is a significant environmental trigger and is potentially harmful to the child, even if the parent "smokes outside"

✔ Failure to send the patient home with a written action plan. It can provide guidance and help avoid an unnecessary ED visit

References

1. Ben-Ziv Z, Lam C, Hoffman J, et al. An evaluation of the initial treatment of acute asthma. *Pediatrics* 1982;70:348–353.
2. Bloom B, Cohen RA, Vickerie JL, Wondimu EA. Summary health statistics for U.S. children: National Health Interview Survey, 2001. National Center for Health Statistics. *Vital Health Stat* 2003;216:2003.
3. Bradding P, Freezer NJ, Sheffer AL, et al. Asthma. In: Frank MM, Austen KF, Claman HN, et al, eds. *Samter's immunologic diseases*, 5th ed. Boston: Little, Brown and Company, 1995:1293–1327.

4. Ciarallo L, Brousseau D, Reinert S. Higher-dose intravenous magnesium therapy for children with moderate to severe acute asthma. *Arch Pediatr Adolesc Med* 2000;154:979–983.
5. Ellul-Micallef R, French FF. Effect of intravenous prednisolone in patients with diminished adrenergic responsiveness. *Lancet* 1975;2:1269–1271.
6. Ferrer A, Roca J, Wagner PD, et al. Airway obstruction and ventilation-perfusion relationships in acute severe asthma. *Am Rev Respir Dis* 1993; 147:579–584.
7. Fortenberry JD, Del Toro J, Jefferson LS, et al. Management of pediatric acute hypoxemic respiratory insufficiency with bilevel positive pressure (BiPAP) nasal mask ventilation. *Chest* 1995;108:1059–1064.
8. Fuglsang G, Pederson S, Borgstrom L. Dose-response relationships of intravenously administered terbutaline in children with asthma. *J Pediatr* 1989; 114:315–320.
9. Green SM, Johnson NE. Ketamine sedation for pediatric procedures: part 2, review and implications. *Ann Emerg Med* 1990;19:1033–1046.
10. Hess DR, Acosta FI, Ritz RH, et al. The effect of heliox on nebulizer function using a beta-agonist bronchodilator. *Chest* 1999;115:184–189.
11. Howton JC, Rose J, Duffy S, Zoltanski, Levitt MA. Randomized, double-blind, placebo-controlled trial of intravenous ketamine in acute asthma. *Ann Emerg Med* 1996;27:170–175.
12. Kerem E, Levison H, Schuh S, et al. Efficacy of albuterol administered by nebulizer versus spacer device in children with acute asthma. *J Pediatr* 1993;123:313–317.
13. Kudukis TM, Manthous CA, Schmidt GA, et al. Inhaled helium-oxygen revisited: effect of inhaled helium-oxygen during the treatment of status asthmaticus in children. *J Pediatr* 1997;30:217–224.
14. Lagerstrand L, Bylin G, Hedenstierna G, et al. Relationships among gas exchange, spirometry and symptoms in asthma. *Eur J Med* 1992;1:145–152.
15. Louridas G, Kakoura M, Galanis N, et al. Bronchodilatory effect of inhaled versus oral salbutamol in bronchial asthma. *Respiration* 1983;44:439–443.
16. National Center for Health Statistics. Asthma Prevalence, Health Care Use and Mortality, 2000–2001. http://www.cdc.gov/nchs/products/pubs/pubd/hestats/asthma/asthma.htm.
17. National Heart, Lung, and Blood Institute, National Institutes of Health. Expert panel report 2: guidelines for the diagnosis and management of asthma. NIH Publication No. 97-4051, Bethesda, MD, 1997.
18. National Heart, Lung, and Blood Institute, National Institutes of Health. Expert Panel Report: Guidelines for the Diagnosis and Management of Asthma—Update on Selected Topics 2002. NIH Publication No. 02-5074, Bethesda, MD, 2003.
19. Nelson HS, Spector SL, Whitsett TL, et al. The bronchodilator response to inhalation of increasing doses of aerosolized albuterol. *J Allergy Clin Immunol* 1983;72:371–375.
20. Papo MC, Frank J, Thompson AE. A prospective, randomized study of continuous versus intermittent nebulized albuterol for severe status asthmaticus in children. *Crit Care Med* 1993;21:1479–1486.
21. Petrillo TM, Fortenberry JD, Linzer JF, Simon HK. Emergency department use of ketamine in pediatric status asthmaticus. *Journal of Asthma* 2001;38:657–664.
22. Pierce RJ, Payne CR, Williams SJ, et al. Comparison of intravenous and inhaled terbutaline in the treatment of asthma. *Chest* 1981;79:506–511.
23. Reisman J, Galdes-Sebalt M, Kazim F, et al. Frequent administration by inhalation of salbutamol and ipratropium bromide in the initial management of severe acute asthma in children. *J Allergy Clin Immunol* 1988;81:16–20.
24. Rodrigo GJ. Inhaled therapy for acute adult asthma. *Curr Opin Allerg & Clin Immunol* 2003;3:169–175.
25. Rowe BH, Bretzlaff JA, Bourdon C, Bota GW, Camargo CA Jr. Intravenous magnesium sulfate treatment for acute asthma in the emergency department: a systematic review of the literature. *Ann Emerg Med* 2000;36:181–190.
26. Sarma VJ. Use of ketamine in acute severe asthma. *Acta Anaestesiol Scand* 1992;36:106–107.
27. Scarfone RJ, Fuchs SM, Nager AL, Shane SA. Controlled trial of oral prednisone in the emergency department treatment of children with acute asthma. *Pediatrics* 1993;92:513–518.
28. Schuh S, Johnson DW, Callahan S, et al. Efficacy of frequent nebulized ipratropium bromide added to frequent high-dose albuterol therapy in severe childhood asthma. *J Pediatr* 1995;126:639–645.
29. Schuh S, Parkin P, Rajan A, et al. High- versus low-dose, frequently administered, nebulized albuterol in children with severe, acute asthma. *Pediatrics* 1989;83:513–518.
30. Skoner DS. Asthma. In: Fireman P, Slavin RG, eds. Atlas of allergies. Philadelphia: JB Lippincott Co, 1991:5.1–5.23.
31. Spivey WH, Skobeloff EM, Levin RM. Effect of magnesium chloride on rabbit bronchial smooth muscle. *Ann Emerg Med* 1990;19:1107–1112.
32. Strube PJ, Hallam PL. Ketamine by continuous infusion in status asthmaticus. *Anaesthesia* 1986;40:1017–1119.
33. Wood DW, Downes JJ, Lecks MS. A clinical scoring system for the diagnosis of respiratory failure. *Am J Dis Child* 1972;123:227–228.

Selected Readings

Chipps BE, Chipps DR, A review of the role of inhaled corticosteroids in the treatment of acute asthma. *Clin Pediatr* 2001;40:185–189.
Edmonds ML, Camargo CM, Pollack CV Jr. Rowe BH. The effectiveness of inhaled corticosteroids in the emergency department: a meta-analysis. *Ann Emerg Med* 2002;40:145–154.

CHAPTER 238

Bronchiolitis

Kathy Shaw

Each epidemic season, the emergency physician is faced with evaluating and treating infants and young children with bronchiolitis and determining their disposition. Unlike children with reactive airway disease, their lower respiratory tract symptoms are caused by inflammation of the bronchiolar epithelium by an acute infection. The resultant necrosis of epithelium and plugging of the 75- to 300-μm airways by cellular debris may result in air trapping or atelectasis distal to the obstruction (2). This lower airway pathology may manifest as tachypnea, wheezing, rales, increased work of breathing, and/or hypoxemia.

Respiratory syncytial virus (RSV) is probably the most important respiratory pathogen among young children and may cause serious morbidity and mortality. Annually, it is the leading cause of infant hospitalization (19). More than 50% of infants will acquire RSV infection during the first epidemic that they experience, and 40% will progress from upper to lower respiratory tract illness. Three percent of all children <1 year of age will require hospital admission for bronchiolitis (29). The peak incidence of lower airway disease occurs in infants 2 to 5 months of age (11,12,19,29). Two major subtypes of the virus, strains A and B, circulate concomitantly, with one predominating during a given season. Subtype A is more commonly associated with more severe disease (21). Children in the first few months of life, those with a history of prematurity (≤35 weeks gestational age), children with congenital heart disease (CHD), especially uncorrected pulmonary hypertension, and those who are immunosuppressed or have chronic lung disease are most at risk for severe disease and death (14,15,20,28). Many high risk groups of infants require immunoprophylaxis with palivizumab or RSV immunoglobulin monthly during the RSV season for their first year or two of life (3). Although RSV is the most common pathogen, other viruses, such as parainfluenza, influenza, adenovirus, and rhinoviruses, may cause bronchiolitis (11,17).

CLINICAL PRESENTATION

The presentation of the infant or young child with bronchiolitis ranges from the smiling, interactive child with mild tachypnea and end-expiratory wheezing to the child who presents with severe respiratory distress or failure. Typically, there is a several-day history of upper respiratory tract symptoms of coryza and congestion before the onset of lower respiratory tract symptoms. The parent may have noted that the child started with a cold and now is not as active, is breathing faster, and has difficulty feeding. Although most have tachypnea, cough, wheezing, and increased work of breathing, the young infant may present with lethargy or irritability, apnea or tachypnea, and have few lower respiratory findings (13,28). Fever is often present early in the course of illness, but may be absent or low grade at the time that lower respiratory tract symptoms manifest. Once lower respiratory tract involvement occurs, it usually progresses and peaks within 3 to 5 days. However, resolution of symptoms, including cough, wheezing, and some degree of hypoxemia, may take days to weeks.

DIFFERENTIAL DIAGNOSIS

Because bronchiolitis is so endemic during the winter months, the emergency physician must remember to consider other causes of acute onset of lower respiratory tract distress in infants. Congestive heart failure in the infant is often thought initially to be bronchiolitis during epidemics, as the infant may present with a history of poor feeding and tachypnea, rales, and wheezing on examination. Congenital lesions compromising the airway, such as vascular rings, slings, or teratomas, may appear to have acute onset. Aspiration from gastroesophageal reflux or tracheoesophageal "H-type" fistulas should cause symptoms around feeding. Congenital infections such as chlamydia pneumonia are prevalent throughout the year. Community-acquired bacterial pneumonia should also be considered in children of all ages. Foreign-body aspiration should also be suspected in young children.

In older infants and children, it is often difficult to distinguish bronchiolitis from asthma or reactive airway disease. The first episode of wheezing with upper respiratory tract symptoms in the young child should be considered bronchiolitis. Children with prior episodes of wheezing responsive to bronchodilator therapy, atopy, and a family history of asthma may have reactive airway disease. Repeat episodes of bronchiolitis are not uncommon, even with RSV. Additionally, infants who have had RSV bronchiolitis may be more prone to have repeated episodes of wheezing (30). Whether the viral infection causes pulmonary damage or immunologic changes or the child who develops lower respiratory tract illness has a predisposition to reactive airway disease is the subject of debate.

EMERGENCY DEPARTMENT EVALUATION

No single fact or finding during emergency department (ED) evaluation is sensitive enough to predict which child will develop severe disease (23,28). A combination of historic, physical examination, and laboratory measures must be considered when determining risk for significant morbidity and mortality (Table 238.1). In taking a history, it is important to determine the gestational age at birth and whether there were any perinatal complications, such as chronic lung disease (CLD) (formerly called bronchopulmonary dysplasia). Underlying diseases or anomalies such as congenital heart disease, cystic fibrosis, or immunodeficiencies may put the infant at increased risk. It is also important to determine whether the child is in the first few days of illness, in which the disease will continue to progress, or beyond the 3- to 5-day peak of illness. Social issues, such as the mother's ability to care for a sick infant or return if the disease progresses, are also important to evaluate.

The overall appearance of the child is a sensitive indicator of disease severity. The child's respiratory rate, accessory muscle use for breathing, and air exchange are important to evaluate at presentation and after therapeutic trials. The infant's oxygen saturation, as determined by pulse oximetry, is the single most objective predictor of more severe disease and should be measured on all infants and children presenting to the ED with bronchiolitis (28). Assessment of the child's hydration status by physical examination (moistness of mucous membranes, capillary refill at the fingertip, presence or absence of tears) should also be done, as many have a history of poor oral intake.

Radiographs are indicated in infants or young children with their first episode of wheezing or in children with high fever or severe disease. The majority of radiographs will show some degree of hyperaeration (flattening of the diaphragms on lateral view or increased radiolucency with small heart size on the

TABLE 238.1.   Risk Factors Associated with More Severe Disease (7,12–14,21,23,28)

Moderate Risk	High Risk
HISTORIC FACTORS	
Prematurity 34–36 wks Age < 3 mo First 3 days of illness	Prematurity < 34 wks History of cyanosis or apnea Underlying condition Pulmonary disease Congenital heart disease (pulmonary hypertension, cyanosis) Immunodeficiency
PHYSICAL EXAMINATION FINDINGS	
General appearance: ill, not toxic Moderate accessory muscle use Respiratory rate: 60–70/min	General appearance: toxic Marked accessory muscle use Respiratory rate: > 70/min
TESTING	
Oxygen saturation: 95%–96% Atelectasis on chest radiograph RSV infection, subtype A	Oxygen saturation: < 95%

anterior view) or peribronchial thickening. Atelectasis or infiltrates occur in less than 10% of children presenting for outpatient evaluation (28). Most areas of opacity represent atelectasis, but pneumonia cannot be excluded as a cause.

Evaluation of fever in infants less than 2 or 3 months of age should be performed as per usual practice. For infants over 2 months of age with classic bronchiolitis, fever is unlikely to indicate serious bacterial illness and more likely to indicate early viral illness, pneumonia, or otitis media (4,18). Therefore, routine culture of the blood or urine may be unnecessary. Complete blood cell counts are rarely useful. Microbiologic testing to determine viral etiology is indicated only for those with or at great risk for severe disease (CLD, CHD) or for cohorting purposes for hospital admission.

EMERGENCY DEPARTMENT MANAGEMENT

Children with moderate or severe respiratory distress should be allowed to assume a position of comfort, and 100% oxygen should be delivered. Suctioning of copious nasopharyngeal secretions may relieve some distress caused by airway obstruction. A trial of bronchodilators and/or racemic epinephrine should be delivered. Intubation is required for the child with severe respiratory distress not responding to these measures.

Table 238.2 lists current treatment options for children with bronchiolitis. However, there is no strong or convincing evidence of effectiveness for any treatment for bronchiolitis (1). Most children presenting to the ED with bronchiolitis have mild or moderate severity of illness. Those with mild disease require supportive therapy only. The use and effectiveness of bronchodilators such as nebulized albuterol is controversial (1,6,9,16). A trial of two nebulized treatments of albuterol (0.15 mg/kg per dose) or salbutamol plus ipratroprium bromide given 20 to 30 minutes apart is usually given to infants and young children with moderate-to-severe symptoms. Assessment for objective improvement in oxygen saturation, lowering of the respiratory rate, or improved aeration indicates response. For those without improvement, there is no need or benefit to continue further

TABLE 238.2. Bronchiolitis Treatment Options

Therapy	Indications	Effectiveness
Supportive (suctioning, mist)	Mainstay of therapy for mild or moderate bronchiolitis; suctioning prior to feeding helps infant feed better.	Moistening of inspired air may be as beneficial as β_2 agonists in treatment (1,6)
Oxygen	Oxygen saturation: < 94%	Protects against hypoxia
Antibiotics	Not indicated empirically or for treatment of bronchiolitis	Use only for specific diagnosed bacterial infections, such as otitis media or pneumonia (4,8)
Bronchodilators (β_2 agonists, anticholinergics)	Poor air exchange Respiratory rate > 50/min Marked work of breathing Oxygen saturation: < 97%	Undetermined: probably helps some children; for infants <6 mo, less than half respond (1,5,19,26)
Racemic epinephrine	No response to trial of β_2 agonists and persistent severe symptoms requiring admission	Multiple clinical trials have shown effectiveness for moderate-to-severe disease (22,26)
Cromolyn sodium	To prevent or limit future episodes of wheezing	Undetermined; not indicated at this time (25)
Ribavirin	Not useful in the ED	Probably not effective, even for those hospitalized for severe disease (1,24)
Immunotherapy (RSV-IGIV or palivizumab)	For prevention only	Proven to be beneficial in reducing hospitalization and severity of disease for infants who were premature, have chronic lung disease, or congenital heart disease with cyanosis or pulmonary hypertension (palivizumab only) (3)
Steroids (oral or inhaled)	Moderate to severe episode with prior history of wheezing, but has shown some potential (1,5,10,27)	Not proven or recommended for first episode

treatments (6). Nebulized racemic epinephrine has been more effective than β_2 agonists in several clinical trials and may be tried for those who do not respond and will require hospitalization (22,26). Cromolyn sodium and immunoglobulin therapies are used for preventive care and have no role in the ED (3,25). Ribavirin, an expensive antiviral agent, is probably not effective and also has no role in the ED (3,24). Steroids, either inhaled or oral, may have some potential (1,5,10,27), but require more rigorous study with adequate sized trials. At present, steroids should be reserved for children who have reactive airway disease. Antibiotics are indicated only when a specific bacterial infection has been diagnosed or for neonates with fever (8). Many children with bronchiolitis have or develop bacterial ear infections (4).

CRITICAL INTERVENTIONS

- Use pulse oximetry to identify children with hypoxemia. This is the most specific and objective indicator of more severe disease. Cyanosis that is detectable on physical examination does not occur until the oxygen saturation is less than 85%!
- Suction the infant to help improve airway obstruction
- Keep the infant in the position of comfort as long as possible and avoid agitating the patient

DISPOSITION

Most infants and children with bronchiolitis do not require admission. Clearly, those in respiratory distress or with hypoxia require intervention and admission. Among those with mild or moderate disease, no single factor can predict necessity for admission (1,23,28). Children at high risk for developing more severe disease (see Table 238.1) should be considered for admission or close outpatient observation. Infants less than 2 months of age are at risk for apnea and admission should be strongly considered. Any child who is early in the course of the illness or has moderate severity of illness, not requiring admission, should have follow up arranged in 24 hours.

Children with underlying medical conditions should have their subspecialist physicians consulted about treatment and indications for admission. For example, the pediatric cardiologist can determine whether the child with congenital heart disease has significant uncorrected pathology putting them at higher risk. If the diagnosis of bronchiolitis is not clear, a pediatrician may offer further help with the differential diagnosis or work up.

Children with respiratory failure requiring intubation should be transferred to a facility with a pediatric intensive care unit. Children with underlying medical conditions or at high risk for severe disease or mortality should also be transferred to a facility with pediatric subspecialists and a pediatric intensive care unit.

COMMON PITFALLS

✔ Failure to identify that the child is in the first few days of illness and may get progressively worse. These children who appear to have mild illness may progress over the next hours or days and require close outpatient follow up. The caregiver should be given specific instructions of what to look for and when to return
✔ Failure to identify that the child has an underlying condition or history of prematurity. It is important to ask and document whether the child has risk factors that put him or her at high risk for morbidity and mortality
✔ Persistence in using bronchodilators despite no evidence of response. Less than half of infants with bronchiolitis will respond to bronchodilators. If they have mild disease, they

should be sent home with symptomatic care instructions and follow up arrangements

✔ Use of routine laboratory tests or radiographs. Evaluation of infants and young children with bronchiolitis should be tailored to the individual patient

References

1. Agency for Healthcare Research and Quality. Management of bronchiolitis in infants and children. U.S. Department of Health and Human Services, Evidence Report/Technology Assessment, 2003;69:1–5.
2. Aherne W, Bird T, Court SD, et al. Pathological changes in virus infections of the lower respiratory tract in children. *J Clin Pathol* 1970;23:7.
3. American Academy of Pediatrics, Committee on Infectious Diseases and Committee on Fetus and Newborn. Revised indications for the use of palivizumab and respiratory syncytial virus immune globulin intravenous for the prevention of respiratory syncytial virus infections. *Pediatrics* 2003;112:1447–1452.
4. Andrade MA, Hoberman A, Glustein J, et al. Acute otitis media in children with bronchiolitis. *Pediatrics* 1998;101:617.
5. Csonka P, Kaila M, Laippala P, et al. Oral prednisolone in the acute management of children age 6 to 35 months with viral respiratory infection-induced lower airway disease: a randomized, placebo-controlled trial. *J Pediatr* 2003;143:725–730.
6. Dobson JV, Stephens-Groff SM, McMahon SR, et al. The use of albuterol in hospitalized infants with bronchiolitis. *Pediatrics* 1998;101:361.
7. Eriksson M, Forsgren M, Sjoberg S, et al. Respiratory syncytial virus infection in young hospitalized children: identification of risk patients and prevention of nosocomial spread by rapid diagnosis. *Acta Paediatr Scand* 1983;72:47.
8. Field CMB, Connolly JH, Murtagh G, et al. Antibiotic treatment of epidemic bronchiolitis—a double-blind trial. *BMJ* 1966;1:83.
9. Flores R, Horwitz RI. Efficacy of β2-agonists in bronchiolitis: a reappraisal and meta-analysis. *Pediatrics* 1997;100:233–239.
10. Garisson MM, Christakis DA, Harvey E, Cummings P, Davis RL. Systemic corticosteroids in infant bronchiolitis: a meta-analysis. *Pediatrics* 2000;105:e44.
11. Glezen WP, Denny FW. Epidemiology of acute lower respiratory disease in children. *N Engl J Med* 1973;288:498.
12. Green M, Brayer A, Schenkman KA, et al. Duration of hospitalization in previously well infants with RSV infection. *Pediatr Infect Dis J* 1989;8:601.
13. Hall CB, Kopelman AE, Douglas RG, et al. Neonatal respiratory syncytial virus infection. *N Engl J Med* 1979;300:393.
14. Hall CB, Powell KR, MacDonald WE, et al. RSV infection in children with compromised immune function. *N Engl J Med* 1986;315:77.
15. Horn SD, Smout RJ. Effect of prematurity on respiratory syncytial virus hospital resource use and outcomes. *J Pediatr* 2003;143:S133–S141.
16. Kellner JD, Ohlsson A, Gadomski AM, Wang EEL. Efficacy of bronchodilator therapy in bronchiolitis. A meta-analysis. *Arch Pediatr Adolesc Med* 1996;150:1166.
17. Kim HW, Arrobio JO, Brandt CD, et al. Epidemiology of respiratory syncytial virus in Washington, DC. Importance in different respiratory tract disease syndromes and temporal distribution. *Am J Epidemiol* 1973;98:216.
18. Kuppermann N, Bank DE, Walton EA, et al. Risks for bacteremia and UTI in young febrile children with bronchiolitis. *Arch Pediatr Adolesc Med* 1997;151:1207.
19. Leader S, Kohlhase K. Recent trends in severe respiratory syncytial virus (RSV) among U.S. infants, 1997 to 2000. *J Pediatr* 2003;143:S127–S132.
20. MacDonald NE, Hall CB, Suffin SC, et al. Respiratory syncytial viral infection in infants with congenital heart disease. *N Engl J Med* 1982;307:397.
21. McConnochie KM, Hall CB, Walsh EE, et al. Variation in severity of respiratory syncytial virus with subtype. *J Pediatr* 1990;117:52.
22. Menon K, Sutcliffe T, Klassen TP. A randomized trial comparing the efficacy of epinephrine with salbutamol in the treatment of acute bronchiolitis. *J Pediatr* 1995;126:1004.
23. Opavsky MA, Stephens D, Wang EEL. Testing models predicting severity of respiratory syncytial virus infection on the PICNIC RSV database. *Arch Pediatr Adolesc Med* 1995;149:1217.
24. Randolph AG, Wang EEL. Ribavirin for respiratory syncytial virus lower respiratory tract infection. *Arch Pediatr Adolesc Med* 1996;150:942.
25. Reijonen T, Korppi M, Kuikka L, et al. Anti-inflammatory therapy reduces wheezing after bronchiolitis. *Arch Pediatr Adolesc Med* 1996;150:512.
26. Reijonen T, Korppi M, Pitkakangas S, et al. The clinical efficacy of nebulized racemic epinephrine and albuterol in acute bronchiolitis. *Arch Pediatr Adolesc Med* 1995;149:686.
27. Schuh S, Coates AL, Binnie R, et al. Efficacy of oral dexamethasone in outpatients with acute bronchiolitis. *J Pediatr* 2002;140:27–32.
28. Shaw KN, Bell LM, Sherman NH. Outpatient assessment of infants with bronchiolitis. *Am J Dis Child* 1991;145:151.
29. Shay DK, Holman RC, Newman RD, et al. Bronchiolitis-associated hospitalizations among US children, 1980–1996. *JAMA* 1999;282:1440–1446.
30. Sigurs N, Bjarnason R, Sigurbergsson F, et al. Asthma and immunoglobulin E antibodies after respiratory syncytial virus bronchiolitis: a prospective cohort study with matched controls. *Pediatrics* 1995;95:500.

CHAPTER 239
Cellulitis

Christopher S. Kennedy and Mary E. Moffatt

Cellulitis is a common, acute, rapidly spreading, nonsuppurative inflammation of the epidermis, dermis, and subcutaneous fat that is usually caused by bacterial infection. The age of the child, the history, and the location of the infection all serve as important determinants of the most likely causative bacterial organisms. Cellulitis may occur by local tissue invasion following minor, traumatic skin breaks and bite wounds, or by hematogenous dissemination of a pathogenic organism. It may also be the presenting sign of disease states such as septic arthritis, osteomyelitis, sinusitis, or pyomyositis (5). Neonatal omphalitis, infection of the umbilical stump and surrounding tissues, and neonatal mastoiditis are unique to the newborn period.

In most instances, children with cellulitis recover uneventfully. However, the recent resurgence of invasive group A β-hemolytic *Streptococcus* (GABHS) infection, characterized by bacteremia, toxic shock, and necrotizing fasciitis emphasizes both the potential for serious complications, and the need for accurate diagnosis and appropriate management of pediatric cellulitis. In addition, one must be cognizant of the increasing incidence of nonnosocomial, community-acquired methicillin-resistant *Staphylococcus aureus* (MRSA) skin infections in otherwise healthy children (12).

EPIDEMIOLOGY

During the course of normal play, children routinely incur minor injuries with breaks of the skin. Any injury or skin opening that disrupts the protective barrier of the skin can serve as a portal of entry for pathogens, most commonly GABHS or *Staphylococcus aureus*.

Community-acquired MRSA superficial skin and subcutaneous tissue infections are now being described in several areas of the United States (12). Reasons for this increased frequency are not yet clear, but evidence suggests that some MRSA strains originating within the community are likely as a result of increased selection pressure from antimicrobials. There are many recognized risk factors for MRSA infection in children, one of which is visitation to a hospital emergency room within the previous 6 months.

Puncture wounds by a contaminated object such as a nail penetrating a shoe may predispose to infections with pathogens such as *Pseudomonas* species. Likewise, animal and human bites result in an increased likelihood that *Pasteurella multocida* and *Eikenella corrodens* infections, respectively are the causative organisms.

Omphalitis, infection of the umbilicus, with accompanying erythema of the abdomen, is a diagnosis unique to the newborn period usually occurring in the first few weeks of life. Neonatal mastitis is infection of the breast tissue in prepubertal children, only occurring in the first 2 to 5 weeks of life (7). Female infants are affected twice as often as male infants. Hormonally induced hypertrophy of the glandular tissue facilitates bacterial entry and abscess formation. The most common pathogen is *S. aureus*, however occasionally gram-negative enterics are involved.

The epidemiology of childhood facial cellulitis has changed dramatically since the introduction of the *Haemophilus influenzae* type B vaccine (HbCV) in 1985. *Haemophilus influenzae* type B (HIB) had been the cause of more than 50% of cases of facial cellulitis, but, in the post vaccine era, it has become a rare agent (16). In fact, there has been about a 90% decrease in the incidence of HIB disease (13). Any child who has received the second dose of HbCV more than 7 days prior is unlikely to have HIB disease. Now common organisms include *Streptococcus pneumoniae*, GABHS, and *S. aureus*. As more children become completely immunized with the conjugated pneumococcal vaccine one would anticipate a decrease in cellulitis due to *S. pneumoniae* vaccine serotypes, as well as nonvaccine serotypes. Facial and periorbital infections caused by HIB and *S. pneumoniae* are usually spread by the hematogenous route, and hence can be isolated by blood culture. Primary dental infection may also lead to bacterial seeding of adjacent facial soft tissues, by a variety of aerobic and anaerobic bacteria such as *Bacteroides*, *Prevotella*, *Fusobacterium*, and *Peptostreptococcus* (3).

Important preexisting conditions that may predispose to cellulitis include other traumatic injuries particularly crush injuries, preexisting vascular or lymphatic compromise, chronic cutaneous conditions such as eczema, and immunocompromised states. More recently, there has been an increase in case reports of necrotizing fasciitis due to GABHS infection occurring in conjunction with varicella infection (6).

CLINICAL PRESENTATION

The most reliable way to diagnose cellulitis is to recognize the characteristic clinical features: localized erythema, warmth, edema, and pain. Demarcation between involved and adjacent normal skin may be indistinct. Most often cellulitis involves the extremities, with the leg affected three times as often as the arm (5). There may be associated lymphangitis, appearing as red streaks radiating from the margin of the lesion, and also enlargement and tenderness of regional lymph nodes, particularly with streptococcal infection. The white blood cell (WBC) count is usually normal. In 10% to 20% of cases cellulitis is associated with fever and other systemic symptoms such as chills, malaise, myalgias and even emesis. When fever is present, a concomitant bacteremia should be presumed and leukocytosis expected.

Distinct clinical entities include erysipelas, buccal cellulitis, Ludwig angina, periorbital cellulitis, orbital cellulitis, omphalitis, neonatal mastitis, extremity cellulitis, and necrotizing fasciitis.

Erysipelas is a more superficial cellulitis which predominately affects only the upper dermis. It is characterized by tender, rapidly enlarging, erythematous, indurated plaques with sharply demarcated borders and extensive lymphatic involvement. Patients tend to be young children, and most cases involve the legs and feet (2,4). Symptoms also include toxic appearance with fever and chills (1). Facial erysipelas may occur after streptococcus upper respiratory tract infection (2). GABHS is the most common cause of erysipelas, but other streptococcal groups include group B, C and G. Rarely the infection is due to staphylococci.

Buccal cellulitis presents as a tender swelling of the cheek, which is mildly erythematous in color. It occurs in children aged 6 to 24 months most frequently, and usually there is no history of trauma. Hematogenous seeding of oropharyngeal or middle ear bacteria is suggested as the pathogenesis (13). Previously HIB was by far the most common etiologic agent, with rare cases caused by *S. Aureus* and *S. pneumoniae*. Overall the incidence of buccal cellulitis has decreased, attributable to routine immunization with HbCV (1). Of note, in infants less than 3 months of age, facial cellulitis may be the only presenting sign of GBS bacteremia.

Ludwig angina is a cellulitis of the submandibular and sublingual space. Patients present with rapidly progressive, tense, and painful induration of the neck, along with drooling, dysphonia, high fever, and leukocytosis. It is important to recognize the potential for airway compromise in such patients (1). Predisposing factors include poor dental hygiene, dental extractions, and impacted foreign bodies in the oral cavity. Infection is polymicrobial involving typical oral flora.

Periorbital or preseptal cellulitis, a form of facial cellulitis, is usually seen in children less than 5 years old (13). Infection is contained anterior to the orbital septum by fibrous tissue arising from the periosteum of the skull and continuing onto the eyelids (8). It presents with sudden onset of tender swelling of the eyelid and periorbital area, erythema, normal eye movements and visual acuity, and absence of proptosis. It is usually unilateral in nature (1). More than half of cases are secondary to local extension form a nearby facial wound, infected with either GABHS or *S. aureus*. In general, children are nontoxic in appearance, but bacteremia and leukocytosis may be associated, particularly with infection by *H. influenzae* or *S. pneumoniae*. Periorbital cellulitis secondary to hematogenous seeding is generally more fulminant with rapid progression and systemic toxicity.

By contrast, orbital cellulitis, which is less common than periorbital cellulitis, is post septal in origin with involvement of the orbit itself (8). It presents with painful swelling and erythema of the eye, and the child usually appears toxic. In addition, extraocular movements are painful and may be restricted, visual acuity is reduced, and proptosis may be present. Eyelid edema may be so marked that complete examination of the eye is precluded and orbital computerized tomography (CT) scan is required for diagnosis. The most common cause of orbital cellulitis is by direct extension from an adjacent, ipsilateral sinusitis; thus infection tends to occur in older children. Ethmoid sinusitis is most commonly the source of infection as the ethmoid sinus is separated from the orbit by the rather thin bony structure called the lamina papricia (8).

Omphalitis presents in the newborn as purulent, foul-smelling discharge from the umbilical stump, and erythema of the abdominal wall. However, both of these clinical findings may occur without infection, thus making the diagnosis challenging at times. Suggestive findings include anterior abdominal erythema and circumferential erythema of the umbilicus (7). The cord stump may serve as a portal of bacterial entry for *S. aureus*, GABHS, group B *Streptococci* (GBS), and gram-negative enterics. Infection is clearly indicated when induration and erythema of the anterior abdominal wall are present. Associated fever, temperature instability, lethargy, and irritability may be seen late as signs of sepsis. Laboratory studies such as WBC count will be normal in early localized infections. Fortunately this entity is rare in developed countries because of advances in local cord care practices.

Tender enlargement of the breast bud with warmth, erythema, and purulent discharge from the nipple are the clinical signs of neonatal mastitis (7). Hormonally induced hypertrophy of the breast tissue does not present as erythema or tenderness, and is associated with a milky white discharge only. About one quarter of infants will present with fever and appear ill. The WBC is normal and blood culture negative in most cases as the infection is well localized.

Cellulitis of the extremities is usually preceded by direct trauma to the skin. Wound-related cellulitis is the most common cause, especially in older children and adolescents (1). The area is red, warm, and tender, and systemic signs of fever, chills, and leukocytosis are usually present. Lymphangitic streaking and regional lymphadenopathy are more common than in cases of erysipelas. Children with cellulitis of an extremity may exhibit limitation of movement of the affected limb or refusal to walk due to pain from the infection. Infections tend to be polymycrobial. Offending agents are age related with GBS in infants less than 3 months old, *S. pneumoniae* and HIB in patients aged 6 to 24 months still undergoing primary vaccination series with these agents, and *S. aureus* and GABHS most likely in children older than 24 months (5). In the case of GBS, *S. pneumoniae*, and HIB high fevers, WBC above 15,000, and bacteremia are to be expected.

Necrotizing fasciitis is an uncommon infection of the subcutaneous and fascial tissues, and is a medical/surgical emergency (4). Traumatic skin lesions such as varicella zoster infection, eczema or burns may predispose the child (11). There are two forms: the flesh-eating bacterial syndrome caused by GABHS or rarely streptococci groups B, C, and G, and a polymicrobial infection with both anaerobic and aerobic bacteria. GABHS is the most commonly reported associated organism (1). Necrotizing fasciitis may initially present as a cellulitis, but subsequently there is rapid development of dusky, painful, indurated plaques progressing to purpura, blistering, and finally necrosis. There may be crepitance in the tissues. The infection spreads rapidly along fascial planes between subcutaneous tissue and superficial muscle fascia (11). Initial diagnosis may be difficult due to only modest skin changes, but extreme pain very much out of proportion to the cutaneous findings should raise a high degree of clinical suspicion. The child presents with fever and marked fussiness, and may refuse to bear weight or move the affected limb. Severe systemic toxicity with tachycardia, hypotension, and even multiorgan system failure are common with fulminant disease. The child may be lethargic, disoriented, and in profound hypotensive septic shock. There is a high associated mortality rate especially when necrotizing fasciitis occurs in conjunction with streptococcal toxic shock syndrome (STSS) (11).

Streptococcal toxic shock syndrome may be associated with NF in as many as 50% of cases (2).

The syndrome presents with a generalized, fine, scarlatiniform rash and hyperemia of the conjunctivae or other mucous membranes, along with fever, tachycardia out of proportion to the fever, hypotension, and possibly altered mental status. Gastrointestinal disruption including vomiting and diarrhea, renal and hepatic dysfunction, and respiratory distress are often present. Production of pyrogenic exotoxin A by certain strains of GABHS, along with certain M protein types, is associated with STSS cases (2,11).

A similar toxin-mediated syndrome affecting young children is Staphylococcal Scalded Skin Syndrome (SSSS). Skin manifestations are age related and include the spectrum of bullous impetigo, scarlatiniform eruption, and widespread exfoliation (4). Generalized SSSS, called Ritter disease, usually occurs in patients less than 5 years of age. Older children tend to have more localized infection. After a purulent conjunctivitis, upper respiratory infection, or localized superficial skin infection a generalized orange-red macular erythema resembling sunburn erupts along with fever and irritability. During the subsequent scarlatiniform phase, the skin becomes extremely tender. Within 1 to 3 days, the skin becomes wrinkled and large flaccid bullae develop in flexural areas or around orifices. During this phase Nikolsky sign is present as the epidermis pulls away from the dermis with gentle traction leaving raw, weeping and denuded skin underneath (1). As the skin dries, large flakes are formed leading to widespread desquamation with complete recovery in 10 to 14 days. Dehydration and superinfection may occur due to loss of the protective skin barrier with extensive exfoliation.

DIFFERENTIAL DIAGNOSIS

Any tender, erythematous swelling of the skin and subcutaneous soft tissue may resemble cellulitis. Trauma, insect bites or stings, localized urticarial eruptions, lymphadenitis, swelling overlying a sprain or fracture, or a joint with septic arthritis may all be mistaken for cellulitis. Mosquito bites may induce significant lymphedema surrounding the bite site, which develops over hours. The bites are usually described as pruritic rather than painful. Bee stings and spider bites may also cause significant lymphedema, warmth, and even tenderness, and therefore may be more difficult to distinguish from cellulitis.

"Popsicle panniculitis" can mimic facial cellulitis. Thought to be a cold-induced histamine response from eating ice water, typically the skin involvement begins at the labial crease and spreads outward with a warm mildly tender cheek. Insect bites and stings, panniculitis, and orthopaedic injuries all tend to lack systemic signs such as fever or ill appearance.

Localized, specific soft-tissue infections, such as folliculitis (infection of a hair follicle), furuncles and carbuncles (deep follicular abscess, either solitary or multiseptate and loculated), impetigo (vesiculopustular lesions), ecthyma (impetigo involving the dermis), and others, should be differentiated from cellulitis by their characteristic clinical appearances.

Extremity cellulitis, as mentioned earlier, may cause limitation of movement of the affected limb; for that reason, it may be difficult to distinguish from deeper tissue infection such as osteomyelitis or septic arthritis.

EMERGENCY DEPARTMENT EVALUATION

In most cases cellulitis is a clinical diagnosis. Blood culture and WBC count should be reserved for patients presenting with fever or other signs of associated systemic toxicity, and for those who are immunocompromised. Clinical judgment and age of the patient should be used to decide to perform a lumbar puncture for cerebral spinal fluid (CSF) culture, particularly in the context of cellulitis affecting the head and neck region (13,16). Lumbar puncture should be performed on infants with facial cellulitis who have not received 2 doses of HbCV, and on all children suspected of having meningeal signs (13).

Certain clinical features are specific enough to make a reasonable etiologic assumption. Erysipelas, with its characteristic rapidly advancing, raised, sharply demarcated margin, is usually caused by GABHS. A bluish or violaceous discoloration of the area involved by cellulitis suggests infection by *H. influenzae* or *S. pneumoniae*. Cellulitis in the perineal or buccal area, or cellulitis in an area involving devitalized or necrotic tissue, should raise concern for polymicrobial anaerobic organisms. Cellulitis caused by pet bites is often associated with *Pasteurella multocida*; whereas human bite infections often contain *Eikenella corodens*. Cellulitis due to water-contaminated wounds is usually caused by *Mycobacterium marinum* or *Aeromonas* and *Vibrio* species (10). Systemic symptoms in any patients with cellulitis should suggest the possibility of concurrent bacteremia. Presence of immunocompromised states should alert the clinician to the possibility of atypical infectious agents, and consideration should be given to the presence of neutropenia masking the actual depth and extent of infection.

Invasive GABHS should be considered in children with varicella who have fever on or beyond the fourth day of the exanthem (6). With the reemergence of suppurative GABHS infections, it is important to distinguish early streptococcal necrotizing fasciitis from cellulitis, as necrotizing fasciitis usually requires prompt and aggressive surgical debridement. Necrotizing fasciitis is characterized by diffuse swelling with extreme tenderness at the local site, followed by bulla formation with rapid purplish discoloration and extension into deeper fascial planes.

Although the combination of clinical features and epidemiologic considerations may suggest the etiology of cellulitis, definitive bacteriologic diagnosis requires isolation of the causative organism. In the past, because of the high prevalence of bacteremia with *H. influenzae*, blood cultures were routinely done in children with cellulitis. In the post HbCV era, however, the association of bacteremia with cellulitis in children has been dramatically reduced, and recent studies indicate that the practice of obtaining blood cultures routinely may not be cost effective (15,16). Of note, positive blood cultures are most commonly associated with younger age, active varicella, and deeper tissue infections such as osteomyelitis or septic arthritis.

Needle aspiration of the cutaneous inflammatory lesion, accompanied by prompt gram stain and culture, is a rapid and specific tool to establish a bacteriologic diagnosis. Aspiration is performed by inserting a 22-gauge needle attached to a 1-cc syringe into the advancing edge of the cellulitis. If no material is aspirated, 0.1 ml of normal saline may be injected in to the area, followed by immediate aspiration. The yield of needle aspiration, however, is modest; a positive aspiration rate in different studies varies from 5% to 50% (14).

If underlying deeper trauma or infection is suspected, appropriate imaging should be done. In any patient with periorbital cellulitis, it is particularly important to rule out orbital cellulitis, a much more severe infection that may need surgical intervention. In a patient with orbital cellulitis, unlike periorbital cellulitis, the ocular movements are restricted and painful, and proptosis is usually present. If thorough examination of the eye is not possible secondary to eyelid edema, CT scan of the orbits is useful to delineate the diagnosis. CT scan is also helpful when periorbital inflammation progresses despite optimal antibiotic treatment (9).

Complications of cellulitis should be considered in the evaluation process and may result from direct extension, seeding of an overlying joint space, or hematogenous spread with metastatic effects. Septicemia can develop in patients with severe, suboptimally treated infections. Meningitis, endocarditis, or other serious complications, although rare, may also develop. Immunocompromised patients and younger patients are at the greatest risk for such complications. Patients with cellulitis involving the midface are susceptible to cavernous sinus thrombosis, based on the venous drainage patterns of this area.

EMERGENCY DEPARTMENT MANAGEMENT

Antibiotic therapy, in most cases, except in the mildest form of cellulitis, is warranted. Given the low yield of microbiologic work up, in most situations antibiotic therapy is empiric but should be based on sound clinical judgment. Hospital admission and parenteral antibiotic therapy should be strongly considered in any febrile child. Application of warm compresses to the affected area, elevation of the affected limb, and bed rest are often useful adjunctive therapies. Analgesics may be needed for control of pain, and antipyretics may be required for relief of fever.

All neonates with suspected omphalitis or mastitis should be promptly admitted and started on parenteral antibiotics to cover empirically against *S. aureus*, GABHS, GBS, and gram-negative enterics. In infants less than 3 months of age, facial or extremity cellulitis can be caused by GBS and thus should be treated with parenteral penicillin along with an aminoglycoside, and hospital admission. Between 3 months and 3 years of age, *H. influenzae* or *S. pneumoniae* may be causative organisms, and third-generation cephalosporins (ceftriaxone or cefotaxime) should be administered, plus clindamycin. Vancomycin is required if meningitis is suspected.

Any patient with orbital cellulitis also requires hospital admission. Multispecialty involvement by Otorhinolaryngology, Infectious Diseases, and Ophthalmology is warranted as surgical drainage of abscess formation and/or the sinuses may be required. Patients should be started on intravenous antibiotics to empirically cover against respiratory pathogens; ampicillin with a beta-lactamase inhibitor, such as clavulanic acid, is a reasonable choice (8). Intravenous antibiotics for a total of 7 days, followed by a course of oral antibiotics for 14 days are recommended.

Patients suspected of a severe infection with GABHS, such as NF, should receive parenteral clindamycin in addition to penicillin, intravenous immunoglobulin, a surgical consultation for emergent debridement of necrotic tissue, and close cardiorespiratory monitoring for signs of shock. Liberal fluid resuscitation and management of multi-organ system failure may be required. Radiologic investigations to detect edema infiltrating fascial planes must not delay surgical intervention (2,11).

Immunocompromised patients often develop cellulitis caused by atypical organisms: *Corynebacterium*, *Pseudomonas*, atypical mycobacteria, and even fungi. A microbiologic diagnosis should be vigorously pursued in these patients, particularly when initial empirical therapy fails to show any response.

Beyond age 3 years, patients with well-localized cellulitis and without fever or systemic toxicity may be treated on an outpatient basis with an antistaphylococcal and anti-GABHS oral antibiotic, including penicillinase-resistant penicillins such as amoxicillin clavulanate, or first generation cephalosporins such as cephalexin. Ceftriaxone, with its once-a-day intramuscular dosing, may also be used in appropriate patients. Consider the addition of anaerobic coverage, by an antibiotic such as clindamycin, for cases of bite wounds, infections related to oral flora, or those wounds involving devitalized tissue. The guardians of children who are treated as outpatients require instruction about the necessity of close follow up within 48 hours, and about which signs and symptoms necessitate prompt return to the ED.

Resistance patterns of community-acquired MRSA in children without identified risk factors have been limited to methicillin and erythromycin. Fortunately susceptibility to both clindamycin and trimethoprim-sulfamethaxazole has been retained and either of these agents can be used enterally to treat mild to moderate cellulitis due to such MRSA. In the case of severe infection with community-acquired MRSA, empiric, parenteral vancomycin is recommended (12).

A patient who is diagnosed with cellulitis who shows severe systemic toxicity or does not improve within 48 hours of oral antibiotic therapy, should receive high-dose intravenous broad-spectrum antibiotic therapy covering both streptococci and staphylococci (semi-synthetic penicillins such as oxacillin or nafcillin, or first generation cephalosporin cefazolin).

Patients who respond promptly to parenteral antibiotics may be changed over to oral antibiotics, but, in most cases of cellulitis, total duration of therapy should be a full 10 days.

CRITICAL INTERVENTIONS

- Recognize that patients with necrotizing fasciitis present with pain out of proportion to the physical examination findings
- Patients with cellulitis who are treated on an outpatient basis should have followup within 48 hours
- Mastitis and omphalitis are serious forms of cellulitis in the neonatal period that mandate emergent evaluation and treatment

DISPOSITION

Most children with simple cellulitis can be started on oral antibiotics on an outpatient basis, with follow up arranged at 48-hour intervals. With the decreasing incidence of *H. influenzae* and *S. pneumoniae* cellulitis, and the availability of potent oral antibiotics, more and more patients with cellulitis can be safely managed as outpatients.

Admission should be strongly considered in all infants younger than 6 months old who have cellulitis. Any child who appears to be ill, has extensive lesions, or is immunosuppressed should also be admitted. Patients with facial cellulitis and a fever of more than 38.5°C, or patients with extremity cellulitis and a fever of more than (39°C, and a WBC count of more than 15,000/mL require intravenous antibiotic therapy. The recommendations for hospital admission are essentially based on the risk of bacteremia associated with cellulitis and the consequent need for intravenous antibiotics.

Patients with necrotizing fasciitis in most cases will require surgical debridement in the operating room. Children with severe systemic symptoms, like shock, need aggressive treatment and admission to a pediatric intensive care unit. Wound management in cases of extensive Staphylococcal scalded skin syndrome may be best accomplished in a pediatric burn unit.

COMMON PITFALLS

✔ Failure to recognize that community-acquired MRSA infection in children without identified risk factors is increasing in prevalence nationwide
✔ Failure to include orbital cellulitis in the differential diagnosis of periorbital cellulitis
✔ Failure to recognize that in immunocompromised patients with cellulitis, atypical and opportunistic infections are common, and microbiologic diagnosis should be actively pursued

Acknowledgment

Thanks to the previous edition's chapter author Madhumita Sinha.

References

1. Bhumbra NA, McCullough SG. Skin and subcutaneous infections. *Prim Care* 2003;30:1–24.
2. Bisno A, Stevens DL. Streptococcal infections of skin and soft tissues. *N Engl J Med* 1996;334:240–245.
3. Brook I. Anaerobic infections in children. *Adv Pediatr* 2000;47:395–437.
4. Callahan EF, Adal KA, Tomecki KJ. Cutaneous (non-HIV) infections. *Dermatol Clin* 2000;18:497–508.
5. Danik SB, Schwartz RA, Oleske JM. Cellulitis. *Cutis* 1999;64:157–164.
6. Doctor A, Harper MB, Fleisher GR. Group A β-hemolytic streptococcal bacteremia: historical overview, changing incidence, and recent association with varicella. *Pediatrics* 1995;96:428–433.
7. Fleisher GR. Infectious disease emergencies. In: Fleisher GR, Ludwig S, eds. *Textbook of Pediatric Emergency Medicine.* 4th ed. Philadelphia: Lippincott Williams & Wilkins, 2000;763–768.
8. Givner LB. Periorbital versus orbital cellulitis. *Pediatr Infect Dis J* 2002;21:1157–1158.
9. Goldberg F, Berne AS, Oski FA. Differentiation of orbital cellulitis from preseptal cellulitis by computed tomography. *Pediatrics* 1978;62:1000–1005.
10. Gottlieb T, Atkins BL, Shaw DR. Soft tissue, bone and joint infections. *Med J Aust* 2002;176:609–615.
11. Jackson MA, Colombo J, Boldrey A. Streptococcal fasciitis with toxic shock syndrome in the pediatric patient. *Orthop Nurs* 2003;22:4–8.
12. Metry D, Katta R. New and emerging pediatric infections. *Dermatol Clin* 2003;21:269–276.
13. Powell KR. Orbital and periorbital cellulitis. *Pediatr Rev* 1995;16:163–167.
14. Sachs MK. Cutaneous cellulitis. *Arch Dermatol* 1991;127:493–496.
15. Sadow KB, Chamberlain JM. Blood cultures in the evaluation of cellulitis. *Pediatrics* 1998;101:E4.
16. Schwartz GR, Wright SW. Changing bacteriology of periorbital cellulitis. *Ann Emerg Med* 1996;28:617–620.

CHAPTER 240
Congenital Heart Disease, Congestive Heart Failure, and Other Cardiac Presentations

Ann M. Dietrich and Leslie Mihalov

Children may present to the emergency department with a variety of cardiac disorders or complications of cardiac disease. It is imperative that undiagnosed cardiac disease be recognized as early as possible to facilitate medical and surgical management of the disease process (11,13). Congenital heart disease occurs in nearly 1% of live-born infants. The emergency care required by a child with cardiac disease may be quite variable, and symptoms are usually based on the underlying etiology (congenital heart defects, arrhythmias, cardiomyopathies). This potentially broad range of presentations makes definitive diagnosis and treatment a complex topic (7). This chapter will divide cardiac lesions by presentation: cyanosis, poor perfusion/acidosis/shock (low cardiac output), cardiac dysrhythmias and congestive heart failure.

CYANOSIS

Cyanosis is a relatively infrequent complaint in pediatric patients. Cyanosis results from one of three mechanisms: (1) obstruction of blood flow to the pulmonary circulation, (2) return of the deoxygenated systemic blood back to the systemic circulation without going through the lungs resulting in severe oxygen desaturation or (3) inability of pulmonary venous blood return to the left atrium due to anomalous return of all pulmonary veins to a systemic venous structure. Most commonly, cyanosis is secondary to lung disease rather than heart disease. It is important to differentiate between peripheral cyanosis (discoloration of the extremities which is particularly common in a neonate or a cold child), and central cyanosis. Almost one-third of all infants with critical heart lesions present during the first week of life at the time of closure of the ductus arteriosus (24). A useful bedside test to determine the etiology of a child's cyanosis (respiratory vs cardiac) is a hyperoxia test. This test is conducted through use of arterial blood gases (ABGs) and 100% oxygen. With application of 100% oxygen an increase in $pO_2 > 220$ mm Hg suggests lung disease, a pO_2 of 100 to 220 mm requires an evaluation for congenital heart disease, a $pO_2 < 100$ mm suggests cyanotic congenital heart disease and a $pO_2 < 40$ to 50 mm would be likely due to transposition of the great arteries (TGA) with poor mixing (19). If an ABG is not available, the test can also be performed by measuring the oxygen saturation before and after application of 100% oxygen. The oxygen saturation should increase by at least 10% in the presence of a pulmonary process. The most common causes of cyanotic congenital heart disease are Tetralogy of Fallot, tricuspid atresia, TGA, truncus arteriosus, total anomalous pulmonary venous return and pulmonary atresia or stenosis.

Tetralogy of Fallot (TOF)

The four defects associated with this anomaly include ventricular septal defect, pulmonary stenosis, right ventricular hypertrophy and overriding aorta. Clinically these patients typically present within the first 12 weeks of life. The child may present with isolated cyanosis or older children may have clubbing, squatting and poor growth. These patients may also have a history of hypercyanotic ("TET") spells, which are acute, severe episodes of dyspnea and hypoxemia that may occur spontaneously or following prolonged crying. Occasionally, a child with TOF may present, in the newborn period, with acidosis due to low cardiac output as a result of closure of a ductus arteriosus. The chest radiograph may be particularly helpful in patients with Tetralogy of Fallot and reveal a heart with a "boot-shaped" appearance.

Transposition of the Great Arteries

Transposition of the great arteries is the second most common congenital cardiac abnormality (17). In a heart with the D-transposition of the great vessels the pulmonary and systemic systems are isolated, making a connection between the two systems (atrial or ventricular) critical for survival. Radiographically, transposition of the great arteries may present with cardiomegaly or a narrowed mediastinum with an "egg on a string" appearance.

Management focuses on stabilization, a prostaglandin E$_1$ infusion to improve oxygenation, and palliative or definitive surgery.

Tricuspid Atresia

This cardiac lesion is the third most common cause of cyanotic heart disease and has a mortality rate of 50% by 6 months of age without surgical intervention. Children with tricuspid atresia usually present within the first 4 weeks of life with cyanosis. If the atrial septal defect or patent foramen ovale is restrictive, an urgent balloon atrial septostomy or atrial septectomy may be required for survival.

Total Anomalous Pulmonary Venous Return

Total anomalous pulmonary venous return is a cyanotic congenital defect in which all the pulmonary veins drain to the right atrium, directly or by way of systemic veins. Since an interatrial communication is required for survival, restriction of the atrial connection will result in cyanosis and circulatory collapse. These patients may present in severe distress, with tachypnea, metabolic acidosis, low cardiac output, and central cyanosis.

The chest radiograph generally demonstrates a heart that is either normal or small in appearance, with pulmonary edema. Patients with supracardiac TAPVR may demonstrate a "snowman sign," due to the ascending vertical vein.

Treatment generally requires aggressive support including prostaglandin E$_1$ infusion (permits right ventricular blood to be shunted by way of the PDA to systemic circulation), inotropic support and immediate intervention, which may include balloon atrial septostomy, balloon dilation at the site of obstruction, or surgical repair or palliation.

Pulmonary Atresia or Stenosis

Pulmonary valve stenosis with an intact ventricular septum occurs in 8% to 10% of infants with congenital heart defects and is associated with a mortality rate as high as 42% without intervention (6). Neonates with severe pulmonary stenosis typically present from 1 to 4 weeks after delivery and have signs and symptoms of severe right heart failure (tachypnea, cyanosis) (5).

TABLE 240.1.   Etiology of Cyanosis Based on Radiographic Findings
NORMAL/LARGE HEART WITH DECREASED PVMS
Tetralogy of Fallot
Double-outlet right ventricle with pulmonary stenosis
Pulmonary atresia, severe pulmonary stenosis
Transposition of great arteries with VSD and PS
Tricuspid atresia
Ebstein anomaly of the tricuspid valve
SMALL HEART WITH PULMONARY EDEMA
Total anomalous pulmonary venous return with obstruction, often below the diaphragm to the portal system
LARGE HEART WITH INCREASED PVMS
Transposition of the great arteries
Total anomalous pulmonary venous return
Truncus arteriosus
Double-outlet right ventricle
Single ventricle
PVMs, pulmonary vascular markings; PS, pulmonary stenosis; VSD ventricular septal defect.

Therapy initially focuses on stabilization with prostaglandin E$_1$ therapy followed by balloon pulmonary valvulotomy.

Radiographic Findings

Table 240.1 lists radiographic findings in patients with cyanotic congenital heart disease.

ECG Findings

Electrocardiographically, these patients may have right ventricular hypertrophy (tetralogy of Fallot, double-outlet right ventricle, pulmonary stenosis, transposition of the great arteries, or Ebstein anomaly) or decreased right ventricular forces (tricuspid atresia and pulmonary atresia). This becomes more pronounced the older the infant is at presentation. If the QRS axis is negative with right atrial enlargement, then tricuspid atresia should be considered.

EMERGENCY DEPARTMENT MANAGEMENT

Any child who presents with cyanosis should be carefully evaluated and close attention should be paid to assessment and management of the ABCs. If the child is suspected of having a ductal-dependent lesion (usually a child presenting at less than 2 weeks of age), then a prostaglandin E$_1$ infusion should be initiated at a rate of 0.05 mcg/kg/min to 0.1 mcg/kg/min. Adverse effects associated with prostaglandin E$_1$ infusions include apnea (12%), fever, hypotension, and seizures. Intubation should be considered prior to initiation of the PGE$_1$ infusion, because of the frequent occurrence of apnea associated with use of this medication (23).

In patients with TOF and a hypercyanotic spell, the treatment of choice includes oxygen and sedation. When possible, the mother should be allowed to hold the child, and the patient adequately sedated with low-dose morphine (0.05 to 0.1 mg/kg intravenously or intramuscularly) or, in some cases, ketamine (1 mg/kg intravenously or 2 mg/kg intramuscularly). In addition, maneuvers such as "knee-to-chest" positioning and volume administration are performed to increase systemic vascular resistance. In refractory cases, alpha agonists (e.g., phenylephrine) should be considered to increase systemic vascular resistance and promote pulmonary blood flow by diminishing the right-to-left shunt.

POOR PERFUSION, ACIDOSIS AND SHOCK (LOW CARDIAC OUTPUT)

The severity of symptoms in patients with low cardiac output may vary depending on the cardiac lesion and degree of ductal closure. Patients may have tachypnea with or without distress, pallor or mottling of the extremities, peripheral cyanosis, diminished or asymmetric pulses and oliguria and/or acidosis (26). The differential diagnosis should include sepsis however, the distinguishing features of absent lower extremity pulses and blood pressures, heart murmur and S$_3$ gallop and enlarged heart on chest radiograph will help identify heart lesions (19).

The pathophysiology of low cardiac output in the pediatric cardiology patient generally falls into three categories: (1) left-sided obstructive lesions, (2) poor myocardial function, and (3) poor ventricular filling (Table 240.2).

Left-Sided Obstructive Lesions

The timing of presentation of a left-sided obstructive lesion is variable and is dependent on the degree of obstruction. The most common lesions that present in the emergency setting are critical aortic stenosis, critical coarctation of the aorta, hypoplastic left heart syndrome (HLHS), and interrupted aortic arch (IAA).

Critical Aortic Stenosis and Critical Coarctation of the Aorta

The patient with severe aortic stenosis may present in early infancy and have very little murmur due to the small orifice of a unicuspid aortic valve and associated diminished cardiac output. These patients may appear cyanotic due to right-to-left shunting across a patent ductus arteriosus (PDA), their main source of systemic blood flow. Alternatively, they may present obtunded with severe acidosis following spontaneous ductal closure. Infants with a critical coarctation, generally present at 2 weeks of age due to progressive ductal closure, while older children with less severe coarctations may present with hypertension. Unlike patients with aortic stenosis and HLHS, who present

---

TABLE 240.2. Etiology and Pathophysiology of Low Cardiac Output

LEFT-SIDED OBSTRUCTION

Aortic stenosis
Hypoplastic left heart
Coarctation of the aorta
Interrupted aortic arch

POOR MYOCARDIAL FUNCTION

Cardiomyopathy
Myocarditis
Glycogen storage diseases
Coronary artery anomaly

POOR VENTRICULAR FILLING

Congenital mitral stenosis
Tachyarrhythmias
Pulmonary venous obstruction

---

with diminished pulses throughout, patients with coarctation of the aorta and IAA have asymmetric upper and lower extremity pulses. Pulse oximetry may also be a valuable adjunct for patients with a severe aortic coarctation and a PDA. Simultaneous pulse oximetry readings in the right hand and a foot will show significantly lower oxygen saturation in the foot (23).

Both of these lesions lead to obstruction of left ventricular outflow and subsequent left atrial dilatation and pulmonary venous congestion. The systemic circulation is maintained through the ductus arteriosus which is the reason for circulatory collapse with ductal closure. The radiographic findings of patients with left-sided obstructive lesions vary. Infants with coarctation of the aorta who present in failure may have cardiac dilatation; however, older children may have a normal heart size with visible indentation at the coarctation site and evidence for collateral blood vessels, characterized by rib notching.

Hypoplastic Left Heart Syndrome

Infants with hypoplastic left heart syndrome (HLHS) have hypoplastic left-sided cardiac structures and hypertrophied right-sided structures. Left-to-right shunting typically occurs at the atrial level through a patent foramen ovale (27). Similar to patients with preductal coarctation of the aorta and critical aortic stenosis, systemic perfusion depends on a patent ductus arteriosus. The closure of the ductus results in rapid, progressive cardiogenic shock and circulatory collapse (27). However, infants with HLHS may, surprisingly, have normal radiographic findings.

ECG Findings

Electrocardiographic (ECG) findings vary considerably. In most of these lesions, the ECG may be normal. As the patient develops evidence of ventricular failure, evidence of left ventricular (LV) hypertrophy and lateral T-wave inversion may arise. Patients with coarctation often have evidence of right ventricular hypertrophy, characterized by a Q wave in the anterior precordial leads.

EMEGENCY DEPARTMENT MANAGEMENT

The initial management should focus on stabilization of the child's airway, breathing and circulation. Once a diagnosis of congenital heart disease is suspected, a call to the tertiary care center pediatric ED or pediatric cardiologist is appropriate. Because 100% oxygen accelerates ductal closure, in some congenital heart defects (e.g., HLHS), it is acceptable to decrease the F$_i$O$_2$ to 21% to increase pulmonary vascular resistance and promote systemic blood flow across the PDA (27). Controlled hypoventilation and positive end-expiratory pressure may also be utilized to augment systemic perfusion by increasing pulmonary vascular resistance (20). If there is concern regarding a *left-sided obstructive lesion*, initiation of prostaglandin E$_1$(PGE$_1$) at 0.05 mcg to 0.1 mcg/kg/min may keep the PDA open until the baby may be moved to a pediatric cardiologist. Remember to secure the airway prior to initiation of the prostaglandin drip (may accelerate apnea) and to have inotropic support available to maintain systemic blood flow. Sodium bicarbonate and sodium nitroprusside (to decrease systemic vascular resistance) may also be required. A prompt referral to a pediatric cardiologist or pediatric cardiovascular surgeon is indicated for evaluation and treatment. Treatment may include staged or definitive surgery or interventional cardiac catheterization. Balloon angioplasty of coarctation of the aorta has been shown to be highly effective (20). Aortic stenosis may also be managed by interventional catheterization. Patients with HLHS are dependent on heart transplantation or a palliative Norwood procedure.

POOR MYOCARDIAL FUNCTION

Clinical signs of diminished cardiac output may occur in patients with poor myocardial function due to a cardiomyopathy or myocarditis. A cardiomyopathy may occur as a result of ischemia due to a coronary anomaly, a glycogen storage disease, a previous viral infection, a muscular dystrophy, or an inherited or idiopathic myopathy. The degree of symptomatology is usually related to the degree of cardiac dysfunction. The patient with mild dysfunction may present with only mild cardiomegaly on a routine chest radiograph, while the patient with an end-stage cardiomyopathy may present in florid congestive heart failure requiring emergent resuscitation. Likewise, the child with acute myocarditis may present with severe cardiac dysfunction and an associated tachyarrhythmia (e.g., polymorphic ventricular tachycardia) or bradyarrhythmia (e.g., complete atrioventricular [AV] block).

Radiographic Findings

The classic radiographic findings in these patients include cardiomegaly and, frequently, pulmonary edema.

ECG Findings

Patients with a "dilated," poorly functioning hypertrophic cardiomyopathy may have evidence of increased voltages throughout the precordium, with evidence of ST-segment or T-wave changes. Children with glycogen storage diseases, such as Pompe disease, may have evidence of a short PR interval with very large precordial QRS voltages. Decreased amplitudes, manifested as a *low-voltage QRS* (less than 5 mm total in each frontal lead), suggest the presence of myocarditis with decreased contractility or restrictive disease. Patients with an anomalous left coronary arising from the pulmonary artery will have evidence of an LV infarct with an abnormal Q wave in leads aVL and I, as well as T-wave and ST-segment changes laterally (15).

EMERGENCY DEPARTMENT MANAGEMENT

If the etiology of the low cardiac output appears to be due to poor myocardial function, then the initial focus should be on maximizing oxygenation and improving cardiac output through inotropic support, including afterload reduction. One series showed a reduction in mortality in children with dilated cardiomyopathy treated with angiotensin converting enzyme inhibitors (21). ACE inhibitors also have been shown in some series to provide stabilization and clinical improvement (25). Beta-blockers have also been suggested to provide some clinical benefit in patients with dilated cardiomyopathy (26). Although not an ED therapy, one study has suggested that children who receive intravenous gamma globulin early in the course of viral myocarditis were more likely to achieve normal left ventricular function within the first year of presentation (8). These measures are used to reduce cardiac work in an attempt to improve cardiac output. The use of steroids in myocarditis is controversial.

POOR VENTRICULAR FILLING

Diminished cardiac output may occur in children with poor ventricular filling as a result of congenital or rheumatic mitral valve stenosis, pulmonary venous obstruction, and tachyarrhythmias. These children may not only present with evidence of poor systemic blood flow, but also, in the most severe cases, often have evidence of pulmonary edema and right heart failure, manifested by hepatomegaly and peripheral edema.

Radiographic Findings

Radiographically, these patients will have evidence of cardiac enlargement and pulmonary edema. Patients with mitral stenosis have the classic radiographic findings of left atrial enlargement, with pulmonary edema and dilation of the pulmonary vasculature. In patients with pulmonary venous obstruction, the left atrium is usually small, with pulmonary edema and right heart enlargement. In particular, the pulmonary blood vessels may be massively dilated due to chronic pulmonary hypertension. Patients with sustained tachyarrhythmias usually have cardiac enlargement as a result of LV failure and, as such, demonstrate LV enlargement on the chest radiograph.

ECG Findings

Patients with congenital mitral stenosis have electrocardiographic evidence of left atrial enlargement and LV voltages, while patients with tachyarrhythmias tend to have retrograde P waves.

EMERGENCY DEPARTMENT MANAGEMENT

In patients with poor ventricular filling as the etiology of poor cardiac output, oxygen administration and diuretics are usually indicated. If symptomatic, many patients may also require correction of a severe metabolic acidosis. If obstruction is significant, these patients can become severely ill in a short period of time. Although administration of PGE_1 may promote systemic blood flow via a patent ductus, prompt referral to a pediatric cardiovascular surgeon is required for surgical repair or palliation.

If the patient has a tachyarrhythmia, conversion either by adenosine (0.1 mg/kg per dose) or, if hemodynamically compromised, synchronized cardioversion (0.5 to 2.0 J/kg) is indicated (22). Calcium channel blockers in children, particularly in infants, are contraindicated. They are negative inotropes as well as peripheral vasodilators and, as such, can produce dramatic hemodynamic compromise and, in some cases, cardiac arrest.

CONGESTIVE HEART FAILURE

Congestive heart failure (CHF) is defined as the inability of the heart to pump enough blood to meet the metabolic demands of the body (14). Ninety percent of the cases of CHF in children occur before the end of the first year of life (29). Infants with congestive heart failure, typically present with tachypnea, tachycardia, and diaphoresis (2). Because the majority of work performed by infants and small children occurs during feeding, many of these children will also have feeding intolerance and failure to thrive. Toddlers and older children usually have tachycardia, tachypnea, fatigue, and exercise intolerance. In older children peripheral edema and venous distension may be apparent. Physical examination findings of CHF may include hepatomegaly, and a diastolic gallop. A chest radiograph may show cardiac enlargement with or without pulmonary edema.

Dividing the differential by age group facilitates ED management. CHF in the first day of life is usually secondary to cardiac muscle dysfunction from hypoxia, hypoglycemia, hypocalcemia, myocarditis or sepsis. During the first 6 weeks of life CHF is usually secondary to decompensation of a congenital heart lesion with ductal closure (HLHS, aortic stenosis, TAPVR and

TABLE 240.3. Etiology and Pathophysiology of Congestive Heart Failure[a]

PATHOPHYSIOLOGY

Increased pulmonary blood flow
Pulmonary interstitial edema
Volume overload (dilation)

CONGENITAL DEFECTS

Ventricular septal defects
Atrioventricular canal
Patent ductus arteriosus
Atrial septal defects
Aortopulmonary window
Truncus arteriosus

[a] Stiff lungs, large heart, and increased pulmonary vascular markings.

pulmonary stenosis) or a coarctation syndrome. At 6 to 8 weeks of age, significant left-to-right shunts, such as large VSDs and AV canal defects, typically present following the normal physiologic decrease in pulmonary vascular resistance which permits pulmonary overcirculation (23). Children presenting later in life should be suspected of having an acquired rather than a congenital heart disease.

The pathophysiology of congestive heart failure in these children is increased pulmonary blood flow, pulmonary interstitial edema, and volume overload. The congenital heart defects most commonly associated with congestive heart failure are those that result in pulmonary recirculation via a large left-to-right shunt (Table 240.3).

Radiographic Findings

The clinical findings of "stiff, wet lungs" and a large heart correlate with the radiographic findings. Typically, there is cardiac enlargement and increased pulmonary vascular markings, with pulmonary edema.

ECG Findings

The electrocardiographic findings may be nonspecific, depending on the level of the shunt; however, a QRS axis of –30 degrees to –120 degrees in an infant, particularly one with trisomy 21, is consistent with an AV canal.

EMERGENCY DEPARTMENT MANAGEMENT

The treatment, in general, includes respiratory support and inotropic support. In children with a structural heart defect, medical therapy is used as temporizing therapy pending surgical correction. In the acute care setting dopamine, dobutamine, and the phosphodiesterase inhibitors, amrinone and millrinone have been successfully used (14). Dopamine and dobutamine are the most appropriate inotropes in the immediate management of CHF and should be initiated as continuous infusions at 2 to 20 mcg/kg/min. Two issues regarding these agents should be considered when selecting the initial agent. Dobutamine has less arrhythmogenic potential and reduces afterload by its vasodilatory effect when compared to dopamine, however, there is some data to question the efficacy of dobutamine in children less than 1 year of age (13). Therefore, in children older than 1 year of age dobutamine would be the initial agent of choice and in children less than 1 year of age with hypotension,

dobutamine may be more appropriate as an adjunct rather than as the primary inotrope. Agents such as epinephrine and norepinephrine should be avoided in the patient with ventricular dysfunction because they may aggravate the sympathetic overstimulation in fulminant CHF.

Digoxin may be the mainstay of medical therapy for stable children in CHF, but the length of time required to reach a therapeutic serum level makes it not an optimum choice for the acute care setting. Diuretic therapy also has a role in the management of CHF by promoting diuresis. Furosemide may be given intravenously as a bolus of 1 mg/kg. Evidence from adult studies regarding the use of ACE inhibitors shows a clear improvement in symptomatology and longevity in adults with CHF (17). Unfortunately the majority of adult studies focused on ischemic cardiomyopathy therefore providing little information for the pediatric population. Several small studies have shown clinical improvement in children treated with an angiotensin converting enzyme inhibitor (21,25). Beta-blockers have been shown in two nonrandomized trials to improve left ventricular function in pediatric patients with idiopathic, drug-induced or inherited dilated cardiomyopathy (16,28).

CARDIAC DYSRHYTHMIAS

Pediatric patients present with three basic categories of rhythm disturbances—fast, slow, or absent. Asystole and bradyarrhythmias are primarily seen in resuscitation settings and are discussed in Chapter 206. Other dysrhythmias unique to pediatric patients are discussed below.

SUPRAVENTRICULAR TACHYCARDIA

Paroxysmal supraventricular tachycardia (SVT) is the most common pediatric tachydysrhythmia and children may present in an emergency department setting at almost any age. In general SVT is well tolerated. Patients may demonstrate symptoms of tachypnea and feeding intolerance or in more severe cases mottling or cyanosis. Older children may have chest pain, palpitations, syncope, fatigue, and dyspnea. The longer the SVT continues, in general, the more severe the symptoms.

The etiology of the SVT varies by age group. In infants more than 50% are idiopathic, 24% have associated conditions (infection, fever or drug exposure), 23% have congenital heart disease (usually corrected transposition of the great vessels, Ebstein anomaly) and 22% Wolff-Parkinson-White syndrome (13). Older children are more likely to have WPW, concealed bypass tracts, or congenital heart disease. Young infants are more likely to present with CHF.

ECG Findings

A typical ECG of a patient with SVT will show a rapid rate, a narrow QRS complex and invisible p waves. The tachycardia is usually characterized by a regular rate of 220 to 320 beats per minute for an infant and 150 to 250 beats per minute for an older child.

EMERGENCY DEPARTMENT MANAGEMENT

Most children are able to tolerate SVT for prolonged periods of time (hours to days) without developing significant clinical symptoms. In an asymptomatic hemodynamically stable patient, vagal maneuvers followed by pharmacologic cardioversion are indicated as an initial approach. The success of vagal maneuvers have been shown to be related to the age of the patient, with the success rate lower in infants and young children (10,12). Although, vagal maneuvers may not have a high success rate in the younger child, the occasional conversion justifies their initial trial. For infants and young children the application of a bag of crushed ice to the face (induces diving reflex), for up to 30 seconds, is an effective vagal stimulus. Older children may have a trial of a vagal maneuver, with an effective Valsalva maneuver requiring cooperation and usually a sustained duration of 15 seconds of effort. Ocular compression is not a recommended form of vagal maneuver because of the risk of retinal detachment.

The majority of SVTs are reentrant and therefore respond to intravenous adenosine (20). The initial recommended dose for adenosine is 0.1 mg/kg as a rapid bolus, followed by a rapid push of 5 to 10 mL of normal saline. Following adenosine therapy, the patient may have a short break in tachycardia, with early recurrence requiring additional doses. An infant may require up to 0.3 mg/kg by rapid intravenous push in a peripheral intravenous line, preferably positioned in the right arm. Usually, the adenosine dose required is lower if central venous access is obtained. In general, calcium channel blockers are contraindicated in infants and children (9). An ECG should be obtained prior to and during the conversion to document the underlying rhythm. If preexcitation is present, digoxin and calcium channel blockers are contraindicated for chronic therapy. Additionally, intravenous beta blockers are almost never required in infants and children for conversion from a reentrant arrhythmia. In all cases, chronic therapy in an infant should be decided after consultation with a pediatric cardiologist.

If the patient is hemodynamically unstable, immediate synchronized cardioversion with 0.5 to 1 J/kg should be attempted. Cardioversion may not be successful in the presence of hypoxia or an acid-base disorder, so careful attention to correction of airway breathing and circulatory issues should be initiated simultaneously.

COMPLETE HEART BLOCK

Complete heart block may be congenital or acquired. Complete heart block may be associated with structural heart defects or occur postoperatively following repair of a CHD (VSD).

Maternal collagen vascular disease may also result in transmission of maternal immunoglobins across the placenta that result in an abnormal fetal conduction system. Infants typically present with bradycardia and a ventricular rate that is usually less than 75 beats per minute. The clinical presentation for infants may range from asymptomatic to CHF. Older children may have syncope, fatigue and decreased exercise tolerance. In unstable patients, management focuses on stabilization of the ABCs, and consideration of an infusion of isoproterenol (0.02 to 0.5 mcg/kg/min) or epinephrine (0.05 to 0.5 mcg/kg/min) pending pacemaker placement.

VENTRICULAR DYSRHYTHMIAS

Isolated premature ventricular contractions may occur in up to 15% of normal newborns, 33% of normal adolescents and 66% of patients with repaired heart disease (TOF, VSD, AV canal defects, transposition of the great vessels, and aortic stenosis) (1). Sustained ventricular tachycardia is very uncommon in a healthy heart. Although uncommon, hemodynamically unstable arrhythmias require immediate and aggressive therapy. Patients with ventricular tachycardia who are hemodynamically compromised require immediate DC cardioversion. Electrolyte abnormalities should be considered in patients who are refractory to cardioversion. Patients with a history of intoxication (e.g., with cocaine) may require pharmacologic therapy in addition to cardioversion, such as with lidocaine or beta blockers. In patients with a history of digoxin toxicity, DC cardioversion should be avoided, and treatment with digoxin-specific Fab fragments initiated. These patients require cardiopulmonary resuscitation while managing their malignant dysrhythmia in order to avoid permanent central nervous system injury.

ATRIAL FIBRILLATION

In patients with atrial fibrillation and Wolff-Parkinson-White syndrome, there may be rapid conduction to the ventricles (3). Electrocardiographically, this may mimic rapid ventricular tachycardia (Fig. 240.1). However, these patients may be surprisingly hemodynamically stable initially and then deteriorate rapidly if they remain in this dysrhythmia. Again, synchronized cardioversion is the treatment of choice; however, if the patient

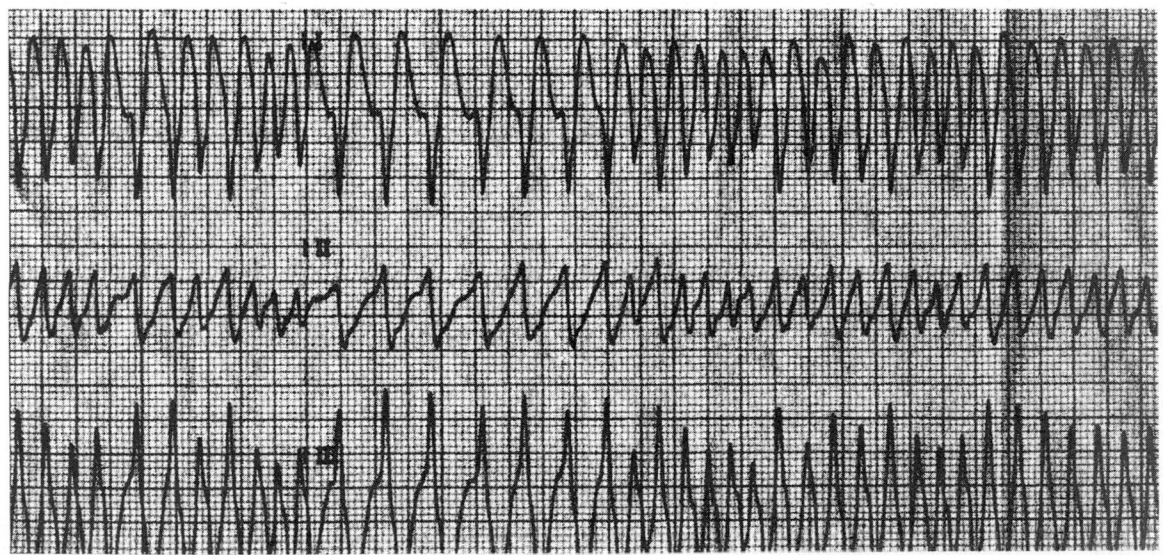

Figure 240.1.   Atrial fibrillation with rapid conduction via an accessory pathway in a child with Wolff-Parkinson-White syndrome. There was no response to adenosine.

appears stable, infusion with intravenous procainamide or ibutilide may be tolerated. In general, treatment with adenosine will not result in any dysrhythmia change. Because digoxin and calcium channel blockers may increase accessory pathway conduction, resulting in ventricular fibrillation, these medications are contraindicated whenever this dysrhythmia is suspected.

CRITICAL INTERVENTIONS

- Differentiate respiratory from cardiac disease; use the hyperoxia test
- Consider sepsis in a child with poor perfusion and cyanosis
- Stabilize ABCs
- For ductal dependent lesions use prostaglandin E1. Be prepared to intubate as apnea may occur as a side effect
- For patients in congestive heart failure who require inotropic support, dopamine or dobutamine are good initial agents

COMMON PITFALLS

✔ Infants with cardiogenic shock and septic shock can present similarly with poor perfusion and metabolic acidosis. However, it is an important distinction to make, because septic shock requires fluid resuscitation and cardiogenic shock often requires the use of prostaglandin E1 infusions

✔ A chest radiograph should be considered for any "first-time wheezer" less than three months of age to exclude cardiomegaly. Hyperinflation from bronchiolitis should result in a normal or small cardiac silhouette. Cardiomegaly in a child with wheezing suggests "cardiac asthma" due to myocarditis, anomalous left coronary from the pulmonary artery, or other cardiac etiologies

✔ Intravenous calcium channel blockers are almost always contraindicated in infants and small children

References

1. Alexander ME, Berul CJ. Ventricular arrhythmias: When to worry. *Pediatr Cardiol* 2000;21:532–541.
2. Barkin RM. Congestive heart failure in children. *J Emerg Med* 1986;4:379–382.
3. Binder LS, Boeche R, Atkinson D. Evaluation and management of supraventricular tachycardia in children. *Ann Emerg Med* 1991;20:51–54.
4. Bromberg BI, Lindsay BD, Cain ME, et al. Impact of clinical history and electrophysiologic characterization of accessory pathways on management strategies to reduce sudden death among children with Wolff-Parkinson-White syndrome. *J Am Cardiol Coll* 1996;27:690–695.
5. Burton DA, Cabalka AK. Cardiac evaluation of infants. The first year of life. *Pediatr Clin North Am* 1994;41:991–1015.
6. Coles J, Freedom R, Olley P, et al. Surgical management of critical pulmonary stenosis in the neonate. *Ann Thorac Surg* 1984;38:458–465.
7. Daliento L, Fasoli G, Mazzucco A. Anomalous origin of the left coronary artery from the anterior aortic sinus: role of echocardiography. *Int J Cardiol* 1993;38:89–91.
8. Drucker NA, Colan SD, Lewis AB, et al. Gamma-globulin treatment of acute myocarditis in the pediatric population. *Circulation* 1994;89:252–257.
9. Epstein ML, Kiel EA, Victorica BE. Cardiac decompensation following verapamil therapy in infants with supraventricular tachycardia. *Pediatrics* 1985;75:737–740.
10. Fulton D, Grodin M. Pediatric cardiac emergencies. *Emerg Med Clinics North America* 1983;1:45–61.
11. Fyler DC. Trends. In: Fyler DC, ed. *Nadas pediatric cardiology.* Philadelphia: Hanley & Belfus, 1992;273–280.
12. Garson A, Gillette P, Mcnamara D. Supraventricular tachycardia in children: Clinical features, response to treatment, and long-term follow-up in 217 patients. *J Pediatr* 1981;98:875–882.
13. Gewitz M, Vetter V. Cardiac Emergencies. In: Fleisher GR, Ludwig S, (eds.): *Textbook of pediatric emergency medicine, 4th ed.* Philadelphia: Lippincott, Williams and Wilkins, 2000;659–700.
14. Gupta ML, Lantin-Hermoso MR, Rao PS. What's new in pediatric cardiology. *Indian Journal of Pediatrics* 2003;70:41–48.
15. Gutgesell HP, Barst RJ, Humes RA, et al. Common cardiovascular problems in the young. Part I. Murmurs, chest pain, syncope and irregular rhythms. *Am Fam Physician* 1997;56:1825–1830.
16. Ishikawa Y, Bach JR, Minami R. cardioprotection for Duchenne's muscular dystrophy. *Am Heart J* 1999;137:895–902.
17. Kambam J. Transposition of the great arteries. In: Kambam J, (ed.): *Cardiac Anesthesia for Infants and Children.* St Louis: Mosby, 1994;229–241.
18. Kay JD, Colan SD and Graham TP. Congestive heart failure in pediatric patients. *Am Heart J* 2001;142:923–928.
19. Krishnan US. Approach to congenital heart disease in the neonate. *Indian Journal of Pediatrics* 2002;69:501–505.
20. Lee C, Mason LJ. Pediatric cardiac emergencies. *Anesth Clin North Am* 2001;19:287–307.
21. Lewis AB, Chabot M. The Effect of treatment with angiotensin-converting enzyme inhibitors on survival of pediatric patients with dilated cardiomyopathy. *Pediatr Cardiol* 1993;14:9–12.
22. Losek JD, Endom E, Dietrich A, et al. Adenosine and pediatric supraventricular tachycardia in the emergency department: multicenter study and review. *Ann Emerg Med* 1999;33:185–191.
23. McCollough M, Sharieff GQ. Common Complaints in the first 30 days of Life. *Emerg Med Clin North Am* 2002;20:27–48.
24. Moller JH, Neal WA. Fetal neonatal and infant cardiac disease. Norwalk, CT: Appleton & Lange, 1989.
25. Montigny M, Davignon A, Fouron JC, et al. Captopril in infants for congestive heart failure secondary to a large ventricular left-to-right shunt. *Am J Cardiol* 1989;63:631–633.
26. Prasodo AM. Management of congenital heart disease. *Paediatr Indones* 1989;29:78–90.
27. Rao P, Streipe V, Merrill W. Hypoplastic left heart syndrome. In: Kambam J, (ed.): *Cardiac Anesthesia for Infants and Children.* St Louis: Mosby, 1994;296–309.
28. Shaddy RE, Tani LY, Gidding SS, et al. Beta-blocker treatment of dilated cardiomyopathy with congestive heart failure in children: a multi-institutional experience. *J Heart Lung Transplant* 1999;18:269–274.
29. Talner N, McGovern J, Carboni M. Congestive Heart Failure. In: Moller J, Hoffman J, (eds.): *Pediatric Cardiovascular Medicine, ed 1.* Philadelphia: Churchill Livingstone, 2000;817–832.

CHAPTER 241
Croup and Other Airway Disorders

Timothy G. Givens

Croup is a clinical syndrome characterized by a barklike cough, hoarseness, inspiratory stridor, and respiratory distress of variable severity. The two most common forms are viral laryngotracheobronchitis (LTB) and spasmodic croup. The former is due to infection with parainfluenza viruses types 1, 2, and 3; respiratory syncytial virus; influenza virus type A; or adenovirus (8). The virus causes inflammation of the subglottic tissues and sometimes of the tracheal mucosa. The supraglottic structures are normal.

Spasmodic croup is of uncertain etiology, although seen more commonly in patients with a family history of asthma, allergies, or recurrent episodes of croup. The peak incidence of LTB is during late fall and early winter. It can occur in all age groups but is most often seen during the second year of life. There is a 2:1 male-to-female ratio, with a recurrence rate of 5%. Most cases of croup are mild to moderate in severity and are self-limited.

Epiglottitis, in contrast, is an acute bacterial process that is life-threatening. While the epiglottis and the aryepiglottic folds become inflamed and swollen, the glottis and subglottis remain normal. Epiglottitis is usually caused by *Haemophilus influenzae* type B (HIB) (8,21). Its incidence has fallen dramatically since the introduction of HIB vaccination (6,19). Epiglottitis occurs throughout the year. It traditionally afflicts preschool children (2 to 6 years old) but can present in almost any age group, including adults. Because of widespread HIB vaccination, cases are now more often seen in older children and adolescents. Epiglottitis does not recur after the first infection. The onset of epiglottitis is usually rapid, with a fulminant course that leads to respiratory arrest from either complete airway obstruction or fatigue associated with a partial airway obstruction. If properly managed, the signs and symptoms of the acute infection resolve within 24 to 72 hours.

Another croup variant is bacterial tracheitis, also known as pseudomembranous croup. This relatively uncommon illness occurs in children between 6 months and 8 years of age. Its distinguishing feature is the presence of thick, mucopurulent secretions. Although most commonly caused by *Staphylococcus aureus*, other pathogens, such as *Haemophilus influenzae*, α-hemolytic streptococcus, pneumococcus, and *Moraxella catarrhalis*, have been associated with bacterial tracheitis (3).

CLINICAL PRESENTATION

Inspiratory stridor, a barking cough, and hoarse voice with mild-to-moderate respiratory distress are the common presenting symptoms of LTB. One to 2 days of coryza with a low-grade fever is the usual prodrome. The symptoms peak by 2 to 3 days, with improvement and resolution noted by 5 to 7 days (8). Respiratory distress worsens when the patient cries or becomes agitated. Some patients may present with wheezing, tachypnea, and stridor. These patients have a combined illness of bronchiolitis and croup. A clinical scoring system may assist the physician in assessing the degree and progression of respiratory distress. In spasmodic croup, the same barking cough, stridor, and labored breathing are observed, but the patient is afebrile and does not have the upper respiratory symptoms that precede LTB. Patients with spasmodic croup are usually responsive to cool, humidified air and often improve by time they reach the emergency department (ED).

Patients with epiglottitis usually have the abrupt onset of sore throat, high fever, and one or more of the four Ds: dysphagia, dysphonia, drooling, and distress. Inspiratory stridor may be audible, but there is usually no cough. Secretions, laryngospasm, and fatigue can further compromise breathing. Classically, patients assume a tripod sitting position, with the mandible extended forward in an effort to maintain airway patency. Patients appear very apprehensive and often toxic because of sepsis (21).

Bacterial tracheitis lies between croup and epiglottitis on the clinical spectrum. Similarly to patients with LTB, patients may have a viral prodrome for a few days, and then rapidly deteriorate, appearing toxic with high fever and signs of upper airway obstruction. As opposed to those with epiglottitis, those patients with bacterial tracheitis often cough, are able to lie flat with relative comfort, and do not have problems handling their secretions. They often fail to respond to standard treatment for croup, such as racemic epinephrine and steroids (3).

DIFFERENTIAL DIAGNOSIS

With a typical presentation of croup, the diagnosis is clinical, and laboratory and radiographic studies are unnecessary (8). Atypical clinical features should prompt other considerations. Occasionally, a child with LTB caused by parainfluenza or influenza virus will present with stridor and wheezing and is diagnosed as having bronchiolitis. Epiglottitis is differentiated by its more acute and fulminant presentation (Table 241.1). A

TABLE 241.1. Comparison between Epiglottitis and Laryngotracheobronchitis

Characteristic	LTB	Epiglottitis
Age	6 mo–3 yr	2–6 yr
Onset	Gradual	Rapid
Etiology	Viral	Bacterial
Swelling site	Subglottic	Supraglottic
Symptoms		
Cough-voice	Hoarse cough	No cough Muffled voice
Posture	Any position	Sitting
Mouth	Closed; nasal flaring	Open-chin forward, drooling
Fever	Absent to high	High
Appearance	Often not acutely ill	Anxious, acutely ill
Radiograph	Narrow subglottic area	Swollen epiglottis and supraglottic structures
Palpation larynx	Nontender	Tender
Recurrence	May recur	Rarely recurs
Seasonal incidence	Winter	None

(From Backofen JE, Rogers MC. Upper airway disease. In: Rogers MC, ed. *Textbook of pediatric intensive care*, vol. 1. Baltimore: Williams & Wilkins, 1987.)

history of HIB vaccination does not rule out epiglottitis. Ludwig angina (a rapidly spreading inflammation of the sublingual, submandibular, and submaxillary spaces) and retropharyngeal and peritonsillar abscesses are suspected based on inspection of the oral cavity. If membranes are noted in the oropharynx, diphtheria and infectious mononucleosis must also be considered. Bacterial tracheitis may be suspected when there is no response to the standard management for LTB, or when the patient's symptoms worsen. If the patient is afebrile or has a history of choking, the possibility of aspiration of a foreign object should be investigated, using noninvasive techniques such as inspiratory and expiratory chest radiographs, fluoroscopy, or computed tomography scanning. Direct visualization by laryngobronchoscopy may be required (21). For recurrent or persistent stridor or a clinical presentation of LTB during an atypical time of year, the following also should be considered: congenital airway anomalies, acquired tracheal stenosis secondary to previous intubations, congenital heart disease with associated vascular anomalies, tracheal hemangiomas, or recurrent angioneurotic edema.

EMERGENCY DEPARTMENT EVALUATION

The child in respiratory distress should not be separated from parental comfort unless respiratory arrest is imminent (8). Minimal manipulation is necessary so as not to increase the child's work of breathing and worsen the respiratory distress. The physical examination consists of inspection and observation at a comfortable distance from the patient. Oxygen can be delivered in a manner tolerable to the child. Venipuncture should be deferred to avoid distressing the patient. When epiglottitis is highly suspected, immediate arrangements must be made to transport the patient to an operating room in order to secure placement of an artificial airway. Further evaluation of the airway by direct visualization can then be done with the patient anesthetized. A physician experienced in airway management must accompany the child during transport to the operating room.

If the history and physical examination suggest LTB, the physician may apply a clinical scoring system to assess the

TABLE 241.2.   Clinical Croup Score

	0	1	2
Inspiratory breath sounds	Normal	Harsh with rhonchi	Delayed
Stridor	None	Inspiratory	Inspiratory and expiratory
Cough	None	Hoarse cry	Barking cough
Retractions/flaring	None	Flaring, suprasternal retractions	As in 1 plus subcostal/intercostal retractions
Cyanosis *or*	None	In room air	In 40% O2
PaO$_2$ (mm Hg)	70–100	< 70	< 70
CNS function	Normal	Depressed/agitated	Coma

(Modified with permission from Downes JJ, Raphaely R. Pediatric intensive care. Anesthesiology 1975;43:242.)

patient's degree of compromise (Table 241.2). Sequential scoring is done after each intervention. If the diagnosis is in doubt and the child is stable, an inspiratory soft-tissue lateral neck radiograph and chest radiograph may be helpful (Figs. 241.1 through 241.3). Classic radiographic signs of epiglottitis include the thumb sign (enlarged epiglottis), swelling of the aryepiglottic folds, blunting of the vallecula, and obliteration of the piriform sinuses. In LTB, the steeple sign (a gradual narrowing at the subglottic area) may be observed, but all supraglottic structures should appear normal. In bacterial tracheitis, the tracheal air column may appear hazy due to the presence of pseudomembranes. Radiographic widening of the soft tissue between the air column and cervical vertebrae points to retropharyngeal abscess or cellulitis.

EMERGENCY DEPARTMENT MANAGEMENT

Maintenance or provision of an adequate airway is the first priority in any illness in which airway obstruction is possible. Each institution must establish an epiglottitis protocol that can be rapidly activated. Once the diagnosis of suspected epiglottitis is made, appropriate personnel must be mobilized. The patient must be taken to the operating room immediately, where inhalation anesthesia is given with the patient in a sitting position. The hypopharynx is then visualized, and rapid intubation is performed with an endotracheal tube 0.5 to 1.0 mm smaller in diameter than that predicted for the patient's age and weight. A surgeon skilled in pediatric tracheostomy should be prepared to perform an emergency tracheostomy, if necessary. Intravenous access and laboratory studies are obtained at the discretion of the anesthesiologist, usually after induction of anesthesia. In the case where bacterial tracheitis is suspected, the management is the same as for suspected epiglottitis.

Patients with LTB who have a clinical score of 7 or greater and who do not respond quickly to initial therapeutic maneuvers may also be candidates for endotracheal intubation. Continuous pulse oximetry monitoring may reveal early deterioration in the patient's oxygenation status in a noninvasive fashion (23). Ventilatory failure should be suspected if the patient loses head control or becomes lethargic. Because of airway narrowing, an endotracheal tube size smaller in diameter than that predicted for the child's age and weight should be used if intubation becomes a necessity.

For patients who present to the emergency department with impending or complete respiratory arrest, the airway must be addressed immediately. Bag-valve-mask ventilation with 100% oxygen should be initiated. Higher positive pressures are sometimes necessary, requiring a two-handed technique to obtain an adequate chest rise. If these measures are unsuccessful within 15 to 30 seconds, a rapid oral intubation should be attempted. Tips for intubating children with epiglottitis include using a smaller size endotracheal tube, using a stylet, and looking for an air bubble at the glottic opening while someone compresses the chest.

If intubation is impossible, emergency cricothyrotomy must be done. A large-bore (14-gauge) angiocatheter is inserted

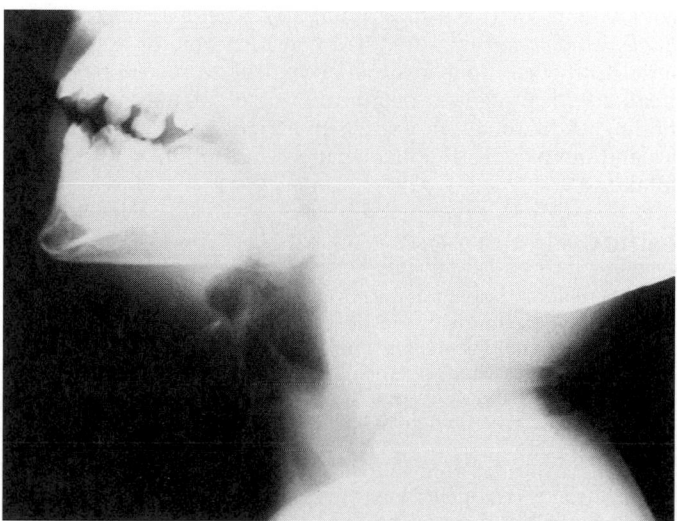

Figure 241.1.   Normal inspiratory soft-tissue lateral neck radiograph.

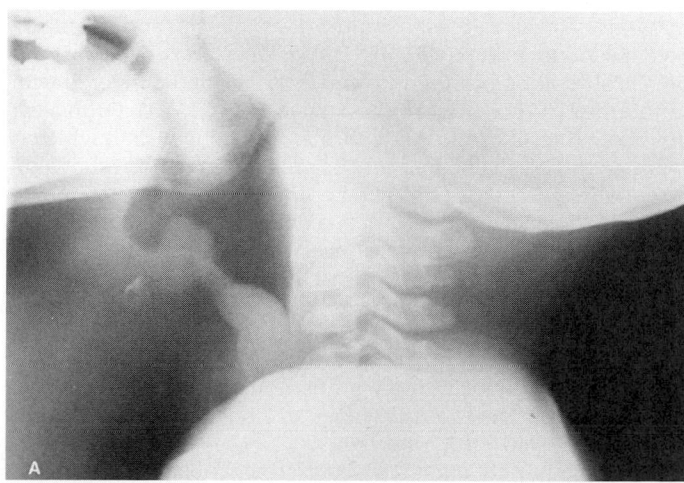

Figure 241.2.   Epiglottitis on inspiratory soft-tissue lateral neck radiograph. Supraglottitis.

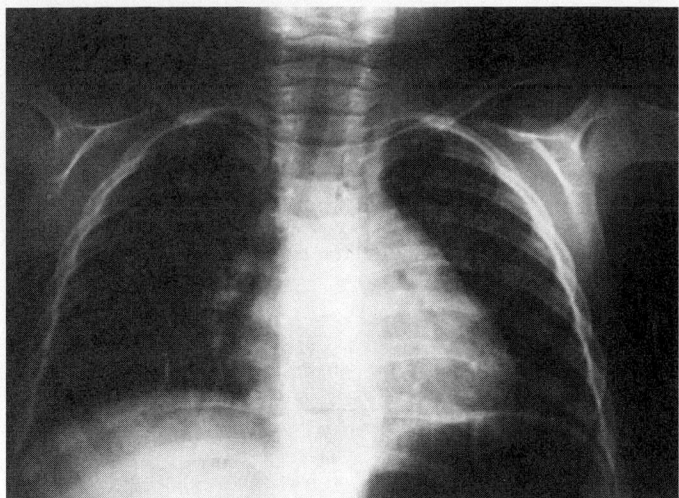

Figure 241.3.   Croup. Steeple sign on a soft-tissue neck radiograph.

through the cricothyroid membrane at a caudad angle and attached to a 3.0 endotracheal tube. This maneuver may provide a temporary open airway for bag ventilation or direct connection to a pressurized continuous-flow oxygen source (21). A pediatric surgeon or otolaryngologist should be consulted for emergency tracheostomy. Complications associated with the disease, as well as the artificial airway placement, include pulmonary edema, tension pneumothorax, subcutaneous emphysema, pneumomediastinum, bleeding, endotracheal tube plugging, accidental extubation, and bronchospasm (21).

In LTB, therapy is provided commensurate with the patient's level of respiratory distress. In mild cases (croup score less than 4), a trial of humidification therapy may be offered. Cool, humidified air is thought to work by moistening the inflamed airway and thinning secretions to facilitate clearance, activating mechanoreceptors in the larynx to produce reflex slowing of the respiratory rate, or by reducing patient anxiety and associated hyperventilation as the parent holds the child close to administer the mist (8,17). However, no significant benefit to cool mist therapy has ever been proven, and a recent randomized, controlled trial of children with moderate croup failed to demonstrate effectiveness of mist therapy in improving the clinical symptoms of croup (17). Croup tents, which may actually interfere with observation of the patient or increase anxiety, have become passé (8).

Patients with LTB who have a clinical score of 4 or greater or inspiratory stridor at rest should receive oxygen and nebulized racemic epinephrine (0.05 mL/kg per dose [max dose, 0.5 mL] of a 2.25% solution diluted in 3 mL of saline and delivered with humidified oxygen, repeated as necessary) (8,16,21). Equivalent doses of either racemic epinephrine or L-epinephrine, which is more readily available and less expensive, have been shown to be equally efficacious (25). The l-epinephrine dose is 0.5 ml/kg of a 1:1000 concentration to a maximum of 5 ml/dose. There should be almost immediate clinical improvement due to reduction of the edema and vasoconstriction of the inflamed mucosa through the stimulation of the α-adrenergic receptors. Parents should be encouraged to deliver the nebulized treatment in a nonthreatening manner. Heart rate should be monitored during treatment with nebulized sympathomimetics. The treatment should be stopped when the heart rate exceeds 200 beats per minute or if dysrhythmias occur.

Previously, patients who received nebulized epinephrine were admitted to the hospital because of a possible rebound effect, a clinical worsening due to vasodilation, and increased mu-

cosal edema as the adrenergic effects abate. This phenomenon usually occurs within 2 to 4 hours after epinephrine treatment. Recently, the need for hospitalization has been reassessed. Several studies suggest that discharge from the emergency department is safe following epinephrine therapy if, after 2 to 4 hours of observation, the patient has no stridor at rest and has normal air entry, normal color, and normal level of consciousness (8,13,14,18).

There is now ample evidence to suggest that corticosteroids are of benefit to patients with moderate-to-severe croup (10,22). Steroids promote resolution of laryngeal edema through antiinflammatory activity. Dexamethasone (Decadron), 0.15 to 0.6 mg/kg, administered either orally or as a single intramuscular injection, has been shown to reduce the severity of symptoms (1,4,9,24), rate of hospital admissions (4), need for subsequent nebulized epinephrine treatments (24) and duration of hospital stay or observation in the ED (4,5). Dexamethasone has a half-life of 54 hours, so one dose is usually sufficient. Inhaled budesonide has been shown to have a rapid onset (within 2 to 4 hours) and to be effective in mild-to-moderate croup (7,11,12). Whether treatment with dexamethasone is necessary in mild croup is still uncertain. However, two studies–one comparing 0.6 mg/kg of oral dexamethasone to a comparable dose of nebulized dexamethasone or placebo;(15); and a second trial comparing a smaller 0.15-mg/kg oral dose of dexamethasone with placebo (5)—have both shown that treatment with dexamethasone reduces the number of return visits to the ED and speeds the resolution of symptoms in children with mild croup that were discharged home.

Both oral and intramuscular routes of administration have been shown to be effective compared with placebo (20), and a recent randomized clinical trial comparing equivalent doses of intramuscular and oral dexamethasone showed no difference between the two in terms of clinical efficacy (2). The ease of administration of oral dexamethasone over nebulized or intramuscular agents makes the oral route preferable in most cases (22). The other routes become options in complicated croup requiring admission or associated with vomiting. As effects from corticosteroid treatment take 6 hours, early use is most beneficial. All patients who require epinephrine therapy should also receive steroids.

Antibiotics are unnecessary for patients with LTB. Patients with epiglottitis or bacterial tracheitis should receive intravenous antibiotics beginning in the operating room. Epiglottitis treatment options include ceftriaxone (100 mg/kg/d at 12-hour intervals), cefuroxime (150 mg/kg/d at 8-hour intervals), cefotaxime (150 mg/kg/d at 8-hour intervals), or chloramphenicol (100 mg/kg/d at 6-hour intervals). Adequate coverage for *Staphylococcus aureus* should be a consideration in cases of bacterial tracheitis. Bronchospasm secondary to secretions can be treated with β₂-agonist nebulization (e.g., albuterol) and suctioning. Additional supportive treatment includes antipyretics and intravenous fluids for patients with compromised oral intake.

CRITICAL INTERVENTIONS

- The child in respiratory distress should not be separated from parental comfort unless respiratory arrest is imminent
- Oxygen should be delivered in a manner tolerable to the child
- Venipuncture should be deferred in patients with respiratory distress to avoid distressing the patient
- Have airway equipment at the bedside in a child with respiratory distress
- Use BVM ventilation with 100% oxygen as the initial airway maneuver in patients with impending complete respiratory compromise

DISPOSITION

Intubated patients (including all epiglottitis patients) must be admitted to a pediatric intensive care unit, accompanied by personnel skilled in pediatric airway placement. LTB patients with a clinical score of 4 or greater (significant respiratory distress), those with persistent stridor at rest, and those with minimal to no response to nebulized adrenergic treatment should be admitted. Instructions to parents whose children are sent home include monitoring the child's work of breathing (respiratory rate, retractions, and agitation), implementing a method of rapid and easy communication access between physician and family, and ensuring minimal stimulation.

COMMON PITFALLS

✔ Separating children from parents during initial assessment or during administration of nebulized medications or oxygen
✔ Underestimating the degree of respiratory distress
✔ Increasing agitation and respiratory distress by performing medical procedures (vital signs, laboratory and x-ray studies)
✔ Obtaining radiographic studies when the diagnosis by history and clinical presentation is clear
✔ Delaying the establishment of an artificial airway or not having the appropriate equipment readily available
✔ Failure to have a physician skilled in establishing artificial airways accompany the child during transport
✔ Using too large an endotracheal tube during intubation

References

1. Cruz MN, Stewart G, Rosenberg N. Use of dexamethasone in the outpatient management of croup. *Pediatrics* 1995;96:220–223.
2. Donaldson D, Poleski D, Knipple E, et al. Intramuscular versus oral dexamethasone for the treatment of moderate-to-severe croup: a randomized, double-blind trial. *Acad Emerg Med* 2003;10:16–21.
3. Donaldson JD, Maltby CC. Bacterial tracheitis in children. *J Otolaryngol* 1989;18:101–104.
4. Geelhoed GC. Sixteen years of croup in a Western Australian teaching hospital: effects of routine steroid treatment. *Ann Emerg Med* 1996;28:621–626.
5. Geelhoed GC, Macdonald WBG. Oral dexamethasone in the treatment of croup: 0.15 mg/kg vs. 0.3 mg/kg vs. 0.6 mg/kg. *Pediatr Pulmonol* 1995;20:362–368.
6. Gorelick MH, Baker MD. Epiglottitis in children, 1970–1992. Effects of *Haemophilus influenzae* type b immunization. *Arch Pediatr Adolesc Med* 1994; 148:47–50.
7. Husby S, Agertoft L, Mortensen S, et al. Treatment of croup with nebulised steroid (budesonide): a double blind, placebo controlled study. *Arch Dis Child* 1993;68:3:352–355.
8. Kaditis AG, Wald ER. Viral croup: current diagnosis and treatment. *Pediatr Infect Dis J* 1998;17:827–834.
9. Kairys SW, Olmstead EM, O'Connor GT. Steroid treatment of laryngotracheitis: a meta-analysis of the evidence from randomized trials. *Pediatrics* 1989;83:683–693.
10. Klassen TP. Croup. A current perspective. *Pediatr Clin North Am* 1999;46:1167–1178.
11. Klassen TP, Feldman ME, Watters LK, et al. Nebulized budesonide for children with mild-to-moderate croup. *N Engl J Med* 1994;331:285–289.
12. Klassen TP, Watters LK, Feldman ME, et al. The efficacy of nebulized budesonide in dexamethasone-treated outpatients with croup. *Pediatrics* 1996;97:463–466.
13. Kunkel NC, Baker MD. Use of racemic epinephrine, dexamethasone, and mist in the outpatient management of croup. *Pediatr Emerg Care* 1996;12:156–159.
14. Ledwith CA, Shea LM, Mauro RD. Safety and efficacy of nebulized racemic epinephrine in conjunction with oral dexamethasone and mist in the outpatient management of croup. *Ann Emerg Med* 1995;25:331–337.
15. Luria JW, Gonzalez del Rey JA, DiGiulio GA, et al. Effectiveness of oral or nebulized dexamethasone for children with mild croup. *Arch Pediatr Adolesc Med* 2001;155:1340–1345.
16. McDonogh AJ. The use of steroids and nebulised adrenaline in the treatment of viral croup over a seven year period at a district hospital. *Anaesth Intensive Care* 1994;22:175–178.
17. Neto GM, Kentab O, Klassen TP, Osmond MH. A randomized controlled trial of mist in the acute treatment of moderate croup. *Acad Emerg Med* 2002;9:873–879.
18. Prendergast M, Jones JS, Hartman D. Racemic epinephrine in the treatment of laryngotracheitis: can we identify children for outpatient therapy? *Am J Emerg Med* 1994;12:613–616.
19. Progress toward eliminating *Haemophilus influenzae* type b disease among infants and children—United States, 1987–1997. *MMWR* 1998;47:993–998.
20. Rittichier KK, Ledwith CA. Outpatient treatment of moderate croup with dexamethasone: intramuscular versus oral dosing. *Pediatrics* 2000;106:1344–1348.
21. Rogers MC. *Textbook of pediatric intensive care*, vol 3 Baltimore: Williams & Wilkins, 1996:69–70.
22. Rowe BH. Corticosteroid treatment for acute croup. *Ann Emerg Med* 2002;40:353–355.
23. Stoney PJ, Chakrabarti MK. Experience of pulse oximetry in children with croup. *J Laryngol Otol* 1991;105:295–298.
24. Super DM, Cartelli NA, Brooks LJ, et al. A prospective randomized double-blind study to evaluate the effect of dexamethasone in acute laryngotracheitis. *J Pediatr* 1989;115:323–329.
25. Waisman Y, Klein BL, Boenning DA, et al. Prospective randomized double-blind study comparing *l*-epinephrine and racemic epinephrine aerosols in the treatment of laryngotracheitis (croup). *Pediatrics* 1992;89:302–306.

CHAPTER 242
Dermatologic Disorders

Atima Chumpa Delaney

The sudden onset of a rash, particularly with fever, is a frequent cause of emergency department (ED) visits in children. Definitive diagnosis may not be possible in the ED in some cases. Most patients have a nonspecific, self-limited viral illness requiring only supportive care, however, it is important to identify diseases that are life-threatening and those that require specific therapy, or have public health implications. This chapter describes a number of pediatric dermatologic disorders commonly presenting to the ED and the classic childhood exanthems.

Exanthems are generalized erythematous eruptions that occur with many viral or bacterial infections. Certain exanthems have characteristic morphology and presentation. Patient history should establish the initial location, spread, duration, and changes in appearance of the rash. Any fever or other associated symptoms, such as sore throat, cough, vomiting, headache, and neck pain, should be noted. A history of recent exposure to a highly contagious disease is often helpful. Recent medication use may suggest a drug reaction. If either the patient or a household contact is a neonate, pregnant, or immunocompromised, the management of an otherwise benign illness may be altered.

Physical examination should focus on assessing the general severity of illness (e.g., irritability, state of hydration) and should thoroughly characterize skin and mucous membrane lesions. Complications such as otitis media, cellulitis, pneumonia, and encephalitis should also be sought.

DISEASES WITH MACULOPAPULAR ERUPTIONS

Nonspecific viral eruptions commonly have maculopapular lesions, often resembling the classic childhood diseases. Differentiating features of illnesses with characteristic maculopapular eruptions are shown in Table 242.1.

TABLE 242.1.   Differentiating Features of Selected Diseases with Maculopapular Eruptions

Disease	Ages Most Affected	Typical Seasons	Type/Distribution of Skin and Oral Lesions	Common Associated Symptoms/Signs	Complications
Measles	Children, young adults	Winter, spring	Skin—purple-red maculopapules spreading from the hairline downward, confluent on face and neck Oral mucosa—Koplik's spots	Prodrome of high fever, coryza, cough, conjunctivitis	Common: otitis media, pneumonia Rare: encephalitis, severe laryngotracheitis
Rubella	Children, young adults	Winter, spring	Skin—discrete, pink-red maculopapules spreading from face downward Soft palate—Forchheimer's spots	Children—lymphadenopathy, minimal fever Adolescent/adult—febrile prodrome, joint pains	Common: arthritis in older patients Very rare: encephalitis, purpura Prenatal exposure: congenital rubella syndrome
Roseola infantum	6 mo to 3 yr	Spring, fall, summer	Discrete, small rose-pink macules spreading from trunk to rest of body	High fever for 3–4 days before rash, mild pharyngitis, otitis, and adenopathy	Common: febrile seizures Very rare: encephalitis
Erythema infectiosum	2 to 12 yr	Late winter, spring	1st stage—"slapped-cheek" malar rash 2nd stage—truncal/extremity, rash, fading in lacelike pattern 3rd stage—recurrence of rash with stimuli	Asymptomatic or mild fever	Rare: arthritis (especially in adults), hemolytic anemia, encephalitis, fetal loss
Scarlet fever	3 to 12 yr	Winter, spring	Skin—face flushed with circumoral pallor, trunk/extremities with "sandpapery," blanching pinpoint red rash most prominent in creases, Pastia lines Mucosa—pharyngitis/tonsillitis, palatal petechiae, strawberry tongue	Fever, sore throat, vomiting, abdominal pain, tender anterior cervical nodes	Early: otitis media, peritonsillitis, cervical adenitis Late: rheumatic fever, glomerulonephritis

CLINICAL PRESENTATION OF SPECIFIC DISEASES

Measles

Measles is caused by a paramyxovirus. The incidence of measles has declined greatly since the measles vaccine was first licensed more than 40 years ago. The data reported by the CDC in recent years showed that measles is no longer endemic in the United States (31). A large number of measles cases in the United States have been due to importation from other countries with the majority of these cases occurring in patients older than 20 years of age.

Measles has a 3- to 4-day prodrome, characterized by fever, malaise, and the "3 C's"—cough, coryza, and conjunctivitis. A pathognomonic enanthem known as Koplik spots precedes the rash and consists of small red patches capped by bluish-white specks (resembling sprinkles of salt), seen first on the buccal mucosa opposite the molars, with subsequent spread and coalescence within the mouth. Koplik spots resolve by the second or third day of rash and have often disappeared by the time the patient is seen. The rash appears on the third or fourth day of illness, and consists of purplish-red maculopapules that begin at the hairline and spread downward, tending to be confluent on the face and neck.

A comparison of the progression of skin findings in measles, rubella, and scarlet fever is shown in Figure 242.1. The child with full-blown measles appears miserable ("measly"), with high fever, impressive conjunctivitis, marked cough, and rhinorrhea. The severity of symptoms peaks on the second day of the rash, with subsequent rapid recovery in uncomplicated cases. Measles is highly contagious, with infectivity from about 2 days before onset of illness to 4 days after the rash appears. The virus is transmitted by direct contact with infectious droplets and, less commonly, by airborne. The incubation period is 8 to 12 days from exposure to onset of illness. Immunocompromised patients frequently have atypical presentation and may present with no rash (24).

Otitis media, diarrhea, dehydration, pneumonia, and croup are common complications of measles. Pneumonia is the most common fatal complication of measles. Severe laryngotracheobronchitis has also been reported (42). Encephalitis is a rare complication. However, risks of severe complications such as encephalitis and pneumonitis are much higher in immunocompromised patients (24). While measles is seldom fatal in the United States, it remains one of the leading causes of death worldwide. Mortality rates increase in children younger than 5 years old, immunocompromised patients and those with severe malnutrition.

Rubella

Rubella (German measles) is a mild disease caused by *Rubivirus*. Its major significance is the ability to cause severe illness and birth defects in prenatally infected infants. Since vaccination began, the incidence of rubella and congenital rubella syndrome has declined significantly. The epidemiology of rubella in the United States changed in the past decade. By the end of the 1990s, there was an increase in the number of adult cases, particularly those who were foreign-born, while the incidence in children decreased (40). Likewise, the majority of congenital rubella syndrome infants were born to foreign-born mothers.

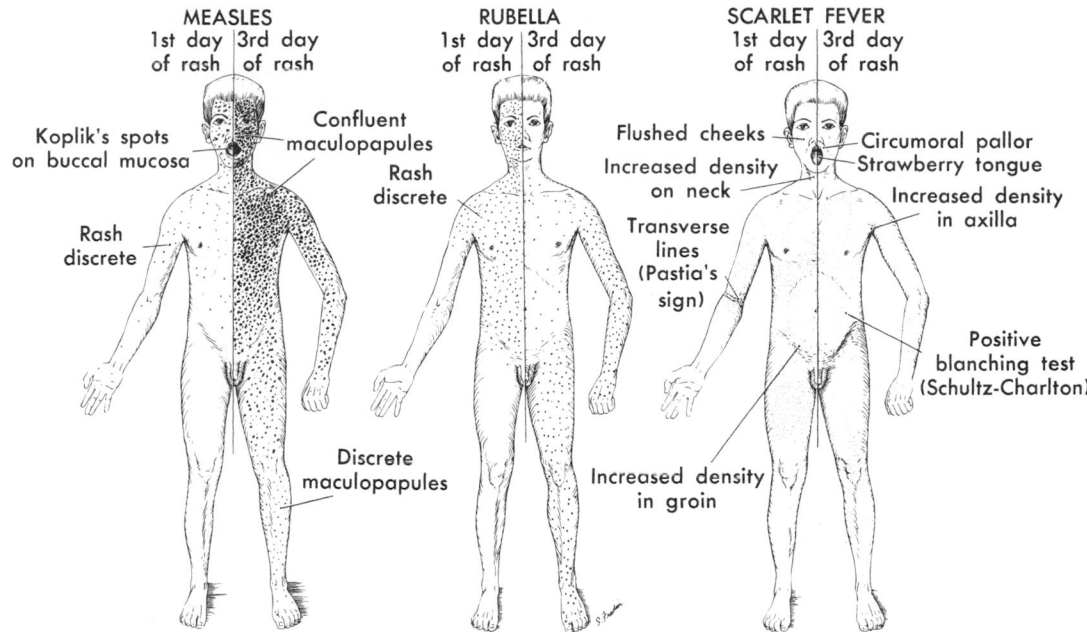

Figure 242.1.   Differences in appearance and progression of rashes in measles, rubella, and scarlet fever. (From Krugman S, et al. *Infectious diseases of children,* 8th ed. St. Louis: CV Mosby, 1985, with permission.)

Symptoms consist of mild fever and acute onset of rash that begins with discrete pink-red maculopapules on the face that rapidly spread downward (see Fig. 242.1). A nonspecific enanthem of small reddish dots on the soft palate (Forchheimer spots) may be seen. The rash often coalesces on the trunk and usually fades within 3 days. Generalized lymphadenopathy, particularly postauricular, suboccipital, and cervical, is typical. Arthralgia and arthritis are rare in children, but can commonly occur in adolescent and adult females. Serious complications, such as encephalitis or thrombocytopenia, are extremely rare. First-trimester prenatal infection may cause miscarriage, still birth or severe congenital anomalies and illness in the fetus, including congenital heart disease, deafness, cataracts, microcephaly or mental retardation, hepatosplenomegaly, and purpura.

Roseola

Roseola infantum (exanthem subitum) is a mild exanthematous illness that occurs most commonly in children between 6 months to 2 years of age (6). Human herpesvirus 6 (HHV-6) is the primary etiologic agent, although human herpesvirus 7 (HHV-7) can cause a similar illness (13). HHV-6 accounts for a significant number of children with acute febrile illness in infants and young children presenting to the ED, especially among those 6 to 12 months of age (20,38). However, approximately 20% of HHV-6 infections present as typical roseola (20).

Classic roseola has a characteristic history of high fever (39–40.5°C) for 3 to 5 days, followed by sudden defeverescence that coincides with the onset of rash. The rash usually appears within 24 to 48 hours of defeverescence and consists of small, discrete, rose-pink macules or maculopapules distributed primarily on the trunk before spreading to the rest of the body. The rash usually resolves within 1 to 2 days. Other associated symptoms and findings include diarrhea, cough, a bulging fontanel, edematous eyelids, erythematous papules on the soft palate and base of the uvula (6). Febrile seizures occur in approximately 10% to 15% of primary HHV-6 infections. Serious complications such as encephalitis are rare.

Erythema Infectiosum

Erythema infectiosum (fifth disease), a common childhood exanthem, is caused by human parvovirus B19. Erythema infectiosum (EI) typically affects school-aged children in epidemics during late winter or early spring. The symptoms begin with a mild, nonspecific illness consisting of fever, malaise, and headache approximately 7 to 10 days before the onset of rash. The skin findings appear in three stages. A bright red raised macular rash on the cheeks that spares the nasal bridge and mouth appears first, giving the child a distinctive "slapped-cheek" appearance. The second stage begins about 1 day later with a symmetric maculopapular rash on the trunk and extremities, which becomes lacy-appearing as confluent areas clear. During the third stage, lasting weeks to months, the rash may reappear with various stimuli, such as bathing, temperature extremes, or local irritation. Adolescent patients can develop transient arthralgia and arthritis, which may occur as a complication of EI or as the primary manifestation of infection.

Parvovirus B19 infections are ubiquitous. In addition to EI, patients with parvovirus B19 infection may have asymptomatic infection, a mild respiratory tract illness with no rash or a rash atypical for EI. Moreover, it can also cause myriad illnesses including aplastic crisis in patients with chronic hemolytic anemia (e.g., sickle cell anemia), chronic anemia in immunocompromised persons, and arthritis. Maternal infection, particularly in the first half of pregnancy, may result in fetal anemia, hydrops, and fetal demise.

Parvovirus B19 is transmitted via respiratory droplets, percutaneous exposure to blood or blood products and vertical transmission from mother to fetus. Patients with EI are most infectious before onset of the rash and unlikely to be contagious after onset of the rash.

Scarlet Fever

Scarlet fever (scarlatina) is a rash seen in association with group A beta-hemolytic streptococcal (GABHS) infections caused by strains producing an erythrogenic toxin. Scarlatiniform rash may also be caused by other organisms, including *Staphylococcus aureus* and *Arcanobacterium haemolyticum*. Scarlet fever is most common in school-aged children in the winter and spring and is more prevalent in temperate or colder climates. The rash occurs most commonly in association with pharyngitis. Other than the occurrence of rash, the epidemiologic features, symptoms, sequelae, and the treatment of scarlet fever are the same as those of streptococcal pharyngitis. The symptoms begin with abrupt onset of fever, headache, vomiting and sore throat. The skin lesions appear within 1 to 2 days, beginning on the trunk and spreading rapidly. The skin has red, blanches, and has fine punctate bumps that feel like sandpaper. The face is often flushed with circumoral pallor. The rash is prominent in skin folds and can exhibit transverse areas of hyperpigmentation with a petechial character in the antecubital fossae, axillary folds and inguinal regions (Pastia lines) (see Fig. 242.1). Desquamation after resolution of symptoms is characteristic.

Exanthems Caused by Other Agents

Many other agents cause nonspecific maculopapular eruptions. Nonspecific cutaneous reactions to viral infection are those that do not have unique clinical presentation of classic childhood exanthems. Nonspecific viral exanthems usually present as diffuse blanchable erythematous macules and papules on the trunk and extremities. Common causes include nonpolio enteroviruses (e.g., coxsackievirus, echovirus, and enterovirus) and respiratory viruses (e.g., adenovirus, rhinovirus, parainfluenza virus, influenza virus, and respiratory syncytial virus). Exanthems associated with Epstain-Barr Virus infection in children are usually maculopapular. Morbilliform erythematous or copper-colored macules and papules may develop in patients with infectious mononucleosis who receive amoxicillin or ampicillin. *Mycoplasma pneumoniae* infections have a wide variety of associated cutaneous eruptions, including maculopapular and urticarial rashes.

DIFFERENTIAL DIAGNOSIS

Many other conditions are associated with maculopapular skin lesions, including drug reactions, rheumatic diseases, and Kawasaki disease. Scarlatiniform rashes can be seen in streptococcal and staphylococcal toxic shock syndromes. Differentiation of viral exanthems from other life-threatening infections, such as meningococcemia and Rocky Mountain spotted fever, which can occasionally present with a benign-appearing rash, is crucial. These possibilities should be considered in the child with severe or unusual symptoms.

EMERGENCY DEPARTMENT EVALUATION

The presumptive diagnosis of viral exanthems is usually made clinically. Specific viral tests may be necessary in some cases when definitive diagnosis is needed such as immunocompromised patients. The results, however, are often not readily available for ED management. The child's overall degree of illness is the most important assessment. A throat culture or rapid strep test (with confirmatory culture if negative) should be obtained if the child has a sore throat or suspected scarlet fever (8). Antibody titers may be useful for confirming suspected cases of measles, rubella, and parvovirus B19 exposure (pregnant contacts). White blood cell counts and blood cultures are helpful in evaluating the ill-appearing child who is suspected of having complications or a more serious disease. Further work up should be aimed at confirming clinically suspected complications such as pneumonia or encephalitis.

EMERGENCY DEPARTMENT MANAGEMENT

A child with an uncomplicated, presumably viral illness should be treated symptomatically with acetaminophen or ibuprofen and oral fluids, antibiotics should be reserved for secondary bacterial infection. Scarlet fever requires antimicrobial treatment to prevent serious acute rheumatic fever. Penicillin is the drug of choice (1,8). The dose of penicillin V is 250 mg given orally 2 to 3 times per day for children weighing less than 27 kg and 500 mg for older children and adolescents. The treatment should be given for 10 days to prevent acute rheumatic fever. A single dose of intramuscular penicillin G benzathine is an alternative to ensure compliance. Erythromycin and azithromycin are alternatives for those allergic to penicillin.

Children with suspected measles or rubella should be isolated within the ED and reported to the health department. Vitamin A deficiency is associated with increased morbidity and mortality from measles (12). Treatment with vitamin A should be considered for selected children with measles, such as children 6 months to 2 years of age hospitalized with complications, and children older than 6 months with immunodeficiency, impaired intestinal absorption, malnutrition, or recent immigration from areas with high measles mortality rates (1).

Live-virus vaccine, if given within 72 hours of measles exposure, will provide protection in some cases. Immune Globulin can be given to prevent or modify measles in a susceptible person within 6 days of exposure. Immune Globulin is indicated for susceptible household contacts of patients with measles, particularly those younger than 1 year of age, pregnant women, and immunocompromised persons. The standard dose is 0.25 ml/kg intramuscularly and 0.5 ml/kg for immunocompromised children (1).

DISPOSITION

A pediatrician or infectious disease specialist should be consulted if the patient appears to have a serious complication, is a neonate, or is immunosuppressed, or if a potentially serious disease is under consideration. Indications for hospitalization include dehydration, pneumonia, measles, croup, encephalitis, and clinical toxicity.

Obstetric follow up should be arranged for pregnant patients who may have been exposed to rubella or parvovirus B19. Children with erythema infectiosum need not be isolated or restricted from school or daycare attendance, because they have already passed their period of infectivity.

Patients discharged home should follow up with their primary care physician or the ED if their illness worsens or does not resolve within the expected time course. Occasionally, the physician or parent may be uncomfortable with a diagnosis of "nonspecific viral exanthem." If the child is not acutely ill, outpatient consultation is appropriate.

Transfer to a tertiary pediatric facility should be considered if the child needs a higher level of care or expertise (e.g., intensive care or sub-specialists) that is not available at the treating facility.

DISEASES WITH VESICULAR OR PUSTULAR LESIONS

Viral vesicular rashes and enanthems are frequently distinctive, allowing a presumptive diagnosis in many cases. The basic approach to the history and physical examination is described earlier in this chapter.

CLINICAL PRESENTATION OF SPECIFIC DISEASES

Varicella

Varicella (chickenpox) is a common childhood exanthematous disease caused by the varicella-zoster virus. Most cases occur in children, but adolescents and adults tend to have a severe course, with more frequent complications. Varicella is most common in late winter and spring. The incidence of varicella has declined in recent years as a result of increased use of varicella vaccine.

Signs and symptoms of varicella in healthy children include mild systemic symptoms, fever, and rash following an incubation period of 10 to 21 days. The skin lesions appear in crops, beginning as macules that rapidly progress to papules, then vesicles that eventually rupture and crust. The classic early vesicle is small and surrounded by erythema, resembling a dewdrop on a rose petal. The first lesions often develop on the face and scalp.

As the rash spreads, lesions of all stages (papules, vesicles, crusts) are characteristically present within a single affected area. Shallow ulcers often occur in the mouth but may also be seen on other mucous membranes. The number of skin lesions generally correlates with the height of fever and severity of symptoms. Pruritus is common, and scarring may result if the lesions are traumatized by severe scratching or become infected. The patient is contagious from 1 day before onset of the rash until all of the lesions are crusted, or until 6 days from the onset of rash.

Secondary bacterial skin infections, usually caused by group A beta-hemolytic streptococcus (GABHS) or *Staphylococcus aureus*, are the most common complications seen in children. In the past decade, there have been increased reports of invasive group GABHS infections associated with chickenpox, including necrotizing fasciitis and streptococcal toxic shock syndrome (11,28). GABHS infection should be suspected in children with varicella who develop localized skin swelling, warmth, redness, or pain, and in those with fever persisting beyond the fourth day of illness or who have recurrence of fever after becoming afebrile (3).

Other serious complications in children include acute cerebellar ataxia, encephalitis, postviral transverse myelitis and Reye's Syndrome. Varicella pneumonia is relatively common in adolescent and adult patients but is less common in immunocompetent children.

Patients with altered cell-mediated immunity, such as children with leukemia receiving chemotherapy, are susceptible to disseminated varicella with hemorrhagic lesions, pneumonitis, and encephalitis. Children with HIV infection can develop chronic or recurrent varicella, with new lesions appearing for months. Severe varicella has also been reported in healthy children receiving intermittent courses of corticosteroids for treatment of asthma or other illnesses (14).

Herpes Zoster

Herpes zoster (shingles) is caused by reactivation of latent varicella-zoster virus in sensory ganglia. Children are less commonly affected than are adults, and younger patients tend to have a less painful course and little postherpetic neuralgia. The characteristic findings include grouped, vesicular lesions in a dermatomal distribution, accompanied by pain and tenderness along the pathway of the nerves involved. The most common sites of zoster infection are the areas supplied by trigeminal nerve and the thoracic ganglia. Fever and local lymphadenopathy are common. The presence of lesions on the tips of the nose signals possible eye involvement.

Herpes Simplex

Primary infection with herpes simplex viruses (HSV) in childhood is extremely common and often asymptomatic. The most common presentation in the ED is acute herpetic gingivostomatitis, usually caused by HSV type 1. It primarily affects children aged 1 to 4 years. Symptoms include high fever, irritability, and reluctance to eat or drink. The child looks uncomfortable, drools, and has marked gingival redness, swelling, and friability. Ulcerations or plaques may be seen on the tongue, buccal mucosa, palate, and pharynx. Vesicles may be present on the lips, and there is tender cervical adenopathy. Lesions can occasionally be seen on the fingers or genitalia from autoinoculation. Dehydration is not uncommon. Symptoms may last 1 to 2 weeks.

Other primary and recurrent herpes infections, including herpes labialis, herpetic whitlow, and herpes keratoconjunctivitis, may be seen in children. Children with atopic dermatitis may develop extensive herpes simplex infection on eczematized areas (eczema herpeticum). Although herpetic vulvovaginitis can be a rare manifestation of innocently acquired primary herpes simplex infection in young children, the possibility of sexual abuse must be strongly considered.

Enteroviruses

Nonpolio enteroviruses are a frequent cause of febrile illnesses and exanthems. Pathogens include group A and B coxsackieviruses, echoviruses, and enteroviruses. Epidemics occur during the summer and fall, affecting primarily 1- to 4-year-old children.

Hand-foot-and-mouth disease is a distinctive clinical syndrome, usually caused by coxsackie A16 and enterovirus 71. Children have fever and lesions on the oral mucosa and tongue that progress from small red macules to vesicles on an erythematous base to discrete ulcers. The exanthem occurs shortly after the enanthem. The skin lesions are oval or linear vesicles (about 3 to 7 mm) surrounded by erythema. They occur on the dorsum of the hands and feet, the interdigital areas, and the palms and soles. Some patients have mild diarrhea or cervical adenopathy.

Cases in which cutaneous findings are absent are referred to as herpangina due to the resemblance to herpes gingivostomatitis. Herpangina presents with fever, sore throat, and dysphagia. Examination discloses small vesicles or punched-out ulcers involving the tonsillar pillars, tonsils, pharynx, and soft palate. The illness resolves in 5 to 6 days.

Clinical manifestations of enteroviral infections can include nonspecific febrile illness, upper respiratory tract infection, stomatitis, exanthem, myopericarditis, vomiting and diarrhea. Aseptic meningitis, encephalitis and paralysis have been reported in children with hand-foot-mouth disease and herpangina (23).

DIFFERENTIAL DIAGNOSIS

Classic varicella is usually easily recognized and laboratory testing is usually not needed. Early cases may require a meticulous search to find the first vesicles. Herpes zoster and herpes simplex infections can overlap in presentation, and viral vesiculopustular lesions are sometimes confused with impetigo. Herpetic gingivostomatitis may be confused with herpangina, Vincent angina, or aphthous stomatitis. Herpetic whitlow is often misdiagnosed as a paronychia. Many other disorders may present with vesicular lesions.

EMERGENCY DEPARTMENT EVALUATION

ED evaluation includes assessment of the child's degree of clinical toxicity, state of hydration, and ability to take oral fluids. Laboratory evaluation is indicated for suspected complications, when the diagnosis is in question, and in high-risk patients in whom definitive diagnosis is necessary. There are numerous testing methods available (e.g., enzyme immunoassay, latex agglutination, indirect fluorescent antibody, fluorescent antibody-to-membrane antigen); the practitioner should consult with the laboratory and pertinent specialists (i.e., infectious diseases), if necessary, to determine the best available methods. Immunofluorescent staining of vesicle scrapings, using monoclonal antibodies, can distinguish between herpes simplex virus and varicella-zoster virus. Tzanck preparation from vesicle scrapings demonstrates multinucleated giant cells with inclusion in both varicella-zoster and herpes simplex infections. While it is a rapid diagnostic test, it has low sensitivity and accuracy.

The diagnosis of enteroviral exanthem can usually be made clinically without laboratory tests. When a specific diagnosis is needed, specimens from the throat, stool, and rectal swabs can be obtained for viral isolation.

EMERGENCY DEPARTMENT MANAGEMENT

Symptomatic therapy for varicella includes acetaminophen and measures to decrease itching and discomfort. Children with varicella should not receive aspirin because of the increased risk of Reye's syndrome. A number of reports found an association between nonsteroidal antiinflammatory drug (NSAID) use and invasive GABHS infections in children with varicella (36,50). A recent multicenter study (29) showed that the use of ibuprofen did not increase the risks of necrotizing GABHS infection, although an association between nonnecrotizing invasive GABHS infection and ibuprofen use was observed. However, the data also showed that ibuprofen was given to children with high fever and severe illness, which identified children at high risk for invasive GABHS infection. Topical measures, such as cool baths, calamine lotion, and colloidal oatmeal baths, may help alleviate pruritus. Oral antihistamines may be helpful for severe itching; topical antihistamines are less desirable because of the risks of sensitization and excessive systemic absorption through nonintact skin.

Antiviral medications have a limited window of opportunity in treatment of varicella-zoster infection. The administration of antiviral medication within 24 hours after the onset of rash results in a modest decrease in symptoms. Oral acyclovir is not recommended for routine use in otherwise healthy children with varicella (1). Oral acyclovir treatment (80 mg/kg/day in 4 divided doses for 5 days; maximum dose, 3200 mg/day) beginning within 24 hours of rash onset should be considered for otherwise healthy children at risk of moderate-to-severe varicella (> 12 years of age, chronic skin or pulmonary disorders, chronic salicylate therapy, and recent treatment short, intermittent, or aerosolized courses of corticosteroids). Intravenous acyclovir is recommended for treatment of immunocompromised patients with varicella-zoster infections and should be initiated early in the course of illness, especially within 24 hours of the onset of the rash. Current recommended dosing regimens for acyclovir and other antiviral agents are best referenced in the American Academy of Pediatrics Red Book (1). Airborne and contact precautions are recommended for patients with varicella for a minimum of 5 days after onset of the rash and as long as vesicular lesions are present. Postexposure prophylaxis includes either Varicella-Zoster Immune Globulin within 96 hours for high risk, susceptible persons or varicella vaccine within 72 hours after varicella exposure for susceptible children.

The use of antiviral medication for nongenital herpes in immunocompetent hosts remains controversial. Limited data are available in pediatric patients. One study showed therapeutic benefits for herpetic gingivostomatitis in children when oral acyclovir was administered within the first three days of the onset (4). Children with frequent recurrent herpes labialis may benefit from continuous oral acyclovir therapy for 1 year (80 mg/kg/day in 3 divided doses; maximum 1 g/day) (1).

Children with oral lesions, especially those with herpetic gingivostomatitis, may refuse to drink. Cold substances such as Popsicles, ice cream, and nonirritating fluids are often accepted. Acetaminophen or ibuprofen usually suffices for symptomatic relief in mild cases. However, children with severe mouth pain may require narcotic analgesia. Oral anesthetics (e.g., viscous lidocaine) are seldom helpful in children with widespread stomatitis and should be used sparingly to avoid toxicity. Intravenous hydration may be required. Antibiotics should be given only for secondary bacterial infections.

DISPOSITION

Children with chickenpox who have significant or rapidly progressing cellulitis should be hospitalized for intravenous antibiotics and carefully observed for the development of necrotizing fasciitis. Neonates or immunocompromised patients with suspected varicella-zoster or herpes simplex infection should be referred to a specialist in infectious disease, oncology, neonatology, or pediatrics. These patients usually require hospitalization for intravenous acyclovir. An ophthalmologist should be consulted when herpes keratoconjunctivitis is suspected.

Children with uncomplicated viral stomatitis or rash are discharged on symptomatic therapy, with outpatient follow up scheduled if further symptoms develop or the child does not improve within a few days.

Transfer to a tertiary pediatric facility should be considered if the child is seriously ill or needs intensive care, or when subspecialty consultation is indicated.

IMPETIGO

Impetigo, a bacterial infection of the superficial layers of the epidermis, is a common bacterial skin infection in children. It is highly contagious and usually transmitted by direct contact. Impetigo affects the entire pediatric population, predominantly in preschool-age children. It is more prevalent during warm, humid summer months in temperate climates, but year round in more tropical climates.

Impetigo is caused by either *Staphylococcus aureus* or group A beta-hemolytic streptococci (*S. pyogenes*), or both. Within the past decade, *S. aureus* has become the predominant pathogen causing impetigo (9,33,43).

CLINICAL PRESENTATION

Two distinct clinical forms have been described; nonbullous and bullous impetigo. Classic or nonbullous impetigo, accounting for approximately 70% of cases, is caused by either *S. aureus* or GABHS or both. Generally, bacterial invasion occurs through a break in the skin traumatized by a scratch, abrasion, or insect bite. The nares and perioral region are most often involved. The lesion begins as a discrete papule or vesicle that erodes and forms a thick, honey-colored crust, but may coalesce with progression of infection. When the crust is removed, a cloudy serous fluid exudes from a moist erythematous base. Bullous impetigo is generally caused by toxin-producing strains of *S. aureus*. The lesions of bullous impetigo are flaccid bullae filled with a cloudy fluid. The bullae are often ruptured before presentation, leaving a shiny, lacquered, erythematous base with peeling edges. The lesions of bullous impetigo develop on intact skin and favor moist intertriginous regions such as neck folds, axilla, anogenital area and buttocks.

The lesions of both forms of impetigo are usually not painful. Fever and systemic involvement are rare, although nonbullous impetigo frequently is accompanied by lymphadenopathy. When treated, impetigo heals completely without scarring. The neonate with bullous impetigo is at risk for systemic involvement. The source of infection is often the nursery where the baby was born. When the possibility of bullous impetigo secondary to *S. aureus* occurs in a neonate in the period 2 weeks post discharge from the nursery, the emergency department should alert the newborn nursery of the possibility of a *S. aureus* epidemic.

Many skin conditions in children become impetiginized, especially varicella, scabies, and atopic dermatitis. Patients with atopic dermatitis have been noted to have an increasing incidence of streptococcal impetigo in addition to increased colonization of *S. aureus* (2).

Acute poststreptococcal glomerulonephritis, a major complication of nonbullous impetigo, has an incidence of 1% to 5%, with higher occurrences during epidemic infections. Patients between 3 and 7 years of age are most commonly affected with a latent period averaging 18 to 21 days. Treatment with antibiotics does not prevent the development of acute glomerulonephritis. Anti-DNAase B titers are often elevated following streptococcal impetigo whereas antistreptolysin-O titers are minimally elevated or absent. Rheumatic fever has not been established as a sequel of impetigo. Other rare but possible complications of impetigo include cellulitis, regional adenitis, osteomyelitis, and sepsis.

DIFFERENTIAL DIAGNOSIS

The diagnosis of impetigo is commonly made on the basis of the typical appearance of the lesions. The differential diagnosis of nonbullous impetigo includes other vesicular or crusted dermatologic conditions or thermal burns. Occasionally, impetigo may be mistaken for cigarette burns, but cigarette burns are usually deeper, more punched-out-appearing lesions and do not have the distribution characteristic of bullous impetigo. Chickenpox is distinguished by the appearance of a macular, papular erythematous rash, which then turns into vesicles. The rash and vesicles start centrally and progress peripherally, appear in crops, may be present on mucous membranes, and are often accompanied by systemic symptoms of illness. Herpes zoster is distinguished by its characteristic dermatomal distribution. Herpes simplex should be suspected when the vesicles have a grouped or tightly coalesced appearance. The child may complain of itching, burning, or pain, and there may be a history of previous occurrences at the same site. Hand-foot-and-mouth disease is usually caused by a coxsackievirus infection. The vesicles are individual, firm, and oval and are most often located on the palms and soles and in the mouth. Scabies is frequently vesicular or pustular in children. Helpful points in differentiation of scabies are its characteristic distribution on the wrists and in the web spaces of the fingers and toes, complaints of intense pruritus, and presence of similar lesions in other family members. Contact dermatitis such as

poison ivy can be vesicular or crusted. There is usually a history of exposure, and the lesions are pruritic and grouped in streaks. Occasionally, tinea corporis may be mistaken for impetigo when the lesions are crusted. Bullous impetigo on the buttocks can be difficult to differentiate from suspected child abuse due to submersion scald burns. Other differential diagnosis of bullous impetigo includes Stevens-Johnson syndrome, necrotizing fasciitis, bullous erythema multiforme and bullous pemphigoid.

EMERGENCY DEPARTMENT EVALUATION

Impetigo can usually be identified by the characteristic appearance of its lesions, and cultures are not indicated routinely. The diagnosis can be confirmed by gram stain and bacterial culture from the lesions. All patients with impetiginized skin conditions need to be treated with antibiotics.

EMERGENCY DEPARTMENT MANAGEMENT

Localized, superficial impetigo with a few lesions to one area of the body can be treated with topical mupirocin (10). Mupirocin should be applied three times daily for 7 to 10 days. Impetigo with multiple lesions or impetigo in multiple family members, child care groups, or athletic team should be treated with systemic antibiotic (1). Because lesions of nonbullous impetigo due to GABHS or *S. aureus* cannot be distinguished clinically, these patients should be treated with antibiotic active against both organisms. Recommended antibiotics include penicillinase-resistant beta-lactam drugs, such as cloxacillin, dicloxacillin, or first- or second-generation cephalosporins. For penicillin-allergic patients, trimethoprim-sulfamethoxazole or clindamycin can be used. Macrolides may be an alternative in individuals who are allergic to penicillin. However, it should not be used as first-line therapy because of emerging erythromycin-resistant *S. aureus*. Infants with bullous impetigo may need admission and intravenous antibiotic therapy if systemic signs of illness are present.

DISPOSITION

Consultation with a dermatologist or infectious disease specialist is generally not required. Rarely does a child need to be admitted to the hospital, except in cases of extensive disease, immunocompromised states, or infants with bullous impetigo with systemic involvement. In most cases, follow up is not indicated unless a satisfactory clinical response is not achieved in 7 days, at which point, a culture of the site is recommended to evaluate for resistance.

SCABIES

Scabies is a highly contagious, pruritic skin rash caused by the mite *Sarcoptes scabiei*. The gravid female mite burrows beneath the skin while laying two to three eggs per day. Eggs hatch after 3 to 4 days, and the larvae migrate toward the surface of the skin, where they mature from the nymph stage into adults in 2 weeks. These adult mites then repeat the cycle. After mating, the adult female migrates more deeply into the skin, continuing the mite's life cycle. The adult female mite, measuring 0.4 mm in length, is barely visible to the human eye. The male, which is much smaller, dies shortly after mating.

Transmission usually occurs via skin-to-skin contact and is common among family members. The incubation period is 10 to 30 days. Symptoms may be delayed up to 3 weeks with initial infestation however, symptoms develop within 1 to 3 days with subsequent infestations. The highest prevalence is in young children.

CLINICAL PRESENTATION

Patients usually present with persistent generalized pruritus which occurs secondary to host sensitization to the mites, its eggs and feces. Itching is typically worse at night and may precede the actual rash. Two typical types of scabies lesions include burrows and erythematous papules. The burrows are most commonly found on the hands, wrists, and genitalia. Other common sites include axillae, umbilicus, buttocks and nipples. The burrow, which is several millimeters in length, consists of serpiginous, gray-white lines. The mite may be visible as a black dot at the leading end. The erythematous papules are most often found on the trunk. The lesions commonly occur on the face and scalp in infants and young children, while these locations are spared in adults. Excoriations are common and may alter the appearance of primary lesions, which can become secondarily infected leading to pustule formation.

Other variations of scabies are less common. Crusted or Norwegian scabies presents with gross scaling, especially of the hands, feet, scalp, and pressure-bearing areas. Pruritus is variable and may be minimal. This form is more likely to be seen in the immunocompromised or debilitated patients. Norwegian scabies is extremely contagious.

DIFFERENTIAL DIAGNOSIS

Atopic dermatitis can be difficult to differentiate from scabies, but it tends not to involve the web spaces, axilla, or wrists. Hand-foot-mouth disease is usually seen with fever and mucosal lesions. Dyshidrotic eczema may manifest as vesicles on the sides of the fingers. Lesions of papular urticaria may resemble those of scabies, but these lesions are self-limited and do not spread over time. Acropustulosis of infancy consists of recurring crops of pruritic papules, vesicles, and pustules. Other considerations in the differential diagnosis include contact dermatitis, dermatitis herpetiformis, syphilis, folliculitis, pityriasis rosea, impetigo, seborrhea, nodular lymphoma, psoriasis, lichen planus, fiberglass exposure, histiocytosis X, and keratosis follicularis.

EMERGENCY DEPARTMENT EVALUATION

Intense pruritus should raise the suspicion of scabies, especially when nocturnal exacerbation of pruritus is present and when similar history is reported in family members. The diagnosis is confirmed by identification of the mite, or its eggs or feces from the scrapings of intact burrows or papules. Mineral oil, microscopic immersion oil, or water applied to the skin facilitates the collection. Scraping can be obtained using a number 15 scalpel. The scrapings and oil are then transferred to a glass slide and examined under low power.

EMERGENCY DEPARTMENT MANAGEMENT

Standard treatment of scabies includes lotion or cream containing a scabicide, which should be applied over the entire body below the head. In infants and young children, the treatment of the entire head, neck and body is required, as the infestation can occur in these locations in this population. The drug of choice, particularly for infants and young children, is 5% permethrin cream (1). Permethrin (5%) cream was found to be effective and less toxic when compared to other agents (45,46). It should be removed by bathing 8 to 14 hours after the application. Alternative drugs include lindane (1%) cream or lotion and crotamiton (10%). Lindane should be removed by bathing after 8 to 12 hours. Crotamiton is applied once a day for 2 days followed by a bath 48 hours after the last application. Central nervous system toxicity including seizure has been reported in children treated with lindane (34). Lindane should not be used in patients with crusted scabies or extensive dermatitis, persons with seizure disorders or hypersensitivity to the product, women who are pregnant or breastfeeding and young infants. Ivermectin has been reported to be effective in treatment of severe or crusted scabies (30,32). Ivermectin should be considered for patients with refractory symptoms or those who cannot tolerate topical therapy (1). However, it is currently not licensed by the US Food and Drug Administration for the treatment of scabies.

Response to treatment is not dependent on the number of lesions present. Pruritus may persist for 1 to 2 weeks and can be treated with oral antihistamines or topical corticosteroids. Antibiotic treatment is indicated for secondary bacterial infection.

DISPOSITION

Follow up with the patient's primary care physician should suffice in most cases. Dermatology consultation may be prudent in severe cases or in immunocompromised patients. Children may return to school or child care after treatment has been completed. All clothing, bedding, and towels contacted within the 2 days prior to treatment should be either washed in hot water, dry cleaned, or stored for 1 week. Household members should be treated simultaneously regardless of symptoms to prevent reinfestation.

HEAD LICE

Head lice (Pediculosis capitis) infestation is common in children. Although it can affect persons in all ages and socioeconomic groups, it is most common among children 3 to 12 years of age, in girls and less common in blacks. The head louse infests only human head and feeds by sucking blood. The female lays approximately 10 eggs per day. The eggs (nits) are firmly attached to the hair shaft close to the scalp with glue-like saliva injected by the lice. This saliva may cause scalp pruritus as a result of sensitivity reaction. The eggs are initially translucent, after hatching the nymphs separate from the egg cases. The empty egg cases, 1 mm long, become white and more visible. After 9 to 12 days, the nymph grows to an adult size of a sesame seed, which is 3 to 4 mm long. Nits remain firmly attached to the hair shaft, moving away from the shaft as the hair grows. Transmission occurs through direct head-to-head contact. Transmission through sharing combs, hairbrushes or hats is much less likely, but cannot be excluded (17).

CLINICAL PRESENTATION

Itching is the most common presentation, although many children are asymptomatic. Adult lice or nits can be found in the hair. Excoriations and crusting secondary to bacterial infection may occur and are often associated with regional lymphadenopathy.

DIFFERENTIAL DIAGNOSIS

Conditions with scalp pruritus or irritation such as tinea capitis, seborrheic dermatitis should be considered.

EMERGENCY DEPARTMENT EVALUATION

A history of exposure and/or intense pruritus should prompt a suspicion of head lice infestation. The gold standard for diagnosing head lice is finding a live louse on the head (17). This is often difficult as adult lice can move rapidly. The nits may be easier to find, especially at the nape of the neck or behind the ears. However, finding nits alone is not an indication for infestation. Most children with nits alone did not become infested in one study (49) and nits may persist for months after successful treatment (41). Using a fine-toothed detection comb may aid in finding the lice and nits (41).

EMERGENCY DEPARTMENT MANAGEMENT

Several pediculocides are available for treatment of head lice. Permethrin (1%) is currently the recommended treatment of choice (17); it has a lower toxicity, high cure rate and possible ovicidal activity. It is available without prescription in a cream rinse that is applied to the scalp and hair. The cream is left on for 10 minutes and then rinsed off. Although its activity continues for 2 weeks or longer after the application, most experts recommend that a second application be done 7 to 10 days after the first (1).

Pyrethrin-based products are available in shampoos without prescription. The shampoos are applied to dry hair and left on for 10 minutes before rinsing out. Ovicidal activity is low and a repeat application 7 to 10 days later is necessary to kill newly hatched lice.

Malathion (0.5%) is an organophosphate available by prescription as a lotion. It is applied to the hair, left air dry, and then rinsed off after 8 to 12 hours. Malathion is highly effective, however a second application in 7 to 9 days is recommended if lice are still seen at that time. Malathion has high alcohol content; therefore it is highly flammable and can cause severe respiratory depression if accidentally ingested. It is contraindicated in neonates and infants.

Lindane (1%) is indicated primarily for patients who have not responded to or are intolerant to other therapies (1). It is available by prescription as a shampoo that should be left on no longer than 10 minutes. Ovicidal activity is low and repeat application in 7 to 10 days is recommended.

Resistance has been reported with lindane, pyrethrins, and permethrin (37). Other agents found to be effective in treatment of head lice include Sulfamethoxazole/Trimethoprim in combination with 1% permethrin (21) and ivermectin (16). These agents, however, are not licensed by the US Food and Drug Administration for the treatment of head lice.

DISPOSITION

Children may return to school on the day after treatment regardless of the presence of nits (1,41). Nit removal after treatment with a pediculicide is not necessary to prevent spread (17). It may be done for aesthetic reason or to decrease diagnostic confusion. Household and close contacts should be examined. Those with live lice or nits within 1 cm of the scalp should be treated. Bedmates should be treated prophylactically. Although fomite transmission is less likely than direct head-to-head transmission, parents should clean hair care items and bedding. Hair care items can be washed with a pediculicide shampoo or soaked in hot water. Bedding can be washed in hot water and machine dried in hot cycle. Detection of living lice on scalp 24 hours or more after the treatment suggests incorrect use of pediculicide, a very heavy infestation, reinfestation, or resistance to the pediculicide.

ENTEROBIASIS (PINWORMS)

Pinworm infestation is caused by a small nematode, *Enterobius vermicularis*. The prevalence is greatest in preschool and school-aged children, family contacts and institutionalized population. Infestation often clusters in families and does not equate with poor home sanitary measures.

E. vermicularis is an obligate parasite, with humans as the only natural host. Fecal–oral contamination via fomites, such as toys and clothes, is a common method of infestation. After ingestion, eggs usually hatch in the duodenum within 6 hours. Worms mature in as little as 2 weeks. Adult worms normally inhabit the terminal ileum, cecum, vermiform appendix, and proximal ascending colon. The worms live free in the intestinal lumen, and little evidence exists to support invasion of healthy tissue under normal conditions. The female worm migrates to the rectum after copulation. If not expelled during defecation, she migrates to the perineum usually at nighttime to release eggs and then dies. The movement of the female worms and the eggs cause intense local pruritus.

CLINICAL PRESENTATION

The majority of patients with pinworm infestation are asymptomatic, while those with symptoms have pruritus ani, restlessness at night, and rarely pruritus vulvae and vulvovaginitis. Vulvovaginitis in prepubertal girls, presenting with vaginal discharge of several weeks' or months' duration, is a result of migration of the adult worm from the perineum or the secondary bacterial infection from repeated scratching of the perineum that spreads to the vulvovaginal area.

DIFFERENTIAL DIAGNOSIS

Other diagnoses to consider include cervicitis, dermatitis, contact dermatitis, giardiasis, inflammatory bowel disease, appendicitis, roundworm or tapeworm infestation, and vulvovaginitis.

EMERGENCY DEPARTMENT EVALUATION

Patients often have excoriation or erythema of the perineum and/or vulvae, but the infestation can occur without these signs. The diagnosis is made when the adult worms are visualized on the patient's perineum at night. Alternatively, a wide transparent tape pressed against the perineum in the morning before the patient washes can be used to search for the eggs. Diagnosis is made by identifying eggs under the low-power lens of the microscope, using a slide to which dilute sodium hydroxide or toluene is added.

EMERGENCY DEPARTMENT MANAGEMENT

Treatment of pinworms is via family education and medications administered as an outpatient. Fear and guilt are common parental reactions to parasitic worm infestation. Many families come to the emergency department with misconceptions about pinworms. It is helpful to inform them that infestation occurs in spite of proper child and household hygiene. Families also should be counseled to avoid overreaction through aggressive sanitary measures. The drugs of choice are pyrantel pamoate (11 mg/kg; maximum, 1 gram as suspension or capsule), mebendazole (100 mg as a chewable tablet), and albendazole (400 mg), given in a single dose with a repeat treatment in 2 weeks (1). Symptomatic relief of pruritus can be obtained by applying topical antipruritic ointments or creams (1% hydrocortisone) to the perianal region.

DISPOSITION

Consultation and admission are generally not required unless more serious conditions cannot be ruled out. Because asymptomatic infestation of other members in a household is frequent, treatment of the entire household is recommended. The family should be informed that repeat infestations are common. If reinfestation occurs, it should be treated in the same fashion as an initial infestation. Measures such as clipping fingernails, washing hands frequently, showering daily in the morning, and normal laundering of linen weekly can prevent recurrence.

TINEA CAPITIS

Tinea capitis is a fungal infection of the scalp, mostly affecting school-aged children. The incidence is higher in African-American children. Most cases of tinea capitis in the United States are caused by *Trichophyton tonsurans*, and less commonly by *Microsporum canis* and *Microsporum audouinii*. Spread occurs as a result of person-to-person transmission.

CLINICAL PRESENTATION

Tinea capitis has variable presenting features. The patient may have one of the following presentations:

- "Seborrheic" type: patches of dandruff-like scaling, with subtle or extensive hair loss. This is the usual form of tinea capitis caused by *T. tonsurans* (60% of cases).
- "Black dot" type: swollen stubs of broken off hairs within the discrete areas of alopecia
- Numerous discrete pustules with little hair loss or scaling
- Kerion: boggy, localized swelling surrounded by follicular pustules often accompanied by fever and cervical lymphadenopathy.

Dermatophytid or id reaction, a hypersensitivity response to the fungus, may be observed in patients with tinea capitis. The id reaction presents as pruritic, small papules or scaling papules, usually more intense on the face and the upper torso.

DIFFERENTIAL DIAGNOSIS

Differential diagnosis of tinea capitis includes alopecia areata, dandruff, seborrheic dermatitis, atopic dermatitis, folliculitis, impetigo and trichotillomania. Diffuse pustular tinea capitis is often incorrectly treated with antibiotic. Although there may be bacterial colonization in diffuse pustular type, the main pathogen is the dermatophyte. Kerion is commonly misdiagnosed as cellulitis or abscess of the scalp.

EMERGENCY DEPARTMENT EVALUATION

Once the clinical diagnosis of tinea capitis is suspected, it can be confirmed with potassium hydroxide wet mount examination and culture of scalp scale and broken off hair. Samples can be obtained by gentle scraping with blunt scalpel, toothbrush, moistened cotton swab or tweezers. Potassium hydroxide wet mount examination is a rapid method; in *T. tonsurans* infection, numerous arthroconidia can be found within the hair shaft, while spores surrounding the hair shaft are found in *Microsporum* infection. A potassium hydroxide preparation can be difficult to interpret and may be falsely negative in early or inflammatory lesions. The ultimate diagnosis is made by culture. Wood lamp examination reveals a bright green fluorescence when the infection is due to *Microsporum*, but not in the case of *T. tonsurans* infection, and therefore it is not a helpful diagnostic tool in most cases.

EMERGENCY DEPARTMENT MANAGEMENT

Tinea capitis requires systemic antifungal therapy. Topical antifungal therapy is ineffective due to its inability to penetrate the hair shaft to clear the infection. The current standard treatment of tinea capitis is griseofulvin. The treatment options include microsize griseofulvin 15 to 20 mg/kg/day given orally once daily or ultramicrosize griseofulvin 5 to 10 mg/kg/day once daily (1). Treatment is recommended for 4 to 6 weeks and it should be continued 2 weeks beyond the clinical resolution. Concerns that the pathogens are less sensitive to griseofulvin have increased and most specialists use doses of 20 to 25 mg/kg/day for 6 to 8 weeks (19). Oral itraconazole, fluconazole and terbinafide are effective for treatment of tinea capitis (18,19), however these medications have not been licensed by the US Food and Drug Administration for treatment of tinea capitis. In kerion, systemic corticosteroid therapy, consisting of prednisone or prednisolone 1.5 to 2 mg/kg/day given orally for 2 weeks, may be added to griseofulvin therapy (1). The doses should be tapered toward the end of therapy. Adjunctive therapy with selenium sulfide shampoo is effective in reducing the shedding of the organism and the spread of the disease. Personal hair items should not be shared by family members.

ATOPIC DERMATITIS

Atopic dermatitis is a highly pruritic chronic inflammatory skin disease that usually presents during early infancy and childhood, with onset before 7 years of age in 80% to 90% of the cases. Though commonly referred to as eczema, atopic dermatitis is a disease among a group of eczematous diseases including nummular dermatitis, seborrheic dermatitis and hand eczema. The estimated lifetime prevalence is 10% to 20% in children (44). The frequency of atopic dermatitis has also increased substantially during the recent decades. Interactions between susceptibility genes, the host's environment, pharmacologic abnormalities, and immunologic factors contribute to the pathogenesis of atopic dermatitis. There are clear associations between atopic dermatitis and other allergic disorders including asthma (15). Among these are elevated serum IgE and peripheral eosinophilia found in patients with atopic dermatitis as well as other allergic diseases. Atopic dermatitis is frequently the first manifestation of an atopic diathesis and up to 80% of children with atopic dermatitis will eventually developed allergic rhinitis or asthma later in childhood (15). Atopic dermatitis is a familial transmitted disease; it also shares genetic determinants with asthma (15).

Exacerbating factors of atopic dermatitis include xerosis (dry skin), irritants, aeroallergens, food, infections, psyche, temperature and climate.

CLINICAL PRESENTATION

The essential features of atopic dermatitis include pruritus, typical morphology and distribution in facial and extensor areas in infants and children, flexural lichenification in adolescence, chronic or relapsing dermatitis, and personal or family history of atopic diseases (e.g., asthma, allergic rhinitis, and atopic dermatitis). The character and the distribution of the skin lesions often vary with age of the patient. In infants, the symptoms usually begin between 6 weeks to 6 months of age. The eruption starts on the face and scalp and consists of intensely pruritic erythematous papules associated with excoriation and serous exudates, it then spreads to the trunk and extensor surface of extremities. The eruption in children and adolescents usually consists of ill-defined, erythematous, scaly patches and usually distributes on flexural folds of extremities. Lichenification develops secondary to persistent scratching and rubbing. Many patients with atopic dermatitis may also develop bacterial, viral or fungal infections exacerbating and complicating their disease. Flares of atopic dermatitis often are associated with bacterial infection, predominantly *Staphylococcus aureus*, and the lesions have honey-crusted weeping pustules presentation.

DIFFERENTIAL DIAGNOSIS

Seborrheic dermatitis is the disease most often confused with atopic dermatitis. However, seborrheic dermatitis typically has onset at birth or before 6 weeks of age. It also involves the intertriginous areas and is usually not pruritic. Contact dermatitis may be confused with atopic dermatitis. The lesions of contact dermatitis are less intensely pruritic and involve the area of contact with the responsible agent. Patients with scabies may present with severely pruritic eczematous dermatitis. The linear papulovesicular lesions are characteristic of scabies. Wiskott-Aldrich syndrome and Hyper-IgE syndrome should be considered in patients with severe eczematous eruptions. These patients usually have severe or recurrent infections.

EMERGENCY DEPARTMENT EVALUATION

The diagnosis of atopic dermatitis in the ED can be made clinically, based on the history and clinical manifestation. The essential features mentioned above can distinguish atopic dermatitis from other skin disorders. Family history of atopic diseases should raise a high suspicion of atopic dermatitis in children who present with a pruritic rash. Specific diagnostic testing may be needed to rule out other differential diagnoses such as scabies. Culture from the lesions should be sent in patients with bacterial or viral infections.

EMERGENCY DEPARTMENT MANAGEMENT

Treatment of atopic dermatitis involves several approaches including skin care, avoiding exacerbating factors, and pharmacologic treatment. Hydration is essential in treatment. Patients should be advised to limit the frequency and length of bathing and to use mild, moisturizing soaps or nonsoap cleanser. Emollients should be applied to the skin within a few minutes after bathing and throughout the day. Avoidance of irritants such as wool clothing, excessive heat and perspiration is important. Topical corticosteroids are the mainstay treatment of atopic dermatitis and are used for acute flare-ups. Suggested topical corticosteroids include hydrocortisone 1% ointment or cream for mild disease and fluticasone propionate 0.005% ointment or 0.05% cream, mometasone furoate 0.1% cream, or prednicarbate 0.1% cream for moderate to severe disease (39). Most corticosteroids can be applied thinly over the affected area twice daily for 7 to 14 days. The use of higher potency topical corticosteroids and prolonged treatments are associated with complications such as skin atrophy, telangiectasia, bruising, infection, and suppression of the hypothalamic-pituitary-adrenal axis. Low potency corticosteroids should be used for the face because of the risk of developing telangiectasia in this area. Ointment is generally preferred over cream because of its occlusive property, which results in better penetration of corticosteroids. Although existing data suggested that histamine is not a major pruritogen in atopic dermatitis without urticaria (47) and some data suggested that nonsedating antihistamines were not beneficial in treatment of pruritus in patients with atopic dermatitis (7,25), both nonsedating and sedating antihistamines may be beneficial for controlling pruritus in individual patients. Sedating antihistamine such as hydroxyzine and diphenhydramine can be used at bedtime for sedative effect. Oral antibiotics may be necessary when bacterial infection is causing or complicating the acute flare. Penicillin-resistant *Staphyloccus aureus* is the most common causative organism. Dicloxacillin or first generation cephalosporins may be used as first line therapy. Erythromycin and clindamycin can be used in patients with penicillin allergy.

EMERGENCY DEPARTMENT DISPOSITION

Patients with severe symptoms or those who do not respond to short course topical steroids should be referred to allergists or dermatologists. In addition, patients with moderate to severe symptoms should also be evaluated for specific allergens. A significant percentage of patients have symptomatic food allergy.

PITYRIASIS ROSEA

Pityriasis rosea is typically seen in adolescents and young adults.

CLINICAL PRESENTATION

Although the etiology is unknown, patients may report a prodrome of pharyngitis and lymphadenopathy. Most cases present with a single scaly patch approximately 2 to 5 cm in diameter which is known as the "herald patch." Secondary small oval patches then appear on the trunk parallel to the skin's cleavage line, forming a "Christmas tree" pattern. The face and extremities are typically not involved. The herald patch resolves before the other lesions which can take up to 3 months to completely disappear. Patients also may complain of itching.

DIFFERENTIAL DIAGNOSIS

While the herald patch may be mistaken for tinea corporis, nummular eczema and drug eruptions, the most important look-alike lesion is that of secondary syphilis. Sexually active patients should undergo serologic testing.

EMERGENCY DEPARTMENT MANAGEMENT

After secondary syphilis is excluded, management of pityriasis rosea is symptomatic. Sunlight, topical lubricants as well as antihistamines help with the pruritus.

DIAPER DERMATITIS

Diaper dermatitis is a nonspecific term used to describe a variety of dermatologic conditions that occur in the diaper area. Diaper dermatitis is the most common dermatologic problem seen in infants and children, with a peak incidence at 9 to 12 months of age.

The cause of diaper dermatitis can be complex. Several factors contribute to the pathophysiology of diaper dermatitis. These include friction, prolonged contact between the skin and diaper, moisture, and contact with urine and feces and their degradation products.

The practice of using disposable diapers has become commonplace, and use of the traditional cloth diaper has become relatively uncommon in the United States. The disposable diaper, with its exterior plastic film, maintains humidity and heat between the skin and the diaper, predisposing to the growth of *Candida albicans* and bacteria. The modern superabsorbent disposable diapers containing absorbent gelling materials, which absorb fluid many times their weight and store away the absorbed fluid from the skin, reduce the frequency and severity of diaper dermatitis (35).

Alterations in gastrointestinal flora due to viral infections or antibiotic use contribute in particular to the development of candidal dermatitis with satellite lesions. The most frequently seen diaper rash occurs after onset of diarrhea caused by gastroenteritis or associated with antibiotic therapy. The usual sequence of skin changes following the onset of diarrhea is an initial hyperemia to the skin covered by the diaper, with development of candidal colonization within 3 days. As the diarrhea continues, the initial candidal colonization may progress to development of satellite *C. albicans* lesions. The infant may experience pain due to the irritation of cleaning solutions or commercially prepared wipes, or the skin may become excoriated and secondarily infected with bacteria.

CLINICAL PRESENTATION

The infant is usually brought for medical attention because the diaper rash has been prolonged or unresponsive to over-the-counter preparations or is worsening in severity and extent.

Diaper rash due to irritation is common and may be divided into causes such as mechanical, intertrigo, miliaria, and contact irritation. Mechanical irritation is caused by constant friction of the wet, excessively hydrated skin of the diaper area against both the diaper and skin folds. It is aggravated by frequent over vigorous cleansing. The infant's diaper area appears chafed, with shiny, erythematous patches that tend to wax and wane in severity. Any diaper dermatitis induced by other factors can be aggravated by mechanical irritation.

Intertrigo occurs in areas where skin surfaces are apposed, such as the groin or intergluteal cleft. It is produced when heat, moisture, and sweat retention combine to cause maceration and irritation. Intertrigo is characterized by red denuded areas in the skin folds.

Miliaria rubra, or prickly heat, is the result of contact of the hot, moist diaper with the infant's skin. It is characterized by small, clear superficial vesicles that are nonerythematous in the newborn, or by small erythematous papules and pustules in the older infant.

There are two types of contact irritation: allergic and primary irritant. Allergic contact diaper dermatitis is caused by the development of sensitivity to detergents, chemicals in the diaper, or creams and medications used in the diaper area. The rash of contact dermatitis usually begins with tiny erythematous vesicles that rupture and adopt an eczematous appearance. The distribution of the rash is characteristic and involves skin surfaces in contact with the diaper, such as the convexities of the buttocks, the medial thighs, and scrotum, while the skin folds are spared.

Primary irritant contact dermatitis is thought to be caused by the effect of noxious components of urine and feces on skin that is already sensitive or irritated from other causes (5). Primary irritant dermatitis is most often described as a parchment-like erythema, resembling a scald that involves the convex surfaces. In boys, inflammation of the urethral meatus is common.

C. albicans is commonly found in the gastrointestinal tract of infants and is frequently implicated as a cause of diaper rash. The rash consists of small, beefy-red papules that may be coalesced centrally but appear to spread outward as small satellite lesions. Usually, the perianal area and skin folds are spared. Candida may be introduced to the diaper area from gastrointestinal tract via oral candidiasis (thrush) consisting of white plaques on the buccal mucosa, tongue and gingivae.

DIFFERENTIAL DIAGNOSIS

Numerous other skin conditions that are not directly caused by diaper wearing have a predilection for the diaper area. Seborrheic dermatitis is common in infancy and appears at 3 or 4 weeks of age. Most cases subside spontaneously by 3 to 4 months of age. Seborrheic dermatitis is characterized by a sharply demarcated zone of erythema that commonly starts in the skin folds and spreads out over convex skin areas. It may be accompanied by small papules that are similar in appearance to the satellite lesions of *C. albicans*. Seborrheic dermatitis can be distinguished from intertrigo by the involvement of other areas of the body, such as the axilla, face, and scalp. Lesions of scabies may be prominent in diaper area. Herpes simplex infection is usually either congenitally acquired or caused by sexual abuse. The lesions are small singular, coalescing, or grouped vesicles that rupture to form small crusted ulcers on an erythematous base. Staphylococcal scalded skin syndrome has sudden onset of rash which is rapidly spreading and painful to touch or with voiding and stooling.

Other less common causes of diaper rash should be considered when clinical presentation varies or response to therapy is not adequate. These include syphilis, Letterer-Siwe disease, psoriasis, Langerhans cell histiocytosis (histiocytosis X), granuloma gluteale infantum and nutritional disorders.

EMERGENCY DEPARTMENT EVALUATION

The diagnosis can usually be established on the basis of history and physical examination. The history should include the use of creams and medications, especially antibiotics that may alter gastrointestinal flora and any recent gastroenteritis with accompanying diarrhea. Diagnostic errors occur because of failure to do a full physical examination to rule out underlying conditions that may present as a diaper rash.

Diaper dermatitis is common and usually easily diagnosed and treated. Because more serious clinical entities must be differentiated, several clinical caveats are in order:

- Seborrheic dermatitis in an infant younger than 6 months of age that does not respond to conventional therapy should alert the physician to the possibility of Letterer-Siwe disease.
- Diaper dermatitis may be secondarily infected with yeast or bacteria and should be treated accordingly.
- When sexually transmitted disease such as herpes simplex virus is the cause of diaper rash, the possibility of congenital infection or sexual abuse must be entertained.
- Psoriasis presents after the resolution of another primary skin condition and may lack the typical thick, silvery scale.

EMERGENCY DEPARTMENT MANAGEMENT

The management of diaper rash begins with a discussion of the pathophysiology of the rash in terms that the parents can understand. The ED physician must explain the effects that infrequent diaper changes, prolonged exposure of the skin to urine and stool, diarrhea, and antibiotic use have on the production of diaper rashes.

The prevention and treatment of diaper dermatitis aim to keep the skin dry and protected. Removing the diaper takes away the friction, occlusion and overhydration. The infant should be allowed to sleep on an open diaper and the diaper area should be exposed to air as long as possible. Frequent diaper changes with the superabsorbent disposable diapers are recommended. The application of water-repellent emollient is recommended at each diaper change as a barrier from skin overhydration and irritants; these include over-the-counter paste, cream and ointment containing zinc oxide and petrolatum. Topical steroids should be limited to the lowest effective strength given for the short course. 1% Hydrocortisone cream or ointment is usually effective in mild irritant diaper dermatitis.

Infection with *C. albicans* is common and may be treated with a topical clotrimazole, miconazole, or nystatin cream twice daily. The preparation containing combination of antifungal and mid-to-high potency topical corticosteroids is not recommended for use in infants and children (27). Systemic and local adverse effects of these topical steroids such as skin atrophy, hirsutism, growth retardation, and Cushing's syndrome have been observed in children (27). If thrush is a consideration, oral nystatin suspension, 1 mL three times a day for 5 to 7 days, is prescribed.

CRITICAL INTERVENTIONS

- Avoid potentially toxic preparations such as oral viscous lidocaine or topical diphenhydramine
- Children with benign, nonspecific febrile exanthems do not need lengthy diagnostic evaluation unless they are ill-appearing
- Explain to parents the innocent acquisition of most childhood infections, to avoid confusion and anxiety particularly if the term *herpes infection* is used
- Children with vesicular skin infections or stomatitis are often uncomfortable, and their parents are frequently frustrated. Give reassurance and careful explanations about the expected course, communicability, and self-limited nature of the disease
- Antibiotics should be prescribed only for the infrequent superimposed bacterial infection
- Do not prescribe repeated courses of lindane, due to its cumulative neurotoxicity

COMMON PITFALLS

✔ Overlooking the subtle signs of scarlet fever, especially in children with minimal pharyngitis

✔ Failing to differentiate impetigo from burns due to child abuse
✔ Failing to recognize that bullous impetigo in neonates may be related to a staphylococcal nursery epidemic
✔ Giving inadequate anticipatory guidance. It is important to inform the patient and family that pruritus may not subside for several weeks despite successful treatment
✔ Failure to treat all household contacts of patients with scabies simultaneously can result in reinfestation
✔ Failure to recognize secondary infection in patients with diaper dermatitis
✔ Overuse of potent corticosteroids in the perineal area

Acknowledgments

Thanks to the previous edition's chapter authors Lindsey Alan Johnson, Mary A. Hegenbarth, Jeffrey G. Michael and Jane F. Knapp, R. Wayne Wolfram, Kevin R. Kowaleski, Eugene Izsak, and Amy S. Spangler.

References

1. AAP. Red Book: 2003 Report of the Committee on Infectious Diseases. Elk Grove Village, IL, 2003.
2. Adachi J, Endo K, Fukuzumi T, Tanigawa N, Aoki T. Increasing incidence of streptococcal impetigo in atopic dermatitis. *J Dermatol Sci* 1998;17:45–53.
3. American Academy of Pediatrics. Committee on Infectious Diseases. Severe invasive group A streptococcal infections: a subject review. *Pediatrics* 1998; 101:136–140.
4. Amir J, Harel L, Smetana Z, Varsano I. Treatment of herpes simplex gingivostomatitis with aciclovir in children: a randomised double blind placebo controlled study. *BMJ* 1997;7097:1800–1803.
5. Andersen PH, Bucher AP, Saeed I, et al. Faecal enzymes: in vivo human skin irritation. *Contact Dermatitis* 1994;30:152–158.
6. Asano Y, Yoshikawa T, Suga S, et al. Clinical features of infants with primary human herpesvirus 6 infection (exanthem subitum, roseola infantum). *Pediatrics* 1994;93:104–108.
7. Berth-Jones J, Graham-Brown RA. Failure of terfenadine in relieving the pruritus of atopic dermatitis. *Br J Dermatol* 1989;121:635–637.
8. Bisno AL, Gerber MA, Gwaltney JM, Jr. , Kaplan EL, Schwartz RH. Practice guidelines for the diagnosis and management of group A streptococcal pharyngitis. Infectious Diseases Society of America. *Clin Infect Dis* 2002;35:113–125.
9. Bisno AL, Stevens DL. Streptococcal infections of skin and soft tissues. *N Engl J Med* 1996;334:240–245.
10. Britton JW, Fajardo JE, Krafte-Jacobs B. Comparison of mupirocin and erythromycin in the treatment of impetigo. *J Pediatr* 1990;117:827–829.
11. Brogan TV, Nizet V, Waldhausen JH, Rubens CE, Clarke WR. Group A streptococcal necrotizing fasciitis complicating primary varicella: a series of fourteen patients. *Pediatr Infect Dis J* 1995;14:588–594.
12. Butler JC, Havens PL, Sowell AL, et al. Measles severity and serum retinol (vitamin A) concentration among children in the United States. *Pediatrics* 1993;91:1176–1181.
13. Caserta MT, Hall CB, Schnabel K, Long CE, D'Heron N. Primary human herpesvirus 7 infection: a comparison of human herpesvirus 7 and human herpesvirus 6 infections in children. *J Pediatr* 1998;133:386–389.
14. Dowell SF, Bresee JS. Severe varicella associated with steroid use. *Pediatrics* 1993;92:223–228.
15. Eichenfield LF, Hanifin JM, Beck LA, et al. Atopic dermatitis and asthma: parallels in the evolution of treatment. *Pediatrics* 2003;111:608–616.
16. Elgart GW, Meinking TL. Ivermectin. *Dermatol Clin* 2003;21:277–282.
17. Frankowski BL, Weiner LB. Head lice. *Pediatrics* 2002;110:638–643.
18. Friedlander SF, Aly R, Krafchik B, et al. Terbinafine in the treatment of Trichophyton tinea capitis: a randomized, double-blind, parallel-group, duration-finding study. *Pediatrics* 2002;109:602–607.
19. Friedlander SF. The evolving role of itraconazole, fluconazole and terbinafine in the treatment of tinea capitis. *Pediatr Infect Dis J* 1999;18:205–210.
20. Hall CB, Long CE, Schnabel KC, et al. Human herpesvirus-6 infection in children. A prospective study of complications and reactivation. *N Engl J Med* 1994;331:432–438.
21. Hipolito RB, Mallorca FG, Zuniga-Macaraig ZO, Apolinario PC, Wheeler-Sherman J. Head lice infestation: single drug versus combination therapy with one percent permethrin and trimethoprim/sulfamethoxazole. *Pediatrics* 2001;107:E30.
22. Ho VC, Gupta A, Kaufmann R, et al. Safety and efficacy of nonsteroid pimecrolimus cream 1% in the treatment of atopic dermatitis in infants. *J Pediatr* 2003;142:155–162.
23. Huang CC, Liu CC, Chang YC, et al. Neurologic complications in children with enterovirus 71 infection. *N Engl J Med* 1999;341:936–942.
24. Kaplan LJ, Daum RS, Smaron M, McCarthy CA. Severe measles in immunocompromised patients. *JAMA* 1992;267:1237–1241.
25. Klein PA, Clark RA. An evidence-based review of the efficacy of antihistamines in relieving pruritus in atopic dermatitis. *Arch Dermatol* 1999;135:1522–1525.

26. Kristal L, Klein PA. Atopic dermatitis in infants and children. An update. *Pediatr Clin North Am* 2000;47:877–895.

27. La Grenade L VA, Luke MC. Adverse Effects of Lotrisone Cream Used in Infants. *Pediatrics* 2000;106:1519.

28. Laupland KB, Davies HD, Low DE, et al. Invasive group A streptococcal disease in children and association with varicella-zoster virus infection. Ontario Group A Streptococcal Study Group. *Pediatrics* 2000;105:E60.

29. Lesko SM, O'Brien KL, Schwartz B, Vezina R, Mitchell AA. Invasive group A streptococcal infection and nonsteroidal antiinflammatory drug use among children with primary varicella. *Pediatrics* 2001;107:1108–1115.

30. Marliere V, Roul S, Labreze C, Taieb A. Crusted (Norwegian) scabies induced by use of topical corticosteroids and treated successfully with ivermectin. *J Pediatr* 1999;135:122–124.

31. Measles–United States, 2000. *MMWR Morb Mortal Wkly Rep* 2002;51:120–123.

32. Meinking TL, Taplin D, Hermida JL, Pardo R, Kerdel FA. The treatment of scabies with ivermectin. *N Engl J Med* 1995;333:26–30.

33. Misko ML, Terracina JR, Diven DG. The frequency of erythromycin-resistant Staphylococcus aureus in impetiginized dermatoses. *Pediatr Dermatol* 1995;12:12–15.

34. Nordt SP, Chew G. Acute lindane poisoning in three children. *J Emerg Med* 2000;18:51–53.

35. Odio M, Friedlander SF. Diaper dermatitis and advances in diaper technology. *Curr Opin Pediatr* 2000;12:342–346.

36. Peterson CL, Vugia DJ, Meyers HB, et al. Risk factors for invasive group A streptococcal infections in children with varicella: a case-control study. *Pediatr Infect Dis J* 1996;15:151–156.

37. Pollack RJ, Kiszewski A, Armstrong P, et al. Differential permethrin susceptibility of head lice sampled in the United States and Borneo. *Arch Pediatr Adolesc Med* 1999;153:969–973.

38. Pruksananonda P, Hall CB, Insel RA, et al. Primary human herpesvirus 6 infection in young children. *N Engl J Med* 1992;326:1445–1450.

39. Raimer SS. Managing pediatric atopic dermatitis. *Clin Pediatr* 2000;39:1–14.

40. Reef SE, Frey TK, Theall K, et al. The changing epidemiology of rubella in the 1990s: on the verge of elimination and new challenges for control and prevention. *JAMA* 2002;287:464–472.

41. Roberts RJ. Clinical practice. Head lice. *N Engl J Med* 2002;346:1645–1650.

42. Ross LA, Mason WH, Lanson J, Deakers TW, Newth CJ. Laryngotracheobronchitis as a complication of measles during an urban epidemic. *J Pediatr* 1992;121:511–515.

43. Sadick NS. Current aspects of bacterial infections of the skin. *Dermatol Clin* 1997;15:341–9.

44. Schultz Larsen FHJ. Epidemiology of atopic dermatitis. *Immun Allerg Clin North Am* 2002;22:1.

45. Schultz MW, Gomez M, Hansen RC, et al. Comparative study of 5% permethrin cream and 1% lindane lotion for the treatment of scabies. *Arch Dermatol* 1990;126:167–170.

46. Taplin D, Meinking TL, Chen JA, Sanchez R. Comparison of crotamiton 10% cream (Eurax) and permethrin 5% cream (Elimite) for the treatment of scabies in children. *Pediatr Dermatol* 1990;7:67–73.

47. Wahlgren CF. Itch and atopic dermatitis: an overview. *J Dermatol* 1999;26:770–779.

48. Wahn U, Bos JD, Goodfield M, et al. Efficacy and safety of pimecrolimus cream in the long-term management of atopic dermatitis in children. *Pediatrics* 2002;110:e2.

49. Williams LK, Reichert A, MacKenzie WR, Hightower AW, Blake PA. Lice, nits, and school policy. *Pediatrics* 2001;107:1011–1015.

50. Zerr DM, Alexander ER, Duchin JS, Koutsky LA, Rubens CE. A case-control study of necrotizing fasciitis during primary varicella. *Pediatrics* 1999;103:783–790.

CHAPTER 243
Diabetic Ketoacidosis

Timothy G. Givens

Diabetic ketoacidosis (DKA) is caused by either an absolute or a relative insulin deficiency accompanied by increased action of four counterregulatory hormones: glucagon, epinephrine, cortisol, and growth hormone (16,19). Counterregulatory hormone activity increases the patient's insulin resistance, thus compounding the effects of insulin deficiency. The results of this imbalance are hyperglycemia, dehydration, ketosis, and acidosis.

Precipitating events for this cascade include acute infection, inflammatory reactions, trauma, psychological stress, or medical noncompliance in patients known to have insulin-dependent diabetes mellitus (IDDM). Recurrent DKA is almost always due to insulin omission (8,9). Approximately 30% of cases of new-onset IDDM present as DKA (19); a high index of suspicion is required to make the diagnosis in infants and children. Mortality in DKA is primarily due to the development of cerebral edema (20), the risk of which is significantly higher in children than in adults (1,18).

CLINICAL PRESENTATION

Children with DKA have a variable clinical picture, and the diagnosis may be difficult, particularly in patients not known to have IDDM. Acutely, the child may appear moderately dehydrated and be misdiagnosed as having viral gastroenteritis or a urinary tract infection. Presenting symptoms include nausea, vomiting, abdominal pain, hyperpnea, fruity breath odor, dehydration, and lethargy or coma. Polyuria, polydipsia, and polyphagia—three classic features of diabetes—as well as weight loss should signal the physician to consider DKA.

DIFFERENTIAL DIAGNOSIS

Because new-onset IDDM presenting as DKA may be mistaken for gastroenteritis or a urinary tract infection, a history of polyuria and polydipsia should be sought in every case of a child who is vomiting, particularly in very young children. Occasionally, dehydrated children with gastroenteritis will have hyperglycemia and glucosuria due to stress and do not have IDDM (2); they are usually nonketotic.

It is unclear whether patients with stress-induced hyperglycemia are at risk for future development of IDDM (22). If the history is obscure or unavailable in a child who presents with altered mental status, the differential diagnosis widens to include intoxication, inborn errors of metabolism, Reyes syndrome, sepsis, meningoencephalitis, nonketotic hyperglycemic coma, or hypoglycemic coma (19). In children with known IDDM, the differential diagnosis includes precipitants for the development of DKA, such as bacterial infections, viral gastroenteritis, appendicitis, pancreatitis, or other acute intraabdominal disorders.

EMERGENCY DEPARTMENT EVALUATION

The initial evaluation of a child who presents as described previously consists of:

1. Establishing the diagnosis of DKA
2. Assessing and correcting dehydration and electrolyte imbalance
3. Providing adequate insulin to restore normal metabolism
4. Searching for the precipitating event for DKA
5. Avoiding complications of therapy (cerebral edema, hypoglycemia, hypokalemia)

Hyperglycemia (serum glucose is typically greater than 300 mg/dL), ketonuria, and metabolic acidosis (venous pH less than 7.3 or serum bicarbonate less than 15 mEq/L) confirm the diagnosis of DKA (19,21).

The physical examination should focus, as always, on the ABCs first. Next, attention is directed toward establishing the degree of dehydration, as well as identifying processes that may have precipitated DKA. Because the extracellular fluid of children with DKA is hyperosmolar, the percentage of dehydration is commonly underestimated when relying on physical signs that correlate with extracellular volume (e.g., hydration of mucous membranes, skin turgor, and temperature). In general, one should assume at least 10% dehydration in all patients with DKA (15,21).

Measurement of serum electrolyte levels may assist in assessment but must be interpreted in light of the physiologic derangements that accompany DKA. The measured sodium level is often low because of the dilutional effects of water flowing into the vascular compartment to compensate for hyperosmolarity generated by high plasma glucose levels. Treatment of this "pseudohyponatremia" with administration of excessive sodium is not required, as the sodium level should rise as the glucose level falls with treatment for DKA. Serum potassium is usually elevated—despite the fact that the patient's total body potassium stores are depleted—because intracellular potassium ions are exchanged for extracellular hydrogen ions in the presence of acidosis. Low-normal potassium levels in DKA indicate extreme total-body potassium depletion. Continuous electrocardiographic monitoring for evidence of cardiac dysrhythmias is necessary in DKA, particularly in patients with alterations in their serum potassium concentrations.

EMERGENCY DEPARTMENT MANAGEMENT

Fluid replacement and correction of dehydration should begin as soon as possible. Formerly, volume expansion with a bolus of isotonic fluid such as normal saline, 20 mL/kg, was recommended during the first 1 to 2 hours of therapy. Because overly vigorous administration of fluids may precipitate a rapid fall in plasma osmolarity and predispose to the development of cerebral edema, pediatric treatment protocols now advise more conservative fluid replacement, on the order of 5 to 10 mL/kg over the first hour (1,4,18). Unless the patient is hemodynamically compromised, larger fluid boluses should be avoided. Lactated Ringer solution is less commonly used, due to a theoretical risk of hyperchloremic acidosis (8).

After the first hour, fluids are adjusted to correct the remainder of the patient's water deficit (10% dehydrated = 100 mL/kg) over the next 48 hours. Again, slow correction of hyperosmolarity is desirable. Maintenance fluids are calculated in the usual manner (100 mL/kg for the first 10 kg, 50 mL/kg for the second 10 kg, and 20 mL/kg for every additional kg) and added to estimates of ongoing losses and rehydration fluids to calculate an infusion rate (see Chapter 221, "Dehydration"). This calculation can be accomplished with a solution of 0.45% sodium chloride (which closely approximates the fluid lost in DKA), with the addition of 40 mEq/L of potassium as the chloride and/or phosphate salt. Some authors suggest that isotonic saline is the most appropriate fluid for the first 24 hours of therapy (4). The use of higher sodium concentrations may prevent the development of cerebral edema during the treatment of DKA (12), although this theory has not been proven (20). In any case, the guiding precept is the gradual correction of fluid and electrolyte deficits, with frequent monitoring of serum chemistries (4,13). Dextrose is added to fluids when the plasma glucose level approaches 300 mg/dL; the desired goal is maintenance of a glucose level between 200 and 300 mg/dL.

Hypophosphatemia and deficiency of 2,3-diphosphoglycerate are well-known features of DKA. They occur because of osmotic diuresis and phosphate competition with glucose for reabsorption at the renal tubules. Potassium phosphate has thus been proposed as an alternative to potassium replacement with the chloride salt. Correction of phosphate homeostasis, however, has not been shown to clinically benefit children with DKA (14,19). Its use should be limited to those patients with extremely low serum phosphate concentrations (less than 1 mg/dL) or when potassium concentrations in the intravenous fluid > 40 mEq/L are needed.

Once hyperglycemia and ketosis confirm the diagnosis of DKA, insulin administration should be begun. While insulin administration has been effective using intramuscular or subcutaneous routes, continuous low-dose intravenous infusion allows for slower, more even correction of hyperglycemia and fewer episodes of hypoglycemia than do other forms of insulin administration (3,19), and is preferable in children. There is no evidence that an initial bolus of intravenous insulin is helpful, and it may be harmful (1,19). Rather, a continuous infusion of intravenous insulin at a rate of 0.05–0.1 U/kg/h is the current recommendation. When mixing the insulin for infusion, the concentration of insulin should be at least 0.5 U/mL, and the infusion line should be primed to overcome insulin binding to the intravenous infusion equipment.

The use of bicarbonate is highly controversial in the treatment of DKA, largely because its reported benefits and risks have been unproven (10,15,16,21). The potential advantages of bicarbonate are improved myocardial function; reduction of potential for dysrhythmias; decreased insulin resistance; and through avoidance of hypochloremia, a more rapid correction of acidosis. Major disadvantages of bicarbonate use are its potential for generation of paradoxical central nervous system acidosis, due to increased diffusion of carbon dioxide across the blood–brain barrier; increased hemoglobin affinity for oxygen (increased tissue hypoxia, due to reduced off-loading); and promotion of hypokalemia. Recent data indicate that bicarbonate administration provides no benefit in terms of reduction of the severity of acidosis, improvement in mental status, or in correction of hyperglycemia in DKA (23). Rapid infusion of bicarbonate may produce hypokalemia and exacerbate the degree of hyperosmolarity, and its use has been associated with an increased incidence of cerebral edema in children (6,18). Hence, if bicarbonate is used at all, it should be reserved for severe and refractory acidosis or life-threatening hyperkalemia only.

Plasma glucose levels should be monitored hourly. Serum electrolyte concentrations and venous blood gases should be monitored every 2 to 4 hours, and calcium and phosphate concentrations should be checked every 8 hours. The rate of decrease in glucose should be no faster than 50 to 100 mg/dL/h (15,19).

In spite of improvements in DKA management, mortality due to cerebral edema has not changed (11,19). Data suggest that a large percentage of patients in DKA have subclinical cerebral edema on computed tomography scans (17); however, clinically significant cerebral edema is reported in less than 1% of cases of DKA (5,12,20). Typically, signs of increased intracranial pressure present several hours into therapy, as the patient experiences a sudden decline in sensorium, headache, sluggish pupillary reflexes, or change in vital signs despite an apparent improvement in metabolic and other clinical parameters.

Thus, cerebral edema is thought to be the result of overly vigorous treatment for DKA (5,11,12,13,15,19,20). Although specific mechanisms remain elusive, children with new-onset IDDM and/or a prolonged period of untreated DKA (i.e., lower partial pressure of carbon dioxide and higher blood urea nitrogen on presentation, suggesting more severe acidosis and dehydration) appear to be at increased risk (6,7,19,20).

Once clinically apparent, cerebral edema leads to mortality in 60% to 80% of cases, with long-term neurologic morbidity in most of the remaining patients. Hence, if cerebral edema becomes clinically evident, the patient should receive rapid, aggressive intervention with intravenous mannitol (1 g/kg), or 2–3 mL/kg of 3% saline (1,20). Intubation and hyperventilation should be considered. Because of the devastating outcomes in patients who develop this complication, the need for frequent neurologic reassessment and early intervention must be underscored.

CRITICAL INTERVENTIONS

- A history of polyuria and polydipsia should be sought in every case of a child who is vomiting, particularly in very young children
- Pediatric treatment protocols now advise more conservative fluid replacement, on the order of 5 to 10 ml/kg over the first hour
- Unless the patient is hemodynamically compromised, larger fluid boluses should be avoided
- An initial bolus of intravenous insulin should not be administered as it may be harmful. Rather, a continuous infusion of intravenous insulin at a rate of 0.05–0.1 u/kg/h is the current recommendation

DISPOSITION

Children in moderate-to-severe DKA should be admitted to a pediatric intensive or intermediate care unit because of the frequency and extent of monitoring that is required (1). Patients with new-onset IDDM should be admitted to a facility where age-appropriate diabetes education can be given.

Patients who can retain oral intake without vomiting and who are not significantly dehydrated or acidotic (pH greater than 7.25) may be discharged home from the emergency department if appropriate follow up care can be arranged. Follow up includes frequent telephone contact over the ensuing 24 hours with an individual knowledgeable in diabetes management.

COMMON PITFALLS

✔ Failure to administer adequate insulin, which may result from errors in insulin dilution or infusion. Concerns about therapy-related hypoglycemia are addressed by adding dextrose to the fluid replacement, not by slowing or stopping the insulin infusion
✔ Failure to treat the precipitating process. Patients with refractory DKA should be thoroughly reexamined for a source of infection or intraabdominal disorder, such as pancreatitis or appendicitis
✔ Inadequate volume expansion from failure to monitor the patient's fluid input and output
✔ Too-rapid correction of the hyperosmolarity may lead to cerebral edema and brainstem herniation
✔ Inadequate potassium replacement during correction of acidosis, which leads to a shift of potassium into the cells and resultant hypokalemia

References

1. Bohn D, Daneman D. Diabetic ketoacidosis and cerebral edema. *Curr Opin Pediatr* 2002;14:287–291.
2. Boulware SD, Tamborlane WV. Not all severe hyperglycemia is diabetes. *Pediatrics* 1992;89:330–332.
3. Butkiewicz EK, Leibson CL, O'Brien PC, et al. Insulin therapy for diabetic ketoacidosis. *Diabetes Care* 1995;18:1187–1190.
4. Carlotti APCP, Bohn D, Halperin ML. Importance of timing of risk factors for cerebral oedema during therapy for diabetic ketoacidosis. *Arch Dis Child* 2003;88:170–173.
5. Duck SC, Wyatt DT. Factors associated with brain herniation in the treatment of diabetic ketoacidosis. *J Pediatr* 1988;113:10–14.
6. Edge J, Hawkins MM, Winter DL, Dunger DB. The risk and outcome of cerebral edema developing during diabetic ketoacidosis. *Arch Dis Child* 2001;85:16–22.
7. Glaser N, Barnett P, McCaslin I, et al. for the Pediatric Emergency Collaborative Research Committee of the American Academy of Pediatrics. Risk factors for cerebral edema in children and adolescents with diabetic ketoacidosis. *N Engl J Med* 2002;344:264–269.
8. Glasgow AM, Weissberg-Benchell J, Tynan WD, et al. Readmissions of children with diabetes mellitus to a children's hospital. *Pediatrics* 1991;88:98–104.
9. Golden MP, Herrold AJ, Orr DP. An approach to prevention of recurrent diabetes ketoacidosis in the pediatric population. *J Pediatr* 1985;107:195–200.
10. Green SM, Rothrock SG, Ho JD, et al. Failure of adjunctive bicarbonate to improve outcome in severe pediatric diabetic ketoacidosis. *Ann Emerg Med* 1998;31:41–48.
11. Harris GD, Fiordalisi I. Physiologic management of diabetic ketoacidemia: a 5-year prospective pediatric experience in 231 episodes. *Arch Pediatr Adolesc Med* 1994;148:1046–1052.
12. Harris SD, Fiordalisi I, Harris WL, et al. Minimizing the risk of brain herniation during treatment of diabetic ketoacidemia: a retrospective and prospective study. *J Pediatr* 1991;117:22–31.
13. Inward CD, Chambers TL. Fluid management in diabetic ketoacidosis. *Arch Dis Child* 2002;86:443–444.
14. Keller U, Berger W. Prevention of hypophosphatemia by phosphate infusion during treatment of diabetic ketoacidosis and hyperosmolar coma. *Diabetes* 1980;29:87–95.
15. Klekamp J, Churchwell KB. Diabetic ketoacidosis in children: initial clinical assessment and treatment. *Pediatr Ann* 1996;25:387–393.
16. Krane EJ. Diabetic ketoacidosis: biochemistry, physiology, treatment and prevention. *Pediatr Clin North Am* 1987;34:935–960.
17. Krane EJ, Rockoff MA, Wallman JK, et al. Subclinical brain swelling in children during treatment of diabetic ketoacidosis. *N Engl J Med* 1985;312:1147–1151.
18. Lawrence S, Pacaud D, Dean H, et al. Pediatric diabetic ketoacidosis. *CMAJ* 2003;169:278–279.
19. Rogers MC. *Textbook of pediatric intensive care,* vol. 3. Baltimore: Williams & Wilkins, 1996:1261–1272.
20. Rosenbloom AL. Intracerebral crises during treatment of diabetic ketoacidosis. *Diabetes Care* 1990;13:22–33.
21. Rosenbloom AL, Schatz DA. Diabetic ketoacidosis in childhood. *Pediatr Ann* 1994;23:284–288.
22. Vardi P, Shehade N, Etzioni A, et al. Stress hyperglycemia in childhood: a very high risk group for the development of type 1 diabetes. *J Pediatr* 1990;117:75–77.
23. Viallon A, Zeni F, Lafond P, et al. Does bicarbonate therapy improve the management of severe diabetic ketoacidosis? *Crit Care Med* 1999;27:2690–2693.

Ear Infections

Noel S. Zuckerbraun and Robert W. Hickey

Earache can be caused by infections or from referred pain from sore throat, toothache, external otitis, parotitis, impacted ear cerumen or a foreign body in the ear canal. Infections of the ear can involve the outer ear (otitis externa), middle ear (otitis media) and mastoid air cell system (mastoiditis).

OTITIS EXTERNA

Otitis Externa (OE) is an acute inflammation or infection of the external ear canal. It is commonly caused by recurrent exposure of the external ear canal to water while swimming (swimmer's ear). The recurrent moisture causes maceration of the canal wall lining and bacterial overgrowth. Although swimming is the most common precipitant, a break in the epithelial lining from any cause (e.g. trauma, foreign body, and eczematous skin disorder) can result in OE. The most common bacterial pathogens are *Pseudomonas aeruginosa* followed by *Staphylococcus aureus* (23). *Staphylococcus epidermis*, *Enterobacter*, *Proteus* and *Klebsiella* species are less common pathogens. Fungal OE (*Aspergillus and Candida* species), seen predominantly in tropical climates, is rare in the United States (<1%) (23).

CLINICAL PRESENTATION

Otalgia (ear pain), otorrhea (drainage) and pruritis are the most common presenting complaints. The key exam finding is tenderness elicited by manipulation of the tragus or pinna. Canal wall erythema, edema and a scant discharge are present. Canal wall edema may progress to obstruction, trapping debris and secretions in the proximal canal. The infection may spread to the surrounding soft tissue resulting in a periauricular cellulitis and perichondritis. Bone infections can occur with spread to the mastoid or cranium. Necrotizing (malignant) OE is a rare, but aggressive infection (usually caused by *Pseudomonas* species) associated with systemic invasion. It is more common in patients with diabetes or immunosuppression (12).

DIFFERENTIAL DIAGNOSIS

The differential diagnosis includes middle ear infections, other external ear canal disorders (furunculosis, herpes zoster oticus) and mastoiditis. OE and acute otitis media (AOM) can often be distinguished clinically by the presence or absence of pain with manipulation of the outer ear. However, if an episode of AOM is complicated by tympanic membrane perforation, the purulent drainage can cause a secondary OE. *Furunculosis* is a localized abscess in the skin of the external auditory canal that responds well to drainage and antistaphylococcal antibiotics. Ramsay Hunt syndrome is a *Herpes-zoster* infection in the distribution of the facial nerve that can present with vesicles in the external auditory canal or auricle, facial nerve paralysis, hearing loss and vertigo. Finally, *mastoiditis* may be difficult to distinguish from OE with postauricular cellulitis, and may require diagnostic imaging to clarify the diagnosis.

EMERGENCY DEPARTMENT MANAGEMENT

Management consists of controlling inflammation and infection, and it is important for the appropriate topical otic agents to reach the inflamed, edematous canal. In mild OE, secretions can be dry mopped with rolled tissue or swabs prior to antibiotic administration. In severe OE with near-obstruction of the canal, a wick can be inserted. The topical antibiotic is then dripped onto the absorbent wick allowing delivery of the medication to the obstructed portion of the canal. If the wick does not fall out on its own as the canal edema decreases, it should be removed in 2 to 3 days. Oral antibiotics are less effective than topical antibiotics in clearing OE, and are thus reserved for cases with signs of invasive infection such as fever and periauricular cellulitis (25). Classes of ototopicals currently used to treat OE include acidifying agents, antiseptics, antibiotics and steroids. Topical acidic solutions inhibit bacterial growth, but are not commonly used because they cause local burning and irritation. Topical antimicrobials aimed at treating the leading causative organisms (*P. aeruginosa* and *S. aureus*) are the mainstay of therapy (25) (Table 244.1). Polymixin B-neomycin-hydrocortisone agents have been used extensively for years with good results; however, they have been associated with hypersensitivity and ototoxicity (4). The recently introduced topical fluoroquinolones (ofloxacin and ciprofloxacin) are as effective as the traditional agents and have decreased risk of ototoxicity, hypersensitivity, and burning (more neutral pH) (15,21). A disadvantage of the fluoroquinolones is cost, with the price being approximately double that of the neomycin-polymixin B-hydrocortisone preparations. The two flouroquinolones differ in that the ciprofloxacin preparation contains hydrocortisone whereas the ofloxacin preparation does not. Two studies have examined the additional benefit of a topical steroid, and the results suggest that clinical symptoms improve sooner when a steroid-containing agent is used (21–22), Fungal OE treatment includes cleansing with acidifying agents and antifungal drops, such as clotrimazole (12). Eczematous OE treatment is the same as for the primary disorder.

DISPOSITION

In the absence of an accompanying cellulitis with systemic symptoms, children can be managed at home. Re-evaluation should occur if symptoms do not improve in 72 hours. Follow up is also recommended in severe cases when complete examination of the external canal and tympanic membrane is not possible or when an ear wick is placed. Prophylaxis against recurrent swimmer's ear includes application of drops containing equal parts vinegar and alcohol (to alter pH and dry the canal, respectively) immediately after swimming. The use of earplugs for prevention of OE is controversial. Earplugs will keep the canal dry only when properly fitted and may cause local irritation and impaction of debris/cerumen.

COMMON PITFALLS

- ✔ Failure to diagnose a concurrent AOM
- ✔ Failure to use a wick in severe cases
- ✔ Failure to recognize complicating conditions (periauricular cellulitis and necrotizing OE) that require systemic antibiotics

TABLE 244.1.   Ototopical Antibiotics for Treatment of Otitis Externa

Antibiotic	Product Name (s)	Antiseptic	Acid	Steroid	Dose	Duration
Polymyxin B/neomycin	Cortisporin Suspension	+	−	+	3 gtts tid–qid	10 days
	Pediotic	+	−	+	3 gtts tid–qid	10 days
	Cortisporin Solution	+	+	+	3 gtts tid–qid	10 days
	Otocort	−	−	+	3 gtts tid–qid	10 days
Ofloxacin	Floxin Otic	+	+	−	1–12 y: 5 gtts bid	10 days
					>12 y: 10 gtts bid	10 days
Ciprofloxacin	Cipro Otic	+	+	+	3 gtts bid	7 days

ACUTE OTITIS MEDIA

Acute otitis media (AOM) is the leading reason for acute care visits and antibiotic prescriptions in children (19). Children are prone to develop AOM secondary to their eustachian tube (ET) anatomy (short, narrow, horizontal and floppy) and their frequent acquisition of viral upper respiratory infections (URIs). URIs cause ET dysfunction via inflammation/edema and decreased ciliary activity. This prevents physiologic drainage of middle ear secretions into the nasopharynx, and creates a negative pressure that draws bacteria from the nasopharynx into the middle ear. Accordingly, the peak incidence of AOM correlates with susceptibility to URIs (children 6–18 mo of age) and day care attendance (10). Other risk factors include smoke exposure, prone sleeping position, pacifier, lack of breast-feeding, allergies, and craniofacial anomalies (e.g. Down Syndrome, cleft palate) (14).

The most common pathogens in order of decreasing frequency are *Streptococcus pneumoniae*, *Haemophilus influenzae* and *Moraxella catarrhalis*. Less common pathogens include *Streptococcus pyogenes* (group A) and *S. aureus*. In children with tympanostomy tubes, *S. aureus* and *P. aeruginosa* are also common, entering the middle ear via the external ear canal (18). Infants under 8 weeks of age with AOM most often have the same pathogens, but can also have *Group B streptococcus* and gram-negative bacilli (29). Injudicious use of antibiotics (e.g., use of antibiotics for viral URIs) has lead to an increased incidence of drug-resistant pathogens. Recent studies have reported up to 50% of *S. pneumoniae* are penicillin (PCN) nonsusceptible (13). Similarly, 30% of *H. influenzae* and nearly 100% of *M. catarrhalis* are beta-lactamase producers (14). Furthermore, although the mechanisms of drug-resistance are phenotypically distinct and antimicrobial specific (mutations of penicillin-binding protein, beta-lactamase production, ribosomal mutations and a macrolide efflux pump that extrudes drug from the organism), several are frequently found within the same bacteria because of selective pressure from antibiotic exposure. Thus, it is not surprising that in the setting of recent antibiotic use, *S. pneumoniae*, the most common AOM pathogen, is often multi-drug resistant (17).

The rising rate of antimicrobial-resistant infections can be attenuated by the use of stringent criteria for diagnosis of AOM (see below) and avoidance of antimicrobials for patients with uncomplicated viral URIs or middle ear effusion without signs of inflammation (otitis media with effusion) (10,20).

CLINICAL PRESENTATION

Otalgia and otorrhea are fairly specific symptoms of AOM. Nonspecific signs and symptoms include fever, irritability, anorexia, vomiting and diarrhea. Although ear pulling can be a sign of AOM, it is frequently found in the absence of AOM.

Examination of the tympanic membrane (TM) is facilitated by using the largest speculum that fits comfortably in the canal to allow proper visualization, and most importantly, to provide a tight seal to assess TM mobility. If the tympanic membrane cannot be visualized because of cerumen, the cerumen can be removed with a curette or by gentle irrigation with warm water. Ceruminolytics can be instilled before irrigation. A normal TM is intact, neutrally positioned (not retracted or bulging), pearly grey, translucent and moves easily with gentle positive and negative insufflating pressure. Middle ear effusions (MEE) can change the appearance and mobility of the TM. The color of the TM can change to white, yellow, or amber. Air-fluid levels and bubbles may be visualized behind the TM or the TM may appear opaque. In addition, TM mobility may be diminished or absent. MEE signifies either AOM or OME. AOM is distinguished by the acute onset and presence of middle ear inflammation. When the signs and symptoms of acute inflammation are absent, OME is diagnosed (Fig. 244.1) (10,11). It is important to note that although redness of the TM can represent inflammation, it can also be secondary to vascular engorgement caused by fever or crying. Relying on TM redness alone will result in the overdiagnosis of AOM. Bulging is a discriminatory sign of AOM. Bullous myringitis is a form of AOM in which inflammation is severe and intensely painful bullous lesions form within the layers of the TM.

Adjunctive Diagnostics

Tympanometry and *acoustic reflectometry* are noninvasive diagnostic tools that can supplement pneumatic otoscopy as objective means to diagnose MEE. Both use electromagnetic impedance and sound waves, respectively, to distinguish between air and fluid-filled spaces. They can supplement pneumatic otoscopy, but cannot confirm signs of inflammation and thus, can not differentiate AOM from OME (20). *Tympanocentesis*, needle aspiration of MEE, is useful to establish a bacterial diagnosis. It should be considered in neonates and patients with immunosuppression, persistent treatment failure and/or suppurative complications (20).

Complications of Acute Otitis Media

Complications *within the middle ear* include cholesteatoma (a white cystic mass behind or involving the TM) and peripheral facial nerve palsy. Nerve palsy is secondary to inflammation of the facial nerve as it traverses the inner and middle ear, and is treated by emergent myringotomy and tube placement. AOM can extend *laterally* out of the middle ear space causing TM perforation and otorrhea. *Posterior* spread causes acute mastoiditis. *Inferior* spread can cause mastoid tip rupture and the formation of an abscess deep in the sternocleidomastoid muscle. *Medial* spread can cause labyrinthitis. Rare, but potentially life-threatening, *superior* spread can cause intracranial complications

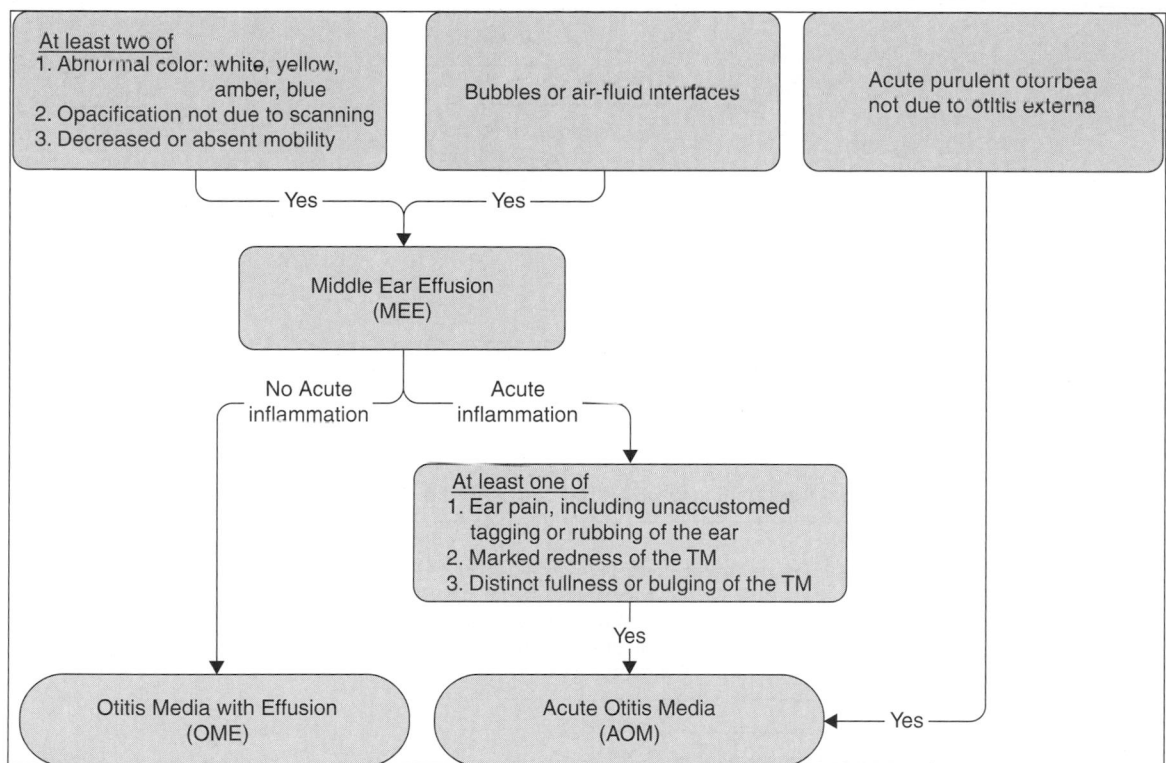

Figure 244.1. Approach to distinguishing between AOM and OME. (From Hoberman A, Marchant CD, Kaplan SL, et al. Treatment of acute otitis media consensus recommendations. *Clin Pediatr* 2002;41:373–390). (From Hoberman A, Paradise JL. Acute otitis media: diagnosis and management in the year 2000. *Pediatr Ann* 2000;29:609–620, with permission.)

that include sphenoid sinus thrombosis, intracranial abscess, and meningitis (2).

DIFFERENTIAL DIAGNOSIS

When AOM is not present, the most likely cause of otalgia is referred pain from infection or trauma in regions with shared innervation, namely the pharynx, nares and teeth. Eustachian tube dysfunction causing negative pressure and temporal-mandibular joint pathology can also cause otalgia.

EMERGENCY DEPARTMENT MANAGEMENT

The primary goals of treatment are to relieve symptoms and prevent complications. Appropriate management decisions are based upon the child's age, allergies, recent antibiotic exposure, and the severity of the infection (Fig. 244.2). Refer to Table 244.2 for drug dosages. Febrile or irritable neonates require hospitalization for parenteral antibiotics.

First-Line Antimicrobial Therapy

Because *S. pneumoniae* is the most common pathogen and the least likely to spontaneously resolve, initial therapy is directed at this organism (7).

Based upon prevalence, spontaneous clearance rates (80%, 50%, and 20% for, *M. catarrhalis, H. influenzae, and S. pneumoniae,* respectively) and drug resistance patterns, amoxicillin should fail to treat AOM in only 8% to 10% of cases (16). Risk factors identified for the presence of bacterial species likely to be resistant to amoxicillin include attendance at child care, recent receipt of antibiotics (<30 days) and age younger than 2 years. Thus, although amoxicillin remains the antibiotic of choice for first-line therapy,

it is now recommended at high dose (HD), 80 to 90 mg/kg/day in two divided doses. Higher doses of amoxicillin are necessary to overcome the mechanism of *S. pneumoniae* penicillin resistance (mutations of the PCN-binding protein resulting in less efficient binding kinetics) (7,10). Recently published guidelines from the American Academy of Pediatrics recommend a strategy of treatment based on the severity of the AOM episode and anticipated microbiologic flora likely to be present (1). For children with nonsevere AOM (mild otalgia or fever < 39°C), HD amoxicillin is the recommended initial agent. For children with severe AOM (moderate to severe otalgia or fever > 39°C) and in those for whom additional coverage for beta-lactamase positive *M. catarrhalis and H. influenzae* is desired, HD amoxicillin-clavulanate is the recommended initial agent (1). HD amoxicillin-clavulanate is an ES (extra strength) preparation which allows HD amoxicillin dosing (90 mg/kg/day based on the amoxicillin component, divided BID) while keeping the clavulanate portion in a range less likely to cause diarrhea and other side-effects. HD amoxicillin-clavulanate is preferred for patients with concomitant conjunctivitis because of the association of nontypeable H. influenzae with conjuncitivits-otitis (3).

Second-Line Anti-Microbial Therapy

If signs and symptoms fail to improve after 48 to 72 hours, or if the patient was treated with an antibiotic in the preceding month, second-line therapy should be started (7). Second-line therapy should take into consideration the spectrum of the "failed" antibiotic, in order to provide coverage against the most likely organism(s) untreated by this regimen. Treatment failure with HD amoxicillin suggests beta-lactamase producing organisms; thus, options include HD amoxicillin-clavulanate, selected second-generation cephalosporins (cefdinir, cefuroxime or cefpodoxime) and ceftriaxone (7,13). Of these oral agents, HD

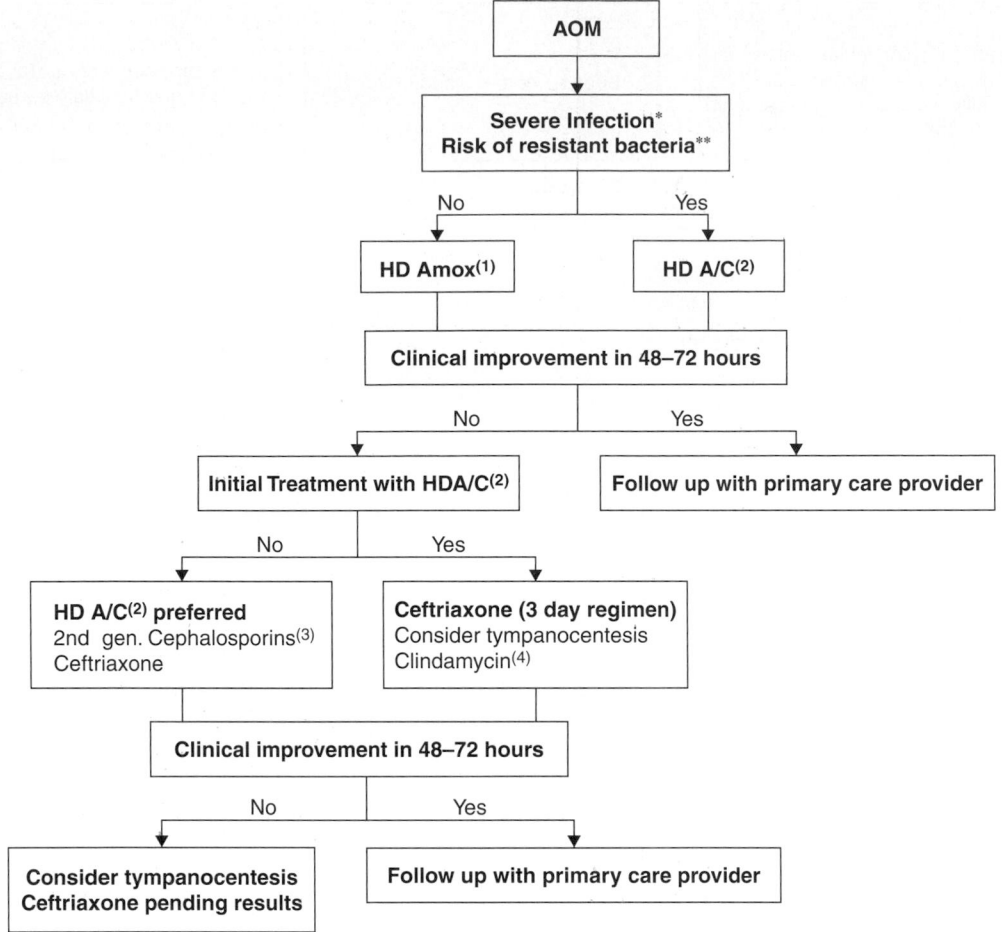

Figure 244.2. Algorithm for antibiotic choice in AOM. *Severe infection refers to patients with severe otalgia or high fever (see text); [1]HD Amox, high dose amoxicillin (see text); [2]HD A/C, high dose amoxicillin-clavulanate (see text); [3]Selected 2nd generation cephalosporins, including cefuroxime, cefpodoxime and cefdinir; [4]Clindamycin should only be used if *S. pneumoniae* is highly suspected or confirmed by tympanocentesis. (From American Academy of Pediatrics and American Academy of Family Physicians, Subcommittee on Management of Acute Otitis Media. Clinical Practice Guideline: Diagnosis and Management of Acute Otitis Media. *Pediatrics* 2004;113:1451–1465, with permission.)

TABLE 244.2. Oral Antibiotic Treatment Options for AOM

Antibiotic	Dosage
High-Dose Amoxicillin	90 mg/kg/day divided BID
High-Dose Amoxicllin-Clavulanate	90 mg/kg/day divided BID based on amoxicillin component, using ES preparation, see text
Cefuroxime	30 mg/kg/day divided BID
Cefpodoxime	10 mg/kg/day divided QD or BID
Cefdinir	14 mg/kg/day divided QD or BID
Azithromycin	10 mg/kg loading dose, then 5 mg/kg QD
Clarithromycin	15 mg/kg/day divided BID
Erythromycin-Sulfasoxazole	40 mg/kg/day divided Q 6–8 hours
Trimethoprim-Sulfamethoxazole	10 mg/kg/day divided BID

*Standard duration of therapy is 10 days for all except azithromycin which is 5 days.
**For those older than 6 years who have nonsevere illness, a 5–7 day course is acceptable.[1]

amoxicillin-clavulanate is preferred because it is more biologically potent than the second-generation cephalosporins (1,10). Although a single injection of ceftriaxone (50 mg/kg IM) can be used for first-line therapy in patients that are vomiting or who cannot take oral antibiotics, a three dose (three day) regimen is recommended if the AOM was unresponsive to initial antibiotic therapy (1,7). Treatment failure with HD amoxicillin-clavulanate suggests PCN-resistant *S. pneumoniae*; thus, options include three day ceftriaxone therapy or consideration of tympanocentesis for definitive diagnosis. Clindamycin may be used if *S. pneumoniae* is strongly suspected or confirmed by tympanocentesis (7).

PCN Allergic Patients

Most maculopapular rashes, often mislabeled "penicillin allergy," are not mediated by IgE. Patients with reactions that are not mediated by IgE can be safely given PCN-containing (β-lactam) drugs and should be considered for standard first-line AOM therapy (27). On the other hand, patients with a true IgE-mediated PCN allergy (anaphylaxis, urticaria) should not be given PCN-containing drugs or cephalosporins (due to their potential cross-reactivity with β-lactams). For these patients, options include clarithromycin, azithromycin, erythromycin/sulfisoxazole or trimethoprim sulfamethoxazole, and if *S. pneumoniae* is strongly suspected or can be confirmed, clindamycin (7,10).

Watchful Waiting Strategy

A management strategy of "watchful waiting" with the avoidance of antibiotics is standard therapy in the Netherlands and has recently gained support in the United States (1,24,28). Proponents argue that the rate of spontaneous cure is high and avoidance of antibiotics will reduce the prevalence of drug-resistant bacteria. Opponents of watchful waiting argue that the supportive evidence is flawed and insufficient (7,10,30). Recently published guidelines from the American Academy of Pediatrics include an "observation option" for selected children (1). Observation is an option for those 6 months to 2 years of age with non-severe illness (defined above) and when the diagnosis of AOM is "uncertain." For those over the age of 2 years, observation is an option regardless of whether the diagnosis of AOM is "certain" or "uncertain," as long as the illness is nonsevere. For all patients being observed, follow up must be assured and antibiotics must be able to be initiated if symptoms worsen or fail to improve within 48 to 72 hours.

Topical Antibiotics

Children with AOM and otorrhea secondary to acute TM perforation are managed similarly to patients without a perforation. However, some clinicians advocate the concomitant use of ototopical agents (Table 244.1) to hasten the resolution of AOM and prevent the development of OE (2). Because the perforation may seal before sterilization of the middle ear, topical agents cannot be used as monotherapy.

There is no standard therapy for children with tympanostomy tubes and otorrhea from AOM. Systemic antimicrobials are effective in reducing the duration of otorrhea and bacterial growth (26). However, monotherapy with topical agents is as effective for the typical pathogens and is also effective for P. aeruginosa, a common pathogen in this setting for which no oral systemic antibiotic is approved for children (5,6,9). In addition, topical agents do not lead to bacterial resistance, have fewer side effects, and are more convenient for the patient compared with systemic therapy (5). Pumping the tragus after the installation of ear drops can improve delivery through the tube. Concomitant treatment with systemic antibiotics is advocated by some clinicians for those children with systemic signs and symptoms or with copious exudate that may interfere with the administration of topical agents. In these cases, use of an agent with additional staphylococcal coverage, such as HD amoxicillin-clavulanate, is useful as *S. aureus* is common in those with chronic drainage. Although routine culture of otorrhea is unnecessary, careful culturing with appropriately sized swabs after cleaning the ear canal can be helpful in those with persistent infection.

Analgesics

Pain relief is an important part of therapy for AOM. Options include systemic agents such as acetaminophen or ibuprofen, or benzocaine-containing topical agents. Topical analgesics should only be used in the presence of an intact TM. Other adjunctive medications, namely decongestants, antihistamines and systemic steroids, are not beneficial and are associated with increased side effects.

DISPOSITION

If no evidence of serious systemic infection is present, children may be managed as outpatients. A follow up appointment with the primary care physician should occur in 2 to 3 weeks to monitor recovery of the MEE. Instruction should be given for patients to seek care sooner if symptoms, including fever, do not resolve in 48 to 72 hours or signs of worsening infection develop. Children with toxicity, other serious systemic infections, intracranial complications, clinically significant immunodeficiencies and febrile neonates should be hospitalized and placed on parenteral antibiotics.

COMMON PITFALLS

✔ Over diagnosis of AOM secondary to failure to remove cerumen from ear canal
✔ Diagnosis based solely upon redness of the TM
✔ Failure to use pneumatic otoscopy to assess middle ear effusion
✔ Failure to distinguish OME from AOM
✔ Failure to consider other more serious coexisting diagnosis, such as sepsis or meningitis

CRITICAL INTERVENTIONS

- For children with nonsevere AOM, high-dose amoxicillin should be the initial agent
- For children with severe AOM, high-dose amoxicillin-clavulanate is the preferred initial agent

MASTOIDITIS

Mastoiditis is a suppurative complication of AOM. It predominantly affects younger children with 50% of cases seen in children < 3 years old (2). Mastoiditis is a spectrum of disease ranging from infectious inflammation of mastoid air cells to abscess development and subsequent spread to contiguous areas.

CLINICAL PRESENTATION

Acute Mastoiditis (AM) without periosteitis or osteitis is the initial subclinical stage involving inflammation of the lining of the mastoid air cells. Because the mastoid is directly connected to the middle ear, almost all episodes of AOM are thought to be associated with some inflammation of the mastoid. Diagnosis of this stage is often made incidentally when cranial imaging, obtained for other reasons, reveals cloudy mastoids without evidence of bony erosion. There are no specific clinical signs or symptoms of mastoiditis in this stage, and no special treatment is required (2).

AM with periosteitis occurs when the infection spreads into the periosteum. Signs and symptoms of AOM are present, as well as postauricular edema, erythema, and tenderness. The postauricular crease may be absent. In younger children the pinna may be displaced downward and outward, whereas in older children it is usually displaced upward and outward. Rarely, signs and symptoms of AOM are absent. This will occur when the middle ear infection resolves but granulation tissue or edema obstruct the narrow tube connecting the middle ear to the mastoid thus preventing drainage and resolution of the mastoiditis. The most common bacterial pathogens are *S. pneumoniae* and *S. pyogenes*, *S. aureus* and *P. aeruginosa* (8). If symptoms are severe or toxicity is present, a CT scan of the temporal bones and intracranial cavity should be performed to determine if osteitis is present (2).

AM with osteitis occurs when the infection results in erosion of the bony septae that separate the mastoid air cells, resulting in an empyema. Some children may appear toxic. If the infection continues to spread, signs and symptoms associated with spread to the contiguous areas will be present. Infection can spread laterally creating a postauricular subperiosteal abscess, anteriorly creating a preauricular abscess, inferiorly towards the sternocleidomastoid muscle, medially into the petrous air cells and inner ear labyrinth, or posteriorly into the calvarium. A CT scan of the temporal bones and intracranial cavity may reveal the destruction and coalescence of the mastoid air cells or intracranial infection, respectively (2).

Chronic mastoiditis is most commonly a manifestation of chronic suppurative otitis media (otitis with perforation and persistent otorrhea) that has failed outpatient therapy. However, it can occur in a child with ineffectively treated AM.

DIFFERENTIAL DIAGNOSIS

The differential diagnosis of AM includes OE with postauricular cellulitis, perichondritis of the pinna and postauricular lymphadenitis. In each of these, middle ear disease is usually absent, and with perichondritis of the pinna and postauricular lymphadenitis, the posterior auricular crease usually remains intact. Postauricular lymphadenitis is usually seen in the presence of scalp infection or inflammation.

EMERGENCY DEPARTMENT MANAGEMENT

Although some clinicians treat all patients with AM with admission for parenteral antibiotics and surgical drainage (8), others will manage patients with early, mild cases of AM with periosteitis with outpatient antibiotic therapy and close follow up (2). HD amoxicillin or HD amoxicillin-clavulanate will treat the most common pathogens, with the exception of *P. aeruginosa*. Fluoroquinolones are relatively contraindicated in young children because of theoretic, but unproven, concerns about cartilage toxicity. When *Pseudomonas* is suspected, tympanocentesis can be helpful in directing therapy. Any patient with AM presenting with fever, ill-appearance or osteitis should be admitted for parenteral antibiotics, otolaryngology consultation, tympanocentesis and myringotomy with or without tympanostomy tube placement (2). Ampicillin-sulbactam or second- and third- generation cephalosporins are acceptable for initial antibiotic therapy. Vancomycin may be added if there is a suspicion of PCN resistant *S. pneumoniae*. If *P. aeruginosa* is suspected, initial, empiric antipseudomonal coverage with ceftazidime or piperacillin-tazobactam can be used. Subsequent therapy can be modified based upon culture results from tympanocentesis. Surgical mastoidectomy is often required for patients with CT evidence of bony destruction (osteitis) or abscess.

Chronic mastoiditis may be treated with a parenteral antipseudomonal antibiotic. Otolaryngology consultation is advised as mastoidectomy is necessary for patients that do not improve with medical management.

DISPOSITION

Patients early, mild cases of AM with periosteitis may be managed as outpatients using antibiotic therapy combined with close follow up. All other cases require hospital admission, parenteral antibiotics and otolaryngology consultation.

COMMON PITFALLS

✔ Failure to recognize AM or distinguish AM from OE with cellulitis, perichondritis of the pinna or postauricular lymphadenitis
✔ Failure to consider concurrent intracranial complications of AM such as meningitis and brain abscess

CRITICAL INTERVENTIONS

- Admit all patients with acute mastoiditis presenting with fever, ill-appearance or osteitis for parenteral antibiotics

Acknowledgments

The authors gratefully acknowledge the contributions of Katalin I. Koranyi, who wrote the previous version of this chapter, as well as Ellen Wald and Alejandro Hoberman for their review of the current chapter.

References

1. American Academy of Pediatrics and American Academy of Family Physicians, Subcommittee on Management of Acute Otitis Media. Clinical practice guideline: diagnosis and management of acute otitis media. *Pediatrics* 2004;113:1451–1465.
2. Bluestone CD, Klein JO. Otitis media in infants and children. Philadelphia: WB Saunders Company, 2001.
3. Bodor FF. Conjunctivitis-otitis syndrome. *Pediatrics* 1982;69:695–698.
4. Dohar JE. Evolution of management approaches for otitis externa. *Pediatr Infect Dis J* 2003;22:299–305.
5. Dohar JE, Garner ET, Nielsen RW, et al. Topical ofloxacin treatment of otorrhea in children with tympanostomy tubes. *Arch Otolaryngol Head Neck Surg* 1999;125:537–545.
6. Dohar JE, Kenna MA, Wadowsky RM. Therapeutic implications in the treatment of aural Pseudomonas infections based on in vitro susceptibility patterns. *Arch Otolaryngol Head Neck Surg* 1995;121:1022–1025.
7. Dowell SF, Butler JC, Giebink GS, et al. Acute otitis media: management and surveillance in an era of pneumococcal resistance–a report from the Drug-resistant Streptococcus pneumoniae Therapeutic Working Group. *Pediatr Infect Dis J* 1999;18:1–9.
8. Ghaffar FA, Wordemann M, McCracken GH, Jr. Acute mastoiditis in children: a seventeen-year experience in Dallas, Texas. *Pediatr Infect Dis J* 2001;20:376–380.
9. Goldblatt EL. Efficacy of ofloxacin and other otic preparations for acute otitis media in patients with tympanostomy tubes. *Pediatr Infect Dis J* 2001;20:116–119.
10. Hoberman A, Marchant CD, Kaplan SL, et al. Treatment of acute otitis media consensus recommendations. *Clin Pediatr* 2002;41:373–390.
11. Hoberman A, Paradise JL. Acute otitis media: diagnosis and management in the year 2000. *Pediatr Ann* 2000;29:609–620.
12. Hughes E, Lee JH. Otitis externa. *Pediatr Rev* 2001;22:191–197.
13. Jacobs MR, Bajaksouzian S, Lin G, et al. Susceptibility of Streptococcus pneumoniae, Haemophilus influenzae, and Moraxella catarrhalis to oral agents: results of a 1998 US outpatient surveillance study. Presented at: 39th International Conference on Antimicrobial Agents and Chemotherapy; September 26, 1999; San Francisco, California. 1999.
14. Jacobs MR, Dagan R, Appelbaum PC, et al. Prevalence of antimicrobial-resistant pathogens in middle ear fluid: multinational study of 917 children with acute otitis media. *Antimicrob Agents Chemother* 1998;42:589–595.
15. Jones RN, Milazzo J, Seidlin M. Ofloxacin otic solution for treatment of otitis externa in children and adults. *Arch Otolaryngol Head Neck Surg* 1997;123:1193–1200.
16. Klein JO, Bluestone CD. Management of otitis media in the era of managed care. *Adv Pediatr Infect Dis* 1996;12:351–386.
17. Leibovitz E, Raiz S, Piglansky L, et al. Resistance pattern of middle ear fluid isolates in acute otitis media recently treated with antibiotics. *Pediatr Infect Dis J* 1998;17:463–469.
18. Mandel EM, Casselbrant ML, Kurs-Lasky M. Acute otorrhea: bacteriology of a common complication of tympanostomy tubes. *Ann Otol Rhinol Laryngol* 1994;103:713–718.
19. McCaig LF, Hughes JM. Trends in antimicrobial drug prescribing among office-based physicians in the United States. *JAMA* 1995;273:214–219.
20. Pichichero ME. Acute otitis media: Part I. Improving diagnostic accuracy. *Am Fam Physician* 2000;61:2051–2056.
21. Pistorius B, Westberry K, Drehobl M. Prospective, randomised, comparative trial of ciprofloxacin otic drops, with or without hydrocortisone, vs. polymyxin B-neomycin-hydrocortisone otic suspension in the treatment of acute diffuse otitis externa. *Infect Dis Clin Pract* 1999;8:387–395.

22. Roland PS, Kreisler LS, Reese B, et al. Topical ciprofloxacin/dexamethasone otic suspension is superior to ofloxacin otic solution in the treatment of children with acute otitis media with otorrhea through tympanostomy tubes. *Pediatrics* 2004;113:E40–E46.
23. Roland PS, Stroman DW. Microbiology of acute otitis externa. *Laryngoscope* 2002;112:1166–1177.
24. Rosenfeld RM, Vertrees JE, Carr J, et al. Clinical efficacy of antimicrobial drugs for acute otitis media: metaanalysis of 5400 children from thirty-three random-ized trials. *J Pediatr* 1994;124:355–367.
25. Rowlands S, Devalia H, Smith C, et al. Otitis externa in UK general practice: a survey using the UK General Practice Research Database. *Br J Gen Pract* 2001;51:533–538.
26. Ruohola A, Heikkinen T, Meurman O, et al. Antibiotic treatment of acute otorrhea through tympanostomy tube: randomized double-blind placebo-controlled study with daily follow-up. *Pediatrics* 2003;111:1061–1067.
27. Salkind AR, Cuddy PG, Foxworth JW. The rational clinical examination. Is this patient allergic to penicillin? An evidence-based analysis of the likelihood of penicillin allergy. *JAMA* 2001;285:2498–2505.
28. Takata GS, Chan LS, Shekelle P, et al. Evidence assessment of management of acute otitis media: I. The role of antibiotics in treatment of uncomplicated acute otitis media. *Pediatrics* 2001;108:239–247.
29. Turner D, Leibovitz E, Aran A, et al. Acute otitis media in infants younger than two months of age: microbiology, clinical presentation and therapeutic approach. *Pediatr Infect Dis J* 2002;21:669–674.
30. Wald ER. Acute otitis media: more trouble with the evidence. *Pediatr Infect Dis J* 2003;22:103–104.

CHAPTER 245
Eye Disorders

Janet G. Alteveer and Kathryn McCans

A complete pediatric eye examination includes inspection of the eyelids, conjunctivae, pupil, and iris; evaluation of the ex-traocular muscles; funduscopy; and testing of visual acuity. This examination is an essential part of the evaluation in any child presenting with primarily ophthalmologic conditions such as conjunctivitis, periorbital edema, visual change or loss, trauma, or neurologic complaints.

Inspection of the eyelids and conjunctivae should document the presence of erythema, ecchymosis, edema, proptosis, or masses. The cornea should be evaluated for normal contour and clarity. A bulging or hazy cornea in a neonate may indicate con-genital glaucoma. The cornea should be stained using topical anesthetic drops and fluorescein test strips, after the rest of the examination is completed so as not to interfere with visual acuity testing. Shining a Wood light on the cornea in a darkened room will reveal stain adherent to corneal defects caused by an abra-sion, herpetic infection, or ulcer. The pupil should be assessed for contour, bilateral symmetry and reactivity to light. An abnor-mally shaped or reactive pupil may indicate defects in the iris or disruption of the afferent or efferent nerve pathways to the eye.

Extraocular muscle testing can be accomplished by 4 months of age. By this age, a normal, full-term infant should be able to fixate on and follow a small, brightly colored toy held 6 to 12 in. from the baby's face. By 5 to 6 months, the infant should fixate and follow an object through the full range of motion. By 2 to 3 years of age, most children, with gentle encouragement, will follow a light or finger (3).

Evaluation of the posterior chamber via direct ophthal-moscopy is dependent on the child's age and cognitive devel-

TABLE 245.1. Visual Acuity by Age

Age	Visual Acuity
6 mo	20/60 to 20/100
3 yr	20/25 to 20/30
5–7 yr	20/20 to 20/25
By 8 yr	20/20

opment, becoming easier as cooperation increases. The use of a short-acting topical parasympatholytic such as tropicamide (Mydriacyl 0.5%), will facilitate the examination of the retina. To encourage the child to look beyond the examiner and away from the direct light, use a brightly colored toy or have the parent wave at the child from directly behind the examiner. The mini-mal examination in an infant is the documentation of a normal red reflex. The presence of an abnormal red reflex (leukocoria), which could indicate a cataract or intraocular tumor, mandates formal consultation with a pediatric ophthalmologist.

The corneal light reflex, or Hirschberg test, is useful in de-tecting strabismus or an ocular muscle palsy. It is conducted by shining a penlight, held 3 ft (1 m) away, centrally onto the child's face. In a normal child, the light will reflect centrally on both pupils when the child is fixated on the light or a small toy held in front of the face. If the light reflex is eccentric on one eye, a strabismus or palsy is present (3).

Visual acuity testing is an extremely important aspect of the complete eye examination. The manner of testing is dependent on the age and cognitive ability of the child. Visual acuity also varies by age (Table 245.1). To assess an infant, have the baby fixate (on a bright toy or light) and cover one eye gently with your thumb. If the uncovered eye has normal vision, the child will continue to fixate on the object. If the uncovered eye has poor vision, the child may lose interest, push the covering thumb away, or protest (7).

By 3 years of age, depending on developmental and cognitive ability, more objective visual testing can be achieved. The Allen chart, HOTV matching test, or "Tumbling E" game can be used. By 5 years of age, most cognitively normal children can use the Snellen chart. Testing with the Snellen, Tumbling E, or HOTV chart should be performed at a distance of 20 ft (6 m). The Allen test can be performed at 10 ft (3 m) (3).

In all of these charts, letters or objects are presented as a group. Children with poor vision have increased difficulty identifying objects when presented as a group (the crowding phenomenon) and will perform better when objects are presented singly (3).

THE RED EYE

Children frequently present to the emergency department (ED) with a complaint of one or both eyes being reddened. The most common diagnosis will be conjunctivitis due to bacterial or vi-ral infection, chemical, or allergic exposure. Rarely, the red eye will be due to keratitis (from HSV or HVZ infection) or anterior uveitis (formerly called iritis). The etiologies of infectious con-junctivitis after the neonatal period are nontypable *H. influenzae,* *Streptococcus pneumoniae, Moraxella catarrhalis,* herpesvirus, and adenovirus (27). *N. meningitides and N. gonorrhea* are uncommon pathogens (27). Infrequently, gonococcal conjunctivitis may oc-cur after the neonatal period and in the prepubescent child, who is not sexually active. Sexual abuse must be excluded; however, cases of transmission from an infected caregiver who is not abus-ing the child have been reported (2).

The syndrome of conjunctivitis–otitis was first described in 1966 by Coffey, et al. Nontypable *H. influenzae* will commonly cause concomitant otitis and conjunctivitis. Additionally, as many as 60% of children presenting with conjunctivitis without clinical findings or symptoms of otitis will develop an otitis within 2 weeks (29).

Herpesviruses can cause ocular involvement during primary or recurrent infections. Herpes simplex virus (HSV) is ubiquitous and is transmitted from person to person during primary and recurrent infections that may or may not be symptomatic. Periocular inoculation can occur from the HSV-1 perioral infections so common in children. Herpes zoster represents a reactivation of latent varicella-zoster virus. When it occurs in the dermatomal distribution of the trigeminal nerve, it can cause a keratitis with conjunctivitis (2).

Five percent of uveitis in the United States presents in children less than 16 years old and 41% of cases are associated with juvenile rheumatoid arthritis. Toxoplasmosis accounts for approximately 10% of cases. HSV and HVZ may also cause uveitis. Uveitis in children is a chronic disease with a high incidence (up to 20%) of developing blindness in one eye (10).

Adenoviral conjunctivitis may be associated with two distinct clinical syndromes: pharyngoconjunctival fever and epidemic keratoconjunctivitis. Pharyngoconjunctival fever is caused by adenovirus types 3 and 7. It is most commonly spread by person-to-person contact, but has also been reported to be spread through swimming; thus, the infection may be referred to as "swimming pool" conjunctivitis. Adenovirus types 8, 19, and 37 cause epidemic keratoconjunctivitis. This entity is transmitted by direct contact with infected people or contaminated instruments and is often iatrogenic. Attention to frequent hand washing prevents transmission (27).

Infectious neonatal conjunctivitis is caused by *Neisseria gonorrhoeae*, *Chlamydia trachomatis*, and, less commonly, HSV. The infant is infected at birth during passage through the birth canal. The incubation period for gonococcal conjunctivitis (ophthalmia neonatorum) is 2 to 7 days. Neonatal prophylaxis for ophthalmia neonatorum with a 1% silver nitrate solution, 0.5% erythromycin ophthalmic ointment, or 1% tetracycline ophthalmic ointment is recommended universally in the United States. Only silver nitrate solution is effective in prevention of infection by a penicillinase-producing gonococcus. Neonatal chlamydial conjunctivitis develops a few days to several weeks after birth. Fifty percent of infants born to infected women acquire *C. trachomatis*, and, of those, 25% to 50% develop conjunctivitis. Neonatal ophthalmic prophylaxis is not effective in the prevention of chlamydial conjunctivitis. Neonatal HSV infection occurs in 1 per 3,000 to 1 per 20,000 live births. The infant is most at risk if the mother has a primary infection at the time of delivery. The risk to an infant born to a mother with a recurrent infection is much lower. Neonatal infections are of three types: generalized infection, localized central nervous system (CNS) infection, or disease localized to the skin, eye, and mouth (SEM) (2).

The most common cause of allergic conjunctivitis in children is seasonal rhinoconjunctivitis. The symptoms are caused by a localized IgE-mediated hypersensitivity reaction to airborne allergens, with resultant release of histamine and other products from mast cells. Pollens and grasses are the most common allergens. In up to 25% of children, ocular findings may be the sole manifestation. The findings are caused by the release of products from mast cells, predominantly histamine (5,23).

Chemical conjunctivitis is most often caused by ocular medications. Neomycin has the greatest incidence of contact sensitivity. Silver nitrate is a common cause in the neonate. Accidental environmental exposure to a toxin, such as cleaning agents, is also common.

CLINICAL PRESENTATION

The clinical presentation, while not completely specific, may help the clinician determine the etiology of conjunctivitis. Bacterial conjunctivitis is most often bilateral and occurs predominantly in infants and preschool-aged children. A conjunctival papillary response is consistent with bacterial disease (27). There is usually a mucopurulent exudate, and the palpebral and bulbar conjunctivae are erythematous but not hemorrhagic. Eyelid erythema and swelling may be present, and the child may be febrile. *N. meningitides* and *N. gonorrhea* cause copious purulent exudates in all age groups. A neonate with ophthalmia neonatorum may appear toxic, with a copious purulent discharge. *C. trachomatis* infection causes a beefy red conjunctiva (2).

Viral conjunctivitis, on the other hand, is often bilateral and occurs in school-aged children. A mucopurulent discharge may be present, but the presence of a conjunctival inflammatory membrane is diagnostic. The discharge is often copious and clear. Marked periorbital edema can be present, leading to a false diagnosis of periorbital cellulitis. Pharyngoconjunctival fever is manifested by pharyngitis, fever to 40°C (104°F), and conjunctivitis. Conjunctival findings may persist from 4 days to 2 weeks. Epidemic keratoconjunctivitis lacks upper respiratory symptoms and fever. Corneal involvement predominates, with an early keratitis that causes photophobia and a foreign-body sensation. Subepithelial opacities develop 7 to 10 days after onset, which may cause a temporary mild decrease in visual acuity. These opacities resolve without scarring of the cornea (27).

HSV infection of the eye is of the SEM type; however, skin and mouth lesions may not be present at the time of presentation. The conjunctiva is erythematous, and keratitis may be present. Characteristic dendritic keratitis may be seen with fluorescein staining for both varicella-zoster virus and herpes simplex virus. Varicella-zoster infection of the first division of the trigeminal nerve affects the eye. There may be characteristic vesicular lesions on the forehead and eyelid. The conjunctivae are usually injected. Herpes zoster is a unilateral infection, and, often, periorbital pain precedes the appearance of the vesicles (2).

Anterior uveitis classically presents with eye pain, a constricted pupil and perilimbic injection of the conjunctiva (injection that is limited to the area of the conjunctiva surrounding the cornea). Visual acuity may be reduced as well.

Allergic conjunctivitis is bilateral, with variable conjunctival injection and watery eye discharge. Other allergic symptoms, such as boggy nasal turbinates, watery nasal discharge, and allergic shiners (dark circles around the eye), may or may not be present.

Chemical conjunctivitis presents with conjunctival injection and, often, a burning sensation.

DIFFERENTIAL DIAGNOSIS

The differential diagnosis of the red eye includes conjunctivitis, periorbital cellulitis, corneal abrasion, Kawasaki syndrome, glaucoma, dry-eye syndromes, blepharitis, dacryocystitis and Parinaud oculoglandular syndrome (a syndrome of cat scratch disease involving the conjunctiva and ipsilateral preauricular lymph node).

EMERGENCY DEPARTMENT EVALUATION

The ED evaluation of the red eye begins with a detailed history and physical, including a complete age-appropriate eye examination. A slit-lamp examination in an older child who is cooperative is helpful. Outside of the neonatal period, conjunctival cultures are rarely obtained. Fluorescein staining should be considered, especially with severe photophobia or corneal changes. A gram stain should be obtained if the discharge is copious, suggesting *neisseria* infection.

All young infants in whom the diagnosis of ophthalmia neonatorum or SEM secondary to HSV is being considered require a full evaluation for disseminated disease. In addition to blood and cerebrospinal fluid (CSF) studies (complete blood count, chemistries, blood culture, CSF culture for bacteria and viruses, glucose, protein, Gram stain), conjunctival cultures for bacteria and viruses should be obtained. In suspected gonococcal infection, a Gram stain of the eye is helpful in early confirmation of the diagnosis (27). A Tzanck preparation may be helpful in herpetic infections. A conjunctival scraping for epithelial cells is more sensitive than swab cultures (27). When a chlamydial infection is suspected, cultures or specimens for rapid antigen testing of the conjunctiva and nasopharynx should be obtained using a Dacron swab (2). A chemical conjunctivitis is suggested when a history of ocular exposure to a toxin or ophthalmic medication is elucidated in the presence of conjunctival injection.

Anterior uveitis is diagnosed with the slit lamp: showing cells (leucocytes) and flare (protein) in the anterior chamber.

EMERGENCY DEPARTMENT MANAGEMENT

The management of conjunctivitis is dependent on the suspected etiology and the age of the child. Treatment ranges from supportive care to hospital admission for parenteral antibiotics. Bacterial conjunctivitis, although a self-limited disease, is most frequently treated with topical ophthalmic antibiotics as this results in a bacterial cure and hastens clinical improvement (27). Trimethoprim–polymyxin B or polymixin-bacitracin are appropriate first line treatments. Trimethoprim–polymyxin B eradicates *H. influenzae* most effectively (29), is inexpensive and has few side effects (27). The topical agent is administered every 4 hours, while the patient is awake, for 5 to 7 days. Sulfonamides are no longer recommended because of increasing bacterial resistance and significant discomfort on instillation. Fluoroquinolones, while providing excellent broad spectrum coverage, are expensive and should be reserved for patients who do not respond to first line therapy (6).

In the instance of conjunctivitis–otitis syndrome, oral therapy with an appropriate antibiotic to treat *H. influenzae,* such as amoxicillin–clavulanate, will cure both the otitis and the conjunctivitis. Oral therapy for conjunctivitis without otitis has been shown to decrease the occurrence of otitis in the ensuing 2 weeks (29). Further data are needed to substantiate the efficacy of oral treatment of conjunctivitis. Meningococcal conjunctivitis is treated with systemic antibiotics.

Table 245.2 lists the etiologies of neonatal conjunctivitis with the indicated treatment.

Localized herpesvirus infections involving the eye should be treated with intravenous acyclovir 60 mg/kg/d in three divided doses for children less than 1 year of age, and for older children, 1500 mg/m^2/d in three divided doses for 7 to 10 days. Higher dosing is used for disseminated or CNS disease (2). Acyclovir-resistant Herpes virus (an issue usually only with HIV infected children previously exposed to acyclovir) is treated with foscarnet, 80 to 120 mg/kg/day in two or three divided doses (2).

Adenoviral conjunctivitis is treated with supportive therapy. To prevent the spread of infection to other family members, the family should be counseled to wash hands frequently and to avoid sharing wash cloths. The infected child should be kept away from immunocompromised persons and neonates, because this group is at increased risk for severe disease. The child should also be kept home from school or day-care for 5 to 7 days.

TABLE 245.2. Etiology of Neonatal Conjunctivitis and Therapy

Organism	Medications	Other Therapy
N. gonorrhea	Ceftriaxone 25–50 mg/kg i.v. or i.m., not to exceed 125 mg; given once *or* Cefotaxime 100 mg/kg i.v. or i.m.	Frequent eye irrigation with saline
C. trachomatis	Erythromycin 50 mg/kg/d divided q.i.d. PO for 14 d	
Herpes simplex virus	Acyclovir 60 mg/kg/d i.v. divided q8h Duration: 14 to 21 d *and* 1% to 2% trifluridine, 1% iododeoxyuridine, or 3% vidarabine, applied topically	Ophthalmologic consultation

Data from American Academy of Pediatrics (2).

The treatment of allergic conjunctivitis is avoidance of the allergen and topical therapy with antihistamines, vasoconstrictors, or nonsteroidal antiinflammatory agents, mast cell stabilizers, or combination products (23). Cool compresses may also be soothing.

Corticosteroid-containing eye drops have no place in the treatment of acute conjunctivitis. They may be necessary in the treatment of uveitis or severe keratitis, but should be used only after consultation with an Ophthalmologist. Long-term use of steroid drops can endanger vision by causing cataracts or glaucoma. Short-term use may inhibit the hosts' ability to limit infection and prolong viral shedding in contagious conjunctivitis. Corticosteroid/antibiotic combinations may also promote or increase the severity of fungal keratitis.

DISPOSITION

Bacterial conjunctivitis outside of the neonatal period is an outpatient disease. Follow up with a primary care provider should be recommended. Children do not need to be isolated and may return to school immediately, as bacterial conjunctivitis is not very contagious (27).

If large corneal defects or defects involving the visual axis are detected, emergent ophthalmologic evaluation by a provider skilled in pediatric ophthalmology is necessary. All cases of suspected ophthalmia neonatorum, HSV, and varicella-zoster ophthalmic infection as well as anterior uveitis should be referred to a pediatric ophthalmologist emergently. The risk for ocular damage and permanent visual loss is high.

Neonatal, herpetic, meningococcal, and gonococcal conjunctivitis requires inpatient therapy at a facility well versed in pediatric care and with pediatric ophthalmologic resources. When chlamydial infection is suspected, consultation with a pediatrician is helpful.

COMMON PITFALLS

✔ Failure to recognize herpetic infection of the eye. Delay in treatment can often lead to visual loss, CNS disease, or systemic disease

✔ Failure to recognize that minor infections in the immunocompromised host can result in major complications and possible visual loss

✔ Failure to recognize otitis in association with conjunctivitis

✔ Inappropriate use of corticosteroid containing eye drops, unless discussed with an ophthalmologist

THE SWOLLEN EYE

Children with a swollen, red eye represent a relatively common problem in the ED. In the past 5 years it has become increasingly evident that Periorbital (POC) and Orbital (OC) cellulitis are distinct clinical entities with different pathogenesis and treatment (13). *Periorbital cellulitis* is defined as an inflammatory or infectious process superficial to the orbital septum. If untreated, it has the potential to spread via blood vessels to the CNS. *Orbital cellulitis* is defined as inflammation or infection deep to the orbital septum. OC may involve the ocular structures, causing abscess formation and loss of vision. It may also spread to the CNS via the cavernous sinus, causing cavernous sinus thrombosis or meningitis.

The mean age of children with POC is 21 months. The pathogenesis of POC may occur via two different routes. The skin barrier near the eye may be broken by local trauma, an insect sting, or the lesions of varicella or herpes zoster, with local spread of infected material to the periorbital tissues. Alternatively, there may be seeding of periorbital tissues from bacteremia (26). OC on the other hand occurs as a complication of sinusitis with extension of infected material into the orbit, or as the result of direct penetrating injury to the orbit. The most common sinus involved is the Ethmoid. The mean age for OC is 12 years (13).

A bacterial pathogen in POC/OC is identified in only up to 30% of cases, with most of these, in the past, identified by blood culture. Prior to the introduction of the *H. influenzae* vaccine (HIB), 50% of the cultures were positive for *H. influenzae*. Widespread usage of the vaccine has resulted in a 90% decrease in the incidence of *H. influenzae*-related PO/OC (4,13). The most common organisms, currently, are *S. aureus*, group A *Streptococcus* species, and *S. pneumoniae*. The heptavalent Pneumococcal vaccine was introduced in the United States in February of 2000. In children under 2 years this resulted in a 69% reduction in the rate of invasive Pneumococcal disease and a rate of decline of disease caused by vaccine serotypes of 78% (30). It is expected that the incidence of *S. pneumoniae* bacteremia and thus the incidence of bacteremia-related POC and sinusitis in the young child also will decline (13). *S. aureus* and group A *Streptococcus* are more likely to be involved when there is a history of local trauma or a wound. Anaerobic bacteria and *M. catarrhalis* should be considered in the older child with documented sinusitis (13). *H. influenzae* should still be considered in the child who has not received, or not completed, the primary series of HIB vaccination (2, 4, 6 months) (24).

CLINICAL PRESENTATION

The thin skin and loose connective tissue of the eyelid allow for easy and rapid accumulation of fluid. A child with POC/OC may often present within hours of onset with a red and swollen eyelid. Ninety-five percent of cases are unilateral, with the actual color of the lid described as violaceous or purple. Seventy-five percent of children are febrile. Two-thirds will have an upper respiratory infection; one-third, a history of minor trauma; one-fourth, an acute otitis media; and one-fifth, an associated conjunctivitis (26).

In POC, palpation of the periorbital tissues will elicit tenderness, but the eye itself should move freely and painlessly. In advanced OC, the eye may be proptotic and extremely painful to voluntary movement of the extraocular muscles, and visual acuity may be reduced. There may be diplopia on upward gaze. The child may appear "toxic" or irritable, with early meningeal signs.

DIFFERENTIAL DIAGNOSIS

The most common differential diagnoses to consider are local allergic reactions, blunt trauma, swelling secondary to an underlying sinusitis and bulbar or retrobulbar neoplasms. The history of an insect bite, the presence of loose swelling and itching, and the absence of systemic symptoms should aid in the diagnosis of a local allergic reaction. Likewise, the history of recent trauma to the area surrounding the eye, the presence of a "shiner," or the dissection of hematoma downward from a frontal contusion should be obtainable on careful questioning of the parent and child. Sinusitis is thought to cause swelling by obstruction of venous drainage from the overlying skin. The swelling is usually painless and not erythematous, but it sometimes may be difficult to distinguish from true PO. The time course for neoplasms of the lids and orbit is usually much more insidious. While retrobulbar tumors may cause proptosis and decreased vision, the lid swelling and periorbital cellulitis are usually not present.

EMERGENCY DEPARTMENT EVALUATION

The ED evaluation begins with a careful history and physical. The rapidity of onset; the history of trauma, insect bite, or skin lesions; the presence of an upper respiratory infection or sinusitis; and immunization status, particularly HIB and Pneumococcal vaccines, must be ascertained. The examination of the eye must include not only gentle palpation of the periorbital area, but also an assessment of whether the globe is proptotic, the function of the extraocular muscles, and whether there is any pain with movement of the eye. Visual acuity, pupillary function and confrontation visual fields must be assessed, if necessary, with the use of lid retractors. Specialists in the care of POC/OC currently use a staging process of I to IV with Stage I being POC and Stage II through IV reflecting increasingly severe levels of OC (26).

Laboratory studies are of limited value, although a white blood cell count greater than 15,000 may suggest bacteremia. Cultures of any wounds near the eye should be obtained; however, conjunctival or nasopharyngeal swabs are generally not helpful (26). Blood cultures have been reported to be positive in up to 30% of children; however 70% to 80% of these were *H. influenzae* in the prevaccine era (4,13,24). It seems likely that blood cultures will identify fewer and fewer organisms. In the pre-HIB era, lumbar puncture (LP) was considered almost mandatory in the young child because of the invasive and virulent character of *H. influenzae* bacteremia. Currently, most authors reserve LP for children less than 1 year of age (increased risk of *S. pneumoniae* bacteremia) (13), those who are "toxic" or irritable, or those who have not yet received or completed the HIB and Pneumococcal vaccination series.

Computerized tomography (CT) of the orbit may be useful in delineating sinusitis, orbital involvement, proptosis, abscess, or foreign body. It should be reserved for the child who presents with proptosis, pain on extraocular movement, decreased visual acuity, or inability to conduct a full eye examination (13).

EMERGENCY DEPARTMENT MANAGEMENT

After appropriate cultures have been obtained, an intravenous line should be started and antimicrobial therapy initiated with a third-generation cephalosporin:

Ceftriaxone 50 to 75 mg/kg intramuscularly or intravenously q24h, *or*

Cefotaxime 50 mg/kg per dose intravenously q6h

plus Clindamycin 10 mg/kg per dose q8h, or nafcillin 100 to 200 mg/kg/d q6h (26), *or*

Augmentin/Sulbactam 200 mg/kg/d in 4 divided doses *plus*

Vancomycin 60 mg/kg/d in 4 divided doses if suspicious for highly resistant *S. pneumoniae*

DISPOSITION

All children with OC and many children with POC should be admitted to the hospital. The inpatient unit should have the capability to care for children and have an ophthalmologist available for urgent consultation. Immediate consultation with an ophthalmologist and/or otolaryngologist should be undertaken if there are any physical findings suggestive of orbital involvement (proptosis, pain on eye movement, or decreased visual acuity), if there is difficulty obtaining an adequate eye examination, or if there has been failure to respond to parenteral antimicrobial therapy. Surgical evacuation is currently recommended for those patients who develop optic nerve findings such as decreasing visual acuity, afferent pupillary defect or visual field deficits; or who do not respond to 24 to 36 hours of medical management (13).

Recently, certain selected children with POC have been managed on an outpatient basis. There are several criteria that need to be met before the child can be discharged: there must be *no* orbital involvement (proptosis, ophthalmoplegia, decreased visual acuity), the child should be well-appearing, and the support system should be such that, not only are the parents willing and able to take the child home, but also willing and able to return the child immediately should there be a worsening in the child's condition. In uncomplicated posttraumatic POC (i.e., no purulent draining wound) treatment should be directed against gram-positive organisms with oral cephalexin, dicloxacillin or clindamycin (13) and next day follow up. In nontraumatic cases, after appropriate cultures are taken, an initial dose of ceftriaxone 50 mg/kg intramuscularly or intravenously (not to exceed 1 g) is given, followed by ampicillin–clavulanate 45 mg/kg/d in 2 divided doses orally for 7 to 10 days (13). In the penicillin-allergic child, give azithromycin 12 mg/kg (max, 500 mg/d) once a day for 5 days (15). The choice of outpatient antibiotics should reflect the level of *S. pneumoniae* and group A *Streptococcus* antibiotic resistance within the community. The child should be brought back for daily examinations to document and follow resolution, until blood cultures are negative (usually 48 hours) (24,26).

COMMON PITFALLS

✔ Failure to conduct a thorough eye examination, thus missing signs of orbital involvement

✔ Failure to consider an LP in a child less than 12 months of age

✔ Failure to consult an ophthalmologist early in cases of orbital involvement, which could result in a poor outcome, possible visual impairment, or loss of the eye

✔ Discharging a child who does not meet all of the criteria for outpatient management, resulting in a poor outcome from OC or abscess or spread to the CNS

ABNORMAL VISION

Children with complaints related to vision rarely present to the ED. When they do, the visit is prompted by their own complaints of abnormal vision or complaints from their parents, teachers, or school nurses. Occasionally, the ED physician, during the course of an examination, discovers a particular finding that necessitates urgent ophthalmologic referral. The complaints and etiologies for visual loss can vary greatly with the age of the child.

Cataracts, glaucoma, intraocular tumors, optic nerve problems, and nystagmus may all present in infancy. The incidence of congenital cataracts is one to four of 10,000 live births in industrialized countries and five to 15 of 10,000 births in the developing world. Cataracts usually present in the newborn nursery (12). However, with home births and the easy movement of populations between developing countries and the industrialized world, it is conceivable that the first presentation may be in the ED. Cataracts are strongly associated with several chromosomal abnormalities (trisomy 13, 18, 21), perinatal infections (rubella, toxoplasmosis, or varicella-zoster), and inborn errors of metabolism (12). Infantile glaucoma has an incidence of less than 1 in 10,000 live births. The sclera of an infant is more elastic than that of an older child. Increased intraocular pressure results in a gradual expansion of the globe. While the predisposition is congenital, the term *infantile* is used to express the variability in the time of onset from birth to clinically apparent disease (19).

Cortical visual impairment, defined as bilateral visual impairment in the presence of normal ocular structures, pupillary light reflex and absence of nystagmus, has increased in the United States in the last decade to become one of the most common causes of childhood blindness. The most common cause is perinatal hypoxia, however many other entities such as CNS infections, CNS malformations, epilepsy, malignancy, drugs and head trauma may result in cortical visual impairment (1).

Retinoblastoma is the most common intraocular malignancy. The average age of presentation is 18 months, with most occurring prior to 3 years of age. One-third of tumors are bilateral and present earlier than unilateral tumors. The underlying genetic defect is felt to be associated with changes to the Rb gene on chromosome 13q14 (9,25).

Nystagmus in childhood may be congenital or acquired. The etiologies of congenital nystagmus are essentially the same as those that cause visual impairment in infancy. Nystagmus that develops in the older child is usually either drug-induced or associated with severe visual loss or intracranial neoplasm (22).

By far, the most common complaint in the toddler and preschool-age child that is seen in the primary care office is strabismus, or ocular malalignment. The prevention of amblyopia (abnormal vision in an anatomically normal eye) is the major visual concern in this age group. If not detected and treated appropriately, the child may be left with a functionally blind eye (14,19).

Visual loss in childhood may result from compression of the optic nerve by tumor, inflammation of the optic nerve, and heredodegenerative conditions. Ten percent of rhabdomyosarcomas occur in the eye, arising from the intraocular muscles. The peak incidence is at age 8, with 75% occurring before age 10 (9,19). Optic neuritis in the child is felt to be a postviral autoimmune phenomenon. The most common preceding infections are measles, mumps, varicella, pertussis, mononucleosis, and postimmunization. Optic neuropathy has been reported in a few children with Lyme disease. There is a weaker association with multiple sclerosis than in young adults (9,22). In a 19-year follow up of 79 cases, 19% developed MS (21).

Optic gliomas and craniopharyngiomas are the two most common tumors that compress the optic nerve. Optic gliomas

TABLE 245.3.   Differential Diagnosis of Abnormal Vision[a]

Physical Finding	Age	Differential Diagnosis
Leukocoria	Infant	Cataract
	Older child	Retinoblastoma
		Other tumor
Tearing	Neonate	Congenital nasal lacrimal duct obstruction
		Glaucoma
Failure to fix or follow	2–3 mo	Abnormal visual development
		Any cause of decreased vision
		Strabismus
Nystagmus	Infant	Benign
	Older child	Any cause of decreased vision
		Tumor
		Amblyopia
		Drug-induced
Decreased visual acuity (monocular)	Infant	Cataract
		Glaucoma
		Tumor
		Refractive errors
	Child	Amblyopia
		Refractive errors
		Tumor
		Orbital cellulitis
	Older child	Optic neuritis
	Adolescent	Tumor
		Trauma
		Refractive errors
Decreased visual acuity (binocular)	Variable ages	Glaucoma
		Retinoblastoma
		Optic neuritis
		Refractive errors
		Cortical Visual Loss
Proptosis	All ages	Rhabdomyosarcoma
		Other tumor
		Retrobulbar infiltrative process
Strabismus	All ages	Amblyopia
		Muscle palsy
		Large unilateral refractive error

[a]This table is intended as a guide to the more common diagnoses and is not comprehensive.

are intrinsic tumors of the optic nerve. They usually occur between 4 and 8 years of age. There is a strong association with neurofibromatosis. Craniopharyngiomas are the third most common brain tumor of childhood, representing 10% of all tumors in childhood. They arise from the embryonic rests of Rathke pouch near the sella turcica. Craniopharyngiomas affect visual acuity by compressing the optic chiasm or the optic nerve (22).

CLINICAL PRESENTATION

The clinical presentation of visual loss varies with age and ability to express oneself. The infant may be brought to the ED because the parents have noted unilateral swelling of the globe or haziness of the cornea. The parents may complain that the 2- to 3-month-old infant does not seem able to fix on and follow objects. There may be no complaints at all, and the physician may discover one of these findings or note an abnormal red reflex or the presence of nystagmus.

The parents of a preverbal child may bring him or her to the ED because of perceived strabismus or a persistent head tilt. Intraocular tumors may present with decreasing visual acuity, leukocoria (absent red reflex), strabismus, or gradually increasing proptosis and corneal edema (14). Rhabdomyosarcoma may present explosively, with rapid development of proptosis and decreased visual acuity (9). Craniopharyngiomas may present with advanced visual defects, with or without headache, and

sometimes with an unusual vertical "see-saw" nystagmus (22). By contrast, optic neuritis presents with sudden, severe visual loss, often bilateral. There may be a history of an antecedent viral infection. On examination, there is reduced vision, nonreactive pupils, and swollen optic nerves. Hemorrhages and exudates may be seen on the optic disc (22).

There are certain behaviors that are typical, though not pathognomonic of low visual acuity. These include poor visual attention, photo aversion or the opposite, light gazing, rocking, head-nodding, exaggerated finger play and the oculo-digital reflex. The latter is vigorous eye rubbing that triggers ganglion cell action potentials which in turn create flashes of light and suggest retinal pathology (28). Table 245.3 lists the differential diagnoses of abnormal vision.

EMERGENCY DEPARTMENT EVALUATION

A complete history is very important to help narrow the differential diagnosis. The second most important step is a methodic and complete, age-appropriate eye examination. When a tumor is suspected, neuroimaging, beginning with a CT scan, is imperative. Particularly, any finding of proptosis, with or without decreased vision, necessitates an urgent CT scan. The evaluation of optic neuritis includes magnetic resonance imaging and an LP. The LP usually reveals a monoclonal pleocytosis and mild protein elevation (22).

EMERGENCY DEPARTMENT MANAGEMENT

The emphasis in management, in the majority of these conditions, should be on recognition of the potential severity of the problem; timely neuroimaging, when applicable; and prompt, sometimes emergent, referral.

Therapy for optic neuritis is based on randomized clinical trials conducted in adults. The ONTT (Optic Neuritis) trial showed that IV steroids resulted in a more rapid improvement in vision, a benefit that was lost at 12 months. There was, however, a significant reduction in progression in adults to multiple sclerosis at 2 years, but this also was lost at 5 years. Oral steroids (prednisone) alone were conclusively shown to be detrimental. The decision to treat with IV steroids remains somewhat controversial, but is frequently offered by ophthalmologists to children with bilateral disease, because of a worse prognosis for visual recovery (18,21). The steroid therapy of choice is methylprednisolone 15 to 30 mg/kg/d for 10 to 14 days (18,21). This is followed by a slow prednisone taper over 1 to 2 months. Too rapid a taper has been associated with a recurrence of optic neuritis and compounded visual loss (22).

DISPOSITION

Tumors, glaucoma, cataracts, and optic neuritis often involve urgent admission to the hospital. The facility, as well as the consultant, should be experienced in pediatric eye disorders. Because the growth of some tumors, such as rhabdomyosarcoma, can be explosive, consultation with an experienced ophthalmologist is emergent.

The presence, in an infant, of leukocoria or a swollen anterior chamber requires urgent referral to an ophthalmologist comfortable with the treatment of pediatric cataracts, tumors, or glaucoma. The treatment of these conditions is largely surgical. Because infancy represents a critical period in normal visual maturation, failure to remove the obstruction to clear vision could result in a functionally blind eye.

Because nystagmus can represent a structural lesion as well as amblyopia, referral on a semiurgent basis to an ophthalmologist should be done.

The finding of strabismus in the preverbal or preschool child mandates outpatient referral to an ophthalmologist.

COMMON PITFALLS

✔ Failure to perform an age-appropriate, complete eye examination
✔ Failure to refer a time-dependent process urgently to an appropriate ophthalmologist

CORNEAL ABRASION IN INFANTS

Corneal abrasion occurs in infants as a result of known or occult trauma. Infants under 1 year of age are more likely to present without a history of trauma and without any physical findings that point to the eye (20).

CLINICAL PRESENTATION

Infants may present, as with older children, with eye pain, tearing, photophobia, blepharospasm, conjunctival injection, eye-rubbing, and lid edema. On the other hand, they may present with only excessive crying or irritability. The infant may present only with grunting respirations, without any evidence of respiratory compromise (20).

DIFFERENTIAL DIAGNOSIS

In the infant who presents with injection, tearing, and blepharospasm, the differential diagnosis includes other etiologies of the "red eye." In the infant who presents with crying, irritability, or grunting, the differential needs to include systemic causes, such as respiratory insufficiency, sepsis, and meningitis.

EMERGENCY DEPARTMENT EVALUATION

A history and full eye examination should be done in infants with physical findings pointing to the eye. A corneal abrasion is diagnosed by staining the cornea with fluorescein-impregnated strips and shining a Wood light on the surface of the eye. An abrasion will stand out as a stained defect on the surface of the cornea. Both eyelids should be everted to search for a retained foreign body.

In the infant who presents with excessive crying, irritability, or grunting, a drop of topical anesthetic may be diagnostic as well as therapeutic (20). The infant may calm down almost immediately.

EMERGENCY DEPARTMENT MANAGEMENT

Treatment of corneal abrasions includes the use of a lubricating antibiotic ointment, such as erythromycin, bacitracin, or polysporin. Cyclopentolate 1% drops may be used if significant pain or ciliary spasm is present. Patching the affected eye may also be comforting to the infant. Any contact lenses should be removed.

DISPOSITION

Immediate consultation with an ophthalmologist should be sought if penetration past the superficial layers of the cornea is suspected. The abrasion should be followed daily until resolution of symptoms. This can be accomplished by the ED physician or primary care physician. If the abrasion is large or central (involving the visual axis), the infant should be referred to an ophthalmologist for examination within 24 hours.

COMMON PITFALLS

✔ Failure to recognize a deep abrasion or corneal ulcer, which could result in corneal scarring or deep infection of the eye
✔ Failure to consider corneal abrasion in the infant with otherwise unexplained crying or irritability

CONGENITAL NASOLACRIMAL DUCT OBSTRUCTION AND DACRYOCYSTITIS

Congenital nasolacrimal duct obstruction (CNLDO) is a common problem of infancy, with 20% of children exhibiting some symptoms within the first year of life (19). Canalization of the nasolacrimal duct may not be complete at birth. In most of these children, a membranous obstruction is the etiologic factor; however, a nasolacrimal duct cyst may also result in obstruction (16). Ninety-six percent of infants with CNLDO show spontaneous resolution of the obstruction by the first birthday (19).

Dacryocystitis, or infection of the nasolacrimal duct, may be acute or chronic. It may occur as a complication of CNLDO or of acquired nasolacrimal duct obstruction (ANLDO). In the neonatal period, dacryocystitis is rare, occurring in less than 2% of infants with CNLDO. However, if a duct cyst is the etiology of the obstruction, the risk of dacryocystitis is greater, with earlier presentation, usually by 2 weeks of age (16). The causative organisms are most often *S. aureus, S. epidermidis,* and alpha-hemolytic streptococci. *Corynebacterium* diphtheria and Epstein-Barr virus have also been reported (8). The risk of bacteremia is higher in the neonatal period than in the older infant or child. ANLDO may occur as the result of ethmoidal sinusitis or maxillary fracture through the wall of the nasolacrimal duct (8).

CLINICAL PRESENTATION

Symptoms of CNLDO may be present at birth or may be delayed for several weeks, until normal tear production develops. Signs include excessive tear lake, tear overflow, or a mucoid discharge that is produced by the lacrimal sac. There may be crusting or stickiness of the eye; however, the conjunctivae are clear, the eye is neither red nor swollen, and fever should not be present. The tearing is often distressing to the parent (19).

Dacryocystitis is characterized by erythematous and swollen skin over the lacrimal sac and purulent drainage from the punctum. Fever may be present, and periorbital or orbital cellulitis may develop as a complication of dacryocystitis (8).

DIFFERENTIAL DIAGNOSIS

The differential diagnosis includes corneal abrasion, conjunctivitis of various etiologies, local insect bite, or local trauma with resultant infection.

EMERGENCY DEPARTMENT EVALUATION

A careful history and physical examination should differentiate CNLDO from dacryocystitis. In the latter case, cultures of any purulent drainage, as well as blood cultures, need to be obtained. A complete blood count may be helpful, a high white blood cell count indicating a higher risk of bacteremia. In the infant who is 1 month old or younger, a full sepsis work up, including LP, should be done.

EMERGENCY DEPARTMENT MANAGEMENT

In dacryocystitis, antibiotics to cover *Staphylococcus* and *Streptococcus* species should be started immediately after cultures are obtained. The choice of particular antibiotics should reflect *Staphylococcus* and *Streptococcus* resistance within each community.

Suggested choices include the following:

Nafcillin 150 mg/kg/d intravenously in four divided doses
Cefuroxime 150 mg/kg/d intravenously in three divided doses
In the penicillin-allergic infant or child, vancomycin can be used.

DISPOSITION

All patients with acute dacryocystitis should be admitted to the hospital, on the service of a pediatrician capable of dealing with the potential complications of sepsis and/or meningitis. Immediate consultation with an ophthalmologist is needed, because

early nasolacrimal duct probing is important to the successful treatment of acute dacryocystitis. Because neonatal dacryocystitis is often associated with a nasolacrimal duct cyst, a complete intranasal examination at the time of surgery and marsupialization of any cyst are imperative to prevent recurrence (16).

The treatment of chronic or "low-grade" dacryocystitis is primarily surgical, with duct probing within several weeks. Systemic antibiotics are not necessary, although some consultants recommend a topical antibiotic ointment such as polymixin B (8).

Dacryocystitis after facial fracture or sinusitis requires referral to the appropriate specialist; ophthalmology; ear, nose, and throat; or plastics (8).

Conservative management of CNLDO includes warm-water compresses (to remove the mucoid discharge) and nasolacrimal duct massage. The latter is performed by occluding the common canaliculus with the index finger and then stroking firmly downward. This maneuver increases the hydrostatic pressure in the nasolacrimal sac, with the ultimate goal of overcoming the membranous obstruction. The massage should be repeated 5 to 10 times, 4 to 6 times a day. Erythromycin ophthalmic ointment applied 4 times a day is recommended; however, its efficacy in speeding recovery has not been proved. Referral to an ophthalmologist is recommended for those cases that do not resolve with conservative management. Probing will cure 90% of these infants (8). Newer, minimally invasive techniques such as balloon dacryocystoplasty, lacrimal stents, conjunctivoplasty and endoscopic dacryocystorhinostomy are continually being refined and may be offered in individual cases.

COMMON PITFALLS

✔ Failure to consider bacteremia, sepsis, or meningitis in the neonate or young infant
✔ Failure to consult an ophthalmologist early in cases of acute dacryocystitis

PARASITIC INFESTATION OF THE EYELASHES

Lice infestation of the eyelashes is caused by the genus *Phthirus,* otherwise known as the crab or pubic louse. Transmission may occur via the hand from infestation in the genital area, but it may also occur from contaminated towels and bedding. Infants may become infected as a result of close contact with an infested caretaker.

The adult lice feed on the host's blood, depositing their excrement at the base of the lashes. The females lay eggs (nits), which are firmly cemented in groups to the lashes. Exposure to the lice saliva and feces results in a dermal hypersensitivity reaction, causing severe pruritus. The intense desire to scratch often results in excoriations of the eyelids and, often, secondary bacterial infections.

CLINICAL PRESENTATION

Patients present with a history of itching and irritation of the eyes and eyelids, often of several weeks' duration. The lids may appear reddened, with a brownish crust at the base of the lashes. Close observation may reveal adult lice as well as clusters of nits on the upper and lower lashes. The nits appear as small, pearly, oval structures cemented to the base of the lashes. The palpebral conjunctiva may be red and inflamed. The cornea is rarely involved. There may be preauricular node swelling, reflecting secondary bacterial involvement (11).

DIFFERENTIAL DIAGNOSIS

Bacterial, viral, or allergic conjunctivitis represents the main differential diagnoses. Identification of adult lice and nits should effectively rule these out.

EMERGENCY DEPARTMENT EVALUATION

Slit-lamp examination should reveal, in addition to adult lice and nits, a brownish granular crust at the bases of the lashes (lice feces). Blue spots (maculae ceruleae) on the lid margins are characteristic of lice infestation and represent bite marks. A full eye examination, including fluorescein staining of the cornea to rule out concomitant corneal abrasion, should be done.

EMERGENCY DEPARTMENT MANAGEMENT

Eliminating lice infestation involves several management issues: killing adult lice, removing existing nits, and preventing reinfestation. In the cooperative patient, mechanical removal can be accomplished by using a slit-lamp, cotton swabs, and fine-toothed forceps. This needs to be followed by medical treatment aimed at killing the lice when they hatch. Several ophthalmic preparations have been endorsed over the years. The only clearly nontoxic preparation is petroleum jelly, applied to the eyelashes several times a day for 8 days, in order to suffocate the organisms (11). Yellow mercuric oxide ointment is pediculicidal, but a case of mercury poisoning has been reported in a 4-month-old infant. Physostigmine ointment likewise kills the lice, but it may cause such unwanted side effects as miosis and ciliary spasm. The argon laser has been used to kill lice and nits, but its use requires a cooperative patient as well as a skilled operator.

DISPOSITION

The patient needs to be evaluated for infestation of other body sites, and appropriate therapy instituted. If genital infestation is found, the possibility of sexually transmitted diseases needs to be addressed and treated. In order to prevent reinfestation, the caretaker needs to be educated on the sterilization of bedding, towels, and clothing, as well as the discarding of any cosmetic products used about the eye. Evaluation of potential infestation in the parent, especially in the case of an infant, should also be done (11).

COMMON PITFALLS

✔ Failure to entertain the diagnosis of louse infestation in the eyelashes
✔ Failure to educate the caretaker on the necessary measures needed to prevent reinfestation

SUPERGLUE IN THE EYE

Superglue (cyanoacrylate glue) in the eye usually occurs as the result of an accidental "squirt" while using the glue to repair an object, or by mistaking the bottle for an ophthalmic preparation and directly instilling glue in the eye. Cyanoacrylates form strong bonds between opposing surfaces within seconds. In the eye, they may form a layer covering the conjunctival and corneal surfaces, or they may tightly seal the lids and lashes together. They may also cause corneal abrasions, eyelid skin excoriation, and loss of eyelashes (17).

CLINICAL PRESENTATION

The clinical presentation is usually that of eyelids firmly glued together. If the cyanoacrylate has seeped into the eye, there may be pain, photophobia, tearing, and decreased vision. A film of glue may be adherent to the corneal surface of the eye, or there may be fragments under the lids.

DIFFERENTIAL DIAGNOSIS

Corneal abrasions present with similar symptoms, and may result from glue in the eye.

EMERGENCY DEPARTMENT EVALUATION

When the eyelids are firmly sealed together, the condition of the underlying eye needs to be inferred indirectly from complaints of pain, foreign-body sensation, tearing, and ability to move the globe without pain. As complete an examination as possible should be carried out.

EMERGENCY DEPARTMENT MANAGEMENT

Eyelids that are firmly bonded together are generally allowed to separate on their own, which will occur in 1 to 4 days. Trimming the involved eyelashes may facilitate separation of the lids. If the lashes are not pulled out, they should grow back normally. In the case of glue that is adherent to the cornea, the treatment is the same as for a corneal abrasion, with antibiotic preparations, mydriatic agents, and possible eye patching. Pain medication should be administered as needed.

DISPOSITION

Reexamination in 24 hours is recommended to evaluate for any signs of infection. The appearance of purulent drainage necessitates ophthalmologic consultation and surgical separation of the lids in order to evaluate fully the cornea and the globe. In the case of glue that is adherent to the cornea, followup evaluation often reveals spontaneous separation of the glue from the cornea, with a resultant epithelial defect. This corneal abrasion is usually superficial and requires continued therapy with antibiotic drops and mydriatics (17).

CRITICAL INTERVENTIONS

- Visual Acuity determination
THE RED EYE
  - Fluorescein staining
  - Gram stain if copious purulent discharge
  - Full septic work up in the young infant and neonate—particularly with suspected gonococcal infection
THE SWOLLEN EYE
  - Extraocular muscle examination
  - CT scan if the diagnosis of OC is being considered
ABNORMAL VISION
  - Urgent referral to an Ophthalmologist in the case of rapid visual loss

COMMON PITFALLS

✔ Unnecessary, early surgical separation of the lids, with pulling and subsequent loss of eyelashes

✔ Application of "home remedies" or chemicals that are potentially harmful to the eye, in an effort to "unbond" the lids

References

1. Afshari MA, Afshari NA, Fulton AB. Cortical visual impairment in infants and children. *Int Ophthalmol Clin* 2001;41:159–169.
2. American Academy of Pediatrics. Chlamydial infections, gonococcal infections, herpes simplex, and varicella zoster. In: Pickering LK, ed. *2003 Red book: report of the Committee on Infectious Diseases.* 26th ed. Elk Grove Village, IL: *American Academy of Pediatrics* 2003:235–237, 285–291, 344–353, 672–686, 730.
3. Bacal DA, Rousta ST, Hertle RW. Why early vision screening matters. *Contemp Pediatr* 1999;16:155– 156, 159–163, 167.
4. Barone SR, Aiuto LT. Periorbital and orbital cellulitis in the *Haemophilus influenzae* vaccine era. *J Pediatr Ophthalmol Strabismus* 1997;34:293–236.
5. Bielory L, Wagner RS. Allergic and immunologic pediatric disorders of the eye. *J Investig Allergol Clin Immunol* 1995;5:309–317.
6. Block SL, Hedrick J, et al. Increasing bacterial resistance in pediatric acute conjunctivitis (1997–1998). *Antimicrob agents Chemother* 2000;44:1650–1654.
7. Broderick P. Pediatric vision screening for the family physician. *Am Fam Physician* 1998;58:691–700, 703–704.
8. Campolattaro BN, Lueder GT, Tychsen L. Spectrum of pediatric dacryocystitis: medical and surgical management of 54 cases. *J Pediatr Ophthalmol Strabismus* 1997;34:143–153.
9. Castillo BV Jr, Kaufman L. Pediatric tumors of the eye and orbit. *Pediatr Clin North Am* 2003;50:149–172.
10. de Boer J, Wulffraat N, Rothova A. Visual loss in uveitis of childhood. *Br J Ophthalmol* 2003;87:879–884.
11. Dornic DI. Ectoparasitic infestation of the eyelashes. *J Am Optom Assoc* 1985;56:716–719.
12. Foster A, Gilberr C, Rahi J. Epidemiology of cataract in childhood: a global perspective. *J Cataract Refract Surg* 1997;23[Suppl 1]:601–604.
13. Givner LB. Periorbital versus orbital cellulitis. *Pediatr Infect Dis J* 2002;21:1157–1158.
14. King RA. Common ocular signs and symptoms in childhood. *Pediatr Clin North Am* 1993;40:753–766.
15. Langtry HD, Balfour JA. Azithromycin: a review of its use in paediatric infectious diseases. *Drugs* 1998;56:273–297.
16. Leuder GT. Neonatal dacryocystitis associated with nasolacrimal duct cysts. *J Pediatr Ophthalmol Strabismus* 1995;32:102–106.
17. Maitra AK. Management of complications of cyanoacrylate adhesives. *Br J Clin Pract* 1984;38:284–286.
18. Morales DS, Siatkowski RM, Howard CW, Warman R. Optic Neuritis in children. *J Pediatr Ophthalmol Striabismus* 2000;7:254–259.
19. Olitsky SE, Nelson LB. Common ophthalmologic concerns in infants and children. *Pediatr Clin North Am* 1998;45:993–1012.
20. Poole SR. Corneal abrasion in infants. *Pediatr Emerg Care* 1995;11:25–26.
21. Purvin V. Optic Neuritis. *Curr Opin Ophthalmol* 1998;9:3–9.
22. Repka MX. Common pediatric neuro-ophthalmologic conditions. *Pediatr Clin North Am* 1993;40:777–788.
23. Sabbah A, Marzetto M. Azelastine eye drops in the treatment of seasonal allergic conjunctivitis or rhino conjunctivitis in young children. *Curr Med Res Opin* 1998;14:161–170.
24. Schwartz GR, Wright SW. Changing bacteriology of periorbital cellulitis. *Ann Emerg Med* 1996;28:617–620.
25. Shields JA, Shields CL. Pediatric ocular and periocular tumors. *Pediatr Ann* 2001;30:491–501.
26. Starkey CR, Steele RW. Medical management of orbital cellulitis. *Pediatr Infect Dis J* 2001;20:1002–1025.
27. Teoh DL, Reynolds S. Diagnosis and management of pediatric conjunctivitis. *Pediatr Emerg Care* 2003;19:48–55.
28. Thompson L, Kaufman LM. The visually impaired child. *Pediatr Clin North Am* 2003;50:225–239.
29. Wald ER. Conjunctivitis in infants and children. *Pediatr Infect Dis J* 1997; 16[2 Suppl]:S17–S20.
30. Whitney CG, et al. Decline in invasive Pneumococcal disease after introduction of protein-polysaccharide conjugate vaccine. *NEJM* 2003;348:1737–1746.

CHAPTER 246
Foreign Bodies

Lance Brown

The emergency department management of foreign bodies can be quite rewarding. The history is typically as straightforward as the declaration that a foreign body is present and the management of foreign bodies is conceptually simple. Attempted removal, reassurance, and consultation are the basic management plans, each of which is implemented based on the clinical presentation, body cavity, and type of foreign body. Fortunately, few truly emergent or urgent conditions related to foreign bodies exist.

CLINICAL PRESENTATION

Ear – A wide range of pediatric ages present with ear canal foreign bodies. From studies of emergency department patients, the age range has been reported to be from 1.4 years to 17.6 years (1,4) with a median of 6 years. The literature is conflicting regarding presenting complaints as one study reported that 90% of patients presented with pain or discomfort (1), while another study reported that nearly half were asymptomatic (4). In both studies, however, decreased hearing was seen in about 30% and bleeding was seen in fewer than 10% of cases. A wide range of objects has been identified as ear foreign bodies. These include insects, paper, beads, seeds, eraser tips, earring parts, and toy parts (1). One concerning presentation is that of an ear canal disk or button battery. The destructive nature of the chemicals released from button batteries can cause an intense localized inflammation that can be quite similar to otitis externa in clinical appearance (3). If not identified and managed promptly, the destructive process will spread locally and lead to significant cosmetic and functional problems.

Nose – When compared to ear foreign bodies, nasal foreign bodies tend to present in younger children with a reported median age of 2 to 3 years (1,4,13). Children with nasal foreign bodies are reported to be asymptomatic about half of the time (4,13). Less common complaints include a foul odor, pain or discomfort, and bleeding. The presentation with unilateral nasal discharge deserves special emphasis. In about 10% of cases of nasal foreign bodies, unilateral nasal discharge is present and may be the sole presenting complaint for these toddlers (4,13). A wide range of small objects may be found in the noses of children. These most commonly include beads, plastic toy parts, corn kernels, and beans (1,13). Although bilateral nasal foreign bodes are uncommon, bilateral nasal magnets adherent across the nasal septum have been described (5,17). These children usually present with pain and if the magnets are not identified and removed promptly, septal necrosis may ensue.

Airway – Aspirated foreign bodies are seen most commonly in toddlers. In one study, nearly 80% of the children who had aspirated foreign bodies identified on bronchoscopy were younger than 3 years of age (2). Aspirated foreign bodies are not common. Even large tertiary care pediatric centers accepting patients in transfer from other facilities can expect to see only one or two cases a month (6). The literature tends to consist of retrospective case series that span years or even decades. The reported frequency of various signs and symptoms, therefore, vary widely.

The most commonly reported symptoms include choking or coughing in 25% to 75% of cases (6). Other relatively common signs and symptoms include dyspnea, fever, and wheezing. Stridor, hemoptysis, and the absence of symptoms are uncommon. The most commonly reported aspirated objects are foods, with peanuts seen in about one-third of cases (6). In one study that reviewed consumer products over a 20-year time period, there were fewer than 25 deaths per year due to aspiration in the entire United States (20). Balloons were the most common objects that caused death (20).

Gastrointestinal – Swallowed foreign bodies are relatively common. In the year 2000, there were more than 77,000 pediatric foreign body ingestions reported to poison control centers in the United States (16). The true number is probably much greater as parents may not be aware of many benign ingestions or may not seek medical attention even when a foreign body ingestion occurs (10). Ingested foreign bodies that make it past the esophagus seem to pass through the intestines and exit the body with the stool in about 99% of cases with normal anatomy (8,18). Developmentally delayed children may ingest large or sharp foreign bodies, present in an atypical fashion, or provide a limited history due to language difficulties (8). Most children with subdiaphragmatic foreign bodies are asymptomatic including those that ingest batteries (6,15). The ingestion of multiple magnets may cause pressure necrosis as the wall of the intestines is trapped between magnets. The child may present with abdominal pain without fever (17). The most widely studied esophageal foreign bodies are coins (6). More than 90% of children with esophageal coins are symptomatic before or at the time of presentation to the emergency department (9). Symptoms of esophageal foreign bodies include drooling, substernal pain, or a foreign body sensation. Few children with esophageal coins are asymptomatic.

Genitourinary – Genitourinary foreign bodies are quite unusual in children. For boys, there is a single case of a teen male putting a chain through his urethra up into his bladder (6). Vaginal foreign bodies are unusual in prepubertal girls. Objects that have been described include coins, safety pins, hair pins, fruit pits, small toys, and pen tops (6,21). The most common intravaginal material may be toilet paper in girls of toilet training age (21). The most common symptoms of intravaginal foreign bodies are vaginal bleeding or discharge in a prepubertal girl.

Rectal – Rectal foreign bodies in children are very unusual (7). There are old reports of broken or retained glass rectal thermometers in infants (14).

DIFFERENTIAL DIAGNOSIS

Ear – The appearance of a foreign body in the ear canal is usually quite distinct. If the pinna and canal are markedly inflamed it may be difficult to distinguish a retained button battery in the ear canal from typical otitis externa on physical examination alone (3). Impacted wax may be confused with foreign material in the ear canal. Rare ear canal masses may be mistaken for foreign bodies.

Nose – Unilateral nasal discharge that is somewhat chronic may be mistakenly treated for the highly unlikely condition of "unilateral sinusitis." Young children with unilateral nasal discharge should be treated as if they have a nasal foreign body until proven otherwise regardless of how adamantly the parents deny that a foreign body is present (6). Nasal polyps may be mistaken for foreign bodies. In addition to a nasal foreign body, children who have a foul odor emanating from the mouth and nose may have halitosis, purulent pharyngitis, sinusitis, or a dental infection.

Airway – The signs and symptoms of aspirated foreign bodies are neither sensitive nor specific (24). As many as 10% of children

who have a history of aspirated foreign body do not reveal a foreign body on bronchoscopy (24). The symptoms associated with aspirated foreign bodies are nonspecific and include choking, coughing, wheezing, fever, dyspnea, and stridor. Any of a myriad of respiratory conditions including viral upper respiratory tract infections, bronchiolitis, croup, asthma, pneumonia, and hydrocarbon aspiration can all present with at least some of these symptoms.

Gastrointestinal – The vast majority of children with subdiaphragmatic foreign bodies are asymptomatic. If symptomatic, abdominal pain or rectal bleeding may be present (19). Conditions such as appendicitis, intussusception, Meckel diverticulum, intestinal polyps, or other rarer causes of abdominal pain in this age group may be considered in the differential diagnosis of abdominal pain in these young children.

Genitourinary – Vaginal discharge and bleeding in a prepubertal girl may be indicative of sexual abuse. There is a single study of 12 girls with vaginal foreign bodies, most of whom also met the criteria for sexual abuse including 2 girls with concurrent sexually transmitted diseases (11).

Rectal – Occasionally a rectal polyp will emerge from the anus. The unsuspecting physician may confuse this bright red, fleshy mass with a foreign body.

EMERGENCY DEPARTMENT EVALUATION

Ear – The emergency department evaluation of a suspected ear foreign body is almost always straightforward and involves visual inspection of the ear canal with an otoscope. If a button battery is suspected in the setting of an otitis externa, radiography should easily identify this metallic foreign body.

Nose – Often a nasal foreign body can be identified by simply tipping the child's head back and visually inspecting the nasal passages. A well directed overhead lamp or a hand held otoscope and expanding the nasal opening with a pediatric nasal speculum will offer a better view.

Airway – Definitively determining whether or not a child who had an abrupt choking or coughing episode has an aspirated foreign body can be difficult. If the object is radiopaque, a 2-view chest x-ray can clearly reveal the location of the foreign body in the trachea or a bronchus. Unfortunately, about 85% of aspirated foreign bodies are radiolucent. Therefore, alternative techniques are usually needed. A commonly used approach is to perform inspiratory and expiratory chest x-rays. If the radiology technologist can time it properly, inspiratory and expiratory chest x-rays may reveal a relatively normal and symmetric inspiratory radiograph, but relative hyperinflation on the side with the foreign body on an expiratory radiograph. This is thought to be due to a ball-valve effect whereby the inspired air can move past an intrabronchial foreign body when the bronchus expands during the negative pressure of inspiration, but cannot be expelled when the bronchus collapses around the foreign body during expiration. Because it can be difficult to time these films properly, this same principle can be applied to bilateral lateral decubitus films. Normally the mediastinum shifts down with gravity when a child is placed in the lateral decubitus position. If there is air trapping due to an intrabronchial foreign body, the mediastinum will fail to shift down toward the side with the foreign body. There is essentially no literature to support this time-honored approach (6). A more definitive diagnostic approach is to have a child for whom there are persistent symptoms or a high degree of suspicion for an aspirated foreign body undergo bronchoscopy which can be both diagnostic and therapeutic (2).

Gastrointestinal – A traditional approach to evaluating a child with an ingested foreign body is to obtain x-rays from the nasopharynx to the bottom of the pelvis looking for radiopaque foreign bodies. If a foreign body is identified, the critical question is whether or not the foreign body is esophageal as these typically require treatment. If a child is asymptomatic, can eat and drink without apparent pain or difficulty, and has a negative set of x-rays, a subdiaphragmatic radiolucent foreign body is assumed. If the child has persistent foreign body sensation or pain in the substernal area or neck and the x-rays are unrevealing, the child may need to undergo esophagoscopy to evaluate for esophageal abrasions or radiolucent retained esophageal foreign bodies.

Genitourinary – For young girls with vaginal discharge or bleeding, the first step is to perform a visual inspection of the area. If sexual abuse is suspected after this visual exam or if an intravaginal foreign body is suspected, coordination with a forensic pediatrician or pediatric gynecologist is prudent. If an intravaginal procedure or examination is required, sedation should be strongly considered. Pelvic x-rays may reveal a radiopaque foreign body (6).

EMERGENCY DEPARTMENT MANAGEMENT

Appropriate ENT equipment and restraint or sedation is essential for appropriate evaluation and foreign body removal. This may include ENT microscopes, foreign body removal devices, and lighting or irrigation devices.

Ear – Most ear canal foreign bodies can be removed by emergency physicians in the emergency department (1,4). There are multiple techniques that have been successfully used and described in the literature (1,4,6). The most commonly described techniques involve grasping the object with forceps, using a hook, loop, or curette to drag the object out of the ear canal, and irrigation to wash the object out (1,4,6). Irrigation should only be undertaken if the tympanic membrane is intact. This may be difficult to determine on clinical exam due to the foreign object obscuring the view of the tympanic membrane. The depth of the object in the canal and the object shape may help in risk stratifying these patients with regard to the likelihood of tympanic membrane injury. Because working on the ear canal may be both loud and painful, and because the bony ear canal tends to bleed quite easily, procedural sedation with an agent such as ketamine seems to improve the chances of successful removal in the emergency department (4). Urgent removal is indicated if a button battery is the suspected or confirmed foreign body as continued tissue destruction will occur if the battery is not removed promptly (3).

Nose – The vast majority of nasal foreign bodies can be managed in the emergency department by emergency physicians (1,4,13). Fewer of these cases seem to require sedation than ear foreign bodies, but sedation may be helpful in uncooperative children with large or adherent foreign bodies (4). The techniques for removal are similar to those used for ear foreign bodies (6). These techniques include grasping the object with forceps, using a hook, loop, or curette to drag the object forward, and suction applied directly to the foreign body. Because of the communication with the mouth, there are 2 additional techniques that can be employed. One is a positive pressure technique whereby the parent applies pressure to the contralateral nostril to close it and then blows into the mouth. The intended consequence is that the foreign body will be expelled. The other technique is to insert a balloon catheter (such as a 6 French silicon Foley catheter) past the foreign body, inflate the balloon, and then withdraw the catheter with the balloon inflated. This process sweeps the nasal cavity and is a good choice for large round smooth objects that are difficult to grasp and friable, fragmented materials such as clay that fall apart when grasped. Although there is a theoretical risk that a nasal foreign body could be dislodged posteriorly

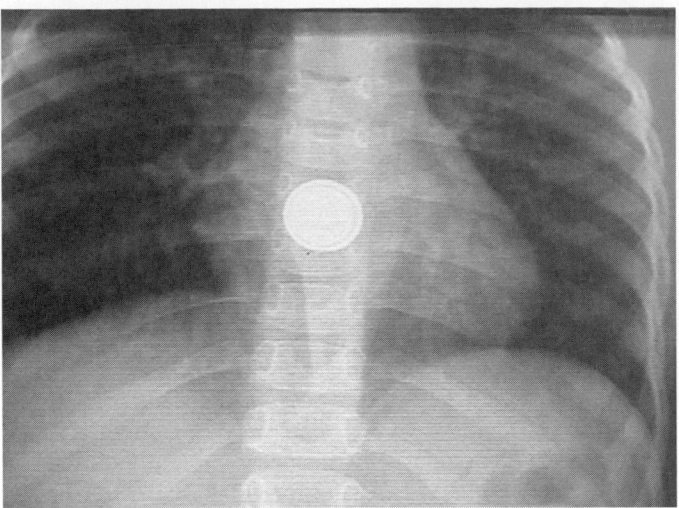

Figure 246.1. Radiograph of a large, flat disc battery in the distal esophagus of a young child. Note the faint circular area of relative radiolucency near the periphery of the object shadow. This characteristic target appearance distinguishes this object from the more homogeneous appearance of an ingested coin. (*Photograph by Lance Brown, MD MPH*)

and subsequently aspirated, there are no reported cases of aspirated nasal foreign bodies in the medical literature. Bilateral nasal magnets adherent across the nasal septum may be atraumatically removed by sequentially placing the metal handle of a pair of forceps in the nostrils to break the magnetic attraction and individually remove the magnets (5).

Airway – Once an aspirated foreign body has been identified or is strongly suspected based on radiographic studies, appropriate consultation for bronchoscopy is indicated. A variety of pediatric specialists perform this procedure including pulmonologists, intensivists, and surgeons.

Gastrointestinal – The vast majority of subdiaphragmatic foreign bodies require only reassurance and will pass on their own (8,18). Although it has been historically recommended that parents sift through stools until the foreign body is identified as having been passed, this process does little more than punish the parents. Regardless of the transit time, nearly all subdiaphragmatic foreign bodies pass spontaneously. Exceptions include very large or very sharp objects typically ingested by developmentally delayed older school-aged children, children with abnormal gastrointestinal anatomy (e.g., an ileostomy), children with multiple magnets in the intestines (17), children with intestinal batteries that appear to be fragmenting on x-ray (15), and symptomatic children. Esophageal foreign bodies, especially button batteries, tend to need removal to avoid esophageal erosion (6) (Fig. 246.1).

Genitourinary – There is no evidence-based emergency department (ED) management approach to pediatric genitourinary foreign bodies. Young girls with a suspected foreign body may need an examination under sedation or general anesthesia if an intravaginal foreign body is suspected. Referral for sexual abuse assessment may be needed for prepubertal girls with intravaginal foreign bodies and vaginal discharge or bleeding (11).

Rectal – Rectal foreign bodies are unusual in children and management must be individualized.

CRITICAL INTERVENTIONS

- Urgent removal of button batteries in the ears, nose, or esophagus
- Urgent removal of bilateral nasal magnets adherent across the nasal septum

- Use of sedation to remove ear foreign bodies if not accomplished easily on first attempt
- Surgical consultation for the ingestion of multiple magnets
- Consideration of sexual abuse in prepubertal girls with intravaginal foreign bodies

DISPOSITION

Ear – Essentially all ear foreign bodies can be managed in the ED with or without sedation (4). In the event that a foreign body cannot be removed in the ED, outpatient referral to an ear, nose, and throat (ENT) surgeon is appropriate in all cases except button batteries.

Nose – Essentially all nose foreign bodies can be managed in the ED with or without sedation (4). If a foreign body cannot be removed in the ED, outpatient referral to an ENT surgeon is appropriate in all cases except button batteries and magnets adherent across the nasal septum.

Airway – Aspirated foreign bodies and children with a clinical picture suspicious for aspirated foreign bodies should be admitted to the hospital and undergo urgent bronchoscopy.

Gastrointestinal – The vast majority of ingested foreign bodies, especially those that have been confirmed to be subdiaphragmatic can be managed expectantly at home without further intervention unless symptoms such as vomiting, bloody stools, or abdominal pain develop. An exception is multiple magnets that can become adherent to each other across the bowel wall and cause necrosis. These children typically require admission to a surgeon and laparotomy for magnet removal (17). Children with esophageal foreign bodies may require admission for removal (6) or removal may be attempted on a sedated child in the ED (12). Children with acute (less than 24 hour) mid-esophageal and distal esophageal coins may be observed for 24 hours with the prospect that the coin will pass spontaneously obviating the need for endoscopy (22). If on repeat next day radiographs, the coin is still in the esophagus, then the coin should be removed (23).

Genitourinary – Young girls with intravaginal foreign bodies without other indications for admission can probably be managed as outpatients. Prepubertal girls suspected of being victims of sexual abuse may need admission to the hospital for social indications.

Rectal – Removal of rectal foreign bodies in adults can be accomplished in the emergency department under procedural sedation. Whether this approach is appropriate for most children must be determined on an individual case basis.

COMMON PITFALLS

✔ Delaying management of a disk battery or multiple magnets
✔ Relying on a single chest x-ray to rule out an aspirated foreign body
✔ Not considering unilateral nasal discharge to be a foreign body
✔ Not using procedural sedation and appropriate equipment to manage ear foreign bodies

Acknowledgment

Thanks to the previous edition's chapter author Linda L. Settle.

References

1. Baker MD. Foreign bodies of the ears and nose in childhood. *Pediatr Emerg Care* 1987;3:67–70.
2. Black RE, Johnson DG, Matlak ME. Bronchoscopic removal of aspirated foreign bodies in children. *J Pediatr Surg* 1994;29:682–684.
3. Bhisitkul DM, Dunham M. An unsuspecting alkaline battery foreign body presenting as malignant otitis externa. *Pediatr Emerg Care* 1992;8:141–142.
4. Brown L, Denmark TK, Wittlake WA, et al. Procedural sedation use in the emergency department management of pediatric ear and nose foreign bodies. *Am J Emerg Med* 2004;22:310–314.
5. Brown L, Tomasi A, Salcedo G. An attractive approach to magnets adherent across the nasal septum. *Can J Emerg Med* 2003;5:356–358.
6. Brown L, Dannenberg B. A literature-based approach to the identification and management of pediatric foreign bodies. *Pediatr Emerg Med Reports* 2002;7:93–104.
7. Busch DB, Starling JR. Rectal foreign bodies: Case reports and a comprehensive review of the world's literature. *Surgery* 1986;100:512–519.
8. Cheng W, Tam PK. Foreign-body ingestion in children: Experience with 1,265 cases. *J Pediatr Surg* 1999;34:1472–1476.
9. Conners GP, Chamberlain JM, Ochsenschlager DW. Symptoms and spontaneous passage of esophageal coins. *Arch Pediatr Adolesc Med* 1995;149:36–39.
10. Conners GP, Chamberlain JM, Weiner PR. Pediatric coin ingestion: a home-based survey. *Am J Emerg Med* 1995;13:638–640.
11. Herman-Giddens ME. Vagianl foreign bodies and child sexual abuse. *Arch Pediatr Adolesc Med* 1994;148:195–200.
12. Hostetler MA, Barnard JA. Removal of esophageal foreign bodies in the pediatric ED. Is ketamine an option? *Am J Emerg Med* 2002;20:96–98.
13. Kadish HA, Corneli HM. Remoaval of nasal forcign bodies in the pediatric population. *Am J Emerg Med* 1997;15:54–56.
14. Lau JTK, Ong GB. Broken and retained rectal thermometer in infants and young children. *Aust Paediatr J* 1981;17:93–94.
15. Litovitz T, Schmitz BF. Ingestion of cylindrical and button batteries: An analysis of 2382 cases. *Pediatrics* 1992;89:747–757.
16. Litovitz TL, Klein-Schwartz W, White S, et al. 2000. Annual Report of the American Association of Poison Control Centers Toxic Exposure Surveillance System. *Am J Emerg Med* 2001;19:337–395.
17. McCormick S, Brennan P, Yassa J, Shawis R. Children and mini-magnets: an almost fatal attraction. *Emerg Med J* 2002;19:71–73.
18. Pellerin D, Fortier-Beaulieu M, Gueguen J. The fate of swallowed foreign bodies: experience of 1250 instances of sub-diaphragmatic foreign bodies in children. *Progr Pediatr Radiol* 1969;2:286–302.
19. Pinero MA, Fernandez-Hernandez JA, Carrasco PM, et al. Intestinal perforation by foreign bodies. *Eur J Surg* 2000;166:307–309.
20. Rimell FL, Thome A, Stool S, et al. Characteristics of objects that cause choking in children. *JAMA* 1995;274:1763–1766.
21. Sanfilippo JS, Wakim NG. Bleeding and vulvovaginitis in the pediatric age group. *Clin Obstet Gynecol* 1987;30:653–661.
22. Soprano JV, Fleisher GR, Mandl KD. The spontaneous passage of esophageal coins in children. *Arch Pediatr Adolesc Med* 1999;153:1073–1076.
23. Sharieff G, Brousseau T, Bradshaw J, et al. Acute Esophageal Coin Ingestions-Is Immediate Removal Necessary? *Pediatr Radiol* 2003;10–11.
24. Zarella JT, Dimler M, McGill LC, Pippus KJ. Foreign body aspiration in children: value of radiography and complication of bronchoscopy. *J Pediatr Surg* 1998;33:1651–1654.

CHAPTER 247
Genitourinary Disorders

Brianna Enriquez and Marianne Gausche-Hill

FEMALE GENITOURINARY DISORDERS

The genitourinary and gynecologic evaluations of pediatric patients pose specific challenges to practitioners. The physician must incorporate knowledge about stages of development, likely diagnoses for different age groups, and the patient's specific history to tailor an appropriate and thorough examination. Any child presenting with abdominal pain must undergo a genitourinary exam. In addition, the emergency department (ED)

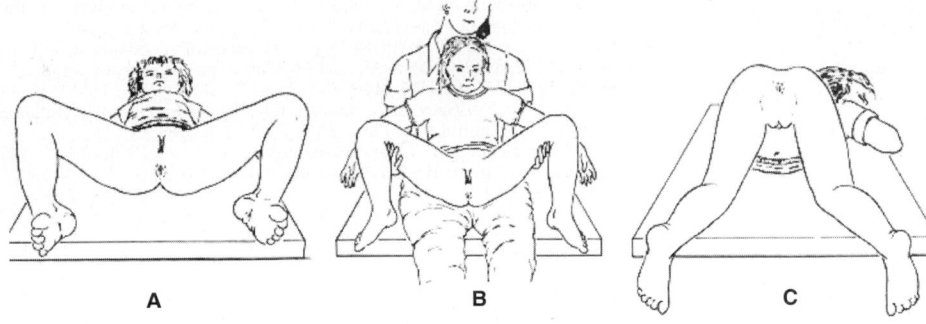

Figure 247.1. Positions for genitourinary examination of the female child: **(A and B)** Frog-leg position and **(C)** knee-chest position.

physician must always maintain a high index of suspicion for sexual abuse as children who are abused may present with unusual or vague complaints.

The response of the premenarchal patient to the genitourinary exam depends upon their stage of development. A younger child will generally cooperate easily while older children tend to be more private, especially in the early stages of puberty. Putting the child at ease to make the evaluation as atraumatic as possible is crucial. Infants can be examined in a parents lap instead of on the examination table. Older girls must be evaluated on the examination table. Two positions commonly used in the evaluation of the female child are the frog-leg position, and for girls older than four-years-old, the knee-chest position. In the frog-leg position, the child is supine on the table with her heels together, while her knees and hips are flexed (Fig. 247.1). With gentle lateral and caudal traction on the labia majora, the hymen and introitus can be seen. The knee-chest position generally affords a better view of the vaginal vault. The child is instructed to get on her hands and knees, fold her arms, rest on her elbows and then place her head on her arms.

The premenarchal patient should be examined in the frog-leg position and if possible knee-chest position. A rectal exam is required for complaints of abdominal pain and abdominal mass. A thorough examination under anesthesia or with procedural sedation is necessary in young children. This examination is necessary only if vaginal bleeding is indicated with no obvious source on external examination, suspected vaginal foreign body, or if significant trauma is also suspected. For most complaints in this age group, a careful history and physical with thorough evaluation of the external genitalia and cultures of any vaginal discharge is adequate.

When evaluating an adolescent with a genitourinary complaint or abdominal pain, the history must include age of menarche, menstrual history, sexual activity, pregnancies, history of sexually transmitted diseases, and contraception. The adolescent must be interviewed alone to enable a full and accurate history. A virginal female may also be evaluated as a premenarchal patient. However, every postmenarchal girl must have a pregnancy test. A sexually experienced female requires a full gynecologic evaluation, due to the high rates of pregnancy and sexually transmitted disease in this age group. The physician should use the encounter as an opportunity to address pregnancy, disease, violence prevention and provide health care resources.

PEDIATRIC VULVOVAGINITIS

CLINICAL PRESENTATION

Inflammation of the vulva and vagina is the most common gynecologic complaint in the prepubertal female (6). Vaginitis is also the most common chief complaint for adolescents in obstet-

rics and gynecology offices (14). The premenarchal genitourinary area has several risk factors that make it prone to inflammation. There is an absence of labial fat pads and pubic hair for protection and there is a low estrogen level, which keeps the vaginal epithelium atrophied and the pH of vagina more alkaline. In addition, the proximity to the anus and poor local hygiene place the patient at risk for inflammation. There is no physiologic vaginal discharge from approximately one month of age until prepuberty. Therefore, a prepubertal girl with the chief complaint of vaginal discharge warrants an evaluation. Patients may also present with vaginal bleeding, pruritis, and odor. The postpubertal female will present with a change in vaginal discharge, pruritis, or pain. Frequency and dysuria can be associated symptoms.

DIFFERENTIAL DIAGNOSIS

The differential diagnosis varies depending upon the age and risk factors of the patient. An infant is more likely to have neonatal leukorrhea, diaper dermatitis, impetigo, chemical/mechanical irritation, seborrheic dermatitis, or a genitourinary malformation. A chronic irritation may be secondary to lichen sclerosis, labial adhesions, molluscum contagiosum, enterobiasis (discussed below), or a vaginal foreign body.

The etiology of vulvovaginitis in pediatrics is usually divided into two groups, specific and nonspecific. The specific pathogens include *Candida albicans, Neisseria. gonorrhoeae, Shigella, Streptococcus pyogenes,* and *Trichomonas vaginalis.* Nonspecific vaginitis remains a diagnosis of exclusion and is usually attributed to poor hygiene, chemical irritation, and tight fitting clothing.

EMERGENCY DEPARTMENT EVALUATION

Premenarchal patients with visible discharge on examination must have vaginal cultures for bacteria, cytology, and yeast. Cultures may be obtained with a moist swab placed in the introitus. A culture for Chlamydia is usually only sent if other cultures are negative. Urine tests are now available for gonorrhea and chlamydia and is used to screen for disease, however culture remains the only FDA approved and court-permissible proof of infection in children (4). Postmenarchal patients must undergo a pregnancy test and a complete speculum and bimanual examination with sexually transmitted disease (STD) screening if they have ever been sexually active.

EMERGENCY DEPARTMENT MANAGEMENT

The diagnosis of specific vulvovaginitis must be culture proven with targeted antimicrobial treatment. See Table 247.1 for specific treatments. The treatment of nonspecific vaginitis is focused on proper hygiene (i.e., front to back wiping), and avoidance of

TABLE 247.1.   Treatment of Vulvovaginitis*

Organism	Treatment
Trichomonas	Metronidazole 2 g PO in single dose, or 500 mg PO BID for 7 days, or 15 mg/kg/24 hours divided tid for 7 days
Candida albicans	Butoconazole 2% cream 5 g intravaginally for 3 days, or
	Butaconazole1-sustained release 2% cream 5 g intravaginally as single dose, or
	Clotrimazole 500 mg tablet intravaginally in single dose, or
	Ticonazole 6.5% ointment 5 g intravaginally as single dose
Chlamydia trachomatis	
<45 kg	Erythromycin base 50 mg/kg/day PO divided QID for 14 days
>45 kg, <8 years	Azithromycin 1 g PO as single dose
> 8 years	Azithromycin 1 g PO as single dose, or
	Doxycycline 100 mg PO BID for 7 days
Neisseria gonorrhea	
<45 kg	Ceftriaxone 125 mg IM in single dose
>45 kg	Ceftriaxone 125 mg IM in single dose, or
	Ciprofloxacin 500 mg PO in single dose, or
	Ofloxacin 400 mg PO in single dose, or
	Levofloxacin 250 mg PO in single dose
Penicillin allergic	Spectinomycin 2 g IM in single dose if >45 kg, or 40 mg/kg IM in single dose

*Treatments per CDC sexually transmitted diseases treatment guidelines 2002.

irritation. A diagnosis of candidal vaginitis in a prepubertal patient is unusual, and the patient should have an additional work up for diabetes or other immunodeficiencies.

DISPOSITION

All patients require follow up to ensure the cultures are followed and that the organism was properly treated. It is recommended that patients are appropriately referred if there is a possibility of immunosuppression or a dermatologic condition.

PINWORMS

CLINICAL PRESENTATION

Enterobius vermicularis infection is a common finding in children even in industrialized countries. Those at increased risk are children living in crowded places, institutions, and where sanitation is poor. Males and females may be affected. Children become infected by ingesting the eggs of the worm. The eggs hatch in the stomach and migrate to the cecum where they mature. At night, female worms travel to the anus and deposit eggs in the perianal area. The ensuing pruritis causes the infected child to scratch the perianal area, thus eggs are lodged under the fingernails to pass to others. The eggs can also be passed onto clothing and bedding. The eggs remain viable for twenty days.

Patients usually present with anal pruritis, noted to be worse at night and in the early morning. Symptoms may be vague however, such as sleeplessness, anorexia, abdominal pain, and weight loss. Infected persons may be asymptomatic. Pinworms have been found in the vagina and intraabdominal sites. They have caused appendicitis, salpingitis, and perianal granulomas.

DIFFERENTIAL DIAGNOSIS

The differential diagnosis for pinworms includes causes of perianal pruritis, vaginitis, abdominal pain and weight loss.

EMERGENCY DEPARTMENT EVALUATION

The diagnosis is established by recovery of eggs or worms. The best collection time is early morning, and clear tape should be repeatedly pressed against the perianal region. The tape is placed on a glass slide for evaluation under a microscope. An alternate method of detection is the evaluation of stool for adult pinworms. Fingernail scrapings examined microscopically demonstrate eggs 60% of the time (5). Pinworms do not produce eosinophilia.

EMERGENCY DEPARTMENT MANAGEMENT

The patient should be fully examined to rule out other causes of presenting symptoms. All infected individuals should be treated. In addition, family members should be evaluated for symptoms and treated simultaneously. Treatment is albendazole 400 mg PO or mebendazole 100 mg PO with a repeat dose in two weeks. A third option is pyrantel pamoate 11 mg/kg PO (max 1 g/dose) repeated every two weeks twice.

IMPERFORATE HYMEN

CLINICAL PRESENTATION

There are two periods in development in which the female with imperforate hymen is generally diagnosed: infancy and menarche. In the neonate the circulating maternal hormones stimulate vaginal mucus secretion. The imperforate hymen is often not recognized at birth and thus presents within days to weeks of life. Due to the outlet obstruction the vagina becomes distended resulting in hydrocolpos or mucocolpos. If the distension extends to the uterus it is referred to as hydrometrocolpos. The infant may present with a lower abdominal mass, urinary retention secondary to extrinsic obstruction, or constipation. The parents may have noted a mass at the introitus. In severe cases, the patient may have evidence of compression of the inferior vena cava or respiratory compromise. Only 0.1% of term female infants (9) have an imperforate hymen.

Girls who remain undiagnosed in childhood will present during or after menarche when the vagina fills with blood resulting in hematocolpos or hematometrocolpos. They will be noted to have normal pubertal development with primary amenorrhea. The chief complaint may be lower abdominal pain that may or may not be monthly, a pelvic mass or urinary retention.

DIFFERENTIAL DIAGNOSIS

The diagnosis of imperforate hymen is generally made upon examination of the external genitalia. However, other causes of vaginal obstruction must be considered. Transverse vaginal septum, labial adhesions, pelvic mass, agenesis of the vagina, testicular feminization, and Gartner duct cysts should be included as possible diagnoses. Sexual or physical abuse could also mimic the presentation of imperforate hymen.

EMERGENCY DEPARTMENT EVALUATION

A thorough history and physical should lead to the diagnosis. In infants, a whitish bulging membrane is common. Infants should be evaluated for the complications of the mass effect of the collected fluid. This includes evaluation for respiratory distress, inferior vena cava compression and hydronephrosis. A urinalysis should be sent if symptoms warrant evaluation. A bulging membranous dark blue mass at the introitus is the classical description of hematocolpos. An adolescent with severe pain may require an ultrasound evaluation as case reports of ruptured hematosalpinx have been documented (2).

EMERGENCY DEPARTMENT MANAGEMENT

The treatment for imperforate hymen is surgical incision and resection. The emergency department physician must determine the speed with which this should be accomplished. Any patient with complications requires emergent repair. If there are no complications these patients can be followed up as outpatients.

DISPOSITION

If the patient is stable and not experiencing complications, a referral for outpatient management should be made. Asymptomatic infants and prepubertal children can be scheduled for elective repair. Adolescents with hematocolpos should undergo surgical treatment promptly. The patient should be carefully evaluated for other genitourinary, rectal, and spinal anomalies and referred for work up as indicated. In addition, all female siblings should undergo an external examination as familial occurrences have been reported (19).

URETHRAL PROLAPSE

CLINICAL PRESENTATION

Urethral prolapse is a disorder seen in prepubertal girls and postmenopausal women. In children, the diagnosis is commonly seen in African-American girls from 2- to 10-years-old (20). The patient presents with painless vaginal bleeding or a vaginal mass. Upon inspection, the mass is generally swollen, purple or deep red, and doughnut-shaped. A central depression representing the lumen of the urethra may or may not be evident. The area may have evidence of thrombosis and necrosis. The patient may report dysuria, vaginal bleeding, or perineal discomfort; however, it can go unrecognized by the patient and can be found on routine examination. A recent history of coughing or straining may be reported.

DIFFERENTIAL DIAGNOSIS

The differential diagnoses are those that can present as a hymenal mass. Urethral processes that can present similarly are urethral polyps, prolapsed ureterocele, and rarely a urethral carcinoma. Dermatologic causes include condylomata and hemangiomas. Accidental and nonaccidental trauma can cause a hematoma that mimics prolapse. Imperforate hymen and hair tourniquets are other possibilities. An important entity on the differential that must be excluded is botryoid sarcoma, as it requires immediate referral.

EMERGENCY DEPARTMENT EVALUATION

A complete physical examination that properly establishes the anatomy of the mass is diagnostic. If the origin of the mass remains in doubt, a catheter can be passed through the mass to verify the diagnosis. A urinalysis can be performed which will likely be positive for erythrocytes but sterile.

EMERGENCY DEPARTMENT MANAGEMENT

If the prolapse is small and without evidence of necrosis, sitz baths or warm moist compresses can be recommended. A topical estrogen cream applied twice a day for two weeks may aid in resolution. If there is evidence of extreme congestion or necrosis, a surgical evaluation is indicated for reduction and excision.

DISPOSITION

The uncomplicated urethral prolapse will generally resolve in approximately two weeks. Follow up should be given to all patients to ensure resolution has occurred. Patients with necrosis at presentation or those that fail to resolve need surgical referral.

VAGINAL FOREIGN BODY

CLINICAL PRESENTATION

Four percent of prepubertal girls presenting with genitourinary complaints are subsequently found to have a vaginal foreign body (16). The classic presentation is vaginal bleeding or brown discharge with a foul-smelling odor. They may also report perineal or lower abdominal pain. A prepubertal girl with chronic vaginal discharge should have a thorough work up for vaginal foreign body. Multiple episodes in the same child have been reported (8). Items found in prepubertal girls include toilet paper, cotton balls, hair, and a myriad of other small items. Adolescents are more likely to present with retained tampons and condoms.

DIFFERENTIAL DIAGNOSIS

The presenting symptoms of a patient with a vaginal foreign body include vaginal bleeding, discharge, and abdominal/pelvic pain. Thus, the emergency physician must maintain a broad differential. Vulvovaginitis, urethral prolapse, dysfunctional uterine bleeding, labial adhesions, tumor, and urinary tract infection can all present similarly.

EMERGENCY DEPARTMENT EVALUATION

The patient should undergo a full genitourinary evaluation. The knee-chest position with a good light source will provide the best evaluation of a premenarchal vaginal area. The use of an otoscope or anoscope placed carefully into the hymen enhances the evaluation. If a vaginal foreign body is highly likely but not visualized with the above methods, an exam under anesthesia or with procedural sedation may be indicated. Postmenarchal patients can undergo a speculum and bimanual exam. A roentgenogram or ultrasound can be considered, although the objects found are generally not radioopaque.

EMERGENCY DEPARTMENT MANAGEMENT

With evidence or strong suspicion of a vaginal foreign body a gentle vaginal lavage should be performed. A 50cc syringe should be attached to a catheter that is inserted in the introitus. The plunger should be removed from the syringe and normal saline poured into the syringe providing a continuous flow. If this procedure is not tolerated or fails to remove object, a gynecologist can perform vaginoscopy under anesthesia.

DISPOSITION

The relationship between vaginal foreign bodies and sexual abuse has not been well studied or described in the literature. A retrospective case review suggests a possible connection in some cases (8). All patients with genitourinary complaints should be questioned about and screened for signs of sexual abuse.

LABIAL ADHESIONS

Labial adhesions are another common entity encountered in the pediatric patient. They are an acquired fusion of the labia minora due to low levels of estrogen in prepubescent girls that causes the epithelium of the labia to be thin and prone to irritation. The two medial edges of the labia minora become inflamed, stick together resulting in fusion. It is estimated that the incidence in prepubertal girls is 1.8% to 3.3% (11). Most patients are between 1- and 6-years-old. The child presents to the physician after the parents note the vagina appears to be closing. They may also present with urinary symptoms, recurrent urinary tract infections, or be found on exam. The diagnosis is generally made by examination, with a central line or raphe obstructing the view of the introitus and hymen. The characteristic central thickened line differentiates the diagnosis from possible malformations.

Significant debate over the treatment of labial adhesions persists in the literature with proponents for both conservative management and manual separation (15). The natural progression is for labial adhesions to resolve in early puberty when estrogen levels rise. Thus, asymptomatic patients do not require treatment. If the patient is having complications or recurrences, estrogen cream can be applied sparingly to the adhesions at bedtime for two weeks. After separation, zinc oxide or Vaseline should be applied at bedtime for an additional two weeks. Patients should be followed closely for failure of separation and recurrence. At that time manual separation may be performed.

COMMON PITFALLS

✔ An incomplete sexual history is taken due to inaccurate assumptions of risk
✔ Failing to recognize that candidal infections in prepubertal patients are unusual and may be associated with diabetes or an immune disorder
✔ Pediatric patients with recurrent or chronic vaginitis must be thoroughly evaluated for a vaginal foreign body

MALE GENITOURINARY DISORDERS

As with females, any male with abdominal or genitourinary complaints must undergo a complete exam. This section will focus on common pediatric causes of testicular pain and masses. A useful designation is summarized in Table 247.2 in which diagnoses are divided into painful and nonpainful scrotal swellings.

TESTICULAR TORSION

CLINICAL PRESENTATION

Testicular torsion is a critical diagnosis to make in the emergency department. It is common during adolescence, 62% of cases occur between the ages of 12 and 18, and has an incidence of one in 160 males before the age of 25 (21). Although it has been reported at any age from in utero through adulthood. An additional peak is seen in the neonatal period and is associated with a poor salvage rate.

Patients classically present with acute onset unilateral scrotal pain and swelling. However, the pain can be more insidious and may even be bilateral. It is common for patients to have associated nausea and vomiting. The cremasteric reflex is usually absent, however its absence is not pathognomonic. The presence of a cremasteric reflex is highly suggestive that torsion is not the correct diagnosis, however, its presence in patients with torsion has been reported (12). Patients with an undescended testis have a higher incidence of torsion and may present with abdominal pain (7).

Torsion in adolescence is due to improper attachment of the testicle to the tunica vaginalis resulting in the "bell clapper"

TABLE 247.2. Causes of Scrotal Swelling and Masses

Painful	Generally Painless
Testicular torsion	Inguinal hernia
Torsion of appendix testis	Hydrocele
Epididymitis	Varicocele
Incarcerated hernia	Tumor
Trauma	Henoch-Schonlein pupura
Edema	

deformity. The result is a free hanging testicle, with a transverse lie that leaves the spermatic cord susceptible to twisting. The abnormal attachment is usually bilateral.

DIFFERENTIAL DIAGNOSIS

The two primary competing diagnoses are epididymitis and torsion of the testicular appendage. Epididymitis generally has a slower onset of symptoms, an intact cremasteric reflex, a normal riding testis, and a reduction of pain with elevation of the scrotum (Prehn sign). Despite these tendencies, none of these findings are diagnostic for epididymitis. Torsion of the testicular appendage is diagnosed on exam. A firm tender nodule can be palpated and a "blue-dot sign" visualized. Missed or late diagnoses of testicular torsion result in loss of the testicle and therefore testicular torsion must be considered in any patient that presents with scrotal pain. Table 247.2 lists other causes of painful scrotal swelling.

EMERGENCY DEPARTMENT EVALUATION

If the patient presents with a history and physical examination consistent with torsion, immediate urologic evaluation is warranted without further studies. Only if the diagnosis of torsion is uncertain should imaging be performed. The two imaging modalities used to evaluate the acute scrotum are radionuclide scanning (technetium-99 pertechnetate or scintigraphy) and color Doppler ultrasonography. Radionuclide scanning requires time for preparation, intravenous access, and is difficult to perform in smaller children. Radionuclide studies are often not available 24 hours a day. Color Doppler ultrasonography is often available 24 hours a day and requires no intravenous access, however it is limited in prepubertal boys due to low blood flow and can result in indeterminate findings. Studies comparing the two modalities in the literature show similar results. A literature review of 400 cases reported 95% accuracy when radionuclide scanning was used. Color Doppler ultrasonography demonstrated an accuracy of 88% with 7% indeterminate studies (7). A recent prospective study comparing color Doppler sonography and scintigraphy in forty-six boys with acute scrotal pain demonstrated each modality had a sensitivity of 78.6% for the diagnosis of testicular torsion with 91.3% and 87% accuracy respectively (13). Thus, the decision for mode of imaging is based on availability and ease of the test in specific institutions with the caveat that both methods can have indeterminate scans and false-negative results.

Additional information that may aid in diagnosis is a urinalysis. If significant pyuria is demonstrated, a diagnosis of epididymitis becomes more likely. However, patients with testicular torsion can also have pyuria.

EMERGENCY DEPARTMENT MANAGEMENT

Testicular torsion is a surgical emergency. If the diagnosis is likely, emergent urologic evaluation should be obtained immediately. Imaging studies should not delay this evaluation. Aggressive pain control is also vital. The survival of the testis is correlated with duration of symptoms. Manual detorsion can be attempted to increase blood flow to the testis. Sedation and pain medication should be administered prior to the procedure. Classically this maneuver is performed by facing the patient and the testicle rotated outward like opening a book: the left testis is rotated clockwise and the right counterclockwise until the symp-

toms improve. A recent review by Sessions demonstrated that the degree of rotation ranged from 180 to 1080 degrees, with a median of 540 degrees. However, it was also noted that the medial rotation that is classically reported only occurred in two-thirds of patients (17). Manual detorsion remains only a temporizing measure, emergent surgical exploration is the goal.

DISPOSITION

The patient with testicular torsion must undergo surgical exploration of both testes and bilateral orchiopexy. The survival of the testis is inversely correlated with duration of symptoms. Orchidectomy is recommended if necrosis is present.

EPIDIDYMITIS

CLINICAL PRESENTATION

Acute epididymitis is a common cause of acute scrotal pain. The pain of epididymitis is usually gradual in onset. It is associated with swelling of the scrotum, fever, vomiting and urinary symptoms. It is more common in adolescent males, however, prepubertal boys with genitourinary anomalies and urinary retention are susceptible to epididymitis. The tenderness is generally posterior and lateral to the testis. The cremasteric reflex is usually intact, however this reflex can be absent in epididymitis.

DIFFERENTIAL DIAGNOSIS

The main entity that must be distinguished from epididymitis is testicular torsion. Patients with testicular torsion generally have a more acute onset of symptoms, no fever, fewer urinary complaints, and may have increased pain with elevation of the scrotum (Prehn sign), although this sign has not be shown to be reliable.

EMERGENCY DEPARTMENT EVALUATION

A urinalysis should be performed which usually demonstrates white blood cells. However, torsion can have similar findings. A urine culture should be sent. The complete blood count may show an elevated white blood cell count. If the patient is sexually active the patient must be screened for *Gonorrhea* and *Chlamydia*, and serologies for syphilis sent. If the diagnosis of torsion cannot be excluded but the probability is low, then imaging studies should be done to support the diagnosis of epididymitis and rule out torsion. Either color Doppler ultrasonography or nuclear scan can be obtained, both of which will show increased flow/activity in epididymitis.

EMERGENCY DEPARTMENT MANAGEMENT

The treatment for acute epididymitis depends upon the age of the patient. Younger children may be treated for urinary tract infection organisms (*Escherichia Coli*, *Klebsiella pneumoniae*, and *Pseudomonas aeruginosa*), although viruses may also cause epididymitis (see Chapter 267, "Urinary Tract Infections") for treatment of urinary tract infection. A child less than one month old should be admitted for inpatient antibiotics. In children less than 2 years old, admission should be considered for patients whom appear ill. The causes of infection in adolescents are sexually transmitted diseases thus treatment should focus on *Neisseria gonorrhoeae* and *Chlamydia trachomatis* (Table 247.1).

DISPOSITION

The patient should be prescribed analgesics, sitz baths, and scrotal elevation. Antibiotics should be prescribed as outlined above, with a low threshold for admitting young patients. Prepubertal boys or any episode associated with a urinary tract infection necessitates an ultrasound and voiding cystourethrogram to evaluate for genitourinary anomalies. Postpubertal boys with a urinary tract infection should have an abdominal computed tomography to rule out nephrolithiasis. Older boys should be questioned about voiding symptoms to determine if urologic evaluation is needed to rule out dysfunctional voiding (3). All patients should have urologic follow up.

HYDROCELE

CLINICAL PRESENTATION

Hydroceles are common findings in infants and young children. The child is noted to have a painless swollen scrotum that tends to increase in size throughout the day and decrease when supine. The fluid collection located in the space surrounding the testis may appear after coughing or straining. A simple hydrocele is defined as presence of this fluid collection without a patent processus vaginalis. A communicating hydrocele has a patent processus vaginalis and generally has greater fluctuation in size. Communicating hydroceles may have an associated indirect inguinal hernia.

DIFFERENTIAL DIAGNOSIS

See Table 247.2 for the differential diagnosis of nonpainful scrotal swelling. To aid in distinguishing a hydrocele from an inguinal hernia, it should be noted that the spermatic cord above the hydrocele should not feel thickened.

EMERGENCY DEPARTMENT EVALUATION

Palpation of the scrotum should elucidate a normal testis and normal spermatic cord above the mass. The mass, which is fluid filled should transilluminate. If the testis cannot be palpated adequately, ultrasound evaluation is recommended.

EMERGENCY DEPARTMENT MANAGEMENT

If the hydrocele is tense or painful, the patient must undergo a surgical evaluation. If the mass fluctuates in size rapidly or the exam is consistent with a communicating hydrocele, a surgical referral should be performed to rule out an inguinal hernia.

DISPOSITION

A small, uncomplicated hydrocele can be managed conservatively as most resolve spontaneously. Failed resolution at age two years warrants a surgical referral for repair (10). Any communicating hydrocele with an associated hernia needs surgical

closure. It is recommended that parents be counseled on the signs and symptoms of incarceration.

TESTICULAR TUMORS

CLINICAL PRESENTATION

Testicular tumors present as an abnormally large testis or mass that is discovered by the patient, parent, or on routine exam. They are painless scrotal masses although they may have associated abdominal pain. Lymphadenopathy may also be reported or discovered on examination.

DIFFERENTIAL DIAGNOSIS

A mass within the testis should be evaluated under the assumption that it is a malignancy (18) (Table 247.2).

EMERGENCY DEPARTMENT EVALUATION

A full physical evaluation should be performed examining carefully for lymphadenopathy and location of the mass. If the mass is within the testis, surgical exploration is warranted. The scrotum should be transilluminated to determine if the mass is cystic or solid. If cystic the likely etiologies are hernia, hydrocele, hematocele, varicocele, or spermatocele. If unable to establish location of mass or palpate the testis fully, an ultrasound evaluation should be performed. Solid extratesticular masses require surgical exploration. If malignancy is suspected alpha-fetoprotein can be sent which may be elevated, however levels are elevated early in life.

EMERGENCY DEPARTMENT MANAGEMENT

Solid extratesticular masses and any intratesticular mass requires surgery. A urine pregnancy test can be performed and will occasionally be positive in some germ cell testicular tumors. A computed tomography of the chest and retroperitoneum may aid in staging.

DISPOSITION

All patients with a testicular tumor should be admitted for evaluation by an oncologist and surgeon.

INGUINAL HERNIA

Approximately 15 in 1,000 births result in an abdominal hernia, with a higher incidence in premature infants. Inguinal hernias are more common in males, with bimodal peaks before 1 year of age and then again after 40. An indirect inguinal hernia occurs when the processus vaginalis does not obliterate in infancy and abdominal contents invaginate through this patent sac. These hernias are more common on the right side. Entrapment of mesentery, bowel, intraperitoneal organs, and the hernial sac can occur and are more common with small hernias. If the contents of the hernia can be returned to their anatomic position, then the hernia is reducible; if it remains entrapped, then it is incarcerated or irreducible. Hernias that remain incarcerated can result in strangulation, with resultant bowel necrosis.

CLINICAL PRESENTATION

Patients with incarcerated hernias may present with pain, edema extending to the scrotum, nausea, vomiting and low-grade fever. Physical examination may reveal bowel sounds in the scrotal sac. If the inguinal mass can be palpated separately from the testes, then it is possible to diagnose an inguinal hernia clinically. Rarely, the incarcerated and strangulated hernia can present as a tense, blue mass in the scrotum.

EMERGENCY DEPARTMENT MANAGEMENT AND DISPOSITION

The patient should be placed in the Trendelenburg position with an ice pack placed on the groin to reduce swelling; sedation may be necessary before reduction. Slow gentle pressure should be applied to reduce the hernia. If the hernia cannot be reduced or strangulation is suspected (fever, overlying cellulitis), the patient should receive fluid resuscitation, broad-spectrum parenteral antibiotics, and a surgical consult.

Patients who are found to have a hernia on routine examination and are without symptoms suggestive of incarceration or strangulation should be referred for surgical repair because incarceration can occur in the first year of life. If the hernia cannot be reduced or strangulation is suspected (fever, overlying cellulitis), the patient should receive fluid resuscitation, broad-spectrum parenteral antibiotics, and a surgical consult.

Patients who are found to have a hernia on routine examination and are without symptoms suggestive of incarceration or strangulation should be referred for surgical repair because incarceration can occur in the first year of life.

PHIMOSIS

Phimosis is defined as the inability to retract the distal foreskin or prepuce over the glans. When caused by normal physiologic adhesions it is called primary phimosis. Phimosis is normal in infants and young children with resolution generally by six years of life. Secondary phimosis may occur due to scarring of the foreskin following inadequate circumcision, irritation, and infection. Patients generally are asymptomatic. However, in some patients, the constricted opening causes interference with voiding, urinary tract infection, and local infection of the foreskin and glans.

Physical examination establishes the diagnosis. If symptoms of a UTI are present, urinalysis, urine culture and renal function tests are warranted. A renal ultrasound is recommended.

No treatment is needed for asymptomatic patients less than 6 years of age. Secondary phimosis can be treated with topical betamethasone valerate 0.6% cream twice daily for six weeks. Steroid treatment has been shown to be effective in 75% to 88% of boys (1). Symptomatic patients should receive urologic referral for circumcision.

PARAPHIMOSIS

Paraphimosis is a condition seen in uncircumcised males when the foreskin is retracted over the glans and becomes caught in that position. This leads to edema and venous congestion of the foreskin and impedes blood flow to the glans. The patient presents with impressive swelling and severe pain.

Treatment requires reduction of the foreskin to restore its normal position over the glans. This is best accomplished with effective pain control. The physician should then place both thumbs on the glans with the index and middle fingers on the distal end of the foreskin. Simultaneous persistent pressure is applied to the glans with the thumbs and to the rolled edge of the foreskin by the fingers to return the foreskin to its proper position. If the patient is experiencing additional pain, a penile block can be performed followed by ice pack application for 10 to 15 minutes prior to further reduction attempts. If the physician is not able to achieve reduction, emergent surgical reduction by an urologist may be required. If reduction in the emergency department is accomplished then urologic follow up is recommended for possible circumcision.

BALANITIS/BALANOPOSTHITIS

A break in the foreskin caused by local trauma or poor hygiene can lead to posthitis. Extension of the cellulitis or inflammation to the glans is referred to as balanoposthitis. The patient presents with swelling, erythema, and penile pain. A penile discharge may be associated. The diagnosis is made clinically, systematically ruling out paraphimosis and hair tourniquet. A swab of discharge may be sent for identification and proper antibiotic treatment.

Classically the causative organisms are skin flora (i.e., *stapholococcus* and *streptococcus*). Treatment includes sitz baths and topical antibiotics. In severe cases, cephalexin (25–50 mg/kg/day divided three times daily for 7 days) can be added. Follow up is recommended as treatment failures, repeat episodes, and scarring can lead to phimosis. Patients with recurrent episodes of candidal balanitis/balanoposthitis should be checked for diabetes mellitus.

CRITICAL INTERVENTIONS FOR MALE GU DISORDERS

- Obtain immediate urologic evaluation without further studies in patients with suspected testicular torsion
- Younger children diagnosed with epididymitis need further evaluation for genitourinary abnormalities
- Hydroceles can be associated with testicular tumors therefore if adequate palpation of the testis cannot be performed, ultrasound evaluation is indicated
- Obtain an emergent urologic consultation for patients with paraphimosis that cannot be reduced

COMMON PITFALLS

✔ Failing to perform a complete abdominal and GU exam on all adolescent males with a complaint of abdominal pain or GI symptoms even when the patient denies GU symptoms or testicular swelling or pain

✔ Performing imaging studies and delaying surgical consultation in a patient with suspected testicular torsion

✔ Failing to consider testicular torsion in patients with undescended testis who present with abdominal pain

✔ Assuming that transillumination excludes underlying genitourinary pathology

Genitourinary emergencies are common in children. A thorough history and physical examination along with the identification of specific genitourinary signs and symptoms can distinguish minor conditions easily treated in the emergency department, such as epididymitis or urethral prolapse, from serious conditions leading to significant morbidity and mortality, such as testicular torsion or sexual abuse.

References

1. Ashfield JE, Nickel KR, Siemens DR, MacNeily AE, Nickel JC. Treatment of phimosis with topical steroids in 194 children. *J Urol* 2003;169:1106–1108.
2. Bakos O, Berglund L. Imperforate hymen and ruptured hematosalpinx: a case report with a review of the literature. *J Adolesc Health* 1999;24:226–228.
3. Bukowski TP, Lewis AG, Reeves D, Wacksman J, Sheldon CA. Epididymitis in older boys: dysfunctional voiding as an etiology. *J Urol* 1995;154:762–765.
4. Centers for Disease Control and Prevention. Sexually transmitted diseases treatment guidelines 2002. *MMWR* 2002;51(No. RR-6):1–78.
5. Elston DM. What's eating you? Enterobius vermicularis (pinworms, threadworms). *Cutis* 2003;71:268–270.
6. Farrington PF. Pediatric vulvo-vaginitis. *J Pediatr Adolesc Gynecol* 1997;40:135–140.
7. Haynes BE, Bessen HA, Haynes VE. The diagnosis of testicular torsion. *JAMA* 1983;249:2522–2527.
8. Herman-Giddens ME. Vaginal foreign bodies and child sexual abuse. *Arch Pediatr Adolesc Med* 1994;13:236–237.
9. Kahn R, Dumean B, Bowes W. Spontaneous opening of congenital imperforate hymen. *J Pediatr* 1975;87:768–770.
10. Kapur P, Caty MG, Glick PL. Pediatric hernias and hydroceles. *Pediatr Clin North Am* 1998;45:773–789.
11. Leung A, Robson W, Tay-Uyboco J. The incidence of labial fusion in children. *J Paediatr Child Health* 1993;29:235.
12. Nelson CP, Williams JF, Bloom DA. The cremasteric reflex: a useful but imperfect sign in testicular torsion. *J Pediatr Surg* 2003;38:1248–1249.
13. Nussbaum AR, Bulas D, Shalaby-Rana E, et al. Color Doppler sonography and scintigraphy of the testis: a prospective, comparative analysis in children with acute scrotal pain. *Pediatr Emerg Care* 2002;18:67–71.
14. Nyirjesy P. Vaginitis in the adolescent patient. *Pediatr Clin North Am* 1999;46:733–745.
15. Omar HA. Management of labial adhesions in prepubertal girls. *J Pediatr Adolesc Gynecol* 2000;13:183–185.
16. Paradise JE, Willis ED. Probability of vaginal foreign body in girls with genital complaints. *Am J Dis Child* 1985;139:472–476.
17. Sessions AE, Rabinowitz R, Hulbert WC, Goldstein MM, Mevorach RA. Testicular torsion: direction, degree, duration, and disinformation. *J Urol* 2003;169:663–665.
18. Skoog SJ. Benign and malignant pediatric scrotal masses. *Pediatr Clin North Am* 1997;44:1229–1250.
19. Stelling JR, Gray MR, Davis AJ, Cowan JM, Reindollar RH. Dominant transmission of imperforate hymen. *Fertil Steril* 2000;74:1241–1244.
20. Valerie E, Gilchrist BF, Frischer J, et al. Diagnosis and treatment of urethral prolapse in children. *Urology* 1999;54:1082–1084.
21. Williamson RC. Torsion of the testis and allied conditions. *Br J Surg* 1976;63:465–76.

CHAPTER 248

Glomerulonephritis and the Nephrotic Syndrome

Kathy W. Monroe and Annalise Sorrentino

ACUTE GLOMERULONEPHRITIS

Acute glomerulonephritis (AGN) is a disease that is a result of immunologic effects on the glomerular tissue. It is described as a clinical syndrome that typically presents as acute onset of proteinuria, hematuria, and red cell casts. This is often seen in combination with edema, hypertension, and renal insufficiency (7). In the United States, glomerulonephritis most often occurs between the ages of 5 and 15 years with only 10% occurring in patients older than 40 years. There is a male to female ratio of 2:1. In the pediatric population (younger than 20 years old), glomeru-

lonephritis is the most common cause of hematuria accounting for up to 50% of all cases.

There are three broad categories of acute glomerulonephritis: postinfectious, renal, and systemic disease (Table 248.1).

Poststreptococcal acute glomerulonephritis (PSAGN) is one of the most common causes and has a peak incidence between the ages of 2 and 6 years. PSAGN is known to follow infections of the skin (impetigo) or upper respiratory tract with certain nephrogenic strains of group A β-hemolytic streptococci. It can occur as sporadic disease (usually associated with pharyngitis), or may be part of an epidemic (more common with skin infections). PSGN is associated with pharyngitis more often during the winter months and with pyoderma more often during the summer. Pyoderma-related AGN is typically seen more in the southern regions of the United States and may account for as many as 60% to 70% of the cases (3). Characteristically there is a latent period between the onset of the streptococcal infection and the onset of nephritis (8–14 days for pharyngitis and 14–21 days for skin infections) (3). In PSGN, there is evidence to suggest that immune complexes formed with streptococcal antigens localize on the glomerular capillary wall, activate the complement system then initiate a proliferative and inflammatory response.

NEPHROTIC SYNDROME

The nephrotic syndrome is a clinical condition characterized by proteinuria (greater than 40 mg/m2/day or urine dipstick greater than 2+) and hypoalbuminemia (usually less than 2.5 gm/dl) often associated with edema and hypercholesterolemia. A small number of patients may also have hypertension, hematuria and reduced glomerular filtration rate. This combination of clinical findings may be found alone, or in association with a number of systemic illnesses (10). The primary abnormality is increased permeability of the glomerular capillary wall to plasma proteins leading to an excessive albuminuria (8).

The incidence of nephrotic syndrome is 2 to 7 new cases per 100,000 children (18 years of age and younger) annually. The peak age of onset is 2 to 3 years, and 75% of children are less than 10 years old (10). There is a male to female ratio of 2:1.

The nephrotic syndrome is categorized into primary (> 90% of cases) and secondary forms (see Table 248.2). Minimal change nephrotic syndrome, commonly called "nil" disease, is the most common primary form seen in pediatrics accounting for 80% to 85% of primary nephrotic cases, followed by focal segmental glomerulosclerosis and membranoproliferative glomerulonephropathy (10). In these patients, renal biopsy reveals minimal glomerular abnormalities. These patients have a much better prognosis than other forms of nephrotic syndrome. Ninety-two percent of patients with minimal change syndrome will respond to a course of corticosteroid therapy (12).

CLINICAL PRESENTATION

AGN

The clinical presentation varies as does the intensity of the disease but many patients are not ill appearing. Hematuria and edema are the most common complaints. Gross hematuria (tea-colored urine) has been reported in 30% of patients and microscopic hematuria is present in virtually all children with the disease. The initiating streptococcal infection usually has resolved by the time of presentation, with a latent period of approximately three weeks. Onset of glomerulonephritis less than a week after streptococcal infection is highly suggestive of preexisting renal disease (7).

TABLE 248.1. Causes of Glomerulonephritis

Postinfectious	Renal	Systemic
Streptococcus GAS *Other bacteria:* Staphylococcus, mycobacteria, salmonella *Viral:* CMV, coxsackie, EBV, hepatitis, rubella, mumps *Fungal:* Coccidioides immitis *Parasite:* *Plasmodium spp, Schistosoma mansoni, Toxoplasma gondii,* filariasis, trichinosis, trypanosomes	*Membranoproliferative glomerulonephritis* Type I and II *IgA nephropathy* (Berger disease) *Idiopathic rapidly progressive glomerulonephritis* Type I: antiglomerular basement membrane disease Type II: mediated by immune complexes Type III: antineutrophil cytoplasmic antibodies	*Wegener granulomatosis* *Hypersensitivity vasculitis* *Cryoglobulinemia* *Systemic lupus erythematosus* *Polyarteritis nodosa* *Henoch Schönlein Purpura* *Goodpasture Syndrome*

Hypertension is present in more than 75% of patients, but usually does not require treatment with antihypertensive medication. It typically resolves with treatment of the fluid retention. Edema is the presenting symptom in many patients, and is present in the majority (~90%). This is typically noted in the face and upper extremities, but can manifest as anasarca. Table 248.3 lists the clinical manifestations in PSAGN in order of frequency. A variety of laboratory and radiologic abnormalities may be seen in these patients.

Patients who are presenting with underlying systemic diseases may present with specific symptoms that aid in the diagnosis. Goodpasture syndrome often has hemoptysis. Systemic lupus erythematosus and Henoch-Schönlein purpura are distinguished by arthralgias and characteristic rashes. A triad of sinusitis, glomerulonephritis, and pulmonary infiltrates suggests Wegener granulomatosis.

Nephrotic Syndrome

It is important to differentiate between AGN and nephrotic syndrome because the management may be entirely different. Regardless of the histopathologic abnormalities, edema is the most prominent clinical manifestation of the nephrotic syndrome in most children. The edema may be initially seen in the periorbital area and often follows a flu-like illness so it may often be confused with allergies or sinusitis. It is pitting in nature, and typically seen in dependent areas, so facial swelling may be observed in the morning, while lower extremity edema exhibited in the evenings. Oliguria may be seen, but is more common in relapses (13). Other symptoms such as anorexia, abdominal pain (thought to be due to bowel wall edema), vomiting, diarrhea, and fatigue can also be present. With anasarca and abdominal distention, patients may have respiratory distress, umbilical and inguinal hernias and/or rectal prolapse. Pleural effusions and less often pericardial effusions may be present. Ascites has also been described, and can serve as a site of infection if the child presents with fever. On rare occasions, a child may present with signs of thrombosis as a result of the hypercoagulable state (13).

The initial episode and subsequent relapses may follow a viral upper respiratory infection. Microscopic hematuria occurs in approximately 20% of children with minimal change nephrotic syndrome and in 50% of those with membranoproliferative disease. The presence of macroscopic hematuria should prompt investigation for underlying causes (2). Blood pressure is usually normal in minimal change nephrotic syndrome but in up to

TABLE 248.2. Etiology of Nephrotic Syndrome

PRIMARY/MINIMAL CHANGE

Congenital
Steroid-responsive
Steroid-resistant

SECONDARY

Associated with systemic disease:
SLE
HSP
Sickle cell disease
Diabetes mellitus
Lymphoma
Berger's disease/IgA nephropathy
Postinfectious glomerulonephritis
Syphilis
Malaria
HIV
CMV
Toxoplasmosis
Hepatitis
Amyloidosis
Associated with medications:
NSAIDS
Penicillin
Heroin
Gold salts
Tridione
Associated with toxins/allergens:
Bee sting
Poison oak
Vaccinations
Food allergy

TABLE 248.3. Clinical Symptoms of Glomerulonephritis

Most Frequent	Less Frequent
Edema Periorbital most common *Hematuria* Microscopic to gross *Hypertension* Mild-moderate *Oliguria* *Nonspecific systemic symptoms* Anorexia, nausea, fever, malaise, abdominal pain *Pallor*	*Urinary tract syndrome* Flank pain, dysuria, frequency *Circulatory congestion* Mild congestive heart failure, pulmonary edema *Hypertensive encephalopathy* *Acute renal failure*

TABLE 248.4. Laboratory and Radiographic Findings in PSAGN

Urine	Biochemistry	Serology	Hematology	Radiographs
Hematuria	Nl to high BUN	Rising ASO titer	Nl to low Hct	Cardiomegaly
Red blood cell casts	Nl to high creatinine	+ anti-Dnase B		Pulmonary congestion
Hyaline granular casts	Nl to low sodium	Low C3		Pleural effusion
Proteinuria	Nl to high potassium			
	Nl to low albumin			

*Nl = normal; Hct = hematocrit.

13% of patients, hypertension (above the 98th percentile for age) has been reported. Persistent hypertension is uncommon and should suggest a syndrome other than minimal change nephrotic syndrome (1).

Primary laboratory findings diagnostic of the nephrotic syndrome include the following:

1. Proteinuria: Greater than 40 mg/m2/d (greater than 2+ on urine dipstick) and spot urine protein to creatinine ratio greater than 2
2. Hypoproteinemia: serum albumin less than 2.5 gm/dL
3. Hyperlipidemia: elevated serum levels of triglycerides, cholesterol and total lipids
4. Normal serum creatinine
5. Normal or slightly elevated serum BUN
6. Increased hemoglobin (seen frequently due to hemoconcentration)

Secondary findings can include hypocalcemia (with a normal ionized fraction), hyperkalemia, hyponatremia, and hypercoagulability (13).

DIFFERENTIAL DIAGNOSIS

A number of illnesses may mimic the presentation of PSAGN and many can be seen in Table 248.1. It is often impossible to make a final causal diagnosis in the emergency department. It is more important to recognize that the patient has nephritis and to be aware of possible life-threatening complications such as hypertension and hyperkalemia.

The differential diagnosis of nephrotic syndrome is listed in Table 248.2). Although nephrosis may be the presenting manifestation in the secondary forms, there is usually other clinical evidence of the underlying disorder.

EMERGENCY DEPARTMENT EVALUATION

AGN

Many patients with AGN are asymptomatic and will be diagnosed only by examination of the urine. At the other extreme is the child with severe disease manifested by edema, hypertension, oliguria and azotemia. The history should include questions regarding previous illnesses such as a preceding impetigo or pharyngitis. Patients who have unstable vital signs should be started on cardiac monitoring while evaluation proceeds.

Hematuria is the most consistent urinary abnormality in AGN but the urinalysis can be normal (3). In two-thirds of patients, the hematuria is microscopic. The sediment may reveal red blood cell casts. Urine will be dark with specific gravity greater than 1.020 with proteinuria usually in subnephrotic range. In a small number of patients, there is profound azotemia with elevations of blood urea nitrogen (BUN) and serum creatinine. Hyponatremia, hyperkalemia and metabolic acidosis also can occur, related to

transient hyporeninemic states. The CBC may reveal anemia which is usually due to dilutional effect. Rising antistreptolysin-O titers suggest previous recent streptococcal infection; however the ASO may not rise after pyoderma therefore, antiDNase B is the best single test to detect recent streptococcal infection. The C3 complement level is decreased in most patients (11), but returns to normal in six to eight weeks. Complement levels, as well as antinuclear antibody tests, may be helpful if a diagnosis of underlying systemic disease is being entertained (7). Culture from the throat and skin should be sent in an effort to isolate a nephrogenic strain of Streptococcus. Chest radiographs may reveal cardiomegaly, pulmonary edema, pleural effusions, and edema of the soft tissues. A summary of the laboratory and clinical findings can be seen in Table 248.4.

The four major problems seen in newly diagnosed patients with nephrotic syndrome include edema, hypovolemia, infection, and thrombotic phenomena. Many children with nephrotic syndrome are apparently healthy and have edema as their only obvious presenting abnormality. A thorough physical examination is indicated however, to assess for respiratory difficulties which may develop secondary to ascites and pleural effusions. The presence of edema can be deceptive, giving the impression of fluid overload when, in fact, many patients are intravascularly volume-depleted secondary to their hypoproteinemia. The child with tachycardia and hypotension may require prompt fluid resuscitation.

Children with nephrotic syndrome are prone to serious infections and fever in such a child warrants careful evaluation. Coagulation abnormalities and thrombotic tendencies are infrequently observed but common sites for thrombosis include cerebral veins and arteries, renal veins and pulmonary and femoral arteries.

Initial laboratory investigations necessary to establish the diagnosis include total serum protein, serum albumin, spot urine protein to creatinine ratio and a urinalysis. Baseline laboratory data that should be obtained include: complete blood cell count, serum electrolytes, calcium, phosphorus, BUN, creatinine, cholesterol, triglycerides, and complement.

Depending on the clinical findings, other laboratory studies may be performed such as antinuclear antibodies, antistreptolysin O titer, syphilis serology, Hepatitis B surface antigen, testing for the human immunodeficiency virus and skin testing for tuberculosis. There are no radiographic studies routinely recommended, but a chest x-ray may be helpful in evaluating for pleural effusions.

EMERGENCY DEPARTMENT MANAGEMENT

AGN

In most cases of PSAGN, there is no specific therapy that influences healing of the glomerular lesions, and much of the treatment is supportive. Antibiotics do not alter the course of the disease but may decrease the spread of nephrogenic strains of

Streptococcus in patients with positive cultures, and therefore penicillin should be administered to the nonallergic patient. Appropriate therapy is indicated promptly for the child with acute renal failure, hypertension or hyperkalemia. This may include fluid restriction or diuretics (7). As many as 60% of these patients will have hypertension with up to 10% having hypertensive encephalopathy (3). Symptoms suggestive of hypertensive encephalopathy consist of headache, nausea, vomiting, seizures and transient cortical blindness. For hypertensive emergencies in children with PSAGN, therapy should be gradual and controlled. In hypertensive encephalopathy, there is a sense of urgency to decrease the blood pressure, however, overly vigorous therapy can cause decreased perfusion of vital organs (4). Many drugs are available such as diazoxide, hydralazine, labetalol, loop diuretics, and calcium channel blockers. The calcium channel blockers are becoming the drugs of choice due to their modest effect on blood pressure and quick onset of action.

In patients with glomerulonephritis that is nonstreptococcal, the use of steroids or cytotoxic agents may be indicated. The decision to use these drugs should be made in conjunction with the nephrology consultant.

Nephrotic Syndrome

Typically, the treatment of the initial presentation of nephrotic syndrome is not an emergency, however, children are admitted to the hospital for therapy and further testing. Patients who have relapsed may present to the emergency department (ED) but not require admission. General measures to treat the edema of nephrotic syndrome include salt restriction (no added salt diet) and occasionally diuretics. Furosemide (Lasix) is the diuretic of choice for nephrotic patients with severe discomfort due to fluid retention. It is given orally or intravenously in a dose of 1 to 2 mg/kg and may require giving an infusion of salt poor albumin for optimal benefit. A useful regimen is to give furosemide intravenously then 1g/kg of 25% salt poor albumin solution intravenously over 2 hours followed by a second dose of furosemide at the end of the infusion. Patients should be observed closely for hypotension or hypertension. Diuretics should be used cautiously as the risk of intravascular volume depletion and thrombosis is high in these patients. Some patients will require thoracentesis for relief of respiratory distress secondary to pleural effusions. Paracentesis should only be performed for ascites that impairs respirations, as there is risk of causing peritonitis with this procedure.

It is not uncommon for the nephrotic patient to present to the ED in hypovolemic shock. Clinically this can be a difficult diagnosis, since the patient is edematous. Treatment consists of prompt fluid resuscitation and hospital admission. Albumin, when available is the preferred fluid for intravascular resuscitation.

Infections and related complications account for up to 70% of deaths in patients with childhood nephrotic syndrome. Because their immune system is altered, there is a high incidence of invasive infections such as septicemia, pneumonia, cellulitis and peritonitis caused by *Streptococcus pneumoniae*. These patients are also susceptible to gram-negative organisms such as *Escherichia coli*, *Pseudomonas*, and *Haemophilius influenzae*. Any child with nephrotic syndrome and fever should be evaluated thoroughly and admitted to the hospital with broad spectrum antibiotic coverage, taking into account the emergence of penicillin resistant *S pneumoniae* in some regions (6). Pneumococcal vaccine is indicated for patients who have experienced relapse (13). Because of their altered immune system, children with the nephrotic syndrome are particularly at risk for severe varicella infections. Treatment with acyclovir and or varicella zoster immune globulin may be indicated in these patients. Consultation

with a pediatric infectious disease specialist should be obtained in this circumstance (9).

Total serum calcium is decreased in patients with nephrotic syndrome. Hypoalbuminemia leads to a decrease in protein-bound calcium but ionized calcium levels can also be decreased due to excessive loss of vitamin D-binding protein in the urine, leading to decreased absorption of calcium. Symptomatic hypocalcemia is rare, although bone demineralization and osteomalacia may occur. Occasionally a patient will present to the Emergency Department with tetany or muscle cramps. Such a patient should be placed on a cardiac monitor and given an initial dose of 0.5 to 1.0 ml/kg of a 10% solution of calcium gluconate intravenously over 3 to 5 minutes. Calcium gluconate is preferable to calcium chloride as it is less sclerosing to the patient's veins. When symptoms are relieved, calcium gluconate may be added to the intravenous solution at a dose of 100 mg elemental calcium/kg/day or calcium may be administered orally (10% calcium gluconate contains 9 mg elemental calcium/100 mg of the salt).

A serious complication of the nephrotic syndrome is the increased risk of vascular thromboses. Thromboses have been demonstrated in all the major arteries and veins and may occur more commonly in children than is recognized by clinical symptoms and signs. Many reasons for this susceptibility to thromboses have been proposed. Nephrotic patients have increased levels of plasma fibrinogen and coagulation factors V and VIII. A decrease in the circulating level of antithrombin III has been observed and the platelets of some patients show an increase in spontaneous aggregation. Hyperviscosity of the plasma resulting from hyperfibrinogenemia and volume depletion may increase the likelihood of thromboses. The value of routine anticoagulant and antiplatelet therapy has not been adequately assessed. Since clinically apparent thrombosis is fairly rare, routine anticoagulation is generally not recommended. However, if a patient has evidence for thrombosis or has additional risk factors (e.g., prolonged immobility) most nephrologists would give anticoagulant medication. Renal vein thrombosis should be suspected in a patient with acute flank pain, renal enlargement, hematuria, unexplained deterioration in renal function, oliguria and renal failure.

The cornerstone of treatment of nephrotic syndrome is corticosteroid therapy. This is initiated after contraindications to the use of high-dose steroids are eliminated, such as active bacterial infection or positive tuberculin skin test (10). The typical starting dose is 2 mg/kg/d for the first 4 to 6 weeks. The majority of patients (~90%) will experience complete clearing of their urine on this regimen. Maintenance therapy (with slow tapering of the steroid dose) is then continued for a total of about 28 weeks. Typical side effects of corticosteroids (cushingoid facies, increased appetite, and hirsutism) are often seen in the initial 6 weeks of therapy, but tend to subside with decreasing dose (13). Studies suggest that the greatest benefit of steroids comes from a longer duration of treatment rather than an increased dose in terms of relapse (5). However, with longer duration of steroid administration comes a higher risk of complications, such as growth arrest, obesity, osteoporosis, hypertension, and adrenal insufficiency (13). Nonsteroidal agents, such as cyclophosphamide or cyclosporine, are sometimes used in steroid-resistant patients (10).

DISPOSITION

AGN

When the diagnosis of AGN has been made, consultation with a nephrologist should be obtained. Because of the possible complications, such as hypertension, hyperkalemia and acute renal failure, most consultants choose to admit these children or to ensure close follow up. The decision to discharge a patient with possible AGN should not be made without consulting a specialist in nephrology. The acute phase of PSAGN generally resolves within 6 to 8 weeks but persistent microscopic hematuria may persist for 1 to 2 years. Biopsy should be considered in cases of acute renal failure and in cases that are persistent for more than 2 months. Biopsy is also considered in cases where no evidence of recent streptococcal infection can be found.

Nephrotic Syndrome

Overall, the long-term prognosis for PSAGN is good, with more than 98% of patients asymptomatic at 5 years. Other causes of AGN have varying outcomes. Complications from acute glomerulonephritis are rare, but can occur. They can range from persistent microscopic hematuria to renal failure (7). The most common long term complication is mild hypertension.

Most children with new onset nephrotic syndrome are admitted to the hospital for initiation of steroid therapy and aggressive education of the patient and family. A thorough history regarding tuberculosis exposure and a CXR should be performed in the ED. If these are negative, steroid therapy may be initiated. Children presenting with a relapse may be discharged home if stable. Children older than 6 years of age, those with hypertension, hematuria or evidence of impaired renal function should be admitted for further evaluation to elucidate the underlying cause of their disease. Mild edema is treated with salt restriction at home. Discharge instructions should include warnings regarding fever, tachypnea, abdominal pain, chest pain, vomiting, increasing edema and decreasing urine output. Patients and caregivers should be advised to call their primary physician if exposed to measles or varicella.

CRITICAL INTERVENTIONS

- Patients with nephritis may have signs of fluid overload and should be fluid restricted. Diuretics should be used in the management of circulatory congestion
- Patients with nephrotic syndrome may present with edema despite being intravascularly volume depleted. The use of diuretic agents in nephrotic syndrome should be done with great caution as this may lead to severe hypovolemia
- It is important to remember that too rapid a correction of the elevated blood pressure can be dangerous and the patient must be monitored closely during treatment. A continuous infusion of nitroprusside or labetalol allows cautious titration for desired effect

COMMON PITFALLS

✔ Mistakenly diagnosing a urinary tract infection in AGN. Hematuria is the most common urinary abnormality but the presence of polymorphonuclear leukocytes and renal epithelial cells may be the only abnormalities early in the disease
✔ Not considering AGN in the differential, especially in the presence of other, potentially subtle clinical signs such as edema
✔ Incorrectly diagnosing patients with periorbital edema due to nephrotic syndrome as allergy-related or sinusitis. It is advisable to perform a urinary dipstick to check for proteinuria. Patients may present with periorbital edema as the only obvious manifestation of nephrotic syndrome
✔ Aggressively treating edema in the patient with nephrotic syndrome in the absence of respiratory compromise. Profound hypotension may result
✔ Treating hyponatremia too aggressively in patients with nephrotic syndrome. These patients have excess water as the cause of hyponatremia and should not be treated with significant sodium infusions to correct low sodium values
✔ Not taking fever or other signs of infection seriously. Children with nephrotic syndrome are relatively immunocompromised, even before the initiation of steroid therapy. Fever or other signs of infection should be taken very seriously in these patients

Acknowledgments

The authors would like to thank Mark Benfield for his assistance in writing this manuscript. The authors gratefully acknowledge the contributions of Asad Tolaymat and Anne Schaefer who wrote a previous version of this chapter.

References

1. Barratt TM, Clark G. Minimal change nephrotic syndrome and focal segmental glomerulosclerosis. In: Holliday MA, Barratt T, Avner ED, eds. *Pediatric nephrology*, 3rd ed. Baltimore: Williams & Wilkins, 1994:767.
2. Bothner J. Nephrotic Syndrome. In: Reisdorf E, Roberts M, Wiegenstein J, eds. *Pediatric emergency medicine*. Philadelphia: WB Saunders Company, 1993:400–405.
3. Davis I, Avner E, Behrman RE, Kliegman R, Jensen HB. Conditions particularly associated with hematuria. In: Nelson's Pediatrics. 17th ed. Philadelphia: WB Saunders Company, 2004:1734–1735.
4. Demby BL. Renal and Genitourinary System. In: Reisdorf E, Roberts M, Wiegenstein J, eds. *Pediatric emergency medicine*, Philadelphia: W.B. Saunders Company, 1993:395–400.
5. Hodson EM, et al. Corticosteroid therapy in nephrotic syndrome: a meta-analysis of randomized controlled trials. *J Pediatr* 2001;138(1):143–145.
6. Ilyas M, et al. Serious infections due to penicillin resistant *Streptococcus pneumoniae* in two children with the nephrotic syndrome. *Pediatric Nephrology* 1996;10:639–641.
7. Kazzi AA. Glomerulonephritis, Acute. www.emedicine.com. Cited October 16, 2003.
8. Nash MA, Edelmann CM Jr, Burnstein J, et al. The nephrotic syndrome. In: Edelmann CM Jr, ed. *Pediatric kidney disease*, 2nd ed. Boston: Little Brown and Company, 1992;1247.
9. *Red Book report of the Committee of Infectious Disease 1997*, 24th ed. Dallas: American Academy of Pediatrics, 1997:573–585.
10. Roth KS, et al. Nephrotic Syndrome: Pathogenesis and management. *Pediatrics in Review*. 2002;23:237–248.
11. Travis L. Acute Poststreptococcal Glomerulonephritis. www.emedicine.com. Cited August 28, 2002.
12. Travis LB. The nephrotic syndrome. In: Rudolph AM, ed. *Rudolph's Pediatrics*, 20th ed. Norwalk CT: Appleton & Lange, 1996:1366.
13. Travis L. Nephrotic Syndrome. www.emedicine.com. Cited October 16, 2003.

CHAPTER 249
Human Immunodeficiency Virus (HIV)

Joseph A. Church and Jeffrey F. Linzer

In the early 1980s children were identified with clinical features similar to severe combined immunodeficiency (SCID), but with distinct epidemiologic and pathological findings. These first cases of pediatric acquired immunodeficiency syndrome (PAIDS) were reported in 1982. By 1983 the causative agent of AIDS was identified as human immunodeficiency virus (HIV).

TABLE 249.1.   Pediatric AIDS Defining Conditions*

Lymphoid interstitial pneumonitis
Specified opportunistic infections (abbreviated list):
   Pneumocystis carinii pneumonia (PCP)
   Myobacterium avium complex (MAC/MAI)
   Disseminated *Mycobacteria tuberculosis*
   Histoplasmosis
   Candidiasis (esophageal or pulmonary)
Severe bacterial infections (multiple or recurrent ≥2 over 2 years)
Specified lymphomas
Wasting syndrome
Encephalopathy

   *CDC. MMWR 1994;43(No.RR-12):1–10.

HIV is a RNA retrovirus that selectively infects T-Cells and cells of the monocyte lineage. The host cell targets of HIV are critical components of the immune system. When confronted with pathogens, these cells normally produce a coordinated, protective effector response. The molecular signals that activate normal cell responses to pathogens are read by the HIV proviral DNA as signals to initiate replication.

Three pathologic consequences of HIV infection induce recognizable patterns of clinical disease: progressive immunologic attrition and immune deficiency, central nervous infection, and uncontrollable immune activation. Because functional CD4+ T-cells are required for the generation of protective, antigen-specific T-cell and antibody responses, T-cell loss and impaired T-cell production eventually induce an acquired severe immune deficiency and progressive susceptibility to opportunistic infections. Neurons in the central nervous system are not specific targets for HIV, although it infects and activates local microglial cells. These activated macrophage-like cells generate a variety of cytokines that cause activation-induced programmed cell death of adjacent neurons resulting in signs and symptoms of neuroencephalopathy. HIV may also induce an inappropriate and uncontrolled activation of infected target cells, producing a variety of proliferative disorders such as lymphoid interstitial pneumonitis, lymphadenopathy, hepatosplenomegaly, and systemic features of chronic infection, including fatigue, fever, and wasting.

The term "acquired immunodeficiency syndrome," AIDS, refers to the most serious clinical consequences of HIV infection as defined by the Centers for Disease Control and Prevention (CDC) (Table 249.1). The CDC also has developed a specific classification system to describe the immunologic (Table 249.2) and clinical features of the disease in children. These categories are combined to provide a pediatric HIV classification (Table 249.3). The classification system defines patients at their worst clinical and immunologic states, and the assigned class would not be upgraded even if a patient improves with treatment.

Between 1982 and 2001, 9,074 cases of PAIDS were reported to the CDC, with many more HIV-infected children who have not had an AIDS defining condition. Of the reported cases with PAIDS, 91% were children born to HIV-infected mothers. Currently, this "vertical transmission" accounts for all but a few isolated cases of new pediatric HIV infections. In the United States, children born to untreated HIV-infected mothers have approximately a 20% to 25% chance of being infected. With recent recommendations for universal HIV screening of pregnant women and effective pre- and postnatal prophylaxis, the transmission rate has been reduced to below 5% and the number of new cases of PAIDS reported each year has fallen from a peak of over 900 in 1992 to 175 in 2001.

CLINICAL PRESENTATION

The initial presentation and assessment of an HIV-infected child may differ depending upon whether or not the diagnosis of HIV infection has been made previously. The child with perinatally-acquired HIV may appear to be growing normally and to have no more than the usual number of routine childhood infections. Therefore, previously undiagnosed HIV-infected children may present through the emergency department (ED) with their first clinical manifestations of HIV-associated disease, and a degree of suspicion must be kept for HIV even in relatively healthy older children.

Additionally, as teens engage in high-risk behavior, they too may present to the ED with complications of previously undiagnosed HIV infection.

HIV infection should be considered in children who present with unexplained poor growth or developmental delay, or with recurrent or chronic infections. Recurrent infections do not need to be severe or debilitating, and the most common infections seen early in the course of HIV-associated immunodeficiency are frequent otitis media, sinusitis and bacterial pneumonia as well as adenitis and diarrhea. Any opportunistic infection (OI) immediately suggests an underlying immune deficiency. The most common presenting physical findings in previously undiagnosed HIV-infected children are lymphadenopathy (LAD) especially involving cervical and axillary lymph nodes, and hepatic or splenic enlargement. Parotid gland enlargement may also be seen. The presence of recurrent or chronic oral candidiasis especially in a child over one year of age suggests immune deficiency. Common hematologic findings in HIV-infected children include anemia, neutropenia, and in approximately 5% of undiagnosed HIV-infected children "idiopathic" thrombocytopenia. Blood chemistry abnormalities may include nonspecific liver enzyme elevations, hypoalbuminemia and hyperproteinemia with an increased globulin fraction. The erythrocyte sedimentation rate is often markedly elevated.

Acute manifestations of an OI may be the initial presenting process in a child with undiagnosed HIV. *Pneumocystis carinii* pneumonia (PCP) remains the most common presenting OI in undiagnosed children. Although typically presenting at less than

TABLE 249.2.   CDC Immunologic Categories Based on Age-Specific CD4+ T-Lymphocyte Counts and Percent of Total Lymphocytes for HIV-Infected Children < 13 Years of Age

| | Age of Child | | | | | |
| | < 12 mos | | 1–5 yrs | | 6–12 yrs | |
Immunologic Category	cells/cc	(%)	cells/cc	(%)	cells/cc	(%)
1: No evidence of suppression	≥ 1,500	(≥ 25)	≥ 1,000	(≥ 25)	≥ 500	(≥ 25)
2: Evidence of moderate suppression	750–1,499	(15–24)	500–999	(15–24)	200–499	(15–24)
3: Severe suppression	< 750	(< 15)	< 500	(< 15)	< 200	(< 15)

   CDC. *MMWR* 1994;43(No.RR-12):4.

TABLE 249.3.   CDC Classification System for HIV-Infected Children <13 Years of Age

Immunologic Category	Clinical Categories*			
	N: No Signs/ Symptoms	A: Mild Signs/ Symptoms	B: Moderate Signs/ Symptoms	C: Severe Signs/ Symptoms
1: No evidence of suppression	N1	A1	B1	C1
2: Evidence of moderate suppression	N2	A2	B2	C2
3: Severe suppression	N3	A3	B3	C3

*For definitions of mild, moderate and severe symptoms see CDC. *MMWR* 1994;43(No.RR-12):1–10.

2 years of age, PCP may occur in a child at any time and depends upon the status of an individual patient's T-cells. Symptoms of PCP include dyspnea, tachypnea, cough, and fever that may be slowly progressive over several weeks. Physical examination often reveals clear lung sounds and disproportionate hypoxemia. The severity of symptoms may range from a mild repetitive cough to severe respiratory distress. Chest radiograph shows a diffuse interstitial pattern often disproportionately mild compared to the patient's hypoxemia and respiratory distress. Lymphoid interstitial pneumonitis (LIP) and pulmonary lymphoid hyperplasia (PLH) also cause respiratory symptoms and may mimic infection or reactive airway disease. In contrast to PCP, LIP and PLH often have radiographic findings worse than respiratory symptoms would suggest. Children with this process often have generalized lymphadenopathy and hepatosplenomegaly, and may display digital clubbing. The most common organisms causing respiratory infections in HIV-infected children remain the typical pediatric respiratory pathogens such as *S. pneumonia*, *H. influenzae* and *M. catarrhalis*.

Children with profound immune deficiency may present to the ED with a variety of other OIs. *Mycobacterium avium* complex (MAC), presents with prolonged fevers, night sweats, chronic diarrhea, abdominal pain, and weight loss. Chronic oral thrush is common and esophageal candidiasis should be suspected in a child with oral thrush accompanied by dysphagia, irritability, and weight loss. Diarrhea is common. Although at times related to persistent gastrointestinal infections with "routine" organisms such as salmonella, shigella, and campylobacter, HIV-infected children are particularly at high risk for *C. difficile*, *Giardia*, cryptosporidium and cytomegalovirus (CMV) enteritis. Disseminated toxoplasmosis, histoplasmosis, and cryptococcosis, although uncommon, may be seen in children. Herpes virus infections (herpes simplex virus (HSV), varicella-zoster virus (VZV) and CMV), are often particularly severe and may present as disseminated disease. CMV retinitis, a common cause of vision loss in adult HIV patients, is uncommon in children, but can occur with advanced disease and may present to the ED as acute blurry vision. Malignancies, especially B-cell lymphomas, occur at an increased rate with HIV infection and may occur in the central nervous system (CNS) or gastrointestinal tract. Kaposi sarcoma is rare in children. Acute cardiac and renal manifestations are uncommon, but cardiomyopathy with congestive heart failure and acute renal failure has been described. Chronic HIV-associated encephalopathy and developmental delay are common in untreated children, and acute CNS manifestations such as infection, space occupying lesions and thromboembolic events may occur. Infected children are at risk for sepsis and meningitis with the usual pediatric pathogens, and patients may be particularly susceptible because of compromised ability to respond to routine immunizations.

Less acute but common presentations to the ED include infectious skin eruptions, such as molluscum, verrucae, and drug eruptions. The child with HIV-associated immune compromise is at greater risk for severe HSV and VZV infections and may present with recurrent or persistent chicken-pox, varicella zoster, or mucocutaneous herpes simplex infections. Oral aphthous ulcers are common and present as painful, shallow oropharyngeal ulcers, which often result in decreased oral intake, weight loss and at times dehydration. Aphthous ulcers need to be differentiated from oral HSV lesions, as corticosteroids are useful in the treatment of the former and contraindicated in the later.

Children known to be infected with HIV often present to the ED with a different constellation of chief complaints. Patients who are adherent to their highly active antiretroviral therapy (HAART) are very unlikely to develop an opportunistic infection, and acute infections most often reflect routine childhood illnesses. More commonly, ED visits are associated with adverse effects of patients' treatment regimens. Acute pancreatitis can be seen with several antiretroviral agents and can be severe and life-threatening. Drug eruptions ranging from mild nonspecific erythroderma and urticaria to overwhelming Stevens-Johnson syndrome may be seen with agents used for PCP prophylaxis (trimethoprim-sulfamethoxazole (TMP-SMX)) or antiretroviral agents (for example abacavir and nevirapine). Nausea, vomiting, and liver function abnormalities are commonly seen in patients on HAART. Drug-induced hematologic abnormalities that may present to the ED include thrombocytopenia-associated bleeding, anemia-associated congestive heart failure, and granulocytopenia-associated secondary infections, such as those caused by *Staphylococcus aureus* and *Pseudomonas aeruginosa*.

DIFFERENTIAL DIAGNOSIS

Any of the SCID syndromes may present identically to HIV. Children with either autosomal recessive or X-linked SCIDs often present with overwhelming infections within the first six months of life, although later presentation may occur. Patients with DiGeorge syndrome may develop OIs but these patients usually have conotruncal congenital heart disease, hypocalcemia or typical facial dysmorphisms. Primary antibody deficiencies including X-linked agammaglobulinemia and common variable immune deficiency typically present with recurrent upper and lower respiratory tract infections caused by encapsulated bacteria. *Giardia* and enteroviral disease are also commonly seen in these patients.

Lymphoma, leukemia, and other malignancies can present with weight loss, organomegaly, LAD, cytopenias and OIs. Cystic fibrosis may also present with recurrent pneumonias, sinus disease, chronic diarrhea, and poor weight gain. Autoimmune diseases such as systemic lupus erythematosus and systemic juvenile rheumatoid arthritis, and metabolic and mitochondrial diseases may present with features suggestive of immune

TABLE 249.4.   Indications for HIV Testing in Children Presenting to the Emergency Department

History of parental HIV infection
Signs of congenital viral infection
Suspected opportunistic infection
History of recurrent, severe, bacterial infections
Hepatosplenomegaly, lymphadenopathy
Unexplained wasting, myopathy, hepatitis, carditis, nephritis,
   developmental regression, neuropathy, encephalopathy

deficiency. Many chronic conditions may be associated with secondary immunodeficiency including protein calorie malnutrition, zinc deficiency, nephrotic syndrome, inflammatory bowel disease and protein-losing enteropathies.

In infants less than three months of age TORCH infections (toxoplasmosis, rubella, CMV, HSV, syphilis) may present with features similar to HIV.

EMERGENCY DEPARTMENT EVALUATION

Assessment in the ED will depend upon whether the patient is known to be infected with HIV or is presenting with a suspected but undiagnosed immune deficiency. A careful physical examination and history should assess factors listed in Table 249.4. However, absence of known risk factors should not override clinical suspicion for HIV. A child with findings strongly suggestive of immune deficiency should be considered for hospitalization for comprehensive evaluation. The recent approval of a simple, point-of-service test for HIV antibodies allows rapid and accurate HIV diagnosis in acute settings. Use of the OraQuick® rapid HIV testing device provides highly sensitive and highly specific results in 20 minutes, and may be performed at the bedside. The clinical management of the patient presenting with a complica-

tion possibly related to HIV will be dramatically enhanced by the availability and use of this type of testing.

For the child with known HIV infection, ED evaluation should address the presenting problems in the context of the patient's immunologic status (Fig. 249.1). The risk of OI is related to the degree of immune deficiency and adherence to a HAART regimen. In general, children who are in CDC category 1 (no evidence of immune suppression) may receive the same evaluation as a non-infected child with similar clinical symptoms. Children in more advance categories are at higher risk of serious illness and more intensive evaluations are indicated.

Although potentially a sign of underlying malignancy, fever is usually an indication of secondary infection. In most children a routine complete blood count (CBC), appropriate cultures and indicated radiographs should be performed. In children with severe immune compromise, blood cultures should also be obtained for acid-fast bacilli, CMV and adenovirus. Pulse oximetry or blood gases are indicated for patients with cough, wheeze or respiratory distress. Nasal pharyngeal washings for rapid viral diagnostic assessment should be sent and sputum should be obtained in older children. For acute diarrheal disease, stool examinations are indicated for routine bacterial and rotavirus infections, ova, and parasites, *Giardia* and *C. difficile*. In children with advanced HIV disease, evaluation for cryptosporidium, acid-fast bacilli, CMV, and adenovirus would be added to this list. Where dehydration is a consideration, serum electrolytes, calcium and magnesium levels should be monitored. For children presenting with acute abdominal pain, serum amylase and lipase and tests of liver function should be ordered. Abdominal imaging may be indicated for patients with severe or persistent pain. For acute rashes suggestive of drug-hypersensitivity, a history of recent medication changes should be sought. Skin lesions appearing infectious in origin should be cultured. Children with acute CNS symptoms should have appropriate imaging and lumbar puncture if deemed safe and appropriate.

HIV infection is often associated with generalized LAD. Differentiation from chronic parotid gland involvement is

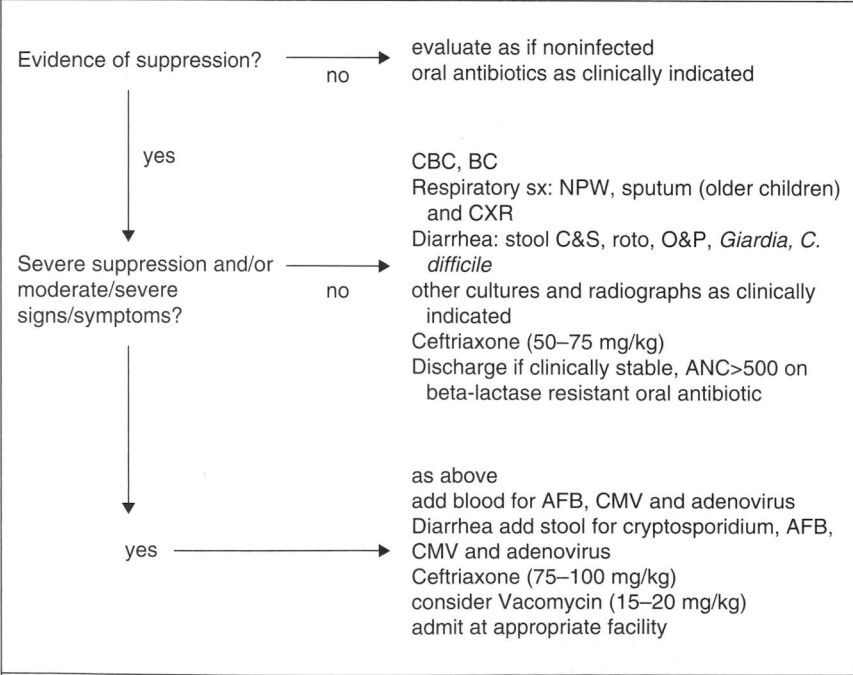

Key. CBC = complete blood count, BC = blood culture, NPW = nasal pharyngeal wash for virus analysis, CXR = chest radiograph, C&S = culture and sensitivity, roto = rotozyme assay, O&P = ova and parasite, ANC = absolute neutrophil count, AFB = acid fast bacillus, CMV = cytomegalovirus

Figure 249.1.   Fever evaluation and treatment in HIV-infected children.

TABLE 249.5.   Primary Side Effects Associated with Antiretroviral Agents

Antiretroviral Class/Agent	Primary Side Effects and Toxicities
Nucleoside Reverse Transcriptase Inhibitors (NRTIs)	
Zidovudine (Retrovir®; ZDV; AZT)	Anemia, neutropenia, nausea, headache, insomnia, muscle pain, and weakness
Lamivudine (Epivir®; 3TC) Emtricitabine (Emtriva®)	Abdominal pain, nausea, diarrhea, rash, and pancreatitis
Stavudine (Zerit®; d4T)	Peripheral neuropathy, headache, diarrhea, nausea, insomnia, anorexia, pancreatitis, increased liver function tests (LFTs), anemia, and neutropenia
Didanosine (Videx®; ddI) Zalcitabine (Hivid®; ddC)	Pancreatitis, lactic acidosis, neuropathy, diarrhea, abdominal pain, and nausea
Abacavir (Ziagen®; ABC)	Nausea, diarrhea, anorexia, abdominal pain, fatigue, headache, insomnia, and hypersensitivity reactions
Tenofovir (Viread®; TNV)	Nausea, diarrhea, vomiting
Nonnucleoside Reverse Transcriptase Inhibitors (NNRTIs)	
Nevirapine (Viramune®; NVP)	Rash (including case of Stevens-Johnson syndrome), fever, nausea, headache, hepatitis, and increased LFTs
Delavirdine (Rescriptor®; DLV)	Rash (including case of Stevens-Johnson syndrome), nausea, diarrhea, headache, fatigue, and increased LFTs
Efavirenz (Sustiva®; EFV)	Rash (including cases of Stevens-Johnson syndrome), insomnia, somnolence, dizziness, trouble concentrating, and abnormal dreaming.
Protease Inhibitors (PIs)	
Indinavir (Crixivan®; IDV)	Nausea, abdominal pain, nephrolithiasis, and indirect hyperbilirubinemia
Nelfinavir (Viracept®; NFV)	Diarrhea, nausea, abdominal pain, weakness, and rash
Ritonavir (Norvir®; RTV)	Weakness, diarrhea, nausea, circumoral paresthesia, taste alteration, and increased cholesterol and triglycerides
Saquinavir (Fortovase®; SQV)	Diarrhea, abdominal pain, nausea, hyperglycemia, and increased LFTs
Amprenavir (Agenerase®; APV) Fos-Amprenavir (Lexiva®)	Nausea, diarrhea, rash, circumoral paresthesia, taste alteration, and depression
Lopinavir/Ritonavir (Kaletra®; LPV/r)	Diarrhea, fatigue, headache, nausea, and increased cholesterol and triglycerides
Atazanavir (Rayataz®; ATV)	Jaundice, hyperbilirubinemia, nausea, vomiting, headache, diarrhea, rash
Entry Inhibitor	
Enfuvirtide (Fuzeon®; T-20)	Injection site reactions; household exposure to contaminated needles/syringes

sometimes difficult. Acute infectious lymphadenitis or focal bacterial parotitis may complicate long-term LAD or parotid gland swelling. HIV-associated B-cell lymphoma may present as a rapidly growing local adenopathy in a patient irrespective of T-cell level.

Adverse medication reactions are very common in HIV patients and may develop acutely or after prolonged exposure to various drugs. The primary side effects associated with antiretroviral agents are listed in Table 249.5. The long-term adverse impact of antiretroviral agents on metabolism and bone is increasingly being seen. Many agents may cause acute, severe lactic acidosis. HIV-associated lipodystrophy known to affect adults is now being seen more commonly in children and is associated with increased abdominal girth, dorsocervical fat accumulation and peripheral fat loss characterized by thinning of the face, extremities, and buttocks. Metabolic complications may include insulin resistance leading to frank diabetes, hyperlipidemia with elevated cholesterol and triglyceride levels which may be associated with early coronary artery disease, and osteopenia with increased risk for spinal compression and extremity fractures. Antiretroviral agents, particularly the protease inhibitors, have pharmacologic interactions with many other agents. Of particular concern in the ED is the prolongation of activity of midazolam

(Versed®). Many other drug interactions exist and care must be taken in adding new drugs to any HIV-infected patient's current treatment regimen.

EMERGENCY DEPARTMENT MANAGEMENT

Three principles guide ED management of children with HIV: HIV is not spread by routine clinical contact with patients or their families; the risk of any acute process being a serious one is inversely related to the patient's T-cell count; close communication with the patient's HIV specialist is crucial.

Presenting illness in an HIV-infected child with intact T-cells can generally be managed in a manner similar to that of the same process in a noninfected child. For other HIV-infected children the degree of T-cell deficiency needs to be considered when ED management is initiated. Importantly, ED identified physical or laboratory abnormalities may be known to the primary HIV healthcare provider as chronic conditions, and the primary service may be aware of psychosocial factors unique to the patient and family which need to be incorporated into ED management.

The insight of the patient's HIV provider will help guide the empiric antibiotic treatment of a child presenting to the ED with fever. Children with advanced HIV disease require a more aggressive diagnostic assessment and earlier antibiotic intervention. The specific antibiotic regimen is based on the source of infection, likely organisms and degree of T-cell compromise. Parenteral ceftriaxone followed by a course of oral antibiotics effective against beta-lactamase positive agents is a good choice for community-acquired pneumonia, acute otitis media or sinusitis in a patient with mild immunologic suppression but stable T-cell numbers. Children with normal T-cells may be treated with oral antibiotics alone. Fever with granulocytopenia, which may develop at any time as a complication of antiretroviral therapy, requires broad-spectrum antibiotic coverage, as does the patient with fever and an indwelling central venous catheter.

Although HIV-positive infants less than 1 year of age may develop PCP at any T-cell level, older patients with severe T-cell suppression are at particular risk for this complication, particularly if adherence to prescribed prophylaxis is inconsistent. Patients with PCP usually present with a history of progressive cough, tachypnea, shortness of breath, dyspnea and intermittent fever, which may be low-grade. Auscultation of the chest often reveals an expiratory grunt without other adventitious sounds. Hypoxemia is demonstrable with pulse oximetry and may be exacerbated with simple exercise. Chest radiograph may show only minimal changes; marked interstitial infiltration reflects vary advance disease and a guarded prognosis. Any patient suspected of having PCP should be hospitalized at a center familiar with the management of this disorder. Bronchoalveolar lavage (BAL) is particularly useful in confirming the diagnosis. TMP-SMX is the antibiotic of choice, and systemic corticosteroids are indicated as adjunctive therapy in these patients. HIV-infected children, even those with T-cells sufficient to avoid opportunistic infections, are at increased risk for pneumonias and other respiratory tract infections with "routine" organisms including *S. pneumoniae*, *M. catarrhalis*, and *H. influenzae*. They are also at risk for reactive airway disease and over 30% of patients require bronchodilators or more intense therapy for asthma. Differentiation between an acute asthma attack and a serious acute infectious process is essential.

The most common cause of diarrhea in HIV-infected children is their antiretroviral therapy. Dietary changes and loperamide are usually sufficient to control symptoms. Dehydration is treated with oral or intravenous rehydration depending on severity. Because of the increased risk for infectious enteritis, HIV-positive children presenting to the ED with diarrhea should be screened for salmonella, shigella, campylobacter, and parasitic infections with *Giardia lamblia* and cryptosporidium. *C. difficile* and intestinal candidiasis may be complications of long-term prophylactic antibiotics. Nonspecific enteritis commonly seen in children with long-term HIV disease may be associated with electrolyte imbalance, malabsorption and wasting.

It is not appropriate to institute or make changes in an individual's antiretroviral therapy, prophylactic therapy or other chronic medical treatment in the ED. Any such changes should be made only after discussion with patient's HIV healthcare provider.

CHEMOPROPHYLAXIS AFTER EXPOSURE TO HIV

Children may present to the ED after exposures which put them at risk for HIV infection. Examples include accidental puncture wounds during play with discarded needles or from needles in the home, and sexual abuse. If the source is known to be HIV-infected, recommendations for chemoprophylaxis are based on the type of exposure (percutaneous, mucous membrane, nonintact skin) and source material (blood, other infectious body fluids such as semen or vaginal secretions). Larger volume or area of exposure, higher HIV level and prolonged contact all increase the risk of transmission. Often the HIV status of the contact source is not known. In these cases recommendations for chemoprophylaxis must be made on a case-by-case basis. Prophylaxis should be *recommended* for children with high-risk exposure, *offered* to children with low but nonnegligible exposure and *not offered* for exposures with negligible risk such as contact with urine or saliva. The CDC has made detailed recommendations regarding the initiation of postexposure prophylaxis (Table 249.6). In general combination drug therapy is recommended when the risk is high. In most cases the combination should include zidovudine (AZT) combined with one or two other drugs. When possible, postexposure prophylaxis should be started after consultation with an expert in antiretroviral therapy, and should be initiated as soon as possible after exposure preferably within 1 to 2 hours. It is unlikely that postexposure prophylaxis started 48 hours after exposure would be effective. The optimal duration of postexposure prophylaxis is unknown, but should be administered for at least 4 weeks if tolerated or until the source of the

---

TABLE 249.6.   Recommended Post-Exposure Prophylaxis (Pep) in the Healthcare Setting*

Percutaneous Injuries

Exposure Type	HIV Status of Source		
	HIV+ "Class 1"[1]	HIV+ "Class 2"[2]	HIV Status Unknown
"Less Severe" (solid needle, superficial injury)	2-drugs	3-drugs	Generally n/a[3], "consider" 2-drugs
"More Severe" (large bore, hollow needle, deep puncture, visible blood on device, or needle used in patient's artery or vein)	3-drugs	3-drugs	Generally n/a, "consider" 2-drugs

Mucous Membrane or Nonintact Skin Exposures

Exposure Type	HIV Status of Source		
	HIV+ "Class 1"	HIV+ "Class 2"	HIV Status Unknown
"Small volume" (few drops)	"consider" 2-drugs	2-drugs	Generally n/a, "consider" 2-drugs
"Large volume" (major blood splash)	2-drugs	3-drugs	Generally n/a, "consider" 2-drugs

*CDC. *MMWR* 2001;50(No. RR-11):1–42.
[1]Class 1 – asymptomatic or known low viral load.
[2]Class 2 – symptomatic, AIDS, acute seroconversion, known high viral load.
[3]n/a – not advisable.

exposure is shown to be HIV negative. The child should be tested for HIV antibodies at the initiation of postexposure prophylaxis to confirm the absence of preexisting HIV infection. Postexposure prophylaxis should be offered in conjunction of appropriate counseling as to the risks and benefits of antiretroviral therapy and the infectious risk of the exposure, and after arrangements are made for ongoing counseling and followup testing.

DISPOSITION

As with any chronic disorder, children with HIV are best followed by a primary service experienced in the multidisciplinary management of the disease. Children who are suspected of having undiagnosed HIV and who do not have compelling clinical findings should be referred to a pediatric infectious disease or other HIV specialist for urgent consultation. Discussion with the consultant prior to discharge from the ED can help assess whether the child can be safely discharged and to arrange follow up. Known HIV-infected children who are manageable at home may be discharged from the ED after consultation with the primary HIV healthcare service and arrangement for follow up.

Children requiring hospitalization should be carefully evaluated to determine if admission to an intensive care or regular inpatient unit is required. If the hospital is not equipped to manage seriously ill HIV-infected children, or if the necessary specialists are not available, the patient should be transported to an appropriate center by qualified transport personnel.

CRITICAL INTERVENTIONS

- Patients suspected of having an immune deficiency should not be given a live virus vaccine; all blood products required by such patients should be irradiated and CMV-negative
- Fever in an HIV-infected patient suggests infection and appropriate investigations (such as complete blood count, blood culture, chest radiograph, urinalysis, lumbar puncture) are indicated

COMMON PITFALLS

- ✔ The clinical latency from infection to manifestation of HIV disease may be years. Perinatally infected children may present with their first complications at ten years of age or older
- ✔ Many parents do not know their HIV status so the diagnosis of a child's HIV infection is often the index for an entire family
- ✔ Not all parents will volunteer that their child is HIV-infected, and others may deny their own risk factors. Decisions to test or treat a child as HIV-infected may need to be based on clinical suspicion alone
- ✔ In any suspected immune deficient patient under one year of age, the presence of tachypnea and hypoxia suggest PCP and empiric therapy should not be withheld while waiting for a definitive diagnosis. Children prescribed appropriate PCP prophylaxis may develop the disease if they are nonadherent to their prophylaxis regimen
- ✔ Any child over a year of age with persistent or recurrent oral thrush should be considered to be immune deficient
- ✔ In an HIV-infected patient, the risk for a more serious disease is inversely related to the patient's T-cell count. Immune-suppressed children should receive more intensive evaluation and treatment intervention than immunologically normal children

- ✔ A child at risk for HIV by either history or suggestive clinical findings should be offered rapid HIV testing and managed accordingly
- ✔ The HIV-infected patient's primary service should be contacted for final disposition. Effective outpatient followup will minimize the need for future ED care

Acknowledgment

The authors wish to thank Ronald M. Ferdman, who helped write the previous version of this chapter.

Bibliography

Centers for Disease Control and Prevention. 1994 Revised classification system for human immunodeficiency virus infection in children less than 13 years of age. *MMWR* 1994;43(No.RR-12):1–10.

Centers for Disease Control and Prevention. Updated U.S. Public Health Service Guidelines for the Management of Occupational Exposures to HBV, HCV, and HIV and recommendations for postexposure prophylaxis. *MMWR* 2001;50(RR-11):1–42.

Committee on Pediatric AIDS and Committee on Infectious Diseases, American Academy of Pediatrics. Issues related to human immunodeficiency virus transmission in schools, childcare, medical settings, the home and community. *Pediatrics* 1999;104:318–324.

McNicholl IR, Peiper L. Database of antiretroviral drug interactions. http://hivinsite.ucsf.edu/arvdb?page = ar-00-02.

Merchant RC, Keshavarz R. Human immunodeficiency virus postexposure prophylaxis for adolescents and children. *Pediatrics* August 2001;108:e38.

National Pediatric and Family HIV Resource Center. http://www.pedhivaids.org/.

Shearer WT, Hanson IC, eds. Medical management of AIDS in children. Philadelphia; Saunders, 2003.

U.S. Department of Health and Human Services. Guidelines for the use of antiretroviral agents in Pediatric HIV infection. 2004. http://aidsinfo.nih.gov/.

CHAPTER 250
Immunizations

Marla J. Friedman and Javier A. Gonzalez del Rey

Immunizations have been instrumental in reducing the incidence, morbidity, and mortality of preventable diseases throughout the world. Consequently, disease prevention through vaccination has become a major public health concern. Childhood immunization has been a cornerstone of pediatric health care since the American Academy of Pediatrics (AAP) first policy statement on immunization practices was released in 1977 (13). Despite recommendations of universal immunization, only 77.2% of children in the United States less than 3 years of age have received their basic immunization series (3). Immunization rates drop to 60% for children who are poor, live in inner-city or rural areas, or are members of a racial or ethnic minority (3,30). If these children have many siblings and a young mother who did not graduate from high school, their risk of being unimmunized is even greater (32). Although most routine immunizations are administered in a primary health care setting, many view an emergency department (ED) visit by an underimmunized child as an opportunity to vaccinate (14,15,21,35,36).

High |

Sickle
Immu
Chror
Diabe
Cochl

Mode

Childr
Childr
Africar
Low so
Home
Chron
Histor

PCV7
coccal
most |
vaccin
bacter
of pne
  PC
for chi
mende
risk of
large s
invasiv
coccal
have a:
are ber
fered f
all dos
  Mil
injectic
cinatio

Polio

Disease
the Un
vaccina
associa
United
which
the rou
VAPP |
(6). The
Unted
with for
lifelong
  IPV i
Althoug
of neon
traindic
antimic

Varice

The liv
United
age whe

benefit-to-cost ratio. A negative guaiac should not be used to exclude the diagnosis, yet a positive stool guaiac should reduce the threshold for further evaluative and management decisions. When symptoms are brief and the child appears nontoxic and well hydrated, blood chemistries and a hemogram are not warranted. However, a complete blood count, serum electrolytes, blood urea nitrogen, creatinine, and urinalysis may facilitate decision making concerning a child who appears to be volume depleted. A blood sugar is required for the child with altered mental status. The child who appears septic should have cultures of blood, urine, stool, and cerebrospinal fluid (20).

A variety of abdominal imaging procedures can be utilized for a provisional diagnosis of intussusception (21–23). Those who advocate plain films suggest acquiring supine and upright or supine and left lateral decubitus radiographs of the abdomen (7,10). Depending on the time course at presentation, age of the patient, and presence of a lead point, films may be normal or reveal nonspecific findings such as localized air–fluid levels or reduced intestinal air. The presence of a mass, inability to visualize the liver tip or obliteration of usual gas shadows of the colon is suggestive of intussusception (26). The presumed diagnosis can be confirmed only by plain film findings if the head of the intussusception is clearly visible in the bowel lumen. Those with nonspecific or suggestive findings should undergo either a barium or an air contrast enema (25). Those patients with radiographic evidence of complete bowel obstruction, intraperitoneal air, ascites, or pneumatoses intestinalis should not be subjected to contrast enema.

Ultrasound also is excellent for showing intussusception and is used in place of contrast enemas in some institutions depending on pediatric radiologic expertise (9,22,24). Suggestive findings are created by the edematous head of the intussusception (3). Findings include a "target" or "donut" sign on transverse section and a "pseudokidney" sign viewed on longitudinal section (10,22,24).

In children whom a pathologic lead point is suspected, a computed tomography scan may be of utility (16).

EMERGENCY DEPARTMENT MANAGEMENT

The uncomplicated patient with intussusception should not require airway intervention or respiratory support. Fluid depletion may occur as a result from vomiting, diarrhea, bowel wall ischemia or hemorrhage. Fluid resuscitation may be necessitated for frank obstruction, bowel wall necrosis, pneumoperitoneum with peritonitis or sepsis. Monitoring should be initiated that is appropriate for the degree of patient instability. Those who evidence mild-to-moderate dehydration should be given a normal saline bolus, followed by polyionic intravenous fluids pending serum electrolyte results. Although not universally performed, pending imaging procedures, a nasogastric tube is recommended. All patients should be placed NPO.

If imaging is to be carried out beyond the emergency department (ED), provide information to the radiologist and surgeon. A decision must be made concerning whether there are contraindications to nonoperative attempts at reduction of the intussusception. For patients without contraindication, the surgeon and radiologist can determine whether air inflation or barium or ultrasonography should be employed. Attempts at reduction should be done with the consent of the surgeon, who must accept the responsibility of operating if the reduction is unsuccessful or if the patient sustains a perforation. If either hydrostatic pressure or pneumatic reduction techniques fail to reduce the intussusception, sedation of the patient, with repeated efforts at nonoperative reduction or operative interventions, is an option (4,10).

DISPOSITION

Whether under ultrasonographic or fluoroscopic guidance, both air and barium reductions have success rates ranging from 65% to 90% (4,14). Recurrence of nonsurgically reduced intussusception within 1 to 3 days following pneumatic or hydrostatic reduction may occur in approximately 10% of patients (4,14). It is not possible to establish which patients are likely to have recurrent intussusception based on presenting signs and symptoms, age, or sex. Therefore, admission for a 24-hour period may be customary at many institutions but considered unnecessary at others. If the child is discharged home, the emergency physician must ascertain that parents know the indications that warrant a return for further medical attention.

COMMON PITFALLS

✔ Obstacles to accurate diagnosis include failure to recognize the typical history, failure to perform a rectal examination, reluctance to accept the diagnosis in a well-appearing child with a prolonged history, and failure to consider the disease in older children

✔ Marked variation from the classic picture may lead to misdiagnosis. The absence of pain, lack of a mass, the presence of bright red rectal bleeding, or neurologic aberrations should not dissuade one from the diagnosis

✔ A normal plain abdominal radiograph should not deter performance of the reduction techniques or further imaging studies

✔ An inopportune hour of the patient encounter should not prevent recruitment of the radiologist or the surgeon

References

1. Bergdahl S, Hugosson C, Lauren T, et al. Atypical intussusception. *J Pediatr Surg* 1972;7:700.
2. Birkhahn R, Fiorini M, Gaeta TJ. Painless intussusception and Altered Mental Status. *Am J Emerg Med* 1999;17:345–347.
3. Buchert GS. Abdominal pain in children: an emergency practitioners guide. *Emerg Med Clin North Am* 1989;7:497.
4. Champoux AN, Del Beccaroma, Nazar Stewart V. Recurrent intussusception: risks and features. *Arch Pediatr Adolesc Med* 1994;148:174.
5. Eins S, Stephens C. Intussusception: 354 cases in 10 years. *J Pediatr Surg* 1971; 6:16.
6. Fanconi S, Berger D, Rickham P. Acute intussusception: a classic clinical picture? *Helv Paediatr Acta* 1982;37:345.
7. Felter RA. Nontraumatic surgical emergencies in children. *Emerg Med Clin North Am* 1991;9:589.
8. Gierup J, Jorulf H, Livaditis A. Management of intussusception in infants and children: a survey based on 288 consecutive cases. *Pediatrics* 1972;50:535.
9. Harrington L, Connolly B, Hu X, et al. Ultrasonographic and clinical predictors of intussusception. *J Pediatr* 1998;132:836.
10. Irish MS, Pearl RH, Katy MG, et al. The approach to common abdominal diagnoses in infants and children. *Pediatr Clin North Am* 1998;45:729.
11. Losek JD. Intussusception: don't miss the diagnosis! *Pediatr Emerg Care* 1993;9:46.
12. Luks FI, Yazbeck S, Perreault G, et al. Changes in the presentation of intussusception. *Am J Emerg Med* 1992;10:574.
13. McCabe J, Singer J, Love T, et al. Intussusception: a supplement to the mnemonic for coma. *Pediatr Emerg Care* 1987;3:118.
14. McLario D, Rothrock SG. Understanding the varied presentation and management of children with acute abdominal disorders. *Pediatr Emerg Med Rep* 1997;Nov:111–122.

15. Orenstein J. Update on intussusception. *Contemporary Pediatrics* 2000;17:180–191.
16. O'Ryan M, Lucero Y, Pena A, Valenzuela MT. Two year review of intestinal intussusception in six large public hospitals of Santiago, Chile. *Pediatr Infect Dis J* 2003;22:217–21.
17. Ravitch M. Considerations of errors in the diagnosis of intussusception. *Am J Dis Child* 1952;84:17.
18. Shteyer E, Koplewitz, BZ, Gross E, Granot E. Medical treatment of recurrent intussusception associated with intestinal lymphoid hyperplasia. *Pediatrics* 2003;111:682–685.
19. Singer J. Altered consciousness as an early manifestation of intussusception. *Pediatrics* 1979;64:93.
20. Singer J. Acute abdominal conditions that may require surgical intervention. In: Strange G, ed. *A comprehensive study guide in pediatric emergency medicine.* New York: McGraw-Hill 1998:313–319.
21. Smith DS, Bonadio WA, Losek JD, et al. The role of abdominal x-rays in the diagnosis and management of intussusception. *Pediatr Emerg Care* 1992;8:325.
22. Swischuk LE. Imaging techniques for abdominal emergencies. Clinical Pediatric Emergency Medicine 2002;3:45–54.
23. Swischuk L. Acute vomiting and abdominal pain in an infant. *Pediatr Emerg Care* 1986;2:201.
24. Swischuk LE, Hayden CK, Boulden T. Intussusception : Indications for ultrasonography and an explanation of the donut and pseudokidney signs. *Pediatr Radiol* 1985;15:388–391.
25. Tamanaha K, Winbish K, Talwalker Y, et al. Air reduction of intussusception in infants and children. *J Pediatr* 1987;111:733.
26. Teitelbaum JE, Fishman SJ, Leichtner AM, Tunnessen WW. "Read my lips": Abdominal pain in a 14-year-old. *Contemporary Pediatrics* 1999;16:31–41.
27. Yamamoto LG, Morita SY, Boychuk RB, et al. Stool appearance in intussusception: assessing the value of the term "currant jelly." *Am J Emerg Med* 1997;15:293.

CHAPTER 252
Kawasaki Disease

James A. Wilde

Kawasaki disease (KD), also known as mucocutaneous lymph node syndrome, was first described in Japan in 1967 (5) and reported in the United States literature in 1974 (6). Although initially thought to be a new disease, KD was soon recognized to be clinically indistinguishable from infantile periarteritis nodosa (7). The disease is primarily a vasculitis that affects the coronary arteries most significantly, but can also produce pathology in the central nervous system, liver, gallbladder, lungs, and digits.

Three to five thousand cases of Kawasaki Disease are estimated to occur in the United States annually (1). Children less than 5 years of age account for 80% of cases, although the disease has also been reported in young adults (12,13). Peak incidence is the second year of life. Intense efforts to identify the causative agent have failed to yield an etiology, although certain clinical and epidemiologic features favor an infectious cause.

There is no diagnostic assay that can definitively identify a case of KD, so cases must be diagnosed presumptively based on characteristic clinical features and laboratory findings. Some children have been described with an incomplete form of KD that does not fit the classic case definition, thereby making identification more difficult (2,4,8). These children are also at risk for development of significant cardiac sequelae. Twenty-five percent to 30% of KD patients will develop coronary artery aneurysms without therapy, while only 5% to 8% do so with the current recommended regimen of intravenous immune globulin (IVIG) and aspirin (10). The overall mortality rate is 1% to 3% in untreated KD (9), but, with recommended therapy, may be as low as 0.08% (17).

CLINICAL PRESENTATION

Classic KD is diagnosed by clinical criteria as originally described by Dr. Kawasaki, with only slight modifications. These criteria include fever of at least 5 days' duration, at least four of five physical findings, and no other explanation for the illness (Table 252.1). A diagnosis of KD can be made in a patient with less than 5 days' fever if all the remaining clinical criteria are met (11). The fever is generally over 39°C, spiking, remittent, and prolonged in untreated patients, with some children remaining febrile for 2 to 4 weeks. Another commonly reported finding is extreme irritability in excess of that seen in other childhood febrile illnesses (11).

The conjunctivitis is primarily bulbar, spares the area around the limbus, and is not associated with an exudate. Changes in the lips may include erythema, bleeding, dryness, and fissuring. The oral mucosa may show erythema with a strawberry tongue, but exudates and oral ulcerations are not found. Hands and feet may show edema, erythema, or both, primarily on the palms and soles, with characteristic desquamation 1 to 2 weeks after the onset of the illness. The rash can be quite variable, but it is most commonly diffuse, maculopapular, and erythematous.

Cervical lymphadenopathy is usually unilateral, is nonfluctuant, and is defined by a node diameter of at least 1.5 cm. Each of the clinical criteria is found in approximately 90% of cases, with the exception of the cervical lymphadenopathy, which occurs in only 50% to 75% of cases. Multiple organ system involvement has been reported, including pericarditis, myocarditis, arthritis, cerebrospinal fluid pleocytosis (3), peripheral extremity gangrene (14), pulmonary infiltrates, and hydrops of the gallbladder (11). A desquamated, erythematous, perineal rash in the first 3 to 4 days is an early finding that can be helpful in making the diagnosis, although it is not specific for KD (15).

Approximately 1 to 2 weeks after the onset of the acute symptoms, resolution of the fever, rash, and lymphadenopathy can be expected, although the conjunctival injection often persists. It is during this subacute stage that desquamation of the digits occurs. This is also the stage at which coronary artery aneurysms develop and the risk of sudden death is at its highest.

Incomplete KD, or atypical Kawasaki disease (AKD), was first described in a number of case reports and case series in the early 1980s (2). Most of these patients were under 6 months of age, but cases in older children have also been reported (8). AKD is a febrile illness that does not meet the case definition for KD but that can result in similar cardiac sequelae. In most cases reported to date, one to three of the physical findings typical of KD have been present, but several cases of AKD have been manifested solely by fever. Indeed, one investigator has suggested that AKD be considered in any child with prolonged fever of unknown etiology (8).

TABLE 252.1. Diagnostic Criteria for Kawasaki Disease

Fever of at least 5 days' duration
Presence of four out of five physical findings:
    Bilateral, nonpurulent conjunctival injection
    Inflammatory changes of the lips and oral mucosa
    Erythema or swelling of the hands or feet
    Nonvesicular rash, primarily truncal
    Cervical lymphadenopathy, usually unilateral
Illness not explained by other known disease

DIFFERENTIAL DIAGNOSIS

There are several diseases that can mimic KD, but careful attention to the clinical criteria, as outlined, can help to avoid misdiagnosis. Among these diseases are scarlet fever, measles, toxic shock syndrome, Stevens-Johnson syndrome, leptospirosis, and Rocky Mountain spotted fever. Tonsillar exudates help to differentiate KD from an illness caused by group A streptococci, such as scarlet fever, as does the characteristic scarlet fever rash. Prominent respiratory symptoms, particularly cough, should suggest measles. Many of the symptoms of toxic shock are similar to those of KD, but hypotension is an uncommon finding in KD unless heart failure secondary to severe carditis is present.

Recent exposure to inciting drugs, the presence of oral lesions, an exudative conjunctivitis, and the typical "target lesion" rash can serve as clues to the diagnosis of Stevens-Johnson syndrome. The centripetal spread of a petechial rash that begins on the hands or feet, severe myalgias, and seasonal and epidemiologic clues might point to Rocky Mountain spotted fever. Chills, myalgia, and abdominal pain may lead to the diagnosis of leptospirosis. Serologic tests are of limited value in the acute stage of any of these illnesses, but they can be helpful during the recovery phase for retrospective diagnoses.

In the emergency department (ED), the diagnosis of KD is usually one of exclusion and is often not considered until the patient has presented to a clinic or emergency setting multiple times.

EMERGENCY DEPARTMENT EVALUATION

Immediate work up of a suspected case of KD should include a complete blood count and differential, platelet count, blood cultures, erythrocyte sedimentation rate (ESR), and a chemistry panel including serum transaminases, total protein, and albumin. White blood cell counts are usually elevated, with polymorphonuclear cell predominance; leukopenia is uncommon. Platelet counts are usually normal in the acute stage, but after a week increase markedly, often rising to above 1 million per microliter. The ESR is virtually always elevated during the acute stage (11).

Serum transaminases are often 2 to 3 times the normal value. Marked rises in serum immunoglobulin levels in the acute stage may result in an elevation in the serum protein level. Lumbar puncture may reveal aseptic meningitis (3), and urinalysis may reveal a sterile pyuria.

Further work up should include a baseline electrocardiogram to search for evidence of myocarditis or pericarditis. A baseline echocardiogram should also be obtained but should not delay therapeutic interventions.

EMERGENCY DEPARTMENT MANAGEMENT

Uncomplicated presentations require no more than supportive management in the emergency department: an antipyretic for fever and intravenous fluids for rehydration and maintenance. Cardiovascular decompensation must be treated as appropriate, and may require inotropic support.

DISPOSITION

Children with a presumptive diagnosis of Kawasaki disease should ideally be admitted to a tertiary care pediatric center with pediatric cardiologists and infectious disease consultants available. Therapy to be instituted in the hospital includes high-dose IVIG at 2 g/kg over a 10-hour period. IVIG has been shown to substantially reduce the incidence of serious cardiac sequelae, particularly coronary artery aneurysms, if administered early in the course of the disease (10). High-dose aspirin therapy at 100 mg/kg is also begun on admission and is continued until the acute phase has resolved. Corticosteroids are not currently recommended and may lead to higher rates of aneurysm formation. Transfer to a pediatric intensive care unit should be considered for patients with signs of cardiac decompensation.

CRITICAL INTERVENTIONS

- Include a baseline electrocardiogram to search for evidence of myocarditis or pericarditis
- Recognize that a child may have Kawasaki Disease based on clinical presentation
- Ensure timely initiation of high dose IVIG and aspirin therapy
- Perform a full fever evaluation even if you suspect that the fever is due to KD

COMMON PITFALLS

✔ Failure to consider KD in the differential diagnosis of prolonged fever in young children
✔ Failure to consider AKD in prolonged fever in children
✔ Failure to monitor for or identify cardiac decompensation
✔ Failure to use certain laboratory screening tests, such as ESR, to help differentiate KD from common childhood viral exanthems
✔ Failure to recognize the importance of early admission and institution of therapeutic interventions such as IVIG and aspirin and cardiology consultation

References

1. American Academy of Pediatrics. Kawasakii Syndrome. In: Pickering LK, ed. *Red Book: 2003 Report of the Committee on Infectious Diseases.* 26th ed. Elk Grove Village, IL: American Academy of Pediatrics 2003:392–395.
2. Burns JC, Wiggins JW, Toews WH, et al. Clinical spectrum of Kawasaki disease in infants younger than 6 months of age. *J Pediatr* 1986;109:759–763.
3. Dengler LD, et al. Cerebrospinal fluid profile in patients with acute Kawasaki disease. *Pediatr Infect Dis J* 1998;17(6):478–481.
4. Fukushige J, Takahashi N, Ueda Y, et al. Incidence and clinical features of incomplete Kawasaki disease. *Acta Paediatr* 1994;83:1057–1060.
5. Kawasaki T. Acute febrile mucocutaneous lymph node syndrome: clinical observation of 50 cases. *Jpn J Allergy* 1967;16:178.
6. Kawasaki T, Kosaki F, Okawa S, et al. A new infantile acute febrile mucocutaneous lymph node syndrome (MLNS) prevailing in Japan. *Pediatrics* 1974;54:271–276.
7. Landing BH, Larson EJ. Are infantile periarteritis with coronary artery involvement and fatal MLNS the same: comparison of 20 patients from North America with patients from Hawaii and Japan. *Pediatrics* 1977;59:651–662.
8. Levy M, Koren G. Atypical Kawasaki disease: analysis of clinical presentation and diagnostic clues. *Pediatr Infect Dis J* 1990;9:122–126.
9. Morens DM, Anderson LJ, Hurwitz ES. National surveillance of Kawasaki disease. *Pediatrics* 1980;65:21–25.
10. Newburger JW, Takahashi M, Beiser AS, et al. Single infusion of intravenous gamma globulin compared to four daily doses in the treatment of acute Kawasaki syndrome. *N Engl J Med* 1991;324:1633–1639.
11. Rowley AH, Shulman ST. Kawasaki syndrome. *Pediatr Cardiol* 1999;46:313–329.
12. Rowley A, Taubert K, et al. (Barron KS, Shulman ST, co-eds). Report of the National Institutes of Health workshop on Kawasaki disease. *J Rheumatol* 1999;26:170–190.
13. Taubert KA. Epidemiology of Kawasaki disease in the United States and worldwide. *Prog Pediatr Cardiol* 1997;6:181–185.
14. Tomita S, Chung K, et al. Peripheral gangrene associated with Kawasaki disease. *Clin Infect Dis* 1992;14:121–126.
15. Urbach AH, McGregor RS, Malatack JJ, et al. Kawasaki disease and perineal rash. *Am J Dis Child* 1988;142:1174.
16. Yamamoto LG. Kawasaki Disease. *Pediatr Emerg Care* 2003;19:422–424.
17. Yanagawa H, Nakamura Y, Yashiro M, et al. Update of the epidemiology of Kawasaki disease in Japan: from the results of the 1993–1994 nationwide survey. *J Epidemiol* 1996;6:148–157.

Lymphadenitis and Neck Masses

Mobeen H. Rathore and Sabiha Hussain

Lymph nodes are commonly palpated in children's necks. Cervical nodes greater than 10 mm are considered abnormal and are often referred to as lymphadenopathy (6). The most common cause of a benign neck mass in children is cervical adenopathy secondary to an upper respiratory tract infection, usually of viral origin. Lymphadenitis is one type of lymphadenopathy. Although some define *lymphadenitis* as broadly as an "inflammation of a lymph node," others restrict the definition to include only bacterial infections of the lymph gland (6,19).

After invading regional tissues, microorganisms enter the lymphatic system, where they are trapped and destroyed by phagocytes. This, in conjunction with the lymphocytic proliferation and transformation that occurs, results in swelling of the node. Abscess formation ensues when neutrophils accumulate (6,8).

Group A β-hemolytic streptococci and *Staphylococcus aureus* are the most frequent pathogens of bacterial lymphadenitis. Children with staphylococcal infections generally have a longer history of symptoms and an increased incidence of fluctuance, compared with those with streptococcal infections (6,8,15).

CLINICAL PRESENTATION

Cervical lymphadenitis presents most commonly in children between 1 and 4 years of age, and there is no significant difference in incidence between genders. It is helpful to determine whether the cervical lymphadenitis developed in an acute, subacute, or chronic manner. The acute bacterial nodal enlargement usually develops rather quickly and unilaterally. These nodes are typically very tender and sometimes feel fluctuant. Erythema of the overlying skin is occasionally noted. Affected children often experience malaise and irritability and may be febrile. Frequently, a concurrent pharyngitis, otitis media, upper respiratory tract infection, dental abscess, or adjacent skin infection can be detected, or a recent history of infection can be elicited. Subacute or chronic lymphadenitis develops over 2 to 3 weeks and tends to be relatively painless. It may be caused by cat-scratch disease, atypical mycobacteria, or tuberculosis.

There are rarely significant sequelae when adenitis is managed appropriately. Of particular concern is the possibility of misdiagnosing and consequently mismanaging another more serious problem (2). It is sometimes difficult to distinguish lymphadenopathy or adenitis from a true neck mass. Neck masses may be congenital or acquired, infectious or neoplastic, benign or malignant. In children, the incidence of neoplastic lesions is low compared to adults. In neither group does the neck mass commonly present as an acutely emergent or life-threatening problem.

DIFFERENTIAL DIAGNOSIS

Obtaining a careful history and performing a complete examination can often differentiate the disorders most commonly confused with adenitis (2). See Table 253.1.

Viral Lymphadenopathy

Viral infections, especially those that produce viremia, are the most common cause of lymphadenopathy in children and usually subside within a few days to 2 weeks. Often bilateral, causative agents include respiratory viruses such as adenovirus, Epstein-Barr virus (EBV), cytomegalovirus (CMV), human herpesvirus 6, coxsackievirus, rubella, rubeola, and varicella (6,8).

Bacterial Lymphadenitis

The presence of erythema, warmth, and tenderness overlying a node typically indicates the acute inflammatory response of pyogenic bacterial lymphadenitis. Most acutely infected nodes in children are rubbery or firm in consistency and are freely mobile. Left untreated, these nodes, often unilateral, tend to suppurate and may rupture onto the skin or, less commonly, dissect into the underlying soft tissues (6,8,15).

Infectious Mononucleosis

EBV causes infectious mononucleosis. It often presents as acute or subacute cervical lymphadenopathy. These nodes tend to be posterior cervical, bilateral, and moderately painful (8). Associated findings include malaise, fever, tonsillopharyngitis, hepatosplenomegaly, and generalized lymph node enlargement. A positive heterophil test (Monospot) confirms the diagnosis. In children less than 4 years of age the heterophil test is unreliable and specific EBV titers should be done. Treatment is supportive. The patient should be instructed to avoid contact sports for several months after the illness because of the risk of splenic rupture. Rarely, cervical lymphadenopathy in infectious mononucleosis is associated with respiratory distress because of extremely enlarged ("kissing") tonsils and this may require hospitalization and steroid use.

Cat-Scratch Disease

Most cases of cat-scratch disease are caused by *Bartonella henselae*. In approximately 50% of cases, there is a primary lesion at the site of a 7- to 14-day-old scratch or bite by a cat. This lesion begins as an indurated erythematous papule and later may become vesicular or pustular. It resolves within 10 to 20 days. Cat-scratch disease usually presents subacutely. Several days to weeks later, the lymph nodes draining this area become progressively enlarged. These nodes are typically only moderately tender, but, occasionally, they will suppurate. Sometimes, patients are febrile and may experience headache, myalgia, or malaise. Other complications, such as encephalitis, hepatosplenic abscesses, and osteolytic lesions, are uncommon. Although the diagnosis is usually made on clinical grounds, it can be confirmed serologically. Antibiotics are often not needed, and the adenopathy generally resolves in 6 to 8 weeks, with supportive treatment only. However, azithromycin is recommended by some experts for the treatment of cat scratch disease lymphadenopathy (4). Fluctuant nodes often need surgical intervention (6,9,10,17).

Mycobacterial Lymphadenitis

Atypical mycobacterial cervical lymphadenitis usually presents as subacute or chronic unilaterally enlarged lymph nodes that

TABLE 253.1.   Differential Diagnosis of Lymphadenitis

Differential Diagnoses	Causative Agents	Comments
Viral Lymphadenopathy	*Adenovirus* *EBV* *CMV* *Human herpesvirus 6* *Coxsackie* *Rubella* *Rubeola* *Varicella (5,7)*	Lymphadenopathy usually resolves within a few days to two weeks Often bilateral Respiratory viruses commonly involved
Bacterial Lymphadenitis	*Group A beta hemolytic streptococcus* *Staphylococcus aureus*	Erythema, warmth and tenderness overlying a node typically indicates bacterial lymphadenitis Rubbery or firm in consistency and freely mobile Often unilateral Untreated nodes tend to suppurate and may rupture onto the skin or dissect into underlying soft tissues
Infectious Mononucleosis	*EBV*	Often presents as acute or subacute cervical lymphadenopathy Nodes tend to be posterior cervical, bilateral and moderately painful Associated findings include malaise, fever, tonsillopharyngitis, hepatosplenomegaly and generalized node enlargement Positive heterophil (Monospot) confirms the diagnosis except in children younger than four years for whom EBV titers should be done Treatment is supportive; avoid contact sports for several months
Cat-Scratch Disease	*Bartonella henselae*	In approximately 50% of cases, primary lesion is at the site of a 7- to 14-day-old scratch or bite by a cat Begins as indurated erythematous papule and later may become vesicular or pustular; resolves in 10 to 20 days Days to weeks later, the nodes draining this area become enlarged Nodes are typically only moderately tender but occasionally suppurate Associated symptoms include fever, headache, myalgia or malaise Complications such as encephalitis, hepatosplenic abscess, and osteolytic lesions are uncommon Consider azithromycin to shorten the clinical course
Atypical Mycobacterial Lymphadenitis	*Nontuberculous mycobacteria*	Subacute or chronic unilaterally enlarged lymph nodes Does not respond to antibiotics Infected nodes tend to be relatively painless Systemic symptomatology is uncommon Tuberculin skin testing is unreliable Treatment of choice is excisional biopsy
Kawasaki Disease	*Unknown*	Also known as mucocutaneous lymph node syndrome Diagnosed in the presence of fever plus four of the diagnostic criteria including cervical lymphadenopathy, rash, oral exanthem, conjunctival injection and swelling and redness of palms and soles Exclusion of other illnesses is necessary Cervical lymphadenopathy is only found in 50% of cases Nodes are usually unilateral and confined to the anterior triangle Early diagnosis is critical because treatment can prevent coronary aneurysm
Tuberculous Lymphadenitis	*Mycobacterium tuberculosis*	Rare Diseased nodes are similar to those of nontuberculous mycobacterial adenitis Work up includes history of TB exposure, a TB skin test and chest x-ray Tuberculous lymph nodes should never be aspirated because this could lead to sinus development Antituberculous drugs are effective in treating this condition Infection should be reported to public health authorities
Group B Streptococcal Cellulitis-Adenitis Syndrome	*Group B streptococcus*	This syndrome occurs in neonates Abrupt onset of fever and facial or submandibular erythema and swelling Symptoms include irritability, poor feeding and toxicity About 80% have ipsilateral otitis media Meningitis may accompany lymphadenitis Organism can be isolated from blood and lymph node or cellulitis aspirates Complete sepsis workup should be performed, admission and IV antibiotics
Toxoplasmosis	*Toxoplasma gondii*	May present as single, enlarged, posterior cervical node that may or may not be tender Nodes vary in size but do not suppurate The diagnosis can be made by performing serial toxoplasma titers Pharmacologic therapy should be withheld unless fever or a complication such as pneumonitis, myocarditis, meningitis, or encephalitis ensues

do not respond to antibiotics (6,11). Nontuberculous mycobacterial lymphadenitis generally occurs in early childhood. Infected nodes tend to be relatively painless but are sometimes tender and may even suppurate and drain. Systemic symptomatology is uncommon. Tuberculin skin testing is unreliable. Antituberculous drugs are not recommended, and excisional biopsy is both diagnostic and therapeutic (12).

Tuberculous lymphadenitis is rarely seen in the United States (7,17,18). Diseased nodes are similar to those of nontuberculous mycobacterial adenitis. To exclude the diagnosis, the family should be questioned about exposure to tuberculosis, a tuberculin skin test should be done, and a chest radiograph should be ordered. Tuberculous lymph nodes should never be aspirated, because this could lead to sinus development. Antituberculous drugs are effective in treating this condition. Infection should be reported to public health authorities.

Kawasaki Disease

Also known as mucocutaneous lymph node syndrome, Kawasaki disease is diagnosed in the presence of fever, plus four of the five diagnostic criteria (cervical lymphadenopathy, rash, oral exanthem, conjunctival injection, and swelling and redness of palms and soles) and exclusion of other illnesses. Cervical lymphadenopathy is found in only 50% of cases. Nodes are usually unilateral and confined to the anterior triangle, moderately tender, nonfluctuant, and firm, with or without overlying erythema. The early diagnosis of Kawasaki disease is critical, because treatment with salicylates and intravenous immunoglobulin can prevent the most serious complication, namely, coronary aneurysm (17) (see Chapter 252, "Kawasaki Disease").

Group B Streptococcal Cellulitis–Adenitis Syndrome

The group B streptococcal cellulitis–adenitis syndrome occurs in neonates (16). The neonate presents with the abrupt onset of fever, facial or submandibular erythema and swelling, irritability, poor feeding, and toxicity. About 80% have an ipsilateral otitis media. Meningitis may accompany lymphadenitis. The organism can be isolated from blood and from aspirates of the lymph node or the cellulitis. A complete sepsis workup should be performed, and the infant must be admitted to the hospital for intravenous antibiotic therapy (1,16,17).

Toxoplasmosis

Acquired toxoplasmosis sometimes presents as a single, enlarged, posterior cervical node that may or may not be tender (6,13,20). These nodes tend to vary in size but do not suppurate. The diagnosis can be made by performing serial toxoplasma titers. Pharmacologic therapy should be withheld unless fever or a complication such as pneumonitis, myocarditis, meningitis, or encephalitis ensues.

Other Infectious Etiologies

Other uncommon causes of cervical lymphadenopathy include *Pasteurella multocida, Yersinia pestis,* histoplasmosis, and CMV.

Rheumatologic Lymphadenopathy

A number of rheumatologic illnesses can cause cervical lymphadenopathy, chief among them is juvenile rheumatoid arthritis.

Neoplasms

Neoplasms are rare in children, occurring in 1.4% of patients younger than 17 years of age with a superficial lump on any part of the body. Careful follow up of all lymphadenopathy is mandatory, especially if it is associated with fever or weight loss or if it fails to resolve (5,6,10).

Benign neoplasms in children that present as neck masses include hemangiomas, lymphangiomas, fibromas, neurofibromas, and lipomas. Malignant neck neoplasms in children tend to be single, nontender, immobile and fast-growing, and are located in the posterior triangle of the neck. Age is a key element in the occurrence of the various malignant neck neoplasms. From ages 1 to 5, neuroblastoma, rhabdomyosarcoma, histiocytic lymphoma, and Hodgkin disease are more common. In the older child, histiocytic lymphoma and Hodgkin disease occur equally often. The adolescent most commonly acquires Hodgkin disease. Rhabdomyosarcoma is the most common solid tumor of the head and neck in childhood and is one of the most common tumors in children under age 6. It is less common in non-Whites. Rhabdomyosarcoma presents with rapid growth in the orbit, nasopharynx, ear, mastoid, face, or tongue. Neuroblastoma is the most common solid tumor in children overall, but it presents as a neck mass only about 5% of the time.

Congenital and Other Neck Masses

A few other entities may be confused with adenopathy or adenitis. These include dermoid cysts, thyroglossal duct cysts, branchial cleft defects, cystic hygromas, and hematomas (5). About 6% of neck masses are congenital. Thyroglossal duct cysts and dermoid cysts present as midline neck masses; branchial cleft cysts and cystic hygromas (lymphangiomas) typically as lateral neck masses.

Thyroglossal duct cyst is the most common benign congenital neck mass. The thyroglossal duct is a microscopic thread of undifferentiated epithelial cells, a remnant of the embryogenic development of what becomes the pyramidal lobe of the thyroid gland. It descends from the base of the tongue, through the hyoid bone to the inferior neck, where it fuses with the lateral aspects of the thyroid gland. The cyst tends to be fluctuant, smooth, rounded, well defined, and nontender. Although the size is usually 1 to 2 cm, it may fluctuate in size and can become infected. The majority occur between 1 and 9 years of age, with a peak incidence between 3 and 5 years. An infrahyoid position and history of inflammation and fluctuating size are helpful in differentiating between a thyroglossal duct cyst, an epidermoid cyst, and a midline enlarged lymph node. Surgical excision of the cyst and tract is necessary to prevent recurrent infection.

An **epidermoid cyst** is a nontender midline cervical mass that moves with the overlying skin and tends not to fluctuate in size or become inflamed. The submental and infrahyoid areas are the most common locations. Dermoid cysts are more common in children under 5 years of age, but may be acquired at any age as a result of a prior puncture wound. Serious complications or emergencies associated with dermoid cysts are rare, and the treatment is surgical excision.

Branchial anomalies may present as cysts, sinuses, or fistulas. The second branchial cleft is responsible for most anomalies, of which cysts are the most common. Cysts lie anterior to and in the middle third of the sternocleidomastoid muscle. The cyst may develop at any age, although it may be more common in adults. When the cyst does develop in childhood, it occurs more often in the early school years. The cyst typically is rounded, nontender, slightly mobile, and of variable firmness. It may gradually increase in size, and may appear to enlarge with upper respiratory tract infections. Infections of the cyst are uncommon. Branchial sinuses are relatively uncommon. They may open internally or externally. Branchial sinuses are usually noted at birth, with the external sinus opening anterior to the lower third of the sternocleidomastoid muscle. The treatment is elective surgical excision of the cyst, sinus, or fistula.

Cystic hygromas and lymphangiomas are congenital masses of lymphatic tissue thought to arise from lymphatic sacs. Most are located in the posterior triangle of the neck. Sixty-five percent are present at birth, 80% are noted in the first year of life, and 90% are found before the end of the second year. The masses can be smooth, rounded or lobulated, soft, and compressible, and can be transilluminated. An increase in size may occur with an upper respiratory tract infection. They tend to be asymptomatic but rarely become large enough to cause difficulty with swallowing or breathing due to compression of the trachea.

Another congenital lateral neck mass is the **hemangioma,** a vascular anomaly present at birth that usually regresses spontaneously. The hemangioma is a bluish, nonpulsatile mass with a "bag of worms" texture located in the area of the parotid gland (15). Airway compromise can occur if the mass reaches sufficient size to encroach on the upper airway.

Other uncommon congenital neck masses include thyroid cysts, parotid gland cysts, and thymus remnants.

EMERGENCY DEPARTMENT EVALUATION

Many of the aforementioned diagnoses can be made simply by taking a complete history and performing a thorough examination. The following points should be addressed when questioning the family: duration of adenopathy or mass, history of an adjacent skin lesion, earache, upper respiratory tract infection, sore throat, or dental problem; presence of fever or weight loss; exposure to tuberculosis; contact with cats; and travel (6,8). When attempting to determine whether a neck mass may be a lymph node, it is important to recognize the location of the normal chain of cervical lymph nodes. The size, consistency, mobility, and tenderness of each affected node must be noted (6,15). Marking the dimensions with ink and recording them in the emergency department (ED) record can be helpful to the next physician who evaluates the patient. The head, ears, eyes, nose, oropharynx, and neck are examined, and the child is evaluated for hepatomegaly, splenomegaly, and other adenopathy (6).

Useful studies include a complete blood cell count, erythrocyte sedimentation rate, a Monospot or EBV serology, a throat culture for group A *Streptococcus*, and a tuberculin skin test. It is, however, unnecessary to order all of these tests on every patient. They prove most helpful when the cause of the adenopathy is unknown. A blood culture should be obtained if the patient appears toxic. Older children with cervical adenitis are rarely bacteremic, but neonates often are and must be evaluated for possible sepsis (1). Additional studies may be needed in the older child, depending on the history and physical examination (e.g., serology for cat-scratch disease or EBV). Sometimes, a definitive diagnosis is not made until a biopsy is performed and results evaluated.

Needle aspiration is useful both diagnostically and therapeutically, and any fluctuant node should be aspirated if tuberculous lymphadenitis can be excluded. An ultrasound can help determine whether a node or mass is cystic or solid, if necessary (14). The largest, most fluctuant node is selected, the overlying skin is cleansed, a 20-gauge needle attached to a 20-mL syringe is inserted into the fluctuant region, and aspiration is done. If pus is not obtained, 1 to 2 mL of sterile, nonbacteriostatic saline is injected into the node, which is reaspirated. The aspirate is sent

TABLE 253.2. Management of Bacterial Lymphadenitis

Outpatient Therapy (3, 6, 13)	Inpatient Therapy (3, 6, 13)
1. Cefodroxil 30 mg/kg/day divided q12h PO	1. Cefazolin 100 mg/kg/day divided q8h iv
2. Clindamycin 20 mg/kg/day divided q6h PO	2. Clindamycin 40 mg/kg/day divided q6h to q8h iv
3. Cefuroxine 20 mg/kg/day divided q12h PO	3. Nafcillin 125 mg/kg/day divided q6h iv

*Failure to respond to oral antibiotics does not necessarily mean that the cause of adenitis is not bacterial; parenteral antibiotics may be required.
**If the lymphadenitis is associated with dental disease, anaerobic infection needs to be considered, and the following agents are recommended: (3,5)
Amoxicillin-clavulanate (Augmentin) 45 mg/kg/day divided q12h PO
*** Treatment should last at least 10 days. (5, 12) After a good response to parenteral antibiotics is observed, oral agents can be substituted (5).

for Gram stain and cultures for aerobic and anaerobic bacteria, mycobacteria, and fungi (6,8,15).

EMERGENCY DEPARTMENT MANAGEMENT

If bacterial cervical lymphadenitis is suspected, treatment with antibiotics effective against the principal bacterial pathogens, group A β-hemolytic *Streptococcus* and *S. aureus*, is started. Analgesics and warm compresses may also be helpful (6). Outpatient and inpatient therapy is outlined in Table 253.2 (3,6,13). Failure to respond to oral antibiotics does not necessarily mean that the cause of adenitis is not bacterial; parenteral antibiotics may be required. If the lymphadenitis is associated with dental disease, anaerobic infection needs to be considered (3,6).

CRITICAL INTERVENTIONS

- Take a detailed history including travel and animal contact to differentiate lymphadenitis from other disorders
- Encourage or arrange follow up for all lymphadenitis cases, especially for those with large nodes, fever, weight loss or other concerning systemic signs

DISPOSITION

Most children can be managed successfully as outpatients. They should be reevaluated, to monitor their progress, within 2 to 3 days of the ED visit. Follow up is very important and is done best by the patient's primary care physician, who should reexamine the child serially until the node regresses.

Admission for intravenous antibiotics is warranted if the child appears toxic, if the lymphadenitis is severe (e.g., node diameter greater than 3 to 4 cm, or high fever), if the lymphadenitis fails to respond to oral medications, or if the patient is a neonate or cannot tolerate oral antibiotics (13). Admission for further evaluation is recommended if there is mediastinal lymphadenopathy on the chest radiograph, weight loss, fever for more than 1 week, or a suspicion of Kawasaki Disease or malignancy (10).

Biopsy is indicated if the node increases in size or does not decrease in 4 to 6 weeks or return to normal in 8 to 12 weeks (10). Particularly worrisome findings are weight loss, persistent fever, or fixation to adjacent tissues or overlying skin (4,6,8).

COMMON PITFALLS

✔ Treating patients with severe lymphadenitis orally and delaying an inevitable admission for intravenous antibiotics

✔ Failure to consider atypical mycobacterial lymphadenitis, Kawasaki disease, and cat-scratch disease in the differential diagnosis

Acknowledgment

Thanks to the previous edition's chapter author Nizar F. Maraqa.

References

1. Albanyan EA, Baker CJ. Is lumbar puncture necessary to exclude meningitis in neonates and young infants: lessons from the group B streptococcus cellulitis-adenitis syndrome. *Pediatrics* 1998;102:984.
2. Armstrong WB, Giglio MF. Is this lump in the neck anything to worry about? *Postgrad Med* 1998;104:63.
3. Barone MA, ed. *The Harriet Lane handbook.* St. Louis: Mosby–Year Book, 1996.
4. Bass J, Freitas B, Alexande D, et al. Prospective randomized double blind placebo-controlled evaluation of azithromycin for treatment of cat-scratch disease. *Pediatr Infect Dis* 1998;17:447–452.
5. Brown RL, Azizkhan RG. Pediatric head and neck lesions. *Pediatr Clin North Am* 1998;45:889.
6. Chesney PJ. Cervical adenopathy. *Pediatr Rev* 1994;15:277.
7. Kanlikama M, Gokalp A. Management of mycobacterial cervical lymphadenitis. *World J Surg* 1997;21:516.
8. Kelly CS, Kelly RE. Lymphadenopathy in children. *Pediatr Clin North Am* 1998;45:875.
9. Klein JD. Cat scratch disease. *Pediatr Rev* 1994;15:349.
10. Knight PJ, Mulne AF, Vassy LE. When is lymph node biopsy indicated in children with enlarged peripheral nodes? *Pediatrics* 1982;69:391.
11. Losurdo G, et al. Cervical lymphadenitis caused by nontuberculous mycobacteria in immunocompetent children: clinical and therapeutic experience. *Head Neck* 1998;20:245.
12. Makhani S, et al. Atypical cervicofacial mycobacterial infections in childhood. *Br J Oral Maxillofac Surg* 1998;36:119.
13. Marcy SM. Cervical adenitis. *Pediatr Infect Dis* 1985;4:523.
14. Na DG, et al. Differential diagnosis of cervical lymphadenopathy: usefulness of color Doppler sonography. *AJR* 1997;168:1311.
15. Rathore MH, Barton LL. Cervical adenitis. In: Koplan SL, ed. *Current therapy in pediatric infectious diseases.* St. Louis: Mosby–Year Book, 1993:20–21.
16. Rathore MH. Group B streptococcal cellulitis and adenitis associated with meningitis. *Clin Pediatr* 1989;28:411.
17. *Red book: report of the Committee on Infectious Diseases,* 26th ed. 2003; American Academy of Pediatrics, Elkgrae, IL.
18. Smith MHD, Marquis JR. Tuberculosis and other mycobacterial infections. In: Feigin RD, Cherry JD, eds. *Textbook of pediatric infectious diseases.* Philadelphia: WB Saunders, 1987:1342.
19. *Stedman's medical dictionary,* 24th ed. Baltimore: Williams & Wilkins, 1982.
20. Wilson CB, Remington JS. Toxoplasmosis. In: Feigin RD, Cherry JD, eds. *Textbook of pediatric infectious diseases.* Philadelphia: WB Saunders, 1987:2067.

CHAPTER 254
Meningitis and Encephalitis

James A. Wilde

Central nervous system (CNS) infections are a source of significant morbidity and mortality, and are often included in the differential diagnosis of a febrile child. Bacterial meningitis and viral disease presenting as meningitis, encephalitis, or meningoencephalitis are the most common forms of CNS infection in children. They present a formidable challenge to the emergency physician, both diagnostically and therapeutically, because of their relative rarity, often subtle presenting signs and symptoms, and, sometimes, fulminant course.

The organisms that are most commonly isolated in cases of bacterial meningitis vary with the age of the patient. Among neonates, group B *Streptococcus* (GBS) is, by far, the most commonly isolated bacterium. Other less common but significant organisms include *Listeria monocytogenes* and gram-negative enteric bacilli such as *Escherichia coli, Klebsiella* and *Enterobacter* spp., *Citrobacter diversus,* and *Salmonella* spp. GBS and *L. monocytogenes* typically present as "late-onset" meningitis at 1 to 12 weeks of life, while meningitis due to the gram-negative enteric bacteria often presents during the first 2 weeks. Beyond the age of 3 months, *Streptococcus pneumoniae* and *Neisseria meningitidis* are the major pathogens, with *S. pneumoniae* predominating from 1 to 23 months and *N. meningitidis* predominating from 2 to 18 years (41). Meningitis due to *Haemophilus influenzae* type B (HIB) is now rare in the United States because vaccines have improved.

The leading pathogens caused an estimated 2,800 cases of bacterial meningitis in U.S. children younger than 18 years in 1995 (41). This represents a dramatic decline, resulting from the near disappearance of HIB meningitis over the preceding decade. While two-thirds of patients with bacterial meningitis in 1986 were between 1 month and 5 years of age, by 1995 meningitis in this age group had dropped by 87%, and the median age of bacterial meningitis cases rose from 15 months to 25 years.

Bacterial meningitis is almost always preceded by a hematogenous spread of bacteria. The mechanism whereby bacteria gain access to the intravascular space is unclear, although some data indicate that a breach of the normal mucosal barriers may be caused by viral upper respiratory infections (32). It is also unclear how bacteria gain access to the CNS from the bloodstream.

One point that is clear is that most instances of bacteremia do not progress to invasion of the CNS (12). Once in the CNS, bacteria can initially multiply relatively unimpeded because of poor immunologic defenses in normal cerebrospinal fluid (CSF) (28). It is only after local release of bacteria-associated chemotactic factors that a significant defense is mounted in the CNS. The resulting inflammation, edema, and CNS dysfunction are manifested as severe headache, nuchal rigidity, photophobia, or seizures (i.e., classic symptoms of meningitis). A patient with fever can be anywhere on this continuum, but in the absence of CSF for evaluation, it is impossible to state definitively that the child has reached the meningitic stage. Bacterial meningitis can also result from direct invasion of the CNS after trauma or erosion through an infected sinus, but this is a much less common mechanism.

Several infectious or noninfectious agents can cause aseptic meningitis, that is, meningitis without evidence of a bacterial pathogen detectable in CSF. Among the most common infectious etiologies are the enteroviruses (ECHO and coxsackievirus) and mumps virus.

Encephalitis is an inflammation of the brain that can occur as the primary pathologic event, as in arbovirus encephalitis, or as a simultaneous event with primary meningitis. The latter is more correctly termed *meningoencephalitis,* and is common in bacterial meningitis. Among the many viral causes of encephalitis are the enteroviruses, arboviruses (La Crosse strain of the California encephalitis virus [CEV], St. Louis encephalitis), herpes simplex virus (HSV), varicella virus, and mumps virus (44). Infections due to enteroviruses and arboviruses occur primarily during the warmer months, with the latter paralleling mosquito activity. Infection by CEV is typically seen in young boys exposed to hardwood forests or small pools of stagnant water, where mosquitoes breed (15). HSV encephalitis can occur at any age, including a neonatal form that presents during the second to third week of life.

CLINICAL PRESENTATION

Due to the protean clinical manifestations of bacterial meningitis in infants and young children, physicians must maintain a high index of suspicion for the disease. Inflammation of the meninges can be manifested by headache, nausea and vomiting, fever, photophobia, mental confusion and lethargy, or excessive irritability in children. Clinical findings indicative of CNS dysfunction, such as seizures, focal neurologic signs (hemiparesis, quadriparesis, cranial nerve palsies, visual field defects), and ataxia suggest meningitis, but no single sign is pathognomonic. The symptoms and signs of meningitis vary and depend, in part, on the patient's age, the duration of illness, and the host's response to the infection (20). Clinical findings may be subtle, especially in neonates and young children, and may include only nonspecific manifestations such as disinterest in feeding, lethargy, respiratory distress, or jaundice. Fever is commonly not present in neonates with bacterial meningitis (7).

A change in the child's affect or state of alertness is one of the most important signs of bacterial meningitis. In one study, 36% to 60% of children with this diagnosis were described as toxic or moribund, and 73% to 100% lethargic or comatose, depending on the age of the patient (47). These findings were generally not present in infants younger than 3 months in this study. *Lethargy* refers to a decreased level of consciousness with an inappropriate response to stimuli, bordering on unconsciousness. A child who is sleepy is not necessarily a child who is lethargic. True lethargy is an ominous finding and warrants further investigation. A febrile child who is playful, smiling, or interactive is unlikely to have bacterial meningitis in the absence of other signs or symptoms suggestive of the disease.

Seizures are found at presentation in 20% to 30% of children with bacterial meningitis (39). However, seizures are rarely the sole manifestation of meningitis in febrile children; most children with seizures secondary to bacterial meningitis will have a significant, prolonged alteration in their level of consciousness or focal findings on physical examination (22). This is in marked contrast to children with simple febrile seizures, who, after a short postictal period, usually return quickly to their baseline mental status and have no neurologic deficits on examination.

Bacterial meningitis in infants and children can present insidiously over several days or acutely in a fulminant fashion. The prognosis may be worse for the second group (24), a group that is generally not difficult to recognize at presentation. Delays are common in diagnosing those with an insidious presentation, despite the best efforts of physicians. It is unclear whether these delays contribute to the subsequent morbidity or mortality (10,19,23,37). Enteroviral infection is typically insidious in onset and may have a biphasic course extending over ten days or more. The patient with enteroviral meningitis does not usually appear seriously ill unless the infection occurs during the neonatal period (14).

Differentiating HSV infection of the CNS from bacterial meningitis may be difficult because the nonspecific symptoms just described are found in both. Helpful clues include the absence of bacteria on CSF Gram stain, negative cultures of blood and CSF, the presence of focal seizures, and difficult-to-control seizures. Cutaneous vesicles are found at presentation in only 30% to 50% of infants with neonatal HSV, and are uncommon at any stage of HSV encephalitis in older children. St. Louis encephalitis and La Crosse encephalitis can present either in a mild form, consisting of a 2- to 3-day prodrome of low-grade fever,

headache, malaise, and vomiting with subsequent development of higher fever, lethargy, and meningeal signs, or a severe form, characterized by the abrupt onset of fever and headache, followed rapidly by generalized or focal seizures, focal neurologic signs, and coma (44). HSV encephalitis in the older child may be similar to this severe form of arboviral encephalitis.

An altered state of consciousness is apparent in most children with encephalitis due to inflammation of the brain parenchyma. This may be manifested by only lethargy or delirium, but in severe cases, the lethargy may progress to a stuporous state or frank coma.

DIFFERENTIAL DIAGNOSIS

Although not always apparent at presentation, nuchal rigidity is probably the one clinical sign that physicians most consistently associate with meningitis. However, nuchal rigidity may be associated with a variety of illnesses (45):

- Infections: meningitis, encephalitis, brain abscess, epidural abscess, Guillain-Barré syndrome, transverse myelitis, acute cerebellar ataxia, poliomyelitis, tetanus, cervical adenitis, retropharyngeal abscess, vertebral body osteomyelitis, discitis, epiglottitis, trichinosis, tonsillitis, otitis media, pyelonephritis, mumps, hepatitis, shigellosis, malaria, typhoid fever
- Vascular abnormalities: subarachnoid hemorrhage, intracranial venous thrombosis
- Neoplasms: meningeal leukemia, intracranial and brainstem tumors, tumors of the cervical vertebrae (osteoid osteoma, eosinophilic granuloma)
- Metabolic disorders: infantile Gaucher disease, maple syrup urine disease, kernicterus
- Toxins: phenothiazines, strychnine, lead
- Bony or muscular disorders: vertebral anomalies; subluxations, dislocations, and fractures of the cervical spine; myositis; fibromyositis; congenital torticollis
- Miscellaneous causes: juvenile rheumatoid arthritis, black widow spider bite, effects of lumbar puncture (LP), Arnold-Chiari malformation.

Children with common, self-limited viral infections may present with symptoms that mimic meningitis. Headache, somnolence, and decreased activity are common symptoms in childhood infectious diseases. Children with these non-CNS infections may appear toxic on initial presentation but often become alert and playful if the fever responds to antipyretics. Symptoms of bacterial meningitis generally do not abate with antipyretics alone.

EMERGENCY DEPARTMENT EVALUATION

History

A careful history can help to differentiate a child with a serious systemic bacterial infection such as sepsis or meningitis from one with a self-limited viral infection. It is important to remember that the overwhelming majority of children with fever do not have bacterial meningitis; less than 1,500 children under two years of age are diagnosed with this disease each year in the United States (43). If each child in this age group had only one febrile illness per year of life, the expected rate of bacterial meningitis would be less than one case per 4,000 febrile episodes. Most children in this age group have more than one febrile illness per year, so the actual rate is much less than one case per 4,000 febrile episodes. Information gathered from the history and physical

TABLE 254.1. Indications for Lumbar Puncture and/or Immediate Empiric Treatment for Meningitis

Recommended	Strongly Consider
Unexplained fever and:	**Unexplained fever and:**
Lethargy	Seizure in child under 18 mo or over 5 yr of age
Coma	Severe headache
Shock	No obvious source for fever, child under 3 mo of age
Extreme irritability in infant	Poor feeding in infant
Age < 1 mo	Increased sleep in infant
New neurologic deficit	Petechial or purpuric rash
Nuchal rigidity	Any afebrile, toxic-appearing child with symptoms from either column
Photophobia	
Uncontrolled seizure	
Seizure in child under 6 mo of age	
New-onset focal seizure	

examination can help the physician to decide who requires LP for further evaluation (Table 254.1).

Bacterial meningitis leads to inflammation of the brain and meninges, which causes symptoms such as extreme irritability, photophobia, vomiting, headache, lethargy, and seizures. In infants, excessive sleep or poor feeding may result. The emergency department (ED) physician should initially focus on these elements of the history in the assessment of a febrile child. Their absence does not rule out meningitis but does make it less likely. Conversely, their presence should heighten suspicions for meningitis.

In addition, questions should be directed toward establishing a source for the fever. Are there any ill contacts with fever? Are there signs or symptoms that are temporally related to the fever and that together constitute a self-limited viral illness? Prior or current antibiotic administration is another important historic item to ascertain.

In the evaluation of a neonate with fever, the mother should be questioned about infections during pregnancy or at delivery. The physician should ask about pruritic or burning vaginal lesions, antibiotic use during pregnancy, ingestion of raw dairy products during pregnancy (listeriosis), parental history of or exposure to HSV, perinatal complications in the mother or child, prolonged care in the nursery after delivery, the mother's GBS status at the time of delivery, and any antibiotic use in the child since birth.

In all febrile children, a history of exposure to someone with HIB or *N. meningitidis* should be sought. Travel history and animal contact are important factors to consider when dealing with the less common causes of CNS infections. Mosquito bites may suggest an arbovirus infection.

A history of lethargy should be cause for concern. However, parents tend to use the word *lethargic* to describe their children when, in fact, true lethargy is not present. A child who is less playful or more sleepy than usual is not necessarily a lethargic child. These symptoms are almost universally present in young children with febrile illnesses. Questions should be directed toward establishing the presence or absence of true lethargy.

Physical Examination

A complete physical examination is critical in the evaluation of a febrile child to detect a CNS infection or to establish a reasonable alternative explanation for the fever. An abnormal blood pressure or prolonged capillary refill time in the absence of

dehydration suggests a potentially life-threatening bacterial infection. Does the child have symptoms of an acute upper respiratory infection? Does the child have an obvious pharyngitis, or oral lesions consistent with herpangina or herpetic gingivostomatitis? Is there a rash consistent with a clear etiology, such as varicella or the sandpaper rash of scarlet fever? Does the child have conjunctivitis or otitis?

Examine the chest, abdomen, and extremities to search for other foci of infection such as pneumonia, myopericarditis, hepatitis, pyelonephritis, arthritis, cellulitis, or osteomyelitis. Look for the presence of a bulging anterior fontanelle in infants in the seated position, an indication of increased intracranial pressure (ICP). Although the funduscopic examination is usually normal in acute CNS infections, the presence of papilledema should raise concern for a brain abscess, subdural empyema, or venous sinus thrombosis. A complete neurologic examination is important to determine the presence and severity of a CNS insult and to document a baseline against which the response to therapy can be monitored.

In all patients with suspected CNS infection, signs of meningeal irritation are sought by examining for nuchal rigidity and Kernig and Brudzinski signs. Especially in a very young child who is frightened by the emergency department setting, forceful flexion of the neck can be misleading, because the child's natural tendency is to resist the examiner. A toy or flashlight placed at the sitting child's umbilicus usually causes the child to flex the neck spontaneously, and may be more helpful in excluding nuchal rigidity. Kernig sign is positive when pain is elicited by extension of the knee from its initial flexed position, with the patient supine and the leg flexed at the hip. The Brudzinski sign consists of spontaneous flexion of the lower extremities after passive flexion of the neck. Meningeal signs are almost invariably present at the time of diagnosis in children older than 13 months with bacterial meningitis, but are only rarely present in children younger than 6 months (47).

Careful attention to the child's affect or state of alertness is critical to distinguish those who should undergo LP for further evaluation from the vast majority who need no further invasive tests. The emergency physician should carefully document the general appearance of the child.

Laboratory Evaluation

The definitive diagnosis of meningitis requires CSF analysis, generally after performance of an LP. This procedure should include an opening pressure, if available, cellular analysis, glucose (including simultaneous serum glucose) and protein determinations, Gram-stained smear, and appropriate cultures. Viral, mycobacterial, and fungal cultures should be reserved for special circumstances, and are not considered routine in otherwise healthy children.

LP should be delayed in the presence of cardiopulmonary instability, signs of significantly increased ICP, evidence of bacterial infection in or around the LP site, coma, focal seizures, and new focal neurologic deficits, or if there are signs or a history of a bleeding disorder. These situations may warrant immediate therapeutic interventions aimed at saving the child's life, or radiologic procedures to assess for increased ICP.

If the LP is to be delayed, blood cultures are obtained and empiric antibiotics administered immediately; lifesaving therapy takes priority over diagnostic procedures. The laboratory diagnosis of bacterial meningitis rests on demonstration of bacteria or inflammation in the CSF. While early antibiotics may prevent the isolation of bacteria in subsequent CSF culture, obvious laboratory markers of inflammation persist for days to weeks in most cases (8). In addition, bacteria can be isolated from blood culture in up to 80% of patients with bacterial meningitis

TABLE 254.2.   Typical Cerebrospinal Fluid in Infants and Children[a]

Component	Normal Children	Normal Newborn	Bacterial Meningitis	Viral Meningitis	Herpes Meningitis
Leukocytes/μL	0–6	0–30	> 1,000	100–500	10–1,000
Neutrophils (%)	0	2–3	> 50	< 40	< 50
Glucose (mg/dL)	40–80	32–121	< 30	> 30	> 30
Protein (mg/dL)	20–30	19–149	> 100	50–100	> 75
Erythrocytes/μL	0–2	0–2	1–10	0–2	10–500

[a]The values shown should be used only as a guide to diagnosis, because there is considerable overlap in CSF values for the different etiologic categories.

Modified from Wubbel L, McCracken GH. Management of bacterial meningitis 1998. *Pediatr Rev* 1998; 19:78–84.

(9). The various rapid antigen diagnostic tests, including countercurrent immunoelectrophoresis, latex particle agglutination, and enzyme-linked immunosorbent assay, also may be helpful in establishing the etiologic agent if antibiotics have already sterilized the CSF.

A head computed tomography (CT) scan is not necessary before performance of LP (27,29) if the clinical scenario is consistent with uncomplicated meningitis or encephalitis. However, if the patient has focal neurologic findings, has signs of a severe increase in ICP, or is comatose (making neurologic examination unreliable), a brain imaging study such as a contrast-enhanced CT would be prudent to determine the advisability of performing an LP.

Results of CSF analysis can give important clues to the etiology of the CNS infection (Table 254.2). However, in approximately 1% of cases of bacterial meningitis, CSF cell counts, glucose, and protein are normal, and there are no organisms on Gram stain (43). A "normal" CSF profile does not rule out the possibility of bacterial meningitis, but it does render this diagnosis very unlikely. Viral infections of the CNS are typically associated with fewer than 500 white blood cells per microliter in the CSF and a lymphocytic predominance. CSF Glucose and protein concentrations are usually normal. However, the initial CSF examination in a child with acute enterovirus meningitis may reveal a predominance of polymorphonuclear leukocytes, and the cell count may rarely exceed 1,000/μL (2).

Interpretation of a traumatic tap is difficult, and previous recommendations for estimating the number of white cells based on the ratio of white to red cells in peripheral blood may be inaccurate (11).

In addition to blood culture and CSF analysis, the minimum laboratory evaluation should also include a complete blood count with differential and platelet count, coagulation studies if thrombocytopenia is present, serum electrolytes, urine sodium concentration, urinalysis, and, in some cases, a chest radiograph.

In suspected cases of encephalitis, helpful additional studies include viral cultures of CSF and mucosal surfaces, specific viral detection in CSF by polymerase chain reaction, electroencephalogram, and brain imaging studies (30,40).

EMERGENCY DEPARTMENT MANAGEMENT

Supportive care and stabilization are of the utmost importance with CNS infections. Among the initial complications encountered are septic shock with its associated metabolic derangements, coagulopathy, intracranial hypertension, seizures, and hyponatremia resulting from the syndrome of inappropriate antidiuretic hormone (SIADH) secretion. The ED physician must be prepared to support the patient with acute meningitis and manage complications until transfer to an intensive care unit (ICU) setting can be arranged for definitive care.

Septic Shock

Simultaneous shock and cerebral edema present a theoretic therapeutic dilemma, because the treatment of one may adversely affect the other. However, treatment of systemic hypotension must take priority, and fluid resuscitation is an integral part of the management of septic shock. Massive amounts of crystalloid or colloid may be required, but if there is no response after intravenous infusion of 40 to 60 mL/kg, pharmacologic support should be instituted with pressor agents such as dopamine. Patients who require this level of intervention should ideally be managed in an ICU setting, with a central venous pressure line, Foley catheter, and cardiorespiratory monitors.

Previous recommendations for the fluid management of children with meningitis have stressed fluid restriction to avoid cerebral edema resulting from SIADH (13). New data, however, have led to the hypothesis that an elevated ADH and the concomitant increase in extracellular water may be part of a compensatory mechanism to overcome elevated ICP and maintain adequate cerebral blood flow (36,42). A study in children with acute bacterial meningitis demonstrated poorer survival among those who received restricted fluids (42). Further studies are required to determine optimal fluid management in these patients (18), but restriction of fluids should no longer be considered standard (48). If the patient is not dehydrated and the cardiovascular system is stable, maintenance fluids can be initiated, using a solution containing one-fourth to one-half normal saline in 5% dextrose.

Increased Intracranial Pressure

The upper limit of normal for ICP is about 50 mm H_2O in neonates and 85 mm H_2O in older infants and children, but it can be much higher in CNS infections (19,21). In patients with suspected intracranial hypertension, the head of the bed is elevated 15 to 30 degrees (49). Although the practice is somewhat controversial, some physicians use mannitol (0.25 to 1.0 g/kg infused over 10 minutes), with or without diuretics, to treat intracranial hypertension. Hyperventilation is another effective means of decreasing ICP in the severely affected patient. If hyperventilation is utilized, the $PaCO_2$ should be maintained at 25 to 30 mm Hg (17). ICP should be monitored continuously in patients requiring hyperventilation and mannitol infusions.

Several clinical trials have advocated the use of adjunctive dexamethasone therapy for bacterial meningitis, particularly in disease due to HIB (26,35). However, a recent large multicenter study failed to demonstrate any improvement in neurologic or developmental outcome in children who received steroids for bacterial meningitis (46). Other authors have pointed out that, in light of the low incidence of side effects and the potential benefits, administration of steroids is appropriate (31), particularly if CSF Gram stain or epidemiologic clues point to a likely case of HIB meningitis. The AAP Committee on Infectious Diseases has suggested the use of dexamethasone in suspected bacterial meningitis but has stopped short of recommending it as routine therapy, unless disease is due to HIB (3). If dexamethasone is used, it should be given only to children over age 6 weeks with suspected bacterial meningitis, at a dose of 0.15 mg/kg intravenously just before the first parenteral dose of antibiotic.

Seizures

Early seizure activity occurs in 20% to 30% of patients with bacterial meningitis. Effective anticonvulsants include diazepam or lorazepam acutely, and phenobarbital or phenytoin as maintenance. Seizures associated with hyponatremia require infusion of hypertonic sodium solutions. Generally 4 cc/kg of 3% NaCl is infused over 10 minutes; repeat doses may be necessary (37).

Disseminated Intravascular Coagulation

Treating the underlying disease process and correcting the shock and metabolic derangements constitute the best approach to reversing disseminated intravascular coagulation (DIC). If the patient is actively bleeding from peripheral sites or from the gastrointestinal or urinary tract, treatment options include platelet transfusions to raise the count above 50,000/μL, vitamin K to correct a prolonged prothrombin time, and infusions of fresh-frozen plasma to correct a prolonged activated partial thromboplastin time. In the setting of DIC and thrombotic manifestations, heparin therapy may be considered, although its use in this setting is controversial.

Antimicrobial Therapy

Table 254.3 lists the antibiotics and dosages suggested for the initial therapy of suspected bacterial meningitis (20,37). Because penicillin- and cephalosporin-resistant pneumococci have been reported throughout the United States, vancomycin should be added to the regimen any time infection due to *S. pneumoniae* is suspected (25). Previous concerns about reduced penetration of vancomycin into the CNS after administration of dexamethasone appear to be unwarranted (1). If HSV encephalitis is strongly

suspected, acyclovir therapy is instituted at 10 mg/kg every 8 hours.

DISPOSITION

Pediatric infectious disease consultation is suggested for the management of CNS infections in children. Neurosurgical consultation for placement of an ICP monitoring device may also be required.

All patients with bacterial meningitis or HSV encephalitis require immediate hospitalization with intensive monitoring. CNS infections of probable enteroviral or arboviral origin may require hospitalization for diagnostic purposes or for supportive care. Sometimes, the results of the initial CSF examination do not distinguish between a bacterial and a viral process. If patients have been pretreated with antibiotics, are younger than 6 months, or are clinically unstable, they should initially be managed as if bacterial meningitis were present.

If clinical signs and symptoms and laboratory analysis of CSF suggests viral meningitis, outpatient management may be appropriate (34). Some authors suggest observation for 4 to 8 hours followed by a second LP to help confirm the diagnosis (48). If the second CSF analysis reveals lymphocyte predominance, no significant worsening of pleocytosis, normal glucose and protein, and continued absence of bacteria on Gram stain, bacterial meningitis is highly unlikely.

According to the report of the Task Force on Diagnosis and Management of Meningitis, "It is advisable to manage infants and children with meningitis in a hospital that has specialized equipment and staff with expertise in caring for infants and children who are critically ill. The staff should include physicians who are capable of managing the complications of meningitis" (20). Therefore, transport to a pediatric referral center should be strongly considered for any child with meningitis. If LP has been performed, an aliquot of the CSF should be sent with the patient, along with documentation of clinical management up to the point of transfer.

PREVENTION

If meningitis is due to *N. meningitidis* or HIB, rifampin chemoprophylaxis should be considered for the child's household contacts (4,5). The dosage regimen is 10 mg/kg (maximum dose, 600 mg) every 12 hours for four doses, and 20 mg/kg (maximum dose, 600 mg) once daily for 4 days, respectively. Chemoprophylaxis is given to household contacts of children with HIB meningitis only if there is at least one unvaccinated household member younger than 48 months. Rifampin should not be given to a pregnant patient. Medical personnel exposed to a case of meningococcal infection need chemoprophylaxis only if that exposure was intimate (e.g., mouth-to-mouth resuscitation). The use of appropriate isolation precautions (mask and gown, hand-washing) for suspected cases of meningococcal disease eliminates any need for prophylaxis in most situations.

RISK MANAGEMENT

Failure to diagnose meningitis is one of the leading causes of malpractice litigation among physicians who care for children (16). While failure to diagnose and treat meningitis in a patient with a fulminant presentation probably does constitute a breach of the standard of care, failure to recognize meningitis in a child with an insidious presentation may not. Consider a 10-month-old

Age	Drug	Dosage (mg/kg)
Newborn–30 d	Ampicillin *and*	50–75
	Gentamicin *or*	2.5
	Cefotaxime	50
30 d–3 mo	Ampicillin *and*	50–75
	3rd-generation cephalosporin	
	• Ceftriaxone	80–100
	• Cefotaxime	50–75
> 3 mo	Ceftriaxone or cefotaxime *and*	
	Vancomycin	15

TABLE 254.3. Initial Antimicrobial Therapy for Suspected Bacterial Meningitis

child who presents to Doctor "A" on day 2 of a febrile illness. If the child is not toxic, has no nuchal rigidity or photophobia, is alert, has good state variation (cries when examined but is easily consolable when left with the mother), and has symptoms consistent with a viral illness, few (if any) physicians would perform an LP.

If the child is then diagnosed with bacterial meningitis later in the course of the illness, a reasonable explanation is that the child had not yet seeded the meninges when seen by the first physician. However, that physician may still find him- or herself the defendant in a lawsuit. The physician can do substantial harm to the case by failing to fully document the aforementioned findings, particularly the general appearance of the patient. After good medical care, good documentation is the best defense against malpractice litigation. Finally, careful follow up instructions, including specific symptoms or circumstances that should prompt the parent to seek immediate care, are a part of good medical practice and also serve to protect the physician who may be a target in malpractice litigation.

CRITICAL INTERVENTIONS

- Consider bacterial meningitis and perform an LP in lethargic, irritable infants, even in the absence of classic signs of meningitis
- Consider repeat LP if the clinical setting suggests meningitis, even if a CSF culture obtained hours or days earlier was negative
- Always obtain a blood culture before instituting antibiotic therapy for suspected bacterial meningitis
- Always reassess a child with a positive blood culture. LP should be considered if the febrile illness persists or if any suggestions of meningitis are present

COMMON PITFALLS

✔ Failure to consider meningitis in infants with fever without a source

✔ Failure to consider CNS infection in febrile or afebrile, vomiting children, with or without diarrhea

✔ Excluding the diagnosis of bacterial meningitis in the presence of strong clinical clues simply because the CSF white cell count is normal or the Gram-stained smear is negative for bacteria

✔ Failure to always obtain a Gram-stained smear of the CSF when bacterial meningitis is suspected

✔ Not considering the possibility of a CNS infection in a child who has had a simple febrile seizure. Although LP is not mandatory, it should be considered in a child less than 18 months of age, especially if the child has not returned to baseline mental status

✔ Failure to document the physical examination thoroughly, particularly the general appearance of the child

✔ Failure to provide adequate discharge instructions, especially reasons for immediate return to the emergency department

Acknowledgment

The author gratefully acknowledges the contribution of William J. Barson, who wrote a previous version of this chapter.

References

1. Ahmed A. A critical evaluation of vancomycin for treatment of bacterial meningitis. *Pediatr Infect Dis J* 1997;16:895–903.

2. Akasu Y. Outbreak of aseptic meningitis due to ECHO-9 in northern Kyushu Island in the summer of 1997. *Kurume Med J* 1999;46:97–104.

3. American Academy of Pediatrics. Dexamethasone therapy for bacterial meningitis in infants and children. In: Peter G, ed. *1997 Red book: report of the Committee on Infectious Diseases*, 24th ed. Elk Grove Village, IL: American Academy of Pediatrics, 1997:620–623.

4. American Academy of Pediatrics. *Haemophilus influenzae* infections. In: Peter G, ed. *2003 Red book: report of the Committee on Infectious Diseases*, 26th ed. Elk Grove Village, IL: American Academy of Pediatrics, 2003:293–301.

5. American Academy of Pediatrics. Meningococcal infections. In: Peter G, ed. *2003 Red book: report of the Committee on Infectious Diseases*, 26th ed. Elk Grove Village, IL: American Academy of Pediatrics, 2003:430–436.

6. Archer BD. Computed tomography before lumbar puncture in acute meningitis: a review of the risks and benefits. *Can Med Assoc J* 1993;148(6):961–965.

7. Bell AH, Brown D, Halliday HL, et al. Meningitis in the newborn—a 14 year review. *Arch Dis Child* 1989;64:873–874.

8. Blazer S, Berant M, Alon U. Bacterial meningitis: effect of antibiotic treatment on CSF. *Am J Clin Pathol* 1983;80:386.

9. Bohr V, Rasmussen N, Hansen B, et al. Eight hundred seventy-five cases of bacterial meningitis: diagnostic procedures and the impact of preadmission antibiotic therapy. *J Infect* 1983;7:193–202.

10. Bonadio WA. Medical-legal considerations related to symptom duration and patient outcome after bacterial meningitis. *Am J Emerg Med* 1997;15:420–423.

11. Bonadio WA, Smith DS, Goddard S, et al. Distinguishing CSF abnormalities in children with bacterial meningitis and traumatic LP. *J Infect Dis* 1990;162:251.

12. Bratton L, Teele DW, Klein JO. Outcome of unsuspected pneumococcemia in children not initially admitted to the hospital. *J Pediatr* 1977;90:703–706.

13. Brown LW, Feigin RD. Bacterial meningitis: fluid balance and therapy. *Pediatr Ann* 1994;23:93–98.

14. Cherry JD. Enteroviruses. In: Feigin RD, Cherry JD, eds. *Textbook of pediatric infectious diseases*. Philadelphia: WB Saunders, 2004:1984–2041.

15. Cherry JD, Shields WD. Encephalitis and meningoencephalitis. In: Feigin RD, Cherry JD, eds. *Textbook of pediatric infectious diseases*. Philadelphia: WB Saunders, 2004:505–517.

16. Committee on Medical Liability. Liability issues in diagnosing meningitis. In: Robertson WO, Lockhart JD, eds. *Medical liability for pediatricians*. Elk Grove Village, IL: American Academy of Pediatrics, 1995:99–103.

17. Dacey RD. Monitoring and treating increased ICP. *Pediatr Infect Dis J* 1987;6:1161.

18. Duke T. Fluid management of bacterial meningitis in developing countries. *Arch Dis Child* 1998;79:181–185.

19. Feigin RD, Kaplan SL. Commentary. *Pediatr Infect Dis J* 1992;11:698–699.

20. Feigin RD, McCracken GH, Klein JO. Diagnosis and management of meningitis. *Pediatr Infect Dis J* 1992;11:785–814.

21. Goitein KJ, Tamir I. Cerebral perfusion pressure in central nervous system infections of infancy and childhood. *J Pediatr* 1983;103:40–43.

22. Green SM, Rothrock SG, Clem KJ, et al. Can seizures be the sole manifestation of meningitis in febrile children? *Pediatrics* 1993;92(4):527–534.

23. Kallio MJT, Kilpi T, Anttila M, et al. The effect of a recent previous visit to a physician on outcome after childhood bacterial meningitis. *JAMA* 1994;272:787–791.

24. Kilpi T, Anttila M, Kallio M, et al. Severity of childhood bacterial meningitis and duration of illness before diagnosis. *Lancet* 1991;338:406–409.

25. Klugman KP, Friedland IR, Bradley JS. Bactericidal activity against cephalosporin resistant *Streptococcus pneumoniae* in cerebrospinal fluid of children with acute bacterial meningitis. *Antimicrob Agents Chemother* 1995;39:1988–1992.

26. Lebel MH, Freij BJ, Syrogiannopoulos GA, et al. Dexamethasone therapy for bacterial meningitis. Results of two double-blind, placebo-controlled trials. *N Engl J Med* 1988;319:964.

27. Lipton JD, Schafermeyer RW. Pediatric meningitis [Letter]. *Ann Emerg Med* 1994;24:118.

28. Lipton JD, Schafermeyer RW. Evolving concepts in pediatric bacterial meningitis. Part I: pathophysiology and diagnosis. *Ann Emerg Med* 1993;22:1602–1615.

29. Lipton JD, Schafermeyer RW. Evolving concepts in pediatric bacterial meningitis. Part II: current management and therapeutic research. *Ann Emerg Med* 1993;22:1616–1629.

30. Lukeman FD, Whitley RJ, National Institute of Allergy and Infectious Diseases Collaborative Antiviral Study Group. Diagnosis of herpes simplex encephalitis: application of polymerase chain reaction to cerebrospinal fluid from brain-biopsied patients and correlation with disease. *J Infect Dis* 1995;171:857.

31. McIntyre PB, Berkey CS, King SM, et al. Dexamethasone as adjunctive therapy in bacterial meningitis. *JAMA* 1997;278:925–931.

32. Michaels RH, Myerowitz RL. Viral enhancement of nasal colonization with *Haemophilus influenzae* type b in the infant rat. *Pediatr Res* 1983;17:472–473.

33. Nichols DG, Yaster M, Lappe DG, et al. In: Shock and fluid resuscitation, eds. *Golden hour, the handbook of advanced pediatric life support*. St. Louis: Mosby–Year Book, 1991:88.

34. Nigrovic LE, Kuppermann N, Malley R. Development and validation of a multivariable predictive model to distinguish bacterial from aseptic meningitis in children in the post-*Haemophilus influenzae* era. *Pediatrics* 2002;110:712–719.

35. Odio CM, Faingezicht I, Paris M, et al. The beneficial effects of early dexamethasone administration in infants and children with bacterial meningitis. *N Engl J Med* 1991;324:1525.

36. Powell KR, Sugarman LI, Eskenazi AE, et al. Normalization of plasma arginine vasopressin concentrations when children with meningitis are given maintenance plus replacement fluid therapy. *J Pediatr* 1990;117:515–522.

37. Quagliarello VJ, Scheld WM. Treatment of bacterial meningitis. *N Engl J Med* 1997;336:708–716.

38. Radetsky M. Duration of symptoms and outcome in bacterial meningitis: an analysis of causation and the implications of a delay in diagnosis. *Pediatr Infect Dis J* 1992;11:694–698.

39. Rosman NP, Peterson DB, Kaye EM, et al. Seizures in bacterial meningitis: prevalence, patterns, pathogenesis, and prognosis. *Pediatr Neurol* 1985;1:278–285.

40. Schroth G, Gawehn J, Thron A, et al. Early diagnosis of *Herpes simplex* encephalitis by MRI. *Neurology* 1987;37:179.

41. Schuchat A, Robinson D, Wenger JD, et al. Bacterial meningitis in the United States in 1995. *N Engl J Med* 1997;337:970–976.

42. Singhi SC, Singhi PD, Srinivas B, et al. Fluid restriction does not improve the outcome of acute meningitis. *Pediatr Infect Dis J* 1995;14:495–503.

43. Sivakmaran M. Meningococcal meningitis revisited: normocellular CSF. *Clin Pediatr* 1997;36:258–262.

44. Tsai TF. Arboviral diseases of North America. In: Feigin RD, Cherry JD, eds. *Textbook of pediatric infectious diseases.* Philadelphia: WB Saunders, 1992:1390–1423.

45. Tunnessen WW. Nuchal rigidity. In: Tunnessen WW, ed. *Signs and symptoms in pediatrics.* Philadelphia: JB Lippincott Co, 1988:259.

46. Wald ER, Kaplan SL, Mason EO, et al. Dexamethasone therapy for children with bacterial meningitis. *Pediatrics* 1995;95:21.

47. Walsh-Kelly C, Nelson DB, Smith DS, et al. Clinical predictors of bacterial versus aseptic meningitis in childhood. *Ann Emerg Med* 1992;21:910–914.

48. Wubbel L, McCracken GH. Management of bacterial meningitis 1998. *Pediatr Rev* 1998;19:78.

49. Yatsiv I. Central nervous system support techniques. In: Holbrook PR, ed. *Textbook of pediatric critical care.* Philadelphia: WB Saunders, 1993.

CHAPTER 255
Metabolic and Endocrine Disorders

Kenneth T. Kwon

Metabolic disorders comprise a variety of entities which cause derangement in normal physiology and metabolism and can be acquired or congenital. These include diseases related to electrolyte imbalances, endocrine dysfunction, or inborn errors of metabolism. This chapter focuses on the general approach to pediatric patients with metabolic disorders in the emergency department (ED) setting.

Metabolic diseases can vary as much in clinical presentation as they can in classifications. Because the symptomatology of these disorders is also associated with a variety of nonmetabolic diseases, many metabolic conditions are missed in the ED. Initial consideration of a metabolic disease in the differential diagnosis is important, especially in previously healthy neonates with acute deterioration. Definitive diagnosis is frequently not possible or necessary in the ED, but proper initial management based on probable diagnosis can be life-saving or reduce permanent neurologic sequelae. Those disorders which are responsive to ED treatment will be highlighted.

CLINICAL PRESENTATION

Children with metabolic disorders frequently present with non-specific symptoms similarly seen with other infectious, neurologic, and toxicologic emergencies. Differences in presentation can be subtle, especially in the neonatal period. Vomiting, alterations in neurologic status and feeding difficulties are perhaps the most prominent features of metabolic diseases. Characteristic clinical manifestations of specific disorders are discussed below.

DIFFERENTIAL DIAGNOSIS

Laboratory Entities

Hypoglycemia

The definition of hypoglycemia is somewhat controversial and age-dependent. In children, infants, and term neonates older than 1 to 2 days of life, hypoglycemia is usually defined as a serum glucose concentration less than 40 to 45 mg/dL (4,5). The laboratory value should be interpreted in the context of the clinical presentation, as symptoms may occur within a continuum of low glucose levels. Thus, glucose levels of 50 to 60 mg/dL with symptoms of hypoglycemia may warrant treatment. Glucose is the main energy substrate for the brain. Its levels represent a balance between exogenous supply and endogenous gluconeogenesis and glycogenolysis. Mobilization and use of glucose is mediated by hormones, primarily insulin. Insulin stimulates glucose uptake in cells and glycogen synthesis, and its actions are opposed by glucagon, cortisol, epinephrine, and growth hormone. Hypoglycemia can occur when imbalances exist between exogenous and endogenous substrate supply which may involve these hormonal abnormalities. Causes of hypoglycemia in the pediatric population are listed in Table 255.1. Important etiologies in the ED include infection, adrenal insufficiency, inborn errors, and medication-induced.

TABLE 255.1.   Causes of Hypoglycemia

DECREASED PRODUCTION/AVAILABILITY OF GLUCOSE

Low glycogen stores
  Small for gestational age, prematurity
Malnutrition/fasting
Malabsorption/diarrhea

INCREASED UTILIZATION OF GLUCOSE

Hyperinsulinemic states
  Infant of diabetic mother
  Nesidioblastosis
  Islet cell adenoma/hyperplasia
  Beckwith-Wiedemann syndrome
Stress
  Infection/sepsis

COMBINED OR OTHER MECHANISM

Inborn errors of metabolism
Hormone deficiency
  Adrenal (glucocorticoid) insufficiency
  Growth hormone deficiency
  Glucagon deficiency
Iatrogenic
  Insulin/oral hypoglycemic therapy
  Poisoning (ethanol, propanolol, salicylates)
  Reye's syndrome

Symptoms of hypoglycemia generally fall into two categories: those associated with activation of the autonomic nervous system (adrenergic), and those associated with decreased cerebral glucose utilization (neuroglycopenic). Adrenergic symptoms are usually seen early with a rapid decline in blood glucose and include tachycardia, tachypnea, vomiting, and diaphoresis. Because most patients are hypoglycemic prior to ED arrival, these symptoms are frequently absent. More familiar are the neuroglycopenic symptoms, which are usually associated with slower or prolonged hypoglycemia. These symptoms include poor feeding, altered mental status, lethargy, and seizures. These classic symptoms are usually evident in older children and adults, but in infants the presentation may be subtle and include only hypotonia, hypothermia, or feeding difficulties. Early detection of hypoglycemia is critical, particularly in newborns and infants, as permanent brain damage may begin shortly after symptoms develop. Hypoglycemia is also associated with increased mortality in children requiring resuscitative care (13).

Hyponatremia

Hyponatremia is reported as one of the most common electrolyte abnormalities in hospitalized children (8). It is typically defined as a serum sodium level less than 125 to 130 mEq/L, although treatment is based on the presence and severity of symptoms. Hyponatremia can be caused by salt-losing states, such as vomiting/diarrhea, diuretic excess, and adrenal insufficiency, or by excess total body water states, such as infection-induced SIADH, nephrotic syndrome, and cirrhosis. Factitious, or pseudo-hyponatremia, can occur with hyperglycemia, hyperlipidemia, or hyperproteinemia. In children, hyponatremia is commonly due to excess GI loss from prolonged vomiting or diarrhea, or from inappropriately diluted formulas.

Symptoms include altered mental status, lethargy, vomiting, diarrhea, seizures, and circulatory collapse. Vomiting can be both a cause and a manifestation of hyponatremia. The presence of symptoms is dependent in part on the rate of change in serum sodium. Gradual or chronic progression of hyponatremia may not become clinically evident even at levels below 110 mEq/L; conversely, less severe hyponatremia may be symptomatic if the decline in serum sodium is rapid. Treatment should be geared toward the underlying disorder, and aggressive treatment with hypertonic saline should be initiated if significant symptoms are present. Central pontine myelinolysis is a potential complication of hypertonic saline use, although it has been less well described in children than adults (8). This may reflect the fact that hyponatremia in the pediatric population tends to occur acutely rather than chronically.

Metabolic Acidosis

The presence of metabolic acidosis has important diagnostic considerations depending on the classification of acidosis as either normal anion gap or increased anion gap. The anion gap is calculated as the difference between serum sodium and the sum of serum chloride and bicarbonate [$Na^+ - (Cl^- + HCO_3^-)$]. A normal anion gap range is somewhat age-dependent but in children is 12 ± 4, thus an anion gap of greater than 16 is considered increased. Causes of metabolic acidosis based on anion gap are listed in Table 255.2.

Clinical manifestations of metabolic acidosis are nonspecific and include altered mental status, vomiting, and poor perfusion. An important sign that can alert the ED physician of metabolic acidosis in children is tachypnea, which is a compensatory mechanism creating a respiratory alkalotic response. Breathing can range from mild shallow tachypnea to deep Kussmaul respirations of severely acidotic patients. Treatment is geared toward appropriate fluid resuscitation and specific therapy of the underlying cause of the acid-base disturbance.

TABLE 255.2. Causes of Metabolic Acidosis

NORMAL ANION GAP

Gastroenteritis/diarrhea
Renal tubular acidosis
Adrenal (mineralocorticoid) insufficiency

INCREASED ANION GAP

MUDPILES
  Methanol, uremia, DKA, paraldehyde, iron or INH, lactic acidosis, ethanol or ethylene glycol, salicylates
Inborn errors
  Carbohydrate, amino acid, or fatty acid metabolism
Starvation
Chronic renal insufficiency

Diagnostic Entities

Adrenal Insufficiency

Adrenal insufficiency can be acquired or inherited and is due to primary adrenal disease or secondary to pituitary suppression. Congenital adrenal hyperplasia is an important cause of primary adrenal insufficiency in the newborn period, while Addison disease is a more common etiology in children and adolescents. Secondary adrenal insufficiency is more common in older children and almost always involves exogenous steroid use. Acute adrenal insufficiency or crisis occurs when the adrenal glands fail to produce adequate glucocorticoid and mineralocorticoid in response to stress. The common ED presentation involves a patient previously on corticosteroid treatment for a chronic disease such as asthma, who has recently discontinued the medication and is exposed to a precipitating stressor such as infection. A careful history eliciting previous steroid use is the key to diagnosis in these patients with unexplained electrolyte abnormalities or hypotension.

Congenital adrenal hyperplasia (CAH) refers to a group of inherited autosomal recessive disorders with defects in adrenal biosynthesis of the glucocorticoid cortisol. The low cortisol production stimulates pituitary production of ACTH which causes the characteristic hyperplasia of the adrenal cortex. Depending on the affected enzyme, the synthesis of other steroids such as mineralocorticoids (aldosterone) and androgens may also be affected, and clinical expression will vary depending on the accumulated biosynthetic precursors. Deficiency of 21-hydroxylase (21-OH) accounts for up to 95% of CAH cases, and discussion here will be limited to this particular form of CAH. This disorder occurs in 1 in 10,000–15,000 live births worldwide (14). Up to 75% of affected newborns have the "classic" salt-losing virilizing variant, which is associated with aldosterone deficiency and androgen overproduction (17-hydroxyprogesterone); up to 25% have the nonsalt-losing virilizing type. The degree of virilization and other clinical signs are usually greater in the salt-losing variant.

Many states now screen newborns for CAH, however these results may not be available for several weeks, allowing for an acute adrenal crisis to occur during this time. Males are particularly prone to missed diagnosis, as their genitalia may appear normal at birth; females will usually exhibit some degree of ambiguous genitalia. Another physical examination sign is hyperpigmentation, which may be present in the axilla and scrotal/labial areas and is due to the accumulation of a corticotropin precursor which stimulates melanocytes. With the classic salt-losing type, symptoms may begin 1 to 2 weeks after birth and include weight loss, poor feeding, vomiting, polyuria and dehydration. Progression can occur rapidly, particularly in the setting of infection or trauma, to altered mental status, hypotension, or death.

Acute adrenal insufficiency, whether acquired or from classic CAH, is associated with hyponatremia, hyperkalemia, and hypoglycemia. A normal anion gap metabolic acidosis is often seen due to aldosterone deficiency. Unexplained hypotension unresponsive to intravenous (IV) fluids is another sign of steroid deficiency. Treatment should be geared toward aggressive fluid resuscitation and rapid stress doses of corticosteroids. Prior to treatment, if possible, blood should be collected for nonemergent testing of specific endocrine hormones and metabolites.

Thyroid Disorders

Hyperthyroidism in children is almost always due to Graves' disease (diffuse toxic goiter), an autoimmune disorder which produces TSH-receptor antibodies causing increased thyroid hormone release. Nearly 5% of all patients with hyperthyroidism are less than 15 years old, with the majority being adolescents. Unlike adults, children with hyperthyroidism usually have an indolent progression of symptoms over months, although it may occur more abruptly. Personality or emotional disturbances may be the earliest symptoms, followed by the classic symptoms of weight loss, heat intolerance, diaphoresis, palpitations, diarrhea and amenorrhea. A goiter is present in nearly 100% of cases, and exophthalmos, tachycardia, and hypertension are common (18). Thyroid storm can occur in the pediatric population and consists of extreme signs and symptoms of hyperthyroidism combined with a high fever and altered mental status; it is life-threatening and treatment should be aggressive and similar to adult management.

Neonatal thyrotoxicosis, also called congenital hyperthyroidism, is due to in utero passage of thyroid-stimulating immunoglobulins from mother to fetus. In most cases, it is due to maternal Graves' disease, occurring in up to 10% of infants born to these mothers (20). Euthyroid mothers treated for hyperthyroidism are still at risk for having a newborn with thyrotoxicosis. These infants are commonly born preterm with low birthweight, microcephaly, and craniosynostosis. They usually present within a few days of life but can sometimes be delayed ten days or more. Symptoms are transient and last less than 6 to 12 weeks, the duration of which is dependent on the persistence of maternally-transmitted immunoglobulins. Symptoms include vomiting, diarrhea, poor feeding, weight loss, sweating, and irritability. Most will have a goiter, and many will also have exophthalmos, hyperthermia, tachycardia, hepatomegaly and jaundice. Although transient, neonatal thyrotoxicosis can be life-threatening, with a reported mortality of up to 20%, usually from heart failure (15).

Hypothyroidism does not occur with acute signs or symptoms and is rarely classified as an emergent condition. Congenital hypothyroidism, however, may occasionally be missed due to laboratory errors in newborn screening, and early ED detection and treatment within the first few weeks of life are important to prevent irreversible brain damage. Classic symptoms include prolonged jaundice, poor feeding, constipation, somnolence, and hypothermia. Classic signs include coarse puffy facies, large fontanelles, macroglossia, hypotonia, jaundice, and distended abdomen with umbilical hernia.

Inborn Errors of Metabolism (IEMs)

These diverse hereditary disorders involve gene mutations, usually of an enzyme or transport system, causing clinically significant blocks in metabolic pathways and accumulation of toxic metabolites. Due to the large number and complexity of IEMs, the reported incidence of these disorders varies greatly, ranging from 1 in 1,000 to 200,000 live births (7,19). It is now possible to screen for many of these defects even prior to birth. Many IEMs manifest clinically in the newborn period or shortly thereafter, and failure of early diagnosis may lead to permanent brain damage and death if specific treatment is not initiated. Although collectively numerous, only a handful of IEMs are amenable to treatment. The most common emergent clinical manifestations in the neonatal period include vomiting, neurologic abnormalities, metabolic acidosis, and hypoglycemia (2,10). These nonspecific findings can mimic other disorders like sepsis, but an IEM should be considered in a previously normal neonate with acute clinical deterioration. Conversely, the presence of infection does not exclude the possibility of an IEM, as these patients frequently deteriorate and become septic quickly. Standard laboratory values, particularly blood ammonia, electrolytes, and urinalysis can be helpful in further classifying the IEM and tailoring treatment in the ED (see Fig. 255.1).

IEMs can be divided into disorders of amino acid metabolism (phenylketonuria, nonketotic hyperglycinemia), fatty acid oxidation/metabolism (acyl-CoA dehydrogenase deficiency, primary carnitine deficiency), energy metabolism (primary lactic acidemias), and carbohydrate metabolism (glycogen storage diseases, galactosemia). Organic acidemias (methylmalonic, propionic, and isovaleric acidemias, maple syrup urine disease) refer to a specific group of disorders of amino and fatty acid metabolism in which high levels of nonamino organic acids accumulate in serum and urine.

Most patients with IEMs exhibit symptoms as newborns after feedings have been initiated, but a minority may go undetected into childhood with only psychomotor delay until a stressor causes acute deterioration. Recurrent vomiting, dehydration, and acute metabolic encephalopathy are common clinical manifestations. Neurologic symptoms can range from hypotonia to seizures to frank coma. Intractable seizures are characteristic of nonketotic hyperglycinemia and pyridoxine-dependent seizures. Hepatomegaly is a common physical exam finding and can be pronounced in glycogen storage diseases and galactosemia. Risk of infection, particularly *E. coli* sepsis, and liver failure are also increased in patients with galactosemia. A peculiar odor in body fluids can be associated with specific disorders and may offer an invaluable aid to diagnosis. Maple syrup urine disease is named for its characteristic sweet sugar odor, isovaleric acidemia is associated with a "sweaty feet" scent, and methylmalonic and propionic acidemias can exude a fruity ketotic odor similar to that of diabetic ketoacidosis. Metabolic acidosis with an increased anion gap is common in many IEMs. Hypoglycemia is also common and can be pronounced, particularly in glycogen storage diseases and defects of fatty acid oxidation (16). Hyperammonemia is most commonly seen in organic acidemias and urea cycle defects.

Urea cycle defects are a specific classification of IEMs which lead to hyperammonemia due to the inability to detoxify ammonia to urea. Common disorders include ornithine transcarbamylase (OTC) deficiency, arginase deficiency (argininemia), and argininosuccinic acid synthetase deficiency (citrullinemia). Clinical manifestations parallel those seen in other IEMs. Neonates frequently present after a few days of protein feeding of either breast milk or formula; older infants and children may present with recurrent vomiting, ataxia, or developmental delay. Tachypnea is common due to stimulation of the respiratory center by ammonia. The level of hyperammonemia tends to be higher than that seen in organic acidemias. Blood ammonia is usually above 200 μmol/L (normal is <35–50 μmol/L), with some complete enzyme defects reaching levels greater than 500–1000 μmol/L (1,12). Although sicker infants tend to have higher ammonia levels, no strict correlation exists between ammonia levels and clinical findings. The degree of neurologic impairment is thought to be related more to the rate and duration of ammonia rise. Blood urea nitrogen (BUN) is usually low, but a normal BUN does not exclude a urea cycle defect. Metabolic acidosis does not

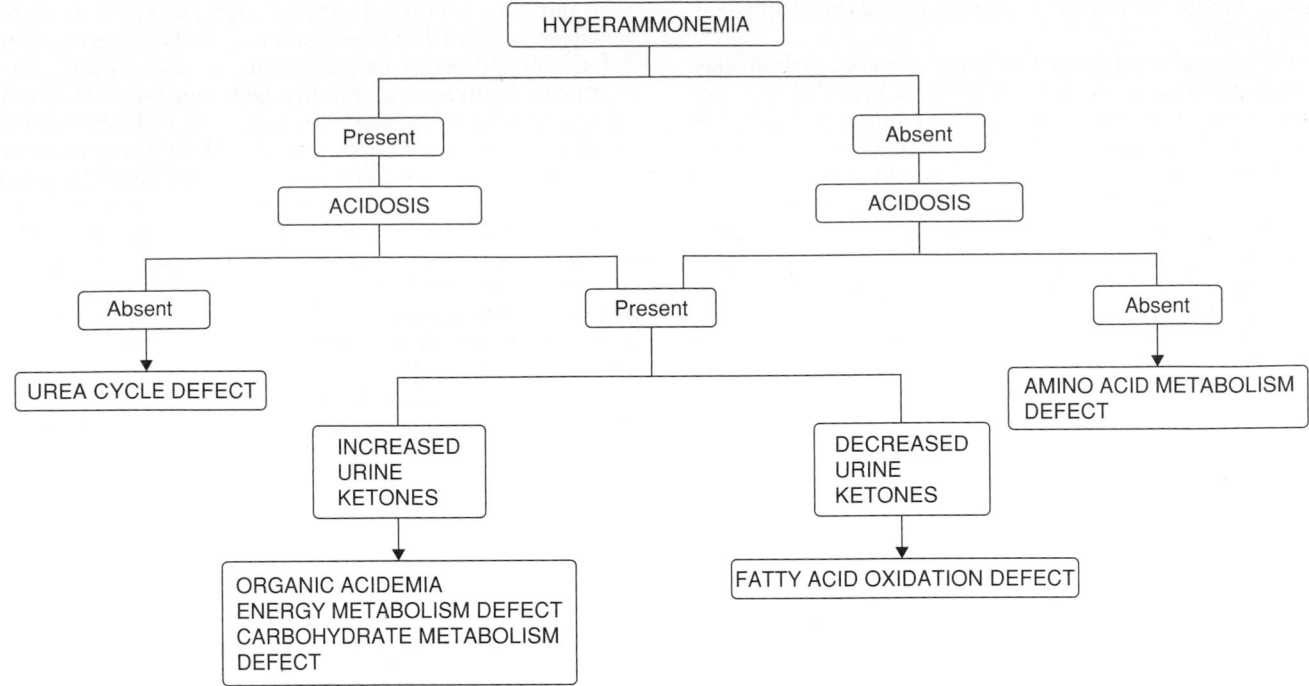

Figure 255.1.   Diagnostic pathway for inborn errors. Modified from Brousseau T, Sharieff G. The critically ill newborn. *Critical decisions in emergency medicine* 2003;18:1–7.

occur with these disorders, thus the lack of acidosis is helpful in differentiating urea cycle defects from many of the other IEMs.

EMERGENCY DEPARTMENT EVALUATION

Careful history may reveal important clues suggestive of metabolic disease. Questions about prenatal care and maternal medications may elucidate an endocrine disorder. A history of consanguinity or sudden infant death in the immediate family is suspicious for an IEM. Feeding difficulties, weight loss, or association of symptoms with dietary intake or particular types of food are important inquiries, especially in newborns. Vomiting is a prominent feature in most metabolic disorders, both as a primary symptom as well as a compensatory mechanism by which excess body acid is eliminated via the gastrointestinal tract.

Physical examination should focus on the patient's neurologic and circulatory status. Alterations in consciousness can range from mild lethargy to seizures and coma. Hypotonia with poor suck and Moro reflexes are frequently seen. Dehydration with tachycardia, poor perfusion, or hypotension should be recognized early and treated aggressively. Tachypnea is a characteristic sign in acidotic patients, and the degree of tachypnea frequently correlates with the severity of acidosis. Unusual or peculiar body fluid odors suggest IEMs. Hepatomegaly and jaundice may be prominent, especially in glycogen storage diseases and galactosemia.

Emergent diagnostic testing should begin with bedside glucose testing which should be verified by standard laboratory testing. Electrolytes with calculation of anion gap are important for diagnostic classification (see Table 255.2). Acid-base status can be more precisely measured with an arterial blood gas, although in the absence of hypoxia, a venous or capillary measurement may be adequate and less invasive to the patient. Serum calcium, magnesium, and liver function tests should also be obtained. Urinalysis will reveal the presence or absence of ketones, which can help to differentiate particular metabolic disorders; the lack of an

appropriate ketonuric response to metabolic acidosis is indicative of a fatty acid oxidation defect. The pH of urine is normally less than 5 in organic acidemias, while the most common urea cycle defect ornithine transcarbamylase deficiency may contain urinary orotic acid crystals. Urine reducing substances is indicative of galactosuria and presumptive galactosemia. Urine electrolytes and osmolality can better classify a hyponatremic disorder. Serum osmolality, both measured and calculated, along with drug screens and levels, can help to exclude a toxicologic cause. Concurrent with these studies should be standard investigations for infection, including a complete blood count (CBC), cerebrospinal fluid studies, and body fluid cultures.

Blood ammonia level should be obtained in any altered patient in whom metabolic disease is suspected. Ammonia is significantly elevated in urea cycle defects and many of the organic acidemias. Of note is that mild transient elevation of ammonia is common in asymptomatic neonates, especially premature infants. Lactate and pyruvate levels can be of use. While both acids can be elevated in sepsis and IEMs, the lactate-to-pyruvate ratio tends to be increased in sepsis (greater than 10:1), whereas in many IEMs such as primary lactic acidosis, the ratio is usually normal. Because stat thyroid function testing is now available in many laboratories, these tests should be initiated in the ED when indicated. Although variable studies exist, essential testing should include levels for thyroid-stimulating hormone (TSH) and free thyroxine (T_4).

Additional archival body fluid samples should be appropriately collected and stored if an undiagnosed metabolic disease is considered in the ED, and preferably prior to initiation of any therapy. For adrenal insufficiency and CAH, additional blood studies to consider include cortisol, ACTH, 17-hydroxyprogesterone, aldosterone, renin, insulin, and growth hormone. For organic acidemias and other defects in amino acid and fatty acid metabolism, quantitative blood amino acids and urinary amino and organic acids will aid in definitive diagnosis. Although these tests are nonemergent, the ED physician may on occasion be requested to order these studies by a consultant.

EMERGENCY DEPARTMENT MANAGEMENT

Initial ED management should begin with the standard ABCs approach. Poorly perfusing or hypotensive patients require standard intravenous fluid replacement, and antibiotics should be administered promptly when suspecting sepsis.

Acute treatment for hypoglycemia begins with glucose bolus replacements. The recommended bolus amount ranges from 0.25 to 1 gm/kg; thus a mid-level range of 0.4–0.5 gm/kg glucose translates to approximately 4 ml/kg of 10%, 2 ml/kg of 25%, or 1 ml/kg of 50% dextrose-containing solution. Generally, a 10% solution is used in neonates and infants (to minimize vascular injury), 25% solution in toddlers and children, and 50% solution in adolescents and adults. Continuous glucose infusion should follow bolus administration to maintain normal glucose homeostasis, especially in neonates. Normal glucose requirement in a neonate is 8 to 10 mg/kg/min, which is roughly equivalent to an infusion of 10% dextrose-containing solution at $1^1/_2$ times maintenance rate. Glucose levels should be rechecked frequently (every 1–2 hours) and the infusion rate adjusted accordingly. If hypoglycemia persists despite boluses and infusions in an infant, a hyperinsulinemic state should be considered. Glucagon 0.1 to 0.2 mg/kg (up to 1 mg) parenterally can be given for refractory hypoglycemia. Because it can be given intramuscularly, glucagon can be particularly helpful when IV access is difficult or delayed. Glucagon will not be effective in patients lacking adequate glycogen stores such as those with inherited storage diseases [17]. Hydrocortisone 2 to 3 mg/kg or 25 to 50 mg/m² can also be considered for refractory hypoglycemia [11].

Hyponatremia should be treated with 3% hypertonic saline (514 mEq/L) only if significant symptoms exist, such as seizures or coma. A dose of 5 ml/kg over 10 to 15 minutes should raise the sodium level by approximately 5 mEq/L; smaller additional doses of 2 to 3 ml/kg can be considered if no clinical improvement is seen. The exact sodium deficit can be calculated as follows: mEq Na⁺ needed = 0.6 × weight (kg) × (Na⁺ desired – Na⁺ measured). Acute correction to 125 mEq/L should alleviate symptoms in most cases. After acute correction for symptoms, the goal is to raise the sodium level slowly at a rate of 0.5 mEq/L per hour (maximum 12 mEq/L per day) by using 0.9% normal saline infusion. If SIADH is suspected, consider fluid restriction to 2/3 maintenance and administration of furosemide 1 to 2 mg/kg.

Acute adrenal insufficiency is treated with stress doses of corticosteroids. Table 255.3 lists various options. Hydrocortisone is the steroid of choice as it has equal glucocorticoid and mineralocorticoid effects; cortisone is an alternative but cannot be given intravenously. The stress dose of hydrocortisone is 50 mg/m² (approximately 2–3 mg/kg), which is 3 to 4 times the physiologic dose. Dexamethasone has no mineralocorticoid effect but is ad-

vocated by some over hydrocortisone in normotensive patients with an unconfirmed diagnosis due to its noninterference with diagnostic ACTH stimulation testing. An oral mineralocorticoid such as fludrocortisone can be started after initial stabilization with IV fluids and glucocorticoids.

Neonatal hyperthyroidism and thyroid storm have many therapeutic options. Beta-adrenergic blockade can be achieved with propanolol 0.01 mg/kg/dose IV and titrated to clinical effect; alternative oral dosing is 2 mg/kg/d in 3 to 4 divided doses. Thyroid hormone synthesis can be blocked using propylthiouracil 5 to 10 mg/kg/d or methimazole 0.5 to 0.7 mg/kg/d, both in 3 divided oral doses. Iodine can be given in the form of Lugol solution (8 mg iodine/drop) 1 to 3 drops daily. Iodine should be started at least 1 hour after administering an antithyroid drug like propylthiouracil to avoid increasing thyroid gland stores before the antithyroid effect occurs. Glucocorticoid treatment with hydrocortisone or prednisone may also be helpful in severe cases.

Treatment for IEMs consists of general measures as well as specific medications if a probable type of IEM is suspected. All dietary intake should be withheld and feedings only re-introduced after consultation with a specialist. Metabolic acidosis unresponsive to IV fluids should be treated with sodium bicarbonate boluses of 1 to 2 mEq/kg. Although controversial for other diseases, bicarbonate use for IEMs is indicated, but standard calculations of bicarbonate requirements will underestimate actual needs due to ongoing production of acidic metabolites [1,9]. Correction of severe acidosis will often require large doses of bicarbonate up to 20 mEq/kg in some organic acidemias [3]. Liberal use of bicarbonate, however, should be done in consultation with a metabolic specialist. The rapid removal of toxins may be life-saving in some cases, particularly with severe hyperammonemia; hemodialysis is more effective than peritoneal or other extracorporeal routes [1,6]. Temporizing empiric therapy with arginine with or without sodium benzoate/phenylacetate can reduce ammonia levels acutely in most urea cycle defects. Table 255.4 lists specific therapies to consider when suspecting particular IEMs.

CRITICAL INTERVENTIONS

- Bedside glucose testing and frequent glucose monitoring (every 1–2 hours based on diagnosis)
- Recognizing the signs and symptoms of thyrotoxicosis or thyroid storm in an infant
- Sodium bicarbonate if severe refractory metabolic acidosis is present and IEM suspected
- Rapid treatment of severe hyperammonemia with arginine and emergent hemodialysis

TABLE 255.3. Corticosteroids for Adrenal Insufficiency

Drug	Dose	Potency Effect (per mg)	
		Glucocorticoid	Mineralocorticoid
Glucocorticoid			
Hydrocortisone	50 mg/m² IV/IM or Infant: 25 mg Child: 50 mg Teen: 75 mg	1	1
Cortisone	1 mg/kg IM	0.8	1
Dexamethasone	0.1–0.2 mg/kg IV/IM	40	none
Mineralocorticoid			
Fludrocortisone	0.1 mg PO daily	15	400

TABLE 255.4.   Specific Therapies for Inborn Errors of Metabolism

Drug	Dose	Indication
Arginine HCL 10%[a]	300–600 mg/kg IV	Urea cycle defects
Biotin	10 mg IV or PO	Organic acidemias
Carnitine	50–100 mg/kg IV or PO	Fatty acid defects, organic acidemias
Pyridoxine	50–100 mg IV	Pyridoxine-dependent seizures
Sodium benzoate[a] and/or phenylacetate[a]	250 mg/kg IV	Urea cycle defects
Thiamine	25–100 mg IV	MSUD, primary lactic acidosis

[a] can infuse over 1–2 hours in dextrose-containing solution.
Data from Burton (1), de Baulny (6), Ozand (16), and Yudkoff (19).

DISPOSITION

Most symptomatic patients with a known or suspected metabolic disorder will require hospitalization, usually in an intensive care setting for frequent monitoring of metabolic parameters and neurologic status. Prompt consultation should be initiated with a pediatric endocrinologist or metabolic specialist. If appropriate resources are unavailable, transfer should be arranged with a pediatric center skilled in managing metabolic disorders. This should be done expeditiously after resuscitation and empiric treatment for suspected disorders have been started. In the event of a failed resuscitation or imminent death in a patient with suspected IEM, permission for autopsy and specimen testing should be thoughtfully discussed with parents. Perimortem samples to consider include frozen blood and urine specimens, skin biopsy, and needle liver biopsy (1,3).

COMMON PITFALLS

✔ Failure to consider a metabolic disorder in the differential diagnosis in a previously healthy infant with acute clinical deterioration
✔ Delayed recognition and treatment of hypoglycemia and hyperammonemia
✔ Failure to recognize acute adrenal insufficiency in a patient with refractory hypotension

References

1. Burton BK. Inborn error of metabolism in infancy: a guide to diagnosis. *Pediatrics* 1998;102:e69.
2. Calvo M, Artuch R, Macia E, et al. Diagnostic approach to inborn errors of metabolism in an emergency unit. *Pediatr Emerg Care* 2000;16:405–408.
3. Chakrapani A, Cleary MA, Wraith JE. Detection of inborn errors of metabolism in the newborn. *Arch Dis Child Fetal Neonatal Ed* 2001;84:F205–F210.
4. Cornblath M, Hawdon JM, Williams AF, et al. Controversies regarding definition of neonatal hypoglycemia: suggested operational thresholds. *Pediatrics* 2000;105:1141–1145.
5. Cowett R, Loughead J. Neonatal glucose metabolism: differential diagnoses, evaluation, and treatment of hypoglycemia. *Neonatal Netw* 2002;21:9–19.
6. de Baulny HO. Management and emergency treatments of neonates with a suspicion of inborn errors of metabolism. *Semin Neonatol* 2002;7:17–26.
7. Greene CL, Goodman SI. Catastrophic metabolic encephalopathies in the newborn period. *Clin Perinatol* 1997;24:773–786.
8. Gruskin AB, Sarnaik A. Hyponatremia: pathophysiology and treatment, a pediatric perspective. *Pediatr Nephrol* 1992;6:280–6.
9. Hazard PB, Griffin JP. Calculation of sodium bicarbonate requirement in metabolic acidosis. *Am J Med Sci* 1982;283:18–22.
10. Henriquez H, el Din A, Ozand PT, Subramanyam SB, al Gain SI. Emergency presentations of patients with methylmalonic acidemia, propionic acidemia and branched chain amino acidemia (MSUD). *Brain Dev* 1994;16:S86–S93.
11. Kappy MS, Bajaj L. Recognition and treatment of endocrine/metabolic emergencies in children: part 1. *Adv Pediatr* 2002;49:245–272.
12. Leonard JV, Morris AA. Inborn errors of metabolism around time of birth. *Lancet* 2000;12:583–587.
13. Losek JD. Hypoglycemia and the ABC's (sugar) of pediatric resuscitation. *Ann Emerg Med* 2000;35:43–46.
14. Merke D, Kabbani M. Congenital adrenal hyperplasia: epidemiology, management and practical drug treatment. *Pediatr Drugs* 2001;3:599–611.
15. Ogilvy-Stuart AL. Neonatal thyroid disorders. *Arch Dis Child Fetal Neonatal Ed* 2002;87:F165–F171.
16. Ozand, PT. Hypoglycemia in association with various organic and amino acid disorders. *Semin Perinatol* 2000;24:172–193.
17. Pollack CV Jr. Utility of glucagon in the emergency department. *J Emerg Med* 1993;11:195–205.
18. Saladino RA. Endocrine and metabolic disorders. In: Barkin RM, Caputo GL, Jaffe DM, Knapp JF, Schafermeyer RW, Seidel JS, eds. *Pediatric emergency medicine: concepts and clinical practice*. St. Louis: Mosby-Year Book, Inc., 1997:755–773.
19. Yudkoff M. Metabolic emergencies (inborn errors of metabolism). In: Fleisher GR, Ludwig S, Henretig FM, Ruddy RM, Silverman BK, eds. *Textbook of pediatric emergency medicine*. Philadelphia: Lippincott Williams and Wilkins, 2000:1117–1127.
20. Zimmerman D. Fetal and neonatal hyperthyroidism. *Thyroid* 1999;9:727–733.

CHAPTER 256
Newborn Problems

Robert D. Kregenow and David M. Jaffe

Newborn infants less than 28-days-old are especially challenging to evaluate in the emergency department (ED) due to anatomic and physiologic characteristics specific to the transition from the fetal to infant state, vulnerability to environmental and microbial insults, and limited behavioral repertoire. Newborns with serious medical conditions may have limited or subtle signs and symptoms.

Newborns must accomplish and transition between the controlled environment of the uterus and the stressful extra uterine environment. The early newborn period is often defined as the first 7 days post birth, and late newborn life is 7 to 28 days (18). Infection, hypoxia, or hypothermia and acquired or genetic congenital disorders can greatly alter the newborn's orderly transition process and sometimes threaten life. Two-thirds of all deaths in the first year of life occur in the neonatal period (4).

Another challenge is that caregivers must provide all of the historical information. Caregivers are often inexperienced and have only had a short period of time to learn their own newborn child's behavior patterns. The history is based on a very short time period and should always include the prenatal period.

NEWBORN PHYSIOLOGY AND PATHOPHYSIOLOGY

While in the uterus, the fetus is entirely dependent on the utero-placental blood flow. The placenta facilitates gas exchange, nutrient and electrolyte exchange, nutrition, hormone production, and antibody transmission. Oxygenated blood leaves the placenta at approximately 80% oxygen saturation. It travels through the umbilical vein, and a large portion traverses the ductus venosus to the inferior vena cava. This blood mixes with deoxygenated blood from the lower limbs and again with blood from the superior vena cava. The majority of the blood then traverses the foramen ovale into the left atrium. The blood again mixes in the left ventricle with a small amount of deoxygenated blood from the lungs and from the pulmonary arteries by way of the ductus arteriosis. The resulting oxygen saturation is approximately 58% (17).

In utero, the pulmonary vascular resistance is high, resulting in the right to left shunting of blood across the foramen ovale and the ductus arteriosis, and only a small amount of blood flowing through the lungs (17). At birth, clamping of the umbilical cord prompts respirations by the infant and increased oxygenation in the blood. These actions result in a dramatic drop in the pulmonary vascular resistance and closure of foramen ovale, the ductus venosus, and the ductus arteriosus, leading to a dramatic decrease in the right to left shunt. Stressors in the first week of life can result in regression to the fetal circulatory pattern.

Lung development begins early in gestation, but only 15% to 20% of the eventual adult alveoli are formed at birth. The majority of the alveoli are formed during the next 1 1/2 years, and the lungs reach adult development in late childhood (16). Respiratory drive at birth depends on both CO_2 and O_2 tensions, and does not change to a more CO_2-dependent system until 4 weeks of age (18). Newborns are at risk to develop atelectasis and hypoxemia because of the relative parity of alveoli, lack of lung elasticity and weak respiratory musculature. The newborn is an obligate nose breather with a small mouth, large tongue, small chin, anterior upper airway, large flat epiglottis, small subglottic diameter and less rigid trachea. These factors along with large occiput, which tends to flex the airway, result in an airway that obstructs easily, particularly in a state of decreased tone or unconsciousness.

Vascular resistance increases soon after birth, but systemic vascular resistance is heavily dependent on cardiac output. The increased sensitivity to vagal stimuli and the decreased level of cardiac contractility compared to older children result in a higher heart rate to maintain cardiac output. Cardiac output and blood pressure are highly dependent on heart rate and preload (15).

Thermoregulation is difficult for newborns. Because of the increased surface to body mass ratio, large head, minimal heat reserve, lack of adipose tissue for insulation, and the inability to generate heat spontaneously, the newborn is particularly susceptible to hypothermia. The infant also lacks a convectional heat loss mechanism, and is susceptible to hyperthermia.

Renal function depends on renal blood flow, glomerular filtration, and reabsorption of electrolytes and water. At birth, renal blood flow is 5% of total cardiac output, and it increases to 10% at 1 week of life. Fractional excretions of sodium and creatinine clearance also improve during the first two weeks as the kidneys and hormonal receptors develop. Newborns are highly susceptible to water intoxication and dehydration (16).

The immaturity of the newborn immune system results in increased susceptibility to infection and inability to localize infection. Neutrophils demonstrate decreased chemotaxis, adherence, transendothelial migration, deformability, and bactericidal activity (6). Monocytes also have decreased chemotaxis, and

there is a deficient secretion of interferon gamma (18). Lymphocytic germinal centers in the spleen and lymph nodes are poorly developed until four to eight weeks. Splenic T cells are predominately suppressor type, inhibiting B cell antibody production. Neonatal B cells cannot respond to polysaccharides without T cell help. Natural killer cell activity against herpes virus infected cells is immature (6). Full-term newborns also have slightly diminished classic and moderately diminished alternative complement pathways.

Maternal IgG accounts for the majority of the newborn's immunoglobulin, and is proportional to the gestational age at birth. Because IgG is both passively and actively transported across the placenta, infant IgG levels are 10% higher than maternal levels. IgG levels decrease during the first few months and reach a nadir between 4 to 6 months. Maternal IgG assists in protecting against viruses such as varricella, rubella, measles, mumps, polio, and bacteria such as tetanus diphtheria, *H. influenza* type B, and group B *Streptococcus*. All other sub classes of immunoglobulin are in low quantities at full-term birth, making infants susceptible to enteric and mucosal infections. IgM levels begin to increase at 25 days and reach adult levels by age two years (6).

Newborns are at an increased risk for hypoglycemia as a result of increased glucose consumption and decreased reserve. As compared to adults who consume 2 to 4 mg/kg/min, newborns consume 6 to 8 mg/kg/min of glucose, and even more when under stress. Low glycogen stores and muscle mass result in a small glucose reserve, making the newborn dependent on feeding to maintain normal glucose levels.

NORMAL PHYSIOLOGIC FUNCTION OF THE NEONATE

Respiratory

Normal newborns have a characteristic pattern of periodic breathing seen after the first 2 days of life. The pattern consists of rapid breathing for 10 to 15 seconds followed by a pause for 5 to 15 seconds with no cyanosis or significant hypoxia. Periodic breathing has been attributed to an imbalance of the central and peripheral chemoreceptors. For further discussion, see Chapter 216, Apnea/ALTE for further information. Pathologic apnea is generally defined as lasting longer than 20 seconds, and/or having associated cyanosis or significant hypoxemia.

Cardiovascular

The heart rate of newborns is noticeably faster than adults, ranging from 95 to 160 beats per minute. While an infant is sleeping, the normal heart rate may fall below ninety. Normal post birth systolic blood pressure ranges from 65 mm Hg to 95 mm Hg and is dependent on gestational age, weight, and height. The systolic blood pressure increases during the first month to range from 80 mm Hg to 105 mm Hg. Normal post birth diastolic blood pressure ranges from 40 mm Hg to 75 mm Hg and does not change much during the first month of life (10).

Feeding and Weight Gain

Feeding is the major form of energy expenditure in the newborn. It is normal for term infants to lose up to 10% of their weight during the first few days of life, but they should regain their birth weights by 7 to 10 days of life. Normal caloric intake for a term newborn is 100 to 120 kcal/kg/day. While it is difficult to quantify volume intake precisely in breastfed newborns, some general feeding parameters do apply. The newborn should be feeding every 2 to 4 hours, or 6 to 10 times in 24 hours. The mother should feel full breasts prior to feeding, there should be a good latch and suck mechanism. Bottle fed infants generally start at 30 ml per meal and increase to 60 to 90 ml every 3 to 4 hours at 5 to 10 days of life. During the first few days, these patterns can be variable, and may not normalize until 1 to 2 weeks of life. Weight gain should approximate 30 grams per day by the end of the second week.

Voiding and Stooling

Voiding patterns vary among infants, but in general should produce 6 to 10 wet diapers daily. Most newborns should void at least once in the first 24 hours, and pass meconium within the first 48 hours. Stool patterns can also vary. Breast fed newborns generally stool more frequently than those that are bottle fed. Normal stool patterns can range from once every 2 to 3 days to 8 to 10 times a day. Stool appearance can also vary in color and consistency, from loose watery yellow or green to more solid brown. Absent bowel movements up to 7 days can be normal in newborns and does not necessarily signify constipation.

Developmental and Neurologic

Newborns sleep an average of 16 hours per day, generally in 2- to 3-hour segments. These segments tend to lengthen to 2.5 to 3.5 hours by 1 month of age (4). Infants can typically fixate on a parental face at birth, but they do not start to track objects until 6 to 8 weeks. They have an exaggerated startle reflex, and will often demonstrate myoclonic jerks while sleeping. At birth, newborns have certain primitive reflexes, such as the Moro, suckling, rooting, palmar grasp, and toe grasp reflexes. By two weeks of age, the infant should demonstrate the fencer position. Tone can be evaluated by ventral suspension. With the infant draped prone over the examiner's hand, the head should be in a slightly flexed position and the trunk mildly convex (20).

ESSENTIAL HISTORY AND EVALUATION

Certain components of the history are specific to the newborn period. Prenatal history should include infections, group B *Streptococcus* status, exposures, fetal movement, and complications. The birth history includes the number of gestational weeks, vaginal delivery versus cesarean section, APGAR scores, and birth weight. The immediate postnatal history includes the length of hospital stay, neonatal intensive care support, antibiotic usage, feeding problems, first void and passage of meconium, voiding and stool patterns, and any abnormal physical findings. The remainder of the postnatal history includes types of nutrition, feeding patterns, length and effort of feeding, weight gain, exposures to sick contacts, activity and movement, interaction with caregivers, and voiding and stool patterns.

Ask about family history of childhood deaths or illnesses, the number of siblings and their health status, and genetic evaluations. Inquire about the living situation, the parental coping skills, the level of stress, the local support network, who is caring for the newborn, and screen for maternal depression and domestic violence.

The physical examination of the newborn begins with a quick assessment of the airway, breathing, and circulation. A patent airway can be ascertained by the presence of an audible cry, absence of stridor, and normal respirations. Normal breathing is characterized by symmetric chest rise, absence of intercostal and subcostal retractions, and the lack of nasal flaring. Circulation can quickly be assessed by peripheral skin color and temperature, central capillary refill time, and the quality of brachial or femoral pulses. After the initial cardiopulmonary assessment, complete the general physical examination. Head circumference, weight, and length are plotted on growth curves. Cranial sutures should be open and mobile to palpation, and the anterior and posterior fontanels should be open, flat, and soft. The eyes should have a red reflex bilaterally. The palate should be intact, and the infant should demonstrate strong suck and swallow mechanisms on a bottle or gloved finger. The abdominal examination includes evaluation of the umbilicus. The genitourinary examination should note any concerns for abnormal or ambiguous genitalia and a normal appearing anus.

Whenever the rectal temperature is greater than 38°C (100.4F) or the child is toxic appearing, a full sepsis evaluation should be initiated. Laboratory studies include a complete blood count with a differential cell count, a basic metabolic panel (electrolytes, blood urea nitrogen, creatinine, glucose, and calcium), blood culture, catheterized urine microscopy and analysis, urine culture, and cerebrospinal fluid analysis for glucose, protein, cell count, gram stain and culture. Intravenous antibiotics should be administered to provide broad spectrum coverage of the typical neonatal pathogens including *Listeria*, such as the combination of cefotaxime and ampicillin (see Table 256.1 for doses). If neonatal herpes is suspected, acyclovir should be added, and a Herpes Simplex Virus (HSV) polymerase chain reaction (PCR) on the cerebrospinal fluid should be ordered. Always check the blood glucose level.

CRYING AND IRRITABILITY

CLINICAL PRESENTATION

The crying and irritable newborn can be a great challenge in the ED. Inconsolability or paradoxical irritability (irritability increases with holding and movement) raises serious concern for meningitis or peritonitis (see Chapter 220, "Crying, Fussy Infant").

Colic is best defined as an otherwise healthy, well-fed newborn who has paroxysmal (excessive, full force) crying episodes lasting more than three hours a day and occurring on more than three days in any one week (12). It generally begins in the third to fourth week, and will resolve by the third to fourth month. The episodes usually occur in the evening and can cause withdrawal of the infant's legs as if in pain, but with no obvious bowel malfunction (13).

DIFFERENTIAL DIAGNOSIS

Causes of crying are listed on Table 256.2.

EMERGENCY DEPARTMENT EVALUATION

The specific history should include the time span, time of day, patterns, and context of the crying. Disrobe and evaluate the newborn from head to toe. Examine the eyes and stain with Fluorescein® to detect any corneal abrasions or foreign bodies. Examine the abdomen for distention or masses, the genitourinary area for any evidence of injury, and the extremities for signs of inflammation or hair tourniquet. Palpate the skull for tenderness or deformities, and the fontanel for fullness or sunken appearance. Examine the skin for bruising, bites, or abnormal markings.

For patients with suspected colic, obtain a detailed description of the newborn's day, have the parents demonstrate their soothing techniques, and look for parental anxieties or family stressors (12).

TABLE 256.1.   Formulary: Common Newborn Pharmacological Agents (10)

Medicine	Indication/Age	Dose
Ceftriaxone IV/IM	Gonococcal opthalmia	25–50 mg/kg/dose × 1
	Bacteremia	50–75 mg/kg/24 hours divided q12–24 hrs
	Meningitis	100 mg/kg/24 hours divided q12 hrs
		Maximum dose: 4 gm/24 hrs
Cefotaxime IV/IM	Bacteremia: age ≤ 7 days	
	<2000 gm	100 mg/kg/24 hours divided q12 hrs
	>2000 gm	100–150 mg/kg/24 hours divided q8–12 hrs
	Bacteremia: age ≥ 7 days	
	< 1200 gm	100 mg/kg/24 hours divided q12 hrs
	>1200 gm	150 mg/kg/24 hours divided q8 hrs
	Meningitis	200 mg/kg/day divided q6 hrs
		Maximum dose: 12 gm/24 hrs
Ampicillin IV/IM; Methicilin IV (for Staphylococcal Conjunctivitis)	Bacteremia: age ≤ 7 days	
	<2000 gm	50–100 mg/kg/24 hrs divided q12 hrs
	>2000 gm	75–150 mg/kg/24 hrs divided q8 hrs
	Bacteremia: age ≥ 7 days	
	< 1200 gm	50–100 mg/kg/24 hrs divided q12 hrs
	>1200 gm – 2000 gm	75–150 mg/kg/24 hrs divided q8 hrs
	>2000 gm	100–200 mg/kg/24 hrs divided q6 hrs
	Severe infections	200–400 mg/kg/24 hrs divided q4–6 hrs
		Maximum dose: 12 gm/24 hrs
Gentamicin IV/IM	< 7 days	2.5 mg/kg/dose q12 hrs
	> 7 days	2.5 mg/kg/dose q8 hrs
Vancomycin IV	Bacteremia	40 mg/kg/24 hrs divided q6–8 hrs
	Meningitis	60 mg/kg/24 hrs divided q6 hrs
		Maximum dose: 1 gm/dose
Metronidazole PO/IV	Anaerobic infections	30 mg/kg/24 hours divided q6 hrs
		Maximum dose: 4 gm/24 hrs
Oxacillin IV	Omphalitis	100–200 mg/kg/24 hrs divided q4–6 hrs
		Maximum dose: 12 gm/24 hrs
Acyclovir IV	Neonatal HSV encephalitis	60 mg/kg/24 hrs divided q8 × 21 days
Erythromycin PO (multiple forms)	Chlamydia conjunctivitis and pneumonia	50 mg/kg/24 hrs divided q6 × 14 days
Nystatin	Thrush	Suspension 1 ml (100,00 units) to each side of mouth QID
	Diaper rash	Apply ointment q diaper change
Phenobarbital IV	Status epilepticus	Load 15–20 mg/kg/dose
		May give additional 5 mg/kg/dose q30 min
		Maximum dose: 30mg/kg
Fosphenytoin IV	Status epilepticus	Load 15–20 mg/kg/dose
		Maximum dose: 1500 mg/24 hrs
Alprostadil (PGE$_1$)	To open ductus arteriosum	Usual dose: 0.05–0.1 micrograms/kg/min
Furosemide IV	Diuesis	0.5–2 mg/kg/dose q6–12 hrs
		Maximum dose: 6mg/kg/dose
Racemic Epinephrine (2.25% Nebulized)	Stridor, airway edema	0.05 ml/kg/dose in 3 ml saline nebulized q1 hr
		Maximum dose: 0.5 ml/dose
Dexamethasone IV/PO	Croup	0.6 mg/kg/dose × 1 IV/IM/PO
Prednisolone PO/	Croup	0.5–2 mg/kg/24 hrs divided qd-bid
Prednisone PO	Croup	0.5–2 mg/kg/24 hours divided qd-bid
Hydrocortisone IV	Adrenal insufficiency	50 mg/m^2 IV bolus followed by 25–100 mg/m^2/24 hrs IV as continuous infusion
Calcium Gluconate IV	Hypokalemia (cardiac arrest)	100 mg/kg/dose over 10 minutes or greater
	Hypocalcemia	200–500 mg/kg/24 hours divided q6 hrs
Sodium Bicarbonate	Hyperkalemia	1 me/kg q10 min prn
Kayexolate®	Hyperkalemia	1 gram/kg/dose q6 hrs prn

Modified from (10).

EMERGENCY DEPARTMENT MANAGEMENT

If no obvious source of the crying is found, the onset is acute, and the newborn is inconsolable, then a full sepsis evaluation should be considered. If there are respiratory complaints, a chest radiograph is obtained. If there are abdominal findings, a flat plate and/or upright abdominal radiograph is obtained. If there appears to be increased pain with movement of the extremities, then radiographs of the limb and a bone scan should be obtained. If intentional injury is suspected, obtain a computed tomography (CT) scan of the head, request a skeletal survey to evaluate for other fractures, and an ophthalmologic examination. Care-

fully describe and photograph all physical findings suggestive of intentional injury.

DISPOSITION

If colic is the suspected cause after appropriate evaluation, then reassure the parents, acknowledge that the crying is more than average, and discuss parental anxieties that arise. Assist the parents with soothing techniques and encourage unnecessary handling. Encourage close follow up with the primary care physician.

TABLE 256.2.   Differential Diagnosis of Crying Fussy
Newborn (7,19)

Hunger
Infantile colic
Gastroesophageal reflux
Constipation
Otitis media
Anal fissure
Unrecognized fracture
Drug withdrawal
Meningitis
Sepsis
Urinary tract infection
Gastroenteritis
Testicular torsion
Incarcerated hernia
Bowel obstruction
Intussusception
Excess gastric air
Hair tourniquet (digit or penis)
Congenital glaucoma
Corneal abrasion (foreign body/eyelash in eye)
Increased intracranial pressure
Cow milk protein allergy
Urinary retention
Shaken baby/child abuse
Osteomyelitis
Arthritis
Hypercalcemia/hypernatremia/hypoglycemia
Insect bites

Modified from (7,19).

CARDIORESPIRATORY SYSTEM SYMPTOMS AND SIGNS

CLINICAL PRESENTATION

Tachypnea in a newborn can have pulmonary, cardiac, upper airway, neuromuscular, and metabolic causes. Tachypnea constitutes 10% to 20% of hospital ED visits, and 20% to 30% of hospital admissions (7). Normal respiratory rate varies from 30 to 60 breaths per minute and can be periodic. Resting respiratory rates greater than 60 usually signify pathology. Accessory muscle use (nasal flaring, intercostal and supraclavicular retractions and paradoxical abdominal breathing) is a sign of respiratory distress and requires immediate interventions. Infants are obligate nose breathers until 4 months of age, so nasal congestion is a common cause of respiratory symptoms.

DIFFERENTIAL DIAGNOSIS

See Table 256.3 for differential diagnosis and (see also Chapter, 238, "Bronchiolitis," Chapter 240, "Congenital Heart Disease, Congestive Heart Failure, and Other Cardiac Presentations," and Chapter 261, "Pneumonia").

EMERGENCY DEPARTMENT EVALUATION

The history should include the newborn's age, length, and progression of the tachypnea, birth history, weight gain, feeding patterns, presence of cyanosis, and evidence of noisy breathing. Obtain a chest radiograph and an anterior/posterior and lateral neck radiograph if stridor is present. If the cardiac examination is abnormal, obtain an electrocardiogram and echocardiogram. If metabolic disturbances are suspected, obtain serum ammonia, lactate, amino acids, and urine organic acids in your laboratory studies. Analyze arterial or capillary blood gases to help differentiate a respiratory or metabolic pathology. If neurologic abnormalities are evident, obtain a noncontrast head CT. If abdominal pathology is suspected, obtain a flat plate and upright abdominal radiograph looking for obstruction or perforation.

EMERGENCY DEPARTMENT MANAGEMENT

Emergency management begins with rapid cardiopulmonary assessment and immediate interventions to correct oxygenation and ventilation. Monitor heart and respiratory rates continuously. If fatigue, decreased level of consciousness, or other signs of respiratory failure are present, then provide assisted ventilation using bag mask technique or endotracheal intubation

TABLE 256.3.   Differential Diagnosis of Tachypnea in the Newborn (7,19)

Pulmonary	UPPER AIRWAY	Choanal atresia, nasal congestion, foreign body, macroglossia, micrognathia, congenital craniofacial anomalies, laryngomalacia, hemangioma, papilloma, vocal cord paralysis, tracheomalacia/stenosis, TE fistula,
	LOWER AIRWAY	Bronchiolitis, broncomalacia, brochogenic cyst, broncopulmonary dysplasia, congenital emphysema, congenital adenomatoid malformations, aspirations, pneumonia (viral and bacterial), pulmonary hypoplasia, atelectasis
Cardiovascular	CONGENITAL	Structural defects, arrhythmias, congestive heart failure
	ACQUIRED	Myocarditis, pericardial effusions/tamponade, mediastinal masses, congestive heart failure
Central Nervous System	CENTRAL	Hydrocephalus, mass, cerebral agenesis, hypo/hyperventilation, seizures, spinal muscular atrophy, cerebral palsy
	PERIPHERAL	Phrenic nerve dysfunction, congenital myasthenia gravis, botulism, muscular/myotonic dystrophies, mitochondrial defect
Chest Wall Intrathoracic		Foreign body, pleural effusion, diaphragmatic hernia, great vessel abnormality, intrathoracic mass, pectus excavatum/carinatum, congenital bone/muscle deformity, rib fracture
Metabolic/Endocrine	ACIDOSIS	Fever, hypothermia, dehydration, sepsis, shock, inborn error of metabolism, liver disease, kidney disease
	HYPERAMMONEMIA	Inborn error of metabolism, liver failure
	ELECTROLYTES	hyper/hypokalemia, hyper/hypocalcemia, hypophosphatemia, hyper/hypomagnesemia
	ENDOCRINE	Hyper/hypoglycemia, hyper/hypothyroidism, congenital adrenal hyperplasia, hyper/hypoparathyriodism
Hematologic		Anemia, hemoglobinopathy, carboxyhemoglobin
Gastrointestinal	DISTENSION/PAIN	Necrotizing enterocolitis, mass, obstruction, perforation, colitis

Modified from (7,19).

(see Chapter 205, "Newborn Resuscitation," and Chapter 206, "Pediatric Resuscitation." If bag mask ventilation is performed or abdominal distention develops, place a nasogastric tube to decompress the stomach. Intravenous or intraosseous access should be obtained (see Chapter 208, "Shock and Vascular Access in Children").

When respiratory symptoms are less severe, a history and physical examination will help guide management. Apply supplemental oxygen as needed to correct hypoxemia. In situations where no identifiable cause has been identified, a sepsis evaluation should be initiate.

DISPOSITION

Since respiratory distress can easily progress to respiratory failure in newborns, admission and observation are necessary both to evaluate for sepsis and to provide supportive care. Establish continuous cardiorespiratory monitoring and pulse oximetry on the patient as part of the initial hospital care until the diagnosis is made and/or the patient's cardiorespiratory stability is restored.

CYANOSIS

CLINICAL PRESENTATION

Cyanosis is always a concerning symptom in a newborn infant. The two main systems causing cyanosis in newborns are cardiac and respiratory, but polycythemia and methemoglobinemia should also be considered. Cyanosis occurs when oxygen saturations reach 85% or when the total deoxygenated blood exceeds 5 g/100 ml (7). Peripheral cyanosis can occur in newborns secondary to acrocyanosis or cold exposure, and is generally not concerning. Congenital heart defects occur in 8 in 1000 live births (15). Although most congenital heart lesions will be discovered in the nursery, some will present to the ED within the newborn period. Cyanotic heart lesions appearing in the first few days of life are generally ductus arteriosum dependent. Cyanosis appears as the duct closes causing decreased mixing of oxygenated and deoxygenated blood. Examples include Tetralogy of Fallot, transposition of the great vessels, truncus arteriosis, tricuspid atresia, and total anomalous pulmonary venous drainage. Those that can appear later in the first month are generally the result of hemodynamic and pressure gradient changes that result in a right to left shunt, such as large atrial septal defects, large ventricular septal defects, atrioventricular canal, or aortic stenosis (see Chapter 240, "Congenital Heart Disease, Congestive Heart Failure, and Other Cardiac Presentations").

DIFFERENTIAL DIAGNOSIS

See Tables 256.4 through 256.6 for the differential diagnosis of cyanosis in the newborn. See Table 256.7 for common cyanotic congenital heart defects.

EMERGENCY DEPARTMENT EVALUATION

When a newborn arrives in the ED with cyanosis, rapid cardiopulmonary assessment should be initiated immediately. Obtain a 12 lead ECG and portable chest radiograph. If a cardiac lesion is suspected, perform an echocardiogram as soon as possible, obtain blood pressures in all four extremities, and pulse oximetry of the right hand and either lower limb. Low systolic blood pressure in the lower extremities or diminished

---

TABLE 256.4.   Life-Threatening Causes of Cyanosis in the Newborn (7,15)

Respiratory
  Upper Airway Obstruction
  Decreased Inspired O_2
  Tension Pneumothorax
  Restrictive Chest Wall
  Congenital Lung Disease
  Pneumonia
Cardiovascular
  Cyanotic Congenital Heart Defect
  Congestive Heart Failure
  Cardiogenic Shock
  Pulmonary Hypertension
  Pulmonary Hemorrhage
  Pulmonary Embolism
Other
  Septic Shock
  Neurologic Cause of Respiratory Depression
  Oxygen Displacement (CO, Cyanide)
  Methemoglobinemia

  Modified from (7,15).

---

femoral pulses suggest coarctation of the aorta. Obtain an arterial blood gas, preferably prior to administration of 100% oxygen. Assess carboxyhemoglobin and methemoglobin levels. The oxygen-challenge test can help to distinguish between cardiac and pulmonary etiologies. A rise of the PaO_2 greater than 100 mm Hg after 100% oxygen under an oxygen hood for 10 minutes suggests pulmonary rather than cardiac pathology.

Evaluate the history of weight gain since birth, feeding habits, and developmental patterns. Listen for murmurs, irregular heart rate, and irregular rhythm. Palpate the liver edge and peripheral pulses. Examine the lung for stridor, rales, or decreased breath sounds. Check pre- and postductal PaO_2. A difference of 10 to 25 mm Hg is suggestive of a right to left shunt (15).

EMERGENCY DEPARTMENT MANAGEMENT

If a cardiac lesion is suspected and the newborn is in the first 14 days of life, intravenous Prostaglandin E_1 (refer to formulary in Table 256.1) may be life-saving by opening the ductus arteriosus. Because Prostaglandin E_1 may reduce the systemic vascular resistance, if the patient becomes hypotensive stop the Prostaglandin E_1. Inotropic support may improve cardiac function and assist in correcting left to right flow. Correction of acidosis, hypocalcemia, and hypoglycemia may also improve cardiac function. Administer oxygen by mask or endotracheal tube to improve cardiac function and decrease pulmonary vascular resistance. Assist preload with gentle intravenous fluid boluses of normal saline at 10 ml/kg. Administer furosemide for diuresis in cases of pulmonary edema secondary to congestive heart failure, but watch closely for hypotension.

TABLE 256.5.   Common Causes of Cyanosis in the Newborn (7,15)

Peripheral cyanosis
  Acrocyanosis
  Cold exposure
Generalized cyanosis
  Respiratory dysfunction
  Congenital heart disease

  Modified from (7,15).

TABLE 256.6. Differential Diagnosis of Cyanosis in the Newborn (7,15)

Respiratory	Upper airway	Congenital anomalies (vascular malformation, anatomical defects causing airway obstruction, laryngomalacia, trachoemalacia, foreign body
	Lower Airway	Bronchiolistis, pneumonia, bronchopulmonary dysplasia, hypoplastic lung
Cardiovascular	Heart Defect	Tetralogy of Fallot (first 12 weeks)
		Transposition of the great vessels (first week)
		Truncus arteriosis (first week)
		Pulmonary atresia/stenosis (first hours to week)
		Tricuspid atresia (first to fourth)
		Double outlet right ventricle
		Ebstein anomaly (first week)
		Total anomalous pulmonary venous drainage (first week)
		Atrioventricular canal defect (birth to 2 weeks)
	Pulmonary	Pulmonary hypertension, persistent pulmonary hypertension of the newborn, pulmonary edema
	Peripheral	Cold exposure, shock
Neurologic		Spinal muscular atrophy, seizures
Hematologic		Polycythemia, methemoglobinemia
Infectious		Sepsis, pneumonia

Modified from (7,15).

In the case of persistent pulmonary hypertension of the newborn (PPHN), correct hypoglycemia, hypomagnesemia, hypoglycemia, polycythemia, or hypothermia. Administer oxygen, monitor vital signs, and minimize handling and external stimuli.

DISPOSITION

If true central cyanosis is present, admit for observation, monitoring, and definitive care. Cardiology consultation should be obtained early if a cardiac defect is suspected.

STRIDOR

CLINICAL PRESENTATION

Stridor is defined as an audible sound heard with respirations. It is caused by turbulent air flow in narrowed large airways. Stridor is usually inspiratory but may also be expiratory or biphasic. It can be either low pitched or high pitched. Stridor can be acute or chronic, febrile or afebrile, positional or fixed.

DIFFERENTIAL DIAGNOSIS

See Tables 256.8 and 256.9 for the differential diagnosis of stridor.

EMERGENCY DEPARTMENT EVALUATION

Note whether stridor is acute or chronic and whether fever is present. Determine if the stridor is inspiratory, expiratory, biphasic, or positional (weak airway structure). Stridor is associated with laryngeal or subglottic obstructions. Stridor is a low-pitched noise signifying nasopharyngeal obstruction. Note changes in phonation or cry, increased drooling, and difficulty feeding. Obtain an esophogram for evaluating vascular rings, slings, and masses that compress the esophagus. Direct laryngoscopy may assist in diagnosing unclear cases.

EMERGENCY DEPARTMENT MANAGEMENT

If the airway appears obstructed or respiratory failure is present, an immediate definitive airway must be established. Since paralytic agents may worsen the airway if there are floppy structures or vocal cord paralysis, attempts should be made to avoid using them during intubation. In less severe cases, nebulized racemic epinephrine 2.25% (Table 256.1) may improve stridor. Treat hypoxia with humidified oxygen by hood or mask. Consider giving dexamethasone or prednisolone (Table 256.1). Position change may also assist with breathing. In most cases of stridor in newborns, consultation with an otolaryngologist may be helpful.

TABLE 256.7. Common Cyanotic Heart Defects (15)

Cardiac Defect	Radiograph Finding	ECG Finding	Examination Finding
Tetralogy of Fallot	Boot-shaped heart 25% with right aortic arch	RVH	Long systolic murmur ULSB Neonate also with pulmonary atresia have soft continuous murmur
Total anomalous pulmonary venous return	Snowman sign Pulmonary venous congestion	RVH, Q wave in V1	No murmur Rales +/−
Transposition of the great arteries	Egg on a string	Normal or RVH	Usually no murmur Murmur if VSD Signs of CHF Single S2
Tricuspid atresia	Boot-shaped heart	Superior QRS axis	Murmur of VSD or PDA
Ebstein anomaly	Globular heart Oligometric lung fields	RAH, WPW, First degree block	S3 and S4 Soft TR murmur

Modified from (15).

TABLE 256.8.   Differential Diagnosis of Acute Stridor in the Newborn (7)

Acute	Cause	Type	Presentation
Febrile	URI with anatomic defect	Inspiratory	Usually preceding upper respiratory infection, degree of severity is dependent on type of defect
	Bacterial tracheitis	Expiratory	Indistinguishable from croup in early phase, does not improve, thick, purulent tracheal secretions, usually due to *Streptococcus aureus*, child appears toxic
	Exacerbation of congenital anomaly	Either	If congenital or anatomical anomaly is present, a mild upper respiratory infection can exacerbate it.
	Diphtheria		Rare, fever, hoarseness, serous or serosanginous nasal discharge, cervical adenopathy
	Epiglottitis	Inspiratory	Rare, especially in infants, sudden onset, increased secretions, stridor not always seen
Afebrile	Foreign body	Usually inspiratory, could be expiratory	Unusual, unless parents giving solids or sibling inserts a foreign body
	Trauma	Either	Fall, strangle, MVA with improper restraint
	Caustic/thermal injury	Either	Unusual unless sibling induced or abuse
	Laryngeal Spasm		Due to hypocalcemic tetany

Modified from (7).

DISPOSITION

Most newborns with stridor should be admitted to the hospital for observation or definitive diagnosis and management. However, newborns with laryngomalacia, who are not in respiratory distress, may be managed safely as outpatients.

GASTROINTESTINAL TRACT SYMPTOMS AND SIGNS

CLINICAL PRESENTATION

Vomiting is one of the most common complaints in the ED. While it often signifies a benign gastrointestinal infection, vomiting in the newborn can be the first sign of a more serious problem. Most congenital fixed defects that cause obstruction such as esophageal or intestinal stenosis and meconium plugs will present during the first few days of life. Pathologic defects that can lead to obstruction such as malrotation with volvulus, enteric duplication, and incarcerated hernia may occur at any time during the newborn period. Distal obstructions such as Hirschsprung disease or imperforate anus are usually recognized early because of failure to pass meconium. Pyloric stenosis is associated with projectile vomiting and increased hunger after emesis. It is more common in males and usually appears during the latter part of the first month. Symptoms of gastroesophageal reflux can be similar, but vomiting is not usually projectile, the history is more chronic, and the child is well appearing and typically gains weight. Bloody stools with vomiting can be signs of necrotizing enterocolitis or cow milk allergy. Vomiting and cyanosis with feeding suggest a tracheoesophageal (TE) fistula.

See Tables 256.10 and 256.11 for the differential diagnosis of vomiting and distention in the newborn.

Vomiting has many nongastrointestinal causes: increased intracranial pressure (hydrocephalus, trauma), meningitis, sepsis, pneumonia, metabolic disorders (urea cycle defect, amino acid defect, organic acid defect galactosemia, and fructose intolerance), congenital adrenal hyperplasia, hepatitis, uremia, obstructive uropathy, and urinary tract infection.

EMERGENCY DEPARTMENT EVALUATION

The history should include frequency, time course, and relationship of vomiting to feeding. Note the presence of bile or fecal matter. Look for diarrhea, bowel pattern, abdominal distension, flatulence, and feeding coordination. Ask about

TABLE 256.9.   Differential Diagnosis of Chronic Stridor in the Newborn (7)

Chronic Cause	Type	Presentation
Laryngomalacia	Inspiratory	Stridor is more significant supine, absent with crying
		Results from collapse of loose immature tissue
Subglottic stenosis	Inspiratory	Present from birth, may be secondary to prolonged intubation, exacerbated with URI
Vascular ring/aberrant vessels	Expiratory or biphasic	Most commonly are double aortic arch, anomalous innominate artery, aberrant subclavian artery, usually worsens as child grows
Omega-shaped epiglottis (floppy epiglottis)	Inspiratory	Worse in supine position
Laryngeal web, cyst, laryngocele	Inspiratory or biphasic	Usually present at birth
Hemangioma	Either	If present at birth, then may appear in newborn period, otherwise will start to grow after first month
Laryngeal paralysis		May be one cord (laryngeal nerve injury) or both (central nervous system), may present at birth or later on, weak cry or high pitched
Laryngeal papilloma		Unusual in newborn period, due to vertical transmission of papilloma virus
Tracheal stenosis		Congenital small cartilaginous ring, may also be from external compression (thymus, thyroid, esophagus, mediastinal mass)

Modified from (7).

TABLE 256.10.   Causes of Vomiting and Abdominal Distention in a Newborn (7,8,14)

Gastrointestinal
  Congenital gastrointestinal stenosis/atresia
  Intestinal obstruction
  Malrotation with volvulus
  Anal atresia
  Meconium ileus/plug
  Hirschsprung disease
  Necrotizing enterocolitis
  Pyloric stenosis
  Incarcerated hernia
  Gastroesophageal reflux
Neurologic
  Mass lesion
  Hydrocephalus
  Kernicterus
Renal
  Uremia
Infection
  Sepsis
  Meningitis
  Pneumonia
  Urinary tract infection
Metabolic
  Inborn error in metabolism
  Congenital adrenal hyperplasia

Modified from (7,8,14).

extra-gastrointestinal symptoms such as fever, lethargy, voiding pattern, cough, increased work of breathing, feeding pattern, type of feeding, and weight gain.

Examine the abdomen for firmness, bowel sounds, tenderness, masses, or organomegaly. Examine the genitourinary and anal areas for abnormalities. If abdominal distention is present, obtain flat plate and upright abdominal radiographs. Obtain a basic metabolic panel to evaluate for electrolyte abnormalities. If the newborn is ill or septic appearing, evaluate arterial blood gases to investigate a metabolic or respiratory cause and initiate an evaluation for sepsis.

EMERGENCY DEPARTMENT MANAGEMENT

If obstruction or perforation is suspected, consult the surgical service. Begin intravenous fluid infusion to correct dehydration and electrolyte abnormalities. Place a nasogastric tube to decompress the stomach and to improve ventilation if the abdomen is distended. In many cases, a bladder catheter should be inserted to monitor urine output. In suspected peritonitis or perforation, start broad spectrum antibiotics such as ampicillin, gentamicin and metronidazole (Table 256.1).

DISPOSITION

When surgery is required, close observation and postoperative care will be necessary. For gastroesophageal reflux, parental reassurance and follow up visits with the primary physician are recommended. "Reflux precautions" (small, frequent feeds, keep upright 20 minutes after feeds, elevate the head of the bed 30 degrees) are sometimes recommended but have no proven benefit. For nonsurgical causes of vomiting, such as gastroenteritis, the need for admission is determined by assessing hydration status and parental competence. If the etiology is unclear after the evaluation, admission for observation and diagnosis may be appropriate.

DIARRHEA

CLINICAL PRESENTATION

Diarrhea is defined as the increase in volume of loose watery stools. In newborns, the gastrocolic reflex will often result in the passage of stool after many meals; however, normal stool frequency and consistency can be quite variable. It is important to ascertain the infant's normal bowel habit. Parental misconceptions regarding normal bowel patterns prompt many consultations about diarrhea. Most causes of true diarrhea are infectious, but some noninfectious causes can also occur.

DIFFERENTIAL DIAGNOSIS

Common viral infectious etiologies of diarrhea in the United States include rotavirus, adenovirus, Norwalk virus, enterovirus, and astrovirus. Bacterial etiologies include: *Campylobacter, Shigella, Salmonella, Escherchia Coli, and Yersinia. Clostridium difficile* should be considered if antibiotics have been used, but it also can occur without previous antibiotic use. Also consider *Giardia lamblia, Echerchia histolytica,* and *Cryptosporidium* in special circumstances such as drinking contaminated water, travel, or known epidemics (2). Many pathogens can cause bloody stools. Noninfectious causes of hematochezia include necrotizing enterocolitis, milk allergies (rare), and intussusception. Rare causes of nonbloody diarrhea include lactose intolerance, carbohydrate malabsorption, familial chloride diarrhea, and congenital villous atrophy. Partial obstructions can result in persistent unformed stools. Pancreatic exocrine deficiencies and cystic fibrosis can result in fatty loose stools. Metabolic disorders such as galactosemia, tyrosinemia, and Wolman disease can cause diarrhea. Finally, diarrhea can be caused by over feeding or excessive glucose loads from juice.

EMERGENCY DEPARTMENT EVALUATION

Document the number of stools, color, and appearance of the stools. Note the feeding patterns, milk or formula composition, weight change, associated vomiting, fever, blood or mucus in stool, and recent antibiotic use. Also note infectious contacts. Evaluate the abdomen for distention and abnormal bowel sounds, and collect stool for culture when possible. Document fever and initiate a full sepsis evaluation if present. If *Clostridium dificile* is suspected, order a *C. dificle* toxin analysis of the stool. If an abnormal abdominal examination is noted, obtain flat plate and upright abdominal radiographs to detect necrotizing enterocolitis or bowel obstruction. If blood is noted, examine the rectal area for fissures. Test the stool for reducing substances if a metabolic disorder is suspected.

EMERGENCY DEPARTMENT MANAGEMENT

If the neonate is ill appearing or dehydrated, initiate a sepsis evaluation and begin fluid resuscitation. Bacterial enteritis should be treated with systemic parenteral antibiotics because the risk of systemic bacteremial infection is high in the newborn period (10). In most cases, the combination of ampicillin and cefotaxime (Table 256.1) should cover most organisms, but stool cultures should be obtained.

TABLE 256.11.   Gastrointestinal Causes of Vomiting and Abdominal Distention in a Newborn (7,8,14)

Possible Gastrointestinal Cause	Presentation	Radiographic Test
Normal physiologic reflux	Effortless spitting up of milk, usually small amounts, can be exacerbated by incorrect burping, overfeeding	None needed
Esophageal stenosis/atresia	Present in first few hours of life , immediate return of undigested food	CXR with NG placed shows curling, lack of air in bowel if no fistula present
Intestinal stenosis, atresia, web of duodenum, jejunum, ileum, colon	Present early with bilious vomiting, +/− abdominal distension, +/− jaundice, +/− respiratory difficulties	Obstruction series Double bubble in duodenal atresia
Hirschsprung disease	Failure to pass meconium in first 24 hours, constipation, abdominal distention, bilious emesis	Barium enema shows transition zone of narrowing with distal and proximal bowel
Meconium plug	Associated with small left colon syndrome, diabetic mother, cystic fibrosis, maternal drug abuse, magnesium therapy for pre-eclampsia, presents like obstruction	UGI with small bowel follow through show obstruction with micro-colon
Meconium ileus	95% have cystic fibrosis, can result in bowel perforation	Obstruction series shows distended bowel loops with thickened bowel
Imperforated anus	Most diagnosed soon after birth	Obstruction series shows small and large bowel distention
Enteric duplication	Abdominal pain and melena, may also have vomiting, hematemasis, abdominal distention	Contrast will enhance duplication
Malrotation of the bowel with or without volvulus	40% present in first week, 50% present in first month Bilious vomiting, abdominal distention, peritonitis from bowel ischemia	UGI contrast will show "coiled" duodenum to the right. Cutoff "beak" sign suggest obstruction
Necrotizing enterocolitis	Can present in a full-term infant Associated with congenital heart disease, perinatal asphyxia, hypoglycemia, polycythemia, maternal cocaine use, maternal pre-eclampsia. Present with feeding intolerance, abdominal distention, jaundice, abdominal tenderness, bilious vomiting, grossly bloody stools, septic appearing	Obstruction series shows ileus, pneumotosis intestinalis, +/− portal vein gas, +/− gasless abdomen, pneumoperitoneum
Cow milk allergy	Rare, abdominal distention, flatulence, non bilious emesis, bloody stools	
Incarcerated inguinal hernia	Inguinal mass, abdominal distention, vomiting, decrease bowel movements	Obstruction series shows small bowel obstruction
Pyloric stenosis	Projectile non-bilious vomiting, males > females by 5:1, present after 2–3 weeks, often family history, usually hungry after feed	Ultrasound shows pyloric muscle thickness equal or greater than 4 mm UGI shows filling defect in distal stomach with a string of contrast through the pylorus
Tracheoesophageal fistula	Choking, coughing, and cyanosis with feeds	Contrast will show fistula Bronchoscopy will show fistula If no communication with distal esophagus, then lack of air in stomach

Modified from (7,8,14).

DISPOSITION

If a bacterial source cannot be excluded, admit the child for intravenous antibiotic administration and observation. If the neonate appears well, no bacterial etiology is suspected by laboratory results or history, and the parents are competent and comfortable, the child may be discharged with close evaluation by the primary physician.

JAUNDICE

CLINICAL PRESENTATION

Neonatal hyperbilirubinemia is the result of elevated levels of production and/or a diminished ability to excrete and conjugate bilirubin. Newborn red blood cells have a high rate of destruction and a short life span. Preterm infants are at even higher risk of jaundice. Physiologic jaundice occurs in the first few days to week of life. Levels greater than 17 mg per deciliter in full term infants are considered abnormal (5). Common clinical risk factors for severe hyperbilirubinemia are listed in Table 256.12.

The adverse consequence of hyperbilirubinemia is the development of kernicterus, which in turn can cause neurologic and

TABLE 256.12.   Clinical Risk Factors for Hyperbilirubinemia (1)

Blood group incompatibility
Jaundice in first 24 hours
Visible jaundice before discharge
Previous jaundice sibling
Gestational age 35–38 weeks
Exclusive breastfeeding
East Asian race
Bruising/cephalohematoma
Maternal age ≥ 25 years
Male sex

developmental problems. Many factors can affect the risk of kernicterus including: stability of the blood brain barrier (affected by infection, acidosis, hypoxia, prematurity, and hyperosmolarity), percentage of bilirubin bound by albumin, and total level of bilirubin. Under normal physiologic conditions, the bilirubin should rise on day 2, peak by day 4 or 5, and then slowly decrease over the next few weeks. Elevated conjugated bilirubinemia is generally defined as a level greater than 30% of the total bilirubin.

DIFFERENTIAL DIAGNOSIS

See Table 256.13 for causes of unconjugated and Table 256.14 for causes of conjugated hyperbilirubinemia.

EMERGENCY DEPARTMENT EVALUATION

Obtain an unconjugated and conjugated bilirubin, complete blood count with differential count and peripheral smear, a reticulocyte count, and a Coombs test. Examine the smear for elliptocytes, spherocytes, and helmet or fragmented cells seen in microangiopathic hemolytic anemia. Test for G6PD deficiency if the family history is suggestive. Initiate a full sepsis evaluation if the child appears toxic. If there is an elevation in the direct bilirubin, then obtain hepatic enzymes, coagulation studies, ammonia, albumin and total protein levels.

TABLE 256.13.   Common Causes of Unconjugated Hyperbilirubinemia in the Newborn (5)

Risk Factor	Causes
MATERNAL FACTORS	
Pregnancy complications	Diabetes mellitus
	Rh incompatibility
	ABO incompatibility
Breast milk	Competitive inhibitor of hepatic uridine diphosphate glucuronosyltransferase
PERINATAL FACTORS	
Birth trauma	Cephalohematoma
	Ecchymosis
Infection	Bacterial
	Viral
	Protazoal
NEONATAL FACTORS	
Prematurity	
Genetic Factors	Gilbert Disease
	Crigler-Najjaar syndrome
	G6PD
	Pyruvate kinase deficiency
	Hexokinase deficiency
	Congenital erythropoetic porphyria
Erythrocyte destruction	Spherocytosis
	Elliptocytosis
	Autoimmune hemolytic anemia
	Microangiopathic hemolytic anemia
	Drug-induced hemolytic anemia
	Polycythemia
Drugs	Streptomycin
	Chloramphenicol
	Benzyl alcohol
	Sulfisoxazole
Poor intake	Leading to increased enterohepatic circulation
	Dehydration
	Secondary to bowel obstruction

Modified from (5).

TABLE 256.14.   Differential Diagnosis of Conjugated Hyperbilirubinemia in the Newborn (7,19)

Hepatic disorders	Biliary atresia
	Intrahepatic biliary hypoplasia
	Idiopathic hepatocellular cholestasis
	Ischemic hepatitis
Perinatal infections	Bacterial sepsis
	Urinary tract infection
	Toxoplasmosis
	Rubella
	Cytomegalovirus
	Varicella
	Herpes simplex
	Coxsackievirus
	Leptospirosis
Metabolic disorders	Galactosemia
	Galactokinase deficiency
	Hereditary fructose intolerance
	α1-antitrypsin deficiency
	Cystic fibrosis
Biliary tree disorder	Bile duct perforation
	Choledochal cyst

Modified from (7,19).

EMERGENCY DEPARTMENT MANAGEMENT

American Academy of Pediatrics guidelines suggest starting phototherapy with phototherapy lights and possible phototherapy blanket at the following levels: 15 mg/dL at 24 to 48 hours, 18 mg/dL at 49 to 72 hours, and 20 mg/dL > 72 hours (10). These guidelines should be applied in the context of patient-specific clinical information. If there are other potential risk factors, or the rate of rise in the bilirubin level is dramatic, then phototherapy should be initiated earlier. When phototherapy is not able to prevent bilirubin levels from exceeding 20 mg/dL, consider double exchange transfusion. Intravenous fluid should be given if there is evidence of dehydration or poor feeding, oral feeding can be continued as tolerated. Phototherapy may result in an excess loss of fluid, requiring additional isotonic saline containing 5% glucose. Start antibiotics if there is evidence of infection. If there is an elevated direct bilirubin and the child otherwise is well-appearing, prompt referral to a pediatric gastroenterologist if indicated is recommended.

DISPOSITION

The disposition will depend on the laboratory values, the age of the child, other risk factors, and the appearance of the child. In some cases, home phototherapy can be arranged. Patients with jaundice may be discharged from the ED if bilirubin levels are below the guideline levels for age, have normal physical examinations, have good follow up with a physician, and have the availability of repeat bilirubin levels in 12 to 24 hours.

NEUROLOGIC SYMPTOMS AND SIGNS

CLINICAL PRESENTATION

Neonatal seizures can present in subtle ways such as jittery movements, apnea, subtle eye deviations, lip smacking, tongue thrusting, or chewing movements. Hypoxic ischemic encephalopathy causes 50% to 60%, hemorrhages cause 15%, and inborn errors in metabolism cause approximately 10% of newborn seizures (13).

TABLE 256.15.   Common Causes of Newborn Seizures (13)

Hypoxic ischemic encephalopathy
Trauma (shaken baby)
Intracranial/intraventricular hemorrhage
Infection (bacterial, HSV)
Hypoglycemia
Hypocalcemia
Hypomagnesemia
Hyponatremia
Drug withdrawal
Inborn errors of metabolism
Congenital anomalies or developmental brain disorders

Modified from (13).

DIFFERENTIAL DIAGNOSIS

See Table 256.15 for causes of newborn seizures.

EMERGENCY DEPARTMENT EVALUATION

Obtain a prenatal and perinatal history including: maternal infections, maternal laboratory studies, maternal drug exposures, birth complications. If the infant is formula fed, evaluate the process of formula preparation. Examine for cutaneous lesions such as petechiae, herpes vesicles, café au lait spots, hair swirl patterns, or areas of hyperpigmentation. Smell for unusual odors as a clue for inborn errors of metabolism. Laboratory studies include serum glucose, CBC and blood culture, urine analysis and culture, spinal fluid studies as well as a HSV PCR, electrolytes, glucose, calcium, magnesium, phosphorous. If inborn error of metabolism is suspected, send additional blood for amino acids, lactate, pyruvate, ammonia and urine for organic acids. Image the head by head ultrasound and/or CT.

EMERGENCY DEPARTMENT MANAGEMENT

In addition to basic life-support measures, benzodiazepines are used for initial seizure management, followed by a loading dose of phenobarbital or fosphenytoin (Table 256.1). Administer broad spectrum antibiotics and acyclovir (Table 256.1) after studies have been obtained. Admit the patient and monitor pulse oximetry, respiratory rate, and the cardiac rhythm, looking for signs of seizure activity. Consult a neurologist at the earliest convenience.

FLOPPY INFANT

CLINICAL PRESENTATION

Floppy infants are infants with decreased tone or strength. Hypotonia is defined functionally as diminished resistance to movement as the limb is passively moved through a range of motion. Hypotonia and weakness can present as decreased activity, poor suck or choking, weak cry, respiratory distress, constipation, decreased head movement, or decreased eye movement.

DIFFERENTIAL DIAGNOSIS

Some of the common causes are in Table 256.16.

TABLE 256.16.   Common Causes of the Floppy Newborn (19)

Brain	Hypoxic ischemic encephalopathy
	Cerebral hemorrhage
	Lissencephaly
	Brain malformations
Spinal cord	Spinal cord injury
	Meningomyelocele
	Unrecognized spina bifida
Lower motor	Spinal muscular atrophy
Peripheral nerve	Brachial plexus injury
Motor junction	Infantile botulism
	Neonatal myasthenia
Muscular	Muscular dystrophy
	Mitochondrial diseases
Infection	Sepsis
	Congenital TORCHS infections
Syndromes	Down syndrome
	Prader willi
Other	Electrolyte disturbance (Ca, Mg, K)
	Hypothyroidism
	Metabolic disorders

Modified from (19).

EMERGENCY DEPARTMENT EVALUATION

Begin with assessment of the respiratory function and strength. Tone can be evaluated by ventral suspension. With the infant draped prone over the examiner's hand, the head should be in a slightly flexed position and the trunk mildly convex. Muscle strength is more difficult to evaluate. Hold the child with the hand under the axilla to test the shoulder girdle. Strength of the palmer grasp is another indicator. Evaluation of the infant reflexes may also give a clue to weakness. Obtain laboratory studies looking for electrolyte disturbances or evidence of infection.

EMERGENCY DEPARTMENT MANAGEMENT/DISPOSITION

Respiratory distress or insufficiency may require assisted ventilation and continuous monitoring of vital signs. Intravenous access should be obtained if the infant is unable to feed adequately. Obtain a computed tomogram of the head to exclude trauma or obvious brain abnormalities. If the child is stable, consult a neurologist as soon as possible.

INFECTIOUS DISEASE SYMPTOMS AND SIGNS

The immune system of the newborn is immature and infectious exposures can occur in the uterus during both the pre- and postnatal periods. Determination of the timing of prenatal exposure is important because timing of prenatally acquired infection can affect the type and severity of the disease. Perinatal and postnatal infections are more likely to be causes of problems seen in the ED, because most in utero infections will have been diagnosed in the first few days of life. See congenital infections (Table 256.17). Maternal viral illness during the immediate perinatal period is associated with serious infections in the neonate because passive immunity is low and viremic levels in the mother are high. Systemic manifestations of perinatally acquired viral disease can be life threatening. Viruses to consider are hepatitis B virus, hepatitis C virus, varicella zoster virus, HSV, and human immunodeficiency virus (HIV).

TABLE 256.17. Prenatal Newborn Infections (3)

Prenatal	Clinical Presentation	Diagnosis	Treatment
CMV 0.4%–2.5% of births	Most have no apparent signs 10% will have systemic signs (petechiae, hepatosplenomegaly, IUGR) Neurologic findings (microcephaly, chorioretinitis, hearing loss, hypo/hypertonia)	Amniotic fluid cell culture Urine viral culture CMV IgM Head US: Periventricular calcifications	Gancyclovir 6 mg/kg every 12 hours for 6 weeks
Toxoplasma gondi 0.8–10 per 10,000 births	Exposure to cat feces, undercooked meat 40% have symptoms jaundice, splenomegaly, hepatomegaly, fever, anemia, hydrocephalus, chorioretinitis	Serologic studies Head CT: Parenchyma calcifications	Sulfadiazine Pyrimethamine
Rubella 0.1/100,000	Cataracts, retinopathy, micro-opthalmia, microcephaly, sensorineural hearing loss, meningoencephalitis, osteopathy, pneumonitis, hepatitis, thrombocytopenia	Serology Viral culture from nasal secretion, urine, CSF	none
Herpes simplex virus	Skin vesicles, chorioretinitis, microcephaly, micro-opthalmia, IUGR	Viral culture or PCR from vesicle fluid Viral sample from CSF, conjunctiva, rectum, oropharynx Ophthalmology examination Head CT: calcifications in the basal ganglia and thalami, diffuse hemispheric cystic lesions, lissencephalic like appearance of the cerebral cortex	Acyclovir 60 mg/kg/d for 21 days
Varicella	VZV before 20 weeks gives a 2% risk of fetal varicella syndrome (limb hypoplasia, chorioretinitis, cataracts, microopthalmia, cutaneous scarring) Neurologic (microcephaly, hydrocephalus, seizures, paralysis)	Head CT: intracranial calcifications, cortical dysplasia, hydranencephaly	Not helpful
Syphilis	IUGR, rash, hepatosplenomegaly, jaundice, lympadenopathy	Radiograph: osteochondritis Quantitative treponemal and non treponemal assays of serum, VDRL of CSF CBC Long bone radiographs	Procaine Penicillin G 50,000 U/kg every day for 10 days

Modified from (3).

Bacterial Infections

Group B Beta-hemolytic Streptococcus (GBS), *Escherichia coli*, and *Listeria monocytogenes* comprise 70% of newborn bacterial disease. *E. coli*, the most common of these, can cause meningitis, urinary tract infection and sepsis syndrome throughout the neonatal period. GBS and *L. monocytogenes* both have early (first week) and late onset (2nd to 12th week) forms. Early onset disease generally results from transplacental or ascending infections from the maternal genital tract. The pretreatment of maternal GBS prior to delivery has reduced the incidence of early onset neonatal GBS. It is important to ask about pretreatment. Late onset disease is transmitted by the mother or nosocomially. Meningitis occurs more often in late than early onset disease (6,9). Immediately start empiric therapy with ampicillin and an aminoglycoside (Table 256.1) for early onset disease and ampicillin and cefotaxime (Table 256.1) for late onset disease. High dose ampicillin should be administered in cases of meningitis (Table 256.1).

Human Immunodeficiency Virus

Manifestations of interuterine human immunodeficiency virus (HIV) infections will appear at birth but postnatal infections typically cause symptoms after the neonatal period. It has been shown that HIV can infect the fetus in utero and during the process of birth. Postnatal transmission occurs through breast feeding. The use of zidovudine (AZT®), at the time of birth has greatly reduced the number of infected infants. The clinical manifestations of HIV infections include sepsis, interuterine growth restriction (IUGR), failure to thrive, chronic pneumonitis, chronic diarrhea, and thrombocytopenia. Always consider HIV when the newborn is ill-appearing or has signs of infection without a clear diagnosis (6).

Fever

Fever in the newborn period is usually considered greater than or equal to 100.4°C measured rectally. Parental reports of fever should be taken seriously. Bundling has been shown to increase surface temperature but rarely raises core temperature above the threshold for fever. Neonates with fever should receive an evaluation for sepsis. During the appropriate season send an enteroviral PCR on the cerebrospinal fluid and a nasal pharyngeal swab for seasonal viruses (respiratory syncytial virus [RSV], adenovirus, parainfluenza A and B). Ampicillin and cefotaxime are the most common antibiotics used (Table 256.1). If there is evidence of meningitis, the doses of antibiotics are increased and acyclovir (Table 256.1) is added, until results of cultures of blood, urine and cerebrospinal fluid are available.

ENDOCRINE/METABOLIC DISORDER

CONGENITAL ADRENAL HYPERPLASIA

Congenital adrenal hyperplasia (CAH) is a family of inherited disorders of adrenal steroidogenesis transmitted by mutated autosomal recessive genes that encode enzymes essential for cortisol biosyntheses. Cortisol production is decreased and ACTH secretion is increased. This causes overproduction of the precursor steroid in the defective pathway, and also of other adrenal steroids. Specific syndromes depend on the specific genetic defect and enzyme deficiency. Deficiency of 21 hydroxylase causes more than 90% of all congenital adrenal hyperplasia. Aldosterone deficiency (salt wasting form) may or may not accompany cortisol deficiency. Excess adrenal androgen secretion is stimulated by increased ACTH.

The peak age for developing symptoms of adrenal crisis is 3 weeks but the range is 1 to 4 weeks. Symptoms include: poor feeding, lethargy, weak cry, vomiting, diarrhea, dehydration, hypotension, weight loss and failure to thrive. Untreated cardiovascular collapse and death may occur. Diagnosis in affected girls is often made at birth because the virilizing effect of excess androgens in utero causes ambiguous external genitalia. Boys, however, develop symptoms and signs of adrenal crisis.

Evaluation and Management

Assess vital signs and degree of dehydration. Examine genitalia for signs of abnormal virilization in girls. Obtain plasma electrolyte and blood glucose values as soon as possible. Hyperkalemia and hyponatremia are characteristic of adrenal crisis with CAH. Try to obtain blood for adrenal steroid profile (17-OH progesterone, dehydroepiandrosterone (DHEA), andeostenedione, and testosterone). Begin fluid resuscitation with normal saline 20 ml/kg during the first hour, but faster if shock is present. Administer hydrocortisone 25 mg intravenous bolus, and then 50 mg/meter squared per 24 hours as an intravenous infusion or 25 mg of hydrocortisone acetate by intramuscular injection every 24 hours. Volume restoration and hydrocortisone will also begin to treat hyperkalemia but fludrocortisone 0.1 mg can be added by oral or nasal route. Treat associated life-threatening cardiac arrhythmia with sodium bicarbonate, calcium gluconate, and the carbon exchange resins Kayexolate® (Table 256.1). Treat hypoglycemia with glucose 0.25 mg/kg. Note that 20 ml/kg of D5NS contains one gram of glucose per kilogram. Acidosis does not require specific treatment but low serum bicarbonate may take several days to correct.

OTHER ENDOCRINE PROBLEMS

Other endocrine emergencies that present in the neonatal period include hypoglycemia, and thyroid irregularities.

Hypoglycemia should be considered in any ill appearing or irritable infant. It can be caused by sepsis, adrenal insufficiency, abnormal glycogen synthesis pathways, abnormal gluconeogenic or glycogenolysis pathways, hyperinsulinemia, or fatty acid oxidation defects. Management includes a sepsis evaluation and correction of hypoglycemia. Consultation with an endocrinologist can be useful in determining the definitive diagnosis (4).

Undiagnosed thyroid abnormalities are rare with the advent of newborn screening, but symptoms can occur prior to the results being available. Neonatal thyrotoxicosis occurs in 1% to 5% of mothers with hyperthyroidism. These infants usually have a goiter and exophthalmos. Other symptoms and signs include failure to thrive, tachycardia, and congestive heart failure. Undetected congenital hypothyroidism is rare since neonatal screening has been implemented. Symptoms may be subtle in the first month. In severe cases, there will be large posterior fontanel, hypothermia, poor feeding, constipation, and prolonged jaundice. Large tongue, coarse facies, and hoarse cry may or may not occur. Laboratory evaluation includes a TSH, T_4, T_3 and thyroid binding capacity (4).

OTHER

Circumcision

There is a decrease in the number of circumcisions being done in the United States, but they still range from 64% to 82% in various ethnic and racial groups. The most common complications are bleeding and infection. Other complications can include: phimosis, skin bridges, and inclusion cysts. Obtain the history of the number of days since circumcision, quantity of bleeding, and voiding problems. Test coagulation studies if there is excessive bleeding. Bleeding can generally be controlled by direct pressure. Gel Foam® may be helpful in severe cases of bleeding. Once bleeding is controlled, application of Vaseline gauze may protect the site from repeated trauma. Signs of infection should prompt administration of intravenous antibiotics effective against gram-positive organisms (11).

Conjunctivitis

Ophthalmia neonatorum, or neonatal conjunctivitis, is the most common eye complaint. It is characterized as redness and chemosis of the conjunctiva, edema of the eyelid, and purulent discharge. The most common forms of neonatal conjunctivitis are *Chlamydia trachomatis* appearing between 5 to 14 days, *Neisseria gonorrhoeae* appearing between 2 to 5 days, chemical (silver nitrate) appearing between 6 to12 hours. *Staphylococcus aureus* can appear any time during the neonatal period. Other causes are kerititis (Herpes simplex), viral (adenovirus, ECHO virus, Coxsackievirus), foreign body (eye lash), dacrocytitis (*S. aureus*), and congenital dacrocystocele. Because it is sometimes difficult to differentiate these causes by clinical appearance and time of onset, laboratory studies will help guide management. If it is beyond 48 hours, an infectious cause should be investigated. Gram stain and culture of the discharge should be obtained. Direct fluorescent antibody testing, conjunctiva tissue culture, and immunofluorescent staining for chlamydia should be done.

The neonate with a gram stain showing gram-negative diplococci should be hospitalized and undergo a full septic work up. Treatment consists of ceftriaxone (Table 256.1) along with eye irrigation. The treatment for chlamydia is 14 to 21 days of oral erythromycin (Table 256.1) in order to treat the 20% risk of chlamydia pneumonia. For Staphylococcal infections, treatment includes: admission, parenteral methicillin (Table 256.1) and irrigation (4).

Umbilical Cord Complaints

Umbilical cord problems are common in the newborn period. The cord area should be kept dry. Overzealous cleaning with antiseptic agents can inhibit the normal degradation that is assisted by normal flora. Cord separation at greater than 4 to 6 weeks should prompt a work up for immune deficiencies. Treat persistent granulomas with topical silver nitrate. If there is purulent drainage or urine like drainage, obtain prompt surgical evaluation for an abscess or patent urachus. Omphalitis is a medical emergency because of its high mortality rate. Omphalitis appears as erythema of the skin immediately surrounding the umbilical cord. Administer parenteral gentamicin and oxacillin for *S. aureus* and *E. coli* coverage, and admit to the hospital.

Thrush

Oral mucus membrane *Candida* infections occur in approximately 2% to 5% of normal newborns. The characteristic white plaques on erythematous base of *Candida* may be acquired during delivery and can cause colonization. It may develop as early as 7 days of age, but can appear at anytime during the newborn period. The plaques may occur on the lips, buccal mucosa, tongue, and palate. Removal of a plaque may produce a small amount of bleeding, which can be suggestive of thrush. The newborn is generally asymptomatic but can have pain, fussiness, and difficulty feeding (2). Treatment includes application of nystatin suspension with a cotton swab to the affected areas. Bottle supplies should be washed in hot water. Breast feeding mothers may also need to apply nystatin cream to the nipple area. Affected newborns are at an increased risk of developing *Candida* diaper dermatitis.

Diaper Rash

Diaper rashes occur frequently during the newborn period. The moisture resulting from wet diapers provides an environment of both skin irritation and growth of *Candida albicans*. Contact dermatitis appears as simple redness in the diaper area with distinct borders at the diaper edges and sparing of the skin folds. For contact dermatitis, more frequent diaper changes plus a protective agent such as zinc oxide ointment is usually sufficient. For severe cases, use a brief course of hydrocortisone ointment (0.5% or 1.0%).

Candida diaper rash has a well-defined erythematous appearance with satellite lesions and small pustules, and it generally involves the skin folds. Nystatin ointment applied to affected areas with each diaper change will generally cure most cases. Remember to also treat any oral *Candida* infections.

MANAGEMENT OF THE SEPTIC OR ILL-APPEARING NEONATE

The septic-appearing infant always requires immediate attention. Although there can be many causes, overwhelming bacterial or viral infection are the most common. These should be investigated and treated first. Other causes of this syndrome include: viremia, inborn errors of metabolism and other metabolic disorders, electrolyte abnormalities, endocrine disorders, cardiac disorders both congenital and acquired, congenital pulmonary pathologies, congenital and acquired gastrointestinal pathologies, seizures, encephalitis, and trauma secondary to child abuse. A mnemonic that can aid in determining the etiology of disease are: " THE MISFITS" (13)

T-Trauma
H-Heart disease, hypovolemia
E-Electrolyte abnormalities (hypoglycemia)_
M-Metabolic disorders (congenital adrenal hyperplasia, thryroxocosis)
I-Inborn errors of metabolism
S-Sepsis
F-Formula problems (over or underdilution)
I-Intestinal catastrophes
T-Trauma secondary to child abuse
S-Seizures

Emergency management of the ill-appearing infant requires rapid treatment of abnormalities of cardiopulmonary function and simultaneous efforts to reach a specific diagnosis.

Nonspecific but vital therapeutic interventions typically require rapid application of supplemental oxygen, support for airway and breathing, establishment of intravenous access and administration of fluid with NS 10 ml/kg over 20 to 30 minutes to support circulation. Monitor vital signs and oxygen saturation and determine bedside glucose. Sick infants often become hypoglycemic because of inadequate glycogen stores.

Physical examination should be directed at detecting signs of focal infection or clues to the diagnosis such as petechial or purpuric rash or skin ulcers indicative of HSV infection. In addition to the complete sepsis laboratory evaluation, obtain arterial or capillary blood gases, coagulation studies, and complete metabolic panel, including liver enzyme levels. Lumbar puncture and computerized head tomography should be done, but should not delay administration of antibiotics (ceftriaxone, ampicillin) and antivirals (acyclovir). Chest radiography should also be obtained. Other laboratory studies should be selected based on the specific signs and symptoms. These patients usually require admission to a facility with expertise in pediatric intensive care.

CRITICAL INTERVENTIONS

- Check serum glucose in all ill-appearing or lethargic infants
- Perform a full-septic work up in infants, initiate antibiotics and hospitalize all infants less than 28 days of age with a temperature greater than 38°C

COMMON PITFALLS

✔ Unfamiliarity with normal newborn behavior and body functions
✔ Failure to include congenital malformations in differential diagnosis
✔ Failure to consider child abuse
✔ Failure to consider inborn errors of metabolism in a sick infant
✔ Failure to assess growth parameters
✔ Failure to appreciate subtle signs and symptoms of serious illness

Acknowledgments

Thanks to the previous edition's chapter authors Michael O. Gayle and Niranjan Kissoon.

References

1. American Academy of Pediatrics. *Neonatal jaundice and kernicterus.* Pediatrics. 2001;108:763–765.
2. American Academy of Pediatrics. *Report of the Committee on Infectious Disease.* Elk Grove Village, Illinois, 2003.
3. Bale JF. Congenital infections. *Neurol Clin* 2002;20:1039–1060.
4. Behrman LJ, Kleigman RM, Arvin AM, eds. *Nelson textbook of pediatrics,* 16th ed. Philadelphia: W.B. Saunders, 2000.
5. Dennery PA, Seidman DS, Stevenson DK. Drug therapy: neonatal hyperbilirubinemia. *New Engl J Med* 2001;344:581–590.
6. Feigen RD, Cherry JD, eds. *Textbook of pediatric infectious diseases,* 2nd ed. Philadelphia, W.B. Saunders, 1987.
7. Fleisher GR, Ludwig S, eds. *Textbook of pediatric emergency medicine,* 4th ed. Philadelphia, Lippincott Williams & Wilkins, 2000.
8. Garcia, EA. Intestinal obstruction in infants and children. *Clin Ped Emerg Med* 2002;3:14–21.
9. Gotoff SP. Group B Streptococcal Infections. *Pediatrics (in review)* 2002;23:381–386.
10. Gunn VL, Nechyba C, eds. *The Johns Hopkins Hospital Harriet Lane Handbook,* 16th ed. Philadelphia, Mosby, 2002.
11. Lerman SE, Laio JC. Neonatal circumcisions. *Pediatr Clin N Am* 2001;48:1539–1557.
12. Levine DL, Carey WB, Crocker AC, Ruth TG, eds. *Developmental-behavioral pediatrics,* 1st ed. Philadelphia: W.B. Saunders, 1983.

13. McCollough M, Sharieff GQ. Common complaints in the first 30 days of life. *Emerg Med Clin North Am* 2002;20:27–48.
14. Okada PJ, Hicks B. Neonatal surgical emergencies. *Clin Ped Emerg Med* 2002; 3:3–13.
15. Park MK, Troxler RG, eds. *Pediatric cardiology for practitioners,* 4th ed. St. Louis, Mosby, 2002.
16. Polin RA, William WF, eds. *Fetal and neonatal physiology,* 2nd ed. Philadelphia: WB Saunders, 1998.
17. Sadler TW. *Langman's medical embriology,* 7th ed. Baltimore: Williams & Wilkins, 1995.
18. Taeusch HW, Ballard RA, eds. *Avery's disease of the newborn,* 7th ed. Philadelphia: WB Saunders, 1998.
19. Tunnessen WW, Roberts KB, eds. *Signs and symptoms in pediatrics,* 3rd ed. Philadelphia: Lippincott Williams & Wilkins, 1999.
20. Zitelli BJ, Davis HW, eds. *Atlas of pediatric physical diagnosis,* 3rd ed. St Louis: Mosby-Wolfe, 1997.

CHAPTER 257

Nursemaid's Elbow

Cynthia C. Hoecker

CLINICAL PRESENTATION

Nursemaid's elbow (radial head subluxation) is a common orthopaedic injury occurring in early childhood. The peak incidence is in the toddler years; however, the condition also occurs in the first year of life and has been described as late as age six (3,5,6). The left arm is more commonly affected, as are females (2,3,6,7).

Many theories have been proposed to explain this condition but the evidence suggests that it is caused by distraction of the radiocapitellar joint in pronation followed by the upward slip of the annular ligament upon the radial head (1). The most commonly described mechanism of injury is that of axial traction on the extended arm usually occurring when an adult pulls up or swings a child by the arm (2,4–6). This pulling mechanism, however, may not be elicited in up to half the cases (4–6). Occasionally the history of a fall may be provided (5).

Children with Nursemaid's elbow present because of disuse of the affected arm and will be noted to hold the arm at their side with the forearm in a pronated position. Because of their young age they are often unable to localize their pain. The examiner often has difficulty detecting any point of tenderness but will note that the child resists and has pain with any movement at the elbow joint. It is important to note that patients with Nursemaid's elbow do not have swelling, warmth or ecchymosis about the elbow. If these findings are present Nursemaid's elbow is unlikely to be the cause.

DIFFERENTIAL DIAGNOSIS

The differential diagnosis of decreased arm use in a child includes, but is not limited to, fractures of the clavicle, humerus or forearm, septic joint, osteomyelitis and brachial plexus injury. The presence of fever, swelling, bruising or other skin changes involving the affected arm is an indication for radiography.

EMERGENCY DEPARTMENT EVALUATION

The history elicited from the caregiver should include the timing and mechanism of injury, the presence of fever and any prior episodes of a similar problem with the arm. Any history of chronic medical conditions predisposing the child to bone or joint disease should also be sought (e.g., hemophilia, sickle cell anemia, osteogenesis imperfecta, immune disorders) as this may indicate another more likely cause of the child's arm pain or disuse.

During examination of the upper extremity, it is often helpful to have the child placed on the parent's lap in a sitting position facing the examiner. Before touching the child, produce a toy or colorful object to see if the child will reach for it with each arm. Visually inspect the arm for any swelling, skin changes or signs of trauma. It may be helpful to compare one arm to the other. Begin with palpation of the bones beginning with the clavicle and working downward towards the hand noting any areas of particular tenderness or warmth. Assess distal pulses and perfusion. Sensation and motor function should also be assessed if the child is able to cooperate with a neurosensory examination. Once it is decided that Nursemaid's elbow is the most likely diagnosis the next step is to attempt a reduction maneuver.

Radiographs should be performed prior to reduction attempts in cases in which aspects of the history (e.g., witnessed direct trauma to the upper extremity) and examination findings (e.g., swelling, bruising, warmth over the joint) suggest that infection or fracture are more likely than radial head subluxation. Patients who present with a history and exam findings consistent with nursemaid's elbow need not undergo radiography prior to reduction attempts. When Nursemaid's elbow is present, radiographs are generally not helpful as abnormal findings are either not present or very subtle in this condition (1). Not uncommonly, a child with a Nursemaid's elbow who is sent for radiographs of the arm will undergo an incidental reduction in the radiology suite during the repositioning of the arm for the study.

EMERGENCY DEPARTMENT MANAGEMENT

There are two different methods commonly used for reducing a Nursemaid's elbow. Prospective studies comparing the two methods reveal that the hyperpronation technique has a significantly higher initial success rate than the supination/flexion technique (2,3). Furthermore, the former method may result in less pain to the patient (3). Both techniques are described in this chapter.

Hyperpronation Technique

The hyperpronation method involves the examiner cradling the child's elbow with one hand (with thumb or forefingers overlying the radial head) while the examiner's other hand is used to hyperpronate the child's forearm by holding and turning the child's hand into a hyperpronated position (Fig. 257.1). With successful reduction a "click" will be felt about the child's elbow by the examiner. The child usually experiences some momentary discomfort during the procedure.

Supination/Flexion Technique

The supination/flexion technique involves the examiner cradling the child's elbow with one hand (again with thumb or forefingers over the radial head) and with the other hand supinating the patient's hand completely until the palm faces

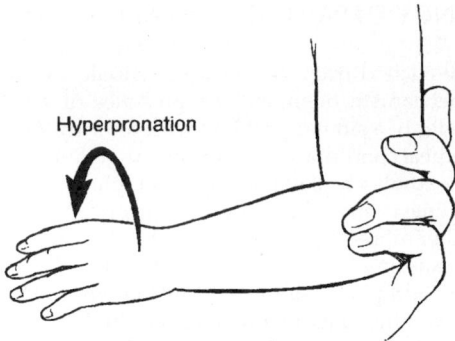

Figure 257.1. Hyperpronation technique. Pronation at the wrist. (From Macias CG, Bothner J, Wiebe R. A comparison of supination/flexion to hyperpronation in the reduction of radial head subluxations. *Pediatrics* 1998;102:e10, with permission.)

the ceiling. The examiner then fully flexes the child's elbow by bringing the supinated hand up toward the shoulder (Fig. 257.2). With successful reduction a "click" will be felt near the elbow. The child usually experiences momentary discomfort at the time of the procedure.

Regardless of which reduction technique is used, it may be as long as 15 minutes before the child begins to use the arm normally again. It is often helpful for the examiner to leave the room following the procedure while the parent distracts the child and encourages use of the arm again. A failed reduction attempt should be followed by a second attempt using either the same or alternate technique. This second attempt often meets with success (2). Following two or three failed reduction attempts radiographs of the upper extremity should be obtained to help exclude fracture or other pathology as the cause of the child's symptoms.

DISPOSITION

The child with a successfully reduced Nursemaid's elbow does not need specific follow up with the primary care giver unless symptoms (pain or disuse of the arm) return. Parents and caregivers should be cautioned about refraining from any activity that involves pulling on the child's arm as the condition recurs

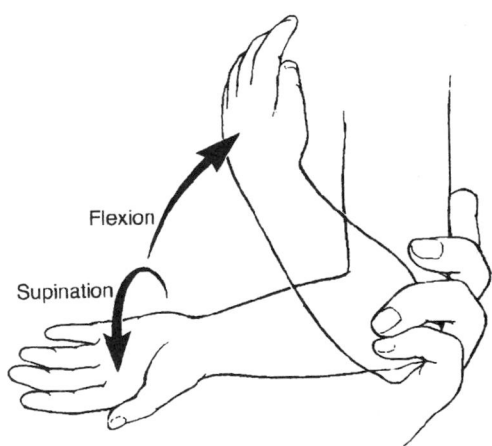

Figure 257.2. Supination/flexion technique. Supination at the wrist followed by flexion at the elbow. (From Macias CG, Bothner J, Wiebe R. A comparison of supination/flexion to hyperpronation in the reduction of radial head subluxations. *Pediatrics* 1998;102:e10, with permission.)

in about a quarter of children who have experienced at least one episode (7).

The patient who does not respond to Nursemaid's elbow reduction attempts will require close primary care follow up and possibly orthopaedic consultation if the cause of the patient's pain and disuse of the arm cannot be determined at the time of the emergency department visit.

COMMON PITFALLS

✔ Do not attempt a nursemaid reduction in any child that has swelling, ecchymosis or deformity of the extremity as these findings are not consistent with a Nursemaid's elbow and manipulation could result in further injury and unnecessary pain to the patient

✔ Do not assume that a patient cannot have a Nursemaid's elbow simply because there is not a clear history of a pull on the child's arm; this history will be lacking in a large percentage of the cases (6)

Acknowledgments

Thanks to the previous edition's chapter author Julide Ayse Ozan.

References

1. Bretland PM. Pulled elbow in childhood. *Br J Radiol* 1994;67:1176–1185.
2. Macias CG, Bothner J, Wiebe R. A comparison of supination/flexion to hyperpronation in the reduction of radial head subluxations. *Pediatrics* 1998;102:e10.
3. McDonald J, Whitelaw C, Goldsmith LJ. Radial head subluxation: Comparing two methods of reduction. *Acad Emerg Med* 1999;6:715–718.
4. Sachetti A, Ramoska EE, Glasgow C. Nonclassic history in children with radial head subluxations. *J Emerg Med* 1990;8:151–153.
5. Schutzman SA, Teach S. Upper-extremity impairment in young children. *Ann Emerg Med* 1995;26:474–479.
6. Shunk JE. Radial head subluxation: epidemiology and treatment of 87 episodes. *Ann Emerg Med* 1990;19:1019–1023.
7. Teach ST, Schutzman SA. Prospective study of recurrent radial head subluxation. *Arch Pediatr Adolesc Med* 1996;150:164–166.

CHAPTER 258
Osgood-Schlatter Disease

Todd Wylie

In 1903, Osgood and Schlatter each described, in separate papers, a disturbance of the tibial tuberosity in adolescents, which came to be known as Osgood-Schlatter disease (11,14). The condition is thought to be a traction apophysitis of the tibial tubercle resulting from repeated normal stresses or overuse (12). Generally, the pathology is considered to be a result of partial avulsion of developing ossification centers and overlying cartilage from the anterior surface of the tibial apophysis (9). Radiologic studies have demonstrated changes in the patellar tendon at the insertion on the tibial tuberosity, suggesting that patellar tendinitis may be a significant source of the clinical symptoms seen in patients with Osgood-Schlatter disease (13). Both Magnetic resonance imaging and ultrasound of the knee have been shown to be superior to plain radiographs in demonstrating soft tissue changes and early stages of disease (2,7). Neither of these studies, however, is necessarily indicated in the emergency department's assessment of Osgood-Schlatter disease.

Patients are usually between 10 to 15 years of age at onset of Osgood-Schlatter disease (9). Boys are affected more often than girls. The condition is usually unilateral, but it may be bilateral in 35% to 56% of boys and approximately 18% of girls (5,8). It is usually a self-limiting condition but should be distinguished from a fracture, tumor, or infection.

CLINICAL PRESENTATION

Osgood-Schlatter disease rarely presents as an acute complaint. The pain may have been present intermittently for a period of time before the patient seeks medical attention. Common complaints include knee pain that is exacerbated by running, kneeling, squatting, and climbing or descending stairs (12). Children almost always point specifically to the tibial tubercle as the site of discomfort. There may also be a history of relief of pain with rest or cessation of strenuous activities.

Physical findings include localized swelling and tenderness over the tibial tuberosity at the site of patellar tendon insertion. Effusion and other abnormalities of the joint should be absent. The pain is reproducible by extending the knee against resistance.

EMERGENCY DEPARTMENT EVALUATION

A reasonably certain diagnosis can be made from the history and physical examination. If Osgood-Schlatter disease is suspected from the history, the diagnosis usually can be confirmed by having the patient sit on the edge of the examination table, hang his or her legs off the table, and point to the site of greatest tenderness. If the patient points to the tibial tubercle, the diagnosis is reasonably certain.

Radiographs are not necessary in all cases of Osgood-Schlatter disease. Radiographs may help confirm the diagnosis but are more helpful in ruling out other disorders, such as fractures and occult bone tumors. Anteroposterior knee radiographs usually appear normal. A lateral knee radiograph is best for demonstrating abnormalities, which may include areas of calcification in the tibial tubercle region, separate ossicles from the anterior border of the tubercle, and prominence of the tubercle (12).

EMERGENCY DEPARTMENT MANAGEMENT

Treatment of Osgood-Schlatter disease is usually symptomatic. Restriction of vigorous activities for 2 to 4 months is recommended, based on the severity of symptoms. Resolution of symptoms may take up to 12 to 18 months (4). Total restriction from all athletic activities is generally not necessary. Stretching exercises for the quadriceps and hamstrings are advisable. Icing after sporting activities and use of nonsteroidal antiinflammatory agents may be helpful. Corticosteroid injections are not recommended and may actually cause complications (15,16). Immobilization is not generally recommended except in severe or persistent cases.

DISPOSITION

Patients with Osgood-Schlatter disease should be referred to their primary care physicians for follow up care. Orthopedic referral may be indicated in persistent or severe cases. Symptoms usually resolve with conservative treatment. In almost all cases, resolution of symptoms is final at skeletal maturity, when the apophysis of the tibial tubercle fuses to the metaphysis of the tibia. Occasional patients develop chronic pain, associated with a discrete ossicle in the patellar tendon. Surgical treatment can provide relief in the majority of these chronic cases (1,6,10).

COMMON PITFALLS

✔ Radiographs may be incorrectly interpreted as an acute fracture
✔ Do not forget to stress the importance of activity restriction to the patient, parents, and the child's school

References

1. Binazzi R. Surgical treatment of unresolved Osgood-Schlatter lesion. *Clin Orthop Rel Res* 1993;289:202.
2. DeFlavis L, Nessi R, Scaglione P, et al. Ultrasonic diagnosis of Osgood-Schlatter and Sinding-Larsen-Johansson diseases of the knee. *Skeletal Radiol* 1989;18:193.
3. Dunn JF. Osgood-Schlatter disease. *Am Fam Physician* 1990;41:173.
4. Duri ZA, Patel DV, Aichroth PM. The Immature Athlete. *Clin Sports Med* 2002;21:461.
5. Ehrenborg G. The Osgood-Schlatter lesion. A clinical and experimental study. *Acta Chir Scand (Suppl)* 1962;288:1.
6. Flowers MJ, Bhadreshwar DR. Tibial tuberosity excision for symptomatic Osgood-Schlatter diseaes. *J Pediatr Orthop* 1995;15:292.
7. Hirano A, Fukubayashi T, Ishii T, Ochiai N. Magnetic resonance imaging of Osgood-Schlatter disease: the course of the disease. *Skeletal Radiol* 2002;31:334.
8. Kujala UM, Kvist M, Heinonen O. Osgood-Schlatter's disease in adolescent athletes. Retrospective study of incidence and duration. *Am J Sports Med* 1985;13:236.
9. Morrissy RT, ed. *Lovell and Winter's pediatric orthopaedics*, 4th ed. Philadelphia: Lippincott–Raven Publishers, 1996.
10. Orava S, Malinen L, Karpakka J, et al. Results of surgical treatment of unresolved Osgood-Schlatter lesion. *Ann Chir Gynaecol* 2000;89:298.
11. Osgood RB. Lesions of the tibial tubercle occurring during adolescence. *Boston Med Surg J* 1903;148:114.
12. Rockwood CA, ed. *Fractures in children*, 4th ed. Philadelphia: Lippincott–Raven Publishers, 1996.
13. Rosenberg ZS, et al. Osgood-Schlatter lesion: fracture or tendinitis? Scintigraphic, CT, and MR imaging features. *Radiology* 1992;185:853.
14. Schlatter C. Veletzungen des schnabelfermigen Fertsatzeo der oberon Tibiaepiphyse. *Bruns Beitr Klin Chir* 1903;38:874.
15. Smith JB. Knee problems in children. *Pediatr Clin North Am* 1986;33:1439.
16. Wojtys EM. Sports injuries in the immature athlete. *Orthop Clin North Am* 1987;18:689.

CHAPTER 259

Pertussis

Roger M. Barkin

Pertussis is a respiratory illness, occurring symptomatically primarily in unprotected infants and children. The risk of disease is highest in children under 5 years of age. Mortality and hospitalization rates are greater in preterm and unimmunized infants younger than 6 months of age (4). Neonatal pertussis is particularly severe with maternal peripartum pertussis as the usual source. The incidence of pertussis has decreased markedly since the institution of the pertussis vaccine. However, the increasing incidence of pertussis in those > 10 years is probably the result of waning immunity (4).

Bordetella pertussis, a gram-negative, pleomorphic bacillus is the causative agent. However, less frequently, a parallel disease can be caused by *Bordetella parapertussis.* The descriptive name of the disease, "whooping cough," is derived from the characteristic sound of the inspiratory effort that follows the paroxysmal coughing. The source of infection is usually an infected older sibling or adult who has mild or asymptomatic infection (4,7). Transmission is by respiratory droplets, with extremely high attack rates (70% to 100%) for susceptible hosts. The incubation period is 6 to 20 days, with a mean of 7 to 10 days (2). During the catarrhal phase, patients are most infectious.

Although immunization reduces the incidence and mortality of pertussis, it is neither complete nor permanent. There is no evidence of a causal relationship between pertussis vaccine and brain damage (1). Natural immunity to pertussis could be lifelong although many believe that this is waning as well (5,6). In patients 12 years after vaccination, 95% of the vaccinees are susceptible to pertussis (9). Susceptible hospital staff can acquire the infection easily, and although most of these infections are mild. they serve to maintain immunity following these subclinical episodes.

CLINICAL PRESENTATION

The clinical manifestation of pertussis depends on age and previous immunization or infection. The classic illness, which lasts for 6 to 10 weeks, occurs as a primary infection in unimmunized children and is generally divided into three stages: catarrhal, paroxysmal, and convalescent. The course of the disease may be atypical (10).

The **catarrhal stage** is characterized by rhinorrhea, lacrimation, mild cough, and low-grade or no fever. This stage lasts 1 to 2 weeks, and the diagnosis is usually not suspected, yet patients are most contagious in this stage.

In the **paroxysmal stage,** episodes of coughing increase in severity and number. A characteristic repetitive series of six to 12 forceful coughs during a single expiration is followed by a sudden, massive inspiratory effort that produces the classic whoop as air is inhaled forcefully against a narrow glottis. Cyanosis, bulging eyes, protrusion of the tongue, salivation, lacrimation, and distention of the neck veins may occur during episodes of coughing. The paroxysms are frequently precipitated by a variety of events, such as feeding, crying, or even hearing another person cough.

Physical examination during this stage may reveal conjunctival hemorrhages and petechiae over the neck and head. Some patients can have diffuse rhonchi and rales on auscultation. In very young infants, the paroxysm and whoop are often absent. Infants usually present with choking spells, apnea, bradycardia, cyanosis, and unresponsiveness. The majority of fatal cases occur in infancy. Infants who were victims of "sudden infant death syndrome" may have positive tests for *B. pertussis.*

In the **convalescent stage,** which usually lasts 1 to 2 weeks, but can persist for up to 6 to 10 weeks, symptoms gradually abate, but the cough may persist for several months.

Complications of pertussis include otitis media, seizures, pneumonia, encephalopathy (risk, 1: 12,000), and death. Pneumonia, seizures and encephalopathy occurred in 22%, 2% and < 0.5%, respectively, in infants under 12 months of age with pertussis. The case fatality rate is 1% in those under 2 months of age and < 0.5% in infants 2 to 11 months of age. Premature infants are at especially increased risk for severe disease. Pneumonia can be due to *B. pertussis* or to secondary bacterial infection. Apnea may be a serious complication, commonly in children under 6 months of age. Other complications include interstitial or subcutaneous emphysema, atelectasis, ulcer of the tongue frenulum, epistaxis, melena, subdural hematoma, rectal prolapse, syndrome of inappropriate antidiuretic hormone secretion, and nutritional disturbances.

DIFFERENTIAL DIAGNOSIS

In classic disease, the clinical diagnosis of pertussis can be made without difficulty. Other infectious agents that cause similar illness include *Mycoplasma pneumoniae, Chlamydia trachomatis, Chlamydia pneumoniae,* adenoviruses, respiratory synctical virus and other respiratory viruses. *B. parapertussis* and *B. bronchiseptica* occasionally produce a pertussis-like syndrome.

Spasmodic attacks of coughing may be observed in infants and children with bronchiolitis, bacterial pneumonia, cystic fibrosis, tuberculosis, an airway foreign body, and other diseases that cause lymphadenopathy and extrinsic compression of the trachea and bronchi. This can also occur in patients with sinusitis.

Difficulty in recognizing pertussis occurs in the catarrhal stage, in mild illness, and in adults or very young infants. Pertussis should be included in the differential diagnosis of infants presenting with choking or apneic episodes and in children who present with a history of severe, spasmodic coughing or posttussive emesis.

EMERGENCY DEPARTMENT EVALUATION

A child or infant suspected to have pertussis should be observed for signs and symptoms of respiratory distress. Paroxysmal coughing episodes should be documented. These attacks may be triggered by eating, drinking, yawning, sneezing, or other physical activities. Between attacks, patients may appear normal and are usually in no distress. It is important to remember that young infants require hospitalization and close observation, in spite of looking well in between paroxysms.

Evaluation of the white blood cell count may be helpful. Leukocytosis of 20,000 to 60,000 cells/mL with an absolute lymphocytosis is characteristic in severe disease. The degree of elevation of the white blood cell count reflects the severity of the cough.

Nasopharyngeal secretion culture remains the gold standard for diagnosis. Dacron (polyethylene terephthalate) or calcium alginate swabs are used to collect the specimen. A selective medium such as Bordet-Gengou should be rapidly inoculated (within 1 to 2 hours) for optimal isolation of the organism. Recovery of *B. pertussis* from nasopharyngeal secretions is highest during the catarrhal stage. Direct immunofluorescent assay (DFA) of nasopharyngeal secretions has a low sensitivity and a variable specificity, and is not reliable for laboratory confirmation (2,7). Culture confirmation is usually appropriate. In the interim following a positive DFA, DNA amplification methods such as polymerase chain reaction assay (PCR) is sensitive and rapid if available. Chest radiograph findings are nonspecific and may include perihilar infiltrate, atelectasis, a "shaggy" heart border or emphysema.

EMERGENCY DEPARTMENT MANAGEMENT

Treatment is mostly supportive and can be managed at home for older children and those with mild disease. Young infants or children with severe disease require hospitalization, and often admission to an intensive care unit, for close observation.

In the emergency department (ED), if the patients are unable to handle the mucoid secretions, they should be placed in a head-down position (45 to 60 degrees) to take advantage of gravity. Suction of the oropharynx with a catheter large enough to permit flow of tenacious secretions is required during paroxysms. In a severely ill child, oxygen may be needed. Hydration must be monitored and maintained, as well as caloric intake. Apneic infants may require active airway and ventilation management. Children less than 6 months of age are more likely to be hospitalized, tend to have longer hospitalization, and are more likely to require intensive care monitoring.

The paroxysmal coughing episodes may prove to be exhausting, and avoidance of factors that provoke such attacks may be helpful. Patients with severe paroxysms should be monitored to ensure early recognition of hypoxia or bradycardia. Corticosteroids and albuterol may reduce the frequency and severity of symptoms, but before they can be recommended, further studies are required to establish their safety and efficacy. Maintenance of hydration and nutritional status is of utmost importance for optimal recovery, especially in infants with severe disease or posttussive vomiting.

Antimicrobial agents, if given early during the course of illness, may ameliorate the symptoms. However, once paroxysmal coughing is established, antibiotics have no discernible effect on the course of illness, but they are recommended to limit the spread of the organism to other susceptible individuals. Nasopharyngeal cultures usually test negative for *B. pertussis* within 5 days after beginning therapy.

The first choice for treatment is oral erythromycin. The dosage for children is 40 to 50 mg/kg/d, given every 6 hours (maximum, 2 g/d) for 7 to 14 days to prevent bacteriologic relapse (7). Azithromycin dihydrate 10 to 12 mg/kg/d in 1 dose for 5 days, or clarithromycin 15 to 20 mg/kg/d in two divided doses (maximum, 1 g/d), are likely to be effective and are thus alternatives for patients who cannot tolerate erythromycin. Erythromycin has been associated with infantile hypertrophic pyloric stenosis when administered to children younger than 2 months of age. Trimethoprim-sulfamethoxazole (8/40 mg/kg/d in two divided doses) is an acceptable alternative.

In addition to standard precautions, droplet precautions are recommended for 5 days after initiation of effective antimicrobial therapy. Chemoprophylaxis with erythromycin, 40 to 50 mg/kg/d, given every 6 hours (maximum, 2 g/d) for 14 days, is recommended for all household contacts, irrespective of age and immunization status (2). Clarithromycin and azithromycin may be alternatives if erythromycin is not tolerated. Close contacts who are less than 7 years of age who are unimmunized or received less than 4 doses of pertussis vaccine should have pertussis immunization initiated or continued.

DISPOSITION

Patients with severe disease and those younger than 6 months of age with significant clinical evidence of pertussis should generally be hospitalized because of the high rate of complications in this age group. The immunization history of siblings should always be reviewed. Older children and those with milder forms of illness may be discharged home after appropriate evaluation and initiation of antimicrobials. Parents should be instructed to call if breathing difficulties occur, there is any evidence of cyanosis, restlessness or if sleeplessness develops, fluid intake decreases, or medicines are not tolerated.

COMMON PITFALLS

- ✔ Failure to recognize and diagnose pertussis, especially when presenting in an atypical fashion
- ✔ Assuming that infants younger than 6 months of age will have a benign illness
- ✔ Failure to administer chemoprophylaxis to contacts
- ✔ Incorrect specimen collection and delay in plating secretions on appropriate media
- ✔ Failure to diagnosis pertussis in adolescents who present with an aura of suffocation followed by coughing episodes
- ✔ Failure to know that there is no effective transplacental immunity

Acknowledgments

The author gratefully acknowledges the contributions of Samier Midani and Hanif Kamal, who wrote the previous version of this chapter.

References

1. American Academy of Pediatrics. Committee on Infectious Diseases. The relationship between pertussis vaccine and brain damage. *Pediatrics* 1991;88:397–400.
2. American Academy of Pediatrics. Pertussis. In: Pickering LK ed. *2003 Red book: report of the Committee on Infectious Diseases*, 26th ed. Elk Grove Village, IL: American Academy of Pediatrics, 2003.
3. Beiter A, Lewis K, et al. Unrecognized maternal peripartum pertussis with subsequent fatal neonatal pertussis. *Obstet Gynecol* 1993;82:691–693.
4. Center for Disease Control and Prevention, Pertussis – United States, 1997–2000. *MMWR Morb Mortal Wkly Rep*, 2002;51:73–76.
5. Cherry JD. The science and fiction of "resurgence" of pertussis. *Pediatrics* 2003;112:405–406.
6. Cherry JD. Epidemological, clinical and laboratory aspects of pertussis in adults. *Clin Infect Dis* 1999;28:S112–S117.
7. Friedman RL. Pertussis: the disease and new diagnostic methods. *Clin Microbiol Rev* 1998;1:365–376.
8. Halperin SA, Bartoluss R, Langley JM, et al. Seven days of erythomycin estolate is as effective as fourteen days for the treatment of *Bordetella pertussis* infection. *Pediatrics* 1997;100:65.
9. Lambert HJ. Epidemiology of small pertussis outbreak in Kent County, Michigan. *Publ Health Rep* 1992S;80:365–339.
10. Yaari E, Yafe-Zimerman Y, Schwartz SB, et al. Clinical manifestations of *Bordetella pertussis* infection in immunized children and young adults. *Chest* 1999;115:1254.

CHAPTER 260
Pharyngitis and Rheumatic Fever

Martha S. Wright

Sore throat is a common chief complaint among pediatric patients presenting to the emergency department (ED). Most of these children will have acute pharyngitis. Many infectious agents cause acute inflammation of the tonsils and pharynx, including Epstein-Barr virus (EBV), adenovirus, parainfluenza virus, group A and other β-hemolytic streptococci, and *Mycoplasma pneumoniae* (3,4,8). Nonbacterial agents are the cause of pharyngitis in 70% to 85% of patients, especially in adolescents and in children less than 2 years of age (3).

The most important agent for diagnostic, treatment, and public health considerations remains group A, β-hemolytic *Streptococcus* (GABHS) (3,4). As a result, the clinician's primary goal is to identify those cases of acute pharyngitis that are caused by GABHS. While pharyngeal infection with most other common organisms will resolve without intervention, infection with GABHS can lead to suppurative complications, including peritonsillar and retropharyngeal abscesses, otitis media, mastoiditis and cervical adenitis, as well as the nonsuppurative complication of acute rheumatic fever (ARF), if inadequately treated. Acute rheumatic fever continues to be the leading cause of acquired valvular heart disease in the world (14) and is especially prevalent in the developing world. Although the incidence of ARF has declined dramatically in the United States during the past half century, regional outbreaks among American children in the 1980s and 1990s (10,21) serve as reminders to clinicians of the need for appropriate diagnosis and treatment of GABHS pharyngitis, as well as familiarity with the clinical presentation of ARF.

ACUTE PHARYNGITIS

CLINICAL PRESENTATION

Most children with acute pharyngitis present with one or more subjective complaints in addition to sore throat. Those with GABHS infection typically report the sudden onset of throat pain associated with fever, headache, abdominal pain, and/or vomiting (3,4). On physical examination, patients with streptococcal pharyngitis usually have pharyngeal erythema, patchy tonsillar exudate, palatal petechiae and tender anterior cervical adenopathy (3,4,17). If the infection is caused by a toxin-producing GABHS strain, a fine, diffusely papular erythroderma ("sandpaper" or scarlatiniform rash) may be present. While there is considerable overlap between the findings in children with GABHS and those with other etiologies, diarrhea or upper respiratory symptoms such as hoarseness, rhinorrhea and cough and physical findings of conjunctivitis or discrete ulcers in the posterior pharynx are more suggestive of viral causes (4). The exception is for toddlers with GABHS infection, in whom copious, purulent rhinorrhea is common and pharyngeal exudates are rare (3,17).

DIFFERENTIAL DIAGNOSIS

While the diagnosis of acute pharyngitis is readily made from historical and physical exam findings, the challenge for the clinician is in differentiating GABHS pharyngitis from other etiologies and in recognizing associated complications. Although patients infected with GABHS often have more significant pharyngeal inflammation, prominent exudates and tender anterior cervical lymphadenopathy than those patients with viral etiologies, these findings are not reliably predictive. Numerous studies have demonstrated that clinicians can differentiate GABHS from non-GABHS pharyngitis with only 50% to 75% accuracy (22). There are certain signs or symptoms that may be more suggestive of nonstreptococcal causes (3). *Mycoplasma* often presents with a history of prolonged cough or pneumonia/bronchitis. Ebstein-Barr virus may present with extreme fatigue, significant pharyngeal exudate, or an enlarged spleen (see chapter on mononucleosis). Adenoviral pharyngitis is typically accompanied by nonpurulent conjunctivitis and preauricular adenopathy. Coxsackie pharyngitis is associated with the discrete posterior pharyngeal ulcers of herpangina. Parainfluenza virus causes croup or laryngitis in older children.

Acute pharyngitis may be accompanied by more serious infectious entities, such as peritonsillar, parapharyngeal and retropharyngeal abscesses. Clinically, patients with deep tissue abscesses secondary to bacterial pharyngitis are ill-appearing, highly febrile and have localized pain. A patient with a peritonsillar abscess will present with trismus, a muffled ("hot potato") voice, and unilateral swelling of the soft palate with deviation of the uvula. Parapharyngeal abscesses are frequently associated with tender, unilateral neck swelling on the side of the abscess. Younger children with acute pharyngitis may develop retropharyngeal lymphadenitis that can suppurate into the retropharyngeal space. The diagnosis of retropharyngeal abscess should be considered in a toxic-appearing toddler with dysphagia, drooling, airway obstruction, and pain with neck movement.

EMERGENCY DEPARTMENT EVALUATION

In the ED, the pediatric patient with pharyngitis should initially be evaluated for conditions that require acute intervention. These include airway compromise, pain, and dehydration. Edematous tonsils may cause upper airway obstruction, resulting in respiratory distress or sleep apnea. Often, children refuse to drink because of pain and can become significantly dehydrated. Secondarily, the patient should be evaluated for suppurative complications and for the presence or absence of GABHS as the etiology of the acute symptoms. If a deep tissue abscess is suspected, a computed tomography scan of the neck with intravenous contrast can confirm the diagnosis as well as assess the airway for compromise and localize the pus collection for possible surgical intervention.

The patient should be evaluated for GABHS using a rapid antigen detection test, if available. Rapid antigen detection tests (RADTs) provide quick and highly specific identification of the GABHS antigen and have been shown to increase appropriate care of patients with GABHS pharyngitis in the emergency department (12). In contrast to diagnostic recommendations for adults with sore throat, a confirmatory culture should be performed in children and adolescents with a negative RADT because of the higher pediatric incidence of streptococcal infection and ARF (4). False-Negative RADTs are usually related to inadequate tonsillar or pharyngeal secretions on the specimen swab. To minimize false-negative results, the specimen should be obtained from the posterior pharynx and tonsillar pillars (1).

EMERGENCY DEPARTMENT MANAGEMENT

In the symptomatic pediatric patient with pharyngitis, a variety of acute interventions may be necessary. For airway obstruction secondary to enlarged tonsils, a nasopharyngeal airway should restore airway patency. Intravenous fluid resuscitation and analgesics may be used to treat acute dehydration and pain. Most often, routine analgesics such as acetaminophen or ibuprofen in association with cold fluids will provide adequate comfort. Older children may use over-the-counter analgesic throat sprays. There is debate in the literature regarding the efficacy of dexamethasone for pain relief in children with acute pharyngitis (5).

If GABHS is identified as the responsible organism by laboratory testing, antibiotic therapy is indicated. Therapy can be postponed up to 9 days from initial symptoms and still safely prevent both suppurative and nonsuppurative sequelae, such as ARF, so empiric therapy is not recommended (1,3). Penicillin, an inexpensive drug with a narrow spectrum of activity and proven efficacy and safety, remains the drug of choice for GABHS initial therapy (1,3,4). A 10 day course of oral penicillin V is recommended at 400,000 U (250 mg) 2 to 3 times daily for children weighing less than or equal to 27 kg (60 lb) or 800,000 U (500 mg) for those who weigh more. In patients that may not complete a 10-day course, benzathine penicillin G, 600,000 U intramuscularly should be given to children less than 27 kg (60 lb) and 1.2 million U in larger children (1,4). Use of amoxicillin for 10 days at the doses described above is equivalent to penicillin and as it is more palatable in suspension may improve compliance.

In penicillin-allergic patients, erythromycin ethylsuccinate (40 mg/kg/d) or erythromycin estolate (20 to 40 mg/kg/d) in 2 to 4 divided doses for 10 days is recommended (1,4), although GABHS resistance to macrolides has recently been reported (16). An alternative for penicillin-allergic patients who do not have immediate hypersensitivity-type reactions to penicillin is a 10 day course of a first generation cephalosporin such as cefadroxil or cephalexin (1). While there are now a number of once-daily and short course antibiotic regimens that have been FDA approved for treatment of streptococcal pharyngitis, these regimens use unnecessarily broad-spectrum antibiotics, have not been rigorously studied and are not cost effective when compared to penicillin (4).

DISPOSITION

Most children with pharyngitis can be evaluated and managed as outpatients. For patients with airway obstruction or deep tissue abscesses, admission to monitored settings is recommended. Patients with abscesses should additionally be evaluated by an otolaryngologist to assess the need for surgical drainage. Admission should also be considered for those children who continue to refuse oral intake after rehydration.

ACUTE RHEUMATIC FEVER

CLINICAL PRESENTATION

Acute rheumatic fever is a multisystem, postinfectious inflammatory disorder that follows an acute GABHS pharyngeal infection. While the pathogenic mechanisms underlying the development of ARF are incompletely understood, it appears that certain rheumatogenic strains of GABHS display antigens that are similar to those found in myosin (19). During infection with one of these streptococcal strains, host antibodies are produced that attack both the bacterial organism as well as human myosin, valvular endothelium and other host proteins.

ARF occurs most commonly in school-aged children and adolescents. The characteristic febrile illness typically develops 2 to 4 weeks after an acute GABHS pharyngitis and is associated with one or more of the following symptoms: arthritis, carditis, rash, subcutaneous nodules and/or chorea. Often patients with symptoms suggestive of ARF may not recall a recent sore throat, so the clinician must have a high index of suspicion for the condition based on the clinical findings (21).

Arthritis is the most common and often earliest manifestation of ARF (2,18). Classically described as a "migratory polyarthritis," multiple larger joints, such as knees, ankles, and wrists develop painful swelling, warmth and erythema. As the onset of individual joint involvement is variable, the arthritis appears to "migrate" from one joint to another. The joint findings are self-limited, resolving spontaneously within 2 to 4 weeks if untreated. The typical pattern of migration may not be observed in those patients who have been treated with antiinflammatory medications, as the joint symptoms typically resolve within a day or two after the beginning of therapy.

Carditis is the second most common manifestation and may present clinically with signs and symptoms of pericarditis, myocarditis and/or valvulitis (18). The initial physical findings may be as subtle as mild tachycardia or chest pain or the patient may exhibit more suggestive findings such as a pericardial friction rub or a new or changing murmur, usually from mitral regurgitation (20). Heart failure is an exceedingly rare initial presentation.

The other characteristic signs of ARF include subcutaneous nodules, erythema marginatum and Sydenham chorea (2,11,18). Subcutaneous nodules are firm, painless lumps over bony prominences and extensor surfaces near tendons. They are most often seen in patients with carditis. Subcutaneous nodules resolve spontaneously, usually within a week of presentation. The classic rash of ARF, erythema marginatum, is described as an evanescent, nonpruritic, reddish-pink eruption with an irregular, "serpiginous" border. Erythema marginatum is most often found on the trunk and is also seen primarily in patients with carditis. Chorea is an uncommon manifestation of ARF, present in only 10% of rheumatic fever patients, most commonly in girls (15). It may occur in isolation of other signs of ARF and is presumably due to deposition of autoantibodies in the basal ganglia. Chorea is characterized by involuntary, tic-like and purposeless movements of the extremities and face. Gait and speech disturbances may result. Muscular weakness, especially of the hands, can result in a characteristic finding known as the "milking sign" in which the patient's grip relaxes and tightens in a nonrhythmic fashion. Emotional lability and other psychiatric disturbances like obsessive-compulsive disorder, depression and anxiety may accompany the disordered movements or may be the only symptoms (15). In contrast to the other manifestations of ARF, chorea is a late finding and may not present for several months after the initial pharyngitis.

DIFFERENTIAL DIAGNOSIS

Acute rheumatic fever should be considered in the differential diagnosis of any febrile child with acute arthritis or a new or changing heart murmur. Making the diagnosis can be a challenge, however, as there is no definitive laboratory test to confirm the diagnosis and it shares common characteristics with a number of pediatric disease entities. Other etiologies of acute pediatric arthritis include primarily rheumatologic and infectious causes. Rheumatologic conditions such as systemic onset juvenile rheumatoid arthritis (JRA) may resemble ARF on initial presentation, as fever, rash and arthritis are common characteristics. While polyarticular JRA involves multiple joints, these are often small joints in the hand. Patients with pauciarticular JRA will manifest arthritis in 4 or fewer large joints but the pattern of involvement is symmetric and nonmigratory. In all forms of JRA, the joint pain tends to be less severe than that of ARF, but lasts longer and does not respond as quickly to antiinflammatory therapy. Systemic lupus erythematosus may present with arthritis but other aspects of the illness typically differentiate it from ARF. Henoch-Schönlein purpura may rarely present with isolated arthritis, the development of the purpuric rash on the lower extremities confirms the diagnosis.

Infectious causes of pediatric arthritis include septic arthritis which tends to be monoarticular and accompanied by high fever. Arthritis can accompany a number of viral infections including rubella, mumps, mononucleosis, varicella and Hepatitis A and B. Lyme disease may mimic ARF as the characteristic rash, erythema chronicum migrans, may be mistaken for erythema marginatum. The associated signs and symptoms that accompany these systemic infections often easily differentiate these conditions. The same is true for Kawasaki disease, which has diagnostic criteria that may partially overlap those of ARF, and inflammatory bowel disease which may present in up to 20% of cases with acute arthritis. Finally, reactive arthritis may follow a number of infectious diseases including those caused by streptococci, staphylococci, gonococci, salmonella, shigella, brucella, yersinia and Campylobacter. Acute poststreptococcal reactive arthritis (PSRA) is a particularly perplexing entity. There is significant controversy in the literature as to whether this condition, which usually follows an acute streptococcal infection by 1 to 2 weeks and is associated with an arthritis that is not particularly responsive to antiinflammatory medication, is actually a variant of ARF, requiring the same prophylactic interventions as classic ARF (2,18).

In the child with a new or changing murmur or new-onset heart failure, bacterial endocarditis, infectious myocarditis, pericarditis, or cardiomyopathy should be considered (see Chapter 240, "Congenital Heart Disease, Congestive Heart Failure, and Other Cardiac Presentations"). The most common cause of acquired chorea in children is ARF, although it has been reported in children taking methylphenidate, phenothiazines, amphetamines, antihistamines, phenytoin and lithium.

EMERGENCY DEPARTMENT EVALUATION

In a patient with evidence of a preceding streptococcal infection, the presence of two major criteria or one major and two minor criteria as first described by Jones in 1944 (11) is adequate to make the diagnosis of ARF (Table 260.1) (2). The validity of the Jones criteria has recently been reconfirmed (2,7). The major criteria include the clinical entities described above. The minor criteria include fever > 39°C, arthralgias (which cannot be applied if the patient has arthritis), elevated acute phase-reactants such as C-reactive protein (CRP) and/or erythrocyte sedimentation rate (ESR) and a prolonged PR interval on electrocardiogram. While there are no confirmatory laboratory tests, laboratory findings can be used to support the diagnosis as well as to rule out other entities.

Evidence of recent streptococcal pharyngitis is a diagnostic requirement. This may be ascertained by a positive throat culture or RADT, or an elevated streptococcal antibody titer. Most patients with ARF will not have a positive throat culture or RADT as the disease occurs several weeks after the acute pharyngitis so elevation of antistreptolysin-O (ASO), anti-DNAse B, anti-DNAse or antihyaluronidase antibodies is most commonly used to document a prior infection.

TABLE 260.1. The Jones Criteria

Two major or one major and two minor criteria plus evidence of a prior streptococcal infection* indicate a high probability of an initial attack of acute rheumatic fever

MAJOR

Carditis
Arthritis
Chorea
Subcutaneous nodules
Erythema marginatum

MINOR

Clinical Findings
Arthralgia
Fever

Laboratory Findings
Elevated acute-phase reactants
　Erythrocyte sedimentation rate
　C-reactive protein
Prolonged PR interval

PLUS

Supporting evidence of antecedent group A streptococcal infection
　Positive throat culture or rapid streptococcal antibody titer
　Elevated or rising streptococcal antibody titer

　*Note: Chorea may be used as the sole diagnostic criteria for the diagnosis of ARF. Evidence of preceding streptococcal infection is not required in this circumstance.
　(Adapted from American Heart Association. Guidelines for the diagnosis of rheumatic fever. Jones criteria, 1992 update. JAMA 1992;268(15):2069–2073.)

Adjunctive tests may include a chest x-ray to evaluate heart size and echocardiography, which can be used to confirm the presence and severity of valvulitis (9,20). An electrocardiogram should be performed in any patient with concern for ARF to evaluate the patient for conduction abnormalities that may be associated with pancarditis. Obtaining a complete blood count, blood culture, ANA, complement levels and/or rheumatoid factor may be useful to rule out other diseases. Aspiration of joint fluid is not indicated unless the alternative diagnostic concern is septic arthritis.

EMERGENCY DEPARTMENT MANAGEMENT

In the ED, the focus for patients with ARF is on recognition, diagnostic evaluation, treatment of streptococcal pharyngitis and assurance of appropriate follow up. In exceedingly rare cases a pediatric patient may require acute intervention for heart failure, severe arthritis or chorea.

When the diagnosis of ARF is made in the ED, treatment for GABHS pharyngitis, using the regimens described above (1,4), is indicated even if the RADT is negative. The mainstay of treatment for carditis and arthritis is high-dose aspirin at doses of 80 to 100 mg/kg/day (18). While patients with moderate to severe carditis are often treated with corticosteroids or intravenous immunoglobulin, there is no evidence in the literature that these modalities improve outcome over aspirin therapy alone (6). Nonsteroidal antiinflammatory drugs (NSAIDs) are an alternative treatment for arthritis. Treatment of Sydenham chorea may require haloperidol, valproic acid, or carbamazepine (15).

All patients diagnosed with ARF require antibiotic prophylaxis following their acute course of antibiotic treatment. Current prophylactic regimens for patients with ARF include Penicillin

V 250 mg twice a day, benzathine penicillin G 1.2 million units every 3 to 4 weeks or sulfadiazine 500 mg for children < 27 kg and 1000 mg for children > 27 kg once per day (1). Prophylaxis should be continued until the patient is at least 21 years old (1), although many experts recommend continuing prophylaxis for life (18).

CRITICAL INTERVENTIONS

> **Acute Pharyngitis and Acute Rheumatic Fever**
> - Assess and manage airway patency, hydration status, and pain
> - Always look closely (even in the uncooperative child) for oropharyngeal abcesses
> - Diagnose and treat GABHS pharyngitis with appropriate antibiotics
> - Consider ARF in the diagnosis of any febrile school-aged child with arthritis or a new or changing heart murmur

DISPOSITION

Most patients with ARF are now managed as outpatients with the severity of carditis or arthritis determining need for admission (13). Follow up with the child's primary care physician should be assured so that salicylate therapy can be monitored, prophylaxis ensured and evaluation of family members for GABHS be performed. For patients with severe carditis or heart failure, cardiology consultation and admission to an intensive care setting is indicated. If the diagnosis of chorea is unclear or the patient is severely symptomatic, neurology consultation will be helpful in clarifying the evaluation and treatment options.

COMMON PITFALLS

Acute Pharyngitis

✔ Do not treat nonbacterial pharyngitis with antibiotics
✔ Do obtain an adequate throat swab for RADT or culture to prevent false negative results
✔ Do send a confirmatory throat culture if RADT is negative
✔ Do not forget to evaluate and document the airway examination

Acute Rheumatic Fever

✔ Do consider the diagnosis of ARF even in the absence of a history of pharyngitis
✔ Do perform a thorough physical examination on any pediatric patient with arthritis looking for other major or minor criteria for ARF
✔ Do consider chorea in the differential diagnosis of emotional lability

Acknowledgments

Thanks to the previous edition's chapter authors Karen Camasso-Richardson, Robert D. Schremmer and Jane F. Knapp.

References

1. American Academy of Pediatrics. Group A streptococcal infections. In: Pickering LK, ed. The Red Book: *2003 Report of the Committee on Infectious Diseases. 26th ed.* Elk Grove Village, IL: American Academy of Pediatrics, 2003:573–584.
2. American Heart Association. Guidelines for the diagnosis of rheumatic fever. Jones criteria, 1992 update. *JAMA* 1992;268:2069–2073.
3. Bisno AL. Acute pharyngitis. *N Engl J Med* 2001;344:205–211.
4. Bisno AL, Gerber MA, Gwaltney JM, Kaplan EL, Schwartz RH. Practice guidelines for the diagnosis and management of Group A Streptococcal pharyngitis. *Clin Infect Dis* 2002;35:113–125.
5. Bulloch B, Kabani A, Tenenbein M. Oral dexamethasone for the treatment of pain in children with acute pharyngitis: a randomized, double-blind, placebo-controlled trial. *Ann Emerg Med* 2003;41:601–608.
6. Cillers AM, Manyemba J, Saloojee HJ. Anti-inflammatory treatment for carditis in acute rheumatic fever (Cochrane Methodology Review). In: The Cochrane Library, Issue 4, 2003. Chichester, UK: John Wiley and Sons, Ltd.
7. Ferrieri P and the Jones Criteria Working Group. Proceedings of the Jones criteria workshop. *Circulation* 2002;106:2521–2523.
8. Glezen WP, Clyde WA, Senior RJ, Sheaffer CI, Denny FW. Group A streptococci, mycoplasmas and viruses associated with acute pharyngitis. *JAMA* 1976;202:119–124.
9. Hilario MO, Andrade JL, Gasparian AB, et al. The value of echocardiography in the diagnosis and followup of rheumatic carditis in children and adolescents: a 2 year prospective study. *J Rheumatol* 2000;27:1082–1086.
10. Hoffman TM, Rhodes LA, Pyles LA, et al. Childhood acute rheumatic fever: comparison of recent resurgence areas to cases in West Virginia. *WV Med J* 1997;93:260–263.
11. Jones TD. The diagnosis of rheumatic fever. *JAMA* 1944;126:481–484.
12. Lieu TA, Fleisher GR, Schwartz JS. Clinical evaluation of a latex agglutination test for streptococcal pharyngitis: performance and impact on treatment rates. *Pediatr Infect Dis J* 1988;7:847–854.
13. Loeffler AM, et al. Identification of cases of acute rheumatic fever managed on an outpatient basis. *Pediatr Infect Dis J* 1995;14:975–978.
14. Marcus RH, Sareli P, Pocock WA, Barlow JB. The spectrum of severe rheumatic mitral valve disease in a developing country. Correlations among clinical presentation, surgical pathologic findings, and hemodynamic sequelae. *Ann Intern Med* 1994;120:177–183.
15. Marques-Dias, MJ, Mercandante MT, Tucker D, Lombroso P. Sydenham's chorea. *Psychiatr Clin North Am* 1997;20:809–820.
16. Martin JM, Green M, Barbadora KA, Wald ER. Erythromycin-resistant group A streptococci in schoolchildren in Pittsburgh. *N Engl J Med* 2002;346:1200–1206.
17. Schwartz RH. Pharyngeal findings of group A streptococcal pharyngitis. *Arch Pediatr Adolesc Med* 1998;152:927–928.
18. Stollerman GH. Rheumatic fever. *Lancet* 1997;349:935–942.
19. Van de Rijn I, Zabriske JB, McCarty M. Group A streptococcal antigens cross-reactive with myocardium: purification of heart-reactive antibody and isolation and characterization of the streptococcal antigen. *J Exp Med* 1977;146:579–599.
20. Vasan RS, Shrivastava S, Vijayakumar M, et al. Echocardiographic evaluation of patients with acute rheumatic fever and rheumatic carditis. *Circulation* 1996;94:73–82.
21. Veasy LG, Wiedmeier SE, Orsmond GS, et al. Resurgence of acute rheumatic fever in the intermountain area of the United States. *N Engl J Med* 1987;316:421–427.
22. Wald ER, Green MD, Schwartz B, Barbadora K. A streptococcal score card revisited. *Pediatr Emerg Care* 1998;14:109–111.

CHAPTER 261
Pneumonia

Ian McCaslin

Pneumonia is an inflammatory process of the pulmonary parenchyma that results from infection in the outpatient setting, typically caused by bacteria, including *Mycoplasma pneumoniae*, by viruses, and by *Chlamydia* spp. Although mortality rates from childhood pneumonia in the United States have declined markedly over the past half century, acute lower respiratory tract infections are a major cause of morbidity and mortality in children worldwide, killing an estimated 4 million children each year (6). Respiratory tract infections are common in children, with attack rates for lower tract pathogens ranging from 2.2 to 4.7 infections/100 children/year in studies from Chapel Hill (5) and Seattle (7). Younger children tend to have higher attack rates for pneumonia, with the peak incidence in the first year of life, diminishing progressively with age through adolescence.

Low socioeconomic status, poor nutrition, underlying disease, crowded living conditions, and smoke exposure have all been implicated in increased risk of pneumonia. Children who are immunocompromised for a variety of reasons, including malignancy, sickle cell disease, HIV, and genetic disorders demonstrate a particularly increased risk. Seasonal epidemics of respiratory illness are familiar to practicing physicians. In particular, late fall and winter peaks of lower respiratory illness due to viruses such as respiratory syncytial virus (RSV) and influenza tend to predominate, whereas pneumonia caused by bacteria exhibit less marked seasonal variation.

PATHOGENESIS AND ETIOLOGY

Transmission of viral agents of lower respiratory disease is generally accomplished by means of droplet spread between close contacts, often within household, school, or day care settings. After inoculation, replication of virus and direct extension into the lower respiratory tract ensue, causing loss of the ciliated epithelium, mucus production, and migration of mononuclear cells at the site of tissue damage. The accumulation of dead cells and inflammatory exudate lead to narrowing of terminal airways, expiratory obstruction, air trapping, and atelectasis.

Bacterial pneumonia occurs when the lung tissue is invaded by an aspirated pathogen. The normal upper respiratory tract barriers that screen, filter, engulf, and kill bacteria are presumably neutralized by recent viral infection, but firm evidence for this theory is lacking. Infection results in an acute inflammatory response characterized by neutrophil and macrophage infiltration, exudation of edema fluid, and deposition of fibrin, all of which result in diminished air flow and gas exchange.

Pneumonia may be divided into bacterial and other etiologies (i.e., viruses, fungi, or parasites), but in the majority of cases a microbiologic agent is not identified. Children do not produce sufficient sputum to obtain an adequate sample for culture, differentiation of infection from colonization is problematic, and nasopharyngeal culture is rarely useful in cases of presumed bacterial pathogen. Most infections do not produce enough pleural fluid from which to obtain an organism, and neither pleural biopsy nor needle aspiration are recommended in the outpatient management of community-acquired pneumonia. Rapid, reliable diagnostic methods are rarely available to the practicing physician. Thus the emergency provider must base decision-making on likely etiology based upon such factors as age, clinical setting, and season of presentation.

Large prospective studies performed on ambulatory children with community-acquired pneumonia in Finland (9) and Dallas (24) using combinations of serology, culture, and PCR have identified an etiologic agent in from 43% to 66% of patients. Regardless of age and severity, *Streptococcus pneumoniae* was responsible for 25% to 30% of cases, followed by viruses (20%–25%), *Mycoplasma pneumoniae* (7%–22%), and *Chlamydia pneumoniae* (6%–14%). The most common viral agent was RSV, and evidence of coinfection of *S. pneumoniae* with RSV was common, particularly in younger children. Rates of mixed infection of *S. pneumoniae* with either *M. pneumoniae* or *C. pneumoniae* were relatively frequent in older children, suggesting that the historical classification of clinical pneumonia into "typical" and "atypical" categories should be discouraged. Since infections with *C. pneumoniae* are often subclinical, its role as a primary lower respiratory tract pathogen has been questioned (8,15,16); however, evidence of its presence in children with radiographically proven pneumonia has been demonstrated (3).

Overall, both the Finland and Dallas studies confirmed the importance of *S. pneumoniae* as the primary agent responsible for the majority of cases of bacterial pneumonia across all age groups beyond the newborn period. Viruses cause relatively more disease in younger infants and children, and mycoplasmal and chlamydial infections become more prevalent in the school-aged population. In newborns and infants Group B *Streptococcus* and gram-negative enteric bacilli, such as *E. coli*, can cause severe infections, including sepsis and meningitis, in addition to pneumonia. Invasive disease caused by *Haemophilus influenzae* type b has been virtually eliminated following introduction of a conjugate vaccine.

Staphylococcus aureus causes abrupt and severe disease, primarily in infants and young children, immunocompromised hosts, and following influenzal infections, but is rarely encountered. *Mycobacterium tuberculosis* may cause pneumonia in healthy children, and presents with findings similar to bacterial disease. Nontypable *H. influenzae, Moraxella catarrhalis, Bordetella pertussis*, and even *Neisseria meningitidis* occasionally can cause pneumonia. Anaerobic bacteria may be implicated in a host who is susceptible to aspiration, particularly if there is evidence of abscess formation. *Legionella* spp. and the hantaviruses cause serious disease more frequently in adults than children. Preliminary data from Toronto suggest that severe acute respiratory syndrome (SARS) is a relatively mild and nonspecific respiratory illness in previously healthy young children, whereas adolescents may present with the more severe illness characteristic of adults (2).

Pneumonia in the immunocompromised host is often caused by common viral and bacterial pathogens but may also be caused by opportunistic organisms. Children with agamma- or hypogammaglobulinemia are susceptible to repeated bacterial pneumonias and may develop bronchiectasis. These children are also at risk for infections with *Aspergillus* or *P. carinii*. Children with cancer and chemotherapy-induced neutropenia or anergy and decreased T-cell lymphocyte function are also susceptible to viral pneumonias due to cytomegalovirus (CMV), herpesvirus and varicella-zoster. Fungal infections with Candida may also occur. Children with lymphomas are susceptible to infections with *Toxoplasma gondii* and *Cryptococcus neoformans*. In children with the acquired immunodeficiency syndrome (AIDS), pneumonia may be caused by *P. carinii*, CMV, and mycobacteria in addition to typical bacterial organisms.

CLINICAL PRESENTATION

Symptoms and signs of pneumonia in children vary with age, duration of illness, and underlying condition rather than by bacterial vs. viral etiology. Many children with early pneumonia do not have specific respiratory complaints and do not appear particularly ill. The "classic" presentation of sudden onset of fever, chills, chest pain, and productive cough is very rare. In fact, studies have shown that febrile children ultimately found to have pneumonia often present with nonspecific findings on both history and physical examination (1,16,20). Infants under 2 months of age may present with fever and tachypnea and no signs of pulmonary consolidation, or with findings consistent with sepsis. Young children usually are found to exhibit some combination of fever, tachypnea, rales and/or wheezes following a chief complaint of cough, URI symptoms, decreased activity, and poor intake (10). The majority of older children demonstrate a short period of prodromal symptoms, including rhinitis, low-grade fever, decreased appetite, and decreased activity. The proportion of cases of pneumonia due to *M. pneumoniae* and *C. pneumoniae* increases in children after 5 years of age (3,9,24), and wheezing with crackles rather than signs of consolidation are more often noted on examination. Cases of bacterial pneumonia which present with abdominal pain, vomiting, and dehydration may be mistaken for acute appendicitis.

Few findings on physical examination exhibit uniform inter-observer reliability. Fever, respiratory rate, and pulse oximetry are objective, reproducible parameters that help guide examiners in the clinical diagnosis of pneumonia. Virtually all children with either bacterial or viral pneumonia exhibit some fever by history or examination (21,23). The World Health Organization has developed guidelines based primarily upon the presence of tachypnea and retractions (17), but the low specificity of these findings limits their applicability in patients with asthma or during bronchiolitis season. Definition of tachypnea varies with age and conservatively is suggested with a respiratory rate > 60 per minute in infants, a rate of > 40 per minute in toddlers, and a rate > 25 per minute in older children. The majority of infants and young children with pneumonia will demonstrate tachypnea on careful examination. The presence of hypoxemia can be difficult to detect on physical examination alone (14); pulse oximetry is a noninvasive means of demonstrating diminished arterial oxygenation, defined as saturation less than 92%.

Certain combinations of clinical findings are characteristic of more complicated lower respiratory tract disease. Grunting respirations with fever are nonspecific but should prompt further investigation. Rales, retractions, and localized diminished breath sounds are highly correlated with parenchymal disease. Presence of an associated pleural effusion is suggested by unilateral decreased breath sounds and dullness to percussion.

DIFFERENTIAL DIAGNOSIS

Other conditions that may be mistaken for community-acquired pneumonia should be considered. Lower respiratory illness characterized by cough, rhinitis, fever, and either wheezing or dry crackles on examination of children less than two years of age is characteristic of bronchiolitis. Caused principally by RSV, bronchiolitis is not improved with antibiotics, and can run a protracted course over 1 to 2 weeks. More severe disease can present with cyanosis and signs of respiratory failure, particularly in infants with underlying medical conditions such as congenital heart disease. Reactive airways disease affects nearly 10% of children, and acute episodes of difficulty breathing and cough, particularly at night, are commonly triggered by viral respiratory infections. Many children with acute exacerbations of underlying asthma or reactive airways disease are diagnosed with pneumonia and treated with antibiotics rather than bronchodilators and steroids. A past history of similar recurrent episodes suggestive of reactive airways disease should be carefully sought.

Primary tuberculosis (TB) pneumonia is more common in urban or lower socioeconomic areas, in recent immigrants to the United States, and in children exposed to contacts with TB. Usual findings of pneumonia are common, with lobar consolidation, frequently hilar adenopathy and, less frequently, cavitary lesions or pleural effusion. PPD placement should be considered for all patients with newly diagnosed pneumonia. The pertussis syndrome (whooping cough), caused principally by *Bordetella pertussis*, is an infection of the lower respiratory tract characterized by upper respiratory symptoms progressing to prolonged paroxysms of cough which can result in hypoxemia, cyanosis, and respiratory compromise. Findings on examination are nonspecific, the breath sounds are usually clear, and vital signs are normal between paroxysms. The diagnosis is suggested clinically, and patients should be treated empirically while awaiting laboratory confirmation. Careful consideration should be given to hospitalization in a monitored setting for all children less than 1 year of age with suspected pertussis (see Chapter 259, "Pertussis").

Foreign-body aspiration, gastroesophageal reflux with aspiration, congenital heart disease, hydrocarbon aspiration, and other conditions may be mistaken for infectious pneumonia in the outpatient setting. History of a choking episode should be sought in all young children presenting with suspected pneumonia. Congenital heart disease is suggested by evidence of either diminished peripheral perfusion or congestive heart failure on examination. Depending upon the specific defect, cardiomegaly on chest radiography or diminished pulse oximetry readings that do not respond to oxygen administration is often supportive of the diagnosis. Diagnosis of hydrocarbon aspiration is normally made by history and clinical findings. Tachypnea, high fever, oxygen requirement, and pulmonary consolidation are predictive of significant exposure and need for hospitalization. Cystic fibrosis should be considered in the child with recurrent pneumonia associated with chronic diarrhea and failure to thrive.

EMERGENCY DEPARTMENT EVALUATION

The emergency physician will usually suspect the diagnosis of pneumonia based upon the history and physical examination alone. A chest radiograph is not required but is often helpful in establishing the diagnosis and excluding noninfectious concerns. Specific patterns of findings can guide the clinician in appropriate treatment and subsequent management. While extreme dehydration or early illness may produce a falsely negative study, a normal chest radiograph provides reassurance that acute bacterial pneumonia is unlikely to be the source of fever. Empiric radiographs obtained for a "rule/out sepsis" evaluation of the highly febrile child with no obvious source on examination and an elevated WBC count will frequently reveal an occult infiltrate (1).

Chest radiography is not helpful in establishing the specific etiology of pneumonia in children (24). Diffuse peribronchial thickening with hyperinflation of the lungs from air trapping is, however, more consistent with bronchiolitis and a viral etiology in the younger child, whereas focal lobar consolidation and pleural effusion in the older child would suggest *S. pneumoniae* or less likely *M. pneumoniae* (Fig. 261.1). Decubitus chest radiography is particularly useful in identification of complications associated with pneumococcal pneumonia, including pleural effusion, empyema, necrosis, and lung abscess. These more complicated cases are occurring with increasing frequency, particularly in white children more than 5 years of age (22).

Both blood culture and CBC with differential should be obtained for the hospitalized patient, but are not routinely indicated in the outpatient management of pneumonia. Blood cultures are

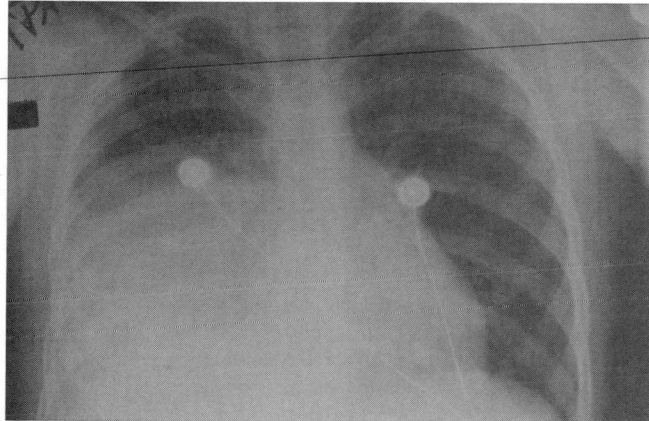

Figure 261.1. Right lower lobe infiltrate with moderate pleural effusion in a child with fever, cough, and localized decreased breath sounds found to have pneumococcal pneumonia. *(Courtesy of John Kanegaye)*

SECTION XXI PEDIATRICS

very rarely positive (11,12), and management of pneumococcal pneumonia is not altered by demonstration of the organism in the bloodstream. The CBC does not reliably differentiate the specific etiology of pneumonia, although bacterial disease is suggested by a peripheral WBC of > 20,000/mm^3. Likewise, neither specific therapy nor consideration for admission is generally aided by knowledge of the peripheral WBC at time of presentation (21,24). Thoracentesis for analysis and culture of pleural effusion should be reserved for ill-appearing children who require critical care admission, immunocompromised children, and in cases where chest tube drainage is under consideration for suspected empyema or abscess. From the perspective of the emergency physician, diagnostic techniques such as serology, antigen assay, PCR, and nasopharyngeal swab for culture can be considered investigational and of little benefit in clinical decision-making in the outpatient setting (15,16,19).

EMERGENCY DEPARTMENT MANAGEMENT

After careful history and physical examination and judicious use of radiography and laboratory, the emergency physician's primary tasks are to initiate necessary therapy and determine the need for hospitalization. Ill-appearing patients should be placed on continuous cardiorespiratory monitoring while in the ED. Significantly dehydrated or vomiting patients with pneumonia should be given a saline fluid bolus of 20 cc/kg intravenously. Initial pulse oximetry readings of < 92% on room air or ill clinical appearance prompt oxygen administration by non-rebreather mask until response to therapy can be determined. Many children with a large pleural effusion or an underlying medical condition will require supplemental oxygen for several days. A trial of bronchodilator aerosols and steroids may be considered for patients with associated wheezing or history of reactive airways, but antitussives are contraindicated.

Infants below three months of age with pneumonia should be treated intravenously in the hospital with both ampicillin (50 mg/kg) and cefotaxime (50 mg/kg) after cultures of blood, urine, and CSF are obtained. For older patients requiring hospitalization, parenteral antibiotic therapy may be initiated with cefuroxime (50 mg/kg, maximum 3 gm) or ceftriaxone (50 mg/kg, maximum 2 gm) (4,18). These recommendations apply despite reports of increasing rates of antibiotic resistance for isolates of *S. pneumoniae* in the United States (13); however, emergency providers should maintain awareness of regional antimicrobial susceptibility reports.

CRITICAL INTERVENTIONS

- Early pulse oximetry determination, and oxygen supplementation if < 92%
- Intravenous fluids for significant dehydration or persistent vomiting
- Chest radiography
- Consideration of parenteral antibiotics

DISPOSITION

Most children with pneumonia can be managed as outpatients. Antibiotic therapy is not indicated for the patient with suspected bronchiolitis or if findings are consistent with viral syndrome. Sudden onset of high fever and signs of pneumonia after several days of nonspecific viral illness may represent bacterial superinfection and likely warrant antibiotics. Preschool patients and infants beyond three months of age with suspected pneumonia

may be treated with high dose Amoxicillin (80–100 mg/kg/day divided tid) (4). High dose Amoxicillin/clavulanate (Amoxicillin component 80–100 mg/kg/day divided tid) is another option. In penicillin-allergic patients and for school age children where *M. pneumoniae* and perhaps *C. pneumoniae* are possible etiologic agents, macrolides including azithromycin (10 mg/kg initial single dose followed by 5 mg/kg daily as a single dose for 4 days) or erythromycin (40 mg/kg/day divided qid) represent acceptable options. Children who appear more ill or for whom fluid intake is a concern may be given parenteral ceftriaxone (50 mg/kg as a single dose) for coverage of the initial 24 hours of therapy (4).

Printed language-appropriate discharge instructions should be reviewed with caretakers prior to discharge from the ED. Attention to adequate hydration, fever control, medication compliance, and observation for worsening condition should be emphasized. The emergency physician may wish to communicate directly with the primary care provider prior to patient discharge. All children diagnosed with pneumonia in the emergency department should be re-evaluated within 24 hours. Fever often persists for 48 hours into the course of treatment of bacterial pneumonia (21).

Indications for admission include: age < 3 months, respiratory compromise, persistent oxygen requirement, inability to retain oral fluids or medication, concerning underlying medical condition, and uncertain home environment. Patients with immune compromise, large pleural effusion, respiratory distress, or concerning blood gas findings should be admitted to an intensive care unit or transferred to a facility where appropriate monitoring and critical intervention is ensured.

COMMON PITFALLS

✔ Failure to obtain pulse oximetry in respiratory illness despite "well" clinical appearance
✔ Missing a patient with foreign-body aspiration or congenital heart disease
✔ Treating for pneumonia instead of reactive airway disease in the young wheezing child
✔ Failure to ensure understanding of discharge instructions, including follow up in 24 hrs

References

1. Bachur R, Perry H, Harper MB. Occult pneumonias: empiric chest radiographs in febrile children with leukocytosis. *Ann Emerg Med* 1999;33:166–173.
2. Bitnun A, Allen U, Heurter H, et al. Children hospitalized with severe acute respiratory syndrome-related illness in Toronto. *Pediatrics* 2003;112:e261–268.
3. Block S, Hedrick J, Hammerschlag MR, Cassell GH, Craft JC. *Mycoplasma pneumoniae* and *Chlamydia pneumoniae* in pediatric community-acquired pneumonia: comparative efficacy and safety of clarithromycin vs. erythromycin ethylsuccinate. *Pediatr Infect Dis J* 1995;14:471–477.
4. Bradley JS. Management of community-acquired pediatric pneumonia in an era of increasing antibiotic resistance and conjugate vaccines. *Pediatr Infect Dis J* 2002;21:592–598.
5. Denny FW, Clyde WA. Acute lower respiratory tract infections in nonhospitalized children. *J Pediatr* 1986;108:635–646.
6. Dowell SF, Kupronis BA, Zell ER, Shay DK. Mortality from pneumonia in children in the United States, 1939 through 1996. *N Engl J Med* 2000;342(19):1399–1407.
7. Foy HM, Cooney MK, Maletzky AJ, Grayston JT. Incidence and etiology of pneumonia, croup, and bronchiolitis in pre-school children belonging to a pre-paid medical care group over a four-year period. *Am J Epidemiol* 1973;97:80–92.
8. Hammerschlag MR. Pneumonia due to *Chlamydia pneumoniae* in children: epidemiology, diagnosis, and treatment. *Pediatr Pulmonol* 2003;36:384–390.
9. Heiskanen-Kosma T, Korppi M, Jokinen C, et al. Etiology of childhood pneumonia: serologic results of a prospective, population-based study. *Pediatr Infect Dis J* 1998;17:986–991.
10. Jadavji T, Law B, Lebel MH, et al. A practical guide for the diagnosis and treatment of pediatric pneumonia. *Can Med Assoc J* 1997;156(suppl):S703–711.
11. Hickey RW, Bowman MJ, Smith GA. Utility of blood cultures in pediatric patients found to have pneumonia in the emergency department. *Ann Emerg Med* 1996;27:721–725.

12. Juven T, Mertsola J, Waris M, et al. Etiology of community-acquired pneumonia in 254 hospitalized children. *Pediatr Infect Dis J* 2000;19:293–298.

13. Kaplan SL, Mason EO, Barson WJ, et al. Outcome of invasive infections outside the central nervous system caused by *Streptococcus pneumoniae* isolates nonsusceptible to ceftriaxone in children treated with beta-lactam antibiotics. *Pediatr Infect Dis J* 2001;20:392–396.

14. Maneker AJ, Petrack EM, Krug SE. Contribution of routine pulse oximetry to evaluation and management of patients with respiratory illness in a pediatric emergency department. *Ann Emerg Med* 1995;25:36–40.

15. McCracken GH. Etiology and treatment of pneumonia. *Pediatr Infect Dis J* 2000; 19:373–377.

16. McIntosh K. Community-acquired pneumonia in children. *N Engl J Med* 2002; 346:429–437.

17. Mulholland EK, Simoes EA, Costales MO, McGrath EJ, Manalac EM, Gove S. Standardized diagnosis of pneumonia in developing countries. *Pediatr Infect Dis J* 1992;11:77–81.

18. Nelson JD. Community-acquired pneumonia in children: guidelines for treatment. *Pediatr Infect Dis J* 2000;19:251–253.

19. Neuman MI, Harper MB. Rapid antigen assay for the diagnosis of pneumococcal bacteremia in children: a preliminary study. *Ann Emerg Med* 2002;40:399–404.

20. Rothrock SG, Green SM, Fanelli J, Cruzen E, Costanzo KA, Pagane J. Do published guidelines predict pneumonia in children presenting to an urban ED? *Pediatr Emerg Care* 2002;17:240–243.

21. Tan TQ, Mason EO, Barson WJ, et al. Clinical characteristics and outcome of children with pneumonia attributable to penicillin-susceptible and penicillin-nonsusceptible *Streptococcus pneumoniae*. *Pediatrics* 1998;102:1369–1375.

22. Tan TQ, Mason EO, Wald ER, et al. Clinical characteristics of children with complicated pneumonia caused by *Streptococcus pneumoniae*. *Pediatrics* 2002;110:1–6.

23. Waites KB. New concepts of *Mycoplasma pneumoniae* infections in children. *Pediatr Pulmonol* 2003;36:267–278.

24. Wubbel L, Muniz L, Ahmed A, et al. Etiology and treatment of community-acquired pneumonia in ambulatory children. *Pediatr Infect Dis J* 1999;18:98–104.

CHAPTER 262
Psychosocial and Behavioral Emergencies

Cynthia Jacobstein and Jill M. Baren

Mental health disorders in children have become a significant health problem. It is estimated that 1 of every 5 children in the United States between the ages of 9 and 17 years have a "diagnosable mental or addictive disorder" with at least some small impairment (15). While the mental health needs of children are quite large, there are many barriers to accessing mental health services for pediatric patients. These barriers include lack of insurance, insufficient numbers of caregivers who specialize in the care of children with mental health problems, the stigma that accompanies mental health disorders, and a mental health delivery system with suboptimal structure to provide necessary care (14,16).

The most recent epidemiologic data indicate that over a 6-year period from 1993 to 1999 over 3 million ED pediatric mental health visits were made with an annual average of approximately 400,000 patients (15). Depressive disorders, anxiety and unspecified neurotic disorders were the 3 most common groups of diagnoses. Although visits increased on the whole, ED visits made for suicide attempts, self-injury, and psychoses remained constant over this time interval suggesting that the ED has become a site for the evaluation of nonlife threatening mental health problems

as well. The highest visit rate was from adolescents, with females utilizing the ED more commonly than males. Children younger than 6 years of age had the lowest visit rates.

CLINICAL PRESENTATION

Depression/Suicidality

Emergency physicians should be skilled at recognizing the signs and symptoms of depression/suicidality, as it is the leading serious cause for an ED visit. Depression is defined as a chronic, recurrent, familial illness that frequently presents in childhood or adolescence (4). Although sadness is often a predominant feature, children may manifest other signs such as irritability, boredom, anhedonia, or mood swings. Suicide is very closely associated with depression and there are multiple risk factors for suicide, which have been published extensively but may not be that useful for any given individual patient (1,4,14). Depression is often initially diagnosed and treated by primary care as well as psychiatric physicians, but emergency physicians may also be the first to suspect the disorder. When depression/suicidality is suspected, the initial step in management is to establish a contract for safety with the patient. This is often referred to as the "no-suicide contract." Inability to establish this automatically indicates the need for further consultation with a mental health consultant and possibly admission to a psychiatric facility.

Anxiety/Obsessive Compulsive Disorder/Post Traumatic Stress Disorder

Anxiety disorders, such as panic disorder, separation anxiety, phobias, posttraumatic stress, or obsessive-compulsive disorder, are the most prevalent type of mental health disease in children and adolescents (17). A complete discussion of all of these disorders is beyond the scope of this chapter (see Chapter 122). However, there are a few important points regarding this group of mental health disorders that the emergency physician should keep in mind when evaluating pediatric patients for possible anxiety complaints. Patients with anxiety often have comorbid mental health issues, including the coexistence of depression. One important risk factor for the completion of suicide is the presence of "significant anxiety" (17). Thus, it is essential for the emergency physician to screen for depression and suicidality when a patient presents with an anxiety-related complaint. Anxiety in children is often manifested by nonspecific physical complaints. Therefore, the history related to such complaints must be extremely thorough in order to separate organic disease from anxiety-related disorders.

Neurobehavioral

There are numerous visits to the ED by children with known neurobehavioral disorders such as attention-deficit hyperactivity disorder (ADHD). In general, the management of these disorders occurs in the outpatient setting but it is important for the emergency physician to have some knowledge of potential complications associated with these disorders. Children with ADHD are frequently prescribed medications for the treatment of this disorder. As with almost all medications, the potential for adverse effects exists with ADHD medications, and the emergency physician should have easy access to this information in order to best evaluate patients. For example, use of stimulant medications for ADHD can lead to loss of appetite and weight loss. A controversial problem associated with stimulant medication is that of rebound- the increase of symptoms of ADHD when the stimulant medication is wearing off (9). Thus, it is vital to get a detailed history related to the timing of medication and onset of worsening symptoms. Other potential problems include noncompliance with stimulant medications or abuse of medications for the purpose of weight loss, to experience euphoria, or selling or trading them to others (9). Children with ADHD or other behavioral disorders often present to the ED for routine emergency complaints. Their underlying disorder(s) or baseline medications may complicate evaluation, medical management, sedation, or therapeutic options.

DIFFERENTIAL DIAGNOSIS

When considering the potential etiologies of a pediatric mental health emergency, emergency physicians must recognize that many medical disorders can present as acute behavioral disturbances. For example, acute delirium from an intracranial lesion or a metabolic disturbance can be confused with an acute psychiatric disorder; acute drug withdrawal presenting as acute delirium can be missed when a history of drug abuse is unobtainable. The differential diagnosis of medical disorders that present with psychiatric symptoms in children is extensive and includes illnesses in every disease category. Symptoms that are often part of the presentation of chronic medical diseases, such as infectious mononucleosis and Lyme disease, may mimic depression (7). Patients with these disorders may present with changes in sleep and eating patterns. Other diagnoses that have been confused with psychiatric disorders in children include: head injury, epilepsy, endocrinopathies, autoimmune diseases, medication use (steroids, birth control pills), drug overdose, abuse and neglect, and sepsis.

When differentiating between organic and psychiatric etiologies of psychosis, the following factors are helpful but not absolute in establishing the underlying cause. New onset of symptoms (no previous psychiatric history), sudden onset of symptoms, altered level of conscious, abnormal vital signs, abnormal neurologic examination, and abnormal physical examination all support an organic etiology (11).

EMERGENCY DEPARTMENT EVALUATION

The history is perhaps the most critical portion of the ED encounter when dealing with a pediatric mental health problem. Some authors have referred to the concept of gathering "collateral" information (10). Children, especially younger ones, are usually unable to provide a clear history of past and current problems so the ED physician must rely on information from other people in the child's environment. Key informants are individuals such as parents, siblings, other relatives, teachers, youth leaders, social workers, and other health care providers. While many of these individuals may not be available at the time of the ED encounter, every effort should be made to obtain such information, via telephone or by using another staff member or mental health consultant.

A standard medical history should be performed and in addition questions should explore the circumstances for the ED visit (escalation of a behavioral problem, threat to self or others, change in affect or school performance). Questions should be directed at the patient if appropriate, and the caretaker, affording privacy. While it would probably not be appropriate to separate a 5-year old from his/her parents, a 15-year old should be interviewed with extreme attention to privacy and confidentiality. A detailed medication and substance use history is also important. If a patient is already prescribed a psychotropic medication, it is important to inquire about compliance and side effects, as issues surrounding medication use may prompt many ED mental

TABLE 262.1.	Components of the Psychosocial Assessment of Adolescents
HEADSS	**SHADSSS**
Home	**S**chool
Education	**H**ome
Activities	**A**ctivities
Drug use and abuse	**D**epression/self-esteem
Sexual behavior	**S**ubstance abuse
Suicidality and depression	**S**exuality
	Safety

health visits. Physical examination may be focused for the vast majority of mental health complaints. However, when a toxicologic problem is suspected or when potential injury is an inciting factor for the visit, a complete physical examination is recommended. ED physicians should be aware that many organic etiologies can easily be mistaken for psychiatric illness; therefore especially with the first presentation of psychiatric symptoms, organic etiologies must be considered.

Adolescents are a special group of patients who, in addition to a general medical history, require a thorough psychosocial assessment particularly when evaluating a mental health complaint. Several structured approaches have been widely accepted as a template for gathering information on all aspects of teenage life (5,6). The areas to cover are contained in one of two mnemonics HEADSS or SHADSSS. The components of these mnemonics are detailed in Table 262.1 and include home life, school activities, extracurricular activities, sexuality, substance use, suicidality, depression, and safety issues. The structured interview progresses from the least sensitive topics to the most sensitive in order to give the patient an opportunity to become more comfortable in the discussion (5,6). Prior to the start of the psychosocial interview, it is imperative that the emergency physician clarifies when confidentiality will be upheld and when it could be breached (possibility of harm to patient or others or in circumstances where abuse is occurring) (12).

Although an abbreviated form of the psychosocial assessment may be performed if the ED complaint does not appear relevant, the majority of encounters with adolescents and mental health issues will require this approach. In particular, substance abuse is often a comorbid condition with underlying psychiatric disease and the only mechanism for obtaining this information is through a detailed psychosocial assessment (3,4,7,14). Other important information such as the existence of firearms in the home or sexual orientation issues could also be revealed in this manner. Both of these have been linked to the diseases of suicidality and depression (1,4,14,17).

A team approach to the ED evaluation of pediatric mental health disorders is considered optimal. Physicians, nurses, social workers, child life personnel, ED technicians, security personnel, and mental health consultants all play a role in establishing an effective evaluation, treatment plan, and safe disposition. However, it is recognized that many EDs will not have these comprehensive resources. It is recommended that if pediatric specific mental health resources are not available at a particular location, that EDs have already established referral patterns and a mechanism for transfer and/or hospitalization. Other potential resources for families with children with mental health needs include primary care physicians, the school system, clergy, support groups and community-based mental health centers.

The ED evaluation of mental health complaints must be tailored to the specific problem. In some instances, no laboratory or radiologic imaging will be required such as in the case of a patient with a known history of depression and an exacerbation of suicidal thoughts but no actions. In contrast, any patient without a well-delineated history of mental health disease, any patient with change in mental status not otherwise accounted for by psychiatric disease, or any patient with generalized medical or traumatic complaints, should undergo a complete evaluation. For the undifferentiated patient, laboratory and radiologic evaluation might include: CBC, electrolytes, BUN and creatinine, fingerstick glucose, urine HCG in females, head CT, lumbar puncture, ECG, CXR, liver function tests, ammonia level, thyroid function tests, and other serologic tests such as ANA. The signs and symptoms of the individual patient determine the degree of testing. In addition, acetaminophen and salicylate levels should be obtained on all patients with suspected or admitted ingestion. Testing for alcohols and other substances can be left to the discretion of the emergency physician.

Serum and urine toxicologic screens are often a focus of testing in the ED. Specific agents included on available hospital laboratory screens will differ by location and ED physicians must be aware of these local variations. A general approach in children is to obtain a drug screen to confirm or document a reported ingestion or substance exposure. Many inpatient psychiatric facilities will require such testing prior to admission. It is worth noting that drug testing should never be forced upon a patient simply for parental or caretaker request. There should be a definite medical or psychiatric indication for doing so (12). Often parental requests for drug testing stem from a more serious communication problem with the child and that should become the focus of the ED evaluation instead (12). The American Academy of Pediatrics has a policy statement that supports this practice (3).

EMERGENCY DEPARTMENT MANAGEMENT

The ED management of pediatric mental health disorders varies according to the specific disorder. The ED physician's role is one of advocacy and protection and usually involves ruling out organic disease as discussed above and deciding on the need for consultation and the need for transfer as a potential disposition. Rarely in the ED will medication be needed except in cases of extreme agitation. Psychoses are exceedingly rare in childhood. If psychosis is suspected, an exhaustive medical evaluation should be performed first, to exclude organic causes.

In the setting of acute psychiatric or behavioral crisis, the need to provide for safety of patients and caregivers and to the limit disruption to the care of others is paramount. Although rarely necessary in children, physical and chemical restraints are important elements of safety and often complement each other. A show of force may elicit cooperation from a disruptive, violent child, but if restraints become necessary, appropriate policies and procedures must be followed.

The AAP statement on the use of physical restraints calls for documentation of the reasons for use of restraint, specific orders (verbal or written) with attempt to define time limits of use, assessment that restraints are being used properly (not causing physical harm to patient) with close monitoring, and for possible release from restraints when acute crisis has abated and safety can be assured (2). The practice of patient restraint is carefully regulated by the Joint Commission for Accreditation of Health Care Organizations (JCAHO). It emphasizes that physical and chemical restraint must be used as a last resort when other methods to control the patient have failed. JCAHO also requires that each health care facility have a written policy and procedure in place to ensure appropriate use (13).

Chemical restraint may be needed when a patients continues to be agitated while in physical restraints. Some patients may vol-

TABLE 262.2. Medications for Control of Acute Agitation

	Pediatric Dose	Route	Interval
Lorazepam	0.05 0.1 mg/kg (max 2 mg)	PO/IM/IV	Q 4–8 hrs
Haloperidol (> 12 years)	2–5 mg 1–15 mg	IM PO	Q 1 hr prn Q 1 hr prn
Diphenhydramine	1.25 mg/kg	PO/IM/IV	Q 6 hrs

untarily take medications to avoid physical restraint. In children, the most commonly used medications for chemical restraint are benzodiazepines and butyrophenones (8). These drugs are useful in the control of agitated behavior and have a long duration of action. An alternative sedative is diphenhydramine, which can cause paradoxical excitement (8) (Table 262.2).

CRITICAL INTERVENTIONS

- Perform an exhaustive medical evaluation first to exclude organic causes before making the diagnosis of psychosis
- Consider depression in children who present with a change in their behavior
- Question adolescents with privacy and confidentiality
- Document the reason for restraints

DISPOSITION

In patients who are considered to be at immediate risk for suicide, one to one observation by an ED staff member should be initiated and maintained throughout the ED stay. All pediatric patients who are actively suicidal should have consultation with a mental health provider. Patients with a clear plan of suicidal intent are considered very high risk. The safest course of action in these cases is hospitalization. If hospitalization is recommended by either the emergency physician or mental health consultant, it is preferred that the parent/patient consent to admission. Rarely will caretakers refuse this treatment plan, as they are often the reason that the patient was brought to the ED in the first place. In cases when the patient is a mature minor and refuses hospitalization, an involuntary commitment order may need to be applied if the patient is considered to be at risk for harm to self or others. An emergency physician or mental health physician is authorized to apply such a commitment. The specifics of involuntary commitments vary from state to state.

Depressed patients who are not considered high risk, have responsible caretakers, and establish a contract for safety, may be discharged with urgent outpatient follow up. Emergency physicians should take extra precautions to insure that this follow up is prearranged at the time the patient leaves the ED and that an alternative plan is in place if follow up fails (i.e., primary care visit, return to the ED).

COMMON PITFALLS

✔ Depression can often masquerade as nonspecific somatic complaints. Studies have shown that many depressed and suicidal patients have visited a physician shortly before attempting suicide. Any nonspecific complaint in a child or adolescent that does not seem to have a rational basis should be aggressively explored for the possibility of depression/suicide. Use of the psychosocial assessment structured interviews may help uncover risk factors and precipitating factors for depression/suicide

✔ When making a disposition on a pediatric patient with depression, current or past suicidal ideation or attempt, inquire about the presence of firearms in the home or access to firearms in general. Presence of firearms in the home is considered a highly lethal risk factor for completion of suicide. Parents and caretakers should be counseled to remove firearms from the home under these circumstances

✔ Emergency physicians should establish a verbal or written contract for safety with pediatric patients who are suicidal at the outset of the ED encounter and again prior to disposition. This may also be done for patients undergoing an evaluation for behavioral disturbances, particularly aggression

✔ Many medical conditions have presenting symptoms that may mimic psychiatric disorders. Specifically, metabolic, infectious, and toxicologic problems may present with acute mental status changes. The ED approach to a patient with an acute change in behavior should assume an organic etiology particularly in the case of a first episode or in a younger patient and in the absence of a known psychiatric or behavioral disorder

References

1. American Academy of Pediatrics, Committee on Adolescence. Suicide and suicide attempts in adolescents. *Pediatrics* 2000;105:871–874.
2. American Academy of Pediatrics, Committee on Pediatric Emergency Medicine. The use of physical restraint interventions for children and adolescents in the acute care setting. *Pediatrics* 1997;99:497–498.
3. American Academy of Pediatrics, Committee on Substance Abuse. Testing for drugs of abuse in children and adolescents. *Pediatrics* 1996;98:305–307.
4. Brent DA, Birmaher B. Adolescent depression. *N Engl J Med* 2002;347:667–671.
5. Clark LR, Ginsburg KR. How to talk to your teenage patients. *Contemp Adol Gynecol* 1995;Winter:23–27.
6. Cohen E, Mackenzie RG, Yates GL. HEADSS–a psychosocial risk assessment instrument: Implications for designing effective intervention programs for runaway youth. *J Adol Health* 1991;12:539–544.
7. Elliott GR, Smiga S. Depression in the child and adolescent. *Pediatr Clin North Am* 2003;50:1093–1106.
8. Lee C, Nechyba C, Gunn VL. Drug doses. In: Gunn VL, Nechyba C, eds. *The Harriet Lane handbook: a manual for pediatric house officers*. 16th ed. Philadelphia: Mosby, 2002.
9. Greydanus DE, Pratt HD, Sloane MA, Rappley MD. Attention-deficit/hyperactivity disorder in children and adolescents: interventions for a complex costly clinical conundrum. *Pediatr Clin North Am* 2003;50:1049–1092.
10. Halamandaris PV, Anderson TR. Children and adolescents in the psychiatric emergency setting. *Psychiatr Clin North Am* 1999;22:865–874.
11. Hodas GR, Sargent J. Psychiatric emergencies. In: Fleisher GR, Ludwig S, eds. *Textbook of Pediatric Emergency Medicine*. 4th ed. Philadelphia: Lippincott Williams and Wilkins, 2000;1705–1734.
12. Jacobstein CR, Baren JM. Emergency department treatment of minors. *Emerg Med Clin North Am* 1999;17:341–352.
13. Joint Commission on Accreditation of Healthcare Organizations. *Comprehensive accreditation manual for hospitals*. Oakbrook Terrace, Ill.: Joint Commission on Accreditation of Healthcare Organizations, 1999.
14. Sampson SM, Mrazek DA. Depression in adolescence. *Curr Opin Pediatr* 2001;13:586–590.
15. Sills MR, Bland SD. Summary statistics for pediatric psychiatric visits to US emergency departments, 1993–1999. *Pediatrics* 2002;110:e40.
16. Stephenson J. Children with mental problems not getting the care they need. *JAMA* 2000;284:2043–2044.
17. Varley CK, Smith CJ. Anxiety disorders in the child and teen. *Pediatr Clin North Am* 2003;50:1107–1138.

CHAPTER 263
Pyloric Stenosis

Ronald A. Furnival

Hypertrophic pyloric stenosis is the most common surgical etiology for the young infant presenting to the emergency department (ED) with nonbilious vomiting. The Ramstedt extramucosal pyloromyotomy, first reported in 1912, continues as the standard surgical therapeutic procedure to this day.

Pyloric stenosis occurs in approximately 3 of every 1,000 infants, affecting 4 males for every female. The etiology of pyloric stenosis is likely multifactorial, with a number of genetic, biochemical, and environmental associations. For example, erythromycin treatment during the first 2 weeks of life, has been associated with a 6- to10-fold increased risk for developing pyloric stenosis (8,19). Regardless of the underlying cause, the pathologic gastric outlet obstruction results from hypertrophy of the pyloric muscle, leading to the subsequent vomiting, dehydration, poor weight gain, and eventual hypochloremic metabolic alkalosis of the 'classic' presentation.

CLINICAL PRESENTATION

The typical infant with pyloric stenosis presents at an average age of 3 weeks, with a 1- to 2-week history of gradually worsening nonbilious vomiting. Pyloric stenosis is relatively rare among newborns younger than 1 week of age, or infants older than 3 to 4 months of age. A number of authors note that this condition is currently being diagnosed at an earlier age than 20 or 30 years ago, with fewer infants developing the 'classic' findings of hypochloremic alkalosis, weight loss, and a palpable pyloric muscle mass or 'olive' in the right epigastrium (4,5,17,23). The progressive vomiting of pyloric stenosis is often characterized as 'projectile' in nature, which unfortunately does not adequately distinguish it from parental descriptions of gastroesophageal reflux (24). The infant with pyloric stenosis may also have a history of blood-streaked or 'coffee-grounds' emesis from gastritis, weight loss or poor weight gain relative to the birth weight, or physiologic jaundice (in 2%–9% of cases.)

As infants with pyloric stenosis present at an earlier age, often without significant complications, their physical examination findings have become correspondingly more subtle. These infants may appear continuously hungry, even after vomiting an attempted feeding. With more advanced cases, the infant may appear thin-limbed and cachectic, with reduced subcutaneous fat stores, weight loss, and evidence of dehydration in up to 30% of cases (14). Visible peristaltic waves may be noted in the epigastrium, moving from the left side toward the pylorus on the right. Palpation of the hypertrophied pylorus or 'olive' is diagnostic, and is noted on exam in 25% to 75% of recent reports, depending on the duration of symptoms (12,17,20,23,24,26). The infant should be calmed with a sugar water-soaked pacifier, or even a small feeding after NG tube placement, if necessary. Several methods for palpation of the 'olive' have been described, including an approach with the infant in a ventral decubitus position, but most authors prefer to keep the infant supine, with the legs fully flexed to relax the abdominal wall musculature (3,9,14,15). Gentle and deep palpation under the liver margin, directed toward just right of midline should reveal a firm nodule

1 cm to 2 cm in diameter. Presence of the 'olive' on examination is diagnostic, and directs care to surgical consultation and hospitalization, without need for additional imaging or diagnostic studies.

Nasogastric (NG) tube placement may aid the physical examination as mentioned, but may also serve as a simple diagnostic aid. In the infant suspected to have pyloric stenosis, who has been kept NPO for at least one hour, NG aspiration of greater than 5cc of gastric contents is highly sensitive (91%) and specific (88%) for the diagnosis (20). However, the authors of that NG tube study did confirm the aspiration findings with a diagnostic imaging study (20).

DIFFERENTIAL DIAGNOSIS

The most common cause of nonbilious vomiting in the otherwise healthy infant is gastroesophageal reflux. The infant with reflux may have a history of overfeeding, positional variation in symptoms, or respiratory complications in the more advanced cases. Other common medical conditions presenting with nonbilious vomiting include viral gastroenteritis or an occult urinary tract infection, although both usually would have a history of shorter duration, with fever or other associated symptoms. Central nervous system disorders (hydrocephalus, intracranial hemorrhage, meningitis) may present with vomiting, but seldom without neurologic findings in a healthy appearing infant. Less common medical causes of nonbilious vomiting during infancy include congenital adrenal hyperplasia, inborn errors of metabolism, or renal insufficiency, which may present with characteristic electrolyte abnormalities (i.e., hyponatremia and hyperkalemia with the salt-wasting form of adrenal hyperplasia) or specific diagnostic laboratory findings (21).

While pyloric stenosis is the most common surgical consideration associated with nonbilious vomiting in early infancy, other surgical conditions (intestinal malrotation/volvulus, intussusception, Hirschsprüng disease, tracheoesophageal fistulas, esophageal or duodenal webs, duodenal atresia or stenosis, appendicitis, incarcerated hernia) must also be considered. Most infants with pyloric stenosis are initially well, gradually developing progressive vomiting with time. Congenital abnormalities of the upper gastrointestinal tract generally present early in the newborn period, and without a progressive history of feeding difficulty. The infant with abdominal pain, abdominal distention, or bilious (either yellow- or green-stained) emesis has a possible emergent condition. Immediate imaging studies should be performed for diagnosis, and surgical consultation should be arranged.

EMERGENCY DEPARTMENT EVALUATION

If the infant's history and physical examination raises the possibility of pyloric stenosis, carefully attempt to palpate the 'olive' for diagnosis. If the 'olive' can be felt, no further diagnostic work up is usually required and the surgeon can be notified. However, if the abdominal examination is not diagnostic, place an NG tube as described above for gastric content aspiration, give a small feeding of sugar water, and try another examination. An imaging evaluation may be needed if the abdominal examination does not reveal the diagnosis.

Although a number of authors recommend surgical referral for an abdominal examination as the next step (1,3,26), recent reports also note that abdominal imaging is performed in 70% to 90% of infants with pyloric stenosis, including those with a palpable 'olive' (1,7,26). While an increased use of imaging is credited with the earlier diagnosis and improved clinical con-

dition of today's infants with pyloric stenosis, imaging should be reserved for those with a nondiagnostic examination. Several studies have compared ultrasound (US) to the upper gastrointestinal series (UGI) for pyloric stenosis. US has the advantage of allowing direct visualization of the hypertrophied pyloric muscle, without the risk of radiation or aspiration of radiographic contrast associated with the UGI (1,7,12,20,25). UGI has the advantage of reducing the overall cost of imaging for a patient population, with slightly better sensitivity (~100% vs. ~95%) for pyloric stenosis when compared to US, and with the ability to identify other causes of vomiting not recognized by US, such as gastroesophageal reflux, malrotation, etc (11,12,16,20,22). Many authors feel the risk of UGI is overemphasized, with an epidemiologic risk of radiation exposure in the long term, and an exceedingly low risk of aspiration in experienced hands. UGI is also the recommended next diagnostic step when the US does not reveal a hypertrophied pylorus, thus necessitating 2 studies for some infants. Whether the diagnosis of pyloric stenosis is made on clinical examination, or with US or UGI, the infant should be hospitalized for preoperative fluid resuscitation and pyloromyotomy.

EMERGENCY DEPARTMENT MANAGEMENT

Once the diagnosis of pyloric stenosis is clear, an NG tube should be placed for gastric decompression, intravenous (IV) access should be obtained, and the infant should remain NPO. Blood should be obtained for measurement of serum glucose and electrolytes. The primary goals of preoperative care are IV fluid resuscitation and correction of any electrolyte and acid-base imbalances. Electrolyte abnormalities, ranging from metabolic acidosis early on, to the 'classic' hypochloremic metabolic alkalosis with more advanced illness, are uncommon (present in < 15% of cases) with earlier recognition of the condition (17,23). Infants presenting with elevated serum bicarbonate (> 25 mEq/L) and severe hypochloremia (< 99 mEq/L) generally had a longer duration of vomiting, more severe dehydration, greater weight losses, and longer hospitalizations (5). Preoperative fluid resuscitation should consist of 1 or 2 initial 20 ml/kg IV boluses of normal saline, followed by 5% Dextrose and 1/2 normal saline at 1.5 times the infant's maintenance rate. If the serum potassium is not elevated, 20 mEq/L of KCl may be added to the IV infusion (9,14). Twelve hours is generally adequate for complete fluid resuscitation, although more severely dehydrated infants may require 24 to 48 hours of IV fluids prior to surgery (17,23).

CRITICAL INTERVENTIONS

- The dehydrated infant suspected to have pyloric stenosis should begin receiving IV normal saline 20 ml/kg boluses, and have a serum glucose and electrolyte panel sent to the lab, while awaiting surgical consultation or imaging studies
- Adjust the IV fluid infusion to 5% Dextrose and 1/2 normal saline at 1.5 times the maintenance rate after the initial boluses
- Place an NG tube to decompress the stomach, and keep the infant NPO

DISPOSITION

The infant with diagnosed pyloric stenosis must be hospitalized for surgical intervention. The Ramstedt extramucosal pyloromyotomy remains the standard approach, with excellent cosmetic and functional outcomes, minimal morbidity, and essentially no

(<0.5%) mortality (3,9,14). Given the remarkable success and longevity of the open procedure, laparoscopic pyloromyotomy has only recently begun to see widespread interest (2,6,10,13). After an initial learning period, laparoscopy appears to result in similar outcomes, with perhaps slightly less postoperative vomiting than the open pyloromyotomy (2,6,10,13). Early postoperative feeding protocols have reduced the total hospital length-of-stay for the average pyloric stenosis infant to 24 to 48 hours, with few complications. Postpyloromyotomy vomiting is common, with coexisting gastroesophageal reflux occurring in 10% to 15% of infants. This vomiting should resolve within 1 to 2 weeks after surgery; persistent vomiting may represent the very rare failed pyloromyotomy. Nonsurgical medical therapy with IV atropine for pyloric stenosis has been reported, but requires a longer hospital stay than the rapidly effective pyloromyotomy and is rarely used (18).

COMMON PITFALLS

✔ Assuming that bilious vomiting in the infant < 2 months of age is pyloric stenosis. Bilious emesis mandates an immediate UGI for possible malrotation and volvulus

✔ Fluid resuscitation with IV solutions of lower chloride concentrations than normal saline, or 1/2 normal saline after an initial IV bolus, may not correct the infant with hypochloremic metabolic alkalosis. The kidneys will continue to absorb Na+ with HCO3-, causing persistent alkalosis, rather than absorbing Na+ with Cl−, until the serum chloride level is normal

Acknowledgments

Thanks to the previous edition's chapter authors Maureen Campbell and Lisa Horton.

References

1. Abbas AE, Weiss SM, Alvear DT. Infantile hypertrophic pyloric stenosis: delays in diagnosis and overutilization of imaging modalities. *Am Surg* 1999;65:73–76.
2. Alain JL, Grousseau D, Longis B, Terrier G. Laparoscopic pyloromyotomy for infantile hypertrophic stenosis [letter; comment]. *J Pediatr Surg* 1996;31:1197–1198.
3. Barksdale EM.Pyloric stenosis. In: MM Ziegler; RG Azizkhan, TR Weber, eds. *Operative Pediatric Surgery.* New York: McGraw-Hill Companies; 2003:583–588.
4. Breaux CW, Jr., Georgeson KE, Royal SA, Curnow AJ. Changing patterns in the diagnosis of hypertrophic pyloric stenosis. *Pediatrics* 1988;81:213–217.
5. Breaux CW, Jr., Hood JS, Georgeson KE. The significance of alkalosis and hypochloremia in hypertrophic pyloric stenosis. *J Pediatr Surg* 1989;24:1250–1252.
6. Campbell BT, McLean K, Barnhart DC, Drongowski RA, Hirschl RB. A comparison of laparoscopic and open pyloromyotomy at a teaching hospital. *J Pediatr Surg* 2002;37:1068–1071; discussion 1068–1071.
7. Chen EA, Luks FI, Gilchrist BF, Wesselhoeft CW, Jr., DeLuca FG. Pyloric stenosis in the age of ultrasonography: fading skills, better patients? [see comments]. *J Pediatr Surg* 1996;31:829–830.
8. Cooper WO, Griffin MR, Arbogast P, et al. Very early exposure to erythromycin and infantile hypertrophic pyloric stenosis. *Arch Pediatr Adolesc Med* 2002;156:647–650.
9. Dillon PW, Cilley RE.Lesions of the stomach. In: KW Ashcraft, ed. *Pediatric Surgery.* Philadelphia, PA: W.B. Saunders Company; 2000:391–405.
10. Downey EC, Jr. Laparoscopic pyloromyotomy. *Semin Pediatr Surg* 1998;7:220–224.
11. Foley LC, Slovis TL, Campbell JB, et al. Evaluation of the vomiting infant. *Am J Dis Child* 1989;143:660–661.
12. Forman HP, Leonidas JC, Kronfeld GD. A rational approach to the diagnosis of hypertrophic pyloric stenosis: do the results match the claims? *J Pediatr Surg* 1990;25:262–266.
13. Fujimoto T, Lane GJ, Segawa O, Esaki S, Miyano T. Laparoscopic extramucosal pyloromyotomy versus open pyloromyotomy for infantile hypertrophic pyloric stenosis: which is better? *J Pediatr Surg* 1999;34:370–372.
14. Garcia VF, Randolph JG. Pyloric stenosis: diagnosis and management. *Pediatr Rev* 1990;11:292–296.
15. Hoekelman RA. Pyloric stenosis is a pediatrician's diagnosis. *Pediatr Ann* 1994;23:181–182.
16. Hulka F, Campbell JR, Harrison MW, Campbell TJ. Cost-effectiveness in diagnosing infantile hypertrophic pyloric stenosis. *J Pediatr Surg* 1997;32:1604–1608.
17. Hulka F, Campbell TJ, Campbell JR, Harrison MW. Evolution in the recognition of infantile hypertrophic pyloric stenosis. *Pediatrics* 1997;100:E9.
18. Kawahara H, Imura K, Nishikawa M, Yagi M, Kubota A. Intravenous atropine treatment in infantile hypertrophic pyloric stenosis. *Arch Dis Child* 2002;87:71–74.
19. Mahon BE, Rosenman MB, Kleiman MB. Maternal and infant use of erythromycin and other macrolide antibiotics as risk factors for infantile hypertrophic pyloric stenosis. *J Pediatr* 2001;139:380–384.
20. Mandell GA, Wolfson PJ, Adkins ES, et al. Cost-effective imaging approach to the nonbilious vomiting infant. *Pediatrics* 1999;103:1198–1202.
21. Nadel FM, Weinzimer SA. The case of the missing olive. *Pediatr Ann* 2000; 29:119–122.
22. Olson AD, Hernandez R, Hirschl RB. The role of ultrasonography in the diagnosis of pyloric stenosis: a decision analysis [see comments]. *J Pediatr Surg* 1998;33:676–681.
23. Poon TS, Zhang AL, Cartmill T, Cass DT. Changing patterns of diagnosis and treatment of infantile hypertrophic pyloric stenosis: a clinical audit of 303 patients. *J Pediatr Surg* 1996;31:1611–1615.
24. Smith GA, Mihalov L, Shields BJ. Diagnostic aids in the differentiation of pyloric stenosis from severe gastroesophageal reflux during early infancy: the utility of serum bicarbonate and serum chloride. *Am J Emerg Med* 1999;17:28–31.
25. van der Schouw YT, van der Velden MT, Hitge-Boetes C, Verbeek AL, Ruijs SH. Diagnosis of hypertrophic pyloric stenosis: value of sonography when used in conjunction with clinical findings and laboratory data. *AJR Am J Roentgenol* 1994;163:905–909.
26. White MC, Langer JC, Don S, DeBaun MR. Sensitivity and cost minimization analysis of radiology versus olive palpation for the diagnosis of hypertrophic pyloric stenosis [see comments]. *J Pediatr Surg* 1998;33:913–917.

CHAPTER 264
Sickling Syndromes

B. Nazeema Khan and Paul A. Pitel

Sickle cell anemia is an autosomal recessive hemoglobinopathy characterized by hemolytic anemia, recurrent vasoocclusion, and end-organ dysfunction. The heterozygous state (AS), sickle cell trait, is found in 8% to 10% of African-Americans. The homozygous state (SS), sickle cell anemia, occurs in one in 400 to 600 newborns. The disease is seen less commonly in the Hispanic, southern European, and Middle Eastern populations.

The molecular basis of the disease is the substitution of glutamine for valine at the sixth position of the globin beta chain. This permits the crystallization of the hemoglobin molecules in conditions of relative hypoxemia. The cell becomes irreversibly sickled, leading to premature cell destruction (hemolysis) and blood vessel obstruction.

Hemoglobin electrophoresis permits the accurate diagnosis of sickle cell anemia, sickle cell trait, hemoglobin sickle cell disease, and other sickle variants as early as the newborn period. The sickle cell prep (Sickledex) is inaccurate before age 4 to 6 months. In the older infant or child with sickle cell anemia, the hemoglobin averages 8 g/dl, the hematocrit 24%, and the reticulocyte count 10%, with an elevated platelet count and a white count of 13,000 to 17,000/cubic mm.

Today, most children with sickle cell anemia are diagnosed through state-mandated newborn screening programs. However, unexplained anemia in an African-American children should raise the suspicion of a hemoglobinopathy. The presence of any sickle forms on a peripheral blood smear is presumptive evidence of sickle cell anemia. Children with sickle cell trait have normal hematologic values.

The emergency department (ED) evaluation depends on the patient's presentation or sickle cell crisis. Clinical symptoms may begin as early as 3 to 4 months of age, when significant amounts of hemoglobin S become present. Referral for ongoing treatment and parent education, preferably through a sickle cell center, is vital.

DACTYLITIS (HAND–FOOT SYNDROME)

The hand–foot syndrome is the most common presentation of the child with sickle cell anemia from age 6 to 24 months. Painful swelling of the hands or feet, or both, results from symmetric infarction of the metacarpals and metatarsals. Low-grade fever (less than 101.5°F) is common, and no significant changes in hematologic values are noted. Radiographs initially show only soft-tissue swelling, but osteolytic and periosteal changes are seen 2 to 3 weeks after the onset of symptoms. The presentation is often classic but must be differentiated from osteomyelitis (either unifocal or multifocal) and trauma. Therapy consists of hydration at 150% to 200% maintenance (oral or intravenous fluids) and analgesia. Pain and swelling commonly require 2 to 5 days to resolve. Recurrence is not rare, but the syndrome generally ends by age 2 as the vascular supply to these bones collateralizes.

INFECTION

Bacterial infection is the most common cause of serious morbidity and mortality in children with sickle cell anemia (13,16). The primary pathogens are the encapsulated organisms *Streptococcus pneumoniae* and *Haemophilus influenzae*, but *Salmonella* osteomyelitis and severe *Mycoplasma pneumoniae* infections are also seen. The primary cause is functional asplenia secondary to autoinfarction, which may occur as early as 5 months of age but is routine by age 5 years. Defects in complement and opsonization are also noted in sickle cell patients.

Bacterial meningitis and septicemia are more than 600 times more common in children with sickle cell anemia than in normal children (21,22). Bacterial pneumonia is 100 times more common in these children. Pneumococcal sepsis in sickle cell patients carries a 14% mortality, often within hours of presentation, even when recognized and treated. Pneumococcal disease is most common before age 6 and is particularly common in the first 2 to 3 years of life (21,22).

Prophylactic daily penicillin should be started at age 2 to 3 months and continued until at least 5 years of age. In children less than 3 years the dose is 125 mg orally twice daily (10,17). A dose of 250 mg orally twice daily is given from ages 3 to 5 years. Also, *H. influenzae* type B (HIB) and pneumococcal (Pneumovax) vaccines are given routinely. The effectiveness of the 23- valent pneumococcal polysaccharide vaccine among children with sickle cell disease is 80% to 90% (1,7), with data on the newer vaccines being more limited. Educating the family about the signs and risks of infections is critical.

Despite optimal treatment, children with sickle cell anemia may present with fever and potential bacterial infections. Initial evaluation should include:

- A careful history of the present illness. Bacteremia is more likely to be of only several hours' duration and associated with a fever above 103°F.
- A careful review of the medical history, including penicillin prophylaxis and possible missed doses.
- A careful physical examination. Focal sites of infection can coexist with bacteremia.

- For fever above 101.5°F, a complete blood count with differential, a reticulocyte count, and a blood culture are probably minimal requirements. Marked leukocytosis (above the baseline 13,000 to 17,000/cubic mm) or a left shift is usually seen. Lumbar puncture and chest radiographs may be indicated. The erythrocyte sedimentation rate and C-reactive protein assessment are unreliable.

Children less than age 1 year with fever are routinely admitted for appropriate intravenous antibiotics. In selected cases, older children with a fever below 103°F and no focal source of infection may be discharged home after obtaining appropriate cultures and giving ceftriaxone 75 mg/kg intramuscularly (23). Reliable follow up must be assured. A repeat dose of ceftriaxone should be administered 24 hours later. With a focal source, blood cultures and ceftriaxone should be followed up with appropriate oral antibiotics. Children with a temperature above 103°F should routinely be admitted and observed on appropriate antibiotic coverage. Antibiotic choice should depend on local patterns of bacterial sensitivity; however, coverage of both *H. influenzae* and *S. pneumoniae* is necessary in the young child. The emergence of resistant or partially resistant *S. pneumoniae* must be considered. Children older than 8 or 9 years can often be managed with penicillin alone.

VASOOCCLUSIVE EPISODES

The hallmark of sickle cell anemia is the painful "crisis" caused by arterial occlusion by irreversibly sickled cells. Vasoocclusion may be precipitated by dehydration, hypoxia, acidosis, or infection, but it often occurs without ready explanation. Symptoms vary according to the location of vascular obstruction, but pain secondary to tissue hypoxemia is common. Pain episodes commonly involve the extremities or abdomen, but head pain (calvarial) or chest wall pain (rib, sternal) is common in older children. Low-grade fever is often noted.

Therapy consists of aggressive hydration (twice maintenance) and analgesics. For mild pain, ibuprofen or acetaminophen may be adequate. For moderate pain, intravenous or intramuscular morphine sulfate or meperidine may be appropriate, followed by hydration and transfer to oral agents such as acetaminophen with codeine (3,24,25). Severe pain requires intravenous morphine sulfate, fluids, and hospitalization (24,25). Ketorolac, IV or IM, can also be used in the ED setting for acute pain management. Pain may be the prodrome to the development of acute chest syndrome, and incentive spirometry may be useful to avoid this complication.

Hydroxyurea, has been shown to reduce the number of hospitalizations and vasoocclusive crises in sickle cell patients (6,26).

CEREBROVASCULAR ACCIDENT

About 7% of sickle cell patients suffer a central nervous system event, often a stroke. In the younger child, the event is usually thrombotic; in the adolescent or adult, it may be hemorrhagic (2). These events are unpredictable, although many can now be predicted with the use of transcalvarial Doppler ultrasound evaluation. They routinely involve major cerebral arteries and can be devastating. In the ED, any untoward neurologic event in a sickle cell patient is considered a cerebrovascular accident until proven otherwise.

Initial evaluation should include a careful history for precipitating events, a formal neurologic examination, insertion of an intravenous line, and measurement of baseline laboratory values. Computed tomography scanning without contrast is needed routinely. Neurology and hematology consultations are obtained. Arteriography is usually not needed and can precipitate further sickling in the untransfused patient.

Acute therapy usually includes intravenous hydration and exchange transfusion to decrease the percentage of hemoglobin S to below 30%. Prompt recognition and treatment in an intensive care setting usually results in a gratifying outcome (14). Long-term treatment necessitates hypertransfusion for several years to reduce the 66% chance of a recurrent cerebrovascular accident (9,12,20). Hydroxyurea therapy has also been shown to be effective for prevention of recurrent stroke in sickle cell patients (19).

ACUTE SPLENIC SEQUESTRATION

Splenic sequestration is a life-threatening condition seen in young children before the onset of autoinfarction of the spleen. Over a period of hours, a significant portion of the circulating blood volume is sequestered in the spleen because of vasoocclusion in the splenic vein. Thus, the patient develops hypovolemia, pallor, massive splenomegaly, and, occasionally, shock and death. Families should be educated in splenic palpation. Evaluation demonstrates splenomegaly (often massive), anemia, and reticulocytosis.

Treatment is aimed at sustaining blood volume until the condition spontaneously reverses, releasing the sequestered blood. Careful monitoring and, often, a transfusion of 10 mL/kg of packed red blood cells may be required (11,20). Overtransfusion should be avoided, as the condition will reverse.

APLASTIC CRISIS

The term *aplastic crisis* refers to acute anemia that may be superimposed on sickle cell patients by episodes of marrow hypoplasia. The severely decreased red cell survival in these patients necessitates a marked reticulocytosis (greater than 10%) to maintain baseline hemoglobin levels. Episodes of erythroid hypoplasia, manifested by progressive anemia with reticulocytopenia (less than 1%), occur both sporadically and epidemically in association with the human parvovirus B19 (15). Packed red blood cell transfusion may be necessary until erythroid production returns, usually within a few weeks. Patients with aplastic crisis require close monitoring because their hemoglobin may fall to 4% or lower within a few days. Hydroxyurea has been shown to reduce the occurrence of aplastic crisis (6,26).

ACUTE CHEST SYNDROME

Episodes of cough, chest pain, fever, and pulmonary infiltrates are common. In younger children, the cause is usually infection, and in older children and adolescents, infarction. A syndrome of progressive infection and infarction may develop, with diffuse lung involvement. Acute chest syndrome is the second most common cause for admission in sickle cell patients, and is now the leading cause of death (4,18). *M. pneumoniae* can produce severe and unusual patterns of infection in these patients. Treatment focuses on appropriate antibiotic coverage. Oxygen supplementation, transfusion, or both, may be indicated. In addition, hydroxyurea has been shown to reduce the occurrence of acute chest syndrome (6,26).

PRIAPISM

Priapism is painful, involuntary penile erection. Sickling within the penile cavernous sinuses is most common in adolescents and young adults. Any episode lasting more than 3 hours is unlikely to resolve spontaneously and requires intravenous hydration and narcotic analgesia. Hematologic consultation regarding transfusion or exchange transfusion should be considered. Episodes persisting more than 24 hours require surgical intervention. Pseudoephedrine may be a useful prophylactic drug. Physiologic sexual impotence commonly occurs from chronic scarring of the erectile tissue (5).

CRITICAL INTERVENTIONS

- Rapid administration of antibiotics for all febrile sickle cell patients, especially those less than 2 years of age
- Hospitalization of infants less than 1 year of age with fever and also older children with a temperature greater than 103°F
- Hydration and analgesia for patients presenting with vasoocclusive crises
- Recognition of acute chest syndrome and hypoxia with close monitoring for deterioration
- Consider exchange transfusion for patients with priapism and cerebrovascular accidents

DISPOSITION

Most children with sickle cell disease are monitored by a pediatric hematologist and a primary care physician (8). It is essential that these physicians be advised of the patient's emergency visit and consulted regarding the discharge plan.

COMMON PITFALLS

✔ Failing to recognize that any sickled cell on peripheral smear is presumptive evidence of sickle cell anemia
✔ Failing to appreciate the immune status of the sickle cell patient. The febrile sickle cell child requires careful evaluation and often hospitalization and intravenous antibiotics
✔ Failing to recognize that sickle cell anemia can be diagnosed in the newborn period; symptoms may begin by age 3 to 4 months. Many states have mandatory newborn screening programs
✔ Failing to recognize that the sickle prep is inaccurate before 4 to 6 months of age
✔ Failing to consider a cerebrovascular accident when evaluating any untoward neurologic event in a sickle cell patient
✔ Failing to consider aplastic crisis and acute splenic sequestration in the acutely anemic sickle cell patient

Acknowledgment

Thanks to the previous edition's chapter author James L. Harper.

References

1. Adamkiewicz TV, Sarnaik S, Buchanan GR, et al. Invasive pneumococccal infections in children with sickle cell disease in the era of penicillin prophylaxis, antibiotic resistance, and 23-valent pneumococcal polysaccharide vaccination. *Journal of Pediatrics* 2003;143:438.
2. Adams RJ. Stroke prevention and treatment in sickle cell disease. *Archives of Neurology* 2001;58:565.
3. American Academy of Pediatrics, Committee on Genetics. Health supervision for children with sickle cell diseases and their families. *Pediatrics* 1996;98: 467.
4. Claster S, Vichinsky EP. Managing sickle cell disease. *BMJ* 2003;327:1151.

5. Emond A, Holman R, Hayes R, et al. Priapism and impotence in homozygous sickle cell disease. *Arch Intern Med* 1980;140:1434.

6. Ferster A, Tahriri P, Vermylen C, et al. Five years of experience with hydroxyurea in children and young adults with sickle cell disease. *Blood* 2001;97:3628.

7. Fiore AE, Levine OS, Elliott JA, Facklam RR, Butler JC. Effectiveness of Pneumococcal polysaccharide vaccine for preschool-age children with chronic disease. *Emerging Infectious Disease* 1999;5:828.

8. Frush K, Ware RE, Kinney T. Emergency department visits by children with sickle hemoglobinopathies: factors associated with hospital admission. *Pediatr Emerg Care* 1995;11:9.

9. Harmatz P, Butensky E, Quirolo K, et al. Severity of iron overload in patients with sickle cell disease receiving chronic red blood cell transfusion therapy. *Blood* 2000;96:76.

10. Hord J, Byrd R, Stowe L, Windsor B, Smith-Whitley K. Streptococcus pneumoniae sepsis and meningitis during the penicillin prophylaxis era in children with sickle cell disease. *J Pediatr Hematol Oncol* 2002;24:470.

11. Kinney TR, Ware RE, Schultz WH, Filstron HC. Long term management of splenic sequestration in children with sickle cell disease. *Journal of Pediatrics* 1990;117:194.

12. Pegelow CH, Adams RJ, Mckie V, et al. Risk of recurrent stroke in patients with sickle cell disease treated with erythrocyte transfusions. *Journal of Pediatrics* 1995;126:896.

13. Platt OS, Dover GJ. *Hematology of infancy and childhood*. Philadelphia: WB Saunders/Harcourt Brace Jovanovich, 1993:732.

14. Platt OS, Thorington BD, Brambilla DJ, et al. Pain in sickle cell disease: rates and risk factor. *N Engl J Med* 1991;325:11.

15. Serjeant GR, Serjeant BE, Thomas PW, et al. Human parvovirus infection in homozygous sickle cell disease. *Lancet* 1993;15:1237.

16. Serjeant GR. *Sickle cell disease* Oxford: Oxford University Press, 1985:326.

17. Teach SJ, Lillis KA, Grossi M. Compliance with penicillin prophylaxis in patients with sickle cell disease. *Arch of Pediatr Adoles Med* 1998;152:274.

18. Vichinsky EP, Styles LA, Colangelo L, et al. Acute chest syndrome in sickle cell disease: clinical presentation and course. Cooperative study of sickle cell disease. *Blood* 1997;89:1787.

19. Ware R, Zimmerman S, Schultz W. Hydroxyurea as an alternative to blood transfusions for the prevention of recurrent stroke in children with sickle cell disease. *Blood* 1999;94:3022.

20. Wayne AS, et al. Transfusion management of sickle cell disease. *Blood* 1993;81:1109.

21. West TB, West DW, Ohene-Frempong K. The presenatation, frequency, and outcome of bacteremia among children with sickle cell disease and fever. *Pediatr Emerg Care* 1994;10:141.

22. West DC, Andrada E, Azari R, Rangaswami AA, Kuppermann N. Predictors of bacteremia in febrile children with sickle cell disease. *J Pediatr Hematol Oncol* 2003;24:279.

23. Wilimas JA, Flynn P, Harris S, et al. A randomized study of outpatient treatment with ceftriaxone for selected febrile children with sickle cell disease. *N Engl J Med* 1993;329:472.

24. Yaster M, Kost-Byerly S, Maxwell LG. The management of pain in sickle cell disease. *Pediatr Clin North Am* 2000;47:699.

25. Zimmerman SA, Ware RE, Kinney TR. Gaining ground in the fight against sickle cell disease. *Contemp Pediatr* 1997;14:154.

26. Zimmerman SA, Schultz WH, Davis JS. Sustained long-term hematologic efficacy of hydroxyurea at maximum tolerated dose in children with sickle cell disease. *Blood* 2004;15:2039.

CHAPTER 265

Sinusitis

Kelli A. Maiers and Daniel J. Isaacman

The maxillary, ethmoid, frontal and sphenoid sinuses comprise the paranasal sinuses. These sinuses develop as outpouchings of the nasal chamber, and their mucosal lining is continuous with that of the nose. The maxillary and ethmoid sinuses develop during the third to fourth month of gestation and are therefore present at birth. The ethmoid sinuses consist of both anterior and posterior cells, totaling 3 to 18 in number. These are the most commonly involved sinuses in childhood sinusitis. The frontal sinuses develop from an anterior ethmoid cell and become supraorbital between 4 and 6 years of age. They continue to grow and reach full adult size during adolescence, when they become clinically important. The sphenoid sinuses pneumatize by age 5, but are rarely an isolated site of infection. They may be involved in pansinusitis (16).

The mucosal lining of the paranasal sinuses consists of pseudostratified ciliated columnar epithelium with goblet cells. The epithelium is covered by a blanket of mucus, which is continually moved towards the ostium of each sinus and into the nasopharynx by the beating of the cilia (8). The maxillary ostium sits high on the medial wall of the sinus, and therefore secretions must drain against gravity. The ostium for each individual anterior ethmoid cell is very narrow, and is easily obstructed. The shape, length and course of the ostia of the frontal sinuses are variable. Each of these sinuses drains into the middle meatus. This area and the surrounding structures comprise the osteomeatal complex, a key structure in the pathophysiology of sinusitis. The posterior ethmoid cells and the sphenoid sinus drain into the superior meatus (8,16).

Interference with paranasal sinus drainage is a key factor in the development of sinusitis. Contributing factors include ostial obstruction, abnormal mucociliary apparatus function, and either increased production or viscosity of mucus. Ostial obstruction may be caused either by mechanical obstruction or mucosal swelling. Certain underlying diseases may cause decreased ciliary action, but there are also some respiratory viruses that have a direct cytotoxic action on the cilia (16).

The most common predisposing factor in the development of acute sinusitis is an upper respiratory infection (URI) (12). Children average approximately 6 to 8 URIs per year in the first few years of life. These infections cause ostial obstruction secondary to mucosal swelling, abnormal mucociliary function, and increased mucus production, which increases the risk for secondary bacterial infection. It is estimated that 5% to 13% of childhood URIs evolve into acute bacterial sinusitis (1,6,8,19). Children in daycare have a higher risk of developing sinusitis than those in home care (4).

The second most common predisposing factor in the development of childhood acute sinusitis is allergic rhinitis (2). Asthma is frequently associated with sinusitis, (13). and many children with asthma have shown improvement in their symptoms after recognition and treatment of sinusitis. Other predisposing conditions include cystic fibrosis, immune disorders, conditions associated with abnormal ciliary function (such as ciliary dyskinesia), chronic indwelling nasogastric tubes, and anatomic obstruction (16).

ETIOLOGY

The most common organisms causing acute bacterial sinusitis in children are the same as those that cause acute otitis media: *Streptococcus pneumoniae,* nontypeable *Haemophilus influenza,* and *Moraxella catarrhalis.* Other organisms that may contribute to acute bacterial sinusitis are group A streptococci, group C streptococci, viridans streptococci, peptostreptococci, other Moraxella species, and Eikenella corrodens. Isolates of respiratory viruses, including adenovirus, parainfluenza, influenza, and rhinovirus may be found in some patients with a clinical diagnosis of acute sinusitis (16). Anaerobes and staphylococci are not common causes of acute disease but may be found in children with chronic sinusitis (12). Fungal sinusitis is rare in children but may occur, especially in immunocompromised patients. Children with cystic fibrosis often have *Pseudomonal* sinusitis (12).

CLINICAL PRESENTATION

Children with acute bacterial sinusitis will present with upper respiratory symptoms that are either persistent or severe. Most viral URIs last approximately 5 to 7 days, and almost all are resolved or at least improving by 10 days. Children that have symptoms beyond 10 days without improvement should be considered to have acute bacterial sinusitis (2,15). The most common symptoms include nasal discharge and cough. The nasal discharge may be of any quality ranging from clear to purulent, thin to thick. The cough may be either "wet" or "dry," and is usually present in the daytime but may worsen at night (6). Malodorous breath without signs of poor dental hygiene or pharyngitis is commonly reported by parents of preschool-aged children (16,20). Fever, headache, facial pain or swelling, and sore throat may be present, especially in older children, but occur less commonly than in adults (21).

Children that present with severe upper respiratory symptoms and high fever should also be considered to have acute bacterial sinusitis (6). In the usual course of a viral URI, fever may be present during the first 48 hours, but then usually disappears, and purulent nasal discharge does not usually develop until later in the illness. In contrast, children with the severe onset of acute bacterial sinusitis present with concurrent high fever ($>39°C$) and purulent nasal discharge for 3 to 4 consecutive days, and are ill-appearing. In addition, they may complain of intense headache above or behind the eye or present with periorbital swelling (16).

Subacute sinusitis is defined as persistent mild to moderate respiratory symptoms lasting between 30 and 90 days, whereas chronic sinusitis is defined as symptoms persisting beyond 90 days. The most common symptoms are nasal discharge and cough. Sore throat may also be present secondary to mouth breathing (16).

Recurrent acute bacterial sinusitis is defined as 3 episodes in 6 months or 4 episodes in 12 months. Patients are completely free of symptoms between episodes (2).

COMPLICATIONS AND DIFFERENTAL DIAGNOSIS

Complications of acute bacterial sinusitis occur rarely but can be serious and life-threatening. The differential diagnosis of sinusitis is similar to its complications and may involve the orbit or the central nervous system via direct extension through the thin bones of the paranasal sinuses. Orbital complications include periorbital (or preseptal) cellulitis, subperiosteal abscess, orbital abscess or orbital cellulitis. Periorbital (or preseptal) cellulitis results from passive venous congestion and infection is confined to the sinuses—it is neither a true orbital complication nor a true cellulitis (See Chapter 245). Central nervous system complications include cavernous sinus thrombosis, osteomyelitis of the frontal (Pott's puffy tumor) or maxillary bones, meningitis, subdural empyema, epidural abscess and cerebral abscess (12,15,16,21,22).

DIAGNOSIS

Physical Examination

There are no physical examination findings that are specific for sinusitis, as children with uncomplicated URI will often have similar exam findings (2,12,16). However, careful attention should be paid to abnormalities that may suggest an orbital or intracranial complication. These include periorbital swelling or erythema, proptosis, abnormal extraocular movements, decreased visual acuity, pain with eye movement, frontal swelling (Pott's puffy tumor), nuchal rigidity, abnormal mental status, signs of increased intracranial pressure or toxic appearance. Transillumination is inaccurate in children and therefore not helpful (2,8,12).

Laboratory

There are no specific lab tests that aid in the diagnosis of acute sinusitis. White blood cell count and acute-phase reactants may be elevated, or may be normal. Cultures of the throat and nasopharynx have poor correlation with maxillary sinus aspirates and are not recommended (20). Although the gold standard of diagnosis is culture of aspirated fluid from the affected sinus, this is not necessary in uncomplicated cases of acute sinusitis.

Radiology

Plain films that may be used in the diagnosis of sinusitis include the Caldwell (AP) view for the frontal and ethmoid sinuses, Waters (occipitomental) view for the maxillary sinuses, and lateral and submentovertex views for the sphenoid sinus (10). Findings that may help to confirm a diagnosis of sinusitis include air-fluid levels, complete sinus opacification, and mucosal thickening (3–5 mm) (2). However, these radiographs can be technically difficult to perform, especially in young children, and may under or overestimate sinus disease (10). In one study, 80% of children with a history of persistent symptoms had abnormal sinus radiographs (88% for those under 6, and 70% for those ages 6 and older). When maxillary sinus aspiration was performed, bacteria were recovered in high density in 75% of cases (18). Another study found 23 of 30 children (77%) with persistent symptoms and abnormal radiographs to have positive sinus aspirates (20). Finally, a more recent study showed that 92.5% of children with persistent symptoms had abnormal radiographs (15). Because there is such a high correlation between persistent symptoms, abnormal radiographs, and positive sinus aspirates, it is not necessary to perform further testing in children with a history consistent with sinusitis. The American Academy of Pediatrics, the American College of Radiology, and the Sinus and Allergy Health Partnership do not recommend the use of radiography in the diagnosis of acute uncomplicated sinusitis in children. Instead, it should be reserved for children that do not improve with therapy, or that worsen during therapy (2). A Water's view alone may be sufficient in comparison to a complete sinus series for most cases of acute sinusitis in children (14).

CT scans should be reserved for patients with complications, multiple recurrences, anatomic abnormalities, failure of response to therapy, and in those being considered for surgical treatment. MRI is used for patients with suspected intracranial complications (22).

EMERGENCY DEPARTMENT MANAGEMENT

Antibiotics are the mainstay of treatment for acute bacterial sinusitis. Many children will spontaneously improve without the use of antibiotics; however, several studies have shown more rapid improvement with the use of antibiotics. Children that are treated with antibiotics should show reduction in symptoms and overall general improvement within 48 to 72 hours (2).

The antibiotic chosen should have adequate coverage for the most common causative organisms of acute bacterial sinusitis, which include *Streptococcus pneumoniae*, nontypeable *Haemophilus influenzae*, and *Moraxella catarrhalis*. Resistance of

S. pneumoniae to penicillins has been increasing, and attention should be paid not only to local resistance patterns, but also to factors that increase the risk that a child harbors a resistant strain. These factors include day care attendance, age less than 2 years, and antibiotic use within 90 days. In areas of low resistance and in children without risk factors, amoxicillin at a usual dose (45 mg/kg/day in 2 divided doses) or high dose (90 mg/kg/day in 2 divided doses) may be used as first-line therapy. Although amoxicillin does not adequately cover beta-lactamase producing organisms, approximately 80% of children without risk factors for resistance will respond to treatment with amoxicillin. This is because *S. pneumoniae* is the most common causative organism, and many cases of sinusitis caused by *H. influenzae* and *M. catarrhalis* will resolve spontaneously. In children that are allergic to penicillins, the following options exist: cefdinir (14 mg/kg/day in 1 or 2 doses), cefuroxime (30 mg/kg/day in 2 divided doses) or cefpodoxime (10 mg/kg/day in 1 dose). In children that have had anaphylactic reactions to penicillins, clarithromycin (15 mg/kg/day in 2 divided doses) or azithromycin (10 mg/kg/day on day 1 and 5 mg/kg/day × 4 more days, given once daily) can be used. It should be noted that the FDA has not approved the use of azithromycin for the treatment of sinusitis. A final option in the allergic patient is clindamycin (30–40 mg/kg/day in 3 divided doses) (2).

In areas of high resistance, and in children with risk factors for resistance, first-line therapy should be initiated with high dose amoxicillin-clavulanate (80–90 mg/kg/day of amoxicillin component in 2 divided doses). Alternatives again include cefdinir, cefuroxime, or cefpodoxime. A single dose of IM or IV ceftriaxone (50 mg/kg) may be used for children that are vomiting, followed by completion of the treatment course with an oral antibiotic starting 24 hours later (2).

Recent studies have shown significant resistance of *S. pneumoniae* to trimethoprim-sulfamethoxazole and erythromycin-sulfisoxazole, and therefore these antibiotics are not appropriate for the treatment of sinusitis (5,9).

Current recommendations for length of treatment vary from 10 to 28 days of antibiotics. In most cases, treatment for 7 days beyond the time when the patient becomes symptom-free results in adequate treatment (2,16). Most patients will become symptom-free by 3 days of treatment, so that 10 days of treatment will usually suffice. A good recommendation for emergency department treatment is to treat the patient for 10 days, and to have patients with longer symptomatic periods follow up with their primary care physician for continuation of antibiotics.

Topical steroids, topical decongestant-antihistamines, and oral decongestant-antihistamines have all been suggested as therapies that may add some benefit in the treatment of acute sinusitis (7). However, there are only a few studies that have specifically addressed these options in children. In one study looking at the use of intranasal budesonide spray in addition to antibiotics, a significant improvement in symptoms of cough and nasal discharge was noted in the treatment group (3). Another study compared the addition of an oral decongestant-antihistamine to placebo (in addition to amoxicillin) and found similar treatment response in both groups (11).

Any child suspected of having an orbital or central nervous system complication should be treated aggressively. This includes imaging, IV antibiotics, and emergent consultation with either an ophthalmologist, otolaryngologist or neurosurgeon, as well as an infectious disease specialist. Antibiotic treatment should be with either ceftriaxone (100 mg/kg/day in 2 divided doses) or ampicillin-sulbactam (200 mg/kg/day in 4 divided doses), or an antibiotic with equivalent antimicrobial spectrum. Vancomycin (60 mg/kg/day in 4 divided doses) should be added if *S. pneumoniae* resistance is suspected (2).

CRITICAL INTERVENTIONS

- The diagnosis of sinusitis in children can be made based on clinical criteria: either persistent upper respiratory symptoms without improvement (>10 days) or severe upper respiratory symptoms (high fever and purulent nasal discharge for 3–4 days)
- Careful physical examination is important to rule out potential orbital and central nervous system complications
- Imaging should be reserved for toxic-appearing patients, those suspected of having complications, or those that have failed treatment
- Amoxicillin or amoxicillin-clavulanate should be used as first-line therapy for children with uncomplicated acute bacterial sinusitis. Options for children allergic to penicillins include second generation cephalosporins, macrolides, or clindamycin. Trimethoprim-sulfamethoxazole and erythromycin-sulfisoxazole should not be used. Initial treatment course should be ten days
- Patients suspected of having orbital or central nervous system complications need aggressive treatment, including IV antibiotics, imaging, emergent consultation with the appropriate subspecialist and hospital admission

DISPOSITION

Children diagnosed with uncomplicated acute bacterial sinusitis may be discharged from the emergency department with appropriate antimicrobial treatment. They should follow up with their primary care physician if their symptoms have not improved within 72 hours, or if they have not completely resolved at the end of their treatment course. Furthermore, caregivers should be informed about the potential complications of sinusitis and instructed to seek medical attention immediately if any worrisome signs or symptoms develop.

Children that are toxic in appearance or suspected to have orbital cellulitis or intracranial complications should be admitted to the hospital, with appropriate antimicrobial treatment, imaging, and subspecialty consultation (2).

COMMON PITFALLS

✔ Not completing a thorough neurologic examination and missing the associated intracranial or suppurative complications of sinusitis
✔ Relying on radiographs to make the diagnosis of sinusitis in children. Pneumatization of the sinuses is variable in children

Acknowledgments

Thanks to previous edition's chapter authors Elizabeth A. Wedemeyer and Vinay M. Nadkarnu.

References

1. Aitken M, Taylor JA. Prevalence of clinical sinusitis in young children followed up by primary care pediatricians. *Arch Pediatr Adolesc* 1998;152:244.
2. American Academy of Pediatrics Subcommittee on Management of Sinusitis and Committee on Quality Improvement. Clinical practice guideline: Management of sinusitis. *Pediatrics* 2001;108:798.
3. Barlan IB, Erkan E, Bakir M, et al. Intranasal budesonide spray as an adjunct to oral antibiotic therapy for acute sinusitis in children. *Ann All Asthma Imm* 1997;78:598.
4. Celedon JC, Litonjua AA, Weiss ST, et al. Day care attendance in the first year of life and illnesses of the upper and lower respiratory tract in children with a familial history of atopy. *Pediatrics* 1999;104:495.
5. Doern GV, Pfaller MA, Kugler K, et al. Prevalence of antimicrobial resistance among respiratory tract isolates of *Streptococcus pneumoniae* in North America: 1997 results from SENTRY antimicrobial surveillance program. *Clin Infect Dis* 1998;27:764.

6. Fireman P. Diagnosis of sinusitis in children—emphasis on the history and physical examination. *J Allergy Clin Immunol* 1992;90:433.

7. Hopp R, Cooperstock M. Medical management of sinusitis in pediatric patients. *Curr Porbl Pediatr* 1997;27:178.

8. Isaacson G. Sinusitis in childhood. *Pediatr Clin North Am* 1996;43:1297.

9. Jacobs MR, Bajaksouzian S, Zilles A, et al. Susceptibilities of *Streptococcus pneumoniae* and *Haemophilus influenzae* to 10 oral antimicrobial agents based on pharmacodynamic parameters: 1997 US Surveillance study. *Antimicrob Agents Chemother* 1999;43:1901.

10. Lazar R, Younis R, Parvey L. Comparison on plain radiographs, coronal CT, and intraoperative findings in children with chronic sinusitis. *Otolaryngol Head Neck Surg* 1992;107:29.

11. McCormick DP, John SD, Swischuk LE, et al. A double-blind, placebo-controlled trial of decongestant-antihistamine for the treatment of sinusitis in children. *Clin Ped* 1996;35:457.

12. Newton D. Sinusitis in children and adolescents. *Prim Care* 1996;23:701.

13. Ott NL, O'Connell EJ, Hoffman AD, et al. Childhood Sinusitis. *Mayo Clin Proc* 1991;66:1238.

14. Ros SP, Herman BE, Azar-Kia B. Acute sinusitis in children: is the Water's view sufficient? *Pediatr Radiol* 1995;25:306.

15. Ueda D, Yoto Y. The ten-day mark as a practical diagnostic approach for acute paranasal sinusitis in children. *Pediatr Infect Dis J* 1996;15:576.

16. Wald ER. Sinusitis. *Pediatr Ann* 1998;27:811.

17. Wald ER. Sinusitis in children. *N Engl J Med* 1992;326:319.

18. Wald ER, Chiponis D, Ledesma-Medina J. Comparitive effectiveness of amoxicillin and amoxicillin-clavulanate potassium in acute paranasal sinus infections in children: a double-blind, placebo-controlled trial. *Pediatrics* 1986;77:795.

19. Wald ER, Guerra N, Byers C. Upper respiratory infections in young children: duration of and frequency of complications. *Pediatrics* 1991;87:129.

20. Wald ER, Milmoe GJ, Bowen A, et al. Acute maxillary sinusitis in children. *N Engl J Med* 1981;304:749.

21. Wald ER, Pang D, Milmoe GJ, et al. Sinusitis and its complications in the pediatric patient. *Pediatr Clin North Am* 1981;28:777.

22. Younis, RT, Anand VK, Davidson B. The role of computed tomography and magnetic resonance imaging in patients with sinusitis with complications. *Laryngoscope* 2002;112:224.

CHAPTER 266
Torticollis

Gregory G. Gaar

The word *torticollis* is derived from the Latin words *tortus*, meaning "twisted," and *collum*, meaning "neck." Medically, *torticollis* is defined as "a contraction, often spasmodic, of the muscles of the neck, chiefly those supplied by the spinal accessory nerve; the head is drawn to one side and usually rotated so that the chin points to the other side" (13) It is a manifestation of illness, not a disease in itself, which means the etiology and pathophysiology can be very wide-ranging. As many as 80 different etiologies have been documented in the medical literature (12).

CLINICAL PRESENTATION

The clinical presentation of torticollis in the newborn is often a firm, nontender, unilateral enlargement in the sternocleidomastoid muscle, which is noticed shortly after birth (5). Older children and adults present with the head rotated on the neck, tilted to the affected side, with the chin pointed to the opposite direction.

DIFFERENTIAL DIAGNOSIS

The most commonly accepted categories of torticollis are congenital and acquired, depending on the etiology and time of onset and recognition.

Congenital Torticollis

The congenital causes can be subdivided into those caused by malformations and those caused by deformations. Malformations are caused by a defect during morphogenesis, whereas deformations occur secondary to intrauterine postures and crowding.

Malformations can develop in the cervical spine, the cervical musculature, or the central nervous system. Rare cervical spine anomalies cause torticollis: odontoid hypoplasia, cervical spine fusions (Klippel-Feil syndrome), hemivertebrae, spina bifida, or congenital scoliosis (1,15). Hypertrophy or absence of the cervical musculature is one etiology (15). An arteriovenous fistula at the craniocervical junction has been reported (2).

Pseudotumor of infancy and congenital muscular torticollis are reported with an incidence of 0.4% to 1.3%, respectively (6). The condition results from a unilateral fibrous contraction of the sternocleidomastoid muscle (1,4,6). It usually appears at ages younger than 1 month and resolves by the age of 6 months (4). Physical examination often reveals a firm, nontender, immobile mass in the sternocleidomastoid muscle (5). The exact etiology is unknown. There is a higher prevalence in breech and difficult deliveries assisted by forceps. Although most cases resolve spontaneously, some 10% to 20% of the cases will develop progressive torticollis (4).

Congenital ocular disturbances can be a cause of torticollis that presents later in life. In one series, 4% of the total number of children with torticollis had ocular abnormalities. These were usually a fourth nerve palsy with resultant strabismus (1).

Deformations of the spine leading to torticollis can happen in the presence of uterine tumors, oligohydramnios, and multiple fetuses (15). These cases of torticollis secondary to intrauterine postures are usually transient and resolve within a few months.

Brachial plexus palsies due to birth trauma can also cause torticollis (1).

Acquired Torticollis

The causes of acquired torticollis are extremely varied. Often, the cause is associated with involvement of the cervical spine. Trauma to the cervical spine, resulting in subluxations or fracture and dislocations, is one cause. This trauma can be relatively minor, such as the hyperflexion or hyperextension of a "whiplash" injury. Onset of symptoms can be delayed by several months (15). The most common areas affected are the atlantoaxial area and C-2 on C-3 (15). Ligamentous laxity in the atlantoaxial region is commonly a cause of subluxation, which can present as torticollis. These cases are often associated with underlying disorders, such a trisomy 21 (Down syndrome), mucopolysaccharidosis, and invasive erosion from surrounding soft-tissue infections (1,11). Infections of the cervical spine, such as osteomyelitis and discitis, can present as torticollis (15), as can metastatic or primary osteomas (11).

Other causes of torticollis do not involve the cervical spine. Clavicle fractures, with resultant splinting of that area because of pain, has been recognized as a cause (1,11). Infections of the surrounding soft tissues, such as nasopharyngeal abscesses, retropharyngeal abscesses, cervical adenitis, tonsillitis, mastoiditis, and sinusitis, have been reported in the literature as etiologic agents (1,15). In one recent study, 37% of patients with radiography confirmed retropharyngeal abscess presented with physical examination findings of torticollis (8). The twisting of the neck found on physical examination in these cases is felt to be due to pain from underlying cervical muscle spasms and not from an underlying spinous abnormality. If the infection is extensive, erosion of paraspinous ligaments has been reported, with subsequent rotatory subluxation in the atlantoaxial region (15). Pseudotumor cerebri can present as torticollis in older children as well (14).

Torticollis appearing later in childhood can be due to compensation for underlying strabismus or diplopia (1,11).

Paroxysmal torticollis of infancy is due to vestibular dysfunction. It typically presents between the ages of 2 and 8 months (9). This episodic torticollis often is associated with vomiting, pallor, ataxia, or irritability (10). It is usually a self-limiting disease that resolves by age 2 to 3 years (3).

Dystonic reactions to medication can present as torticollis. These are most commonly caused by phenothiazine ingestions. Differentiation, in these instances, is usually made by the presence of ocular symptoms suggestive of oculogyric crisis.

The nuchal rigidity of bacterial meningitis can be confused with torticollis in younger patients. The mental status, behavioral, and physiologic changes that accompany meningitis are the key to differentiation.

EMERGENCY DEPARTMENT EVALUATION

Careful historic questioning concerning the location, severity, and onset of pain and abnormal posture of the neck is important. Patients should be asked about radiation of any pain. In classic cases of torticollis, there is unilateral neck pain. The pain may radiate to the ipsilateral shoulder but no further. Historic information about fever and constitutional signs and symptoms is important in determining infectious or inflammatory causes of torticollis. The possibility of phenothiazine exposure should be explored.

In older children and adults, acute torticollis often presents after trauma. Even with seemingly mild trauma, careful evaluation of the cervical spine, including appropriate radiographs, is necessary to rule out cervical spine fractures or subluxations. In the absence of such fractures, a thorough examination of the head, eyes, ears, nose, and throat should be performed to search for inflammatory causes. Careful physical examination should distinguish torticollis from the nuchal rigidity of bacterial meningitis. Palpation of the clavicles is necessary to isolate bony pain or crepitus. On neurologic examination, there should be no motor or sensory deficit in congenital muscular torticollis or that due to muscle spasm. There should be no sign of papilledema.

In infants, especially those less than 1 month of age, historic data concerning the birth should be collected. Information concerning birth presentation and the use of forceps may be found only by review of the birth medical records. Careful physical examination in these cases is likely to find the mass in the sternocleidomastoid, which helps to make the diagnosis of pseudotumor of infancy. Signs consistent with brachial plexus palsy are diagnostic of torticollis due to that etiology.

The evaluation of chronic torticollis differs if it is episodic or static in nature. For patients with recurring episodes, the emergency physician should perform a careful history of drug usage and a careful neurologic examination. Torticollis that is constant requires careful ophthalmologic and neurologic examination for strabismus and subtle cerebellar or other neurologic signs, which might be indicative of central nervous system lesions.

EMERGENCY DEPARTMENT MANAGEMENT

Patients who are younger than 1 month and present with a physical examination consistent with pseudotumor of infancy or brachial plexus palsy from a birth injury can be referred to their pediatricians for further work up and follow up. Similarly, those whose history and examination are consistent with an intrauterine deformity due to multiple births, uterine tumor, or oligohydramnios can be referred for follow up.

All other patients who present with an acute onset of torticollis that is not chronic and paroxysmal in nature, and those who present to be evaluated for the first time with a history of static torticollis, should have radiographs of their cervical spines after proper immobilization. This is necessary to rule out fracture or subluxation. It must be remembered that ligamentous instability from a congenital cause can often present as the result of a minor injury received several months prior to the emergency department visit. When no radiographic fracture or subluxation is identified, further history and physical examination will help to uncover the underlying etiology of the torticollis.

The management then follows based on the etiology and pathophysiology. If there are any abnormalities on neurologic examination, computerized tomography of the brain or magnetic resonance imaging is indicated. If there are signs and symptoms of an infection or inflammatory process, appropriate diagnostic studies should be obtained prior to institution of antibiotic therapy. If the torticollis is felt to be related to phenothiazine use, diphenhydramine [2 mg/kg IV (50 mg maximum)] can be given to counteract the dystonic reaction. Careful evaluation of the optic nerves should help in establishing the diagnosis of pseudotumor cerebri in older children (14).

Depending on the etiology, consultation with neurosurgery, neurology, or radiology colleagues should be considered.

CRITICAL INTERVENTIONS

- Obtain a good birth history in newborns with torticollis
- Obtain a cervical spine films to rule out a fracture or subluxation in the patient with potential traumatic etiology

DISPOSITION

Neurosurgical consultation and admission should be obtained for all patients with evidence of cervical spine fractures, subluxation, or dislocation. Ambulatory follow up by the primary care pediatrician is sufficient in those infants with pseudotumor or congenital muscular torticollis. In some cases, conservative therapy in the form of manual stretching is all that is necessary (7). Some children eventually require surgical treatment (7).

Appropriate treatment for the underlying cause of the torticollis is the mainstay of good therapy.

COMMON PITFALLS

✔ Failure to consider the myriad nonmuscular causes of torticollis
✔ Failure to immobilize the neck
✔ Failure to consider phenothiazine side effects, even when used in an appropriate therapeutic dosage
✔ Failure to consider infectious causes such as retropharyngeal abscesses and retropharyngeal cellulitis

References

1. Ballock RT, Song KM. The prevalence of nonmuscular causes of torticollis in children. *J Pediatr Orthop* 1996;16:500.
2. Bayraker B, Aysun S, Firat M. Arteriovenous fistula: a cause of torticollis. *Pediatr Neurol* 1999;20:146.
3. Bratt HD, Menelaus MB. Benign paroxysmal torticollis of infancy. *J Bone Joint Surg Am* 1992;74:449.
4. Bredenkamp JK, Hoover LA, Berke GS. Congenital muscular torticollis: a spectrum of disease. *Arch Otolaryngol Head Neck Surg* 1990;116:212.
5. Chandler FA, Altenberg A. "Congenital" muscular torticollis. *JAMA* 1944; 125:476.
6. Cheng JCY, Au AW. Infantile torticollis: a review of 624 cases. *J Pediatr Orthop* 1994;14:802.
7. Cheng JCY, Tang SP, Chen TMK. Sternocleidomastoid pseudotumor and congenital muscular torticollis in infants: a prospective study of 510 cases. *J Pediatr* 1999;134:712.
8. Craig FW, Schunk JE. Retropharyngeal abscess in children: clinical presentation, utility of imaging, and current management. *Pediatrics* 2003;111:1394.
9. Deonna T, Martin D. Benign paroxysmal torticollis in infancy. *Arch Dis Child* 1981;56:956.
10. Hanukoglu A, Somekh E, Fried D. Benign paroxysmal torticollis in infancy. *Clin Pediatr* 1984;23:272.
11. Kahn ML, Davidson R, Drummond DS. Acquired torticollis in children. *Orthop Rev* 1991;20:667.
12. Kiwak KJ. Establishing an etiology for torticollis. *Postgrad Med* 1984;75:126.
13. Spraycar M, ed. *Stedman's medical dictionary*, 26th ed. Baltimore: Williams & Wilkins, 1995.
14. Straussberg R, Harrel L, Amir J. Pseudotumor cerebri manifesting as stiff neck and torticollis. *Pediatric Neurology* 2002;26:225.
15. Suchowersky O, Caine DB. Non-dystonic causes of torticollis. *Adv Neurol* 1988; 50:501.

CHAPTER 267
Urinary Tract Infections in Children

Kathleen Brown

Urinary tract infections (UTIs) are the most common serious bacterial infections in infants and young children. Estimates of the true incidence of urinary tract infection depend on rates of diagnosis and investigation. At least 8% of girls and 2% of boys will have a urinary tract infection in childhood, and between 30% and 40% will have another episode within 2 years (24). A high index of suspicion is necessary to diagnose UTI in infants as they often present with nonspecific symptoms. Accurate diagnosis, prompt therapy and appropriate follow up studies are thought to be more important in infants and young children because they are at higher risk for vesicoureteral reflux (VUR) and renal scarring (1). Renal scarring is thought to be associated with a greater risk of hypertension and renal failure.

CLINICAL PRESENTATION

The clinical presentation of children with UTI varies with age. Children younger than age 2 years, usually present with fever alone, or nonspecific symptoms such as vomiting, diarrhea, failure to thrive, irritability and jaundice. Preschool children may present with more specific symptoms of suprapubic pain, ur-

gency, dysuria, and frequency. However children in this age group may also present with only nonspecific symptoms such as fever, generalized abdominal pain, and diarrhea. Parental report of foul smelling urine has not been shown to be associated with infection (25). Enuresis in a previously continent child may be an indicator of possible infection. In the school-age child with a UTI, symptoms associated with the urinary tract are usually present. Fever may or may not be present and although it suggests upper tract disease, it can be present in patients with cystitis, and may be absent in a patient with significant renal involvement. In this age group, the overwhelming majority of patients are girls, with a higher risk among white girls.

The cumulative risk for a primary symptomatic UTI to occur in a child from age one to eleven years is 1.1% for a boy and 3% for a girl, with the highest risk occurring during infancy and decreasing with increasing age. Several factors affect the risk for UTI in children. In neonates the prevalence rate in patients presenting with fever is highest, reported as 7.5% to 13.6%. In this age group the reported rate of prevalence for boys is 5 to 8 times that in girls (3,16). In febrile children 2 months to 2 years of age with no apparent source of fever, the overall prevalence of UTI is approximately 3% to 5% (8,22). This rate varies due to a number of known factors including age, race, sex, and in males, whether they have been circumcised. The prevalence of UTI in febrile girls age 2 months to 2 years is more than twice that in boys (relative risk, 2.27). The prevalence of UTI in girls younger than 1 year of age is 6.5%; in boys, it is 3.3%. The prevalence of UTI in girls between 1 and 2 years of age is 8.1%; in boys it is 1.9%. Recurrence rates are also higher in girls, reaching 40%. White race and a fever of 39° Celcius also raise the risk of a UTI in children under 2 years (12,22). Reported rates of UTI in uncircumcised boys are 5 to 20 times higher than in circumcised boys (21). The presence of an identifiable "source" for fever may also be a factor. Patients with bronchiolitis have been shown to have a relatively decreased risk of UTI (14). However patients in this age group who present with an upper respiratory infection or otitis media and fever have not been shown to have a lower prevalence of UTI (22). Therefore, while patients with bronchiolitis and fever may not need to undergo a full septic work up, a urinalysis and urine culture should usually be obtained in these infants.

Clinical presentation does not reliably differentiate cystitis from pyelonephritis nor predict those with associated bacteremia. The large majority of children under age 5 years with UTIs have renal parenchymal involvement seen by technetium-99m dimercaptosuccinic acid (DMSA) renal scan. In this age group, all UTIs should be presumed to be pyelonephritis. Two recent studies have compared the use of a serum procalcitonin level to the CRP as a marker for pyelonephritis. These studies suggest that procalcitonin may be a more specific marker for pyelonephritis.

DIFFERENTIAL DIAGNOSIS

In infants, UTI should be included in the differential diagnoses of fever, irritability, gastroenteritis, failure to thrive, and sepsis. When the preschool-age and older child present with urgency, dysuria, or frequency, the differential diagnosis for this complex of symptoms should include urethritis, pinworms, vaginitis, and child abuse. Physical examination of the genitalia is necessary to assess for the presence of these problems. Children with constipation are at increased risk of UTIs, and the diagnosis should also be considered in these patients. In the adolescent patient the presence of sexually transmitted diseases needs to be considered.

EMERGENCY DEPARTMENT EVALUATION

When evaluating a pediatric patient with a possible UTI in the ED the overall condition of the patient and the need for supportive therapy such as hydration should be assessed. The presence and risk for short term complications such as sepsis or meningitis need to be evaluated especially in the young infant. The overall risk of bacteremia in children less than 5 years old with UTI is 5%, with the highest prevalence in those less than 6 months of age (8%). Laboratory studies to assess renal function may be indicated in the neonate or infant or those with appropriate signs and symptoms.

When considering diagnostic testing for UTI in pediatric patients a number of issues arise. These include: who should be screened for UTI; how should specimens be collected; and which screening tests should be employed?

Who Should be Screened for UTI?

As discussed above, children less than 2 years usually present with nonspecific signs and symptoms. All children less than 2 months with fever or unexplainable symptoms should be screened for UTI. The American Academy of Pediatrics (AAP) strongly recommends screening girls and uncircumcised males greater than 2 months but less than 2 years with unexplained fever. In circumcised males greater than 1 year of age the prevalence of both UTI and VUR is lower and thus it is not cost effective to pursue invasive diagnostic procedures in this group for unexplained fever unless empiric antibiotic therapy is to be given (1). Gorelick and Shaw attempted to define a decision rule for obtaining cultures on febrile girls younger than 2 years old. They found that the presence of two of five high risk criteria predicted a positive culture with a sensitivity of 0.95 (0.85–0.99) and specificity of 0.31 (0.28–0.34). The high-risk criteria were: age less than 12 months, white race, temperature of 39° Celsius or higher, fever for 2 days or more and absence of another source of fever on exam (5). In older children, testing can usually be reserved for those with more specific signs and symptoms, but may still be indicated in those with unexplained fever, especially if antibiotics are to be given empirically.

How Should Specimens be Collected?

In children who are continent of urine and able to produce a clean catch sample with the help of an adult, this is an acceptable means of obtaining a specimen for culture and screening tests. However in children who are not yet continent of urine, which includes those less than 2 years of age, the age group in which testing is most often indicated, other methods of collection must be utilized. Urine collected by a bag affixed to the perineum is likely to yield an unacceptably high rate of false-positive results no matter how well the perineum is cleaned. It has been estimated that a positive culture obtained from urine collected by a bag applied to the perineum will be a false result 85% of the time when the prevalence rate of UTI is 5%. In a population with a lower prevalence rate, the false positive rate is even higher, and up to 99% in circumcised boys (1).

Urine obtained by suprapubic aspiration (SPA) or transurethral catheterization is unlikely to be contaminated and therefore is the preferred specimen for documenting UTI. SPA has been considered the "gold standard" for obtaining urine for detecting bacteria in bladder urine accurately. Urine obtained by transurethral catheterization of the urinary bladder for urine culture has a sensitivity of 95% and a specificity of 99% compared with that obtained by SPA. Both techniques have limited risks but require some skill and experience, particularly in small infants,

girls, and uncircumcised boys. In boys with moderate or severe phimosis or girls with extensive vaginal adhesions, catheterization may be difficult or impossible. Variable success rates for obtaining urine by SPA have been reported (23% to 90%).

Many physicians and parents perceive these procedures as unacceptably invasive and are therefore tempted to use a specimen collected in a bag affixed to the perineum as a "screening" test. If this option is used, the bag specimen should be sent for UA or other screening test. If that test is negative and antimicrobial therapy is not otherwise indicated, further testing can be avoided. However, if the screening test suggests presence of a UTI, a specimen must be collected by suprapubic aspiration or catheterization for culture. This option will often result in a longer ED stay as in many cases two specimens will need to be collected and analyzed. This may be an acceptable practice in a situation where immediate or empiric antibiotic therapy is not indicated. However if antimicrobial therapy is initiated before obtaining a specimen of urine for culture that is unlikely to be contaminated, the opportunity may be lost to confirm the presence or establish the absence of UTI. Therefore, in the situation in which antimicrobial therapy will be initiated, SPA or catheterization is required to establish the diagnosis of UTI.

What Screening Tests Should be Ordered?

The urine culture is considered the gold standard for diagnosis of UTI in both children and adults. However in the ED setting these results are rarely available when making treatment decisions. In the adult population treatment is often based on screening tests or the presence of symptoms. In children, symptoms are often absent or nonspecific and screening tests may be less reliable. In addition the consequences of delaying treatment in an infant with a UTI may be more important.

Multiple studies have compared the various available screening tests for UTI for accuracy. These have often yielded conflicting results. The AAP practice parameter released in 1999 reviewed the studies available at that time. They suggested using the urinalysis (UA) as a screen for treatment while awaiting culture results. They stated that the presence of >5 wbc/hpf, a positive LE or nitrite test and the presence of bacteria on an unspun gram stain were all suggestive but not diagnostic of UTI. The estimated sensitivity and specificity of tests based on available data at that time are reproduced in Table 267.1.

A meta-analysis of the accuracy of screening tests by Gorelicjk and Shaw was also published in 1999. These authors concluded that both gram stain of an uncentrifuged specimen and dipstick analysis for either nitrite and leukocyte esterase (LE), perform similarly in detecting UTI in children and are superior to microscopic analysis for pyuria (6). They reported a sensitivity and false-positive rate (FPR) for the gram stain as 0.93 and 0.05 respectively. The urine dipstick had a sensitivity of 0.88 for the presence of either LE or nitrite and an FPR of 0.04 for the presence of both LE and nitrite. Other studies also suggest that the use of a gram stain may be more sensitive and specific than a microscopy in this age group (4,17). A more recent metaanalysis by Huicho et al, concluded that pyuria > 10 WBC/hpf or 10 WBC/mm^3 and bacteriuria (any) are best suited for assessing the risk of UTI in children (13). An "enhanced urinalysis" that consists of an unspun urine sample using a standardized hemocytometer and a gram stain has been reported to have a sensitivity of up to 96% (9). However this test is not available in most ED settings and is more expensive than urine dipstick testing. A cost effectiveness analysis of 3873 children less than 2 years who had urine collected by catheterization, found that while the enhanced urinalysis was most sensitive (94%), the most cost-effective strategy was to perform cultures on all patients and begin treatment on those who had a dipstick positive for LE or nitrite (23).

TABLE 267.1. Sensitivity and Specificity of Components of the Urinalysis

Source	*AAP Practice Parameter	**Gorelick and Shaw
TEST	Sensitivity/Specificity (Range)	
NITRITE	53 (15–82)/98 (90–100)	50 (16–72)/98 (95–100)
LE	83 (67–94)/78 (64–92)	83 (64–89)/84 (71–95)
NITRITE OR LE	93 (90–100)/72 (58–91)	88 (71–100)/93 (76–98)
NITRITE AND LE		72 (14–83)/96 (95–100)
MICROSCOPY		
> 10 WBC/HPF		77 (57–92/89 (37–95)
> 5 WBC/HPF	73 (32–100)/81 (45–98)	67 (55–88)/79 (77–84)
BACTERURIA (ANY)	81 (16–99)/83 (11–100)[#]	93 (80–98)/95 (87–100)[##]
ENHANCED URINALYSIS[&]	Not Reported	95/89 (No Range Given)

Not stated whether specimens were gram stains.
Gram-stained specimens.
[&] UA plus unspun gram stain.
*Modified from: Practice parameter: the diagnosis, treatment, and evaluation of the initial urinary tract infection in febrile infants and young children. American Academy of Pediatrics. Committee on Quality Improvement. Subcommittee on Urinary Tract Infection, Pediatrics. 1999 Apr;103(4 Pt 1):843–52. Erratum in: 2000 Jan;105(1 Pt 1):141. Pediatrics 1999 May;103(5 Pt 1):1052, 1999 Jul;104(1 Pt 1):118.
**(Modified from Pediatrics 104 (5):1117–1118.)

EMERGENCY DEPARTMENT MANAGEMENT

When deciding on a management plan for pediatric patients in the ED with a possible UTI, the overall condition of the patient and the presence of associated conditions such as dehydration or possible sepsis need to be considered. The need for pain control should also be addressed. When deciding to treat a patient with antibiotics based on the results of preliminary clinical and laboratory assessments, a number of questions arise. These include; who should be treated empirically? Which of these patients require parenteral therapy? What drug should be used and how long should therapy be continued? Finally the ED physician needs to be able to interpret the results of urine cultures in patients who are referred or who have left the ED with or without antibiotic therapy.

Who Should Be Treated in the ED?

The gold standard for diagnosing a UTI in a pediatric patient is the urine culture obtained by the appropriate method as discussed above. However the emergency physician must often decide on treatment prior to availability of the culture results. Therefore screening tests become important in deciding who should be treated empirically. The discussion of screening tests above demonstrates that there is no one "best" test. In the youngest infants in whom it would be most harmful to miss the diagnosis of UTI, the most sensitive test available should be employed. The gram stain performed on unspun urine and the "enhanced UA" as discussed above meet these criteria. However they are not available in all EDs and are generally more expensive. A strategy of sending a culture for confirmation on all patients and treating only those with a positive UA for LE or nitrite has been proposed as the most cost-effective strategy by Shaw et al (23).

Who Should Receive Parenteral Antibiotics?

In the past it has been recommended that all infants with a UTI be hospitalized for IV antibiotic therapy. More recent studies indicate that it may be safe to treat otherwise healthy infants greater than 1 month of age with a presumptive UTI who do not appear toxic, are tolerating oral fluids and likely to be compliant with oral antibiotics. Hoberman et al, looked at outpatient management of children greater than 1 month of age, using oral cefixime (16 mg/kg administered in the ED, followed by 8 mg/kg/d for 13 additional days), and found outcomes similar to a 3-day course of intravenous cefotaxime followed by oral cefixime (11). Reasons to consider intravenous therapy include age less than 1 month, toxic appearance, need for hydration, inability to tolerate oral medication, or need for intravenous pain control.

Which Antibiotic Should You Use?

Antibiotic coverage depends on the age of the child. For febrile infants younger than 2 months of age, broad-spectrum intravenous antibiotic coverage with ampicillin and gentamicin or ampicillin and a third-generation cephalosporin is appropriate until culture results are available. In older infants and children who require IV therapy a third generation cephalosporin or aminoglycoside is appropriate (ceftriaxone (75 mg/kg/d divided q24h), cefotaxime (150 mg/kg/d divided q6h) gentamycin (7.5 mg/kg/d divided q8h). In patients with compromised renal function, the use of potentially nephrotoxic antimicrobials (e.g., aminoglycosides) requires caution, and serum creatinine and peak and trough antimicrobial concentrations need to be monitored. The change to an appropriate oral drug may be made after clinical response usually within 24–48 hours. Choice of drug should be based on culture sensitivity and resistance data and continued to complete a 7- to 14-day course of therapy.

In children to be treated with oral therapy, initially the main consideration in choosing an antibiotic is regional and local resistance patterns. Recent data demonstrate that resistance to many drugs traditionally used to treat UTIs in children are unacceptably high and increasing. Reported rates of resistance in pediatric UTI isolates are as high as 78%, 60% and 82% for amoxicillin, trimethoprim–sulfamethoxazole and cefazolin respectively. Most of this data is from international reports and resistance rates are thought to vary widely by geographic region (2,15,18,20). Reported resistance rates to amoxicillin-clavulanate are lower (3%–24%) but still may be significant in some communities. Reported rates of resistance to Ceftin remain low (< 5%). Cefixime, which has been used effectively as pediatric UTI therapy, is no longer manufactured. Knowledge of current rates of resistance in your community is essential to choosing effective therapy.

How Long Should You Treat?

Recommendations on the duration of therapy vary. Because short-course and single-dose therapies have been successful with

TABLE 267.2.   Interpretation of Urine Culture Results

Method of Collection	Colony Count (cfu/ml of Single Organism)*	Probability of Infection	ED Management
Suprapubic aspiration (either sex)	Any gram-negative bacilli Other organism > 1000	99%	Treat
Catheterization (either sex)	$> 10^5$	95%	Treat
	10^4–10^5	Likely	Treat
	10^3–10^4	Suspicious	Repeat test
	$< 10^3$	Unlikely	—
Clean catch /girl	$> 10^5 \times 3$ cultures	95%	Treat
	$> 10^5 \times 2$ cultures	90%	Treat
	$> 10^5 \times 1$ cultures	80%	Treat
	10^4–$10^5 \times 5$ cultures	Suspicious	Repeat test
	$< 10^4$	Unlikely	—
Clean catch boy	$> 10^4$	Likely	Treat

women, short-course regimens may be acceptable for uncomplicated cystitis in adolescent girls. Because studies of short-course therapy in children have yielded conflicting results and it is often difficult to differentiate uncomplicated cystitis from pyelonephritis in younger children most experts still recommend a 7- to 10-day course of antibiotics in prepubertal children with cystitis and up to 14 days when pyelonephritis is suspected. However a recent metaanalysis comparing short course (2–4 days) and standard duration (7–14 days) therapy for uncomplicated cystitis in children did not find a difference in the frequency of positive cultures either at the end of treatment or at follow up 1 to 15 months after treatment. They concluded that in children with clear evidence of uncomplicated cystitis short course therapy may be acceptable (19).

How Do You Interpret Culture Results?

The emergency physician is often asked to interpret culture results and decide on treatment for patients who have been discharged from the ED. In adult patients with symptoms of UTI or pyelonephritis the presence of greater than 10^5 cfu per ml of a urinary tract pathogen is a widely accepted standard for documenting a UTI. In pediatric patients interpretation of urine culture results is dependent on gender and method of collection of the specimen. In children as in adults the identification of the isolated organism is also significant. Organisms such as lactobacillus species, coagulase negative staphylococci and corneybacterium species are not usually clinically relevant. Hellerstein first outlined criteria for pediatric patients, based on method of collection, gender of the patient, and the number of cfu/ml of urinary tract pathogens isolated by culture. Similar criteria were endorsed by the AAP practice parameter on UTIs. This information is summarized in Table 267.2.

CRITICAL INTERVENTIONS

- Screen for UTI in all girls and uncircumcised boys less than 2, and all boys less than 1 with unexplained fever
- Always obtain a specimen for culture in this age group if you are planning to treat with empiric antibiotics for suspected sepsis
- Obtain culture by appropriate method SPA or catheterization (not urine bag) in incontinent children
- Assess all children with suspected UTI for presence of dehydration, sepsis or renal failure
- Treat children with suspected UTI or pyelonephritis promptly with antibiotics known to have a low rate of resistance in your locality
- Make sure caregivers of young children understand the importance of follow up and the possible need for repeat urine culture and anatomic evaluation

DISPOSITION

Hospital admission is indicated for all infants younger than age 1 month and should be strongly considered in those less than 1 year of age. As noted previously, clinical judgment may be used for those infants who do not appear ill, who are more than 1 month old, and who will comply with oral antibiotics and recommended follow up in 24 hours. In any patient managed as an outpatient, an initial dose of antibiotic should be given in the ED either orally or parentally.

The 1999 AAP practice parameter recommends that infants and young children 2 months to 2 years of age with UTI who do not demonstrate the expected clinical response within 2 days of antimicrobial therapy should undergo ultrasonography promptly, and either voiding cystourethrography (VCUG) or radionuclide cystography (RNC) should be performed at the earliest convenient time. Infants and young children who have the expected response to antimicrobials should have a sonogram and either VCUG or RNC performed at the earliest convenient time. Although these studies would not be performed in the ED the emergency physician must be cognizant of the fact that referral for these studies is considered standard of care by many experts. The reasoning behind this recommendation is that UTI in young children serve as a marker for abnormalities of the urinary tract. Identification of such abnormalities including VUR may allow for treatment that prevents further renal scarring. However evidence of their value in altering management or improving outcomes is limited. In fact in recent years many have published studies that question these guidelines. Studies of infants with intrauterine dilatation of the urinary tract show that many children previously thought to have incurred kidney damage after an infection actually have congenital renal damage. The importance of VUR in the pathogenesis of acute pyelonephritis has been downgraded with the recognition of the frequency with which kidney infection occurs in the absence of VUR. Some infants with intrauterine VUR and no history of UTI have impaired kidney function or hypertension secondary to renal hypoplasia or dysplasia (7,10).

COMMON PITFALLS

✔ Failure to consider UTI as a source of fever in otherwise asymptomatic children leads to missed or incorrect diagnoses. Mild respiratory and gastrointestinal symptoms do not preclude UTI as the source of fever in the young child
✔ Failure to obtain an appropriate collected urine culture before administering antibiotics may lead to delay in diagnosis
✔ Failure to recognize local antibiotic resistance patterns may lead to inappropriate treatment

✔ Failure to arrange adequate follow up for radiographic studies and repeat cultures may result in failure to find treatable causes of renal disease

Acknowledgments

The author gratefully acknowledges the contribution of Thomas G. Mcloughlin, Jr. who wrote the previous version of this chapter.

References

1. Anonymous. Practice parameter: the diagnosis, treatment, and evaluation of the initial urinary tract infection in febrile infants and young children. American Academy of Pediatrics. Committee on Quality Improvement. Subcommittee on Urinary Tract Infection. *Pediatrics* 1999;103:843–852.
2. Byington CL, Rittichier KK, Bassett KE, et al. Serious bacterial infections in febrile infants younger than 90 days of age: the importance of ampicillin-resistant pathogens. *Pediatrics* 2003;111:964–968.
3. Crain EF, Gershel JC. Urinary tract infections in febrile infants younger than 8 weeks of age. *Pediatrics* 1990;86:363–367.
4. Dayan PS, Bennett J, Best R, et al. Test characteristics of the urine Gram stain in infants. *Ped Emerg Care* 2002;18:12–14.
5. Gorelick MH, Shaw KN. Clinical decision rule to identify febrile young girls at risk for urinary tract infection. *Arch Ped Adolesc Med* 2000;154:386–390.
6. Gorelick MH, Shaw KN. Screening tests for urinary tract infection in children: A meta-analysis. *Pediatrics* 1999;104:e54,
7. Hellerstein S. Long-term consequences of urinary tract infections. Current Opinion in *Pediatrics* 2000;12:125–128.
8. Hoberman A, Chao HP, Keller DM, et al. Prevalence of urinary tract infection in febrile infants. *J Pediatr* 1993;123:17–23.
9. Hoberman A, Wald ER, Penchansky L, Reynolds EA, Young S. Enhanced urinalysis as a screening test for urinary tract infection. *Pediatrics* 1993;91:1196–1199.
10. Hoberman A, Charron M, Hickey NW, et al. Imaging studies after a first febrile urinary tract infection in young children. *NEJM* 2003;348:195–202.
11. Hoberman A, Wald ER, Hickey RW, et al. Oral versus initial intravenous therapy for urinary tract infections in young febrile children. *Pediatrics* 1999;104:79–86.
12. Hoberman A, Wald ER. Urinary tract infections in young febrile children. *Pediatr Infect Dis J* 1997;16:11–17.
13. Huicho L, Campos-Sanchez M, Alamo C. Metaanalysis of urine screening tests for determining the risk of urinary tract infection in children. *Pediatr Infect Dis J* 2002;21:1–11.
14. Kupperman N, Bank DE, Walton EA, et al. Risks for bacteremia and urinary tract infections in young febrile children with bronchiolitis. *Arch Pediatr Adolesc Med* 1997;151:1207–1214.
15. Ladhani S, Gransden W. Increasing antibiotic resistance among urinary tract isolates. *Archives of Disease in Childhood.* 2003;88:444–445.
16. Lin DS, Huang SH, Lin CC, et al. Urinary tract infection in febrile infants younger than eight weeks of Age. *Pediatrics* 2000;105:E20.
17. Lockhardt G, Lewander W, Cimini D, Josephson S, Linakis J. Use of urinary gram stain for detection of urinary tract infection in infants. *Ann Emerg Med* 1995;25:31–35.
18. McLoughlin TG, Joseph MM. Antibiotic resistance patterns of uropathogens in pediatric emergency department patients. *Acad Emerg Med* 2003;10:347–351.
19. Michael M, Hodson EM, Craig JC, Martin S, Moyer VA. Short compared with standard duration of antibiotic treatment for urinary tract infection: a systematic review of randomised controlled trials. *Arch Dis Child* 2002;87:118–123.
20. Prais D, Straussberg R, Avitzur Y, et al. Bacterial susceptibility to oral antibiotics in community acquired urinary tract infection. *Arch Dis Child* 2003;88:215–218.
21. Schoen EJ, Colby CJ, Ray GT. Newborn circumcision decreases incidence and costs of urinary tract infections during the first year of life. *Pediatrics* 2000;105:789–793.
22. Shaw KN, Gorelick M, McGowan KL, Yakscoe NM, Schwartz JS. Prevalence of urinary tract infection in febrile young children in the emergency department. *Pediatrics* 1998;102:e16.
23. Shaw KN, McGowan KL, Gorelick MH, Schwartz JS. Screening for urinary tract infection in infants in the emergency department: which test is best? *Pediatrics* 1998;101:E1.
24. Stark H. Urinary tract infections in girls: the cost-effectiveness of currently recommended investigative routines. *Pediatr Nephrol* 1997;11:174–177.
25. Struthers S. Scanlon J. Parker K. Goddard J. Hallett R. Parental reporting of smelly urine and urinary tract infection. *Arch Dis Child* 2003;88:250–252.

CHAPTER 268
Ventricular Shunt Problems

Erin Doherty Phrampus and Christopher King

Cerebral ventricular shunts are the most widely accepted treatment for hydrocephalus in pediatric patients. In fact, the placement of these devices has become one of the most common procedures performed by pediatric neurosurgeons. Despite ongoing advances in the development of improved shunt "hardware," however, complications associated with ventricular shunts, which can cause significant morbidity and even mortality, remain relatively common. For this reason, emergency physicians must be familiar with the clinical presentations of common shunt problems—which is no small feat, as the signs and symptoms can be subtle and often mimic a variety of benign illnesses (otitis media, viral syndrome, etc.) Additionally, the emergency physician must understand the primary management principles for these patients regarding stabilization and initial treatment in the emergency department (ED). It should be noted that while this is typically a presentation of pediatric patients, adults with ventricular shunt complications will occasionally require management in the ED as well. As is often the case, adults are more likely than children to demonstrate the expected "classic" findings, such as fever, headache, neck pain, vomiting, and visual changes.

Hydrocephalus, an abnormal accumulation of cerebrospinal fluid (CSF) within the central nervous system (CNS), may be either congenital or acquired. Among the congenital abnormalities associated with hydrocephalus are congenital cysts, intraventricular hemorrhage associated with prematurity and congenital malformation of the brain. Acquired conditions that can lead to hydrocephalus include neoplasm, infection, and trauma. If untreated, the natural history of hydrocephalus is, initially, neurologic deficits resulting from elevated intracranial pressure (ICP), followed by profound, irreversible brain injury, and eventually death (5). The purpose of a ventricular shunt is to allow CSF to drain, through a series of catheters and valves, from areas of increased accumulation in the brain. By far the most common indication for placement of a shunt is hydrocephalus, although occasionally shunts are used to prevent elevated ICP in patients with pseudotumor cerebri (4).

All modern ventricular shunts are entirely subcutaneous and have the following components: (1) a proximal catheter that drains one of the cerebral ventricles; (2) an extracranial one-way valve; and (3) a distal catheter. Some shunts also have a single- or double-reservoir system located adjacent to the opening in the skull that can be "pumped" to rapidly drain CSF or accessed percutaneously with a needle to obtain a CSF specimen. The catheters and valves are impregnated with radiopaque markings to provide radiographic visualization. The distal catheter is tunneled through the subcutaneous tissue and terminates in the peritoneal cavity (the most common site), subclavian vein, pleura, or gall bladder (4).

The evaluation of a patient with a suspected ventricular shunt abnormality includes a detailed history, a thorough physical examination (with particular attention given to the neurologic examination), and imaging studies. In some cases, laboratory studies will also be necessary. As mentioned previously, children and adults with shunt complications present with similar symptoms, although adults are usually diagnosed earlier because they are better able to verbalize their complaints. The most common presenting symptom for an adult is headache.

Complications with ventricular shunts can be divided into *malfunction* (failure) and *infection*. Obstruction, the most common cause of shunt malfunction, can be further categorized based on the site of occlusion: (1) proximal obstruction caused by occlusion of the ventricular catheter, (2) obstruction of the valve and (3) obstruction at the terminal end of the distal catheter. Other important causes of shunt failure include disconnection, which usually results from improper use of connectors distal to the valve, and fracture of the shunt tubing. Less commonly, complications can occur within the structures where the distal tubing terminates, e.g., pneumothorax and hydrothorax with shunts that drain in the pleura; pulmonary hypertension and endocarditis with atrial shunts; and cholecystitis and fistula formation with shunts draining in the gall bladder. Rarely, failure of a shunt valve to function properly can lead to excessive drainage of CSF rather than inadequate drainage. Slit ventricle syndrome, orthostatic hypotension, subdural fluid collections, craniosynostosis, ventricular compartmentalization, and cerebellar tonsillar herniation are all reported complications of this type of shunt malfunction (6).

As with other types of artificial devices implanted in the body, ventricular shunt infection primarily occurs when the shunt hardware becomes a locus for bacterial growth through direct contamination or hematogenous seeding. The potential consequences of a shunt infection are similar to those of other bacterial CNS infections (meningitis, brain abscess) and include severe neurologic injury and death. Shunt infection can be broadly defined as any infection of the shunt hardware, the overlying wound, or the distal site. The reported incidence ranges from 1% to 41%, with an average of 10% to 15% (6). Risk factors for infection include patient age younger than 6 months, placement of the shunt within the previous 6 months, and a history of prior shunt infections. The bacteria which most commonly cause ventricular shunt infections are *Staphylococcus epidermidis* and *Staphylococcus aureus*.

CLINICAL PRESENTATION

In addition to the presenting complaints, the history for a patient suspected of having a ventricular shunt problem should include a description of prior events related to the shunt itself. Parents are often very knowledgeable about their child's medical history and can sometimes provide a detailed account of such events from memory. In fact, a parent may well be able to educate the physician about a rare disorder that caused the child to develop hydrocephalus. Yet whenever possible, information from the patient's medical record should also be carefully reviewed to ascertain key information such as the indication for shunt placement, the date of the procedure, complications during the postoperative course, and any history of shunt infections or revisions.

Presenting symptoms of a child with a shunt infection include fever, headache, nausea, vomiting, drowsiness, and redness at the shunt site. Furthermore, progressively worsening abdominal pain may be reported if a patient with a ventriculoperitoneal shunt has infection of the distal tubing (in the peritoneum) leading to formation of a pseudocyst. Indeed, some experts contend that a child with a ventriculoperitoneal shunt who develops significant abdominal pain and signs of peritonitis has an infected shunt until proved otherwise.

Shunt malfunction typically causes symptoms of increased ICP (headache, nausea, vomiting, focal neurologic deficits, etc.) When a child with a ventricular shunt presents with seizures, elevated ICP due to shunt failure should be suspected. Atypical presentations include hemiparesis, cranial nerve palsies, and visual impairment (1). Patients may even have subtle behavioral changes, such as a decline in school performance or incontinence (5). Once again, information obtained from caregivers can be very helpful in such instances, as no neurologic abnormality may be apparent in the ED. As mentioned previously, slit ventricle syndrome, named for the characteristic finding on head CT scan of severely narrowed ventricles, can occur when shunt valve malfunction results in overdrainage of CSF. Interestingly, these patients often present with the very same symptoms described by those with shunt obstruction and elevated ICP, (i.e., headaches, nausea, and vomiting). Physical findings consistent with a shunt malfunction include a tense fontanelle, split sutures, or swelling at the shunt site. Warmth, erythema, and swelling over the shunt hardware are all suggestive of a shunt infection. It is important to remember that a patient can have both shunt malfunction *and* shunt infection at the same time, so that all of the described signs and symptoms may be present.

DIFFERENTIAL DIAGNOSIS

Many symptoms that occur with shunt infection and shunt malfunction overlap with symptoms due to common, benign childhood illnesses like otitis media and gastroenteritis. The child with acute otitis media can present with fever and headache, just as a child with a shunt infection can present with fever and a headache. Whenever there is doubt in such situations, it is generally prudent to assume the presence of a shunt problem until there is sufficient evidence to the contrary. Missing a case of otitis will rarely harm a patient; missing a shunt infection, on the other hand, can quickly lead to life-threatening complications. Clinicians should therefore have a low threshold for performing whatever actions are necessary to definitively exclude a shunt problem from the list of potential diagnoses.

EMERGENCY DEPARTMENT EVALUATION

The first step in the ED evaluation of a child with a potential ventricular shunt complication is to perform a thorough history and physical examination. As mentioned previously, parents and the medical records are usually the most important sources of information, although an older child with good verbal skills may be capable of providing additional historical details, assuming the patient has an intact mental status and is not in significant distress.

The most important aspects of the physical examination are an overall assessment of the condition of the patient (airway/breathing/circulation, vital signs, level of consciousness) and a complete neurologic examination (including a fundoscopic examination to detect papilledema). In addition, the shunt itself should be examined for any signs of infection (warmth, tenderness, erythema) or malfunction (broken tubing, subcutaneous collection of CSF, improper valve function).

As mentioned previously, the typical path of a ventricular shunt starts within the ventricle and exits through a hole in the skull, then travels in the subcutaneous tissue of the scalp inferiorly behind the ear, and continues down the neck to the chest. At this point, the path traveled depends on the location of the terminal portion of the shunt tubing. For a ventriculoatrial shunt, the tubing passes posterior to the clavicle, enters the subclavian vein, and ends in the right atrium of the heart. For a ventriculoperitoneal shunt, the tubing travels anterior to the clavicle, passes through the subcutaneous tissue overlying the chest wall, and ultimately enters the peritoneal cavity (4). Other types of shunts follow analogous pathways leading to the specific terminal structure (pleura, gall bladder, etc.). Wherever the shunt tubing has been tunneled through the superficial subcutaneous tissue (scalp, neck, chest wall), it can be easily seen and palpated. Once the tubing "descends" into the intrathoracic or intraperitoneal spaces, it can no longer be examined externally. Of note, when inspecting shunts that have been recently placed, it is always important to carefully examine any incision sites for evidence of infection.

Digital compression of the shunt reservoir(s) is traditionally described as part of the assessment for possible obstruction. The advantages of this technique are that it is not dangerous, it is straightforward to perform, and it does not require any special equipment. In normally functioning shunts, reservoirs should be easily compressed and should refill rapidly. Difficulty compressing the pump mechanism suggests a possible distal obstruction. A pump that does not refill after compression may indicate a proximal obstruction. Unfortunately, however, the sensitivity, specificity, and predictive values of assessments based on this type of shunt pumping are unacceptably low, and additional studies are always indicated to properly evaluate shunt function (4).

The standard radiographic imaging studies performed in the ED for patients with suspected shunt failure are a shunt series and a noncontrast computed tomography (CT) scan of the head. A shunt series is simply a set of plain radiographs showing the entire course of the shunt tubing (skull, neck, chest and, when necessary, abdomen). A shunt series may reveal a fracture or dislocation of the tubing, fluid collections, or migrated catheters. The head CT scan is used primarily for assessing ventricular size. Ideally, prior CT scans will be available for comparison, since many of these patients have abnormally large ventricles at baseline. Occasionally, an abdominal ultrasound may be used to diagnose complications such as an intraperitoneal fluid collection or a pancreatic pseudocyst. Overall, proximal (intracranial) shunt malfunction due to ventricular catheter occlusion remains the most common cause of obstruction. The proximal catheter can become occluded if the fenestrations are clogged with choroids plexus, if the tip is embedded in the ventricular ependyma, or if the tip migrates to a nondraining space.

For emergency physicians, it is always advisable to consult with a neurosurgeon before performing a diagnostic puncture and aspiration ("tap") of a ventricular shunt. For patients who are not critically ill, a shunt tap is performed to measure the opening pressure and to obtain CSF for laboratory analysis (cell count, protein, glucose, Gram's stain, and culture). If the shunt is infected, the CSF will typically demonstrate a marked pleocytosis and a low glucose. Rarely, a patient with a ventricular shunt may present to the ED with signs of imminent cardiorespiratory arrest due to elevated intracranial pressure (unilateral fixed and dilated pupil, posturing, apnea, etc.). In an effort to save the life of the child, in may be appropriate in such circumstances for the emergency physician to perform a therapeutic shunt tap without first consulting a neurosurgeon.

EMERGENCY DEPARTMENT MANAGEMENT

As outlined previously, the standard approach to a child who presents in the ED with a potential shunt problem includes: (1) a thorough history and physical examination, (2) a shunt series and noncontrast head CT scan, and (3) evaluation by a neurosurgeon. Other diagnostic tests (blood culture, serum electrolytes, etc.) should also be obtained as appropriate.

A good rule of thumb is that any patient with a suspected ventricular shunt problem should be seen by a neurosurgeon while still in the ED regardless of the results of the diagnostic tests. An experienced neurosurgeon may be alerted to a higher level of concern by a subtle finding that might be difficult to convey in a telephone conversation. Indeed, it is not uncommon for a neurosurgeon to perform a shunt tap to measure the opening pressure because of a lingering suspicion for a shunt malfunction, even when the shunt series and head CT scan show no acute changes. In situations where evaluation by a neurosurgeon in the ED is not possible, transferring the patient to another facility where such services are available is virtually always the best option.

Patients with a confirmed shunt infection should be started on an appropriate regimen of antibiotics that will eradicate both gram-positive and gram-negative organisms. The combination of a third generation cephalosporin (e.g., ceftriaxone) and vancomycin would be an acceptable choice for initial therapy. If the patient is found to have a shunt malfunction, surgical revision will be necessary. The timing of the surgery is determined by the neurosurgeon based on the condition of the patient—patients with severe symptoms require immediate repair, while patients with mild symptoms seen late at night can usually have their surgery delayed until the following morning.

For the critically ill child who is suspected of having impending respiratory or cardiovascular decompensation due to a shunt problem, appropriate monitoring modalities should be initiated (pulse oximetry, cardiac monitoring) and all necessary advanced life-support procedures should be performed. If elevated ICP from a shunt malfunction is believed to be causing cardiorespiratory instability, then vigorous hyperventilation ($pCO_2 = 20$–25 mmHg) and administration of furosemide would generally be appropriate as temporizing measures until a more definitive intervention can be performed. For patients who require transport, any invasive procedures that are likely to become necessary (endotracheal intubation, central line placement, etc.) should ideally be performed while the patient is still in the ED, where space and personnel advantages greatly increase the chances for success.

CRITICAL INTERVENTIONS

- Obtain a detailed history of the indication for shunt placement, date of placement, and prior complications/infections
- Obtain a shunt series and non contrast CT
- Review prior CT scans
- Consult a neurosurgeon and request that the patient be examined in the ED
- Perform any appropriate advanced life-support procedures for the critically ill patient
- Transport the patient as necessary to a facility where proper evaluation and care will be provided

DISPOSITION

Any child with infection or malfunction of a ventricular shunt will require hospital admission. As mentioned previously, a shunt infection is treated with intravenous antibiotics, and a shunt malfunction usually necessitates operative revision or replacement of the shunt by a neurosurgeon. A child with a suspected shunt problem can be safely discharged from the ED if the diagnostic work up is negative and the patient is examined and cleared by a neurosurgeon. Close follow up for these patients must always be assured.

COMMON PITFALLS

✔ Failure to recognize the presence of shunt malfunction or infection due to nonspecific patient complaints. In other children, complaints such as "decreased activity" or "poor appetite" might well be a simple viral illness; but in patients with a ventricular shunt, such symptoms warrant further investigation for other potential manifestations of a shunt abnormality
✔ Failure to review previous head CT scans
✔ Failure to obtain a neurosurgical consultation

References

1. Barnes NP, Jones SJ, Hayward RD, Harkness WJ, Thompson D. *Arch Dis Child* 2002;87:198–201.
2. Drake JM, Kestle JRW, Tuli, S. CSF shunts 50 years on- past, present and future. *Child's Nerv Syst* 2000;16:800–804.
3. Iskandar BJ, Tubbs S, Mapstone TB, et al. Death in shunted hydrocephalic children in the 1990s. *Pediatr Neurosurg* 1988;28:173–176.
4. Naradzy JFX, Browne BJ, Rolnick MA, Doherty RJ. Cerebral ventricular shunts. *J Emerg Med* 1999;17:311–322.
5. Sood S, Ham SD, Canady AI. Current Treatment of Hydrocephalus. *Neurorsurg Quarterly* 2001;11:36–44.
6. Weprin BE, Swift DM. Complications of Ventricular Shunts. In: Honeycutt J, Boop R, eds. *Techniques in Neurosurgery* 2002;7(3):224–242.

PART V

Administrative and Clinical Issues

CHAPTER 269
Pediatric Sedation and Pain Management

William F. Coombs

Appropriate relief of pain and anxiety should always be a priority in the overall management of the acutely ill or injured child. Historically, the medical profession has done a poor job of alleviating such symptoms, preferring to focus on the diagnostic evaluation (16). This attitude has been especially prevalent in the care of children (15).

Dramatic advances in procedural sedation techniques, along with a greater understanding of the pharmacodynamics of available sedatives and analgesics, have led to safer, more effective sedation and analgesia in children. The Agency for Health Care Policy and Research, noting the widespread inadequacy of pain management, has stated in its guidelines that it is the physician's "ethical obligation to manage pain and relieve the patient's suffering" and that such pain management should be at the core of every health-care professional's commitment (1).

GUIDELINES FOR PEDIATRIC SEDATION AND ANALGESIA

The first attempts at developing uniform guidelines for children requiring sedation or analgesia for diagnostic or therapeutic procedures occurred in 1985, when the National Institutes of Health (NIH) and the American Academy of Pediatrics (AAP) published consensus documents on procedural sedation (3). These guidelines discussed appropriate patient selection, monitoring and equipment needs and attempted to define the different levels of sedation and analgesia. Subsequent revisions have focused on more accurately defining these various states of sedation. In 1996, the American Society of Anesthesiologists (ASA) Task Force on Sedation and Analgesia by Non-Anesthesiologists published their own guidelines, which were, in essence, a compromise of those proposed by the various subspecialty societies (4). The ASA rejected the term *conscious sedation* and offered the following definitions, stressing that these states represent different points on a continuum and that movement along this continuum can occur in any direction at any time:

Analgesia: Relief of perception of pain without intentional production of a sedated state.
Sedation–analgesia: Medically induced state of depressed consciousness, during which there is a margin of safety wide enough to have a reasonable expectation that the patient:

1. Will be easily aroused
2. Will maintain intact protective reflexes
3. Will maintain patent airway independently
4. Will have appropriate responses to stimulation, commands

Deep sedation: Medically induced state of depressed consciousness, during which it is reasonable to expect that the patient:

1. May not be easily aroused
2. May developed partial or complete loss of protective reflexes
3. May lose ability to maintain independent airway
4. May be unable to respond appropriately to physical stimulation or verbal commands

General anesthesia: Medically induced state of unconsciousness, during which the patient has

1. Complete loss of protective reflexes
2. Inability to maintain independent airway
3. Inability to respond to any stimulation or command

Although most practitioners would undoubtedly feel more comfortable with the idea of sedation-analgesia, the reality is that the nature of procedures performed in the emergency department (ED) often necessitates deep sedation to ensure an appropriate level of analgesia and cooperation. It is important to note that these guidelines are not absolute rules but rather recommendations that may be adopted, modified, exceeded, or rejected according to clinical needs and constraints (7). The Joint Commission on Accreditation of Hospital Organizations (JCAHO) does not recommend a specific set of guidelines, but mandates that hospitals develop institution-specific policies and procedures regarding procedural sedation that ensure all patients receive "one standard of care," regardless of what area of the hospital it occurs in (7). This mandate should not be misinterpreted as requiring *identical* care in all areas of the hospital.

PATIENT SELECTION AND MONITORING

Administration of sedatives–analgesics should occur in a facility suitable for appropriate evaluation and monitoring of

TABLE 269.1.   Equipment

Positive-pressure oxygen delivery system
Suction apparatus
Blood pressure and CR monitor
Pulse oximeter
Emergency crash cart

TABLE 269.3.   Documentation

Monitor	Document
Oxygenation	Consent
Ventilation	Vital signs
Airway	Oxygen saturation
Level of consciousness	Medications
	Untoward events
	Recovery

the patient and for the performance of emergency resuscitative measures if needed. Monitoring and emergency equipment suitable for children of all ages and sizes must be available (Table 269.1). It should include a positive-pressure oxygen delivery system, suction apparatus, blood pressure monitor, pulse oximeter, and an emergency crash cart. Reversal agents should be readily available. Ideally the practitioner responsible for administering the sedative and monitoring the patient must be someone other than the one performing the diagnostic or therapeutic procedure, and should be appropriately trained and certified.

A full evaluation of the patient's health and medical history should be performed, with consideration given to the physiologic reserve of the patient's major organ systems, as defined by the ASA physical status classification (Table 269.2). Patients who are ASA class I or II are usually considered appropriate candidates for sedation–analgesia or deep sedation in the ED. Patients in ASA class III or IV present special problems that require additional and individual considerations (4).

Evaluation of the patient's recent food and fluid intake is also recommended. Although there is no evidence supporting a relationship between preprocedure fasting and a decreased incidence of adverse outcomes from procedural sedation, specific NPO guidelines have been proposed:

1. Infants less than 6 months: no milk or solids for 4 hours prior to procedure
2. Infants greater than 6 months: no milk or solids for 6 hours prior to procedure
3. All patients, regardless of age, are allowed to ingest clear liquids up until 2 hours prior

In emergent circumstances, in which NPO guidelines cannot be followed, sound clinical judgment should be exercised and the risks of aspiration versus the benefits of the procedure should be weighed very carefully.

Most guidelines dictate that the following parameters be monitored carefully: oxygenation, ventilation, airway, and level of consciousness. Proper documentation calls for the person who administers sedation to obtain appropriate informed consent from the parents and to record the patient's vital signs, oxygen saturation, medications given, and any remarkable or unexpected events (Table 269.3). The frequency of documentation varies with the level of sedation. It is recommended that the

heart rate, respiratory rate, blood pressure, and oxygen saturation be recorded prior to the sedation, every 15 minutes during sedation–analgesia, every 5 minutes for deep sedation, and once again prior to discharge. After the procedure is terminated and sedation is no longer desired, monitoring and recording should be continued until the patient has recovered sufficiently to meet the following discharge criteria:

1. Cardiovascular function and airway patency are satisfactory and stable.
2. The patient can be easily aroused, and protective reflexes are intact.
3. The patient can talk and sit up (age-appropriate).
4. Hydration is adequate.

For the very young or special-needs child who is incapable of the usual expected responses, the presedation level of responsiveness or a level as close as possible to the child's baseline should be achieved. Appropriate discharge instructions include anticipatory guidance regarding sleep, diet, and activity, as well as specific instructions on how to access care in the event of untoward effects or unexpected complications.

PHARMACOLOGIC THERAPY

There is currently no single agent available that possesses all the qualities desired for optimal procedural sedation and analgesia in children. There are, however, many existing drugs that when used alone or in combination for the right indications, are very effective and relatively safe (Table 269.4).

In selecting an agent, the physician must consider the effects desired, the risks and benefits, and the logistics of administration for each situation (Table 269.5). When pure sedation is the desired end-point, agents such as benzodiazepines, barbiturates and propofol should be considered. These agents do not inhibit perceptions of pain and should never be used as the sole agent for pain management. Purely sedative agents however can be used for painful procedures in conjunction with other agents to provide sedation as an adjunct to analgesia. Sedative analgesics such as narcotics, nitrous oxide and ketamine, on the other hand, are excellent choices for painful procedures. Although they have varying degrees of sedation, they should rarely be used as a single agent for providing control for a painless diagnostic study. Combining different classes of agents is a way to produce an effect not present in either agent alone. Such combinations must be used with caution, because they enhance not only desired responses, but also adverse effects.

PURE ANALGESICS (NONNARCOTICS)

Indications: Relief of mild-to-moderate pain
Complications: Gastritis, peptic ulcer disease

TABLE 269.2.   American Society of Anesthesiologists Physical Status Classification

Class I	A healthy patient
Class II	A patient with mild systemic disease
Class III	A patient with severe systemic disease
Class IV	A patient with severe systemic disease that is a constant threat to life
Class V	An ill patient not expected to survive without an operation

TABLE 269.4. Pharmacologic Therapy

	SEDATIVES			
	Midazolam	Pentobarbital	Thiopental	Methohexital
Class	Benzodiazepine	Short-Acting Barbiturate	Ultrashort-Acting Barbiturate	Short-Acting Barbiturate
Peds dose	0.1–0.2 mg/kg IV 0.2 mg/kg IM 0.5–0.7 mg/kg PO	2–6 mg/kg IV	4–6 mg/kg IV	1 mg/kg IV
Adult dose	0.025–0.05 mg/kg Usual dose 2.5–5.0 mg, 10 mg max	—	0.5–1.0 mg/kg	—
Onset	0.5–5.0 min IV 5–20 min PO	1–5 min	30 s	1–5 min
Duration	15–80 min	30–60 min	3–5 min	3–10 min
Effects	Hypotension Apnea Skeletal muscle relaxation Anticonvulsant	Hypoxia Apnea Hypotension Decreased ICP	Hypotension Apnea Decreased ICP Bronchospasm	Fewer cardiorespiratory effects than thiopental

Note: Reversal Agents: *Naloxone (Narcan)*. Dose: 0.01–0.1 mg/kg; how supplied: 1-mg/mL, 0.4-mg/mL, 0.02-mg/mL vials.
Flumazenil (Mazicon). Dose: 0.01 mg/kg (maximum 0.2 mg) repeated every 1 min to maximum of 3 mg; supplied as: 0.1 mg/mL in 5- and 10-mL vials.

Specific Agents

Acetaminophen: Pure analgesic agent with antipyretic properties. The standard dose is 15 mg/kg every 4 hours, can be given orally or rectally, and can be combined with narcotics such as oxycodone and hydrocodone.

Ibuprofen: Nonsteroidal antiinflammatory agent with analgesic and antipyretic properties. The standard dose is 10 mg/kg by mouth every 6 hours.

Ketorolac: Nonsteroidal antiinflammatory agent best suited for relief of biliary and renal colic. The standard dose is 0.4 to 1.0 mg/kg intravenously (IV) or intramuscularly (IM).

PURE SEDATIVES

Indications: Sedation for nonpainful diagnostic or therapeutic procedures

Complications: Dose-dependent respiratory depression, hypotension, "paradoxical" (disinhibitory) effects

Specific Agents

Benzodiazepines

Midazolam: Potent sedative with amnesic and anxiolytic properties, a rapid onset, and short duration of action. The stan-

TABLE 269.5. Clinical Applications

Desired Effect	Age	Options
Moderate-to-severe painful condition	Infant, child, and adolescent	Morphine 0.1–0.2 mg/kg IV
Painless diagnostic study	Infant	Pentobarbital 2–6 mg/kg IV
	Child and adolescent	Midazolam 0.1 mg/kg IV or 0.5 mg-0.7 mg/kg PO
Sedation-analgesia	Infant and child	Ketamine 3–5 mg/kg IM or 1–2 mg/kg IV
	Child and adolescent	Fentanyl 1–2 µg/kg and midazolam 0.1 mg/kg IV (titrate to effect), or Nitrous oxide inhalation

dard dose is 0.02 to 0.1 mg/kg IV, 0.5 to 0.7 mg/kg orally, and 0.3 mg/kg intranasally. When titrating intravenously, remember that the onset of sedation may take 2 to 5 minutes. Children younger than 5 years of age can become excited and agitated when given midazolam (18). Whether this represents a paradoxical or disinhibitory effect and whether higher doses would eliminate the effect are not known. For this reason, the use of midazolam as a single agent for sedation in this age group should be reconsidered.

Barbiturates

Pentobarbital: Sedative agent best used intravenously for nonpainful diagnostic studies. The onset of action is within 1 to 2 minutes, with duration of 30 to 60 minutes and the standard dose is 2 to 6 mg/kg IV. It is recommended to start with an initial dose of 2 mg/kg and titrate to effect with subsequent doses of 1 to 2 mg/kg every 30 seconds as needed.

Thiopental: Ultrashort-acting agent that can cause profound respiratory depression and hypotension. Standard dose is 3 to 5 mg/kg IV or 25 mg/kg rectally.

Methohexital: Ultrashort-acting agent with dose-dependent respiratory depression and apnea but minimal associated cardiovascular side effects. Standard dose is 1 mg/kg IV.

Others

Etomidate: Ultrashort-acting sedative hypnotic with onset of action less than 1 minute and duration of 3 to 5 minutes; it has minimal cardiorespiratory effects. Standard dose is 0.1 to 0.3 mg/kg IV. There is minimal experience with this drug for pediatric procedural sedation although a recent observational retrospective study showed positive results (5).

Propofol: Ultrashort-acting sedative hypnotic with no analgesic or amnestic properties. It has an onset of action within one circulation time following IV infusion and an effective duration of action of less than 5 to 10 minutes. Standard initial dose is 0.5 to 3 mg/kg, followed by either repeated boluses or a constant infusion at 1 to 3mg/kg/hour. It can cause pain at the site of infusion, has potent respiratory depressant effects and can produce significant hypotension. There are very few published studies regarding the use of propofol for pediatric procedural sedation. In one prospective, randomized study comparing propofol with ketamine sedation, propofol scored better by all evaluators, with recovery and total observation time significantly shorter than ketamine (10). In another study involving 91 patients, propofol

TABLE 269.4.   Pharmacologic Therapy (Continued)

	SEDATIVES		SEDATIVE-ANALGESICS	
	Etomidate	Propofol	Fentanyl	Ketamine
Class	**Nonbarbiturate Hypnotic**	**Nonbarbiturate Hypnotic**	**Synthetic Apiate**	**Dissociative Anesthetic**
Peds dose	0.3–0.4 mg/kg IV	0.5–3.0 mg/kg IV	1–2 μg/kg IV	1–2 mg/kg IV
			10 mg/kg PO	3–5 mg/kg IM
Adult dose	0.1–0.3 mg/kg	0.5–1.0 mg/kg	0.5–1.0 μg/kg	0.5–1.0 mg/kg
Onset	30 s	30 s	30 s	30 s
Duration	5 10 min	5–10 min	30–60 min	5–15 min IV
				20–40 min IM
Effects	Relative cardiovascular and respiratory stability	Hypotension Apnea	Bradycardia Apnea Antiemetic	Increased heart rate and blood pressure Airway reflexes intact
	Myoclonus Adrenal suppression	Myoclonus Anaphylaxis with soy and egg allergy	Hypotension (less than morphine) Chest wall rigidity	Bronchodilation Increased IOP & ICP Emergence reaction

used in combination with morphine for closed fracture reductions was shown to have essentially equivalent efficacy and complication rates compared with midazolam/morphine but with a much faster time to recovery (11). Despite these promising reports, further study is needed before propofol can be routinely recommended for procedural sedation in children.

Chloral Hydrate: Sedative hypnotic with a long history of safety in pediatrics. The onset of sedation is unpredictable and can be as long as 40 to 60 minutes. Recovery time is also prolonged and highly variable, limiting its use in the emergency setting. The standard dose is 25 to 100 mg/kg orally or rectally with a maximum of 1 gram for infants and 2 grams for older children.

SEDATIVE ANALGESICS

Indications: Moderate-to-severe pain management, painful procedures
Complications: Respiratory depression, nausea, vomiting

Specific agents

Narcotics

Morphine: The gold standard against which all other narcotics are compared. The standard dose is 0.1 to 0.2 mg/kg IV.

Fentanyl: The most potent of the commonly used narcotics, it has a rapid onset of action (1 to 10 minutes) and a relatively brief duration of 30 to 60 minutes. It has fewer respiratory and cardiovascular depressive effects than other narcotics but can cause severe respiratory depression and apnea when combined with benzodiazepines. The standard dose is 1 to 2 μg/kg IV administered slowly. Rapid boluses have been associated with chest wall rigidity and should be avoided (14). Although available in transmucosal form as a lollipop, the high incidence of nausea and vomiting has limited its acceptability (6).

Nonnarcotics

Ketamine: Ketamine is unique among the sedative analgesics in that it produces a dissociative state between the thalamus and limbic systems, which is characterized by four features: sedation, analgesia, amnesia, and catalepsis. It possesses positive inotropic and bronchodilatory effects, with preservation of spontaneous respirations and protective airway reflexes. These qualities make it an ideal choice for outpatient procedures, with

an excellent safety and efficacy record documented in over 11,000 children (9). The standard dosages are 1 to 2 mg/kg IV, 3 to 5 mg/kg IM, and 10 mg/kg PO. The clinical state produced by ketamine differs from that of other sedatives in that the patient's eyes often remain open but with a disconnected stare and marked nystagmus. This "lights on, nobody home" look can be disconcerting to parents, and they should be forewarned prior to administration of the drug. Potential side effects of ketamine include increased salivary and tracheobronchial secretions and emergence reactions (9). Increased secretions can be ameliorated by adding atropine (0.01 mg/kg; min: 0.1mg, max: 0.5 mg) or glycopyrrolate (0.005 mg/kg; max: 0.25 mg). Emergence reactions are uncommon in children under 8 years of age. Whether the frequency of emergence reactions can be reduced by premedication with a benzodiazepine (midazolam 0.05 mg/kg) is controversial. A recent study concluded that the incidence of emergence phenomena was not affected by the addition of midazolam (13). Laryngospasm following administration of ketamine has been documented in small infants (less than 3 months) with respiratory tract infections, and use of ketamine is therefore contraindicated in this patient population. Other contraindications include: conditions associated with increased intracranial or intraocular pressure, hypertension, thyroid disease, and porphyria.

Inhalation Agents

Nitrous Oxide: This is the only inhalation agent in common use, usually in concentrations of 30% to 70% N₂O. It is a safe, effective sedative–analgesic with a rapid onset and short duration of action upon withdrawal. Nitrous oxide is inexpensive and easy to administer by experienced hands. It is very operator-dependent, with a substantial learning curve. As with hypnosis, suggestion is very important, and the patient must be well prepared in regard to expectations. This method of sedation is best used in older children and adolescents who are more likely to cooperate.

REVERSAL AGENTS

Reversal agents that are available for narcotics and benzodiazepines are:

Naloxone (Narcan): Narcotic antagonist; dose: 0.01 mg/kg to 0.1 mg/kg IV or IM

Flumazenil (Mazicon): Benzodiazepine antagonist; dose: 0.01 mg/kg IV (maximum 0.2 mg), repeated every 1 min to a maximum of 3 mg.

NONPHARMACOLOGIC THERAPY

The involvement of child life specialists in the management of pain and anxiety in the pediatric patient can be invaluable. By providing the patient with age-appropriate information regarding the procedures to be undertaken and teaching appropriate coping strategies, these specialists often succeed in lessening the child's fear and anxiety, thereby reducing and occasionally eliminating the need for pharmacologic intervention. Distraction techniques such as listening to music with headsets, singing, or imagery can also be powerful coping strategies. Finally, parental support at the bedside can play a significant role in reducing the child's distress (2).

COMMON PITFALLS

✔ Inappropriate monitoring during and after procedural sedation

✔ Electing a sedative agent without analgesia before painful procedure

✔ Not giving enough medication because of time factors or fears about side effects, especially respiratory depression

✔ Selecting an agent that titrates too slowly and fails to produce the desired state

✔ Not having reversal agents readily available

✔ Not anticipating disinhibitory effects with the use of benzodiazepines in small children

✔ Not preparing the parents for the nystagmus and catalepsy seen with ketamine

References

1. Agency for Health Care Policy and Research. Clinical practice guideline: acute pain management: operative or medical procedures and trauma. U.S. Department of Health and Human Services, AHCPR Pub. No. 92-0032, Rockville, MD, 1992.
2. Algren JJ. Sedation and analgesia for minor pediatric procedures. *Pediatr Emerg Care* 1996;12:435–440.
3. American Academy of Pediatrics, Committee on Drugs. Guidelines for monitoring and management of pediatric patients during and after sedation for diagnostic and therapeutic procedures. *Pediatrics* 1992;89:1110–1115.
4. American Society of Anesthesiologists. Practice guidelines for sedation and analgesia by non-anesthesiologist. *Anesthesia* 1996;84:459–470.
5. Vinson DR. Etomidate for procedural sedation in emergency medicine. *Ann Emerg Med* 2002;39:592–598.
6. Cote CJ. Sedation for the pediatric patient—a review. *Pediatr Clin North Am* 1994;41:31–59.
7. Green SM, Whittaker WA. Meeting the guidelines and standards for pediatric sedation and analgesia. *Emerg Med Rep* 1997;2:67–78.
8. Green SM, Nakamura R, Johnson NE. Ketamine sedation for pediatric procedures. Part 1: a prospective series. *Ann Emerg Med* 1990;19:1024–1032.
9. Green SM, Johnson NE. Ketamine sedation for pediatric procedures. Part 2: review and implications. *Ann Emerg Med* 1990;19:1033–1046.
10. Vardi A. Is Propofol safe for procedural sedation in children? *Crit Care Med* 2002;30:1231–1235.
11. Havel CJ. A clinical trial of propofol vs midazolam for procedural sedation in a pediatric emergency department. *Acad Emerg Med* 1999;6:989–997.
12. Krauss BS, Shannon M,. Guidelines for pediatric sedation. *Am Coll Emerg Physicians* 1995.
13. Wathen, JE. Does Midazolam alter the clinical effects of Intravenous Ketamine sedation in children? *Ann Emerg Med* 2000;36:579–588.
14. Sachetti A, Schafermeyer R, et al. Pediatric analgesia and sedation. *Ann Emerg Med* 1994;23:237–250.
15. Selbst SM, Clark M. Analgesic use in the emergency department. *Ann Emerg Med* 1990;1010–1013.
16. Wilson JE, Pendelton JM. Oligoanalgesia in the emergency department. *Am J Emerg Med* 1989;7:620–623.
17. Wright SW, Chudnofsky CR, Dronen CR, et al. Midazolam use in the emergency department. *Am J Emerg Med* 1990;8:97–100.
18. Vander Bijl P, Roelofse JA. Disinhibitory reactions to benzodiazepines—a review. *J Oral Maxillofac Surg* 1991;49:519–523.

CHAPTER 270
Dealing with Death or Catastrophic Illness in Children

Phyllis L. Hendry and Mardi Steere

Emergency physicians and prehospital care providers often face the task of telling a family that their child has died or has a catastrophic illness. Dealing with death in the emergency department (ED) is difficult for many reasons. The hectic surroundings and the lack of acquaintance with the family or patient make a difficult situation even worse. Deaths in infants or children differ from those in adults in etiology and in the emotions they create in family and staff members.

EPIDEMIOLOGY OF INFANT AND PEDIATRIC DEATH

Half of all infant deaths are attributable to the 4 leading causes: congenital malformations, disorders relating to prematurity and low birth weight, sudden infant death syndrome (SIDS), and complications of pregnancy (Table 270.1) (3). Infant mortality in the United States has declined by 46% since 1980 and between 1995 and 2001, the overall infant mortality rate declined by 10.5 percent (3,14). Many infant deaths occur in the neonatal period,

TABLE 270.1. Top Ten Causes of Infant Mortality in the United States

Cause of Infant Death	Percentage
Congenital malformations	20%
Prematurity and low birth weight	16%
SIDS	8.1%
Newborn affected by maternal pregnancy complications	5.4%
Newborn affected by placenta, cord & membrane complications	3.7%
Respiratory distress of newborn	3.7%
Accident/unintentional injuries	3.5%
Bacterial sepsis of newborn	2.5%
Diseases of circulatory system	2.3%
Intrauterine hypoxia/birth asphyxia	1.9%

(Adapted from Arias, E, MacDorman, MF, Strobino, DM and Guyer, B. Annual Summary of Vital Statistics—2002. Pediatrics 2003;112(6):1215.)

often before the infant goes home from the hospital. Birth weight is one of the most important predictors of infant mortality (3).

Death due to suspected SIDS is commonly encountered by the emergency physician. SIDS deaths are particularly tragic: a family puts a happy, well baby down for a nap and faces unanticipated death hours later. The emergency physician should be knowledgeable about the epidemiology and differential diagnosis of SIDS. Many states have death review teams for unexplained infant deaths. Deaths due to carbon monoxide poisoning, asphyxia in mechanically unsafe sleeping environments, and overlying (smothering) are often initially labeled as possible SIDS. Fortunately, after slow declines during the 1980s, SIDS rates dropped by almost 40% between 1992 and 1998 and have continued to decline since then, subsequent to the American Academy of Pediatrics recommendation to place infants on their backs or sides to sleep (2,6,8,16). Medical reporting practices have also contributed to decreases in death rates for SIDS as physicians have begun to use other terms that result in classification of these deaths to a different ill-defined or undetermined category as the cause of death (3).

The physical examination of infants who present with sudden, unexplained death or arrest should include a search for signs of abuse, metabolic disorders, and congenital syndromes. Child abuse can be a great imitator of medical and traumatic disease. About 2,000 children die each year of abuse or neglect; 50% of these victims are less than 1 year old (3,16).

After the infant year, the death rate of children decreases. Injury (usually from motor vehicle accidents) is the most common cause of death in children older than 1 year. For all children the leading causes of death in 2001 were accidents (43.5%) and assault (10.2%) (3). Leading causes of fatal injury among American children aged under 15 years are motor vehicle collisions, suffocations and drownings (4). Pedestrian accidents, falls, bicycle injuries, and house fires are other common causes of lethal injury. In adolescents, an adult pattern is seen, with the leading three causes of death being unintentional injuries (49% of all deaths), homicide (14%) and suicide (12%) (3). In some western and southern states, drowning is the leading cause of death in children over age 1 year (8,11).

Most pediatric deaths are sudden and unexpected. Malignancy, congenital malformations, congenital heart disease, and asthma are the more common preexisting disorders seen in pediatric sudden deaths (3). HIV/AIDS is a less common cause, with the annual number of children who died with HIV infection decreasing by 81% to between 1994 and 1999 (19).

GRIEF REACTIONS

In general, society reacts to pediatric death or terminal illness with disbelief, helplessness, and, often, anger. Children are expected to remain healthy and reach adulthood. The high infant mortality rates of past decades are no longer accepted. Parents and family members will usually express guilt feelings, especially when the death was a result of accidental injury. If the death was associated with inadequate parental supervision, family members may blame one another. Hostility among family members may be increased in cases of divorced or separated parents.

Infants and children have often had a recent primary care visit before a sudden death occurs, and parents commonly express anger at the last physician who treated the child. An example is a SIDS death in an infant who recently received immunization shots. Parents may ask the emergency physician why their regular physician failed to see that something was wrong with the child.

Cultural and religious background should be taken into consideration when responding to a parent's grief. Physicians

Religion	Death Practices
Buddhism	The body is left as it is found in death, gently covered with a sheet.
Catholicism	Before or after the time of death, a priest should administer the sacrament of anointing the sick.
Hinduism	Death should be peaceful, and the body must be attended until cremation.
Islam	After the death, the eyes are closed, the mouth is closed with a bandage, and the arms and legs are straightened.
Judaism	The burial is arranged within 24 hours. The body must be attended until the burial. Cremation is not acceptable.

TABLE 270.2. Common Burial Traditions

should be aware of the most common cultural and religious beliefs and respect these traditions (12) (Table 270.2).

SUPPORT AND COUNSELING

Interventions for helping survivors cope with grief are reviewed in Chapter 125. Parental guilt must be addressed soon after the news of death or illness is given to the family. Assure parents that guilt feelings are an expected reaction, and praise them for the positive things they did for their child. Avoid statements such as, "At least you have other children," after a pediatric or neonatal death or a miscarriage. When SIDS is suspected, inform the family that SIDS is a diagnosis of exclusion and that other investigation is required.

EDs should have a plan addressing notification of family, burial arrangements, organ donation, autopsy requests, and family support. The support team may include physicians, nursing staff, social workers, chaplains, the primary care physician, and other local support groups. An example of an emergency department death protocol is shown in Fig. 270.1. (1,6,7,13). Encourage, but do not force, family members to view the body or spend time saying goodbye to the child. Providing a quiet room, privacy, blankets, or a rocking chair can enhance this experience. Many EDs provide foot- or handprints, a lock of hair, or photographs. This is especially applicable in neonatal or infant deaths, when no pictures of the child have been taken before death. These well-meaning acts may be prohibited by local law enforcement policies or in suspicious or abuse-related deaths.

A followup support plan should be in place when the parents leave the emergency department; in one study 70% of the parents reported that it took 3 to 4 years to put their children's death into perspective and continue with their own lives (7,15). Thus it is important to offer support services, although they may not be accepted for days or weeks after the death. National support organizations are listed in Table 270.3.

SIBLING AND CHILDHOOD BEREAVEMENT

The emergency physician should also be knowledgeable about the grieving process in surviving children. The American Academy of Pediatrics recommends addressing the following questions:

1. What is death?
2. What made the person die?
3. Where is the person?
4. Can it happen to me?
5. Who will take care of me?

PROCEDURE: Pediatric Death In The ED
Support For Survivors

Physician Responsibilities

1. Notify chaplain early, as soon as death appears inevitable. Ask clerk or nurse to page chaplain via operator
2. Talk with family (listen!)
   Intervene early and report progress
   Answer specific questions to the best of your ability
   Assure the family that medical care was complete
   Allay parental guilt
   Take PA/Nursing staff with you
   Remember: Doing nothing is doing something! Some people just cannot be consoled or reached acutely
3. Allow family to view or hold their child.

Nursing Responsibilities

1. Assign consistent nurse to the family
2. Facilitate ED phase
3. Accompany physician and chaplain
4. Provide a quiet room and rocking chair
5. Complete ED checklist
6. Personally ensure paperwork forwarded to ED Nurse Manager's office
7. Attach letter requesting medical examiner's report to Notice of Death worksheet

Follow-Up Phase

1. Chaplain phone call to parents 1-2 weeks after death to coordinate support group participation
2. Patient relations to coordinate physician/survivor meeting to review autopsy findings or answer questions

Checklist for Pediatric Deaths

Patient name _____ Unit # _____ Date _____

Relative name _____ Address _____

Phone # _____ Account # _____

Initial Emergency Department Phase

_____ Staff person assigned to family members, who?
_____ Ask family if patient has had a primary physican or medical clinic
_____ If so, who?
_____ Medical examiner notifed
_____ Family notification of death and tentative cause (essential family members present in emergency department)
_____ Family permitted to see baby/tangible evidence of death offered (eg, lock of hair), special requests honored, if so, what?
_____ Family allowed to express grief; respond to individual needs
_____ Family members understand how they may receive autopsy report
_____ Family informed of follow-up procedures and given a phone number to call if they have questions
_____ ED chart completed (including ED form)
_____ Copy of chart enclosed
_____ Organ donation

EMS Office Phase
Family physician/clinic notified of death on _____ Phone # _____

Copy of checklist retained in EMS office? _____ Yes _____ No

Comments _____

Chaplain's Phase
Phone call to family (3–5 days after death) on _____ by _____

Comments _____

Phone call to family (2–3 weeks after death) on _____ by _____

Comments _____

Support group offered on _____ by _____

Comments _____

Patient Relations Phase
Autopsy results requested on _____ by _____

Appointment made for follow-up with physician on _____ by _____

Appointment date _____ Physician _____

Comments _____

Physician/EMS office Phase
Physician's comments after meeting _____

Checklist/chart returned to Chaplain's office by EMS office on _____ by _____

Chaplain's Phase
Call made to family (6 months following death) on _____ by _____

Comments _____

Checklist/chart returned to EMS office for final filing on _____ by _____

Comments _____

Figure 270.1. Example of emergency department death protocol.

TABLE 270.3. National Support Organizations

The Compassionate Friends Inc. (www.compassionatefriends.org)
P. O. Box 3696
Oak Brook IL 60522-3696
Ph: 630-990-0010; Toll Free: 877-969-0010
Support for bereaved parents, siblings, and grandparents;
  chapters in all states.

American SIDS Institute (www.sids.org)
2480 Windy Hill Road, Ste #380
Marietta, GA 30067
Ph: (770) 612-1030; Toll Free: (800) 232-SIDS
Provides crisis phone counseling, grief literature and referrals.

SIDS Alliance (www.sidsalliance.org)
1314 Bedford Avenue, Suite 210
Baltimore, MD 21208
Ph: (410) 653-8226; Toll Free: 1-800-221-SIDS
Provides support to those affected by an infant death.

Pregnancy and Infant Loss Center (www.bloomington.in.us/
  socserv/mit/PREGNANCY_AND_INFANT_LOSS_CENTER.html)
1421 East Wayzata Blvd., Suite 30
Wayzata, MN 55391
(612) 473-9372

Offers support, resources, and education on miscarriage, stillbirth,
  and newborn death. Literature, keepsake items, and sympathy
  cards available.

Table 270.4 lists manifestations of grief in children by age and developmental level. The child's pediatrician or primary care physician should be involved in monitoring the grief process (1).

AUTOPSY

The ED staff should be aware of state and local requirements for reporting deaths and for organ donation. Postmortem examinations by state medical examiners are often required in all sudden deaths of patients in apparently good health. The jurisdiction of medical examiners varies among states but usually includes death as a result of accident, homicide, suicide, or suspected SIDS. Autopsies in infant deaths are strongly encouraged, to find evidence of familial genetic disease, infection, public health threats, or child abuse and neglect.

This subject is difficult to approach. Advise parents that an autopsy allows them and their physician to understand why the child died and how other or future children might be affected. Autopsy results should be made available to the parents in lay terms.

Pediatric autopsies require expertise in pediatrics, pathology, child abuse, and forensic pathology. The fact that many jurisdictions do not have such experts may lead to underreporting, misclassification, and mismanagement of pediatric deaths.

Regarding organ donation, one study suggests that a delay in initiating brain death protocols appears to increase willingness to participate in organ donation and that attending physician involvement is important for families. A delay provides an opportunity for family members to deal with the shock of the initial trauma, and organ donation may be better broached in the environs of the Pediatric ICU (21).

EMERGENCY DEPARTMENT STAFF CONCERNS

A review by Schmidt and Tolle (18) found that emergency physicians responded to a mean of 17 patient deaths per year and were exposed to a much higher death rate than were other specialties. Pediatric deaths usually make up a very low proportion of these deaths, but the exposure to death varies, depending on the patient population, the number of shifts worked, and other factors. Most emergency physicians feel uncomfortable dealing with death and giving bad news to families, and historically they have received little training in this area. The most recent Pediatric Advanced Life Support (PALS) and Advanced Pediatric Life Support (APLS) courses now include modules on the death of a child. Recent literature suggests that physicians involved in the resuscitation of a child should attempt to meet caregivers during the resuscitation when possible to establish contact prior to informing them of the death of their child. This approach may ease both the discomfort of notification and the grieving of the caregivers (12). Parental presence during the resuscitation process has also been advocated and would be preferred by some families, although a recent survey found that only 32% of emergency physicians and 41% of emergency nurses believed that parents should be present for a major resuscitation (5).

TABLE 270.4. Manifestations of Grief in Children

Young Children (<3 yr of age)	Preschool Children	School-Age Children	Adolescents
Regression	Increased activity	Deterioration of school performance caused by loss of concentration, disinterest, lack of motivation, failure to complete assignments, and day dreaming in class	Depression
Sadness	Constipation	Resistance to attending school	
Fearfulness	Encopresis	Crying spells	Somatic complaints
Anorexia	Enuresis	Lying	Delinquent behavior
Failure to thrive	Anger and temper tantrums	Stealing	Promiscuity
Sleep disturbance	"Out-of-control" behavior	Nervousness	Suicide attempts
Social withdrawal	Nightmares	Abdominal pain	Dropping out of school
Developmental delay	Crying spells	Headaches	
Irritability		Listlessness	
Excessive crying		Fatigue	
Increased dependency			
Loss of speech			

Adapted from American Academy of Pediatrics. The pediatrician and childhood bereavement. Committee on Psychosocial Aspects of Child and Family Health. Pediatrics 1992;89:516.

Pediatric deaths are particularly stressful for staff members; staff should be observed for signs of depression, hostility, burnout, or substance abuse. A crisis intervention team should be considered if an unusual number of pediatric deaths occur or if a mass-casualty incident exposes the staff to many deaths at one time. Death policies and crisis counseling skills should be part of the orientation program for new emergency department staff members (10,18,20,23).

COMMON PITFALLS

✔ Do not assume that unexplained infant deaths are due to SIDS without looking for signs of abuse, congenital disorders, or sepsis
✔ Do not handle deaths on a haphazard, day-to-day basis; have an organized plan or protocol
✔ Do not ignore the grieving of the ED staff
✔ Do not ignore grief reactions in siblings
✔ Remember to contact the primary care physician

References

1. American Academy of Pediatrics. The pediatrician and childhood bereavement. Committee on Psychosocial Aspects of Child and Family Health. *Pediatrics* 1992;89:516.
2. American Academy of Pediatrics. Distinguishing SIDS from child abuse fatalities. Committee on Child Abuse and Neglect. *Pediatrics* 1994;94:124.
3. Arias E, MacDorman MF, Strobino DM, Guyer B. Annual Summary of Vital Statistics—2002. *Pediatrics* 2003;112:1215–1230.
4. Ballesteros MF, Schieber RA, Gilchrist J, Holmgreen P, Annest JL. Ranking of causes of fatal versus non-fatal injuries among US children. *Inj Prev* 2003;9:173–176.
5. Beckman AW, Sloan BK, Moore GP, et al. P50 (Parental Presence during Painful Pediatric Procedures) Research Group. Should parents be present during emergency department procedures on children, and who should make that decision? A survey of emergency physician and nurse attitudes. *Acad Emerg Med* 2002;9:154–158.
6. Corey TS, McCloud LC, Nichols GR, et al. Infant deaths due to unintentional injury. *Am J Dis Child* 1992;146:968.
7. Edlich RF, Kubler-Ross E. On death and dying in the emergency department. *J Emerg Med* 1992;10:225.
8. Emery JL. Child abuse, SIDS, and unexpected infant death. *Am J Dis Child* 1993;147:1097.
9. Greenberg LW, Ochsenschlager D, Cohen GJ, et al. Counseling parents of a child dead on arrival: a survey of emergency departments. *Am J Emerg Med* 1993;11:225.
10. Greenberg LW, Ochsenschlager D, O'Donnell R, et al. Communicating bad news: a pediatric department's evaluation of a simulated intervention. *Pediatrics* 1999;103;1210.
11. Keeling JW, Knowles SA. Sudden death in childhood and adolescence. *J Pathol* 1989;159:221.
12. Knazik SR, Gausche-Hill M, Dietrich AM, et al. The death of a child in the emergency department. *Ann Emerg Med* 2003;42:519–529.
13. Krahn GL, Hallum A, Kime C. Are there good ways to give bad news? *Pediatrics* 1993;91:578.
14. Mathews TJ, Menacker F, MacDorman MF. Infant mortality statistics from the 2001 period linked birth/infant death data set. *Natl Vital Stat Rep* 2003;52:1–28.
15. Murphy SA, Johnson LC, Wu L, Fan JJ, Lohan J. Bereaved parents' outcomes 4 to 60 months after their children's deaths by accident, suicide, or homicide: a comparative study demonstrating differences. *Death Stud* 2003;27:39–61.
16. Reece RM. Fatal child abuse and SIDS: a critical diagnostic decision. *Pediatrics* 1993;91:423.
17. Schmidt TA, Norton RL, Tolle SW. Sudden death in the ED: educating residents to compassionately inform families. *J Emerg Med* 1992;110:643.
18. Schmidt TA, Tolle SW. Emergency physicians' responses to families following patient death. *Ann Emerg Med* 1990;19:125.
19. Selik RM, Lindegren ML. Changes in deaths reported with human immunodeficiency virus infection among United States children less than thirteen years old, 1987 through 1999. *Pediatr Infect Dis J* 2003;22:635–641.
20. Smith TL, Walz BJ, Smith RL. A death education curriculum for emergency physicians, paramedics, and other emergency personnel. *Prehosp Emerg Care* 1999;3:37.
21. Vane DW, Sartorelli KH, Reese J. Emotional considerations and attending involvement ameliorates organ donation in brain dead pediatric trauma victims. *J Trauma* 2001;51:329–331.
22. Walsh-Kelly CM, Lang KR, Cheevako EL, et al. Advance directives in a pediatric emergency department. *Pediatrics* 1999;1103:826.
23. Wolfram RW, Timmel DJ, Doyle CR, et al. Incorporation of a "coping with the death of a child" module into the pediatric advanced life support (PALS) curriculum. *Acad Emerg Med* 1998;5:242.

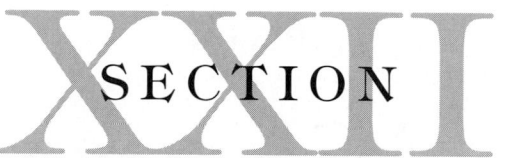

SECTION XXII

Section Editors: Christopher H. Linden and
Jeffrey R. Suchard

Toxicology

PART I

General Considerations

CHAPTER 271

Approach to the Poisoned Patient

Christopher H. Linden and William A. Watson

Poisoning refers to the occurrence of dose-related adverse effects following exposure to a foreign chemical (xenobiotic), including those of animal and plant origin. The principal objectives in the evaluation and treatment of the poisoned or potentially poisoned patient are listed in Table 271.1.

Treatment is determined by both existing and predicted toxicity. Current effects are assessed by the physical examination and routine ancillary studies. Predicting toxicity requires information that may not always be available: an accurate history and knowledge of the chemical's mechanism of action, toxicokinetics (biological disposition), and toxicodynamics (dose-response and concentration-response relationships) (13,20).

The mechanism of action of a chemical depends on its molecular size, structure, charge, and intrinsic chemical reactivity, which determine whether effects are local (limited to the site or surface of exposure) or systemic. Local effects result from exposure to highly reactive chemicals and result from nonspecific chemical reactions such as tissue desiccation, oxidation, protein denaturation, and salvation (see Chapter 307, "Corrosives and Chemical Burns"). In contrast, systemic effects are caused by chemicals that have low intrinsic reactivity and selectively interact with specific targets (e.g., enzymes or membrane receptors), whose function and distribution determine the nature of effects.

Absorption, distribution and, in some cases, biotransformation are prerequisites for systemic poisoning. Because absorption follows first-order kinetics (i.e., the rate of absorption is proportional to the concentration or dose), effects tend to begin sooner and peak later after an overdose than after a therapeutic one. Gastric emptying and the solubility of a substance in gastrointestinal (GI) fluids are rate-limiting steps in enteral absorption. Agents that slow GI motility can have erratic and prolonged absorption. The same is true for overdoses of solid dosage forms because they must first undergo disintegration and dissolution. The rate of tissue distribution, also a first-order process, usually remains unchanged after overdose, but the extent or volume of distribution may increase. This may caused by the presence of more free drug (i.e., the binding capacity of plasma proteins is exceeded) or changes in pH, which can increase the amount of un-ionized drug available to diffuse across cell membranes.

The occurrence and severity of poisoning depend on the concentration of a substance at its target tissue and this depends on the exposure dose: the larger the dose, the greater the tissue concentration, and hence the effect. To paraphrase Paracelsus, the dose makes the poison. Blood concentrations accurately correlate with toxicity only if tissue distribution (or redistribution) occurs faster than absorption (or elimination). If not, blood levels may be higher than tissue levels during absorption and distribution (and lower than tissue levels during elimination and redistribution). Hence, the rate and phase of disposition should always be considered when interpreting blood levels.

Elimination is usually accomplished by metabolic (mainly hepatic) inactivation and renal excretion. Regardless of whether elimination is constant (zero-order), concentration-dependent (first-order), or saturable (Michaelis-Menten equation), it takes longer to eliminate a substance as the dose increases. Hence, the duration of effects is longer following an overdose than after a therapeutic dose. When the rate of elimination is or becomes constant (i.e., is saturable), overdose results in a proportionately greater (i.e., nonlinear) increase in the time for elimination and hence the duration of effects.

The disposition and effect of a of chemical depend on many other factors: the structure, activity, and integrity of external and internal membrane barriers to chemical translocation; body water, fat, and muscle content (which depend on age, sex, and habitus); serum protein levels and organ function (which depend on age and state of health); genetic influences (e.g., target enzyme or receptor polymorphism); and prior chemical exposures (e.g., metabolic enzyme induction or inhibition, target receptor up- or downregulation, and tolerance). The reversibility of poisoning depends on the functional reserve and regenerative capacity

TABLE 271.1. Goals of Patient Evaluation and Management in Poisoning

Evaluation	Management
Recognition of poisoning	Provision of supportive care
Identification of the poison	Prevention of poison absorption
Prediction of toxicity	Administration of antidotes
Assessment of severity	Enhancement of poison elimination
	Prevention of reexposure

of the target organ or tissue (which depends on age and health status) and its importance to overall body function as well the dose and mechanism of action of a chemical. Because host factors are variable and distributed within the population according to a normal (gaussian) curve, disposition and response cannot be precisely predicted, even when the dose and mechanism of action are known.

CLINICAL PRESENTATION

Poisoning most frequently occurs after ingestion (23). Dermal, inhalational, ophthalmic, envenomation (bites and stings), and parenteral injection exposures are also common. Rarely, poisoning may result from rectal, vaginal, urethral, or other routes of exposure. Acute exposures (those that occur over a short period) are more common than chronic ones (those that occur repeatedly or over a prolonged period).

Unintentional poisoning may result from misidentification of a substance (the label may be misread, not read, or missing), its misuse or abuse, therapeutic misadventures, or true accidents, such as unforeseen exposures in adults or children. Misuse can apply to either unintentional exposure (due to carelessness or ignorance) or intentional exposure (excessive self-dosing to achieve a greater or faster response). Abuse is the intentional use of a substance for its psychotropic effects. Therapeutic misadventures may result from dosing errors or may simply be an adverse reaction to an appropriate dose. Intentional poisoning usually implies attempted (or successful) suicide with a chemical agent. It may also refer to the use of substances to harm another person (e.g., attempted murder, child abuse, and chemical warfare).

The agents most frequently involved in reported exposures are pharmaceuticals (particularly analgesics and cough or cold preparations), cleaning products, cosmetics, plants, and hydrocarbons. Ingestion of substances available in the home by children under age 6 is, by far, the most common scenario. Serious or fatal poisoning usually occurs in suicidal adults but is increasingly reported in teenagers and the elderly. Agents commonly implicated in poisoning fatalities include alcohols and glycols, analgesics, anticonvulsants, antidepressants, antihistamines, antipsychotics, carbon monoxide, other gases and fumes, cardiovascular drugs, iron, muscle relaxants, sedative–hypnotics, stimulants, and automotive and cleaning products.

Poisoned patients may present with a wide variety of signs and symptoms (13,16). Manifestations may be local, systemic, or both. Systemic effects may be behavioral, biochemical, cognitive, or physiologic. Subjective complaints may occur without objective findings. The severity of poisoning may range from minor to life-threatening. Patients who eventually become severely poisoned may be relatively asymptomatic on presentation. They can suddenly and precipitously deteriorate with little or no warning.

A history of exposure may be absent when the victim is confused, comatose, unaware of an exposure or its relation to harmful effects (e.g., victims of animosity, chronic or insidious poisoning, and therapeutic misadventures), or unable or unwilling to admit to an exposure (e.g., infants and toddlers, those who have attempted self-abortion or suicide, body packers and stuffers—those attempting to conceal or smuggle illicit drugs in body cavities (21), drug addicts, recreational users of illicit drugs, patients with or proxy to Münchhausen syndrome). The history is notoriously unreliable, with respect to both the identity and amount of substance ingested, in patients with intentional overdose.

Poisoning should always be suspected in patients with a sudden or unexplained illness or injury; those with a history of psychiatric problems or a recent change in behavior, health, economic status, or social relations; those who use chemicals at work or for hobbies; and those who become ill soon after arriving from a foreign country or being arrested or incarcerated for criminal activity (suspect illicit drugs concealed in a body cavity), or after ingesting food, drink (especially ethanol), or medications.

DIFFERENTIAL DIAGNOSIS

Because the signs and symptoms of poisoning are usually nonspecific, the diagnosis may be missed unless it is included in virtually every differential diagnosis. In the absence of a history of exposure, the clinical course may suggest this diagnosis. Poisoning typically evolves more rapidly than other disorders: effects usually begin within 30 to 60 minutes of acute exposure, peak within several hours, and resolve over hours to days. When the history of exposure is unknown or unreliable, a progressive pathophysiological "pattern recognition" approach can help narrow the differential diagnosis (Table 271.2). The first step is to characterize the overall physiological state as stimulated, depressed, mixed, or normal, on the basis of the vital signs and neuromuscular status. The next step is to evaluate the magnitude and pattern of vital sign and neuromuscular abnormalities, other physical findings, and the results of routine ancillary tests and attempt to identify the underlying cause (pathophysiological condition or toxidrome). Grading the severity of physiological abnormalities (Tables 271.3 and 271.4) is also useful for following the clinical course and assessing the response to treatment. The final step is to attempt to identify the particular agent responsible for a condition or toxidrome by looking for unique or relatively poison-specific pathognomonic findings. This approach to the differential diagnosis of poisoning is summarized in the following paragraphs. Further details regarding specific toxidromes and poisonings can be found in subsequent chapters.

Physiological stimulation is characterized by increased pulse, blood pressure, respiratory rate, temperature (8), and neuromuscular activity. It can be caused by four toxidromes: sympathomimetic, anticholinergic, hallucinogen poisoning, and drug withdrawal (Table 271.2). Other features are noted in Table 271.3. Anticholinergic poisoning is distinguished by the presence of hot, dry, flushed skin, decreased bowel sounds, and urinary retention. Myoclonus and choreoathetoid movements can also be seen. Other causes of flushing include boric acid, monosodium glutamate, rifampin, or scombroid poisoning or to a disulfiram-ethanol or niacin reaction. The remaining stimulant toxidromes cause sympathetic hyperactivity resulting in diaphoresis, pallor, tremors, fasciculations, and increased bowel activity with varying degrees of nausea, vomiting, abdominal distress, and occasionally diarrhea. Markedly increased vital signs and organ ischemia suggest sympathomimetic poisoning, since theses agents are the most potent and direct (peripherally acting) physiological stimulants. In contrast, relatively mild increases in vital signs suggest hallucinogen poisoning or drug withdrawal,

---

TABLE 271.2. Manifestations of Stimulant Poisoning

Severity	Signs and Symptoms
Grade 1	Hyperreflexia, irritability, mydriasis, tremors
Grade 2	Confusion, fever, hyperactivity, hypertension, tachycardia, tachypnea
Grade 3	Delirium, mania, hyperpyrexia, tachydysrhythmias
Grade 4	Coma, convulsions, cardiovascular collapse

(Adapted from Espelin DE, Done AK. Amphetamine poisoning: effectiveness of chlorpromazine. N Engl J Med 1968;278:1361.)

TABLE 271.3.   Manifestations of Depressant Poisoning

Severity	Signs and Symptoms
Grade 1	Lethargic; able to answer questions and follow commands
Grade 2	Comatose; responsive to pain; brain stem and deep tendon reflexes intact
Grade 3	Comatose; unresponsive to pain; most reflexes absent; respiratory depression
Grade 4	Comatose; unresponsive to pain; all reflexes absent; cardiovascular and respiratory depression

(Adapted from Reed CE, Driggs MF, Foste CC. Acute barbiturate poisoning: a study of 300 cases based an a physiological system of classification of the severity of intoxication. Ann Intern Med 1952;37:290.)

which cause indirect (CNS-mediated) sympathetic hyperactivity. Mydriasis, a characteristic feature of all stimulant toxidromes, is most marked in anticholinergic poisoning, where pupils are minimally responsive to light and accommodation. Seizures sug-gest a sympathomimetic, anticholinergic with membrane-active properties (e.g., cyclic antidepressants, orphenadrine, and phe-nothiazines), or withdrawal syndrome. Drug- or class-specific findings include reflex bradycardia from selective a-adrenergic stimulants (e.g., decongestants), hypotension from selective β-adrenergic stimulants (e.g., asthma therapeutics), limb is-chemia from ergot alkaloids, cardiac conduction disturbances from high doses of cocaine and some anticholinergic agents (e.g., antihistamines, cyclic antidepressants, and antipsychotics), and intractable vomiting and focal seizures from theophylline. Of the physiological stimulants, only phencyclidine and ketamine cause nystagmus (which can be rotary and vertical as well as horizontal). A bizarre back and forth ("ping pong") gaze can be seen in monoamine oxidase inhibitor poisoning.

Physiological depression is characterized by decreased pulse, blood pressure, respiratory rate, temperature, and neuromus-cular activity (2) (Table 271.4). It, too, can be caused by four toxidromes: sympatholytic, cholinergic, opioid, and sedative-hypnotic poisoning (Table 271.2). Included in the sympatholytic group are agents that decrease cardiac function and vascu-lar tone by nonadrenergic mechanisms. Cholinergic poisoning

TABLE 271.4.   Differential Diagnosis of Poisoning Based on Vital Signs and Mental Status

Physiologic Stimulation	Physiologic Depression	Mixed Physiologic Effects	Absent Physiologic Effects
Sympathomimetics Amphetamines β-Adrenergic agonists Caffeine/theophylline Catecholamines Cocaine Decongestants (oral) Ergot alkaloids MAO inhibitors Thyroid hormones	**Sympatholytics** Adrenergic blockers Antidysrhythmics Antipsychotics ACE inhibitors Calcium channel blockers Clonidine Cyclic antidepressants (late) Digitalis Imidazoline decongestants	**Asphyxiants** Carbon monoxide Cyanide Hydrogen sulfide Inert gases Inhaled irritants Methemoglobinemia Nitrophenol herbicides	**Slow Absorption** Carbamazepine Digitalis preparation Dilantin Kapseals Enteric-coated pills Lomotil Salicylates Sustained-release preparations Valproic acid
Anticholinergics Antihistamines Belladonna alkaloids Cyclic antidepressants (early) Cyclobenzaprine Drugs for Parkinson disease GI/GU antispasmodics Mydriatics (topical) Nonprescription sleep aids Orphenadrine Phenothiazines Plants/mushrooms	**Cholinergics** Bethanecol Carbamate insecticides Drugs for myasthenia gravis Edrophonium Organophosphate insecticides Physostigmine Pilocarpine Nicotine	**CNS Syndromes** Disulfiram Extrapyramidal reactions Isoniazid Lithium Neuroleptic malignant syndrome Serotonin syndrome Strychnine Volatile hydrocarbons	**Slow Distribution** Digitalis preparations Heavy metals Lithium Salicylates **Active Metabolite** Acetaminophen Chloramphenicol Chlorinated hydrocarbons Ethylene glycol L-Thyroxine Methanol Paraquat Some methemoglobin inducers Some organophosphates Thyroxine
Hallucinogens Ketamine LSD and its analogs Marijuana Mescaline and its analogs Phencyclidine Psilocybin mushrooms	**Opioids** Analgesics Heroin Lomotil (diphenoxylate) Tramodol	**Membrane-Active Agents** Amantadine Antidysrhythmic agents Antimalarial agents β-Adrenergic blockers Cyclic antidepressants (late) Fluorides Heavy metals Local anesthetics Meperidine Neuroleptic agents Propoxyphene	**Metabolic Inhibitors** Anticancer agents Antiviral agents Colchicine Disulfiram Fluoride Immunosuppressive drugs Inhibitors of thyroid hormone synthesis MAO inhibitors Mushrooms (amatoxins) Podophyllin Salicylates
Drug Withdrawal Antidepressants β-blockers Clonidine Ethanol Opioids Sedative–hypnotics	**Sedative–Hypnotics** Alcohols Anticonvulsants Barbiturates Benzodiazepines Bromide Ethchlorvynol Hydrocarbons Gamma-hydroxybutyrate (GHB) Glutethimide Methyprylon Muscle relaxants	**Metabolic Acidosis (Low Lactate; High Anion Gap)** Alcoholic ketoacidosis Ethylene glycol Iron Methanol Formaldehyde/paraldehyde Salicylate Sulfur/sulfate Toluene Valproic acid	**Inhibitors of Nucleic Acid Synthesis** **Nontoxic Exposure** **Psychogenic Illness** **Toxic Time-Bombs**

ACE, angioteusin-converting enzyme; CNS, central nervous system; MAO, monoamine oxidase.

is distinguished from other depressant toxidromes by the presence of excessive secretions (lacrimation, salivation, bronchorrhea, and wheezing, diaphoresis), increased bowel and bladder activity (resulting in nausea, vomiting, diarrhea, abdominal cramps, and incontinence of feces and urine), and fasciculations. Relatively more cardiovascular depression than central nervous system (CNS) or respiratory depression suggests a direct or peripherally acting sympatholytic. In contrast, relatively greater CNS and respiratory depression suggest opioid and sedative-hypnotic poisoning, since the cardiovascular effects of these agents are primarily caused by brainstem cardiovascular center depression (or respiratory center depression and consequent hypoxemia) and do not usually occur until the patient is deeply comatose (grade 3 or 4 physiological depression, Table 271.3). Reflex tachycardia may be seen in poisoning by some antihypertensive drugs (e.g., α-adrenergic blockers, nitrates, and direct-acting vasodilators). Most physiological depressants cause miosis, which is most pronounced in cholinergic, opioid, and phenothiazine poisoning. Exceptions include tricyclic antidepressants, class Ia antiarrhythmics, meperidine, and Lomotil, which can cause mydriasis. Nystagmus is characteristic of sedative-hypnotic poisoning. Cardiac dysrhythmias and conduction disturbances suggest antidysrhythmic, β-blocker, calcium channel blocker, digitalis, propoxyphene, and cyclic antidepressant poisoning. Cyclic antidepressants, cholinergic agents, meperidine, and propoxyphene can cause seizures.

The mixed physiological state is characterized by abnormal pulse, blood pressure, respiratory rate, temperature, or neuromuscular activity, but these parameters change direction over time or are discordant (i.e., some are increased and others are decreased). Again, there are four major causes: asphyxiants, CNS syndromes, membrane-active agents (i.e., sodium and potassium channel blockers), and low-lactate increased anion gap metabolic acidosis (Table 271.2). Initial physiological stimulation is followed by depression in asphyxiant poisoning, whereas vital sign and neuromuscular findings are discordant with other etiologies. Except with extrapyramidal reactions and strychnine, the mental status or level of consciousness is abnormal. Marked neuromuscular dysfunction without significant cardiovascular or respiratory abnormalities suggests a CNS syndrome. Membrane-active agents can cause simultaneous coma, seizures, hypotension, and tachydysrhythmias (14). Coma with seizures can also occur in cyanide, isoniazid, and lithium poisoning. Seizures caused by hypoglycemia can be focal. Tachypnea, with relatively mild changes in other physiological parameters, is characteristic of poisoning by agents that cause low-lactate increased anion gap metabolic acidosis. Hyperthermia suggests nitrophenol or salicylate poisoning and the neuroleptic malignant and serotonin syndromes (8). These syndromes also cause pronounced muscular rigidity. Lithium causes tremors, hyperreflexia, vomiting, and nystagmus. Vomiting is also a prominent in arsenic, fluoride, mercury, salicylate, and strychnine poisoning. Brown, gray, or purple cyanosis that is unresponsive to oxygen suggests methemoglobinemia. Hair loss, nail growth abnormalities, mucosal pigmentation, and skin lesions suggest chronic metal poisoning.

The normal physiologic state may be a result of nontoxic exposure, psychogenic illness, or "toxic time-bombs": agents with characteristically delayed or slowly progressive toxicity because of slow absorption, slow distribution, active metabolites, or disruption of metabolic processes (Table 271.2). These conditions usually cannot be diagnosed without a suitable period of observation. Ancillary testing may also be necessary. Criteria for a nontoxic exposure are listed in Table 271.5. Psychogenic illness typically presents as an anxiety reaction (fear of poisoning), often in the form of mass hysteria (3). It can be indistinguishable from low-grade poisoning by stimulants (Table 271.3)

TABLE 271.5. Criteria for Nontoxic Ingestion

1. Time of ingestion and the amount and identity of each and every substance ingested are known with reasonable certainty.
2. Amount ingested relative to patient weight is less than the smallest dose known or predicted to cause toxicity.
3. Time elapsed since ingestion is greater than the longest known or predicted interval between ingestion and peak toxicity.
4. Detailed history and physical examination reveal that the patient is without symptoms and signs of toxicity.

and agents or conditions that caused mixed physiologic dysfunction. This diagnosis should be considered when symptoms occur after a nonexistent or nontoxic exposure or are inconsistent with those expected from a known exposure. Toxic time-bombs include acetaminophen, carbon tetrachloride, colchicine, digoxin, ethylene glycol, heavy metals, methanol, mushrooms, opioids (especially Lomotil), salicylates, and slow- or sustained-release medications (e.g., carbamazepine, cardiovascular drugs, enteric-coated tablets, lithium, phenytoin, theophylline) (4).

The odor of a chemical or the breath or vomitus of a poisoned patient may sometimes suggest the identity of the offending agent (11). Agents with recognizable odors include acetone, ammonia, arsenic (garlic), camphor, chloral hydrate, cyanide (bitter almond), ethanol, ethchlorvynol (vinyl), hydrogen sulfide (rotten egg), isopropyl alcohol, marijuana, methyl salicylate (oil of wintergreen), naphthalene and paradichlorobenzene (mothballs), organophosphate insecticides (garlic), paraldehyde, petroleum distillates, phenol, phosphine (fishy), and thallium (garlic).

Routine laboratory findings, particularly the anion gap, acid–base status, serum lactate level, and osmolal gap, can also be useful in the differential diagnosis (Fig. 271.1) (1,18). The anion gap—the difference between the serum sodium concentration and the sum of the chloride and bicarbonate concentrations (sodium [chloride + bicarbonate])—is normally 13 (±4) mEq/L, the serum lactate level is normally less than 2 mEq/L, and the osmolal gap—the difference between the serum osmolality measured by freezing point depression (but not the vapor pressure or head space method) and that calculated from the serum sodium, glucose, and blood urea nitrogen (BUN) ([2 × sodium] + [glucose/18] + [BUN/3])—is normally 5 (±7).

An increased anion-gap metabolic acidosis (AGMA) is an important finding because it suggests advanced ethylene glycol, methanol, or salicylate poisoning, conditions that require early, specific therapy to prevent progressive toxicity and irreversible tissue damage. An increased AGMA can also be caused by asphyxiants and other agents (Table 271.2) and by any poisoning that results in hepatic, renal, or respiratory failure, seizures, or shock. The serum lactate concentration is low (or significantly less than the anion gap) in the methanol, ethylene glycol, and salicylate poisoning and high (nearly equal to the anion gap) in most other conditions. An abnormally low anion gap can be caused by elevated blood levels of bromide, calcium, iodide, lithium, magnesium, or nitrate.

The osmolal gap can be useful in differentiating ethylene glycol and methanol poisoning from salicylate poisoning. It may be increased when high levels of ethylene glycol and methanol are present but is normal in salicylate poisoning. The osmolal gap also may be increased by when high levels of acetone, alcohols (benzyl, ethanol, isopropanol, methanol), glycols (diethylene, ethylene, propylene), or ethers (ethyl, glycol), "unmeasured" cations (calcium, magnesium), or sugars (glycerol, mannitol, sorbitol) are present. It can be used to estimate the serum concentration of these agents when direct measurement is not immediately available by multiplying the concentration

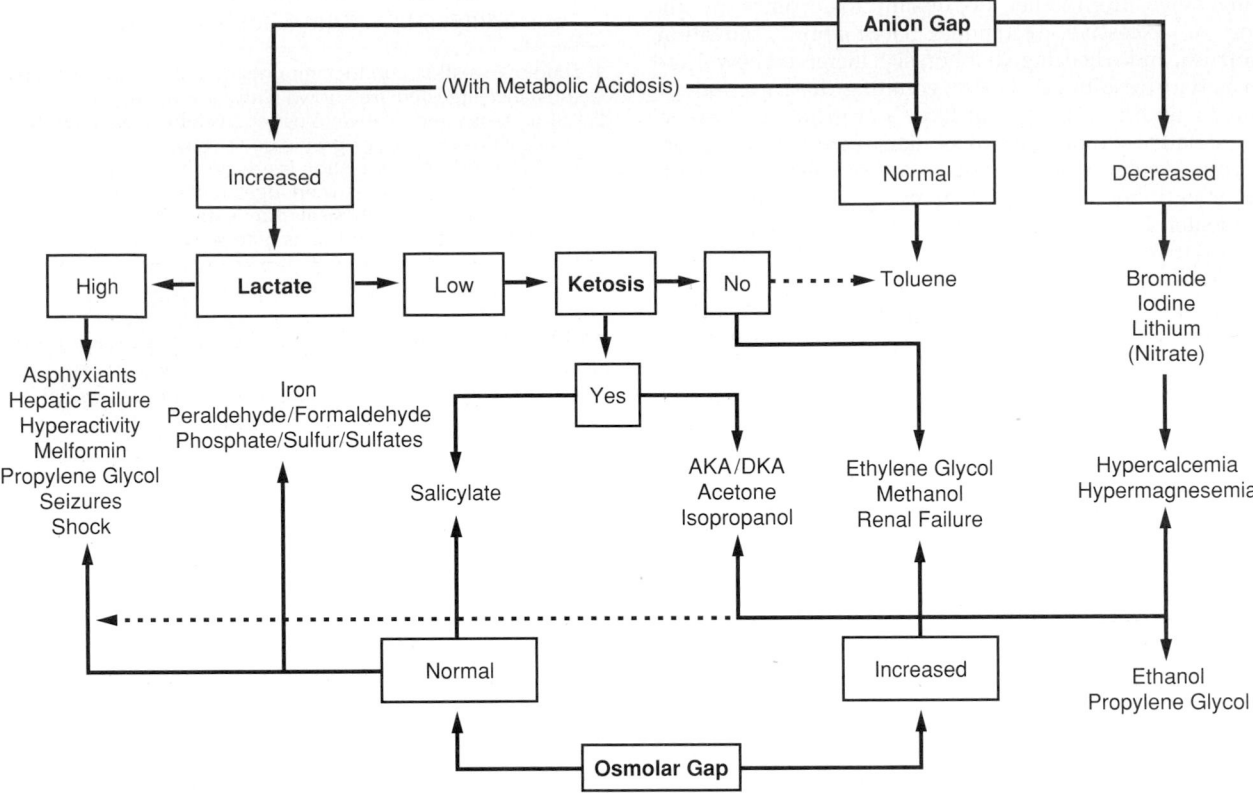

Figure 271.1. Use of routine laboratory findings and calculated gaps in the differential diagnosis of poisoning.

equivalent to 1 mOsm/kg by the osmolal gap (Table 271.6). Other findings that can help differentiate ethylene glycol, methanol, and salicylate poisoning include back pain, crystalluria, hypocalcemia, and renal dysfunction (ethylene glycol), visual symptoms (methanol), and tinnitus or hearing loss, hypoglycemia, ketosis, and a mixed acid–base disorder (salicylate).

Crystalluria can also be caused by acyclovir, felbamate, indinavir, oxalate, primidone, and sulfadiazine, and hypocalcemia can also be seen in fluoride and oxalate poisoning. Other causes of hypoglycemia include β-blocker, ethanol, hypoglycemic agent, and quinine intoxication. Hyperglycemia may be seen with acetone, β-agonist, caffeine, calcium channel blocker,

iron, and theophylline intoxication. Ketosis can also be caused by the presence of acetone (and its parent isopropyl alcohol). An elevated serum creatinine with a normal blood urea nitrogen (BUN) suggests acetone or isopropyl alcohol poisoning, because acetone interferes with the colorimetric assay for creatinine. A falsely elevated creatinine can also be caused by barbiturates, cephalosporins, creatine, flucytosine, ketoacids, levodopa, nitromethane, and vitamin C. Acute renal failure may result from dehydration, shock, and other nephrotoxins (e.g., acetaminophen, anti-tumor agents, carbon tetrachloride, immunosuppressants, metals, and nonsteroidal antiinflammatory agents. Hypokalemia can be caused by barium, β-agonists, caffeine, diuretics, theophylline, and toluene; hyperkalemia suggests poisoning by an α-adrenergic agonist, β-blocker, cardiac glycoside, fluoride, or lithium (5).

An oxygen saturation gap (a difference between the oxygen saturation calculated from the PO_2 and that measured directly by co-oximetry) indicates the presence of abnormal hemoglobin, such as carboxyhemoglobin or methemoglobin. When these hemoglobins are present, the oxygen saturation measured by pulse oximetry will be higher than the true value (falsely elevated) but less than normal and lower than calculated value. Heme (orthotoluidine)–positive urine in the absence of red blood cells suggests hemoglobinuria or myoglobinuria caused by hemolysis or rhabdomyolysis, respectively. Clear serum with a decreased hematocrit, increased unconjugated bilirubin level, and abnormal red blood cell morphology is seen in the former; pink serum with increased creatine kinase, aldolase, and lactate dehydrogenase levels is present in the latter. Agents that cause hemolysis include arsine gas, antibiotics (in patients with glucose-6-phosphate dehydrogenase deficiency), and oxidizing compounds (which also cause methemoglobinemia). Rhabdomyolysis is characteristic of the neuroleptic

TABLE 271.6.   Amount of Solute That Increases Serum Osmolality by 1 mOsmol/kg

Solute	Serum Concentration (mg/dL)[a]
Alcohols, glycols, and ketones	
Acetone	5.8
Ethanol	4.6
Ethylene glycol	5.2
Isopropanol	6.0
Methanol	2.6
Propylene glycol	7.6
Electrolytes	
Calcium	4
Magnesium	2.4
Sugars	
Mannitol	18
Sorbitol	18

[a]Equivalent to 2 mmol/L of electrolyte and 1 mmol/L of other solutes.

malignant and serotonin syndromes. It can occur in patients with high grade physiologic stimulation or depression of any cause.

The electrocardiogram (ECG) may also provide clues to the diagnosis. QRS- and QT-interval prolongation suggests hyperkalemia or poisoning by membrane active agent (Table 271.2). Bradycardia and atrioventricular (AV) block can be caused by α-adrenergic agonists, antidysrhythmics, β-blockers, calcium channel blockers, cardiac glycosides, cholinergics (Table 271.2), clonidine, lithium, magnesium, and tricyclic antidepressants. Ventricular tachydysrhythmias may be caused by the agents that cause hyperkalemia, anticholinergics (e.g., diphenhydramine, orphenadrine), cardiac glycosides, chloral hydrate, membrane active agents, solvents (e.g., aliphatic and chlorinated hydrocarbons), and sympathomimetics (Table 271.2). Torsades de pointes (polymorphous ventricular tachycardia) suggests a prolonged Q-T interval as the underlying cause.

Radiologic studies are occasionally useful in the differential diagnosis. Pulmonary edema without cardiomegaly (acute respiratory distress syndrome) suggests carbon monoxide, cyanide, opioid, paraquat, sedative–hypnotic, or salicylate poisoning; irritant gas, fume, or vapor inhalation (acids and alkali, ammonia, aldehydes, chlorine, hydrogen sulfide, isocyanates, metal oxides, mercury, nitrogen oxides, phosgene, and polymers); or hydrocarbon aspiration. Pulmonary edema and aspiration pneumonitis can also be seen in patients with coma, seizures, or prolonged shock of any cause. Radiopaque densities in the GI tract suggest the ingestion of chlorinated hydrocarbons (e.g., chloral hydrate and carbon tetrachloride); heavy metals (e.g., arsenic, iron, lead, mercury, and thallium); iodinated compounds; packets of drugs; Play-Doh; psychotherapeutics (e.g., cyclic antidepressants, lithium, and phenothiazines); enteric-coated tablets; salicylates; and salts (e.g. calcium, magnesium, potassium, and sodium compounds) (22). CHIPES is a mnemonic for these agents. Ingested drug packets appear as uniform oval or round, marble-sized densities (21). A double gastric bubble, representing an air–fluid and fluid–fluid interfaces, may be seen with hydrocarbon ingestions, as these compounds are less dense than and immiscible in water and layer on top of the gastric contents.

Antidotes can be diagnostic as well as therapeutic tools. Prompt resolution of mental status and vital sign abnormalities after the intravenous administration of dextrose, naloxone, or flumazenil is virtually diagnostic of hypoglycemia, opioid poisoning, and benzodiazepine (or zolpidem) intoxication, respectively. Occasionally, poisoning by clonidine (and other imidazoline) and valproate respond to naloxone. Rapid reversal of an acute dystonic (extrapyramidal) reaction after the intravenous administration of benztropine or diphenhydramine implicates a drug etiology. A change in urine color after deferoxamine can confirm but not exclude iron poisoning. A therapeutic response to physostigmine is suggestive but not diagnostic of anticholinergic poisoning, because this agent can cause nonspecific arousal in patients with CNS depression of any cause. Details of antidotal therapy are described in chapters that pertain to the corresponding poison.

EMERGENCY DEPARTMENT EVALUATION

Objectives in the evaluation of the poisoned or potentially poisoned patient are listed in Table 271.1. The history in patients with a known exposure should include the time, route, dose, location (e.g., home or work), surrounding circumstances, and intent. The specific name and amount (weight, volume, concentration, or duration of contact) of all substances involved should be determined. The time of onset, nature, and severity of symptoms; the type of first aid undertaken; and the victim's medical and psychiatric history should also be noted.

If the history is vague or of questionable reliability, an attempt should be made to obtain or verify as much information as possible from paramedics, police, family, and friends. Communicating with the patient's employer, pharmacist, or physician may also be valuable. A search of the patient's clothes, home, or place of discovery may reveal a suicide note, pill bottle, or chemical container. All available chemicals or other evidence of exposure or intent should be brought to the hospital for identification.

The label of a commercial product may provide a clue to the nature and severity of potential poisoning. Products containing locally acting chemicals may be labeled with the words "weak irritant," "strong irritant," or "corrosive," depending on whether exposure can cause mucosal irritation, mucosal and skin irritation, or severe burns with permanent tissue damage or death, respectively. Those containing substances that cause systemic poisoning may be labeled with the words "danger," "warning," or "caution," if they are extremely, highly, or moderately toxic, corresponding to an oral LD_{50} (median lethal dose) of less than 1 mg/kg, 1 to 50 mg/kg, and 50 to 500 mg/kg, respectively.

If the exposure involves a chemical or product whose ingredients are unknown, consultation with a regional poison control center or poison information reference may provide the desired data. Drugs can be identified by the pill or tablet imprint code (now required by law) or by their street slang names. The composition of a brand-name product may also be determined from reference sources or by calling the manufacturer. The odor or use of an unknown chemical may also suggest its identity. Local nurseries, horticultural and mycologic societies, botany departments of academic institutions, and field guides may help to identify an unknown plant. Similarly, pet stores, zoos, veterinarians, entomologists, herpetologists, and zoologists may help to identify unknown insects, reptiles, snakes, and other potentially poisonous animals.

A complete physical examination is necessary in all patients. It should begin with vital signs and initially be directed toward assessment of cardiovascular, respiratory, and neuromuscular function. Vital signs should include measurement of the oxygen saturation and neurologic evaluation should include a mental status examination. The respiratory rate should be measured over a full minute) to detect subtle abnormalities. Although often delayed or neglected, core (rectal) temperature measurement is essential in critically ill patients. Odors, eye findings (e.g., nystagmus, papilledema, and pupil size and reactivity), bowel and bladder activity (e.g., bowel sounds, distention, and incontinence), the condition of the skin and mucosa (e.g., color, warmth, moisture, burns, bullae, pressure sores, and puncture marks), and urine color should be noted. Vital signs and physical examination should initially be repeated frequently in patients who present soon after exposure and when abnormal findings are noted.

Evidence of underlying illness and coexisting trauma, especially head injury, also should be sought. With few exceptions (e.g., dystonic reactions, focal seizures caused by theophylline, and hypoglycemic agents), neuromuscular disturbances caused by poisoning are almost always generalized. Hence, focal neurologic abnormalities should prompt evaluation for a structural CNS lesion. When the history suggests the possibility of illicit drug concealment, all orifices and body cavities should be visually or digitally examined for the presence of drug packages.

Unless the exposure is clearly trivial, continuous monitoring the cardiac rhythm is prudent. Laboratory studies in symptomatic patients, particularly those with unreliable histories, should include a complete blood count, determination of electrolyte, BUN, creatinine, and glucose levels, and a urinalysis.

In asymptomatic patients, blood and urine samples can be obtained on presentation and saved for later (baseline) analysis in the event of subsequent deterioration.

Patients with an abnormal cardiac rhythm, low oxygen saturation, cardiorespiratory complaints, or grade 2 or greater physiological dysfunction (Tables 271.3 and 271.4) should have a 12-lead ECG and chest radiograph. Those with grade 2 or greater physiologic dysfunction should have also have serum amylase, calcium, magnesium, creatine phosphokinase, and liver function testing. Serum osmolality and ketone levels, urinalysis for crystalluria, and arterial blood gas analysis may be useful in patients with unexplained increased AGMA. A methemoglobin level should be measured in patients with cyanosis despite a normal PO_2.

Toxicology screening—the qualitative analysis of urine, blood, and, sometimes, gastric contents, or a sample of the chemical itself—may confirm or rule out a suspected diagnosis (6,12). Comprehensive screening is expensive and generally requires 2 to 6 hours to perform. It is of greatest value in patients with severe and unexplained findings, such as acid–base disturbances, abnormal cardiac conduction or rhythm, cardiovascular instability, coma, seizures, respiratory failure, and multiple-organ dysfunction. In these patients, the results may prompt a significant change in treatment but usually not in disposition. Selective ordering of an anticonvulsant, hallucinogen, depressant (coma), stimulant, or drugs of abuse screen may increase the speed and utility of qualitative testing. Routine screening is neither clinically useful nor cost effective in patients who are asymptomatic or have clinical findings consistent with the reported history. Despite increased diagnostic certainty and specificity, only rarely do the results lead to a change in treatment or disposition, particularly in mildly poisoned patients. Because of their ready availability, delayed onset of toxicity, and need for specific therapy, acetaminophen and salicylate are exceptions, and levels of these drugs should generally be measured in all patients with intentional overdose.

Optimal use of the toxicology laboratory requires knowledge of the tests (e.g., thin-layer, gas–liquid, high-performance liquid chromatography; colorimetric, enzymatic, fluorometric, and immunologic assays; gas chromatography; and mass spectrometry) used for screening and subsequent confirmation, and their sensitivity (i.e., limit of detection) and specificity. Personal communication with laboratory personnel is recommended in all cases; it is essential when laboratory results do not agree with clinical findings. A negative screen should never be interpreted as excluding a diagnosis of poisoning: It may indicate only that the suspected agent cannot be detected by the test used, that a chemical is present but cannot be positively identified, or that its concentration is too low for detection in the specimen submitted.

In many cases, obtaining a quantitative serum level of a specific chemical may be more appropriate than a ordering a toxicology screen. The results of quantitative analyses are often available within 1 hour. Acetaminophen, acetone, alcohols (ethylene glycol as well as ethanol, isopropanol, and methanol), antidysrhythmics, antiepileptics, barbiturates, carbon monoxide, digoxin, electrolytes, heavy metals, lithium, salicylate, and theophylline are agents whose quantitative measurement is necessary for optimal patient management.

EMERGENCY DEPARTMENT MANAGEMENT

The management of the poisoned or potentially poisoned patient depends on the actual or predicted toxicity and the time of presentation relative to the time of exposure (10,19). The time of presentation is important, because it reflects the phase of chemical disposition and allows a more refined prediction of toxicity based on knowledge of kinetic data.

During the preclinical or *induction phase*, the time between exposure and the onset of poisoning, decontamination (see subsequent text and Chapter 272, "Gastrointestinal Decontamination") is the top priority. Early and effective decontamination may prevent absorption and subsequent toxicity, or at least reduce its severity and duration. Regardless of the method used, the sooner decontamination is performed, the more effective it is. The history determines whether or not decontamination is indicated. A worse case scenario should be assumed. All missing pills or contents of commercial products should be assumed to have been ingested by the child who is found with an open container and every ingestion in a suicidal adult should be assumed to be potentially serious. When a reliable history is available, the maximum possible severity should be estimated from either previously reported exposures or predicted blood levels. If a poison causing delayed toxicity or irreversible damage is suspected, blood and urine should be sent for toxicologic analysis. Serial blood levels may be necessary. High levels of agents whose metabolites are more toxic than the parent compound (acetaminophen, ethylene glycol, or methanol) may indicate the need for additional interventions (antidotes or dialysis). If the history suggests the potential for significant poisoning, it is prudent to establish intravenous access and initiate cardiac monitoring. Unless toxicity is expected to be negligible or the predicted time of peak effect has passed without incident, a period of observation is necessary. Most patients who remain or become asymptomatic 4 to 6 hours after ingestion will not develop subsequent toxicity and can be discharged safely. Longer observation may be necessary for patients who have ingested toxic time-bombs (Table 271.2).

During the *toxic phase*, the time from the beginning of poisoning until its peak, supportive care is the top priority. The interventions that are necessary depend primarily on the severity of poisoning as assessed by the physical examination. If vital signs are unstable, the history and physical examination should initially be concurrent with resuscitation. Unless toxicity is minimal and expected to remain so, all symptomatic patients should have an intravenous line, cardiac monitoring, supplemental oxygen, continuous observation, and baseline laboratory, ECG, and radiographic evaluation. Those with severe poisoning should have comprehensive toxicology testing. Patients with altered mental status, particularly coma or seizures, should be checked or empirically treated for hypoglycemia. Thiamine should be given along with intravenous dextrose. Patients with respiratory depression should receive intravenous naloxone. The use of other antidotes may be indicated. Unless it is likely that absorption is complete, decontamination measures should be considered. Enhancement of elimination therapies may also be appropriate (see subsequent text).

During the *resolution phase*, the time from peak toxicity to the time of full recovery, supportive care, based primarily on the severity of poisoning, is again the top priority. Supportive care and monitoring should continue until the patient is awake and alert and laboratory and electrocardiographic abnormalities have resolved. Clinical relapse can occur when previously depressed GI function returns and poison still present in the gut is absorbed. A prolonged or cyclic clinical course suggests the possibility of a gastric drug bezoar or concretion. This can occur with bupropion, ethchlorvynol, glutethimide, iron and other metals, lithium, meprobamate, and salicylate. Further decontamination may be indicated in such cases. Continued antidotal therapy and measures to enhance poison elimination may also be appropriate. As in the preclinical phase, some patients may require additional therapy solely because of a potentially toxic dose or blood level.

Decontamination

Topical Exposures

Immediate flushing with water, saline solution, or any other readily available, clear, drinkable liquid is the initial treatment for topical exposures, particularly those that involve local irritants and corrosives. If possible, particulate material should be manually removed before irrigation. A hand-held vacuum is useful for removing dry or powdered chemicals from the skin. Caregivers should use gloves to avoid contamination. A triple wash (flushing, followed by a soap scrub, and repeat flushing) is suggested for dermal decontamination.

Saline solution is the preferred fluid for eye irrigation. Buffered solutions are better tolerated than unbuffered ones. One or 2 L is usually sufficient. If ophthalmic exposure involves an acidic or alkaline chemical, the tear pH should be determined, although searching for pH paper should never delay treatment. The goal of treatment is a neutral pH (7.0). Tears, not the irrigation fluid, must be tested; the pH of unbuffered normal saline solution averages 5.5.

Patients with inhalational exposures should be rapidly removed from the exposure scene and treated with fresh air or supplemental oxygen. A rescuer should never enter a hazardous gas, vapor, fume, or dust environment without adequate eye, skin, and respiratory protection. Liquid chemicals can be removed from body cavities (e.g., vagina or rectum) by irrigation. Accessible solids (e.g., drug packets and pills) should be removed manually under visual guidance.

Ingestions

Decontamination is accomplished by inducing the evacuation of GI contents either orally or rectally. Activated charcoal, gastric lavage, and syrup of ipecac are the methods most commonly used. Whole-bowel irrigation (WBI) and endoscopic or surgical removal of the ingested poison are reserved for special situations. Cathartics and dilution are used in conjunction with other modalities but are not, by themselves, effective methods of GI decontamination. These measures are discussed in detail in the following chapter.

Supportive Care

The goal of supportive therapy is to maintain physiologic homeostasis until detoxification is accomplished. It is also necessary to prevent or treat secondary complications such as aspiration, bedsores, cerebral and pulmonary edema, pneumonia, rhabdomyolysis, renal failure, sepsis, thromboembolic disease, and generalized organ dysfunction caused by prolonged hypoxia or shock. Only those aspects of supportive care of particular importance in the management of poisoned patients are discussed.

Respiratory Care

Intubation and mechanical ventilation may be indicated for the prevention of aspiration and to facilitate therapeutic sedation or paralysis as well as for the treatment of respiratory depression and hypoxia. Aspiration is common in patients with CNS depression or seizures and increases morbidity and mortality (24). The gag reflex is not a reliable indicator of the need for intubation. Many healthy people have an absent gag reflex, and many comatose patients will gag with sufficient stimulation. Similarly, patients may be able to maintain a patent airway while being stimulated but not if left unattended. Hence, those who cannot respond to and by voice, or who cannot sit up and drink fluids without assistance, are best managed by prophylactic intubation. Because clinical assessment of respiratory function is often inaccurate, arterial blood gas analysis can be helpful in questionable cases. A short-acting sedative or muscle relaxant is useful in facilitating intubation in patients with low-grade coma. Intubation and mechanical ventilation may be indicated in patients with high-grade physiologic excitation to allow for the pharmacologic control of seizures or behavioral agitation and to prevent or limit the extent of complications (e.g., hyperthermia, acidosis, and rhabdomyolysis).

The initial treatment of pulmonary edema in poisoned patients should also include early endotracheal intubation. The use of positive end-expiratory pressure is often beneficial. Profound CNS depression and cardiac conduction abnormalities suggest a cardiac etiology. Iatrogenic fluid overload often contributes to pulmonary edema in hypotensive patients with myocardial depression. In such cases, an inotropic vasopressor (e.g., dopamine) is the treatment of choice. Only when the blood pressure has been normalized should a diuretic be given. In some cases, measurement of pulmonary artery pressure may be necessary to establish etiology and direct appropriate therapy. Extracorporeal measures (membrane oxygenation, venoarterial perfusion, and cardiopulmonary bypass), partial liquid (perfluorocarbon) ventilation, and hyperbaric oxygen therapy should be considered for patients with severe but reversible respiratory failure.

Cardiovascular Care

Supraventricular tachycardia associated with generalized physiologic stimulation is usually not hemodynamically compromising and requires only observation or nonspecific sedation (e.g., a benzodiazepine). However, if chest pain, electrocardiographic evidence of ischemia, or extreme hypertension is present, specific therapy is indicated. The use of a nonselective adrenergic blocker (e.g., labetalol) or both a β-blocker and a vasodilator (e.g., esmolol or propranolol and nitroprusside) is preferred for patients with sympathetic hyperactivity. Physostigmine is the treatment of choice for those with anticholinergic poisoning.

Lidocaine is generally safe to use for ventricular tachyarrhythmias of any etiology. Procainamide and other class IA antiarrhythmics should be avoided in patients with poisoning by membrane-active agents because of their similar (and hence additive) electrophysiologic effects. Bicarbonate may be therapeutic for dysrhythmias caused by these agents. Torsades de pointes and ventricular tachydysrhythmias secondary to digitalis poisoning may respond to magnesium. Overdrive pacing (by isoproterenol or electricity) may be necessary in those with prolonged Q-T intervals. Antibody therapy as well as pacing should be considered for dysrhythmias caused by digitalis.

Bradydysrhythmias associated with hypotension should initially be treated with atropine, isoproterenol, and intravenous fluids. In patients with β-blocker and calcium-channel blocker poisoning, the administration of calcium and glucagon may obviate the need for cardiac pacing. The treatment of bradycardia secondary to hypertension or increased intracranial pressure should be directed at the primary cause. In patients with any dysrhythmia, underlying metabolic abnormalities and extremes of temperature must be corrected.

Hypotension in poisoned patients is more often caused by loss of vascular tone than by cardiac depression. It should initially be treated with crystalloids. If vasopressors are subsequently required, direct-acting agents (e.g., norepinephrine or high-dose dopamine) are preferred. Advanced cardiovascular and pulmonary supportive measures, such as extracorporeal membrane oxygenation, intraaortic balloon pump counterpulsation, and partial cardiopulmonary bypass pump assistance, should also be considered in severe but reversible poisoning.

Neurologic Care

Seizures and muscular hyperactivity can lead to hyperthermia, lactic acidosis, and rhabdomyolysis, each of which can lead to additional complications, and should be treated aggressively (25). When caused by excessive sympathetic stimulation (e.g., sympathomimetic or hallucinogen poisoning and drug withdrawal) or decreased activity of inhibitory γ-aminobutyric acid (GABA) or glycine receptors (e.g., isoniazid and strychnine poisoning, respectively), GABA enhancers such as benzodiazepines or barbiturates are the treatment of choice. Because benzodiazepines and barbiturates act by slightly different mechanisms (the former increases the frequency and the latter increases the duration of chloride channel opening in response to GABA), therapy with both may be effective when neither is effective alone. Seizures caused by isoniazid, which inhibits the synthesis of GABA, may require high doses of pyridoxine (which facilitates the synthesis of GABA). Those caused by membrane active agents may require a membrane-active anticonvulsant such as phenytoin as well as GABA enhancers. For neuromuscular stimulation caused by excessive dopaminergic activity (e.g., phencyclidine poisoning), a dopamine antagonist (e.g., haloperidol) is appropriate. For that caused by the serotonin syndrome, a serotonin antagonist (e.g., cyproheptadine) may be beneficial. In anticholinergic and cyanide poisoning, specific antidotal therapy may be necessary. The treatment of seizures secondary to cerebral ischemia, edema, or metabolic abnormalities should include correction of the underlying cause. Neuromuscular paralysis is indicated in refractory cases. When therapeutic paralysis is used, electroencephalographic monitoring and treatment of electrical seizure activity with anticonvulsants are also necessary.

Antidotal Therapy

Antidotes are chemicals that counteract the effects of poisons. They act by a variety of mechanisms: neutralization by antibody–antigen reactions, chelation, or chemical binding; physiologic antagonism by blocking or reversing the interaction of a chemical and its target site; activation or inhibition of an opposing division of the nervous system; and altered disposition by enhancing or inhibiting metabolism, excretion, or secretion. Although antidotes can reduce morbidity and mortality, relatively few poisons and toxic syndromes have antidotes (Table 271.7). Antidotes can themselves be toxic, so their indiscriminate use should be avoided. Details regarding the use of specific antidotes can be found in the corresponding poisoning chapters.

Enhancement of Elimination

Although the elimination of many chemicals can be accelerated by various therapeutic interventions (Table 271.8), the clinical efficacy of such interventions is often insignificant or unknown. Clinical efficacy implies a shortened duration of toxicity and improved patient outcome. In most instances, if vital signs can be adequately supported, the poison will be intrinsically detoxified and full recovery will follow. Hence, the decision to use an active removal procedure should be based on the actual or predicted maximal severity of the poisoning and the risk (i.e., invasiveness or complications) of the procedure. In addition, invasive procedures are expensive and require technical expertise and specialized equipment. Diagnostic certainty, usually by way of laboratory confirmation, is, therefore, a prerequisite.

The use of extracorporeal procedures should be limited to patients who would not otherwise have a favorable outcome: those with severe clinical or laboratory toxicity who do not respond to

TABLE 271.7.   Chemicals and Related Syndromes with Specific Antidotes

Acetaminophen
Anticholinergics
Anticoagulants
Benzodiazepines
β-Blockers
Calcium channel blockers
Carbon monoxide
Cyanide
Digitalis
Ethylene glycol
Envenomations
Fluoride
Heavy metals
Hydrogen sulfide
Hypoglycemics
Isoniazid
Methanol
Methemoglobinemia
Opioids
Sympathomimetics
Vacor (PNU)

supportive care and noninvasive elimination therapy; those with blood levels predictive of a significant risk of severe, irreversible, or prolonged toxicity, particularly if an invasive procedure is the only or most effective method of enhancing elimination; those who lack the capacity for self-detoxification because of liver or kidney failure; and those who have serious underlying illnesses or complications of poisoning that would adversely affect recovery.

Gastrointestinal dialysis refers to the use of whole bowel irrigation (see Chapter 272, "Gastrointestinal Decontamination") to enhance the elimination of chemicals rather than to prevent their absorption. There are few data on its efficacy in this regard. Multiple-dose activated charcoal is discussed in the following chapter. Chelation therapy is covered in the chapters on metal poisoning. Hyperbaric oxygenation is addressed in the chapters on carbon monoxide, hydrogen sulfide, and cyanide poisoning and methemoglobinemia.

Enhanced Urinary Excretion

Diuresis and ion trapping by altering the urinary pH may prevent the passive renal tubular reabsorption of chemicals that enter the urine by glomerular filtration and active tubular secretion, and thus increase their excretion (9,17). Because biologic membranes are more permeable to un-ionized molecules than

TABLE 271.8.   Methods of Enhancing Chemical Elimination

Chelation therapy
Extracorporeal techniques
  Peritoneal dialysis
  Hemodialysis
  Hemoperfusion
  Hemofiltration
  Plasmapheresis
  Exchange transfusion
Cholinergics
Forced diuresis
Gastrointestinal dialysis
Hyperbaric oxygenation
Multiple-dose activated charcoal
Urine pH manipulation

to their ionized counterparts, acidic (low pK_a) chemicals are ionized and trapped in an alkaline urine, and basic chemicals are ionized and trapped in an acid urine. Saline diuresis can enhance the excretion of alcohols, bromide, calcium, chromium, isoniazid, lithium, meprobamate, potassium, and thallium. Alkaline diuresis can enhance the renal elimination of chlorphenoxyacetic acid herbicides (i.e., 2,4-D and 2,4,5-T), chlorpropamide, diflunisal, fluoride, mecroprop, methotrexate, phenobarbital (and probably other long acting barbiturates), sulfonamides, and salicylates. Acid diuresis, although it enhances the excretion of amphetamines, chloroquine, cocaine, local anesthetics, phencyclidine, quinine, quinidine, strychnine, tricyclic antidepressants, and tocainide, is not recommended, because the risks are significant and clinical efficacy has not been established. Indeed, barbitures and salicylates are the only agents for which is the clinical benefit of these procedures is widely accepted.

The goal of diuresis is a urine flow of at least 3 mL/kg/hour; that of alkalinization is a urine pH of 7.5 or greater. An intravenous alkaline diuresis solution can be prepared by adding one to three ampules (44 to 132 mEq) of sodium bicarbonate to 1 L of appropriately hypotonic fluid so that the final solution is roughly isotonic. The carbonic anhydrase inhibitor acetazolamide should not be used to alkalinize the urine, because it may produce a concomitant acidemia and enhance the tissue distribution of acidic chemicals. Acid–base, fluid, and electrolyte parameters as well as clinical response must be carefully monitored during therapy. Contraindications include congestive heart failure, kidney failure, and cerebral or pulmonary edema.

Extracorporeal Elimination

Extracorporeal techniques (see Table 271.6) theoretically can remove any diffusible chemical from the bloodstream (17). Dialysis is most effective in enhancing the elimination of agents with a low molecular weight (less than 500 daltons), high water solubility, low protein binding, small volume of distribution (less than 1 L/kg), slow intrinsic elimination (i.e., long half-life), and high dialysis clearance relative to total body clearance. The efficacy of other extracorporeal procedures is not limited by molecular weight, water solubility, or protein binding.

Chemicals considered dialyzable with respect to both kinetic and clinical efficacy include acetone, atenolol, bromide, barbiturates, chloral hydrate, ethanol, ethylene glycol, isopropyl alcohol, lithium, methanol, procainamide, theophylline, salicylates, and possibly heavy metals. Although hemoperfusion may be more effective in removing some of these poisons, it does not readily correct associated acid–base and electrolyte abnormalities. Hemoperfusion is the preferred technique for enhancing the elimination of carbamazepine, carbon tetrachloride, chloramphenicol, dapsone, disopyramide, sedative–hypnotics (e.g., barbiturates, ethchlorvynol, glutethimide, meprobamate, and methaqualone), methotrexate, and mushrooms containing amatoxins, paraquat, phenytoin, procainamide, theophylline, and valproate. Both techniques require central venous access and systemic anticoagulation, and may cause hypotension and bleeding complications. Hemoperfusion may also result in hemolysis, hypocalcemia, and thrombocytopenia.

Cardiovascular deterioration upon initiating hemodialysis (and hemoperfusion) is common in poisoned patients and deserves emphasis. In contrast to the usual patient undergoing these procedures, who is typically fluid overloaded, hypertensive, and stable, those with poisoning are often volume depleted, hypotensive, and unstable. Priming the pump with saline prior to initiating such therapy and bolusing the patient with saline at the time it begins may prevent decompensation. Being prepared and treating it aggressively is critical.

Peritoneal dialysis is less effective, but it may be used when other extracorporeal procedures are unavailable, contraindicated, or technically difficult (e.g., in infants). Exchange transfusion is also less effective, but it may be used in the same situations, as well as for poisons that cause severe hemolysis or methemoglobinemia. The role of other extracorporeal techniques has not been defined. After the termination of any invasive elimination procedure, clinical relapse or a rebound increase in the blood level of a chemical may occur as it undergoes tissue redistribution.

DISPOSITION

After evaluation, treatment, and an appropriate observation period, asymptomatic patients may be discharged from the emergency department. The disposition of symptomatic patients depends on the actual or predicted severity and the need or potential need for therapeutic interventions. Most patients develop only mild toxicity and can be observed in the emergency department or comparable facility until asymptomatic. Those with significant (grade 2 or greater) physiologic stimulation or depression (Tables 271.3 and 271.4), hypoxia, hypercarbia, acid–base disturbances, metabolic abnormalities, extremes of temperature, and cardiac conduction or rhythm abnormalities should be admitted to an intensive care unit (10,15). Patients who require close monitoring of antidotal therapy or high-risk elimination procedures, those showing progressive clinical deterioration, and those with significant underlying medical problems are also candidates for the intensive care unit. Lack of resources for the continuous observation of suicidal patients may require a higher level of care than is medically necessary.

Consultation with a poison control center or toxicologist is recommended whenever the treating physician is not completely familiar with the specific agent(s) involved in a given exposure or poisoning. Consultation with other specialists is dictated by the nature of poisoning and its actual or potential severity.

The possibility of re-exposure and its prevention must be addressed before discharge. Suicidal patients require psychiatric assessment, disposition, and followup. Prescriptions given to depressed or psychotic patients should be written for a limited amount of the drug and a limited number of refills. Such patients also require close monitoring for compliance with and response to therapy. Drug abusers should be referred for counseling and given the opportunity for rehabilitation.

Advising that the environment of children be poison-proofed is recommended. Parents and other caretakers should be instructed to store alcoholic beverages; medications; all automotive, cleaning, cosmetic, fuel, painting, and pet care products; nonedible plants; vitamins; and toiletries above or out of the child's reach or in cabinets with locks or childproof latches. Safety caps are always advisable, but are not necessarily sufficient to prevent access by children. Adults with accidental home exposures should be instructed regarding the safe use of drugs and other chemicals, advised to read the instructions on labels carefully, and to avoid circumstances that caused the current problem. Notifying the appropriate governmental agency (e.g., Environmental Protection Agency [EPA], Occupational Safety and Health Administration [OSHA], National Institute for Occupational Safety and Health [NIOSH], the local health department) should be considered in cases of environmental or workplace exposure. Unsafe working conditions should also be brought to the attention of the employer. Assistance with the administration of medications should be arranged for confused patients with accidental exposures caused by dosing errors. Preventive education and evaluation and correction of system flaws are important when a health-care provider causes a dosing error.

COMMON PITFALLS

✔ Failure to consider the diagnosis of poisoning in patients with unexplained signs and symptoms of any nature

✔ Failure to appreciate that the dose determines whether or not an exposure results in poisoning

✔ Failure to appreciate that treatment is determined by the time since exposure and the clinical status of the patient as well as the details of exposure (agent, dose, and route)

✔ Failure to appreciate that the history is notoriously unreliable in patients with intentional (suicidal) overdose

✔ Failure to appreciate the limitations of toxicology testing

✔ Failure to appreciate that supportive care is the mainstay of treatment and to consider invasive artificial circulatory and respiratory assistance measures in critically ill patients

✔ Failure to consider "toxic time-bomb" exposure and to address prevention of re-exposure prior to discharge or psychiatric disposition

CRITICAL INTERVENTIONS

- Consult a regional poison center or toxicologist if not completely familiar with the toxicology of exposure agent
- Establish intravenous access, institute continuous cardiac monitoring, and frequently re-evaluate the vital signs and clinical status of patients with actual or potential systemic poisoning
- Carefully assess the risks as well as the benefits of therapy prior to performing gastrointestinal decontamination, administering antidotes, and utilizing enhanced elimination procedures

References

1. Aabakken L, Johansen KS, Rydningen EB, et al. Osmolal and anion gaps in patients admitted to an emergency medical department. *Hum Exp Toxicol* 1994;13:131.
2. Ashton CH, Teoh R, Davies DM. Drug-induced stupor: some physical signs and their pharmacological basis. *Adverse Drug React Acute Poison Rev* 1989;8:1.
3. Bartholomew RE, Wessely S. Protean nature of mass sociogenic illness: from possessed nuns to chemical and biological terrorism fears. *Br J Psychiatry* 2002;180:300.
4. Bosse GM, Matyunas NJ. Delayed toxidromes. *J Emerg Med* 1999;17:679.
5. Bradberry SM, Vale JA. Disturbances of potassium homeostasis in poisoning. *Clin Toxicol* 1995;33:295.
6. Brett AS. Implication of discordance between clinical impression and toxicology analysis in drug overdose. *Arch Intern Med* 1988;148:437.
7. Brett AS, Rothschild N, Gray R, et al. Predicting the clinical course of intentional drug overdose: implications for utilization of the intensive care unit. *Arch Intern Med* 1987;147:133.
8. Chan TC, Evans SD, Clark RF. Drug-induced hyperthermia. *Crit Care Clin* 1997;13:785.
9. Garrettson LK, Geller RJ. Acid and alkaline diuresis: when are they of value in the treatment of poisoning? *Drug Saf* 1990;5:220.
10. Goldberg MJ, Spector R, Park GD, et al. An approach to the management of the poisoned patient. *Arch Intern Med* 1986;146:1381.
11. Goldfrank LR, Weisman R, Flomenbaum N: Teaching the recognition of odors. *Ann Emerg Med* 1982;11:684.
12. Hepler BR, Sutheimer CA, Sunshine I. Role of the toxicology laboratory in the treatment of acute poisoning. *Med Toxicol* 1986;1:61.
13. Klaassen CD (ed). Casarett & Doull's toxicology: The basic science of poisons, 6th edition. New York: McGraw-Hill, 2001.
14. Kolecki PF, Curry SC. Poisoning by sodium channel blocking agents. *Crit Care Clin* 1997;13:829.
15. Kulling P, Persson H. Role of the intensive care unit in the management of the poisoned patient. *Med Toxicol* 1986;1:375.
16. Olson KR, Pentel PR, Kelley MT. Physical assessment and differential diagnosis of the poisoned patient. *Med Toxicol* 1987;2:52.
17. Pond SM. Diuresis, dialysis and hemoperfusion: indications and benefits. *Emerg Med Clin North Am* 1984;2:29.
18. Smithline N, Gardner KD. Gaps: anionic and osmolal. *JAMA* 1976;236:1594.
19. Spyker DA, Minocha A. Toxicodynamic approach to the management of the poisoned patient. *J Emerg Med* 1988;6:117.
20. Sue YJ, Shannon M. Pharmacokinetics of drugs in overdose. *Clin Pharmacokinet* 1992;23:93.
21. Traub SJ, Hoffman RS, Nelson LS. Body packing—the internal concealment of illicit drugs. *N Engl J Med* 2003;349:2519.
22. Wason S, Dalsey W, Billmire ME, et al. Radiological case of the month: Play-Doh in the gastrointestinal tract: modify CHIP to CHIPPED. *Am J Dis Child* 1985;139:1149.
23. Watson WA, Litovitz TL, Rodgers GC, et al. 2002 Annual Report of the American Association of Poison Control Centers Toxic Exposure Surveillance System. *Am J Emerg Med* 2003;21:353.
24. Wright N. Common errors in the management of poisoning. *J Royal Coll Phys* 1980;14:114.
25. Zaccara G, Muscas GC, Messori A. Clinical features, pathogenesis, and management of drug induced seizures. *Drug Saf* 1990;5:109.

CHAPTER 272
Gastrointestinal Decontamination

Joshua G. Schier and Robert S. Hoffman

The poisoned patient may present to the emergency department in a variety of ways. The patient's presentation, type of substance or drug ingested, and time elapsed since ingestion all affect decisions regarding the method of gastrointestinal decontamination (GID) utilized. Evaluating the appropriateness of any of the GID techniques begins with a thorough understanding (including advantages and disadvantages) of the different techniques, a complete assessment of the patient, and knowledge of the potential severity of the poisoning. The basic principle of GID is that toxin removed from the gastrointestinal tract cannot be absorbed. Removing even a fraction of available drug from the gastrointestinal tract may convert a fatal poisoning to a severe, but nonfatal one. Regional poison control centers can be contacted to assist in the decision-making process for the most appropriate GID technique(s).

There are five GID techniques that may be employed by the clinician: orogastric lavage (OGL), induced emesis with syrup of ipecac (SOI), administration of single- or multiple-dose activated charcoal (AC), whole-bowel irrigation (WBI), and cathartics (24).

The term "gastric emptying" generally refers to either OGL or ipecac-induced vomiting. The utility of either method depends on the inherent risk to the patient posed by the ingestion, a risk-benefit assessment of the procedure, the likelihood of removing a clinically significant amount of toxin, and the availability of alternative methods of treatment, such as antidotes (24). It would probably be inappropriate to perform a gastric emptying procedure (GEP) on a patient with a benign overdose who is expected to do very well with minimal treatment, whereas a patient who has just ingested numerous extended release verapamil tablets has an inherently higher risk of severe toxicity and may benefit from a GEP. The ability to remove a clinically significant portion of toxin by a GEP depends on a number of factors, including drug pharmacokinetics and elapsed time from ingestion (9). Generally, beyond 2 to 5 hours after ingestion, there is little likelihood of removing any drug from the stomach, with the exception of drugs that can slow gastrointestinal mobility (e.g. anticholinergics, opioids, and sedative-hypnotics) (11,12,24). Occasionally, concretions of partially digested drug tablets may form in the stomach and serve as a reservoir for continued and delayed absorption. Drugs implicated in forming such concretions or bezoars include salicylates, meprobamate, phenobarbital, and iron (7,15,16,24). The availability of alternative GID techniques, or therapies such as antidotes (e.g. N-acetylcysteine for acetaminophen toxicity), also influences the decision to use a GEP.

Gastric emptying can remove the drug from the stomach and decrease drug absorption (10,12,24,25). However, there is considerable controversy as to whether gastric emptying affects clinical outcome. Only a few studies have examined the clinical benefit of GEPs in poisoned patients (17,19,21). Limitations of these studies include excluding the sickest patients from enrollment, excluding cases involving agents with significant inherent toxicity, and extrapolating the results to unsupported conclusions (17,19,21). However, studies that are well-designed and well and appropriately conducted, can show clinical benefit from GID. For example, multiple-dose activated charcoal (MDAC) given for yellow oleander poisoning reduced deaths and cardiac dysrhythmias significantly when compared to placebo (13).

The current literature supports beneficial effect on outcome if OGL is performed for the sickest patients within one hour of ingestion (17,21). This literature neither supports nor refutes the utility of OGL in other situations, and it may benefit in the scenarios mentioned previously. In the majority of patients, those who present more than one hour after ingestion or who are asymptomatic, a GEP is unlikely to add any benefit to AC administration alone, since there is little residual material in the stomach (8). In general, a GEP should be strongly considered for ingestion of a life-threatening or difficult-to-treat poison (such as the tricyclic antidepressants, calcium channel blockers, and β-adrenergic blockers), and for severely ill patients who present within one hour of ingestion (8,17,24). Other factors that may make gastric emptying appropriate include a relatively recent ingestion (less than 2 hours), an ingested amount that exceeds the adsorptive capacity of AC, the ingested agent is poorly adsorbed to activated charcoal, ineffective or nonexistent antidotal therapy, and the possibility that the ingested agent may form concretions in the stomach (24). General contraindications to GEP include nontoxic ingestions, if performing the act would cause unnecessary danger (e.g., increasing aspiration risk after a hydrocarbon ingestion), and if the risks outweigh the benefits (24). For patients who are not candidates for a GEP, the use of single- or multiple-dose activated charcoal should be strongly considered.

The choice of which GEP to use, if one is indicated, can be a difficult one. Although there is currently no definitive evidence to support one method over the other, ipecac-induced emesis is essentially obsolete (6,22,23). Thus, the real question is whether or not to perform orogastric lavage.

OROGASTRIC LAVAGE

OGL refers to the use of a 36 to 40 French tube inserted through the mouth to evacuate the contents of the stomach. "Nasogastric lavage" is a misnomer, since nasal tubes are much smaller (14 to 18 French) and can not remove pills, pill fragments, or other particulate matter as easily (3,24). OGL is probably best considered for patients ingesting a potentially life-threatening amount of a poison when the procedure can be undertaken within 60 minutes of ingestion (3,24). This time frame is based on data

obtained from very small studies of patients with low acuity and should be used as a general guideline rather than an absolute cutoff (3,24). OGL is contraindicated in patients with altered mental status if the airway is not protected and if utilization increases the risk or potential severity of aspiration (3,24). Other factors to be considered include conditions predisposing to perforation, such as esophageal pathology or recent surgery (3,24). Complications of OGL are numerous; they include aspiration pneumonia, laryngospasm, tension pneumothorax, charcoal empyema, esophageal perforation, atrial and ventricular ectopic beats, and conjunctival hemorrhage (3,24). Although there are no absolute indications for OGL, the procedure should be strongly considered in any patient with a life-threatening ingestion in whom there is a reasonable expectation that toxin may be present in the stomach. This is especially true when the clinical situation has already mandated endotracheal intubation, or if the toxin is not adsorbed to activated charcoal.

OGL should be performed only if the patient's airway is secure. In an awake, oriented patient, when no imminent deterioration is expected, the procedure should be explained completely to the patient and consent documented in the medical record. The length of tube to be inserted should be estimated externally and marked prior to insertion, and the patient should be placed in the left lateral decubitus position. In normal-sized adults, a 36 to 40 French tube should be used, whereas in children there is considerably more variation and generally nothing larger than a 24 to 28 French tube is needed. The lubricated tube should be inserted into the mouth and through the esophagus, taking care to not force it if significant resistance is encountered. Placement should be confirmed by auscultation of insufflated air over the stomach. Lavage should be conducted with small amounts (adults, 200 to 300 mL; children, 10 mL/kg) of warmed normal saline and care should be taken to try to remove most of the administered fluid before giving more. It is reasonable to repeat the procedure until the fluid reclaimed from the stomach no longer has any particulate matter (3). The airway should be protected by endotracheal intubation if OGL is to be used in any scenario other than an awake, alert patient who is not in danger of developing airway compromise during the procedure. After completion of the procedure, a dose of AC should be administered while the tube is in place, after which the tube is removed.

SYRUP OF IPECAC

Emetine and cephaeline are the two main alkaloids in SOI that are responsible for its emetic effects, which are induced both through local stimulation of receptors in the gastrointestinal tract and by direct activation of the central vomiting center (14). SOI has historically been used mainly in the home setting, with extremely limited applicability as a GID technique in the hospital, mostly because of delayed patient presentation. In 2003, the American Academy of Pediatrics completed its review of available evidence and no longer recommends that syrup of ipecac be used routinely for home treatment of poisoning (6). The first action in the treatment of a poisoned or potentially poisoned child is to call the regional poison control center (6). This recommendation is likely to affect the overall availability of syrup of ipecac to the public in the future.

ACTIVATED CHARCOAL

The pyrolysis of any carbonaceous material such as wood or peat results in the formation of charcoal. Treatment with an oxidizing agent such as steam or carbon dioxide activates charcoal by greatly increasing the adsorptive surface area through the formation of pores within the material (14). Adsorption is believed to occur through a variety of different interactions, including hydrogen bonding, ion-ion, dipole, and van der Waals forces (14). There must be physical contact between the ingested poison and charcoal for adsorption to occur, and this will prevent systemic absorption (14,24). AC decreases the systemic absorption of many drugs, although its efficacy, much like the other GID techniques, decreases when administration is delayed and depends significantly on the particular drug ingested (14,20,24). Certain drugs are not very well bound by activated charcoal; examples include alcohols, caustics, and most metals (14,20). The presence of food decreases AC's effectiveness (14). Patients who ingest drugs in controlled-release formulations may benefit from activated charcoal beyond the immediate postingestion period. These preparations usually contain a larger amount of total drug per unit dose but are designed to release a controlled amount of drug for absorption over an extended period.

AC is most likely to prevent absorption if it is administered within 1 hour after ingestion of a toxin (4,14,24). It may still be used to enhance elimination later in the patient's course (1,14,18). Although there is very limited evidence to support the notion that a single dose of AC confers clinical benefit in all poisonings beyond one hour of ingestion, the same methodological concerns expressed earlier apply. Logic suggests that in the majority of poisonings, the potential benefits of adsorbing any residual toxin by AC even beyond one hour of the ingestion outweigh most of the associated risks.

The risks associated with single-dose AC administration are generally few. Emesis, nausea, vomiting, and respiratory problems are reported (4,14,24). The complication of greatest concern is pulmonary aspiration, which may be fatal (14,24). Aspiration is usually a result of inappropriate administration or inadequate airway control prior to administration (24). Although it is important to recognize that even endotracheal intubation does not provide an absolute guarantee against aspiration, proper administration (defined as through a correctly placed nasogastric or orogastric tube or orally in an awake, alert patient) in the correct setting does not increase the risk of pulmonary aspiration (24).

The ideal dose of AC is relative and varies with the patient and the ingested agent. Generally, a 10:1 ratio of charcoal to drug or 1 g/kg patient body weight (whichever is larger) should be administered (1,4,14,24). The 10:1 ratio may be easily achievable in some ingestions when the amount ingested per unit dose is small (e.g., clonidine, 0.2 mg, or levothyroxine, 0.3 mg) but may be more difficult with other toxins. Ingestions with very large amounts per unit dose (e.g., aspirin 325 mg, or theophylline 300 mg) should be treated with a higher initial dose of AC, but not exceeding, 1.5 to 2.0 g/kg (14,24). The use of nasogastric tubes and antiemetics is encouraged to facilitate AC administration when appropriate.

Multiple doses of activated charcoal (MDAC) can reduce intensive care unit (ICU) admissions and fatalities in select circumstances (1,13,14,20). Volunteer studies and some clinical studies demonstrate that MDAC enhances elimination of the following drugs (although a clinical benefit has not been confirmed in all of these mentioned): carbamazepine, dapsone, phenobarbital, quinine, theophylline, phenylbutazone, digitoxin, digoxin, salicylate, cyclosporine, propoxyphene, nortriptyline, amitriptyline, phenytoin, sotalol, nadolol, piroxicam, and disopyramide (1,14). Some ingestions may particularly benefit from administration of MDAC, including controlled-release formulations, agents that form concretions in the stomach (e.g., salicylate), large ingestions where a 10:1 ratio of AC to drug cannot be achieved with a single dose, or if the agents undergo enteroenteric or enterohepatic cycling (1,14,18,20,24). Drugs that undergo entero-enteric recirculation have increased exposure time to blood vessels in the gastrointestinal tract. When AC is present in the gastrointestinal tract, unbound drug diffuses down its concentration gradient and into the lumen; this process is referred to as "gut dialysis" (1,14,24). Enterohepatic recirculation occurs with drugs that are miscible in bile salts and are secreted with them into the gastrointestinal lumen (14,24). Once in the lumen of the intestine, the drug is accessible to intraluminal charcoal for binding and excretion.

There is no single optimal dosing regimen for MDAC. Reported dosing regimens vary from 0.25 g/kg every 1 to 6 hours to 60 g (in adults) every 1, 2, 4. or 6 hours (1,14). Clinicians should follow the guidelines for single-dose activated charcoal for the first dose, and total doses administered should generally not exceed 3 or 4 (1,4,14). A reasonable dosing regimen for most ingestions that meet the criteria for using MDAC is to administer 1 g/kg of activated charcoal as the initial dose and follow it with 0.5 g/kg every 3 to 4 hours for a total of 3 additional doses. Complications of MDAC are similar to those of single dose AC, with the addition of intestinal obstruction. Contraindications to MDAC administration are also similar, with the addition of patients with decreased peristalsis as a relative contraindication (1,4,14).

WHOLE-BOWEL IRRIGATION

The goal of WBI is to flush any unabsorbed toxin rapidly through the intestinal tract so as to prevent absorption. In the past, different types of solutions were tried for this purpose (including normal saline and specific electrolyte preparations), many of which led to systemic electrolyte imbalances. Polyethylene glycol electrolyte lavage solution (PEG-ELS, available as Go-Lytely and others) is the currently recommended preparation for WBI, as it causes minimal water and electrolyte shifts (5,14).

Most drugs are relatively rapidly absorbed from the gastrointestinal tract, and effective GID can be performed with single dose AC. However, certain drug formulations are designed specifically not to dissolve immediately and completely, but rather to dissolve at a predesignated rate. These drug formulations are generally referred to as "controlled-release." Many of the cardiovascular drugs currently available are packaged as once- or twice-a-day formulations designed to enhance patient compliance. The controlled-release formulations of β-blockers and calcium channel blockers are good examples of drugs that are good candidates for WBI (5,14). Patients who ingest carefully packaged units of illegal drugs and swallow them for the purpose of transporting them across international borders (i.e., body-packers) are also good candidates for WBI (5,14). Finally, WBI enhances the elimination of certain metals such as iron, lead and arsenic, which are not well adsorbed to activated charcoal and have significant associated toxicity (5,14).

Although WBI may enhance toxin elimination from the gut, it has not been shown to confer clinical benefit. However, it is logical to assume that if ingested drug is forced out of the gastrointestinal tract before absorption, it cannot be absorbed systemically and cause toxicity. Whole bowel irrigation should be performed only with PEG-ELS and should be administered orally or through an oro- or nasogastric tube (5,14). The recommended dosing regimen is 0.5 L/hours for small children and 1.5 to 2 L/hours for adolescents and adults (5,14). Treatment should continue until all ingested drug has passed or until the rectal effluent is clear (5,14). Contraindications to WBI include known or suspected gastrointestinal disease or dysfunction (ileus, perforation, obstruction, and hemorrhage), an unprotected airway, hemodynamic instability, absent bowel sounds or intractable vomiting (5,14).

CATHARTICS

The use of cathartics originates from the notion that if drug is forced through the gastrointestinal tract, it cannot be systemically absorbed. Cathartics generally cause a watery stool to be passed within 1 to 3 hours of administration (2,14). They are discussed primarily because of their familiarity to clinicians, rather than for any proven clinical benefit. Cathartic administration generally does not result in reduction of peak or total drug absorption equivalent to that achieved with activated charcoal alone (2,14). In fact, the administration of a cathartic together with activated charcoal is not consistently more efficacious than activated charcoal alone (2,21).

The complications of the generally available cathartics (e.g., sorbitol, saline, and other) are similar: dehydration, electrolyte imbalance (from absorption of salts in saline cathartics or volume depletion), metabolic alkalosis (from dehydration), vomiting, abdominal cramps, nausea, vomiting, diaphoresis, frequent stools, transient hypotension, hypermagnesemia, hyperphosphatemia, and hypokalemia (2,14).

Contraindications to cathartic use include absent bowel sounds, intestinal obstruction or perforation, recent gastrointestinal surgery, hypotension, preexisting electrolyte imbalance, caustic ingestion, nontoxic ingestion, renal insufficiency or failure (saline cathartics), and patient age less than 1 year (2,14).

Because there are no definite indications for the general use of cathartics in poisoned patients and only a few indications for cathartic use in selected overdoses, their routine administration with activated charcoal is discouraged (2,14).

CRITICAL INTERVENTIONS

- Consider the time since ingestion, potential severity of poisoning, and complications and contraindications of the intervention before performing gastrointestinal decontamination
- Assess the patient's ability to protect the airway and the potential for deterioration prior to performing gastrointestinal decontamination
- Consult a poison center or toxicologist regarding the choice of procedure and necessity for performing gastrointestinal decontamination in questionable cases

COMMON PITFALLS

✔ Failure to appreciate that gastrointestinal decontamination is likely to be effective only if performed within an hour or two of ingestion
✔ Failure to secure the airway prior to gastrointestinal decontamination in patients with CNS depression
✔ Failure to appreciate that activated charcoal alone is the most appropriate method of gastrointestinal decontamination for most ingestions
✔ Failure to appreciate that MDAC can enhance the elimination of some toxins
✔ Failure to consider WBI for ingestions of controlled-release formulations or agents that are slowly absorbed

Acknowledgments

Thank you to previous edition chapter authors William A. Watson and Christopher H. Linden.

References

1. American Academy of Clinical Toxicology. Position statement and practice guidelines on the use of multi-dose activated charcoal in the treatment of acute poisoning. *J Toxicol Clin Toxicol* 1999;37:731–751.
2. American Academy of Clinical Toxicology. Position statement: Cathartics. 1997;35:743–752.
3. American Academy of Clinical Toxicologists. Position statement: Gastric lavage. *J Toxicol Clin Toxicol* 1997;35:711–9.
4. American Academy of Clinical Toxicology. Position Statement: Single-dose activated charcoal. *J Toxicol Clin Toxicol* 1997;35:721–741.
5. American Academy of Clinical Toxicology. Position statement: Whole bowel irrigation. *J Toxicol Clin Toxicol* 1997;35:753–762.
6. American Academy of Pediatrics, Committee on Injury, Violence, and Poison Prevention. Poison treatment in the home. *Pediatrics* 112:1182–1185.
7. Bogacz K, Caldron P. Enteric-coated aspirin bezoar: elevation of serum salicylate level by barium study. Case report and review of medical management. *Am J Med* 1987;83:783–786.
8. Bond GR. The role of activated charcoal and gastric emptying in gastrointestinal decontamination: A state-of-the-art review. *Ann Emerg Med* 2002;39:273–286.
9. Bond GR, Requa RK, Krenzelok EP, et al. Influence of time until emesis on the efficacy of decontamination using acetaminophen as a marker in a pediatric population. *Ann Emerg Med* 1993;22:1403–1407.
10. Bosse GM, Barefoot JA, Pfeifer MP, et al. Comparison of three methods of gut decontamination in tricyclic antidepressant overdose. *J Emerg Med* 1995;13:203–209.
11. Comstock EG, Boisaubin EV, Comstock BS, et al. Assessment of the efficacy of activated charcoal following orogastric lavage in acute drug emergencies. *J Toxicol Clin Toxicol* 1982;19:149–165.
12. Comstock EG, Faulkner TP, Boisaubin E, et al. Studies on the efficacy of gastric emptying as practiced in a large metropolitan hospital. *J Toxicol Clin Toxicol* 1981;18:581–597.
13. De Silva HA, Fonseka MMD, Pathmeswaran A, et al. Multiple-dose activated charcoal for treatment of yellow oleander poisoning: a single-blind, randomized, placebo-controlled trial. *Lancet* 2003;361:1935–1938.
14. Howland MA.Antidotes in depth: syrup of ipecac, activated charcoal, cathartics, whole bowel irrigation. In: Goldfrank LR, Flomenbaum NE, Lewin NA, et al., eds. *Goldfrank's toxicologic emergencies*, 7th ed. New York, 2002: 465–479.
15. Jenis EH, Payne RJ, Goldbaum LR. Acute meprobomate poisoning: A fatal case followed by a lucid interval. *JAMA* 1969;207:361–365.
16. Johnson WE. Massive Phenobarbital ingestion with survival. *JAMA* 1967;202:1106–1109.
17. Kulig K, Bar-Or D, Cantrill SV, et al. Management of acutely poisoned patients without gastric emptying. *Ann Emerg Med* 1985;14:59–64.
18. Lim DT, Singh P, Nourtsis S, et al. Absorption inhibition and enhancement of elimination of sustained-release theophylline tablets by oral activated charcoal. *Ann Emerg Med* 1986;15:1303–1307.
19. Merigian KS, Woodard M, Hedges JR, et al. Prospective evaluation of gastric emptying in the self-poisoned patient. *Am J Emerg Med* 1990;8:479–483.
20. Neuvonen PJ. Clinical pharmacokinetics of oral activated charcoal in acute intoxications. *Clin Pharmacokinet* 1982;7:465–489.
21. Pond SM, Lewis-Driver DJ, Williams GM, et al. Gastric emptying in acute overdose: a prospective randomized controlled trial. *Med J Aust* 1995;163:345–349.
22. Saetta JP, March S, Gaunt ME, et al. Gastric emptying procedures in the self-poisoned patient: Are we forcing gastric content beyond the pylorus? *J R Soc Med* 1991;84:274.
23. Saetta JP, Quinton DN. Residual gastric content after orogastric lavage and ipecacuanha induced emesis in self-poisoned patients: An endoscopic study. *J R Soc Med* 1991;84:35–38.
24. Smilkstein MJ. Techniques used to prevent gastrointestinal absorption of toxic compounds. In: Goldfrank LR, Flomenbaum NE, Lewin NA, et al., eds. *Goldfrank's toxicologic emergencies*, 7th ed. New York, 2002: 44–57.
25. Tandberg D, Diven BG, McLeod JW. Ipecac-induced emesis versus orogastric lavage: A controlled study in normal adults. *Am J Emerg Med* 1986;4:205–209.

PART II

Alcohol-Related Agents and Conditions

CHAPTER 273
Ethanol

Tri C. Tong and Binh T. Ly

Ethanol, or ethyl alcohol, is a 2-carbon chain alcohol with the chemical formula CH_3CH_2OH. Although often simply referred to as "alcohol," this expression can be misleading since other alcohols such as methanol and ethylene glycol have unique properties and impart significant and individual toxicities. Ethanol's use and abuse is ubiquitous throughout the world, and it is undoubtedly a leading cause of morbidity across cultures. Although ethanol-containing drinks are used frequently in recreational settings, inappropriate use and addiction has resulted in tremendous costs to the individual and to society.

Following ingestion, ethanol is rapidly absorbed from the gastrointestinal tract with approximately 80% to 90% of a full dose absorbed within 60 minutes (16). Twenty percent of ingested ethanol is absorbed in the stomach, whereas the remainder is absorbed by the small intestine. Absorption is enhanced by rapid gastric emptying, intake without food, and the dilution of the ethanol solution (a solution of 20% ethanol is absorbed most readily). Absorption may be delayed by spasm of pyloric sphincter, which can be induced by high concentrations of ethanol, food in the stomach, coingestion of drugs, or it may vary simply from individual differences (1).

A typical drink contains about 14.4 g of ethanol. This is the amount of ethanol found in 1.5 ounces of 80 proof liquor (40% alcohol by volume), 5 ounces of wine (12% alcohol), or 12 ounces of beer (5% alcohol). Ethanol is also a constituent in varying proportions of many other commercially available products, including mouthwashes, after-shaves, cooking ingredients (e.g., vanilla extract), and pharmaceutical agents (e.g., elixirs). Theoretically, one standard drink will elevate the blood ethanol level by about 35 mg/dL, assuming instantaneous and complete absorption and no distribution or metabolism (12). In reality, ingested alcohol is absorbed over time and distributed and metabolized during absorption, resulting in peak blood levels that are one-half or two thirds of the theoretical level, about 18 mg/dL and 23 mg/dL, depending on whether the stomach is full or empty, respectively.

Although only a small proportion of ethanol is excreted unchanged in the urine, greater than 90% is eliminated via enzymatic oxidation in the liver (3). Although there are at least three enzymatic pathways through which ethanol is metabolized in the liver, the principle route of elimination is through breakdown by the alcohol dehydrogenase (ADH) pathway. Metabolism of ethanol by ADH begins shortly after initial ingestion and even prior to systemic absorption. When ethanol contacts the gastric mucosa, it is oxidized by a subtype of ADH located in the stomach, resulting in decreased of amounts of ethanol available for absorption into the systemic circulation. This process is more notable in men than in women and more in tolerant than intolerant individuals (5).

Once absorbed, ethanol follows a conversion process that begins with the metabolism of ethanol to acetaldehyde catalyzed by a second class of ADH. Acetaldehyde is then transformed to acetate by aldehyde dehydrogenase (ALDH). Acetate is ultimately converted to carbon dioxide and water. Individuals with a point mutation in mitochondrial ALDH can exhibit a decreased ability to metabolize acetaldehyde. The prevalence of this mutation varies among different ethnic populations. As a result of acetaldehyde accumulation, nearly 30% of Caucasians, 40% of Asians, and 80% of Native Americans may exhibit significant flushing reactions similar to those exposed to ethanol while using disulfiram, which inhibits ALDH (4). Disulfiram is now rarely used for the deterrence of ethanol use, reserved mainly for motivated alcoholics when other measures have failed.

Another common and significant drug interaction occurs when ethanol is used in conjunction with other sedative-hypnotic agents. When ethanol is coingested it may add to the sedative effects of these agents and may increase morbidity by worsening CNS and respiratory depression. This effect appears to be independent of any alteration in the pharmacokinetics of the sedative-hypnotic drug itself (10,15). Agents that may contribute to ethanol's added sedation when co-ingested include benzodiazepines, phenothiazines, barbiturates, cyclic antidepressants, antihistamines, and opioids, among others.

In the process of oxidizing ethanol to acetaldehyde, ADH uses nicotinamide adenine dinucleotide (NAD^+) as a hydrogen acceptor. Nicotinamide adenine dinucleotide is then reduced to NADH. Similarly, the conversion of acetaldehyde to acetate reduces NAD^+ to NADH, resulting in further accumulation of reducing potential in the form of NADH. Increased NADH

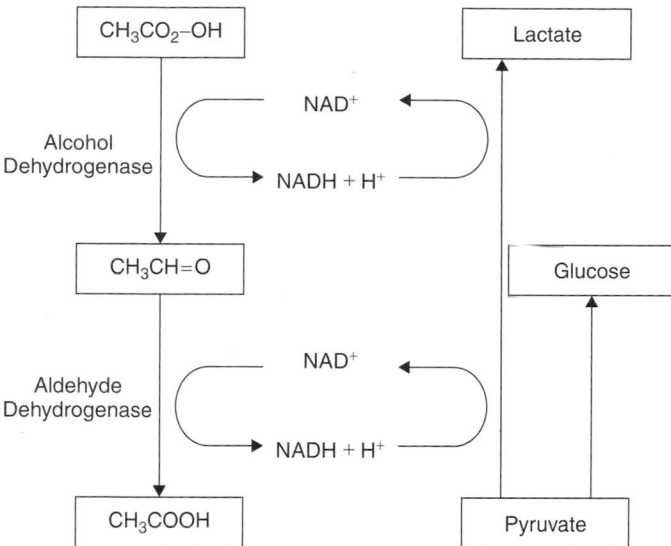

Figure 273.1. Mechanism of ethanol-induced hypoglycemia. During the course of ethanol metabolism, the formation of NADH favors the conversion of pyruvate to lactate rather than to glucose.

impairs the cell's ability to perform oxidative reactions and can lead to numerous metabolic abnormalities, including alteration of fatty acid metabolism resulting in ketoacidosis (see Chapter 277, "Alcoholic Ketoacidosis"). Accumulation of NADH may also lead to the impairment of gluconeogenesis (Fig. 273.1). Although this has minimal consequences in normal adults, it may lead to clinically significant hypoglycemia in individuals with limited glycogen stores particularly children and malnourished alcoholics (11).

The ADH pathway for metabolism and elimination of ethanol is saturable at relatively low levels of ethanol (less than 10 mg/dL) (9). With saturation, elimination converts from first-order to zero-order kinetics, which describes a state in which the elimination rate ceases to be concentration-dependent. In this state, higher dosages will prolong the period of elimination. The average-sized (70 kg) adult male metabolizes 7 to 10 g of alcohol per hour, corresponding to an hourly decrease of the blood ethanol level by approximately 15 to 20 mg/dL/hour. The tolerant individual may increase this clearance of ethanol to 30 mg/dL/hour (6). Intuitively, rates of elimination will vary among individuals by as much as 5 to 6 mg/dL/hour, although the average rate is approximately 20 mg/dL/hour (2).

Although much of the kinetics and metabolism of ethanol has been elucidated, its exact mechanism of inebriation is still the subject of much debate. Current theories postulate that ethanol acts upon a variety of neurotransmitters. In particular, it appears that ethanol is an agonist at γ-aminobutyric acid subtype A (GABA$_A$) receptors while blocking the N-methyl-D-aspartate (NMDA) subtypes of excitatory glutamate receptors (8,13). Ethanol's agonism of inhibitory receptors and inhibition of excitatory receptors mediate its primary role as a central nervous system (CNS) depressant (8). At times, ethanol may appear to function as a CNS stimulant when it selectively depresses inhibitory mechanisms in the brain.

CLINICAL PRESENTATION

Clinical manifestations following acute ethanol consumption can vary considerably. Although determinations of serum ethanol concentrations are now readily available in most hospitals, caution must be employed when trying to attribute clinical manifestations to any particular level. Effects of ethanol at any particular concentration will vary from individual to individual. At lower dosages, ethanol's depression of inhibitory cortical pathways in the brain may create the appearance of CNS stimulation caused by disinhibition. These effects may be most pronounced in mildly to moderately intoxicated individuals who engage in functions requiring higher degrees of cortical integration. Individuals may exhibit euphoria, gregariousness, verbosity, or emotional lability. Often times, disinhibited behavior may strongly reflect the individual's basic personality, and boisterous or aggressive behavior may ensue. Other manifestations may include ataxia, nystagmus, and impaired reactions.

With deeper intoxication, disinhibition and impairment of cognitive integration will progress. Overt displays of hostility and aggressiveness may emerge. Finally, with higher dosages of ethanol, severe intoxication will ensue, thereby leading to deep CNS depression hearkened by coma and respiratory depression. In this state, the risk of significant morbidity rises as concomitant loss of protective reflexes develops.

Because gluconeogenesis is impaired by NADH produced during ethanol metabolism, clinically significant hypoglycemia may develop, particularly in the malnourished adult or the young child. With acute ethanol ingestion, abdominal pain with possible nausea and vomiting may be present and may be due to either direct gastric irritation by ethanol or secondary processes such as pancreatitis or ethanol-induced hepatitis.

Only small amounts of ethanol may induce an adverse reaction in a patient taking disulfiram. Often times, the source of ethanol may be elusive since ethanol-containing products in the home are ubiquitous. Signs and symptoms of the disulfiram-ethanol reaction (DER) include flushing of the face and body, sensations of warmth, urticaria, pruritus, light-headedness, headache, nausea, and vomiting. Complaints of palpitations, chest pain, and shortness of breath are common. A sulfur or garlic odor of the breath may be noted. Findings of tachycardia and hypotension can also be seen. ECG findings consistent with myocardial ischemia are less common and are usually associated with severe hypotension. In general, deaths attributable to DERs are extremely rare. Disulfiram-ethanol reactions usually begin within 30 minutes of ethanol exposure. Symptoms may last for several hours.

Of note, acute disulfiram overdose in the absence of ethanol is rare and generally well-tolerated. Early symptoms such as nausea, vomiting, and general abdominal pain may occur within the first 12 hours after ingestion, but typically subside after the first 24 hours. Severe adverse effects from chronic use may involve the liver, skin, and central nervous system, but are uncommon.

DIFFERENTIAL DIAGNOSIS

Because presentations of acute ethanol intoxication can be quite protean, ranging from CNS depression to excitation, patients with acute altered mental status in the setting of ethanol use must be carefully evaluated for other causes of altered sensorium unrelated to ethanol intoxication. In the appropriate setting, head trauma causing acute intracranial hemorrhage, CNS infections, and encephalopathy (e.g., Wernicke or hepatic) related to chronic ethanol use merit consideration as sources of cognitive alteration. Intentional ingestion of other drugs with sedating properties can also lead to CNS depression. Exposure to other more toxic alcohols (e.g., methanol, ethylene glycol; see Chapters 274 ["Ethylene Glycol] and 275 ["Methanol"]) may create a similar picture of inebriation, but failure to recognize and treat their separate toxicities may have negative consequences for the patient.

An acutely intoxicated patient may present with classic features that include flushed skin, diaphoresis, tachycardia,

TABLE 273.1. Substances That Potentially Induce Disulfiram-Like Reactions Following Ethanol Exposure

MUSHROOMS	*Coprinus* species mushrooms
CHEMICALS	Carbon disulfide
	Carbon tetrachloride
	Tetramethylthiuram (thiram)
	Trichloroethylene
MEDICATIONS	Antimicrobials
	Cephalosporins
	Cefamandole
	Cefmenoxime
	Cefoperazone
	Cefotetan
	Metronidazole
	Trimethroprim-sulfamethoxazole
	Chloramphenicol
	Griseofulvin
	Nitrofurantoin
	Oral hypoglycemics (sulfonylureas)
	Chlorpropamide
	Tolbutamide
	Chloral hydrate

hypothermia, hypoventilation, vomiting, nystagmus, dysarthria, and incoordination. However, it is important for the clinician to recognize covert signs of concomitant medical processes, even in the presence of overt signs of ethanol intoxication. Hypoglycemia can complicate ethanol ingestion in the malnourished patient or the young child. Abdominal pain in acute alcohol ingestion may simply be related to gastric mucosal irritation, ethanol-induced hepatitis, or pancreatitis, but the clinician should be aware of more serious complications such as esophageal rupture and perforated peptic or duodenal ulcers. Ophthalmoplegia, ataxia, and characteristic mental status alterations suggest Wernicke's encephalopathy.

A number of natural and synthetic compounds may induce a reaction similar to the DER in the presence of ethanol (Table 273.1). Similar signs and symptoms can be caused by reactions to niacin, monosodium glutamate, rifampin, and vancomycin, and by boric acid and scombroid poisoning.

EMERGENCY DEPARTMENT EVALUATION

Often times, obtaining an accurate and thorough history may be impossible because the patient is intoxicated. In the lucid, co-operative patient, information regarding the type, amount, and time of last ethanol use should be gathered, in addition to basic medical history. Clues from friends, family members, or witnesses may be helpful in assessing the risk of trauma or other organ system involvement. Such sources can also be helpful in identifying other substances that might have been ingested.

Clinicians should avoid complacency when performing a physical examination, as biased assessments of uncomplicated inebriation may occur with recurrent presentations. Key features of the examination include assessments of airway protective reflexes, mental status, neurological function, gastrointestinal disturbances, and cardiopulmonary status. Frequent monitoring of vitals signs should be performed for tachycardia, hypothermia, and hypotension. In the patient who is unable to offer history, clinicians must be vigilant when performing a physical examination for evidence of concomitant trauma and consider other diagnostic adjuncts such as computed tomography of the head or abdomen and laboratory testing to assess for the presence of associated pathology.

The necessity of absolute, objective determination of the presence of ethanol remains debatable in the patient who

presents with an uncomplicated clinical presentation consistent with acute ethanol intoxication. The subjective perception of the presence or absence of ethanol on a patient's breath is often an unreliable means of assessing whether an individual has or has not recently used ethanol. This has been proven true even under optimum laboratory conditions (13). An initial breath-alcohol level may be helpful in confirming the presence of ethanol, although an accurate level often depends on patient compliance. Alternatively, the absence of ethanol or the presence of an inconsequential ethanol level should prompt the clinician to pursue other diagnostic possibilities for conditions that may mimic ethanol intoxication. Factors that interfere with breath-alcohol analyses include recent use of ethanol-containing products (e.g., inhaled bronchodilators within 15 to 30 minutes), recent belching or vomiting, obstructive pulmonary disease, or poor technique (7). Blood ethanol levels should be obtained in the severely intoxicated patient because a sufficient history may not be available. An accurate blood ethanol level can help the clinician estimate a reasonable time for observation while the patient metabolizes ethanol. Comatose patients with inappropriately low blood ethanol levels should be considered for more aggressive diagnostic evaluation that may include head computed tomographic imaging and lumbar puncture. All patients with significantly depressed mental status should have an early point-of-care screening for hypoglycemia to rule out this rapidly reversible process.

In addition to ethanol levels, other blood tests that may be helpful include a complete blood count, serum electrolytes, blood urea nitrogen (BUN), creatinine, ketones, acetone, lipase, liver enzymes, a coagulation profile, ammonia levels, calcium, and magnesium. The decision to initiate these tests will depend upon specific scenarios. An anion gap metabolic acidosis and elevated serum ketones may signify acute alcoholic ketoacidosis (see Chapter 277, "Alcoholic Ketoacidosis"). It also warrants measurement of serum osmolality (by freezing point depression) and calculation of the osmolal gap (the difference between the measured and the calculated osmolality). Ethanol's contribution to the osmolality can be estimated by dividing the serum ethanol level in milligrams per deciliter by 4.6. Ethanol-like intoxication in a patient with an osmolal gap unexplained by the amount of ethanol present should raise suspicion of acetone, isopropanol, methanol, or ethylene glycol ingestion and prompt measurement of these agents. Analysis of a urine specimen for drugs of abuse is often not needed, but may be helpful if certain drugs of abuse are suspected to be contributing to the patient's clinical condition.

Similar considerations apply to the evaluation of patients with DERs. Those with chest complaints or abnormal vital signs should also have an ECG and cardiac marker measurements, and further evaluation as clinically indicated.

Although blood-ethanol levels may not reliably predict clinical intoxication, they do define driving while under the influence. In October 2000, the United States Congress established a blood-alcohol concentration (BAC) of 0.08 g/dL as the national standard for impaired driving. Since then, nearly 30 states have adopted this level as the legal limit above which it is illegal to drive a motor vehicle because of the influence of alcohol; other states have used a higher limit of 0.10 g/dL (14). When an individual's blood ethanol level is at or above the legal limit, driving is considered illegal regardless of the degree of impairment on his ability to operate a vehicle. The BAC is a measure of ethanol in whole blood, rather than in serum. Because ethanol more readily distributes into aqueous solutions, serum ethanol concentrations (the standard measurement in most medical institutions) are generally 15% to 20% higher than BACs because of the higher water content in serum compared to whole blood. An individual who is not tolerant to ethanol often exhibits impaired driving ability at blood ethanol concentrations as low as 20 mg/dL (17). An average nontolerant adult with a blood-alcohol level of greater than 300 to 350 mg/dL will often be comatose.

EMERGENCY DEPARTMENT MANAGEMENT

As with all patients who present to the emergency department (ED) with acute mental status changes, reversible causes must first be identified and addressed. An inappropriately comatose patient should be checked for possible hypoglycemia and treated with intravenous dextrose if necessary. If co-ingestion of opioid drugs is suspected, naloxone should be considered. Thiamine (100 mg i.v.) should also be given as clinically indicated for suspicion or prevention of Wernicke's encephalopathy. Agitated or combative patients should be restrained with physical and then chemical means. Intravenous benzodiazepines (e.g., lorazepam) or haloperidol are recommended for chemical sedation.

Fluid and electrolyte abnormalities should be corrected. Because the chronic alcoholic patient's principle source of caloric intake (ethanol) is deficient in essential nutrients, supplemental administration of multivitamins with folate can be considered in those patients suspected of severe malnutrition. Such supplements may be given either orally or parenterally if an intravenous line has already been established. Significant cost savings may result if oral repletion is possible. Vigilant and repeated assessments should be performed while the acutely intoxicated patient is in the ED to monitor for signs of deterioration. Patients who do not respond appropriately as they metabolize the absorbed ethanol should be subjected to further diagnostic examinations and possible therapeutic interventions such as advanced airway management.

Treatment of DERs is also supportive. Intravenous crystalloids should be administered. Antiemetics can be given for nausea and vomiting. Antihistamines such as diphenhydramine (H_1 subtype) may help alleviate cutaneous flushing.

CRITICAL INTERVENTIONS

- Perform a fingerstick blood sugar determination to rule out hypoglycemia as a cause of altered mental status in patients with alcohol ingestion
- Obtain a computed tomographic scan of the brain and rule out infection, metabolic disturbances, and other ingestants in patients whose mental status and level of consciousness are not consistent with the ethanol level
- Administer thiamine (100 mg i.v.) to alcoholic patients with altered mental status
- Utilize physical and chemical restraints to facilitate the evaluation and treatment of agitated or combative patients

DISPOSITION

A patient with uncomplicated intoxication can generally be discharged from the ED after a period of observation until the patient is deemed clinically sober enough to make sound decisions. Because clinical sobriety may not correlate with measured ethanol levels, particularly in the chronic alcoholic with tolerance, a repeat ethanol level is usually not necessary. However, repeat assessments of ambulation status and cognition should be made to avoid prematurely discharging a patient who is still clinically intoxicated. When a safe destination with a responsible adult is available, discharge may be considered for a patient who is still clinically intoxicated but stable and improving with intact protective reflexes. Such patients should not be allowed to leave until after they have been fully evaluated.

Indications for hospitalization are often self-evident in a complicated case of ethanol intoxication and include prolonged and inappropriate depressed mental status, metabolic derangements not correctable in an appropriate time-period, persistently abnormal vital signs, associated major trauma, severe withdrawal, mixed overdose, and concomitant medical processes such as gastrointestinal bleeding, pancreatitis, or severe acute hepatitis. A lower threshold for admission should be applied to those patients who lack social support, are indigent, or who have baseline organic brain syndromes that may be related to chronic ethanol abuse.

Most DERs can be managed in the emergency department. Patients can be discharged once they become asymptomatic and vital signs normalize, provided there are no cardiac complications or further evaluation of chest complaints is not indicated.

COMMON PITFALLS

- ✔ Failure to appreciate that alcohol intoxication can mask or mimic medical and traumatic conditions and to obtain a blood-ethanol level when the history is unclear or inconsistent with clinical findings
- ✔ Failure to recognize signs of ethanol withdrawal and to appreciate that withdrawal can develop in patients with an elevated blood ethanol level
- ✔ Failure to monitor and re-evaluate the intoxicated patient until clinically sober, even those with an initially benign examination
- ✔ Failure to refer intoxicated patients for counseling or detoxification

Acknowledgments

Thank you to previous edition chapter authors Susan S. Fish and Edward P. Krenzelok.

References

1. Adinoff B, Gone GH, Linnoila M. Acute ethanol poisoning and the ethanol withdrawal syndrome. *Med Toxicol Adverse Drug Exp* 1988;3:172–196.
2. Brennan DF, Betzelos S, Reed R, et al. Ethanol elimination rates in an ED population. *Am J Emerg Med* 1983;12:294–296.
3. Crab DW, Bosrom WF, Li TF. Ethanol metabolism. *Pharmacol Ther* 1987;34:59–73.
4. Dohmen K, Baraona E, Ishibashi H, et al. Ethnic differences in gastric–alcohol dehydrogenase activity and ethanol first-pass metabolism. *Alcohol Clin Exp Res* 1996;20:1569–1576.
5. Frezza M, DiRadova C, Pozzato G, et al. High blood alcohol levels in women: The role of decreased gastric alcohol dehydrogenase activity and first pass metabolism. *N Engl J Med* 1990;322:95–110.
6. Gershman H, Steper J. Rate of clearance from the blood of intoxicated patients in the emergency department. *J Emerg Med* 1991;9:307–311.
7. Gomez HF, Moore L, McKinney P, et al. Elevation of breath ethanol measurements by metered-dose inhalers. *Ann Emerg Med* 1995;25:608–611.
8. Kalant H. Ethanol and the nervous system: experimental neurophysiological aspects. *Int J Neurol* 1974;9:111–120.
9. Keiding S, Johansen S, Midtboll I, et al. Ethanol elimination kinetics in human liver and pig liver in vivo. *Am J Physiol* 1979;237:E316–324.
10. Kuitunen T, Mattila MJ, Seppala T. Actions and interactions of hypnotics on human performance: single doses of zopiclone, triazolam and alcohol. *Int Clin Psychopharmacol* 1990;[Suppl 2]:115–130.
11. Laminpaa A. Alcohol intoxication in childhood and adolescence. *Alcohol* 1995;30:5–12.
12. Lands WE. A review of alcohol clearance in humans. *Alcohol* 1998;15:147–160. Review.
13. Moskowitz H, Burns M, Ferguson S. Police officer's detection of breath odors from alcohol ingestion. *Accid Anal Prev* 1999;31:175–180.
14. National Highway Safety Administration. Setting limits, saving lives, the case for 0.08 BAC laws. 2001. Press release.
15. van Steveninck AL, Gieschke R, Schoemaker RC, et al. Pharmacokinetic and pharmacodynamic interactions of bretazenil and diazepam with alcohol. *Br J Clin Pharmacol* 1996;41:565–573.
16. Wilson PK. Pharmacokinetics of ethanol: a review. *Alcohol Clin Exp Res.* 1980;4:6–21.
17. Zador PL. Alcohol-related relative risk and fatal driver injuries in relation to driver age and sex. *J Stud Alcohol* 1991;52:302–310.

CHAPTER 274
Ethylene Glycol

Michael Joseph Burns

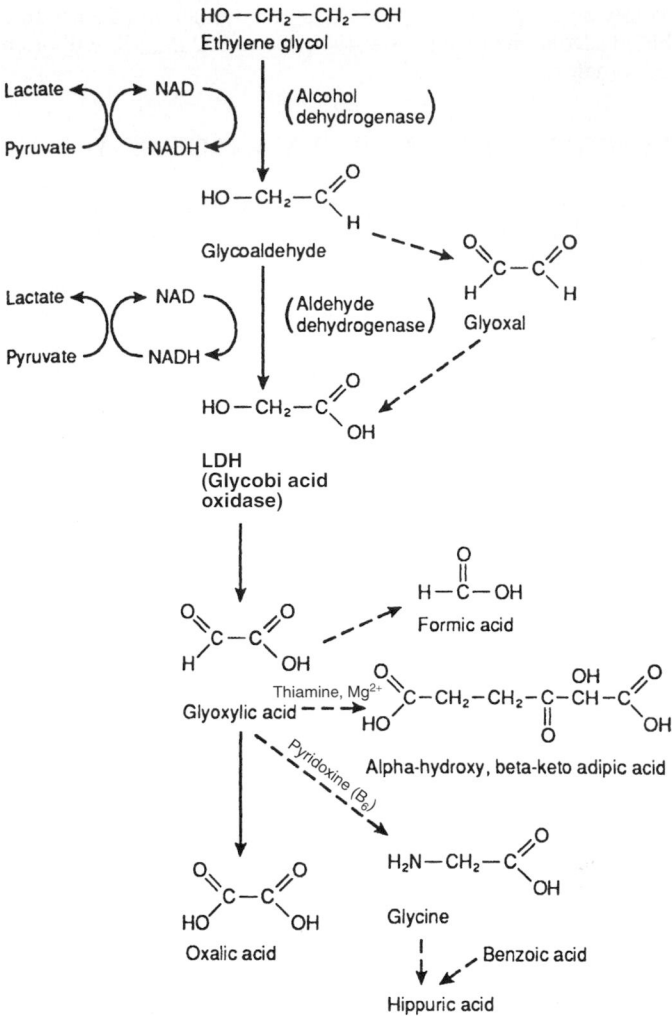

Ethylene glycol (EG; 1,2-ethanediol) is a colorless, odorless, sweet-tasting, water-soluble liquid that has a wide variety of household and commercial uses (1). Because of its low freezing point (~13°C) and high boiling point (198°C), EG is commonly used as an antifreeze–coolant. Automotive antifreeze contains about 95% EG and is the source of most EG poisonings. EG may also be found in adhesives, brake and hydraulic fluids, cosmetics, de-icers, detergents, fire extinguishers, inks, lacquers, paints, pesticides, polishes, and some windshield-washer fluids. The majority of exposures occur unintentionally through misuse or by accident (23). Intentional ingestion of EG for purposes of inebriation or suicide accounts for a minority of exposures but the most fatalities. In 2002, 6,077 exposures to EG were reported to United States poison centers, including 40 fatalities. Intentional ingestion with suicidal intent accounted for 15% of EG exposures yet 90% of fatalities (23). Widespread availability, interesting color, and pleasant, bittersweet taste likely account for its ingestion by alcoholics seeking an ethanol substitute and by children.

Unmetabolized EG produces about the same degree of central nervous system (CNS) depression as ethanol. Other effects (anion gap metabolic acidosis, coma, seizures, cardiopulmonary dysfunction, and acute renal failure) result largely from accumulation of the toxic metabolites, glycolic and oxalic acids (1,4,6,8,10).

EG is rapidly absorbed from the gastrointestinal tract and distributed throughout total body water (0.6 L/kg). Peak blood concentration occurs about 2 hours after enteral administration (9). About 20% to 50% of EG is excreted unchanged in the urine (9). The remaining EG is metabolized in the liver to a variety of compounds with varying toxicities (Fig. 274.1). In patients with normal renal function and alcohol dehydrogenase activity, EG elimination is first order with a half-life of 2.5–4.5 hours (1,8,9,18,19).

The first step in the metabolism of EG is its oxidation to glycoaldehyde by alcohol dehydrogenase (ADH) (8,9). Because ADH has a much higher affinity for ethanol and fomepizole (a synthetic ADH inhibitor) than for EG, these substrates are preferentially bound when present along with EG. Their presence inhibits the metabolism of EG sixfold and prevents the formation of toxic metabolites (1,2,5,8,9,20).

When formed, glycoaldehyde is rapidly metabolized by aldehyde dehydrogenase to glycolic acid, which is further metabolized slowly by glycolic acid oxidase to glyoxylic acid (1,8–10). Glycolic acid oxidation is rate-limiting; for this reason, it tends to accumulate (4,10,14). Glycolic acid accumulation correlates with the increased anion gap, decreased arterial pH, development of renal injury, and mortality associated with advanced EG poisoning (2,4,6,9,10,11). Once formed, glyoxylic acid is rapidly oxidized to one of several different metabolites. Its principal metabolite, oxalic acid, rapidly precipitates as calcium oxalate crystals in various organs and tissues (1,8–10).

Calcium oxalate crystal deposition is responsible for much of the end-organ injury that results from serious EG poisoning (e.g., nephrotoxicity, meningoencephalitis, and cerebral and pulmonary edema) (1,8–10). Crystal accumulation within proximal renal tubules leads to physical blockage and compression of tubular lumen and, subsequently, to the development of acute

Figure 274.1. Metabolism of ethylene glycol. *Solid lines,* known pathways of metabolism; *dotted lines,* postulated pathways of metabolism.

tubular necrosis and renal insufficiency (8–10). Renal tubular toxicity is also the result of direct cytotoxicity (cell membrane and oxidative cellular injury) produced by the oxalate ion and calcium oxalate crystals (12,13). Although some evidence suggests that glycoaldehyde and glyoxylic acid are also highly nephrotoxic (16), their contribution to renal tubular injury in EG poisoning is probably negligible because they are rapidly metabolized (1,8–10,12).

Significant systemic toxicity from EG occurs only after ingestion (1,9). Skin exposure may cause minor irritation, and direct eye contact may result in conjunctivitis, chemosis, and iridocyclitis (21). Due to the high boiling point of EG, toxicity from vapor inhalation does not occur. The toxic and lethal doses of EG after acute ingestion vary. Death has been reported in two men who shared 60 mL of 95% EG, but one patient survived after ingesting about 2 L of EG (20,24). Because as little as 0.1 mL/kg of pure EG may result in potentially toxic blood concentrations, the ingestion of even a mouthful of EG should be considered hazardous. Conversely, although the oral lethal dose is approximately 1.5 mL/kg, the correlation between the amount consumed and prognosis is usually poor (5,8,9,18).

CLINICAL PRESENTATION

With EG poisoning, three distinct stages of organ system involvement—CNS, cardiopulmonary, and renal—have been classically described, but the onset, progression, and confluence of these stages vary widely (1,5,9). Thirty minutes to 12 hours after ingestion, CNS signs and symptoms predominate. Initially, slurred speech, ataxia, nystagmus, and lethargy occur. The patient may appear drunk but lacks the breath odor of ethanol; instead, a faint, sweet, or aromatic odor may be detected. Nausea, vomiting, and abdominal pain may also be present.

During this early stage, the presence of an elevated osmolal gap may provide a clue to the diagnosis of EG poisoning (5,8,9,18). Because of its low molecular weight (62 g/mol), high concentrations of EG (and other low molecular weight solutes, see Chapter 271, "Approach to the Poisoned Patient") increase the serum osmolality. This results in an increase in the osmolal gap, the difference between the serum osmolality measured by the freezing-point depression (but not the vapor pressure method) and the calculated osmolarity ([2 × sodium] + [glucose/18] + [blood urea nitrogen/2.8] + [serum ethanol concentration/4.6]). Normally, serum osmolality ranges from 280 to 300 mOsmol/kg H_2O, with a corrected osmolal gap of -2 ± 6 mOsmol/kg (7). Measurement of EG in serum or urine will confirm the diagnosis.

Following a latent period of 3 to 12 hours, the signs and symptoms caused by accumulated toxic metabolites develop. CNS depression progresses to stupor and coma. Hyperreflexia, tremors, tetany, and seizures (both focal and generalized) may occur. Severe CNS disturbances may reflect the development of cerebral edema and meningoencephalitis (8–10). Decreased serum bicarbonate and increased anion gap metabolic acidosis may be seen as early as 3 hours following EG ingestion (1,2,5). Hyperventilation occurs as a compensatory response to acidemia. Present in approximately 80% of patients, anion gap metabolic acidosis is the most frequently reported laboratory abnormality associated with EG poisoning (2,11). The normal anion gap (serum sodium minus chloride and bicarbonate) is 12 ± 2 mEq/L and represents unmeasured anions in the serum. In EG poisoning, glycolic acid is the unmeasured anion that increases the anion gap. The absence of metabolic acidosis suggests early presentation, an insignificant ingestion, or the co-ingestion of ethanol, which blocks the metabolism of EG. In the late stages of poisoning, when most or all EG has been metabolized, measuring the serum glycolic acid level may be the only way to confirm the diagnosis.

Cardiopulmonary signs and symptoms, such as hypertension, tachycardia, dysrhythmias, and pulmonary edema, develop 12 to 36 hours after the ingestion of EG. During this stage, tachypnea and Kussmaul respirations reflect a progressively worsening anion gap metabolic acidosis.

Urinalysis may provide additional evidence of EG poisoning. Proteinuria and microscopic hematuria may be seen in over 60% of cases (2,8–10,18). Calcium oxalate crystalluria, highly suggestive of EG poisoning, is present on admission in over 40% of patients; this percentage increases with serial urinalysis and delayed presentation (2,9,11,18). Calcium oxalate is often excreted as needle-shaped monohydrate crystals that may be misidentified as hippuric or uric acid crystals (5,9). At higher urinary concentrations, calcium oxalate is also excreted in an envelope-shaped dihydrate form (8–10). The formation of calcium oxalate may cause hypocalcemia with myoclonic jerks or tetanic contractions (1,8–10). The presence of hematuria and oxaluria is not predictive of acute renal failure (18). Because fluorescein is added to many commercial antifreeze preparations, fluorescence of urine or gastric contents with a Wood lamp supports EG poisoning early after ingestion (25). Fluorescence is insensitive and nonspecific, however, and should not be relied on to make or exclude the diagnosis of EG poisoning (3,22). Death is most common during the cardiopulmonary stage and results from cerebral edema and infarction, multiple organ failure, and irreversible shock (1,8–10,11,17). Even with conventional treatment, mortality rates of 5% to 17% are still described (2,11). The time elapsed between ingestion and treatment and the degree of metabolic acidosis at the initiation of treatment are the factors most closely correlated with survival (9,11). Rapid diagnosis and treatment prevents EG bioactivation and lethality, regardless of the initial plasma EG concentration (9,11). EG plasma concentrations are not predictive of renal failure and not correlated with mortality (18).

Patients who survive may complain of severe flank pain and develop costovertebral angle tenderness and acute renal insufficiency 18 to 48 hours after ingestion (1,8–10). Renal dysfunction is seen in nearly 70% of cases and is characterized by oliguria, proteinuria, and urine with a low specific gravity and sodium content (acute tubular necrosis); renal dysfunction may be noted within 9 hours of ingestion (2,11). The high frequency of renal injury reflects delayed presentation and delayed diagnosis and treatment (18). The degree of metabolic acidosis or glycolic acid accumulation at the initiation of treatment is closely correlated with the subsequent development of renal injury (2,9,11,18). In one retrospective study of 41 patients with EG poisoning, an initial glycolic acid level of greater than 8 mmol/L, anion gap of greater than 20 mmol/L, or arterial pH of less than 7.30 were highly predictive of acute renal failure (18).

Conversely, patients who have an initial glycolic acid level of less than 8 to 10 mmol/L, arterial pH of greater than 7.30, or have normal renal function upon initiation of appropriate treatment are very unlikely to develop acute renal insufficiency (2,18,19). Although most patients treated for EG poisoning have a complete recovery, some may have protracted renal insufficiency that requires months of hemodialysis. Uncommonly, cranial neuropathies and bilateral basal ganglia and brainstem infarction may develop 2 to 18 days after acute poisoning (1,8–10).

DIFFERENTIAL DIAGNOSIS

EG intoxication can mimic a large variety of poisonings or disease states, depending on the amount of EG ingested and the degree of EG metabolism at presentation. Diagnostic clues include drunkenness without the odor of ethanol, a delay between ingestion and significant illness, hyperventilation on physical examination, increased osmolal or anion gaps, metabolic acidosis, calcium oxalate crystalluria, and hypocalcemia. The differential diagnosis includes alcoholic, diabetic, and starvation ketoacidosis; lactic acidosis; renal failure; methanol poisoning; and advanced, untreated acetaminophen or salicylate poisoning. If the history is not suggestive of lactic acidosis or ketoacidosis, a high osmolal gap with anion gap metabolic acidosis strongly points toward EG or methanol poisoning (5,8–10). In methanol intoxication, crystalluria is absent and visual complaints and an abnormal eye examination may be present. Although a large osmolal gap (particularly if greater than 25) is suggestive of toxic alcohol poisoning, a small gap (less than 10), however, cannot be used to exclude significant EG poisoning, particularly in the later stages of poisoning, when significant metabolism has already occurred (1,5,7–9,18). The presence of glycolate can cause artifactual elevation of the plasma lactate level with lactate analyzers that use the reagent L-lactate oxidase, and lead to a misdiagnosis of lactic acidosis (15). Previously unrecognized disorders of organic acid metabolism should be considered in the differential diagnosis of young children with an increased anion gap metabolic acidosis.

EMERGENCY DEPARTMENT EVALUATION

The history should include the time of ingestion, the volume and concentration of the ingested product, and the onset, nature, and progression of symptoms. The ingestion of any other substance, particularly ethanol, and the details of such events should be documented. Patients should be specifically asked about symptoms of ethanol-like intoxication, shortness of breath, flank pain, and urinary dysfunction.

Initially, the physical examination should focus on the neurologic status and cardiopulmonary function. A complete physical with documentation of any abdominal and back tenderness should then be performed. In symptomatic patients, evaluation should include a complete blood count; measurement of serum electrolytes, blood urea nitrogen, creatinine, glucose, amylase, calcium, ketones, and lactate; serum osmolality; arterial blood gas analysis; toxicologic screen; urinalysis; electrocardiogram; and a chest radiograph.

A quantitative serum EG concentration should be obtained in all patients to confirm the diagnosis, preferably by gas chromatography and mass spectrometry (GC/MS). Semiquantitative, alcohol oxidase reagents (enzymatic assays) should not be used to confirm or exclude the presence of EG; they are insensitive and nonspecific for this purpose (15). In all patients with intentional ingestion, a serum ethanol concentration should also be obtained. In addition, since many antifreeze products also contain methanol or propylene glycol, serum concentrations of these agents should be ordered if the identity of the ingested substance cannot be confirmed. Propylene glycol or propionic acid may rarely be misinterpreted as EG by GC/MS. Occasionally, glycolic acid quantification by special GC/MS techniques may be necessary for those patients that present very late (e.g., renal failure and no detectable EG) (2,14,18).

If EG analysis is not readily available, the serum level (mg/dL) can be estimated by multiplying the osmolal gap by 6.2 (mg/dL per mOsm of EG). When interpreting the osmolal gap and using it in calculations, the contribution of ethanol (1 mOsm for each 4.6 mg/dL of serum ethanol), if present, must first be subtracted (8–10,18).

EMERGENCY DEPARTMENT MANAGEMENT

Airway protection and respiratory and circulatory support with cardiac and hemodynamic monitoring, should be instituted as necessary. Initially, intravenous fluids should be liberally administered to maintain an adequate urine output; a large urine flow increases the urinary excretion of EG in those without renal failure (8,9). If the patient has ingested EG within 4 hours, gastric aspiration, with or without lavage, via a nasogastric tube should be performed immediately. Activated charcoal adsorbs EG but may be clinically ineffective because EG is rapidly absorbed and the capacity of charcoal to bind EG is exceeded when moderate amounts of EG are ingested. Regardless, the administration of activated charcoal is recommended, particularly if a co-ingestant is suspected.

Specific treatment for EG poisoning consists of sodium bicarbonate to correct metabolic acidosis, calcium to correct symptomatic hypocalcemia, ethanol or fomepizole to inhibit production of toxic metabolites, hemodialysis to remove EG and its toxic metabolites, and cofactors (e.g., magnesium, pyridoxine, and thiamine) to theoretically enhance endogenous clearance of toxic metabolites (1).

Correction of metabolic acidosis may require the use of large amounts of intravenous sodium bicarbonate (NaHCO$_3$): $0.7 \times$ kg $\times$ (24 $-$ actual [HCO$_3^-$]), where 0.7 is the volume of distribution of bicarbonate in acidemia, 24 is the desired [HCO$_3^-$], and kg is the lean body weight. NaHCO$_3$ should be given in 1 mEq/kg increments (1,8–10). Increasing the serum pH increases the fraction of ionized acid metabolites, thereby minimizing their tissue redistribution and while maximizing their renal clearance through ion trapping. The acid–base status should be frequently reevaluated to assess the response to therapy. Hypocalcemia may be worsened by sodium bicarbonate administration (1,8–10).

Serum calcium levels should be monitored frequently. Symptomatic hypocalcemia (e.g., cardiac dysrhythmias, tetany, and seizures) should be treated initially with intravenous calcium chloride or gluconate (7 to 14 mEq for adults and 1 to 7 mEq for children). The 10% calcium chloride solution contains 1.4 mEq of calcium per milliliter, whereas the 10% calcium gluconate solution contains 0.46 mEq/mL. Calcium is not recommended for those with asymptomatic hypocalcemia, since its administration could theoretically enhance calcium oxalate tissue precipitation and overall EG toxicity. Seizures should otherwise be treated with standard drugs (diazepam, lorazepam, or a barbiturate).

Traditionally, ethanol has been used to inhibit the alcohol dehydrogenase–mediated metabolism of EG. Fomepizole (4-methylpyrazole, 4-MP; Antizol) is a potent, long-acting, competitive alcohol dehydrogenase inhibitor that appears to be a safe, easy, and effective alternative to ethanol (1,2,4,6,9,19). Unlike ethanol, fomepizole is approved by the U.S. Food and Drug Administration (FDA) for the treatment of EG and methanol poisoning. Fomepizole has been shown to both attenuate and prevent metabolic acidosis and renal failure in humans and animals poisoned by EG by halting the accumulation of glycolic and oxalic acids, respectively (1,2,4,6,18). Fomepizole offers several advantages over ethanol, which include a higher potency, longer duration of action, and easier dosing regimen (1,2,8). Unlike treatment with ethanol, fomepizole treatment does not require frequent monitoring and adjustment of plasma concentrations. In addition, fomepizole does not produce adverse effects commonly associated with ethanol therapy, such as CNS depression, hypoglycemia, gastritis, pancreatitis, fluid overload, and habituation (1,2,4,6,8).

Potential disadvantages of fomepizole include its high acquisition cost ($\sim$$1,000 U.S. per 1.5-g vial) and incompletely established safety profile. Although likely safe, fomepizole has been associated infrequently with dizziness, eosinophilia, headache, nausea, rash, transient hepatic transaminase elevation, and seizures in humans (1,2,8). The higher acquisition cost of fomepizole, however, is balanced by greater patient safety and the decreased cost of monitoring patients as compared to ethanol. Since its introduction, fomepizole has become the preferred antidote to ethanol in the United States (8,23).

Regardless of which antidote is used, both ethanol and fomepizole preferentially bind alcohol dehydrogenase and prevent further EG metabolism. Once administered, EG can then be eliminated by urinary excretion or hemodialysis. Indications for treatment with ethanol or fomepizole include a documented history of significant recent EG ingestion when a serum EG concentration is not immediately available, particularly if the osmol gap is elevated; strong suspicion of EG ingestion based on abnormal clinical or laboratory findings (e.g., unexplained anion gap metabolic acidosis or elevated corrected osmolar gap, or a combination thereof; oxalate crystalluria); or a measured serum EG concentration greater than 20 mg/dL (1,2,8–10).

For ethanol therapy, the therapeutic goal is a serum ethanol concentration of at least 100 mg/dL (8,9). Theoretically, a serum ethanol concentration of 100 mg/dL is sufficient to prevent metabolism of EG at a serum concentration of 546 mg/dL (9). Oral or intravenous ethanol loading is possible; intravenous administration is preferred since it provides a more rapid and constant serum concentration (1,8,9). An intravenous loading dose of 10 mL/kg of 10% ethanol (preferably in a glucose-containing solution, such as D5W to avoid hypoglycemia) over 30 to 60 minutes, followed by a maintenance infusion of 1.5 mL/kg/hour, generally produces a serum ethanol concentration of slightly greater than 100 mg/dL (8,9). Alternatively, 5 mL/kg of 20% (40 proof) ethanol may be administered orally or via nasogastric tube to achieve the desired loading dose; the hourly maintenance oral dose is similar to that for intravenous administration

(1.5 mL/kg/hour of 10% ethanol). (1,8,9). Serum ethanol and glucose concentrations should be monitored and the dose of ethanol adjusted, as necessary, to maintain a therapeutic ethanol concentration.

For fomepizole, a loading dose of 15 mg/kg i.v. should be administered, followed by doses of 10 mg/kg i.v. every 12 hours thereafter (2). All doses are diluted in 100 mL of 5% dextrose in water or normal saline and are administered by slow intravenous infusion over 30 minutes (2). Like ethanol, fomepizole is also effective following oral administration (1). Antidotal therapy is continued until EG concentrations fall below 20 mg/dL (2).

Hemodialysis rapidly removes both EG and glycolic acid (8–10,14). Elimination half-lives are reduced to approximately 3 hours for each, as compared with 19 and 10 hours, respectively, during alcohol dehydrogenase inhibitor therapy alone (1,2,10,14,19). Indications for hemodialysis include significant metabolic acidosis (arterial pH less than 7.30), renal insufficiency (serum creatinine greater than 1.2 mg/dL), as well as deterioration in these parameters or clinical status despite conventional treatment (1,2,8,9,18).

Traditionally, hemodialysis has also been recommended for a serum EG concentration greater than or equal to 50 mg/dL (5,8,9). This concentration, however, does not define toxicity, predict prolonged elimination, or correlate with patient outcome. Recent evidence suggests that patients who present before the development of metabolic acidosis and renal impairment can be effectively and safely managed with fomepizole monotherapy (no hemodialysis) regardless of initial EG concentration (1,2,18). For these patients, EG is excreted by the kidneys, with an approximate half-life of 18 hours (1,2,18,19). For patients who present with elevated serum creatinine, however, EG elimination half-life is prolonged to approximately 49 hours and hemodialysis is recommended (2,19). These patients will also likely require hemodialysis based on the presence of a significant metabolic acidosis. When initiated, hemodialysis should be continued until acid–base and metabolic abnormalities are corrected and serum EG concentrations are below 50 mg/dL (2,8,9).

During hemodialysis, the infusion rate of ethanol should be increased to 3 mL/kg/hour to compensate for increased clearance (1,8,9). Because fomepizole is also dialyzable, dosing frequency should be increased to every 4 hours during hemodialysis (2). If hemodialysis is unavailable or technically difficult (e.g., in infants), peritoneal dialysis can be used, although this method is considerably less effective than hemodialysis.

Pyridoxine, thiamine, and magnesium are cofactors in the degradation of EG to less toxic products (Fig. 274.1). Their administration may preferentially shunt metabolism of glyoxylic acid away from oxalic acid. Pyridoxine and thiamine should both be given intravenously in doses of 100 mg four times daily (8,9).

Recently, novel agents have been identified that could decrease nephrotoxicity associated with EG poisoning. Treatment of cultured human proximal renal tubular cells with ethylenediaminetetraacetic acid (EDTA) to solubilize calcium oxalate crystals or with aluminum citrate to prevent crystal precipitation significantly reduces cytotoxicity associated with calcium oxalate (13).

CRITICAL INTERVENTIONS

- Administer ethanol or fomepizole to patients with signs, symptoms, or laboratory evidence of EG poisoning
- Administer intravenous sodium bicarbonate to patients with acidemia
- Arrange hemodialysis for patients with methanol poisoning that is severe or refractory to other treatment

DISPOSITION

Patients with EG poisoning almost always require admission to an intensive care unit. Early consultation with a toxicologist or local poison center is encouraged to aid in patient care and to determine the availability of EG concentrations. The need for hemodialysis should always be anticipated, and the patient should be transferred if such treatment is unavailable.

COMMON PITFALLS

- ✔ Failure to consider EG as a cause of ethanol-like intoxication and increased anion gap metabolic acidosis
- ✔ Failure to appreciate that a normal osmolal or anion gap does not exclude the presence of potentially toxic amounts of EG
- ✔ Failure to observe and monitor all patients with known or suspected ethylene EG ingestion until an EG level can be obtained or until the time of expected toxicity has passed without incident
- ✔ Failure to appreciate the importance of fully correcting acidemia
- ✔ Failure to appreciate that ethanol and fomepizole are removed by hemodialysis and to adjust their dosing during this procedure accordingly

Acknowledgment

Thank you to previous edition chapter author Francis P. Renzi.

References

1. Barceloux DG, Krenzelok EP, Olsen K, et al. American Academy of Clinical Toxicology practice guidelines on the treatment of ethylene glycol poisoning. *J Toxicol Clin Toxicol* 1999;37:537–560.
2. Brent J, McMartin K, Phillips S, et al. Fomepizole for the treatment of ethylene glycol poisoning. *N Engl J Med* 1999;340:832–838.
3. Casavant MJ, Shah MN, Battels R. Does fluorescent urine indicated antifreeze ingestion by children? *Pediatrics* 2001;107:113–114.
4. Clay KL, Murphy RC. On the metabolic acidosis of ethylene glycol intoxication. *Toxicol Appl Pharmacol* 1977;39:39–49.
5. Eder AF, McGrath CM, Dowdy YG, et al. Ethylene glycol poisoning; toxicokinetic and analytic factors affecting laboratory diagnosis. *Clin Chem* 1998;44:168–177.
6. Grauer GF, Thrall MA, Henre BA, et al. Comparison of the effects of ethanol and 4-methylpyrazole on the pharmacokinetics and toxicity of ethylene glycol in the dog. *Toxicol Lett* 1987;35:307–314.
7. Hoffman RS, Smilkstein MJ, Howland MA, Goldfrank LR. Osmolal gaps revisited: normal values and limitations. *J Toxicol Clin Toxicol* 1993;31:81–93.
8. Jacobsen D, McMartin KE. Antidotes for methanol and ethylene glycol poisoning. *J Toxicol Clin Toxicol* 1997;35:127–143.
9. Jacobsen D, McMartin KE. Methanol and ethylene glycol poisonings: mechanisms of toxicity, clinical course, diagnosis and treatment. *Med Toxicol* 1986;1:309–334.
10. Jacobsen D, Ovrebo S, Ostborg J, et al. Glycolate causes the acidosis in ethylene glycol poisoning and is effectively removed by hemodialysis. *Acta Med Scand* 1984;216:409–416.
11. Karlson-Stiber C, Persson H. Ethylene glycol poisoning: experiences from an epidemic in Sweden. *J Toxicol Clin Toxicol* 1992;30:565–574.
12. McMartin KE, Cenac TA. Toxicity of ethylene glycol metabolites in normal human kidney cells. *Ann NY Acad Sci* 2000;919:315–317.
13. McMartin KE, Guo C. Inhibition of cellular toxicity of oxalate by EDTA and citrate. *J Toxicol Clin Toxicol* 2003;41:694–695.
14. Moreau CL, Kerns II W, Tomaszewski CA, et al. Glycolate kinetics and hemodialysis clearance in ethylene glycol poisoning. *J Toxicol Clin Toxicol* 1998;36:659–666.
15. Morgan TJ, Clark C, Clague A. Artifactual elevation of measured plasma L-lactate concentration in the presence of glycolate. *Crit Care Med* 1999;27:2177–2179.
16. Poldelski V, Johnson A, Wright S, et al. Ethylene glycol-mediated tubular injury: identification of critical metabolites and injury pathways. *Am J Kidney Dis* 2001;38:339–348.
17. Pons CA, Custer RP. Acute ethylene glycol poisoning: a clinicopathologic report of 18 fatal cases. *Am J Med Sci* 1946;211:544–552.
18. Porter WH, Rutter PW, Bush BA, et al. Ethylene glycol toxicity: the role of serum glycolic acid in hemodialysis. *J Tox Clin Toxicol* 2001;39:607–615.

19. Sivilotti M, Burns M, McMartin K, Brent J. Toxicokinetics of ethylene glycol during fomepizole therapy: implications for management. *Ann Emerg Med* 2000;36:114–125.
20. Stokes JB, Aueron F. Prevention of organ damage in massive ethylene glycol ingestion. *JAMA* 1980;243:2065–2066.
21. Sykowski P. Ethylene glycol toxicity. *Am J Ophthalmol* 1951;34:1599.
22. Wallace KL, Suchard JR, Curry SC, Reagan C. Diagnostic use of physicians' detection of urine fluorescence in a simulated ingestion of sodium fluorescein-containing antifreeze. *Ann Emerg Med* 2001;38:49–54.
23. Watson WW, Litovitz TL, Rodgers GC, et al. 2002 annual report of the American Association of Poison Control Centers Toxic Exposure Surveillance System. *Am J Emerg Med* 2003;21:353–421.
24. Widman C. A few cases of ethylene glycol intoxication. *Acta Med Scand* 1946;126:294–306.
25. Winter ML, Ellis MD, Snodgrass WR. Urine fluorescence using a Wood's lamp to detect the antifreeze additive fluorescein: a qualitative adjunctive test in suspected ethylene glycol ingestions. *Ann Emerg Med* 1990;19:663–667.

CHAPTER 275
Methanol

Dag Jacobsen

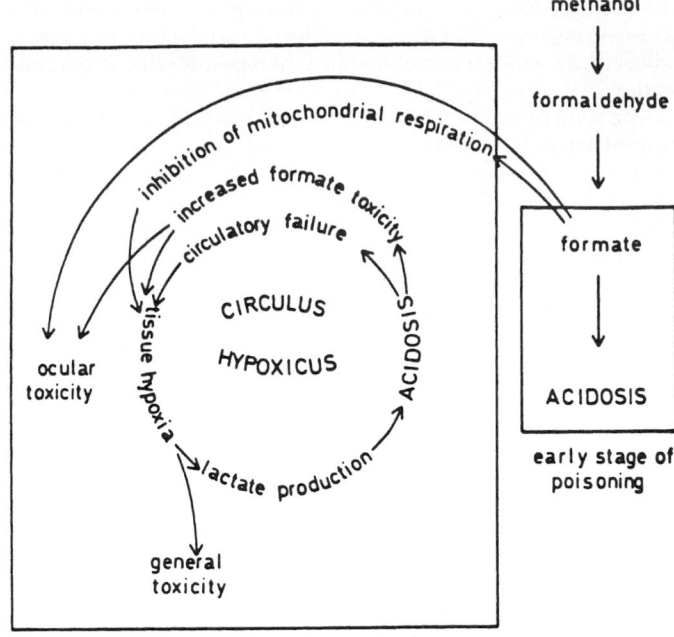

Figure 275.1.   The "circulus hypoxicus" resulting from methanol ingestion.

Methanol (methyl alcohol, "colonial spirit," "wood alcohol," "solvent alcohol") is a colorless, volatile, highly flammable liquid with a density of 0.81 g/mL and a weak smell that resembles that of ethanol. Methanol is widely used industrially as a solvent and in the production of formaldehyde and methylated compounds. It is found in commercial products such as gasoline, antifreeze, gasohol, windshield washer fluid, copy machine fluid, canned heat (Sterno), paint, shellac, and solvents for removing wood finishes. Poisoning may occur after the accidental or intentional ingestion of such products. Although most cases are isolated, epidemics of poisoning may occur when methanol is mistakenly substituted for ethanol by, for instance, alcoholics, or when methanol contaminates other alcoholic beverages, such as wine or moonshine whisky.

Methanol is rapidly absorbed after ingestion and distributes in the total body water compartment (about 0.6 L/kg). It is metabolized first to formaldehyde and then to formic acid, which is responsible for the toxic effects in methanol intoxication (10). The metabolism of formate depends on the folate pool (10). Primates have a small folate reserve and are the only species that accumulate formate and, thus, suffer from methanol toxicity (10). The metabolism of methanol by alcohol dehydrogenase, which accounts for 90% of its elimination, is zero order, with a rate of 8.5 mg/dL/hour in one case (11). Small amounts are excreted in expired air and urine.

In the early stages of poisoning, toxicity is caused by the central nervous system (CNS) depressant effect of methanol and to metabolic acidosis caused by the accumulation of formic acid (10). In late stages, when more formate is accumulated, the toxicity is mainly caused by the histotoxic effects of formate as it inhibits the mitochondrial respiration within the cell. This leads to lactate production and worsening acidosis, as well as increasing the toxicity of formate as it becomes more protonated and thereby penetrates the blood–brain barrier more easily (5). Thus, a vicious *circulus hypoxicus* is initiated (Fig. 275.1) (8). Why the eye, and later the basal ganglia, are the primary targets for methanol's toxic effects is unknown (10,14,15,18,20). The lethal dose of methanol is variably given as 30 to 240 mL, with 1 g/kg

(1g = 1.2 mL) as the best estimate (10,19). The minimum dose that can cause permanent visual defects is unknown.

Ethanol and fomepizole bind to alcohol dehydrogenase with a higher affinity than does methanol, and hence block the production of toxic metabolites. Ethanol is metabolized by alcohol dehydrogenase, but fomepizole is not. When these antidotes are present, the elimination half-life of methanol increases to 30 to 60 hours (6,10).

CLINICAL PRESENTATION

Usually 6 to 24 hours elapse from the time of ingestion to the occurrence of symptoms. It takes this much time for sufficient amounts of formic acid to be produced by methanol metabolism. This latent period may be longer if ethanol is coingested because ethanol competitively inhibits methanol metabolism by alcohol dehydrogenase. A latent period up to 90 hours has been reported when ethanol is coingested (9).

Methanol itself has few direct effects. Mild ethanol-like CNS depression has been reported (10). Methanol is about half as potent than ethanol in this regard. With concentrated methanol solutions, nausea, vomiting, and abdominal pain may develop shortly after ingestion. During the early stages of poisoning, the diagnosis is confirmed by measuring the serum methanol level but levels are often not readily available or rapidly obtainable. Because of its low molecular weight (32 g/mol), high concentrations of methanol (and other low-molecular-weight solutes, see Chapter 271, "Approach to the Poisoned Patient") increase the serum osmolality. The diagnosis may, therefore, be suggested by an increased osmolal gap, the difference between the measured osmolality and the calculated osmolality (2 × sodium [mEq/L]+ blood urea nitrogen [mg/dL]/3 + glucose [mg/dL]/18). The "normal" range for the osmolal gap is 5 ± 7 mOsm/kg H$_2$O (mean ± SD) (1). An osmolal gap above 19 indicates exogenous osmoles of some kind (10). The serum methanol level can be estimated (in mg/dL) by multiplying the excess osmolal gap by 2.6, the amount of methanol that increases the osmolality by 1 mOsm/kg H$_2$O. In early stages, when the highest methanol levels and osmolal gap are present, significant metabolic acidosis is absent as metabolism to formate is just beginning.

Clinical features during the intermediate stage of poisoning include anorexia, headache, nausea, and vomiting, accompanied or followed by increasing hyperventilation as a result of progressive increased anion gap metabolic acidosis (10,18,19). The "normal" range for the anion gap ($[Na + K] - [Cl + HCO_3]$) is 13 ± 4 mEq/L (mean $\pm$ SD) (1). Visual symptoms (blurred vision, decreased acuity, halo vision, tunnel vision, photophobia, and "snowfields") may precede or accompany the aforementioned symptoms. Objective signs such as dilated pupils that are partially reactive or nonreactive to light and funduscopy showing optic disk hyperemia with blurring of the margins occur later. During this stage, the diagnosis is confirmed by detecting methanol or formate in the serum; the osmolal gap may or may not be elevated. Occasionally, patients may present with an acute abdomen, probably because of acute pancreatitis (10,11).

Without treatment, coma and respiratory and circulatory failure may ensue. A few patients may also develop methemoglobinemia with cyanosis, probably because of an interaction between formate and the ferric part of hemoglobin. In the late stages of methanol poisoning, when most or all methanol is metabolized to formate, the anion gap is elevated but the osmolal gap is normal, and methanol may or may not be detectable. When methanol is undetectable, measuring the serum formate level is the only way to confirm the diagnosis. Toxic effects on basal ganglia do not lead to immediately detectable signs and symptoms because they are concealed by pronounced CNS depression. Survivors may later manifest a Parkinson-like syndrome with necrosis in the basal ganglia seen on cerebral computed tomography (CT) or magnetic resonance imaging (MRI) (12,20).

DIFFERENTIAL DIAGNOSIS

Other causes of metabolic acidosis and increased serum osmolality should be considered in the differential diagnosis (Fig. 275.2), particularly when the history unclear and quantitative methanol and formate levels are not readily available. Increased anion and osmolal gaps also occur in ethylene glycol poisoning. Differentiating the two may be difficult, but the treatments are essentially the same. Visual complaints suggest methanol poisoning, whereas hypocalcemia, seizures, and urine oxalate crystals indicate ethylene glycol poisoning (10).

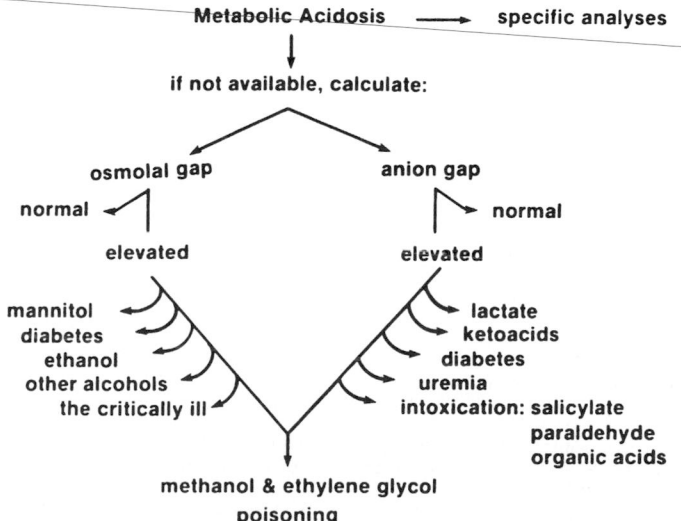

Figure 275.2.   Causes of an increased anion and osmolal gap.

EMERGENCY DEPARTMENT EVALUATION

The history should include the amount, concentration, and time of methanol ingestion; the nature and onset of symptoms; and whether ethanol was co-ingested. Patients should be questioned carefully about the presence or absence of visual complaints, gastrointestinal (GI) symptoms, and a feeling of intoxication. The physical examination should focus on vital signs (especially respiratory rate) and the neurologic, visual, and cardiopulmonary status. Visual acuity and funduscopic examinations should be documented. Laboratory evaluation should include arterial blood gas analysis; complete blood count; measurement of electrolytes, blood urea nitrogen, creatinine, glucose, and amylase; urinalysis; and quantitative serum methanol or formic acid level. A chest radiograph and an electrocardiogram are obtained if clinical toxicity is pronounced.

If the diagnosis is based on the osmolal and anion gaps, osmometry must be performed by the freezing-point depression technique and not by the vapor pressure technique, as the latter does not detect the increased osmolality caused by volatile alcohols. A computed tomographic scan or MRI of the brain should be performed on patients with coma or persistent neurologic dysfunction.

EMERGENCY DEPARTMENT MANAGEMENT

General treatment measures include intensive supportive care and GI decontamination. If the patient is seen soon after ingestion (within 2 hours) immediate gastric aspiration, preferably with a nasogastric tube, is recommended. Emesis induction and activated charcoal alone are probably of limited value because of slow onset and limited binding, respectively.

Specific treatment of methanol poisoning includes intravenous (i.v.) sodium bicarbonate for metabolic acidosis, antidotal therapy with ethanol or fomepizole, to inhibit methanol metabolism to formate, and hemodialysis to remove methanol and formate. Folinic acid (leucovorin), 1 mg/kg i.v. up to 50 mg every 4 hours, may be of value in increasing the metabolism of formate (17). If folinic acid is unavailable, folic acid, in the same dose, can be used.

Metabolic acidosis should be aggressively treated by infusing enough sodium bicarbonate ($NaHCO_3$) to fully correct acidemia: $NaHCO_3$ dose $= 0.7 \times$ kg $\times (24 - $ actual $[HCO_3^-])$, where 0.7 is the volume of distribution of bicarbonate in acidemia, 24 is the desired $[HCO_3^-]$, and kg is the lean body weight. $NaHCO_3$ should be given in 1 mEq/kg increments. As much as 400 to 600 mEq of $NaHCO_3$ may be required during the first few hours. It is important to realize that bicarbonate treatment also decreases the amount of undissociated formic acid, resulting in less access of formate to the CNS, and thereby less toxicity (5,10). Hence, metabolic acidosis resulting from methanol poisoning, in contrast to other causes of metabolic acidosis, should *always* be treated with bicarbonate. Frequent re-assessment of acid–base, clinical, and electrolyte status is necessary during and after such therapy.

Alkali treatment must be accompanied by administration of ethanol or fomepizole; otherwise, the acidosis becomes bicarbonate-resistant, as more formic acid will be produced from the metabolism of methanol. If a methanol poisoning is suspected and a level cannot readily be obtained, ethanol or fomepizole therapy should be started in any patient with an increased osmolal gap, acidosis, symptoms, or a potentially toxic ingestion by history. Antidotal treatment can be discontinued when the methanol level drops below 20 mg/dL, provided that the acid–base status is normal and there are no complications.

Most authors recommend a therapeutic blood ethanol level of at least 100 mg/dL. However, the amount of ethanol necessary to block methanol metabolism depends on the concomitant methanol level because there is a dynamic competition for the enzyme alcohol dehydrogenase in the liver. If the blood methanol level is known, the molar–ethanol concentrations should be at least one fourth of the molar–methanol concentration (10,13).

A blood ethanol level of 100 mg/dL may be achieved by giving a bolus dose of 0.6 mg/kg, followed by 66 to 154 mg/kg/hour intravenously or orally, with the higher maintenance dose for heavy drinkers. Mixing 50 mL of absolute ethanol with 500 mL isotonic glucose yields a 10% solution if a 10% ethanol solution for intravenous use is unavailable. With this solution, a bolus of 10 mL/kg (over 0.5 hour), followed by 1.5 mL/kg/hour, will produce the desired ethanol concentration. The maintenance infusion should be increased or decreased according to frequently measured ethanol levels. Monitoring the blood–ethanol level is important, especially during hemodialysis, as this procedure also removes ethanol. As a rule of thumb, the maintenance dose of ethanol should be doubled during hemodialysis. If not, methanol metabolism can resume when the ethanol level drops, resulting in worsening toxicity despite hemodialysis.

Fomepizole (4-methylpyrazole; Antizol) can be used instead of ethanol (3,4,7,16). A loading dose of 15 mg/kg i.v. is followed by doses of 10 mg/kg i.v. every 12 hours thereafter. If hemodialysis is begun, fomepizole dosing frequency should be increased to every 4 hours. The dosing of fomepizole and therapeutic considerations are the same as for ethylene glycol (see Chapter 274, "Ethylene Glycol"). The author favors fomepizole over ethanol (2). However, it is much more expensive than ethanol. If diagnosis is uncertain (methanol level not readily available), the osmolal gap is only mildly elevated (less than 30 to 40 mOsm/kg), and visual disturbances are absent, ethanol may be preferable, since the methanol level will likely be low and prolonged ethanol therapy, which requires labor intensive monitoring and frequent dosage adjustments, will not likely be necessary.

Hemodialysis effectively removes methanol and formate and also counteracts metabolic acidosis (6,10). The only absolute indication for hemodialysis is visual impairment of any degree in a patient with metabolic acidosis or a detectable methanol level. Other indications include severe acidemia (particularly if unresponsive to bicarbonate and ethanol therapy), a blood methanol level above 50 mg/dL (because of the very slow elimination of methanol during antidotal therapy), and ingestion of more than 1 g/kg of methanol. Because of the advent of fomepizole use for methanol poisoning, the situation is somewhat different. In most patients (i.e., those with no visual disturbances), dialysis is now only indicated to shorten the duration of fomepizole treatment. In the severe poisoning, however, with pronounced acidemia (base deficit greater than 20 to 25 mEq) and visual disturbances, hemodialysis should be performed to remove formate as well as methanol. Hemodialysis should be continued until the blood methanol level is below 20 mg/dL and acidemia is corrected. If methanol analyses are unavailable, hemodialysis should be continued for at least 8 hours or until the osmolal gap is normal (possible osmolal contribution from ethanol must be subtracted). Peritoneal dialysis may also remove methanol but not as effectively as hemodialysis. Hemoperfusion is ineffective.

CRITICAL INTERVENTIONS

- Administer ethanol or fomepizole to patients with signs, symptoms, or laboratory evidence of methanol poisoning
- Administer intravenous sodium bicarbonate to patients with acidemia
- Arrange hemodialysis for patients with methanol poisoning that is severe or refractory to other treatment

DISPOSITION

Consultation with a poison center or toxicologist is strongly recommended if the physician is unfamiliar with the management of methanol poisoning. In addition, information on where to obtain methanol or formate levels may be provided. When the diagnosis of methanol poisoning is made or suspected, a nephrologist should be consulted, as many patients ultimately require hemodialysis, especially when admitted in a late stage. If hemodialysis is unavailable, the patient who needs it, or will probably need it, should be transferred to a facility with this capability. Bicarbonate and antidotal therapy (if available) should be given prior to and during transport.

If a methanol level is immediately unavailable, asymptomatic patients with known or suspected methanol ingestion and a normal anion and osmolar gap should be observed or admitted for to the hospital and have clinical and acid–base reevaluation every 4 hours until the methanol level becomes known. All patients with signs, symptoms, or laboratory evidence of methanol intoxication should be admitted, usually to an intensive care unit because of the frequency of monitoring required. They should also have an initial and followup examination by an ophthalmologist.

COMMON PITFALLS

✔ Failure to consider methanol poisoning in the differential diagnosis of metabolic acidosis of unknown origin
✔ Failure to consider the possibility of multiple victims when the source of methanol is unknown or is known to be contaminated ethanol
✔ Failure to appreciate that the absence of early symptoms and the presence of normal anion and osmolal gaps do not exclude a potentially toxic methanol level
✔ Failure to observe and monitor all patients with known or suspected methanol ingestion until a methanol level can be obtained or until the time of expected toxicity has passed without incident
✔ Failure to appreciate the importance of fully correcting acidemia
✔ Failure to appreciate that ethanol and fomepizole are removed by hemodialysis and to adjust their dosing during this procedure accordingly
✔ Failure to have the visual function of patients with poisoning formally assessed by an ophthalmologist

References

1. Aabakken L, Johansen KS, Rydningen EB, et al. Osmolal and anion gaps in patients admitted to an emergency medical department. *Hum Exp Toxicol* 1994;13:131.
2. Barceloux DG, Bond GR, Krenzelok EP, et al. American Academy of Clinical Toxicology practice guidelines on the treatment of methanol poisoning. *J Toxicol Clin Toxicol* 2002;40:415.
3. Brent J, McMartin KE, Phillips S, et al. Fomepizole for the treatment of methanol poisoning. *N Engl J Med* 2001;344:424.
4. Burns MJ, Graudins A, Aaron CK, et al. Treatment of methanol poisoning with intravenous 4-methylpyrazole. *Ann Emerg Med* 1997;30:829.
5. Herken W, Rietbrock N, Henschler D. Zum mechanismus der Methanol-Vergiftung. Toxisches Agens und Einfluss der Sure-Basenstatus auf die Giftwirkung. *Arch Toxicol* 1969;24:214.
6. Hovda KE, Froyshov S, Urdal P, Jacobsen. P, Severe methanol poisoning treated with fomepizole and hemodialysis. *J Toxicol Clin Toxicol* 2003;41:473.
7. Jacobsen D. New treatment for ethylene glycol poisoning. *N Engl J Med* 1999;340:879.
8. Jacobsen D. *Studies in methanol and ethylene glycol poisonings: acidosis—kinetics—management.* Thesis, University of Oslo, 1985.
9. Jacobsen D, Jansen H, Wiik-Larsen E, et al. Studies on methanol poisoning. *Acta Med Scand* 1982;212:5.
10. Jacobsen D, McMartin KE. Methanol and ethylene glycol poisonings: mechanism of toxicity, clinical course, diagnosis and treatment. *Med Toxicol* 1986;1:309.
11. Jacobsen D, Webb R, Collins TD, et al. Methanol and formate kinetics in late diagnosed methanol intoxication. *Med Toxicol* 1988;3:418.

12. Kuteifan K, Oesterele H, Tajahmady T, et al. Necrosis and haemorrhage of the putamen in methanol poisoning shown on MRI. *Neuroradiology* 1998;40:158.
13. Makar AB, Tephly TR, Mannering GJ. Methanol metabolism in the monkey. *Mol Pharmacol* 1968;4:471.
14. Martinasevic MK, Green MD, Baron J, et al. Folate and 10-formyltetra-hydrofolate dehydrogenase in human and rat retina: relation to methanol toxicity. *Toxicol Appl Pharmacol* 1996;141:373.
15. McKellar MJ, Hidajat RR, Elder MJ. Acute ocular methanol toxicity: clinical and electrophysiological features. *Aust N Z J Ophthalmol* 1997;25:225.
16. Megarbane B, Borron SW, Trout H, et al. Treatment with acute methanol poisoning with fomepizole. *Int Care Med* 2001;27:1370.
17. Osterloh JD, Pond SM, Grady S, et al. Serum formate concentrations in methanol intoxication as criterion for hemodialysis. *Ann Intern Med* 1986;104:200.
18. Roe O. The metabolism and toxicity of methanol. *Pharmacol Rev* 1955;7:399.
19. Roe O. Species differences in methanol poisonings. *CRC Crit Rev Toxicol* 1982;10:275.
20. Server A, Hovda KE, Nakstad PH, et al. Conventional and diffusion-weighted MRI in the evaluation of methanol poisoning. *Acta Radiologica* 2003;44:691.

CHAPTER 276
Isopropanol, Acetone, and Other Glycols

Jeffrey R. Suchard

Although methanol (Chapter 275, "Methanol") and ethylene glycol (Chapter 274, "Ethylene Glycol") are potentially more dangerous, exposure to other alcohols and closely related chemicals occurs much more frequently. In 2001, more than 30,000 exposures to isopropanol and over 4,000 exposures to acetone were reported to U.S. poison centers. More than 5,000 of these patients were evaluated in healthcare facilities, without any fatalities. In contrast, methanol and ethylene glycol were involved in just over 8,000 exposures, with 49 reported deaths (10).

Isopropanol (2-propanol, isopropyl alcohol) is used as a disinfectant, solvent, cleaner, and de-icing agent. Rubbing alcohol is the most common household source, typically containing 70% isopropanol by volume. Despite a slightly bitter taste and distinctive, pungent smell, isopropanol is the most commonly ingested nonbeverage alcohol. Other routes of exposure include inhalation and transdermal absorption, particularly among small children (22,23). Isopropanol is rapidly absorbed from the stomach, and peak serum levels can be measured within 30 minutes of ingestion (9,15). Clinical effects are evident within 0.5 to 1.5 hours (19). Isopropanol is a CNS depressant with a potency about twice that of ethanol in rats (24).

The primary route of isopropanol clearance is through metabolism by alcohol dehydrogenase (ADH) to acetone (Fig. 276.1). Ketonemia and ketonuria caused by the presence of acetone occurs rapidly after exposure to isopropanol (9,22).

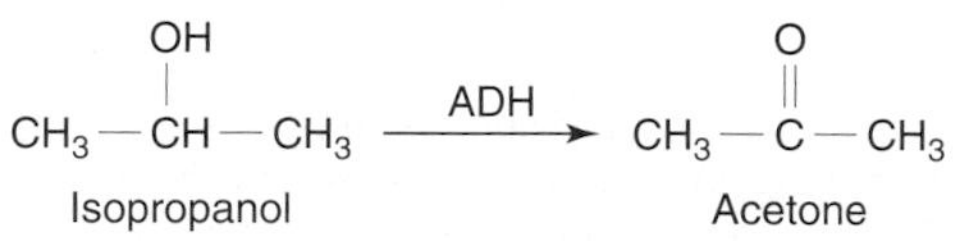

Figure 276.1. Isopropanol metabolized to acetone.

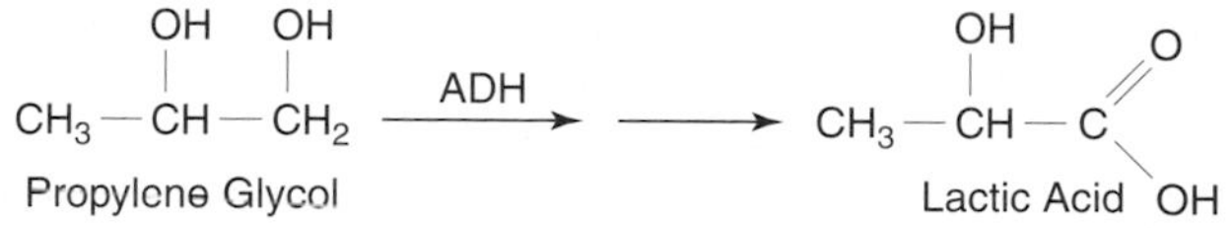

Figure 276.2. Propylene glycol metabolized to lactic acid.

Unlike methanol and ethylene glycol, no organic acid metabolites are produced and an elevated anion-gap metabolic acidosis is not expected. If acidosis is present, it is likely a result of isopropanol-induced hypotension, as may occur with severe toxicity, and consequent accumulation of lactate (22). Isopropanol clearance follows first-order elimination kinetics. The reported serum half-life varies, ranging from 2.5 to 5.8 hours (12,15,16,23) and even up to 9.6 hours in neonates (22). The intoxicating effects of isopropanol tend to be longer lasting than ethanol because of isopropanol's slower metabolism and the subsequent accumulation of acetone, which has similar CNS depressant effects and an even longer elimination phase (18).

Acetone (2-propanone, dimethyl ketone), a metabolite of isopropanol (6,7), is also used as a solvent in industry and the home; one of the most common methods of domestic acetone exposure is ingestion of fingernail polish remover (3). Acetone is rapidly absorbed, and then is mainly excreted unchanged by the renal and pulmonary routes (7). Reports of acetone's elimination half-life vary widely in the literature (6), but it is clearly more prolonged than that of isopropanol, and probably in the range of 17 to 31 hours (3,6,7). Propylene glycol (1,2-propanediol, PG) is a solvent and CNS depressant found in many foods, cosmetics, and drugs. Roughly 50% of PG is excreted unchanged into the urine, and the remainder is metabolized via ADH and aldehyde dehydrogenase (AldDH) into lactic acid (Fig. 276.2).

Diethylene glycol (DG), another solvent and CNS depressant, is composed of two ethylene glycol molecules connected by an ether bond (Fig. 276.3). Although the ether bond is not metabolized in humans to release free ethylene glycol, diethylene glycol poisoning produces a clinical syndrome similar to ethylene glycol. Epidemics of renal failure have occurred when DG has been used as a drug excipient (13).

Glycol ethers are compounds that consist of a glycol, usually ethylene glycol, is connected to an alkyl group by an ether bond. Ethylene glycol butyl ether (2-butoxyethanol), a typical glycol ether, is shown in Figure 276.3. Glycol ethers are used as industrial solvents, as glass and surface cleaners, and in automobile brake fluid. Acute ingestions of glycol ethers cause a clinical syndrome similar to ethylene glycol. Poisoning is caused by metabolism by ADH and AldDH, resulting in the formation of toxic organic acid metabolites. Because the molecular weights of glycol ethers are higher than that of the other alcohols, toxic levels of glycol ethers do not significantly elevate the osmolal gap (4).

CLINICAL PRESENTATION

Isopropanol poisoning is characterized by CNS depression, ketosis, an elevated osmolal gap without metabolic acidosis, and gastrointestinal effects. The two most common scenarios for

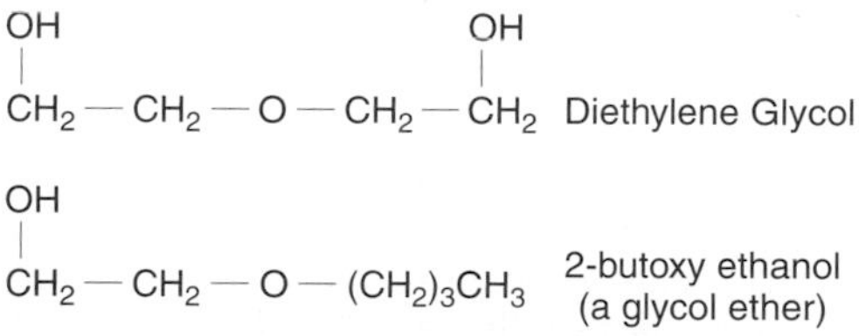

Figure 276.3. Other glycols.

isopropanol poisoning are chronic alcoholics seeking an alternate intoxicant when deprived of ethanol (5,21), and ingestions by children (12,16,19). It is difficult to correlate the degree of intoxication with serum isopropanol levels (8), probably because of cross-tolerance to isopropanol in alcoholics or to intoxicant naiveté among children. Additionally complicating the issue is the ubiquitous presence of acetone, an isopropanol metabolite that is also a CNS intoxicant.

Signs and symptoms of isopropanol and acetone intoxication are very similar to that from ethanol, with a few exceptions. The disinhibited phase that may be seen with early ethanol intoxication has not been reported with isopropanol, but the CNS depressant effects are otherwise the same, ranging from mild inebriation, to ataxia, dysarthria, lethargy, and coma, depending on the amount ingested. Patients ingesting isopropanol are often found to have higher levels of acetone than isopropanol by the time of presentation (5,12). Some cases suggest that acetone causes most of the CNS depressant effects seen in isopropanol ingestion (16), but this conclusion is not consistent in all reports. The duration of isopropanol intoxication is longer than occurs with ethanol because of the slower metabolism and the fact that the acetone metabolite is itself a CNS depressant (18).

Gastrointestinal effects are common and include nausea, vomiting, abdominal pain, and hemorrhagic gastritis. Vomiting is the most common symptom of any type seen among ninety-one children ingesting isopropanol, and occurred among all patients in this series demonstrating any CNS effects (19).

Acetone produces a characteristic fruity or ethereal odor to the breath. Serum acetone levels following ingestion of isopropanol or acetone often greatly exceed those found in diabetic ketoacidosis, so this olfactory clue may be even more obvious than usual. The presence of ketonemia and ketonuria occur rapidly after isopropanol or acetone poisoning (9). Vapor exposures to acetone and isopropanol are irritating to the mucous membranes and may produce a burning sensation, tearing, coughing, and erythema to exposed areas.

Most reported cases of PG toxicity occur iatrogenically among hospitalized patients, particularly in association with the use of high doses of intravenous benzodiazepines (17,20,25). PG poisoning can also result from acute ingestion of PG-containing household products such as cosmetics and automotive antifreezes (sold as safer alternatives to ethylene glycol). Signs and symptoms include CNS depression, hyperosmolality, lactic acidosis, and renal insufficiency.

Diethylene glycol and glycol ether poisoning may result in CNS depression, metabolic acidosis, renal failure, hepatitis, and pancreatitis. Glycol ethers can also cause hemolysis, hypotension, hypoglycemia, hematuria, and acute respiratory distress syndrome (ARDS) (4,11,14).

DIFFERENTIAL DIAGNOSIS

The differential diagnosis of isopropanol and acetone exposure obviously includes any of the other CNS depressants, and other medical or surgical conditions that alter mental status, including intracranial trauma, CNS infection or tumors, hypoglycemia and other severe metabolic derangements.

The primary exogenous substances in the differential diagnosis of isopropanol or acetone toxicity are other alcohols. Patients ingesting any of the short-chain alcohols typically present with a similar clinical picture of CNS depression and an elevated osmolal gap. Without quantitative toxicologic evaluation, differentiating the early stages of intoxication with any of these agents may be difficult. Fortunately, the most commonly ingested alcohol is ethanol, which can be rapidly quantified by most clinical laboratories. Patients presenting later in their clinical course might be differentiated by the presence of an anion-gap metabolic acidosis

(methanol and ethylene glycol), renal insufficiency (ethylene glycol), visual symptoms (methanol), hyperlactatemia (propylene glycol), and the smell of acetone on the breath (isopropyl alcohol or acetone). Patients who present with ethanol-like CNS effects, an elevated osmolal gap, a normal anion gap, and who smell like acetone may presumptively be diagnosed with isopropanol or acetone toxicity pending laboratory confirmation. Concurrent ingestion of isopropanol and ethanol or another "toxic alcohol" is not uncommon (8,15,21).

Ketones from isopropanol or acetone ingestion may falsely elevate measurements of serum creatinine (5), and an elevated creatinine with a normal BUN suggests this diagnosis. Renal insufficiency from ethylene glycol should occur in conjunction with an increased BUN and a significant anion-gap metabolic acidosis. Other causes of ketosis to consider include diabetic ketoacidosis (DKA) and alcoholic ketoacidosis (AKA), both of which also elevate the osmolal gap, and starvation ketosis. If measured, elevated serum acetone levels will be found in patients with ketoacidosis. Because of the high NADH–NAD ratio seen with DKA, acetone can be reduced to isopropanol, falsely suggesting a toxic ingestion (1). The quantitative acetone and isopropanol levels seen in such cases, however, are often far lower (usually less than 50 mg/dL) than seen with isopropanol ingestion and are not associated with significant hyperglycemia. Theoretically, patients with AKA may similarly test positive for isopropanol and acetone in the absence of a toxic ingestion.

Although fingernail-care product ingestion is a common and usually benign source of acetone exposure, care should be taken to confirm the history and product ingredients in such cases. The ingestion of artificial nail remover (as opposed to nail polish remover) containing acetonitrile, rather than acetone, has resulted in fatal cyanide toxicity.

Propylene glycol–induced lactic acidosis, especially among already hospitalized patients, may be confused with many other potential causes of lactic acidosis, including hypoxia, hypotension, and sepsis. A thorough medical evaluation is necessary before ascribing hyperlactatemia solely to PG toxicity.

The close chemical structural relationship between ethanol, isopropanol, and acetone can cause analytical interference when employing breath ethanol tests (6) and enzymatic ethanol assays using ADH (21). Even gas chromatography, the preferred testing method for isopropanol and acetone, is not completely foolproof, as propylene glycol can be mistaken for ethylene glycol (2).

EMERGENCY DEPARTMENT EVALUATION

The history should include identification of the substance(s) involved, concentration, route(s) of exposure, estimated volume ingested, and time elapsed since exposure. Any history of potential co-ingestants or trauma should be elicited. Early definitive product identification can help rule out potential disasters, such as acetonitrile-containing nail-care products in children or methanol and ethylene glycol ingestion by chronic alcoholics deprived of ethanol. Physical examination should initially address the patient's mental status, airway control, and vital signs. Concomitant trauma should be excluded.

If signs and symptoms of intoxication are present, laboratory tests should include a quantitative level of the substance involved (if available), routine serum chemistries (to rule out anion gap metabolic acidosis), a rapid serum glucose determination (to rule-out hypoglycemia as the cause of any altered mental status), and an ethanol level. Arterial blood gas analysis and measurement of serum and urinary ketones may also be helpful, especially in severe cases or where the diagnosis is not clear by history.

Determination of the serum osmolal gap (OG) can be helpful as a screening tool for detecting the presence of exogenous low-molecular-weight alcohols or glycols. A serum osmolality measured by freezing-point depression exceeding the calculated osmolality ($2[Na] + [BUN]/2.8 + [Glucose]/18 + [Ethanol]/4.2$) suggests the presence of isopropanol, acetone, methanol, ethylene glycol, or propylene glycol. If the identity of the substance is known, its serum concentration in mg/dL can be roughly estimated by multiplying the OG by the substance's molecular weight and dividing by ten. The molecular weight of isopropanol is 60 g/mol, acetone is 58 g/mol, and propylene glycol is 76 g/mol. For example, if a patient with an acetone ingestion has an OG of 20, the estimated serum acetone concentration is $(20 \times 58)/10 = 116$ mg/dL.

EMERGENCY DEPARTMENT MANAGEMENT

Treatment of isopropanol or acetone toxicity is primarily supportive, with most patients only requiring observation. Patients presenting early after exposure should be observed for clinical deterioration, as signs of toxicity should manifest within the first few hours of exposure. Absorption occurs rapidly, so gastrointestinal decontamination is not generally indicated. Furthermore, activated charcoal does not bind these toxins well, unless given in very large doses. Patients with CNS depression should be endotracheally intubated if not adequately protecting their airway. Hypotension, if present, should be treated with intravenous saline and, if necessary, vasopressor agents.

Hemodialysis can greatly enhance isopropanol and acetone elimination (18). Hypotension refractory to treatment with intravenous saline is the primary indication for hemodialysis. Because acetone is not substantively more toxic than isopropanol, treatment with ethanol or fomepizole to inhibit ADH is not recommended. Patients with abdominal pain or heme-positive emesis may have a hemorrhagic gastritis, and should be evaluated for gastrointestinal bleeding and anemia.

The treatment of severe toxicity from diethylene glycol, propylene glycol, or glycol ethers should include ethanol or fomepizole, and hemodialysis, with similar doses and protocols as used with methanol (Chapter 275, "Methanol") or ethylene glycol (Chapter 274, "Ethylene Glycol") toxicity (4,11,14,17,20).

CRITICAL INTERVENTIONS

- Evaluate and support the airway and respiratory function in patients with CNS depression
- Administer intravenous fluids and pressors for hypotension
- Consult a poison center or toxicologist and a nephrologist regarding hemodialysis for patients with profound CNS depression, refractory hypotension, metabolic acidosis, or renal failure
- Administer ethanol or fomepizole to patients with severe diethylene glycol, propylene glycol, and glycol ether poisoning

DISPOSITION

Patients with minor exposures to isopropanol or acetone, as often occurs with pediatric nonintentional ingestions, will need only a few hours of observation to assure they do not develop CNS depression. Patients who remain or become asymptomatic after a 4 to 6 hour observation period and have no comorbid conditions may be discharged. Patients with altered mental status, hypotension, metabolic disturbances, or organ toxicity should be admitted to an intensive care unit; these patients may also benefit from hemodialysis, so consultation with a poison center, toxicologist, and nephrologist should also be obtained.

COMMON PITFALLS

✔ Assuming that isopropanol and acetone exposures are benign because they are not metabolized into organic acids
✔ Assuming that toxicity has peaked by the time the patient is examined and failure to monitor and reevaluate both asymptomatic and intoxicated patients
✔ Failure to appreciate that the serum osmolality is useful for estimating acetone, isopropanol, and propylene glycol concentrations only if it is measured by the freezing-point depression method
✔ Failure to appreciate that acetone causes falsely elevated serum creatinine levels, and diagnosing renal failure when the BUN is normal
✔ Failure to appreciate that diethylene glycol, propylene glycol, and glycol ethers can cause toxicity similar to that from ethylene glycol

Acknowledgment

Susan S. Fish was the author of a similar chapter in the previous edition.

References

1. Bailey DN. Detection of isopropanol in acetonemic patients not exposed to isopropanol. *J Toxicol Clin Toxicol* 1990;28:459–466.
2. DeWitt C, Pamer R, Phillips S, Dart RC. False positive ethylene glycol level [abstract]. *J Toxicol Clin Toxicol* 2003;41:736.
3. Gamis AS, Wasserman GS. Acute acetone intoxication in a pediatric patient. *Pediatr Emerg Care* 1988;4:24–26.
4. Gualtieri JF, DeBoer L, Harris CR, Corley R. Repeated ingestion of 2-butoxyethanol: Case report and literature review. *J Toxicol Clin Toxicol* 2003;41:57–62.
5. Hawley PC, Falko JM. "Pseudo" renal failure after isopropyl alcohol intoxication. *South Med J* 1982;75:630–631.
6. Jones AW. Driving under the influence of acetone. *J Toxicol Clin Toxicol* 1997;35:419–421.
7. Jones AW. Elimination half-life of acetone in humans: Case reports and review of the literature. *J Anal Toxicol* 2000;24:8–10.
8. Kelner M, Bailey DN. Isopropanol ingestion: Interpretation of blood concentrations and clinical findings. *J Toxicol Clin Toxicol* 1983;20:497–507.
9. Lacouture PG, Heldreth DD, Shannon M, Lovejoy FH. The generation of acetonemia/acetonuria following ingestion of a subtoxic dose of isopropyl alcohol. *Am J Emerg Med* 1989;7:38–40.
10. Litowitz TL, Klein-Schwartz W, Rodgers GC, et al. 2001 Annual report of the American Association of Poison Control Centers Toxic Exposure Surveillance System. *Am J Emerg Med* 2002;20:391–452.
11. McKinney PE, Palmer RB, Blackwell W, Benson BE. Butoxyethanol ingestion with prolonged hyperchloremic metabolic acidosis treated with ethanol therapy. *J Toxicol Clin Toxicol* 2000;38:787–793.
12. Mydler TT, Wasserman GS, Watson WA, Knapp JF. Two-week-old infant with isopropanol intoxication. *Pediatr Emerg Care* 1993;9:146–148.
13. O'Brien KL, Selanikio JD, Hecdivert C, et al. Epidemic of pediatric deaths from acute renal failure caused by diethylene glycol poisoning. *JAMA* 1998;279:1175–1180.
14. Osterhoudt KC. Fomepizole therapy for pediatric butoxyethanol intoxication. *J Toxicol Clin Toxicol* 2002;40:929–930.
15. Pappas AA, Ackerman BH, Olsen KM, Taylor EH. Isopropanol ingestion: A report of six episodes with isopropanol and acetone serum concentration time data. *J Toxicol Clin Toxicol* 1991;29:11–21.
16. Parker KM, Lera TA. Acute isopropanol ingestion: Pharmacokinetic parameters in the infant. *Am J Emerg Med* 1992;10:542–544.
17. Parker MG, Fraser GL, Watson DM, Riker RR. Removal of propylene glycol and correction of increased osmolar gap by hemodialysis in a patient on high dose lorazepam infusion therapy. *Intensive Care Med* 2002;28:81–84.
18. Rosansky SJ. Isopropyl alcohol poisoning treated with hemodialysis: Kinetics of isopropyl alcohol and acetone removal. *J Toxicol Clin Toxicol* 1982;19:265–271.
19. Stremski E, Hennes H. Accidental isopropanol ingestion in children. *Pediatr Emerg Care* 2000;16:238–240.
20. Tayar J, Jarbour G, Saggi SJ. Severe hyperosmolar metabolic acidosis due to a large dose of intravenous lorazepam. *N Engl J Med* 2002;346:1253–1254.
21. Vasiliades J, Pollock J, Robinson CA. Pitfalls of the alcohol dehydrogenase procedure for the emergency assay of alcohol: A case study of isopropanol overdose. *Clin Chem* 1978;24:383–385.
22. Vicas IMO, Beck R. Fatal inhalational isopropyl alcohol poisoning in a neonate. *J Toxicol Clin Toxicol* 1993;31:473–481.
23. Vivier PM, Lewander WJ, Martin HF, Linakis JG. Isopropyl alcohol intoxication in a neonate through chronic dermal exposure: A complication of a culturally based umbilical care practice. *Pediatr Emerg Care* 1994;10:91–93.

24. Wallgren H. Relative intoxicating effects in rats of ethyl, propyl, and butyl alcohols. *Acta Pharmacol Toxicol* 1960;16:217–222.

25. Yorgin PD, Theodorou AA, Al-Uzri A, Davenport K, Boyer-Hassan LV, Johnson MI. Propylene glycol-induced proximal renal tubular cell injury. *Am J Kid Dis* 1997;30:134–139.

CHAPTER 277
Alcoholic Ketoacidosis

Sage W. Wiener and Robert S. Hoffman

Americans consume 6.8 l of pure alcohol per capita each year, equivalent to over 30 gallons of beer. A total of 15 to 20 million are problem drinkers, and alcohol is responsible for the death of 100,000 people each year in the United States (13). Alcohol dependency commonly results in malnutrition and toxicity to multiple organ systems. When alcohol-dependent patients become ill and are unable to tolerate oral intake, they are at greater risk than other patients because of their underlying disease. Alcoholic ketoacidosis (AKA) is a common result.

The chronic consumption of ethanol leads to substantial metabolic derangements. Unlike most drugs and toxins, ethanol is itself an energy source, and alcoholic patients may come to depend on this source for as much as half of their daily caloric intake (13). This leads to nutritional deficiencies, most notably of vitamin B_1 (thiamine). Furthermore, since the two-carbon molecule of ethanol cannot be utilized for anything other than energy production or fatty acid synthesis (20), these patients become glycogen-deficient.

Alcoholic ketoacidosis is a condition that results from these derangements, typically during a period of ethanol abstinence that immediately follows a drinking binge. As in diabetic ketoacidosis (DKA), the lack of glucose substrate leads to the production of the "ketone bodies" acetoacetate, and β-hydroxybutyrate as alternate energy sources. Unlike in DKA, however, the underlying problem is not the absence of insulin preventing glucose utilization (although relative insulin deficiency may play a role), but rather the absence of glucose substrate because of malnutrition and lack of glycogen. In addition, ethanol metabolism shifts the redox state of the body toward a more reduced state by generating NADH (Fig. 277.1). High levels of NADH cause the equilibrium between lactate and pyruvate to shift, favoring lactate (Fig. 277.2). Thus, gluconeogenesis is inhibited in alcoholics, further limiting available glucose, because pyruvate is the initial substrate (20). Low glucose levels lead to low levels of insulin, so hormone-sensitive lipase is disinhibited. The result is lipolysis

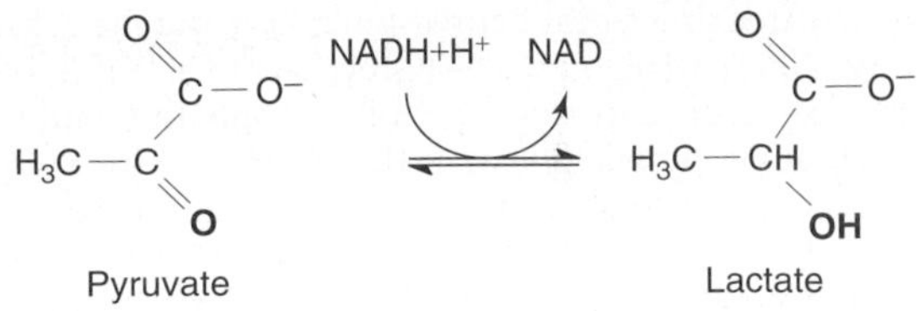

Figure 277.2.   The relative concentrations of pyruvate and lactate are also governed by the redox state (the ratio of NAD to NADH). When the body is reduced (high levels of NADH), there is insufficient pyruvate for gluconeogenesis.

with release of free fatty acids that are broken down to acetyl CoA, subsequently forming ketone bodies (3,10,12,13).

Although significant morbidity may result from coexisting medical disorders (6,7), AKA generally responds well to therapy once recognized and has a low mortality rate in the hospital. However, a Danish prospective study of medicolegal autopsies in alcoholics found that 7% of deaths in their population could be attributed to AKA (21). This suggests that overall mortality from this disorder is higher than previously thought, possibly because many patients do not come to medical attention.

CLINICAL PRESENTATION

Patients generally present with nausea and vomiting, and have abdominal pain suggestive of gastritis or pancreatitis. Vital signs are significant for tachypnea, tachycardia, and orthostatic hypotension. Patients tend to have significant volume depletion (several liters or more) caused by decreased oral intake, vomiting, osmotic diuresis from ketone bodies and increased insensible losses from tachypnea, a compensatory response to metabolic acidosis (10). Their breath may have a characteristic fruity odor of ketosis. Although metabolic acidosis with an elevated anion gap (caused by the presence of unmeasured ketoacid anions) is always present, the serum pH may be normal or even elevated (25). This is because mixed acid-base disorders are common, including metabolic alkalosis from vomiting, contraction alkalosis from volume depletion, and compensatory respiratory alkalosis (10). Severe acidemia with a serum pH as low as 6.70 has been reported in fatal cases (6). Serum or urine ketones are typically only weakly positive, even in severe AKA (6). This is because the nitroprusside reaction used to measure ketones can only detect the functional ketone group of acetone or acetoacetate. β-Hydroxybutyrate is not a true ketone, and is missed by this test (Fig. 277.3). As in the case of the lactate–pyruvate ratio discussed earlier, the reduced redox state of the alcoholic patient causes the equilibrium between the ketone bodies to favor β-hydroxybutyrate. As patients improve with treatment, the NADH/NAD$^+$ ratio shifts to favor the production of acetoacetate, and ketones may actually appear to rise (3).

Electrolyte abnormalities are also common, particularly hypomagnesemia, hypophosphatemia, hypocalcemia, and hypokalemia (3,10,15,25). Other abnormalities on laboratory evaluation (e.g., liver enzymes and amylase) while common, are

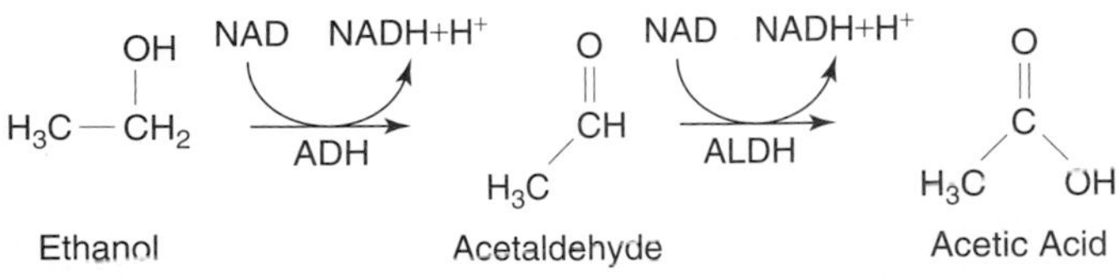

Figure 277.1.   Ethanol is oxidized by alcohol dehydrogenase (ADH) and aldehyde dehydrogenase (ALDH) to acetic acid, generating reduced NADH.

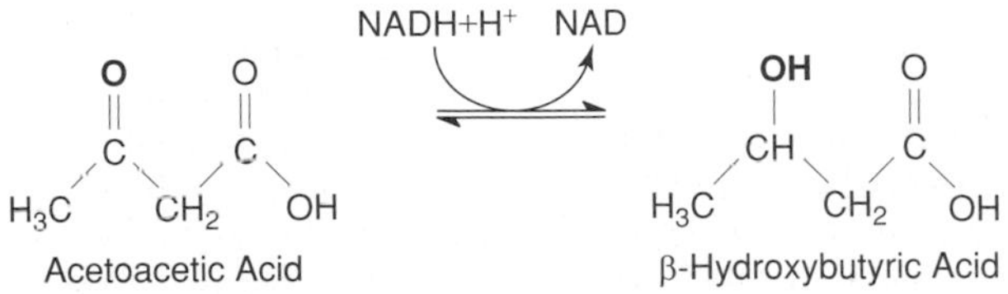

Figure 277.3.   The relative concentrations of the "ketone bodies" acetoacetate and β-hydroxybutyrate depend on the redox state (the ratio of NAD$^+$ to NADH) of the body. Note that β-hydroxybutyrate is not a true ketone.

typically a result of associated illness, rather than being primary manifestations of AKA.

DIFFERENTIAL DIAGNOSIS

The differential diagnosis of anion gap metabolic acidosis in the alcoholic patient is extensive. The familiar, although incomplete, "MUDPILES" mnemonic for causes of anion gap acidosis includes: methanol, metformin, uremia, DKA and other ketoacidoses, such as starvation ketosis and AKA (18), paraldehyde, phenformin, iron, isoniazid, ibuprofen, lactate, ethylene glycol, and salicylates. Common causes of acidosis in the alcohol-dependent population include lactic acidosis, AKA, and (much less frequently) toxic alcohols like methanol and ethylene glycol.

Lactic acidosis, a marker of anaerobic metabolism, may be produced by many disorders including infections, ischemia, or hypoxia, which can lead to decreased oral intake and precipitate AKA. Illnesses such as pancreatitis, pneumonia, sepsis, Wernicke encephalopathy and hepatic dysfunction are associated with an elevated lactate. In fact, lactic acidosis is one of the most common causes of metabolic acidosis in the alcoholic, as in other patients (8).

The distinction between alcoholic and other ketoacidosis is primarily based on history. A history of diabetes mellitus in the setting of ketoacidosis suggests DKA. Serum glucose elevation also suggests DKA, although hyperglycemia has been reported in AKA and DKA may rarely present with euglycemia (9). Significant acidosis caused by starvation is uncommon in the modern world, and is usually a result of hyperemesis gravidarum, hunger strikes, or other similar causes of prolonged decrease in oral intake. A history of ethanol dependence should immediately suggest a diagnosis of AKA in the ketotic patient. Rubbing alcohol (isopropanol) ingestion also causes ketosis because it is metabolized to acetone. However, because acetone does not undergo further metabolism to an organic acid, isopropanol ingestion does not cause a metabolic acidosis. (See Chapter 276, "Isopropanol, Acetone, and Other Glycols").

Methanol and ethylene glycol (see Chapters 275 and 274) are metabolized to the carboxylic acids formate, glycolate and oxalate, and thus may cause an anion-gap metabolic acidosis in the alcohol-dependent patient. Late findings in methanol poisoning include visual changes ranging from blurred vision to total blindness. In ethylene glycol poisoning, renal failure is the feared late complication. Unless the patient presents late enough to have end-organ toxicity or there is a known history of ingestion of these substances, this diagnosis is difficult to make, because timely levels are not available in most hospitals.

The serum ethanol level provides important information, but is frequently misinterpreted. Most importantly, an undetectable ethanol level does not exclude a diagnosis of AKA, and in fact supports it. This is because patients generally do not develop AKA until oral intake ceases. In contrast, the presence of any significant ethanol level (~100 mg/dL or more) almost excludes toxic alcohols as a source of metabolic acidosis, by blocking alcohol dehydrogenase and preventing the metabolism of toxic alcohols to their carboxylic acid metabolites. Except in the rarely reported event of a patient drinking a toxic alcohol, waiting several hours and then drinking ethanol before presenting, patients with significant ethanol levels should not be able to generate a metabolic acidosis.

A further source of confusion is the osmolal gap, a screening test for toxic alcohols. The serum osmolality can be significantly elevated in AKA, and an elevated osmolal gap does not necessarily indicate the presence of a toxic alcohol (1,19). Toxic alcohol poisoning should be considered if there is a known history of ingestion, if there are signs of end-organ toxicity with acidosis (although temporary blindness has also been reported in association with AKA), or if other causes of an increased anion gap have been excluded.

Rapid improvement following intravenous fluids and dextrose is typical of AKA and the anion gap generally returns to baseline after several hours (7,10,25). Such a response does not occur in toxic alcohol poisoning and most other conditions causing anion gap acidosis (except lactate). Without specific therapy, the anion gap would be expected to rise after toxic alcohol ingestion.

EMERGENCY DEPARTMENT EVALUATION

The history should include the time, amount, duration, and pattern of prior alcohol consumption, circumstances that prevented continued consumption, the time of onset, nature, and severity of symptoms, prehospital treatment, and past medical history. The physical examination should focus on the vital signs and cardiopulmonary and neurologic status as well as assessment of the abdomen and hydration status. If the patient's mental status is abnormal, as occurs in 15% of AKA patients (10), the fingerstick glucose should be checked early, because alcohol inhibits gluconeogenesis and is frequently associated with hypoglycemia (11,14). Electrolytes, including calcium, magnesium and phosphate, and an ethanol level should be sent and a urinalysis performed.

AKA is usually first considered once the electrolytes reveal an elevated anion gap (4,16,17,24). The next step is to send a blood gas with lactate, because lactate is the most common cause of metabolic acidosis. The blood gas is usually performed on arterial samples, although a venous sample is probably adequate (2). If the lactate does not account for the anion gap elevation, then urine or serum ketones should be checked. If urine ketones are trace or negative and AKA is suspected, a few drops of hydrogen peroxide can be added to a sample of urine to oxidize the β-hydroxybutyrate to acetoacetate. A repeat dipstick analysis on this sample is often positive.

Once the diagnosis of alcoholic ketoacidosis is made, it is important to look for any precipitating factors that led to the patient's condition. Further evaluation should be guided by the patient's signs and symptoms, and may include stool guaiac, chest radiography, serum lipase, liver enzymes, urine and blood cultures, and lumbar puncture.

EMERGENCY DEPARTMENT MANAGEMENT

Advanced life support measures should be instituted as needed. Airway and breathing difficulties are rarely caused by AKA, although associated ethanol withdrawal, or severe respiratory infections may warrant endotracheal intubation. Specific therapy includes fluids, glucose, and thiamine administration. Intravenous crystalloids should be given to restore intravascular volume and to promote the renal clearance of ketones from the blood (3). In severely ill patients, a central venous catheter may be helpful in assessing volume status and response to treatment, particularly in those with underlying cardiac, hepatic, or renal disease.

Glucose is given to correct the underlying cause of AKA, notably the lack of glucose and glycogen stores, and relative insulin deficiency. It provides energy substrate and stimulates insulin release from the pancreatic β-islet cells (6,7,10,12). Insulin, once released, inactivates hormone-sensitive lipase. This leads to decreased release of free fatty acids, the substrates for ketogenesis. Thus, glucose is able to stop ketone formation. In the rare cases of AKA with significant hyperglycemia, dextrose may be withheld, but the fingerstick glucose should be followed closely and insulin should be considered (9). Glucose should initially be given intravenously as 5% dextrose. Food should given as soon as tolerated.

Thiamine is required for the utilization of glucose in the Krebs cycle (20), and the chronic administration of dextrose without thiamine has been reported to precipitate or worsen acute Wernicke encephalopathy (23). A dose of 200 mg should be administered parenterally, since alcohol-dependent patients do not absorb oral thiamine well (22).

Associated problems may require additional therapy. Abnormal electrolytes (potassium, phosphate, and magnesium) should be corrected. Although patients may have significant acidosis, sodium bicarbonate is unnecessary and should be avoided. The acidosis typically resolves rapidly once fluids and glucose are replete (6,7,15,25). Insulin is also an unnecessary intervention, unless the patient has a known history of diabetes mellitus or persistent hyperglycemia (which would suggest relative insulin deficiency and thus impaired clearance of ketones) (6,7,10,25). Treatment of underlying or intercurrent medical problems should be instituted.

CRITICAL INTERVENTIONS

- Administer intravenous crystalloids to correct dehydration
- Administer intravenous dextrose to provide nutritional substrate and reverse ketosis unless the patient is severely hyperglycemic; feed patients who are able to eat
- Administer parenteral thiamine (200 mg)
- Correct electrolyte abnormalities such as hypokalemia, hypomagnesemia, and hypophosphatemia
- Avoid the use of sodium bicarbonate and insulin
- Identify and treat associated precipitating medical illness (e.g., infectious pancreatitis, alcoholic hepatitis)

DISPOSITION

In the hospital, AKA has low morbidity and mortality, and responds well to treatment. The symptoms and metabolic derangements of mild AKA may often be corrected in a short time in the emergency department. Because of this, some authors have advised that most patients can be safely discharged with close followup. In one series, only 54% of patients with AKA were admitted (25). However, AKA occurs only in patients with a significant degree of alcohol dependence and nutritional deprivation. These patients are at high risk and by definition cannot be relied upon to followup appropriately. Furthermore, as discussed earlier, coexisting medical illness is common. We believe that rapid discharge from the emergency department without an evaluation for precipitating factors is potentially dangerous. In the absence of severe electrolyte abnormalities, however, most patients can safely be admitted to low-acuity beds.

COMMON PITFALLS

- ✔ Failure to appreciate that patients with AKA may have an undetectable serum ethanol level and trace or absent serum and urine ketones
- ✔ Failure to identify and treat associated or precipitating medical illness (e.g., infection, pancreatitis, and hepatitis)
- ✔ Underestimating the degree of dehydration
- ✔ Failure to administer supplemental dextrose
- ✔ Failure to recognize that the normal anion gap is diminished in hypoalbuminemia
- ✔ Misdiagnosing AKA as DKA, usually because of incomplete history
- ✔ Failure to administer thiamine or failure to appreciate that thiamine may not be absorbed by the oral route in patients with AKA

- ✔ Inappropriately using insulin or sodium bicarbonate to treat AKA

References

1. Almaghams AM, Yeung CK. Osmolal gap in alcoholic ketoacidosis. *Clin Nephrol* 1997;48:52.
2. Brandenburg MA, Dire DJ. Comparison of arterial and venous blood gas values in the initial emergency department evaluation of patients with diabetic ketoacidosis. *Ann Emerg Med* 1998;31:459–465.
3. Dubose TD, Cogan MG, Rector FC. Acid-base disorders. In: Brenner BM, ed. *Brenner & Rector's the kidney*, 5th ed. Philadelphia: WB Saunders, 1996:964–969.
4. Emmett M, Narins RG. Clinical use of the anion gap. *Medicine (Baltimore)* 1977;56:38–54.
5. Figge J, Jabor A, Kazda A, Fencl V. Anion gap and hypoalbuminemia. *Crit Care Med* 1998;26:1807–1810.
6. Fulop M, Hoberman HD. Alcoholic ketoacidosis. *Diabetes* 1975;24:785–790.
7. Fulop M. Alcoholism, ketoacidosis, and lactic acidosis. *Diabetes Metab Rev* 1989;5:365–378.
8. Gabow PA, Kaehny WD, Fennessey PV, et al. Diagnostic importance of an increased serum anion gap. *N Engl J Med* 1980;303:854–858.
9. Gill G, Yong A. Recurrent alcoholic ketoacidosis with hyperglycaemia in a nondiabetic patient. *Hosp Med (London)* 2000;61:506–507.
10. Höjer J. Severe metabolic acidosis in the alcoholic: differential diagnosis and management. *Human Exp Toxicol* 1996;15:482–488.
11. Jain H, Beriwal S, Singh S. Alcohol induced ketoacidosis, severe hypoglycemia and irreversible encephalopathy. *Med Sci Monit* 2002;8:CS77–9.
12. Jenkins DW, Eckel RE, Craig JW. Alcoholic ketoacidosis. *JAMA* 1971;217:177.
13. Lieber CS. Medical disorders of alcoholism. *N Engl J Med* 1995;333:1058–1065.
14. Marinella MA. Alcoholic ketoacidosis presenting with extreme hypoglycemia. *Am J Emerg Med* 1997;15:280–281.
15. Miller PD, Heinig RE, Waterhouse C. Treatment of alcoholic acidosis. The role of dextrose and phosphorus. *Arch Intern Med* 1978;138:67–72.
16. Oh MS, Carroll HJ. Current concepts: the anion gap. *N Engl J Med* 1977;297:814–817.
17. Salem MM, Mujais SK. Gaps in the anion gap. *Arch Intern Med* 1992;152:1625–1629.
18. Schade DS, Eaton RP. Differential diagnosis and therapy of hyperketonemic state. *JAMA* 1979;241:2064–2065.
19. Schelling JR, Howard RL, Winter SD, Linas SL. Increased osmolal gap in alcoholic ketoacidosis and lactic acidosis. *Ann Intern Med* 1990;113:580–582.
20. Stryer L. *Biochemistry*, 3rd ed. New York, NY: W.H. Freeman and Company, 1988:389–390.
21. Thomsen JL, Simonsen KW, Felby S, Frohlich B. A prospective toxicology analysis in alcoholics. *Forensic Sci Int* 1997;90:33–40.
22. Thomson AD, Baker H, Leevy CM. Patterns of 35S-thiamine hydrochloride absorption in the malnourished alcoholic patient. *J Lab Clin Med* 1970;76:34–45.
23. Watson AJS, Walker JF, Tomkin GH, et al. Acute Wernicke's encephalopathy precipitated by glucose loading. *Ir J Med Sci* 1981;150:301–303.
24. Winter SD, Pearson JR, Gabow PA, et al. The fall of the serum anion gap. *Arch Intern Med* 1990;150:311–313.
25. Wrenn KD, Slovis CM, Minion G, Rutkowski R. The syndrome of alcoholic ketoacidosis. *Am J Med* 1991;91:119.

CHAPTER 278
Alcohol Withdrawal

Mark Su

Alcohol is the most commonly abused drug in the world. Alcohol abuse is one of the largest health problems in the United States, causing approximately 200,000 deaths annually and implicated in 50% of motor vehicle collisions, 67% of homicides, and 37% of suicides (23). In a recent study performed in a primary care setting, 15% to 20% of patients reported problems with alcohol use (11). The comprehension of the effects of alcohol and its association with clinical syndromes is well known. On the contrary, problems associated with acute alcohol abstinence and improved treatment of consequent withdrawal have only been recently elucidated. Alcohol withdrawal is not the most common presenting chief complaint of the ethanol-dependent patient, but is potentially fatal if untreated. Emergency department physicians must, therefore, be able to recognize the various clinical manifestations of the alcohol withdrawal syndromes and their appropriate treatment.

Although alcohol is often classified as a sedative-hypnotic, it is likely to have multiple effects on the central nervous system. As with other sedative-hypnotic agents, the enhancement of inhibitory tone by alcohol is mediated via gamma-aminobutyric acid (GABA) agonism. With chronic alcohol use, the GABA receptor undergoes downregulation, leading to the development of tolerance (14). *Tolerance* is the pharmacologic effect whereby either increasing doses or increasing frequency of alcohol intake is required to achieve the same physiologic effect. Tolerance to alcohol is necessary for withdrawal to occur. *Dependence* is the altered physiologic state resulting from chronic alcohol use, and is also a prerequisite for the development of withdrawal. Continued alcohol use is also associated with inhibition of the excitatory glutaminergic pathways and subsequent upregulation of the *N*-methyl-D-aspartate (NMDA) receptors occurs (18). When alcohol intake is abruptly stopped, excess excitatory tone and sympathetic stimulation result. Although the exact mechanism has not been fully elucidated, this is in large part because of decreased inhibition (GABA effects) and increased excitation (glutamate effects). Increased dopaminergic activity may contribute to hallucinations (6).

CLINICAL PRESENTATION

Alcohol withdrawal may present with a wide spectrum of clinical signs and symptoms. For classification purposes, there are four distinct withdrawal syndromes: alcoholic tremulousness, alcoholic hallucinosis, alcoholic withdrawal seizures, and delirium tremens (20). These four clinically distinct entities may occur in isolation or simultaneously in any combination (Fig. 278.1).

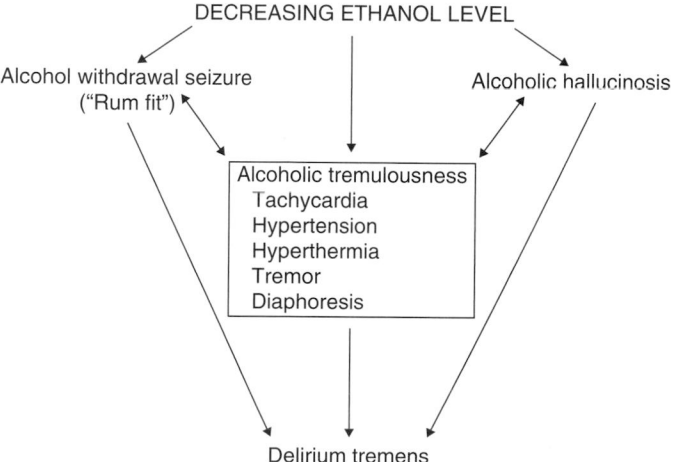

Figure 278.1.   Representation of alcohol withdrawal. As ethanol levels fall, patients may develop alcohol withdrawal seizures ("rum fits"), alcoholic hallucinosis, or alcoholic tremulousness. Following this state, the patient can recover, develop another early manifestation of withdrawal, or progress to delirium tremens. (Adapted from Hamilton RJ. Substance withdrawal. In: Goldfrank L (ed). *Goldfrank's toxicologic emergencies*, 7th edition. New York: McGraw-Hill Professional Publishing, 2002, with permission.)

Alcoholic tremulousness is characterized by catecholamine excess that results from abstinence. Patients present to the emergency department with hypertension, tachycardia, diaphoresis, tremor, fasciculations, mild hyperthermia, agitation, and insomnia (17). The patient appears to be extremely uncomfortable but usually has a normal mental status. Symptoms may begin as early as 6 hours after the last drink and most patients will be symptomatic within 24 to 48 hours after the last intake of alcohol (20). A small percentage of patients will develop symptoms after up to 7 days of abstinence (20).

Alcoholic hallucinosis is characterized by hallucinations that are either visual or auditory and may be persecutory in nature. Formication, the sensation of insects or snakes crawling on the skin, may also occur. The onset is often within a few hours of cessation of alcohol intake and no other manifestations, including abnormal vital signs, are necessarily present (20).

Alcohol withdrawal seizures, or "rum fits," are the acute onset of a single seizure or a brief flurry of seizures that peaks within 24 hours after the last drink. More than 60% of patients will have a single seizure characterized by a brief post-ictal state; status epilepticus is rare (21). As with alcoholic hallucinosis, other signs of alcohol withdrawal may concomitantly occur either before or after the seizures. Furthermore, about one third of patients with seizures who are untreated will progress to delirium tremens (21).

Delirium tremens is the most severe form of alcohol withdrawal. It includes all of the manifestations of the acute withdrawal syndrome in combination with delirium. Only 5% of patients with alcohol withdrawal will progress to delirium tremens. Signs of delirium tremens include extreme autonomic hyperactivity and alteration in sensorium. Delirium tremens usually occurs within 24 to 96 hours after the last drink and has a typical duration of 3 to 7 days (20). In the past, mortality from delirium tremens was reportedly in the range of 15% to 20% secondary to fluid and electrolyte abnormalities, seizures, and/or infection. Today, the mortality rate is significantly less (approximately 5%) in properly treated patients (17).

DIFFERENTIAL DIAGNOSIS

The differential diagnosis of alcohol withdrawal is extremely broad because of the varying clinical manifestations that occur in isolation or simultaneously and the progression of the condition if left untreated. Furthermore, because patients often may also have other illnesses, the diagnosis of alcohol withdrawal may be initially overlooked. Consequently, it is crucial for health care providers to be aware of other etiologies that may mimic the spectrum of alcohol withdrawal (Table 278.1).

EMERGENCY DEPARTMENT EVALUATION

The clinical presentation of alcohol withdrawal may be extremely diverse depending on the particular patient. Hospital staff may become very familiar with patients who are repeatedly brought to emergency departments for alcohol intoxication. When these patients present to the hospital with signs and symptoms of alcohol withdrawal, they are easy to identify. However, in those patients who are not readily identifiable as being "alcoholic," the diagnosis is easy to overlook. Moreover, when patients are identified as having an alcohol withdrawal syndrome, it is crucial to determine the underlying reason for alcohol abstinence. Most alcohol-dependent patients do not intentionally stop drinking without a concurrent medical illness or social barrier prohibiting continued consumption.

TABLE 278.1. Differential Diagnosis of Major Withdrawal Symptoms

Tremor	Seizures	Hallucinations	Delirium

Withdrawal
  Ethanol
  Sedative–hypnotics
Intoxications
  Theophylline
  Caffeine
  Beta agoists
  Mercury
  Lithium
  TCAs
  Phenytoin
Metabolic
  Hypoglycemia
  Thyrotoxicosis
Structural
  Cerebellar disease
Other
  Parkinsonism
	Withdrawal
	  Ethanol
	  Sedative–hypnotics
	Intoxications
	  Cocaine
	  Anticholinergics
	  Phenothiazines
	  TCAs
	  Theophylline
	  Camphor
	  Isoniazid
	  Phencyclidine
	  Lidocaine
	  Organophosphates
	Infectious
	  Meningitis
	  Encephalitis
	Metabolic
	  Hypoglycemia
	  Hypoxia
	  Hypothyroidism
	  Thyrotoxicosis
	  Hypocalcemia
	  Hyperosmolar state
	  Hepatic failure
	  Uremia
	Structural
	  Head trauma
	  CNS hemorrhage
	  Tumor
	  CVA
	Other
	  Idiopathic epilepsy
	  Posttraumatic epilepsy
	  Degenerative disease
		Withdrawal
		  Ethanol
		  Sedative–hypnotics
		Intoxications
		  LSD
		  Mescaline
		  Mushrooms
		  Peyote
		  Phencyclidine
		  Anticholinergics
		  Ergot
		  Nutmeg
		Infectious
		  Meningitis
		  Encephalitis
		  Sepsis
		Metabolic
		  Hypoglycemia
		  Hypoxia
		Structural
		  CNS hemorrhage
		  Tumor
		Psychiatric
		  Schizophrenia
		  Bipolar disorder
		Other
		  Seizures
		  Heat-related illness
			Withdrawal
			  Ethanol
			  Sedative–hypnotics
			Intoxications
			  Cocaine
			  Amphetamine
			  Phencyclidine
			  Anticholinergics
			  LSD
			Infectious
			  Meningitis
			  Encephalitis
			  Sepsis
			Metabolic
			  Thyrotoxicosis
			  Hypoglycemia
			  Hyperglycemia
			  Hypocalcemia
			  Hypoxia
			  Thiamine
			    deficiency
			Structural
			  Head trauma
			  CNS hemorrhage
			  Tumor
			Psychiatric
			Other
			  Seizures
			  Heat-related illness

TCAs, tricyclic antidepressants; CVA, cerebrovascular accident.

All patients should have a fingerstick glucose and oxygen saturation analysis performed. The physician must obtain a complete history of substance abuse, previous withdrawal episodes, and all current and former medications. If possible, family, friends, and prehospital personnel are interviewed to gain additional information. All vital signs, including rectal temperature, are recorded and closely monitored. Examination of the skin, abdomen, eyes, and pulse rate may help to distinguish an anticholinergic toxidrome (dry skin, decreased bowel sounds, urinary retention, mydriasis, and tachycardia) from a sympathomimetic toxidrome (moist skin, normal bowel sounds, no urinary retention, mydriasis, and tachycardia). Attention should be made to any stigmata of chronic liver disease or evidence of intravenous drug use.

Because substance abusers are at high risk for concomitant trauma, traumatic injury should always be considered, especially in patients with an altered sensorium. Furthermore, these patients should also be evaluated for other complications of ethanol and drug abuse, such as pneumonia, skin abscesses, bacterial endocarditis, acquired immunodeficiency syndrome, pancreatitis, liver disease, and gastrointestinal bleeding.

Laboratory studies should include a complete blood count; measurement of electrolytes, glucose, blood urea nitrogen, and serum creatinine; aminotransferases; coagulation studies, and ethanol concentration. Ethanol concentrations are likely to be negligible or low in most patients in withdrawal; however, measurable serum ethanol concentrations in patients experiencing alcohol withdrawal correlate with the severity of symptoms (22). Patients believed to have delirium tremens should undergo computed tomography of the brain and, if negative, a subsequent lumbar puncture to rule out organic CNS pathology as the cause of their altered mental status.

EMERGENCY DEPARTMENT MANAGEMENT

In any patient who presents with an altered sensorium, the diagnosis of a toxin-related condition is always a possibility. Administration of intravenous dextrose is indicated if the patient has numerical hypoglycemia (usually less than 60 mg/dL). Chronic alcohol use is commonly associated with hypoglycemia for several reasons. Alcoholics are often nutritionally depleted and may have insufficient glycogen stores secondary to liver dysfunction. Furthermore, chronic ethanol use leads to an impaired redox potential due to the accumulation of NADH and subsequent depletion of pyruvate, one of the major precursors of gluconeogenesis.

Thiamine (vitamin B_1) is also indicated in the "coma cocktail" for patients with an altered sensorium and patients with a history of alcohol abuse because of the possibility of Wernicke encephalopathy (triad of ataxia, dementia, or confusion and ophthalmoplegia). This condition is rare but it may occur secondary to nutritional deficiency. The standard initial dose is 100 mg intravenously. For patients who are known alcoholics, other multivitamin preparations and magnesium sulfate may also be administered, but their benefit is unproven (24).

Administration of intravenous fluids is often necessary and an important part of the treatment of alcohol withdrawal, because alcohol induces a diuresis and leads to volume depletion. Furthermore, precipitation of alcohol withdrawal is often caused by some underlying medical condition (e.g., pneumonia, pancreatitis, or head trauma) that prevents the patient from their usual intake of alcohol. These patients may require aggressive volume resuscitation in the treatment of this concurrent condition.

Significantly agitated patients may need to be physically restrained to prevent injury, establish intravenous access, and facilitate sedation. Soft restraints should be used. Prolonged use of restraints is discouraged, because continued struggling may lead to rhabdomyolysis, hyperthermia, and metabolic acidosis. Once intravenous access is obtained and chemical sedation has been achieved, physical restraints should be discontinued.

The goal of therapy for the agitated alcohol withdrawal patient is sedation. Benzodiazepines are, therefore, the cornerstone of therapy (7). Benzodiazepines, like alcohol, are classified as sedative-hypnotics and exert their pharmacologic effect via the GABA receptor.

Benzodiazepines are effective in the treatment of alcohol withdrawal because of their ability to enhance and often restore inhibitory tone because of their *cross tolerance* with alcohol. Nevertheless, case reports exist of patients requiring massive doses of intravenous benzodiazepines for treatment (15,25). Patients whose conditions are refractory to benzodiazepines may be treated with a different GABA agonist, such as a barbiturate. "Anesthetic" barbiturates have direct effects on the GABA receptor and together with benzodiazepines exert a synergistic effect (17,19). Patients with severe refractory alcohol withdrawal who do not respond to benzodiazepines may be given a propofol infusion. Propofol is an ideal agent to treat alcohol withdrawal because in addition to being a GABA agonist, it is an NMDA antagonist. Propofol has also been shown in several case reports to be efficacious in the treatment of alcohol withdrawal (5,13). It should be noted that if either barbiturates or propofol are used, the patient will likely require airway protection because of their potential to cause respiratory depression. Although experimental NMDA antagonists have been shown to be efficacious in the treatment of alcohol withdrawal in animal models, no current pure NMDA antagonists are clinically used in humans yet.

Although many regimens are advocated for the administration of benzodiazepines for the treatment of alcohol withdrawal, symptom-triggered therapy is recommended. Symptom-triggered therapy consists of the administration of intravenous benzodiazepines when the patient's symptoms exceed a threshold of severity, and benzodiazepines are given as often as necessary until the patient's symptoms are adequately controlled. This is in contrast to the fixed-dose regimen where the patients are given a set amount of benzodiazepine at regular intervals with a subsequent taper after the patient's symptoms are under control. The symptom-triggered method is by far the better technique and has been demonstrated to decrease the total amount of benzodiazepines administered, decrease the duration of treatment and decrease the incidence of delirium tremens when compared to the fixed-dose regimen (9,16).

There are many choices of benzodiazepines that may be used, including diazepam (Valium®), chlordiazepoxide (Librium®), and lorazepam (Ativan®). These are the most commonly used agents for alcohol withdrawal and can also be used for sedative–

TABLE 278.2. Pharmaceutical Management of Ethanol and Drug Withdrawal

ETHANOL OR SEDATIVE–HYPNOTIC WITHDRAWAL

1st Choice: Diazepam
  5 mg i.v. bolus q5–15 min until sedated
  May increase dose to 20 mg q5–15 min in refractory cases
  Total over 24-h period may >1,000 mg
  Do not exceed 5 mg/min
2nd Choice: Lorazepam
  1–2 mg i.v. bolus q5–15 min until sedated
  Not as long-acting as diazepam
  Preferable in cases of hepatic failure or recurrent seizures
3rd Choice: Pentobarbital
  100 mg i.v. bolus
  Continued titration to sedation or 600 mg total
  Potential for more respiratory depression than benzodiazepines
  Do not exceed 50 mg/min
Alternatives:
  Chlordiazepoxide, secobarbital, phenobarbital

hypnotic withdrawal. These agents are preferred over benzodiazepines with shorter half-lives, because they require less frequent dosing as they allow gradual drug elimination over several days. (See Table 278.2 for dosing recommendations for various benzodiazepines.)

Compared with short-acting agents, long-acting agents may be more effective in preventing withdrawal seizures and may contribute to smoother withdrawal with fewer rebound symptoms (12). Active metabolites of diazepam and chlordiazepoxide prolong their therapeutic effect. In elderly patients and those with hepatic dysfunction, lorazepam, which has no active metabolites, may be preferred. In other cases, lorazepam does not appear to offer any distinct advantage over diazepam or chlordiazepoxide (3).

Intravenous dosing is preferred in all but the mildest cases of ethanol withdrawal. Agitation may preclude oral administration, and gastritis may impair drug absorption. Intravenous therapy can be readily titrated. Lorazepam (but not diazepam or chlordiazepoxide) is predictably absorbed intramuscularly. This route is recommended in the wildly agitated patient who has not had intravenous access established.

Patients who have alcohol abstinence seizures should be given standard supportive therapy as well as benzodiazepines to stop seizure activity. Phenytoin is proven to be of no use for the treatment of alcohol withdrawal seizures and should not be given unless the patient has a known seizure focus and was previously taking this drug prior to presentation (1). Other anticonvulsants, such as carbamazepine and valproic acid, have also been advocated (10). They have both been shown to be mildly efficacious in certain settings, but these agents have limitations because of potential hepatic and hematologic complications that may exacerbate some alcohol related conditions. Furthermore, they have not been studied in an emergency department setting or in patients with delirium tremens. Consequently, it is currently unknown whether these anticonvulsant therapies have any role in the acute treatment of patients with significant signs and symptoms of alcohol withdrawal.

Historically, some additional agents have been used for the treatment of alcohol withdrawal. These include β-adrenergic antagonists, clonidine, and antipsychotics (phenothiazines and butyrophenones) (2,4,8). None of these agents exert their primary effects through GABA. As a result, although they may appear to be efficacious in controlling certain clinical manifestations, their efficacy in improving outcomes in alcohol withdrawal has not been demonstrated, and occasionally harm has occurred. The routine use of these agents is discouraged.

CRITICAL INTERVENTIONS

- Identify and treat alcohol withdrawal early; treatment becomes increasingly more difficult as the disease progresses
- Identify and treat comorbid illness; concurrent infectious illness is often the precipitant for ethanol abstinence and subsequent withdrawal

DISPOSITION

Depending on the particular withdrawal syndrome, the reason for cessation of alcohol intake, and the severity of alcohol withdrawal signs and symptoms, the disposition of patients with alcohol withdrawal is extremely variable. For mild alcoholic tremulousness, as long as there are no potentially critical medical conditions that will prevent the patient from resuming his normal his normal activities, they may be safely discharged with treatment and referred to a detoxification program.

Patients with more severe signs and symptoms of alcohol withdrawal, including alcohol withdrawal seizures and alcoholic hallucinosis, will require hospital admission. Patients with delirium tremens will require admission to an intensive care unit for close cardiac and hemodynamic monitoring. Patients who are not adequately sedated with conventional doses of benzodiazepines may require more potent GABA-ergic agents, also necessitating intensive care unit admission for respiratory monitoring and subsequent endotracheal intubation, if necessary.

COMMON PITFALLS

✔ Not considering alcohol withdrawal as a potential cause of altered sensorium and autonomic instability
✔ Failure to perform computed tomography of the brain and a lumbar puncture to exclude organic CNS pathology in patients diagnosed with delirium tremens
✔ Using a fixed-dose schedule of benzodiazepines to treat ethanol withdrawal in the emergency department; escalating doses or symptom-triggered therapy is preferred

Acknowledgment

Thank you to previous edition chapter author Paul M. Wax.

References

1. Alldredge BK, Lowenstein DH, Simon RP. Placebo-controlled trial of intravenous diphenylhydantoin for short-term treatment of alcohol withdrawal seizures. *Am J Med* 1989;87:645–648.
2. Baumgartner GR, Rowen RC. Clonidine vs. chlordiazepoxide in the management of acute alcohol withdrawal syndrome. *Arch Intern Med* 1987;147:1223–1226.
3. Bird RD, Makela EH. Alcohol withdrawal: what is the benzodiazepine of choice? *Ann Pharmacother* 1994;28:67–71.
4. Blum K, Eubanks JD, Wallace JE, Hamilton H. Enhancement of alcohol withdrawal convulsions in mice by haloperidol. *Clin Toxicol* 1976;9:427–434.
5. Coomes TR, Smith SW. Successful use of propofol in refractory delirium tremens. *Ann Emerg Med* 1997;30:825–828.
6. Heinz A, Schmidt K, Baum SS, Kuhn S, Dufeu P, Schmidt LG, Rommelspacher H. Influence of dopaminergic transmission on severity of withdrawal syndrome in alcoholism. *J Stud Alcohol* 1996;57:471–474.
7. Holbrook AM, Crowther R, Lotter A, Cheng C, King D. Meta-analysis of benzodiazepine use in the treatment of acute alcohol withdrawal. *Can Med Assoc J* 1999;160:649–655.
8. Horwitz RI, Gottlieb LD, Kraus ML. The efficacy of atenolol in the outpatient management of the alcohol withdrawal syndrome. *Arch Intern Med* 1989;149:1089–1093.
9. Jaeger TM, Lohr RH, Pankratz VS. Symptom-triggered therapy for alcohol withdrawal syndrome in medical inpatients. *Mayo Clin Proc* 2001;76:695–701.
10. Kosten RD, O'Connor PG. Management of drug and alcohol withdrawal. *N Engl J Med* 2003;348:1786–1795.
11. Manwell LB, Fleming MF, Johnson K, Barry KL. Tobacco, alcohol, and drug use in a primary care sample: 90-day prevalence and associated factors. *J Addict Dis* 1998;17:67–81.
12. Mayo-Smith MF. Pharmacological management of alcohol withdrawal. A meta-analysis and evidence-based practice guideline. American Society of Addiction Medicine Working Group on Pharmacological Management of Alcohol Withdrawal. *JAMA* 1997;278:144–151.
13. McCowan C, Marik P. Refractory delirium tremens treated with propofol: a case series. *Crit Care Med* 2000;28:1781–1784.
14. Morrow AL, Suzdak PD, Karanian JW, Paul SM. Chronic ethanol administration alters (-aminobutyric acid, pentobarbital and ethanol-mediated $^{36}Cl^-$ uptake in cerebral cortical synaptoneurosomes. *J Pharmacol Exp Ther* 1988;246:158–164.
15. Nolop KB, Natow A. Unprecedented sedative requirements during delirium tremens. *Crit Care Med* 1985;13:246–247.
16. Saitz R, Mayo-Smith MF, Roberts MS, et al. Individualized treatment for alcohol withdrawal. A randomized double-blind controlled trial. *JAMA* 1994;272:519–523.
17. Trevisan LA, Boutros N, Petrakis IL, Krystal JH. Complications of alcohol withdrawal. Pathophysiological insights. *Alcohol Health Res World* 1998;22:61–66.
18. Tsai G, Gastfriend DR. Coyle JT. The glutamatergic basis of human alcoholism. *Am J Psychiatry* 1995;152:332–340.
19. Twyman RD. Rogers CJ, Macdonald RL. Differential regulation of γ-aminobutyric acid receptor channels by diazepam and phenobarbital. *Ann Neurol* 1989;25:213–220.
20. Victor M, Adams, RD. The effect of alcohol on the nervous system. *Res Pub Assoc Res Nerv Ment Dis* 1953;32:526–573.
21. Victor M, Brausch C. The role of abstinence in the genesis of alcoholic epilepsy. *Epilepsia* 1967;8:1–20.
22. Vinson DC, Menezes M. Admission alcohol level: a predictor of the course of alcohol withdrawal. *J Fam Pract* 1991;33:161–177.
23. West LJ, Maxwell DS, Noble EP, Solomon DH. Alcoholism. *Ann Intern Med* 1984;100:405–416.
24. Wilson A, Vulcano B. A double blind, placebo-controlled trial of magnesium sulfate in the ethanol withdrawal syndrome. *Alcohol Clin Exp Res* 1984;8:542–545.
25. Woo E, Greenblatt DJ. Massive benzodiazepine requirements during acute alcohol withdrawal. *Am J Psychiatry* 1979;136:821–823.

CHAPTER 279
Other Complications of Chronic Ethanol Abuse

Cynthia K. Aaron and Ivan E. Liang

Few diseases or comorbid conditions are as pervasive, if not unavoidable, in the emergency department as is chronic alcohol abuse and dependence (the currently preferred term for addiction). Alcohol abuse is a maladaptive pattern of substance use leading to clinically significant impairment or distress, as manifested by recurrences of one (or more) of the following, within a 12-month period: use resulting in failure to fulfill major role obligations at work, school, or home; use in situations in which it is physically hazardous; alcohol-related legal problems; continued use despite alcohol exacerbated interpersonal problems (3). Alcohol dependence is defined by the occurrence of three or more of the following over 1 year: tolerance (increased consumption to achieve same effect); withdrawal (use to avoid a withdrawal syndrome); consumption in larger amounts than intended; persistent desire or unsuccessful attempts to control substance use; excessive time related to obtaining or recovering from alcohol use; forgoing of important social, occupational, or recreational activities; continued use despite an understanding of the physical and psychological harm of alcohol (3).

About 44% of the adult population of the United States consumes alcohol. The current prevalence of alcohol abuse and dependence is estimated to be between 7.4% and 9.7%, with lifetime prevalence between 13.7% and 23.5%, and 43% of adults reporting alcoholism in their families (17,20). Recent research reveals alcoholism as a mounting problem in both younger and older populations; 40% of adult alcoholic patients demonstrated symptoms from age 15 to 19 years (4). Greater than one half of high school students in one study reported themselves to have been "drunk" in the last month, and a quarter had been "drunk" seven times or more (9). Among a study group of subjects aged 55 and older, 38% had used alcohol in the past month, 9% reported binge drinking (five or more drinks on the same occurrence), and 2% reported heavy use (five or more drinks on five or more days of the week). Late-onset drinkers (starting at age 50 and older) comprise approximately one third of older patients diagnosed with alcohol dependence, often starting after a traumatic event or loss (21).

Alcohol is the leading contributor to death in people between ages of 15 and 45 years and contributes to 85% of the 11,000 deaths per year from liver disease (12). Alcohol dependence has both a genetic and familial predisposition and is associated with immunosuppression, myocardial disease, and an increased propensity toward oral, pharyngeal, laryngeal, esophageal, and liver cancers (2). Studies suggest that women are risk for ethanol-related morbidity at lower levels of ingestion than men, perhaps because ethanol has less pre-hepatic metabolism and a lower volume of distribution in women.

It can be difficult to recognize alcoholism. Despite the recent impetus to increase physician participation in recognition and treatment of the alcoholic patient, as many as 50% of patients with alcoholism go undiagnosed and untreated by their general practitioners (17). Despite its role in trauma, 45% of trauma centers do not screen patients for alcohol abuse (22). Detection and treatment are often delayed for women, perhaps because of cultural and social value systems in which it may be less acceptable for a woman to have an alcohol or substance abuse disorder.

Criteria that mandate a diagnosis of alcoholism include alcoholic hepatitis, blackouts, drinking despite social contraindications, and withdrawal symptoms. A number of simple questionnaires can be used to rapidly identify high-risk patients in the emergency department (see Appendix, Tables 279.A1 through 279.A5) (8). High-risk groups include adolescents, patients involved in violent activity or trauma (especially single-car crashes), caretakers accused of child abuse, spouses of known alcoholics, suicidal patients, and those presenting with neuropsychiatric disturbances (19). Other risk factors include male sex, unemployment, homelessness, polysubstance use or abuse, and tobacco use (25). The great majority of emergency department patients who present with ethanol levels of 300 mg/dL or greater score high in response to two or more CAGE questions (see Table 279.A1). Yet even when the CAGE questionnaire is successfully utilized, it is often unclear what clinical approach to take with patients identified at risk, beyond responding to the chief complaint that initially brought them to the emergency department (20).

Chronic alcohol consumption can result in several metabolic complications. The oxidation of ethanol acetaldehyde is accomplished via three separate pathways (10,11). The two minor pathways are via catalase and the microsomal ethanol oxidiz-

ing system (MEOS). The simplest pathway, via catalase, generates H_2O from H_2O_2. Metabolism through the MEOS oxidizes the reduced cofactor nicotinamide adenine dinucleotide phosphate (NADPH) to $NADP^+$. This reaction generates free radicals, which then interact with glutathione, eventually leading to glutathione depletion and possibly contributing to hepatotoxicity.

The principal metabolic pathway involves alcohol dehydrogenase (ADH) with nicotinamide adenine dinucleotide (NAD^+) as a cofactor. During this reaction, NAD^+ is reduced to NADH. The conversion of NADH back to NAD^+ requires large amounts of oxygen. When excessive amounts of ethanol are metabolized, oxygen requirements in the centrilobular areas of the liver exceed those delivered. The relative hypoxia that results in these areas is believed to contribute to hepatic damage.

Increased oxygen demand also shifts the redox potential of the cell. The result of this shift is an increased ratio of lactate to pyruvate, which favors glycolysis and depletes available glycogen stores. The increase in free hydrogen ions (H^+) tends to favor ketone formation and fatty acid generation. Excess H^+ depresses the citric acid cycle and decreases the use of free fatty acids as an energy source. This favors hypercholesterolemia and fatty liver formation (17). Ethanol-induced metabolic derangements, especially in the setting of poor nutritional intake, increase the patient's risk of developing ketoacidosis and hypoglycemia. Renal magnesium wasting, secondary to ethanol's inhibitory effect on magnesium resorption, combined with intestinal malabsorption of magnesium, make the chronic alcoholic prone to hypomagnesemia. Thiamine deficiency, usually secondary to poor nutrition, can lead to life-threatening lactic acidosis. Thiamine is a water-soluble nutrient with limited body stores: roughly a 10-day supply. Pyruvate, which is normally converted to acetyl coenzyme A using thiamine as a cofactor, is converted instead to lactate (18).

Perhaps the most commonly associated condition with long-term alcohol consumption is hepatic cirrhosis. Alcoholic liver injury can range from acute inflammation to steatosis to fibrotic cirrhosis. The complications of cirrhosis are more thoroughly discussed in Section VIII, Chapter 65, "Hepatic Failure and Cirrhosis." Two common emergency department presentations of alcohol-induced cirrhosis are variceal bleeding (although alcohol itself can also cause upper gastrointestinal bleeding from gastritis) and hepatic encephalopathy. Chronic alcohol abuse will also lead to chronic pancreatitis, although the pathophysiology of this disease is not at well understood (16). Current research debates whether chronic pancreatitis is a separate entity from acute pancreatitis, or is the cumulative result from recurrent acute episodes.

Nutritional deficiencies become important in patients who chronically substitute alcohol for a balanced diet. Most classically associated with chronic alcohol abuse is thiamine (vitamin B_1) deficiency, which leads to Wernicke-Korsakoff syndrome (23). Wernicke's encephalopathy is the triad of altered mental status, ataxia, and ophthalmoplegia. Progression will lead to the irreversible Korsakoff psychosis, characterized by memory impairment and confabulation. Chronic alcoholism is also linked to syndromes of vitamin B_{12} and folate deficiency.

Alcohol is also a direct cardiotoxin. "Holiday heart," resulting from binge drinking (often over a weekend or holiday), is a paroxysmal, usually atrial, dysrhythmia that represents an acute exacerbation of chronic cardiac toxicity and may be an early indication of ventricular dilation and interstitial fibrosis (24). Studies have demonstrated that patients with alcohol-induced atrial fibrillation are less likely to complain of palpitations than are patients with atrial fibrillation from another cause (24).

Chronic cardiomyopathy requires a relatively constant high intake of alcohol over an extended period. Studies have demonstrated that alcohol has direct toxic effects on skeletal and cardiac muscle. Chronic cardiomyopathy is associated with the ingestion of at least 90 g per day of absolute ethanol (approximately eight shots of hard liquor or eight bottles of beer) for 5 years (15). Cardiomyopathy usually lingers subclinically for years before presenting with acute decompensation. Asymptomatic cardiomyopathy is usually associated with ventricular wall dilation and thinning and diastolic dysfunction. Acute decompensation will present with signs and symptoms of congestive heart failure and systolic dysfunction (15).

Recent investigations have identified chronic alcohol abuse as a significant risk factor for development of acute respiratory distress syndrome. The mechanism of lung injury is not clear, but current research is focused on decreased levels of glutathione in the alveolar space associated with chronic alcohol exposure (13).

CLINICAL PRESENTATION

Clinical findings suggestive of alcohol abuse are listed in Table 279.1. An alcoholic who is still able to function socially or occupationally may present with chief complaints of memory difficulties, gastrointestinal (GI) dysfunction (including abdominal pain, diarrhea, vomiting, hematemesis, and hepatitis), respiratory complaints, frequent infections, weakness, polysubstance use, withdrawal, or recurrent trauma. Electrolyte imbalances (hypokalemia, hypomagnesemia, and hypocalcemia) are

TABLE 279.1. Clinical Manifestations of Alcohol Abuse

CNS	HEMATOLOGIC
Inebriation	Myelosuppression
Seizures	Coagulopathies
Dementia	Microcytic anemia
Coma	Megaloblastic anemia
Wernicke-Korsakoff psychosis	Thrombocytopenia
Polyneuropathy	
	INFECTIOUS
CV	
	Pneumonia
Autonomic dysfunction	Meningitis
Alcoholic congestive myopathy	Endocarditis
"Holiday heart"	Cellulitis
	Bacteremia
GI	Spontaneous bacterial peritonitis
Alcoholic hepatitis	
Alcoholic cirrhosis	**METABOLIC**
Peptic ulcer disease	
GI bleeding	Ketoacidosis
Pancreatitis	Electrolyte abnormalities
Pancreatic pseudocyst	Vitamin deficiencies
Varices and hemorrhoids	Hypothermia
Ascites	
Malabsorption and malnutrition	**MUSCULOSKELETAL**
Cancers of the GI tract	
	Myopathies
GU	Gout
	Rhabdomyolysis
Uric acid nephropathy	
Acute tubular necrosis	**PULMONARY**
Hepatorenal syndrome	
	Sleep apnea
BEHAVIORAL	Chronic respiratory insufficiency
	TB
Anxiety, insomnia	
Irrational behaviors	
Polysubstance abuse	
Sexual dysfunction	

more common in the chronic alcoholic, but may occur in the setting of acute intoxication as well (5,17).

Adolescents may present to the emergency department with myriad nonspecific complaints, none of which may directly point to alcohol abuse as a possible underlying etiology. Obtaining a history from family members can be invaluable. The adolescent may have recently undergone significant changes in personality, behavior, or peer contacts and peer relations. College-age alcoholics, who may use the emergency department as their only source of health care, can present with vague flu-like symptoms, headache, insomnia, chest palpitations, trauma, GI disturbances, or psychiatric complaints.

Young, otherwise healthy males presenting with chest palpitations, showing paroxysmal atrial fibrillation, atrial tachycardia, or frequent atrial extrasystoles, should be questioned regarding their history of ethanol use. Female alcoholics may present with symptoms of anxiety, increased fatigue, insomnia, depression, or irregular menses (19). Geriatric alcoholics may be brought to the department by their families with complaints of altered mental status, daytime sleepiness, and irrational behavior.

DIFFERENTIAL DIAGNOSIS

Because alcoholic patients may have myriad nonspecific complaints, they represent a complex diagnostic challenge. The indigent or homeless alcoholic may present as a marked contrast to the affluent alcoholic. There is the danger of the emergency physician developing negative attitudes toward the acutely intoxicated patient because of prior poor interactions. It is important not to overlook potentially lethal or devastating pathology by negatively stereotyping alcoholic patients.

Ethanol use can have serious deleterious effects on virtually all organ systems and tissues (10,12,24). The differential diagnosis can include hypoglycemia, sepsis, drug or other toxin exposures, carbon monoxide poisoning, Wernicke-Korsakoff syndrome, tumors, blunt trauma, meningitis, epidural or subdural hematoma, subarachnoid hemorrhage, dementia, and a host of others (5,10,19). There is always the danger that an alcoholic may ingest other, potentially lethal intoxicants such as isopropyl alcohol, methanol, ethylene glycol, alcohol-containing products (e.g., colognes, medicinal elixirs, and mouthwash), or drugs, particularly when deprived of access to ethanol.

EMERGENCY DEPARTMENT EVALUATION

The initial evaluation of the alcoholic is identical to the evaluation of any other potentially ill patient. Advanced cardiac life support measures should be instituted as needed. Obtain a full set of vital signs, including core temperature and oxygen saturation, and continuously monitor or frequently reevaluate them. The patient should be disrobed and carefully examined for signs of trauma. Signs of trauma may become apparent as the patient becomes less intoxicated.

Patients with abnormal vital signs and cardiorespiratory or nonspecific constitutional symptoms should have continuous electrocardiographic monitoring and a 12-lead electrocardiogram (ECG) to evaluate for ischemia and dysrhythmias (especially atrial arrhythmias). Those with altered mental status require a rapid bedside fingerstick blood glucose determination. Patients should also be evaluated for hematologic and metabolic abnormalities.

An alcoholic presenting with respiratory complaints or altered mental status should also be evaluated for pneumonia and tuberculosis. Chest radiography may be prudent even if signs of infection are absent. Complaints of vomiting or GI distress warrant an evaluation for gastritis, ulcers, esophageal varices,

TABLE 279.2. Laboratory and Radiographic Evaluation

LABORATORY	RADIOLOGIC
CBC	Chest radiograph
Cell counts for evaluation of marrow function	Pneumonitis
Indices for folate, iron, pyridoxine, B_{12} deficiencies	Aspiration
Electrolytes/BUN/creatinine/glucose	Tuberculosis
Anion gap	Pneumothorax
Hypoglycemia or hyperglycemia	Fractured ribs/trauma
Renal failure	Cardiac size
Electrolyte imbalance	Abdominal radiograph
Calcium/magnesium/phosphorus	Pancreatic calcifications
Hypocalcemia	Free air
Hypomagnesemia	Ileus
Hypophosphatemia	Limb radiograph
Hyperphosphatemia	Fractures
Coagulation profile	Dislocations
Hepatic insufficiency reflected in elevated PT and aPTT and abnormal liver function tests	Osteomyelitis
Arterial blood gas with co-oximeter	Foreign bodies
Hypoxemia	CT scan
Acid-base disturbances	Extraaxial hemorrhage
Carbon monoxide exposure	Intracerebral hemorrhage
Therapeutic drug monitoring	Intracerebral contusion
Anticonvulsant levels	Intraabdominal trauma
ECG	
Arrhythmia	
Evidence of electrolyte abnormalities	
Ischemia	
Osborn waves (hypothermia)	
Urinalysis	
Crystalluria	
Myoglobinuria	
Hemoglobinuria	
Liver function tests	
GGT elevation	
AST elevation	
ALT elevation	

electrolyte abnormalities, and pancreatitis. Table 279.2 summarizes some of the important aspects of the laboratory and radiologic assessment. When alcoholism is suspected, obtaining liver function tests and determining red cell mean corpuscular volume may be supportive in making the diagnosis.

Because alcohol intoxication can mimic as well as mask disease and injury, a blood or breath ethanol level should be obtained to assess the contribution of alcohol in all patients with systemic complaints. The serum ethanol level can be expected to fall by 10 to 30 mg/dL/hour, depending, in part, on individual variables and the timing of the ethanol ingestion, allowing the physician to estimate if or when the patient will be functionally (or legally) sober (1,6). In chronic alcoholics, sobriety typically occurs at blood levels of 100 to 300 mg/dL. Such levels may even be accompanied by signs and symptoms of withdrawal. Once meeting clinical criteria of sobriety, the patient may be safely discharged. If the patient fails to improve within a reasonable time, or if there is a disparity between the patient's clinical examination and their blood alcohol level, further investigation is mandatory in order to exclude occult head trauma or another severe comorbidity (5,7,10,12).

Chronic alcoholism, itself, can be difficult to diagnose. A number of laboratory abnormalities have been linked to chronic alcohol intake, but sensitivities and specificities vary from study to study. γ-Glutamyl transferase, the most sensitive indicator of hepatic injury, rises in patients who have had more than five drinks a day for several weeks. Also readily available is an ele-

vated mean red blood cell corpuscular volume. A carbohydrate-deficient transferrin test (if possible) is highly sensitive and specific for detecting alcohol abuse (11).

EMERGENCY DEPARTMENT MANAGEMENT

In the prehospital setting, the patient with altered mental status should receive 50 to 100 mL of 50% dextrose solution intravenously (or have a fingerstick blood sugar) and high-flow oxygen (or pulse oximetry to rule-out hypoxia). If opiate use is suspected, parenteral naloxone 0.1 mg to 2.0 mg may be indicated for respiratory depression. If trauma is suspected, full spinal immobilization may be required until the patient is sober and can cooperate with a thorough examination (10).

In the emergency department, chronic alcoholics, particularly those who are malnourished, should receive parenteral thiamine (100 mg) and intravenous hydration with an electrolyte solution containing glucose (e.g., D5NS or D5½NS), folate (1 mg), multiple (B complex) vitamins (1 ampule), and magnesium sulfate (2 g). Alternatively, they can be given fluids and vitamins orally. Those who are frequent emergency department patients do not need vitamins on every visit. Glucose supplementation, however, remains important, as many alcoholics have inadequate glycogen stores and will become hypoglycemic with stress (11).

Intoxicated patients frequently are uncooperative, belligerent, or violent. Judicious use of chemical and physical restraints may be necessary to protect emergency department staff and other patients. The risks associated with chemical or physical restraint are far outweighed by the benefit of controlled, thorough, serial examinations that can assess for subtle injury or pathology. Concomitant medical or surgical problems are treated through standard measures. Treatment of ethanol withdrawal (see Chapter 278, "Alcohol Withdrawal") may also be required.

CRITICAL INTERVENTIONS

- Obtain a fingerstick blood sugar on intoxicated patients with confusion or an altered level of consciousness
- Obtain a complete blood count (CBC), routine serum chemistries, liver function tests, ECG, chest X-ray, and head CT on patients with alcohol abuse or dependence who have unexplained constitutional complaints
- Administer thiamine, glucose, folate, multiple vitamins, and magnesium to patients with alcohol dependence who are potentially malnourished
- Advise or arrange for counseling or detoxification in patients with suspected alcohol abuse or dependence

DISPOSITION

The decision to admit or discharge the patient depends on the nature and severity of comorbid illness or injury as well as the patient's ability to care for him or herself. If the patient is admitted, the potential for ethanol withdrawal needs to be considered.

Legal precedents suggest that the patient can be discharged when no longer clinically intoxicated, although no specific criteria exist to determine clinical sobriety. In the United States, per se laws define "driving under the influence" as a breath or whole blood alcohol level of 0.08 g%, equivalent to a serum ethanol of 94 mg/dl. Observing an alcoholic until his or her blood level is below this limit risks iatrogenic withdrawal. In general, if a patient is functionally sober and demonstrates no signs of injury or comorbidity, he or she can be safely discharged. It is important, as always, to accurately document relevant aspects of the physical and neurologic examination on the patient's chart.

The inebriated patient who wishes to leave the emergency department against medical advice (either before or after evaluation and treatment) should be considered analogous to a patient with altered mental status who requests discharge. It is the emergency department's responsibility to protect patients who do not have the capacity to make competent decisions for themselves. Documentation of a blood ethanol level greater than the per se limit offers support for the emergency physician's decision that the patient was not competent. Psychiatric consultation may also be helpful if there is any question concerning the patient's competency. When in doubt, it is prudent to err on the side of safety by holding the patient in the emergency department.

Prior to discharge, the patient should be offered any available social assistance, and arrangements should be made for medical followup. Patients should be offered medical detoxification or an appropriate referral, and such arrangements and discussions should be documented on the patient's chart.

COMMON PITFALLS

✔ Failure to consider the possibility of alcohol abuse and dependence in adolescents, the elderly, and those of medium or high socioeconomic status

✔ Failure to appreciate that altered mental status in an intoxicated patient may be caused by something other than ethanol intoxication

✔ Failure to consider the possibility of a concomitant psychiatric disorder

✔ Failure to obtain a complete set of vital signs and to fully undress and examine the alcoholic patient

✔ Failure to evaluate the alcoholic with constitutional symptoms for metabolic abnormalities and occult infection

✔ Failure to reevaluate the patient frequently and prior to discharge, and to document the findings

Acknowledgment

Thank you to previous edition chapter author Thomas A. Brunell.

References

1. Brennan DF, et al. Ethanol elimination rates in an ED population. *Am J Emerg Med* 1995;13:276–280.
2. Brown C. Alcohol. *Ann Emerg Med* 1986;15:989.
3. Diagnostic and Statistical Manual IV. The American Psychiatric Association.
4. Enoch M, Goldman D. Problem drinking and alcoholism: diagnosis and treatment. *Am Fam Phys* 2002;65:441–448.
5. Gentilello LM, Donovan DM, Dunn CW, et al. Alcohol interventions in trauma centers: current practice and future directions. *JAMA* 1995;274:1043–1048.
6. Gershman H, Steeper J. Rate of clearance of ethanol from the blood of intoxicated patients in the emergency department. *J Emerg Med* 1991;9:307–311.
7. Gibb K. Serum alcohol levels, toxicology screens, and use of the breath alcohol analyzer. *Ann Emerg Med* 1986;15:349.
8. Kitchens JM. Does this patient have an alcohol problem? *JAMA* 1994;273:1782.
9. Lewinsohn PM, Rohde P, Seeley JR. Alcohol consumption in high school adolescents: frequency of use and dimensional structure of associated problems. *Addiction* 1996;91:375–390.
10. Lieber CS. Medical disorders of alcoholism. *N Engl J Med* 1995;333:1058–1065.
11. Lieber CS. Microsomal ethanol-oxidizing system (MEOS): the first 30 years (1968–1998)—a review. *Alcohol Clin Exp Res* 1999;23:991–1007.
12. Martinez R. Alcoholism and society. *Emerg Med Clin North Am* 1990;8:904–909.
13. Moss M, Burnham EL. Chronic alcohol abuse, acute respiratory distress syndrome, and multiple organ dysfunction. *Crit Care Med* 2003;31[4 Suppl]:S207–212.
14. O'Connor PG, Schottenfeld RS. Patients with alcohol problems. *N Engl J Med* 1998;338:592–602.
15. Piano MR. Alcoholic cardiomyopathy: incidence, clinical characteristics, and pathophysiology. *Chest* 2002;121:1638–1650.
16. Pitchumoni CS. Pathogenesis of alcohol-induced chronic pancreatitis: facts, perceptions, and misperceptions. *Surg Clin North Am* 2001;81:379–390.
17. Ragland G. Electrolyte abnormalities in the alcoholic patient. *Emerg Med Clin North Am* 1990;8:761–773.
18. Romanski SA, McMahon MM. Metabolic acidosis and thiamine deficiency. *Mayo Clin Proc* 1999;74:259–263.
19. Ross SM, Chappel JN. Diagnostic dilemmas. Part II: substance use disorders—difficulties in diagnoses. *Psychiatr Clin North Am* 1998;21:803–828.
20. Samet J, Rollnick S, Barnes H. Beyond CAGE: a brief clinical approach after detection of substance abuse. *Arch Intern Med* 1996;156:2287–2293.
21. Sattar SP, Petty F, Burke WJ. Diagnosis and treatment of alcohol dependence in older alcoholics. *Clin Geriatr Med* 2003;19:743.
22. Schermer CR, Gentilello LM, et al. National survey of trauma surgeons' use of alcohol screening and brief intervention. *J Trauma* 2003;55:849–856.
23. Thomson AD, Cook CC, Touqet R, Henry JA. The Royal College of Physicians report on alcohol: guidelines for managing Wernicke's encephalopathy in the accident and emergency department. *Alcohol* 2002;37:513–521.
24. Urbano-Marquez A, Estruch R, Navarro-Lopez F, et al. The effects of alcoholism on skeletal and cardiac muscle. *N Engl J Med* 1989;320:409–415.
25. Whiteman PJ, Cerinich M, Hoffman RS, et al. Alcoholism in the emergency department: an epidemiologic study [abstract]. *Vet Hum Toxicol* 1994;36:350.

APPENDIX

TABLE 279.A1.   CAGE Questionnaire[a]

1. Have you felt you should **C**ut down on your drinking?
2. Have people **A**nnoyed you by criticizing your drinking?
3. Have you felt bad or **G**uilty about your drinking?
4. Have you ever had a drink first thing in the morning to steady your nerves or get rid of a hangover (**E**ye-opener)?

[a] Positive answers to two or more questions indicate a high likelihood of alcoholism.

TABLE 279.A2.   TACE Questionnaire[a]

T How many drinks does it **take** to get you high? (More than two suggests tolerance)
A Have people **annoyed** you by criticizing your drinking?
C Have you ever felt you ought to **cut down** on your drinking?
E Have you ever had a drink first thing in the morning to steady your nerves? (**eye-opener**)

[a] Positive test (a score ≥1) identifies at-risk drinking in pregnant women.

TABLE 279.A3.   Michigan Alcoholism Screening Test (MAST)

No.	Points	Question
1	2	*Do you feel you are a normal drinker?
2	2	Have you ever awakened the morning after some drinking the night before and found that you could not remember a part of the evening before?
3	1	*Does your spouse or parents ever worry or complain about your drinking?
4	2	Can you stop drinking without a struggle after one or two drinks?
5	1	*Do you ever feel bad about your drinking?
6	2	*Do friends or relatives think you are a normal drinker?
7	2	*Are you always able to stop drinking when you want to?
8	5	*Have you ever attended a meeting of Alcoholics Anonymous?
9	1	Have you gotten into fights when drinking?
10	2	*Has drinking ever created problems with you and your spouse?
11	2	Has your spouse or other family member ever gone to anyone for help about your drinking?
12	2	Have you ever lost friends or girlfriends/boyfriends because of your drinking?
13	2	*Have you ever gotten into trouble at work because of drinking?
14	2	Have you ever lost a job because of drinking?
15	2	*Have you ever neglected your obligations, your family, or your work for 2 or more days in a row because you were drinking?
16	1	Do you ever drink before noon?
17	2	Have you ever been told you have liver trouble? Cirrhosis?
18	2	Have you ever had delirium tremens (DTs), severe shaking, heard voices, or seen things that weren't there after heavy drinking?
19	5	*Have you ever gone to anyone for help about your drinking?
20	5	*Have you ever been in a hospital because of your drinking?
21	2	Have you ever been a patient in a psychiatric hospital or on a psychiatric ward of a general hospital where drinking was part of the problem?
22	2	Have you ever been seen at a psychiatric or mental health clinic or gone to a doctor, social worker, or clergyman for help with an emotional problem in which drinking had played a part?
23	2	*Have you ever been arrested, even for a few hours, because of drunk behavior?
24	2	*Have you ever been arrested for drunk driving or driving after drinking?

*These questions are included in the short form of the MAST
0–3 points   Not alcohol-dependent
4–5 points   Probably alcohol-dependent
>5 points   Definitely alcohol-dependent

TABLE 279.A4. SADD Questionnaire

1. Do you find difficulty in getting the thought of a drink out of your mind?
2. Is getting drunk more important than your next meal?
3. Do you plan your day around when and where you can drink?
4. Do you drink in the morning, afternoon, and evening?
5. Do you drink for the effect of alcohol without caring what the drink is?
6. Do you drink as much as you want no matter what you are doing the next day?
7. Given that many problems might be caused by alcohol, do you still drink too much?
8. Do you know that you won't be able to stop drinking once you start?
9. Do you try to control your drinking by giving it up completely for days or weeks at a time?
10. The morning after a heavy drinking session, do you need your first drink to get yourself going?
11. The morning after a heavy drinking session, do you wake up with a definite shakiness in your hands?
12. After a heavy drinking session, do you wake up and retch or vomit?
13. The morning after a heavy drinking session, do you go out of your way to avoid people?
14. After a heavy drinking session, do you see frightening things that you later realize were imaginary?
15. Do you go drinking and the next day find that you have forgotten what happened the night before?

Questions are answered with never (0 points), sometimes (1 point), often (2 points), and nearly always (3 points). The point total is utilized to guide treatment.
From Gentilello LM, Donovan DM, Dunn CW, et al. Alcohol interventions in trauma centers: current practice and future directions. *JAMA* 1995;274(13):1043–1048.

TABLE 279.A5. The Ten-Item AUDIT Questionnaire

1. How often do you have a drink containing alcohol?
2. How many drinks do you have on a typical day when you are drinking?
3. How often do you have 6 or more drinks on one occasion?
4. How often during the last year have you found that you were not able to stop drinking once you had started?
5. How often during the last year have you failed to do what was normally expected from you because of drinking?
6. How often during the last year have you needed a first drink in the morning to get yourself going after a heavy drinking session?
7. How often during the last year have you had a feeling of guilt or remorse after drinking?
8. How often during the last year have you been unable to remember what happened the night before because you had been drinking?
9. Have you or someone else been injured as a result of your drinking?
10. Has a relative or friend or a doctor or other health worker been concerned about your drinking or suggested you cut down?

Questions are answered and scored on a 0- to 4-point scale, and the total is used as a guideline for therapy.
From Saunder JB, Aasland OG, Babor TF, et al. Development of the Alcohol Use Disorders Identification Test (AUDIT): WHO Collaborative Project on Early Detection of Persons with Harmful Alcohol Consumption-II, 1194. *Addiction* 1993;88:791–804.

Analgesics and Related Conditions

CHAPTER 280
Acetaminophen

Jeffrey Brent and Robert Palmer

Acetaminophen (*N*-acetyl-p-aminophenol, or APAP) is the most commonly used analgesic/antipyretic in the world. Given its widespread availability, poisoning with acetaminophen is commonplace. Because many lay people underestimate its toxicity, suicide gestures may result in actual suicides. In 2002, over 119,000 potential APAP poisonings and 285 deaths as a result of acetaminophen alone and in combination with other agents were reported to U.S. poison centers. These figures represent only a fraction of the total number of incidents.

Acetaminophen itself has a very low intrinsic toxicity. It is almost entirely metabolized in the liver by the pathways shown in Fig. 280.1. About 94% of an ingested dose of APAP is metabolized to the nontoxic glucuronide (52%) or sulfate (42%) conjugates which are excreted in the urine (11). Of the remaining 6% of the dose, about half is excreted unchanged in the urine and a similar amount undergoes oxidative metabolism primarily by the 2E1 isozyme of the hepatic P-450 system (CYP2E1) to form a highly reactive intermediate, *N*-acetyl-para-benzoquinoneimine (NAPQI) (11,13). With therapeutic APAP dosing, the small amount of NAPQI produced is rapidly conjugated by glutathione and excreted as the nontoxic mercapturate conjugate plus other minor metabolites (11,21). Toxicity occurs when hepatic glutathione stores are depleted by about 70%, which renders the hepatocytes vulnerable to the effects of NAPQI (7,11). In the setting of inadequate glutathione stores, NAPQI is conjugated by hepatic macromolecules resulting in hepatocyte death. Histologically, necrosis occurs at centrilobular (zone III; perivenular) portions of the hepatic lobule (9). The histologic specificity of APAP-induced hepatic damage is a result of the highest concentrations of CYP2E1 being present in the centrilobular portion of the lobule.

Although the clinical picture of APAP overdose is predominantly one of hepatotoxicity, some patients also have nephrotoxicity (24). Rarely, renal damage has been reported to occur in the absence of substantial hepatotoxicity. The nephrotoxicity is most likely a result of renal APAP biotransformation to the toxic NAPQI metabolite by renal CYP2E1. Additionally, renal failure is an occasional concomitant complication of severe APAP-induced hepatotoxicity as a result of the hepatorenal syndrome.

CLINICAL PRESENTATION

The evolution of APAP toxicity can be divided into four sequential stages (Table 280.1). The first stage of APAP poisoning is a relatively subtle period characterized by nausea, vomiting, and general malaise. In this phase, sometimes referred to as phase I, APAP is being absorbed and metabolized and glutathione stores are being consumed. Although hepatotoxicity is beginning, it will often not be apparent clinically or in laboratory results. Phase I typically lasts less than 24 hours. Interventions to blunt the evolving hepatotoxicity are most effective during this early phase and are almost 100% effective in preventing hepatotoxicity if initiated within 8 hours of ingestion.

The second phase is entirely different. During this period, the onset of which is usually late on the day of the ingestion, some resolution of the gastrointestinal effects of phase I is seen and low or nondetectable concentrations of APAP are found in the plasma. The hepatotoxic effects of NAPQI, which has not been inactivated by glutathione, begin to manifest during this time and the predominant clinical picture becomes one of hepatotoxicity from hepatocellular destruction. As toxicity evolves cholestatic features may occur. However primary cholestatic injury is not caused by APAP.

Phase III of acetaminophen toxicity is the reported time of maximum hepatotoxicity. During this phase, transaminases will peak and then decline but effects on coagulation may worsen. Patients who present in stage II or III may have right upper quadrant pain, nausea, vomiting, jaundice, bleeding, encephalopathy, and symptoms of fulminant hepatic failure. Associated with this is a progressive increase in bilirubin, alanine aminotransferase (ALT), and aspartate aminotransferase (AST) levels, and prothrombin time. The magnitude of these liver function abnormalities can be dramatic with ALT and AST levels of 10,000 to 20,000 IU/L frequently seen. In most cases, these abnormalities peak in 48 to 96 hours (stage III) and gradually resolve.

In the final phase (IV), there will be either recovery or fulminant hepatic failure. The occasional patient with severe, untreated APAP toxicity exhibits a pattern of rising prothrombin time and bilirubin and ammonia levels as the AST and ALT decline. This pattern signifies fulminant hepatic failure. However, most patients, even those with severe hepatotoxicity, eventually recover, with normal livers. It is not expected that patients who recover from APAP hepatotoxicity will suffer any residual liver abnormalities.

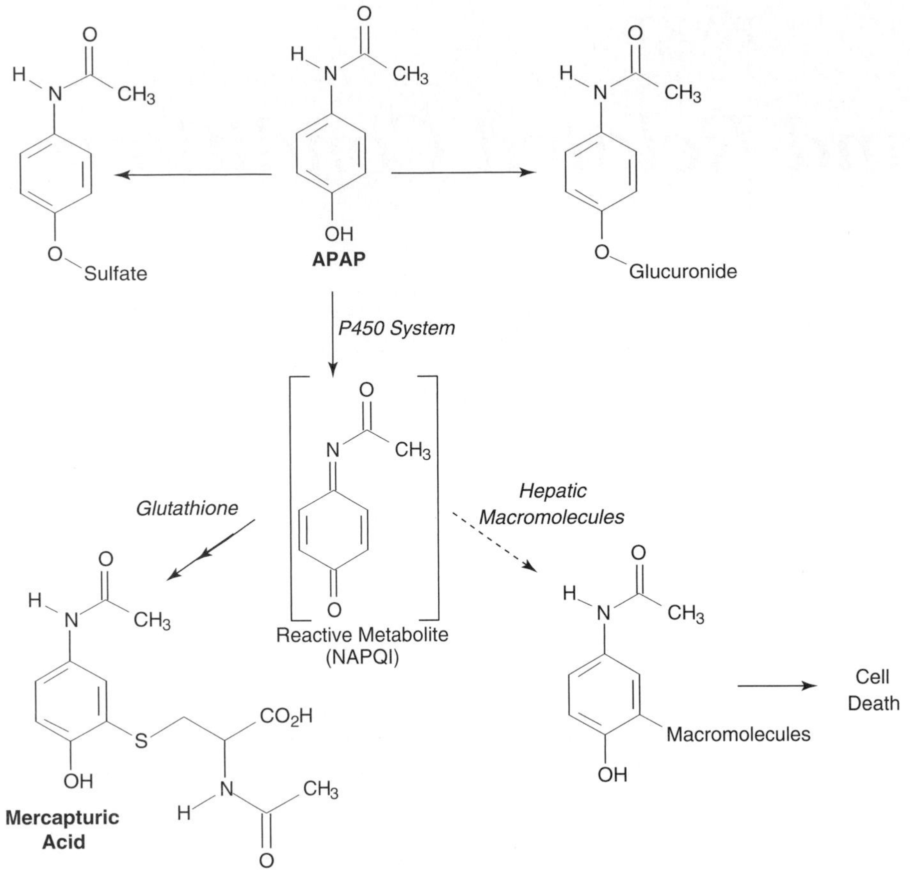

Figure 280.1. Metabolic pathways for acetaminophen metabolism.

The relationship between the plasma concentration of APAP, the time after ingestion, and the potential for toxicity is described by the nomogram developed by Rumack and Matthew (Fig. 280.2) (16). The nomogram stratifies patients into risk categories of "probable" or "possible" hepatotoxicity. Its utility was confirmed in a national multicenter study (23). Toxicity has not been demonstrated to occur in the "possible risk" area, which represents a 25% margin of safety to account for possible errors in establishing the time of ingestion, and is traditionally considered an indication for antidotal treatment in the United States. In most other countries, treatment is given only when the APAP level is in the probable toxicity area. The practice of treating patients with possibly toxic APAP levels has been questioned (1)

and some toxicologists and poison centers in the United States are now treating otherwise healthy patients only if the level falls in the probable toxicity area of the nomogram.

The nomogram begins at 4 hours after ingestion and extends to 24 hours. Plasma APAP concentrations determined obtained before this time—during the absorption and distribution phases—are difficult to interpret. However, early APAP concentrations of less than 100 µg/mL suggest a lack of toxicity risk (7). The nomogram cannot be used to assess potential toxicity of plasma concentrations obtained beyond 24 hours from the ingestion. Both nomogram lines have a slope equivalent to a 4-hour half-life. By remembering that they start at 150 and 200 ug/mL, the level at each subsequent 4-hour time can be calculated by dividing the previous one by two.

The APAP nomogram is based on presenting plasma concentrations. Repeat levels offer no further useful information and should not be routinely obtained. Although this has been recommended for delayed release APAP overdose (e.g., Tylenol Extended-Relief, Tylenol Arthritis Pain), the value of this practice for determining risk of hepatotoxicity has been studied only in a very small case series (5). Based on the known volume of distribution of APAP of 0.9 to 1.0 L/kg, an ingestion of 10.5 g APAP in a 70-kg adult, or 150 mg/kg in a child, may cause toxic concentrations. The current nomogram is derived solely from adult cases. Children with toxic plasma levels appear to be less susceptible to APAP toxicity than are adults (18). Because there have been no reported cases of APAP-induced hepatotoxicity in infants following a single overdose, the utility of the nomogram in this population is unknown and some toxicologists and poison centers do not routinely treat such infants.

Patients who have ingested a potentially toxic dose of APAP and have a history of alcoholism, chronic liver disease, or malnutrition may be more susceptible to APAP hepatotoxicity because of decreased glutathione stores. Conversely, patients with

TABLE 280.1. Stages in the Clinical Course of Acetaminophen Toxicity

Stage	Time after Ingestion	Characteristics
I	$1/2$–24 h	Anorexia, nausea, vomiting, malaise, pallor, diaphoresis
II	24–48 h	Resolution of above; right upper quadrant abdominal pain and tenderness; elevated bilirubin, prothrombin time, hepatic enzymes; oliguria
III	72–96 h	Peak liver function abnormalities; anorexia, nausea, vomiting, malaise may reappear
IV	4 d–2 wk	Resolution of hepatic dysfunction or fulminant hepatic failure

Modified from Linden CH, Rumack BH. Acetaminophen Overdose. *Emerg Med Clin North Am* 1984;2:103.

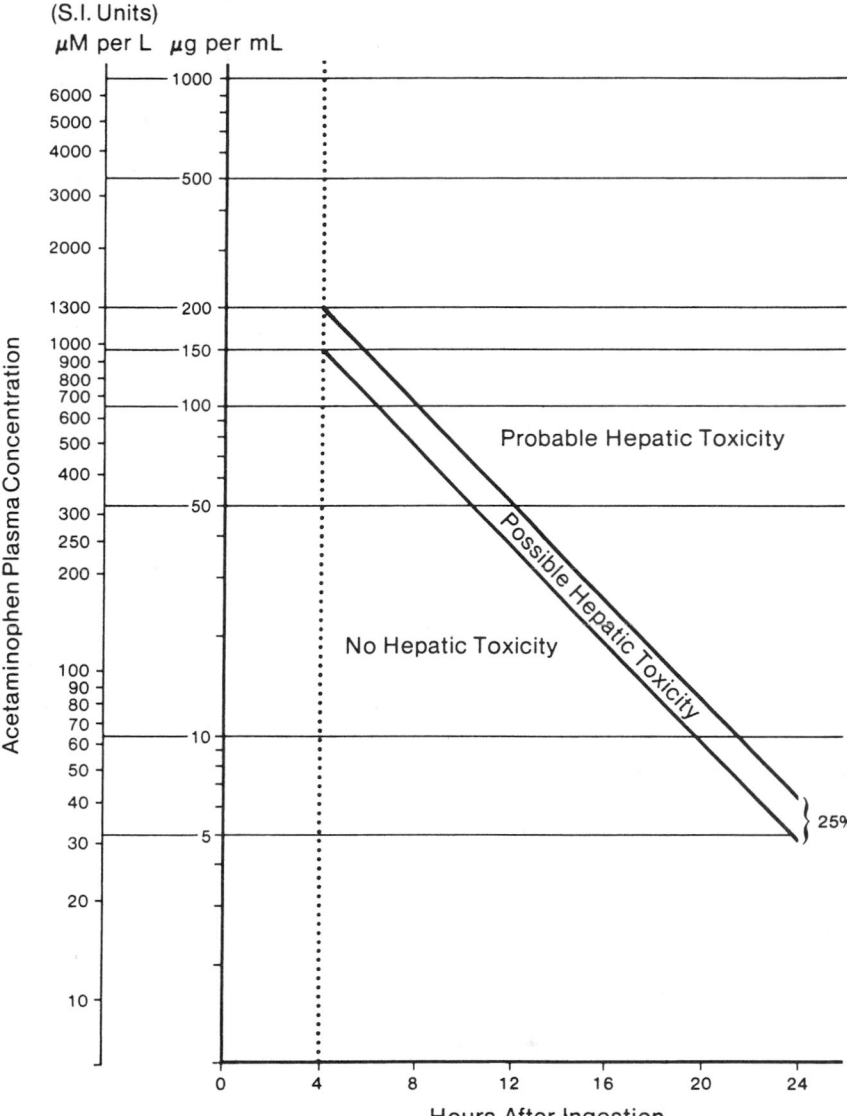

Figure 280.2. Rumack–Matthew nomogram for acetaminophen poisoning. Relation between plasma APAP levels and toxicity correlated with time after exposure. (From Rumack BH. *Pediatr Clin North Am* 1986;33 : 691, with permission.)

cirrhotic liver disease, and, consequently, poorly functioning cytochrome P450 enzyme systems may be relatively protected because of inability to generate the toxic metabolite. Nonetheless, in acute overdose, these patients should also be evaluated using the standard nomogram. Ethanol is an inducer of CYP2E1, the enzyme responsible for generation of the toxic metabolite. Alcoholics without liver disease, who have both induced CYP2E1 systems and depressed hepatic glutathione stores, may be more susceptible to the hepatotoxic effects of APAP in overdose. The same situation may occur in patients with acute illnesses associated with poor oral food intake (e.g., acute starvation). However, given the large therapeutic index for APAP, these populations are not expected to be at enhanced risk for hepatotoxicity with normal therapeutic doses.

DIFFERENTIAL DIAGNOSIS

In the earliest stage of APAP poisoning, the diagnosis is made by a history suggestive of overdose. No consistently reliable or pathognomonic signs or symptoms can be expected. Therefore, the physician must consider the possibility of occult APAP poisoning when confronted with any overdose or chronic pain patient. The finding of any APAP in the plasma must alert the clinician to the possibility of a toxic APAP ingestion.

The patient who presents in stage II, III, or IV of APAP toxicity is another kind of diagnostic challenge. By this time, there may be little or no detectable APAP in the serum, so the diagnosis depends on the history and clinical suspicion.

The differential diagnosis of hepatic injury includes most commonly, viral, autoimmune or chemical etiologies. Virtually any drug can cause hepatotoxicity as an idiosyncratic reaction. The correct diagnosis requires an astute history supplemented by laboratory studies. One particularly difficult diagnostic quandary is distinguishing between Reye's syndrome and APAP toxicity in the child given acetaminophen for an antecedent viral syndrome. The chemistry profiles typically seen with the different types of hepatitis are shown in Table 280.2. As shown in Fig. 280.3, liver function test results may not rise dramatically until a day after the ingestion, although LFT elevations are often seen within the first day (20).

EMERGENCY DEPARTMENT EVALUATION

The amount, formulation, and time(s) of APAP or other drug ingestion should be noted. The history should address acute or chronic alcohol use, preexisting liver disease, and chronic malnutrition or acute starvation. The physical exam should focus

TABLE 280.2.   Laboratory Values in the Common Acute Hepatitides:
Viral, Alcoholic, Acetaminophen

Hepatotoxin	Acute Viral Studies	AST (IU/L)	AST (IU/L)
Viral	Usually positive	Hundreds to low thousands	Variable but less than AST
Alcohol	Negative	Usually <300 or 10 × normal	Usually 100 and ALT/AST >2
APAP	Negative	May be very high	Much less than AST

AST, aspartate aminotransferase; ALT, alanine aminotransferase.

on the vital signs and assessment of cardiovascular, gastrointestinal, and neurological function and hydration status. An APAP level should be obtained and compared to the nomogram. If the level is potentially toxic or the time of ingestion is unknown and APAP is present, baseline liver function tests (AST, ALT, and total bilirubin levels and prothrombin time) and renal function tests (plasma urea nitrogen and creatinine concentrations and urinalysis) should be obtained.

EMERGENCY DEPARTMENT MANAGEMENT

Advanced life-support measures should be provided if necessary (e.g., for coingested agents). Intravenous fluids may be required for patients with vomiting and dehydration. Treatment of acute APAP overdose is directed toward preventing absorption and administering *N*-acetylcysteine (NAC) when indicated. Although the common and preferred method of gastric decontamination is activated charcoal (AC), the efficacy of this procedure for altering clinical course or outcome has not been firmly established. There is evidence that early administration of single dose of AC, if given within 2 hours after ingestion may decrease measured plasma APAP concentrations, the single metric relied on for the determination of the need for therapy (3). Thus, it is advisable to administer AC it can be done within 2 hours of ingestion.

Although charcoal binds NAC, charcoal therapy does not have a clinically significant effect on plasma NAC concentrations. Therefore, it is unnecessary to increase the NAC dose when the patient is receiving both of these therapies (2). However, charcoal and NAC should not be mixed together before administra-

tion. The routine use of gastric emptying, by syrup of ipecac or lavage, has little role and should be avoided.

The most effective treatment for patients with a potentially toxic APAP level is NAC (3,15,17,22,23). NAC is metabolized by hepatocytes to cysteine, a precursor of glutathione. NAC also enhances APAP sulfation, potentially leaving less APAP available to the hepatic P450 system (see Fig. 280.1). NAC therapy is almost 100% effective in preventing APAP toxicity if it is started within 8 hours of the ingestion, independent of the plasma APAP concentration (23). Delay in starting therapy beyond this time results in a progressive diminution of its effectiveness (17,23). If a plasma APAP concentration is unavailable by 8 hours after ingestion, a history (or suspicion) of APAP overdose is sufficient to warrant the initiation of NAC therapy until the plasma APAP levels are known. If APAP is present and the time of ingestion is unknown or liver function tests are abnormal and possibly as a result of APAP poisoning, NAC therapy should be instituted regardless of the APAP level.

Three protocols have been used for the treatment of APAP overdose (see Table 280.3). It is now common practice to treat patients with NAC until plasma APAP concentrations are undetectable and to discontinue therapy at that time if transaminase levels and prothrombin time remain normal or are falling and approaching normal values (6). The duration of NAC therapy by this method is frequently less than 48 hours, although the doses and dosing frequency are the same.

Intravenous NAC has long been the standard therapy outside the United States. It was finally approved for use in the United States in 2004. Even before formal approval, many U.S. toxicologists and poison centers were giving oral NAC intravenously and considered it to be first-line therapy (8,14). Although NAC given intravenously is easier to administer than oral NAC, intravenous administration is associated with a relatively high (up to 20%) incidence of anaphylactoid reactions (primary itching and rash but also bronchospasm and hypotension). Debate continues regarding which route and dosing protocol is the most effective, cost-effective, and favorable in terms of risk-benefit profile (4).

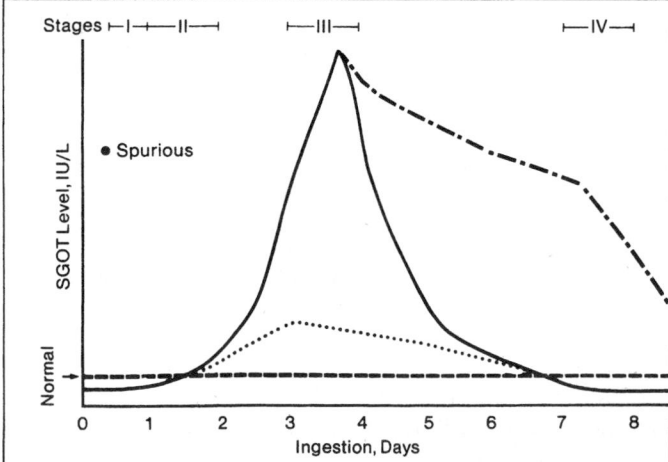

Figure 280.3. *Dotted line:* the course of those who received acetylcysteine. *Solid line:* those with natural a course. *Dotted–dashed line:* those with a severe course. (From Rumack BH, et al. Acetaminophen overdose. *Arch Intern Med* 1981;141:380, with permission.)

TABLE 280.3.   Protocols for *N*-Acetylcysteine Administration

Route of Administration	Loading Dose	Subsequent Doses	FDA Approved
Oral	140 mg/kg	70 mg/kg q4h	Yes
Intravenous	150 mg/kg over 30 minutes	50 mg/kg over 4 hours, followed by 100 mg/kg over 16 hours	Yes
Intravenous	140 mg/kg over 30 minutes	70 mg/kg q4h	No

TABLE 280.4. Transplantation Criteria for Patients with APAP-Induced Fulminant Hepatic Failure

---

- Arterial pH < 7.25–7.30 after adequate fluid resuscitation
  OR all of the following
- Prothrombin time of >100–180 seconds, and
- Serum creatinine >3.4 mg/dL, and
- Grade III–IV encephalopathy

Giving oral NAC can be challenging. Because it tastes and smells like rotten eggs, it is poorly tolerated. Emesis after NAC ingestion is common; if it occurs within an hour of the dose, the dose should be repeated in full. NAC is available as the mucolytic agent Mucomyst in a 10% or 20% solution. Before administration, it should be diluted to 5% in a soft drink to increase its palatability. It is also helpful to have the patient drink it through a straw from a closed container to prevent the unpleasant vapors from causing emesis. Adding ice is helpful as it will decrease the vapor pressure of NAC. If emesis occurs during NAC administration, standard antiemetics such as metoclopramide (Reglan; 0.1–1.0 mg/kg), promethazine (Phenergan; 12.5–25 mg i.v.), ondansetron (Zofran, 0.15 mg/kg i.v.) or another 5HT$_3$ antagonist (e.g., granisetron, dolasetron) may be given and repeated as necessary. If emesis continues, it is best to switch to i.v. administration to assure adequate and timely therapy. Increases in hepatic transaminase may rarely occur with ondansetron, which can obscure the assessment of APAP hepatotoxicity.

APAP crosses the placenta, so when a pregnant patient overdoses on APAP, fetal hepatotoxicity is possible. However, NAC also appears to cross the placenta (10). If spontaneous delivery occurs while the mother is being treated, NAC could be given to the newborn. However, the necessity for NAC administration to the neonate has not been established because their immature P450 system may not cause significant quantities of NAPQI to be formed.

A particularly perplexing group of patients are those who have taken a potentially toxic cumulative amount of APAP but have done so by ingesting multiple excessive doses over a period of time (19). One approach is to treat for potential APAP toxicity if the patient has ingested more than 10.5 g or 150 mg/kg during the preceding 24 hours and has an APAP level above the therapeutic range or detectable APAP and elevated transaminase levels. All patients with a potentially toxic plasma APAP level based on the time since the last dose should be treated with NAC.

The management of patients with APAP-induced hepatic or renal failure consists of NAC and supportive care (12). Patients who appear to have fulminant hepatic failure may be candidates for transplantation. However, transplantation should not be done simply on the basis of an elevated transaminase level, because this does not portend a poor prognosis. The single best indicator of a poor outcome is increasing prothrombin time. The most commonly used transplantation criteria are given in Table 280.4.

CRITICAL INTERVENTIONS

- Obtain a serum APAP level on all patients with a known or suspected drug overdose or hepatotoxicity of unknown cause
- Administer NAC if the APAP level is potentially toxic by the nomogram, if APAP is present and the time of an acute overdose is unknown, and if the APAP level is elevated or liver function tests are abnormal after chronic excessive dosing

---

DISPOSITION

Any patient who has a potentially toxic APAP level by the nomogram requires admission and treatment. Patients who present more than 24 hours after acute APAP ingestion or who have taken repeated supratherapeutic doses and have abnormal liver function test results, should receive NAC therapy until the hepatotoxicity resolves (12). A toxicologist or poison center should be consulted regarding the evaluation and treatment of patients with other presentations. All intentional overdose patients should a psychiatric evaluation before discharge.

COMMON PITFALLS

✔ Failure to consider an occult APAP overdose in all patients with intentional overdose, chronic pain, or unexplained hepatitis

✔ Withholding AC because of concern about its effect on NAC therapy

✔ Delaying NAC treatment beyond 8 to 10 hours while waiting for APAP levels and not starting NAC therapy in the emergency department when indicated

✔ Failure to appreciate that NAC has beneficial effects in patients with hepatotoxicity

References

1. Brandwene E, Williams SR, Tunget-Johnson C, et al. Refining the level of anticipated hepatotoxicity in acetaminophen poisoning. *J Emerg Med* 1996;14:691–695.
2. Brent J. Are activated charcoal/N-acetylcysteine interactions of clinical significance? *Ann Emerg Med* 1993;22:1860.
3. Buckley NA, Whyte IM, O'Connell DL, et al. Activated charcoal reduces the need for n-acetylcysteine treatment after acetaminophen (paracetamol) overdose. *J Toxicol Clin Toxicol* 1999;37:753–757.
4. Buckley NA, Whyte IM, O'Connell DL, et al. Oral or intravenous N-acetylcysteine: which is the treatment of choice for acetaminophen (paracetamol) poisoning? *J Toxicol Clin Toxicol* 1999;37:759–767.
5. Cetaruk E, Dart RC, Hurlbut KM, et al. Tylenol extended relief overdose. *Ann Emerg Med* 1997;30:104–108.
6. Clark D, Ruck B, Jennis T, et al. Compliance with PCC recommendations: discontinuation of NAC. *J Toxicol Clin Toxicol* 2001;39:485.
7. Douglas DR, Smilkstein MJ, Rumack BH. APAP levels within 4 hours: are they useful? *Vet Hum Toxicol* 1994;36:350.
8. Falk JL. Oral N-acetylcysteine given intravenously for acetaminophen overdose: we shouldn't have to, but we must. *Crit Care Med* 1998;26:7.
9. James O, Roberts SH, Douglas AP, et al. Liver damage after paracetamol overdose: comparison of liver function tests, testing serum bile acids, and liver histology. *Lancet* 1975;2:579.
10. Johnson D, Simone C, Koren G. Transfer of N-acetylcysteine by the human placenta. *Vet Hum Toxicol* 1993;35:365.
11. Jollow DG, Thorgelrsson SS, Potter WZ, et al. Acetaminophen-induced hepatic necrosis. IV. Metabolic disposition of toxic and nontoxic doses of acetaminophen. *Pharmacology* 1974;12:251–71.
12. Keays R, Harrison PM, Wendon JA, et al. Intravenous acetylcysteine in paracetamol-induced fulminant hepatic failure: a prospective controlled trial. *BMJ* 1991;303:1026.
13. Mitchell JR, Jollow DJ, Potter WZ, et al. Acetaminophen-induced hepatic necrosis. I. Role of drug metabolism. *J Pharmacol Exp Ther* 1973;187:185.
14. Perry HE, Shannon MW. Efficacy of oral versus intravenous N-acetylcysteine in acetaminophen overdose: results of an open-label, clinical trial. *J Pediatr* 1998;132:149–152.
15. Prescott LF, Illingworth RN, Critchley JAJH, et al. Intravenous N-acetylcysteine: the treatment of choice for paracetamol poisoning. *BMJ* 1979;2:1097.
16. Rumack BH, Matthew II. Acetaminophen poisoning and toxicity. *Pediatrics* 1975;55:871.
17. Rumack BH, Peterson RG, Koch GC, et al. Acetaminophen overdose: 662 cases with evaluation of oral acetylcysteine treatment. *Arch Intern Med* 1981;141:380.
18. Rumack BH. Acetaminophen overdose in young children; treatment and effects of alcohol and other additional ingestants in 417 cases. *Am J Dis Children* 1984;138:428.
19. Schiodt FV, Rochling FA, Casey DL, et al. Acetaminophen toxicity in an urban county hospital. *N Engl J Med* 1997;337:1112–1127.
20. Singer AJ, Carracio TR, Mofenson HC. The temporal profile of increased transaminase levels in patients with acetaminophen-induced liver dysfunction. *Ann Emerg Med* 1995;26:49–54.

21. Slattery JT, Knapp JR, Levy G. Acetaminophen pharmacokinetics after over-dose. *J Toxicol Clin Toxicol* 1981;18:111.
22. Smilkstein MJ, Bronstein AC, Linden C, et al. Acetaminophen overdose: a 48-hour intravenous N-acetylcysteine treatment protocol. *Ann Emerg Med* 1991;20:1058.
23. Smilkstein MJ, Knapp GL, Kulig KW, et al. Efficacy of oral N-acetylcysteine in the treatment of acetaminophen overdose. Analysis of the national multicenter study (1976–1985). *N Engl J Med* 1988;319:1557.
24. Wilkinson SP, Moodle H, Arrogo VA, et al. Frequency of renal impairment in paracetamol overdose compared with other causes of acute liver damage. *J Clin Pathol* 1977;30:141.

TABLE 281.1. Ergot Alkaloids

Bromocriptine
Dihydroergotamine
Dihydroergocornine[a]
Dihydroergocristine[a]
Dihydroergocryptine[a]
Ergotamine
Ergonovine
Methylergonovine
Methysergide

[a]Dihydroergotoxine (ergoloid) derivatives.

CHAPTER 281
Ergot Alkaloids

Leslie S. Carroll and Steven Guillen

Ergot alkaloids are natural and semisynthetic derivatives of compounds produced by parasitic fungi of the genus Claviceps, most classically *Claviceps purpurea*. Various flowering grasses and grains, particularly rye, are susceptible to fungal infestation during warm, wet weather. Historically, epidemics of ergotism resulted from the ingestion of bread made from contaminated grain. In the Middle Ages, ergotism was known as holy fire (ignis sacer) or St. Anthony's fire; victims claimed that a pilgrimage to the Shrine of St. Anthony in France relieved their symptoms. Because the mold Claviceps did not infect rye in the area of the shrine, spontaneous cures probably did result (2). Today, ergot poisoning is caused almost exclusively by medicinal preparations.

Ergot alkaloids are derivatives of the tetracyclic compound 6-methylergoline, a compound structurally similar to the amine neurotransmitters dopamine, norepinephrine, and serotonin. There are three classes of ergot alkaloids: the naturally occurring forms with amine groups, the naturally occurring forms with amino acid groups, and the synthetic dihydrogenated groups. The naturally occurring ergot alkaloids consist of a lysergic acid base; the amine alkaloids contain amine side chains, and the amino acid alkaloids contain polypeptide side chains. The synthetic ergot alkaloids contain a lysergic acid base that has been dihydrogenated. Individual agents are listed in Table 281.1. The structural similarity between the lysergic acid nucleus of ergot alkaloids and the endogenous amines dopamine, norepinephrine and serotonin accounts for their pharmacologic activity. Effects are complex and may include simultaneous stimulation and blockade of peripheral and central neuroreceptors (2).

Physiologic effects are variable and depend on the particular alkaloid's affinity and specificity for receptors, the dose of the drug, individual sensitivity, the route of administration, underlying disease states, and preexisting vascular tone. For instance, ergotamine produces both partial α-adrenergic agonist and partial α-adrenergic antagonist effects. Additionally, ergotamines mediate vasoconstrictor action by direct agonism at serotonin (5-HT) receptors. There are 7 classes of 5-HT receptors (5-HT$_{1-7}$). Ergots agonize multiple 5-HT receptors including 5-HT$_{1A}$, 5HT$_{1B}$, 5-HT$_{1D}$, 5-HT$_{1F}$, 5-HT$_{2A}$, 5-HT$_{2C}$, and 5-H$_{T4}$.

Ergots may also induce vasodilatation secondary to central vasomotor center depression. The net clinical effect may be vasoconstriction or vasodilation, depending on the dose taken and preexisting vascular tone (2). Clinically, vasoconstriction predominates, which can produce unexpected complications, such as acute myocardial infarction (MI) (11).

Ergotamine, the classic ergot prototype drug, is the agent most commonly involved in poisoning. It has been used for migraine and other vascular headaches because of its cranial vasoconstrictive effect, and it can be given orally, sublingually, rectally, parenterally, and by inhalation. Suppository formulations of ergotamine combined with caffeine and other products are popular and are implicated in many cases of iatrogenic ergotism. The usual recommendations for rectal ergotamine use (2 mg rectally at the beginning of a headache, not to exceed 10 mg a week) may be grossly exceeded and may produce true physical dependency with withdrawal headaches, prompting more ergotamine use (19). Although severe vasospasm has been reported with single-dose use of ergotamine, it is the setting of cyclic and increasing self-dosing with ergotamine by any route that usually precedes vasospastic toxicity (8).

Methylergonovine (0.2 mg three to four times daily) or ergonovine (0.2–0.4 mg two to four times daily) may be prescribed for a 2- to 7-day period to control postpartum bleeding and maintain uterine contraction. Bromocriptine is used in the treatment of hyperprolactinemia and Parkinson's disease. Because of cardiovascular toxicity, bromocriptine must be used with caution when prescribed for the suppression of postpartum lactation. Usual adult doses range from 1.25 to 7.5 mg two to six times a day and vary with the condition being treated.

Sumatriptan was approved for the treatment of acute migraine headache in 1992. Multiple other triptans are now available. These agents are structurally similar to the indole serotonin but do not have the tetracyclic structure particular to the ergots. The side effect profile, however, is similar to the ergots as a result of vasoconstrictive properties. The triptans are "cleaner" pharmacological agents than ergots in that they possess receptor specificity primarily at the 5-HT$_{1B}$ and 5-HT$_{1D}$ receptors. Agonism at the 5-HT$_{1B/1D}$ receptors results in extracranial vasoconstriction and resultant resolution of migraine headache (22). Triptans and ergots should be avoided in patients with risk factors for vascular diseases.

CLINICAL PRESENTATION

Two major forms of toxicity—gangrenous and convulsive—have historically been described after ingestion of contaminated grain products. The most recent natural outbreak of ergotism was the gangrenous form, which occurred in Ethiopia from 1977 to 1978 as a consequence of the ingestion of ergot-infested wild oats (13).

In the gangrenous form of natural ergotism, clinical progression begins with paresthesias of the extremities, then vomiting and diarrhea, and finally, excruciating extremity pain, heralding the onset of gangrene. The convulsive form terminates in painful spasms of limb muscles, culminating in epileptic-like activity.

Toxicity from an acute overdose of ergot alkaloids is unusual. A 13-month-old child survived a dose of 15 mg of ergotamine (plus 1 g of phenobarbital), whereas a dose of 12 mg of ergotamine (plus 1.2 g of caffeine) was fatal to a 14-month-old child (14). Seven cases of acute neonatal toxicity resulted from inadvertent intramuscular administration of ergotamine (0.25–0.5 mg), which culminated in reversible encephalopathy, seizures, peripheral vasoconstriction, and occasional oliguria (5). An obese man who ingested 120 mg of ergotamine (plus 3 g of cyclizine and 6 g of caffeine) developed myocardial ischemia and peripheral arterial spasm (14). Symptoms of acute toxicity may include nausea, vomiting, diarrhea, severe thirst, formication (skin tingling), chest pain, bradycardia or tachycardia, hypotension, confusion, convulsions, or coma. Overdose in a gravid female may result in fetal death (1).

Chronic ergot toxicity may present with a multitude of neurologic, gastrointestinal, and vascular symptoms. Neurologic complications include lassitude, impaired mental function, headaches, vertigo, psychosis, convulsions, and coma. Nausea, vomiting, diarrhea, and abdominal pain may occur. As in the acute overdose, abortions may occur. Vascular effects predominate and may involve both venous and arterial circulations. Angiography has shown spasm, formation of collaterals, and intravascular thrombi. Vascular involvement may be unilateral or bilateral, and virtually any vascular distribution may be involved. The legs are most often involved; signs and symptoms include pallor, numbness, progressive pain, progressive loss of pulses, demarcation of ischemic areas and, finally, frank gangrene. Other complications include angina, MI and stroke. Factors that may accelerate ergot toxicity include tobacco smoking, concomitant use of β-blocker medications, sepsis, and hepatic or renal disease (14).

Clinical ergotism continues to appear in the literature secondary to drug interactions. Ergots are metabolized in the liver by the cytochrome P450 (CYP) system. Ergots are substrates for CYP3A4. Inhibitors of CYP3A4 (see Table 281.2) including macrolide antibiotics, protease inhibitors, and antifungal agents have resulted in clinical ergotism when combined with ergot

preparations (6). One patient, stabilized on protease inhibitor therapy, received three caffeine/ergotamine tablets over a 48-hour period for a migraine headache and succumbed to a cerebral death. Autopsy revealed "global hypoxic ischemic encephalopathy" (23). Another patient on ritonavir self-administered only 1 mg of ergotamine-tartrate and developed ischemic feet (16). The low doses of ergotamine ingested by these patients usually do not produce toxicity. However, the combination of a CYP3A4 inhibitor and an ergotamine substrate will produce elevated concentrations of ergotamines and subsequent toxicity. Ergot preparations should be avoided in all patients on CYP3A4 inhibitors.

Bromocriptine poisoning may result in nausea, vomiting, dizziness, lethargy, confusion, hallucinations, and either hypertension or hypotension (15).

Vasoconstrictive effects of triptans can result in chest tightness (21), MI (17), and ventricular dysrhythmias (3).

DIFFERENTIAL DIAGNOSIS

The diagnosis of ergotism should become readily apparent when the history reveals the use of an ergot derivative. Unfortunately, however, patients may be reluctant to admit to self-use of ergot preparations, and the entire range of causes of vasoocclusive disease may need to be considered. Included in the differential are arteriosclerosis, compartmental and entrapment syndromes, Raynaud's disease, thromboangiitis obliterans, thromboembolic disease, vasculitides, and drug-induced vasospasm (e.g., ingestion of amphetamines, cocaine, and other sympathomimetics).

EMERGENCY DEPARTMENT EVALUATION

Details regarding the use, abuse, and accidental or suicidal ingestion of ergot preparations should be noted. Physical examination should include a careful evaluation of central nervous system function, cardiovascular and peripheral vascular status, and potential pregnancy, in addition to a meticulous general examination. Doppler-technique pulse measurements, digital pulse monitoring, skin temperature recordings, and magnetic resonance or traditional angiography should be considered in patients with ischemic complications. Plasma drug levels are unavailable for routine use and are probably not clinically helpful (14). Laboratory assessment of renal and hepatic function, baseline coagulation tests, pregnancy testing, drug screens to rule out other agents, and an electrocardiogram are indicated.

EMERGENCY DEPARTMENT MANAGEMENT

Advanced life-support measures are instituted as necessary. In the acute overdose, gastrointestinal decontamination with activated charcoal (AC) should be performed. In chronic presentations, all ergot preparations, and caffeine and nicotine, must be discontinued. No current evidence supports the efficacy of extracorporeal removal procedures (hemodialysis and hemoperfusion) or repeated oral doses of AC. Immediate attention is directed toward treating emergent catastrophes such as acute MI, seizures, and threatened abortion.

The management of ergot-induced vasospasm is requires consideration of multiple modalities and consultation with a vascular surgeon. Ischemic extremities must be protected from trauma and should be warmed but not overheated. The mainstay of therapy consists of vasodilators combined with

---

TABLE 281.2. CYP3A4 Inhibitors

Macrolide antibiotics
 Clarithromycin
 Erythromycin
Antifungal agents
 Clotrimazole
 Fluconazole
 Itraconazole
 Ketoconazole
Protease inhibitors
 Amprenavir
 Indinavir
 Nelfinavir
 Ritonavir
 Saquinavir
Antidepressants
 Nefazodone
Other
 Cyclosporin
 Grapefruit juice

anticoagulants. Numerous drugs have been recommended to reverse vasospasm, including nitroprusside (the current drug of choice for severe spasm) (25), nitroglycerin (10), and nifedipine (12). Prostaglandin E1 analogs infused intra-arterially (9) and intravenously (18) have restored arterial patency. Heparin and antiplatelet agents are recommended to prevent thrombi as a result of vascular stasis. Intraarterial thrombolytics (4) have been utilized to dissolve thrombi. Invasive procedures including intraarterial balloon dilation (20) and thrombectomy (24) have been used successfully. The serotonin antagonist cyproheptadine (see Chapter 322, "Serotonin Re-uptake Inhibitors") may be beneficial in combating the vasospastic properties of the ergots (7).

Bromocriptine overdoses require supportive care, with attention to reversal of hypotension with fluids and protection from self-injury if confusion and agitation are present (15).

CRITICAL INTERVENTIONS

- Establish intravenous access, institute cardiac and oxygen saturation monitoring, and obtain an ECG on patients with signs or symptoms of ergot poisoning
- Administer vasodilators, heparin, and antiplatelet agents and consult a vascular surgeon for patients with ergot-related vascular compromise

DISPOSITION

Asymptomatic patients with acute overdoses are observed for 4 to 6 hours. Those who become symptomatic and those with vasospastic sequelae are admitted. The management of ergot-induced vasospasm requires an interdisciplinary approach. Patients with vasospastic sequelae should be admitted to a facility that can perform interventional vascular diagnostic and therapeutic procedures including arteriography, intraarterial infusions, and intraarterial balloon dilatation. Medical intensivists should be consulted for pharmaceutical interventions. Vascular surgeons need to be available to perform invasive procedures. After the toxic episode resolves, consideration must be given to continuing care of headache symptomatology.

COMMON PITFALLS

✔ Failure to inform patients of the toxic effects of ergot preparations and to recognize important drug interactions, which place patients on ergots at risk
✔ Failure to consider ergot poisoning in the differential diagnosis of vaso-occlusive disease and to discontinue ergot therapy in patients with signs or symptoms of vascular insufficiency
✔ Failure to appreciate that almost any vascular bed may be affected by ergot, potentially giving rise to diverse clinical presentations

Acknowledgments

We dedicate this chapter to the late Donald B. Kunkel—our esteemed colleague, mentor, and friend, who was coauthor of previous versions of this chapter.

References

1. Au KL, Woo JSK, Wong VCW. Intrauterine death from ergotamine overdose. *Eur J Obstet Gynecol Reprod Biol* 1985;19:313–315.
2. Bigal ME, Tepper SJ. Ergotamine and dihydroergotamine: a review. *Curr Pain Headache Rep* 2003;7:55–62.
3. Curtin T, Brooks AP, Roberts JA. Cardiorespiratory distress after sumatriptan given by injection. *BMJ* 1992;305:713–714.
4. D'Amore MJ, Borge MA, Messersmith RN. Limb-threatening lower extremity ischemia successfully treated with intra-arterial infusion. *Angiology* 1999;50:233–237.
5. Dargaville PA, Campbell NT. Overdose of ergometrine in the newborn infant: acute symptomatology and long-term outcome. *J Paediatr Child Health* 1998;34:83–89.
6. Dresser GK, Spence DJ, Bailey DG. Pharmacokinetic-pharmacodynamic consequences and clinical relevance of cytochrome P450 3A4 inhibition. *Clin Pharmacokinet* 2000;38:41–57.
7. Graudins A, Stearman A, Chan B. Treatment of the serotonin syndrome with cyproheptadine. *J Emerg Med* 1998;16:615–619.
8. Harrison TE. Ergotaminism after a single dose of ergotamine tartrate. *J Emerg Med* 1984;2:23–25.
9. Horstmann R, Daum H, Heller M, Schroder A. Critical limb ischemia caused by ergotism: Treatment with intraarterial prostaglandin E1 infusion. *Dtsch Med Wochenschr* 1993;118:1067–1071.
10. Hussun B, Metz P, Rasmusen J. Nitroglycerin infusion for ergotism. *Lancet* 1979;2:794–795.
11. Iffy L, Ten Hove W, Frisoli G. Acute myocardial infarction in the puerperium in patients receiving bromocriptine. *Am J Obstet Gynecol* 1986;155:371–372.
12. Kemerer VF, Dagher FJ, Pais SO. Successful treatment of ergotism with nifedipine. *Am J Roentgenol* 1984;143:333–334.
13. King B. Outbreak of ergotism in Wollo, Ethiopia. *Lancet* 1979;1:1411.
14. Jones EM, Williams B. Two cases of ergotamine poisoning in infants. *Br Med J* 1966;5485:466.
15. Mack RB. Bromocriptine (Parlodel) overdose. *N C Med J* 1988;49:17–18.
16. Montero A, Giovannoni AG, Tvrde PL. Leg ischemia in a patient receiving ritonavir and ergotamine. *Ann Int Med* 1999;130:329–330.
17. Ottervanger JP, Paalman HJA, Boxma GL, et al. Transmural myocardial infarction with sumatriptan. *Lancet* 1993;341:861–862.
18. Piquemal R, Emmerich J, Guilmot JL, et al. Successful treatment of egotism with Iloprost. *Angiology* 1998;49:493–497.
19. Saper JR, Jones JM. Ergotamine tartrate dependency: features and possible mechanisms. *Clin Neuropharmacol* 1986;9:244–256.
20. Shifrin E, Perel A, Olschwang D, et al. Reversal of ergotamine-induced arteriospasm by mechanical intra-arterial dilatation. *Lancet* 1980;2:1278–1279.
21. Stricker BH. Coronary vasospasm and sumatriptan. *BMJ* 1992;305:118.
22. Tepper SJ, Rapoport AM, Sheftell FD. Mechanisms of action of the 5-HT receptor agonists. *Arch Neurol* 2002;59:1084–1088.
23. Tribble MA, Gregg CR, Margolis DM, et al. Fatal ergotism induced by an HIV protease inhibitor. *Headache* 2002;42:694–695.
24. Vila A, Mykietiuk A, Bonvehi P, Temporiti E, Uruena A, Herrera F. Clinical ergotism induced by ritonavir. *Scand J Infect Dis* 2001;33:788–789.
25. Wells KE, Stead DL, Zajko AB, Webster MW. Recognition and treatment of arterial insufficiency from Cafergot. *J Vasc Surg* 1986;4:8–15.

CHAPTER 282
Nonsteroidal Antiinflammatory Drugs

Marco L. A. Sivilotti

Nonsteroidal antiinflammatory drugs (NSAIDs) are a heterogeneous group of agents that have antiinflammatory, analgesic, and antipyretic activity. Excluding salicylates (discussed in Chapter 284, "Salicylates"), there are a variety of NSAIDs, which can be classified by target specificity and structure (Table 282.1). With widespread use and over-the-counter availability of some NSAIDs, it is not surprising that NSAIDs constitute one of the most common medications encountered in intentional overdose.

TABLE 282.1. Pharmacokinetics of NSAIDS after Therapeutic Doses

Drug	Brand Name	Time to Peak Level (h)	Half-life (h)	Maximum Recommended Daily Adult Dose (mg)
NONSELECTIVE COX INHIBITORS				
Acetic acids				
Diclofenac sodium[a]	Voltaren	2–3	1.2–1.8	225
Diclofenac potassium	Cataflam	0.3–2.0	1.2–1.8	150
Etodolac[a]	Lodine	1–2	7.3	1,200
Indomethacin[a,b,c]	Indocin	1–2	4.5–6.0	200
Ketorolac[c]	Toradol	0.5–1.0	2.4–8.6	IM 120; PO 40
Nabumetone[d]	Relafen	2.5–4.0	22–30	2,000
Sulindac[e]	Clinoril	1–2	7.8	400
Tolmetin	Tolectin	0.5–1.0	1.1–1.5	2,000
Fenamic acids				
Mefenamic acid	Ponstel	1–3	2–4	1,000
Meclofenamate	Meclomen	0.5–2.0	2	400
Oxicams				
Meloxicam[f]	Mobicox	5–6	20	22.5
Piroxicam	Feldene	3–5	30–60	20
Propionic acids				
Fenoprofen	Nalfon	1–2	2–3	3,200
Flurbiprofen	Ansaid, etc.	1–2	3–4	200
Ibuprofen[b]	Motrin, Advil, Nuprin	0.5–2.0	1.8–2.5	3,200
Ketoprofen[a]	Orudis, etc.	0.5–2.0	1.5–4.0	300
Naproxen[a,b]	Naprosyn, Aleve	2–4	12–15	1,500
Naproxen sodium[a]	Anaprox	1–2	12–15	1,375
Oxaprozin	Daypro	3–5	42–50	1,800
Carprofen	Rimadyl			1,200
Pyrazolones				
Oxyphenbutazone	Oxalid		27–72	600
Phenylbutazone	Azolid, Butazolidin	1–4	50–100	600
Salicylates				
Acetylsalicylic acid	Aspirin, etc.	1–2	2–30	4,000
Diflunisal	Dolobid	1–2	5–20	1,500
SELECTIVE COX-2 INHIBITORS				
Celecoxib	Celebrex	2–4	11	400
Rofecoxib	Vioxx	2–3	17	50
Parecoxib	Dynastat	2 (IM)	8	IV/IM 40
Valdecoxib	Bextra	8		40
Etoricoxib	Arcoxia		22	120

[a] Available as a sustained-release product.
[b] Available as a liquid formulation.
[c] Also available as parenteral formulation.
[d] Prodrug metabolized to 6-methoxy-2-naphthylacetic acid (6 MNA).
[e] Prodrug metabolized to sulindac sulfide (half-life 16.4 hr).
[f] Preferential COX-2 inhibitor, but selectivity lost at therapeutic doses.

Three-fourths of these ingestions involve ibuprofen, the first non-salicylate NSAID to be approved for over-the-counter use in the United States. Despite their frequency, most NSAID overdoses result in minimal symptoms, and death is rare. Major complications such as gastrointestinal (GI) bleeding during therapeutic use are a much greater health problem.

The primary pharmacologic effects of NSAIDs result from the inhibition of cyclooxygenase (COX), the enzyme family involved in the initial step of prostaglandin (PG) synthesis. Two isoforms of COX have been identified: COX-1, constitutively present in platelets, endothelium, gastric mucosa, and the kidney; and COX-2, induced by inflammatory mediators and suppressed by glucocorticoids. Because the antiinflammatory properties of NSAIDs appear to result from COX-2 inhibition, NSAIDs with selective COX-2 inhibition have recently been developed, with the promise of reduced side effects (8). The significance and conservation of COX-2 selectivity in overdose are unknown.

Inhibition of COX may result in increased shunting of arachidonic acid to leukotrienes, at times precipitating severe allergic reactions. The adverse GI effects of gastritis and ulceration are as a result of the inhibition of PGD_2, PGE_2, and $PGF_{2\alpha}$, which maintain the gastric mucosal barrier, inhibition of platelet thromboxane A_2 production and hence platelet aggregation, and direct irritation. The salt and water retention and acute renal failure that can occur with NSAID ingestion are attributed to inhibition of PGI_2 and PGE_2, which have vasodilatory and natriuretic activity in the kidney (5).

NSAIDs are rapidly and almost completely absorbed (3,17). They are weak acids with pKa values ranging from 3.5 to 5.6, have small volumes of distribution (0.08–0.4 L/kg; celecoxib, at 6 L/kg, is an exception), and are highly protein bound (more than 90%) (3,17). Elimination depends on hepatic metabolism primarily via the CYP2C subfamily of cytochrome P-450 enzymes, with subsequent renal excretion of metabolites conjugated with glucuronide. As much as 50% of ketorolac and 30% of indomethacin are excreted in the urine unchanged (3). Only small quantities (less than 10%) of other NSAIDs are excreted unchanged in the urine, limiting the utility of urinary alkalinization in promoting elimination. Indomethacin, sulindac, etodolac, phenylbutazone, meloxicam, and piroxicam undergo enterohepatic recirculation (17). The renal clearance of naproxen and oxaprozin is increased at high plasma concentrations as a result of saturated protein binding (17). Only phenylbutazone exhibits dose-dependent Michaelis-Menten elimination (17). Pharmacokinetic data are summarized in Table 282.1.

Except for pyrazolones and fenamic acids, NSAIDs seldom cause serious toxicity, even in large doses (4,16). There is inadequate information to determine the minimum toxic or lethal dose for most NSAIDs. In a series of ibuprofen overdoses, all children who ingested less than 100 mg/kg remained asymptomatic, whereas those who ingested more than 400 mg/kg were at risk of developing significant toxicity (7). In adults, the correlation between the amount ingested and subsequent development of symptoms was poor, with those ingesting between 6 and 54 g of ibuprofen at risk for potentially serious toxicity. In contrast, seizures have been reported with mefenamic acid ingestions of as little as 2.5 g in a 12-year-old child (4). Phenylbutazone has caused death with as little as 2 g in a 1-year-old child and 2.5 g in an alcoholic adult (4,15).

CLINICAL PRESENTATION

Most patients remain asymptomatic or develop only mild GI or neurologic symptoms following acute overdose. Specific signs and symptoms are summarized in Table 282.2. Death is rare and usually results from secondary complications such as aspiration or sepsis. In the absence of acute renal failure or secondary complications, full recovery can be expected within 6 to 24 hours. The elderly have an increased propensity to develop adverse effects with therapeutic doses and toxicity with overdoses. There is relatively little information regarding acute toxicity of the new selective COX-2 inhibitors, but they are presumed to resemble the nonselective agents in overdose.

In contrast, the pyrazolones and fenamic acids can cause severe toxicity. Phenylbutazone and its active metabolite oxyphenbutazone can cause coma, seizures, dysrhythmias, cardiogenic shock, respiratory alkalosis, and metabolic acidosis (4,16). Tinnitus, deafness, and a rash may be present. Hepatic necrosis, without other symptoms, may develop 24 hours after overdosage. A red discoloration of the urine caused by the metabolite rubazonic acid may be observed. Mefenamic acid has a propensity to cause muscle twitching and tonic–clonic

---

TABLE 282.2.   Signs and Symptoms of NSAID Overdose

Gastrointestinal: nausea, vomiting, anorexia, abdominal pain, diarrhea, gastritis, gastrointestinal bleeding, occasional hepatocellular injury, rare cholestasis
Neurologic: dizziness, nystagmus, diplopia, blurred vision, headache, tinnitus, restlessness, lethargy, ataxia, confusion, coma, muscle fasciculations, seizures
Respiratory: hyperventilation, respiratory depression with cyanosis, apnea, diaphoresis
Cardiovascular: hypotension, bradycardia, occasional tachycardia, rare cardiac arrest
Renal: sodium retention and edema, proteinuria, hematuria, acute oliguric or nonoliguric renal failure
Hematologic: decreased platelet aggregation, prolongation of prothrombin time and partial thromboplastin time
Other: occasional metabolic acidosis, rare electrolyte imbalance

---

seizures. In one series, 15 of 54 patients had muscle twitching, and 11 of these progressed to grand mal seizures (1). One 12-year-old patient seized after taking 2.5 g of mefenamic acid, and four adult patients seized after ingesting less than 5 g (4). The time between ingestion and onset of seizures varies between 0.5 and 12 hours. Both cardiac and respiratory arrest may follow seizures.

Propionic and acetic acid derivatives are associated with relatively low toxicity. Of these agents, fenoprofen appears to be the most toxic (4). Metabolic acidosis after ibuprofen overdose is probably related to high levels of acidic drug and metabolites (9,10). Indomethacin frequently causes headaches, even in therapeutic doses. It is also more often associated with tinnitus than are other NSAIDs.

After piroxicam overdose, dizziness with blurred vision and brief coma are reported (4). Because of the long elimination half-life of piroxicam, overdose symptoms can be prolonged (11,13). Multisystem toxicity (with GI, neurologic, renal, hepatic, and hematopoietic effects) was noted in a 2-year-old who ingested 100 mg of piroxicam (12). Experience in the overdose of other NSAIDs with long half-lives (oxaprozin and nabumetone) is limited, but prolonged toxicity should be anticipated. NSAID plasma levels are not routinely available and are not necessary for the treatment of acute ingestion; however, a rough correlation between ibuprofen plasma levels and clinical toxicity has been noted (7).

DIFFERENTIAL DIAGNOSIS

Because GI symptoms, neurologic symptoms, and respiratory depression are common to many drug ingestions and medical illnesses, NSAID overdose cannot be diagnosed by clinical findings alone. The diagnosis is made primarily on the basis of history and the exclusion of other etiologies. The possibility of acetaminophen, colchicine, and salicylate ingestion should be considered in patients with overdose of an unknown arthritis medication.

The central nervous system (CNS) depression that occurs with NSAID overdose is usually mild; coma unresponsive to stimulation is uncommon. Deep coma, marked hypotension, and severe respiratory depression suggest the presence of other drugs. The metabolic acidosis caused by ibuprofen is relatively mild and short-lived compared with that caused by salicylates, isoniazid, ethylene glycol, and methanol (10).

EMERGENCY DEPARTMENT EVALUATION

A detailed history, including all medications available in the household, should be obtained, and may provide the only clue to NSAID overdose. The amount and time of ingestion, and the onset, nature, and progression of symptoms should be noted. The physical examination should include complete vital signs, oxygen saturation measurement, and assessment of mental status and cardiorespiratory function. Evaluation for occult GI bleeding should be considered for patients with abdominal pain.

A complete blood count (CBC), electrolytes, blood urea nitrogen, creatinine, glucose, and urinalysis should be obtained in all symptomatic patients, those with underlying kidney dysfunction, and the elderly. Etodolac may cause a false-positive urine bilirubin and a false-positive urine ketone test when dipstick methods are used. Although the time of onset of renal failure varies and is poorly defined, it has been recommended that these tests be performed in all adults with ibuprofen overdoses of more than 6 g (6). Arterial blood gases should be monitored in patients with significant mental status changes or respiratory depression. In patients with pyrazolone overdose, liver function tests should also be obtained.

Urine and blood samples should be sent for a toxicology screen in cases of altered sensorium of unknown cause. NSAIDs are difficult to detect and correctly identify using common screening procedures. Hence, a negative screen does not necessarily rule out overdose of these agents. Toxicology analysis may also help to rule out other drugs that cause similar symptoms.

EMERGENCY DEPARTMENT MANAGEMENT

Initial management consists of standard supportive care and GI decontamination. Mechanical ventilation may be necessary in severe poisonings. Hypotension can be managed with intravenous crystalloids. Vasopressors are seldom necessary. Atropine may be used for symptomatic bradycardia, and benzodiazepines are indicated for seizures. Sodium bicarbonate should be given to patients with significant metabolic acidosis. GI bleeding should be treated by standard measures. Coagulopathy can be corrected by administering fresh-frozen plasma and vitamin K_1.

Activated charcoal is the preferred method of GI decontamination. It should be considered in all patients with recent intentional overdose of more than 10 therapeutic doses, and children who present within 4 hours of accidentally ingesting more than five adult doses (16). Fenamic acids or pyrazolones may cause serious toxicity with even a two-fold overdose, and decontamination is appropriate for all these patients. Multiple-dose activated charcoal (MDAC) therapy has not been studied with most NSAIDs. Although the elimination half-life of therapeutic doses of phenylbutazone was decreased by 30% using MDAC (14), the clinical efficacy of this treatment is likely to be minimal, even for NSAIDs that undergo enterohepatic recirculation. Because most NSAIDs are highly protein bound and rapidly metabolized, diuresis or dialysis is not expected to remove a significant amount of active drug. Charcoal hemoperfusion may benefit patients with severe phenylbutazone poisoning (2).

CRITICAL INTERVENTIONS

- Establish intravenous access, initiate cardiac monitoring, and provide supportive care as clinically indicated
- Obtain a CBC, electrolytes, blood urea nitrogen, creatinine, glucose, and urinalysis in symptomatic patients, those with underlying kidney dysfunction, and the elderly
- Exclude the possibility of occult acetaminophen and salicylate ingestion in patients with intentional ingestions

DISPOSITION

Patients should be observed for 4 to 6 hours after ingestion, or until minor symptoms resolve (6,16). Following the ingestion of fenamic acids or pyrazolones, symptomatic patients should be monitored for at least 12 hours. Patients with significant toxicity such as coma, respiratory depression, seizures, or renal failure should be admitted to a medical intensive care unit.

Patients with an abnormal urinalysis or underlying renal dysfunction should have follow-up kidney function tests. A complete blood count and kidney and liver function tests should be repeated 24 to 48 hours after pyrazolone overdose. Follow-up liver function tests should be obtained in symptomatic piroxicam overdose patients.

Transfer should not ordinarily be necessary. If acute renal failure develops, a nephrologist should be consulted. All intentional ingestions should be evaluated for ongoing suicidality.

COMMON PITFALLS

✔ Failure to consider the possibility of other ingestions in patients with intentional overdose, significant CNS depression, metabolic acidosis, or vital sign abnormalities
✔ Failure to consider colchicine ingestion in the differential diagnosis of poisoning by an unknown arthritis medicine
✔ Failure to appreciate that only phenylbutazone and mefenamic acid commonly cause serious toxicity following overdose
✔ Failure to recognize that a negative toxicology screen does not necessarily exclude NSAID poisoning

Acknowledgment

The author thanks Paula L. Townsend who wrote previous editions of this chapter.

References

1. Balali-Mood M, Proudfoot AT, Critchley JAJH, et al. Mefenamic acid overdosage. *Lancet* 1981;1:1354.
2. Berlinger WG, Spector R, Flanigan MJ, et al. Hemoperfusion for phenylbutazone poisoning. *Ann Intern Med* 1982;96:334.
3. Brater DC. Clinical pharmacology of NSAIDs. *J Clin Pharmacol* 1988;28:518.
4. Court H, Volans GN. Poisoning after overdose with nonsteroidal antiinflammatory drugs. *Adverse Drug React Acute Poisoning Rev* 1984;3:1.
5. Dunn MJ. Nonsteroidal antiinflammatory drugs and renal function. *Annu Rev Med* 1984;35:411.
6. Hall AH, Rumack BH. Treatment of patients with ibuprofen overdose [Letter]. *Ann Emerg Med* 1988;17:184.
7. Hall AH, Smolinske SC, Conrad FL, et al. Ibuprofen overdose. 126 cases. *Ann Emerg Med* 1986;15:1308.
8. Hawkey CJ. COX-2 inhibitors. *Lancet* 1999;353:307.
9. Lee CY, Finkler A. Acute intoxication due to ibuprofen overdose. *Arch Pathol Lab Med* 1986;110:747.
10. Linden CH, Townsend PL. Metabolic acidosis after acute ibuprofen overdosage. *J Pediatr* 1987;111:922.
11. Lo GCC, Chan JYW. Piroxicam poisoning. *BMJ* 1983;287:798.
12. Macdougall LG, Taylor-Smith A, Rothberg AD, et al. Piroxicam poisoning in a 2-year-old child. *S Afr Med J* 1984;66:31.
13. Mosvold J, Mellem H, Stave R, et al. Overdosage of piroxicam. *Acta Med Scand* 1984;216:335.
14. Neuvonen P, Elonen E. Effect of activated charcoal on absorption and elimination of phenobarbitone, carbamazepine and phenylbutazone in man. *Eur J Clin Pharmacol* 1980;17:51.
15. Okonek S, Reinecke H. Acute toxicity of pyrazolones. *Am J Med* 1983;75(5A):94.
16. Vale JA, Meredith TJ. Acute poisoning due to nonsteroidal anti-inflammatory drugs: clinical features and management. *Med Toxicol* 1986;1:12.
17. Verbeeck RK, Blackburn JL, Loewen GR. Clinical pharmacokinetics of nonsteroidal anti-inflammatory drugs. *Clin Pharmacokinet* 1983;8:297.

CHAPTER 283
Opioids

Patricia Murphy and R. Brent Furbee

The term opioid applies to all agonists and antagonists with morphine-like activity, including both naturally occurring and synthetic compounds (Table 283.1). Additional agonists include levomethadyl, levorphanol, sufentanil and the methadone derivative L-α-acetylmethadol (LAAM). Buprenorphine is an additional agonist–antagonist. Dextromethorphan is an opioid agonist which is used as an antitussive. It is low in potency, but also binds to NMDA receptors and increases serotonin neurotransmission (1). The distinction between different opioids is important from the standpoint of therapeutic effectiveness (potency), side effects, duration of action, and detectability by drug screens.

Abuse of, and poisoning by, opioids is relatively common and increasing, particularly in the adolescent age group. Recent data from the Drug Abuse Warning Network (DAWN) on hospital emergency department (ED) visits as a result of drug abuse reported by shows that heroin/morphine were the third most commonly reported substances of abuse, after alcohol and cocaine. In

2000, the number of exposures to heroin/morphine was 97,287, an increase of 15% over 1999. Oxycodone and hydrocodone exposures increased 108% and 53% respectively. The prevalence of heroin use among 8th to 12th graders is two to three times higher now than in 1991. Injecting or ingesting the contents of fentanyl patches is another recently recognized trend.

Heroin/morphine rank among the top three drugs cited by DAWN in their substance related deaths (accompanied by alcohol and cocaine). Narcotic analgesics including methadone, codeine, hydrocodone, and oxycodone frequently ranked in the top ten drugs mentioned by medical examiners. In the past, fentanyl resulted in hundreds of fatal overdoses in intravenous heroin users who purchased it as "synthetic heroin" or "China White."

Opioids are rapidly absorbed by all routes. Those with high lipid solubility can even be absorbed transdermally. Most opioids are metabolized by hepatic conjugation, with 90% excreted in the urine as inactive compounds. Significant first-pass metabolism results in lesser effects after oral administration than after parenteral administration of the same dose. Opioids have a large volume of distribution (1 to 4 L/kg) and variable penetration of the blood–brain barrier. The rate of metabolism of opioids does not accelerate with ongoing usage.

Opioids act by binding to and activating specific receptors in the central nervous system (CNS) and peripheral nervous system. Three major opioid receptor classes have been described: μ, κ, and δ, some of which have been divided into subtypes. Two additional receptor types, ε and ζ have been discovered but are not characterized in humans. The σ receptor, originally

TABLE 283.1.   Comparison of Common Opioids

Drug	Dose and Route	T$_{1/2}$	Duration of Action	Equiv. Dose (10 mg of MSO4)
NATURAL				
Codeine	60 mg PO	2.9 h	4–6 h	120 mg
Morphine sulfate	2–10 mg IM/IV	1.5–2.0 h	4–5 h	10 mg
	60 mg PO			
SEMISYNTHETIC				
Heroin	3 mg IM/IV	as MSO4	3–4 h	3 mg
Hydrocodone	5–10 mg IM/IV	3.8 h	4–8 h	—
	25–30 mg PO			
Hydromorphone	1–2 mg IM/IV	2.6 h	4–5 h	1.5 mg
	2 mg PO			
	3 mg per rectum			
Oxycodone	5 mg PO	—	3–4 h	10 mg
Oxymorphone HCl	0.5–1.0 IM/IV	—	3–6 h	1.1 mg
SYNTHETIC				
Diphenoxylate	5 mg PO	12–14 h	6–8 h	—
Fentanyl	0.05 mg IM/IV	2–4 h	30–60 min IV	0.125 mg
Meperidine	50–100 mg IM/IV	3.5 h	2–4 h	80–100 mg
Methadone	5–15 IM/IV	15 h	36–48 h	—
Propoxyphene	65–100 mg PO	3.5 h	2–4 h	240 mg
Tramadol	50–100 mg PO	6.3 h	4–6 h	—
AGONIST–ANTAGONIST				
Butorphanol	1 mg IV	3–4 h	3–4 h	—
	2 mg IM			
	1 mg intranasally			
Nalbuphine	10 mg IM/IV	5 h	3–6 h	—
Pentazocine	30 mg IM/IV	2 h	2–3 h	—
	50 mg PO	3.6 h		

TABLE 283.2.   CNS Opioid Receptors

Receptor	Effects
Mu1 (μ1)	Supraspinal analgesia
	Peripheral analgesia
	Euphoria
	Prolactin release
Mu2 (μ2)	Spinal analgesia
	Respiratory depression
	Physical dependence
	Gastrointestinal dysmotility
	Miosis
	Pruritus
	Bradycardia
Kappa1 (κ1)	Spinal analgesia
	Miosis
Kappa2 (κ2)	Psychotomimesis
	Dysphoria
Kappa3 (κ3)	Supraspinal analgesia
Delta (Δ)	Spinal analgesia
	Modulation of μ-receptor function
	Modulation of dopaminergic neurons

described as an opioid receptor, has been reclassified because actions mediated via this receptor are not reversed by the opiate antagonist naloxone. Endogenous peptides such as enkephalins, β-endorphin, and dynorphin A are opioid receptor agonists.

Stimulation of opioid receptors activates G-proteins, which modify specific effector systems such as phospholipase C and adenylate cyclase. Blockage of voltage-gated calcium channels, activation of potassium efflux channels and hyperpolarization of the nerve terminal with suppression of neurotransmitter release effectively dampens nociceptive transmission. Alpha$_2$ (α_2) adrenergic receptors modulate production of cyclic AMP, which is necessary for operation of the potassium and calcium channels. Alpha$_2$ (α_2) agonists are capable of decreasing some neural transmission, which at least partially explains the similarities between opioid and α2 agonist activity (20). Opioid receptors also have inhibitory effects at postsynaptic sites, interrupting pain sensations at afferent nerves (14).

Effects resulting from opioid receptor stimulation are summarized in Table 283.2. All opioid receptors are involved in analgesia. Mu (μ) receptors mediate most supraspinal analgesic effects and euphoria, sedation, and respiratory depression. Delta (Δ) and κ receptors exert most of their action at the spinal cord. Dysphoric reactions and psychosis appear to be as a result of σ receptor stimulation.

Opioid-induced respiratory depression results from diminished sensitivity to hypercapnia and depressed ventilatory response to hypoxia. The risk of respiratory depression increases after 60 years of age with therapeutic application of opioids (3). Heroin-related noncardiogenic pulmonary edema (NCPE) appears to be a neurogenic process initiated by CNS hypoxia. Patients who have not been comatose and apneic do not appear to be at risk for this complication (23). NCPE can occur with any route of exposure. Although historically, retrospective case series described a NCPE rate of 48% to 80%, recent case studies indicate that NCPE is an infrequent complication of patients (0.8–2.4%) who present with an acute heroin overdose. The decrease in NCPE in patients with nonfatal overdose may be related to better prehospital care and to regular administration of naloxone.

Interstitial lung disease associated with the injection of oral opioid preparations results from the injection of insoluble binding agents such as talc, cornstarch, or cellulose. The pathologic result is microscopic pulmonary emboli and inflammation

progressing to interstitial fibrosis and pulmonary hypertension. Clinically this results in emphysema and chronic respiratory failure. Historically the oral opioid most cited in pulmonary talcosis is pentazocine (often used in conjunction with methylphenidate). There are however cases of interstitial lung disease associated with methadone, meperidine, codeine, and oxycodone injection (17,18). Similarly, excipient retinopathy can result from the injection of oral medications.

Opioids increase venous capacitance which may cause a slight decrease in both systolic and diastolic pressures. Opioids may cause bradycardia secondary to decreased CNS stimulation. Nonspecific histamine release may cause hypotension. Propoxyphene may produce sodium channel blockade in myocytes causing QRS prolongation, ventricular dysrhythmias, and hypotension. Methadone and LAAM inhibit delayed potassium rectifier currents thereby increasing QT intervals (10,11,16). Prolonged QT syndrome and its sequelae of torsades de pointes is most likely when high dose methadone is used (16).

The mechanisms responsible for seizures as a result of propoxyphene, tramadol, and meperidine are not completely elucidated. Propoxyphene causes seizures in animals although its metabolite, norpropoxyphene, does not. Inhibition of the reuptake of serotonin and norepinephrine is postulated as the etiology for tramadol associated seizures. Meperidine's metabolite normeperidine may cause excitatory neurotoxicity (8) and serotonin syndrome as it blocks the reuptake of serotonin (1). Seizures in the setting of opioid overdose may also result from hypoxia.

Severe, acute parkinsonism occurring after the illicit use of a meperidine analogue synthesized in a clandestine laboratory was found to be a result of a metabolite of the contaminant MPTP (1-methyl-4-phenyl-1,2,3,6-tetrahydropyridine) (12). MPTP selectively destroys dopamine-containing substantia nigra cells through inhibition of oxidative phosphorylation. Affected individuals were known as "frozen addicts."

It is not fully understood why physical dependence or behavioral addiction develop. Theories regarding dependence are developed from neurobiologic evidence and data from studies of learning behavior (2). Animal models implicating the μ receptor as knockout mice lacking the μ receptor neither exhibit the behavioral effects induced by opioids nor become physically dependent when given opioids (2). The dopamine pathway is also thought to be involved in dependence as opioids indirectly stimulate dopamine release.

There are three possible pharmacodynamic mechanisms for tolerance, in which steadily increasing doses of opioid and/or increasing frequency of usage are required to produce the same physiologic response with the prolonged use of opioids. First, consistent agonist exposure may result in removal of receptors from the cell surface (downregulation). Second, chronic exposure could lead to decreased synthesis and/or release of endorphins (22). Finally, continued exposure may reduce the ability of opioid agonists to activate G proteins.

Tolerance is most pronounced in the euphoric, analgesic, and sedative effects of opioids (6). Respiratory tolerance has also been reported in the setting of large therapeutic doses of morphine. The delivery of up to 1,000 mg/hour of morphine for pain control without concomitant respiratory depression has been reported. Tolerance is developed to pharmacological doses of opioids and cross-tolerance with synthetic and natural opioids has also been shown (22).

Withdrawal symptoms are the result of an interaction between opioid and other neurotransmitter systems. During withdrawal, decreased dopamine levels are found in the parts of the brain associated with neural reward circuits (2). Amounts of endogenous opioids are insufficient to provide inhibition to adrenergic pathways resulting in over-activation (6). Unlike benzodiazepine, barbiturate, or alcohol withdrawal, opioid withdrawal is generally not lifethreatening. Withdrawal seizures can, however, occur in neonates (4).

Methadone is the most commonly prescribed agent involved in opioid maintenance treatment. Methadone maintenance treatment (MMT) involves the daily administration of oral methadone, a long acting agonist that eliminates withdrawal symptoms for 24 to 36 hours. It is designed to decrease overdoses, decrease infectious disease transmission, and to improve the overall health of injection drug users. Furthermore, once daily administration decreases the patient's need to be frequently seeking a "fix" and diminishes the chaotic lifestyle associated with opioid addiction. Patients involved in MMT are still at risk for overdose, especially in the setting of ongoing illicit drug use, and do experience withdrawal symptoms if scheduled maintenance doses are missed. Emerging alternatives to methadone include the longer acting LAAM and the agonist-antagonist buprenorphine. There are programs in the UK, Netherlands, and the United States in which injectable-heroin maintenance treatment has been successful at decreasing illicit heroin use and crime.

The goal of rapid and ultra-rapid opioid detoxification programs is to provide same-day detoxification for opioid addicted individuals. High-dose opioid antagonists are given to patients under anesthesia so that they undergo acute withdrawal but are spared the conscious experience. The patient awakens without opioid dependency and is started on oral naltrexone; subsequent and persistent symptoms are treated symptomatically with benzodiazepines, clonidine, and antidiarrheals. Complications include treatment failures (relapse) and pulmonary edema associated with naloxone.

CLINICAL PRESENTATION

Poisoning may occur after intravenous, intramuscular, intranasal, inhalational, oral, subcutaneous, intradermal, or transdermal exposure. Unintentional poisoning in addicts or recreational users and intentional use in suicide attempts is frequently encountered. In the setting of injection, inhalational, and intranasal drug use, poisoning typically occurs in novice users, during binging, or when an experienced user obtains an unfamiliar supply of heroin and accidentally miscalculates the dose as a result of differences in purity. The possibility of an intentional self-overdose or attempted homicide must also be considered. Unintentional exposure is most common in children, although iatrogenic poisonings do occur. Children may ingest pills or apply or ingest transdermal patches (that sometimes become stuck on the roof of the mouth). Elderly patients, particularly those on chronic opioid therapy for pain control of systemic illness, also constitute a high-risk group for unintentional poisoning.

The onset of symptoms is nearly immediate after injection, inhalation, and nasal insufflation. Although effects are usually noted within 30 minutes of ingestion, absorption can be erratic and delayed, particularly in children and with sustained-release formulations. Lomotil (diphenoxylate and atropine) is particularly notorious for causing delayed toxicity, perhaps because both constituents can inhibit gastrointestinal (GI) motility (19). The effects of transdermal medications also begin about 30 minutes after application. They can, however, develop or progress after the patch is removed. Intravenous injection and oral ingestion of fentanyl patches deliver the entire drug content of the patch at one time rather than the ongoing absorption of small aliquots of fentanyl.

TABLE 283.3. Atypical Presentations of Opioid Poisoning

Agent	Prominent/Atypical Features
Propoxyphene (Darvon)	Rapid, sudden onset of opioid effects
	Seizures, psychosis (unresponsive to naloxone)
	Hypotension
	Prolongation of PR, QRS, and ventricular tachycardia
	Delayed onset of membrane depressant effects
	Low dose is life-threatening (11 mg/kg)
	Higher doses of naloxone needed to antagonize narcotic effects
Diphenoxylate (Lomotil)	Initial anticholinergic features
	Delayed onset of opioid effects
	Children at high risk for toxicity
Meperidine (Demerol)	Mydriasis
	Prolonged half-life of metabolite
	Seizures
	Increased muscle tone; serotonin syndrome
Pentazocine (Talwin)	Higher doses of naloxone needed to antagonize effects
Tramadol (Ultram)	Seizures unresponsive to naloxone
	Serotonin syndrome

CNS depression, miosis, and respiratory depression are the three hallmark signs of opioid poisoning, although atypical presentations can occur (Table 283.3). CNS effects range from drowsiness to deep coma. In some cases, however, paradoxic excitation may be seen. Seizures can occur in a pure opioid overdosage, particularly in children, but are most common in propoxyphene, tramadol (14,24), and meperidine (8) poisoning. Increased muscle tone, tremors, or twitching may be seen with meperidine, and muscle rigidity has been associated with fentanyl.

Miosis is present in most cases of opioid poisoning (7). Mydriasis or midrange pupils do not rule out this diagnosis, however, as they can be seen with Lomotil, meperidine, hypoxic injury, hypoglycemia, a postictal state, or co-intoxicant.

Initially, the rate (but not the depth) of respirations is decreased. With increasing severity, cyanosis and extreme bradypnea are noted. Respiratory decompensation from NCPE typically develops within minutes to several hours after respiratory depression but radiographic evidence may be delayed up to 24 hours (21). Rapid, shallow respirations may be noted and arterial blood gas analysis reveals hypoxemia, hypercarbia, and a respiratory acidosis (5). Manifestations include copious pink, frothy sputum and rhonchi, rales, or wheezes. Central venous pressure is normal or low. Hence, jugular venous distention and an S3 gallop are absent. Chest radiograph findings include a normal-size heart and a variable pattern of pulmonary edema ranging from unilateral localized infiltrates to classic hilar-based bilateral infiltrates. As a result of the CNS depressant effects of opioids, aspiration pneumonitis must also be considered as the cause of abnormal pulmonary findings on examination and radiograph (5). These entities may be difficult to differentiate in the emergency department. Aspiration is more likely the cause when the chest radiograph abnormalities do not resolve within 48 hours.

Opioids may cause a slight decrease in both systolic and diastolic pressures. In the supine patient, this effect often goes unnoticed. Except for propoxyphene, meperidine, and pentazocine, opioids have no direct inotropic or chronotropic effects (24). Although significant hypotension can occur in propoxyphene poisoning and as a consequence of nonspecific histamine release, it is usually secondary to hypoxia, a co-intoxicant, or shock from other etiologies. Likewise, although rhythm disturbances can occur in propoxyphene poisoning (24), they otherwise suggest hypoxia or a co-ingestant. Propoxyphene can cause QRS widening, ventricular ectopy, decreased contractility, and hypotension (24). Other electrocardiographic (ECG) abnormalities include right bundle-branch block, left bundle-branch block, first-degree atrioventricular block, ventricular bigeminy, and ventricular fibrillation. A murmur in an intravenous abuser should raise the possibility of endocarditis. Pulmonary hypertension with cor pulmonale may result from the injection of adulterants or contaminants.

GI side effects of opioids include nausea and vomiting, decreased bowel sounds, and abdominal distention. Genitourinary complications of opioid use include urinary retention as a result of increased sphincter tone. Other complications pressure necrosis, compartment syndrome, rhabdomyolysis, hypoglycemia, and hypothermia in the patient who has been comatose.

DIFFERENTIAL DIAGNOSIS

Opioid poisoning should be considered in any patient with altered mental status (including seizures), miosis, and respiratory depression. Anticonvulsant, antidepressant, antihistamine, ethanol, muscle relaxant, neuroleptic, and sedative–hypnotic intoxication should be included in the differential diagnosis. Pontine hemorrhage, cholinergic agents, clonidine, and other imidazolines, phencyclidine, and phenothiazines may cause also cause miosis. In pontine hemorrhage, the patient exhibits tachypnea (central neurogenic hyperventilation) and hypertension. Cholinergic agents (e.g., organophosphate insecticides) may cause a diagnostic dilemma initially, because the patient may appear to have pulmonary edema (profuse oral secretions, wheezing, and rales). The GI tract is stimulated rather than depressed, however, resulting in hyperactive bowel sounds, recurrent vomiting, and diarrhea. Overdose of clonidine and other imidazolines (e.g., tetrahydrozoline, guanabenz) may result in bradycardia, hypotonia, and bradypnea. Phencyclidine intoxication is usually accompanied by tachycardia, hypertension, and muscle rigidity or tremor. In phenothiazine poisoning, hypotension and tachycardia occur in conjunction with coma. Hypothermia, encephalopathy, postictal state, CNS trauma or infection, cerebral vascular accident, and metabolic or electrolyte abnormalities, including hypoglycemia, hypercalcemia, hyponatremia, and hypernatremia, should also be considered in the differential diagnosis.

EMERGENCY DEPARTMENT EVALUATION

The history should attempt to include the identity of the opioid and any co-intoxicants and the amount, time, intent, and route of exposure. The physical examination should initially focus on assessing the patency of the airway and the adequacy of ventilation. Patients should be placed on a cardiac monitor and have continuous oxygen saturation monitoring and/or an arterial blood gas analysis. Intravenous access should be established and blood obtained for determination of glucose (at the bedside for patients with altered mental status), electrolytes, blood urea nitrogen, and creatinine. A chest radiograph and ECG should be obtained in patients with unstable vital signs, hypoxia, or abnormal findings on cardiopulmonary examination. An ECG should also be performed in patients with propoxyphene ingestions or abnormal rhythm or conduction intervals on cardiac monitoring. Creatine kinase and urine for myoglobin should be checked in patients with altered mental status. Toxicology testing is appropriate to exclude co-intoxicants such as acetaminophen (found in combination with opioids in many prescription medications) in cases of oral overdose. Urine screening and comprehensive toxicology testing for drugs of abuse can detect some, but not all, opioids. Hence, a negative toxicology screen does not rule out opioid poisoning. A positive toxicology screen confirms exposure but not toxicity from opioids. In contrast, a lack of response to opioid antagonists virtually excludes this diagnosis. A positive response to opioid antagonists, although usually diagnostic, must be interpreted with caution, as poisoning with clonidine and valproate (and rarely benzodiazepines, ethanol, and chlorpromazine) sometimes responds to naloxone.

EMERGENCY DEPARTMENT MANAGEMENT

Supplemental oxygen and assisted ventilation should be provided, as necessary. With the expeditious use of opioid antagonists and ventilation temporarily provided by bag-valve-mask, endotracheal intubation can often be avoided. The application of four-point restraints should be considered before antagonist administration, because the patient may become uncooperative and combative. Suction equipment should be set up in advance, because vomiting may occur after naloxone administration (25).

Opioid antagonists are indicated primarily for the treatment of respiratory depression. They may also be effective for opioid-induced seizures and can be used for diagnostic purposes in patients with altered mental status of unknown etiology (7). In suspected addicts, a low initial dose of naloxone (0.1–0.4 mg intravenously) should be administered to avoid precipitating a severe withdrawal reaction. This dose may be repeated every minute until a total of 2 mg has been given or respiratory depression is reversed and the patient awakens. Because some opioid overdoses (e.g., propoxyphene and methadone) are relatively resistant to naloxone, increments of 2 mg every 2 to 5 minutes, up to a total of 10 mg, should be given if there is little or no response to the initial 2-mg bolus (7). If the patient is not a suspected addict, 0.4 to 2.0 mg of naloxone can be given as the initial bolus. The dose of nalmefene is essentially the same as for naloxone (9). Although longer acting than naloxone (4–8 hours vs. 30–100 minutes), this antagonist is more expensive. Naltrexone, an oral opioid antagonist, is only used for abstinence maintenance.

If intravenous access cannot be obtained, naloxone may be administered intramuscularly, subcutaneously, or endotracheally. The time to response after intramuscular administration is about the same as that required to start an intravenous line and give the drug intravenously. Indeed, because intramuscular administration has less risk of needlestick injury (and attendant potential for infections such as hepatitis and the human immunodeficiency virus) to health care workers than attempting to start an intravenous line in an uncooperative patient or in one with sclerosed veins from injection drug use, this route is preferred by many, particularly prehospital care providers.

Because naloxone has a shorter duration of action—shorter than almost all of the opioid agents it antagonizes—opioid toxicity can recur (primarily after oral overdose and particularly with diphenoxylate and methadone), and repeat doses of naloxone may be necessary. A continuous naloxone drip may be appropriate in such situations. An infusion of two-thirds of the initial dose of naloxone required to reverse respiratory depression, given every hour, should maintain arousal. It may be necessary to give one-half of the original dose as an additional bolus 15 to 20 minutes after initiation of the drip (13). Health care providers must be diligent in monitoring patients placed on a naloxone drip.

A partial response to naloxone requires a careful search for other accompanying illness, injury, or intoxicants. Endotracheal intubation is necessary in patients with hypercarbia, hypoxia, or an inability to protect their airway. A neuromuscular blocking agent (e.g., succinylcholine) may be needed to perform an atraumatic intubation in some patients. Fluid restriction and positive end-expiratory pressure are also useful in the treatment of noncardiac pulmonary edema, but morphine and diuresis are inappropriate. Seizures unresponsive to naloxone should be treated with intravenous benzodiazepines (diazepam or lorazepam) or phenobarbital. Ongoing seizures suggest a cause other than pure opiate poisoning.

Hypotension should be managed initially with a crystalloid fluid bolus and an aggressive search for another cause (6). Propoxyphene, however, may necessitate aggressive use of vasopressors such as dopamine (24). Dysrhythmias as a result of propoxyphene are similar to those of the tricyclic antidepressants and may require sodium bicarbonate therapy (see Chapter 318, "Cyclic Antidepressants"). Naloxone will not reverse propoxyphene cardiotoxicity. Although naloxone only partially inhibits tramadol-mediated analgesia, it reverses respiratory depression and coma as a result of this agent. Patients with oral overdoses should receive activated charcoal if they are awake and alert. Delayed gastric emptying may slow drug absorption and make gastric decontamination efforts effective many hours after ingestion.

CRITICAL INTERVENTIONS

- Administer naloxone to patients with altered mental status and respiratory depression
- Begin with small doses of naloxone in opioid addicts with unintentional poisoning
- Give large doses of naloxone to those with intentional overdose and to children with accidental ingestions
- Admit all patients who require naloxone after oral overdose and all children with possible opioid ingestions

---

DISPOSITION

Careful observation is required for any patient who has demonstrated clinical evidence of opioid poisoning requiring naloxone administration. Although it is often recommended that patients with intravenous overdose be observed for a minimum of 6 hours for evidence of relapse or the development of noncardiac pulmonary edema, this may not be necessary. Such patients usually have taken only slightly more heroin than necessary to achieve the desired effect. Additionally, complications, if they develop, are usually evident soon after presentation. In contrast, all patients who require naloxone after an oral overdose should be admitted to an intensive care unit with cardiac and respiratory monitoring (and suicide precautions, as needed). They should not be discharged until they are symptom-free for 12 hours. Adults who are or become asymptomatic during a 6-hour observation period after oral overdose may be discharged, whereas all children with an oral overdose should be admitted to the hospital for observation and monitoring for 12 to 24 hours. Psychiatric or social work follow-up must be arranged for all intentional or pediatric poisonings. Asymptomatic patients who have been treated with narcotic antagonists should be monitored.

COMMON PITFALLS

✔ Failure to consider opioid overdose in patients who present with altered mental status, including seizures or combativeness, and CNS depression

✔ Failure to apply restraints, thereby risking injury to staff, before giving naloxone to suspected addicts

✔ Failure to evaluate for pulmonary complications, aspiration, and concomitant traumatic and medical illness

✔ Failure to examine thoroughly for medication patches (e.g., Fentanyl)

References

1. Browne B, Linter S. Monoamine oxidase inhibitors and narcotic analgesics. A critical review of the implications for treatment. *Br J Psychiatry* 1987;151:210–212.
2. Cami J, Farre M. Drug addiction. [see comment]. *N Engl J Med* 2003;349:975–986.
3. Cepeda MS, Farrar JT, Baumgarten M, Boston R, Carr DB, Strom BL. Side effects of opioids during short-term administration: effect of age, gender, and race. *Clinical Pharmacology & Therapeutics* 2003;74:102–112.
4. Doberczak TM, Kandall SR, Wilets I. Neonatal opiate abstinence syndrome in term and preterm infants. *J Pediatr* 1991;118:933–937.
5. Duberstein JL, Kaufman DM. A clinical study of an epidemic of heroin intoxication and heroin-induced pulmonary edema. *Am J Med* 1971;51:704–714.
6. Goldfrank L, Bresnitz E, Weisman R. Clinical aspects of drug intoxication: opioids and opiates. *Heart Lung* 1983;12:114–122.
7. Hoffman JR, Schriger DL, Luo JS. The empiric use of naloxone in patients with altered mental status: a reappraisal. *Ann Emerg Med* 1991;20:246–252.
8. Kaiko RF, Foley KM, Grabinski PY, et al. Central nervous system excitatory effects of meperidine in cancer patients. *Ann Neurol* 1983;13:180–185.
9. Kaplan JL, Marx JA. Effectiveness and safety of intravenous nalmefene for emergency department patients with suspected narcotic overdose: a pilot study. *Ann Emerg Med* 1993;22:187–190.
10. Katchman AN, McGroary KA, Kilborn MJ, Kornick CA, Manfredi PL, Woosley RL, Ebert SN. Influence of opioid agonists on cardiac human ether-a-go-go-related gene K(+) currents. *Pharmacol Exp Ther* 2002;303:688–694.
11. Krantz MJ, Martell BA, Arnsten JH, et al. Medications that prolong the QT interval. [comment]. *JAMA* 2003;290:1025; author reply 1026.
12. Langston JW, Irwin I. MPTP: current concepts and controversies. *Clin Neuropharmacol* 1986;9:485–507.
13. Lewis JM, Klein-Schwartz W, Benson BE, Oderda GM, Takai S. Continuous naloxone infusion in pediatric narcotic overdose. *Am J Dis Child* 1984;138:944–946.
14. Lewis KS, Han NH. Tramadol: a new centrally acting analgesic. *Am J Health Syst Pharm* 1997;54:643–652.
15. Lutz RA, Pfister HP. Opioid receptors and their pharmacological profiles. *J Recept Res* 1992;12:267–286.
16. Martell BA, Arnsten JH, Ray B, Gourevitch MN. The impact of methadone induction on cardiac conduction in opiate users. *Ann Intern Med* 2003;139(2):154–155.
17. O'Brien RJ, Schroedl BL. Talc retinopathy. *Opto Vis Sci* 1991;68:54–57.
18. Padley SP, Adler BD, Staples CA, et al. Pulmonary talcosis: CT findings in three cases. *Radiology* 1993;186:125–127.
19. Rumack BH, Temple AR. Lomotil poisoning. *Pediatrics* 1974;53:495–500.
20. Sarne Y, Fields A, Keren O, et al. Stimulatory effects of opioids on transmitter release and possible cellular mechanisms: overview and original results. *Neurochem Res* 1996;21:1353–1361.
21. Sey MJ, Rubenstein D, Smith DS. Accidental methadone intoxication in a child. *Pediatrics* 1971;48:294–296.
22. Simon E. *Opiates: neurobiology*. Baltimore: Lippincott, Williams & Wilkins, 1997.
23. Sporer KA, Dorn E. Heroin-related noncardiogenic pulmonary edema: a case series. *Chest* 2001;120:1628–1632.
24. Strom J. Acute propoxyphene self-poisoning–with special reference to propoxyphene cardiotoxicity and treatment. *Dan Med Bull* 1989;36:316–336.
25. Yealy DM, Paris PM, Kaplan RM, et al. The safety of prehospital naloxone administration by paramedics. *Ann Emerg Med* 1990;19:902–905.

CHAPTER 284
Salicylates

Christopher H. Linden

The incidence of pediatric salicylate poisoning has declined steadily since 1965 as a result of safety packaging, legislation limiting the number of tablets in bottles of children's aspirin, and decreased use because of the association between aspirin use and Reye's syndrome. Similarly, the increased use of non-salicylate nonsteroidal antiinflammatory drugs (NSAIDs) has resulted in a reciprocal decrease in the incidence of adult salicylate poisoning. Despite these trends, however, salicylate continues to be a major cause of poisoning morbidity and mortality, with thousands of exposures and dozens of deaths reported in the United States each year. Additionally, salicylate poisoning is misdiagnosed and mistreated with alarming frequency (1,19). Aspirin is available in tablet, capsule, and suppository formulations, often in combination with anticholinergic, antihistamine, muscle-relaxing, narcotic, and neuroleptic agents. The recommended analgesic, antiinflammatory, and antipyretic dose is 10 to 15 mg/kg every 4 to 6 hours, not to exceed 80 mg/kg/d. Much lower doses (e.g., 80 mg/d) inhibit platelet aggregation. Aspirin acts primarily by inhibiting cyclo-oxygenase (COX), also known as prostaglandin G/H synthase, which converts arachidonic acid to prostaglandins and thromboxanes (22). Analgesic, antiinflammatory, and antipyretic effects result from inhibition of the COX-2 isoform, which is ubiquitous, induced by a variety of inflammatory mediators (e.g., cytokines, endotoxin, growth factors, hormones, and tumor promoters), and suppressed by glucocorticoids. Antipyretic effects may also be as a result of decreased pyrogen production. Adverse effects (e.g., gastric inflammation and ulceration, decreased renal blood flow and glomerular filtration) are mediated by primarily by the COX-1 isoform, constitutionally present in platelets, endothelium, gastric mucosa, and the kidney. Inhibition of COX may result in increased lipoxygenation of arachidonic acid to leukotrienes. This effect appears to be responsible for allergic reactions, especially prevalent in adults with asthma and nasal polyps.

Aspirin (acetylsalicylic acid) is unique in that it acetylates a serine residue near the active site of COX, thereby irreversibly inhibiting COX. In contrast, the effect of nonaspirin salicylates and other NSAIDs is reversible and transient. This difference is most notable in platelets, which have limited synthetic ability and in which thromboxane A_2, a product of COX-1, is essential for normal function. Aspirin inhibits platelet aggregation and prolongs the bleeding time for up to 1 week (pending the production of new platelets) whereas other agents do not have clinically significant platelet effects. Similarly, salicylates are unique among NSAIDs in that at high doses, they can inhibit the hepatic synthesis of clotting factor VII and, to some degree, factors IX and X, and thus prolong the prothrombin time. This effect appears to be a result of interference with the activity of vitamin K and can be reversed by administration of phytonadione (vitamin K_1).

Aspirin, a weak acid (pKa 3.5), is mostly nonionized (absorbable) but poorly soluble at gastric pH. Hence, most absorption occurs in the small intestine. After absorption, aspirin is rapidly hydrolyzed by plasma esterases, with a half-life of about 15 minutes, to the active metabolite salicylic acid (16,22). Salicylic acid (salicylate) is also available from other sources

TABLE 284.1. Nonaspirin Sources of Salicylate

Formulation (Brand Name)	Percentage of Salicylate
Aspirin	75
Bismuth subsalicylate (Pepto-Bismol)	37
Choline and magnesium salicylate (Trilisate)	76
Choline salicylate (Arthropan)	56
Homomenthyl salicylate (sunscreen)	51
Magnesium salicylate (Doan's; Magan)	90
Methyl salicylate (oil of wintergreen)	89
Salicylic acid (topical keratolytic)	100
Salicylsalicylic acid (Disalcid; Salsalate)	96
Sodium salicylate (Pabalate)	84

(Table 284.1). Benorylate and diflunisal are conjugates of salicylic acid. Only benorylate is metabolized to free salicylate, but diflunisal may cause a false-positive result on blood or urine salicylate testing.

After a single oral dose, pharmacologic effects begin within 30 minutes, peak in 1 to 2 hours, and last for about 4 hours. Peak blood levels of 10 to 20 mg/dL occur 1 to 2 hours after ingestion. Therapeutic concentrations range from 10 to 30 mg/dL. High therapeutic levels, required for maximal antiinflammatory effects, are achieved only with chronic dosing. Salicylic acid is extensively (up to 90%) bound to serum proteins, predominantly albumin. The apparent volume of distribution is small (0.15 L/kg), not only because of high protein binding, but also because, at physiologic pH, salicylic acid (pKa 3.0) is greater than 99% ionized, and hence poorly diffusible across cell membranes. Salicylate is primarily eliminated by hepatic metabolism to inactive metabolites with a half-life of 2 to 3 hours (Table 284.2). Metabolites are excreted unchanged or after further metabolism, in the urine. Salicylates readily cross the placenta and enter breast milk. Elimination in the fetus or infant may be prolonged because of immature metabolic pathways and renal function. It may also be delayed in patients with liver or renal disease.

Salicylate kinetics differ markedly after the ingestion of multiple therapeutic doses or a single large overdose (16,21,22). After an overdose, gastric emptying is slowed and salicylate tablets may form concretions, resulting in delayed and prolonged absorption. This is particularly true of enteric-coated and sustained-release formulations. As serum levels increase, protein binding decreases (to 50% or less) and both free salicylate concentrations and the volume of distribution increase to more than 0.35 L/kg. In the presence of acidemia, as occurs in poisoning, the fraction of nonionized (diffusible) salicylate also increases, leading to further tissue distribution. Because of increased

TABLE 284.2. Elimination of a Single Dose of Salicylic Acid

Pathway	Product(s)	Percentage
Conjugation with glycine	Salicyluric acid	75*
Conjugation with glucuronic acid	Salicyl phenolic glucuronide	10*
Hydroxylation	Gentisic acid	5
Urinary excretion	Salicylic acid	1
		10

*Saturable pathways.
(From Flower RJ, et al. Analgesic–antipyretics and antiinflammatory agents. In: Goodman and Gilman's the pharmacological basis of therapeutics, 7th ed. New York: Macmillan, 1985:674.)

distribution, tissue salicylate levels increase proportionately more than serum drug levels.

The two main pathways of hepatic metabolism (see Table 284.2) become saturated when salicylate levels reach or exceed the high therapeutic range and elimination changes from first order (proportional to the level) to zero order (constant), as described by the Michaelis-Menton equation. Hence, with chronic dosing, the salicylate "half-life" increases to 6 to 12 hours, and a small increase in dose results in a much (proportionately) greater increase in serum and tissue salicylate levels, with the potential for chronic intoxication. For the same reason, the salicylate "half-life" may increase to 20 to 40 hours after a large acute overdose.

When hepatic metabolism becomes saturated, urinary excretion becomes the major route of salicylate elimination (16,21,22). The amount of salicylate excreted depends on the balance among glomerular filtration of nonionized salicylate, active proximal tubular secretion of ionized salicylate (by the organic anion active membrane transport system), and passive distal tubular reabsorption of nonionized drug. Increasing urine flow increases glomerular filtration and tubular secretion and decreases reabsorption. Raising the urine pH decreases reabsorption by way of ion trapping (conversion of urinary salicylate to the ionized, nondiffusible form). These mechanisms are the rationale for alkaline diuresis in the treatment of salicylate poisoning. Raising the serum pH also increases the ionized fraction and limits tissue distribution. Alkaline diuresis can increase the renal elimination of salicylate by a factor of 20 or more. Conversely, low urine output and pH, which may occur with illnesses associated with fever, dehydration, and aciduria, decrease salicylate excretion and predispose to salicylates toxicity. Similar conditions, which develop as a result of salicylate poisoning itself (discussion follows), may lead to increased severity and duration of poisoning.

The mechanisms underlying salicylate poisoning are complex (4,10,21–23,25). When salicylate concentrations exceed therapeutic levels, direct stimulation of the medullary chemoreceptor trigger zone and respiratory center causes nausea and vomiting, and hyperventilation (respiratory alkalosis), respectively. Vomiting may occur shortly after salicylate ingestion as a consequence of direct gastric irritation and increased carbon dioxide production may contribute to respiratory stimulation. These effects result in dehydration, not only from gastrointestinal (GI) and insensible fluid losses, but also from the bicarbonate diuresis (and consequent alkaluria) that occurs as a compensatory response to hyperventilation-induced alkalemia. Because sodium and potassium are excreted with bicarbonate (in exchange for hydrogen ion reabsorption), there is concomitant depletion of these electrolytes. Alkalosis may also cause functional hypocalcemia (decreased ionized calcium) with cardiac irritability, tetany, and seizures.

As toxicity progresses, the accumulation of intracellular salicylate causes uncoupling of mitochondrial oxidative phosphory-lation, inhibition of Krebs cycle enzymes (aminotransferases and dehydrogenases) and amino acid metabolism, and stimulation of gluconeogenesis, glycolysis, and lipid metabolism. These derangements result in increased but ineffective metabolism, with increased glucose, lipid, and oxygen consumption and increased amino acid, carbon dioxide, glucose, ketoacid (acetoacetic and β-hydroxybutyric), and lactic and pyruvic acid production. The accumulation of these organic acids, with a small additional contribution from salicylic acid and its metabolites, leads to an increased anion gap metabolic acidosis (2,18). The associated diaphoresis, fever, and osmotic diuresis cause further electrolyte and fluid losses and consequent dehydration. The renal excretion of organic acids results in aciduria.

When high salicylate levels are sustained, progressive metabolic derangements and increasing levels of organic acids may cause increased pulmonary capillary permeability, central nervous system (CNS) and respiratory depression, cerebral and pulmonary edema, cardiovascular collapse, and acute renal failure (acute tubular necrosis).

Acute salicylate poisoning may result from a single ingestion of more than 150 mg/kg of aspirin. Ingestions of 150 to 300 mg/kg may cause mild toxicity, those of 300 to 500 mg/kg may cause moderate toxicity, and those of more than 500 mg/kg may result in severe or fatal poisoning (4,23). Salicylate levels may be quite high during the first 6 to 18 hours after an acute overdose without significant clinical or laboratory evidence of toxicity. Conversely, minimally elevated or even "therapeutic" salicylate levels may be seen with severe poisoning after chronic overdose or late in the course of an acute overdose. Hence, the severity of poisoning is defined by clinical and metabolic findings, not by the salicylate level, and decisions regarding management should be based on direct assessments of severity rather than the Done nomogram. This nomogram, which relates severity to a timed (postingestion) salicylate level, is not applicable to chronic poisoning and sustained-release aspirin overdose, and it has poor predictive value in acute overdoses (9,25). Salicylate poisoning may also result from the topical (skin or gum) application of methyl salicylate or salicylic acid (4,21). It may occur in breast-fed infants and in the newborns of mothers taking therapeutic doses of aspirin.

CLINICAL PRESENTATION

Mild or early salicylate poisoning is characterized by respiratory alkalosis with alkalemia and alkaluria (urine pH > 6) (Table 284.3) (4,10,21–24). It typically develops 3 to 8 hours after acute overdose but can occur days after chronic overdose. Signs and symptoms include nausea, vomiting, abdominal pain, headache, hearing loss, tinnitus (may occur at therapeutic levels), tachypnea or hyperpnea, ataxia, dizziness, agitation, and lethargy. Mild to moderate dehydration is invariably present.

TABLE 284.3.   Stages and Treatment of Salicylate Poisoning

Stage/Severity	Plasma pH	Urine pH	Intravenous Solution	NaHCO$_3$* (mEq/L)	Potassium* (mEq/L)
Early/mild	>:7.4	>6	D$_5$ NS	50	20
Intermediate/moderate	≥7.4	<6	D$_5$ ½ NS	100	40
Late/severe	<7.4	<6	D$_5$ W	150	60–80

* Added to intravenous solution.
(Adapted from Linden CH, Rumack BH. The legitimate analgesics: aspirin and acetaminophen. In: Hanson W Jr, ed. Toxic emergencies. New York: Churchill Livingstone, 1984:118.)

Tachypnea and hyperpnea can be subtle. Hearing loss is typically mild and symmetrical. Tinnitus is often described as a continuous high pitch sound. Functional hypocalcemia (a decrease in ionized calcium) and tetany may result from respiratory alkalosis. Minor increases or decreases in serum glucose, potassium, and sodium levels may be noted. Blood urea nitrogen (BUN), creatinine, sodium, and potassium levels may remain normal despite total body fluid and electrolyte deficits.

Moderate poisoning is characterized by metabolic acidosis with respiratory alkalosis, alkalemia, and "paradoxical" aciduria (Table 284.3) (4,10,21–24). It usually occurs 6 to 18 hours after an acute overdose and days after chronic overdose. The anion gap may be elevated or normal. GI effects persist and dehydration and neurologic symptoms become more pronounced. Fever, asterixis, diaphoresis, deafness, pallor, confusion, slurred speech, disorientation, hallucinations, tachycardia, tachypnea, and mild or orthostatic hypotension may be present. Leukocytosis, thrombocytopenia, increased or decreased glucose and sodium levels, hypokalemia, hypocalcemia, and increased BUN, creatinine, ketone, and lactate levels may be seen on laboratory evaluation.

Severe or late salicylate poisoning is characterized by an increased anion gap metabolic acidosis, acidemia, and aciduria (see Table 284.3) (4,6,10,21–24). It usually develops 12 to 24 hours after acute overdose and longer after chronic overdose. Hyperventilation (respiratory alkalosis) or hypoventilation (respiratory acidosis) and hypoxemia may be present. Other manifestations include coma, seizures, cerebral edema, papilledema, respiratory depression, hypothermia or hyperthermia, hypotension, pulmonary edema, congestive heart failure, dysrhythmias, and profound dehydration with oliguria. The laboratory abnormalities described above become more pronounced. The chest radiograph may show pulmonary edema with a normal-size heart, and a computed tomography (CT) scan of the head may reveal cerebral edema and hemorrhage. Electrocardiographic (ECG) abnormalities may result from direct cardiotoxicity, fluid and electrolyte abnormalities, or coingestants. Sinus tachycardia is common and can be extreme. Other dysrhythmias occur primarily as a terminal event. Asystole is the most common cause of cardiac arrest but ventricular tachycardia and ventricular fibrillation can also occur (6,24). When cardiac arrest occurs, death appears to be inevitable. Successful resuscitation in this situation has yet to be reported.

GI bleeding, hepatic toxicity, pancreatitis, proteinuria, abnormal urinary sediment, an increased prothrombin time, and a low serum uric acid level (as a result of salicylate's uricosuric effect) may be also be present. These effects can occur with therapeutic and toxic doses. Clinically significant bleeding, GI perforation, blindness, and inappropriate antidiuretic hormone secretion are rare complications of acute poisoning. Intrauterine fetal demise resulting from poisoning during pregnancy has been described (19). The ingestion of methyl salicylate (oil of wintergreen, also present in a variety Chinese propriety medicines) or salicylic acid (e.g., Compound W) may cause concomitant corrosive injury to the GI tract (3). Magnesium and bismuth (Pepto-Bismol) salts and enteric-coated or sustained-release formulations of salicylate may be seen as radiopaque densities on abdominal radiographs.

Poisoning as a result of acute methyl salicylate ingestion can progress more rapidly than described above, presumably because of liquid nature and higher lipid solubility of this formulation. Poisoning in children tends to progress faster than in adults whereas adults appear to be more prone to pulmonary complications (1,10,11,25). The onset and progression of toxicity may be delayed, with peak drug levels occurring up to 5 days after overdose, with enteric-coated or sustained-release formulation ingestions (25).

Morbidity is higher in chronic poisoning than in acute poisoning, and when the presentation or diagnosis is delayed (10). Although the overall mortality rate is low (less than 0.01%), fatality rates of 15% to 50% have been reported in those with severe poisoning (6,18,21,23). Persistent neurological dysfunction has been noted in those who recover from severe poisoning (6).

DIFFERENTIAL DIAGNOSIS

Although an increased anion gap metabolic acidosis is said to be pathognomonic of salicylate poisoning, it is seen in only 15% to 20% of adults with such poisoning (6,10). Metabolic acidosis with respiratory alkalosis is the most common acid–base abnormality, occurring in 50% to 61% of poisoned adults. Respiratory alkalosis is the sole acid-base disturbance in 20% to 25% and a combined respiratory and metabolic acidosis is seen in 5%. Metabolic acidosis is more common and respiratory alkalosis less common (and often absent) in children than in adults. Metabolic acidosis is also more common in patients with large acute ingestions, chronic intoxication, and delayed presentation or treatment. Additionally, the anion gap is rarely above 20 mEq/L, even in advanced poisoning (10). It is therefore more appropriate to conclude that abnormal acid–base status is the hallmark of salicylate poisoning.

Salicylate poisoning should be considered in any patient with an unexplained acid–base disturbance. The diagnosis is initially (sometimes fatally) missed in 25% to 60% of patients with salicylate poisoning, particularly those chronically taking the drug for therapeutic purposes (1,10,18). These patients are often elderly, have been taking nonaspirin salicylates, and have serious underlying medical problems. Signs and symptoms of salicylate poisoning have been mistakenly attributed to anxiety, cardiopulmonary disease, cerebrovascular disease, chronic obstructive pulmonary disease, dementia, encephalopathy, alcohol intoxication, ketoacidosis and withdrawal, viral encephalitis and meningitis, pancreatitis, psychiatric disorders, and sepsis (1,2,13,15,18). Salicylate poisoning in children may be indistinguishable (clinically and by routine laboratory evaluation) from Reye's syndrome. A low (subtherapeutic) cerebrospinal fluid salicylate level, high serum alanine, glutamine, and lysine levels, and fatty infiltration of the liver (by CT, ultrasound, or biopsy) indicate Reye's syndrome rather than salicylate poisoning. In infants and children, salicylate poisoning may also be confused with inborn errors of metabolism.

Other poisons that cause an anion gap metabolic acidosis include methanol and ethylene glycol, but lactic acidosis may occur in any poisoning that is complicated by hypoxia, seizures, or shock (see Chapter 271, "Approach to the Poisoned Patient"). A persistently normal metabolic workup (arterial blood gas analysis and determination of serum levels of electrolytes) in a patient who remains symptomatic many hours after an unknown overdose rules out salicylate poisoning.

EMERGENCY DEPARTMENT EVALUATION

The history should include the time(s), amount(s), and formulation of salicylate ingested. The physical examination should focus on vital signs, neurologic status, and cardiorespiratory function. Attention should be given to accurately measuring the respiratory rate (e.g., counted for a full minute) and temperature (e.g., rectal) and to assessing the degree of dehydration. If possible, orthostatic measurements of pulse and blood pressure should be performed. The fundi should be examined for papilledema, the abdomen should be examined for peritoneal signs, and vomitus and stool should be tested for occult blood.

In all cases of intentional ingestion and in those in which the history is uncertain, a serum salicylate level should be obtained. Not infrequently, aspirin is confused with (misidentified as) acetaminophen and vice versa. Unless the product (or its container) is available for positive identification or the history can be confirmed by a third party, serum levels of both drugs should be obtained when the ingestion of either is reported, particularly in those with intentional overdose. If the patient is symptomatic or the salicylate level is elevated, an arterial blood gas, serum electrolytes, glucose, BUN, and creatinine, and a urinalysis should be obtained. If acid–base abnormalities are present, further evaluation should include serum calcium, magnesium, and ketone levels, liver function tests, complete blood count, coagulation profile, ECG, and chest radiograph. Patients who are unresponsive should have a CT scan of the brain to assess for cerebral edema. A toxicology screen may be useful to rule out the coingestion of other detectable poisons.

Because of delayed and prolonged absorption, serial salicylate levels should be obtained until levels are noted to be declining. A nontoxic salicylate level soon after ingestion does not rule out a significant overdose, particularly with ingestions of enteric-coated or sustained-release formulations. If levels continue to rise, repeated metabolic evaluation is necessary.

The ferric chloride spot test can be used for the rapid detection of aspirin in the urine. Several drops of 10% ferric chloride added to 1 mL of urine turns purple if acetylsalicylic acid is present. This test can confirm exposure but not overdose because positive results are seen with therapeutic doses of aspirin. False-positive reactions may be caused by acetoacetic acid, phenylpyruvic acid, phenothiazines, and phenylbutazone.

EMERGENCY DEPARTMENT MANAGEMENT

Advanced life-support measures should be instituted as needed. In patients who require endotracheal intubation, maintaining hyperventilation before, during, and after this procedure is critical because worsening acidemia (as a result of an increase in the pCO_2) enhances toxicity by increasing the fraction of nonionized salicylic acid available for tissue distribution. Failure to adequately hyperventilate patients who are intubated can result in rapid deterioration and death (13,25). Because artificial ventilation is accompanied by increased airway resistance and dead space, mechanical hyperventilation is unlikely to be as effective spontaneous hyperventilation and an increase in the pCO_2 (and decrease in serum pH) following intubation is inevitable in patients with a pCO_2 of less than 20 mm Hg. It is therefore recommended that prophylactic sodium bicarbonate (1 mEq/kg over 2–5 minutes) be given at the time of induction (sedation and paralysis) of patients with acidemia or a pCO_2 less than 20 mm Hg.

Because CNS hypoglycemia may occur despite a normal serum glucose in patients with salicylate poisoning, 50 mL of 50% dextrose in water (D50W) should be given to those with altered mental status (unless the glucose level is known to be elevated) (4,25). Anticonvulsants (e.g., benzodiazepines, phenytoin, and barbiturates) and supplemental glucose should be given to patients with seizures. It is also advisable to administer sodium bicarbonate (0.5 mEq/kg i.v. over 2–5 minutes) and calcium (0.1–0.2 mL/kg of 10% calcium chloride or gluconate i.v. over 2–5 m) as acidemia is likely to preexist and worsen after a seizure and seizures can be as a result of hypocalcemia. This dose of calcium can be safely given even if the serum calcium level is normal (e.g., in functional hypocalcemia) and is the preferred treatment for tetany as a result of hyperventilation (respiratory alkalosis). Paper-bag breathing is not recommended because an increase in

the pCO_2 can worsen concomitant acidemia. This is also true regarding the use of sedatives for the treatment of agitation. Similarly, should an antiemetic be necessary a nonsedating agent such as ondansetron is preferred. Patients who are unresponsive or becomes so after a seizure should be assumed to have cerebral edema. This complication should be treated with head elevation, hyperventilation, and possibly mannitol, furosemide, and dexamethasone. Diuretics should be used cautiously in patients with hypovolemia.

The degree of dehydration is often underestimated. Treatment should begin with 1 to 3 L (20 mL/kg) of intravenous 5% dextrose in normal saline (D5NS) or 5% dextrose in one-half normal saline (D5 $^1/_2$NS) with 1 ampule (44–50 mEq) of sodium bicarbonate (NaHCO$_3$) per liter, with or without potassium (10–20 mEq/L), over the first hour (23). Two i.v. lines are often necessary. Such therapy is contraindicated in patients with cerebral or pulmonary edema and should be monitored closely in those with renal dysfunction. Because its efficacy is best determined by urine output, bladder catheterization is indicated for monitoring purposes. The use of a dextrose-containing solution is important because of the potential for occult CNS hypoglycemia. In patients with hypernatremia, a more hypotonic solution should be used. Furosemide may also be used in an attempt to reverse oliguric renal failure unresponsive to volume replacement.

Central venous or pulmonary artery pressure monitoring may be necessary for optimal treatment of patients with hypotension or oliguria, especially if there is evidence of heart failure or pulmonary edema. Congestive heart failure can be treated by standard measures, but patients with noncardiac pulmonary edema should be treated with intubation or mask ventilation with positive end-expiratory pressure (PEEP) rather than diuretics. Again, preventing increased acidemia by maintaining hyperventilation is critical in patients with compromised pulmonary function.

Acidemia should be treated aggressively. As noted above, it promotes salicylate tissue distribution and enhances toxicity. Treatment includes artificial ventilation for respiratory acidosis and intravenous sodium bicarbonate (NaHCO$_3$) for metabolic acidosis. Calculating the dose of NaHCO$_3$ for metabolic acidosis in salicylate poisoning is more complicated than for other causes of metabolic acidosis because respiratory alkalosis is usually present and in salicylate poisoning, it is a concomitant primary acid–base disturbance, not just a compensatory response to academia. Hence, the administration of bicarbonate is unlikely to blunt the respiratory drive (increase the pCO_2), which would otherwise limit the increase in serum pH. Additionally, the goal of therapy is to limit the tissue distribution of salicylates by increasing the pH to 7.45, not to correct the base deficit.

Calculating the dose of bicarbonate needed to bring the pH to 7.45 in patients with acidemia and underlying metabolic acidosis and respiratory alkalosis requires two steps. First, using the law of mass action equation, $[H+] = 24 \times (pCO_2/[HCO_3-])$, and the fact that a pH of 7.45 corresponds to a $[H+]$ of 36 (nEq/l or nmol/L), calculate the serum $[HCO_3-]$ necessary to produce a $[H+]$ of 36: desired $[HCO_3-] = (24 \times pCO_2)/36 = 0.67 \times pCO_2$. Next, calculate the amount of NaHCO$_3$ necessary to produce the desired $[HCO_3-]$: NaHCO$_3$ dose = $0.7 \times kg \times$ (desired $[HCO_3-]$ - actual $[HCO_3-]$), in which 0.7 is the volume of distribution of bicarbonate in acidemia and kg is lean body weight. Two examples are illustrative. To achieve a pH of 7.45, a 70-kg person with a pH of 7.32, pCO_2 of 30 mm Hg, and $[HCO_3-]$ of 15 mEq/L needs an $[HCO_3-]$ of 20 mEq/L ($= 0.67 \times 30$) and the dose of NaHCO$_3$ necessary to achieve is about 245 mEq ($\approx 0.7 \times 70 \times [20$-$15]$). In a 70-kg person with a pH of 7.20, pCO_2 of 18 mm Hg, and $[HCO_3-]$ of 10 mEq/L, the desired $[HCO_3-]$ is 12 mEq/L ($= 0.67 \times 18$)

and the dose of $NaHCO_3$ required is 98 mEq/L ($= 0.7 \times 70 \times$ [12-10]). Note that the dose of $NaHCO_3$ does not necessarily correlate with the severity of acidemia and that increasing the serum $[HCO_3^-]$ to the normal range of 24 to 32 mEq/L (i.e., correcting the base deficit) would cause potentially dangerous alkalemia.

As with rehydration therapy, the dose of $NaHCO_3$ necessary to achieve a pH of 7.45 should be given over the first hour. It can be given as an infusion or in aliquots of 0.5 to 1 mEq/kg (over 2–5 minutes) every 10 minutes. Potassium supplementation will also be necessary because patients are typically potassium depleted and the serum potassium decreases by about 1 mEq/L for every increase in the pH of 0.1. As a general guideline, 10 to 20 mEq of potassium will be necessary for each 50 mEq of $NaHCO_3$ administered. An alternative (empiric) approach to the treatment of acid–base derangements in salicylate poisoning is to administer the intravenous fluid shown in Table 284.3. Depending on severity, 1 to 3 liters should be over the first hour. Potential complications of $NaHCO_3$ administration include excessive alkalemia, hypocalcemia, hypokalemia, hypernatremia, and fluid overload with cerebral and pulmonary edema, particularly in the elderly and those with severe poisoning. Hence, regardless of the method used, cardiac monitoring, frequent evaluation of vital signs, mental status, cardiorespiratory function, urine output, and laboratory parameters (arterial blood gas analysis, serum calcium and electrolytes) should be performed during and after such therapy. Relative contraindications to giving $NaHCO_3$ for acidemia include oliguric renal failure, congestive heart failure, and cerebral or pulmonary edema.

Hyperthermia should be treated with cooling blankets, ice packs, and evaporative methods. Acetaminophen is unlikely to be effective and NSAIDs should be avoided. The presence of peritoneal signs necessitates evaluation for surgical complications. Vitamin K should be given for coagulation abnormalities. Those with overt bleeding should also receive fresh-frozen plasma. Underlying metabolic derangements should be corrected. Insulin is unnecessary for nondiabetics with hyperglycemia and may be dangerous, particularly if there is coexisting hypokalemia. Similarly, hyperkalemia does not usually require specific therapy and usually resolves with fluid administration and correction of acidosis.

GI decontamination should be done in patients with accidental ingestions of more than 150 mg/kg and in all patients with intentional overdoses (4,8,21,22,25). Charcoal alone is superior to ipecac followed by charcoal in simulated overdose patients (7) and is the preferred method in those with mild-to-moderate overdoses. Because charcoal binds neutral agents better than ionized ones, salicylate may desorb from charcoal in the alkaline milieu of the small intestine (6). Therefore, at least two doses of charcoal should be given. Gastric lavage should be considered for large ingestions (500 mg/kg). Even in patients with spontaneous vomiting, large amounts of salicylate have been recovered as long as 18 hours after ingestion, hence the adage, "It's never too late to aspirate with salicylate." Optimal decontamination for large overdoses may be to give a dose of charcoal before and after gastric lavage (5). Whole-bowel irrigation should be considered in patients with large ingestions of enteric-coated or sustained-release preparations (25). Serial salicylate levels should be obtained to assess the efficacy of GI decontamination. Levels that continue to rise despite decontamination measures therapy suggest gastric drug concretion or bezoar formation. Evaluation and treatment of this complication by endoscopy should be considered if drug levels become markedly elevated or clinical toxicity is severe or progressive.

Salicylate elimination can be enhanced by repeated oral doses of activated charcoal, alkaline diuresis, and extracorporeal removal (4,12,13,20–25). The administration of glycine (or

N-glycylglycine), a cofactor for one of the salicylic acid pathways subject to saturation (see Table 284.2), can also enhance the elimination of salicylate but clinical experience is limited and this therapy should be considered experimental. Although data from experimental studies are conflicting, multiple-dose charcoal (MDAC) shortened the salicylate half-life to 2 to 4 hours in patients with salicylate levels as high as 66 mg/dL after acute overdosage (12). In this study, the brand of charcoal used (Medicoal) was an effervescent preparation containing bicarbonate which may have ionized and trapped salicylate in the gut (decreased its absorption) or been absorbed and caused concomitant urinary alkalinization (enhanced its elimination). Although other brands of charcoal may not be as effective, MDAC therapy is recommended for all patients with clinical or laboratory evidence of salicylate poisoning or a salicylate level greater than 30 mg/dL after an acute overdose.

Alkaline diuresis can shorten the salicylate half-life to 6 to 12 hours in acute overdose patients with salicylate levels less than 70 mg/dL (20). Although urinary alkalinization alone was more effective than either diuresis alone or alkaline diuresis, patients in the "alkalinization alone" group actually received substantial amounts of fluid (i.e., they were treated with diuresis as well as urinary alkalinization)—about 375 to 500 mL/h over the treatment period. Animal studies have shown that both alkalinization and diuresis are effective. Indications for alkaline diuresis are the same as for MDAC. Contraindications include cerebral and pulmonary edema, oliguric renal failure, and a serum pH above 7.55. It should be performed with caution in patients with a history of cardiac failure. Adequate hydration (urine output) should be established before initiating this therapy.

The goal of alkaline diuresis is a urine pH of 7.5 or more and a brisk (3–6 mL/kg/h) urine output. If academia has been corrected, alkaline diuresis can usually be accomplished by administering fluid therapy for early or mild poisoning (Table 284.3) at a rate equal to the desired urine output. Alternatively, the empiric fluid therapy as described for the correction of academia can initially be used. Although counterintuitive, alkaline diuresis is indicated during early or mild intoxication, when the serum and urine pH are both alkaline, because respiratory alkalosis with compensatory renal bicarbonate and fluid excretion account for these findings. If left untreated, this can lead to dehydration and more severe metabolic acidosis during later stages of poisoning. Carbonic anhydrase inhibitors (e.g., acetazolamide) should not be used to alkalinize the urine because they can cause acidemia, which increases ionized drug fraction and enhances its tissue distribution. This may result in increased CNS salicylate levels and clinical deterioration, and increased mortality (25). Because potassium reabsorption occurs at the expense of bicarbonate reabsorption and hydrogen ion excretion, it is often stated that alkalinization of the urine is impossible until potassium deficits are corrected. Whether this is true or not is controversial (25). In one study, no correlation was found between serum potassium levels and urinary pH (16). Although correction of hypokalemia is clearly indicated, doing so should not delay instituting alkaline diuresis. Complications, precautions, and monitoring during alkaline diuresis are the same as those noted when giving bicarbonate for the correction of acidemia. Additionally, patients treated with alkaline diuresis should have hourly monitoring of fluid intake, urinary output, and urine pH. If intake persistently exceeds output, diuresis may be enhanced by giving furosemide.

Hemodialysis is the treatment of choice for patients with severe poisoning (4,8,14,22–25). A reduction in the salicylate half-life to 2 to 3 hours can be achieved. Although hemoperfusion is slightly more effective in removing salicylate, it is technically more difficult and does not correct associated acid–base, fluid, and electrolyte abnormalities (14). Peritoneal dialysis (with

5% albumin added to compete with serum proteins for salicylate binding) and exchange transfusion are less effective and should be used only if hemodialysis is unavailable, contraindicated, or technically impossible (e.g., in infants or in patients with active or recent bleeding complications) (4,17).

Indications for hemodialysis include coma, seizures, cerebral or pulmonary edema, renal failure, and clinical or metabolic deterioration (or failure to improve) despite other therapies (4,8,14,21,23–25). Although hemodialysis is often recommended if the salicylate level is greater than 100 mg/dL after an acute ingestion, it may not be necessary in the absence of severe or progressive clinical and metabolic toxicity (e.g., as a result of early presentation and aggressive treatment with other measures). Conversely, patients with moderate toxicity that progresses or fails to improve with other treatment (e.g., those with underlying cardiopulmonary disease or limited reserves because of advanced age or co-existing illness) should be considered for hemodialysis even if the salicylate level is not markedly elevated.

In contrast to the usual dialysis patient with chronic renal failure, fluid overload, and hypertension, patients with salicylate poisoning are often hemodynamically compromised or tenuously stable because of underestimated or undertreated dehydration and cardiac dysfunction. As such, they are prone to cardiovascular decompensation on initiation of hemodialysis. Hypotension is common and dysrhythmias can occur. Priming the dialysis circuit with normal saline and administering a fluid bolus prior to and during dialysis are recommended as prophylactic measures, along with correction of volume deficits and metabolic abnormalities, if possible. To facilitate the treatment and prevention of acidemia, and also to enhance the trapping and removal of salicylate, the dialysate bath should contain a high concentration of bicarbonate (32 mEq/L).

CRITICAL INTERVENTIONS

- Maintain hyperventilation during and after endotracheal intubation and administer sodium bicarbonate prior to this procedure in patients with acidemia
- Perform frequent clinical and laboratory re-evaluation and obtain serial salicylate levels to assess the progression and severity of poisoning and the efficacy of decontamination and enhanced drug elimination therapies
- Consult a nephrologist regarding hemodialysis for patients with severe clinical or metabolic manifestations of salicylate poisoning or progressive deterioration despite other treatments
- Administer a fluid bolus, prime the pump with saline, and attempt to correct fluid and metabolic abnormalities prior to hemodialysis

DISPOSITION

Patients with mild or absent clinical and laboratory toxicity after acute overdose can often be treated in the emergency department if the peak salicylate level is less than 60 mg/dL. Patients with chronic poisoning, higher levels, underlying medical problems, and moderate or severe toxicity should be admitted to an intensive care unit. A nephrologist should be consulted if poisoning is severe. If hemodialysis is unavailable, patients with severe poisoning or moderate poisoning with very high (or rising) salicylate levels should be transferred to a facility in which such treatment is available. Unless the patient has oliguria, alkaline diuresis should be continued during dialysis.

COMMON PITFALLS

✔ Failure to ask specifically about salicylate ingestion and to obtain a serum salicylate level on patients with unexplained acid–base disturbances, particularly in those with altered mental status

✔ Failure to obtain quantitative levels of both aspirin and acetaminophen in patients who report an overdose of either agent

✔ Failure to obtain serial salicylate levels to rule out delayed absorption

✔ Failure to appreciate the differences between acute and chronic salicylate poisoning

✔ Failure to monitor for complications of salicylate poisoning and its treatment

✔ Failure to recognize the limitations of salicylate levels and the salicylate nomogram and to base treatment on clinical and laboratory findings, not drug levels

References

1. Bailey RB, Jones SR. Chronic salicylate intoxication: a common cause of morbidity in the elderly. *J Am Geriatr Soc* 1989;37:556.
2. Bartels PD, Lund-Jacobsen H. Blood lactate and ketone body concentrations in salicylate intoxication. *Hum Toxicol* 1986;5:363.
3. Botma M, Colquhoun-Flannery W, Leighton S. Laryngeal oedema caused by accidental ingestion of Oil of Wintergreen. *Int J Pediatr Otorhinolaryngol* 2001;58(3):229–232.
4. Brenner BE, Simon RR. Management of salicylate intoxication. *Drugs* 1987; 24:335.
5. Burton BT, Bayer MJ, Barron L, et al. Comparison of activated charcoal and gastric lavage in the prevention of aspirin absorption. *J Emerg Med* 1984;1:411.
6. Chapman BJ, Proudfoot AT. Adult salicylate poisoning: deaths and outcome in patients with high plasma salicylate concentrations. *Q J Med* 1989;72:699.
7. Curtis RA, Barone J, Giacon N. Efficacy of ipecac and activated charcoal/cathartic: prevention of salicylate absorption in a simulated overdose. *Arch Intern Med* 1984;144:48.
8. Dargan PI, Wallace CI, Jones AL. An evidence based flowchart to guide the management of acute salicylate (aspirin) overdose. *Emerg Med J* 2002;19(3):206–209.
9. Dugandzic RM, Tierney ME, Dickinson GE, et al. Evaluation of the validity of the Done nomogram in the management of acute salicylate poisoning. *Ann Emerg Med* 1989;18:1186.
10. Gabow PA, Anderson RJ, Potts DE, et al. Acid–base disturbances in the salicylate-intoxicated adult. *Arch Intern Med* 1978;138:1481.
11. Gaudrealt P, Temple AR, Lovejoy FH. The relative severity of acute vs. chronic salicylate poisonings in children: a clinical comparison. *Pediatrics* 1982;70:566.
12. Hillman RJ, Prescott LF. Treatment of salicylate poisoning with repeated activated charcoal. *BMJ* 1985;291:1472.
13. Greenberg MI, Hendrickson RG, Hofman M: Deleterious effects of endotracheal intubation in salicylate poisoning. *Ann Emerg Med* 2003;41(4):583–4.
14. Jacobsen D, Wiik-Larsen E, Bredesen JH. Haemodialysis or haemoperfusion in severe salicylate poisoning? *Hum Toxicol* 1988;7:161.
15. Leatherman JW, Schmitz PG. Fever, hyperdynamic shock, and multiple system organ failure: a pseudo-sepsis syndrome associated with chronic salicylate poisoning. *Chest* 1991;100:1391.
16. Levy G. Comparative pharmacokinetics of aspirin and acetaminophen. *Arch Intern Med* 1981;141:279.
17. Manikian A, Stone S, Hamilton R, et al: Exchange transfusion in severe infant salicylism. *Vet Hum Toxicol* 2002;44(4):224–227.
18. McGuigan MA. A 2-year review of salicylate deaths in Ontario. *Arch Intern Med* 1987;147:510.
19. Palatnick W, Tenenbein M: Aspirin poisoning during pregnancy: increased fetal sensitivity. *Am J Perinatol* 1998;15(1):39–41.
20. Prescott LF, Balali-Mood M, Critchley JAJH, et al. Diuresis or urinary alkalinization for salicylate poisoning? *BMJ* 1982;285:1383.
21. Proudfoot AT. Toxicity of salicylates. *Am J Med* 1983;75:99.
22. Roberts LJ, Morrow JD. Analgesic-antipyretic and antiinflammatory agents and drugs employed in the treatment of gout. In: Hardman JG, Limbird LE, Gilman AG, eds. *Goodman and Gilman's: the pharmacological basis of therapeutics*, 9th ed. New York, McGraw-Hill, 2001:687.
23. Temple AR. Acute and chronic effects of aspirin toxicity and their treatment. *Arch Intern Med* 1981;141:364.
24. Thisted B, Krantz T, Strom J, et al. Acute salicylate poisoning in 177 consecutive patients treated in ICU. *Acta Anaesthesiol Scand* 1987;31:312.
25. Yip L, Dart RC, Gabow PA. Concepts and controversies in salicylate toxicity. *Emerg Med Clin North Am* 1994;12:351.

CHAPTER 285
Complications of Injection Drug Use

James A. Feldman, Michael K. Tibbles,
and Susan S. Fish

An estimated 1.1 to 1.8 million people in the United States currently use nonprescribed drugs by intravenous, subcutaneous, and other routes of injection, and another 2.5 million have self-injected drugs at least once. The lifestyle associated with drug use increases the risk of trauma, and numerous infections including HIV, hepatitis, tuberculosis, and sexually transmitted diseases. Injection drug use (IDU) brings with it the risk of complications directly related to the local or systemic effects of the substances injected, the use of nonsterile methods of injection, and other aspects of injection practices (Table 285.1). Complications from unsafe injection methods are the most common reason IDU patients present to the emergency department (15).

Cutaneous and superficial soft-tissue infections, particularly abscesses often occur at the site of injection. The bacteriology of abscesses in IDU patients is more likely to be mixed aerobic–anaerobic infections than in non-IDU patients (20). Although *S. aureus* is the most common organism (36%–50%), flora of the oropharynx are often isolated. Cutaneous abscesses of the neck may lead to respiratory complications such as airway obstruction, laryngeal edema, and vocal cord paralysis (14).

Wound botulism has been increasingly reported since 1982, with 35 cases identified in California during a recent 26-month study period (17). IDU-related tetanus has also been increasingly reported. Of the 67 cases of tetanus reported in California from 1987 through 1997, 40% occurred in IDU patients (21). Skin lesions or small abscesses that appear innocuous may harbor *C. botulinum* or *C. tetani*. Injection drug users are also at risk for more serious and deeper soft-tissue infections, including necrotizing fasciitis (see Chapter 136, "Skin and Soft-Tissue Infections"), myositis, and pyomyositis. Broken needles at the site of intravenous injection are usually an incidental finding noted on radiograph. Such retained needle fragments rarely embolize centrally. However, pericarditis with pericardial effusion secondary to central migration has been reported (11).

Vascular complications related to IDU include unintentional intraarterial injection, with resultant vasospasm or thrombosis and limb ischemia; venous and arterial pseudoaneurysm formation; development of infected hematoma; and venous thrombosis and septic thrombophlebitis. IDU is a major risk factor for deep vein thrombosis (DVT) especially among those who injected in the femoral veins.

Mycotic aneurysms involving central arteries, such as the hepatic, mesenteric, cerebral, and pulmonary arteries, and large vessel occlusive emboli may occur in the context of endocarditis (see Chapter 47, "Infectious Endocarditis"). The bacteriology of both arterial and venous mycotic aneurysm is polymicrobial in up to 40% of cases. *S. aureus*, frequently β-lactam–resistant, is often cultured from the wound or blood. Anaerobic organisms have been reported in up to 20% of some series.

"Pocket shooting," or injection into the supraclavicular fossa to access the jugular, subclavian, or brachiocephalic veins, often leads to pneumothorax, hemothorax, hydropneumothorax, or

---

TABLE 285.1.   Medical Complications of Injection Drug Use by Organ System

CUTANEOUS

Needle foreign body
Abscess
Necrotizing fasciitis
Gas gangrene
Cellulitis

VASCULAR

Septic phlebitis
Thrombophlebitis
Pseudoaneurysm
Infected hematoma
Intraarterial injection

MUSCULOSKELETAL

Vertebral osteomyelitis
Septic arthritis
Compartment syndrome
Pyomyositis

PULMONARY

Pneumothorax
Hemothorax
Talcosis
Septic pulmonary embolus
Pneumonia

NEUROLOGIC

Peripheral nervous system
    Puncture injuries
    Compression injuries
    Plexitis/plexopathy
Central nervous system
    Infections
    Meningitis
    Abscesses: cerebral, epidural, spinal
    Mycotic aneurysm
    Transient ischemic attacks
    Mucormycosis
    Stroke

INTERNAL ORGANS

Heart
    Endocarditis
    Myocardial infarction, ischemia
Liver
    Hepatitis
Spleen
    Abscess
Kidney
    Nephrotic syndrome
    Glomerulonephritis
    Abscess
    Infarct
Intestine
    Mesenteric ischemia, infarction

GENERAL/OTHER

Cotton fever
Septicemia
HIV infection
Tetanus
Wound botulism
Endophthalmitis
Malaria

pyopneumothorax. In one review of 525 cases of pneumothorax, 20% were related to IDU. Of these, 19% were complete collapse or tension pneumothorax (two were bilateral), 43% were large, 32% moderate or small, and 6% had only an apical cap (4).

Injection of solubilized tablets and capsules can lead to pulmonary dysfunction from injected particulate matter that deposit in the lung. Tablets are usually crushed, dissolved in water or other liquid, sometimes heated. Then the solution is drawn up into a syringe either directly or filtered through cotton. The fillers in the tablet consist usually of talc, cornstarch, or cellulose. Talc is well known to induce granulomas in and around the arterioles and capillaries of the lung, and it can also deposit in retinal vessels; this condition is referred to as "talcosis"(16). Both restrictive and obstructive pulmonary dysfunction can be seen, and pulmonary hypertension and cor pulmonale. Although cornstarch is not associated with granuloma formation, the resultant bland pulmonary thromboses can lead to pulmonary hypertension.

Osteomyelitis and septic arthritis secondary to IDU may result from direct contamination or hematogenous spread. Vertebral osteomyelitis is the most common form of skeletal infection in IDU patients (12). The sites of vertebral involvement reported are lumbar (54%), cervical (27%), and thoracic (4%). The increased frequency of cervical involvement noted in IDU patients is an important variation in the distribution of vertebral osteomyelitis, compared with the general population.

The sacroiliac, sternoclavicular, costochondral, and pubic symphysis synchondroses are frequent sites of septic arthritis in IDU patients. Although these axial fibrocartilaginous joints are the most common sites of septic arthritis in IDU patients (1), other joints, including the knees, hips, and shoulders, may be involved. Although *Pseudomonas aeruginosa* and *Serratia marcescens*, in the past, had been the most common cause of osteoarticular infections, *S. aureus* has more recently replaced gram-negative bacilli and Candida as the primary cause of these infections (3).

IDU patients are at increased risk of central nervous system (CNS) infections, including fungal and bacterial meningitis, cerebritis, and spinal, epidural, and brain abscesses (7). Indolent CNS aspergillosis, cerebral mucormycosis, and anterior spinal artery syndrome with subsequent paraplegia have been reported. A syndrome of cerebral mucormycosis has been well described in IDU patients who were seronegative for the human immunodeficiency virus (HIV) (9). Fungal endophthalmitis, caused by such organisms as Aspergillus and Fusarium, has been described in patients with IDU as the only identified risk factor for these uncommon infections (24). Peripheral nerve injuries may result from needle-induced trauma, extrinsic compression, and direct toxic or hypersensitivity reactions to injected materials.

Systemic infections may result from exposure to skin contaminants, contaminated apparatus, contaminated injection mixture, and blood-borne pathogens transmitted by the practice of needle sharing. HIV and hepatitis B, C, and δ infections are discussed in other chapters. Infection with the HTLV virus (types I and II) is associated with injection drug use (5). Hepatitis GB virus type C (HGBV-C), an important cause of fulminant non–A-E hepatitis, is also more commonly identified in IDU patients (22). The lifetime seroconversion rate for hepatitis B in IDU patients is 80% to 90%, and the incidence of bacterial endocarditis is 5% (2). A number of uncommon infections have also been described. A syndrome of disseminated candidiasis, characterized by scalp, ocular, and osteoarticular involvement, was attributed to the use of lemon juice in the preparation of brown heroin for injection (3). Malaria, both falciparum and vivax, endophthalmitis, and tick-borne relapsing fever have been reported.

In IDU patients presenting with fever, 64% had readily identifiable major illnesses such as pneumonia, cellulitis, or endo-carditis; another 4% of patients had major illnesses that were not clinically apparent on initial evaluation (18). An acute but self-limited pyrogenic reaction induced by intravenous injection of foreign material from cotton balls used to filter injected solution is another common cause of fever. The history, physical examination, and laboratory testing can not reliably differentiate "cotton fever" or other minor conditions from more serious causes of fever (13).

CLINICAL PRESENTATION

Patients with superficial abscesses complain of localized pain. Fever and systemic complaints may also be present. The classic signs and symptoms of warmth, redness, tenderness, swelling, and fluctuance may be absent in IDU patients. As many as 25% of patients with cutaneous abscesses do not have fluctuance.

Tetanus presents as increased muscle tone, spasm, or trismus. Patients with wound botulism usually present with neurologic complaints such as cranial palsies or descending symmetrical paralysis. Atypical signs, including asymmetric or unilateral cranial nerve weakness and peripheral motor weakness, may be present (10). Atypical presentations and false-positive edrophonium tests have caused patients to be misdiagnosed with Eaton-Lambert syndrome or myasthenia gravis, resulting in prolonged delays in appropriate therapy.

Deep soft-tissue infections can have a subtle initial presentation but can rapidly progress to limb and life threatening illness. Myositis and pyomyositis may present initially with only mild erythema of the overlying skin but will rapidly develop pain, significant edema and crepitus. Sometimes a brown discoloration of the skin or purplish blebs may develop. When the infection has progressed enough to cause marked cutaneous changes the patient will frequently develop septic shock.

Broken needle fragments at injection sites may be asymptomatic or patients may have localized complaints of pain as a result of the needle itself or to infectious complications. Patients may present with concerns about the risks of a retained needle fragment. They may also be unaware of its presence or fail to mention it unless asked.

Inadvertent intraarterial injection causes immediate severe pain, hyperemia, numbness, weakness, distal swelling, cyanosis, and motor deficit and, often, sensory abnormalities. Distal ischemia may progress to gangrene, myonecrosis, and associated complications. The use of crushed oral medications and the lower extremity as a site of injection appears to be associated with more severe complications.

Venous pseudoaneurysms are most commonly noted in the groin. Pain, swelling, and purulent drainage may be noted. Some patients may appear clinically septic, with minimal localized complaints. In these patients, either pulmonary complaints or symptoms referable to sites of metastatic septic involvement may be more prominent.

Any mass over a vascular territory may actually be a pseudoaneurysm and should be approached with caution. Arterial mycotic aneurysms usually present as an indurated mass with local pain, and swelling. The mass is pulsatile in approximately 50% cases, and a bruit is often heard over the swelling (25). Fever and leukocytosis are common, but bleeding, although occasionally massive, is usually intermittent, minor, or absent. Claudication, paresthesias, or compression neuropathy can occur. Signs and symptoms of distal embolic phenomenon, including cutaneous purpura, may be present and may precede systemic manifestations. Although upper and lower extremity arteries are most commonly involved, mycotic aneurysms of the subclavian and carotid arteries have been reported following attempted central venous injections.

IDU patients with infective endocarditis usually have fever but a new heart murmur, Roth's spots, Osler's nodes, Janeway lesions, splinter hemorrhages, or embolic phenomena are rare. The history and physical exam have a poor sensitivity and specificity for detecting infective endocarditis (23).

Patients with pneumothorax typically present with a history of recent neck injection, dyspnea, and pleuritic chest pain (4). Particulate-induced pulmonary dysfunction frequently presents as progressive dyspnea. Chest radiograph can show a micronodular pattern; over time, the pattern changes to show large homogenous opacities, usually in the perihilar regions and upper lobes (16). Retinoscopy can show talc depositions (small, whitish, glistening dots) and may have a higher diagnostic yield than either chest radiograph or pulmonary function tests.

Skeletal infections often present as localized pain and tenderness. IDU patients commonly develop septic arthritis and osteomyelitis at sites rarely seen in the general population including the sternum, sacroiliac joints, and pubic symphysis. Almost 20% of patients with vertebral osteomyelitis related to IDU have had pain for more than 3 months at the time of diagnosis. About 15% report a history of minor blunt back trauma, such as a fall or kick, a factor that may contribute to delayed diagnosis. Fever is usually absent or of low grade. Neurologic signs and symptoms occur infrequently (less than 15%) and are usually transient. Routine laboratory studies are usually normal. The erythrocyte sedimentation rate (ESR) usually is elevated but can be normal. Plain x-rays may demonstrate disc space narrowing (82%) or paravertebral shadows, suggesting abscess (12%), but magnetic resonance imaging (MRI) is diagnostic.

Patients with septic arthritis associated with IDU are similar in presentation to other patients with septic arthritis, except for the prominence of fibrocartilaginous joint involvement. Local signs of inflammation and fever, leukocytosis, and elevated ESR are usually noted. Asymptomatic HIV infection has been reported in one-third of IDU patients with septic arthritis (1).

A patient with fungal endophthalmitis usually presents with decreased vision, photophobia and ocular pain, which develop slowly. The infection may occur in one or both eyes. White vitreal exudates may be seen on ophthalmic exam. Bacterial endophthalmitis has a similar but more rapidly progressing presentation.

Patients with cerebral mucormycosis usually have headache, fever, and rapidly developing cranial nerve and motor deficits. Basal ganglia lesions on computed tomography (CT) scan should suggest this diagnosis. Cotton fever may cause dyspnea, palpitations, headache, and rigors.

Patients who inject drugs are also at risk for systemic drug or drug-contaminant toxicity (see Chapters 283, "Opioids," Chapter 290, "Muscle Relaxants and Other Sedative–Hypnotic Agents," Chapter 324, "Cocaine," and Chapter 328, "Sympathomimetics"), withdrawal syndromes (see Chapter 333, "Drug Withdrawal"), and CNS infections (see Chapter 138, "Meningitis and Encephalitis").

DIFFERENTIAL DIAGNOSIS

The most important requirement for developing an appropriate differential diagnosis is obtaining the history of IDU. Biases can easily enter into the physician's decision to obtain this information. It may be necessary to consider the possibility of IDU, even if denied by the patient. In such cases, a urine screening test for drugs of abuse may be helpful.

Unless the history of IDU is routinely obtained or considered, conditions such as vertebral osteomyelitis and epidural abscess may not be considered in the differential diagnosis of complaints such as back pain. Consider botulism, endocarditis, or intracranial abscesses and mycotic aneurysms in the IDU patient presenting with stroke symptoms. What appears to be an abscess in an IDU may actually be a pseudoaneurysm and a simple incision and drainage might have disastrous consequences. The IDU patient who develops a fever or flu-like symptoms is much more likely to have an infection requiring hospital admission than is a non-IDU patient who presents with similar complaints. Infective endocarditis should be in the differential diagnosis of all IDU patients with fever, even if another source of fever is found.

EMERGENCY DEPARTMENT EVALUATION

The possibility of IDU, recent or remote, should be included in the standard "screening history." A nonthreatening question such as, "Do you smoke cigarettes, or use alcohol or other drugs?" should be routinely asked of all patients. Patients with IDU should be asked about the specifics of drug type, amount, needle sharing, skin preparation (alcohol wipes), and whether they have a history of hepatitis, endocarditis, HIV, pain at injection sites, recent fever, and nonprescribed antibiotic self-treatment. Because many IDU patients will not reveal their drug use, track marks or a positive urine toxicology screen may be the only clue to the diagnosis.

The physical examination of a patient with recognized IDU should include a careful review of vital signs, particularly an accurate temperature. Examination of the skin for signs of endocarditis, jaundice, infection at injection sites, and markers of HIV infection, such as oral thrush, should be performed in addition to a complaint-oriented examination. Evidence of opiate withdrawal, such as diaphoresis, lacrimation, yawning, pupillary dilation, and piloerection, should also be sought.

Routine laboratory tests are of limited use. Drug screens provide little information that will affect decisions, except possibly to suggest drug use when it is denied. Although the complete blood count (CBC) and ESR lack sufficient sensitivity and specificity to guide disposition decisions, if infection is suspected or present, a very high or low white blood cell count might prompt admission, even for a simple abscess.

The use of ultrasonography may identify occult abscesses that require drainage that otherwise would have been missed on physical exam alone. Cutaneous abscesses with associated systemic complaints should be cultured. A radiograph should be routinely considered in patients with cutaneous complaints of pain and tenderness at injection sites to exclude retained needle foreign bodies and to identify gas-forming infections. Suspected deep soft tissue infections such as myositis or pyomyositis should be evaluated with MRI or CT scan. Ultrasound may identify a perivascular abscess but is not very sensitive for detecting pseudoaneurysms. Although digital subtraction angiography may be a useful diagnostic modality, color-flow duplex scans may be the diagnostic study of choice (25). Arteriography may be necessary to confirm the diagnosis.

Patients in whom endocarditis is suspected should have three sets of blood cultures, a chest radiograph and cardiac ultrasonography. Pocket shooters and those with respiratory complaints should have a chest radiograph and oxygen saturation.

Patients with joint pain and effusion should have two sets of blood cultures and aspiration, Gram stain, and culture of affected joints. Septic synchondroses may be safely aspirated in the emergency department and should be evaluated similarly. Two sets of blood cultures and an MRI should be obtained for suspected vertebral osteomyelitis or epidural abscess. Consider an MRI on all IDU patients presenting with back pain given that history, physical exam and all other diagnostic testing lack significant sensitivity and specificity.

Patients with complaints that suggest a CNS process (headache, weakness, ataxia) require a detailed neurologic examination, CT scan or MRI, and a lumbar puncture to identify cerebrovascular complications of IDU use, opportunistic CNS infections, or malignancy (related or unrelated to HIV infection). Patients with complaints of visual loss require a complete eye examination, usually dilation with indirect funduscopy. In patients with fever, three sets of blood cultures, chest radiograph, urinalysis, and urine culture should be obtained.

EMERGENCY DEPARTMENT MANAGEMENT

All patients with IDU-related infections should be given tetanus prophylaxis as needed. Except for patients with uncomplicated cutaneous abscesses, an infectious disease specialist should be consulted. Localized cutaneous abscesses without vascular involvement may be managed with routine incision and drainage. If there is a possibility of vascular involvement, needle aspiration should be performed first. Patients with localized infections involving the neck, groin, or vascular structures and those with suspected deep soft tissue infections such as myositis or pyomyositis should be evaluated by a surgeon. Although antibiotics and hospitalization are not routinely required for cutaneous abscesses that have been drained, patients with HIV infection, neutropenia, vascular involvement, deep space infections, or possible sepsis should be admitted and given parenteral antibiotics. Extensive extremity infections should be explored in the operating room, as inadequate drainage may prolong hospitalization.

Initial antibiotic therapy for soft tissue infections should include a penicillinase-resistant synthetic penicillin such as nafcillin. Clindamycin 600 mg i.v. q 8h or cephazolin 1–2 gm i.v. q 8h are alternatives for nonmethicillin-resistant *S. aureus* (MSRA). In areas with MRSA, vancomycin (1–2 gm i.v. q 12h) should be used until culture results are available. An antipseudomonal regimen including an aminoglycoside (APAG) such as gentamicin (traditional dosing 1–2 mg/kg i.v. q 8–24 hrs with the frequency dependant upon renal function and high dose 5–7 mg/kg i.v. q 24h) combined with an agent such as ceftazidime (2 g i.v. q 8h) or cefepime (1–2 gram i.v. q 12h) should also be given if enteric organisms or Pseudomonas has been identified as part of the "IDU" flora. Patients with gas-forming or necrotizing infections require *immediate* operative intervention and combination broad spectrum antibiotic therapy that might include clindamycin, high-dose penicillin G, and an APAG as well as consideration of such adjunctive therapy as intravenous immunoglobulin (IVIG) and hyperbaric oxygen therapy. Such antibiotics as Pipericillin/Tazobactam (3/0.375 g i.v. q 4–6h) or imipenim (1 g i.v. q 6–8h) can also be considered. Where available, infectious disease consultation should be considered to aid in antibiotic selection and adjunctive therapy for such complex soft tissue infections as necrotizing fascitis or myonecrosis associated with Clostridium (see Chapter 136, "Skin and Soft Tissue Infections").

Early administration of antitoxin is important in patients with wound botulism. In a retrospective case series, 57% patients who received antitoxin within 12 hours of presentation required mechanical ventilation for a median duration of 11 days whereas 85% of those who received antitoxin 12 hours after presentation required mechanical ventilation for a median of 54 days (19).

When associated with infection or vascular injury, needle fragments require urgent removal. Patients with retained needle foreign bodies without these complications may be given appropriate discharge instructions and referral to a surgeon for elective removal (11). In general, removal of fractured needle fragments should not be attempted by emergency physicians. Even if palpable, finding them may be difficult, important neurovascular structures nearby may be injured, and migration may occur despite the use of a proximal tourniquet.

Patients with signs and symptoms of intraarterial injection require aggressive management because of the potential for distal limb ischemia. Treatment should include antibiotics and anticoagulation with heparin. Consultation with a general or vascular surgeon is essential. Measurement of extremity compartment pressures should also be considered. Some authors suggest the use of dextran 40 (20 mL/h) give intravenously and dexamethasone (4 mg every 6 hours) or the intraarterial injection of a vasodilator such as papaverine (40–60 mg) or phentolamine (2 mg). Favorable results have been reported from the use of Iloprost, a prostacyclin analogue, and intraarterial thrombolysis (25).

Patients with pseudoaneurysms require blood cultures, preoperative laboratory testing, including blood typing, and consultation with a general or vascular surgeon. Hospitalization is usually indicated. Hemorrhage control with direct pressure may be required. Local drainage should not be attempted in the emergency department, as life-threatening hemorrhage may result.

In IDU patients admitted with fever and suspected endocarditis, oral antibiotics may be an acceptable alternative to intravenous therapy. Ciprofloxacin (750 mg p.o. bid) and rifampin (300 mg p.o. bid) can be given to the stable patient in whom intravenous access is extremely difficult or high risk pending culture results (8). However, *S. aureus* may be resistant to fluoroquinolones. A more in depth discussion on endocarditis management is covered in Chapter 47, "Infectious Endocarditis."

The management of pneumothorax is discussed in Chapters 37, "Spontaneous Pneumothorax and Pneumomediastinum" and Chapter 183, "Penetrating Chest Trauma." Pulmonary dysfunction from other causes is treated by supportive measures.

Vertebral osteomyelitis and septic arthritis should be treated with vancomycin and an APAG. Consultation with an orthopedic surgeon should be obtained. The management of CNS infections is covered in Chapter 138, "Meningitis and Encephalitis" and endophthalmitis is covered in Chapter 21, "Acute Eye Infections."

Patients with cotton fever require only supportive care. This illness usually resolves within 12 to 24 hours. However, given the possibility that a serious medical condition is the etiology of fever, inpatient observation is recommended until the patient is well and the results of blood cultures are known.

CRITICAL INTERVENTIONS

- Consult an infectious disease specialist or admit IDU patients with infectious complications or fever
- Consult a general or vascular surgeon for IDU patients with deep soft tissue infections, retained needle fragments, limb ischemia, or masses in the neck or groin
- Consult an orthopedic surgeon for IDU patients with vertebral osteomyelitis and septic arthritis
- Consult an ophthalmologist for IDU patients with visual complaints

DISPOSITION

Patients with cutaneous abscesses who are otherwise asymptomatic and healthy may be discharged with appropriate instructions and referral for follow-up in 24 to 48 hours. Patients with retained needle foreign bodies can be referred for elective surgery on an outpatient basis unless there are signs of infection. The ability of a patient to comply with outpatient therapy and follow-up should be considered. Most patients with other infectious complications require admission. Concomitant HIV infection should lower the threshold for admission.

Patients should also be educated about secondary prevention and "harm reduction," practices that have been shown to reduce the morbidity and mortality from injection drug use. They should be referred for substance abuse treatment and, if available, to needle-exchange, hepatitis, influenza, and pneumococcal vaccination programs and for HIV, hepatitis, and sexually transmitted disease screening. Patients who continue to use injection drugs may benefit from teachings about prevention practices, such as antiseptic skin preparation prior to injection, the use of bleach for cleaning needles and syringes, and the use of condoms to prevent sexually transmitted disease. Innovative programs such as the San Francisco Wound and Abscess Clinic, which combines medical care with public health services, have reduced emergency department visits by 40%, surgical admissions by 43%, and operating room procedures by 71% (6).

COMMON PITFALLS

✔ Failure to ask about IDU in all patients, including adolescents and older adults

✔ Failure to consider the possibility of undiagnosed HIV infection

✔ Labeling patients with IDU as "pain medication seekers" and allowing a judgmental attitude toward patients who use injection drugs to interfere with a careful medical evaluation

✔ Failure to appreciate that IDU patients with back pain as a result of vertebral infections may give a history of minor trauma and have a normal neurologic examination

✔ Attributing fever in an IDU to a trivial illness or to cotton fever

✔ Attempting to drain a soft-tissue mass in proximity to a major blood vessel

✔ Failure to consider the possibility of arterial injection, compartment syndrome, deep-space infection, or nerve injury in patients with limb complaints

✔ Failure to appreciated that extensive abscesses cannot be adequately drained in the emergency department

References

1. Brancos MA, Peris P, Miro JM, et al. Septic arthritis in heroin addicts. *Semin Arthritis Rheum* 1991;21:81–87.
2. Brettle RP. Infection and injection drug use. *J Infect* 1992;25:121–131.
3. Cherubin CE, Sapira JD. The medical complications of drug addiction and the medical assessment of the intravenous drug user: 25 years later [see comments]. *Ann Intern Med* 1993;119:1017–1028.
4. Douglass RE, Levison MA. Pneumothorax in drug abusers. An urban epidemic? *Am Surg* 1986;52:377–380.
5. Garfein RS, Vlahov D, Galai N, et al. Viral infections in short-term injection drug users: the prevalence of the hepatitis C, hepatitis B, human immunodeficiency, and human T-lymphotropic viruses. *Am J Public Health* 1996;86(5):655–661.
6. Harris HW, Young DM. Care of injection drug users with soft tissue infections in San Francisco California. *Arch Surg* 2002;137(11):1217–1222.
7. Haverkos H, Lange W. Serious infections other than human immunodeficiency virus among intravenous drug abusers. *J Infect Dis* 1990;161:894.
8. Heldman AW, Hartert TV, Ray SC, et al. Oral antibiotic treatment of right-sided staphylococcal endocarditis in injection drug users: prospective randomized comparison with parenteral therapy. *Am J Med* 1996;101(1):68–76.
9. Hopkins RJ, Rothman M, Fiore A, et al. Cerebral mucormycosis associated with intravenous drug use: three case reports and review [see comments]. *Clin Infect Dis* 1994;19:1133–1137.
10. Horowitz BZ, Swensen E, Marquardt K. Wound botulism associated with black tar heroin. *JAMA* 1998;280:1479–1480.
11. Kulaylat MN, Barakat N, Stephan RN, et al. Embolization of illicit needle fragments. *J Emerg Med* 1993;11:403–408.
12. Lohr KM. Rheumatic manifestations of diseases associated with substance abuse. *Semin Arthritis Rheum* 1987;17:90–111.
13. Marantz PR, Linzer M, Feiner CJ, et al. Inability to predict diagnosis in febrile intravenous drug abusers. *Ann Intern Med* 1987;106(6):823–828.
14. Myers EM, Kirkland LS Jr, Mickey R. The head and neck sequelae of cervical intravenous drug abuse. *Laryngoscope* 1988;98:213–218.
15. Palepu A, Tyndall MW, Leon H, et al. Hospital utilization and costs in a cohort of injection drug users. *CMAJ* 2001;165(4):415–420.
16. Pare JP, Cote G, Fraser RS. Long-term follow-up of drug abusers with intravenous talcosis. *Am Rev Respir Dis* 1989;139(1):133–241.
17. Passaro DJ, Werner SB, McGee J, et al. Wound botulism associated with black tar heroin among injecting drug users. *JAMA* 1998;279:859–863.
18. Samet JH, Shevitz A, Fowle J, et al. Hospitalization decision in febrile intravenous drug users. *Am J Med* 1990;89:53–57.
19. Sandrock CE, Murin S. Clinical predictors of respiratory failure and long-term outcome in black tar heroin-associated wound botulism. *Chest* 2001;120(2):562–566.
20. Summanen PH, Talan DA, Strong C, et al. Bacteriology of skin and soft-tissue infections: comparison of infections in intravenous drug users and individuals with no history of intravenous drug use. *Clin Infect Dis* 1995;20[Suppl 2]:S279–S282.
21. Talan DA, Moran GJ. Tetanus among injecting-drug users—California 1997. *Ann Emerg Med* 1998;32:385–386.
22. Thomas DL, Nakatsuji Y, Shih JW, et al. Persistence and clinical significance of hepatitis G virus infections in injecting drug users. *J Infect Dis* 1997;176:586–592.
23. Weisse AB, Heller DR, Schimenti RJ, et al. The febrile parenteral drug user: a prospective study in 121 patients. *Am J Med* 1993;94(3):274–280.
24. Weishaar PD, Flynn HW Jr, Murray TG, et al. Endogenous Aspergillus endophthalmitis. Clinical features and treatment outcomes. *Ophthalmology* 1998;105:57–65.
25. Woodburn KR, Murie JA. Vascular complications of injecting drug misuse. *Br J Surg* 1996;83:1329–1334.

Anticonvulsants and Sedative–Hypnotics

CHAPTER 286

Barbiturates

Beth H. Manning

Barbiturates reversibly depress excitable tissues, particularly those of the central nervous system (CNS). They are used as sedative–hypnotics, for the induction of anesthesia, and as anticonvulsants. Based on their pharmacologic properties and clinical use, barbiturates are often divided into 4 distinct categories: ultra-short acting, short acting, intermediate acting, and long acting barbiturates (Table 286.1). Ultra-short acting barbiturates are highly lipid soluble and rapidly penetrate into the CNS, making

their primary use as anesthesia induction. They are only available as intravenous formulations and overdoses are usually as a result of iatrogenic error.

Short-acting barbiturates were widely prescribed in the 1960s and 1970s for sedation and hypnosis. In the late 1970s nearly 70% of all suicides by drug ingestion were as a result of barbiturates (8). Their use has declined enormously over the last 20 years because they have a lower therapeutic index than the benzodiazepines, tolerance occurs more frequently, the potential for abuse is greater and the number of drug interactions is considerable (10).

Intermediate-acting barbiturates are most commonly found in combination analgesic medications such as Fiorinal®, which contains butalbital. Amobarbital and butabarbital are rarely used, largely as a result of replacement by benzodiazepines. Long acting barbiturates such as phenobarbital and primidone are still commonly used to treat epilepsy.

Pharmacokinetic data are summarized in Table 286.1. Barbiturates are well absorbed from the intestinal tract, except for

TABLE 286.1. Barbiturate Kinetic Data

Drug	Usual Adult Dose (mg)	Onset (h)	Peak (h)	Duration (h)	Half-life (h)	Percentage Protein Binding	Volume of Distribution (L/kg)
ULTRA SHORT ACTING							
Thiopental	50–75	<0.1	<0.1	<0.5	3–11	72–86	1.4–6.7
Methohexital	50–120	<0.2	<0.2	<0.5	1–4	83	1–2.6
SHORT ACTING							
Pentobarbital	50–200	0.25	0.5–2	>3–4	15–50	45–70	0.5–1
Secobarbital	100–200	0.25	1–6	>3–4	19–34	45–70	1.5–1.9
INTERMEDIATE ACTING							
Amobarbital	65–200	<1	2	>4–6	10–40	59	0.9–1.4
Aprobarbital	40–160	<1	12	>4–6	14–34	20	
Butabarbital	100–200	<1	0.5–1.5	>4–6	66–140	26	
Butalbital	100–200		2		61		
LONG ACTING							
Mephobarbital	50–100	0.5–2		>6–12	10–70	40–60	2.6
Phenobarbital	100–320	<0.1	0.5–2	>6–12	80–120	20–50	0.5–0.9
Primidone	300–1,000				3.3–12	20–30	0.4–1.0

mephobarbital which is about 71% to 75% absorbed. The onset of action varies from 10 to 60 minutes depending on the agent and formulation. Food in the stomach decreases the rate of absorption but not the total amount absorbed. In overdose, the onset and peak of symptoms may be delayed. Ultra–short-acting barbiturates are administered intravenously with initial effect seen within 1 minute and duration of effect 10 to 30 minutes. With the short- and intermediate-acting barbiturates, symptoms usually begin with 1 hour of ingestion and peak effects seen within 4 to 6 hours. Long-acting barbiturates have a lower lipid solubility than that of short-acting barbiturates causing them to accumulate more slowly in tissue and delay peak effects for several hours. Onset of symptoms usually occurs within 1 to 2 hours and the peak effect may occur more than 10 hours postingestion. Short-acting barbiturates are almost entirely metabolized in the liver to inactive metabolites that are excreted in the urine as glucuronides. Liver metabolism of barbital, phenobarbital, primidone, and PEMA is limited because of lower lipid-water partition coefficients and urinary excretion accounts for 95%, 25% to 35%, 15% to 42%, and 95% of the elimination of these agents, respectively. Phenobarbital undergoes enterohepatic recirculation, which contributes to its long half-life.

Barbiturates are weak acids with pK_as ranging from 7.2 to 8.5. Increasing the urine pH increases the fraction of ionized drug in the urine, and thus decreases the amount of un-ionized drug available for passive tubular reabsorption. With alkalinization of the urine, the renal clearance of phenobarbital may be increased up to ten times and its half-life shortened by one-half to two-thirds. The elimination of phenobarbital is also enhanced by multiple oral doses of activated charcoal (MDAC) (3).

Barbiturates induce cytochrome p-450 isozymes, including CYP2C9, CYP2C19, CYP2C8, and CYP3A4, and can enhance the elimination of other drugs metabolized by these enzymes (21). Although phenobarbital is a strong inducer of cytochrome p-450, it does not induce its own metabolism and appears to have a longer half-life with chronic use (22). Barbiturates also increase production of δ-aminolevulinic acid, a precursor of porphobilinogen, and may precipitate attacks of acute intermittent porphyria; thus, porphyria is a contraindication to barbiturate use.

Barbiturates act by enhancing γ-aminobutyric acid (GABA) inhibition in excitable tissues of the CNS, skeletal muscle, smooth muscle and heart (10,13,16). GABA opens chloride channels, hyperpolarizing the cells and thereby inhibiting depolarization. Phenobarbital also decreases the paroxysmal firing of nerve cells by an unknown mechanism different from GABA inhibition. Ethanol and barbiturates have synergistic effects. This has been demonstrated in rats, with a significant decrease in the LD_{50} of short acting barbiturates when given in combination with ethanol (9). Chronic use of barbiturates leads to tolerance, physical dependence, and withdrawal symptoms when discontinued (6,23). Barbiturate withdrawal is discussed in Chapter 333, "Drug Withdrawal."

CLINICAL PRESENTATION

Mild to moderate barbiturate intoxication will commonly present with lethargy, slurred speech, ataxia, and nystagmus. At higher doses, coma, respiratory depression, and hypotension may be seen. In deep coma the pupils are usually small or mid-position, all reflex activity may disappear, the electroencephalogram (EEG) may show no brain activity and the patient may appear to be brain dead (8). About 40% of patients who present with severe toxicity develop aspiration pneumonia (12). Drug-induced dilatation of capacitance vessels (venous circula-

tion) with a consequent pooling of blood and reduction in effective vascular volume can lead to shock (8). In patients who have been comatose for a prolonged period, hypothermia and venous thromboembolism occur. Other complications include rhabdomyolysis and acute tubular necrosis secondary to shock. Blisters of the skin occur in about 6% of acute intoxications (1). Methohexital, which is only given intravenously for anesthesia induction, is the only barbiturate associated with an increased risk of seizures from acute overdose (24). Recovery may take 1 to 2 days for short-acting barbiturates and 3 to 7 days for long-acting barbiturates.

Common laboratory abnormalities include hypoglycemia and electrolyte disturbances. Alterations in acid–base and fluid balance may be present. The creatine phosphokinase (CPK) may be elevated if the patient has been comatose and immobile for a prolonged period. A chest radiograph may show aspiration pneumonia or pulmonary edema. The electrocardiogram (ECG) is usually normal. The EEG shows diffuse slowing during barbiturate-induced coma.

The amount of drug required to produce toxic symptoms can vary significantly depending on patient tolerance. The therapeutic doses for common barbiturates are given in Table 286.1. For nonaddicted patients, the toxic dose for short acting barbiturates is about 3 to 6 g (5–8 mg/kg in pediatrics) and phenobarbital is about 6 to 9 g (8mg/kg in pediatrics). Barbiturate addicts may tolerate higher doses. Geriatric patients may be much more sensitive to the drug effects and present with significant findings at even lower doses (11).

Barbiturate blood levels may be significantly elevated but are unreliable in predicting duration or severity of an overdose. Plasma barbiturate levels may not accurately reflect brain concentrations as tissue solubility changes with fluctuations in pH. Chronic abusers may also develop tolerance to the drug, thus exhibiting very few symptoms at levels that would cause severe intoxication in naïve patients (7). Butalbital may cross react with some enzyme multiplied immunoassay technique (EMIT) assays for phenobarbital quantification, particularly following large ingestions (15).

DIFFERENTIAL DIAGNOSIS

A similar clinical picture may be produced by overdosage of other sedative–hypnotics, benzodiazepines, γ hydroxybutyric acid (GHB), alcohol, narcotics, clonidine, imidazoline decongestants (e.g., oxymetazoline), skeletal muscle relaxants, trazodone, phenothiazines, neuroleptics, or carbon monoxide. Sometimes phencyclidine, cyclic antidepressants, or methyl bromide may also present with a similar clinical picture. Drug-induced coma must be differentiated from hypoglycemia, electrolyte abnormalities, head trauma, cerebrovascular insults, CNS infections, and other medical causes.

EMERGENCY DEPARTMENT EVALUATION

Initial history should focus on the identity of the drug, time of ingestion, treatment at the scene, known medical or psychiatric illnesses, and current drug therapy, especially use of other CNS depressant medications or treatment for epilepsy. The physical exam should focus on the vital signs, including rectal temperature and pulse oximetry, and the degree of CNS depression. Absence of bowel sounds signifies ileus and suprapubic percussion may reveal a distended urinary bladder.

Routine laboratory tests should be ordered including a complete blood count, serum electrolyte panel, blood urea nitrogen, creatinine, glucose and urinalysis, including a drugs-of-abuse screen. Serum alcohol and barbiturate concentrations should be quantified if possible. Patients with abnormal vital signs or significant CNS depression should have a chest radiograph, electrocardiogram, arterial blood gas, liver function tests, and CPK level. Patients in deep coma and those with focal neurologic findings should have a computed tomography scan of the head to rule out cerebral edema and structural causes of coma. A lumbar puncture may be necessary to rule out meningitis.

EMERGENCY DEPARTMENT MANAGEMENT

The treatment of acute barbiturate poisoning is primarily supportive, including intravenous access, administration of oxygen, cardiac monitoring, intubation, and mechanical ventilation as necessary. As part of the general treatment of a comatose patient, hypoglycemia and opiate intoxication should be considered and treated as necessary with intravenous glucose and naloxone. Depending on the patient's level of consciousness and gag reflex, intubation should be performed to protect the patient from aspiration and may be needed to provide respiratory support. Intravenous fluid therapy may be adequate to resuscitate patients presenting with mild hypotension, although refractory hypotension may require intravenous vasopressors and more invasive monitoring, as with a pulmonary artery catheter. The goal of therapy is to maintain a systolic blood pressure of 90 mm Hg with adequate tissue perfusion. Mild or moderate hypothermia is treated with warm blankets to prevent further heat loss. For treatment of more severe hypothermia, see Chapter 351, "Hypothermia."

After resuscitation and stabilization, patients with a recent suspected ingestion should undergo gastrointestinal (GI) decontamination. Administration of activated charcoal (AC) is the procedure of choice (4). For a massive recent ingestion of a long acting barbiturate, gastric lavage should also be considered, after protecting the patient's airway. Patients with long-acting barbiturate overdose may also benefit from MDAC (see Chapter 272, "Gastrointestinal Decontamination") (see Chapter 271, "Approach to the Poisoned Patient"). MDAC enhances the elimination of phenobarbital (2,3), even when the drug is given intravenously (2), and is superior to alkaline diuresis for enhancing phenobarbital elimination (5,14,19). In one study, the combination of alkaline diuresis and MDAC was less effective in enhancing phenobarbital elimination than MDAC alone (14), and the clinical efficacy of either procedure remains controversial. One study found that although serum phenobarbital levels declined more rapidly with MDAC therapy, there was no significant difference in the duration of coma or time until extubation criteria were met (18), but another found that the time to mental alertness and to extubation were significantly less in patients treated with MDAC than with alkaline diuresis or combined therapy (14). Whether or not MDAC is effective for other barbiturates is unknown. It should not be given to patients without bowel activity. Urinary alkalinization is contraindicated in patients with renal failure and cerebral or pulmonary edema.

Charcoal hemoperfusion and high flux hemodialysis will also enhance the elimination of all barbiturates. Because of high protein binding, hemoperfusion is generally viewed as more effective than hemodialysis. However, recent case reports indicate that hemodialysis with a high-efficiency dialyzer and a high blood flow rate may be superior to hemoperfusion (17,20). Given the limited availability of hemoperfusion, high flux hemodialysis may be a useful alternative. These procedures are invasive and accompanied by inherent risks. Their use should be reserved for patients with pulmonary edema, cerebral edema, or shock unresponsive to supportive measures.

CRITICAL INTERVENTIONS

- Establish intravenous access and institute cardiac and oxygen saturation monitoring
- Provide airway protection and respiratory support as needed
- Treat hypotension with intravenous fluids and vasopressors, if necessary
- Administer MDAC (if tolerable) to patients with long-acting barbiturate poisoning
- Consult a nephrologist regarding hemoperfusion or hemodialysis for patients with pulmonary edema, cerebral edema, or shock

DISPOSITION

A poison control center or toxicologist should be consulted if the treating physician is not familiar with the management of barbiturate intoxication. Nephrology consultation should be obtained when hemodialysis or hemoperfusion is being considered. Psychiatric consultation is indicated for all suspected suicide attempts as soon as the patient is alert enough to be interviewed.

Awake patients who have ingested short-acting barbiturates may be observed for 4 to 6 hours and then discharged if symptoms are mild and not progressing. For patients who have ingested long-acting barbiturates, the observation period should be based on barbiturate levels and clinical symptoms. If quantitative serum levels are available, as with phenobarbital, serial levels should be obtained and the patient observed until levels peak and are decreasing. Patients with abnormal vital signs or significant CNS depression should be admitted to an intensive care unit. Patients who require intensive care monitoring or extracorporeal elimination measures may need to be transferred if such facilities are unavailable. Advanced life-support measures and GI decontamination should be performed prior to transfer.

COMMON PITFALLS

- ✔ Failure to consider barbiturate withdrawal in patients with seizures
- ✔ Misinterpreting an isoelectric EEG as evidence of brain death in patients with severe barbiturate toxicity
- ✔ Failure to protect the airway in a somnolent patient, putting the patient at risk for aspiration, especially when giving AC
- ✔ Failure to consider extracorporeal drug removal in patients with severe poisoning

Acknowledgment

The author thanks previous edition chapter author Margaret M. McCarron.

References

1. Allen GE, Hadden DR. Barbiturate coma and blisters. *Lancet* 1972;1(7756):904.
2. Berg MJ, Berlinger WG, Goldberg MJ, et al. Acceleration of the body clearance of phenobarbital by oral activated charcoal. *N Engl J Med* 1982;307:642–644.
3. Boldy DAR, Vale JA, Prescott LF. Treatment of phenobarbitone poisoning with repeated oral administration of activated charcoal. *Q J Med* 1986;235.997.
4. Chyka PA, Seger D. Position statement: single-dose activated charcoal. American Academy of Clinical Toxicology: European Association of Poisons Centres and Clinical Toxicologists. *J Toxicol Clin Toxicol* 1997;35:721–741.

5. Frenia ML, Schauben JL, Wears RL, et al. Multiple-dose activated charcoal compared to urinary alkalinization for the enhancement of phenobarbital elimination. *J Toxicol Clin Toxicol* 1996;34(2):169–175.
6. Gallerani M, Zanotti C, Menozzi L, et al. Barbiturate, analgesic and caffeine withdrawal. *Am J Emerg Med* 1994;12(5):603–605.
7. Goldberg MJ, Berlinger WG. Treatment of phenobarbital overdose with activated charcoal. *JAMA* 1982;247(17):2400–2401.
8. Goldfrank L, Osborn H. The barbiturate overdose. *Hosp Physician* 1977;9:30–34.
9. Gupta RC, Kofoed J. Toxicological statistics for barbiturates, other sedatives, and tranquillizers in Ontario: a 10-year survey. *Can Med Assoc J* 1966;94:863–865.
10. Hardman JG, Limbird LE, eds. *Goodman and Gilman's: the pharmacological basis of therapeutics,* 10th ed. McGraw-Hill, 2001.
11. Irvine RE et al: The effect of age on the hydroxylation of amylobarbitone sodium in man. *Br J Clin Pharmacol* 1974;1:41.
12. McCarron M, Schulze B, Walberg C, et al. Short-acting barbiturate overdosage. *JAMA* 1982;248(1):55–61.
13. Mendelson WB, Davis T, Paul SM, et al. Do benzodiazepine receptors mediate the anticonflict actions of phenobarbital? *Life Sci* 1983;32:2241.
14. Mohammed Ebid AH, Abdel-Rahman HM. Pharmacokinetics of Phenobarbital durin certain enhanced elimination modalities to evaluate their clinical efficacy in management of drug overdose. *Ther Drug Monit* 2001;23(3):209–215.
15. Nordt SP. Butalbital cross-reactivity to an emit assay for phenobarbital. *Ann Pharmacother* 1997;31:254–255.
16. Olsen RW. GABA-benzodiazepine-barbiturate receptor interactions. *J Neurochem* 1981;37:1.
17. Palmer BF. Effectiveness of hemodialysis in the extracorporeal therapy of Phenobarbital overdose. *Am J Kidney Dis* 2000;36(3):640–643.
18. Pond SM, Olson KR, Osterloh JD, et al. Randomized study of the treatment of Phenobarbital overdose with repeated dose of activated charcoal. *JAMA* 1984;251(23):3104–3108.
19. Proudfoot AT, Krenzelok EP, Vale JA. Position Paper on urine alkalinization. *J Toxicol Clin Toxicol* 2004;42(1):1–26.
20. Quan DJ, Winter ME. Extracorporeal removal of phenobarbital by high-flux hemodialysis. *J Appl Ther Res* 1998;2(1):75–79.
21. Raucy JL, Mueller L, Duan K, et al. Expression and induction of CYP2C P450 enzymes in primary cultures of human hepatocytes. *J Pharmacol Exp Ther* 2002;302(2):475–482.
22. Viswanathaen CT, Booker HE, Welling PG. Pharmacokinetics of phenobarbital following single and repeated doses. *J Clin Pharmacol* 1979;19:282.
23. Wesson D, Smith D. Barbiturate toxicity and the treatment of barbiturate dependence. *J Psychedelic Drugs* 1972;5(2):158–165.
24. Zink B, Darfler K, Salluzzo R, et al. The efficacy and safety of methohexital in the emergency department. *Ann Emerg Med* 1991;20(12):1293–1298.

CHAPTER 287
Benzodiazepines

Thomas R. Carraccio, Howard C. Mofenson, and Robin B. McFee

Benzodiazepines are widely used as anxiolytics, muscle relaxants, and anticonvulsants. Twenty-one different benzodiazepines are marketed in the United States (Table 287.1). Some of the newer ones are primarily used as anticonvulsants or neuroleptics. Emerging data suggest a role for γ aminobutyric acid (GABA) neurotransmission in depression and schizophrenia, and benzodiazepines may someday play a role in the treatment of these illnesses (4).

Although the incidence of benzodiazepine abuse and overdose is second only to that of alcohol, serious toxicity and fatalities are seldom encountered unless benzodiazepines are combined with other central nervous system (CNS) depressants (3,10). Benzodiazepines may be prescribed for panic disorder and anxiety, conditions that may increase the risk of overdose (4,8,13). Additionally, benzodiazepines increase the risk of falling, particularly in the elderly.

Benzodiazepines (BZD) potentiate the inhibitory action of (GABA) neurotransmission at postsynaptic GABA$_A$ receptor sites (15,16). BZDs enhance chloride ion permeability, rendering the postsynaptic sites less excitable. Several benzodiazepine receptor sites have been identified in the CNS that modulate anxiolytic, hypnotic, neuroleptic, and anticonvulsant properties. Receptor antagonists, such as flumazenil, may be useful in the treatment of benzodiazepine poisoning.

Gastrointestinal (GI) absorption is rapid and complete for most benzodiazepines, but absorption by the intramuscular route is sometimes erratic and delayed. The rate of GI absorption, rather than lipophilicity, determines the onset of action. Diazepam, alprazolam, and triazolam are the most rapidly absorbed oral agents; prazepam is the slowest. Peak levels occur in 1 to 3 hours, but ethanol enhances absorption and may cause the peak level to be doubled at 1 hour. The volume of distribution (Vd) for diazepam is 0.95 to 2.0 L/kg, lorazepam Vd = 1.3 L/kg, chlordiazepoxide Vd = 0.3 to 6.0 L/kg. The range for other drugs in the class is 0.26 to 6 L/kg (Table 287.1). The benzodiazepines are highly protein bound (85% to 99%).

The more lipophilic benzodiazepines, such as diazepam and midazolam, have a shorter duration of action after a single dose than do less lipid soluble derivatives, such as lorazepam and chlordiazepoxide, because increasing lipophilicity enhances drug distribution into peripheral sites (adipose tissue). This leads to the rapid egress of the drug out of blood and brain into inactive storage sites, thus diminishing its effects on the CNS. Hepatic metabolism is their primary route of elimination. The two principal pathways involve either hepatic microsomal oxidation (*N*-dealkylation or aliphatic hydroxylation) or glucuronide conjugation (Fig. 287.1). Benzodiazepines are substrates for CYP 2C19 and CYP 3A4 hepatic enzymes. CYP 3A4 is the predominant P450 enzyme for xenobiotic metabolism, and is inducible by a variety of drugs, including rifampin, phenobarbital, and phenytoin (13). Elimination half-life can be increased by microsomal enzyme inhibitors, thus producing a potentially hazardous interaction, especially with midazolam. Examples of inhibitors include clotrimazole, erythromycin, estrogens, isoniazid, and ketoconazole. The elimination half-life is prolonged in elderly men owing to unknown mechanisms. The elimination half-life is also prolonged in obese patients because of an increased volume of distribution and in patients with hepatic dysfunction because of impaired metabolism. Pharmacokinetic parameters and duration of action are summarized in Table 287.1 (7).

Massive overdoses of benzodiazepines, up to 2,000 mg of chlordiazepoxide and 1,400 mg of diazepam, have limited toxic effects and recovery is rapid and complete with proper supportive care (6). A lethal dose for benzodiazepines has not been established; BZD-associated deaths most often occur in the presence of other CNS depressants that enhance sedation and respiratory depression. Rapid intravenous administration may result in apnea and hypotension. The propylene glycol vehicle used in the parenteral BZD formulations may be the cause of cardiovascular toxicity. Dose adjustments should be considered in the elderly, as dosing requirements decrease with age (5). Concerns about the ability to produce abuse, dependence, and delayed withdrawal reactions have led to restricting the range of indications for dispensing these agents (11). Dependence on diazepam is produced by a dosage of 60 mg/day for 40 days; dependence on chlordiazepoxide is produced by a dosage of 200 mg/day for 60 days.

Flunitrazepam (Rohypnol), known on the street as "roofies," "Mexican valium," "parachute," and "roach 2," is a long-acting benzodiazepine agonist sold by prescription in over 60 countries

TABLE 287.1. Benzodiazepines Dosage and Kinetics

Agent	Dosage Oral Adult mg/day Child mg/kg/24h	Peak Plasma Concentration Hours	Half-life (hrs)	Major Active Metabolites (t1/2 hrs)	PB %	Vd L/kg
ANXIOLYTICS						
Alprazolam (Xanax)	0.75–4 (1.0) 0.25,0.5,1 tabs	0.7–1.6	6–26	yes	68–80	0.7–1
Clobazam (Frisium)*	20–80	1–3	11–77	n-desmethyl-clobazam	NA	NA
Chlordiazepoxide (Librium)	15–100 (25) 0.5 mg/kg/24h 5,10,25 mg tabs	2–4 Total 2–5 days***	5–30	Desmethyl CPZ demoxepam, desmethyl DZP (0–100 hrs)	95	0.3
Chlorzepate (Tranxene)	15–60 (15) 3.75,7.5,15 mg tabs	1–2.5+ Total 2–4 days***	1.1–2.9	Desmethyl DZP (50–100 hrs) Elimination	NA	0.1–0.8
Diazepam (Valium)	6–40 (10)** 0.12–0.8 mg/kg/24h 2,5,10,15 mg tabs	1–2 Total 2–4 days***	14–100	Desmethyl DZP (50–100 hrs) Oxazepam (active)	98	0.9–1.1
Halazepam (Paxipam)	60–160 (40) 20,40 mg tabs	1–3 Total 2–4 days***	1.6–5.3	3-Hydroxy desmethyl DZP (50–100 hrs)	NA	3.4
Lorazepam (16) (Ativan)	2–6 (2) 0.05–0.2 mg/kg/dose 0.5,1.2 tabs	2–5 IV*	10–20	None	85–95	NA
Oxazepam (Serax)	30–120 (30) 10,15,30 tabs	1–2	8–25	None Elimination	97	0.6–2
Prazepam (Centrax)	20–60 (10) 5,10 mg tabs	6 Total 2–4 days***	0.6–2	3-Hydroxy desmethyl DZP	NA	9–19
HYPNOTICS						
Estazolam (Pro-Som)	1–2 mg 1,2 mg tabs	1–2	12–15	1-oxo-estazolam	NA	NA
Flurazepam (Dalmane)	15–60 (30) 15,30 tabs	0.5–2	1.6–5.3 2–4 days***	desalky l FZP (50–100 hrs)	NA	1–1.3
Midazolam (Versed)	5–30 (7.5–15) PO >6 yrs syrup 0.25–1.0 mg/kg	20–50 min 3–5 min after IV dose	1.2–12.3	a-hydroxy	97	0.8–1.7
Quazepam (Doral)	15 7.5, 10 mg	2	39	N-Dealkkylqzp	95	NA
Temazepam (Restoril)	15–30 (20) 15,30 tabs	2–3	10–20	None	96	0.7–1.5
Triazolam (Halcion)	0.125–0.5 (0.5) for debilatated or elderly max dose 0.25 mg 0.125,0,25,0.5 mg	0.5–1.5	2–5 (2–5)	None	90	0.8–1.3
Nitrazepam (Mogadon)*	5–10 (10)	2	24–29	No data Not currently available	NA	NA
Flunitrazepam (Rohypnol)*	1–2	<1	24	7-Aminoflu-nitrazepam (23) N-desmethyl flunitrazepam (31)	NA	NA
Zolpidem (Ambien)+	5–20 mg 5,10 mg tabs	1–2	1.5–2.5	3 inactive		92%
ANTICONVULSANTS						
Clonazepam (Klonopin)	1.5–20 (2) 0.1–0.2 mg/kg/24h 0.5,1,2 tabs	1–4	18–50 2–3 days***	desmethyl DZP (50–100 hrs)	74–80	3.2
Diazepam	See above					

Key to table: IV = Intravenous, **Average dose in parenthesis (), ***Half-lives include active metabolites, PB = protein binding, Vd = volume distribution. Half-lives vary; some include the metabolites half-life. + Not a benzodiazepine chemically but an imidazopyridine which is selective benzodiazepine-1 receptor agonist.

worldwide, but not legally available in the United States. Flunitrazepam is sold illegally in the United States, and abused as a "date rape" drug because of the antegrade amnesia it causes (1). The drug readily mixes with alcohol-containing beverages, although the manufacturer (Roche) has produced tablets that will breakdown into small particles and turn the beverage blue. It is touted as a remedy for the depression that often follows a stimulant high, hence the street name "parachute." The pharmacokinetics include an onset of effects within 1/2 to 2 hours, peak effect 2 hours after oral ingestion, a duration of action of 8 hours or more after a 2 mg dose, and an elimination half-life of 20 to 30 hours (4). Flunitrazepam can be identified in urine from 4 to 30 days after ingestion. Although routine drug screens check for several benzodiazepines, they usually can not detect

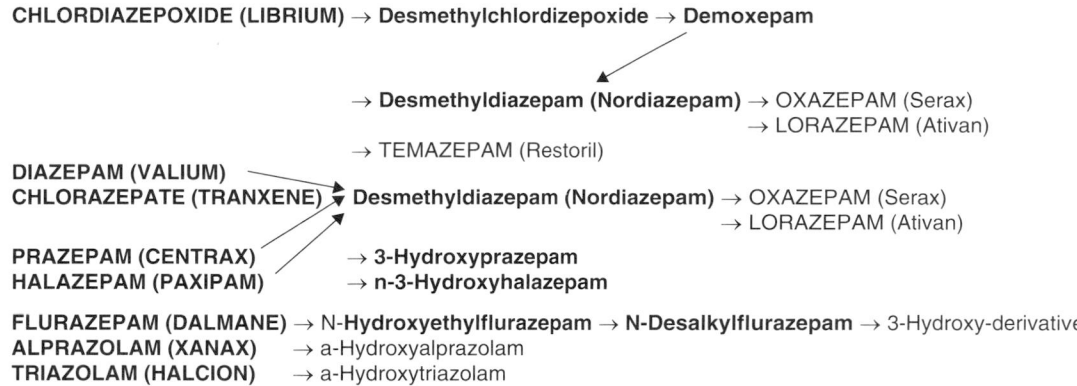

Figure 287.1.   Metabolism of Benzodiazepines. Compounds in **CAPITAL BOLD** have active metabolites. Compounds in CAPITAL nonbold are active drugs without active metabolites. Compounds in noncapital **bold** are active metabolites. Compounds in nonbold, noncapital are not clinically significant active metabolites.

flunitrazepam. However, Hoffman-LaRoche has made available a free testing service in cases in which "date rape" drugs are suspected (see Chapter 93, "Sexual Assault"). For testing authorization, emergency departments, rape crisis centers, and law enforcement agencies can call 1(800) 608-6540. National Medical Services (1-800-522-6671 or 1-215-657-4900) also has a date rape drug-testing service. They test for flunitrazepam, ketamine, or γ hydroxybutyric acid (GHB). There is a fee charged for this service.

Quantitative drug levels are useful only for diagnostic confirmation, not for evaluation or management. Tolerance, drug co-ingestion, active metabolites, and distant tissue binding sites result in poor correlation between blood concentrations and clinical effects. Although diazepam levels of 5 to 20 μg/ml are often associated with toxicity and levels over 20 μg/ml may be seen in lethal cases, chronic daily consumption of large doses may result in blood concentrations of 5 to 6 μg/ml without signs of toxicity.

Zolpidem (Ambien®) is a nonbenzodiazepine, imidazopyridine sedative–hypnotic drug (17). Imidazopyridines are thought to interact with the same GABA receptor/chloride channel complex as the BZDs by high affinity with the "central-type" benzodiazepine receptors (4). Zolpidem is approved only for short-term treatment of insomnia. It is rapidly absorbed from the gastrointestinal tract, with a Vd of 0.54 L/Kg, 92.5% protein binding, and serum peak concentrations being reached in 1 to 2 hours. It is metabolized in the liver, and has a half-life of 2.5 hours, which is prolonged in the elderly (4). Like the benzodiazepines, zolpidem overdose usually does not produce severe respiratory depression unless other agents are co-ingested. However, caution should be exercised in patients with obstructive sleep apnea. Adverse effects are headache, nausea, diarrhea, miosis, and next-day drowsiness. Although zolpidem produces some psychomotor and memory impairment over the first few hours after administration, it has few next-day effects (including effects on daytime well-being and morning coordination) (4). Confusion in the elderly can occur at doses over 20 mg. Cases of zolpidem withdrawal and tolerance have been reported (9).

Zaleplon (Sonata®) is a pyrazolopyrimidine derivative GABA_A benzodiazepine receptor agonist (11,18). It is another nonbenzodiazepine recently introduced for clinical use, for the short-term treatment of insomnia. Zaleplon appears to possess reduced risk of tolerance compared to triazolam, is less likely to potentiate the effects of ethanol, and is unlikely to produce

amnestic effects. Zaleplon is rapidly absorbed and undergoes extensive presystemic metabolism. The compound has a plasma half-life of approximately one hour and is metabolized primarily via the aldehyde oxidase system (4,11,12). CYP3A may also contribute to metabolism. Therefore care should be taken when used with CYP inhibitors or inducers as there may be at least a theoretical risk of altered effect in zaleplon or the other drugs. A few patients presenting comatose after zaleplon overdose had blue-green coloration of urine (12). Studies in patients with a history of drug abuse suggest that the abuse potential of zaleplon (at doses above the therapeutic dose range) is similar to that seen with triazolam (11). Zaleplon has a quick onset of action and undergoes rapid elimination, which results in a better safety profile than previously available agents. Rebound insomnia and other withdrawal effects have not been demonstrated with zaleplon, and the drug is well tolerated in both young and elderly patients. These characteristics may be clinically advantageous for patients who should not receive BZDs (14).

CLINICAL PRESENTATION

Manifestations of benzodiazepine poisoning include ataxia, lateral nystagmus, hypotonia, drowsiness, slurred speech, and coma (2). Even when benzodiazepines are given in large doses, a resultant deep coma causing cardiorespiratory depression and loss of deep tendon reflexes is rare. The ultrashort-acting agents are important exceptions, however. Triazolam has been reported to produce apnea and coma within one hour after doses of 2 to 5 mg. (19). Two fatal poisonings have also been associated with temazepam overdose (17). The toxic dose of flunitrazepam for a child is 0.1 mg/kg (22). This agent is approximately ten times as potent as diazepam.

Paradoxical excitement, including hallucinations, hostility, and seizures, has been reported to result from benzodiazepine overdose (19). Triazolam has been noted to produce delirium and psychosis. The elderly and very young children are more susceptible to the CNS depressant action of benzodiazepines. In rare instances, the adult respiratory distress syndrome has developed after a 30-mg intravenous dose of chlordiazepoxide and massive flurazepam ingestion (23). Most patients with acute benzodiazepine poisoning recover without sequelae within 24 hours. Patients with preexisting medical conditions such as hepatic disease may be more susceptible to toxicity.

drug's influence. GHB and flunitrazepam (Rohypnol®) are common agents among the list of sedatives that have been used for this purpose. In addition to the characteristics mentioned, the presence of vomiting, myoclonus, hyper-reflexivity, bradycardia, and sudden loss of muscle control with an inability to resist the attacker's assault is more consistent with GHB over other agents used to facilitate sexual assault (18). However, these patients typically arrive to medical care after the acute effects of the drug have dissipated. Clinically determining the specific sedative involved rarely alters patient management; however, forensic evaluation requires focused differentiation utilizing knowledge of the unique symptom patterns, the pharmacokinetic time course along with the availability of analytic confirmation for this class of agents.

The differential diagnosis of emergence agitation and delirium includes intoxication with cocaine, sympathomimetics, hallucinogens, and anticholinergic agents, as well as withdrawal from GHB, ethanol, barbiturates, benzodiazepines, and other sedative–hypnotics.

EMERGENCY DEPARTMENT EVALUATION

The history should focus on the identity of the drug, time of ingestion, treatment at the scene, known medical or psychiatric illnesses, and current drug therapy, especially use of ethanol and other CNS depressants. The physical exam should focus on the vital signs and assessment of cardiopulmonary and neurological function. Special attention should be given to evaluating airway patency and protective reflexes and the adequacy of ventilation in comatose patients. Pulse oximetry monitoring is advised for all GHB-overdosed patients. The adequacy of ventilation can be assessed from measurement of the arterial blood gasses. Frequent monitoring of vital signs and clinical status is necessary.

Laboratory studies should include a serum ethanol level, drug of abuse screen, electrolytes, blood urea nitrogen, creatinine, glucose, and urinalysis to assist in ruling out or confirming other possible etiologies or co-ingestants. Patients with agitated delirium should have a serum creatine kinase level to check for rhabdomyolysis. GHB is not detected on routine drug screening tests although GHB serum and urine testing is available at reference laboratories. Results may take several days to obtain and rarely play a role in aiding a prompt diagnosis, because most patients recover and are discharged from the emergency department. Documentation for victims of drug-facilitated assault should follow established chain-of-custody procedures (see Chapter 93, "Sexual Assault"). GHB blood levels are undetectable within 6 hours as a result of the drug's short half-life (19). GHB may be detected in the urine up to 12 hours after use (19,20), thus prompt specimen collection is essential for detection.

EMERGENCY DEPARTMENT MANAGEMENT

The mainstay of treatment is maintaining a patent airway, ensuring adequate oxygenation and taking measures to prevent aspiration of gastric contents. Respiratory depression (e.g., pCO_2 level >60 mm Hg) or the loss of airway reflexes are indications for endotracheal intubation and assisted ventilation; however, the majority of GHB overdose victims do not require these interventions. Gastrointestinal decontamination is rarely indicated, because GHB is typically ingested as a small volume of liquid that is rapidly absorbed. Induction of emesis and gastric lavage are contraindicated, because both procedures are unlikely to be beneficial and may significantly increase the risk of aspiration. Activated charcoal (AC) may be considered in situations of an unclear diagnosis, other co-ingested agents, or a very large recent ingestion; however, AC is rarely indicated for patients presenting with a pure GHB overdose already experiencing significant central nervous system (CNS) depression.

Bradycardia is often asymptomatic and rarely requires any intervention. Hypotension, when present, is most commonly associated with co-ingestion of ethanol and the presence of bradycardia. Intravenous fluids, atropine, and vasopressors such as dopamine or norepinephrine are effective in managing these situations, but are rarely necessary. The few cases of atrial fibrillation to date have resolved spontaneously without any intervention.

There is no specific antidote to reverse the effects of GHB in overdose. In one animal study, naloxone was shown to partially reverse some of GHB's effect on the CNS (21); however, naloxone has not been shown to reverse the effects of GHB poisoning in humans (5,10). It is reasonable to empirically administer naloxone in any comatose patient, because narcotics may be a contributing factor of CNS depression. Physostigmine has been reported to improve the level of consciousness or even arouse comatose patients who tested positive for GHB. However, in addition to testing positive for GHB, these patients also tested positive for one or more of the following co-ingestants: tetrahydrocannibinoids (THC), opiates, pseudoephedrine, amphetamines, methamphetamines, or methylenedioxymethamphetamine (22,23). It is important to note that physostigmine is an analeptic agent that causes nonspecific CNS arousal from many etiologies and therefore is not a specific "antidote" for GHB intoxication. The use of physostigmine in this setting is unwarranted, because mechanistic evidence is lacking, potentially dangerous side effects are possible (e.g., asystole, seizures) and patients have an excellent prognosis with supportive care alone.

Treatment of "agitated or emergence delirium" is best managed with the use of nonpharmacologic modalities to allow continued monitoring of the patient's mental status. It is best to minimize stimulation and, if possible, place the patient in a quiet, nonthreatening area while he or she becomes reoriented. In some patients it is necessary to use soft physical restraints to prevent self-injury. Rarely, these measures are ineffective and benzodiazepines are needed to calm the patient. Because benzodiazepine therapy may prolong the course of altered sensorium, a short-acting agent such as midazolam should be used.

Initial management of patients chronically dependent on GHB who present after GHB overdose is the same as with a naïve overdosed patient, but it is important to observe these patients for the onset of withdrawal symptoms, typically seen within 6 hours of awakening. Treatment of GHB withdrawal is the same as that for ethanol and other sedative–hypnotic withdrawal syndromes (see Chapter 278, "Alcohol Withdrawal" and Chapter 333, "Drug Withdrawal").

CRITICAL INTERVENTIONS

- Perform endotracheal intubation in patients who are unable to protect their airway or have respiratory depression or pulmonary edema
- Administer intravenous fluids and vasopressors for hypotension; give atropine for concomitant bradycardia
- Use calming measures, physical restraints, and, if necessary, midazolam, for the treatment of agitated delirium

DISPOSITION

The duration of GHB's effects is remarkably short. The majority of GHB poisoned patients, even those with coma requiring intubation, typically recover fully within 6 hours and may be discharged from the ED. Complications requiring prolonged observation and care are usually evident within this time frame. Patients who have complications, those who have ingested multiple agents, those who require sedation for agitation and emergence delirium, and those at risk for GHB withdrawal may require an extended observation period or admission. Intensive care unit admission is advised for any patient suffering from pulmonary edema, aspiration pneumonia, profound respiratory depression, or atrial fibrillation. Dependent patients with severe withdrawal symptoms may also require admission to an intensive care unit. Chronic GHB users should be referred for substance abuse counseling and treatment.

COMMON PITFALLS

✔ Overlooking the possibility of criminal assault in patients with GHB overdose

✔ Failure to appreciate that a negative urine toxicology screen does not rule out GHB exposure

✔ Administering excessive sedation to patients with agitation as a result of emergence delirium

✔ Failure to observe chronic GHB users for signs and symptoms of withdrawal and to appreciate that withdrawal can begin within hours after recovering from acute overdose

✔ Failure to consider the possibility of ethanol or other substance dependence in chronic GHB users

Acknowledgments

We thank the National Institute of Drug Abuse DA 14935-01 for research grant support.

References

1. Zvosec DL, et al. Adverse events, including death, associated with the use of 1,4-butanediol. *N Engl J Med* 2001;344(2):87–94.
2. DAWN. The DAWN Report—trends in drug-related emergency department visits, 1994–2002: at a glance 2003. Rockville, Maryland: Office of Applied Studies, SAMHSA, Drug Abuse Warning Network.
3. Borgen LA, et al. The influence of gender and food on the pharmacokinetics of sodium oxybate oral solution in healthy subjects. *J Clin Pharmacol* 2003;43(1):59–65.
4. Chin RL, et al. Clinical course of gamma-hydroxybutyrate overdose. *Ann Emerg Med* 1998;31(6):716–722.
5. Li, J, Stokes SA, Woeckener A. A tale of novel intoxication: seven cases of gamma-hydroxybutyric acid overdose. *Ann Emerg Med* 1998;31(6):723–728.
6. Chin MY, Kreutzer RA, Dyer JE. Acute poisoning from gamma-hydroxybutyrate in California. *Western J Med* 1992;156(4):380–384.
7. Zvosec DL, Smith SW, Anderson D. Agitation as a common manifestation of GHB intoxication (gamma hydroxybutyrate). *J Toxicol Clin Toxicol* 2002;40(5):619.
8. Grove-White IG, Kelman GR. Effect of methohexitone, diazepam and sodium 4-hydroxybutyrate on short-term memory. *Br J Anaesth* 1971;43(2):113–116.
9. Sturman P. Drug assisted sexual assault 2000. London, UK: Home Office of the Metropolitan London Police: 1–123.
10. Ross TM. Gamma hydroxybutyrate overdose: two cases illustrate the unique aspects of this dangerous recreational drug. *J Emerg Nurs* 1995;21(5):374–376.
11. Li, J, Stokes SA, Woeckener A. A tale of novel intoxication: a review of the effects of gamma-hydroxybutyric acid with recommendations for management. *Ann Emerg Med* 1998;31(6):729–736.
12. Metcalf DR, Emde RN, Stripe JT. An EEG-behavioral study of sodium hydroxybutyrate in humans. *Electroencephalography Clin Neurophysiology* 1966;20(5):506–512.
13. Dyer JE, Haller CA. GHB Related Fatalities. *J Toxicol Clin Toxicol* 2001;39(5):518.
14. Poldrugo F, et al, Ethanol potentiates the toxic effects of 1,4-butanediol. *Alcohol Clin Exp Res* 1985;9(6):493–497.
15. Serebryakov LA, Effect of Sodium Gamma-Hydroxybutyrate Combined with Anesthetics. *Farmakologiyai Toksikologiya* 1964;27(3):275–277.
16. McCabe ER, et al, Synergy of ethanol and a natural soporific—gamma hydroxybutyrate. *Science* 1971;171(969):404–406.
17. Multistate outbreak of poisoinings associated with illicit use of gamma hydroxy buyrate. *Morb Mortal Wkly Rep* 1990;39(47):861–863.
18. Schwartz RH, Milteer R, LeBeau MA. Drug-facilitated sexual assault ('date rape'). *South Med J* 2000;93(6):558–561.
19. Hoes MJ, Vree TB, Guelen PJ. Gamma-hydroxybutyric acid as hypnotic. Clinical and pharmacokinetic evaluation of gamma-hydroxybutyric acid as hypnotic in man. *Encephale* 1980;6(1):p 93–9.
20. Stephens BG, Baselt RC. Driving under the influence of GHB?. *J Anal Toxicol* 1994;18(6):357–358.
21. Feigenbaum JJ, Howard SG. Naloxone reverses the inhibitory effect of gamma-hydroxybutyrate on central DA release in vivo in awake animals: a microdialysis study. *Neurosci Lett* 1997;224(1):p 71–4.
22. Caldicott DG, Kuhn M. Gamma-hydroxybutyrate overdose and physostigmine: teaching new tricks to an old drug?. *Ann Emerg Med* 2001;37(1):99–102.
23. Yates SW, Viera AJ. Physostigmine in the treatment of gamma-hydroxybutyric acid overdose. *Mayo Clin Proc* 2000;75(4):401–402.

CHAPTER 290
Muscle Relaxants and Other Sedative–Hypnotic Agents

Barbara Insley Crouch and Fred M. Henretig

Muscle relaxants are used to treat muscle spasms and muscle spasticity. They include baclofen, chlorzoxazone, cyclobenzaprine, dantrolene, metaxalone, methocarbamol, orphenadrine, and tizanidine. Nonbarbiturate, nonbenzodiazepine sedative–hypnotic agents are used for the relief of anxiety and as sleeping aids; these include buspirone, chloral hydrate, meprobamate, zaleplon, zolpidem, and zopiclone. Zopiclone is not currently available in the United States. Ethchlorvynol, glutethimide, and methaqualone are sedative–hypnotic agents that are no longer available for medicinal use in the United States; however, reports of abuse and overdose still occur infrequently.

Adverse and toxic effects from these drugs are primarily an extension of their pharmacologic activity. The sedative–hypnotic agents produce central nervous system (CNS) depression when taken alone or in combination with alcohol and other CNS depressants. The older nonbarbiturate sedative–hypnotic agents have a lower margin of safety than the benzodiazepines and the newer members of this class, such as buspirone, zaleplon, and zolpidem. As a class, sedative–hypnotics are notorious for their abuse potential. Given their propensity to cause tolerance and dependence, abstinence from sedative–hypnotic agents may cause severe effects, including a delirium tremens–like syndrome and convulsions. Methaqualone in particular had such a high abuse potential that it was made a class I agent and withdrawn from the United States market in 1983. Although there is limited experience with zolpidem and zaleplon to date, there is evidence that these drugs have some abuse potential as well.

The muscle relaxants are a diverse group of pharmacologic agents. Drowsiness and dizziness are the most commonly reported adverse effects with therapeutic use of all these agents. The use of baclofen, dantrolene, and tizanidine are primarily limited to patients with spasticity related to severe chronic disease, such as multiple sclerosis. Baclofen is also used intrathecally, and a withdrawal syndrome is noted in patients who abruptly discontinue baclofen by either the oral or intrathecal route.

TABLE 290.1. Summary of Pharmacokinetic Data for Nonbarbiturate, Nonbenzodiazepine Sedative–Hypnotic Agents and Muscle Relaxants

	$t_{1/2}$ (h)	PB (%)	VD (L/kg)	Renal (%)	Active Metabolite	Th	Blood Levels	
							T (µg/mL)	L
Buspirone	2	95	6–7	1	Pyrimidinyl piperazine	NA	NA	NA
Carisoprodol	8	NA	NA	Trace	Meprobamate	2.5–4.0	30	110
Chloral hydrate	8–35[a]	40[a]	0.6	0	TCE	10	100	250
Chlorzoxazone	1.1	NA	0.4	<1	None	9–20	NA	NA
Cyclobenzaprine	24–36 .050	93	NA	1	NA	30	0.03	0.35–0.50
Ethchlorvynol	1–3/10–25[b]	35–50	3–4	10	None	5	20	150
Glutethimide	10–12	35–59	>TBW	<1	4-HEPG	0.2	19	30–100
Meprobamate	6–16	20	0.75	10–12	None	10	80–120	200
Metaxalone	2–3	NA	NA	0	NA	0.9	NA	19–39
Methaqualone	10–40	70–90	2.4–6.4	<1	None	5	10–30	30
Methocarbamol	0.9–2	46–50	NA	10–15	NA	25.8	NA	257–525
Orphenadrine	14–20	20	4.3–7.8	8	nororphenadrine	0.150	3.1	20
Tizanidine	2–4	30	2.4	<2	None		0.004–0.015	NA
Zaleplon	1	60	1.4	<1	None	0.015	NA	NA
Zolpidem	2	92	0.54	<1	None	0.2	>0.5	1.6–7.7

PB, protein binding; VD, volume of distribution; renal, percentage eliminated unchanged; TBW, total body water; 4-HEPG, 4-hydroxy-2-ethyl-2-phenylglutarimide; TCE, trichloroethanol; Th, therapeutic; T, toxic; L, lethal; NA, data not available.
[a]Data for TCE
[b]Distribution of $t_{1/2}$ of 1–3 hr, with elimination $t_{1/2}$ of 10–25 hr.

Dantrolene is used infrequently, as it is associated with muscle weakness. Tizanidine is an α-2 adrenergic agonist, similar to clonidine, which may be used to treat tension headaches and trigeminal neuralgia in addition to muscular spasticity. The remaining agents (carisoprodol, chlorzoxazone, cyclobenzaprine, metaxalone, methocarbamol, orphenadrine) are all sedative agents. Their efficacy as muscle relaxants is in significant part as a result of their sedative properties. Abuse potential varies by drug and is noted to be high with carisoprodol.

All sedative–hypnotics and muscle relaxants are metabolized in the liver. Several undergo oxidation by cytochrome p450 enzymes, making drug interactions a significant concern. Pharmacokinetic data for these agents are summarized in Table 290.1. A list of important drug metabolizing enzyme substrates are summarized in Table 290.2.

The majority of sedative–hypnotic agents are well absorbed and onset of effect occurs within 30 minutes to 1 hour after ingestion, sooner for zaleplon. Orphenadrine has a slower onset of effects as a result of its significant anticholinergic properties. The onset of action for baclofen is several days, although peak concentrations occur within 2 to 3 hours. The absorption of dantrolene is also slow and bioavailability is approximately 40%. The onset of effect from tizanidine is also slow with initial response for spasticity taking several weeks.

Buspirone, an azaspirodecanedione derivative, is an antianxiety agent that is a partial agonist at the serotonin 1A (5-HT1A) receptor (3). Unlike other sedative agents, it does not seem to interact with the benzodiazepine–γ-aminobutyrate (GABA) receptor complex. Chloral hydrate is one of the oldest known hypnotics. It was first synthesized in 1832 and used as a hypnotic as early as 1869 (22). The first cases of poisoning were reported in 1890. Chloral hydrate use in adults has declined considerably in recent years, but it is still popular for procedural sedation in children at doses ranging from 50 to 100 mg/kg. The toxic dose in adults is 5 to 10 g. As little as 1.5 g has resulted in significant toxicity in a toddler. The half-life of its active metabolite trichloroethanol is 8 hours at therapeutic doses, but may be prolonged to 12 to 35 hours after overdose. The combination of alcohol and chloral hydrate ("Mickey Finn") is particularly potent, as these agents not only have additive CNS depressant effects, but also inhibit each other's metabolism.

Carisoprodol, chlorzoxazone, cyclobenzaprine, metaxalone, and methocarbamol are all CNS depressants with both sedative and muscle relaxant properties, although the exact mechanism of these actions is not known. Carisoprodol is metabolized to meprobamate, another sedative–hypnotic agent (see below) that contributes to carisprodol's effects. The usual dose is 350 mg given three times a day. Chlorzoxazone is not a commonly prescribed muscle relaxant. The usual dose is 250 mg given three to four times a day. However, up to 750 mg per dose can be administered. Cyclobenzaprine is structurally similar to the cyclic antidepressants, and has significant anticholinergic properties. The usual dose is 20 to 40 mg daily in 2 to 4 divided doses. Metaxalone is available in 400-mg tablets and the usual dose is 800 mg three to four times daily. Methocarbamol is available as both an oral and parenteral preparation. The usual oral dose is 1.5 g given four times daily. Ethchlorvynol and glutethimide are older sedative–hypnotic agents that were discontinued by their manufacturers between 1999 and 2000. Although they are no longer available as prescription medications, toxic exposures may continue.

Meprobamate, originally synthesized and used as a muscle relaxant in the late 1940s, was introduced in the United States for use as an anxiolytic agent in 1955. Although still used today for this purpose, there is little evidence that it is effective. It is available in 200-mg and 400-mg tablets. Meprobamate is structurally related to the skeletal muscle relaxants carisoprodol, methocarbamol, and chlorphenesin, and to the anticonvulsant felbamate.

TABLE 290.2. Drug Metabolizing Enzymes

Drug	Cytochrome Substrate	Inducer/Inhibitor
Buspirone	CYP 3A3/4	
Carisoprodol	CYP 2C19	
Chloral hydrate	CYP 2E1	
Chlorzoxazone	CYP 2E1	
Cyclobenzaprine	CYP 1A2, 2D6, 3A3/4	
Orphenadrine	CYP2B6, 2D6, 3A3/4	CYP 2B6 inhibitor
Zaleplon	CYP 3A3/4 (minor)	
Zolpidem	CYP 3A3/4	

Meprobamate itself has anticonvulsant and skeletal muscle relaxant properties. Its mechanism of action is similar to that of barbiturates, although it is thought to be more selective in its depression of areas in the cerebral cortex. It also suppresses polysynaptic reflexes in the spinal cord, which probably contributes to its skeletal muscle relaxation properties. The therapeutic dose of meprobamate for adults is usually 1.2 to 1.6 g daily, in three or four doses; the maximal daily dose is 2.4 g. Toxic effects may occur after ingestions of as little as 2 to 4 g. Death has been reported with as little as 12 g, but survival has been reported after ingestions of up to 40 g (1). Drug concentrations do not correlate well with clinical effects, although concentrations above 100 μg/mL are associated with severe toxicity. Methaqualone, a quinazoline derivative, was introduced in 1965 as a nonaddicting substitute for the barbiturates and rapidly became popular as a drug of abuse. Abused for its purported euphoric and aphrodisiac effects, methaqualone was nicknamed the "love drug."

Orphenadrine is a centrally acting anticholinergic agent that is used to treat acute musculoskeletal disorders. It is structurally similar to diphenhydramine. The usual dose is 100 mg twice daily. It is also available in a 25 mg tablet in combination with aspirin 385 mg and caffeine 30 mg and a 50 mg tablet with aspirin 770 mg and caffeine 60 mg. Central anticholinergic effects are not uncommon with overdose.

Zaleplon and zolpidem, are nonbenzodiazepine hypnotic agents that selectively bind to the central benzodiazepine receptor subtype BZ_1 located in the $GABA_A$ receptor complex. Zopiclone also works by binding to the benzodiazepine receptor complex and enhancing the activity of GABA. Because they act via the benzodiazepine receptor, more details regarding these agents may also be found in Chapter 287, "Benzodiazepines." Unlike benzodiazepines, these agents do not appear to possess significant anticonvulsant or muscle relaxant properties. Both zaleplon and zolpidem have significant first-pass metabolism, reducing the oral bioavailability to 30% and 70% respectively. They are rapidly absorbed, and the onset of effect is 15 to 30 minutes. Ingestions of up to 300 mg of zolpidem without the development of symptoms have been reported (17). However, a 44-year-old man developed coma and respiratory failure after the ingestion of 200 mg of zolpidem (10). An ingestion of 1,000 mg resulted in tachycardia and agitation only (8). Deaths related to zolpidem are not common and usually involve coingestants.

CLINICAL PRESENTATION

The onset of toxicity is expected to occur within 1 to 2 hours for most of these sedative–hypnotic agents and skeletal muscle relaxants. Delays may be possible, especially with those agents that have significant anticholinergic properties such as orphenadrine and cyclobenzaprine. CNS depression is the most common toxic effect associated with these agents. The extent of the CNS depression depends on the potency of the agent, the dose ingested, and the presence of alcohol or other central nervous system depressants.

Baclofen overdose is associated with profound CNS depression. Coma, hypotonia, hyporeflexia, and respiratory depression requiring mechanical ventilation were present in 100% of pediatric patients reported in one study (4). Autonomic disturbances (e.g., bradycardia or tachycardia, hypotension, or hypertension) occur less frequently. Pupillary response is inconsistent, and both mydriasis and miosis have been reported. Seizures and cardiac dysrhythmias can occur and do not necessarily correlate with serum concentrations (18). Elimination of baclofen is slow following an overdose. In a series of adolescents with acute baclofen toxicity, mechanical ventilation was required for up to 60 hours after ingestion (18). Death has been reported following the ingestion of 1 to 1.8 gm (7).

Seizures have been described 36 hours after the ingestion of 420 mg of buspirone (3). The serotonin syndrome (see Chapter 322, "Serotonin Re-uptake Inhibitors") has been reported in patients concurrently taking buspirone and fluoxetine or St. John's Wort (5,15).

Carisoprodol primarily produces CNS depression in overdose. Myoclonic encephalopathy was reported in a 39-year-old man who ingested 35 g of carisoprodol in a self-harm attempt. The patient remained unresponsive with muscle rigidity for 2 days following the overdose (20). Physical dependence can occur following chronic use, and withdrawal can occur following abrupt discontinuation.

Manifestations of chloral hydrate overdose resemble those as a result of barbiturates, with coma, miosis, and hypotension (22). Chloral hydrate is also a GI irritant and commonly causes nausea and vomiting. Hemorrhagic gastritis and gastric necrosis occur rarely. As a halogenated hydrocarbon, it can also cause hepatic injury, renal failure, and cardiotoxicity. It reduces myocardial contractility, shortens the refractory period, sensitizes the myocardium to circulating catecholamines, and can precipitate cardiac dysrhythmias (see Chapter 310, "Hydrocarbons").

Cyclobenzaprine produces profound CNS depression and also significant anticholinergic effects. Although it is structurally similar to amitriptyline, serious cardiovascular (CV) effects have not been noted. In a retrospective review of cyclobenzaprine exposures reported to five regional poison centers, the most common toxic effects in patients greater than 10 years of age were lethargy and tachycardia (23).

Prolonged coma is the predominant effect of severe ethchlorvynol and glutethimide overdose (14,25). Glutethimide also has anticholinergic properties that contribute to toxicity. Ocular and neurologic signs associated with glutethimide can be dramatic: papilledema; nystagmus; unilateral or bilateral pupillary dilation; ataxia; tonic spasms and seizures; coma progressing to loss of deep tendon, corneal, gag, and pupillary light reflexes; and an isoelectric electroencephalogram. Meprobamate often causes hypotension (1). The observation that hypotension may occur without respiratory depression suggests a direct myocardial depressant effect. Tachycardia is also common. Miosis, mydriasis, nystagmus, respiratory depression, disconjugate gaze, seizure activity, hallucinations, and hypothermia have also been reported. Meprobamate pills have a tendency to clump in the stomach forming a pharmacobezoar.

Methaqualone commonly causes muscle hyperactivity, including hyperreflexia, twitching, and clonus, in addition to CNS depression (16). Hypotension and respiratory depression occur infrequently. Dysrhythmias and myocardial infarctions have been noted in a few patients. Fixed drug eruptions have been noted in methaqualone abusers; lesions resolved once the drug was withdrawn. Bleeding tendencies, believed to be caused by coagulopathy and abnormal platelet count or aggregation, have been reported, with retinal hemorrhage being described in one case.

Orphenadrine overdose commonly results in both peripheral and central anticholinergic effects (9,24). Generalized seizure activity is reported commonly. Ventricular tachycardia and prolongation of the QRS interval have been reported, and are likely the result of sodium channel blockade (6).

Zolpidem overdose appears to be relatively benign. In a series of 35 patients, 51% developed no symptoms (17). The remainder had mild CNS effects, including dizziness, slurred speech, and lethargy. Four patients complained of nausea, vomiting, and abdominal discomfort. Only two patients in this series had deep sedation. Of 344 cases reported to a poison center, 28% of patients remained asymptomatic, and over half of those with symptoms had concomitant drug ingestions (8). Of patients who ingested zolpidem alone, the majority experienced only drowsiness. Limited experience is available with zaleplon and zopiclone, but toxic effects are likely to primarily involve CNS depression. In addition to coma, two patients had bluish-green urine following an overdose of zaleplon (11).

Toxic effects from chlorzoxazone, metaxalone, and methocarbamol are primarily CNS depression. Miosis has been noted with chlorzoxazone (19).

DIFFERENTIAL DIAGNOSIS

Poisoning by alcohols, anticonvulsants, barbiturates, benzodiazepines, β blockers, calcium channel blockers, centrally acting antihypertensives, cyclic antidepressants, opioids, and skeletal muscle relaxants can cause similar signs and symptoms. Hypotension out of proportion to the degree of CNS depression suggests meprobamate, a CV agent, or a cyclic antidepressant. Cyclic coma suggests glutethimide ingestion or formation of a gastric pharmacobezoar. CNS infection and trauma, hypoglycemia, hypernatremia, hypercalcemia, and hypermagnesemia should also be considered. Anticholinergic effects can occur following ingestion of plants, mushrooms, and many different nonprescription and prescription medications.

EMERGENCY DEPARTMENT EVALUATION

The history should include the time and amount of drug(s) ingested, the time of onset and the nature of symptoms, and medical history, including the pattern and extent of muscle relaxant or sedative–hypnotic drug use. The physical examination focuses on vital signs and the neurologic and cardiopulmonary status.

Symptomatic patients should have baseline laboratory testing as indicated by clinical severity; such testing may include oxygen saturation or arterial blood gas analysis, complete blood count, determination of electrolytes, blood urea nitrogen, creatinine, and glucose concentrations, urinalysis, an electrocardiogram (ECG), a chest radiograph, and liver function tests. Patients with deeper comas should also be evaluated for possible rhabdomyolysis by serum creatine phosphokinase and urine myoglobin tests. Comprehensive urine toxicology screening tests may confirm the presence of some muscle relaxants and sedative–hypnotic agents. Drugs-of-abuse immunoassays will not detect these agents. In general, quantitative serum drug levels are neither readily available nor clinically useful.

EMERGENCY DEPARTMENT MANAGEMENT

Generally, therapy involves stabilization and support of vital signs and gut decontamination, with the administration of activated charcoal (AC) being the preferred modality. Patients normally respond well to good supportive measures. If a patient starts to deteriorate after apparent recovery, or is deteriorating despite good supportive care, a pharmacobezoar should be suspected. Endoscopy can be both diagnostic and therapeutic in such cases. Gastrotomy has been used for meprobamate pharmacobezoar removal (21). If hypotension fails to respond to fluids, or if the patient is already fluid-overloaded, a trial of agents with positive inotropic activity, such as dopamine and epinephrine, is indicated. Unless hypoxic injury is present, full recovery can be expected once these drugs have been eliminated. Invasive CV support (e.g., partial or full cardiopulmonary bypass and intraaortic balloon pump therapy) should be considered for hemodynamically unstable patients.

Patients with methaqualone poisoning may require pharmacologic paralysis for control of neuromuscular hyperactivity. The benzodiazepine antagonist, flumazenil has been reported to re-

verse CNS depression as a result of zolpidem, zaleplon, and chlorzoxazone (2,11,19). Routine use of flumazenil in the management of overdoses due to these agents requires caution, as detailed in the discussion of its role in treatment of benzodiazepine toxicity (see Chapter 287 "Benzodiazepines"). Sodium bicarbonate should be the first line therapy for dysrhythmias or conduction disturbances associated with orphenadrine. Physostigmine may be useful to control severe anticholinergic effects associated with orphenadrine.

The anticholinergic properties of cyclobenzaprine, glutethimide, and orphenadrine may slow absorption and lead to delayed gastric emptying. Decontamination may therefore be useful many hours after ingestion. Repeated doses of AC may also be helpful, given the prolonged and fluctuating degree of intestinal absorption. Fluids should be given with caution in treating the hypotensive effects of meprobamate, because its myocardial depressant properties increase the risk of pulmonary edema. Hemodialysis, resin, and charcoal hemoperfusion, and continuous arteriovenous hemoperfusion (CAVHP) have been used successfully in the treatment of life-threatening meprobamate overdoses (12,13). These methods should be reserved for patients who are unresponsive to supportive measures. Proponents of CAVHP note its efficacy in hypotensive patients, and its potential availability in smaller community hospitals.

Ventricular dysrhythmias as a result of chloral hydrate are often refractory to treatment (22). Lidocaine, magnesium (especially for torsades de pointes), β blockers, and overdrive pacing have been used with success. Excess patient manipulation or excitement, and catecholamine pressor agents should be avoided, if possible, to decrease the risk of precipitating refractory dysrhythmias. Hemodialysis may be considered in extremely severe cases of chloral hydrate toxicity with profound hypotension and unstable dysrhythmias. The use of extracorporeal methods for enhancing the elimination of ethchlorvynol is controversial. Plasma half-life can be decreased with hemodialysis. Resin hemoperfusion, although not widely available, is even more efficacious (25). Such therapy should be considered only for patients with life-threatening toxicity unresponsive to intensive supportive care.

CRITICAL INTERVENTIONS

- Establish intravenous access, institute cardiac monitoring, and assess and maintain airway patency and respirations with endotracheal intubation and mechanical ventilation as necessary
- Administer inotropic vasopressors such as dopamine and epinephrine for hypotension refractory to intravenous crystalloid
- Administer intravenous sodium bicarbonate for dysrhythmias or conduction disturbances as a result of orphenadrine
- Consider invasive hemodynamic support and enhanced elimination measures (e.g., cardiopulmonary bypass, intraaortic balloon pump, hemodialysis) in severe poisoning refractory to standard therapy

DISPOSITION

Patients with mild symptoms may be observed in the emergency department until asymptomatic. Patients with moderate or severe symptoms require admission, because prolonged close monitoring and supportive care are necessary. Intensive care unit admission is advisable. Patients with unstable vital signs should be transferred to a facility that is capable of targeted intensive care for poisoning victims. Advanced life-support equipment and staff should accompany the patient during transfer.

COMMON PITFALLS

✔ Failure to consider the possibility of gastric drug bezoar and continuing drug absorption in patients with progressive, prolonged or cyclic coma, particularly that as a result of glutethimide and meprobamate, and to consider interventions such as endoscopy and multiple-dose charcoal

✔ Failure to appreciate that meprobamate can cause hypotension in the absence of severe CNS depression

✔ Failure to appreciate that buspirone, methaqualone, and agents with anticholinergic properties such as cyclobenzaprine, glutethimide, and orphenadrine can cause neuromuscular hyperactivity or seizures in addition to CNS depression

✔ Failure to monitor for pulmonary edema, especially in patients who require fluid resuscitation for hypotension

✔ Failure to perform toxicology testing to rule out occult coingestants (e.g., acetaminophen), especially in comatose patients

✔ Failure to anticipate and treat withdrawal syndromes in patients chronically taking muscle relaxants and sedative–hypnotics

✔ Failure to consider the use of flumazenil in selected cases as a reversal agent for depression as a result of zolpidem, zaleplon, and chlorzoxazone

✔ Failure to appreciate that chloral hydrate-induced ventricular dysrhythmias are exacerbated by endogenous and exogenous catecholamines and may respond to β-blocker therapy

References

1. Bailey DN. The present status of meprobamate ingestion: a 5-year review of cases with serum concentrations and clinical findings. *Am J Clin Pathol* 1981;75:102.
2. Burton JH, Lyon L, Dorfman T, Tomassoni AJ. Continuous flumazenil infusion in the treatment of zolpidem (Ambien®) and ethanol coingestion. *J Toxicol Clin Toxicol* 1998;36:743–744.
3. Catalano G, Catalano MC, Hanley PF. Seizures associated with buspirone overdose: case report and literature review. *Clin Neuropharmacol* 1998;21:347–350.
4. Chapple D, Johnson D, Connors R. Baclofen overdose in two siblings. *Pediatr Emerg Care* 2001;17:110–112.
5. Dannawi M. Possible serotonin syndrome after combination of buspirone and St. John's Wort. *J Psychopharmacol* 2002;16:401.
6. Danze LK, Langdorf MI. Reversal of orphenadrine-induced ventricular tachycardia with physostigmine. *J Emerg Med* 1991;9:453–457.
7. Fraser AD, MacNeil W, Isner AF. Toxicological analysis of a fatal baclofen (Lioresal) ingestion. *J Forensic Sci* 1991;36:1596–1602.
8. Garnier R, Gueralt E, Muzard D, et al. Acute zolpidem poisoning—analysis of 344 cases. *J Toxicol Clin Toxicol* 1994;32:391–404.
9. Garza MB, Osterhoudt KC, Rutstein R. Central anticholinergic syndrome from orphenadrine in a 3 year old. *Pediatr Emerg Care* 2000;16:97–98.
10. Hamad A, Sharma N. Acute zolpidem overdose leading to coma and respiratory failure. *Intensive Care Med* 2001;27:1239.
11. Hojer J, Salmonson H, Sundin P. Zaleplon-induced coma and bluish-green urine: possible antidotal effect by flumazenil. *J Toxicol Clin Toxicol* 2002;40:571–572.
12. Hoy WE, Rivero A, Marin MG, et al. Resin hemoperfusion for treatment of a massive meprobamate overdose. *Ann Intern Med* 1980;93:455.
13. Lawson AAH, Brown SS. Acute methaqualone (Mandrax) poisoning. *Scott Med J* 1967;12:63.
14. Lin JL, Lim PS, Lai BC, et al. Continuous arteriovenous hemoperfusion in meprobamate poisoning. *J Toxicol Clin Toxicol* 1993;32:645.
15. Maher JF, Schreiner GE, Nestervelt FB. Acute glutethimide intoxication. I. Clinical experience (22 patients) compared to acute barbiturate intoxication (63 patients). *Am J Med* 1962;33:70.
16. Manos GH. Possible Serotonin Syndrome Associated with Buspirone Added to Fluoxetine. *Ann Pharmacother* 2000;34:871–874.
17. Mercurio M, DeRoos F, Hoffman RS. Zolpidem (Ambien): exposure assessment of a new nonbenzodiazepine GABA agonist. *Vet Hum Toxicol* 1994;36:371.
18. Perry HE, Wright RO, Shannon MW, Woolf AD. Baclofen overdose: drug experimentation in a group of adolescents. *Pediatrics* 1998;101:1045–1048.
19. Roberge RJ, Atchley B, Ryan K, Krenzelok EP. Two chlorzoxazone (parafon forte) overdoses and coma in one patient: reversal with flumazenil. *Am J Emerg Med* 1998;16:393–395.
20. Roth BA, Vinson DR, Kim S. Carisoprodol-induced myoclonic encephalopathy. *J Toxicol Clin Toxicol* 1998;36:609–612.
21. Schwartz HS. Acute meprobamate poisoning with gastrotomy and removal of a drug-containing mass. *N Engl J Med* 1976;295:1177.
22. Sing K, Erickson T, Amitai Y, et al. Chloral hydrate toxicity from oral and intravenous administration. *J Toxicol Clin Toxicol* 1996;34:101–106.
23. Spiller HA, Winter ML, Mann KV, et al. Five-year multicenter retrospective review of cyclobenzaprine toxicity. *J Emerg Med* 1995;13:781–785.
24. Van Herreweghe I, Mertens K, Maes V, et al. Orphenadrine poisoning in a child: clinical and analytical data. *Intensive Care Med* 1999;25:1134–1136.
25. Yell RP. Ethchlorvynol overdose. *Am J Emerg Med* 1990;8:246–250.

CHAPTER 291
Phenytoin

Thomas E. Kearney

Phenytoin, formerly called diphenylhydantoin, is an anticonvulsant belonging to the chemical class known as hydantoins, which also includes mephenytoin and ethotoin. It is effective for a variety of seizure disorders, including generalized tonic–clonic, partial-complex, and other focal seizures. However, phenytoin is probably ineffective for toxin-induced seizures and alcohol withdrawal. Phenytoin has also been used in the management of trigeminal neuralgia and as a type IB antiarrhythmic, especially for digitalis- and tricyclic antidepressant–induced conduction defects and ventricular dysrhythmias.

Phenytoin, a weak acid with a pKa of 8.5, is readily soluble only in a highly alkaline medium, and therefore requires formulation in a special diluent (40% propylene glycol and 10% ethanol) and adjustment of pH (to 12) with alkali (sodium hydroxide) for parenteral administration. Although this preparation may precipitate if added to acidic parenteral solutions, it may be added to normal saline if properly diluted and used immediately. Intramuscular injection may result in erratic absorption, muscle pain, and necrosis.

Another parenteral preparation and phosphate ester prodrug of phenytoin, fosphenytoin (Cerebyx®), has a more neutral pH (8.6–9.0) and greater water solubility. It is compatible with common intravenous preparations and lacks the cardiotoxic diluent propylene glycol and the high alkalinity responsible for local soft-tissue injuries; additionally, it may be administered intramuscularly. Because of its higher cost, however, fosphenytoin has not replaced parenteral phenytoin. Fosphenytoin is dosed in phenytoin equivalents or PEs (1.5 mg fosphenytoin = 1.0 mg phenytoin) to avoid conversion errors, and is metabolized to phenytoin in 6 to 16 minutes.

Oral preparations include extended-release and prompt-release capsule formulations of sodium salt, chewable tablets, and suspension of the free acid. Phenytoin poisoning commonly results from acute accidental ingestion by children or from suicidal ingestion and even illicit use by adolescents and adults (11,16,19). Additionally, therapeutic misadventures and iatrogenic poisonings frequently result from drug–drug or drug–disease interactions that affect its distribution, protein binding, and clearance; excessive dosing, with administration of a daily amount of phenytoin greater than the patient's metabolic capacity for elimination; therapeutic dosing in patients with a polymorphism and deficiency of phenytoin metabolic enzymes, CYP2C9; or improper parenteral administration (9).

Toxicity may also result from improper mixing of phenytoin suspensions before use and switching between products with different absorption characteristics. Non–dose-related, idiosyncratic, or hypersensitivity-type toxic effects may be associated with its therapeutic use, particularly in patients with neurologic deficits or occult neurologic lesions, and receiving concomitant radiotherapy (14,19).

As an anticonvulsant, phenytoin is essentially devoid of hypnotic effects at therapeutic levels. It prevents the spread of abnormal neuronal discharges by stabilizing neuronal membranes. This effect is achieved by altering fluxes of sodium, calcium, and potassium ions in neuronal conducting membranes and by reducing the posttetanic potential of synaptic transmission. It may also deplete folate in the central nervous system (CNS), red blood cells, and bone marrow. Additionally, phenytoin may have an excitatory effect on Purkinje cell discharge in the cerebellum that, in turn, activates GABA-ergic inhibitory pathways in the cerebral cortex. Phenytoin may, however, produce or unmask focal neurologic deficits in patients with GABA receptor supersensitivity resulting from hypoxic or ischemic insults. Serotonergic and dopaminergic activity may also be enhanced by phenytoin, as evidenced by its precipitation of movement disorders.

Phenytoin's effects on the myocardium parallel those of lidocaine. It inhibits sodium channels, decreases the effective refractory period and automaticity in Purkinje fibers, and has little or no effect on the QRS and action potential duration.

Phenytoin's anticonvulsant and antiarrhythmic effects are usually achieved at plasma levels in the range of 10 to 20 μg/mL. This level can be quickly attained with an intravenous loading dose of 15 to 20 mg/kg of phenytoin or PE (phenytoin equivalent) units of fosphenytoin. Because of potential toxicity from the propylene glycol diluent (cardiac dysrhythmias and hypotension), phenytoin should be given no faster than 50 mg/min (13).

Fosphenytoin, despite its lack of propylene glycol, may be associated with similar cardiovascular toxicity if administered at high infusion rates and doses. Hence, the rate of fosphenytoin administration should not exceed 150 PE units/min in adults (3 mg/kg/min in children). Phenytoin concentrations should not be monitored until conversion of fosphenytoin to phenytoin is complete, 2 hours and 4 hours after intravenous infusion and intramuscular administration, respectively. The maintenance dose of phenytoin is usually 4 to 6 mg/kg/d as single or divided doses. Neonates may require higher loading doses (15–20 mg/kg) and maintenance doses (5 to 8 mg/kg/d) (5).

Phenytoin is poorly soluble, and hence sparingly absorbed, in the acid milieu of the stomach. Absorption from the duodenum and lower gastrointestinal (GI) tract is extremely variable and depends on the oral dosage form, gastric emptying time, and bowel motility. Peak serum levels are observed at 2.6 to 8.9 hours after a single dose of extended-release capsule (e.g., Dilantin). After overdosage with this formulation, absorption has continued for up to 12 days. This lengthy absorption period may be as a result of its high lipophilicity and slow dissolution rate, the formation of a slowly disintegrating mass of capsules (pharmacobezoar) or decreased GI motility (22).

Phenytoin is metabolized predominantly in the liver. Up to 70% of a given daily dose is converted by parahydroxylation to 5-(p-hydroxyphenyl)-5-phenylhydantoin (HPPH), which is then conjugated with glucuronide into a more water-soluble metabolite and excreted renally. About 1% to 5% of phenytoin is excreted unchanged in the urine. Phenytoin is actively secreted into the gut and undergoes enterohepatic recirculation.

The cytochrome P-450 enzyme system responsible for parahydroxylation of phenytoin is "saturable" at plasma levels around 10 μg/mL. Below this level, phenytoin follows first-order elimination kinetics, with an average half-life of 22 hours (range, 7–55 hours) in adults. Above this level, it follows zero-order kinetics, resulting in a much longer half-life. There are 2 key cytochrome P-450 enzymes, CYP2C9 (accounting for approximately 80% of metabolism) and CYP2C19 (minor pathway) (9). These metabolic enzymes are subject to inhibition or induction by other drugs or may be deficient because of inherited genetic traits or liver disease (Table 291.1). Cytochrome P-450 enzyme systems may also be responsible for the formation of toxic metabolites and adverse effects such as hypersensitivities and gingival hyperplasia (14,25).

Phenytoin has a relatively low volume of distribution (0.6 L/kg in adults) and preferentially distributes to the cerebellum and brainstem (8). It is 90% bound to plasma protein, mostly albumin. Decreased protein binding, resulting from competition with protein receptors by endogenous or exogenous substrates or reduced albumin levels, increases free (pharmacologically active) drug levels and the volume of distribution. Because only total serum phenytoin levels are routinely monitored, decreased protein binding results in therapeutic and toxic effects at lower-than-usual serum concentrations (see Table 291.1). Reagent kits to monitor free phenytoin levels are commercially available and may be useful in patients with altered protein binding (uremia, liver disease, hypoalbuminemia) (7).

Toxic effects result from exaggerated pharmacologic activity, nutritional deficiencies (folate, vitamin D and K depletion), altered collagen metabolism, idiosyncratic, and hypersensitivity reactions, and propylene glycol toxicity with parenteral

---

TABLE 291.1. Factors Influencing Phenytoin Kinetics

Pharmacokinetic Effects	Condition or Concomitant Drug Use	Pharmacologic Effect
Decreased protein binding	Acidosis Age (neonates) Uremia Hepatitis Hypoalbuminemia Valproic acid Nonsteroidal antiinflammatory agents	Increased risk for phenytoin toxicity Higher free fraction of circulating phenytoin
Decreased clearance	Metabolic inhibitors (e.g., amiodarone, SSRIs [fluoxetine]) Tamoxifen, isoniazid, disulfiram, ticlopidine Genetic deficiency of liver enzyme system (CYP2C9 & CYP2C19 polymorphisms)	Increased; risk for phenytoin toxicity Accumulation of phenytoin during chronic dosing caused by prolonged half-life
Increased clearance	Hepatic enzyme inducers (e.g., phenobarbital, carbamazepine) Ciprofloxacin, ethanol Pregnancy	Decreased loss of efficacy with risk for breakthrough seizures Shortened half-life results in less accumulation during chronic dosing

administration. Numerous teratogenic effects (fetal hydantoin syndrome in 10% to 30% of exposed pregnancies) have also been reported (4).

Acute poisoning may result from single ingestions of 20 mg/kg or more. Death is rare but has been reported in children aged 3 to 7 years with ingestions of 100 to 220 mg/kg (11,18). The cause of death is CNS depression with respiratory insufficiency and hypoxia-related sequelae. Survival has been noted after acute ingestion of 249 mg/kg in a 2.5-year-old child, who had a level of 112 µg/mL at 70 hours (23). Reported cases of adult phenytoin poisoning have demonstrated moderate CNS toxicity with recovery after ingestion of 12 to 25 g, with the highest recorded level of 130 µg/mL at 96 hours after ingestion (3).

CLINICAL PRESENTATION

Because tolerance to phenytoin has not been described, dose- and level-related toxic effects are similar for both acute and chronic overdosage (5). Phenytoin initially affects cerebellar and vestibular function, with cerebral depression occurring later. At serum levels of 20 to 40 µg/mL, signs and symptoms of mild intoxication include dizziness, ataxia, tremors, lethargy, nausea, vomiting, slurred speech, diplopia, blurred vision, normal-to-dilated pupils, and nystagmus (coarse, horizontal, or vertical) (10). An initial excitatory phase has also been reported. At levels of 40 to 90 µg/mL, confusion, psychosis, hallucinations (visual, auditory, and tactile; also occasionally observed at therapeutic levels), and progressively deeper CNS depression with suppression of nystagmus and sluggish ocular and deep tendon reflexes may be noted (2). Levels above 90 µg/mL are associated with severe toxicity and manifest by coma with respiratory depression (23).

Note that all of the above serum phenytoin levels and corresponding toxic effects were based on total levels (bound and free). Free phenytoin levels are approximately 10% of total in patients with normal protein binding (but may increase to over 30% in patients with altered protein binding) and dose-related toxicity is not anticipated or minor with free phenytoin levels less than 2 µg/mL.

"Paradoxical intoxication" with increased seizure frequency, dystonias, dyskinesias, choreoathetoid movements, and decerebrate rigidity may be noted in patients with underlying seizure disorders (16). Additionally, those with focal neurologic lesions may develop contralateral deficits (e.g., hemianopia, hemianesthesia, and hemiparesis). Other etiologies should be considered for seizures that occur in phenytoin-intoxicated patients without preexisting seizure or neurologic disorders. Laboratory abnormalities are generally limited to hyperglycemia and decreased thyroxine levels (24). The electroencephalogram characteristically shows slowing of a-wave activity. With severe intoxication, brainstem evoked potentials may be absent.

Unless complications as a result of anoxia or sepsis ensue, recovery is usually complete once the drug is eliminated. Depending on the phenytoin level, elimination may take longer than a week. In rare cases, chronic poisoning has resulted in encephalopathy and cerebellar degeneration with persistent ataxia (8).

With chronic use, folate depletion may occur and result in megaloblastic anemia and peripheral neuropathy. Additionally, altered collagen metabolism may lead to gingival hyperplasia, hirsutism, and hypertrichosis. The mechanism may involve the formation of reactive metabolites as a result of cytochrome P-450 in gingival tissue (25). Vitamin D deficiency and altered calcium homeostasis, and direct effects on osteoblasts, may result in osteomalacia and osteoporosis (20).

Idiosyncratic and hypersensitivity reactions may have multisystem involvement and include fever, rash, eosinophilia, hematologic abnormalities (thrombocytopenia, leukopenia, aplastic anemia, agranulocytosis), dermatological (erythema multiforme, Stevens-Johnson syndrome, toxic epidermal necrolysis), hepatitis, lupus-like syndrome, lymphadenopathy, myositis, rhabdomyolysis, nephritis, vasculitis, and hemolytic anemia (19). The hypersensitivity reaction has been termed the "Anticonvulsant Hypersensitivity Syndrome" and may be attributed to the formation of arene oxide metabolites of aromatic anticonvulsants (phenytoin, phenobarbital, and carbamazepine), thereby accounting for the cross-sensitivity between these anticonvulsants. There may be variation in the latency (weeks to months) and organ systems involved, patch testing may be unpredictable, and a more severe syndrome may occur in patients receiving concomitant radiotherapy (6,14).

The rapid infusion of propylene glycol (at phenytoin rates above 50 mg/min) may result in bradycardia, hypotension, ventricular fibrillation and asystole, conduction defects, congestive heart failure, and respiratory arrest (13). These effects are usually transient and seldom persist for more than 1 hour after the infusion is stopped. The rapid infusion of high doses (5 to 10 times the recommended dose) of fosphenytoin has also resulted in severe cardiovascular (CV) toxicity in infants with status epilepticus (12). CV effects and dysrhythmias have not been reported with phenytoin toxicity associated with ingestions. Phenytoin may induce the "purple glove syndrome" (limb edema, discoloration, and pain) after peripheral intravenous administration (17). It can occur hours after infusion, in the absence of clinical signs of extravasation, and can lead to limb ischemia and necrosis from a compartment syndrome. This has not been observed with fosphenytoin and risk factors may include: elderly patients receiving large multiple doses, use of small i.v. catheters, high infusion rates, and same catheter site for 2 or more i.v. push doses (21).

DIFFERENTIAL DIAGNOSIS

The differential diagnosis of phenytoin intoxication includes intoxication with other anticonvulsants, sedative–hypnotics, and CNS depressants; seizure disorders; postictal states; CNS trauma and tumors; and extrapyramidal disorders. Phenytoin poisoning may also mimic ketotic and nonketotic hyperglycemic coma (19). Although it has been stated that nystagmus is pathognomonic of phenytoin toxicity, this finding is neither sensitive nor specific. It can be present with therapeutic levels and absent with toxic levels, and may be present in a variety of other conditions and intoxications.

EMERGENCY DEPARTMENT EVALUATION

The history should include the time, amount, and preparation of phenytoin taken; the onset and nature of symptoms; chronic medications; and past and current medical problems. The clinician should also note previous use of phenytoin and preexisting seizure disorders.

The physical examination should focus on vital signs, cardiopulmonary findings, and a detailed neurologic assessment. Serum phenytoin and glucose levels and an electrocardiogram (ECG) should be included in the initial evaluation. Other routine laboratory studies, toxicology screening, and a chest radiograph should be obtained as clinically indicated. Because phenytoin absorption and elimination may be greatly prolonged after overdosage, two (or more) serum levels taken several hours apart, along with serial clinical evaluations, are necessary to assess the degree and progression of toxicity.

Patients with the purple glove syndrome should be evaluated for limb ischemia; intracompartmental pressure measurement may be useful in guiding therapy in those with manifestations of arterial insufficiency.

EMERGENCY DEPARTMENT MANAGEMENT

Advanced life-support measures should be instituted as necessary. Patients with a preexisting seizure disorder should be placed on seizure preventives because of the possibility of paradoxical seizures during the acute intoxication phase and breakthrough seizures if serum levels drop too low. Although CV toxicity has not been reported after oral overdose, cardiac monitoring is advisable for patients with severe CNS toxicity and during intravenous administration.

In addition to stopping the infusion, it may be necessary to administer crystalloids to patients who develop hypotension during intravenous administration. Dysrhythmias usually resolve spontaneously on stopping the infusion but can be treated according to advanced cardiac life-support guidelines, if necessary.

Seizures caused by phenytoin toxicity require discontinuation of the drug and treatment instead with another agent, such as diazepam or a barbiturate. Hyperglycemia usually resolves with discontinuation of phenytoin and seldom requires insulin unless the patient has diabetes.

Administration of activated charcoal is the preferred method of GI decontamination. Multiple oral doses of activated charcoal (MDAC) can enhance the elimination of phenytoin after systemic absorption (15). Controlled evidence is lacking, however, that MDAC therapy shortens the duration of toxicity or improves outcome. For patients taking phenytoin for therapeutic purposes, an extended observation period may be necessary to ensure that phenytoin levels do not become subtherapeutic.

Because of phenytoin's high degree of protein-binding and hepatic elimination, procedures such as forced diuresis with ion trapping, hemodialysis, and peritoneal dialysis have not been beneficial (23). Although hemoperfusion has resulted in a minimal increase in clearance in one reported case (1), patients with phenytoin poisoning usually have a favorable outcome with good supportive care alone. Hence, the risk of hemoperfusion usually outweighs its possible benefit.

Idiosyncratic or hypersensitivity reactions and complications of chronic therapy are treated by drug withdrawal and supportive measures. A vascular surgeon should be consulted for the management of patients with purple glove syndrome who have signs of vascular compromise.

CRITICAL INTERVENTIONS

- Obtain serial phenytoin levels after acute overdose as drug absorption and elimination may be prolonged
- Discontinue phenytoin and fosphenytoin infusion if CV toxicity occurs

DISPOSITION

Asymptomatic patients who accidentally ingest less than 20 mg/kg of phenytoin, do not have a preexisting neurologic disorder, and are not taking phenytoin chronically can be observed at home and followed by telephone contact. All other patients should be evaluated at a health care facility.

Nonsuicidal patients with mild-to-moderate toxicity (those who can sit up, feed themselves, and walk with assistance) can be discharged with home observation after documentation of declining drug levels. Suicidal patients, those with severe toxicity or rising drug levels after several measurements, and those without responsible friends or relatives to assist and observe them at home should be admitted. Inpatient level of care (floor vs. intensive care unit) should be determined by the degree and progression of toxicity and underlying medical problems. Any facility that can provide intensive respiratory therapy should be able to manage uncomplicated cases of phenytoin poisoning. Patients who are transferred should be accompanied by personnel trained in advanced life support.

COMMON PITFALLS

✔ Failure to recognize that nystagmus is of limited value in the diagnosis of phenytoin poisoning

✔ Failure to consider alterations in protein binding when interpreting phenytoin levels and potential utility in monitoring free levels

✔ Failure to appreciate that CV toxicity is as a result of propylene glycol and occurs only with high infusion rates and not with ingestions

✔ Failure to appreciate that phenytoin can exacerbate preexisting neurologic problems

✔ Failure to consider the risks and unproven benefit of using ipecac, flumazenil, and MDAC therapy in patients with seizure disorders and phenytoin toxicity

✔ Failure to appreciate that patients with uncomplicated phenytoin poisoning do well with supportive care and that extracorporeal drug removal measures are ineffective or unnecessary

✔ Failure to appreciate that purple glove syndrome may occur hours after peripheral intravenous administration of phenytoin and that risk factors for this complication include advanced ages, high infusion rates and doses, and use of small catheters and the same infusion site

✔ Failure to recognize early symptoms of an anticonvulsant hypersensitivity syndrome (fever, rash, lymphadenopathy) and the common cross-reactivity between aromatic anticonvulsants

References

1. Baechler RW, Work J, Smith W, et al. Charcoal hemoperfusion in the therapy for methsuximide and phenytoin overdose. *Arch Intern Med* 1980;40:1466.
2. Benatar MG, Sahin M, Davis RG. Antiepileptic Drug-induced Visual Hallucinations in a Child. *Pediatr Neurol* 2000;23:439–441.
3. Blair AAD, Hallpike JF, Lascelles PT. Acute diphenylhydantoin and primidone poisoning treated by peritoneal dialysis. *J Neurol Neurosurg Psychiatry* 1968;31:520.
4. Bodendorfer TW. Fetal effects of anticonvulsant drugs and seizure disorders. *Drug Intell Clin Pharm* 1978;12:14.
5. Borofsky LG, Louis S, Kutt H, et al. Diphenylhydantoin efficacy, toxicity and dose-serum relationships in children. *J Pediatr* 1972;81:995.
6. Choi TS, Doh KS, Kim SH, et al. Clinicopathological and genotypic aspects of anticonvulsant-induced pseudolymphoma syndrome. *Br J Dermatology* 2003;148:730–736.
7. Dasgupta A. Clinical Utility of Free Drug Monitoring. *Clin Chem Lab Med* 2002;40(10):986–993.
8. Luef G, Burtscher J, Kremser C, et al. Magnetic resonance volumetry of the cerebellum in epileptic patients after phenytoin overdosages. *Eur Neurol* 1996;36:273–277.
9. Kidd RS, Curry TB, Gallagher S, et al. Identification of a null allele of CYP2C9 in an African-American exhibiting toxicity to phenytoin. *Pharmacogenetics* 2001;11:803–808.
10. Kutt H, Winters W, Kokenge R. Metabolism of diphenylhydantoin, blood levels and toxicity. *Arch Neurol* 1964;11:642.
11. Laubscher FA. Fatal diphenylhydantoin poisoning. *JAMA* 1966;198:1120.
12. Lieber BL, Snodgrass WR. Cardiac arrest following large intravenous fosphenytoin overdose in an infant. *J Toxicol Clin Toxicol* 1998;36:473(abst).
13. Louis S, Kutt H, McDowell F. The cardiocirculatory changes caused by intravenous Dilantin and its solvent. *Am Heart J* 1967;74:523.
14. Maldonado R, Tello S, Garcia-Baquero R, et al. Anticonvulsant hypersensitivity syndrome with fatal outcome. *Eur J Dermatology* 2002;12(5):503–505.

15. Mauro LS, Maruo VF, Brown DL. Enhancement of phenytoin elimination by multiple-dose activated charcoal. *Am J Emerg Med* 1987;16:1132.
16. Murphy JM, Motiwala R, Devinsky O. Phenytoin intoxication. *South Med J* 1991;84:1199.
17. O'Brien TJ, Cascino GD, So EL, et al. Incidence and clinical consequence of the purple glove syndrome in patients receiving intravenous phenytoin. *Neurology* 1998;51:1034–1039.
18. Petty CS, Muelling RJ, Sindell HW. Accidental poisoning with diphenylhydantoin (Dilantin). *J Forensic Sci* 1957;2:279.
19. Powers NG, Carson SH. Idiosyncratic reactions to phenytoin. *Clin Pediatr (Phila)* 1987;26:120.
20. Rogvi-Hansen B, Gram L. Adverse effects of established and new antiepileptic drugs: An attempted comparison. *Pharmacol Ther* 1993;68:425–434.
21. Spengler RF, Arrowsmith JB, Kilarski DJ, et al. Severe soft-tissue injury following intravenous infusion of phenytoin. *Arch Intern Med* 1988;148:1329–1333.
22. Stevenson CM, Kim J, Fleisher D. Colonic absorption of antiepileptic agents. *Epilepsia* 1997;38(1):63–67.
23. Tenckhoff H, Sherrard DJ, Hickman O, et al. Acute diphenylhydantoin intoxication. *Am J Dis Child* 1968;116:422.
24. Wagner KJ, Zeil M, Leiken JB. Metabolic effects of phenytoin toxicity. *Ann Emerg Med* 1986;15:509.
25. Zhou LX, Pihlstrom B, Hardwick JP, et al. Metabolism of phenytoin by the gingival of normal humans: possible role of reactive metabolites of phenytoin in the intiation of gingival hyperplasia. *Clin Pharmacol Ther* 1996;60:191–198.

CHAPTER 292
Valproic Acid

Gregory G. Gaar

Valproic acid (VPA), valproate sodium, and divalproex sodium are used either alone or in combination with other anticonvulsants primarily in the treatment of absence seizures, both simple and complex. Although not currently included in the labeling approved by the Food and Drug Administration, they are also used to treat temporal lobe seizures, myoclonic seizures, and generalized tonic–clonic seizures. They are now approved for use in prophylaxis and treatment of migraine headaches, in the manic phase of bipolar illness, and for neuropathic pain.

The compounds are carboxylic acid derivatives that differ structurally from any of the other commercially available anticonvulsants (19). Although valproate's mechanism of action has not been fully elucidated, it is believed to exert some effects through modulation of regional levels of γ-aminobutyric acid (GABA), an inhibitory central nervous system (CNS) neurotransmitter. Hyperammonemia is as a result of effects on renal and hepatic metabolism. Valproate blocks renal glutamine synthesis resulting in increased ammonia production. VPA metabolites inhibit hepatic carbamoxyl phosphate synthetase, the enzyme involved in the first step of the urea cycle, thereby inhibiting the metabolism of ammonia.

In the United States, forms for oral use include capsules of VPA (250 mg), a solution of valproate sodium (250 mg VPA per 5 mL), a "sprinkle capsule" containing coated granules of divalproex sodium (equivalent to 125 mg of VPA), and enteric-coated tablets of divalproex sodium (equivalent to 125, 250, and 500 mg of VPA) (19). Depakene and Depakote are the most widely used brands of valproate sodium and divalproex sodium, respectively. The initial starting dosage is 15 mg/kg/d (maximum, 600 mg/d). Once weekly, the dosage may be increased by 5 to 10 mg/kg/d until adequate seizure control is established or adverse effects necessitate smaller dosages. The manufacturer does not recommend a dosage of more than 60 mg/kg/d. Although definite therapeutic or toxic serum levels have not been established, it is generally accepted that therapeutic concentrations are in the range of 50 to 100 µg/mL (19).

Absorption of VPA is rapid and complete from either capsule or solution formulation. Although valproate sodium must be converted to VPA to be absorbed, this reaction occurs rapidly in the stomach. Peak plasma concentrations occur within 1 to 4 hours of a single oral dose of valproic acid. Food in the gastrointestinal (GI) tract decreases the rate of absorption but not the total amount (19). When enteric-coated tablet or granule preparations are used, the compound must dissociate into valproate in the jejunum before absorption can occur. The enteric coating slows this process, so the peak plasma level occurs later, usually within 3 to 5 hours of a single oral dose (8,19). The volume of distribution ranges from 0.1 to 0.4 L/kg.19 Therefore, distribution is mostly into plasma and extracellular water. Protein-binding is significant in the therapeutic range; at concentrations of 80 µg/mL, almost 90% is bound to proteins (8,19). At concentrations above 100 µg/mL, saturation of these proteins occurs and the percentage of drug bound to plasma protein decreases (19). Accordingly, after the acute ingestion of toxic amounts, the percentage of circulating "free" drug increases markedly (11). At serum levels >300 µg/mL, only 35% of the drug is protein-bound (12,15). The elimination half-life ranges from 7 to 15 hours (8,19). VPA is metabolized by the liver; the metabolites are usually conjugated with glucuronide and then eliminated in the urine. Small amounts of drug are excreted unchanged in the urine and feces (19). Other antiepileptic drugs used concomitantly can alter the half-life of valproic acid, usually reducing it (8). In contrast, concomitant use of valproate may inhibit the metabolism of phenobarbital and increase phenobarbital levels (16).

VPA can be toxic both after acute overdoses and during chronic therapy. In acute ingestion, there are no absolute guidelines for predicting toxicity based on the amount ingested. A 19-month-old infant survived an ingestion of 204 mg/kg, with a serum drug level of 185 µg/mL, and adults have recovered from ingesting as much as 75 g (13,18,21). In one large series, patients were likely to be unconscious only after ingesting more than 200 mg/kg (13). Death from complications of pneumonia has been reported after an ingestion of 15 g (705 mg/kg) in a 20-month-old boy (23).

Toxic manifestations have occurred during chronic use at therapeutic dosages. Blood levels above 100 µg/mL may cause unusual neurologic effects or potentiate seizures. Dosages of 2.2 to 2.5 g/d have caused CNS effects (7).

CLINICAL PRESENTATION

The predominant symptoms and signs of toxicity after acute overdosage with VPA relate to the CNS. Drowsiness, confusion, and change in mental status are the most common (7,18). Coma may ensue, with subsequent respiratory failure (13,18,23). In one multi-center case series, 100% of patients with levels greater than 850 µg/mL were comatose (24). Seizures and myoclonic movements have been reported (13). Pupils may be pinpoint and sluggishly reactive to light (1). Cerebral edema has been reported. GI toxicity includes nausea, vomiting, and diarrhea. Hyperammonemia can occur in the absence of hepatotoxicity. Patients with markedly elevated VPA levels can also have an increased anion gap metabolic acidosis as a result of elevated lactate and/or valproic acid levels (each 144 ug/ml of valproate equals 1 umole/mL and represents 1 mEq/L of unmeasured VPA anion). Cardiovascular toxicity is often manifest by tachycardia after acute overdosage (24). Hypotension and cardiorespiratory arrest are rare (23,24).

Toxicity during chronic VPA usage includes mental status changes such as drowsiness, confusion, and social withdrawal (7). Cerebral edema has been reported. Nausea, emesis, and abdominal pain have been observed. Elevated liver enzyme levels, hepatocellular necrosis, and fatal cholestatic hepatitis are rare (6). Hyperammonemia and hyperglycinemia have occurred independent of hepatotoxicity (17). Thrombocytopenia and impaired platelet aggregation have been reported. Acute pancreatitis is rare (3).

DIFFERENTIAL DIAGNOSIS

The differential diagnosis of a patient with impaired mental status as a result of the acute ingestion of a toxic amount of VPA includes trauma, hypoglycemia, hypoxia, other CNS depressant drugs (see Chapter 271, "Approach to the Poisoned Patient"), CNS infection, metabolic disorders (diabetic ketoacidosis and Reye syndrome), intracranial tumors, and the postictal state. An elevated serum valproate level and the exclusion of other causes confirm the diagnosis.

EMERGENCY DEPARTMENT EVALUATION

The history should include the amount and preparation of valproate ingested, other substances available for ingestion in the patient's environment, and the time of the ingestion (or the last time the patient was in his or her usual state of health). The patient's preexisting health status should be noted. Events that occurred between the time of the ingestion and presentation to the emergency department should be documented.

The physical examination should initially focus on cardiorespiratory function and the CNS. Cardiorespiratory monitoring and pulse oximetry should be instituted in patients with a known ingestion of toxic amounts or in patients demonstrating toxic effects. A quantitative valproate level should be ordered to confirm the diagnosis. Serial levels are necessary after an acute overdose. As most patients with seizure disorders have access to multiple medications, an "anticonvulsant screen" is often useful. Full toxicology testing should be considered in patients with intentional overdoses. In symptomatic patients, routine laboratory evaluation includes a complete blood count (CBC); measurement of serum electrolytes, blood urea nitrogen, creatinine, and glucose; hepatic function tests and serum ammonia. A chest radiograph, arterial blood gas analysis, and serum lactate level should be obtained in patients with signs of severe toxicity.

For patients on chronic VPA therapy, monitoring should include a CBC with differential, a platelet count, liver function tests (including serum ammonia), and serum electrolyte measurements.

EMERGENCY DEPARTMENT MANAGEMENT

Advanced cardiac life-support measures should be instituted as necessary. In patients with coma of unknown cause, appropriate doses of naloxone, glucose, and thiamine should be given. In case reports, naloxone has reversed CNS depression secondary to valproate poisoning (1), but no study of a series of patients has replicated this finding, and responses have been inconsistent.

Prevention of absorption is the next consideration. In patients who present within 1 hour of ingestion, single dose activated charcoal (AC) is the preferred method of preventing absorption

of VPA if no contraindications exist (2). Charcoal adsorbs valproate (21). Emesis with syrup of ipecac is not recommended. Gastric lavage should be reserved for patients who are comatose and present within 30 minutes to 1 hour after the ingestion. In patients who have ingested large amounts of enteric-coated tablets, whole-bowel irrigation might, theoretically, be advantageous (2). Hemodialysis and hemoperfusion have been beneficial in enhancing the elimination of VPA in both adults and children (10,12,15,20). Given the complications of these procedures and the fact that toxicity is usually responsive to good supportive care, extracorporeal removal is not routinely recommended. It should be reserved for those with hemodynamic instability, which has not responded to aggressive supportive care (14,24,25). Forced diuresis is ineffective.

L-carnitine appears to be beneficial in the prevention and treatment of hyperammonemia. It has been recommended as a prophylactic supplement in certain patients on valproate therapy (9), as therapy for symptomatic hepatotoxicity or hyperammonemia, and following acute overdosage to prevent cerebral edema and encephalopathy associated with hyperammonemia (5,9). It's mechanism of action is unknown and its efficacy following acute overdosage remains speculative. However, as a result of the favorable safety profile of *L*-carnitine, some experts are recommending it for acutely poisoned patients with hyperammonemia and coma (150 mg/kg/day intravenously, with maximum of 3 grams) (22,25).

Most patients recover fully. Sequelae are rare, although a report of visual disturbances has been published (4).

CRITICAL INTERVENTIONS

- Obtain serial drug levels in patients with acute VPA overdose
- Obtain hepatic function tests and serum ammonia in patients with signs and symptoms of VPA poisoning or elevated drug levels
- Check acid–base status and serum lactate levels in patients with severe VPA poisoning

DISPOSITION

All patients with changes in mental status or respiratory function after an acute overdose of VPA should be hospitalized in a facility capable of providing continuous cardiorespiratory monitoring. Appropriate consultation from physicians trained in clinical toxicology, intensive care, and pulmonary medicine may be indicated, depending on the clinical course. If intensive care necessitates transfer to another facility, stabilization—including appropriate airway management, intravenous access, and maintenance of circulatory status—should precede advanced cardiac life-support–capable transport to the appropriate institution.

Patients who have ingested rapidly absorbed products should have valproate levels monitored for at least 6 hours after the overdose; those who have ingested enteric-coated preparations should be monitored for 8 to 10 hours. If drug levels are decreasing and there are no clinical signs of toxicity, they can be discharged. Psychiatric consultation should be obtained before discharge on all patients with intentional overdose.

COMMON PITFALLS

✔ Failure to appreciate that the onset of toxicity may be delayed after acute overdose and that an extended period of observation is necessary, particularly after overdose of enteric-coated or granule formulations of divalproex sodium

✔ Failure to obtain serial drug levels after an acute overdose, to determine whether further observation is necessary

✔ Failure to appreciate that hyperammonemia can occur in the absence of other evidence of hepatotoxicity in patients with VPA poisoning

✔ Failure to appreciate that although therapy is primarily supportive and depends on the clinical condition, not the drug level, extracorporeal elimination procedures may be useful in the comatose patient with hemodynamic instability

References

1. Alberto G, Erickson T, Popiel R, et al. CNS manifestations of a valproic acid overdose responsive to naloxone. *Ann Emerg Med* 1989;18:889.
2. American Academy of Clinical Toxicology and European Association of Poison Centres and Clinical Toxicologists. Position statements on gastrointestinal decontamination. *J Toxicol Clin Toxicol* 1997;7:695.
3. Anderson GO, Ritland S. Life threatening intoxication with sodium valproate. *J Toxicol Clin Toxicol* 1995;33:279.
4. Bigler D. Neurological sequelae after intoxication with sodium valproate. *Acta Neurol Scand* 1985;72:351.
5. Bohan TP, Helton E, McDonald I, et al. Effect of L-carnitine treatment for valproate-induced hepatotoxicity. *Neurology* 2001;56:1405.
6. Bryant AE, Dreifuss FE. Valproic acid hepatic fatalities. III. US. experience since 1986. *Neurology* 1996;46:465.
7. Chadwick DW, Cumming WJK, Livingston I, et al. Acute intoxication with sodium valproate. *Ann Neurol* 1979;6:552.
8. Davis R, Peters DH, McTavish D. Valproic acid: a reappraisal of its pharmacological poperties and clinical efficacy in epilepsy. *Drugs* 1994;47:332.
9. DeVivo DC, Bohan TP, Coulter DL, et al. L-carnitine supplementation in childhood epilepsy: Current perspectives. *Epilepsia* 1998;39:1216.
10. Dharnidharka VR, Fennel RS, Richard GA. Extracorporeal removal of toxic valproic acid levels in children. *Pediatr Nephrol* 2002;17:312.
11. Farrar HC, Herold DA, Reed MD. Acute valproic acid intoxication: enhanced drug clearance with oral activated charcoal. *Crit Care Med* 1993;21:299.
12. Franssen EJ, van Essen GG, Portman AT et al. Valproic acid toxicokinetics: Serial hemodialysis and hemoperfusion. *Ther Drug Monit* 1999;21:289.
13. Garnier R, Boudignat O, Fournier PE. Valproate poisoning. *Lancet* 1982;2:97.
14. Graeme K, Higgins T, Curry S, et al. Markedly elevated valproate levels do not serve as an indication for hemodialysis or hemoperfusion. *J Toxicol Clin Toxicol* 1999;37:636.
15. Kane SL, Constantiner M, Staubus AE, et al. High-flux hemodialysis without hemoperfusion is effective in acute valproic acid overdose. *Ann Pharmacother* 2000;34:1146.
16. Keys PA. Valproic acid: interactions with phenytoin and phenobarbital. *Drug Intell Clin Pharm* 1982;16:737.
17. Kulick SK, Kramer DA. Hyperammonemia secondary to valproic acid as a cause of lethargy in a postictal patient. *Ann Emerg Med* 1993;22:610.
18. Lakhani M, McMurdo MET. Survival after severe self-poisoning with sodium valproate. *Postgrad Med J* 1986;62:409.
19. AHFS Drug information 2004. McEvoy GK, Miller J, Snow EK, et al (eds). Bethesda, MD: American Society of Health-System Pharmacists, 2004:2152.
20. Mortensen PB, Hansen HE, Pedersen B, et al. Acute valproate intoxication: biochemical investigations and hemodialysis treatment. *Int J Clin Pharmacol Ther Toxicol* 1983;21:64.
21. Neuvonen PJ, Kannisto H, Hirvisalo EL. Effect of activated charcoal on absorption of tolbutamide and valproate in man. *Eur J Clin Pharmacol* 1983;24:243.
22. Perez A, McKay CA. Role of carnitine in valproic acid toxicity. *J Toxicol Clin Toxicol* 2003;41:899.
23. Schnabel R, Rambeck B, Janssen F. Fatal intoxication with sodium valproate. *Lancet* 1984;1:221.
24. Spiller HA, Krenzelok EP, Klein-Schwartz W, et al. Multicenter case series of valproic acid ingestion: Serum concentrations and toxicity. *J Toxicol Clin Toxicol* 2000;38:755.
25. Sztajnkrycer MD. Valproic acid toxicity: Overview and management. *J Toxicol Clin Toxicol* 2002;40:789.

CHAPTER 293
Other Anticonvulsants

Walter H. Mullen

Epilepsy is one of the most common neurologic disorders and includes a variety of seizure disorders that affect approximately 2 million people in the United States. The lifetime incidence of epilepsy at some point in a person's life is approximately 3% (5). The toxicology of the anticonvulsants is particularly important because epileptic patients have a tenfold greater incidence of suicide (11.5%) compared to the general population (1.1%–1.2%) (11).

This chapter will focus on the toxicology of the newer anticonvulsants (Table 293.1), each of which possesses its own unique pharmacology and toxicologic considerations. Historically, 25% to 30% of epilepsy patients continued to have seizures despite optimal therapy with the older, standard agents (6). The newer agents have decreased the number of epilepsy patients with refractory seizures. In addition to their anticonvulsant properties, several possess pharmacologic properties useful for a variety of other disorders and are becoming frequently prescribed for nonanticonvulsant uses. One of them, gabapentin (Neurontin®), was the twenty-ninth most frequently dispensed drug in the United States in 2002 and was the twelfth leading drug in total sales dollars in 2002 (24).

Newer anticonvulsants are an increasingly encountered overdose in the emergency department. Data from the American Association of Poison Control Centers Toxic Exposure Surveillance System (TESS) shows that exposures reported by health care facilities to United States poison centers increased over the last decade from 242 in 1994 to 10,100 patients in 2002 (16,25). Although these agents are generally lower in toxicity than the older standard agents, they still possess potential for serious harm in overdose. Although 70% of the 10,100 exposures reported to TESS in 2002 resulted in no or minimal symptoms, 772 were classified as having a major outcome (defined as life-threatening or resulting in significant residual disability or disfigurement) and there were 31 deaths (0.003% fatality rate).

Felbamate (Felbatol®), a dicarbamate structurally related to the muscle relaxant methocarbamol, was approved by the United States Food and Drug Administration (FDA) in 1993 and was the first of the newer anticonvulsants. Felbamate was originally approved as a first-line agent in adults for treatment of partial seizures and for treatment of multiple types of seizures associated with Lennox-Gastaut syndrome in children. Initial enthusiasm for this new agent was soon tempered by reports of fatal hepatic failure and aplastic anemia (18). Felbamate is now only indicated for patients with severe, refractory seizure disorders in whom the benefits of the drug outweigh the potential risks. Felbamate interacts with several sites in the brain. It inhibits voltage-sensitive sodium channels and decreases their firing rate. It also blocks voltage-sensitive calcium channels and potentiates GABA (γ-aminobutyric acid, an inhibitory neurotransmitter) activity. Felbamate also has a novel site of action compared to other anticonvulsants. It is thought to interact with N-methyl-D-aspartate (NMDA) receptors, resulting in decreased excitatory amino acid neurotransmission (12). Felbamate has poor water solubility and can precipitate as crystals in the urine.

Gabapentin (Neurontin®), a structural analog of GABA approved by the FDA in 1993 for the adjuvant treatment of partial

TABLE 293.1. Anticonvulsants Introduced in the United States Since 1993

Drug	Indications	Dosage Range	Pharmacokinetics	Drug Interactions	Side Effects	Toxic Dose	Toxic Effects
Felbamate (Felbatol®, FBM) Approved 1993 Chemical class: dicarbamate	Adjunctive treatment of partial seizures and Lennox-Gastaut syndrome	Adults: 1,200–3,600 mg/d Pediatric: 15–45 mg/kg/d	Oral bioavailability: 90% $T_{1/2}$, 11–23 hr, Vd, 0.7–1.0 L/kg Fb, 0.25 40% hepatically metabolized and 40% to 50% excreted as unchanged drug	Increases levels of phenytoin, phenobarbital, valproic acid Decreases carbamazepine levels Carbamazepine, phenobarbital, and phenytoin induce decrease felbamate clearance May decrease oral contraceptive effectiveness	Black box warning for aplastic anemia and hepatic failure Most common: anorexia, nausea, vomiting, insomnia, headache, dizziness, and somnolence Dystonia reported in two pediatric cases	Not known A 12 g intentional overdose in an adult was tolerated with no serious effect	Drowsiness, ataxia, nystagmus Crystalluria and renal failure have been reported EKG abnormalities possible per product info
Gabapentin (Neu-ontin®, GBP) Approved 1993 Chemical class: GABA analog	Adjunctive treatment of partial seizures and postherpetic neuralgia Unlabeled uses include neuropathic pain, bipolar disorder, and migraine prophylaxis	Adults: 900–3,600 mg/d Pediatric: 10–50 mg/kg/d	Oral bioavailability: 27%–60% (decreases with increasing dose) $T_{1/2}$, 5–9 hr (increased in renal impairment) Vd, 0.8–1.3 L/kg, Fb, <0.03 not metabolized; excreted unchanged in the urine (75% to 80%) and feces	Hydrocodone and morphine decrease gabapentin clearance	Most common: somnolence, dizziness, ataxia, fatigue, nystagmus Pediatric: emotional lability, hostility	Not known Acute overdose of 108 g has been tolerated without serious effects	Coma and respiratory depression reported hemodialysis patients Drowsiness, ataxia, nystagmus, diplopia, diarrhea
Lamotrigine (Lamictal®, LTG) Approved 1994 Chemical class: phenyltriazine	Adjunctive treatment of partial seizures and Lennox-Gastaut syndrome	Adults: 25–500 mg/d Pediatric: 0.15–15 mg/kg/d	Oral bioavailability: 98% $T_{1/2}$, 12–62 hr; Vd, 0.9–1.3 L/kg Fb, 0.55 extensively hepatically metabolized and renally excreted primarily as glucuronide conjugates	Decreases carbamazepine and valproic acid levels APAP, carbamazepine, oral contraceptives, oxcarbazepine, phenobarbital, phenytoin, rifampin, succinimides, and valproic acid, decrease lamotrigine clearance	Black box warning for serious rashes including Stevens-Johnson syndrome Multiorgan failure and blood dyscrasias have been reported Most common: dizziness, ataxia, somnolence, headache, diplopia, blurred vision, nausea, vomiting, and rash	Overdoses up to 15 g have been reported, some fatal	Somnolence, stupor, lethargy, coma, dyskinesia, seizures, hypertonia, conduction disturbances with PR and QRS prolongation, tachycardia, hypokalemia
Topiramate (Topamax®, TPM) Approved 1996 Chemical class: sulfamate-substituted monosaccharide	Adjunctive therapy for partial onset and tonic-clonic seizures and Lennox-Gastaut syndrome Unlabeled uses include cluster headache and infantile spasms	Adults: initial dose 25–50 mg/d, increase 25–50 mg/wk to 400 mg/d Pediatric: initial dose 1–3 mg/kg/d, increase by 1–3 mg/kg/d 1–2 weeks to 5–9 mg/kg/d	Oral bioavailability: 80% $T_{1/2}$, 19–23 hr (increased in renal impairment); Vd, 0.5–0.8 L/kg; Fb, 0.15 Small amount hepatically metabolized; 70% to 97% excreted unchanged in urine	Phenytoin and carbamazepine decrease topiramate clearance Contraindicated with carbonic anhydrase inhibitors May decrease oral contraceptive efficacy	Most common: somnolence, dizziness, ataxia, speech disorders, psychomotor slowing, nystagmus, and paresthesias Other side effects: tremors, confusion, anxiety, nervousness, depression, weight loss, fatigue	Ingestions of 20 to 40 g have caused seizures, acidosis, and coma Doses up to 1,600 mg/d were tolerated in clinical trials	Coma, generalized seizures, nonanion-gap metabolic acidosis Inhibition of carbonic anhydrase believed the mechanism of nonanion gap acidosis

Drug	Indication	Dose	Pharmacokinetics	Drug interactions	Adverse effects	Overdose experience	Signs/symptoms of overdose
Tiagabine (Gabitril®, TIA) Approved 1997 Chemical class: nipecotic acid derivative	Adjunctive therapy for partial onset seizures	Adults: 4–56 mg/d Pediatric: >12 yrs, 4–32 mg/d (not approved <12 years)	Oral bioavailability: >95% $T_{1/2}$, 4–9 hr; Vd, 0.8–2.1 L/kg; Fb, 0.96; extensive hepatic metabolism and primarily excreted in the feces	Carbamazepine, phenobarbital, phenytoin, and valproic acid decrease tiagabine clearance	Most common: dizziness, asthenia, somnolence, nausea, nervousness, irritability, tremor, abdominal pain, difficulty with concentration or attention	Not known Eleven patients in clinical trials took single doses up to 800 mg and recovered with supportive care	Coma, somnolence, agitation, confusion, dysphagia, hostility, depression, weakness, myoclonus
Levetiracetam (Keppra®, LEV) Approved 1999 Chemical class: pyrrolidine analog	Adjunctive therapy for partial onset seizures	Adults: 500–3,000 mg/d Pediatric: no pediatric dose	Oral bioavailability: 100% $T_{1/2}$: 6–8 hr; Vd, 0.7 L/kg; Fb, <0.10 95% excreted in urine (66% unchanged drug and 24% hydrolyzed drug)	No known significant interactions	Most common: somnolence, coordination difficulties, nervousness, headache, personality changes and cognitive dysfunctions	Not known	Coma, respiratory depression, somnolence, agitation, aggression, depressed level of consciousness
Oxcarbazepine (Trileptal®, OXC) Approved 2000 Chemical class: iminostilbene derivative	Treatment of partial seizures in adults and adjunctive therapy in the treatment of partial seizures in children	Adults: 600–2,400 mg/d Pediatric: 8–10 mg/kg/d, increase to 900 to 1,800 mg/d depending on patient weight	Oral bioavailability: >95% $T_{1/2}$, OXC 1–3 hr; MHD (active metabolite) 11–15 hr; Vd, OXC 3–15 L/kg; MHD 0.7 L/kg Fb, 0.40; extensively hepatically metabolized and eliminated in urine	Inhibits the metabolism of phenobarbital and phenytoin Carbamazepine, phenytoin, and phenobarbital increase oxcarbazepine clearance May decrease oral contraceptive efficacy	Most common: dizziness, somnolence, diplopia, fatigue, nausea, vomiting, ataxia, abnormal vision, abdominal pain, tremor, dyspepsia, abnormal gait	Not known A 24-g overdose recovered with supportive care	Coma, somnolence, lethargy, diplopia, tinnitus, bradycardia, hypotension
Zonisamide (Zonegran®) Approved 2000 Chemical class: sulfonamide	Adjunctive therapy in the treatment of partial seizures	Adults: 100–600 mg/d	Oral bioavailability: >90% $T_{1/2}$, 63 hr; Vd, 1.45 L/kg; Fb, 0.40. Eliminated in urine and in feces as unchanged drug and as acetylated and conjugated metabolites	Carbamazepine and phenytoin increase zonisamide clearance	Warnings for fatalities from severe rash and hematologic toxicity with sulfonamides Kidney stones reported in 4% of zonisamide patients Most common: somnolence, anorexia, dizziness, headache, nausea, and agitation	Not known	Coma, respiratory depression, bradycardia, hypotension, seizures, dysrhythmias, cardiopulmonary arrest

$T_{1/2}$, serum half-life; Vd, volume of distribution; Fb, fraction of drug bound to serum proteins.

seizures and postherpetic neuralgia, has also become a common agent for a number of unlabeled uses such as neuropathic pain and bipolar disorder. Despite being a structural analog of GABA, gabapentin has no direct action on GABA receptors nor does it block GABA uptake or metabolism. The mechanism of anticonvulsant action is not known but is believed to involve an intracellular site, because the maximal anticonvulsant effect is delayed 2 hours after an intravenous dose. The most favored theory involves an interaction with an as yet undescribed receptor protein linked with the L-system amino acid transporter protein (22). Of note, because gabapentin is eliminated primarily be urinary excretion, the half-life increases dramatically in renal failure and the dose must be adjusted downward with decreasing creatinine clearance. In one hemodialysis patient the serum half-life was reported as being over 2,200 hours (2).

Lamotrigine (Lamictal®), a phenyltriazine structurally unrelated to other currently available anticonvulsants, was approved by the FDA for adjunctive treatment of partial seizures and Lennox-Gastaut syndrome in 1994. Although lamotrigine's exact mechanism of action is not known, in vitro studies suggest it inhibits voltage-dependent sodium channels, thereby stabilizing neuronal membranes and modulating presynaptic release of excitatory neurotransmitters (e.g., glutamate and aspartate). Lamotrigine has been associated with fatalities from severe rashes including Stevens-Johnson syndrome and toxic epidermal necrolysis. As a result of the possibility of severe rash, it is recommended that lamotrigine be discontinued at the first sign of rash, unless the rash is clearly not drug related.

Topiramate (Topamax®), a sulfamate-substituted monosaccharide structurally similar to the carbonic anhydrase inhibitor acetazolamide, was approved by the FDA for adjunctive therapy of partial onset and tonic-clonic seizures and for treatment of Lennox-Gastaut syndrome in 1996. Topiramate is believed to exert its anticonvulsant effect by blocking sodium channels, potentiating the activity of the inhibitory neurotransmitter GABA and antagonizing the ability of kainate to activate the kainate/AMPA subtype of excitatory amino acid (glutamate) receptor.

Tiagabine (Gabitril®), a nipecotic acid derivative, was approved by the FDA for adjunctive therapy of partial seizures in 1997. Tiagabine is a potent and selective inhibitor of both neuronal and glial GABA uptake, resulting in an increase in GABAergic mediated inhibition in the brain. Tiagabine lacks significant affinity for other neurotransmitter receptor binding and uptake sites.

Levetiracetam (Keppra®), a pyrrolidine analog, was approved by the FDA for adjunctive therapy in the treatment of partial onset seizures in 1999. The precise mechanism of anticonvulsant action is not known. It does not work through any of the commonly recognized anticonvulsant mechanisms. Studies of epileptiform activity from the hippocampus have shown that levetiracetam inhibits burst firing without affecting normal neuronal excitability, suggesting that it may selectively prevent hypersynchronization of epileptiform burst firing and propagation of seizure activity.

Oxcarbazepine (Trileptal®), an iminostilbene derivative, is the 10-keto analogue of the antiepileptic drug carbamazepine. Oxcarbazepine is a prodrug. The primary metabolite, 10-hydroxycarbazepine, is the active agent. Oxcarbazepine, approved by the FDA in 2000, is indicated for monotherapy or adjunctive therapy in the treatment of partial seizures in adults and children over 4 years of age. The major mechanism of anticonvulsant activity is believed to be through blockade of voltage-sensitive sodium channels, stabilizing hyperexcited neural membranes, inhibiting repetitive firing and diminishing propagation of synaptic impulses. Increased potassium conductance and modulation of high-voltage activated calcium channels may contribute to the anticonvulsant effects.

Zonisamide (Zonigran®), a sulfonamide, was approved by the FDA for adjunctive therapy in the treatment of partial seizures in 2000. The precise mechanism of anticonvulsant activity of zonisamide is unknown. Studies suggest that it blocks sodium channels and reduces voltage-dependent, transient inward currents (T-type Ca^{++} currents), stabilizing neuronal membranes and suppressing neuronal hypersynchonization. Zonisamide's labeling includes a warning for potential fatal reactions to sulfonamides and a warning for oligohidrosis and hyperthermia in pediatric patients. The manufacturer advises there have been 40 reported cases.

CLINICAL PRESENTATION

Because anticonvulsants exert their pharmacologic benefits in the CNS, the toxicity of newer anticonvulsants is primarily involves the CNS. Although their chemistry and pharmacology is heterogeneous, all cause a similar picture of mild to moderate CNS depression following overdose, with somnolence, lethargy, dizziness, ataxia, nystagmus, and diplopia being the most common symptoms.

There are few published reports of felbamate overdose. A 15-year-old female developed only minor drowsiness after ingesting 6.9 g (17). A 20-year-old female developed acute renal failure secondary to massive felbamate crystalluria following the ingestion of 18 g. She was treated with intravenous fluids and fully recovered (21).

Gabapentin overdose in otherwise normally healthy patients is generally benign. In one series, drowsiness, dizziness, nausea/vomiting, tachycardia, and hypotension were the only symptoms noted and no patient required hospital admission for medical treatment (13). Respiratory depression and coma have been reported in hemodialysis patients receiving therapeutic doses (2,4,10).

Overdose of lamotrigine can cause serious toxicity including death (15). CNS effects include somnolence, stupor, transient coma, lethargy, choreatic dyskinesia, seizures, nystagmus and ataxia. Generalized tonic-clonic seizures, tremor, muscle weakness, and hypertonia occurred in a 2-year old with ingestion of 800 mg (3). Cardiac conduction disturbance with QRS and PR interval prolongation, tachycardia, and hypokalemia have been reported (19).

There is limited data on topiramate overdose. Two patients became comatose and had generalized convulsive status epilepticus after ingesting 20 and 40 g (7). Both recovered within 2 days but each had a persistent nonanion-gap metabolic acidosis that lasted for 5 to 6 days. Their urine pH remained alkaline although the serum remained acidotic, possibly because of inhibition of carbonic anhydrase (7).

Overdose information on tiagabine is also limited. One patient became comatose after ingestion of 320 mg tiagabine and 400 mg phenytoin. Recovery was rapid without sequelae (14). The manufacturer reports that patients who ingested single doses of up to 800 mg experienced somnolence, agitation, confusion, dysphagia, hostility, depression, weakness, and myoclonus and that all recovered fully with supportive care.

Only one case of levetiracetam overdose has been reported. A 38-year-old woman became obtunded with respiratory depression requiring intubation after ingesting 30 g. She was extubated the following day and recovered without sequelae (1). The manufacturer reports that somnolence, agitation, aggression, depressed level of consciousness, respiratory depression, and coma have been observed after overdose.

Published reports of oxcarbazepine overdose are rare. Somnolence, lethargy, diplopia, tinnitus, bradycardia, and hypotension occurred in a 38-year-old female on 2,100 mg/day who accidentally took an extra 1,200 mg (9). A 23-year-old male who took oxcarbazepine 8.7 g, risperidone 60 mg and atenolol 1.4 g developed coma, bradycardia, and hypotension but recovered fully (20). The manufacturer states that patients with overdoses of up to 24 g have recovered with supportive treatment.

There is limited overdose experience with zonisamide. Multiple tonic-clonic seizures and cardiopulmonary arrest with asystole that converted to a wide-complex tachycardia were reported in an 18-year-old female after the ingestion of 4.8 g (8). A computed tomography (CT) scan 24 hours later revealed massive cerebral edema with tonsillar herniation. A postmortem drug screen also revealed the presence of mirtazapine, diphenhydramine metabolites, and caffeine, making the cause of death unclear (23). The manufacturer reports that coma, respiratory depression, bradycardia, and hypotension can occur after overdose.

DIFFERENTIAL DIAGNOSIS

CNS depression similar to that caused by newer anticonvulsants can be caused by older anticonvulsants (carbamazepine, phenobarbital, phenytoin, and valproic acid), cyclic antidepressants (e.g., amitriptyline and trazodone), antihistamines (e.g., diphenhydramine), asphyxiants (e.g., carbon monoxide), benzodiazepines, β-blockers, barbiturates, calcium channel blockers, clonidine and similar centrally- acting antihypertensives, ethanol, and other alcohols, γ hydroxybutyric acid (GHB), isoniazid, neuroleptics, opioids, sedative–hypnotics, and skeletal muscle relaxants. Drug-induced CNS depression must also be differentiated from medical causes such as hypoglycemia, electrolyte abnormalities, trauma, infection, and cerebrovascular accidents.

EMERGENCY DEPARTMENT EVALUATION

The history should include the time and amount of drug(s) taken, treatment in the field, if any, the onset and nature of symptoms, known medical or psychiatric problems, and current drug therapy, particularly if the patient is on multiple medications for epilepsy. The physical exam should focus on the vital signs, including temperature and pulse oximetry, cardiopulmonary status, and a neurologic assessment. A stat fingerstick or serum glucose concentration should be obtained. Arterial blood gases, chemistry panel, complete blood count, toxicology testing, ECG, and chest radiograph should be obtained when clinically indicated. Cardiac conduction intervals should be evaluated in patients with lamotrigine and zonisamide overdose. Those with felbamate overdose should have a urine sample examined for crystals. Serum levels of the newer anticonvulsants are generally not available, and their clinical utility is unclear.

EMERGENCY DEPARTMENT MANAGEMENT

The treatment of overdose of the newer anticonvulsant agents is supportive. Advanced cardiac life-support measures should be instituted as needed. Coma and/or respiratory depression may require endotracheal intubation for airway protection and mechanical ventilation. Hypotension usually responds to intravenous crystalloids. Intravenous sodium bicarbonate (see Chapter 318, "Cyclic Antidepressants") should be given for cardiac dysrhythmias if the QRS interval is prolonged. Seizure precautions should be implemented for patients with a preexisting seizure disorder. Status epilepticus from topiramate has responded to benzodiazepines. Hydration and monitoring for

development of crystalluria for a minimum of 12 hours is advisable after felbamate overdose.

Decontamination with oral activated charcoal (AC) should be considered for recent ingestion or when other potentially toxic agents have been co-ingested. The low fatality rate of these agents makes invasive decontamination procedures such as gastric lavage likely to be of more risk than benefit and should be reserved for suspected ingestions of seriously toxic co-ingestants. There is no known role for repeated doses of activated charcoal.

Hemodialysis can enhance the elimination of gabapentin with hemodialysis and levetiracetam, oxcarbazepine and topiramate have pharmacokinetic profiles favorable to removal by hemodialysis. This intervention might be useful for severe poisoning by one of these agents that does not respond to supportive care.

CRITICAL INTERVENTIONS

- Provide airway protection and respiratory support when indicated
- Administer intravenous fluids for hypotension
- Administer intravenous sodium bicarbonate for dysrhythmias associated with a prolonged QRS interval
- Administer benzodiazepines for seizures

DISPOSITION

A poison control center or toxicologist should be consulted if the treating physician is not familiar with the management of newer anticonvulsant overdose. Patients with newer anticonvulsant overdose who remain or become asymptomatic after an observation period of 4 to 6 hours may be discharged, except with felbamate, in which evaluation for crystalluria should continue for at least 12 hours. Patients with CNS or respiratory depression, hemodynamic instability or cardiac conduction disturbances should be admitted to an intensive care unit. A psychiatric consult should be obtained for all suspected suicidal ingestions.

COMMON PITFALLS

✔ Failure to appreciate that, although rare, significant CNS depression can occur after overdose with newer anticonvulsants
✔ Failure to appreciate that most patients with newer anticonvulsant overdose do well with supportive care and that giving syrup of ipecac or using invasive decontamination measures puts the patient at unnecessary risk for complications of treatment
✔ Failure to appreciate that topiramate and zonisamide can cause seizures
✔ Failure to appreciate that cardiac conduction disturbances can occur after lamotrigine and zonisamide overdose
✔ Failure to evaluate patients with felbamate overdose for crystalluria and renal dysfunction

References

1. Barrueto F, Williams K, Howland MA, et al. A case of levetiracetam (Keppra) poisoning with clinical and toxicokinetic data. *J Toxicol Clin Toxicol* 2002;40:881–884.
2. Bassilios N, Launay-Vacher V, Khoury N et al. Gabapentin neurotoxicity in a chronic haemodialysis patient. *Nephrol Dial Transplant* 2001;16:2112–2113.
3. Briassoulis G, Kalabalikis P, Tamiolaki M, et al. Lamotrigine childhood overdose. *Pediatr Neurol* 1998;19:239–242.
4. Butler TC, Rosen RM, Wallace AL, et al. Flumazenil and dialysis for gabapentin-induced coma. *Ann Pharmacother* 2003;37:74–6.
5. Chang BS, Lowenstein DH. Epilepsy. *N Engl J Med* 2003;349:1257–1266.
6. Dichter MA, Brodie MJ. New antiepileptic drugs. *N Engl J Med* 1996;334:1583–1590.

7. Fakhoury T, Murray L, Seger D, et al. Topiramate overdose: clinical and laboratory features. *Epilepsy Behav* 2002;3:185–189.

8. Huang EE, Sztajnkrycer MD, Bond GR. Seizures, dysrhythmia and death after zonisamide overdose. *J Toxicol Clin Toxicol* 2002;40:611(abst).

9. Jolliff HA, Fehrenbacher N, Dart RC. Bradycardia, hypotension and tinnitus after accidental oxcarbazepine overdose. *J Toxicol Clin Toxicol* 2001;39:316–317(abst).

10. Jones H, Aguila E, Farber HW. Gabapentin toxicity requiring intubation in a patient receiving long-term hemodialysis. *Ann Intern Med* 2002;137:74.

11. Jones JE, Hermann BP, Barry JJ et al. Rates and risk factors for suicide, suicidal ideation and suicide attempts in chronic epilepsy. *Epilepsy Behav* 2003;S31:8.

12. Kleckner NW, Glazewski JC, Chen CC et al. Subtype-selective antagonism of N-methyl-D-aspartate receptors by felbamate: insights into the mechanism of action. *J Pharmacol Exp Ther* 1999;289:886–894.

13. Klein-Schwartz W, Shepard JG, Gorman S, et al. Characterization of gabapentin overdose using a poison center case series. *J Toxicol Clin Toxicol* 2003;41:11–15.

14. Leach JP, Stolarek I, Brodie MJ. Deliberate overdose with the novel anticonvulsant tiagabine. *Seizure* 1995;4:155–157.

15. Levine B, Jufer RA, Smialek JE. Lamotrigine distribution in two postmortem cases. *J Anal Toxicol* 2000;24:635–637.

16. Litovitz TL, Felberg L, Soloway RA et al 1994 annual report of the American Association of Poison Control Centers Toxic Exposure Surveillance System. *Am J Emerg Med* 1995;13:551–597.

17. Nagel TR, Schunk JE. Felbamate overdose: a case report and discussion of a new antiepileptic drug. *Pediatr Emerg Care* 1995;11:369–371.

18. O'Neil MG, Perdun CS, Wilson MB, et al. Felbamate-associated fatal hepatic necrosis. *Neurology* 1996;46:1457–1459.

19. Paopairochanakorn C, White S, Malafa MJ. Cardiac and neurotoxicity from lamotrigine ingestion. *J Toxicol Clin Toxicol* 2002;40:620(abst).

20. Raja M, Azzoni A. Oxcarbazepine, risperidone and atenolol overdose with benign outcome. *Int J Neuropsychopharmacol* 2003;6:309–310.

21. Rengsdorff DS, Milstone AP, Seger DL, et al. Felbamate overdose complicated by massive crystalluria and acute renal failure. *J Toxicol Clin Toxicol* 2000;38:667–669.

22. Rose MA, Kam PC. Gabapentin: pharmacology and its use in pain management. *Anaesthesia* 2002 May;57:451–462.

23. Sztajnkrycer MD, Huang EE, Bond GR. Acute zonisamide overdose: a death revisited. *Vet Hum Toxicol* 2003;45:154–156.

24. Vaczek D. Top 200 drugs of 2002. *Pharmacy Times*. April 2003,Vol. 20, Issue 3.

25. Watson WA, Litovitz TL, Rodgers GC, et al. 2002 annual report of the American Association of Poison Control Centers Toxic Exposure Surveillance System. *Am J Emerg Med* 2003;21:353–421.

PART V

Anti-Infective Agents and Biocides

CHAPTER 294
Antimalarial Drugs

Timothy E. Albertson, Kathy Marquardt,
and Judith Alsop

Malaria continues to be a major contributor to the world disease burden with 300 to 500 million new cases and as many as a million childhood deaths each year. Because of the lack of indigenous malaria, only about 1,000 new cases are reported each year in the United States associated with immigration and travel (10).

The treatment and prophylaxis for malaria has changed significantly with the evolution of drug-resistant organisms. Much of the world now has chloroquine-resistant Plasmodium falciparum requiring very different strategies for chemoprophylaxis and treatment than in years past. The reduced availability of quinine and the lack of availability in the United States of some agents such as the Artemisin (ginhaosu) derivatives, including artesunate and artemether, further limits choices (10). Table 294.1 summarizes the current common malaria chemoprophylaxis and treatment options.

As a result of resistance, fixed combinations of drug therapy have become more common (11). The potential for toxicity is now more likely to be seen from these newer drugs because the older drugs are being used less frequently, and thus are less available for accidental or purposeful overdosing. Little toxicological data exists on many of these newer drugs particularly in combination overdoses. Extension and enhancement of the therapeutic side effect profiles are frequently all that has been reported to date.

The classification of agents used as antimalarials includes quinoline derivatives, dihydrofolate reductase inhibitors, antibacterials, Artemisin derivatives, and ubiquinone analogs (see Table 294.2). Most antimalarial poisonings are the result of accidental childhood exposures or intentional adolescent and adult suicide attempts.

Quinine, hydroxychloroquine, and chloroquine are quinoline derivatives known to cause severe toxicity in overdoses (9,17). The antimalarial quinine is an alkaloid derived from the bark of the cinchona tree (22). Quinine has been used as an antipyretic, an adulterant for street cocaine and heroin, a muscle relaxant, and is found in small amounts in tonic water (1). Quinoline derivatives have an undeserved reputation as abortifacients (1,22). Chloroquine and hydroxychloroquine are also used for the treatment of rheumatoid arthritis and lupus erythematosus.

Quinine has local anesthetic and irritant effects, some skeletal muscle blocking action, vasodilates, and acts centrally to cause emesis (1). Chloroquine and hydroxychloroquine share these properties and act as respiratory depressants as well. Quinoline derivatives have several electrocardiac effects, causing negative cardiac inotropism, slowing depolarization and conduction, increasing action potential duration, and in overdose lengthening the effective refractory period (1,9). Both chloroquine and hydroxychloroquine are associated with hypokalemia.

Oral quinine and chloroquine are rapidly absorbed in the small intestine, with 80% to 90% bioavailability and peak levels occurring 1 to 3 hours after ingestion (24). The apparent volume of distribution (Vd) is 1.6 to 1.8 L/kg for quinine and 116 to 285 L/kg for chloroquine, with plasma protein binding of 89% and 55% respectively (22). The Vd for hydroxychloroquine is about 63 L/kg (17). The elimination of quinine is primarily by hepatic microsomal oxidation, but 20% is excreted unchanged in the urine (1). With a pKa of 8.4, urinary quinine excretion increases as the pH falls. However, urinary flow rate may be more important than pH in determining clearance (1). The elimination half-life ($t^{1}/_{2}$) of quinine is 10 to 12 hours. It increases to 16 to 18 hours in malaria patients as a result of reduced hepatic elimination and an increase in drug distribution (9). In overdose, the $t^{1}/_{2}$ increases to 26 to 34 hours, because of saturable metabolism. Chloroquine is eliminated by slow hepatic degradation, and 55% is excreted in the urine (9). The $t^{1}/_{2}$ for chloroquine and for hydroxychloroquine are 75 to 278 hours and 15.5 to 31 hours respectively (9,17). The toxic effects of quinoline derivatives are caused by their cardiac, cytotoxic, and irritant properties. Oculotoxicity develops in 17% to 42% of patients with quinine poisoning and appears to be caused by a direct toxic effect on the photoreceptor and ganglion cell layers of the retina (1,6). Constriction of retinal arterioles also occurs and has been the focus of many unsuccessful therapies.

The toxic dose of quinine in adults ranges from 1.8 g to 4.0 g (9). Chloroquine has a narrow margin of safety, with toxicity occurring at doses as low as 1.0 g to 1.5 g, or 20 mg/kg (9). Doses greater than 2 g in adults are almost always associated with toxic effects, and doses greater than 5 g are usually lethal. Correlation exists between plasma quinine and chloroquine concentrations and the development of toxicity. Quinine levels as low as 2 μg/mL are associated with mild, reversible hearing loss. More toxic effects are seen with levels of 6 to 15 μg/mL. Levels of 10 μg/mL are often tolerated in malaria patients because of enhanced drug protein binding. Cardiac dysrhythmias,

TABLE 294.1.   Common Chemoprophylaxis for and Treatment of Malaria

Drugs	Usage	Prophylaxis	Treatment	Safe in Pregnancy	Contradictions
Chloroquine (Aralen)	Sensitive *Plasmodium falciparum* *Plasmodium vivax* *Plasmodium ovale* *Plasmodium malaria*	(+)	(+)	(+)	Hepatic disease, persons with visual changes
Hydroxychloroquine sulfate (Plaquenil)	Chloroquine-sensitive *P. falciparum* and non-*falciparum* species	(+)	(+)	(+)	Hepatic disease, persons with visual changes
Mefloquine (Lariam)	Chloroquine-resistant *P. falciparum*	(+)	(+)	(+)	Seizure disorders, conduction disturbance, or history of significant psychiatric disease
Doxycycline (Vibramycin)	Chloroquine resistant *P. falciparum*	(+)	(+)	(−)	Lactating females and children if patient <8 yr should be taken with food
Atovaquone/proguanil (Malarone)	Chloroquine-resistant *P. falciparum* and probably chloroquine-resistant non-*falciparum* species	(+)	(+)	(−)	Severe renal failure, (CrCl 30 mL/min), should be taken with food
Primaquine (Palum)	Prolonged exposure to *P. vivax* or *P. oval*	(+)	(+)	(−)	G6PD deficiency
Quinine dihydrochloride	Chloroquine-resistant *P. falciparum* and probably non-*falciparum* species	(−)	(+)	(−)	Limited use in United States for malaria
Quinidine	Chloroquine-sensitive *P. falciparum* and non-*falciparum* species when parenteral drug needed	(−)	(+)	(?)	Conduction disorders
Artemether	Chloroquine-sensitive *P. falciparum*	(−)	(+)	(?)	Not available in United States
Artesunate	Chloroquine-sensitive *P. falciparum*	(−)	(+)	(?)	Not available in United States

Adapted from References: 4,10,11,16,20,25

TABLE 294.2.   Classification of Antimalarials

Quinoline derivatives
  Methanol quinolones
    Quinine
    Mefloquine
    Amino-4-quinolines
    Chloroquine
    Hydroxychloroquine
  Amino-8-quinolines
    Primaquine
Dihydrofolate reductase inhibitors
  Proguanil
  Pyrimethamine
    (Pyrimethamine/Dapsone [Maloprim])
    (Pyrimethamine/sulfadoxine [Fansidar])
  Sulfonamides
  Dapsone
Antibacterials
  Doxycycline
Artemisin derivates (qinhaosu)
  Artemether
  Artesunate
Ubiquinone Analog–α-hydroxy-1,4-naphthoquinone
  Atovaquone
    (Atovaquone/proquanil (Malgrone)

irreversible blindness, and death are reported with levels greater than 15 μg/mL. Survival has occurred with levels as high as 23.5 μg/mL, but concentrations higher than 13 μg/mL at 5 hours and 6 μg/mL at 20 hours postingestion predict severe toxicity. Blood chloroquine levels greater than 3 μg/mL are usually toxic and death is likely if the level is greater than 8 μg/mL (9). Hydroxychloroquine plasma concentration from 0.6 to 9.9 μg/mL have been associated with severe toxicity (17). Chloroquine and hydroxychloroquine poisonings are associated with high fatality rates, but are infrequent in the United States (17).

Mefloquine, a methanol quinoline, has a similar structure to chloroquine but has activity against many drug resistant strains of Plasmodium falciparum. About 11% to 17% of users note incapacitating complaints but withdrawal rates are similar to other regimens (21). Severe neuropsychiatric reactions have been reported with mefloquine use in 1 in 15,000 to 20,000 users at prophylactic doses (15). Rapid oral absorption is seen. The protein binding is 98% with a very large Vd of between 13 to 29 L/kg and a t$\frac{1}{2}$ of 9 to 13 days. Hepatic biotransformation using the CYP3A4 enzyme system is its primary elimination.

Artemisin or qinghaosu (its Chinese name) derivatives are sesquiterpene lactones isolated from the plant *Artemisa annua* (sweet wormwood). Artemisin and its antimalarial derivatives artesunate and artemether are well-tolerated in both adults and children (19). Sesquiterpene alkaloids have been associated with allergic dermatoses and liver toxicity.

Artemether is oil-soluble and available as an oral and intramuscular form. The drug is well absorbed orally, highly protein bound with a Vd of 5.4 to 8.6 L/kg. It is metabolized by the liver to the antimalarial dihydroartemisinin. Artemisinin has a $t^1/_2$ between 1 and 7 hours while the active dihydroartemisinin's $t^1/_2$ is approximately 2 hours. Intramuscular artesunate has a $t^1/_2$ of approximately 45 minutes (13,23). Adverse effects of artemether and Artemisin derivatives include bradycardia, dizziness, gastrointestinal (GI) disturbances (oral route), rash, and fever. Human poisonings have been rare with the potential for GI, liver, and cardiac toxicity.

CLINICAL PRESENTATION

In quinine overdose, cinchonism is the most common early feature, occurring in about 75% of patients. It usually occurs within 4 hours of ingestion but may appear as early as 2 hours and as late as 8 to 12 hours after ingestion (6). Cinchonism can be seen with acute and chronic poisoning and is characterized by tinnitus, hearing loss, nausea, vomiting, vertigo, ataxia, diaphoresis, headache, flushing, lethargy, and hypotension (1,7,9).

Cardiac toxicity after quinine is typically mild, with sinus tachycardia and minor electrocardiographic (ECG) changes. However, ventricular dysrhythmias, including torsades de pointes, significant conduction disturbances, and complete atrioventricular dissociation have been reported (1). Specific ECG abnormalities include prolonged P-R and Q-T intervals, ST- and T-wave changes, U waves, bundle-branch blocks, and QRS interval widening. With massive exposures, convulsions, coma, respiratory depression, adult respiratory distress syndrome, and cardiac arrest may occur.

Visual disturbances can be delayed for 6 to 24 hours after ingestion, and may present with progressive blurring of vision or sudden blindness. Dilated pupils that become fixed before vision loss occurs have been reported. Peripheral visual field defects, color misperceptions, diplopia, and poor dark adaptation can precede the development of total blindness or can be transient (1,7). The fundus usually is normal at the onset of visual defects, but retinal arteriole constriction, macular edema, and a cherry-red macular spot can develop within hours, evolving into optic atrophy in these cases (1). Laboratory findings may include hypoglycemia, hypokalemia, and thrombocytopenia (9). The hypoglycemia may occur as a result of quinine-induced insulin secretion (1). Quinine seldom induces abortion but has been associated with fetal abnormalities and maternal deaths (22).

Chloroquine toxicity differs in presentation by producing rapid onset of symptoms, severe cardiovascular (CV) effects, greater respiratory depression, marked hypokalemia, and milder and transient ocular and auditory toxicity (9). Cardiovascular collapse is common within 2 hours in serious overdoses and is as a result of marked myocardial depression and ventricular dysrhythmias (9). Toxicity can be predicted by a prolonged QRS interval and by the degree of hypokalemia, which is probably caused by intracellular shifts (9). Toxic effects are usually short-lived, despite persistently high plasma levels of the drug.

Other quinoline derivatives, such as primaquine, are not associated with severe CV toxicities, but they are associated with gastrointestinal distress, hemolytic anemia, and methemoglobinemia (9).

In the few mefloquine overdose cases reported, neuropsychiatric manifestations including headache, dizziness, vertigo, seizures, affective disorder, anxiety, hearing loss, and sleep disturbances have occurred along with prolongation of the QTc interval (14). Nausea, vomiting, diarrhea, abdominal pain, and transient elevations in transaminase levels have been reported. These effects may be a posthepatic syndrome caused by drug-induced liver damage coupled in some to thyroid inhibition (4). Because of the prolonged $t^1/_2$, these adverse events can persist for weeks. Two cases in which mefloquine (Lariam) was dispensed in error to patients who had been prescribed terbinafine (Lamisil) for onychomycosis resulted in overdose and prolonged symptoms (14).

Of the dihydrofolate reductase inhibitors, pyrimethamine is the most toxic and may cause ataxia, seizures, coma, blindness, and deafness, and folate deficiency with megaloblastic anemia (9). Proguanil, another dihydrofolate reductase inhibitor, is one of the safest antimalarial drugs with limited examples of poisoning (9). GI distress with vomiting, diarrhea, and abdominal pain coupled with headaches, nausea, and hematuria have been reported with ingestions of 1 g or more. Therapeutic doses of proguanil have been associated with mouth ulcerations, gastrointestinal distress, rash, and anemia.

Dapsone, another dihydrofolate reductase inhibitor, may also cause acute methemoglobinemia and hemolytic anemia (9). A series of five HIV patients developed methemoglobinemia while on primaquine and dapsone.

Massive doxycycline overdoses have been associated with precipitation of calcium and hypocalcemic death in animals. In humans, precipitation of calcium can lead to staining of the teeth in children under 8 years of age. Doxycycline has been associated with Sweet's syndrome characterized by nonpruritic, painful, reddish modules on the head, neck, chest, or upper limbs usually with fever, general malaise, and leukocytosis (12). Phototoxicity and esophageal ulcerations have also been reported with doxycycline (4).

Atovaquone, a novel hydroxynaphthoquinone, has produced minimal effects with overdoses up to 31.5 grams. In one case, methemoglobinemia was reported but an unknown amount of dapsone was also ingested (8).

DIFFERENTIAL DIAGNOSIS

Quinoline derivative toxicity may resemble other agents that cause visual, auditory, or cardiac effects. Methanol, ergot derivatives, and heavy metals (e.g., lead and mercury) are in the differential diagnosis of visual disturbances from an unknown agent. Unlike the quinolones, methanol is usually associated with a marked anion gap acidosis and osmolal gap. Manifestations of cinchonism are similar to those of salicylate toxicity, but the latter also causes an elevated anion gap, acid–base imbalances, and no visual effects. Quinidine, an isomer of quinine, causes similar cardiac effects but no visual deficits (9). Many drugs such as the cyclic antidepressants can cause similar CV and electrocardiographic effects but are not linked to auditory or visual changes.

EMERGENCY DEPARTMENT EVALUATION

In the overdose or toxic patient who presents with visual, auditory, neuropsychiatric, and CV symptoms of unknown cause, a history of use or availability of antimalarial agents will be significant. Attempted abortion by quinine should be suspected in a pregnant patient with these complaints. Physical examination and evaluation of the vital signs, cardiac rhythm, auditory and visual acuity, pupillary size and reactions, funduscopic findings, visual field testing, and cerebellar status are important. Studies to assist in the differential include determination of quinine, quinoline, salicylate, electrolyte, glucose, liver enzyme, blood urea nitrogen, and creatinine levels along with a complete blood count. An ECG should also be obtained. If available, electroretinograms and visual evoked response testing may detect signs of retinal damage in quinine overdose (7).

EMERGENCY DEPARTMENT MANAGEMENT

A suspected ingestion of antimalarials requires immediate attention to the vital signs, cardiac monitoring, and gastric decontamination. Prevention of absorption is probably only effective in the first 2 to 3 hours, but if done early can reduce peak plasma levels. Activated charcoal (AC) binds very effectively to chloroquine and quinine, and its immediate use is more likely to be efficacious than induced emesis or gastric lavage (18). The $t^{1}/_2$ in healthy volunteers taking a therapeutic dose of quinine was reduced by 50% and, in overdoses, was shortened from over 24 hours to 8 hours by repeated doses of activated charcoal. However, clinical outcome improvement has not been documented. Both gastric emptying procedures and the use of AC may be complicated by rapid onset of central nervous system (CNS) depression, particularly with chloroquine overdose.

Hypotension usually responds to intravenous fluids but may require a vasopressor (e.g., dopamine or norepinephrine) and inotropes (e.g., dobutamine) (1,9). Hypotension, ventricular dysrhythmias, and cardiac conduction abnormalities are also likely to respond to serum alkalization to a pH of 7.5 (5,9). This may be accomplished by sodium bicarbonate administration, hyperventilation, or a combination (see Chapter 318, "Cyclic Antidepressants"). Lidocaine has been used but may potentate the dysrhythmias. Class 1A and 1C antidysrhythmics should be avoided. Torsades de pointes can be treated with intravenous magnesium and isoproterenol or overdrive pacing (see Chapter 317, "Neuroleptics").

Benzodiazepines, combined with mechanical ventilation and inotropes, have improved chloroquine overdosed patients (9). High doses of diazepam (0.5–3 mg/kg i.v.) may counteract the hemodynamic and ECG changes associated with chloroquine toxicity. This benefit may derive from its anticonvulsant and sedating effects. The use of other sedating and anticonvulsant agents, such as the barbiturates have been suggested but may risk exacerbation of the hypotension seen in severe chloroquine toxicity (3). Because the cardiac toxicity seen is similar to that caused by hyperkalemia, potassium replacement is not advised unless it is severe (9).

Despite its theoretical potential for enhanced quinoline derivative elimination, acidification of the urine is unproven and potentially increases cardiac toxicity. Resin and charcoal hemoperfusion, hemodialysis, peritoneal dialysis, plasmapheresis, and exchange transfusion have all been tried in attempts to enhance drug elimination. However, because of protein binding and high volumes of distribution, these techniques remove only a small portion of the total body drug load, and clinical improvements are more likely as a result of the natural course of recovery (1,2,9,21). Methylene blue should be given for methemoglobinemia (see Chapter 315, "Methemoglobinemia").

Attempts at reversal of retinal arteriolar vasospasm by way of stellate ganglion block, anterior chamber paracentesis, retrobulbar injections, and systemic vasodilators have not been effective and can produce significant complications (6,9). Hyperbaric oxygenation therapy has been promoted on the premise that retinal hypoxia secondary to arteriolar vasoconstriction contributes to visual loss. However, the reported benefit may again represent natural recovery.

Recovery from quinoline overdose is usually gradual and complete, but visual defects from quinine may not completely resolve (6,9).

CRITICAL INTERVENTIONS

- Establish i.v. access, institute cardiac monitoring, and obtain an ECG
- Protect the airway and assist ventilation in patients with seizures or significant CNS depression
- Administer i.v. benzodiazepines and sodium bicarbonate to patients with severe chloroquine toxicity
- Administer i.v. dopamine or norepinephrine to patients with hypotension unresponsive to i.v. fluids

DISPOSITION

Patients suspected of ingesting a toxic amount of a quinoline derivative should be observed for 6 to 8 hours. Symptomatic patients and any with cardiac conduction abnormalities should be admitted to an intensive care unit. Early consultation with a medical toxicologist or the regional poison center should be considered. An ophthalmologist should be consulted in patients with visual symptoms.

COMMON PITFALLS

✔ Failure to consider antimalarial poisoning in patients with auditory, visual, cardiac, and neuropsychiatric abnormalities of unknown cause
✔ Failure to appreciate that rapid neurologic and CV deterioration can occur after chloroquine overdose
✔ Failure to appreciate that benzodiazepines can prevent dysrhythmias and seizures in patients with chloroquine overdose
✔ Failure to perform prompt gastrointestinal decontamination and to consider multiple-dose AC therapy
✔ Failure to appreciate that potassium replacement could exacerbate chloroquine-induced cardiac toxicity

Acknowledgment

We thank previous edition chapter author J. Ward Donovan.

References

1. Bateman DN, Dyson EH. Quinine toxicity. *Adverse Drug React* 1986;5: 215–233.
2. Boereboom FT, Ververs FF, Meulenbelt J, et al. Hemoperfusion is ineffectual in severe chloroquine poisoning. *Crit Care Med* 2000;28:3346–3350.
3. Clemessy JL, Taboulet P, Hoffman JR, et al. Treatment of acute chloroquine poisoning: a 5-year experience. *Crit Care Med* 1996;24:1189–1195.
4. Croft AM, Whitehouse DP, Cook GC, et al. Safety evaluation of the drugs available to prevent malaria. *Expert Opin Drug Saf* 2002;1:19–27.
5. Curry SC, Connor DA, Clark RF, et al. The effect of hypertonic sodium bicarbonate on QRS duration in rats poisoned with chloroquine. *J Toxicol Clin Toxicol* 1996;34:73–76.
6. Dyson EH, Proudfoot AT, Prescott LF, et al. Death and blindness due to overdose of quinine. *Br Med J (C ResEd)* 1985;291:31–33.
7. Guly U, Driscoll P. The management of quinine-induced blindness. *Arch Emerg Med* 1992;9:317–322.
8. Haile LG, Flaherty JF. Atovaquone: a review. *Ann Pharmacother* 1993;27:1488–1494.
9. Jaeger A, Sauder P, Kopferschmitt J, et al. Clinical features and management of poisoning due to antimalarial drugs. *Med Toxicol* 1987;2:242–273.
10. John CC. Drug treatment of malaria in children. *Pediatr Infect Dis J* 2003;22:649–651.
11. Jong EC, Nothdurft HD. Current drugs for antimalarial chemoprophylaxis: a review of efficacy and safety. *J Travel Med* 2001;8:S48–S56.
12. Khan Durani B, Jappe U. Drug-induced Sweet's syndrome in acne caused by different tetracyclines: case report and review of the literature. *Br J Dermatol* 2002;147:558–562.
13. Lee IS, Hufford CD. Metabolism of antimalarial sesquiterpene lactones. *Pharmacol Ther* 1990;48:345–355.
14. Lobel HO, Coyne PE, Rosenthal PJ. Drug overdoses with antimalarial agents: prescribing and dispensing errors. *JAMA* 1998;280:1483.
15. Luzzi GA and Peto TE. Adverse effects of antimalarials. An update. *Drug Saf* 1993;8:295–311.
16. Magill AJ. The prevention of malaria. *Prim Care* 2002;29:815–842.

17. Marquardt K and Albertson TE: Treatment of hydroxychloroquine overdose. *Am J Emerg Med* 2001;19:420–424.
18. Neuvonen PJ, Kivisto KT, Laine K, et al. Prevention of chloroquine absorption by activated charcoal. *Hum Exp Toxicol* 1992;11:117–120.
19. Price RN. Artemisinin drugs: novel antimalarial agents. *Expert Opin Investig Drugs* 2000;9:1815–1827.
20. Re VL 3rd, Gluckman SJ. Prevention of malaria in travelers. *Am Fam Physician* 2003;68:509–514.
21. Schlagenhauf P. Mefloquine for malaria chemoprophylaxis 1992–1998: a review. *J Travel Med* 1999;6:122–133.
22. Smit JA, McFadyen ML. Quinine as unofficial contraceptive—concerns about safety and efficacy. *S Afr Med J* 1998;88:865–866.
23. White NJ. Clinical pharmacokinetics and pharmacodynamics of artemisinin and derivatives. *Trans R Soc Trop Med Hyg* 1994;88(Suppl 1):S41–S43.
24. White NJ. Clinical pharmacokinetics of antimalarial drugs. *Clin Pharmacokinet* 1985;10:187–215.
25. Whitty CJ, Rowland M, Sanderson F, et al. Malaria. *BMJ* 2002;325:1221–1224.

CHAPTER 295
Herbicides

Christopher H. Linden and William J. Lewander

Herbicides are chemicals that kill or inhibit the growth of plants. Although there are hundreds of herbicides with a variety of chemical structures and mechanism of actions, this chapter will focus on the three classes most commonly involved in human poisoning: bipyridyls (paraquat, diquat), chlorophenoxy acids, and organic phosphorus compounds (glyphosate, glufosinate).

Paraquat (1,1'-dimethyl-4,4'-bipyridilium) and diquat (1,1'-ethylene-2,2'-dipyridilium) are relatively nonselective, rain-fast, foliage-applied, contact herbicides (9,17,21,22). These quaternary ammonium compounds are available as a dibromide, dichloride, or dimethyl salts. Commercial paraquat preparations contain about 20% (wt/wt) cation, and household products, 0.2% (wt/wt). Common brand names include Herbaxone, Gramoxone, Gramonol, Preglone, and Weedol. Diquat is available as Aquacide, Reglone, Reglox, and Weedtrim.

Herbicidal activity is as a result of interference with electron transfer during photosynthesis. The resulting inhibition of the reduction of nicotinamide–adenine dinucleotide phosphate (NADP) to NADPH leads to the production of superoxide and peroxide radicals, reactive forms of oxygen, which destroy lipid cell membrane components. Although these agents form inert complexes with most types of soil and become rapidly harmless in the environment, they are extremely toxic when ingested. Mortality has been estimated at 20% to 50% from accidental ingestion and is probably greater after intentional ingestion.

Only 1% to 5% of paraquat is absorbed from the gastrointestinal (GI) tract. Peak concentrations are achieved within 2 hours. Although dermal absorption is minimal unless the skin is abraded, fatal cutaneous exposures have been reported after a single or chronic application of commercial concentrates (22). Inhalation of paraquat spray is unlikely to cause systemic toxicity because its low vapor pressure and large spray droplets prevent its absorption. The smoking of paraquat-sprayed marijuana results in minimal absorption, estimated at 0.03% to 0.2%. Nevertheless, an estimated 60% to 70% of the paraquat in marijuana is converted to biperiden when smoked, and this is a direct respiratory irritant.

Paraquat has a large volume of distribution (2–8 L/kg). Although it is distributed to all major organ systems, it selectively accumulates in the lungs. Its pulmonary toxicity may be accounted for by lung tissue concentrations 10 to 15 times greater than plasma levels. Peak lung concentrations are achieved 4 to 5 days after ingestion. Paraquat is not metabolized. Most of an oral dose is eliminated by glomerular filtration and active tubular secretion within 48 hours, but 20% to 30% that may remain tissue-bound is excreted over 2 to 3 weeks.

Although not fully understood, the mechanism of human toxicity of bipyridyl herbicides is believed to be as a result of the formation of free radical metabolites that damage cells directly or through the generation and reduction-oxidation cycling of other free radicals (e.g., superoxide). The lung is the site of greatest toxicity in paraquat poisoning. Pathologic changes in the lung include alveolar epithelial destruction, with pulmonary hemorrhage and congestion progressing to intraalveolar and obliterative fibrosis. Oxygen potentiates the paraquat-induced pulmonary fibrosis (8). Diquat is much less likely to cause respiratory failure than paraquat and it has not been reported to cause pulmonary fibrosis (9). Toxicity involving the central nervous system, kidneys, liver, heart, and adrenal glands can occur with either agent. The more concentrated the herbicide solution, the greater the corrosive effect. Depending on the route of exposure, burns may involve the eyes, respiratory tract, and skin, and the oropharynx, esophagus, and stomach.

The ingestion of less than 20 mg/kg of paraquat and 1 g of diquat ion results in a mild poisoning with GI symptoms, possible renal dysfunction, and full recovery. Moderate-to-severe poisoning follows ingestions of 20 to 40 mg/kg, with corrosive GI injury and slowly progressive renal failure and pulmonary fibrosis (over days to weeks). An acute fulminant course with corrosive effects and multisystem organ failure occurs within hours to days after the ingestion of more than 40 mg/kg (22). Death can occur within days but is usually delayed 2 to 3 weeks. Similar toxicity is seen in adults with ingestions of less than 1, 1 to 12, and greater than 12 g of diquat ion, respectively (9). Death occurs in about a third of those with moderate-to-severe poisoning and in all fulminant cases.

Chlorophenoxy acid herbicides act as plant hormones (auxins) to limit the growth of broadleaf and woody vegetation (2,5,17). Examples are 2,4-D (2,4-dichlorophenoxyacetic acid), 2,4,5-trichlorophenoxyacetic acid (2,4,5-T), 4-chloro-2-methylphenoxypropionic acid (MCPA, MCPP, or mecoprop), 4-chloro-2-methylphenoxyacetic acid (2,4,-DP, DCPP, or dichlorprop), and 2-(2,4,5-trichlorophenoxy)propionic acid (2,4,5-TCPPA or silvex). 2,4-D and 2,4,5-T were used extensively as defoliants in the Vietnam War, and referred to by the colors of the drums that contained them. Agent Orange was a 50:50 mixture of the *N*-butyl esters of 2,4-D and 2,4,5-T, whereas agents Green, Pink, and Purple were primarily 2,4,5-T. All contained the contaminant 2,3,7,8-tetrachlorodibenzo-p-dioxin (TCDD, or dioxin), known to be carcinogenic and teratogenic in animals, with analogous toxicity suspected in humans. Only 2,4-D is currently available for general use in the United States, and its TCDD concentrations are quite low. Brand names include Aqua-Kleen, Chloroxine, Esterom, Salvo, Weedar, Weed-B-Gone, and Weedone.

The GI absorption chlorophenoxy acids is slow; peak blood levels may not occur for 12 hours or longer (1). 2,4-D has an apparent volume of distribution (Vd) of about 0.1 L/kg, with the highest concentrations found in the blood and heart. Elimination occurs mainly by renal excretion of unchanged 2,4-D, with a half-life of about 12 hours after low doses. With overdose, the volume of distribution and half-life appear to be much greater. Elimination is prolonged in the presence of renal failure. Because it is a weak acid (pKa 3.3), alkaline diuresis shortens the half-life by a factor of 10 or more (4,14).

It is unclear how chlorophenoxy acid herbicides cause toxicity in humans. Interference with cell membrane lipid structure and function, formation of acetyl-Co-A analogs and choline esters with disruption of metabolic pathways and neurotransmission, and uncoupling of oxidative phosphorylation may be involved. Myotonia and rhabdomyolysis may be as a result of increased activity of skeletal muscle mitochondrial enzymes. Neuronal demyelinization and rhabdomyolysis are pathologic findings.

Serious poisoning almost always results from suicidal ingestion of concentrated solutions. 2,4,-D doses of roughly 50 mg/kg produce mild toxicity, those of 100 mg/kg cause severe poisoning, and those of 250 mg/kg or more may be fatal (2,5,14). Pulmonary absorption is possible but unlikely to cause systemic toxicity. Although skin absorption is low but chronic dermal exposure may result in systemic toxicity.

Glyphosate and glufosinate are phosphorylated glutamic acid analogs that inhibit plant enzymes involved in amino acid metabolism (17,21). Glyphosate (N-phosphonomethyl glycine) is sold in the United Sstates under the brand names Glifonox, Glycel, Rodeo, Rondo, and Roundup. Glufosinate (2-amono-4-hydroxymethylphosphonyl butanoic acid) is marketed as Basta, Challenge, Finale, Hayabusa, and Ignite. Bialaphos (phosphenothricin-alanyl-alanine), which is metabolized to glufosinate in plants, is available outside the United States (e.g., Herbiace).

These herbicides have limited oral and poor dermal absorption, undergo negligible metabolism, and are eliminated by urinary excretion. Glyphosate has a Vd of about 0.3 L/kg and a half-life of 2 to 3 hours. Glufosinate has a larger Vd (about 1.4 L/kg) and longer half-life (about 10 h). Elimination is decreased in renal failure.

It is unclear how or if glyphosate causes human toxicity. Although ingestion of commercial formulations clearly causes poisoning and uncoupling of oxidative phosphorylation has been suggested, it appears that polyoxyetheneamine, a nonionic surfactant with cationic (corrosive) effects, is actually responsible for GI, cardiovascular (CV), and pulmonary toxicity (11,15,21). Neurotoxic effects of glufosinate may be as a result of stimulation of excitatory N-methyl-D-aspartate (NMDA) receptors or inhibition of glutamine acid decarboxylase and consequent decreased synthesis of the inhibitory neurotransmitter γ-aminobutyric acid (GABA) whereas CV toxicity appears to be as a result of the anionic surfactant (sodium polyoxyethylene alkyl ether sulfate) component (21). In an adult, the ingestion of 50 to 100 mL of an undiluted organic phosphorus herbicide-surfactant formulation is likely to cause mild poisoning, 100 to 200 mL may result in moderate to severe poisoning, and 200 to 300 mL or more is potentially fatal.

CLINICAL PRESENTATION

The toxicity of paraquat and diquat depends on the dose, which primarily relates to the concentration of the solution involved (9,17,21,22). Exposure to dilute solutions (e.g., commercial concentrates that have been diluted for use) usually cause only local toxicity such as dermatitis, conjunctivitis, cough, sore throat, and burning in the mouth and throat. Concentrated solutions can cause dermal and corneal burns. Stomatitis, epistaxis, and bronchial irritation have been reported after inhalation. Ingestion causes oropharyngeal pain, dysphagia, substernal chest pain, abdominal cramps, diarrhea, and vomiting. Examination may reveal hemorrhagic mucositis and ulcerations of mouth, larynx, trachea, esophagus, stomach, and even small intestine. Paralytic ileus with third-spacing of fluid, esophageal perfora-

tion with mediastinitis, and hypovolemic shock may also occur. The time of symptom onset also correlates with the dose. Of note, onset may be delayed many hours after the ingestion of dilute solutions or small amounts of concentrate.

Systemic effects usually occur only after ingestion and include coma, seizures, pulmonary fibrosis (paraquat only), acute proximal renal tubular necrosis, centrilobular hepatic necrosis, myocarditis and necrosis, pancytopenia, and adrenal hemorrhage. In fulminant cases, severe corrosive effects are accompanied by multiorgan failure, with death occurring within hours to days from pulmonary edema (ARDS), seizures, and cardiogenic shock. Intracerebral hemorrhages have been reported in diquat poisoning.

Pulmonary dysfunction may result in dyspnea, chest pain, tachypnea, and cyanosis. The chest radiograph may demonstrate pulmonary infiltrates, atelectasis, pneumothorax, and pleural effusions. Pulmonary function testing may reveal low compliance and decreased lung volumes and diffusing capacity. Blood gas analysis reveals hypoxemia, with respiratory alkalosis and metabolic acidosis. Respiratory failure and pulmonary fibrosis from paraquat usually progress relentlessly. Patients who survive may be left with restrictive lung disease.

Renal involvement may result in uremia, proteinuria, and oliguria or anuria. Signs of hepatotoxicity include right upper quadrant tenderness and elevated serum bilirubin and transaminase levels. Those with cardiac involvement may have chest pain and electrocardiogram (ECG), serum cardiac enzyme, or imaging evidence of ischemia or myocarditis. Ventricular tachycardia and fibrillation can occur. Renal and hepatic toxicity are potentially reversible. An elevated serum creatinine, low serum potassium, and metabolic acidosis on presentation are associated with the development of renal failure and death within 48 hours. Coma, early onset renal failure, abnormal urinalysis, elevated serum transaminases, ileus, pancreatitis, alveolar-arterial oxygen gradient, need for mechanical ventilation, oxygen requirement, cardiac dysrhythmias, and an Apache II score of more than 20 are also predictive of mortality.

The ingestion of concentrated chlorophenoxy acid herbicides may cause a burning sensation in the pharynx, chest, and abdomen (2–5,16,17,21,25). Vomiting occurs early and may be persistent. Within a few hours, neurologic abnormalities such as agitation, confusion, headache, dizziness, lethargy, coma, and seizures may develop. Cyanosis, flushed skin, and diaphoresis have been reported. Pupils tend to be small but reactive. Deep tendon reflexes and muscle tone may be increased, decreased, or normal. Opisthotonus, myoclonus, fasciculations, and muscle tenderness have been described. Dyspnea and tachypnea are often present. In severe cases, progressive tachycardia, hypotension, and hyperthermia may ensue. Early death may be as a result of ventricular fibrillation. Eye, skin, and respiratory tract irritation may follow exposure by these routes.

Laboratory abnormalities include an increased anion gap metabolic acidosis, hypoxia, hyperkalemia, hypocalcemia, leukocytosis, evidence of rhabdomyolysis (increased creatine phosphokinase level and myoglobinuria), mildly elevated hepatic enzyme levels, and renal function disturbances (elevated BUN and creatinine levels, proteinuria, and glycosuria). The ECG may show flat or inverted T waves. Although pulmonary edema and aspiration have been reported, the chest radiograph usually is normal. Nerve conduction and electromyographic studies may show evidence of peripheral neuropathy and myopathy.

In mild-to-moderate chlorophenoxy acid intoxication, recovery usually occurs within 2 to 3 days; in severe cases, it may take longer than 1 week. Coma and acidemia are poor prognostic signs (4). Neuritis and myopathy with limb pain, paresthesias, twitching, tenderness, and weakness may be delayed in onset and persist for several months (12).

The ingestion of concentrated solutions of organophosphorus-surfactant herbicides can cause acute GI and pulmonary injury, delayed CV toxicity, and secondary hepatic and renal dysfunction (10,11,15,17,20,21). Glufosinate also causes neurological toxicity, which can be delayed (4–36 hours postingestion) in onset and progressive (over 24–48 hours) (19,24). Neurological findings include ataxia, confusion, disconjugate gaze, nystagmus, tremors, CNS depression ranging from drowsiness to coma with central hypoventilation and apnea, and seizures. Seizures are generalized, invariably preceded by coma, typically recurrent, and can last for several days. Complications include hyperthermia, acidosis, and rhabdomyolysis.

Signs and symptoms of GI, pulmonary, CV, hepatic, and renal toxicity are similar to those described for bipyridyl and chlorophenoxy acid herbicides. Hypovolemic shock may result from GI fluid losses and sequestration. Cardiogenic shock can occur subsequently. Severe GI injury, respiratory failure, and cardiogenic shock are associated with a fatal outcome. Patients with coma or seizures can have prolonged amnesia, encephapathy, and myopathy with recovery taking weeks. Exposure to organophosphorus-surfactant herbicides that have been diluted for use may cause eye, skin, and mucosal irritation but systemic toxicity is unlikely.

DIFFERENTIAL DIAGNOSIS

Herbicide poisoning should be suspected in a patient who presents with signs and symptoms of corrosive ingestion, cardiopulmonary toxicity, and hepatorenal dysfunction of unknown etiology. The initial presentation may resemble that of other corrosive exposures (see Chapter 307, "Corrosives and Chemical Burns"). Paraquat poisoning is distinguished by progressive pulmonary failure. Diquat is less corrosive than paraquat but appears to be more likely to cause acute renal failure and paralytic ileus (17). Colchicine, podophyllin, fluoride, iron, and heavy-metal ingestion can cause multisystem organ toxicity and corrosive GI effects. Except with glufosinate, the CNS depression caused by herbicides is not associated with respiratory depression. Other causes of CNS depression include trauma, infection, hypoglycemia, asphyxiant, opioid, and sedative–hypnotic poisoning.

Severe 2,4-D and glufosinate poisoning, with coma, seizures, tachycardia, hypotension, fever, rhabdomyolysis, and metabolic acidosis, may be confused with septic shock, diabetic ketoacidosis, severe stimulant poisoning (e.g., amphetamines, cocaine, theophylline), and intoxication by methanol, ethylene glycol, and salicylates. Other uncouplers of oxidative phosphorylation, such as the dinitrocresol and dinitrophenol herbicides and the pentachlorophenol fungicides, may produce a similar clinical picture. Cresylic and phenolic herbicides may stain the skin yellow and cause dark-colored urine. Other herbicides to consider when the product ingested is unknown include amides (e.g., alachlor, propanol); aniline and arsenic derivatives; carbamates, thiocarbamates, and dithiocarbamate; chlorates; nitriles (e.g., dichlobenil, ioxynil), and triazenes and triazoles (e.g., atrazine, propazine). Toxicologic analysis of the blood may be necessary for a definitive diagnosis.

EMERGENCY DEPARTMENT EVALUATION

The history should include the concentration, amount, and route of herbicide exposure, and the time of onset and nature of symptoms. Determining whether or not the product was diluted prior to exposure and estimating the exposure dose are particularly important. Commercial products containing concentrated herbicide (e.g., 15% to 50% solutions) are highly toxic whereas signifi-

cant poisoning is unlikely once these products have been diluted for use (typically by a factor of 100). Vitals signs should include measurement of the oxygen saturation. The physical examination should include inspection of exposed surfaces for evidence of corrosive injury. Patients with eye exposures should have fluorescein and slit-lamp examinations. Patients with GI signs and symptoms should also have an ECG, chest radiograph, arterial blood gas analysis, pulmonary function tests, complete blood count (CBC), electrolytes, blood urea nitrogen (BUN), creatinine, glucose, amylase, liver function tests, cardiac enzymes, and urinalysis. Endoscopy is recommended for those with evidence of corrosive injury to the airway or upper GI tract (see Chapter 307, "Corrosives and Chemical Burns"). Nerve conduction studies and electromyography may be helpful in those with persistent paresthesias or weakness.

Unless drug co-ingestion is suspected, toxicology screening tests are not helpful because herbicides are not detected by the methods used. The detection and quantitation of herbicides usually requires sending a blood specimen to a reference laboratory. Although results can confirm exposure, they will not be immediately available and, except for paraquat, they have no prognostic value and will not help with making treatment decisions. Plasma paraquat concentrations above 2.0, 0.9, 0.3, 0.16, and 0.10 g/mL at 4, 6, 10, 16, and 24 hours after ingestion, respectively, are predictive of death (7), and a potentially lethal level may warrant the use of unproven but potentially beneficial therapies. Arrangements for a quantitative paraquat level can be made by calling Zeneca Ag Products (800-327-8633). A qualitative urine test detects paraquat concentrations greater than 1 g/mL and confirms exposure but is not prognostic. It may be performed by adding 1 mL of a 1% solution of sodium dithionite in 2N sodium hydroxide to 10 mL of urine. A blue color indicates the presence of paraquat (7).

EMERGENCY DEPARTMENT MANAGEMENT

Contaminated skin should be flushed with copious amounts of water. Material splashed in the eyes should be removed by prolonged irrigation with water. Immediate and aggressive GI decontamination is critical, even when small amounts have been ingested. Unless the risk of esophageal perforation is great (e.g., the patient is unable to swallow and many hours have passed since the time of ingestion), GI decontamination should be performed. Because the absorption of chlorophenoxy acids is slow, decontamination may be effective much longer after ingestion (possibly as long as 18 hours) than usual. Activated charcoal (AC) is the preferred method. Fuller's earth and bentonite suspensions (15 and 7.5% w/v, respectively, in the same dose as AC) are also effective in binding paraquat. Preceding AC by gastric aspiration or following it with gastric lavage and another dose of AC should be considered in those with potentially lethal ingestions. Multiple dose activated charcoal therapy is also recommended.

Advanced life-support measures and supportive care should be instituted as necessary. In severe cases, endotracheal intubation and fluid resuscitation may be required. When intubating patients with chlorophenoxy acid poisoning, a nondepolarizing neuromuscular blocker (e.g., rocuronium) may be preferable to succinylcholine because the muscle effects of succinylcholine are similar to those caused by these herbicides. Benzodiazepines, muscle relaxants, or therapeutic paralysis should be used for the treatment agitation, fasciculations, myoclonus, or muscle rigidity, particularly those with hyperthermia or rhabdomyolysis. Propofol, which has antioxidant activity, should be considered for intubated patients with paraquat poisoning. Active external cooling measures may be necessary in patients with hyperthermia. Because salicylates can cause uncoupling of oxidative phosphorylation, their use should be avoided. Urinary alkalinization and diuresis may be helpful in patients with rhabdomyolysis. These measures also enhance the elimination of chlorophenoxy acid herbicides (see sodium bicarbonate administration below).

Supportive care should include monitoring for and treatment of hepatic, renal, cardiac, and pulmonary dysfunction, and fluid and electrolyte abnormalities. With the exception of oxygen therapy in paraquat poisoning, standard therapies are employed. Because oxygen increases the pulmonary toxicity of paraquat, concentrations greater than 21% should be used only when the Po_2 falls below 50 mm Hg. Positive end-expiratory pressure may improve arterial oxygenation while obviating the need for increasing the inspired oxygen concentration.

The administration of sodium bicarbonate is indicated to correct acidemia and enhance herbicide elimination in patients with chlorophenoxy acid poisoning (2,5,14,25). It also appears to improve survival (4). Chlorophenoxy acids have pKa values between 1.9 and 4.8, the pH at which the concentration of ionized and unionized forms are equal. Because only the nonionized fraction is diffusible across cell membranes, increasing the pH increases the ionized fraction and traps these compounds in the blood and urine, thereby preventing their tissue distribution and enhancing their renal excretion. Sodium bicarbonate should be given as a bolus to correct acidemia and as a constant infusion to alkalinize the urine. Alkaline diuresis decreases the half-life of 2,4,-D by about 50%. Urine pH must be increased to 8.0 to enhance excretion significantly. Infusing a solution of two ampules (88 mEq) of sodium bicarbonate per liter of dextrose 5% in sodium chloride 0.45% at a rate of 3 to 6 ml/kg/h is usually necessary. Adjustments in the rate and the amount of bicarbonate should be made on the basis of urine flow and pH.

Extracorporeal elimination therapies are indicated for patients with severe paraquat, diquat, and chlorophenoxy acid poisoning or potentially lethal ingestions and progressive clinical toxicity. Charcoal or resin hemoperfusion are the procedure of choice for bipyridyls although hemodialysis is preferred for chlorophenoxy acids. Although these measures are effective in removing glyphosate and glufosinate, they are unlikely to remove significant amounts of surfactant, and a clinical benefit has not been demonstrated.

Early, prolonged hemoperfusion appears to be useful in removing paraquat and limiting systemic toxicity when started within 10 hours of ingestion (15–20 hours in the presence of renal failure) and performed 8 hours daily or continuously for 2 to 3 weeks until paraquat can no longer be detected in the urine or blood (14,22). Clinical efficacy has been questioned, particularly if initial plasma concentrations exceed 3 mg/L (6). Hemodialysis and continuous arteriovenous hemofiltration also enhance the elimination of paraquat and may be useful if hemoperfusion is unavailable (13). Hemodialysis may also be indicated for the treatment of renal failure. Data is limited regarding the use of hemoperfusion in diquat poisoning. The efficacy of hemodialysis in enhancing 2,4-D elimination is about the same as inducing alkaline diuresis (2,3,5,25).

A variety of free radicals scavengers and antioxidants have been used in an attempt to prevent pulmonary fibrosis paraquat poisoning but their efficacy remains unproven (2,5,17,18). Given the lethality of this condition, however, the following treatments should be considered in patients with severe poisoning or progressive deterioration in pulmonary function: corticosteroids (methylprednisolone, 15 mg/kg/d i.v. in divided doses, with or without dexamethasone., 0.2–0.3 mg/kg/d i.v. in divided doses), cyclophosphamide (15 mg/kg i.v. up to a maximum of 1 g in 200 mL of 5% dextrose infused over 2 hours for 2 days, in conjunction with corticosteroids), N-acetylcysteine (same dose as for acetaminophen poisoning), vitamin C (4 g/d p.o. or i.v.),

and vitamin E (250 mg/d p.o.). S-carboxymethylcysteine (Loviscol, 20 mg/kg p.o. q.i.d) has been used when n-acetylcysteine is unavailable. If a patient survives more than 3 weeks and has end-stage respiratory failure, single and bilateral lung transplantation should be considered. Most patients who have had this procedure still die; only one case has been successful (23). Nitric oxide inhalation and ECMO (extracorporeal membrane oxygenation) might be useful as an interim measures.

CRITICAL INTERVENTIONS

- Estimate the dose of herbicide before making treatment and disposition decisions
- Obtain a serum paraquat level, administer oxygen only if absolutely necessary (e.g., Po2 <50 mm Hg), arrange for hemoperfusion, and consider antioxidant therapy in patients with significant paraquat poisoning
- Correct acidemia, institute alkaline diuresis, and consider hemodialysis in patients with chlorophenoxy acid herbicide poisoning

DISPOSITION

A toxicologist or regional poison center should be consulted in all cases of herbicide poisoning. The National Pesticide Telecommunications Network also provides 24-hour-a-day consultation services (800-858-7378). All patients with symptoms after herbicide ingestion and dermal burns from paraquat should be admitted. Unless the exposure is minor and the severity of poisoning is mild, transfer to a tertiary care center and admission to an intensive care unit are advised. Patients who remain or become asymptomatic after trivial ingestions or exposure by other routes, can be discharged, after evaluation and decontamination. Patients with ingestions should be observed for 4 to 6 hours (6–12 hours for chlorophenoxy acid herbicides) prior to discharge. Consultation with gastroenterologist or ophthalmologist is recommended for those with evidence of corrosive injury to the GI tract or eyes. A nephrologist or pulmonologist should be consulted for patients with renal or pulmonary dysfunction.

COMMON PITFALLS

✔ Underestimating the potential toxicity of herbicides, particularly in those with intentional ingestions of concentrated solutions

✔ Failure to appreciate that although concentrated herbicide formulations are highly toxic, the likelihood of serious toxicity is greatly diminished once they have been diluted for use

✔ Failure to perform decontamination and to appreciate that because the absorption of chlorophenoxy acid herbicides is slow, GI decontamination may be effective many hours ingestion

✔ Failure to appreciate that prolonged observation is necessary to rule out toxicity in patients with ingestions of dilute herbicide and significant skin exposures to paraquat

✔ Failure to evaluate symptomatic patients for multisystem organ dysfunction, including metabolic disturbances and rhabdomyolysis

✔ Failure to appreciate that the pulmonary toxicity of paraquat is potentiated by oxygen and that the lowest possible concentration of supplemental oxygen should be administered

✔ Failure to appreciate that extracorporeal removal can enhance the elimination of paraquat, diquat, and chlorophenoxy acid herbicides

References

1. Arnold EK, Beasley R. The pharmacokinetics of chlorinated phenoxy acid herbicides: a literature review. *Vet Hum Toxicol* 1989;31:121.
2. Bradberry SM, Watt BE, Proudfoot AT, Vale JA. Mechanisms of toxicity, clinical features, and management of acute chlorophenoxy herbicide poisoning: a review. *J Toxicol Clin Toxicol* 2000;38(2):111–122.
3. Durakovic Z, Durakovic A, Durakovic S, et al. Poisoning with 2,4-dichlorophenoxyacetic acid treated by hemodialysis. *Arch Toxicol* 1992;66(7):518–521.
4. Flanagan RJ, Meredith TJ, Ruprah M, et al. Alkaline diuresis for acute poisoning with chlorophenoxy herbicides and ioxynil. *Lancet* 1990;335:454.
5. Friesen EG, Jones GR, Vaughan D. Clinical presentation and management of acute 2,4-D oral ingestion. *Drug Saf* 1990;5:155.
6. Hampson ECGM, Pond SM. Failure of haemoperfusion and haemodialysis to prevent death in paraquat poisoning: a retrospective review of 42 patients. *Med Toxicol* 1988;3:64.
7. Hart TB. A statistical approach to the prognostic significance of plasma paraquat concentrations. *Lancet* 1984;2:1222.
8. Hoet PH, Demedts M, Nemery B. Effects of oxygen pressure and medium volume on the toxicity of paraquat in rat and human type II pneumocytes. *Hum Exp Toxicol* 1997;16:305.
9. Jones GM, Vale JA. Mechanisms of toxicity, clinical features, and management of diquat poisoning: a review. *J Toxicol Clin Toxicol* 2000;38(2):123–128.
10. Koyama K, Andou Y, Saruki K: Delayed and severe toxicities of a herbicide containing glufosinate and a surfactant. *Vet Hum Toxicol* 1994;36(1):17–18.
11. Lee HL, Chen KW, Chi CH. Clinical presentations and prognostic factors of a glyphosate-surfactant herbicide intoxication: a review of 131 cases. *Acad Emerg Med* 2000;7:906–910.
12. O'Reilly JF. Prolonged coma and delayed peripheral neuropathy after ingestion of phenoxyacetic acid weed killers. *Postgrad Med J* 1984;60:76.
13. Pond SM, Johnston SC, Schoof DD, et al. Repeated hemoperfusion and continuous arteriovenous hemofiltration in a paraquat-poisoned patient. *J Toxicol Clin Toxicol* 1987;25:305.
14. Prescott LF, Park J, Carrien I. Treatment of severe 2,4-D and mecoprop intoxication with alkaline diuresis. *Br J Clin Pharmacol* 1979;7:111.
15. Sawada Y, Nagai Y, Ueyama M, et al: Probable toxicity of surface-active agent in commercial herbicide containing glyphosate. *Lancet* 1988;1(8580):299.
16. Schmoldt A, Iwersen S, Schluter W: Massive ingestion of the herbicide 2-methyl-4-chlorophenoxyacetic acid (MCPA). *J Toxicol Clin Toxicol* 1997;35(4):405–408.
17. Stevens JT, Sumner DD.Herbicides. In: Hayes WJ, Laws ER, eds. *Handbook of Pesticide Toxicology.* San Diego: Academic Press, 1991:1317.
18. Suntres ZE. Role of antioxidants in paraquat toxicity. *Toxicology* 2002;180:65–77.
19. Tanaka J, Yamashita M, Yamashita M. Two cases of glufosinate poisoning with late onset convulsions. *Vet Hum Toxicol* 1998;40:219–222.
20. Talbot AR, Shiaw MH, Huang JS. Acute poisoning with a glyphosate-surfactant herbicide ('Round-up'): a review of 93 cases. *Hum Exp Toxicol* 1991;10:1–8.
21. Tominack RL, Pond SM.Herbicides. In: Goldfrank LR, Flomenbaum NE, Lewin NA, et al, eds. *Goldfrank's toxicological emergencies,* 7th ed. New York: McGraw-Hill, 2002:1393.
22. Vale JA. Paraquat poisoning: clinical features and immediate general management. *Vet Hum Toxicol* 1987;6:41.
23. Walder B, Brundler MA, Spilopoulos A, et al. Successful single-lung transplantation after paraquat intoxication. *Transplantation* 1997;64:789.
24. Watanabe T, Sano T: Neurological effects of glufosinate poisoning with a brief review. *Hum Exp Toxicol* 1998;17:35–39.
25. Wells WDE, Wright N, Yeoman WB. Clinical features and management of poisoning with 2,4-D and mecoprop. *J Toxicol Clin Toxicol* 1981;18:273.

CHAPTER 296
Isoniazid

Alan D. Woolf

Isoniazid (isonicotinic acid hydrazide, INH), a derivative of vitamin B_3 (nicotinamide), has been used for the prophylaxis and treatment of tuberculosis since 1952. With the resurgence of tuberculosis has come an increasing incidence in isoniazid poisoning (17). There were 415 isoniazid poisonings reported by the American Association of Poison Control Centers in 2002 (23). The incidence of self-poisoning is greatest among those adult populations with a high prevalence of both tuberculosis and depression (e.g., Native Americans, immigrant populations) (3,18). INH is rapidly absorbed from the small intestine within 30 to 60 minutes after ingestion. Therapeutic doses are 5 to 10 mg/kg (maximum, 300 mg) daily, given orally or by intramuscular injection (2). Peak INH serum levels (therapeutic range, 5 to 8 μg/mL) are reached within 1 to 2 hours (24). The drug is minimally bound to plasma proteins and has a small apparent volume of distribution (0.6 L/kg) (24). INH can be detected in such diverse bodily fluids as saliva, cerebrospinal fluid (CSF), and breast milk. Up to 36% of the drug may be excreted unchanged in urine (12). Metabolism by acetylation in the liver yields inactive metabolites that are predominantly excreted in the urine. People with normal renal function excrete 50% to 80% of a therapeutic dose of INH within 24 hours (4).

There is great genetic variability in the metabolism of INH. Between 45% and 75% of Caucasians are "slow acetylators" and have a mean serum INH half-life of about 5 hours. By contrast, 95% of Inuit are "fast acetylators" and have an average serum half-life of 80 minutes (13). These differences are therapeutically important: slow acetylators can achieve sustained bactericidal drug levels on every-other-day dosage regimens, whereas fast acetylators may have inadequate levels unless they receive the drug daily (12).

Various mechanisms are responsible for the toxic effects of INH. In acute overdoses, INH decreases the conversion of glutamic acid to γ-aminobutyric acid (GABA) by inhibiting the pyridoxal phosphate–dependent enzyme glutamic acid decarboxylase (GAD). Because GABA is an inhibitory neurotransmitter, seizures may ensue (25). With chronic therapy, INH hydrazone analogues, which arise spontaneously *in vivo* (especially in slow acetylators), and form rapidly excreted complexes with pyridoxine, leading to a pyridoxine deficiency. INH hydrazones also inhibit pyridoxine kinase, thereby decreasing the conversion of pyridoxine to its active cofactor form, pyridoxal phosphate.

INH is structurally similar to nicotinic acid and may substitute for it in the synthesis of nicotinamide adenine dinucleotide (NAD), producing an inactive coenzyme. Inhibition of NAD-dependent Krebs cycle enzymes may result in hyperglycemia, and inhibition of NAD-mediated conversion of lactate to pyruvate may contribute to the profound lactic acidosis that typically accompanies seizures.

Patients who are malnourished, pregnant, alcoholic, elderly, diabetic, or uremic may be at particularly high risk for pyridoxine deficiency during chronic INH therapy (15). In the absence of supplemental doses of pyridoxine (e.g., 10 mg/d), pyridoxine deficiency may develop and lead to peripheral neuropathies, anemia, and a lowered seizure threshold. Pyridoxine depletion can also inhibit the activity of pyridoxine-dependent decarboxylases and transaminases (leading to decreased catecholamine synthesis), cytochrome P-450 enzymes (leading to decreased drug metabolism), histaminase, and monoamine oxidase (MAO).

CLINICAL PRESENTATION

Seizures may be seen after acute overdoses of INH as low as 35 mg/kg in adults. Severe toxicity has been noted with ingestions of 5 to 7 g (80 to 150 mg/kg); death has resulted after the ingestion of as little as 3 g (21). Although ingestions of more than 12 g in an adult have a high fatality rate, survival has been reported after the ingestion of as much as 25 g (22). Poisoning is associated with an INH serum concentration above 30 μg/mL, although such laboratory assays for INH are not routinely available.

The initial symptoms of acute poisoning, which may occur as soon as 30 to 120 minutes after ingestion, include nausea, vomiting, slurred speech, blurred vision, and disorientation. Anticholinergic signs (e.g., mydriasis, tachycardia, and urinary retention) and hyperreflexia or areflexia may also be prominent. In severe poisonings, seizures appear abruptly and precede the development of a profound metabolic acidosis and coma, the triad of which forms the classic clinical picture. An arterial pH as low as 6.49 was recorded in an adolescent who survived INH poisoning with no sequelae (11). Other patients with INH-induced seizures and arterial pH <6.99 have survived with full recovery after receiving pyridoxine (1).

Multiple seizures over a short time period are the hallmark of INH poisoning. Other symptoms and signs of acute poisoning include confusion or hallucinations, garbled speech, hyperpyrexia, and respiratory depression. Laboratory findings include lactic acidosis, ketosis, hyperglycemia, an increased anion gap, hyperkalemia, peripheral blood leukocytosis, CSF pleocytosis, and renal defects (e.g., glycosuria, albuminuria, and oliguria). An elevated creatine phosphokinase as a result of rhabdomyolysis may precede myoglobinuria and renal failure. An electroencephalogram (EEG) often demonstrates diffuse slowing or paroxysmal electrical activity compatible with subclinical seizures. A chest radiograph may reveal aspiration pneumonia. The clinical course of the untreated patient with a massive INH overdose is often unremitting seizures, resulting in death from acidosis and cardiovascular and respiratory collapse.

Hepatic damage, manifested by elevated liver enzyme levels, has an incidence of 20.7 cases per 1,000 patients treated chronically with INH (5). Such hepatotoxicity appears transient in most cases, even with continued use of the drug (19,20). Rarely, patients go on to develop acute liver necrosis, liver failure, and death (5,9,20). Toxic effects of chronic INH use also include euphoria, tinnitus, ataxia, impaired memory, encephalopathy, and optic neuritis. Progressive lethargy, garbled speech, confusion, and coma were described in a man who mistakenly treated his tuberculosis with 1,200 mg of INH daily for 6 weeks (15).

Allergic manifestations, such as rashes, eosinophilia, vasculitis, arthralgias, and a positive antinuclear antibody test, have also been described (10). By inhibiting P450 series cytochromes, INH can interfere with drug clearance and increase the toxicity of such agents as phenytoin, carbamazepine, theophylline, and warfarin (16). INH's action as a weak MAO inhibitor may result in symptoms (e.g., headache, flushing, nausea, vomiting, palpitations) in patients consuming foods containing tyramine or histamine (16). Pure red cell aplasia was described in two siblings who were started on isoniazid prophylaxis at 15 mg/kg/day for

6 months (14). Other hematological abnormalities such as neutropenia, thrombocytopenia, sideroblastic anemia, and autoimmune hemolytic anemia have also been described in association with exposure to isoniazid.

Patients with underlying impaired renal function or hepatic disease do not metabolize INH well, have a prolonged serum half-life, and are at greater risk for intoxication. Those with a preexisting seizure disorder are at higher risk for neurotoxic effects.

DIFFERENTIAL DIAGNOSIS

INH overdose should be strongly considered in the patient who presents with seizures refractory to conventional anticonvulsants and a high anion gap metabolic acidosis, especially within the context of a history of a depression, suicidal ideation, and tuberculosis, with access to INH. A diagnostic clue to INH poisoning is the prompt termination of seizure activity after the administration of intravenous pyridoxine.

Agents that can cause a clinical picture similar to that of INH overdose include salicylates, cyanide, carbon monoxide, other hydrazines (e.g., monomethylhydrazine-containing mushrooms), anticholinergics, and sympathomimetics. Neurotoxins such as pesticides, camphor, lead, narcotics, strychnine, and tricyclic antidepressants must also be considered (6). Other medical conditions, such as meningitis with sepsis, diabetic ketoacidosis, uremia, meningoencephalitis, and head trauma, should also be included in the differential of patients presenting with seizures, coma, and acidosis (6,8).

EMERGENCY DEPARTMENT EVALUATION

If known, the time, dose, and intent of ingestion, the time of onset, nature, and severity of symptoms, prehospital care, and medical and psychiatric history should be noted. The physical examination should focus on vital signs and the neurologic status, including assessment for hyperreflexia, focal neurologic deficits, abnormal thought processes, and CNS depression. Cardiac monitoring should be instituted. Laboratory evaluation should include determination of serum electrolytes, glucose, blood area nitrogen, creatinine, and arterial pH and blood gases. A toxicology screen of blood and urine should also be obtained. In severe or chronic cases, creatine kinase and liver function tests should be obtained. A chest radiograph can diagnose aspiration, and an EEG may be helpful in patients with coma.

EMERGENCY DEPARTMENT MANAGEMENT

Advanced life-support measures should be instituted as necessary. Pyridoxine (vitamin B_6) is the specific antidote for seizures; it should be given in gram-for-gram equivalency to the estimated total amount of INH ingested (17,22). If the total ingested dose of INH is unknown, 5 g of pyridoxine can be given empirically by slow intravenous push and repeated in 20 minutes if there is no clinical response. Typically, the seizures abate and the patient's level of consciousness slowly improves. Diazepam (5–10 mg intravenously) may be used as an adjunct to control seizures. Additional pyridoxine is sometimes necessary for the resolution of INH-induced coma.

The use of adequate doses of diazepam and pyridoxine has essentially eliminated the need for barbiturates, paralyzing agents, anesthesia, dialysis, or exchange transfusion in the management of INH overdose. Chronic pyridoxine overdosing can cause a peripheral sensory neuropathy. Multiple large doses should be avoided because of pyridoxine's neurotoxic potential; only gram-for-gram replacement is recommended in INH poisoning.

Although severe metabolic acidosis should be treated with sodium bicarbonate given intravensouly, large doses are usually unnecessary, because the acidosis is secondary to seizures and resolves shortly after seizures have been controlled (7,21). Diuresis is not of proven benefit in INH overdose. After stabilization, instillation of activated charcoal into the gut should be done in all early presenting, acute overdose patients to prevent further absorption of INH or other coingestants.

CRITICAL INTERVENTIONS

- Administer intravenous pyridoxine along with benzodiazepines for INH-induced seizures
- Obtain an ABG and administer i.v. sodium bicarbonate to patients with severe acidemia

DISPOSITION

Asymptomatic or mildly symptomatic patients can be observed in the emergency department for 6 hours. A toxicologist or poison control center can be helpful to the clinician. Such consultants can give advice in assessing the patient with seizures and acidosis of unknown cause, in managing patients with complex INH-related toxicity, and in locating supplies of pyridoxine.

Moderately or severely symptomatic patients should be admitted to an intensive care unit. Patients with refractory seizures, severe respiratory depression, or renal failure should be transferred to a hospital with intensive care capabilities if they are not locally available.

COMMON PITFALLS

✔ Failure to consider INH poisoning in patients with seizures refractory to conventional anticonvulsants and a high anion gap metabolic acidosis

✔ Failure to appreciate that asymptomatic patients may rapidly deteriorate

✔ Failure to give pyridoxine early after a known overdose

✔ Giving excessive doses of sodium bicarbonate for the treatment of metabolic acidosis, which spontaneously resolves when convulsions cease

References

1. Alvarez FG, Guntupalli KK. Isoniazid overdose: four case reports and review of the literature. *Intensive Care Med* 1995;21:641.
2. American Thoracic Society. Treatment of tuberculosis and other mycobacterial diseases. *Am Rev Respir Dis* 1983;127:790.
3. Blanchard P, Yao J, McAlpine D, et al. Isoniazid overdose in the Cambodian population of Olmstead County, Minnesota. *JAMA* 1986;256:3131.
4. Bowersox DW, Winterbauer RH, Stewart GL, et al. Isoniazid dosage in patients with renal failure. *N Engl J Med* 1973;289:84.
5. Centers for Disease Control. Severe isoniazid-associated hepatitis—New York 1991 to 1993. *MMWR* 1993;42:545.
6. Chang YD, Yang CC, Lin TJ, et al. Acute isoniazid intoxication: a case report. *Chin Med J (Taipei)* 1996;57:152.
7. Chin L, Sievers M, Herrier R, et al. Convulsions as the etiology of lactic acidosis in acute isoniazid toxicity in dogs. *Toxicol Appl Pharmacol* 1979;49:377.
8. Ehsan T, Malkoff MD. Acute isoniazid poisoning simulating meningoencephalitis. *Neurology* 1995;45:1627.
9. Gal A, Klatt E. Fatal isoniazid hepatitis in a child. *Pediatr Infect Dis* 1986;5:490.
10. Goldman A, Braman S. Isoniazid: review with emphasis on adverse effects. *Chest* 1972;62:71.
11. Hankins DG, Saxena K, Faville RJ, et al. Profound acidosis caused by isoniazid ingestion. *Am J Emerg Med* 1987;5:165.
12. Hughes H, Schmidt L, Biehl J. The metabolism of isoniazid: its implications in therapeutic use. Transactions of the 14th Conference on the Chemotherapy of Tuberculosis. Washington, DC: Virginia Department of Medicine and Surgery, 1976:276.
13. Jeanes C, Schaefer O, Eidus L. Inactivation of isoniazid by Canadian Eskimos and Indians. *CMAJ* 1972;106:331.
14. Marseglia GL, Locatelli F. Isoniazid-induced pure red cell aplasia in two siblings. *J Pediatr* 1998;132:898.
15. Salkind AR, Hewitt CC. Coma from long-term overingestion of isoniazid. *Arch Intern Med* 1997;157:2518.
16. Self TH, Chrisman CR, Baciewicz AM, Bronze MS. Isoniazid drug and food interactions. *Am J Med Sci* 1999;317:304.
17. Shah BR, Santucci K, Sinert R, et al. Acute isoniazid neurotoxicity in an urban hospital. *Pediatrics* 1995;95:700.
18. Sievers M, Cynamon M, Bittker T. Intentional isoniazid overdosage among Southwestern American Indians. *Am J Psychiatry* 1975;132.662.
19. Stuart RL, Grayson ML. A review of isoniazid-related hepatotoxicity during chemoprophylaxis. *Aust NZ J Med* 1999;29:362.
20. Stuart RL, Wilson J, Grayson ML. Isoniazid toxicity in health care workers. *Clin Infect Dis* 1999;28:895.
21. Terman D, Teitelbaum D. Isoniazid self-poisoning. *Neurology* 1970;20:299.
22. Wason S, Lacouture P, Lovejoy F. Single high-dose pyridoxine treatment for isoniazid overdose. *JAMA* 1981;246:1102.
23. Watson WA, Litovitz TL, Rodgers GC, Klein-Schwartz W, et al. 2002 annual report of the American Association of Poison Control Centers Toxic Exposure Surveillance System. *Am J Emerg Med* 2003;21:353.
24. Weber W, Hein D. Clinical pharmacokinetics of isoniazid. *Clin Pharmacokinet* 1979;4:401.
25. Wood J, Peesker S. A correlation between changes in GABA metabolism and isonicotinic acid hydrazide-induced seizures. *Brain Res* 1972;45:489.

CHAPTER 297
Organophosphate and Carbamate Insecticides

Jeanmarie Perrone

Organophosphates (OP) and carbamates are most commonly encountered during their use as pesticides (Table 297.1). Human exposures most often occur inadvertently in the agricultural setting or from intentional ingestion of products used to control pests around the home. OPs are a very common cause of completed suicide attempts in developing countries such as India (9). World health statistics estimate that 3 million serious pesticide poisonings occur worldwide annually (7). Rarely, pesticide residues on crops have led to multiperson outbreaks of cholinergic poisoning (6). Unintentional pediatric and occasional adult exposures occur when these toxic products are left in open or unmarked containers and are ingested. Poison center data reveal that at least 2,600 patients were evaluated in health care facilities and four deaths occurred secondary to OP or carbamate exposures in 2002 (19).

OP and carbamates are also used as pharmaceuticals and chemical warfare agents (see Chapter 331, "Chemical Warfare Agents"). Malathion (Ovide), used topically for the treatment of head lice, and echothiophate a long-acting topical miotic utilized in the treatment of glaucoma, and the nerve gas agents soman, sarin, and tabun are OPs. Pyridostigmine and neostigmine, used for myasthenia gravis, and rivastigmine, galantamine and donepezil, newer agents for treatment of Alzheimer disease, are carbamates.

TABLE 297.1. Toxicity of Selected Carbamate and Organophosphate Insecticides (17)

Name	Trade Names	Carbamate (C) or Organophosphate (OP)	Toxicity High (H) Moderate (M)
Aldicarb	Temik	C	High
Carbofuran	Furadan, Crisfuran	C	High
Aminocarb	Matacil	C	High
Methomyl	Lannate, Nudrin	C	High
Promecarb	Carbamult	C	Moderate
Methiocarb	Mesurol, Draza	C	Moderate
Propoxur	Baygon, Aprocarb	C	Moderate
Pirimicarb	Pirimor, Aphox, Rapid	C	Moderate
Carbaryl	Sevin, Dicarbam	C	Moderate
Bufencarb	Bux, Metalkamate	C	Moderate
Tetraethyl pyrophosphate (TEPP)	Bladan, Kilmite 40, Tetron, Vapatone	OP	High
Mevinphos	Phosdrin, Duraphos	OP	High
Sulfotep	Bladafum, Dithione, Thiotepp	OP	High
Methyl parathion	E-601, Penncap-M	OP	High
Ethyl parathion	Parathion, E-605, Thiophos	OP	High
Methamidophos	Monitor	OP	High
Bomyl	Swat	OP	High
Leptophos	Phosvel	OP	Moderate
Dichlorvos	DDVP, Vapona, No Pest Strip	OP	Moderate
Chlorpyrifos	Lorsban, Dursban, Brodan	OP	Moderate
Fenthion	Baytex, Entex, Tiguvon	OP	Moderate
Dichlofenthion	Mobilawn, Bromex, Nemacide	OP	Moderate
Diazinon	Spectracide, Diazide, Gardentox	OP	Moderate
Trichlorfon	Dylox, Dipterex, Neguvon	OP	Moderate
Acephate	Orthene	OP	Moderate
Merphos	Folex, Easy off-D	OP	Moderate
Malathion	Cythion	OP	Moderate
Temephos	Abate, Abathion	OP	Moderate
Ronnel	Korlan, Fenchlorphos	OP	Moderate

OPs and carbamates are rapidly absorbed from the skin and respiratory and gastrointestinal (GI) tracts. They are acetylcholinesterase inhibitors and potentiate acetylcholine at sites of cholinergic neurotransmission in the parasympathetic, sympathetic, and central nervous systems (CNS) and at the neuromuscular junction (Figs. 297.1 and 297.2). OPs inactivate the acetylcholinesterase enzyme by phosphorylation; the resulting enzyme complex is stable, and thus binding is irreversible. Carbamates bind to the acetylcholinesterase enzyme but form an unstable complex, which spontaneously hydrolyzes within 24 to 48 hours, regenerating acetylcholinesterase and limiting toxicity. Acetylcholine released into the synapse in the presence of either type of acetylcholinesterase inhibitor is prevented from degradation, and excess acetylcholine activates postsynaptic receptors.

Cholinesterase inhibition usually occurs rapidly. Following acute exposure, a 50% decrease in enzyme activity is associated with mild symptoms, and a 90% decrease with severe poisoning.

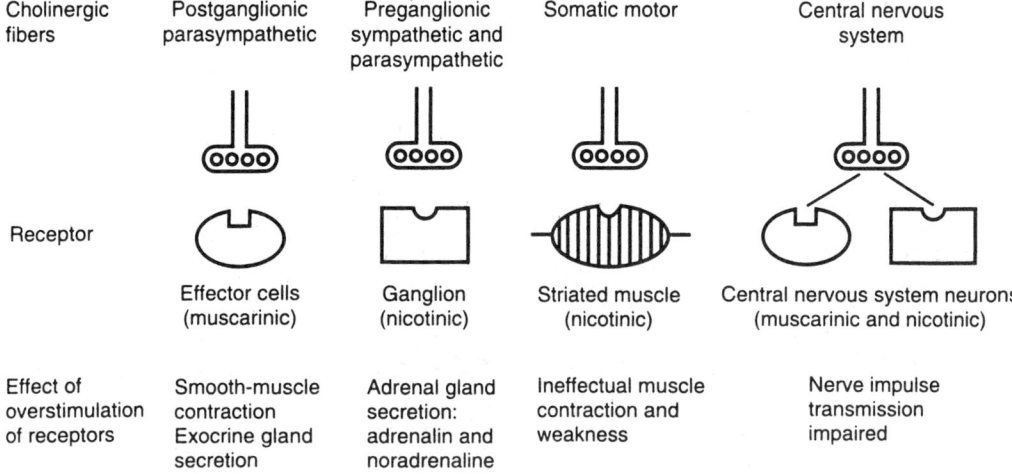

Figure 297.1. Acetylcholine (depicted as open circles) released by cholinergic nerve endings combines with four different groups of receptors to produce characteristic effects in different organs. OP poisoning leads to decreased destruction of acetylcholine and overstimulation of the receptors (cholinergic crisis). (From Bardin PG, van Eeden SF, Moolman JA, et al. Organophosphate and carbamate poisoning. *Arch Intern Med* 1994;154:1435, with permission.)

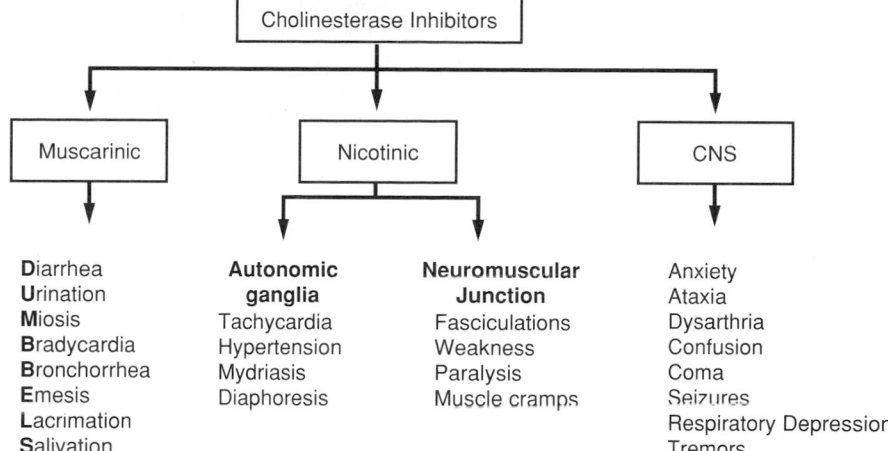

Figure 297.2. Cholinergic toxidrome.

Plasma or pseudocholinesterase activity may remain depressed for days to weeks, and red blood cell (RBC) cholinesterase activity for 1 to 3 months following organophosphate exposure. In carbamate poisoning, activity may return to normal within minutes to hours.

CLINICAL PRESENTATION

Acute Toxicity

Patients with acute organophosphate poisoning are often critically ill (2,10,13,16). Cholinergic findings (see Fig. 297.2) may be subtle or obvious, depending on the exposure. Vital signs may be unstable, including depressed respirations and heart rate. Respiratory failure may result from excess pulmonary and oropharyngeal secretions, CNS depression and neuromuscular weakness. CNS toxicity may include altered mental status, confusion, lethargy, seizures, and coma. Overstimulation of postsynaptic receptors at the neuromuscular junction results initially in fasciculations and then muscle fatigue and weakness. In the autonomic nervous system, parasympathetic effects predominate as muscarinic cholinergic nerve fibers are stimulated. The mnemonic DUMBBELS (see Fig. 297.2) is helpful in describing the cholinergic muscarinic findings as a result of parasympathetic stimulation of hollow viscous organs and glands. Sympathetic ganglia effects may result in hypertension and tachycardia. Diaphoresis occurs commonly as a result of direct cholinergic stimulation of sympathetic sweat glands. Pancreatitis and rhabdomyolysis are relatively common complications.

The severity and extent of cholinergic toxicity is dependent on dose, agent, and route of exposure. The onset of symptoms is generally most rapid after inhalation and most delayed after skin exposure. Symptoms have been reported as early as 5 minutes after ingestion but usually occur by 12 to 24 hours. Highly fat soluble agents such as fenthion may cause delayed or prolonged toxicity (4,12). Generally, toxicity is less with carbamate exposures. The OPs are a widely variable class, and some may produce protean cholinergic effects, although others may produce selected toxicity. The nerve gas agents (Sarin, Soman) characteristically produce more CNS effects and fewer peripheral signs of cholinergic toxicity. Therefore, muscarinic findings (DUMBBELS) may be absent in patients with significant nerve gas poisoning. The elderly are at especially high risk for complications, including aspiration and pneumonia, severe neurologic toxicity, and prolonged weakness. Patients with myasthenia gravis who intentionally or inadvertently develop toxicity from their own medications, such as pyridostigmine, may develop more severe cholinergic findings as a result of their compromised acetylcholine neurotransmission at baseline.

Intermediate Syndrome

In 1987, a syndrome of recrudescent organophosphate neurotoxicity was described in a series of patients 1 to 4 days following acute organophosphate poisoning (18). Although all had initially improved following therapy with atropine and pralidoxime, cranial nerve palsies and a progressive truncal and proximal limb weakness became evident; 40% of the affected patients required intubation. Symptoms lasted 5 to 15 days, and one patient died. Subsequent prospective studies have demonstrated that this syndrome occurs frequently following exposure to highly fat soluble OPs and is related to prolonged cholinesterase inhibition (5). It is proposed that redistribution of OPs from tissue reservoirs causes recrudescent toxicity at a time when atropine and oxime (pralidoxime) therapy have been completed (3).

Delayed Peripheral Neuropathy

A distinct polyneuropathy may occur 1 to 3 weeks following organophosphate exposure. This syndrome was first described in 1930, when an estimated 40,000 persons became symptomatic as a result of contamination of an alcoholic beverage by tri-ortho-cresyl phosphate (15). The debilitating distal flaccid paresis resulting from the neuropathy was termed the Jamaican ginger paralysis after the contaminated beverage, a ginger extract imported from Jamaica. The neuropathy resulting from organophosphate-induced inhibition of the enzyme, neuropathy target esterase, is characterized by axonal degeneration followed by myelin degeneration, with the large distal neurons affected first (1). Patients with underlying medical problems such as alcoholism or nutritional deprivation may be at higher risk for developing delayed peripheral neuropathy. Recovery is incomplete in many cases, and motor symptoms are often persistent.

DIFFERENTIAL DIAGNOSIS

Identical manifestations can be seen in patients poisoned with direct-acting cholinergic agonists such as bethanechol or pilocarpine. Digitalis, clonidine, calcium- or β-receptor antagonist poisoning, myocardial ischemia, or conduction disease should be considered in patients who present with altered mental status and bradycardia, without other obvious signs of cholinergic toxicity. Miosis, bradycardia, lethargy, and respiratory depression are also seen in opioid poisoning. Lethargy and prominent sialorrhea or salivation may occur with certain neuroleptic agents, such as clozapine and risperidone. OP-induced bronchorrhea and pulmonary edema may be difficult to distinguish from any other etiology of pulmonary edema. Patients with nicotine poisoning as a result of ingestion of tobacco products or harvesting wet tobacco may have similar findings, including vomiting, diarrhea, fasciculations, weakness, altered mental status, and autonomic instability.

Pseudocholinesterase activity can be reduced in advanced liver disease, chronic alcoholism, dermatomyositis, malnutrition, and pregnancy, and following exposure to birth control pills, carbon disulfide, ciguatoxin, and organic mercury compounds. Activity is genetically lower than the norm in about 3% of the population. RBC cholinesterase activity is reduced in those with decreased red cell lifespan, such as in patients with hemolytic anemia and sickle cell disease.

EMERGENCY DEPARTMENT EVALUATION

The history should document the amount, time, and route of exposure and the identity of the agent involved if known. A regional poison center can assist in product identification and characterization of anticipated toxicity. Continuous cardiac monitoring and pulse oximetry are crucial because of potential cardiac and respiratory toxicity. The physical examination should focus on the vital signs and assessment of cardiopulmonary and neuromuscular function, especially motor strength and respiratory effort. Cholinergic signs, particularly respiratory tract secretions, should be noted. Arterial blood gas (ABG) analysis and forced vital capacity (FVC) should be obtained to help quantify respiratory dysfunction. An electrocardiogram, chest radiograph, and routine blood work, including complete blood count, electrolytes, blood urea nitrogen, creatinine, glucose, creatine phosphokinase, amylase, and liver function tests, should be obtained on symptomatic patients.

The diagnosis is confirmed by documenting decreased plasma or RBC cholinesterase activity. RBC cholinesterase activity is more specific, but plasma (pseudo) cholinesterase activity tests are less expensive and more widely available. Although results are usually unavailable in a clinically relevant time frame, they can be helpful in cases in which the diagnosis is uncertain and in the evaluation of occupationally exposed patients. Specimens should be obtained prior to the administration of pralidoxime, because this antidote can increase measured enzyme activity. Interpretation of results may be difficult as a result of the variability in baseline values, which are subject to a variety of factors. In some cases (e.g., chronic or occupational exposures), serial activity levels, showing a return to baseline with time, may be necessary. Specific pesticides can also be identified by detecting certain compounds and metabolites in the urine.

EMERGENCY DEPARTMENT MANAGEMENT

Health care providers should wear protective gear when treating patients with potential organophosphate poisoning because significant dermal contamination may be present and can lead to secondary poisoning. Nitrile or neoprene gloves, impervious gowns, masks, and head and shoe covers are recommended. Self-contained breathing devises and chemical suits are necessary for rescuers responding to chemical spills and or nerve agent incidents.

Advanced life-support measures should be instituted as needed. This may require endotracheal intubation by emergency medical services in the field or soon after arrival in the emergency department (ED). Atropine may be initiated prehospital in patients with bronchorrhea and/or bradycardia, because this may be effective in decreasing respiratory compromise. GI and skin decontamination should be undertaken as soon as the patient is stabilized. Activated charcoal is the preferred method for GI decontamination.

Patients who require intubation in the emergency department should undergo a rapid-sequence protocol. The duration of effect of succinylcholine may be much longer than usual as a result of the concomitant inhibition of cholinesterases that degrade succinylcholine (17). An alternative, short-acting, nondepolarizing neuromuscular blocking agent such as mivacurium may be preferable.

Patients with muscarinic findings, particularly excessive pulmonary secretions, should be given intravenous atropine (1–4 mg in adults and 0.02–0.05 mg/kg in children). Atropine acts by competitively blocking acetylcholine at muscarinic receptors, thereby reversing the excessive parasympathetic stimulation. It is only partially effective in treating CNS symptoms and has a variable effect on seizures and altered mental status. It has no effect on nicotinic receptors and, therefore, will not reverse muscle weakness or sympathetic ganglionic effects. Repeated doses of atropine may be needed to decrease bronchorrhea and oropharyngeal secretions. Atropine should be titrated to the drying of secretions, and not to irrelevant end points such as mydriasis or tachycardia. Very often, tachycardia is a result of dyspnea and inadequate atropine dosing. Atropine may be repeated every 5 to 15 minutes, with consideration of an atropine infusion (0.02–0.08 mg/kg/h) if frequent doses are needed. Atropine requirements are highly variable; patients with significant poisoning may require as much as 40 mg/d; one reported case describes a patient requiring 1,000 mg of atropine in a 24-hour period (16).

Any patient who requires treatment with atropine should also receive pralidoxime (2-PAM). Pralidoxime may be infused as a bolus therapy (1–2 g in saline and administered over 30 minutes in adults; 20–40 mg/kg to a maximum of 1 g per dose in children), repeated in 1 to 2 hours if fasciculations are still present, and then given at 6- to 12-hour intervals for 24 to 48 hours. Alternatively, it may be administered as a continuous infusion of 500 mg/h (in adults). Pralidoxime initially binds to cholinesterase enzymes and then to the inhibitor. The inhibitor–pralidoxime complex detaches from the acetylcholinesterase enzyme, returning it to a functional state. Pralidoxime is effective in diminishing nicotinic effects, and it is synergistic with atropine at muscarinic receptors. Improvement in muscle strength is usually noted within 10 to 40 minutes. Although it is not thought to cross the blood–brain barrier, pralidoxime may reverse some CNS effects (8,16). Benzodiazepines may be needed for neurotoxic effects such as agitation and seizures.

Certain OPs have "aging" properties, which refer to their ability to bind permanently to acetylcholinesterase and not respond to pralidoxime. Although many OPs share this capability, aging occurs at different rates. Nerve gas chemical warfare agents age quickly, rapidly becoming resistant to any antidotal intervention (see Chapter 331, "Chemical Warfare Agents"). Because carbamates undergo spontaneous hydrolysis from the acetylcholinesterase enzyme, the need and safety of treating carbamate poisoned patients with 2-PAM has been questioned. Recent data support treating any poisoned patient requiring atropine with 2-PAM, regardless of the anticholinesterase agent (11).

Therapy for the intermediate syndrome includes additional pralidoxime and, possibly, atropine, and supportive care. No specific therapy exists for peripheral neuropathy.

CRITICAL INTERVENTIONS

- Monitor oxygen saturation, evaluate airway patency, and obtain ABGs and FVC to assess oxygenation and ventilation
- Monitor the cardiac rhythm and obtain an ECG
- Administer atropine to patients with increased secretions and bronchospasm
- Intubate early if inadequate improvement with atropine or if significant CNS depression
- Administer pralidoxime to patients who require atropine

DISPOSITION

Patients with an unintentional exposure who remain asymptomatic following at least 6 hours of observation may be discharged home with a family member. Those requiring treatment with atropine or pralidoxime and those with evolving toxicity should be admitted to an intensive care unit (ICU) for close observation and monitoring. If the patient needs to be transferred to an ICU for admission, advance cardiac life-support (ACLS) personnel should accompany the patient. Prophylactic intubation prior to initiating transport may be advisable in patients with borderline respiratory status. Consultation with a regional poison control center or medical toxicologist is advised for all exposures. Even asymptomatic patients need follow-up with their family doctor, because peripheral neuropathy can occur even in the absence of initial cholinergic manifestations (14).

COMMON PITFALLS

✔ Failure to decontaminate the skin of patients with dermal exposures and to take appropriate precautions to prevent secondary exposure to health care workers
✔ Failure to appreciate that tachycardia may be as a result of respiratory dysfunction and to give atropine to patients with tachycardia and dyspnea resulting from excessive respiratory tract secretions or bronchospasm
✔ Failure to appreciate that atropine therapy should be titrated to drying of secretions rather than to heart rate or pupil size, and that doses far exceeding standard ACLS recommendations may be necessary
✔ Failure to treat all patients requiring atropine with pralidoxime to prevent "aging" of the cholinesterase inhibitor-enzyme complex and to decrease atropine requirements
✔ Failure to appreciate that highly fat-soluble OPs may cause delayed, prolonged, or recurrent toxicity

Acknowledgment

The author thanks previous edition chapter author Stephanie B. Abbuhl.

References

1. Abou-Donia MB, Lapadula DM. Mechanisms of organophosphorus ester induced delayed neurotoxicity: type 1 and type II. *Ann Rev Pharmacol Toxicol* 1990;30:405.
2. Bardin PG, van Eeden SF, Moolman JA, et al. Organophosphate and carbamate poisoning. *Arch Intern Med* 1994;154:1433.
3. Benson B, Tolo D, McIntire M. Is the intermediate syndrome in organophosphate poisoning the result of insufficient oxime therapy? [Editorial]. *J Toxicol Clin Toxicol* 1992;30:347.
4. Borowitz SM. Prolonged organophosphate toxicity in a 26-month-old child. *J Pediatr* 1988;112:302–304.
5. De Bleecker J, Van Den Neucker K, Colardyn F. Intermediate syndrome in organophosphorus poisoning: a prospective study. *Crit Care Med* 1993;21:1706–1711.
6. Green MA, Heumann MA, Wehr M, et al. An outbreak of watermelon-borne pesticide toxicity. *Am J Public Health* 1987;77:1431–1434.
7. Jayaratnam J. Acute pesticide poisoning: a major global health problem. *World Health Stat Q* 1990;43:139–144.
8. Lotti M, Becker C. Treatment of acute organophosphate poisoning: evidence of a direct effect on central nervous system by 2-PAM (pyridine-2-aldoxime methyl chloride). *J Toxicol Clin Toxicol* 1982;19:121–127.
9. Malik GM, Mubarik M, Romshoo GJ. Organophosphorous poisoning in the Kashmir Valley 1994–1997. *N Engl J Med* 1998;338:1078.
10. Marrs TC. Organophosphate poisoning. *Pharmacol Ther* 1993;58:51.
11. Mercurio-Zappala M, Hack J, Salvador A, et al. Carbaryl poisoning: 2-PAM or not 2-PAM. *J Toxicol Clin Toxicol* 1998;36:428(abst).
12. Merril D, Milton F. Prolonged toxicity of organophosphate poisoning. *Crit Care Med* 1982;10:550–551.
13. Minton NA, Murray VSG. A review of organophosphate poisoning. *Med Toxicol* 1988;3:350.
14. Moretto A, Lottei M. Poisoning by organophosphorus insecticides and sensory neuropathy. *J Neurol Neurosurg Psychiatry* 1998;64:463–468.
15. Morgan JP. The Jamaica ginger paralysis. *JAMA* 1982;248:1864–1867.
16. Namba T, Nolte C, Jackrel J, et al. Poisoning due to organophosphate insecticide. *Am J Med* 1971;50:475.
17. Selden BS, Curry SC. Prolonged succinylcholine-induced paralysis in organophosphate insecticide poisoning. *Ann Emerg Med* 1987;16:215–217.
18. Senanayake N, Karalliedde L. Neurotoxic effects of organophosphorus insecticides. An intermediate syndrome. *N Engl J Med* 1987;316:761–763.
19. Watson WA, Litovitz TL, Rodgers GC, et al. 2002 Annual report of the American Association of Poison Control Centers Toxic Exposure Surveillance System. *Am J Emerg Med* 2003;21:353–421.

CHAPTER 298
Other Insecticides

William K. Chiang and Richard Y. Wang

Nicotine, the primary alkaloid of tobacco, is a naturally occurring pesticide obtained from *Nicotiana tabacum*, *N. rustica*, and other plants. It is also used in gum, nasal inhalers, and transdermal patches to aid in the cessation of smoking. Nicotine binds to nicotinic cholinergic (acetylcholine) receptors in the sympathetic and parasympathetic ganglion cells, neuromuscular junction, adrenal medulla, and the central nervous system (CNS) (20). An initial transitory stimulation of nicotinic receptors is followed by a more persistent depression and paralysis as a result of desensitization. Clinical symptoms may reflect receptor stimulation, depression, or both.

Absorption occurs through intact skin, the gastrointestinal tract, and the respiratory tree. Nicotine has a pKa of 8.5 and is not well absorbed in the acid milieu of the stomach; alkalinization markedly increases absorption (8). The volume of distribution is approximately 1 L/kg. Protein binding is 20%. Once absorbed, 80% to 90% of the chemical is detoxified into cotinine by the liver and 20% is excreted unchanged by the kidneys. The elimination half-life is 0.8 hours in smokers and 1.3 hours in nonsmokers. Elimination is complete in about 16 hours.

Tobacco leaves contain 1% to 6% nicotine; a cigarette contains 15 to 20 mg of nicotine, with one-fourth remaining in the butt; snuff contains 4.6 to 15.0 mg of nicotine per gram of moist material; chewing tobacco contains 2.5 mg of nicotine per gram of dry material; a cigar contains 15 to 20 mg of nicotine. Nicotine gum (e.g., Nicorette) contains 2 mg of nicotine buffered to a pH of 8.5 to enhance absorption. Transdermal nicotine patches (Habitrol, Nicoderm, Nicotrol, Prostep) release 7 to 21 mg of nicotine per day. However, the total nicotine content may range from 8.3 mg to 114.0 mg per patch. Nicotine nasal spray contains 10 mg of nicotine per mL.

The toxic dose of nicotine varies. As little as 4 mg can cause symptoms; 40 to 60 mg is potentially fatal in an adult. In a small child, 1 mg of nicotine may cause symptoms (10). Ingestion of one cigarette, three cigarette butts, one cigar butt, or any amount of nicotine chewing gum or patch should be considered potentially toxic in a child.

Pyrethrins and pyrethroids are widely used as bug sprays because of their rapid incapacitating ("knock-down") effects on insects. Most are formulated in petroleum distillates for spray applications; many are marketed in pressurized cases. Synergists such as piperonyl butoxide, N-octyl-bicycloheptene dicarbonimide, and sesame oil derivatives are commonly added to inhibit the metabolism of pyrethrins and thus increase their efficiency. Pyrethrins and pyrethroids are also used for the treatment of head lice and scabies and as insect repellents (Table 298.1).

Pyrethrins are naturally occurring insecticides extracted from chrysanthemum flowers; they are esters of pyrethric and chrysanthemic acid (16). Pyrethroids (e.g., permethrin, deltamethrin) are synthetic pyrethrins that are more stable (resist photolysis) in the natural environment and have greater insecticide potency than do pyrethrins. They can be separated into two classes based on their chemical structures: Type II agents contain a cyano group at the a carbon, and type I agents do not (5).

In insects, pyrethrins and pyrethroids rapidly cause death by paralyzing the nervous system. They inactivate sodium channels in nerve axons by binding and prolonging the opened state. Other potential mechanisms of toxicity include the inhibition of adenosine triphosphatases and direct effects on membrane integrity. Type II pyrethroids also antagonize inhibitory chloride channels at the GABA binding site (5). Because type II pyrethroids cause more prolonged opening of the sodium channels, they are generally more toxic than type I agents.

These compounds are rapidly degraded and leave almost no residuum in the environment. They are considered less toxic to mammals than any other major class of insecticides. Human toxicity is limited by factors such as a large first-pass effect by the liver, poor bioavailability, and rapid metabolic breakdown by ester hydrolysis, followed by hepatic oxidation (14). Furthermore, the diversity of the α-subunits of the sodium channels in humans are less susceptible to pyrethroid toxicity than insects (14). Ingestion of amounts up to 5 mg/kg is unlikely to cause significant toxicity. The toxic oral dose is estimated to be more than 100 to

---

TABLE 298.1. Common Pyrethrin/Pyrethroid Preparations

SHAMPOOS FOR HEAD LICE

Elimite
Nix-Creme Rinse
Rid

ENVIRONMENTAL SPRAYS

Ambush	Pounce
Anvil	Pydrin
Atroban	Pynamin
Cesso 7c	Rondo
Dragon	Scourge
Insectiban	Time Mist
	Torpedo

TABLE 298.2. Chlorinated Hydrocarbon Insecticides

Insecticide	Brand/Trade Name
Aldrin	Aldrex, Aldrite, Drinox
Chlorobenzilate	Acaraben, Folbex, Kop-Mite
Chlordane	1068, Belt, Chlor Kill, Niran
Chlordecone	Depone, Tat Ant Trap
DDT	Anofex, Dinocide, Pentech
Dieldrin	Albit, Dorytox, Octalox
Endrin	Agrine, Endrex, Hexadrin
Heptachlor	Velaicol, 53-CS-17
Lindane	Agrocide, Isotox, Kwell
Methoxychlor	DMDT, Marlate, Moxie
Mirex	Dechlorane, Ferriamide
Toxaphene	Alltox, Camphoclor, Motox

1,000 mg/kg, with a lethal dose estimated to be 10 to 100 g (3). Synergists also have low human toxicity (7).

Organochlorine insecticides are low-molecular-weight, fat-soluble aliphatic, aromatic, and complex hydrocarbons that contain chlorine (Table 298.2) (7,15,19). The U.S. Environmental Protection Agency banned the use of many of these pesticides in the 1970s and 1980s because they are stored indefinitely in human tissue and are felt to be ecologically harmful (19). Chlordane and toxaphene are still available, but their use is restricted. Other available agents include methoxychlor, dicofol, and the miticide and scabicide lindane (γ hexachlorocyclohexane).

Organochlorines can be absorbed from the skin, lungs, and GI tract. Enteral absorption is efficient and increased in the presence of animal or vegetable fat. To a lesser extent, they are absorbed across pulmonary membranes, but only 10% or less of a dermally applied dose (e.g., lindane) is absorbed. Different compounds exhibit different tissue-storage and hepatic elimination rates. Many (e.g., chlordane, dieldrin, and heptachlor) can induce hepatic enzymes.

As the body stores decrease, their half-lives markedly increase, as a result of either altered lipoprotein binding or lessened chemical concentration gradient across body compartments. It may require months to years to eliminate mirex, kepone, DDT, and β-hexachlorocyclohexane; weeks to months for aldrin, dieldrin, heptachlor, and hexachlorobenzene; and hours to several days for endrin, chlordane, toxaphene, endosulfan, methoxychlor, and chlorobenzilate. Most residents of the United States have detectable organochlorine residues in their bodies, especially in fat. These compounds are excreted in the feces and can be found in breast milk.

Toxicity is due primarily to interference with the axonal transmission of nerve impulses. Organochlorines interfere with the normal flow of sodium and potassium ions across the axon membrane as nerve impulses pass (19). Unlike organophosphate (OP) insecticides, they do not depress cholinesterase enzymes.

The acute toxic potential of organochlorines varies with the different compounds and their rates and routes of absorption. The highest risk occurs from endrin, dieldrin, aldrin, chlordane, and toxaphene (15). Intermediate-risk products include kepone, endosulfan, heptachlor, mirex, and DDT. The lowest risk products are methoxychlor, perthan, kelthane, chlorobenzilate, and hexachlorobenzene. Lindane is potentially toxic with multiple applications to the skin (11). Dermal and inhalational exposures most commonly occur in workers who spray organochlorine insecticides. Oral exposure may result from the ingestion of contaminated food or drinking water (4). The estimated oral lethal dose in adults is 3 to 7 g for aldrin, 6 g for chlordane (less than 2 g can cause stupor and seizures), 1 to 5 g for dieldrin, and 10 to 30 g for lindane (as little as 1.6 g can cause seizures in children) (15).

CLINICAL PRESENTATION

Poisoning from nicotine can occur from any of the following: exposure to nicotine sulfate insecticides; percutaneous absorption of nicotine in tobacco harvesters who pick and brush up against wet tobacco leaves (green tobacco sickness) (6); ingestion of tobacco products, such as cigarettes, snuff, chewing tobacco, and cigars; chewing or ingestion of nicotine chewing gum; and improper use or ingestion of nicotine patches (24). Infants and young children are most susceptible to nicotine poisoning because of their small body size and the lack of tolerance. Similarly, tobacco harvesters are more likely to be symptomatic in the beginning of the harvesting season and workweek because of the lack of nicotine tolerance. Nonsmokers are also more susceptible to nicotine toxicity than smokers (22). Many nonsmoking tobacco harvesters resort to tobacco chewing as a mean to develop nicotine tolerance. Overall, nicotine-related fatalities are rare because of its decreasing usage as a pesticide.

Onset of toxicity is rapid and can be seen within 15 minutes of exposure. Initial signs and symptoms include nausea, vomiting, salivation, bronchorrhea, abdominal pain, and diarrhea from parasympathetic stimulation; and tachycardia, hypertension, and diaphoresis as result of sympathetic and adrenal stimulation. Early CNS effects include dizziness, headache, confusion, agitation, incoordination, and seizures. Muscular fasciculations may result from neuromuscular junction stimulation.

As the symptoms progress, hypotonia, muscle paralysis, respiratory failure, coma, bradycardia, and hypotension may ensue (1,13). Because of both stimulatory and inhibitory effects on multiple systems, the signs and symptoms vary by the time, dose, and route of exposure. In severe cases, such as nicotine pesticide poisoning, the progression from stimulation to inhibition of the various systems may be rapid (10).

In mild nicotine poisoning, symptoms can last for several hours. In severe cases, clinical toxicity can endure for 18 to 24 hours or more. Severe cases involve seizures and coma within 30 minutes, with respiratory arrest and death within 1 hour or less, especially with concentrated nicotine products. Patients who survive the first 4 hours usually recover fully. Radiographic and electrocardiographic (ECG) findings are nonspecific. Nicotine can be detected in the urine by chromatographic drug assays. Leukocytosis and glycosuria may be noted.

Direct toxicity from pyrethrins and pyrethroids is uncommon. Adverse effects, when they occur, are usually as a result of allergic hypersensitivity and include bronchospasm, vasomotor rhinitis, contact dermatitis, and, rarely, anaphylaxis (23). Following inhalation, the most common presentation is a stuffy nose with clear discharge and a "scratchy" throat. In rare cases, sudden bronchospasm, swelling of the laryngeal mucosa, and shock (anaphylaxis) can occur. Patients allergic to ragweed have a higher risk of developing allergic reactions to pyrethrins. Synthetic pyrethroids are less likely to cause these reactions than natural pyrethrins.

Direct dermal exposure to pyrethrins can produce a contact dermatitis consisting of redness, blisters, burning, stinging, and numbness. Ocular exposure to hydrocarbon propellants can cause eye irritation and corneal abrasions. Large exposure to type II pyrethroids can cause tremors, salivation, paresthesia, ataxia, choreoathetosis, and seizures. Similar exposure to type I agents can result in tremors, agitation, and hyperthermia (5).

The onset of symptoms following exposure to organochlorine insecticides may vary from minutes to hours, depending on the route and method of exposure and the physicochemical properties of the agent (4). Nausea, vomiting, and diarrhea can occur as soon as 45 minutes after acute ingestion. Initial CNS effects include apprehension, headache, dizziness, tremors, ataxia, and disorientation. Stupor, coma, and seizures with respiratory depression may be seen in severe cases. Dysrhythmias may result from increased myocardial sensitivity to catecholamines.

Aspiration of formulations containing a petroleum distillate can result in a chemical pneumonitis. CNS toxicity, including seizures, can also occur in children following prolonged or excessive topical lindane exposures during the treatment of lice or scabies (11). In severe cases, potential complications include lactic acidosis, rhabdomyolysis, and disseminated intravascular coagulation.

Chronic exposure to organochlorines can cause hepatomegaly. Extensive or prolonged dermal contact can result in skin irritation. Chronic ingestion of hexachlorobenzene has been associated with cutaneous porphyria. Cases of leukemia have been associated with the use of chlordane or heptachlor to control termites in homes.

DIFFERENTIAL DIAGNOSIS

Without a history of exposure, there are no pathognomonic signs of nicotine poisoning. It could be confused with acetylcholinesterase inhibitor poisoning, such as OP or carbamate insecticides, and carbamate drugs (edrophonium, physostigmine). In nicotine poisoning, however, there is no depression of the red blood cell cholinesterase.

Direct-acting cholinomimetic agents such as bethanechol, carbachol, methacholine, and pilocarpine can also produce cholinergic effects similar to those of nicotine. However, because these agents have minimal effects on nicotinic receptors (except for carbachol), they produce minimal or no sympathetic or muscular symptoms (20). Central and peripheral sympatholytics (a-adrenergic and β-adrenergic receptor blockers, clonidine, guanabenz, topical decongestant imidazoline derivatives, and calcium blockers) can mimic the later stages of nicotine poisoning. These agents will not produce any muscarinic symptoms or neuromuscular weakness. Tree tobacco (*Nicotiana glauca*), native to the temperate regions of America, contains the alkaloid anabasine, an isomer of nicotine that can cause similar symptoms (12). Other substances to consider are the insect repellent diethyltoluamide; Veratrum and sabadilla plants; Clitocybe and Inocybe mushroom species; and poison hemlock (*Conium maculatum*).

Pyrethrins and pyrethroids should be included in the differential diagnosis of patients who present with an apparent hypersensitivity reaction of the skin or respiratory system when exposed to flora, insecticides, or insect bites. Because almost all of the insecticides containing these compounds are in a hydrocarbon base, the risk of hydrocarbon pneumonitis must be considered in humans ingesting these products.

Acute organochlorine insecticide poisoning must be distinguished from any condition that produces "gastroenteritis" with an altered mental status, especially ataxia, tremors, and seizures. CNS disease, drug withdrawal, stimulant intoxication (e.g., from sympathomimetics, xanthines, anticholinergics, hallucinogens, and isoniazid), and infectious etiologies should be considered. In locations outside of the United States, the clinician must be more aware of organochlorine exposures because these insecticides are still being used (17).

EMERGENCY DEPARTMENT EVALUATION

The history should document the time, agent, dose, route, intent, and duration of exposure and the nature and course of symptoms. A complete physical examination should be performed, with particular attention to assessing cardiovascular, respiratory, and neurologic function. Patients with vital sign abnormalities should have an ECG. Symptomatic patients should have cardiac and oxygen saturation monitoring. Chest radiographs, oxygen saturation measurement or arterial blood gas analysis, and pulmonary function tests can help to assess respiratory function and possible aspiration in patients with wheezing, dyspnea, cough, and fever. Blood chemistries and hematologic analysis should be obtained based on clinical severity.

No specific laboratory tests are diagnostic. The presence of nicotine in the urine of a nonsmoker is supportive. Plasma nicotine levels are not useful. Chlorinated hydrocarbons can be measured in the serum by using gas chromatography, but levels are not useful for clinical management (9). However, in a patient with a suspicious exposure for DDT, a high DDT to DDE ratio confirms that the exposure was recent (18).

EMERGENCY DEPARTMENT MANAGEMENT

GI, skin, and eye decontamination should be performed. Activated charcoal (AC) is the preferred method of GI decontamination. Pyrethrins and pyrethroids are lipophilic, so milk, cream, or substances that contain animal or vegetable fats should not be administered. Except for recent ingestion (less than an hour) of large quantities of a nicotine pesticide, gastric aspiration or lavage would not likely provide additional benefit. Because emesis is usually rapid and spontaneous, ipecac is not advised. Additionally, seizures and coma can occur rapidly, and emesis increases the risk of aspiration. If present, any transdermal patches should be removed.

Exposed skin areas should be washed with soap and water. Exposed eyes should be irrigated with copious amounts of water for 15 minutes. Powder contaminating the skin should first be vacuumed off. Contaminated clothing should be removed, and the skin, hair, and nails scrubbed.

The patient should be closely monitored for the first few hours after exposure. Supportive care, including oxygen, endotracheal intubation, and assisted ventilation, should be instituted as necessary. Intravenous access and cardiac monitoring are indicated for all but mild intoxications. Seizures should be treated with intravenous benzodiazepines such as diazepam (for adults, 5–10 mg initially, repeated every 5–10 minutes as necessary, up to 30 mg; for children, 0.25–0.4 mg/kg per dose) or lorazepam (0.05–0.1 mg/kg; may be repeated twice every 15 minutes as necessary). If seizures cannot be controlled with diazepam or lorazepam, a barbiturate (such as phenobarbital or pentobarbital) or propofol may be given. Phenytoin may be less effective than barbiturates and may actually increase the incidence of seizures in organochloride insecticide poisoning (21).

Excess parasympathetic stimulation (e.g., marked bronchial secretions) from nicotine and type II pyrethroids can be controlled by atropine (Adults, 0.5–1 mg intravenously, repeated every 5 minutes as necessary; Children, 0.01–0.02 mg/kg intravenously). Hypotension should be treated initially with administration of intravenous fluids; if it fails, dopamine or norepinephrine may be added. Artificial ventilation and oxygen therapy may be necessary. Mecamylamine (Inversine), an older antihypertensive agent, is a specific nicotine antagonist; it is available only in tablets, however, and is not a practical form of therapy in a patient who is vomiting, convulsing, or hypotensive.

Anaphylaxis should be treated as usual (see Chapter 131, "Anaphylaxis"). The management of hydrocarbon aspiration is supportive (see Chapter 310, "Hydrocarbons"). Respiratory distress as a result of bronchospasm is managed with inhaled bronchodilators and humidified oxygen. Parenteral administration of adrenergic amines (e.g., epinephrine) is not recommended in organochlorine insecticide poisoning because myocardial irritability may be enhanced. Contact dermatitis may be treated with topical corticosteroids.

Because organochlorine compounds have an extensive enterohepatic recirculation, repeat doses of AC are recommended to enhance their elimination. Multiple doses of cholestyramine resin are also effective, but cholestyramine is less well tolerated than charcoal. Extracorporeal procedures are not effective in enhancing organochlorine elimination. Multiple-dose charcoal (MDAC) has not been evaluated in nicotine and pyrethrin poisoning, nor have hemodialysis and hemoperfusion.

CRITICAL INTERVENTIONS

- Establish i.v. access and institute cardiac monitoring
- Secure the airway and assist ventilation as necessary in patients with neurotoxicity
- Administer benzodiazepines, and if necessary, barbiturates and propofol for seizures
- Administer atropine to treat excess parasympathetic stimulation
- Treat hypersensitivity reactions to pyrethrins/pyrethroids the same as any other allergic reaction

DISPOSITION

Patients who remain or become asymptomatic after a 6-hour period of observation following an acute exposure may be discharged with appropriate follow-up. Patients with allergic reactions can usually be discharged after treatment. Those with chronic organochlorine insecticide exposures can generally be treated as outpatients. All others should be admitted to the hospital, observed, and treated supportively. Because the cardiorespiratory system requires monitoring, intensive care unit admission is advised. If such facilities are unavailable, the patient should be transferred. Advanced life-support measures and anticonvulsants should be available during transport. If necessary, consultation can be obtained by calling a regional poison control center (1-800-222-1222) or the National Pesticide Telecommunications Network (1-800-858-7378). If the exposure occurred at the workplace, the proper health agency should be notified to prevent further occurrences.

COMMON PITFALLS

- ✔ Failure to discover a nicotine patch unintentionally stuck to the skin of an infant or toddler with altered mental status because they were not completely undressed
- ✔ Failure to properly decontaminate patients with dermal exposures
- ✔ Failure to diagnose and treat respiratory failure, the primary cause of death in nicotine poisoning
- ✔ Failure to appreciate that administering antacids for GI symptoms may increase the absorption of ingested nicotine
- ✔ Failure to recognize and treat anaphylactic reactions from pyrethrins/pyrethroids
- ✔ Failure to consider the possibility of aspiration (hydrocarbon) pneumonitis in patients with respiratory symptoms after ingestion

✔ Mistaking organochlorine insecticides for OP insecticides (and vice versa), resulting in incorrect treatment

✔ Failure to administer MDAC for organochlorine insecticides ingestions

Acknowledgment

We thank Ronald B. Mack for his contribution to the previous edition of this chapter.

References

1. Borys DJ, Setzer DJ, Ling LJ. CNS depression after ingestion of tobacco. *Vet Hum Toxicol* 1988;30(1):21.
2. Boulton M, Stanbury M, Wade D, et al. Nicotine poisoning after ingestion of contaminated ground beef—Michigan 2003. *MMWR* 2003;52:413.
3. Casida JE, Kimmel EC, Elliott M, et al. Oxidative metabolism of pyrethrins in mammals. *Nature* 1971;230:326.
4. Chugh SN, Dhawan R, Agrawal N, et al. Endosulfan poisoning in Northern India: a report of 18 cases. *Int J Clin Pharmacol Ther* 1998;36:474.
5. Dorman DC, Beasley R. Neurotoxicology of pyrethrin and pyrethroid insecticides. *Vet Hum Toxicol* 1991;33:238.
6. Gehlbach SH, Williams WA, Perry LD, et al. Green tobacco sickness. *JAMA* 1974;229:14.
7. Hayes WJ Jr. Pesticides studied in man. Baltimore, MD: Lippincott, Williams & Wilkins, 1982.
8. Ivey KJ, Trigg EJ. Absorption of nicotine in the human stomach and its effect on gastric ion fluxes and potential difference. *Am J Dig Dis* 1978;23:809.
9. Kutz FW, Strassman SC, Sperling JF, et al. A fatal chlordane poisoning. *J Clin Toxicol* 1983;20:167.
10. Lavoie FW, Harris TM. Fatal nicotine ingestion. *J Emerg Med* 1991;9:133.
11. Lee B, Groth P. Scabies: transcutaneous poisoning during treatment. *Pediatrics* 1977;59:643.
12. Mellick LB, Makowski T, Mellick GA, et al. Neuromuscular blockade after ingestion of tree tobacco (Nicotiana glauca). *Ann Emerg Med* 1999;34:101.
13. Mensch AR, Holden M. Nicotine overdose after a single piece of nicotine gum. *Chest* 1984;86:801.
14. Miyamoto J. Degradation, metabolism and toxicity of synthetic pyrethroids. *Environ Health Perspect* 1976;14:15.
15. Morgan DP. Solid organochlorine pesticides. In: *Recognition and management of pesticide poisoning*. Publication EPA-540/9–80–005. Washington, DC: US Environmental Protection Agency, 1982:14.
16. Ngowi AV, Maeda DN, Partanen TJ. Assessment of the ability of health care providers to treat and prevent adverse health effects of pesticides in agricultural areas of Tanzania. *Int J Occup Med Environ Health* 2001;14:349.
17. Radomski JL, Astolfi E, Deichmann WB, Rey AA. Blood levels of organochlorine pesticides in Argentina: occupationally and nonoccupationally exposed adults, children and newborn infants. *Toxicol Appl Pharmacol* 1971;20:186.
18. Ray DE. Pesticides derived from plants and other organisms. In: Hayes WJ Jr, Law ER, eds. *Handbook of pesticide toxicology*. San Diego: Academic Press, 1991:585.
19. Sharp DS, Eskenazi B, Harrison R, et al. Delayed health hazards of pesticide exposure. *Annu Rev Publ Health* 1986;8:441.
20. Taylor P. Agents acting at the neuromuscular junction and autonomic ganglia. In: Hardman JG, Limbird LE, Molinoff PB, et al, eds. *Goodman & Gilman's: the pharmacological basis of therapeutics*, 9th ed. New York: McGraw-Hill, 1996:192.
21. Tilson HA, Hong JS, Mactutus CF. Effects of 5,5 diphenylhydantoin on neurobehavioral toxicity of organochlorine pesticides and permethrin. *J Pharmacol Exp Ther* 1985;233:285.
22. Trape-Cardoso M, Bracker A, Grey M, et al: Shade tobacco and green tobacco sickness in Connecticut. *J Occup Environ Med* 2003;45:656.
23. Wax PM, Hoffman RS. Fatality associated with inhalation of a pyrethrin shampoo. *J Toxicol Clin Toxicol* 1994;32:457.
24. Woolf A, Burkhart K, Caraccio T, et al. Self-poisoning among adults using multiple transdermal nicotine patches. *J Toxicol Toxicol* 1996;34:691.

CHAPTER 299
Rodenticides

Richard D. Shih and Robert S. Hoffman

A large number of chemically distinct compounds with varied mechanisms of action and toxicities are utilized as rodenticides (Table 299.1). Fortunately, medically significant, unintentional rodenticide exposures are uncommon in the United States. Most occur in children, especially those under 6 years old, involve an oral anticoagulant and result in minimal or no toxicity (16,20,22,24). Adults with intentional ingestions, however, often develop significant morbidity and mortality.

Alpha-naphthylthiourea (ANTU) causes pulmonary toxicity but its mechanism of action is unknown.

Oral anticoagulants are the most commonly used rodenticides in America (5,8,24). They are either hydroxycoumarin or indandione derivatives. Toxicity results from inhibition of the cyclic regeneration of vitamin K, a cofactor required for the activation of coagulation factors II, VII, IX, and X (23). Although vitamin K depletion occurs almost immediately, no anticoagulant effect is seen until the activity of at least one clotting factor is diminished to below 25% of normal (8). Because factor VII has the shortest half-life among the clotting factors affected ($t^1/_2 = 5$ hours), at least three half-lives (15 hours) are usually required before any toxicity is manifested.

Conventional anticoagulant rodenticides contain low concentrations of warfarin (0.025%–0.05% or 100 to 200 mg in a pound of bait). These products were designed to kill rodents who ingest this bait daily over a period of several weeks. Their widespread use resulted in rodents becoming resistant to their effects. Thus, higher-potency agents (superwarfarins), which

---

TABLE 299.1.   Rodenticides

HIGHLY TOXIC

(LD_{50} <50 mg/kg in rats)
Arsenic
Oral anticoagulants ("superwarfarin" types)
Sodium monofluoracetate
Strychnine
Tetramine
Thallium
Vacor
Yellow phosphorus
Zinc phosphide

MODERATELY TOXIC

(LD_{50} 50–500 mg/kg in rats)
α-Naphthylthiourea
Cholecalciferol

LOW TOXICITY

(LD_{50} 500–5000 mg/kg in rats)
Norbormide
Red squill
Oral anticoagulants ("non-superwarfarin" types)

Adapted from Goldfrank L, Flomembaum N, Weisman RS. Rodenticides. *Hosp Physician* 1981;17:87.

cause prolonged coagulopathy ingestions of smaller doses, were developed.

Arsenic compounds, used more commonly in the past, were a leading cause of rodenticide-related deaths in the 1950s and 1960s. Professional exterminators may still have access to this compound depending on local laws. Arsenic causes rapid onset of toxicity by combining with and inhibiting sulfhydryl-containing enzymes (see Chapter 305, "Arsenic and Mercury").

Cholecalciferol is a vitamin D analog.

Cholinesterase inhibitors include organophosphate (OP) and carbamate compounds, which are used as primarily are insecticides (see Chapter 297, "Organophosphate and Carbamate Insecticides"). Although they are not sanctioned for use as rodenticides in the United States, foreign manufacturers may use them for this purpose, and these products may reach the United States (14).

Norbormide is relatively nontoxic in humans, but, in rodents, it causes diffuse vasoconstriction and ischemia. Although the mechanism is not entirely understood, rodent smooth muscle has a specific norbormide receptor that, when stimulated, leads to these effects.

Red squill is a cardiac glycoside derived from the plant Urginea maritima. Its toxicity relates to its ability to block sodium–potassium-ATPase similar to digoxin. This toxin is poorly absorbed in humans because of its potent emetic effects. In rodents, however, whose vomiting mechanism is less well developed, the toxin is fairly effective.

Sodium monofluoroacetate (SMFA) is a white, odorless, tasteless, water-soluble salt typically available as a powder. Once absorbed, SMFA (and the closely related compound fluoroacetamide) rapidly enters the Krebs cycle, in which it is converted to fluorocitric acid, which inhibits the Krebs cycle, blocking aerobic metabolism.

Strychnine, a natural alkaloid derived from the native Indian tree *Strychnos nux-vomica*, has been used as a rodenticide since the 1600s. It is a potent neurotoxin that acts by competitively inhibiting glycine at postsynaptic receptors. Because glycine is the predominant inhibitory neurotransmitter in the spinal cord, its inhibition results in muscular hyperexcitability.

Tetramine is not sanctioned for use as a rodenticide in the United States. However, it is utilized for this purpose in Asia. Tetramine is an extremely potent picrotoxin-like agent that blocks γ-aminobutyric acid receptors in the brain.

Thallium is an odorless, tasteless, highly toxic heavy metal. Although it can penetrate intact skin, it is more readily absorbed when ingested. Thallium, like arsenic, binds to and inhibits sulfhydryl-containing enzymes. Unlike arsenic, however, it preferentially affects mitochondria.

When first introduced, Vacor was thought to have no human toxicity. After numerous cases of severe poisoning occurred, it was voluntarily withdrawn from the market in 1979. Vacor is selectively toxic to pancreatic β islet cells, producing a chemically induced form of insulin-dependent diabetes mellitus. The exact mechanism for the islet cell destruction is unclear, but it may be as a result of Vacor's ability to deplete β islet cells of nicotinamide adenine dinucleotide (NAD) (7,17). Yellow phosphorus has a garlic-like odor, is soluble in oils, and is usually sold as a paste. It is often mixed with molasses or peanut butter and spread on bread for rodents to eat. Because it resembles food, the risk of unintentional childhood exposure is high. When yellow phosphorus comes into contact with moisture, it often ignites. Additionally, this toxin is a protoplasmic poison that uncouples oxidative phosphorylation, primarily in the gastrointestinal (GI) tract, liver, kidneys, and bone.

Zinc phosphide and aluminum are degraded to zinc or aluminum and phosphine gas in the presence of water and stomach acid. Phosphides are dark gray powders and phosphine has a "rotten fish" odor. The mechanism of action of phosphine is unclear but may involve inhibition of cytochrome oxidase.

CLINICAL PRESENTATION

ANTU ingestion can result in dyspnea, cough, and pleuritic chest pain but effects are not typically life-threatening. With large, acute exposures, however, acute lung injury or pulmonary edema (ARDS) can occur (18).

The majority of patients with oral anticoagulant exposures involve unintentional ingestions in children less than 6 years of age (16,20,21,24). Acute, single, unintentional ingestions of conventional anticoagulants are unlikely to cause toxicity because of their low warfarin concentrations. Similarly, children who unintentionally ingest superwarfarins are unlikely to develop toxicity. In contrast, adults with intentional ingestions or children with repeated ingestions often develop a coagulopathy within 24 or, at the latest, 48 hours (20,22). If this goes untreated, bleeding complications may develop. The most common sites of bleeding are the GI and genitourinary tracts (5,9). Patients with acute ingestions of arsenic may have a garlic-like odor on their breath and present with severe vomiting and diarrhea, dehydration, ventricular dysrhythmias, and central nervous system (CNS) and cardiovascular (CV) depression (see Chapter 305, "Arsenic and Mercury").

Cholecalciferol is relatively nontoxic in acute exposures, but with large doses, symptoms consistent with hypervitaminosis D (see Chapter 341, "Vitamins") and hypercalcemia might occur. These symptoms include GI complaints such as nausea, vomiting, constipation, and abdominal pains; mental status depression; and rare cardiac dysrhythmias. Despite numerous exposures in children and adults, not a single case of hypercalcemia has been reported from these products.

Cholinesterase inhibitor poisoning can occur by the oral, dermal, or inhalational routes. Signs and symptoms include salivation, lacrimation, urination, defecation, nausea, vomiting, GI cramping and/or pain, diarrhea, mental status change, seizures, muscle fasciculations, or weakness (see Chapter 297, "Organophosphate and Carbamate Insecticides") (11,14). No human fatalities have been reported from norbormide and the only complaints following exposure seem to be headache and weakness related to mild hypotension.

If large amounts of red squill are ingested, a presentation similar to digoxin poisoning may occur; patients may have GI symptoms, cardiac dysrhythmias, and hyperkalemia (see Chapter 304, "Cardiac Glycosides").

Although SMFA toxicity can occur by inhalation, ingestion is the most common route of severe poisoning. Initial symptoms include nausea and apprehension, followed shortly by severe lactic acidosis, pulmonary edema, coma, hypokalemia, hypocalcemia, seizures, and dysrhythmias. A poor prognosis is associated with hypotension, the early onset of acidosis, and increased creatinine levels (4).

Strychnine ingestion may result in opisthotonos, facial spasm (risus sardonicus), and decorticate posturing Patients are often mistakenly described as having "seizures," but their mental status is usually normal. Prolonged muscle activity can lead to hyperthermia, rhabdomyolysis, lactic acidosis, and death, often from respiratory dysfunction (15).

Tetramine ingestion can cause rapid onset seizures that progress to status epilepticus. Based on experience for China and a single case report in the United States, this toxin has a high fatality rate, and may be associated with residual neurological injury in survivors (1).

The effects of thallium may be delayed 12 to 24 hours after ingestion. Initially, GI symptoms such as nausea, vomiting, diarrhea, constipation, and abdominal pain predominate. Characteristically, extremely painful paresthesias then develop in the extremities and are unique in their intensity. In severe cases, dysrhythmias occur and can cause death. Respiratory failure has also been described. Survival is characterized by a period of alopecia and neurologic findings such as neuropathies, paresis, ataxia, choreiform movements, and optic nerve atrophy (19).

Patients who ingest Vacor may develop rapid loss of glucose control and severe diabetic ketoacidosis (DKA). Along with DKA, patients often present with abdominal pain from acute pancreatitis, autonomic instability, and peripheral paresthesias (17). Survivors of Vacor exposure are characterized by brittle insulin-dependent diabetes and accelerated microvascular diabetic disease (7).

Dermal exposures to yellow phosphorus can result in second- and third-degree burns. After ingestion, the clinical manifestations of poisoning occur in three stages (25). Initially, there is a rapid onset of severe GI symptoms, including nausea, vomiting, hematemesis, diarrhea, and abdominal pain. The stool and vomitus often have a garlicky odor and a luminescent appearance ("smoking stools") (21). If death occurs at this stage, it is typically from CV collapse. The second stage constitutes a relatively asymptomatic phase lasting 2 to 3 days. In the third stage, hepatorenal syndrome develops, and CNS symptoms such as altered mental status and coma.

Although inhalational toxicity has been reported, zinc and aluminum phosphide poisoning usually results from ingestion, which may result in the rapid development of profuse, black vomitus and abdominal pain. Phosphine gas formed in the stomach is then inhaled and absorbed by the lungs, causing acute lung injury, liver and renal damage, dysrhythmias, and circulatory collapse (6).

DIFFERENTIAL DIAGNOSIS

Exposure to an unknown rodenticide is not uncommon. In such cases, it is useful to classify rodenticides clinically, based on their time of onset and symptoms (Table 299.2). When the time of symptom onset and the nature of the symptoms are considered, a presumptive diagnosis can be established. Patients exposed to rodenticides with a rapid onset of action can be expected to

---

TABLE 299.2. Time of Symptom Onset in Rodenticide Poisoning

EARLY ONSET

α-Naphthylthiourea
Arsenic
Cholinesterase inhibitors
Norbormide
Red squill
Sodium monofluoroacetate
Strychnine
Tetramine
Thallium*
Yellow phosphorus
Zinc and aluminum phosphide

LATE ONSET

Oral anticoagulants
Cholecalciferol
Vacor

*Symptoms can also be delayed in onset.

---

manifest symptoms within 6 hours of ingestion. Those with exposure to rodenticides that have a delayed onset typically manifest symptoms beginning 12 hours or more after ingestion.

When symptoms are rapid in onset, cholinergic findings suggest OP poisoning; muscular hyperactivity suggests strychnine; seizures, coma, and metabolic acidosis suggest SMFA or tetramine; severe GI symptoms suggest arsenic or yellow phosphorus; respiratory manifestations suggest ANTU or zinc phosphide; hyperglycemia suggests Vacor; GI symptoms with cardiac dysrhythmias suggest red squill.

Lack of symptoms during the first 6 hours after exposure to an unknown rodenticide suggests either a nontoxic exposure to a rapidly acting agent or a potentially toxic exposure to a rodenticide with a delayed onset of toxicity (e.g., an oral anticoagulant or thallium). The most common cause of delayed rodenticide poisoning is superwarfarin anticoagulants (24).

The odor may also serve as a clue to the diagnosis. Arsenic and yellow phosphorus smell like garlic. Zinc and aluminum phosphide (phosphine) smells like rotten fish. Vacor smells like peanuts, and patients with Vacor-induced DKA have the fruity odor of ketones on their breath.

EMERGENCY DEPARTMENT EVALUATION

The history should include the amount and time of ingestion and the identity of the product involved. When a patient presents with an unknown rodenticide exposure, the most useful piece of information is the precise name and manufacturer of the ingested product. A family member should be asked to return home and try to get this information if the product is not brought along with the patient. The actual container or list of active ingredients is preferred over the commercial name, because many commercial names have been used for several products with different active ingredients.

If this information is unavailable, the time of symptom onset (see Table 299.1) and clinical manifestations may suggest the identity of the offending agent. Although the diagnostic evaluation is proceeding, consideration and institution of therapy (discussion follows) must occur simultaneously, as many of these poisons cause rapid and potentially fatal toxicity.

The initial assessment should address the airway, breathing, and circulation. Although uncommon, respiratory distress may be a problem with the toxins that have pulmonary effects, such as zinc or aluminum phosphide and ANTU. Strychnine may cause respiratory failure secondary to tonic muscle contractions and inability to ventilate. Toxicity from several of the other rodenticides can evolve rapidly to produce CV collapse.

Vital signs should be obtained immediately. Hyperthermia may occur with strychnine poisoning, as a result of increased muscle activity, or from yellow phosphorus, secondary to the uncoupling of oxidative phosphorylation. Clinical clues from the physical examination include specific odors associated with the different toxins and the quality and amount of emesis or diarrhea. Signs of bleeding in the GI or genitourinary tract may indicate oral anticoagulant exposure, although these findings would be delayed in onset.

Blood chemistries and a complete blood count are rarely useful in the absence of clinical findings. A low serum bicarbonate concentration might be found in symptomatic patients with SMFA, yellow phosphorus, strychnine, tetramine, or Vacor exposures. An elevated serum glucose level, especially in association with a metabolic acidosis, would indicate Vacor-induced DKA. A prothrombin time (PT) should be obtained in patients with remote (more than 24 hours) or repeated anticoagulant ingestions. If obtained shortly after a single ingestion, it should be normal. In chronic anticoagulant exposures or in patients who present several days after exposure with active bleeding, this test may be diagnostic.

The need for radiographic assessment should be guided by the toxin involved. Exposure to agents that produce pulmonary toxicity (e.g., ANTU, zinc phosphide) mandate a chest radiograph. Abdominal radiography may help detect opacities in the gut in recent ingestions of the metal toxins (arsenic, thallium, zinc, or aluminum phosphide). If a sample of an unidentified rodenticide is obtained, a radiograph of it may help to determine its heavy-metal content (13).

EMERGENCY DEPARTMENT MANAGEMENT

Treatment begins with stabilization of vital signs; advanced life-support measures are instituted, as appropriate. Once the patient is stable, gastric decontamination should be considered. For the asymptomatic patient who has ingested an unknown rodenticide, activated charcoal (AC) is the preferred method. Syrup of ipecac–induced emesis is contraindicated because numerous toxins can cause rapid decompensation. Orogastric lavage may be used in any patient giving a history of recent ingestion (within 2–4 hours) of a highly toxic rodenticide. Although little data exist on the efficacy of orogastric lavage, this intervention seems justified given the severe toxicity and lack of effective antidotes for most of the compounds in the highly toxic group. AC should be given following lavage.

Management of asymptomatic patients with unknown ingestions involves daily follow-up with PT testing to see if anticoagulant toxicity has manifested. A normal PT at 48 hours postingestion excludes significant anticoagulant toxicity (10). Prophylactic therapies with vitamin K_1 or AC is neither needed nor recommended in these cases. It is important to note that vitamin K_1 will not prevent toxicity which might last for a month, and thus only delays detection (10).

The treatment of ANTU, cholecalciferol, nobormide, tetramine, and yellow phosphorus poisoning is entirely supportive. Management of arsenic poisoning also includes chelation therapy (see Chapter 305, "Arsenic and Mercury") and that for cholinesterase inhibitor poisoning also includes atropine and pralidoxime (see Chapter 297, "Organophosphate and Carbamate Insecticides"). Red squill poisoning is treated the same as cardiac glycoside toxicity from other causes; digoxin specific Fab fragments can be used (see Chapter 304, "Cardiac Glycosides").

Coagulopathy without significant bleeding is treated with vitamin K_1. Not all vitamin K preparations are effective; phytonadione (AquaMEPHYTON, vitamin K_1) is recommended for this purpose. The dose needed, and the duration of treatment, varies with the type and amount of anticoagulant ingested and the patient's rate of toxin metabolism. Obtaining serial levels of the toxin to determine its elimination curve may help guide the duration of treatment necessary (2). Doses of up to 100 mg/d of vitamin K_1 for as long as 10 months have been necessary for superwarfarin poisoning (12). In patients with life-threatening bleeding, fresh-frozen plasma should also be administered.

Suggested antidotal treatments for SMFA toxicity include the use of glycerol monoacetate and ethanol, although neither approach has been well studied. Glycerol monoacetate is theorized to work by bypassing the site of blockage in the Krebs cycle. Ethanol may inhibit the conversion of SMFA to fluorocitrate and allow for excretion of the nontoxic parent compound (3). Given the availability and relative safety of ethanol administration and the severe toxicity of SMFA, ethanol administration appears warranted.

Treatment of muscle overactivity, the main problem that leads to the life-threatening complications in strychnine poisoning, includes high doses of benzodiazepines and, if necessary, neuromuscular paralysis. If the patient is hyperthermic, aggressive rapid cooling (see Chapter 353, "Heat-Related Illness") is the most important intervention.

The management of thallium poisoning is controversial. There are limited data on the efficacy of proposed treatments. Prussian blue (ferric ferrocyanide) (19) multiple dose activated charcoal (MDAC), and hemodialysis or hemoperfusion have been used. Although it is unclear which form of treatment is beneficial, we recommend MDAC and Prussian blue (250 mg/kg/d with a cathartic in divided doses), both of which bind thallium and may enhance its elimination and prevent its absorption, as the main therapeutic measures.

Niacinamide (nicotinamide) is an effective antidote for Vacor in experimental animals, and the earlier the antidote was given after exposure, the better the outcome. Niacin is not an effective substitute. Niacinamide (500 mg initially, followed by 100–200 mg every 4 hours for 2 days) is recommended for all patients with Vacor ingestion. Because an intravenous formulation is not available, it should be given orally. Patients who develop DKA are managed like other diabetic patients.

The treatment phosphine poisoning includes measures to prevent the generation of this gas when ingested zinc and aluminum phosphide enters the acid and aqueous environment of the stomach. Alkalinization of the stomach with oral bicarbonate, antacid, and H_2 antagonists is recommended, although the efficacy of these modalities is unclear.

CRITICAL INTERVENTIONS

- Positively identify the rodenticide's active ingredients whenever possible
- Arrange a 48-hour follow-up PT for asymptomatic superwarfarin or unknown rodenticide exposures

DISPOSITION

For symptomatic patients exposed to any rodenticide in the highly toxic group (see Table 299.1), hospital admission to a monitored setting is warranted. Because of the relative rarity of these exposures, consultation with a medical toxicologist or poison center is recommended early in the presentation.

Patients with unintentional exposures who remain asymptomatic after a period of observation (6 hours) can be discharged. For patients exposed to superwarfarin or long-acting oral anticoagulants, follow-up coagulation studies are needed at 48 hours after ingestion. These studies may be performed in the outpatient setting for patients with unintentional ingestions, if adequate family and social supports are in place. All other patients, including those with intentional ingestions, are best managed as inpatients.

COMMON PITFALLS

✔ Failure to obtain a sample or container for identifying the ingested agent
✔ Misidentification of the rodenticide because an identical or similar brand or market name is used for more than one agent
✔ Failure to consider ingestion of an agent with delayed onset of action in a patient with an unknown rodenticide exposure who remains asymptomatic after a period of observation
✔ Using the wrong type of vitamin K to treat oral anticoagulant toxicity
✔ Failure to confirm the diagnosis of superwarfarin toxicity by laboratory testing before beginning vitamin K treatment

References

1. Barrueto Jr F, Furdyna PM, Hoffman RS, et al. Status epilepticus from an illegally imported Chinese rodenticide: "Tetramine." *J Toxicol Clin Toxicol* 2003;41:991.
2. Bruno GR, Howland MA, McMeeking A, et al. Long acting overdose: brodifacoum kinetics and optimal vitamin K dosing. *Ann Emerg Med* 2000;36:262.
3. Chenoweth MB, Kandel A, Johnson LB, et al. Factors influencing fluoroacetate poisoning—practical treatment with glycerol monoacetate. *J Pharmacol Exp Ther* 1951;102:31.
4. Chi CH, Chen KW, Chan SH, et al. Clinical presentation and prognostic factors in sodium monofluoroacetate intoxication. *J Toxicol Clin Toxicol* 1996;34:707.
5. Chua JD, Friedenberg WR. Superwarfarin poisoning. *Arch Intern Med* 1998;158:1929.
6. Chugh SN, Aggarwal, Mahajan SK. Zinc phosphide intoxication symptoms: analysis of 20 cases. *Int J Clin Pharmacol Ther* 1998;36:406.
7. Feingold KR, Lee TH, Chung MY, et al. Muscle capillary basement membrane width in patients with Vacor-induced diabetes mellitus. *J Clin Invest* 1986;78:102.
8. Freedman MD. Oral anticoagulants: pharmacodynamics, clinical indications, and adverse effects. *J Clin Pharmacol* 1992;32:196.
9. Hoffman RS, Smilkstein MJ, Goldfrank LR. Evaluation of coagulation factor abnormalities in long-acting anticoagulant overdose. *J Toxicol Clin Toxicol* 1988;26:233.
10. Ingels M, Lai C, Tai W, et al. A prospective study of acute, unintentional, pediatric superwarfarin ingestions managed without decontamination. *Ann Emerg Med* 2002;40:73.
11. Lima JS, Reis CA. Poisoning due to illegal use of carbamates as a rodenticide in Rio De Janeiro. *J Toxicol Clin Toxicol* 195;33:687.
12. Lipton RA, Klass EM. Human ingestion of a "superwarfarin" rodenticide resulting in a prolonged anticoagulant effect. *JAMA* 1988;252:3004.
13. Meggs WJ, Hoffman RS, Shih RD, et al. Malicious thallium poisoning: rapid diagnosis by x-ray, laboratory and clinical evaluation. *Vet Hum Toxicol* 1993;35:317.
14. Nelson LS, Perrone J, DeRoos F, et al. Aldicarb poisoning by an illicit rodenticide imported into the United States: tres pasitos. *J Toxicol Clin Toxicol* 2001;39:447.
15. Palatnick W, Meatherall R, Sitar D, et al. Toxicokinetics of acute strychnine poisoning. *J Toxicol Clin Toxicol* 1997;35:617.
16. Parsons BJ, Day LM, Ozanne-Smith J, et al. Rodenticide poisoning among children. *Aust NZ J Public Health* 1996;20:488.
17. Pont A, Rubino JM, Bishop D, et al. Diabetes mellitus and neuropathy following Vacor ingestion in man. *Arch Intern Med* 1979;139:185.
18. Richter CP: The development and use of alpha-napthyl-thiourea (ANTU) as a rat poison. *JAMA* 1945;129:927.
19. Hoffman RS: Thallium toxicity and the role of Prussian blue in therapy. *Toxicol Rev* 2003;22:29–40.
20. Shepherd G, Klein-Schwartz W, Anderson BD. Acute, unintentional pediatric brodifacoum ingestions. *Pediatr Emerg Care* 2002;18:174.
21. Simon FA, Pickering LK. Acute yellow phosphorus poisoning: "smoking stool syndrome. " *JAMA* 1980;244:148.
22. Smolinske SC, Scherger DL, Kearns PC, et al. Superwarfarin poisoning in children: a prospective study. *Pediatrics* 1989;84:490.
23. Sutie JW. Warfarin and vitamin K. *Clin Cardiol* 1990;13:16.
24. Watson WA, Litovitz TL, Rogers GC, et al. 2002 annual report of the American Association of Poison Control Centers Toxic Exposure Surveillance System. *Am J Emerg Med* 2003;21:353.
25. Winek CL, Collom WD, Fusia EP. Yellow phosphorus ingestion—three fatal poisonings. *J Toxicol Clin Toxicol* 1973;6:541.

PART VI

Cardiovascular Drugs

CHAPTER 300
Antidysrhythmic Drugs and Local Anesthetics

S. Rutherfoord Rose and James E. Cisek

This chapter focuses on Vaughn-Williams classes I and III antidysrhythmic agents (Table 300.1). Local anesthetics, whose mechanism and toxic effects are similar to lidocaine, are also discussed. β-adrenergic blockers (Vaughn-Williams class II) and calcium-channel blockers (Vaughn-Williams class IV) are covered in Chapter 302, "Beta Blockers" and Chapter 303, "Calcium Channel Antagonists," respectively.

Class I antidysrhythmics decrease the influx of sodium through fast channels in myocardial cell membranes during depolarization (phase zero of the action potential), thereby slowing the rate of rise of the action potential (Vmax) in myocardial cells. This action results in decreased conduction velocity and increased QRS duration. Class I drugs are further divided into A, B, and C subclasses based on their respective rates of dissociation from fast sodium channels. Class IC agents dissociate slowly and therefore produce the greatest degree of QRS prolongation, even at therapeutic doses. Class IB drugs quickly dissociate from binding sites and produce no QRS prolongation at therapeutic concentrations. Lidocaine, also frequently used as a local anesthetic agent, is a class IB antidysrhythmic. Class IA drugs have intermediate dissociation constants and cause mild QRS prolongation with therapeutic dosing.

Class IA drugs also have variable a-adrenergic blocking effects, and disopyramide has relatively potent negative inotropic and anticholinergic effects. Propafenone has relatively weak β-adrenergic activity, which may be clinically important in patients on high doses or in the approximately 7% of patients who poorly metabolize propafenone to an active metabolite, which has class IC-like properties.

Amiodarone, sotalol, dofetilide, and ibutilide are examples of class III drugs that are currently available. Class III drugs prolong repolarization and the refractory period in all cardiac tissue by blocking the outward potassium channels. Amiodarone has vasodilating and weak β-adrenergic blocking properties; however, i.v. administration results in pharmacologic effects consis-

tent with all four Vaughn-Williams classes. Sotalol is a nonselective β-adrenergic blocker that also prolongs the refractory period throughout the conduction system, including bypass tracts. Dofetilide prolongs the action potential duration and effective refractory period without affecting conduction velocity. It does not affect sodium channels or adrenergic receptors. Dofetilide is available only to hospitals and physicians who have received appropriate dosing and treatment education as the risk of inducing dysrhythmias is significant. Dofetilide toxicity can be minimized by giving careful attention to pretreatment QT intervals and renal function. Ibutilide is structurally related to sotalol but does not affect β-adrenergic receptors. Ibutilide's pharmacologic effects are related to activation of slow sodium channels (low doses) in addition to blocking potassium (delayed rectifier) channels in higher doses.

Class IA drugs are used to treat a wide variety of dysrhythmias of both ventricular and supraventricular origin, including reentry tachycardias and Wolff-Parkinson-White syndrome. The efficacy of these drugs in preventing reentry dysrhythmias is probably as a result of a change from unidirectional to bidirectional block resulting from slowed conduction. Class IC drugs have very narrow therapeutic windows and are primarily used for maintenance of sinus rhythm in patients with atrial fibrillation. The Cardiac Arrhythmia Suppression Trial study demonstrated increased mortality in patients given encainide or flecainide after myocardial infarction. Encainide was subsequently withdrawn from the U.S. market in 1991; however, it may be obtained directly from the manufacturer for patients with life-threatening dysrhythmias who have previously responded to the drug. Flecainide is typically reserved for treatment of refractory supraventricular tachycardias. The class III drugs have assumed more prominent roles as initial therapy for both ventricular and supraventricular rhythm disturbances.

Overdose with antidysrhythmic drugs is rare, compared with other cardiovascular (CV) drugs (e.g., β blockers or calcium channel blockers). Most overdoses occur in adults and are accidental. Adverse effects are common and occur in 20% to 50% of patients on chronic therapy.

The salt forms of these drugs are well absorbed orally. Peak plasma levels following ingestion of immediate-release dosage forms usually occur within 1 to 3 hours, except with amiodarone (typically 4 to 6 hours, but up to 10 hours) and with disopyramide (as a result of its anticholinergic effects). Metabolites of quinidine, encainide, propafenone, and amiodarone have varying degrees of pharmacologic activity and probably contribute to overall effects. These metabolites are not monitored clinically. The principal metabolite of procainamide, N-acetylprocainamide (NAPA), is approved under orphan drug status for patients with procainamide-induced lupus, and most closely resembles

TABLE 300.1. Classification of Antidysrhythmic Drugs[a]

Class	Actions	Examples
I A	Sodium channel inhibition Increased APD Increased ERP Slowed conduction	Quinidine, Disopyramide, Procainamide
B	Little/no decrease in APD Increased ERP in diseased tissue May increase conduction velocity	Lidocaine, Tocainide, Phenytoin, Mexiletine
C	Variable effect on APD Small increase in ERP Markedly slowed conduction	Encainide, Flecainide, Propafenone
II	β-adrenergic blockade	Atenolol, Metoprolol, Propranolol, Acebutolol, Bisoprolol, Sotalol
III	Prolonged repolarization	Amiodarone, Bretylium, Dofetilide, Ibutilide, Sotalol, N-acetylprocainamide
IV	Calcium channel inhibition	Diltiazem, Nifedipine, Verapamil, Bepridil

[a]APD, action potential duration; ERP, effective refractory period.

class III drugs because of its ability to prolong repolarization. Amiodarone is unique in that it has a very prolonged elimination half-life (50 days), and serum levels may continue to rise for a month after starting therapy.

The toxic effects of antidysrhythmics result from exaggerated therapeutic activity. Dose-dependent delays in conduction lead to varying degrees of atrioventricular block and, eventually, asystole. High drug levels also result in myocardial depression (classes IA, IC, and III) and peripheral vasodilatation (classes IA and III), which can result in profound hypotension. Central nervous system (CNS) effects appear to be independent of cardiac effects unless shock is present.

There are insufficient data to determine the minimum toxic doses for most antidysrhythmic drugs. For class IA drugs, toxicity may be expected after acute ingestions of 1 g or more. Ingestions of more than 2.5 to 3.0 g may result in serious toxicity. Survival has been reported following acute doses of up to 20 g and peak serum levels of 21.4 μg/mL (quinidine) and 77 μg/mL (procainamide). However, 2 g of disopyramide resulted in cardiopulmonary arrest in a 16-year-old girl, and fatalities have been reported following estimated doses as low as 3.6 to 6.8 g in adults and 600 mg in a child, and serum levels of 8.3 μg/mL (1,8).

Class IC drugs appear to be more toxic than class IA drugs. Severe toxicity has been reported in a 6-month-old child who ingested a 25-mg encainide tablet (12). A healthy 46-year-old man ingested 3.0 to 3.5 g of encainide and suffered seizures, hypotension, bradycardia, and coma (16). Ingestion of 1.8 g of flecainide was fatal in an 18-year-old, and 1.5 g produced seizures and polymorphous ventricular tachycardia (VT) (9). An acute overdose of 1.8 g (133 mg/kg) of propafenone in a 2-year-old child resulted in hypotension, seizures, and a prolonged QT interval (13). Ingestion of 8.1 g of propafenone caused seizures, coma, hypotension, and prolonged QRS interval in an adult with a propafenone serum level of 3.2 μg/mL (10). An overall mortality of 22.5% was reported in a retrospective review of propafenone, flecainide, ajmaline, and prajmaline toxicity (11). About half of the patients became nauseated within 30 minutes of ingestion, and severe cardiac toxicity (atrioventricular block, bradycardia, pulseless electrical activity, asystole) occurred within 30 to 120 minutes after ingestion.

There is considerably less information about the acute toxicity of class III drugs. Amiodarone doses of 2.6 to 8.0 g have produced mild bradycardia, prolonged QT interval, and a brief episode of nonsustained VT, all with a delayed onset of 12 to 48 hours (5).

Sotalol toxicity may also result in QT prolongation and cardiac dysrhythmias (see Chapter 302, "Beta Blockers").

Excessive dosing or impaired excretion of these compounds frequently leads to toxic levels during chronic therapy. Clinical toxicity at a relatively lower serum concentration may be expected during chronic therapy as a result of prior saturation of tissue stores and the likelihood of preexisting cardiac disease.

Local anesthetics act by decreasing neuronal permeability to sodium ions (a similar mechanism to the cardiac antidysrhythmics), thereby preventing transmembrane depolarization and subsequent propagation of the action potential. Lidocaine, also sometimes called lignocaine, is the most commonly utilized local anesthetic and was introduced in 1940. Lidocaine is a group II (amide-type) local anesthetic. Other members of group II include bupivicaine, mepivicaine, prilocaine, dibucaine, and etidocaine. A common mnemonic device states that the local anesthetics with two letter "i"s in the generic name are all in the amide class.

The group I local anesthetics contain esters of benzoic acid, p-aminobenzoic acid, and meta-aminobenzoic acid; this group includes cocaine (see Chapter 324, "Cocaine"), tetracaine, procaine (Novocaine), proparacaine, butethamine, and benzocaine. Patients with a reported allergy to a local anesthetic are typically allergic to all agents of the same group (amide or ester), but may be safely given an anesthetic from the other group.

Lidocaine is well absorbed through mucous membranes and the gastrointestinal (GI) tract. Peak plasma concentrations are reached within 2 minutes of i.v. administration, within 10 minutes of endotracheal administration, and within 30 to 60 minutes of ingestion. Following i.v. injection, lidocaine is rapidly distributed to well-perfused tissue (brain and heart), with subsequent slower distribution to less well perfused tissues (skeletal muscle and fat). The initial distribution serum half-life is approximately 10 minutes. The peak serum concentration, which depends on the rate of administration, then rapidly declines. Because of this biphasic pattern of distribution, an infusion is required to maintain therapeutic serum concentrations following intravenous bolus for an antidysrhythmic effect. A standard i.v. dosing regimen is 1.0 to 1.4 mg/kg, followed in 10 minutes by an additional bolus of 0.7 mg/kg and a maintenance infusion of 1 to 4 mg/min (20 to 50 μg/kg/min for children).

Lidocaine is metabolized to two active compounds: monoethylglycinexylidide (MEGX) and glycine xylidide (GX). These metabolites achieve peak concentrations in 1 to 2 hours after an oral dose. The plasma elimination half-life of lidocaine ranges from 1.5 to 2.0 hours. The elimination half-lives of MEGX and GX are 3 and 5 hours, respectively. Only 5% to 10% of the parent drug is excreted unchanged into the urine along with its metabolites. High concentrations of MEGX may produce toxic effects even when serum lidocaine concentrations are low (17). The risk of lidocaine toxicity is increased in patients with hepatic dysfunction, congestive heart failure, and shock as a result of alterations of metabolism, hepatic blood flow, and volume of distribution. The volume of distribution of lidocaine in patients with congestive heart failure can be decreased by 30%. Conversely, in patients with chronic hepatic disease, an increase of parent drug in the circulation and a decrease in α-1 glycoprotein may increase the volume of distribution by 30% to 40%.

CLINICAL PRESENTATION

The onset of symptoms following acute oral antidysrhythmic overdose usually occurs within 4 hours, and often within 1 to 2 hours. However, drug absorption may continue for many hours following the ingestion of massive amounts, sustained-release preparations, or agents with anticholinergic effects. Delayed onset of toxicity has been observed following amiodarone overdose (5).

Extracardiac manifestations of acute toxicity include dizziness, visual disturbances, psychosis, anticholinergic symptoms (disopyramide), hypoglycemia (disopyramide), hyperglycemia (encainide), hypokalemia, and hypersensitivity reactions (e.g., fever, rash, urticaria) (7,19). Thrombocytopenia and a lupus-like syndrome (arthralgias, fever, myocarditis) with antinuclear antibodies have been well documented during chronic quinidine and procainamide therapy. The use of amiodarone is increasing despite the risk of numerous adverse effects, including corneal microdeposits, photosensitivity, hepatic dysfunction, myopathy, pulmonary fibrosis, hypo- or hyperthyroidism, and peripheral neuropathies.

Hypotension, bradycardia, CNS depression, seizures, metabolic acidosis, and CV collapse can occur in severe poisoning. Patients with disopyramide overdose may demonstrate early loss of consciousness, apnea, or cardiac failure. Seizures appear to be more prevalent with class IC drugs. Disopyramide has resulted in acute congestive heart failure at therapeutic doses in patients with heart disease. Clinical effects associated with quinidine include seizures, immune-mediated hemolytic anemia, syncope, and cinchonism. Syncope is due primarily to torsades de pointes (discussion follows), but may also be associated with adrenergic blockade (orthostasis) or, rarely, idiosyncratic reactions. Cinchonism (see Chapter 294, "Antimalarial Drugs") is associated with chronic therapy and does not appear to be dose-related. Procainamide and quinidine can predictably produce hypotension if given by too-rapid i.v. infusion. Death can result from refractory dysrhythmias or CV collapse.

Disturbances in cardiac conduction and rhythm are the electrocardiographic (ECG) hallmarks of antidysrhythmic agent poisoning. Excessive prolongation of the QT interval is almost always present in severe poisoning. With class IA agents, this results from prolongation of the QRS interval, whereas with class IC and III agents, it is due primarily to QRS and QT prolongation, respectively. In general, an increase of the QRS or QT interval by 25% is considered therapeutic, and widening by 50% or more suggests toxicity. The PR interval may also be prolonged if there is sinus activity. Conduction disturbances and myocardial depression contribute to a host of supraventricular and ventricular dysrhythmias, including sinus bradycardia, atrioventricular dissociation, VT or fibrillation, slow idioventricular rhythm, and asystole. Torsades de pointes is a triggered (early after depolar-

ization) polymorphous VT resulting from excessive QT prolongation, most commonly associated with class IA and III drugs (e.g., quinidine, amiodarone, dofetilide, ibutilide).

All antidysrhythmic drugs can aggravate existing dysrhythmias or induce new ones in patients being treated for supraventricular or ventricular dysrhythmias (i.e., antidysrhythmics may be pro-arrhythmic). The incidence of proarrhythmia is estimated at 5% to 20% and most often is associated with initiation of therapy or a dosage increase (12). The induction of dysrhythmias should always be suspected in patients on antidysrhythmic drugs who present with syncopal episodes.

The correlation of serum levels with clinical effects depends on previous exposure to the drug, the presence of heart disease, and the degree of absorption, metabolite formation, and elimination. In general, serum levels exceeding 7, 8, and 15 μg/mL for quinidine, disopyramide, and procainamide (NAPA), respectively, should be considered toxic. Flecainide levels of 1.48 to 3.7 μg/mL have been observed in patients with prolonged QT intervals, bradycardia, hypotension, ventricular dysrhythmias, and seizures, and levels of 13.0 to 16.3 μg/mL have been reported in fatal cases (21). Lower levels may result in toxicity in patients who ingest other CV agents. Patients on chronic therapy who take an acute overdose appear to be at greater risk for severe intoxication.

Although lidocaine toxicity can result from all routes of administration (2,14), it most frequently occurs during intravenous infusion (3,4). Manifestations involve the CNS and the CV system. CNS effects have been reported in up to 47% of patients receiving i.v. lidocaine. Initial symptoms, such as lightheadedness, dizziness, drowsiness, and euphoria, may occur at therapeutic concentrations. At higher concentrations, more serious symptoms include confusion, hearing loss, dysarthria, visual disturbances, ataxia, agitation, and muscle twitching, which may lead to seizures and coma. Seizures may be prolonged (3,4). CV toxicity is rare and usually occurs from rapidly administered intravenous infusions. When serum concentrations are above 11 μg/mL, the refractory period is decreased, automaticity and myocardial contractility are depressed, and hypotension and bradycardia ensue (18). Conduction abnormalities include sinus bradycardia, atrioventricular block, complete heart block, and sinus arrest. Conduction defects may be more common in patients with preexisting bundle-branch abnormalities.

Mucosal absorption bypasses hepatic first-pass metabolism, making the drug more bioavailable than by intestinal absorption. Seizures have been reported several times in children following mucosal application of 2% to 4% viscous lidocaine (4,14). Topical or oral lidocaine for the treatment of painful oral lesions in children, therefore, should be used cautiously if at all.

Seizures have also been reported following lidocaine infiltration. During laceration repair, the total dose for infiltration of lidocaine without epinephrine should not exceed 4.5 mg/kg, nor should the dose exceed 7.0 mg/kg of lidocaine with epinephrine. The standard 1% lidocaine solutions stocked in the emergency department (ED) contain 10 mg/mL of lidocaine; thus, the maximal volumes used for local infiltration in a 70-kg adult patient are roughly 30 mL without epinephrine and 50 mL with epinephrine. Fortunately, most wounds repaired in the ED will only require smaller volumes of anesthetic.

The neurologic and cardiac toxicities of other local anesthetics are similar to that of lidocaine. For example, many patients referred to the ED from a dental office are experiencing CNS toxic effects as a result of injection of procaine or other local anesthetics for dental procedures. Several local anesthetics have also been reported to cause methemoglobinemia (see Chapter 315, "Methemoglobinemia"), especially benzocaine. Benzocaine is found in over-the-counter infant teething gels and adult oral anesthetics, and is also used in the clinical setting as a topical anesthetic to aid in endotracheal or gastric intubation and for various endoscopic procedures.

DIFFERENTIAL DIAGNOSIS

Similar bradyarrhythmias may be caused by β blockers, calcium antagonists, cholinergic agents (carbamate and organophosphate insecticides), digitalis, clonidine, lithium, and cyclic antidepressants. QRS and QT interval prolongation may result from poisoning with antihistamines, phenothiazines, cyclic antidepressants, lithium, magnesium, or potassium. Ventricular tachyarrhythmias may occur in poisoning with sympathomimetics.

Stimulants, hypoglycemia, hypoxia, and metabolic disturbances should be considered in the differential diagnosis of patients with CNS manifestations. Patients presenting with apprehension, anxiety, or other neurologic symptoms after very recent dental work, medical procedures on the upper aerodigestive tract, or wound repair would strongly suggest the possibility of local anesthetic toxicity. Methemoglobinemia should be considered in a patient who becomes cyanotic and is responding poorly to oxygen therapy after exposure to local anesthetics.

EMERGENCY DEPARTMENT EVALUATION

The history should include the exact product and strength (immediate- or sustained-release), the amount ingested, the time ingested, and treatment before arrival. Any history of CV disease should be elucidated. Mechanisms for chronic toxicity, such as excessive dosing, exacerbation of congestive heart failure, or change in renal function, should be investigated.

The physical examination should focus on vital signs, with attention to CV stability and respiratory and neurologic status. A 12-lead ECG should be obtained as soon as possible to check for conduction blockade and dysrhythmias. In most patients with local anesthetic toxicity, an extensive metabolic work-up will not be necessary. Patients suspected of having toxicity from antidysrhythmic drugs are often taking these agents therapeutically, and often have significant underlying disease. For them, laboratory evaluation should include a blood glucose level; electrolyte analysis; blood urea nitrogen, creatinine, and magnesium measurement; liver function tests; and appropriate serum drug levels, if available. Procainamide and NAPA levels should always be ordered concurrently. Chest radiography and arterial blood gas analysis are included for patients with depressed levels of consciousness or serious dysrhythmias. If methemoglobinemia is suspected, venous or arterial blood should be sent for a methemoglobin level.

EMERGENCY DEPARTMENT MANAGEMENT

Advanced life-support measures should be instituted, as necessary. All patients suspected of antidysrhythmic drug toxicity should have an i.v. line, continuous cardiac monitoring, and pulse oximetry. Unstable patients must have close hemodynamic monitoring, supplemental oxygen and airway management as indicated clinically. Acid–base, electrolyte, and magnesium derangements should be corrected. Potassium should be replaced cautiously, because hypokalemia may protect against cardiotoxicity as a result of quinidine (and possibly other agents). Seizures are treated with standard doses of intravenous benzodiazepines and barbiturates.

Hypotension is initially treated with i.v. normal saline. Infusions of sodium bicarbonate can reverse hypotension associated with class IA and IC drugs. Patients with compromised left ventricular function must not be overly fluid resuscitated. Hypotension refractory to volume expansion may require the use of direct acting vasopressors or inotropes (epinephrine, norepinephrine, dopamine), aortic balloon counterpulsation, or cardiopulmonary bypass pump support (7,19,20).

Sodium bicarbonate (2 mEq/kg i.v. bolus) should be given to patients with hypotension, prolonged QRS intervals, PVCs, and monomorphic VT if Class I antiarrhythmic toxicity is suspected. Sodium bicarbonate has beneficial affects by increasing the serum sodium level to help offset the sodium channel antagonism, increasing serum protein binding (decreased free drug) in a more alkalotic serum, and by driving drugs off the sodium channels. Symptomatic bradycardia or atrioventricular dissociation will probably require ventricular pacing if there is inadequate response to atropine or sodium bicarbonate. Successful pacemaker capture may require concomitant epinephrine therapy (10).

After sodium bicarbonate, lidocaine is the drug of choice for ventricular ectopy (except, of course, for patients with lidocaine toxicity). Other antidysrhythmic drugs in the same class are obviously contraindicated for treatment of dysrhythmias. Torsades de pointes usually responds to isoproterenol infusion (1–6 μg/min) and atrial or ventricular overdrive pacing (19). A heart rate of 150 beats/min is usually required. Intravenous magnesium sulfate (1–4 g over several minutes to 1 hour, depending on the hemodynamic stability) may also be effective.

Once the patient has been stabilized, activated charcoal should be administered to decontaminate the GI tract in patients with recent ingestions. If present and causing symptomatology, methemoglobinemia may be treated with supplemental oxygen and methylene blue (see Chapter 315, "Methemoglobinemia").

Patients whose vital signs can be supported during endogenous drug elimination usually recover fully. Efforts to enhance elimination of these compounds have had variable success. Patients should be adequately hydrated to maintain renal perfusion. Extracorporeal elimination may have a role in the treatment of procainamide and NAPA toxicity. In the presence of renal failure, hemodialysis can increase the clearance of NAPA fourfold and procainamide twofold.

CRITICAL INTERVENTIONS

- Establish intravenous access, initiate cardiac monitoring, and obtain a 12-lead ECG on patients with potential toxicity from antidysrhythmic agents and local anesthetics
- Administer sodium bicarbonate to patients with hypotension, prolonged QRS intervals, PVCs, and monomorphic VT as a result of Class I antiarrhythmic poisoning
- Administer magnesium sulfate intravenously and induce sinus tachycardia with isoproterenol or overdrive pacing in patients with torsades de pointes

DISPOSITION

Patients with local anesthetic exposures can be discharged once free of neurologic and cardiac toxic effects, often within just a few hours. Those with persistent CNS symptoms or an abnormal ECG after should be admitted to a monitored setting.

Patients who remain asymptomatic following antidysrhythmic agent ingestions and have a normal ECG after 6 hours of observation can usually be safely discharged. A 12-hour observation period is recommended if a sustained-release preparation is involved. Patients with amiodarone overdose should be admitted for prolonged observation. Patients who are symptomatic or exhibit ECG evidence of cardiotoxicity from either acute or chronic intoxication need admission to a monitored bed. Those with CV instability should be admitted to an intensive care unit. A regional poison center or toxicologist can help with disposition and management decisions. A cardiologist should be consulted if pacing is required. Patients with severe toxicity should be admitted or transferred to a facility with cardiopulmonary bypass (CPB) and aortic balloon counterpulsation capabilities. Patients presenting after intentional overdose should undergo psychiatric evaluation before discharge.

COMMON PITFALLS

- ✔ Failure to appreciate that severe toxicity can result from therapeutic doses of antidysrhythmic agents
- ✔ Failure to consider the possibility of drug-induced dysrhythmias as a cause of syncope and weakness in patients taking antidysrhythmic agents
- ✔ Failure to appreciate that drug-induced dysrhythmias may resemble the ones for which the drug was prescribed and to check drug levels before treating them with more drug
- ✔ Failure to consider sodium bicarbonate and magnesium for the treatment of dysrhythmias
- ✔ Failure to consider invasive CV supportive therapies, such as pacing, aortic balloon counterpulsation, and CPB in patients with severe poisoning
- ✔ Failure to check the dose and concentration of local anesthetic solutions and to adhere to recommended dosing guidelines, resulting in iatrogenic poisoning
- ✔ Failure to perform cardiac monitoring on patients receiving intravenous regional local anesthetics and large doses of local anesthetics by infiltration
- ✔ Failure to appreciate that local anesthetics can cause CNS excitation and depression
- ✔ Failure to appreciate that multiple doses of oral viscous lidocaine can be toxic and to warn patients and parents of children that it should not be swallowed

Acknowledgment

We thank Donna Seger for her contributions to previous versions of this chapter.

References

1. Accornero F, Pellanda A, Ruffini C, et al. Prolonged CPR during acute disopyramide poisoning. *Vet Hum Toxicol* 1993;35:231.
2. Alfaro SN, Leicht MJ, Skiendzielewski JJ. Lidocaine toxicity following subcutaneous administration. *Ann Emerg Med* 1984;13:465.
3. Brown DL, Skiendzielewski JJ. Lidocaine toxicity. *Ann Emerg Med* 1980;9:627.
4. Bryant CA, Hoffman JR, Nichtes LS. Pitfalls and perils of intravenous lidocaine. *West J Med* 1983;139:528.
5. Goddard CJR, Whorwell PJ. Amiodarone overdose and its management. *Br J Clin Pharmacol* 1989;43:184.
6. Gosselin B, Mathieu D, Chopin C, et al. Acute intoxication with disopyramide: clinical and experimental study by hemoperfusion on Amberlite XAD 4 resin. *J Toxicol Clin Toxicol* 1980;17:439.
7. Holt DW, O'Keeffe B, Marshall CB, et al. Successful management of serious disopyramide poisoning. *Postgrad Med J* 1980;56:256.
8. Hutchison A, Kilham H. Fatal overdose of disopyramide in a child. *Med J Aust* 1978;2:335.
9. Kennedy A, Thomas P, Sheridan DJ. Generalized seizures as the presentation of flecainide toxicity. *Eur Heart J* 1989;10:950.
10. Kerns W, English B, Ford M. Propafenone overdose. *Ann Emerg Med* 1994;24: 98–103.
11. Koppel C, Oberdisse U, Heinemeyer G. Clinical course and outcome in class IC antiarrhythmic overdose. *J Toxicol Clin Toxicol* 1990;28(2):433.
12. McCollam PL, Parker RB, Beckman KJ, et al. Proarrhythmia: a paradoxic response to antiarrhythmic agents. *Pharmacotherapy* 1989;9.144.
13. McHugh TP, Perina DG. Propafenone ingestion. *Ann Emerg Med* 1987;16:437.
14. Mofenson HC, Caraccio TR, Miller H, et al. Lidocaine toxicity from topical mucosal application. *Clin Pediatr (Phila)* 1983;22:190.
15. Mortensen ME, Bolon CE, Kelley MT, et al. Encainide overdose in an infant. *Ann Emerg Med* 1992;21:998.
16. Pentel PR, Goldsmith SR, Salerno DM, et al. Effect of hypertonic sodium bicarbonate on encainide overdose. *Am J Cardiol* 1986;57:878.
17. Pieper JA, Slaughter RL, Anderson GD, et al. Lidocaine: clinical pharmacokinetics. *Drug Intell Clin Pharm* 1982;16:291.
18. Promisloff RA, Dupont DC. Death from ARDS and cardiovascular collapse following lidocaine administration. *Chest* 1983;3:585.
19. Shub C, Gau GT, Sidell PM, et al. The management of acute quinidine intoxication. *Chest* 1978;73:173.
20. Villalba-Pimentel L, Epstein LM, Sellers EM, et al. Survival after massive procainamide ingestion. *Am J Cardiol* 1973;32:727.
21. Wood DM, Angel T, Dargan PI, et al. Flecainide toxicity: a case report with toxicokinetic data. *Br J Clin Pharmacol* 2003;55:431.

CHAPTER 301
Centrally Acting Antihypertensive Agent

James R. Roberts and Rachel Haroz

Centrally acting antihypertensives include clonidine, guanabenz, guanfacine, methyldopa, and reserpine. Clonidine hydrochloride is available in tablet form (Catapres: 0.1 mg, 0.2 mg, 0.3 mg), in combination with the diuretic chlorthalidone (Combipres), or as a transdermal patch (Catapres TTS) designed to be worn for a week and to slowly release 0.1 mg, 0.2 mg, or 0.3 mg per day. Significant amounts of clonidine may remain in used patches, and children have mistaken discarded patches for Band-Aids or stickers, resulting in clonidine toxicity from transdermal absorption, oral ingestion, or mouthing of patches. Although it has no known teratogenicity in humans, clonidine use in pregnancy has been associated with transitory hypertension in neonates and hyperactivity and sleep disturbances in children; therefore, this drug is not recommended for use during pregnancy.

In addition to its use as an antihypertensive agent, clonidine has been used to ameliorate the symptoms associated with alcohol, narcotic, nicotine, and gamma-hydroxybutyrate (GHB) withdrawal (19). The drug is titrated to control symptoms, particularly tremor, tachycardia, and agitation; a suggested starting dose is 5 to 8 µg/kg/d (divided into three to four doses), tapered over 5 to 10 days. Excessive sedation and orthostatic hypotension are the main side effects, limiting outpatient use. Not surprisingly, withdrawal symptoms can also occur after the abrupt cessation of long-term clonidine therapy.

Other clinical applications include use as an adjunct to pain management, including nerve block and intrathecal administration; to reduce postmenopausal flushing; as migraine headache prophylaxis; for acute pancreatitis, and to control postoperative nausea and vomiting (1,8). Clonidine has been increasingly used to treat both attention deficit disorder in children and Tourette's. The use of clonidine for opiate addiction has led to its increased use among addicts primarily for its withdrawal amelioration and for its sedative properties (2).

Clonidine, an imidazole first used as a nasal decongestant, is the prototype of a group of centrally acting agents (including guanabenz and methyldopa) that produce their antihypertensive effect through a complex interaction between α2-adrenergic and imidazoline receptors in the rostral ventrolateral medulla resulting in a decreased sympathetic outflow from the central nervous system (CNS) (3,17,22). This is thought to be modulated both by inhibition of norepinephrine and indirect action on gamma-aminobutyric acid (GABA), serotonin and opioid interneurons (22). Although clonidine is primarily a central α2-adrenergic agonist, it also possesses some peripheral α1-adrenergic receptor agonist properties. This accounts for the paradoxical hypertension sometimes seen in the early phase of overdose. The therapeutic effect of clonidine is attributed primarily to a reduction in heart rate and cardiac output rather than to a significant reduction in total peripheral resistance. The withdrawal syndrome results from an unbalancing of central adrenergic activity; as clonidine's inhibitory effect at α2-adrenergic receptors is removed, upregulated α1-adrenergic receptors and elevated catecholamine levels operate to increase sympathetic outflow.

After absorption from the gastrointestinal tract, clonidine is 20% to 40% protein bound and highly lipid soluble, with excellent CNS penetration. Forty percent to 60% of the drug is excreted unchanged in the urine, and the remainder undergoes hepatic metabolism. Onset of action is 30 to 60 minutes, peaking in 2 to 3 hours. The elimination half-life is 5 to 13 hours, with minimal accumulation in renal failure. There are no known pharmacologically active metabolites. The volume of distribution is 3.2 to 5.6 L/kg.

Except for one poorly documented fatality attributed to a massive ingestion in a child, deaths have not been reported from clonidine poisoning alone. In fact, a 1,000-fold increase in dose in a 5-year-old child as a result of an error was successfully managed supportively with no sequelae (18). A recent retrospective study examined over 10,000 clonidine exposures in children over a 7-year period and found that major effects occurred in only 2% of children and that there was only one fatality (13). Deaths have been reported when clonidine has been taken with other drugs in suicide attempts (20). A combined overdose of clonidine and methylphenidate, drugs used to treat attention deficit disorder, has anecdotally been associated with sudden death.

Guanfacine (Tenex) and guanabenz (Wytensin) are structurally and pharmacologically similar to clonidine and produce similar toxicity (9). The usual adult dose is 1 to 2 mg for guanfacine and 2 to 4 mg for guanabenz. Proprietary preparations may also contain thiazide diuretics. There are no known deaths related to a pure guanabenz or guanfacine overdose. Mild withdrawal symptoms have been noted after abrupt cessation of maintenance therapy.

Methyldopa (Aldomet) is metabolized α-methylnorepinephrine, which may stimulate α2-adrenergic receptors, indirectly reduce plasma renin activity, or act as a "false" (i.e., inactive) neurotransmitter. Peripheral vascular resistance is decreased, as cardiac output is maintained. The usual adult dose is 250 to 500 mg, which can be given intravenously and orally. Methyldopa preparations commonly include a thiazide diuretic. A mild rebound syndrome (mainly hypertension) has been associated with the abrupt cessation of maintenance therapy.

The pharmacologic effects of reserpine (and other rauwolfia alkaloids) are attributed to a depletion of catecholamine and serotonin in the brain and adrenal medulla. The usual adult dose of reserpine ranges from 0.1 to 0.25 mg. Most preparations also contain a thiazide diuretic. As a result of the high incidence of adverse side effects, its current use is limited. No fatalities have been reported after overdose. As with other centrally acting antihypertensive agents, abrupt cessation of therapy can lead to withdrawal symptoms.

CLINICAL PRESENTATION

Clonidine overdose can result in significant respiratory and cardiovascular instability. CNS depression is common in overdose, even after a few pills. In adults, significant clinical toxicity occurs after the ingestion of 1 to 2 mg of clonidine. A specific lethal dose has not been determined. Children seem to be particularly susceptible to even small doses of clonidine, and serious symptoms have been precipitated by ingestion of a single adult therapeutic dose (0.1 to 0.3 mg) (11,25). Toxicity has been reported in children who have sucked on a used transdermal patch containing residual clonidine (10).

Signs and symptoms of toxicity usually occur within 30 to 60 minutes after ingestion, producing a clinical scenario that resembles a narcotic overdose, consisting of bradycardia, respiratory depression, lethargy, coma, and miosis. With serious toxicity, hypotension, hypothermia, and hyporeflexia are common. Hypertension may be seen in the initial phases of clonidine overdose and is associated with high plasma drug levels. This phase is transient, resolves spontaneously, and is quickly and precipitously followed by prolonged or serious hypotension. Hypertensive crisis, seizure, and anterior myocardial infarction (MI) has been described after a massive subcutaneous dose of 12.24 mg (6). A peculiar intermittent apnea, responsive to physical or auditory stimuli, has been noted in children. Clonidine interacts with other CNS depressants, such as alcohol and barbiturates, and the concomitant ingestion of these substances or sedative–hypnotics can increase CNS depression. Seizures are rare after overdose and are likely related to hypoxia rather than a direct effect. Rebound hypertension and other withdrawal symptoms may subsequently develop 2 to 4 days after an overdose if the patient has been on maintenance clonidine therapy.

A more obscure complication has been described in two patients who were receiving elevated doses of clonidine given intravenously for delirium tremens. These patients both developed colonic pseudoobstruction (Ogilvie's syndrome) 2 to 5 days after initiation of therapy (23). Long-term sequelae are rare. Permanent brain damage occurred in a child administered high doses of clonidine by the mother as a result of Munchausen by proxy (24).

Maintenance therapy with clonidine may be associated with dry mouth, fatigue, sedation, constipation, sexual dysfunction, and nonpostural dizziness. In children, maintenance therapy has been reported to rarely cause bradycardia and heart block (5). Skin reactions including erythema, vesiculation and induration have been associated with transdermal patches.

The clonidine withdrawal syndrome is characterized by varying degrees of rebound hypertension, tachycardia, tremulousness, insomnia, anxiety, sweating, and palpitations (7). Although usually mild and not life-threatening, significant cardiac dysrhythmias and hypertensive crises have been reported, and one case of MI thought to have resulted from acute clonidine withdrawal (16).

There are few reports of overdose involving other centrally acting antihypertensive agents. Significant guanabenz or guanfacine ingestion may produce lethargy, bradycardia, and hypotension (9). With methyldopa overdose, a benign clinical course is generally seen (14). Drowsiness, lethargy, bradycardia, hypotension, and atrioventricular conduction abnormalities have been reported. Significant reserpine ingestion may cause drowsiness, lethargy, hypotension, and bradycardia (15).

Side effects of guanabenz and guanfacine are similar to those of clonidine. Sedation is also a prominent side effect encountered during methyldopa therapy. A positive direct Coombs' test develops in about 25% of patients taking methyldopa, but hemolysis is seldom a clinical problem. Hepatitis occurs in 6% of patients using methyldopa. Depression, increased gastrointestinal motility, nasal congestion, and parkinsonian-like effects are relatively common during reserpine therapy. Signs and symptoms of guanabenz, guanfacine, methyldopa, and reserpine withdrawal are similar to but less pronounced than with clonidine.

DIFFERENTIAL DIAGNOSIS

Clonidine, guanabenz, and guanfacine poisoning may be clinically indistinguishable from toxicity caused by other $\alpha2$-adrenergic and imidazoline receptors agonists such as naphazoline, oxymetazoline (Afrin), tetrahydrozoline (Visine), and xylometazoline. These compounds are found in nasal decongestant and topical ophthalmic preparations. In children, the ingestion or topical application of such preparations has resulted in signs and symptoms that are identical to clonidine poisoning. Centrally acting antihypertensive agent poisoning may also resemble overdose from other substances, particularly narcotics, β-adrenergic blockers, calcium channel blockers, digitalis, and sedative–hypnotics. Hypoglycemia, sepsis, hypothermia, cerebrovascular accident, and head trauma should also be considered in the differential diagnosis.

EMERGENCY DEPARTMENT EVALUATION

The evaluation of patients with known or suspected centrally acting antihypertensive agent overdose includes close clinical observation, frequent vital sign determinations, and continuous electrocardiographic (ECG) monitoring. Special attention should be directed toward the clinical assessment of airway and breathing abnormalities, cardiovascular status, and evaluation for concomitant trauma.

The diagnosis of poisoning is based on the history and clinical findings. There are no laboratory or clinical tests that are of specific diagnostic or therapeutic value. These agents are not detected on routine drugs of abuse screening. Quantitative levels are unavailable in the clinical setting and are of no value in management. If the diagnosis is certain, ancillary studies will be of no additional value. Radiographic imaging, routine laboratory tests, and toxicologic analysis are useful only to rule out or confirm concomitant pathology.

EMERGENCY DEPARTMENT MANAGEMENT

Prehospital care is supportive. The routine administration of naloxone and evaluation or treatment for hypoglycemia are warranted in symptomatic patients. Because of the rapidity of onset of clonidine toxicity, prehospital or hospital use of ipecac should be avoided. Gastric lavage has no proven benefit and is generally not performed. It may be considered in a polydrug overdose including clonidine or in a recent massive ingestion, but such relevant clinical information is usually not readily available to the clinician. Activated charcoal alone is the preferred form of gastrointestinal decontamination. In the case of clonidine patch ingestion there may be a role for whole bowel irrigation. Continuous ECG monitoring and intravenous access should be maintained during the prehospital care and emergency department evaluation.

Treatment is primarily supportive and symptomatic, with therapy aimed at reversing specific derangements in cardiovascular and respiratory status. Hypotension usually responds

to crystalloid infusion. Occasionally, vasopressors, such as dopamine and norepinephrine, are required. Bradycardia secondary to clonidine usually responds to intravenous atropine, with repeated doses titrated against heart rate and blood pressure. Dopamine, epinephrine, and cardiac pacing are of theoretic benefit, but their use in clonidine poisoning has not been described. Respiratory depression is a serious consequence of clonidine overdose, and tracheal intubation and assisted ventilation may be required. In the unusual case in which transient hypertension is noted, antihypertensive treatment should generally be avoided because of the potential for subsequent serious and prolonged hypotension (4). Hypertension usually requires only observation, although, occasionally, a short-acting antihypertensive such as nitroprusside may be warranted. Hypothermia and coma are treated with supportive care. Clinical recovery is usually noted within 24 to 48 hours. Hemodialysis, charcoal hemoperfusion, and forced diuresis are of no proven value. Because clonidine is excreted unchanged in the urine, adequate urine output should be assured. Antacid therapy has been recommended to counter hyperchlorhydria during reserpine overdose.

There are no proven antidotes for centrally acting antihypertensive agent overdose. Naloxone has been used to reverse clonidine toxicity, but the response is inconsistent and unproven. The occasional anecdotal improvement in mental status and hemodynamic parameters noted after naloxone has been explained on the basis of a reversal of clonidine's opiate-like activity in the CNS. Its use is acceptable as a therapeutic trial in patients with depressed mental status. The optimal dose is unknown, but doses similar to those used for narcotic poisoning have been suggested. Both hypertension and hypotension have been temporally associated with the use of naloxone to reverse clonidine overdose. Patients who are given naloxone should be closely observed for potential hemodynamic deterioration.

Tolazoline, a central and peripheral α-adrenergic blocking agent, was once touted as an antidote for clonidine toxicity (21). Because its efficacy is based on sporadic case reports and it has potentially serious side effects (e.g., hypotension, tachycardia, and dysrhythmia), its use is not recommended.

Yohimbine, a centrally acting α_2-adrenergic antagonist, may be expected to have clinical activity opposite that of clonidine. Yohimbine has been suggested as a possible antidote for clonidine overdose, but little evidence is available to support its use, and no clinical guidelines are available.

The clonidine withdrawal syndrome is best treated by the reinstitution of clonidine therapy and tapering the dose over 5 to 10 days. A similar approach can be used the treatment of withdrawal from other agents.

CRITICAL INTERVENTIONS

- Establish intravenous access and institute continuous respiratory and cardiac monitoring in patients with acute overdose or significant CNS or cardiovascular manifestations following chronic exposure
- Make sure that advanced life support airway equipment and cardiovascular drugs are readily available

DISPOSITION

If vital signs are normal and the patient remains or becomes asymptomatic within 4 to 6 hours of ingestion, he or she may be discharged from the emergency department with appropriate psychiatric or social service follow-up. Symptomatic patients require admission to a unit capable of continuous cardiac and respiratory monitoring. A toxicology consultant or the drug and poison information center may be helpful in providing advice regarding the use of particular antidotes or final disposition. There is no known cyclical nature to clonidine overdose, and improvement is not followed by relapse. Patients may be safely transferred to another facility with paramedic-level transportation.

COMMON PITFALLS

✔ Failure to appreciate that clonidine poisoning may result in CNS and respiratory depression and cardiovascular depression

✔ Misdiagnosis of clonidine poisoning as narcotic overdose because of clinical similarities

✔ Overly aggressive treatment of early but transient hypertension, especially with long-acting agents

✔ Reliance on unproved antidotes rather than supportive care in the treatment of toxicity

✔ Failure to consider the possibility of child abuse or attempted homicide in children with overdose and to address psychiatric issues in patients with suicide attempts

Acknowledgments

We thank J. Frank Bonfiglio, David G. Hassard, and Sharona Bryant for their contributions to previous editions of this chapter.

References

1. Baumgartner GR, Rower RC. Clonidine vs chlordiazepoxide in the management of acute alcohol withdrawal syndrome. *Arch Intern Med* 1987;147: 1223.
2. Beuger M, et al. Clonidine use and abuse among methadone program applicants and patients. *J Subst Abuse Treat* 1998;15(6):589–593.
3. Bousquet P, Feldman J, Tibirica E, et al. New concepts on the central regulation of blood pressure: alpha-2-adrenoreceptors and imidazoline receptors. *Am J Med* 1989;87[Suppl 3C]:3C–10S.
4. Campbell BC, Reid JL. Regimen for the control of blood pressure and symptoms during clonidine withdrawal. *Int J Clin Pharmacol Res* 1985;5:215.
5. Cantwell DP, Swanson J, Connor DF. Case Study: adverse response to clonidine. *J Am Acad Child Adolesc Psychiatry* 1997;36(4):539–544.
6. Frye CB. Vance MA. Hypertensive crisis and myocardial infarction following massive clonidine overdose. *Ann Pharmacother* 2000;34(5):611–615.
7. Geyskes GG, Boer P, Mees EJD. Clonidine withdrawal: mechanism and frequency of rebound hypertension. *Br J Clin Pharmacol* 1979;7:55.
8. Gold MS, Pottash AL, Sweeney DR, et al. Efficacy of clonidine in opiate withdrawal. *Drug Alcohol Depend* 1980;6:201.
9. Hall AH, Smolinske SC, Kulig KW, et al. Guanabenz overdose. *Ann Intern Med* 1985;102:787.
10. Harris J. Clonidine patch toxicity. *DICP (Ann Pharmacol)* 1990;24:1191.
11. Heideman S, Sarnaik A. Clonidine poisoning in children. *Crit Care Med* 1990;18:618.
12. Klein-Schwartz W, Gorman R, Oderda GM, et al. Central nervous system depression from ingestion of non-prescription eyedrops. *Am J Emerg Med* 1984;2:217.
13. Klein-Schwartz W. Trends and toxic effects from pediatric clonidine exposures. *Archives of Pediatrics and Adolescent Medicine* 2002;156(4):392–396.
14. Lawson DH, Glass D, Jick H. Adverse reactions to methyldopa with particular reference to hypotension. *Am Heart J* 1978;96:572.
15. Loggie JMH, Saita H, Kahn I, et al. Accidental reserpine poisoning: clinical and metabolic effects. *Clin Pharmacol Ther* 1967;8:692.
16. Nakagawa S, Yamamoto Y, Koiwaya Y. Ventricular tachycardia induced by clonidine withdrawal. *Br Heart J* 1985;53:654.
17. Oster J, Epstein M. Use of centrally acting sympatholytic agents in the management of hypertension. *Arch Intern Med* 1991;152:1638.
18. Romano MJ, Dinh A. A 1000-fold overdose of clonidine caused by a compounding error in a 5 year old child with attention-deficit/hyperactivity disorder. *Pediatrics* 2001;108(2):471–472.
19. Rosenberg MH, Deerfield LJ, Baruch EM. Two cases of severe gamma-hydroxybutyrate withdrawal delirium on a psychiatric unit: recommendations for management. *Am J of Drug & Alcohol Abuse* 2003;29(2):487–496.
20. Sanklecha M, Jog A, Raghavan J. Clonidine casualty. *Indian J Pediatr* 1993;60:611.
21. Schieber RA, Kaufman ND. Use of tolazoline in massive clonidine poisoning. *Am J Dis Child* 1981;135:77.
22. Seger D. Clonidine Toxicity Revisited. *J Toxicol Clin Toxicol* 2002;40(2):145–155.
23. Stieger DS. Cantieni R. Frutiger A. Acute colonic pseudoobstruction (Ogilvie's syndrome) in two patients receiving high dose clonidine for delirium tremens. *Intensive Care Med* 1997;23(7):780–782.
24. Tessa C, et al. Permanent brain damage following acute clonidine poisoning. *Neuropediatrics* 2001;32(2):90–92.
25. Wiley J, Wiley C, Torrey S, et al. Clonidine poisoning in young children. *J Pediatr* 1990;116:654.

CHAPTER 302
Beta Blockers

Fermin Barrueto, Jr.

β-Adrenergic blocking agents (β-blockers) are primarily used for the treatment of acute coronary syndromes, cardiac dysrhythmias, congestive heart failure, and hypertension, and to decrease morbidity and mortality after myocardial infarction (MI). They are also used to treat glaucoma, migraines, pheochromocytoma, portal hypertension, tremors, and thyrotoxicosis. More than 14,000 exposures to β-blockers were documented by U.S. poison centers in 2002, making this the most common class of cardiovascular (CV) drugs associated with poisoning (25).

β-Blockers competitively block β-adrenergic receptors. These receptors are part of the sympathetic nervous system and have three main subtypes (β_1, β_2, and β_3) which regulate physiology in various locations in the body (Table 302.1) (5). Their blockade results in a decrease in the intracellular concentration of cyclic adenosine monophosphate (cAMP), a secondary messenger that mediates the cellular effects of β-stimulation.

β-Blockers vary in regard to β-receptor selectivity, α-receptor blocking activity, lipophilicity, intrinsic sympathomimetic (β-receptor agonist) activity, and membrane stabilizing activity (Table 302.2). β_1-Selectivity is preferred for cardiovascular therapy so as to avoid the detrimental effects of β_2-blockade, such as bronchoconstriction. Labetalol and carvedilol antagonize α-adrenergic receptors, although not as prominently as β-receptors, and may exacerbate hypotension as a result of vasodilation. β-Blockers with membrane stabilizing activity (MSA) inhibit fast sodium channels, which can lead to QRS prolongation and ventricular dysrhythmias. In overdose, selective activity is often lost and only a few β-blockers have unique toxicological profiles.

TABLE 302.1. Beta-Receptor Location and Function

	Anatomic Location	Effect of Receptor Agonism
β_1	Heart	Increase inotropy and chronotropy
	Eye	Increase aqueous humor production
	Kidney	Increase renin secretion
β_2	Smooth muscle	Relaxation around bronchi and vasculature
	Skeletal muscle	Glycogenolysis, K+ uptake
	Liver	Glycogenolysis and gluconeogenesis
β_3	Adipose	Lipolysis

TABLE 302.2. Beta-Blocker Properties and Selectivity

	Receptor Selectivity	Lipophilicity	Intrinsic Sympathomimetic Activity	Membrane Stabilizing Activity
Acebutolol	β_1	Low	+	++
Atenolol	β_1	Low	−	−
Betaxolol	β_1	Low	−	++
Bisoprolol	β_1	Low	−	−
Carteolol	β_1, β_2	Low	+	−
Carvedilol	$\alpha_1, \beta_1, \beta_2$	High	−	−
Esmolol	β_1	Low	−	−
Labetalol	$\alpha_1, \beta_1, \beta_2$	Mod	−	+
Metoprolol	β_1	Mod	−	+
Nadolol	β_1, β_2	Low	−	−
Oxprenolol	β_1, β_2	High	+	++
Pindolol	β_1, β_2	Mod	+	+
Propranolol	β_1, β_2	High	−	++
Sotalol	β_1, β_2	Low	−	−
Timolol	β_1, β_2	Mod	−	−

β-Blockers also vary with respect to protein binding, volume of distribution, route of elimination, and half-life (Table 302.3). They are generally well absorbed following ingestion, with peak levels and effects occurring 1 to 2 hours after a therapeutic dose. Because their duration of action is relatively short (6 hours or less), extended-release formulations were developed, allowing for less frequent dosing.

CLINICAL PRESENTATION

Most β-blocker overdoses are relatively minor and do not result in significant toxicity (23,25); however, large doses or the combination of a β-blocker with another cardioactive medication (e.g., calcium channel blockers) can result in significant morbidity and mortality (11). Patients who remain asymptomatic for 6 hours from the time of ingestion are unlikely to develop toxicity unless sotalol or an extended-release preparations was ingested. Sotalol has produced symptoms, QT prolongation, and other dysrhythmias up to 20 hours from the time of ingestion (13). With extended-release preparations, prolonged and erratic absorption may result in delayed toxicity.

Bradycardia and hypotension are the most common effects after overdose (4). Nausea and vomiting can occur. The skin may be pale and clammy. Lethargy and decreased mental status may result from hypoperfusion of the central nervous system. Hypoperfusion can lead to myocardial infarction, mesenteric ischemia, renal insufficiency, and stroke. Highly lipophilic agents and those with membrane-stabilizing effects can cause altered mental status in the face of a normal blood pressure. Delirium, coma, and seizures may occur in severe poisoning.

The electrocardiogram (ECG) may reveal AV nodal dysfunction with PR interval prolongation and AV block (10). If the SA node is affected, sinus bradycardia may progress to sinus pauses or arrest. Negative inotropic effects add to cardiotoxicity, particularly with β-blockers that have MSA (17). β-Blockers that have MSA can cause delayed depolarization with QRS prolongation and ventricular tachyarrhythmias (10,11). Sotalol is unique in that also blocks delayed rectifier potassium channels which results in delayed repolarization with QT prolongation, and can cause torsade de pointes (polymorphic) ventricular tachycardia and other lethal ventricular dysrhythmias (1,7,13).

In overdose, all β-blockers can cause β2-antagonism resulting in bronchospasm. This scenario may be more prominent

TABLE 302.3. Pharmacokinetics of Beta Blockers

Agent	Dose (mg)*	Absorption (%)	First-Pass Metabolism	Protein Binding (%)	Volume of Distribution (L/kg)	Route of Elimination	Half-Life (h)
Acebutolol	200–400	70	Yes	25	2.3	Renal	6
Atenolol	50–100	50	No	15	0.7	Renal	6–9
Betaxolol	10–40	100	Yes	50	6.1	Hepatic	14–22
Bisoprolol	5–40	90	No	30–36	2.7–3.1	Hepatic	11
Carvedilol	2.5–10	>90	Yes	98	1.6	Hepatic	7–10
Carteolol	3.125–25	80	No	23–30	4	Renal	6
Esmolol	IV only	NA	NA	55	3.4	Serum esterase	0.15
Labetalol	200–400	>90	Yes	50	10.0	Hepatic	3–4
Metoprolol	50–400	>90	Yes	12	5.5	Hepatic	3–4
Nadolol	40–320	30	No	30	2.1	Renal	14–24
Penbutolol	20–80	100	No	80–98	32–42	Hepatic	5
Pindolol	2.5–30	>90	No	57	2.0	Renal	5–12
Propranolol	20–120	>90	Yes	93	3.6	Hepatic	3–6
Sotalol	80–480	70	No	0	0.23	Renal	5–12
Timolol	20–60	>90	No	10	1.5	Renal	4–5

*Single oral adult dose.

and dangerous in patients with a history of asthma or chronic obstructive pulmonary disease (23). Hypoglycemia and hyperkalemia are distinct metabolic derangements that result from β-receptor blockade, although they are usually mild and not clinically significant (23). Hypoglycemia may be more common in children.

DIFFERENTIAL DIAGNOSIS

Diseases that cause bradycardia include sick sinus syndrome, inferior wall MI, hypothermia, severe sepsis, and carotid sinus hypersensitivity. Toxic causes include calcium channel blockers, cardiac glycosides, cholinergic agents, α₂-agonists, opioids, and sedative–hypnotics.

Like β-blockers, diltiazem and verapamil have strong negative inotropic and chronotropic effects. Dihydropyridine calcium channel blockers (e.g., nifedipine, nimodipine, and amlodipine) more typically cause reflex tachycardia in response to vasodilation and hypotension. In severe overdose, bradycardia is possible. Unlike β-blocker overdose, the mental status is often surprisingly normal. Also, in contrast to β-blockers, calcium channel blockers cause hyperglycemia rather than hypoglycemia. Cardiac glycoside (e.g., digoxin) poisoning usually does not cause hypotension until a nonperfusable dysrhythmia occurs. Additionally, cardiac glycoside overdose induces characteristic electrocardiographic patterns that differentiate this condition from β-blocker overdose. Vomiting is a more predominant feature, especially acute exposures. Like β blockers, cardiac glycosides can cause hyperkalemia, confusion, and lethargy.

Cholinergic agents (e.g., organophosphorus insecticides) cause diarrhea, lacrimation, urination, miosis, and vomiting along with bradycardia, bronchorrhea, and bronconstriction. Overdose with opioids, sedative hypnotics, and α₂-agonists may lead to mild bradycardia and hypotension associated with a depressed mental status but cardiac conduction disturbances are not usually seen.

EMERGENCY DEPARTMENT EVALUATION

The history should include the time and amount of drug(s) taken, treatment in the field (if any), the time of onset and nature of symptoms, known medical or psychiatric problems, and current drug therapy. Determining if the β-blocker was a sustained-release preparation or if there were any coingestants with CV effects is particularly important.

The physical exam should focus on the vital signs, cardiopulmonary system, and neurologic status. A 12-lead electrocardiogram should be a priority, along with continuous cardiac monitoring. A stat fingerstick or serum glucose concentration should be obtained, particularly in patients whose mental status is abnormal. Arterial blood gases, chemistry panel, complete blood count, toxicology testing, ECG, and chest radiograph should be obtained when clinically indicated.

EMERGENCY DEPARTMENT MANAGEMENT

Advanced cardiac life support measures should be instituted as needed. Once the airway, breathing, and circulation have been stabilized, gastrointestinal decontamination should be performed. Activated charcoal is the preferred method. If a sustained-release preparation has been ingested, multiple-dose activated charcoal or whole bowel irrigation should be considered.

Should the patient become bradycardic or hypotensive, a stepwise approach is recommended, in which interventions, each employed to a maximal degree, are successively applied and the hemodynamic response assessed. In severely poisoned patients, multiple therapies must be instituted and maintained simultaneously. Patients with bradycardia need only close monitoring if the blood pressure is normal. Hypotension can initially be treated with intravenous fluids. If bradycardia is also present, atropine, 1 mg intravenously (0.02 mg/kg; minimum dose, 0.1 mg in children), repeated in 5 minutes if necessary, can initially be given.

Glucagon (5 mg intravenously over 5 minutes; 50–100 ug/kg in children) may be effective for hypotension, even when it occurs in the absence of bradycardia. If there is no effect after 10 to 15 minutes, the dose should be repeated. Patients who respond should then be given an infusion of glucagons at a rate of 1 to 5 mg/hr (50 ug/kg/hr in children). Glucagon bypasses the β-blockade by activating a G protein bound to adenylate cyclase and activating the cascade indirectly to increase intracellular cAMP (Fig. 302.1). Glucagon often causes vomiting. Animal studies show that it has a positive chronotropic effect in β-blocker overdose but has minimal effect on mean arterial pressure (8,14,20,21). One animal study showed improved survival (8). Although there are no controlled trials, glucagon is widely accepted as effective in humans (2).

Intravenous calcium has been shown to assist with inotropy in animal β-blocker toxicity (12) and has been successful in reversing hypotension in humans (3,16). The dose is the same as for calcium channel blocker poisoning (see Chapter 303, "Calcium Channel Antagonists"). Vasopressors are often necessary. Although there are no human data to state if one pressor is more efficacious than the other, theoretically isoproterenol would be the ideal agent (23). However, this pressor can exacerbate hypotension and dysrhythmias. There is minimal clinical experience with isoproterenol. Dobutamine, epinephrine, and dopamine have all been used, but the dose is often much higher than what is traditionally used (23). If a vasopressor must be added to the treatment regimen, invasive cardiac monitoring or echocardiography should be performed to identify the agent that brings the appropriate response and to titrate to the desired effect, especially if the patient ingested other cardioactive drugs.

If the patient requires vasopressors, hyperinsulinemia-euglycemia (insulin and glucose) therapy should be considered.

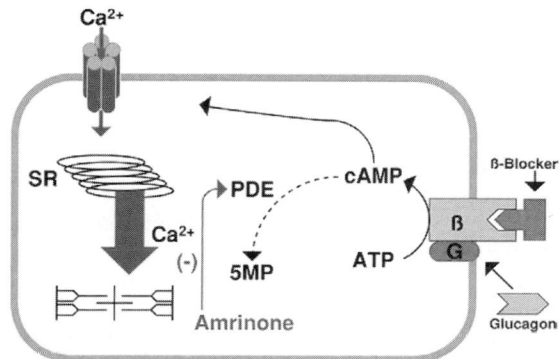

Figure 302.1. The Effects of Amrinone and Glucagon on cAMP. Extracellular Ca²⁺ influx will cause the SR (Sarcoplasmic Reticulum) to release Ca²⁺ exponentially to bind the excitation-contraction apparatus, made of actin and myosin filaments. cAMP increases intracellular Ca²⁺ and is created by an adenylate cyclase that is part of the β receptor and broken down by PDE (Phosphodiesterase). Glucagon can activate the G protein, bypass the β receptor if blocked and increase cAMP. Amrinone inhibits PDE thus also increasing cAMP.

The same protocol as in calcium channel blocker poisoning (see Chapter 303, "Calcium Channel Antagonists") should be used. In canine propranolol poisoning, this therapy was superior to glucagon and epinephrine. Hyperinsulinemia-euglycemia therapy may work by maximizing myocardial glucose utilization, augmentating cytosolic calcium concentrations, or possibly a direct inotropic effect (8). The response may be delayed 15 to 60 minutes, so other therapies must be continued.

A phosphodiesterase inhibitor such as inamrinone may also be effective (Fig. 302.1) This drug has a propensity to cause vasodilation, is difficult to titrate, and often does not assist with the negative chronotropy seen in β-blocker exposure (9,15,20,21,24). Hence, it should only be used in conjunction with other therapies.

Should pharmacological therapy be ineffective, invasive procedures such as cardiac pacing, artificial circulatory assistance, and extracorporeal drug removal should be considered. Intravenous cardiac pacing can be used to treat bradycardia; however, little improvement in cardiac output and difficulty with capture should be expected. Some authors have reported a decrease in blood pressure, which may be caused by loss of atrial contraction and/or impaired ventricular relaxation (23). Intraaortic balloon pump counterpulsation and partial or complete cardiac bypass pump support have been utilized in severe poisoning (14,18). Hemodialysis has been used with apparent success in the treatment of atenolol and sotalol overdose; charcoal hemoperfusion might be effective for removing water-soluble β-blockers that have a low volume of distribution (e.g., (19,22)). However, patients who would benefit from extracorporeal elimination measures are already hypotensive, making these procedures technically difficult and potentially hazardous. Continuous veno-venous hemodialysis is another alternative but it has never been studied and is time consuming.

In patients with sotalol poisoning, hypokalemia and hypomagnesemia should be corrected. The treatment of recurrent torsade de pointes should include overdrive pacing and magnesium infusions (1,6,7,13). Bradycardia and hypotension are treated the same as with other β-blockers.

CRITICAL INTERVENTIONS

- Institute a step-wise approach to managing cardiovascular toxicity: start with intravenous fluids for hypotension and atropine for bradycardia; if hypotension and bradycardia persist, administer glucagon, calcium, vasopressors, hyperinsulinemia-euglycemia therapy, and phosphodiesterase inhibitors; if still unstable, try transvenous pacing, intraaortic balloon pump counterpulsations, extracorporeal circulatory support measure, and consider hemodialysis or hemoperfusion

DISPOSITION

Patients with β-blocker ingestions who remain or become asymptomatic 6 hours after ingestion can be discharged or medically cleared for a psychiatric disposition. If sotalol or a sustained-release preparation was ingested, a 12- to 24-hour observation period is recommended. Patient who have abnormal vital signs, mental status, or ECG findings require continuous cardiac monitoring and frequent vital signs to assess the progression of toxicity. This usually necessitates admission to an ICU. The hospital's supply of glucagon should be ascertained, as many pharmacies are not prepared to administer the large doses required to treat β-blocker exposures. Transfer of the patient to a tertiary care facility should be considered in cases of severe poisoning or if the institution does not have sufficient

glucagon. Psychiatric consultation should be obtained for patients with intentional ingestions prior to discharge. Education in poison prevention, particularly in the pediatric population, should also be provided prior to discharge.

COMMON PITFALLS

✔ Failure to determine whether the drug ingested was an immediate- or extended-release formulation, particularly when making treatment and disposition decisions

✔ Failure to appreciate that β-blockers can cause hypoglycemia and to check a fingerstick blood sugar in patients with altered mental status

✔ Failure to appreciate that β-blockers with membrane stabilizing activity have sodium channel blocking activity and can cause delayed depolarization, cardiac conduction disturbances (QRS prolongation), and ventricular tachyarrhythmias

✔ Failure to appreciate that sotalol has potassium channel blocking effects and can cause delayed repolarization with prolonged QT intervals and torsades de pointes

✔ Failure to appreciate that patients with severe poisoning are likely to require invasive monitoring and multiple pharmacological treatments and mechanical hemodynamic support

Acknowledgments

The author thanks Walter Barrueto of BarruetoDesign for illustrating Fig. 302.1, Linda Kesselring for assisting with the technical writing and editing, and Christopher H. Linden for his contribution to the previous version of this chapter.

References

1. Arstall MA, Hii JT, Lehman RG, et al. Sotalol-induced torsade de pointes: management with magnesium infusion. *Postgrad Med J* 1992;68:289–290.
2. Bailey B. Glucagon in β-blocker and calcium channel blocker overdoses: a systematic review. *J Toxicol Clin Toxicol* 2003;41:595–602.
3. Brimacombe JR, Scully M, Swainston R. Propranolol overdose: a dramatic response to calcium chloride. *Med J Aust* 1991;155:267–268.
4. DeLima LGR, Kharasch ED, Butler S. Successful pharmacologic treatment of massive atenolol overdose: sequential hemodynamics and plasma atenolol concentrations. *Anesthesiology* 1995;83:204–207.
5. Enocksson S, Shimizu M, Lonnqvist F, et al. Demonstration of an in vivo functional beta 3-adrenoceptor in man. *J Clin Invest* 1995;95:2239–2245.
6. Gustavsson CG, Vinge E, Norlander BO, et al. Pharmacokinetic evaluation of a case of massive sotalol intoxication. *Ann Pharmacother* 1997;31:856–859.
7. Hohnloser SH, Woosley RL. Sotalol. *N Engl J Med* 1994;331:31–38.
8. Kerns W, Schroeder D, Williams C, et al. Insulin improves survival in a canine model of acute [beta]-blocker toxicity. *Ann Emerg Med* 1997;29:748–757.
9. Kollef MH. Labetalol overdose successfully treated with amrinone and alpha adrenergic receptor agonists. *Chest* 1994;105:626–627.
10. Love JN, Enlow B, Howell JM, et al. Electrocardiographic changes associated with β-blocker toxicity. *Ann Emerg Med* 2002;40:603–610.
11. Love JN, Howell HM, Litovitz TL, et al. Acute beta blocker overdose: factors associated with the development of cardiovascular morbidity. *J Toxicol Clin Toxicol* 2000:38:275–281.
12. Love JN, Hanfling D, Howell JM. Hemodynamic effects of calcium chloride in a canine model of acute propranolol intoxication. *Ann Emerg Med* 1996;28:1–6.
13. McVey FK, Cork CF. Extracorporeal circulation in the management of massive propranolol overdose. *Anaesthesia* 1991;46:744–746.
14. Love JN, Leasure JA, Mundt DJ, et al. A comparison of amrinone and glucagon therapy for cardiovascular depression associated with propranolol toxicity in a canine model. *J Toxicol Clin Toxicol* 1992;30:399–412.
15. Neuvonen PJ, Elonen E, Vuorenmaa T, et al. Prolonged Q-T interval and severe tachyarrhythmias, common features of sotalol intoxication. *Eur J Clin Pharmacol* 1981;20:85–89.
16. Pertoldi F, D'Orlando L, Mercante WP. Electromechanical dissociation 48 hours after atenolol overdose: usefulness of calcium chloride. *Ann Emerg Med* 1998;31:777–781.
17. Reith DM, Dawson AH, Epid D, et al. Relative toxicity of beta blockers in overdose. *J Toxicol Clin Toxicol* 1996;34:273–278
18. Rooney M, Massey KL, Jamali F, et al. Acebutolol overdose treated with hemodialysis and extracorporeal membrane oxygenation. *J Clin Pharmacol* 1996;36:760–763.

19. Saitz R, Williams BW, Farber HW. Atenolol-induced cardiovascular collapse treated with hemodialysis. *Crit Care Med* 1991;19:116–119.
20. Sato S, Tsuji MH, Okubo N, et al. Combined use of glucagon and milrinone may not be preferable for severe propranolol poisoning in the canine model. *J Toxicol Clin Toxicol* 1995;33:337–342.
21. Sato S, Tsuji MH, Okubo N, et al. Milrinone versus glucagon: comparative hemodynamic effects in canine propranolol poisoning. *J Toxicol Clin Toxicol* 1994;32:277–289.
22. Salhanick SD, Wax PM. Treatment of atenolol overdose in a patient with renal failure using serial hemodialysis and hemoperfusion and associated echocardiographic findings. *Vet Hum Toxicol* 2000;42:224–225.
23. Taboulet P, Cariou A, Berdeaux A, et al. Pathophysiology and management of self-poisoning with beta-blockers. *J Toxicol Clin Toxicol* 1993;31:531–551.
24. Travill CM, Pugh S, Noble MIM. The inotropic hemodynamic effects of intravenous milrinone when reflex adrenergic stimulation is suppressed by beta-adrenergic blockade. *Clin Ther* 1994;16:783–792.
25. Watson WA, Litovitz TL, Rodgers GC Jr, et al. 2002 annual report of the American Association of Poison Control Centers Toxic Exposure Surveillance System. *Am J Emerg Med* 2003;21:353–421.

CHAPTER 303
Calcium Channel Antagonists

Matthew D. Sztajnkrycer and G. Randall Bond

Calcium channel antagonists (CCAs) are a structurally diverse group of drugs that are used in the treatment of supraventricular tachyarrhythmias, hypertension, angina, heart failure, and subarachnoid hemorrhage, and in the prevention of migraine headaches. The term calcium channel blocker is inaccurate, as these agents cause the channel to favor a closed state rather than physically blocking them. Ten CCAs are currently approved for use in the United States: verapamil, diltiazem, nifedipine, nicardipine, felodipine, isradipine, amlodipine, nisoldipine, nimodipine, and bepridil.

The divalent calcium cation is critical for biological function of the cell, involved in such diverse tasks as myocyte excitation-contraction coupling, intracellular second messenger signaling, release of neurotransmitters and hormones, and initiation and propagation of the action potential. Intracellular calcium is largely sequestered within the sarcoplasmic reticulum, and released through direct receptor activation or through second-messenger mediated systems. Calcium channels are found in the membranes of many cells, including vascular smooth muscle, the myocardium, and the specialized pacemaker and conducting fibers of the heart. Three general classes of calcium channel have been identified, based on mechanism of activation: voltage-operated calcium channels (VOCCs), receptor-operated calcium channels, and second messenger-operated calcium channels. VOCCs have been subcategorized into six distinct channel subtypes: L, N, P, Q, R, and T (22). Membrane depolarization leads to the influx of calcium ions by way of voltage-operated calcium channels. In contrast to skeletal muscle in which sodium entry and voltage changes trigger calcium release from the intracellular sarcoplasmic reticulum, myocardium and vascular smooth muscle are both dependent on extracellular calcium entry through VOCCs for excitation-contraction coupling. In the pacemaker cells of the sinoatrial (SA) and atrioventricular (AV) nodes, the influx of calcium by way of slow channels during phase 4 of the action potential accounts for spontaneous depolarization. In His-Purkinje cells, calcium influx by way of slow channels contributes to phase 2 (plateau) and to phase 4 of the action potential.

Currently available CCAs act by depressing the activation, inactivation, and recovery of L-type (slow) VOCCs, and are thus classified as class IV antiarrhythmics. Cardiovascular (CV) responses to therapeutic doses vary considerably (Tables 303.1 and 303.2).

CCAs are well absorbed after oral administration. With immediate release preparations, effects are typically noted within 2 to 3 hours of oral administration. Effects are delayed 6 to 8 hours after the ingestion of sustained release preparations, and delays as long as 15 hours postingestion have been reported. CCAs are significantly protein-bound (80% to 98%), have a moderate volume of distribution (1.4–4.3 L/kg), are extensively metabolized by the liver, and are excreted in the urine and bile. Verapamil, diltiazem, and bepridil have active metabolites. The elimination half-life for most CCAs is 2 to 9 hours in therapeutic doses. Amlodipine and bepridil have longer half-lives, ranging from 24 to 60 hours. After overdose, the half-life of diltiazem remains unchanged, although those of verapamil and nifedipine increase slightly (5,11,12,17).

Most of the CCA clinical toxicology experience is based on four agents: verapamil, diltiazem, nifedipine, and amlodipine (19). Nicardipine, felodipine, nisoldipine, isradipine, and nimodipine are members of the same class as nifedipine and amlodipine (dihydropyridines) and can be expected to have similar toxicity. Bepridil is a unique agent, with sodium and potassium channel antagonism in addition to CCA effects. Toxic CV effects of CCAs are in large part an exaggeration of their therapeutic effects. Peripheral vascular resistance is always decreased, but cardiac output may be normal, increased, or decreased. With the exception of nimodipine, CCAs do not penetrate the blood–brain barrier. Central nervous system (CNS) effects are secondary to hypoperfusion. Both hypoperfusion and impaired carbohydrate metabolism may lead to lactic acidosis. Impaired

TABLE 303.1. Cardiovascular Response to Drug Therapy

	Verapamil	Diltiazem	Nifedipine and Other Dihydrophyridines	Bepridil
Heart rate (sinoatrial node)	↑ or ↓	↓	↑	↓
Atrioventricular nodal conduction	↓↓	↓	↑	↓
Smooth-muscle tone	↓↓	↓	↓↓↓	↓
Blood pressure	↓	↓	↓↓	↓
Contractility (*in vivo*)	↓↓	↓	↑ or ↓	↓

TABLE 303.2.   Therapeutic Doses of Calcium Channel Blockers

Drug	Trade Name	Usual Dose	Therapeutic Range
Verapamil	Calan, Isoptin, Verelan		
Oral		80–160 mg t.i.d.	15–100 ng/mL
Intravenous		5–10 mg	
Diltiazem	Cardizen, Dilacor	30–90 mg q.i.d.	30–130 ng/mL
Nifedipine	Adalat, Procardia	10–40 mg t.i.d.	25–100 ng/mL
Nicardipine	Cardene	20–40 mg q.i.d.	28–50 ng/mL
Nimodipine	Nimotop	60 mg q4h	7–96 ng/mL
Felodipine	Plendil	5–20 mg qd	0.7–8.0 ng/mL
Isradipine	DynaCirc	2.5–10.0 mg b.i.d.	2–8 mg/mL
Nisoldipine	Sular	20–40 mg qd	
Amlodipine	Norvasc	2.5–10.0 mg qd	5–15 mg/mL
Bepridil	Vascor	200–400 mg qd	

calcium-dependent insulin release and peripheral insulin resistance may cause hyperglycemia (14). With overdosage, the drug-specific effects noted in Table 303.1 are often lost (15,20). Because people ingest drugs that are readily available to them, an unusually large percentage of CCA poisoning occurs in older people. Most of these are intentional, but some result from confusion or failing vision. Toxic doses are at least one to two times the usual total daily dose (20). Death has been reported after ingestion of a single tablet of nifedipine by a child (16). The elderly are susceptible to lower toxic doses (20). Toxicity can also be seen when these agents are used in therapeutic doses with other myocardial depressants, such as β-adrenergic antagonists and quinidine-like agents.

CLINICAL PRESENTATION

Signs and symptoms of toxicity usually develop within 30 minutes of ingestion but may be delayed as long as 15 hours after overdose of sustained-released preparations. Findings include hypotension, bradycardia, thready pulse, and peripheral cyanosis. Reflex tachycardia has been reported, especially with dihydropyridine ingestion. Older patients may experience chest pain and myocardial ischemia and infarction. Inadequate perfusion may also result in cerebral, renal and bowel ischemia or infarction in patients of all ages. In severe cases, coma, seizures, and respiratory distress associated with cardiogenic and non-cardiogenic pulmonary edema are described. The electrocardiogram (ECG) often shows decreased rate and first-, second-, or even third-degree AV block, and may have changes indicative of ischemia or infarction (20). QT-prolongation may be noted with bepridil ingestion, and torsades de pointes has been reported (18). Chest radiography may show pulmonary edema. Laboratory abnormalities include metabolic acidosis and hyperglycemia. Serum drug levels are not readily available and have not proved useful in the management of these patients.

Toxic effects typically last 24 to 36 hours. Duration may be longer after ingestion of bepridil, amlodipine, and sustained-release preparations. Complications have required longer hospitalizations in many patients.

DIFFERENTIAL DIAGNOSIS

Patients with primary myocardial infarction, and those with overdosage of β-adrenergic antagonists, cardiac glycosides, clonidine, guanabenz, imidazolines, angiotensin converting enzyme inhibitors, cholinergic agents (nicotine, organophosphate and carbamate insecticides, and agents to treat myasthenia gravis), tricyclic antidepressants, α-methyldopa, and veratrum alkaloids, may present similarly to those with CCA ingestion. B-adrenergic blocking agents are more likely to cause hypoglycemia, and CCAs are more likely to cause hyperglycemia. With cholinergic agents salivation, nausea, vomiting, diarrhea, and weakness dominate the presentation. Tricyclic antidepressant (TCA) overdosage infrequently presents with heart block and bradycardia. Although both TCA and CCA ingestions may result in prolonged QRS complexes (the latter as a result of ventricular escape rhythms), TCA-intoxicated patients often manifest evidence of antimuscarinic toxidrome and CNS depression in normotensive or hypertensive patients.

EMERGENCY DEPARTMENT EVALUATION

The history should include time of ingestion and all other substances ingested or available to the patient. Physical examination should focus on cardiopulmonary and CNS status. All patients should have cardiac monitoring, an ECG, and frequent monitoring of blood pressure. Those with symptoms, abnormal vital signs, or an abnormal ECG should have arterial blood gas analysis and determination of serum electrolytes, glucose, blood urea nitrogen, and creatinine. Continuous peripheral and pulmonary artery pressure monitoring may be necessary in patients with hemodynamic compromise.

EMERGENCY DEPARTMENT MANAGEMENT

Advanced life-support measures should be initiated as necessary. Intravenous access should be established in all patients. Early management should include gastrointestinal decontamination. Activated charcoal is the preferred method. Multiple-dose activated charcoal and whole bowel irrigation is recommended for ingestions of sustained release preparations.

Mild hypotension may respond to a fluid challenge with 1 to 2 L of saline solution (10–20 mL/kg in children). When bradycardia, with or without AV block, is also present, atropine (1.0 mg i.v., 0.02 mg/kg in children) can be tried. Response is infrequent but may be improved following calcium administration (9,20). Hypotension and symptomatic bradycardia should also be treated with calcium chloride (1 g i.v. slow push; 10–20 mg/kg in children) (20). Calcium gluconate (3 g i.v. slow push; 30–60 mg/kg in children) may be given if calcium chloride is unavailable. This dose may be repeated every 10 to 15 minutes up to 3 times in patients who show incomplete, transient, or no response (4,7,10,15). Care must be taken to avoid extravasation, which can result in severe tissue damage. A continuous infusion at a rate of 0.2 to 0.4 cc/kg/hr (10% calcium chloride) or 0.6 to 1.2 cc/kg/hr (10% calcium gluconate) may be used to support heart rate and blood pressure in patients who relapse after an initial bolus (22). Although calcium administration is frequently ineffective, proponents argue that this is as a result of inadequate dosing. Doses as high as 30 g of calcium gluconate in 12 hours have been used with success (4). Calcium levels should be monitored in patients receiving more than two doses, but very high serum calcium levels are not a reason to discontinue treatment. Response and survival have been associated with dosing that resulted in a peak serum calcium level of 23.8 mg/dL (4) In another patient who responded to high-dose calcium, irreversible hypotension occurred when calcium gluconate was discontinued, solely because the serum calcium level had reached 17.7 mg/dL (15).

Hemodynamically significant bradycardia or heart block unresponsive to atropine and calcium may respond to an infusion of glucagon or isoproterenol, but a pacemaker is often required (2,19,20,23). In a prospective study, electrical capture occurred in only 50% of patients (22). Heart rate is improved more than blood pressure.

Hypotension unresponsive to fluids and calcium should be treated with pressors. Dopamine, dobutamine, norepinephrine, isoproterenol, and combinations of these have been used with success. Glucagon may also be of benefit for hypotension, but it should not be used until the effects of traditional pressors are optimized (2). Inamrinone has produced additive effects, with isoproterenol in one case report and glucagon in another (6,23).

Exogenously supplied insulin, in the form of hyperinsulinemia–euglycemia (HIE) therapy, significantly improved hemodynamics and survival in an animal model of CCA intoxication and reversed catecholamine-unresponsive shock in a series of 5 patients (13,24). It is recommended for patients with inadequate response to the measures above. Insulin has been noted to have positive inotropic effects in conditions of myocardial stress. During myocardial toxicity, the metabolism of the myocardial cells is shifted away from fatty acid oxidation, toward carbohydrate dependence. The result is a decrease in net ATP production but improved oxygen utilization. However, in cases of severe CCA toxicity hyperglycemia is frequently noted. The etiology is multifactorial, reflecting both impaired insulin release and peripheral resistance (14). The result is that the CCA-intoxicated myocardium is further impaired as a result of limited cellular glucose uptake at a time of glucose dependence. The aim of HIE therapy is to reverse this state.

Published experience suggests the following HIE protocol (3,22). Patients with serum glucose levels less than 200 mg/dL should receive one 50 mL ampule of 50% dextrose (0.25 g/kg in children), followed by frequent glucose measurements and supplemental glucose as required. Due to potential insulin mediated effects on serum potassium, patients with serum potassium concentrations less than 2.5 mEq/L should receive 40 mEq of potassium (1mEq/kg in children, maximum 20–40 mEq/dose) as an oral supplement or i.v. potassium 10–20 mEq (0.10–0.30 mEq/kg in children) administered over the course of 1 hour. A bolus of 1.0 IU/kg regular insulin is recommended, followed by an infusion of 0.5 to 1.0 IU/kg/hr, titrated to clinical effect (systolic BP >100 mm Hg, HR > 50/min). Fluid and glucose support with D10 $\frac{1}{2}$NS at 80% maintenance is recommended. Serum glucose should be checked every 20 minutes for the first hour and hourly thereafter. Serum potassium should be checked hourly during HIE therapy.

The use of an intraaortic balloon pump should be considered in patients who are unresponsive to pharmacologic therapies. Cardiopulmonary bypass was also used to sustain a child until hepatic metabolism of verapamil occurred (8). Full recovery can be expected, unless prolonged shock has resulted in irreversible end-organ damage.

Limited information exists regarding the use of multiple-dose charcoal to enhance CCA elimination in the overdose setting,

but when used it has not been shown to be of benefit (21). Although enhanced elimination using charcoal hemoperfusion was described in a patient with diltiazem overdose, it should not be regarded as standard therapy (1). If supportive measures can maintain a pulse and blood pressure sufficient to allow hemoperfusion, there is little to be gained from this procedure.

CRITICAL INTERVENTIONS

- Admit or observe asymptomatic patients with overdoses of sustained preparations for an extended period of time
- Administer i.v. fluids and calcium for hypotension and bradycardia
- Administer i.v. chronotropic agents, pressors, glucagons, and hyperinsulinemia-euglycemia therapy for refractory hypotension and bradycardia

DISPOSITION

Asymptomatic patients should be observed for 4 to 6 hours after ingestion of standard formulations and 18 to 24 hours following ingestion of sustained-release ones. Those who remain asymptomatic may be discharged or referred for psychiatric evaluation. Symptomatic patients should be admitted to an intensive care unit. A regional poison center or a toxicologist should be consulted if the physician is unfamiliar with the management of CCA overdose. Transfer may be necessary if an intensive care unit bed is unavailable and should be arranged as soon as the ingestion is recognized, because CV performance may rapidly deteriorate. The patient should be transferred in an advanced life-support unit with an adequate supply of CV drugs, including calcium chloride and glucagon, on hand.

COMMON PITFALLS

✔ Failure to consider CCA poisoning in patients with hypotension, bradycardia, or AV block, particularly when hyperglycemia is present

✔ Failure to appreciate that ingestion of a single pill may be lethal in a toddler

✔ Failure to consider whole bowel irrigation and multiple-dose charcoal for patients with overdoses of sustained preparations

✔ Failure to administer chronotropic agents and pressors to patients with myocardial ischemia secondary to hypoperfusion

✔ Failure to consider invasive hemodynamic monitoring and CV support in patients with refractory shock

References

1. Anthony T, Jastremski M, Elliot W, et al. Charcoal hemoperfusion for the treatment of a combined diltiazem and metoprolol overdose. *Ann Emerg Med* 1986;15:1344.
2. Bailey B. Glucagon in β-Blocker and Calcium Channel Blocker Overdoses: A Systematic Review. *J Toxicol Clin Toxicol* 2003;41:595–602.
3. Boyer EW, Duic PA, Evans A. Hyperinsulinemia therapy for calcium channel blocker therapy. *Pediatr Emerg Med* 2002;18:36–37.
4. Buckley N, Whyte I, Dawson H. Overdose with calcium channel blockers [Correspondence]. *BMJ* 1994;308.1639.
5. Ferner RE, Monkman S, Riley S, et al. Pharmacokinetics and toxic effects of nifedipine in massive overdose. *Hum Exp Toxicol* 1990;9:309–311.
6. Goenen M, Col J, Compete A, et al. Treatment of severe verapamil poisoning with combined amrinone-isoproterenol therapy. *Am J Cardiol* 1986;58:1142.
7. Haddad LM. Resuscitation after nifedipine overdose exclusively with intravenous calcium chloride. *Am J Emerg Med* 1996;14:602–603.
8. Hendren WG, Schieber RS, Garrettson LK. Extracorporeal bypass for the treatment of verapamil poisoning. *Ann Emerg Med* 1989;18:984–987.
9. Howarth DM, Dawson AH, Smith AJ, et al. Calcium channel blocking drug overdose: an Australian series. *Hum Exp Toxicol* 1994;13:161–166.

10. Isbister GK. Delayed asystolic cardiac arrest after diltiazem overdose; resuscitation with high dose intravenous calcium. *Emerg Med J* 2002;19:355–357.
11. Jablowski AT, Mizgala HF. Effect of diltiazem overdose. *Am J Cardiol* 1987;60:932
12. Kivisto K, Neuvonen PJ, Tarssanen L. Pharmacokinetics of verapamil in overdose. *Hum Exp Toxicol* 1997;16:35–37.
13. Kline JA, Tomaszewski CA, Schroeder JD, et al. Insulin is a superior antidote for cardiovascular toxicity induced by verapamil in the anesthetized canine. *J Pharmacol Exp Ther* 1993;267:744–750.
14. Kline JA, Raymond RM, Schroeder JD, et al. The Diabetogenic Effects of Acute Verapamil Poisoning. *Toxicol Appl Pharmacol* 1997;145:357–362.
15. Koch AR, Vogelaers DP, Decruyenaere JM, et al. Fatal intoxication with amlodipine. *J Toxicol Clin Toxicol* 1995;33:253–256.
16. Lee DC, Greene T, Dougherty T, et al. Fatal nifedipine ingestions in children. *J Emerg Med* 2000;19:359–361.
17. Malcolm N, Callegari P, Goldberg J, et al. Massive diltiazem overdosage: clinical and pharmacological observations. *Drug Intell Clin Pharm* 1986;20:888.
18. Oshawa M, Tanaka F, Kunugita F, et al. A case of sick sinus syndrome that developed torsades de pointes, pacing failure and sensing failure during administration of bepridil. *Jpn Heart J* 2003;4:783–788.
19. Ramoska EA, Spiller HA, Myers A. Calcium channel blocker toxicity. *Ann Emerg Med* 1993;22:196–200.
20. Ramoska EA, Spiller HA, Winter M, et al. A one-year evaluation of calcium channel blocker overdoses. Toxicity and treatment. *Ann Emerg Med* 1993;22:196–200.
21. Roberts D, Honcharik N, Sitar DS, et al. Diltiazem overdose. Pharmacokinetics of diltiazem and its metabolites and effect of multiple dose charcoal therapy. *J Toxicol Clin Toxicol* 1991;29:45–52.
22. Salhanick SD, Shannon MW. Management of calcium channel antagonist overdose. *Drug Saf* 2003;26:65–79.
23. Wolf LR, Spadafora MP, Otten EJ. Use of amrinone and glucagon in a case of calcium channel blocker overdose. *Ann Emerg Med* 1993;22:1225–1228.
24. Yuan TH, Kerns WP II, Tomaszewski CA, et al. Insulin-glucose as adjunctive therapy for severe calcium channel antagonist poisoning. *J Toxicol Clin Toxicol* 1999;37:463–474.

CHAPTER 304
Cardiac Glycosides

John S. Kashani and Richard D Gerkin

TABLE 304.1. Sources of Cardiac Glycosides

Genus and Species	Common Name	Part Used
Digitalis purpurea	Purple foxglove	Leaf
Digitalis lanata	Grecian foxglove	Leaf
Strophanthus kombé		Seed
Strophanthus gratis		Seed
Urginea maritima (squill)	Sea onion	Bulb
Nerium oleander	Oleander	All parts
Thevetia neriifolia	Yellow oleander	All parts
Convallaria majalis	Lily of the valley	All parts
Bufo spp.	Toad	Skin

Cardiac glycosides (CGs) are a closely related group of chemicals having a common effect on the myocardium. CGs are found in a variety of plants, including oleander, foxglove, red squill, and lily of the valley, and in the skin, salivary glands and venom glands of Bufo genus toads (Table 304.1). CGs have also been found in some herbal preparations, sometimes as an unintentional ingredient. The term "digitalis" is often used as a generic term referring to any substance containing CGs. Digoxin (Lanoxin, Digoxin, Digitek) is the only preparation for routine therapeutic use in the United States. Digoxin is used in the treatment of congestive heart failure, atrial fibrillation, atrial flutter and paroxysmal atrial tachycardia. As a result of its narrow therapeutic window, digoxin has historically been implicated as one of the most common causes of adverse drug reactions. Digitalis toxicity occurs in upwards of 20% of people treated with digitalis drugs, and 30% of those taking CGs who are admitted to the hospital exhibit some degree of toxicity (11).

CGs inhibit the sodium-potassium adenosine triphosphatase (ATPase) membrane pump found in cardiac cells (3). Normally, depolarization follows the opening of the fast sodium channels. The rise in the intracellular potential opens voltage gated calcium channels causing the influx of calcium. The rise in intracellular calcium causes further calcium release from the sar-

coplasmic reticulum, producing contraction. Extracellular movement of sodium in exchange for potassium and sequestering of calcium by the sarcoplasmic reticulum results in repolarization of the cell. In the presence of CGs, the sodium-potassium ATPase is blocked, causing a relative intracellular hypernatremia. Intracellular sodium is exchanged for calcium, raising cytoplasmic calcium levels, which promotes interaction between actin and myosin and results in an increased inotropic effect. In addition to the inotropic effects, automaticity is increased, there is shortening of the time for repolarization of the atria and ventricles, conduction through the SA and AV node is slowed, and vagally-mediated parasympathetic tone is increased.

The therapeutic daily dose of digoxin ranges from about 0.005 mg/kg in premature infants to as much as 0.75 mg in adults. Digoxin is 40% to 90% intestinally absorbed, with a range of onset of action from 1.5 to 6 hours. High blood levels occur early after ingestion, before the drug has time to redistribute to tissues. The actual volume of distribution ranges from 4 to 7 L/kg in adults and 10 to 16 L/kg in children. Digoxin is 25% protein bound, predominantly renally eliminated with a half-life upwards of 1.6 days. Dosing adjustments based on creatinine clearance and a decrease in the dose amount and frequency must be considered in the renal failure patient (7). Both serum (total) and free digoxin levels may be measured. The most common method of obtaining a level is by fluorescence polarization immunoassay (FPIA). Therapeutic serum digoxin levels are 0.5 to 2.0 ng/mL. Patients with a serum concentration above 2.0 ng/mL measured at least 6 hours postingestion may have CG toxicity, although the patient may not have signs or symptoms (1). Some patients, however, may exhibit toxicity in the therapeutic range. After an acute ingestion, before the drug has equilibrated between the serum and the tissues in which it exerts its effects, the serum digoxin level will only verify that ingestion has occurred, and will not predict the degree of clinical toxicity.

Ingestion of oleander or Bufo toxins can result in an apparent or false positive digoxin level. This is a result of the partial cross reactivity in the assay, but the measured digoxin levels do not correlate with toxicity. Other nondigoxin cardiac glycosides may or may not cross react with digoxin immunoassays. Another source of false positive digoxin assays are substances called endogenous digoxin-like steroidal substances (EDLS). These substances may be present in patients with renal insufficiency, hepatic disease, hypertension, agonal states, pregnancy, cor pulmonale, myocardial infarction, mucocutaneous lymph node syndrome, subarachnoid hemorrhage, congestive heart failure, and in both premature and full-term infants (8). Levels are usually low, but have occasionally been measured above 2.0 ng/mL.

ECG changes occur frequently. It is important to understand that, in the absence of significant dysrhythmias, ECG changes indicate the presence of digoxin, but do not correlate with toxicity. The "digitalis effect" refers to four typical ECG findings (10). These ECG changes can be seen at levels within therapeutic range. The first finding includes T wave abnormalities, with

TABLE 304.2.   Conditions Contributing to Digoxin Toxicity

Advanced age
Renal impairment
Hypoxia
Myocardial ischemia
Hypothyroidism
Hypokalemia
Hypomagnesemia
Hypercalcemia

inversion or elevation that may mimic acute ischemia or pericarditis. Peaking of the terminal of the T wave may occur. The second finding is a shortened QT interval. The third finding is scooping or sagging of the ST-segment with concomitant ST-segment depression (more pronounced in the lateral leads). Lastly, there may be an increase in the U-wave amplitude.

Digoxin toxicity is the result of exaggeration of therapeutic effects. Ectopy results from increased automaticity and bradycardia and atrioventricular block result from depressed cardiac conduction. The mortality rate from CG toxicity varies by study, but is roughly 10%. The mortality rate is higher 13 to 25% (11) in suicidal and accidental ingestions. Ventricular tachycardia (VT) in the setting of CG toxicity has an associated 50% mortality rate. Risk factors associated with a poor prognosis include advanced age, heart disease, male sex, high-degree AV block, and hyperkalemia (4). Hypokalemia tends to exacerbate tachydysrhythmias (12). Many other factors are known to contribute or predispose to toxicity (Table 304.2).

CLINICAL PRESENTATION

Toxicity may occur in the acute or chronic setting. Acute toxicity is most often in a younger population as an accidental or intentional ingestion. Chronic toxicity usually occurs in the elderly population. In healthy adults, single acute doses of less than 5 mg of digoxin seldom cause toxicity. Fatal doses are almost always greater than 10 mg. As a result of the narrow therapeutic range of digoxin, toxicity can occur with only two to three times the therapeutic dose in patients on chronic therapy.

Patients with digoxin toxicity will often present with nausea and vomiting. Chronic toxicity is more likely to present with central nervous system (CNS) findings, including confusion, lethargy, depression, fatigue, headache, paresthesias, weakness, scotomata and disturbances of color vision, especially xanthopsia (yellow vision). Digoxin toxicity may present as a fulminant psychiatric disturbance as its sole manifestation (5).

Virtually any dysrhythmia may develop as a result of toxicity, although rapid atrial fibrillation or atrial flutter are rare (see Table 304.3) (10). Most commonly PVCs, either unifocal or multifocal, occur. The three classically described dysrhythmias include paroxysmal atrial tachycardia with block (considered to be pathognomonic of digitalis toxicity), junctional (AV nodal) tachycardia, and VT. The presence of any tachydysrhythmia with

TABLE 304.3.   Digitalis-Induced Dysrhythmias

Bradyarrhythmias	Tachyarrhythmias
Sinus exit block or sinus arrest	Atrial tachycardia with block
Sinus bradycardia	Junctional tachycardia
Atrioventricular nodal block first degree; second degree type 1; third degree	Ventricular premature beats
	Ventricular tachycardia especially bidirectional
	Ventricular fibrillation

block (e.g., paroxysmal atrial tachycardia with block, atrial fibrillation with a regular ventricular response as a result of AV block with a junctional escape rhythm) is highly suggestive of CG toxicity. Any slowing of the ventricular response to atrial fibrillation in a patient on digoxin also suggests toxicity. Atrioventricular conduction blocks ranging from first degree to third degree may occur, although Mobitz type II is rare (10). Additionally, sinus bradycardia, from increased vagal tone, and other bradydysrhythmias are common. Hypotension suggests a hemodynamically significant dysrhythmia, loss of vasomotor regulation, or the presence of coingestant(s). Complications resulting from inadequate perfusion include hypoxic seizures, encephalopathy, and acute renal tubular necrosis.

In 150 patients with acute ingestions, life-threatening complications were high-grade AV block (53%), refractory VT (46%), hyperkalemia (37%), and ventricular fibrillation (33%) (2). After acute overdose, the most common ECG abnormalities are sinus bradycardia and varying degrees of AV block; ventricular dysrhythmias are less frequently seen. Chronic intoxication is more commonly associated with ventricular dysrhythmias, atrial tachycardia, and junctional tachycardia. Hyperkalemia is common after acute overdose whereas hypokalemia, probably related to concurrent diuretic use, is more common in chronic poisoning.

DIFFERENTIAL DIAGNOSIS

Intoxications that can cause CG-like bradydysrhythmias include those from class 1B antidyshythmics, baclofen, β adrenergic blockers, calcium channel antagonists, cholinergic agonists and cholinesterase inhibitors, clonidine, guanabenz, and ingested imidazoline decongestants, and nicotine. CG-like tachydysrhthythmias can be caused by poisoning with class 1A, IC, and III antidysrhythmics, antihistamines, baclofen, cyclic antidepressants, fluoride, heavy metals, local anesthetics, meperidine, neuroleptics, propoxyphene, quinine and related antimalarials, and sympathomimetics. Plants cause similar cardiotoxicity include *Phoradendron tomentosum* (American mistletoe), Remijia and Rhododendron species, *Schoenocaulon officinalis* (sabadilla), *Stylophorum diphyllun*, Veratrum species (e.g., American hellebore), and *Zanthoxylum brachycanthum*. Worsening cardiomyopathy and congestive heart failure, CNS hemorrhage/ischemia, electrolyte abnormalities, myocardial ischemia/infarction, myocarditis, pericarditis, pheochromocytoma, preexitation syndromes, thyroid dysfunction should also be considered in the differential diagnosis of CG-like cardiotoxicity.

Intoxications that can cause CG-like visual disturbances include those from carbon disulfide, ergot alkaloids, ethambutol, heavy metals, methanol, quinine and antimalarials, salicylates, and tamoxifen. The differential diagnosis of visual disturbances also includes diseases such as cataracts, cerebrovascular disease, corneal disease, diabetes, glaucoma, macula degeneration, migraine, optic neuritis, retinal detachment, vasculitis, and vitreous hemorrhage.

EMERGENCY DEPARTMENT EVALUATION

The history should include the amount, route, duration, and intent of exposure. Because CGs may be present in herbal supplements (13), the medication history should include herbal supplement use. Vital signs should include pulse oximetry. The patient should be specifically examined for signs consistent with congestive heart failure and decreased peripheral perfusion. The patient should be placed on continuous cardiac monitoring and a 12-lead ECG should be obtained. Routine laboratory studies should be ordered, including determination of serum electrolytes, calcium, magnesium, blood urea nitrogen, and serum creatinine. Digoxin levels should be obtained and serum levels should checked every 3 to 4 hours after an acute ingestion. A chest radiograph should be obtained in patients with cardiac dysrhythmias, hypotension, underlying cardiac disease, or hypoxia. Patients with chronic intoxication should have liver function tests.

EMERGENCY DEPARTMENT MANAGEMENT

Advanced cardiac life support (ACLS) measures should be instituted as necessary. Intubation should be considered in patients with an altered mental status. Acid–base abnormalities, hypoxia, fluid, and electrolyte imbalances should be corrected. Although hypokalemia can exacerbate digoxin toxicity, caution is advised when replacing potassium in the renal failure patient. Similarly, although intravenous calcium is commonly used to treat hyperkalemia, it should be avoided in the setting of digoxin toxicity, as hyperkalemia may be as a result of impaired intracellular pumping of potassium, in which case cells are already relatively hypercalcemic. Intravenous sodium bicarbonate, inhaled β-adrenergic agonists, insulin and glucose can be used to treat hyperkalemia but because this condition may reflect transmembrane shifts not total body overload, exchange resins that deplete potassium should be avoided. Antidigoxin Fab fragments may also be indicated for hyperkalemia as a result of acute CG poisoning.

The preferred method of gastrointestinal decontamination following acute ingestion is activated charcoal. Repeat doses of activated charcoal are effective in shortening the half life of digoxin, digitoxin, and probably other CGs. Multiple dose activated charcoal, for instance, has been useful in the setting of CG toxicity secondary to yellow oleander (6). Vagal effects associated with emesis and gastric lavage may worsen bradycardia and hypotension. Resin binders (cholestyramine) are no more effective than charcoal. Neither forced diuresis, hemodialysis, peritoneal dialysis, nor hemoperfusion enhances elimination.

Antidotal therapy with antidigoxin Fab fragment antibodies is the treatment of choice for hemodynamically compromising or life-threatening bradydysrhythmias and tachydysrhythmias and for hyperkalemia (serum potassium greater than or equal to 5.5 mEq/L) after an acute overdose (14). An elevated serum digoxin level is merely confirms an overdose, and the degree of elevation should not be used to guide the administration of Fab fragments. The use of prophylactic Fab therapy in the setting of nonlife-threatening dysrhythmias and associated risk factors for toxicity remains to be proven (14).

Atropine (0.5 mg i.v.) can also be given for bradydysrhythmias. Antibody therapy appears to be more effective and safer than electrical cardiac pacing (14). Although pacing may sometimes be necessary, irritation by the pacing wire in a digoxin poisoned heart can precipitate ventricular tachydysrhythmias, and this therapy should not delay definitive therapy with antibody therapy.

Standard therapy for CG-induced ventricular tachydysrhythmias includes intravenous phenytoin (25 mg/min until a desired effect is achieved or a total of 15 mg/kg has been given) and lidocaine (1 mg/kg), and magnesium sulfate (2–3 g i.v. over 1 min) (10). Such therapy may be necessary if antidigoxin antibodies are unavailable, while waiting for an effect, and when antibody therapy is unsuccessful. Refractory cardiac tachydysrhythmias induced by digoxin have responded to magnesium infusions (2 g/h for 4–5 hours) (11). Pulseless rhythms require defibrillation or cardioversion. Cardioversion may precipitate ventricular fibrillation. If possible, medical management should be used initially. When cardioversion is necessary, initial settings should be at reduced power settings (5–10 joules).

Antidigoxin Fab fragments are prepared by immunizing sheep, purifying their antibodies, and cleaving off the Fc fragments with papain. Hence, those with a history of allergy to sheep or papaya may be at risk for an allergic reaction. Two antibody preparations are commercially available, DigiBind® (Glaxo Wellcome) and DigiFab® (Protherics Inc.), which are virtually identical therapeutically. Antibody fragments possess a greater affinity for digoxin than does sodium-potassium ATPase and lower the extracellular unbound digoxin concentration. Further equilibration of receptor-bound digoxin with the fluid in the extracellular space leads to an eventual release of digoxin from its receptor sites (15). The drug-antibody complex is renally excreted, with a half life of 16 hours in normal renal function and up to 4 days in patients with renal failure.

Antidigoxin Fab fragments are given intravenously over 30 minutes unless the patient is in cardiac arrest, when it can be given as a bolus. If the quantity of digoxin ingested is known, the dose (in vials) of DigiBind or DigiFab can be calculated. The ingested dose in milligrams is divided by 0.6 mg/vial. Each vial of DigiBind contains 38 mg of Fab fragments, which will bind 0.5 mg of digoxin, although each vial of DigiFab contains 40 mg of Fab fragments. The usual dose for acute overdose is 5 to 10 vials. In chronic toxicity, the body load in milligrams can be estimated by multiplying the steady state serum concentration of digoxin by 5.6 times the patients weight in kilograms divided by 1,000. The usual dose of Fab fragments in the setting of chronic toxicity is 1 to 2 vials. Resolution of the digoxin-induced dysrhythmias and hyperkalemia are usually noted within 30 minutes of Fab fragment administration, but it may take several hours for a maximal effect. In the setting of CG toxicity secondary to oleander or bufo toxins, larger doses of Fab fragments may be required, because of weak cross-reactivity.

Serum digoxin assays measure both bound and unbound drug. After administration of antidigoxin Fab fragments the serum digoxin level will rise as the drug is pulled from the tissues and is sequestered with the antibody in the serum. Free digoxin levels, measured by equilibrium dialysis or ultrafiltration will be low if the proper amount of Fab fragment drug is given. A rebound rise in serum digoxin levels within 24 hours of antibody administration is seen in patients with normal renal function, and may be seen in up to 8 days in patients with renal failure. This is presumably as a result of metabolic degradation of the antigen antibody complex. Recurrent clinical toxicity is rare (6).

CRITICAL INTERVENTIONS

- Administer antidigoxin antibody Fab fragments for hemodynamically compromising or potential lethal dysrhythmias, and for hyperkalemia (K > 5.5 mEg/L) after acute overdose
- Avoid using calcium and exchange resins to treat hyperkalemia
- Begin with low power settings when cardioverting tachydysrhythmias

DISPOSITION

Intensive care unit admission is advised for acutely symptomatic patients or patients who have elevated digoxin levels and dysrhythmias. When the use of antidigoxin Fab fragment therapy is considered, consultation with a poison center, toxicologist, and cardiologist is advised. Chronically poisoned patients that are hemodynamically stable and do not require active treatment may be admitted to a telemetry unit. If Fab fragments or pacemaker therapy is not available, the patient should be transferred (by ACLS personnel) to the nearest facility that has these modalities.

COMMON PITFALLS

✔ Failure to consider plant products such as herbals or teas in the differential diagnosis of CG-like cardiotoxicity

✔ Failure to appreciate that a serum digoxin level drawn less than 8 hours after ingestion does not reflect toxicity or need for treatment

✔ Failure to appreciate that digoxin assays may not yield a measurable digoxin level with ingestions of CGs from plants or Bufo toads

✔ Failure to appreciate the differences between acute and chronic CG poisoning

✔ Failure to appreciate that pacemaker wires can irritate the myocardium and precipitate ventricular tachydysrhythmias in patients with CG poisoning

✔ Failure to appreciate that intravenous phenytoin and magnesium may be useful for the treatment of CG-induced tachydysrhythmias

Acknowledgment

We thank previous edition chapter author Thomas J. Higgins, Jr.

References

1. Abad-Santos F, Carcas AJ, Ibanez C, et al. Digoxin level and clinical manifestations as determinants in the diagnosis of digoxin toxicity. *Ther Drug Monit* 2000;22(2):163–168.

2. Bayer MJ. Recognition and management of digitalis intoxication: implications for emergency medicine. *Am J Emerg Med* 1991;9[Suppl]:29.

3. Bigger JT. Digitalis toxicity. *J Clin Pharmacol* 1985;25:514

4. Bismuth C. Hyperkalemia in acute digitalis poisoning: prognostic implications and therapeutic implications. *J Toxicol Clin Toxicol* 1973;6:153.

5. Brubacher JR, Ravikumar PR, Bania T, et al. Treatment of toad venom poisoning with digoxin-specific Fab fragments. *Chest* 1996;110(5):1282–1288.

6. De Silva HA, Fonseka MM, Pathmeswaran A, et al. Multiple-dose activated charcoal for treatment of yellow oleander poisoning: a single-blind, randomised, placebo-controlled trial. *Lancet* 2003;361(9373):1935–1938.

7. Fenton F, Smally AJ, Laut J. Hyperkalemia and digoxin toxicity in a patient with kidney failure. *Ann Emerg Med* 1996;28(4):440–441.

8. Jortani S, Valdes R. Digoxin and Its Related Endogenous Factors. *Crit Rev Clin Lab Sci* 1997;34(3):226–274.

9. Kinlay S, Buckley NA. Magnesium sulfate in the treatment of ventricular dysrhythmias due to digoxin toxicity. *J Toxicol Clin Toxicol* 1995;33(1):55–59.

10. Ma G, Brady WJ, Pollack M, et al. Electrocardiographic manifestations: digitalis toxicity. *J Emerg Med* 2001;20(2):145–152.

11. Mauskopf JA, Wenger TL. Cost-effectiveness analysis of the use of digoxin immune Fab (ovine) for treatment of digoxin toxicity. *Am J Cardiol* 1991;68:1709.

12. McDonough AA, Wang J, Farley RA. Significance of sodium pump isoforms in digitalis therapy. *J Mol Cell Cardiol* 1995;27(4):1001–1009.

13. Scheinost ME. Digoxin toxicity in a 26-year old woman taking a herbal dietary supplement. *J Am Osteopath Assoc* 2001;101(8):444–446.

14. Taboulet P, Baud FJ, Bismuth C. Clinical features and management of digitalis poisoning—rationale for immunotherapy. *J Toxicol Clin Toxicol* 1993;31(2):247.

15. Valdes R Jr, Jortani SA. Monitoring of unbound digoxin in patients treated with anti-digoxin antigen-binding fragments: a model for the future? *Clin Chem* 1998;44(9):1883–1885.

16. Varriale P, Mossavi A. Rapid reversal of digitalis delirium using digoxin immune Fab therapy. *Clin Cardiol* 1995;18(6):351–352.

17. Wenger TL. Experience with digoxin immune Fab (ovine) in patients with renal impairment. *Am J Emerg Med* 1991;9[Suppl]:21.

18. Yound IS, Goh EMS, McKillop UH, et al. Magnesium status and digoxin toxicity. *Br J Clin Pharmacol* 1991;32:717.

PART VII

Chemicals, Gases, and Metabolic Poisons

CHAPTER 305

Arsenic and Mercury

Jay L. Schauben

Arsenic can be found in rodenticides, insecticides, herbicides, paints, veterinary medicinals, folk remedies, and naturally in the earth's crust. It is also present in drinking water and seafood, is used in the production of glass, metals, and computer chips and can be found as a chemical intermediate in the manufacture of many products. An estimated 1.5 million exposures to arsenic occur each year. It is the most common cause of acute heavy-metal poisoning and is second only to lead as a cause of chronic intoxication. Arsine gas is formed when arsenic compounds interact with acids.

Arsenic most commonly exists in trivalent (arsenite) and pentavalent (arsenate) forms. The average dietary intake is about 2 mg/d in adults. The trivalent form exhibits rapid gastrointestinal (GI) absorption, with more than 80% of the ingested dose absorbed. The pentavalent form is even more readily absorbed. Blood arsenic levels may be as high as 60 μg/L in normal people, with urine arsenic concentrations ranging from 10 to 300 μg/L. A seafood dinner can transiently elevate arsenic urine levels to 20 to 1,700 μg/L.

Arsenic is an intracellular toxin that appears to act by combining with sulfhydryl groups of enzymes and proteins involved in the Krebs cycle, thereby interfering with oxidative phosphorylation processes. It has also been postulated that arsenic is capable of substituting itself for the phosphate moiety in many cellular reactions, resulting in the loss of high-energy bonds. The pentavalent form appears less toxic than the trivalent form but may be converted to it at the cellular level. An acute dose of 100 to 200 mg is potentially fatal, whereas larger cumulative doses can be tolerated when exposure is chronic. Organoarsenicals are generally considered to be nontoxic.

In poisoned patients, blood arsenic levels usually exceed 100 μg/L, with urine concentrations ranging from several hundred to several thousand μg per L. Arsenic levels tend to remain elevated with chronic exposure but decrease rapidly over a period of several days after acute exposure. Long-term occupational exposure to arsenic has been associated with an increase in cancer of the buccal cavity, pharynx, lung, kidney, bone, large intestine, and rectum (23).

Rare instances of chronic arsenic toxicity have been reported when chromated copper arsenate-treated wood is burned in fireplaces or stoves (11). Even though the manufacturers moved to voluntarily withdraw the use of chromated copper arsenate in 2003, there has been no evidence that chromated copper arsenate-treated wood presents any threat to health with normal use, especially if a sealant has been applied.

The major route of arsenic elimination is renal excretion, with small amounts excreted in bile, feces, and saliva. The elimination curve is biphasic, apparently because of protein binding and redistribution of arsenic into the extravascular compartment.

Mercury was used as a folk remedy for GI problems, an antiseptic, an antisyphilitic, an unguent, a purgative, and a cure for adynamic ileus during the latter half of the nineteenth century. It is still used medically in dental amalgam and as a germicide, bactericide, diuretic, and laxative. In industry, it is used as a chemical intermediate, in the manufacture of electrical apparatus, and as an antifouling agent, a paint pigment, an instrument fluid, a fungicide, and a catalyst in the production of plastics and paper.

Mercury is found in elemental, inorganic, and organic forms. Toxic effects vary considerably with the chemical form of the metal, and the duration and intensity of exposure. There is evidence that *in vivo* conversion exists between the various forms of the metal, and that these forms may accumulate in tissue by binding to proteins. Mercury crosses the placenta and can be secreted into breast milk. Normal blood mercury levels may be 20 μg/L or higher as a result of its presence in the diet (e.g., seafood consumption). Urine concentrations are normally less than 50 μg/L.

Elemental mercury exposure commonly results from the accidental ingestion of the contents of a broken thermometer (0.1 mL), suicidal ingestion, rupture of mercury-containing balloons used for GI procedures, inhalation of mercury vapor, or i.v. or s.c. injection. Although mercury is present in dental amalgam, there is little evidence that mercury-containing restorations are hazardous to health (4,19). Elemental mercury volatilizes slowly at room temperature (more rapidly with heat), producing mercury vapor that is absorbed through the lungs. Elemental mercury is poorly absorbed from the GI tract or through intact skin. The solubility of the lipophilic elemental form, and therefore its potential to cause toxicity, depends on its oxidation to the mercuric ion. This conversion is enhanced with exposure to heat, acids, and strong oxidants. As is true of arsenic, the ionic form of mercury combines with the sulfhydryl groups of various proteins, leading to the inhibition of enzyme systems. Excretion is primarily through the urine and feces, with a half-life of up to 60 days. What constitutes a toxic dose is poorly defined.

In general, bivalent inorganic mercuric salts (e.g., sulfide, chloride, and oxide) are more soluble and more toxic than monovalent ones (e.g., mercurous chloride or calomel). They are irritating, occasionally producing dermatitis with or without vesication, discoloration of the nails, and burns of mucous membranes. The potentially fatal acute oral dose is about 100 mg. Percutaneous absorption can also result in systemic toxicity (24). Once absorbed, inorganic salts are converted to the mercuric form and are concentrated in the kidneys. They do not penetrate the blood–brain barrier to any significant extent, consistent with its limited central nervous system (CNS) effects. Excretion is mainly through the urine and feces, with a half-life of about 40 days.

Exposure to organic mercury compounds (merbromin, Merthiolate, thimerosal, methylmercury, ethylmercury, and phenylmercuric salts) is most often as a result of the ingestion of contaminated fish, shellfish, or grain and to the inhalation of vaporized organomercurials. Consumption of seafood from Minamata Bay, which contained high levels of methylmercury, resulted in an outbreak of chronic organic mercury poisoning (Minamata disease). Mass poisoning has also resulted from the ingestion of grain treated with methylmercury fungicide. Organic forms of mercury are well absorbed by the GI and respiratory tracts, but the potential for dermal absorption appears low.

Alkyl mercury compounds (e.g., methyl and ethylmercury) are highly lipid-soluble, become distributed widely throughout the body, become concentrated in the blood and CNS, and easily pass the placental barrier. Long-chain aryl and alkyl compounds (e.g., phenyl and methoxyethyl mercury) are converted *in vivo* to the inorganic form. The shorter chain alkyl agents undergo enterohepatic recirculation, with final excretion in the feces and a half-life approaching 70 days. The potentially fatal acute oral dose of organic mercurials is about 1 g.

CLINICAL PRESENTATION

Manifestations of acute arsenic poisoning begin 30 minutes to 2 hours after ingestion and usually consist of violent gastroenteritis, with vomiting, profuse diarrhea, colicky abdominal pain, and, in severe cases, GI hemorrhage. Rapidly progressive toxicity, with hypotension, renal failure, QT prolongation with ventricular dysrhythmias (e.g., torsades de pointes), rhabdomyolysis, and CNS depression may occur (2). Severe, generalized capillary damage can lead to massive third-spacing, resulting in cardiovascular (CV) collapse, adult respiratory distress syndrome, and massive proteinuria.

Delayed neurologic, dermatologic, and hematologic effects can occur after acute arsenic poisoning and are similar to the manifestations of chronic intoxication. Symmetric polyneuropathy, involving both sensory and motor nerve fibers, is common. Symptoms can resemble those of the Landry-Guillain-Barré syndrome (8). Histologic studies demonstrate axonal degeneration of large myelinated fibers. However, evidence supports a demyelinating polyradiculopathy, evolving to an axonal degeneration neuropathy (16). Recovery is slow (as long as 6 years) and often incomplete. An encephalopathy resembling Wernicke's or one characterized by prominent disinterest and lack of awareness of peripheral neurologic deficits can be seen. Dermatologic manifestations may include diffuse exfoliative dermatitis, pal-

mar hyperkeratosis, and Mees' lines (transverse white bands on the nails). Normochromic, normocytic anemia, leukopenia, and thrombocytopenia may develop. Chronic exposure may also cause edema, sore throat, stomatitis, pruritus, coryza, alopecia, lacrimation, salivation, weakness, and restrictive or obstructive lung disease (15).

Symptoms of arsine gas inhalation include abdominal pain, headache, weakness, malaise, nausea, and vomiting. Laboratory manifestations include hemolysis, renal failure, hyperkalemia, and anemia. These findings may be delayed up to 24 hours after milder exposures.

Elemental mercury is relatively nontoxic when ingested, as a result of poor GI absorption and slow oxidation to a more absorbable form. The oral LD_{10} for humans has been reported to be in the range of 1,429 mg/kg, or about 100 g in a 70-kg adult (24), although patients who remained asymptomatic after ingesting 500 grams have been reported (21). With ileus or leakage of mercury into the peritoneal cavity, mercuric oxide or sulfide salts may form, be absorbed, and cause systemic inorganic mercury poisoning. Without an ileus or GI perforation, systemic absorption is unlikely, and the elemental mercury usually passes uneventfully per rectum. Dermal contact with elemental mercury, as with the contents of a broken thermometer, should not cause toxicity.

Aspiration of elemental mercury into the lungs can cause acute respiratory distress, pneumonitis, hemoptysis, cyanosis, tachycardia, hypotension, hematuria, and bloody diarrhea. This type of exposure may also lead to chronic respiratory and systemic problems (13).

Intravenous injection of elemental mercury has caused abscess and granuloma formation at the injection site, hemoptysis, pulmonary embolization of mercury with consequent pulmonary dysfunction, and elevated blood and urine mercury levels (17,25). Systemic manifestations include weeping dermatitis, leukopenia, anemia, diarrhea, salivation, liver damage, and kidney damage.

S.c. injection has also caused local inflammation, abscess and granuloma formation, elevated mercury concentrations, and rarely death (5). The tissue reactions seen include both early and late reaction patterns. Initially necrosis, acute inflammatory reactions and aseptic abscess formation are witnessed, followed by foreign-body giant cell reactions, fibrosis, granuloma formation, and membranous fat necrosis (5).

Exposure to elemental mercury within a confined space may cause toxicity as a result of inhalation of fumes. Heat and oxidative processes accelerate the formation of mercury vapor (mercuric oxide). Symptoms usually begin within a few hours of exposure and include cough, dyspnea, chills, fever, weakness, salivation, nausea, vomiting, diarrhea, and a metallic taste. Respiratory symptoms may subside or progress to interstitial pneumonitis with patchy bilateral infiltrates, pulmonary edema, atelectasis, pneumothorax, necrotizing bronchiolitis, and, possibly, death. The onset of acute lung injury may be delayed up to 24 to 72 hours. Systemic effects similar to those of inorganic mercury poisoning and CNS depression can occur. Fumes can also cause skin and mucous membrane irritation, with manifestations similar to the mucocutaneous lymph node syndrome (Kawasaki disease) (1).

Chronic exposure to mercury vapor can result in mild-to-moderate CNS dysfunction, including increased irritability, emotional instability, memory loss, and insomnia (19). GI complaints, renal failure, chronic pneumonitis, constriction of visual fields, discoloration of the lens capsule, dermatitis, anorexia, and tremor may also be present. Hyperthyroidism and autonomic findings similar to those seen with pheochromocytoma have been described (12). Findings typically associated with chronic inorganic mercury poisoning (acrodynia) have also been reported.

Acute exposure to the inorganic mercury salts may cause tachycardia, hypotension or hypertension, and sudden CV collapse. The corrosive nature of such salts often causes nausea, vomiting, abdominal pain, bloody diarrhea, edema, and necrosis of the GI tract. Symptoms may progress over 1 to 3 days to include mercurial stomatitis (glossitis and ulcerative gingivitis), loosening of teeth, jaw necrosis, proximal renal tubular necrosis resulting in transient polyuria, albuminuria, urine cast formation, hematuria, anuria, and acidosis (24). Hepatic necrosis can also occur.

Chronic exposure to inorganic mercury salts may result in acrodynia ("pink disease"). Originally reported in children exposed to elemental mercury or teething powders containing calomel, it is characterized by redness of the palms and soles, edema of the hands and feet, rashes, diaphoresis, tachycardia, hypertension, photophobia, irritability, and anorexia.

Poisoning by organic mercurials is usually much more insidious than that which results from inorganic mercury. Symptoms may not occur for as long as several weeks after exposure. Nausea, vomiting, diarrhea, and abdominal pain are common GI complaints. Phenylmercury (and other aryl compounds), however, can cause acute malaise and myalgias, and the alkylmercurials (methylmercury and ethylmercury) are irritating to skin and mucous membranes, possibly resulting in burns, papular or papulovesicular rash and dermatitis. Neurologic effects range from paresthesias, confusion, hallucinosis, irritability, sleep disturbances, ataxia, memory loss, slurred speech, auditory defects, narrowing of the visual fields, emotional instability, and inability to concentrate to stupor, coma, and death. Chronic exposure to organic mercurials can result in similar neurotoxicity.

DIFFERENTIAL DIAGNOSIS

Arsenic or mercury poisoning should be suspected in patients with acute or chronic GI and neurologic symptoms and multiple organ dysfunction of unknown etiology. Similar GI symptoms may be caused by viral or bacterial pathogens or the ingestion of other heavy metals (e.g., iron, thallium), food-borne toxins, and a variety of plants, mushrooms, and toxic agents (e.g., theophylline, ricin, abrin, cholinergics, corrosives, lithium, laxatives, alcohol, hydrocarbons, and fluoride). Solvents, hydrocarbons, other heavy metals, alcohol, and vitamins, and the possibility of organic disease, should be considered in the differential diagnosis of neurotoxicity. Multiple organ failure can occur after the ingestion of antimetabolites, colchicine, or other heavy metals and exposure to carbon monoxide or cyanide.

EMERGENCY DEPARTMENT EVALUATION

The history should include identification of the product and the route, dose, and duration of exposure. For ingestions, the physical examination should focus on vital signs, assessment of hydration, the abdomen, the CV system, and neurologic function. The mucosa should be checked for corrosive injury, and airway patency should be confirmed. For mercury inhalation or injection, the examination should also focus on respiratory function.

Ancillary studies include cardiac monitoring, electrocardiogram (ECG), chest radiograph, abdominal radiographs (for ingestions), oxygen saturation or arterial blood gas analysis, complete blood count (CBC), serum electrolytes, blood urea nitrogen (BUN), creatinine, glucose, liver function tests, coagulation profile, creatine phosphokinase (CPK), and urinalysis. Blood and 24-hour urine arsenic or mercury levels (with or without chelation, depending on the presence or absence of acute symptoms) should be obtained.

EMERGENCY DEPARTMENT MANAGEMENT

Advanced life-support measures are instituted, as necessary. Patients with acute ingestions of arsenic or inorganic mercury salts and those with arsine gas inhalation commonly require aggressive intravenous fluid resuscitation. Maintenance fluids should be sufficient to sustain a brisk urine output. Central venous pressure monitoring and bladder catheterization with urine-output monitoring may be necessary. Exposure to elemental mercury fumes may necessitate endotracheal intubation.

For acute ingestions of arsenic and inorganic or organic mercurials, gastric aspiration and lavage may be the preferred initial methods of GI decontamination if the patient presents within one hour of the exposure. Consideration should be given to the corrosive effects of the inorganic mercury salts. Activated charcoal should be considered for arsenic and inorganic mercury salt ingestions if these present within 1 to 2 hours postexposure. Whole-bowel irrigation presents a good alternative for large ingestions or cases in which abdominal radiographs show the persistent presence of radiopaque material in the GI tract. In patients with progressive toxicity and persistent metal present on x-ray despite these interventions, endoscopic or surgical removal may be warranted. GI decontamination is not recommended for acute elemental mercury ingestion or chronic exposures. The patient exposed to arsine gas should have dermal decontamination performed.

Cases of s.c. injections of elemental mercury should receive surgical debridement of all readily accessible subcutaneous areas in which mercury is located (5,22). Historically, the management of i.v. injections involved close observation and symptomatic treatment for emboli resulting from the i.v. administration of the mercury. Delayed systemic toxicity can arise from the formation of mercury oxides. The use of chelating agents such as BAL and DMSA (17), and DMPS (25), have been suggested for these cases.

Chelation therapy is warranted in acutely symptomatic patients and possibly in asymptomatic patients who present to the emergency department early after a significant exposure to arsenic and inorganic or aryl mercury compounds. Dimercaprol (BAL in peanut oil) should be initiated with an i.m. loading dose of 3 to 5 mg/kg and followed by doses of 2.5 to 3.0 mg/kg every 4 to 6 hours during the first 2 days, then every 8 to 12 hours thereafter. If the integrity and function of the gut are intact, DMSA (succimer, dimercaptosuccinic acid; Chemet), an oral chelator, may also be given. The use of D-penicillamine has fallen out of favor (11). The dose of DMSA is 10 mg/kg every 8 hours for 5 days, and then the same dose every 12 hours. Some investigators have advocated an optimal adult DMSA dose of 30 mg/kg/d for 5 days (3,6,10). The duration of the initial chelation course varies, depending on the severity of the exposure. A 5- to 7-day course may be adequate in mild intoxications, but it seems prudent with severe exposures to continue the initial course for 10 to 14 days. Thereafter, 24-hour urine arsenic levels should be followed, with repeat 5- to 14-day courses of chelation therapy prescribed until the 24-hour urine arsenic or mercury level falls below 50 μg/L. Courses of therapy should be interrupted by a 5- to 10-day abstinence period to allow for redistribution of arsenic from peripheral tissues into the blood and more effective subsequent chelation.

Hemolysis caused by arsine gas exposure is usually not responsive to dimercaprol therapy, but exchange transfusion or blood replacement may help. Alkalinization of the urine may benefit patients with significant rhabdomyolysis and hemoglobinuria. The use of chelation therapy in organic and elemental mercury poisoning is controversial, although DMSA, DMPS and N-acetyl-D, L-penicillamine have shown some promise in the treatment of elemental mercury exposures.

DMSA therapy is also indicated for asymptomatic patients with an elevated arsenic or mercury body burden (as indicated by blood and urine levels) or for patients exhibiting very mild symptoms who can be treated on an outpatient basis. They may be given in the same dosages described previously. The course may be repeated on the basis of the measurement of urine arsenic or mercury excretion after a 10- to 14-day abstinence period. Dimercaprol should be used instead of DMSA if the latter cannot be taken orally, if significant renal impairment is evident, or if the patient is allergic to DMSA, but it is contraindicated in organic mercury exposures.

Dimercaprol can cause a dose-dependent rise in blood pressure accompanied by tachycardia. Other adverse reactions include pain at the injection site, urticaria, hyperpyrexia, CNS stimulation, headache, nausea, vomiting, conjunctivitis, a burning sensation around the mouth and throat, blepharospasm, and diaphoresis. Because dimercaprol undergoes biliary excretion, it can be used in patients with renal impairment.

Although DMSA is approved by the Food and Drug Administration (FDA) only for the treatment of lead poisoning in children, it is now advocated for the management of mercury or arsenic toxicity in children or adults (3,6,9,10,18). DMSA has the advantage of being relatively nontoxic. GI complaints are among the most common adverse effects. Mild and transient elevations in serum transaminase levels have been reported, so it is prudent to monitor liver function tests during therapy. Thrombocytosis, eosinophilia, and dysrhythmias occur infrequently. Pharyngitis, rhinorrhea, nasal congestion, rash, and mucocutaneous eruptions have also been reported. Because it is primarily eliminated in the urine, it should be used with caution in patients with renal impairment.

N-acetyl-D, L-penicillamine, an investigational oral chelator, appears to be more specific for chelating mercury than is D-penicillamine. It has been effective in reversing neurotoxicity as a result of chronic elemental and inorganic mercury exposures (14). The dosage regimen for adults is 250 to 500 mg four times a day (children, 30 mg/kg/d) for 6 to 10 days.

Dimercaptopropane sulfonate (DMPS) is an effective chelator of arsenic, elemental mercury, and inorganic mercurial salts. It has been used in Europe and is not readily available (not FDA approved) in the United States. It can be given by a variety of parenteral routes (intravenous, intramuscular, subcutaneous) and orally. For chronic arsenic chelation, an oral regimen of 100 mg, administered three times a day for 3 weeks, has been used for up to 9 months. For the management of mercury exposures, 5 mg/kg of a 5% solution has been administered intramuscularly or subcutaneously three to four times within the first 24 hours, two to three times a day on day 2, and then one to two administrations daily on subsequent days.

N-acetylcysteine has also shown some promise in the treatment of arsenic and inorganic mercury salt exposures (7,20). It could be used in the same doses as for acetaminophen poisoning. Limited experience suggests that hemodialysis (in conjunction with chelation therapy) performed within the first 24 hours of acute arsenic or mercury poisoning may remove a significant percentage of the ingested toxin before distribution into tissues, possibly averting, or at least minimizing, the toxic effects. It is ineffective later in the course, when there is relatively little metal in the blood. Hemodialysis is, however, indicated for the removal of chelated mercury or arsenic when renal dysfunction impairs its clearance.

CRITICAL INTERVENTIONS

- Obtain a CBC, serum electrolytes, BUN, creatinine, glucose, liver function tests, coagulation profile, CPK, urinalysis, ECG, and blood and 24-hour urine arsenic and mercury levels in patients with arsenic or mercury poisoning
- Obtain an abdominal radiograph to check for opaque material in the GI tract in patients with acute arsenic or mercury ingestions, particularly those who are symptomatic
- Obtain a CBC and urinalysis to check for hemolysis in patients with arsine gas exposure
- Administer i.v. fluids to patients with acute inorganic arsenic or mercury poisoning
- Consult a poison center or toxicologist regarding the interpretation of arsenic and mercury levels and the use of chelation therapy

DISPOSITION

Patients with acute poisoning after ingesting inorganic arsenic or mercury salts and long-chain aryl organic mercurials, or inhaling arsine or elemental mercury should be admitted. Patients with significant chronic toxicity should also be admitted for initial therapy. The level of care (intensive care unit or floor bed) should be dictated by the clinical presentation. The asymptomatic patient should be observed for 6 to 8 hours before discharge, with arrangements made for next-day follow-up. Patients who present with asymptomatic exposures or mild-to-moderate chronic toxicity may be treated as outpatients.

Consultation with a regional poison control center or a clinical toxicologist and a nephrologist should be part of the treatment plan. Although chelation therapy is not technically difficult, the details of treatment must be individualized, and optimal management requires the guidance of an experienced consultant. If antidotes and experts are not available locally, transfer of the patient to a tertiary care facility may be necessary. Patients with intentional exposures require psychiatric evaluation prior to discharge.

COMMON PITFALLS

✔ Failure to consider the possibility of acute arsenic or mercury poisoning in patients with intense abdominal pain and violent gastroenteritis of unknown cause
✔ Failure to appreciate that acute poisoning by inorganic arsenic or mercury salts can be rapidly progressive and result in CV collapse
✔ Failure to appreciate that the ingestion of liquid elemental mercury is usually benign, whereas inhalation of elemental mercury vapor may result in severe acute toxicity
✔ Failure to treat poisoning by long-chain aryl organomercurials the same as for inorganic salts, because the former is converted to the latter *in vivo*
✔ Failure to appreciate that the type of exposure, clinical severity, GI and renal function, and potential side effects of therapy influence the choice of chelating agent

References

1. Adler R, Boxtein D, Schaft P, et al. Metallic mercury vapor poisoning simulating mucocutaneous lymph node syndrome. *J Pediatr* 1982;101:967.
2. Beckman KH, Bauman JL, Pimental PA, et al. Arsenic-induced torsades-de-pointes. *Crit Care Med* 1991;19:290.
3. Bond GR, Bloom A, Pinar A, et al. Use of succimer to enhance elimination of mercury in 6 human beings. *Vet Hum Toxicol* 1992;34:353.

4. Dodes JE. The amalgam controversy. An evidence-based analysis. *JADA* 2001;132:348.
5. Ellabban MG, Ali R, Hart NB. Subcutaneous metallic mercury injection of the hand. *Br J Plastic Surgery* 2003;56:47.
6. Fournier L, Thomas G, Garnier R, et al 2,3-Dimercaptosuccinic acid treatment of heavy metal poisoning in humans. *Med Toxicol* 1988;3:499.
7. Girardi G, Elias MM. Effectiveness of N-acetylcysteine in protecting against mercuric chloride-induced nephrotoxicity. *Toxicology* 1991;67:155.
8. Goddard MJ, Tanhehco JL, Dau PC. Chronic arsenic poisoning masquerading as Landry-Guillain-Barré syndrome. *Electromyogr Clin Neurophysiol* 1992;32:419.
9. Graziano JH. Role of 2,3-dimercaptosuccinic acid in the treatment of heavy metal poisoning. *Med Toxicol* 1986;1:1051.
10. Graziano JH, Cuccia D, Friedheim E. Potential usefulness of 2,3-dimercaptosuccinic acid for the treatment of arsenic poisoning. *J Pharmacol Exp Ther* 1978;207:1051.
11. Hall AH. Chronic arsenic poisoning. *Toxicol Lett* 2002;128:69
12. Henningsson C, Hoffman S, McGonigle L, et al. Acute mercury poisoning mimicking pheochromocytoma in an adolescent. *J Pediatr* 1993;122:252.
13. Janus C, Klein B. Aspiration of metallic mercury: clinical significance. *Br J Radiol* 1982;55:675.
14. Markowitz L, Schaumburg NH. Successful treatment of inorganic mercury neurotoxicity with N-acetyl-penicillamine despite an adverse reaction. *Neurology* 1980;30:1000.
15. Mazumder DNG, Gupta JD, Santra A, et al. Chronic arsenic toxicity in West Bengal—the worst calamity in the world. *J Indian Med Assoc* 1998;96:4.
16. McFall TL, Richards JS, Matthews G. Rehabilitation in an individual with chronic arsenic poisoning medical, psychological, and social implications. *J Spinal Cord Med* 1998;21:142.
17. McFee RB, Caraccio TR. Intravenous mercury injection and ingestion: clinical manifestations and management. *J Toxicol Clin Toxicol* 2001;39:733
18. Muckter H, Liebl B, Reichl F, et al. Are we ready to replace dimercaprol (BAL) as an arsenic antidote? *Human Exp Toxicol* 1997;16:460.
19. Ratcliffe HE, Swanson GM. Human exposure to mercury: a critical assessment of the evidence of adverse health effects. *J Toxicol Environ Health* 1996;49:221.
20. Shum S, Skarbovig J, Habersang R. Acute lethal arsenic poisoning in mice: effect of treatment with N-acetylcysteine, d-penicillamine and dimercaprol on survival time. *Vet Hum Toxicol* 1981;23[Suppl 1]:39.
21. Singh S, Wig N, Kumari S. Massive metallic mercury ingestion without toxicity. *JAPI* 1997;45:897.
22. Soo TM, Wong CH, Griffith JF, et al. Subcutaneous injection of metallic mercury. *Human Exp Toxicol* 2003;22:345.
23. Thomas DJ, Styblo M, Lin S. The cellular metabolism and systemic toxicity of arsenic. *Toxicol Appl Pharmacol* 2001;176:127.
24. Von Burg R. Inorganic mercury. *J Appl Toxicol* 1995;15:483.
25. Winker R, Schaffer AW, Konnaris C, et al. Health consequences of an intravenous injection of metallic mercury. *Int Arch Occup Environ Health* 2002;75:581.

CHAPTER 306
Carbon Monoxide

Kent R. Olson

Carbon monoxide (CO) is a colorless, odorless gas produced by the combustion of any carbon-containing material. It is found in automobile exhaust and in gas and coal heaters, and it is an important toxin in smoke inhalation victims of fires (see Chapter 316, "Smoke Inhalation") (5,14,15). CO is also produced *in vivo* by the metabolism of inhaled methylene chloride (6). In the 10-year period from 1979 through 1988, a total of 56,133 deaths in the United States were attributed to CO poisoning. Of these, 25,889 were suicides, 15,523 were associated with severe burns or house fires, and 11,547 were classified as unintentional (1). When fire-related CO exposures were excluded, the National Center for Health Statistics estimated that approximately 516 deaths per year are attributable to CO poisoning (7). Three-fifths of these were caused by automobile exhaust; the other common sources were natural gas-based heating systems, charcoal grills, and camp stoves and lanterns. In 2002, 15,904 cases of CO poisoning were reported to the American Association of Poison Control Centers (AAPCC) Toxic Exposures Surveillance System (TESS), with 184 cases experiencing serious but nonfatal toxicity and 31 deaths (18).

CO produces toxicity by three possible mechanisms: hypoxemia, ischemia, and cellular asphyxia (10). It combines with hemoglobin with an affinity approximately 250 times greater than that of oxygen. Thus, at even low levels, significant saturation of hemoglobin-binding sites may occur, decreasing the oxygen-carrying capacity of the blood. Additionally, CO binding to hemoglobin alters the shape of the oxygen–hemoglobin dissociation curve, effectively shifting it to the left, resulting in further lowering of intracellular oxygen concentrations. CO may also produce toxicity by decreasing cardiac output and causing hypotension, resulting in ischemic organ damage (4). Finally, it has been proposed that CO may bind to intracellular cytochromes, interfering with oxygen utilization (14,22). Following the exposure, reperfusion injury may occur with release of reactive oxygen species from neutrophils adhering to the brain microvascular endothelium.

The dose required to produce toxicity varies, depending on the rate of ventilation, the underlying health of the victim, and the presence of other toxins. Equilibrium is reached more rapidly in people who perform vigorous physical activity. As little as 0.1% CO (1,000 ppm) may produce potentially fatal 50% saturation of hemoglobin at equilibrium, although this might require several hours of exposure. The exposure limit in the workplace is 25 ppm as an 8-hour time-weighted average. The level considered immediately dangerous to life or health is 1,200 ppm. People with underlying pulmonary or cardiovascular (CV) disease may not be able to tolerate hypoxia produced by even mild or moderate CO levels. Infants and fetuses are more susceptible to CO poisoning, because fetal hemoglobin has an even higher affinity for CO (12).

CO is rapidly absorbed from the lungs. After removal from exposure, CO slowly leaves hemoglobin, with an apparent half-life in room air of about 4 to 5 hours (10,14). The apparent half-life of CO produced by methylene chloride metabolism is substantially longer.

CLINICAL PRESENTATION

The signs and symptoms of CO poisoning are highly variable and nonspecific. At low levels, headache, dizziness, nausea, vomiting, and diarrhea are common. With higher levels, confusion, syncope, shortness of breath, and angina pectoris may occur. Severe poisoning may cause coma, seizures, hypotension, cardiac dysrhythmias, and death (Table 306.1) (4,8,9,10,14). Although the severity of intoxication usually parallels the CO–hemoglobin level, there are reports of patients with severe intoxication with relatively low levels and of patients with high levels but minimal symptoms (2). Survivors of severe poisoning are often left with permanent neurologic injury, which may be gross (blindness, deafness, seizures, parkinsonism, or vegetative state) or subtle (memory loss or personality changes) (4,9,10,14,21).

The physical examination may reveal cherry-red coloration of the skin, mucous membranes, and venous blood, owing to the bright red color of the CO–hemoglobin complex. However, this finding is inconsistently noted in patients with CO poisoning, and its presence or absence cannot be considered diagnostic; it is more likely to be noted at autopsy than in patients with sub-lethal poisoning (10). Retinal hemorrhage may be present.

Carboxyhemoglobin Level (%)	Signs & Symptoms
0–10	Usually none
10–20	Headache, dyspnea with minimal exertion, angina in patients with coronary disease
20–30	Moderate headache, dyspnea, nausea, dizziness
30–40	Severe headache, vomiting, fatigue, poor judgment
40–50	Confusion, syncope, tachypnea, tachycardia
50–60	Syncope, seizures, coma
60–70 or higher	Coma, hypotension, dysrhymthias, death

TABLE 306 1. Signs and Symptoms of Carbon Monoxide Poisoning[a]

[a] This table is intended only as a general guide, as symptoms and signs are quite variable and may not correlate with measured levels.

Neurologic examination usually reveals altered mental status, which may rapidly improve after the patient is removed from the poisoned atmosphere and oxygen is administered. Cerebellar ataxia has been found to be an important predictor of severity of intoxication (19). Arterial blood gas analysis and serum electrolyte levels often reveal metabolic acidosis, which is caused by tissue hypoxia–ischemia. The arterial PO_2, and hence the calculated oxygen saturation, are usually normal, because dissolved oxygen in the serum is not affected by CO. Although the oxygen saturation measured directly by co-oximetry is less than that calculated from the PO_2 (by an amount roughly equal to the percent CO–hemoglobin), the oxygen saturation measured by pulse oximetry is typically falsely normal (17). Signs of myocardial ischemia are frequently present on the electrocardiogram (ECG), and, occasionally, myocardial infarction (MI) occurs.

DIFFERENTIAL DIAGNOSIS

Other causes of coma and altered mental status should be sought, such as hypoglycemia, head trauma, stroke, meningitis, and drug or alcohol intoxication. Many suicidal patients ingest medications and alcohol as they poison themselves with CO. Other toxic gases should be considered in any patient with smoke inhalation. Cyanide, hydrogen sulfide, agents that cause methemoglobinemia, and other toxins may produce symptoms and signs of systemic hypoxia that are similar to those of CO (4,10,15).

EMERGENCY DEPARTMENT EVALUATION

Immediate evaluation in the emergency department should include rapid neurologic assessment and determination of the specific carboxyhemoglobin saturation (this may be performed on a venous or arterial blood sample). History that may be helpful in raising suspicion of CO poisoning includes being found in a car with the engine running, riding in the back of a pick-up truck, multiple victims found in a common room, smoke inhalation, and use of paint strippers or solvents that contain methylene chloride in a poorly ventilated area. Depending on severity, arterial blood gas analysis (using a co-oximeter), routine laboratory evaluation, ECG, and chest radiography may be indicated. Patients with suspected trauma should have a computed tomography scan of the head.

EMERGENCY DEPARTMENT MANAGEMENT

Advanced life-support measures should be instituted as needed. Decontamination is performed by removing the victim from the toxic environment; the rescuer should take care not to become exposed during the rescue (a self-contained breathing apparatus is recommended). Oxygen should be provided through a nonrebreather mask with an oxygen reservoir bag or by way of an endotracheal tube. Oxygen decreases the half-life of carboxyhemoglobin: the higher the inspired oxygen concentration, the shorter the half-life. A nonrebreather mask with a reservoir delivers 60% oxygen at flow rates greater than 10 L/min. 100% oxygen, which can only be delivered by endotracheal tube, decreases the carboxyhemoglobin half-life to 40 to 80 minutes. If the patient is hypotensive, 1 to 2 L of crystalloid solution should be administered. ECG, arterial blood gases, and the carboxyhemoglobin level should be monitored. Mild-to-moderate metabolic acidosis (i.e., serum pH 7.2 to 7.3) should not be treated with sodium bicarbonate, because acidosis may facilitate oxygen delivery to the tissues by moving the oxygen–hemoglobin dissociation curve to the right.

Hyperbaric oxygen (HBO), 100% oxygen provided under pressures greater than 1 atm, can further decrease the half-life of carboxyhemoglobin, to 20 minutes or less (10,14,20). Some clinicians believe that HBO may also drive CO from intracellular sites, although this has not been proven. Animal studies suggest a potential protective effect of HBO against CO-induced postischemic reperfusion injury, although this benefit may be nonspecific.

Controversy remains about which patients should receive HBO treatment. Most hospitals do not have ready access to a hyperbaric chamber, which means that unstable patients may require transport over long distances at a time when dysrhythmias and hypotension are more likely to occur. Because the half-life of CO–hemoglobin in 100% oxygen at 1 atm is less than 1 hour, in most cases, the level has already dropped to low levels by the time the HBO chamber is ready. Despite numerous case reports and uncontrolled case series supporting the use of HBO, its value has not been settled. Proponents of HBO argue that it may provide protection against late neurologic sequelae, but this claim has never been proven (14,16,20). Up until recently, no randomized controlled studies were available to compare HBO with normobaric oxygen (NBO). In a study that failed to show a benefit of HBO compared with 100% oxygen at normal pressure, only patients without a reported loss of consciousness were randomized, a subgroup that has an expected good outcome anyway (11). Although a greater incidence of delayed neuropsychiatric sequelae was observed in another study of patients who received NBO compared with HBO, all patients reportedly had resolution of their symptoms within 77 days (14). Moreover, this and other previous studies did not blind patients and health care providers to the treatment received.

Recently, two double-blind, randomized, and placebo-controlled ("sham" HBO) studies were completed, and found conflicting results (13,19). Both studies randomized all patients regardless of severity. Scheinkestel found no benefit from HBO compared with NBO, whereas Weaver found a marginal but statistically significant benefit in a subset of neuropsychiatric tests (19). Weaver also reported that patients with cerebellar findings on admission were more likely to suffer neurological sequelae.

Despite the lack of conclusive scientific data, HBO is often recommended for patients with coma (including a history of loss of consciousness or syncope), CV dysfunction (including ECG evidence of ischemia), pulmonary edema, significant acidosis, CO–hemoglobin level greater than 30% to 40%, symptoms that persist despite NBO therapy, or delayed-onset neuropsychiatric complaints. Weaver recommends that HBO be considered for patients with any of the following: age greater than 50 years; metabolic acidosis; history of loss of consciousness; or COHgb level greater than 25% (19).

Pregnant women and infants pose a special problem in CO poisoning, because fetal hemoglobin has a greater affinity for CO than does normal hemoglobin (12,14). Prolonged oxygen therapy and a lower threshold for HBO are often recommended, although, once again, studies are lacking.

The prognosis after severe CO poisoning is unpredictable but grim. As many as 40% of victims have permanent neurologic injury. Patients with an abnormal computed tomography, SPECT scan, or magnetic resonance imaging scan on admission appear to be at higher risk for permanent sequelae (3,21).

CRITICAL INTERVENTIONS

- Administer oxygen at 10 to 15 L/min by nonrebreather mask with an oxygen reservoir bag or 100% by endotracheal tube to all patients with possible carbon monoxide poisoning
- Consult a poison center, toxicologist, or hyperbaric medicine specialist regarding HBO therapy for patients with a history of loss of consciousness or syncope, CV depression or ischemia, carboxyhemoglobin fractions 25% to 40% or higher, significant acidemia, symptoms that persist despite NBO therapy, extremes of age, pregnancy, or delayed-onset neuropsychiatric complaints

DISPOSITION

All patients with loss of consciousness or with seizures should be admitted to the hospital, as should those with evidence of MI or ischemia. Similarly, infants, young children, and pregnant women require intensive or prolonged treatment and should be admitted. Most authorities would also automatically admit any patient with a CO–hemoglobin level greater than 25%, regardless of symptoms. A neuropsychiatric screening protocol may help determine which patients with low CO levels should be admitted for aggressive therapy (7).

A poison center or medical toxicologist may provide assistance with the decision to use HBO and may also know the location of nearby HBO chambers. If the patient is experiencing cardiac dysrhythmias or hypotension, a critical care nurse or physician should accompany the patient during transport to an HBO facility. Once the acute episode of poisoning has resolved, patients should be referred for follow-up neuropsychiatric evaluation. Those discharged from the emergency department should be instructed to return to the emergency department if any neurological symptoms develop.

COMMON PITFALLS

✔ Failure to consider the diagnosis of CO poisoning in patients presenting with headache, altered mental status, and symptoms of gastroenteritis or upper respiratory infection, particularly in cold climates or seasons
✔ Failure to consider the ingestion of alcohol or other drugs in patients with suicidal exposure to carbon monoxide
✔ Failure to appreciate that the arterial blood gas PO_2, calculated oxygen saturation, and pulse oximetry oxygen saturation are usually normal despite severe CO poisoning
✔ Failure to appreciate that the severity of poisoning depends on the duration of exposure and that carboxyhemoglobin levels may not correlate with the severity of poisoning
✔ Failure to warn patients about the possibility of delayed neurological toxicity and to return if symptoms develop

References

1. Cobb N, Etzel RA. Unintentional carbon monoxide-related deaths in the United States 1979 through 1988. *JAMA* 1991;266(5):659.
2. Davis SM, Levy RC. High carboxyhemoglobin level without acute or chronic findings. *J Emerg Med* 1984;1:539.
3. Gale SD, Hopkins RO, Weaver LK, et al. MRI, quantitative MRI, SPECT, and neuropsychological findings following carbon monoxide poisoning. *Brain Inj* 1999;13(4):229–243.
4. Ginsberg MD. Carbon monoxide intoxication: clinical features, neuropathology, and mechanisms of injury. *J Toxicol Clin Toxicol* 1985;23:281.
5. Hampson NB, Norkool DM. Carbon monoxide poisoning in children riding in the back of pickup trucks. *JAMA* 1992;267(4):22,538.
6. Horowitz BZ. Carboxyhemoglobinemia caused by inhalation of methylene chloride. *Am J Emerg Med* 1986;4:48.
7. Mah JC. US Consumer Product Safety Commission: non-fire carbon monoxide deaths associated with the use of consumer products: 1998 annual estimates. Available at http://www.cpsc.gov/library/co01.pdf. Accessed February 26, 2004.
8. Messier LD, Myers RA. A neuropsychological screening battery for emergency assessment of carbon-monoxide-poisoned patients. *J Clin Psychol* 1991;47(5):675.
9. Mofenson HC, Caraccio TR, Brody GM. Carbon monoxide poisoning. *Am J Emerg Med* 1984;2:254.
10. Olson KR. Carbon monoxide poisoning: mechanism, presentation, and controversies in management. *J Emerg Med* 1984;1:233.
11. Raphael JC, Elkharrat D, Jars-Guincestre MC, et al. Trial of normobaric and hyperbaric oxygen for acute carbon monoxide intoxication. *Lancet* 1989;2(8660):414.
12. Rudge FW. Carbon monoxide poisoning in infants: treatment with hyperbaric oxygen. *South Med J* 1993;86(3):334.
13. Scheinkestel CD, Bailey M, Myles PS, et al. Hyperbaric or normobaric oxygen for acute carbon monoxide poisoning: a randomised controlled clinical trial. *Med J Aust* 1999;170(5):203–210.
14. Thom SR, Keim LW. Carbon monoxide poisoning: a review. Epidemiology, pathophysiology, clinical findings, and treatment options including hyperbaric oxygen therapy. *J Toxicol Clin Toxicol* 1989;27(3):141.
15. Thom SR. Smoke inhalation. *Emerg Med Clin North Am* 1989;7(2):371.
16. Thomson LF, Mardel SN, Jack A, et al. Management of the moribund carbon monoxide victim. *Arch Emerg Med* 1992;9(2):208.
17. Vegfors M, Lennmarken C. Carboxyhaemoglobinaemia and pulse oximetry [see comments]. *Br J Anaesth* 1991;66(5):625.
18. Watson WA, Litovitz TL, Rodgers GC Jr, et al. 2002 annual report of the American Association of Poison Control Centers Toxic Exposure Surveillance System. *Am J Emerg Med* 2003;21:353–421.
19. Weaver LK, Hopkins RO, Chan KJ, et al. Hyperbaric oxygen for acute carbon monoxide poisoning. *N Engl J Med* 2002;347(14):1057–1067.
20. Weiss LD, Van Meter KW. The applications of hyperbaric oxygen therapy in emergency medicine. *Am J Emerg Med* 1992;10(6):558.
21. Zagami AS, Lethlean AK, Mellick R. Delayed neurological deterioration following carbon monoxide poisoning: MRI findings. *J Neurol* 1993;240(2):113.
22. Zhang J, Piantadosi CA. Mitochondrial oxidative stress after carbon monoxide hypoxia in the rat brain. *J Clin Invest* 1992;90(4):1193.

CHAPTER 307

Corrosives and Chemical Burns

Larissa I. Velez and Collin S. Goto

Most corrosive injuries involve acids or alkalis. Acids (pH < 7) are proton donors that dissociate into conjugate bases and free hydrogen ions (H^+) in solution. Alkalis (pH > 7) accept protons, resulting in the formation of conjugate acids and free hydroxide ions (OH^-). The tissues are injured when these excess ions are neutralized. These reactions are exothermic, and may be explosive or produce excessive gas, resulting in further tissue damage.

TABLE 307.1. Approximate pH of Some Common Solutions

Solution	pH
1.0 M HCl	0
Battery acid (1% solution)	1.4
Acid toilet cleaner (1%)	2.0
Citrus juices	1.8–4
Wines	2.8–3.8
Black coffee	5.0
Rainwater	6.5
Water (25°C)	7.0
Bleach (1% solution)	9.5–10.2
Automatic dishwasher detergents	10.4–13
Laundry detergents	11.6–12.6
Ammonia cleaners (<10%)	11.9–12.4
Alkaline drain cleaners	13.3–14
1.0 M NaOH	14
Saturated ammonia solution	15

Substances with a pH less than 3 or greater than 11 have the most potential to cause significant corrosive injury (Table 307.1). Other corrosives damage tissues by various mechanisms, including oxidation, reduction, vesication, desiccation, metabolic inhibition, or cellular poisoning. Hydrofluoric acid is discussed in Chapter 309, "Fluoride and Hydrofluoric Acid" and chemical warfare agents are discussed in Chapter 331, "Chemical Warfare Agents."

The pKa, which is equal to the pH of a solution in which half of the acid has dissociated, is a measure of the ease with which the acid donates a proton. Strong (easily dissociated) acids and alkalis are those with a pKa of less than 0 and greater than 14, respectively (Table 307.2). Another measure of corrosive potential is called the titratable reserve. It is expressed as the amount of sodium hydroxide or hydrochloric acid required to neutralize an acid or alkali, respectively.

Acids denature proteins and generally cause coagulation necrosis. The formation of a firm coagulum or eschar often limits the penetration of injury. Alkalis cause liquefaction necrosis, which dissolves proteins dissolve and saponifies fats. The injured tissues slough, allowing for deeper injury compared to acids.

The extent, location, and severity of gastrointestinal (GI) injury depend on the physical state of the corrosive or chemical agent, the amount ingested, the duration of tissue contact, the presence of food, and the tonicity of the pyloric sphincter. Solid compounds dissolve on contact with body fluids, producing highly concentrated solutions, which may result in severe localized damage. Solids and solutions of high viscosity tend to adhere to tissues and frequently result in proximal rather than distal involvement. Acids often have a strong odor and result in immediate pain and smooth muscle spasm, often limiting the amount ingested. Alkalis often are odorless and do not cause immediate pain after contact. Cell death results from the disruption of cellular membranes and is exacerbated by small vessel thrombosis (23). Sloughing of tissue after liquefactive necrosis may assist the penetration of alkalis to deeper levels. These characteristics cause alkali ingestions to be of larger volumes and thus more dangerous.

The subsequent injury and repair steps are similar for both acids and alkali. There is bacterial invasion after 24 to 48 hours, an inflammatory response, and development of granulation tissue. Because collagen deposition may not begin until the second week, tensile strength of the healing tissue is low during the first 3 weeks (23). Scar retraction begins in the third week, commonly continuing for months, and may result in stricture formation and shortening of the involved segment of the GI tract. Finally, mucosal repair can take weeks to months (7). Ocular damage is most severe following alkali burns as a result of early disruption of the corneal epithelium, liquefaction necrosis, and rapid tissue penetration. Although acids can also cause severe ocular burns, the overall severity is generally less than that seen with alkalis. As with ingestions, the coagulation necrosis caused by acids tends to prevent deeper tissue penetration and damage. Most hydrocarbons are considered only irritants. In reality, ocular damage following hydrocarbon exposure ranges from mild to severe. In general, aliphatic (straight-chain) hydrocarbons tend to cause only mild conjunctival irritation, aromatic (ring structure) hydrocarbons cause mild corneal damage, and halogenated hydrocarbons can cause severe corneal damage.

Dermal injuries caused by corrosives differ in several important ways from thermal burns. The initial severity of the injury may be underestimated because direct tissue penetration of the chemical may be deeper than anticipated by visual inspection, and also because tissue penetration and damage may continue for several hours to days. Furthermore, absorption of the chemical may result in systemic toxicity. The majority of these injuries occur in young adults in the occupational or household setting (19). As with ingestions, the severity of the injury is dependent on several factors including the specific mechanism of toxicity of the agent, the concentration, duration of exposure, surface area exposed, depth of penetration. Patient factors such as age, preexisting condition of the skin, and concurrent illnesses also play a role in determining the severity of the injury.

TABLE 307.2. pK$_a$ of Acids and Alkalis

Acids	Formula	pK$_a$	Alkalis	Formula	pK$_a$
Perchloric	HClO$_4$	−8	Calcium carbonate	CaCO$_3$	5.7
Hydrochloric	HCl	−3	Hydrazine	N$_2$H$_4$	8
Chromic	CrO$_3$	0.3	Ammonia	NH$_3$	9.3
Bromic	HBrO$_3$	<1	Ammonium hydroxide	NH$_4$OH	9.3
Nitric	HNO$_3$	<1	Ethanolamine	NH$_2$C$_2$H$_4$OH	9.5
Oxalic	C$_2$H$_2$O$_4$	1.5	Magnesium hydroxide	H$_2$MgO$_2$	10
Sulfuric	H$_2$SO$_4$	1.9	Zinc hydroxide	Zn(OH)$_2$	11
Phosphoric	H$_2$P$_2$O$_7$	2.1	Calcium hydroxide	Ca(OH)$_2$	11.6
Arsenic	H$_3$AsO$_4$	2.3	1,6-Hexane-diamine	(NH$_2$)$_2$C$_6$H$_{12}$	11.8
Nitrous	HNO$_2$	3.3	Lithium hydroxide	LiOH	>14
Hydrofluoric	HF	3.4	Potassium hydroxide	KOH	>14
Acetic	H$_3$C$_2$OOH	4.8	Sodium hydroxide	NaOH	>14
Sulfurous	HSO$_3$	6.9	Calcium oxide	CaO	>14
Hydrogen sulfide	H$_2$S	7.0	Sodium carbonate	Na$_2$CO$_3$	>14
Boric	H$_3$BO$_3$	9.2	Potassium carbonate	K$_2$CO$_3$	>14
Hydrogen peroxide	H$_2$O$_2$	11.6	Sodium hypochlorite	NaClO	>14

CORROSIVE INGESTIONS

CLINICAL PRESENTATION

Sites commonly affected by corrosive ingestion are the oropharynx, esophagus, and stomach, although sites as distal as the proximal jejunum may be injured (25). The areas most damaged generally represent areas of stagnation of luminal contents or anatomic narrowing (7).

Systemic toxicity may sometimes accompany severe GI injuries and is usually secondary to tissue inflammation, perforation, acidosis, infection, and necrosis. Fluid and electrolyte shifts accompanying extensive burns can result in hypovolemic shock. Some corrosives can be dangerous when systemically absorbed.

Patients usually present with oral, throat, chest, or abdominal pain. Dysphagia, drooling, and vomiting are common. Children may refuse to drink, cry excessively, or be unable to swallow their secretions. Stridor, hoarseness, hematemesis, and melena occur less frequently (11). Tachypnea can occur from aspiration of the corrosive with resultant pneumonitis, or as a compensation for a metabolic acidosis. Metabolic acidosis may reflect tissue necrosis or the systemic absorption of ingested acids (5). Superficial burns of the oropharynx are often covered with a pale membrane. Deeper burns are black, hemorrhagic, or friable. The presence or absence of burns in the oropharynx, however, does not reliably predict more distal injuries (6,10,11,25). Full-thickness injuries to the esophagus or stomach are at risk of perforation and fistula formation into the trachea, mediastinum, or peritoneum (25). Mediastinitis presents with chest pain, respiratory distress, fever, subcutaneous emphysema, pleural rub, and Hamman's sign. Chest radiographic findings may include mediastinal widening, pleural effusion (usually left-sided), pneumomediastinum, and pneumothorax.

The abdominal examination is an unreliable indicator of the severity of the injury (22), but frank peritonitis is an ominous sign. Peritonitis may result from viscus perforation or the extension of severe gastric burns to surrounding abdominal organs. Patients with peritonitis may have marked third-spacing of fluids, resulting in abdominal distention and hypotension.

The late presentations after a corrosive ingestion include dysphagia, nausea, and vomiting as a result of the formation of strictures. Esophageal strictures develop in up to 70% of patients with deep esophageal ulcers and in nearly all patients with areas of necrosis (25). Ulceration superficial to the muscularis mucosa layer does not lead to stricture formation (1,8,12). Half of all esophageal strictures develop during the initial hospitalization, and 80% are evident within 2 months. Esophageal carcinoma, a late sequela of alkali ingestion, has been diagnosed after a latency period of about 40 years (3,23). This complication has not been associated with acid burns except in a few cases.

Ocular injury most commonly results from splash exposures at home or in the work environment. The severity of these injuries ranges from transient irritation to severe disabling ocular damage and blindness (17). Manifestations include immediate eye pain, photophobia, blepharospasm, lacrimation, conjunctival injection or hemorrhage, and decreased visual acuity. With more significant involvement, chemosis and corneal edema, opacification, sloughing, ulceration, and necrosis occur. Ischemia and corneal opacification are ominous signs. The pupils may be nonreactive as a result of severe iritis. Intraocular pressure rises with damage to the trabecular meshwork, resulting in glaucoma. If penetration is deep enough, retinal damage occurs. Ultimately, inflammation leads to fibrosis, synechiae, and cataract formation.

Dermal exposure usually results in immediate pain, but the onset of pain can sometimes be delayed for several hours. Petroleum distillates, weak NaOH solutions, and cement typically do not produce burns unless allowed to remain in contact with the skin for prolonged periods. Such exposures may initially appear trivial but can progress to full-thickness burns.

The depth of dermal injury can be difficult to assess. Chemical burns rarely blister and the affected skin is usually dark, insensate, and firmly attached regardless of the burn depth. Burns from hydrochloric, sulfuric, and nitric acid may have a green, gray, or yellow hue, respectively. With time, the skin hardens and cracks, exposing the underlying dermis or subcutaneous tissue. Healing usually takes longer than for thermal burns.

DIFFERENTIAL DIAGNOSIS

With ingestions, the most important diagnosis to exclude is the potential coingestion of other agents. If shock or altered mental status are present soon after ingestion, other causes should be sought. Hematemesis and esophageal perforation can result from protracted vomiting of any cause. Gastroenteritis as a result of the corrosive effects of ingested heavy metals and hydrocarbons can cause similar symptoms. Allergic reactions may present with some of the features of corrosive ingestion if the hypopharynx or larynx is involved. Infections such as epiglottitis, croup, retropharyngeal abscess, and mucosal ulceration as a result of herpesvirus or coxsackievirus should be considered in children.

The differential diagnosis of corrosive injury to the eye includes traumatic corneal abrasion or ulceration, foreign body, allergic reactions, infectious processes such as viral or bacterial conjunctivitis, iritis, iridocyclitis, acute narrow-angle glaucoma, and exposure to fumes, vapors, and sensitizing agents.

Considerations in the differential diagnosis of dermal injuries include thermal burns, radiation burns including sunburns, mechanical irritation or trauma, allergic reactions and drug eruptions (such as Steven-Johnson syndrome or toxic epidermal necrolysis), contact dermatitis, infections, and bacterial toxin-mediated conditions such as Staphylococcal scalded skin syndrome or toxic shock syndrome.

EMERGENCY DEPARTMENT EVALUATION

The identity, concentration, and amount of chemical or product involved and the time and circumstances of exposure should be determined. Product labels should be examined for ingredients and signal words. The signal words caution, warning, and danger identify a product as a weak irritant (to eyes, nose, and throat), strong irritant (to skin and mucous membranes), or corrosive (capable of causing permanent of fatal tissue damage), respectively. If a sample is available, the pH should be measured. A pH meter is more accurate than pH paper (e.g., pHydrion paper, which is also used for testing amniotic fluid) but is not generally available.

In patients with corrosive ingestion, attention should initially be directed to airway patency, because obstruction may develop with progressive mucosal edema. In the absence of clinical indications for immediate endotracheal intubation, patients with respiratory symptoms should have the upper airway assessed by direct fiberoptic laryngoscopy. Patients suspected of having a significant corrosive injury should also have an electrocardiogram, arterial blood gas analysis, complete blood count, type and cross-match, prothrombin time, and electrolyte, glucose, and liver and renal function tests. Radiologic studies should include an upright chest radiograph whenever the patient has respiratory symptoms and an acute abdominal series if perforation is suspected.

Endoscopy of the upper GI tract is the gold standard for the diagnosis of corrosive injury (20). It should be performed in all symptomatic patients. A complete lack of symptoms or signs usually indicates that significant injuries, i.e., those that require treatment or are likely to lead to complications, are absent and that endoscopy is not necessary (6,11). Nevertheless, endoscopy should still be considered for apparently asymptomatic patients who have intentionally ingested a strong acid or alkali, or if the history is unreliable. Because injuries may progress over a period of several hours, endoscopy is optimally performed 12 to 24 hours after exposure (25). If undertaken earlier, the full extent of injury may not be apparent; if performed later, the risk of perforation may be increased by the procedure (7). Esophageal and gastric burns are graded in a similar fashion as dermal burns. Grade 1 burns just have erythema of the mucosa (25). Grade 2 burns have partial thickness submucosal lesions, ulceration, and exudates. Some authors divide grade 2 burns into categories 2a and 2b. The 2a burns are noncircumferential and the 2b are near-circumferential. Grade 3 burns are deep, full thickness burns with ulcers and necrosis into the periesophageal tissues (10,11). In a study of 1296 patients with caustic ingestions, those with third-degree burns had 85% incidence of stricture development. The best predictor for the development of strictures is the severity of the initial injury (1). Contrast esophagography is less sensitive than endoscopy in assessing burn injury, although it is useful for the detection of perforation. A water-soluble contrast agent (gastrograffin) should be used whenever perforation is suspected. Cine-esophagography can detect esophageal motility disorders, which are predictive of stricture formation.

The evaluation of patients with eye exposures should be deferred until after decontamination if significant pain is present. A complete eye examination including measurement of visual acuity and conjunctival pH and a slit-lamp examination should then bee performed. If injury to the anterior chamber is suspected, intraocular pressure should be measured.

The assessment of dermal injuries is similar to that for thermal burns. Location, size, color, texture, and neurovascular status should be noted. If the affected area is greater than 15% of total body surface area or if systemic toxicity is possible, a complete physical examination and routine laboratory testing should be performed.

EMERGENCY DEPARTMENT MANAGEMENT

Airway management is the first priority in patients with corrosive ingestion. Any patient with respiratory distress, stridor, or inability to speak should undergo immediate endotracheal intubation. If laryngoscopy reveals laryngeal edema, prophylactic intubation is also advised.

The efficacy of GI decontamination is limited. The mouth should be rinsed liberally with water in patients with oral burns. Emesis is contraindicated because it re-exposes the esophagus to the corrosive agent and increases the risk of aspiration. For this reason, antiemetics should be given to patients with persistent nausea or vomiting. The placement of a nasogastric tube for stomach emptying may be considered in recent, large volume ingestions. Activated charcoal is contraindicated because it obscures the endoscopists's view, and most corrosives are not significantly adsorbed by charcoal. Dilution by giving oral fluids may be beneficial, although the current evidence is inconclusive. If dilution is to be used, it should be limited to very recent exposures (within minutes), patients with normal airway and mental status, without significant nausea, vomiting or pain, and patients who are able to speak and cooperate. The amount swallowed should be limited to 5 mL/kg to avoid inducing emesis.

Although corticosteroids reduce the incidence and severity of esophageal strictures in animal studies, their value in humans is controversial. In human trials in which steroids were not given until up to 24 hours after exposure, there have been conflicting conclusions and several points of general agreement (13,16). Patients with first-degree esophageal burns do not require steroids,

because strictures do not develop in this group (1,12,13). Steroids do not appear to alter the development of esophageal strictures in patients with extensive areas of deep ulceration or necrosis (grade 3 burns) and may actually increase the rate of complications such as infection, hemorrhage or perforation (1,12). For patients between these two extremes, whose injuries consist of circumferential or extensive superficial ulceration or small areas of deep ulceration or necrosis, steroids are of potential benefit (1,13). The decision to use steroids is based on the grading of the burns, which highlights the importance of early endoscopic evaluation.

Recommended dosages of methylprednisolone are 2 mg/kg/d in children and 40 mg every 8 hours in adults. This therapy is continued for 14 to 21 days, followed by a taper (16). The concomitant use of antibiotics is recommended whenever steroids are being used (16). The antibiotics of choice are penicillin, ampicillin, or clindamycin. Although they are of no proven benefit in promoting healing or reducing complications, antacids, sucralfate, H2-blockers, and analgesics can provide symptomatic relief (7). Oral medications and feedings should be withheld until the results of endoscopy are known, and then they should be given only to patients with injuries limited to mucosal inflammation or small areas of superficial ulceration. These patients may be given oral fluids when they are able to swallow their own secretions. Those with more severe injuries should receive i.v. fluids and nothing by mouth (16). Surgical exploration is indicated if perforation is confirmed by radiographs or endoscopy, when there is persistent hypotension, or in the presence of abdominal rigidity. It has also been recommended in patients who are at high risk of perforation, sepsis, necrosis, or hemorrhage. Because endoscopy cannot fully evaluate the depth of the burns (e.g., the status of the serosal surface), exploration has also been proposed for patients with grade 2 or 3 burns, in order to overcome this limitation (8). In a recent study, a serum pH less than 7.22 and a base excess more than −12.0 were predictors of severe injury requiring an emergency salvage operation (5).

Immediate irrigation is the single most important intervention in the management of eye exposures (4). The severity of ocular damage at the time of presentation is a good predictor of the ultimate outcome, as are timeliness and adequacy of irrigation. Ideally, irrigation will have been performed immediately at the time of exposure in the home or workplace, and continued en route to the hospital. Any drinkable liquid can be used if water is not available. If the patient has significant pain, irrigation again be performed in the emergency department. Irrigation will be aided greatly by the application of topical anesthetic solution and use of eyelid retractors. Intravenous analgesics or sedatives may be required. Acceptable irrigation solutions include tap water, normal saline, Ringer's lactate, or D5W (14). Initially, the eyelids should be everted and any particulate matter removed with a cotton swab. Continuous irrigation of the eye is made easier with use of a scleral lens with inflow channel (Morgan Therapeutic Lens). If this device is not available, simply irrigate manually with i.v. tubing connected to a liter of irrigation solution, beginning with 1 L and irrigate at least 20 minutes. For high corrosive substances, especially alkali exposures, prolonged irrigation of at least an hour is recommended (21).

After initial irrigation is complete, the pH of the inferior cul-de-sac should be tested with litmus or pH paper. If a neutral pH of 7 to 8 has not yet been achieved, then continued irrigation is warranted. Once a neutral conjunctival pH is achieved, the pH should be checked every 30 minutes for 2 hours because corrosive material may be slowly released from corneal tissue for several hours. A subsequent change in pH indicates the need for further irrigation.

Standard treatment for corneal injuries includes topical antibiotics, steroids, cycloplegics, and mydriatics (18). Topical timolol maleate and oral acetazolamide may be required if intraocular pressure is elevated. Tetanus prophylaxis and analgesics should be administered if needed.

Initial management of dermal injuries should is also directed at rapid decontamination. Copious irrigation of the skin surface with water is the decontamination method of choice for most exposures. Any drinkable liquid can be used if water is not available. Ideally, irrigation will have been initiated immediately at the scene and continued en route to the hospital (15). Delayed decontamination can result in increased tissue damage and deeper penetration of the offending agent (24). In industrial accidents, rescuers should wear appropriate protective gear such as gloves, gowns, masks, and eye shields. All contaminated clothing, footwear, jewelry, and contact lenses should be removed from the victim. In experimental alkali burns, irrigation of the skin with 5% acetic acid (household vinegar) decreases the severity of the injury (2). Clinical studies are needed to confirm this effect in humans, and it must be emphasized that immediate irrigation with water or should never be delayed as one searches for the specific irrigation solution. Irrigation should continue for at least 20 minutes. A longer period of irrigation lasting up to several hours is required for alkalis and other serious exposures. Adherent materials may be removed by gentle scrubbing with soapy water. Appropriate analgesia and tetanus prophylaxis should be provided and wounds should be treated with topical antibiotic cream and protective dressings.

Irrigation should not be performed for burns caused by elemental forms of alkali metals such as sodium, potassium, lithium, cesium, and rubidium. These elements react with water to form hydroxides, strong bases that will significantly increase tissue damage. Furthermore, ignition or explosion occurs when water contacts pure magnesium, sulfur, strontium titanium, uranium, yttrium, zinc, and zirconium. These two groups of substances should be covered with mineral oil to isolate them from water. Any solid particles that are removed from the victim must be stored in mineral oil to prevent further reactivity. These special agents are not readily available and thus seldom encountered. Patients with such exposures may come to the emergency department with Material Safety Data Sheets (MSDS) from their workplace. These data sheets provide specific information about the agent and the proper decontamination techniques.

CRITICAL INTERVENTIONS

- Consult a gastroenterologist for the endoscopic evaluation of all patients with GI symptoms or suicidal corrosive ingestion
- Consult a surgeon for patients with radiographic evidence of perforation, endoscopic evidence of severe GI injury, peritoneal signs, hypotension, or metabolic acidosis after corrosive ingestion
- Evaluate the airway in patients with ingestions or facial skin exposures and perform immediate endotracheal intubation in patients with respiratory distress, stridor, or inability to speak
- Begin irrigation immediately and continue it for at least 20 minutes in symptomatic patients with eye and skin exposures
- Consult an ophthalmologist for patients who have evidence of corneal injury or persistent pain after eye exposure
- Consult or refer patients with significant dermal injury to a plastic surgeon or regional burn center

DISPOSITION

Patients with ingestions who are asymptomatic or become asymptomatic after oral rinsing and dilution may be discharged from the emergency department after an observation period (23). It is generally agreed that asymptomatic patients after unintentional ingestions will have normal endoscopies (11). A gastroenterologist or surgeon should be consulted regarding endoscopy. If endoscopy or surgical consultation is unavailable, patients should be transferred to an appropriate facility. A regional poison control center can be consulted regarding current treatment recommendations. All patients with confirmed or suspected suicidal ingestions require psychiatric evaluation. Finally, nonaccidental injuries must be considered in all pediatric cases (23). Patients with no visible injury on endoscopy and those with injuries limited to mucosal inflammation or small areas of superficial ulceration may be discharged or referred for psychiatric care, as long as they are able to tolerate oral fluids (1,8,12). Patients with persistent symptoms or inconclusive findings at endoscopy should be admitted for observation. If symptoms persist, endoscopy should be repeated.

Patients with chemical conjunctivitis can be referred to an ophthalmologist for follow up the next day. Immediate ophthalmology consultation should be obtained for those with evidence of corneal injury or persistent pain. All patients with significant eye injuries should be admitted to the hospital for further management, assessment of injury progression and the need for surgical intervention, and to ensure initial compliance with the medical regimen.

Consultation with a general surgeon, plastic surgeon, or regional burn center is recommended for patients with significant dermal injuries. Patients with minor injuries may be discharged if the patient is reliable and follow-up the next day can be arranged. Those with systemic toxicity, second- or third-degree burns, extensive first-degree burns (greater than 15% of body surface area), burns to the face, eyes, ears, perineum, hands and feet, and high-risk patients such as those with significant preexisting illness, the elderly, and psychiatric or otherwise noncompliant patients should usually be admitted (9).

COMMON PITFALLS

✔ Failure to positively identify the substance ingested, test its pH, or seek information on its potential for corrosive injury
✔ Administering syrup of ipecac or unintentionally inducing vomiting by giving excessive amounts of oral fluid for dilution
✔ Failure to appreciate that activated charcoal is not indicated for acid or alkali ingestion and will obscure endoscopic evaluation
✔ Assuming that the absence of oropharyngeal burns precludes the presence of significant GI injury in patients with ingestions
✔ Failure to evaluate for and treat systemic toxicity
✔ Failure to continue eye irrigation long enough, as determined by conjunctival pH testing
✔ Underestimation of the severity of the dermal injury

Acknowledgments

We thank Robert P. Dowsett and Christopher H. Linden for their contributions to the previous edition of this chapter.

References

1. Anderson KD, Rouse TM, Randolph JG. A controlled trial of corticosteroids in children with corrosive injury of the esophagus. [comment]. *N Engl J Med* 1990;323(10):637–640.
2. Andrews K, Mowlavi A, Milner SM. The treatment of alkaline burns of the skin by neutralization. *Plast Reconstr Surg* 2003;111:1918–1921.
3. Appelqvist P, Salmo M. Lye corrosion carcinoma of the esophagus: a review of 63 cases. *Cancer* 1980;45(10):2655–2658.
4. Burns FR, Paterson CA. Prompt irrigation of chemical eye injuries may avert severe damages. *Occup Health Saf* 1989;Apr:33–36.
5. Cheng YJ, Kao EL. Arterial blood gas analysis in acute caustic ingestion injuries. *Surg Today* 2003;33(7):483–485.
6. Crain EF, Gershel JC, Mezey AP. Caustic ingestions. Symptoms as predictors of esophageal injury. *Am J Dis Child* 1984;138(9):863–865.

7. de Jong AL, Macdonald R, Ein S, et al. Corrosive esophagitis in children: a 30-year review. *Int J Pediatr Otorhinolaryngol* 2001;57(3):203–211.
8. Estrera A, Taylor W, Mills LJ, et al. Corrosive burns of the esophagus and stomach: a recommendation for an aggressive surgical approach. *Ann Thorac Surg* 1986;41(3):276–283.
9. Fitzpatrick KT, Moylan JA. Emergency care of chemical burns. *Postgrad Med* 1985;78:189–192.
10. Gaudreault P, Parent M, McGuigan MA, et al. Predictability of esophageal injury from signs and symptoms: a study of caustic ingestion in 378 children. *Pediatrics* 1983;71(5):767–770.
11. Gorman RL, Khin-Maung-Gyi MT, Klein-Schwartz W, et al. Initial symptoms as predictors of esophageal injury in alkaline corrosive ingestions. *Am J Emerg Med* 1992;10(3):189–194.
12. Hawkins DB, Demeter MJ, Barnett TE. Caustic ingestion: controversies in management. A review of 214 cases. *Laryngoscope* 1980;90(1):98–109.
13. Howell JM, Dalsey WC, Hartsell FW, et al. Steroids for the treatment of corrosive esophageal injury: a statistical analysis of past studies. *Am J Emerg Med* 1992;10(5):421–425.
14. Kompa S, Schareck B, Tympner J, et al. Comparison of emergency eye-wash products in burned porcine eyes. *Graefe's Arch Clin Exp Ophtlmol* 2002;240:308–313.
15. Leonard LG, Scheulen JJ, Munster AM. Chemical burns: effect of prompt first aid. *J Trauma* 1982;22:420–424.
16. Mamede RC, de Mello Filho FV. Treatment of caustic ingestion: an analysis of 239 cases. *Dis Esophagus* 2002;15(3):210–213.
17. Nelson JD, Kopietz LA. Chemical injuries to the eyes: emergency, intermediate, and long term care. *Postgrad Med* 1987;81:62–75.
18. Pfister RR, Koski J. Alkali burns of the eye: pathophysiology and treatment. *South Med J* 1982;75:417–422.
19. Ricketts S, Kimble FW. Chemical injuries: the Tasmanian burns unit experience. *ANZ J Surg* 2003;73:45–48.
20. Rigo GP, Camellini L, Azzolini F, et al. What is the utility of selected clinical and endoscopic parameters in predicting the risk of death after caustic ingestion? *Endoscopy* 2002;34(4):304–310.
21. Saari KM, Leinonen J, Aine E. Management of chemical eye injuries with prolonged irrigation. *Acta Ophthalmol Suppl* 1984;161:52–59.
22. Sarfati E, Gossot D, Assens P, et al. Management of caustic ingestion in adults. *Br J Surg* 1987;74(2):146–148.
23. Wilsey MJ Jr, Scheimann AO, Gilger MA. The role of upper gastrointestinal endoscopy in the diagnosis and treatment of caustic ingestion, esophageal strictures, and achalasia in children. *Gastrointest Endosc Clin N Am* 2001;11(4):767–787.
24. Yano K, Hata Y, Matsuka K, et al. Experimental study on alkaline skin injuries—periodic changes in subcutaneous tissue pH and the effects exerted by washing. *Burns* 1993;19:320–323.
25. Zargar SA, Kochhar R, Mehta S, et al. The role of fiberoptic endoscopy in the management of corrosive ingestion and modified endoscopic classification of burns. *Gastrointest Endosc* 1991;37(2):165–169.

CHAPTER 308
Cyanide

Alan H. Hall

Acute cyanide poisoning is a rare, potentially fatal but treatable condition (9). It may be encountered in a variety of settings: smoke inhalation, chemical exposures, thermal degradation or acid contact with chemical compounds (e.g., cyanogen, cyanogen halides, calcium cyanide), and metabolic release after systemic absorption of laetrile, amygdalin, other cyanogenic glycosides of plant origin (e.g., apricot, cherry, and peach pits) and aliphatic nitrile compounds (3,5,7,10,20). Sodium nitroprusside therapy at high doses may sometimes cause elevated blood cyanide levels (8).

Of the 303 cases of cyanide exposure reported to poison centers in the United States during 2001, there were 14 deaths (19). Although 116 patients developed some signs or symptoms, only 7 who had severe cyanide poisoning survived. Antidotal treatment with amyl nitrite was administered in 13 cases, sodium nitrite in 27 cases, and sodium thiosulfate in 57 (19).

Cyanide produces intracellular hypoxia by complexing with the ferric iron of mitochondrial cytochrome oxidase, inhibiting the electron transport chain and oxidative phosphorylation, and causing anaerobic metabolism with decreased adenosine triphosphate and increased lactic acid production (3). Tissues with the greatest oxygen demand (myocardium and brain) are most profoundly and rapidly affected. Initial central nervous system (CNS) and cardiovascular (CV) stimulation is followed by depression.

Human cyanide toxicokinetics are poorly understood, but the volume of distribution is probably between 0.4 and 0.5 L/kg, and the initial half-life between 30 minutes and 1 hour. Systemic absorption by the ingestion route is nearly complete, but only a small percentage of a dose is excreted unchanged in the urine (2,9). Whole blood cyanide levels in acute ingestion poisoning decrease rapidly after specific antidote treatment, but they may remain elevated for prolonged periods when antidotes are not administered (9). Except in rare cases, patients with whole blood cyanide levels greater than 3.0 µg/mL have not survived unless specific antidote therapy was administered (9,10).

Although a number of specific antidotes are in clinical use worldwide, only the amyl nitrite, sodium nitrite, and sodium thiosulfate combination (the Cyanide Antidote Kit) is available in the United States. Hydroxocobalamin, available in some countries, is much less toxic and equally efficacious (2,3,6,8). Oxygen has an antidotal effect of its own and having synergistic action with certain specific cyanide antidotes, perhaps because oxidized cytochrome oxidase resists inactivation by cyanide to a greater extent than does reduced cytochrome oxidase.

CLINICAL PRESENTATION

Inhalation of high concentrations of hydrogen cyanide gas may cause sudden loss of consciousness after only a few breaths (9). With ingestion of alkaline cyanide salts (calcium cyanide, potassium cyanide, sodium cyanide), the onset of life-threatening symptomatology may occur in 30 minutes to 1 hour (9). In fatal cases, rapid progression to coma, seizures, dysrhythmias, intractable hypotension, apnea, and death is common.

Onset of symptoms may be delayed with exposure to cyanogens such as laetrile and cyanogenic glycosides from plant sources (up to 1.5 hours), or aliphatic nitrile compounds, such as acetonitrile in artificial glue-on nail removers (up to 6 to 12 hours) (5,7,10). Systemic poisoning may occur after dermal hydrogen cyanide exposure (21).

Initial signs and symptoms include CNS stimulation (giddiness, headache, and anxiety), hyperpnea, mild hypertension, and palpitations (9). Later manifestations include nausea, vomiting, hypotension, generalized seizures, coma, apnea, mydriasis, noncardiogenic pulmonary edema, and a variety of cardiac effects (tachycardia or bradycardia, supraventricular and ventricular dysrhythmias, atrioventricular blocks, ischemic electrocardiographic changes, and, eventually, asystole) (3,9). Patients with significant cyanide poisoning have elevated serum lactate levels and an elevated anion gap metabolic acidosis (2,9). Cyanosis is a late sign, noted only at the stage of apnea and circulatory collapse. The retinal veins and arteries may appear nearly equally red, as a result of the inability of tissues to extract oxygen from the blood. Development of a diabetes insipidus–like condition secondary to severe brain damage following acute cyanide poisoning is an ominous prognostic sign (22).

During high-dose nitroprusside infusion, whole blood cyanide levels may become elevated. However, even when this occurs, clinical signs of cyanide poisoning (e.g., elevated lactate levels, metabolic acidosis) are not necessarily present (18). Cyanide poisoning in this setting can be prevented by the concomitant administration of hydroxocobalamin or sodium thiosulfate (4,18).

DIFFERENTIAL DIAGNOSIS

Early symptoms may be confused with anxiety or hyperventilation, which are common after nontoxic exposures. Development of more serious clinical signs differentiates these benign conditions from true cyanide poisoning. Hydrogen sulfide and sodium azide poisoning may cause similar findings, and diabetic decompensation has been initially suspected in patients who were later found to have ingested cyanide.

Cyanide poisoning should be suspected in patients with rapid development of unexplained coma, seizures, elevated anion gap metabolic acidosis, and intractable hypotension.

The following laboratory values may suggest the diagnosis when no history is available: elevated plasma lactate level, elevated anion gap metabolic acidosis, relatively normal pO2 in ventilating patients, and an elevated peripheral venous pO2 (greater than 40 mm Hg) or decreased arteriovenous O2 saturation difference (central venous or mixed pulmonary artery O2 saturation greater than 70% with a relatively normal co-oximeter–measured arterial O2 saturation), owing to decreased tissue oxygen extraction from the blood. Hydrogen sulfide and sodium azide poisoning can also cause this combination of laboratory findings (9,14,15). Patients exposed to hydrogen sulfide may have the odor of sulfur or "rotten eggs" on the body or clothes or in a freshly drawn tube of blood (14).

EMERGENCY DEPARTMENT EVALUATION

Whenever possible, the history should include the specific compound involved, route of exposure, any decontamination measures already undertaken, possible dose, time since ingestion or exposure, and any preexisting allergies or chronic medical conditions. Initial physical examination should focus on vital signs (monitored frequently and serially) and the respiratory system, CV system, and CNS. The cardiac rhythm should be continuously monitored.

Determination of serum electrolytes (with calculation of the anion gap), blood glucose levels, pulse oximetry, arterial blood gas analysis, chest radiography, and 12-lead electrocardiography should be done initially and monitored frequently if clinical signs or symptoms of cyanide poisoning are present. Whole blood cyanide levels can be measured, but these determinations usually take hours or days to obtain, and thus cannot be used to guide emergent diagnosis or treatment. They are useful only to document exposure.

EMERGENCY DEPARTMENT MANAGEMENT

Rescuers must not enter areas of potential cyanide gas exposure without a self-contained positive-pressure breathing apparatus (9). Mouth-to-mouth resuscitation should be avoided, if at all possible. If it is unavoidable, rescuers must be careful not to inhale the victim's expired air. Prehospital care consists of airway management, administration of 100% supplemental oxygen, cardiac monitoring, placement of at least one large-bore i.v. line, administration of sodium bicarbonate if hypotension (and, presumably, metabolic acidosis) is present, decontamination of

exposed skin or eyes, and administration of standard anticonvulsant or antiarrhythmic medications, if indicated. If i.v. access cannot be established or in severe poisoning cases, amyl nitrite pearls may be given by inhalation (broken in gauze and held close to the nose and mouth of spontaneously breathing patients or placed into the lips of the face mask or inside the ventilation bag in apneic patients) for 30 seconds out of each minute, using a fresh pearl every 3 to 4 minutes (9).

Exposed skin or eyes should be copiously flushed with water. Contaminated clothing should be removed and isolated. Induced emesis must be avoided, because rapid progression to coma or seizures with potential pulmonary aspiration of gastric contents may occur. Activated charcoal has decreased mortality in experimental cyanide poisoning (17), and 1 g may bind as much as 35 mg of cyanide (1). An activated charcoal dose of 1 g/kg should be administered to patients who have ingested cyanide.

Supportive measures alone may be satisfactory treatment for some patients, although supportive therapy and specific antidotes have resulted in survival with higher whole blood cyanide levels (11). Standard anticonvulsant and antiarrhythmic medications should be administered when clinically indicated. Pulse oximetry or arterial blood gases should be monitored and metabolic acidosis corrected with sodium bicarbonate. Pulse oximetry may be unreliable following administration of methemoglobin-inducing nitrite antidotes.

Patients with coma, seizures, apnea, acidosis, or hypotension should be administered specific antidotes. Once i.v. access has been established, amyl nitrite inhalation should be discontinued and sodium nitrite administered intravenously. The dose is one 10-mL ampule (300 mg) of a 3% solution for adults and 0.12 to 0.33 mL/kg (3.6–9.9 mg/kg) for children. Sodium nitrite is a potent vasodilator; rapid administration may result in severe hypotension, which can be avoided by slow i.v. infusion over absolutely no less than 5 minutes. It can be diluted in 50 to 100 mL of 5% dextrose in water. The infusion is begun slowly, with frequent blood pressure monitoring, and then increased to the most rapid infusion rate not causing hypotension. Rarely, sodium nitrite may induce excessive methemoglobinemia. Methemoglobin levels should be monitored, especially if multiple doses of sodium nitrite are required, and should be kept to less than 30% of total hemoglobin.

Sodium nitrite should be followed by sodium thiosulfate given intravenously in a dose of one 50-mL ampule (12.5 g) of a 25% solution for adults or 1.65 mL/kg for children. When used as a cyanide poisoning antidote, no significant adverse effects as a result of sodium thiosulfate infusion have been reported.

Second doses of sodium nitrite and sodium thiosulfate at one-half the initial amounts may be given 30 minutes later if there is incomplete clinical response. Continued metabolic release of cyanide from cyanogenic glycosides or aliphatic nitrile compounds may cause prolonged poisoning, necessitating multiple antidote doses (7,9). Repeated doses or a continuous infusion (1 g/h) of sodium thiosulfate (without further sodium nitrite) should be considered in such cases (7,13).

When available, hydroxocobalamin is administered in a dose of 4 to 5 g intravenously over 20 to 30 minutes (2,3,6,10). Sodium thiosulfate in the preceding doses may be infused after hydroxocobalamin is given (8). Hyperbaric oxygen (HBO) therapy may be useful in patients unresponsive to supportive and antidotal therapy (3,12,20). Smoke inhalation victims (see Chapter 316, "Smoke Inhalation") may have significant cyanide and carbon monoxide poisoning (2). Inducing methemoglobinemia could be dangerous in this setting. When HBO therapy is available, it is suggested that sodium thiosulfate be given first, with administration of sodium nitrite only as the smoke inhalation victim is receiving HBO therapy. Extracorporeal elimination procedures such as hemodialysis and hemoperfusion have no place in the treatment of acute cyanide poisoning.

CRITICAL INTERVENTIONS

- Administer sodium nitrite and sodium thiosulfate intravenously to patients with coma, seizures, apnea, acidosis, or hypotension
- Monitor methemoglobin levels in patients receiving sodium nitrite, especially in children or when multiple doses are given

DISPOSITION

Consultation with a clinical toxicologist or regional poison center can be invaluable in guiding therapy. Physicians admitting cyanide-poisoned patients should be skilled in intensive care medicine.

Asymptomatic cyanide-exposed patients should be observed in a controlled setting for a minimum of 4 to 6 hours. With aliphatic nitrile and cyanogenic glycoside exposure, the observation period should be extended to 12 hours (7,9). Mildly symptomatic patients can be observed in the emergency department (ED) until symptoms resolve. Those requiring antidote administration should be admitted to an intensive care unit until all symptoms have resolved, or for a minimum of 24 hours.

A few survivors of acute cyanide poisoning have developed parkinsonian-like states or more subtle neuropsychiatric deficits (9,16). Outpatient follow-up should be arranged for patients with significant acute toxicity to screen for these rare sequelae.

If transfer is necessary, the most rapid means available should be used. Accompanying personnel should be able to initiate i.v. access, perform endotracheal intubation and mechanical ventilation, and administer specific antidotes and sodium bicarbonate and standard anticonvulsant and antiarrhythmic medications.

COMMON PITFALLS

✔ Failure to stock an in-date cyanide antidote kit in the ED or other readily available location
✔ Failure to consider the diagnosis of cyanide poisoning in patients with sudden-onset coma, CV collapse, or lactic acidosis of unknown etiology
✔ Inappropriate antidote administration to a hemodynamically stable, conscious patient
✔ Rapid administration of sodium nitrite, resulting in hypotension
✔ Administration of adult doses of cyanide antidotes to children
✔ Failure to consider HBO therapy in patients unresponsive to supportive and antidotal therapy

Acknowledgment

I thank Dr. Barry H. Rumack: teacher, colleague, fellow pilot, and friend who wrote the initial version of this chapter.

References

1. Anderson AH. Experimental studies on the pharmacology of activated charcoal. *Acta Pharmacol* 1946;2:69–78.
2. Baud FJ, Barriot P, Toffis V, et al. Elevated blood cyanide concentrations in victims of smoke inhalation. *N Engl J Med* 1991;325:1761–1776.
3. Beasley DMG, Glass WY. Cyanide poisoning: pathophysiology and treatment recommendations. *Occup Med* 1998;48:427–431.
4. Cottrell JE, Casthely P, Brodie JD, et al. Prevention of nitroprusside-induced cyanide toxicity with hydroxocobalamin. *N Engl J Med* 1978;298:809–811.
5. Espinoza OB, Perez M, Ramirez MS. Bitter cassava poisoning in eight children: a case report. *Vet Hum Toxicol* 1992;34:65.
6. Forsyth JG, Mueller PD, Becker CE, et al. Hydroxocobalamin as a cyanide antidote: safety, efficacy and pharmacokinetics in heavily smoking normal volunteers. *J Toxicol Clin Toxicol* 1993;31:277–294.
7. Geller RJ, Ekins BR, Iknoian RC. Cyanide toxicity from acetonitrile-containing false nail remover. *Am J Emerg Med* 1991;9:268–270.
8. Hall AH, Rumack BH. Hydroxycobalamin/sodium thiosulfate as a cyanide antidote. *J Emerg Med* 1987;5:115–121.
9. Hall AH, Rumack BH. Cyanide and related compounds. In: Haddad LM, Shannon MW, Winchester JF, eds. *Clinical management of poisoning and drug overdose*, 3rd ed. Philadelphia: WB Saunders, 1998:899–905.
10. Hall AH, Linden CH, Kulig KW, et al. Cyanide poisoning from laetrile: role of nitrite therapy. *Pediatrics* 1986;78:269–272.
11. Hall AH, Rumack BH, Schaffer MI, et al. Clinical toxicology of cyanide. In: Ballantyne B and Marrs TC, eds. *Clinical toxicology of cyanide*. Bristol, UK: Wright, 1987:312–333.
12. Hart GB, Strauss MB, Lennon PA, et al. Treatment of smoke inhalation by hyperbaric oxygen. *J Emerg Med* 1985;3:211–215.
13. Heintz B, Bock TA, Kierdorf H, et al. Cyanid-intoxikation: Behandlung mit Hiperoxigenation und Natriumthiosulfat. *Dtsch Med Wochenschr* 1990;115:1100–1103.
14. Hoidal CR, Hall AH, Robinson MD, et al. Hydrogen sulfide poisoning from toxic inhalations of roofing asphalt fumes. *Ann Emerg Med* 1986;15:826–830.
15. Johnson RP, Mellors JW. Arteriolization of venous blood gases: a clue to the diagnosis of cyanide poisoning. *J Emerg Med* 1988;6:401–404.
16. Kales SN, Dinklage D, Dickey J, et al. Paranoid psychosis after exposure to cyanide. *Arch Environ Health* 1997;52:245–246.
17. Lambert RJ, Kindler BL, Schaeffer DJ. The efficacy of superactivated charcoal in treating rats exposed to a lethal oral dose of potassium cyanide. *Ann Emerg Med* 1988;17:595–598.
18. Linakis JG, Lacouture PG, Woolf A. Monitoring cyanide and thiocyanate concentrations during infusion of sodium nitroprusside in children. *Pediatr Cardiol* 1991;12:214–218.
19. Litovitz TL, Klein-Schwartz W, Rodgers GC, et al. 2001 Annual Report of the American Association of Poison Control centers Toxic Exposure Surveillance System. *Am J Emerg Med* 2001;20:391–452.
20. Meyer GW, Hart GB, Strauss MB. Hyperbaric oxygen therapy for acute smoke inhalation injuries. *Postgrad Med* 1991;89:221–223.
21. Steffens W, Leng G, Pelster M. Percutaneous hydrocyanic acid poisoning. Abstract. *J Toxicol Clin Toxicol* 2003;41:483.
22. Yen D, Tsai ZJ, Wang L-M, et al. The clinical experience of acute cyanide poisoning. *Am J Emerg Med* 1995;13:524–528.

CHAPTER 309

Fluoride and Hydrofluoric Acid

Kennon Heard

Fluoride is the most electronegative of all anions. It binds strongly to divalent serum cations such as calcium and magnesium, which precipitate as fluoride salts resulting in hypocalcemia and hypomagnesemia (20). Fluoride inactivates enzymes required for cellular metabolism, and may activate intracellular second messengers (25). Fluoride also interferes with Na^+/K^+-ATPase and activates calcium-dependent potassium channels in cell membranes, causing potassium to enter into the extracellular space, with potential hyperkalemia. Hypocalcemia, hypomagnesemia, and most importantly, hyperkalemia, contribute to cardiac dysrhythmias. Hypocalcemia inhibits calcium-dependent clotting factors and can cause coagulopathy.

Hydrofluoric acid (HF) is a relatively weak acid (pKa = 3.8). Low concentration exposures may not cause an initial caustic injury but can still cause significant tissue damage and pain. High concentration exposures may cause life-threatening systemic poisoning and classic caustic injury.

Hydrofluoric acid is found in products used for glass etching and silicon chip manufacturing. It is also used in household and commercial rust removal products. Although fluoride is found in many household dental products (e.g., toothpaste), exposure to these products rarely results in serious effects (2). However, exposure to prescription sodium fluoride does have the potential to result in serious toxicity. Sodium fluoride has been used as a pesticide. Ammonium fluoride and ammonium bifluoride have been used as wheel cleaners in the past, but these products were pulled from the market following several cases of severe accidental poisoning (16).

CLINICAL PRESENTATION

Dermal hydrofluoric acid exposures are the most commonly encountered fluoride exposure in the emergency department. The main manifestation of these exposures is pain. At low concentrations ($< 20\%$ HF), symptoms may be delayed more than 24 hours (7). Dermal findings may be minimal initially, but can progress to full thickness injury. With lower concentration exposures, dermal findings range from normal skin to full thickness burns. In one series of low concentration exposures, just over half of the patients had erythema and swelling, 5% developed blisters and 23% had normal skin (7). Burns from high concentration ($> 50\%$ HF) may appear similar to other caustic injuries. Exposure of more than 1% of the body surface area to a 50% HF product may result in systemic poisoning (9,15).

Ocular exposures to low concentration products may result in eye pain and corneal injury (22), and animal models suggest that exposure to concentrations over 20% will cause immediate corneal edema and opacification (19).

Oral exposures may be deceptive in that patients may have minimal or no findings suggestive of caustic exposure. Fatal intoxication has been reported without significant gastrointestinal (GI) symptoms (5,13). When present, GI symptoms include abdominal pain, vomiting and hematemesis (13). Effects following inhalation may range from mild pulmonary irritation (17) to hemorrhagic pulmonary edema and delayed multisystem organ failure (4). Systemic absorption of fluoride may occur following inhalational exposure (4).

Manifestations of systemic fluoride poisoning include headache, paresthesias, visual complaints, and signs of hypocalcemia such as carpopedal spasm, Chvostek's and Trousseau's signs, hyperreflexia, tetany, and prolongation of the QT interval on the electrocardiogram. Coma, seizures, shock, dysrhythmias, and death may occur in severe cases. Lethal dysrhythmias include refractory ventricular tachycardia, ventricular fibrillation, and pulseless idioventricular rhythm. Hypocalcemia is often severe (serum calcium level < 5 mEq/L). Metabolic acidosis, hypomagnesemia, hyperkalemia, and coagulopathy can also occur.

DIFFERENTIAL DIAGNOSIS

The diagnosis of HF acid exposure should be entertained when a patient with a chemical exposure presents with severe pain and minimal dermal findings. Other diseases with similar findings would include other chemical burns, Raynaud's syndrome, local ischemia, or sensory neuropathy. Systemic fluoride poisoning should be considered for the patient that presents with cardiovascular (CV) instability and hypocalcemia. Other potential causes of this presentation would include acute hypoparathyroidism and hyperphosphatemia.

EMERGENCY DEPARTMENT EVALUATION

Important factors in the history include the route of exposure, product involved, the use of protective equipment and whether decontamination was performed. Signs and symptoms and their time of onset with respect to exposure should be noted. The physical examination should initially be focused on the site of exposure. Patients with facial burns should have conjunctival pH determined and a full eye exam performed.

Patients with small ($<5\%$ body surface area) dermal exposures to HF products with a concentration of less than 10% do not require any laboratory testing or monitoring. Patients with more extensive dermal exposures, dermal exposure to higher concentration products or ingestion of HF products should have continuous cardiac monitoring, an electrocardiogram, and serum calcium determinations. Those with hypocalcemia should have a complete blood count, serum electrolytes, magnesium, blood area nitrogen, and creatinine. Chest radiographs are indicated for symptomatic patients with inhalational exposure.

EMERGENCY DEPARTMENT MANAGEMENT

The first step in management of dermal exposure is immediate irrigation with water. In an older case series of over 400 dermal exposures (most involving 40% HF) treated with immediate water irrigation, no patient developed deep tissue necrosis and all recovered within days (10). Irrigation should be performed for a minimum of 20 minutes. If symptoms have not resolved, irrigation should be continued. Recently, hexafluorine, a proprietary product that binds fluoride much more effectively than calcium, has been advocated (18). However, hexafluorine offers no clear advantage over water irrigation.

Patients that have continued pain despite irrigation or that present several hours out from exposure should be treated in a stepwise fashion. Topical calcium is the standard first-line therapy. The most effective way to deliver the calcium is to mix 10% calcium chloride with methylcellulose to form a gel with a final calcium concentration of 2.3 to 2.5%. If methylcellose is not available, a water-based lubricant (e.g., KY jelly) may be used. The mixture is then applied topically to the affected area. Exposures involving the digits are best treated by having the patient wear a tight-filling glove filled with the gel. The glove is worn for at least 30 minutes after the pain resolves. Fingernail removal is not advocated, and patients with exposure that involves the nail beds are best treated with region perfusion (see below). Patients that have relief may be discharged with additional gel and told to apply the gel every 4 to 6 hours or sooner if needed, for the next 24 hours (6).

Patients that have continued pain despite topical calcium therapy should be treated with calcium injection or regional perfusion. Local subcutaneous injection of calcium gluconate is best suited for areas in which the tissue can expand to accommodate the fluid. The dose is 0.5cc of 10% calcium gluconate per cm^2 of involved skin. Calcium chloride should not be used as it may cause tissue injury. The injection is performed with a small (27 g or smaller) needle. Successful treatment results in immediate improvement in symptoms (1). Use of a local anesthetic is not recommended as relief of pain is used as an indication of the success of therapy. Patients may then be discharged with a plan to use topical therapy as described in the previous paragraph.

Often, the skin on the hand and foot cannot comfortably accommodate the volume of fluid injected during these injections. These areas are best treated by regional perfusion. This may be accomplished by either direct arterial injection or using intravenous injection with Bier's technique. Arterial perfusion requires placing an arterial catheter. After confirming intraarterial placement by either waveform or arteriography, 100 cc of a 2.5% calcium gluconate solution is infused over 60 minutes (23). An alternative to arterial infusion is regional venous calcium infusion using a Bier block. With this technique, an i.v. catheter is placed in the hand or foot and the extremity is exsanguinated by elevation (with or without application of an elastic bandage). A pneumatic tourniquet is applied proximal to the burn, and inflated to 100 mg above systolic blood pressure. Once the tourniquet is inflated, 10 cc of a 10% calcium gluconate diluted with 40 cc of saline is infused into the catheter in the affected extremity. After 15 to 25 minutes, the tourniquet is deflated slowly over 5 minutes (8). Most patients will require parenteral analgesia to tolerate the tourniquet.

Ocular exposures should be treated with immediate water irrigation. As with any caustic exposure to the eye, the ocular pH should be monitored. There is no evidence that irrigation with calcium or magnesium-containing solutions offers any advantage, and any delay that occurs while these solutions are obtained is likely to be detrimental. Although animal models suggest that severe injury is possible (22), reported cases have gone on to good recovery (3,19). One report suggested that calcium gluconate drops may be a useful adjunctive therapy after decontamination, but this is not routinely recommended (3).

Nebulized calcium gluconate has been recommended for inhalational exposures, but the evidence is anecdotal and limited, so this therapy cannot be considered standard (17).

Patients with ingestions of fluoride-containing products should rinse their mouth and ingest 50 to 100 cc of water to dilute the caustic effects. Charcoal does not adsorb fluoride and should not be administered unless life-threatening coingestion is strongly suspected. Oral decontamination by administration of calcium-containing solution is of unproven value. One animal model of oral HF exposure was not able to demonstrate a protective effect from oral calcium administration in a 1:1 equivalent ratio (11). A second study did show a survival benefit, but only when the ratio of calcium to fluoride exceeded a 1:1 equivalent ratio (14). This would translate to more than 3 grams of calcium chloride for each gram of fluoride ingested.

Accidental exposures to most nonprescription dental products that contain fluoride do not result in serious toxicity although patients may develop gastrointestinal symptoms. Patients with small (suspect less than 30 cc ingested), accidental exposures to low concentration HF products or dental sodium fluoride products almost always do well (13).

Asymptomatic patients with small ingestions (e.g., a sip) should have venous access obtained and be placed on a cardiac monitor. Baseline ionized calcium measurements should be obtained. If the serum calcium is below the normal range, it is reasonable to administer 1 gm of calcium gluconate over 30 minutes and then immediately repeat the calcium level. Persistent hypocalcemia suggests that there was a significant exposure and the patient should be treated similar to deliberate exposures as outlined below.

Patients with deliberate ingestions (or accidental ingestions suspected to involve more than 30 cc) of low concentration HF products or sodium fluoride may benefit from prophylactic treatment with intravenous calcium. Animal models suggest that such treatment improves survival (12). The author recommends that any patient that presents after deliberate ingestion of an HF product should be treated with prophylactic calcium

gluconate (at a rate of 3 gm/hour) while baseline calcium studies are measured. Calcium chloride may be used, but it must be given through a well-functioning line, as extravasation may cause extensive tissue injury. If the initial serum calcium is normal, the infusion may be stopped, but serum calcium levels should be measured every 30 minutes for at least 3 hours, and if calcium levels are decreasing, the infusion should be restarted.

Patients that develop hypocalcemia or manifest CV effects must be treated very aggressively. Survival following cardiac arrest from fluoride poisoning has always been associated with very aggressive calcium therapy. One report describes a patient that suffered cardiac arrest and survived following the administration of over 110 mEq of calcium chloride (approximately 9 gm) during a resuscitation (24). Interestingly, this patient presented again after ingesting the same amount a few weeks after her initial treatment. At this presentation she was treated with 65 mEq of calcium prior to developing symptoms and had an uncomplicated course. Although only suggestive, this case suggests that early administration may prevent CV collapse.

Patients that have or develop hypocalcemia, hyperkalemia, cardiac dysrhythmias, hypotension, coma or seizures should have central venous access obtained, the calcium infusion should be changed from calcium gluconate to calcium chloride (which contains 3 times as much calcium per gram) and continued at the same rate using the central venous access. The serum calcium should be measured every 30 minutes, and if hypocalcemia persists, the calcium infusion rate should be doubled. Fluids should also be administered for hypotension. Cardiac dysrhythmias and hyperkalemia do not respond to usual therapies. Magnesium and potassium levels should also be monitored and magnesium should be administered to maintain a normal serum level. Consideration should also be given a sodium bicarbonate infusion to achieve a serum pH of 7.45 to 7.50, as systemic alkalosis improves survival in animal models (21).

CRITICAL INTERVENTIONS

- Immediately irrigate dermal or ocular exposures with water or saline
- Administer topical or s.c. calcium gluconate, followed by intravenous regional or intraarterial calcium gluconate infusion, for patients who have skin findings or persistent pain after dermal exposure
- Establish venous access, institute cardiac rhythm (and QT interval) monitoring, obtain a serum calcium level, and give prophylactic intravenous calcium gluconate to patients with intentional ingestions or large dermal, inhalational, or oral exposure
- Establish central venous access and administer intravenous calcium chloride to patients with hypocalcemia or QT interval prolongation

DISPOSITION

Patients that present with dermal exposures that have no symptoms following irrigation may be discharged with instructions to return or begin topical calcium therapy if pain develops. Similarly, patients that present with pain and respond well to topical or intradermal therapy in the emergency department may be discharged with topical therapy every 4 to 6 hours and a 24-hour follow-up. If visible burns are noted, a burn or hand surgeon should be consulted. Patients that require regional infusions are likely to require repeat therapy and should be admitted for 24-hour observation. Intraarterial administration is an indication for ICU admission (primarily for monitoring of the arterial line).

Patients that have no symptoms and a normal exam following irrigation for ocular exposures may be discharged with next day follow-up. An ophthalmologist should be consulted and see all patients with persistent symptoms or an abnormal ocular exam emergently. Patients with ingestions of HF products who have no symptoms and normal serum calcium levels after 6 hours may be discharged or referred for psychiatric evaluation. Those who require intravenous calcium should be admitted to an intensive care unit for ongoing monitoring and treatment. A poison center or toxicologist should be consulted if the physician is not familiar with the evaluation and management of fluoride and HF poisoning.

COMMON PITFALLS

✔ Failure to appreciate that patients with dermal HF injury may have pain without abnormal skin findings
✔ Failure to appreciate that systemic fluoride poisoning may occur in the absence of gastrointestinal symptoms following ingestion
✔ Failure to appreciate that severe systemic fluoride poisoning may result from large dermal and inhalational exposures
✔ Failure to appreciate that large doses of calcium and magnesium may be required in patients with systemic fluoride poisoning

Acknowledgment

The author thanks previous edition chapter author, Andis Graudins. Kennon Heard was supported by an American Geriatric Society Jahnigen Career Scholars Award.

References

1. Anderson WJ, Anderson JR. Hydrofluoric acid burns of the hand: mechanism of injury and treatment. *J Hand Surg [Am]* 1988;13:52–57.
2. Augenstein WL, Spoerke DG, Kulig KW, et al. Fluoride ingestion in children: a review of 87 cases. *Pediatrics* 1991;88:907–912.
3. Bentur Y, Tannenbaum S, Yaffe Y, et al. The role of calcium gluconate in the treatment of hydrofluoric acid eye burn. *Ann Emerg Med* 1993;22:1488–1490.
4. Braun J, Stoss H, Zober A. Intoxication following inhalation of hydrogen fluoride. *Arch Toxicol* 1984;56:50–54.
5. Chan KM, Svancarek WP, Creer M. Fatality due to acute hydrofluoric acid exposure. *J Toxicol Clin Toxicol* 1987;25:333–339.
6. Chick LR, Borah G. Calcium carbonate gel therapy for hydrofluoric acid burns of the hand. *Plast Reconstr Surg* 1990;86:935–940.
7. El Saadi MS, Hall AH, Hall PK, et al. Hydrofluoric acid dermal exposure. *Vet Hum Toxicol* 1989;31:243–247.
8. Graudins A, Burns MJ, Aaron CK. Regional intravenous infusion of calcium gluconate for hydrofluoric acid burns of the upper extremity. *Ann Emerg Med* 1997;30:604–607.
9. Greco RJ, Hartford CE, Haith LR, et al. Hydrofluoric acid induced hypocalcemia. *J Trauma* 1988;28:1593–1596.
10. Hamilton M. OH Congress. Hydrofluoric acid burns. Occupational Health (London) 1975;27:468–70.
11. Heard K, Delgado J. Oral decontamination with calcium or magesium salts does not improve survival following hydrofluoric acid ingetsion. *J Toxicol Clin Toxicol* 2003;41:789–792.
12. Heard K, Hill RE, Cairns CB, et al. Calcium decreases fluoride bioavailability in a lethal model of fluoride poisoning. *J Toxicol Clin Toxicol* 2001;39:349–353.
13. Kao WF, Dart RC, Kuffner E, et al. Ingestion of low-concentration hydrofluoric acid: an insidious and potentially fatal poisoning. *Ann Emerg Med* 1999;34:35–41.
14. Kao WF, Deng JF, Chiang SC, et al. A simple, safe, and efficient way to treat severe fluoride poisoning—oral calcium or magnesium. *J Toxicol Clin Toxicol* 2004;42:43–50.
15. Kirkpatrick JJ, Enion DS, Burd DA. Hydrofluoric acid burns: a review. *Burns* 1995;21:483–493.
16. Klasner AE, Scalzo AJ, Blume C, et al. Ammonium bifluoride causes another pediatric death. *Ann Emerg Med* 1998;31:525.
17. Lee DC, Wiley JF 2d, Synder JW 2d. Treatment of inhalational exposure to hydrofluoric acid with nebulized calcium gluconate. *J Occup Med* 1993;35:470.
18. Mathieu L, Nehles J, Blomet J, et al. Efficacy of hexafluorine for emergent decontamination of hydrofluoric acid eye and skin splashes. *Vet Hum Toxicol* 2001;43:263–265.
19. McCulley JP, Whiting DW, Petitt MG, et al. Hydrofluoric acid burns of the eye. *J Occup Med* 1983;25:447–450.
20. McIvor ME. Acute fluoride toxicity: pathophysiology and management. *Drug Saf* 1990;5:79–85.
21. Reynolds KE, Whitford GM, Pashley DH. Acute fluoride toxicity: The influence of acid-base status. *Toxicol Appl Pharmacol* 1978;45:415–427.
22. Rubinfeld RS, Silbert DI, Arentsen JJ, et al. Ocular hydrofluoric acid burns. *Am J Ophthal* 1992;114:420–423.
23. Siegel DC, Heard JM. Intra-arterial calcium infusion for hydrofluoric acid burns. *Aviat Space Environ Med* 1992;63:206–211.
24. Stremski ES, Grande GA, Ling LJ. Survival following hydrofluoric acid ingestion. *Ann Emerg Med* 1992;21:1396–1399.
25. Wittinghofer A. Signaling mechanistics: aluminum fluoride for molecule of the year. *Curr Biol* 1997;7:R682–R685.

CHAPTER 310
Hydrocarbons

Sophia Dyer

The term "hydrocarbon" refers to compounds with both hydrogen and carbon as integral to the structure of the compound. Petroleum distillates are hydrocarbons isolated from crude oil. The distillation process uses columns that separate components based on their volatility. Some distillation products are more or less pure compounds, although others are mixtures of several compounds. Examples include gasoline, mineral spirits, naphtha, various fuel oils, xylene, toluene, and benzene. Both aromatic (cyclic) and aliphatic (straight-chain) petroleum products can be produced by distillation.

Aromatic hydrocarbons represent a large family of compounds used in an extensive array of products. The unifying factor is their structure, based on a 6-carbon benzene ring. The aromatic hydrocarbons include toluene, xylene, cresols, styrene, and phenols. Many products contain aromatic hydrocarbons, ranging from shoe polish, glues, and mothballs to industrial pesticides.

Halogenated hydrocarbons include the aliphatic and aromatic hydrocarbons to which halogen atoms (bromine, chlorine, fluorine, or iodine) have been added. Many solvents, for example, are halogenated hydrocarbons. Other sources of patient exposure to halogenated hydrocarbons are fire extinguishers, fumigants, and refrigerants.

Terpenes comprise a class of aliphatic cyclic hydrocarbons that occur naturally as plant oils and resins. Familiar examples include camphor, pine oil, and turpentine. Each has a distinctive smell that is often easily recognizable. Old-style mothballs were comprised of camphor but most mothballs are now made from para-dichlorobenzene, a nonterpene aromatic hydrocarbon. Pine oil is found in varying concentrations in a number of commercial products such as Pine Sol® cleaner.

Aromatic and aliphatic hydrocarbons up to 16 carbons in length are well absorbed following inhalation. Aliphatics greater than 16 carbons long, on the other hand, are not. Oral absorption also depends on the size of the hydrocarbon molecule. Lower molecular weight aliphatic and aromatic hydrocarbons are readily absorbed via the gastrointestinal (GI) tract, but aromatic hydrocarbons of 9 carbons or more and aliphatic of greater than 28 carbons are poorly absorbed after ingestion.

Many hydrocarbons cause pulmonary toxicity if aspirated and the risk of aspiration risk correlates with the viscosity of the hydrocarbon. Viscosity is measured in Saybolt seconds universal (SSU) units. If the value for SSU is 60 or less, the chance of aspiration if the hydrocarbon is ingested is greater. Mineral seal oil (contained in many furniture polishes), gasoline and kerosene possess SSU values of less than 60. Other petroleum distillates, such as fuel oil and long-chain aliphatic hydrocarbons, have a viscosity greater that 100 SSU and present less of an aspiration risk. Volatility, as measured by the vapor pressure of the substance, also affects the likelihood of a hydrocarbon producing toxicity. More volatile hydrocarbons have a greater chance of pulmonary absorption and thus of affecting the central nervous system. High lipid solubility increase the potential for central nervous system (CNS) effects.

The majority of hydrocarbon exposures are accidental. Ingestion is common in children less than 6 years of age. Volatile hydrocarbons, especially aromatic and other volatile hydrocarbons, can be intentionally abused for euphoric effects, a situation encountered most frequently in adolescent populations. Direct neurotransmitter effects have been described. For example, toluene and trichloroethane are believed to stimulate GABAA activity (3,4). The mechanics of inhalant abuse are simple. "Sniffing" involves inhalation from an open container. A cloth saturated with the chemical is placed over the nose and mouth for inhalation in "huffing." Spraying or pouring a volatile hydrocarbon into a plastic or paper bag for inhalation of the vapors is called "bagging."

The long-term effects of inhalant abuse include diffuse CNS demyelination of subcortical white matter (12). Toluene and probably other aromatic agents can cause renal toxicity. Intravenous hydrocarbon exposures, for abuse or suicide attempts, are also occasionally reported.

Skin contact is another potential route of exposure to hydrocarbons. Hydrocarbons with similar water/lipid partition coefficients are well absorbed. As expected, the degree of systemic absorption will vary with the amount of surface area and duration of exposure. Dermal exposure to hydrocarbons may produce varying degrees of a chemical "burn." Long-chain hydrocarbons such as bitumen and tar are not significantly absorbed, but can be difficult to remove from the skin and cause thermal burns when the product is hot.

CLINICAL PRESENTATION

The nature of toxicity depends on multiple variables including the class of hydrocarbon (aromatic, halogenated, terpene or petroleum distillate), the route and duration of exposure, and the presence of other substances such as metals or pesticides in the hydrocarbon product. For example, inhalation of leaded gasoline has been associated with lead toxicity (16).

Acute hydrocarbon inhalation can cause euphoria, hallucinations, agitation, CNS depression, and syncope. Coma can occur in severe cases. Dysrhythmias and "sudden sniffing death" syndrome are most often seen with chlorinated hydrocarbons and aromatic hydrocarbons (2,8). Victims are frequently noted to exhibit agitation and to have engaged in physical activity such as running prior to collapse. Myocardial depression can also occur (1).

Chronic inhalation can lead to cognitive impairment, cerebellar ataxia, oculomotor and corticospinal abnormalities. Patients who chronically inhale toluene may present with nausea, vomiting, dehydration, and weakness as a result of metabolic acidosis, hypokalemia, and hypophosphatemia resulting from distal renal tubular acidosis (i.e., bicarbonate wasting). Both increased anion gap metabolic acidosis and hyperchloremic normal anion

gap metabolic acidosis can be seen. Rhabdomyolysis may also be present. Goodpasture's syndrome, renal calculi, and reversible renal failure have been described. Traumatic injury can result from impaired judgment and burns may results from unintentional ignition of hydrocarbons.

Two unique syndromes can be seen after inhalational exposure to hydrocarbons in the occupational setting. 'Chloracne' is acneiform eruption that sometimes occur after chronic exposure to chlorinated aromatic hydrocarbons (dioxins and polychlorinated biphenyls). It can last for months. "Degreaser's flush" refers to the generalized erythema that can occur after the ingestion of ethanol in those with chronic exposure to chlorinated hydrocarbons, most notably trichloroethylene. It is transient and represents a disulfiram-like reaction.

Pulmonary toxicity can occur after inhalational exposure, but it more commonly results from aspiration during ingestion. Choking, coughing, or gagging suggests aspiration. Vomiting is common after hydrocarbon ingestion and is a risk factor for aspiration (11). Signs and symptoms of aspiration pneumonitis include dyspnea, tachypnea, nasal flaring, grunting, rhonchi, rales, and agitation (secondary to hypoxia). Lack of tachypnea in the patient presenting after hydrocarbon exposure has a high negative predictive value for aspiration (18). Symptoms usually begin within 30 minutes of exposure and typically worsen over the course of 1 to 5 days. In severe cases, pulmonary edema, hemoptysis, pleural effusions, pneumothorax can occur. Radiographic abnormalities may lag behind clinical presentation. Other findings on chest radiograph include infiltrates, increased bronchovascular markings, and pneumomediastinum.

Fever and leukocytosis are frequently demonstrated in a chemical pneumonitis induced by aspiration of hydrocarbons (9).

Ingestion of petroleum distillates and most other hydrocarbons are associated with some degree of gastrointestinal symptoms. Oral mucosal irritation, nausea, vomiting and diarrhea are common. An abdominal radiograph may demonstrate a "double bubble" sign with hydrocarbon layering over stomach contents (6).

The ingestion of camphor and other terpenes can cause CNS toxicity. Agitation, restlessness, and seizures can occur as soon as 4 minutes after camphor ingestion (14). Ingestions of less than 50 mg/kg of camphor do not generally cause significant toxicity (7). Turpentine can cause CNS depression after ingestion, but seizures are infrequent. It has also been reported to induce thrombocytopenic purpura (17). Lethargy and ataxia are the most common symptoms after pine oil ingestion (5). Methylene chloride, found in many paint strippers, is metabolized by the liver to carbon monoxide. Ingestion or inhalation can cause carbon monoxide poisoning (see Chapter 306, "Carbon Monoxide") (15). Carbon tetrachloride can cause hepatic and renal toxicity which may not be evident until 2 to 3 days after ingestion. Naphthalene ingestion can cause methemoglobinemia and associated hemolytic anemia.

Intravenous injection of hydrocarbons, although rare, is associated with systemic and local effects. Local inflammation, sterile abscess formation, tissue necrosis, thrombophlebitis, myositis are all reported effects of attempts to inject various hydrocarbons, and a pneumonitis may result as well (10,13).

DIFFERENTIAL DIAGNOSIS

The odor of a hydrocarbon or hydrocarbon product (for example, that of pine oil) could assist in narrowing the differential diagnosis of hydrocarbon exposure. Intoxication by ethanol, carbon monoxide, gamma hydroxybutyrate and other sedative-hypnotics, opiates and centrally acting pharmaceuticals such as phenothiazines, antihistamines and tricyclic antidepressants) can have effects on the central nervous system similar to those hydrocarbons. Changes in mental status can also resemble those from traumatic head injury or infection (either systemic or directly related to the central nervous system). Like camphor, isoniazid and tricyclic antidepressant can cause the rapid development of seizures after toxic exposure. Although petroleum distillates are poorly absorbed after ingestion, pulmonary aspiration and resultant hypoxia can lead to CNS depression.

Other potential etiologies of anion or non-anion gap metabolic acidosis include methanol, ethylene glycol, salicylates, and iron poisoning, which should be considered in the differential diagnosis of chronic aromatic hydrocarbon inhalation.

GI symptoms following hydrocarbon ingestions could resemble those of a host of other etiologies, including other toxic ingestions (such as caustics) or more common entities, such as food-borne or infectious gastroenteritis.

The respiratory symptoms of hydrocarbon aspiration can mimic reactive airway disease, pulmonary infection or pulmonary embolism. A delay in radiographic changes associated the hydrocarbon aspiration frequently complicates the immediate diagnosis. Pulmonary infiltrates, fever and leukocytosis secondary to aspiration of hydrocarbons may mimic an infectious process.

Tachydysrhythmias that result from aromatic and halogenated hydrocarbon inhalation can also be seen with electrolyte derangements, myocardial ischemia, or other toxic exposures (see Chapter 271, "Approach to the Poisoned Patient"). Pulmonary aspiration and resultant hypoxia secondary to petroleum distillate ingestion could also lead to CV toxicity.

EMERGENCY DEPARTMENT EVALUATION

Pertinent points of history include the name of product, identity of ingredients, manufacturer (if possible to assist poison control specialists in locating the product), time and route of exposure, and time of onset and nature of symptoms. If the substance could pose an inhalational or dermal hazard to the emergency department staff or other patients, the patient should be disrobed and decontaminated prior to entering the emergency department. The history should include a respiratory, neurological and gastrointestinal review of symptoms. If the historian is a parent who suspects an ingestion in a child, they should be asked a about the occurrence of vomiting, coughing, and other respiratory symptoms. The possibility of concomitant trauma should also be considered.

All suspected hydrocarbon-exposed patients should receive complete vital signs including determination of oxygen saturation. Cardiac monitoring should be initiated and an electrocardiogram obtained to evaluation for conduction abnormalities and tachydysrhythmias. A complete blood count and chest radiography are indicated for patients with respiratory symptoms. Arterial blood gas should be considered in any patient with suspected aspiration of petroleum distillates who presents with respiratory symptoms. Liver function tests should be obtained in those exposed to chlorinated hydrocarbons, such as carbon tetrachloride. Patients with altered mental status, weakness, dehydration, or chronic inhalational abuse should a serum electrolytes, creatinine, blood area nitrogen, and creatine kinase and urinalysis to screen for renal tubular acidosis and rhabdomyolysis. Concomitant use of alcohol or other central acting drug of abuse can be evaluated by serum and urine toxic screens if necessary. If the history is uncertain, a trauma evaluation should be performed, particularly computerized tomography (CT) of the brain in those with altered mental status. Patients with persistent neurological dysfunction and a normal CT should have an magnetic resonance imaging (MRI) of the brain, which is the best diagnostic tool for detecting CNS demyelination.

EMERGENCY DEPARTMENT MANAGEMENT

Advanced cardiac life support measures should be instituted as needed. If the patient is stable presents a risk of contamination to the health care providers—for example, a patient with dermal hydrocarbon exposure containing a pesticide—decontamination with soap and water washing and rinsing should be performing prior entering the emergency department. If this is not possible, health care providers should wear gloves and protective clothing. Flammability is also a potential hazard of many hydrocarbons, especially if the situation calls for the use of medical devices such as a defibrillator.

Any patient with respiratory symptoms should receive oxygen therapy. Consideration should be given to early endotracheal intubation, especially if the patient is to be transferred to another facility and is demonstrating respiratory distress. Bronchodilators can be given for bronchospasm secondary to pulmonary aspiration. Alternative methods of ventilation such as high-frequency jet ventilation, partial liquid ventilation or extracorporeal membrane oxygenation should be considered in patients with refractory hypoxemia.

Seizure activity can be managed with benzodiazepine therapy. Because tachydysrhythmias appear related to sensitization of the myocardium to endogenous catecholamines, β-adrenergic blockers such as propranolol may be the best treatment. Lidocaine in standard doses may also be used. Adrenergic agents, such as epinephrine, may be deleterious in such situations.

The issue of gastric decontamination in the case of ingested hydrocarbons is controversial. Because the risk of aspiration increases with maneuvers that manipulate the GI tract, gastric decontamination should only be considered when potentially toxic amounts of agents with systemic toxicity (e.g., aromatic, halogenated, and terpene hydrocarbons or pesticides and metals in a hydrocarbon vehicle). It is not indicated for the ingestion of petroleum distillates. A poison center or toxicologist should be consulted if the need for gastric decontamination is unclear. Generally, if decontamination is attempted, gastric aspiration using a small nasogastric tube is preferred over traditional lavage with large orogastric tube. As most hydrocarbons are not well absorbed by activated charcoal, this method of decontamination is only indicated for coingestants and agents with systemic toxicity.

CRITICAL INTERVENTIONS

- Obtain a chest radiograph in patients with coughing, gagging, vomiting, tachypnea, abnormal pulmonary exam, or low oxygen saturation after hydrocarbon ingestion
- Obtain serum electrolytes, creatinine, blood urea nitrogen, creatine kinase, and urinalysis in patients with altered mental status, weakness, dehydration, or chronic inhalational abuse
- Admit patients with persistent tachypnea, hypoxemia, or abnormal pulmonary exam as a result of suspected hydrocarbon aspiration even if the chest radiograph is normal

DISPOSITION

Any patient presenting with known or suspected cardiac dysrhythmia (by history of syncope) should be admitted for cardiac monitoring. Patients with significant metabolic abnormalities, renal dysfunction, or potential hepatoxicity should also be admitted (16). Those with persistent neurologic should be

EMERGENCY DEPARTMENT EVALUATION

Despite loss of consciousness at the scene, patients may be asymptomatic or minimally symptomatic on arrival at the emergency department (1,5,7,17). Initial history is directed toward confirming H_2S exposure and the severity of symptoms prior to arrival. Important historical information includes location and actions preceding symptom onset, duration of exposure, time course of any alterations in level of consciousness, and any unusual odors noted. The possibility of coexistent trauma should be also be addressed.

After evaluation of vital signs, the physical examination should focus on assessment for irritant (ocular, dermal, mucus membrane, pulmonary) and systemic (cardiovascular and neurological) effects. Presence of an alert mental status does not preclude the existence of significant underlying CNS dysfunction. A thorough neurological examination, including mental status testing, should be performed to evaluate for evidence of subtle neurological dysfunction. If available, neuropsychiatric screening batteries should be administered.

Patients with limited irritant symptoms, normal vital signs, and normal physical examinations, require no further laboratory assessment. Those patients with evidence of systemic toxicity should have a chest radiograph, electrocardiogram, and arterial blood gas analysis for evaluation of oxygenation and acid–base status. Additional testing may include routine hematology and chemistry profiles. Patients with prolonged loss of consciousness, persistent alteration in level of consciousness, or focal neurological deficits may additionally require radiologic imaging to evaluate for cerebral ischemic insult and occult trauma.

EMERGENCY DEPARTMENT MANAGEMENT

Initial management involves removing the patient from the source of exposure. Survivors frequently improve simply with this intervention (3,5). Rescuers should not attempt to enter the environment of exposure without wearing self-contained breathing apparatus (SCBA). Numerous reports document the incapacitation of rescue parties attempting to remove an isolated victim from environments with high H_2S concentrations (5,8,13,17). As systemic toxicity does not result from dermal exposure, protective clothing is not required. However, decontamination should include removal of grossly contaminated clothing and cleansing with soap and water, to limit local irritant effects. Ocular decontamination requires the removal of contact lenses and copious irrigation with normal saline.

Supportive care is the mainstay of treatment for systemic toxicity, with specific attention to advanced life support modalities, and management of altered mental status, pulmonary edema, hypotension, acidosis, and concomitant trauma. One hundred percent oxygen should be administered to enhance oxygen delivery and increase endogenous sulfide metabolism (16). Laboratory studies have demonstrated that endogenous sulfide detoxification is so rapid that minimal cytochrome-bound sulfide would be expected by the time of patient arrival in the emergency department. As a result, specific data regarding antidotal therapy remains sparse and controversial.

Similarities with cyanide intoxication led to the use of sodium nitrite in severe H_2S intoxication. The resultant methemoglobinemia was thought to limit cytochrome-sulfide binding, by acting as a sulfide scavenger and preferentially generating sulfide-methemoglobin complexes (sulfmethemoglobin), or by further catalyzing sulfide oxidation (2). Anecdotal reports and pretreatment animal models have demonstrated improvement with nitrite therapy (14,18,19). However, no convincing evidence exists that nitrite administration improves patient outcome or changes clinical course. *In vitro* time-course studies indicate that nitrite must be administered within minutes of exposure in order to be effective (3). Additionally, the induction of methemoglobinemia, further impairing oxygen transport, may potentially worsen the clinical situation. Nitrite therapy remains recommended for patients with severe H_2S intoxication who do not rapidly improve on removal from the source. Ideally, the nitrite should be administered within 1 hour of exposure. The dose of sodium nitrite is identical to that used for cyanide (adults, 10 mL of 3% sodium nitrite intravenously over 5 minutes; children 0.2 to 0.33 mL/kg, up to 10 mL). Sodium thiosulfate is not recommended, as rhodanese does not appear to be involved in H_2S detoxification.

Improvement with hyperbaric oxygen (HBO) therapy has been reported, even in nitrite-refractory H_2S poisoning (15,16,23). Animal studies have suggested an outcome benefit from the use of HBO therapy, with the best outcome occurring in an experimental group receiving both sodium nitrite and HBO at 3 ATA (4). However, the efficacy of HBO in H_2S poisoning remains to be established. HBO may be considered for severely intoxicated patients with persistent neurological abnormalities, especially those patients unresponsive to supportive care or nitrite therapy, given the documented potential for delayed and persistent neuropsychiatric sequelae.

CRITICAL INTERVENTIONS

- Wear SCBA when extricating the victim from the source
- Administer 100% oxygen to all patients and consider sodium nitrite given intravenously and HBO therapy in patients with persistent neurological abnormalities
- Search for concomitant trauma

DISPOSITION

Consultation with a medical toxicologist or regional poison control center is recommended if the physician is unfamiliar with the management of H_2S poisoning. Asymptomatic patients presenting after a minor H_2S exposure may be discharged after a 4 to 6 hour observation period. Patients with toxicity limited to dermal or ocular irritation may be managed as outpatients. Patients with significant exposure (including loss of consciousness) or local airway irritation should be monitored for at least 24 hours. Patients with abnormal vital signs, cardiopulmonary and neurological examinations should be admitted to an intensive care unit. Patients with initial loss of consciousness should be followed up within 1 week for examination for delayed neuropsychiatric sequelae. Transfer of severely intoxicated patients should be considered if intensive care admission or antidotal therapy is indicated but unavailable.

COMMON PITFALLS

✔ Failure to consider the possibility of H_2S poisoning in otherwise healthy patients who suddenly collapse at work
✔ Failure to appreciate that the lack of an odor does not imply safety, as a result of olfactory paralysis at dangerous levels
✔ Failure to consider the possibility of other victims and perform a scene search when an index case is found
✔ Failure to appreciate the potential for delayed pulmonary injury in the minimally symptomatic patient

Acknowledgments

The author thanks Daniel R. Douglas and Martin J. Smilkstein for their contributions to a previous edition of the chapter.

References

1. Audeau FM, Gnanaharan C, Davey K. H$_2$S poisoning associated with pelt processing. *N Z Med J* 1985;98:145–147.
2. Beauchamp RO Jr, Bus JS, Popp JA, et al. A critical review of the literature on H$_2$S toxicity. *Crit Rev Toxicol* 1984;13:25–97.
3. Beck JF, Bradbury CM, Connors AJ, et al. Nitrite as an antidote for acute H$_2$S intoxication? *Am Ind Hyg Assoc J* 1981;42:805–809.
4. Bitterman N, Talmi Y, Lerman A, et al. The effect of hyperbaric oxygen on acute experimental sulfide poisoning in rat. *Toxicol Appl Pharmacol* 1986;84:325–328.
5. Burnett WW, King EG, Grace M, et al. Hydrogen sulfide poisoning: review of 5 years' experience. *Can Med Assoc J* 1977;117:1277–1280.
6. Costigan MG. Hydrogen Sulfide: UK occupational exposure limits. *Occup Environ Med* 2003;60:308–312.
7. Gabbay DS, De Roos F, Perrone J. Twenty-foot fall averts fatality from massive hydrogen sulfide exposure. *J Emerg Med* 2001;20:141–144.
8. Gunn B, Wong R. Noxious gas exposure in the outback: two cases of hydrogen sulfide toxicity. *Emerg Med (Fremantle)* 2001;13:240–246.
9. Hendrickson R, Hamilton RJ, Greenberg MI. Epidemiology of U.S. workplace hydrogen sulfide fatalities—an immediately fatal toxin with multiple casualties [Abstract]. *J Toxicol Clin Toxicol* 2000;38:544.
10. Hoidal CR, Hall AH, Robinson MD, et al. Hydrogen sulfide poisoning from toxic inhalations of roofing asphalt fumes. *Ann Emerg Med* 1986;15:579–582.
11. Lindell H, Jappinen P, Savolainen H. Determination of sulfide in blood with an ion-selective electrode by preconcentration of trapped sulfide in sodium hydroxide solution. *Analyst* 1988;113:839–840.
12. Park CM, Nagel RL. Sulfhemoglbinemia: clinical and molecular aspects. *N Engl J Med* 1984;310:1579–1584.
13. Peters JW. Hydrogen sulfide poisoning in a hospital setting. *JAMA* 1981;246:1588–1589.
14. Ravizza AG, Carugo D, Cerchiari EL. The treatment of hydrogen sulfide intoxication oxygen vs nitrites. *Vet Human Toxicol* 1982;24:241–242.
15. Schneider JS, Tobe EH, Mozley PD, et al. Persistent cognitive and motor deficits following acute hydrogen sulphide poisoning. *Occup Med* 1998;48:255–260.
16. Smilkstein MJ, Bronstein AC, Pickett HM, et al. Hyperbaric oxygen therapy for severe hydrogen sulfide poisoning. *J Emerg Med* 1985;3:27–30.
17. Smith RP, Gosselin RE. Hydrogen sulfide poisoning. *J Occup Med* 1979;21:93–96.
18. Smith RP, Kruszyna R, Kruszyna H. Management of acute sulfide poisoning: effects of oxygen, thiosulfate, and nitrite. *Arch Environ Health* 1976;31:166–169.
19. Stine RJ, Slosberg B, Beacham BE. Hydrogen sulfide intoxication. *Ann Intern Med* 1976;85:756–758.
20. Vathenen AS, Emberton P, Wales JM. Hydrogen sulphide poisoning in factory worker (Letter). *Lancet* 1988;1:305.
21. Warenycia MW, Goodwin LR, Benishin CG, et al. Acute H2S poisoning—demonstration of selective uptake of sulfide by the brain stem by measurement of brain sulfide levels. *Biochem Pharmacol* 1989;38:973–981.
22. Warencyia MW, Smith KA, Blashko CS, et al. Monoamine oxidase inhibition as a sequel of hydrogen sulfide intoxication: increases in brain catecholamine and 5-hydroxytryptamine levels. *Arch Toxicol* 1989;63:131–136.
23. Whitcraft DD, Baily TD, Hart GB. Hydrogen sulfide poisoning treated with hyperbaric oxygen. *J Emerg Med* 1985;3:23–25.

CHAPTER 312

Iron

Jeffrey R. Suchard and Steven C. Curry

Although iron poisoning occurs in all age groups, it is the leading cause of accidental poisoning death from pharmaceutical agents among young children. The American Association of Poison Control Centers reported over 30,000 iron ingestions annually in 2001 and 2002 (9,10). Household sources of iron are commonplace, making them readily available for impetuous ingestions.

TABLE 312.1. Iron Compounds and Their Percent Elemental Iron Content

Compound	Percent Elemental Iron by Weight
Ferrous carbonate, anhydrous	48
Ferrous fumarate	33
Ferrous gluconate	12
Ferrous phosphate	37
Ferrous pyrophosphate	12
Ferrous sulfate	16
Ferrocholinate	12
Ferroglycine sulfate	16
Ferric pyrophosphate	12

Parental iron supplements of these preparations are often found in homes with young children; many of these preparations appear nearly identical to candy, and some are even candy-coated. Chewable multivitamins with iron are specifically designed to appeal to young children.

The amount of iron in each preparation varies, and toxicity after acute ingestion depends on the amount of elemental iron ingested (Table 312.1). Toxic doses are difficult to define, given the frequently unreliable histories surrounding accidental ingestions. In general, the ingestion of more than 20 mg of elemental iron per kilogram of body weight produces significant gastroenteritis; doses above the 40- to 60-mg/kg range are potentially fatal. Although confirmatory epidemiology studies are lacking, many physicians believe that the ingestion of children's chewable multiple vitamins with iron rarely causes severe iron poisoning, and that toxicity from such exposures is less than expected on the basis of elemental iron ingested per body weight (8). Some poison centers choose to observe asymptomatic or only mildly symptomatic children at home after ingesting such preparations, even when the estimated ingestion exceeds 20 mg/kg of elemental iron.

About 10% of ingested iron, mainly the ferrous (Fe^{2+}) state, is absorbed each day from the small intestine. Because free, unbound iron is toxic to tissues, the body has many mechanisms to keep iron bound to proteins or other macromolecules. After absorption, iron changes to the ferric (Fe^{3+}) state and is stored in the intestinal mucosa complexed to ferritin. Transport to other tissues occurs with iron bound to transferrin. The total amount of iron that transferrin can bind is termed the total iron-binding capacity (TIBC). Normal serum iron concentrations vary from 50 to 150 μg/dL, although normal TIBCs can range from 300 to 450 μg/dL. Because the TIBC is far in excess of the iron concentration, there normally is no circulating unbound iron.

Excessive iron is corrosive to the gastrointestinal (GI) tract, resulting in gastroenteritis, with the potential for hemorrhage, hypovolemia, and perforation. If enough iron is absorbed, systemic and metabolic consequences of iron poisoning develop. Iron accumulates mainly in the liver after overdose but can have toxic effects in almost any organ. Iron is concentrated in mitochondria, in which it disrupts oxidative phosphorylation and catalyzes the formation of oxygen free radicals, leading to lipid peroxidation and cell death. Toxic amounts of iron also produce venodilation and increase capillary permeability. The metabolic acidosis seen in iron poisoning is as a result of several factors, including hypovolemia, tissue hypoperfusion, a shift to anaerobic metabolism as mitochondrial function is impaired, and the hydration of the ferric ion with generation of hydrogen ions: [Fe^{3+} + 3H$_2$O → Fe(OH)$_3$ + 3H$^+$].

Coagulopathy may occur, even before the onset of hepatic dysfunction, from iron's ability to inhibit serine proteases, such as thrombin, and other coagulation factors. Isolated liver damage may occur, but multiple organ system failure is typical in severe iron poisonings (5,12,14).

CLINICAL PRESENTATION

Clinical effects of iron poisoning are usually considered in stages (5,12,14). It is important to remember, however, that the time frame for staging is imprecise, patients present at variable times after ingestion, and distinguishing between stages can be difficult as a result of overlapping signs, symptoms, and laboratory manifestations, and because of rapid progression. Patients can die in any stage of iron poisoning, but for different reasons.

The first stage of iron poisoning develops within the first few hours after ingestion. It is as a result of the direct corrosive effects of iron on the GI tract, and is characterized by abdominal pain, vomiting, and diarrhea. Diarrhea may be the only manifestation in patients who ingest multiple vitamins with iron, particularly preparations intended for children. Hematemesis or melena may occur if significant GI bleeding is present. Patients with serious toxicity develop lethargy, shock, and metabolic acidosis as a result of hypovolemia, anemia, and tissue hypoperfusion. Serum iron concentrations may be normal or elevated.

The second stage is characterized by resolution of GI symptoms, despite continued absorption of toxic amounts of iron and increasing tissue iron burden. Sometimes unseen, this stage may last until about 24 hours after ingestion. Patients frequently lie quietly and clinically appear improved, but this can be falsely reassuring. If laboratory studies are obtained, they are likely to show elevated serum iron levels and a progressive metabolic acidosis.

In the third stage, systemic iron poisoning becomes clinically evident. This may occur early in patients with severe poisoning (bypassing stage 2). Toxic amounts of iron have now moved from blood into tissues, disrupting cellular metabolism, causing third-spacing of fluids and producing venous pooling of blood. Shock and metabolic acidosis in this stage can result from hypovolemia, anemia, hepatic dysfunction, impaired oxidative phosphorylation, heart failure, and renal failure. Fulminant hepatic failure with hypoglycemia, hyperammonemia, and coagulopathy may occur, although significant hepatic injury is unusual when peak serum iron levels remain below 500 μg/dL.

The fourth stage is characterized by gastric outlet or small-bowel obstruction. GI obstruction is an unusual occurrence but may develop several weeks after the acute toxicity has resolved, as a result of scarring produced by iron's corrosive effects.

Elevated serum iron levels obtained within the proper time frame are helpful in confirming the diagnosis of iron poisoning. Serum iron concentrations usually peak 2 to 6 hours after ingestion. Because iron in tissue produces systemic toxicity, a patient may be seriously ill and have a normal serum iron level many hours after ingestion. On the other hand, a serum iron level drawn early after ingestion may be misleadingly low if absorption is still occurring. Therefore, a normal serum iron concentration very early or many hours after ingestion does not exclude iron poisoning.

Clinical and laboratory test such as white blood cell count and serum glucose concentrations are not of sufficient sensitivity to be of much assistance in assessing the severity of acute iron poisoning (6,7,13). The "deferoxamine challenge" test, in which the presence of vin rosé-colored urine after giving a dose of deferoxamine was considered an indication for chelation therapy, is no longer recommended because this color change is unreliable (18). A kidney–ureter–bladder (KUB) radiograph may demonstrate radiopacities in the GI tract, a finding often present in patients who develop serious poisoning. However, a normal KUB radiograph does not exclude the possibility of a significant ingestion. Even when iron tablets are noted initially, they are usually no longer visible at 24 hours.

DIFFERENTIAL DIAGNOSIS

The differential diagnosis of patients presenting with GI symptoms includes poisoning by acetaminophen, salicylate, hepatotoxic mushrooms, arsenic, caffeine and theophylline, caustics, copper salts, and mercurial salts. Infectious gastroenteritis, medical and surgical intraabdominal conditions, or sepsis may cause vomiting, diarrhea, acidosis, and shock. Acute iron poisoning, however, is not accompanied by fever unless a complication such as aspiration or bowel infarction develops.

EMERGENCY DEPARTMENT EVALUATION

The history should include the time and amount of ingestion, the identity of the iron preparation ingested, and the nature, severity, time of onset, and progression of symptoms. The physician should specifically ask about abdominal pain, vomiting, and diarrhea, and whether blood was noted. The amount of elemental iron ingested, in mg per kg, should be calculated. The physical examination should focus on vital signs, overall appearance, and the abdomen.

Patients who have had only one or two episodes of vomiting or diarrhea and are subsequently asymptomatic should have a complete blood count (CBC) and measurement of serum electrolytes, glucose, blood urea nitrogen, creatinine, and iron levels. Those with more pronounced or persistent GI symptoms, evidence of hypovolemia, or lethargy should also have a prothrombin time, liver function studies, arterial blood gas analysis, and a KUB radiograph. A TIBC is not helpful in the evaluation of iron toxicity and should not be ordered. It does not assist in the treatment decisions, and several laboratory methods to measure the TIBC are inaccurate in the setting of iron overload.

EMERGENCY DEPARTMENT MANAGEMENT

In general, all symptomatic patients and those who ingested more than 20 mg/kg of elemental iron less than 6 hours earlier are referred by poison control centers to emergency departments for evaluation. Prehospital care of symptomatic patients includes adequate oxygenation and intravenous hydration for patients with hypotension or other evidence of hypovolemia.

Gastric decontamination measures are of questionable value in iron ingestion, especially if vomiting has already occurred. Activated charcoal does not effectively bind iron, and its use should be limited to cases in which coingestion of other substances that bind to charcoal is known or suspected. If activated charcoal is administered, cathartics should be withheld, especially in patients who already have gastroenteritis, as this may exacerbate hypovolemia. Syrup of ipecac is not recommended. Gastric lavage has not been shown to be of clinical benefit, possibly because most iron tablets are too large to evacuate by this method. The decision to employ lavage is made on an individual basis. Simulated overdose studies suggest that oral magnesium oxide (Milk of Magnesia, 60 mL/g of elemental iron ingested) (17) or a slurry of charcoal mixed with deferoxamine (3) can reduce iron absorption, but the utility of such treatments in actual overdose patients is unknown. There are no data supporting lavage with sodium bicarbonate solutions or administration of phosphates to prevent iron absorption. Lavage with deferoxamine solutions is not recommended because of the tremendous amounts required and because only a small portion of the ingested iron is absorbed. Whole-bowel irrigation with polyethylene glycol–electrolyte lavage solutions (16) and gastrotomy to remove iron pills (2) have also been reported, but such recommendations are based on anecdotal data. Whether they are more effective than supportive care alone has not been studied in controlled trials.

Patients who remain completely asymptomatic (including no lethargy) for 6 hours after ingestion and who have a normal physical examination do not require treatment. Those who ingested more than 20 mg/kg of elemental iron but are seen within 6 hours might possibly benefit from GI decontamination. If the serum iron concentration in an asymptomatic patient is lower than 350 µg/dL, and a repeat study documents no rise in the iron level, the patient can be released. On the other hand a KUB radiograph demonstrating numerous tablets suggests that serum iron concentrations will be rising. Patients who have suffered only a single emesis or diarrheal stool but who have remained asymptomatic for several hours and have a normal physical examination, KUB, and laboratory evaluation do not require treatment.

Patients who present with or develop more than two episodes of emesis or diarrhea, have evidence of hypovolemia, or exhibit lethargy require treatment with fluids and chelation therapy with deferoxamine mesylate. In patients with significant symptoms, treatment should not be delayed to wait for results of a serum iron determination, because the therapy is indicated regardless of the serum iron concentration. In contrast, iron ingestion can raise the serum iron level above the normal range, and an elevated iron level does not constitute an indication for deferoxamine or admission in the absence of clinical signs of toxicity.

With rare exceptions, all symptomatic patients are hypovolemic. Fluid challenges of 20 mL/kg of lactated Ringer's or normal saline are given to restore fluid volume and ensure a normal urine output. Patients commonly require maintenance infusions at twice normal rates to keep up with GI losses and third-spacing.

Deferoxamine mesylate can remove iron from tissues and nontransferrin-bound iron from plasma. Deferoxamine binds to iron to form ferrioxamine, which is excreted in the urine over days to weeks. Ferrioxamine occasionally imparts a vin rosé color to the urine, but this color change is unreliable and inconsistent and should not be used to determine the need for additional treatment (12,18). Deferoxamine mesylate can be mixed in any crystalloid and should be continuously infused at 15 mg/kg/h. Higher infusion rates are recommended in severe cases by some authorities. Rapid i.v. administration is sometimes associated with hypotension, presumably from histamine release, but this is not usually a problem with infusion rates below 45 mg/kg/h. Intramuscular deferoxamine is not recommended.

Many statements in the manufacturer's package insert for deferoxamine do not reflect currently accepted treatment practices. Deferoxamine is not contraindicated for the treatment of acute iron poisoning in pregnancy. Animal data and human experience strongly suggest that toxic amounts of maternally ingested iron, deferoxamine, and ferrioxamine do not cross into the fetal circulation (1,11). Fetal death, therefore, results from maternal demise, and a pregnant woman should be treated the same as any other person. At 15 mg/kg/h, many patients receive well over 6 g deferoxamine mesylate each day; this is safe for the short-term treatment of iron poisoning.

Deferoxamine causes falsely low serum iron concentrations (4). Because tissue iron, not serum iron, is responsible for toxicity, a normal or low serum iron concentration by itself cannot be used to justify stopping deferoxamine. Intravenous deferoxamine should be continued until clinical toxicity has resolved, serum iron levels are normal or low, and vin rosé-colored urine

(if present) disappears (12). A urinary iron assay, which theoretically might define when to stop deferoxamine therapy, has also been described, but its clinical utility has not been proved (18). Most patients require 12 to 24 hours of deferoxamine infusion, but occasional patients with very large overdoses require therapy for longer periods.

In renal failure, deferoxamine should be continued but at much lower infusion rates. Assuming that therapeutic deferoxamine levels have been obtained, anuric patients should continue to receive infusions at about 1.5 mg/kg/h, based on the known prolonged half-life in renal failure (12). The use of prochlorperazine (Compazine) and deferoxamine together has produced coma in humans that has been reproduced in animals. This drug combination should therefore be avoided. The treatment of complications (e.g., liver failure, GI bleeding) is the same as for any other patient.

CRITICAL INTERVENTIONS

- Obtain a CBC, serum electrolytes, glucose, blood urea nitrogen, creatinine, and iron levels, prothrombin time, liver function studies, arterial blood gas analysis, and a KUB radiograph on patients with significant GI symptoms, hypotension, or lethargy
- Administer normal saline intravenously and deferoxamine to patients with significant GI symptoms, hypotension, or lethargy

DISPOSITION

Patients who remain completely asymptomatic and those with a normal physical examination, KUB, and laboratory evaluation who have had only one or two episodes of emesis or diarrhea and then become asymptomatic 6 hours after ingestion can be discharged.

Patients with mild symptoms should have repeat labs demonstrating no rise in the serum iron level and no evidence of metabolic acidosis prior to discharge. Symptomatic patients should be admitted. The level of monitoring and treatment required usually necessitates intensive care. If the necessary laboratory and treatment services are not available, the patients should be transferred to a facility in which such services are available. A poison center or toxicologist can be consulted for assistance with management.

COMMON PITFALLS

✔ Failure to administer adequate amounts of i.v. fluids
✔ Waiting for the result of the serum iron level before treating symptomatic patients with deferoxamine
✔ Using the TIBC for evaluation and treatment decisions
✔ Assuming that a "nontoxic" serum iron concentration excludes the diagnosis of iron poisoning or the need for treatment in a symptomatic patient
✔ Sending a patient home during the second stage of poisoning because they appear improved
✔ Assuming a normal serum glucose, white blood cell count, and KUB x-ray excludes significant iron poisoning
✔ Failure to appreciate that deferoxamine may falsely lower serum iron concentration

References

1. Curry S, Bond GR, Raschke R, et al. An ovine model of maternal iron poisoning in pregnancy. *Ann Emerg Med* 1990;19:632.
2. Foxford R, Goldfrank L. Gastronomy—a surgical approach to iron overdose. *Ann Emerg Med* 1985;14:1223.

3. Gomez HF, McClafferty HH, Flory D, et al. Prevention of gastrointestinal iron absorption by chelation from an orally administered premixed deferoxamine/charcoal slurry. *Ann Emerg Med* 1997;30:587.
4. Helfer RE, Rodgerson DO. The effect of deferoxamine on the determination of serum iron and iron-binding capacity. *J Pediatr* 1966;68:804.
5. Jacobs J, Greene H, Gendel BR. Acute iron intoxication. *N Engl J Med* 1965;273:1124.
6. Knasel AL, Collins-Barrow MD. Applicability of early indicators of iron toxicity. *J Natl Med Assoc* 1986;78:1037.
7. Lacouture PG, Wason S, Temple AR, et al. Emergency assessment of severity in iron overdose by clinical and laboratory methods. *J Pediatr* 1981;99:89.
8. Linakis JG, Lacouture PG, Woolf A. Iron absorption from chewable vitamins with iron versus iron tablets: implications for toxicity. *Pediatr Emerg Care* 1992;8:321.
9. Litovitz TL, Klein-Schwartz W, Rodgers GC Jr, et al. 2001 Annual report of the American Association of Poison Control Centers Toxic Exposure Surveillance System. *Am J Emerg Med* 2002;20:391.
10. Watson WA, Litovitz TL, Rodgers GC Jr, et al. 2002 annual report of the American Association of Poison Control Centers Toxic Exposure Surveillance System. *Am J Emerg Med* 2003;21:3353.
11. McElhatton PR, Roberts JC, Sullivan FM. The consequences of iron overdose and its treatment with desferrioxamine in pregnancy. *Hum Exp Toxicol* 1991;10:251.
12. Mills KC, Curry SC. Acute iron poisoning. *Emerg Med Clin North Am* 1994;12:397.
13. Palatnick W, Tenebein M. Leukocytosis, hyperglycemia, vomiting, and positive x-rays are not indicators of severity of iron overdose in adults. *Am J Emerg Med* 1996;14:454.
14. Robotham J, Lietman P. Acute iron poisoning. *Am J Dis Child* 1980;134:875.
15. Siff JE, Meldon SW, Tomassoni AJ. Usefulness of the total iron binding capacity in the evaluation and treatment of acute iron overdose. *Ann Emerg Med* 1999;33:73.
16. Tenenbein M. Whole bowel irrigation as a gastrointestinal decontamination procedure after acute poisoning. *Med Toxicol* 1988;3:77.
17. Wallace KL, Curry SC, LoVecchio FL, et al. Effect of magnesium hydroxide on iron absorption following simulated mild iron overdose in human subjects. *Acad Emerg Med* 1998;5:961.
18. Yatscoff RW, Wayne EA, Tenenbein M. An objective criterion for the cessation of deferoxamine therapy in the acutely iron-poisoned patient. *J Toxicol Clin Toxicol* 1991;29:1.

CHAPTER 313
Irritant Gas Inhalation

Philip A. Edelman

The airway serves as a conduit, allowing the passage of fresh and waste gases. Extrapulmonary forces (muscles) effect inhalation, but the elastic recoil of the lung is primarily responsible for normal exhalation (bellows function). The lungs provide a large surface area for diffusion of gases between the alveolar spaces and the bloodstream. The upper airways are responsible for humidifying inspired air to prevent drying and irritation of lower airway surfaces. Lung compliance is dynamic, and contractile elements (smooth muscles), particularly those of the lower airways, respond to various stimuli by relaxing or contracting. The lung is also a metabolic and immunologically active organ. Mucous secretion (from goblet cells and mucous glands), combined with ciliary motion, is responsible for clearing particles from the airways. Any of the lung's functions may be affected by inhalation of an irritant gas (23).

The response of the nose to inhalation of irritants may vary from rhinitis or sinusitis to septal perforation (e.g., with chronic chromate exposure). The trachea and bronchi may respond by bronchoconstriction (immediate or delayed) and the develop-

ment or exacerbation of asthma or acute tracheobronchitis. The responses of lung parenchyma include allergic alveolitis, pulmonary edema, emphysema, acute alveolitis, bronchiolitis, bronchoconstriction, and interstitial fibrosis. The exact pathology depends on the nature, intensity, and duration of the exposure and the actual properties of the inhaled irritant.

Although asthma may be exacerbated by exposure to irritant chemicals, chemical exposure may also produce de novo asthma. Chemically induced asthma is known as reactive airway dysfunction syndrome (RADS). RADS is defined as symptoms of asthma, primarily cough, wheezing, and dyspnea, beginning within 24 hours of a single high level irritant exposure (usually, but not exclusively, the result of an industrial accident or workplace exposure) and persisting for at least 3 months (1). Other criteria for a diagnosis of RADS include the presence of airflow obstruction and bronchial hyperreactivity to methacholine on pulmonary function testing and the absence of preexisting atopy, cigarette smoking (for 10 years), eosinophilia (peripheral or pulmonary), lymphocytic inflammation on bronchoalveolar lavage or lung biopsy, and other pulmonary disease (3).

Acute changes in lung function caused by irritant inhalation can be detected by several types of tests. Air flow capacity is best determined by spirometry, especially a flow-volume loop. The peak flowmeter is a simple device useful in determining the presence and severity of bronchoconstriction. In motivated and carefully trained patients, it may be a reliable indicator of the need for, and response to, treatment. However, it has not been demonstrated to be an effective screening tool for patients with subtle changes in small airways resulting from early or mild exposures. The flow-volume loop provides additional information about the status of the smaller airways and is better for this evaluation.

Reversibility of bronchospasm can be assessed by the use of a bronchodilator and repeat testing. Changes in alveolar–capillary permeability can be measured by the single-breath carbon monoxide diffusing capacity (D_LCOSB or D_LCO). A chest radiograph is also useful, particularly for visualizing inflammatory reactions of the parenchyma. Arterial blood gas analysis can assist in the assessment of blood oxygenation (PO_2) and ventilation (PCO_2). Ventilation–perfusion scanning does not usually provide significant additional information, except to rule out other processes, such as pulmonary emboli. Most important, careful physical examination may demonstrate pathology not detected by these studies, such as fine wheezes in subtle or early asthma and fine crackles in early pulmonary edema.

Toxic gases can also injure internal organs after inhalation. Absorption of gases by routes other than inhalation is usually minimal compared with the dose delivered by inhalation.

The physical characteristics of the inhalant are extremely important in determining the site and depth of lung penetration and systemic absorption, and local effects of the exposure. A gas is a material without a defined shape when unconstrained at room temperature under ambient conditions. A fume is a small, solid particulate dispersion formed by the coalescence of gases volatilized during an oxidative process such as combustion. Fumes are usually submicronic particles that can penetrate deeply into the lung. Mists are suspended liquid droplets generated by the condensation of gases or the breaking up of liquids (e.g., by splashing, atomization, or related actions). A vapor is the gaseous phase of a material that is normally a liquid at room temperature. Its concentration depends on the liquid's vapor pressure and temperature. Various other definitions apply to fogs, aerosols, smokes, and dusts (see Chapter 316, "Smoke Inhalation").

The deposition and absorption of a gas or vapor in the respiratory tract are primarily governed by its water solubility. Highly soluble gases are absorbed in the upper airways, whereas less soluble materials reach the lower airways. The deposition of particulates, such as dusts, is a function of their size. Particles 5 μm or smaller reach the lower airways. Larger particles are deposited more proximally; those of submicron size may pass in and out of the airways without substantial impaction or deposition.

These concepts are important in determining the likely signs and symptoms of a person exposed to airborne irritants. Highly water soluble airway irritants usually cause upper airway (eye, nose, and throat) irritation. Materials that are less water soluble may reach the lower airways and alveolar membrane, causing bronchospasm and pulmonary edema.

Although not generally considered chemical warfare agents (see Chapter 331, "Chemical Warfare Agents"), toxic industrial chemicals (TICs), particularly irritant gases, fumes, and vapors, pose a significant threat to the public as potential weapons of mass destruction. Many of these chemicals are produced, shipped, and stored in large volumes and high concentrations, in highly populated areas, and are readily available for terrorist exploitation.

CLINICAL PRESENTATION

Primary Pulmonary Irritants

The signs and symptoms of irritant inhalation may be immediate or delayed in onset. Primary irritants include corrosive, acid, or alkaline materials that may become airborne and inhaled. Irritant substances may also adsorb to the surfaces of otherwise inert particles, causing deeper penetration and persistence in the lungs. For example, the products of combustion in a plastics fire may include highly irritant aldehydes and organic acids that may adsorb to the carbonaceous particulates in smoke (see Chapter 316, "Smoke Inhalation").

Signs and symptoms vary with the nature of the exposure. Low-level, long-term (months to years) exposures may contribute to the development of chronic bronchitis or related lung disease. Exposure to high levels of irritants for short periods, may cause irritation of the eyes, nose, and throat, leading to lacrimation, rhinorrhea, conjunctivitis, pharyngitis, dyspnea, chest tightness, and, possibly, dysphonia. If the exposure is great enough, tracheobronchitis and stridor may occur. Chest tightness, wheezing, decreased inspiration–expiration ratio, and increased sputum production may result. Arterial blood gas analysis frequently demonstrates altered ventilatory mechanics consistent with acute airway obstruction. Pulmonary function studies, especially a prebronchodilator and postbronchodilator flow-volume loop, usually demonstrate reversible abnormalities.

In severe exposures, pulmonary edema may occur. The diffusing capacity as evaluated by the D_LCO is decreased with pulmonary edema. The chest radiograph may be normal, especially at the earlier phases of injury, or it may show signs of interstitial edema. Arterial blood gas analysis may demonstrate hyperventilation with hypoxemia, or it may be normal. Bronchiolitis obliterans has been infrequently reported after these exposures but may be underdiagnosed. This is an elusive diagnosis, and although a high resolution thin cut computer tomography scan of the lung may be helpful, the diagnosis often requires open lung biopsy.

Tear gases (see Chapter 331, "Chemical Warfare Agents") can cause severe upper and lower respiratory tract irritation, and asphyxia with prolonged or high-dose exposure (e.g., in a confined space) (2).

Chloropicrin is used as an additive to fumigants such as methyl bromide (see later discussion) because it is a strong lacrimatory agent. Mercaptans and thiophene are used to odorize natural gas; they are slightly irritating in high doses, but they are generally known for their particular offensive sulfur odors.

Oxides of sulfur react with water in the air to form sulfuric (or sulfurous) acid vapor or mists. These gases (e.g., SO_2) and vapors are responsible for urban air pollution resulting from fossil fuel combustion, smelting, and paper and rubber manufacturing. They are also used in bleaching, brewing, fumigation, tanning, preserving, and refrigeration (6). Oxides of nitrogen and sulfur are the principal causes of acid rain.

Ozone is a by-product of bleaching, water purification, and processes that generate a spark or electric arc in the presence of oxygen (e.g., welding, mercury vapor lamps, photocopiers, and x-ray generators) (18). It is also found in the atmosphere, and higher levels are found at higher altitudes; flight at altitudes above 35,000 feet may result in transient toxicity.

Isocyanates, classically toluene diisocyanate, can cause chemically induced (occupational) asthma (4,20). After long-term, low-level exposures, a worker may develop increasing symptoms of asthma. Alternatively, short-term, high-level exposures may produce the same problem. As there may be a delay of several hours between the exposure and the asthma (delayed hypersensitivity reaction), careful questioning for sources of exposure may be necessary. Isocyanates are used in the production of urethane foams for insulation, packaging, and the sealing and potting of electrical equipment. They are also used in many paints and finishes. Some chemicals in this class have different physiochemical and toxicologic properties—for instance, the more toxic methyl isocyanate was responsible for the deaths at Bhopal. It is important to distinguish between the monomeric form and polymeric forms that have less volatility and toxicity.

Oxides of nitrogen (NO, NO_2, N_2O_3, N_2O_4) are generated in many oxidative processes, including welding, fires, and industrial applications such as dye, fertilizer, celluloid, and lacquer manufacturing (19). The accidental introduction of organic materials into nitric acid may cause combustion and release of nitrogen oxides. They may also evolve during the decomposition of plants with a high nitrate content, as in silo filler's disease. The color of the gas varies according to the exact species, but it may be clear, orange-brown, or red (bromine may have a similar appearance, but chlorine is more yellow). Symptoms usually occur immediately after inhalation. Any portion of the respiratory tract may be involved, but frequently, only lower airway effects are noted. Pulmonary edema may be delayed for 12 hours. Asthma may develop immediately or over the first few days and may be severe, even in the nonasthmatic patient. After resolution of a moderately severe, acute reaction, relapse may occur 3 weeks later and can be more serious than the original episode.

Phosgene (carbonyl chloride, $COCl_2$) is a classic inducer of delayed pulmonary edema (10). The main chemical warfare agent used in World War I, it is used in various chemical processes (drug, dye, insecticide, and isocyanate manufacturing). It is most frequently encountered in situations of combustion or pyrolysis when carbon, oxygen, and chlorine are available to react (e.g., burning plastics, chlorinated hydrocarbons, or carbons along with hydrochloric acid vapors). A haylike, musty odor may be noted. In contrast to past decades, many companies using phosgene now produce it on site in limited quantities as needed. This reduces the hazard of storage and transportation.

Formaldehyde is a reactant or by-product in many chemical processes, such as embalming, cosmetic and resin manufacture, and sterilizing. It may evolve spontaneously from plastics, resins, insulation material, and many other occult sources (14,16). Formaldehyde has been noted to be a carcinogen in limited rodent studies and is suspected as a human carcinogen, although no confirmatory human studies have been completed.

Inorganic acids cause immediate irritation or corrosion of tissues, depending on the concentration and the agent. Sulfuric acid is also a desiccating agent, and chromic acid is a strong oxidizer. Although most acids do not cause systemic poisoning, chromates are hepatotoxic and nephrotoxic, and hydrofluoric acid (or hydrogen fluoride) may cause systemic fluoride poisoning (hypocalcemia and hypomagnesemia as principal effects). Acid vapor inhalation usually causes upper airway irritation with ocular and nasopharyngeal inflammation. If the acid forms a mist, deeper pulmonary penetration may occur, resulting in pulmonary edema, bronchiolitis obliterans, or asthma.

Chlorine is a heavier-than-air, water-soluble, yellow-green gas that is irritating to the mucous membranes (8). The warning properties of chlorine are usually adequate to alert the person to the presence of the material and afford time for escape. However, when a person is caught in a confined space or an overwhelming cloud, inhalation may cause irritation of the lower airways. Chlorine is used in many chemical industries and processes (e.g., sanitation of water) and can be generated by the action of an acid on hypochlorite, as found in bleaches. For example, the inappropriate mixing of bleach with an acidic cleanser can generate chlorine during the cleaning of toilet bowls (15). Mixing hypochlorite with ammonia-based cleaners can produce chloramine, another gaseous irritant (12).

Ammonia is highly water soluble and very irritating to the upper airways (7). In solution as ammonium hydroxide, its vapors can produce an immediate reaction. Although the odor of ammonia provides excellent warning of its presence, sudden overwhelming exposures, large clouds of the gas, or confined-space exposures can cause severe corrosive burns to the skin or eyes (with potential blindness). The oropharynx is readily burned, and hoarseness is common. Deeper injury to the lung can cause severe pulmonary dysfunction that is usually transient but can be permanent after severe exposures. The effects are rapid; "delayed" effects are usually the result of the progression of burns to the mucous membranes. Ammonia is used in various chemical processes, such as cleaning, fertilization, and refrigeration, and evolves during the combustion of a number of products.

Hydrocarbons comprise a wide variety of compounds. Although the irritancy of these gases or vapors cannot easily be generalized, the ketones, aldehydes, acid anhydrides, and halogenated compounds are most irritating. Aromatic compounds (e.g., benzene, xylene, and toluene) are more irritating than aliphatic ones (pentane, hexane, and butane). Additionally, hydrocarbons are often systemic poisons, with central nervous system (CNS) effects predominating.

Epoxy resins, catalysts, and hardeners frequently produce vapors that can cause irritation or allergic sensitization of the airways. Styrene is used in the manufacture of boats, bathtubs, and many other products (polystyrene).

Pulmonary Irritants With Systemic Toxicity

Gases and vapors may gain entry to the body through the lungs and may inflict serious injury on a target organ remote from the portal of entry. The internal dose depends on the solubility of the gas, blood flow through the lungs (more important with materials with low blood solubility), gas distribution in the lungs, and ventilatory rate (as affected by activity). Delivery to the target organ depends on similar factors, including tissue perfusion, tissue penetration (especially lipid solubility for the liver, brain, and other organs), binding materials in the blood, and pH. Uptake into a temporary depot may occur, allowing the chemical to be redistributed to the target organ over a more protracted period (seen with highly fat soluble materials).

Arsine (AsH_3, arsenic trihydride) may be generated when arsenic-containing materials contact acids (e.g., during the processing of metals in which arsenic may be a natural contaminant, in sewer gases, and in laboratories) (11). Arsine gas is also commonly used in the manufacture of computer chips. It has a garlic odor. In addition to its irritant effects, inhalation of arsine in high doses can cause immediate death from CNS toxicity. Classically, however, arsine combines with hemoglobin, causing intravascular hemolysis. Onset is usually rapid but may be delayed several hours depending on dose. Symptoms include nausea, vomiting, abdominal pain, fatigue, and weakness. The hematocrit may drop by 50% in a matter of minutes. Examination may reveal brownish skin, hepatosplenomegaly, tachycardia, tachypnea, and dark urine. Renal failure may ensue from the effects of the free plasma hemoglobin, the sludging of red cells, and the direct effects of the arsine–hemoglobin complex on the renal cells. Anemia may result in secondary ischemic complications such as congestive heart failure. Systemic toxicity as a result of inorganic arsenic poisoning may ensue (see Chapter 305, "Arsenic and Mercury"). The urine arsenic level may confirm exposure but is usually unavailable acutely. The arsine-hemoglobin complex is not dialyzable, and although dialysis may be needed for renal failure, exchange transfusion has been reported to remove the arsenic-hemoglobin.

Ethylene oxide is a colorless gas with an indistinct odor or taste (9). For gas sterilization, it is frequently supplied with a halogenated hydrocarbon in a nonflammable 12:88 mixture, but, at higher concentrations, it is flammable. In addition to mucosal irritation, ethylene oxide may cause CNS depression, seizures, skin and pulmonary burns, allergic reactions, and mild chemical hepatitis with transient lymphocytosis after acute exposure. It can also cause peripheral neuropathies, is a suspected human carcinogen, and is considered a reproductive hazard. It is used in many chemical industries and in hospitals (e.g., gas sterilization of products that cannot be steam-autoclaved).

Phosphine gas (PH_3, phosphorous trihydride) is used in fumigation (of grains), in silos and ship holds, in the electronics industry, and in the production of acetylene (22). Phosphine can cause severe gastrointestinal (GI) and CNS toxicity, and immediate or delayed pulmonary edema. Symptoms are usually mild: headache, nausea, chest tightness, and lethargy. Coma, seizures, and shock may be seen in severe cases. Although there is no specific biologic test for exposure, a fishy or garlic odor may suggest the presence of zinc or aluminum phosphide (both of which generate phosphine in the presence of water) and phosphine, respectively. Phosphine is not considered a primary irritant, but is cytotoxic resulting is delayed pulmonary effects that lead to pulmonary edema.

Methyl bromide is used as a fumigant (13). When pumped into tented structures, the concentrations of gas are usually lethal. Intractable seizures, coma, and severe neurologic sequelae can result from exposure to this material. Severe acidosis may occur, presumably secondary to seizure activity. Mild exposure results in a flulike syndrome that is often delayed in onset. For fumigation, chloropicrin (a lacrimatory agent) is usually added to methyl bromide to provide olfactory warning of its presence. Serum bromide levels above 5 mg/dL are probably consistent with exposure. If a lumbar puncture is performed to evaluate seizures or coma, determination of the bromide level in the cerebrospinal fluid may also be useful.

Sulfuryl fluoride, marketed as Vikane, is a fumigant that is primarily an irritant, although recent reports have suggested systemic toxicity (5).

Ethylene dibromide was commonly used as a fumigant for soil, fruit, and other foods before 1984. Deaths have occurred after high-level exposure to this chemical as the result of combined dermal and inhalation absorption. Although symptoms are mainly limited to the respiratory and GI tracts, severe illness with acidosis and renal failure has been reported (17). Because of its potential carcinogenicity, its use is now restricted.

Inhalation of cryogenic materials (e.g., liquid nitrogen, volatile hydrocarbons such as ethyl chloride) can cause severe respiratory tract and lung injury. Polymer fume fever (from the pyrolysis of polytetrafluoroethylene (PTFE or Teflon®) and metal fume fever typically from zinc fume, cause a delayed (about 12 hours) self-limited pulmonary reaction with chest tightness, dyspnea and fever.

DIFFERENTIAL DIAGNOSIS

Respiratory symptoms after irritant gas exposure are nonspecific. Similar findings may be caused by cardiac, allergic, infectious etiologies, and intrinsic lung diseases. Although the onset is usually acute with toxic gas exposure, it may be delayed. Additionally, a low-grade fever and leukocytosis may be present in patients with pneumonitis. Irritant-induced pulmonary edema is almost always noncardiogenic, as is that caused by severe narcotic and sedative–hypnotic poisoning. Bronchospasm may result from an exacerbation of asthma or chronic obstructive pulmonary disease as a result of other or unknown factors. Only a careful exposure (environmental or occupational) history will identify the correct cause.

EMERGENCY DEPARTMENT EVALUATION

The history includes medical history, previous exposures, and details of the presenting illness, such as the nature, progression, and severity of symptoms and antecedent activities. History of an exposure should include activity of the patient at the time, physical processes (burning, heating, grinding), immediate reactions, and the use of any protective equipment or special ventilation systems. When possible the product label or the Material Safety Data Sheet should be reviewed.

The physical examination is directed, but not limited, to the skin, eyes, nose, mouth, and chest. All patients should have oxygen saturation measured and, if capable, bedside spirometry. Depending on clinical findings, response to bronchodilator inhalation, arterial blood gas analysis, chest radiography, D_LCO, and ventilation–perfusion scanning may be necessary to assess the nature and severity of signs and symptoms. Patients with respiratory distress should have an electrocardiogram, particularly those with or at risk for cardiac disease. Laboratory evaluation may be indicated in patients with poisoning by systemic toxins (e.g., arsine and methyl bromide), as noted previously.

EMERGENCY DEPARTMENT MANAGEMENT

Removal from the exposure, decontamination, and supportive care are the mainstays of prehospital treatment. A rescuer should never enter an area in which an irritant gas is potentially present without adequate skin, eye, and respiratory protection. Along with provision of supplemental oxygen, thorough flushing of irritated surfaces (skin and eyes) with water (preferably saline) may be required. Eye irrigation is especially important with acid fume, ammonia, chlorine, alkalies, and tear gas exposure.

Respiratory therapy should include humidified oxygen, bronchodilators, and mechanical measures (intubation, assisted ventilation, continuous positive airway pressure, positive end-expiratory pressure (PEEP), and suctioning), as clinically indicated for bronchospasm or pulmonary edema. A course of high-dose corticosteroids to reduce inflammation is theoretically beneficial and should be considered in patients with moderate, severe, or progressive symptoms. Animal experiments suggest that inhaled corticosteroids decrease pulmonary vascular resistance and improve lung compliance and survival. However, the benefit may depend on rapid treatment (21).

With arsine-induced hemolysis, exchange transfusion may be necessary when the resulting anemia is severe and free

hemoglobin levels are high (greater than 1.5 g/dL). Chelation therapy may also be indicated if urine arsenic levels are elevated (see Chapter 319, "Dystonic Reactions"). Supportive therapies may be indicated for coexisting toxicity, such as anticonvulsant therapy for seizures and dialysis for renal failure.

CRITICAL INTERVENTIONS

- Measure oxygen saturation in all patients with irritant gas exposure and perform bedside spirometry in those able to cooperate
- Administer oxygen and bronchodilators to patients with cough, dyspnea, or wheezing; consider corticosteroid therapy in those with severe or persistent symptoms
- Administer positive airway pressure by mask or perform endotracheal intubation and provide PEEP-assisted ventilation in patients with pulmonary edema or respiratory distress unresponsive to bronchodilator therapy

DISPOSITION

The decision to admit or discharge depends primarily on the severity and progression of clinical and laboratory manifestations. Young, otherwise healthy patients who become asymptomatic or mildly symptomatic after 4 hours of emergency department observation and treatment may be discharged. Those with moderate, severe, or worsening symptoms or abnormal spirometry, arterial blood gas analysis, or chest radiograph should be admitted, especially if they are elderly or have underlying cardiac, respiratory, or other significant medical problems. If delayed toxicity is possible, patients who have persistent symptoms of any degree of severity should be admitted. If the physician is unfamiliar with the toxicity of a certain agent and its treatment, a poison center, toxicologist, or toxicology text should be consulted.

Patients who are discharged should be instructed to return if symptoms recur or worsen. Those with persistent symptoms should be referred to a pulmonologist or have formal pulmonary function testing. Discharged patients should also be advised to avoid circumstances that resulted in exposure.

COMMON PITFALLS

- ✔ Failure to use adequate protective equipment (in prehospital treatment) so that additional casualties are avoided
- ✔ Failure to take an environmental or occupational exposure history and to recognize that a toxic exposure has occurred
- ✔ Failure to consider the possibility of systemic poisoning after irritant gas exposure
- ✔ Failure to obtain additional information and advice when unfamiliar with the toxicity and management of a particular exposure
- ✔ Failure to instruct patients to avoid circumstances that led to exposure
- ✔ Failure to instruct discharged patients to return immediately if delayed symptoms develop or mild symptoms worsen
- ✔ Failure to document discharge instructions

References

1. Bardana EJ. Reactive airways dysfunction syndrome (RADS): guidelines for diagnosis and treatment and insight into likely prognosis. *Ann Allergy Asthma Immunol* 1999;83:583.
2. Beswick FW. Chemical agents used in riot control and warfare. *Hum Toxicol* 1983;2:247.

3. Brooks SM, Weiss MA, Bernstein IL. Reactive airways dysfunction syndrome (RADS): persistent asthma after high level irritant exposures. *Chest* 1885;88:376.
4. Brugsch HG, Elkins HB. Toluene diisocyanate (TDI) toxicity. *N Engl J Med* 1963;268:353.
5. Centers for Disease Control and Prevention. Fatalities resulting from sulfuryl fluoride exposure after home fumigation. *MMWR* 1987;36:602.
6. Charan NB, Myers CG, Lakshminarayan S, et al. Pulmonary injuries associated with sulfur dioxide inhalation. *Am Rev Respir Dis* 1979;119:555.
7. Close GL, Cattin FI, Cohn AM. Acute and chronic effects of ammonia burns of the respiratory tract. *Arch Otolaryngol* 1980;106:151.
8. Das R, Blanc PD. Chlorine gas exposure and the lung: a review. *Toxicol Indust Health* 1993;9:439.
9. Deschamps D, Rosenberg N, Soler P, et al. Persistent asthma after accidental exposure to ethylene oxide. *Br J Indust Med* 1992;49:523.
10. Diller WF. Medical phosgene problems and their possible solution. *J Occup Med* 1975;20:189.
11. Fowler BA, Weissberg JB. Arsine poisoning. *N Engl J Med* 1974;291:1171.
12. Gapany-Gapanavicius M, Molko M, Tirosh M. Chloramine-induced pneumonitis from mixing household cleaning agents. *BMJ* 1982;285:1086.
13. Greenberg JO. The neurological effects of methyl bromide poisoning. *Indust Med* 1977;27:959.
14. Harris JC, Rumack BH, Alrich FD. Toxicology of urea formaldehyde and polyurethane foam insulation. *JAMA* 1981;245:243.
15. Jones FL. Chlorine poisoning from mixing household cleaners. *JAMA* 1972;222:1312.
16. L'abbe KA, Hoey JR. Review of the health effects of urea formaldehyde foam insulation. *Environ Res* 1984;35:246.
17. Letz GA, Pond SM, Osterloh JD, et al. Two fatalities after occupational exposure to ethylene dibromide. *JAMA* 1984;252:2428.
18. Nasr ANH. Ozone poisoning in man: clinical manifestations and differential diagnosis. *J Toxicol Clin Toxicol* 1971;14:461.
19. Tse RL, Bockman AD. Nitrogen dioxide toxicity: report of four cases in firemen. *JAMA* 1970;212:1341.
20. Vandenplas O, Malo JL, Saetta M, et al. Occupational asthma and extrinsic alveolitis due to isocyanates: current status and perspectives. *Br J Indust Med* 1993;50:213.
21. Wang J, Zhang L, Walther, SM. Inhaled budesonide in experimental chlorine gas lung injury: Influence of time interval between injury and treatment. *Intensive Care Medicine* 2002:28:352.
22. Wilson R, Lovejoy FH, Jaeger RJ, et al. Acute phosphine poisoning aboard a grain freighter. *JAMA* 1980;244:148.
23. Witschi HR, Last JA. Toxic responses of the respiratory system. In: Klaassen CD (ed), *Casarett and Doull's toxicology: the basic science of poisons,* 6th ed. New York: McGraw-Hill, 2001:515.

CHAPTER 314
Lead

Steven M. Marcus

Lead is a heavy metal that exists in elemental, inorganic, and organic forms and as a contaminant of other metals. More than 900 hobbies and occupations involve contact with lead, such as metal extracting and refining, plumbing, pottery production, soldering, and painting. Children develop lead poisoning by eating chips of paint from surfaces painted with lead-based pigments or by ingesting dust, which contains lead. Data suggest that lead-contaminated house dust is, currently, the major source of lead exposure for children living in the United States. Adult lead poisoning is primarily the result of occupational exposure. The potential for developing lead poisoning from the leaching of lead from imported lead-glazed cookware, dinnerware, and glassware and from the use of folk remedies such as azarcon, "pay-loo-ah," and maha yogran guggula by Mexican, Hmong, and Asian Indian immigrants, respectively, foot powder imported from the Dominican Republic (litargirio),

from imported candies and even window blinds has received much publicity (4,7,14). Lead is principally absorbed through the gastrointestinal (GI) tract and the lungs. Although there is minimal or no absorption through the skin, absorption of lead from bullets lodged in joints (synovial fluid) or the spinal cord (cerebrospinal fluid) has been reported (9). The degree of absorption depends on the particle size and concentration. Lead has a melting point of 327°C and a vapor pressure of 1.77 mm Hg at 1,000°C. Thus, lead becomes volatilized and airborne at relatively low temperatures. Gaseous lead and particulate lead with a diameter of less than 5 μm are nearly completely absorbed through pulmonary alveoli. Inhaled lead dust particles of larger size are usually trapped by cilia or in the tracheobronchial mucus and are cleared without being absorbed.

The absorption of ingested lead depends on factors such as the concentration, coincidental or previously ingested food, the status of the metal transfer protein, and age (8,12). In laboratory animals and humans, the younger the age, the greater the percentage of absorption of ingested lead. Iron and calcium deficiencies appear to promote absorption of lead, as does the coincidental ingestion of high-fat, low-protein, and low-phosphate meals. Unabsorbed lead is excreted in the stool.

Once absorbed, lead is principally carried on the red blood cell membrane, distributed to all parts of the body, and stored in bones. The calculated, apparent, volume of distribution is quite high (18). The average blood lead level in United States residents is currently less than 4 μg/dL (6). Lead is not required for normal body function, nor is it metabolized. Lead is primarily eliminated by urinary excretion, with a small proportion excreted in bile and eliminated with stool. The total body elimination half-life of lead is greater than 18 months.

Lead is a protean poison that affects sulfhydryl-containing enzyme systems throughout the body—virtually all enzymes and organ systems are affected. Chief among the enzyme systems affected are those that involve heme synthesis. Inhibition of δ-aminolevulinic acid dehydratase levels has been associated with CNS symptoms. Interference with ferrochelatase, the enzyme that promotes the incorporation of iron into protoporphyrin to produce heme, results in deficits in heme synthesis and thus any metabolic process which requires heme, and because there is lack of synthesis feedback, elevated free protoporphyrin levels (17).

Acute lead poisoning occasionally occurs from exposure to high concentrations of organic lead (e.g., tetraethyl lead). Although symptoms may suggest acute intoxication, poisoning from metallic and inorganic lead is usually as a result of chronic or subacute exposure, and the insidious onset of symptoms before presentation can be elicited by taking a careful history.

Chronic lead exposure has been associated with abnormality of semen quality, sperm morphology and physiology, hearing deficits, defects in reaction time (specifically the central component [decision slowing]), decreased numbers of CD16+ cells, chronic nephropathies associated with hypertension (11,19), gout, Fanconi syndrome (years after treatment with chelators), and a possible association with various cancers.

CLINICAL PRESENTATION

Patients with lead poisoning may present with such nonspecific symptoms such as headache, fatigue, malaise, abdominal pain, constipation, and vomiting. The abdominal pain is usually colicky and not responsive to standard analgesics. There may be complaints of peripheral paresthesias or hypoesthesias and occasional frank neurologic symptoms (e.g., wrist or ankle drop). Muscle weakness may also be noted. Depression and other affective disorders have been reported in lead-poisoned adults (1).

Hyperactivity, delayed development, or loss of recently acquired skills may be seen in children (12,15). In severe cases, coma and seizures may be noted.

Physical examination is generally unrevealing, although the blood pressure may be elevated. Occasionally, in adults with poor dental care, a dark bluish-black discoloration of the gingiva at the dental border (lead lines) may be present. This finding is seldom present in children and in those with good dental hygiene. If increased intracranial pressure accompanies lead encephalopathy, examination of the optic fundi may show papilledema. Cardiac dysrhythmias such as premature ventricular contractions have been reported.

An abdominal radiograph may reveal radiopaque foreign bodies in patients with pica or accidental lead ingestion. In developing children, long-bone radiographs may show an increased density of metaphyseal growth plates as a result of disordered calcium deposition resulting in "lead lines." This finding is seldom present in adults although it may persists into later childhood or adolescence.

The laboratory evaluation usually reveals a hypochromic microcytic anemia. Lead may produce a nonautoimmune hemolytic anemia with increased red cell fragility and an elevated reticulocyte count. Basophilic stippling and eosinophilia are less often noted. Proteinuria, glycosuria, a Fanconi syndrome (with aminoaciduria and renal tubular acidosis), and increased blood urea nitrogen and creatinine levels may be seen in patients with lead nephropathy. Because lead reduces the excretion of uric acid, patients with lead toxicity are prone to develop gout.

The definitive diagnosis of lead poisoning depends on the measurement of whole-blood lead and free erythrocyte protoporphyrin (FEP). The former indicates exposure and the latter is evidence of poisoning, because it is the result of lead's effect on ferrochelatase. Lead levels as low as 5 μg/dL have been reported to produce biochemical abnormalities, and levels between 10 and 20 μg/dL may be associated with clinical pathology (e.g., decreased intelligence and neurobehavioral problems in children) (6). Lead levels above 10 μg/dL in children are currently considered to be evidence of increased lead absorption, and lead levels above 40 μg/dL in adults are considered evidence of lead poisoning serious enough to warrant intervention. Although the importance of FEP levels has been de-emphasized over the last decade, levels above 15 μg/dL are uncommon in healthy people and in the absence of iron deficiency suggest chronic lead exposure. Although FEP levels over 20 μg/dL may be seen with either iron deficiency or lead poisoning, FEP levels above 35 μg/dL usually indicate lead poisoning (17).

DIFFERENTIAL DIAGNOSIS

Lead poisoning shares symptomatology with other heavy metal poisonings. The peripheral neuropathy from lead poisoning tends to be more motor then sensory. Additionally, unlike poisoning with arsenic, the peripheral neuropathy from lead is associated with decreased sensitivity; with arsenic, there are painful paresthesias. The "hallmark" of thallium poisoning, is burning paresthesias and hair loss. Both lead and mercury poisoning are characterized by personality changes. Mercury intoxication is characterized by erythrism and rapid changes in affect, with outbursts of anger alternating with happiness. Lead poisoning is more often accompanied by depressive disorders. Urinary heavy metal analysis may be necessary for differentiation.

EMERGENCY DEPARTMENT EVALUATION

Patients who present to the emergency department with multisystem complaints, particularly chronic abdominal symptoms that have not responded to standard conservative therapy, should be suspected of having lead poisoning. The patient's occupation, hobbies, or living conditions may suggest exposure to lead. The physician should ask about subtle changes in bowel habits, behavior, mood, and cognitive function, and headaches, weakness, and paresthesias.

In addition to vital signs and a general physical examination, a detailed neurologic examination should be performed. The physician should specifically check for papilledema and gingival pigmentation. If recent lead ingestion is suspected, an abdominal radiograph may be helpful. In children, long-bone radiographs (knee and wrist) may suggest chronic lead exposure. The laboratory evaluation should include a complete blood count, whole-blood lead and FEP levels, serum blood urea nitrogen and creatinine levels, and a urinalysis.

Elevated blood lead levels should usually be confirmed before initiating treatment. Asymptomatic patients with mildly elevated lead levels (20–44 μg/dL in children, 40–60 μg/dL in adults) may be evaluated with the calcium disodium EDTA lead mobilization test (discussion follows) (15).

EMERGENCY DEPARTMENT MANAGEMENT

Cerebral edema should be treated by hyperventilation, elevation of the head, and restriction of fluids. Seizures should be controlled with pharmacologic agents such as diazepam, barbiturates, and phenytoin. In patients with acute encephalopathy (with or without coma or seizures), chelation therapy should be initiated before obtaining confirmatory laboratory data, because the long-term outcome is related to the length of time the vital organs are exposed to elevated lead levels. GI decontamination should be performed if there is radiopaque material in the intestine. Decontamination should not delay definitive parenteral chelation therapy but oral chelation should not be attempted if there is evidence of lead within the intestinal lumen.

Chelation therapy is usually indicated for children with lead levels above 45 μg/dL, for adults with levels above 80 μg/dL, and for patients with lower levels who have a positive lead mobilization test or evidence of lead-associated symptoms or signs (discussion follows) (16). Dimercaprol (British Anti-Lewisite [BAL]) crosses the blood–brain barrier and forms a tight bond with lead; in patients with lead encephalopathy, it is the initial therapy of choice. An oil-based solution of dimercaprol is given intramuscularly in a usual dose of 3 to 5 mg/kg every 4 to 6 hours. Dimercaprol is painful when injected and foul-smelling, and it may produce adverse local and systemic reactions. Sterile abscesses may occur at the site of dimercaprol injection, and febrile responses are not unusual. Many patients complain of a terrible taste in their mouths and of lightheadedness.

Calcium disodium EDTA (CaNa$_2$EDTA) is water soluble and can be given intramuscularly or intravenously. The lead–EDTA bond is very strong and stable at a physiologic pH. However, in acid urine, the bond is less stable, and there is the potential for release of free lead into the renal tubule and subsequent renal tubular damage. The main side effects of EDTA are phlebitis (with concentrations of greater than 0.5 mg/mL) and potential renal toxicity. Because intramuscular injections are extremely irritating and produce elevations of creatine phosphokinase, intravenous administration is preferred (20). If the intramuscular route is used, procaine or lidocaine is usually added to produce an 0.5% concentration of the local anesthetic.

CaNa$_2$EDTA is given in a dose of 50 mg/kg/d. Intravenous CaNa$_2$EDTA is given as a continuous drip. At a concentration of 0.5 mg/mL, a large amount of fluid must be infused. However, if the patient can tolerate the fluid load, the incidence of side effects, particularly renal dysfunction, may be decreased. Intramuscular CaNa$_2$EDTA is given in divided doses every 4 to 24 hours. Because the use of CaNa$_2$EDTA alone may liberate bone lead and transiently raise brain lead levels and increase symptoms (2,3), it may be advisable to start with a dose of dimercaprol in all symptomatic patients and those with high blood lead levels (greater than 55 µg/dL in children and 100 mg/dL in adults).

The dose of CaNa$_2$EDTA for a diagnostic lead mobilization test is 1 g for adults and 25 mg/kg in children, infused over 1 to 2 hours with 250 to 1,000 mL of normal saline solution. The bladder is initially emptied, fluid intake is encouraged, and the urine is collected for 24 hours (3 days in patients with abnormal renal function) and analyzed for its lead content. If the amount of lead excreted (in micrograms) exceeds the amount of CaNa$_2$EDTA given (in milligrams), therapeutic chelation therapy may be indicated. In children, the challenge dose of CaNa$_2$EDTA can be given intramuscularly and the urine collected for 8 hours. With this regimen, chelation therapy is indicated if the urinary lead excretion (in micrograms) exceeds 60% of the dose of CaNa$_2$EDTA (in milligrams).

Oral chelation with dimercaptosuccinic acid or succimer (Chemet) is indicated for children with lead levels above 45 µg/dL and is as effective in clearing lead as the combination of dimercaprol and EDTA (5). The side-effect spectrum is minimal, with a small incidence of skin rash, transaminase elevations, and GI discomfort (13). Although not officially licensed for use in adults, its effectiveness, combined with its low order of toxicity, argues for its use in this population (10). The published dosage in children may be used safely in adults—10 mg/kg/dose every 8 hours for 5 days, followed by 10 mg/kg per dose every 12 hours for an additional 14 days. Patients should be monitored for toxicity with weekly blood counts, chemistry profiles, and urinalysis. The presence of ketones in the urine may be used as a measure of compliance, because it is a very common accompaniment of successful treatment. A mild rash or mild transaminitis is usually not a reason to abandon therapy, but requires closer observation, with more frequent laboratory investigation. It is important to insure that no further exposure to lead occur while on oral chelation.

Another oral chelator, d-penicillamine, a derivative of penicillin, is given orally at a dosage of 30 mg/kg/d, with the average adult dose of about 1.0 to 1.5 g/d (12,20). It is usually used only for adults with mild or no symptoms but high lead levels. Side effects include diarrhea, renal toxicity, leukopenia, and, occasionally, a rash. Penicillamine is less effective than dimercaprol or CaNa$_2$EDTA (21).

If renal toxicity develops as a result of antidotal therapy, fluid input should be increased in an attempt to dilute the lead content of the urine. Alkalinization of the urine may also be helpful.

Therapy should be continued until the lead level drops below 20 µg/dL in children and 40 µg/dL in adults. Maximum lead excretion occurs during the first 3 days of chelation therapy and falls off rapidly. After 5 days of therapy, it is unlikely that there will be further significant plumburesis without a rest period to allow lead to redistribute from tissue compartments to the blood. Hence, chelation therapy is usually limited to a 5-day course of parenteral drug, followed by a treatment-free interval of 2 to 7 days. Oral succimer therapy is usually discontinued after 19 total days of therapy. Additional courses of therapy are indicated if symptoms persist or blood lead levels remain elevated. Repeat lead levels should be evaluated, initially, at least weekly Reinstitution of therapy, depending on the rebound in lead level, should be considered. Children with lead levels below 20 µg/dL and adults with levels below 40 µg/dL should be managed by preventing further exposure by environmental and educational interventions (see discussion in next section). Follow-up evaluation and periodic monitoring are required.

The vast majority of lead-poisoned patients survive. The final neurologic outcome may not be known for many weeks or months after treatment. Patients with cerebral edema have a poor prognosis.

CRITICAL INTERVENTIONS

- Consult a poison center or lead-poisoning expert for management advice in patients with suspected or confirmed lead poisoning
- Admit patients with lead encephalopathy and administer dimercaprol (BAL) intermuscularly and calcium disodium EDTA intravenously

DISPOSITION

All patients with evidence of encephalopathy should be admitted. Although chelation with CaNa$_2$EDTA, penicillamine, and succimer can be done on an outpatient basis, it is advisable to admit all patients who are symptomatic or who have markedly elevated lead levels (requiring dimercaprol therapy). However, because blood lead levels are not immediately available at the time of initial evaluation, patients who are not acutely ill can be discharged and admitted later if blood lead analysis or an CaNa$_2$EDTA mobilization test confirms the suspected diagnosis.

Further exposure to lead must be prevented. Environmental and occupational investigations should be performed to determine the most likely source of lead so that it can be eliminated. Involvement of the public health department, primarily in dealing with a child with lead poisoning, is imperative. The Occupational Safety and Health Administration may be helpful in investigating cases of occupational lead exposure. Many states also have active divisions of occupational and environmental health that may be helpful in the long-term treatment of patients.

Although chelation therapy is not difficult, some of the nuances are appreciated only after treating many patients. Hence, the physician unfamiliar with the evaluation and therapy of lead exposure and poisoning is advised to consult an experienced toxicologist, usually available through a regional poison control center (1-800-222-1222).

All patients should be seen within 2 weeks of chelation therapy for repeat lead and FEP levels, because lead will be mobilized from storage sites and blood levels will rebound after treatment. It is not uncommon for the lead level at 2 weeks after therapy to equal or exceed the initial level.

COMMON PITFALLS

✔ Failure to consider the diagnosis of lead poisoning in patients with cognitive dysfunction, neurologic symptoms, and GI complaints
✔ Failure to appreciate that elevated lead levels without coincidental elevations in FEP may be seen with recent exposures and to treat the patient with an extremely high lead level regardless of the FEP level
✔ Failure to appreciate that, in many states, lead poisoning is a reportable illness, and both state and local health officials must be notified
✔ Failure to identify the source of lead and to prevent reexposure

References

1. Baker EL, Feldman RG, White RF, et al. The role of occupational lead exposure in the genesis of psychiatric and behavioral disturbances. *Acta Psychiatr Scand* 1983;67[Suppl]:38.
2. Chisolm JJ. Mobilization of lead by calcium disodium edetate—a reappraisal. *Am J Dis Child* 1987;141(12):1256–1257.

3. Cory-Slechta DA, Weiss B, Cox C. Mobilization and redistribution of lead over the course of Ca-EDTA therapy. *J Pharmacol Exp Ther* 1987;243:804.
4. FDA Talk Paper. "FDA Warns Consumers About Use of "Litargirio"—Traditional Remedy That Contains Dangerous Levels of Lead." Washington, DC: Food and Drug Administration, T-03-67. October 2, 2003. http://www.fda.gov/bbs/topics/ANSWERS/2003/ANS01253.html. Accessed January 3, 2005.
5. Graziano JH, Sins ES, Lolacono N, et al. 2,3-Dimercaptosuccinic acid as an antidote for lead intoxication. *Clin Pharmacol Ther* 1985;37:431.
6. Harvey B. Should blood lead screening recommendations be revisited? *Pediatrics* 1994;93:201.
7. Hasegawa S, Nakayama K, Iwakiri K, et al. Herbal medicine-associated lead intoxication. *Intern Med* 1997;36(1):56–58.
8. Johnson NE, Tenuta K. Diets and lead blood levels of children who practice pica. *Environ Res* 1979;18:369.
9. Kilkano GE, Strange KC. Lead poisoning in a child after a gunshot injury. *J Fam Pract* 1992;34:498.
10. Lifshitz M, Hashkanazi R, Phillip M. The effect of 2,3 dimercaptosuccinic acid in the treatment of lead poisoning in adults. *Ann Med* 1997;29(1):83–85.
11. Lin JL, Ho HH, Yu CC. Chelation therapy for patients with elevated body lead burden and progressive renal insufficiency. A randomized, controlled trial. *Ann Intern Med* 1999;130(1):7–13.
12. Mahaffey K, Michaelson A. Interactions between lead and nutrition. In: Needleman HL, ed. *Low-level lead exposure: the clinical implications of current research.* New York: Raven Press 1980:159.
13. Marcus SM. Experience with d-penicillamine in treating lead poisoning. *Vet Hum Toxicol* 1982;24:18.
14. Natelson EA, Fred HL. Lead poisoning from cocktail glasses: observations of two patients. *JAMA* 1976;236:2527.
15. Needleman HL, Gunnoe CG, Leviton A, et al. Deficits in psychological performance and classroom behavior in children with elevated dentine lead levels. *N Engl J Med* 1979;300:689.
16. Piomelli S, Rosen JF, Chisolm JJ, et al. Management of childhood lead poisoning. *J Pediatr* 1984;105:523.
17. Piomelli S, Seaman C, Zullow D, et al. Threshold for lead damage to have synthesis in urban children. *Proc Natl Acad Sci U S A* 1982;79:3335.
18. Rabinowitz MB, Wetherill GW, Kopple JD. Kinetic analysis of lead metabolism in healthy humans. *J Clin Invest* 1976;58:260.
19. Sanchez-Fructusos AI, Torralbo A, Arroyo M, et al. Occult lead intoxication as a cause of hypertension and renal failure. *Nephrol Dial Transplant* 1996;11(9):17775–17780.
20. Santiago M, Charnock R, Whitehead B, et al. Toxicity of EDTA in treating lead poisoning: IM vs IV. Platform session, American Association of Poison Control Centers, American Academy of Clinical Toxicologists, American Board of Medical Toxicologists, annual meeting, Boston 1983. *Vet Hum Toxicol* 1983;25[Suppl 1]:67.
21. Vitale LF, Rosalinas-Bailon A, Brennan JF, et al. Oral penicillamine therapy for chronic lead poisoning in children. *J Pediatr* 1973;83:1041.

CHAPTER 315
Methemoglobinemia

David A. Tanen and Michael J. Matteucci

Normal hemoglobin (oxyhemoglobin and deoxyhemoglobin) contains four heme groups, each with a ferrous (Fe^{2+}) ion capable of binding oxygen. Oxidative stress within the red cell produces methemoglobinemia. When the iron in reduced hemoglobin is oxidized to the ferric state (Fe^{3+}), methemoglobin is formed. Under normal conditions, methemoglobin levels are less than 1% to 2% of total heme pigments (12). Higher fractions are termed methemoglobinemia.

Oxidative stress within the red cell can also lead to the denaturation of red cell proteins, splenic sequestration of damaged erythrocytes, and hemolysis. Damaged erythrocytes may appear as "bite cells," pie shaped red cells with a bite taken out of the edge, on peripheral blood smear. Denatured proteins or Heinz bodies can not being visualized by the standard Wright stain, but

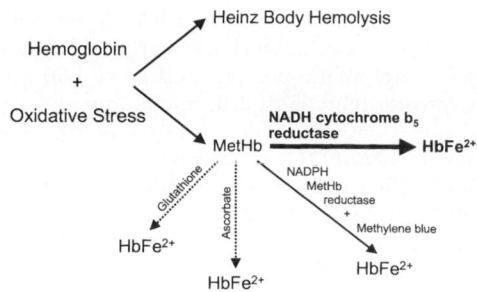

Figure 315.1. Pathways of hemoglobin oxidation and methemoglobin reduction.

appear as dark dots within the erythrocyte with special (Heinz body) staining of the blood.

Oxyhemoglobin is red and methemoglobin is dark brown and may possess a characteristic "chocolate brown color." Cyanosis typically requires 5 g/dL blood of reduced (ferrous) hemoglobin. However, in methemoglobinemia, only 1.5 g/dL of ferric heme produces noticeable discoloration. Therefore, cyanosis may be produced in nonanemic patients with 10% to 20% methemoglobin. Methemoglobin cannot transport oxygen and results in a functional anemia. The presence of ferric heme groups impairs the unloading of oxygen by oxygenated (ferrous) heme, producing a leftward shift in the oxyhemoglobin dissociation curve (3,12). Taken together, the physiologic consequences of methemoglobinemia are secondary to decreased tissue oxygenation. Metabolic acidosis develops secondary to functional hypoxia.

Hemoglobin is slowly oxidized to methemoglobin under normal conditions. The erythrocyte contains enzymes that can catalyze the reduction of methemoglobin back to reduced hemoglobin (Fig. 315.1). More than 95% of methemoglobin reduction is accomplished by the transfer of electrons from NADH (the reduced form of nicotinamide-adenine dinucleotide, which is generated in glycolysis) to cytochrome-b_5 and then to methemoglobin by way of the enzyme variously known as NADH-dependent methemoglobin reductase, diaphorase I, and, most recently, NADH cytochrome-b_5 reductase (6,12).

In normal persons, enzymatic reduction of methemoglobin occurs at a rate 200- to 300-fold greater than its spontaneous formation. However, congenital deficiencies in NADH cytochrome-b_5 reductase (12) or in cytochrome-b_5 itself (6) can cause methemoglobinemia, or can greatly predispose a person to developing methemoglobinemia. Neonates, especially those with a metabolic acidosis (17), are at increased risk for developing methemoglobinemia after oxidant stress (e.g., drugs, toxins, sepsis) because they have lower levels of NADH cytochrome-b_5 reductase and cytochrome-b_5 until they reach 4 months of age (3,6,12).

A second enzyme, NADPH (the reduced form of nicotinamide-adenine dinucleotide phosphate) methemoglobin reductase, can facilitate the reduction of methemoglobin by transferring electrons from NADPH (produced in the hexose monophosphate shunt) to an intermediate compound and then to methemoglobin (3,12). There is no known endogenous cofactor for this enzyme, and consequently it has little or no physiologic role in maintaining methemoglobin levels at low or normal concentrations. However, exogenously administered methylene blue has been demonstrated to act as an intermediate for electron transfer and greatly increase the activity of this enzyme.

People with depressed levels of erythrocytic NADPH (e.g., glucose-6-phosphate dehydrogenase [G6PD] deficiency) or a congenital lack of the NADPH-dependent reducing enzyme do not normally suffer from and are not predisposed to developing

TABLE 315.1. Some Methemoglobin-Producing Agents

Acetanilid	Food additives	Phenacetin
Amyl nitrite	Hydrazines	Phenols
Aniline dyes	Hydroxylamine	Phenylazopyridine
Arsine	Inks	Prilocaine
Benzocaine	Lidocaine	Primaquine
Bismuth sulfate	Local anesthetics	Pyridine
Chlorates	Methylene blue	Quinones
Chromates	Metoclopramide	Riluzole
Cyclophosamide	Mushrooms	Shoe dye or polish
Dapsone	Naphthalene	Sulfonamides
Dinitrophenol	Nitrates	Sulfones
Dinitrotoluene	Nitrites	Toluidine
EMLA	Nitrobenzene	Trinitrotoluene
Flutamide	Nitroglycerin	

methemoglobinemia. However, if these patients who are functionally G6PD deficient do develop methemoglobinemia, treatment with methylene blue would be ineffective and may even trigger massive hemolysis (11).

Exposure to a variety of agents may result in acquired methemoglobinemia (Table 315.1). Not all of the compounds are direct oxidants, implying that their metabolites or oxidizing intermediates (e.g., free radicals) are responsible for producing methemoglobin in some cases. The most commonly reported therapeutic agents that cause methemoglobinemia are local anesthetics, which may be injected or applied topically (e.g. infant teething gels and benzocaine sprays). Other commonly prescribed medications frequently implicated in methemoglobinemia include metoclopramide (Reglan), phenazopyridine (Pyridium), and diaminodiphenylsulfone (Dapsone) (3,4).

Environmentally, there are numerous exposures that can lead to the induction of methemoglobinemia. Aniline and related aromatic amines are some of the most common, along with exposure to nitrates that are converted to nitrites by bacteria in the gastrointestinal (GI) tract. Fatal cases of methemoglobinemia have been reported in infants who ingested well water high in nitrites. Bacteria colonizing burn wounds treated with silver nitrate have been also reported to oxidize nitrate to nitrite and produce methemoglobinemia (3). The recreational use of inhalable nitrites such as isobutyl nitrite has resulted in large numbers of recent cases of methemoglobinemia (7). Other toxins such as chlorates and arsine may not only cause methemoglobinemia but are frequently responsible for inducing massive hemolysis (2,15).

CLINICAL PRESENTATION

Nonanemic patients with 10% to 20% methemoglobinemia usually present with unexplained cyanosis and no other symptoms. Headache, dyspnea on exertion, tachypnea, tachycardia, and mild hypertension usually are not noted until the methemoglobin levels reach 15% to 35%. Higher fractions can result in confusion, coma, seizures, apnea, ventricular dysrhythmias, bradyarrhythmias, hypotension, and lactic acidosis. Death is frequently seen with methemoglobin fractions above 70%.

Patients with underlying cardiovascular or cerebrovascular disease are more susceptible to the effects of hypoxia. Those with preexisting anemia or with concomitant Heinz body hemolytic anemia suffer greater toxicity at a given methemoglobin level, because the remaining functional hemoglobin concentration is lower. Also, cyanosis may not be apparent in the anemic patient because a greater percentage of methemoglobin would be needed to reach the 1.5 g/dL threshold of cyanosis as compared

to the nonanemic patient. Hence, anemic patients can suffer from significant methemoglobinemia without exhibiting cyanosis.

The cyanosis of methemoglobinemia is refractory to the administration of oxygen. The arterial PO_2 is normal or elevated. The oxygen saturation by pulse oximetry is falsely elevated with respect to the true value but less than the value calculated from the PO_2. Metabolic acidosis may be present in severe cases. Venous blood may have a brown hue. A low hemoglobin and hematocrit, bite cells on peripheral blood smear, Heinz bodies with this stain, and increased serum haptoglobin and pink plasma from hemoglobinemia may be noted in severe cases of hemolysis. The electrocardiogram (ECG) may reveal tachycardia, bradycardia, ventricular dysrhythmias, and changes suggestive of myocardial ischemia.

DIFFERENTIAL DIAGNOSIS

Cyanosis as a result of methemoglobinemia may be differentiated from that as a result of hypoxia by the presence of a normal PO_2 and by the fact that it is unresponsive to oxygen. The cyanotic patient whose arterial blood gas reveals a normal PO_2 and a normal percentage of oxyhemoglobin (percentage saturation) may be confusing. This situation arises from the fact that most blood gas instruments do not directly measure oxyhemoglobin fractions, but rather, calculate and report what the percentage hemoglobin saturation should be based on the oxygen tension. These calculations assume the absence of methemoglobin, carboxyhemoglobin, and sulfhemoglobin, and further that there is no shift in the dissociation curve from changes in erythrocytic 2,3-diphosphoglycerate concentrations. A co-oximeter is required to directly measure the true percentage saturation and other hemoglobin pigments. Co-oximeters measure the total hemoglobin concentration and percentages of oxyhemoglobin, methemoglobin, and carboxyhemoglobin. Sulfhemoglobin is usually recognized as methemoglobin by these instruments. The difference between the percentage of hemoglobin saturation calculated by the blood gas analyzer and the saturation measured by the co-oximeter is called the oxygen saturation gap. A large oxygen saturation gap in arterial blood is almost always as a result of carboxyhemoglobin or methemoglobin. To interpret blood gas reports accurately, the emergency physician must know whether reported percentage saturations on arterial blood gas samples are determined by co-oximetry.

Pulse oximeters (e.g., ear or finger oximeters) usually measure only oxyhemoglobin and deoxyhemoglobin. They do not predictably or accurately recognize the presence of methemoglobin or carboxyhemoglobin. Therefore, a pulse oximeter can report a falsely normal or factitious percentage hemoglobin oxygen saturation in the presence of methemoglobinemia or carboxyhemoglobinemia (8). Hyperlipidemia, such as that seen after infusions of lipid emulsions (e.g., Intralipid, Liposyn) or in patients with diabetes mellitus, interferes with the measurement of hemoglobin pigments by co-oximeters, resulting in falsely elevated methemoglobin concentrations (13). In these instances, the patient with a normal hemoglobin concentration and without cyanosis does not have serious methemoglobinemia.

A peculiar and poorly characterized cyanosis may also be seen in some cases of hydrogen sulfide or tellurium poisoning. Both carbon monoxide and sulfhemoglobinemia produce a noticeable saturation gap with a normal arterial PO_2. Sulfhemoglobinemia, a rare cause of cyanosis, causes noticeable discoloration at only 0.5 g/dL blood. Most co-oximeters measure sulfhemoglobin as methemoglobin. Fortunately, sulfhemoglobin is rarely (if ever) severe enough to cause life-threatening symptoms. Generalized bluish discoloration from excessive administration of methylene blue may also be confused with cyanosis (5).

EMERGENCY DEPARTMENT EVALUATION

A careful history should be taken from the patient and family regarding medications, occupational exposures to chemicals, family history of methemoglobinemia, recreational drug use, and, in the case of children, any substances in the house that could have been ingested. The physical examination should focus on vital signs, skin color, and any evidence of cerebral or myocardial hypoxia.

Besides determining the methemoglobin fraction, the physician should also seek evidence of hemolysis (2,15). Therefore, a hemoglobin–hematocrit, Heinz body stain, serum haptoglobin, and plasma free hemoglobin concentration should be ordered if hemolysis is suspected. Additional evaluation should include a complete blood count, serum electrolytes, blood urea nitrogen, creatinine, and glucose, arterial blood gas analysis, urinalysis, and ECG.

If accurate determination of methemoglobin concentration by co-oximetry is unavailable, the oxygen saturation gap can be used to estimate the methemoglobin fraction. Alternatively, a drop of the patient's blood can be placed on filter paper and allowed to dry. If the blood appears obviously brown, as compared with a drop of blood from a healthy person, then a level of at least 15% methemoglobin is present, assuming a normal total hemoglobin concentration (3). Furthermore, venous blood from a healthy person becomes bright red when shaken in the air as oxyhemoglobin is formed. Venous blood that contains elevated methemoglobin concentrations will remain dark brown after shaking.

EMERGENCY DEPARTMENT MANAGEMENT

Patients with methemoglobinemia should be placed on oxygen to maximize the oxygen delivery of the residual normal hemoglobin. Intravenous access should be established, and the patient should be placed on a cardiac monitor.

Most patients with mild methemoglobinemia (<30%) are blue but asymptomatic and do not require treatment (3). Once exposure to the offending agent is terminated, methemoglobin levels usually return to normal within 12 to 36 hours. Patients with symptoms unrelieved by oxygen, those with methemoglobin fractions above 30%, those with ECG changes, or those with a metabolic acidosis should receive antidotal therapy with methylene blue, provided there is no history of G6PD deficiency. Methylene blue is usually available as a 1% solution (10 mg/mL) and should be given intravenously over 3 to 5 minutes at an initial dose of 2 mg/kg (0.2 mL/kg of a 1% solution) (3). A dramatic response with resolution of cyanosis is usually noted within 15 minutes. If the patient is seriously symptomatic and no response is noted within 15 minutes, or if the patient remains moderately symptomatic after 15 to 30 minutes, repeat doses of 1 mg/kg (0.1 mL/kg of 1% solution) can be given. If methemoglobin levels are readily available, repeat determinations of methemoglobin concentration should be performed before repeat doses of methylene blue are given, because large doses of methylene blue themselves might produce methemoglobinemia and can cause discoloration of skin (3,5). The total dose of methylene blue during the first 2 to 3 hours should not exceed 5 to 7 mg/kg (3).

Adverse effects of methylene blue include dysuria, substernal chest pain, and anxiety (10). Urine frequently turns blue and then green as the drug is excreted. Single doses of methylene blue as low as 5 mg/kg has been shown to induce methemoglobinemia in animals (9).

Methylene blue is contraindicated in patients with G6PD deficiency. These patients have low erythrocytic NADPH concentrations, making augmentation of the NADPH-dependent, methemoglobin-reducing enzyme by methylene blue impossible. More important, methylene blue may trigger massive hemolysis in such patients, further compromising oxygen delivery to tissues (11). About 15% of African American males are thought to be deficient in G6PD; men and women of Mediterranean ancestry also have an increased incidence of this enzyme deficiency.

As soon as time allows, GI and skin decontamination should be performed to limit continued absorption of the offending agent. This is particularly important after acute dermal exposures to chemicals or after intentional ingestions of toxic agents. Dermal decontamination can be performed with a triple wash (water rinse, soap scrub, water rinse). GI decontamination is discussed in Chapter 272, "Gastrointestinal Decontamination."

If the drug or chemical causing methemoglobinemia cannot be readily eliminated from the body (e.g., dapsone), methemoglobinemia may continually recur for hours or days despite successful initial treatment with methylene blue. In this instance, serial measurements of methemoglobin levels are required, and a constant intravenous infusion of methylene blue at a rate of 0.1 mg/kg/h has been used to maintain methemoglobin concentrations at a safe level (1). Repeated oral doses of activated charcoal may also enhance the elimination of dapsone. Additionally, high-dose cimetidine given intravenously has been shown to lessen dapsone-induced methemoglobin production. Renal failure is a relative contraindication to using a constant infusion or frequently repeated doses of methylene blue, because the drug is mainly renally excreted.

Treatment with hyperbaric oxygen (HBO) or exchange transfusions should be considered for patients with G6PD deficiency or for those who do not respond satisfactorily to methylene blue. HBO can provide enough dissolved oxygen to support life in the presence of severe methemoglobinemia.

Symptomatic hemolytic anemia may require treatment with blood transfusions. Because massive hemolysis may cause hyperkalemia and acute renal failure, efforts should be made to maintain a good rate of urine flow.

Ascorbic acid also reduces methemoglobin to hemoglobin (nonenzymatically). A dose of 0.5 to 1.0 g ascorbic acid every 6 hours may be given intravenously or orally in conjunction with methylene blue. However, ascorbic acid works too slowly to be useful in the treatment of acute, acquired methemoglobinemia (3). Although N-acetylcysteine has been proposed as a possible adjunct in the treatment of methemoglobinemia, it has not been shown to reduce elevated methemoglobin levels in a human model of methemoglobinemia (14,16).

CRITICAL INTERVENTIONS

- Administer 100% oxygen to patients with suspected or diagnosed methemoglobinemia
- Measure methemoglobin levels with a co-oximeter, if available
- Obtain Heinz body blood stain, serum haptoglobin, and plasma free hemoglobin concentration in patients with a low hemoglobin–hematocrit
- Administer methylene blue to patients with signs of cardiac ischemia, dyspnea, metabolic acidosis, or methemoglobin levels > 30%

DISPOSITION

Patients with methemoglobinemia should be admitted after emergency department evaluation and management. Patients are best managed at a facility in which methemoglobin concentrations can be measured easily and quickly. Physicians unfamiliar with the management of methemoglobinemia should consult a toxicologist or hematologist or the regional poison center. If transfer is necessary, advanced life-support services should be provided and should include a supply of methylene blue. In the case of an accidental or intentional poisoning, the physician must evaluate and treat other toxic effects of methemoglobin-producing agents. All patients who receive methylene blue should be observed for recurrence of symptomatic methemoglobinemia and for adverse effects such as hemolysis.

An asymptomatic and otherwise healthy patient who has been cyanotic for several days although taking therapeutic doses of an offending drug does not necessarily require admission if the total hemoglobin concentration is normal (e.g., no significant hemolysis), the methemoglobin level is below 20%, exposure to the offending agent is terminated, and reliable follow-up is available. Methemoglobin concentrations will return to normal in these patients as the offending drug is cleared from the body. A wise and conservative approach would be to admit all young children and elderly patients for observation, serial methemoglobin concentrations, and, when indicated, serial ECGs.

Any patient who unexpectedly develops methemoglobinemia after ingestion of therapeutic doses of drugs should be referred to a hematologist for evaluation of possible NADH cytochrome-b5 reductase deficiency. Any patient with methemoglobinemia that is unresponsive to treatment with methylene blue should be evaluated, after full recovery, for G6PD deficiency or, much less commonly, NADPH methemoglobin reductase deficiency.

COMMON PITFALLS

✔ Failure to consider the diagnosis of methemoglobinemia in patients with cyanosis unresponsive to oxygen

✔ Failure to appreciate that a normal arterial Po_2 and normal oxygen saturation (as measured by pulse oximetry or calculated from arterial blood gases) do not rule out methemoglobinemia

✔ Failure to appreciate that resolution of cyanosis in a patient with methemoglobinemia may be as a result of accompanying hemolysis, with actual worsening of oxygen delivery to tissues

✔ Failure to appreciate that methylene blue is contraindicated in patients with G6PD deficiency

Acknowledgment

We thank Steven Curry, who contributed to this chapter in previous editions.

References

1. Berlin G, Brodin B, Hilden J-O. Acute dapsone intoxication: a case treated with continuous infusion of methylene blue, forced diuresis, and plasma exchange. *J Toxicol Clin Toxicol* 1985;22:537.
2. Chan TK, Mak LW, Ng RP. Methemoglobinemia Heinz bodies and acute massive intravascular hemolysis in Lysol poisoning. *Blood* 1971;38:739.
3. Curry S. Methemoglobinemia. *Ann Emerg Med* 1982;11:214.
4. Gibson GR, Hunter JB, Raabe DS, et al. Methemoglobinemia produced by high-dose intravenous nitroglycerin. *Ann Intern Med* 1982;96:615.
5. Goluboff N, Wheaton R. Methylene blue-induced cyanosis and acute hemolytic anemia complicating the treatment of methemoglobinemia. *J Pediatr* 1961;58:86.
6. Hegesh E, Hegesh J, Kaftory A. Congenital methemoglobinemia with a deficiency of cytochrome b5. *N Engl J Med* 1986;314:757.
7. Horne MK III, Waterman MR, Garriott JC, et al. Methemoglobinemia from sniffing butyl nitrite. *Ann Intern Med* 1982;91:417.
8. Kulick RM. Pulse oximetry. *Pediatr Emerg Care* 1987;3:127.
9. Lovejoy FH. Methemoglobinemia. *Clin Toxicol Rev* 1984;6:1.
10. Nadler JE, Green H, Rosenbaum A. Intravenous injection of methylene blue in man with reference to its toxic symptoms and effect on the ECG. *Am J Med Sci* 1934;188:15.
11. Rosen PJ, Johnson C, McGehee WG, et al. Failure of methylene blue treatment in toxic methemoglobinemia; association with glucose-6-phosphate dehydrogenase deficiency. *Ann Intern Med* 1971;75:83.
12. Schwartz JM, Reiss AL, Jaffe ER.Hereditary methemoglobinemia with deficiency of NADH cytochrome b5 reductase. In: Stanbury JB, Wyngaarden JB, Fredrickson DS, et al, eds. *The metabolic basis of inherited disease*, 5th ed. New York: McGraw-Hill, 1983.
13. Spurzem JR, Bonekat HW, Shigeoka JW. Factitious methemoglobinemia caused by hyperlipemia. *Chest* 1984;86:84.
14. Tanen DA, Lovecchio F, Curry SC. Failure of intravenous N-acetylcysteine to reduce methemoglobin produced by sodium nitrite in human volunteers: a randomized controlled trial. *Ann Emerg Med* 2000;35:369.
15. Teunis BS, Leftwich El, Pierce LA. Acute methemoglobinemia and hemolytic anemia due to toluidine blue. *Arch Surg* 1971;101:527.
16. Wright RO, Magnani B, Shannon MW, et al. N-acetylcysteine reduces methemoglobin in vitro. *Ann Emerg Med* 1996;26:499.
17. Yano SS, Danish EH, Hsia YE. Transient methemoglobinemia with acidosis in infants. *J Pediatr* 1982;100:415.

CHAPTER 316
Smoke Inhalation

Heather Long

Smoke inhalation is the number one cause of death from fire and is the most likely cause of acute inhalation injury seen in the emergency department (20). In the 1990 Happy Land Social Club fire in New York City, all 87 deaths were as a result of smoke inhalation (11). Furthermore, the combination of smoke inhalation with burns results in much greater morbidity and mortality: acute respiratory failure develops in 12% with burn injuries, but jumps to 61% in those with both smoke inhalation and burn injuries (21,24). The overall mortality rate from burns listed with American Burn Injury Patient Registry is 4.1%, but among those with concomitant smoke inhalation injury, mortality is 29.4% (22). The mortality rate from smoke inhalation ranges from 5% to 8%; however, this represents 50% to 80% of deaths as a result of fire (6,14,21). Smoke is a mixture of heated air, gases, fumes, aerosols, vapors, and solid and liquid particles in suspension. Smoke toxicity depends on the composition of the fuel, the availability of oxygen, the completeness of combustion, and the heat intensity generated (13). Even within the same building, smoke composition can vary considerably with duration of the fire and location. In addition to the major toxic threats posed by carbon monoxide, oxygen depletion, and heat, toxic combustion products (TCP) from naturally occurring materials and synthetic polymers found in the modern environment contribute to smoke toxicity (1). See Table 316.1 for TCPs and their common sources.

TCPs are categorized as either simple asphyxiants, chemical asphyxiants, or irritant toxins (see Table 316.2). Simple asphyxiants displace oxygen from the ambient environment; they generally have no inherent toxicity. The process of combustion itself depletes oxygen from the environment as well.

Chemical asphyxiants inhibit cellular respiration, either by inhibiting mitochondrial electron transport or by impairing oxygen delivery. Agents inhibiting mitochondrial electron transport include carbon monoxide (see Chapter 306, "Carbon Monoxide"), hydrogen cyanide (see Chapter 308, "Cyanide") and hydrogen sulfide (see Chapter 311, "Hydrogen Sulfide"). Carbon monoxide and oxides of nitrogen, by inducing carboxyhemoglobin formation or methemoglobinemia (see Chapter 315, "Methemoglobinemia"), respectively, impair oxygen transport

TABLE 316.1. Common Toxic Products of Combustion and Their Sources

Product of Combustion	Common Sources
Acids/aldehydes	Cellulose acetate (film), cotton, paper polystyrene, polyvinyl acetate, wood
Acrolein	Acrilan (carpet), acrylic, celluloid, cellulosics, polyolefins
Ammonia	Nylon, resins (melamine, phenolic), silk, wood
Carbon monoxide/dioxide	All organic material
Chlorine/hydrochloric acid/phosgene	Chlorinated acrylics and hydrocarbons (fire extinguishers and retardants)
Cyanide/hydrogen cyanide	Acrylonitriles, nylon, paper, polyurethane, nitrocellulose (film), resins, silk, wool
Halogen acids and gases (Br, F)	Halogenated hydrocarbons, films, resins, flame retardants and extinguishers
Isocyanates	Polyurethane
Nitrogen oxides	Celluloid, cellulose nitrate fabrics, paper, petroleum products, wood
Styrene	Polystyrene
Sulfur oxides/ hydrogen sulfide	Hair, hides, meat, petroleum products, rubber, wool

and delivery to tissues. Carbon monoxide, produced by the incomplete combustion of any carbon-containing compound such as wood, charcoal and propane, is still the major toxicant in modern fires (1).

Among the 87 people who died in the Happy Land Social Club fire, carboxyhemoglobin concentrations ranged from 37% to 93% with a mean of 77%; 97% had a carboxyhemoglobin concentration greater than 50% (11). Frequently however, carboxyhemoglobin fractions in those who succumb to smoke inhalation are lower than 50%. Animal studies have demonstrated that an oxygen-poor environment when combined with even sublethal levels of carbon monoxide significantly reduces the time to death (1). Blood ethanol concentrations have been found to correlate strongly with the carboxyhemoglobin fraction (7). This suggests that ethanol intoxication impairs the ability to recognize and escape danger, with consequent prolongation of smoke exposure.

Cyanide is produced from the combustion of nitrogen-containing products such as wool, silk, nylon, plastics, polyurethane, nitrocellulose, and synthetic rubber. Cyanide is present in appreciable amounts in air samples from fires and in blood

TABLE 316.2. Toxic Combustion Products (TCPs)

Simple Asphyxiants	Chemical Asphyxiants	Irritants
Carbon dioxide	Carbon monoxide	Highly water soluble
Helium	Hydrogen cyanide	Acrolein
Methane	Hydrogen sulfide	Ammonia
Natural gas	Oxides of nitrogen	Formaldehyde
Nitrogen		Hydrogen chloride
Noble gases		Sulfur dioxide
Oxygen-deprived environment		
Propane		Intermediate water solubility
		Chlorine
		Isocyanates
		Poorly water soluble:
		Oxides of nitrogen
		Phosgene

from fire victims and is thought to have an additive, even synergistic effect, on smoke toxicity (1). Cyanide levels greater than 0.1 mg/L are considered abnormal.

Combustion of nitrogen-containing materials also generates oxides of nitrogen. These oxides are capable of inducing methemoglobinemia; also, they may directly oxidize cells of the respiratory tract or generate free radicals that induce delayed damage to the respiratory epithelium. Methemoglobinemia has infrequently been reported in smoke inhalation victims (16). Combustion of nitrocellulose, a major component of radiographic film, resulted in 125 deaths as a result of cyanide and nitrogen dioxide poisoning in the 1929 fire in the Cleveland Clinic radiology department (12).

Irritant toxins are a varied group of chemically reactive compounds that ultimately exert their toxic effects through damage to the respiratory tract (see Chapter 313, "Irritant Gas Inhalation"). Mechanisms by which the gases produce damage vary with the different agents; some, like the lipid-soluble acrolein, penetrate cell membranes and denature proteins and nucleic acids. Ammonia, hydrogen chloride, and sulfur dioxide react with the moisture of respiratory mucosa to yield the caustic agents ammonium hydroxide, hydrochloric acid, and sulfurous acid respectively. Chlorine and phosgene generate free radicals, mediating oxidative stress on cellular membranes.

Water solubility is the chemical property most important in determining where along the respiratory tract an irritant toxin exerts its damage. Highly water-soluble irritants dissolve on initial contact with mucus membranes resulting in damage to the upper airway, mouth, and eyes. Poorly soluble gases like phosgene are able to penetrate the lung parenchyma in which they react slowly, resulting in delayed toxicity.

Inhalation of soot and aerosols results in enhanced delivery of irritant gases to respiratory tract. As soot deposits, adsorbed gases are able to react with the moist mucosal surface. Size of the soot particle determines where it is deposited; particles 1 to 3 microns are able to reach the alveoli. Particles generated from building fires predominantly range from 3 to 5 microns (20).

Unless the victim is exposed to steam, direct heat injury is confined to the upper airway because of its marked ability to dissipate heat (8). Steam, however, has approximately 4,000 times the heat carrying capacity of hot air, and steam inhalation may be rapidly fatal as a result of laryngeal and glottic edema, thermal tracheitis, and hemorrhagic edema of the bronchial mucosa (4).

Smoke inhalation injury is a product of the inherent toxicity of the TCPs delivered, the victim's minute ventilation and the duration of exposure. Duration of exposure may be prolonged by factors inherent to a fire situation including anxiety, confusion, impaired visibility as a result of darkness, tearing, smoke, and physical obstacles. Symptoms resulting from TCP exposure and a low ambient oxygen concentration, including respiratory distress, altered cognition, and impaired awareness and mobility as a result of drug and alcohol intoxication, physical handicaps, and extremes of age, may all prolong duration of exposure.

Among firefighters, the type of oxygen mask used influences the risk of smoke inhalation. If oxygen is supplied via a demand valve requiring negative inspiratory pressure, smoke inhalation may occur if the mask does not fit tightly. With continuous positive-pressure devices, smoke inhalation will not occur unless the oxygen supply, which typically lasts 20 to 30 minutes, runs out. If either type of mask is removed during clean-up activities after the flames are extinguished, smoke inhalation may still occur.

Fires and explosions that give rise to smoke inhalation injuries pose significant potential for mass casualties. Although no deaths occurred, a train hauling hydrochloric acid, hydrofluoric acid, and acetic acid derailed in Baltimore, Maryland in July 2001, causing a fire that burned for 5 days and sent hundreds of people to local emergency departments (17). In November, 2000, 155 people died, most of them from smoke inhalation, after a fire broke out in a cable car traveling through a tunnel in Austria (2).

CLINICAL PRESENTATION

Respiratory signs and symptoms are the primary clinical manifestations of smoke inhalation toxicity. Clinical effects range from transient respiratory tract irritation to severe upper airway compromise and respiratory failure. Cough is often the first symptom. Other initial responses include increased mucus secretion and sneezing. Manifestations of upper airway involvement include hoarseness and stridor. With injury to the lower respiratory tract, crackles and/or wheezing may be auscultated. Breath sounds may be inaudible in cases of severe bronchospasm. Important signs of potential inhalation injury include cough, dyspnea, hoarseness, carbonaceous sputum, singed nasal hair, edema of the posterior pharynx, burns to the face, and any major burn to the body.

Smoke inhalation may cause systemic manifestations as well. Examination of the eye may reveal the irritant effects of increased tearing, conjunctival injection, and blepharospasm. Progressive airway compromise and toxicity from agents with systemic effects, notably carbon monoxide, will produce signs and symptoms of hypoxia—tachycardia, tachypnea, dizziness, headache, nausea and vomiting, chest pain, and deteriorating mental status manifesting as agitation, confusion and ultimately seizures, coma, and death.

Laboratory evaluation may reveal hypoxemia, metabolic (lactic) acidosis, and elevated carboxyhemoglobin and methemoglobin fractions and whole blood cyanide levels. The ECG may reveal dysrhythmias or evidence of myocardial ischemia or infarction.

DIFFERENTIAL DIAGNOSIS

Patients with smoke inhalation may have concomitant dermal burns, traumatic injuries, drug or alcohol intoxication, and may be victims of arson, attempted murder, or attempted suicide. For patients presenting with coma and shock, head computed tomography scanning, whole-blood cyanide levels, toxicology screening tests, and invasive hemodynamic measurements (e.g., central venous and pulmonary artery pressures) may be necessary to define the etiology.

EMERGENCY DEPARTMENT EVALUATION

Significant smoke inhalation injuries may not manifest early after exposure; factors associated with inhalation injury should be noted. History of entrapment, fire within an enclosed space, and altered consciousness at the scene should all raise the suspicion of inhalation injury. Key risk factors associated with inhalation injury are in Table 316.3. In addition to eliciting the patient's complaints, the history should address the nature of burning material, presence of steam, evidence of trauma or suicidality, and, among rescuers presenting as patients, the type of mask used.

Examination begins with obtaining vital signs and oxygen saturation. An important caveat regarding measurement of oxygen saturation is that transcutaneous pulse oximetry is unreliable in victims of smoke inhalation because it overestimates the true oxygen saturation in the presence of carboxyhemoglobin and methemoglobin (6,10). Co-oximetry accurately measures oxygen saturation even in the presence of these dyshemoglobinemias. A trauma survey and a skin survey with attention to signs associated with increased risk of smoke inhalation including

TABLE 316.3.   Key Factors Associated With Inhalation Injury

Initial Exposure Associated With:	Symptoms	Signs
Entrapment	Cough	Carbonaceous sputum
Fire in an enclosed space	Shortness of breath	Singed nasal hair
Loss of consciousness at the scene	Hoarseness	Pharyngeal edema
		Facial or neck burns; any major burn
		Stridor
		Crackles/wheezing
		Altered mental status

facial burns, singed facial hair, soot in the nasal passages and airway, and burns involving extensive body surface area (greater than 15%) should follow. The eyes should be examined with the aid of fluorescein staining to detect corneal burns and lacerations in comatose patients or those with eye complaints. Repeat examinations should focus on respiratory status and alterations in mental status.

Carboxyhemoglobin and methemoglobin fractions should be measured by co-oximetry. An elevated carboxyhemoglobin fraction in a fire victim is an indicator of significant exposure to combustion products and is associated with a markedly increased risk of smoke inhalation injury and toxicity (9). The converse, however, is not true: a low or undetectable carboxyhemoglobin concentration does not rule out the possibility of developing even severe inhalation injury (23).

Obtaining whole blood cyanide levels does not affect the acute management of the smoke inhalation victim because there is no timely confirmatory test. A more practical test is the plasma lactate concentration. A lactate concentration of greater than 10 mmol/L refractory to adequate ventilation, oxygenation, and perfusion in the right clinical setting is a surrogate marker of cyanide toxicity (3). The methemoglobin fraction should be determined in the initial laboratory assessment of symptomatic patients, particularly in those with cyanosis that does not improve with supplementary oxygen (see Chapter 308, "Cyanide" and Chapter 315, "Methemoglobinemia").

Arterial blood gas (ABG) measurements should also be obtain to assess arterial oxygenation, alveolar ventilation, and for metabolic acidosis. Initially, the ABG of even a significantly injured patient may be normal; serial measurements are recommended.

An ECG and chest radiograph are recommended in symptomatic patients, especially in those with preexisting cardiovascular or pulmonary disease. Chest radiographs may appear normal early in the course of smoke inhalation and therefore lack sensitivity as indicators of inhalation injury (9). Early findings, if present, are subtle: perivascular cuffing, bronchial wall thickening, and subglottic edema (18). Serial chest radiographs, however, may be very useful in monitoring disease progression. Common complications that do not typically manifest radiographically until more than 24 hours after the initial insult include acute lung injury/acute respiratory distress syndrome, aspiration, volume overload, and infection.

EMERGENCY DEPARTMENT MANAGEMENT

Prehospital directives include the rapid, safe removal of victims from the scene by those with adequate training and protection. Basic and advanced life support measures are instituted as indicated, and attention is given to cervical spine immobilization. Supplemental oxygen is indicated for all patients. The decision of whether a patient should be transported to a burn center, trauma center, or hyperbaric facility is determined by local practice guidelines. Intravenous access and cardiac monitoring may be established en route.

On arrival to the emergency department, upper airway patency must be determined immediately. Airway compromise may be present initially, rapidly ensue, or develop insidiously over the next few hours. Failure to appreciate the potential for rapid decline in airway status is the major pitfall in managing the smoke inhalation patient. Early endotracheal intubation, performed in a controlled setting before edema makes it impossible, may be life-saving and should be undertaken when there are obvious oropharyngeal burns or edema, full-thickness circumferential neck burns, stridor, or coma. In the patient with the edematous or difficult airway, fiberoptic laryngoscopy, flexible intubation guides, intubation laryngeal masks, retrograde intubation, transtracheal jet ventilation, and ultimately cricothyroidotomy may assist with establishing tracheal intubation (20). Aggressive rehydration of the burn victim may also cause airway edema and early intubation may also be indicated in these patients.

Although not typically performed in the emergency department setting, fiberoptic bronchoscopy is considered the gold standard for diagnosis and evaluation of inhalation injury. It may also assist in clearing debris from the respiratory tract, and permits fiberoptically assisted intubation if required. Early consult for fiberoptic bronchoscopy should be considered if there is suspicion of significant inhalation injury.

β_2 adrenergic agonists may be useful in improving airflow. Corticosteroids, although of benefit in the asthma patient with refractory bronchospasm, are not indicated in the management of patients with inhalation injury as they are associated with increased incidence of bacterial pneumonia and mortality (19). Prophylactic antibiotics also have no demonstrated benefit in the treatment of inhalation injury (15). Fever and leukocytosis that develop 2 days or more after injury do suggest infection, and empiric antibiotic treatment that covers *S. aureus* and gram-negative organisms should be instituted until culture results become available. Progressive respiratory failure and the development of pneumonitis, acute lung injury/adult respiratory distress syndrome or other complications may require mechanical ventilation, continuous positive airway pressure, positive end-expiratory pressure, and frequent suctioning of pulmonary secretions.

Trauma-related injuries as a result of falls or explosions and burns must be managed concurrently with inhalation injury. The approach to the patient with altered mental status and coma should include administration of hypertonic dextrose, thiamine and naloxone and work-up of other causes. Drug and ethanol intoxication should be excluded.

Until the carboxyhemoglobin fraction is known, all patients with a history of potential smoke inhalation should receive supplemental oxygen via high-flow, nonrebreather mask or endotracheal tube. Hyperbaric oxygen (HBO) therapy, if available, should be considered in patients with a history of loss of consciousness, coma, acute coronary syndrome, pregnancy, focal neurological deficits, or a carboxyhemoglobin fraction greater than 25% (see Chapter 306, "Carbon Monoxide"). Patients with low carboxyhemoglobin concentrations who do not meet any of these criteria, or those for whom hyperbaric therapy is not available or not a practical option as a result of hemodynamic instability or life-threatening injury, may be treated with 100% normobaric oxygen.

Treatment options for cyanide poisoning include oxygen administration and supportive care and administration of all or part of the Cyanide Antidote Kit (see Chapter 308, "Cyanide"). When oxygen transport is already compromised, as in a patient with concomitant carbon monoxide poisoning, further impairment by the inducement of methemoglobinemia may exacerbate cellular hypoxia. Sodium thiosulfate administration alone may enhance cyanide detoxification, and can safely be given even to the critically ill smoke inhalation victim with associated carbon monoxide toxicity. A reasonable approach in the smoke inhalation patient with suspected cyanide toxicity, particularly the seriously ill patient with a lactate level greater than 10 mmol/L refractory to resuscitation with i.v. fluids and oxygen supplementation, is to administer 12.5 g of sodium thiosulfate (50 mL of a 25% solution for adults, pediatric dose 1.65 mL/kg).

Symptomatic methemoglobinemia and/or concentrations greater than 20% to 30% should be treated with methylene blue (0.1–0.2 mL/kg of a 1% solution). A second dose of methylene blue may be required if no improvement is seen within 1 hour of administration and alternative diagnoses may need to be considered (see Chapter 315, "Methemoglobinemia").

CRITICAL INTERVENTIONS

- Perform endotracheal intubation in patients with oropharyngeal burns or edema, full-thickness circumferential neck burns, stridor, coma, or hypoxemia or respiratory distress unresponsive to oxygen administration
- Obtain a carboxyhemoglobin fraction, ABG, chest radiograph, and ECG and administer oxygen to patients with significant smoke exposure or respiratory symptoms

DISPOSITION

Indications for admission for observation and further treatment are listed in Table 316.4. Severity of illness and the presence of concomitant burns or traumatic injuries should guide the decision to admit to an intensive care unit, telemetry unit, or floor bed. Patients with carbon monoxide poisoning may require transfer for HBO therapy (see Chapter 306, "Carbon Monoxide"), and those with significant surface burns or physical injuries may require transfer to a burn or trauma center. Advanced life-support capability should be available during transfer.

Patients in good general health who are asymptomatic (on arrival or after a short period of oxygen therapy) and have a normal physical examination including pulse oximetry, arterial blood gas results (while breathing room air), ECG, chest radiograph, and carboxyhemoglobin level may be discharged. It is generally advised that these patients be observed for at least 3 or 4 hours before making a discharge disposition. Discharged patients should be instructed to return immediately if any respiratory symptoms develop. Scheduled follow-up at 24 hours may be prudent.

TABLE 316.4. Indications for Admission Following Smoke Inhalation

---

Facial or nasal burns
Persistent respiratory symptoms (including cough and chest tightness)
Crackles or wheezing on auscultation
Altered mental status
History of loss of consciousness
Abnormal ABG, CXR, or ECG
History of chronic cardiopulmonary disease

COMMON PITFALLS

✔ Failure to anticipate deterioration despite an initially normal initial physical examination, laboratory evaluation, and chest radiograph and to frequently re-evaluate the respiratory status

✔ Failure to evaluate and treat for coexisting carbon monoxide poisoning, drug or alcohol intoxication, traumatic injuries, and psychiatric problems

✔ Failure to give oxygen to all patients (including those with chronic obstructive pulmonary disease)

✔ Failure to fluid-resuscitate patients with trauma or surface burns for fear of exacerbating the edema of inhalation injury

✔ Failure to recognize the potential hazards of inappropriate corticosteroid, antibiotic, and cyanide antidote administration

Acknowledgment

The author thanks previous edition chapter author Christopher H. Linden.

References

1. Alarie Y. Toxicity of fire smoke. *Crit Rev Toxicol* 2002;32:259–89.
2. Anonymous. Trial in deadly cable car fire resumes in disarray. *Jefferson City News Tribune.* Jefferson City, Missouri. January 13, 2003.
3. Baud FJ, Barriot P, Toffis V, et al. Elevated blood cyanide concentrations in victims of smoke inhalation. *N Engl J Med* 1991;325:1761–66.
4. Balakrishnan C, Tijunelis AD, Gordon DM, et al. Burns and inhalation injury caused by steam. *Burns* 1996;22:313–5.
5. Barker SJ, Tremper KK. The effect of carbon monoxide inhalation on pulse oximetry and transcutaneous PO2. *Anesthesiology* 1987;66:677–9.
6. Bowes PC. Casualties attributed to toxic gas and smoke at fires: a survey of statistics. *Med Sci Law* 1976;16:104–10.
7. Birky MM, Clarke FB. Inhalation of toxic products from fires. *Bull NY Acad Med* 1981;57:997–1013.
8. Cahalane M, Demling RH. Early respiratory abnormalities from smoke inhalation. *JAMA* 1984;251:771–3.
9. Clark WR, Bonaventura M, Weyers W. Smoke inhalation and airway management at a regional burn unit: 1974–1983. *J Burn Care Rehabil* 1989;10:52–62.
10. Eisencraft JB. Pulse oximeter desaturation due to methemoglobinemia. *Anesthesiology* 1988;68:279–82.
11. Gill JR, Goldfeder LB, Stajic M. The happy land homicides: 87 deaths due to smoke inhalation. *J Forensic Sci* 2003;48:161–3.
12. Gregory KL, Malinoski VF, Sharp CR. Cleveland Clinic fire survivorship study 1929–1965. *Arch Environ Health* 1969;18:508–15.
13. Hartzell GE. Overview of combustion toxicology. *Toxicology* 1996;115:7–23.
14. Harwood B, Jall JR. What kills in fires: smoke inhalation or burns? *Fire J* 1989;84:29–34.
15. Herndon DN, Thompson PB, Traber DL. Pulmonary injury in burned patients. *Crit Care Med* 1985;1:79.
16. Hoffman RS, Sauter D. Methemoglobinemia resulting from smoke inhalation. *Vet Hum Toxicol* 1989;31:168–70.
17. Hsu EB, Grabowski JG, Chotani RA, et al. Effects on local emergency departments of large-scale urban chemical fire with hazardous materials spill. *Prehospital Disaster Med* 2002;17:196–201.
18. Lee MJ, O'Connell DJ. The plain chest radiograph after acute smoke inhalation. *Clin Radiol* 1988;39:33.
19. Moylan JA, Chan C. Inhalation injury—an increasing problem. *Ann Surg* 1977;188:34–7.
20. Miller K, Chang A. Acute inhalation injury. *Emerg Med Clin North Am* 2003;21:533–57.
21. Rocker GM. Acute respiratory distress syndrome: different syndromes, different therapies? *Crit Care Med* 2001;29:202–19.
22. Saffle JR, Davis B, Williams P, et al. Recent outcomes in the treatment of burn injury in the United States: a report from the American Burn Association Patient Registry. *J Burn Care Rehabil* 1994;16:219–32.
23. Sokal JA, Kralkowska E. The relationship between exposure duration, carboxyhemoglobin, blood glucose, pyruvate and lactate and the severity of intoxication in 39 cases of acute carbon monoxide poisoning in man. *Arch Toxicol* 1985;57:196–9.
24. Thompson PB, Herndon DN, Traber DL, et al. Effects on mortality of inhalation injury. *J Trauma* 1986;26:163–65.

Psychotherapeutic Agents and Related Conditions

CHAPTER 317
Antipsychotic Agents

Christopher H. Linden

Neuroleptics, also known as antipsychotic agents and major tranquilizers, are used to treat schizophrenia, the manic phase of bipolar disorders, and agitated behavior. They are also used for nausea, vomiting, sedation, hiccoughs, and tics. The older or classic agents are mainly effective for treating the positive symptoms of schizophrenia (e.g., agitation, delusions, disorganized behavior, hallucinations), whereas the newer or atypical antipsychotic agents are also effective for treating negative symptoms (e.g., alogia, avolition, flattened affect, social withdrawal) and cognitive deficits (4,8). Whether the more costly atypical agents are more effective than traditional ones remains a matter of debate.

Neuroleptics are a structurally diverse group of compounds containing two to five aliphatic, aromatic, or heterocyclic rings (Table 317.1). Formulations include tablets, capsules, liquids, sustained-release preparations, suppositories, and injectable solutions. Their mechanism of action is complex and incompletely understood. Neuroleptics block α-adrenergic (α_1 and α_2), dopamine (primarily D_2, but also D_1 and D_4), histamine (H_1), muscarinic (primarily M_1), and serotoninergic (primarily $5-HT_{1A}$, $5-HT_{2A}$, and $5-HT_{1C}$) receptors (4,8). Antipsychotic activity, extrapyramidal effects, and the neuroleptic malignant syndrome (NMS) appear to result from interference with central nervous system (CNS) (cortical, limbic, basal ganglia) D_2 neurotransmission. Antiemetic activity and disordered temperature regulation and increased prolactin secretion also appear to result from inhibition of D_2 receptors (in the chemoreceptor trigger zone of the medulla and in the hypothalamus, respectively). Most neuroleptics are much more potent H_1 blockers than diphenhydramine. Anticholinergic (M_1) potency correlates directly with sedative activity and inversely with the incidence of extrapyramidal reactions. Chlorpromazine, chlorprothixene, and thioridazine have potent sedative effects, whereas fluphenazine, haloperidol, trifluoperazine, and triflupromazine are commonly associated with extrapyramidal side effects.

The atypical agents have lower and more selective (mesolimbic) D_2 potency and higher M1 and/or $5-HT_{2A}$ antagonist activity than the traditional agents (4,8). Although higher doses are required for antipsychotic effect, they are less likely to cause acute dystonia and tardive dyskinesia and have minimal or no effect on prolactin secretion. Only clozapine, olanzapine, and quetiapine have significant anticholinergic activity. Risperidone can cause extrapyramidal effects. For reasons that are unclear, all atypical antipsychotics can cause hyperglycemia. In 2003, the labeling of these agents was amended to include a black box warning regarding this effect and the recommendation that diabetics and those at risk for diabetes (e.g., obese patients and those with a family history of diabetes) be monitored for this complication at the start of therapy.

Hypotension and miosis appear to be as a result of peripheral α-adrenergic blockade and central effects. Hypotensive effects are primarily orthostatic and systolic in nature and tend to correlate in incidence and severity with sedative potency. Concomitant therapy with β agonists (e.g., epinephrine) or β blockers (e.g., propranolol) may result in severe hypotension. Neuroleptics, particularly chlorpromazine, clozapine, and loxatine, lower the seizure threshold and can induce epileptiform encephalogram (EEG) discharge patterns, possibly because of inhibition of γ-aminobutyric acid receptors or norepinephrine reuptake.

Neuroleptics also have a variety of dose-related effects on excitable membrane ion channels (4,6–8,11). Phenothiazines, particularly chlorpromazine, thioridazine and its metabolite mesoridazine, block both voltage- and frequency-dependent sodium channels and have local anesthetic and quinidine-like (class 1a) antidysrhythmic, negative dromotropic, and myocardial depressant effects. These effects are potentiated by the tachycardia that results from cholinergic receptor antagonism and include delayed depolarization with conduction disturbances, most notably QRS prolongation. Droperidol, haloperidol, sertindole (Serlect), thioridazine, most atypical antipsychotics, and probably other neuroleptics block delayed rectifier, voltage-gated potassium channels resulting in delayed repolarization with JT interval prolongation. Electrocardiogram (ECG) changes such as prolonged P-R and Q-T intervals, ST-segment depression, T-wave abnormalities (biphasic, blunting, inversion, notching, widening), and increased U waves may be seen with both therapeutic and excessive doses (6). QT prolongation is usually as a result of an increased JT interval rather than to QRS prolongation. In 2001, reports of QT prolongation leading to torsades de pointes (polymorphic) ventricular tachycardia (VT) and death associated

TABLE 317.1.   Neuroleptic Agents

Structural Class	Generic Name	Trade Name	Oral Dose (Adult, mg)
Traditional Antipsychotics			
Benzamide	Trimethobenzamide	Tigan	250–300
Butyrophenone	Droperidol	Inapsine	2.5–10.0[c]
	Haloperidol	Haldol	0.5–2.0
Dibenzoxazepine	Loxapine	Loxitane	10–50
Diphenylbutylpiperidine	Pimozide	Orap	0.5–1
Indole	Molindone	Moban	5–25
Phenothiazine	Chlorpromazine	Thorazine	25–50
	Fluphenazine	Prolixin	2.5–10
	Mesoridazine	Serentil	25–100
	Perphenazine	Trilafon	4–16
	Prochlorperazine	Compazine	5–10
	Promazine	Sparine	25–100
	Promethazine[a]	Phenergan	25–50
	Thiethylperazine[a]	Torecan	10–30
	Thioridazine	Mellaril	25–100
	Trifluoperazine	Stelazine	2–5
	Triflupromazine	Vesprin	5–15[c]
	Trimeprazine[b]	Temaril	2.5
Thioxanthene	Chlorprothixene	Taractan	25–50
	Thiothixene	Navane	2–15
Atypical Antipsychotics[d]			
Benzisoxazole	Risperidone	Risperdal	1–3
Dibenzodiazepine	Clozapine	Clozaril	200–600
Dibenzothiazepine	Quetiapine	Seroquel	50–250
Piperazine	Ziprasidone	Geodon	20–80
Quinolone	Aripiprazole	Abilify	5–30
Thienobenzodiazepine	Olanzapine	Zyprexa	10–15

[a]Used only as antiemetic.
[b]Used only as antipruritic.
[c]Parenteral dose.
[d]Atypical agents available outside the United States include raclopride, remoxipride, sertindole, sulpiride, and ziprasidone.

with the i.v. administration of droperidol prompted a black box warning that an ECG be obtained prior to its use, that it not be given to those with QT prolongation (> 440 msec in males and 450 msec in females), and that cardiac monitoring be performed during and for 2 to 3 hours after its use. The reasonableness and necessity of these recommendations remains highly controversial. Haloperidol, pimozide, thioridazine, mesoridazine, and possibly other agents also block calcium channels. Ventricular dysrhythmias or asphyxia as a result of aspiration or respiratory depression resulting from seizures have been postulated as the cause of sudden death in patients taking therapeutic doses of neuroleptics, particularly phenothiazines (12,21).

Gastrointestinal (GI) absorption is relatively slow and unpredictable, with peak levels occurring 2 to 4 hours after ingestion. Bioavailability after parenteral administration is two to ten times greater than with oral dosing because presystemic (GI and hepatic) metabolism occurs following ingestion. Hence, therapeutic i.v. or i.m. doses are substantially less than oral ones. Neuroleptics are highly bound to plasma proteins (90%–99%). Because they are highly lipophilic, volumes of distribution are large (10–40 L/kg), therapeutic serum levels are low (1 to several hundred ng/mL), and drug accumulates in the brain and fat and readily crosses the placenta.

The neuroleptic dose–response curve is relatively flat. Hence, therapeutic doses vary widely (see Table 317.1) and are adjusted on the basis of clinical response and side effects, not by monitoring drug levels. Pharmacologic effects generally last 24 hours or more, allowing once-a-day dosing. Elimination oc-

curs slowly by hepatic metabolism, with serum concentration half-lives averaging 20 to 40 hours. Small amounts (1%–3%) are excreted unchanged by the kidney. As a rule, hepatic metabolism yields multiple metabolites, some of which are pharmacologically active (e.g., mesoridazine is an active metabolite of thioridazine). Metabolites are eliminated by urinary and, to some extent, by biliary excretion and can be detected in the urine for a month or more after cessation of chronic therapy. Concomitant use of agents that inhibit or stimulate hepatic cytochrome oxidases (CYP isoenzymes) can increase or decrease, respectively, the blood level and effect of these agents (4,8). Toxic effects result from exaggerated pharmacologic activity. Poisoning may result from accidental or intentional overdosage. It has also been reported in infants treated with topical promethazine cream (21). Side effects of therapeutic doses include the anticholinergic syndrome (see Chapter 323, "Anticholinergic Agents"), extrapyramidal syndromes, the NMS, hypotension, and sedation (4,8). Clozapine can cause agranulocytosis, myocarditis, and cardiomyopathy.

Antipsychotic agents have a high therapeutic index. Of the thousands of overdoses reported each year, only 1% to 2% of patients develop serious toxicity; only about 1 in 50 overdoses proves fatal. Thioridazine (because of its tricyclic antidepressant–like cardiotoxicity) or mixed overdoses are involved in most successful suicides (4,6–8,21). Toxic doses are not well established. In general, acute ingestion of the maximal therapeutic will result in significant side effects, particularly in a nontolerant person, and ingestion of five to ten times this amount can result in serious toxicity in adults and potentially fatal poisoning in a child. Many patients, however, have survived much larger ingestions.

CLINICAL PRESENTATION

Although nausea and vomiting may develop soon after acute overdose, CNS depression and cardiovascular (CV) effects dominate the clinical picture (1,3,5–9,11,13,17,18,21,25). Manifestations of mild poisoning include ataxia, confusion, lethargy, slurred speech, tachycardia, and diastolic or orthostatic hypotension. Miosis is common but mydriasis can also occur. Anticholinergic signs and symptoms (Chapter 323, "Anticholinergic Agents") and hyperreflexia may be present. Prolonged P-R and Q-T intervals and nonspecific ST-segment, T-wave, and U-wave abnormalities (see Introduction) may be seen, particularly with sertindole, thioridazine and mesoridazine.

Moderate poisoning is characterized by low-grade coma (responsive to voice or tactile stimulation), with or without respiratory depression, and systolic hypotension accompanied reflex tachycardia. Hypothermia (occasional) and hyperthermia (rare) may be present. Paradoxical agitation, delirium, and tachypnea have been reported. Sialorrhea may be seen following clozapine overdose.

In severe poisoning, deep coma with loss of brainstem and deep tendon reflexes, apnea, hypotension, tachycardia and cardiac dysrhythmias (especially with thioridazine and mesoridazine) are seen. Bradyarrhythmias include all degrees of atrioventricular block, bundle-branch block, QRS widening, and asystole. Tachyarrhythmias include ventricular premature beats, VT and fibrillation, and polymorphic VT (torsades de pointes). Cardiac conduction delays and tachyarrhythmias are common in thioridazine and mesoridazine poisoning. Q-T interval prolongation and torsades de pointes have also been reported after haloperidol, loxapine, phenothiazine, pimozide quetiapine, risperidone, sertindole, and ziprasidone overdose, and during high-dose intravenous droperidol and haloperidol therapy (20,24). Pulmonary edema can occur (14). Seizures are rare, except with loxapine, which can cause severe, prolonged convulsions, leading to rhabdomyolysis and subsequent renal failure (19).

The onset of poisoning occurs within 1 to 2 hours of acute ingestion, with maximal severity usually apparent in 2 to 6 hours. The presentation is the same regardless of age and whether the overdose is acute or chronic. Children appear more susceptible to toxicity than adults. Recovery can be expected within several hours to several days, depending on the severity. The mortality rate from acute poisoning is less than 1%.

Extrapyramidal side effects may occur early (within days), or late (after 3 months) after beginning neuroleptic therapy, increasing the dose, or changing the agent (4). Dyskinesia or acute dystonic reactions (see Chapter 319, "Dystonic Reactions"), akathisia, the NMS, and parkinsonism (see Chapter 119, "Parkinsonism and Other Movement Disorders") occur early whereas tardive dyskinesia or dystonia, and the "rabbit syndrome" occur late. These idiosyncratic reactions are most common with older high-potency agents. Akathisia, a subjective sensation of motor restlessness, occurs in about 20% of patients treated with traditional neuroleptics and is sometimes associated with severe parkinsonism (see Chapter 119, "Parkinsonism and Other Movement Disorders"). Transient akathisia has been observed in up to 50% of those treated with intravenous droperidol or prochlorperazine for headache, nausea, and vomiting. Women are affected more often than men. Patients complain of feeling restless, jittery, and tense; they cannot sit or stand still, and when standing may shift their weight from foot to foot as if walking in place. Vital signs remain normal. Semi-purposeful or purposeless limb movements (especially of the lower extremities), frequent shifting of body position, and tremors, and myoclonic jerking may be noted. Rabbit syndrome, also known as focal perioral tremor, is a rhythmic vertical motion of the mouth and lips, resembling the chewing movements of a rabbit. In contrast to oral tardive dyskinesia, tongue movements do not occur in rabbit syndrome.

The NMS can be precipitated by intercurrent illness, surgery, dehydration, heat stress, acute agitation, and, very rarely, by acute overdose (2,10,16). It is estimated to occur in about 1% of patients treated with neuroleptics for psychiatric conditions, and appears to be more common with parental therapy and in those with bipolar disorder, dementia, and concurrent treatment with lithium and anticholinergic agents (e.g., benztropine). The NMS is characterized by fever (> 38°C or 100.4°F), altered mental status, autonomic dysfunction, increased motor activity, and laboratory abnormalities. Mental status changes range from confusion and delirium to coma. Awake patients may be mute. Seizures are rare. Autonomic disturbances include hypertension (> 150/100 mm Hg; diastolic or systolic blood pressure increased 20 or 30 mm Hg above baseline, respectively), tachycardia (heart rate > 90–100 or increased by 30/min), increased respiratory rate (alternatively dyspnea, hypoxemia, of respiratory failure), diaphoresis (often profuse), and incontinence. Increased salivation and drooling may be seen. Hypotension, rather than hypertension, sometimes occurs. Although "lead pipe" rigidity is the classic motor finding, lesser increases in muscle tone, akinesia, dystonia, dyskinesia, tremor, choreiform movements, opisthotonus, and parkinsonism (cogwheel rigidity) may be present. Hyperactivity of pharyngeal muscles may result in dysarthria, dysphagia, dysphonia, and trismus. Laboratory abnormalities include leukocytosis (WBC > 14,000/mm³ without a left shift), rhabdomyolysis (CPK > 500 IU/ml or 3 × normal), and decreased serum iron (< 60 ug/dl or 10 umol/L). Markedly elevated WBCs and CPKs are not uncommon. Hyponatremia, hypernatremia, hypokalemia, and SIADH may be present. Onset is typically insidious and resolution occurs slowly, sometimes taking up to 2 weeks. Complications include aspiration pneumonia and other infections, coagulopathy, renal failure and metabolic disturbances from rhabdomyolysis, myocardial infarction, heart failure, dysrhythmias, and venous thromboembolism. The mortality rate ranges from 12% to 20% and is primarily related to complications. Sequelae include dysarthria, dysphagia, myoclonus, and weakness.

DIFFERENTIAL DIAGNOSIS

Antidysrhythmic, anticholinergic, anticonvulsant, opioid, and sedative–hypnotic overdose may cause CNS or CV effects similar to those seen in neuroleptic poisoning. The veterinary tranquilizer xylazine also has similar toxicity. It may be impossible to distinguish tricyclic antidepressant from neuroleptic poisoning, particularly that as a result of thioridazine or mesoridazine, without toxicology testing. Of note in this regard, quetiapine, in therapeutic as well as overdose amounts, can cause a false positive result on tricyclic antidepressant immunoassays. CNS infection, infarction, and trauma should also be considered in the differential diagnosis of neuroleptic poisoning.

Akathisia may be misdiagnosed as anxiety or agitation related to an underlying psychiatric disorder. Other causes of the NMS include beginning or increasing therapy with non-neuroleptic dopamine antagonists (e.g., hydroxyzine, metoclopramide, reserpine) or other, possibly synergistic, psychotherapeutic agents (e.g., benzodiazepines, carbamazepine, lithium, monoamine oxidase inhibitors, phenytoin, tricyclic antidepressants), and discontinuing or decreasing therapy with a dopamine agonist (e.g., amantadine, bromocriptine, carbidopa, levodopa, lithium, pergolide, pramipexole, ropinirole) or an inhibitor of its metabolism (e.g., catechol-o-methyltransferase inhibitors such as entacapone and tolcapone). The differential diagnosis of the NMS also includes dystonic reactions, lithium, monoamine oxidase inhibitor, salicylate, stimulant, and strychnine poisoning, heat stroke, malignant (lethal) catatonia, malignant hyperthermia (MH), encephalitis, meningitis, and systemic infection, pheochromocytoma, serotonin syndrome (SS), tetanus, thyrotoxicosis, and withdrawal states.

Distinguishing the NMS from MH and the SS (see Chapter 322, "Serotonin Re-uptake Inhibitors") is particularly difficult. Because clinical features are almost identical, the diagnosis relies primarily on the drug exposure history. Onset after general anesthesia or ketamine administration implicates MH but psychiatric patients are often on multiple medications which have both dopaminergic and serotonergic effects. The SS begins more abruptly and resolves more quickly than the NMS (over hours rather than days), neuromuscular hyperactivity is less sustained than in NMS, and myoclonus, hyperreflexia, and shivering, which are rare in NMS, are often present.

And finally, although specific criteria have been proposed for the diagnosis of the NMS, the required elements are not universally agreed on, and patients can have the NMS without manifesting a classic or characteristic feature (e.g., fever or rigidity). Diagnosing the NMS in patients with attenuated forms (forme frustes) of NMS relies primarily on the history (antecedent setting and drug exposure).

EMERGENCY DEPARTMENT EVALUATION

A complete history should be obtained from the patient and, to corroborate the patient's history, from the person who either found or brought the patient to the emergency department. The name, quantity, and time of ingestion should be determined. In patients taking neuroleptics for therapeutic purposes, determining whether there was a recent medication or dosage change, illness, or surgery is important.

The physical examination should focus on the vital signs, CV system, and neurologic function. An initial rhythm strip and subsequent 12-lead ECG should be evaluated. Arterial blood gas analysis and a chest radiograph should be ordered in patients with severe poisoning. Because phenothiazines can be radiopaque, abdominal radiographs may be useful if the identity of the overdose agent is unknown. However, the lack of x-ray visualization does not rule out an ingestion and does not necessarily imply successful gastric decontamination. Routine laboratory evaluation should include a complete blood count and measurements of electrolytes, blood urea nitrogen, creatinine, and glucose to rule out concomitant abnormalities. In patients with seizures or hyperthermia, the laboratory evaluation should also include urinalysis (routine and for myoglobin); measurement of serum muscle enzymes (creatine phosphokinase, aldolase, alkaline phosphatase), calcium, magnesium, and phosphate; and a coagulation profile. Toxicologic analysis of the urine and serum by chromatography or immunoassay may be useful to confirm the identity of the agent and rule out other ingestants. Quantitative drug levels are not helpful in predicting clinical toxicity or in guiding treatment. Although neither sensitive nor specific, the Forest, Mason, and Phenistix colorimetric urine tests may be positive with phenothiazine ingestions and can be used to rapidly screen for these agents.

EMERGENCY DEPARTMENT MANAGEMENT

As always, supportive care is the top priority and mainstay of treatment. The tempo and sequence of interventions depend on clinical severity. Advanced life-support measures should be instituted as necessary. All patients require cardiac and respiratory monitoring and intravenous access. Those with hyperthermia or hypothermia should have continuous (rectal or axillary probe) temperature monitoring. Patients with altered mental status or seizures should receive supplemental oxygen and empiric therapy with naloxone, dextrose (or a rapid fingerstick glucose determination), and thiamine. Endotracheal intubation may be required for respiratory or CNS depression. Because succinylcholine (and other depolarizing neuromuscular blockers) can cause MH, using only a nondepolarizing agent such as pancuronium (0.06 to 0.1 mg/kg i.v.) or vecuronium (0.08 to 0.1 mg/kg i.v.) has been recommended. Although the manifestations of MH and NMS are similar, the underlying pathophysiology is different and there is no clinical data to support this recommendation.

Hypotension should initially be treated with intravenous crystalloids. Norepinephrine and high-dose dopamine are the drugs of choice for refractory hypotension. Unstable tachyarrhythmias should be treated with electrical cardioversion (15). Unsynchronized defibrillation should be used for ventricular fibrillation and nonperfusing monomorphic or polymorphic VT. Stable VT can be treated with lidocaine or amiodarone. If the QRS complex is wide prior to onset or after termination, sodium bicarbonate (1 mEq/kg intravenously) may be effective (see Chapter 300, "Antidysrhythmic Drugs and Local Anesthetics," and Chapter 318, "Cyclic Antidepressants"). Type Ia (disopyramide, quinidine, procainamide) and II (β blockers) antidysrhythmic drugs should be avoided. If the QT interval (specifically the JT portion) was or is prolonged or torsades de pointes is observed, magnesium (50–100 mg/kg i.v. over 1 hour) or overdrive pacing using isoproterenol or electricity are preferred. Increasing the heart rate shortens the Q-T interval and is recommended for preventing the recurrence of torsades de pointes. β blockers (e.g., esmolol, propranolol), which inhibit the afterdepolarizations that can trigger this dysrhythmia have also been used as preventive therapy. Hypotension may complicate isoproterenol therapy. Bradyarrhythmias should be treated according to current Advanced Cardiac Life Support (ACLS) protocols. Complete heart block may require temporary cardiac pacing. Underlying metabolic abnormalities should be corrected.

Seizures should be treated with incremental doses of lorazepam (initial dose 0.05 mg/kg i.v.) or diazepam (initial dose 0.1 mg/kg i.v.), followed by a loading dose of phenytoin (18 mg/kg i.v.; maximal rate, 50 mg/min) and then a barbiturate (e.g., amobarbital 10 to 15 mg/kg i.v., maximal rate 100 mg/min; or phenobarbital 20 mg/kg i.v., maximal rate 30 mg/min), if necessary. Refractory convulsions may require a pharmacological paralysis prevent complications such as hyperthermia and rhabdomyolysis. Treatment of seizures, as indicated by continuous or serial EEG monitoring, should be continued during the period of paralysis. Diuresis and alkalinization of the urine may prevent myoglobinuric renal failure in patients with rhabdomyolysis. Physostigmine can be given to control agitation and delirium as a result of the anticholinergic syndrome if cardiac conduction intervals are normal (see Chapter 323, "Anticholinergic Agents").

Muscular hyperactivity and hyperthermia in patients with the NMS is treated similarly, initially with benzodiazepines, therapeutic paralysis for refractory cases, and alkaline diuresis for patients with rhabdomyolysis (10,16). Early and aggressive treatment appears to improve outcome. The dopamine agonists bromocriptine (5 mg p.o. q.i.d.), amantadine (100 mg p.o. b.i.d.), and carbidopa/levodopa (25/100 mg, 1–2 tablets p.o. q.i.d.) are theoretically attractive and can also be given. Because their onset of action is slow (up to 3 days), they should be used as adjunctive rather than primary therapy (23). In contrast, although dantrolene (2.5–10 mg i.v., repeated as necessary, up to four times a day) has been used with success to treat the NMS, there is no clinical data or theoretical reason suggesting that it is better than any other skeletal muscle relaxant. Although the release of calcium from endoplasmic reticulum is involved in the pathogenesis of MH and inhibited by dantrolene, it does not cause or contribute to the NMS. Cooling blankets, ice packs, and evaporative cooling methods should also be applied to patients with hyperthermia. Antipyretics are unlikely to be effective. Obviously, neuroleptic therapy must be discontinued.

After stabilization, treatment should focus on GI decontamination in cases of acute oral overdosage. Activated charcoal and gastric lavage are preferred. Drug-induced decreased GI motility may allow for effective decontamination many hours after the overdose. Measures to enhance the elimination of neuroleptic agents, such as diuresis, dialysis, and hemoperfusion, have not been shown to be effective. Repeated oral doses of activated charcoal are of potential but unproven benefit.

Patients with extrapyramidal syndromes who require continued neuroleptic therapy can be managed by reducing the dose, switching to an agent of lower potency, or giving an anticholinergic agent (e.g. benztropine or diphenhydramine). Benzodiazepines, clonidine, propranolol, and short-acting barbiturates have been used with moderate success. These syndromes do not respond to treatment with dopamine agonists. Patients who develop akathisia after a single therapeutic dose of neuroleptic (e.g., for migraine or vomiting) should be reassured that symptoms will resolve within 24 hours. Pretreatment with diphenhydramine may prevent this complication.

CRITICAL INTERVENTIONS

- Establish intravenous access, institute cardiac monitoring, obtain an ECG, and frequently re-evaluate the vital signs and clinical status of patients with actual or potential neuroleptic poisoning
- Treat hyperthermia, muscle hyperactivity, and seizures aggressively with benzodiazepines, therapeutic paralysis for refractory cases, physical cooling measures for hyperthermia, and alkaline diuresis for rhabdomyolysis
- Administer sodium bicarbonate to patients with monomorphic VT refractory to lidocaine
- Administer magnesium and isoproterenol or overdrive pacing to patients with torsades de pointes refractory to lidocaine

DISPOSITION

Physicians unfamiliar with the details of the evaluation and management of neuroleptic poisoning or the NMS should consult a poison center or toxicologist for advice. Asymptomatic patients with an acute overdose should be observed for 6 hours. Symptomatic patients should be observed until alert. Those with significant CNS depression, hypotension, seizures, or dysrhythmias should be admitted to an intensive care unit (ICU) or a similarly equipped observation area. Alert patients with a history of overdose and abnormal ECG findings present a difficult disposition problem, because ECG abnormalities can be seen with therapeutic doses, yet they have been implicated as a cause of sudden death. It seems safest to admit these patients for 24 hours of cardiac monitoring.

Except for NMS, extrapyramidal syndromes, although worrisome to the patient, are not life-threatening and do not require admission. Medication adjustment may be appropriate but this should be done in consultation with the patient's psychiatrist. Patients with NMS require ICU admission. Patients requiring transfer to a facility capable of providing intensive care should be accompanied by advanced life-support personnel and should have cardiac monitoring en route.

COMMON PITFALLS

- ✔ Failure to appreciate that neuroleptics can prolong the prolonged QRS, JT, and QT intervals cause cardiac dysrhythmias
- ✔ Failure to appreciate that atypical antipsychotics, although less likely to cause extrapyramidal side effects than traditional agents, are more sedating and cause similar CV toxicity
- ✔ Failure to appreciate that loxapine can cause intractable seizures leading to rhabdomyolysis and renal failure
- ✔ Failure to appreciate that attenuated forms of the NMS can occur and to discontinue neuroleptic therapy in patients with any manifestation of NMS
- ✔ Failure to obtain an accurate temperature and CPK in patients with suspected NMS (altered mental status, autonomic dysfunction and muscle hyperactivity)
- ✔ Failure to appreciate that dopamine agonists are not as effective as routine supportive measures in the treatment of the NMS

References

1. Acri AA, Henretig FM. Effects of risperidone in overdose. *Am J Emerg Med* 1998;16:498.
2. Baker PB, Merfian KS, Roberts JR, et al. Hyperthermia, hypertension, hypertonia, and coma in a massive thioridazine overdose. *Am J Emerg Med* 1988;6:346.
3. Balit CR, Isbister GK, Hackett LP, et al. Quetiapine poisoning: a case series. *Ann Emerg Med* 2003;42:751–758.
4. Baldessarini RJ, Tarazi FI. Drugs and the treatment of psychiatric disorders: psychosis and mania. In: Hardman JG, Limbird LE, Gilman AG, eds. *Goodman & Gilman's the pharmacological basis of therapeutics*, 10th ed. New York: McGraw-Hill, 2001:485.
5. Biswas AK, Zabrocki LA, Mayes KL, et al. Cardiotoxicity associated with intentional ziprasidone and bupropion overdose. *J Toxicol Clin Toxicol* 2003;4:101–104.
6. Buckley NA, White IM, Dawson AH. Cardiotoxicity more common in thioridazine overdose than with other neuroleptics. *J Toxicol Clin Toxicol* 1995;33:199.
7. Buckley NA, Sanders P. Cardiovascular adverse effects of antipsychotic drugs. *Drug Saf* 2000;23:215–228.
8. Burns MJ. The pharmacology and toxicology of atypical antipsychotic agents. *J Tox Clin Toxicol* 2001;39:1.
9. Capel MM, Colbridge MG, Henry JA. Overdose profiles of new antipsychotic agents. *Int J Neuropsychopharmacol* 2000;3:51–54.
10. Carbone JR. The neuroleptic malignant and serotonin syndromes. *Emerg Med Clin North Am* 2000;18:317.
11. Elkayan U, Frishman W. Cardiovascular effects of phenothiazines. *Am Heart J* 1980;100:397.
12. Haddad PM, Anderson IM. Antipsychotic-related QTc prolongation, torsade de pointes and sudden death. *Drugs* 2002;62:1649.
13. LeBlaye I, Donatoni B, Hall M, et al. Acute overdosage with clozapine: a review of the available clinical experience. *Pharm Med* 1992;6:169.
14. Li C, Gefter WB. Acute pulmonary edema induced by overdose of phenothiazines. *Chest* 1992;101:102.
15. Nelson LS. Toxicological myocardial sensitization. *J Toxicol Clin Toxicol* 2002;40:867.
16. Nierenberg D, Disch M, Manheimer E, et al. Facilitating prompt diagnosis and treatment of the neuroleptic malignant syndrome. *Clin Pharmacol Ther* 1991;50 (5 Pt 1):580.
17. O'Malley GF, Seifert S, Heard K, et al. Olanzepine overdose mimicking opioid intoxication. *Ann Emerg Med* 1999;34:279.
18. Palenzona S, Meier PJ, Kupferschmidt H, et al. The clinical picture of olanzapine poisoning with special reference to fluctuating mental status. *J Toxicol Clin Toxicol* 2004;42:27.
19. Peterson C. Seizures induced by acute loxapine overdose. *Am J Psychiatry* 1981;138:1089.
20. Richards JR, Schnier AB. Droperidol in the emergency department: is it safe? *J Emerg Med* 2003;24:441.
21. Shawn DH, McGuigan MA. Poisoning from dermal absorption of promethazine. *Can Med Assoc J* 1984;130:1460.
22. Trenton A, Currier G, Zwemer F. Fatalities associated with therapeutic use and overdose of atypical antipsychotics. *CNS Drugs* 2003;17:307.
23. Ward A Chafman MO, Sorkin EM. Dantrolene: a review of pharmacodynamic and pharmacokinetic properties and therapeutic use in malignant hyperthermia, the antipsychotic malignant syndrome, and an update of its use in muscle spasticity. *Drugs* 1986;32:130.
24. Wilt JL, Minnema AM, Johnson RF, et al. Torsade de pointes associated with the use of intravenous haloperidol. *Ann Intern Med* 1993;119:391.
25. Zaratzian VL. Psychotropic drugs—neurotoxicity. *J Toxicol Clin Toxicol* 1980;17:231.

CHAPTER 318
Cyclic Antidepressants

Keith K. Burkhart

The availability of cyclic antidepressants (CAs) has provided a major therapeutic adjunct for the successful treatment of depression since the 1950s. Additional therapeutic use has included attention deficit disorder, anorexia nervosa, obsessive-compulsive disorder, phobias, chronic pain syndromes, migraine headaches, enuresis, and peptic ulcer disease. The term, cyclic antidepressants, refers to a family of drugs that have similar pharmacology and toxicity (Table 318.1). Serious CA poisoning continues to account for significant numbers of intensive care unit (ICU) admissions (6,8). In a pediatric series many of the CA cases resulted from therapeutic misadventures either taking extra pills or a teenage friend loaning some medication for a headache (6). A child who presented with ten seizure admissions was recently reported to be a case of Munchausen by proxy (19). In the 1980s another group of antidepressants, the selective serotonin reuptake inhibitors (SSRIs, see Chapter 322, "Serotonin Re-uptake Inhibitors"), was introduced. This class of antidepressants offers a wider margin of safety, with less central nervous system (CNS) and cardiovascular (CV) toxicity, compared with the CAs (8). During the 1990s and 2000s the atypical antipsychotic agents (see Chapter 317, "Antipsychotic Agents") have grown in popularity. This class of drugs is also being used to treat depression, especially in association with psychotic disorders. The toxicity profile of the atypical antipsychotics is not uniform, because of differing pharmacological actions within the class, but shares many aspects that resemble CA poisoning, including coma, tachycardia, delirium, QTc prolongation, and cardiac dysrhythmias. Even with these alternative drug classes, CAs are still commonly used and hundreds of CA deaths still occur every year in the United States (15).

The pharmacologic properties of the CAs contribute to their toxicity in overdose. CAs are highly lipophilic, with large volumes of distribution (Vd = 10 to 50 L/kg), and are highly protein-bound (>95%). CAs typically manifest a rapid onset of toxicity, because they are rapidly absorbed and quickly distributed to the target organs. Most CAs are tertiary or secondary amines. Tertiary amines (e.g., amitriptyline and imipramine) are metabolized to their respective secondary amines (e.g., nortriptyline and desipramine), which are also active drugs. Tertiary amines block norepinephrine and serotonin reuptake, although secondary amines primarily block norepinephrine reuptake. Tertiary amines have more anticholinergic and antihistaminic effects than the secondary amines. CAs have half-lives greater than 24 hours. Early reports described delayed recovery from toxicity. Improved supportive care, including alkalinization therapy and the administration of activated charcoal (AC), is probably responsible for a better outcome today (11). Most CA-poisoned patients that are provided with good supportive care make a full recovery within one to three days.

Therapeutic doses of CAs are typically less than 5 mg/kg. Tolerance does develop in chronically dosed patients. Toxicity is generally seen with ingestion greater than 10 mg/kg, although greater than 15 mg/kg may result in severe, potentially fatal ingestions.

The CNS and CV toxicity of CAs result from their pharmacologic actions. These properties include quinidine-like cardiac conduction disturbances from sodium-channel blockade, initial sympathomimetic, and late sympatholytic actions resulting from the blockade of norepinephrine reuptake, and anticholinergic, antihistaminic, $GABA_A$ receptor channel, and α_1-adrenergic blocking properties. Some CAs produce predominantly CNS or cardiac toxicity. Amoxapine produces seizures, including status epilepticus, but cardiac conduction disturbances do not generally occur. The relative absence of quinidine-like effects, catecholamine reuptake blockade, and anticholinergic effects of the SSRIs is responsible for their increased margin of safety, although some of the atypical antipsychotics do have these actions and may produce similar toxicity to the CAs.

CLINICAL PRESENTATION

The presentation of CA poisoning may rapidly change from asymptomatic to cardiopulmonary arrest (7). An alert patient may become comatose, have seizures, or develop hemodynamic and cardiac instability within minutes. Although CA-induced seizures tend to be short-lived, they may deteriorate into status epilepticus (5,23). Status myoclonic activity is seen with severe poisoning. Patients may initially be tachycardic and mildly hypertensive (as a result of the blockade of norepinephrine reuptake and anticholinergic effects), or they may be hypotensive (from α_1 blockade). The metabolism of norepinephrine may lead to a catecholamine depletion state resulting in hypotension, bradycardia, and finally cardiogenic shock. Most patients recover in less than 24 hours with careful supportive care.

Cardiac dysrhythmias may include supraventricular tachydysrhythmias and ventricular dysrhythmias. Intraventricular

TABLE 318.1.   Antidepressant Agents

Class	Drug	Trade Name(s)
TRICYCLICS		
Tertiary Amines		
	Amitriptyline	Amitid, Amitril, Elavil, Endep, Etrafon, Triavil
	Clomipramine	Anafranil
	Doxepin	Adapin, Sinequan
	Imipramine	Janimine, Presamine, SK-Pramine, Tofranil
	Trimipramine	Surmontil
Secondary Amines		
	Desipramine	Norpramin, Pertofrane
	Nortriptyline	Aventyl, Pamelor
	Protriptyline	Vivactil
TETRACYCLICS		
	Maprotiline	Ludiomil
	Mianserin	Bolvidon, Norval
DIBENZOXAZEPINE		
	Amoxapine	Ascendin
SELECTIVE SEROTONIN REUPTAKE INIBITORS		
	Fluoxetine	Prozac
	Sertraline	Zoloft
	Paroxetine	Paxil
	Fluvoxamine	Lunox, Faverin, Celexa, Cipramil, Seropram
	Citalopram	
	Escitalopram	Lexapro, Cipralex

conduction disturbances often make it difficult to distinguish a ventricular tachycardia (VT) from a supraventricular tachycardia with aberrant conduction. Polymorphous VT (torsades de pointes) has also been reported. Aspiration pneumonia is relatively common in comatose patients, and adult respiratory distress syndrome may occur. Rhabdomyolysis and compartment syndrome are additional potential complications.

Patients with ingestions of less than 15 mg/kg may display a predominant anticholinergic syndrome without cardiac conduction effects. Anticholinergic effects can also occur during recovery from severe poisoning and may last for days. Typical signs and symptoms include absent bowel sounds, ileus, and urinary retention. Other anticholinergic effects, such as dilated pupils, flushed hot skin, and dry mucous membranes, however, are more variable. Central anticholinergic findings may vary from agitation to psychosis to coma. Additional neurologic manifestations include choreoathetosis, ataxia, myoclonus, status epilepticus, and coma.

DIFFERENTIAL DIAGNOSIS

The differential diagnosis of coma, seizures, and cardiac dysrhythmias includes hypoxia, metabolic abnormalities, and intrinsic neurologic and cardiac disease. Other drugs with toxicities that can appear similar to CAs include the antidysrhythmics, antihistamines, antimalarials, atypical antipsychotics, β-blockers, calcium channel blockers, carbamazepine, phenothiazines, and propoxyphene. Anticholinergic agents, camphor, cocaine, chloral hydrate, isoniazid, lithium, sympathomimetic poisoning and drug withdrawal should also be considered.

EMERGENCY DEPARTMENT EVALUATION

The history should be obtained from the patient, family, friends, or prehospital personnel. If possible, the time, amount, and identity of all agents ingested should be determined. When known, the amount of CA ingested often helps anticipate the potential for deterioration. The therapeutic dose of 5 mg/kg should be tolerated by all, including children (17). Observation without intervention would be the best approach for these patients. On the other hand, patients who ingest 15 mg/kg (roughly one gram for a 70 kg adult) have the potential for serious poisoning.

The physical examination should focus on the vital signs and CV, pulmonary, and neurological function. The potential for rapid deterioration requires that i.v. access and continuous cardiac and oxygenation monitoring be initiated immediately. Vital signs and neurologic status should initially be evaluated every 15 minutes, and a limb lead QRS duration (discussion follows) should be checked every 30 minutes.

Early into the evaluation, an electrocardiogram (ECG) should be performed. A QRS duration greater than 100 milliseconds is associated with seizures, although a QRS duration greater than 160 milliseconds is associated with ventricular dysrhythmias. Patients with a QRS duration greater than 120 msec who have a seizure are at great risk for rapid CV toxicity including CV collapse (23). More subtle, early ECG changes include a rightward axis of the terminal 40 milliseconds of the QRS in the frontal plane. This manifestation can be quickly assessed by looking for the presence of a widened S wave in leads 1 and aVL, and an R wave in lead aVR (Fig. 318.1). These terminal 40 millisecond changes are good indicators for sodium channel blockade, as seen with CA poisoning, but they do not absolutely confirm or exclude the diagnosis (25).

Other than a lactic acidosis secondary to seizures or shock, CAs are not known to produce biochemical disturbances. How-

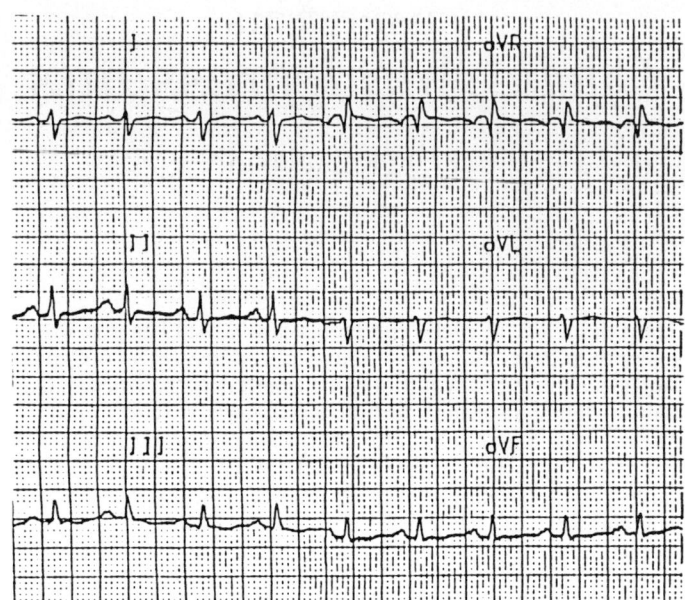

Figure 318.1.   Terminal QRS changes in CA poisoning.

ever, evaluation of patients with altered mental status or cardiotoxicity includes assessment of serum electrolytes, blood urea nitrogen, creatinine, and glucose; a serum osmolality should also be obtained in patients with metabolic acidosis. An arterial blood gas, creatine phosphokinase, calcium, magnesium, phosphorus, liver chemistries, and a chest radiograph should be considered for patients with abnormal vital signs, significant CNS depression, seizures, or an abnormal ECG.

Drug screening for CAs has very little impact on the management of the CA-poisoned patient. Qualitative screens may identify the presence of CAs in urine, although quantitative screens provide drug levels. Although serum levels greater than 1,000 ng/mL generally correlate with significant toxicity, levels do not assist in emergency management. Monitoring the changes on the ECG and the patient's mental status are more clinically useful indicators of ongoing CA toxicity.

EMERGENCY DEPARTMENT MANAGEMENT

Prehospital care for patients with coma, seizures, hypotension, and dysrhythmias includes endotracheal intubation, administration of anticonvulsants, intravenous crystalloids, and serum alkalinization with parenteral sodium bicarbonate boluses. Most, but not all paramedic training programs have lecture time dedicated to CA poisoning (4).

Parenteral benzodiazepines such as diazepam or midazolam (5–10 mg), or lorazepam (2–4 mg) are the agents of choice for the prevention and treatment of seizures. They should be administered to any patient with severe poisoning. Repeat doses may be required. When intubation is required, parenteral benzodiazepines may be useful for sedative and anticonvulsant effects. If benzodiazepines do not completely control seizures, phenobarbital or propofol should be considered (18). Phenobarbital or propofol may be necessary for the treatment of myoclonus. In the intubated patient, a phenobarbital loading dose of 18 mg/kg is usually sufficient. The dose for propofol sedation of the intubated patient begins with a bolus infusion of 0.3 mg/kg. The dose is titrated to the desired sedation level in increments of 0.3 to 0.6 mg/kg/hr every 5 to 10 minutes. Propofol's rapid onset and offset make it ideal for the management of these ventilated CA-poisoned patients. Seizures will rapidly produce a lactic acidosis that may further compromise the cardiac and hemodynamic status (23). Hence, an i.v. bolus of 1 to 2 ampules (44–100 mEq) of hypertonic sodium bicarbonate is recommended as adjunctive treatment for seizures. Neuromuscular paralysis with a short-acting agent should be considered for neuromuscular toxicity that does not respond to the above treatment.

Hypotension should be treated with intravenous crystalloid boluses up to 20 mL/kg. This treatment should overcome hypotension secondary to α-adrenergic blockade and mild dehydration. For more seriously poisoned patients, vasopressors may be needed. Dopamine and norepinephrine have been used successfully; however, some cases have been refractory to dopamine. Because dopamine partially acts as an indirect sympathomimetic agent, causing catecholamine release from sympathetic nerve terminals, it may lose some of its effectiveness when norepinephrine stores are depleted following CA poisoning. High infusion rates of dopamine may be tried initially. The dose should be greater than or equal to 10 μg/kg/min, to provide direct α-adrenergic agonism. Lower doses of dopamine have relatively more β-adrenergic effects that could cause vasodilation and actually worsen hypotension. If there is an inadequate response, norepinephrine should be given (substituted for or added to dopamine). Patients usually respond to low infusion rates of 1 μg/kg/min. In patients unresponsive to these measures, the insertion of a pulmonary artery catheter may be useful to guide additional fluid and vasopressor management.

Cardiac dysrhythmias can be terminated with the administration of sodium bicarbonate (20). Many reports have described the important role for serum alkalinization therapy in the management of CA poisoning. Sodium and bicarbonate have proven to be beneficial treatments for toxins that have quinidine-like, sodium-channel blocking actions. In experimental models of amitriptyline toxicity, sodium loading and pH elevation improved cardiac conduction, but both treatments together produced the greatest improvement (20,21). The use of hypertonic saline, 7.5% in dextran, without bicarbonate in a swine model has also been shown to dramatically elevate blood pressure and narrow the QRS interval following nortriptyline poisoning (16). The use of hypertonic saline has not gained widespread popularity as a clinical practice standard, however. The use of sodium bicarbonate boluses and normal saline infusions are usually sufficient. In fact these therapies require careful monitoring as they have resulted in patients developing severe hypernatremia and alkalemia. In refractory ventricular dysrhythmias, lidocaine and phenytoin should be considered, but type 1A antidysrhythmics, such as procainamide, and β-blockers, should be avoided.

Dysrhythmias should be treated with at least one or two ampules (44–100 mEq) of sodium bicarbonate (1 mEq/kg for pediatric patients). Sodium bicarbonate has acutely terminated VT and wide complex tachycardia. The QRS duration shortens, and the terminal 40-millisecond changes become less evident (11). Respiratory alkalosis is advocated by many clinicians, but the pH elevation is not as instantaneous as with bolus bicarbonate administration and sustained respiratory alkalosis, which will lead to compensatory renal bicarbonate excretion, resulting in a relative deficiency state. The target pH for alkalinization is 7.45 to 7.55. Caution is also needed when sodium bicarbonate is given because of the potential to overshoot the desired pH or cause hypernatremia or ionized hypocalcemia. Additionally, the administration of large amounts of bicarbonate for a number of hours may lead to respiratory acidosis and hypoventilation. Overdrive pacing including the use of β-agonist infusions and also magnesium therapy (2) warrant consideration for refractory ventricular dysrhythmias.

The administration of Fab antibody fragments specific for CAs has resulted in hemodynamic improvement and decreased mortality in animal models (3,12,13). The use of ovine antibody (Fab fragment) in a 48-year-old amitriptyline-poisoned patient resulted in clinical CNS and cardiac improvements, but these antibody fragments are not commercially available yet (10). Extracorporeal removal techniques play no role in the management of the CA-poisoned patient.

Because benzodiazepines can be therapeutic, flumazenil is contraindicated for patients with coma and a history or ECG suggestive for moderate or severe CA poisoning. Physostigmine may be effective in reversing anticholinergic toxicity (see Chapter 323, "Anticholinergic Agents") but it has resulted in asystole when used to treat cardiac dysrhythmias as a result of CA poisoning, especially if concomitant treatment with atropine has occurred. It is therefore contraindicated for patients with a prolonged QRS interval or dysrhythmias suggestive of CA cardiotoxicity. Physostigmine may be beneficial in patients with the anticholinergic syndrome after mild overdose or in the recovery phase of severe poisoning (22). Concomitant use of benzodiazepines is always recommended. Benzodiazepines alone do not effectively control anticholinergic delirium unless heavily sedating doses are used, which may extend the lengths of stay for many patients (1).

Gastrointestinal decontamination should be accomplished following the institution of any necessary life-support measures. AC in a dose of 1 g/kg is the method of choice, when safe to administer. A clinical benefit from multiple doses of AC (MDAC), however, has not been clearly demonstrated and therefore is not recommended. Care should be taken to avoid aspiration of charcoal into the lung, which can dramatically prolong hospital stays; MDAC may only increase this risk (9). Syrup of ipecac is contraindicated in the setting of CA poisoning. Patients may become comatose, lose their gag reflex, and have seizures before or during emesis, resulting in airway compromise or aspiration pneumonitis. Gastric lavage may benefit some CA poisoned patients who present early (within an hour) after the ingestion (14). An example of the usual futility of gastric lavage in CA overdose is demonstrated by Watson et al (24). Despite many liters of gastric lavage fluid in 13 patients, the amount recovered ranged from two to at most 342 mg. This amount of drug recovery would not be expected to have a significant effect on clinical outcome measures. Therefore, gastric lavage with its associated risk of complications is no longer routinely recommended.

CRITICAL INTERVENTIONS

- Establish i.v. access and initiate continuous cardiac and oxygen saturation monitoring
- Administer benzodiazepines and sodium bicarbonate to patients with seizures, coma, hypotension, dysrhythmias, and cardiac conduction disturbances
- Administer intravenous fluids and high-dose dopamine or norepinephrine for hypotension
- Administer phenobarbital or propofol for refractory seizures or myoclonus

DISPOSITION

The maximal severity of CA poisoning is usually apparent within 2 to 6 hours of an overdose. Patients who develop coma, hypotension, seizures, or dysrhythmias require intensive care unit admission. Those who remain or become asymptomatic after 6 hours of observation can be medically cleared for discharge or psychiatric evaluation (a requirement for all intentional ingestions). Patients with persistent but mild symptoms, such as lethargy or tachycardia, will require prolonged monitoring and observation. Emergency department observation units or intermediate care units are appropriate.

A regional certified poison information center or medical toxicologist can be consulted for treatment and disposition decisions. Critically ill and complicated poisoned patients are best served at a regional poison treatment center or tertiary care facility. When indicated, transfer requires either an air ambulance or an advanced cardiac life support–equipped crew, accompanied by a nurse or physician.

COMMON PITFALLS

✔ Failure to appreciate that awake and stable appearing patients with recent CA overdose may rapidly deteriorate

✔ Failure to recognize the subtle electrocardiographic changes consistent with cyclic antidepressant poisoning

✔ Failure to aggressively treat seizures and to correct the resultant metabolic acidosis

✔ Inappropriate use of antidotes such as flumazenil and physostigmine

References

1. Burns MJ, Linden CH, Graudins A, et al. A comparison of physostigmine and benzodiazepines for the treatment of anticholinergic poisoning. *Ann Emerg Med* 2000;35:374–381.
2. Citak A, Soysal D, Ucsel R, et al. Efficacy of long duration resuscitation and magnesium sulphate treatment amitriptyline poisoning. *Eur J Emerg Med* 2002;9:63–66.
3. Dart RC, Sidki A, Sullivan JB, et al. Ovine desipramine antibody fragments reverse desipramine cardiovascular toxicity in the rat. *Ann Emerg Med* 1996;27:309–315.
4. Davis CO, Cobaugh DJ, Leahey NF, et al. Toxicology training of paramedic students in the United States. *Am J Emerg Med* 1999;17:138–140.
5. Ellison DW, Pentel PR. Clinical features and consequences of seizures due to cyclic antidepressant overdose. *Am J Emerg Med* 1989;7:5–10.
6. Farrar HC, James LP. Characteristics of pediatric admissions for cyclic antidepressant poisoning. *Am J Emerg Med* 1999;17:495–496.
7. Frommer DA, Kulig KW, Marx JA, et al. Tricyclic antidepressant overdose: a review. *JAMA* 1987;257:521–526.
8. Graudins A, Dowsett RP, Liddle C. The toxicity of antidepressant poisoning: is it changing? A comparative study of cyclic and newer serotonin-specific antidepressants. *Emerg Med* 2002;14:440–446.
9. Harris CR, Filandrinos D. Accidental administration of activated charcoal into the lung: aspiration by proxy. *Ann Emerg Med* 1993;22:1470–1473.
10. Heard K, O'Malley GF, Dart RC. Treatment of amitriptyline poisoning with ovine antibody to tricyclic antidepressants. *Lancet* 1999;354:1614–1615.
11. Hoffman JR, Votey SR, Bayer M, et al. Effect of hypertonic sodium bicarbonate in the treatment of moderate-to-severe cyclic antidepressant overdose. *Am J Emerg Med* 1993;11:336–341.
12. Hursting MJ, Opheim KE, Raisys VA, et al. Tricyclic antidepressant-specific Fab fragments alter the distribution and elimination of desipramine in the rabbit: a model for overdose treatment. *J Toxicol Clin Toxicol* 1989;27:53–66
13. Keyler DE, LeCouteur DG, Pond SM, et al. Effects of specific antibody fragments on desipramine pharmacokinetics in the rat in vivo and in the isolated perfused liver. *J Pharmacol Exp Ther* 1995;272:1117–1123.
14. Kulig K, Bar-Or D, Cantrill SV, et al. Management of acutely poisoned patients without gastric emptying. *Ann Emerg Med* 1985;14:562–567.
15. Litovitz TL, Klein-Schwartz W, Rodgers GC, et al. 2001 Annual report of the American Association of poison control centers toxic exposure surveillance system. *Am J Emerg Med* 2002;20:391–452.
16. McCabe JL, Menegazzi JJ, Cobaugh DJ, et al. Recovery from severe cyclic antidepressant overdose with hypertonic saline/dextran in a swine model. *Acad Emerg Med* 1994;1:111–115.
17. McFee RB, Mofenson HC, Caraccio TR. A nationwide survey of the management of unintentional-low dose tricyclic antidepressant ingestions involving asymptomatic children: implications for the development of an evidence-based clinical guideline. *J Toxicol Clin Toxicol* 2000;38:15–19.
18. Merigian KS, Browning RG, Leeper KV. Successful treatment of amoxapine-induced refractory status epilepticus with propofol (Diprivan). *Acad Emerg Med* 1995;2:128–133.
19. Mullins ME, Cristofani CB, Warden CR, et al. Amitriptyline-associated seizures in a toddler with Manchausen-by-proxy. *Pediatr Emerg Care* 1999;15:202–205.
20. Nattel S, Mittleman M. Treatment of ventricular tachyarrythmias resulting from amitriptyline toxicity in dogs. *J Pharmacol Exp Ther* 1984;231:430–435.
21. Sasyniuk BI, Jhamandas V. Mechanism of reversal of toxic effects of amitriptyline on cardiac Purkinje fibers by sodium bicarbonate. *J Pharmacol Exp Ther* 1984;231:387–394.
22. Suchard JR. Assessing physostigmine's contraindication in cyclic antidepressant ingestions. *J Emerg Med* 2003;25:185–191.
23. Taboulet P, Michard F, Muszynski J, et al. Cardiovascular repercussions of seizures during cyclic antidepressant poisoning. *J Toxicol Clin Toxicol* 1995;33:205–211.
24. Watson WA, Leighton J, Guy J, et al. Recovery of cyclic antidepressants with gastric lavage. *J Emerg Med* 1989;7:373–377.
25. Wolfe TR, Caravati EM, Rollins DE. Terminal 40-ms frontal plane QRS axis as a marker for tricyclic antidepressant overdose. *Ann Emerg Med* 1989;18:348–351.

CHAPTER 319
Dystonic Reactions

Anthony S. Manoguerra

Dystonic reactions are seldom life-threatening, but the pain and discomfort of the bodily contortions that develop often prompt the victim to seek help in the emergency department (ED). Additionally, iatrogenic dystonic reactions and akathisia are not infrequent in the ED setting, particularly in association with the administration of antiemetic and antipsychotic medications. These effects appear early and are reversible with reduction or discontinuation of the offending agent. Tardive dyskinesia refers to the sometimes irreversible involuntary movements that develop later (20). Primary dystonia, abnormal movements that occur spontaneously in the absence of drug treatment, is a separate diagnosis with similar manifestations. Dystonias may begin during infancy, childhood, adolescence, or adulthood for both the primary and secondary or environmentally produced types (8).

Dystonias of all types probably result from an abnormality of neurotransmitter function in the basal ganglia. Several specific mechanisms have been proposed for those that are drug-induced. According to one theory, they are due to direct blockade of central dopaminergic receptors. Another theory proposes that the underlying mechanism involves both dopamine and acetylcholine, with an imbalance of neurotransmitters resulting in excessive cholinergic activity. A third theory holds that acute dystonic reactions may be caused by a combination of dopamine blockade and dopamine activation in the nigrostriatal system (17). The delay in onset of acute dystonias after the administration of antipsychotic medication may be explained by this mechanism. Dopamine synthesis and release have been shown to increase in response to an initial blockade of dopamine receptors. A single dose of an antipsychotic drug has also produced supersensitivity of dopamine receptors 24 to 48 hours after drug administration. This occurs at a time when plasma and red-cell drug concentrations are actually falling. Therefore, enhanced dopamine release, occurring simultaneously with the unblocking of supersensitive receptors, may result in acute dystonias (16).

The true incidence of dystonia is unknown, but it occurs in about 2% of patients treated with phenothiazines and in about 25% of patients treated with haloperidol and the depot phenothiazines. Most acute dystonias occur within 5 days of starting therapy with neuroleptics or other agents (4). Such reactions are more common in men than in women (19).

The patient who presents to the emergency department with a drug-induced dystonic reaction will probably be a young male (2), manifesting a buccolingual or torticollar reaction (19). The presence of a piperazine side chain attached to the phenothiazine nucleus increases the likelihood that a compound will produce a dystonic reaction. Symptoms seem to develop earlier with haloperidol than with other neuroleptics. The development of a dystonic reaction depends more on individual susceptibility than on the chemical structure, milligram potency, dosage, or duration of treatment. The drugs currently known or suspected to produce acute dystonic reactions and for which there is reasonable supportive evidence in the literature are listed in Table 319.1.

Patients under age 15 and those with a family history of dystonia are at greatest risk of developing drug-induced dystonias (1,2), although acute dystonias are also seen in the elderly (16). Another factor that may predispose a patient to dystonic reactions is a history of drug or alcohol use (10,11,15).

TABLE 319.1. Drugs Reported or Suspected to have Caused Acute Dystonic Reactions

Generic Name	Brand Name
Amitriptyline	Elavil®
Amoxapine	Asendin®
Azatadine	Optimine®
Bupropion	Zyban®, Wellbutrin®
Chlorpromazine	Thorazine®
Chlorprothixene	Taractan®
Cimetidine	Tagamet®
Cisapride	Propulsid®
Cocaine	
Clomipramine	Anafranil®
Clozapine	Clozaril®
Cyclizine	Marezine®
Dextromethorphan	
Diazepam	Valium®
Diphenhydramine	Benadryl®
Doxepin	Sinequan®
Etomidate	Amidate®
Fluoxetine	Prozac®
Fluphenazine	Prolixin®
Fluvoxamine	Luvox®
Haloperidol	Haldol®
Imipramine	Tofranil®
Ketamine	Ketalar®
Loxapine	Loxitane®
Mesoridazine	Serentil®
Methohexital	Brevital®
Metoclopramide	Reglan®
Olanzapine	Zyprexa®
Paroxetine	Paxil®
Perphenazine	Trilafon®
Phenelzine	Nardil®
Phenytoin	Dilantin®
Pimozide	Orap®
Prochlorperazine	Compazine®
Promazine	Sparine®
Promethazine	Phenergan®
Propofol	Diprivan®
Quetiapine	Seroquel®
Ranitidine	Zantac®
Risperidone	Risperdal®
Sertraline	Zoloft®
Thiethylperazine	Torecan®
Thiopental	Pentothal®
Thioridazine	Mellaril®
Thiothixene	Navane®
Tiagabine	Gabitril®
Tranylcypromine	Parnate®
Trifluoperazine	Stelazine®
Triflupromazine	Vesprin®

Akathisia is an uncomfortable condition of motor restlessness and agitation, which occurs in association with the same drugs that may induce dystonic reactions and probably has the same pathophysiology. Prochlorperazine, often used as an antiemetic and for benign headache syndromes, commonly induces akathisia and is the most well-studied drug in the ED setting regarding this complication. When patients are carefully monitored for signs and symptoms, prochlorperazine induces akathisia in 44% of patients within one hour of administration and in a few percent more in a delayed fashion up to 48 hours later (7). The rate of i.v. administration (15-minute infusion vs. 2-minute bolus) does not appear to significantly affect the incidence of akathisia (5). The use of adjuvant diphenhydramine (50 mg i.v.) in association with prochlorperazine (10 mg i.v.) reduced the incidence of akathisia from 36% to 14%, but was also associated with an increase in sedation scores (21).

CLINICAL PRESENTATION

Any striated muscle group may be involved in a dystonic movement. Blepharospasm, progressing to oculogyric crisis, is the most common form of dystonia in the upper face. It usually begins with increased blinking of the eyelids. The muscles of the lower jaw most commonly involved are those of the pharynx and tongue. The term oromandibular dystonia describes the involvement of any combination of these muscles. Specifically, mandibular dystonia is manifested as a pulling down or up of the jaw. Lingual dystonia may present as either a sustained protrusion of the tongue or an upward deflection so that the tongue curves and touches the hard palate. In the neck region, torticollis is most common, although retrocollis and anterocollis may also occur. In most cases, the shoulder is elevated on the side toward which the chin is pointing. Jerking, rhythmic movements of the head may also occur. When the trunk is involved, twisting movements and postures such as lordosis, scoliosis, kyphosis, tortipelvis, and opisthotonos develop. Dystonic movements may begin as focal but become segmental as they spread in a contiguous manner. Generalized dystonia refers to involvement of the leg plus other body parts, with or without the trunk. Dystonic movements are usually continual, repetitive, and twisting, varying in speed from rapid to slow and being sustained from seconds to minutes at the height of the involuntary contraction (9).

The prognosis is excellent for patients with drug-induced dystonias when correctly treated. However, cardiorespiratory arrest and death have been linked to metoclopramide in a case in which diagnosis and treatment were delayed (18).

DIFFERENTIAL DIAGNOSIS

Dystonic reactions have been misdiagnosed as tetanus, hysterical conversion, and even seizure disorders. Children with such abnormal movements have been thought to have encephalitis or meningitis (12,14). Strychnine poisoning and the choreiform movements sometimes seen with sympathomimetic abuse ("crack dancing") or with rheumatic fever may appear similar to dystonic reactions as well.

EMERGENCY DEPARTMENT EVALUATION

The patient, family, or friends should be asked about the recent use of medications. Physical examination is remarkable for abnormal posturing or movements. Urinalysis may provide information about recent drug use in a patient who is unable or unwilling to provide a history.

EMERGENCY DEPARTMENT MANAGEMENT

As dystonic reactions are not usually associated with an acute drug overdosage (13), gastrointestinal decontamination procedures are not necessary. Induction of emesis, administration of activated charcoal, or gastric lavage could lead to airway compromise in the patient with abnormal head or neck posturing or swallowing difficulty. If activated charcoal administration is thought to be indicated, as in the case of a multiple drug ingestion, it should be administered once the acute dystonic reaction has been treated and the dystonia has subsided.

Administration of an anticholinergic medication rapidly reverses the symptoms, presumably because of restoration of the cholinergic–dopaminergic balance in nigrostriatal neurons. Diphenhydramine (Benadryl®) and benztropine mesylate (Cogentin®) are used more often than biperiden (Akineton®) or trihexyphenidyl (Artane®). I.v. administration is preferable to i.m. or oral administration. Symptoms typically abate within 2 minutes and completely resolve within 15 minutes when the i.v. route is used. Muscle relaxation begins in 30 minutes but may not be complete for 90 minutes when the antidote is given i.m. or orally. Benztropine has been advocated over diphenhydramine because of fewer side effects and more rapid improvement of both objective and subjective findings, regardless of route (14). One report describes a patient who responded minimally to multiple doses of diphenhydramine but completely to a subsequent dose of benztropine (3). Diphenhydramine should be used in children under the age of 3, as benztropine is considered contraindicated in this age group as children may be more sensitive to the effects of anticholinergic medications. Drowsiness should be anticipated as a side effect of anticholinergic drug administration, especially with diphenhydramine.

After reversal of the reaction, treatment should continue with an oral agent for 72 hours to prevent a relapse (6).

The usual dose of benztropine is 1 to 2 mg for adults and 0.02 to 0.05 mg/kg for children age 3 years or older, given i.v. over 2 minutes, followed by the same dose given orally twice a day for 3 days. The dose of diphenhydramine is 50 to 100 mg for adults and 1 to 2 mg/kg for children, given i.v. over 2 minutes, followed by 12.5 to 50.0 mg orally three or four times a day for 3 days. Some patients may require more than one dose of i.v. medication to control the reaction.

CRITICAL INTERVENTIONS

- Recognize acute dystonia as an adverse drug reaction, rather than due to other medical or psychiatric causes
- Treat dystonic reactions with anticholinergic medications (benztropine or diphenhydramine)

DISPOSITION

The patient may be discharged after the acute dystonia resolves. Consultation with the prescribing psychiatrist is advisable if the patient is to remain on neuroleptic medication. When anticholinergics are prescribed, patients should be advised not to drive or perform potentially dangerous activities for 72 hours. They should be instructed to return if symptoms recur.

COMMON PITFALLS

✔ Dystonic reactions may be delayed in onset 12 to 24 hours from the time of drug ingestion
✔ The timely administration of an anticholinergic medication may prove to be diagnostic as well as therapeutic
✔ Dystonic reactions are not usually the result of an overdose; because of their delayed onset, gastrointestinal decontamination is seldom indicated and may be dangerous in patients with head or neck involvement
✔ Prescribing oral anticholinergic medication for 3 days after acute treatment may prevent relapses

Acknowledgment

The author would like to thank previous edition chapter author Mary A McCormick.

References

1. Addonizio G, Alexopoulos GS. Drug-induced dystonia in young and elderly patients. *Am J Psychiatry* 1988;145:869–871.
2. Ayd FJ Jr. A survey of drug-induced extrapyramidal reactions. *JAMA* 1961;175:1054–1060.
3. Bailie GR, Nelson MV, Krenzelok EP, et al. Unusual treatment response of a severe dystonia to diphenhydramine. *Ann Emerg Med* 1987;16:705–708.
4. Ballerini M, Bellini S, Niccolai C, et al. Neuroleptic-induced dystonia: incidence and risk factors. *Eur Psychiatry* 2002;17:366–368.
5. Collins RW, Jones JB, Waithall JD, et al. Intravenous administration of prochlorperazine by 15-minute infusion versus 2-minute bolus does not affect the incidence of akathisia: a prospective, randomized, controlled trial. *Ann Emerg Med* 2001;38:491–496.
6. Corre K, Niemann J, Bessen H. Extended therapy for acute dystonic reactions. *Ann Emerg Med* 1984;13:194–197.
7. Drotts DL, Vinson DR. Prochlorperazine induces akathisia in emergency patients. *Ann Emerg Med* 1999;34:469–475.
8. Fahn S, Jankovic J. Practical management of dystonia. *Neurol Clin* 1984;2:555–569.
9. Fahn S. The varied clinical expressions of dystonia. *Neurol Clin* 1984;2:541–454.
10. Felser JM, Orban DJ. Dystonic reaction after ketamine abuse. *Ann Emerg Med* 1982;11:673–675.
11. Freed E. Alcohol-triggered-neuroleptic-induced tremor, rigidity and dystonia. *Med J Aust* 1981;2:44–45.
12. Goel R, Misra PK. Phenothiazine induced dyskinesia in children. *Indian Pediatr* 1981;18:203–207.
13. Goldfrank, L Flomenbaum N, Weisman R. Management of overdose with psychoactive medications. *Emerg Med Clin North Am* 1984;2:63–76.
14. Lee AS. Treatment of drug-induced dystonic reactions. *JACEP* 1979;8:453–457.
15. Lutz EG. Neuroleptic-induced akathisia and dystonia triggered by alcohol. *JAMA* 1976;236:2422–2423.
16. Magnuson TM, Roccaforte WH, Wengel SP, et al. Medication-induced dystonias in nine patients with dementia. *J Neuropsychiatry Clin Neurosci* 2000;12:219–225.
17. Marsden C, Jenner P. The pathophysiology of extrapyramidal side effects of neuroleptic drugs. *Psychol Med* 1980;10:55–72.
18. Pollera CF, et al. Sudden death after acute dystonic reaction to high-dose metoclopramide. *Lancet* 1984;2(8400):460–461.
19. Swett C Jr. Drug-induced dystonia. *Am J Psychiatry* 1975;132:532–534.
20. Tarsy D. Neuroleptic-induced extrapyramidal reactions: classification, description, and diagnosis. *Clin Neuropharmacol* 1983;6 Suppl 1:S9–S26.
21. Vinson DR, Drotts DL. Diphenhydramine for the prevention of akathisia induced by prochlorperazine: a randomized, controlled trial. *Ann Emerg Med* 2001;37:125–131.

CHAPTER 320
Lithium

Kenneth W. Kulig

TABLE 320.1.   Severity of Lithium Poisoning

Grade 1 (mild): Nausea, vomiting, tremor, hyperreflexia, agitation, muscle weakness, ataxia

Grade 2 (moderate): Confusion, dysarthria, rigidity, hypertonia, hypotension, stupor

Grade 3 (severe): Convulsions, myoclonic jerking, coma, cardiovascular collapse

The primary use of lithium is in the treatment of bipolar disorders. Other uses have included the treatment of drug and alcohol abuse, episodic aggression, anorexia nervosa, Huntington's chorea, tardive dyskinesia, SIADH, neutropenia, and Felty syndrome (1).

In the United States, lithium is available as lithium carbonate tablets in regular (300 mg; 8.12 mEq) or slow-release (450 mg; 12.18 mEq) form, and as lithium citrate syrup (8 mEq/5 mL). Common adult daily doses are 900 to 2,400 mg. Numerous adverse drug reactions and drug–drug interactions have been reported, and serum levels must be monitored carefully to avoid toxicity. Therapeutic lithium levels vary slightly from one laboratory to another but are generally cited as being within the range of 0.5 to 1.5 mEq/L.

The exact mechanism of action of lithium in the treatment of bipolar disorders is unknown. Therapeutic doses have no psychotropic effect in humans who do not have a bipolar disorder. Although lithium can replace sodium in supporting a single action potential in a nerve cell, it cannot maintain membrane potentials. Its ability to substitute for other cations, such as potassium, calcium, and magnesium at the cell membrane, has uncertain physiologic effects. Changes in the release or reuptake of norepinephrine and serotonin or modified hormonal responses mediated by adenyl cyclase have been postulated.

Understanding the kinetics of lithium, particularly its distribution, is important in the proper management of lithium overdose patients. Lithium ions are completely absorbed from the gastrointestinal (GI) tract. Absorption, which is rapid after therapeutic doses, may be delayed after large overdoses, in the presence of food, or if the patient has decreased intestinal motility from coingestants. Slow-release preparations result in lower peak concentrations, which occur at a later time (3,8,9). Lithium is initially distributed into the extracellular space and then more slowly into tissues, including the primary target organ of toxicity, the brain. After an acute overdose, the patient may initially appear well, with a high serum level, but deteriorate as the levels fall. The blood is not a target organ but is only an indirect measure of the total body burden of lithium. Invasive measures to remove lithium, such as hemodialysis or venovenous hemofiltration, may be more effective during the distribution phase in select patients, when the drug is still found in the intravascular compartment (13,14). The volume of distribution is about that of body water—0.8 to 1.2 L/Kg.

Lithium is entirely eliminated by renal excretion. The renal handling of lithium is similar to that of sodium; it is filtered and reabsorbed by the proximal tubule. Reabsorption is enhanced and toxicity is more likely in the setting of hyponatremia, volume depletion, renal hypoperfusion, and diuretic use (1). Lithium, itself, may be nephrotoxic (11,20). After a single dose, the serum half-life is 9 to 13 hours. At steady state, the half-life may be 30 to 58 hours. After an overdose, the serum half-life depends on how much lithium has been distributed into tissues; the figure is meaningful only after absorption is complete.

CLINICAL PRESENTATION

Toxic effects depend on the dose, the time since ingestion, underlying medical conditions such as renal disease or dehydration, concomitant ingestions, and the patient's age. It is sometimes useful to classify the overdose as acute (single ingestion), acute on top of chronic therapy, or chronic. Because the latter situation is likely to result in the greatest lithium distribution into tissues, it is the most dangerous. There can be overlap among these categories. The clinical classification given in Table 320.1 (12) is valuable in the initial assessment. One poison center reported a mortality rate of 1% (5).

Patients may move from one category to another with time, depending primarily on the tissue distribution of lithium, which is not accurately measured by the serum level (3,8,21,25). Electrocardiographic (ECG) changes are nondiagnostic and may occur in patients with therapeutic levels who are not clinically toxic (20). Common changes include nonspecific ST-T wave changes, first-degree atrioventricular block, mild intraventricular conduction delay, and prolonged Q-T interval. These ECG changes may be responsible for the common misconception that lithium is primarily toxic to the heart, when the brain is the primary target organ. Cardiovascular collapse generally occurs only as a result of severe central nervous system (CNS) toxicity.

Permanent neurologic sequelae (e.g., encephalopathy) can result from lithium intoxication (2,6,24,28). Neuroleptic malignant syndrome (NMS) with fever, tachypnea, muscle rigidity, rhabdomyolysis, acute renal failure, confusion, and elevated creatine kinase has been described in one patient beginning 7 days after an acute overdose, despite dialysis (10).

DIFFERENTIAL DIAGNOSIS

The classic painless rigidity, tremor, and hyperreflexia may not be present early in the clinical course. Neurologic manifestations might mimic a cerebrovascular accident, a postictal state, metabolic disorders such as hypercalcemia or hyperthyroidism, or meningitis. The common nausea and vomiting seen after an acute overdose may be easily confused with gastroenteritis or another intraabdominal process. Particularly in the elderly, parkinsonism or tardive dyskinesia should be considered. Coingestants should be considered, especially other psychiatric medications such as antipsychotics, antidepressants, and carbamazepine and sodium valproate, which are also used to treat bipolar illness.

EMERGENCY DEPARTMENT EVALUATION

Attention should focus on the mental status and neurologic examination, searching particularly for tremor, myoclonus, hyperreflexia, and stiffness. Hydration status, renal function, and diuretic use should be assessed. When lithium toxicity is suspected, serum electrolytes should be measured, paying particular attention to the serum sodium. Blood urea nitrogen, creatinine, and urine output should be assesses. A lithium level should be taken when the patient has symptoms or signs consistent with lithium toxicity or if an acute overdose is suspected. Lithium levels are not included in broad toxicology screens and must be ordered separately. The toxicology screen is indicated if the patient is ill enough to require admission to the hospital or will assist in the psychiatric assessment of the patient. More than one lithium level separated by several hours should be drawn if the patient has taken an acute overdose (22–24), particularly if the preparation is of the sustained-release type (3,8).

An ECG should be performed to serve as a baseline and to help rule out coingestants such as the tricyclic antidepressants. ST-T abnormalities are common with therapeutic dosing and do not necessarily mean cardiotoxicity (17). Obtaining the patient's pill bottles or calling the pharmacy where the patient gets the medications can also help to rule out coingestants. Medications such as acetaminophen, which do not cause early symptoms, should also be considered.

Vital signs, including temperature, should be measured often. Serial neurologic examinations, including a mental status examination, should be performed. Neurotoxicity is the most important manifestation of lithium toxicity (19). A Foley catheter to monitor urine output should be placed if the patient exhibits moderate or severe toxicity.

EMERGENCY DEPARTMENT MANAGEMENT

Advanced life-support measures are instituted as necessary. An i.v. line of normal saline should be started, and the patient should be rehydrated aggressively. However, once euvolemia and normal urine output have been established, there may be little added advantage to aggressive saline diuresis. Fluid overload may occur from overly aggressive saline administration.

The use of ipecac should be avoided, as it is unlikely to remove significant quantities of drug.

Ipecac also interferes with patient assessment, because vomiting is an early sign of lithium toxicity. Lavage is also unlikely to remove much lithium from the stomach and should probably be considered only if the patient presents very soon after an acute ingestion. Activated charcoal does not bind lithium, but it should be given if coingestants are suspected. If only lithium was ingested, or if the patient is chronically lithium-intoxicated without other drugs involved, activated charcoal is unnecessary.

There is experimental evidence that sodium polystyrene sulfonate (Kayexalate), an ion-exchange resin usually used to treat hyperkalemia, can both prevent absorption of lithium and enhance its removal once absorbed (7,16,26). The clinical efficacy of this therapy is unproved, and it is probably best reserved for patients who have taken a massive overdose, have high or rising levels, or are otherwise severely ill. The optimum dose and dosing intervals have not been defined; 15 to 50 g orally or by nasogastric tube every 4 to 6 hours might be a reasonable starting point. Kayexalate can cause nausea, vomiting, and constipation. The serum potassium level should be carefully monitored to prevent hypokalemia.

Whole-bowel irrigation has also been recommended as a GI decontamination measure for lithium overdose (15,23). It is uncertain whether this technique is as effective as using Kayexalate, or whether, in fact, either approach is necessary.

Hemodialysis is the most efficient method of removing lithium from the intravascular compartment, allowing lithium to redistribute into it from the brain (1,13,14). Because this redistribution is relatively slow, however, clinical improvement lags behind the fall in serum lithium levels. A significant rebound of

the serum lithium level usually occurs, which may necessitate a second or third round of dialysis in the sickest patients. It may take days or longer for toxicity to resolve, despite hemodialysis.

Hemodialysis is recommended for patients with severe or progressive lithium toxicity. It is difficult to give a precise lithium level above which all patients need to be hemodialyzed. Patients on chronic therapy may manifest some toxicity even though their levels may be within the therapeutic range. Other patients may be relatively asymptomatic with levels higher than 5 mEq/L (same as mmol/L) following acute overdose (14,22). Clinical judgment, preferably by a physician experienced in the treatment of lithium-poisoned patients, is necessary in making these important decisions. Consulting a regional poison center or toxicologist can be very helpful in this regard. In general, serum lithium levels above 3 meq/L (mmol/L) in any patient are a warning that the patient could deteriorate. Levels less than that could still result in serious illness in some patients, particularly those who are dehydrated, hyponatremic, have renal insufficiency, or other serious chronic disease.

Whether hemodialysis can prevent the persistent cognitive deficits that sometimes occur after physical recovery in patients with severe poisoning is unclear. One study has suggested that hemodialysis may be somewhat ineffective in altering outcome (4), although one death was attributed to the lack of hemodialysis. Peritoneal dialysis is much less effective and is not usually considered for the treatment of severe lithium intoxication. Continuos venovenous hemofiltration has been proposed as an alternative to hemodialysis in some patients (18,27).

CRITICAL INTERVENTIONS

- Administer normal saline intravenously for rehydration and hyponatremia; establish and maintain a normal urine output
- Consult a poison center or toxicolist and a nephrologist regarding hemodialysis in patients with significant clinical toxicity and high lithium levels

DISPOSITION

A patient with an acute lithium overdose cannot usually be medically cleared on the basis of a single lithium level, unless it is zero or very near zero and it has been hours since the reported ingestion. In most cases, a second level should be measured several hours later to ensure that delayed absorption is not occurring which may be clinically important. In all cases of overdose with suicidal intent, psychiatric consultation should be obtained before discharge.

Patients should be admitted if they have any neurologic symptoms from lithium, such as altered mental status, new and significant tremor, new and significant hyperreflexia, or stiffness. If patients are dehydrated, are in renal failure, or have a high or rising lithium level, they should be admitted to an intensive care unit. Consultation with a poison center or toxicologist, and a nephrologist is also recommended. Although hemodialysis may not be necessary and is not usually performed in the emergency department, nephrology consultation can result in the dialysis team being mobilized more quickly when needed.

COMMON PITFALLS

✔ Failure to consider the possibility of lithium toxicity, and to obtain a serum lithium level in patients taking lithium who develop hyponatremia, dehydration, or renal compromise

✔ Failure to consider the kinetics of lithium and whether toxicity is acute, acute on chronic, or chronic when interpreting serum lithium levels; relatively lower serum lithium levels in a chronic scenario may be more dangerous than higher levels from a single acute overdose

✔ Failure to obtain serial lithium levels in patients with acute overdose, especially with a sustained release lithium preparation

✔ Failure to appreciate the degree of dehydration

✔ Failure to appreciate that severe lithium poisoning can lead to permanent neurologic impairment, and that aggressive treatment is warranted

References

1. Amdisen A. Clinical features and management of lithium poisoning. *Med Toxicol Adverse Drug Exp* 1988;3:18.
2. Apte SN, Langston JW. Permanent neurological deficits due to lithium toxicity. *Ann Neurol* 1983;13:453.
3. Astruc B, Petit P, Abbar M. Overdose with sustained-release lithium preparations. *Eur Psychiatry* 1999;14:172–174.
4. Bailey B, McGuigan M. Comparison of patients hemodialyzed for lithium poisoning and those for whom dialysis was recommended by PCC but not done: what lesson can we learn? *Clin Nephrol* 2000;54:388–392.
5. Bailey B, McGuigan M. Lithium poisoning from a poison control center perspective. *Ther Drug Monit* 2000;22:650–655.
6. Barth L, Marksteiner J, Bauer G, et al. Persistent cognitive deficits associated with lithium intoxication: a neuropsychological case description. *Cortex* 2002;38:743–752.
7. Belanger DR, Tierney MG, Dickinson G. Effect of sodium polystyrene sulfonate on lithium bioavailability. *Ann Emerg Med* 1992;21:1312.
8. Bosse GM, Arnold TC. Overdose with sustained-release lithium preparations. *J Emerg Med* 1992;10:719.
9. Branger B, Peyriere H, Zabadani B, et al. [Voluntary lithium salt poisoning: risks of slow released forms] *Nephrologie* 2000;21:291–293.
10. Gill J, Singh H, Nugent K. Acute lithium intoxication and neuroleptic malignant syndrome. *Pharmacotherapy* 2003;23:811–5.
11. Gitlin M. Lithium and the kidney. *Drug Saf* 1999;20:231–243.
12. Hansen HE, Amdisen A. Lithium intoxication: report of 23 cases and review of 100 cases from the literature. *Q J Med* 1978;47:123.
13. Hazouard E, Ferrandiere M, Rateau H, et al. Continuous veno-venous haemofiltration versus continuous veno-venous haemodialysis in severe lithium self-poisoning: a toxicokinetics study in an intensive care unit. *Nephrol Dial Transplant* 1999;14:1605–1606.
14. Jaeger A, Sauder P, Kopferschmitt J, et al. When should dialysis be performed in lithium poisoning? A kinetic study in 14 cases of lithium poisoning. *J Toxicol Clin Toxicol* 1993;31:429.
15. Kirshenbaum LA, Mathews SC, Sitar DS, et al. Whole bowel irrigation versus activated charcoal in sorbitol for the ingestion of modified-release pharmaceuticals. *Clin Pharmacol Ther* 1989;46:264.
16. Linakis JG, Eisenberg MS, Lacoutre PG, et al. Multiple-dose sodium polystyrene sulfonate in lithium intoxication: an animal model. *Pharmacol Toxicol* 1992;70:38.
17. Mateer JR, Clark MR. Lithium toxicity with rarely reported EKG manifestations. *Ann Emerg Med* 1982;11:208.
18. Menghini VV, Albright RC Jr. Treatment of lithium intoxication with continuous venovenous hemodiafiltration. *Am J Kidney Dis* 2000;36:E21.
19. Oakley PW, Whyte IM, Carter GL. Lithium toxicity: an iatrogenic problem in susceptible individuals. *Aust N Z J Psychiatry* 2001;35:833–840.
20. Rose SR, Klein-Schwartz W, Oderda GM, et al. Lithium intoxication with acute renal failure and death. *Drug Intell Clin Pharm* 1988;22:691.
21. Sadosty AT, Groleau GA, Atcherson MM. The use of lithium levels in the emergency department. *J Emerg Med* 1999;17:887–891.
22. Sawyer D, Kulig K. Lithium overdose superimposed on chronic therapy—lack of indication for dialysis. *Vet Hum Toxicol* 1983;25:273 (abstract).
23. Smith SW, Ling LW, Halstenson CE. Whole bowel irrigation as a treatment for acute lithium overdose. *Ann Emerg Med* 1991;20:536.
24. Strayhorn JM, Nash JL. Severe neurotoxicity despite therapeutic serum lithium levels. *Dis Nerv Syst* 1977;38:107.
25. Timmer RT, Sands JM. Lithium intoxication. *J Am Soc Nephrol* 1999;10:666.
26. Tomaszewski C, Musso C, Pearson JR, et al. Lithium absorption prevented by sodium polystyrene sulfonate in volunteers. *Ann Emerg Med* 1992;21:1308.
27. VanBommell EF, Kalmeijer MD, Ponssen HH. Treatment of life-threatening lithium toxicity with big volume continuous venovenous hemofiltration. *Am J Nephrol* 2000;20:408–411.
28. Von Hartitzch B, Hoenich NA, Leigh RJ, et al. Permanent neurological sequelae despite hemodialysis for lithium intoxication. *BMJ* 1972;4:757.

CHAPTER 321
Monoamine Oxidase Inhibitors

Michael Joseph Burns

The monoamine oxidase (MAO) inhibitors have been available for the treatment of major depression since the 1950s (4,19). Although effective, MAO inhibitors are infrequently prescribed because of their risk for producing dangerous food and drug interactions and serious toxicity following overdose. These agents are generally reserved for the management of atypical, drug-resistant, neurotic, or reactive depression (4). MAO inhibitors are also occasionally used to treat anxiety states, bulimia, hypertension, migraine headaches, narcolepsy, obsessive-compulsive disorder, Parkinson's disease, and phobias (4). Newer selective, reversible inhibitors of MAO have a lower propensity for adverse effects (1,4,7,8,10). These agents block the oxidative deamination of endogenous and exogenous monoamines by means of MAO, a flavin-containing enzyme located in the outer mitochondrial membranes of most tissues (4,19). Two subtypes of MAO exist (MAO-A and MAO-B), which differ in their substrate and inhibitor specificities and tissue distribution (4,7,12,15,19,25). MAO-A is found in the brain (monoaminergic neurons), peripheral sympathetic postganglionic neurons, intestinal mucosa, and liver. MAO-B is located in the brain (glial cells and some serotonergic neurons), platelets, liver, and intestinal mucosa (4).

Noradrenergic neurons contain predominantly MAO-A; serotonergic neurons contain both MAO-A and MAO-B. Substrates primarily deaminated by MAO-A include epinephrine, metanephrine, norepinephrine (NE), and 5-hydroxytryptamine (5-HT, or serotonin). Substrates metabolized primarily by MAO-B include β-phenylethylamine, methylhistamine, phenylethanolamine, and benzylamine (4). Many substrates are metabolized by both enzymes, including tyramine, dopamine (DA), octopamine, and tryptamine. Substrate specificity is not absolute and is primarily dependent on the relative concentrations of substrate and MAO subtype in a particular anatomic location. Inhibition of MAO-A is necessary for therapeutic efficacy in the treatment of depression (4,19). MAO enzymes function to maintain low body concentrations of monoamines (4,6,7,19,25). Hepatic and intestinal MAOs prevent the absorption of and systemic effects from dietary monoamines (e.g., tyramine) (4). Intraneuronal MAO maintains a low cytoplasmic concentration of monoamine neurotransmitters that allows for net reuptake and termination of effect of extracellular monoamines (4,7,19). Glial cell MAO scavenges monoamines and prevents their accumulation within the central nervous system (CNS) (4,7). All MAO inhibitors are false substrates for the MAO enzyme; they bind competitively (with respect to natural amine substrate) to the active site of MAO and prevent it from further activity (1,4,19). MAO inhibitors may be classified by their differential selectivity for MAO subtypes, reversibility of MAO binding (inhibition), or by chemical structure (Table 321.1). The oldest MAO inhibitors in use are nonselective, irreversible ("suicide") inactivators of MAO. Initially, they bind reversibly to the flavin active site of MAO but are subsequently oxidized to a reactive intermediate, which forms an irreversible covalent bond with the enzyme (4).

TABLE 321.1.   Classification of Monoamine Oxidase Inhibitors

Agent (Trade Name)	Inhibition	Selectivity	Structure
Befloxatone	Reversible	MAO-A	Oxazolidinone
Brofaromine	Reversible	MAO-A	Piperidylbenzofuran
Clorgyline	Irreversible	MAO-A	Acetylenic agent
Iproniazid (Marsilid)	Irreversible	Nonselective	Hydrazine (Hydrazide)
Isocarboxazid (Marplan)	Irreversible	Nonselective	Hydrazine (Hydrazide)
Linezolid (Zyvox)	Reversible	Nonselective	Oxazolidinone
Moclobemide (Aurorix)	Reversible	MAO-A	Benzamide
Nialamide (Niamid)	Irreversible	Nonselective	Hydrazine
Pargyline (Eutonyl)	Irreversible	MAO-B	Acetylenic agent
Phenelzine (Nardil)	Irreversible	Nonselective	Hydrazine
Procarbazine (Matulane)	Irreversible	Nonselective	Hydrazine
Rasagiline	Irreversible	MAO-B	Acetylenic agent
Selegiline, l-deprenyl (Eldepryl)	Irreversible	MAO-B	Acetylenic agent
Toloxantrone (Humoryl)	Reversible	MAO-A	Oxazolidinone
Tranylcypromine (Parnate)	Irreversible	Nonselective	Cyclopropylamine

New enzyme must be synthesized before the function of MAO returns to normal.

Currently, only irreversible inhibitors of MAO are available for clinical use in the United States (4). Nonselective inhibitors include isocarboxazid, phenelzine sulfate, and tranylcypromine sulfate. Selegiline is a selective inhibitor of MAO-B used to treat Parkinson's disease (4,10,16,19). It is not associated with dangerous food and drug interactions at doses used clinically (4). Its specificity for MAO-B, however, is dose-dependent and lost at supratherapeutic doses (4). Certain pharmaceuticals (e.g., linezolid, procarbazine) and herbal preparations (e.g., St. John's Wort, yohimbe alkaloids) have also been noted to have MAO inhibitor activity (4,9,16,20,21). These agents are all weak, reversible, nonselective inhibitors of MAO but still have the potential for adverse drug and food interactions.

Reversible selective inhibitors of MAO-A (befloxatone, brofaromine, cimoxatone, moclobemide, and teloxantrone), often termed RIMAs, have been developed and are used clinically outside the United States (1,4,7,8,10). With these agents, MAO inhibition is short-lived (enzyme activity commonly restored within 24 hours) and may be overcome by increasing levels of amine substrate. Initial experience with these agents has demonstrated greater safety following overdose and a significant reduction of adverse effects when combined with other pharmaceutical agents or dietary amines (1,4,7,8,10). MAO inhibitors may also be classified by chemical structure into hydrazines (iproniazid, isocarboxazid, and phenelzine), acetylenic agents (clorgyline, pargyline, selegiline), cyclopropylamines (tranylcypromine), benzamide derivatives (moclobemide, lazabemide), piperidyl-benzofurans (brofaromine), and oxazolidinones (cimoxatone, teloxantrone) (4,12,13,19,25). Most MAO inhibitors are structurally similar to amphetamines and other sympathomimetic agents, illustrating the concept that structure begets function (4,19). In fact, both selegiline and tranylcypromine are partly metabolized to amphetamine and methamphetamine (3,13,17,19). MAO inhibitors exert their pharmacologic and toxic effects by increasing neuronal and synaptic concentrations of biogenic amines (see Fig. 321.1) (4,18,19). By decreasing the degradation of MAO substrates, MAO inhibitors result in expansion of cytosolic and vesicular storage pools of NE, DA, and 5-HT in presynaptic nerve terminals. Increased presynaptic neurotransmitter concentrations increase their quantal release from vesicles during normal neurotransmission, cause spontaneous spill-over into the synaptic cleft independent of nerve activity, and decrease concentration-dependent reuptake by nerve-ending amine transporters (4,7,19,25). Spontaneous hypertensive episodes that occur in patients taking therapeutic doses of MAO inhibitors (in the absence of dietary indiscretions or drug interactions) likely result from the spontaneous release of NE from nerve terminals (13,15,19,25). As amphetamine congeners and indirect-acting sympathomimetics themselves, MAO inhibitors further enhance the release of cytoplasmic amines from the nerve ending in the absence of vesicle exocytosis (4,13,19). They bind competitively to the amine uptake transporter and prevent reuptake of natural amine neurotransmitters. When the MAO inhibitor is transported into the neuron, reverse transport of cytosolic biogenic amines occurs that further increases their synaptic concentrations. MAO inhibitors similarly prevent uptake from glial cell transporters that scavenge extracellular (synaptic) monoamines (4,7).

Overdose of MAO inhibitors produces an exaggeration of these neuronal effects and may result in profound hyperadrenergic, hyperdopaminergic, and hyperserotonergic states. The delayed appearance of signs and symptoms following overdose is attributed to initial reversible binding with MAO and the time required for significant enzyme inhibition and cumulative effects to occur (e.g., neuronal accumulation of NE, DA, 5-HT) (4,13,15). Although effects from NE and DA contribute significantly, the neuromuscular abnormalities (e.g., rigidity, myoclonus), hyperthermia, and unusual ocular movements associated with MAO overdose appear to be mediated primarily by enhanced serotonergic neurotransmission in the brainstem and spinal cord (12,18). Stimulation of 5-HT1A receptors from raphe bulbospinal neurons results in myoclonus and rigidity. These neuromuscular effects combined with stimulation of 5-HT2 receptors in the diencephalon result in hyperthermia. Enhanced raphe serotonergic neurotransmission, which controls saccadic eye movements, may produce an unusual "ping-pong" gaze in patients with severe MAO inhibitor toxicity (6,12). These effects are also seen in the serotonin syndrome (Chapter 322, "Serotonin Re-uptake Inhibitors").

The most serious adverse reactions associated with MAO inhibitor therapy result from drug and food interactions and are also the result of exaggerated neuronal effects (16). The administration or ingestion of any agent that increases CNS dopamine, norepinephrine, or serotonin levels may result in potentially life-threatening toxicity (4,16). Enhanced serotonergic neurotransmission, known as the serotonin syndrome (see Chapter 322, "Serotonin Re-uptake Inhibitors"), occurs

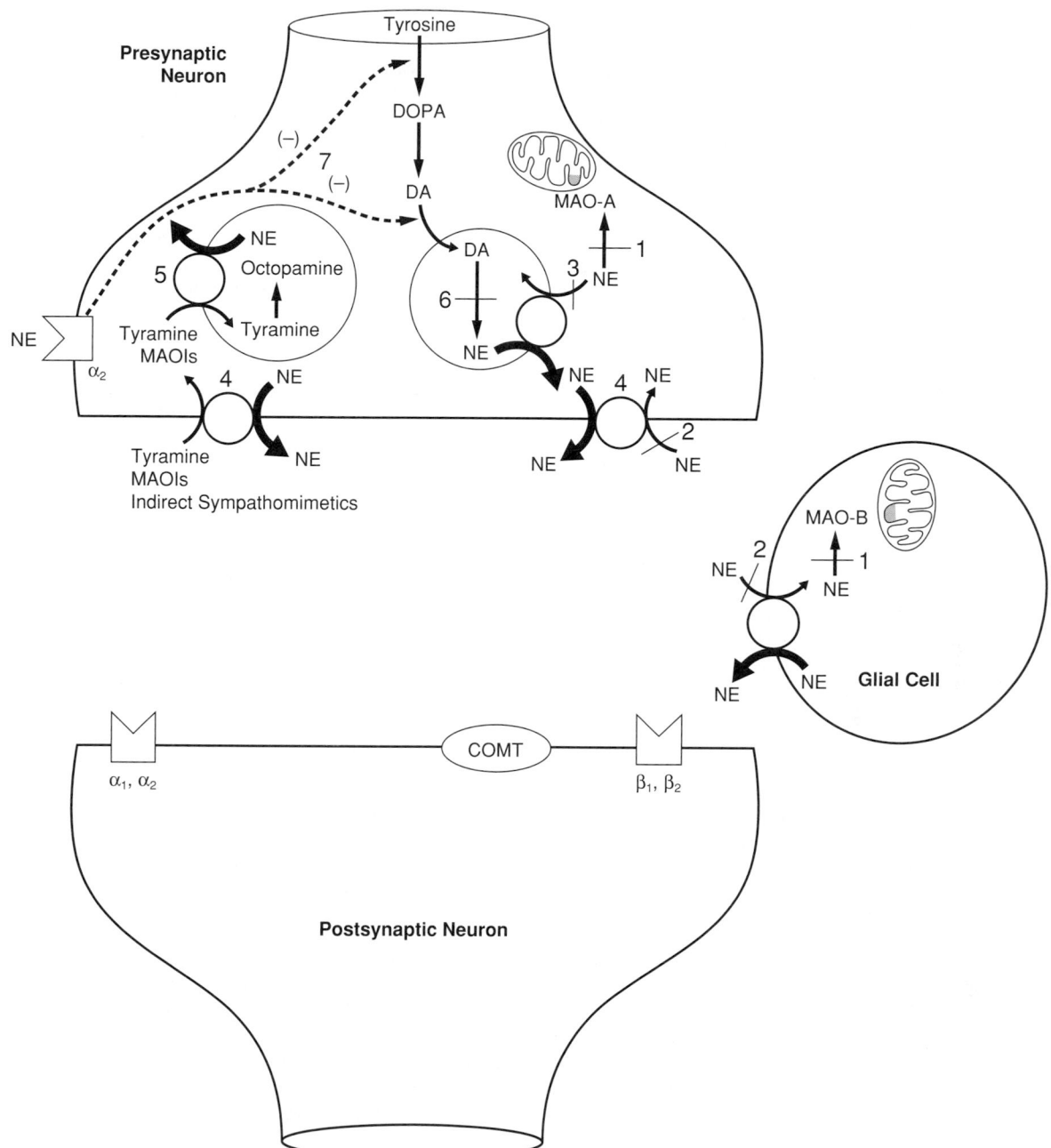

Figure 321.1. Diagram of a noradrenergic synapse illustrating the mechanisms underlying monoamine oxidase inhibitor (MAOI) toxicity: (1) Inhibit MAO to prevent norepinephrine (NE) degradation; (2) inhibit NE reuptake by monoamine transporter; (3) inhibit NE reuptake by vesicles; (4) promote reverse transport of NE from nerve ending; (5) promote reverse transport of NE from vesicles; (6) block dopamine (DA) β-hydroxylase; (7) indirectly inhibit enzymes necessary for production of NE. Similar mechanisms operate at dopaminergic and serotonergic nerve endings. α and β refer to adrenergic receptors; COMT = catechol-o-methyltransferase, another enzyme that degrades catecholamines.

when MAO inhibitors are combined with agents that enhance synthesis (e.g., *L*-tryptophan), promote release (e.g., methylene-dioxymethamphetamine, fenfluramine), or block reuptake (e.g., selective serotonin reuptake inhibitors, tricyclic antidepressants, lithium, meperidine) of serotonin (4,12,16,18,25). The use of indirectly acting sympathomimetic agents (e.g., amphetamine, cocaine, ephedrine, phenylpropanolamine, methylphenidate), which act primarily by causing the release of NE from the presynaptic nerve terminal, may result in the release of the expanded pool of NE and signs and symptoms of catecholamine poisoning (hypertensive crisis) (13–16,25). Most of these agents also

enhance release and block reuptake of dopamine to further potentiate the sympathomimetic effects.

A similar adverse sympathomimetic effect, called the "cheese reaction," may occur when foods containing large amounts of tyramine (e.g., aged cheeses; aged, pickled, or smoked meats; certain beers; red wines; and yeast extracts) and other indirectly acting monoamines (e.g., ephedrine, phenylethylamine, phenylethanolamine, pseudoephedrine, octopamine, reserpine, and tryptamine) are ingested (14,16). Inhibition of MAO in the liver and intestinal mucosa allows for systemic absorption of these amines. Like other indirect-acting amines, they may precipitate a rapid, massive release of NE when taken up into noradrenergic nerve endings.

Chronic MAO inhibition increases intraneuronal concentrations of false monoamine neurotransmitters (e.g., tyramine, phenylethylamine, octopamine), which are normally present in very small amounts. With the scavenging function of hepatic and intestinal MAO blocked, dietary monoamines gradually accumulate within noradrenergic nerve endings and displace NE from synaptic vesicles (see Fig. 321.1) (4,14,19,25). Stimulation of sympathetic neurons results in release of these false neurotransmitters, which have minimal postsynaptic effect. Functional blockade of sympathetic neurotransmission is manifested clinically by orthostatic hypotension. This hypotensive effect is potentiated by other adaptive responses that result from chronic MAO inhibition and include upregulation of inhibitory presynaptic receptors and downregulation of postsynaptic receptors (14,19,23). Orthostatic hypotension occurs in up to 47% of patients treated chronically with MAO inhibitors (4).

Additionally, MAO inhibitors, through feedback inhibition and via direct effects, inhibit tyrosine hydroxylase, *l*-amino acid decarboxylase, and DA decarboxylase, enzymes necessary for the production of catecholamine neurotransmitters (14,19,25). These pharmacologic effects likely contribute to the profound sympatholytic phase that follows an initial sympathomimetic phase in severe MAO inhibitor poisoning (13). After the initial massive catecholamine release, neuronal stores of these neurotransmitters are depleted, and there is the inability to rapidly regenerate new neurotransmitter. Hypotension and cardiovascular (CV) collapse result.

The acute and chronic toxic effects of MAO inhibitors are mediated by several additional mechanisms. MAO inhibitors interfere with the production, activation, supply, and function of pyridoxine and γ-amino butyric acid (GABA) by binding to and inhibiting pyridoxine, pyridoxine phosphokinase, *l*-amino acid decarboxylase, and the GABA$_A$ receptor (19,22). These effects may mediate seizures and peripheral neuropathy that are occasionally associated with acute overdose and chronic use of MAO inhibitors, respectively.

Hydrazine MAO inhibitors inhibit diamine oxidase, an enzyme that, in addition to MAO, metabolizes histamine (13,22). Flushing and hypotension may result from these effects. Hydrazine MAO inhibitors are also occasionally associated with the development of severe hepatotoxicity (4,16). Iproniazid was withdrawn from the market because of this (19,22). Hepatic injury is likely mediated by a toxic metabolite that binds irreversibly to hepatocellular macromolecules.

Several MAO inhibitors also inhibit hepatic cytochrome P-450 enzymes, and thus may potentiate the effects of alcohol, antihistamines, barbiturates, opioids, neuroleptics, anticonvulsants, benzodiazepines, and warfarin (3,4,15,16,19,22). Additionally, the hypoglycemic effects of insulin and oral antidiabetic drugs may be potentiated by MAO inhibitors (4,15,16). Currently, MAO inhibitors are available in oral formulation only (3,4). Recently developed transdermal delivery systems may enhance the safety of MAO inhibitors because parenteral drug administration preserves the activity of intestinal and hepatic MAO-A enzyme, thus avoiding sensitivity to dietary tyramine (2).

Following ingestion, MAO inhibitors are rapidly and completely absorbed from the gastrointestinal (GI) tract, with peak plasma concentrations ranging from 1 to 4 hours after ingestion (1,3,4,8,13,17). Plasma elimination for these agents is also rapid, with half-lives ranging from 1 to 3 hours (3,4). For the irreversible MAO inhibitors, plasma drug concentrations do not correlate with level of MAO inhibition, and toxic plasma concentrations have not been defined (13,15,22). Maximal inhibition of MAO occurs after 5 to 10 days of therapy with these agents (3,4,22). For reversible inhibitors, however, maximal MAO inhi-

bition is achieved within a few hours after the first dose (1,4,7,8). MAO inhibitors are extensively metabolized in the liver, often by many different enzymes (1,3,4,8,17). Hydrazines are partly inactivated by acetylation (3,4). Individuals with a reduced capacity to acetylate drugs ("slow acetylators") may be more likely to experience hyperadrenergic effects with therapeutic doses of MAO inhibitors. With irreversible MAO inhibitors, the potential for drug or dietary interactions may last for 2 to 3 weeks after discontinuation of treatment (14,15,16,19,22). For reversible agents, MAO activity is restored within 24 hours after the last dose, and the potential for drug and dietary interactions is much less (1,8). The ingestion of 2 to 3 mg/kg or more of an irreversible MAO inhibitor should be considered potentially life-threatening (13,15). Fatal amounts have been reported to be 4 to 6 mg/kg (13). Death has been reported after the ingestion of 170 to 650 mg of tranylcypromine and 375 to 1,500 mg of phenelzine (13). Survival after larger ingestions has also been reported (13,22).

CLINICAL PRESENTATION

Drug or food interactions with MAO inhibitors are common, with hypertensive crisis occurring in 1% to 8% of those taking MAO inhibitors therapeutically (4,15). The clinical presentation may include headache, hypertension, tachycardia (or reflex bradycardia), diaphoresis, agitation, hypertonicity, hyperreflexia with myoclonus, rigidity, seizures, and coma (14,15). Hyperpyrexia, intracranial hemorrhage, and death may occur (14). Toxicity begins within 30 to 90 minutes of the ingestion or administration of sympathomimetic amines (4). The duration of effect is variable but often resolves within a few hours.

MAO inhibitor overdose follows a distinctly different time course (5,6,13). The absence of early symptomatology is typical with nonselective irreversible agents. Onset of toxicity is usually delayed from 6 to 12 hours after the overdose, peaks from 24 to 48 hours for severe cases, and may last for 72 to 96 hours (13,23). A latent period as long as 29 hours has been described following tranylcypromine overdose (4,25). During the latent phase, the patient usually appears well or mildly sedated (4,5,13). Poisoning is characterized by alterations in behavior, cognition, autonomic nervous system function, and neuromuscular activity and may be classified as mild, moderate, or severe (Table 321.2) (13). Signs and symptoms vary greatly in their onset, severity, and duration. Patients with early or mild toxicity may demonstrate mild lethargy or restlessness, dysarthria, nausea, headache, ataxia, palpitations, flushing, shivering, sweating, tremor, nystagmus, incoordination, or hyperreflexia. Signs and symptoms of moderate toxicity may include confusion, hallucinations, disorientation, agitated delirium, mutism, salivation, diarrhea, marked diaphoresis, myoclonus, fasciculations, trismus, writhing movements, and mild-to-moderate elevations of temperature, pulse, respiratory rate, and blood pressure. Severe toxicity may be characterized by unresponsive coma; fixed, dilated pupils; "ping-pong" gaze; pathologic reflexes; generalized rigidity; seizures; hyperpyrexia (temperature greater than 104°F); marked tachypnea or respiratory depression; extreme sinus tachycardia or bradycardia; malignant cardiac dysrhythmias; hypotension; and death (4–6,13,22). Death from CV collapse is most likely to occur in patients with severe hyperpyrexia (5,13).

Although seizures may occur following MAO overdose, they are uncommon and can be confused with neuromuscular hyperactivity produced by these agents (4,5,12). Secondary complications may occur in patients with moderate-to-severe toxicity and include aspiration pneumonitis, adult respiratory distress syndrome, rhabdomyolysis, acute renal failure, metabolic acidosis, and disseminated intravascular coagulation (DIC) (13). The

TABLE 321.2.   Clinical Course of Monoamine Oxidase Inhibitor Poisoning

Phase-Severity[a]	Time after Ingestion[a]	Cognitive-Behavioral Dysfunction	Autonomic Dysfunction	Neuromuscular Dysfunction
0-Latent	0–24 h	Mild lethargy	Absent	Absent
I-Mild	6–12 h	Mild lethargy Dysarthria Ataxia Headache Anxiety Insomnia	Nausea Flushing Diaphoresis Shivering Irritability	Mild tremor Hyperreflexia Incoordination Nystagmus Mydriasis
II-Moderate	10–24 h	Confusion Disorientation Agitated delirium Mumbling/rambling speech Mutism Hyperactivity	Mild hyperthermia (temperature <104°F) Marked diaphoresis Salivation Piloerection Hypertension Sinus tachycardia (P <150 beats/min) Hyperventilation	Myoclonus Fasciculations Trismus Facial grimacing Writhing extremities
III-Severe	16–72 h	Incomprehensible speech Coma Seizures	Hyperventilation to respiratory arrest Extreme sinus tachycardia to sinus bradycardia Malignant dysrhythmias (VT, VF, bradyasystole) Hypotension Pale, clammy, mottled skin Severe hyperthermia (temperature <104°F)	Generalized rigidity Opisthotonus Fixed, dilated pupils "Ping-pong" gaze Pathologic reflexes (decorticate, decerebrate, Babinski)
IV-Complications	24–96 h	Aspiration pneumonitis Adult respiratory distress syndrome	Anion gap metabolic acidosis Hemolysis	Rhabdomyolysis Acute renal failure Disseminated intravascular coagulation Hepatic failure

[a] Signs and symptoms vary greatly in their onset, severity, and duration.

likelihood of secondary complications (e.g., rhabdomyolysis, DIC) and death is related to the degree and duration of hyperthermia. Patients with severe toxicity can manifest fixed, dilated pupils; posturing; and extensor plantar response yet make a complete neurologic recovery (4–6,12,23).

When taken alone, reversible inhibitors of MAO-A appear to have a benign course following acute overdose. Ingestion of doses as high as 20.5 g has resulted in only mild to moderate toxicity (8). Large overdoses are characterized by mild CNS depression, agitation, tachycardia, hypertension, and mydriasis (8). Although death is rare following overdose with moclobemide alone, mixed-drug overdoses are more serious. Many fatalities have been reported from the serotonin syndrome when moclobemide has been combined with other serotonin-potentiating drugs (e.g., citalopram, clomipramine, methylenedioxymethamphetamine, paroxetine, and sertraline) (8,11,24). Chronic use of irreversible nonselective inhibitors has been associated with hyperadrenergic adverse effects similar to the chronic use of amphetamines. These effects include agitation, confusion, hallucinations, hyperhidrosis, hypomania, insomnia, tremors, and seizures (4).

DIFFERENTIAL DIAGNOSIS

Amphetamine, cocaine, and sympathomimetic (including over-the-counter appetite suppressants) overdose may produce a clinical picture similar to the hypertensive reactions associated with MAO inhibitors and dietary and drug monoamines. The clinical presentation anticholinergic, hallucinogen (e.g., lysergic acid diethylamide, phencyclidine), lithium, salicylate, sympathomimetic (e.g., amphetamines, cocaine), and strychnine poisoning may be similar to that of MAO inhibitor overdose. MAO inhibitor toxicity may be confused with the neuroleptic malignant syndrome and withdrawal from alcohol or sedative–hypnotic agents. Clinical features of the serotonin syndrome are nearly identical to those following overdose with MAO inhibitors. Medical emergencies such as hypoglycemia, malignant hyperthermia, intracranial hemorrhage, meningitis, encephalitis, pheochromocytoma, septicemia, tetanus, and thyrotoxicosis may present in a similar manner.

EMERGENCY DEPARTMENT EVALUATION

The history should include the time, dose, and duration of exposure; the time of onset, nature, and severity of symptoms; the type of first aid undertaken; and the medical and psychiatric history. Accurate and complete historical data are essential in differentiating the toxic syndromes related to MAO inhibitors. The physical examination should focus on the vital signs and CV and neurologic function. Except for "ping-pong" gaze, there are no pathognomonic physical findings or laboratory abnormalities. Initial testing for patients with suspected intentional overdose should include an electrocardiogram and measurements of routine serum chemistries. Patients who present with signs and symptoms of toxicity should also have a complete blood count; prothrombin and partial thromboplastin times; creatine phosphokinase, calcium, magnesium, and liver function tests; and a urinalysis. Patients with altered mental status should have a bedside fingerstick glucose determination and appropriate intervention, as necessary. A lumbar puncture and computed tomography scanning may be necessary to differentiate drug intoxication from intracranial hemorrhage, meningitis, and encephalitis.

Toxicology screening may be useful to exclude other intoxications (e.g., acetaminophen and salicylate), but it rarely detects MAO inhibitors because of their low concentrations in blood and urine samples (13). Overdose of selegiline or tranylcypromine, however, may produce a positive qualitative screen for amphetamines (13,17,19). Quantitative MAO inhibitor levels are not generally available and have not been shown to correlate with the severity of poisoning (13,15). Similarly, the degree of MAO enzyme activity inhibition does not correlate with clinical toxicity.

EMERGENCY DEPARTMENT MANAGEMENT

Supportive care is the primary treatment for MAO inhibitor overdose. Advanced life-support measures should be instituted, as necessary. The administration of glucose, oxygen, naloxone, and thiamine should be considered for patients with altered mental status. Activated charcoal is the preferred method of GI decontamination for recent acute MAO inhibitor overdose. Before any drug or food is given, the potential for an adverse interaction with MAO inhibitors must be considered.

Agitation, neuromuscular hyperactivity, and seizures should be treated promptly with liberal doses of benzodiazepines (e.g., diazepam, lorazepam) or barbiturates (e.g., phenobarbital) (13). Phenytoin is unlikely to be as effective for seizures associated with MAO inhibitors. Pyridoxine administration (see Chapter 296, "Isoniazid") is recommended for seizures that occur following overdose with a hydrazine MAO inhibitor.

Rapid cooling is essential to minimize patient morbidity and mortality from hyperthermia. Because hyperthermia is almost invariably associated with CNS agitation and neuromuscular hyperactivity, initial treatment with benzodiazepines or barbiturates is recommended. In conjunction with these initial pharmacologic measures, evaporative and convective cooling methods, using wet sheets or cool mist sprays and fans, are recommended (13). Antipyretics and cooling blankets are generally ineffective. If these initial maneuvers do not provide rapid patient cooling, neuromuscular paralysis is strongly recommended (5,6,13).

Evidence from animal studies and human case reports suggests that neuromuscular paralysis is effective for the treatment of severe hyperthermia (5,6). Cooling times of less than 1 hour have been achieved with this method of treatment. Although dantrolene (2.5 mg/kg orally or intravenously every 6 hours) has also been reported to be effective (23), it is itself toxic and does not terminate muscular rigidity and hyperthermia as rapidly as paralyzing agents. Because the pathophysiology of serotonin syndrome overlaps considerably with MAO inhibitor overdose, nonspecific serotonin receptor antagonists (e.g., cyproheptadine, methysergide; see Chapter 322, "Serotonin Re-uptake Inhibitors") could be of benefit (11). Because there is no clinical data in this regard, such therapy cannot currently be recommended.

Severe hypertension may be treated with the intravenous administration of rapid-onset, short-acting agents such as sodium nitroprusside or phentolamine (13,15,22). Phentolamine (2–10 mg i.v.) is pharmacologically attractive because it can block α-adrenergic receptors and antagonize the effects of NE. It has proven effective for the treatment of hypertension associated with the "cheese reaction"(14). Long-acting agents (tolazoline, clonidine) also have been used but are not recommended, as hypertension is often followed by severe hypotension (13).

β-adrenergic antagonists are not recommended for the control of hypertension because of the potential for unopposed α-adrenergic vasoconstriction and worsened hypertension.

Hypotension should initially be treated with fluid resuscitation. When pressors are required, direct-acting agents (e.g., epinephrine, NE) are recommended (13,15). The use of indirect-acting agents (e.g., DA), which require the release of intracellular amines for their pressor effect, may either precipitate a hypertensive crisis or be ineffective on account of depleted stores of catecholamines (4). Additionally, MAO inhibition is less likely to potentiate the effects of exogenously administered, direct-acting pressors, which circulate extracellularly and are primarily metabolized by catechol-o-methyltransferase. Regardless, low doses of direct-acting pressors should be used initially to minimize the risk of an exaggerated pressor response. Phenylephrine, a direct-acting agent, has been associated with an exaggerated pressor response and is not recommended for the treatment of hypotension in MAO inhibitor poisoning (14).

Ventricular dysrhythmias and severe bradycardias, usually premorbid signs, should be treated according to current advanced cardiac life-support protocols. Bretylium, however, is not recommended for the treatment of refractory ventricular dysrhythmias; it has initial catecholamine-releasing effects that may potentiate the cardiotoxic effects of MAO inhibitors (13,15).

Diuresis, urinary acidification, hemodialysis, and hemoperfusion play no role in the management of MAO inhibitor poisoning (3,13,15).

CRITICAL INTERVENTIONS

- Admit all patients with known or suspected MAO inhibitor overdose to an intensive care unit for 24-hour monitoring
- Treat neuromuscular hyperactivity with benzodiazepines or barbiturates; if severe or accompanied by hyperthermia or rhabdomyolysis, institute neuromuscular paralysis
- Rapidly and aggressively cool patients with hyperthermia
- Administer a direct-acting pressor (e.g., norepinephrine) for hypotension unresponsive to fluid administration

DISPOSITION

All patients with suspected MAO inhibitor overdose should be admitted for extended observation (24 hours) in a monitored setting. Symptomatic patients and those with abnormal vital signs should be admitted to an intensive care unit. If intensive care is unavailable, patients should be transferred to an institution with this capacity.

Patients who present with drug or dietary interactions may not require hospital admission if the clinical response has been mild. Patients with severe reactions, those with persistent symptoms after a 4- to 6-hour observation period, and those with symptoms that necessitate active intervention should be admitted. The level of in-hospital care required (intensive care or floor) depends on the severity of symptoms. For patients well enough to eat, an MAO inhibitor diet (e.g., low tyramine) should be ordered.

COMMON PITFALLS

✔ Failure to check for or recognize MAO inhibitor use before prescribing sympathomimetics or giving pain medications, particularly meperidine

✔ Failure to appreciate that the history is key to differentiating acute overdose from drug and food interactions, including the serotonin syndrome

✔ Failure to appreciate that the onset of toxicity may be delayed and gradual in onset after MAO inhibitor overdose

✔ Failure to appreciate that early sympathetic stimulation may be followed by catecholamine depletion and CV collapse in patients with acute MAO inhibitor overdose

References

1. Amrein R, Allen SR, Guentert TW, et al. The pharmacology of reversible monoamine oxidase inhibitors. *Br J Psychiatry* 1989;155[Suppl 6]:66.
2. Amsterdam JD. A double-blind, placebo-controlled trial of the safety and efficacy of selegiline transdermal system without dietary restrictions in patients with major depressive disorder. *J Clin Psychiatry* 2003;64:208–214.
3. Baker GB, Urichuk LJ, McKenna KF, et al. Metabolism of monoamine oxidase inhibitors. *Cell Mol Neurobiol* 1999;19:411–426.
4. Baldessarini RJ. Drugs and the treatment of psychiatric disorders. In: Hardman JG, Limbird LE, Gilman AG, eds. *Goodman & Gilman's: the pharmacological basis of therapeutics,* 10th ed. New York, McGraw-Hill, 2001:447–483.
5. Ciocatto E, Gagiano G, Bava GL. Clinical features and treatment of overdosage of monoamine oxidase inhibitors and their interaction with other psychotropic drugs. *Resuscitation* 1972;1:69.
6. Erich JL, Shih RD, O'Connor RE. "Ping-pong" gaze in severe monoamine oxidase inhibitor toxicity. *J Emerg Med* 1995;13:653.
7. Finberg JPM. Pharmacology of reversible and selective inhibitors of monoamine oxidase type A. *Acta Psychiatr Scand* 1995;91[Suppl 386]:8.
8. Fulton B, Benfield P. Moclobemide: an update of its pharmacological properties and therapeutic use. *Drugs* 1996;52:450.
9. Hammerness P, Parada H, Abrams A. Linezolid: MAOI activity and potential drug interactions. *Psychosomatics* 2002;43:248–249.
10. Hartmann D, Cesura AM, Schmid-Burgk W, et al. Relevance of reversible inhibitors of monoamine oxidase type A and reuptake inhibition for noradrenaline turnover. *Acta Psychiatr Scand* 1995;91[Suppl 386]:14.
11. Hojer J, Personne M, Skagius AS, et al. Serotonin syndrome: several cases of this often overlooked diagnosis. *Tidsskr Nor Laegeforen* 2002;122:1660–1663.
12. Lieberman JA, Kane JM, Reife R. Neuromuscular effects of monoamine oxidase inhibitors. *Adv Neurol* 1986;43:231.
13. Linden CH, Rumack BH. MAO inhibitor overdose. *Ann Emerg Med* 1984;13:1137.
14. Lippman SB, Nash K. MAO inhibitor update: potential adverse food and drug interactions. *Drug Saf* 1990;5:195.
15. Lipson RE, Stern TA. Management of monoamine oxidase inhibitor-treated patients in the emergency and critical care setting. *J Intensive Care Med* 1991;6:117.
16. Livingston MG, Livingston HM. Monoamine oxidase inhibitors. An update on drug interactions. *Drug Saf* 1996;14:219–227.
17. Mallinger AG, Smith E. Pharmacokinetics of MAO inhibitors. *Psychopharmacol Bull* 1991;27:493.
18. Marley E, Wozniak KM. Interactions of non-selective monoamine oxidase inhibitors, tranylcypromine and nialamide, with inhibitors of 5-hydroxytryptamine, dopamine, or noradrenaline uptake. *J Psychiatr Res* 1984;18:191.
19. McDaniel KD. Clinical pharmacology of monoamine oxidase inhibitors. *Clin Neuropharmacol* 1986;9:207.
20. Miller LG. Herbal medicinals: selected clinical considerations focusing on known or potential drug-herbal interactions. *Arch Intern Med* 1998;158:2200–2211.
21. Patel S, Robinson R, Burk M. Hypertensive crisis associated with St. John's Wort. *Am J Med* 2002;112:507–508.
22. Tollefson GD. Monoamine oxidase inhibitors: a review. *J Clin Psychiatry* 1983;44:280.
23. Verrilli MR, Salanga VD, Kozachuk WE, et al. Phenelzine toxicity responsive to dantrolene. *Neurology* 1987;37:865.
24. Vuori E, Henry JA, Ojanpera I, et al. Death following ingestion of MDMA (ecstasy) and moclobemide. *Addiction* 2003;98:365–368.
25. Wells DG, Bjorksten AR. Monoamine oxidase inhibitors revisited. *Can J Anaesth* 1989;36:64.

CHAPTER 322
Serotonin Re-uptake Inhibitors

Andis Graudins

The serotonin re-uptake inhibitor antidepressants are a widely prescribed group of agents used for the treatment of depression and numerous other psychiatric disorders. They have largely replaced the cyclic antidepressants as first-line therapy for depression. This group includes the selective serotonin re-uptake inhibitors (SSRIs); fluoxetine, sertraline, paroxetine, citalopram, and fluvoxamine and the serotonin norepinephrine re-uptake inhibitors (SNRIs); venlafaxine and nefazodone. In general, these drugs have relatively safe side effect profiles when compared to the cyclic antidepressants and do not cause significant cardiac or neurologic toxicity in overdose. The most significant form of toxicity seen with this group is the serotonin syndrome, which is a syndrome of serotonergic excess resulting from either drug interactions between two serotonergic agents or following overdose of SSRIs or other serotonergic drugs.

All antidepressants potentiate monoaminergic neurotransmission in the central nervous system (CNS), which is responsible for the therapeutic effects of these drugs. The majority of clinically used antidepressants either attenuate the reuptake of serotonin (5-HT) and/or norepinephrine (NE), as is the case with SSRIs, or inhibit the metabolism of these neurotransmitters, as occurs with monoamine oxidase inhibitors (22). The biochemical effects of inhibiting biogenic amine re-uptake and metabolism are immediate and readily demonstrable in both experimental animals and man, but there is a 2- to 6-week delay in the onset of the clinical therapeutic effect. SSRIs and SNRIs exert their effect primarily by inhibiting the re-uptake of amine neurotransmitters into the presynaptic nerve terminal.

All the SSRI agents are well absorbed from the gastrointestinal (GI) tract with peak serum concentrations occurring 6 to 12 hours postingestion of therapeutic doses. These agents are highly protein bound with large volume of distribution and extensively metabolized by hepatic microsomal enzymes, in particular CYP-2D6 (22). The SSRIs also inhibit various other hepatic microsomal enzymes, which may result in significant interactions with other pharmaceutical agents and increase the risk of development of serotonin syndrome from drug interactions, particularly with the older MAO-inhibitors (20). Fluoxetine is metabolized to an active metabolite, norfluoxetine, with an elimination half-life greater than the parent compound (fluoxetine $t_{1/2} = 1$–3 days, norfluoxetine $t_{1/2} = 4$–16 days). A substantial wash-out period should be observed when changing a patient from fluoxetine to another serotonergic antidepressant to avoid the risk of serotonergic complications such as serotonin syndrome. The half-life of other agents is significantly shorter than that of fluoxetine (sertraline and paroxetine $t_{1/2} = 20$ hrs, venlafaxine $t_{1/2} = 6$–12 hours) (1).

SSRI and SNRI antidepressants are much safer following overdose than the traditional cyclic antidepressants and irreversible monoamine oxidase (MAO) inhibitors (13, 25). The most common toxic effect seen following overdose is the serotonin syndrome. This may occur in up to 10% of overdoses with SSRIs (13). Despite this, SSRI overdose commonly results in a shorter

TABLE 322.1. Drugs Affecting Central Nervous System Serotonin Concentrations with the Potential to Produce Serotonin Syndrome[a]

Increased serotonin production Increased presynaptic serotonin release	L-tryptophan Amphetamines MDMA Cocaine
Decrease serotonin breakdown by monoamine oxidase	*Irreversible inhibitors of MAO-A and MAO-B* *Phenelzine, tranylcypromine, isocarboxazid* *Reversible inhibitors of MAO-A* Moclobemide *Reversible inhibitors of MAO-B* Selegiline
Inhibition of serotonin reuptake	*Serotonin-specific reuptake inhibitors* fluoxetine, citalopram, paroxetine, sertraline, fluvoxamine, cyclic antidepressants, meperidine, dextromethorphan *Serotonin-noradrenaline reuptake inhibitors* Venlafaxine, nefazodone
Direct agonists of postsynaptic receptors	Bromocriptine, lithium, levo-DOPA, electroconvulsive therapy

From (Gillman PK. Ecstasy, serotonin syndrome and the treatment of hyperpyrexia. *Med J Aust* 1997;197:109–110, Mills KC. Serotonin Syndrome. *Crit Care Clin* 1997;13;763–783) with permission.

length of hospital stay, a lesser need for intensive care unit admission or endotracheal intubation and a lower incidence of coma, seizures, or cardiac toxicity than seen with cyclic antidepressants (13). The exception to this is venlafaxine, which has the potential to produce seizures in overdose and cardiac conduction delays (QRS > 100 milliseconds) and ventricular tachycardia in large overdoses (> 5–8 grams) (25). Venlafaxine blocks sodium channels in cardiac myocytes in the resting state. This is unlike the cyclic antidepressant effect of sodium channel blockade during the inactivated phase of the sodium channel cycle (17).

The serotonin syndrome is the result of pharmacologic overstimulation of CNS 5-hydroxytryptamine (5-HT) or serotonin receptors. It may result from drug interactions during therapeutic dosing or from overdose with one or multiple serotonin-specific antidepressant agents. Most reports of the syndrome are either single case reports or small case series. There is no obvious gender or age preference. In a study of 204 patients exposed to serotonergic antidepressants, there was a 10% incidence of serotonin syndrome. Seventy percent of these cases were the result of overdose; the remainder were a result of therapeutic drug interactions. A single agent was involved in 50%, and two were involved in 45% (6). Drug interactions often result from substituting a new antidepressant for one with a long elimination half-life (e.g., fluoxetine) or duration of action (e.g., a MAO inhibitor; see Chapter 321, "Monoamine Oxidase Inhibitors") without an adequate wash-out period. Drug interactions also may be precipitated by the addition of a second serotonergic antidepressant. Finally, patients may be taking an antidepressant and unknowingly be given another medication with serotonergic activity (e.g., meperidine or dextromethorphan in a patient taking an MAOI or serotonergic antidepressant) (5,8,24). The severe hyperthermic response sometimes seen following methylenedioxymethamphetamine (MDMA, "ecstasy") abuse may also be as a result of the serotonergic hyperstimulation (10).

Serotonin is a neurotransmitter found widely throughout the body. Large amounts are stored in the enterochromaffin cells of the gastrointestinal tract (greater than 90% of body stores), in which it produces stimulation of vascular and GI smooth muscle contraction. Lesser amounts (8% of body stores) are found in platelets. The CNS contains a relatively small amount of serotonin (2% of body stores). Its main action is the inhibition of

excitatory neurotransmission. Animal models of serotonin syndrome suggest that excessive stimulation of brainstem $5HT_{1A}$ and cortical $5HT_2$ receptors is responsible for the serotonin syndrome (11). Various drugs and mechanisms of action may be involved (Table 322.1).

CLINICAL PRESENTATION

In most instances, an isolated ingestion of an SSRI agent in overdose will not result in significant toxicity. Common symptoms include mild nausea, occasional vomiting, and transient drowsiness. Seizures may be seen following venlafaxine overdose, particularly in doses greater than 3 grams (25) and cardiac conduction delays (increased QRS duration) and ventricular dysrhythmias have been reported, particularly with ingestions over 5 to 8 grams (2,21,25). The onset of toxicity can be delayed by several hours if the sustained-release formulation of venlafaxine has been ingested. Seizures and electrocardiographic QRS-duration prolongation have also be reported following overdose with fluoxetine (3,15).

Serotonin syndrome remains the most common significant complication following SSRI overdose. The signs and symptoms of this can be divided into three major categories: altered mental status, autonomic nervous system instability, and neuromuscular hyperactivity (Table 322.2). Milder forms of the syndrome may present with abnormalities in only one or two of these categories. A review of 127 cases of the serotonin syndrome found that the most common clinical findings were myoclonus, hyperreflexia, confusion, hyperthermia, diaphoresis, and sinus tachycardia (19). The diagnosis remains one of exclusion and should be considered in patients with a history of recent exposure to serotonergic agents and findings in any of the major categories.

The time of onset of symptoms following exposure to serotonergic agents is variable. Symptoms are often reported to develop within 1 to 2 hours of ingestion (7,14). The syndrome has also been reported to occur after several days following gradual increases in dosing of antidepressant medications (4). There appears to be no relationship between the amount of drug ingested and the risk of serotonin syndrome, as it can occur both with therapeutic dosing and in overdose. Reported serum

TABLE 322.2.   Summary of Potential Clinical Findings Associated with Serotonin Syndrome

Autonomic Instability	Altered Mental Status	Neuromuscular Hyperactivity
Tachycardia	Anxiety	Myoclonus
Fluctuating blood pressure	Confusion	Hyperreflexia
Diaphoresis	Drowsiness	Muscle rigidity
Flushed skin	Hallucinations	Tremor
Hyperthermia	Coma	Agitation
Tachypnea	Insomnia	Restlessness
Mydriasis	Dizziness	Ataxia
Unreactive pupils		Nystagmus
Diarrhea		Trismus
Abdominal pain		Opisthotonus
Excessive salivation		

levels of drugs measured in patients with the serotonin syndrome have been either at therapeutic or below therapeutic levels in up to 90% of cases (19).

DIFFERENTIAL DIAGNOSIS

Meningitis, encephalitis, septicemia, hypoglycemia, and neurotrauma should be considered in the differential diagnosis of patients presenting with mental status changes, seizures, autonomic instability, or hyperthermia. Intoxication with amphetamines, cocaine, or hallucinogens and withdrawal from alcohol and benzodiazepines should be considered when agitation, hallucinations, and sympathetic excess are present. In these conditions, the characteristic neuromuscular features of serotonin syndrome are usually absent.

Neuromuscular hyperactivity may be seen in dystonic reactions, tetanus, strychnine poisoning, and lithium intoxication. Lithium toxicity and tetanus may have additional features suggestive of the serotonin syndrome. The most similar condition, however, is the neuroleptic malignant syndrome (NMS; see Chapter 317, "Antipsychotic Agents"). In contrast to patients with the serotonin syndrome, those with NMS have a history of recent commencement of, or increase in, dosage of neuroleptic medications. Symptoms tend to develop (and later resolve) over days rather than hours; muscular hyperactivity is characterized by sustained "lead pipe" rigidity rather than by myoclonus; and hyperreflexia is rarely, if ever, seen (19).

In patients presenting with obtundation and cardiac QRS-conduction delay, hypotension and/or seizures other poisonings should be considered. This should include cyclic antidepressants, Class 1a and 1c antiarrhythmic agents, and first generation antihistamines such as diphenhydramine, chloroquine, and venlafaxine.

EMERGENCY DEPARTMENT EVALUATION

In patients presenting with a clinical picture suggestive of serotonin syndrome the history should focus on drug use. Specifically, any evidence of drug overdose and use of multiple serotonergic medications, drugs of abuse, and over-the-counter medications containing dextromethorphan should be sought. The time course of onset and progression of symptoms is important in discriminating between NMS and serotonin syndrome.

Both the history and physical examination should focus on excluding other causes of the clinical picture. Vital signs should include an accurate temperature. A thorough search for evidence

of trauma should be made. Patients should be questioned about the presence of visual or auditory hallucinations and examined for neuromuscular features of serotonin syndrome. Features of serotonin syndrome that are present should be documented. The vital signs should be repeated frequently, as autonomic instability can result in fluctuating blood pressure and pulse. A finger-stick blood sugar should be performed on patients with altered mental state. A 12-lead electrocardiogram should be performed to exclude cardiac conduction disturbances that may be the result of venlafaxine overdose.

Laboratory investigation should focus on excluding other causes of the clinical picture and evaluating for potential complications of the serotonin syndrome. A complete blood count, electrolytes, glucose, blood urea nitrogen, creatinine, and urinalysis and creatine kinase (to rule out rhabdomyolysis) are suggested. A coagulation profile, liver function tests, cultures, chest radiograph, head computed tomography scan, and lumbar puncture may be necessary in severely ill or hyperthermic patients to exclude sepsis, cranial trauma, meningitis, and complications such as multiorgan failure and coagulopathy (disseminated intravascular coagulation). Although toxicology testing is unlikely to be of any benefit in the acute management, detecting a serotonergic agent can support the diagnosis when a history of drug ingestion cannot be obtained.

EMERGENCY DEPARTMENT MANAGEMENT

First and foremost, the management of SSRI poisoning and serotonin syndrome consists of supportive care. Advanced life-support measures should be instituted, as necessary. Airway control and assisted ventilation may be required in obtunded patients with severe forms of the syndrome to maintain oxygenation and prevent aspiration pneumonia. Agitation, myoclonus, hypertonia, or hyperpyrexia should initially be treated with intravenous benzodiazepines, crystalloids, and external cooling measures. If no response is observed, chemical neuromuscular paralysis with sedation should be used to reduce muscle tone and decrease hyperthermia (7,9).

Venlafaxine-induced cardiac conduction delays may respond to hyperventilation and serum alkalinization with hypertonic sodium bicarbonate in view of the mechanism of action at the voltage-gated sodium channel. Unfortunately, no clinical data exist regarding the efficacy this therapy in this setting. Ventricular dysrhythmias should be treated utilizing standard advanced cardiac life-support guidelines.

Seizures resulting from serotonin syndrome or venlafaxine toxicity should be treated with intravenous benzodiazepines and barbiturates. Continuous electroencephalographic monitoring should be considered in paralyzed patients with suspected seizures. In milder forms of serotonin syndrome, benzodiazepines should be given to reduce anxiety, restlessness, and tremor, but they may be ineffective on their own (19). Serotonergic medications must be discontinued and avoided. GI decontamination, using activated charcoal, should be considered for patients with acute overdose presenting within 1 to 2 hours of ingestion. In patients who have ingested a sustained-release formulation of venlafaxine, GI decontamination with whole-bowel irrigation should be considered.

Serotonin-receptor antagonists can be considered as an adjunctive therapy in the treatment of serotonin syndrome. Cyproheptadine (Periactin), a first-generation antihistamine with $5HT_{1A}$ and $5HT_2$ receptor-blocking effects, has been used in a number of cases of serotonin syndrome with apparent success (14,18,23). It appears to be relatively free of potential major adverse effects. The initial adult dose is 4 to 8 mg, orally or by gastric tube, with repeat doses every 2 to 4 hours until a response is noted. It is then continued at a dose of 4 mg every 6 to 8 hours for a period of 24 hours. The maximum recommended dose is 32 mg in 24 hours. In patients with signs and symptoms of mild-to-moderate severity, a response is typically noted in 1 to 2 hours (14). Cyproheptadine may not produce an obvious response in severe cases. Sublingual administration has been previously suggested in patients who have been given activated charcoal. In a pharmacokinetic study of oral vs. sublingual cyproheptadine absorption it was found that sublingual absorption is negligible (16).

Chlorpromazine, a nonspecific serotonin receptor antagonist, has been used successfully in doses of 50 to 100 mg i.v. and i.m. (9,12). Administration should be preceded by adequate intravenous fluid hydration to prevent hypotension. Other side effects include anticholinergic effects and dystonic reactions. The use of chlorpromazine in patients with NMS wrongly diagnosed as serotonin syndrome has the potential to worsen this condition.

CRITICAL INTERVENTIONS

- Establish i.v. access, institute cardiac monitoring, and obtain an ECG in patients with SSRI overdose or suspected serotonin syndrome
- Administer benzodiazepines and crystalloids intravenously, and provide cooling measures as necessary in patients with agitation, myoclonus, hypertonia, or hyperpyrexia as a result of the serotonin syndrome; institute neuromuscular paralysis with continued sedation therapy in refractory cases

DISPOSITION

Patients ingesting SSRIs can be observed in the emergency department for 6 hours and medically cleared if asymptomatic at that time. Patients ingesting sustained-release formulations of venlafaxine should be observed for delayed signs of toxicity or serotonin syndrome in a monitored setting for 24 hours.

Most patients with serotonin syndrome require admission and 12 to 24 hours of close observation and cardiac monitoring in a telemetry or intensive care unit symptoms and signs resolve. Severe cases or those with evidence of complications require intensive care. In mild forms of the syndrome, symptoms may resolve spontaneously, or following use of a specific serotonin antagonist such as cyproheptadine, in a shorter time. All patients with a history of intentional overdose require psychiatric assessment prior to discharge. The risk of recurrent serotonin syndrome must be weighed against the benefits of therapy and alternative treatments when considering reinstitution of serotonergic medications.

COMMON PITFALLS

✔ Prescribing meperidine for pain relief or dextromethorphan as a cough suppressant to patients taking serotonergic medications, particularly MAOIs
✔ Failure to obtain a temperature and to recognize the serotonin syndrome in patients with agitation, myoclonus, and hypertonia and to exclude other conditions causing similar signs and symptoms
✔ Failure to appreciate the variety of drugs with serotonergic activity and to take a detailed history of recent drug exposure
✔ Failure to appreciate that supportive care is the primary treatment for SSRI poisoning and the serotonin syndrome
✔ Failure to consider hyperventilation and serum alkalinization with hypertonic sodium bicarbonate for venlafaxine-induced cardiac conduction delays
✔ Failure to appreciate that serotonin-specific antagonists such as cyproheptadine and chlorpromazine can be used as adjunctive therapies in serotonin syndrome but may be ineffective in severe forms of the condition

References

1. Baumann P. Pharmacokinetic-pharmacodynamic relationship of the selective serotonin reuptake inhibitors. *Clin Pharmacokinet* 1996;31:444–469.
2. Blythe D, Hackett LP. Cardiovascular and neurological toxicity of venlafaxine. *Hum Exp Toxicol* 1999;18:309–313.
3. Braitberg G, Curry SC. Seizure after isolated fluoxetine overdose. *Ann Emerg Med* 1995;26:234–237.
4. Brodribb TR, Downey M, Gilbar PJ. Efficacy and adverse effects of moclobemide (letter). *Lancet* 1994;343:475.
5. Chan BS, Graudins A, Whyte IM, et al. Serotonin syndrome resulting from drug interactions. *Med J Aust* 1998;169:523–525.
6. Chan BS, Graudins A, Braitberg G, et al. A survey of serotonin syndrome by the New South Wales Poison Information Centre. *Proceedings of the Australasian Society of Experimental and Clinical Pharmacologists* 1997;4:63.
7. Francois BP, Marquet ADesachy, et al. Serotonin syndrome due to an overdose of moclobemide and clomipramine. A potentially life-threatening association. *Intensive Care Med* 1997;23:122–124.
8. Gillman PK. Possible serotonin syndrome with moclobemide and pethidine. [letter]. *Med J Aust* 1995;162:554.
9. Gillman PK. Successful treatment of serotonin syndrome with chlorpromazine. (letter). *Med J Aust* 1996;165:345.
10. Gillman PK. Ecstasy, serotonin syndrome and the treatment of hyperpyrexia. *Med J Aust* 1997;197:109–110.
11. Goodwin GM, DeSouza RJ, Green AR. The pharmacology of the behavioural and hypothermic responses of rats to 8-hyroxy2-(di-n-propylamino)tetralin (8-OH-DPAT). *Psychopharm* 1987;91:506–511.
12. Graham PM. Successful treatment of the toxic serotonin syndrome with chlorpromazine. (letter). *Med J Aust* 1997;166:166–167.
13. Graudins A, Dowsett RP, Liddle C. The toxicity of antidepressant poisoning: is it changing? A comparative study of cyclic and newer serotonin-specific antidepressants. *Emergency Med* 2002;14:440–446.
14. Graudins A, Stearman A, Chan B. Treatment of the serotonin syndrome with cyproheptadine. *J Emerg Med* 1998;16:615–619.
15. Graudins A, Vossler C, Wang R. Fluoxetine-induced cardiotoxicity with response to bicarbonate therapy. *Am J Emerg Med* 1997;15:501–503.
16. Gunja N, Collins M, Graudins A. A comparison of the pharmacokinetics of oral and sublingual cyproheptadine. *J Toxicol Clin Toxicol* 2004;42:1–5.
17. Khalifa M, Daleau P, Turgeon J. Mechanism of sodium channel block by venlafaxine in guinea pig ventricular myocytes. *Journal of Pharmacology & Experimental Therapeutics* 1999;291:280–284.
18. Lappin RI. Auchinschloss EL. Treatment of serotonin syndrome with cyproheptadine. (letter). *N Engl J Med* 1994;331:1021–1022.
19. Mills KC. Serotonin Syndrome. *Crit Care Clin* 1997;13:763–783.
20. Mitchell PB. Drug interactions of clinical significance with selective serotonin reuptake inhibitors. *Drug Saf* 1997;17.
21. Peano C, Leikin JB, Hanashiro PK. Seizures, ventricular tachycardia, and rhabdomyolysis as a result of ingestion of venlafaxine and lamotrigine. *Ann Emerg Med* 1997;30:704–708.
22. Popik P. Preclinical Pharmacology of Citalopram. *J Clin Psychopharmacol* 1999;19:4S–22S.
23. Sternbach H. The serotonin syndrome. *Am J Psychiatry* 1991;148:705–713.
24. Weiner AL, Tilden FF Jr, McKay CA Jr. Serotonin syndrome: case report and review of the literature. *Conn Med* 1997;61:717–721.
25. Whyte IM, Dawson AH, Buckley NA. Relative toxicity of venlafaxine and selective serotonin reuptake inhibitors in overdose compared to tricyclic antidepressants. *QJM* 2003;96:369–374.

Stimulants and Hallucinogens

CHAPTER 323
Anticholinergic Agents

Andis Graudins

Anticholinergic syndrome (ACS) is a common side effect of many pharmaceutical agents, natural remedies, and plants both after therapeutic doses and overdose. Toxic effects result from inhibition of normal muscarinic-cholinergic transmission in the peripheral and central nervous system. Symptoms and signs may range from mild manifestations of the syndrome (e.g., dry mouth and blurred vision) to severe anticholinergic delirium with agitation, hallucinations and aggressive behavior. Some of the many pharmaceuticals and toxins capable of causing the ACS are listed in Table 323.1.

Agents with anticholinergic side effects are often abused for their ability to produce hallucinations. This may include pure anticholinergics agents such as benztropine, older or first generation histamine-1 receptor blockers, and botanical agents such as Jimsonweed (*Datura stramonium*). Commonly implicated antihistamines include diphenhydramine, promethazine, and pheniramine. ACS may also occur as a side effect following overdose of pharmaceuticals with other mechanisms of toxicity such as cyclic antidepressants and antipsychotics. Finally, it may be seen as an iatrogenic complication of therapy with medications that have anticholinergic properties; this is particularly the case in susceptible populations such as infants and the elderly.

Histamine-1 receptor blockers are a class of pharmaceuticals widely available both in prescription and over-the-counter formulations. They are used for multiple purposes in the control and treatment of allergic conditions, as sleep aids, and as antiemetics. This group can be further divided into the "first generation" agents which tend to be more lipophilic and are more sedating, and the "second generation" or nonsedating agents. These agents are available in their pure forms or combined with multiple other substances (e.g., analgesics, sympathomimetics, caffeine, anticholinergic compounds), which can significantly alter the clinical presentation in overdose (5). The H_2-receptor antagonists are primarily used in the treatment of peptic ulcer disease and gastroesophageal reflux but are also used in conjunction with H_1 antagonists in the treatment of severe allergic reactions.

TABLE 323.1. Substances That May Result in the Production of Anticholinergic Delirium

Pharmaceuticals	Anticholinergic Agents	Atropine
		Benzhexol
		Benztropine
		Scopolamine
	Cyclic antidepressants	Amitriptyline
		Imipramine
		Dothiepin
		Doxepin
	Antipsychotics	Phenothiazines
		Clozapine
		Risperidone
	First generation H_1 receptor blockers	Cetirizine
		Cyproheptadine
		Dexchlorpheniramine
		Diphenhydramine
		Diphenylpyraline
		Hydroxyzine
		Methdilazine
		Pheniramine
		Promethazine
		Trimipramine
	Others	Amantadine, cyclobenzaprine
		Carbamazepine, orphenadrine
		Chinese herbal medicines
Botanicals		*Datura spp.*
		Jimsonweed or thorn apple
		Datura sawolens- Angel's trumpet
		Atropa belladona – deadly nightshade
		Hyoscyamus niger- Black henbane

The incidence of antihistamine overdose increased markedly following the approval of over-the-counter sale for brompheniramine, chlorpheniramine, and diphenhydramine in 1983. In 1997 antihistamines represented 4.9% of all exposures reported to poison control centers in the United States (16). This number appears to be rising with each year and may be related to the increasing availability of these agents over the counter. Half of all exposures occurred in children under 6 years of age. Half the ingestions were with over-the-counter medications and half involved the use of diphenhydramine. There were 25 reported deaths with H_1 receptor antagonist ingestions but none from

H_2 receptor antagonists (16). H_1 blockers are reversible competitive pharmacologic antagonists of histamine at H_1 receptor sites. They decrease vascular permeability, reduce pruritus, and relax smooth muscle in the respiratory and gastrointestinal (GI) tracts. The older, or first-generation, H_1 blockers are lipophilic, readily penetrate the blood–brain barrier, and cause sedation. These agents may also have anticholinergic, antiserotonergic, and α-sympathetic receptor blocking effects, which can become more apparent in overdose. Some of the newer second-generation agents also reduce the release of mediators of inflammation from mast cells. They are much less sedating as a result of less central nervous system (CNS) penetration and lack many of the unwanted side effects of the older agents (22). H_1 blockers can also block sodium channels in excitable tissues and have local anesthetic effects and antiarrhythmic effects similar to class IA antiarrhythmics (e.g., quinidine, procainamide, disopyramide; see Chapter 300, "Antidysrhythmic Drugs and Local Anesthetics"). In particular, diphenhydramine and cyproheptadine are notable for prolonging cardiac muscle action potential duration (6). Astemizole and, the no longer marketed, terfenadine prolong myocardial repolarization by blockade of potassium rectifier currents during myocardial repolarization. This may result in QT-interval prolongation on the electrocardiogram and polymorphic ventricular tachycardia (VT) (2,24). Fexofenadine, an active metabolite of terfenadine, has replaced its parent compound as a therapeutic antihistamine in view of its lack of cardiac toxicity. To date, there are no reports of human overdose in the literature.

Antihistamines are rapidly and extensively absorbed from the GI tract, with peak levels occurring in 2 to 4 hours. In overdose, peak levels may be delayed as a result of anticholinergic gastric stasis. All antihistamines are affected by extensive first-pass metabolism with bioavailability of 40% to 60%. Some of these agents may form active metabolites; for instance, hydroxyzine is metabolized to cetirizine, a second-generation agent (22). Protein-binding is highly variable, ranging from 20% for cimetidine to 99% for diphenhydramine. Volumes of distribution range from 1 L/kg for cimetidine to 3 to 7 L/kg for diphenhydramine. First-generation H_1 blockers are quite lipophilic and readily cross the blood–brain barrier. Most agents are metabolized in the liver and the metabolites are excreted renally. Some of the newer agents are excreted unchanged in the urine (cetirizine, a metabolite of hydroxyzine) or fecally (astemizole) (22). Elimination half-lives are variable for the antihistamines. Most of the first-generation H_1 antagonists have half-lives of 2 to 6 hours. The half-lives of the second-generation H_1 blockers tend to be longer, allowing once-daily dosage (22). In the elderly, those with hepatic dysfunction, and patients with overdoses, elimination may be slower.

CLINICAL PRESENTATION

The patient presenting with ACS may exhibit peripheral or central manifestations of the syndrome, or both (Table 323.2). Usually, peripheral stigmata of ACS predominate, with some central features. Mydriasis, tachycardia, dry skin and mucous membranes, fever, and altered mentation are common. These features provide the basis for the mnemonic "hot as a hare, mad as a hatter, red as a beet, dry as a bone." Although this describes many of the features of the ACS, it ignores tachycardia, one of the most consistent and reliable clinical findings. However, in infants, the elderly, alcoholics with autonomic neuropathy, and patients taking β blockers or calcium channel blockers, tachycardia may be absent. Hence, the absence of tachycardia does not rule out the ACS. Central effects vary with the ability of

TABLE 323.2.   Anticholinergic Symptoms and Signs

Peripheral Muscarinic Effects	Central Nervous Effects
Tachycardia	Fever
Mydriasis	Delirium
Loss of accommodation	Seizures
Dry skin and mucous membranes	Coma
	Agitation
Flushed skin	Psychotic behavior
Decreased bowel motility	Extrapyramidal signs
Ileus	Respiratory depression
Urinary retention	Cardiovascular collapse
Constipation	

an agent to penetrate the CNS. Central manifestations of the ACS have been colorfully described in patients who were found confused and inappropriately and scantily dressed after ingesting alcoholic beverages adulterated with scopolamine eye drops. Impaired perception of the environment may result in behavior which could injure the patient.

Patients with a severe ACS can present with extreme findings such as seizures, hypotension, rhabdomyolysis, and respiratory or cardiac arrest (23). It is unclear whether these complications are direct anticholinergic effects, are the end result of severe physiologic stimulation, or are as a result of other pharmacologic properties of the agents involved. Most patients have a self-limited course, the extent and duration of which are determined by the amount and nature of the agent. Finally, in patients who present to hospital several hours following poisoning with an anticholinergic agent, the peripheral features of the troxidone may be absent (9,12).

Although tricyclic antidepressants can predominantly cause the ACS when taken in small overdoses, the clinical presentation of large overdoses of these agents is usually dominated by hypotension, seizures, and cardiac conduction delay resulting from nonanticholinergic effects.

Toxicity resulting from H_1-receptor blockers can be divided into CNS, cardiovascular (CV), and anticholinergic effects. CNS depression (drowsiness, ataxia, coma) is common in adults following overdose of first-generation agents (13). In children, CNS excitation is more common as a result of their sensitivity to the anticholinergic effects. Tremors, confusion, hyperpyrexia, agitation, and seizures are often seen with significant overdose (18). Children and the elderly may develop anticholinergic toxicity or encephalopathy following exposure to topical antihistamines, especially if these are used on broken skin (8,21). There have also been rare reports of anisocoria and diplopia and dystonias after diphenhydramine overdosage.

The most common CV effect is sinus tachycardia, as a result of cholinergic blockade. Conduction disturbances can occur with significant overdoses. Diphenhydramine can cause QRS interval prolongation and ventricular dysrhythmias (6,18). Astemizole can cause Q-T prolongation, atrioventricular block, VT, and ventricular fibrillation following overdose (11,15).

After large H_1-receptor blocker exposures, coma and seizures may occur within 30 minutes of ingestion. Patients with these findings have an increased risk of death (18). In children less than 2 years old, seizures have occurred with doses as little as 150 mg diphenhydramine. Fatal doses in adults may range from 20 to 40 mg/kg; in children as little as 500 mg may result in death.

Significant toxicity following isolated H_2-antagonist overdose is rare (14,16). Sinus bradycardia, atrioventricular block, and Q-T segment prolongation have been reported in patients on oral or parenteral cimetidine and ranitidine (7).

DIFFERENTIAL DIAGNOSIS

The ACS should be included in the differential diagnosis of any patient who presents with altered mental status, fever, urinary retention, tachycardia, or seizures. Given the clinical features of the ACS, it may easily be misdiagnosed as a CNS infection, dehydration, psychiatric disorder, or sepsis. Intoxications with sympathetic stimulants, hallucinogens, and drug withdrawal should also be considered in the differential diagnosis.

The history and physical examination are often crucial in this regard. The history should focus not only on prescribed medications, but also on over-the-counter agents, plant or mushroom ingestions, anticholinergic eye drops, antihistamine-containing skin lotions, or circumstances in which illegitimate use of these agents may be a possibility. Often overlooked exposures include anticholinergic drops used to treat infantile colic and as mydriatics for funduscopic examination (13,19). The history alone can be misleading, and the clinician should consider ACS in patients with characteristic signs and symptoms such as delirium and hallucinations, tachycardia, mydriasis, dry skin, decreased bowel sounds, and a distended bladder, even without a supporting history.

Antihistamines are widely available as over-the-counter preparations and as such are often abused or used in suicide gestures. The diagnosis antihistamine poisoning should be considered in any patient presenting with ACS, CNS depression, psychosis, encephalopathy, and cardiac dysrhythmias and conduction disturbances. Other agents capable of producing similar toxicity include antiarrhythmics, cyclic antidepressants, neuroleptics, anticholinergic medications, and plant ingestions such as jimsonweed, henbane, and deadly nightshade. Antihistamine poisoning must be differentiated from varicella encephalitis in children with altered mental status who have chickenpox and have been treated with topical or oral antihistamines.

EMERGENCY DEPARTMENT EVALUATION

A detailed history and complete physical examination are essential in the evaluation of ACS or antihistamine poisoning. The physical examination should specifically search for the features of an ACS. Flushing of the skin may also be present as a result of excessive ingestion of anticholinergic agents, but this occurs infrequently. Cardiac monitoring and a 12-lead electrocardiogram (ECG) should be obtained on all patients, particularly in the presence of tachycardia. If seizures or altered mentation are present, a neurologic evaluation, including a cranial compute tomography (CT) scan and a lumbar puncture, is required if it cannot be proven that these effects are secondary to anticholinergic poisoning. The administration of physostigmine (see below) may be useful distinguishing between suspected ACS and a CNS infection and can obviate the need for the investigations mentioned above (4). In patients with significant ACS or intentional overdoses, routine laboratory evaluation should include electrolytes, blood urea nitrogen, creatinine, glucose, and creatine kinase. Serum levels of acetaminophen and salicylate should be obtained to rule out co-ingestion of these agents.

Toxicology screens are rarely helpful in defining the agents that may be implicated in producing ACS. Many of the medications and all of the plants that cause the ACS are not detected by routine toxicology screens. Antihistamines are not detected by standard immunoassay tests for drugs of abuse. They can be detected by thin-layer and gas chromatography, but these techniques are unavailable in most hospital laboratories. As a result,

the diagnosis must be made predominantly by the history and physical examination.

EMERGENCY DEPARTMENT MANAGEMENT

The mainstay of therapy for poisoning with anticholinergic agents is supportive care. Patients with ACS require a safe environment in which they cannot do themselves any harm. Comatose or hypoventilating patients should have appropriate airway intervention on arrival. Hypotension should be treated initially with i.v. crystalloid boluses. Hypotension refractory to fluids may necessitate the use of pressor agents such as norepinephrine. Agitation and seizures can be controlled using parenteral benzodiazepines in the first instance. Barbiturates may be considered in refractory cases of seizure activity.

GI decontamination should be performed with a single dose of oral activated charcoal in most instances. The benefit of activated charcoal in patients presenting with minimal or no signs of toxicity more than 2 hours following ingestion, however, is questionable. In patients presenting with significant toxicity the administration of charcoal after this time may prevent absorption of substances unabsorbed in the GI tract as a result of the presence of an anticholinergically- induced ileus. Enhancing the elimination of antihistamines by extracorporeal methods or multiple-dose activated charcoal are ineffective in view of their large volumes of distribution and high protein binding.

The short-acting, reversible acetylcholinesterase inhibitor physostigmine has been used in the management and diagnosis of anticholinergic agitation and delirium (1,4,17). Physostigmine rapidly reverses anticholinergic delirium and may prevent the need for escalating doses of benzodiazepines to control agitation. Physostigmine should never be used in patients with suspected acute cyclic antidepressant poisoning and ECG evidence of cardiac conduction delay because of the risk of precipitating sinus bradycardia, cardiac conduction delays and asystole (20). Other contraindications include patients with bowel obstruction, significant cardiac or peripheral vascular disease, asthma, chronic obstructive pulmonary disease, and preexisting urinary tract obstruction.

When using physostigmine, patients require continuous cardiac monitoring. An initial test dose 0.5 mg is followed by one to two mg over the next 2 to 3 minutes in an adult (0.02 mg/kg in a child to a maximum of 0.5 mg). A partial response may necessitate further 0.5 to 1.0 mg boluses. Clinical effects may last from 30 to 120 minutes and dosing may be repeated as needed for recurrence of symptoms. In true anticholinergic poisoning, dramatic resolution of the syndrome is expected to occur within minutes of physostigmine administration. The ideal response to physostigmine is complete or near-complete reversal of abnormal mental status, in which the patient can verbally confirm overingestion of an anticholinergic agent and denies symptoms consistent with alternative diagnoses (e.g., preceding fever, headache, and neck stiffness). A lack of a response should cause the diagnosis of ACS to be questioned. The presence of excessive cholinergic symptoms following physostigmine administration can be reversed by atropine (atropine dose in this case is half the dose of physostigmine that precipitated cholinergic effects).

In cases in which the diagnosis of ACS is questionable, agitation may be controlled with parenteral benzodiazepines. Neuroleptic agents such as phenothiazines or butyrophenones should be avoided because of their associated anticholinergic effects.

Wide-complex tachycardia associated with massive diphenhydramine overdose may respond to serum alkalinization and sodium bicarbonate infusion given intravenously (18). Torsades de pointes associated with astemizole overdose may respond to intravenous magnesium sulfate and overdrive pacing (15). Phenytoin and bretylium may be useful in refractory cases. Class IA antiarrhythmics (e.g., procainamide) and class III agents (e.g., sotalol) should be avoided as they can promote dysrhythmias as a result of prolongation of cardiac muscle cell repolarization (10). Conduction disturbances and ventricular dysrhythmias astemizole are often self-limiting and may require only ECG monitoring.

CRITICAL INTERVENTIONS

- Rapidly control agitation or violent behavior from the ACS with physostigmine or benzodiazepines given intravenously in order to prevent injury to the patient or staff and complications such as rhabdomyolysis and hyperthermia
- Obtain an ECG and ensure that cardiac conduction delays are not present prior to the administration of physostigmine
- Alkalinize the serum with intravenous sodium bicarbonate and hyperventilation in patients with cardiac conduction delays and ventricular tachydysrhythmias as a result of antihistamine poisoning

DISPOSITION

Patients with a significant ACS should be observed until the clinical signs, including tachycardia, resolve and the patient has a normal mental state examination. This often requires admission to a monitored unit. The duration of anticholinergic delirium may be from 12 hours to several days depending on the agent and dose ingested.

With regards to patients with antihistamine poisoning, those who become or remain asymptomatic after a 4- to 6-hour observation period may be discharged. Patients with hallucinations, agitation, coma, seizures, or CV instability should be admitted to the intensive care unit. Patients with persistent but mildly depressed levels of consciousness and stable vital signs may be monitored in a telemetry unit until symptoms have resolved. All patients with intentional overdoses should have a psychiatric evaluation before discharge.

COMMON PITFALLS

- ✔ Failure to consider the diagnosis of the ACS in patients with altered mental status (particularly agitated delirium), tachycardia, urinary retention, fever, or seizures
- ✔ Failure to appreciate that patients with the ACS may have isolated central or peripheral manifestations
- ✔ Using physostigmine without adequate monitoring and resuscitation capability
- ✔ Using neuroleptics to treat agitation and hallucinations as a result of the ACS

- ✔ Giving a class IA or 1C (e.g., procainamide, flecainide) or class III (e.g., sotalol, amiodarone) antidysrhythmic agent to patients with ventricular tachyarrhythmias as a result of antihistamines

Acknowledgments

The author thanks previous edition chapter authors Jeffrey Brent and Kenneth W. Kulig.

References

1. Beaver KM, Gavin TJ. Treatment of acute anticholinergic poisoning with physostigmine. *Am J Emerg Med* 1998;16:505–507.
2. Berul CI, Morad M. Regulation of potassium channels by nonsedating antihistamines. *Circulation* 1995;91:2220–2225.
3. .Brunner GA, Fleck S, Pieber TR. Near fatal anticholinergic intoxication after routine fundoscopy. *Intensive Care Med* 1998;24:730–731.
4. Burns MJ, Linden CH, Graudins A, et al. Acomparison of physostigmine and benzodiazepines for the treatment of anticholinergic poisoning. *Ann Emerg Med* 2000;35:374–481.
5. Cetaruk EW, Aaron CK. Hazards of non-prescription medications. *Emerg Med Clin North Am* 1994;12:483.
6. Clark RF, Vance MV. Massive diphenhydramine poisoning resulting in a wide-complex tachycardia: successful treatment with sodium bicarbonate. *Ann Emerg Med* 1992;21:318–321.
7. Cohen ND, Modai A, Golik, et al. Cimetidine-related cardiac conduction disturbances and confusion. *J Clin Gastroenterol* 1989;11:68.
8. Danze LK, Langdorf MI. Reversal of orphenadrine-induced ventricular tachycardia with physostigmine. *J Emerg Med* 1991;9:453.
9. Feinberg M. The problems of anticholinergic adverse effects in older patients. *Drugs Aging* 1993;3:335–348.
10. Feroze H, Suri R, Silverman DI. Torsade de pointes from terfenadine and sotalol given in combination. *Pacing Clin Electrophysiol* 1996;19:1519–1521.
11. Heidemann SM, Sarnaik AP. Arrhythmias after astemizole overdose. *Pediatr Emerg Care* 1996;12:102–104.
12. Koppel C, Hopfe T, Menzel J. Central anticholinergic syndrome after ofloxacin overdose and therapeutic doses of diphenhydramine and chlormezanone. *J Toxicol Clin Toxicol* 1990;28:249–253.
13. Koppel C, Ibe K, Tenczer J. Clinical symptomatology of diphenhydramine overdose: an evaluation of 136 cases in 1982 to 1985. *J Toxicol Clin Toxicol* 1987;25:53–70.
14. Krenzelok EP, Litovitz T, Lippold KP, et al. Cimetidine toxicity: an assessment of 881 cases. *Ann Emerg Med* 1987;16:1217–1221.
15. Leor J, Harman M, Rabinowitz B, et al. Giant U waves and associated ventricular tachycardia complicating astemizole overdose: successful therapy with intravenous magnesium [letter]. *Am J Med* 1991;91:94–97.
16. Litovitz TL, Klein-Schwarz W, Dyer KS, et al. 1997 Annual reports of the American Association of Poison Control Centers Toxic Exposure Surveillance System. *Am J Emerg Med* 1998;16:443–498.
17. Mendelson G. Pheniramine aminosalicylate overdosage. Reversal of delirium and choreiform movements with tacrine treatment. *Arch Neurol* 1977;34:313.
18. Mullins ME, Pinnick RV, Terhes JM. Life-threatening diphenhydramine overdose treated with charcoal hemoperfusion and hemodialysis. *Ann Emerg Med* 1999;33:104–107.
19. Myers JH, Moro-Sutherland D, Shook JE. Anticholinergic poisoning in colicky infants treated with hyoscyamine sulfate. *Am J Emerg Med* 1997;15:532–535.
20. Pentel P, Peterson CD. Asystole complicating physostigmine treatment of tricyclic antidepressant overdose. *Ann Emerg Med* 1980;9:588–590.
21. Reilly JF Jr, Weisse ME. Topically induced diphenhydramine toxicity. *J Emerg Med* 1990;8:59–61.
22. Rimmer SJ, Church MK. The pharmacology and mechanism of action of histamine H1 antagonists. *Clin Exp Allergy* 1990;20:3.
23. Winn RE, McDonnell KP. Fatality secondary to massive overdose of dimenhydrinate. *Ann Emerg Med* 1993;22:1481.
24. Woosley RL, Chen Y, Freiman JP, et al. Mechanism of the cardiotoxic actions of terfenadine. *JAMA* 1993;269:1532–1536.

CHAPTER 324
Cocaine

Richard D. Shih and Judd E. Hollander

Cocaine (benzoylmethylecgonine) has been used for social, religious, and medicinal purposes for many centuries. Over the past several decades, its illicit use as a drug of abuse has risen dramatically. An estimated 23 million Americans have used cocaine at least once, and approximately 5 million use it regularly (18). Further, among visits to emergency departments as a result of drugs of abuse, cocaine is the most commonly involved drug (15).

Cocaine is well absorbed on contact with mucous membranes or by pulmonary inhalation. It is derived from the *Erythroxylum coca* plant, which is found in abundance in Central America, South America, the West Indies, and Indonesia. In the manufacturing process, leaves are initially dissolved in hydrochloric acid to form the cocaine hydrochloride salt. This is the form most often abused via nasal insufflation or i.v. injection. Crack cocaine or cocaine free base are the alkaloid forms of cocaine that are produced by an extraction process utilizing a basic solution, a solvent (usually ether), and heat. The free-base form is close to 100% purity, while crack approximates 75%. These forms are heat stable, and thus can be smoked and absorbed by the lungs.

By the i.v. or inhalational routes, cocaine is rapidly distributed throughout the body and central nervous system (CNS), with peak effects in 3 to 5 minutes. With nasal insufflation, absorption is slower and effects peak at approximately 20 minutes. Although not a typical route of abuse, oral ingestion delays absorption even further, with peak effects occurring at 40 to 60 minutes.

Cocaine has a half-life of 0.5 to 1.5 hours. It is predominantly metabolized to the active metabolites ecgonine methyl ester and benzoylecgonine (BE) by hydrolysis. These two metabolites account for approximately 80% of cocaine metabolism. They have half-lives of 4 to 8 hours and many effects similar to their parent compound, cocaine. Other metabolites include cocaethylene, ecgonine, and norcocaine. Urine drug tests typically test for BE, and this cocaine metabolite is typically present for 48 to 72 hours after use (1).

Cocaine has a number of pharmacologic effects peripherally and in the central nervous systme (CNS). It acts to augment the peripheral sympathetic system, producing such findings as tachycardia, hypertension, diaphoresis, arterial vasoconstriction, and dilated pupils. Additionally, cocaine has local anesthetic effects. In the amide group of topical anesthetic agents, it is the only one that has vasoconstrictive effects, which help control secretions and bleeding. Because of these properties, it is used for otolaryngology procedures and wound repair. The central effects of cocaine are very complex and not completely understood. It has effects on a number of neurotransmitters in the CNS. However, the net effect is the augmentation of the sympathetic nervous system.

"Body stuffers" and "body packers" are individuals who have ingested containers of an illicit drug (most commonly cocaine and heroin) (6). These containers can be plastic bags, plastic vials, elastic wraps, elastic condoms, or other packaging material. A "stuffer" is someone who hastily ingests containers just prior to being arrested by police in order to conceal the evidence (20). A packer, or "mule," is an individual who ingests a large number of carefully wrapped containers of highly pure drug as a means of concealing and smuggling it into the United States from a foreign country or into jail.

CLINICAL PRESENTATION

Cocaine toxicity can be manifested in a number of different organ systems. The most commonly seen manifestations in the emergency department involve the cardiovascular (CV) and neurologic systems (3). Signs and symptoms of mild cocaine intoxication include normal or minimally increased blood pressure, pulse, respiratory rate, and temperature; agitation; anxiety; euphoria; headache; hyperreflexia; nausea; vomiting; mydriasis; pallor; diaphoresis; tremors; and twitching. Moderate intoxication may result in hypertension, tachycardia, dyspnea, tachypnea, hyperthermia, confusion, hallucinations, marked hyperactivity, increased muscle tone and deep tendon reflexes, abdominal cramps, formication, and generalized but brief tonic-clonic seizures. Severe intoxication may be manifested by hypotension, tachycardia (or preterminal bradycardia), ventricular dysrhythmias, Cheyne-Stokes respirations, apnea, cyanosis, severe hyperthermia, coma, flaccid paralysis, and status epilepticus.

Chest pain is a common chief complaint associated with cocaine use. Myocardial infarction (MI) as a result of cocaine is well established (9,10) and occurs in approximately 6% of patients presenting with this complaint (24). Cocaine causes coronary ischemia through coronary artery vasoconstriction (13), in situ thrombus formation, platelet activation, and inhibition of endogenous fibrinolysis, and triggering an increase in the myocardial oxygen demand through generation of tachycardia and hypertension (9). Chronic users develop premature atherosclerosis and left ventricular hypertrophy, which can further exacerbate the oxygen supply–demand mismatch (9). Other less common but equally important CV complications of cocaine use include atrial and ventricular dysrhythmias, both systolic and diastolic congestive heart failure, coronary and aortic dissection, dilated cardiomyopathy, and ischemia in other vascular beds (e.g., intestinal, renal, etc.).

Euphoria, the impetus for the recreational use of cocaine, is typically short-lived and without serious sequelae. The stimulatory effects of cocaine can lead to seizures, both bland and hemorrhagic cerebral infarction, and subarachnoid hemorrhage. Severe, persistent lethargy with an altered mental status can occur following prolonged and intense cocaine usage and has been termed the cocaine wash-out syndrome. This diagnosis should be made only after exclusion of the aforementioned neurologic catastrophes (i.e., after a normal computerized tomography (CT) of the head and lumbar puncture, if indicated). The syndrome is thought to be a result of such excessive cocaine usage that essential neurotransmitters are depleted. Symptoms will generally abate within 12 to 24 hours.

Rhabdomyolysis is another common manifestation of cocaine toxicity (12). Cocaine's stimulatory effects lead to severe agitation and marked muscular agitation and rigidity. Ischemia of the skeletal muscle beds may also contribute. Profound elevations in creatinine kinase (CK) may be seen. Concurrent development of severe hyperthermia and acute renal failure can be life-threatening (5). Hyperthermia is most commonly as a result of a combination of environmental exposure and heat production from excessive muscle activity (5). Renal failure is as a result of muscle breakdown and renal tubular precipitation of the released muscle myoglobin.

Cocaine has a number of direct and indirect effects on the lungs. Many of the effects of cocaine are as a result of the method of abuse rather than direct toxin effects. Asthma exacerbations have been frequently reported with crack cocaine usage. This is most likely as a result of particulate by-products of combustion. Further, crack usage is typically associated with deep Valsalva maneuvers to maximize drug delivery. This can cause pneumothorax, pneumomediastinum, and noncardiogenic pulmonary edema. Other less common effects on the lung include pulmonary infarction, bronchiolitis obliterans, pulmonary artery hypertrophy, and alveolar hemorrhage. Treatment of these conditions follows standard management protocols, whether they are related to cocaine, or not.

The intestinal vascular system is very sensitive to the effects of cocaine. Acute intestinal vascular infarction has been associated with all routes of administration. Although oral ingestion is not a common route of abuse, local intestinal and systemic effects can occur when containers of cocaine leak or rupture in body stuffers and packers. Body packers most often present asymptomatically, having been discovered by customs officers.

Habitual cocaine usage during pregnancy is associated with low birth weight, small head circumference, developmental problems, and a number of birth defects. Acute toxicity can also cause the induction of premature labor, eclampsia, and abruptio placentae. After delivery, neonates exposed to cocaine *in utero* are at risk for the development of neonatal withdrawal. This diagnosis of exclusion is manifested as irritability, jitteriness, and poor eye contact.

DIFFERENTIAL DIAGNOSIS

Similar toxicity can be caused by a variety of physiologic stimulants (see Table 270.4). A sympathomimetic toxidrome can also be seen with hypoglycemia, environmental and malignant hyperthermia, pheochromocytoma, psychiatric conditions, status epilepticus, and thyroid storm. Patients with persistent altered mental status need to be evaluated for possible meningitis and CNS lesions. Table 324.1 lists the differential diagnosis of chest pain related to cocaine use.

EMERGENCY DEPARTMENT EVALUATION

The diagnostic evaluation of patients manifesting cocaine toxicity relies on a history of cocaine use, recognition of signs and symptoms consistent with a sympathomimetic toxidrome, and evaluation of specific organ system complaints. The history should include the total amount and time of cocaine use in relation to symptom onset. Friends (or witnesses) of confused patients should be questioned about a history of seizures or syncope and antecedent activities. New-onset seizures, epistaxis, hypertension, MI, intracranial hemorrhage, or psychiatric illness, especially in young patients, should suggest the possibility of cocaine use. Many patients deny cocaine use unless approached with reassurance and compassion or confronted with a positive urine test.

The physical examination should include a complete set of vital signs and a detailed examination of the cardiac, pulmonary, and neurologic systems. Patients should initially have continuous cardiac monitoring.

When the history is clear and symptoms are mild, laboratory evaluation is unnecessary. In contrast, if the history is absent or unreliable or the patient manifests moderate or severe toxicity, routine laboratory evaluation should include a complete blood count; determination of electrolyte, glucose, blood urea nitrogen, and creatinine levels; arterial blood gas analysis; urinalysis; and CK. Qualitative toxicologic analyses of blood and urine can confirm the diagnosis and rule out other intoxicants. Toxicology testing is indicated only when confirmation of drug use would change management, counseling, or referral patterns.

A chest radiograph and electrocardiogram (ECG) should be obtained in patients with chest pain or moderate-to-severe toxicity. Those with prolonged, unexplained pain should have serial ECG and cardiac marker measurements to rule out MI. Many of the clinical parameters to assess ischemia or infarction are not as reliable as when they are used for patients with traditional coronary artery disease (7). The ECG is less sensitive and specific for identifying ischemia or infarction in this setting, the CK is often elevated as a result of associated rhabdomyolysis, and false elevations in the MB fraction can occur. Cardiac troponin I testing can help distinguish true-positive from false-positive CK-MB elevations (11).

Persistent headache despite normalization of blood pressure requires evaluation by CT scan and lumbar puncture to rule out intracranial hemorrhage. Patients with severe abdominal or back pain must be evaluated for intestinal or renal infarction. The urine should be inspected and the CK level determined, because myoglobinuric renal failure may develop.

Occult infections must be excluded in patients with fever, even though fever can be due solely to cocaine toxicity. A brief seizure clearly related (temporally) to cocaine use in an otherwise healthy person should be evaluated with CT to exclude serious underlying pathology, but it does not require further workup, provided the patient is alert and coherent, has no headache, and has a normal neurologic examination. Patients suspected of body packing or stuffing should be evaluated by abdominal radiographs (including contrast imaging) and cavity searches (digital or visual examination of the rectum or vagina). Toxicity lasting for more than 4 hours suggests continued drug absorption and should prompt a similar workup.

The route of administration may influence the patient's chief complaint or which organ system is affected. Intravenous users may present with fever and malaise secondary to infectious complications such as cellulitis, endocarditis, hepatitis, pneumonia, and the acquired immunodeficiency syndrome. Chronic nasal use may lead to rhinitis, septal perforation, and epistaxis. Inhalational use may produce dyspnea, cough, or hemoptysis from reactive airway disease, "crack lung" pneumonitis, or pulmonary edema, or may result in pulmonary barotrauma (e.g., pneumothorax, pneumomediastinum, pneumopericardium) as a result of the Valsalva maneuver or from blowing smoke into the mouth of a partner. Patients with barotrauma may also complain of neck and chest pain and demonstrate tachypnea, subcutaneous emphysema, or Hamman's sign.

Behavioral disorders (e.g., agitation, combative behavior), headache, back pain (renal infarction or aortic dissection), abdominal pain (mesenteric ischemia), altered level of consciousness, or cardiopulmonary arrest are other common presentations that may follow the use of cocaine by any route. Patients may present as victims of trauma, because of the violent, irrational, and risk-taking behavioral associated with drug use. Delayed CV complications can sometimes occur. Myocardial infarction has been reported in the first few days after cocaine use. MI has been reported 1 to 2 weeks after last use (17).

Manifestations of chronic cocaine abuse include anorexia, insomnia, formication, depression, impotence, weight loss, paranoia, and psychosis. Halo vision (lights around objects) and "snow lights" (flashes in the peripheral fields) have also been described.

TABLE 324.1.   The Differential Diagnosis of Cocaine-Associated Chest Pain

Aortic dissection	Pericarditis
Bacterial endocarditis	Pleurisy
Bronchospasm	Pneumonia
Esophageal illnesses	Pneumomediastinum
Gastrointestinal illnesses	Pneumothorax
Musculoskeletal injury	Pulmonary emboli
Myocardial infarction	Pulmonary infarction
Myocardial ischemia	
Myocarditis	

EMERGENCY DEPARTMENT MANAGEMENT

Management depends on the specific complaint and presentation (Table 324.2). Patients presenting with a sympathomimetic toxidrome are at risk for hyperthermia and rhabdomyolysis (5,12). After initial attention to the airway and CV status, management should focus on lowering core body temperature, halting further muscle agitation and heat production, and giving i.v. fluids to ensure a good urinary output. The agents of choice for muscle relaxation in this setting are benzodiazepines (4). Supranormal cumulative doses may be necessary in severely agitated individuals.

Patients with severe hypertension or tachycardia necessitating pharmacologic measures can usually be safely treated with

TABLE 324.2.   Treatment of Specific Cocaine-Related Medical Diseases[a]

Medical Problem	Treatments
Dysrhythmias	
Sinus tachycardia	observation
	oxygen
	diazepam 5–10 mg i.v. or lorazepam 2–4 mg i.v. titrated to effect
Supraventricular tachycardia	oxygen
	diazepam 5 mg i.v. or lorazepam 2–4 mg i.v.
	diltiazem 20 mg i.v. or verapamil 5 mg i.v.
	adenosine 6 mg or 12 mg i.v. for AV node reentry
	digoxin 0.5 mg i.v.
	Consider verapamil, 5–10 mg i.v.
	cardioversion if hemodynamically unstable
Ventricular dysrhythmias	oxygen
	sodium bicarbonate
	lidocaine 1.5 mg/kg i.v. bolus followed by 2 mg/min infusion
	defibrillation if hemodynamically unstable
	diazepam 5 mg i.v. or lorazepam 2–4 mg i.v.
Ischemic chest pain	oxygen
	diazepam 5–10 mg i.v. or lorazepam 2–4 mg i.v.
	soluble aspirin 325 mg
	nitroglycerin 1/150 sublingual × 3 every 5 minutes followed by a drip titrated to a mean arterial pressure reduction of 10% or relief of chest pain.
	morphine sulfate 2 mg i.v. titrated to pain relief
	phentolamine 1 mg i.v.; repeat in 5 m
	verapamil 5–10 mg i.v.
	heparin 60–70 unit/kg (maximum of 5,000 units) followed by continuous infusion of 12–15 units/kg/h (maximum 1,000 units per hour)
	mechanical reperfusion (angioplasty)
	thrombolytic therapy
Hypertension	observation
	diazepam 5–10 mg i.v. or lorazepam 2–4 mg i.v. titrated to effect
	phentolamine 1 mg i.v.; repeat in 5 m
	nitroglycerin or nitroprusside drip titrated to effect
Pulmonary edema	lasix 20–40 mg i.v.
	morphine sulfate 2 mg i.v. titrated to pain relief
	nitroglycerin drip titrated to blood pressure or respiratory status
	consider phentolamine or nitroprusside
Hyperthermia	Cool environment with minimal activity
	Sedation with benzodiazepines
	Tepid water with fans, cool water, or ice baths
Neurologic symptoms	
Anxiety and agitation	diazepam 5–10 mg i.v. or lorazepam 2–4 mg i.v. titrated to effect
Seizures	diazepam 5–10 mg i.v. or lorazepam 2–4 mg i.v. titrated to effect
	phenobarbital 25–50 mg/m up to 10–20 mg/kg.
Intracranial hemorrhage	neurosurgery consult
Rhabdomyolysis	Serial potassium determination
	i.v. hydration to maintain urine output at 3cc/kg/h
	sodium bicarbonate titrated to an alkaline urine
	hemodialysis, as necessary for renal failure
Cocaine washed out syndrome	supportive care
Body packers	Activated charcoal
	Whole bowel irrigation
	Admission to monitored setting even if asymptomatic
	Laparotomy or endoscopic retrieval for obstruction or symptoms

[a] From Hollander JE, Hoffman RS. Cocaine. In: Goldfrank LR, Flomenbaum NE, Lewin NA, et al., eds. *Goldfrank's Toxicologic Emergency*, 6th edition. Stamford, Connecticut: Appleton and Lange, 1998:1071–1089) with permission.

benzodiazepines. When large doses of benzodiazepines are not effective, intravenous nitroprusside or phentolamine should be considered. B antagonists or compounds with partial β-blocking effects are contraindicated; the use of β antagonists in the setting of cocaine intoxication can lead to unopposed α stimulation, with resultant marked increases in hypertension and worsening coronary vasoconstriction (9,14,21).

Patients with suspected cocaine-induced ischemia or MI should be treated similarly to those with traditional acute coronary syndromes (ACS), with some notable exceptions (9,14). Aspirin, nitroglycerin, and heparin remain important initial therapies. Intravenous benzodiazepines should be provided as early management (2). They will decrease the central stimulatory effects of cocaine, thereby indirectly reducing the CV toxicity of cocaine (4,9). B antagonists should are contraindicated, as they exacerbate cocaine-induced coronary artery vasoconstriction (14,21). Another management difference in the setting of cocaine use relative to patients with traditional ACS is a preference for percutaneous interventions (angioplasty) over fibrinolysis. Fibrinolysis in the setting of cocaine-associated MI has no proven efficacy, a possible reduced safety profile, and an increased likelihood of being administered to patients who are not sustaining an acute infarction (because young patients with recent cocaine use have a high prevalence of early repolarization and "false-positive" ST-segment elevations on the ECG). Such therapy should, therefore, be used with caution. Finally, there are anecdotal reports of the safety and efficacy of phentolamine, an α antagonist, for treatment of cocaine-associated ACSs (8,9). Verapamil reverses cocaine-induced vasoconstriction (19), but several animal experiments suggest that it exacerbates CNS toxicity. Therefore, it may have a role in patients with continued ischemia who do not have signs of central stimulation from cocaine.

Supraventricular dysrhythmias may be difficult to treat. Adenosine can be administered, but its effects may be temporary. Use of calcium channel blockers in association with benzodiazepines appear to be most beneficial. B blockers should be avoided (9).

Ventricular dysrhythmias may be a result of excess adrenergic tone or cocaine's sodium channel blocking effects. Management with benzodiazepines, lidocaine, and/or sodium bicarbonate appears to be most useful (9,22). Bicarbonate is preferred when patients have dysrhythmias directly following the use of cocaine. In this setting, the dysrhythmias are presumably related to the type I antiarrhythmic effects of cocaine. Bicarbonate reverses cocaine-associated QRS widening. Lidocaine can be used when dysrhythmias appear to be related to cocaine-induced ischemia. ECG evidence for the type I effects of cocaine has often disappeared by the time symptomatic ischemia develops.

Cocaine-induced seizures are typically brief and self-limited. For refractory cases, benzodiazepines and phenobarbital are the first- and second-line agents, respectively. Phenytoin is not recommended.

Patients with suspected cerebrovascular infarctions and hemorrhage should be treated the same as other patients with these conditions. Intracranial and systemic hypertension necessitating treatment is accomplished using standard therapies, except that β blockers should not be utilized.

The main concern in asymptomatic body stuffers and packers is eliminating the packages out of the GI system. Whole-bowel irrigation with subsequent radiologic verification of passage of all drug-filled containers may be warranted.

Body stuffers who manifest clinical signs of toxicity should be treated similarly to other cocaine-exposed individuals. Additionally, GI decontamination with activated charcoal should be administered liberally (23).

Symptomatic body packers should be treated more aggressively, because rapid deterioration and severe toxicity can result from their potentially massive exposures. Immediate surgical removal of the ruptured package(s) may be lifesaving. Aggressive supportive care with activated charcoal and benzodiazepines is warranted as preparation for surgery occurs (16).

CRITICAL INTERVENTIONS

- Assess patients with cocaine toxicity for myocardial ischemia/MI, dysrhythmias, hyperthermia, and rhabdomyolysis
- Administer intravenous benzodiazepines for CNS and CV toxicity

DISPOSITION

Patients with severe agitation, hyperthermia, and possible rhabdomyolysis need to be admitted. Patients with cocaine-associated chest pain need to be assessed for risk of CV events. Criteria for patients with a low risk of CV events that are safe for emergency department (ED) discharge after a brief observation period include: lack of ischemic changes on EKG; normal serial cardiac troponin I values; no dysrhythmias, or recurrent symptoms during a 9 to 12 hour observation period (25). Most patients with ED cocaine-associated chest pain (~ 70%) will meet these criteria (25).

The disposition of patients with neurologic complications is the same as for other patients with these conditions. The likelihood of compliance with outpatient follow-up should be considered when contemplating the discharge of patients who may need further evaluation. If definitive care cannot be provided at the site of presentation, transfer may be necessary. Personnel with advanced life-support training should accompany patients requiring transfer. All patients should be referred for substance abuse counseling and treatment.

COMMON PITFALLS

✔ Failure to consider cocaine toxicity in the differential diagnosis of patients with chest pain, seizures, agitation, altered mental status, and dysrhythmias
✔ Failure to recognize the limitations of the electrocardiogram in the evaluation of cocaine-related chest pain
✔ Failure appreciate the differences between the management of cocaine-related chest pain and tradition therapy for ACSs
✔ Failure to recognize the dangers of using β-adrenergic antagonists to treat cocaine toxicity
✔ Failure to ensure the rectal passage of cocaine-filled packages in body stuffers and body packers prior to discharge

Acknowledgments

We thank William A. Watson and Christopher H. Linden for their contributions to previous chapters and this chapter.

References

1. Ambre J. The urinary excretion of cocaine and metabolites in humans: a kinetic analysis of published data. *J Anal Toxicol* 1985;9:241–245.
2. Baumann DM, Perrone J, Hornig SF, et al. Randomized, double-blind, placebo-controlled trial of diazepam, nitroglycerin, or both for treatment of patients with potential cocaine-associated acute coronary syndromes. *Acad Emerg Med* 2000;7:878–885.
3. Brody SL, Wrenn KD, Wilber MM, et al. Predicting the severity of cocaine associated rhabdomyolysis. *Ann Emerg Med* 1990;19:1137–1143.
4. Catravas JD, Waters IW. Acute cocaine intoxication in the conscious dog: studies on the mechanism of lethality. *J Pharmacol Exp Ther* 1981;217:350–356.
5. Crandall CG, Vongpatanasin W, Victor RG. Mechanism of cocaine-induced hyperthermia in humans. *Ann Int Med* 2002;136:785–791.

6. Gill JR, Graham SM. Ten years of "body packers" in New York City: 50 deaths. *J Forensic Sci* 2002;47:843–846.

7. Gitter MJ, Goldsmith ER, Dunbar DN, et al. Cocaine and chest pain: clinical features and outcome of patients hospitalized to rule out myocardial infarction. *Ann Intern Med* 1991;115:277–282.

8. Hollander JE, Carter WC, Hoffman RS. Use of phentolamine for cocaine-induced myocardial ischemia. *N Engl J Med* 1992;327:361.

9. Hollander JE. Management of cocaine-associated myocardial ischemia. *N Engl J Med* 1995;333(19):1267–1272.

10. Hollander JE, Hoffman RS, Burstein J, et al, and the Cocaine Associated Myocardial Infarction Study (CAMI) Group. Cocaine associated myocardial infarction. Mortality and complications. *Arch Intern Med* 1995;155:1081–1086.

11. Hollander JE, Levitt MA, Young GP, et al. The effect of cocaine on the specificity of cardiac markers. *Am Heart J* 1998;135(2):245–252.

12. Horowitz BZ, Panacek EA, Jouriles NJ. Severe rhabdomyolysis with renal failure after intranasal cocaine use. *J Emerg Med* 1997;15:833–837.

13. Lange RA, Cigarroa RG, Yancy CW, et al. Cocaine-induced coronary-artery vasoconstriction. *N Engl J Med* 1989;321:1557–1561.

14. Lange RA, Cogarroa RG, Flores ED, et al. Potentiation of cocaine-induced coronary vasoconstriction by beta-adrenergic blockade. *Ann Intern Med* 1990;112:897–903.

15. MacDonald DI. Cocaine leads emergency department drug visits. *JAMA* 1987;258:2029.

16. McCarron MM, Wood JD. The cocaine body packer syndrome. *JAMA* 1983;250:1417–1420.

17. Nademanee K, Gorelick DA, Josephson MA, et al. Myocardial ischemia during cocaine withdrawal. *Ann Intern Med* 1989;111:876–880.

18. 1999 National Household Survey on Drug Abuse: summary findings. Rockville, Md: Substance Abuse and Mental Health Services Administration, 2000.

19. Negus BH, Willard JE, Hillis LD, et al. Alleviation of cocaine induced coronary vasoconstriction with intravenous verapamil. *Am J Cardiol* 1994;73:510–513.

20. Roberts J, Price D, Goldfrank L. The body stuffer syndrome: a clandestine form of drug overdose. *Am J Emerg Med* 1986;4:21–27.

21. Sand IC, Brody SL, Wrenn KD, et al. Experience with esmolol for the treatment of cocaine associated cardiovascular complications. *Am J Emerg Med* 1991;9:161–163.

22. Shih RD, Hollander JE, Hoffman RS, et al, and the Cocaine Associated Myocardial Infarction Study (CAMI) Study Group. Clinical safety of lidocaine in cocaine associated myocardial infarction. *Ann Emerg Med* 1995;26:702–706.

23. Tomaszewski C, McKinney P, Phillips S, et al. Prevention of toxicity from oral cocaine by activated charcoal in mice. *Ann Emerg Med* 1993;22:1804–1806.

24. Weber JE, Chudnofsky CR, Boczar M, et al. Cocaine-associated chest pain: how common is myocardial infarction? *Acad Emerg Med* 2000;7:873–877.

25. Weber JE, Shofer FS, Larkin GL, et al. Validation of a brief observation period for patients with cocaine-associated chest pain. *N Eng J Med* 2003;348:510–517.

CHAPTER 325
Hallucinogens

Howard A. Greller and Lewis S. Nelson

Hallucinogens are a diverse class of compounds that have as their primary effect the alteration of sensory perception and interpretation, without the alteration of orientation. Commonly, they are referred to as "psychedelics." In order to categorize the effects of these compounds, it helps first to define a few terms. Hallucination is the perception of phenomena or objects that have no basis in reality (e.g., the pink elephants of ethanol withdrawal). Visual hallucinations tend to be a result of toxic-metabolic causes, whereas auditory hallucinations tend to be primarily psychiatric or organic. Psychotomimetic describes a substance that produces psychological and behavioral changes resembling psychosis. Hallucination contrasts with illusion, in which a sensory perception misinterpretation occurs (e.g., a coat hanging in a dark room is perceived as being a person). The term hallucinogen is also used as the medico-legal descriptor for this group of related compounds. An entactogen is a compound or substance that enhances feelings of empathy, love, and emotional closeness and facilitates expression of emotions (e.g. methylene-dioxy-methamphetamine [MDMA], or ecstasy). A synesthesia is a mixed perception (e.g., hearing color or seeing taste) (5,15).

It has been proposed that the primary ideas behind religious thought, the concept of deity and spirit, were direct results of the use of hallucinogens (4,9,20,21,25). The compounds found naturally in plant and animal species have been used in a variety of religious, spiritual, ordeal and other practices for centuries. The Rig-Veda, an Indian text more than 3,000 years old, praises soma, believed today to be the mushroom *Amanita muscaria*, containing the psychoactive compound muscimol. The Aztecs were known to use a number of hallucinogens, including Psilocybe mushrooms ("flesh of the gods") and ololiuqui (morning glory seeds) (20,21).

The modern era of the hallucinogens had its origins when Albert Hofmann, working for Sandoz Laboratories, synthesized lysergic acid diethylamide-25 (LSD, the twenty-fifth compound he isolated) in 1938. On April 16, 1943, he was unintentionally exposed to LSD and developed unexpected hallucinations ("...there surged upon me an uninterrupted stream of fantastic images of extraordinary plasticity and vividness and accompanied by an intense, kaleidoscope-like play of colors")(23). He confirmed the response with re-exposure and reported the results to his superiors (25). A few years later, Sandoz began marketing the product as Delysid®, for use in the psychiatric community as a therapeutic adjunct for psychotherapy. As with most compounds that have effects that alter perception, LSD found its way into recreational use in the 1960s. The use of this and related agents was popularized by the promotion of concepts such as the "fifth freedom" by figures such as Timothy Leary, Albert Hoffmann, and others. As a result of concerns over birth defects and other toxicity, federal law in the mid-1960s banned LSD. Hallucinogens as a class are currently classified as FDA schedule I agents, meaning that they have no proven medical value, and are therefore illicit (5).

Teens and young adults primarily use LSD and other hallucinogens. In one report concerning adolescent LSD users, it ranked only behind alcohol and marijuana as the third most commonly ingested drug (15). LSD use has declined somewhat, and its annual prevalence was 6.6% in 2001 (12). Although the use of LSD has declined among secondary school students, it has resurged in popularity among older adolescents and others exposed to the "rave" scene. There has also been a rise in the use of other hallucinogenic compounds, such as "foxy" (5-methoxy-*N*,*N*-diisopropyltryptamine), Psilocybe mushrooms, PCP, and ketamine (5,15,22).

The mechanism by which the hallucinogens produce their effects is not fully understood. Although they are derived from very different sources, and although they are from chemically distinct classes of chemicals, most share a structural similarity to serotonin. The tryptamine derivatives share the pyrrole structure of the indole ring. The amphetamine derivatives typically considered "hallucinogenic," such as MDMA, share the methoxylated or methylenedioxylated catechol ring. Each of these structural features appears to be essential to hallucinogenic activity (Fig. 325.1) (8,10,24). Current theory proposes that the similarity of LSD and other hallucinogenic compounds to serotonin provides them with agonist activity at the 5-HT2 receptor. Specifically, the 5-HT2A receptor subtype found predominantly on a population of postsynaptic neurons in the cerebral cortex, has been implicated by functional studies in the modulation of hallucinations (19,24). Additional mechanisms for the generation of hallucinations include agonism at the kappa opioid receptor, as in the case of Salvia divinorum and ibogaine (5,18).

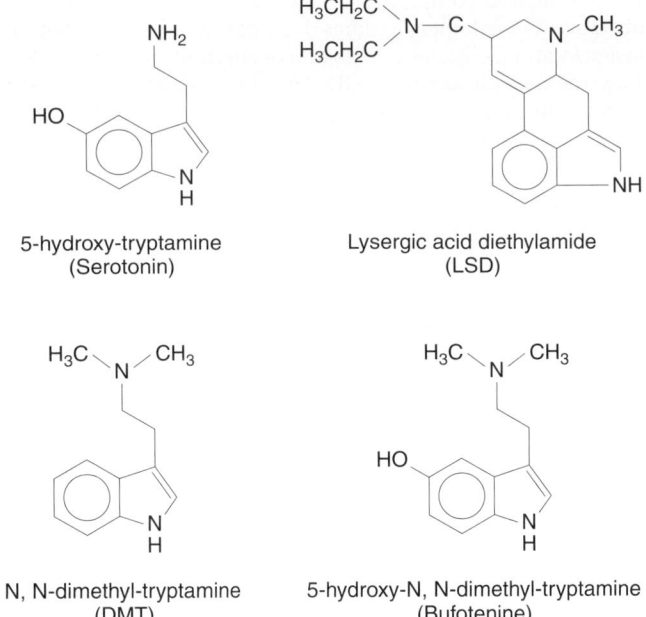

5-hydroxy-tryptamine
(Serotonin)

Lysergic acid diethylamide
(LSD)

N, N-dimethyl-tryptamine
(DMT)

5-hydroxy-N, N-dimethyl-tryptamine
(Bufotenine)

Figure 325.1. Hallucinogenic compounds and their structural similarity to serotonin.

LSD is a semi-synthetic compound derived from the ergot fungus *Claviceps purpurea*. There are other naturally occurring analogues of LSD found in the seeds from plants of the morning glory family (Convolvulaceae), including the South American morning glory, the Mexican morning glory, and Hawaiian woodrose (7,20,21).

LSD is very potent, with hallucinogenic doses in the range of a few hundred micrograms. It is most commonly administered through the oral route, generally as fancifully designed blotter paper. The perforated paper defines a dosing unit, and the designs provide "branding." Other forms include impregnated gelatin ("window panes") or microdots (small pills or tablets), and LSD is occasionally found as a liquid.

Mescaline, or 3,4,5-trimethoxyphenylethylamine, is an amphetamine-like compound that is derived from the cactus *Lophophora williamsii*, also known as the peyote cactus. Although mescaline can be isolated from the peyote cactus, this is a difficult process, and most of the time, the compound is ingested in its "natural" form. Typically, a few of the small cactus crowns or "buttons" are removed, dried, and then ingested (15).

There are many structural analogues of mescaline. Although the primary clinical effects of recreational doses of MDMA or ecstasy (see Chapter 328, "Sympathomimetics"), do not involve hallucinations, they may occur at very high doses. It is structurally related to mescaline. The seeds of nutmeg (*Myristica fragrans*) are known to contain myristicin and elemicin, two mescaline-like substituted amphetamines with hallucinogenic properties (20,21). Large amounts of the ground spice need to be ingested (up to 20 grams) in order to produce the hallucinatory effects.

Psilocybin (4-phosphoryloxy-N, N-dimethyltryptamine) and psilocin (4-hydroxy-N, N-dimethyl-tryptamine) are two compounds of the indolalkylamine class isolated from mushrooms of the Psilocybe genus (4,19,20,21). The two most common species are *P. semilanceata* (also known as the "liberty cap") and *P. cubensis*. These mushrooms are readily available through a variety of sources and are often homegrown from spores. Being a natural product, the amount, and type of hallucinogenic compound contained within any singular mushroom varies widely and therefore there is no "typical" dose.

Foxy, also known as "foxy methoxy," and α-methyltryptamine (AMT) are tryptamine derivatives (5,14,15). Both are available as capsules filled with powder and are orally bioavailable.

Secretions of the modified parotid gland of the Colorado River toad, *Bufo alvarius*, contain a mixture of chemicals designed to protect the toad from predators. They include catecholamines, cardioactive steroids, and 5-methoxy-N, N-dimethyltryptamine (5-MeO-DMT, or bufotenine), a potent hallucinogenic compound. People engage in the practice of "toad-licking" in attempts to experience the psychedelic properties of this chemical (16).

N, N-dimethyl-tryptamine (DMT) is a tryptamine derivative of the Yakee plant (*Virola calophylla*). It is not orally bioavailable and therefore is most often smoked (5,14,15).

Ayahuasca is a psychotropic plant that is used as a tea throughout the Amazon basin in traditional medicine, and shamanistic practices. It is made by steeping the pounded stems of the vine *Banisteriopsis caapi*, alone or in combination with the leaves of *Psychotria viridis*. This combination is ethnopharmacologically interesting because *P. viridis* contains N, N-dimethyltryptamine (DMT) and *B. caapi* contains alkaloids such as harmine and tetrahydroharmine; the latter improves the oral bioavailability of the former. This occurs because DMT is metabolized by gastrointestinal (GI) monoamine oxidase (MAO) and harmine and the other β-carboline alkaloids are MAO-inhibitors (17,20,21).

A more recently popularized hallucinogen is *Salvia divinorum*, a member of the mint family. The active compound is a neoclerodane diterpene, salvinorin A. This plant has been used for centuries by the Mazatecs of Oaxaca, Mexico. It is taken orally, in which it has rapid oral mucosal absorption, and by inhalation (5,18).

Ibogaine is derived from the root of the *Tabernanthe iboga* plant, found primarily in West African nations. It has gained recent attention as a potential treatment for addiction to compounds such as cocaine and heroin, and is under investigation by the FDA for such purposes. Ibogaine is taken orally (3,5,15,20,21).

CLINICAL PRESENTATION

Unlike many other drugs of abuse, most users of hallucinogens rarely present acutely to the health care provider (5,15). Hallucinogens in general have few significant adverse side effects and patients generally present to the emergency department for secondary reasons (e.g., trauma) or for "bad trips." The unique nature of hallucinogens defines their clinical presentation. Unless combined with other drugs, patients should be alert and fully oriented and able to give a history of use. For those without knowledge of their ingestion or exposure, the finding of a clear sensorium is a key historical and examination point suggesting the use of LSD. This contrasts with drug-induced delirium, such as that associated with phencyclidine (PCP) use, in which, by definition, their orientation is altered.

Hallucinations or illusions are alterations in the perception of time and body image, and changes in the interpretation of sensory information. Hallucinogenic experiences are commonly referred to as a "trip," and the experience tends to be an extremely personal one. The perceptual changes that users perceive can affect any of the senses; hearing, taste, smell, touch, sight. They can experience exaggeration, diminution, or mixing (synesthesias) of their sensory perception. The users' sense of time may be altered, generally slowed, as may their sense of space. Body dysmorphisms are common, in which personal physical features take on abnormal proportions. Events can be perceived as hyper-religious, or evil (4,23). Additional clues to the diagnosis include the identification of the sympathomimetic effects of some of the compounds involved, although these

TABLE 325.1. Common Hallucinogenic Compounds

Common Name	Name	Onset (hrs)	Duration (hrs)
DMT	N, N-dimethyl-tryptamine	Rapid	0.5 to 1
Salvia divinorum	Salvinorin A	Rapid	1 to 2
Foxy	5-methoxy-N, N-dipropyltryptamine	Rapid	3 to 6
Psilocybin	4-phosphoryloxy-N, N-dimethyltryptamine	0.5	4 to 6
LSD	Lysergic acid diethylamide	Few	4 to 12
Mescaline	3,4,5-trimethoxyphenylethylamine	4 to 6	6 to 12
Nutmeg	5-allyl-1,2,3-trimethoxybenzene	1 to 4	12 to 24
AMT	Alaha-methyltryptamine	Rapid	12 to 24
Ibogaine	Ibogaine	4 to 8; 10 to 20	12 to 24

effects may be mild. Common physical signs and symptoms of acute intoxication include mydriasis, diaphoresis, piloerection, tremors, and mildly elevated blood pressure, pulse, respiratory rate, and temperature. These findings, however, may be masked by the co-ingestion of ethanol or other sedative–hypnotic agent.

Injury is the predominant adverse event related to hallucinogen use and generally results from the acute behavioral effect of the drug. There are few, if any, directly concerning physiologic effects of the drugs themselves. The psychological effects can be overwhelming, and occasionally the hallucinations can be perceived as frightening or threatening. Panic, paranoia, catatonia, and homicidal and/or suicidal behaviors on this basis have been reported (23).

There is no reported withdrawal syndrome from hallucinogens, although tolerance and cross-tolerance between compounds can occur.

The time of onset and duration of effect can help determine the identity of the hallucinogen (Table 325.1). Long-acting agents include LSD, mescaline, and nutmeg. Medium-acting agents include psilocybin and psilocin, Foxy, AMT, and Bufo species toad toxins. Short-acting hallucinogens include DMT, ibogaine, and salvinorin A. Associated side effects can also be a clue to the identity of the agent involved.

Hallucinatory effects of LSD typically begin within a few hours, and last anywhere from 4 to 12 hours. Although generally considered pleasant, as noted above there are occasionally "bad trips," which can include paranoia, acute psychosis, panic, and significant depression. Suicide and unintentional death have been reported (6,7,15,23).

The hallucinogen persisting perception disorder (HPPD), commonly known as "flashbacks," associated with the use of LSD should not be confused with prolonged sensory perception (afterimages), also known as palinopsia. Patients with HPPD characteristically experience recurrent perceptual disturbances similar to those encountered during acute intoxication in the absence of drug. HPPD is often triggered by stress, illness or other challenges. It can occur after a single use of the drug and may last for a prolonged period (up to years) (1). HPPD is associated with the use of phenothiazine antipsychotics to control the acute behavioral symptoms of acute intoxication, suggesting that sedatives such as benzodiazepines, rather than antipsychotics should be used for this purpose. Proposed therapies for HPPD include clonazepam, carbidopa, and psychotherapy (11,13). Another rarely reported adverse effect of LSD is permanent psychosis (1,11,23).

Mescaline use is associated with significant, unpleasant, side effects. Initial signs and symptoms include nausea, vomiting, abdominal pain, diaphoresis, nystagmus, and ataxia. These symptoms typically resolve within an hour or two of ingestion, and precede the onset of the hallucinations, which begin within 4 to 6 hours. The effects typically last for 6 to 12 hours (15).

Hallucinogenic doses of nutmeg cause severe side effects, such as dizziness, flushing, tachycardia, nausea, vomiting, con-

stipation and panic. As a result of the relative severity of the side effects, it is not a popular means of producing hallucinations. When ingested, the hallucinations begin within 1 to 4 hours and last 12 to 24 hours. Many users report an extended period of sleep after use (upwards of 16 hours).

Ingestion of psilocybe mushrooms is typically associated with nausea and sometimes vomiting. Onset of effect is approximately 30 minutes and their duration is typically 4 to 6 hours. The effects are typically described as being "less intense" and more illusionary than those produced by LSD (4,19,20,21). AMT has a longer duration of effect (approximately 12–24 hours) than that of Foxy (between 3 and 6 hours). Toad-licking has resulted in digoxin-like bradycardia and significant adverse effects from other components of toad secretions (16).

Smoking DMT leads to effects that typically begin within minutes and last between 30 and 60 minutes. Rapid onset and short duration of action has earned DMT the moniker "the businessman's lunch," because the user can experience a "trip" in the time allotted for a meal (5,14,15). Following the ingestion of Ayahuasca, DMT also has a rapid onset of action and short duration of effect (17,20,21).

The ingestion of *S. divinorum* produces effects that begin in 5 to 10 minutes and last approximately 1 to 2 hours. When the vapor is inhaled, or the plant is smoked, effects begin in seconds and last about 30 minutes (5,18). Ibogaine ingestion can cause both early (4–8 hours after ingestion) and late (10–20 hours after ingestion) hallucinations (3,5,15,20,21).

Other abused agents that can cause hallucinations include sympathomimetics, anticholinergics, and dissociative anesthetic agents and related compounds. Cocaine and amphetamines are associated with psychosis at high doses or following binges. Patients characteristically develop a delusional state that does not always involve clear hallucinations. Symptoms may last for several days, but typically respond to antipsychotic medications. Anticholinergic agents (e.g., scopolamine and atropine) may produce dramatic epidemic hallucinations when teenagers discover Jimsonweed (*Datura stramonium*) and ingest the seeds. Patients generally have other manifestations of the anticholinergic syndrome and are always delirious. Dissociative anesthetic agents, such as PCP and ketamine, and the related compound dextromethorphan produce hallucinations that are generally described as dysphoric. Clinical features include delirium and prominent nystagmus. Autonomic manifestations are usually more prominent than hallucinations in each of these conditions. In contrast, with traditional hallucinogens such as LSD, hallucinations are prominent and autonomic effects are usually mild.

Hallucinations have been reported as idiosyncratic reactions to almost all medications. Street-drug adulterants (e.g., cyanide, local anesthetics, quinine, quinidine, caffeine, theophylline, and strychnine) should also be considered in the differential of the cause of toxic effects of alleged hallucinogens. Because central nervous system (CNS) structural, infectious, and psychiatric conditions can cause hallucinations, the use of a hallucinatory compound should be a diagnosis of exclusion. With or without the history of hallucinogen exposure, these conditions should be considered in the differential diagnosis.

EMERGENCY DEPARTMENT EVALUATION

The history should include the name or description of the hallucinogen, the time of ingestion, amount(s) taken, the route of exposure, and the nature and time of onset of hallucinations and other symptoms. Slang names may provide a presumptive identity if the chemical name is not known. A regional poison control center (1-800-222-1222) can assist with identification and provide information on local drug use trends. A history of previous drug use, psychiatric problems, and medical conditions, particularly cardiovascular disease, should be documented. The clinician should specifically ask about the possibility of concomitant traumatic injuries.

The physical examination should focus on the mental status, neurologic evaluation, and cardiovascular system. A full set of vital signs is documented and repeated frequently. The patient should be examined carefully for evidence of trauma, underlying disease, and heat- related illness.

Ancillary testing is neither necessary nor useful in patients with mild hallucinogen intoxication, except to rule out other diagnoses. Patients with moderate or severe symptoms (e.g., excessive agitation and significantly abnormal vital signs) should have a chest radiograph; cardiac monitoring and a 12-lead ECG; complete blood count; determination of electrolyte, glucose, blood urea nitrogen, creatinine, and creatine kinase levels; and urinalysis (including myoglobin). Routine toxicology screening may be useful for detecting or excluding other agents. Specific assays of the urine are usually necessary to confirm the presence of hallucinogens. Quantitative blood (or urine) hallucinogen levels are not clinically useful or routinely available.

Significant psychomotor agitation can occur with a variety of perceived stimuli, and rhabdomyolysis should be considered.

EMERGENCY DEPARTMENT MANAGEMENT

Management is supportive. Standard life support measures should be instituted as needed. The focus of care should then be to provide a calm, quiet environment for the patient. Providers should attempt to reduce the patient's anxiety, help to provide a foundation for reality testing, and provide continued, empathetic reassurance. In cases in which the experience is causing the patient significant agitation or distress, pharmacologic sedation with a benzodiazepine should be provided. Phenothiazines should be avoided because they have been implicated in HPPD (11,13,23).

Although activated charcoal can bind most, if not all, of these compounds, the efficacy of this intervention is undefined. Because consequential morbidity is exceedingly rare, and because GI decontamination may be particularly unpleasant for a patient who is hallucinating, its use should be limited to patients with significant co-ingestions or hallucinogen "overdose."

CRITICAL INTERVENTIONS

- Provide a calm, quiet environment with continuous observation and repeated reassurance
- Administer benzodiazepines for persistent or severe agitation or psychological distress

DISPOSITION

For the majority of patients presenting after use of a hallucinogen, their disposition will be discharge. In the absence of any adverse sequelae (e.g., trauma, rhabdomyolysis, electrolyte abnormality, etc.) the patient should be watched until reality testing is assured, and appropriate referral to a psychiatrist or substance abuse program can be provided. Admission is warranted only for persistence of psychosis or if the patient has a concomitant medical or surgical issue that makes this necessary.

COMMON PITFALLS

- ✔ Failure to obtain a complete set of vital signs, especially an accurate core temperature
- ✔ Failure to differentiate between hallucinations and delirium; patients with drug-induced hallucinations have clear orientation with altered content
- ✔ Failure to make safety of the patient and staff a priority
- ✔ Failure to consider metabolic, structural, infectious, traumatic, psychiatric etiologies of the hallucinatory state
- ✔ Failure to screen for occult conditions caused by the behavioral abnormalities of these compounds, such as rhabdomyolysis
- ✔ Failure to consider co-ingestants, or nonclassical hallucinogen producing compounds (i.e. anticholinergic agents), and their specific toxicities

Acknowledgment

We thank previous edition chapter author Christopher H. Linden.

References

1. Abraham HD, Aldridge AM. Adverse consequences of lysergic acid diethylamide. *Addiction* 1993;88:1327–1334.
2. Blaho K, Merigian K, Winbery S, et al. Clinical pharmacology of lysergic acid diethylamide: Case reports and review of the literature. *Am J Ther* 1997;4:211–221.
3. Deecher DC, Teitler M, Soderlund DM, et al. Mechanism of action of ibogaine and harmaline congeners based on radioligand binding studies. *Brain Res* 1992;571:242–247.
4. de Rios MD, Grob CS, Baker JR. Hallucinogens and redemption. *J Psychoactive Drugs* 2002;34(3):239–248.
5. Drug Enforcement Agency (DEA). LSD. DEA Web site. From http://www.dea.gov/. Accessed on November 30, 2003.
6. Forest JAH, Tarala RA. 60 hospital admissions due to reactions to lysergide (LSD). *Lancet* 1973;2:1310.
7. Gertsch JH, Wood C. Case report: an ingestion of Hawaiian Baby Woodrose seeds associated with acute psychosis. *Hawaii Med J* 2003;62(6):127–129.
8. Goldrank LR, Flomenbaum NE, Lewin NA, et al, eds. *Goldfrank's Toxicologic Emergencies*, 7th ed. New York: McGraw Hill, 2002;1046–1053.
9. Goodman N. The serotonergic system and mysticism: Could LSD and the nondrug-induced mystical experience share common neural mechanisms? *J Psychoactive Drugs* 2002;34(3):263–72.
10. Hardman JG, Limbird LE, eds. *Goodman & Gilman's the pharmacological basis of therapeutics*, 10th ed. New York: McGraw Hill, 2001;260–290.
11. Halpern JH, Pope HG Jr. Hallucinogen persisting perception disorder: What do we know after 50 years? *Drug Alcohol Depend* 2003;69(2):109–119.
12. Johnston LD, O'Malley PM, Bachman JG. *Monitoring the future: national survey results on drug use 1975–2001*. Volume 1. NIH Publication No. 02–5106. Bethesda, MD: National Institute on Drug Abuse, 2002.
13. Lerner AG, Gelkopf M, Skladman I, et al. Clonazepam treatment of lysergic acid diethylamide-induced hallucinogen persisting perception disorder with anxiety features. *Int Clin Psychopharmacol* 2003;18(2):101–105.
14. Long H, Nelson LS, Hoffman RS. Alpha-methyltryptamine revisited via easy Internet access. *Vet Hum Toxicol* 2003;45(3):149.
15. National Institute on Drug Abuse (NIDA). Acid/LSD. NIDA Web site. From http://www.drugabuse.gov/drugpages/acidLSD.html. Accessed on November 30, 2003.
16. Ott J. Pharmanopo-psychonautics: human intranasal, sublingual, intrarectal, pulmonary and oral pharmacology of bufotenine. *J Psychoactive Drugs* 2001;33(3):273–281.
17. Riba J, Valle M, Urbano G, et al. Human pharmacology of Ayahuasca: subjective and cardiovascular effects, monoamine metabolite excretion, and pharmacokinetics. *J Pharmacol Exp Ther* 2003;306(1):73–83.

18. Roth BL, Baner K, Westkaemper R, et al. Salvinorin A: a potent naturally occurring nonnitrogenous? opioid selective agonist. *Proc Natl Acad Sci* 2002;99(18):11934–11939.
19. Sadzot B, Baraban JM, Glennon RA, et al. Hallucinogenic drug interactions at human brain 5-HT2 receptors: implications for treating LSD-induced hallucinogenesis. *Psychopharmacology* 1989;98(4):495–499.
20. Schultes RE. The plant kingdom and hallucinogens (part I). *Bull Narc* 1969;21(3):3–16.
21. Schultes RE. The plant kingdom and hallucinogens (part II). *Bull Narc* 1969;21(4):15–27.
22. Schwartz RH. LSD: its rise, fall, and renewed popularity among high school students. *Pediatr Clin North Am* 1995;42(2):403–413.
23. Taylor RL, Maurer JI, Tinklenberg JR. Management of "bad trips" in an evolving drug scene. *JAMA* 1970;213(3):422–425.
24. Titeler M, Lyon RA, Glennon RA. Radioligand binding evidence implicates the brain 5HT$_2$ receptor as a site of action for LSD and phenylisopropylamine hallucinogens. *Psychopharmacology* 1988;94(2):213–216.
25. Ulrich RF, Patten BM. The rise, decline, and fall of LSD. *Perspect Biol Med* 1991;34(4):561–579.

CHAPTER 326
Methylxanthines

Pierre Gaudreault

Methylxanthines, methylated derivatives of xanthine, include theophylline, caffeine, diphylline, pentoxifylline, and theobromine. Theophylline (1,3-dimethylxanthine) is used to treat asthma, apnea of premature infants, and chronic obstructive pulmonary disease (COPD), and as an analgesic adjunct. It is available as anhydrous theophylline or as a variety of salts (Table 326.1).

Aminophylline is theophylline ethylenediamine, and oxtriphylline is 7-choline theophyllinate. Available formulations include i.v. solutions of aminophylline and suspensions, capsules, tablets, and sustained-release formulations for oral use. Therapeutic oral doses range from 13 to 24 mg/kg/d, usually administered in divided doses.

Caffeine (1,3,7-trimethylxanthine) is a naturally occurring alkaloid contained in beverages such as coffee (60–180 mg/5 oz), tea (20–60 mg/5 oz), chocolate milk (2–7 mg/8 oz), and cola soft drinks (45 mg/12 oz) and in chocolate candy bars (7 mg per bar). It is also contained in analgesic preparations and over-the-counter diet and stimulant ("wake-up" or "stay awake" pills) formulations in doses of 15 to 100 mg. Street-drug capsules that contain caffeine, phenylpropanolamine, and ephedrine are sold as stimulants. These products are called "look-alikes" because they are usually prepared to resemble prescription amphetamines (8). Since 1983, it has been illegal in the United States to market products that contain combinations of caffeine and ephedrine, pseudoephedrine, or phenylpropanolamine.

Methylxanthines are rapidly absorbed after ingestion, with peak blood levels occurring in 1 to 2 hours. With sustained-release preparations, peak levels are maintained for 6 to 24 hours. Absorption is prolonged, and peak blood levels are delayed after overdosage, particularly with sustained-release preparations. Theophylline is 60% protein-bound, and caffeine is 35% protein-bound, mainly to albumin. Protein binding decreases with acidemia (resulting in increased free drug) and increases with alkalemia. The volume of distribution averages 0.5 L/kg (range, 0.3–0.7 L/kg) for theophylline and 0.4 L/kg for caffeine. Therapeutic serum levels are 10 to 20 μg/mL. Caffeine levels ranging from 12 to 36 μg/mL are effective in preventing neonatal apnea, but levels are only 3 to 10 μg/mL following usual adult doses.

Theophylline is eliminated by hepatic metabolism (90%) and urinary excretion of unchanged drug (10%). The half-life is age-dependent and influenced by concomitant drug therapy and illnesses. It averages 20 hours in newborns, 6 to 7 hours in infants, 3 to 5 hours in ages 6 months to 18 years, and 4 to 6 hours for adults. Hepatic elimination is increased by β agonists, smoking, rifampin, and antiepileptic drugs (carbamazepine, phenobarbital, and phenytoin) and is decreased by allopurinol, β blockers (nonselective), calcium channel blockers, cimetidine, congestive heart failure, fever, influenza virus vaccine, interferon, liver disease, macrolide antibiotics, mexiletine, oral contraceptives, and quinolones. Active metabolites include 3-methylxanthine, caffeine, and theobromine. Metabolism is saturable at serum theophylline levels near or above 20 μg/mL, resulting in a prolonged half-life after overdose. Metabolites may also contribute to overdose toxicity. The kinetics of caffeine are similar, with half-lives ranging from 2 to 12 hours in infants, children, and adults. In newborns, the half-life of caffeine is about 4 days, because up to 85% is excreted unchanged in the urine.

Therapeutic, adverse, and toxic effects of methylxanthines are a result of adenosine antagonism, resulting in central nervous system (CNS) stimulation, reduction of the ventricular fibrillation (VF) threshold, smooth muscle relaxation, and gastric acid and pepsin secretion. Cardiovascular (CV) effects also result from epinephrine and norepinephrine release (low theophylline concentrations) and inhibition of phosphodiesterase, leading to increased cyclic adenosine and guanosine monophosphate (high theophylline concentrations) (9). Tachydysrhythmias may result from a decrease of the VF threshold, a nonuniform increase in the cardiac conduction velocity that favors reentry phenomena, and the liberation of catecholamines. Hypokalemia and a reduced oxygen delivery in the face of increased demand by the myocardium seen with theophylline overdoses might also be contributory. Caffeine, the most potent CNS stimulant of the methylxanthines, stimulates the cortex (increases alertness and enhances performance), increases the spontaneous activity of the reticular formation and directly stimulates the respiratory center located in the medulla, and increases its sensitivity to the stimulatory effects of carbon dioxide. Theophylline and caffeine cause peripheral vasodilation, yet cerebral vasoconstriction. The latter effect may be involved in the pathogenesis of CNS toxicity.

Poisoning may result from chronic (therapeutic) oral overdose, acute ingestion of more than 10 mg/kg, or excessive intravenous dosing. The chronic use of caffeine can lead to a dependence syndrome. Abrupt withdrawal in dependent persons is characterized by headache, lethargy, and depression.

TABLE 326.1. Theophylline Salts

Drug	Anhydrous Theophylline (%)
Aminophylline, anhydrous	84–86
Aminophylline, dihydrate	78–82
Oxtriphylline	62–66
Theophylline calcium salicylate	48–50
Theophylline monohydrate	91
Theophylline olamine	73–75
Theophylline sodium acetate	55–65
Theophylline sodium glycinate	49

CLINICAL PRESENTATION

Initial symptoms of poisoning include nausea, vomiting, and abdominal pain. Diarrhea and gastrointestinal (GI) bleeding may develop later. Spontaneous vomiting may limit drug absorption, especially with caffeine ingestions. However, serum drug levels may continue to rise despite vomiting, particularly when sustained-release preparations have been ingested. Additional signs and symptoms may include headache, insomnia, agitation, delirium, tinnitus, tremors, motor hyperactivity and hypertonicity, jitteriness, hyperventilation, polyuria, seizures, coma, GI bleeding, hyperthermia, and ventricular and supraventricular tachyarrhythmias (9,15,18). At low doses, theophylline induces a mild and transitory hypertension. At high doses, the direct effect of theophylline on the β_2 adrenoreceptors reduces the total peripheral resistance, inducing hypotension. This may partly explain why hypotension is seen with acute, but not chronic, overdose. Laboratory evaluation may reveal leukocytosis, hyperglycemia, hypokalemia, hypophosphatemia, ketosis, metabolic acidosis, and respiratory alkalosis (9,15,16). Decreased serum calcium and magnesium levels, elevated serum amylase and uric acid levels, and evidence of dehydration (elevated blood urea nitrogen and creatinine levels) or rhabdomyolysis (elevated creatine phosphokinase level and myoglobinuria) may be noted (19).

The risk of tachydysrhythmias depends on the duration of exposure, drug concentration, and age. After an acute overdose (single ingestion), patients aged 6 months to 60 years may develop life-threatening dysrhythmias or seizures when serum concentrations exceed 80 μg/mL (9). For the same age group, serious toxic manifestations can occur with serum concentrations above 60 μg/mL with chronic intoxication. Patients younger than age 6 months or older than age 60 years may experience serious toxic manifestations with serum concentrations above 30 μg/mL, regardless of the type of intoxication. Patients over age 40 are at risk of developing serious cardiac dysrhythmias when serum concentrations are above 35 μg/mL. In contrast, serum concentrations higher than 50 μg/mL are necessary to induce serious dysrhythmias in healthy younger patients (age 40 or less) (11).

Seizures are usually generalized but can be focal. The neurotoxicity of theophylline seems to be dose-dependent, but other factors also influence the development of neurotoxicity. Indeed, patients younger than age 6 months or older than age 60 years who are chronically intoxicated or have a history of neurologic problems (e.g., seizures, cerebrovascular insufficiency) are at greater risk of seizing (7,15). Permanent neurologic damage (e.g., encephalopathy) is not uncommon in patients with prolonged coma or intractable seizures and appears to correlate with their duration.

DIFFERENTIAL DIAGNOSIS

Because the clinical effects of methylxanthine poisoning can be characterized as a "β-adrenergic storm," poisoning by direct-acting β agonists (e.g., albuterol, terbutaline and related bronchodilators) can cause a similar clinical picture. Poisoning by amphetamines, sympathomimetics, anticholinergics, hallucinogens, monoamine oxidase inhibitors, and epinephrine should also be considered in the differential diagnosis. Agitated psychiatric states, drug withdrawal, and medical conditions such as CNS infection, electrolyte disturbance, hypoglycemia, hypocalcemia, pheochromocytoma, and thyroid storm may cause similar signs and symptoms.

EMERGENCY DEPARTMENT EVALUATION

The history should include the time, amount, and formulation of theophylline or caffeine ingested; past or recent therapeutic use of these agents; and routine medical history. Symptoms before arrival should be noted. The maximum possible serum drug level (micrograms per milliliter) can be estimated by doubling the acutely ingested dose (milligrams per kilogram).

The physical examination should focus on vital signs, mental status and neurologic evaluation, cardiorespiratory status, and GI function. Vomitus and stool should be checked for overt or occult blood. Laboratory evaluation should include a quantitative theophylline or caffeine level; complete blood count; determination of electrolyte, glucose, blood urea nitrogen, and creatinine levels; and urinalysis. Drug levels should be repeated every 2 to 4 hours following acute ingestions, until the level is no longer rising. Patients with elevated theophylline levels and moderate or severe clinical toxicity should also have measurements of serum amylase, calcium, creatine phosphokinase, ketones, magnesium, and phosphorus levels, urine myoglobin, and arterial blood gas analysis.

Cardiac monitoring and an electrocardiogram (ECG) should be obtained on all patients. Patients with respiratory symptoms, an abnormal pulmonary examination or ECG, or coma or seizures should have a chest radiograph.

EMERGENCY DEPARTMENT MANAGEMENT

Advanced life-support measures are instituted, as necessary. Activated charcoal (AC) significantly reduces the absorption of theophylline and is the preferred method of GI decontamination. The repetitive administration of activated charcoal also enhances the total body clearance of theophylline (2). The effects of charcoal on the absorption and elimination of other methylxanthines are predicted to be similar. Because serum concentrations may not peak for many hours after ingestion (up to 24 hours with slow-release preparations), every patient with an oral theophylline overdose should receive activated charcoal, regardless of the alleged time of ingestion. A dose of 0.5 to 1.0 g/kg of body weight should be given every 2 to 4 hours until drug levels are in the therapeutic range. If the patient cannot tolerate charcoal because of persistent vomiting, the administration of smaller but more frequent doses (by continuous infusion by way of nasogastric tube, if necessary), metoclopramide (up to 10 mg i.v.), ranitidine (50 mg i.v.), droperidol (2.5 mg intravenously), or ondansetron (8 to 32 mg i.v.) may be used (1,10,13).

Gastric drug bezoar formation has been reported after sustained-release theophylline overdose (3). Endoscopic evaluation and drug mass removal, if necessary, should be considered in patients with rising drug levels and severe poisoning. Although often recommended, whole-bowel irrigation did not add to the benefit of multiple-dose activated charcoal in an experimental sustained-release theophylline overdose (6).

Seizures should be treated aggressively. Diazepam or lorazepam should be given first. If the seizures do not stop rapidly or if they recur, phenobarbital (15–20 mg/kg) should be administered intravenously. If seizures do not stop within 20 to 30 minutes, thiopental should be given; a loading dose of 3 to 5 mg/kg, followed by an infusion of 2 to 4 mg/kg/h is usually efficacious, but these doses can be increased, if necessary. Phenytoin or fosphenytoin are ineffective in controlling methylxanthine–induced seizures (5). Neuromuscular paralysis (e.g., pancuronium) may be necessary to stop muscle contractions, facilitate ventilation, and prevent hyperthermia and rhabdomyolysis.

Electroencephalographic monitoring and continued treatment of seizures are necessary during paralysis. Treatment should also include correction of accompanying acidemia, as this may promote dysrhythmias.

β-adrenergic antagonists (e.g., propranolol, esmolol) are the drug of choice to treat supraventricular and ventricular dysrhythmias after acute overdose. Intravenous doses of propranolol (1 mg in adults or 0.02 mg/kg in children) should be given slowly and repeated every 5 to 10 minutes until dysrhythmias stop, or to a maximal dose of 0.1 mg/kg (4). Although propranolol is normally contraindicated in patients with asthma or COPD, it has been used without adverse effects in asthmatics with acute theophylline poisoning. In such patients, the short-acting β antagonist esmolol has been used and may be preferable to propranolol (14). However, because esmolol is selective for β_1 receptors, it could theoretically worsen hypotension resulting from β_2 stimulation. Clinical evidence of bronchospasm is an absolute contraindication to the use of β blockers. Lidocaine, at standard doses, may also be used for ventricular dysrhythmias. In patients with atrial tachyarrhythmias exacerbated by theophylline intoxication, verapamil has been effective (10). Correction of hypoxemia, acidemia, hypokalemia, and other metabolic abnormalities is also important. Because hypokalemia is a result of an intracellular shift of potassium rather than a total body deficit, overly aggressive therapy for this condition may result in hyperkalemia as toxicity resolves and should be avoided. Hyperglycemia is transitory and well tolerated and usually does not necessitate insulin therapy.

Hypotension is initially treated with fluid administration. Persistent hypotension may be treated with pressors (e.g., phenylephrine or norepinephrine) or propranolol (because of its β_2 blocking effect) (4). Hyperthermia and rhabdomyolysis should be treated with standard measures.

Charcoal hemoperfusion can enhance the elimination of theophylline and should be considered for patients with the following criteria: persistently unstable hemodynamic parameters; seizures; or theophylline serum concentrations above 80 to 100 μg/mL after an acute ingestion, above 60 μg/mL after chronic ingestion, and above 40 μg/mL after an acute or chronic intoxication if age is less than 6 months or above 60 years or there is severe underlying CV disease (9–11,17). Similar parameters should be used in patients with caffeine poisoning.

Hemodialysis also enhances the elimination of theophylline and should be used if hemoperfusion is not immediately available. A tandem set-up (in-line hemodialysis and hemoperfusion) can be used for patients with severe metabolic abnormalities and high drug levels. Exchange transfusion has also been used in neonates with caffeine intoxication when hemoperfusion is technically difficult (12).

CRITICAL INTERVENTIONS

- Obtain quantitative drug levels every 2 to 4 hours following acute overdose, until the level is no longer rising
- Administer AC for GI decontamination and to enhance drug clearance; give antiemetics, if necessary
- Administer benzodiazepines and barbiturates intravenously for seizures
- Administer β-adrenergic antagonists (e.g., propranolol, esmolol) for supraventricular and ventricular tachydysrhythmias unless concomitant bronchospasm is present
- Consult a poison center or toxicologist and a nephrologist regarding charcoal hemoperfusion and/or hemodialysis for patients with seizures, hypotension, tachydysrhythmias, progressive clinical toxicity, or theophylline serum concentrations above 40 μg/mL

DISPOSITION

Patients with a serum theophylline concentration above 35 μg/mL should be admitted to a monitored bed. Those with severe neurologic or cardiotoxic manifestations or serum concentrations above 50 μg/mL should be admitted to an intensive care unit. Those with levels under 35 μg/mL and mild symptoms can usually be treated in the emergency department and discharged when they become asymptomatic. A poison center or toxicologist and a nephrologist should be consulted for patients who meet or are approaching criteria for extracorporeal elimination therapy. If ICU and extracorporeal treatment are not available, the patient should be transferred to a facility with these capabilities.

COMMON PITFALLS

✔ Failure to consider the effects of age, underlying disease, and potential drug interactions on drug kinetics and dosing when prescribing theophylline
✔ Failure to appreciate that patients with chronic exposures develop toxicity at lower drug levels than those with acute or acute-on-chronic overdose
✔ Failure to consider the patient's age, the type of intoxication (acute vs. chronic), and underlying diseases (previous neurologic or cardiac problems) when interpreting theophylline serum concentrations
✔ Failure to appreciate that hypotension (not hypertension) is characteristic of severe, acute (but not chronic) caffeine or theophylline poisoning
✔ Failure to appreciate that seizures can result in acidemia, hyperthermia, rhabdomyolysis, and permanent neurologic damage

References

1. Amitai Y, Yeung AC, Moye J, et al. Repetitive oral activated charcoal and control of emesis in severe theophylline toxicity. *Ann Intern Med* 1986;105: 386–387.
2. Berlinger WG, Spector R, Goldberg MJ, et al. Enhancement of theophylline clearance by oral activated charcoal. *Clin Pharmacol Ther* 1983;33:351–354.
3. Bernstein G, Jehle D, Bernaski E, et al. Failure of gastric emptying and charcoal administration in fatal sustained-release theophylline overdose: Pharmacobezoar formation. *Ann Emerg Med* 1992;21:1388–1390.
4. Biberstein MP, Ziegler MG, Ward DM. Use of beta-blockade and hemoperfusion for acute theophylline poisoning. *West J Med* 1984;141:485–490.
5. Blake KV, Massey KL, Hendeles L, et al. Relative efficacy of phenytoin and phenobarbital for the prevention of theophylline-induced seizures in mice. *Ann Emerg Med* 1988;17:1024–1028.
6. Burkhart KK, Wuerz RC, Donovan JW. Whole-bowel irrigation as adjunctive treatment for sustained-release theophylline poisoning. *Ann Emerg Med* 1992;21:1316–1320.
7. Covelli HD, Knodel AR, Heppner BT. Predisposing factors to apparent theophylline-induced seizures. *Ann Allergy* 1985;54:411–415.
8. Garriott JC, Simmons LM, Poklis A, et al. Five cases of fatal overdose from caffeine-containing "look-alike" drugs. *J Anal Toxicol* 1985;9:141–143.
9. Gaudreault P, Guay J. Theophylline poisoning: pharmacological considerations and clinical management. *Med Toxicol* 1986;1:169–191.
10. Minton NA, Henry JA. Treatment of theophylline overdose. *Am J Emerg Med* 1996;14:606–612.
11. Olson KR, Benowitz NL, Woo OF, et al. Theophylline overdose: Acute single ingestion versus chronic repeated overmedication. *Am J Emerg Med* 1985;3: 386–394.
12. Perrin C, Debruyne D, Lacotte J, et al. Treatment of caffeine intoxication by exchange transfusion in a newborn. *Acta Paediatr Scand* 1987;76:679–681.
13. Sage TA, Jones WN, Clark RF. Ondansetron in the treatment of intractable nausea associated with theophylline toxicity. *Ann Pharmacother* 1993;27: 584–585.
14. Seneff M, Scott J, Friedman B, et al. Acute theophylline toxicity and the use of esmolol to reverse cardiovascular instability. *Ann Emerg Med* 1990;19: 671–673.
15. Sessler CN. Theophylline toxicity: clinical features of 116 consecutive cases. *Am J Med* 1990;88:567–576.
16. Shannon M. Hypokalemia, hyperglycemia, and plasma catecholamine activity after severe theophylline intoxication. *J Toxicol Clin Toxicol* 1994;32:41–47.

17. Shannon MW. Comparative efficacy of hemodialysis and hemoperfusion in severe theophylline intoxication. *Acad Emerg Med* 1997;4:674–678.
18. Shum S, Seale C, Hathaway D, et al. Acute caffeine ingestion fatalities: management issues. *Vet Hum Toxicol* 1997;39:228–230.
19. Wrenn KD, Oschner I. Rhabdomyolysis induced by a caffeine overdose. *Ann Emerg Med* 1989;18:94–97.

CHAPTER 327
Phencyclidine and Ketamine

Cyrus Rangan

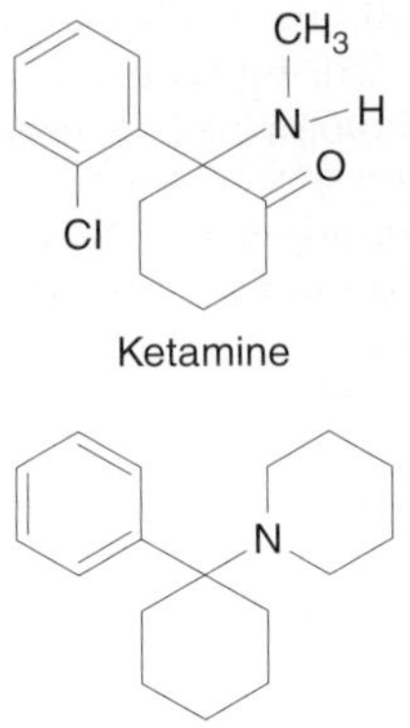

Figure 327.1. The chemical structures of PCP and ketamine account for similarities in clinical effects and cross-reaction on the PCP urine immunoassay.

Phencyclidine (PCP, 1-(1-phenylcyclohexyl)-piperidine) was first synthesized in 1926, after the reaction of Grignard reagents with 1-piperidinocyclohexanecarbonitrile, a cyanide precursor (13). Powerful analgesic properties, with minimal respiratory depression, made it an intriguing general anesthetic (Sernyl®) in the 1950s (7). Such use ceased in 1965 secondary to the high frequency of emergence reactions, although its use as a veterinary anesthetic (Sernylan®) continued until 1979, after which all U.S. production of PCP was stopped (22). PCP became a popular street drug in the late 1960s. As an illicit psychoactive substance, PCP is known by the street names "Angel Dust," "DOA," "Goon," "Horse Tranquilizer," "Loveboat," "Lovely," "Ozone," "Paz," "Peace Pill," "Peep," "Pig Killer," "Polvo de Angel," "Puffy Hog," "Purple Rain," "Rocket Fuel," and "Wack." When smoked with tobacco, parsley, mint, oregano, or marijuana, it may be known as "Crystal," "Krystal," "Killerjoints," "Supergrass," "Sherm," "Sherman Sticks," or "Sherman Tanks." Absorption of PCP is rapid via ingestion, snorting, injection, or smoking. Recreational use ranges from 1 mg to 10 mg per dose, and toxic psychosis is usually seen after about 5 mg. PCP is eliminated via hepatic metabolism, with very little parent drug cleared by the kidney (10).

Ketamine (2-(2-chlorophenyl)-2-methylaminocyclohexanone) was synthesized from PCP derivatives in the 1960s, and has been used primarily as a pediatric and veterinary anesthetic since 1970. The 1980s saw the first well-documented cases of abuse in the United States, with multiple reports of theft from veterinary facilities. Still a legally manufactured drug (Ketalar®), ketamine is a popular hallucinogenic at rave parties, and is also a recognized "date-rape" drug (1,22). Ketamine is known by the street names "Cat Valium," "Green," "Honey Oil," "Jet," "K," "K-blast," "Ket," "Ketter," "Kit-Kat," "Lady K," "Special K," "Special LA Coke," "Super Acid," "Super C," and "Vitamin K." Its pharmacodynamic effects are quite similar to those of PCP, with substantially reduced potency, volume of distribution, half-life, and duration of action. Absorption of ketamine is rapid, via ingestion, snorting, injection, or smoking. Recreational use ranges from 10 mg to 500 mg per dose. The liver metabolizes ketamine to the active metabolite norketamine, which is eliminated by the kidney (4).

PCP and ketamine have similar chemical structures (Fig. 327.1), and bind to the same receptors in the nervous system. At the N-methyl-D-aspartate (NMDA) receptor, they act as noncompetitive antagonists by blocking calcium influx via stimulation of the PCP binding site, accounting for their dissociative anesthetic effects (12). At sympathetic nerve terminals, they act as catecholamine reuptake inhibitors, leading to sympathomimetic effects in vital signs and mental status (16). In higher doses, they bind to sigma opioid receptors, in which they cause lethargy, obtundation, or coma (17). They variably stimulate muscarinic, dopaminergic, GABAergic, and nonsigma opioid receptors, possibly by modulation of potassium conductance (9).

CLINICAL PRESENTATION

The effects of PCP and ketamine begin within minutes after administration, and tend to last 8 to 24 hours for PCP and 30 minutes to 4 hours for ketamine. Patients with impaired hepatic or renal function experience longer durations of toxicity. Psychological dependence and tolerance are described with both drugs. Despite sedative effects, neither drug diminishes respiratory drive significantly, and deaths resulting from direct drug toxicity are rare (5,18,19,25). Associated traumatic injury is common (19).

The most prominent clinical manifestations of PCP intoxication are psychiatric, including euphoria, severe auditory hallucinations, and short-term memory impairment. Some patients may experience visual distortions, increased strength and aggressiveness, and feelings of disconnection from reality. Curiously, they undergo rather extreme behavioral swings between catatonia and excessive agitation, in which severe violence, combativeness, and "super-human strength" are commonly described (18). Children, however, tend to exhibit mostly motor effects as opposed to aggressive behavior (21). Acute psychotic reactions to PCP may be clinically indistinguishable from schizophrenia (24).

Neurologic signs include ataxia, dystonic reactions, seizures, and hypertonia. Nystagmus occurs in over 50% of PCP overdoses, and may be horizontal, vertical, or rotatory. Hypertension from PCP intoxication may lead to intracranial hemorrhage, giving rise to other neurologic symptoms (2). Sympathomimetic findings tend to be moderate and include tachycardia, hypertension, diaphoresis, and agitation. Less than 5% of cases develop hyperthermia, secondary to excessive muscular rigidity, hyperactivity, or sustained seizures. Pupils are paradoxically small, and patients may lacrimate and hypersalivate, secondary to stimulation of opioid and cholinergic nerve fibers (19). Rhabdomyolysis may ensue secondary to increased tone and muscular activity from agitation. It may be exacerbated by crush injury induced by hard leather restraints, although these restraints may be necessary to control the patient initially (14).

Ketamine intoxication is very similar but less severe. The clinical picture is characterized by dose-dependent disturbances in perception with less agitation and violent behavior than in PCP intoxication (25). Patients often describe a "floating" feeling. Although signs and symptoms tend to be more short-lived than those of PCP, severe overdoses may result in a prolonged effect, described by the user as a numbing, out-of-body experience with the perception of paralysis, also known as a "K-Hole" (5). Smaller doses result in diminished attention span, pain perception, and memory, via NMDA receptor antagonism. Mild tachycardia and hypertension may result from sympathomimetic effects. Miosis, nystagmus, ataxia, mumbling speech, delirium, and hallucinations are also common. Although ketamine is a known clinical bronchodilator, it also induces bronchorrhea and sialorrhea (25).

DIFFERENTIAL DIAGNOSIS

Phencyclidine intoxication should be suspected in any patient with acute onset of schizophrenic or psychotic behavior (especially with fluctuating mental status changes). Violent behavior, indifference to painful stimuli, and difficulty restraining the patient are useful clues.

Signs and symptoms of PCP and ketamine intoxication are similar to those seen with several other drug intoxications and disease processes. PCP and ketamine can mimic the effects of sympathomimetics (16) (see Chapter 328, "Sympathomimetics"), anticholinergic agents (9) (see Chapter 323, "Anticholinergic Agents"), and opiate derivatives (9,17) (see Chapter 283, "Opioids"). Patients with sympathomimetic and anticholinergic poisoning have tachycardia and hypertension but miosis, nystagmus, and salivation are typically absent. Withdrawal from PCP or ketamine (violence, muscle rigidity, convulsions, coma, and psychosis) can mimic withdrawal from ethanol and sedative–hypnotic agents (18,19) (see Chapters 278, "Alcohol Withdrawal" and 333, "Drug Withdrawal").

Because PCP or ketamine may be taken with any number of other drugs, additional signs or symptoms may also be present (22). Cyanide poisoning should be considered in PCP-intoxicated patients who have been smoking the drug (15) (see Chapter 308, "Cyanide"). The possibility of occult traumatic injury should also be considered (19).

EMERGENCY DEPARTMENT EVALUATION

The history should include the time, amount, and route of exposure, and the circumstances and events prior to arrival. Details should be obtained from sources other than the patient, if necessary. A general physical examination and mental status examination should be performed, with a search for focal neurologic findings and evidence of trauma, aspiration pneumonia, and other complications. Substance abuse patients should be evaluated for complications of injection drug use (see Chapter 285, "Complications of Injection Drug Use").

Quantitative serum or urine determinations for PCP or ketamine are not practical in the emergency department setting; drug levels do not correlate with severity of symptoms, and such levels are not likely to return before symptoms have resolved. Qualitative analysis via urine drug rapid immunoassay may be useful to confirm the presence of PCP, although many hospital-based drug screens do not routinely test for PCP. False-negative results for PCP are very common, because

urinary PCP excretion often falls below the limit of immunoassay detection (11). False-positive results have occurred with both ketamine and dextromethorphan (3). Ketamine detection is not a component of commercially available rapid drug screens. Urine may be sent for high performance liquid chromatographic analysis for PCP or ketamine, although symptoms are likely to resolve long before these results return (20). Urinalysis may be positive for hemoglobin, suggesting the presence of myoglobin and rhabdomyolysis (14). Lethargic, comatose, or extremely violent patients will also benefit from determinations of serum electrolytes, complete blood count, arterial blood gas, hepatic transaminases, renal function studies, creatinine phosphokinase, and serum ethanol level. Computed tomography scan of the brain is indicated if signs of cranial trauma are present (2).

EMERGENCY DEPARTMENT MANAGEMENT

Advanced life support measures should be instituted as necessary. Symptomatic care is mainstay the treatment. Patients with coma should receive empiric therapy with glucose (or have a rapid bedside glucose determination), thiamine, and naloxone. Because naloxone does not bind to sigma opioid receptors, the opioid effects of PCP and ketamine are not directly reversible (23).

Agitation and psychosis may initially require physical restraints. As soon as possible, intravenous diazepam (0.1 mg/kg/dose) or lorazepam (0.1 mg/kg/dose) should be given. The dose may be repeated every 5 to 10 minutes if necessary. Haloperidol 5 to 10 mg i.v./i.m. (0.5 mg for children) every 30 to 60 minutes is very effective, but should be used with caution, because butyrophenones may exacerbate hypertonia (6,18). Anecdotal evidence suggests agitation may be further decreased by placing the patient into a darkened room with minimal sensory stimulation. Phenothiazines are not recommended because they may lower the seizure threshold, exacerbate hyperthermia, contribute to systemic acidosis, and induce hypotension. Neuromuscular paralysis may be necessary in refractory cases of violent psychosis (18).

Seizures should also initially be treated with benzodiazepines: diazepam 0.1 to 0.2 mg/kg/dose i.v., lorazepam 0.05 to 0.1 mg/kg i.v., or midazolam 0.1 to 0.2 mg/kg i.v.. Refractory seizures may be treated with phenobarbital 10 to 15 mg/kg i.v. Phenytoin has not been shown to be effective in seizures induced by PCP or ketamine.

Severe hypertension is generally short-lived. Severe and persistent hypertension may be treated with esmolol 0.025 to 0.1 mg/kg/min i.v. or nitroprusside 2 to 10 mcg/kg/min i.v.. Hyperthermia should be treated with evaporative cooling, sedation, and chemical paralysis in refractory cases (see Chapter 353, "Heat-Related Illness"). Patients with rhabdomyolysis should be given intravenous saline to restore and maintain adequate urine flow. Mannitol 0.5 g/kg i.v. may also be of some benefit. Deposition of myoglobin into renal tubules may be decreased by alkalinization with sodium bicarbonate 100 mEq/L of 5% dextrose solution. Hemodialysis may be indicated if myoglobin-induced oliguria or anuria occur (14).

In patients with PCP or ketamine ingestion, activated charcoal should be administered once the patient is stabilized. Gastrointestinal decontamination is not indicated for other routes of administration. Because PCP is secreted into the stomach, continuous gastric suctioning and multiple-dose activated charcoal therapy can theoretically enhance its elimination. These practices are not routinely indicated because very little drug is secreted into the stomach, and neither therapy significantly increases drug clearance or shortens the duration of symptoms (18).

Although urinary acidification with ammonium chloride can enhance excretion of PCP (and ketamine) and turn a false-negative immunoassay into a true-positive, this practice is not recommended. It has not been shown to shorten the duration of toxicity, will worsen acidemia, and may promote renal failure by increasing myoglobin precipitation in renal tubules (11). Although not currently available, monoclonal Fab fragments are another potential treatment option (8). Hemodialysis and hemoperfusion are not recommended for enhancing PCP or ketamine elimination because high protein binding and large volumes of distribution limit their efficacy.

CRITICAL INTERVENTIONS

- Obtain a core temperature, ABG, and serum creatine kinase to assess for hyperthermia, acidosis, and rhabdomyolysis in patients with agitation, psychosis, and seizures
- Administer benzodiazepines or haloperidol intravenously for agitation and psychosis requiring physical restraint
- Administer benzodiazepines and barbiturates intravenously for seizures and neuromuscular hyperactivity resulting in hyperthermia or rhabdomyolysis
- Treat hyperthermia with evaporative cooling, sedation, and neuromuscular paralysis in refractory cases
- Administer saline intravenously, with or without mannitol and sodium bicarbonate, to patients with rhabdomyolysis
- Administer esmolol or nitroprusside intravenously for severe and persistent hypertension

DISPOSITION

Neurosurgical and orthopaedic consultation may be necessary in cases of physical trauma associated with PCP or ketamine intoxication. Patients with altered mental status beyond 4 to 6 hours, major trauma, or hemodynamic instability should be admitted or transferred to a critical care setting. Patients with persistent psychiatric symptoms after resolution of drug toxicity should be referred to a psychiatrist. All patients should be referred to substance abuse counseling.

COMMON PITFALLS

✔ Failure to consider the possibility of intracranial hemorrhage and concomitant trauma in patients with altered mental status
✔ Excluding PCP or ketamine intoxication on the basis of a negative drug screen
✔ Failure to appreciate that ketamine and dextromethorphan can result in a false positive result on PCP immunoassays
✔ Inappropriate acidification of the urine to enhance drug elimination or produce a positive immunoassay result

Acknowledgment

The author thanks previous edition chapter author Andis Graudins.

References

1. Bobo WV, Miller SC. Ketamine as a preferred substance of abuse. *Am J Addict* 2002;11:332–334.
2. Boyko OB, Burger PC, Heinz ER. Pathological and radiological correlation of subarachnoid hemorrhage in phencyclidine abuse. *J Neurosurg* 1987;67:446–448.
3. Budai B. Dextromethorphan can produce false positive phencycldine testing with HPLC. *Am J Emerg Med* 2002;20(1):61–62.
4. Clements JA, Nimmo WS, Grant IS. Bioavailability, pharmacokinetics, and analgesic activity of ketamine in humans. *J Pharm Sci* 1982;71(5):539–542.
5. Curran HV, Monaghan L. In and out of the K-hole: a comparison of the acute and residual effects of ketamine in frequent and infrequent ketamine users. *Addiction* 2001;96(5):749–760.
6. Giannini AJ, Underwood NA, Condon M. Acute ketamine intoxication treated by haloperidol: a preliminary study. *Am J Ther* 2000;7:389–391.
7. Greifenstein FE, Devault M, Yoshitake J, et al. A study of a 1-aryl cyclo hexyl amine for anesthesia. *Anesth Analg* 1958;37(5):283–294.
8. Hardin JS, Wessinger WD, Proksch JW, et al. Pharmacodynamics of a monoclonal antiphencyclidine Fab with broad selectivity for phencyclidine-like drugs. *J Pharmacol Exp Ther* 1998;285:1113–1122.
9. Hustveit O, Aurset A, Oye I. Interaction of chiral forms of ketamine with opioid, phencyclidine, sigma, and muscarinic receptors. *Pharmacol Toxicol* 1995;77(5):355–359.
10. Jackson JE. Phencyclidine pharmacokinetics after massive overdose. *Ann Intern Med* 1989;111(7):613–615.
11. Kaul B, Davidow B. Application of radioimmunoassay screening test for detection and management of phencyclidine intoxication. *J Clin Pharmacol* 1980;20 (8–9):500–505.
12. Kemp JA, Foster EC, Wong HF. A comment on the classification and nomenclature of phencyclidine and sigma receptor sites. *Trends Neurosci* 1988 Sep;11(9):388–3899.
13. Koetz A, Merkel P. Zür kenntnis Hydroaromatischer alkamine. *J Prakt Chem* 1926;113(1):49–76.
14. Lahmeyer HW, Stock PG. Phencyclidine intoxication, physical restraint, and acute renal failure: case report. *J Clin Psychiatry* 1983;44:184–185.
15. Lue LP, Scimeca JA, Thomas BF, et al. Pyrolytic fate of piperidinocylcohexanecarbonitrile, a contaminant of phencyclidine, during smoking. *J Anal Toxicol* 1988;12:57–61.
16. Massamiri T, Duckles SP. Interations of sigma and phencyclidine receptor ligands with the norepinephrine uptake carrier in both rat brain in rat tail artery. *J Pharmacol Exp Ther* 1991;256(2):519–524.
17. Mendelsohn LG, Kalra V, Johnson BG. Sigma opioid receptor: characterization and co-identity with the phencyclidine receptor. *J Pharmacol Exp Ther* 1985;233(3):597–602.
18. McCarron MM, Schulze BW, Thompson GA, et al. Acute PCP intoxication: clinical patterns, complications, and treatment. *Ann Emerg Med* 1981;10:290–297.
19. McCarron MM, Schulze BW, Thompson GA, et al. Acute PCP intoxication: incidence of clinical findings in 1000 cases. *Ann Emerg Med* 1981;10:237–242.
20. Moore KA, Sklerov J, Levine B, et al. Urine concentrations of ketamine and norketamine following illegal consumption. *J Anal Toxicol* 2001;25:583–588.
21. Schwartz RH, Einhorn A. PCP intoxication in seven young children. *Pediatr Emerg Care* 1986;2(4):238–241.
22. Siegel RK. Phencyclidine and ketamine intoxication: a study of four populations of recreational users. *NIDA Res Monogr* 1978;(21):119–147.
23. Tam SW. Naloxone-inaccessible sigma receptor in rat central nervous system. *Proc Natl Acad Sci USA* 1983;80(21):6703–6707.
24. Vollenweider FX, Geyer MA. A systems model of altered consciousness: integrating natural and drug-induced psychoses. *Brain Res Bull* 2001;56(5):495–507.
25. Weiner AL, Vieira L, McKay CA, et al. Ketamine abusers presenting to the emergency department: a case series. *J Emerg Med* 2000;18(4):447–451.

CHAPTER 328
Symptomimetics

Christine Haller

Sympathomimetics include the amphetamines and other phenylethylamines that are structural analogues of catecholamines and have the ability to stimulate adrenergic receptors. These drugs are less rapidly metabolized than catecholamines and have adequate bioavailabilities and sufficiently long half-lives to make oral administration feasible. They are also commonly smoked, snorted, and injected intravenously for abuse purposes. The Substance Abuse Mental Health Services Administration's (SAMHSA) Drug Abuse Warning Network (DAWN) reports that emergency department visits related to stimulant use has increased steadily from 1995 to the present (24).

Methamphetamine use remains geographically concentrated in the western United States although admission rates to substance abuse treatment facilities for methamphetamine have increased 250% from 1993 to 1999 in 14 states. In SAMHSA's 2002 National Survey on Drug Use and Health, 1.2 million Americans age 12 and older reported current illicit stimulant use, and an additional 676,000 reported current use of methylenedioxymethamphetamine (MDMA) or ecstasy (24).

The activity of sympathomimetics at various adrenergic receptors varies and, in part, explains their clinical uses (Table 328.1). α-mediated vasoconstriction of the nasal mucosa is responsible for decongestion. β_2 stimulation causes bronchodilation. Anorectic effects are centrally mediated, and may be as a result of reduced taste and olfactory acuity or direct suppression of the appetite center in the hypothalamus. The dopaminergic action of amphetamines may be an important determinant of amphetamine abuse. MDMA's mild hallucinogenic effects are attributed to its actions on CNS serotonin. The cardiovascular (CV) toxicity of sympathomimetics is largely as a result of α- and β_1-agonist activity.

Several sympathomimetics occur as optical isomers. Dextroamphetamine is a more potent central nervous system (CNS) stimulant than racemic or l-amphetamine. Ephedrine is a more effective bronchodilator than its isomer, pseudoephedrine. Phenylpropanolamine (PPA) is a racemic mixture of *d*- and *l*-norephedrine. Despite structural similarities, sympathomimetics differ significantly in potency, and therefore, literature regarding these compounds must be interpreted cautiously.

Over-the-counter (OTC) sympathomimetics are usually safe when taken by healthy people in recommended doses, but their therapeutic index is low. Although dose-response relations for toxicity are not well documented, available data suggest that ingestion of as little as four or five times the usual dose may produce toxicity (6,16). PPA was voluntarily withdrawn from the U.S. market in 2000 after a published case control study reported an increased risk of hemorrhagic stroke in women (but not men) taking PPA as a weight loss aid (but not as a decongestant) (12).

One explanation for these findings is that women using PPA for weight loss may have surreptitiously taken excessive doses.

Patients with orthostatic hypotension as a result of autonomic neuropathy exhibit marked sensitivity to the pressor effect of both prescription and OTC sympathomimetics, even in subtherapeutic doses, and should avoid these drugs. Concurrent use of monoamine oxidase (MAO) inhibitors and pharmaceuticals such as venlafaxine, which block central norepinephrine reuptake can lead to catecholamine excess, and exaggerated adverse effects of sympathomimetics. When used as decongestants, sympathomimetics are frequently formulated in combination with antihistamines, anticholinergics, and analgesics. Each of these additional drugs may add to the toxicity of sympathomimetic overdose by increasing heart rate, contributing to cardiac dysrhythmias, or lowering seizure threshold.

Ephedrine and related isomers are active constituents in Ephedra species, the source of the Chinese herbal medicine called ma huang. Combinations of ma huang and plant-derived caffeine (e.g., kola nut and guarana), and other herbs, such as ginseng and willow bark, are marketed as herbal weight loss aids and sold as dietary supplements. These products have been widely promoted and used to stimulate weight loss, increase energy, and enhance athletic performance. Ephedrine alkaloids taken as ma huang have similar pharmacological effects as synthetic compounds. Although drug combinations of caffeine with ephedrine or PPA are banned because of adverse effects and the potential for abuse, herbal ephedrine in combination with caffeine and multiple other ingredients is allowed under provisions of the Dietary Supplement Health and Education Act (DSHEA) of 1994. Since 1993, the Food and Drug Administration (FDA) has received more than 2000 reports of adverse events associated with the use of ephedra-containing dietary supplements. Adverse events ranged in severity from insomnia and nervousness to seizures, strokes, cardiac dysrhythmias, and death (9). Because of these adverse events, several states began restricting or eliminating sales of ephedra-containing dietary supplement products, and the FDA ultimately banned such products in late 2003. Other plants that are natural sources of sympathomimetics, such as Citrus aurantium (contains synephrine, octopamine, and *N*-methyl-tyramine), are increasingly being substituted for ephedra in herbal weight loss and athletic performance-enhancing products. The effects of these herbal stimulants in humans are not well described.

Prescription sympathomimetics, particularly amphetamines, may be abused for their stimulant properties. Toxicity results from excessive doses or prolonged periods of use. OTC stimulants are often sold illicitly to buyers who think they are getting amphetamine or cocaine. Because their CNS actions are weak compared with amphetamine or cocaine, unpleasant peripheral effects (tremors and tachycardia) or toxicity is common when these drugs are abused for their weak stimulant properties. Sympathomimetic overdose may also result from excessive use of diet pills, inadvertent use of several different OTC products that all contain sympathomimetics, or suicidal ingestion.

Various other forms of, or derivatives of, sympathomimetics are also subject to abuse. "Ice," relatively pure crystalline methamphetamine hydrochloride, is volatile enough that it can be smoked (18). The leaves of the Catha edulis plant are commonly chewed in East Africa for the euphoric effects of cathinone, and this stimulant drug is known as khat (11). A derivative, methcathinone (CAT) is a drug of abuse that is growing in use and popularity in the United States and has been classified as a schedule I substance (8). Many other "designer drug" derivatives of amphetamine have been synthesized; which are psychoactive at lower doses, but may produce sympathomimetic effects in higher doses. Life-threatening adverse effects of MDMA, a popular "Club" or "Rave" drug, include hyperthermia and

---

TABLE 328.1.   Sympathomimetics

Drug	Common Uses
Prescription	
Amphetamine	Narcolepsy, attention deficit disorder
Dextroamphetamine	Narcolepsy, attention deficit disorder
Methamphetamine	Narcolepsy, attention deficit disorder
Methylphenidate	Attention deficit disorder
Pemoline	Narcolepsy, Attention deficit disorder
Diethylpropion	Anorectic agent
Dexfenfluramine	Withdrawn from U.S. market in 1997
Fenfluramine	Withdrawn from U.S. market in 1997
Mazindol	Anorectic agent
Phendimetrazine	Anorectic agent
Phenmetrazine	Anorectic agent
Phentermine	Anorectic agent
Albuterol	Bronchodilator
Terbutaline	Bronchodilator, tocolytic
Nonprescription	
Ephedrine	Decongestant, bronchodilator; FDA ban 2003
Phenylpropanolamine	Withdrawn from U.S. market in 2000
Pseudoephedrine	Decongestant
Dietary Supplements	
Ephedra	Anorectic agent
Citrus aurantium	Anorectic agent

profound hyponatremia leading to cerebral edema. Paramethoxyamphetamine (PMA), a highly potent illicit amphetamine similar to MDMA, has also been associated with severe hyperthermia, seizures, coma, and several fatalities (14).

With chronic use of prescription sympathomimetics such as amphetamine or methylphenidate, considerable tolerance may develop. Chronic effects of sympathomimetic drug abuse include weight loss, paranoia and cardiomyopathy. When chronic use is discontinued, users may demonstrate fatigue, hunger, and dysphoria. Unlike withdrawal from sedative–hypnotics, this syndrome poses no medical risk except for the possibility of suicidal depression. Prolonged use of fenfluramine or dexfenfluramine in combination with phentermine ("fen-phen") has been associated with increased risk of valvular fibrosis and pulmonary hypertension (4).

Sympathomimetic toxicity is typically greatest 1 to 4 hours after oral drug ingestion and lasts for 4 to 8 hours, but sustained-release formulations may alter this time course. Onset of toxicity with intravenous use is within minutes. Ephedrine, pseudoephedrine, and PPA are eliminated almost entirely by renal excretion (25). Because these drugs are weak bases, excretion is quickest when the urine pH is low. At the usual urine pH (5.0 to 6.5), half-lives are about 3 to 6 hours (15). Renal failure or alkaline urine could prolong the duration of toxicity. Amphetamine undergoes both hepatic and renal elimination, and metabolites may contribute to toxicity. The elimination half-life of amphetamine and methamphetamine is 4 to 5 hours when the urine is acidic but considerably longer (up to 20 hours for amphetamine) when it is alkaline (7).

Sympathomimetic toxicity is primarily mediated by excessive adrenergic stimulation. Hypertension is due primarily to α-mediated vasoconstriction and may be aggravated by concomitant β_1-mediated increases in heart rate and cardiac contractility. Hypertension caused by PPA alone is usually accompanied by reflex bradycardia or atrioventricular block; however, co-ingestion of drugs such as anticholinergic agents that increase heart rate may aggravate hypertension by preventing the reflex slowing of heart rate (21). Most other sympathomimetics have more β_1 activity than does PPA, and hypertension is usually accompanied by sinus tachycardia. Atrial tachyarrhythmias, premature ventricular beats, and ventricular tachycardia (VT) are presumably as a result of excessive β_1 stimulation. Acute coronary syndromes may be as a result of coronary vasospasm or to sympathomimetic-induced platelet aggregation superimposed on focal coronary artery disease (3).

The mechanisms by which sympathomimetics produce CNS toxicity are less clear. Symptoms of CNS stimulation, including insomnia, agitation, mania, psychosis, and seizures, may result from sympathomimetic triggered release of dopamine and other neurotransmitters in the brain. Hyperthermia is associated with increased heat production caused by agitation or seizures, and impaired heat loss is caused by cutaneous vasoconstriction. Toxicity may rarely result from contaminants of illicitly synthesized drugs, as in one episode of lead poisoning from methamphetamine (1).

CLINICAL PRESENTATION

Acute peripheral manifestations of sympathomimetic intoxication include sweating, tremor, muscle hyperactivity, tachycardia, and hypertension. The most common life-threatening toxic effect of sympathomimetics is hypertension. If severe, hypertension may result in headache, hypertensive encephalopathy, or intracerebral hemorrhage (5,13). However, hypertension may be asymptomatic, even at highly elevated blood pressures. Patients with sympathomimetic overdose usually do not have chronic

hypertension, and therefore have not developed an autoregulatory shift in cerebral blood flow that allows patients with chronic hypertension to tolerate very high blood pressures. Encephalopathy or intracerebral hemorrhage may therefore develop with blood pressures as low as 170 mm Hg systolic or 110 mm Hg diastolic.

Dysrhythmias include sinus or supraventricular tachycardia, premature ventricular beats, and VT (23). Patients may present with palpitations or with hypotension as a result of hemodynamic compromise. Sympathomimetic overdose may also produce chest pain, ischemic electrocardiographic (ECG) changes, and elevation of cardiac enzymes (CK-MB, troponin), simulating myocardial infarction (22).

CNS toxicity of amphetamine overdose includes euphoria, anxiety, agitation, confusion, psychosis, and seizures (19). Psychotic behavior usually occurs during drug use but has been noted to persist during abstinence in chronic amphetamine abusers. Seizures have been reported when overdoses of OTC sympathomimetics are taken in combination with antihistamines or caffeine (20). Patients may present with focal neurologic signs or symptoms, most commonly caused by intracerebral hemorrhage. Several cases of ischemic stroke with angiographic changes suggestive of cerebral vasculitis have been reported in patients taking amphetamine or PPA (17). Pupils may be dilated or normal. Patients who have been "clubbing" or "raving" may present with altered mental status as a result of hyponatremia or cerebral edema resulting from excessive fluid ingestion.

Hyperthermia may occur in patients who are agitated, physically active, or seizing. Rhabdomyolysis, myoglobinuric renal failure, and encephalopathy may ensue from these severe manifestations. Death as a result of sympathomimetic poisoning is most often caused by ventricular dysrhythmia, intracerebral hemorrhage, or status epilepticus.

Chronic, high-dose use of sympathomimetics has been associated with cardiomyopathy and heart failure (10). Chronic amphetamine abuse has also been associated with renal, cerebral, or systemic vasculitis, mimicking polyarteritis nodosa (2). The mechanisms of these toxic effects are unknown.

DIFFERENTIAL DIAGNOSIS

Sympathomimetic toxicity should be considered in patients with unexplained hypertension, cardiac dysrhythmias, hyperthermia, or CNS stimulation. Differentiation of hypertension due sympathomimetic overdose to from essential hypertension is important, because patients with sympathomimetic overdose are at risk for intracerebral hemorrhage at blood pressures much lower than those of patients with accelerated or malignant hypertension of other causes (see Emergency Department Management). Essential hypertension can be distinguished by history or the finding of funduscopic changes indicative of long-standing hypertension. Patients with ischemic stroke may have secondary hypertension. These patients may be recognized by the finding of focal neurological deficits, or focal lesions on a brain computed tomography (CT) scan. Diagnosis of stroke is important, because treatment of hypertension in patients with ischemic stroke may worsen the neurological deficit, and may be contraindicated. Headache is a common, nonspecific finding in patients with sympathomimetic-induced hypertension, but it may also be as a result of intracerebral hemorrhage. Seizures may occur as a direct toxic stimulant effect, or as an indirect complication of a primary CNS insult such as intracerebral hemorrhage, or hypoperfusion of cardiac origin.

Other causes of drug-induced hypertension, tachycardia, and agitation include anticholinergic, cocaine, and phencyclidine poisoning, MAO inhibitor interactions with drugs or food, serotonin syndrome, and withdrawal from alcohol, clonidine (or, rarely, overdose), GHB, or sedative–hypnotics. Nondrug-induced causes that should be considered in the differential diagnosis of sympathomimetic intoxication include brain tumor, infection, thyroid storm, and neurological and psychiatric illnesses.

EMERGENCY DEPARTMENT EVALUATION

The history should include the time, dose, and route of exposure, surrounding circumstances, and intent. The time of onset, nature, and severity of symptoms; the type of first aid undertaken; and the victim's medical and psychiatric history should also be noted. The physical examination should focus on vital signs and CV and neurological function. It should include evaluation of the optic fundi and testing for focal neurologic changes. Blood pressure monitoring is essential. Core body temperature should be measured immediately. A 12-lead ECG should be obtained and continuous cardiac monitoring instituted. If intracerebral hemorrhage is suspected because of focal neurologic findings, seizures, depressed level of consciousness, severe headache, or headache that persists after hypertension resolves, a head CT scan is indicated. Other tests including an electroencephalogram (EEG), echocardiogram, and cardiac catheterization may be indicated, depending on the clinical presentation. Laboratory tests should include electrolytes, blood urea nitrogen, creatinine, glucose, creatine kinase, urinalysis and urine toxicology testing. Most sympathomimetics can be detected in urine by thin-layer chromatography or enzyme-multiplied immunoassay technique (EMIT). Methods for measuring serum concentrations are not usually available.

EMERGENCY DEPARTMENT MANAGEMENT

Initial management is directed at treating severe hypertension, life-threatening dysrhythmias, seizures, and hyperthermia. This should take precedence over gastric decontamination or a head CT scan. A blood pressure exceeding 170/110 mm Hg should be treated emergently, with a goal of lowering the blood pressure within 15 minutes. This can often be accomplished by administering a benzodiazepine (e.g., diazepam 0.1–0.2 mg/kg, lorazepam 0.05–0.1 mg/kg, midazolam 0.02–0.05 mg/kg) i.v.. If this is ineffective, nitroprusside (0.5–5.0 μg/kg/min) or phentolamine (1- to 5-mg bolus initially, repeated at 5- to 10-minute intervals as needed) can be given intravenously. If intravenous access cannot be established rapidly, "sublingual" or chewed nifedipine is an alternative. Propranolol is not recommended as a single agent for treatment of hypertension caused by sympathomimetics, because paradoxical worsening of the hypertension may result from blockade of β_2-mediated vasodilatation, with unopposed α_1-adrenergic vasoconstriction. Supraventricular tachycardia seldom requires therapy. Premature ventricular beats or VT may be treated with the short-acting β_1-selective blocker esmolol (loading dose 500 μg/kg; maintenance dose 50–100 μg/kg/min i.v.). Reflex bradycardia or atrioventricular block in patients with PPA overdose is a normal response that serves to limit hypertension; reversal of the bradycardia (e.g., with atropine) can worsen hypertension and is not recommended.

Hyperthermia should be managed with sedation or muscle paralysis, if necessary, to decrease heat production, and external evaporative cooling measures by applying cool, but not cold, water to the skin, optimally, with a mechanical fan directed at the patient. Ice baths should be avoided because resultant shivering and cutaneous vasoconstriction are countereffective.

Agitation or psychotic behavior may be managed with benzodiazepines given intravenously in the same doses as noted above, with a goal of calming the patient but not obscuring the neurological examination. Benzodiazepines are also the first-line therapy for sympathomimetic drug-induced seizures.

Gastric decontamination is best accomplished with oral activated charcoal. Gastric lavage may be indicated for patients with massive, recent ingestions, but it should be performed only after initial treatment to lower the blood pressure. Urine acidification is not recommended, because the normal urine pH is usually optimal for elimination of weak bases, and because toxic effects are more appropriately managed with the previously mentioned measures. Moreover, if rhabdomyolysis occurs, acidification of the urine may aggravate myoglobin-induced renal injury. Because of their large volumes of distribution and rapid elimination, there is little benefit from hemodialysis or hemoperfusion for elimination of sympathomimetic drugs.

CRITICAL INTERVENTIONS

- Treat sympathomimetic-induced hypertension (> 170/110 mm Hg in a previously normotensive person) urgently with parenteral benzodiazepines, nitroprusside, or phentolamine
- Obtain a CT scan of the brain to rule out intracranial hemorrhage in patients with persistent headache or other neurological signs or symptoms after blood pressure is controlled
- Obtain a creatine kinase level to check for rhabdomyolysis in patients with agitation, seizures or hyperthermia; if elevated administer i.v. hydration
- Institute core body temperature monitoring and rapidly cool patients with hyperthermia

DISPOSITION

Patients with mild signs or symptoms may be monitored in the emergency department because the duration of toxicity is often brief. Observation and monitoring of vital signs and cardiac rhythm is advised for a minimum of 6 hours. When acute toxicity resolves, admission is indicated only for evaluation or management of concurrent psychiatric diagnoses. Patients with headache or neurological signs that persist when hypertension resolves may need an urgent CT scan of the head and consultation with a neurologist. Patients with persistent or severe hypertension, dysrhythmias, or CNS stimulation should be monitored in a medical intensive care unit. Hospitalization for several days may be required if significant rhabdomyolysis and renal failure ensues. Long-term skilled nursing care has been needed in cases of severe sympathomimetic drug-induced encephalopathy.

COMMON PITFALLS

- ✔ Failure to inquire about the use of herbal remedies or dietary supplements as part of the medication history
- ✔ Failure to differentiate sympathomimetic-induced hypertension from essential hypertension
- ✔ Failure to obtain a temperature in a timely manner in patients with agitation, hyperactivity, seizures, and other vital sign abnormalities
- ✔ Failure to appreciate that headache, even without focal signs or symptoms, may be as a result of intracerebral hemorrhage
- ✔ Failure to appreciate that a blood pressure above 170/110 mm Hg in a previously normotensive person should be treated urgently
- ✔ Failure to appreciate that bradycardia or atrioventricular block in patients with hypertension as a result of PPA is a normal (reflex) response that serves to limit hypertension and

that treatment with atropine could aggravate hypertension and be harmful

Acknowledgment

The author thanks previous edition author Paul R. Pentel.

References

1. Anonymous. Lead poisoning associated with intravenous methamphetamine use—Oregon 1988. *MMWR* 1989;38:830.
2. Bashour TT. Acute myocardial infarction resulting from amphetamine abuse: a spasm-thrombus interplay? *Amer Heart J* 1994;128(6 Pt 1):1237–9.
3. Citron BP, Halpern M, McCarron M, et al. Necrotizing angiitis associated with drug abuse. *N Engl J Med* 1970;283:1003.
4. Connolly HM, Crary JL, McGoon MD, et al. Valvular Heart Disease Associated With Fenfluramine-Phentermine. *N Engl J Med* 1997;337:581–8.
5. Delaney P, Estes M. Intracranial hemorrhage with amphetamine abuse. *Neurology* 1980;30:1125.
6. Drew CDM, Knight GT, Hughes DTD, et al. Comparison of the effects of D-(—) ephedrine and L-(pl)-pseudoephedrine on the cardiovascular and respiratory systems in man. *Br J Clin Pharmacol* 1978;6:221.
7. Gunne LM, Anggard E. Pharmacokinetic studies with amphetamines—relationship to neuropsychiatric disorders. *J Pharmacokinet Biopharm* 1973;1:481.
8. Gygi MP, Gibb JW, Hanson GR. Methcathinone: an initial study of its effects on monoaminergic systems. *J Pharmacol Exp Ther* 1996;276(3):1066–1072.
9. Haller CA, Benowitz NL. Adverse cardiovascular and central nervous system events associated with dietary supplements containing ephedra alkaloids. *N Engl J Med* 2000;343:1833–8.
10. Jacobs LJ. Reversible dilated cardiomyopathy induced by methamphetamine. *Clin Cardiol* 1989;12:725–727.
11. Kalix P. Catha edulis, a plant that has amphetamine effects. *Pharm World Sci* 1996;18(2):69–73.
12. Kernan WN, Viscoli CM, Brass LM, et al. Phenylpropanolamine and the Risk of Hemorrhagic Stroke. *N Engl J Med* 2000;343:1826–32.
13. Kizer KW. Intracranial hemorrhage associated with overdose of decongestant containing phenylpropanolamine. *Am J Emerg Med* 1986;2:180.
14. Ling LH, Marchant C, Buckley NA, et al. Poisoning with the recreational drug paramethoxyamphetamine ("death"). *Med J Aust* 2001;174:453–455.
15. Lonnerholm G, Grahnen A, Lindstrom B. Steady-state kinetics of sustained-release phenylpropanolamine. *Int J Clin Pharmacol Ther Toxicol* 1984;22:39.
16. MacNab MW, Seaman JJ, Schumann PR, et al. Phenylpropanolamine HCl and blood pressure. *Clin Pharmacol Ther* 1988;43:163(abst).
17. Matick H, Anderson D, Brumlik J. Cerebral vasculitis associated with oral amphetamine overdose. *Arch Neurol* 1983;40:253.
18. Meng Y, Dukat M, Bridgen DT, et al. Pharmacological effects of methamphetamine and other stimulants via inhalation exposure. *Drug Alcohol Depend* 1999;53(2):111–120.
19. Mueller SM. Neurologic complications of phenylpropanolamine use. *Neurology* 1983;33:650.
20. Mueller SM, Solow EB. Seizures associated with a new combination "pick-me-up" pill. *Ann Neurol* 1982;11:322.
21. Pentel PR, Mikell F. Reaction to phenylpropanolamine-chlorpheniramine-belladonna compound in a woman with unrecognized autonomic dysfunction. *Lancet* 1982;1:274.
22. Pentel PR, Mikell FL, Zavoral JH. Myocardial injury after phenylpropanolamine ingestion. *Br Heart J* 1982;47:51.
23. Peterson RB, Vasquez LA. Phenylpropanolamine-induced arrhythmias. *JAMA* 1973;233:324.
24. www.samhsa.gov/oas
25. Wilkinson GR, Beckett AH. Absorption, metabolism and excretion of the ephedrines in man. I. The influence of urinary pH and urine volume output. *J Pharmacol Exp Ther* 1968;162:139.

CHAPTER 329

Thyroid Hormones

Milton Tenenbein

Thyroid hormones are used as replacement therapy for hypothyroid states and as pituitary suppressants in the treatment or prevention of euthyroid goiters. The two available types are tetraiodothyronine (thyroxine, or T_4) and triiodothyronine (T_3). A given preparation may be of natural (beef or pork thyroid extract) or synthetic origin and contain one or both of these hormones (Table 329.1).

In addition to regulating growth and development, thyroid hormones increase heat production and oxygen consumption by body tissues and stimulate the cardiovascular (CV) system. The usual daily adult replacement dose is 100 to 300 µg of T_4, 25 to 75 µg of T_3, and 60 to 180 mg of thyroid extract or its liotrix equivalent. The normal serum concentration is 4 to 12 µg/dL for T4 and 110 to 250 ng/dL for T_3. T_3 is well absorbed from the stomach (greater than 90%), but the absorption of T_4 is less efficient (50%–90%). Peripheral tissues convert T_4 to T_3, the metabolically active thyroid hormone. More than 99% of circulating thyroid hormones are metabolized by deiodination; most of the remainder are conjugated before excretion, with some being excreted intact. The half-life of a therapeutic dose of T_4 is 4 to 7 days; it is about 1 day for T_3.

Acute oral overdose of thyroid hormones seldom produces serious toxicity, and no deaths have been reported. Thus, the minimal toxic and lethal doses are unknown, and there is no correlation between serum T_4 concentration and clinical severity. Children are resistant to the effects of large overdoses (20). Elderly patients with compromised CV function may be more sensitive, but there are no data to support this speculation.

To assess toxic risk, it is important to differentiate between the different types of thyroid hormone supplements. Because T_3

TABLE 329.1. Thyroid Hormone Preparations

Levothyroxine, L-thyroxine (T_4) – Synthetic	
Levo-T	(Mova Pharmaceuticals)
Levothroid	(Forest Pharmaceuticals)
Levoxyl	(King Pharmaceuticals)
Synthroid	(Abbott Laboratories)
Unithroid	(Jerome Stevens Pharmaceuticals)
Liothyronine (T_3) – Synthetic	
Cytomel	(King Pharmaceuticals)
Liotrix (T_4 & T_3) – Synthetic	
Thyrolar	(Forest Pharmaceuticals)
Natural Thyroid Drugs (T_4 & T_3) – all are porcine-derived	
Armour Thyroid	(Forest Pharmaceuticals)
Bio-Throid	(BIO-TECH Pharmacal)
Nature-throid	(Western Research Laboratories)
Westhroid	(Western Research Laboratories)

is the active thyroid hormone, acute toxicity would be predicted. Only one case of its ingestion has been reported (4), and although the onset of toxicity was within a few hours, it was minor and of brief duration (12 hours) despite a documented serum concentration 50 times normal. Eighty tablets were ingested (or 80 therapeutic doses); this patient co-ingested significant amounts of an antidepressant and an antihistamine, which may have contributed to the observed toxicity.

In contrast, T_4 overdose is relatively common (6,8,10,11, 13,14,17,20). There has been no evidence of toxicity in children who have ingested up to 1.5 mg of T_4 (14). Ingestions of up to 30 mg have produced negligible toxicity (20), as have serum T_4 concentrations of 84.720 and 90 μg/dL (17). Thus, there is a large tolerance for acute massive ingestion of levothyroxine. Several factors contribute to this inherent low toxicity. Conversion of T_4 to T_3 takes several days, and is regulated by a negative-feedback loop. The presence of excess T_4 inhibits endogenous secretion of this hormone, inhibits the peripheral conversion of T_4 to T_3 (2), increases the disposal rates of both T_4 and T_3 (2), and down-regulates the T_3 nuclear receptors (19). Also, elevation of serum concentrations of reverse T_3 (an inhibitor of thyroid hormones) has been observed in two T_4 overdose patients (11,16). Therefore, it is expected that the occurrence of toxicity would be less likely and its onset later (several days).

The only reported case of serious toxicity occurred in a 2-year-old boy who took 18 mg of levothyroxine (10). At about 6 hours after ingestion, his serum thyroxine concentration was 117.4 μg/dL, and he had two seizures 7 days later. There have been reports of minor toxicities such as asymptomatic tachycardia, low-grade fever, diarrhea, and hyperactivity (6,8,13,14).

The ingestion of products that contain both T_3 and T_4 may theoretically result in biphasic toxicity with early (within hours) and late (after several days) phases. In fact, only one of the six reported patients with acute combined overdose developed significant toxicity (5,9,12). This 15-month-old boy was seriously ill within 6 hours, but asymptomatic by 24 hours (12).

The repeated ingestion of excessive amounts of thyroid hormones on a daily basis (chronic overdose or abuse) will probably produce toxicity. Overt hyperthyroidism and even death may occur (1,7,15,18). Such patients may be abusing thyroid hormones to lose weight or because of emotional instability or frank psychiatric illness. They often deny thyroid ingestion.

CLINICAL PRESENTATION

Most patients with acute thyroid overdoses are asymptomatic on presentation, and it is uncommon for signs and symptoms to develop. The few patients who manifest toxicity have the features of hyperthyroidism (fever; tachycardia; warm, moist skin; diarrhea; restlessness; and anxiety). For T_4, the onset is between many hours and several days; for T_3, the onset is within a few hours. However, chronic rather than acute overdose is more likely to produce this picture. Such patients may have virtually all the signs of hyperthyroidism except for exophthalmos.

DIFFERENTIAL DIAGNOSIS

The differential diagnosis of chronic thyroid hormone abuse includes metabolic conditions (e.g., pheochromocytoma and hypoglycemia), central nervous system infection, organic brain syndrome, overdose with psychoactive drugs (e.g., amphetamine, cocaine, anticholinergics, and hallucinogens), acute withdrawal states, and acute psychotic illness. For patients with elevated serum T_4 concentrations, the chief differentiation is from endogenous hyperthyroidism, in which the serum thyroglobulin

concentration is elevated. It is depressed in patients with exogenous hyperthyroidism (15).

EMERGENCY DEPARTMENT EVALUATION

The history includes the identity of the ingestant, the dose, the time of ingestion, symptoms of hyperthyroidism, the reason for ingestion, and prior medical conditions. The identity of the hormones involved is important because of their differing clinical courses after overdose. The physical examination is directed toward eliciting the findings of hyperthyroidism. In the case of acute ingestions, the T_4 concentration is measured 4 to 6 hours after ingestion if the patient has ingested more than 2 mg of levothyroxine or its equivalent. This amount identifies patients who require follow-up; this measurement should be done in all patients with chronic thyroid overdose.

EMERGENCY DEPARTMENT MANAGEMENT

Supportive measures are instituted as necessary. Gastrointestinal (GI) decontamination should be considered for patients who have ingested more than 2 mg of thyroxine or its equivalent. For the uncommon patient who develops symptoms after acute ingestion, acetaminophen for fever and propranolol (20–40 mg q.i.d for adults and 0.25–0.5 mg/kg q.i.d. for children) for sympathetic hyperactivity may be necessary (6,8,13). The oral administration of iopanoic acid (Telepaque, 125 mg per day in a 2.5-year-old), an iodine-containing radiocontrast agent that inhibits the conversion of T_4 to T_3, has also been used with apparent success (3). The use of prophylactic therapy (cholestyramine, prednisone, propylthiouracil, and propranolol) in asymptomatic patients is controversial, but experience has demonstrated that it is unnecessary (6,11,14,20). For the symptomatic patient with chronic thyroid ingestion, thyroid supplements should be discontinued, and the patient should be treated as for endogenous hyperthyroidism and thyroid storm. Enhanced elimination by extracorporeal removal has not been shown to be of benefit (20).

CRITICAL INTERVENTIONS

- Admit or observe patients with large T_3 overdoses for 12 to 24 hours
- Arrange for daily outpatient follow-up for a week after acute overdose of T_4 in patients with T_4 levels over 25 μg/dL
- Administer propranolol to patients with clinically significant sympathetic hyperactivity

DISPOSITION

Patients with significant T_3 overdoses (20 therapeutic doses or more) should be admitted to an observation or inpatient unit. Vital signs, cardiac rhythm, and clinical status should be monitored for 12 to 24 hours. Because patients with acute T_4 overdose are at risk only for delayed toxicity, immediate inpatient observation is unnecessary. Toxicity after acute T_4 overdose has not been reported with serum concentrations under 25 μg/dL; daily assessment for the next 10 days is required if this value is exceeded. Symptomatic patients should be treated, as necessary. Patients who present with hyperthyroidism as a result of chronic abuse usually require admission. Consultation with an endocrinologist is advisable.

COMMON PITFALLS

✔ Failure to differentiate between T_3 and T_4 overdose
✔ Failure to differentiate between acute and chronic overdose
✔ Failure to appreciate that acute overdose can result in delayed toxicity
✔ Overzealous, unnecessary, and potentially harmful use of antithyroid drugs and extracorporeal removal in asymptomatic patients

References

1. Bhasin S, Wallace W, Lawrence JB, et al. Sudden death associated with thyroid hormone abuse. *Am J Med* 1981;71:887.
2. Braverman LE, Vagenakis A, Downs P, et al. Effects of replacement doses of sodium l-thyroxine on the peripheral metabolism of thyroxine and triiodothyronine in man. *J Clin Invest* 1973;52:1010.
3. Brown RS, Cohen JH, Braverman LE. Successful treatment of massive thyroid hormone poisoning with iopanoic acid. *J Pediatr* 1998;132:903.
4. Dahlberg PA, Karlsson FA, Wide L. Triiodothyronine intoxication. *Lancet* 1979;2:700.
5. Gerard P, Malvaux P, de Visscher M. Accidental poisoning with thyroid extract treated by exchange transfusion. *Arch Dis Child* 1972;47:980.
6. Golightly LK, Smolinske SC, Kulig KW, et al. Clinical effects of accidental levothyroxine ingestion in children. *Am J Dis Child* 1987;141:1025.
7. Gorman CA, Wahner HW, Tauxe WN. Metabolic malingerers: patients who deliberately induce or perpetuate a hypermetabolic or hypometabolic state. *Am J Med* 1970;48:708.
8. Gorman RL, Chamberlain JM, Rose SR, et al. Massive levothyroxine overdose: high anxiety—low toxicity. *Pediatrics* 1988;82:666.
9. Jahr HM. Thyroid "poisoning" in children. *Nebr State Med J* 1936;21:388.
10. Kulig K, Golightly LK, Rumack BH. Levothyroxine overdose associated with seizures in a young child. *JAMA* 1985;254:2109.
11. Lehrner LM, Weir MR. Acute ingestions of thyroid hormones. *Pediatrics* 1984;73:313.
12. Levy RP, Gilger WG. Acute thyroid poisoning. *N Engl J Med* 1957;256:459.
13. Lewander WJ, Lacouture PG, Silva JE, et al. Acute thyroid ingestion in pediatric patients. *Pediatrics* 1989;84:262.
14. Litovitz TL, White JD. Levothyroxine ingestions in children: an analysis of 78 cases. *Am J Emerg Med* 1985;3:297.
15. Mariotti S, Martino E, Cupini C, et al. Low serum thyroglobulin as a clue to the diagnosis of thyrotoxicosis factitia. *N Engl J Med* 1982;307:410.
16. Nystrom E, Lindstedt G, Lindbert PA. Minor signs and symptoms of toxicity in a young woman in spite of massive thyroxine ingestion. *Acta Med Scand* 1980;207:135.
17. Roesch C, Becker PG, Sklar S. Management of a child with acute thyroid ingestion. *Ann Emerg Med* 1985;14:1114.
18. Rose E, Sanders TP, Webb WL Jr, et al. Occult factitial thyrotoxicosis—thyroxine kinetics and psychological evaluation in three cases. *Ann Intern Med* 1969;71:309.
19. Samuels HH, Stanley F, Shapiro LE. Dose-dependent depletion of nuclear receptors by l-triiodothyronine: evidence for a role in induction of growth hormone synthesis in cultured GH1 cells. *Proc Natl Acad Sci USA* 1976;73:3877.
20. Tenenbein M, Dean HJ. Benign course after massive levothyroxine ingestion. *Pediatr Emerg Care* 1986;2:15.

PART X

Miscellaneous Agents and Conditions

CHAPTER 330
Biological Warfare Agents

Jeffrey R. Suchard

Biological weapons are microorganisms, or toxins derived from microorganisms, that are intentionally used to cause death, disability, or damage to humans, animals, or plants. Although small-scale biological warfare has been practiced since antiquity, it is only in the last several decades that such weapons could be mass-produced and hold the potential to cause widespread casualties (8). Even limited releases of biological warfare agents can have major public health impact, as occurred with the 2001 outbreak from anthrax spore-contaminated mail (2,3,10,16,19,21). Biological weapons may hold particular appeal to terrorists, because the investment required is less than for other weapons of mass destruction, although the potential morbidity and mortality remain high.

Biological warfare (BW) agents fall into three general categories: bacteria, viruses, and toxins. The first two categories are infectious agents, although the diseases they generate may be rarely encountered in clinical medicine (e.g., anthrax, plague, Q fever, viral equine encephalitis) or no longer occur naturally (e.g., smallpox). Some fungi could potentially be used as infectious BW agents, but have not been weaponized to date. Although most of the diseases caused by infectious BW agents can not be contracted by interaction with the patient, some are able to cause secondary casualties (e.g., pneumonic plague, smallpox, viral hemorrhagic fevers), necessitating careful precautions and patient isolation to prevent uncontrolled outbreaks. Toxins are not transmissible, because they can not reproduce, effectively making them chemical weapons from a biological source. Biological warfare agents share many characteristics with chemical warfare agents, including intent of use, dispersion methods, and defensive measures, although key differences exist (Table 330.1) (12).

The most efficient method of producing mass casualties from BW agents is by aerosol inhalation. A likely clinical scenario fol-

lowing BW agent exposure would be an epidemic of persons with an acute respiratory syndrome (i.e., fever and cough). The ideal aerosol particle size to promote deposition in the respiratory tract is 1 to 5 μm, which corresponds to the size of individual bacteria or spores and would not be detectable by sight, smell, or taste.

Although chemical weapons produce acute symptoms (within minutes to hours), the effects from BW agents may take many hours, days, or sometimes weeks to manifest (depending on the incubation period of the agent involved). Thus, the epidemic curve of case incidence will be more difficult to detect than for chemical weapons, as patients will present less tightly clustered in time and location. An obvious ploy for BW agent users to avoid early detection would be to release an agent causing an endemic infection (or disease resembling an endemic infection) during its season of peak incidence. In some areas, a few cases of bubonic plague may not attract undue attention, and an intentional release of *Yersinia pestis* may elude detection until many more cases develop. Similarly, the early symptoms of inhalational anthrax could easily be missed during influenza season, and it would not be until unusually high morbidity was evident that a biological weapons attack was detected. On the other hand, even a single case of smallpox or a viral hemorrhagic fever in a nonendemic area would immediately raise suspicion of a BW attack.

The potential BW agents have been categorized by their risk of causing a mass-casualty outbreak (6). High-risk agents include smallpox, anthrax, plague, botulism, tularemia, and several hemorrhagic fever viruses. They are easily disseminated or transmitted from person to person, cause high mortality with the potential for major public health impact, and may cause panic and social disruption requiring special action for public health preparedness. Moderate-risk agents include Q fever, brucellosis, the viral equine encephalitis viruses, ricin, and staphylococcal enterotoxin B. Many other biological agents could potentially be used as weapons (Table 330.2). This chapter focuses on agents of greatest concern for causing mass casualties.

Bacillus anthracis is a spore-forming gram-positive rod. Anthrax spores are found in the soil in many parts of the world and mostly cause disease among grazing animals. Human anthrax cases generally occur in farmers, ranchers, and among workers handling animal carcasses, hides, hair, and bones. Different clinical forms of anthrax occur depending on the route of exposure. Cutaneous anthrax results from direct inoculation of spores into the skin via abrasions, and accounts for approximately 95% of human cases. Gastrointestinal anthrax results from the ingestion

TABLE 330.1. Biological and Chemical Weapons: Comparison and Contrast

Similarities
  Agents most effectively dispersed in aerosol or vapor forms
  Delivery systems frequently similar
  Movement of agents highly subject to wind and weather conditions
  Appropriate personal protective equipment prevents illness

Differences	Chemical Warfare Agents	Biological Warfare Agents
Rate at which attack results in illness	Rapid, usually minutes to hours	Delayed, usually days to weeks
Identifying release of agent	Easier, because of Rapid effects Possible chemical odor Chemical detectors available	More difficult Delayed effects Lack of color, odor, taste Lack of real-time detectors
Agent persistence	Variable Liquids semipersistent to persistent Gases nonpersistent	Generally nonpersistent; most degraded by sunlight, heat, and desiccation (exception, anthrax spores)
Victim distribution	Near and downwind from release point	Victims may be widely dispersed by the time disease is apparent
First responders	Emergency medical technicians (EMTs), hazmat teams, firefighters, law enforcement officers	Emergency physicians and nurses, primary care practitioners, infectious disease physicians, public health officials
Decontamination	Critically important in most cases	Not needed for delayed presentations; less important for acute exposures
Medical treatment	Chemical antidotes, supportive care	Antibiotics, vaccines, supportive care
Patient isolation	Unnecessary after decontamination	Crucial for easily communicable diseases; however, many biological warfare (BW) agents are not easily transmissible

of insufficiently cooked meat of infected animals. Inhalational anthrax results from exposure to aerosolized spores. The spores are taken up into the lymphatic system, where they germinate, reproduce, and cause swelling of the mediastinal lymph nodes. Although this form of anthrax is very rare, it is so closely associated with occupational exposures that it has been called *woolsorter's disease*. Inhalational anthrax is the most likely form of the disease in a BW attack, because the spores would be most effectively disseminated by aerosol. In the 2001 anthrax attack in the United States, 11 cases were inhalational (all 5 fatalities were in this group) and 12 were cutaneous (7,15). A previous inhalational anthrax outbreak in 1979 caused by an unintentional release of spores from a Soviet military research facility caused at least 66 fatalities (20).

Y. pestis is the gram-negative bacillus that causes plague. Like anthrax, plague occurs in different clinical forms. Bubonic plague is the most common naturally-occurring form of the disease, resulting from the bites of infected fleas. Pneumonic plague may be secondary to septicemic cutaneous plague seeding the lungs, or it may occur primarily from the inhalation of infected respiratory droplets or an intentionally disseminated BW aerosol. Primary pneumonic plague is the expected form of the disease from an aerosol BW agent release, and should occur in the absence of cases of bubonic plague (14). When plague-infected fleas are released, rather than a bioaerosol, more cases of bubonic plague would be expected.

Francisella tularensis is a small, aerobic, gram-negative coccobacillus. Tularemia may occur in ulceroglandular or typhoidal forms, depending on the route of exposure. Ulceroglandular tularemia is more common, occurring after skin or mucous membrane exposure to infected animal blood or tissues. Exposure to aerosolized bacteria may result in typhoidal tularemia with prominent respiratory symptoms.

Variola virus is a large DNA-bearing orthopoxvirus with a host range limited to humans. Naturally-occurring smallpox was eradicated by a global vaccination campaign in the 1960s and 1970s, yet stocks of the virus are known to remain in labs in the United States, Russia, and possibly elsewhere. Smallpox remains a significant potential BW threat, because a large portion of the current population has not been immunized and the degree of immunity conferred by remote vaccination is not clear. Transmission typically occurs through inhalation of droplets or aerosols, but may also occur through contaminated fomites.

Several taxonomically diverse RNA viruses produce viral hemorrhagic fever (VHF), an acute febrile illness with increased vascular permeability that can result in bleeding manifestations in the more severely affected. VHF agents of greatest concern are those that are infectious by viral inhalation and can therefore be intentionally disseminated by an aerosol route. They include the Marburg, Ebola, and Hanta viruses and those causing Lassa fever, yellow fever, Rift Valley fever, and Crimean-Congo hemorrhagic fever.

Botulinum toxin would most likely be disseminated through food contamination or by aerosol. Either method would result in the clinical syndrome of botulism (see Chapter 335, "Botulism"). Inhalation botulism from laboratory accidents has occurred rarely.

Several clinical syndromes may occur from exposure to BW agents. Because inhalation of an aerosol is the most likely method of exposure to any of these agents, development of an acute respiratory syndrome is common to many agents. Other syndromes include influenza-like illnesses, cutaneous lesions or ulcerations, fever with lymphadenopathy or arthralgias, acute neurologic syndromes (with or without fever), and hemorrhagic diathesis. An individual case of illness from BW agent exposure may be very difficult to detect, because many commonly occurring diseases also fit into such clinical syndromes. It is quite likely that a BW agent attack will be detected by the presence of an unusual epidemiologic curve, when a cluster of patients with unusual findings or with a fulminant clinical course present within a short period of time.

CLINICAL PRESENTATION

The clinical presentation of patients exposed to BW agents will obviously vary depending on the agent. The most likely scenarios, however, involve patients without actual disease, i.e., victims

TABLE 330.2.   Potential Biological Warfare Agents

Infectious Agents	Bacteria
Bacteria	
Anthrax	*Bacillus anthracis*
Brucellosis	*Brucella suis* or *Brucella melitensis*
Cholera	*Vibrio cholerae*
Glanders	*Burkholderia mallei*
Legionellosis	*Legionella pneumophila*
Leptospirosis	*Leptospira interrogans*
Melioidosis	*Burkholderia pseudomallei*
Plague	*Yersinia pestis*
Psittacosis	*Chlamydia psittaci*
Q Fever	*Coxiella burnetii*
Rocky Mountain Spotted Fever	*Rickettsia sickettsii*
Salmonellosis (Typhoid Fever)	*Salmonella* species
Shigellosis	*Shigella* species
Tularemia	*Francisella tularensis*
Typhus	*Rickettsia* species
Viruses	
Crimean-Congo Hemorrhagic Fever	Bunyavirus
Dengue Fever	Flavivirus
Ebola virus	Filovirus
Encephalitis viruses	Alpha- and flaviviruses
Hantavirus	Bunyavirus
Lassa Fever	Arenavirus
Marburg virus	Filovirus
Nipah virus	Paramyxovirus
Omsk Hemorrhagic Fever	Flavivirus
Rift Valley Fever	Bunyavirus
Smallpox (*Variola major*)	Orthopoxvirus
Yellow Fever	Flavivirus
Fungi	
Blastomycosis	*Blastomyces dermatitis*
Coccidioidomycosis	*Coccidioides immitis*
Toxins	
Abrin	Plant toxin from *Abrus precatorius*
Aflatoxins	Fungal toxin from *Aspergillus* species
Botulinum toxin	Bacterial toxin from *Clostridium botulinum*
Domoic Acid	Algal toxin from *Nitzschia pungens*, causes Amnestic Shellfish Poisoning
Ricin	Plant toxin from *Ricinus communis*
Saxitoxin	Algal toxin from *Alexandrium* species and others, causes Paralytic Shellfish Poisoning
Staphylococcal Enterotoxin B	Bacterial toxin from *Staphylococcus aureus*
Tetrodotoxin	Toxin from bacteria found in some marine animals
Trichothecene	Fungal toxins from several mold species

of a BW hoax (5), or those who are worried that they have contracted a disease from a biological weapon. This latter group of patients may either have a somatization disorder, or they may interpret the signs and symptoms of some alternate disease as resulting from a BW agent.

Cutaneous anthrax results in a black eschar with significant surrounding edema forms at the site of entry. Most lesions will heal spontaneously, although 10% to 20% of untreated cases progress to septicemia and death. Cutaneous anthrax fatalities are rare with antibiotic therapy. Gastrointestinal anthrax causes nausea, vomiting, fever, abdominal pain, and mucosal ulcers,

which can cause hemorrhage, perforation, and sepsis; mortality is high (15).

Inhalational anthrax has an incubation period of 1 to 6 days. Patients then develop fever, malaise, fatigue, nonproductive cough, and mild chest discomfort. Symptoms may abruptly progress to severe respiratory distress with dyspnea, diaphoresis, stridor, and cyanosis. Bacteremia, shock, metastatic infection (meningitis occurs in approximately 50% of cases), and death follow within 24 to 36 hours. Inhalational anthrax is a mediastinitis, rather than a pneumonia. Chest radiography and computed tomography typically shows mediastinal widening and pleural effusions, although pneumonic infiltrates are also reported (15).

Historically, the mortality rate from inhalational anthrax was nearly 100% once symptoms develop, even with antibiotics. Experience from the 2001 outbreak in the United States, however, shows that just over half of the patients with inhalational anthrax survived with aggressive supportive care and antibiotic therapy (15.) Earlier hospitalization appeared to correlate with improved outcome (3,16,19).

Bubonic plague has an incubation period of 2 to 10 days preceding the onset fever, malaise, and painful, enlarged regional lymph nodes (buboes). Septicemia may occur and can be accompanied by disseminated intravascular coagulation and acral gangrene. Necrosis of the digits and nose seen with septicemic plague is the likely origin of the term "black death" associated with the second plague pandemic (14).

Pneumonic plague has in incubation period of 2 to 3 days. The onset of disease is acute and often fulminant. Patients develop fever, malaise, and cough productive of bloody sputum, rapidly progressing to dyspnea, stridor, cyanosis, and cardiorespiratory collapse. Plague pneumonia is almost always fatal unless treatment is begun within 24 hours of symptom onset.

Ulceroglandular tularemia is characterized by local skin ulceration and associated lymphadenopathy, fever, chills, headache, and malaise. Typhoidal tularemia presents with fever, prostration, and weight loss without adenopathy. Exposure to aerosolized bacteria should result in typhoidal tularemia with prominent respiratory symptoms like a nonproductive cough and substernal chest discomfort. Chest radiographs may show infiltrates, mediastinal lymphadenopathy, or pleural effusions. Fatalities may occur, yet development of a temporarily incapacitating infection is more likely.

Smallpox has a 12- to 14-day incubation period. Initial symptoms include fever, malaise, and prostration with headache and backache. Oropharyngeal lesions appear first, shedding virus into the saliva. Two to three days after the onset of fever, a papular rash develops on the face and spreads to the extremities. The fever continues as the rash becomes vesicular and then pustular. The pustules scab over and eventually separate, leaving pitted and hypopigmented scars. Deaths usually occur during the second week of the illness.

VHF is characterized by fever, malaise, prostration, and hemorrhagic rash. Clinical features, such as the extent of renal, hepatic, and hematologic involvement, vary according to the agent involved. Mortality rates also vary, from less than 1% for Rift Valley fever up to 50% to 90% for the Ebola virus.

Botulism results in multiple bulbar nerve palsies and a symmetric descending paralysis, with death occurring from respiratory failure (see Chapter 335, "Botulism"). Onset of symptoms can occur within 24 to 36 hours or take several days.

DIFFERENTIAL DIAGNOSIS

Familiarity with the expected clinical syndromes produced by BW agents will aid in the differential diagnosis. An acute respiratory syndrome with fever may occur with inhalational

DISPOSITION

All cases of suspected exposure to BW agents should be reported local public health and law enforcement authorities. Unless the patient contracted their illness through unintentional exposure in a research laboratory, each case is potential evidence of a criminal bioterrorist act, requiring contact also with law enforcement agencies such as the local Federal Bureau of Investigation field office. Consultation with a physician familiar with BW agents, such as an infectious disease specialist, military physician, toxicologist, or poison center, is also recommended. Other potential resources include the CDC (770-488-7100) and the U.S. Army Medical Research Institute for Infectious Diseases (1-888-USA-RIID) which have 24-hour hotline services to assist physicians with biological agent inquiries.

Patients with known or suspected acute exposures to infectious BW agents are likely to be asymptomatic and require no emergent interventions. Such patients require initiation of appropriate postexposure prophylactic antibiotics and/or vaccinations, depending on the agent involved. Asymptomatic patients acutely exposed to anthrax or plague may, for example, be discharged home with antibiotic prescriptions if adequate follow-up can be arranged through the local public health agency or their private physicians.

Patients exposed to smallpox may require quarantine, which should be coordinated with the assistance of public health and law enforcement agencies. Patients acutely exposed to toxin weapons might be asymptomatic at presentation but still require admission for a period of observation depending on the agent involved. Botulinum toxin exposure, for example, mandates admission to monitor for development of respiratory failure.

Unless part of a mass-casualty incident, all patients known or suspected to have illness from BW agent exposure should be admitted, with the level of care dependent on clinical severity. Outpatient management of cutaneous anthrax may be considered for patients without systemic toxicity, who can tolerate oral antibiotics, and for whom outpatient follow-up can be assured. Isolation precaution will be necessary for patients with pneumonic plague, smallpox, and many of the viral hemorrhagic fevers. In mass-casualty situations, admission may need to be more selective and reserved for patients who can not tolerate outpatient therapy but who are not moribund.

COMMON PITFALLS

✔ Lack of familiarity with likely BW agents and the clinical syndromes they produce
✔ Failure to appreciate that some BW agents are transmissible and others are not and that isolation requirements may or may not be necessary
✔ Failure to institute appropriate postexposure prophylaxis among patients with plausible exposure scenarios

Acknowledgments

We thank previous edition chapter authors Michael Joseph Burns and Christopher H. Linden.

References

1. Arnon SS, Schechter R, Inglesby TV, et al. Botulinum toxin as a biological weapon: medical and public health management. *JAMA* 2001;285:1059–1070.
2. Barakat LA, Quentzel HL, Jernigan JA, et al. Fatal inhalational anthrax in a 94-year-old Connecticut woman. *JAMA* 2002;287:863–868.
3. Borio L, Frank D, Mani V, et al. Death due to bioterrorism-related inhalational anthrax: report of 2 patients. *JAMA* 2001;286:2554–2559.
4. Borio L, Inglesby T, Peters CJ, et al. Hemorrhagic fever viruses as biological weapons: medical and public health management. *JAMA* 2002;287:2391–2405.
5. CDC. Bioterrorism alleging use of anthrax and interim guidelines for management—United States 1998. *MMWR Morb Mortal Wkly Rep* 1999;48:69–74.
6. CDC. Biological and chemical terrorism: strategic plan for preparedness and response. *MMWR Morb Mortal Wkly Rep* 2000;49(RR-04):1–14.
7. CDC. Suspected cutaneous anthrax in a laboratory worker—Texas 2002. *MMWR Morb Mortal Wkly Rep* 2002;51:279–281.
8. Christopher GW, Cieslak TJ, Pavlin JA, Eitzen EM. Biological warfare: a historical perspective. *JAMA* 1997;278:412–417.
9. Dennis DT, Inglesby TV, Henderson DA, et al. Tularemia as a biological weapon: medical and public health management. *JAMA* 2001;285:2763–2773.
10. Freedman A, Afonja O, Chang MW, et al. Cutaneous anthrax associated with microangiopathic hemolytic anemia and coagulopathy in a 7-month-old infant. *JAMA* 2002;287:869–874.
11. Friedlander AM, Pittman PR, Parker GW. Anthrax vaccine: evidence for safety and efficacy against inhalational anthrax. *JAMA* 1999;282:2104–2106.
12. Henderson DA. The looming threat of bioterrorism. *Science* 1999;283:1279–1282.
13. Henderson DA, Inglesby TV, Barlett JG, et al. Smallpox as a biological weapon: medical and public health management. *JAMA* 1999;281:2127–2137.
14. Inglesby TV, Dennis ST, Henderson DA, et al. Plague as a biological weapon: medical and public health management. *JAMA* 2000;283:2281–2290.
15. Inglesby TV, O'Toole T, Henderson DA, et al. Anthrax as a biological weapon 2002: updated recommendations for management. *JAMA* 2002;287:2236–2252.
16. Jernigan JA, Stephens DS, Ashford DA, et al. Bioterrorism-related inhalational anthrax: the first 10 cases reported in the United States. *Emerg Infect Dis* 2001;7:933–944.
17. Keim M, Kaufmann AF. Principles for emergency response to bioterrorism. *Ann Emerg Med* 1999;34:177–182.
18. Kuehnert MJ, Doyle TJ, Hill HA, et al. Clinical features that discriminate inhalational anthrax from other acute respiratory illnesses. *Clin Infect Dis* 2003;36:328–336.
19. Mayer TA, Bersoff-Matcha S, Murphy C, et al. Clinical presentation of inhalational anthrax following bioterrorism exposure: report of 2 surviving patients. *JAMA* 2001;286:2549–2553.
20. Meselson M, Guillemin J, Hugh-Jones M, et al. The Sverdlovsk anthrax outbreak of 1979. *Science* 1999;266:1202–1208.
21. Mina B, Dym JP, Kuepper F, et al. Fatal inhalational anthrax with unknown source of exposure in a 61-year-old woman in New York City. *JAMA* 2002;287:858–862.

CHAPTER 331
Chemical Warfare Agents

Michael Joseph Burns and Christopher H. Linden

Chemicals have been used to impede, incapacitate, or kill the opposition throughout history. It is only within the past decade, however, that chemical weapons have attracted global attention. Although international treaties (e.g., 1925 Geneva Protocol, 1997 Chemical Weapons Convention) ban the development, production, stockpiling, and use of chemical weapons, Iraq is known to have used both nerve and blistering agents in its war with Iran and against Kurdish civilians in the 1980s (5). More recently, Russian military used a gas thought to contain a fentanyl derivative and halothane to subdue Chechen rebels in a Moscow theater (4,22).

Of greater concern is that chemical warfare agents (CWA) may be used by terrorists. CWA are easy to acquire, synthesize, and use; fairly inexpensive; and readily hidden (5). On three occasions, the terrorist group, Aum Shinrikyo, released nerve agents (sarin and VX) in Japan (10,12–14). The Tokyo subway incident in 1995 resulted in 12 deaths and over 5,000 civilian casualties (14). In 1996, the Defense Against Weapons of Mass Destruction

TABLE 331.1. Chemical Warfare Agents

Classification	Military Code	Chemical Name/Common Name
Lethal Agents		
Blood agents	AC	Hydrogen cyanide
	CK	Cyanogen chloride
	SA	Arsenic trihydride/arsine
Choking agents	CL	Chlorine
	CG	Carbonyl chloride/phosgene
	DP	Trichloroethyl chloroformate/diphosgene
Vesicating agents		
Mustards	HD	bis(2-chloroethyl)sulfide/distilled mustard
Nitrogen mustards	HN-1	2,2-dichlorotriethylamine
	HN-2	2,2-dichloro-N-methylethylamine
	HN-3	2,2,2-trichlorotriethylamine
Arsenicals	MD	Methyldichloroarsine
	PD	Phenyldichloroarsine
	ED	Ethyldichloroarsine
	L	Dichloro (2-chlorovinyl)arsine/lewisite
Oximes	CX	Dichloroform oxime/phosgene oxime
Mixes	HL	None/ML mix (mustard-lewisite mixture)
	HT	None/HT mix (mustard-T mixture)
(Not produced)	Q	4,bis(methylchloroethyl sulfide)/Q
	T	bis(2-chloroethyl sultide)monoxide/T
Nerve agents	GA	Ethyl *N,N*-dimethyl phosphoamicocyanidate/Tabun
	GB	Isopropyl methyl phosphonofluoridate/Sarin
	GD	Pinacolyl methyl phosphonefluoridate/Soman
	GF	Cyclohexyl-methyl phosphonofluoridate/Cyclosarin
	VR	O-isobutyl S-(2-diethylamino)ethyl)methylphosponothioate
	VX	Ethyl S-2-diisopropyl aminoethyl methylphosphonothiolate/VX
Nonlethal Agents		
Vomiting agents	DA	Diphenylchlorarsine
	DC	Diphenylcyanoarsine
	DM	Diphenylaminochloroarsine/adamsite
Lacrimating agents	CA	Bromobenzeneacetonitrile/camite
	CN	2-chloro-1-phenylethanone/chloroacetophenone
	CNB	None/chloroacetophenone, carbon tetrachloride, benzene mix
	CNC	None/chloroacetophenone chloroform mix
	CNS	None/chloroacetophenone, chloroform, chloropicrin mix
		CR dibenz-1,4-oxazepine
	CS	*o*-chlorobenzlidene malonitrile/CS (tear gas)
		Capsaicin/pepper gas
Incapacitating agents	BZ	3-quinuclidinyl benzilate
		Opioids (alfentanil, carfentanil, fentanyl, remifentanil, sufentanil)

Act directed the U.S. Department of Defense to establish a domestic preparedness program to improve the ability of local, state, and federal agencies to respond to chemical and biologic incidents (3,5).

CWA generally fall into one of seven major categories: chemical choking agents, vesicating or blister agents, lacrimating agents, nerve agents, vomiting agents, systemic asphyxiants, and incapacitating agents (Table 331.1) (25). They are classified as lethal or nonlethal, depending on whether they are intended to either stun or kill. The "code" refers to their U.S. military designation. Lacrimating agents are currently used for personal protection and by police for crowd dispersal and incapacitation of criminal suspects. Because the Chemical Weapons Convention permits the use of chemical agents for "law enforcement," other nonlethal weapons (e.g., incapacitating agents) may soon become available for domestic riot control and hostage rescue (4,22).

CWA can be delivered in multiple ways. They may be aerosolized as a spray from handheld or vehicle-mounted pressurized tanks, low-flying aircraft, crop-dusters, cruise missiles, and spray bottles or be dispersed as liquid droplets or vapor from low-flying aircraft, artillery, missiles, detonated bombs, and hand-held devices. Sarin was dispersed by evaporation from punctured plastic bags left on subway cars in the Tokyo incident (14). Although highly toxic agents could be added to the enemy's water supply or food source, aerosolization is most likely to cause the maximum number of casualties and thus be used by terrorists and military groups (5,25).

Blood agents, incorrectly labeled as such by the military, include the systemic asphyxiant gases cyanogen chloride, hydrogen cyanide (see Chapter 308, "Cyanide"), and hydrogen sulfide (see Chapter 311, "Hydrogen Sulfide"), and the hemolytic gas arsine (see Chapter 305, "Arsenic and Mercury") (25). Another asphyxiant, sodium monofluoroacetate (see Chapter 299, "Rodenticides,"), could potentially be used in food or drink. Hydrogen cyanide (prussic acid) and cyanogen chloride are clear liquids with a bitter almond odor which readily volatilize at temperatures above 26°F (1). As warfare agents, efficacy is limited by nonpersistence in open air and low toxicity compared with nerve agents (25).

The choking agents, introduced in World War I, include chlorine, phosgene, and diphosgene and are pulmonary irritants (see Chapter 313, "Irritant Gas Inhalation"). Chlorine, a dense, water soluble, yellow-green gas that smells like concentrated bleach, reacts with tissue water to form hydrochloric acid and oxygen free radicals, which produce corrosive and cytotoxic effects. Toxicity is proportional to the gas concentration, duration of contact, and water content of exposed tissue.

Phosgene (carbonyl chloride) is thought to have been responsible for more than 80% of all chemical agent fatalities in World War I (25). It is a colorless gas that is poorly soluble in water and heavier than air. Its propensity to settle into low-lying areas, such as trenches, led to its tactical success. Phosgene smells like freshly mown hay but odor is not a reliable indicator of exposure. Because it is only mildly irritating to the eyes and upper respiratory tract on initial contact; exposure may temporarily go unnoticed (25). Phosgene hydrolyzes with terminal bronchial and alveolar mucosal water to produce hydrochloric acid. This and other toxic by-products of phosgene stimulate the synthesis of leukotrienes and other inflammatory products, which leads to pulmonary edema. The rate and extent of pulmonary injury depend on the concentration and duration of exposure, but it typically occurs slowly over hours.

Diphosgene (trichloroethyl chloroformate), created shortly after World War I, is simply phosgene with chloroform attached to it (25). The chloroform moiety allowed it to penetrate crude chemical filters. Diphosgene causes a more immediate irritation than does phosgene, as a result of its higher chlorine content.

Vesicating agents, which cause blistering of exposed surfaces, include mustard gases and organic arsenicals. Sulfur mustard (2,2,-dichlorodiethyl sulfide) was used in World War I and in the Iran–Iraq war (5,15,25). Most of injuries were disabling but nonfatal; mortality during World War I was less than 2%; rates of 3% to 4% were reported in the Iran–Iraq war (2,15,20). Street clothing offers no protection, but military protective garments (chemical-resistant suit) can provide up to 6 hours of protection following exposure (2). Low volatility results in persistence (for several days in temperate climates), thereby restricting enemy use of contaminated equipment and terrain (5,25).

Sulfur mustard is an oily amber liquid that smells like burning garlic or mustard. Upon tissue contact, it spontaneously forms highly reactive and unstable episulfonium compounds, which irreversibly alkylate nucleic acids and cellular proteins within 2 minutes of exposure (2,15). This leads to DNA strand breaks and inhibition of DNA replication, protein synthesis, and enzyme function. In the process of cellular DNA repair, depletion of nicotinamide adenine dinucleotide (NAD^+) occurs, glycolysis is inhibited, cellular proteases are released, and cell death occurs (2,15). Toxicity may also be a result of binding to and depletion of the free radical scavenger glutathione, which results in an inactivation of sulfhydryl-containing enzymes, loss of calcium homeostasis, lipid peroxidation, cellular membrane breakdown, and cell death. Blister formation occurs subsequent to the destruction of anchoring filaments in the epidermal-dermal junction (2,15).

Nitrogen mustards (HN) have identical cytotoxicity. They are used medically in the intravenous form as alkylating chemotherapeutic agents and can cause severe local tissue damage if, inadvertently, extravasation occurs. Because mustards are alkylating agents, they may be mutagenic and carcinogenic (2,15).

Lewisite (2-chlorovinyldichloroarsine), the best known organic arsenical, was developed in 1918 to complement sulfur mustard as a semipersistent blistering agent (25). Its vapor is about seven times heavier than air and will flow into lower terrain (25). It has low water solubility and persists in the environment for up to 24 hours under temperate conditions (5). Many countries have large stockpiles of lewisite, but its actual use in combat is not well documented (20,25).

Lewisite is an amber, oily liquid that smells like geraniums. It is rapidly absorbed after vapor inhalation and penetrates intact skin within 15 minutes, more rapidly than mustard agents, as a result of higher lipid solubility (25). In the dermis, it hydrolyzes to hydrochloric acid and chlorovinylarsenious oxide, the vesi-

cating agent. The organic arsenical moiety binds to the dithiol component of pyruvate dehydrogenase, prevents formation of acetyl coenzyme A from pyruvate, and produces systemic toxicity similar to other arsenicals (see Chapter 305, "Arsenic and Mercury"). Increased capillary permeability and extensive interstitial fluid losses may result in hypovolemia or "lewisite shock" (25). Inhalation may result in severe pulmonary edema (25).

Nerve agents are similar in structure and function to organophosphorus pesticides (see Chapter 297, "Organophosphate and Carbamate Insecticides") but are more potent and typically have a more rapid onset and shorter duration of action symptoms. The "G" (German) agents Tabun (GA), Sarin (GB), and Soman (GD), were developed in Germany between 1936 and 1944 (1,6,9,16,19,25). The fourth, VX, with the "V" standing for "viper," was synthesized in 1952 in England (1,25). Newer compounds include GF and VR (18). Although commonly referred to as gases, these agents are colorless, odorless liquids under temperate conditions (6,9,19,25). Vapors are heavier than air and, thus, will concentrate closer to the ground. Lethality is directly correlated to the product of vapor concentration and time of exposure (LCt) (6,9,19,25). The G agents are moderately volatile, evaporate within several hours, and are environmentally nonpersistent (9,19,25). The human lethal inhaled dose of the G agents is estimated to be 1 mg (19,25). VX, an oily liquid that is much less volatile, persists for several weeks after dispersion (19,25). It is the most potent nerve agent, with a LCt_{50} (vapor concentration–time product necessary to kill 50% of an unprotected population) of 10 mg a minute per m3, which is 5, 10, 40, and 500 times less than for soman, sarin, tabun, and hydrogen cyanide, respectively (9,19,25).

Nerve agents can also be absorbed through the skin. Time of onset and severity are determined by the dose, agent, and skin integrity/location (9,25). The longer the time interval between the exposure and onset of symptoms, the less severe the effects will be (9). Clothing will offer a protective barrier if it remains dry (9). The dose of VX necessary to kill one half of unprotected victims through percutaneous exposure is 6- to 10-mg, or 10, 100, and 170 times less than that of soman, tabun, and sarin, respectively (9,19,25). VX also has a slower rate of elimination than G agents and would be expected to have a longer duration of action.

Toxicity results primarily from phosphorylation and inactivation of acetylcholinesterase (AChE) at its serine active site (see Chapter 297, "Organophosphate and Carbamate Insecticides"). Acetylcholine accumulates at nerve terminals, initially stimulating, then paralyzing, cholinergic neurotransmission at both central and peripheral nicotinic and muscarinic receptors. Once inactivated, AChE may undergo three processes. The phosphorylated enzyme may spontaneously reactivate via endogenous hydrolysis, be reactivated by nucleophilic oximes, or become incapable of reactivation. Endogenous hydrolysis is insignificant, as a result of tight binding of nerve agents to AChE. Reactivation of AChE occurs if an oxime binds the phosphate moiety of the nerve agent more avidly than the serine residue of AChE. Reactivation is impossible once dealkylation ("aging") of the phosphorylated cholinesterase occurs, and de novo AChE synthesis is required for enzyme replenishment. The rate of aging varies among the nerve agents. It occurs within 2 minutes after Soman exposure, 5 to 8 hours after Sarin exposure, and more than 40 hours after Tabun or VX exposure (9,19,25).

There is poor correlation between clinical toxicity and AChE activity (6). Agonist activity at nicotinic receptor sites (G agents), blockade of nicotinic receptor ionic channels (VX), direct stimulation of cardiac muscarinic receptors, antagonism of inhibitory GABA neurotransmission, and stimulation of excitatory glutamate N-methyl-d-aspartate receptors may be additional mechanisms of toxicity produced by nerve agents (6,25). Effects on central nervous system (CNS) neurotransmission may contribute to seizures and CNS neuropathology and explain why some compounds that are neuroprotective do not reactivate AChE and why CNS-active oximes (e.g., Pro-2-PAM) are not more effective than oximes that do not reach the brain (19).

Vomiting agents are arsenic-based compounds used for riot control (25). They are normally solids that are vaporized by heating and then condense to form aerosols, which produce rapid irritation of exposed tissues. Systemic arsenic toxicity is also possible (see Chapter 305, "Arsenic and Mercury").

Lacrimating agents, also known as irritant incapacitants, tear gas, and riot-control or harassing agents, include o-chlorobenzylidenemalonitrile (CS), ω-chloroacetophenone (CN or mace), dibenz-1,4-oxazepine (CR), and oleoresin capsaicin (OC or pepper spray). Except for capsaicin, toxicity results from SN2 alkylation and inhibition of sulfhydryl-containing enzymes. It may also be as a result of chlorine effects and their ability to generate bradykinin. Capsaicin is a lipid-soluble alkaloid that first stimulates release of substance P from nociceptive neurons and then blocks its synthesis and transport. Substance P depolarizes neurons to produce dilatation of blood vessels, stimulation of smooth muscle, and activation of sensory nerve endings that mediate pain. With repeated application, nociceptive fiber response and number are decreased (desensitization). This forms the basis for the medicinal use of capsaicin as a topical analgesic (counterirritant).

CN and CS are usually delivered as a vapor or cloud of suspended solid particles (a smoke) produced by a thermal grenade. CS is the riot-control agent of choice in the United States. It is about ten times more potent as a lacrimator than CN but is much less corrosive to tissues (25). Newer CS formulations consist of an unheated micropulverized powder (CS1, CS2) that can remain active in the environment for several weeks. CS powders were used by the U.S. military during the Vietnam War. CR is the most potent and least corrosive lacrimator currently available but is not commonly used because it must be delivered as a mist and it persists longer in the environment. OC is used frequently by civilians for personal protection and by law enforcement personnel for immobilization of assailants. "Pepper Mace" can contain CS, oleoresin of capsicum, or both.

Incapacitating agents include stimulants (e.g., amphetamines), depressants (e.g., opioids), psychedelics (e.g., d-lysergic acid diethylamide), and deliriants (e.g., anticholinergics) (25). Historically, the anticholinergic agent, 3-quinuclidinyl benzilate (BZ), was the only incapacitating agent considered feasible for use by the US military (25). BZ is a potent, glycolate, anticholinergic agent that exists as a crystalline solid under normal atmospheric conditions but would likely be dispersed as a vapor or liquid aerosol by military personnel or terrorists (25). Although ultrapotent fentanyl derivatives (alfentanil, carfentanil, remifentanil, and sufentanil) show promise, preliminary data suggest that these agents have unpredictable effects as a result of high lipid solubilities and large volumes of distribution (21,22). Like other chemical agents, they are most likely to be delivered as an aerosol of fine particles. The unpredictable nature of these agents is evidenced by the tragic end to the October 2002 Moscow hostage crisis in which 127 of 800 hostages were fatally poisoned by a fentanyl-halothane gas intended to incapacitate its victims (4,22).

CLINICAL PRESENTATION

Choking Agents

Clinical symptoms begin within minutes after significant chlorine exposure and include lacrimation, conjunctival irritation, rhinorrhea, cough, sore throat, chest burning, dyspnea, sputum production, nausea, headache, and respiratory failure. Corneal abrasions and cutaneous burns may result from eye and skin exposure, respectively. Following significant chlorine exposures, pulmonary edema may develop within 2 to 4 hours and peaks at 12 to 24 hours (25). The chest radiograph may be normal or may display noncardiogenic pulmonary edema. After a typical latency period of 4 to 6 hours (range, 1–24 hours), patients with significant phosgene exposure present with dyspnea, chest tightness, cyanosis, hemoptysis, hypotension, and pulmonary edema. Chest radiographic findings of pulmonary edema are rather late and nonspecific, occurring 6 to 8 hours after exposure. Diphosgene produces identical signs and symptoms. Following significant pulmonary agent exposure (e.g., chlorine gas), patients may subsequently develop reactive airways dysfunction syndrome, a chronic asthma-like condition.

Vesicating Agents

After mustard exposure, there is typically a latency period of 4 to 12 hours before the onset of symptoms. The latency period is shorter with high concentrations and long exposures, with increased ambient temperature and humidity, and in victims previously exposed to or innately susceptible to mustard (2,15,20,25). Sites of injury principally involve the skin, eye, and respiratory tract and may follow vapor or liquid exposure. Heavy exposure may lead to systemic effects such as bone marrow depression and sloughing of intestinal mucosa.

Cutaneous injury resulting from mustard exposure ranges from erythema to vesication and skin necrosis. The moist, thinner skin of the neck, axilla, and groin is more severely affected. After an asymptomatic period of 4 to 12 hours, erythema and edema develop. Vesication typically starts within 24 hours and evolves over several days. Vesicles coalesce into blisters, and skin necrosis occurs over 24 to 72 hours (20,25). Blister fluid does not contain active mustard and is not toxic (20,25). Skin denudation occurs over 6 to 9 days, and healing may take 4 to 10 weeks.

The eye is the organ most sensitive to sulfur mustard. Tissue injury occurs rapidly, but symptoms develop gradually over 4 to 8 hours and include eye pain, lacrimation, photophobia, and blurred vision (2,25). Physical findings include blepharospasm, eyelid edema, conjunctival injection and edema, chemosis, anterior chamber cellular infiltrates, and decreased vision. Corneal edema begins within 1 hour after exposure, and the corneal epithelium vesicates and sloughs within 4 to 36 hours (15,20,25). Resolution of injury depends on the severity of exposure and typically takes 1 to 2 weeks. About 90% of victims are visually disabled for 10 days with conjunctivitis, photophobia, and corneal swelling. The remaining 10% are severely affected and are at risk for permanent blindness from corneal opacification, scarring, and ulceration (15,20,25).

Respiratory epithelial damage occurs several hours after exposure. Victims may develop rhinitis, nasal bleeding, sinus discomfort, hoarseness, sore throat, cough, sputum production, and dyspnea of increasing severity. Hemorrhagic inflammation and erosions of the upper airway mucosa are followed by fibrinous pseudomembrane formation and sloughing of necrotic, ulcerated mucosa. Bronchospasm and partial airway obstruction result. After high-dose exposures, severe bronchitis, secondary bronchopneumonia, and respiratory failure may develop within 24 to 48 hours (2,15,25). Pulmonary edema is not a characteristic finding, as mustard does not typically affect the pulmonary parenchyma.

In the presence of high concentration or prolonged exposure, bone marrow and gastrointestinal (GI) mucosal toxicity may be seen. Leukopenia develops within 5 to 7 days, with the white cell nadir occurring 10 days after exposure. Thrombocytopenia and anemia typically follow. The development of hematologic effects from mustard poisoning is a grave prognostic sign (15,25). Respiratory failure, bone marrow suppression, or superimposed bacterial infection are the most common causes of death from sulfur mustard poisoning (1,2).

The clinical manifestations of lewisite poisoning are similar to those of sulfur mustard, although lewisite causes immediate severe pain on contact with the skin, eyes, and nasal mucosa. Vapor condensing on the skin causes erythema within 30 minutes and blister formation within 2 to 3 hours (20,25). The eyes are very sensitive to lewisite, and permanent blindness from corneal destruction may result if decontamination is not initiated within 1 minute. Inhalation of lewisite vapor can result in death within 10 minutes from rapid respiratory mucosal sloughing and bleeding, leading to asphyxiation.

Nerve Agents

Clinical manifestations of nerve agent exposure are described in detail in Chapter 297, "Organophosphate and Carbamate Insecticides." Toxicity may occur after inhalation of vapor, skin contact with vapor or liquid, or ingestion. The rate of onset and severity of effects are determined by the route of exposure and dose (6). At high ambient temperature, skin absorption is rapid, and increasing amounts of the agent are volatilized, leading to increased inhalation (19). Small amounts of vapor causes miosis, rhinorrhea, mild dyspnea, cough, and wheezing (6,19,25). This can occur within seconds to minutes. Symptoms include eye pain, blurred and dim vision, headache, and dizziness (14). As the dose of vapor increases, nausea and vomiting, increased respiratory difficulty, progressive muscular weakness, and agitation develop. A high vapor concentration causes rapid loss of consciousness, seizures, flaccid paralysis, and respiratory arrest within seconds to minutes. Following Sarin vapor exposure in the Tokyo incident, the most common manifestations were miosis (99%), headache (75%), dyspnea (63%), nausea (60%), eye pain (45%), blurred vision (40%), and vomiting (37%) (14). Tachycardia and hypertension were also common, but bradycardia and bronchorrhea were not. Electrocardiographic manifestations may include supraventricular and ventricular dysrhythmias, ischemic ST-T changes, atrioventricular conduction disturbances, and QTc interval prolongation (9,19). Seizures may be single and brief or multiple and persistent; status epilepticus will often occur in severely poisoned patients (9,12,14). Death is primarily as a result of respiratory failure secondary to depression of the central respiratory drive (6,9,16,25). Respirations cease before significant neuromuscular blockade or bronchoconstriction occurs.

Victims of vapor exposure are unlikely to deteriorate once removed from exposure (6,14). In contrast, those with dermal exposure may subsequently worsen. Skin absorption of a lethal dose may occur within 1 to 2 minutes, yet symptoms are commonly delayed and develop after a latency period of 30 minutes to 18 hours (2,6,9,25). Skin exposure may produce local sweating and twitching or fasciculations before systemic toxicity (9,19,25). Conversely, serious effects may also occur abruptly, without antecedent local or mild symptoms after dermal exposure (9,12). In contrast to vapor exposure, miosis is absent early following skin exposure (6,12). Miosis may be present for weeks after exposure and does not readily respond to systemic treatment (9,16,19).

Lacrimating Agents

Lacrimating agents cause intense eye discomfort, blepharospasm, lacrimation, stinging and burning of the mouth and nose, salivation, rhinorrhea, irritation of the respiratory tract and stomach with coughing and vomiting, and skin irritation leading to burning pain and erythema within seconds to minutes of exposure (25). They are miscible in sweat, and skin irritation is amplified in areas of increased sweat, such as the axilla, popliteal and antecubital areas, inguinal region, and buttocks.

Skin effects are heightened following concentrated liquid spray or aerosol exposures, in warm, moist environments, and in those with preexisting skin conditions. Toxic effects following exposure to tear agents typically resolve within 20 to 30 minutes (25). High-concentration, enclosed space exposures, however, may result in significant respiratory effects that include acute laryngotracheobronchitis, pulmonary edema, and death. Pulmonary edema can be delayed 4 to 8 hours; peak effects should be evident by 12 hours.

Prolonged or repeated exposures to lacrimating agents may produce malaise, skin blistering, chest tightness, coughing, wheezing, hemoptysis, shortness of breath, and a feeling of suffocation. Reactive airways dysfunction (RADS) and allergic contact dermatitis have been described in sensitized individuals. A severe dermatitis, labeled Hunan hand syndrome, has been described after prolonged skin exposure to capsaicin.

Incapacitating Agents

Manifestations of BZ and fentanyl derivative poisoning are described in detail in Chapters 322, "Anticholinergic Agents," and Chapter 283, "Opioids," respectively. BZ poisoning may occur after inhalation of vapor or liquid aerosol, intravenous or intramuscular injection, or, to a small degree, skin contact with liquid. Following exposure by all routes (except skin), the onset of effects take 1 hour, peaks at 8 hours, and gradually subsides over 24 to 72 hours (25). Effects may be delayed up to 24 hours after dermal exposure. Doubling the dose produces incapacitation within 1 hour but prolongs recovery an additional 48 hours. It is expected that wide variability in the onset, severity, and duration of effects will occur after BZ deployment by aerosol or vapor (25). The rate of onset and duration of clinical effects after inhalation of aerosolized fentanyl derivatives has not been fully elucidated (22). The gas mixture utilized in the Moscow hostage crisis produced effects within 15 minutes of exposure; toxicity lasted days in some survivors (4,22).

DIFFERENTIAL DIAGNOSIS

Deliberate release of chemicals by terrorists is likely to involve substances that cannot be immediately identified. Thus, the diagnosis is likely to be made by history, physical examination, and initial diagnostic testing (7). Diagnosis is also strongly suggested by the complete reversal of toxic effects following empiric antidotal therapy (12,14,22).

CWA poisoning should be suspected when a group of patients present with the abrupt onset of a similar constellation of signs or symptoms, particularly if they involve the exposed mucosal or skin surfaces, the respiratory tract, or sudden systemic effects (7). Following a chemical attack, clinical effects will occur within minutes to hours, and large numbers of symptomatic patients will present to medical facilities within a short period of time (3,5,7). In contrast, following a bioagent attack, clinical effects are delayed as a result of the incubation period of the illness (see Chapter 330, "Biological Warfare Agents") (7). After several days, patients will present insidiously, often with nonspecific signs and symptoms. It is often difficult to identify the release site of the weapon, and the geographic distribution of patients may be wide by the time symptomatic disease develops.

Irritant or corrosive gas inhalation, hydrocarbon aspiration, and vesicating agent and high-dose lacrimating agent exposures may produce pulmonary signs and symptoms similar to those caused by choking agents. Exacerbations of asthma and chronic obstructive pulmonary disease and allergic or infectious pneumonitis may present similarly. The vesiculobullous skin lesions that result from vesicating agents may mimic those resulting from Stevens-Johnson syndrome, toxic epidermal necrolysis, pemphigus vulgaris, bullous pemphigoid, scalded skin syndrome, thermal and chemical burns, and hypersensitivity reactions. Nerve agent poisoning is nearly identical to organophosphate and carbamate pesticide poisoning. Other agents and conditions that can produce similar clinical effects are botulism; nicotine; cholinergic drugs such as bethanechol, carbachol, edrophonium, methacholine, neostigmine, pilocarpine, physostigmine, pyridostigmine, and succinylcholine, and muscarine-containing mushrooms.

Nerve agent, cyanide, or fentanyl derivative exposure should be suspected if victims of a suspected chemical weapons incident become comatose within minutes of exposure (7,19,25). Although the presence of coma, miosis, and respiratory depression is likely following exposure to opioid and nerve agents alike, the additional presence of a seizure, fasciculations, and/or cholinergic findings strongly suggest intoxication with a nerve agent (12). Although a seizure may be present following exposure to cyanide and nerve agents alike, the presence of intractable hypotension and acidemia despite adequate oxygenation suggests severe cyanide toxicity (7,19,25). BZ will produce effects identical to other anticholinergic agents (25). In the absence of history, unintentional atropine poisoning following use of a nerve agent autoinjector cannot be differentiated from BZ toxicity. Lacrimating agents cause effects similar to those of irritant gas and lewisite exposure. Anxiety and hysterical reactions must also be considered in the differential diagnosis of patients exposed to warfare agents.

EMERGENCY DEPARTMENT EVALUATION

An attempt should be made to document the amount, time, nature, and duration of exposure. The color and odor of the toxic agent may provide clues to its identity. The time of onset, nature, progression, and severity of symptoms should be noted. Ideally, all patients should have continuous cardiac and oxygen saturation monitoring, but priority must be given to the most severely affected patients in mass-casualty situations.

Physical examination should first focus on vital signs and an assessment of neuromuscular and cardiopulmonary function, and then on the eyes, skin, and GI tract. Patients with eye symptoms should have fluorescein and slit-lamp examinations. If signs and symptoms of cyanide, choking, vesicating, or lacrimating agent toxicity are present, ancillary studies should include a chest radiograph, electrocardiogram (ECG), and arterial blood gas analysis, depending on the severity of symptoms. Additional laboratory evaluation after exposure to cyanide or a vesicating agent should include baseline complete blood count and serum electrolyte, blood urea nitrogen, creatinine, and glucose levels. Measurements of whole blood or plasma cyanide confirm cyanide poisoning but are rarely readily available. High blood lactate concentrations, a large anion gap metabolic acidosis, and high venous blood oxygen content, however, are rapidly available surrogate markers for cyanide poisoning.

Patients with signs and symptoms of nerve agent toxicity should have a chest radiograph, ECG, arterial blood gas analysis, routine admission laboratory studies, and measurement of peak expiratory flow rate and plasma or red blood cell cholinesterase activity (see Chapter 297, "Organophosphate and Carbamate Insecticides"). Cholinesterase activity, however, will not be available in time to be useful in making treatment decisions and it does not always correlate with the severity of disease (6,25). In the Tokyo Sarin attack, 27% of patients with clinical manifestations of moderate poisoning had plasma cholinesterase levels in the normal range (14).

Routine toxicology testing will not identify CWA. The diagnosis of CWA poisoning is confirmed by detecting chemical agents and their degradation products or cellular macromolecule adducts in environmental or body fluid samples. Unambiguous identification of CWAs should utilize gas or liquid chromatography in combination with mass spectrometry (GC or LC/MS) (11). Rapid detection kits may soon become available for clinical use.

EMERGENCY DEPARTMENT MANAGEMENT

In the event of a chemical weapon attack, emergency field personnel will be responsible for performing on-scene triage, decontamination, and initial treatment prior to patient transport. Although the nature of the exposure may not be immediately known, the release site of the weapon ("hot zone") is quickly discoverable and should be cordoned off. Emergency field personnel should wear appropriate personal protective equipment (PPE) until patients can be decontaminated and the threat of secondary exposure is no longer present. If the hazardous substance is unknown, this consists of an encapsulated, vapor-impermeable, and chemical-resistant suit; chemical-resistant gloves and boots; and a positive-pressure self-contained breathing apparatus (level A PPE) (1,3,7). The importance of first-responder personal protection was illustrated in the Matsumoto and Tokyo Sarin gas attacks in which 10% to 35% of rescuers developed mild toxicity (10,14). In each incident, patients were not decontaminated, and rescuers wore standard work clothing without respiratory protection. Mouth-to-mouth rescue breathing should be avoided as 10% of inhaled nerve agents are expired and could result in rescuer toxicity (16).

Initial victim management includes establishing and maintaining the airway, breathing, and circulation, and gross decontamination (brushing off chemical powder, removal of clothing and jewelry, and of the patient from the contaminated environment). Rapid dermal decontamination is critical following exposure to the liquid or aerosolized formulations but less important following exposure to vapor (3,6). Patient decontamination was inadequately performed in the Tokyo Sarin gas exposure (vapor), yet secondary injury to hospital staff was minimal and did not necessitate treatment (13). Clothing should be removed and discarded in impervious plastic bags, particularly leather items (e.g., shoes, watchbands), which can absorb chemicals and act as a depot. Clothing removal eliminates 85% to 90% of a contamination hazard (7,9). Skin should be decontaminated with a triple wash, which includes initial irrigation with tepid water, followed by 0.5% hypochlorite solution (household bleach diluted 1:10 with water) or alkaline soap, and then repeated, thorough water rinsing (3,25). The waste water should be collected and isolated, if possible. If exposed, the eyes should be irrigated with copious amounts of water or saline. A topical anesthetic may be used, if available. For inhalation exposure, initial treatment includes administration of 100% humidified oxygen, assisted ventilation, as necessary, and removal from the vapor source.

Police, fire department, emergency medical, and HAZMAT (hazardous materials) personnel should inform hospital personnel of the nature and magnitude of exposure, the number and severity of casualties, and the manifestations of illness. On recognition of a mass-casualty incident, emergency physicians must implement the hospital disaster plan and establish a well-demarcated decontamination area outside the emergency department for patients that arrive without prior decontamination (3). Details of disaster planning and management are discussed in Chapter 362, "Disaster Planning and Management." Emergency department personnel treating a patient exposed to an unknown chemical agent should wear a chemical-resistant suit, gloves, and boots, and an external SCBA or positive-pressure supplied air respirator (level B PPE) until the threat of secondary exposure is no longer viable (1,3).

Choking Agents

Treatment of choking agent poisoning consists of copious saline irrigation of exposed skin and eyes, humidified oxygen, bronchodilators, ventilatory support, intravenous crystalloids for hypotension, and antibiotic administration for secondary infection (25). Nebulized 2% sodium bicarbonate may provide symptomatic relief following acute chlorine gas exposure (7). Although sometimes recommended for chlorine and phosgene exposure, corticosteroids have no proven benefit. Animal studies suggest that tomelukast, a leukotriene-receptor antagonist, and N-acetylcysteine, an antioxidant, may limit the development of pulmonary edema following phosgene exposure.

Vesicating Agents

Because of rapid and irreversible binding to tissues, immediate decontamination is the best form of treatment for mustard agent exposure (2,15,25). Exposure to tissue or vesicle fluid will not produce secondary injury to health care personnel (1). The recommended method of decontamination is to wash with standard 5% household bleach, diluted 1:10, or copious amounts of soap and water (2). Water alone is ineffective, as mustard is relatively water-insoluble. Bleach produces "free" chlorine, which inactivates the mustard compound. Dry decontamination can be performed by applying absorbent powders (flour, baking soda [sodium bicarbonate], talcum powder, activated charcoal, or Fuller's earth) to the skin and wiping off with moist paper towels (2). Skin can also be decontaminated by irrigating with 10% sodium thiosulfate. Copious water or saline irrigation is the favored method of ocular decontamination.

Treatment is otherwise supportive. Skin burns should be treated with topical antibiotics such as silver sulfadiazine. Blisters and necrotic skin should be débrided. Ocular injury requires urgent ophthalmologic consultation. Treatment may include topical anesthetics, antibiotic ointment to prevent infection, and mydriatic or cycloplegic medication to prevent adhesions between iris and cornea (2,25). Respiratory care is the same as for choking agents.

Potential antidotes for system sulfur mustard poisoning including mustard scavengers (glutathione, N-acetylcysteine, thiosulfate), antioxidants (vitamin E), NAD$^+$-level stabilizers (niacin and nicotinamide), antiinflammatory drugs (corticosteroids, indomethacin), and nitric oxide synthase inhibitors (l-nitroarginine methyl ester) (15,25). Bone marrow suppression may respond to granulocyte colony-stimulating factor.

Treatment of lewisite exposure involves washing the skin with water, soap and water, or solutions of dilute chlorine bleach (0.5%) or baking soda (sodium bicarbonate) (25). Dry decontamination may also be efficacious. Neither scrubbing nor hot water is appropriate, because both enhance lewisite absorption and toxicity. Blisters, shown to contain arsenic, should be opened and drained of fluid. Treatment is otherwise identical to that of thermal burns.

Historically, systemic lewisite poisoning has been treated by intramuscular British antilewisite (BAL, 2,3-dimercaptopropanol, or dimercaprol), an arsenic chelator antidote, along with supportive care (see Chapter 305, "Arsenic and Mercury"). BAL has also been used topically as a 5% ointment for skin lesions and as a 5% to 10% oil solution for ocular symptoms. Newer, less toxic dithiol analogs of BAL, meso-dimercaptosuccinic acid (DMSA, marketed as Succimer or Chemet) and 2,3-dimercapto-1-propan-sulfonic acid (DMPS) can be given orally (DMSA) or intravenously (DMPS) and have equal efficacy (see Chapter 305, "Arsenic and Mercury" and Chapter 314, "Lead Poisoning").

Nerve Agents

Self-protection minimally involves a well-sealed respirator with a charcoal filter and heavy butyl rubber gloves (6). Victims of vapor exposure pose little threat to hospital personnel once clothing has been removed. Patients with liquid contamination of skin and clothing, however, pose a significant vapor and skin contact risk to rescuers (6,25). Skin should be decontaminated with a triple wash—irrigation with tepid water, followed by 0.5% hypochlorite solution or alkaline soap, and repeated, thorough water rinsing (3,6,19,25). U.S. military decontamination kits contain towelettes impregnated with a hypochlorite solution. Scrubbing should be avoided because abrading the skin can increase absorption. Water alone will not hydrolyze nerve agents but it will dilute them. Eye decontamination involves copious saline irrigation. Hypochlorite should not be used in the eye.

Intubation, mechanical ventilation, and the use of muscarinic antagonists (e.g., atropine), oximes (e.g., pralidoxime), and benzodiazepines (e.g., diazepam) may be necessary. The use of succinylcholine to assist intubation may result in prolonged neuromuscular blockade as a result of nerve agent–induced plasma cholinesterase inhibition (6). If endotracheal intubation is necessary, a nondepolarizing neuromuscular blocker such as rocuronium (0.6–1.0 mg/kg i.v.) is recommended. Antidotal therapy is discussed in Chapter 297, "Organophosphate and Carbamate Insecticides." Initially, atropine should be administered intravenously at a dose of 2 mg every 3 to 5 minutes (0.02–0.05 mg/kg in children) until respiratory secretions clear, bronchospasm resolves, and ventilation is normal (1,9,16). Heart rate and pupil size are poor clinical indicators of adequate atropinization (9,14,25). U.S. soldiers carry three atropine autoinjectors, each containing 2 mg, for rapid intramuscular self-injection. Cumulative atropine doses of 10 to 20 mg are usually adequate over the first 2 to 3 hours, with little or no therapy required thereafter (6,14,19,25). This differs from organophosphate pesticide poisoning, which may require significantly greater amounts of atropine and a longer duration of therapy. In the Tokyo Sarin attacks, only 19% of poisoned patients required more than 2 mg of atropine; severely poisoned patients required 1.5 to 15.0 mg of atropine (mean, 6 mg) (10,13,14). Topical mydriatic–cycloplegic eye drops (e.g., tropicamide) may be used for patients with intractable eye pain as a result of ciliary spasm. Eye drops are not recommended for those patients with miosis as their only ocular finding.

Oxime therapy is recommended for all cases of nerve agent poisoning. Because nerve agents age extremely rapidly, pralidoxime must be given as soon as possible after exposure to be effective. Initially, 1 to 2 g of pralidoxime should be administered as an intravenous bolus over 10 minutes (20–50 mg/kg in children), followed by a continuous infusion of 500 mg per hour (10–20 mg/kg/hr in children) (1,9,16). Toxicity from pralidoxime includes hypertension and tachycardia. U.S. soldiers also carry three pralidoxime autoinjectors, each containing 600 mg of the oxime to be injected intramuscularly along with each atropine injection (25). Pralidoxime is dosed until signs and symptoms of intoxication have resolved or stabilization of RBC cholinesterase levels has occurred (9). In the Tokyo Sarin attacks, severely poisoned patients required 1 to 36 g pralidoxime (mean, 11 g) (10,13,14).

Seizures should be aggressively treated with high-dose benzodiazepines, such as intravenous diazepam 10 mg (0.2–0.4 mg/kg) or midazolam (0.1–0.3 mg/kg), in addition to standard therapy with an antimuscarinic and oxime agents (9,16,18,19). Both antimuscarinic agents and benzodiazepines are effective in treating nerve agent seizures in experimental animals; trihexyphenidyl and midazolam are the most potent and rapidly acting agents; and seizure control protects against acute lethality and brain pathology (6,18,25). Military physicians recommend diazepam prophylaxis for all severely exposed victims (20,25). U.S. soldiers carry 10-mg diazepam autoinjectors for intramuscular use following nerve agent exposure. In primates poisoned with Sarin, administration of the glutamate antagonist, GK-11 (gacyclidine), prevented seizures, mortality, and delayed neuropathology and accelerated clinical recovery (8).

Conventional oximes (pralidoxime preparations, obidoxime, trimedoxime) are not clinically useful against Soman. Newer H-series oximes (named after their inventor, Inge Hagedorn) are superior in their ability to reactivate unaged Soman-inhibited AChE. They also have direct antimuscarinic and antinicotinic (ganglia-blocking and nondepolarizing neuromuscular-blocking) actions but do not protect from nerve agent-induced seizures (17,25). HI-6 is effective against all nerve agents and no significant side effects from its use have been reported in human studies (18,25). HI-6 is given intramuscularly at an adult dose of 250 to 500 mg every 6 hours. Efficacy is enhanced when it was used with atropine. The dioxime, HLö 7, is more effective than HI-6 in animals (24).

Pretreating those at risk with a reversible AChE inhibitor, such as the carbamates physostigmine or pyridostigmine, is also effective against Soman, in which enzyme aging is rapid and pralidoxime alone is unlikely to be effective (25). The intent is to carbamylate or bind 20% to 40% of AChE and limit subsequent nerve agent binding. Carbamylated cholinesterase then spontaneously reactivates or is regenerated with oxime therapy, leaving the victim with enough AChE to function normally. Pyridostigmine pretreatment does not protect against Sarin and VX, in which aging is slower and pralidoxime is effective. During the Persian Gulf war, U.S. soldiers were given pyridostigmine bromide in blister packs containing twenty-one 30-mg tablets (9,25). Pyridostigmine was taken orally every 8 hours without causing impaired performance. Side effects were minimal, but they can mimic those of mild nerve gas poisoning.

Pyridostigmine does not cross the blood–brain barrier and offers no protection from CNS toxicity (19,23). Pretreatment with physostigmine and hyoscine (agents that penetrate the CNS) provides better protection than pretreatment with pyridostigmine against the lethal and incapacitating effects of nerve agents in experimental animals (23). Other promising treatments include human monoclonal antibodies, which provide passive protection before exposure, and pretreatment with excess cholinesterase, which presumably scavenges nerve agent.

A dermal topical protective agent containing a 50:50 mixture of perfluoroalkylpolyether and polytetrafluoroethylene has been developed for protection against all CWA. It is known as "serpacwa" (skin exposure reduction paste against chemical warfare agents) and is applied to the skin of military personnel when chemical agent exposure is deemed possible (9).

Lacrimating Agents

Treatment of lacrimating agent exposure is frequently unnecessary because effects resolve quickly. Symptomatic patients may require decontamination and supportive care. Health care personnel should wear rubber gloves; if contamination is heavy, airway protection may also be necessary. Skin should be washed thoroughly with soap and water or a mild alkaline solution such as 6% sodium bicarbonate or 1% benzalkonium chloride (25). Ambulatory patients can be bathed in a shower. Contact dermatitis may respond to topical corticosteroids and antipruritics. Tearing usually irrigates the eyes adequately, but topical anesthetics and saline irrigation may be helpful. Chemical conjunctivitis may require symptomatic treatment with topical vasoconstrictors (see Chapter 17, "The Red Eye"). Corneal injuries are treated with cycloplegics, topical antibiotics, and ophthal-

mologic referral (see Chapter 18, "Corneal Abrasion and Foreign Bodies"). Patients exposed to high concentrations of aerosols, as in enclosed spaces or near exploding tear gas canisters, should be observed for 12 to 24 hours because of delayed pulmonary effects (25). Treatment of pulmonary toxicity consists of humidified oxygen, bronchodilators, and assisted ventilation, as needed.

Incapacitating Agents

Treatment of incapacitating agent toxicity includes supportive care and the administration of antidotes. Standard doses of physostigmine (initial dose, 30 to 45 mcg/kg i.v.) are usually effective in reversing the anticholinergic effects of BZ (see Chapter 323, "Anticholinergic Agents") (25). For unclear reasons, however, physostigmine is ineffective if administered during the first 4 to 6 hours after the onset of clinical effects (25). The treatment fentanyl derivative poisoning is similar to that recommended for other opioids (see Chapter 283, "Opioids"). Because these agents bind with high affinity to opiate receptors, large doses of naloxone may be required for complete reversal of toxic effects. As a result of high lipophilicity, fentanyl derivatives will redistribute from tissue stores to the CNS and likely produce recurrent opioid effects (22). Based on animal studies, antagonist redosing will likely be necessary for a period of 2 to 24 hours (22).

CRITICAL INTERVENTIONS

- Decontaminate victims of CWA exposure by removing and discarding all clothing and washing the skin with copious amounts of soap and water
- Wear level B PPE (e.g., chemical-resistant suit, gloves, boots, SCBA) when the CWA is unknown
- Notify local law enforcement authorities, the FBI, and local or state health departments when CWA poisoning is suspected
- Activate the hospital disaster plan and establish a decontamination area outside the emergency department for mass casualty incidents
- Administer oxygen, bronchodilators, and artificial ventilation to patients with respiratory symptoms following choking, vesicating, and lacrimating agent exposure
- Administer antidotal therapy to victims with cyanide, nerve agent, anticholinergic, and opioid poisoning

DISPOSITION

Consultation with a toxicologist, regional hazardous materials (HAZMAT) specialist, poison center, or experienced military physician is recommended for all CWA poisoning except civilian exposures to the lacrimating agents. Suspected CWA poisoning should prompt an immediate call to local law enforcement authorities, the local Federal Bureau of Investigation (FBI) field office, and local or state health department and laboratory. An ophthalmologist or plastic surgeon should be consulted for patients with corneal or skin burns.

Asymptomatic patients with choking agent exposure should be observed and monitored for at least 6 hours. Mild to moderately symptomatic patients may be discharged safely after several hours of observation if symptoms have improved or resolved with treatment. Some recommend that all patients with a history of phosgene exposure should be admitted and closely observed because of phosgene's varying latency period and high potential morbidity. Asymptomatic patients with vesicating agent exposure should be observed and monitored for 12 hours. Following exposure to nerve agent vapor, patients with signs and symptoms confined to the eyes may be discharged safely after a short period of observation (6,14). Those with skin exposure to nerve agents (liquid or aerosolized droplets) should be observed for 24 hours. Victims of lacrimating agents may be treated and released if there is no significant pulmonary toxicity.

All patients with systemic symptoms, pulmonary toxicity, and severe or extensive dermal injury should be hospitalized. As a result of the long duration and recrudescent nature of clinical effects from incapacitating agents, all symptomatic victims should be observed for a minimum of 24 hours. The appropriate level of care will depend on clinical severity.

COMMON PITFALLS

✔ Failure to protect rescuers and medical personnel from secondary contamination
✔ Failure to decontaminate victims of chemical agent exposure in a timely fashion
✔ Failure to appreciate that effects can be delayed and progressive and to observe asymptomatic victims for appropriate periods of time
✔ Failure to administer antidotes in a timely manner

References

1. Bozeman WP, Dilbero D, Schauben JL. Biologic and chemical weapons of mass destruction. *Emerg Med Clin North Am* 2002;20:975–993.
2. Borak J, Sidell FR. Agents of chemical warfare: sulfur mustard. *Ann Emerg Med* 1992;21:303–308.
3. Brennan RJ, Waeckerle JF, Sharp TW, et al. Chemical warfare agents: emergency medical and emergency public health issues. *Ann Emerg Med* 1999;34:191–204.
4. Enserink M, Stone R. Questions swirl over knockout gas used in hostage crisis. *Science* 2002;298:1150–1151.
5. Henderson DA. The looming threat of bioterrorism. *Science* 1999;283:1279–1282.
6. Holstege CP, Kirk M, Sidell FR. Chemical warfare: nerve agent poisoning. *Crit Care Clin* 1997;13:923–942.
7. Kales SN, Christiani DC. Acute chemical emergencies. *N Engl J Med* 2004;350:800–808.
8. Lallement G, Clarencon D, Masqueliez C, et al. Nerve agent poisoning in primates: antilethal, anti-epileptic and neuroprotective effects of GK-11. *Arch Toxicol* 1998;72:84–92.
9. Leikin JB, Thomas TGH, Walter R, et al. A review of nerve agent exposure for the critical care physician. *Crit Care Med* 2002;30:2346–2354.
10. Morita H, Yanagisawn, Nakajima T, et al. Sarin poisoning in Matsumoto, Japan. *Lancet* 1995;346:290–293.
11. Noort D, Benschop HP, Black RM. Biomonitoring of exposure to chemical warfare agents: a review. *Toxicol Appl Pharmacol* 2002;184:116–126.
12. Nozaki H, Aikawa N, Gujishima S, et al. A case of VX poisoning and the difference from sarin. *Lancet* 1995;346:698–699.
13. Nozaki H, Aikawa N, Shinozawa Y, et al. Sarin poisoning in Tokyo subway [Letter]. *Lancet* 1995;345:980–981.
14. Okumura T, Takasu N, Ishimatsu S, et al. Report on 640 victims of the Tokyo subway sarin attack. *Ann Emerg Med* 1996;28:129–135.
15. Papirmeister B, Feister AJ, Robinson SI, et al. *Medical defense against mustard gas: toxic mechanisms and pharmacological implications*. Boca Raton, FL: CRC Press, 1991.
16. Rotenberg JS, Newmark J. Nerve agent attacks on children: diagnosis and management. *Pediatrics* 2003;112:648–658.
17. Shih T-M, Whalley C, Valdes J. A comparison of cholinergic effects of HI-6 and pralidoxime-2-chloride (2-PAM) in Soman poisoning. *Toxicol Lett* 1991;55:131–147.
18. Shih T-M, Duniho SM, McDonough JH. Control of nerve agent-induced seizures is critical for neuroprotection and survival. *Toxicol Appl Pharmacol* 2003;188:69–80.
19. Sidell FR, Borak J. Chemical warfare agents: nerve agents. *Ann Emerg Med* 1992;21:865–871.
20. Smith WJ, Dunn MA. Medical defense against blistering chemical warfare agents. *Arch Dermatol* 1991;127:1207–1213.
21. Van Bever WF, Niemegeers CJ, Schellekens KH, et al. N-4-substituted 1-(2-arylethyl)-4-piperidinyl-N-phenylpropanamides, a novel series of extremely potent analgesics with unusually high safety margin. *Arzneimittel-Forschung* 1976;26:1548–1551.
22. Wax PM, Becker CE, Curry SE. Unexpected "gas" casualties in Moscow: a medical toxicology perspective. *Ann Emerg Med* 2003;41:700–705.
23. Wetherell J, Hall T, Passingham S. Physostigmine and hyoscine improves protection against the lethal and incapacitating effects of nerve agent poisoning in the guinea-pig. *Neurotoxicology* 2002;23:341–349.
24. Worek F, Widmann R, Knopff O, et al. Reactivating potency of obidoxime, pralidoxime, HI 6 and HLö 7 in human erythrocyte acetylcholinesterase inhibited by highly toxic organophosphorus compounds. *Arch Toxicol* 1998;72:237–243.
25. Zajtchuk R, Bellamy RD, eds. *Textbook of military medicine: medical aspects of chemical and biological warfare. Part I.* Washington, DC: Office of the Surgeon General, US. Dept of the Army, 1997.

CHAPTER 332
Complications of Parenteral Drug Therapy

Jennifer A. Oman and Scott E. Rudkin

Parenteral drug therapy includes administration by the intravenous (i.v.), intramuscular (i.m.), intradermal (i.d.), intraosseous (i.o.), intraarterial (i.a.), intrathecal (i.t.), intracardiac (i.c.), and subcutaneous (s.q.) routes. Benefits of parenteral therapy include rapid onset of effect, titratable effect, and improved efficacy but such therapy is not without risk. Infrequent but serious complications can occur. The annual cost associated with complications of i.v. drug therapy is estimated at greater than $112 million annually (8).

Complications of parental drug therapy include injection site pain, ecchymosis, itching, inflammation, infection, infiltration, extravasation, nerve injury, vascular injury, inadvertent intraarterial or venous injection, and anaphylaxis. Complications are more common with certain therapeutic agents and/or their diluent. Categorizing them as local or systemic aids the clinician in both diagnosis and treatment (Table 332.1).

CLINICAL PRESENTATION

Local complications usually involve the digits or extremities and are injection-site dependent. Usually, these injuries are caused by s.q., i.m., or i.v. routes and are located at the site of administration. Symptoms such as pain at the site of the i.v. catheter or increased pain after local injection is completed are common. Pain and phlebitis of the vein used for i.v. injections may also occur. Drugs that often cause pain and phlebitis include cations (potassium, calcium and magnesium) chemotherapeutic agents, glucagon (phenol diluent), phenytoin, hypertonic solutions, adenosine, propofol, and ethanol.

Phlebitis may present as redness, warmth, pain and swelling or induration along the course of the vein and may or may not be associated with thrombosis. Signs of thrombosis may include a palpable cord along the course of the vein or swelling. Local inflammation or infection with the common signs of redness, warmth, and induration can accompany i.m. or s.q. injections.

Signs of venous extravasation include swelling, paleness or cyanosis, cool temperature, blistering, frank necrosis, and pain (both immediate and delayed) to the affected area. Pain may initially occur distal to injection site and subsequently progress

TABLE 332.1. Adverse Effects of Parenteral Drug Administration

LOCAL

Pain (all routes)
Infiltration/extravasation (IV)
Phlebitis/thrombosis/thrombophlebitis (IV)
Cellulitis (all routes)
Abscess (all routes)
Granuloma (IM, SQ)
Allergic (all routes)
Nerve injury (all routes)
Vascular injury (all routes)
Ischemia (all routes)
Inadvertent IV injection (IM, SQ)
Inadvertent IA injection (all routes)
Tissue irritation/necrosis (all routes)

SYSTEMIC

Noninfectious febrile reactions (all routes)
Sepsis (all routes)
Anaphylaxis (all routes)
Fluid overload (IV)
Diluent toxicity (IV)

TABLE 332.2. Common Parenteral Drugs Containing Propylene Glycol (Trade Name/Generic Name)

Amidate/etomidate
Apresoline/hydralazine
Bactrim/trimethoprim–sulfamethoxazole
Berocca PN/multivitamins
Brevibloc/esmolol
Dilantin/phenytoin
Dramamine/dimenhydrinate
Dramocen/dimenhydrinate
Konakion/phytonadione
Lanoxin/digoxin
Lanoxin Pediatric/digoxin
Librium/chlordiazepoxide
Loxitane/loxapine
Luminal sodium/phenobarbital
MVC9 Plus/multivitamins
MVI-12/multivitamins
Nitro-BID/nitroglycerin
Nembutal/pentobarbital
Nitrostat/nitroglycerin
Nitroglycerin
Pentobarbital sodium
Phenobarbital sodium
Phenytoin sodium
Septra/trimethoprim–sulfamethoxazole
Tridil/nitroglycerin
Valium/diazepam

either proximally or distally (25). Although extravasation injury can occur with any medication or fluid, certain agents (e.g., vasopressors, phenytoin, chemotherapeutic agents, TPN, calcium chloride and gluconate, promethazine, lipid solutions, and antibiotics) frequently cause extravasation injury.

Drugs that can cause skin necrosis following extravasation are chemotherapeutic agents, hypertonic agents (e.g., 10%, 25%, and 50% dextrose, and mannitol), sodium bicarbonate, calcium gluconate and chloride, potassium salts, nafcillin, norepinephrine, dopamine, epinephrine, radiologic dyes, and methylene blue (2). Damage from phenytoin extravasation can range from mild to devastating. It is unclear whether the damage results from the phenytoin itself, the alkaline pH of intravenous formulations, or the propylene glycol diluent; the mechanism of damage is poorly described but may result from thrombosis of vessels and subsequent tissue necrosis (3,18).

Accidental i.a. injection may result in injury, infarction or gangrene of the area supplied by artery. Agents frequently described as causing arterial injury with accidental i.a. injection include penicillin, antiinflammatory drugs, barbiturates, benzodiazepines, phenothiazines, phenytoin, and TPN (19,22). Accidental injection of epinephrine (e.g., from an auto-injection device such as the Epi-Pen) into a digit can result in digital ischemia with pain, pallor, coolness, paresthesia, and pulselessness.

Numbness, tingling or "shooting" pain, especially along the course of a nerve, and neuropathy may occur if a peripheral nerve is injured by i.v./i.m. or s.q. injection (6,7,12,17). Delayed neuropathy without pain is less common. Often times, symptoms will be difficult to discriminate from the patients underlying condition (12). The most common nerve injury involves the sciatic and radial nerves from i.m. injections (17).

Pruritus, urticarial rash, erythema and swelling may occur in the area of drug administration or along the intravenous route of drug administration from local allergic reaction or from histamine release caused by drugs such as morphine and protamine.

Serious systemic reactions may occur if a drug intended for i.m. or s.c. injection is inadvertently given intravenously or intraarterially. Such reactions include hypotension, rapid heart rate, dysrhythmia, seizures, and cardiovascular collapse. Addi-

tional systemic reactions include anaphylaxis, fluid overload, electrolyte disturbances, and sepsis.

Systemic reactions may also result from the vehicle or solvent in which a drug is delivered. Propylene glycol has been linked to central nervous system (CNS) depression, seizures, hypotension, cardiac dysrhythmias, hemolysis, and lactic acidosis. Propylene glycol toxicity has been associated with the intravenous administration of benzodiazepines, etomidate, nitroglycerin, phenytoin and other medications at high doses or rates of infusion (Table 332.2) (1). Alcohol intoxication has resulted from excessive coadministration of ethanol with nitroglycerin infusions.

DIFFERENTIAL DIAGNOSIS

The differential diagnosis for complications from parenteral injection is limited when the presentation is immediate and temporally related to the injection. Trauma, thermal or chemical burn, catheter breakage or embolization also must be considered in patients presenting with a possible extravasation injury. Compartment syndrome, deep venous thrombosis (DVT), cellulitis and phlebitis should be considered in any patient with a swollen limb related to i.v. infiltration or extravasation injury. Cellulitis, abscess or local allergic reaction should also be considered in patients with a history of i.m. or s.q. injection. Osteomyelitis, fracture, and local cellulitis should be considered in patients with i.o. lines. Parenteral therapy can cause nerve injury from direct nerve damage, mechanical nerve root impingement, neuronal ischemia from compartment syndrome, disc herniation, occult vascular injury, or cerebrovascular accident.

When a complication of parenteral drug therapy is delayed, the differential diagnosis becomes more broad. Many of these patients may be recently discharged from the emergency department (ED) or hospital or receiving chemotherapy. If the patient denies a history of parenteral therapy, snake bite, insect, Raynaud's phenomenon, mechanical trauma, thermal burn, infection, gangrene, and topical chemical injury should be considered.

EMERGENCY DEPARTMENT EVALUATION

Evaluation should include a complete history and physical exam. Pertinent historical factors include time of onset, route of injection (s.q., i.m., i.v.), injected agent, amount injected, and symptom progression. The effected extremity should be examined thoroughly with attention to neurological, vascular, and integumentary involvement.

A plain radiograph can help exclude catheter breakage or embolization as most catheters are radiopaque; radiography should be considered for those patients who present with a history of a recent i.v. in an affected area. Ultrasound for a catheter breakage or embolization has an unclear role. If significant swelling or neurovascular compromise is suspected, a compartment syndrome or DVT should be excluded with compartment pressure measurement or ultrasonography of the involved vessels, respectively. If a nerve injury is suspect from direct injury from injection, nerve conduction studies can be useful to identify the extent of injury. If systemic signs are present (e.g., alteration in oxygenation, heart rate, or blood pressure), the patient should undergo cardiac monitoring and pulse oximetry. Arterial blood gases, complete blood count (CBC), serum chemistries, and drug or diluent levels may be indicated in patients with systemic reactions.

EMERGENCY DEPARTMENT MANAGEMENT

Prevention is central to reducing parenteral drug therapy complications. Placement and proper i.v. access should always be verified; blood aspiration may help aid in confirming placement, but is not diagnostic. Digital pressure should be placed over the skin at the tip of the inserted catheter and the i.v. flow rate of normal saline observed. If the cannula is in the vein, the i.v. infusion will stop with compression at the distal tip of the catheter/vein. If the i.v. solution continues despite digital pressure, the i.v. is infiltrating and should be removed (5).

Some medications cause pain on injection based on their high lipid content, acidity, or osmolarity. Pain may be minimized in these situations by first administering 1 mL of 1% lidocaine through the i.v. line, as in the case of propofol, or by slowing the rate of infusion for calcium or potassium infusions. Extremities with arteriovenous fistulas for hemodialysis, fractures or extremities (upper or lower) with lymph node dissection should not be used for i.v. access.

Complications from i.m. injections may be minimized by administering injections in the upper outer quadrant of the buttock or in children less than 3 years of age in the vastus lateralis muscle of the thigh. Aspiration of blood prior to i.m. injection should result in relocation of the injection to avoid inadvertent intraarterial or i.v. medication deposition. However, aspiration of blood is not always reliable in signifying intravessel location especially with prepackaged medications/Tubex syringes (22). S.q. or i.m. injections containing epinephrine should be avoided in areas with end arterioles such as the fingers, toes, penis, nose, and ears.

Treatment of superficial venous phlebitis and thrombophlebitis consists of warm compresses, elevation and nonsteroidal antiinflammatory medications. Antibiotics are not indicated unless there is evidence of an infection.

Intravenous extravasation requires removal of the catheter. A neurovascular assessment of the involved extremity should be performed especially if a large volume of fluid has infiltrated. If there is no evidence of neurovascular compromise, therapy consists of elevation of the extremity and range of motion exercises (5).

Therapy for digital ischemia from accidental discharge from an epinephrine auto-injector should start with submersion of the affected digit in warm water or wrapping the digit in a warm compress, especially if the exposure occurred just prior to initiation of therapy. Topical 2% nitroglycerin (no more than 4 mm/kg in infants) or local infiltration of dilute terbutaline solution (1mg in 1 mL of sterile normal saline [NS]) may be considered, although their effectiveness is controversial (16,21,25). The use of nitroglycerin may result in hypotension and should be used with caution. Phentolamine in low doses (0.5mg or 2.5mg) may be injected either by digital block or locally into the digit near the initial puncture site and along the line of ischemic demarcation (9,14,15,21). The amount of phentolamine injected is limited by the physical space of the finger and the possibility of inducing compartment syndrome (14,15,21).

Treatment of vasopressor extravasation can be treated in the same manner as the accidental epinephrine auto-injection. However, because of the severity of the exposure, conservative management with warm compresses or warm water submersion should be bypassed so that more aggressive therapies can be initiated without delay. Intravenous phentolamine (5mg in 10mL NS) (20,21) is traditionally recommended but terbutaline (1:1 dilution) can also be used (20,21). If a compartment syndrome is suspected, consultation with a general, vascular, orthopaedic, or plastic surgeon is warranted. If there is evidence of necrosis, plastic surgery consultation should be obtained.

There is no well described treatment for phenytoin extravasation. Heparin has been proposed but its use is not well described in the literature (18). Infiltration of the affected site with hyaluronidase (15–150 units) may increase the absorption of extravasated aminophylline, chemotherapeutic agents, hyperosmolar solutions (mannitol, TPN, 10% calcium or dextrose, 30% urea), nafcillin, and potassium (13). Most extravasation injuries involving chemotherapeutics can be managed expectantly in coordination with a plastic surgeon (11).

Papaverine, phentolamine, nitroprusside, or blocks of the stellate or brachial plexus have been used in intraarterial injection of phenytoin. Consultation with a vascular surgeon should be obtained if intraarterial injection is suspected (19).

If nerve contact is suspected during needle insertion or drug injection, the procedure should be stopped immediately because frequently the medication injected compounds the mechanical injury to the nerve (4). The treatment of peripheral nerve injury consists of pain medications and possible immobilization and consultation with an orthopaedic, hand, or neurological surgeon (4,23).

Local or systemic histamine reactions may be treated with stopping or slowing the infusion, and oral or parenteral antihistamines and corticosteroids. Systemic reactions should be treated with supportive measures such as supplemental oxygen or intubation, i.v. fluids or cardioactive medications as indicated by the clinical picture. Anaphylaxis, abscesses, cellulitis, and sepsis are treated as usual (see Chapter 131, "Anaphylaxis," Chapter 135, "Bacteremia, Sepsis, and Septic Shock," and Chapter 136, "Skin and Soft-Tissue Infections").

CRITICAL INTERVENTIONS

- Consult a general, vascular, orthopaedic, or plastic surgeon if a compartment syndrome is suspected
- Consultation a vascular surgeon for patients with manifestations of limb ischemia
- Consult a plastic surgeon for patients with evidence of skin necrosis
- Consult an orthopedist, neurologist, or neurosurgeon for patients with signs and symptoms of peripheral nerve injury

DISPOSITION

Patients with minor extravasation injuries, cellulitis, drained abscess, phlebitis, or thrombosis, and local allergic reactions may be discharged home if appropriate follow-up can be arranged. Those with more significant local injuries should have specialist consultation, with disposition guided by the specialist's recommendations. Admission is recommended for patients with severe of persistent systemic reactions.

COMMON PITFALLS

✔ Lack of knowledge of proper injection techniques
✔ Failure to recognize local and systemic complications from parenteral drug therapy
✔ Failure to consider the use of medications, which may reverse or limit the damage from extravasated agents

References

1. Bedichek I, Kirschbaum B. A case of propylene glycol toxic reaction associated with etomidate infusion. *Arch Intern Med* 1991;151:2297.
2. Dufresne RG. Skin necrosis from intravenously infused materials. *Cutis* 1987;39:197–198
3. Edwards JJ, Bosek V. Extravasation injury of the upper extremity by intravenous phenytoin. *Anesth Analg* 2002;94:672–673.
4. Edwards WC, Fleming LL. Radial nerve palsy at elbow following venipuncture—case report. *J Hand Surg [Am]* 1981;6:468–469.
5. Fabian B. Intravenous complication: infiltration. *J Intraven Nurs* 2000;23:229–231.
6. Frederick HA, Carter PR, Littler JW. Injection injuries to the median and ulnar nerves at the wrist. *J Hand Surg [Am]* 1992;17A:645–7.
7. Gentili F, Hudson AR, Hunter D. Clinical and experimental aspects of injection injuries of peripheral nerves. *Can J Neurol Sci* 1980;7:143–151.
8. Halpern MT, Yabroff KR, Sloan EP. Costs of medical resource use associated with complications of IV drug therapy. *Formulary* 1997;32:944.
9. Hinterberger JW, Kintzi HE. Phentolamine reversal of epinephrine-induced digital vasospasm: how to save an ischemic finger. *Arch Fam Med* 1994;3:193–195.
10. Kumar MM, Sprung JS. The use of hyaluronidase to treat mannitol extravasation. *Anesth Analg* 2003;97:1199–2000.
11. Langstein HN, Duman H, Seelig D, et al. Retrospective study of the management of chemotherapeutic extravasation injury. *Ann Plast Surg* 2002;49:369–374.
12. Linskey ME, Segal R. Median nerve injury from local steroid injection in carpal tunnel syndrome. *Neurosurgery* 1990;26:512–515.
13. MacCara ME. Extravasation: a hazard of intravenous therapy. *Drug Intell Clin Pharm* 1983;17:713.
14. Maguire WM, Reisdorff EJ, Smith D, et al. Epinephrine-induced vasospasm reversed by phentolamine digital block. *Am J Emerg Med* 1990;8:46–7.
15. Markovchick V, Burkhart KK. The reversal of the ischemic effects of epinephrine on a finger with local injections of phentolamine. *J Emerg Med* 1991;9:323–324.
16. Mvros R, Anderson BD, Krenzelok. BD, Accidental injury of epinephrine from an autoinjector: Invasive treatment not always required. *Vet Hum Toxicol* 2001;43:366–369.
17. Preston D, Logigian E. Iatrogenic needle-induced peroneal neuropathy in the foot. *Ann Intern Med* 1988;109:921–2.
18. Rao VK, Feldman PD, Dibbell DG. Extravasation injury to the hand by intravenous phenytoin. *J Neurosurg* 1988;68:967–969.
19. Sintenie JB, Tuinebreijer WE, Kreis RW, et al. Digital gangrene after accidental intra-arterial injection of phenytoin. *Eur J Surg* 1992;158:315–316.
20. Siwy BK, Sadove AM. Acute management of dopamine infiltration injury with Regitine. *Plast Reconstr Surg* 1987;80:610–612.
21. Stier PA, Bogner MP, Webster K, et al. Use of subcutaneous terbutaline to reverse peripheral ischemia. *Am J Emerg Med* 1999;17:91.
22. Stoller KP, Losey R. Inadvertent intra-arterial injection of penicillin: an unseen danger. *Pediatrics* 1985;75:785.
23. Thrush DN, Belsoe R. Radial nerve injury after routine peripheral vein cannulation. *J Clin Anesth* 1995;7(2):160–2.
24. Turco SJ. Hazards associated with parenteral therapy. *Bull Parenter Drug Assoc* 1974;28(4):197.
25. Wong AF, McCulloch LM, Solo A. Treatment of peripheral tissue ischemia with topical nitroglycerin ointment in neonates. *J Pediatr* 1992;121:980.

CHAPTER 333
Drug Withdrawal

Paul M. Wax

Anticipating and recognizing the early signs of withdrawal allow for timely treatment and may help prevent the development of serious withdrawal manifestations. Ethanol withdrawal is the most common withdrawal syndrome (see Chapter 278, "Alcohol Withdrawal"). A severe, potentially life-threatening withdrawal syndrome similar to that as a result of ethanol can occur on cessation of use or decrease in the dose of other sedative–hypnotics such as benzodiazepines, barbiturates, chloral hydrate, and meprobamate (Chapter 290, "Muscle Relaxants and Other Sedative–Hypnotic Agents"), which enhance the activity of the inhibitory neurotransmitter gamma-aminobutyric acid (GABA) at the GABA$_A$/benzodiazepine receptor/chloride-channel complex. More recently, withdrawal from gamma hydroxybutyrate (GHB) and its congeners (e.g., 1,4-butanediol), which also stimulate the GABA$_A$/benzodiazepine receptor/chloride-channel complex has been reported. Ethanol-like withdrawal symptoms may also occur after the abrupt cessation of baclofen (Chapter 290, "Muscle Relaxants and Other Sedative–Hypnotic Agents"), a GABA$_B$ receptor agonist that is used to treat muscle spasms in spinal cord injury and multiple sclerosis patients.

Withdrawal symptoms from opioids (Chapter 283, "Opioids"), antidepressants (Chapter 318, "Cyclic Antidepressants," Chapter 321, "Monoamine Oxidase Inhibitors," and Chapter 323, "Anticholinergic Agents"), and cocaine (Chapter 324, "Cocaine") are less severe than those as a result of ethanol and sedative–hypnotic withdrawal and have unique features. Somatic and psychological symptoms have been reported after sudden cessation or tapering the dose of monoamine oxidase inhibitors (MAOIs), tricyclic antidepressants (TCAs) and serotonin selective reuptake inhibitors (SSRIs) (11).

Physical tolerance and dependency are a prerequisite for the development of a withdrawal syndrome. The dose of the drug, duration of effect, frequency of administration, and duration of abuse all contribute to the development of dependency. More severe withdrawal phenomena may be associated with a longer period of abuse or a history of previous withdrawal episodes. Sporadic use of a drug does not generally alter pharmacodynamic and pharmacokinetic responses required for the development of withdrawal symptoms. In all withdrawal scenarios, the precipitant is a decrease in the dose of the dependent drug. Complete abstinence and a serum drug level of zero are not required. It is important to realize that abuse (i.e., use simply for pleasurable CNS effects) is not a prerequisite for withdrawal and that physiological dependence dose not require excessive doses. It may occur after prolonged treatment with therapeutic doses.

Withdrawal from sedative–hypnotics is characterized by intense sympathetic stimulation. The underlying mechanism has not been fully elucidated, but it may result, in part, from unopposed compensatory central nervous system (CNS) mechanisms that counteract the depressant effects of sedative–hypnotics. Contributory mechanisms may involve changes in GABA and glutamate receptor activity. Chronic benzodiazepine use results in down-regulation of the GABA receptor complex. Benzodiazepine withdrawal results excitatory effects because there is less baseline GABA inhibition. The "excitotoxicity" associated with sedative–hypnotic withdrawal may also be a result of upregulation in *N*-methyl-D-aspartate (NMDA) glutamate receptors, thereby increasing calcium flux through these receptors (23).

Withdrawal from opioids may also involve an increase in sympathetic discharge, but by a different mechanism. Decreased opioid receptor stimulation increases catecholamine release in the locus ceruleus of the CNS. Severe catecholamine storm, however, is not observed during opioid withdrawal.

CLINICAL PRESENTATION

The clinical presentation of drug withdrawal varies significantly among patients. Some patients underreport their substance use although others overreport it. Patients who present with withdrawal symptoms (e.g., seizures) may or may not admit to drug use. They may present with medical and surgical complications of drug abuse, such as pneumonia, endocarditis and skin abscess, or an unrelated problem, such as a myocardial infarction or motor vehicle accident, and develop withdrawal symptoms while in the emergency department (ED) or after admission. Others present to the ED because they desire detoxification.

Sedative–hypnotic withdrawal may be indistinguishable from ethanol withdrawal except for differences in the time course (Table 333.1). Because many benzodiazepines have a much longer elimination half-life than ethanol and have active metabolites, withdrawal manifestations may be delayed after cessation of drug use. Withdrawal symptoms after lorazepam discontinuation may begin within 2 days of the last dose. Following diazepam cessation a week or more may pass before the onset of significant symptoms. More severe withdrawal appears associated with high doses or short-acting benzodiazepines (20).

The clinical presentation of sedative–hypnotic withdrawal varies in intensity and duration. Mild withdrawal symptoms include anxiety, apprehension, irritability, dysphoria, and insomnia (20). Other symptoms may include anorexia, nausea, and vomiting. Mild autonomic and CNS hyperactivity is characterized by tachycardia, hypertension, irritability, and hyperreflexia. Unlike patients with severe withdrawal, patients with mild withdrawal have a clear mental status. Most patients with mild withdrawal recover uneventfully after a few days, but some may develop more serious withdrawal manifestations.

Hallucinations, delusions, myoclonus, seizures, and agitation may appear with more severe withdrawal. Tachycardia, hypertension, tachypnea, hyperthermia, diaphoresis, and mydriasis may develop, as may tachyarrhythmias. At times, a new-onset seizure heralds the onset of sedative–hypnotic withdrawal. These patients may or may not have tremulousness and other sympathetic hyperactivity before seizure activity begins. Seizures tend to be of the generalized tonic–clonic type.

They may occur singly or as a brief flurry with normal sensorium between seizures. Status epilepticus is uncommon. Severe withdrawal symptoms, including seizures, may occur after the administration of flumazenil to patients chronically taking benzodiazepines. Symptoms from long-acting benzodiazepine withdrawal may persist for as long as 3 weeks.

Withdrawal from GHB, or its congeners gammabutyrolactone (GBL) or 1,4 butanediol, may also produce severe withdrawal manifestations (15). Frequent users of GHB ingest it multiple times per day (17). Initial symptoms may include anxiety and tremor. More severe GHB withdrawal is characterized by severe agitation requiring physical restraints, tachycardia, hypertension, auditory and visual hallucinations, and delirium. The onset of symptoms may appear as early as 1 to 6 hours after the last dose and the symptoms may persist for as long as 5 to 15 days. Deaths from GHB withdrawal have been reported (4).

Withdrawal from oral or intrathecal baclofen may also be quite problematic (7). Withdrawal symptoms generally start 12 to 72 hours after the last dose. Typical symptoms of withdrawal include sleeplessness, confusion, agitation, hallucinations, delusions, hyperthermia, and hypertonia. Interestingly, seizures may occur in the setting of either baclofen toxicity or withdrawal. Abrupt withdrawal from intrathecal baclofen (ITB) therapy, sometimes precipitated by unrecognized pump failure, may also cause similar symptoms that may be life-threatening (3). In some cases profound muscle rigidity develops resembling neuroleptic malignant syndrome or malignant hyperthermia (21).

Symptoms of mild opioid withdrawal include lacrimation, rhinorrhea, yawning, diaphoresis, anxiety, restlessness, and dysphoria. Piloerection is particularly characteristic. The patient may exhibit mild elevations in pulse, blood pressure, and respiratory rate, but these changes are usually not very significant. More severe opioid withdrawal is characterized by vomiting, diarrhea, abdominal pain, and dehydration. Unlike sedative–hypnotic withdrawal, severe agitation, seizures (except in neonatal withdrawal), mental status changes, and hyperthermia are not seen with opioid withdrawal.

The severity and time course of the opioid withdrawal syndrome depends on the pharmacokinetics of the opioid. Shorter-acting agents (e.g., heroin) tend to have a more intense course than longer-acting agents (e.g., methadone). Heroin withdrawal usually begins within 4 to 8 hours after the last dose, peaking by 36 to 72 hours. In contrast, the onset of methadone withdrawal may be delayed 36 to 72 hours after the last dose, and symptoms may persist for up to 2 weeks (5). At comparable doses, the severity and duration of withdrawal appears greater in patients who inject heroin compared to those who smoke heroin (22).

The sudden onset of opioid withdrawal may occur after an opioid antagonist such as naloxone is given to an unsuspected opioid-dependent patient. As a result of naloxone's short half-life, withdrawal symptoms do not usually persist beyond 20 to 60 minutes. Treatment with additional opioid to reverse these effects is not indicated. Giving opioids with agonist–antagonist properties, such as pentazocine (Talwin), nalbuphine (Nubain), and butorphanol (Stadol), to the opioid-dependent patient may also precipitate withdrawal symptoms. Opioid withdrawal from the long-acting opioid antagonists naltrexone and nalmefene may result in a markedly prolonged withdrawal period lasting upwards of 1 to 2 days.

Antidepressant withdrawal may result in anxiety, insomnia, lethargy, nausea, vomiting, headache, problems with balance, sensory abnormalities, and possibly aggressive and impulsive behavior. In most cases these symptoms are mild and transient (9). Withdrawal from cocaine may result in lethargy, dysphoria, and depression.

TABLE 333.1. Withdrawal Syndromes Seen in the Emergency Department

Type of Withdrawal	Onset of Symptoms
Ethanol	6–8 h
Sedative–hypnotic (e.g., benzodiazepines, barbiturates)	3–7 d (long acting drugs)
GHB	Hours to days
Baclofen	12–72 h
Opioids	4–8 h (heroin); 36–72 h (methadone)
Cocaine	Within hours after binge
Antidepressants	Few days

DIFFERENTIAL DIAGNOSIS

The differential diagnosis of the withdrawal state is broad and includes many other serious conditions that may require different therapy (Table 333.2). Because drug-dependent patients are particularly prone to develop many of these conditions, careful exclusion of other etiologies is critically important. Examination of the skin, abdomen, eyes, and pulse rate may help to distinguish an anticholinergic toxidrome (dry skin, decreased bowel sounds, urinary retention, mydriasis, tachycardia) from a sympathomimetic toxidrome (moist skin, normal bowel sounds, no urinary retention, mydriasis, tachycardia).

Sedative–hypnotic withdrawal may be particularly difficult to distinguish from an underlying anxiety disorder. Differentiating withdrawal seizures from other types of seizures may also be difficult. Other common causes include preexisting idiopathic epilepsy, posttraumatic epilepsy, and other complications of drug abuse (e.g., hypoglycemia, hypomagnesemia, hyponatremia, head trauma). Poor anticonvulsant compliance with underlying seizure disorders may add to the diagnostic confusion. In the setting of baclofen use, a seizure could result from either overdose or withdrawal.

Opioid withdrawal must be distinguished from ethanol and other sedative–hypnotic withdrawal because of the significant differences in therapy. Symptoms of significant sedative–hypnotic withdrawal, such as confusion, agitation, and seizures, are not generally seen with opioid withdrawal; opioid withdrawal symptoms such as piloerection, yawning, lacrimation, and rhinorrhea are not seen with ethanol and sedative–hypnotic withdrawal. Some patients, however, may be withdrawing from both substances. Gastrointestinal (GI) manifestations of opioid withdrawal must be differentiated from other causes of gastroenteritis.

EMERGENCY DEPARTMENT EVALUATION

Patients presenting with drug withdrawal require a comprehensive assessment. All patients initially should have cardiac monitoring. A fingerstick glucose and oxygen saturation analysis should also be performed. The physician must obtain a complete history of substance abuse, previous withdrawal episodes, and all current and former medications. If possible, family, friends, and prehospital personnel are interviewed to gain additional information.

Physical examination should focus on vital signs, including rectal temperature, cardiovascular, neurological, and pulmonary systems, the skin, abdomen, and eyes. Close attention should be directed to any stigmata of chronic liver disease or evidence of i.v. drug use. A full assessment for obvious and occult traumatic injury should be done. Patients should also be evaluated for other complications of drug abuse, such as pneumonia, skin abscesses, bacterial endocarditis, acquired immunodeficiency syndrome, pancreatitis, liver disease, and GI bleeding.

Laboratory studies should include a complete blood count; measurement of electrolytes, glucose, blood urea nitrogen, and creatinine levels; liver function tests; coagulation profile; and ethanol level. A urine drug screen may be positive or negative for the offending agent. Screening urine drug screens using immunoassays techniques may not detect synthetic opioids such

TABLE 333.2. Differential Diagnosis of Major Withdrawal Symptoms

Tremor	Seizures	Hallucinations	Delirium
Withdrawal	**Withdrawal**	**Withdrawal**	**Withdrawal**
Ethanol	Ethanol	Ethanol	Ethanol
Sedative–hypnotics	Sedative–hypnotics	Sedative–hypnotics	Sedative–hypnotics
Intoxications	**Intoxications**	**Intoxications**	**Intoxications**
Theophylline	Cocaine	LSD	Cocaine
Caffeine	Anticholinergics	Mescaline	Amphetamine
β agonists	Phenothiazines	Mushrooms	Phencyclidine
Mercury	TCAs	Peyote	Anticholinergics
Lithium	Theophylline	Phencyclidine	LSD
TCAs	Camphor	Anticholinergics	**Infectious**
Phenytoin	Isoniazid	Ergot	Meningitis
Metabolic	Phencyclidine	Nutmeg	Encephalitis
Hypoglycemia	Lidocaine	**Infectious**	Sepsis
Thyrotoxicosis	Organophosphates	Meningitis	**Metabolic**
Structural	**Infectious**	Encephalitis	Thyrotoxicosis
Cerebellar disease	Meningitis	Sepsis	Hypoglycemia
Other	Encephalitis	**Metabolic**	Hyperglycemia
Parkinsonism	**Metabolic**	Hypoglycemia	Hypocalcemia
	Hypoglycemia	Hypoxia	Hypoxia
	Hypoxia	**Structural**	Thiamine deficiency
	Hypothyroidism	CNS hemorrhage	**Structural**
	Thyrotoxicosis	Tumor	Head trauma
	Hypocalcemia	**Psychiatric**	CNS hemorrhage
	Hyperosmolar state	Schizophrenia	Tumor
	Hepatic failure	Bipolar disorder	Psychiatric
	Uremia	**Other**	**Other**
	Structural	Seizures	Seizures
	Head trauma	Heat-related illness	Heat-related illness
	CNS hemorrhage		
	Tumor		
	CVA		
	Other		
	Idiopathic epilepsy		
	Posttraumatic epilepsy		
	Degenerative disease		

as methadone or propoxyphene. In patients with significant agitation, a creatine phosphokinase determination may help detect rhabdomyolysis.

An elevated temperature requires a full sepsis workup, including urine and blood cultures, chest radiograph, and, often, a lumbar puncture. Obtaining a head computed tomography scan before lumbar puncture is critical in patients presenting with either focal neurologic deficits or high risk for intracranial hemorrhage. Patients with a first-time seizure in the setting of withdrawal should be evaluated the same as any other patient with a new seizure (see Chapter 231, "Seizures"). Subsequent withdrawal seizures do not usually require extensive reevaluation unless there are extenuating circumstances.

EMERGENCY DEPARTMENT MANAGEMENT

Drug withdrawal syndromes, particularly sedative–hypnotic withdrawal must be recognized and treated in a timely fashion because early treatment can prevent withdrawal from progressing to a more serious stage. A successful treatment strategy must address several basic goals: alleviating symptoms, preventing progression, avoiding complications, and recognizing and treating coexisting medical problems. Planning for long-term rehabilitation and drug independence is usually better done as part of inpatient management.

Initial treatment should be directed at readily correctable causes of altered mental status. Oxygen should be given if the oxygen saturation is low, and an i.v. line should be established. Glucose and thiamine should be administered if there is evidence of hypoglycemia and malnutrition respectively. Volume resuscitation is often necessary, particularly in patients with severe withdrawal manifestations and dehydration.

Significantly agitated patients may initially need to be physically restrained to prevent injury, establish intravenous access, and facilitate sedation. Soft restraints should be used. Prolonged use of restraints is discouraged, because continued struggling against them may lead to rhabdomyolysis, hyperthermia, and metabolic acidosis. Once i.v. access is obtained and chemical sedation has achieved behavioral control, physical restraints should be discontinued.

Achieving adequate sedation is the cornerstone of successful treatment of sedative–hypnotic withdrawal. It may prevent progression to a severe agitated delirium state with its attendant complications. Reinstitution of therapy with the withdrawn drug or a cross-tolerant one is required to achieve proper sedation. Many agents have been used over the years, but benzodiazepines have proven to be the most effective. Compared with other sedative–hypnotic agents, benzodiazepines are safer and produce less respiratory depression. Their dosage is easier to titrate and the effects are more predictable.

Diazepam (Valium), chlordiazepoxide (Librium), and lorazepam (Ativan) are the most commonly used agents for ethanol withdrawal and can also be used for sedative–hypnotic withdrawal. These agents are preferred over benzodiazepines with shorter half-lives, which require frequent dosing, because they allow gradual drug elimination over several days. Compared with short-acting agents, long-acting agents may be more effective in preventing withdrawal seizures and contribute to smoother withdrawal with fewer rebound symptoms (13). Active metabolites of diazepam and chlordiazepoxide prolong their therapeutic effect. In elderly patients and those with hepatic dysfunction, lorazepam, which has no active metabolites, may be preferred. In other cases, lorazepam does not appear to offer any distinct advantage over diazepam or chlordiazepoxide.

Intravenous dosing is preferred in all but the mildest cases of sedative–hypnotic withdrawal: Agitation may preclude oral administration, and gastrointestinal dysfunction may impair drug absorption. Intravenous therapy can be readily titrated. Lorazepam (but not diazepam or chlordiazepoxide) is predictably absorbed intramuscularly. This route may be useful in the wildly agitated patient before intravenous access is established.

The dose of benzodiazepines required to achieve proper sedation must be individualized and varies considerably, depending on the patient's tolerance to the drug. Symptom-triggered therapy is as efficacious as fixed-schedule therapy and decreases both the amount of benzodiazepine used and treatment duration. Frequent i.v. boluses should be given until the patient has achieved a restful state. When using diazepam, 5 to 20 mg can be given every 5 to 15 minutes until the patient is sleepy but arousable. Usually, sedation is obtained before respiratory depression develops, but close airway observation is always required.

Failure to obtain immediate sedation need not prompt switching to an alternative agent. Mixing different drugs or different routes of administration may increase the risk of adverse effects, particularly respiratory depression. However, if a patient does not respond completely to the chosen benzodiazepine, the use of another cross-tolerant agent may be valuable. Intermediate-acting or long-acting barbiturates such as pentobarbital, secobarbital, or phenobarbital are recommended in these situations. Doses of 100 mg of pentobarbital may be given intravenously every 5 to 10 minutes until sufficient sedation is achieved or a total dose of 600 mg is given.

Phenobarbital may also be used, although its onset of action may be delayed. Phenobarbital's long duration of effect, however, requires less frequent dosing and allows gradual self-tapering. Phenobarbital may be particularly helpful in withdrawal patients with idiopathic or posttraumatic epilepsy who require maintenance anticonvulsant levels. The barbiturates are more likely to cause excessive sedation and respiratory depression.

The use of midazolam (a short-acting benzodiazepine) by continuous i.v. infusion has been suggested to treat for withdrawal. This approach, however, requires more vigilant monitoring, especially in the patient who is not intubated, and does not provide the advantages of a long-acting agent. Propofol infusion has been used for refractory delirium tremens in ethanol withdrawal and should be also considered for refractory sedative–hypnotic withdrawal (14).

Withdrawal seizures should also be treated with benzodiazepines or barbiturates. Phenytoin is ineffective in treating or preventing withdrawal seizures. It should be reserved for patients with a history of an underlying chronic seizure disorder who require maintenance phenytoin therapy.

Neuroleptics such as the phenothiazines and butyrophenones (e.g., haloperidol) should never be used as monotherapy in the treatment of sedative–hypnotic withdrawal. Although sometimes used for severe agitation, these neuroleptics are not cross-tolerant with ethanol or sedative–hypnotics and do not prevent or suppress withdrawal. Hypotension, impaired thermoregulation, a lowered seizure threshold, and dystonic reactions may result from their use (1,8). Uncontrolled clinical experience suggests that neuroleptics may be considered as adjunctive therapy for patients with refractory agitation and hallucinations (13). They may also be useful in treating concomitant nausea, vomiting, and GI cramps.

Sympatholytic therapy with β blockers (e.g., propranolol) and central adrenergic agonists (e.g., clonidine) has been used for sedative–hypnotic withdrawal, but these agents have drawbacks. Sympatholytics are not cross-tolerant with sedative–hypnotics and do not prevent agitation, confusion, or seizures. Their ability to normalize vital signs may mask a deteriorating clinical situation.

Once withdrawal is controlled, the dose of sedative–hypnotic should be gradually reduced over a period of 3 weeks to 3 months, depending on the dosage and duration of prior use. In order to avoid precipitating another episode of withdrawal, the dose should be generally be tapered by no more than 10% a day, or 25% every 3 days.

The approach to GHB withdrawal is similar to other sedative–hypnotic withdrawal. Severe cases are often resistant to benzodiazepine treatment and require barbiturates or propofol. Neuroleptics should be avoided if possible (2).

Reinstitution of baclofen is the initial therapy in the management of baclofen withdrawal. For patients exhibiting symptoms and signs of more significant withdrawal, high-dose benzodiazepine treatment given intravenously may be required (3). For patients refractory to benzodiazepines, dantrolene (for muscle relaxation) and cyproheptadine have also been recommended, although such approach have not been subject to clinical trials (3,16).

For acute opioid withdrawal, clonidine may offer symptomatic relief because it decreases sympathetic activity in the locus ceruleus. An initial oral dose of 0.1 to 0.2 mg is recommended. Because hypotension may be particularly problematic after the first dose, the blood pressure should be monitored for 2 hours while the patient remains in the emergency department. A dose of 0.1 to 0.2 mg every 4 to 6 hours may help prevent recurrence of opioid withdrawal symptoms (5). Nonspecific sedation with benzodiazepines is also an option.

For patients who will be hospitalized with other medical problems, methadone may be given to relieve the symptoms of significant opioid withdrawal (6). A dose of 5 to 25 mg intramuscularly or orally blocks most manifestations of physiologic withdrawal. Parenteral administration guarantees absorption in the vomiting patient. Symptomatic improvement usually occurs within 30 to 60 minutes. Daily maintenance doses average 50 mg and range from 25 to more than 150 mg. Shorter-acting opioids such as morphine or meperidine are not recommended.

The implementation of a detoxification program is generally not initiated in the ED and requires referral to an appropriate facility. Federal regulations restrict the use of methadone to Food and Drug Administration–designated programs. Although this legislation does not prohibit the use of methadone in opioid addicts who are admitted for other reasons, unless the facility has an approved treatment program, the use of methadone solely for the treatment of opioid withdrawal is prohibited. Similarly, legislation prohibits prescribing methadone for the outpatient treatment of withdrawal without a specific license.

Buprenorphine, a partial μ-opioid agonist has recently been approved for treatment of opioid dependence (12). Similar to methadone, buprenorphine suppresses opioid withdrawal symptoms and decreases use of illicit drugs. It is used both to manage heroin withdrawal and detoxification as well as to prevent relapse in maintenance therapy. However, unlike methadone, it can be prescribed and dispensed without specific licensing because it has less potential for abuse and is less dangerous in overdose. Nonetheless, respiratory depression and deaths from buprenorphine has been reported (18).

Rapid and ultrarapid opioid detoxification followed by naltrexone maintenance therapy have also been used in recent years (19). These controversial techniques utilize antagonist-precipitated opioid withdrawal as a quick "cure" for opioid dependence. Complications include persistent withdrawal symptoms, pulmonary edema, and death (10).

Reinstitution of drug therapy and gradual tapering of the dose is recommended for antidepressant withdrawal. Benzo-

diazepines can be used for signs and symptoms of adrenergic hyperactivity. The treatment of cocaine withdrawal is supportive.

DISPOSITION

Patients with moderate-to-severe sedative–hypnotic withdrawal should be admitted. Because withdrawal usually persists for several days, admitted patients should be closely monitored for signs of progression and treated as necessary. The level of care necessary depends on clinical severity. Because of potential complications, patients requiring i.v. sedation are best managed in an intensive or intermediate care unit. Patients with less severe withdrawal may be managed and observed on a medical floor, psychiatric floor, hospital-based detoxification unit, or detoxification unit outside of the hospital. Patients with mild withdrawal may also need to be admitted for the evaluation and treatment of concomitant medical problems that have not been adequately addressed in the past as a result of poor use of outpatient services. The inpatient setting also provides a protected environment away from the temptations of illicit drug use.

Outpatient management should be attempted only if the patient can be discharged home with a supportive family member or friend and appropriate outpatient follow-up can be arranged. Supervised withdrawal in the home setting, under the direction of a visiting nurse, may be appropriate in some of these circumstances.

Patients who present to the emergency department with opiate withdrawal may be discharged home if they do not have other concomitant medical problems that require hospital admission and they can tolerate oral fluids. Offering the patient a limited supply of clonidine (if tolerated in the emergency department) may help prevent further withdrawal symptoms. Prescriptions for opioids should not be given. Referral to a detoxification program is strongly recommended.

Social service, detoxification, or substance-abuse counseling and psychiatric referrals should be offered to all patients with a history of substance abuse.

CRITICAL INTERVENTIONS

- Administer diazepam or other long-acting benzodiazepine to patients with sedative–hypnotic withdrawal; administer barbiturates and propofol for refractory cases
- Administer clonidine and buprenorphine to patients with isolated opioid withdrawal
- Administer methadone to patients with opioid withdrawal who have other conditions that require admission or treatment
---

COMMON PITFALLS

✔ Failure to consider the possibility of drug withdrawal in all patients with signs and symptoms of adrenergic hyperactivity
✔ Failure to appreciate that sedative–hypnotic withdrawal is potentially life-threatening, whereas opioid withdrawal, although bothersome, does not usually cause significant morbidity
✔ Failure to appreciate that neuroleptics do not cross-react with sedative-hypnotics and are not indicated as the primary treatment of sedative–hypnotic withdrawal
✔ Failure to appreciate that GHB withdrawal may begin within hours of the last dose and be relatively resistant to treatment

✔ Failure to appreciate that baclofen withdrawal may occur in the setting of intrathecal baclofen pump dysfunction

References

1. Bobolakis I. Neuroleptic malignant syndrome after antipsychotic drug administration during benzodiazepine withdrawal. *J Clin Psychopharmacol* 2000;20:281–283.
2. Bowles TM, Sommi RW, Amiri M. Successful management of prolonged gamma-hydroxybutyrate and alcohol withdrawal. *Pharmacotherapy* 2001;21:254–257.
3. Coffey RJ, Edgar TS, Francisco GE, et al. Abrupt withdrawal from intrathecal baclofen: recognition and management of a potentially life-threatening syndrome. *Arch Physical Med Rehab* 2002;83:735–741.
4. Dyer JE, Roth B, Hyma BA. Gamma-hydroxybutyrate withdrawal syndrome. *Ann Emerg Med* 2001;37:147–153.
5. Freitas PM. Narcotic withdrawal in the emergency department. *Am J Emerg Med* 1985;3:456–460.
6. Fultz JM, Senay EC. Guidelines for the management of hospitalized narcotics addicts. *Ann Intern Med* 1975;82:815–818.
7. Greenberg MI, Hendrickson RG. Baclofen withdrawal following removal of an intrathecal baclofen pump despite oral baclofen replacement. *J Toxicol Clin Toxicol* 2003;41:83–85.
8. Greenblatt DJ, Gross PL, Harris J, Shader RI, Ciraulo DA. Fatal hyperthermia following haloperidol therapy of sedative-hypnotic withdrawal. *J Clin Psychiatry* 1978;39:673–675.
9. Haddad P. Newer antidepressants and the discontinuation syndrome. *J Clin Psychiatry* 1997.
10. Hamilton RJ, Olmedo RE, Shah S, et al. Complications of ultrarapid opioid detoxification with subcutaneous naltrexone pellets. *Acad Emerg Med* 2002;9:63–68.
11. Lejoyeux M, Ades J. Antidepressant discontinuation: a review of the literature. *J Clin Psychiatry* 1997.
12. Lintzeris N, Bell J, Bammer G, et al. A randomized controlled trial of buprenorphine in the management of short-term ambulatory heroin withdrawal. *Addiction* 2002;97:1395–1404.
13. Mayo-Smith MF. Pharmacological management of alcohol withdrawal: a meta-analysis and evidence-based practice guideline. American Society of Addiction Medicine Working Group on Pharmacological Management of Alcohol Withdrawal. *JAMA* 1997;278:144–151.
14. McCowan C, Marik P. Refractory delirium tremens treated with propofol: a case series. *Crit Care Med* 2000;28:1781–1784.
15. McDaniel CH, Miotto KA. Gamma hydroxybutyrate (GHB) and gamma butyrolactone (GBL) withdrawal: five case studies. *J Psychoactive Drugs* 2001;33:143–149.
16. Meythaler JM, Roper JF, Brunner RC. Cyproheptadine for intrathecal baclofen withdrawal. *Arch Physical Med Rehab* 2003;84:638–642.
17. Miotto K, Darakjian J, Basch J, et al. Gamma-hydroxybutyric acid: patterns of use, effects and withdrawal. *Am J Addict* 2001;10:232–241.
18. O'Connor PG, Fiellin DA. Pharmacologic treatment of heroin-dependent patients. *Ann Intern Med* 2000;133:40–54.
19. O'Connor PG, Kosten TR. Rapid and ultrarapid opioid detoxification techniques. *JAMA* 1998;279:229–234.
20. Petursson H. The benzodiazepine withdrawal syndrome. *Addiction* 1994;89:1455–1459.
21. Samson-Fang L, Gooch J, Norlin C. Intrathecal baclofen withdrawal simulating neuroepileptic malignant syndrome in a child with cerebral palsy. *Develop Med Child Neurol* 2000;42:561–565.
22. Smolka M, Schmidt LG. The influence of heroin dose and route of administration on the severity of the opiate withdrawal syndrome. *Addiction* 1999;94:1191–1198.
23. Tsuda M, Shimizu N, Suzuki T. Contribution of glutamate receptors to benzodiazepine withdrawal signs. *Jpn J Pharmacol* 1999;81:1–6.

CHAPTER 334
Food Poisoning

Marc C. Restuccia

Despite improvements in detection of food-borne illnesses and increased regulatory oversight, food-borne illness remains a serious cause of morbidity and mortality throughout the world, including the United States. With the growth in modern mass production farms, importation of foods from countries that may or may not have strict controls for the handling of foods and the steady growth of immense food handling and processing plants, the potential for amplification of food-borne pathogens is great. As a result of concerns that terrorists could contaminate either food or water supplies, Congress enacted the Public Health Security and Bioterrorism Preparedness and Response Act of 2002. The Food and Drug Administration (FDA) was charged with developing guidelines to insure the safety of food produced in this country and imported from outside American borders.

Food-borne illness is common but the exact incidence of is not accurately known (6). Each year, millions of people are affected worldwide (4). Although the majority of persons suffer only temporary discomfort, for the very young, old, and immunocompromised, it can be fatal. In the United States, 76 million persons suffer food-borne illnesses every year resulting in about approximately 5,000 deaths (2).

Improper food handling, leading to fecal contamination of food is the usual cause of most food-borne illnesses. Causative agents include bacteria, viruses, parasites, and toxins. More recently, prions, a new infectious class of agents have been implicated in causing transmissible spongiform encephalopathies (TSEs) (7). Prion-infected beef cattle, found in the United Kingdom and more recently in the United States, have severely disrupted the cattle industry in both countries, with other nations banning the import of British and American beef.

Bacterial food poisoning can be characterized as toxin-induced or invasive. Toxins cause diarrhea by disrupting intestinal sodium absorption in the small intestine. This leads to large amounts of salt and water being presented to the large intestine, which has limited absorptive capacity, and consequent watery diarrhea. Invasive bacteria on the other hand, invade or destroy the mucosal layer of the intestine, leading to inflammatory diarrhea, which contains blood and leukocytes.

CLINICAL PRESENTATION

Alteration of normal gastrointestinal tract function is the hallmark of food poisoning. Almost all types present with similar complaints which include some or all of the following: nausea, vomiting, diarrhea, and abdominal pain. The central nervous system (CNS), the liver and the musculoskeletal system may also be involved (see Tables 334.1 and 334.2). Abdominal pain in food poisoning is most often characterized as colicky, but can be quite severe. Patients with *Salmonella* food poisoning will occasionally present with marked abdominal pain, even peritoneal signs. Pain from *Yersinia* infections can mimic appendicitis.

Fever and dehydration are often present. Signs and symptoms of dehydration include thirst, dry skin and mucous membranes, lethargy, weakness, tachycardia, hypotension, decreased urine

TABLE 334.1. Bacterial Causes of Food Poisoning[a]

Agent	Incubation	Duration	Common Food Sources	Manifestations	Treatment
Bacillus anthracis*	2 d to weeks	Weeks	Insufficiently cooked and contaminated meat	Nausea, vomiting, malaise, bloody diarrhea Acute abdominal pain	PCN,I^st Cipro, 2nd
Bacillus cereus Vomiting	3 h	12 h	Spices and grains such as rice, especially	Fried rice ingestion	Supportive
Diarrhea (Toxin)	10 h	36 h	if inadequate refrigeration	(−) fecal leukocytes	
Campylobacter jejuni	3 d	4 d	unpasteurized milk, dairy products	abdominal pain, fever, diarrhea, biphasic illness (+) fecal leukocytes	FQ, AG, macrolides
Clostridium botulinum (toxin)	30 h	Variable	Improper home canning, unpasteurized honey	Flu-like symptoms, descending weakness or paralysis, ptosis paralysis, may have no GI symptoms	Supportive (horse serum antitoxin)
Clostridium perfringens	12 h	24 h	Meat, meat by-products, poultry (cooked but inadequately refrigerated)	Nonbloody diarrhea (−) fecal leukocytes	Supportive
Cryptosporidium	6 d	6 d	Hand pressed cider, municipal water supplies, public pools	Vomiting, diarrhea, worse if immunocompromised	Supportive
Escherichia coli 0157:H7 (toxin)	48 h	1 wk	Raw or undercooked beef Fast food restaurants	Copious bloody diarrhea, (+) fecal leukocytes, rarely HUS, renal failure	Supportive
Traveler's diarrhea enterotoxigenic (toxin)	12–72 h	24–72 h	Raw vegetables, seafood, improperly cooked food from street vendors, hot pepper sauce, tap water	Watery diarrhea, low-grade fever,(−) fecal leukocytes	Prophylaxis with Bismuth subsalicylate TMS, FQ, treat with FQ, TMS + antidiarrheal(s)
Enteroinvasive (invasive)	12–72 h	24–72 h	Similar to above	Severe cramps, malaise initially watery, then bloody diarrhea, (+) fecal leukocytes	FQ, TMS
Listeria monocytogenes	1–70 d	Variable	Beef, pork, poultry, cheese, (soft, "Mexican style," Swiss) milk, contaminated after pasteurization fruits and vegetables, other dairy products	More severe in pregnancy immunocompromised, usually + fever, may have limited GI symptoms	Ampicillin, TMS, Chloramphenicol
Salmonella (invasive)	24 h	5 d	Dairy products, poultry, eggs, chocolate, coconut, dried foods	Watery, bloody diarrhea, (+/−) fecal leukocytes, possible, possible bacteremia	Immunocomp. Pts. septic pts., Rx with RMS, ceftriaxone FQ, chloramphenicol
Shigella (invasive)	1–3 d	5 d	Any food contaminated with fecal material during processing, ice in developing countries	Copious bloody diarrhea, fever, cramps, rarely; DIC, HUS, sepsis, children may have seizures, usually (+) fecal leukocytes	TMS or FQ
Staphylococcus aureus (toxin)	4 h	20 h	Milk and dairy products, ham, potato salad, custards, pastry	Vomiting, cramps, diarrhea, usually no fever	Supportive
Streptococcus (invasive)	1–3 d	3–5 d	Salads, meats, inadequately refrigerated, fried, boiled rice	Viral type syndrome, pharyngitis, myalgia, fever, chills	Penicillin
Vibrio b Cholerae	24–72 h	3–7 d	Profuse, watery diarrhea and vomiting, can lead to death from severe dehydration	contaminated water, fish, shellfish, street vended food typically Latin America or Asia	Supportive care, rehydr. tetracycline, doxycycline adults, TMS if <8yrs.
Para hemolyticus	2–48 h	2–5 d	Watery diarrhea, abdominal cramps, nausea, vomiting	Undercooked or raw seafood, such as fish, shellfish	Supportive care, in severe cases, TCN, DCN, Gentamicin or cefotaxime
Vulnificus	1–7 d	2–8 d	vomiting, diarrhea, abdominal pain, bacteremia, wound infections, more common if immunocompromised	Undercooked or raw shellfish, especially oysters, other seafood, open wounds	Supportive care, TCN, DCN, ceftazidime
Yersinia enterocolitica	15–24 h	2 wk	Foods contaminated with fecal material during handling (e.g., tofu, bean sprouts, milk, milk products, water supply)	Diarrhea, fever, abdominal pain, vomiting, bloody stools, may be protracted, can lead to appendicitis operations (+) or (−) fecal leukocytes	Antibiotics of value FQ, TMS, AG

[a]AG, aminoglycosides; DIC, disseminated intravascular coagulation; FQ, fluoroquinolones; HUS, hemolytic uremic syndrome; TMS, trimethoprim-sulfamethoxazole; TCN, tetracycline; DCN, doxycycline.
[b]From Diagnosis and management of foodborne illness; a primer for physicians and other health care professionals. MMWR, 2004

TABLE 334.2. Selected Nonbacterial Causes of Food Poisoning[a]

Agent	Incubation	Duration	Common Food Sources	Manifestations	Treatment
Viral					
Norovirus	1–2 d	12–60 h	Undercooked shellfish	Nausea, vomiting, diarrhea	Supportive
Hepatitis A	15–50 d	Wks to mo	Produce, undercooked shellfish, food contaminated during processing or handling	Hepatitis	Vaccine available
Parasitic					
Cryptosporidium parvum	2–10 d	Weeks	Contaminated produce, water	Nausea, vomiting, diarrhea	Supportive
Cyclospora Cayetanensis	1–11 d	Weeks	Contaminated produce, water	Nausea, vomiting, diarrhea	Supportive
Giardia lamblia	1–4 weeks	Weeks	Contaminated water	Nausea, vomiting, diarrhea, Asymptomatic, cysticercosis	Metronidazole
Taenia solium	Variable	Variable	Raw or undercooked pork (especially in immigrants)	Nausea, vomiting, intestinal obstruction, non-GI infection	Praziquantel[a] Albendazole[b]
Toxoplasma gondii	5–23 d	Months	Food contaminated with cat feces, undercooked meat	Influenza-like illness, lymphadenopathy	Pyrimethamine

[a]Adult infection in the intestine
[b]Larval, non-GI infection
[c]From Acheson, Fiore. Preventing foodborne disease—what clinicians can do, *NEJM*. 2004;350(5):437–440, with permission.

output and serum bicarbonate, and increased blood area nitrogen (BUN), creatinine, and hematocrit.

Except with *Shigella*, the mental status remains normal. Complications include bacteremia, septic complications (arthritis, meningitis), disseminated intravascular coagulation, hemolytic-uremic syndrome, and renal failure (Table 334.1).

DIFFERENTIAL DIAGNOSIS

Food-borne illness is usually a clinical diagnosis. Only in multiperson outbreaks is the diagnosis reasonable certain and the cause typically confirmed. Clues to the etiology include the time from ingestion to onset of symptoms (incubation period), type of food (source), and the nature, severity and duration of illness (Tables 334.1 and 334.2) (3,4). Toxin-producing organisms such as enterotoxigenic *E. coli*, *Staphylococcus aureus*, and *Vibrio cholera* often cause profuse watery diarrhea, with symptoms beginning within hours after ingestion. Other causes of watery diarrhea include *Cryptosporidium*, *Cyclospora*, and *Giardia*, but diarrhea begins weeks after exposure to these agents. *Giardia lamblia* is common among hikers, campers, and travelers who are infected through drinking contaminated water. Other parasites such as *Entamoeba histolytica*, *Cryptosporidium*, and *Isospora belli* are seen in male homosexuals or those with HIV infection. Watery diarrhea is also typical in viral gastroenteritis.

In contrast, invasive bacteria (e.g., nonenterotoxigenic *E. coli*, *Campylobacter*, *Salmonella*, *Shigella*, *Yersinia*, and *Vibrio*) tend to cause bloody diarrhea, which contains leukocytes and begins 24 hours or more following ingestion. *Entamoeba histolytica* can also cause bloody diarrhea. Blood loss can be significant with *Salmonella*. Overgrowth of *Clostridium difficile* can cause pseudomembranous colitis with bloody diarrhea, severe abdominal pain, and toxic megacolon in persons taking wide spectrum antibiotics.

Viral gastroenteritis is the most common cause of nausea, vomiting, and diarrhea. Rotavirus infection usually occurs in the winter. Other viruses (e.g., adenovirus, astrovirus, Norwalk, or norovirus and other caliciviviruses, Hepatitis A, parvovirus) have no seasonal predilection. Vomiting is usually more prominent in viral gastroenteritis and toxin-related food poisoning

(e.g., *Bacillus cereus*, *Staphylococcus aureus*) than in other types of food poisoning, in which diarrhea is the predominant symptom.

Contamination of food with pesticides or chemicals can also lead to food-borne illness (1). Other conditions to consider in the differential diagnosis include food intolerance/allergies, biliary tract disease, appendicitis, diverticulitis, inflammatory bowel disease, irritable bowel disease, peptic ulcer disease, urinary tract infection, acute coronary syndromes, gynecologic disorders, and poisoning by heavy metals, mushrooms, organophosphate and carbamate insecticides, and seafood toxins (see Chapter 340, "Seafood Toxins").

EMERGENCY DEPARTMENT EVALUATION

The history should focus on recent meals (out to 2–3 days if possible), what foods were consumed, how were they prepared, in what manner was it kept after being prepared, who else ate the food and their current health. The time of onset, nature and progression of the illness, particularly the character of the diarrhea, should be noted. Patients should be asked about recent travel (especially to regions known for having a high incidence of food-borne infections such as Mexico), camping or hiking, and antibiotic use. Campers and hikers should be questioned about drinking water sources and what measures were taken to make it "safe" (boiling, disinfecting, or filtering of the water). Underlying medical conditions, particularly HIV, sickle cell disease, malignancy, diabetes, cardiac or renal disorders, and immunodeficiency states (including history of organ transplants), should be asked about and documented.

The physical exam should focus on the vital signs, abdomen, and assessment for dehydration. Patients with severe abdominal pain, significant tenderness, or bloody stool should have a rectal exam. Serial exams and vital signs are imperative to insure that any clinical deterioration in the patient is detected quickly.

The extent of the laboratory evaluation will vary from patient to patient. A white blood cell count will not usually be helpful. Although a high white blood cell suggests an inflammatory process, it does little to narrow the possible causes. On the other hand, a hematocrit and hemoglobin may be useful, if followed serially in patients with bloody diarrhea. In the patient who appears well-hydrated, routine chemistries are unlikely to detect significant abnormalities. Patients with significant dehydration, particularly those at extremes of age and who have underlying medical problems, should have serum electrolytes, BUN, creatinine, blood sugar and urinalysis measurements. A urine specific gravity greater than 1.025 or a BUN/creatinine ratio more than 20:1 are consistent with severe dehydration. Likewise, serum bicarbonate below 20mEq/l is consistent with significant dehydration, particularly in children.

Patients with marked abdominal pain or tenderness or a high fever may require more extensive evaluation. Consideration should be given to obtaining liver function tests, a lipase, a complete blood count, bilirubin, and blood cultures. All woman of childbearing age should be tested for pregnancy. In the elderly, infants, and patients with a history of intraabdominal surgery, upright views of the abdomen and chest are indicated to rule out perforation or obstruction. In the elderly, consideration should also be given to abdominal computed tomography imaging, with oral or rectal contrast. In patients with risk factors for or a coronary artery disease, or have a history of heart disease, an ECG and cardiac enzymes may be warranted. In patients who are acutely ill, particularly those with blood in the stool, it may be helpful to send a stool specimen for bacterial culture or toxin assay (e.g., *C. difficile*). Routine stool cultures usually only detect Campylobacter, Salmonella, and Shigella. Other bacteria (e.g., *Bacillus cereus, E. coli, Vibrio* and *Yersinia* species) require special growth media and consultation with laboratory personnel or requesting a specific testing is necessary if one of these agents is suspected. In patients with weeks or months of diarrhea, sending a specimen for ova and parasites is appropriate.

EMERGENCY DEPARTMENT MANAGEMENT

The first priority in treating a patient with suspected food poisoning is to replace fluid and electrolyte losses. Rehydration therapy should be instituted during the evaluation of the patient.

In the mild or moderately ill patient, who is not vomiting and can take fluids by mouth, oral rehydration is acceptable. Examples of acceptable oral replacement formulas include "Sport Drinks" (Gatorade and others, usually diluted with water) or the WHO Rehydration Formula are acceptable. Intravenous access for fluid resuscitation and to obtain blood samples for laboratory evaluation will often be required. Intravenous crystalloid, either Lactated Ringers or Normal Saline, with or without 5% dextrose, is indicated for the moderately to severely ill patient especially if they continue to vomit and/or are seriously dehydrated. The initial bolus should be from 5 to 20 cc/kg depending on the patient's age, cardiovascular status, and degree of dehydration. A maintenance infusion should be initiated and further boluses tailored to the patient's clinical response to treatment. The adequacy of the resuscitation can be judged by subjective response, appearance, urinary output, vital signs, and improvement in lab parameters.

Intravenous, intramuscular, or rectal antiemetics (prochlorperazine or metoclopramide) may be helpful in patients with persistent nausea, vomiting, and abdominal cramping. Although antidiarrheal drugs, (e.g., diphenoxylate [Lomotil] or Loperamide [Imodium]) have traditionally been held to be contraindicated in the treatment of food poisoning, in some situations, such as Traveler's Diarrhea, there use may speed recovery (8). However; in patients with bloody diarrhea they are not appropriate. Their use can prolong symptoms (e.g., with *Shigella*), cause perforation, (with amebiasis) and increase mortality (e.g., with *Campylobacter*).

Additional treatment depends on the cause (Tables 334.1 and 334.2). Antibiotics are usually not indicated. Diarrhea caused by viruses and many bacteria do not improve more rapidly when given antibiotics. Some organisms, such as *Salmonella* may have prolonged colonic colonization when antibiotics are used. In patients who are septic, immunosuppressed, HIV positive, are elderly or have other coexistent, antibiotics may be appropriate.

DISPOSITION

Most patients can be discharged once they are rehydrated and are feeling better. The ability to take fluids orally should be documented before discharge. These patients should be instructed to maintain a generous intake of clear fluids and begin frequent small feedings as soon as tolerated. They should be advised to return to the emergency department or to contact their personal physician if symptoms have not abated by 24 hours or sooner if they cannot maintain a sufficient oral intake, develop a high fever or if abdominal pain persists or worsens. Patients with severe dehydration, suspected bacteremia (e.g., fever, elevated white count, or toxic appearance), and those who do not improve with therapy should be admitted, especially those with significant underlying illness or extremes of age. Likewise, patients in whom the diagnosis is in doubt, those who may not be able to seek further medical care because of social circumstances, or those who cannot tolerate oral intake should be admitted. For most patients needing admission, a floor bed or observation unit will suffice. Occasionally a patient with severe dehydration or underlying disease may require a higher level of care.

Local or State Department(s) of Public Health should be contacted if the suspected food was bought at a store or restaurant and other members of the public may be at risk. This can limit the number of people who will become ill (6). Diagnoses requiring Centers for Disease Control and Prevention (CDC) notification are listed in Table 334.3 (5). State and territorial laws may mandate additional reporting. For information in this regard, contact the Council of State and Territorial Epidemiologists (770-458-3811; http://www.cste.org/reporting%20requirements.htm).

COMMON PITFALLS

✔ Failure to consider the possibility of food poisoning in all patients with nausea, vomiting, diarrhea, and abdominal pain
✔ Failure to obtain a history of antecedent antibiotic use, travel, camping, and diet in patients with nausea, vomiting, diarrhea, and abdominal pain
✔ Failure to consider other causes of abdominal complaints, such as appendicitis, aortic aneurysm, pyelonephritis, cholecystitis, pneumonia, myocardial disease, and pregnancy
✔ Failure to consider the effects of underlying diseases in the management of patients with suspected food poisoning

TABLE 334.3. Foodborne Diseases and Conditions Designated as Notifiable at the National Level, United States, 2000

Bacterial	Viral	Parasitic
Botulism	Hepatitis A	Cryptosporidiosis
Brucellosis		Cyclosporiasis
Cholera		Trichinosis
Escherichia coli 0157-H7		
Hemolytic uremic syndrome, postdiarrheal		
Salmonellosis		
Shigellosis		
Typhoid Fever		

✔ Discharging patients who cannot take oral fluids, especially if they have not been adequately rehydrated

✔ Failure to consider potential public health hazards and to notify public health authorities when appropriate

References

1. Poisonings associated with illegal use of aldicarb as a rodenticide—New York City, 1994–1997. *MMWR* 1997;46(41):41.
2. Acheson DW, Fiore AE. Preventing food borne disease—what clinicians can do. *N Engl J Med* 2004;350(5):437.
3. American Medical Association, American Nurses Association-American Nurses Foundation, Centers for Disease Control and Prevention, Center for Food Safety and Applied Nutrition, Food Safety and Inspection Service, Food and Drug Administration U.S. Department of Agriculture. Diagnosis and management of foodborne illness. *MMWR* 2004;53(RR04):1–89.
4. Bashai WR, Sears CL. Food poisoning syndromes. *Gastroenterol Clin North Am* 1993;3:579.
5. Centers for Disease Control and Prevention. Notice to readers changes in national notifiable diseases data presentation. *MMWR* 1999;48(21):447–448.
6. Keene WE. Lessons from investigations of food borne disease outbreaks. *JAMA* 1999;281(19):1845–1847.
7. Tan, Williams, Khan et al. Risk of transmission of bovine-spongiform encephalopathy to humans in the United States. *JAMA* 1999;281(24):2330–2339.
8. Taylor, DN, Sanchez JL, Candlor W, et al. Treatment of traveler's diarrhea: ciprofloxac in plus loperamide compared with ciprofloxacin alone. *Ann of Int Med* 1991;114;731.

CHAPTER 335
Botulism

Adhi N. Sharma

In the late 1700s, 13 people in southern Germany developed gastrointestinal illness and died after eating smoked blood sausage. The German physician Justinus Kerner published the first complete description of "sausage poisoning" in 1817 and suggested it was the result of a poison (toxin) that developed under anaerobic conditions. Five years later, he suggested this toxin could be used therapeutically in patients with muscle spasticity. In 1870, Müller named the disease botulism after *botulus*, the Latin word for sausage (8). Since that time, botulism has been the term used to describe the illness associated with the consumption of food contaminated with *Clostridium botulinum* and its toxin. The toxin can be preformed or generated after germination of *C. botulinum* within the patient. Human to human transmission does not occur. However, multiple cases occur when patients share the same contaminated food.

C. botulinum is an anaerobic, spore-forming, gram-positive bacillus. The spores are ubiquitous and can be found in soil, water, and air. Spores are usually dormant and can tolerate 2 hours of boiling at 100°C. Germination of the spores requires certain environmental conditions; a pH greater than 4.5 and sodium chloride content less than 3.5%. Unlike the spores, the toxin is heat-labile and can be destroyed by boiling for a few minutes or if heated for 5 minutes at 85°C. Low pH does not inactivate or destroy preformed toxin.

Botulinum toxin is considered the most lethal substance known, with an estimated oral LD_{50} of 1 μg/kg in humans (10). The active form of the toxin is composed of heavy and light

TABLE 335.1. Incidence of Botulism in the U.S. from 1973–1996[b]

Form of Botulism	Total Cases Reported	Median Annual Cases
Foodborne	724	24
Infant botulism	1444	71
Wound botulism	103	3
Undetermined*	39	N/A

[a]Undetermined is also referred to as the adult form of infant botulism.
[b]From Shapiro RL, Hatheway C, Becker J, et al. Botulism surveillance and emergency response: a public health strategy for a global challenge. JAMA 1997;278:433–435, with permission.

polypeptide chains connected by disulfide bonds, with a molecular weight of 150 kDa. Botulinum toxin enters presynaptic nerve terminals via endocytosis, in which it irreversibly prevents the release of acetylcholine by inhibiting calcium-dependent exocytosis (13). The net result is a decrease in the acetylcholine concentration within the synaptic cleft. This affects cholinergic neurotransmission in the autonomic nervous system and at neuromuscular junctions resulting in anticholinergic (muscarinic and nicotinic) effects and flaccid paralysis, respectively.

Seven different serotypes of botulinum toxin have been identified (types A–G). Type A is found predominantly west of the Mississippi, type B predominantly east of the Mississippi, and type E in the Pacific-Northwest, especially in Alaska (6). Types A and B are typically found in improperly processed meats and vegetables. The food usually appears foul and may have an odor. By contrast, type E does not alter the smell or appearance of food. Human intoxications have been well documented with serotypes A, B, E, and rarely F. Type A accounts for more than one-third of the food-borne cases. Types C and D cause disease in birds and mammals and disease with type G has yet to be documented in either humans or animals in the United States (22).

Classically, four distinct diseases have been described that relate to intoxication as a result of *C. botulinum* (Table 335.1). Food-borne (adult) botulism occurs after consumption of preformed toxin. Smoked or salted meats and fish as well as canned vegetables are typical sources. Mortality ranges from 5% to 10%. Infant botulism occurs after ingestion and propagation of *C. botulinum* in the intestinal tract. The vast majority of cases are a result of serotypes A (47%) or B (52%). Almost half the cases reported over the last 30 years have been from California (6). Wound botulism occurs after a wound is contaminated with spores that germinate and produce toxin over time. Botulism of undetermined origin is the adult version of infant botulism, in which no food vehicle can be identified and there is no evidence of wound botulism in a patient over 1 year of age. This type usually results from intestinal colonization in an adult (15).

The World Health Organization describes seven types of botulism. In addition to the four classic or natural forms, inhalational, waterborne, and iatrogenic botulism are possible (2). Inhalational botulism is a potential threat if the toxin is aerosolized as a biological weapon (18). Waterborne botulism is only a theoretical concern as water treatment processes inactivate the toxin. Iatrogenic botulism stems from the administration of botulinum toxin for therapeutic or cosmetic purposes.

CLINICAL PRESENTATION

The initial symptoms of foodborne botulism are predominantly gastrointestinal, including nausea, vomiting, abdominal pain, and distention, and are likely a result of pathogenic agents or toxins in the contaminated food other than *C. botulinum*. Symptoms usually develop within 12 to 36 hours but may develop as early as 4 hours or as late as 10 days. Other initial symptoms are often mild and include fatigue, weakness, and vertigo. Additional symptoms include sore throat, dry mouth, and poor visual accommodation. If the toxin exposure is minimal, patients gradually recover. Otherwise, symmetric, descending flaccid paralysis with prominent bulbar palsies such as diplopia, dysarthria, dysphonia, and dysphagia develops. Physical examination may reveal weakness or paralysis of the upper extremities, dilated, nonreactive pupils, and ophthalmoplegia. The patient may be drooling secondary to dysphagia and may have difficulty phonating. Deep tendon reflexes are preserved and ataxia is absent. Weakness of the extremities and paralysis of respiratory muscles are the most concerning symptoms. Patients maintain a normal mental status and are afebrile. Autonomic instability, such as orthostatic hypotension, may also occur, and may be the predominant or only symptom on presentation, confounding the diagnosis (17).

Infant botulism is characterized by constipation followed by neuromuscular paralysis. Cranial nerves are affected first and paralysis may progress to peripheral and respiratory musculature. The term "floppy infant syndrome" may best describe the presentation. Symptoms can vary from mild lethargy with poor feeding to hypotonia with respiratory compromise. Since 1980, infant botulism has been the most common form of botulism reported. It results from the ingestion of *C. botulinum* with toxin formation and absorption in the gut lumen (16). The gastrointestinal tracts of infants lack some of the bile acids and gastric acids that normally inhibit clostridial growth. Honey and corn syrup have been identified as sources of *C. botulinum* spores (3). Vacuum cleaner dust and soil have also been implicated. In the food samples tested, no preformed toxin has been identified, only clostridium spores. About 70% of cases are in breast-fed infants, presumably these infants have altered gut flora when compared with their formula-fed counterparts.

The neurological symptoms of wound botulism are identical to that of food-borne botulism; however, gastrointestinal symptoms are absent. Wounds are typically in avascular areas or can be the result of crush injuries. Recently, an epidemic of wound botulism has occurred in patients injecting black tar heroin subcutaneously ("skin popping"). In one report, only 1 out of 102 cases of wound botulism did not occur in a drug user (24). As black tar heroin is made in Mexico, most cases are from the Western United States with a preponderance from California.

Iatrogenic cases may vary from mild symptoms to profound respiratory compromise requiring intubation (4,7). Often the history of recent botulinum toxin injection will help make the diagnosis. Botulinum toxin is used therapeutically for spasticity, cervical dystonia, blepharospasm, and hyperhidrosis, as well as for cosmetic purposes.

DIFFERENTIAL DIAGNOSIS

Neurological symptoms are similar regardless of the type of botulism. The diagnosis is easy when large outbreaks occur. However, the majority of cases involve only one patient. As a result, the diagnosis is often missed. Botulism should be considered in a patient presenting with gastrointestinal, autonomic, and cranial nerve dysfunction or in an infant with diminished sucking, feeding, and crying ability. The differential diagnosis for food-borne and infant botulism is listed in Table 335.2. Psychiatric illness should be a diagnosis of exclusion. Misdiagnosis as such has been fatal (10).

The gastrointestinal symptoms of botulism are nonspecific and do not demonstrate a distinctive pattern (i.e., "rice water" stools or "bloody" diarrhea). As such, patients at this stage of the

TABLE 335.2. Differential Diagnosis for Botulism

Foodborne	Infant Botulism
Cerebrovascular ischemia (CVA)	Electrolyte abnormalities
Chemical intoxication	Leigh disease[a]
Carbon monoxide	Meningitis
Barium carbonate	Metabolic encephalopathy
Methyl chloride	Myopathy (congenital)
Methyl alcohol	Reye syndrome
Cholinergic (organophosphate)	Sepsis
agents	Werdnig-Hoffman disease[b]
Diphtheria	
Elapidae envenomation (coral	
snake)	
Food poisoning	
Landry-Guillain-Barré syndrome	
Miller-Fisher variant	
Medication reactions	
(esp. aminoglycosides)	
Multiple sclerosis	
Myasthenia gravis	
Eaton-Lambert syndrome	
Paralytic shellfish poisoning	
Poliomyelitis	
Polymyositis	
Psychiatric disorders	

[a] Subacute necrotizing encephalomyelopathy
[b] Spinal muscular atrophy

disease are often discharged with a diagnosis of food poisoning. Fever is absent in patients with botulism, but can be present in certain types of food poisoning. A history of the consumption of canned foods, especially home-canned foods may be helpful in arriving at the diagnosis. See Chapter 334, "Food Poisoning," for further discussion.

Landry-Guillain-Barré syndrome is an acute inflammatory postinfectious demyelinating polyradiculoneuropathy that usually results in ascending weakness or paralysis. In the Miller-Fisher variant of this syndrome, patients have bulbar palsies (diplopia, dysarthria, dysphonia, and dysphagia) and descending weakness or paralysis, making it extremely difficult to distinguish clinically from botulism. Lumbar puncture may reveal elevated protein without pleocytosis in the former. However, early in Landry-Guillain-Barré syndrome, the spinal fluid may be normal and a slightly elevated spinal fluid protein may be seen in botulism. Of note, gastrointestinal symptoms are lacking in Landry-Guillain-Barré syndrome, unless part of the associated antecedent viral syndrome.

Myasthenia gravis may present as weakness, ptosis and ophthalmoplegia however, gastrointestinal symptoms will be absent. A Tensilon (edrophonium) test may be necessary to differentiate myasthenia gravis from botulism. In this test, 10 mg of edrophonium, an anticholinesterase, is administered slowly as a 1 to 2 mg intravenous bolus, followed by 8 mg given over 5 minutes. Within a minute, patients with myasthenia gravis should demonstrate improved strength that should last up to 5 minutes. As this drug blocks the metabolism of acetylcholine in the synapse, it is less effective in botulism in which there is decreased neurotransmitter release, although some smaller degree of clinical improvement may occasionally be seen.

The Centers for Disease Control and Prevention (CDC) have established definitive criteria for the diagnosis of botulism. It requires a patient who presents with descending paralysis to have one of the following: *C. botulinum* isolated from stool or wound specimens; botulinum toxin in serum, stool, or implicated food samples; or, a compatible illness in a person who is epidemiologically linked to a case confirmed by the above methods (5). Currently, a mouse bioassay is used to detect the presence of botulinum toxin. It is complicated and results are often delayed. However, a new rapid assay is under development that can be used in the field (1). This assay would allow for rapid confirmation of any suspected botulism diagnosis and thereby expedite treatment.

Although not included in the CDC diagnostic criteria, electromyography demonstrating findings typical of botulism may be required prior to the release of antitoxin. Botulism demonstrates a typical pattern on repetitive stimulation test (20–50 Hz) (23). Although this pattern is not pathognomonic for botulism, when it is combined with other clinical data it can be used to make the diagnosis.

EMERGENCY DEPARTMENT EVALUATION

The history should include the time of onset, nature, progression, and severity of symptoms as well as questions concerning diet, crush injuries, skin wounds, and injections as noted above. The physical examination should focus on neurological evaluation with attention to assessment of cranial nerve function, muscle strength, and deep tendon reflexes. Abnormalities of pupil size and reactivity, extraocular motor function, swallowing, and phonation should be documented. As death from botulism is usually the result of respiratory insufficiency, patients should have frequent assessments of vital capacity and negative inspiratory force.

Routine laboratory evaluation of cell counts, serum electrolytes, and plain radiographs are usually normal in patients with botulism, but may be helpful to exclude other diagnoses. Cerebrospinal fluid analysis is also normal, but this distinguishes botulism from other disease states such as meningitis or Landry-Guillain-Barré. Similarly, brain imaging (computed tomography [CT] or magnetic resonance imaging [MRI]) is normal in patients with botulism, but may yield the diagnosis of cerebral or cerebellar infarct.

As noted above, the Tensilon test can help differentiate myasthenia gravis from botulism.

When the diagnosis of botulism is suspected, electromyography should be performed as soon as possible. Stool, serum, or wound cultures should be sent for *C. botulinum*. Serum and stool samples and wound tissue should also be sent for detection of botulinum toxin. In one study, at least one of these laboratory tests was positive in 65% of patients diagnosed with botulism (25). Stool and sera should be refrigerated, but not frozen. Wound specimens should be placed in an anaerobic device. Suspected food should be left in their original containers and placed in sterile unbreakable containers if possible.

EMERGENCY DEPARTMENT MANAGEMENT

Supportive care is the mainstay of treatment. Endotracheal intubation with mechanical ventilation is recommended for patients with a vital capacity less than 30% of predicted (or <12 mL/kg). Fluids should be given to replete any gastrointestinal losses and parenteral analgesics can be given for the pain associated with abdominal distention.

Despite the delay from ingestion of contaminated food to presentation, gastric decontamination should be considered in cases of food-borne botulism. Gastric lavage may help remove any remaining toxin or contaminated food from the stomach. Activated charcoal has been shown to reduce morbidity and mortality in an animal model (11). Magnesium cathartics should not be given as magnesium may exacerbate neuromuscular blockade. Instead a

sorbitol-based cathartic should be used. Although whole bowel irrigation can aid in removal of toxin from the gut, this theory has not been evaluated in a formal study.

Multiple antitoxin preparations are available for treatment. The equine derived antitoxins are available in a monovalent (types A, B, or E), bivalent (AB) and trivalent (ABE) formulation. A heptavalent (A–G) antitoxin is held by the U.S. Army. The trivalent antitoxin is recommended when the exact botulinum serotype has not been identified. It is distributed by the CDC to nine local repositories in the United States and is available by contacting the state health department. Antitoxin is most effective when given within 24 hours of symptom onset and should be administered as soon as the diagnosis of botulism is suspected, without waiting for confirmatory testing. The antitoxin does not reverse symptoms already present on administration. It can only prevent symptom progression, further stressing the necessity of early administration.

The initial dose of antitoxin is one vial given intravenously, slowly over several minutes. Each vial contains 10 mL of trivalent antitoxin and should be diluted in a 1:10 ratio with normal saline. Subsequent doses can be given at 2- to 4-hour intervals based on symptom progression. The benefits of antitoxin therapy must be weighed against the potential adverse effects. Because antitoxin is an animal-derived biologic product, its use can result in anaphylaxis, hypersensitivity reactions, and serum sickness. The rate of adverse reactions is 9% to 17% with a 1.9% incidence of anaphylaxis. Test dosing to assess hypersensitivity is not recommended as botulism can be fatal and antitoxin is the only available therapy. Clinicians should be prepared to handle any adverse reactions and should have medications (e.g., epinephrine) readily available.

A human botulism immune globulin (BIG) is available for infant botulism. BIG is harvested from human donors previously immunized with the pentavalent (A–E) toxoid developed by the Army for laboratory personnel who work with *C. botulinum*. It is only available from the California Department of Health Services Infant Botulism Treatment and Prevention Program. BIG has been shown to be more effective than antitoxin for the treatment of infant botulism (9).

Antibiotics should be administered for wound botulism. Penicillin G is usually the first-line agent, although many antibiotics have been shown to be effective against *C. botulinum* (21). Early surgical consultation should be also obtained for cases of wound botulism as debridement is considered a primary therapeutic intervention (12).

In contrast, antibiotic use in infant botulism is not generally recommended. The use of aminoglycosides has been demonstrated both clinically and experimentally to potentiate neuromuscular blockade (14,19). Use of antibiotics in infant botulism can exacerbate the condition as lysis of intraluminal *C. botulinum* may increase the amount of toxin absorbed (6). The benefit of antibiotic therapy for food-borne botulism has not been demonstrated and is not recommended.

CRITICAL INTERVENTIONS

- Consult an infectious disease specialist, neurologist, poison center, or toxicologist, and the State Department of Health or CDC (770-448-7100) for patients with suspected botulism
- Consult a surgeon regarding debridement in cases of suspected wound botulism
- Assess the vital capacity in patients with suspected botulism
- Perform endotracheal intubation and initiated assisted mechanical ventilation in patients with a vital capacity less than 30% of predicted (<12 mL/kg)
- Administer botulism antitoxin as soon as possible

60 mg/dl in nondiabetic volunteers. Neuroglycopenic symptoms such as dizziness, tingling, blurred vision, difficulty thinking, and faintness begin at glucose levels near 50 mg/dl (9). However, there is a wide variation in the glucose level at which symptoms develop. Some individuals, particularly women and children, can be asymptomatic with glucose levels less than 50 mg/dl and diabetics can develop symptoms of hypoglycemia at a "normal" or elevated glucose level when the level rapidly falls from a higher one. Additionally, concurrent therapy with β-adrenergic blockers or underlying diabetic neuropathy may mask the autonomic symptoms of hypoglycemia.

Focal neurologic deficits can occur with hypoglycemia, and in severe cases, coma or seizures can be seen. Mild hypothermia may develop with prolonged hypoglycemia. Hypokalemia may result from intracellular potassium shifting. Chronic chlorpropamide use is associated with hyponatremia.

Metformin-associated lactic acidosis presents with nonspecific signs and symptoms. Patients may have nausea, vomiting, anorexia, epigastric pain, diarrhea, somnolence, or lethargy. Kussmaul respirations (hyperpnea and tachypnea) represent increased ventilation in response to the metabolic acidosis. Hypotension, hypothermia, and respiratory failure have also been reported. Various cardiac dysrhythmias, including premature ventricular contractions, bradycardia, asystole, and ventricular fibrillation have been reported, probably secondary to severe acidemia (18).

DIFFERENTIAL DIAGNOSIS

Hypoglycemia is a potential etiology for any patient with altered mental status, neurologic findings, or signs of sympathetic stimulation such as diaphoresis or tremor. The differential diagnosis of patients with such findings is large, and includes trauma, stroke, brain tumors, central nervous system infections, severe metabolic disorders, and a wide variety of drug intoxications. Hypoglycemia should be considered as the potential cause for patients presenting with trauma or seizures. Patients particularly at risk are those with a personal or family history of noninsulin-dependent diabetes, as a result of their access to oral hypoglycemic drugs.

Diabetics presenting with an elevated anion-gap metabolic acidosis may have metformin-associated lactic acidosis or diabetic ketoacidosis. These may be differentiated based on the history (e.g., intercurrent illness, recent oral intake, intentional ingestion) and the presence or absence of hyperglycemia, ketosis, and hyperlactatemia. The thiazolidinediones and α-glucosidase inhibitors have no significant acute toxicity in overdose, although hepatic dysfunction may occur with chronic use.

EMERGENCY DEPARTMENT EVALUATION

Assessment of the patient's airway, breathing, and circulation is the first priority. The history should determine whether the patient has taken an overdose or a therapeutic one, the type of medication(s), amount ingested, and time-course of symptoms. Physical examination should pay particular attention to the neurologic status, as hypoglycemia may present with subtle cognitive changes, such as irritability or distractibility, or even focal motor deficits. A rapid bedside glucose test should be performed early in patients with altered mental status.

Laboratory evaluation should include a confirmatory quantitative glucose determination. A serum chemistry panel is also indicated, to check for electrolyte abnormalities and renal insufficiency. Repeat bedside glucose determinations should be performed at least every 1 to 2 hours during the initial evaluation, and immediately whenever the patient shows signs of any altered mental status.

Patients with suspected metformin toxicity need a chemistry panel to evaluate for an anion-gap metabolic acidosis and renal insufficiency, as well as a serum lactate level. If an elevated anion-gap is present, an arterial blood gas analysis will help define the degree of acidosis.

EMERGENCY DEPARTMENT MANAGEMENT

Gastrointestinal decontamination with activated charcoal should be considered for patients presenting early after oral hypoglycemic agent ingestion. The first-line treatment for hypoglycemia is intravenous dextrose. Adults should be given 1 to 2 mL/kg of 50% dextrose (typically 1–2 ampules D50W); children should receive 2 to 4 mL/kg of 25% dextrose. Repeat dextrose boluses may be necessary, as determined by serial serum glucose determinations, and an infusion of 5% to 10% dextrose can be initiated to maintain euglycemia (60–110 mg/dl). If higher dextrose concentrations are required, the infusion should be given via a central venous catheter. The transient hyperglycemia that occurs with bolus dextrose therapy can cause reflex secretion of additional insulin (4), exacerbating the underlying problem and increasing the overall dextrose requirements. Hence, excessive dosing of dextrose should be avoided.

Diazoxide and octreotide are two options for treating refractory or recurrent hypoglycemia as a result of sulfonylurea poisoning. Diazoxide is a direct arterial vasodilator that also inhibits pancreatic insulin release by opening potassium channels. Hypotension is an expected potential side effect, although clinically significant hypotension is rarely reported from diazoxide use for sulfonylurea toxicity (10). Dosing has not been rigorously studied and is based on clinical experience, with a 300-mg i.v. bolus over 1 hour in adults and 1 to 3 mg/kg in children (4). Diazoxide is currently rarely used, either for hypertension or for sulfonylurea toxicity.

Octreotide, a synthetic somatostatin analog that inhibits pancreatic insulin secretion, is rapidly becoming a popular therapy for sulfonylurea-induced refractory hypoglycemia (2,4,8). Octreotide is superior to diazoxide plus glucose and to glucose alone in volunteer sulfonylurea overdose by decreasing hypoglycemia, glucose requirements, and circulating insulin levels (2). In clinical experience, octreotide use significantly decreases recurrent hypoglycemic episodes in patients with sulfonylurea toxicity (8). Dosing of octreotide has not been standardized, and it has been given both s.c. and i.v. for this indication. Suggested dosing is 50–100 μg s.c. or i.v. every 6 to 12 hours for adults, and 4 to 5 μg/kg/day divided every 6 hours in children.

No specific therapy exists for metformin-associated lactic acidosis. Endotracheal intubation and correction of hypotension with intravenous fluids and vasopressors are likely to be needed in severe cases. Severe acidosis has been treated with bicarbonate hemodialysis (5), which will correct acidosis as well as remove lactate and metformin.

CRITICAL INTERVENTIONS

- Obtain serial serum glucose levels on patients with potential sulfonylurea and meglitinide overdose
- Administer intravenous dextrose for hypoglycemia but avoid inducing hyperglycemia
- Administer octreotide to patients with recurrent hypoglycemia
- Obtain a serum lactate level on patients with metabolic acidosis who are taking metformin

DISPOSITION

Patients developing hypoglycemia from sulfonylurea drugs should be treated with dextrose and admitted to the hospital. The half-lives of the sulfonylureas are long enough that recurrent episodes of hypoglycemia should be expected. Admission to a critical care unit is often necessary, as the frequency of glucose determinations (at least every 1–2 hours) may preclude observation on a general medical ward. Also, patients may require frequent adjustments in dextrose infusions or treatment with uncommon medications, such as octreotide or diazoxide. Extended observation in an emergency department holding unit may be considered, depending on local capabilities, if the patient does not suffer from recurrent hypoglycemia requiring repeat dextrose boluses or infusions. Hypoglycemia from meglitinide toxicity theoretically should be of shorter duration than from sulfonylureas; however, as a result of a lack of published evidence that short-term observation is safe, such patients should currently be managed like sulfonylurea-toxic patients and be admitted for serial glucose determinations (6).

Considerable controversy remains regarding the optimal management of asymptomatic patients exposed to oral hypoglycemic medications (3,11,12,15,17). This controversy stems from the fact that many of the patients evaluated for sulfonylurea toxicity are children in whom the history of actual ingestion (vs. mere exposure to the pills) is not entirely clear, who present with normal mental status and glucose levels, and generally have a benign outcome. Nevertheless, because rapid drug detection to confirm actual exposure is not commonly available, these patients need a period of observation to monitor for hypoglycemia; the duration of this observation period is the crux of the controversy. Published evidence generally supports an observation period of 8 hours (15). Patients who develop hypoglycemia are treated and admitted, although those who do not manifest hypoglycemia may be discharged home or referred for psychiatric evaluation as appropriate. Prophylactic treatment of asymptomatic euglycemic patients with glucose should be avoided, as this may mask the development of hypoglycemia and lead to an inappropriate disposition. Cases of delayed hypoglycemia from sulfonylurea agents have occurred when the patients have been given parenteral glucose (15,17). Oral food intake is acceptable (15), and seems less likely to mask hypoglycemic agent toxicity. Because of the required length of observation and the potentially dire consequences of discharging a patient who later becomes hypoglycemic, some authors recommend medical admission and at least 24 hours of observation for all patients with a known or suspected overdose of sulfonylurea drugs (11).

Patients with biguanide-associated lactic acidosis also require admission, usually to an intensive care unit, because the associated mortality is so high and these patients often have significant comorbidities. Patients with an acute biguanide overdose, but without lactic acidosis, should be admitted and have serial serum chemistry determinations.

Patients overdosing with the other oral agents for diabetes are unlikely to require admission, unless concerning coingestants or comorbidities are present. In all cases, consultation with a poison control center or medical toxicologist can assist in determining the optimal patient disposition.

COMMON PITFALLS

✔ Failure to appreciate that the normal glucose level varies from person to person and that the diagnosis of hypoglycemia requires that symptoms be present
✔ Failure to appreciate that hypoglycemia can result in focal neurological deficits and focal seizures
✔ Failure to observe patients with sulfonylurea and meglitinide overdose for at least 8 hours
✔ Administering prophylactic dextrose patients with sulfonylurea and meglitinide overdose who are asymptomatic or euglycemic
✔ Failure to appreciate that excessive glucose administration promotes insulin secretion and can lead to recurrent hypoglycemia in sulfonylurea and meglitinide poisoning

References

1. Bailey GJ, Turner RC. Metformin. *N Engl J Med* 1996;334:574–579.
2. Boyle PJ, Justice K, Krentz AJ, et al. Octreotide reverses hyperinsulinumia and prevents hypoglycemia induced by sulfonylurea overdoses. *J Clin Endocrinol Metab* 1993;76:752–756.
3. Burkhart KK. When does hypoglycemia develop after sulfonylurea ingestion? *Ann Emerg Med* 1998;31:771–772.
4. Harrigan RA, Nathan MS, Beattie P. Oral agents for the treatment of type 2 diabetes mellitus: pharmacology, toxicity, and treatment. *Ann Emerg Med* 2001; 38:68–78.
5. Heaney D, Majid A, Junor B. Bicarbonate haemodialysis as a treatment of metformin overdose. *Nephrol Dial Transplant* 1997;12:1046–1047.
6. Hirschberg B, Skarulis MC, Pucino F, et al. Repaglinide-Induced Factitious Hypoglycemia. *J Clin Endocrinol Metab* 2001;86:475–477.
7. McCartney MM, Gilbert FJ, Murchison LE, et al. Metformin and contrast media—a dangerous combination? *Clin Radiol* 1999;54:29–33.
8. McLaughlin SA, Crandall CS, McKinney PE. Octreotide: an antidote for sulfonylurea-induced hypoglycemia. *Ann Emerg Med* 2000;36:133–138.
9. Mitrakou A, Ryan C, Veneman T, et al. Hierarchy of glycemic thresholds for counterregulatory hormone secretion, symptoms, and cerebral dysfunction. *Am J Physiol* 1991;260:E67–E74.
10. Palatnick W, Meatherall RC, Tenenbein M. Clinical spectrum of sulfonylurea overdose and experience with diazoxide therapy. *Arch Intern Med* 1991;151:1859–1862.
11. Quadrani DA, Spiller HA, Widder P. Five year retrospective evaluations of sulfonylurea ingestion in children. *J Toxicol Clin Toxicol* 1996;34:267–270.
12. Robertson WO. Sulfonylurea ingestions: hospitalization not mandatory. *J Toxicol Clin Toxicol* 1997;35:115–116.
13. Salpeter S, Greyber E, Pasternak G, et al. Risk of fatal and nonfatal lactic acidosis with metformin use in type 2 diabetes mellitus. *Cochrane Database Syst Rev* 2003;(2):CD002967.
14. Shorr RI, Ray WA, Daugherty JR, et al. Individual sulfonylureas and serious hypoglycemia in older people. *J Am Geriatr Soc* 1996;44:751–755.
15. Spiller HA, Villalobos D, Krenzelok EP, et al. Prospective multicenter study of sulfonylurea ingestion in children. *J Pediatr* 1997;131:141–146.
16. Stahl M, Berger W. Higher incidence of severe hypoglycaemia leading to hospital admission in Type 2 diabetic patients treated with long-acting versus short-acting sulphonylureas. *Diabet Med* 1999;16:586–590.
17. Szlatenyi CS, Capes KF, Wang RY. Delayed hypoglycemia in a child after ingestions of a single glipizide tablet. *Ann Emerg Med* 1998;31:773–776.
18. Teale KFH, Devine A, Stewart H, et al. The management of metformin overdose. *Anaesthesia* 1998;53:698–701.
19. Van Staa T, Abenhaim L, Monette J. Rates of hypoglycemia in users of sulfonylureas. *J Clin Epidemiol* 1997;50:735–741.
20. Watson WA, Litovitz TL, Rodgers GC, et al. 2002 Annual report of the American Association of Poison Control Centers toxic exposure surveillance system. *Am J Emerg Med* 2003;21:353–421.
21. Watkins PB, Whitcomb RW. Hepatic dysfunction associated with troglitazone. *N Engl J Med* 1998;338:916–917.
22. Zitzmann S, Reimann IR, Schmechel H. Severe hypoglycemia in an elderly patient treated with metformin. *Int J Clin Pharmacol Ther* 2003;40:108–110.

CHAPTER 337
Mushrooms

Brandon Wills and Steven E. Aks

Poisoning from mushroom ingestion is relatively infrequent. Exposures are often from unintentional ingestion of toxic species from inexperienced foragers, desire for mind-altering effects of some species, or unintentional ingestion by children. Cases are more likely to occur during the spring and fall when fungi are present and being harvested. Mushroom growing seasons will be longer in warmer climates and during summer months in more temperate areas. Identifying poisonous from nonpoisonous species can be difficult even for experts, often requiring microscopic examination of the spores. For the clinician evaluating a patient for suspected poisoning, identifying the fungus in question is even more challenging.

In 2002 there were 8,722 exposures to mushrooms reported to the American Association of Poison Control Centers. Of these the species was not identified in 7,304 cases. There were five deaths from the following mushroom classifications: cyclopeptide-2, hallucinogenic-1, monomethylhydrazine-1, and unknown-1 (23). Of the thousands of mushroom species there are several hundred that are considered toxic and represent a discrete number of responsible toxins (see Table 337.1).

Of all the toxic mushrooms, none are more deadly than the cyclopeptide, or amatoxin-containing Amanita species. Amanita poisoning continues to be a rare event in the United States, however; in European countries fatalities from amatoxin-containing mushrooms can be as high as 50 to 100 per year (3). Amatoxins are classically found in *Amanita phalloides* and *A. virosa* species, but are also found in *Galerina autumnalis*, *G. venenata*, *Lepiota spp.*, and *Conocybe filaris* (15). Amatoxins are bicyclic octapeptides that noncompetitively inhibit RNA polymerase II in the liver and, to a lesser extent the kidney. Protein synthesis is interrupted causing hepatocellular necrosis and acute tubular necrosis. Severe poisoning may result in fulminant hepatic and renal failure (24). Phallotoxins are another cyclopeptide toxin found in amanita species, which is thought to produce the gastrointestinal (GI) symptoms seen 6 to 10 hours after ingestion (7).

Mushrooms containing caprine include members of the Coprinus species, including *C. atramentarius*. Metabolites of caprine may inhibit aldehyde dehydrogenase and result in a disulfiram-like reaction if ethanol is consumed concurrently or within 3 days of the meal (11).

There is a diverse and extensive group of mushrooms, whose toxins are irritants causing primarily GI symptoms. Nausea, vomiting, diarrhea, and abdominal pain usually occur within 2 to 3 hours of the meal and are generally self-limiting. Some representative examples of GI irritants include: *Chlorophyllum molybdates*, *Omphalotus olearius*, *Agaricus spp.*, some *Amanita spp.*, *Boletus spp.*, *Hebeloma spp.*, *Lactarius spp.*, *Lepiota spp.*, some *Tricholoma spp.*, and others.

Amanita Muscaria, *A. pantherine*, and *A. gemmata* contain the toxins ibotenic acid and muscimol. Ibotenic acid is similar to the excitatory neurotransmitter glutamate although muscimol is a gamma-aminobutyric acid (GABA) agonist. Symptoms can be diverse and may include: somnolence, hallucinations, myoclonus, and seizures. Patients may consume *A. muscaria* and *A. pantherine* species intentionally for their hallucinogenic effects (2).

Gyromitra esculenta or "false morel" and other species represent one-third of fatal mushroom poisonings in Eastern Europe; however, they are quite rare in the United States (13). These mushrooms contain gyromitrins, a family of hydrazones that are metabolized to monomethylhydrazine, which is structurally related to isoniazid and some types of rocket fuel. Hydrazines inhibit pyridoxine phosphokinase, which prevents the activation of pyridoxine (vitamin B_6). Activated B_6 is required for GABA synthesis, resulting in decreased GABA production. Ingestion results in delayed GI symptoms, hepatic and renal toxicity, and may include seizures (17).

Muscarine is an alkaloid found in both *Clitocybe* and *Inocybe* genera that is structurally similar to acetylcholine. Symptoms are typically less severe, yet similar to the peripheral muscarinic effects seen in organophosphate/carbamate insecticide exposures (Chapter 297, "Organophosphate and Carbamata Insecticides") (8).

A yet to be identified mycotoxin can cause rhabdomyolysis after the ingestion of *Tricholoma equestre* mushrooms. (1).

Species of *Cortinarius* contain the toxin orellanine, whose metabolites cause damage to renal tubules and result in interstitial nephritis and renal failure several days to weeks after ingestion (11). The majority of these cases have been observed in Europe.

Amanita smithiana mushrooms contain alienic norleucine and pentanoic acid, which can cause renal failure several days after ingestion. Unlike *Cortinarius*, these mushrooms may cause GI effects as early as 2 hours of ingestion (22).

Psilocybe species as well as *Concocybe smithii*, *Gymnopilus spectabilis*, and *Panaeolus subbalteathus* are all known to contain psilocybin. Ingestion of this class of mushroom is often intentional for their hallucinogenic effects. Hallucinogenic mushrooms contain psilocybin, which is converted to psilocin in vivo. Psilocin is an indolalkylamine, which is a class of hallucinogenic tryptamine derivatives. Psilocin is a serotonin agonist that often causes an initial sympathomimetic-like effect including tachycardia, hypertension, mydriasis, and tremor, followed by hallucinations (21).

CLINICAL PRESENTATION

Patients will often present within several hours of a mushroom meal with nonspecific GI symptoms including nausea, vomiting, and diarrhea. Fortunately the majority of these patients will be suffering from GI irritants and will only require supportive care. Patients who have consumed the more toxic mushrooms containing cyclopeptides, orellanin, or monomethylhydrazine will have a delay of 8 to 12 hours before symptom onset. The distinction of time to symptom onset generally allows the clinician to be reassured that patients presenting early will likely have a benign clinical course. A notable exception to this is with *A. smithiana* ingestion; patients ingesting this mushroom will likely have GI symptoms within hours of ingestion, but subsequently develop renal failure over the next 48 hours to several weeks (22). Fortunately *A. smithiana* ingestions are rare, and the only cases reported in the United States have been in the Pacific Northwest. (14,22). Another caveat to this distinction would be those who have consumed a "mushroom salad" that contained both cytotoxic and GI irritant species and thus present with symptoms earlier than 6 to 8 hours.

Each class of toxic mushroom has a distinctive constellation of presenting symptoms, signs, laboratory abnormalities, and

TABLE 337.1. The Presenting Symptoms/Signs, Toxin, Laboratory Abnormalities, and Treatment After Mushroom Ingestion

Presenting Symptoms or Laboratory Abnormality	Associated Features	Mushroom Class/Toxin	Species	Treatment[a]
Hallucinations	Mydriasis, tachycardia, coma, seizures	Psilocin	*Psilocybe and Concocybe sp.*	Benzodiazepines Low-stimulus environment
	Mild hallucinations, coma, myoclonus, seizures	Ibotenic acid/ muscimol	*Amanita muscaria, pantheria, gemmata*	Benzodiazepines Low-stimulus environment
Cholinergic signs	DUMBELS	Muscarine	*Clitocybe and Inocybe sp.*	Atropine for pulmonary symptoms
Disulfiram reaction	N/V/D, flushing, iHR assoc. with ethanol use	Coprine	*Coprinus sp.*	Antihistamines
Renal failure	Delayed GI symptoms	Orellanine+	*Cortinarius sp.*	Dialysis
	Early GI symptoms	Allenic norleucine[b]	*Amanita smithiana*	Dialysis
Rhabdomyolysis	Myalgias, fatigue	Unknown myotoxin[b]	*Tricholoma equestre*	Maintenance of urine output & urinary alkalinization
Early gastrointestinal symptoms (2–3 h)	N/V/D	GI irritants	*Amanita phalloides, virosa Lepiota sp.*	Supportive care only Antiemetics
Delayed gastrointestinal symptoms (>6 h)	Delayed hepatotoxicity Nephrotoxicity	α-amanitin[b]	*Amanita phalloides*	MDAC Pen G? NAC? Silibinin? Consider transplant
	N/V/D, CNS, Hepatic	Gyromitrin+ (monomethyl hydrazine)	*Gyromitra sp.*	Pyridoxine

[a] In addition to supportive care including intravenous fluids and antiemetics, and decontamination if appropriate
[b] Mushrooms that lead to potentially lethal poisoning
[c] DUMBELS, (diarrhea, urination, miosis, bradycardia, bronchorrhea, bronchospasm, emesis, lacrimation); MDAC: multiple-dose activated charcoal; NAC, N-acetylcysteine

end-organ involvement (Table 337.1). Patients who have ingested cyclopeptide or amatoxin-containing mushrooms will typically present 6 to 12 hours after ingestion with nausea, vomiting, abdominal pain, and severe watery diarrhea. Time of symptom onset may predict severity with worse outcomes noted in patients presenting 10.3 hours after ingestion compared to a more benign course in those presenting 12.6 hours after ingestion (6). Hypovolemia and electrolyte disturbances may occur from GI losses. Symptoms may improve 24 to 48 hours into the illness, followed by evidence of hepatic injury marked by elevated transaminases, bilirubin, and often renal dysfunction. Within 2 to 5 days, fulminant hepatic and renal failure may develop with subsequent hepatic encephalopathy, coagulopathy, seizures, and death (3). With intensive supportive therapy, survival may be as high as 90% (4); however, with fulminant hepatic failure orthotopic liver transplant may be lifesaving (3).

Mushrooms containing caprine are typically edible and cause no symptoms. If ethanol is consumed within several hours up to 3 days after the ingestion a disulfiram-like reaction may be seen. Symptoms include nausea, vomiting, facial flushing, hypotension, tachycardia, headache, vertigo, and metallic taste. Symptoms typically last up to several hours (18).

Mushrooms containing GI irritants cause symptoms similar to gastroenteritis, usually beginning 30 minutes to 6 hours after ingestion. Vomiting and diarrhea, sometimes bloody, may last for 48 hours and are typically self-limiting. With severe diarrhea, patients may become significantly dehydrated and have electrolyte abnormalities.

Patients consuming mushrooms containing ibotenic acid and muscimol can have a varied presentation as a result of both GABAergic and glutamate effects. Symptoms usually begin within 30 to 180 minutes of ingestion and may include a combination of: euphoria, mild hallucinations, obtundation, agitation, myoclonus, and seizures (2).

The "false" morel Gyromitra esculenta is often confused with the edible true morel or *Morchella* species and results in signifi-

cant toxicity. Severity of symptoms depends on the amount ingested and method of preparation. Parboiling or drying may eliminate the gyromitrin toxins. Patients often become symptomatic 5 to 8 hours after ingestion and present with nausea, vomiting, and diarrhea. These symptoms may last up to several days and resolve. Central nervous system (CNS) effects including fatigue, headache, ataxia, tremor, and rarely seizures may be seen. After 24 to 72 hours postingestion there may be evidence of hepatic and/or renal damage as well as hemolysis and methemoglobinemia. With more severe cases coma and death may result (9,17).

The onset of symptoms following ingestion of muscarine-containing mushrooms is rapid, usually within 30 minutes. Cholinergic signs and symptoms include those identified by the commonly used mnemonic DUMBELS: diaphoresis, urination, miosis, bronchorrhea, emesis, lacrimation, and salivation. With supportive treatment patients typically recover with no long-standing effects (11,16).

Rhabdomyolysis with myalgias, weakness, and fatigue begins 24 to 74 hours after ingesting *T. equestre* mushrooms (1). Symptoms usually improve over the following 2 weeks but death can occur. Those who die exhibit persistent creatine kinase (CPK) elevations and have evidence of myocardial damage on autopsy.

Toxicity from orellanine-containing *Cortinarius* species is most often seen in Europe and is relatively uncommon in the United States. GI symptoms including nausea, vomiting, diarrhea, and abdominal or flank pain begin 2 to 14 days after ingestion at which time renal damage has already occurred. Progression to end-stage renal failure may ensue in 17% to 41% of poisoned patients depending on the series (9).

Similar to poisoning by *Cortinarius* species, the ingestion of alienic norleucine-containing *A. smithiana* produces renal damage 2 to 4 days after ingestion. One distinguishing feature is that *A. smithiana* often causes GI symptoms within 2 to 12 hours (22).

Abuse of psilocin-containing mushrooms is common in young adults, frequently used concomitantly with alcohol and other illicit drugs (21). Patients often present to the emergency department as a result of severe anxiety from unpleasant hallucinations ("bad trip"). Other signs and symptoms may include: mydriasis, tachycardia, GI symptoms, coma, and seizures (12). Another important feature, similar to LSD and other drug use is the association with high-risk behavior and poor decision making, which may lead to traumatic injuries.

DIFFERENTIAL DIAGNOSIS

Toxic mushroom ingestion should be considered in the differential diagnosis of patients presenting with GI symptoms, hepatic or renal damage, delirium or hallucinations, disulfiram-like reactions, refractory seizures, or rhabdomyolysis. The GI symptoms from both GI-irritant and the more toxic mushrooms will often be indistinguishable from gastroenteritis. Eliciting a history of recent ingestion of wild mushrooms may be the only clue to the diagnosis.

Hepatotoxicity similar to that caused by *Amanita* ingestion can occur with overdose of acetaminophen and iron, chronic INH therapy, and many nontoxicologic etiologies including viral hepatitis. In addition to caprine-containing mushrooms, a large number of chemicals and pharmaceuticals can cause a disulfiram-like reaction when ethanol is consumed (Chapter 273, "Ethanol"). Other hallucinogens, CNS depressants, gamma hydroxybutyrate (GHB), or withdrawal syndromes may cause symptoms similar to those seen after the ingestion of mushrooms containing ibotenic acid and muscimol. Agents causing toxicity similar to hydrazine-containing mushrooms include isoniazid and some types of rocket fuel. Direct muscarinic agonists or acetylcholinesterase inhibitors produce cholinergic toxicity similar to that seen with muscarine-containing mushrooms. Some of these agents include organophosphate or carbamate pesticides, nerve agents, physostigmine, and pilocarpine. The differential diagnosis of renal failure includes prerenal, intrinsic nephrotoxins, and postrenal causes. Conditions that may be confused with psilocin intoxication include LSD, mescaline, morning glory, hallucinogenic amphetamine (e.g., MDMA), and hallucinogenic tryptamine (e.g., DMT) poisoning, alcohol withdrawal, or medical causes of delirium. Other causes rhabdomyolysis include increased muscular activity from myoclonus, rigidity or seizures, trauma, or prolonged immobilization as a result of coma.

EMERGENCY DEPARTMENT EVALUATION

Of greatest importance in the history is the time interval between ingestion of the mushroom and the onset of symptoms. Other information that may be helpful is the quantity consumed, cooked versus raw, fresh versus dried, and if ethanol was consumed within 3 days of the meal. Positive identification of the mushroom involved can be difficult but this may be possible if the patient either brings a sample of the offending mushroom or can provide a detailed description. One method that has been used successfully by the Illinois Poison Center involves taking digital images of the mushroom in three planes, sending the images electronically to the poison center, and obtaining consultation from a mycologist (5). Contacting a regional poison center (800-222-1222) can be helpful in this regard.

The physical examination should focus on the vital signs, assessment of hydration status, cardiopulmonary and neurologic function, and the abdomen, eyes, and skin. Patients with prolonged GI symptoms or clinical evidence of dehydration should have serum electrolyte, blood urea nitrogen, creatinine, and glucose determinations and a urinalysis. Those with possible amatoxin poisoning should have liver function tests and a coagulation profile and those with weakness or myalgias should have a serum CPK. Except for muscarine, which can be identified by thin-layer chromatography, mushroom toxins are not detected by routine toxicology screening.

EMERGENCY DEPARTMENT MANAGEMENT

Supportive care is the mainstay for management of any toxic mushroom ingestion. Most patients will not need therapy other than intravenous fluids and antiemetics. Those exhibiting significant CNS effects, dehydration, seizures, or cardiovascular effects should have an i.v. line placed and have cardiac monitoring. Benzodiazepines should be administered for seizures and severe agitation or hallucinations. GI decontamination should be considered for patients presenting within 1 to 2 hours of ingestion. Activated charcoal is the preferred method.

The search for a potential antidote for amatoxin-containing mushrooms has been extensive. As a result of the infrequent nature of exposures, there are no prospective studies that conclusively demonstrate that any single agent is effective. Multiple-dose activated charcoal has been recommended because the amatoxins are enterohepatically recirculated. Continuous nasoduodenal suctioning has also been used. Charcoal hemoperfusion may also enhance toxin elimination if performed in the first 24 hours. High-dose intravenous penicillin (1 million units per kilogram per day for the first day, followed by 0.5 million units per kilogram per day for 2 more days) appears to have variable efficacy. The mechanism is unknown but it is postulated to prevent or reduce hepatic uptake of amatoxins. Silibinin is thought to reduce hepatic uptake of and interrupt enterohepatic circulation of amatoxins but a pharmaceutical preparation is not available in the United States. Oral silymarin (1.4 to 4.2 g/d), a dietary supplement that contains silibinin and is available in capsules from health food stores has been used as an alternative to intravenous silibinin but the efficacy of this formulation is unknown. The cytoprotective drug amifostine has been investigated as a potential treatment for α-amanitin toxicity, but did not appear to be efficacious (25). N-acetylcysteine (NAC), traditionally used for the treatment of acetaminophen poisoning, may also be effective for nonspecific causes of hepatic injury. A large retrospective review and small case series suggest NAC may be an effective adjunct (4,20). When fulminant hepatic failure occurs, orthotopic liver transplantation is the only successful therapy (3,10).

Patients with caprine-containing mushroom ingestion should be counseled to avoid alcohol. Antihistamines may provide symptomatic relief.

Monomethylhydrazine-containing mushrooms (*Gyromitra spp.*) may manifest with seizures. If benzodiazepine therapy is not immediately successful, the patient should be given intravenous vitamin B_6 (pyridoxine). Gyromitrin causes an inhibition of glutamic acid decarboxylase, similar to isoniazid, and B6 is effective in this setting. Suggested doses are 1 gram for children, and 5 grams for adults.

Muscarine-containing mushrooms (e.g., *Clitocybe spp.*) will generally respond well with supportive care alone. Atropine may be used for severe cholinergic symptoms. Atropine dosing should be targeted to reverse pulmonary symptoms of bronchorrhea and bronchospasm.

Patients with hallucinations should be placed in a quiet, dark, low-stimulus environment, if possible. Haloperidol has also been reported to be effective for severe agitation and hallucinations (19).

The treatment of rhabdomyolysis includes maintenance of urine output via adequate hydration, alkalinization of the urine, and possibly dialysis.

CRITICAL INTERVENTIONS

- Determine the time of onset of symptoms with respect to the time of ingestion
- Consult a regional poison center, toxicologist, or mycologist to assist with mushroom identification and management
- Administer intravenous fluids and antiemetics to patients with GI symptoms and dehydration
- Admit patients with symptoms that begin 6 to 8 hours after ingestion and monitor for liver and renal dysfunction

DISPOSITION

Patients who present with GI symptoms that begin within 2 hours after ingestion, and respond to i.v. fluids and tolerate oral food and fluids, may be discharged unless there is a possibility of *A. smithiana* ingestion. Patients who have ingested hallucinogenic mushrooms may be safely discharged after a period of observation when their mental status returns to normal. Those who develop symptoms 6 to 8 hours after ingestion should be admitted to the hospital, and liver and renal function should be followed. Consultation with regional poison center or toxicologist is generally advised. In the case of hepatotoxicity from *A. phalloides* or other cyclopeptide-containing mushroom, consultation with a gastroenterologist and transfer to a center in which liver transplantation is prudent.

COMMON PITFALLS

✔ Failure to include wild mushroom ingestion in the differential diagnosis of gastroenteritis, altered mental status, and liver or kidney dysfunction of unknown cause
✔ Failure to appreciate that although the accidental ingestion of mushrooms by children is generally benign, intentional ingestion by adults can be fatal
✔ Assuming that a potentially lethal mushroom has not been ingested along with less toxic species because symptoms began soon after ingestion
✔ Failure to appreciate that therapy is based primarily on clinical symptoms and should not be delayed or withheld because the mushroom has not been identified

Acknowledgments

We thank previous edition chapter authors Christopher H. Linden and Robert P. Dowsett.

References

1. Bedry R, Baudrimont I, Deffieux G, et al. Wild mushroom intoxication as a cause of rhabdomyolysis. *N Engl J Med* 2001;345(11):798–802.
2. Benjamin D. Mushroom poisoning in infants and children: the amanita pantherine/ muscaria group. *J Toxicol Clin Toxicol* 1992;30(1):13–22.
3. Broussard C, Aggarwal A, Lacey S, et al. Mushroom poisoning—from diarrhea to liver transplantation. *Am J Gastroentero l* 2001;96:3195–3198.
4. Enjalbert F, Rapior S, Nouguier-Soule J, et al. Treatment of amatoxin poisoning: 20-year retrospective analysis. *J Toxicol Clin Toxicol* 2002;40(6);715–757.
5. Fischbein C, Mueller G, Leacock P, et al. Digital imaging: a promising tool for mushroom identification. *Acad Emerg Med* 2003;10:808–810.
6. Floersheim G, Weber O, Tschumi P, et al. Die klinische knollenblatterpilzvergiftung (amanita phalloides): prognostische faktoren und therapeutische massnagmen. *Schwezerische Medizinische Wochenschrift* 1982;112:1164–1177.
7. Frimmer M. What we have learned from phalloidin. *Toxicol Lett* 1987;35(2-3): 169–182.
8. Hanrahan J, Gordon M. Mushroom poisoning—case reports and a review of therapy. *JAMA* 1984;251(8):1057–1061.
9. Karlson-Stiber C, Persson H. Cytotoxic fungi—an overview. *Toxicon* 2003;42: 339–349.
10. Klein, AS, Hart J, Brems JJ, et al. Amanita poisoning: treatment and the role of liver transplantation. *Am J Med* 1989;86:187–193.
11. Koppel C. Clinical Symptomatology and management of mushroom poisoning. *Toxicon* 1993;31(12):1513–1540.
12. Kunz MW, Rauber-Luthy C, Meier PJ, et al. Acute poisoning with hallucinogenic psilocybe mushrooms in Switzerland. *J Toxicol Clin Toxicol* 2000;38(2):233.
13. Lampe K, McCann M. Differential diagnosis of poisoning by North American mushrooms, with particular emphasis on amanita phalloides-like intoxication. *Ann Emerg Med* 1987;16(9):956–962.
14. Leathem AM, Purssell RA, Chan VR, et al. Renal failure caused by mushroom poisoning. *J Toxicol Clin Toxicol* 1997;35:67–75.
15. Lincoff GH. *The Audobon Society Field Guide to North American Mushrooms.* New York: Alfred A. Knopf, 1988.
16. McCormick D, Avbel A, Gibbons R. Nonlethal mushroom poisoning. *Ann Int Med* 1979;90:332–335.
17. Michelot D, Toth B. Poisoning by gyromitra esculenta-a review. *J Appl Toxicol* 1991;11(4):235–243.
18. Michelot D. Poisoning by coprinus atramentarius. *J Nat Toxins* 1992;1:73–80.
19. Miller PL, Gay GR, Ferris KC, et al. Treatment of acute, adverse psychedelic reactions: "I've tripped and I can't get down." *J Psycho Drug* 1992;24:277–279.
20. Montanini S, Sinardi D, Pratico C, et al. Use of acetylcysteine as the life-saving antidote in amanita phalloides (death cap) poisoning. *Arzneim.-Forsch. Drug Res* 1999;49(II):1044–1047.
21. Schwartz R, Smith D. Hallucinogenic mushrooms. *Clin Pediatr (Phila)* 1988; 27(2):70–73.
22. Warden C, Benjamin D. Acute renal failure associated with suspected amanita smithiana mushroom ingestions: a case series. *Acad Emerg Med* 1998;5:808–812.
23. Watson W, Litovitz T, Rodgers G, et al. 2002 annual report of the American Association of Poison Control Centers toxic exposure surveillance system. *Am J Emerg Med* 2003;21(5):353–421.
24. Wieland T. The toxic peptides from amanita mushrooms. *Int J Pept Protein Res* 1983;22(3);257–276.
25. Wills B, Haller N, Peter D, et al. Cytoprotective effects of intraperitoneal amifostine on α-amanitin toxicity in mice. *Acad Emerg Med* 2003;10:521.

CHAPTER 338
Plants

Judith A. Alsop and Timothy E. Albertson

Exposures to potentially poisonous plants account for about 10% of all calls made to poison control centers in the United States according to the American Association of Poison Control Centers (AAPCC) Toxic Exposure Surveillance System (TESS) (23). Of the almost 85,000 plant exposures reported annually in TESS, about 74% involve accidental ingestions by children under age 6, 11% involve children ages 6 to 19 years, and 14.5% involve adults over 19 years old (23). Intentional abuse or misuse of plants comprises less than 3% of all cases (23).

Plants toxins (phytotoxins) include a large number of different chemicals that can affect any organ system. Almost any sign or symptom may be seen. The most common signs and symptoms seen after plant exposure are referable to the skin, gastrointestinal (GI) tract, and the central nervous system (CNS). Of all plant exposures reported to TESS, 16% were related to dermatitis, 18% were nontoxic plants with no signs and symptoms, 17% were plants that caused GI symptoms, 14% were symptoms from plants in the oxalate category that caused oral irritation, and almost 20% of all exposures occurred from unidentified plants (23). Fortunately, 28% of all plant exposures in TESS resulted in no or only minor symptoms, 1.8% resulted in moderate symptoms, and only 0.1% resulted in major symptoms (23). Over a 13-year period, there were a total of 35 plant-related deaths reported to TESS for an average of 2.7 patient deaths from plants per year. However, in the last year that data was reported to TESS, there were no deaths resulting from exposure to plants (23).

There is no single physical characteristic that differentiates a poisonous plant (Table 338.1) from a nonpoisonous one (Table 338.2). A leaf from a nontoxic plant can lodge in the throat and cause choking, gagging and vomiting. Large amounts of non-toxic plant material may cause vomiting. Because of the variety of plants, actual toxic doses are hard to establish. Alkaloid content of plants can vary by year and by location as a result of factors that affect growth such as soil conditions, fertilizer, amount of rainfall, and amount of sunshine. Therefore it is often impossible to make a definite association between symptoms and severity and specific plant and amount of material ingested (22). In general, houseplants are less toxic than outdoor plants (2). Small accidental tastes of plants by young children are very common and less likely to cause severe problems than are intentional use or misuse of plants by adolescents and adults (2,23).

Patients arriving at the emergency department (ED) after a plant exposure may present as a perplexing puzzle, depending on the age of the patient, the type of plant involved, amount of exposure and the reason for the exposure. A young child who sampled some red berries is clinically different from an adolescent who smoked a plant in hopes of becoming intoxicated. In turn, the adult patient who has brewed a concentrated tea to attempt suicide is clinically different than the previous situations. Each case will present different diagnostic and management challenges.

CLINICAL PRESENTATION

Oxalates are found in many common house and garden plants (2,22). Dieffenbachia is a classic example of an insoluble-oxalate containing plant and rhubarb (leaves) is an example of a soluble-oxalate containing plant. Soluble and insoluble oxalates cause different symptoms requiring different treatments (2). However, both have the ability to cause nausea, vomiting, abdominal pain, and diarrhea. After the plant part (usually the leaf) has been chewed, insoluble calcium and magnesium oxalate crystals will often cause almost immediate local irritation, pain, and edema to the mouth, lips, and tongue (10,22). The throat is rarely involved. Because of the local pain, large ingestions are not likely and systemic effects are rare (15). However, upper airway obstruction from swelling may occur in severe cases.

Soluble (sodium, potassium, and ammonium) oxalate crystals do not tend to produce local irritation and may be eaten in sufficient quantities to produce systemic oxalate toxicity (2,22). Following ingestion of these plants, oxalic acid is formed in the stomach. Bloody emesis and diarrhea may occur with soluble salts. Once oxalic acid is absorbed into the systemic circulation, it can bind with calcium and this potentially leads to hypocalcemia. The oxalate-induced hypocalcemia may lead to bradycardia, hypotension and dysrhythmias. The severity of symptoms varies, depending on both the plant species involved and the amount ingested (22).

Alkaloids and glycosides that are also GI irritants are found in a diverse group of plants. These toxins can cause nausea, vomiting, abdominal cramping, and diarrhea, among other symptoms (2,22). The mechanism of action and toxic concentration differ by genus and phytotoxin. Many of these plants can also cause additional systemic effects such as fluid and electrolyte depletion, GI bleeding, tissue sloughing, and shock. Many plants that cause epithelial irritation and dermatitis also cause GI irritation. Usually the degree of severity depends on the amount ingested (23).

Plants containing a protoanemonin (anemones, buttercups and ranunculus) have a harsh, bitter, and alkaloid taste. A burning sensation in the mouth and throat is common. If protoanemonin are ingested, oral pain, mouth ulcers, excessive salivation, hematemesis, and severe gastroenteritis may occur (2,22). Fortunately, human ingestions producing systemic symptoms are rare. The bad taste and oral pain probably prevent the ingestion of larger amounts.

Grayanotoxin, found in rhododendrons and azaleas, binds to myocardial sodium channels and increases permeability by opening the sodium channels (17). Symptoms include burning of the mouth, perioral numbness and tingling, nausea, vomiting, and diaphoresis. Large exposures may cause hypotension, bradycardia, altered mental status, seizures, and coma (2,18,22). Ingestion of plant parts, contaminated honey, or sucking the nectar from flowers can result in toxicity. Onset of symptoms is about 2 hours after ingestion and lasts about 24 hours.

Anticholinergic plants contain various amounts of atropine, hyoscyamine, scopolamine, and mandragorine (17). Plants with anticholinergic toxins cause classic symptoms of dry, red, hot skin; mydriasis; dry mucous membranes; tachycardia; hyperthermia; decreased GI motility; urinary retention; delirium; and hallucinations (see Chapter 323, "Anticholinergic Agents") (2,12,17,22). Large exposures can result in CNS depression. Most patients recover but death has been reported, especially after abuse.

Jimson weed (*Datura stramonium*) intoxication is the classic example of anticholinergic poisoning. All parts are toxic and it can be ingested, smoked, or made into a tea (11,12). Depending on the formulation (raw plant material vs. a concentrated tea vs. smoking), onset of symptoms may occur rapidly or may be delayed. As a result of decreased GI motility and delayed GI emptying, symptoms may persist for a period of several days.

Solanine-containing plants (e.g., black nightshade and the green parts of tomatoes, potatoes, and eggplant) also cause nausea, vomiting, diarrhea, headache, and drowsiness (2,17,22). From animal studies, inhibition of cholinesterase activity with cardiac glycoside effects is thought to be the mechanism of action (17). However, symptoms of hypotension, bradycardia, muscle cramps, increased salivation, paresthesias, and dyspnea are rare, but have been reported. Onset of symptoms is within 2 to 24 hours. Diarrhea may last 3 to 6 days. Some plants that contain solanine may also contain anticholinergic substances as well. This may lead to a confusing and contradictory patient presentation. However, in plants containing a mix of solanine and anticholinergic toxins, solanine symptoms usually dominate.

Plants containing cardiac glycosides, such as oleander and foxglove, inhibit sodium-potassium ATPase and cause signs and symptoms that are similar to those in digoxin poisoning (Chapter 304, "Cardiac Glycosides") (2,5,17,22). GI symptoms are usually seen before cardiotoxicity and CNS dysfunction. Yellow vision changes may occur but are rare. Accidental taste ingestions by children rarely result in toxicity. Digoxin radioimmunoassays can be used to detect digitalis glycosides. Interpretation of quantitative results for plant cardiac glycosides is limited, and the results should only be used as a qualitative marker (2,17).

Symptoms of cyanide poisoning (Chapter 308, "Cyanide") are associated with ingestion of large amount of chewed seeds and pits that contain cyanogenic glycosides (amygdalin) These compounds, when mixed with water and plant enzymes, are hydrolyzed and release cyanide (17,22). The amount of glycoside is usually small, and the liberation of cyanide is a slow, incomplete process. Initial symptoms include nausea, vomiting, diarrhea, weakness, lightheadedness, dyspnea, and cyanosis, followed by seizures, disorientation, paralysis, coma, and cardiovascular collapse (2,17,22). Fortunately, cyanide poisoning

TABLE 338.1. Toxic Plants

Common Name	Botanical Name	Toxins/Effects
Acacia, black	*Robinia pseudoacacia*	Toxalbumin
Acorn	*Quercus* spp	GI, hepatotoxic, dermatitis
Agapanthus	*Agapanthus* spp	Dermatitis
Akee	*Blighia sapida*	CNS stimulants, GI
Almond, bitter	*Prunus dulcis*	Cyanogenic glycoside
Aloe vera	*Aloe vera*	Gastrointestinal
Amaryllis	*Hippeastrum* spp	Gastrointestinal irritant
Amaryllis belladonna	*Amaryllis* spp	Gastrointestinal irritant
American bittersweet	*Celastrus scandens*	Gastrointestinal irritant
Anemone	*Anemone* spp	Protoanemonin
Angel's trumpet	*Brugmansia* spp	Anticholinergic
Angel's trumpet	*Datura* spp	Anticholinergic
Anthurium	*Anthurium* spp	Oxalates, insoluble
Apple (chewed seeds)	*Malus* spp	Cyanogenic glycosides
Apricot (chewed pits)	*Prunus armeniaca*	Cyanogenic glycosides
Arrowhead vine	*Syngonium podophyllum*	Oxalates, insoluble
Arum	*Arum* spp	Oxalates, insoluble
Autumn crocus	*Colchicum autumnale*	Colchicine
Azalea	*Rhododendron genus*	Grayanotoxin
Baneberry	*Actaea* spp	Protoanemonin
Barbados nut	*Jatropha curcas*	Toxalbumin, severe derm
Barberry	*Berberis* spp	Gastrointestinal irritant
Belladonna	*Atropa belladonna*	Anticholinergic
Black cohosh	*Cimicifuga racemosa*	Gastrointestinal irritant
Black henbane	*Hyoscyamus niger*	Anticholinergic
Black lily	*Dracunculus vulgaris*	Oxalates, insoluble
Black locust	*Robinia pseudoacacia*	Toxalbumin
Black nightshade	*Solanum nigrum*	Solanine
Black snakeroot	*Zygadenus venenosus*	GI, bradycardia, hypotension
Black snakeroot	*Cimicifuga racemosa*	Gastrointestinal irritant
Bleeding heart	*Dicentra formosa*	Dermatitis
Bloodroot	*Sanguinaria canadensis*	GI, CNS depressant
Boston ivy	*Parthenocissus tricuspidata*	Oxalates, soluble
Boxwood	*Buxus sempervirens*	Severe GI, dermatitis
Bracken fern	*Pteridium aquilinum*	Potential carcinogen
Broom, Scotch	*Cytisus scoparius*	Cytisine
Broom, Spanish	*Spartium junceum*	Cytisine
Buckeye	*Aesculus* spp	GI, CNS depressant
Buckthorn	*Karwinski humboldtiana*	Ascending paralytic neuropathy
Buckthorn	*Rhamnus cathartica*	Gastrointestinal, nephrotoxic
Burning bush	*Dictamnus albus*	Dermatitis
Buttercup	*Ranunculus* spp	Protoanemonin
Caladium	*Caladium* spp	Oxalates, insoluble
Calla lily	*Zantedeschia* spp	Oxalates, insoluble
Candlenut	*Aleurites moluccana*	Severe GI, dermatitis
Carolina allspice	*Calycanthus* spp	CNS stimulant (Strychnine-like)
Cassava (raw root)	*Manihot esculenta*	Cyanogenic, Severe GI, dermatitis
Castor bean	*Ricinus communis*	Toxalbumin
Catnip	*Nepeta cataria*	GI, mild hallucinogen
Century plant	*Agave americana*	Dermatitis, gastrointestinal
Cherry (chewed pits)	*Prunus* spp	Cyanogenic glycosides
Chili pepper	*Capsicum* spp	Dermatitis, GI irritant
Chinaberry	*Melia azedarach*	GI, CNS depressant
Chokecherry	*Prunus virginiana*	Cyanogenic glycosides
Christmas rose	*Helleborus niger*	GI, dermatitis, CNS stimulant
Chrysanthemum	*Chrysanthemum* spp	Dermatitis
Coffeeberry	*Rhamnus californica*	Gastrointestinal
Coral bean	*Erythrina* spp	Cyanogenic glycosides
Coral berry	*Actaea spicata*	Protoanemonin
Coriaria	*Coriaria* spp	CNS stimulant (picrotoxin-like)
Coyotillo	*Karwinski humboldtiana*	Ascending paralytic neuropathy
Creeping charlie	*Glechoma hederacea*	Gastrointestinal irritant
Croton	*Croton tiglium*	Severe GI, dermatitis
Croton	*Codiaeum* spp	Dermatitis, gastrointestinal
Crown of thorns	*Euphorbia milii*	Severe GI, dermatitis
Cyclamen	*Cyclamen* spp	Gastrointestinal irritant

(continued)

TABLE 338.1.   (Continued)

Common Name	Botanical Name	Toxins/Effects
Daffodil (bulb)	*Narcissus* spp	GI; oxalates, insoluble
Daisy	*Chrysanthemum* spp	Dermatitis, GI irritant
Daphne	*Daphne* spp	GI, dermatitis, CNS depression
Datura	*Datura* spp	Anticholinergic
Deadly nightshade	*Atropa belladonna*	Anticholinergic
Deadly nightshade	*Solanum* spp	Solanine
Death camas	*Zigadenus nuttallii*	GI, cardiotoxic
Delphinium	*Delphinium* spp	GI, parasthesias, dysrythmias
Devil's ivy	*Epipremnum aureum*	Oxalates, insoluble
Devil's ivy	*Scindapsus aureus*	Oxalates, insoluble
Dieffenbachia	*Dieffenbachia* spp	Oxalates, insoluble
Dolls-eyes	*Actaea spicata*	Protoanemonin
Dragon plant	*Dracunculus vulgaris*	Oxalates, insoluble
Dragon root	*Arisaema* spp	Oxalates, insoluble
Dumbcane	*Dieffenbachia* spp	Oxalates, insoluble
Dusty miller	*Senecio* spp	Pyrrolizidine alkaloids
Eggplant (green parts)	*Solanum melongena*	Solanine
Elderberry	*Sambucus* spp	Gastrointestinal irritant
Elephant's ear philodendron	*Philodendron hastatum*	Oxalates, insoluble
Elephant's ear	*Colocasi* OR *Caladium*	Oxalates, insoluble
English ivy	*Hedera helix*	Gastrointestinal, dermatitis
English laurel	*Prunus laurocerasus*	Cyanogenic glycoside
Eucalyptus	*Eucalyptus* spp	Gastrointestinal irritant
False hellebore	*Veratrum* spp	GI, bradycardia, hypotension
False parsley	*Cicuta maculata*	CNS stimulant
False parsley	*Aethusa cynapium*	CNS stimulant
Flag	*Iris* spp	Dermatitis, GI irritant
Flax olive	*Daphne* spp	GI, derm, CNS depressant
Fool's parsley	*Aethusa cynapium*	CNS stimulant
Four o'clock	*Mirabilis jalapa*	GI, dermatitis, possible hallucinogen
Foxglove	*Digitalis purpurea*	Cardiac glycosides
Garden sorrel	*Rumex acetosa*	Oxalates, soluble
Ginkgo	*Ginkgo biloba*	Dermatitis, Chronic: increased bleeding time
Golden chain tree	*Laburnum* spp	Cytisine
Gopher plant	*Euphorbia lathyrus*	Severe GI, dermatitis
Gordoloba	*Achillea millefolium*	Gastrointestinal, dermatitis
Groundsel	*Senecio* spp	Pyrrolizidine alkaloids
Heath/Heather	*Calluna vulgaris*	Grayanotoxin
Heliotrope	*Heliotropium* spp	Pyrrolizidine
Hemlock, poison	*Conium maculatum*	CNS stimulant/ CNS depression
Hemlock, water	*Cicuta maculata*	CNS stimulant
Henbane	*Hyoscyamus niger*	Anticholinergic
Holly (berry)	*Ilex* spp	GI, CNS depression
Hops, wild	*Bryonia* spp	Dermatitis, GI irritant
Horse chestnut	*Aesculus* spp	GI, CNS depressant
Horsetail	*Equisetum* spp	Nicotine-like, dermatitis
Hyacinth (bulb)	*Hyacinthus orientalis*	Gastrointestinal, dermatitis
Hydrangea	*Hydrangea* spp	Gastrointestinal, dermatitis, poss. cyanogenic glycosides
Indian currant	*Symphoricarpos* spp	Gastrointestinal irritant
Indian tobacco	*Lobelia inflata*	GI, CNS stimulant, cardiotoxic
Inkberry	*Phytolacca americana*	Gastrointestinal irritant
Iris	*Iris* spp	Gastrointestinal, dermatitis
Ivy	*Hedera* spp	Dermatitis, GI irritant
Ivy bush	*Kalmia latifolia*	Grayanotoxin
Jack-in-the-pulpit	*Arisaema triphyllum*	Oxalates, insoluble; derm
Jalapeno peppers	*Capsicum annuum*	Dermatitis, GI irritant
Jasmine, Carolina	*Gelsemium sempervirens*	CNS stimulant, (Strychnine-like)
Jequirity bean	*Abrus precatorius*	Toxalbumin
Jessamine, yellow	*Gelsemium* spp	CNS stimulant, (Strychnine-like)
Jessamine, day blooming	*Cestrum diurnum*	Solanine, anticholinergic
Jessamine, poet's	*Jasminum officinale*	Dermatitis
Jimson weed	*Datura stramonium*	Anticholinergic
Juniper	*Juniperus* spp	Dermatitis, GI, Chronic: renal toxicity

(continued)

TABLE 338.1.   (Continued)

Common Name	Botanical Name	Toxins/Effects
Kentucky coffee tree	*Gymnocladus dioica*	Cytisine
Lady slipper	*Cypripedium* spp	Dermatitis
Lantana	*Lantana camara*	Anticholinergic, GI, CNS depressant
Larkspur	*Delphinium*	GI, parasthesias, dysrhythmia
Licorice, wild	*Glycyrrhiza* spp	Chronic: glucocorticoid effects
Licorice, wild	*Abrus precatorius*	Toxalbumin
Lily-of-the-valley	*Convallaria majalis*	Cardiac glycosides
Lily-of-the-valley bush	*Pieris japonica*	Grayanotoxin
Lobelia	*Lobelia berlandieri*	GI, CNS stimulant, cardiotoxic
Locoweed	*Datura stramonium*	Anticholinergic
Locoweed	*Cannabis sativa*	Hallucinogen
Locust, black or yellow	*Robinia pseudoacacia*	Toxalbumins
Marble queen pothos	*Epipremnum aureum*	Oxalates, insoluble
Marijuana	*Cannabis sativa*	Hallucinogen
Marsh marigold	*Caltha palustris*	Protoanemonin
Mate	*Ilex paraguariensis*	Caffeine
Mayapple	*Podophyllum peltatum*	GI, dermatitis, CNS depressant
Meadow crocus	*Colchicum autumnale*	Colchicine
Mescal bean	*Sophora secundiflora*	Cytisine
Mescal button	*Lophophora williamsii*	Hallucinogen, CNS stimulant, GI
Milkweed	*Asclepias* spp	Cardiac glycoside, CNS depressant, GI
Mistletoe, American	*Phoradendron flavescens*	Gastrointestinal irritant
Mistletoe, European	*Viscum album*	Hemoagglutination, seizures, gastrointestinal
Mock azalea	*Adenium* spp	Cardiac glycosides
Mock orange	*Prunus caroliniana*	Cyanogenic glycosides
Monkshood	*Aconitum napellus*	GI, parasthesias, dysrhythmia
Moonflower	*Ipomoea alba*	Dermatitis
Moonflower	*Datura inoxia*	Anticholinergic
Moonseed	*Menispermum* spp	CNS stimulant
Mormon tea	*Ephedra* spp	CNS stimulant
Morning glory (seeds)	*Ipomoea* spp	Hallucinogen
Mountain laurel	*Kalmia latifolia*	Grayanotoxin
Naked lady	*Amaryllis belladonna*	Gastrointestinal irritant
Narcissus	*Narcissus* spp	Gastrointestinal irritant
Nectarine (chewed pits)	Prunus spp	Cyanogenic glycosides
Nephthytis	*Syngonium podophyllum*	Oxalates, insoluble
Nicotine, ornamental	*Nicotiana longiflora*	Nicotine
Nightshade, black	*Solanum nigrum*	Solanine
Nightshade, common	*Solanum nigrum*	Solanine
Nightshade, deadly	*Solanum nigrum*	Solanine
Nightshade, deadly	*Atropa belladonna*	Anticholinergic
Nightshade, poisonous	*Solanum dulcamara*	Solanine
Nightshade, woody	*Solanum dulcamara*	Solanine
Nutmeg	*Myristica fragrans*	Hallucinogen, anticholinergic
Oak	*Quercus* spp	GI, hepatotoxic, dermatitis
Oleander, common	*Nerium oleander*	Cardiac glycosides
Oleander, yellow	*Thevetia peruviana*	Cardiac glycosides
Ornamental crabapple (chewed seeds)	*Malus floribunda*	Cyanogenic glycosides
Ornamental pepper	*Capsicum annuum*	Dermatitis, GI irritant
Ornamental pepper	*Solanum pseudocapsicum*	Solanine
Ornamental plum (chewed seeds)	*Prunus* spp	Cyanogenic glycosides
Paper white narcissus	*Narcissus tazetta*	Gastrointestinal irritant
Paradise tree	*Melia azedarach*	Gastrointestinal, CNS depressant
Parsley	*Petroselinum crispum*	Dermatitis
Parsley, false	*Cicuta maculata*	CNS stimulant
Parlsey, wild	*Cicuta maculata*	CNS stimulant
Parsnip	*Pastinaca sativa*	Dermatitis
Pasque flower	*Anemone* spp	Protoanemonin
Peach (chewed pits)	*Prunus* spp	Cyanogenic glycosides
Pear (chewed seeds)	*Pyrus* spp	Cyanogenic glycosides
Pennyroyal	*Mentha pulegium*	Multi-system failure

(continued)

TABLE 338.1. (Continued)

Common Name	Botanical Name	Toxins/Effects
Periwinkle	*Vinca rosea*	Vincristine, vinblastine
Periwinkle, rose	*Catharanthus roseus*	Vincristine, vinblastine
Persian lilac	*Melia azedarach*	GI, CNS depressant
Peyote; mescal	*Lophophora williamsii*	Hallucinogen, CNS stimulant, GI
Philodendron	*Philodendron* spp	Oxalates, insoluble
Plum (chewed seeds)	*Prunus* spp	Cyanogenic glycosides
Poison ivy/oak/sumac	*Toxicodendron* spp	Dermatitis
Pokeweed	*Phytolacca americana*	Gastrointestinal irritant
Poppy, common	*Papaver somniferum*	Opiates
Potato (unripe, leaves)	*Solanum tuberosum*	Solanine
Potato vine	*Solanum jasminoides*	Solanine
Pothos	*Scindapsus aureus*	Oxalates, insoluble
Pothos	*Epipremnum aureum*	Oxalates, insoluble
Prayer bean	*Arbus prectorius*	Toxalbumin
Prickly poppy	*Argemone* spp	GI, CNS depressant
Privet	*Ligustrum* spp	Gastrointestinal irritant
Purge nut	*Jatropha curcas*	Toxalbumin, severe dermatitis
Queen Anne's lace	*Daucus carota*	Dermatitis
Ragwort	*Senecio* spp	Pyrrolizidine alkaloids
Ranunculus	*Ranunculus* spp	Protoanemonin
Rattlebox	*Crotalaria* spp	Pyrrolizidine alkaloids
Rattlebox	*Daubentonia* spp	Pyrrolizidine alkaloids
Rhododendron	*Rhododendron genus*	Grayanotoxin
Rhubarb (leaves)	*Rheum* spp	Oxalates, soluble; dermatitis
Rosary bean/pea	*Abrus precatorius*	Toxalbumin
Rosary beads/pearls	*Senecio* spp	Pyrrolizidine alkaloids
Sagebrush	*Artemisia* spp	CNS stimulant/CNS depressant, GI
Sesbania	*Sesbania* spp	Pyrrolizidine alkaloids
Shamrock	*Oxalis* spp	Oxalates, soluble
Skunk cabbage	*Symplocarpus foetidus*	Oxalates, insoluble
Skunk cabbage	*Veratrum* spp	GI, cardiotoxic
Snakeroot	*Eupatorium rugosum*	Pyrrolizidine alkaloids
Snakeroot	*Aristolochia serpentaria*	Nephrotoxic, hepatotoxic
Snakeroot	*Cicuta maculata*	CNS stimulant
Snowberry	*Symphoricarpos* spp	GI, CNS depressant
Sorrel	*Oxalis* spp	Oxalates, soluble
Sorrel	*Rumex* spp	Oxalates, soluble
Spathiphyllum	*Spathiphyllum* spp	Oxalates, insoluble
Split leaf philodendron	*Monstera deliciosa*	Oxalates, insoluble
Spurge flax	*Daphne* spp	GI, dermatitis, CNS depressant
Squill	*Urginea maritima*	Cardiac glycosides
Star-of-Bethlehem	*Ornithogalum* spp	Cardiac glycosides
Star-of-Bethlehem	*Laurentia longiflora*	Nicotine
Star-of-Bethlehem	*Hippobroma longiflora*	CNS stimulant, GI
String of pearls/beads	*Senecio* spp	Pyrrolizidine
Strychnos nux-vomica	*Strychnos nux-vomica*	Strychnine
Sweet clover	*Melilotus* spp	Warfarin
Tansy	*Tanacetum* spp	Acute: Dermatitis Chronic: Nephrotoxic
Taro	*Alocasia macrorrhiza*	Oxalates, insoluble
Taro	*Colocasia esculenta*	Oxalates, insoluble
Texas umbrella tree	*Melia azedarach*	GI, CNS depressant
Thornapple	*Argemone mexicana*	GI, CNS depressant
Thornapple	*Datura stramonium*	Anticholinergic
Tobacco	*Nicotiana* spp	Nicotine
Tobacco, wild	*Lobelia inflata*	CNS stimulant, GI
Tomato (leaves, stems)	*Lycopersicon* spp	Solanine
Tonka bean	*Dipteryx odorata*	Coumarin, CNS depression
Toyon (leaves)	*Photinia arbutifolia*	Cyanogenic glycosides
Tree tobacco	*Nicotiana glauca*	Nicotine
Tulip (bulb)	*Tulipa* spp	Dermatitis
Tung nut	*Aleurites fordii*	Severe GI, dermatitis
Umbrella leaf	*Podophyllum peltatum*	GI, CNS depressant dermatitis
Umbrella plant	*Cyperus alternifolius*	Acute: Gastrointestinal; Chronic: renal toxicity
Virginia creeper	*Parthenocissus* spp	Oxalates, soluble
Walnut (green shells)	*Juglans* spp	Dermatitis
Water hemlock	*Cicuta maculata*	CNS stimulant

(continued)

TABLE 338.1.   (Continued)

Common Name	Botanical Name	Toxins/Effects
Wild carrot	*Daucus carota*	Dermatitis
Wild carrot	*Cicuta maculata*	CNS stimulant
Wild parsnip	*Pastinaca sativa*	Dermatitis
Wild parsnip	*Cicuta maculata*	CNS stimulant
Wild parsnip	*Heracleum mantegazzianum*	Dermatitis
Wild parsnip	*Angelica archangelica*	Dermatitis
Wisteria	*Wisteria* spp	Gastrointestinal irritant
Wood rose	*Merremia tuberosa*	Hallucinogen
Wood rose, Hawaiian	*Merremia tuberosa*	Hallucinogen
Wood rose, Hawaiian baby	*Argyreia nervosa*	Hallucinogen
Wormwood	*Artemesia* spp	CNS stimulant/CNS depressant, GI
Yarrow	*Achillea millefolium*	Gastrointestinal, dermatitis
Yellow oleander	*Thevetia peruviana*	Cardiac glycosides
Yew	*Taxus* spp	Cardiotoxic, respiratory depressant
Yohimbine	*Corynanthe yohimbe*	Cardiac glycosides, mild hallucinogen

as a result of acute accidental ingestion of these plants is rare. However, amygdalin has long been touted as a "natural" cancer cure, suggesting that cancer cells selectively absorb the cyanide and die, leaving only healthy cells. Patients who ingest large amounts of bitter almonds or apricot seeds chronically may develop true cyanide toxicity.

The jequirity bean (*Abrus prectorious*) and the castor bean (*Ricinus communis*) plants contain toxalbumins or toxic albumins (2,8,18,22). Toxalbumins are composed of two subunits, the A and the B chains linked by a single disulfide chain. The A chain inhibits protein synthesis and leads to cell death. The B chain binds to cell surface glycoproteins that affect entry of the toxin into the cell. The toxalbumin structure is similar to insulin and the toxins associated with botulism, tetanus, cholera, and diphtheria (17).

Toxalbumins cause severe irritation and lesions to the oropharynx, esophagus, or stomach with hematemesis, tenesmus, and tissue sloughing. These symptoms may occur about 2 to 6 hours after exposure. Symptoms are similar to alkaline caustic burns. The patient may experience a relatively asymptomatic period and then develop late cytotoxic effects. Two to 5 days after exposure, liver, kidneys, adrenal glands, and CNS involvement may occur. This may reflect variations in toxicity of the seeds or poor GI absorption (2,22). The severity of symptoms depends on the degree of chewing. If the seeds are swallowed whole, symptoms are much less likely to occur (18).

Acute large ingestions of plants containing pyrrolizidine alkaloids (e.g., ragwort, heliotrope, and the senecio species) produce liver disease (2,3,22). Toxicity may also result from subacute and chronic exposures (17). Veno-occlusive disease is the primary symptom seen in humans. Patients may present with vomiting and severe abdominal pain. Hepatomegaly, right upper quadrant abdominal tenderness, and ascites follow. Jaundice may be seen as well. Onset of symptoms may be days or weeks after ingestion making diagnosis difficult. In children, toxicity may be confused with Reye's syndrome.

CNS stimulation may be caused by a variety of plants with various mechanisms of action. Cicutoxin, found in water hemlock, is thought to cause status epilepticus from overstimulation of the cholinergic pathways (17). Seizures may occur as suddenly as 5 minutes after ingestion, but may be delayed up to 1 to 2 hours (9). Postictal states following seizures may mislead the clinician into thinking that a depressant drug has been ingested. Other symptoms may include excessive salivation, vomiting, diarrhea, mydriasis, tachycardia, hallucinations, amnesia, muscle rigid-

ity, acidosis, renal failure, and rhabdomyolysis (14,17,22). Death from strychnine-like effects and cardiac arrest has occurred.

CNS depression may range from mild to severe, depending on the type of plant involved and the amount of plant material ingested. Mechanisms of action vary with the plant type (17,22). Generally, large ingestions are required to produce significant CNS depression.

Sudden onset of unconsciousness is seen after ingestion of monkshood, hellebore, or death camus. Ingestion of nicotiana, lantana, and large quantities of mescal beans may cause delayed CNS depression. Anticholinergic plants such as jimson weed or belladonna may cause hallucinations and delirium, along with CNS stimulation or depression. Marijuana causes a sedating or tranquilizing effect (4).

Plants containing cytisine such as the golden chain tree, Kentucky coffee tree, and mescal bean cause symptoms similar to nicotine poisoning but are less severe. (2,22). The onset of symptoms is rapid, within 15 to 60 minutes. Symptoms include pallor; mydriasis; persistent, profuse vomiting; drowsiness; headache; incoordination; delirium and hallucinations; hypotension; and tachycardia (2,17,19). Large doses may produce fasciculations and seizures, followed by a curare-like muscle paralysis and coma. Although cytisine acts as a respiratory stimulant, death is usually a result of respiratory failure secondary to muscle paralysis.

Well-known hallucinogenic or perception-altering plants include marijuana and peyote (2,17,22). Other hallucinogenic plants include the morning glory, Hawaiian wood rose (1), four o'clock, and nutmeg (22). However, usually large amounts are required to result in any effect. Anticholinergic plants, such as jimsonweed and belladonna, also produce hallucinations (17). The associated vomiting and other adverse effects prevent more widespread abuse. Keep in mind that *Amanita muscaria* and *A. psilocybe* mushrooms are also used intentionally for their psychoactive properties.

Dermal exposure can cause skin irritation as a result of mechanical, chemical, or allergic reactions, photodermatitis, or a combination of these. Severity of symptoms depends on the amount of exposure, the individual sensitivity and the part of the body exposed (17). Most cases are self-limiting and resolve within 14 to 21 days.

An allergic reaction is a true sensitization of an individual to the allergen contained in the plant. After the first exposure, the patient's next exposure has a 5- to 7-day latency period before the immunological response develops. Allergic contact

TABLE 338.2.   Nontoxic Plants

Common Name	Botanical Name	Common Name	Botanical Name
African violet	*Saintpaulia ionantha*	Dusty miller	*Lynchnis coronaria*
Aglaonema	*Aglaonema* spp	Easter lily	*Lilium longiflorum*
Ajuga	*Ajuga* spp	Elephant's ear	*Enterolobium cyclocarpum*
Albizia	*Albizia*	Elephant's ear	*Bergenia cordifolia*
Aluminum plant	*Pilea cadierei*	Elephant's ear fern	*Platycerium angolense*
Alyssum	*Alyssum* spp	Elephant's foot	*Dioscorea elephantipes*
Angel's tears	*Soleirolia soleirolii*	Emerald fern	*Asparagus densiflorus sprengeri*
Areca palm	*Areca lutescens*		
Artillery plant	*Pilea* spp	Emerald ripple peperomia	*Peperomia caperata*
Asparagus fern	*Asparagus sprengeri*	Escallonia	*Escallonia* spp
Aspidistra	*Aspidistra* spp	Evening primrose	*Oenothera caespitosa*
Aster, Chinese	*Callistephus chinensis*	Exacum	*Exacum affine*
Astilbe	*Astilbe japonica*	False aralia	*Dizygotheca elegantissima*
Aucuba	*Aucuba japonica*	Fittonia	*Fittonia* spp
Baby's breath	*Gypsophila* spp	Flaming sword	*Vriesea splendens*
Baby's tears	*Soleirolia soleirolii*	Forget-me-not	*Myosotis* spp
Bachelor buttons	*Centaurea cyanus*	Forsythia	*Forsythia* spp
Bamboo palm	*Chamaedorea erumpens*	Freesia	*Freesia* spp
Bamboo, common	*Phyllostachys aurea*	Friendship plant	*Pilea involucrate* OR *Billbergia nutans*
Bee balm	*Monarda didyma*		
Bee balm	*Melissa officinalis*	Fruitless mulberry	*Morus* spp
Bell flower	*Platycodon grandiflorus*	Fuchsia	*Fuchsia* spp
Bell flower	*Campanula* spp	Gardenia	*Gardenia* spp
Bird's nest fern	*Asplenium* spp	Gerbera daisy	*Gerbera jamesonii*
Bishop's cap	*Astrophytum myriostigma*	Ghost plant	*Graptopetalum paraguayense*
Bleeding heart	*Clerodendrum* spp	Glory of the snow	*Chionodoxa luciliae*
Boston fern	*Nephrolepsis exalta*	Glory pea	*Clianthus* spp
Bottlebrush	*Callistemon* spp	Gloxinia	*Sinningia speciosa*
Bromeliad king	*Vriesea hieroglyphica*	Godetia	*Godetia* spp
Bromeliad, blushing	*Neoregelia carolinae*	Goldfish plant	*Hypocyrta* spp
Butterfly bush	*Buddleia davidii*	Good luck plant	*Cordyline terminalis* OR *Kalanchoe daigremontiana*
Butterfly palm	*Chrysalidocarpus lutescens*		
Button fern	*Pellaea rotundifolia*	Gourd	*Cucurbitaceae* spp
Calendula	*Calendula officinalis*	Grape hyacinth	*Muscari* spp
California poppy	*Eschscholzia californica*	Hare fern	*Davallia fejeensis*
Camellia	*Camellia* spp	Hawaiian good luck plant	*Cordyline terminalis*
Canna lily	*Canna* spp	Hawthorne	*Crataegus* spp
Canterbury-bell gloxinia	*Gloxinia perennis*	Hearts entangled	*Ceropegia woodii*
Cardinal flower	*Rechsteineria cardinalis*	Hearts-on-a-string	*Ceropegia woodii*
Cardinal flower	*Sinningia cardinalis*	Hen and chickens fern	*Asplenium bulbiferum*
Cast iron plant	*Aspidistra elatior*	Hen and chicks	*Echeveria* spp
Catalpa	*Catalpa* spp	Hibiscus	*Hibiscus* spp
Chandelier plant	*Kalanchoe tubiforum*	Hollyhock	*Althaea rosea*
Chenille plant, maroon	*Echeveria derenbergii*	Honey locust	*Gleditsia triacanthos*
China doll	*Leea* spp	Ice plant	*Lampranthus* spp
China doll	*Radermachera* spp	Ice plant	*Aptenia cordifolia*
China rose	*Hibiscus* spp	Impatiens	*Impatiens* species
Chinese evergreen	*Aglaonema modestum*	Inch plant	*Zebrina pendula*
Chocolate soldier	*Episcia cupreata*	Inch plant	*Callisia* spp
Christmas cactus	*Schlumbergera bridgesii*	Indian hawthorne	*Raphiolepsis indica*
Cockscomb	*Celosia* spp	Iron plant	*Aspidistra* spp
Coleus	*Coleus* spp	Jacaranda tree	*Jacaranda* spp
Coneflower	*Echinacea angustifolia*	Jade plant	*Crassula* spp
Coral bells	*Kalanchoe uniflora*	Japanese aralia	*Fatsia japonica*
Coral bells	*Heuchera sanguinea*	Kalanchoe	*Kalanchoe* spp
Coral berry	*Ardisia crenata*	Kangaroo vine	*Cissus antartica*
Coreopsis	*Coreopsis* spp	Lady palm	*Rhapis* spp
Corn plant	*Dracaena fragrans*	Lamb's tail	*Sedum morganianum*
Cornflower	*Centaurea cyanus*	Lavender	*Lavandula officinalis*
Cosmos	*Cosmos* spp	Liatris	*Liatris* spp
Crape myrtle	*Lagerstroemia indica*	Lilac	*Syringa* spp
Crataegus	*Crataegus* spp	Lipstick vine	*Aeschynanthus* spp
Creeping charlie	*Plectranthus australis*	Liquidamber	*Liquidamber orientalis*
Creeping charlie	*Pilea nummulariifolia*	Live forever	*Sedum telephium*
Creeping jenny	*Lysimachia nummularia*	Lucky bamboo	*Dracaena sanderiana*
Crocus, spring blooming	*Crocus* spp	Madagascar dragon tree	*Dracaena marginata*
Cupid's bower	*Achimenes erecta*	Madagascar lace plant	*Aponogeton senetralis*
Dahlia	*Dahlia* spp	Magnolia	*Magnolia* spp
Dandelion	*Taraxacum officinale*	Maiden's tears	*Silene acaulis*
Day lily	*Hermocallis* spp	Maid fern	*Adiantum decorum*
Donkey tail	*Sedum morganianum*	Maidenhair vine	*Muehlenbeckia complexa*
Dracaena	*Cordyline* spp OR *Dracaena* spp	Manzanita	*Arbutus* spp
		Manzanita, wooly	*Arctostaphylos tomentosa*

(continued)

TABLE 338.2. (Continued)

Common Name	Botanical Name	Common Name	Botanical Name
Maranta	*Calathea* spp	Rosary vine	*Ceropegia woodii*
Matilija poppy	*Romneya coulteri*	Rose moss	*Portulaca grandiflora*
Mimosa	*Albizia julibrissin*	Rose of Sharon	*Hibiscus syriacus*
Mock orange	*Philadelphus* spp	Sand dollar cactus	*Astrophytum asterias*
Mock orange	*Pittosporum tobira*	Santolina	*Santolina* spp
Mock strawberry	*Duchesnea indica*	Sedum	*Sedum* spp
Money plant	*Lunaria annua*	Sensitive plant	*Mimosa pudica*
Monkey plant	*Ruellia makoyana*	Shrimp plant	*Beloperone guttata*
Mosquito plant	*Pelargonium citrosum*	Shrimp plant	*Justicia brandegeana*
Mother fern	*Aspelenium* spp	Silk tree	*Albizia julibrissin*
Mother of thousands	*Saxifraga stolonifera*	Silver king	*Aglaonema* spp
Mother of thousands	*Kalanchoe pinnata*	Silver net plant	*Fittonia argyroneura*
Mother-of-pearl plant	*Graptopetalum paraguayense*	Silver queen	*Aglaonema* spp
Nerve plant	*Fittonia* spp	Slipper plant	*Calceolaria* spp
Norfolk Island pine	*Araucaria heterophylla*	Snapdragon	*Antirrhinum majus*
Orchid	*Cattleya* spp	Snow bush	*Breynia disticha*
Orchid	*Oncidium* spp	Snowball bush	*Viburnum* spp
Orchid	*Epidendrum* spp	Spanish moss	*Tillandsia usneoides*
Oregon grape	*Mahonia aquifolium*	Sparaxis	*Sparaxis* spp
Parlor palm	*Chamaedorea elegans*	Spider plant	*Chlorophytum comosum*
Passion vine, purple	*Gynura aurantiaca*	Spirea	*Spirea* spp
Peacock plant	*Calathea makoyana*	Star jasmine	*Trachelospermum jasminoides*
Peacock plant	*Kaempferia roscoeana*	Starfish flower	*Stapelia* spp
Peperomia	*Peperomia* spp	Stargazer lily	*Lilium* spp
Persian violet	*Exacum affine*	Statice	*Limonium* spp
Petunia	*Petunia* spp	Strawberry tree	*Arbutus unedo*
Phlox	*Phlox* spp	Strawflower	*Helichrysum bracteatum*
Photina	*Photina fraseri*	String of hearts	*Ceropegia woodii*
Piggyback plant	*Tolmiea menziesii*	Swedish ivy	*Plectranthus australis*
Pilea	*Pilea* spp	Sweet alyssum	*Lobularia maritima*
Pittosporum	*Pittosporum* spp	Sweet flag	*Acorus* spp
Plane tree	*Platanus occidentalis*	Sweet woodruff	*Asperula odorata*
Plush vine	*Mikania apiifolia*	Sword fern	*Nephrolepsis* spp OR
Poinsettia	*Euphorbia pulcherrima*		*Polystichum munitum*
Polka dot plant	*Hypoestes phyllostachya*	Tahitian bridal veil	*Tradescantia multiflora*
Pony tail plant	*Beaucarnea recurvata*	Teddy bear vine	*Cyanotis kewensis*
Portulaca	*Portulaca oleracea*	Temple bells	*Smithiantha cinnabarina*
Potentilla	*Potentilla* spp	Ti plant	*Cordyline terminalis*
Prayer plant	*Maranta leuconeura*	Torch lily	*Kniphofia* spp
Pregnant plant	*Kalanchoe pinnata*	Transvaal daisy	*Gerbera jamesoni*
Propeller plant	*Crassula cultrata*	Urn plant	*Aechmea fasciata*
Protea	*Protea* spp	Velvet plant	*Gynura* spp
Purslane	*Portulaca oleracea*	Veronica	*Veronica* spp
Queen of the night	*Epiphyllum oxypetalum*	Viburnum	*Viburnum* spp
Queen's jewels	*Antigonon leptopus*	Watsonia	*Watsonia* spp
Queen's tears	*Billbergia nutans*	Wax plant	*Hoya carnosa*
Queen's wreath	*Antigonon leptopus*	Weigela	*Weigela* spp
Quince, common	*Cydonia oblonga*	Xylosma	*Xylosma* spp
Quince, flowering	*Chaenomeles* spp	Yucca	*Yucca* spp
Rabbit's foot fern	*Davallia fejeensis*	Zebra plant	*Aphelandra squarrosa*
Red bud	*Cercis canadensis*	Zebra plant	*Calathea zebrine*
Resurrection lily	*Kaempferia* spp	Zebra plant	*Cryptanthus zonatus*
Rosary bead plant	*Ceropegia woodii*	Zinnia	*Zinnia* spp
Rosary vine	*Crassula rupestris*		

dermatitis presents with pruritis and vesiculation. The affected area may be erythematous, edematous, and develop large bullae. Weeping and crusting of the affected areas may occur (17). Most people are sensitized to toxicodendrol (or urushiol), the oily substance seen on the leaves of poison oak, poison ivy, and poison sumac.

Peppers (e.g., chili, jalapeno, cayenne) contain capsaicin alkaloids (24). These alkaloids are thought to deplete nerve terminals of substance P that stimulates sensory nerve endings resulting in pain and burning. Nettle plants have "hairs" that inject the skin with histamine, acetylcholine, and serotonin resulting in wheals, pruritis, and burning at the sting (17,22).

Photodermatitis may result after exposure to plants such as parsnips and limes, which contain oils that intensify the skin's sensitive to sunlight (17,22). Onset occurs within hours but can be delayed for up to 48 hours. A rash similar to sunburn occurs, but only skin that has both been in contact with the plant and exposed to the sun is affected. Exposure to the sun after exposure to may result in photodermatitis.

Mechanical trauma after exposure to the thorns, spines, and barbs of any plant species can occur (16,22). Spines or thorns breaking off in the skin may cause secondary infections and wound ulceration. Symptoms may resemble bone lesions. Granulomas may also develop up to weeks after exposure. Cacti, century plants, roses, and pyracantha are examples of plants with thorns and spines.

EMERGENCY DEPARTMENT EVALUATION

A history of exposure is critical in alerting the clinician to the possibility of plant toxicity. Questions concerning the use of or contact with plants should be asked when a patient presents with an illness of uncertain cause. Additionally, patients should be asked about the ingestion of homemade tea used to treat themselves or their sick children.

In children, even if ingestion was not witnessed, questions should be asked about plant availability. Evidence of plant exposure may include plant material on a child, missing parts on a plant in or around the home, or plant material in the stool or vomitus. If possible, any suspect plant (or a sample) should be brought with the patient to the ED for identification (2,13,22).

Many plants have multiple common and scientific names. Keep in mind that some plants sharing common names may include both toxic and nontoxic species. If the patient provides a common name of a plant, the correct identity should be confirmed by the proper scientific Latin name, as well as a botanic description (6,13,22). Ideally this description should include leaf and flower shape and color, fruits, and general size and shape (22). Because few emergency physicians have the expertise to identify plants, groups such as garden clubs, botanic gardens, floral or garden shops, park rangers, and university agricultural departments may be of value (20,22). Poison control centers may also help with information on plant toxicity and treatment options.

Depending on the patient's signs and symptoms, a complete or focused physical examination is appropriate. All patients should have a complete set of vital signs, including temperature. Depending on the history and physical findings, a rhythm strip or electrocardiogram interpretation may be indicated to evaluate for cardiac toxicity (2,17,22). Laboratory testing may be necessary for the assessment of fluid and electrolyte, hematologic, liver, or renal function abnormalities. With few exceptions (e.g., cardiac-glycoside plants), specific toxicology testing is unlikely to be helpful (22).

EMERGENCY DEPARTMENT MANAGEMENT

Supportive care and GI and skin decontamination are the primary treatment modalities (17,22). Although rarely necessary, advanced life-support measures should be instituted when appropriate. Supportive therapy includes replacement of volume deficits with intravenous crystalloids and correction of electrolyte abnormalities. Patients with CNS depression may require airway protection and ventilatory support. Patients manifesting seizures and CNS stimulation usually respond to treatment with benzodiazepines. Refractory seizures can be treated with benzodiazepines and phenobarbital. Allergic reactions and hematologic, liver, and renal toxicity are treated with standard measures (2,17,22).

Local pain and irritation from the ingestion of plants containing insoluble oxalate crystals can be treated with age-appropriate cold foods or liquids such as juice bars, ice cream, yogurt, milk, or ice cubes, which decrease mouth pain and help alleviate any localized oral swelling. The pain usually lasts 15 to 30 minutes and other treatment is usually not needed (15).

Decontamination varies with the route and nature of the exposure. Dilution with small amounts of clear liquids or milk is usually sufficient for the ingestion of plants that only cause gastroenteritis. Because many plant toxins are large molecules, activated charcoal should be effective and is the preferred method of GI decontamination for recent ingestions of agents with potential systemic toxicity (2,5,22).

Skin and eye exposures are treated with thorough irrigation. Some cactus spines can be removed with tweezers or forceps (16). Fine spines have been removed with tape, facial masks, glue mixtures, and wood pastes applied to the skin and then peeled off. Oily materials, such as the toxicodendrol oils, should be washed thoroughly with soap and water to prevent spread to other parts of the body, clothing, or to emergency room staff (18).

Antihistamines, antiinflammatory agents (e.g., topical or oral systemic steroids), and analgesics for itching and pain may be required for some dermal exposures. Topical antiseptics and tetanus prophylaxis may be useful if there are puncture wounds.

There are few antidotes for plant poisonings (2,5,7,17,21). When an antidote is considered useful, it is generally similar in effectiveness and dosage to a nonplant exposure to the same toxic substance. For example, cardiac glycoside poisoning may be treated with digoxin-specific Fab-fragment antibodies (Chapter 304, "Cardiac Glycosides"), although calculating a dose is challenging (5). Severe anticholinergic plant poisoning is potentially treatable with physostigmine (Chapter 323, "Anticholinergic Agents") (21). Patients with symptomatic cyanogenic glycoside poisoning should be treated with specific cyanide antidotes (Chapter 308, "Cyanide").

CRITICAL INTERVENTIONS

- Obtain complete vital signs, including temperature, on all patients with suspected plant ingestions
- Obtain an accurate name of the plant including the common and scientific name
- Evaluate patients with plant ingestions for possible upper airway obstruction
- Provide supportive care as clinically necessary

DISPOSITION

Although the vast majority of patients with plant exposures can be treated at home or discharged from the ED, patients with acute ingestions of a potentially toxic plant should be observed until symptoms have resolved. Those with irritant and oxalate ingestions may be discharged as soon as their discomfort is under control, they can take fluids orally, and there is no evidence of airway edema. Patients who are symptomatic after ingesting plants containing cardiac glycoside and CNS toxins should be admitted for close observation, monitoring, and treatment. The level of care should be dictated by clinical severity. If severe, patients with fluid and electrolyte imbalance, allergic reactions, and hematologic, liver, or renal toxicity may also require admission.

COMMON PITFALLS

✔ Failure to appreciate that plant poisoning can affect virtually any organ system
✔ Failure to inquire about plant exposure in patients with unexplained complaints, particularly GI and CNS symptoms and rashes
✔ Failure to appreciate that different plants may have the same common name, which may include both toxic and nontoxic plant species

✔ Failure to appreciate that some edible plants also have toxic components

✔ Failure to appreciate that specific antidotes are available for the treatment of anticholinergic, cardiac glycoside, and cyanogenic glycoside plant poisoning

Acknowledgments

We thank previous edition chapter author David G. Spoerke.

References

1. Al-Assmar SE. The seeds of the Hawaiian baby woodrose are a powerful hallucinogen. (Letter). *Arch Intern Med* 1999;159:2090.
2. Alsop JA. Plants. In: Olson KR, ed. *Poisoning & drug overdose*, 4th Ed. New York: Lange Medical Books/McGraw-Hill, 2004;309–319.
3. Bach N, Thung SN, Schaffner F. Comfrey herb tea-induced hepatic veno-occlusive disease. *Am J Med* 1989;87:97–99.
4. Brown JL, Malone MH. Legal highs-constitutes activity, toxicology, and herbal folklore. *Clin Toxicol* 1978;12:1.
5. DiSilva HA, Foneska MMD, Pathmeswaran A, et al. Multiple—dose activated charcoal for treatment of yellow oleander poisoning: a single-blind, randomized, placebo-controlled trial. *Lancet* 2003;361:1935–1938.
6. DiTomaso JM. Problems associated with the use of common names in the identification of poisonous plants. *Vet Hum Toxicol* 1993;35:465–466.
7. Eddleston M, Persson H. Acute plant poisoning and antitoxin antibodies. *J Toxicol Clin Toxicol* 2003;41:309–315.
8. Fernando C. Poisoning due to Abrus prectorious (jequirity bean). *Anaesthesia* 2001;56:1178–1180.
9. Frank BS, Michelson WB, Panter KP, Gardner DR. Ingestion of poison hemlock (Conium maculatum). *West J Med* 1995;163:573–574.
10. Gardner DG. Injury to the oral mucus membranes caused by the common houseplant. *Oral Surg Oral Med Oral Pathol Oral Radiol Endod* 1994;78:631–633.
11. Gopel C, Laufer C, Marcus A. Three cases of angel's trumpet tea-induced psychosis in adolescent substance abusers. *Nord J Psychiatry* 2002;56:49–52.
12. Guharoy SR. Atropine intoxication from the ingestion and smoking of jimson weed (Datura stramonium). *Vet Hum Toxicol* 1991;33:588–589.
13. Harchelroad F, Scalise JA, Dean BS, et al. Identification of common houseplants in the emergent care setting. *Vet Hum Toxicol* 1988;30:161–163.
14. Heath KB. A fatal case of apparent water hemlock poisoning. *Vet Hum Toxicol* 2001;43:35–36.
15. Krenzelok EP, Jacobsen RD, Aronis JM. A review of 96,659 dieffenbachia and philodendron exposures (abstract). *J Toxicol Clin Toxicol* 1994;36:601.
16. Lindsey D, Lindsey WE. Cactus spine injuries. *Am J Emerg Med* 1988;6:362–369.
17. Palmer M, Betz JM. Plants. In: Goldfrank LR, Flomenbaum NE, Lewin NA, et al. (eds). *Goldfrank's toxicologic emergencies*, 7th Ed. New York: McGraw-Hill 2002;1150–1182.
18. Rauber A, Heard J. Castor bean toxicity re-examined: a new prospective. *Vet Hum Toxicol* 1985;27:498–502.
19. Richards HGH, Stephens A. A fatal case of laburnum seed poisoning. *Med Sci Law* 1970;10:260–266.
20. Rondeau-Studer E, Everson G, Savage W, et al. Plant nurseries—a reliable resource for plant identification? *Vet Hum Toxicol* 1992;34:544–546.
21. Salen P, Shih R, Sierzenski P, et al. Effect of physostigmine and gastric lavage in a Datura stramonium-induced anticholinergic poisoning epidemic. *Am J Emerg Med* 2003;21:316–317.
22. Spoerke D, Evans B, Linaburg B.*The hidden hazards in house and garden plants.* Missoula, Montana: Pictorial Histories Publishing Co. Inc., 1991.
23. Watson WA, Litovitz TL, Rodgers GC, et al. 2002 Annual report of the American association of poison control centers toxic exposure surveillance system. *Am J Emerg Med* 2003;21:353–421.
24. Williams SR, Clark RF, Dunford JV. Contact dermatitis associated with capsaicin: Hunan hand syndrome. *Ann Emerg Med* 1995;25:713–715.

CHAPTER 339
Dietary Supplements and Herbal Medications

Richard J. Geller

Dietary supplements (DS) are regularly taken by millions of Americans, and represent a huge industry with estimated annual sales of $16 billion. Herbal medications with annual sales volume in excess of $200 million include echinacea, ginseng, Ginkgo biloba, and St. John's wort (2). Although the use of DS is generally safe, it is neither absolutely safe nor predictably safe. Consumers often have a naive belief that these therapies pose no risk at all, a position often propounded by herbal therapists.

Until 1994, DS were regulated by the U.S. Food and Drug Administration (FDA) under the 1958 Food Additive Amendments to the Federal Food, Drug and Cosmetic Act. Although the Nutrition Labeling and Education Act of 1990 gave the FDA the power to require DS manufacturers to prove both safety and health claims before a product could be marketed, the Dietary and Supplements Health and Education Act of 1994 (DSHEA) limited FDA authority to regulate this industry, shifting responsibility for ensuring the safety of DS products to manufacturers. Unlike pharmaceuticals, however, DS manufacturers are not required to document either the safety or the effectiveness of their products and the FDA has the burden to prove that a product is dangerous if it wants to restrict use of a product or to remove a product from the marketplace. The banning of ephedra-containing products in December 2003 was the first time FDA used its administrative authority to remove a DS from the market (24).

According to DSHEA, a DS is a product taken by mouth that contains a "dietary ingredient" intended to supplement the diet. Dietary ingredients include vitamins (see Chapter 341, "Vitamins"), minerals, herbs or other botanicals, amino acids, and substances such as enzymes, organ tissues, glandulars, and metabolites. Minerals are chemical elements required for numerous biological and physiological processes that are necessary for the maintenance of health. Examples include calcium, magnesium, sodium, potassium, sulfur, and chlorine. Those that are required in amounts less than 100 mg per day (such as iron, iodine, copper, manganese, zinc, molybdenum, selenium, and chromium) are called trace elements. A botanical is a product made from any part of a plant, and this category includes herbal products, which are made from the leaves and stems of plants, but often used when referring to any botanical product. Amino acids are a family of small organic molecules that contain an amino group (NH2) and are used for protein synthesis. Glandulars are extracts from animal glands, a subset of animal extracts, which are derived from any animal tissue.

Comprehensive data regarding the toxicity of DS is sparse. Fewer than 1% of adverse reactions from dietary supplements are identified by current surveillance systems (23). In 1 year, products containing ephedra alkaloids (also called ma huang) accounted for 64% of all adverse reactions to herbs reported in the United States, yet accounted for only 0.82% of herbal product sales (2). Caffeine-containing guarana is often added to ephedra in supplements. Ma Huang contains ephedrine as well as pseudoephedrine, phenylpropanolamine, methylephedrine, methylpseudoephedrine, and norpseudoephedrine (10). Clinical outcomes thought to be "definitely or probably related to the use of supplements containing ephedra alkaloids" include hypertension, seizures, hemorrhagic stroke, myocardial infarction (MI), and cardiac arrest (11).

The FDA has recently issued warnings concerning specific DS including hepatoxicity from comfrey and kava, renal failure from Chinese herbs containing aristolochic acid, and stroke and MI from tiratricol, a potent thyroid hormone. According to the FDA, there is no legitimate evidence supporting a therapeutic role for glandulars, which can be dangerous because organ concentrates may contain chemicals that livestock come in contact with, such as antibiotics, growth hormones, pesticides, and fertilizers.

As with all substances possessing pharmaceutical properties, exaggeration of desired clinical effect with excessive dosing can cause toxicity. Drug–herb interactions are often poorly characterized, but have the same potential for harm as drug–drug or drug–dietary interactions.

Lack of dose standardization with herbal medications can lead to toxicity. A given weight of plant does not yield a standard amount of desired compound. In the mid-nineteenth century practice, in which extract of the colchicum plant was used to treat gout, it was very difficult to give enough of the extract to relieve symptoms without creating gastrointestinal (GI) side effects. As with pharmaceuticals, DS exhibit a broad range of therapeutic margin, and may have toxic effects related (and unrelated) to the desired effect of the substance. Aconite (*Aconitum* species), a plant encountered in Chinese herbal practice, is inherently toxic.

Geographic and seasonal variability of plant constituents can also lead to poisoning. *Senecio longilobus* from Gardner Canyon, Arizona, has been found to contain up to 18% hepatotoxic pyrrolizidine alkaloids whereas the usual content is 0.5%. Cyanide poisoning has occurred after ingesting a grass harvested on the shore of San Francisco which was found to produce cyanogenic glycosides at certain times of the year.

Misidentification of herbs is another potential cause of poisoning. Substitution of *Aristolochia fangchi* for *Stephania tetrandra* led to poisoning in 70 people including 30 cases of terminal renal failure, as a result of aristolochic acid (25). Mistaking foxglove (*Digitalis purpurea*) for comfrey has resulted in death as a result of cardiac glycoside poisoning.

Contamination is also a potential problem. Contaminants in L-tryptophan were believed to be responsible for the eosinophilia-myalgia syndrome. Clam shell powder has been contaminated with lead (12). *Salmonella arizonae bacteremia*, especially in immuno-compromised patients, has resulted from ingestion of contaminated dried rattlesnake meat, a common Hispanic folk remedy sold as a DS (15).

DS, particularly Asian patent and Chinese herbal medicines, are occasionally adulterated or misrepresented (13,14,16). Aplastic anemia occurred after ingesting Gan Mao Tong Pian adulterated with phenylbutazone and aminopyrone (20). Arsenic and mercury have been found in Chinese herbal balls (8). A Chinese patent medicine called "Diankexing" used for treatment of seizures was found to contain phenobarbital and mephobarbital (4). Other substances found in Asian patent medicines include chlorpheniramine, acetaminophen, pulegone, lead, ephedrine, pseudoephedrine, and dipyrone (5). In 2000, the owner of a DS company was sentenced to prison and fined $2,325,000 for misrepresentating a product to which pharmaceutical grade ephedrine and caffeine was added as "all-natural."

The ingestion of herbals intended for topical use can also cause poisoning. Death from liver failure secondary to the pulegone component of pennyroyal oil can occur when this agent is ingested (1). Similarly, the ingestion of a topical "aphrodisiac"

containing cardiac glycosides from toads of the Bufo species has resulted in death (7).

The use of herbal medications in place of established therapies (e.g., for cancer, HIV, diabetes, and hypertension) can result in less than optimal outcomes. Self medication with herbs may also lead to delays in the use of more effective therapies, as patients engage in self-diagnosis (17). A recent evidence-based review of the 10 most commonly used herbs found inconclusive evidence for efficacy in 6 out of 10 (echinacea, ginseng, goldenseal, aloe, Siberian ginseng, and valerian), "probable" benefit in 2 (garlic for reduction of blood pressure and lipids and saw palmetto for benign prostatic hyperplasia) and benefit in only 2 of 10 (St. John's wort for moderate depression and Ginkgo biloba for dementia) (17).

The risks of DS with respect to breast-feeding, carcinogenicity, and teratogenicity are poorly characterized in many cases. The nephrotoxic acids in *Aristolochia* species and the volatile oil in *Sassafras albidum* have also been found to be carcinogenic (6,18).

TABLE 339.1. Toxic Presentations of Dietary Supplements

Allergic reactions: alfalfa, chamomile (*Chamomilla* species), dandelion (*Taraxacum officinale*), echinacea (*Echinacea pallida*), garlic (*Allium sativum*), ginger (*Zingiber officinale*), propolis

Anticholinergic poisoning: burdock root (*Arctium lappa*), jimson weed (*Datura stramonium*), lobelia (*Lobelia inflata*), mandrake (*Mandragon officinarum*)

Coagulopathy: melilot (*Melilotus officinalis*), tonka beans (*Coumarouna oppisitifolia*), woodruff (*Galium odoratum*)

Cardiovascular depression: astragalus, codopsis, cardiac glycosides, goldenseal (*Hydratis canadensis*), prunella, sage (*Salvia species*), hellebore (*Veratrum species*), juniper (*Juniper communis*), monkshood or wolfsbane (*Aconitum napellus;* also found in many Chinese medicines), passion flower (*Passiflora caerulea*), snakeroot (*Rauwolfia serpentina*)

Cardiovascular stimulation: figwort or xuan shen (*Scrophularia species*), khat (*Catha edulis*), monkshood or wolfsbane (*Aconitum napellus;* also found in many Chinese medicines), ma-juang (*Ephedra sinica*), mormon tea (*Ephedra nevadensis*), yohimbine (*Corynanthe yohimbe*)

CNS depression: kava-kava (*Piper methysticum*), peony, peppermint (*Mentha pulegium*), snakeroot (*Rauwolfia serpentina*), St. John's wort (*Hypericum perforatum*), tang-kuei, valerian root (*Valeriana species*)

CNS stimulation: absinthe (wormwood, mugwort; *Artemisia* species), eucalyptus, ginseng (*Panax quinquefolium*), hyssop (*Hyssopus officinalis*), juniper (*Juniper communis*), khat (*Catha edulis*), majuang (*Ephedra sinica*), mormon tea (*Ephedra nevadensis*), passion flower (*Passiflora caerulea*), periwinkle (*Vinca species*), sage (*Salvia species*), yohimbine (*Corynanthe yohimbe*)

Gastroenteritis: common; can be severe with buckthorn (*Hipthothae rhamnoides*), poke root (*Phytolacca americana*), and senna (*Cassia angustifolia*)

Hematologic suppression: goldenseal (Hydratis canadensis), podophyllin (*Dysosmia pleianthum, Podophyhyllum* species)

Hepatitis: chaparral (*Covillea tridentata, Larrea tridenta, L. divaricata*), germander (*Teucrium chamaedrys*), jin bu huan (traditional Chinese medicine), kombucha, ma-juang (*Ephedra species*), pennyroyal (*Hedeoma pugelioides* or mentha pulegium), periwinkle (Vinca species)

Hepatic venoocclusive disease: coltsfoot (*Tussilago farfara*), comfrey (*Symphytum officinale*), Crotalaria species, gordolobo (*Senecio longilobus*), groundsel (*Senecio vulgaris*), Heliotropium species, maté (*Ilex paraguayensis*), tansy ragwort (*Senecio jacobea*), t'u-san-chi (*Gynura segetum*)

Nephrotoxicity: aloe, astragalus, burdock, dandelion, juniper (*Juniper communis*), licorice (*Glycyrrhiza species*), peony

Obstructive airway disease: betel nut (*Areca catechu*), sabah (*Sauropus androgynus*), wild or squirting cucumber (*Ecbolium elaterium*)

TABLE 339.2.   Dietary Supplement/Herbal—Drug Interactions[a]

Dietary Supplement/Herb	Drug	Interaction
Coenzyme Q	Warfarin	May reduce anticoagulant effect.
Dong quai (*Angelica sinensis*)	Warfarin	May increase anticoagulant effect.
Evening Primrose Oil	Warfarin	May increase anticoagulant effect.
Garlic (*Allium sativum*)	Warfarin	May increase anticoagulant effect. Should not be used with other anticoagulant drugs such as aspirin and other NSAIDs.
Ginkgo (*Ginkgo biloba*)	Antiplatelet drugs	May increase effects.
	MAOIs	May potentiate effect of MAOIs.
Ginseng, American (*Panax quinquefolius*)	MAOIs	May cause headaches and manic episode.
Ginseng, Chinese (*Panax ginseng*)	MAOIs	May cause headaches and manic episode.
	Insulin	Hypoglycemic effects may be additive.
	Stimulant drugs	May potentiate effect.
	Warfarin	May decrease effectiveness.
Glucosamine	Diabetes medicines	May increase insulin resistance.
Kava Kava (*Piper methysticum*)	Sedative hypnotics	May potentiate.
St. John's Wort (*Hypericum perforatum*)	HIV drugs, digoxin, blood thinners, chemotherapy agents, theophylline.	May decrease effectiveness.
	SSRIs	Increased serotonergic effect.
Valerian (*Valeriana officinalis*)	Alcohol and sedative hypnotics.	Potentiates effects.
Yohimbine	α_2 blockers	Increased α-adrenergic blockade.
	Tricyclics	Hypertension.
	MAOIs	Additive effects.

[a] Report to the Chairman: Special Committee on Aging: US Senate. *Health products for seniors. "Anti-aging" products pose potential for physical and economic harm.* Washington, DC: US General Accounting Office, 2001. GAO-01–1129.

CLINICAL PRESENTATION

Toxic effects of DS include allergic reactions, anticholinergic poisoning, coagulopathy, cardiovascular depression, cardiovascular stimulation, CNS depression or stimulation, gastroenteritis, hematologic suppression, hepatitis, hepatic veno-occlusive disease, nephrotoxicity, and obstructive airway disease (Table 339.1). The potential dangers of ephedra use are discussed in detail in Chapter 328, "Sympathomimetics" (11). Interactions between commonly used DS and pharmaceutical agents are listed in Tables 339.1 and 339.2. More extensive listing of interactions may be found elsewhere (Table 339.3) (19,21).

DIFFERENTIAL DIAGNOSIS

The clinical presentations of dietary supplement related illnesses are protean. Because poisoning with DS can affect every organ system, DS-related illness should be suspected when a patient presents with unexplained signs, symptoms, or organ dysfunction. The differential diagnostic include a wide variety of organic illnesses and toxic conditions.

EMERGENCY DEPARTMENT EVALUATION

Physicians should routinely inquire about the use of DS because this information is often not disclosed unless specifically asked. Eliciting a history of exposure is critical in alerting the clinician to the possibility of poisoning. Adults should be asked whether they have taken any homeopathic or folk remedies over the past few weeks. In children, even if an ingestion was not observed, questions should be asked about natural medicine availability.

Herbal products may have multiple common and scientific names. Obtaining the actual product used may aid identification. New dietary supplements are coming on the market constantly.

Many have internet web sites. However, the quality of information found there may be unreliable, and clinicians should use internet information with caution in making treatment decisions. Poison control centers are resources for identifying products as well as for treatment advice.

Guided by the history, a focused toxicologic physical examination should be performed. Careful and serial attention to the vital signs, including pulse oximetry and mental status, may help suggest a toxic syndrome. Examination of pupillary size, mucous membrane hydration status, skin, heart, and lungs and of the abdomen for bowel sounds and right upper quadrant tenderness are particularly important. Depending on the history and physical findings, cardiac rhythm strip or 12-lead electrocardiogram interpretation may be indicated to evaluate for cardiovascular toxicity. Laboratory testing may be appropriate for the assessment of fluid and electrolyte status, liver or renal function abnormalities, infections, or hematologic problems. With few exceptions (e.g., cardiac glycoside and heavy-metal poisoning), toxicology testing per se is unlikely to be helpful. Any elevation in liver function studies should prompt an acetaminophen level. Assays used to measure digoxin may cross react with cardiac glycosides in herbs and plants, but cannot be interpreted in quantitative fashion.

EMERGENCY DEPARTMENT MANAGEMENT

The treatment of a patient with an adverse reaction or an overdose from a dietary supplement or herbal product is mainly supportive. If there is any possibility that a DS is the cause of a patient's illness, advise that use be discontinued. GI decontamination should be considered if a serious ingestion is known to have occurred within a time frame in which decontamination would be expected to still be useful (generally within an hour of ingestion). Antidotal therapy seldom has a role in treating overdoses of dietary or herbal products. Rare exceptions might be certain heavy metals and cardiac or cyanogenic glycosides.

TABLE 339.3. Summary of Drug-Herb Interactions of Commonly Used Drug.[a]

Drug	Interaction
Alprazolam	Excessive sedation may result if used concomitantly with kava.
Corticosteroids	The immunostimulating effects of *Echinacea*, *Astragalus*, licorice, alfalfa sprouts, vitamin E, and zinc may offset the immunosuppressive effects of corticosteroids.
Cyclosporine	The immunostimulating effects of *Echinacea*, *Astragalus*, licorice, alfalfa sprouts, vitamin E, and zinc may offset the immunosuppressive effects of cyclosporine.
Digoxin	Additive effects possible with herbs containing cardiac glycosides; hawthorn purportedly potentiates digoxin; licorice may cause hypokalemia, hence predisposing the patient to digoxin's toxic effects; plantain may be adulterated with foxglove, hence elevating digoxin blood levels; Siberian ginseng and kyushin may interfere with digoxin assays; uzara root may exert additive digoxin-type cardiac effects.
Diuretics	Sodium-sparing herbal aquaretics (e.g., dandelion, uva-ursi) may offset antihypertensive effects of diuretics (e.g., hydrochlorothiazide and furosemide); gossypol may exacerbate hypokalemia secondary to diuretics (e.g., hydrochlorothiazide and furosemide).
Hypoglycemics (e.g., sulfonylureas)	Chromium may decrease insulin requirements; karela has been shown to decrease dosage requirements for chlorpropamide.
Iron	Tannin-containing herbs (e.g., chamomile, feverfew, St. John's wort) may interact with iron, hence inhibiting iron absorption.
Levothyroxine	Horseradish and kelp may suppress thyroid function.
Nonsteroidal Antiinflammatory Drugs	Additive gastrointestinal irritation may be encountered with herbs known to irritate the gastrointestinal tract (e.g., gossypol and uva-ursi).
Phenelzine (and Other MAO-Inhibitors)	Concomitant use with ginseng, yohimbine, and *Ephedra* may result in insomnia, headache, and tremulousness; St. John's wort and licorice may have MAO inhibitor activity and should not be used concomitantly with known MAO inhibitors.
Phenobarbital	Thujone-containing herbs (e.g., wormwood and sage) may lower seizure threshold, hence increasing anticonvulsant dosage requirements; gamolenic acid-containing herbs (e.g., evening primrose oil and borage) lower seizure thresholds and may increase anticonvulsant dosage requirements.
Phenytoin	Same as for Phenobarbital plus Shankhapushpi may shorten the half-life and diminish effectiveness of phenytoin.
Spironolactone	Licorice may offset the effects of spironolactone.
Warfarin	Garlic, ginger, Ginkgo, and feverfew may augment the anticoagulant effect of warfarin; ginseng may decrease the effectiveness of warfarin.

[a]From Miller LT. Herbal medicinals: Selected clinical considerations focusing on known or potential drug-herb interactions. *Arch Intern Med* 1998; 158(20): 2200–2211, with permission.

CRITICAL INTERVENTIONS

- Ask all patients with unexplained signs, symptoms, or organ dysfunction about the use of dietary supplements
- Advise that use of dietary supplements be discontinued whenever a toxic reaction or interaction is suspected

DISPOSITION

Disposition is based on the nature and severity of illness. Deliberate overdose requires psychiatric evaluation before discharge. It is generally advisable to consult a poison center whenever toxicity from a DS is suspected or encountered. The poison center can also assist in determining whether a DS product represents a public health hazard and if so, in notifying federal, state and local health authorities.

COMMON PITFALLS

✔ Failure to appreciate that DS, although generally safe, can cause life-threatening toxicity
✔ Failure to include DS toxicity in the differential diagnosis of organ-system dysfunction
✔ Failure to appreciate that DS product labels may be inaccurate with respect to the identity of contents, that ingredients may vary in potency, and that adulteration and contamination can occur
✔ The exact ingredients of ingested herbal and dietary products are often unknown, forcing the clinician to care for an intoxication without complete information. Fortunately, meticulous supportive care usually suffices

Acknowledgments

We thank previous chapter versions by Andrew R. Topliff, William Banner, Jr., Newell E. McElwee, and David G. Spoerke.

References

1. Anderson IB, Mullen WH, Meeker JE, et al. Pennyroyal toxicity: measurement of toxic metabolite levels in two cases and review of the literature. *Ann Intern Med* 1996;124:726–734.
2. Bent S, Tiedt TN, Odden MC, et al. The relative safety of ephedra compared with other herbal products. *Ann Intern Med* 2003;138(6):468–471.
3. Blendon RJ, DesRoches CM, Benson JM, et al. Americans' views on the use and regulation of dietary supplements. *Arch Intern Med* 2001;161(6):805–810.
4. Boyer EW, Kearney S, Shannon MW, et al. Poisoning from a dietary supplement administered during hospitalization. *Pediatrics* 2002;109(3):E49.
5. Cohen MR. Herbal and complementary and alternative medicine and therapies for liver disease. A focus on Chinese traditional medicine in Hepatitis C virus. *Clin Liver Dis* 2001;5(2):461–478.
6. De Smet PA. Health risks of herbal remedies. *Drug Saf* 1995;13(2):82–93.
7. Deaths associated with a purported aphrodisiac—New York City, February 1993–May 1995. *MMWR Morb Mortal Wkly Rep* 1995;46:853–861.
8. Espinoza EO, Mann MJ, Bleasdell B. Arsenic and mercury in traditional Chinese herbal balls. *N Engl J Med* 1995;333(12):803–804.
9. Fugh-Berman A. Herb-drug interactions. *Lancet* 2000;355:134–138.
10. Gurley BJ, Wang P, Gardner SF. Ephedrine-type alkaloid content of nutritional supplements containing Ephedra sinica (Ma-huang) as determined by high performance liquid chromatography. *J Pharm Sci* 1998;87:1547–1553.
11. Haller CA, Benowitz NL. Adverse cardiovascular and central nervous system events associated with dietary supplements containing ephedra alkaloids. *N Engl J Med* 2000;343:1833–1838.
12. Hill GJ, Hill S. Lead poisoning due to hai ge fen. *JAMA* 1995;273(1):24–25.
13. Huang WF, Wen KC, Hsiao ML. Adulteration by synthetic therapeutic substances of traditional Chinese medicines in Taiwan. *J Clin Pharmacol* 1997;37:344–350.
14. Kang-yum E, Oransky SH. Chinese patent medication as a potential source of mercury poisoning. *Vet Hum Toxicol* 1992;34:235–238.
15. Kelly J, Hopkin R, Rimsza ME. Rattlesnake meat ingestion and Salmonella Arizona infection in children: case report and review of the literature. *Pediatr Infect Dis J* 1995;14(4):320–322.

16. Ko RJ. Adulterants in Asian Patent Medicines. *N Engl J Med* 1998;339(12):847.

17. Mar C, Bent S. An evidence-based review of the 10 most commonly used herbs. *West J Med* 1999;171(3):168–171.

18. Nortier JL, Vanherweghem JL. Renal interstitial fibrosis and urothelial carcinoma associated with the use of a Chinese herb (Aristolochia fangchi). *Toxicology* 2002;181–182:577–580.

19. *Physician's Desk Reference for Herbal Medications*, 2nd ed. Montvale, New Jersey: Medical Economics Company, 2000.

20. Ries CA, Sahud MA. Agranulocytosis caused by Chinese herbal medicines: dangers of medications containing aminopyrine and phenylbutazone. *JAMA* 1975;231:352–355.

21. Therapeutic research faculty. Stockton, California: Natural Medicines Comprehensive Database, 2000.

22. Tierra M.The way of herbs. New York: Pocket Books (Simon & Schuster), 1998.

23. Office of the Inspector General. *Adverse Event Reporting for Dietary Supplements: An Inadequate Safety Valve*. Washington, DC: U.S. Dept of Health and Human Services, 2001. http://oig.hhs.gov/oei/reports/0ei-01-00-00180.pdf.

24. Report to the chairman: special committee on aging: U.S. Senate. *Health products for seniors. "Anti-aging" products pose potential for physical and economic harm*. Washington, DC: U.S. General Accounting Office, 2001. GAO-01–1129.

25. Vanhaelen M, Vanhaelen-Fastre R, But P, et al. Identification of aristolochic acid in Chinese herbs. *Lancet* 1994;343(8890):174.

CHAPTER 340
Seafood Toxins

Robert P. Dowsett

Seafood poisoning results from the ingestion of seafood that contain toxic substances. Often, these toxins originate from dinoflagellates and many are closely related. Dinoflagellates, which form the major component of phytoplankton, are unicellular eukaryotic marine algae of the division *Pyrrophyta*. Other toxins are endogenously produced or result from bacterial action.

Some dinoflagellates proliferate under certain conditions, resulting in the discoloration of seawater known as a "red tide" or algae bloom. Other species live below the water, attached to macroalgae; their growth is not as obviously affected by the environment. All dinoflagellates lie at the bottom of a food chain of which humans may be the ultimate consumers. Dinoflagellate toxins are concentrated in the viscera of filter feeders such as shellfish, herbivorous fish, and crustaceans, often causing them no harm. They are among the most potent natural toxins known.

Ciguatera, paralytic shellfish, tetrodotoxin, and scombroid poisoning are relatively well known. Neurotoxic shellfish, diarrheic shellfish, hallucinatory fish, clupeotoxic fish, fish roe, palytoxin, domoic acid (mussel), red whelk poisoning, and Haff disease are less commonly recognized and reported. However, expanding international tourism, the importation of exotic seafood, and the harvesting of seafood from more remote waters, as coastal fishing grounds are exhausted, are likely to increase the frequency of seafood poisoning seen in domestic health facilities.

Ciguatera poisoning results from eating tropical or subtropical fish contaminated with toxins produced by dinoflagellates living in coral reef waters. *Gambierdiscus toxicus* and several other species produce toxins that accumulate in fish feeding on algae. *G. toxicus* and related species are found in coral reef waters between 35° south and 35° north latitude. The toxins they produce are passed up the food chain from herbivores to their predators and eventually to humans. Ciguatoxin is a heat-stable, lipid-soluble, highly oxygenated polyether. They are concentrated in the visceral organs of fish, particularly the liver and gonads, and can remain for several years after accumulation. Environmental factors such as water temperature, salinity, and light affect the growth of *G. toxicus*. Large-scale environmental disruptions such as storms, earthquakes, underwater dredging, pollution, and global climatic changes are also thought to influence toxic dinoflagellate populations.

Ciguatera poisoning is endemic in Australia and the Caribbean and South Pacific islands; French Polynesia has the highest prevalence (10). Outbreaks have been reported worldwide, and over 400 species of fish, mostly reef fish, have been implicated. Barracuda, grouper, red snapper, amberjack, eel, sea bass, and Spanish mackerel are most commonly involved. Fish larger than 2 kg are more likely to be contaminated with significant quantities of toxin. Ciguatoxin is colorless and tasteless and is not destroyed by cooking or gastric acid. It is detectable in affected fish by mouse biologic assay or immunoassay. Ciguatoxin acts by increasing sodium permeability through neuronal voltage-gated sodium channels, resulting in prolonged refractoriness and decreased conduction velocity (7).

Palytoxin poisoning is most common in the South Pacific after ingestion of fish (mackerels, triggerfish, filefish, butterfly fish) and xanthrid crabs that feed on coral (13). Palytoxin is a thermostable terpenoid toxin produced by zoanthid coral of the genus *Palythoa*. It may also be found in dinoflagellates. The livers of affected fish have a high palytoxin content. Palytoxin binds to the ouabain receptor site on Na^+/K^+-ATPase, allowing the influx of sodium and resulting in depolarization of nerves and muscles. Although clinical effects are similar to those seen in ciguatera poisoning, additional toxicity results from norepinephrine release, vasoconstriction, and sustained contraction of skeletal and smooth muscle (13).

Neurotoxic shellfish poisoning also results in a ciguatera-like syndrome. It is caused by brevetoxins from *Ptychodiscus brevis*, a dinoflagellate found off the coast of southeastern North America and western Europe during algae blooms. The toxins are accumulated by clams and oysters. Brevetoxins A, B, and C are polycyclic ethers that bind to the Na^+ channel near the binding site for ciguatoxin. They are toxic to some marine life and birds, causing extensive wild life losses. Brevetoxins can be aerosolized by wave action and carried several kilometers inland, resulting in respiratory irritation.

Paralytic shellfish poisoning results from the ingestion of bivalve and gastropod mollusks (mussels, clams, oysters, scallops, and cockles) and occasionally some univalve mollusks, starfish, crustaceans, and fish, (including pufferfish which are more commonly associated with tetrodotoxin) (1). These creatures become toxic when dinoflagellates, especially *Gonyaulax* spp., multiply explosively, causing red tides. Toxic shellfish are commonly found in the cold, temperate waters of North America, the western coast of Europe, and the coastal waters of Japan, but are increasingly reported in warmer climates. Saxitoxin, gonyautoxins, and neosaxitoxin have been identified. The toxins do not affect shellfish but are concentrated in viscera and can take several weeks to be eliminated. Seabirds, several fish species, and mammals are susceptible to poisoning. Saxitoxin, a potent, heat-stable, water-soluble neurotoxin, acts by blocking fast sodium channels in nerve and muscle during depolarization, resulting in a conduction block that principally affects motor neurons and muscle. There is no reliable taste, smell, or color to identify contaminated shellfish. Saxitoxin can be detected in shellfish meat by a mouse bioassay. A level above 80 μg of purified saxitoxin per 100 g of raw shellfish meat is considered toxic.

Tetrodotoxin is a heat-stable, water-soluble neurotoxin chemically similar to saxitoxin found in the skin and viscera of puffer fish (saltwater and freshwater varieties), porcupine fish, sunfish, toadfish, the blue-ringed octopus, some species of sala-manders, and Atelopid frogs. A dinoflagellate or bacterial origin has been suggested, but remains unproven. It has been identified in a dinoflagellate (*Alexandrium tamarense*), which also contain saxitoxin. Puffer fish, the most common source of tetrodotoxin, is eaten in some Asian countries. Because inadvertent overdose may be fatal, chefs must be licensed in the preparation of this "delicacy."

Although tetrodotoxin is concentrated in the fish's skin and internal organs, all parts of the fish may contain it. Like saxi-toxin, tetrodotoxin inhibits fast sodium channels during depo-larization, but at a separate site. The major effect of tetrodotoxin is to reduce conduction of peripheral motor, sensory, and auto-nomic nerves. Tetrodotoxin also acts on the medulla, stimulat-ing the chemoreceptor trigger zone and possibly depressing the respiratory and vasomotor centers. In high doses, it may have direct effects on cardiac conduction, vascular smooth muscle, and skeletal muscle. Tetrodotoxin can be detected in fish by a bioassay and in serum or urine by gas chromatography or mass spectrometry.

Clupeotoxinism is a poorly documented but severe poison-ing that is more lethal than other forms of seafood poisoning. It is caused by fish of the order *Clupeiformes* (herrings, anchovies, and sardines), particularly those caught in summer, offshore of tropical islands after heavy rains or floods. The identity of the toxin, which primarily affects the central nervous system (CNS), is unknown. A phytoplankton origin has been postulated. It appears to be thermostable and concentrated in the viscera of fish. Toxicity does not depend on the size of the fish or its fresh-ness (11).

Scombroid poisoning is associated with ingestion of fish of the family *Scombridae* such as mackerel, skipjack, bonito and tuna. It also occurs in other fish with dark flesh, such as dolphin fish (mahi mahi), bluefish, amberjack (yellowtail), herrings, sardines and anchovies and may be referred to as histamine fish poison-ing. The muscles of all these fish contain large amounts of free histidine. Fish become toxic when left unrefrigerated (> 20°C), allowing bacteria, particularly *Proteus morganii*, to decarboxylate histidine to histamine. This effect can occur during harvesting, transportation, storage, processing, or preparation for consump-tion (4).

Ingested histamine is normally metabolized by the intesti-nal mucosa and has little systemic effect. Other toxins isolated from contaminated fish, putrescine and cadaverine, both short-chain aliphatic diamines, may facilitate the absorption of in-gested histamine or compete for its metabolism by diamine oxidase. The histamine content of spoiled flesh can vary con-siderably throughout a fish, being highest near the gut cavity. Individual sensitivity to scombroid also varies considerably; fe-males are suggested to be more susceptible.

Scombroid toxins are heat-stable. Affected fish can appear spoiled and have a peppery or sharp taste, but these findings are not always present (8). Symptoms are consistent with the known systemic effects of histamine and resemble IgE-mediated food allergies. The histamine content of dark fish flesh is normally less than 5 mg/100 g of flesh. Toxicity can occur at levels above 20 mg/100 g, although the Food and Drug Administration has set a hazard action level of 50 mg/100 g.

Diarrheic shellfish poisoning is caused by consumption of shellfish, particularly mussels, that have eaten dinoflagellates of *Dinophysis* or *Prorocentrum* species. Toxins have been identified as dinophysistoxins (okadaic acid and derivatives), pectenotox-ins, and yessotoxins and have predominantly gastrointestinal (GI) effects.

Hallucinatory fish poisoning has been described following the ingestion of reef fish from the South Pacific and the In-dian Ocean. Toxins similar to indole compounds from the algae *Microcoleus lyngbyaceus* have been implicated as a source of the poisoning.

Outbreaks of GI and neurologic toxicity have occurred on the eastern coast of Canada following the consumption of mussels contaminated by domoic acid produced by *Nitzschia pungens*, a phytoplankton associated with algae blooms (19). Domoic acid is a heat-stable neuroexcitatory amino acid that is structurally related to glutamic acid but is 40 to 100 times more potent. Aza-spiracid poisoning has occurred following the ingestion of con-taminated mussels in Europe. A dinoflagellate species *Protoperi-dinium*, has been identified as the origin of azaspiracids, which cause mainly a GI illness (12).

Raw carp bile is eaten in rural Asia in the belief that it im-proves visual acuity and treats hypertension and rheumatism. Five species of carp are known to be poisonous. Fish longer than 1 m or heavier than 3 kg are considered more likely to be toxic. Bile salts are thought to be responsible for toxicity (16).

Fish roe poisoning may result from eating the eggs of numer-ous species of freshwater and saltwater fish during the repro-ductive cycle (spring and early summer). The nature of the toxin is unclear, but it does not appear to be destroyed by cooking (14).

Red whelk (*Neptunea antiqua*) and related species, except the common whelk (*Buccinum undatum*), contain tetramine, a heat-stable neurotoxin found in their salivary glands (9).

Hypervitaminosis A (see Chapter 341, "Vitamins") may oc-cur following the ingestion of the liver of marine mammals and several species of shark (11).

Haff disease is a neuromyodystrophic disease that occurs af-ter ingestion of carp from the Baltic Sea and lakes in Scandinavia and Russia, although several cases have been reported in the United States. The causative toxin is heat-stable and is thought to originate from a species of blue-green algae (21).

CLINICAL PRESENTATION

Symptoms and signs of ciguatera poisoning typically occur 6 to 12 hours after ingestion, with a range of 30 minutes to 30 hours. GI and neurologic symptoms predominate, typically beginning with vomiting, diarrhea, and myalgias. These are followed by circumoral and peripheral paresthesias, vertigo, and ataxia (10). Patients may present initially with only neurologic symptoms; these may be delayed up to 72 hours after ingestion or may oc-cur without GI symptoms. Hypotension is common and may be a result of fluid loss, bradycardia, peripheral vasodilatation, or myocardial depression (2). Symptoms vary between patients and depend on where the fish were caught and what parts were eaten (2). More severe toxicity, especially hypotension and bradycar-dia, occurs in patients previously poisoned by ciguatera.

A classic feature of ciguatera poisoning is erroneously de-scribed as a paradoxical or reversed temperature perception: cold objects feel hot, and hot objects feel cold. This feature is proba-bly a result of hyperstimulation of pain receptors at temperatures below 25°C, manifested by an intense burning sensation on ex-posure to cold. Warmth relieves these dysesthesias, and patients can accurately sense temperature changes (6).

Other common neurologic symptoms include asthenia, pare-sis, tremors, and pain affecting the joints, head, and abdomen (2). Paresthesias are often poorly defined and do not conform to der-matomal or peripheral nerve distribution. A sensation of loose-ness of the teeth is another unusual symptom. Insomnia, neu-rosis, depression, and hallucinations may occur. Other features include dyspnea, diaphoresis, salivation, tearing, chills, neck stiffness, pruritus, rashes, and tachycardia (2). In pregnant patients, violent fetal movements have been described. Less commonly, transient blindness, convulsions, rhabdomyoly-sis, polymyositis, or paralysis may occur. Death, although uncommon, may result from severe dehydration or cardiac or respiratory failure.

Symptoms are often exacerbated by the ingestion of nontoxic seafood, nuts, grains, or alcohol and by exercise. Medications containing cyclic ethers, such as opiates, barbiturates, and paraldehyde, may exacerbate symptoms. No specific laboratory abnormalities are characteristic. Electrolyte disturbances may occur secondary to dehydration and rhabdomyolysis. Ventricular extrasystoles and T-wave changes may be seen on the electrocardiogram. GI symptoms usually resolve by 24 to 48 hours, and neurologic symptoms by 3 weeks, but the latter may persist for up to 2 months.

Features of palytoxin poisoning are similar to those of ciguatera and include weakness, sweating, GI distress, paresthesias, muscle spasms, and tremors. Severe poisoning may result in generalized, painful tonic contraction of muscles, mimicking seizures, and in rhabdomyolysis, myoglobinuria, hemolysis, hyperkalemia, respiratory failure, bradycardia, and renal failure (13).

Neurotoxic shellfish poisoning causes a similar but less severe syndrome. Symptoms often begin with circumoral paresthesias, which become more generalized and can be associated with headaches, dilated pupils, tachycardia, and muscle cramps. In severe cases, seizures have occurred, but no cases of paralysis or death have been reported. Symptoms of brevetoxin inhalation include a nonproductive cough, shortness of breath, lacrimation, and irritation of the eyes, nose, and throat. Patients with asthma may develop bronchospasm.

Symptoms of paralytic shellfish poisoning begin 30 minutes to 2 hours after ingestion and typically include numbness of the fingertips, tongue, and lips, often accompanied by nausea and abdominal pain (19). These symptoms are followed by paresthesias of the face and extremities and progressive muscle paralysis. Bulbar muscles are often affected, causing dysarthria, dysphagia, diplopia, and loss of the gag reflex. Other features include vertigo, ataxia, transient blindness, altered temperature perception, hypotension, headache, and low back pain. Vomiting is not a consistent feature but may result from concomitant bacterial or viral contamination (19). Ingestion of large doses of saxitoxin can lead rapidly to coma, diaphragmatic paralysis, and respiratory failure. Children appear to be more susceptible (19). Patients who survive the first 12 hours generally have a complete recovery after 1 to 3 days. Nonspecific T-wave changes and a rise in creatine kinase and its MB fraction have occurred in the absence of myocardial infarction or other signs of cardiac toxicity.

Patients with tetrodotoxin poisoning usually present 10 to 45 minutes after ingesting a tetrodotoxic fish. Very early or mild poisoning reportedly results in a feeling of exhilaration the reason such fish are eaten. Circumoral paresthesias, salivation, nausea, and vomiting then occur, followed by peripheral paresthesias and numbness. Sensory symptoms subsequently become more generalized, with ascending paralysis of the extremities, although deep tendon reflexes remain intact. Next, ataxia and paralysis of peripheral and bulbar muscles occur. Finally, respiratory muscles are affected resulting in hypoventilation, although patients may still be conscious. In the most severe cases, patients may become unconscious and completely paralyzed, with dilated nonreactive pupils and loss of all brainstem reflexes. Uncommon complications include neurogenic diabetes insipidus and hypertensive cardiac failure. Patients who survive beyond 24 hours have a good prognosis. Recovery occurs over a period of days and, unless complicated by anoxia, is complete. Death is usually a result of paralysis of the respiratory muscles.

Symptoms of clupeotoxin poisoning begin with a sharp, metallic taste, followed by severe GI upset and cardiovascular collapse. Violent headaches, paresthesias, muscle cramps, and progressive muscular paralysis may occur. Seizures and coma

may intervene rapidly, resulting in death within 15 minutes of ingestion.

The clinical presentation of scombroid poisoning is similar to that of IgE-mediated food allergies. Symptoms typically begin within 1 hour of ingestion and are usually mild (3). Common features are flushing of the face and upper trunk, nausea, abdominal cramps, diarrhea, and headache. Pruritus and urticaria, burning sensations of the mouth and throat, fever, and palpitations can occur. Severe reactions, such as bronchospasm, hypotension, and supraventricular tachyarrhythmias, are more likely to occur in patients with preexisting cardiac or respiratory disease. Symptoms usually resolve in 6 to 12 hours (range, 3 to 36 hours).

Diarrheic shellfish poisoning results primarily in GI symptoms.

Symptoms of hallucinatory fish poisoning occur within 2 hours of ingestion and typically include ataxia, hallucinations, chest tightness, and a sense of impending doom (11). GI distress and facial and pharyngeal paresthesias are also common.

Azaspiracid poisoning typically consists of nausea, vomiting, severe diarrhea and stomach cramps with an onset of 6 to 18 hours and a duration of up to 5 days (12).

The ingestion of domoic acid-containing mussel results in vomiting, diarrhea, abdominal pain, and headache, occurring about 6 hours after ingestion (range, 15 minutes—38 hours). Toxic encephalopathy resulting in confusion, disorientation, and memory deficits occurs in one-fourth of patients. Severe poisoning can result in profuse airway secretions, hemiplegia, hypotension, cardiac dysrhythmias, myoclonus, seizures, and coma. Resolution of cognitive deficits can take up to 12 weeks, but memory deficits and peripheral neuropathy appear to be permanent.

Patients poisoned by carp bile present 10 minutes to 12 hours after ingestion, with GI upset and diarrhea, followed by fever, chills, bradycardia, hypotension, hematuria, headache, and oliguria (16). Acute tubular necrosis and toxic hepatitis may occur; both resolve after 2 to 3 weeks.

Symptoms of fish roe poisoning develop within several hours of ingestion, with GI symptoms, hypotension and tachycardia, tinnitus, and weakness (14).

Ingestion of red whelk may result in progressive weakness that may include the respiratory muscles. Also seen are GI symptoms and hypotension as a result of vagal-induced bradycardia and peripheral vasodilatation (9).

Haff disease affects motor neurons of the brain, anterior horn cells of the spinal cord, and myocardial muscle cells. Clinical manifestations also include hypertension, tachycardia, diaphoresis, rhabdomyolysis, myoglobinuria, and renal failure (21).

DIFFERENTIAL DIAGNOSIS

The clinical presentation of ciguatera, neurotoxic shellfish, palytoxin, tetrodotoxin, and paralytic shellfish poisoning may be difficult to distinguish, as all may involve symptoms of paresthesias, weakness, and ataxia. Predominant symptoms and the nature of the fish eaten are used to determine the specific etiology. A common shellfish origin has been found for toxins associated with tetrodotoxin and paralytic shellfish poisoning.

The differential diagnosis of toxic seafood poisoning includes infectious gastroenteritis. Common seafood pathogens are hepatitis A, Norwalk virus, *Vibrio* spp. (*V. cholerae*, *V. parahaemolyticus*, and *V. vulnificus*), *Clostridium botulinum*, *Escherichia coli*, *Giardia lamblia*, and species of *Campylobacter*, *Shigella*, and *Salmonella* (7).

Scombroid poisoning can usually be differentiated from true allergic or anaphylactic reactions by the history of fish ingestion. Rarely, histamine poisoning indistinguishable from that caused by scombroid may result from the ingestion of aged cheese. Symptoms similar to scombroid fish poisoning can result from the ingestion of Japanese Callista clams, the ovaries of which have a high content of choline during the summer spawning season. Additional symptoms include paralysis or numbness of the throat, mouth, and tongue, and recovery takes up to 2 days.

The differential diagnosis of skin flushing also includes poisoning by niacin, vancomycin, rifampin, monosodium glutamate, and ethanol or disulfiram reactions.

EMERGENCY DEPARTMENT EVALUATION

The diagnosis of seafood poisoning is based on exposure history, clinical manifestations, and epidemiologic information. A history of seafood ingestion in the past 48 hours should be sought from patients presenting with GI, allergic, or unusual neurologic symptoms. If possible, the origin of the seafood should be identified; this information may help differentiate poisonings specific to certain regions. Public health officials may be able to assist in this process and provide information about similar cases or known quarantined fishing areas.

The physical examination focuses on vital signs, a neurologic evaluation, and assessment of respiratory function. Patients with weakness and other neurological symptoms should have arterial blood gas and vital capacity measurements. Those with significant GI symptoms should have orthostatic vital signs taken. The skin should be examined for rashes. Peritoneal signs on abdominal examination suggest alternative pathology. Laboratory evaluation includes a complete blood count; measurements of electrolytes, blood urea nitrogen, creatinine, glucose, and creatine kinase; and urinalysis. Unless other diagnoses or complications are considered, additional laboratory tests are of no help. Assays for detecting seafood toxins are not readily available for clinical use but may be used by government agencies for epidemiologic investigations.

EMERGENCY DEPARTMENT MANAGEMENT

Life support measures should be instituted as needed. Patients with bulbar paralysis, respiratory muscle weakness, or depressed consciousness require close observation of airway patency and respiratory function. Intubation and mechanical ventilation may be necessary. The treatment of bradycardia and other cardiac problems should follow standard advanced cardiac life-support guidelines. Dehydration should be treated with intravenous normal saline. Hypotension unresponsive to fluids may require dopamine. Dobutamine is used treat hypotension in paralytic shellfish poisoning. Calcium gluconate (1 g i.v. over 30 minutes, followed by 2 to 4 g/d as a constant infusion) may be effective for hypotension as a result of ciguatera poisoning.

Most seafood toxins are readily absorbed by activated charcoal, and this therapy should be considered in patients who present within 4 hours of ingestion. Control of emesis may be necessary first.

Several specific therapies have been tried for ciguatera poisoning. Mannitol given intravenously as a 20% solution in a dose of 1 g/kg, up to 50 g has been suggested as an effective treatment for control of acute toxicity. Numerous case reports have described neurologic symptoms often responding within minutes and resolving completely within 48 hours (15). A recent randomized controlled trial did not show that mannitol was superior to normal saline in reducing symptoms by 24 hours and it must now be questioned regarding whether it should be utilized (20).

Pralidoxime was originally used because it was erroneously thought that ciguatoxin had anticholinesterase activity. Although pralidoxime can be used to control excessive secretions, it may worsen other symptoms, and its efficacy remains unproved. Amitriptyline, which may act by blocking sodium channels, in doses of 25 to 75 mg/d, usually provides some relief from the chronic neurologic symptoms of ciguatera poisoning. Other agents used with varying degrees of success include fluoxetine, nifedipine, vitamins B_{12} and C, calcium gluconate (1–3 g intravenously over 24 hours), lidocaine, and tocainide. Two patients were treated with gabapentin (400 mg orally three times daily) experienced a rapid improvement with recurrence of symptoms therapy was ceased (17). Indomethacin and cyproheptadine are commonly used to relieve arthralgias and pruritus. Opiates and barbiturates should be avoided. Steroids are ineffective. Seafood, nuts, grains, alcohol, and exercise should be avoided for 3 to 6 months after exposure.

Patients with systemic anaphylactoid reactions secondary to scombroid poisoning should be treated with intravenous epinephrine, inhaled albuterol, and steroids. Less severe reactions can be treated with antihistamines. Type 2 histamine receptor blockers such as cimetidine appear more effective than type 1 blockers such as diphenhydramine (5). Nausea and vomiting may respond to prochlorperazine. Once stabilized, patients with scombroid poisoning can be discharged on oral antihistamines for 48 hours.

Edrophonium and neostigmine have been used to reverse motor paralysis as a result of tetrodotoxin poisoning but have not been studied in controlled trials. Diuresis and transfusion of red cells may be necessary in patients with palytoxin poisoning who have rhabdomyolysis and hemolysis, respectively.

For all toxic seafood poisonings, prevention is the best treatment. In areas in which ciguatera poisoning is endemic, people should avoid eating fish larger than 2 kg or those known to be frequently affected; for instance, the sale of barracuda is banned in Miami. Eating any viscera, especially the liver and gonads, should always be avoided. Outbreaks of paralytic shellfish poisoning are prevented by periodic testing of susceptible mollusks. When toxin levels are high, affected areas are quarantined. In some areas, harvesting of susceptible shellfish is banned during the summer. Quarantines also may be introduced during algae blooms (18). Failure to heed quarantines invites disaster. Puffer fish should be eaten only if prepared by a licensed chef. Scombroid poisoning can be prevented by proper refrigeration of fish. Obviously, any fish that appears spoiled or has an unusual taste should be avoided.

CRITICAL INTERVENTIONS

- Assess ability to protect the airway, obtain arterial blood gas and vital capacity measurements, and perform endotracheal intubation and assisted ventilation as necessary in patients with bulbar paresis, weakness, or altered mental status
- Treat scombroid poisoning the same as anaphylaxis
- Administer intravenous fluids for dehydration and hypotension
- Consult a poison center, toxicologist, or public health for current treatment advice

DISPOSITION

Most patients can be treated in the emergency department and then discharged with outpatient follow-up. Those with abnormal vital signs, persistent or severe dehydration, systemic anaphylactoid reactions, and neurologic symptoms should be hospitalized. The level of care required depends on clinical severity. A toxicologist, poison center, or public health agency can be consulted for current trends and treatment advice. Local or state departments of health should be notified of all cases of suspected seafood poisoning, because timely intervention may prevent additional exposures.

COMMON PITFALLS

✔ Failure to inquire about seafood ingestion, including the identity and source, in patients with gastroenteritis or anaphylactoid reactions

✔ Failure to consider seafood poisoning in patients presenting with unexplained or atypical neurologic symptoms

✔ Failure to prescribe antihistamines to patients who are discharged after treatment for scombroid poisoning

✔ Failure to appreciate that most seafood poisonings are reportable and to report cases of possible seafood poisoning to public health agencies

References

1. Anonymous. Update: neurologic illness associated with eating Florida pufferfish. *MMWR* 2002;19:414.
2. Bagnis R, Kuberski T, Laugier S. Clinical observations on 3009 cases of ciguatera fish poisoning in the South Pacific. *Am J Trop Med Hyg* 1967;28:1067.
3. Bartholomew BA, Berry PR, Rodhouse JC, et al. Scombrotoxic fish poisoning in Britain: features of over 250 suspected incidents from 1976 to 1986. *Epidemiol Infect* 1987;99:775.
4. Becker K, Southwick K, Readon J, et al. Histamine poisoning associated with eating tuna burgers. *JAMA* 2001;285:1327.
5. Blakesley ML. Scombroid poisoning: prompt resolution of symptoms with cimetidine. *Ann Emerg Med* 1983;12:104.
6. Cameron J, Capra MF. The basis of the paradoxical disturbance of temperature perception in ciguatera poisoning. *J Toxicol Clin Toxicol* 1993;31:571.
7. Cameron J, Flowers AE, Capra MF. Electrophysiological studies on ciguatera in man (part II). *J Neurol Sci* 1991;101:93.
8. Dickinson G. Scombroid fish poisoning syndrome. *Ann Emerg Med* 1982;11:487.
9. Fleming C. Case of poisoning from red whelk. *BMJ* 1971;3:520.
10. Gillespie NC, Lewis JL, Pearn JH, et al. Ciguatera in Australia. *Med J Aust* 1986;145:584.
11. Halstead BW. Miscellaneous seafood toxicants. In: Ragelis EP, ed. *Seafood toxins.* Washington, DC: American Chemical Society, 1984.
12. James KJ, Moroney C, Roden C, et al. Ubiquitous 'benign; alga emerges as the cause of shellfish contamination responsible for the human toxic syndrome, azaspiracid poisoning. *Toxicon* 2003;41:145.
13. Kodama Y, Hokama Y, Yasumoto T, et al. Clinical and laboratory findings implicating palytoxin as cause of ciguatera poisoning due to Decapterus macrosoma (mackerel). *Toxicon* 1989;27:1051.
14. Listernick R. Fish roe poisoning in childhood. *J Pediatr (Rio J)* 1987;111:729.
15. Palafax NA, Jain LG, Pinano AZ, et al. Successful treatment of ciguatera poisoning with intravenous mannitol. *JAMA* 1988;259:2740.
16. Park SK, Kim DG, Kang SK, et al. Toxic renal failure and hepatitis after ingestion of raw carp bile. *Nephron* 1990;56:188.
17. Perez CM, Vasquez PA, Perret CF. Treatment of ciguatera poisoning with gabapentin. *N Engl J Med* 2001;344:692.
18. Perl TM, B dard L, Kosatsky T, et al. An outbreak of toxic encephalopathy caused by eating mussels contaminated with domoic acid. *N Engl J Med* 1990;322:1775.
19. Rodrigue DC, Etzel RA, Hall S, et al. Lethal paralytic shellfish poisoning in Guatemala. *Am J Trop Med Hyg* 1990;42:267.
20. Schnorf H, Taurarii M, Cundy T. Ciguatera fish poisoning. A double-blind randomized trial of mannitol therapy. *Neurol* 2002;58:873.
21. Solomon M. Haff disease. *Arch Intern Med* 1990;150:683.

CHAPTER 341
Vitamins

Richard J. Geller

Vitamins are organic substances that are provided in small amounts in the normal diet to sustain the normal metabolic functions of life. These substances differ in chemical structure, biologic action, and, in most cases, dietary sources. The therapeutic use of vitamins includes treatment of vitamin deficiencies, treatment of inborn errors of metabolism, and as self-prescribed dietary supplements. Additionally, vitamins are used as antidotes in medical toxicology, such as vitamin B_6 (pyridoxine) for isoniazid and Gyromitra mushroom poisoning, vitamin K1 (phytonadione) for warfarin-type anticoagulant overdoses, and vitamin B_1 (thiamine) and folate as adjunctive therapy for ethylene glycol and methanol intoxications, respectively. Vitamin B_3 (niacin) is used as adjunctive therapy in lowering cholesterol.

Vitamin preparations may be solid or liquid oral dosage forms, parenteral solutions, and, in some cases, topical preparations. Most vitamins are available as a single entity or combined with other vitamins in multivitamin preparations. The Recommended Daily Allowances (RDA) refers to therapeutic doses promulgated by the Committee on Dietary Allowances, Food and Nutrition Board, National Research Council, and National Academy of Sciences, which were last updated (10th edition) in 1989. Although RDAs have been officially replaced by Dietary Reference Intakes (DRIs; http://www.nal.usda.gov/fnic/etext/000105.html), they continue to be the most widely used reference standard (Table 341.1).

Fat-soluble vitamins include vitamins A, D, E, and K. They are stored in fat and can bioaccumulate. Water-soluble vitamins include B_1 (thiamine), B_2 (riboflavin), B_3 (nicotinic acid), B_5 (pantothenic acid), B_6 (pyridoxine), B_{12} (cyanocobalamin), C (ascorbic acid), biotin, and folic acid. Fat-soluble vitamins typically regulate specific metabolic activities, and water-soluble vitamins function as coenzymes.

In the United States, an estimated 23% of adults regularly use vitamin supplements, with higher proportions among females, Caucasians, and people living on the West Coast (6). Several million people regularly take vitamins in excess of the RDA (11,17). Although such self-therapy may be costly, some vitamins have potent antioxidant-free radical quenching activity, with potential to possibly prevent genetic mutation and carcinogenic activity and other forms of disease secondary to free radical mechanisms (7). A recent meta-analysis, however, failed to find scientific evidence to support the use of antioxidant vitamins for the prevention of cardiovascular disease (20).

The ubiquitous distribution of vitamins results in a relatively large number of acute poisonings, both accidental and intentional. United States poison centers reported 57,313 human exposures to vitamins in 2002 (21). Approximately 79% involved children under age 6, 92% were unintentional, and 10% were treated in a health care facility. Less than 1% had moderate adverse effects, only 0.11% had major adverse effects, and there were 2 deaths. The majority of adverse reactions were seen in multivitamins that contained significant amounts of iron (see Chapter 312, "Iron").

Data regarding chronic vitamin toxicity consists primarily of isolated case reports of severe toxicity, some resulting from

TABLE 341.1. Recommended Dietary Allowances for Vitamins[f]

Age Group	Fat-Soluble Vitamins				Water-Soluble Vitamins		
	Vitamin A (μg RE)[a]	Vitamin D (μg)[b]	Vitamin E (mg TE)[c]	Vitamin C (mg)	Thiamine (mg)	Niacin (mg NE)[d]	Pyridoxine (mg)
Infant (< 1 yr)	375	7.5–10	3–4	30–35	0.3–0.4	5–6	0.3–0.6
Child (1–10 yrs)	400–700	10	6–7	40–45	0.7–1.0	9–13	1.0–1.4
Male > 10 yrs	1,000	5–10	10	50–60	1.2–1.5	15–20	1.7–2.0
Female > 10 yrs[e]	800	5–10	8	50–60	1.0–1.1	13–15	1.4–1.6

[a] Retinol equivalents, 1 retinol equivalent = 1 μg retinol = 6 μg beta-carotene = 3.3 IU.
[b] As cholecalciferol, 10 μg cholecalciferol = 400 IU of vitamin D.
[c] Alpha-tocopherol equivalents. 1 mg d-alpha-tocopherol = 1 alpha-tocopherol equivalent (1 TE) = 1.49 IU.
[d] Niacin equivalents. 1 niacin equivalent = 1 mg niacin = 60 mg of dietary tryptophan.
[e] Pregnant or lactating women require larger amounts of all vitamins.
[f] From Committee on Dietary Allowances, Food and Nutrition Board, Recommended dietary allowances, 10th ed. (city?): National Research Council, 1989, with permission.

self-prescribed "megadosing." Megadosing has been defined as the daily intake of more than five to ten times the RDA for longer than 4 weeks. However, even at large doses, chronic vitamin toxicity rarely occurs and, when present, is typically secondary to fat-soluble vitamins and to a few water-soluble vitamins.

Vitamin A is one of several closely related compounds, which are biologically active but have different functions. These include retinol, retinal (retinaldehyde), retinyl esters, and retinoic acid. Retinol is the only one which can remedy all symptoms of vitamin A deficiency (4). It is necessary for reproductive processes and prevention of xerophthalmia (19), retinal functions in vision, and retinoic acid in epithelial cell growth and differentiation. Interconversion between these isomers occurs readily in the body. Retinol is largely stored in the liver and is transported to and from tissue by retinol binding protein (RBP). Carotenoids (e.g., β carotene) are precursors of retinol that are rarely associated with toxicity.

Vitamin A toxicity appears to result from exaggeration of retinol's normal physiologic action (10,15). Retinol acts like a hormone, stimulating mitosis and epithelial cell turnover rates. Thus, excess retinol results in eczema, excessive desquamation, alopecia, bony exostoses, metaphyseal flare, decreased bone remodeling, rarefaction of long bones, and congenital defects. It also appears that unbound retinol and retinyl esters may have membranolytic properties; this may occur when RBP becomes saturated. Diseases that alter RBP levels may increase the risk of toxicity. Preexisting liver disease, protein–calorie malnutrition, cystic fibrosis, febrile infection, proteinuria, and pregnancy have been associated with low RBP levels. When RBP levels are low, less retinol is required to saturate binding sites and increase circulating unbound retinol (15). Elevated plasma retinol and plasma retinyl ester levels have also been noted in patients with type V hyperlipoproteinemia (9). Vitamin A has teratogenic activity, and doses significantly greater than the RDA should be avoided by women of childbearing age unless there is evidence of a deficit.

Vitamin D, a steroid-like substance, is formed by ultraviolet light acting to convert 7-dehydroxycholesterol to cholecalciferol. Cholecalciferol is then hydroxylated by the liver to 25-hydroxycholecalciferol (25-OHD), which is then metabolized by the kidneys to a more potent metabolite, 1,25-hydroxycholecalciferol (1,25-OHD). The latter metabolite regulates calcium and phosphorus absorption from the gut and resorption from bone.

The mechanisms of vitamin-D toxicity are related to exaggerated physiologic effects (including increased calcium absorption, increased bone resorption, and increased levels of the metabolite 25-OHD). 25-OHD may saturate normal protein-binding sites and become bound to albumin, allowing increased cellular membrane damage. 1,25-OHD, the metabolite with more potent physiologic activity, does not appear to be responsible for toxicity, and serum levels may be normal or even depressed.

There are at least eight naturally occurring tocopherols, one of which, α-tocopherol, is referred to as vitamin E. α-tocopherol is the most abundant in animal tissue sources and has the greatest biologic activity. Tocopherols function as antioxidants by protecting lipids from oxidation by cellular components. Vitamin E toxicity is minimal, and its mechanism has not been elucidated.

Two naturally occurring substances have vitamin K activity: phytonadione (K_1) and a series of closely related compounds called menaquinones (K_2). The former is found in plants; the latter are synthesized by gram-positive bacteria in the intestinal tract. Menadione (K_3) is a synthetic derivative with vitamin K activity that is available as a water-soluble salt. Vitamin K promotes biosynthesis of clotting factors II, VII, IX, and X. Only vitamin K_1 (phytonadione) is effective in reversing the suppressive effect on clotting factor II, VII, IX and X synthesis caused by coumarin and indanedione derivative poisoning. Vitamin K3 toxicity is caused by the action of menadione as an oxidizing hemolysin (15).

Most water-soluble vitamins are relatively nontoxic and their mechanisms of toxicity are unknown (15,18). Severe toxicity and death from water-soluble vitamins is exceedingly rare, except for hypersensitivity reactions.

Vitamin B_1 (thiamine) is converted by adenosine triphosphate to its active form, thiamine pyrophosphate, which functions as a coenzyme in the decarboxylation of α-keto acids and in the use of pentose in the hexose monophosphate shunt.

Vitamin B_3 (niacin or nicotinic acid) is the functional component of nicotinamide adenine dinucleotide (NAD) and nicotinamide adenine dinucleotide phosphate (NADP). These coenzymes activate several dehydrogenases important to cellular respiration. Nutritional requirements can also be satisfied by nicotinamide (niacinamide) and tryptophan. The vasodilatory effects of nicotinic acid are thought to result from direct action on small blood vessels and histamine release.

Several naturally occurring substances have vitamin B6 (pyridoxine)-related biologic activity, including pyridoxine, pyridoxal, and pyridoxamine. All three forms are converted to pyridoxal phosphate, which acts as a coenzyme for biotransformations of amino acids. The specific biochemical cause of their neurotoxicity has not been identified.

Several substances also have activities similar to vitamin C (ascorbic acid), but ascorbic acid itself is the most potent and the most commonly available. Ascorbic acid is reversibly oxidized to dehydroascorbic acid. Both function in oxidative biochemical reactions.

CLINICAL PRESENTATION

Patients with a single acute exposure to vitamins often present to the emergency department with either no symptoms or mild gastrointestinal (GI) distress, unless other toxic agents have been coingested. Vitamin formulations that contain significant iron (see Chapter 312, "Iron") are most likely to cause GI symptoms and other adverse sequelae. Notable exceptions include hypersensitivity reactions and niacin- or nicotinic acid–induced flushing. Patients with toxicity from chronic megavitamin therapy may present to the emergency department with vague, nonspecific clinical findings. Some patients may deny exposure to vitamins, either because they do not recognize them as drugs or because they perceive megavitamin therapy as unacceptable to physicians.

Acute vitamin A toxicity has been reported in Arctic explorers who have eaten polar bear or husky liver, which contains large amounts of vitamin A secondary to a marine diet. In this country, acute hypervitaminosis A is a syndrome most commonly the result of dietary fads and self administration of dietary supplements in order to treat acne and dry skin. Toxicity from a single large overdose of vitamin A generally requires more than 25,000 IU/kg. Toxicity has occurred after 4 million U in adults and 300,000 U in children. In adults, symptoms include severe headaches, dizziness, vomiting, diarrhea, fatigue and irritability. Cheilitis (inflammation of the lips), hair loss, hepatomegaly and splenomegaly, and long bone tenderness and bleeding manifestations (petechiae and epistaxis) may be seen (19). An erythematous skin reaction can develop within 8 hours. Later, skin typically cracks and peels (15). Increased intracranial pressure (pseudotumor cerebri), which may be related to altered cellular membrane function in the choroid plexus, can occur. This condition is most common in women in their 30s to 40s, who often present with headaches, blurred vision, and diplopia. Neuroimaging and cerebrospinal fluid (CSF) analysis are normal but the subarachnoid opening pressure is increased (usually greater than 20 mm Hg). Hepatic Ito cells also accumulate excess retinol and lipids, leading to fatty liver, enhanced hepatic collagen production, and, eventually, obstruction of sinusoidal blood flow, and cirrhosis.

In infants and children, anorexia, hyperirritability, vomiting, and bulging fontanelles (secondary to increased intracranial pressure) have been occasionally noted. Within a few days, these infants' skin also cracked and peeled. Symptoms resolved in all age categories, with no apparent long-term sequelae.

Chronic vitamin A toxicity is usually associated with 4,000 IU/kg daily for months, although, occasionally, toxicity can develop with lower dosages (30,000–50,000 IU in adults and dosages of ten times the RDA in children) (15). The minimum toxic dose varies between patients, depending on age, health status, and dosage preparation. Skin and mucous membrane effects (e.g., erythema; eczema; pruritus; dry, cracked skin; epistaxis; conjunctivitis; palmar and plantar peeling; and alopecia) are the most common and first signs of toxicity. Musculoskeletal pain and tenderness over the long bones of the upper and lower extremities is common. Epiphyseal cupping and premature epiphyseal fusion may occur in children. Hypercalcemia has been reported but is not consistently present. Crystals in the retina have been noted in patients ingesting carotene for tanning purposes (22).

Neurologic symptoms include frontal headaches, blurred vision, and diplopia. Hepatotoxicity, usually a later stage of toxicity, is manifested by hepatomegaly, splenomegaly, abnormal liver function tests (primarily aminotransferases, bilirubin, and alkaline phosphatase), and, eventually, portal hypertension, cirrhosis, and ascites. Liver biopsies reveal perisinusoidal, central vein sclerosis, and hypertrophy of Ito cells. Normal retinol levels are 30 to 70 μg/dL, and a level greater than 80 μg/dL would be suggestive of toxicity; however, normal levels do not rule out toxicity, as the majority of vitamin A is hepatically stored. Hypercalcemia resistant to saline and diuretic therapy, but responding to corticosteroids, has been observed (2).

Acute vitamin D toxicity is exceedingly rare, even with the consumption of rodenticides containing cholecalciferol. In a huge overdose, hypercalcemia would be expected. Chronic vitamin D toxicity, although more common, is also rare. It may occur in ingestion of the parent compound or the cholecalciferol metabolite. An outbreak of hypervitaminosis D from Vitamin D fortified milk occurred when a Massachusetts dairy inadvertently added 800 times the intended amount of vitamin D to its milk (5). Daily doses above 1250 μg of cholecalciferol may cause toxicity in adults. Patients with diseases such as hypoparathyroidism, vitamin D–resistant rickets, and osteomalacia who are taking physician-prescribed calciferol are at risk. Those with sarcoidosis, mycobacterial infections, and idiopathic hypercalcemia and hypercalciuria may develop toxicity with doses of 25 μg of cholecalciferol daily.

Chronic vitamin D toxicity has been associated with nausea, vomiting, constipation, anorexia, polydipsia, polyuria, weakness, altered mental status, hyperlipemia, hypercalcemia, and hyperphosphatemia. Hypercalcemia may be present without any symptoms, or it may cause pruritus, calcium deposits in soft tissue, and renal calculi (15). Children and infants appear to be more susceptible to toxic effects and can develop cardiovascular, renal, and central nervous system injury.

Acute vitamin E toxicity is virtually nonexistent, with only mild GI complaints expected. Chronic vitamin E toxicity is quite rare, even at dosages of ten times the RDA (3), and many individuals have taken 800 IU or more daily for several years without apparent toxicity. Minor symptoms, such as nausea, fatigue, headaches, diplopia, muscle weakness, creatinuria, and elevated serum creatine kinase levels, can occur with extremely high doses. Large amounts of vitamin E may hinder the absorption of other fat-soluble vitamins and can cause the inactivation of vitamin K, possibly explaining the minor elevation in prothrombin time in individuals on coumadin (3).

E-Ferol, a discontinued parenteral dosage of vitamin E used in neonates, was associated with ascites, hepatomegaly, hyperbilirubinemia, azotemia, and thrombocytopenia, possibly caused by the emulsificants (polysorbate 20 and 80), which were used in the formulation (14).

No adverse effects have been seen after the ingestion of oral vitamin K_1 (phytonadione). Premature infants given menadione (the synthetic analogue, vitamin K_3) in parenteral doses of 5 to 25 μg daily have developed hemolytic anemia, hyperbilirubinemia, or kernicterus, and fatalities have rarely been reported. Patients with glucose-6-phosphate dehydrogenase deficiency and premature infants with hypoglycemia are at increased risk for these hemolytic effects. Intravenous phytonadione administration can acuse chest pain, hypotension and dyspnea, asystole, and seizures and its use by this route should be discouraged. Because the effects of parenteral vitamin K administration take 6 to 8 hours to occur, there is no advantage to giving this drug intravenously versus subcutaneously, the preferred parenteral route. In the setting of overanticoagulation, intermuscular administration can cause hematoma and is also discouraged. Chronic toxicity is not usually a concern, as phytonadione is rarely used long term and is not readily stored.

Single, acute vitamin B_1 (thiamine) ingestions have not resulted in toxicity. With older preparations and multiple dosing, parenteral administration was associated with tachycardia, hypotension, cardiac dysrhythmias, anaphylaxis, vasodilatation, headache, weakness, paralysis, and convulsions. Toxicity would not be expected in doses of 100 mg (or even much larger dosages) given intramuscularly or intravenously over 1 to 2 minutes, such as is commonly administered to the alcoholic patient. It is unlikely that any chronic toxicity exists. Vitamin B$_2$ (riboflavin) is generally thought to be nontoxic.

Most patients who use vitamin B$_3$ (niacin, nicotinic acid) experience flushing. These effects have been noted with oral doses of 100 mg and intravenous doses of 20 mg and are sometimes accompanied by pruritus, headache, and increased intracranial blood flow. These effects are more common in individuals just starting nicotinic acid therapy. High doses may be associated with nausea, diarrhea, and heartburn. Rarely, near syncope is seen. These effects usually subside rapidly, even without treatment. They have not been associated with nicotinamide therapy.

Chronic niacin therapy can cause of hepatotoxicity with centrilobular cholestasis and necrosis. This typically occurs at large dosages (3 g) used to treat hyperlipidemia (up to 100 times the RDA) (8,16). Hepatotoxicity, although rare, also appears to be associated with sustained-release preparations and, possibly, with dose and frequency of use. Nicotinamide appears to be more hepatotoxic than niacin. Acute gouty arthritis has been precipitated secondary to elevated serum uric acid levels. Coagulopathies and hyperglycemia have rarely been reported.

Acute toxicity from vitamin B$_6$ (pyridoxine) is extremely rare. Very large doses (greater than 100 g in adults) can cause dorsal root and sensory ganglia deficits (1,18). Chronic toxicity often results in a nonspecific (primarily sensory) polyneuropathy, which is often, at least partially, reversible with discontinuance. Some studies have suggested that dosages greater than 200 mg/d could be neurotoxic, but toxicity typically occurs with doses of a gram per day or more in adults (18).

The acute ingestion of vitamin C (ascorbic acid) may cause diarrhea, nausea, and abdominal cramps at single doses as low as 1 to 2 g in adults. Ascorbic acid may cause a false-negative test for occult blood in the stool, spurious blood and urine glucose determinations, and inaccurate liver function (enzyme) tests. Massive intravenous dosages (greater than 40 g) of vitamin C can result in oxalate crystal precipitation and subsequent renal failure (12).

With chronic excessive doses of ascorbic acid, excretion of oxalate (an ascorbic acid metabolite) may rarely lead to kidney stones. The risk of nephrolithiasis is increased further by urinary excretion of uric acid and urine acidification, both of which occur with chronic high-dose ascorbic acid therapy.

The effects of vitamin intoxication are usually reversible. GI symptoms usually resolve in a few hours, but the resolution of hepatic, metabolic, and neurologic toxicity may take days to weeks.

DIFFERENTIAL DIAGNOSIS

Given that the symptoms of vitamin toxicity, both acute and chronic, can be quite vague and nonspecific, it is important to consider this etiology in any patient with unexplained complaints. The key to diagnosis is to ask about the use of vitamins and other supplements.

Vitamin A toxicity should be included in the differential diagnosis of dry eczematous skin, hepatic disease, or symptoms consistent with increased intracranial pressure. Pseudotumor cerebri can be caused by or associated with a variety of medications (e.g., corticosteroids, oral contraceptives, tetracyclines, thyroxin) and medical conditions (e.g., hypertension, hyperthyroidism, lupus, obesity, pheochromocytoma, pregnancy, sarcoidosis, ulcerative colitis), and it is also frequently idiopathic. Some cases have been misdiagnosed as acute encephalitis. Signs and symptoms have also been attributed to optic neuritis and psychiatric illness.

The differential of hypercalcemia should include vitamin A and D toxicity, malignancy (osteolytic metastases and malignancies associated with excess production of parathyroid hormone), sarcoidosis, multiple myeloma, milk–alkali syndrome, thyrotoxicosis, adrenal insufficiency, idiopathic hypercalcemia

of infancy, and secondary complications in patients undergoing chronic hemodialysis.

Causes of neuropathy include alcohol, heavy metals, solvents, other toxins, various drugs (e.g., isoniazid, nitrofurantoin, phenytoin), diabetes, collagen vascular diseases, and malignancy, in addition to pyridoxine.

EMERGENCY DEPARTMENT EVALUATION

The history should routinely include asking about over-the-counter medications, dietary supplements, vitamins, and herbal products. A careful history directed toward medications and all over-the-counter products is necessary to ensure that important details are not missed. It is important to note the iron content of multiple vitamin preparations and to evaluate the patient for possible iron poisoning (see Chapter 312, "Iron") if large amounts of iron are present.

A complete physical examination with attention to the abdomen, skin and mucous membranes, and neurological system should be performed. Examination should include funduscopy (for papilledema) in patients with a headache or vitamin A exposure. Serum calcium and liver function tests are recommended those with possible vitamin A and D poisoning. Liver function tests are also indicated in those with gastrointestinal symptoms and chronic exposure to niacin. Long bone or other x-rays may be helpful in patients with musculoskeletal complaints. Cranial CT imaging and CSF analysis and opening pressure measurement may be necessary in patients with papilledema, headache, or other symptoms of vitamin A poisoning. Additional tests may be indicated depending on the presenting complaint. The diagnosis of vitamin poisoning can be confirmed by measuring blood levels of the vitamin in question.

EMERGENCY DEPARTMENT MANAGEMENT

Therapy is primarily supportive. For acute exposures, GI decontamination may be indicated. Charcoal can be administered, depending on clinical likelihood of toxicity, time since ingestion and the presence of coingestants.

Patients with symptoms secondary to chronic exposure require discontinuation of vitamin therapy. Fluids may promote excretion of water-soluble vitamins and should be encouraged. Intravenous therapy may be necessary in patients with dehydration. Hypercalcemia can be treated with intravenous fluids and diuretics. Recent reports suggest that pamidronate (12) may be useful for hypercalcemia secondary to vitamin D intoxication. Prednisone, calcitonin, chelators, and dialysis can be used for severe hypercalcemia. Low-grade pseudotumor cerebri typically resolves spontaneously and does not require therapy. Acetazolamide, furosemide, mannitol, steroids, and daily lumbar punctures or CSF shunting may be required for severe cases. Red cell transfusion and exchange transfusion or dialysis may be needed for neonates with significant hemolysis secondary to parenteral menadione.

CRITICAL INTERVENTIONS

- Check for papilledema, obtain a cranial CT scan, and measure the opening CSF pressure in patients with headache or visual symptoms and vitamin A or retinoid exposure
- Obtain a serum calcium level in patients with possible vitamin A or vitamin D poisoning, particularly those with lethargy, weakness, kidney stones, and gastrointestinal or musculoskeletal complaints
- Check liver function tests in patients with gastrointestinal symptoms and vitamin A, D, or B$_3$ (niacin, nicotinic acid) exposure

DISPOSITION

Most patients can be referred for appropriate outpatient follow-up. Patients with severe hypercalcemia or increased intracranial pressure should be admitted. Women exposed to vitamin A during the first trimester of pregnancy should be referred to an obstetrician. Those with sensory neuropathies should be referred to a neurologist. Patients taking megadose vitamins should be warned about the dangers of chronic toxicity. Those with intentional overdose should be referred for psychiatric evaluation.

COMMON PITFALLS

✔ Failure to appreciate that although water-soluble vitamins are relatively nontoxic, fat-soluble vitamins can cause significant poisoning, particularly with chronic overdose

✔ Failure to determine whether iron is present in the vitamin preparation in cases of acute overdose

✔ Failure to ask about vitamin use and to include vitamin intoxication in the differential diagnosis of unexplained constitutional symptoms, hypercalcemia, and increased intracranial pressure

✔ Failure to consider gastrointestinal decontamination with activated charcoal for acute overdose

✔ Failure to consider alternative diagnoses when a patient with a history of vitamin overdose is critically ill

✔ Failure to warn patients about the dangers of megadose vitamin therapy

Acknowledgment

We thank previous version chapter author Andrew R. Topliff.

References

1. Albin RL, et al. Acute sensory neuropathy-neuronopathy from pyridoxine overdose. *Neurology* 1987;37:1729–1732.

2. Baxi SC, Dailey GE 3rd. Hypervitaminosis A: a cause of hypercalcemia. *West J Med* 1982;137(5):429–431.

3. Bendich A, et al. Safety of oral intake of vitamin E. *Am J Clin Nutr* 1988;48:612–619.

4. Biesalski HK. Comparative assessment of the toxicology of vitamin A and retinoids in man. *Toxicology* 1989;57(2):117–161.

5. Blank S, Scanlon KS, Sinks TH, et al. An outbreak of hypervitaminosis D associated with the overfortification of milk from a home-delivery dairy. *Am J Public Health* 1995;85(5):656–659.

6. Block G, Cox C, Madans J, et al. Vitamin supplement use by demographic characteristics. *Am J Epidemiol* 1988;127:297.

7. Block G, et al. Fruit, vegetables, and cancer prevention: a review of the epidemiological evidence. *Nutr Cancer* 1992;18:1–29.

8. Dalton TA, et al. Hepatotoxicity associated with sustained release niacin. *Am J Med* 1992;93:102–104.

9. Ellis JK, Russell RM, Makrauer FL, et al. Increased risk of vitamin A toxicity in severe hypertriglyceridemia. *N Engl J Med* 1986;105:877.

10. Goodman DS. Vitamin A and retinoids in health and disease. *N Engl J Med* 1984;310:1023.

11. Lawton JM, et al. Acute oxalate nephropathy after massive ascorbic acid administration. *Arch Intern Med* 1985;145:950–951.

12. Lee DC, Lee GY. The use of pamidronate for hypercalcemia secondary to acute vitamin D intoxication. *J Toxicol Clin Toxicol* 1998;36(7):719–721.

13. Hardman JG, Limbird LE. The vitamins. In: *Goodman & Gilman's the pharmacological basis of therapeutics*, 8th ed. New York: Macmillan 1996:1549.

14. Martone WJ, Williams WW, Mortensen ML, et al. Illness with fatalities in premature infants: association with an intravenous vitamin E preparation, E-Ferol. *Pediatrics* 1986;78:591.

15. Miller DR, Hayes KC. Vitamin excess and toxicity. In: Hathcock JN, ed. *Nutritional toxicology*, vol 1. New York: Academic Press 1982:81.

16. Rader JI, et al. Hepatic toxicity of unmodified and time release preparations of niacin. *Am J Med* 1992;92:77–81.

17. Committee on Dietary Allowances, Food and Nutrition Board, National Research Council *Recommended dietary allowances*, 10th ed. Washington, DC: National Academy of Sciences, 1989.

18. Schaumburg H, Kaplan J, Windebank A, et al. Sensory neuropathy from pyridoxine abuse: a new megavitamin syndrome. *N Engl J Med* 1983;309:445.

19. Silverman AK, Ellis CN, Voorhees JJ. Hypervitaminosis A syndrome: a paradigm of retinoid side effects. *J Am Acad Dermatol* 1987;16:1027–1039.

20. Vivekananthan DP, Penn MS, Sapp SK, et al. Use of antioxidant vitamins for the prevention of cardiovascular disease: meta-analysis of randomised trials. *Lancet* 2003;361(9374):2017–2023.

21. Watson WA, Litovitz TL, Rodgers GC, et al. 2002 Annual report of the American Association of Poison Control Centers Toxic Exposure Surveillance System. *Am J Emerg Med* 2003;21(5):353–421.

22. White GL, Beesley R, Thiese SM, et al. Retinal crystals and oral tanning agents. *Am Fam Pract* 1988;37:125.

23. Yen SS, et al. Replacement of DHEA in aging men and women—potential remedial effects. *Ann NY Acad Sci* 1995;774:128–142.

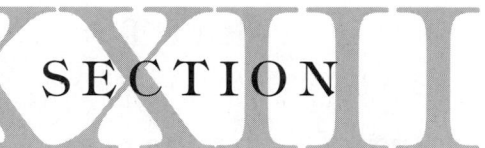

SECTION

XXIII

Section Editors: Christopher H. Linden, and
Jeffrey R. Suchard

Environmental Emergencies

PART

XIII

Bites and Envenomations

CHAPTER 342

Crotaline Snake Envenomation

Richard C. Dart and John B. Sullivan, Jr.

There are several thousand poisonous snakebites in the United States each year, resulting in approximately five deaths (13). Most of these bites involve members of the *Crotalinae* genera: *Crotalus* (rattlesnakes), *Agkistrodon* (copperheads and water moccasins or cottonmouths), and *Sistrurus* (pygmy rattler and massasauga). Although all states except Alaska, Hawaii, and Maine have poisonous snakes, most bites occur in the southeast, southwest, and western regions. The incidence is greatest between March and October, when snakes and victims are the most active.

The crotaline snakes have a temperature (prey)-sensing pit below and in front of the eye (the pupil of which is elliptical)—hence the common name "pit viper." Venom is injected through a pair of fangs attached to the maxilla. Venom is mainly a mixture of digestive enzymes that cause local tissue necrosis and systemic vascular damage, hemolysis, fibrinolysis, and neuromuscular dysfunction. Venom shock and pulmonary injury result from increased vascular permeability and coagulopathy, leading to edema and hemorrhage. Direct cardiac depressant effects may also contribute to shock (15). Venom composition varies with the species.

Up to 25% of bites do not result in envenomation (dry bites) (15). Most envenomations result in a combination of local and systemic effects. However, some populations of Mojave rattlesnakes have a venom (type A) that may cause presynaptic neuromuscular blockade with delayed respiratory failure and mild or absent local effects (3,9,11). Envenomations by Agkistrodon and Sistrurus species tend to be less severe than those of *Crotalus* species.

The size and species of snake, the location and depth of the bite, the victim's size and health, first-aid measures performed, the time to definitive therapy, and the type of therapy influence the severity and outcome. The worst scenario is a small, unwell victim deeply bitten by a large snake in the central body. Improper first-aid measures, delay in arriving at medical care, delayed diagnosis, and inadequate or unnecessary treatment adversely affects the outcome.

Bites by exotic snakes may occur in zoo and pet snake handlers and require specific antivenoms. A regional poison center or zoo can provide information on snake identification, expected toxicity, and antivenom location. Physicians unfamiliar with the management of snake envenomation should consult a toxicologist or regional poison center.

CLINICAL PRESENTATION

Dry bites produce no signs or symptoms other than those of a puncture wound. If envenomation has occurred, the victim (often an intoxicated male) typically notes sudden, severe pain at the bite site, soon followed by progressive swelling and, sometimes, paresthesias.

Examination may show two puncture wounds exuding bloody fluid. However, there are many reports of serious envenomation associated with scratches and single or multiple puncture wounds. Other local findings include erythema, ecchymosis, bullae, and, eventually, necrosis and ulceration. Bites about the face may lead to airway obstruction; those of the extremities may lead to compartment syndrome. Wound infection is a potential complication (10), although this is rarely seen clinically (14).

Systemic effects include nausea, vomiting, diarrhea, perioral paresthesias, salivation, lethargy, and weakness. Severe envenomations may lead to cardiovascular collapse, coma, seizures, dyspnea, respiratory depression, and gastrointestinal and pulmonary hemorrhage. Initial vital signs often show tachycardia and mild hypertension. Laboratory evaluation may reveal hemolysis, anemia, thrombocytopenia, coagulopathy (including severe fibrinolysis), and blood, protein, and glucose in the urine in severe cases. In severe cases, the chest radiograph may reveal pulmonary edema, and the electrocardiogram (ECG) may show dysrhythmias or ischemic changes.

DIFFERENTIAL DIAGNOSIS

Victims at the extremes of age, those with altered mental states, and those who are bitten while reaching into concealed areas may not realize they have been bitten. Snakebite may be misdiagnosed as a nonvenomous bite or sting or as puncture wounds and scratches from thorns and brush. The possible diagnosis of snake venom poisoning can be excluded only by prolonged observation, documenting a lack of progressive local and systemic manifestations.

EMERGENCY DEPARTMENT EVALUATION

On the patient's arrival in the emergency department, vital signs and a rapid patient survey should be performed to determine the patient's clinical stability. The time and circumstances of the bite, the nature and severity of symptoms, the first-aid measures taken before arrival, and any history of allergies, medical problems, previous bites, and antivenom therapy are noted. The bite site should be examined, noting the nature and extent of local findings. Distal neurovascular status should be noted in extremity bites. Initially, the local evaluation should be repeated every 15 minutes. The general examination should focus on the cardiovascular, pulmonary, and neurologic systems.

The clinically relevant characteristics to describe when assessing severity are (a) local manifestations, (b) coagulation abnormalities, (c) systemic effects. The change in these parameters over time is particularly important. An initially mild envenomation may progress over a period of hours to become moderate, severe, or even life-threatening. Coagulation abnormalities may peak as late as 3 days after envenomation. Laboratory tests in questionable or initially mild bites should include complete blood count; serum electrolytes, blood urea nitrogen, and creatinine levels; prothrombin time; platelet count; and urinalysis. In severe cases or in patients who worsen, creatine kinase, fibrinogen, fibrin split products, and arterial blood gas analysis should be obtained. A chest radiograph and an ECG are needed in patients with systemic signs or symptoms.

EMERGENCY DEPARTMENT MANAGEMENT

Advanced life-support measures should be instituted, as necessary. Prehospital personnel should be directed to establish intravenous access, to give oxygen, and to transport victims of venomous snakebites to a medical facility that possesses antivenom. If a tourniquet has been placed, it should not be removed until i.v. access has been established. The limb should be immobilized in a neutral position. Loose (lymphatic) tourniquets, and cooling an extremity may be effective if used within 30 minutes of envenomation, but they are not substitutes for definitive care. Local wound care and tetanus prophylaxis should be provided.

Antivenom is the mainstay of crotaline snakebite treatment. Immunoglobulins in the antivenom neutralize venom proteins by antigen–antibody complex formation. Antivenom therapy has changed with the introduction of *Crotalidae* polyvalent immune Fab (ovine) [FabAV, CroFab]. The primary indication for FabAV therapy is progressive worsening of local injury (e.g., pain, ecchymosis, or swelling), laboratory abnormalities (e.g., worsening platelet count, prolonged coagulation times, decreased fibrinogen), or systemic manifestations (e.g., unstable vital signs or abnormal mental status) (6). If, after several hours, pain and edema remain localized to the bite site and coagulopathy is not progressing, antivenom is unnecessary. Frequent reassessment for worsening of local, systemic and laboratory manifestations cannot be overemphasized. The extent of swelling should be outlined with a marking pen, and the limb circumference should be measured at several sites above and below the bite. If any of these parameters worsen, antivenom therapy is usually warranted.

The initial dose of FabAV for adults or children is 4 to 6 vials (Fig. 342.1). Six vials are used in patients with systemic effects or rapidly progressive local effects. Each vial of FabAV is reconstituted with 10-mL of sterile water. The contents of all vials are then injected into a 250-mL bag of sterile water or saline. A smaller volume is used in children or patients in whom large volumes

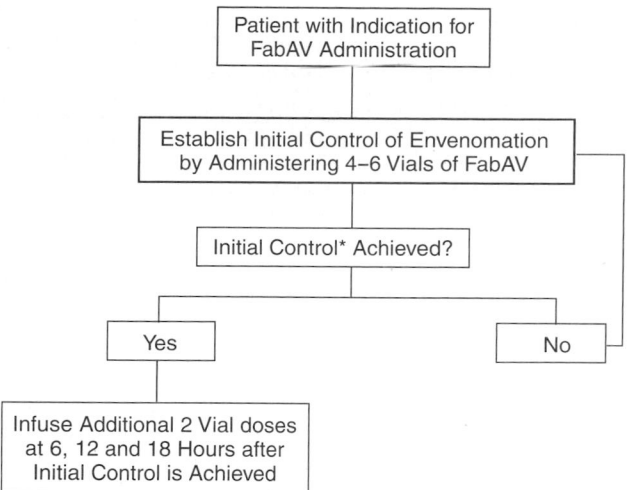

Figure 342.1.   Algorithm for the use of crotaline snake antivenom.

could be detrimental. The initial infusion rate should be slow (e.g., 10–25 mL/hr) and then increased every few minutes, until a rate is reached that will allow for infusion of the entire dose over one hour (e.g., 250 mL/hr). Continuous respiratory and cardiovascular monitoring should be performed. Antivenom should be given only in a critical care setting with epinephrine and antihistamines readily available to treat anaphylaxis, should it occur. Skin-testing is not indicated prior to use of FabAV, as with some other antivenom products.

At the end of the initial infusion, the patient's condition should be re-assessed. If significant clinical and laboratory improvement (e.g., cessation of local progression and improvement in systemic and coagulopathic effects) has not occurred, or the patient continues to worsen, the initial dose of antivenom should be repeated. This process is repeated until initial control has been achieved. Occasionally, with severe envenomation, a large number of vials may be required for control. After initial control has been established, three maintenance doses of FabAV should be given: two vials administered every 6 hours for a total of six vials. In clinical trials, patients receiving scheduled maintenance doses of CroFab had a lower incidence of local recurrence than those assigned to repeat doses on an "as needed" basis (6).

Recurrence is defined as the return of any venom effect after the abnormality had initially resolved. Recurrences occur to some degree with most antivenoms (5). A local recurrence involves return of progressive local swelling after initial control was achieved. Coagulopathy recurrence involves the return of thrombocytopenia, prolonged prothrombin time (PT), or elevated fibrin split products. Local recurrences are uncommon. They usually occur within the 12 to 24 hours of treatment. They should be distinguished from redistribution of blood/edema, secondary infection, venous thrombosis, and other causes of extremity swelling. Typically, local recurrence is managed with another two to four vials of FabAV, followed by regular maintenance infusions.

The recurrence of coagulopathy is more common, and usually does not present until after hospital discharge (developing within 2–3 days). Recurrent coagulopathy is often only partially responsive to further antivenom administration. If given early, further FabAV may be effective in correcting the abnormality. However, the beneficial effect may be mild, and is often transient. Whether additional antivenom should be administered in such circumstances is controversial. Although coagulation tests are often abnormal, the risk of clinically significant hemorrhage is very low. Consequently, current recommendations suggest that recurrent coagulopathy be treated only if it is extreme and involves more than one coagulation abnormality, or there is evidence of significant bleeding (1,17). Most coagulopathy recurrences can be safely managed expectantly with close serial laboratory monitoring and bleeding precautions.

Concomitant supportive care (e.g., fluids and pressors for hypotension, blood component replacement for severe hematologic abnormalities, and respiratory support) is extremely important but often neglected (12). Blood products should be used only if the patient is actively bleeding or cannot receive antivenom (2).

The effectiveness of antivenom in the treatment of snake venom poisoning has been extensively documented. However, fasciotomy and supportive care without antivenom have been proposed in some areas as definitive treatment of snakebite. Experimental evidence in animals shows no beneficial effect (7,8,16). In patients with documented increased intracompartmental pressure unresponsive to limb elevation, mannitol (1–2 g/kg intravenously), and antivenom (four–six vials of FabAV), fasciotomy should be considered. Cultures and antibiotic therapy should be initiated only if clinical signs of infection develop (14).

CRITICAL INTERVENTIONS

- Monitor patients closely for progressive local, systemic, and hematologic effects, which are indications for antivenom therapy
- Perform intensive care unit-level monitoring and have epinephrine and antihistamines (e.g., diphenhydramine) available at the bedside when giving antivenom, as anaphylactic reactions may occur

DISPOSITION

Patients with dry bites who do not develop systemic or local progressive venom effects during an 8- to 12-hour observation period may be discharged. Those with severe or life-threatening bites and those receiving antivenom should be admitted to an intensive care unit. Admission to a floor bed is appropriate for the observation of patients with mild or moderate envenomations. Mobilization of the affected extremity can begin when the progression of swelling has ceased. Discharge is appropriate when swelling is decreasing, any coagulopathy has reversed, and the patient is ambulatory. Outpatient follow-up may be necessary for several days to monitor for infection and serum sickness. Serum sickness may range from a mild viral-like illness to severe urticarial rash, arthralgias, and other complications. In contrast to the immunoglobulin antivenom used in the past, serum sickness is unusual with FabAV (4,5). Most cases can be treated as outpatients, with antiinflammatory analgesics, antihistamines, and corticosteroids.

COMMON PITFALLS

✔ Failure to diagnose envenomation because of a lack of history or inadequate observation of patients with suspicious wounds of unclear cause
✔ Using antivenom unnecessarily, or giving inadequate doses
✔ Failure to provide supportive care and antivenom to patients with severe envenomation

References

1. Boyer LV, Seifert SA, Cain JS. Recurrence phenomena after immunoglobulin therapy for snake envenomations: Part 2. Guidelines for clinical management with crotaline Fab antivenom. *Ann Emerg Med* 2001;37:196.
2. Burgess JL, Dart RC. Snake venom coagulopathy: use and abuse of blood products in the treatment of pit viper envenomation. *Ann Emerg Med* 1991;20:795.
3. Castilonia R, Pattabhiramin T, Russell FE. Neuromuscular blocking effects of the Mojave rattlesnake (Crotalus scutulatus scutulatus) venom. *Proc West Pharmacol Soc* 1980;23:103.
4. Clark RF, McKinney PE, Chase PB, et al. Immediate and delayed allergic reactions to Crotalidae polyvalent immune Fab (ovine) antivenom. *Ann Emerg Med* 2002;39:671.
5. Dart RC, McNally J. Efficacy, safety, and use of snake antivenoms in the United States. *Ann Emerg Med* 2001;37:181.
6. Dart RC, Seifert SA, Boyer LV, et al. A randomized multicenter trial of crotalinae polyvalent immune Fab (ovine) antivenom for the treatment for crotaline snakebite in the United States. *Arch Intern Med* 2001;161:2030.
7. Garfin SR, Castilonia RR, Mubarak SJ, et al. Rattlesnake bites and surgical decompression: results using a laboratory model. *Toxicon* 1984;22:177.
8. Garfin SR, Castilonia RR, Mubarak SJ, et al. The effect of antivenom on intramuscular pressure elevation induced by rattlesnake venom. *Toxicon* 1985;23:677.
9. Glenn J, Straight R, Wolfe M. Geographical variation in Crotalus scutulatus scutulatus (Mohave rattlesnake) venom properties. *Toxicon* 1983;21:119.
10. Goldstein E, Citron D, Gonzales H, et al. Bacteriology of rattlesnake venom and implications for therapy. *J Infect Dis* 1979;140:818.
11. Hardy D. Envenomation by the Mohave rattlesnake (Crotalus scutulatus scutulatus) in Southern Arizona, USA. *Toxicon* 1983;21:111.
12. Hardy D. Fatal rattlesnake envenomation in Arizona: 1969–1984. *J Toxicol Clin Toxicol* 1986;24:1.
13. Langley RL, Morrow WE. Deaths resulting from animal attacks in the United States. *Wilderness Environ Med* 1997;8:8.
14. LoVecchio F, Klemens J, Welch S, et al. Antibiotics after rattlesnake envenomation. *Am J Emerg Med* 2002;23:327.
15. Russell FE. *Snake venom poisoning*. Great Neck, NY: Scholium International 1983.
16. Tanen DA, Danish DC, Clark RF. Crotalidae polyvalent immune Fab antivenom limits the decrease in perfusion pressure of the anterior leg compartment in a porcine crotaline envenomation model. *Ann Emerg Med* 2003;41:384.
17. Yip L. Rational use of Crotalidae polyvalent immune Fab (ovine) in the management of crotaline bite. *Ann Emerg Med* 2002;39:648.

CHAPTER 343
Elapid Snake Envenomation

Richard C. Dart and John B. Sullivan, Jr.

Coral snakes are the only North American snakes belonging to the elapid family. These brightly colored snakes are known for the potency of their venom. Fortunately, few bites occur, because these snakes are usually small, nocturnal, and retiring.

Coral snakes found in the United States include the Eastern coral snake (*Micrurus fulvius fulvius*), the Texas coral snake (*Micrurus fulvius tenere*), and the Arizona (*Sonoran*) coral snake (*Micruroides euryoxanthus*). The Eastern coral snake is found in the deep southeast United States; the Texas and Arizona subspecies are found primarily in the states whose name they bear (3). All these snakes are brightly colored, with black, red, and yellow rings that encircle their bodies. The red and yellow rings touch in coral snakes but are separated by black rings in nonpoisonous snakes, hence the rhyme, "Red on yellow, kill a fellow; red on black, venom lack." Unfortunately, victims may confuse the rhyme, especially when intoxicated (e.g., "Red on yellow, good fellow."). Elapids lack the facial pits seen in pit vipers and have nearly round pupils.

Coral snakes are docile and usually only bite during handling. When biting, they hold on or chew, allowing them to envenomate. Their venom is discharged through grooves on two small, fixed anterior fangs. Their small size makes it difficult, but not impossible, to envenomate humans seriously. The Eastern and Texas subspecies are larger and have seriously envenomated many patients, but the Sonoran coral snake has not caused severe envenomation (3).

CLINICAL PRESENTATION

Coral snake envenomation can be difficult to diagnose and easy to underestimate. The typical bite shows little local damage and few initial systemic symptoms. Minor pain without swelling may be present. This may be followed by numbness and weakness of the affected part as the envenomation syndrome advances. Systemic symptoms, which may take hours to develop, include drowsiness, apprehension, weakness, fasciculation, tremors, difficulty swallowing, dyspnea, salivation, nausea, and vomiting (1).

Physical examination may show fang marks and associated scratches. It is often possible to express a drop of blood. However, the history is particularly important, because significant envenomation without apparent bite marks, despite close examination, has occurred. In such cases, injecting lidocaine under the suspected area may show minute beads of serosanguineous fluid exuding from fang punctures. Signs of systemic toxicity may be delayed in onset and include weakness of extraocular muscles, miotic pupils, bulbar paralysis, ptosis, respiratory depression, and convulsions. An elevated creatine kinase level may be noted.

DIFFERENTIAL DIAGNOSIS

The diagnosis of coral snake envenomation is usually clear, because the snake frequently hangs on to the victim and has bright, identifiable coloring. When the patient cannot clearly communicate, the rapidity of onset distinguishes it from other motor neuron diseases. Laboratory testing may be necessary to rule out poisoning by agents such as botulism, heavy metals, and central nervous system depressant medications.

Envenomation by other members of the elapid family such as the Australian red-bellied Black snake, Ingram's Brown snake, death adder, and cobra, krait, mamba, Taipan, and tiger species may cause similar neurotoxicity. Amateur herpetologists are the typical victims but zookeepers and other professional are occasionally bitten. Specific antivenoms may be available. A poison center should be consulted for assistance in evaluation and management.

EMERGENCY DEPARTMENT EVALUATION

The time and circumstances of the bite, a description of the snake, first-aid treatment before arrival, allergies, previous bites and antivenom therapy, medical history prior to presentation, and the onset, progression, and nature of symptoms should be noted. The physical examination should focus on the neurologic status, particularly cranial motor nerve and respiratory muscle func-

tion. Tidal volume, arterial blood gas analysis, and other studies (laboratory, chest radiograph, electrocardiogram) should be obtained, if clinically indicated. Although positive identification of the offending snake is helpful, it should not delay treatment.

EMERGENCY DEPARTMENT MANAGEMENT

Prehospital care should consist of intravenous line insertion, maintenance of airway, and timely transport to a health care facility capable of full life-support and antivenom therapy. Keeping the bitten extremity still and applying elastic pressure bandages to the extremity to retard venom spread may be useful.

Wound cleansing and tetanus prophylaxis should be provided. Patients who have clearly been bitten or who have developed symptoms or signs of envenomation should be given at least five vials of *M. fulvius* antivenom (equine) by i.v. infusion. It is not advisable to wait for sign of toxicity to develop because the antivenom may not always reverse them or prevent further deterioration. If symptoms progress, the dose of antivenom should be repeated. Allergic reactions can occur and the same precautions as described for crotaline antivenom administration should be taken when giving coral snake antivenom. Although *M. fulvius* antivenom is neither effective nor necessary in Sonoran coral snake envenomation, the aforementioned protocol should be followed unless a positive identification of this species has been made. The elective intubation of patients with bulbar signs or symptoms may prevent aspiration pneumonia (1).

The prognosis is excellent. There is normally no tissue loss or permanent neurologic dysfunction. Even without antivenom treatment, recovery can be expected if appropriate supportive care is provided (2). Hence, patients with allergic reactions to horse serum or antivenom can be managed successfully without antivenom therapy.

CRITICAL INTERVENTIONS

- Admit and monitor all patients with possible coral snake envenomation for neurological dysfunction and hypoventilation
- Administer *M. fulvius* antivenom to patients with known coral snake bites, even before the onset of symptoms

DISPOSITION

All patients in whom the diagnosis of coral snake envenomation is entertained should be admitted to an intensive care area for at least 12 hours of close monitoring of vital signs and neurologic function. This disposition applies to patients with a definite bite, either by history or examination, regardless of whether they are symptomatic. Patients with no evidence of envenomation after 12 hours of observation may be discharged. Those with severe envenomation may require several days of hospitalization.

COMMON PITFALLS

✔ Failure to appreciate that the onset of symptoms after coral snake envenomation may be delayed in onset and slowly progressive
✔ Using antivenom inappropriately in patients with documented Arizona (*Sonoran*) coral snake envenomation and in those with allergic reactions to horse serum or antivenom
✔ Failure to take the same precautions as described for crotaline antivenom when giving coral snake antivenom

✔ Failure to monitor for worsening toxicity after antivenom administration and to provide concurrent supportive care, especially airway protection and ventilatory assistance

References

1. Kitchens CS, Van Mierop LHS. Envenomation by the Eastern coral snake (Micrurus fulvius fulvius). *JAMA* 1987;258:1615.
2. Mosely T. Coral snake bite: recovery following symptoms of respiratory paralysis. *Ann Surg* 1966;163:943.
3. Russell FE. *Snake venom poisoning.* Great Neck, NY: Scholium International, 1983.

CHAPTER 344
Hymenoptera Envenomation

Paul Kolecki

The order *Hymenoptera* ("membrane-winged") includes bees, wasps, hornets, yellow jackets, and ants. Honeybees and bumblebees belong to the family *Apidae*, although wasps, hornets, and yellow jackets belong to the family *Vespidae*. Ants belong to the family *Formicidae*; fire ants are the most medically important species in this family. Anaphylaxis to *Hymenoptera* species affects up to 0.5% of the U.S. population and accounts for about 40 deaths annually (18,21).

Winged *Hymenoptera* species are found throughout the United States, although fire ants are localized mainly in the southern states. Yellow jackets build and live in nests in the ground and in walls, although hornets live in nests built in trees or under branches. Wasps often build nests under roofs, behind shutters, and in dryer vents (1). Domestic honeybees in the United States are generally passive and do not sting unless provoked. Africanized honeybees (also called "killer bees"), indigenous to Central and South America and the southwestern U.S., are notorious for large, aggressive swarms and attacks on animals and humans (16).

The venom of winged *Hymenoptera* insects consists mainly of proteins, enzymes, and vasoactive amines; there is strong cross-reactivity between the venom within families. The venom of Africanized honeybees is very similar to that of domestic honeybees both in composition and amount injected per sting (16), but may cause greater morbidity as a result of a greater likelihood of mass envenomation. Winged *Hymenoptera* species inject their venom quickly, typically causing immediate reactions. The venom of fire ants differs from the other Hymenoptera in that its main constituents are piperidine alkaloids. Fire ants are named as such because of the burning pain inflicted by their unique venom, which they inject more slowly, over seconds to minutes (19). Significant morbidity and even mortality may occur in allergic individuals after a single envenomation by any of the Hymenoptera species.

Reactions to Hymenoptera stings typically are classified by the time of onset and the severity of the clinical reaction.

Classification by time usually is subdivided into immediate and delayed reactions. Immediate reactions occur within minutes to a few hours after an envenomation and are mediated by IgE and vasoactive compounds within the venom. Delayed reactions are much less common than immediate reactions and typically develop several days to a week after the sting. These reactions are non-IgE mediated.

Classification of a Hymenoptera reaction by severity is subdivided into three groups: local, systemic (e.g., anaphylactic), and toxic. Local reactions are common, resulting in swelling, erythema, and a burning sensation at the sting site. These reactions are benign, resolve within hours to a couple of days, and are not predictive of systemic reactions to subsequent stings (1). Large local reactions can occur, perhaps involving an entire extremity. Patients suffering a large local reaction are at minimal risk (approximately 5%) of systemic anaphylaxis from subsequent stings (12).

Systemic reactions to Hymenoptera stings are either generalized or develop at a site remote from the sting site. Systemic reactions that produce life-threatening signs and symptoms are IgE-mediated and commonly are known as anaphylaxis. Potential physiologic effects associated with an immediate and severe systemic reaction include bronchiolar constriction, vasodilation, myocardial depression, increased capillary permeability, and the production of mucous. Most anaphylactic fatalities are a result of laryngeal edema and bronchospasm. An envenomation in someone with no history of a previous systemic reaction results in an anaphylactic reaction less than 1% of the time. However, a negative history of prior systemic reaction does not rule out the possibility of a severe reaction in the future. The risk of anaphylaxis to a subsequent Hymenoptera sting for a patient who has previously suffered venom-induced anaphylaxis is 30% to 60% (17). Again, there is a very strong cross reactivity between the venoms within each *Hymenoptera* family and people sensitized to one species may also react to a sting by another species.

Toxic reactions, also known as direct systemic reactions, typically occur following a massive envenomation and result from the absorption of larger amounts of venom. Africanized honeybees are notorious for large, aggressive swarms and attacks on animals and humans. Depending on the size of the victim, 10 to 50 simultaneous stings may be serious or fatal. The human LD50 for honeybee stings has been estimated to be between 500 to 1,200 stings (22). Toxic reactions may occur immediately or may be delayed, and fatalities typically result from multisystem organ failure (8,22).

CLINICAL PRESENTATION

Local reactions caused by Hymenoptera envenomations are characterized by pain, wheal and flare formation, warmth, and pruritus at the sting site. These types of reactions occur in non-allergic individuals. Reactions to stings by winged species typically begin immediately and last for several hours. Fire ant stings often occur in clusters, and develop into painful vesicles and sterile pustules during the first 24 hours and require up to 10 to 14 days for resolution (1,5). Large local reactions secondary to fire ant envenomations typically are pruritic, erythematous, edematous, and indurated (1).

Persistent swelling, pain, and erythema at the site of the sting manifest local allergic reactions caused by *Hymenoptera* envenomations. These reactions may progress to involve a large area (e.g., an entire extremity) over the first 2 to 3 days and may last for more than a week. Stings after accidental insect inhalation or ingestion by sensitive individuals may result in life-threatening swelling and obstruction of the pharynx, larynx, or esophagus.

Most anaphylactic reactions develop within minutes of envenomation and peak within an hour (3,6,15,18). Rarely, they may be delayed as long as 6 hours after the envenomation. Recurrent reactions may occur for up to 2 days. Mild anaphylactic reactions are characterized by generalized flushing and urticaria, although moderate reactions are characterized by generalized weakness, chest or throat tightness, nausea, vomiting, diarrhea, and generalized angioedema. Cyanosis, dyspnea, stridor, hoarseness, confusion, coma, and collapse are seen in severe cases of anaphylaxis. Physical findings may include hypotension, tachycardia, urticaria, wheezing, and laryngeal and pulmonary edema. Secondary complications associated with severe *Hymenoptera*-induced anaphylaxis include cerebral and myocardial infarction and coagulopathies (9,15,20). Systemic reactions may occur also from fire ant stings; anaphylaxis occurs in 0.6% to 6% of envenomated fire ant victims (19).

Signs and symptoms of direct venom-induced systemic toxicity usually begin within minutes and include vomiting, diarrhea, generalized edema, collapse, loss of consciousness, confusion, headache, muscle spasms, and seizures. Vital signs typically reveal hypotension and tachycardia. Severe cases of direct systemic toxicity may be complicated by hemolysis, thrombocytopenia, disseminated intravascular coagulation (DIC), rhabdomyolysis and acute renal failure, hepatoxicity, and encephalopathy (13,24). Systemic toxicity from mass envenomation may, however, be delayed many hours (8).

Serum sickness is an unusual delayed reaction that typically occurs within 1 week of envenomation (11). Serum sickness is characterized by fever, arthralgia, myalgias, rash, adenopathy, and may include headache, glomerulonephritis, nephrotic syndrome, and necrotizing vasculitis. Delayed atypical hematologic and or neurologic reactions may also occur following envenomations. These types of reactions mainly include hemolytic anemia, thrombocytopenic purpura, Guillain-Barré syndrome, optic neuritis and other neuropathies, parkinsonism, and transverse myelitis (11,15,24).

DIFFERENTIAL DIAGNOSIS

The differential diagnosis for local reactions and anaphylaxis resembling *Hymenoptera* envenomations is extensive. Fortunately, the history of an encounter with a bee, yellow jacket, wasp, or fire ants is typically present.

Virtually any stinging or biting insect may produce limited local reactions of similar appearance. Extensive local reactions must be differentiated from an infectious cellulitis. Progressive extension of the initial reaction beginning shortly after the envenomation usually indicates an allergic component to the reaction. Inflammation, fever, leukocytosis, and lymphangitis beginning more than 24 hours after envenomation suggest a superimposed infection.

Anaphylactic reactions may be caused by a wide variety of drugs, foods, and environmental allergens. Anaphylaxis from *Hymenoptera* envenomation should be considered in any patient discovered outdoors during the spring and summer months with unexplained hypotension, urticaria, wheezing, and or airway obstruction.

Patients who present with delayed reactions should be asked about recent insect stings, illnesses, and medication use within the previous several weeks.

Toxic reactions (e.g., direct systemic reactions or massive envenomation) can be differentiated from anaphylaxis in that systemic toxicity typically progresses more slowly, requires many stings, and causes multiorgan failure. Urticaria, pruritus, and wheezing suggest anaphylaxis and typically these findings are not part of a direct systemic reaction.

Fire ant envenomations typically produce pustules within 24 hours. The differential diagnosis for pustule formation is also extensive, although the history of fire ant exposure is often evident. Risk factors for exposure include outdoor activities in endemic areas, especially when the affected areas are not covered by protective clothing.

EMERGENCY DEPARTMENT EVALUATION

The history should include information pertaining to the time and estimated number of stings, previous *Hymenoptera* reactions, and past medical history. The time of onset, progression, and nature of symptoms should be noted. The physical examination should focus on the vital signs, airway patency, the cardiovascular system, and the skin. Lateral soft-tissue neck radiographs and/or nasopharyngoscopy should be considered for envenomated patients experiencing stridor or voice changes without complete obstruction. Patients with hypotension, loss of consciousness, or who suffer multiple envenomations (ten or more for pediatric patients, fifty or more for adults) should have measurements of the complete blood count (CBC), serum creatine phosphokinase (CPK), liver function tests (LFTs), prothrombin time (PT), partial thromboplastin time (PTT), urinalysis (UA), and a metabolic panel to check for various manifestations of systemic toxicity (8). Measurements of the fibrinogen level and fibrinogen split products (FSP) should be considered for patients with massive envenomation. Patients who experience hypotension, chest pain, or loss of consciousness should have an electrocardiogram (ECG) to rule out myocardial injury, ischemia, or infarction.

EMERGENCY DEPARTMENT MANAGEMENT

The treatment of local reactions includes general wound care and symptomatic therapy for pain, swelling, and pruritus (e.g., analgesics, cool compresses, ice packs, elevation, antihistamines). Envenomation sites should be cleaned and tetanus prophylaxis should be updated, if necessary. Large local reactions can be treated with a short course of antihistamines, analgesics, and steroids. Secondary infections should be treated with appropriate antibiotics to cover skin flora.

With honeybee envenomation, the stingers often remain embedded in the victim's skin, and these should be removed. Previous recommendations often stated that such stingers should be removed by scraping (e.g., with the edge of a needle, scalpel, or credit card) rather than by pinching or use of tweezers, to avoid injecting any remaining contents from the attached venom sacs. However, *in vivo* experiments show that nearly all venom is injected within several seconds, and by the time a patient presents for care, stinger removal by pinching does not increase envenomation effects (23). Bee stinger removal by any method is acceptable.

The treatment for anaphylaxis as a result of *Hymenoptera* stings is very similar to that for anaphylaxis of other etiologies. Advanced life-support measures should be instituted, as necessary. Prehospital personnel should give epinephrine at the first sign of an anaphylactic reaction (2,15). The dose and route of epinephrine depend on the severity of the symptoms and the victim's underlying medical problems; adults usually receive 0.3 mg s.c., but see Chapter 131, "Anaphylaxis," for more details.

Hypotensive patients should receive aggressive volume replacement with intravenous crystalloid. Additionally, envenomated patients suffering anaphylaxis should receive an oral or i.v. antihistamine (e.g., diphenhydramine 0.5–1.0 mg/kg) and steroids (e.g., oral prednisone 0.5–1.0 mg/kg or methyl-prednisolone 1–4 mg/kg i.v.). An H2 blocker (e.g., ranitidine) may also be helpful.

Severe anaphylactic reactions or marked local reactions that involve the nose, mouth, and or throat may require immediate airway control. Because most deaths are as a result of airway obstruction, early airway control by endotracheal intubation may be lifesaving in patients with respiratory distress from upper obstruction and should be strongly considered. A delay in airway control may result in further swelling, an unstable and difficult airway, and the potential need for a surgical airway. The use of inhaled β-1 adrenergic agonists (e.g., nebulized albuterol 2.5 mg) should be considered for envenomated patients who are wheezing or who have decreased lower airway movement.

Recurrent or refractory hypotension may occur following a *Hymenoptera* envenomation. Continuous infusions of vasopressors (e.g., epinephrine, norepinephrine) may be necessary for such patients. Higher-than-usual doses of β-adrenergic agents may be required when treating envenomated patients taking β-adrenergic blocking agents and those patients on chronic β-agonist medications (7).

The treatment of direct toxic reactions associated with multiple or massive envenomation is entirely supportive. These patients need to be monitored closely. These patients are potentially at risk for delayed organ dysfunction. Serial laboratory determinations of CBC, metabolic profile, LFTs, CPK, UA, fibrinogen, and FSP every 6 to 8 hours for 24 hours should be considered (8).

Delayed hypersensitivity reactions typically are treated with analgesics, antihistamines, and a tapering dose of corticosteroids.

Local fire ant reactions can be treated with cool compresses and cleansing with soap and water. Large local reactions may be treated with oral corticosteroids, antihistamines, and analgesics. Secondary infections should be treated with antibiotics. Anaphylactic reactions should be treated in the manner previously described.

CRITICAL INTERVENTIONS

- Administer epinephrine, corticosteroids, antihistamines, and i.v. fluids to patients with anaphylaxis who have abnormal vital signs, oxygen saturation, or dyspnea
- Assess patients with dyspnea for upper airway obstruction and perform endotracheal intubation in patients with severe or progressive signs and symptoms

DISPOSITION

Patients who present immediately after envenomation should be observed for 1 to 2 hours for signs and symptoms of anaphylaxis. Asymptomatic patients may then be discharged. Milder anaphylactic reactions may be delayed and patients should be instructed to return immediately if systemic symptoms ensue. In asymptomatic patients with a history of previous anaphylactic reactions or severe local reactions, a prophylactic 3-day course of antihistamines and corticosteroids, beginning with a dose before discharge, should be considered.

Patients with mild to moderate anaphylaxis should be treated and observed for 4 to 6 hours or until asymptomatic. Patients suffering persistent or recurrent symptoms (excluding isolated urticaria), life-threatening reactions, persistent hypotension, or cardiac complications should be hospitalized with level of care determined by the severity of symptoms. All patients with anaphylactic reactions should be treated with a 3-day course of antihistamines and corticosteroids to prevent a relapse.

Patients with anaphylactic or severe local reactions should be given an epinephrine prescription (e.g., EpiPen or Ana-kit) and instructions for use. They should be cautioned about outdoor work and recreation and should be advised to wear shoes, long-sleeved shirts and pants, and to avoid wearing bright colors and perfumes. The use of insect repellents may be helpful. Referral to an allergist (directly or through the primary care physician) for possible desensitization immunotherapy should also be provided prior to discharge (10). Finally, the patient should be instructed to obtain and wear a hymenoptera allergy identification bracelet.

Patients suffering direct toxic reactions and multiple envenomations need careful observation for delayed end-organ damage. Patients with local or delayed hypersensitivity reactions can be treated as outpatients, with emergency department or primary care follow-up. Atypical reactions may require admission and referral to an allergist.

COMMON PITFALLS

✔ Failure to consider *Hymenoptera*-induced anaphylactic reaction in an unconscious or hypotensive patient found outdoors during the warm seasons
✔ Failure to prescribe antihistamines and corticosteroids for 3 days after anaphylaxis
✔ Failure to prescribe an emergency epinephrine kit for victims of severe local and anaphylactic reactions
✔ Failure to refer patients with severe local and anaphylactic reactions to an allergist

Acknowledgments

We thank previous edition chapter authors Paul A. Janson and Richard J. Iseke.

References

1. Bahna SL. Insect sting allergy: a matter of life and death. *Pediatrics Annals* 2000;29(12):753.
2. Barach EM, Nowak RM, Tennyson LG, et al. Epinephrine for treatment of anaphylactic shock. *JAMA* 1984;251:2118.
3. Barr SE. Allergy to Hymenoptera stings—review of the world literature, 1953–1970. *Ann Allergy Asthma Immunol* 1971;29:49
4. DeShazo RD, Butcher BT, Banks WA. Reactions to the stings of the imported fire ant. *N Engl J Med* 1990;323:462.
5. Ginsberg CN. Fire ant envenomation in children. *Pediatrics* 1984;73:689.
6. Golden DBK, Valentine M. Insect sting allergy. *Ann Allergy Asthma Immunol* 1984;53:444.
7. Ingall M, Goldman G, Page LB. Beta-blockage in stinging insect anaphylaxis [letter]. *JAMA* 1984;251:2118.
8. Kolecki P. Delayed toxic reaction following massive bee envenomation. *Ann Emerg Med* 1999;33:1:114.
9. Levine HD. Acute myocardial infarction following wasp sting. *Am Heart J* 1976;91:365.
10. Li JT, Yunginger JW. Management of insect sting hypersensitivity. *Mayo Clin Proc* 1992;67(2):180.
11. Light WC, Reisman RE, Shimizu M, et al. Unusual reactions following insect stings. *J Allergy Clin Immunol* 1977;59:391.
12. Mauriello PM, Barde SH, Georgitis JW, et al. Natural history of large local reactions from stinging insects. *J Allergy Clin Immunol* 1984;74:494.
13. Mejia G, Arbelaez M, Henao JE, et al. Acute renal failure due to multiple stings by Africanized bees. *Ann Intern Med* 1986;104:210.
14. Muller U, Mosbech H, Henao JE, et al. Emergency treatment of allergic reactions to Hymenoptera stings. *Clin Exp Allergy* 1991;21:281.
15. Ratnoff OD, Nossel HL. Wasp sting anaphylaxis. *Blood* 1983;61:1983.
16. Reisman RE. Insect stings. *N Engl J Med* 1994;331:523.
17. Reisman RE. Natural history of insect sting allergy: relationship of severity of symptoms of initial sting anaphylaxis to re-sting reactions. *J Allergy Clin Immunol* 1992;90:335.
18. Reisman RE. Sting insect allergy. *Med Clin North Am* 1992;76:883.
19. Stafford CT. Hypersensitivity to fire ant venom. *Ann Allergy Asthma Immunol* 1996;77:87.

20. Stan JC, Brasher GW. Wasp sting anaphylaxis with cerebral infarction. *Ann Allergy Asthma Immunol* 1977;39:431.
21. Valentine MD. Anaphylaxis and stinging insect hypersensitivity. *JAMA* 1992;268:2830.
22. Vetter RS, Visscher K, Camazine S. Mass envenomations by honey bees and wasps. *West J Med* 1999;170:223.
23. Visscher PK, Vetter RS, Camazine S. Removing bee stings. *Lancet* 1996;348:301–302.
24. Weizman Z, Mussafi H, Ishay J, et al. Multiple hornets stings with features of Reye's syndrome. *Gastroenterology* 1985;89:1407.

CHAPTER 345
Marine Envenomation

Grant S. Lipman and Paul S. Auerbach

Encounters with venomous marine animals occur predominantly in warm tropical oceans, far from the emergency department. As more people travel internationally for sport diving and marine recreation, emergency physicians everywhere need to become familiar with the unique injuries and illnesses caused by aquatic life. This chapter reviews the most common invertebrate (coelenterate, echinodermata, mollusk) and vertebrate (stingray, scorpionfish) marine envenomations.

Coelenterates exist either as a sedentary polyp or as a free-swimming dome-shaped medusa. Coelenterates dangerous to humans possess venom-bearing stinging cells, called cnidocytes, and are divided into three main groups: (a) hydrozoans, which range from fire coral to the Portuguese man-of-war; (b) scyphozoans, the true jellyfish; and (c) anthozoans, comprised largely of soft corals and anemones. Cnidocytes contain a stinging organelle known as a nematocyst, which is composed of a venom-laden coiled tubule controlled by a single trigger (cnidocil). The cnidocytes are located on the outer tentacles or near the mouth of the creature, and are triggered by either physical contact or chemoreceptors. When the cnidocil is stimulated, the venom-containing tubule is everted with sufficient force to penetrate to the dermis and ensure envenomation. A human encounter with a large Portuguese man-of-war can trigger the discharge of several million nematocysts. Coelenterate venom is a viscous mixture of toxic and antigenic protein fractions that contain histamine, prostaglandins, serotonin, and kinin fractions that can be neurotoxic, cardiotoxic, and dermatonecrotic (1,4,7,11,15).

Echinoderms known to be poisonous to humans include starfish, sea urchins, and sea cucumbers (1). Some starfish are covered with thorny spines of calcium carbonate and produce venom-containing slimes. Of note is the particularly potent crown-of-thorns species with its ice pick-like spines, hardy enough to puncture the neoprene of a diver's wetsuit (2). Sea urchins are protected by a hard shell and regularly arranged spines. Some venomous spines are sharp and brittle, and break off easily; others may be blunt and nonvenom-bearing. Sea urchin venom contains various toxic fractions, including steroid glycosides, hemolysins, proteases, serotonin, and cholinergic substances. Sea cucumbers are worm-like bottom feeders that produce a liquid toxin called holothurin. Holothurin is concentrated in the tentacular organs that can be extended in defense.

Some cucumbers ingest nematocysts and secrete coelenterate venom as well.

Although the majority of mollusk toxicity results from ingestion (11), envenomations can occur; of these, cone shell stings and blue-ringed octopus bites are the most hazardous to humans (8). Cone shells are found in the Indo-Pacific seas. These predators attack by injecting a potent neurotoxin via harpoon-like detachable teeth. The Australian blue-ringed octopuses are small (<20 cm) reclusive creatures with rings that turn an iridescent blue when provoked. A bite releases venom similar to tetrodotoxin, which blocks peripheral nerve conduction (1,20).

Stingrays cause an estimated 2,000 injuries annually in U.S. coastal waters (1). They are reclusive bottom feeders that lie on or submerge themselves in the sand. Injuries usually result from an unsuspecting step on the animal's dorsal surface, causing the barbed caudal appendage ("tail") to whip upward in a reflexive defensive response. The venom mechanism consists of a serrated spine, venom glands, and an enveloping integumentary sheath. As the spine penetrates the victim, the sheath ruptures, releasing venom along with organic debris. Stingray venom consists of heat-labile toxic components, including serotonin, 5′-nucleotidase, and phosphodiesterase.

Scorpionfish (*Scorpionidae*) are found predominantly in the Indian and Pacific oceans and are prized by aquarium enthusiasts for their beauty. There are three groups based on venom organ structure: the mildly venomous lionfishes, the moderately toxic scorpionfishes, and the deadly stonefishes (1,19). The venom apparatus consists of 12 to 13 dorsal, 2 pelvic, and 3 anal spines. Each spine is covered with an integumentary sheath, under which venom runs along grooves from paired glands at the base. Envenomation occurs when a spine punctures the skin, causing the sheath to tear and expose the venom. Scorpionfish venom is composed of multiple toxins, and the potency of the stonefish venom is commonly compared to that of the cobra snake. The principal component (stonustoxin) is a nondialyzable, antigenic, and heat-labile protein. The venom retains full potency for at least 24 to 48 hours after death of the fish (13).

CLINICAL PRESENTATION

Coelenterate envenomation results in three types of reactions—an immediate allergic reaction, an immediate toxic reaction, and a delayed, allergic response (1,4). The most common result of envenomation is localized dermatitis at the point of contact. With hydroids and fire coral, burning or stinging pain occurs immediately. This is followed by pruritus that leads to linear, urticarial, and painful eruptions that can take several days to resolve, occasionally leaving an area of hyperpigmentation.

Jellyfish and the Portuguese man-of-war may have tentacles exceeding 30 meters in length. Severity of envenomation is as a result of the number of nematocysts discharged, and the size and underlying health of the victim. Symptoms range from immediate localized burning to excruciating pain, followed by erythema and urticaria. Further progression leads to vesicular, ulcerative, hemolytic, or necrotizing lesions. Sea bather's eruption, commonly called "sea lice," is a dermatitis caused by larvae of certain thimble jellyfish (9). The eruption occurs a few minutes to 12 hours after contact with ocean water, and predominately affects covered areas of the body, in which the larvae are trapped. The reaction is intensely pruritic, with erythematous wheals, papules, or vesicles that can persist for up to 2 weeks.

Systemic symptoms from coelenterate envenomation, which may appear immediately or be delayed by several hours, include malaise, weakness, ataxia, dizziness, local cramping, muscle spasms, paresthesias, low-grade fever, nausea and vomiting, conjunctivitis, corneal ulcerations, anxiety, tachycardia, and hypotension. Fatal envenomations are attributed to cardiac or respiratory arrest (6), and anaphylaxis (7). The Pacific box-jellyfish (*Chironex fleckeri*) contains the most potent marine toxin known (4), and fatalities have occurred from a sting by this creature within 30 to 60 seconds of envenomation (3). Prevention of jellyfish stings can be best accomplished by keeping exposed skin covered by a protective dive suit. Safe Sea is a new topical sunscreen—jellyfish sting inhibitor that can be applied topically prior to entry into the water.

Envenomation by the spines of starfish, sea urchins, and sea cucumbers causes immediate intense pain, which evolves into local muscle spasm, dermal erythema, and localized edema. The puncture sites often bleed profusely. Sea urchin spines frequently break off and may lodge deeply. Some contain purple or black dye that causes s.c. staining that gives a false impression of retained spines. Embedded spines in or adjacent to a joint or peripheral nerve may cause a severe synovitis or neuropathy (2).

Infrequent systemic symptoms include nausea, vomiting, paresthesias, abdominal pain, syncope, hypotension, and respiratory distress (1,11). A second, delayed reaction can occur

weeks after the injury, consisting of a granuloma surrounding a retained spine fragment, or diffuse inflammation at the puncture site. Puncture-induced infections are common. Holothurin from sea cucumbers has been reported to cause conjunctivitis and blindness (1,14).

Most cone snail stings occur on the fingers or hands. Mild stings produce burning or sharp pain, followed by localized ischemia, cyanosis, and numbness. More serious envenomations produce paresthesias at the wound site, which may become perioral and then generalized. Partial paralysis may progress to respiratory failure. Systemic effects include pruritus, dysphagia, aphonia, and diplopia, with cerebral edema, coma, and cardiopulmonary arrest within a few hours. Victims usually recover within 6 to 8 hours, although some symptoms may take 2 to 3 weeks to resolve completely (16).

Octopus bites usually occur as a result of handling the creature, and consist of one or two small puncture wounds. The initial bite often goes unnoticed. Within 10 minutes, a burning sensation spreads to involve the entire limb, with erythema, swelling, tenderness, warmth, and pruritus. Most often, there is either no

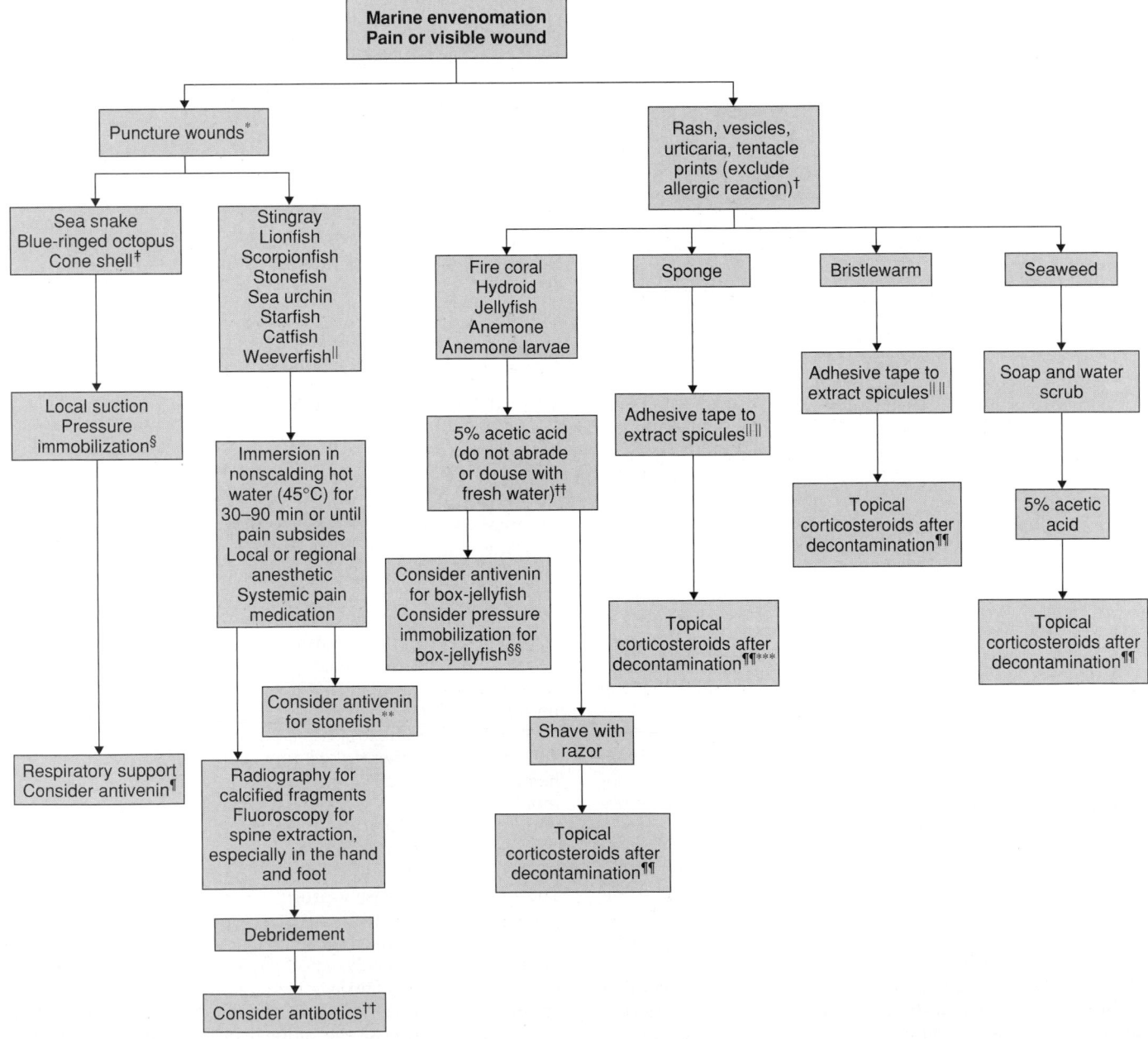

Figure 345.1.   For legend see opposite page.

local reaction or only a tiny blanched area. Within 15 minutes of the bite, the victim may experience neurologic symptoms that include perioral and facial paresthesias, diplopia, aphonia, dysphasia, ataxia, weakness, nausea, vomiting, muscle paralysis, and respiratory failure leading to death (11,20).

A stingray wound can be both an envenomation and a significant traumatic injury. The tail barb may cause a puncture wound or jagged laceration. Although lower extremity wounds are most common, infrequent trunk injuries cause most fatalities (8). Envenomation causes immediate and intense pain, which peaks at 30 to 60 minutes and may last up to 48 hours. A severe wound initially appears cyanotic and rapidly becomes erythematous and hemorrhagic, with possible early necrosis of muscle and fat. Systemic symptoms include weakness, nausea, vomiting, diaphoresis, vertigo, syncope, seizures, fasciculations, paralysis, hypotension, and rarely, dysrhythmias and death.

Scorpionfish and stonefish are well camouflaged, so a sting is usually to the hands or feet of the unwary diver or fisherman who grasps or steps on the animal. Fish handlers and aquarists are also at risk (13). The puncture wound is immediately painful, with radiation proximally up the extremity. Untreated, the pain typically peaks at 60 to 90 minutes, and resolves in 8 to 12 hours. However, pain from a stonefish envenomation may be excruciating and persist for days. The wound is first ischemic, and then becomes cyanotic with surrounding erythema and edema. Vesicles often form, and tissue sloughing with cellulitis may occur within 48 hours (2). Systemic symptoms are similar to coelenterate envenomation. Wound complications include infection, neu-

ropathies, and cutaneous granulomas that may require months to heal.

DIFFERENTIAL DIAGNOSIS

The main considerations in the differential diagnosis are allergic reactions, trauma, infections, and envenomations by other marine animals. Sponges can cause two general syndromes: a pruritic allergic reaction that occurs within a few hours of exposure, or a spicule-induced dermatitis. Erythema multiforme or an anaphylactoid reaction may develop days to weeks after a severe exposure (1).

Sea snakes are found in the warm Pacific and Indian oceans. The venom is similar to that of land snakes, with neurotoxic, hemolytic, and cardiotoxic protein fractions. The bite itself is usually not painful, and may even go unnoticed. Less than 10% of sea snake bites actually inject venom, yet 3% worldwide result in fatalities (8). Symptoms include muscle pain, peripheral weakness, paralysis, and respiratory failure.

EMERGENCY DEPARTMENT EVALUATION

The history should include the identity or description of the suspected envenoming animal, and the time of onset, quality, and progression of symptoms. In cases of recent travel and unknown envenomation, the specific geographic location visited can be

---

Figure 345.1. Algorithmic approach to marine envenomation. (From Auerbach PS. Envenomation by Aquatic Animals. *Wilderness Medicine.* 4th Ed. St. Louis: Mosby, Inc; 2001: 1450–1506, with permission.)

*A gaping laceration, particularly of the lower extremity, with cyanotic edges suggests a stingray wound. Multiple punctures in an erratic pattern with or without purple discoloration or retained fragments are typical of a see urchin sting. One to eight (usually two) fang marks are usually present after a sea snake bite. A single ischemic puncture wound with an erythematous halo and rapid swelling suggests scorpionfish envenomation. Blisters often accompany a lionfish sting. Painless punctures with paralysis suggest the bite of a blue-ringed octopus; the site of a cone shell sting is punctate, painful, and ischemic in appearance.

†Wheal and flare reactions are nonspecific. Rapid (within 24 hours) onset of skin necrosis suggests an anemone sting. "Tentacle prints" with cross-hatching or a frosted appearance are pathognomonic for box-jellyfish (*Chironex fleckeri*) envenomation. Ocular or intraoral lesions may be caused by fragmented hydroids or coelenterate tentacles. An allergic reaction must be treated promptly.

‡Sea snake venom causes weakness, respiratory paralysis, myoglobinuria, myalgias, blurred vision, vomiting, and dysphagia. The blue-ringed octopus injects tetrodotoxin, which causes rapid neuromuscular paralysis.

§If *immediately* available (which is rarely the case), local suction can be applied without incision using a plunger device, such as The Extractor (Sawyer Products, Safety Harbor, Fla.). As soon as possible, venom should be sequestered locally with a proximal venous-lymphatic occlusive band of constriction of (preferably) the pressure immobilization technique, in which a cloth pad is compressed directly over the wound by an elastic wrap that should encompass the entire extremity at a pressure of 9.33 kPa (70 mm Hg) or less. Incision and suction are not recommended.

¶Early ventilatory support has the greatest influence on outcome. The minimal initial dose of sea snake antivenin is one to three vials; up to ten vials may be required.

‖The wounds range from large lacerations (stingrays) to minute punctures (stonefish). Persistent pain after immersion in hot water suggests a stonefish sting or a retained fragment of spine. The puncture site can be identified by forcefully injecting 1% to 2% lidocaine or another local anesthetic agent without epinephrine near the wound and observing the agress of fluid. Do not attempt to crush the spines of sea urchins if they are present in the wound. Spine dye from already-extracted sea urchin spines will disappear (be absorbed) in 24 to 36 hours.

**The initial dose of stonefish antivenin is one vial per two puncture wounds.

††The antibiotics choses should cover *staphylococcus, Streptococcus,* and microbes of marine origin, such as *Vibrio.*

‡‡Acetic acid 5% (vinegar) is a good all-purpose decontaminant and is mandated for the sting from a box-jellyfish. Alternatives, depending on the geographic region and indigenous jellyfish species, include isopropyl alcohol, bicarbonate (baking soda), ammonia, papain, and preparations containing these agents.

§§The initial dose of box-jellyfish antivenin is one ampule intravenously or three ampules intramuscularly.

¶¶If inflammation is severe, steroids should be given systematically (beginning with at least 60 to 100 mg of prednisone or its equivalent) and the dose tapered over a period of 10 to 14 days.

*** An alternative is to apply and remove commercial facial peel materials.

‖‖An alternative is to apply and remove commercial facial peel materials followed by topical soaks of 30 ml of 5% acetic acid (vinegar) diluted in 1 L of water for 15 to 30 minutes several times a day until the lesions begin to resolve. Anticipate surface desquamation in 3 to 6 weeks.

helpful. Tetanus immunization status needs to be documented. The physical exam begins with the skin, looking for wounds, rashes, and signs of infection. Many wounds need to be explored and/or x-rayed for radiopaque foreign bodies. Magnetic resonance imaging (MRI) is probably the most reliable method to identify a foreign body. If there are no clinical signs of infection, wound cultures have not been shown to be useful (1). Patients with abnormal vital signs, systemic symptoms, or altered sensorium should have an electrocardiogram and routine laboratory evaluation, including urine hemoglobin.

EMERGENCY DEPARTMENT MANAGEMENT

An algorithmic approach to managing marine envenomations is depicted in Fig. 345.1. Because both freshwater and saltwater contain an abundance of microbes, wound care is paramount, including irrigation, debridement of devitalized tissues, and removal of foreign bodies. Infected wounds should be cultured for both aerobes and anaerobes. Bacteria of concern to humans include *Aeromonas hydrophilia*, *Bacteroides fragilis*, *Chromobacterium violaceum*, *Clostridium perfringens*, *Erysipelothrix rhusiopathiae*, *Escheria coli*, *Myobacterium marinum*, *Pseudomonas aeruginosa*, *Salmonella enteritidis*, *Staphylococcus aureus*, *Streptococcus* species, and *Vibrio* species. Immunocompromised patients, especially those with hepatic disease, should be empirically started on broad-spectrum antibiotics covering *Vibrio* species. Otherwise, minor wounds can be covered with oral ciprofloxacin, trimethoprim-sulfamethoxazole, doxycycline, or cefuroxime. High-risk wounds (extensive lacerations, deep punctures, joint involvement, or grossly contaminated) require a parenteral third generation cephalosporin, aminoglycoside, or other agent that covers *Vibrio* species. A second antibiotic may be necessary to cover more common organisms, such as *Staphylococcus*. Tetanus prophylaxis should be administered according to the patient's immunization status.

Therapy for coelenterate envenomation includes application of a detoxificant, appropriate analgesia, and general supportive care. If a detoxicant is available (see below), apply it immediately. Otherwise, rinse the wound with normal saline or hypertonic saline. Avoid applying fresh water or rubbing the affected area, both of which are thought to cause discharge of nematocysts. Ice packs (preferably without external moisture) may help alleviate pain. Warm water is generally to be avoided, although recent clinical trials have shown benefit (17). Remove any large tentacles with forceps or while wearing latex gloves.

Vinegar (5% acetic acid) is the treatment of choice to inactivate the nematocysts of box jellyfish or the Atlantic Portuguese man-of-war, although a slurry of isopropyl alcohol and papain (meat tenderizer) has been effective against many other jellyfish species. Other effective detoxicants have included household ammonia, baking soda, and citrus juice. The detoxicant should be continuously applied for at least 30 minutes or until the pain is relieved. Remember that pain may not resolve with nematocyst inhibition (1).

After the detoxicant has been applied, the remaining nematocysts need to be removed. Apply shaving cream, baking soda, or talc to the affected area and shave with a razor. If no medical supplies are available, a paste of sand or mud can be made with seawater and the victim's skin scraped with a sharp edged tool or shell. The envenomed area should be immobilized to decrease venom distribution. For a sting from the box jellyfish, there is anecdotal evidence supporting the use of the pressure-immobilization bandaging technique (12) (a cloth or gauze pad placed over the wound, held in place by a wide bandage applied at venous-lymphatic occlusive pressure, then splinted). The bandage should be applied as soon as possible after tentacle removal

and vinegar dousing, and released once the victim is brought to proper medical attention (1).

Generally, only severe Portuguese man-of-war or box jellyfish stings result in rapid physiological decompensation. Cardiopulmonary supportive care should be given as needed and anaphylaxis should always be anticipated. Box jellyfish attacks have resulted in 67 deaths in Australia (12), and i.v. antivenom must be administered as soon as possible for any severe envenomation (3,7). The initial dose is 20,000 units (one vial) over 5 minutes i.v., or three vials i.m., with standard hypersensitivity precautions. Animal studies have shown benefit from using verapamil in conjunction with the antivenom, but the effectiveness of this in humans is unproven (3). Management may include treatment for the renal sequelae of rhabdomyolysis. Although antibiotics are not always indicated, wounds should be followed for infection. Also, a topical antihistamine or mild corticosteroid may be soothing. A delayed reaction may recur after 1 to 2 months at the area of skin contact, and should be treated with a 10- to 14-day taper of a glucocorticoid.

For starfish, sea urchin, and sea cucumber envenomation, the affected area should immediately be immersed in nonscalding hot water (up to 45°C [113°F]) as tolerated until the pain is relieved. Foreign bodies need to be removed. External percussion to achieve spine fragmentation is contraindicated, and surgical exploration for embedded particles should be delayed until diagnosis can be made by soft tissue radiography or magnetic resonance imaging (MRI) (5). Spines within a joint or adjacent to a neurovascular structure should be referred to a surgeon to extract all fragments as soon as possible. Systemic analgesia is helpful and prophylactic antibiotics should be given for deep puncture wounds. There is no indication for systemic corticosteroids. Sea cucumber envenomation management should include coelenterate detoxification and dermatitis treatment.

No antivenom exists for treatment of cone shell or octopus envenomation, so management is supportive. It is recommended to use the pressure-immobilization bandaging technique to contain the venom (8). Rapid respiratory failure can occur, so it is important to anticipate the need for oxygenation and mechanical ventilatory support. The clinical duration of blue-ring octopus envenomation is 4 to 10 hours, after which a victim who has not suffered significant hypoxia usually begins to show improvement (1,8). Wound management is controversial, with some authors recommending wide excision to remove sequestered toxin, and others favoring irrigation, debridement, and wound observation (1,16,18). There is no compelling evidence that surgical therapy is routinely efficacious.

Treatment of stingray envenomation focuses on inactivating toxin, alleviating pain, and preventing infection. The success of therapy is likely related to the rapidity with which it is initiated (1). The injury should be soaked in hot water (up to 45°C [113°F]) for 30 to 90 minutes. If hot water is unavailable, the wound should be immediately irrigated with water or saline. Visible pieces of the spine or integumentary sheath will continue to envenom the victim and must be excised early. The wound tract needs to be explored, thoroughly débrided, and packed open for delayed primary closure. Prophylactic antibiotics, although controversial, are generally recommended as a result of the high-risk nature of these wounds and high incidence of infections (1,10). Wounds to the abdomen or thorax must be fully evaluated by appropriate imaging studies (11). If the plan is to treat and release, the patient should be observed for 3 to 4 hours for delayed onset of systemic symptoms (1).

The management of scorpionfish envenomation is similar to that for stingray injuries. The wound should immediately be immersed in hot water (up to 45°C [113°F]) for 30 to 90 minutes until symptoms subside. Recurrent pain that occurs after several hours may respond to repeat hot water soaks. Appropriate treatment includes irrigation and thorough wound cleansing to ensure debris removal. Deep puncture wounds may need to be evaluated in the operating room. Stonefish antivenom is available for severe pain or systemic symptoms. It is rarely recommended to use this product for scorpionfish envenomation (1,13). As a rough estimate, one ampule should neutralize two puncture wounds. As with any horse-serum product, the possibility of a hypersensitivity reaction must be anticipated.

Sponge spicules should be removed with adhesive tape or rubber cement, and then the skin soaked briefly with vinegar or isopropyl alcohol. A topical or systemic glucocorticoid may be necessary if there is a significant allergic component.

Treatment of sea snake envenomation includes the pressure-immobilization bandaging technique, early anticipation of respiratory failure, and administration of sea snake antivenom as soon as there is any evidence of envenomation. Patients who remain asymptomatic for 8 hours of observation can be discharged (1,14).

CRITICAL INTERVENTIONS

- Inactivate heat-labile toxins from stingrays and scorpionfish by immersing the affected area in nonscalding hot water
- Administer antivenom for severe systemic toxicity as a result of box jellyfish and stonefish envenomation

DISPOSITION

Some marine envenomations cause delayed onset of symptoms, so a few hours of patient observation may be necessary. Patients with significant systemic signs and symptoms should be admitted to the hospital. Patients need to be educated about wound infection, and follow-up care is essential. A poison center toxicologist can be consulted for treatment advice and access to antivenom.

COMMON PITFALLS

✔ Failure to appreciate that coelenterate envenomation pain can be reduced by vinegar or isopropyl alcohol soaks, and exacerbated by freshwater irrigation
✔ Failure to treat spine-induced envenomation pain with hot water immersion
✔ Failure to consider concomitant traumatic injuries and retained foreign bodies
✔ Failure to consider appropriate antibiotic coverage for marine bacterial infections

Acknowledgment

We thank previous edition chapter author Kenneth W. Kizer.

References

1. Auerbach PS.Envenomation by Aquatic Animals. *Wilderness medicine,* 4th Ed. St. Louis: Mosby, 2001:1450–1506.
2. Auerbach PS. Marine envenomations. *N Engl J Med* 1991;325(7):486–493.
3. Bloom DA, Burnett JW, Hebel JR. Effects of verapamil and CSL antivenom on Chironex fleckeri (box jellyfish) induced mortality. *Toxicon* 1999;37(11):1621–1626.
4. Burnett JW. Jellyfish envenomation syndromes updates. *Ann Emerg Med* 1987:16(9):1000–1005.
5. Burnett JW. Sea urchins. *Cutis* 1999;64(1):21–22.
6. Endean R, Duchemin C, McColm D, et al. A study of the biological activity of toxic material derived from nematocysts of the cubomedusan (Chironex Fleckeri). *Toxicon* 1969;6:179–204.
7. Fenner, PJ. Dangers in the ocean: the traveler and marine envenomation, part 1: jellyfish. *J Travel Med* 1998;5(3):135–141.
8. Fenner, PJ. Dangers in the ocean: the traveler and marine envenomation, part 2: marine vertebrates. *J Travel Med* 1998;5(4):213–216.
9. Freudenthal AR, Joseph PR. Seabather's eruption. *N Engl J Med* 1993;329(8):542–544.
10. Grainger CR. Sting ray injuries. *R Soc Trop Med Hyg* 1985;(79):443–444.
11. Kizer, KW. Marine Envenomations. *J Toxicol Clin Toxicol* 1983 84;21(4-5):527–555.
12. Little M. Is there a role for the use of pressure immobilization bandages in the treatment of jellyfish envenomation in Australia? *Am J Emerg Med* 2002;14(2):171–174.
13. Kizer KW, McKinney HE, Auerbach, PS. Scorpaenidae envenomation. A five-year poison center experience. *JAMA* 1985;253(6):807–810.
14. McGoldrick J. Marine envenomations, part 1: vertebrates. *Am J Emerg Med* 1991;9(6):497–502.
15. McGoldrick J. Marine envenomations, part 2: invertebrates. *Am J Emerg Med* 1991;10(1):71–77.
16. Manowitz NR, Rosenthal RR. Cutaneous systemic reactions to toxins and venoms of common marine organisms. *Cutis* 1979;(23):450–454.
17. Nomura, JT, Sato RL, Ahern RM. A randomized paired comparison trial of cutaneous treatments for acute jellyfish (Carybdea alate) stings. *Am J Emerg Med* 2002;20(7):1–5.
18. Southcott RV. Human injuries from invertebrate animals in the Australian seas. *J Toxicol Clin Toxicol* 1970;(3):617–636.
19. Southcott RV. Australian venomous and poisonous fishes. *J Toxicol Clin Toxicol* 1977;10:291–325.
20. Walker DG. Survival after severe envenomation by the blue-ringed octopus (Hapolochlaene maculosa). *Med J Aust* 1983;2:663–665.

CHAPTER 346
Scorpion Envenomation

Jeffrey R. Suchard and Steven C. Curry

Although nearly 40 scorpion species are found in the United States, *Centruroides sculpturatus* is the only scorpion reported to produce potentially life-threatening illness after a sting. This species, also known as *Centruroides exilicauda*, or the bark scorpion, is found throughout Arizona and in parts of Texas, New Mexico, small areas of California, the northern shore of Lake Mead in Nevada, and northern Mexico (4). *C. sculpturatus* stings may occur elsewhere, as scorpions have been known to stow away in a person's belongings (e.g., shoes, duffel bags) and be transported long distances before encountering their victims. Most other American scorpion stings produce only local pain and inflammation, which respond well to minimal supportive therapy and wound care, although the common striped scorpion, *Centruroides vittatus*, causes mild-to-moderate systemic effects in 20% of cases (13).

C. sculpturatus specimens generally measure about 5-cm (range, 1.3–7.6 cm) long; have a streamlined appearance, with a thin tail and claws; and are a uniform tan, yellow, or light brown. The last (sixth) tail segment, termed a telson, contains a venom apparatus and stinger (Fig. 346.1). *C. sculpturatus* prefers to reside in or near trees, especially sycamore, mesquite, cottonwood, and palm. They may also hide in ground debris, camping equipment, clothing left unattended in natural desert areas, or even in areas long-inhabited by humans. Scorpions spend the daylight hours undercover and are active at night in warm weather, lying quietly while waiting to ambush prey. In defending themselves, they grasp the victim's flesh with pincers and repeatedly sting by thrusting their tails over their bodies.

Although a sting from any scorpion can produce local pain, *C. sculpturatus* venom contains protein neurotoxins that cause

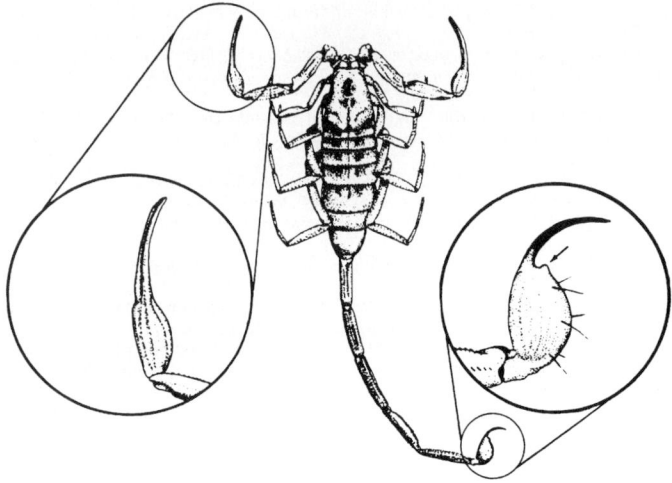

Figure 346.1. The sixth tail segment of *C. sculpturatus* (bark scorpion) contains venom apparatus and stinger.

Grade	Description
I	Local pain and/or paresthesias at site of envenomation
II	Pain and/or paresthesias remote from the site of sting
III	Either cranial nerve or somatic skeletal neuromuscular dysfunction
	Cranial nerve dysfunction: Blurred vision, wandering eye movements, hypersalivation, trouble swallowing, tongue fasciculations, stridor, slurred speech
	Somatic skeletal neuromuscular dysfunction: Jerking of extremity(ies), restlessness, severe involuntary shaking and jerking, which may be mistaken for seizures
IV	Both cranial nerve and somatic skeletal neuromuscular dysfunction

TABLE 346.1. Scorpion Envenomations: Signs and Symptoms

repetitive firing of neurons by binding to sodium channels and preventing channel inactivation during depolarization or after repolarization (4). No destructive enzymes are present in the venom, accounting for lack of inflammation or necrosis. Prolonged and excessive firing of parasympathetic, sympathetic, and somatic motor neurons produces various autonomic effects and uncoordinated and spontaneous activity in voluntary muscle.

Scorpion stings are fairly common in endemic areas. Several thousand stings are reported annually to poison control centers in Arizona. Fortunately, the majority of envenomations are not serious enough to warrant medical attention. Children tend to be more seriously affected by *C. sculpturatus* stings, however, and may require aggressive intervention to avoid morbidity and mortality. Death from direct effects of envenomation has not been reported in Arizona for several years; the lack of recent fatalities probably reflects advances in supportive medical care. One patient, however, recently died following a severe allergic reaction to a scorpion sting (3).

Severe envenomations by *C. sculpturatus* are seen almost entirely in children younger than age 10 and occur in 15% to 20% of this group. In contrast, 95% of envenomations in those older than age 10 result in only mild-to-moderate effects. The life-threatening effects (myocarditis, pulmonary edema, shock) associated with adrenergic storm and caused by the venom from scorpion species found in other parts of the world are not noted after envenomations by *C. sculpturatus*.

CLINICAL PRESENTATION

Scorpion envenomation results in the immediate onset of a painful tingling or burning sensation at the sting site. Tapping the site of the sting may produce severe pain, although no lesion is usually visible. Over minutes to several hours, pain and paresthesias may become generalized. Victims may complain of "thick tongue" and "trouble swallowing," yet lack objective abnormalities on examination. Young children frequently rub their noses, eyes, and ears, and may present with unexplained crying.

Autonomic dysfunction is characterized by tachycardia, excessive secretions, and, occasionally, vomiting and wheezing. Somatic motor abnormalities include roving eye movements, blurred vision, fasciculations (especially of the tongue), and poor control of pharyngeal muscles. Continuous jerking of extremities may be noted and misinterpreted as restlessness, seizures,

or hysteria. The combination of uncoordinated pharyngeal musculature and muscles of respiration, increased secretions, and occasional wheezing may produce stridor, hypoxia, aspiration, and respiratory arrest in severe cases.

Severe envenomations may also be accompanied by metabolic acidosis, respiratory failure, sterile cerebrospinal fluid pleocytosis (9–20 white blood cells per mL), coagulopathy, pancreatitis, and rhabdomyolysis (1,2,4).

Envenomations can be graded on the basis of signs and symptoms (Table 346.1). In serious envenomations, abnormal motor activity may last 10 to 20 hours (4,12). Paresthesias may last up to 2 weeks.

DIFFERENTIAL DIAGNOSIS

Bites or stings from other arthropods should be considered in the differential diagnosis of scorpion envenomation. The pain at the site of envenomation may appear to the observer to be similar to that seen after a black widow spider bite. However, severely ill patients who suffer from scorpion stings appear unable to lie still, whereas those bitten by black widow spiders can maintain a position for short periods of time before moving in an attempt to become comfortable. Black widow envenomations do not produce abnormal eye movements, fasciculations, and paresthesias. Tapping over the site of envenomation produces severe pain in the patient stung by a scorpion, but not in someone bitten by a spider. Black widow spider bites frequently produce a characteristic halo lesion at the site of the bite; no lesion is usually visible after a *C. sculpturatus* sting.

Tachycardia, excessive secretions, wheezing, and respiratory distress accompanying serious scorpion stings may be mistaken for asthma, airway obstruction from a foreign body, or poisoning with cholinergic agents such as organophosphate insecticides. In the absence of a witnessed scorpion sting, other entities to be considered include central nervous system infections, seizures, and intoxication with sympathomimetics, phencyclidine, and nicotine. Methamphetamine toxicity, for instance, is sometimes mistaken for *C. sculpturatus* envenomation when young children from scorpion-endemic areas present with unusual neurologic findings such as agitation or choreiform movements; this has occasionally led to the inappropriate use of antivenom (7,10).

EMERGENCY DEPARTMENT EVALUATION

If a sting was not witnessed, it should be determined whether there are scorpions near where the patient became ill. The physical examination should focus on vital signs, the airway, and neuromuscular function. No specific diagnostic tests are available. Patients with suspected aspiration should have a chest radiograph and consideration given to arterial blood gas analysis. Severe envenomations may rarely cause pancreatitis, rhabdomyolysis, and myocarditis, which would warrant obtaining baseline labs including serum amylase and/or lipase, creatine kinase, and an electrocardiogram.

EMERGENCY DEPARTMENT MANAGEMENT

Advanced life-support measures, with particular attention to airway management, should be instituted as necessary. As with any puncture wound, a primary tetanus immunization or booster should be given, if indicated.

Patients with grade I or II envenomations are treated symptomatically. Application of ice to the sting often provides relief in lower grade envenomations. Oral analgesics are effective in most cases, but parenteral analgesia may sometimes be needed. There are no rational or therapeutic benefits in giving steroids, epinephrine, calcium, or antihistamines to patients with scorpion envenomations. Barbiturates have not been found effective in lessening motor activity or in shortening the course of the illness, and they often produce serious or life-threatening respiratory depression (12). Propranolol has anecdotally been reported to lessen the tachycardia in a severely envenomated child without affecting other neuromuscular abnormalities (11). β-adrenergic blockers are not recommended, because tachyarrhythmias do not cause morbidity, bronchospasm can be seen in severe scorpion envenomations, and such therapy does not correct neurologic abnormalities. Respiratory distress associated with hypersalivation has been treated with atropine, sometimes obviating the need for aggressive airway interventions (14). However, the ideal dosing of atropine has not been determined, nor is this practice considered a standard of care.

Antivenom effective against *C. sculpturatus* is no longer produced within the United States. Until recently, a goat serum antivenom was available for the treatment of severe envenomations in Arizona. This antivenom was very effective in alleviating symptoms of grade III or IV envenomations, reversing severe neurotoxicity usually within 30 to 60 minutes. Abnormal motor activity usually resolves within 60 to 90 minutes (4,5). Patients who do not receive antivenom will continue to have symptoms for 4 to 20 hours. Antivenom is not indicated in the management of grade I or II envenomations. Because antivenom may again become available in the United States, and because it is still used in other countries with serious scorpion envenomation problems, additional details regarding its historical use are discussed here.

Patients with grade III or IV envenomations can be successfully treated with antivenom after the institution of supportive care. Supportive measures include continuous monitoring of the airway, with respiratory assistance as needed; intravenous hydration; and loose restraints to prevent self-harm. One or two vials of antivenom mixed in 50 mL of a crystalloid solution is given intravenously over 20 to 30 minutes. Although skin testing with antivenom is suggested, it is not completely reliable in predicting which patients will suffer allergic reactions (5). The use of β blockers is a relative contraindication to the administration of antivenom, because β-adrenergic blockade complicates the treatment of anaphylaxis, a potential complication of antivenom administration.

Some physicians in scorpion-endemic areas do not use antivenom, but prefer to treat severely envenomated patients with supportive and symptomatic care in the intensive care unit (ICU). Because antivenom is not currently available in the United States, this must necessarily become the primary manner of care. Such treatment requires close respiratory monitoring, as the patients are often given benzodiazepines to control neuromuscular hyperactivity and to induce sedation and amnesia (6), and such therapy has resulted in need for endotracheal intubation and mechanical ventilation. We believe that routine admission unnecessarily increases cost if antivenom is available, and that administering sedatives to patients who already have tenuous airway control unduly increases the risk of respiratory depression and aspiration in those who could potentially be safely discharged home from the emergency department if treated with antivenom (2,9). The main argument against antivenom is that using animal-derived serum products places the patient at risk for potentially serious immunologic reactions. Anaphylactic reactions to antivenom can occur, but they are usually mild and can be reversed with appropriate treatment (2,4,8). Serum sickness occurs in about 60% of patients treated with scorpion antivenom, although the symptoms typically resolve within 3 days when treated with antihistamines and corticosteroids (2,8,9).

CRITICAL INTERVENTIONS

- Airway control is of primary importance. Severely envenomated patients may require airway interventions as a result of hypersalivation and poor control of the oropharyngeal musculature
- ICU admission for close observation is often necessary for patients when antivenom is not available, is contraindicated, or when complications such as aspiration pneumonia have occurred

DISPOSITION

Patients with grade I or II envenomations should be observed for 3 to 4 hours after a sting for evidence of progression of symptoms. Those who do not manifest increased envenomation severity can be discharged home with oral analgesics and follow-up with their personal physician as needed.

Patients with grade III or IV envenomations can be discharged after receiving antivenom if they are asymptomatic and aspiration pneumonia or other complications from envenomation are ruled out. Children with grade III or IV envenomations who have not received antivenom, or who have evidence of a complication after receiving antivenom, should be admitted to an ICU. Adults without respiratory difficulties who require admission for pain control may be admitted to an unmonitored bed. Those with more severe envenomations generally require intensive care.

All patients who receive antivenom should be advised of the signs and symptoms of serum sickness, which could appear 3 to 14 days after the administration of antivenom. Serum sickness is easily controlled with an antihistamine and tapering doses of an oral corticosteroid.

COMMON PITFALLS

- ✔ Mistaking symptoms of severe envenomation for hysterical or uncooperative behavior or for seizures, especially in children
- ✔ Relying on the absence of a visible lesion at the site of the sting to rule out scorpion envenomation
- ✔ Routinely giving sedatives, steroids, epinephrine, antihistamines, or calcium
- ✔ Using antivenom as a substitute for good supportive care
- ✔ Failure to inform patients about potential allergic reactions to antivenom and to monitor for such reactions

References

1. Berg RA, Tarantino MD. Envenomation by the scorpion Centruroides exilicauda (C. sculpturatus): severe and unusual manifestations. *Pediatrics* 1991;87:930.
2. Bond GR. Antivenin administration for Centruroides scorpion sting: risks and benefits. *Ann Emerg Med* 1992;21:788.
3. Boyer L, Heubner K, McNally J, et al. Death from Centruroides scorpion sting allergy [abstract]. *J Toxicol Clin Toxicol* 2001;39:561.
4. Curry SC, Vance MV, Ryan PJ, et al. Envenomation by the scorpion Centruroides sculpturatus. *J Toxicol Clin Toxicol* 1984;21:417.
5. Gateau T, Bloom M, Clark R. Response to specific Centruroides sculpturatus antivenom in 151 cases of scorpion stings. *J Toxicol Clin Toxicol* 1994;32:165.
6. Gibly R, Williams M, Walter F. Continuous intravenous midazolam infusions for Centruroides exilicauda envenomations. *J Toxicol Clin Toxicol* 1998;36:460.
7. Kolecki P. Inadvertent methamphetamine poisoning in pediatric patients. *Pediatr Emerg Care* 1998;14:385.
8. LoVecchio F, Klemens J, Welch S, et al. Prospective study of immediate and delayed hypersensitivity to Centruroides antivenin. *J Toxicol Clin Toxicol* 1998;36:462.
9. LoVecchio F, McBride C. Scorpion envenomation in young children in central Arizona. *J Toxicol Clin Toxicol* 2003;41:937.
10. Nagorka AR, Bergeson PS. Infant methamphetamine toxicity posing as scorpion envenomation. *Pediatr Emerg Care* 1998;14:350.
11. Rachesky IJ, Banner W, Dansky J, et al. Treatment for Centruroides exilicauda envenomation. *Am J Dis Child* 1984;138:1136.
12. Rimsza ME, Zimmerman DR, Bergeson PS. Scorpion envenomation. *Pediatrics* 1980;66:298.
13. Stipetic ME, Lugo A, Brown B, et al. A prospective analysis of 558 common striped scorpion (Centruroides vittatus) envenomations in Texas during 1997. *J Toxicol Clin Toxicol* 1998;36:461.
14. Suchard JR, Hilder R. Atropine use in Centruroides scorpion envenomation. *J Toxicol Clin Toxicol* 2001;39:595.

CHAPTER 347

Black Widow Spider Envenomation

Daniel E. Brooks

The term "black widow spider" (BWS), originally used to describe *L. mactans*, is now used as the generic reference for up to forty species of the genus *Latrodectus* found worldwide (11,14,16,17). BWSs are found in the temperate regions of six continents and are widespread throughout North America. *L. mactans* and *L. hesperus*, the most common species in the western United States, are the classically described black spiders with a red, sometimes yellow, hourglass marking on the ventral abdomen. Several other species are found within the United States, including *L. variolis*, *L. bishopi* (red-legged widow), and *L. geometricus* (brown widow), varying in appearance based on species, maturity, and region (17).

BWSs are commonly encountered in rural and suburban areas, typically in barns, garages, woodpiles, and classically in outhouses. The irregularly shaped webs are usually spun in solitary environments, typically from the underside of low-level structures (e.g., a bench). The spiders, however, can be found anywhere, with some species being arboreal. The female's larger size, up to 15 mm in body length with a 40-mm leg span, allows for larger envenomation apparatus compared to the male, whose fangs and venom glands are too small to injure humans.

The active protein in *Latrodectus* venom, α-atrotoxin, is a potent neurotoxin that causes the release of neurotransmitters (including acetylcholine and norepinephrine) at neuromuscular, central, and pancreatic synapses (8,23). Although the exact mechanism remains unclear, it appears that α-atrotoxin affects several presynaptic membrane receptors and regulatory pathways to initiate exocytosis of secretory vesicles. Depending on the concentration of venom and affected cell type, calcium may or may not be involved in exocytosis (8). Differences in venom structure and lethality have been identified, varying between *Latrodectus* species, geographic location, and seasons (13,14). These differences may be important in human envenomations; for example, a brown widow spider envenomation appears to be less toxic than that of its black-colored counterparts (16). BWSs may be able to control the amount of venom injected, another factor potentially explaining variance in clinical effects (17).

Latrodectism, defined as systemic effects from a BWS envenomation, affects thousands of patients each year and is considered the most important spider-related medical issue worldwide (11). Although the true incidence of human fatality is unknown, previously reported mortality rates of up to 10% are most likely overestimations as a result of selection bias or because the involved cases occurred prior to the development of antivenom. Each year, American poison control centers receive approximately 2,400 reports of human BWS envenomations, yet there has not been a reported fatality in the United States for over 20 years.

CLINICAL PRESENTATION

Envenomations typically occur when the spider feels threatened, often by an unwitting victim. Bites are more common in warmer, summer months. Male gender appears to be the only identifying risk factor among human victims, and approximately 75% of bites occur on extremities (4,6,11). In the past, bites to the genitalia were reported frequently, occurring during the use of outdoor toilets or "outhouses."

The initial bite of a BWS is usually described as a sharp, transient pinprick or burning sensation, but may go unrecognized. The bite site may reveal two small puncture wounds with minimal erythema or inflammation. A pathognomonic "target lesion" is commonly found, described as an erythematous ring, 2 to 6 cm in diameter, with central pallor at the bite site (22). This lesion usually develops within 2 hours of the envenomation and can last up to 24 hours, with varying tenderness. Other signs and symptoms typically begin within 30 to 120 minutes of the envenomation. A severe envenomation will progress to involve localized and then diffuse pain, muscle cramps (typically of the abdomen or back), tachycardia, and hypertension. Diaphoresis and piloerection can occur, sometimes isolated to the bite site.

Additional signs and symptoms include nausea, headache, fever, tremor, and weakness. Rarely reported effects include periorbital edema and ecchymosis, priapism, cardiac dysrhythmias (including reflex bradycardia), and paralysis. Young children may simply present with inconsolable crying or restlessness. Most symptoms peak within several hours and, if untreated, wane over several days. However, peak symptoms can be delayed for up to 24 hours and there are reports of symptoms lasting months (1,9,21,25).

A review of 163 patients treated for BWS envenomation in Arizona reported 56% of patients had generalized abdominal or back pain, 38% had localized or extremity pain, 29% had documented hypertension, 22% experienced diaphoresis, and 11% had nausea or vomiting (4). The average time for the onset of symptoms was 1.2 hours (+/− 1.6 hr), ranging from immediate to 12 hours. Other case series report similar findings, with generalized muscle pain and cramps in 71% to 80%, abdominal pain and cramps in 67% to 71%, pain at the bite site in 67% to 79%, and hypertension in 21% to 60% (15,16). Leukocytosis and an elevated serum creatine phosphokinase are the most commonly reported abnormal laboratory studies (4,17).

The catecholamine surge as a result of uncontrolled release of norepinephrine can compromise patients at age extremes or those with significant, underlying cardiopulmonary disease. Pregnant patients are at risk for uterine contraction, a preeclampsia-like presentation, and fetal compromise, although reported cases document no fetal complications (18,19). Historical reports of spontaneous abortions in women envenomated by BWSs during the nineteenth century are unsubstantiated (18).

DIFFERENTIAL DIAGNOSIS

BWS envenomation can be confused with any illness that produces an acute pain syndrome, such as an acute abdomen or chest pain syndrome (2). Severe abdominal pain has resulted in unnecessary exploratory surgery. In older patients with prolonged chest pain, myocardial ischemia may need to be ruled out, even if a black widow envenomation is known to have occurred. Pain localized to the back or flanks may suggest renal colic or infection, but the urinalysis is normal. Elevated CPK, cramps, and diffuse myalgia can mimic rhabdomyolysis. Leukocytosis may be confused with an infectious process but fever is absent.

Other unwitnessed arthropod or snake envenomations can mimic the associated signs or symptoms of BWS envenomation. Because there is no diagnostic test to confirm a BWS envenomation, a careful history, including activity just prior to the onset of symptoms, may aid in making the correct diagnosis. Inconsolable crying in a child, particularly if starting while playing outside or getting dressed (e.g., putting on shoes that were left outside) should raise the suspicion of BWS envenomation. Patients who suffer BWS envenomation often stay in one position for a few seconds or minutes before moving to a new position. In contrast, severe scorpion envenomation results in constant writhing and abnormal eye movements. Additionally, scorpion stings do not produce halo lesions.

Finally, a significant BWS envenomation may present with little, if any, objective clinical evidence, allowing patients with drug-seeking behavior to use this chief complaint when requesting narcotics or benzodiazepines (20).

EMERGENCY DEPARTMENT EVALUATION

The physician should ask about the circumstances surrounding the suspected bite (e.g., witnessed bite, unexplained crying after a child was placed in a stroller), the description of the spider, and the progression of symptoms.

The physical examination should include a search for minute puncture wounds or halo lesions suggestive of black widow envenomation. The skin should be examined for unexplained diaphoresis, even in areas remote from the bite site. Vital signs should be examined for the presence of hypertension and tachycardia. No laboratory studies specific for BWS envenomations are available. Patients with severe or prolonged muscle pain should have a serum CPK. Evaluation for other causes of pain may be necessary, even in patients with known BWS bites.

EMERGENCY DEPARTMENT MANAGEMENT

After addressing the patient's airway and cardiovascular status, attention should focus on pain relief. Patients with mild to moderate discomfort should be offered oral, opioid-containing analgesics. Prescriptions should be given to manage the resolving pain over the next 24 to 48 hours. Those patients presenting with significant pain should be treated with opioids given intravenously for pain, and if needed, a benzodiazepine.

In adults, an initial aliquot of 4 to 6 mg of morphine (or equivalent dose of another opioid) intravenously is a reasonable starting point, with repeated doses every 2 to 5 minutes as needed. Benzodiazepine, such as lorazepam, given intravenously may be a useful adjunct by inducing sedation and amnesia. Effective amounts can vary tremendously; specific dosing should take into account the patient's weight, mental status, and comorbidities. Frequent reassessment is the key to rapid, effective pain control.

Other pharmacologic interventions have been reported and may occasionally be useful. Patients with adequate analgesia but uncontrolled hypertension should be treated with an antihypertensive medication, preferably an infused, short-acting agent (e.g., nitroglycerin or sodium nitroprusside) that can be weaned off when vital signs normalize. β-blockers, although used successfully in some reports, should not be administered if antivenom administration is being considered, as a result of the theoretical risk of complicating an allergic reaction (24). If the CPK is markedly elevated, serial measurements, i.v. fluids sufficient to maintain a brisk urine output, and alkalinization of the urine with i.v. sodium bicarbonate are appropriate. Although once considered beneficial, there is no objective evidence to support the use of calcium given intravenously or "muscle relaxants" and their use is not recommended.

There are several equine-derived *Latrodectus* antivenoms, each targeted against one species' venom. In the preparation available in the United States, antivenom is targeted against *L. mactans*, yet it is effective in treating envenomation from all North American species (10). The presence of the common, active venom component (α-atrotoxin) in all species allows for clinically useful cross-neutralization, even if the antivenom is produced using the venom of spiders from different continents (5,7).

Clinical experience with latrodectism and recommendations for the use and administration of antivenom vary throughout the world (3,4,10,11,12,15,16). These differences are based on the *Lactrodectus* species, patient presentation, antivenom availability, physician training and expertise. The following recommendations are best suited for the use of *L. mactans* antivenom in the United States. Most importantly, every envenomated patient is unique and a toxicologist or poison center should be consulted before giving antivenom.

Antivenom therapy should be reserved for patients with severe pain or profound hypertension, uncontrolled with opioids and benzodiazepines. A lower threshold for use is indicated for pregnant patients, particularly those with evidence of fetal distress, and patients with known cardiac disease and uncontrolled hypertension. The decision to treat with antivenom should be made as soon as possible, yet there are reports of (varyingly) effective antivenom administration weeks to months after the reported envenomation (1,25).

A known allergy to the antivenom or to horse serum (or other equine-derived antivenoms) is a contraindication to its use. Relative contraindications include a history of severe allergic reactions, severe reactive airway disease (both of which may increase the chance or severity of anaphylaxis), and the use of a β-blockers (which may hinder the management of anaphylaxis). As with all antivenom administration, the patient should be in a high acuity setting (monitored ED bed or ICU), have established i.v. access and a physician available at all times. The manufacturer of the North American *Latrodectus* antivenom recommends routine skin testing; however, this procedure is neither specific for identifying patients at risk for allergic reaction, nor does a negative test rule out potential allergic reactions. Routine skin testing is not absolutely indicated and should not be considered the "standard of care." A single vial of antivenom should be reconstituted in 50 to 100 mL of isotonic crystalloid solution and administered over 30 minutes i.v. Antivenin should be administered in a critical care setting such as the emergency department (ED) or intensive care unit with preparation to immediately treat life-threatening anaphylaxis. The infusion should be started slowly. If no adverse reactions occur, the rate is then increased. Symptoms typically begin to resolve within 30 minutes of antivenom administration, with complete relief within 2 hours. Rarely is a second dose required.

CRITICAL INTERVENTIONS

> • Administer opioids for pain as a result of BWS envenomation, with the route of administration and amount dependent on the clinical severity
> • Administer antivenom for severe envenomations with life-threatening systemic signs and symptoms or severe pain unresponsive to opioids and/or benzodiazepines

DISPOSITION

Asymptomatic patients with a history or suspicion of BWS envenomation can be discharged home after an observation period of 3 to 4 hours. Tetanus immunization status should be addressed and updated as necessary, but prophylactic antibiotics are not indicated. Follow-up instructions should include monitoring for signs of infection, as with any puncture wound.

Patients with mild symptoms typically respond well to oral analgesics and, if needed, benzodiazepines. However, treating physicians should consider the early use of parenteral medications for those with more significant effects. If the presenting pain and discomfort is rapidly relieved with initial i.v. medications, a trial of outpatient oral medications is justified. However, the patient should be monitored for continued relief by oral analgesics prior to discharge.

Patients with severe symptoms, requiring repeated administrations of parenteral analgesics or sedatives, or those with complicating medical conditions (e.g., cardiac disease, malignant hypertension, pregnancy) should be observed longer and considered for admission. If admitted, the patient may benefit from a patient controlled analgesia (PCA) pump.

Patients receiving antivenom can be discharged home if they are asymptomatic without signs of an allergic reaction. These patients should be instructed about the signs and symptoms of serum sickness and the need for follow-up if it occurs. The true incidence of BWS antivenom-induced anaphylaxis and serum sickness are not known, but appear to be low (3,4,16). Furthermore, patients should be counseled that they are at risk for anaphylaxis if reexposed to horse serum-containing medications.

COMMON PITFALLS

✔ Failing to consider BWS envenomation in patients with unexplained pain, muscle cramps, tachycardia, and hypertension

✔ Risking severe anaphylaxis by inappropriately administering antivenom to patients with mild envenomations

✔ Failing to address other medical issues such as acute coronary syndrome or fetal compromise and hypertensive crisis related to the black widow envenomation

✔ Sending patients home with a prescription for oral analgesics without ensuring that they respond to such agents in the ED

Acknowledgments

We thank Thomas Higgins and Steven Curry, who contributed to previous versions of this chapter.

References

1. Banham N, Jelinek G, Finch P. Late treatment with antivenom in prolonged red back spider envenomation. *Med J Aust* 1994;161(6):379.
2. Bush SP. Black widow spider envenomation mimicking Cholecystitis. *Am J Emerg Med* 1999;17(3):315.
3. Clark R, Wethern-Kestner S, Vance M, et al. Clinical presentation and treatment of black widow spider envenomation: a review of 163 cases. *Ann Emerg Med* 1992;21(7):782.
4. Clark R. The safety and efficacy of antivenom latrodectus mactans. *J Toxicol Clin Toxicol* 2001;39(2):125.
5. Daly F, Hill R, Bogdan G, et al. Neutralization of latrodectus mactans and l. hesperus venom by redback spider (l. hasseltii) antivenom. *J Toxicol Clin Toxicol* 2001;39(2):119.
6. Forrester M, Stanley S. Black widow spider and brown recluse spider bites in Texas from 1998 through 2002. *Vet Hum Toxicol* 2003;45(5):270.
7. Graudins A, Padula M, Broady K, et al. Red-back spider (Latrodectus hasseltii) antivenom prevents the toxicity of widow spider venoms. *Ann Emerg Med* 2001;37(2)154.
8. Henkel A, Sankaranarayanan S. Mechanisms of a-latrotoxin action. *Cell Tissue Res* 1999;296:229.
9. Ingram W, Musgrave A. Spider bite (arachnidism): A survey of its occurrence in Australia, with case histories. *Med J Aust* 1933;2:10.
10. Isbister G, Graudins A, White J, et al. Antivenom treatment in arachnidism. *J Toxicol Clin Toxicol* 2003;41(3):291.
11. Jelinek G, Banham N, Dunjey S. Red-back spider bites at Fremantle hospital, 1982-1987. *Med J Aust* 1989;150:693.
12. Jelinek G. Widow spider envenomation (latrodectism): a worldwide problem. *Wilderness Environ Med* 1997;8(4):226.
13. Keegan H, Hedeen R, Whittemore F. Seasonal variations in venom of black widow spiders. *Am J Trop Med Hyg* 1960;10:477.
14. McCrone J. Comparative lethality of several Latrodectus venoms. *Toxicon* 1964;2:201.
15. Moss H, Binder L. A retrospective review of black widow spider envenomations. *Ann Emerg Med* 1987;16(2):188.
16. Müller G. Black and brown widow spider bites in South Africa. *S Afr Med J* 1993;83(6):399.
17. Rauber A. Black widow spider bites. *J Toxicol Clin Toxicol* 1984;21(4&5):473.
18. Russell F, Marcus P, Streng J. Black widow spider envenomation during pregnancy-report of a case. *Toxicon* 1979;17:188.
19. Sherman R, Groll J, Gonzalez D, et al. Black widow spider (Latrodectus mactans) envenomation in a term pregnancy. *Curr Surg* 2000;57(4):346.
20. Spiller H, Schultz O. Envenomations as a novel drug-seeking method. *Vet Hum Toxicol* 2002;44(5):297.
21. Suntornntham S, Roberts J, Nilson G. Dramatic clinical response to the delayed administration of black widow spider antivenom. *Ann Emerg Med* 1994;24(6):1198.
22. Vance M, Curry S, Gerkin R, et al. The "target lesion": a pathognomonic sign of black widow spider (Latrodectus spp.) envenomation. *Vet Hum Toxicol* 1986;28:485.
23. Volkova T, Pluzhnikov K, Woll P, Grishin E. Low molecular weight components from black widow spider venom. *Toxicon* 1995;33(4):483.
24. Weitzman S, Margulis G, Lehmann E. Uncommon cardiovascular manifestations and high catecholamine levels due to "black widow" bite. *Am Heart J* 1977;93(1):89.
25. Wells C, Spring W. Delayed but effective treatment of red-back spider envenomation. *Med J Aust* 1996;164(7):447.

CHAPTER 348
Brown Recluse Spider Envenomation

Gary S. Wasserman

Spiders of the genus *Loxosceles* are distributed throughout the world. *L. reclusa*, the most important species in the United States, is most common in the southern Midwestern states. Depending on the temperature, it prefers living outdoors (under rocks, woodpiles, and debris) or in structures (basements, attics, and storage areas). The name "reclusa" describes its behavior: it is nocturnal, avoids areas of activity, hides its web, and is seldom seen. Bites are most common from April to October, may occur anywhere on the body, and seldom occur unless the spider is disturbed or threatened. Most victims are bitten while asleep, dressing, or working in the yard or house, and they may not initially be aware that envenomation has occurred.

L. reclusa measures 1 to 5 cm leg to leg, is fawn to dark brown, and has on its dorsal cephalothorax a violin- or fiddle-shaped, dark brown marking with the larger end toward the head. The body of a large spider will measure 1 cm in length by 0.5 cm in width. The short-haired body is oval, and the legs are long and slender. Three pairs of eyes, rather than four, is a distinctive but not unique feature of this genus. Although all Loxosceles species are often called "brown," "violin," or "fiddleback" spiders, the recognized common name "brown recluse" should be reserved only for *L. reclusa*.

Loxosceles venom contains at least 11 components, mostly enzymes with cytotoxic activity (e.g., protease, *S*-ribonucleotide phosphohydrolase, hyaluronidase, collagenase, esterase, sphingomyelinase-D), which cause both local and systemic toxicity (7–9,14,17). Dermonecrosis (ulceration) is caused by endothelial cell damage by venom and ischemia secondary to inflammation caused by leukocyte infiltration, hemolysis, complement activation, and intravascular coagulation (4,19).

CLINICAL PRESENTATION

Most bites from the brown recluse spider have a benign clinical course (3). Cutaneous and systemic toxicity (necrotic arachnidism, loxoscelism) may occur, and the systemic reaction is not necessarily proportional to the local reaction. Systemic symptoms may develop before a necrotic lesion appears. Severity relates to the amount of venom injected, the bite location, and the victim's immune status. Children and debilitated victims are at greater risk for severe reaction, but the elderly are often asymptomatic, possibly because of immunity that developed following earlier bites in their lives.

Typically, the bite itself feels like a pinprick that, in a few hours, may itch, tingle, swell, and become tender and red or blanch. Often, a blister or purpuric lesion forms, or both. Necrosis with induration and eschar formation may occur within hours or as late as 2 weeks after the bite; the eschar falls off, leaving an ulceration that may take months to heal. The most severe necrotic lesions occur in fatty areas such as the abdomen, thighs, and buttocks (21). Occasionally, an erythematous or violaceous reaction at the bite site, surrounded by a ring of pallor ("halo," "target," or "bull's eye" lesion), may be seen soon after envenomation. Vast edema may occur to the general bite site, especially on the neck and face. Angioedema of the airway may be life-threatening (11). The inflammatory reaction (pain, redness, induration, swelling, fever, lymphangitis, leukocytosis) can be severe. A rarely seen dermatologic sequelae of loxoscelism is pyoderma gangrenosum with recurrent deep ulcerations (13).

Systemic effects develop within hours after the bite and include fever, chills, headache, malaise, weakness, nausea, vomiting, arthralgia, myalgia, and rash. These signs and symptoms progress after more than 24 to 48 hours and then resolve by 72 to 96 hours postbite. Laboratory findings may include anemia, thrombocytopenia, leukocytosis, and evidence of hemolysis and consumptive coagulopathy. Hemolysis may directly result in hemoglobinuria, renal failure, and shock, or indirectly cause congestive heart failure, coma, convulsions, liver injury, and death as a result of anemic hypoxia (20,21,23). There are a variety of rash presentations. The least seldom-seen rash, a transient, early, diffuse, faint, macular, or speckled erythematous eruption over the trunk and flexural areas, may be a favorable prognostic sign, because it is often observed when a skin lesion suddenly involutes and resolves. The more common scarlatiniform rash may appear within days and persist a few days. This scarlatiniform-like eruption is noted to often represent a toxigenic erythroderma reaction to the venom rather than a *Streptococcus* or *Staphylococcus* infection. Because the spider does not transport bacteria, early infection is very unlikely. Cellulitis, bacteremia, or sepsis is secondary to the victims own flora (usually staph or strep). Envenomation may cause toxic hepatitis, pancreatitis, hematuria, cardiac manifestations, and rarely shock (5,24). Death, although rare, has occurred from multisystem organ failure, especially in young children (25).

DIFFERENTIAL DIAGNOSIS

The differential diagnosis of brown recluse spider bites includes bites and stings from several other arthropods, and many medical conditions (Table 348.1) (24). On further investigation, many cases of necrotic skin wounds presenting with an allegation of a brown recluse spider bite are found to have an alternate etiology. At least five other genera of spiders in the United States have been reported to cause necrotic lesions (2,21). Recent research does not support some of these claims, although there may be regional/country specific differences. Although there are other species of *Loxosceles* spiders in the United States, especially in the southwest, their venom is less potent; the dermal reaction and systemic effects are milder. Erythema that evolves into a violaceous macule distinguishes a necrotic envenomation from a nonnecrotic bite. Additionally, as the macule widens, the edge becomes uneven and the center sinks below skin level; nonnecrotic lesions remain edematous, raised, and red (1). Unless an offending spider is positively identified, a generic diagnosis such as "cutaneous necrosis," "necrotic arachnidism," or "necrotic arthropod bite or sting" should be used rather than a definitive one such as "brown recluse envenomation" or "loxoscelism." Other natural toxins causing hemolysis are *Coelenterata* (Portuguese man-of-war jellyfish), *Hymenoptera* (bees, wasps, hornets), snakes, *Clostridium* infections, and *Streptococcal* and *Staphylococcal* infections (24).

EMERGENCY DEPARTMENT EVALUATION

The history should include the time and circumstances of a bite and a description of the spider (although this information is seldom known), and the nature and progression of signs and symptoms. The skin should be examined closely for typical lesions in patients with acute hemolysis and coagulopathy of unknown

TABLE 348.1. Differential Diagnoses of Loxoscelism[a]

Spiders Common to U.S., Which May Cause Dermonecrosis:
  Argiope (orb weaver)
  Chiracanthium (running or sac spider)
  Loxosceles genera (fiddle or violin)
  Lycosa (wolf spider)
  Phidippus (jumping spider)
  Tegenaria agrestis (northwestern brown spider or hobo spider)

Bites/stings from many marine, flying and crawling creatures causing
  dermonecrosis
Dermatoses of many types
Hereditary hemolytic anemias
Acquired hemolytic anemias

Medical Conditions Causing Dermonecrosis:
  Emboli/thrombi
  Vasculitis/angiitis/periarteritis
  Frost bite
  Ischemic vascular ulcers
  Fat herniation/infarction
  Factitious ulcers (self-inflicted)
  Foreign bodies
  Infectious hemorrhagic lesions (gonococcal, anthrax, pox)
  Traumatic lesions

Other Natural Toxins Causing Hemolysis (and Possibly
    Dermonecrosis):
  Colenterata (Portuguese man-of-war jellyfish)
  Hymenoptera (bees, wasps, fire ants, etc.)
  Snakes (cobra, viper venom)
  Clostridium infections
  Streptococcal/staphylococcal infections

[a] From Wasserman GS. Brown recluse and other necrotizing spiders. In:
Ford MD, Delaney KA, King LJ, Erickson T, eds. *Clinical toxicology.*
Philadelphia: W.B. Saunders, 2001:878;881, with permission.

etiology. The general examination should focus on vital signs, heart, lungs, and neurologic function.

All patients with suspicion of brown recluse envenomation should have a baseline complete blood count and urinalysis. Those with suspected hemolysis or significant systemic reactions may also require plasma and/or urine free hemoglobin levels, a reticulocyte count, coagulation studies (prothrombin time, partial thromboplastin time, fibrinogen, and *d*-dimers), and antiglobulin tests (e.g., Coombs' test). Other helpful tests as indicated include liver function studies (alkaline phosphatase, alanine aminotransferase, aspartate aminotransferase, creatine phosphokinase, and bilirubin); renal function studies (electrolytes, blood urea nitrogen, creatinine); and serum amylase/lipase. Rarely necessary are a serum haptoglobin level/haptoglobin binding capacity, lactase dehydrogenase biopsy, culture, or Gram stain. Hemolysis may be intravascular and/or extravascular. Extravascular hemolysis will not be detectable by finding hemoglobin in blood or urine and should be considered in any patient with a falling hemoglobin/hematocrit and rising reticulocyte count. A specific immunoassay to identify *Loxosceles* venom performed from skin, wound aspirates and hair shafts is sensitive, specific, and reproducible but, at present, is only a research tool (15).

EMERGENCY DEPARTMENT MANAGEMENT

Treatment of necrotic or cutaneous arachnidism should be the same, regardless of the culprit. A "benign neglect" approach nearly always results in an excellent dermal outcome. It is impossible to make an early prediction about which bite will result in a disfiguring lesion. General wound care usually suf-

fices including tetanus prophylaxis, cleansings, and topical antimicrobial ointment. Corticosteroids injected locally or systemically, and vasodilators, have not proved helpful in preventing or decreasing dermonecrosis (1). Antibiotics are not needed routinely, but they may be indicated for secondary bacterial infection. An antipruritic or antianxiety drug is often comforting, and cool compresses (avoid heat, because it may stimulate a toxin produced cascade of inflammatory reactants). Protect the bite site from further trauma but immobilization is not necessary.

Analgesics can be given for pain, but nonsteroidal antiinflammatory drugs that affect platelet functioning are contraindicated because of possible bleeding problems. Early wide excision is ineffective, unnecessary, and expensive; produces complications (such as allowing venom to penetrate deeper into tissues); and may cause disability or worsen scarring. Trimming rapidly enlarging bullae seems to stop their progression but does not necessarily reduce the risk of necrosis within the blister borders (25). Corrective surgery should be delayed for 4 to 8 weeks or longer, when the necrosis is clearly demarcated (21,22). Necrotizing fasciitis or abscess warrants surgical intervention.

The treatment of systemic arachnidism is mainly aggressive, symptomatic, and supportive care. Corticosteroids (methylprednisolone, or equivalent, 0.5-1 mg/kg i.v. every 6 hours) ameliorate hemolysis and are usually required for only 3 to 7 days, with the exception of a tapering dosage schedule if very high doses administered. Alkalinization of the urine and aggressive hydration can protect against renal failure secondary to hemoglobinuria. Anemia and thrombocytopenia should be treated with component therapy (e.g., packed red cells, platelets), as needed. As complement or unknown factors in whole blood and fresh-frozen plasma may react with venom components and contribute to red blood cell destruction, these products are not recommended (12). Blood type and screen/crossmatch may be difficult because of interfering antibodies. In severe cases, consult a hematologist as needed for the most recent coagulopathy therapies such as antithrombin III or recombinant factor VIIa (6).

Some authorities suggest that a polymorphonuclear leukocyte inhibitor such as dapsone (25–100 mg orally twice a day for 1–2 weeks) may prevent ulceration if started early (18). There is no strong evidence supporting dapsone's effectiveness in preventing dermonecrosis. Dapsone, even if theoretically effective, needs to be instituted within hours of envenomation and should be reserved for nonpregnant, healthy adults with rapidly progressive blistering and hemorrhage or impending ulceration in a cosmetic area such as the face or digits, and a strongly suggestive or confirmed history of spider envenomation. Dapsone's adverse effects profile makes it an undesirable agent for children with this envenomation. Glucose-6-phosphate dehydrogenase deficiency is a contraindication for dapsone therapy, and patients treated with this agent must be carefully monitored for drug toxicity (hemolysis, methemoglobinemia, superinfection, leukopenia, rash). There is also no strong evidence supporting the effectiveness of hyperbaric oxygen, although it may be beneficial in a subgroup of patients with a history of poor wound healing (16). Although an antivenom has been produced and used experimentally, it is not commercially available (10).

CRITICAL INTERVENTIONS

- Perform standard wound care for necrotic skin lesions
- Perform serial clinical and laboratory assessments to rule out systemic toxicity
- Treat hemolysis with high-dose parenteral corticosteroids, hydration, and alkalinization of the urine

DISPOSITION

Many claims of a brown recluse or other spider bite have alternate etiologies, and patient disposition will be as per the true underlying disease. In suspect cases, physicians unfamiliar with arachnidism should consult a regional poison control center or toxicologist for advice. A telephone call to an envenomation expert may be necessary. Patients who present immediately after a bite should be followed as outpatients with 24- to 48-hour rechecks for 3 to 5 days postbite. Patients who present with or develop large dermonecrosis/ulcers should be referred to a wound care surgeon for follow-up. Patients with significant systemic symptoms, clinical toxicity, or hematologic abnormalities should be admitted with an appropriate level of monitoring. Those hospitalized and having a benign course with stable physical and laboratory evaluations can be discharged with follow-up in 24 to 48 hours. Liberal admission for observation may be prudent in very young or debilitated patients and in those judged to be unreliable regarding follow-up.

COMMON PITFALLS

✔ Diagnosing "brown recluse spider bite" rather than "necrotic arthropod bite/sting" or "necrotic skin lesion" when positive identification of the offending creature has not been made and alternative diagnoses have not been considered

✔ Failure to appreciate that hemolysis secondary to *L. reclusa* envenomation may be rapid or insidious in onset and be intravascular, extravascular, or both

✔ Failure to perform laboratory evaluations on patients with signs and symptoms, especially skin lesions, highly suspicious for loxoscelism

✔ Failure to discuss therapeutic options and controversies, and to warn patients about potential but unpredictable complications such as hemolysis, coagulopathies, secondary infections, and delayed wound healing, and to arrange for follow-up

References

1. Anderson P. Necrotizing spider bites. *Am Fam Physician* 1982;26:198–203.
2. Atkin J, Wingo C, Sodeman W. Probable cause of necrotic spider bite in the Midwest. *Science* 1957;126:73.
3. Berger R. The unremarkable brown recluse spider bite. *JAMA* 1973;225:1109–1111.
4. Berger R, Adelstein E, Anderson P. Intravascular coagulation—the cause of necrotic arachnidism. *J Invest Dermatol* 1978;61:142–150.
5. Bey TA, Walters FG, Lober W, et al. Loxosceles arizonica bite associated with shock. *Ann Emerg Med* 1997;30.701–703.
6. Chuansumrit A, Chantarojanasiri T, Isarangkura P. Recombinant activated factor VII in children with acute bleeding from liver failure and disseminated intravascular coagulation. *Blood Coagul Fibrinolysis* 2000;11:S101–S105.
7. Forrester L, Barrett J, Campbell B. Red blood cell lysis induced by the venom of the brown recluse spider: the role of sphingomyelinase D. *Arch Biochem Biophys* 1978;187:355–365.
8. Geren C, Chan T, Hewell D, et al. Partial characterization of the low-molecular-weight fractions of the extract of the venom apparatus of the brown recluse spider and its hemolymph. *Toxicon* 1975;13:233–238.
9. Geren C, Chan T, Hewell D, et al. Isolation and characterization of toxins from brown recluse spider venom (Loxosceles reclusa). *Arch Biochem Biophys* 1976;174:90–99.
10. Gomez HF, Mill MJ, Trach JW. Intradermal anti-Loxosceles Fab fragments attenuate dermonecrotic arachnidism. *Acad Emerg Med* 1999;6:1195–1202.
11. Goto CS, Abramo TJ, Ginsburg CM. Upper airway obstruction caused by brown recluse spider envenomation of the neck. *Amer J Emerg Med* 1996;14:660–662.
12. Hardman J, Beck M, Hardman P, et al. Incompatibility associated with the bite of a brown recluse spider (Loxosceles reclusa). *Transfusion* 1983;23:233–236.
13. Hoover EL, Williams W, Koger L. Pseudoepitherliomatons hyperplasia and pyoderma gangrenosum after a brown recluse spider bite. *South Med J* 1990;83:243–246.
14. Hufford D, Morgan P. C-reactive protein as a mediator in the lysis of human erythrocytes sensitized by brown recluse spider venom. *Proc Soc Exp Biol Med* 1981;167:493–497.
15. Krywko DM, Gomez HF. Detection of Loxosceles species venom in dermal lesions: a comparison of 4 venom recovery methods. *Ann Emerg Med* 2002;39:475–480.
16. Maynor ML, Moon RE, Klitzman B et al. Brown recluse spider envenomation: a prospective trial of hyperbaric oxygen therapy. *Acad Emerg Med* 1997;4:184–192.
17. Rees R, Nanney L, Yates R, et al. Interaction of brown recluse spider venom on cell membranes: the inciting mechanism? *J Invest Dermatol* 1984;83:270–275.
18. Rees R, Altenbern P, Lynch J, et al. Brown recluse spider bites: a comparison of surgical excision versus dapsone and delayed surgical excision. *Ann Surg* 1985;202:659–663.
19. Smith C, Micks D. The role of polymorphonuclear leukocytes in the lesion caused by the venom of the brown spider, Loxosceles reclusa. *Lab Invest* 1970;22:90–93.
20. Taylor E, Denny W. Hemolysis, renal failure and death, presumed secondary to the bite of brown recluse spider. *South Med J* 1966;59:1209–1211.
21. Wasserman G, Anderson P. Loxoscelism and necrotic arachnidism. *J Toxicol Clin Toxicol* 1983–84;21:451–472.
22. Wasserman G. Wound care of spider and snake envenomations. *Ann Emerg Med* 1988;17:1331–1335.
23. Wasserman G, Mydler TT, Sharma V. Brown recluse spider envenomation as a cause of hemolysis and hemoglobinuria. *Vet Hum Toxicol* 1991;33:359 (abs).
24. Wasserman GS. Brown recluse and other necrotizing spiders. In: Ford MD, Delaney KA, Ling LJ, Erickson T, eds. *Clinical toxicology*. Philadelphia: WB Saunders Company 2001;878–884.
25. Wasserman GS, Lowry J. Loxosceles spiders. In: Brent J, Burkhart KK, Donovan JW, et al. (eds.). Critical care toxicology: diagnosis and management of the critically poisoned patient. Philadelphia: Mosby, 2004.

CHAPTER 349
Insect, Tick, Mite Bites and Infestations

Michael James Burns

Bites and infestations associated with arthropods that are members of Class *Insecta* (*Hexapoda*; insects) and Class *Arachnida*, subclass *Acari* (ticks and mites) may result in minor annoying local reactions, systemic allergic reactions including anaphylaxis, secondary bacterial infections, and the transmission of a host of serious systemic infectious diseases. Emergency physicians should be familiar with the insect, mite, and tick fauna in their local area. Table 349.1 lists the biting arthropods of medical importance in North America, their geographic distribution, and the diseases they transmit.

Arthropods are invertebrates having an exoskeleton, segmented bodies, jointed appendages, and bilateral symmetry (7). The insects have six legs and three distinct body regions—head, thorax, and abdomen. Some insects have wings (insects are the only arthropods having wings). The insects include cockroaches, termites, lice, the true bugs (bedbugs, wheel bugs, assassin, and kissing bugs), fleas, flies (which include mosquitoes), beetles, ants, wasps, bees, and others. Ticks and mites have eight legs as adults and nymphs, with one disk-shaped body region and no true head (1,7). Tick and mite larvae have six or fewer legs. Adult ticks are pea-size, whereas nymphal ticks and adult mites are about the same size as a grain of sand, or smaller. The arthropods most important to human health are hematophagous, meaning they must feed on warm-blooded vertebrates for blood or

TABLE 349.1. Diseases Transmitted by Biting Arthropods in North America

Arthropod	Geographic Distribution of Arthropod	Disease Transmitted
Conenose bugs ("kissing bugs")	Southwestern U.S., Mexico	American trypanosomiasis
Mosquitoes	Widespread	Malaria, dengue, arbovirus encephalitides
Deer fly	Widespread	Tularemia
Fleas	Widespread	Plague
		Murine (endemic) typhus
		Cat scratch disease
Human body louse (*Pediculus humanus* corporis)	Sporadic	Epidemic typhus
		Trench fever
House mouse mite (*Liponyssoides sanguineus*)	Northeastern U.S.	Rickettsialpox
Ixodes scapularis (deer tick, black legged tick)	Southeast, mid-Atlantic, northeast, upper midwest U.S.	Lyme disease
		Human granulocytic ehrlichiosis
		Babesiosis
Ixodes pacificus (western black legged tick)	Far western U.S. and Canada	Lyme disease
Dermacentor variabilis (American dog tick)	Eastern, midwest U.S., Mexico	Rocky Mountain spotted fever
		Tularemia
		Tick paralysis (neurotoxin)
Dermacentor andersoni (Rocky Mountain wood tick)	Rocky Mountains of U.S. and Canada, Great Basin of U.S.	Rocky Mountain spotted fever
		Tularemia
		Colorado tick fever
		Tick paralysis
Amblyomma americanum (Lone Star tick)	Southeastern, mid-Atlantic U.S.	Human monocytic ehrlichiosis
		Tularemia
		"Southern tick-associated rash illness"
Ornithodoros species (soft ticks)	Mountains of western U.S., Canada, and Mexico	Tick-borne relapsing fever

tissue fluid that is both life-supporting and necessary for growth and gonotrophic development. Their mouth parts are designed for probing and sucking blood and tissue fluids, and their saliva contains substances that counteract host hemostasis. For some species, only the females are hematophagous. They have several different methods of obtaining blood. For example, bedbugs, kissing bugs and fleas obtain blood directly from venules, whereas ticks, black flies, horse and deer flies obtain blood by lacerating blood vessels and feeding from the pool of blood formed.

Most human skin lesions from arthropod bites are produced by hypersensitivity reactions to salivary components or venom; these include wheals, papules, vesicles, and blisters (7). Secondary bacterial infections can occur, and late cutaneous allergic responses may occur in atopic individuals and be confused with many infectious and noninfectious conditions.

CLINICAL PRESENTATION

Bedbugs (*Cimex lectularius*) are blood-sucking insects about 5 mm long (adults), oval shaped and flattened, and smell like rotten raspberries (5,7). The nymphal stages are smaller and also take blood meals. They are found on and in mattresses, in cracks and crevices in walls and floors near beds. Feeding is painless, usually at night, and takes only 5 to 10 minutes. Bedbugs are reported to be increasing recently in the United States, especially in hotel rooms. Bites may produce allergic reactions, consisting of a linear grouping of red blotches or urticarial wheals, or no reaction at all in many persons.

Conenose bugs, also known as kissing, assassin, or reduviid bugs, are 1 to 3 cm long, brown or black in color, with elongated heads and wings, and are good fliers (7). Although usually found in the wild, they can adapt to live in cracks and holes of substandard dwellings, and come out at night to feed on human blood.

Their bites are usually painless, but allergic reactions to their bites can result in papular or nodular lesions.

Wheel bugs (*Arilus cristatus*) are true bugs that bite humans only in self-defense (7). They are 3 cm long and gray, with a small narrow head and a cogwheel-like crest on their thorax. The bite causes immediate intense pain with swelling and inflammation.

Blister beetles are plant-feeding insects, commonly found in the southeastern, central, and southwestern United States, whose body fluids contain a blistering agent, cantharidin, which produces large painless blisters within a few hours after contact with live or dead beetles (7). Mild tingling or burning can occur prior to onset of blistering. The blisters are usually not serious and resolve within several days. Ingestion of beetles or their products may cause vomiting, abdominal cramps, and diarrhea.

Some caterpillars (moth larval stage) have urticating hairs or spines that secrete a toxin when exposed to human skin, causing a burning sensation, swelling, numbness, or intense stabbing pain (7). Other caterpillars may produce a dermatitis by inducing an allergic reaction in human skin when it comes in contact with hairs of the caterpillars.

Centipedes (Class *Chilopoda*), which are not insects or arachnids, can cause a painful "bite," which can become red and swollen (7). The bite is not produced by the mouth parts, but by sharp claws on their first pair of legs, which have attached venom glands. Venom is injected through the claw.

Fleas are small, laterally flattened wingless insects that feed exclusively on blood (7). The cat flea (*Ctenocephalides felis*), which also infests dogs and many other mammals, is the predominant flea species in North America. Fleas are easily recognized by their jumping behavior. Human flea bite lesions are caused by allergic reactions, and often occur in clusters or irregular groups of several to a dozen or more where the flea has explored and probed. In the allergic person, a pruritic wheal forms around each probe site within 5 to 30 minutes. Indurated papules and occasionally vesicular or bullous lesions develop within 12 to 24 hours, accompanied by intense itching, and may last a week or more.

The small female chigoe flea, *Tunga penetrans*, burrows into the skin of persons living or traveling in tropical and subtropical areas of North and South America, the West Indies, and Africa, producing a disorder known as tungiasis. It grows to about 1 cm within 2 weeks and lays eggs beneath the dermis. It commonly infests the legs and feet, including the areas between the toes or under the toenails, and produces intense inflammation and itching. One sees a black dot in the center of a pustule.

Black flies are smaller than mosquitoes, travel in large swarms, and are vicious biters (7). Allergic reactions to the bites result in red itchy papules and nodules with surrounding swelling, and occasionally systemic allergic reactions with fever, wheezing, and diffuse urticaria. Deer and horse flies are large flies whose bites produce deep, painful wounds that often become secondarily infected (7). Bite lesions are solitary or scattered, not grouped or linear. Local and systemic allergic reactions can occur. Stable fly bites produce small papular lesions. Biting midges are so small that they can pass through ordinary screens. Their bites produce small papular lesions with red halos and wheals.

Mosquitoes are also flies. Their bites can result in allergic reactions, producing multiple, scattered lesions that are not linear or grouped (7). A wheal and flare may be seen 30 minutes after the bite, and delayed onset of pruritic papules is common.

Myiasis is an invasion or infestation of the human body by larvae (maggots) of two-winged flies (*Diptera*), which occurs in debilitated or comatose persons or young children (7). It occurs when the female fly lays eggs near a wound, or when the fly deposits freshly hatched larvae directly in a wound. The larvae of some fly species are able to penetrate human skin and invade normal tissues, while others are capable of living only on the surface of the wound. Although usually occurring in wounds, myiasis can also occur in the nose, mouth, sinuses, eyes, anal region, vagina, and bladder.

Furuncular myiasis is a type of myiasis produced by the larva of the human botfly (found in Mexico, Central and South America) and by the Tumbu fly (found in tropical Africa). The larvae burrow into the skin producing painful pruritic nodules called warbles, each with a central opening or punctum. The person sometimes feels something moving. Visitors from developed countries may acquire this disorder while traveling and return home before the maggot completes its development. These lesions are easily mistaken for *Staphylococcal* boils.

Lice are tiny, elongate, soft-bodied, light-colored, wingless insects that feed on blood (7,12,19). Three species infest humans: the human body louse (*Pediculus humanus corporis*), the human head louse (*P. humanus capitis*), and the pubic or crab louse (*Phthirus pubis*). The body louse and the head louse have a similar shape with an elongated body and a pointed head (9). The pubic louse is much wider and shorter and resembles a crab. Lice are transmitted from person-to-person by close body contact (for all), possibly by sharing of hats, combs and brushes (head louse) or by clothing (body louse). Humans infested with lice often develop itchy red papules with excoriated areas that can become secondarily infected. The adult lice are often difficult to see, but the nits of the head louse and pubic louse can be found attached on shafts of hair near the base. Head louse infestation is most common in white schoolgirls, and affects all social and economic backgrounds. Pubic lice can sometimes be found in the eyebrows and eyelashes, in axillary hair, and on the coarse trunk hairs of males, and rarely in the scalp. Bluish-grey macules, known as blue spots, may sometimes be seen on the skin in pubic lice infestation. Persons infested with pubic lice often have other sexually transmitted diseases.

Mites look like tiny small hairy ticks, with one disk-shaped body segment and no true head. Many species bite humans and cause skin lesions due to allergic reactions, but do not live on humans or their clothing. One species, *Sarcoptes scabiei* var. *hominis*, spends its entire life on human skin, causing scabies (3). Chiggers is a condition caused by bites by the larvae of the chigger (or harvest) mite (7). These mites are found in grasses and scrubs, especially at forest edges. Chigger mite larvae, which are tiny (0.2 mm long), round, and red, yellow or orange in color, bite humans and take a meal of tissue juice (not blood). Larval mites inject saliva that dissolves host tissue, then feed on the dissolved tissue. Pruritic macules and wheals develop within 3 to 6 hours, followed by development of intensely pruritic papules and pustules at 10 to 16 hours. Lesions are often linear or grouped. Numerous other species of mites will bite humans, causing painful pruritic red papules. Persons bitten by chicken mites and straw itch mites may have thousands of lesions. Other mites that bite humans include the house mouse mite, tropical rat mite, tropical fowl mite, northern fowl mite, spiny rat mite, and the *Cheyletiella* mite (7). Unlike the scabies mite, none of these mites live on humans.

Scabies, an infestation of the epidermis by *Sarcoptes scabiei* var. *hominis*, is transmitted by close body contact (3,7). The fertilized female mite burrows into the epidermis and lays 2 to 3 eggs daily for 30 days. Larvae hatch in 3 to 4 days and migrate to the skin surface. Maturation from egg to adult takes about 10 to 14 days. The mites feed on cells of the stratum corneum. Their secretions and excretions sensitize the host and produce irritation and itching with pruritic crusted red papules. The incubation period following infestation until symptoms appear is about 4 to 8 weeks for a first infestation, but may be much shorter (as little as 48 hours) in recurrent infestations. A person may be very contagious before there are any symptoms or lesions. There are only 5 to 20 mites on the body in a typical infestation, usually found in burrows on the hands, wrists, elbows, knees, belt line, penis, the breasts of females, and the feet of children, but are especially common in the webs of the fingers and the folds of the wrists. In infants, lesions are frequently found on the scalp, face, palms and soles. Burrows are often difficult to find. Itching commonly occurs in locations where there are no mites present. Extensive excoriations and secondary bacterial infections can cause puzzling skin lesions.

Persons who are immunocompromised (e.g., AIDS) or debilitated (especially elderly or institutionalized persons) may develop a condition known as crusted ("Norwegian") scabies, in which hyperkeratotic crusted nodules and plaques become widespread on the body. Millions of mites may be present in this condition, making it extremely contagious. It is easily misdiagnosed as eczema or another condition. Other closely-related scabies mites infest domestic animals, especially dogs (sarcoptic mange). These mites can bite humans and produce pruritic papular lesions without burrows. They cannot complete their life cycle on humans, so no specific anti-scabies treatment is needed.

Ticks are obligate, blood-sucking, nonpermanent ectoparasites that feed on mammals, birds, reptiles, and occasionally amphibians (1,7,9,13). Among the biting arthropods, ticks are second only to mosquitoes in the number of pathogens transmitted to humans. They are capable of ingesting enormous quantities of blood, lymph or digested tissues. Molting and reproduction is regulated by blood ingestion. There are four stages in the life cycle: egg, larva, nymph, and adult. Larvae have six legs, whereas nymphs and adults have eight legs. Even in highly endemic areas, ticks are not evenly distributed.

There are two major families of ticks: the *Ixodidae* (hard-bodied ticks) and the *Argasidae* (soft-bodied ticks). Hard-bodied ticks include *Ixodes*, *Dermacentor*, and *Amblyomma* species. Prolonged attachment is required before feeding (and disease transmission) begins. Hard ticks will remain attached for 7 to 14 days before dropping off, if not removed (7). When feeding, they excrete large amounts of saliva and feces containing pathogens. In contrast, soft-bodied ticks of the genus *Ornithodoros* (*O. hermsi*, *O. turicata*) bite, feed and drop off within a few minutes. and prefer animal burrows or manmade animal or human shelters (7). Tick bites are usually painless, and there is often no reaction at the bite site after the tick is removed or drops off. Sometimes, a hypersensitivity reaction to the bite occurs or a red nodule may persist at the bite site for weeks to months.

Ixodes scapularis (deer tick or black-legged tick) is most likely to be found in brushy areas at the interface between fields and forests (forest boundaries), whereas *D. variabilis* (American dog tick) prefers meadows and roadsides. They "quest" for host animals by climbing vegetation (few inches to three feet) and passively wait for a host to pass by. Ticks cannot fly, jump or swim. Larvae, nymphs, and adult females (but not adult males) increase in size enormously during feeding. Ticks spend most of their life off their host, usually staying within an area of only a few square feet (other than *D. variabilis*, which may crawl more than a kilometer while questing). Their life is composed of short parasitic periods and extended nonfeeding periods without intake of food or liquid. They are capable of withstanding environmental stresses and adults may live for several years.

Deer ticks nymphs are likely to remain attached undetected for long periods of time because of their small size (about the size of a poppy seed or the head of a pin). Adult deer ticks, which primarily feed on deer, are the size of an apple seed. Dog ticks are larger and usually feed on medium and large mammals. Only adults dog ticks feed on humans.

Soft-bodied ticks live in high mountains of the western United States., Canada, and Mexico and prefer animal burrows or manmade animal or human shelters (7). Humans are typically bitten when they sleep in rodent-infested cabins.

D. variabilis (American dog tick) and *D. andersoni* (Rocky Mountain wood tick) can cause tick paralysis (due to a neurotoxin secreted by the tick). In order for tick paralysis to develop, the tick must remain attached for at least 5 to 6 days. Initial restlessness, irritability, paresthesias, and ataxia, are followed by rapidly progressive ascending flaccid paralysis, with a normal sensory exam, a clear sensorium, and lack of fever. Tick paralysis is especially likely in children and in girls, in whom the ticks are often concealed in long hair at the nape of the neck.

DIFFERENTIAL DIAGNOSIS

Reactions to arthropod bites may be difficult to diagnose since many patients cannot remember any exposure. The pruritic papules, vesicles, pustules, nodules, and bullae resulting from allergic reactions to arthropod bites may easily be misdiagnosed as allergic or irritant reactions to drugs or chemicals, atopic or contact dermatitis, *Herpes simplex*, *Staphylococcal*, and other bacterial infections, or cutaneous fungal infections. Multiple linear papules or vesicles should suggest bites by bedbugs or chigger mites, while irregular groups of papules and vesicles are typical for fleas and chiggers. Lesions caused by mosquitoes are multiple and scattered, not linear or grouped. A deer or horse fly bite that becomes secondarily infected and forms an ulcer could be misdiagnosed as a brown recluse spider bite (see Chapter 348, "Brown Recluse Spider Envenomation").

Arthropod bites and infestations should also be considered in the differential diagnosis of any patient complaining of itching. "Insect bites" should generally not be diagnosed based upon lesions alone. Scabies should be considered in the differential diagnosis of patients presenting with scattered pruritic papules, especially when found on the hands, wrists, elbows, and genital areas. Crusted "Norwegian" scabies should be considered in the differential diagnosis for immunosuppressed or debilitated patients presenting with subacute or chronic widespread hyperkeratotic plaques or eczematous lesions, even in the absence of pruritus. Tick paralysis may be confused with Guillain-Barré syndrome, botulism, or spinal cord compression.

Arthropod-borne infection (Table 349.1) should be considered in the differential diagnosis of persons presenting with an acute febrile illness, even if there is no history of an arthropod bite (2,4). Mosquitoes are the most important arthropod vectors of disease in the world because of their transmission of malaria, yellow fever, dengue, filariasis, and the encephalitis viruses (2).

Several species of the conenose bug group (*Triatoma*, *Rhodnius*) transmit the protozoan parasite *Trypanosoma cruzi* (causative agent of American trypanosomiasis or Chagas' disease). Fleas can transmit plague (*Yersinia pestis*), murine typhus (*Rickettsia typhi*), and cat scratch disease (*Bartonella henselae*). Children who ingest fleas containing the larval stage of the dog and cat tapeworm, *Dipylidium caninum*, may become infected with the adult tapeworm. Deer flies can transmit tularemia, but black, horse, and stable flies, and biting midges do not transmit any diseases in North America. Body lice can transmit epidemic typhus (*R. prowazekii*), trench fever (*Bartonella quintana*), and louse-borne relapsing fever (*Borrelia recurrentis*). The head louse and pubic louse are not known to transmit any diseases. The house mouse mite can transmit rickettsialpox (*R. akari*).

Deer ticks can transmit Lyme disease (*B. burgdorferi*), human granulocytic ehrlichiosis (*Ehrlichia* species), and babesiosis (*Babesia microti*, a protozoan) to humans (1,4,7,22). Lyme disease (see Chapter 141, "Lyme Disease") is most common in the northeastern and upper midwestern U.S. because the primary host for the tick's nymphal stage in these regions, the white-footed mouse, is capable of high rates of spirochetemia and is an excellent transmitter to ticks. The nymph, not the adult tick, most often transmits Lyme disease to humans. Lyme disease transmission requires more than 24 hours of attachment for nymphs and 36 hours for adults. *I. pacificus* (western black-legged tick), found in the western United States, also transmits Lyme disease, but infection rates in the tick are very low due to their feeding behavior. Nymphal deer and *I. pacificus* ticks in the southern and western United States have very low rates of infection with the Lyme disease organism (7). They feed primarily on lizards, which are incapable of infecting ticks and are poor reservoirs of the organism, and they rarely bite humans. Lyme transmission from *I. pacificus* requires over 96 hours of attachment for nymphs.

Dog ticks transmit Rocky Mountain spotted fever (R. rickettsii) in the eastern United States, with disease transmission requiring more than 24 hours of attachment (see Chapter 142, "Rocky Mountain Spotted Fever")(7). Only 1% to 5% of ticks in an endemic area are infected with the rickettsial organism. Dog ticks can also transmit tularemia (*Francisella tularensis*).

D. andersoni (Rocky Mountain wood tick) transmits Rocky Mountain spotted fever in the western United States, tularemia, and Colorado tick fever (*Coltivirus*). *Amblyomma americanum* (Lone Star tick) transmits tularemia, human monocytic ehrlichiosis (*E. chaffeensis*), and "Southern tick-associated rash illness," a newly described Lyme-like disease in the southeastern United States caused by *B. lonestari*, and possibly *R. parkeri*. *A. maculatum* (Gulf coast tick), common in the southeastern U.S., transmits *R. parkeri*, a newly-described agent producing a mild febrile illness accompanied by multiple eschars and a maculopapular eruption (18). Q fever (*Coxiella burnetii*) can be acquired from exposure to hard ticks from inhalation of dead tick parts or feces in dust. Nymph and adult soft-bodied ticks transmit tick-borne relapsing fever (*Borrelia recurrentis*) in the high mountains of the western United States, Canada, and Mexico. Humans are bitten while they sleep. Ticks in other parts of the world transmit a host of diseases which are important to travelers, including rickettsial infections such as Boutonneuse fever and African tick bite fever, as well as arbovirus encephalitis and hemorrhagic fever (2,20).

Patients suffering from delusions of parasitosis have an unwarranted belief that live organisms, such as mites or insects, are present on the body (7,11). The typical patient is a well-educated, responsible, hard-working woman, who may have an excessive preoccupation with cleanliness, and has a single delusion and no other mental disorder. This belief often persists for many years despite numerous physician visits and repeated treatments of the house with pesticides and the patient by medication, usually physician-prescribed. Typical characteristics of the "bugs" include: they change color; they jump; they appear and disappear while being watched; they enter the skin and reappear; they invade the hair; nose and ears; they infest the patient's hair, and can be combed or shaken onto a sheet or towel; and they sometimes come out of common household items (toothpaste, cosmetics) or teeth after brushing. Family members often support the patient, but are never afflicted. Patients typically bring in samples of the supposed pest for examination, which consist of small bits of lint, cloth, dandruff, or scabs. These patients should be referred to a dermatologist to definitively rule out an infestation, as well as to a psychiatrist, although the patients will generally not accept any suggestion that this is "all in their head." Delusions that insects are crawling on the skin are also seen in persons abusing cocaine and amphetamines.

EMERGENCY DEPARTMENT EVALUATION

A complete travel history should be obtained and the patient should be questioned about outdoor activities or any known exposures to biting arthropods (20). Patients complaining of itching or papules in the scalp or genital area should be asked about household or sexual contacts that may have head lice or pubic lice. The skin should be examined carefully for evidence of bites, allergic reactions, adult lice and nits attached to hair shafts, burrows of scabies, secondary bacterial infections, or rashes typical of infections transmitted by arthropods. Ask the patient about medications already used, as these could affect or change the appearance of lesions. Patients found to have pubic lice should be screened for sexually transmitted diseases. The diagnosis of scabies is made by gently scraping burrows with a scalpel blade covered with mineral oil. The mineral oil and scraped material is transferred to a glass slide, a coverslip is applied, and the slide is examined under a microscope for mites, eggs, or feces.

EMERGENCY DEPARTMENT MANAGEMENT

Pruritic skin lesions caused by arthropod bites should be treated with cold compresses, soothing lotions, topical corticosteroids, and systemic antihistamines. Systemic allergic reactions may require treatment with epinephrine, i.v. fluids, systemic corticosteroids, and antihistamines. Secondary bacterial infections, often seen with deer or horse fly bites, or with excoriated mosquito or flea bites, are usually caused by *S. aureus* or *Streptococcus pyogenes*, and should be treated with anti*Staphylococcal* penicillins, first-generation cephalosporins, amoxicillin-clavulanate, clindamycin, or macrolides. Because the incidence of community-acquired methicillin-resistant *S. aureus* (MRSA) infections is rapidly increasing in the United States, empiric therapy for MRSA should be strongly considered. Tetanus immunization status should be determined, and tetanus immunization should be given if needed. Patients who present with undifferentiated fever with or without generalized rash, rash without fever, or signs of encephalitis following an arthropod bite may require investigation for one of the many viral, rickettsial, or bacterial infections transmitted by these creatures (2).

Lesions caused by *Tunga penetrans* should be surgically removed by widening the pustule cavity and removing the flea intact. In myiasis, physical removal of each individual maggot, often surgically, is the only effective treatment. There are no medications or chemicals that will dislodge maggots. When exposed to a chemical insult, maggots retract into the wound, making it more difficult to remove them. In contrast, furuncular myiasis can be treated by applying petroleum jelly which suffocates the maggot, which may come wriggling out backward. "Bacon therapy" is also effective; the punctum is covered with raw meat, and in a few hours the larvae migrate into the meat and are then easily extracted. If these therapies fail, surgical removal of the intact larvae is indicated.

Since resistance of lice to topical pediculicides has increased dramatically (14,19,24), the Centers for Disease Control and Prevention (CDC) recommends treatment of head lice only if live lice are detected or if nits are found attached to hair shafts less than one-quarter inch from the scalp (12). Of the topical agents available for treatment, malathion lotion is the most effective, lindane the least effective, and permethrin and pyrethrins are intermediate in effectiveness (14). If pyrethrins or permethrin are used, a second application should be done 7 to 10 days later. A second application of malathion is not necessary. Use of a fine-toothed comb on wet hair is recommended to remove nits. Lindane should be avoided due to potential for neurotoxicity and high resistance rates. In addition, its sale and use is banned in some states (e.g., California). Mechanical removal of lice with repeated wet combing every 3 to 4 days by parents is an alternative to malathion, which is not recommended in children less than 2 years of age, but is not nearly as effective. "Natural" herbal and chemical products marketed for treatment of lice have not been shown to be effective and may be unsafe. Many schools routinely exclude children for head lice, but this practice is not recommended by the American Public Health Association. Close contacts of patients with head and pubic lice should also be treated.

Scabies should be treated with permethrin cream 5% applied to all areas of the body from the neck down and washed off after 8 to 14 hours. Lindane-resistant scabies is becoming widespread in the United States. Ivermectin 200 mg/kg orally in a single dose for adults is effective in resistant cases (not FDA-approved for this indication). Crusted ("Norwegian") scabies in immunocompromised patients should be treated with topical keratolytic agents followed by total body treatment with permethrin cream; oral ivermectin can also be used (15). An alternative treatment for pregnant and lactating women and children less than 2 months old is precipitated sulfur 6% in petrolatum. Itching may continue for 2 to 3 weeks after curative therapy and is not an indication for repeated treatment. As with lice, those who have had close contact with patients with scabies should also be treated.

To remove an attached adult tick, the tick should be grasped with blunt curved forceps, narrow tweezers, or gloved fingers as close to the point of attachment as possible, then pulled firmly and steadily in the direction of attachment (7,17). Some back-and-forth motion may be needed, but the tick should not be twisted. If the tick's head breaks off in the skin, use tweezers to remove it. Disinfect the bite site and wash hands thoroughly. This method is most effective for the large adults of *Dermacentor* and *Amblyomma* tick species, but may not be effective for adult *Ixodes* ticks or larval ticks of any species, which are much smaller. Application of viscous lidocaine 2% may also be effective (10). Application of isopropyl alcohol, petroleum jelly, a hot match, fingernail polish, or use of sharp forceps should be avoided.

An entomologist should be contacted if it is important to identify a tick or other biting arthropod that has bitten a person.

Routine antimicrobial prophylaxis after a tick bite is not necessary (4,8,21,23). The risk of acquiring Lyme disease or any other tick-borne infection after a tick bite, even in highly endemic areas, is quite low. One study concluded that doxycycline 200 mg orally in a single dose for adults may be effective in preventing Lyme disease in a highly endemic area if the tick is at least partially engorged or attached for more than 72 hours (16). If preventive treatment is prescribed, single dose doxycycline is the preferred agent for nonpregnant adults and children more than 8 years old. Although amoxicillin is an effective treatment for early Lyme disease, and is the preferred agent for pregnant women and children less than 8 years old, there is no evidence that it is an effective preventive agent following a tick bite. There is no evidence that antimicrobial treatment is effective in preventing other tick-borne infections in the United States.

Tick paralysis is treated supportively. Rapid and complete recovery occurs after removal of the tick.

CRITICAL INTERVENTIONS

- Check the skin and scalp for ticks in patients with rapidly progressive ascending flaccid paralysis, particularly children and those with a normal sensory exam, clear sensorium, and no fever
- Treat secondary bacterial infections with *antiStaphylococcal* penicillins, first-generation cephalosporins, amoxicillin-clavulanate, clindamycin, or a macrolide
- Institute infection control measures and offer treatment to those who have had close unprotected contact with patients with lice and scabies

DISPOSITION

Almost all patients suffering from arthropod bites can be discharged, unless they have life-threatening anaphylaxis, serious secondary bacterial infections of skin lesions, or are suspected to have a serious arthropod-borne systemic infectious disease or tick paralysis. Contacting an infectious disease consultant may be quite helpful in the differential diagnosis and initial treatment of patients who might have vector-borne infections.

Patients should be advised to avoid tick-infested areas. If exposure is unavoidable, the use of protective clothing, wearing light-colored clothing (making it easier to spot ticks), daily inspections of the entire body with prompt removal of ticks, and application of tick and insect repellants to skin and clothing is recommended (7). Permethrin aerosol spray is very effective when used on clothing and tents, and should not be applied to the skin. DEET (formerly called *N, N*-diethyl-m-toluamide, now called *N, N*-diethyl-3-methylbenzamide) is the most effective insect repellent that can be applied to the skin (6). Persons who have been bitten by ticks should be advised to promptly seek medical attention if they develop a fever or a skin lesion at the site of the bite up to 30 days later.

COMMON PITFALLS

✔ Failure to obtain a history of travel or exposure to environments where biting arthropods are present
✔ Failure to consider insect bites and infestations in the differential diagnosis of rashes
✔ Failure to recognize that an acute febrile illness, with or without generalized rash, may be caused by an arthropod vector-borne infection
✔ Failure to consider the possibility of other sexually transmitted diseases in persons with pubic lice

Acknowledgment

We thank previous edition chapter author Constance G. Nichols.

References

1. Anderson JF. The natural history of ticks. *Med Clin North Am* 2002;86:205–218.
2. Arboviral encephalitides. Centers for Disease Control and Prevention Web site. Available at http://www.cdc.gov/ncidod/dvbid/arbor/index.htm. Accessed November 15, 2003.
3. Arlien LG. Immunology of scabies. In: Wikel SK, ed. *The Immunology of Host-Ectoparasitic Arthropod Relationships.* Wallingford: CAB International, 1996:232–258.
4. Edlow JA. Lyme disease and related tick-borne illnesses. *Ann Emerg Med* 1999;33:680–693.
5. Elston DM, Stockwell S. What's eating you? Bedbugs. *Cutis* 2000;65:262–264.
6. Fradin MS, Day JF. Comparative efficacy of insect repellents against mosquito bites. *N Engl J Med* 2002;347:13–18.
7. Goddard J. *Physician's guide to arthropods of medical importance,* 4th ed. Boca Raton: CRC Press, 2003.
8. Hayes EB, Piesman J. Current concepts: how can we prevent Lyme disease? *N Engl J Med* 2003;348:2424–2430.
9. Iowa State University Entomology Image Gallery. Iowa State University Web site. Available at http://www.ent.iastate.edu/imagegallery/. Accessed November 1, 2003.
10. Karras DJ. Tick removal [letter]. *Ann Emerg Med* 1998;32:519.
11. Koo J, Lee CS. Delusions of parasitosis: a dermatologist's guide to diagnosis and treatment. *Am J Clin Dermatol* 2001;2:285–290.
12. Lice infestation. Centers for Disease Control and Prevention Web site. Available at http://www.cdc.gov/ncidod/dpd/parasites/lice/default/htm. Accessed November 1, 2003.
13. McGinley-Smith DE, Tsao S. Dermatoses from ticks. *J Am Acad Dermatol* 2003;49:363–392.
14. Meinking TL, Serrano L, Hard B, et al. Comparative in vitro pediculicidal efficacy of treatments in a resistant head lice population in the United States. *Arch Dermatol* 2002;138:220–224.
15. Meinking TL, Taplin D, Herminda JL, et al. The treatment of scabies with ivermectin. *N Engl J Med* 1995;333:26–30.
16. Nadelman RB, Nowakowski J, Fish D, et al. Prophylaxis with single-dose doxycycline for the prevention of Lyme disease after an Ixodes scapularis tick bite. *N Engl J Med* 2001;345:79–84.
17. Needham GR. Evaluation of five popular methods for tick removal. *Pediatrics* 1985;75:997–1002.
18. Paddock CD, Sumner JU, Comer JA, et al. Rickettsia parkeri: a newly recognized cause of spotted fever rickettsiosis in the United States. *Clin Infect Dis* 2004;38:805.
19. Roberts RJ. Head lice. *N Engl J Med* 2002;346:1645–1650.
20. Ryan ET, Wilson ME, Kain KC. Illness after international travel. *N Engl J of Med* 2002;347:505–516.
21. Shapiro ED, Gerber MA, Holabird NB, et al. A controlled trial of antimicrobial prophylaxis for Lyme disease after deer-tick bites. *N Engl J Med* 1992;327:1769–1773.
22. Singh-Behl D, La Rosa SP, Tomecki KJ. Tick-borne infections. *Dermatol Clin* 2003;21:237–244.
23. Wormser GP, Nadelman RB, Dattwyler RJ, et al. Guidelines from the Infectious Diseases Society of America–Practice guidelines for the treatment of Lyme disease. *Clin Infect Dis* 2000;31:1–14.
24. Yoon KS, Gao JR, Lee SH. Permethrin-resistant human head lice: pediculus capitis and their treatment. *Arch Dermatol* 2003;139:994–1000.

Mammal Bites and Associated Infections

Stephen J. Playe

More than a million Americans seek care for animal bites each year, accounting for about 1% of emergency department visits. One percent to 2% of these patients require hospital admission. Ten to 20 fatal dog attacks occur in the United States each year, almost always involving children. Dogs and cats inflict 95% of these animal bites, and they tend to bite the extremities of adults and older children, and the face and scalp of younger children and infants. Infectious complications are often responsible for serious morbidity and mortality.

Bite wounds are unique in several respects. Dog bites are usually crush-type lacerations with devitalized adjacent tissue. About 10% of full-thickness dog bites become infected (1,2). Cat bites tend to be puncture wounds, with an infection rate of up to 50% (1). Human bites are thought to be third most frequent after dog and cat bites. Although occlusional human bites of the extremities or trunk are mechanically similar to dog bites, the epidemiology and microbiology of human bites are different. Occupational exposure can occur in dental professionals, caretakers of the mentally impaired, daycare workers, and medical personnel involved in airway management or the care of seizing or combative patients. "Love bites" can be incurred, often involving the neck, breasts, or genitalia, during passionate sexual encounters. Biting off the tip of the nose as punishment for adultery is reported in some cultures. Teeth marks (wound imprints) have been used by forensic dental pathologists to help identify assailants. Clenched-fist injuries ("fight bites"), which occur when a fist strikes teeth during altercations, are the most serious of human bites. The microbes contained in plaque and deposits around teeth may be carried to deep structures and relatively avascular tissue planes. The patient may present with an innocuous-appearing laceration, initially offer an alternative explanation of the mechanism of injury, and subsequently develop tenosynovitis, septic arthritis, or osteomyelitis. Persistent infections can necessitate amputation. Animal bites may inoculate the site with a host of potentially pathologic microorganisms, including tetanus and rabies viruses, *Staphylococcus* spp., *Streptococcus* spp., *Corynebacterium* spp., and anaerobes (16). Human bite infections are usually polymicrobial and frequently include *S. anginosis*, *S. aureus*, *E. corrodens*, *Fusobacterium nucleatum*, and *Prevotella melaninogenica* (15). Transmission of hepatitis B, hepatitis C, and human immunodeficiency virus (HIV) must also be considered.

Pasteurella species, small gram-negative rods that are part of the normal mouth flora of many animals, have been implicated in up to 50% of infected dog bites (most often *P. canis*) and in up to 75% of infected cat bites (most often *P. multocida* subspecies *multocida* and *septica*) (5,13,16). These organisms typically produce a rapidly developing inflammatory response in the wound, often with purulent drainage, within 24 hours. *Pasteurella* species may also cause cellulitis, abscess, osteomyelitis, septic arthritis, meningitis, and septicemia.

Capnocytophaga canimorsus (DF-2), a fastidious gram-negative bacillus, can infect dog and cat bites and can lead to rapidly fatal bacteremia, disseminated intravascular coagulation, or meningitis. Although more common in immunocompromised patients (17), these infections have been reported in normal hosts (14,18).

The organism thought responsible for cat-scratch disease, *Bartonella henselae*, is a small pleomorphic bacillus identified by Warthin-Starry stain of lymph node or skin biopsies (8). The gram-negative organisms *Streptobacillus moniliformis* and *Spirillum minus* cause rat-bite fever. *Francisella tularensis* is a gram-negative coccobacillus that causes tularemia.

Herpesvirus simiae (B virus) is carried by rhesus and other macaque monkeys. It is spread to humans by bites or scratches and can lead to fatal encephalitis (10).

CLINICAL PRESENTATION

Animal bites can lead to trauma of the skin, tendons, joints, bones, major vessels, viscera, brain, and other organs. Death in immediately fatal cases is usually a result of hemorrhagic shock. Crush lacerations over the dorsum of the proximal phalanges or metacarpophalangeal joints should be presumed to be a result of clenched-fist injuries, even when patients are reluctant to offer this history. Patients who present more than 24 hours after injury frequently have signs of established local or systemic infection, as is often the case with clenched-fist injuries.

Patients with cat-scratch disease present with headache, fever, malaise, and tender regional lymphadenopathy about a week (range, 3 days–6 weeks) after a cat scratch or bite (8). A tender papule that develops at the inoculum site and subsequently blisters and heals with eschar formation or a transient macular or vesicular rash may be noted. A significant number of patients give a history of cat exposure without a wound or primary lesion. Lymph nodes may suppurate and drain spontaneously, or become nontender but remain palpable over a period of weeks to months. Complications and associated conditions include encephalitis, Parinaud syndrome (granulomatous conjunctivitis), mesenteric adenitis without splenomegaly, osteolytic bone lesions, purpura with both normal and low platelet counts, and erythema nodosum.

Patients with rat-bite fever caused by *S. moniliformis* typically develop sudden fever, chills, headache, and myalgias several days (range, 1–22 days) after a bite by a wild, laboratory, or pet rodent or carnivore, or the ingestion of food contaminated by rat excreta (4). A rash (macular, petechial, purpuric, or pustular; centripetal or generalized) and asymmetric polyarthralgia or arthritis may also be present. Complications include soft-tissue and brain abscesses and endocarditis. Patients with *S. minus* infection usually develop relapsing fever, headache (with nausea, vomiting, and photophobia), and signs of nonpurulent local infection with regional lymphangitis and adenopathy several weeks (range, 1–36 days) after the initial healing of the bite wound. A rash (macular, brown or purple) may be noted on the extremities. Endocarditis has been reported.

Patients with tularemia usually present with fever, chills, headache, malaise, myalgias, tender hepatosplenomegaly, wound ulcer, and regional adenopathy 2 to 5 days after a bite or direct or indirect skin contact with virtually any animal (e.g., amphibians, birds, fish, or mammals) (4). Skin inoculation most frequently results from exposure to wild rabbits (usually cottontails) during skinning and preparation for eating and from bites from insect vectors (e.g., ticks, deer flies, mosquitoes). Other animals that commonly harbor *F. tularensis* include beavers, cats, cattle, muskrats, sheep, and squirrels. The initial skin lesion (a bite or puncture wound or contaminated scratch) develops into a well-defined ulcer with a black base and yellow exudate. A macular rash may be present, and lymph nodes may suppurate and drain spontaneously. Contamination of the eye, throat and intestines (ingestion), or lung (inhalation) may also lead to conjunctivitis, pharyngitis, gastroenteritis, or pneumonia, all of which are associated with regional lymphadenopathy. Complications include endocarditis, meningitis, osteomyelitis, pericarditis, and peritonitis.

The presentation of human rabies varies with the time elapsed after exposure. An asymptomatic incubation period (generally 20–60 days) is followed by a prodrome of 2 to 10 days characterized by symptoms that may include pain, paresthesias, or pruritus at the site of the bite and nonspecific symptoms such as fever, headache, nausea, vomiting, and malaise. The ensuing acute neurologic phase lasts 2 to 10 days. In about 80% of cases, the "furious" signs of hyperactivity predominate; these include agitation, hallucinations, thrashing, biting, and the classic hydrophobia caused by an exaggerated respiratory tract protective reflex. In about 20% of cases, paralytic signs predominate; this is termed dumb rabies and is characterized by progressive paralysis with intact sensorium. If patients do not succumb during the acute neurologic phase, they then become comatose and die within 2 weeks (9).

Routine laboratory findings in cat-scratch disease, rat-bite fever, and tularemia are nonspecific (e.g., elevated leukocyte count and erythrocyte sedimentation rate). Cat-scratch disease is confirmed by antigen skin testing or microscopic examination of the primary skin lesion or lymph node. Rat-bite fever is confirmed by culture or antibody response to *S. moniliformis* or examination (Wright's stain or dark-field microscopy) of blood, skin lesion, or lymph node drainage in *S. minus* infections. These infections may result in false-positive syphilis tests. Tularemia is confirmed by serologic response.

DIFFERENTIAL DIAGNOSIS

With the exception of clenched-fist injuries, the history of patients presenting with animal bites is rarely obscure, and the differential diagnosis revolves mostly around determining the presence or absence of concomitant infection and underlying tissue injury.

The differential diagnosis of cat-scratch disease, rat-bite fever, and tularemia is extensive and includes infections such as plague, syphilis, lymphogranuloma venereum, sporotrichosis, anthrax, histoplasmosis, coccidioidomycosis, infectious mononucleosis, toxoplasmosis, brucellosis, bacterial adenitis, and infections with *Mycobacterium*, *Rickettsia*, *Staphylococcus*, and *Streptococcus*. Sarcoid, lymphoma, and cysts and tumors of the neck should also be considered.

Rabies must be differentiated from other infectious causes of encephalitis, including herpes, arboviruses (including West Nile virus), tetanus, malaria, rickettsia, typhoid, poliomyelitis, and botulism. Noninfectious diseases that must be considered include Guillain-Barré syndrome, poisoning, alcohol withdrawal, acute porphyria, and behavioral disorders (9).

EMERGENCY DEPARTMENT EVALUATION

Initial evaluation of acute injuries should include a primary survey, with attention to the basics of trauma care, particularly when a small victim is attacked by a large animal. The history should include details of the biting event: the time, the offending animal and its identity (wild or domestic, immunization and health status, captured or not), and the nature of the attack (provoked or unprovoked). The patient's underlying health status should also be determined.

The patient should be assessed not only for skin wounds, but also for deep-structure injury, particularly of the brain, vessels, viscera, nerves, tendons, joints, bones, and spinal cord. Puncture wounds are particularly prone to cause deep and often undiagnosed injuries. Location of the wound on the hand, wrist, foot, or joint or on the face and scalp of an infant increases the likelihood of deep-structure injury. Because clenched-fist injuries occur in flexion, they must be carefully explored throughout flexion in addition to extension to identify retained tooth fragments or tendon, joint, or bone injury. Radiographs should be obtained.

Local infectious complications include wound infection, cellulitis, abscess, osteomyelitis, prosthesis infection, and septic arthritis (even when the joint is not penetrated). Local wound infections that develop less than 24 hours after the bite are probably caused by either *P. multocida* or *streptococci*. Local infections that develop more than 48 hours after the bite are most frequently caused by *S. aureus*. Systemic complications include bacterial sepsis, meningitis, disseminated intravascular coagulation, cat-scratch disease, rat-bite fever, tetanus, tularemia, and rabies. The risk of infection is high in patients who are very young, very old, or immunocompromised; those who have prosthetic joints or valves; and those who have peripheral vascular or lymphatic compromise. Other risk factors include cat bites; puncture wounds; location on a hand, wrist, foot, or joint; and treatment delay beyond 8 hours.

Although Gram stain and culture of fresh bites do not predict infection, a Gram stain and culture (aerobic and anaerobic) should be obtained in clinically infected wounds. If sepsis is suspected, the Gram stain of the peripheral blood should be examined for evidence of *C. canimorsus*, and blood cultures (anaerobic and aerobic) should be obtained. Complete blood count; determination of blood urea nitrogen, glucose, electrolyte, and creatinine levels; prothrombin time; partial thromboplastin time; fibrin split products; and lumbar puncture with cerebrospinal fluid (CSF) analysis and culture should be obtained, if clinically indicated.

Extremity radiographs are useful to evaluate the possibility of joint penetration, fracture, foreign body, and osteomyelitis. Skull radiographs and computed tomography scanning of the head are indicated for infants with significant face and scalp bites.

The patient who presents with fever, constitutional symptoms, and regional adenopathy should be questioned about animal bites, scratches, or exposures and a history of rash or skin lesions. The extent of adenopathy and tenderness and the size of the lymph nodes, liver, and spleen should be noted. The patient should also be examined for evidence of endocarditis, meningitis, and other complications. Further assessment should include complete blood count, serum electrolyte levels, liver and kidney function studies, blood cultures, and a chest radiograph. Lumbar puncture, peripheral blood smear, lymph node and skin biopsy examination, skin testing, and antibody titers (acute and convalescent) may be necessary.

EMERGENCY DEPARTMENT MANAGEMENT

For acute injuries, prehospital care should initially focus on life-support measures. Wound care should include copious irrigation with sterile saline solution or clean tap water. Wounded extremities should be immobilized and elevated.

In the emergency department, extremity wounds should be assessed for distal function and neurovascular status before local or regional anesthesia. Extremity tourniquets may facilitate exploration and repair. The most important aspect of wound care is copious irrigation with sterile saline solution, 1% povidone–iodine solution (1:10 dilution of the commercial 10% solution), or Pluronic-68. Devitalized tissue should be débrided with a scalpel or fine dissection scissors. Excision of puncture wounds has been recommended but never proved to be effective. Abrasions should be cleansed and treated with topical antibiotics.

Primary closure of animal bite wounds is controversial. When successful, the benefits are early return of function and optimal cosmetic results. As a rule, normal hosts with relatively clean lacerations, especially of the face, can safely be sutured, primarily if seen within a few hours of injury. This practice is supported by a report of 145 sutured mammalian bites that resulted in good cosmetic outcome and a 5.5% infection rate (confidence interval = 1.8%–9.2%) (6). Alternatively, sterile skin tapes may result in a lower incidence of infection. Tissue adhesives have not been studied. Delayed primary closure, often a prudent alternative, and healing by secondary intention are less apt to result in infection. Buried sutures should be avoided whenever possible. All wounded extremities should be immobilized, and strict elevation should be advised.

Clenched-fist bite wounds are best treated by delayed primary closure or secondary intention. In gaping wounds, the edges can be loosely approximated with a minimum of sutures, provided that sufficient space is allowed for drainage. All wounds should be carefully explored, copiously irrigated, splinted, and elevated. Admission to the hand, orthopedic, or plastic surgery service should be considered if there is any injury to the tendon, joint, or bone or if signs of infection are present. Intravenous antibiotics should be administered in all cases. Abscesses and infections that involve deep structures such as tendon sheaths and joints should also be referred to a surgeon, because they may require operative management. Patients may be discharged after consultation and only when reliable, early follow-up can be assured.

Although "prophylactic" antibiotics are often prescribed, there are no prospective controlled studies with sufficient numbers of patients to demonstrate their effectiveness definitively or the superiority of a particular regimen. It seems, however, that antibiotics significantly decrease the incidence of infection in high-risk situations (3,7).

Antibiotics, whether "prophylactic" or as empirical treatment of established infections, should cover *Pasteurella* spp., *streptococci*, *staphylococci*, *C. canimorsus*, and anaerobes. Amoxicillin–clavulanic acid (875 mg twice a day), a second-generation cephalosporin with anaerobic activity (e.g., cefuroxime 500 mg twice a day), or penicillin combined with a first-generation cephalosporin or with a semisynthetic penicillin all offer an appropriately broad spectrum of activity (16). Semisynthetic penicillins or first-generation cephalosporins alone are not sufficiently effective against *P. multocida*. Penicillin-allergic patients can be given the combination of clindamycin (300 mg three times a day) with a fluoroquinolone (e.g., levofloxacin 500 mg daily). A less effective alternative is doxycycline alone (100 mg twice a day for 7 days). Azithromycin (10 mg/kg, up to 500 mg on day 1; then 5 mg/kg, up to 250 mg daily for up to 4 more days) can be used in penicillin-allergic patients who are pregnant, nursing, or less than 9 years of age. Amoxicillin-clavulanate and moxifloxacin have each demonstrated excellent *in vitro* activity against the pathogens most commonly found in infected human bites (15). Intravenous antibiotic administration (e.g., ampicillin–sulbactam 2 g; piperacillin-tazobactam 3.375 g; penicillin G 1 million units, plus nafcillin 1 g; or doxycycline 100 mg; or azithromycin 500 mg) before wound closure, although never formally studied in bites, can produce adequate penetration of the wound coagulum and is advisable in high-risk situations.

If used prophylactically, the course of therapy should be limited to 3 to 5 days, with a follow-up wound check scheduled during this period. Seven to 10 days of oral therapy is usually sufficient for the treatment of superficial wound infections. Close follow-up should be arranged. Deeper infections should be treated initially with intravenous antibiotics. In reliable patients, this can be accomplished on an outpatient basis by scheduling them to return to the emergency department or outpatient clinic. Daily reassessment should be performed until there is improvement, at which time, therapy can be continued with an oral agent and follow-up can be done less frequently.

Septic patients with a history of recent animal bites should be given broad-spectrum intravenous antibiotics initiated in the emergency department as soon as the Gram stain and culture are obtained from wounds, blood, and CSF, if indicated. Meropenem (1 g i.v.) is a reasonable choice for initial therapy pending culture results (3).

Cat-scratch disease resolves spontaneously in 1 to 2 months or can be treated with ciprofloxacin, gentamicin, erythromycin, or trimethoprim–sulfamethoxazole (11). Needle aspiration of fluctuant lymph nodes can alleviate constitutional symptoms and local pain.

Uncomplicated rat-bite fever should be treated with a 10-day course of penicillin, tetracycline, or erythromycin (500 mg orally four times a day).

Treatments of choice for tularemia are streptomycin (10–15 mg/kg i.m. twice a day) or gentamicin (2 mg/kg i.v. for loading dose) for 7 to 10 days. Patients exposed to B-virus (*H. simiae*) should receive prophylactic acyclovir (15 mg/kg i.v. every 8 hours) (10). Bites are tetanus-prone, and immunoprophylaxis should be provided as needed.

Rabies is fatal, and only supportive care can be offered once symptoms develop. Prevention depends on control of exposure, aggressive local wound care, and knowledge of transmission, which is usually by means of saliva contacting a laceration, scratch, abrasion, or mucous membrane. Postexposure prophylaxis is indicated if the offending animal is known or clinically suspected to be rabid or if it is a bat or wild carnivore (e.g., a bobcat, coyote, fox, raccoon, skunk, or wolf) (4,8). The silver-haired bat variant of rabies virus is able to replicate in the superficial dermis and has been associated with several recent cases of human rabies without known history of conventional exposure. For this reason, postexposure prophylaxis is now recommended for persons who may have come in contact with a bat (e.g., an infant or a sleeping adult in a room with a bat, even if a bite or scratch wound is not apparent) (12). Livestock and unprovoked dog and cat bites should be considered individually in consultation with public health officials.

Patients bitten by healthy dogs and cats do not require immunization, provided the animal can be observed for 10 days for signs of illness. Rabbit and rodent (e.g., hamster, mouse, rat, squirrel) bites do not require treatment unless the animal is wild and rabies is endemic in the offending species. Patients who have not been previously immunized should receive both human rabies immune globulin (20 IU/kg), up to half the dose infiltrated at the bite site if anatomically feasible, and the remainder given i.m. (e.g., deltoid), and human diploid cell rabies vaccine (1 mL i.m. on days 0, 3, 7, 14, and 28).

Because hepatitis B can be transmitted by saliva, all human bites must be considered for hepatitis B prophylaxis according to the risk evaluation of the source. Although saliva contains only low concentrations of HIV, there is often admixture of blood in bite situations. This is the case in occlusional bites by persons with friable gingiva or seizing patients who have bitten their tongue. Clenched-fist injuries have significant risk for HIV transmission, especially when a lip laceration was sustained at the time of the altercation. In these situations, postexposure HIV treatment should be offered.

CRITICAL INTERVENTIONS

- Explore all bite wounds for foreign bodies and deep structure injury
- Evaluate small children with dog bites for vital organ injury
- Administer antibiotic therapy for established infections, and postexposure "prophylactic" antibiotics to prevent bacterial infection in fresh bites
- Arrange for a recheck of all but minor animal bite wounds in 24 to 72 hours
- Consider the possibility of viral disease transmission (HIV, hepatitis, rabies) and initiate appropriate treatment in suspect cases

DISPOSITION

Consultation with an infectious disease specialist and a microbiologist (for a careful search for organisms unique to animal bites) is advisable in cases of septicemia. Infectious disease consultation should be considered in cases of possible HIV, hepatitis B, or C transmission. A surgeon (general, hand, plastic, or orthopedic, depending on local practices) should be consulted when there is violation of a deep structure (such as a joint, bone, tendon, or internal organ), extensive facial damage, tissue loss, or a clenched-fist bite. Bites by potentially rabid animals should be reported to state public health officials. All bite wounds should be reported to local agencies.

Patients who sustain major trauma, significant blood loss, or injuries that require operative intervention usually need to be admitted. Those who require i.v. antibiotics (e.g., systemic, central nervous system, hand, joint, or other deep-structure infection or any infection in a high-risk patient) or who cannot receive proper care as outpatients should also be admitted. Clenched-fist injuries with involvement of tendon, joint, or bone should be considered for admission. All patients who do not require admission should be rechecked in 24 to 72 hours for signs of infection. If signs of infection develop, sutures must be removed and the wound left opened for drainage. Transfer to another institution should be arranged whenever appropriate inpatient facilities or consultants are unavailable.

COMMON PITFALLS

✔ Failure to diagnose joint penetration and tendon injury and to refrain from primary closure in clenched-fist bites

✔ Failure to close facial and other wounds that are at low risk for infection
✔ Failure to immobilize and elevate injured extremities
✔ Failure to provide rabies immunization after possible bat exposure
✔ Failure to identify and admit infected immunocompromised patients

Acknowledgment

We thank previous edition chapter author Richard V. Aghababian.

References

1. Aghababian RV, Conte JE. Mammalian bite wounds. *Ann Emerg Med* 1980;9:79.
2. Callaham M. Dog bite wounds. *JAMA* 1980;244:2327.
3. Callaham M. Prophylactic antibiotics in common dog bite wounds: a controlled study. *Ann Emerg Med* 1980;9:410.
4. Callaham ML. Domestic and feral mammalian bites. In: Auerbach PS, Geehr EC, eds. *Management of wilderness and environmental emergencies*, 3rd ed. St. Louis: Mosby, 1995.
5. Chapple CR, Fraser AN. Pasteurella multocida wound infections—a commonly unrecognized problem in the casualty department. *Injury* 1986;17:410.
6. Chen E, Hornig S, Shepherd S, et al. Primary closure of mammalian bites. *Acad Emerg Med* 2000;7(2):157.
7. Cummings PC. Antibiotics to prevent infection in patients with dog bite wounds: a meta-analysis of randomized trials. *Ann Emerg Med* 1994;23:535.
8. Elliot DL, Tolle SW, Goldberg L, et al. Pet-associated illness. *N Engl J Med* 1985;313:985.
9. Fishbein DB. Rabies in humans. In: Baer GM, ed. *The natural history of rabies*. Boca Raton, FL: CRC Press, 1991.
10. Holmes GP, Chapman LE, Stewart JA, et al. Guidelines for the prevention and treatment of B-virus infections in exposed persons. *Clin Infect Dis* 1995;20:421.
11. Margileth AM. Antibiotic therapy for cat-scratch disease: clinical study of therapeutic outcome in 268 patients and a review of the literature. *Pediatr Infect Dis J* 1992;11:6.
12. Morimoto K, Patel M, Corisdeo S, et al. Characterization of a unique variant of bat rabies virus responsible for newly emerging human cases in North America. *Proc Natl Acad Sci U S A* 1996;93:5653.
13. Ordog GJ. The bacteriology of dog bite wounds on initial presentation. *Ann Emerg Med* 1986;15:1324.
14. Pers C, Kristiansen JE, Scheibel JH, et al. Fatal septicemia caused by DF-2 in a previously healthy man. *Scand J Infect Dis* 1986;18:265.
15. Talan DA, Abrahamian FM, Moran GJ, et al. Clinical presentation and bacteriologic analysis of infected human bites in patients presenting to emergency departments. *Clin Infect Dis* 2003;37.
16. Talan DA, Citron DM, Abrahamian EM, et al. Bacteriologic analysis of infected dog and cat bites. *N Engl J Med* 1999;340:85.
17. Underman A. Bite wounds inflicted by dogs and cats. *Vet Clin North Am Small Anim Pract* 1987;17:195.
18. Weber DJ, Hansen AR. Infections resulting from animal bites. *Infect Dis Clin North Am* 1991;5:3.

PART II

Physical Agents

CHAPTER 351
Hypothermia

Andrew K. Chang

Hypothermia is defined as a core temperature less than 35°C (95°F) (3,10,21) and can be classified in different ways. In terms of severity, hypothermia may be classified as mild (35°C–32°C), moderate (32°C–28°C), and severe (less than 28°C). This classification is important because it changes which types of treatment options are used. Hypothermia may also be classified regarding the cause. Primary hypothermia is usually a result of environmental exposure. In contrast, secondary, or "urban," hypothermia occurs in those with predisposing illness, infirmity, intoxication, or extremes of age (3,4). Secondary hypothermia is much more common than primary hypothermia and has a very high mortality rate, approaching 100% in severe cases. In contrast, recovery is the rule for young, healthy adults with primary hypothermia, with case reports of survival from core temperatures as low as 16°C (61°F) (17). In terms of duration, hypothermia of less than 6 hours is classified as acute, although longer durations are considered chronic.

Human temperature is tightly regulated such that the normal diurnal variation is only 1°C around the normal core temperature of 37.2°C to 37.7°C (5). Thermosensors in the skin, spinal cord, and gastrointestinal tract detect changes in body temperature. Afferent impulses are integrated within the spinal cord and transmitted to the hypothalamus, which serves as the central thermoregulatory center. Both neural (vasomotor) and hormonal (e.g., catecholamines, thyroxine) hypothalamic efferents control the balance between heat production and heat loss.

Metabolic activity in the heart and liver contribute most of the endogenous heat production. Newborns can also produce heat by nonshivering thermogenesis, in which specialized adipose tissue (brown fat) can directly transform substrate into heat as a result of the unusually high density of mitochondria (18).

Heat is lost by conduction (direct contact with colder objects, such as ground, snow, and water), convection (air motion across body surfaces), evaporation (from skin, lungs, or wet clothing), and radiation (from exposed surfaces). The rate of heat loss is proportional to the difference between body and environmental temperature. Normal heat dissipation occurs predominantly by radiation, with 90% of heat loss occurring through the skin. The lungs, through evaporation, contribute most of the rest.

Any condition that results in decreased heat production, increased heat loss, or impaired temperature regulation may result in hypothermia (Table 351.1) (3,10,21). Although New York and Pennsylvania had the greatest number of hypothermia related deaths in 1999 (36 each) (14), very low ambient temperatures are not required and hypothermia can occur during all seasons and in all locations (5).

The initial response to cooling includes cutaneous vasoconstriction, shivering, and increased metabolic activity (3,4,10,12,22). Shivering thermogenesis increases heat production from 250 to 1000 kcal per hour (5). Without adequate insulation and intact thermoregulatory mechanisms, exposure to any temperature below 35°C can result in hypothermia. When the core temperature falls below 30°C, the patient becomes poikilothermic and cools to the ambient temperature (5). Neonates are especially at risk because of a relatively large body surface area relative to total mass and ineffective shivering and heat production. The elderly are also at risk as a result of low fat stores, medication effects, lower metabolic rate, relative inability to detect temperature changes, and deteriorating adaptive responses.

Ethanol and drug use may increase heat loss as a result of cutaneous vasodilatation and impaired shivering. Hypothalamic dysfunction and decreased ability to seek shelter from the cold also may contribute. Sepsis, endocrine dysfunction (diabetic ketoacidosis, hypoglycemia, hypothyroidism, hypopituitarism, hypoadrenalism), central nervous system (CNS) disorders (stroke, brain tumors, spinal cord injury), and skin conditions (burns, erythroderma, psoriasis, ichthyosis) are additional predisposing factors. Lengthy exposure times, cool i.v. fluid infusions, and general anesthesia contribute to the hypothermia often seen in trauma victims (4,13,18).

Decreased tissue oxygenation results from hypoventilation, vasoconstriction, increased blood viscosity, ventilation–perfusion mismatch, shifting of the oxyhemoglobin dissociation curve to the left, and volume depletion as a result of cold-induced diuresis. Furthermore, shivering increases lactate production, which, along with poor perfusion of tissues, decreased acid excretion, and impaired hepatic metabolism, contributes to a metabolic acidosis.

CLINICAL PRESENTATION

The physiologic changes that occur during hypothermia are summarized in Table 351.2 (2,3,4,12,21). Mild hypothermia is associated with an initial excitatory response, as reflected by elevations of the pulse, blood pressure, and respirations. Facial

TABLE 351.1. Predisposing Factors in Hypothermia

Decreased Heat Production	Increased Heat Loss
CNS depression (metabolic or traumatic) Immobility (age, neuromuscular disorders) Endocrine failure (adrenal/pituitary/thyroid) Hypoglycemia/malnutrition	Environmental exposure: inadequate clothing/shelter, wind chill, low humidity, perspiration, wet clothing Exfoliative skin disease Vasodilatation Drugs Neuropathy
Hypothalamic Dysfunction	Sepsis Shock Burns
Acidosis/anoxia CNS hemorrhage/infarction Drugs (e.g., phenothiazines) Encephalopathy	Iatrogenic Cooling
	Use of large volumes of cool (<35°C [95°F]) fluids for lavage or i.v. administration; overly aggressive treatment of hyperthermia

immersion in cold water, however, can cause vagally mediated bradycardia (the diving reflex) and apnea. Other manifestations of mild hypothermia include apathy, confusion, lethargy, fatigue, forgetfulness, incoordination, slurred speech, muscle tremor, and shivering. Cessation of shivering occurs at temperatures less than 32°C and this heralds the onset of moderate hypothermia. Pulse, blood pressure, and respirations now become decreased. Disorientation, stupor, inappropriate behavior, ileus, polyuria, rhonchi, and wheezing may be noted. In severe hypothermia, pulse and blood pressure may be undetectable and respirations decreased such that the patient might be presumed to be dead.

After the initial excitatory tachycardia, atropine-resistant bradycardia commonly ensues as a result of decreased spontaneous depolarization of pacemaker cells. Atrial fibrillation is commonly seen and usually converts spontaneously to a sinus rhythm during rewarming. Intervals progressively become prolonged, starting with the PR, then the QRS, and finally the QTc. Other ECG findings include decreased P-wave amplitude, T-wave changes, and premature ventricular contractions. Osborn or J waves, which are present at the junction of the QRS complex and ST segment, may also be seen. It is important to note that Osborn waves are neither pathognomonic nor prognostic in hypothermia (7), and they may also be seen with CNS lesions, focal cardiac ischemia, sepsis, and as a normal variant in young healthy persons (5).

Laboratory findings include respiratory alkalosis in mild hypothermia. Hypoxia, metabolic and respiratory acidosis, increased amylase and hematocrit, and leukopenia, thrombocytopenia, and variable electrolyte abnormalities are seen in moderate and severe hypothermia. Hypothermia can mask potassium-induced changes in the ECG, so potassium levels should be checked frequently, especially if there is concurrent metabolic acidosis, rhabdomyolysis, or renal failure (4). Cold directly inhibits the enzymatic reactions of the coagulation cascade, so hypothermic patients are often coagulopathic despite the presence of normal levels of clotting factors and normal prothrombin and partial-thromboplastin times (4) (these tests are routinely performed only after being warmed to 37°C). Hyperglycemia and, less commonly, hypoglycemia can be seen. The chest radiograph may disclose pulmonary infiltrates characteristic of aspiration or pneumonia. Other abnormalities may be present in patients with coexisting illness or injury.

DIFFERENTIAL DIAGNOSIS

Unless an accurate core (rectal or esophageal) temperature is obtained, hypothermia may be confused with virtually any endocrine, metabolic, toxic, traumatic, or vascular condition causing CNS depression. Even after the diagnosis has been made, it is necessary to distinguish between primary and secondary hypothermia by ruling out predisposing pathology.

The lack of detectable vital signs on physical examination in severe hypothermia may lead to a misdiagnosis of death; careful and prolonged observation, an ECG, intraarterial blood pressure monitoring, core temperature measurement, and reassessment after warming can prevent this error.

EMERGENCY DEPARTMENT EVALUATION

The diagnosis of hypothermia may be suggested by the setting in which the patient was found (e.g., cool or cold, indoor or outdoor

TABLE 351.2. Physiologic Changes During Hypothermia

Stage of Hypothermia	Central Nervous System	Organ System			
		Cardiovascular	Respiratory	Dermatologic/ Neuromuscular	Renal/ Gastrointestinal (GI)
Mild (32.2°C–35.0°C) (Excitation Phase)	Apathy	Tachycardia	Tachypnea	Shivering	Cold-induced diuresis
	Hyperreflexia	Hypertension	Bronchorrhea	Vasoconstriction	Decreased GI motility
Moderate (28.0°C–32.3°C) (Slowing Phase)	Disorientation EEG abnormal	Increased CO Bradycardia	Bronchospasm Bradypnea	Increased tone Decreased shivering	Constipation Ileus
	Hyporeflexia Paradoxical undressing	Hypotension Increased atrial dysrhythmia	Diminished gag Decreased O$_2$ consumption	Spasm	GI erosions Hepatic necrosis/ pancreatitis
Severe (<28°C)	Coma Areflexia	Asystole Ventricular dysrhythmia	Pulmonary edema Apnea	Rigidity Compartment syndrome	Oliguria Decreased renal blood flow
	Flattening EEG				

CO, cardiac output; EEG, electroencephalogram.

environment), although the history obtained from a hypothermic patient may be unreliable (5). The length and conditions of exposure, underlying medical problems, recent illnesses, and medications should be noted. Any patient with altered mental status should have a core temperature measured; the same is true for initially normothermic or hyperthermic patients treated with cooling measures or large volumes of intravenous or lavage solutions.

An esophageal or rectal probe (thermocouple) or a thermometer capable of measuring low temperatures (below the usual 34°C) is required for an accurate diagnosis. The rectal probe should be placed to a depth of 15cm. A false reading can occur if the probe is placed in contact with cold feces (5). Simultaneous esophageal temperature measurements may be helpful in the intubated patient, although probe reliability is often poor if heated inhalational therapy is used (5).

The physical examination initially focuses on vital signs and the neurologic, cardiovascular, and pulmonary systems. In severe cases, observation for 2 minutes or longer may be required to detect a pulse or respirations. Doppler ultrasound may be necessary to locate a pulse and should be supported by continuous ECG monitoring (5). A detailed examination should then be performed, searching for coexisting pathology. An ECG and chest radiograph are usually indicated.

In moderate and severe hypothermia, routine laboratory tests should include arterial blood gas measurement; a complete blood count; measurement of amylase, electrolytes, glucose, blood urea nitrogen, and creatinine; a coagulation profile; and urinalysis. Additional tests, such as bacteriologic cultures; measurement of calcium, magnesium, phosphate, lactate, ketones, cortisol, and cardiac enzymes; liver and thyroid function tests; and toxicology screening, may also be necessary to elucidate concomitant medical problems (21).

The interpretation of arterial blood gas results in hypothermia is controversial. All blood gas samples are first warmed to 37°C. Because the pH increases (0.015 U/°C) and the Pco_2 (4.4%/°C) and Po_2 (7.2%/°C) decrease at temperatures below 37°C as the result of changes in gas solubility, measurement of these parameters in samples warmed to 37°C will result in a falsely decreased pH and increased Pco_2 and Po_2 levels if not corrected for temperature. However, the pH of neutrality increases as temperature decreases. Therefore, the normal pH at room temperature (7.40) is relatively acidic in a hypothermic state, and the uncorrected results of an arterial blood gas analysis may better guide therapy for acid–base disturbances (10,11).

EMERGENCY DEPARTMENT MANAGEMENT

In the prehospital setting, the patient should be protected from further cooling. Wet clothes should be removed, the ambulance should be heated, and the patient should be covered with blankets. All patients should receive oxygen, cardiac monitoring, and an i.v. line should be established. If a pulse is detected, cardiopulmonary resuscitation (CPR) should not be performed because it may precipitate ventricular tachycardia, ventricular fibrillation (VF), or asystole. Ventilation should be assisted by a bag-mask device, and the patient should be moved as little as possible. Hyperventilation should be avoided, as it may induce alkalosis and result in VF.

Emergency department management depends on severity (3,4,10,12,21). Nearly all patients require volume expansion. Normal saline with dextrose is preferable to lactated Ringer's because lactate may not be metabolized by the liver during hypothermia. The volume of fluid should be determined by tissue perfusion and vital signs. If central lines are required, the femoral route may be preferred because guide wires and catheters may precipitate

dysrhythmias if inserted into the right atrium (5) using the internal jugular or subclavian approach. Pulmonary artery catheters should be reserved for complex cases. Room-temperature i.v. fluids are acceptable for mild hypothermia, unless the rapid infusion of large volumes is necessary (e.g., patients with bleeding or severe dehydration). In moderate and severe hypothermia, intravenous fluids should be warmed because room-temperature i.v. fluids are relatively hypothermic compared with most patients suffering from hypothermia. If a blood warmer is unavailable, 1 L of room-temperature i.v. fluid may be warmed in a standard microwave oven (high setting for 1–2 minutes, depending on wattage) (6). Fluids should be warmed to 40°C to 42°C, although some authors suggest that higher temperatures may be safe (5).

Intubation should be performed as needed. In one review, rapid sequence intubation is not recommended in severe and some moderate hypothermic patients because neuromuscular blockade is ineffective at temperatures less than 30°C (86°F) (7). Although intubation is unlikely to induce dysrhythmias (5), it is generally advised that intubation be done with as little airway manipulation as possible. The oral route is preferred as a result of the risk of traumatic bleeding with the nasal route because patients are likely to be coagulopathic. If muscle rigidity of the jaw precludes the oral route and the patient has some spontaneous respirations, then topical vasoconstrictors and a smaller sized endotracheal tube may facilitate blind nasotracheal intubation.

In hypothermic patients, the threshold for VF is decreased as cold temperature causes the myocardium to become irritable. Pulseless rhythms should be treated according to advanced cardiac life-support guidelines, although warming should take precedence, because chemical and electrical treatment of dysrhythmias is usually ineffective at temperatures below 30°C. For many years, bretylium has been considered the drug of choice for VF in hypothermia based on animal studies (15). However, bretylium is no longer listed in the 2000 ACLS guidelines for hypothermia even though it is still available from the manufacturer. Although open cardiac massage in conjunction with mediastinal lavage using warm saline has been advocated for pulseless rhythms, its efficacy remains to be determined. Supraventricular dysrhythmias will generally convert spontaneously during or within 24 hours of rewarming.

Rewarming methods are divided into passive and active techniques. Passive rewarming includes removal of the patient from a cold environment and the use of dry insulating materials (e.g., a warm blanket or an aluminized body cover). Blocking wind results in decreased heat escaping via radiation, convection, and conduction. Passive rewarming is appropriate for adults with mild, primary hypothermia. Warm blankets and shivering will generally increase body temperature by an average of 0.4°C per hour.

Active rewarming involves the direct transfer of exogenous heat to a patient and is usually required in neonates and adults with secondary hypothermia. Because protective mechanisms such as shivering thermogenesis become extinguished at temperatures less than 32°C, active rewarming is also generally indicated in patients with moderate or severe hypothermia. Other indications include cardiovascular instability, inadequate rewarming with other methods, endocrinologic insufficiency, and traumatic peripheral vasodilatation (e.g., spinal-cord injury) (7). Heat from active rewarming can be delivered externally or to the core.

Active external rewarming delivers heat directly to the skin. Examples include hot water bottles, heating pads and blankets, forced air-warming systems such as the Bair Hugger, and immersion in a 40°C water bath. Active core rewarming may be accomplished by providing warm intravenous fluids; humidified air or oxygen (by mask or ventilator) heated to 42°C to 45°C (mouth temperature); peritoneal, gastric, bladder, or colonic lavage with 45°C fluid; blood warming by hemodialysis (with an in-line heat exchanger) or femoral–femoral (partial) cardiopulmonary bypass pump; and warmed pleuromediastinal lavage via thoracostomy or thoracotomy (1–4,9,10,12,19,21).

Inhalational warming, using a cascade humidifier, is safe, easy, and readily available and can increase the core temperature by about 1°C per hour. Gastric, bladder, colonic, and pleuromediastinal lavages are less efficacious. Bath rewarming is more effective than inhalation rewarming but monitoring becomes difficult. Peritoneal lavage can increase the temperature by 2°C to 4°C per hour, whereas extracorporeal techniques can achieve warming rates of up to 10°C per hour. Cardiopulmonary bypass (CB) can support the circulation in lieu of prolonged CPR. Although not as rapid as CB, hemodialysis may be advantageous in the hypothermic patient who also has a coincident drug overdose responsive to dialysis (8).

The optimal rate of rewarming depends on the cardiopulmonary status and the degree of hypothermia. Animal studies suggest that slow rewarming (maintaining an intramyocardial temperature gradient of less than 2°C) minimizes the risk of VF. Hence, invasive procedures should generally be reserved for hemodynamically unstable patients with severe hypothermia. When used in such instances, the most effective techniques available should be employed in order to minimize the rewarming time.

Core temperature afterdrop and rewarming shock are possible complications that can occur with rewarming. Afterdrop is thought to occur either from cold blood that returns to the core after external warming causes peripheral vasodilatation or from continued conduction of heat from the warmer core to the colder periphery. Rewarming shock has generally been attributed to peripheral vasodilation and venous pooling, although some research suggests that cardiac insufficiency and alteration of the peripheral vascular bed may play a role (20). Because there are both central and peripheral thermosensors, afterdrop is theoretically possible with any rewarming technique.

The magnitude and duration of afterdrop appears to be lower with bath rewarming than with spontaneous or inhalation techniques (16). Additionally, metabolic rates are increased with surface rewarming but not by inhalation (8). It thus appears that active surface rewarming is not contraindicated, as previously speculated. Some authors recommend combining truncal active external rewarming with active core rewarming in order to avoid potential side effects (5).

Gastric and bladder catheterization are indicated at temperatures less than 32°C because ileus and fluids shifts are commonly encountered in patients at such temperatures (4).

Additional measures should include correction of underlying metabolic derangements and the treatment of coexisting or secondary medical or surgical problems.

Because the cerebral ischemic tolerance during cardiopulmonary arrest is considerably longer and may be without sequelae in the severely hypothermic patient (7), resuscitation should not be considered unsuccessful until the core temperature has been raised to at least 32°C (19). This gives rise to the commonly used axiom, "the patient is not dead until he is warm and dead."

CRITICAL INTERVENTIONS

- Obtain accurate core body temperature measurements in patients suspected of having hypothermia
- If possible, avoid physical stimulation, airway manipulation, and invasive procedures that may precipitate cardiac dysrhythmias

---

- Treat mild to moderate hypothermia with noninvasive rewarming techniques such as warm forced-air blankets, warmed i.v. fluids, and warmed, humidified air
- Treat severe hypothermia with additional invasive rewarming measures such as warm saline lavage of the stomach, peritoneum, bladder, or pleuromediastinal cavity, and CB
- Replace volume deficits with i.v. fluids and continue resuscitation attempts until the core temperature is at least 32° C

DISPOSITION

Patients with mild hypothermia should be observed until they are asymptomatic and normothermic. Those with extremes of age or coexisting underlying pathology should be admitted for further evaluation and treatment. Patients with moderate or severe hypothermia should be admitted to an intensive care unit. Those with unstable vital signs or a core temperature below 28°C should be transferred by an advanced life-support unit to a facility capable of performing extracorporeal rewarming, if such services are not available at the current facility.

COMMON PITFALLS

✔ Failure to consider the diagnosis of hypothermia in patients with altered mental status
✔ Failure to search diligently for underlying causes of secondary hypothermia
✔ Failure to recognize that chemical and electrical treatment of dysrhythmias is generally ineffective at temperatures below 28°C
✔ Failing to monitor for core temperature after drop

Acknowledgment

The author thanks the contribution of Joseph J. Currier who wrote the previous version of this chapter.

References

1. Baumgartner FJ, Janusz MT, Jamieson WR, et al. Cardiopulmonary bypass for resuscitation of patients with accidental hypothermia and cardiac arrest. *Can J Surg* 1992;35:184.
2. Bolgiano E, Sykes L, Barish RA, et al. Accidental hypothermia with cardiac arrest: recovery following rewarming by cardiopulmonary bypass. *J Emerg Med* 1992;10:427.
3. Curley FJ, Irwin RS. Disorders of temperature control, part III. *J Intensive Care Med* 1986;1:5.
4. Danzl DF, Pozos RS. Accidental hypothermia. *N Engl J Med* 1994;331:26.
5. Danzl DF, Pozos RS, Hamlet MP. Accidental hypothermia. In: Auerbach PS, ed. *Wilderness medicine: management of wilderness and environmental emergencies,* 3rd ed. Mosby, 1995.
6. Gong V. Microwave rewarming of IV fluids in management of hypothermia. *Ann Emerg Med* 1984;13:116.
7. Hanania NA, Zimmerman JL. Accidental Hypothermia. *Critical Care Clinics* 1999;15:235–249.
8. Hernandez E, Praga M, Alcazar JM, et al. Hemodialysis for treatment of accidental hypothermia. *Nephron* 1993;63:214.
9. Ireland KW, Follette DM, Iquidbashian J, et al. Use of a heat exchanger to prevent hypothermia during thoracic and thoracoabdominal aneurysm repairs. *Ann Thorac Surg* 1993;55:534.
10. Jolly B, Ghezzi K. Accidental hypothermia. *Emerg Clin North Am* 1992;10:311.
11. Kofstad J. Blood gases and hypothermia: some theoretical and practical considerations. *Scand J Clin Lab Invest* 1996;56:224.
12. Lazar HL. The treatment of hypothermia. *N Engl J Med* 1997;337:21.
13. Marion DW, Leonov Y, et al. Resuscitative hypothermia. *Crit Care Med* 1996;24:2.
14. National Center for Health Statistics. *Compressed mortality file.* Hyattsville, Maryland: U.S. Dept of Heath and Human Services, CDC, National Center for Health Statistics, 2002.
15. Orts A, Alcaraz C, Delaney KA, et al. Bretylium tosylate and electrically induced cardiac arrhythmias during hypothermia in dogs. *Am J Emerg Med* 1992;10:4.

16. Romet TT, Hoskin RW. Temperature and metabolic response to inhalation and bath rewarming protocols. *Aviat Space Environ Med* 1988;59:630.
17. Sekar T, MacDonnell K, Namsirikul P, et al. Survival after prolonged submersion in cold water without neurologic sequelae. *Arch Intern Med* 1980;140:775.
18. Sessler DI. Mild perioperative hypothermia. *N Engl J Med* 1997;336:24.
19. Steele MT, Nelson MJ, Dessler DI, et al. Forced air speeds rewarming in accidental hypothermia. *Ann Emerg Med* 1996;27:4.
20. Tveita T. Rewarming from hypothermia. New aspects on the pathophysiology of rewarming shock. *Int J Circumpolar Health* 2000;59:260–266.
21. Weinberg A. Hypothermia. *Ann Emerg Med* 1993;22:370.

CHAPTER 352
Cold-Induced Tissue Injuries

Joseph M. Weber and Scott C. Sherman

The first detailed descriptions of cold-induced tissue injury are attributed to Napoleon's surgeon general, Baron Dominique-Jean Larrey. While retreating from Moscow in the winter of 1812–1813, Larrey recognized the ill effects of the freeze-thaw-freeze cycle when he witnessed soldiers thawing their feet by campfires at night, only to march again in the cold the next day. He proposed that the limbs should be rewarmed slowly by rubbing them with wet snow, which became the accepted practice for more than a century. In the 1930s and 1940s, research described the benefits of rapid rewarming (17). In the 1960s, Mills popularized what has become the cornerstone of treatment today—warm the frozen limb in a 40°C to 42°C water bath, avoid additional trauma, and use whirlpool baths to débride necrotic tissue (17). One landmark study from Chicago at Cook County Hospital documented the epidemiology of cold injuries among a mostly indigent patient population. The authors described 1,043 patients over a 10-year period from 1962–1972 who were treated for cold injuries. The most dramatic incidence of injury occurred on New Year's Eve and Day 1968–1969 when the temperature dropped from 31°C to -8°C in less than 9 hours and 38 patients were admitted for cold injury (2).

Today, as a result of better availability of warm shelters among the urban homeless, improved patient awareness, and better protective clothing, the number of cases of frostbite has decreased. Immersion foot, however, is still common, especially among the homeless (25). Recent reports of unusual causes of cold-induced tissue injury remind the clinician that these injuries can occur in any climate. Recreational inhalation of nitrous oxide and fluorinated hydrocarbons have caused frostbite to the face and cold-induced swelling that can compromise the airway (9,10). Another example is frostbite resulting from the inappropriate application of ice packs (16). No matter where they practice, emergency physicians should have an understanding of the pathophysiology and treatment of cold-induced tissue injuries in order to render optimal care.

As tissue temperatures drop to 10°C, cutaneous sensation is lost and capillary blood flow decreases. With temperatures from 3°C to 11°C, cutaneous capillary blood flow is reduced 60% and 5- to 10-minute cycles of vasodilatation and vasoconstriction begin to occur, in order to both preserve core temperatures and to provide blood flow to the extremity. When core temperatures are threatened, however, blood flow to the extremity becomes negligible and skin temperatures may drop as much as 0.5°C per minute.

In frostbite, ice crystals form in the extracellular space at tissue temperatures below 0°C. Frostbite requires ambient temperatures of -6°C to -15°C, as radiation of heat from deeper tissues maintains surface temperatures somewhat above the environment. Irreversible tissue harm begins when extracellular ice crystal formation draws water from intracellular spaces by osmosis, causing intracellular dehydration and enzymatic disruption. With further cooling or rapid freezing (10°C per minute), intracellular ice crystals cause further cellular damage. The endothelium and nerve tissues are more sensitive to cold than muscle, bone, and cartilage, and therefore are the first to be injured.

On rewarming, reperfusion creates an environment of progressive microvascular ischemia. This secondary insult is the result of multiple factors. Fluid extravasates through previously damaged endothelium. The interstitial fluid is rich in inflammatory mediators (prostaglandin and thromboxane) that promote vasoconstriction, and platelet and leukocyte aggregation. Edema formation and endothelial injury may arrest capillary and arteriolar blood flow. Blister formation occurs secondary to vascular injury. Clear blisters form from extracellular exudation of fluid. Hemorrhagic blisters occur when deeper subdermal vessels are disrupted, indicating more severe tissue injury. The end result is arterial thrombosis, ischemia, and ultimately necrosis.

The pathophysiology of nonfreezing cold-induced tissue injuries has many similarities to frostbite. In frostnip, reversible superficial ice crystal formation and intense vasoconstriction occur without tissue destruction. The tissue changes of chilblains result from vascular inflammation and tissue hypoxia secondary to cold-induced vasoconstriction. In patients with immersion foot, the tissues are saturated with water such that the thick stratum corneum of the soles and feet becomes swollen, thickened, and fragmented. There is variable edema of the upper dermis. An inflammatory response ensues, influenced by the water itself in most cases, not a concomitant fungal or bacterial process. The thinner stratum corneum of the dorsum of the foot does not absorb as much water and therefore is less likely to be involved. When exposure to significantly colder water occurs, there is an added insult of vasospasm, intravascular thrombosis, and damage to nerve, fat, and muscle. Thus, the threshold for developing immersion foot is decreased in cold environments. Cold water causes injury in less than 48 hours vs. up to 72 hours in warmer conditions.

The development of frostbite depends on more than ambient temperature: duration of exposure, wind chill, humidity, and wet skin (and clothing) all increase the likelihood of frostbite. Other predisposing factors include alcohol consumption, psychiatric illness, vehicular failure, and drug misuse (23). Greater duration of exposure worsens outcome and is more predictive of injury than the ambient temperature alone (15).

CLINICAL PRESENTATION

Cold-induced tissue injuries present in various forms—frostnip, chilblains, immersion foot, and frostbite. Frostnip is the most mild form and presents with numbness, pain, pallor, and paresthesias to the affected extremity. The distal extremities—fingers, toes, ears, and nose—are most commonly involved. Frostnip usually resolves within 30 minutes, so persistent symptoms suggest an alternate diagnosis.

Chilblains usually occurs in patients with an underlying vasculitis after repeated exposure to dry, above-freezing cold temperatures. Patients present with erythema, edema, pruritus, and a burning sensation. Rarely, ulcerations, vesicles, and bullae may form. The lesions may have a purple or blue appearance. Commonly affected areas include the hands, feet, and pretibial areas. Manifestations occur 12 to 24 hours following cold and damp exposure. The condition is recurrent in some individuals with repeated exposures, and this form is often bilateral and symmetric.

Immersion foot (also known as trench foot) can occur at any temperature, but is more severe when wet exposure is combined with a cold environment. Although a wet environment is a prerequisite, perspiration and absorbent socks may be all that is required. Another common element is time, as immersion foot usually develops slowly over hours to days. Immersion foot is the most commonly encountered cold-induced injury and occurs frequently in the homeless. Numbness and pain are common, and may be so severe that the patient is unable to ambulate. The affected foot is cool, erythematous, and edematous (25). The distinction between immersion foot and the postthaw phase of frostbite may be difficult and therefore, a detailed history is essential.

Frostbite, not unlike frostnip, commonly occurs on the digits, nose, and ear. Initially, the frozen tissue is mottled and violaceous. As rewarming occurs, the tissue becomes hyperemic and the initially insensate extremity regains some sensation. After rewarming, frostbite can be classified into superficial (first and second degree) and deep (third and fourth degree) injury (Table 352.1).

The appearance of first-degree frostbite is of a pale, white epidermis with surrounding erythema. Second-degree frostbite is heralded by clear blister formation with surrounding erythema and edema, and third-degree frostbite consists of hemorrhagic blister formation, indicating deeper tissue injury. Fourth-degree frostbite consists of necrosis and tissue loss. Caution must be exercised, however, as this classification system does not always provide an accurate prognosis, nor does it alter initial management. Poor prognostic indicators include dark fluid-filled blisters, nonblanching cyanosis, and hard, nondeforming skin (indicating loss of dermal viability). Positive prognostic signs include maintenance of pinprick sensation, normal skin color, and large clear blisters (15). In general, patients with superficial frostbite will recover with little or no tissue loss, and patients with deep injury will ultimately have necrosis.

DIFFERENTIAL DIAGNOSIS

The differential diagnosis of frostbite includes the other causes of cold induced injury—frostnip, immersion foot, cold urticaria, and chilblains. Other disease states that are sometimes confused include peripheral vascular disease, cellulitis, and dermatologic conditions such as stasis dermatitis, erysipelas, and bullous diseases. Trauma to an extremity or compartment syndrome may mimic or coexist with a cold-induced injury. Chemical or thermal burns should also be considered if an accurate history cannot be obtained.

EMERGENCY DEPARTMENT EVALUATION

Initial evaluation of the patient with a cold-induced tissue injury begins with a survey of the patient for systemic hypothermia (see Chapter 351, "Hypothermia") and major trauma. Treatment of either of these conditions supersedes care of a frostbitten limb. Once systemic and life-threatening conditions have been addressed, the physician should perform a detailed history and physical examination. Proper treatment and prognosis requires documentation of exposure temperature and duration, wind conditions, and moisture. A history of thawing in the field and any refreezing injury should be documented as it portends a poorer prognosis. A previous history of frostbite doubles the patient's risk for recurrent cold-induced tissue injury in the same body part(s) (4). A history of psychiatric illness or alcohol and drug use should be sought, as many urban emergency department (ED) patients with frostbite will present with one or both. Finally, other risk factors such as peripheral vascular disease, diabetes, and smoking should be ascertained.

Physical examination begins with an accurate core temperature and trauma primary and secondary surveys. This is followed by a thorough examination and description of any

TABLE 352.1. Classification of Frostbite Severity

Severity	Symptoms
First degree: partial thickness	
Erythema, edema, hyperemia	Stinging, burning
No blisters or necrosis	Possible throbbing and aching
Occasional skin desquamation (5–10 d later)	Possible hyperhidrosis
Second degree: full thickness	
Erythema, significant edema	Numbness
Clear vesicles	
Blisters may desquamate and form blackened eschar	
Third degree: involves subcutaneous tissue	Initially insensate; later, shooting pains,
Violaceous/hemorrhagic blisters due to injury to the reticular dermis and subdermal plexus	burning, throbbing, aching
Skin necrosis	
Blue-gray skin	
Fourth degree: involves muscle, tendon, and bone	Possible joint discomfort
Little edema	
Initially mottled, deep red, or cyanotic	
Later dry, black, mummified	

Adapted from Britt L, Dascombe W, Rodriguez A. New horizons in management of hypothermia and frostbite injury. *Surg Clin North Am* 1991;71:345–370.

frostbitten areas. A neurologic and vascular examination should include pulses (by Doppler if necessary), capillary refill, motor movement, and two-point discrimination. Wound description should include skin color and temperature, blister formation and color (clear or hemorrhagic), and soft tissue consistency.

Laboratory studies aid little in the initial evaluation of the frostbitten patient. However, they may be helpful in patients with concomitant illness or associated conditions, and to rule out rhabdomyolysis. Radiographic evaluation is dictated by history or physical examination findings consistent with trauma.

EMERGENCY DEPARTMENT MANAGEMENT

Prehospital care should focus on avoiding mechanical trauma and refreezing injury. A frostbitten extremity should not be rewarmed in the field if there is a risk of refreezing prior to reaching definitive care. A victim who must walk through snow should do so before thawing frostbitten feet. Rubbing the frozen extremity with a warm hand or snow, once thought to be beneficial, does not augment blood flow and causes increased tissue damage (15). On presentation to the ED, general management of any cold-injured patient includes removal of any wet clothing and complete exposure. Treatment begins by addressing hypothermia and dehydration. Thereafter, therapy should be directed to the patient's specific type of tissue injury.

Frostnip usually resolves spontaneously with dry rewarming in ambient temperatures and no further therapy is necessary.

Management of chilblains is also supportive. The affected skin should be rewarmed, washed, dried, and dressed in dry, soft, sterile bandages. Elevation is important to minimize edema that can predispose to infection (15). Nifedipine improves symptoms and helps prevent recurrences in patients with repeated exacerbations. A dose of 20 mg three times a day is recommended as tolerated by its effect on blood pressure (19). Prazosin has also been shown to be effective for both acute exacerbations and prophylaxis. These patients should avoid any further exposure to cold temperatures.

Immersion foot therapy is mainly supportive, consisting of bed rest, elevation of the legs and air-drying at room temperatures (25). In the homeless patient, who is most often affected, this is not easily achieved and admission may be necessary. Nonsteroidal antiinflammatory agents are most useful for pain relief, but parenteral opioid analgesics may be required. Although recovery is usually complete, severe complications such as nerve and muscle injury and gangrene occur infrequently. If the distinction between immersion foot and frostbite is unclear, the patient should be treated for frostbite.

Frostbite therapy is aimed at abating the specific pathophysiologic mechanisms causing tissue destruction. Rapid rewarming of tissues in a warm water bath decreases direct tissue damage created by ice crystal formation and greatly improves frostbitten tissue survival (14). Rapid rewarming is achieved by submersing the frozen extremity in a warm water bath at 40°C to 42°C (104°F–107.6°F) for 15 to 30 minutes. Gentle motion of the extremity may aid in thawing, however rubbing or massaging of the extremity should not be performed, as this will increase tissue damage.

Temperatures below 40°C delay tissue thawing and decrease tissue survival, while temperatures above 42°C can cause a superimposed thermal injury and worsen outcome (11). Maintaining the proper temperature is best achieved with hydrotherapy whirlpools. Because most emergency departments do no have these devices, a warm water bath can be quickly obtained using a mixture of hot and cold tap water from a standard hospital sink. A thermometer should be used to verify the proper temperature because attempts to create the bath without it are inaccurate and potentially dangerous. The water will cool quickly, and the intermittent addition of warm water or complete replacement of the bath will be necessary to maintain the desired temperature. Facial frostbite should be treated with warm water-soaked gauze or washcloths, as immersion is impractical.

The extremity should be rewarmed until tissue becomes pliable and erythematous. This usually occurs in 15 to 30 minutes. Rapid rewarming can be extremely painful, as sensation returns, and parenteral opioid analgesia is usually required. Rapid return of skin warmth, sensation and early formation of large clear blebs are good prognostic signs whereas persistence of cold, anesthetic, cyanotic skin and formation of small dark blebs portend a bad outcome. Compartment syndrome is a rare cause of persistent cyanosis; compartment pressures should be checked in suspect cases, and fasciotomy or escharotomy may be indicated. Postrewarming edema, which occurs within 3 hours of rewarming and persists for up to 5 days, should be treated with limb elevation. Vesicles and bullae appear 6 to 24 hours after rewarming and coincide with a renewed loss of sensation in the extremity. This secondary loss of sensation may persist until complete healing of the tissue (up to 4 years), but may be permanent (15).

Other adjunctive treatments for frostbite aim at preventing secondary tissue loss caused by inflammation and thrombosis. McCauley designed a protocol (12) that has been shown to decrease the progressive microvascular ischemia that occurs in the postthaw period (Table 352.2).

Blister management should follow rapid rewarming. Most authors support the debridement of clear blisters to prevent further contact of prostaglandin and thromboxane containing fluid with the underlying tissues. Hemorrhagic blisters, which indicate deeper damage to subdermal plexus, should be left intact (8,12). Some authors advocate debridement of hemorrhagic blisters, but this practice can lead to tissue desiccation, and therefore is not generally endorsed (4).

Adjunctive measures of proven benefit should be instituted to prevent progressive microvascular ischemia. Topical inhibition of thromboxane and prostaglandin is achieved with aloe vera cream (8,12). Aloe Vera (Dermaide) should be applied to

---

TABLE 352.2. Treatment Protocol for Frostbite[a]

1) Address systemic hypothermia and/or concomitant trauma
2) Rapidly rewarm the frostbitten tissue in warm water at 40–42°C (104–107.6°F) for 15–30 minutes or until thawing is complete.
3) Following rewarming, treat the affected tissue by:
   a. Providing appropriate analgesia in the form of an opioid.
   b. Debridement of clear blisters.
   c. Leave hemorrhagic blisters intact.
   d. Apply aloe vera (Dermaide aloe) every 6 hours to affected parts.
   e. Elevate the affected tissue/extremity and splint as needed.
   f. Administer tetanus prophylaxis (toxoid or Ig) as any other wound.
   g. Administer a non-steroidal anti-inflammatory agent (ibuprofen 400 mg orally every 12 hours).
   h. Administer benzyl penicillin 600 mg every 6 hours for 48–72 hours.
   i. For documentation, obtain photographic records of wounds, if possible.
4) Admit frostbite patient to a specialist unit, if possible
   a. Perform daily hydrotherapy for 30–45 minutes at 40°C
   b. Prohibit smoking

[a]Adapted from McCauley RL, Hing DN, Robson MC, et al. Frostbite injuries: a rational approach based on the pathophysiology. *J Trauma* 1983;23;143–47.

débrided clear blisters and intact hemorrhagic blisters every 6 hours. Systemic inhibition of the arachidonic acid cascade is achieved with oral ibuprofen at a dose of 400 mg every 12 hours (12mg/kg/day) (4,8). Sterile dressings should be applied and the extremity should be elevated to minimize subsequent edema. Edema formation has been shown to increase progressive dermal ischemia and inhibit the skin's bactericidal properties, ultimately predisposing to infection (15). Although there has been no specific randomized clinical trial showing definite benefit, most protocols advocate the use of prophylactic antibiotics in the form of penicillin 500,000 units i.v. every 6 hours for 48 to 72 hours or until edema resolves (12,22). Others advocate i.m. or p.o. antibiotics for the same duration (4,8). One study demonstrated increased efficacy of topical antibacterials (bacitracin and silver sulfadiazine) vs. systemic antibiotics for infection prophylaxis, although again no prospective trials have addressed this topic (23). Finally, frostbite is a tetanus-prone wound and tetanus prophylaxis should be instituted (6).

Many other adjuvant therapies have been studied to prevent progressive microvascular ischemia that occurs in the postthaw phase of frostbite. These agents include low-molecular weight dextran, heparin, thrombolytics, vasodilators, sympathectomy, hyperbaric oxygen, limaprost (a prostaglandin E1 analogue), and pentoxifylline. None of the studies, however, present conclusive evidence supporting their routine use (3,7,13,18,20,21,24).

The natural history of the frostbitten extremity is described by the phrase "frostbite in January, amputate in July." This adage speaks to the delay in demarcation between viable and postviable tissues. Usually about 9 to 15 days after initial injury, severely frostbitten skin develops a black, hard, dry eschar. Mummification forming a line of demarcation between viable and postviable tissue usually occurs at 22 to 45 days postinjury. There have been multiple attempts to define the zone of demarcation earlier, so that tissue in the transition zone may possibly be salvaged through early surgical intervention. Technetium bone scanning has been the main modality used with some success (5). However, one recent case report demonstrates magnetic resonance imaging with magnetic resonance angiography to be superior to bone scans for the early determination of viable tissues (1).

There are multiple late sequelae of frostbite. Residual pain and cold intolerance are the most common sequelae. Vasomotor instability resulting in hyperhydrosis, pigment changes, skin atrophy and posthealing ulcers also occur. Some patients request late amputation of cold injured parts as a result of the severity of these symptoms. Osteoporosis and subchondral bone loss may occur and may result in joint contracture. In children, epiphyseal damage may occur, even without skin loss.

CRITICAL INTERVENTIONS

- Completely undress the patient and address systemic hypothermia and trauma
- Rapidly rewarm frozen tissue in a warm water bath of 40°C to 42°C
- Administer adjuvant therapies as directed in Table 352.1
- Admit all frostbite victims to the hospital

DISPOSITION

Patients with frostnip will rarely present to the emergency department, but if they do, they can be safely discharged after the return of normal sensation. Care should be taken to ensure that they will not re-enter the same environment that exposed them to injury. Patients with chilblains may be discharged to follow-up with a primary care provider. Patients with immersion foot can be discharged if an environment that allows for proper treatment can be provided. Patients with frostbite, on the other hand, should be admitted to the hospital in all but the most superficial cases.

COMMON PITFALLS

✔ Discharging a patient into the same environment that caused the cold-induced injury without arranging proper protection from the elements

✔ Failing to recognize superimposed vascular injury or compartment syndrome after rewarming of a frostbitten extremity

✔ Failure to use a thermometer to accurately measure temperature of the warm water bath. Temperatures of 40°C to 42°C are effective in reducing tissue injury whereas temperatures above 42°C can be harmful

References

1. Barker JR, Haws MJ, Brown RE, et al. Magnetic resonance imaging of severe frostbite injuries. *Ann Plast Surg* 1997;38(3):275–279.
2. Boswick J, Thompson J, Jonas R. The epidemiology of cold injuries. *Surg Gynecol Obstet* 1979;149:326.
3. Bouwman DL, Morrison S, Lucas CE, et al. Early sympathetic blockade for frostbite-is it of value? *J Trauma* 1980;20(9):744–749.
4. Britt DL, Dascombe WH, Rodriguez A. New horizons in the management of hypothermia and frostbite injury. *Surg Clin North Am* 1991;71(2):345–370.
5. Cauchy E, Chetaille E, Lefevre M, et al. The role of bone scanning in severe frostbite of the extremities: a retrospective study of 88 cases. *Eur J Nucl Med* 2000;27(5):497–502.
6. Chan Ty, Smedley FH. Tetanus complicating frostbite. *Injury* 1990;21(4):245.
7. Finderle Z, Cankar K. Delayed treatment of frostbite injury with hyperbaric oxygen therapy: a case report. *Aviat Space Environ Med* 2002;73(4):392–394.
8. Heggers JP, Robson MC, Manavalen K, et al. Experimental and clinical observations on frostbite. *Ann Emerg Med* 1987;16(9):1056–1062.
9. Hwang JC, Himel HN, Edlich RF. Frostbite of the face after recreational misuse of nitrous oxide. *Burns* 1996;22:152–153.
10. Kurbat RS, Pollack CV. Facial injury and airway threat from inhalant abuse: a case report. *J Emerg Med* 1998;16:167–169.
11. Malhotra MS, Mathew L. Effect of rewarming at various water bath temperatures in experimental frostbite. *Aviat Space Environ Med* 1978; July:874–876.
12. McCauley RL, Hing DN, Robson MC, et al. Frostbite injuries: a rational approach based on the pathophysiology. *J Trauma* 1983;23(2):143–147.
13. Miller MB, Koltai PJ. Treatment of experimental frostbite with pentoxifylline and aloe vera cream. *Arch Otolaryngol Head Neck Surg* 1995;121:678–680.
14. Mills WJ, Whaley R, Fish W. Frostbite: experience with rapid rewarming and ultrasonic therapy. Part I, II, III 1960–61. *Alaska Med* 1993;35(1):6–27.
15. Murphy JV, Banwell PE, Roberts AH, et al. Frostbite: pathogenesis and treatment. *J Trauma* 2000;48:171–178.
16. O'Toole G, Rayatt S. Frostbite at the gym: a case report of an ice pack burn. *Br J Sports Med* 1999;33:278–279.
17. Paton BC. A history of frostbite treatment. *Intern J Circumpolar Health* 2000;59:99–107.
18. Purkayastha SS, Bhaumik G, Chauhan SK, et al. Immediate treatment of frostbite using rapid rewarming in tea decoction followed by combined therapy of pentoxifylline, aspirin, and vitamin C. *Indian J Med Res* 2002;116:29–34.
19. Rustin MH, Newton JA, Smith NP, et al. The treatment of chilblains with nifedipine: the results of a pilot study, a double blind placebo controlled randomized study and long term open trial. *Brit J Dermatol* 1989;120:267–275.
20. Saito S, Shimada H. Effect of prostaglandin E1 analogue administration on peripheral skin temperatures at high altitude. *Angiology* 1994;45(6):455–460.
21. Skolnick AA. Early data suggest clot-dissolving drug may help save frostbitten limbs from amputation. *JAMA* 1992;267(15):2008–2010.
22. Smith DJ, Robson MC, Heggers JP. Frostbite and other cold-related injuries. In: Auerbach PS, ed. *Wilderness medicine: management of wilderness and environmental emergencies*, 3rd ed. St. Louis: Mosby, 1995:129–145.
23. Valnicek SM, Chasmir LR, Clapson JB. Frostbite in the prairies: a 12-year review. *Plast Reconstr Surg* 1993;92:633–641.
24. von Heimburg D, Noah EM, Sieckman UP, et al. Hyperbaric oxygen treatment in deep frostbite of both hands in a boy. *Burns* 2001;27(4):404–8.
25. Wrenn K. Immersion foot; a problem of the homeless in the 1990s. *Arch Intern Med* 1991;151:785.

CHAPTER 353
Heat-Related Illness

Eric W. Schmidt and Constance G. Nichols

Heat illness can be defined as the inability of normal regulatory mechanisms to cope with a heat stress. Minor heat-related problems, such as muscle cramps, edema, rash, syncope, and tetany account for significant morbidity. Heat exhaustion and heatstroke are major heat syndromes in that, if left untreated, may cause organ damage or death. Among high school athletes heatstroke is the third leading cause of death (4). In elderly patients mortality has been directly correlated with increased ambient temperature (9). Sunburn and other photodermal ultraviolet (UV) injuries may exacerbate all other heat syndromes or present separately.

Heat cramps are as a result of muscle fatigue combined with water and salt depletion (1). Heat syncope results from vasodilatation usually compounded by volume depletion or the use of drugs that interfere with cardiovascular reflexes. Heat tetany apparatus appears to be a result of hyperventilation-induced respiratory alkalosis resulting in decreased ionized serum calcium. It may be an attempt to compensate for exercise-induced lactic acidosis. Heat rash is caused by the plugging, dilation, and rupture of sweat glands following skin maceration resulting from sweating. The etiology of heat edema is unknown.

Exposed to a variety of temperatures, humans maintain a relatively constant body temperature by balancing heat loss with heat gain. Any condition that increases heat gain or decreases heat loss may result in a major heat illness (Table 353.1). Heat gain may be a result of increased endogenous heat production resulting from basal metabolism and muscle activity or may result from an environmental heat load. For example basal metabolism generates 65 to 85 kcal per hour which may increase five- to six-fold with exertion. Underlying illness or drug ingestion may also increase endogenous heat production. Hot environments decrease heat loss and increase the heat load. The average sunbather may gain 150 kcal/hour. Without heat dissipation, at rest, the average human temperature would increase 1.1°C/hour.

In cool environments heat is lost mainly through passive convection and radiation. As the ambient and body temperatures increase, centrally mediated mechanisms for active heat removal-cutaneous vasodilatation and sweating-begin. Radiational heat loss is first increased as the cardiovascular system adjusts blood flow to the periphery by decreasing the splanchnic and mesenteric flow and increasing heart rate and cardiac output. The second phase of active heat dissipation, sweating, is then brought into play. Sympathetic stimulation releases acetylcholine, which stimulates the sweat glands resulting in evaporative heat loss. Acetylcholine also facilitates the secretion of kallikreins, which facilitate the formation of bradykinin from globin. Bradykinin and other peptides may contribute to superficial vasodilatation. The unacclimatized person can sweat up to 1.5L/hour losing 1.7 kcal/mL of sweat (10).

Heat exhaustion results from dehydration with inadequate fluid and electrolyte replacement. Water or salt depletion or both may be present. Without treatment, heat exhaustion progresses to heatstroke. Heatstroke is a result of severe dehydration with thermoregulatory failure resulting in body temperatures above 40°C (105°F–106°F) and a mortality rate of up to 70%.

TABLE 353.1.   Factors Predisposing to Heat Illness

Increased Heat Gain	
Endogenous Factors	Exogenous Factors
Infection	High ambient temperature
Drugs	Malignant hyperthermia
Stimulants	Sunlight
Hallucinogens	
Increased Activity	
Exercise	
Seizures	
Drug withdrawal	
Psychosis	
Neuroleptic malignant syndrome	
Thyrotoxicosis	

Decreased Heat Loss	
Lack of acclimation	High temperature
Dehydration	High humidity
Hypokalemia	Restrictive clothing
Drugs	Protective garments
Anticholinergics	
Neuroleptics	
Barbiturates	
Anti-Parkinson agents	
Diuretics	
Beta blockers	
Alcohol	
Extremes of Age	
Skin Disorders	
Cystic Fibrosis	
Obesity	
Debilitated/Chronic Disease	
Impaired Voluntary Responses	

Acclimatization is a process of physiologic adaptation to repeated heat stress that occurs over 10 to 60 days. It results in decreased heat production and increased heat loss for a given amount of work. Metabolic function improves by increasing skeletal muscle mitochondria and glycogen stores, thereby enhancing the aerobic work capacity, which produces less heat. Fluid and electrolyte balance is altered by aldosterone secretion, which helps to conserve sodium stores by both sweat and renal mechanisms and by increasing extracellular volume. Cardiac efficiency is improved, with an increase in maximum cardiac output, a decreased peak heart rate, and increased stroke volume. Changes in sweating occur so that the threshold core temperature for sweating is decreased and the volume of sweat is increased. Sweat volumes may decrease with further acclimatization as a result of increased efficiency of the metabolic components. Potassium loss during acclimatization peaks at 8 to 10 days and often increases susceptibility to heat illness (10). Although acclimatization protects against heat illness, as the wet-bulb temperature approaches 30°C (86°F) even young, well-acclimated persons are susceptible during vigorous or prolonged physical activity (2,4). Hand immersion in cold (10°C) water during rest and wearing an ice vest along with hand immersion in cold water increases the time until heat stress limits are reached in those wearing protective garments (7).

Ultraviolet (UV) exposure varies 40- to 80-fold over the course of the year for a given location. Intensity peaks between 10 AM and 2 PM daily. The degree and extent of UV injury is a direct function of the total energy absorbed. UV tissue injury occurs at multiple cellular levels. Initially there is an inflammatory reaction similar to other tissue insults, with a cellular and humoral response involving Langerhans cells, macrophages, lymphocytes,

TABLE 353.2.   Drugs that Increase Direct Phototoxicity and Promote Photoallergy

Drugs that Increase Direct Phototoxicity

Amiodarone
Doxycycline
Furosemide
Naproxen sodium
Phenothiazines
Sulfonamides

Drugs that Promote Photoallergy

Phenothiazines
Sulfonamides
Sunscreens

prostaglandins, interleukins, and multiple cytokines. Individual response ranges from mild transient erythema to urticaria with exacerbation of underlying medical conditions, depending on exposure, skin type, photoallergy, or photodrug reaction (Table 353.2). The maximal response may be delayed up to 30 hours and last for several days.

Phytophotodermatitis is a result of skin exposure to furanocoumarins (psoralens) from fruits and vegetables followed by sun exposure. It is an occupational hazard of harvesters and grocery workers. UVB frequencies (290nm–320nm) are up to 1600 times more injurious than UVA (320nm–400nm), but there is a preponderance of UVA in the environment (6).

CLINICAL PRESENTATION

Heat cramps are painful spasms of heavily used muscle groups. They often occur in acclimatized persons, during or up to several hours after exertion. The victim often has been sweating heavily with insufficient or hypotonic fluid replacement for several days. Serum sodium levels are normal.

Heat edema is manifest by ankle and wrist swelling. It occurs in the first few days of heat exposure and sometimes results in pitting (14).

Heat rash (prickly heat) is most common early in acclimatization, in tropical areas and in those wearing tight clothes. It is an intensely pruritic, red, papular, occasionally vesicular dermatitis. Complications include infection and the formation of large nonpruritic plugs, which take several weeks to desquamate. Persons with advanced heat rash are at risk for heat exhaustion or heatstroke as a result of loss of sweat gland function (4).

Heat syncope is a transient loss of postural tone, with or without brief loss of consciousness occurring early in exposure to a new heat stress. It is often preceded by dehydration or the presence of drugs that affect the body's normal compensatory mechanisms (11). By the time victims are examined, vital signs are usually normal.

Heat tetany presents as carpopedal spasm and is frequently seen in conjunction with other heat syndromes or other causes of hyperventilation. In contrast to heat cramps it does not involve the heavily used proximal muscles. Arterial blood gas analysis may reveal a respiratory alkalosis.

Heat exhaustion usually occurs in nonacclimatized persons who have been working in the heat for several days. It can occur in those wearing protective garments (e.g., in nuclear, biological, and chemical operations) at room temperature or below. Symptoms caused by water depletion include thirst, weakness, dizziness, anxiety, muscular incoordination, agita-

tion, confusion, palpitations, oliguria, and elevated temperature. Those caused by salt depletion include fatigue, weakness, headache, anorexia, vomiting, diarrhea, and skeletal muscle cramps; thirst is absent. Body temperature is usually normal or subnormal in both types of heat exhaustion; the skin is cool and clammy. Tachycardia and hypotension are common. Most victims present with a combined picture of water and salt depletion. Laboratory findings may include hyponatremia, high urinary specific gravity, and mildly elevated serum creatine phosphokinase and liver enzyme levels. Without termination of the heat stressor and immediate treatment heat exhaustion may progress to frank heatstroke (13,14).

Classic heatstroke usually affects the very young or the debilitated elderly and develops over several days, mostly during heat waves (9). The gradual onset may result in severe dehydration and hot, dry skin. Exertional heatstroke usually occurs in an unacclimatized younger person after a few hours of severe heat stress. Victims usually can still sweat. Vital sign abnormalities include hyperthermia (usually > 40°C), tachycardia, tachypnea, and hypotension. Because a high core temperature for a short period of time can produce the same injury as a relatively lower temperature for a longer period, the presenting temperature may not predict severity or outcome.

Widespread damage to almost every organ system, especially the cerebellum, has been described. The central nervous system is one of the first systems involved and the last to recover. Family or witnesses may describe a malaise or flu-like prodrome. Mental confusion begins with a core temperature of 38°C with cessation of brain function at temperatures above 42°C. Coma, seizure activity, and abnormal posturing have been described. The liver is particularly susceptible to heat injury. Serum transaminase levels may initially be in the thousands and peak up to 2 weeks later at more than 10,000. Coagulopathies and hypoglycemia are common. The kidneys are at high risk for acute tubular necrosis. Rhabdomyolysis may contribute to renal injury in victims of exertional heatstroke (13,14). Arterial blood gas measurements usually reveal a respiratory alkalosis. Lactic acidosis may also be seen following heavy exertion (3). Death is usually secondary to disseminated intravascular coagulation, acute renal failure, liver failure, or adult respiratory distress syndrome(5,10,14).

DIFFERENTIAL DIAGNOSIS

The key to diagnosing any heat illness is a history of a heat stress. During a heat wave the diagnosis is easily considered. Vigorous exercise in moderate temperatures, or working in a closed hot environment, may also result in significant heat stress. The clinician should remember the predisposing factors in Table 353.1. Rhabdomyolysis should be excluded in patients with heat cramps. Electrolyte abnormalities should be ruled out in victims of heat cramps and tetany. An extensive evaluation may be necessary to exclude other causes of edema and syncope. The differential diagnosis of heatstroke includes infection, particularly meningitis, thyroid storm, drug intoxication, and the neuroleptic malignant syndrome (malignant hyperthermia). In contrast to heatstroke, patients with the neuroleptic malignant syndrome have muscular rigidity that responds to dantrolene (12).

EMERGENCY DEPARTMENT EVALUATION

The history should include the duration, magnitude, and conditions of heat exposure, recent activity, the nature, progression, and duration of symptoms, medications, drug use, and underlying medical problems. In young healthy victims, a typical history and physical examination that reveals no other pathology is all that is necessary for a diagnosis of minor heat-related problems. Normal laboratory findings will confirm the diagnosis in questionable cases and in those with advanced age or coexisting medical problems.

In victims of heat exhaustion and heatstroke vital signs include orthostatic pulse and blood pressure measurements and a rectal temperature. The temperature should be checked with a rectal thermoresistor temperature probe capable of measuring high temperatures (up to 44°C) if the temperature measured by electronic thermometer approaches its upper limit. Continuous cardiac and oxygen saturation monitoring should be performed. Depending on the severity, laboratory evaluation should include arterial blood gas (ABG) analysis; a complete blood count (CBC); measurements of electrolytes, blood urea nitrogen, creatinine, glucose, creatine kinase and liver enzymes; and urinalysis. Those with elevated levels of creatine kinase, abnormal electrolyte or liver enzyme levels or high temperatures (> 40°C) should also have coagulation studies; calcium, magnesium, phosphorus and uric acid measurements; an ECG and a chest radiograph (14).

EMERGENCY DEPARTMENT MANAGEMENT

Heat cramps are treated with oral or i.v. fluid and salt replacement. Fruit juices or sports drinks by mouth is sufficient for mild cases. Intravenous normal saline is recommended for severe symptoms. Heat edema is self-limited and will resolve with time if the limb is elevated and support hose worn. Patients with heat rash should keep their skin cool and dry and avoid tight clothing. Antihistamines may be given for pruritus but powders should be avoided to prevent further plugging. Desquamating agents (e.g., salicylic acid) and antibiotics effective against staphylococci may be prescribed for secondary infection. Heat syncope is treated with rest, fluids, salt, and gradual return to activity. Heat tetany should resolve with the reversal of hyperventilation (e.g., bag breathing).

The treatment of heat exhaustion centers around replacement of fluid and electrolyte losses with isotonic saline. Orthostatic patients may require 4 L or more of i.v. fluids. Oral fluids can substitute for or supplement i.v. fluid in mild cases. Rare cases will present with severe hyponatremia requiring hypertonic saline infusion (10,13,14).

The cornerstone of heatstroke therapy is rapid cooling. Immersing or covering the patient in ice is not recommended because skin cooling causes both vasoconstriction and shivering and could increase the core temperature. Cooling rates similar to ice immersion can be achieved using immersion in 15°C water. Applying ice packs in the areas of large vessels, such as the groin and axillae, and infusing large volumes of cool i.v. fluids are useful for field management but insufficient for definitive cooling.

Although the fastest cooling rates (0.5°C/minute) have been reported with peritoneal and thoracic lavage using iced dialysate, the combination of evaporative cooling (0.3°C/minute) and iced gastric lavage (0.2°C/minute) with water or saline are more practical and just as effective. Evaporation is maximized without inducing shivering by keeping the patient wet with lukewarm water or wet towels and blowing air over him or her with a fan. Helicopter blade fanning has also been used (12). Cooling blankets may be effective for patients with mild heatstroke. The rectal temperature should be monitored with a probe capable of measuring high temperatures (up to 44°C).

Cooling is continued only until the temperature drops to 38.5°C to 39°C to avoid overshoot hypothermia. Rectal temperature monitoring should be continued, as the patient may rebound hours later and be thermally unstable for days. Along with cooling these patients frequently need sedation and intubation and large volumes of intravenous normal saline. A central venous pressure line and Foley catheter are recommended to monitor fluid therapy. Acid–base, electrolyte, and coagulation abnormalities should be corrected. Alkaline diuresis may be helpful if rhabdomyolysis is present.

Shivering may be treated with chlorpromazine (25 mg i.v.), benzodiazepines, or thiopental. Seizure activity is best treated with diazepam or phenobarbital. Phenytoin is ineffective. Dantrolene sodium has not been proven efficacious in canine studies, although anecdotal reports of success exist. Poor prognostic indicators are a serum glutamic-oxaloacetic transaminase (SGOT) level above 1,000 after 24 hours, a coma that lasts more than 8 hours or a presenting temperature of 42.2°C or higher (13,14).

Prevention of sunburn is the best therapy and can be done by avoiding unnecessary sun exposure (especially between 10 AM and 3 PM); wearing protective clothing, hats, and sunglasses; using broad-spectrum sunscreens with a sun protection factor (SPF) of 15 or higher on exposed areas; and avoiding artificial tanning lights. Treatment is otherwise supportive. Antiinflammatory drugs and topical aloe vera and steroid spray may be useful for mild cases. More severe cases may require therapy similar to that for thermal burns (see Chapter 197, "Burns").

CRITICAL INTERVENTIONS

- Institute continuous rectal temperature monitoring and obtain an ABG, CBC, serum electrolytes, blood urea nitrogen, creatinine, glucose, creatine kinase liver enzymes, and a urinalysis in patients with heatstroke
- Obtain coagulation studies, serum calcium, magnesium, phosphorus and uric acid, and an ECG and chest radiograph in heatstroke patients with elevated levels of creatine kinase, abnormal electrolyte or liver enzyme levels or temperature above 40°C
- Administer large volumes of i.v. fluids and perform evaporative (fan and water) cooling and gastric lavage with iced saline or water in patients with heatstroke

DISPOSITION

Patients with minor heat-related problems may be discharged. Patients with heat exhaustion should be admitted to a floor bed if they have abnormal vital signs or laboratory findings or remain symptomatic after fluid therapy. Patients with heatstroke should be admitted to an intensive care unit. Discharged patients should be advised to avoid the conditions that precipitated their illness. Acclimatization with frequent water breaks and rest periods during hot-weather activity should prevent future problems. Consultation with a dermatologist may be helpful in patients with photosensitivity reactions.

COMMON PITFALLS

✔ Failure to recognize heat-related illness as a result of nonenvironmental causes

✔ Failure to assess carefully for mental status changes in potential heatstroke victims

✔ Failure to obtain a timely and accurate rectal temperature in patients with suspected heat illness

✔ Failing to warn patients to avoid re-exposure until acclimatization has occurred

✔ Prescribing medications that predispose to or exacerbate heat or sun-related illness to patients at risk

References

1. Bergeron MF. Heat cramps: fluid and electrolyte challenges during tennis in the heat. *J Sci Med Sport* 2003;6(1):19–27.
2. Binkley HM, Beckett J, Casa DJ, et al. National Athletic Trainers' Association position statement: exertional heat illnesses. *J Athl Train* 2002;37(3):329–343.
3. Bouchama A, De Vol EB: Acid-base alterations in heat stroke. *Intensive Care Med* 2001;27(4):680–685.
4. Corris EE, Ramirez AM, Van Durme DJ. Heat illness in athletes: the dangerous combination of heat, humidity and exercise. *Sports Med* 2004;34(1):9–16.
5. Hakre S, Gardner JW, Kark JA, et al. Predictors of hospitalization in male Marine Corps recruits with exertional heat illness. *Mil Med* 2004;169(3):169–175.
6. Harber LC. Abnormal responses to ultraviolet radiation: drug induced sensitivity. In: Fitzpatrick T, Eisen A, Wolff K, et al., eds. *Dermatology in general medicine*, 4th ed. New York: McGraw Hill, 1993.
7. House JR, Lunt H, Magnrss A, et al. Testing the effectiveness of techniques for reducing heat stress in Royal Navy nuclear, biological and chemical cleansing stations' teams. *J R Naval Med Serv* 2003;89(1):27–34.
8. Poulton, TJ, Walker, RA. Helicopter cooling of heatstroke victims. *Aviation, Space and Environmental Medicine* 1987;58:358–361.
9. Rajpal RC, Weisskopf MG, Rumm PD, et al. Wisconsin, July 1999 heat wave: an epidemiologic assessment. *WMJ* 2000;99:41–44.
10. Simon, H. Hyperthermia. *N Engl J Med* 1993;329:483.
11. Smalley B, Janke RM, Cole D. Exertional heat illness in Air Force basic military trainees. *Mil Med* 2003;168(4):298–303.
12. Watson J, et al. Exertional heat stroke induced by amphetamine analogues: does dantrolene have a place? *Anaesthesia* 1993;49(12):1057.
13. Weinmann M. Hot on the inside. *Emerg Med Serv* 2003;32(7):34.
14. Wexler RK. Evaluation and treatment of heat-related illnesses. *Am Fam Physician* 2002;65(11):2307–2314.

CHAPTER 354
High-Altitude Illness

David Richardson

Increasing mobility and leisure time have allowed many more people to explore wilderness areas previously experienced only by the privileged few (17). Interest in hiking, camping, rock climbing, mountain biking, alpine and cross-country skiing, and other high-altitude sports has grown dramatically over the past few decades. In the United States alone, tens of millions of athletes and tourists now seek mountainous destinations in every season of the year. High-speed transportation now permits travel from low to high altitudes within hours. Acute mountain sickness is a public health problem and has economic consequences, especially for the ski industry (8).

High-altitude-induced illness, better known as acute mountain sickness (AMS), is a spectrum of disease ranging from subclinical effects to potentially lethal high-altitude pulmonary edema (HAPE) or high-altitude cerebral edema (HACE). Because barometric pressure decreases with increasing altitude, yet the fraction of inspired oxygen in air remains constant at 21%, the PaO2 is reduced. A young, healthy, physically fit nonsmoker will have a PaO2 under 60 mm Hg at 2,500 m (8,100 ft) and under 50 mm Hg at 4,500 m (14,600 ft). Symptomatic AMS is uncommon under 2,500 m but occurs in up to 25% of the population at 2,500 m, 42% at 3,000 m (10,000 ft) and in 75% at 4,500 m (8,10,11). Repeated attacks are common (about 20%), potentially limiting high-altitude activity or requiring prophylactic medications and a slow, controlled ascent.

The incidence, severity, and duration of AMS are proportional to the rate and height of ascent and are modified by individual susceptibility, physical exertion, and sleeping altitude (6,13). Symptoms vary widely but remain consistent on repeated episodes in the same person (13). AMS has been defined as the presence of headache in an unacclimatized person who has recently arrived at an altitude above 2,500 m plus the presence of one or more of the following: gastrointestinal symptoms (anorexia, nausea, or vomiting), insomnia, dizziness and lassitude, or fatigue (18). AMS demonstrates no sexual preference (12), but HAPE is more common in males (13). High-altitude retinal hemorrhage occurs in up to 40% of AMS patients but macular involvement occurs in less than 5% (6,12,13).

On ascent to high altitude, spontaneous diuresis occurs in response to complicated fluid shifts and well-being is proportional to individual diuretic response (6,12). In mild cases, symptoms abate in 3 to 7 days as acclimatization occurs. Chronic mountain sickness, or Monge disease, may develop in some patients who do not acclimatize despite prolonged altitude exposure. It is characterized by persistent hypoxia, polycythemia (hematocrit greater than 60), and development of congestive heart failure (11).

HAPE is a form of noncardiac pulmonary edema associated with pulmonary artery hypertension. A defect in nitric oxide synthesis may be contributory (20). It develops in 0.5% to 15.0% of persons who ascend rapidly to high altitudes, has an overall mortality of 11%, and accounts for most deaths as a result of high-altitude illness (11). HAPE recurs in susceptible persons, thus requiring caution on re-exposure (1).

HACE affects an estimated 1% of travelers to high altitude. Symptoms are as a result of increased intracranial pressure. Although cerebral vessels dilate in response to hypoxia, the exact pathophysiology of this condition is not known (7,11,12,21). Recent findings indicate that the predominant underlying mechanism is vasogenic (extracellular, a result of leakage of fluid and protein through the blood-brain barrier) rather than cytotoxic.

Hypobaric hypoxia can exacerbate preexisting cardiac or pulmonary disease (6). Relative contraindications to high-altitude travel include advanced age, chronic diseases, coronary artery disease, chronic obstructive pulmonary disease, pulmonary hypertension, sickle cell disease, and other diseases that compromise cardiopulmonary function (6,11).

Measures to prevent or reduce AMS in a person who is about to undergo rapid ascent to high altitude (particularly those with previous episodes) include cautious acclimatization and medication.

A staged, gradual ascent is most effective to achieve acclimatization. Either remaining at 2,000 to 3,000 m (6,600–9,800 ft) for 2 to 5 days before going higher, or ascending less than 300 m (1,000 ft) per day above 2,500 m (8,200 ft) can significantly reduce symptomatology (13,19). Climbing high but sleeping low can also be effective in reducing the results of hypobaric hypoxia exacerbated by nighttime hypoventilation (6,7,15). Drinking plenty of fluids, eliminating salt intake, and limiting physical activity may restrict symptom development (6,12,13, 15).

The carbonic anhydrase inhibitor acetazolamide causes a bicarbonate diuresis, resulting in a hyperchloremic metabolic acidosis and a compensatory respiratory alkalosis (7,13). Pretreatment with 250 mg every 6 to 12 hours or with 500 mg of the sustained release formula each day, beginning 1 or 2 days before ascent and continuing at least 48 hours after ascent, mimics the acclimated state of acid–base balance (6,7,12,13,15,20). Some patients may not be helped, but symptoms are lessened in 30% to 50% of patients (13). Side effects include, paresthesias, gastrointestinal distress, somnolence, and dehydration if fluid intake is insufficient (13,15).

Dexamethasone, which stabilizes membranes, reduces vasogenic cerebral edema and AMS symptoms to a greater extent than acetazolamide, with fewer side effects (3,4,13). It does not help with acclimatization, however, and symptoms can return if dexamethasone is discontinued before acclimatization is complete. The dosage is 4 mg every 6 hours, starting 48 hours before ascent and continuing 48 hours after ascent (6,13). Combining it with acetazolamide improves efficacy over either drug alone (23).

CLINICAL PRESENTATION

Early symptoms of AMS are nonspecific and generally develop within 8 to 24 hours of arriving at altitude (range, 6–48 hours) (13). Headache, anorexia, nausea, vomiting, malaise, insomnia, lassitude, shortness of breath, and dyspnea on exertion make up the most common symptom complex (6,12,13,22). The headache is usually throbbing, bilateral, and frontal. It is worse in the morning and when supine, increases with exercise, and may be minimally responsive to aspirin or acetaminophen (13). Sleep is generally poor and often exacerbates symptoms as a result of hypoventilatory hypoxia, so the patient feels worse on waking (6). Findings on physical examination include tachypnea, tachycardia, peripheral or periorbital edema, and rales. Tachypnea and tachycardia serve to maximize oxygenation and oxygen delivery to tissues. Despite having edema, the patient is often dehydrated and hypovolemic, with oliguria, increased hematocrit, and hypercoagulable state (6). Petechiae may indicate disturbed vascular integrity, and papilledema may be present without raised intracranial pressure (12). High-altitude retinal hemorrhage, detectable as flame hemorrhages, is usually asymptomatic and resolves without residua (6,12,13). Macular involvement is manifest by central scotoma (6,12). Laboratory studies may reveal mild leukocytosis and hemoconcentration (6,9).

Manifestations of HAPE include worsening dyspnea, cough, hemoptysis, and cyanosis (6). Complications such as adult respiratory distress syndrome or infection may develop. The chest radiograph reveals a normal-sized heart and diffuse bilateral patchy infiltrates, in contrast to the typical butterfly distribution of alveolar edema (6,12). Arterial blood gas analysis may show hypoxia, hypocapnia, and alkalosis. Pulmonary function tests indicate decreased vital capacity and peak expiratory flow rates (19). Pulmonary hypertension with normal left atrial pressure and normal pulmonary artery wedge pressure are seen if pulmonary artery catheterization becomes necessary (20). The electrocardiogram (ECG) most often shows only sinus tachycardia, but sometimes it shows evidence of right-sided heart strain (6,12).

Signs and symptoms of HACE include increasing headache, nausea, and vomiting, accompanied ataxia, confusion, and poor judgment (6,7,10,11,12,21). Other associated findings may include retinal hemorrhage, cranial nerve palsy, and papilledema. HACE can progress to coma and death if untreated and may leave neuropsychological residua even if promptly recognized and treated (12). White matter edema may be seen on computed tomography (CT) or magnetic resonance imaging of the brain.

DIFFERENTIAL DIAGNOSIS

The differential diagnosis of AMS, HACE, HAPE is shown in Table 354.1. Nonspecific symptoms of early AMS may mimic viral upper respiratory infection or gastroenteritis. Poor central nervous system (CNS) function on environmental exposure can also be caused by hypothermia, hypovolemia, and exhaustion (6). Worsening pulmonary symptoms may also be a result

TABLE 354.1.   Differential Diagnosis of High-Altitude Illness

Acute Mountain Sickness	High Altitude Cerebral Edema (HACE)	High Altitude Pulmonary Edema (HAPE)
Carbon Monoxide Exposure	Drug or Alcohol Ingestion	Asthma
Dehydration	Hypothermia	Bronchitis
Diabetic Ketoacidosis	Hyponatremia	Heart Failure
		MI with CHF
Fatigue/Overexertion	Seizure	Pneumonia
Hangover	Stroke	Pulmonary Embolism
Hypoglycemia	Sepsis	COPD Exacerbation
Hypothermia	CNS Infection	
Migraine		
Viral Syndrome		

of acute exacerbations of chronic respiratory diseases such as asthma or chronic obstructive pulmonary disease (12). Other etiologies of noncardiogenic pulmonary edema should be considered (e.g., medications, neurologic disorders). Low-grade fever and leukocytes expand the differential to more serious infections, including pneumonia and meningitis (12). The differential diagnosis of CNS dysfunction also includes metabolic, psychiatric, toxic, and traumatic disorders (11).

EMERGENCY DEPARTMENT EVALUATION

A history of recent, rapid transit to high altitude or history of similar episodes at altitude should alert the physician to the potential diagnosis of AMS. The rapidity of ascent, altitude, activities and length of stay at altitude, the time of onset, nature and duration of symptoms, and preexisting medical conditions should be noted.

The physical examination should focus on vital signs and evaluation of CNS, cardiac, and respiratory function. A funduscopic examination should also be performed. All patients should have an oxygen saturation measured. Laboratory evaluation of patients with constitutional symptoms of AMS should include a complete blood count, electrolytes, blood urea nitrogen, creatinine, and glucose. Those with tachypnea, hypoxia, altered mental status, or abnormal findings on cardiopulmonary examination should have arterial blood gas analysis, cardiac monitoring, an ECG, and a chest radiograph. A CT scan of the head should be performed in those with an abnormal mental status or severe headache.

EMERGENCY DEPARTMENT MANAGEMENT

The prevention and management of high-altitude illness are summarized in Table 354.2. Descent is the most effective treatment for AMS. Second-line measures include limiting further ascent until symptoms have resolved and pharmacological therapy.

Acetazolamide and dexamethasone are effective for treating mild-to-moderate AMS and preventing it (5). Acetazolamide relieves symptoms, improves arterial oxygenation, and prevents further impairment of pulmonary gas exchange (7). Multiple acetazolamide regimens are effective (2). Administration of 250 mg orally every 8 hours until symptoms of AMS resolve is recommended (7).

Dexamethasone, 4 mg every 6 hours orally, i.m., or i.v. can be given for treatment of AMS. HACE is treated with an initial dose of 8 mg of dexamethasone followed by 4 mg every 6 hours

TABLE 354.2. Prevention and Management of High-Altitude Illness

Prevention	Management
Travelers with history of mild-to-moderate acute mountain sickness who are planning an ascent to high altitude.	A staged, gradual ascent above 2,500 m, ascending less than 300 m per d or give acetazolamide 125 mg–250 mg BID for 24 h prior to rapid ascent and for 48 h at altitude. Dexamethasone 4 mg every 6 h for 48 h before ascent and continuing for 48 h after ascent.
Mild Acute Mountain Sickness	
Mild headache with nausea, dizziness, fatigue, sleep disturbance during first 12 h after rapid ascent to high altitude.	Descend 500 m or more; or stop ascent and acclimatize; or treat with acetazolamide 125 mg or 250 mg p.o. BID for 48 h; treat nausea and headache symptoms with analgesics and antiemetics.
Moderate Acute Mountain Sickness	
Moderate-to-severe nausea, headache, insomnia, dizziness, dyspnea on exertion after 12 h at high altitude	Descent of 500 m or more is primary treatment. If descent impossible, use a portable hyperbaric chamber and/or oxygen 1–2 l/m. If descent and oxygen is unavailable, use acetazolamide 250 mg p.o. BID, dexamethasone 4 mg p.o. or i.m. every 6 h until symptoms resolve.
High-Altitude Pulmonary Edema	
Dyspnea at rest, cough, copious sputum, severe weakness, rales, tachypnea, cyanosis, hemoptysis, tachycardia	Immediate descent. Oxygen 4–6 l/m. Minimize exertion, use a portable hyperbaric chamber and/or nifedipine 10 mg orally and then 30 mg of extended release formulation orally every 12–24 h if immediate descent or evacuation unavailable
High-Altitude Cerebral Edema	
Acute mountain sickness for 24 h, confusion, ataxia, poor judgment, vomiting, seizure, coma	Immediate descent or evacuation. Oxygen 2–4 l/m; use a portable hyperbaric chamber; dexamethasone 8 mg i.v., i.m., or p.o. then 4 mg every 6 h; consider acetazolamide 250 mg p.o. BID if descent or evacuation not available.

orally, i.m., or i.v. (8). Patients with dehydration should be given oral fluids. Those with severe symptoms require descent to a lower altitude. Patients with vomiting should be given antiemetics and hydrated with intravenous saline. Acetaminophen or a nonsteroidal antiinflammatory agent can be given for headache.

Lightweight, portable hyperbaric chambers have become part of the field regimen to treat AMS. The Gamow bag, an inflatable, cylindrical, zippered bag, simulates descent to a lower altitude when pressurized to 100 mm Hg by means of a pop-off valve vent (usually 2 psi). The patient is placed in the bag and air is pumped in. The patient may also be placed on oxygen while in the chamber. Hyperbaric therapy with air is as effective as oxygen for the immediate treatment of AMS (14).

HAPE should be treated initially with oxygen and evacuation to a lower altitude (1,13). Sublingual or oral nifedipine (10 mg every 4 hours until improved, then 30 mg of long-acting preparation every 12–24 hours) has been shown to decrease pulmonary artery pressure, improve oxygenation, and decrease subjective symptoms in patients with HAPE (1,13). It can be used as an emergency measure for patients when descent or evacuation is impossible (13). Nifedipine should not be used prophylactically in HAPE-susceptible subjects, however, because of potential harmful side effects, such as hypotension and consequent myocardial and cerebral ischemia and infarction (13).

CPAP or BiPAP by mask or endotracheal intubation and mechanical ventilation with positive end-expiratory pressure may be necessary for patients with respiratory failure (10,16). Inhaled nitric oxide can also improve arterial oxygenation (19). Diuretics are not helpful and may be harmful in patients with underlying dehydration. On the contrary, fluid therapy may be required for the treatment of dehydration. If recognized early and treated aggressively, nearly all young, physically fit, otherwise healthy patients with all forms of AMS will improve quickly, often with full resolution of symptoms within 24 hours.

CRITICAL INTERVENTIONS

- Administer acetazolamide and dexamethasone to patients with AMS and HACE
- Administer oxygen and positive airway pressure ventilation by mask or endotracheal tube to patients with severe HAPE

DISPOSITION

Young, healthy patients with mild-to-moderate AMS may be discharged with instructions not to resume ascent until after symptoms have subsided and only if preventative measures are taken. Medications should never be used to allow further ascent in light of persistent symptoms. Patients with HAPE, HACE, severe AMS, or moderate AMS with underlying cardiopulmonary or cerebrovascular disease, complications such as chest pain or ECG evidence of ischemia, or other significant medical problems should be admitted. Most such patients will require observation and treatment in an intensive care unit.

COMMON PITFALLS

✔ Failure to consider the diagnosis of AMS in patients who become ill after rapidly ascending to high altitudes
✔ Treating AMS with medications to allow for further ascent or continued exposure

✔ Failure to use adjunctive medications and hyperbaric therapy (if available) when descent is not immediately possible

✔ Giving diuretics and vasodilators to patients with HAPE

References

1. Bartsch P, Maggiorini M, Ritter M, et al. Prevention of high-altitude pulmonary edema by nifedipine. *N Engl J Med* 1991;325:1284.
2. Dickinson JG. Acetazolamide in acute mountain sickness. *BMJ* 1987;295:1161.
3. Ellsworth AE, Larson EB, Strickland D. A randomized trial of dexamethasone and acetazolamide for acute mountain sickness prophylaxis. *Am J Med* 1987;83:1024.
4. Ellsworth AE, Meyer AF, Larson EB. Dexamethasone in the prevention of acute mountain sickness during rapid, active ascent of Mount Rainier. *Clin Res* 1988;36:172a.
5. Ferrazzini G, Maggiorini M, Kriemler S, et al. Successful treatment of acute mountain sickness with dexamethasone. *BMJ* 1987;294:1380.
6. Foulke GE. Altitude-related illness. *Am J Emerg Med* 1985;3:217.
7. Grissom CK, Roach RC, Sarnquist FH, et al. Acetazolamide in the treatment of acute mountain sickness: clinical efficacy and effect on gas exchange. *Ann Intern Med* 1992;116:461.
8. Hackett PH, Roach RC. High-altitude illness. *N Engl J Med* 2001;345:107–114.
9. Hackett PH, Roach RC. High-altitude medicine. In: Auerbach PS, ed. *Wilderness medicine.* St. Louis: Mosby, 2001:2–43.
10. Honigman B, Theis MK, Koziol-McLain J, et al. Acute mountain sickness in a general tourist population at moderate altitudes. *Ann Intern Med* 1993;118:587.
11. Houston CS. Altitude illness. *Postgrad Med* 1983;74(1):231.
12. Houston CS. Altitude illness. *Emerg Med Clin North Am* 1984;2:503.
13. Johnson TS, Rock PB. Current concepts, acute mountain sickness. *N Engl J Med* 1982;73:395.
14. Kasic J, Yaron M, Nicholas R, et al. Treatment of acute mountain sickness: hyperbaric versus oxygen therapy. *Ann Emerg Med* 1991;20:1109.
15. Milledge JS. Acute mountain sickness. *Thorax* 1983;38:641.
16. Olez O, Maggiorini M, Ritter M, et al. Prevention and treatment of high-altitude pulmonary edema by a calcium-channel blocker. *Int J Sports Med* 1992;13:S65.
17. Rennie D. The great breathless mountains. *JAMA* 1986;256:81.
18. Roach RC, Bartsch P, Oelz O, et al.Lake Louise AMS Scoring Consensus Committee: the Lake Louise acute mountain sickness scoring system. In: Sutton JR, Houston CS, Coates G, eds. *Hypoxia molecular medicine.* Burlington, Vt.: Charles S. Houston, 1993:272–274.
19. Scherrer U, Vollenweider L, Delabays A, et al. Inhaled nitric acid for high altitude pulmonary edema. *N Engl J Med* 1996;334:624.
20. Schoene RB. High-altitude pulmonary edema: pathophysiology and clinical review. *Ann Emerg Med* 1987;16:987.
21. Shlim DR. Treatment of acute mountain sickness. *N Engl J Med* 1985;313:891.
22. Tso E. High-altitude illness. *Emerg Med Clin North Am* 1992;10:231.
23. Zell SC, Goodman PH. Acetazolamide and dexamethasone in the prevention of acute mountain sickness. *West J Med* 1988;148:541.

CHAPTER 355
Underwater and Diving Injuries

Brian K. Snyder

Underwater diving, with or without the use of compressed gas, usually takes place without incident. However, injuries that are unique to the underwater environment and diving can occur. These injuries are generally secondary to pressure changes (barotrauma) or the effect of gas bubbles in the vascular system and tissues (arterial gas embolism and decompression sickness) (17). Other injuries associated with compressed air diving include gas toxicity and immersion pulmonary edema.

TABLE 355.1. The Gas Laws

Boyle's Law: Given a constant temperature, the pressure and volume of an ideal gas are inversely related.
Dalton's Law: The total pressure exerted by a mixture of gases is the sum of the partial pressures of each gas.
Henry's Law: At equilibrium, the quantity of a gas in solution in a liquid is proportional to the partial pressure of the gas.

Any discussion of diving injuries requires an understanding of gas physics (Table 355.1). In diving medicine, pressure is commonly referred to in units of atmospheres absolute (ATA) or feet of seawater (fsw) (Table 355.2). Boyle's law states that pressure and volume are inversely related. Changes of volume and pressure in gas-containing organs of the body during descent and ascent lead to barotrauma. According to Dalton's law and Henry's law, compressed gas breathing at depth will lead to an increase of partial pressures of gas within the lung, vascular system, and tissues of the diver. A subsequent decrease in ambient pressure may lead to decompression sickness.

Barotrauma can be divided by whether it occurs during descent (more common) or ascent (more dangerous). Structures potentially injured during descent are the middle and inner ear and the sinuses. The lung is the structure most likely to be injured during ascent, but fortunately, this is uncommon.

Decompression sickness (DCS) or "the bends" is the result of the occlusive and inflammatory effects of inert gas bubbles in the tissues and vascular system (7). Although at depth, inert gas will diffuse into and saturate the tissues. If the ambient pressure decreases too quickly during ascent, gas bubbles will form in the tissue and vascular system. The exact mechanism of bubble formation is unclear, although preexisting micronuclei of gas may serve as the nidus for further bubble growth (4). Given that bubbling often occurs without symptoms, bubbles are necessary but not sufficient to cause DCS, suggesting that there is a threshold above which symptoms occur.

Divers use decompression tables or special diving computers to determine safe dive exposures. Although unusual, DCS can occur even when dives conform to accepted decompression tables or computer algorithms. Factors that may increase the risk of DCS include repetitive dives, rapid ascent, and subsequent altitude exposure.

Bubbles may form in the circulation (usually the low pressure venous system) or directly in tissues. Venous bubbles may cross right-to-left shunts in the heart (e.g., a patent foramen ovale) or the lungs and arterialize, leading to arterial gas embolism (AGE) and ischemia. The pathophysiology of spinal cord DCS appears to be initial bubbling in the venous plexus system causing first a decrease, then complete cessation of venous blood flow from the cord. Decreasing venous blood flow prevents dissolved nitrogen in spinal cord tissues from off-gassing, thereby forming in situ bubbles within the spinal cord (16).

TABLE 355.2. Pressure Units and Equivalents

1 ATM = 760 mm Hg = 14.7 psi = 101.325 kPa = 33 fsw
Therefore at a depth of 66 feet of seawater, total pressure would be 3 ATM: 2 ATM for the pressure exerted by the water column and 1 ATM for the pressure of the atmosphere at sea level.
ATM = atmosphere
mm Hg = millimeters mercury
psi = pounds per square inch
kPa = kilopascal (SI units)
fsw = feet of seawater

Other mechanisms besides direct ischemic effects are prominent in DCS and AGE. The air-blood and air-endothelial interfaces are highly reactive, initiating thrombotic and inflammatory processes. This causes leaky endothelium, leading to third spacing of fluids. Furthermore, adhesion and activation of neutrophils on endothelium leads to the release of reactive oxygen species and other tissue-toxic neutrophil-derived moieties, causing a histopathology similar to an ischemia/reperfusion injury (10).

CLINICAL PRESENTATION

The most common form of barotrauma seen in diving is a middle ear "squeeze." During descent air within the middle ear is contracting as the pressure increases, causing inward movement of the tympanic membrane (TM). If the pressure in the middle ear is not equalized, by opening the Eustachian tube with a Valsalva or other maneuver, the TM can be injured (1). Bleeding can occur within the TM or within the middle ear space leading to a hemotympanum, or the TM may rupture. Similarly, a closed space in the external ear canal from occlusive material (e.g., wax or ear plugs) can bend the TM outward during descent and cause injury. The diver with otic barotrauma will present with a history of difficulty clearing the affected ear, pain, a conductive hearing loss and sometimes vertigo.

Without adequate sinus drainage, during descent pressure will increase in the sinuses, leading to pain and possibly a bloody nasal discharge as the mucosa is stripped from the periosteum.

The inner ear can also be injured secondary to pressure changes. During descent, a forceful Valsalva maneuver can damage the round or oval window of the cochlea, potentially forming a fistula. The diver with inner-ear barotrauma will present with a history of difficulty clearing the ears, the use of a forceful Valsalva maneuver, and sudden onset of vertigo, tinnitus, and hearing loss. On examination the patient will have severe vertigo, a sensorineural hearing loss, and possibly a positive "fistula test." The fistula test involves insufflation of air onto the tympanic membrane. The test is positive if eyes deviate to the contralateral side. The patient with inner ear barotrauma may also exhibit signs of middle-ear barotrauma (1).

During ascent, gas volumes increase as the pressure decreases. Generally, divers have no problems with their ears or sinuses during ascent, because gas leaves the middle ear as the Eustachian tube opens spontaneously or leaves the sinuses through the ostia. Barotrauma of ascent generally involves the lung. The most common scenario leading to pulmonary barotrauma is a panicked, rapid, or out-of-air ascent. If the glottis is closed during ascent, the expanding gas cannot escape, and the lung may rupture. Congenital or acquired gas-trapping pulmonary processes (e.g., a cyst) may also result in lung barotrauma (16). Once the lung ruptures, gas can collect in the mediastinum (pneumomediastinum), interstitium of the lungs (pulmonary emphysema), in the pleural space (pneumothorax), or in the vascular system as an arterial gas embolism (9). Divers with pneumomediastinum or pneumothorax will present with chest pain, dyspnea, and possibly subcutaneous emphysema. A chest radiograph will generally show the abnormal collection of gas.

Although gas from an arterial gas embolism will systemically embolize, the most prominent organ involved is the brain (cerebral arterial gas embolism or CAGE). A diver with CAGE will develop symptoms during ascent or immediately on surfacing. Symptoms include altered level of consciousness, hemiplegia or hemiparesis, seizure, or other cerebral dysfunction; sudden death may occur. If the patient survives, they may spontaneously improve as gas is forced through the cerebral vascular system by a spike in blood pressure. Any neurological symptoms in the setting of pulmonary barotrauma should be thought to be secondary to CAGE and appropriate therapy initiated (16).

Symptoms and classification of DCS depend on the organs affected. Type I DCS ("pain only" DCS) involves the joints, extremities, and skin. Lymphatic obstruction can cause lymphedema, which usually takes days to resolve despite recompression therapy. Type II DCS (or "serious" DCS) includes "neurological DCS" involving the central nervous system (CNS;mainly the spinal cord in compressed air sport divers), vestibular DCS ("staggers"), and cardiopulmonary DCS ("chokes").

The symptoms of DCS usually occur minutes to several hours after surfacing, but cases of DCS symptoms occurring days after diving have been reported. Symptoms from DCS may improve during a subsequent dive (essentially recompression therapy) but can get worse on resurfacing (as the inert gas load increases). Because flying after diving may elicit or worsen DCS symptoms, divers are advised to refrain from flying for at least 12 hours after the last dive (12).

The pain of Type I DCS is typically described as deep, and unrelieved, but not worsened, with movement. Given that divers can injure themselves in other ways (strains, direct trauma), pain from DCS can be confused with or attributed to pain from these injuries. Distention from bubbles in ligaments, fascia, and long bones, or the activation of stretch receptors caused by bubbles in tendons are thought to be mechanism of pain. This mechanism is supported by the rapid improvement of Type I DCS symptoms with recompression. The most common locations for Type I DCS are knees and shoulders, and often only a single joint is involved. Diffuse and difficult to describe back pain may herald the more serious signs of spinal cord DCS.

The classic description of neurologic DCS (type II) begins with this sensation of truncal constriction or girdle-like pain. A wooly feeling may begin in the feet developing into an ascending paralysis. This produces a presentation similar to a transverse myelitis. This form of neurologic DCS is usually rapid in onset and has a tendency to affect the lower cervical and thoracic regions.

In Type II DCS, neurologic deficits do not necessarily follow distinct spinal cord syndromes seen with trauma or ischemia. Furthermore, because lesions are scattered throughout the spinal cord, a definitive "level" will not necessarily be found. Incontinence and sexual dysfunction from autonomic involvement is not uncommon.

Pulmonary DCS, or the chokes, is generally seen only after prolonged, deep exposures. This syndrome is caused by large numbers of pulmonary artery bubbles and manifests itself with cough, hemoptysis, dyspnea, substernal chest pain, or cardiovascular collapse. Vestibular decompression sickness, or the staggers, also usually occurs after deep, long dives, although it is increasingly being reported in sport divers. It manifests itself with vertigo, hearing loss, tinnitus, and dysequilibrium (5). These symptoms are similar to those experienced in inner-ear barotrauma, however historical clues are helpful in distinguishing the two distinct processes.

Inert gas, especially nitrogen, can cause narcosis at depth. Typically, symptoms start at depths of 100 feet or greater if breathing air. Further depth increases symptoms including loss of fine motor skills and high-order mental processes and behavior similar to that seen in alcohol intoxication. Below 300 feet, unconsciousness occurs. Symptoms improve on ascent and may make activities at depth difficult or dangerous.

Oxygen toxicity mainly affects the pulmonary system and the CNS. Pulmonary oxygen toxicity is unusual but can occur at partial pressures of oxygen at or below 1 ATA, as is seen in patients requiring prolonged mechanical ventilation with high fractions of inspired oxygen. Symptoms include dyspnea, chest pain, cough, and decreased pulmonary function.

The CNS effects of oxygen usually begin to occur at depths when the partial pressure of oxygen in the breathing mixture is greater than 1.6 ATA (220 feet of seawater if breathing compressed air). Some divers may breathe oxygen enriched air ("nitrox") with fractions of oxygen of 32% to 36%. Therefore, cerebral oxygen toxicity can occur at lesser depths and actually is the factor that limits diving depth with nitrox. Additionally, there are "oxygen rebreather" systems where the diver breathes in a continuous circuit of gas with more than 95% oxygen. With these systems, cerebral oxygen toxicity can occur at depths as little as 25 feet.

Cerebral oxygen toxicity manifests itself with twitching, nausea, paresthesias, dizziness, and seizures. A seizure may be the initial manifestation of cerebral oxygen toxicity and in the water may cause drowning. Clinical hyperbaric oxygen treatments use oxygen partial pressures up to 3 ATA. Although oxygen toxicity can occur in hyperbaric chambers, it is unusual. Divers are more prone to cerebral oxygen toxicity as they are exerting themselves in a cold, wet environment. Cerebral oxygen toxicity is affected by cerebral blood flow and $PaCO_2$. The mechanism is under investigation but may be caused by an increase in nitric oxide production (3).

Immersion pulmonary edema can occur while diving and swimming. Typical symptoms include dyspnea, chest discomfort, coughing of pink frothy secretions. The mechanism of this condition is unknown. It is not caused by decompression. Hydrostatic forces, thermal stress, and possibly increased capillary permeability may be involved (8).

DIFFERENTIAL DIAGNOSIS

The diver with vertigo may present a diagnostic challenge. Vertigo can be caused by unequal clearing of the ears (leading to unequal vestibular stimulation) or a potentially dangerous processes such as inner-ear barotrauma or vestibular DCS (Table 355.3). The diagnosis can become complicated by combinations of injuries, e.g., a diver sustains inner-ear barotrauma, causing him to panic, leading to a rapid ascent and CAGE. The major confusion in the diagnosis of vertigo is differentiating inner-ear barotrauma from CAGE. Given that hyperbaric oxygen (HBO) treatment for CAGE can worsen inner-ear barotrauma, this distinction is important; however, if one cannot distinguish between the two conditions or both may have occurred, myringotomies can be performed before commencing HBO.

Another sometimes difficult distinction is that between CAGE and DCS. In fact, the two conditions can occur concurrently (Type III DCS) (15). Some authorities do not distinguish between the two entities and call all bubble-related diving injuries decompression illness (DCI). The argument for this approach is that sometimes DCS and AGE cannot be reliably distinguished and the primary treatment is the same. Opponents of the term DCI counter by stating that although sometimes indistinguishable, the two processes can often be separated. Additionally, although primary therapy may be the same, adjunctive therapies may not (e.g., lidocaine in CAGE), and research may be hindered by such a lack of distinction.

CAGE usually occurs immediately or soon on surfacing after a rapid or uncontrolled ascent, and demonstrates mainly cerebral symptoms, such as altered level of consciousness, seizure, or hemiplegia. On the other hand, symptoms of DCS begin minutes to hours after the dive and although cerebral symptoms can occur, neurologic symptoms and signs usually refer to the spinal cord. CNS trauma, near-drowning, and hypothermia should be considered in the differential diagnosis of these conditions.

EMERGENCY DEPARTMENT EVALUATION

The history should include details regarding the dive-profile, symptom latency, severity, and progression, and preexisting health. Vital signs should include measurement of oxygen saturation. The physical exam should focus on the cardiopulmonary and neurological systems, and the ears, nose, and throat. Patients with chest signs and symptoms or altered mental status should have a chest radiograph, electrocardiogram (ECG), and continuous cardiac monitoring. Evaluation for cardiac ischemia or dysfunction should be considered in patients with an abnormal ECG, pulmonary edema, or unexplained chest complaints, particularly those with risk factors for cardiovascular disease. Although routine laboratory studies not helpful in the diagnosis or treatment of diving injury, they should be obtained if clinically indicated.

EMERGENCY DEPARTMENT MANAGEMENT

Patients with uncomplicated barotrauma to the middle ear or sinuses should be treated symptomatically with decongestants and analgesics. Antibiotics can be prescribed in the cases of a perforated tympanic membrane or sinus barotrauma occurring in contaminated water.

Patients with inner-ear barotrauma should sit up and avoid maneuvers that increase intracranial pressure (nose blowing, etc.). Some otolaryngologists advocate conservative treatment

---

TABLE 355.3. Differential Diagnosis of Vertigo in the Diver

Cause of Vertigo	Risk Factors	Onset of Symptoms	Symptoms and Physical Exam Findings
Alternobaric	Unequal clearing of ears	During descent or ascent	Self-limited
Middle-ear barotrauma	Difficulty clearing ears	Occurs during descent	Signs of barotrauma on otoscopic exam, conductive hearing loss
Inner-ear barotrauma	Difficulty clearing ears, forceful Valsalva	Occurs during descent, occurs immediately after attempt to clear ears	Severe vertigo, tinnitus, sensorineural hearing loss, possible fistula test (see text), may have signs of middle-ear barotrauma
Vestibular decompression sickness	Deep, prolonged dives, switching of breathing gas	Occurs after dive completion, usually 15 minutes to hours	May have other signs of DCS
Cerebral arterial gas embolism	Rapid or panic ascent	Occurs on surfacing or within minutes of surfacing	Will have other signs of CAGE (altered or loss of consciousness, hemiplegia) (see text)

with antivertigo and antiemetic drugs, reserving surgical intervention to those who do not improve spontaneously, although others advocate immediate surgical exploration (1).

Patients with pneumomediastinum but with no sign of CAGE can be managed conservatively. Those with a pneumothorax should have it evacuated with a chest tube, especially if HBO therapy is to be employed.

Patients with suspected DCS or CAGE should receive 100% oxygen by nonrebreather face mask or endotracheal tube if necessary to ensure an intact airway. Recompression with HBO should occur as soon as possible, with transfer to a recompression center if necessary. Outcomes seem to correspond to the timeliness of HBO therapy. There are several recompression treatment tables employed in the treatment of DCS or CAGE, the most common being the U.S. Navy Treatment Table 6 (with a maximum treatment pressure of 60 ft or 2.8 ATA), although lesser treatment pressures have been used with good results (11). If symptoms do not fully resolve, some centers will continue HBO treatments daily or twice daily until symptoms plateau. Divers with DCS have responded to HBO days after injury, and therefore this should be instituted even if presentation is delayed.

The beneficial effects of HBO are several. The pressure reduces bubble size. Increased partial pressure of oxygen dissolved in serum creates a gradient causing nitrogen to move from bubbles into serum, increasing off-gassing of inert gas. Oxygen in turn moves into bubbles, but because it is metabolically active, it subsequently moves into cells, leading to further dissolution of bubbles. HBO increases oxygen delivery to ischemic tissues, decreases edema and intracranial pressure, and ameliorates the adherence and activation of leukocytes on vascular endothelium (10).

Historically, patients with suspected AGE were kept in a left lateral Trendelenburg position in order to "trap" air in the right ventricle. The Trendelenburg position increases intracranial pressure and should be avoided. Conversely, divers with CAGE have been known to collapse when sitting or standing, perhaps secondary to redistribution of intravascular air. Therefore divers with CAGE should be kept supine with the head in a neutral position.

Nondextrose containing, isotonic intravenous fluids should be infused in order to preserve tissue perfusion in divers with DCS and CAGE. Various pharmaceutical adjuncts have been used in the treatment of DCS and CAGE, including aspirin, corticosteroids, and heparin. Animal studies and human experience have generally shown no definite benefit (2). Intravenous lidocaine in the treatment of CAGE has been shown to be effective in animal models and in a human study examining neuropsychiatric outcomes after cardiopulmonary bypass (where neuropsychiatric deficits are thought to be secondary to intravascular air) (6,13,14). Typical cardiac doses are generally used.

Oxygen and nitrogen toxicity and immersion pulmonary edema resolve spontaneously. Treatment is primarily supportive. If immersion pulmonary edema is severe or persistent, standard treatments for this condition can be administered (8).

CRITICAL INTERVENTIONS

- Obtain a chest radiograph on patients with cardiopulmonary complaints. If the chest radiograph is normal, consider evaluation for acute coronary syndromes
- Administer oxygen and i.v. fluids and arrange for hyperbaric oxygen therapy in patients with DCS and CAGE
- Remember that medical conditions not related to barotrauma or decompression can occur in or around the water, and the physician must be careful to evaluate for such processes

DISPOSITION

Patients with barotitis or sinus barotrauma should not return to diving until symptoms resolve. Those with a perforated TM must not dive until it heals. Otolaryngology referral in 4 to 6 weeks is warranted. Given that treatment of inner-ear barotrauma is controversial, emergent otolaryngology consultation should be obtained for patients with this condition. Patients with pulmonary barotrauma, but without AGE, should be admitted for observation and treatment. Those with suspected DCS or CAGE should be transferred to a facility capable of providing hyperbaric oxygen therapy. They may require hospitalization or repetitive treatments after initial therapy.

Clinicians unfamiliar with the treatment of underwater diving injuries should consult a diving or hyperbaric medicine specialist or the Divers Alert Network (DAN; phone: 1-919-684-8111; web site: www.diversalertnetwork.org). DAN has staff available 24 hours a day to provide assistance to divers and clinicians and can provide the location of the nearest hyperbaric facility. All divers with DCS or CAGE should be examined by a physician trained in diving medicine before returning to diving. Counseling of divers experiencing immersion pulmonary edema is difficult as it cannot be predicted who will experience another episode.

COMMON PITFALLS

✔ Failure to appreciate that significant barotrauma can occur at shallow depths with breath-holding dives
✔ Failure to appreciate that DCS and CAGE can be delayed in onset, worsen with time, or improve spontaneously and then relapse and that patients may present with these conditions after traveling from remote locations
✔ Failure to consider the possibility of DCS or CAGE in any patient with neurological symptoms after underwater diving
✔ Failure to consult a diving or hyperbaric medicine specialist or the Divers Alert Network for advice, and to consider a diagnostic trial of HBO when the diagnosis is not clear

Acknowledgments

We thank previous edition chapter authors Christopher H. Linden and Christopher J. Degnen.

References

1. Becker GD, Parell GJ. Barotrauma of the ears and sinuses after scuba diving. *Euro Arch Otorhinolaryngol* 2001;258:159–163.
2. Catron PW, Flynn ET. Adjuvant drug therapy for decompression sickness: a review. *Undersea Biomed Res* 1982;9:161–173.
3. Demchenko IT, Boso AE, O'Neill TJ, et al. Nitric oxide and cerebral blood flow responses to hyperbaric oxygen. *J Appl Physiol* 2000;88:1381–1389.
4. Doolette DJ, Mitchell SJ. The physiologic kinetics of nitrogen and the prevention of decompression sickness. *Clin Pharmacokinet* 2001;40:1–14.
5. Doolette DJ, Mitchell SJ. Biophysical basis for inner ear decompression sickness. *J Appl Physiol* 2003;94:2145–2150.
6. Dutka AJ, Mink R, McDermott J, et al. Effect of lidocaine on somatosensory evoked response and cerebral blood flow after canine cerebral air embolism. *Stroke* 1992;23:1515–1521.
7. Dutka AJ, Francis TJ. Pathophysiology of decompression sickness. In: Bove AA. (ed.). *Bove and Davis' diving medicine*, 3rd ed. Philadelphia: WB Saunders Company, 1997:159–177.
8. Hampson NB, Dunford RG. Pulmonary edema of scuba divers. *Undersea Hyper Med* 1997;24:29–33.
9. Harker CP, Neuman TS, Olson LK, et al. The roentgenographic findings associated with air embolism in sport SCUBA divers. *J Emerg Med* 1993;11:443–449.
10. Martin JD, Thom SR. Vascular leukocyte sequestration in decompression sickness and prophylactic hyperbaric oxygen therapy in rats. *Aviat Space Environ Med* 2002;73:565–569.
11. Li RC. The monoplace hyperbaric chamber and management of decompression sickness. *Hong Kong Med J* 2001;7:435–438.
12. Millar I. Post diving altitude exposure. *SPUMS J* 1996;26:135–140.

13. Mitchell SJ, Pellett O, Gorman DF. Cerebral protection by lidocaine during cardiac operations. *Ann Thorac Surg* 1999;67:1117–24.
14. Mitchell SJ. Lidocaine for the treatment of decompression illness: a review of the literature. *Undersea Hyper Med* 2001;28:165–174.
15. Neuman TS, Bove AA. Combined arterial gas embolism and decompression sickness following no-stop dives. *Undersea Biomed Res* 1990;17:429–436.
16. Neuman TS. Arterial gas embolism and decompression sickness. *News Physiol Sci* 2001:17:77–81.
17. Strauss MB, Borer RC. Diving medicine: contemporary topics and their controversies. *Am J Emerg Med* 2001;19:232–238.

CHAPTER 356
Submersion Injuries

Gregory A. Volturo

In 1998, drowning was responsible for 4,406 deaths in the United States (12); this is down from over 8,000 deaths in 1982. Drowning, however, remains the third most common cause of death in children (7). Death rates from drowning are more than five times greater for males than for females, and nearly three times greater for African-Americans than for Caucasians.

The highest incidence occurs between ages 10 and 19. Forty percent of victims are less than 4 years old. More than half of those who drown in swimming pools are under age 10. Most children who have drowned in swimming pools had been reported to be out of sight for less than 5 minutes and in the care of one or both parents (12). Swimming pools, however, account only for 10% of all reported drownings. Drownings are more likely in lakes, rivers, or oceans. Quarries, pits, ornamental pools, spas, and bathtubs also contribute to the toll (8). Toddlers may even become trapped in a bucket when they lean over to play with the water inside. Nonlethal incidents occur an estimated 600 times more often than their fatal counterparts (8). Factors that increase the likelihood of a submersion accident include alcohol and drug use, the inability to swim, seizures, hyperventilation, hypothermia, injury during diving or other water sports, and exhaustion.

Drowning is death from suffocation as a result of submersion in a fluid medium; near-drowning implies survival, at least temporarily, after such suffocation. Wet drowning (when fluid is aspirated) occurs in 85% to 90% of cases, and dry drowning (when fluid is not aspirated) occurs in the remainder. Dry drowning was initially thought to be a result of laryngospasm; however, it is more likely a result of cardiac arrest (CA) and death before aspiration occurs (10). Secondary drowning is death as a result of respiratory failure from the respiratory distress syndrome (RDS) that occurs within 72 hours of initial resuscitation.

RDS results from an influx of proteins and fluid into the alveoli as a result of loss of surfactant and leaky capillary membranes, which results in hypoxia and acidosis. Patients with secondary drowning have subtle respiratory compromise immediately after submersion. About 15% of near-drowning victims who are conscious when admitted to the hospital die of RDS (7). The immersion syndrome is sudden death immediately following immersion in very cold water. It is appears to be as a result of

vagally mediated brady-asystolic CA, or ventricular fibrillation (VF) (5).

Drowning may begin with an initial period of panic, followed by a struggle with breath-holding. Subsequently, apnea occurs, followed by swallowing of large amounts of water, which may be vomited and aspirated. The victim ultimately loses consciousness; shortly thereafter, CA ensues (24). More commonly, however, witnesses report that the victim was just floating on the water and became motionless or disappeared (9).

Theoretically, in fresh-water drowning, aspirated water is hypotonic and should be rapidly absorbed across the alveolar membrane and into the intravascular space, resulting in hemodilution and hypervolemia, with lowering of serum electrolyte and protein levels. In contrast, with hyperosmolar saltwater aspiration, fluid would be expected to diffuse in the opposite direction, resulting in pulmonary edema, hypovolemia, hemoconcentration, and electrolyte abnormalities.

Although such changes may occur in those who are dead at the scene, they are of minor clinical importance in resuscitated patients, who generally have been submerged for a short period and have aspirated a relatively small volume of water (rarely greater than 3 to 4 mL/kg) (7). Although pulmonary injury may occur with aspiration of as little as 2 mL/kg of water, significant changes in intravascular volume are generally not seen with less than 10 mL/kg. Hypermagnesemia has been reported after seawater drowning possibly as a result of both aspiration and ingestion (4). Generally however, more than 22 mL/kg is required before electrolyte changes occur, except for incidents in water with very high solute concentrations, such as the Dead Sea (4).

Noncardiogenic pulmonary edema may occur in both freshwater and saltwater drowning but is less likely with aspiration of fresh water. Hypoxia and the direct effect of aspirated water combine to produce this abnormality in about 5% of near-drowning cases (17). The causes of hypoxia include diffusion abnormalities and decreased lung compliance (a result of the inactivation and dilution of surfactant) and increased intrapulmonary shunting (resulting from atelectasis, bronchospasm, and obstruction of alveoli by water and debris such as vomitus or sand) (7). Chlorine in swimming pools may have an additional deleterious effect on pulmonary tissues. Aspiration of bacteria may also result in pneumonia.

Acidosis is common and is a result of both metabolic and respiratory causes (inadequate ventilation results in anaerobic metabolism with lactic acid production). The acidosis may be worse in warm-water drownings than in cold water (7). Generally, all patients who are acidotic on admission (pH <7.3) do poorly. However, profound acidosis is still compatible with full recovery.

Cardiovascular complications may develop as a result of hypoxia and acidosis. Hypothermia is extremely common in immersion victims and may also contribute to the development of cardiovascular complications. The most common findings are arterial hypotension and CA. VF is rare, particularly in normothermic patients. The diving reflex, a vagally mediated response to cold-water immersion, consisting of apnea, bradycardia, peripheral vasoconstriction, decreased cardiac output, and increased mean arterial blood pressure, may also be responsible for some of the cardiovascular changes seen in drowning victims (25). Although the diving reflex has been thought to have a neuroprotective role in children, it has not been shown to be active in human adults. Hypoxic stimulation of chemoreceptors in the carotid body may result in vagally mediated bradycardia, even to the point of asystole (19).

Renal failure, although uncommon, may be a result of anoxia or to hemoglobin or myoglobin deposition in the renal tubules secondary to hemolysis or rhabdomyolysis (20). Hemolysis can occur in freshwater drownings but is rare. Disseminated intravascular coagulation, also uncommon, may be caused by hypoxia, acidosis, or extensive pulmonary endothelial damage.

Severe neurologic damage occurs in 15% to 25% of near-drowning patients (20). A favorable neurologic outcome is more likely in patients receiving cardiopulmonary resuscitation (CPR) and those with hypothermia (as a result of its protective effect on cerebral metabolism) (3,5).

Neurologic injury is as a result of hypoxia, which is further complicated by metabolic acidosis and secondary cerebral hypoperfusion. As a result, cerebral edema develops and may lead to brainstem herniation and death. The degree of anoxic injury depends on the duration of hypoxia, the water temperature, and the patient's underlying physical condition (5). From 10% to 20% of patients presenting with coma recover completely, despite initially fixed and dilated pupils (14).

CLINICAL PRESENTATION

Victims of near-drowning may be awake, lethargic but arousable, combative, comatose, or in CA on presentation. A history of coughing, choking, or vomiting may be given. In mild cases, the pulse, blood pressure, and respiratory rate may be elevated, but in patients with severe hypoxia, vital signs may be decreased or absent. Hypothermia may be present. Examination may reveal cool, clammy, pale, or cyanotic skin. Aspirated or regurgitated food, water, or other foreign material may be present in the mouth and airway. Rhonchi, rales, or wheezing may be audible on pulmonary examination. Gastric distention is common. In severe cases, decorticate or decerebrate posturing or flaccid paralysis with unreactive pupils and absent cranial nerve, brainstem, and deep tendon reflexes may be observed. Associated traumatic injuries may also be present. Victims of scuba-diving accidents may have signs and symptoms of concomitant barotrauma and decompression sickness (see Chapter 356, "Submersion Injuries").

The electrocardiogram (ECG) may reveal evidence of ischemia, sinus tachycardia or bradycardia, or ventricular ectopy, VF, or asystole. Atrial fibrillation may also occur, primarily in patients with hypothermia. Arterial blood gas analysis may reveal acidosis, hypoxia, and hypercapnia. Although leukocytosis may be present, the hematocrit is usually normal. Except for a decrease in bicarbonate, serum chemistries are usually normal on presentation. Evidence of hemolysis, infection, rhabdomyolysis, and anoxic organ damage (e.g., liver and renal failure, disseminated intravascular coagulation) may appear hours or days after the initial insult.

The chest radiograph may reveal isolated or diffuse patchy infiltrates or frank pulmonary edema. An initially normal radiograph may reveal these findings if repeated several hours later. Pulmonary edema has been reported to develop as long as 12 hours after the submersion incident (16).

DIFFERENTIAL DIAGNOSIS

In patients found unresponsive in water or other fluid, the possibility of trauma (especially head and neck), drug or chemical intoxication, CA, or stroke while swimming, cerebral air embolus (in scuba divers), and attempted suicide, murder, or child abuse or neglect should be considered.

EMERGENCY DEPARTMENT EVALUATION

The history includes details such as submersion time, medium, and temperature; events surrounding the accident; level of consciousness and vital signs at the scene; and signs, symptoms, and treatment before arrival. For children who fall into pails of liquid (e.g., detergent, insecticide), or industrial workers who may be submerged in a medium other than water, the type of liquid and its potential toxicity should be ascertained. An accident near rocks, in heavy surf, or while diving, or an unwitnessed event, should raise suspicion for concomitant traumatic injury.

The physical examination should initially focus on vital signs, cardiopulmonary status, and neurologic findings. To rule out hypothermia, a rectal temperature should be taken using a low-reading thermometer or probe. Serial coma grading (using, for instance, the Glasgow Coma Scale) is helpful in monitoring progress. In all patients, an initial cardiac rhythm and chest radiograph and, subsequently, an ECG, should be obtained. Baseline laboratory evaluation should include an arterial blood gas analysis, complete blood count, platelet count, serum chemistries (electrolytes, glucose, blood urea nitrogen, creatinine), coagulation profile, and urinalysis. Seriously ill patients should also have liver function tests and calcium, magnesium, and creatine phosphokinase measurements. Cardiac enzymes should be obtained in victims who require CPR or who have dysrhythmias or ECG evidence of ischemia. A computed tomography scan of the head should be performed to evaluate for cerebral edema, trauma, and other pathology in those who are comatose.

EMERGENCY DEPARTMENT MANAGEMENT

Rapid prehospital response and early initiation of resuscitation are the most important factors influencing morbidity and mortality. Although artificial ventilation can and should be started immediately in unconscious patients, cardiac compression is impractical and ineffective while the victim is still in the water. Hence, rapid extrication is essential. It is best performed by those trained in, and equipped for, water rescue to prevent additional casualties (e.g., accidental hypothermia or submersion injury in rescuers). C-spine immobilization is an important element in the management of patients truly at risk for C-spine injury. Effective C-spine immobilization may be difficult, especially in the water, and may have adverse effects, making the resuscitation difficult. In a series of 2,244 submersion victims, the incidence of C-spine injury was 0.49%, and occurred only in patients who sustained traumatic injury before or during their submersion. Thus routine C-spine immobilization does not appear to be warranted solely on the basis of a history of submersion. Those individuals who have a history of high impact submersion (water skiing, jet skiing, fall from a height, surfing, etc.), and those individuals with physical evidence of trauma should have backboard and cervical immobilization as soon as possible, and subsequent radiographic studies when stable (23).

After extrication, CPR and advanced cardiac and trauma life-support measures are instituted, as necessary. The airway should be cleared of fluid and vomitus before assisted breathing is started. Except for placing the victim in a head-down position, postural drainage procedures are not recommended, because the risks (loss of airway control, aggravation of spinal and other injuries, aspiration, and interruption of CPR) outweigh the possible but unproven benefits (13,17). The Heimlich maneuver may be used to clear the airway if it is obstructed with particulate matter, but it is of unproven value in removing aspirated fluid. Indiscriminate use in victims with submersion injury may result in vomiting and aspiration of gastric contents.

Immediate therapy is aimed at correcting hypoxemia, pulmonary edema and hypotension, the most common clinical manifestations if near drowning. All victims of submersion injury should receive high-flow oxygen and endotracheal intubation if clinically indicated. Wet clothing should be removed to prevent further cooling and to allow inspection of traumatic injuries. In patients who remain obtunded, cyanotic, or hypotensive despite intubation and fluid resuscitation, and in those who present with cardiac dysrhythmias, acidosis is often present, and $NaHCO_3$ (1–2 mEq/kg i.v.) may be given empirically (20). Caution must be used not to cause an alkalosis, therefore $NaHCO_3$ therapy is best guided by blood gas analysis if rapidly available. Naloxone and 50% dextrose (or a bedside glucose determination) should also be considered in the unconscious patient.

In the emergency department (ED), treatment of hypoxia is of utmost importance. If not intubated on the basis of clinical indications, patients with an arterial PO_2 below 60 mm Hg and a PCO_2 above 50 mm Hg, with an oxygen saturation less than 90% while receiving high-flow O_2 by mask, should be intubated. If only hypoxia is present, continuous positive airway pressure by mask (CPAP) may be useful. In intubated patients with persistent hypoxia, mechanical ventilation with positive end-expiratory pressure (PEEP) will decrease the amount of intrapulmonary shunting, reduce ventilation–perfusion mismatch, and increase the functional residual capacity, resulting in an increased Pao2. Its principal disadvantage is that by diminishing venous return from the head, it may result in worsening cerebral edema (20). The use of extracorporeal membrane oxygenation (ECMO) or partial liquid fluorocarbon ventilation should be considered in patients unresponsive to 100% oxygen and PEEP. Because persistent hypoxia may be a result of aspirated foreign material, aggressive suctioning and bronchoscopy may be necessary. There is no evidence that the use of diuretics improves outcome. Fluid management should be aimed at maintaining hemodynamic stability and urine output. Patient management should follow usual guidelines for the treatment of adult respiratory distress syndrome (ARDS) (2).

Bronchospasm can be treated with aerosolized bronchodilators. The administration of corticosteroids has not been shown to improve outcome and is not indicated in near-drowning (9). Prophylactic antibiotics have not been proven useful in preventing infection after aspiration and are unnecessary, except when aspirated water is known to have been grossly contaminated (e.g., aspiration of sewage) (9).

The initial therapy for hypotension is i.v. fluid replacement with an isotonic crystalloid solution. Monitoring of central venous or pulmonary artery pressures, and urinary output by Foley catheter, may be necessary to guide fluid resuscitation. Adequate fluid resuscitation should be achieved before vasopressors are used. Volume status must be carefully monitored so that the patient is not overloaded with fluid, which may worsen cerebral or pulmonary edema (6,15,20). Severe or persistent metabolic acidosis is treated with i.v. sodium bicarbonate (13).

Gastric decompression by a nasogastric tube is recommended in any symptomatic near-drowning victim to prevent vomiting, aspiration, and further respiratory compromise.

Cerebral resuscitation depends primarily on rapid stabilization and correction of hypoxemia and metabolic abnormalities. Moderate hyperventilation, elevation of the head, osmotic and loop diuretics, and muscle relaxation may be beneficial in patients with increased intracranial pressure. Hyperglycemia may worsen outcome in acute brain injury. It is recommended that in near-drowning patients the blood glucose level be frequently monitored and normoglycemia maintained (22). Pharmacologic treatment of agitation and seizures may also be necessary (15). Mild induced hypothermia (32°C–34°C) for 12 to 24 hours after CA may improve neurological outcome (1,21). Near-drowning patients in whom spontaneous circulation has been restored but who remain comatose should not be actively rewarmed to temperatures of greater than 32°C to 34°C. The 2002 World Congress on Drowning Consensus Statement suggests continuous core temperature monitoring in all near drowning patients both in the ED and intensive care unit settings. They further recommended that rectal temperature be maintained at 33°C to 34°C for the first 12 to 24 hours for patients who remain in coma. For drowning victims who are normothermic and remain in coma, active cooling should be instituted. Following a period of planned hypothermia, passive rewarming at a rate of no greater than 0.5°C to 1.0°C per hour is recommended. Hyperthermia should be prevented at all times in the acute recovery period (11). Treatments such as therapeutic dehydration, induced barbiturate coma, and paralysis are unproved (17).

CRITICAL INTERVENTIONS

- Assess airway patency, oxygenation and ventilation adequacy, and administer oxygen, perform endotracheal intubation, and institute mechanical ventilation as necessary
- Assess for possible traumatic injury
- Maintain normoglycemia and induce mild hypothermia (32°C–34°C) in patients who remain comatose

DISPOSITION

Patients who have been apneic or unconscious; those with extremes of age; those with hypoxia, dysrhythmias, ECG evidence of ischemia, or an abnormal chest radiograph; and those whose symptoms persist after ED evaluation and treatment should be admitted. The level of care (floor or intensive care) depends on the severity and progression of clinical and laboratory findings. Patients who are asymptomatic, or become so after 4 to 6 hours of observation, and have a normal physical examination, room-air arterial blood gas analysis, and chest radiograph may be discharged home with a responsible relative or friend (18). They should be instructed to return immediately if any symptoms develop (e.g., cough, sneezing, dyspnea, fever).

Indications for transfer include lack of intensive care facilities and lack of a pulmonary specialist capable of performing bronchoscopy.

COMMON PITFALLS

✔ Failure to consider the possibility of accidental and nonaccidental trauma, cerebral air embolism, drug intoxication, hypothermia, and medical or psychiatric illness in near-drowning victims

✔ Indiscriminate use of the Heimlich maneuver, which may be useful for clearing the upper airway of particulate matter but is of unproven efficacy in removing aspirated fluid

✔ Failure to appreciate that patients who initially appear moribund may recover completely and that, conversely, those who present with mild symptoms may later deteriorate

✔ Failure to observe patients with a history of near-drowning and normal findings on evaluation for at least 4 to 6 hours

✔ Failure to perform early evaluation and treatment of cerebral edema in order to prevent or minimize neurologic damage

References

1. Bernard SA, Gray TW, Buist MD, et al. Treatment of comatose survivors of out-of-hospital cardiac arrest with induced hypothermia. *N Engl J Med* 2002;346:557–563.
2. Brower RG, Ware LB, Berthiaume Y, et al. Treatment of ARDS. *Chest* 2001;120:1347–1367.
3. Chochinov AH. Recovery of a 62 year old man from prolonged cold water submersion. *Ann Emerg Med* 1998;31:127.
4. Cohen DS, Matthay MA, Cogan MG, et al. Pulmonary edema associated with salt water near-drowning: new insights. *Am Rev Respir Dis* 1992;146:794–796.

5. DeNicola LK. Submersion injuries in children and adults. *Crit Care Clin* 1997; 13:477.
6. Levin DL. Drowning and near drowning. *Pediatr Clin North Am* 1993;40:321.
7. Martin TG. Near-drowning and cold-water immersion. *Ann Emerg Med* 1984;13:263.
8. *Aquatic deaths and injuries—United States. MMWR*, 1982;Aug 13;31(31):417–419.
9. Modell JH. Drowning. *N Engl J Med* 1993;328:253.
10. Modell JH, Bellefleur M, Davis JH. Drowning without aspiration: is this an appropriate diagnosis? *J Forensic Sci* 1999;44:1119–1123.
11. Moon RE, Long RJ. and near-drowning. *Emerg Med (Fremantle)* 2002;14:377–386.
12. National Center for Injury Prevention and Control Injury. *NCIPC Factbook 2001–2.* Atlanta, USA: National Center for Injury Prevention and Control Injury, 2002.
13. Neal JM. Near-drowning. *J Emerg Med* 1985;3:41.
14. Oakes DA, Sherck JP, Maloney JR, et al. Prognosis and management of victims of near-drowning. *J Trauma* 1982;22:554.
15. Olshaker JS. Near drowning. *Emerg Med Clin North Am* 1992;10:339.
16. Orlowski JP. Drowning, near-drowning, and ice-water submersions. *Pediatr Clin North Am* 1987;34:75.
17. Ornato JP. Resuscitation of near-drowning victims. *JAMA* 1986;256(1):75.
18. Pratt FD, Haynes BE. Incidence of secondary drowning after saltwater submersion. *Ann Emerg Med* 1986;15:1084.
19. Redmond AD, Mallikarijun TS. Resuscitation from drowning. *Arch Emerg Med* 1984;2:113.
20. Robinson MD, Seward PN. Submersion injury in children. *Crit Care Med* 1987;3(1):44.
21. The Hypothermia after Cardiac Arrest Study Group. Mild therapeutic hypothermia to improve the neurologic outcome after cardiac arrest. *N Engl J Med* 2002;346:549–556.
22. van den Berghe G, Wouters P, Weekers F, et al. Intensive insulin therapy in the surgical intensive care unit. *N Engl J Med* 2001;345:1359–1367.
23. Watson RS, Cummings P, Quan L, et al. Cervical spine injuries among submersion victims. *J Trauma* 2001;51:658–662.
24. Weinstein MD. Near drowning: epidemiology, pathophysiology, and initial treatment. *J Emerg Med* 1996;14:461.
25. Wittmers LE Jr, Pozos RS, Fall G, et al. Cardiovascular responses to face immersion (the diving reflex) in human beings after alcohol consumption. *Ann Emerg Med* 1987;16:1031.

CHAPTER 357
Electrical Injuries

Scott E. Rudkin and Jennifer A. Oman

Electrocution is an infrequent cause of injury, but when present can damage multiple organ systems. Unlike a thermal burn, where the damage is typically limited to the skin and underlying tissues, electrical injuries have the potential to cause extensive internal injury without any significant sign of external injury. Electrical injuries cause nearly 1,000 deaths annually in the United States, with high-voltage injuries accounting for two-thirds of this total (12). Most adult injuries occur in the workplace; electrical injuries are the fourth leading cause of traumatic, work-related deaths (9). Most fatalities from electrical injuries occur from ventricular fibrillation (VF), asystole, or interruption of the central respiratory control (10). High-voltage injuries account for 5% of all burn unit admissions (6).

Luckily, the majority of household injuries have been mitigated by changes in building codes that require a ground plug for all home outlets. However, misuse or malfunction of home appliances still account for 200 deaths annually (4). Children are typically injured at home and comprise 30% of all electrical injuries. The large majority (60%–70%) of childhood electrical injuries result from inquisitive toddlers who are exposed to electrical cords (4). The amount of injury that is caused by an electrical exposure is related to the voltage, tissue resistance, type of current, duration of exposure, and pathway of electric current. For instance, although a direct lightning strike is an extremely high-voltage source, the extremely short duration of the exposure explains why survival is possible.

Electricity is the flow of electrons through a conductor. The flow of these electrons, the current (I), is measured in amperes and is responsible for tissue damage. The relative force of this electron flow is the voltage (V); impedance to the flow of electrons is called resistance (R) and is measured in ohms (4). All of these variables are interrelated by Ohm's Law, which defines a given current as the voltage divided by the resistance: $I = V/R$, or $V = IR$. By definition, a high-voltage injury is classified as more than 1,000 volts.

Although the voltage is frequently known for an electrical injury, the resistance is usually unknown. The relative resistance of various body tissues explains the relative sensitivities of certain organ systems to electrical injury. Dry, calloused skin has a resistance of 40,000 to 100,000 ohms and is relatively impervious to electrical injury, although wet, thin skin can have a resistance of less than 1,000 ohms and is highly susceptible (10). The least resistance is found in nerves, blood, and mucous membranes, although bones, fat, and tendons have higher resistance (9). The low resistance of nervous tissue explains why the nervous system is frequently injured in electrical injuries. Current travels through and therefore injures those tissues with the lowest resistance. Higher current densities, which are inversely related to the cross-sectional area of the current path, create more heat and more subsequent damage. Appendages, with a smaller cross sectional area, sustain much higher damage with a similar current as the trunk or torso. The amount of heat that is generated is proportional to the current involved, the resistance of the tissue, and the duration of contact (2).

The type of current also determines the ultimate severity of injury. In alternating current (AC), the current flows through the conductor in a back-and-forth fashion. In the United States, the majority of residential electricity is transmitted with AC at 60 Hertz (cycles/second). Although AC is a more efficient means of electrical transmission, it also is three times as dangerous as direct current (DC) (4). AC causes tetanic muscle contraction and prolonged duration of contact. The flexor muscles typically are stronger than the extensors, so that muscle contraction can create a "locked-on" phenomenon where victims cannot release themselves from an electrical source. Additionally, AC is more likely to induce VF (3). DC, as the name implies, moves "directly" along a given circuit in a single direction. Although less efficient for transmission, it is safer than AC since tetanic muscle contraction is limited.

Lightning is a special form of DC; the voltage of a lightning bolt is extremely high (>1,000,000 volts) but the duration of contact is very small (1–2 msec) (10). Lightning causes injury in four ways: direct strike (pathway through the victim), side-flash (lightning first strikes an object, then secondary discharge strikes patient), stride potential (current passes from ground, up one leg and down the other), and flash-over phenomenon (where the current travels outside the body and causes vaporization of surface water) (4). See Chapter 358, "Lightning Injuries" for more details about lightning injuries.

The pathway of the current also determines the severity of injury. A current that traverses the body in the vertical axis is much more deadly than a similar horizontal current since virtually every organ is affected. However, a horizontal pathway from hand to hand can affect the heart or lungs and induce a dysrhythmia or paralysis of the respiratory muscles (4).

Of particular interest for emergency physicians is the utilization of electrical energy by peace officers. "Stun guns" or Taser® devices are employed to deliver a less-than-lethal force to subdue violent suspects. This device deploys two to four metal barbs that are attached to a wire with an effective range of 15 feet. Once the barbs strike an assailant, a high voltage (50,000 volts) but low amperage (3 mA) pulse train is delivered, causing involuntary muscle tetany which effectively paralyzes the assailant. The morbidity and mortality of these devices is low compared to conventional weapons (5,10).

CLINICAL PRESENTATION

Electrical injuries can range from a simple sensation of tingling to multisystem organ failure. Frequently, the cutaneous signs of injury are limited, leading the clinician to underestimate the extent of the electrical injury. Electrical burns are best viewed as crush injuries and not thermal burns (1). Using this analogy helps to reinforce the concept that the multiple systems are involved and that superficial injuries can be deceiving. Given their lower inherent intrinsic resistance, the cardiac and neurologic systems are most commonly injured. Deaths caused by electrical injury are usually VF (low voltage), asystole (high voltage), or respiratory arrest from interruption of the central respiratory center.

The heart is sensitive to electrical injury; one third of electrical injuries have some form of cardiac complication (3). Injury to the myocardium occurs either from direct disruption of normal electrical signal or direct myocardial damage; the latter is more common with high-voltage injuries. Rhythm disturbances can be caused by relatively low currents; only 50 to 100mA (one-half of normal household current) can induce VF in transthoracic injuries (10). In addition to VF and asystole, the more common electrically induced dysrhythmias include sinus tachycardia, nonspecific ST-T wave changes, ventricular tachycardia, ectopic beats and bundle branch blocks (3). Electrical injuries can cause direct myocardial necrosis through the production of heat. Although ST-T wave changes and increased elevation of the CK-MB fraction are common findings, these are usually not indicative of myocardial infarction; the elevation of the CK-MB is usually related to skeletal muscle damage (2,3,13). Patients with upper and lower body locations for entry and exit wound are more likely to have myocardial damage (5). Electrically injured, autopsied heart specimens show scattered areas of myocardial damage with subpericardial micro-hemorrhage (11). However, transmural necrosis is rare and usually related to injury to coronary vessels (8).

The nervous system is also highly sensitive to electrical injury; 70% of electrical injuries have some neurologic component (8). Peripheral nervous system involvement frequently manifests with peripheral neuropathy and motor dysfunction, related to direct electrothermal injury, ischemia from microvascular injury, or compartment syndrome. Central nervous system involvement can present with amnesia, loss of consciousness, confusion, impaired recall, mood lability, anxiety, depression, motor deficits, coma or injury to the respiratory control center with resulting respiratory arrest (9,11). Additionally, visual disturbances, seizures, deafness, and hemi- or quadriplegia may occur (9). In high-voltage injuries, acute insults to the spinal cord can occur from direct electrical injury or associated fractures/ligamentous injuries. Injury at the C4-C8 level is most common with hand-to-hand, transthoracic flow (9). Delayed neurologic symptoms can appear for up to 2 years and may include symptoms that resemble ascending paralysis, amyotrophic lateral sclerosis, transverse myelitis, and incomplete cord transection (2).

The blood functions as an excellent conductor of current, and extensive damage to the vascular system can occur from electrical injuries. Electrical injuries can damage the intima and media of the vessel walls and form thrombi in the blood. Both of these narrow the diameter of given vessels and lead to ischemia and necrosis of those tissues that they supply. Smaller vessels are more sensitive to this damage given their decreased diameter and inherent higher resistance and heat generation. Coagulation necrosis, disseminated intravascular coagulation and delayed vessel rupture can occur (12). Arterial insufficiency and compartment syndrome may occur.

Muscle tissue suffers electrical injury through direct heat damage, ischemia from injured blood vessels, and direct electrical injury (11). Direct heat damage causes rhabdomyolysis, which can also lead to acute renal failure. Additionally, edema and vascular insufficiency can cause a compartment syndrome. Electrically induced tetanic contractions or secondary blunt trauma can cause dislocations and fractures. Long bone, vertebral compression, and scapular fractures are most common, and shoulder dislocations (12).

Injuries to cutaneous tissue can range from asymptomatic lesions to extensive thermal damage. The upper extremities are common locations for entrance wounds, although the exit site is variable, but usually the point nearest to the ground or where the electrical circuit can easiest complete. Injuries at these entrance/exit sites usually have erythema, charring, and edema. The skin can also suffer "flash burns" from electrical arc production, electrothermal burns from electrical conduction, and flame burns from ignition of clothing (9). Of particular note are oral burns in children. Young children may chew on an electrical cord; the mucosa of the mouth has a very low resistance and the current arcs through the lip. This can cause a full thickness burn of the lip with involvement of the mucosa, submucosa, muscle, nerves, and blood vessels (9). The resultant eschar usually falls off in 2 to 3 weeks, and can be associated with significant labial artery bleeding.

Gastrointestinal (GI) tract involvement may be seen, with nausea and vomiting found in 25% and gastric stress ulcers in 13% of electrical injuries (11). Solid organ injuries may result from associated blunt trauma. Paralytic ileus, and hepatic and pancreatic necrosis and bowel perforation can occur from direct electrical injury.

Direct pulmonary injury is rare given the poor conductivity of air. Direct injury to the respiratory drive center can cause respiratory arrest, although diaphragmatic tetany can also lead to respiratory paralysis. Associated blunt trauma can cause rib fractures, hemothoraces, and pneumothoraces.

Although infrequent, cataracts, vitreous and anterior chamber hemorrhage, retinal detachment, macular laceration and central retinal artery occlusion can occur (11). Glaucoma occurs at higher incidence in patients who survive electrical injuries. Irritation of the anterior chamber can cause miosis, Horner's syndrome or mydriasis. This mydriasis can be mistaken as a fixed-pupil, leading to early termination of resuscitation efforts. Rupture of the eardrum is frequently associated with lightning injuries.

Pregnant patients may be completely asymptomatic, yet their fetus may suffer significant morbidity and mortality, as the amniotic fluid is an ideal current conductor. Conduction of this current can cause fetal cardiac arrest and abortion.

DIFFERENTIAL DIAGNOSIS

Unlike other many emergency department entities, the diagnosis of electrical injury is frequently apparent from the initial history. The real challenge is differentiating between damage caused by direct electrical damage and that caused by associated thermal injuries. Electrical sources of thermal injury include electrical arc, flash burns, and ignition of surface clothing. The diagnosis of these thermal burns is relatively straightforward as the extent of the injury can be judged from the signs of external injury. The extent of electrical injuries, however, can be very difficult, as the degree of external injury can underestimate the true extent of damage.

EMERGENCY DEPARTMENT EVALUATION

In the prehospital setting, rescuers must make certain that they do not become victims; secure the electrical source before intervening. The possibility of blunt trauma must be assumed and full cervical-spine precautions utilized in transport. Contrary to frequent misconception, patients who are struck by lightning do not retain a static charge and can receive immediate care. Standard advanced cardiac life support (ACLS) protocols should be followed and all patients should be transported; many apparently deceased patients have had recovery after high-voltage injury.

Electrical injuries can vary from benign to multisystem organ failure; a thorough evaluation is required to help differentiate between these extremes. All patients with high-voltage injuries should be approached as if they may have multisystem failure and concomitant trauma. Cervical spine precautions must be maintained and radiography obtained to exclude cervical fracture. Airway, breathing, and circulation should be immediately assessed on arrival and treated appropriately. The patient must be completely exposed to discover evidence of any secondary blunt trauma. Cardiac monitoring, including electrocardiography, pulse oximetry, and supplemental oxygen should be started. A careful history is required of the patient or emergency personal to help determine the voltage and type (AC vs. DC) of current, and the duration and presumed pathway of the current.

Laboratory studies should be obtained to help determine the extent of injury. An electrocardiogram (ECG) is indicated for all high-voltage injuries and is essential for all cases of transthoracic injury. A complete blood count, arterial blood gas, coagulation studies, serum electrolytes, calcium, creatine, blood urea nitrogen, liver function tests, and urinalysis, including urine myoglobin, should all be obtained in patients with high-voltage injuries. Cardiac enzymes, including isozymes, and a type and cross may also be indicated. Vascular and nerve function should be tested to exclude a compartment syndrome. Ophthalmologic and otologic evaluation is warranted to exclude cataracts and tympanic injuries, respectively.

EMERGENCY DEPARTMENT MANAGEMENT

Maintenance of the ABCs (airway, breathing, and circulation) must be ensured and ACLS and advanced trauma life support algorithms followed. Cervical spine immobilization must be maintained until fracture is excluded. Cardiopulmonary resuscitation should be initiated in the prehospital setting for nonperfusing dysrhythmias and resuscitative efforts should be maintained for extended periods of time; many electrically injured, apparently "dead" patients have been successfully resuscitated (6,11).

The extent of tissue damage is not indicated by the extent of cutaneous injury; extensive internal damage can cause intravascular fluid losses and hypotension. Aggressive hydration through large-bore intravenous catheters is warranted and central venous or arterial catheters should be considered. Urine output should be maintained at a brisk rate to reduce the likelihood

of acute renal failure from rhabdomyolysis. Mannitol (1gram/ kg i.v.) should be utilized if urine output is less than 50 to 100 mL/hour in adults or if dark/pigmented urine is noted. Bicarbonate therapy (1–2 mEq/kg i.v.) should also be initiated for any cases where rhabdomyolysis is suspect; the arterial pH should be kept over 7 (4,5,12).

Serial laboratory testing of electrolytes, liver function tests, creatinine, BUN, and calcium is also warranted to assess ongoing tissue necrosis and injury. Nasogastric decompression will aid in cases of ileus and help to decompress the GI tract. Prophylactic H2-blocker therapy is warranted to prevent stress ulceration. Tetanus status should be evaluated and updated as needed.

CRITICAL INTERVENTIONS

- Consider the potential for rhabdomyolysis in all but the smallest burns
- Admit patients for cardiac monitoring when the patient has experienced a loss of consciousness, has a transthoracic injury pattern, or shows signs of dysrhythmia or external injury
- Provide adequate hydration to reduce risk of renal failure from rhabdomyolysis
- Ensure adequate follow-up for children at risk for labial artery bleeding

DISPOSITION

All cases of high-voltage injury require admission for observation. Given the multisystem nature of injury, transfer to a regional burn center is advisable. Any case of dysrhythmia or signs of myocardial injury require 24-hour cardiac monitoring and serial cardiac enzymes (3). Transthoracic injuries should also be admitted for cardiac monitoring, even in the absence of dysrhythmia. Admission is also warranted for cardiac monitoring for cases of loss of consciousness, dysrhythmia (in the field), abnormal ECG on ED evaluation, or signs of tissue damage (5,14).

Whenever neurovascular compromise is suspected, surgical consultation is warranted to exclude a compartment syndrome. All cases of rhabdomyolysis warrant admission for treatment to reduce the chance of acute renal failure.

For the majority of low-voltage injuries, discharge may be considered assuming that the patient has not had a loss of consciousness, cardiac dysrhythmia, or tissue damage and a thorough ED evaluation has not found evidence of internal injury. Children with oral injury from chewing on electrical cords require special attention. This subset of patients is at high risk for delayed hemorrhage from labial artery bleeding when the eschar sloughs off. Discharge only those patients with reliable follow-up; admit all questionable cases.

COMMON PITFALLS

✔ Failing to recognize that surface injury does not correlate with the extent of internal injury
✔ Trying to remove a patient from an electrical source, prior to stopping the current, and becoming a victim yourself
✔ Failing to examine all patients for compartment syndrome in cases where neurovascular compromise is suspect

Acknowledgment

We thank previous edition chapter author Peter L. Sosnow.

References

1. Artz CP. Electrical injury simulates crush injury. *Surg Gynecol Obstet* 1967;125:1316–1317.
2. Browne BJ, Gaasch WR. Electrical injuries and lightening. *Emerg Med Clin North Am* 1992;10:211–229.
3. Carleton SC. Cardiac problems associated with electrical injury. *Cardiol Clin* 1995;13:263–266.
4. Fahmy SF, Brinsden MD, Smith J, et al. Lightning: the multisystem group injuries. *J Trauma* 1999;46:937–940.
5. Fish R. Electric Shock, part III: deliberately applied electric shocks and the treatment of electrical injuries. *J Emerg Med* 1993;11:599–603.
6. Fontanarosa PB. Electrical shock and lightening strike. *Ann Emerg Med* 1993;22:378–387.
7. Grube BJ, Heimbalch DM, Engrav LH, et al. Neurological consequence of electrical burns. *J Trauma* 1990;30:254–258.
8. James TN, Riddick L, Embry JG. Cardiac abnormalities demonstrated post mortem in four cases of accidental electrocution and their potential significance relative to non fatal electrical injuries of the heart. *Am Heart J* 1990;120:143–157.
9. Koumbourlis AC. Electrical Injuries. *Crit Care Med* 2002;30(11 Suppl):S424–S430.
10. Koscove E. The Taser weapon: a new emergency medicine problem. *Ann Emerg Med* 1985;14:1205–1208.
11. Leibovici D, Shemer J, Shapira SC. Electrical injuries: current concepts. *Injury* 1995;26:623–627.
12. Martinez JA, Nguyen T. Electrical injuries. *South Med J* 2000;93:1165–1168.
13. McBride JW, Kingsley KR, McCoy HG, et al. Is serum creatine-kinase-MB in electrically injured patients predictive of myocardial injury? *JAMA* 1986;255:764–768.
14. Purdue GF, Hunt JL. Electrocardiographic monitoring after electrical injury: necessity or luxury. *J Trauma* 1986;26:166–167.

CHAPTER 358
Lightning Injuries

David F. M. Brown

Lightning injuries are among the leading cause of deaths as a result of environmental phenomena in the United States (5,13,21). Although there is no central agency to collect data, estimates suggest that lightning is responsible for 75 to 300 deaths per year and up to 1,500 nonfatal injuries (2,4,8,11–13,21). The most common victims are people who work or perform recreational activities outside, particularly campers, joggers, farm and construction workers, golfers, and hunters (4,13). Indoor victims are likely to be using the telephone or other household appliances (4). The incidence of lightning injuries parallels the frequency of lightning storms; hence, most injuries occur during the summer months (4,5). Geographically, common areas include the Atlantic seaboard, the Southeast and Southwest, major mountain ranges, and river tidal basins (1,4,9,19). The case fatality rate is between 20% and 32%, and about 75% of survivors suffer permanent sequelae (7,21).

Lightning is produced after warm, moist air rises within a cold high-pressure front, allowing condensation into a cloud. Air currents, ice particles, and water droplets within the cloud create a layering of ionic charges: The uppermost regions have a net positive charge, the lower regions a net negative charge (7). The ground beneath the cloud becomes relatively positively charged, creating a potential difference. Electrical breakdown between positively and negatively charged areas of the atmosphere causes advancement of ionic charges in a downward-branching "stepped leader" or "leader stroke" pattern propagated at 1,000 to 2,000th the speed of light. This causes a path of air to become ionized to a plasma of positive and negative ions that is a better conductor than nonionized air. As the stepped leader pattern of ion propagation nears the ground, a "pilot stroke" or "return stroke" ascends from the ground at about one-tenth the speed of light, completing a channel of ionic movement between the cloud and the ground (7).

Because the stepped leader, which is luminous secondary to the large quantity of ionic movement, is relatively slower than the return stroke, lightning is perceived as traveling from cloud to earth. However, the main electrical discharge is usually from earth to cloud, and it appears as an instantaneous brightening of the ionized pathway (the visible lightning flash) lasting about 0.2 seconds. In rapid succession, multiple secondary leader and return strokes (between 3 and 40) then typically occur until the ionic potential between cloud and ground is eliminated (7).

Thunder results from the rapid expansion of warmed air and its subsequent contraction and implosion. Practically, although not technically, lightning behaves as direct current, with an energy level of 2,000 to 2 billion V and 2,000 to 300,000 A (3,11). This energy is much higher than conventional electricity; however, the distinctly short duration of lightning contact (0.1 to 1.0 milliseconds) usually prohibits cutaneous penetration and commensurate deep-tissue injury (5). Except for direct strikes, most of the lightning current "flashes over" the outside of the victim; only occasionally does enough current leak internally to interfere with cardiac automaticity, respiratory center function, and autonomic stability (10).

There are several major mechanisms of lightning injury. A direct strike occurs when the major pathway of current runs directly through the victim; this results in the highest morbidity and mortality (10). When the lightning current strikes an object in contact with the victim, the injury mechanism approximates a direct strike. With side flash, current splashes or sprays from an object through the air to the victim. Ground current, also known as step voltage or ground potential, occurs when lightning strikes the ground and spreads to involve the victim. The severity of injury as a result of ground current is inversely proportional to the distance from the ground strike (7). If ground resistance is greater than the victim's resistance, current may enter one leg and exit through the other, perhaps accounting for the higher mortality in victims exhibiting leg burns (7). Ground current and side-flash mechanisms often produce multiple casualties.

Associated trauma may result from myotonic extremity or neck contractions, acceleration–deceleration injuries as the victim is thrown, penetrating and blunt injuries from debris, and thermal burns exacerbated by metal jewelry or clothing fasteners or caused by ignition of clothing.

CLINICAL PRESENTATION

Because of the short duration of lightning exposure, current usually passes over the outside of the body ("flashover" phenomenon), commonly producing superficial or partial-thickness burns in a characteristic linear or arborescent pattern (1,2,11,18,19). Although 89% of patients will suffer burns (7), entry and exit burns and deep internal burns with resultant rhabdomyolysis and myoglobinuria are rare (3,8,16,19,20).

The most common cause of death in the lightning victim is cardiopulmonary arrest (CPA) (7–9,21). Internal propagation of the lightning electrical potential acts as a massive direct current countershock, which depolarizes the entire myocardium and causes cardiac asystole (7,8,11–13). As a result of cardiac automaticity, an organized electrical rhythm may occur, restoring spontaneous circulation (8,13,21). However, primary respiratory arrest as a result of lightning-induced paralysis of the medullary center may occur concomitantly and can outlast cardiac arrest (CA) (3,4,8,10,11). The critical factor in determining mortality appears to be the duration of apnea (which may also occur independently) rather than the duration of asystole (19). Without prompt and prolonged ventilatory support, any return of cardiac rhythm and circulation will rapidly deteriorate to hypoxia-induced ventricular fibrillation.(3,7,8,13,19). Survivors of lightning exposure can exhibit a variety of cardiac abnormalities, with dysrhythmias and ST-T wave changes frequently reported (8,13,15). Acute life-threatening (and often reversible) left ventricular dysfunction or pericardial tamponade, as demonstrated by echocardiography, appears to be limited to victims of direct strikes (15).

Myriad neurologic effects of lightning injury are frequently encountered. Usually, the victim falls unconscious immediately (6,17). In the absence of CPA, consciousness eventually returns, occasionally after a prolonged period. The next most common finding is paraplegia, occurring in up to two-thirds of seriously injured patients (8,17). Hemiparesis, hemiplegia, localizing sensory deficits, and autonomic dysfunction may also be found (17).

Virtually all lightning-struck patients have altered mental status and anterograde amnesia; retrograde amnesia is common as well (7,17). Persistent neuropsychological, cognitive and behavioral abnormalities are commonly found (6). When current passes through the brain, intracranial hemorrhage (particularly in the basal ganglia and brainstem), epidural and subdural hematomas, coagulation of brain parenchyma, and thrombosis of vessels can occur (6,7,17). Associated trauma may cause cervical spine fracture with resultant spinal cord injury.

The extremities may initially appear cold, mottled, pulseless, and insensitive secondary to vascular spasm and autonomic instability (5,7,8,11,13,18,19). Normal function usually returns.

Half the patients with lightning injuries have structural eye lesions (4). Cataracts are common and may develop in a few days or up to several years after the injury (3,13,19). Corneal lesions are also common; hyphema, iritis, vitreous hemorrhage, retinal detachment, and optic nerve injury are occasionally seen (5,13). Unreactive, dilated pupil(s) as a result of transient autonomic instability may occur and should not be mistaken for a sign of brain death (5,7,13,17).

Tympanic membrane rupture, the most common otologic injury, occurs in 50% of victims of lightning injury and is thought to be as a result of the shock wave of expanding hot air (thunder) during the strike (7,13,17). Less common findings are hemotympanum, basilar skull fracture, and various acoustic and vestibular sensorineural deficits (13,17).

DIFFERENTIAL DIAGNOSIS

Lightning injuries have been mistakenly diagnosed as a variety of disorders. Neurologic disease processes that can mimic lightning injury include cerebrovascular accidents, seizure disorders, and craniocerebral, spinal cord, or other neurologic trauma (8). Cardiovascular disorders in the differential diagnosis of lightning injury include myocardial infarction, Stokes-Adams attacks, and cardiac dysrhythmias (8). Also in the differential are toxic ingestions, envenomations, and physical assault. Cutaneous injuries may be misdiagnosed as electrical burns.

As in most clinical situations, the history is crucial to making the correct diagnosis. Obtaining information from bystanders is essential when the victim is incapacitated. Important points include a history of thunderstorm and outdoor occurrence of the accident. Physical findings that favor a diagnosis of lightning injury include partial or complete clothing disintegration and superficial linear, punctate, or arborescent burns. Tympanic membrane rupture is also highly suggestive.

EMERGENCY DEPARTMENT EVALUATION

The history should include the time, circumstances, and a description of events at the scene of injury. Any prehospital interventions, and their times, should be documented. Present complaints and medical history prior to presentation should also be noted.

The physical examination should focus initially on vital signs; assessment of the airway, breathing, and circulation; and evaluation for trauma and neurologic dysfunction. Serial neurovascular examinations should be performed in patients with signs of peripheral vascular insufficiency. All patients should have cardiac monitoring, an electrocardiogram (ECG), and oxygen saturation measurement. Laboratory evaluation should include a complete blood count and measurements of serum electrolytes, blood urea nitrogen, creatinine, glucose, and creatine phosphokinase. Urine should be tested for myoglobin. Patients with cardiac dysrhythmias or ischemia, respiratory arrest, or loss of consciousness should have a chest radiograph and cardiac biomarker analysis. Patients with altered mental status or neurologic deficits should also have cervical spine radiographs and a cranial computed tomography scan. Other radiographs and tests should be obtained as indicated by complaints or physical findings.

EMERGENCY DEPARTMENT MANAGEMENT

Lightning injuries may place prehospital health care providers in precarious environmental settings. Although acute medical intervention is paramount to reduce mortality (3,7,11), care should be taken to prevent further injury to the patient and harm to rescuers. Treatment begins with assessment and stabilization of the airway, ventilation, and circulation. Victims should be treated as trauma patients, with special attention given to cervical spine immobilization (5). Triage priorities, in a reversal of the usual dictum, should focus initially on victims in CPA (1,3,5,7,9,11,13,14). This is because virtually all victims of lightning strike who do not suffer CA or respiratory arrest survive (7). Standard advanced life-support (ACLS and ATLS) protocols should be followed. Aggressive, persistent resuscitative efforts are indicated for all victims, especially those with spontaneous cardiac rhythms and prolonged apnea or coma (1,5,11,13). Ventilatory support may be required for several hours, but even in these cases, there is potential for full recovery (3,11). Full support should be continued until cerebral function can be assessed (1).

All patients should initially be given supplemental oxygen, have intravenous access established, and be placed on a cardiac monitor. Intravenous fluids should be minimized to reduce any risk of cerebral edema unless hemorrhage, hypotension, or dehydration is evident or rhabdomyolysis is a concern (e.g., with deep or extensive burns or associated crush injury). Rhabdomyolysis, as indicated by myoglobinuria and elevated serum muscle enzyme levels, may necessitate fluid loading, osmotic diuresis, and urine alkalinization (20). Standard burn and wound care, and tetanus prophylaxis, should be given, if appropriate. Patients with cardiac or neurological abnormalities should have serial ECGs and cardiac biomarker analyses and routine supportive care. All patients require comprehensive and repeated physical and neurological examinations.

CRITICAL INTERVENTIONS

- Give the highest priority to patients in CA or respiratory arrest when making triage decisions in mass casualty incidents involving lightning injury
- Institute advanced cardiac support measures and make a prolonged effort to resuscitate patients found pulseless or apneic after a lightning strike
- Evaluate lightning-stricken patients for traumatic injuries

DISPOSITION

Patients with cardiac or neurological abnormalities require admission for at least 24 to 36 hours of observation and continuous cardiac monitoring. Those with associated trauma, burns, or rhabdomyolysis also may require admission for their injuries (1,3,13). Patients who have sustained CA or respiratory arrest should be admitted to an intensive care unit.

The decision to transfer a patient to another facility depends on the severity of injury and the ability of local resources to provide adequate care. If the necessary services are unavailable, the decision and the timing of transfer should be coordinated with the receiving physician at the nearest appropriate hospital. Emergency personnel with ALS capability should accompany the patient.

COMMON PITFALLS

- Failure to appreciate the difference between lightning and high-voltage injuries
- Misdiagnosing lightning injury as an isolated cutaneous burn or a primary neurologic or cardiovascular event
- Misinterpreting unreactive, dilated pupils as a sign of death in patients struck by lightning
- Failure to appreciate the high incidence of permanent neurologic sequelae from lightning injury and to admit patients with neurologic complaints or deficits for observation

References

1. Amy BW, McManus WF, Goodwin CW, et al. Lightning injury with survival of 5 patients. *JAMA* 1985;253:243.
2. Anonymous. Lightning-associated deaths—United States 1980–1995. *MMWR* 1998;47:391.
3. Apfelberg DB, Masters F, Robinson D. Pathophysiology and treatment of lightning injuries. *J Trauma* 1974;14:453.
4. Blount BW. Lightning injuries. *Am Fam Physician* 1990;42:405.
5. Browne BJ, Gaasch WR. Electrical injuries and lightning. *Emerg Med Clin North Am* 1992;10:211.
6. Cherington M. Neurologic manifestations of lightning strikes. *Neurology* 2003;60:182.
7. Cooper MA. Lightning injuries: prognostic signs for death. *Ann Emerg Med* 1980;9:134.
8. Cooper MA. Emergent care of lightning and electrical injuries. *Semin Neurol* 1995;15:268.
9. Cwinn AA, Cantril SV. Lightning injuries. *J Emerg Med* 1985;2:379.
10. Epperly TD, Stewart JR. The physical effects of lightning injury. *J Fam Pract* 1989;29:267.
11. Fontanarosa PB. Electrical shock and lightning strike. *Ann Emerg Med* 1993;22:378.
12. Graber J, Ummenhofer W, Herion H. Lightning accident with eight victims: case report and brief review of the literature. *J Trauma* 1996;40:288.
13. Jain S, Bandi V. Electrical and lightning injuries. *Crit Care Clinics* 1999;15:319.
14. Kobernick M. Electrical injuries: pathophysiology and emergency management. *Ann Emerg Med* 1982;11:633.
15. Lichtenberg R, Dries D, Ward K, et al. Cardiovascular effects of lightning strikes. *J Am Coll Cardiol* 1993;21:531.
16. Ohashi M, Kitagawa N, Ishikawa T. Lightning injury caused by discharges accompanying flashovers: a clinical and experimental study of death and survival. *Burns* 1986;12:496.
17. Patten BM. Lightning and electrical injuries. *Neurol Clin* 1992;10:1047.
18. Robinson M, Seward P. Electrical and lightning injuries in children. *Pediatr Emerg Care* 1986;2:186.
19. Straser EJ, Davis RM, Menchey JJ. Lightning injuries. *J Trauma* 1977;17:315.
20. Wang X, Jin R, Bartle E, et al. Creatine phosphokinase values in electrical and thermal burns. *Burns* 1987;13:309.
21. Whitcomb D, Martinez JA, Daberkow D. Lightning injuries. *South Med J* 2002;95:1331.

CHAPTER 359
Radiation Injuries

Joe Suyama and Matthew D. Sztajnkrycer

Radiation is defined as the transfer of energy in the form of waves, rays, or particles. Ionizing radiation induces injury by damaging DNA and other subcellular components, generally leading to cell death or dysfunction. Ionizing radiation originates from the decay of inherently unstable radionuclides. Ionizing radiation is emitted in the form of α and β particles, γ rays and x-rays, and neutrons. Positively charged α particles consist of two neutrons and two protons, and do not penetrate further than 0.05 to 0.1 mm tissue depth. However, they demonstrate high linear energy transfer (LET) to tissues. Simplistically, the amount of subsequent cellular damage increases with increasing LET. Internalization of α particles is associated with the potential for significant radiologic damage. Negatively charged β particles are low LET particles with a penetration depth of 5 to 30 mm. Gamma rays and x-rays lack both charge and mass, are low LET rays, but are highly penetrating. Neutrons lack a charge, are deeply penetrating, and are classified as high LET particles. Neutrons do not ionize tissues directly, but rather transfer energy to atoms in tissues, which then create α and β particles, γ rays, and x-rays and subsequent tissue effects.

The amount of energy transferred to tissues per unit mass of the target is quantified by the radiation absorbed dose (rad). One hundred rads equals one Gray (Gy). Potential for tissue injury is dependent on both the dose and radiation quality, which refers to varying biologic effects based on LETs. The rem (radiation equivalent in man) reflects the biological impact of the absorbed radiation dose, and is calculated from the rad and the quality factor (QF) of the specific radioactive type. The rem is expressed as sieverts (Sv) in SI nomenclature, with 100 rem = 1 Sv. A particles, due their large size and strong positive charge, have a QF of 20, resulting in 20 rem from a 1 rad exposure. The QF for β particles, γ rays, and x-rays is 1, resulting in equivalency of rad and rem. The QF for neutrons is variable, ranging from 3 to 20. Radioactive substances can be found in many settings and forms. Naturally occurring background radiation exposure accounts for 300 to 360 mrem dose exposure per year; this and other radiation doses from medical procedures are listed in Table 359.1 (16).

Radioactive materials are found in medical settings, research facilities, industrial sites, and nuclear power plants (22). According to the Department of Energy—Radiation Emergency Assistance Center/Training Site (REAC/TS) Radiation Accidents

TABLE 359.1.   Dose Ranges from Background Radiation Exposures and Selected Medical Procedures

Radiation Exposure	Dose Range	Body Part Affected
Background Radiation	300–360 mrem/yr	Total Body
Smoking 1 PPD/Yr	16000 mrem	Respiratory System, Body
Transcontinental Flight	5 mrem	Total Body
Diagnostic Chest x-Ray Single View	10–15 mrem	Collimated field
Diagnostic Chest x-Ray Two View	60 mrem	Collimated Field
CT Head	1000 mrem	Head
CT Abdomen	2000–5000 mrem	Abdomen
Fluoroscopy	1000 mrem/m	Collimated Field
Bone Scan	5000 mrem	Total Body
Annual Exposure Limit–Public	100 mrem/yr	Total Body
Annual Exposure Limit–Occupational	5000 mrem/yr	Total Body
Annual Exposure Limit–Occupational, Pregnant	500 mrem/yr	Total Body
LD_{50}	450,000 mrem	Total Body

Registry, the majority of radiation accidents occur in the medical, energy production, or industrial settings [1]. Radiation accidents are typically secondary to criticalities, improper use of radiation devices, and improper use of radioisotopes. Between 1944 and 2002, a total of 428 radiation accidents have been documented worldwide resulting in 133,815 persons affected and 134 fatalities. Nearly 90% of these victims were the result of the 1986 Chernobyl nuclear reactor accident. Other recent mass-casualty radiation accidents include the rupture of an Ir source in Venezuela, a Co therapy unit accident in Cuidad Juarez, Mexico, and the theft and subsequent large exposure of a Cs source in Goiania, Brazil [1,2].

Individuals and groups may intentionally use radiological materials for terrorist purposes. Such use may introduce new combinations of radiological injury. A point source of radiation may be deployed by terrorists to cause significant whole body or localized doses over a period of time, such as the reported placement of Cs in a Moscow park by Chechen rebels in November 1995. In contrast, a dirty bomb may combine blast and radiation injury with a radiological dispersion device (RDD) and may disperse radioactive substances, creating a contamination hazard for the environment and individuals resulting in both real and psychological casualties [20]. Initial fatalities from an RDD are anticipated to be minimal and related to blast injuries [14,17]. Computer simulation of a Cs-based RDD detonation in Washington, DC, has suggested contamination of a 1-mile area covering 40 city blocks, including the Capitol, Supreme Court, and Library of Congress [14]. Similarly, simulated detonation of Co at the lower tip of Manhattan would result in a 1,000-square kilometer area of contamination, spanning three states. Direct attacks on nuclear power plants would not yield a nuclear explosion, but intentional meltdown of the core may cause similar environmental and health effects as seen at Chernobyl [23].

Ionizing radiation can produce adverse health effects from either internal or external exposure. Ingestion or inhalation of contaminated materials can cause significant local effects. Incorporation occurs when the body replaces regular components with its radioactive counterpart or similar molecule (e.g., K, C, Ra, I). Radionuclides that are incorporated are difficult to eliminate and have the potential to produce long-term health effects in addition to acute symptoms. Common areas of incorporation include bone and thyroid. External sources can produce local effects from direct skin or clothing contamination, or dose the entire body by irradiation. Simple irradiation from β particles, γ rays, and x-rays, do not create contamination and do not make the target substance radioactive itself. Bombardment with neutrons, however, will cause the target substance to become radioactive and a persistent source for ionizing radiation.

Ionizing radiation initiates a cascade of detrimental chemical reactions by generating free radicals as tissue is energized. Tissue is energized directly by α and β particles. Gamma rays and x-rays excite atoms in the tissue by transferring energy to an electron, which subsequently ionizes other molecules in proximity. Although subcellular damage can occur by structural protein or enzyme degradation, the majority of cellular damage and death occurs through disruption of DNA and the mitotic apparatus. The most radiosensitive cells and tissues are those with high turnover rates, such as hematopoietic, reproductive, GI, and epithelial cells. Radiation-resistant tissues include bone, solid organs, muscle, and neuronal tissues.

Current occupational exposure limits for individuals working with radiation sources are 5 rem per year, and 0.5 rem per year in the pregnant, occupationally exposed individual [4]. For the general public, current limits are 0.1 rem per year.

Four ALARA (As Low As Reasonably Achievable) principles provide the foundation for radiation protection: timing, distance, shielding and quantity. A constant amount of ionizing radiation is emitted per unit time. By determining the dose rate by devices such as the Geiger-Mueller (GM) counter, exposure time can be limited to stay within acceptable safety limits. During lifesaving efforts, the recommended limits for total effective dose range from 25 to 150 rem, or a rate of exposure no higher than 0.1mGy per hour, depending on the radiation organization cited [3,19]. For simplicity, a total body exposure of 50 rem is the National Council of Radiation Protection and Measurements/International Council of Radiation Protection and Measurements (NCRP/ICRP) recommended dose acceptable for preserving life [4]. Workers in this setting should be chosen on the basis of age (older), lowest accumulated lifetime effective doses, and on a volunteer basis. Because the exposure dose decreases in proportion to the square of the distance from the source, the distance from a radiation source should be maximized where feasible. High-density materials such as lead or concrete provide greater relative levels of protection from ionizing radiation than do less dense materials. Most structural elements (e.g., walls, floors, etc.) and personal protective equipment (PPE) will not block high-energy γ rays. PPE will, however, provide a physical barrier to contamination from radioactive fallout and debris from RDDs. PPE is also effective in blocking the effects of α particles and a proportion of β particles as well. The quantity of ionizing radiation can also be limited by removing the radioactive source material from the area.

CLINICAL PRESENTATION

Acute radiation injury to the skin and underlying structures causes changes that clinically resemble thermal burns, with desquamation and blistering. Unlike thermal burns, these signs develop after a period of at least 48 to 72 hours after the contact. The clinical effects of dermal radiation exposure are listed in Table 359.2. Delayed skin effects include carcinogenesis, vascular insufficiency, and chronic nonhealing ulcers.

Whole body radiation exposure clinically manifests as acute radiation sickness (ARS), a progression of systemic effects from derangements of the hematopoietic, GI, and neurological systems. ARS has four general phases—prodromal, latent, illness,

TABLE 359.2.   Cutaneous Manifestations of Radiation Exposure

Musculocutaneous Effect	Radiation Dose Threshold
Early Transient Erythema	200 rads
Temporary Epilation	300 rads
Prolonged Erythema	600 rads
Dry Desquamation	1000 rads
Moist Desquamation	2000 rads
Tissue Necrosis	2000–3000 rads

TABLE 359.4.   Acute Radiation Syndrome: Symptoms and Radiation Dose

Symptoms	Radiation Dose
Prodromal Symptoms	
Anorexia	100 rads
Nausea	140 rads
Vomiting	180 rads
Diarrhea	230 rads
Hematopoietic Syndrome	200–450 rads
Pulmonary Syndrome	500–1000 rads
Gastrointestinal (GI) Syndrome	700–1500 rads
Cerebrovascular Syndrome	900–1700 rads
Acute Encephalopathy	5000–10000 rads

and recovery or death. Depending on the dose rate and total absorbed dose, ARS may progress rapidly to death or be completely asymptomatic (Table 359.3). Larger total body doses correlate with increasing acuity of symptoms and decreasing time interval to onset (6,18). The prodromal phase usually lasts 48 to 72 hours, and manifests as nausea, vomiting, diarrhea, and nonspecific constitutional symptoms. The latent phase, which may last 3 weeks, is characterized by the lack of clinical symptoms and apparent recovery from the prodromal phase (20). The latent phase is followed by the illness or hematopoietic phase, in which initial damage to the bone marrow becomes clinically apparent. Pancytopenia and the subsequent sequelae of immunosuppression, bleeding diathesis, and anemia will likely lead to death from sepsis unless adequately supported. If the patient survives the illness phase, which lasts up to 30 days postexposure, recovery will occur 3 to 6 weeks after initial exposure.

Patients receiving total body doses in excess of 700 rads manifest a distinct entity referred to as the gastrointestinal (GI) syndrome, in addition to the prodromal symptoms (Table 359.4). The GI syndrome results in as significant fluid and electrolyte losses, loss of bowel integrity to enteric bacteria, and subsequent death in over 80% of patients. A pulmonary syndrome is noted at doses of 500 to 1,000 rads, manifesting as pneumonitis, respiratory failure, and subsequent pulmonary fibrosis and cor pulmonale. Patients with total body doses of 900 to 1,700 rads develop a cerebrovascular syndrome, although those receiving more than 5,000 rads develop acute encephalopathy, with rapid (hours to days) progression of cerebral edema, cardiovascular collapse, and 100% mortality.

TABLE 359.3.   Acute Radiation Syndrome and Dose-Related Effects

Whole Body Dose (Rad)	Effect
5–50	No clinical symptoms, minor lymphocyte reductions, potential chromosomal damage
100	Nausea and vomiting within 48 h of exposure (10% of patients)
200	Nausea and vomiting within 24 h of exposure (50% of patients), prominent decreases in lymphocytes and granulocytes
400	Nausea and vomiting within 12 h of exposure (90% of patients), mortality of 50% without medical support
600	Mortality of 100% within 30 d without medical support
1000	Maximum survivable dose with aggressive medical support
5000–10000	CNS and cardiovascular collapse within 24–48 h, mortality of 100%

DIFFERENTIAL DIAGNOSIS

Early symptoms of nausea and vomiting are nonspecific, resembling gastroenteritis or food poisoning. Lymphopenia, immunosuppression, and anemia are not only characteristic of radiation sickness, but can be manifestations of HIV and other viral infections, leukemia, use of chemotherapeutic agents, toxic ingestions, and blood dyscrasias.

The differential for radiation-induced dermal injury includes chemical and thermal burns. In contrast to these entities, radiation-associated dermal injury is typically delayed up to 2 weeks. Other dermal lesions to consider include bullous pemphigoid, necrotic arachnidism, and stasis ulcers.

Concomitant radiation contamination should be suspected in any potential terrorist event. Although extraordinary large doses of radiation can cause rapidly progressive shock, radiation typically does not cause sudden death. It is also unlikely to cause the immediate incapacitation of large numbers of people resulting from weapons of mass destruction incident. Other agents should be suspected should such scenarios arise.

EMERGENCY DEPARTMENT EVALUATION

Because of the extreme rarity and potential calamity of an unexpected radiation exposure, the JCAHO requires every hospital develop a formal plan to deal with such an event. Prudence also dictates that every regional emergency management system include radiation accidents in its disaster management protocol. When notified that a radiation accident may have occurred in which many people were exposed to high levels of radiation, the physician should invoke the hospital and regional plans, following them as closely as the circumstances of the particular incident allow. The hospital's radiation safety officer, and the one employed at the site of the accident (or at the company whose truck has crashed, for instance), must be contacted immediately. Police and fire authorities and a public relations official should be called. The physician should communicate with the scene while the area designated in the hospital to receive patients is prepared.

It must be determined exactly what sort of accident has happened: an exposure to external radiation, contamination by radioactive matter, or possible incorporation of ionizing substances via open wounds or the GI or respiratory tracts. A history of trauma or other toxic exposures and the nature, severity, and time of onset of any symptoms should be elicited. The duration of exposure (partial or whole-body), the nature of and distance from the source, and shielding and dosimeters used, if any, all constitute important data.

Patients will require careful evaluation by a designated radiological emergency response team to minimize contamination of the emergency department (ED) (2). Those with life-threatening illness may be triaged from the scene without any form of decontamination. In one simulated weapons of mass destruction (WMD) event, on-scene surveillance for concomitant radiological contamination did not occur (15). Arriving patients should be undressed in the ambulance, and clothes should be collected and stored at a point distant from the patient care areas.

A designated receiving area large enough to manage the anticipated number of casualties should be established. The decontamination area should be prepared and ready for use for both ambulatory and nonambulatory patients. Areas that are likely to be traversed by contaminated patients and workers should be cordoned off. Paper or plastic sheets should be placed on the floor. Entry points to the radiation treatment areas need to be staffed by radiation officers trained to scan for contamination as workers exit the radiation treatment area, and large amounts of gloves, boots, gowns, and masks need to available for workers entering the area. Strict isolation and double-bagging procedures should be maintained, and a buffer zone established for additional contamination control. No special ventilation controls are currently recommended.

All care providers must wear barrier protection, masks, and eye protection to prevent internal and external contamination. All personnel must also wear a radiation detector to determine the whole body dose accumulated during patient contact. Personal dosimeters with real-time displays are preferred over radiation badges to limit any unnecessary exposure, and determine when to rotate teams of care providers. For routine procedures and care, teams should be rotated once 5 rem have been accumulated. The upper limit to provide lifesaving interventions must be predetermined by the radiation safety officer. Most hospitals accept a one-time exposure dose of 25 to 50 rem as acceptable for circumstances that warrant the increased exposure.

If no life-threatening illness is present, a rapid survey using a "pancake" detector, or a GM counter should be performed. Ideally, survey meters capable of detecting both high-range (up to 500 rem/h) and low-range (up to 20 rem/h) exposures and also common (γ and β) or uncommon (α and neutron) sources should be available. The initial scan should progress rapidly from head to toe, focusing on any open wounds, or obvious debris. For the ambulatory patient, the survey should focus on areas, such as the hair and shoulders, where fallout generally accumulates. If the patient is unstable, critical interventions should be performed in conjunction with the radiation survey.

Anatomic charts should be used to document the location of all radiation emission and the radiation counts. Cotton swabs should be taken of all orifices if external contamination is suspected. The physical examination should include evaluation for concomitant trauma. In all cases of radiation injury, a complete blood count, and differential should be obtained, and a type and screen and serum electrolytes and urinalysis to determine kidney function. Subsequent investigations are driven by the clinical presentation of the patient.

EMERGENCY DEPARTMENT MANAGEMENT

Specific prehospital management guidelines have been developed by REAC/TS, and are available online at www.orau.gov/reacts/manage.htm (2). Emergency medical service (EMS) care providers should be able to survey for radiological material in order to correctly identify contaminated patients. A command post should be established at least 150 feet upwind and uphill of the event. Life-threatening injuries take precedence over assessment of contamination status. Patients are monitored at the established control line only after being stabilized. Prehospital personnel and equipment should not reenter service until

monitored and cleared by the designated radiation safety officer. Likewise, personnel should not eat, drink, or smoke until contamination status is assessed by the designated radiation safety officer.

Decontamination procedures begin with the removal of all clothing. This eliminates 80% to 90% of external contamination (11). As radioactive debris may remain in the hair after removal of grossly contaminated clothing, surgical caps should be placed on the unstable contaminated patient to provide some limited shielding and contamination containment while performing advanced life support procedures. All clothes, debris, and bandages must be properly stored. The hospital radiation safety officer must the properly dispose of the waste once surveyed. When contaminated debris or shrapnel are removed from patients, they should be placed in appropriate lead shielded containers and removed from patient-care areas. Anatomic charts must document the location of all radiation emission, the actual initial radiation counts before and after decontamination. Cotton swabs should be taken of all orifices if external contamination is suspected.

Wounds should be treated as usual and covered with plastic and tape prior to decontamination of intact skin. External decontamination should proceed from the area with the most debris to the area with least. Uncontaminated areas should also be covered and taped. Using tepid water and mild soap or nonionic detergent, very gentle scrubbing should be done for 3 minutes with the patient lying either on a special decontamination table (similar to an autopsy table) or on a makeshift plastic trough placed on a stretcher in slight reverse Trendelenburg. Hot water is avoided as a result of subsequent capillary vasodilation and potential for increased radionuclide absorption. Aggressive scrubbing is likewise avoided as a result of the potential for dermal trauma and increased dermal absorption. Scanning for radioactivity and repeating this procedure as long as counts are decreasing should be done. Gentle brushing under nails and clipping of hair (not shaving, which might leave small open wounds) may be required. All fluids should be collected.

Skin decontamination is accomplished with warm water. Serial measurements of the amount of radiation emission should be performed. Decontamination attempts can stop when the radioactivity level cannot be further reduced.

Most isolated radiation injuries are not medical emergencies and only require supportive care, baseline laboratory testing, and follow up for specialty care such as burns, infectious disease, and hematology/oncology. Specific antidotes and chelation agents are available that may assist in mitigating the effects of the radionuclide burden from internally contaminated patients. These agents do so by decreasing the overall radionuclide burden by dilution, displacement, blockage, or chelation. However, it is difficult to differentiate between radionuclides without scintillators or other advanced laboratory equipment only found in select laboratory settings. If identification is possible, or a likely radionuclide is suspected from the type of radiation accident, antidotes must be administered rapidly or the effectiveness will be limited. Less than 2 hours is available for possibly effective prevention of incorporation after ingestion or inhalation.

Treatment of ingestions should begin with gastric lavage. Whole-bowel irrigation, using a polyethylene glycol bowel prep solution (e.g., GoLYTELY, Colyte) at 0.5 to 2.0 L/h until the rectal effluent is clear, may be beneficial. Activated charcoal is also recommended. Washings should be saved, surveyed, and disposed of by the radiation safety officer. Other methods to reduce GI absorption include administering Prussian blue for thallium, cesium, or rubidium, and barium sulfate or aluminum-based antacids for radium or strontium. Bronchoalveolar lavage may be helpful if radioactive dust has been inhaled, as confirmed by stained or radioactive sputum.

Prussian blue (Radiogardase®) works by increasing fecal elimination of the radionuclide. Prussian blue is taken orally, and will not compete with other treatment agents such as oral potassium iodide (KI). Clinical side effects include constipation and GI upset. Prussian blue is most effective when administered near the time of exposure, but should be administered as soon as cesium or thallium has been identified as the radionuclide in question. In the 137Cs Goiania incident, Prussian blue at doses ranging from 3 to 10 gm/day resulted in a mean 71% dose reduction (13,21).

KI should be administered to those in whom exposure to 131I is likely (5). Such events include an RDD contaminated with medical 131I, release of radioisotopes from a nuclear reactor, and nuclear detonation. Children may benefit most. Residents, childcare facilities, and schools within 10 miles of a nuclear reactor are encouraged to stockpile enough KI to treat their children before the exposure or immediately thereafter. Although KI is available without prescription, local health authorities usually have a supply and will distribute this medication in the event of an accident.

KI works by competition to prevent the incorporation of radioactive iodine by the thyroid gland. It will protect the thyroid from increased risk for cancer but will not mitigate any other forms of acute or long-term radiation effects. The dose of KI is approximately 2 mg/kg. The protective effects of KI last approximately 24 hours and daily dosing for up to 2 weeks, usually at the discretion of the local health department, may be necessary. Short-term treatment of KI at thyroid blocking doses is safe, with side effects of sialadenitis, GI upset, rashes, and allergic reactions being most common. As internal contamination of radioiodine will partition into breast milk, lactating mothers are instructed not to breastfeed their infants until public health authorities have deemed it safe to consume the milk (10).

The initial management of concomitant trauma is the same as usual. Because wound healing is adversely affected by radiation and the likelihood of infection is increased, definitive surgery should be performed within the first 48 hours. If this is not possible, nonemergent procedures such as internal fixation of fractures should be delayed at least 6 to 8 weeks until bone marrow production returns to normal.

Psychological support for those affected is necessary (7,9,12). Physical manifestations of acute stress reaction, including nausea, vomiting, and vague constitutional complaints, can mimic those of acute radiation syndrome and must be differentiated for appropriate disposition of these patients.

CRITICAL INTERVENTIONS

- Notify the hospital radiation safety officer and activate the hospital radiation exposure plan for patients with possible radionuclide contamination
- Use time, distance, shielding, and quantity reduction techniques to minimize exposure
- Wear barrier protection, masks, eye protection, and dosimeter, if available
- Perform resuscitation and stabilization as necessary
- Perform external and internal decontamination and isolate contaminated clothes, debris, and fluids

DISPOSITION

After initial ED management, patients may be discharged for outpatient management depending on extent of prodromal symptoms and absolute lymphocyte count at presentation. Triage guidelines have been developed based on the Chernobyl

TABLE 359.5. Relationship Between Absolute Lymphocyte Count and Outcome After Total Body Radiation Exposure

Outcome	Lymphocyte Count/mm³ at 24 h	Lymphocyte Count/mm³ at 48 h
Normal	1750	>1500
Moderate Injury	1500	1000–1500
Severe Injury	1000	500–1000
Very Severe Injury	500	100–500
Lethal	<100	<100

experience. Onset of prodromal ARS symptoms less than 30 minutes after exposure indicates a total body dose greater than 600 rads, although onset greater than 2 hours after exposure indicates a dose less than 200 rads. Onset of prodromal symptoms more than 24 hours after exposure indicates a dose less than 70 rads (Table 359.4) (6,18). Severe nausea and vomiting indicate a substantial whole body dose, (i.e., 2–10 Gy) that will require inpatient monitoring for supportive care.

Lymphocyte count is routinely used to aid in disposition and management of radiation injuries. If the patient is asymptomatic and has a normal lymphocyte count, early follow-up and frequent complete blood counts may be appropriate. Prognosis is directly tied to the 48-hour lymphocyte count, and is dose dependent (Table 359.5). Lymphocyte counts greater than 1,200/μl indicate a good prognosis, and counts below 300/μl indicate a poor prognosis (8). Individuals with total body doses greater than 1000 rads will likely need admission, and those with doses greater than 3,000 rads may require reverse isolation precautions.

Hematology consultation will be required to administer growth factor therapy, colony stimulating factors, treat anemia and thrombocytopenia, and provide advanced cytokine therapy or cord/placental blood progenitor cells. Burn, infectious disease, and bone marrow transplant consultation may also be necessary.

Questions regarding radiation accidents and exposures can be referred to the U.S. Department of Energy through the Radiation Emergency Assistance Center/Training Site (REAC/TS), Oak Ridge, TN by the web, www.orau.gov/reacts, or by phone, 865-576-1005.

COMMON PITFALLS

✔ Failure to identify presence of radioactive contamination or irradiation injury
✔ Failure to perform disaster training or to perform such drills without including decontamination, use of personal protective equipment, and radiation surveys
✔ Failure to manage concomitant injuries appropriately, and prior to decontamination in critically ill patients
✔ Failure to request appropriate consultations, or to withhold indicated chelation or antidote therapy
✔ Failure to address psychological components of radiation exposure with patients and staff

Acknowledgment

We thank previous edition chapter author Irvin N. Heifetz.

References

1. Anonymous. *DOE-REAC/TS Radiation Accident Registry System*. REAC/TS course material, Oak Ridge Institute for Science and Education, 2003.
2. Anonymous. Guidance for Emergency Accident Management. Oak Ridge Associated Universities Web site. Available at www.orau.gov/reacts/guidance.htm. Accessed October 1, 2003.

3. Anonymous. *Management of terrorist events involving radioactive material.* NCRP report no 138. Bethesda, MD: National Council on Radiation Protection and Measurements, 2001.

4. Anonymous. *Limitations of exposure to ionizing radiation.* NCRP report no 116. Bethesda, MD: National Council on Radiation Protection and Measurements, 1993.

5. US Dept of Health, Center for Drug Evaluation and Research. *Guidance, potassium iodide as a thyroid blocking agent in radiation emergencies: use in radiation emergencies: treatment recommendations.* Food and Drug Administration Web site. Available at http://www.fda.gov/cder/guidance/4825fnl.htm#KI. Accessed December 9, 2003.

6. Barabanova A. *REAC/TS Newsletter.* Oak Ridge, TN: REAC/TS, 1992; (Winter):1–2.

7. Becker, SM. Psychological assistance after environmental accidents: a policy perspective. *Environ Health Perspect* 1997;105(suppl 6):1557–1563.

8. Champlin, RE. Radiation accidents and nuclear energy: medical consequences and therapy. *Ann Intern Med* 1988;109:730.

9. Collins DL. Human responses to the threat of or exposure to ionizing radiation at Three Mile Island, Pennsylvania, and Goiania, Brazil. *Mil Med* 2002;167(2 Suppl):137–138.

10. Committee on Environmental Health, American Academy of Pediatrics. Policy statement, radiation disasters and children. *Pediatrics* 2003;111(6):1455–1466.

11. Cox, RA. Nuclear emergencies: medical preparedness. *Br J Radiol* 1987;60:1180.

12. DiGiovanni C Jr. Domestic Terrorism with chemical or biological agents: psychiatric aspects. *Am J Psychiatry* 1999;156:1500–1505.

13. Farina R, Brandao-Mello CE, Oliveira AR. Medical aspects of 137Cs decorporation: the Goiania radiological accident. *Health Phys* 1991;60:63–66.

14. Federation of American Scientists. Dirty bombs: response to a threat. *FAS Public Interest Report* 2002;55(1):6–10.

15. FitzGerald DJ, Sztajnkrycer MD, Crocco TJ. Chemical weapon functional exercise—Cincinnati: observations and lessons learned from a "typical medium-sized" city's response to simulated terrorism utilizing weapons of mass destruction. *Public Health Rep* 2003;118:205–214.

16. Frame P. *Radiation Fact Sheet.* Oak Ridge, Tenn.: Oak Ridge Institute for Science and Education/Oak Ridge Associated Universities, 1995.

17. Greenberg MI, Farrell TP, Hendrickson RG. Routine Screening for Environmental Radiation by First Responders at Explosions and Fires. *Ann Emerg Med* 2003;41:426–427.

18. Gusev I, Guskova AK, Mettler FA Jr. *Medical management of radiation accidents,* 2nd ed. Boca Raton, FL: CRC Press, 2001.

19. International Commission on Radiological Protection. *1990 Recommendations of the International Commission on Radiological Protection,* vol. 21, No. 1–3 of Annals of the ICRP. Oxford, England: Pergamon Press, 1991;21(60).

20. Jarrett DG. *Medical Management of Radiologic Casualties Handbook,* 1st ed. Armed Forces Radiobiology Research Institute, 1999.

21. Melo DR, Lipsztein JL, de Oliveira CA, et al. 137Cs Internal Contamination Involving a Brazilian Accident, and the Efficacy of Prussian Blue Treatment. *Health Phys* 1994;66:245–252.

22. Mettler FA Jr, Voelz GL. Current concepts: major radiation exposure—what to expect and how to respond. *New Engl J Med* 2002;346(20):1554–61.

23. Weinberg AD, Kripalani S, McCarthy, PL, et al. Caring for survivors of the Chernobyl disaster: what the clinician should know. *JAMA* 1995;274:408–412.

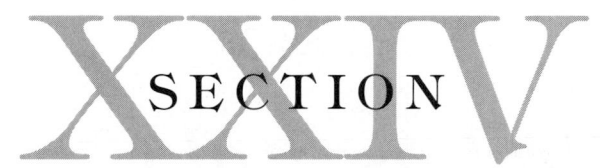

SECTION

XXIV

Section Editor: Carlo L. Rosen

Administrative and Special Clinical Considerations

PART I

Prehospital Care

CHAPTER 360
Emergency Medical Services

Alexander P. Isakov, Marc Restuccia, and
Lawrence Mottley

HISTORICAL PERSPECTIVE

Prior to the rapid evolution of emergency medical services (EMS) in the 1960s and 1970s, only rudimentary systems of prehospital care and patient transport existed. Although hospital-based ambulance services had been functioning in Cincinnati, Ohio, since 1865, and city services were initiated in New York in 1869, private ventures that combined transport services with another trade, such as funeral services, had the greatest market share. Such enterprises delivered prehospital care with little training, regulation, or benchmark for quality (25). The military advanced EMS in its care of wounded soldiers in Vietnam (31). Corpsmen and medics were trained in prehospital intervention and evacuation of the critically wounded to appropriate facilities for prompt surgical attention. The mortality of trauma patients surviving to a medical treatment facility sharply decreased (26).

In 1966, the National Academy of Sciences—National Research Council, which acts as a consulting body to the government, published what has been referred to as the "white paper" of prehospital systems, "Accidental Death and Disability: The Neglected Disease of Modern Society"(26). This document summarized the inadequate delivery of emergency care, the lack of an emergency services infrastructure, and the lack of leadership in this area. It also made specific recommendations for a funded, organized, proactive, prehospital medical delivery system, launching the modern era of civilian EMS in the United States.

The "white paper," along with others showing a rise in accidental deaths, especially on America's highways, prompted Congress to enact the National Highway Safety Act of 1966. This act authorized spending by the newly created Department of Transportation (DOT)/National Highway Traffic Safety Administration (NHTSA) for the improvement of essential prehospital infrastructure, training of personnel, and establishment of practice guidelines. Through this legislation, states developed regional EMS systems with funding for ambulances, personnel, and communication equipment. A nationally recognized curriculum for the training of ambulance attendants (emergency medical technician or EMT-A) was established in 1971.

The success of prehospital cardiac care units in Dublin (35) and of new methods of cardiopulmonary resuscitation (CPR) led EMS programs to expand their focus beyond trauma. The Department of Health, Education and Welfare funded regional EMS demonstration projects in five states, and grants for regional EMS development were offered by the Robert Wood Johnson Foundation. The resulting improved communications, training, and transport capacity in these demonstration projects was viewed favorably in Congress and was followed by the EMS Systems Act of 1973, which legislated further federal funding of comprehensive regional EMS systems; this included money for operations, training, and research. Full-time medical directors and professional prehospital medical providers emerged.

National standards for EMT-A, EMT-I (intermediate level), and EMP-P (paramedic level) training evolved. Because some nonmedical public safety personnel were often the first to arrive at a scene with medical casualties, a first-responder curriculum was developed as well. NHTSA established such curricula, which came to be recognized as national standards.

Communications infrastructure, including 911 access, two-way radio communications, and centralized dispatch were developed and criteria for optimal ambulance design and equipment were established. Regional EMS systems were intended to become financially independent as federal funding was phased out in favor of state discretionary funding of EMS through Preventive Health Block Grants, a product of the Omnibus Budget Reconciliation Act of 1981 (25). The result, however, was deterioration of the movement toward national standards as regional systems yielded to state and local concerns. A multitude of systems developed independently, providing a varied range of skill levels, training, and quality of care, from one community to another. Organizations like the National Association of EMS Physicians emerged to serve as a professional body for consensus in the continuing development of EMS systems. The NHTSA has maintained its leadership role through its EMS division at the federal level (12).

Today, EMS systems operate in an environment of increased fiscal restraint, with an increased demand for objective proof of the efficacy of prehospital interventions. Although these forces may produce more efficient systems, delivering a high quality of care, they could also erode a prehospital infrastructure that took 30 years to develop (30).

EDUCATION

The U.S. DOT first-responder curriculum trains providers to perform basic patient assessment, manage airway obstruction, control external hemorrhage, administer CPR, and apply automatic external defibrillation devices. The length of training is 20 hours. The EMT-A curriculum, historically the minimum level of training required by an ambulance attendant, was revised in 1994, is now known as the basic (EMT-B) curriculum, and currently requires approximately 110 hours of training. The trainee is educated in ambulance operation, communications, documentation, scene assessment, initial patient assessment, triage, patient immobilization, basic airway maneuvers, and CPR. The revised training strategy departed from the traditional diagnosis-based model to an assessment-based model and generated much national debate. Less emphasis was placed on pathophysiology and more emphasis on basic recognition of illness and execution of skills. Automatic external defibrillation was added to the curriculum. Advanced airway training was offered as well.

EMT-I and EMT-P curricula, revised in 1998, are approximately 300 hours and 1,100 hours, respectively, and retain a diagnosis-based strategy for patient evaluation. The EMT-I level requires successful completion of the EMT-B curriculum as a prerequisite and includes additional training in pathophysiology, assessment skills, venous cannulation, and establishment of a patent airway. The EMT-P level includes an anatomy and physiology course, and the EMT-B course as prerequisites, and offers advanced training in pathophysiology, i.v. access, definitive airway control, and the pharmacology and administration of a variety of medications.

Despite national standards for curricula at first-responder, EMT-B, EMT-I, and EMT-P levels, states have variably adopted them in the training and certification of EMS providers in their jurisdictions. As a result, approximately forty levels of EMS providers exist nationwide (11). Each state adopts the curricula, in whole or in part, requires varying hours of formal education, and establishes scopes of practice presumably suited to its own needs. Although this diversity allows for the greatest flexibility to respond to local needs with local resources, it does not foster uniform standards of care and creates confusion regarding interstate reciprocity of privileges. NHTSA sponsored an EMS Education Task Force composed of EMS providers, administrators, educators, and physicians, which authored "EMS Education Agenda for the Future: A Systems Approach" (13). This document calls for more explicitly defined core educational content, scope of practice, and national standards for the education and certification of providers. The Agenda calls for an education system with five primary integrated components: (a) the National EMS Core Content, (b) the National EMS Scope of Practice Model, (c) National EMS Education Standards, (d) National EMS Education Program Accreditation, and (e) National EMS Certification. NHTSA is currently working to develop the National EMS Core Content, which will specify the knowledge and skills necessary for the provision of care in the out-of-hospital environment.

Specialized training programs have been established for EMTs and paramedics who function in settings in which additional education is desirable. Critical care transport specialists may receive training in ventilator, invasive monitoring, and intraaortic balloon pump management. The wilderness curriculum prepares the EMT in search and rescue, environmental injuries, complications of prolonged evacuation and prehospital transport, and basic primary care in remote locations. The EMT-Tactical program prepares providers in comprehensive medical support for law enforcement teams and includes training in medical contingency planning, and in preventive medicine for the tactical team. It also includes medical support of extended operations, including primary care and recognition of performance decrement, hazardous materials (HAZMAT) safety, clinical forensics, and safe management of casualties in an austere, hostile environment. These specialized training programs allow medical directors to fulfill their responsibility, although ensuring that providers are trained to function safely and effectively in unique settings.

The training of physicians for leadership roles in EMS is also developing. Historically, any physician who had an interest and the fortitude would serve as an EMS medical director. No formal training existed. Today, emergency medicine residents are provided some training in EMS systems as part of their core curriculum in postgraduate training (44). EMS experience, however, varies greatly from one training program to another. Postgraduate EMS fellowship training is now available through 1- and 2-year training programs. The 2-year programs concurrently offer a master's degree in public health, hospital administration, business, or other disciplines. Guidelines for a standard curriculum have been endorsed by the Society for Academic Emergency Medicine and the National Association of EMS Physicians (20). The American Board of Emergency Medicine has yet to accept EMS as a certifiable subspecialty.

STRUCTURE

Regardless of the type of EMS system, the necessity for field personnel to obtain adequate clinical exposure cannot be overemphasized. Patient outcomes improve when each medical provider achieves a threshold of patient encounters. Regionalization of EMS systems, as has occurred in the South and West, provides not only economies of scale, but also the ability to rotate personnel to ensure adequate experience, uniform patient treatment protocols, and placement of units based on patient need rather than political boundaries. In the Northeast, in which each city and town often independently maintain their own EMS service, staffing requirements and overall costs are higher, and more personnel almost certainly means diluted experience and loss of skills.

Fire-based Systems

Many fire departments (FDs), especially in the western United States, adopted EMS as part of their mission immediately after the federal legislation was enacted. Fire-based systems allowed dispatch and deployment of EMS units within a currently existing system. In most combined EMS/fire systems, EMS accounts for about three-fourths of the call load. In small cities and towns, existing personnel and facilities may be able to perform EMS duties without adding staff or infrastructure. But because firefighters are usually among the highest-paid employees, larger systems, which need additional staff will incur much higher costs compared with the other EMS models.

Additionally, because the FD's first priority is fire suppression, conflicts of interest may arise and lead to under resourced patient care. As the annual number of fire-suppression calls decreases and cities look more closely at the most efficient use of available resources, more FDs are becoming interested in EMS. Integration of established EMS systems with and under the direction of FDs is a politically charged topic that currently is the subject of heated debate in many cities.

In a full-service EMS system, the FD provides both treatment and transport for all patients. Advanced life-support (ALS) and basic life-support (BLS) ambulances or only ALS ambulances may transport all patients. In a paramedic-only service system, the fire department provides ALS response to all, or a subset, of calls. BLS calls are referred to a private ambulance provider on the basis of either telephone triage or on-scene assessment by paramedics. ALS patients may be transported in an FD ambulance or in a private ambulance accompanied by an FD paramedic. Many FDs now provide first-responder services regardless of the source of ambulance transport, using firefighter personnel trained to respond to immediately life-threatening conditions such as cardiac arrest (CA), respiratory distress, chest pain, and loss of consciousness.

Private Ambulance Services

Private ambulance services often bid for an exclusive contract with a governmental entity to provide EMS services, usually to a city, town, or county. The contract often stipulates that certain indirect measures of quality and performance be met, such as that all units be equipped with defibrillators, that paramedics perform a minimum number of intubations, or that certain response-time parameters be met. The community establishes regulatory control over the private service, with oversight being provided by an EMS agency or a medical director.

Private ambulance services usually provide both ALS and BLS services. To a greater extent than any of the other EMS models, private ambulances depend on efficient management of resources, such as peak-load staffing and system status management, to meet their dual demands: adequate EMS response and being a successful business. Personnel costs for the private sector are usually significantly below those for both the FD and third-service industries. The risk, however, is that the vendor could withdraw from nonlucrative markets, leaving the region or municipality searching for a means to provide uninterrupted service.

Third-service Systems

Third service, simply defined, is an EMS system housed in a municipal department, using municipality-owned and -operated ambulances, and kept separate from police and fire services. Many medium and large cities continue to use municipal hospital–based ambulances as all or part of their EMS systems. Some third services are part of the city's Health Department, and a few are separate city agencies. This model allows for concentration on one mission—patient care—without the distraction of managing, funding, and providing other services. EMT skill maintenance is rarely a problem in these mostly urban systems. A drawback is that the third-service agency must compete with other traditionally well-supported public service agencies for budgetary funding.

Volunteer Systems

Almost three-fourths of all rural EMS providers are volunteers. The tax base cannot support a full-time professional EMS system, and the revenue to attract a private contractor does not exist. The dedication of volunteers is remarkable, as are the challenges they face in finding medical oversight, time for training, the means to maintain their skills, and the financial resources to develop and maintain their systems' infrastructure. Depending on state regulation, some volunteer services may operate without medical direction. Turnover among these providers is high. Rural systems face the same challenge of quality care as urban ones but with drastically different resources.

AMBULANCES

There are five types of ambulances currently used in the United States:

(a) *Type 1*—A truck body with a full hood and box patient care area. These are the largest vehicles with the greatest weight and maximum patient care area. Type 1 ambulances are ideal for busy ALS systems, services with long transport times, and critical care ground transport systems. The disadvantage of such vehicles is higher acquisition costs, higher ongoing maintenance costs, and their size, which can be problematic in tight urban systems.
(b) *Type 2*—A van body on a truck chassis. These ambulances are smaller, lighter, cheaper to acquire, and the most common type. They have a limited patient care area.
(c) *Type 3*—A van front, patient box on a truck chassis. These are intermediate between Types 1 and 2 in acquisition costs. They strike an ideal compromise for many agencies.
(d) *Type 4*—Specialty ambulances. This includes air ambulances (helicopter/airplanes).
(e) *Type 5*—ALS vehicle. These are used to bring ALS capable providers to a patient, and are not generally utilized for patient transport. They are capable of transport in unusual circumstances.

There is increasing pressure to design ambulances that afford EMS personnel and patients maximum protection in the event of a motor vehicle accident. It has become increasingly clear that the vehicles used for EMS operations are not optimally designed for occupant safety (17). Cleared head strike zones, secured equipment, and appropriate restraint of patients and EMS personnel are issues that need to be addressed. Air ambulance services and foreign ambulance manufacturers and EMS agencies have demonstrated leadership in this area. A radical re-design of ambulances can be expected in the future. These "modern" ambulances will likely be smaller, afford better protection for the occupants, have advanced monitoring systems and greatly improve the chance of patients and EMS personnel surviving a traffic accident.

Federal and state laws, which can be extremely detailed, govern the configuration of each vehicle, and its markings. Additionally, each state mandates the minimum and allowable equipment and medications carried on any ambulance, with some latitude afforded to Type-4 vehicles. Despite these regulations, there is wide variation of equipment and medications carried on individual ambulances. These variations reflect not only the medical director's equipment preferences, judgment, and vision for the service, but also those of other personnel and the type and geographic location of the system.

A busy urban EMS system may stock large amounts of consumable equipment to minimize "down time" to restock. Conversely, if all runs end at the base facility, lesser amounts of such items may be required. In contrast, rural EMS agencies may stock every item they may conceivably need during a prolonged transport. Variation in equipment and supplies also reflects the level of service provided. The amount and variability of medical equipment on a BLS ambulance is typically much less than on an ALS vehicle.

MEDICAL OVERSIGHT

Medical oversight of out-of-hospital providers is essential to providing the best medical care. It may take the form of direct or indirect medical control. Direct or online medical control refers to the immediate direction and feedback, usually by radio or telephone that a physician provides to an EMS provider while caring for a patient. Although there is some controversy over whether such communication significantly improves the care provided (19), it gives EMS providers direct access to a physician's level of training and knowledge.

In some systems, online medical control is provided by a specified physician or institution at a single base hospital. In other systems, it is decentralized, with each receiving institution acting as a base station. Medical control physicians must have an in-depth knowledge of the skills and capabilities of the EMS provider on scene and the capabilities and availability of receiving institutions in the area. They must also know applicable state and regional or local protocols and the medicolegal implications of situations such as refusal of treatment or transport and the care of minors, do-not-resuscitate patients, and deceased patients.

Indirect or *off-line* medical control consists of protocol development and implementation, equipment selection, assuring adherence to clinical standards, education of EMS providers, and ongoing quality improvement within the system. Such functions are generally the responsibility of the EMS medical director. The highest functioning EMS agencies are characterized by the triad of commitment to excellence in patient care, dedicated EMS personnel, and actively engaged medical directors. Care must be "patient-centric and physician-directed." Compliance with protocols and standards of care is usually accomplished by reviewing EMS patient care records (charts or "run sheets"). This is accomplished by the EMS medical director or designee reviewing individual cases that were difficult or problematic, or by reviewing the charts of selected conditions (e.g., CAs, pediatric cases, intubations, deaths, refusals of care) or individuals (e.g., new hires, those with whom there may be quality-of-care concerns, those who have just returned from a leave of absence). Additionally, in a highly functional EMS agency, the medical director and other supervisory personnel must spend time "in the field" with their EMTs and paramedics. Chart review can never replace the invaluable experience of seeing how personnel function in their element. EMS agencies must be committed to continuously evaluating the quality of the service delivered and striving to seek ways to improve it.

The initial training and continuing education of EMS providers is a key element in medical direction. The implementation of new medications, interventions, and protocols is an ongoing process. Quality improvement includes not only identifying and correcting deficiencies in current practice, but also identifying areas that, although not necessarily deficient, can be improved (response time, scene time, timely completion of charts, documentation of procedures).

COMMUNICATION

EMS communications is a chain of events that can be best described using queuing theory. The call-taker queue consists of those who dial 911. In the past, most cities and towns had their own emergency call-receiving center, but with the advent of *Enhanced 911* (911E), many have now been consolidated into Public Safety Answering Points (PSAPs) serving one large local jurisdiction, or multiple smaller ones. 911E provides the PSAP call-taker with the physical address of the phone (street address and, in apartment buildings, the apartment number), and the telephone number of the caller. In most jurisdictions, once the last digit of 911 is dialed, the caller cannot disconnect by hanging up. The 911 call can only be released by the Public Safety Dispatcher. This prevents the panicked caller from disconnecting the call before all information is obtained and prearrival instructions are offered. The demographic information allows patients who are unable to speak as a result of illness, injury, or danger, to receive assistance. Protocols may also allow the call-taker to ask a series of yes or no questions that mute callers can answer by pushing the appropriate button (1 or 2). In this way, the correct agency or agencies can respond. Technology is also available to approximate the location of cell phones within a few dozen meters, a feature useful for the location of automobile accidents and that enables the direct routing of a 911 call to the appropriate PSAP.

EMS callers are then placed in the triage queue. Modern EMS systems use written telephone medical triage guidelines, known generically as Emergency Medical Dispatch (EMD), to ensure consistent and appropriate triage and response. More important, by asking only for information that will assist in correctly prioritizing the call, they reduce the amount of time spent questioning the patient prior to dispatch. For example, if the caller is male, over 50 years of age, and has nontraumatic chest pain, no further information is necessary for triaging the call as high priority (potential cardiac etiology). Gathering additional information and attempting to make a presumptive diagnosis is not appropriate and possibly detrimental, because it wastes time and is not relevant to the dispatch decision.

Triage protocols can reduce both type 1 and type 2 errors (over-triage and under-triage). They also protect the call-taker from the abusive retrospective review that can occur after a high-profile adverse event. Because the medical director bears responsibility for the appropriateness of these medical triage guidelines, it is strongly suggested that a nationally recognized EMD product be used. Some of these products are customizable (within limits) to meet local preferences while others require use "as is."

EMS calls are usually triaged into one of three priorities: *Priority One*: life-threatening; *Priority Two*: emergent or unknown; and *Priority Three*: nonemergent. These categories are designed to reflect the instability of an illness or injury and its likelihood of deteriorating in a short period of time. They are not intended to characterize whether the condition justifies the use of an ambulance or how serious it is. For instance, although a fractured hip is serious and appropriate for the use of an ambulance, it is not likely to deteriorate and therefore does not have top priority.

Once the call is prioritized, it enters the dispatch queue. The dispatcher then assigns an ambulance to respond. Assigning the closest ambulance to the call is preferred, but this process is not always straightforward. As the number of ambulances in a system increases, so does the complexity of dispatch. In larger cities, the dispatcher would have to know each street and the location of each ambulance at any given time. Most ambulances are available to be dispatched, or "in-service" 60% to 85% of the time, and they may be located outside their assigned districts, making it difficult to ascertain their position without polling multiple units over the radio.

Automatic Vehicle Locator (AVL) systems can help and are increasingly being used, particularly within the private sector. Using the federal government Global Positioning Satellite (GPS) system, AVLs can locate an ambulance within a few feet, calculate the travel time to a given call, and recommend the nearest units of each appropriate type—first-responder, BLS, and ALS.

EMS demand by time of day is remarkably predictable, especially in systems with a large call volume. System Status Management (SSM) is the process of managing resources based on known patterns of calls in time and place and current demand.

Additional ambulances are placed in service during known periods of higher demand. Available units do not remain static, but are dynamically and proactively redeployed by EMS supervisors when call volume is high in certain areas. The practice of flat staffing, in which the same number of ambulances are on duty 24 hours a day, is less efficient; patients will have to wait longer than necessary during the busier times, and resources will be wasted during slack time.

EMS radio communications primarily utilize four frequency bands: VHF-Low (40–60 MHz), VHF-High (140–170 MHz), UHF (470–490 MHz), and the 800 band (800–900+ MHz). Each has performance characteristics with strengths and weaknesses. The height of the radio antenna is usually one-fourth the wavelength. VHF, especially VHF-Low, has a wavelength a few meters long and travels a great distance, but it is unable to penetrate manufactured obstacles such as buildings. This band is commonly used by agencies similar to the Highway Patrol, covering wide distances with few artificial obstructions. It is not suitable for use in urban or suburban systems.

UHF has good penetration into manufactured objects, and its antenna is of reasonable height for portable use. The 800 band is often used because there are no available channels to be licensed on the UHF frequencies. It has excellent penetration into buildings, but the wavelength is so short that communications are essentially limited to line of sight, meaning poor or nonexistent over-the-horizon reception. This band is ideal for the urban environment, in which one well-placed transmitter can often cover an entire city. It is often used in a "trunking" system.

A trunking radio system usually consists of six to eight actual frequencies but has ten times that number in "virtual frequencies" called channels. For instance, each radio may have channels 1 through 6, and each of these channels may have ten subchannels (e.g., A–J), allowing for 60 discrete channels. Each of these channels and subchannels may have restrictions; that is, channel 1A may be for dispatch, and all users would have the ability to listen while channel 4B might be for medical quality assurance, and only the personnel assigned to that group would have radios with the "privileges" for channel 4B. The central computer controlling the mobile and portable radios senses which radios are tuned to which channels. When a user broadcasts on a given channel, the computer assigns an actual frequency (e.g., 800.435 MHz) and programs only the other radios tuned to this channel to switch to that frequency. A similar process is used for cell phones. The advantage of the trunked system is that it uses bandwidth much more efficiently. The usual public safety radio frequency is actually transmitting less than 10% of the time. Trunking allows this "wasted" air time to be used by others transparently. The disadvantage of trunked systems is that when the system is saturated, users are literally locked out by the computer. Whereas in conventional nontrunked systems a paramedic in trouble can get help by yelling on the radio even if someone else is transmitting, the trunked system does not permit simultaneous transmissions.

Frequencies assigned by the Federal Communications Commission (FCC) for medical control, the "Med Channels," are in the UHF band, thus allowing one radio to serve for both dispatch and hospital communication. There are ten channels in this group, eight for medical control (channels 1–8) and two for EMS dispatch (channels 9 and 10). Receiving hospitals may have permanently assigned med channels that allow medics to call directly, or hospitals may be part of a central medical dispatch (C-MED) system, in which medics call C-MED and are patched into the requested hospital.

Virtually all of the radio frequencies in use for EMS are duplexed; they operate on a pair of frequencies, one to send and another to receive. This setup allows both parties to talk at the same time, so that either the physician or the paramedic can interrupt the other if necessary. Transmissions by field personnel using portable radios are weak and can only be heard directly over a short distance. If desired, the central radio can retransmit these messages with a more powerful transmitter, using the second channel, called a "repeater." This system allows all users to hear all other users.

DISASTER PLANNING

Mass casualty incidents (MCIs) require the response of multiple different public safety and EMS agencies. They threaten to overwhelm the capacity of the out-of-hospital system and the medical facilities supporting them (22). Each EMS agency and hospital must have a plan for dealing with MCIs in their service area. The importance of having a well understood, rehearsed, and commonly recognized plan for responding to an MCI cannot be overemphasized. Practicing implementation of the plan provides training for all participants, prevents needless delays, and identifies areas for improvement. Agencies should have complementary plans and train together to ensure cooperation.

Risk assessment of potential MCI scenarios in a service area should be part of the plan. It involves recognizing and characterizing likely sites of an MCI, such as industrial complexes, airports, residential areas (e.g., high-rise apartments, special-needs facilities), highways and railways, and unique facilities, such as nuclear power plants.

A mechanism for rapidly triaging victims of an MCI should be identified and rehearsed. The objective of patient triage is to do the greatest good for the greatest number of victims. Field triage is based typically on physiologic criteria that assign patients to severity categories identifying those who require treatment and transport to a medical treatment facility most urgently (18). Several triage criteria are published (14). The START (simple triage and rapid transport) system is commonly used (Fig. 360.1). Patient severity is determined in an algorithmic fashion by first assessing ability to ambulate, then airway, respirations, circulation, and mental status. Patients are assigned to five severity categories. *Nonurgent/ambulatory* (green) patients do not have life-threatening injury and will likely do well even if care is withheld several hours or days. Urgent (yellow) patients have a serious injury but will likely not deteriorate with a slight delay in care. *Emergent* (red) patients are critical and will require immediate care. *Expectant* (black) patients are dead or have injuries not compatible with life. The fifth category has been termed *catastrophic* (blue). These patients have life-threatening injuries but might only be saved after receiving extensive and complicated therapy rapidly. These patients will consume extraordinary resources and therefore, in the spirit of doing the greatest good for the greatest number, are treated and transported after patients in red and yellow categories have received care.

Whatever patient triage system is utilized, it must be employed in routine EMS operations to promote familiarity and to insure recognition among emergency service providers at all levels of care, including the medical treatment facility.

A communications plan is essential. Often, however, it is the part of the response that fails most rapidly in an MCI. Overloaded radio channels, cell channels, and phone lines can be expected. Loss of radio towers and telephone wires may occur. The plan should identify ways to minimize the effect of these occurrences.

Mutual aid agreements with EMS, police, and fire services, and medical treatment facilities in contiguous service areas should be in place. The ability to assemble out-of-hospital and hospital assets beyond the affected area is often essential for

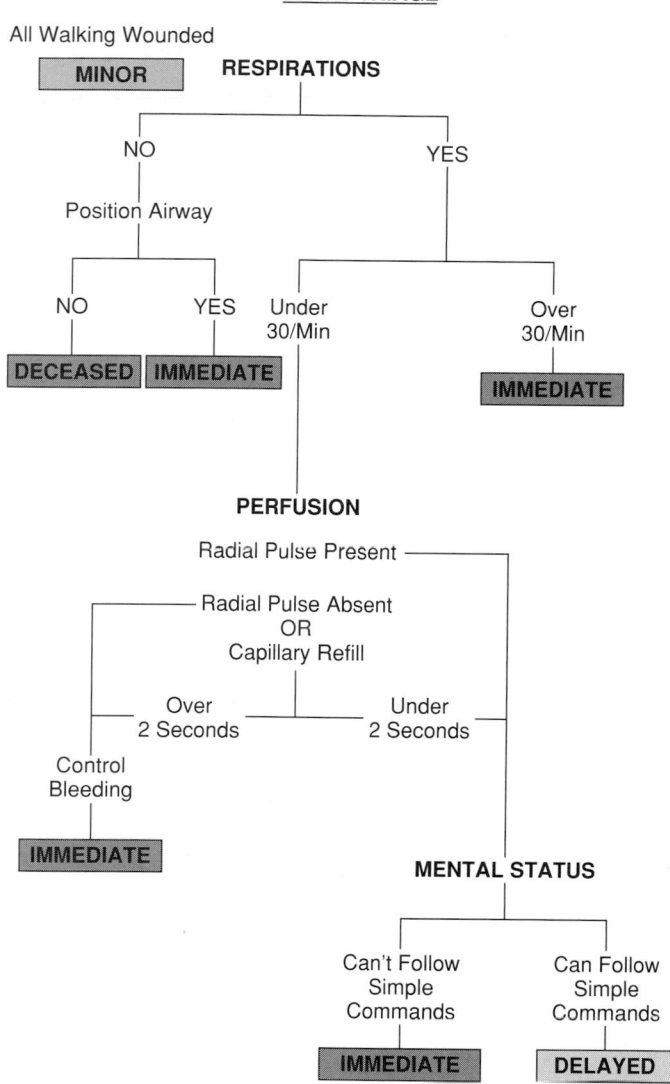

START TRIAGE

All Walking Wounded
MINOR **RESPIRATIONS**

NO · YES

Position Airway

NO · YES · Under 30/Min · Over 30/Min

DECEASED **IMMEDIATE** **IMMEDIATE**

PERFUSION

Radial Pulse Present

Radial Pulse Absent
OR
Capillary Refill

Over 2 Seconds · Under 2 Seconds

Control Bleeding

IMMEDIATE

MENTAL STATUS

Can't Follow Simple Commands · Can Follow Simple Commands

IMMEDIATE **DELAYED**

Figure 360.1. START Triage Algorithm. (Reproduced courtesy of Hoag Presbyterian Memorial Presbyterian Hospital and the Newport Beach Fire Department.)

a timely response to an MCI. The plan should identify the resources, personnel, transport, equipment, and facilities that can be called on.

A clearly defined incident command structure should also be in place. In some states, the highest-ranking fire officer serves as overall "incident commander," with police, EMS, and other agencies functioning as subcommands under Incident Command Rules. All involved must use common nomenclature, practice, and communications protocols. There should be clear direction regarding what freedom of operation prehospital providers might have without resorting to frequent online medical direction. Freedom of operation can be accomplished by having the medical director or designee assume Medical Command at the scene or via radio.

Special planning is required for HAZMAT situations, terrorist activities, weapons of mass destruction, and mass gatherings. Finally, a debriefing plan is necessary to allow for psychological recovery of involved personnel and for the planning to manage future MCIs.

Mass gathering medicine, defined as organized emergency care for mass gathering events, has evolved and become more sophisticated in the last 30 years. The concentration of many

people in a small geographic space can pose significant challenges to proper prehospital management of patients. Recognition of a medical emergency may be difficult and access to the patient may be hindered, delaying care. A mass casualty incident might quickly develop and on-site resources can quickly be overwhelmed. Agreement with the event organizer about what medical resources are required to provide adequate emergency services may be difficult Demands for medical care are often not defined by crowd size alone. Exposure to adverse weather conditions, spectator use of alcohol, inadequate intake of water, consumption of contaminated food, and violent spectator behavior can all increase the likelihood of injury and requirement for medical attention. Rock concerts (0.96–17 per 1,000) have, for example, had a higher incidence or injury than major sporting events (0.3–1.6 per 1,000) (46). The threat of terrorism has also influenced the development of mass gathering medicine. On a national level, an event may be deemed a National Security Special Event because it is high-profile and identified as a possible target of terrorism. In addition to enhanced security measures coordinated by the U.S. Secret Service, medical assets, in the form of Disaster Medical Assistance Teams may be deployed to assist local responders in the event of a mass casualty incident. The Olympics, the Super Bowl, and the World Economic Forum are examples of such events. The National Association of EMS Physicians has developed a position paper describing 15 components of mass gathering medicine planning and offers a planning guide, "Mass Gathering Medical Care: The Medical Director's Checklist" (16).

FINANCING EMERGENCY MEDICAL SERVICES SYSTEMS

The expense of an EMS system is a function of personnel, administration, maintenance, training, equipment, and facilities. Other variables include the level of service provided; response-time requirements; how the cost will be apportioned among patient revenues, tax revenues, and other subsidies; the insurance coverage of the population served; and the cost of medical oversight (32).

Funding of EMS systems varies greatly from system to system but can be divided into four major categories: taxes, fee-for-service billing, subscription program revenues, and special service contracts (32). Local and state tax subsidies can entirely fund an EMS system, in which care is provided as a public service. Most often, this funding comes from general tax revenues and must compete with other public programs for scarce tax dollars.

In some states, the law allows citizens to approve a dedicated tax levy for specific purposes, and voters direct funding for EMS services. Because EMS has a very positive public image, EMS systems tend to enjoy a greater degree of financial support under such a system. In other systems, tax subsidies may simply offset costs that cannot be covered by revenues from EMS billing. Subsidies are often required in small communities that lack economies of scale yet operate a full-service EMS system and in urban and rural settings. It may flow through the budget of a government agency, in the case of third service or FD, or it may be a contractual agreement between a private ambulance provider and a local government. With private contracts, most cities and towns have enjoyed almost a decade of subsidy-free EMS services, as providers have received sufficient revenue from Medicare and Medicaid reimbursement. Changes in reimbursement from these sources have significantly reduced the ability of private ambulances to continue subsidy-free 911 contracts. Systems serving communities with a large number of uninsured indigent patients are particularly in need of funding sources to offset costs that cannot be covered by revenues.

In a service that generates its revenue from a fee-for-service plan, income is derived from emergency and nonemergency patient transports, interfacility transfers, and special-event coverage. To balance the budget, these systems must have adequate economies of scale, a population base that has the means to pay, efficient management, and effective billing. Among the billed entities are Medicare, Medicaid, private insurance companies, and individual patients.

Subscription programs are marketed to the populace by a vendor who essentially enrolls people as an "insurance policy" in case they need ambulance services. This type of system also provides service to unenrolled members but at a charge significantly greater than the enrollment fee. Some arrangements also allow the company to bill third-party payers. Special-events coverage, interfacility transport, air transport, and other contracts can provide added revenue.

EMERGENCY MEDICAL SERVICES FOR CHILDREN

Perhaps no group of patients inspires more angst among EMS providers (and emergency medicine personnel) than ill and injured children. Although they make up only a very small percentage of EMS patient interactions, they are among the most difficult to manage. Children under the age of 18 make up approximately 9% of all EMS calls (42). Half of these calls are for a traumatic condition, with falls and vehicular trauma being the leading causes of injury. Respiratory difficulty, seizures, ingestions, drowning and near-drowning, fever, and altered mental status are common chief complaints. Sick children generate tremendous feelings in the medical professionals who treat them. Being able to simultaneously deal with the needs of the critically ill or injured child and the provider's own emotions (especially if they have children of their own) is a serious challenge to the provider's professionalism. Almost all EMS personnel can relate a particularly ill or injured child who affected them on a visceral level during their career. Finally, children are different from adults. Their anatomy, physiology, and responses to interventions differ from those that can be expected in adults. Thus, when dealing with sick children, EMS providers are treating a group they rarely see, who will affect them emotionally and are different from the vast majority of patients they encounter on a daily basis.

Emergency Medical Services for Children (EMSC) is a federal, state, and local effort to ensure that all children have the same access to high quality EMS care, as do adults. Starting in the 1980s, with federal legislation providing for grant programs based in the U.S. Department of Health and Human Services, EMSC has funded databases, provided grants to the states to study and address the issues experienced by ill or injured children and convened expert panels to enhance the care delivered to children in the out of hospital setting. The EMSC Five Year Plan, 2001–2005 is designed to "serve as a national public blueprint to assist those charged with ensuring healthy futures of our nation's children-futures whereby preventable childhood injuries are diminished and state-of-the-art pediatric emergency medical care is rendered in the face of critical illness or injury"(42).

A key portion of the EMSC initiative is improved education of EMS providers on the special needs and requirements of ill and injured children. Traditionally, EMS providers had little to no experience or training in treating children. EMTs and paramedics would typically receive 1% to 2% of their total training time on the unique aspects of treating pediatric patients. This has been changing. Paramedic training now includes the Pediatric

Advanced Life Support (PALS) course and the new Pediatric Education for Prehospital Providers (PEPP) course. Additionally, many state EMS protocols have specific pediatric protocols, written by emergency physicians and pediatric emergency medicine specialists to guide prehospital providers in treating children. Innovative programs, such as having paramedics spend time in pediatricians' offices, are increasing the comfort levels of both the prehospital providers and the pediatric community. Physicians who provide both online and off-line medical direction are assisting in these developments and are now active participants in furthering the care of pediatric patients.

Special Challenges in Treating Pediatric Patients

Recent literature has challenged the "basic" tenets of treating the injured or ill child. One study questions the benefits of prehospital intubation over noninvasive airway management (15). No difference was demonstrated in the outcome of children managed with an endotracheal tube versus conventional bag-valve-mask ventilation. The study, however, was criticized for having an extremely low rate of success for paramedic field intubations in children and frequent complications of airway management, such as unrecognized esophageal intubations. Medical directors evaluating this study may conclude the "standard of care" is to noninvasively manage pediatric airways. Conversely, proactive EMS medical directors may opt for additional training and oversight of their system's pediatric intubation program. Another study evaluated prehospital intravenous access and found that paramedics performed these procedures rarely, if ever, on pediatric patients (1). Such infrequently used skills are unlikely to be performed as well as procedures performed frequently. The study demonstrated that EMS educational initiatives need to address the maintenance of pediatric skills in prehospital providers.

Prehospital personnel are faced with a unique set of demands and must use a different set of knowledge and skills when dealing with pediatric patients. Children have a relatively larger occiput than adults; this requires that their torsos be elevated to the level of their occiput to achieve an anatomically neutral position during spinal immobilization (23). Smaller children are abdominal breathers and manifest respiratory distress with greater accessory muscle use. Additionally, they can decompensate very rapidly, something an EMT or paramedic with little pediatric experience may fail to anticipate.

EMERGENCY MEDICAL SERVICES AND TRAUMA

The "modern era" of emergency medical services in this country was ushered in as a response to traumatic injury and death on America's highways. Trauma was the catalyst for the drafting of the white paper ("Accidental Death and Disability: The Neglected Disease of Modern Society"), which prompted improvement of essential prehospital infrastructure, training of personnel, and establishment of practice guidelines. In the 40 years since the drafting of the white paper, three basic tenets of trauma patient management in the prehospital setting have clearly evolved. They include, (a) rapid response to the patient, (b) effective management of ventilation, oxygenation, perfusion, and immobilization, and (c) rapid transport to the most appropriate facility.

Rapid response to the patient is determined by multiple factors including recognition of the event, access to the 911 system, the efficiency of the communications center, and the proximity of units available to respond to the scene.

Effective management of ventilation, oxygenation, and perfusion is determined by the quality of the education provided for the responding EMS personnel and the quality of medical oversight enjoyed by the service. Quality adjuncts to the core curriculum of training exist in programs such as Prehospital Trauma Life Support (PHTLS) and Basic Trauma Life Support (BTLS). These programs champion principles of prehospital trauma care, such as scene safety, rapid primary survey, airway control, adequate oxygen delivery and ventilation, control of hemorrhage, management of shock, immobilization, and transport.

Rapid transport of the patient to an appropriate facility is determined by EMS education and medical oversight, but can also be facilitated by regional trauma systems. EMS education and oversight are critical for limiting the scene time, focusing on those interventions which are thought to be life saving in the first few minutes of the EMS response and not wasting precious time on interventions, which could be performed en route or in the hospital. The goal is to preserve as much as possible, the "golden hour" after the injury until arrival at the appropriate medical treatment facility. Regional trauma systems facilitate this tenet of prehospital care by identifying the appropriate trauma centers in a region and establishing guidelines for patient transport to these facilities. The American College of Surgeons, Committee on Trauma publishes guidelines for patient triage to trauma centers (Fig. 360.2) (7). For rural communities, guidelines are also published for the interfacility transfer of trauma patients to appropriate trauma hospitals (8). Air medical transport systems also play a role in regional trauma systems and assist in assuring the rapid transport of injured patients to appropriate medical facilities. Guidelines for the use of air transport are promulgated by the National Association of EMS Physicians and the Air Medical Physicians Association (40).

NHTSA and many other stakeholders in the management of trauma patients have drafted the Trauma System Agenda for the Future (41). Prehospital care is identified as a fundamental component of the trauma care system, along with injury prevention, acute care hospitals, and posthospital care. Challenges to quality prehospital care of trauma patients include isolation of EMS from the injury prevention and acute care hospital components of care, inadequacies of the national 911 system, inequities in distribution of EMS resources, prolonged transport times from rural communities, over and under-triage of patients to trauma centers, and emergency department overcrowding and diversion. Visions for the future include (a) better integration of EMS into injury prevention initiatives and improved dialogue with treatment facilities, (b) standardized protocols and triage, (c) strategic placement of transport vehicles to improve access in rural, underserved communities, and (d) improved communications, including automated collision notification, universal 911 coverage, and enhanced communication with prehospital providers facilitating more accurate triage and delivery of care.

There is a need for prospective randomized controlled clinical trials to resolve the many controversies regarding medical interventions in the prehospital care of the trauma patient. Many available studies attempting to determine the relative value of onscene advanced life support (ALS) are limited by retrospective data collection, small numbers of subjects, lack of comparable control groups, and other challenges (34).

Airway management (oxygenation and ventilation) is a basic tenet of trauma management, yet the means of controlling the airway is debated. In patients with traumatic brain injury (TBI), hypoxemia is associated with an 85% increase in mortality (6). Prehospital endotracheal intubation has been shown to potentially improve outcome in certain trauma patients, especially those suffering from TBI (38,45). A recent study however showed that paramedic rapid sequence intubation protocols, which have been shown to increase the intubation success rate, were associated with an increase in mortality in head-injured patients (9). The question is whether the intubation procedure itself contributes to mortality, or is it some other factor such as transient hypoxia, hypotension, or hyperventilation in the course of patient management. Further research is required to clarify even this most basic tenet of prehospital trauma management.

The issue of prehospital volume resuscitation has also been controversial (21). Debates continue on the value of time spent obtaining i.v. access and outcomes associated with prehospital volume replacement. The management of patients with penetrating torso injuries or other uncontrolled hemorrhage has been influenced by a study that showed that delay of aggressive fluid resuscitation until operative intervention improves outcome (2). Conversely, aggressive volume resuscitation has been recommended for hypotensive patients with TBI. Evidence suggests that patients with hypotension after severe TBI have twice the mortality rate of normotensive patients (43).

The pneumatic antishock garment (PASG) was once universally accepted and widely employed by EMS services as a therapeutic intervention intended to improve outcomes from hypovolemic shock despite the lack of prospective studies demonstrating improved patient survival. A trend toward increased mortality was noted in patients with penetrating chest trauma (24). There was no significant benefit to patients with penetrating abdominal injuries (3). Further study showed that the PASG offered no advantage to blunt trauma patients either (5). The PASG is currently being used to stabilize unstable pelvic fractures and for profound hypotension in systems with prolonged transport times, although its effectiveness has not been established for these indications either.

RESEARCH AND INITIATIVES FOR THE FUTURE

Proper prehospital management requires research, not only to identify which medical interventions have utility, but also to identify those that can cause harm. Rising costs of health care, demands for cost analysis and demonstrated utility of services, and the changing structure of health care delivery all influence EMS system development (28,29). EMS will undoubtedly continue to exist, as access to emergency services has come to be expected by our society. The permissive environment of EMS development and implementation of prehospital interventions without supporting data is coming to a close.

Historically, prehospital cardiac resuscitation research drove much of the training and preparedness of EMS delivery systems. It demonstrates well the success and failure of prehospital research. To its credit, study of CA outcomes required and yielded the development of a standard for uniform reporting of prehospital CA data: the Utstein Style. It demonstrated the effectiveness of early defibrillation in witnessed CA. It fostered the promulgation of CPR and early defibrillation programs as effective means of improving CA outcome. Concurrently, however, there was implementation of many interventions, such as intubation and administration of i.v. medications with scant data describing improved patient outcome. CA represents only 1% of most EMS systems' call volume. Many other interventions have been accepted into prehospital practice with little data to support their use.

Of the 5,842 scientific studies on EMS in MEDLINE between 1985 and 1997, only 54 were randomized controlled trials, only one examined a major outcome, such as survival, and only one other compared the studied intervention with a placebo (4). There is little doubt that the value of EMS systems and the services they provide will come into question in a health care system

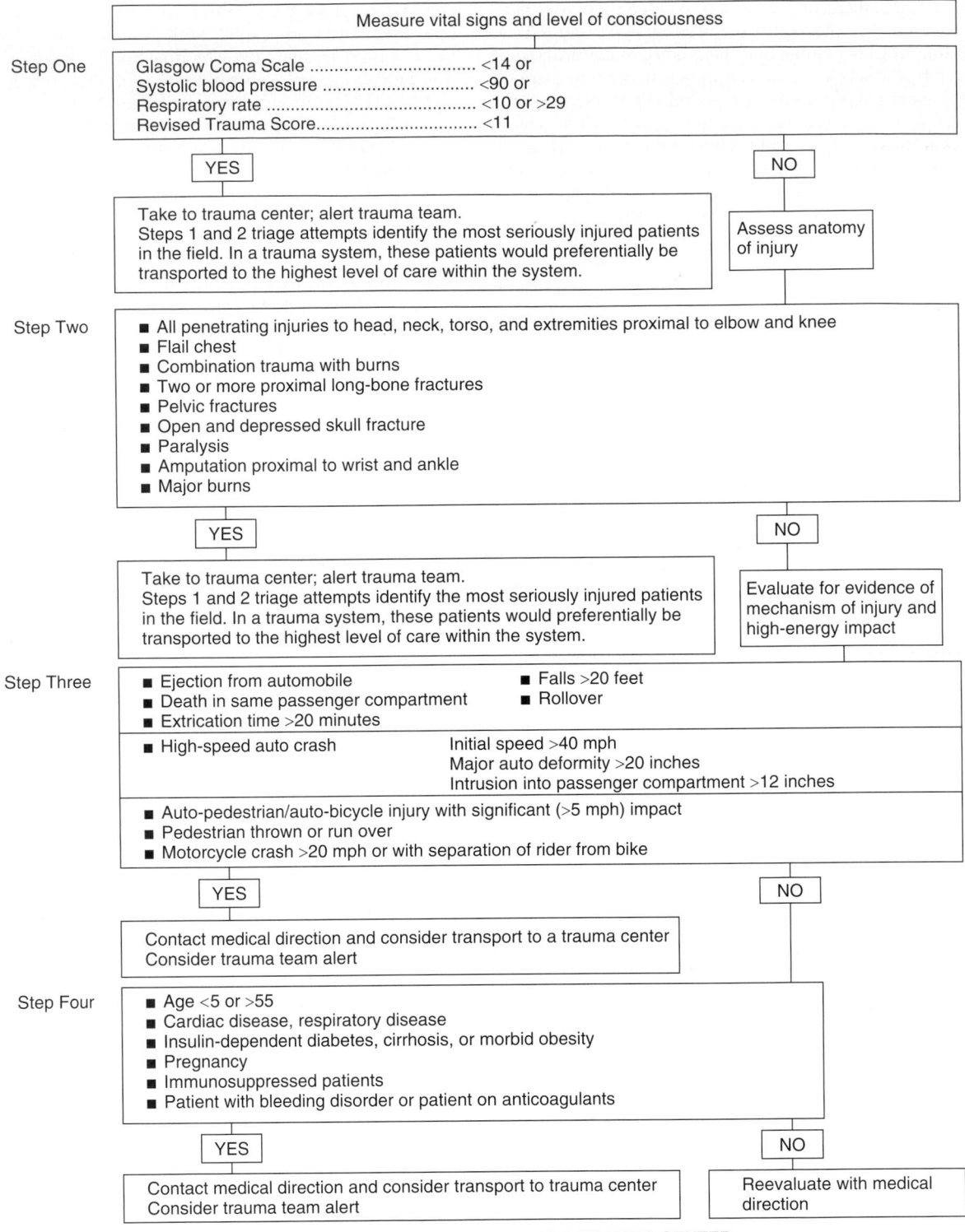

Figure 360.2. Field triage decision scheme. (From the American College of Surgeons Committee on Trauma: resources for optimal care of the injured patient, 1999. Chicago: American College of Surgeons, 1998, with permission.)

under significant financial pressure. Emerging systems may still have a window of opportunity to study these interventions and may, in fact, be obligated to demonstrate improved patient outcome to justify the cost of implementing advanced prehospital services in their areas.

The Ontario Prehospital Advanced Life Support (OPALS) Study is a large prehospital trial attempting to evaluate the efficacy of many of these interventions. The study involves more

than 25,000 CA patients with the intention of evaluating the incremental benefit of rapid defibrillation and prehospital ALS measures for CA survival (39). Phase I of this trial reported the baseline survival status after introduction of an automatic external defibrillation (AED) program in an area in which no AED or ALS services were present (36). Improved survival from CA was associated with younger age and a witnessed event. The authors identified three other areas that are amenable to EMS system optimization: (a) survival may be improved by minimizing EMS response intervals; (b) survival is improved three times if CPR is initiated by a bystander; and (c) survival doubled if initiated by fire or police first responders. Phase II of the trial verified that procedures, which reduced the time to defibrillation significantly improved the survival to hospital discharge rate. An improvement from 72% to 93% for calls responded to within 8 minutes or less by the AED crew resulted in a 33% relative increase in the survival rate (37). Phase III of this study will evaluate ALS intervention to determine the efficacy of endotracheal intubation, intravenous therapy and administration of i.v. drugs.

NHTSA and its partners address the science of prehospital care in its National EMS Research Agenda (27). It identifies five major impediments to the performance of high quality research: (a) A paucity of highly skilled researchers, (b) inadequate funding, (c) failure of EMS professionals to acknowledge the importance of EMS research and its transition into practice, (d) lack of data integration that promotes study of patient outcomes, and (e) difficulty in obtaining informed consent in the prehospital environment. The Agenda offers a strategy to overcome these obstacles.

EMS faces significant challenges. A recent assessment of state systems found a lack of (a) comprehensive EMS legislation and statewide EMS plans, (b) enhanced communication systems, (c) consistent quality-assurance programs for training courses and instructors, (d) enabling legislation for trauma system development, (e) consistent and adequate funding sources, (f) priority for public information and education programs, and (g) effective data collection and evaluation systems (30,33). The EMS Agenda for the Future acknowledges the challenges of the current EMS system and offers a roadmap with recommendations for improvement of 14 EMS attributes: (a) integration of prehospital care with public health, injury prevention and acute care, (b) EMS research, (c) legislation and regulation which will fund essential Federal and state initiatives, (d) system finance to insure proper EMS infrastructure development, (e) human resources to provide a viable career path for prehospital care providers, (f) medical direction with appropriate credentials and sufficient resources, (g) education systems for the development of quality prehospital providers, (h) public education to better inform the community on EMS utilization, (i) injury prevention, (j) public access, (k) EMS communications, (l) prehospital clinical care, (m) information systems, and (n) evaluation of service regarding medical outcomes and cost effectiveness (10,11). Through its unique position in the community as a link to health care access, the "scope of service" of EMS systems may expand to encompass injury prevention and preventive medicine initiatives, complementing and enhancing roles currently served separately and independently by other agencies.

COMMON PITFALLS

✔ Introducing prehospital medical interventions without adequate investigation regarding improvement in patient outcome

✔ Failure to insist on engaged medical direction in the delivery of prehospital medical care

✔ Failure to have a well-understood, rehearsed, and commonly recognized plan for responding to an MCI

✔ Failure to provide an effective plan for communication during an MCI

✔ Failure to adequately plan for HAZMAT situations, terrorist activities, and mass gatherings

✔ Failure to educate EMS providers on the special needs and management of ill and injured children

Acknowledgments

We thank the previous authors of the EMS for Children chapter: Lou E. Romig and Deborah Mulligan-Smith, and also the previous author of the Out-of-Hospital Care and Transport of the Trauma Patient chapter: Juan A. March.

References

1. Babl FE, Vinci RJ, Bauchner H, et al. Pediatric pre-hospital advanced life support in an urban setting. *Pediatr Emerg Care* 2001;17(1):5–9.
2. Bickell W, Wall M, Pepe P, et al. Immediate versus delayed fluid resuscitation for hypotensive patients with penetrating torso injuries. *N Engl J Med* 1994;331(17):1105–1109.
3. Bickell WH, Pepe PE, Bailey ML, et al. Randomized trial of pneumatic antishock garments in the prehospital management of penetrating abdominal injuries. *Ann Emerg Med* 1987;16:653–658.
4. Callaham M. Quantifying the scanty science of prehospital emergency care. *Ann Emerg Med* 1997;30:785–790.
5. Chang FC, Harrison PB, Beech RR, et al. PASG: does it help in the management of traumatic shock? *J Trauma* 1995;39:453–456.
6. Chestnut RM, Marshall LF, Klauber MR, et al. The role of secondary brain injury in determining outcome from severe head injury. *J Trauma* 1993;34:216–222.
7. Committee on Trauma. Resources for optimal care of the injured patient. Chicago, IL: American College of Surgeons, 1998, 1999.
8. Committee on Trauma. Interfacility transfer of injured patients: guidelines for rural communities. Chicago, IL: American College of Surgeons, 2002.
9. Davis DP, Hoyt DB, Ochs M, et al. The effect of paramedic rapid sequence intubation on outcome in patients with severe traumatic brain injury. *J Trauma* 2003;53:444–453.
10. Delbridge TD, Bailey B, Chew JL, et al. EMS agenda for the future: where we are . . . where we want to be. *Ann Emerg Med* 1998;31:251–263.
11. *Emergency medical services agenda for the future.* Washington, DC: NHTSA and the Health Resources and Services Administration, 1996.
12. *Emergency medical services: nHTSA leading the way.* Washington, DC: National Highway Traffic Safety Administration, 1995.
13. *EMS education agenda for the future: a systems approach.* Washington, DC: NHTSA and the Health Resources and Services Administration, 2000.
14. Garner A, Lee A, Harrison K. Comparative analysis of multiple-casualty incident triage algorithms. *Ann Emerg Med* 2001;38:541–548.
15. Gausche M, Lewis RJ, Stratton SJ, et al. Effect of out-of-hospital pediatric intubation on survival and neurological outcome: a controlled clinical trial. *JAMA* YR;283(6)783–90.
16. Jaslow D, Yancey A, Milsten A. National Association of EMS Physicians Standards and Clinical Practice Committee Web site. Mass gathering medical care. Available at http://www.naemsp.org/Position%20Papers/massgathering.pdf. Accessed December 27,2004.
17. Kahn CA, Pirrallo RG, Kuhn EM. Characteristics of fatal ambulance crashes in the United States: an 11 year retrospective analysis. *Prehosp Emerg Care* 2001;5:261–269.
18. Kennedy K, Aghababian R, Gans L, et al. Triage: techniques and applications in decision making. *Ann Emerg Med* 1996;28(2):136–144.
19. Klein KR, et al. Effects of on-line medical control in the prehospital treatment of atraumatic illness. *Prehosp Emerg Care* 1997;1:80–84.
20. Krohmer JR, Swor RA, Benson N, et al. Prototype core content for a fellowship in emergency medical services. *Ann Emerg Med* 1994;23:109–114.
21. Liberman M, Mulder D, Sampalis J. Advanced or basic life support for trauma: meta-analysis and critical review of the literature. *J Trauma* 2000;49:584–599.
22. Lilja GP, Madsen MA, Overton J. Multiple casualty incidents. In: Kuehl AE, ed. *Prehospital systems and medical oversight: National Association of EMS physicians,* 2nd ed. St. Louis: Mosby, 1994.
23. Markenson D, Foltin G, Tunik M, et al. The Kendrick extrication device used for pediatric spinal immobilization. *Prehosp Emerg Care* 1999;3(1):66–69.
24. Mattox KL, Bickell WH, Pepe PE, et al. Prospective MAST study in 911 patients. *J Trauma* 1989;29:1104–1112.
25. Mustalish AC, Post C. History. In: Kuehl AE, ed. *Prehospital systems and medical oversight: National Association of EMS physicians,* 2nd ed. St. Louis: Mosby, 1994.
26. National Research Council. *Accidental death and disability: the neglected disease of modern society.* Washington DC: National Academy of Sciences, 1966.
27. *National EMS research agenda.* Washington, DC: NHTSA and the Maternal and Child Health Bureau, 2004.
28. Neely KW, Drake MER, Moorhead JC, et al. Multiple options and unique pathways: a new direction for EMS? *Ann Emerg Med* 1997;30:797–799.
29. O'Connor RE, Cone DC, DeLorenzo RA. EMS systems: foundations for the future. *Acad Emerg Med* 1999;6:46–53.
30. Page J. Historical perspective in EMS systems. In: Roush WR, ed. *Principles of EMS systems,* 2nd ed. Dallas: American College of Emergency Physicians, 1994.
31. Rice MM, Brown JF. Military systems. In: Kuehl AE, ed. *Prehospital systems and medical oversight: National Association of EMS Physicians,* 2nd ed. St. Louis: Mosby, 1994.
32. Smith JE. Financial considerations in emergency medical services systems. *Emerg Med Clin North Am* 1990;8:155–161.

33. Snyder JA, Baren JM, Ryan SD, et al. Emergency medical service system development: results of the statewide emergency medical service technical assessment program. *Ann Emerg Med* 1995;25:768–775.
34. Spaite DW, Criss EA, Valenzuela TD, et al. Prehospital Advanced Life Support for Major Trauma: critical Need for Clinical Trials. *Ann Emerg Med* 1998;32:480–489.
35. Spaite DW, et al. Emergency medical service systems research: problems of the past, challenges of the future. *Ann Emerg Med* 1995;26:146–152.
36. Stiell IG, Wells GA, DeMaio VJ, et al. Modifiable factors associated with improved cardiac arrest survival in a multicenter basic life support/defibrillation system: OPALS study phase I results. *Ann Emerg Med* 1999;33:44–50.
37. Stiell IG, Wells GA, Field BJ, et al. Improved out-of-hospital cardiac arrest survival through the inexpensive optimization of an existing defibrillation program: OPALS study phase II. *JAMA* 1999;281:1175–1181.
38. Stiell IG, Wells GA, Spaite DW. The Ontario Prehospital Advanced Life Support (OPALS) Study Part II: rational and methodology for trauma and respiratory distress patients. *Ann Emerg Med* 1999;34:256–262.
39. Stiell IG, Wells GA, Spaite, DW. The Ontario Prehospital Advanced Life Support (OPALS) Study: rationale and methodology for cardiac arrest patients. *Ann Emerg Med* 1998;32:180–190.
40. Thomson D, Thomas S. Position paper: guidelines for air medical dispatch. *Prehosp Emerg Care* 2003;7(2):265–271.
41. *Trauma system agenda for the future.* Washington, DC: NHTSA, 2003.
42. Health Resources and Services Administration, Maternal and Child Health Bureau. Five Year plan: Emergency Medical Services for Children 2001–2005. Washington, DC: US Dept of Health and Human Services, 2000.
43. National Institutes of Health. Rehabilitation of persons with traumatic brain injury: NIH Consensus Statement 1998. National Institutes of Health Web site. Available at http://consensus.nih.gov/cons/109/109_intro.htm. Accessed December 27, 2004.
44. Verdile VP, et al. Model curriculum in emergency medical services for emergency medicine residency programs. *Acad Emerg Med* 1996;3:716–722.
45. Winchell RJ, Hoyt DB. Endotracheal intubation in the field improves survival in patients with severe head injury. *Arch Surg* 1997;132:592–597.
46. Yancey AH, Jaslow D. Mass gathering medical care. In: Kuehl AE, ed. *Prehospital systems and medical oversight: National Association of EMS Physicians*, 3rd ed. Dubuque, Iowa: Kendall/Hunt Publishing Company, 2002.

CHAPTER 361
Air Medical Services

Theodore R. Delbridge

Air medical services provide transportation and deliver sophisticated medical care by utilizing rotor or fixed-wing aircraft. They are part of a complex system. Optimally, air medical services are integrated with other regional emergency medical services and the emergency health care system. Emergency physicians should be aware of local air medical service resources, potential advantages and disadvantages of their utilization, flight physiology that may affect patients, and limitations of caring for patients in an aircraft.

HISTORICAL PERSPECTIVE

The 1966 National Academy of Sciences, National Research Council publication, "Accidental Death and Disability: The Neglected Disease of Modern Society" made 29 recommendations for improving the American health care system's capacity to respond to trauma victims. The authors suggested that pilot programs be developed to evaluate automotive and helicopter ambulance services in sparsely populated areas and in regions that lacked hospital facilities adequate for seriously injured persons (28). Currently, there are more than 200 air medical services deploying helicopters throughout the United States. Dozens of other systems utilize fixed-wing aircraft for longer distance transports. Approximately 30% of helicopter medical missions involve response directly to an injury scene (31). The remainder of air medical cases involve the spectrum of seriously ill and injured patients requiring transfer from one medical facility to another.

The genesis of air medical transport can be linked to military conflict. During the Korean Conflict, mortality among wounded U.S. soldiers was less than during World War II. At least part of that reduction was attributed to faster access to surgical care as a result of helicopter use. By the Vietnam War, both helicopters and medical care had become more sophisticated. Wounded soldiers evacuated from the field were now transferred inside a helicopter, and emergency medical care commenced or was continued during transport. Air evacuation of wounded soldiers contributed to lowering the mortality rate to less than 1 per 100 casualties. The average time to reach definitive surgical care decreased from 6 to 12 hours during World War II, to 2 to 4 hours during the Korean Conflict, to 35 minutes during the Vietnam War (21,25,29).

During 1966 and 1967 army helicopters evacuated 40 civilian patients in Alabama and Texas. Between 1967 and 1970 government-funded projects verified the utility of helicopters for civilian air medical missions. They confirmed that helicopters could evacuate rural patients, make safe landings in metropolitan areas, and save valuable time (20). The Military Assistance to Safety and Traffic (MAST) program, initiated in 1970, resulted in average time savings of 53 minutes, when compared to ground ambulances (20).

In 1970 the Maryland State Police also established its med evac program as part of a statewide emergency medical services system (16). Setting up helicopter bases throughout the state resulted in shorter response times to scenes and referring hospitals. The first civilian hospital-based medical helicopter program began operation at St. Anthony Hospital Systems in Denver, Colorado in October 1972.

Many of the same issues that affected earlier air medical programs are still germane. These include maintenance of complex and expensive communications systems. Such systems must provide reliable means of receiving requests for service from various sorts of callers, dispatching helicopters, following the progress of ongoing flights, transmitting and receiving clinical information, and facilitating online medical direction. To be effective, communications must be unhindered across large areas.

Preparation and monitoring of the air medical crew is an obvious concern. As the sophistication of medical care has increased, so has the complexity of patients being transported. Thus, air medical crews must be more familiar than ever with an always expanding potential of therapies and interventions that they might be called on to initiate or continue as part of moving a patient safely to definitive care. Monitoring performance is a clear priority and often a challenge as a result of the relative isolation in which care is delivered. Finally, air medical services have and will continue to struggled with fiscal reality. The balance between the desire to provide service and the associated costs and ability to generate revenue can be delicate. Part of the struggle entails concerns for appropriate utilization.

ADVANTAGES OF AIR MEDICAL SERVICES

Air medical services offer two principal advantages over ground ambulances: speed and the ability to overcome geography. When used appropriately, these advantages can result in significant savings of time to reach a trauma center or other tertiary care facility. In the case of trauma patients, at least one study has suggested that the sooner a patient arrives at the trauma center, the lower the morbidity and mortality (15). For critically ill patients being moved between hospitals, the speed of the helicopter or a fixed-wing aircraft may result in less time outside the more controlled environment of an emergency department or intensive care unit (ICU).

To fully benefit from the potential time savings of air medical transport, it is necessary to consider all of the events that consume time. The aircraft might provide the fastest means to get a patient to his or her destination hospital, but a number of things must occur before the patient is actually on the way. Once dispatched, helicopter liftoff may take several minutes, depending on the organization. Response time to the scene must be considered, and landing might take an additional 3 to 5 minutes. Generally, the more familiar the helicopter crew is with the landing zone and the better prepared it is, the shorter landing time will be. Established helipads provide for the fastest approaches and landings. In many cases, as a result of the difficulties in caring for patients in an aircraft, additional patient preparation must occur prior to initiating transport.

When considering potential time savings of air medical transport, one must weigh the total transit time of the helicopter or fixed-wing aircraft from time of request to arrival at the receiving facility. It is this time that should be compared to ground ambulance transportation (11,37). In general, to optimize time saving effects of air medical services, it should be requested as soon as there is sufficient information to indicate their need.

Medical helicopters often are based at or near the hospital to which patients will be transported. In those cases, the response time to an injury scene or to a referring hospital is the same as the transport time. However, when air medical resources are dispersed, so that helicopter bases are remote from the receiving hospital, response times to the referring scene or hospital may be shorter and the time savings of air medical service utilization may be enhanced (16). Medical helicopters typically offer little advantage in urban areas or when transport distances are short. When the transport distance is longer than 25 miles, and the medical helicopter is readily available, time savings are likely (30,37). Time savings may result for shorter transport distances if the helicopter is dispatched before the patient is ready to go, such as in cases of prolonged extrication at crash sites or when stabilizing measures are ongoing in an emergency department. In these circumstances, the response time of the helicopter becomes negligible (30).

An additional potential benefit of air medical services is the availability of higher levels of care during transport. Air medical service crew configurations typically consist of two clinicians including paramedics, nurses, respiratory therapists, and/or a physician. The crew configuration is the result of local preference and, in some cases, state regulations. In some systems, the crew may be modified for special clinical circumstances. The result is often an air medical crew that is able to manage ongoing or potential problems better than available ground ambulance resources. For this reason, time savings is not always the apparent indication for air medical service utilization.

DISADVANTAGES OF AIR MEDICAL SERVICES

The three principal disadvantages associated with air medical services are logistic considerations, safety, and cost. The disadvantages are appropriate for consideration each time an air medical mission is contemplated.

Logistically, getting a helicopter or fixed-wing aircraft to a scene or referring hospital can be complex. After realizing the need for an air medical service, the first step is notifying a communications center. Calls may arrive at the center from many sources including hospitals, medical control facilities, emergency medical services agencies, law enforcement agencies, fire departments, and other communications centers. The goal then becomes to determine the location, identify the closest available helicopter, and assess whether or not the mission can be completed.

The communications center must coordinate closely with the pilot, who should remain unaware of the clinical situation to avoid biasing decision making. The pilot must assess suitability of the weather and the aircraft for the proposed mission. The location must be translated into information that can be used for navigation, such as latitude and longitude that can be programmed into a global positioning system (GPS). Throughout the mission, the communications center should be continuously in communication with the helicopter to track its progress, convey vital patient information to the medical crew, facilitate updates to the air medical crew from ground based medical providers (and vice versa), and implement contingency plans when necessary. Contingency plans may be necessary in cases of mechanical failure, change in weather, or change in patient condition. While en route, the helicopter should be able to communicate with the ground team to receive updated patient-related information when appropriate and ensure adequate preparation for a safe landing zone.

Requesting a medical helicopter to transport a patient significantly increases the workload for on-scene emergency medical service and public safety workers, and for hospital personnel when the response is to a hospital. Resources at the scene or referring hospital must be sufficient to coordinate the helicopter's arrival without distracting medical personnel from delivering care.

Safety issues should always be at the forefront. Unfortunately, the safety records of U.S. air medical services have been concerning at times. Pilot errors and weather, often in concert, seem to be the greatest factors (8). Medical helicopter operations are inherently more dangerous than other routine helicopter operations. The accident rate is 1.7 times higher for air medical services than it is for helicopter taxi services (34). Although many safety motivated procedural improvements have been made over the past three decades, serious helicopter crashes still occur. A recent 5-year review of National Transportation Safety Board data revealed 47 U.S. medical helicopter crashes, resulting in 40 fatalities of crew members and patients (8). However, the relative safety of air medical services remains uncertain. The crashes that occurred represented hundreds of thousands of patient transport missions involving millions of miles and hours of flight. Some crashes occurred during maintenance procedures not involving actual missions. How this compares to ground ambulances, and their potential for crashes given similar distances traveled, remains unclear.

Nevertheless, each tragic event serves as a reminder that air medical service utilization is not without risk. Safety risks should be considered carefully and weighed against perceived benefits. Strict adherence to safety standards is mandatory for both personnel on the ground and those in the helicopter.

The cost associated with air medical services are considerable. Medical helicopter bases may require $1.5 to $2 million per year to maintain, depending on the helicopter type, personnel qualifications, and abilities to achieve economies of scale. It is predominantly these fixed costs that determine the expense of providing air medical services. The incremental costs for a specific mission (the additional costs for providing service to one more patient) are approximately $800 to $1,000 depending on the aircraft type and distance traveled. Most of that relates to fuel consumption and aircraft maintenance.

Although the cost of providing air medical services may be considerable, they are not necessarily unreasonable when compared to other alternatives. Air medical services, as a system, cost less than providing similar care for interfacility transport through a network of ground ambulances (10). This cost difference relates directly to helicopters' capacities to effectively serve larger geographic areas by virtue of speed and abilities to eliminate geographic barriers. The cost effectiveness of air medical services has previously been determined to be $1,400 to $9,677 per year of life saved (22). Such a cost is consistent with those for other societal health care priorities.

AVIATION ISSUES

Because air medical services are a tool for providing clinical care, it is helpful for physicians to understand some of the inherent aviation issues. The most relevant factors are the limitations of the aircraft and the limitations of the pilot. Weather is a consideration for both.

Medical helicopters are either single- or twin-engine turbine powered aircraft. Twin-engine outnumber single-engine aircraft for air medical use. They are generally felt to be safer by virtue of mechanical redundancy. However, it is not clear that the number of engines greatly affects the safety profiles of air medical services. Nonmedical helicopter crashes, even those with mechanical causes, rarely have to do with engine failure (8). Helicopters generally travel between 100 and 160 miles per hour, with useful loads of 1,500 to 3,000 pounds. The concept of useful load is important; it includes all the medical equipment and helicopter crew. The useful load can also be affected by weather conditions, the amount of fuel on board the helicopter, and the mean sea level altitude of the helipad from which the helicopter will be departing. All of this determines the weight of the patient who can be transported and the equipment, personnel, or family that may accompany him or her. Patients may be heavier if the helicopter crew is lighter, there is less equipment, there is less fuel on board, the weather is cooler and less humid, and the helipad or landing zone is closer to sealevel.

Medical helicopters may not operate in icy conditions; this can be catastrophic if these conditions are not avoided. Thus, operations in some forms of precipitation are not possible. Flight through clouds might not be possible depending on the air temperature.

Most air medical services operate under visual flight rules (VFR), owing to equipment on board the helicopter and pilot qualifications. Visual flight rules require visibility to be 1 mile during the daytime and 2 miles at nighttime, and a cloud ceiling (distance from the ground to the base of clouds) to be 500 feet or higher. Local conditions, including topography, may necessitate that these parameters be more restrictive.

Numerous air medical programs are capable of operating under instrument flight rules (IFR). As the term implies, the pilot flies the aircraft by reference to onboard instruments instead of outside visual cues. The limitation of IFR operations is the necessity to fly from one airport to another one in which there is a bona fide instrument approach developed to facilitate landing in marginal or poor weather conditions. Thus, patients must be first moved to, and then from, an airport to travel via helicopter. This is obviously time-consuming, eliminating some of the benefit of air medical service. Global positioning system technology enables development of instrument approaches to locations other than airports, including hospital helipads. Although these are not widespread, a few air medical services have developed GPS approaches to serve places they often are requested to respond to in suboptimal weather conditions.

The pilot is the lynch pin of air medical service operations, as he or she is ultimately responsible for the safety of the crew and aircraft. Potential for pilot fatigue should be monitored, as it may adversely affect performance. Pilots' decisions regarding aviation issues must be made in the absence of knowledge of clinical circumstances, which may be compelling and inappropriately bias the process. Pilots must maintain the authority and responsibility to make safe decisions, and should not attempt to complete a transport mission in unsafe conditions.

One of the factors thought to make air medical service operations more dangerous is the need to land helicopters at makeshift landing zones. Ground personnel usually have variable experience in setting up landing zones and conveying information about hazards to the helicopter pilot. Pilots may be unfamiliar with the area and surrounding hazards, and may be distracted by adjacent activity and lights. One solution is to develop predesignated landing zones that emergency medical service and public safety agencies preferentially use. The air medical service can then have preexisting knowledge about potential hazards, and the landing zones can be set up systematically when needed. Another advantage is pilots' familiarity, and established locations are easier to identify and navigate to.

In some regions, fixed-wing aircraft may be a valuable component of air medical service resources. They are usually twin-engine propeller or jet engine aircraft, capable of cruise flight between 200 and 400 miles per hour. Their useful loads are generally thousands of pounds, and their range is much longer than helicopters. Another advantage is their ability to fly in more adverse weather conditions than helicopters can. Fixed-wing aircraft fly from airport to airport, necessitating ground transport legs on each end of the patient flight. Thus, a fixed-wing aircraft is used to save time when the transport distance is usually 150 miles or longer. Fixed-wing aircraft often cruise between 14,000 and 30,000 plus feet above the ground. Their cabins are typically pressurized to the equivalent of 5,000 to 8,000 feet above mean sealevel.

MEDICAL ISSUES

Medical issues relate to the interplay between patients' clinical conditions and physiologic effects of flight and the capacity to initiate or continue care during air medical transport. When emergency care practitioners appreciate these issues, they are better able to select appropriate patients for air medical transport and prepare them for that event.

Flight physiology is a discipline unto its own. Its depth and breadth are beyond the scope of this chapter. However, two concepts are particularly germane to ill or injured patients. First, as altitude increases, atmospheric pressure decreases and gases expand. The result is that gas-filled spaces expand. For seriously ill or injured patients, critical spaces might include pneumothoraces and intestines. Additional air-filled spaces that the air medical crew must be cognizant of include patients' middle ears, endotracheal tube cuffs, air splints, i.v. fluid bags, pneumatic antishock garments, and others. Second, as atmospheric pressure decreases, the partial pressure of oxygen decreases. The proportion of oxygen in the air remains constant (approximately 21%). However, because the total atmospheric pressure is less at higher altitudes, so is the pressure of oxygen within the mixture of gases that comprise air. Because the solubility of a gas (i.e., oxygen) within a liquid (i.e., blood) is proportional to the partial pressure of the gas in contact with the liquid (i.e., within the lung alveoli), a patient's ability to remain well-oxygenated decreases at higher altitudes.

Most air medical transports via helicopter are conducted within 2,500 feet of the ground. Thus, the effects of flight physiology are limited. However, by merely ascending 2,000 feet above the ground, patients' oxygen requirements are increased by approximately 8% and air-filled spaces will increase in volume by approximately 8%. If a pneumothorax is known to be present, the referring physician should place a chest tube before transport. Such action greatly diminishes the potential for precipitous deterioration as a result of pneumothorax expansion from the primary injury in conjunction with altitude changes. Additionally, seriously ill and injured patients should receive supplemental oxygen during flight. It is important to understand that if there is difficulty in achieving adequate oxygenation on the ground, the problem will only worsen during air transport. There must always be the capacity to increase the supply of oxygen to patients during air transport, beyond what they were receiving on the ground.

When patients are transported in helicopters operating in IFR conditions or in a fixed-wing aircraft, even more attention must be paid to the physiologic effects of flight. Helicopters operating in IFR conditions are often 5,000 or more feet above the ground and, as noted, fixed-wing aircraft cabin pressures are usually equivalent to 5,000 to 8,000 feet above mean sealevel. Thus, the potential for air-filled spaces to expand and patients' oxygen requirements to increase are significantly greater than during low altitude helicopter operations. One specific group of patients for whom this is a concern is those with dysbarism related to scuba diving. Decreases in the atmospheric pressure to which they are exposed, whether via commercial air travel or air medical transport, can cause precipitous deterioration.

Other important factors include decreased temperature and humidity as altitude increases and effects of vibration. Air medical crews must be cognizant of exposure of the patient to ambient air. Ill patients who might lack intact thermoregulation may be susceptible to rapidly changing air temperature as altitude changes. Crews must also be aware of the need to monitor possible and insensible fluid loss, particularly among patients receiving nonhumidified oxygen. Finally, aircraft vibration and noise are thought to create a potential for autonomic instability in critically ill patients.

The capacity to monitor patients' conditions and initiate and continue care during air medical transport should be a constant concern. It is partly the difficulty in monitoring patients that prompts pretransport placement of thoracostomy tubes for patients with pneumothoraces. In helicopters and many fixed-wing aircraft, breath sounds can be difficult to hear, blood pressures can be difficult to auscultate, weak pulses can be difficult to palpate, and patients can be difficult to communicate with (24,27). Automated equipment, including cardiac monitors, pulse oximetry, noninvasive blood pressure monitors, and capnography, greatly facilitate patient monitoring, but none are entirely foolproof. Air medical crews must continuously assess the quality of data before interpreting and relying on it.

The ability to continue ongoing care is usually a function of its complexity and the qualifications of air medical crews. The most common emergency medicine-related examples relate to airway adjuncts and ventilation. It is necessary to be familiar with the types of airway adjuncts that an air medical crew is trained to use. For example, the crew might lack working knowledge of laryngeal mask airways (LMA) and would not be prepared to manage a patient with an LMA in the event it becomes dislodged. They might not be prepared to continue transtracheal jet ventilation. They might also be limited in their abilities to deliver specific modes of ventilation via mechanical ventilator or continuous positive airway pressure support to a spontaneously breathing patient. In such cases, air medical transport might be inappropriate, or modifications to ongoing care or support might be indicated.

The ability to initiate new care is obviously limited by the available equipment and supplies within the helicopter or fixed-wing aircraft. The close quarters of an aircraft, limited access to the patient, and sometimes cumbersome access to available supplies can make initiating new therapy more difficult in the air than on the ground. Initiating i.v. access and administering i.v. medications are not too difficult. However, providing new airway support, although possible in most cases, is a task best completed on the ground prior to air medical transport. Conditions in a helicopter for tracheal intubation are far from ideal. Adult patients are not easily repositioned, and their heads usually rest between one of the caregiver's legs. Thus, in cases in which a patient's airway stability is in question, the airway should be definitively secured before the patient is loaded into a helicopter, the procedure location of last resort.

Combative or uncooperative patients present a special dilemma. The etiology of their agitation can be multifactorial, but the ability to address it while airborne is quite limited. Additionally, in such a condition, these patients present a significant risk to themselves and the helicopter crew while airborne. Thus, agitation must be dealt with prior to air medical transport. Oversedation may be a concern as a result of difficulties in monitoring patients in a helicopter and barriers to addressing airway instability should it subsequently occur. For these reasons, many agitated patients are best dealt with by sedation, pharmacologic paralysis, and tracheal intubation.

A typical dilemma for an emergency care practitioner who is preparing a patient for air medical transport is how to determine the appropriate amount of preparation. Some clinical situations are best addressed prior to transport. However, not every eventuality can be predicted, nor is it feasible to spend an inordinate amount of time trying. Presumably, air medical transport has been chosen in most cases because of its speed, and there is some urgency in moving a patient from one location to another. It is reasonable to consider the likelihood of potentially serious complications of transport, and do what can be done quickly to attenuate that likelihood. Beyond that, excessive efforts to "stabilize" patients before transport, particularly trauma patients, may do more harm than good by delaying arrival at definitive care. There are times when additional stabilizing interventions are preferred prior to transport. For example, some neonatal or pediatric teams bring their expertise to the patient rather than moving the patient to their expertise. They may be able to provide additional care that improves the safety of transport without delaying the care the patient is being transferred to receive. As each case is a unique event, it must be considered in its own context. However, it is always prudent to think about the amount of patient preparation for transport that is necessary and appropriate.

ADMINISTRATIVE ISSUES

Air medical services administrative issues include a spectrum from mundane to complex. Organizations vary considerably. In the United States, air medical services may be provided by public safety agencies, military services in some cases, hospital-based programs, and independent nonprofit and profit-seeking organizations. Likewise, funding sources for these entities vary. Public safety agencies, for example, receive some or all of their support from taxes or licensing fees. Hospital-based programs attempt to recover costs through revenues from patients and their insurance carriers. However, the hospital may provide a substantial subsidy to support the program. Although the air medical program itself might not be profitable, the patients it brings to its affiliated hospitals may generate significant income for the hospital. Variation in funding sources results in variation in billing procedures and amounts and, at times, some confusion on the part of third-party payers who decide what is appropriate to compensate air medical services.

Selection of aircraft has multiple implications for air medical services. Helicopters routinely adapted for medical transport have varying characteristics; differences exist in terms of size and performance. These result in variation regarding the types of patients and their associated equipment that can be transported and the costs to operate them. The aircraft size affects its interior design. With space at a premium, it is vital to consider equipment and supply needs and their optimal organization to facilitate patient monitoring and treatment. Interior layout among various aircraft even affects abilities to perform CPR (39). Ideally, from a physician's perspective, every aircraft would have an abundance of equipment and supplies, with redundancy, to enable optimal reaction to every eventuality, and have enough interior room to maneuver about the patient. But then the aircraft would have to be so large with performance characteristics that would, for most services, make it prohibitively expensive to operate. Thus, the balance between aircraft performance, size, and cost to operate is important.

As the missions of many air medical services are diverse, so too may be medical direction. The Air Medical Physician Association has prepared a resource for physicians (1). Medical directors evolve from various disciplines, although emergency physicians make up the majority. Nevertheless, transport mission profiles that include neonatal patients, complex pediatric medical cases, cardiac surgery patients with invasive assist devices, and other complicated or special populations often necessitate the appropriate inclusion of multiple physician advisors in the medical direction process. They bring added expertise and support for the service, helping to ensure the delivery of optimal care. Similar to the medical direction of a local emergency medical services system, an air medical service medical director should have working relationships with regional emergency clinicians to ensure adequate quality and volume of communication to assess and improve efforts to provide meaningful service and care.

Paramedics, nurses, respiratory therapists, and physicians serving as medical crew members typically function using extensive protocols and standing orders. However, the communications system must function effectively so that field personnel can request and receive prompt and qualified online medical direction when indicated by clinical circumstances.

The optimal configuration of air medical crews is a point of some controversy. In most cases the medical team is comprised of a flight nurse, accompanied by another flight nurse, paramedic, or respiratory therapist. Part of their sophistication results from intense orientation and continuing education, and from their continual exposure to critically ill and injured patients. Several states allow for medications and procedures by flight nurses and paramedics that are not available to ground-based paramedics (18).

Several hospital-based air medical services have, at one point or another, included a flight physician as part of the crew (6,19,32). More than 10% still do, at least on a part-time basis. Earlier findings suggested that nurse-physician teams reduce mortality from trauma to better than what was predicted, and achieved outcomes that were better than nurse-nurse teams (6). However, these results have not been reproduced (13,14,23). As systems mature, it is possible that nurses and paramedics gain valuable experience to the point that adding a physician adds little significant value (36). Physicians' technical skills rarely augment the proficiency of nonphysician flight teams (32,38). Although physician judgment has been shown to make important contributions to treatments (32,38), it is possible that improved protocols and standing orders and communications systems that enable reliable online medical direction have negated some of that benefit.

Air medical services are called to some special circumstances in which added expertise is probably of some value. Among these are transports involving neonatal or special pediatric populations. Working knowledge and technical competence with the specific needs of such patients seems helpful in effecting safe transport to tertiary care centers. Neonatal and pediatric transport teams, supplementing or supplanting the routine air medical crew, often bring expertise in dealing with small patients, including i.v. access, appropriate medications and doses, and ventilatory support.

Assuring the quality of air medical services is a significant challenge with several facets. There are customer service dimensions involving interfaces between the air medical service and calls for help, emergency medical service and public safety personnel, and hospital personnel. There are aviation-related dimensions focused on aircraft maintenance, pilot proficiency, and safety initiatives. And there are patient care dimensions focused on processes of care and outcomes.

Improving air medical service quality is a community effort. Audits of certain types of cases and events may identify select issues. Reviewing medical crew documentation provides only a limited perspective. However, involving the assessments of many of the people who participated in a case, both before and after the transport, helps to complete an appreciation of the entire event and identify areas for improvement in multiple dimensions. For this reason, many air medical services provide follow-up about patients to referral sources. Additionally, they implement systems or streamline processes that facilitate feedback to the air medical service when either positive or negative events occur, and for receiving hospitals to provide outcomes information that may be used to help assess utilization appropriateness.

UTILIZATION REVIEW

An important aspect of quality improvement activity is utilization review. Again, this should be a community effort to improve appropriate utilization of air medical services. Those who call on air medical services should review cases to determine their appropriateness and provide guidance to their staffs. Air medical services should review their cases to provide guidance and feedback to referring agencies and hospitals.

Ideally, assessment of whether or not utilization of air medical services was warranted is based on some knowledge of the patients for whom it provided a difference. Unfortunately, this is not entirely clear, although intuitively it makes sense in some clinical conditions. The most significant evaluations have been performed regarding trauma patients. Even they suffer from limited sample sizes, selection biases, and confounding factors.

Nevertheless, previous investigations found reduced mortality among severe brain-injured patients when they were transported by a hospital-based helicopter as opposed to advanced life support ambulance (31% vs. 40%) (7). The difference was noted despite the fact that ambulance patients arrived at the trauma center an average of 33 minutes earlier. The reason for the difference is not clear. One factor was, at the time, ground paramedics could only control patients' airways with esophageal obturator airways, whereas physicians in the helicopter could perform endotracheal intubation. Additional medications were also available on the helicopter. The extent to which these affected the outcome is unclear.

Additional studies have noted similar results generalized to the entire trauma population. Among 150 trauma patients transported by helicopter and 150 by ground, mortality was 52% less than predicted in the air group, although it was higher than predicted in the ground group (4). The groups were not homogenous, however. The ground-transported group was urban, and the helicopter-transported group was rural. A physician in the helicopter meant that initial patient to physician contact was sooner for the helicopter-transported group even though their arrival at the trauma center was later.

Among 1,273 patients transported directly from the scene by seven different air medical services, mortality was 21% lower than expected (5). Patients who were more seriously injured, with predicted survival less than 75%, benefited the most. The sicker the patient is, the more opportunity there is to benefit from an intervention. Yet, the factors that reduce mortality remain unclear. Although air medical services seem to provide a survival advantage for many trauma patients, the greatest advantage seems to be for the most seriously injured and those who are transported directly from the scene to a trauma center.

Other studies have documented limited benefit when helicopter and ground-transported trauma patients were compared. When 15,938 helicopter-transported patients were compared with 6,473 ground-transported patients, there was no effect on estimated odds of survival (9). Another investigation yielded similar results after comparing 1,346 helicopter and 17,144 ambulance-transported trauma patients (17). There was a tendency toward improved survival among patients with higher injury scores, but most of the study population had relatively minor injuries.

One reasonable conclusion to draw from the available literature is that air medical transport may positively affect outcome among a subset of trauma patients, those who are injured more severely. Such patients are likely to have lower prehospital trauma scores and lower Glasgow Coma Scale scores. Thus, indicators of severe injury at the scene or community hospital emergency department may be reasonable indications for utilization of air medical services to transport a patient to a trauma center.

The Association of Air Medical Services and the National Association of EMS Physicians have published criteria for appropriate use of air medical services (2,3). For trauma patients, consideration might be given to evidence of injury by virtue of objective scoring systems, anatomic injury, or physiologic derangement; difficulty in accessing the patient by ground; serious mechanism of injury; and a significant increase in transport time. Many emergency medical services systems have adapted these or similar criteria to guide decisions of whether or not to send an air medical service to a scene.

Certain patients, by virtue of the extent of their injuries, are not appropriate for air medical transport. For example, patients who suffer blunt trauma cardiac arrest at the scene will not survive. Transport by helicopter will not change the outcome, but exposes several people to the risk of flying and working around an operating helicopter (26,40).

For nontrauma patients, there is an even greater paucity of information regarding appropriate utilization of air medical services. Locally adapted guidelines might include cardiac patients requiring transport to receive emergency invasive reperfusion therapy, stroke patients being transported to receive emergency reperfusion therapy, neurosurgical patients who are to undergo emergency evaluation for potential craniotomy, high-risk obstetric patients with imminent complications, and tenuous pediatric and neonatal cases. In all such cases, there should be two overriding tenets: (a) the patient requires an emergency evaluation or therapy for a potentially life-threatening problem, and air medical transport saves significant time or (b) the patient has

a life-threatening condition such that ongoing care outside of an ICU is dangerous, and air medical transport significantly reduces the amount of time the patient will spend outside a controlled setting.

One approach to retrospectively assessing utilization appropriateness is to determine what critical interventions occurred during transport. The Therapeutic Intervention Scoring System serves this purpose (35). Previous estimates are that approximately 42% of air medical transports are indicated by virtue of the intensity of care required during transport or on the basis of objective scoring systems (12,37).

Continued evaluation by all stake holders of air medical service utilization helps to ensure the appropriate allocation of resources. Just as some over-triage to trauma centers is expected (less injured patients being taken to trauma centers instead of other hospitals) in order to capture all the patients who might benefit, some over-triage to air medical transport should also be expected. However, to optimize cost effectiveness, it is necessary to keep air medical services busy transporting critically ill and injured patients who might benefit from them, rather than keeping them busy transporting patients for whom there would be no benefit gleaned.

Consensus-created guidelines for utilizing air medical services are not equivalent to proof of effectiveness. However, such proof does not exist for the many patient types routinely transported by helicopter or fixed-wing aircraft. Thus, such guidelines, when developed locally, represent one important basis for evaluating air medical service utilization.Critical Interventions

COMMON PITFALLS

✔ Delaying the request for medical helicopter transportation
✔ Failure to perform tube thoracostomy in patients with pneumothorax prior to transport in a helicopter
✔ Failure to secure the airway prior to transport in patients in whom the airway stability is in question or in combative patients
✔ Delaying helicopter transport by performing excessive efforts to stabilize the patient

Acknowledgment

We thank previous edition chapter author Kenneth A. Williams.

References

1. *Air medical physician handbook.* Salt Lake City: Air Medical Physician Association, 1999.
2. Air Medical Services Committee of the National Association of Emergency Medical Service Physicians. Air Medical Dispatch: guidelines for Service Response. *Prehospital Disaster Med* 1992;7:75–78.
3. Association of Air Medical Services. Position paper on the appropriate use of emergency air medical services. *J Air Medical Transport* 1990;29–33.
4. Baxt WG, Moody P. The impact of a rotorcraft aeromedical emergency care service on trauma mortality. *JAMA* 1983;249:3047–3051.
5. Baxt WG, Moody P, Cleveland HC, et al. Hospital-based rotorcraft aeromedical emergency care services and trauma mortality: a multicenter study. *Ann Emerg Med* 1985;14:859–864.
6. Baxt WG, Moody P. The impact of a physician as part of the aeromedical prehospital team in patients with blunt trauma. *JAMA* 1987;257:3246–3250.
7. Baxt WG, Moody P. The impact of advanced prehospital emergency care on the mortality of severely brain-injured patients. *J Trauma* 1987;27:365–369.
8. Bledsoe BE. Air medical helicopter accidents in the United States: a five-year review. *Prehosp Emerg Care* 2003;7:94–98.
9. Brathwaite CEM, Rosko M, McDowell R, et al. A critical analysis of on-scene helicopter transport on survival in a statewide trauma system. *J Trauma* 1998;45:140–144.
10. Bruhn JD, Williams KA, Aghababian R. True cost of air medical versus ground ambulance systems. *Air Med J* 1993;12:262–268.
11. Burney RE, Fischer RP. Ground versus air transport of trauma victims: medical and logistical considerations. *Ann Emerg Med* 1986;15:1491–1495.

12. Burney RE, Rhee KJ, Cornell RG, et al. Evaluation of hospital-based aeromedical transport programs using therapeutic intervention scoring. *Aviat Space Environ Med* 1988;59:563–566.
13. Burney RE, Passini L, Hubert D, et al. Comparison of aeromedical crew performance by patient severity and outcome. *Ann Emerg Med* 1992;21:375–378.
14. Burney RE, Passini L, Hubert D, et al. Variation in air medical outcomes by crew composition: a two-year followup. *Ann Emerg Med* 1995;25:187–192.
15. Cales RH, Trunkey DD. Preventable trauma deaths: a review of trauma care systems development. *JAMA* 1985;254:1059–1063.
16. Cowley RA, Hudson F, Scanlan E, et al. An economical and general helicopter program for transporting the emergency critically ill and injured patients in Maryland. *J Trauma* 1973;13:1029.
17. Cunningham P, Rutledge R, Baker CL, et al. A comparison of the association of helicopter and ground ambulance transport with the outcome of injury in trauma patients transported from the scene. *J Trauma* 1997;43:940–946.
18. Delbridge TR, Verdile VP, Platt TE. Variability of state-approved emergency medical services drug formularies. *Prehosp Disaster Med* 1994;9:S55.
19. Duke JH, Clarke WP. A university-staff, private hospital-based air transport service. *Arch Surg* 1981;116:703–708.
20. Felix WR. Metropolitan aeromedical service: state of the art. *J Trauma* 1976;16:873–881.
21. Gabram SG, Jacobs LM. The impact of emergency medical helicopters on pre-hospital care. *Emerg Med Clin N Am* 1990;8:85–102.
22. Gearhart PA, Wuerz R, Localio AR. Cost-effectiveness analysis of helicopter EMS for trauma patients. *Ann Emerg Med* 1997;30:500–506.
23. Hamman BL, Cue JI, Miller FB, et al. Helicopter transport of trauma victims: does a physician make a difference? *J Trauma* 1991;31:490–494.
24. Hunt RC, Bryan DM, Whitley TW, et al. Inability to assess breath sounds during air medical transport by helicopter. *JAMA* 1991;265:1982–1984.
25. Jacobs LM, Bennett B. A critical care helicopter system in trauma. *J Nat Med Assoc* 1989;81:1157–1167.
26. Lindbeck GH, Groopman DS, Powers RD. Aeromedical evacuation of rural victims of nontraumatic cardiac arrest. *Ann Emerg Med* 1993;22:1258–1262.
27. Low RB, Martin D. Accuracy of blood pressure measurements made aboard helicopters. *Ann Emerg Med* 1988;17:604–612.
28. National Academy of Sciences, National Research Council. *Accidental death and disability: the neglected disease of modern society.* Washington DC: National Academy Press, 1966.
29. Neel S. Army aeromedical evacuation procedures in Vietnam: Implications in rural America. *JAMA* 1968;204:309–313.
30. Peckler S, Rogers R. Air versus ground transport from the trauma scene: Optimal distance for helicopter utilization. *J Air Medical Transport October* 1989:44.
31. Rau W, Lathrop G. 1998 transport statistics and fees survey. *Air Med J* 1998;4:19–22.
32. Rhee KJ, Strozeski M, Burney RE, et al. Is the flight physician needed for helicopter emergency medical services?. *Ann Emerg Med* 1986;15:174–177.
33. Rhee KJ Baxt WG, MacKenzie JR, et al. Differences in air ambulance patient mix demonstrated by physiologic scoring. *Ann Emerg Med* 1990;19:552–556.
34. Rhee KJ, Holmes EM, Moecke HP, et al. A comparison of emergency medical helicopter accident rates in the United States and the Federal Republic of Germany. *Aviat Space Environ Med* 1990;61:750–752.
35. Savitsky E, Rodenberg H. Prediction of the intensity of patient care in prehospital helicopter transport: use of the revised trauma score. *Aviat Space Environ Med* 1995;66:11–14.
36. Schwartz RJ, Jacobs LM, Lee M. The role of the physician in a helicopter EMS system. *Prehosp Disaster Med* 1990;5:31–37.
37. Smith JS, Smith BJ, Pletcher SE, et al. When is air medical service faster than ground transportation?. *Air Med J* 1993;12:258–261.
38. Snow N, Hull C, Severns J. Physician presence on a helicopter emergency medical service: necessary or desirable? *Aviat Space Environ Med* 1986;57:1176–1178.
39. Thomas SH, Stone CK, Bryan-Berge D. The ability to perform closed-chest compressions in helicopters. *Am J Emerg Med* 1994;12:296–298.
40. Wright SW, Dronen SC, Combs TJ, et al. Aeromedical transport of patients with post-traumatic cardiac arrest. *Ann Emerg Med* 1989;8:721–726.

CHAPTER 362
Disaster Planning and Management

Jonathan L. Burstein

In the past quarter century, disasters worldwide have claimed over 3.4 million lives (11). As world population increases, and population density rises, a single catastrophic event may affect more victims simultaneously. Further, both use of hazardous materials, and population in hazardous environments (flood plains, earthquake zones, etc.) are rising. Disaster planning and response must include not only the ability to care for casualties, but the ability to function in environments rendered dangerous or even actively hostile. The mission of the disaster responder is not only to render aid, but to restore society's homeostasis (3,11,12,23,24).

A "disaster" may be defined as a destructive event that disrupts the normal functioning of a community; it may be natural, technological (e.g., chemical spill), or even deliberate (terrorist act, war). A medical disaster occurs when an event results in casualties that overwhelm the health care resources of the community involved (1). Note that many disasters, such as a jumbo jet crash without survivors, may not in this sense represent a medical disaster, although many slow-evolving events, such as pandemic influenza, may very well represent medical disasters. Response to a disaster may involve all aspects and needs of a community, including restoring food, water, power, communication, and transportation networks. The role of the emergency physician in a response may not be narrowly limited to emergency medical care, as broader public health knowledge and organizational skills may be necessary), requiring emergency physicians to step outside their usual role of individual patient care and take more of a systems-management approach. In the largest scale events, refugees and displaced populations can be both the result and the cause of disasters (6).

As noted above, disasters may be classified by origin. Natural disasters include earthquakes, floods, volcanic eruptions, hurricanes, tornadoes, winter storms, and other geologic and meteorologic phenomena; in this era of electronics, one may add the effects of solar storms disrupting pager and phone systems. Human-caused or technologic disasters include explosions, chemical spills, radiation leaks, biochemical terrorism, transportation accidents, civil disturbances, and armed conflicts. Complex humanitarian emergencies generally include features of both natural and technologic disasters, such as population displacement that results from a combination of drought, famine, and political upheaval.

In a model that is perhaps more useful for the planner, disasters also may be categorized by onset and impact. For example, earthquakes and tornadoes have a rapid onset, with a sudden impact on the community. In contrast, droughts and famines have a more gradual onset and generally have a prolonged impact. Numerous factors may modify the impact of a disaster on a community, including the nature of the event, time of day or year, health and age characteristics of the population affected, and the availability of resources. Planning for a sudden event usually must focus on responding with resources-on-hand, as opposed to the mobilization of resources that can occur in a slower-paced impact (17).

The impact of a disaster also depends on the location where it occurs. For example, an earthquake occurring in a sparsely populated area obviously injures fewer people. In contrast, a similar quake, even one of lesser magnitude, could produce extensive losses of life and property if it occurred in a densely populated region with poor construction or limited medical resources. Additionally, many may be left homeless or without essential services. Even in the acute medical response to an event, a small community hospital could be easily overwhelmed by numbers and types of casualties that might be handled routinely by a large university hospital or metropolitan medical center (4). Hospitals can be resources in a response but also may be severely affected by the impact of a disaster; and the first priority of a hospital or other essential service must be to preserve its function so that it can play its assigned or necessary role in mitigating the disaster.

In the United States, although health care is generally provided by private-sector institutions, governments at all levels have both the responsibility and some capability of supporting disaster medical care. Town or municipal governments often regulate mass-casualty distribution and may coordinate the roles of local hospitals. State governments often serve as providers of funding and equipment, in a support role to local or county agencies, and also provide a conduit to request federal aid. The federal government's main role is to provide funding for response, but there are also directly deployable federal assets (people, mobile hospitals, vehicles) available from the military, the Veterans Administration, and the Department of Homeland Security's National Disaster Medical System (NDMS). The NDMS has over 30 specialty teams throughout the country that can deploy to provide field-hospital capability, including advanced specialty care (burns and pediatrics). These teams can be deployed within 6 to 24 hours of request by a state government. The NDMS also provides or coordinates patient evacuation and mass-fatality management (4,22).

DISASTER PLANNING

Disaster planning must address numerous types of events, ranging in scale from small mass casualty incidents (MCIs), such as motor vehicle collisions with multiple victims, to extensive flooding or earthquake damage, to civil wars. The planning continuum includes advance preparations, and provision for supplies, staff, and training, and actual event management and recovery efforts. Those people and organizations responsible for disaster plans must conduct extensive risk analyses, from the sanitation needs of crowds at mass gatherings to evacuation procedures for buildings and geographic areas, to the threat posed by terrorist or military action that may be directed at the institution or its own personnel (4,12,16).

Risk analysis is an essential feature of disaster planning, in which a comprehensive inventory is created for all existing and potential hazards that are sufficiently likely to be a threat. Hazards may include such items as chemicals used by local industry, transportation elements such as airports and railroad stations, or collections of large groups of people in areas with limited access, such as high-rise office buildings, nursing homes, or sports stadiums. Environmental and meteorologic hazards must also be considered, such as the presence of fault lines and seismic zones and the seasonal risks posed by tornadoes, hurricanes, and snowstorms. Certain types of disasters can even be considered as "planned events" such as mass gatherings for sports or performance events, or political conventions. These events require planning of the same type, although perhaps varying in detail, as do all other disaster responses (18).

Risk analysis should attempt to identify any groups of people at particular risk of injury or death or loss of property from each hazard, and groups with particular needs such as children, the elderly, or the disabled. The estimated risk and patient load may vary by time of day, season, or location within a community. Properly conducted risk analysis necessitates the cooperation of corporate, governmental, and community groups to produce a comprehensive listing of potential hazards (4,13,14). It may be possible to reduce the relative risk posed by some hazards. For example, relocating a chemical depot further away from a school would reduce the risk that children would be exposed to hazardous materials.

The other essential step to take in planning is resource identification. Resources include both human and logistic elements, such as organizations with specialized personnel and equipment (7,21). Disaster preparedness should include assembling lists of medical and paramedical groups, public works and other civic departments, and volunteer agencies, along with phone numbers and key contact personnel for each. Hospital departments should have readily available a complete record of all personnel, including home addresses and telephone numbers, accessible 24 hours a day. Local, state, or federal teams of responders may be available, and a planner must know how this aid can be activated or requested. In the realm of terrorism with weapons of mass destruction, highly trained and extensively equipped specialty teams may be an absolute need for effective disaster mitigation.

Effective disaster planning must occur at all levels, from local institutions to municipal, state and federal governments, including private, volunteer, and international agencies (2). All groups should understand their own capabilities and limitations, and those of the organizations with which interactions are anticipated or intended. The use of a hierarchical management system, such as the Incident Command System (ICS), to coordinate the information and resource management is essential for any large-scale disaster. The ICS is a command system for large-scale firefighting developed by the federal government, which has now been adopted under the name National Incident Management System (NIMS) as the standard system for all U.S. public safety response agencies. Hospitals may choose to use a variant of the Hospital Emergency Incident Command System (a California-developed adaptation of ICS for hospitals) to function within the same structure as all other responding agencies (4). Disaster plans should be both structured and flexible, with provisions made for plan activation and decision making by field-level managers, if indicated (8).

Once a plan has been devised or a strategy outlined, it must be used and tested. Staff must be trained to carry out their roles in the plan. In general the best plans assign to each person a role as close as possible to their everyday job: "do what you always do, but faster." A recurring problem in disaster response is "failure of communications," but this often actually represents failure of coordination; the message may get through but the person getting it doesn't know what to do about it. True communication failures also may result from several conditions, including loss of infrastructure damaged by the disaster itself, and lack of operator familiarity, excessive demands, inadequate supplies, and lack of integration with other communications providers and technologies. Back-up communications systems, such as wireless, hardwire, and cellular telephones, may reduce the impact of disrupted standard communications. However, frequently, even advanced technology has been ineffectual or overloaded during disasters, pointing out the need for personnel to be well-trained in their roles so they can function with minimal outside direction (9).

An essential step in planning and preparedness is the evaluation of the response, both to real events and after drills and exercises. Exercises to test plans are usually "tabletop" drills, in which the responders gather around a tabletop and discuss their theoretical actions. More complex drills may involve activation of communications systems, or transport of supplies or staff to different location. The most complex and helpful "functional exercises" may take the form of full-scale multijurisdictional exercises, using moulaged victims, and requiring vast resources of supplies and personnel. A plan also may be assessed by computer simulations, or seminar sessions focusing on key personnel or limited aspects of the disaster response, but generally this will be of minimal assistance in testing a plan's real value.

The specific goal of any drill should be clearly understood in advance. If drills are to be used as training sessions and evaluations of preparations and response plans, personnel are more likely to make the correct or most appropriate response choices during the drill if they are prepared. Consequently, they will be more likely to take appropriate actions when faced with an unexpected disaster situation in the future. The more realistic the exercise, the more likely it is that useful information about the strengths and weaknesses of both the disaster plan and the responders will be acquired. The factor common to all disasters is a local shortage of available resources; without experiencing at least some of the stress which accompanies that situation, it is unlikely that the disaster plan and response will be taxed at a level that realistically simulates the circumstances of an actual disaster.

Essential features of all effective disaster drills are the inclusion of all parties likely to be involved in the disaster response and a joint critique, with a formal debriefing of all participants following the exercise. This review should consider comments from all individuals, groups, or agencies involved in the drill. It is helpful, and essentially mandatory, to designate observers in advance to assess specific aspects of the plan, such as effectiveness of a phone tree, or accuracy of medication dispensing. The observations and comments should result in modifications of the disaster plan, if necessary (20). A drill that produces no changes in plans or goals likely did not sufficiently stress the system. Any alterations in disaster plans or response procedures must be communicated to all groups involved or affected. Periodic evaluations of disaster plans are essential to ensure that personnel have adequate familiarity with their roles in disaster situations, and to provide for changes in regional emergency response operations, hospital renovations and closings, and other variables. Hospitals have a requirement to conduct at least two disaster-plan exercises per year to maintain compliance with the standards of the Joint Commission on Accreditation of Healthcare Organizations (JCAHO) (4,25).

Mass gatherings provide a unique form of "planned disaster." In general they will occur in a defined location such as a sports stadium, concert hall, waterfront, or field. Planning should include basic sanitation needs, hydration and environmental protection (against sun, heat, or cold exposure), and both routine medical care (acetaminophen and abrasion care), and full emergency care (cardiac resuscitation). Additionally, planning must address the medical response to a mass-casualty event at the scene, such as might be caused by a vehicle accident or terrorist attack. Staffing for a mass gathering is generally composed of a mix of provider types and levels (first aid, EMS, nurses, physicians, security, fire and rescue), a mix of venues (first aid stations, medical tents, ambulances), a mix of roles (on-scene care, evacuation, command and control), and a mix of jurisdictions (private providers, public safety, city authorities, venue staff, state or federal authorities). This complexity makes preplanning critical for success. In terms of types of patient encounters to be anticipated, the best guide is prior experience at the same event, if available

(such as recurring races, sporting events, or concerts). Some data are available in the literature, but the numbers are highly variable. In general, patient volume will be higher in outdoor environments, with younger average crowd age (confounded by event type), and with the increased use of alcohol or other substances in the environment (18,19).

DISASTER MANAGEMENT

The philosophy of disaster management may be summed up in the phrase, "The needs of the many outweigh the needs of the few." Resources may be so limited that stringent rationing of care or supplies is vital to the survival of the maximum number of people. Austere conditions may be alien to responders accustomed to ample quantities of medical supplies, equipment, personnel, and time, but they are commonly encountered with many large-scale disasters. In this setting, difficult triage decisions must be made in order to ensure that all assets are used in the most efficient and pragmatic manner (19).

The goal of disaster management is to provide the most appropriate intervention and assistance based on the most accurate information available in a timely manner. Disaster response includes several phases (Table 362.1) but must begin with recognition that disaster conditions exist. Some disasters, such as hurricanes, may be preceded by a period of time, called the preimpact phase, during which advance information may be gathered about the potential effects of the disaster. The data acquired during the preimpact phase may allow prepositioning of personnel and resources in a strategic location. As a result of a lack of verifiable data, it may be necessary, at times, to begin a response or asset deployment without full intelligence, with efforts made to tailor and modify the response as updated information becomes available (15).

The emergency medical system and hospital responders must be aware that triage in a disaster is devoted to providing the greatest good for the greatest number, rather than maximal effort for each patient. Often, patients in cardiac arrest, who would normally have received a great deal of care, are instead triaged as "expectant" (not resuscitated) so that the personnel and supplies saved may be used to help numerous other salvageable patients. The presence of toxic substances or radioactive materials may also change triage priorities (e.g., severely injured and heavily irradiated patients may be unsalvageable

---

TABLE 362.1.   Components of a Disaster Response

ACTIVATION

Notification and initial response
Scene assessment
Response
Organization of command
Search and rescue
Victim triage, stabilization, and transport

MITIGATION

Definitive management of scene hazards and victims

RECOVERY

Scene withdrawal
Return to normal operations
Debriefing
Updating and improving plans and planning
Drills and exercises

in a disaster setting). There are numerous methods for rapid triage that have been devised, such as the "START" (Simple Triage and Rapid Transport) system, and planners and responders should be familiar with the system in use in their area or institution (4).

Inevitably, in the event of a disaster that produces significant morbidity and mortality, including psychological threats and fears resulting from terrorist actions, the physician on duty in the emergency department will be one of the first people called on to assume a leadership role. The existence of a hospital disaster plan provides a valuable resource, but, ideally, the emergency physician should already be well-versed in the administrative and logistical aspects of the plan and the purely medical functions. The response will evolve more smoothly if the emergency physician understands both the hospital plan and the resources, capabilities, and disaster plans of the first responders and emergency medical services (EMS) system in the region. The physician may be required to coordinate or facilitate the hospital response and to provide direction for numerous aspects of the regional response, and may be looked to as a resource for hospital administrators who want to know "What should I do?" The physician may also be consulted regarding the need for the deployment of agencies and resources from outside the affected region, and will need to know where to direct these inquiries, because they are unlikely to have the knowledge to appropriately answer them. Additionally, emergency department staff should expect to be bombarded with requests for information on all aspects of the disaster and response, from family members, media, and government representatives and from the public at large, and be prepared to refer or respond to such questions. Early in a disaster, the emergency physician and staff will likely be expected to disseminate information about the disaster event, demonstrate expertise and leadership in the response and management efforts, and even make the initial determination that disaster conditions exist. Hospital administrators, social services, and public relations personnel will need to assume their proper roles to allow the ED to continue to provide medical care, and should be notified as soon as a disaster is recognized.

In the case of damaged or destroyed health care facilities or after a large-scale disaster, the physician may also be called on to provide medical care in unconventional settings. In the situation in which field medical care stations must be established, coordinating responses with other agencies is essential. It is important to remember, during the early stage of the disaster, that information available from those at the disaster area (data regarding death, injury, or damage) may not be accurate. Problems with communications are frequently the source of delays and misapplications of disaster resources. The ability of those in a region devastated by a disaster to survey the population and infrastructure may be severely curtailed by damage, such that even initial calls for help may be impossible. It is essential, therefore, that external resources of personnel and equipment be available and accessible if anticipation of potential need for them arises (19). Conversely, as a result of disruption of communications and transportation, it is possible for the effects of the disaster to be overestimated. In order to minimize damage and disruption, expedient decisions must be made, with future consequences of such actions considered as well. Short-term benefits and costs must be weighed against their long-term counterparts. Disasters are costly events, but judicious initial expenditures may result in substantial savings, in both monetary and humanitarian terms, over the long haul. On the other hand, excessive spending by individuals, agencies, or organizations may result in prolonged or delayed recovery from the disaster and may restrict the capability to prepare or respond when the next disaster strikes.

In the case of a disaster that causes substantial destruction of infrastructure, the response may be prolonged, requiring that long-term health care and support services be established. Issues such as nutrition evaluation and ongoing disease surveillance may require the expertise of numerous other health care providers and agencies (10). Additionally, mental health issues must also be considered for the victims and the responders, during both the emergency phase and the recovery. Posttraumatic stress disorder, major depression, generalized anxiety disorder, and substance abuse are frequently reported among disaster survivors who have experienced traumatic bereavement or severe disruption of their lives. Early and voluntary access to mental health workers for evaluation and intervention may reduce the incidence and severity of such reactions (3,5).

COMMON PITFALLS

✔ Failure to prepare for a disaster by identifying potential hazards in the local environment and those hazards that may be brought in, whether by nature or human action
✔ Failure to develop appropriate multiagency and multijurisdictional contingency plans
✔ Failure to properly exercise and update disaster plans
✔ Failure to appreciate that disrupted communication and transportation systems frequently cause problems in assessing and responding to disasters, and that redundancy of equipment, training in its use, and flexibility of use of communication and transportation resources are desirable
✔ Failure to consider the needs of the elderly, children, and other special populations, and to include such things as appropriate medical supplies, diapers, formula, medications, interpreters, and special transportation requirements in disaster planning and response
✔ Failure to appreciate that disaster responders may become casualties themselves, and that they may suffer psychological effects during and after the event, and that personal planning and institutional support is crucial to minimize the impact of disruptions in the personal or professional lives of disaster responders

Acknowledgment

We thank the previous edition chapter author, Lucille Gans.

References

1. Aghababian RV, Lewis CP, Gans L, et al. Disasters within hospitals. *Ann Em Med* 1994;23:771.
2. Al-Madhari AF, Keller AZ. Review of disaster definitions. *Prehosp Disaster Med* 1997;12:17.
3. Auf der Heide E. Disaster planning, part II: disaster problems, issues, and challenges identified in the research literature. *Emerg Med Clin North Am* 1996;14:453.
4. Auf der Heide, Erik. Principles of hospital disaster planning. In: Hogan DE, Burstein JL, eds. *Disaster medicine*. Lippincott, Williams & Wilkins, 2002.
5. Austin LS, Godelski LS. Therapeutic approaches for survivors of disaster. *Psychiatr Clin North Am* 1999;22:897.
6. Burkle FM. Acute-phase mental health consequences of disasters: implications for triage and emergency medical services. *Ann Emerg Med* 1996;28:119.
7. Centers for Disease Control and Prevention. Famine-affected, refugee, and displaced populations: recommendations for public health issues. *MMWR* 1992;41(RR-13):1.
8. Cuny FC. Principles of disaster management. Lesson 2: program planning. *Prehosp Disaster Med* 1998;13:63.
9. De Lorenzo RA. Mass gathering medicine: a review. *Prehosp Disaster Med* 1997;12:68.
10. Garshnek V, Burkle FM. Telecommunications systems in support of disaster medicine: applications of basic information pathways. *Ann Emerg Med* 1999;34:213.
11. Hogan DE, Burstein JL. Basic physics of disasters. In: Hogan DE, Burstein JL, eds. *Disaster Medicine*. Lippincott, Williams & Wilkins, 2002.
12. Koscheyev VS, Leon GR, Greaves IA. Lessons learned and unsolved public health problems after large-scale disasters. *Prehosp Disaster Med* 1997;12:120.

13. Leonard RB, Calabro JJ, Noji EK, et al. SARA (Superfund Amendments and Reauthorization Act), Title III: implications for emergency physicians. *Ann Emerg Med* 1989;18:1212.
14. Leonard RB. Emergency evacuations in disasters. *Prehosp Disaster Med* 1991;6:463.
15. Levitin HW, Siegelson HJ. Hazardous materials: disaster medical planning and response. *Emerg Med Clin North Am* 1996;14:327.
16. Noji EK. Disaster epidemiology. *Emerg Med Clin North Am* 1996;14:289.
17. Noji EK. ed. The public health consequences of disasters. New York: Oxford University Press, 1997.
18. Parillo S. Medical care of mass gatherings. In: Hogan DE, Burstein JL, eds. *Disaster Medicine*. Lippincott, Williams & Wilkins, 2002.
19. Parillo SJ. Medical care at mass gatherings: considerations for physician involvement. *Prehosp Disaster Med* 1995;10:273.
20. Piper PS, Burkle FM, Murray RJ. Constructing a world wide web site for disaster management and humanitarian assistance. *Prehosp Disaster Med* 1997;12:92.
21. Quarantelli EL. Ten criteria for evaluating the management of community disasters. *Disasters* 1997;21:39.
22. Roth PB, Gaffney JK. The federal response plan and disaster medical assistance teams in domestic disasters. *Emerg Med Clin North Am* 1996;14:371.
23. SAEM Disaster Medicine White Paper Subcommittee. Disaster medicine: current assessment and blueprint for the future. *Acad Emerg Med* 1995;2:1068.
24. Waeckerle JF. Disaster planning and response. *N Engl J Med* 1991;324:815.
25. JCAHCO Web site text. Joint Commission on the Accreditation of Healthcare Organizations Web site. Available at www.jcaho.org. Accessed October 30, 2003.

Patient Safety, Ethical, Legal and Regulatory Issues

CHAPTER 363

Errors and Patient Safety

Karen S. Cosby, John Vinen, Christopher B. Beach, and Robert L. Wears

Physicians share a common ethos to offer comfort and healing, and are guided by the Hippocratic injunction to "First, do no harm." But in an era in which incredible progress has been made in medical science and technology, many are shocked to find that intent and desire to do good have proven inadequate to meet these goals.

Medicine has always acknowledged that every treatment and intervention comes with risk. Until the last decade, the focus on iatrogenic harm was directed toward nosocomial infections and unintended side effects of medications, most of which were viewed as the unavoidable consequences of high-tech care. That view began to change with the publication of the Harvard Medical Practice Study (3,13) in 1991, which reported that nearly 4% of hospitalized patients suffer adverse events, many causing permanent injury or death. Although emergency medicine accounted for only a small proportion of injuries, the vast majority of those occurring in the emergency department were thought to be preventable. When this study was replicated (21), and the issue further publicized by the Institute of Medicine (IOM) (11), the conclusions shocked the medical community and the public at large and turned the problem of medical errors into a public health issue. This has led to a movement to better understand the nature of errors in medicine and the injuries that sometimes follow them, and to reform medical practice to make it safer.

SOURCES OF FAILURES IN THE EMERGENCY DEPARTMENT

Traditionally, physicians have viewed successes or failures of care entirely from an individual perspective, or the "person model" (24). This view has three main tenets:

1. adverse events arise from unsafe acts or omissions committed by providers;
2. those acts or omissions are the result of inattention, carelessness, laziness, lack of knowledge or lack of motivation; and
3. failures result from choices made by providers to act safely or unsafely, and are the direct causes of adverse events.

Under the person model, solutions are directed at individuals, in the form of selection, education, exhortation, discipline, blame, punishment, and retraining. No examination of contributing causes is performed, because the person model assumes that physicians should be able to compensate for problematic working conditions, if they would only try hard enough.

There are several difficulties with the person model. It is subject to *hindsight bias* (4,10), in that it fails to note that the course of action that seems so obvious after an adverse event has occurred may not have been so apparent before the fact. Second, failures tend to occur in characteristic patterns, but by dealing with each event as if it resulted from an aberrant individual, the contextual information about the conditions of work that contributed to the error are lost. Not coincidentally, focusing on the individual provider tends to remove questions about management and institutional accountability, which raises questions about the justness of this approach. The focus on punishment and accountability leads to the hiding of information, so that learning is impeded. Finally, the person model does not provide a path to improvement when the workforce is already highly trained and strongly motivated, as is the case with emergency physicians. Berwick has pointed out that if we suspended every doctor who makes an error today, tomorrow's error rates would be exactly the same as today's (1).

An alternative view, the "system model," assumes that providers, no matter how conscientious, well-motivated, and well-trained, will sometimes make mistakes despite themselves, and thus that in order for health care systems to be safe, they must be redesigned to handle these occasional errors without harming patients. Human failures that lead to adverse events are thus seen as the consequences of poor design or bad systems, not as causes in themselves (22).

Additionally, the system model rarely finds a single cause for an adverse event, or even a "root" cause, but rather a set of causal factors that are individually insufficient but jointly necessary for adverse events to occur. It is useful to divide these factors into two broad classes, "active failures" and "latent failures." Active failures are best viewed as triggering events that allow latent failures to become manifest.

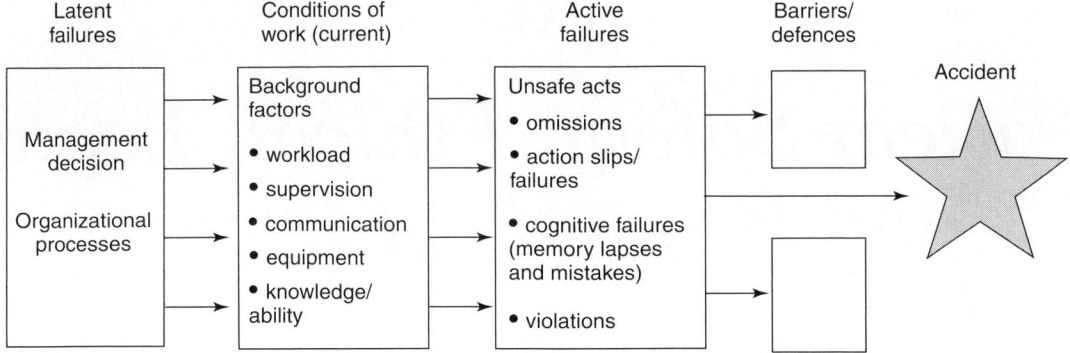

Figure 363.1. Anatomy of a complex accident. (From Vincent C, Taylor-Adams S, Stanhope N. Framework for analysing risk and safety in clinical medicine. *BMJ* 1998;316(7138):1154–1157, with permission.)

Active failures are the unsafe acts or omissions committed by those in direct contact with the patient, at the so-called "sharp end" of the system (5). These can take three forms: (a) action failures, or slips (e.g., writing an order on the wrong chart, or ordering a typical adult dose of a medication for a child); (b) cognitive failures (e.g., memory lapses or misperceptions of a situation); and (c) violations (deviations from safe operating practices, procedures, or rules). Violations are a distinctly different kind of active failure, because they are often (but not always) intentional. Although at first glance it might seem that violations are a problem best suited to the person model, in fact many violations are routine, are generally accepted in the workplace, are viewed as either necessary or at least convenient ways to get the work done, and only come to attention after an adverse event (17). These "work-arounds" and shortcuts are used to improve efficiency and keep the system running smoothly. A classic example of necessary violations comes from air traffic control: when controllers have rigidly followed rules ("worked to rule") in job actions, the normal flow of traffic has been seriously disrupted.

Latent failures are faults created by decisions remote from immediate patient care, at the "blunt end" of the system. Latent failures typically occur at higher levels in the organization. Although any consequences of active failures are immediately apparent, latent failures may lie dormant in the system for quite a long time, becoming evident only when the combined presence of latent failures and local triggering factors (that may include active failures) lead to a system breakdown. Because latent failures typically reside in a system for an extended time before causing a bad outcome, there is a greater opportunity for detection and control than with active failures. Latent failures basically provide the context in which unsafe acts are elicited from providers. In Moray's words (14), "The systems of which humans are a part call forth errors from humans, not the other way around." Examples of latent failures include heavy workloads, inadequate experience or supervision, a stressful environment (e.g., noise or frequent interruptions), production pressure, rapid organizational change, incompatible goals (cost reduction and clinical need), poorly designed or maintained equipment, and so on.

Human factors and safety experts have identified a number of distinct levels at which both active and latent faults can occur, and any investigation of a critical incident should specifically examine all of them, rather than stop prematurely at the first reasonable fault (19). Moving from the lowest to the highest level, one should examine patient factors (complexity of case, communication barriers), task factors (availability and clarity of protocols or procedures), provider factors (fatigue, knowledge, motivation), team factors (team structure and communications), work environment factors (workload, noise, interface design),

organizational factors (financial constraints, safety culture), and the institutional context (the economic and regulatory world of health care organizations) (22,23).

The active and latent failures associated with a critical incident can be arranged in a hierarchy (Fig. 363.1) (16,22,23). Organizational influences and decisions create latent faults in the activities of planning, communication, maintenance, etc. These in turn are realized in departmental and workgroup conditions that favor the commission of errors and violations. Many active faults arise in the course of clinical work, but most are caught by system defenses. Interestingly, the providers themselves are a major system defense, in that they frequently catch their own or their co-workers' errors before harm occurs. In the emergency department, Fordyce (9) has shown that active faults are extremely common (about 1 for every 5 patients), but that only 2% of the errors lead to adverse event; the rest are either caught by the staff or fail to cause any harm. System defenses are not perfect, however, and occasionally (in fact, rarely) an active fault will slip through all the defenses and result in either a near-miss (if no harm occurs) or an adverse event.

This concept of the causal web of events leading to an accident has been immortalized by Reason (18) as the "Swiss cheese" model of accident causation (Fig. 363.2). In this figure, the holes that represent active and latent failures are continually appearing, enlarging, shrinking, and closing. The rare, unfortunate alignment of faults is what leads to an accident. The emphasis here is on the dynamic nature of the system of care; because the system is continually changing its state, assuring safety is a dynamic, active process (25). We can never state that the emergency

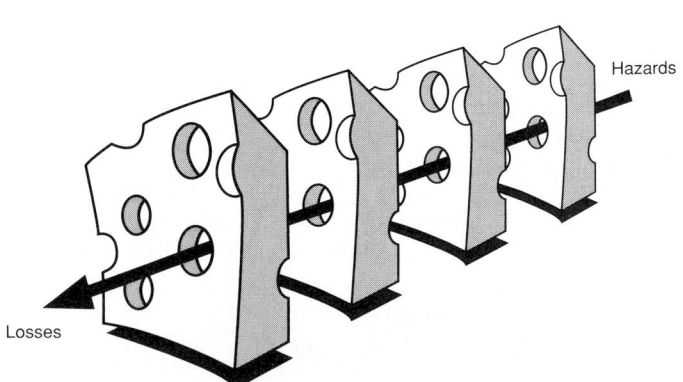

Figure 363.2. The "Swiss cheese" model of accident causation [18]. Taken from BMJ 2000;320:768–770. Reproduced with permission of BMJ Publishing Group.

department "is safe." Rather, we can only say that we are actively and continually managing the system in an attempt to keep it in a safe condition.

EXAMPLES OF SYSTEM FAILURES

The three examples that follow illustrate how system failures can give rise to catastrophic outcomes.

Case #1: An intoxicated patient was given a dose of intravenous magnesium that was tenfold greater than intended. He suffered a respiratory arrest and died. The nurse who administered the medication was fired.

Case #2: A patient with chest pain suffered a cardiac arrest (CA) after a prolonged delay in triage and an inappropriate triage to the emergency department waiting area. A nurse and technician were blamed.

Case #3: A patient was given the seemingly innocuous diagnosis of an ear infection and was discharged home. A few hours later, he returned with an altered mental status, seized, and died. The physician was faulted for not making the diagnosis of brain abscess with increased intracranial pressure.

In each of these cases it seemed clear to the initial investigators that someone had failed in performing their duty to provide a reasonable standard of care. The person model would conclude that they were all incompetent, careless, or lazy. However, a more thorough investigation of each of these cases eventually found that significant system flaws had set the background that made error not only possible, but likely.

In the first case, the hospital had recently changed their supply of magnesium without notifying the medical staff. The packaging on the new preparation was nearly identical to the preparation they had used for years. The only difference was the concentration, and that difference was not apparent from casual inspection. The nurse administered the usual volume, and had no idea that the total dose was excessive.

In the second case, the hospital had a budget shortfall and fell behind in routine equipment maintenance. A broken x-ray machine slowed the flow through the emergency department (ED). Additionally, a staff member called in ill unexpectedly and the most experienced triage nurse was pulled to cover another position. Waiting times for the ED grew and triage personnel were forced to violate standard triage rules.

In the third case, it was later found that critical information regarding the patient's past medical history was never made available to the physician at the time of his encounter with the patient. Communication was never received from a transferring hospital and important records were misplaced.

Health care organizations function in environments of great risk and are often structured in ways that are inherently prone to error. In a simple closed system, it is not difficult to develop well-defined processes. Such systems can be designed to minimize the steps to accomplish a goal, and tightly regulated to detect and correct inaccuracy. But EDs are not simple, closed systems. They are highly complex, and very much subject to the influences of outside variables (15). A failure in any part of the system can affect many other parts in unanticipated ways, and failure in one area may not be immediately visible in other areas and so may not be recognized until an accident occurs.

Complex systems such as EDs or the larger health care organizations in which they operate are also affected by an inadvertent "structural secrecy" that has its roots in the division of labor among professions, among specialties, and between clinicians on the one hand and administrators on the other. This compartmentalization creates a situation in which hospitals cannot learn from their own mistakes, and unfortunately continue to repeat them (8).

TABLE 363.1.   The Joint Commission Patient Safety Goals for 2004[a]

1. Improve the accuracy of patient identification.
2. Improve the effectiveness of communication among caregivers.
3. Improve the safety of high-alert medications.
4. Eliminate wrong-site, wrong-patient, wrong-procedure surgery.
5. Improve the safety of using infusion pumps.
6. Improve the effectiveness of clinical alarm systems.
7. Reduce the risk of health care-acquired infections.

[a]From Joint Commission on Accareditation of Health Care Organizations Web site. Available at http://www.jcaho.org. Accessed December 14, 2003, with permission.

APPROACHES TO IMPROVING SAFETY

The task of improving safety in an industry as large and complex as health care is not easy, nor will it be accomplished quickly. Long-term solutions will require fundamental redesign and reorganization of virtually every part of the health care system. The interventions that ultimately turn out to be the most important will probably not be the ones that are currently experiencing the greatest interest.

There are, however, some short-term interventions which can be useful. Although they should not be confused with more fundamental improvements, emergency physicians can use them to begin to change their practices today.

Medication problems are among the most common of errors noted in hospital organizations. Two interventions that have been incorporated into the Joint Commission's safety goals for 2004 (Table 363.1) were added to remove certain high risk medications (such as concentrated electrolyte solutions) from treatment areas and to require that they be prepared in the pharmacy rather than on the nursing unit. Similarly, organizations are now asked to limit the number of different concentrations of drugs in their formularies in order to reduce the opportunities for inadvertent substitution.

Similarly, many time-honored abbreviations have been shown to be easily confused, especially when hand-written, and institutions are now expected to implement and enforce lists of acceptable and prohibited abbreviations (Table 363.2).

TABLE 363.2.   Dangerous Abbreviations, Acronyms, and Symbols[a]

1. U (for unit)	Confused with zero (0). Write out "unit."
2. IU (for international unit)	Confused with 10. Write "international unit."
3. QD, QOD, QID	Mutually confused. Write "daily," "every other day," or "4 times a day."
4. 1.0 mistaken for 10 .40 mistaken for 40	Avoid trailing zero after a decimal. Use a leading zero before a decimal.
5. MS, MSO4, MgSO4	Mutually confused. Write out full name.
6. μg for microgram	Confused with "mg." Write "mcg."
7. HS, QHS	Mutually confused. Write "half strength" or "at bedtime."
8. TIW	Write "three times weekly."
9. SQ, SC	Write "sub-Q," "subQ," or "subcutaneously."
10. D/C	Write "discharge."
11. cc	Confused with "00." Write "ml."

[a]From Joint Commission on Accreditation of Health Care Organizations Web site. Available at http://www.jcaho.org. Accessed December 14, 2003, with permission.

Ultimately, handwritten medication orders will probably be replaced by computerized physician order entry, and tied to bar coding to prevent errors in the dispensing and administration phases. However, these systems are expensive and not generally available, and run the risk of substituting one kind of failure for another.

ETHICAL CONSIDERATIONS IN PATIENT SAFETY

There is currently an increasing expectation that clinicians will confront their errors honestly and openly. They have the duty to acknowledge error, and a requirement (both legal and ethical) to inform the patient. Although this approach raises fears of litigation, the ethical obligation should outweigh the practical concern; additionally, there is some evidence that such an approach leaves all parties more satisfied and reduces overall costs in the long run (12). An enlightened clinician will report errors and attempt to learn from them, and seek improvements in the systems that have allowed them to emerge. In order for this to occur, hospitals and administrators will have to provide a safe and supportive work culture and environment for reporting, and a commitment to work for productive change.

COMMON PITFALLS

There are three common pitfalls in dealing with patient safety in emergency care.

✔ The first is denial. Many physicians do not believe that the safety problems highlighted by the IOM report (11) are real. Their personal experience leads them to believe that mishaps are uncommon, and from this they infer that the burden of injury must be low. They are correct in their perception, but incorrect in their inference. The upper limit of the IOM estimates for mortality was about 100,000 deaths per year in the United States. Spread over 4,000 acute care hospitals, that is slightly less than one every 2 weeks per hospital. The relationship of those deaths to failures in care is not always obvious, and physicians generally know little about what goes on outside their own departments, so the perception that failure is uncommon is understandable. Although the rate of failure is low, however, the number of opportunities for failure is high (over 100 million ED visits per year)

✔ The second pitfall is *focusing on errors*. Errors are abundant in every human endeavor, and in fact generally arise from the highly adaptive characteristics of the human mind that we would not wish to eliminate even if we could (16). Focusing on errors rather than harm leads to two pernicious traps. First, it focuses attention on changing people, a "virtually bankrupt idea" (2). Second, it is highly vulnerable to *hindsight bias* (10). Judgments regarding the adequacy and quality of care are influenced by knowledge of the outcome. A poor outcome will likely generate a harsh review (4). Investigations that are contaminated by outcome knowledge run the risk of not capturing the complexities and uncertainties facing ED personnel and not understanding why their actions made sense at the time. Human factors professionals have developed specific techniques for reducing the effect of hindsight bias (7), but they are unfamiliar in medicine

✔ The third pitfall is *seeking "silver bullet" solutions that will fix the safety problem once and for all*. These "false gods" include education, technology, and reporting, and although each has

a role to play, it is one that is more limited and problematic than many realize

- *Education.* More (or better, or remedial) training is the most commonly recommended intervention after an adverse event. Obviously education is important, but emergency physicians are already highly educated and intensively trained. Education as an intervention has largely reached its maximum potential benefit in health care
- *Technology.* New technology (particularly computer technology) is another frequently recommended intervention to improve safety. Here again, better technology is clearly part of the solution, but it must be tempered by the knowledge that the introduction of new technology into complex work environments changes the nature of work in fundamental ways, and has invariably been accompanied by unintended and unanticipated consequences (20). Computers and humans have complementary strengths and weaknesses, so the cooperative work between them has great theoretical appeal. However, because we do not have good methods for determining how best to facilitate that cooperation, technological interventions today represent experiments as much as they do solutions (6)
- *Reporting.* A great deal of the initial response to the IOM report focused on reporting systems. At one level, reporting is quite important—you cannot fix what you do not know about. However, reporting as an end in itself accomplishes little; case definitions, categories, and counts have not contributed substantively to the understanding of how safety is created or destroyed in other industries. Reporting coupled with careful investigation, using the appropriate skills from psychology and engineering, is useful to guide improvement. Reporting that loses the narrative of 'what happened and how' is mostly a waste of effort (2)

References

1. Berwick DM. Not again! Preventing errors lies in redesign—not exhortation. *BMJ* 2001;322:247–248.
2. Berwick DM. Patient safety: Lessons from a novice. *Focus on Patient Safety* 2001;4(3):3.
3. Brennan TA, Leape LL, Laird NM, et al. Incidence of adverse events and negligence in hospitalized patients: results of the Harvard Medical Practice Study I. *N Engl J Med* 1991;324(6):370–376.
4. Caplan RA, Posner KL, Cheney FW. Effect of outcome on physician judgments of appropriateness of care. *JAMA* 1991;265(15):1957–1960.
5. Cook RI, Woods DD. Operating at the sharp end: the complexity of human error. In: Bogner MS, ed. *Human Error in Medicine*. Hillsdale, NJ: Lawrence Erlbaum Associates, 1994:255–310.
6. Cook RI. Safety technology: Solutions or experiments? *Nurs Econ* 2002;20(2):80–82.
7. Dekker S. *The field guide to human error investigations*. Aldershot, UK: Ashgate Publishing, 2002.
8. Edmondson AC. Learning from mistakes is easier said than done: Group and organizational influences on the detection and correction of human error. *J Appl Behav Sci* 1996;32(1):5–28.
9. Fordyce J, Blank FSJ, Pekow P, et al. Errors in a busy emergency department. *Ann Emerg Med* 2003;42(3):324–333.
10. Henriksen K, Kaplan H. Hindsight bias, outcome knowledge and adaptive learning. *Qual Saf Health Care* 2003;12(Suppl 2):ii46–ii50.
11. Kohn LT, Corrigan JM, Donaldson MS, eds. *To err is human: building a safer health system*. Washington, DC: National Academy Press, 1999.
12. Kraman SS, Hamm G. Risk management: extreme honesty may be the best policy. *Ann Intern Med* 1999;131(12):963–967.
13. Leape LL, Brennan TA, Laird N, et al. The nature of adverse events in hospitalized patients: Results of the Harvard Medical Practice Study II. *N Engl J Med* 1991;324(6):377–384.
14. Moray N. Error reduction as a systems problem. In: Bogner MS, ed. *Human error in medicine*. Hillsdale, NJ: Lawrence Erlbaum Associates, 1994:67–91.
15. Perrow C. *Normal accidents: living with high-risk technologies*. Princeton, NJ: Princeton University Press, 1999.
16. Reason J. *Human Error*. Cambridge, UK: Cambridge University Press, 1990.
17. Reason J. *Managing the risks of organizational accidents*. Aldershot, UK: Ashgate Publishing, 1997.
18. Reason J. Human error: models and management. *BMJ* 2000;320(7237):768–770.

19. Reason JT. Understanding adverse events: the human factor. In: Vincent C, ed. *Clinical risk management: enhancing patient safety.* London, UK: BMJ Books, 2001.
20. Rochlin GI. *Trapped in the net: the unanticipated consequences of computerization.* Princeton, NJ: Princeton University Press, 1997.
21. Thomas EJ, Studdert DM, Burstin HR, et al. Incidence and types of adverse events and negligent care in Utah and Colorado. *Med Care* 2000;38(3):261–271.
22. Vincent C, Taylor-Adams S, Stanhope N. Framework for analysing risk and safety in clinical medicine. *BMJ* 1998;316(7138):1154–1157.
23. Vincent C, Taylor-Adams S, Chapman EJ, et al. How to investigate and analyse clinical incidents: clinical risk unit and association of litigation and risk management protocol. *BMJ* 2000;320(7237):777–781.
24. Wears RL. Models of error and adverse events. *Harvard Risk Manage Found For* 2001;21(2):13–16.
25. Weick KE. Organizational culture as a source of high reliability. *Califo Manage Rev* 1987;29(2):112–127.

CHAPTER 364
Ethical Issues

James G. Adams

Every patient encounter has ethical dimensions and many encounters result in conflict. Ethical conflict usually surrounds consent and refusal of care, dilemmas near the end of life, lack of information regarding a patient's goals for treatment, questions of decisional capacity, and conflicts between competing interests, such as opposition between individual patient's interests and those of the caregiver or society. This chapter presents specific situations in the emergency department (ED) in which dilemmas are most likely to arise, provides examples of predictable scenarios, and offers frameworks to assist in decision making.

CONSENT ISSUES

It is well accepted that competent adults have the right to make decisions about their own medical treatment. In order for the patient to make informed decisions, the physician must communicate well. The care process is comfortable for all involved when the doctor, nurse, and patient have a rapport, when the patient willingly accepts the treatment suggested, and when there is no unpleasant result. The ethical requirement for all encounters, even in these "good" situations, is to assure that patients are sufficiently informed regarding treatment options, risks and benefits of suggested and alternative courses, enabling the patient to reasonably understand and participate in the process (12). A signed consent form is often obtained as evidence that the discussion has taken place, usually for procedures that entail identifiable risk. It is important to emphasize that informed consent is not the signature on the paper, but the process of effective communication and interaction, resulting in patient understanding. *Informed* means that the treating physician provides a fair and reasonable explanation of the particular procedure or treatment, including risks and benefits (5,10). There are specific elements that must be disclosed to the patient, including the nature of the patient's condition, the proposed treatment or procedure, the risks and benefits of the procedure, and alternatives to the planned procedure, including the risks of the al-

ternative treatments. The physician has a duty to disclose any substantial or material facts about a proposed procedure or treatment.

In routine practice, a global signed consent notes the person's general desire for care. Further, implied consent is present as the person willingly participates in the care. At all times, patients must be provided with material information that is commensurate with the risks involved. Ethically, the quality of communication matters far more than the signed form. As the risk of complications increases, it is wise to document additional informed consent for legal purposes. Informed consent should reflect the patient's autonomous desire, a culmination of communication and understanding. This essence of the process, including content of the discussion, should be documented. The legal standard is that the patient must receive all information about a proposed treatment or procedure that a reasonable and prudent physician knows would be regarded as material by a reasonable and prudent patient. In the case of a relatively risk-free event, such as phlebotomy or physical examination, implied consent is often sufficient. As risk and complexity increase, more information must be shared. It is imperative that the patient and physician understand each other. This takes good communication skills, time, patience, and willingness to work through the inevitable difficulties.

Refusal of Care

Conflict may arise when the patient refuses care or otherwise objects to an element of treatment. Patients can and do refuse care, even when that care is essential to preserve their life or health. A paradox may result. On the one hand, providing unwanted treatment over the objection of a competent patient renders the physician liable for battery. On the other hand, an impulsive or incompletely informed refusal leading to lack of treatment renders the physician liable for negligence. Resolving this paradox at the time of the emergency takes ethical skill.

A valid refusal requires that the person possess decisional capacity (14). Decisional capacity means that the patient is able to understand the medical condition, the treatment suggested, and the risks, benefits, and alternatives (11). Patients must also be able to reason in order to reach a decision in keeping with their goals and values. Whenever a patient refuses care, it is strongly suggested that the patient's decisional capacity be noted on the record, especially reflecting the information, understanding, and ability to reason.

A great challenge for emergency physicians is to expertly assess decisional capacity in order to understand when a refusal is informed and when it is an impulsive gesture of a person who lacks decisional capacity (18,21). Common reasons for lack of capacity include acute psychosis and severe psychiatric illness, overwhelming medical illness and intoxication that impairs reasoning. Importantly, the mere presence of a medical illness, even a life threatening one, does not necessarily mean that the person lacks decisional capacity. It is only the impact of the illness on the person's ability to receive and process information that impairs decisional capacity. Similarly, the presence of intoxicants does not remove a person's ability to make decisions, even risky decisions. The challenge is to ensure that the patient understands the risks and can make a reasoned decision, even if it seems unreasonable to the caregivers. When there is doubt, care should proceed in order to restore decisional capacity. Protecting the patient from a dangerous decision is justifiable when there is doubt about whether the refusal represents a reasoned, durable decision. When treatment is delivered over expressed objection, whether the patient appears to be delirious, intoxicated, or suffering from metabolic, toxic, or infectious conditions, the substantial impairment of decisional capacity should be clearly documented. The critical, necessary skill of the emergency physician is to decide when to respect the patient's expressed desire to refuse and when to treat a seriously ill patient who lacks decisional capacity yet is impulsively refusing care. It is not the responsibility of patients to prove they are competent, it is the responsibility of the physician to identify the impairment. Emergency physicians must begin with the assumption that the patient is autonomous and has the right of self-determination. When there is doubt about the ability of the patient to make informed, autonomous decisions, the physician must deliver care required to restore decisional capacity and access evidence of the patient's enduring wishes in order to guide treatment decisions.

There is an important exception to informed consent, the *emergency rule*, but it is narrowly structured (9). The emergency exception to informed consent, requires two circumstances that must occur simultaneously. The patient must be in actual life-threatening danger and the patient must be unable to give consent. In this situation, the law assumes that the rational patient would consent to care if able. Consent is not waived in this situation; if the physician clearly knows that the patient would not have consented to the proposed lifesaving treatment, it should not be administered.

In the ED, patients in obvious medical crisis often impulsively object to care. A victim of a gunshot wound may curse and yell at the resuscitation team as they provide care. A confused patient with meningitis may tell the nurse to get away, while thrashing and fighting. An intoxicated patient may violently attack the doctor who attempts an examination. Medical conditions such as hypoglycemia, encephalopathy, hypoxemia, and others can make patients impulsive, restless, angry, and antagonistic, so there may be confusion regarding the patient's ability to reason. Some patients without medical concern are angry, antagonistic, and oppose the treatment team. Although the physician must respect autonomy, the objection can, and must, be respected if decisional capacity is present. Limited treatment must proceed when capacity is impaired. Allowing a patient to refuse care when the refusal is not informed may create ethical and legal liability. If there is uncertainty, care must be delivered only to preserve life and health, attempting to optimize decisional capacity.

The criteria for refusal are more strict than those for consent (13,14). Refusal cannot be implied either in fact or in law, because the special knowledge in the situation is held by the physician and not the patient. When a physician "suggests" a medical event (e.g., taking a blood pressure), the patient may give implied consent in fact or in law, because the physician is presumed to be the expert and is therefore in possession of special knowledge that the suggested event is proper and appropriate. The converse is not true. If a physician "suggests" an event and the patient attempts to refuse in any way, that refusal cannot be assumed to be informed. If, for example, the physician asks to take a blood pressure and the patient withdraws his or her arm instead of extending it, a reasonable observer may feel that consent had been refused, but the observer would not likely understand *why* the event was refused. Therefore, only a fully informed patient can refuse suggested treatment. The caregiver must explain. This requires that the patient understand the consequences of the refusal and of failing to follow the recommended course of treatment (11).

Informed refusal may apply to a specific test or treatment (e.g., a rectal examination or lumbar puncture), to any further care (e.g., a patient asking to leave during care or refusing admission to the hospital), or to a portion of the physician's plan of therapy (e.g., follow-up appointments, prescribed medications, or use of seat belts). The discharge of patients from the ED, even if amicable and mutually acceptable, should include a formal process in that the patient must understand the reasonable consequences of refusing to follow the discharge instructions. The information, understanding, and reasoning should be documented.

Physician Liability Related to Consent

Expert testimony is not needed to support claims of lack of informed consent and battery arising out of a medical procedure. If the patient should claim that consent was not obtained, he or she would not need to show that the procedure was the cause of any injury, nor that the procedure was performed in a substandard manner, but only that it was performed at all and had not been consented to. In order to prevail, the physician must be able to show that the patient was informed of and understood known risks and those risks material to the particular patient.

There are exceptions to the informed consent rule, however. A physician does not need to disclose to the patient those risks that are generally known to the public or those risks that are too remote to be considered actual risks and would cause the patient to refuse necessary treatment. In an emergency, as noted previously, the physician may render lifesaving care without obtaining consent, and the physician may not disclose some material facts if he or she believes that the disclosure poses a threat to the patient's well-being.

"Do not Resuscitate" Orders

Often, patients wish to ensure that no unwanted interventions are performed at or near the end of life. In order to enable a refusal of care when patients are no longer competent to do so, "do not resuscitate" (DNR) orders have been implemented. Unfortunately, this has not always promoted clarity. The words DNR have different meanings. American Heart Association (AHA) standards suggest that DNR orders are appropriate for a patient who is "irreversibly, irreparably ill, whose death is imminent; . . ."(3,15). By irreversible, it is meant that there are no known therapeutic measures that would be effective in reversing the course of the illness. Irreparable means the time has been reached when the course of the illness has progressed beyond the capacity of existing knowledge and technique to stem it. Imminent death is defined as death occurring with reasonable probability within 2 weeks of the time that the DNR order is written. This narrow definition is not held by all physicians. Many believe that a patient's instruction to withhold resuscitative efforts should be honored if the patient suffers from any severe impairment. Patient's with Alzheimers disease, progressive cancer, debilitation as a result of advanced age, or a condition that results in significant impairment, may not want resuscitative efforts at the time of their death. If the patient has a clear, valid, applicable directive that specifies what interventions should not be delivered, most physicians would likely honor it, with good ethical justification.

Additional challenges surround portability of directives, because unfamiliar paperwork may be presented to the emergency physician. A photocopy of a DNR directive from the nursing orders of a long term care facility, signed by an unfamiliar physician, may accompany a patient transferred to the ED. Such a directive may have no legal authority, but it may have ethical importance if it reflects the patient's enduring wishes. Many emergency physicians would rightfully take this information as evidence of the patient's desires, confirm the directive with family, and withhold aggressive resuscitation attempts. Some emergency physicians may find the paperwork uncertain and begin life sustaining intervention. The unique details of each situation will dictate what is ethically correct. When there is doubt surrounding patient desires, care should be delivered. When there is good information of enduring, applicable wishes, they should be honored.

Advance Directives

In order to understand and promote the patient's values and goals, health care proxies and other means for expressing personal wishes have been devised. Hospitals are required to have mechanisms in place for patients to express therapy-limiting decisions and to ensure that this information is available to health care providers, even though the utility remains uncertain (16). The tools available to patients and physicians vary by state (6). This can result in problems with legal recognition and portability of documentation. For example, a patient who resides in Minnesota and has a specific, valid living will may be vacationing in Massachusetts, in which living wills are not legally recognized. Another problem, the applicability of a directive, may result from unforeseen circumstances. For example, a cancer patient who made a decision in conjunction with her treating physician to sign a DNR form to forgo cardiopulmonary resuscitation and intubation should her heart stop beating, but who presents to the emergency room unconscious after a motor vehicle accident, presents a dilemma, especially if a relative demands "no heroics." The proper question from an ethical view is whether there is clear, sufficient, valid evidence of what the patient would want for this specific circumstance. If there is doubt, then resuscitative attempts should proceed. As additional information is gained both about the medical condition and the patient's enduring wishes, goals, and values, ongoing treatment can be modified. Decisions might differ whether the patient is found to have an easily correctable condition or injuries that predict an overwhelming risk of imminent death. Relevant information must be incorporated into the decision making process and shared with the patient and family, in order to achieve the best possible resolution.

The *Uniform Durable Power of Attorney Act* permits a competent individual to appoint an "attorney-in-fact," a legally authorized surrogate, for health care decisions (4,17,23,24). The surrogate may then authorize medical treatment if and when the patient becomes incompetent. The Act does not specify whether the surrogate may demand that treatment be withheld or withdrawn, especially if the treatment is arguably beneficial or lifesaving (1). Still, this person may be able to provide evidence of patient wishes if and when there are important questions or concerns.

A legal *health care proxy* enables a named other individual to make medical decisions when the patient is incompetent, often in cooperation with the patient's physician. At the time of emergency, the named proxy may or may not be available. Relying on family members who are not the proxy, but who are present, may be problematic. Family members and significantly involved others often disagree about treatment decisions. The emergency physician should ask if the patient has a legally designated proxy decision-maker, clarify roles and relationships of those expressing opinions, and document the input received. If there is conflict, if the official proxy is unavailable, or if the emergency physician identifies uncertainty because of sudden or unusual medical circumstances, it is appropriate to deliver care so that decision-making can be clarified. Alternatively, if an authorized proxy requests that treatment be withdrawn, this desire can be honored when there is no uncertainty or conflict and when the decision would be concordant with the patient's understood desires.

Living wills are legal instruments in which patients specify desires for the future, in the event that specified medical conditions develop. No proxy decision-maker is necessary, the document can speak for the patient. Nearly all states have enacted some version of a living will statute. Only Massachusetts, Pennsylvania, Michigan, and Nebraska have not yet provided for living wills. Almost all living will statutes include three basic provisions: directive language, immunity clauses, and pregnancy clauses (2,17). In some jurisdictions, a living will is a mandatory directive, and health care providers who fail either to follow a legally authorized living will or to transfer the patient to the care of another provider can be subject to disciplinary action. Immunity clauses are intended to protect the doctor from legal liability for withholding or withdrawing "life-sustaining" or "life-prolonging" treatment from a "terminal" patient or one whose directive is active and applicable. Any person, healthy or ill, can generate a living will, but applicability requires specific medical circumstances. Under the immediacy of an emergency situation, applicability may be uncertain.

Living wills may or may not be relevant in an emergency circumstance. If there is a DNR provision, then the directive might provide useful guidance, but generally phrased living wills are often not helpful, because relevant medical circumstance cannot usually be assured (16). If the patient is unable to participate in the decision-making process and is in the midst of an unusual or unanticipated medical crisis, it may not be clear what treatments to provide. It may take time to clarify the specifics, so treatment may be required. Because this directive stands on its own, without the involvement of a surrogate decision maker, there is potential for controversy when a family members disagrees with specifications in the living will. When the surrogate decision maker disagrees with a plan to limit treatment, most emergency physicians would properly deliver care. Decisions to limit care must be bolstered by clear and absolute information that the patient would not want the specific care in the specific circumstance.

Overcoming Problems with Advance Directives

When a surrogate or paper directive is clear, relevant, and applicable, it should be honored. When there is uncertainty, then attempts must be made to preserve life and health. There is no legal or ethical distinction between withdrawing unwanted care and not initiating the care at all. Although often difficult for caregivers, unwanted interventions can be withdrawn once there is sufficient knowledge regarding the patient's wishes for the circumstance.

The problem of rapidly determining the validity of a variety of legal documents will not be resolved unless and until there is a readily recognizable and standard format adopted. A simple, portable, widely available, clear form (paper or electronic) that is recognizable across health care settings would benefit all. The caregiver would certainly have to validate patient identity and potentially confirm applicability, but format consistency would provide an important step forward toward honoring patient wishes.

COMMUNICATION, PRIVACY, AND CONFIDENTIALITY

Patient privacy, the physical and psychological condition of appropriate separation from others, is both deserved by patients, a challenge for caregivers, and sometimes impossible in a busy, crowded ED. A patient's right to physical, auditory, and visual privacy is violated under the pressing conditions of uncontrollable inflow of ill patients, and physical space limitations. Care is routinely provided in hallways, patients may be separated by inches or feet, and critical medical tasks take priority over important privacy needs. Both patients and caregivers experience stress from crowding, compounding the medical demands. Under such conditions, physical and auditory privacy is easily and frequently undermined. Sometimes, loss of privacy is unavoidable given the physical conditions and environment. Privacy must also be balanced against safety and efficiency. A highly private environment does not allow for visual monitoring by nurses and doctors and may impair efficiency. A balance exists between privacy on the one side and safety and efficiency on the other. Unfortunately, both privacy and safety and efficiency can be compromised at times of excessive crowding. The ED, without limits on the number of patients requiring care, is a relatively unique environment. These circumstances test the caregivers. Can patient privacy be valued in the face of overwhelming demands and a crowded environment? It is easy and perhaps understandable to argue that privacy can be neither expected nor maintained. The better position is to attempt to maintain the value. In the clinical environment, this may require softer voices during patient turnover at shift transitions, lowering voices when communicating with nurses and patients, and attempts to keep curtains fully drawn during examinations. These issues may seem small when lives are at stake, but they are meaningful ways to respect patients and demonstrate high ideals of the profession.

At the same time that patient privacy struggles continue, concerns of patient confidentiality must be addressed. This means that patient information should not be seen by anyone except those with a duty to care for the patient. Federal directive, based on the *Health Insurance Portability and Accountability Act* of 1996, provides specific instruction regarding confidentiality of a person's medical information. This rule applies to any and all who might encounter such information including doctors, nurses, secretaries, clerks, pharmacists, allied providers, insurance agencies, health plans, and businesses with transactional relationships with the health care system. Increased rigor of information management has resulted, affecting virtually every aspect of information sharing. Important attention should continue to be paid to the costs and burdens on health care providers, the ability of health care professionals to use and share full medical information when treating patients, the provision of patient care in a timely and efficient manner, and parents' access to information about the health of their children (7). The directive codifies the U.S. ethical value surrounding individual rights and protection of personal interests. This directive demands confidentiality of records, electronic transactions, and nonmedical use of information. At the same time, sharing information with loved ones at the time of the emergency and accessing critical clinical information from outside medical entities could be necessarily impeded. The patient is required to give permission prior to the sharing of any medical information. This might be impossible given the time constraints and clinical circumstances of emergency care. It is right to invigorate confidentiality, but the consequences are yet to be fully understood.

In the short term, it is prudent to remind all who work in the ED that they have knowledge of the patient's condition only because of their privileged position as a health care worker. Anything that they learn because of this role can never be shared, except with those who have a duty to the patient and a need to know.

TRUTHTELLING AND RELATIONSHIP-BUILDING

It may initially seem simplistic to discuss how to tell patients the truth, but it is not always so easy. The emergency physician and the patient do not have a preexisting relationship, do not know each other well, and may not share a mutual trust. In the busy ED,

it is difficult to spend sufficient time with patients and families so that a productive therapeutic relationship can be established. In the ED, then, first impressions do count. Without a trusting, truthful relationship, the care process breaks down. The truthful relationship begins with proper eye contact, prudent physical contact such as a handshake, attentive body language, and active listening. Elements of this relationship must be established quickly in the ED. The hurried physician may feel there is little time to establish this connection. These elements, however, are the essential core on which a satisfactory relationship is established. A grateful patient, a trusting family, an understanding person, requires at least a minimal amount of relationship building.

These aspects are important under all circumstances but more so when frightening results of diagnostic tests must be communicated or when bad news must be delivered. Perhaps more importantly, the trusting alliance must be established at the same time that information about mistakes are delivered. The patient and family must sense honesty in the language, openness in the posture, and integrity in the practice. Patients can often tolerate mistakes, but they will not tolerate physicians who do not care. Information regarding errors must be explained to the patient in the proper context, but must always be relayed. If the patient is unable or unwilling to engage in a conversation, the attempts should be noted on the record and plans for later communication should be made. Many patients are suspicious, untrusting, demanding, or even violent, even during the typical ED process. Telling of mistakes is all the more risky. It takes expertise to know how and when to communicate properly, a special skill of expert emergency physicians. Human impulse often makes physicians want to hide mistakes and run from adverse events, but if patients and families later find out about mistakes, trust is further eroded. Intellectually, this is obvious, but emotionally, and professionally, the challenge of open and trusting communication is great.

MINORS AND CONSENT

There are special operational and ethical challenges associated with the care of minors. It is important to understand the fundamental principle, namely that parents or legal guardians must consent for the care of the minor, with rare exception. The primary challenge for ED nurses and physicians is to determine when to deliver care without parental consent or before parental consent. Important care must not be delayed, but treatment must not be provided without consent. This paradox is evident daily. Should a teenager with a dislocated shoulder be made to wait until parents arrive? Should a child with a laceration be put on hold? Should the ED respect the wishes of an adolescent who requests that their parent not be told? The answers to each question is "it depends." It depends on the maturity of the minor, the immediacy of harm from delay, the risk of the intervention, the type of illness, and whether the minor is emancipated.

There are several important exceptions to the requirement for prospective parental consent. First is the presence of imminent harm if the minor is not treated. If a delay is dangerous to the life or health of the minor, essential treatment should be provided without delay. Only that care needed to preserve life and health should be administered. Parental contact remains necessary for continued care, even when the care is obviously needed. Second, if the minor is legally emancipated then parental consent is not required. Third, mature minor's opinions and preferences should be taken into account when making treatment decisions, commensurate with the minor's decisional capacity, their ability to understand and appreciate the consequences of their decisions (20,22).

Emancipated minors have a different legal status than that of other minors, as defined by state law. Emancipated minors are able to consent for their own health care because of some condition that warrants their ability to make an independent decision. Although state laws differ, in general, minors are considered emancipated for the following reasons:

- Marital status. The minor is married, divorced, separated, or widowed.
- The nature of his or her physical condition. The patient believes that she is pregnant or he or she believes himself or herself to be suffering from or to have come into contact with any disease defined as a danger to public health, such as a sexually transmitted disease.
- Legal or financial status. The patient is either living on her or his own or is financially independent.
- The minor is a member of the armed forces.
- The minor is a parent.

A special category of minor who may be able to offer limited consent for their own care is the *mature minor*. The mature minor is emotionally and intellectually mature enough to be capable of appreciating the nature of his or her illness or injury and the risks and benefits of proposed treatment. In some cases, a minor originally and incorrectly felt to be emancipated may meet the standards for mature minor status. It is recognized that mature minors may sometimes be able to provide consent, but sometimes also require parental involvement, depending on the nature of the medical condition. Including both the parents and mature minor in medical treatment decisions is optimal. At a time of conflict, the request or refusal of the mature minor must certainly be taken into account. Fundamentally, a minor is not generally able to refuse care, over a parent's objection when substantial harm will result. That said, circumstances could dictate that a mature minor's consent or refusal of essential care should be honored over a parent's objection. In these cases, ethical and legal involvement may be warranted. It is important to note that no unmarried minor can give consent for abortion or sterilization, even if otherwise mature or emancipated, although this is not usually an issue in the ED.

RELIGIOUS BELIEFS AND CONSENT

Some emergency physicians may experience conflict about Jehovah's Witnesses' belief that accepting i.v. blood or blood products is against biblical teaching (8). Under usual circumstances, there should be no difficulty. Jehovah's Witnesses believe that willfully taking blood severs the relationship with God and may eliminate the opportunity to achieve everlasting life. When expressed by an adult with intact decisional capacity, the request should be honored. This should not be misconstrued to mean that they are refusing care. In fact, full care is otherwise required. Ethically, any competent adult has the right to refuse any specific element of medical care, and the competent Jehovah's Witness who refuses necessary blood products is no exception, even if that refusal leads to his or her death. Jehovah's Witnesses value the trusting relationship with a physician, especially because they recognize that many physicians do not share their beliefs, so honest and open dialogue is encouraged.

Certain circumstances do present conflict. For example, competent adults do not have the right to make decisions that will harm their children, even when the decision is consistent with an enduring religious belief. Therefore, when parents refuse to consent to a lifesaving transfusion for their child, the transfusion may have to be administered despite the objection. States are able to intervene on behalf of children when an emergency exists and lifesaving care is being refused by parents. Temporary custody may be taken by the hospital for the duration of the crisis. This is because the state has an overriding interest in protecting the welfare of its citizens, especially those who are unable to care for themselves. Courts have also reasoned that they are unable to interfere in the religious beliefs of parents, but they may interfere with actions that impact minors, given just cause. From the point of view of Jehovah's Witnesses, the involuntary administration of blood is compounded by the violation of the parental bond. There is no easy solution to this dilemma.

RESTRAINTS

Use of physical restraints is common, especially when patients are violent and incoherent. When using restraints, the intent must be to provide for patient and caregiver safety. Restraint cannot be justified because a patient is disruptive, noncompliant, or even hostile. A medical professional can make a determination that a person presents an immediate risk, causing the patient to be restrained, but punitive intent or a decision to exercise control is always improper. Only sound medical indications warrant physical or chemical restraint. Caregivers must understand that the use of restraints, if unwarranted, can represent false imprisonment. This is an intentional tort whereby there is an unlawful (unjustified) restriction of a person's movement. This restriction may be either actual, when the patient is physically unable to move as a result of wrist and ankle restraints, spinal immobilization, or administered medications or apparent, when the patient believes that he or she is unable to move because of verbal warnings, the presence of guards, or a locked room. Because this is an intentional tort, the patient need only show that there was unjustified intent to confine and does not need to show that a damage occurred, as would be required if the suit were based in negligence. Therefore, use of restraints, even those typically thought of as splints or precautions, should be accompanied by justifying documentation.

Proper use of restraints include clear documentation regarding the reasons for use, provision of patient safety so that the person is not injured, and assurance of staff safety. Proper equipment and training is required, and sufficient personnel to maintain patient observation. The degree of care owed to the patient is related to the patient's own ability to provide for his or her own safety. Because restrained persons are unable to care for themselves and are possibly impulsive or delusional, safety must be assured. Most centers administer sedative medication aggressively and remove restraints once the person has demonstrated clearly that they will remain calmed. Often this means that the patient will be asleep. Patients are often uncomfortable with the feeling that they are out of control and, although never expressed during the crisis, often appreciate early medical intervention. Physical restraint heightens the anxiety and tension; they should be used while the patient is being sedated but removed as soon as the physician believes that the patient is acting in a safe manner.

USE OF THE NEWLY DEAD FOR TEACHING PURPOSES

Emergency physicians must develop and maintain expertise in a wide array of procedural skills, some of which are rarely performed. Many training programs taught procedures on patients who were pronounced dead in the ED. In the recent past, it was assumed that there was a broad societal obligation to support the training of physicians and that deceased patients enabled critical training, obtainable in no other way. The tactile accuracy, accessible teaching opportunity, and situational realism enabled the development of expertise for young physicians who would soon have full responsibility to perform the lifesaving skill. For these reasons, the teaching was conducted. In the past, however, the teaching was performed without the awareness or permission of the family. For this reason, discussion, deliberation, and debate regarding the practice has arisen.

Some of the debate surrounding procedural teaching on the recently deceased focused on the type of procedure being taught. Needle insertion, incision, and physical inspection were considered variably acceptable, based primarily on the degree of invasiveness. Therefore endotracheal intubation might be considered relatively more acceptable, because it was not disfiguring, but cricothyrotomy might be deemed unacceptable. Although there may be some merit to such distinctions, the delineation has not been fully satisfactory.

The answer to this dilemma is rooted in the core ethical obligation of the profession. Physicians must maintain the trust of the individual and the public. The transformation of a person from a patient to a teaching tool seems contrary to the requirement to maintain trust. Therefore, family permission is encouraged prior to teaching invasive procedures. The Society for Academic Emergency Medicine (SAEM) has adopted a position that states: "Permission should be obtained from the family or next of kin prior to performing invasive procedures on newly deceased patients in the ED." SAEM goes on to explain, "The profession of emergency medicine is grounded in compassion, trust, integrity, and respect for others. All actions, policies, and positions must support such virtues" (19).

COMMON PITFALLS

✔ Failure to assess and document decisional capacity of patients who refuse care
✔ When encountering an advance directive, failure to ask, "does this represent clear, consistent, and valid evidence of what the patient would want for this specific circumstance?" If there is an affirmative response, the directive should be honored
✔ Failure to supportively communicate in order to optimize treatment for patients whether they consent or refuse care
✔ Failure to document patient's expressed wishes on the medical record
✔ Failure to document justification for the use of physical or chemical restraints

Acknowledgment

We thank previous edition author Abigail R. Williams.

References

1. Durable power of attorney for health care. *Wests Annot Calif Codes Calif* Article 5 Sections 1985;2430–2444.
2. Medicare and Medicaid programs: Advance directives (HCFA), 60 *Federal Register* 123 (1995).
3. National Academy of Sciences—National Research Council. Standards and guidelines for Cardiopulmonary Resuscitation (CPR) and Emergency Cardiac Care (ECC) [published correction appears in *JAMA* 1986;256(13):1727]. *JAMA* 1986;255(21):2905–2989.
4. [No authors listed]. The durable power of attorney for health care. *Ohio Med* 1989;85(11):877–881.
5. Derse AR. Law and ethics in emergency medicine. *Emerg Med Clin North Am* 1999;17(2):307–25, ix.
6. Dixon G. Durable power of attorney for health care. Legislature enacts specific format and guidelines. *Minn Med* 1993;76(7):23–25.
7. Gostin LO. National health information privacy: Regulations under the Health Insurance Portability and Accountability Act. *JAMA* 2001;285(23):3015–3021.
8. Guertler AT. The clinical practice of emergency medicine. *Emerg Med Clin North Am* 1997;15(2):303–313.
9. Hodgkinson DW, Gray AJ, Dalal B, et al. Doctors' legal position in treating temporarily incompetent patients. *BMJ* 1995;311(6997):115–118.
10. *Canterbury v Spence*, 464 F2d 772 (DC Cir 1972).
11. Larkin GL, Marco CA, Abbott JT. Emergency determination of decision-making capacity: Balancing autonomy and beneficence in the emergency department. *Acad Emerg Med* 2001;8(3):282–284.
12. Moskop JC. Informed consent in the emergency department. *Emerg Med Clin North Am* 1999;17(2):327–340, ix–x.
13. Naess AC, Foerde R, Steen PA. Patient autonomy in emergency medicine. *Med Health Care Philos* 2001;4(1):71–77.
14. Palmer RB, Iserson KV. The critical patient who refuses treatment: An ethical dilemma. *J Emerg Med* 1997;15(5):729–733.
15. Paris JJ, Reardon FE. The AMA's guidelines on DNR policy: Conflict over patient autonomy, family consent and physician responsibility. *Clinical Ethics Rep* 1991;5(2):1–7.
16. Schneiderman LJ, Pearlman RA, Kaplan RM, et al. Relationship of general advance directive instructions to specific life-sustaining treatment preferences in patients with serious illness. *Arch Intern Med* 1992;152(10):2114–2122.
17. Siner DA. Advance directives in emergency medicine: Medical, legal, and ethical implications. *Ann Emerg Med* 1989;18(12):1364–1369.
18. Smithline HA, Mader TJ, Crenshaw BJ. Do patients with acute medical conditions have the capacity to give informed consent for emergency medicine research? *Acad Emerg Med* 1999;6(8):776–780.
19. Society for Academic Emergency Medicine, position statement. Procedures on the Newly Deceased. Academic Emergency Medicine 2004;11(9). In press.
20. Sullivan DJ. Minors and emergency medicine. *Emerg Med Clin North Am* 1993;11(4):841–851.
21. Thewes J, FitzGerald D, Sulmasy DP. Informed consent in emergency medicine: Ethics under fire. *Emerg Med Clin North Am* 1996;14(1):245–254.
22. Tsai AK, Schafermeyer RW, Kalifon D, et al. Evaluation and treatment of minors: Reference on consent. *Ann Emerg Med* 1993;22(7):1211–1217.
23. Wencel S. Power of attorney for health care. *Wis Med J* 1990 Oct;89(10):593–5.
24. Winslade WJ, Ross JW, Towers B. California's durable power of attorney for health care. *Mobius* 1984;4(2):83–86.

CHAPTER 365
Legal Issues

Howard A. Peth, Jr.

The interface between law and medicine is never greater than in the specialty of emergency medicine. Because emergency medicine is an ultra-high risk enterprise, the professional liability exposure within the specialty is considerable. This nexus is further underscored by the many federal and state regulations affecting the specialty. It is not necessary or practical for emergency physicians to be experts in the law. On the other hand, there are several predictable legal challenges that emergency physicians face and so it is particularly important to be familiar with the following legal issues: professional liability; emergency consent with an emphasis on the management of treatment refusals; and the law governing the transfer of patients from the emergency department. Chapter 366, "Regulatory Issues," provides more information.

PROFESSIONAL LIABILITY

The emergency department is the hospital entity with the highest incidence of adverse patient events as a result of negligence (1), and emergency medicine is recognized as one of the highest-risk specialties in medicine. The reasons for this are very complex. There are many systems vulnerabilities inherent in the practice of emergency medicine and these systems defects set the stage for a potentially large number of adverse events (2,3,4). Although most of these systems defects are neutralized by human conduct (5), a small percentage of adverse patient events will inevitably occur. The emergency physician is often the final common pathway along a complex cascade of events leading to an adverse patient outcome, which may result in a professional liability action against the physician.

Elements of a Professional Liability Action

The four elements of a professional liability action (medical malpractice claim) against an emergency physician are duty, breach, causation, and damages. In a professional liability action against an emergency physician the plaintiff must prove that (a) the emergency physician owed the patient a duty of reasonable care to conform to a certain standard of conduct; (b) the physician breached that duty; (c) there is a causal connection between the physician's conduct and the resulting injury to the plaintiff (i.e., legal or "proximate" cause); and (d) there is an actual injury (or damages) to the patient (6).

Negligence and Standard of Care

Negligence is defined as the "failure to use such care as a reasonably prudent and careful person would use under similar circumstances; it is the doing of some act which a person of ordinary prudence would not have done under similar circumstances or failure to do what a person of ordinary prudence would have done under similar circumstances" (7). Negligence consists of a breach of the duty to adhere to a concept known as the "standard of care." The traditional measure of the standard of care for physicians was articulated in 1902 and requires that a physician exercise the "average degree of skill, care, and diligence exercised by members of the same profession, practicing in the same or similar locality in light of the present state of medical and surgical science" (8). The "locality" rule has since expanded into a national standard of practice as a result of advances in modern medical education and training, medical journals that now reach a national audience, and continuing medical education courses that operate at the national level.

Negligence is a very complex concept and it is the subject of rather bitter dispute in virtually every professional liability action. The causation element of a professional liability action is also extremely complex and strenuously contested because bad outcomes frequently accompany serious disease processes in the absence of negligence. The courts depend on expert medical opinion testimony to assist the jury in determining whether a physician's conduct was negligent and, if so, in determining whether the alleged negligent conduct was the legal or proximate cause of the patient's injury.

Failure to Diagnose

Most professional liability actions against emergency physicians arise under allegations of a failure to diagnose a serious emergency medical condition in a timely manner. The following ultra-high-risk presentations account for more than 70% of professional liability claims against emergency physicians: chest pain, abdominal pain, febrile infants, headache, and specific high-risk wounds and orthopaedic injuries (9,10,11). Several factors account for the high liability risk associated with these presentations. First, benign and catastrophic conditions commonly share ambiguous signs and symptoms and on initial presentation the seriousness of a patient's complaint may be not be apparent to the emergency physician. Second, many high-risk conditions have atypical presentations that can divert the emergency physician's

focus from the catastrophic diagnosis. Atypical presentations may occur with any disease process but they are particularly prevalent at both extremes of age. As a result of either one or both of the previous factors, the emergency physician may not order a particular diagnostic test that would ordinarily have been routine had the atypical presentation been more classic. Other factors are known to contribute to the delayed critical diagnosis but these are beyond the scope of this chapter. A familiarity with the various atypical manifestations of the high-risk diagnosis can be indispensable to the emergency physician and it is highly worthwhile for the reader to review these presentations in the High-Risk Chief Complaint section of this text, and in the emergency medicine literature (12).

Generic Allegations in Professional Liability Actions

The generic allegations against emergency physicians in professional liability actions (medical malpractice claims) are: (a) a failure to order a particular diagnostic test; (b) a failure to properly interpret the results of a diagnostic test; (c) a failure to obtain a consult; and (d) a failure to admit the patient. In making each of the above allegations, plaintiffs' attorneys are aided by a phenomenon first described by cognitive psychologists known as *hindsight bias*. Hindsight bias describes how knowledge of a particular adverse outcome may bias an observer's perspective of a complex series of events such that a person who has knowledge of the adverse event cannot, in hindsight, maintain an unbiased view of the reasons for the adverse event (13). Hindsight bias creates a "knew it all along" effect in which observers of past events exaggerate what other people should have been able to anticipate in foresight (14). However elusive the patient's diagnosis on initial presentation, it appears deceptively simple to those with knowledge of the adverse event acquired in hindsight. Jurors are prohibited from using knowledge based on hindsight in their deliberations and are so instructed in their jury instructions. However, as a result of the hindsight bias effect inherent in these cases, anyone with knowledge of the adverse outcome will know exactly what diagnostic test or treatment the emergency physician should have ordered and improperly impute that knowledge to the physician. It is a small step for jurors armed with hindsight to proceed to the erroneous conclusion that a physician's failure to order a particular test or treatment course constituted negligence and hold the physician liable to the patient.

CONSENT ISSUES IN EMERGENCY MEDICINE

The General Consent Rule

In general, physicians may proceed with the evaluation and treatment of their patients only after obtaining the patient's permission or consent (15). Justice Benjamin Cardozo first articulated the basis of our modern consent theory nearly 100 years ago as follows: "Every human being of adult years and sound mind has the right to determine what shall be done with his [or her] body" (16). There are five varieties of consent important in medical practice (general consent, specific consent, informed consent, implied consent, and emergency implied consent) and each one has a role to play in the field of emergency medicine.

General consent is the type of consent emergency department clerical personnel obtain when a patient signs in that permits clinical personnel to evaluate the patient. Triage, taking vital signs, connecting the patient to a monitor, obtaining a history and physical, performing basic diagnostic tests (i.e., laboratory tests, electrocardiograms, and x-rays), and initiating noninvasive (or minimally invasive) treatment are all activities covered under a general consent. A general consent is not informed, and very little if any discussion about the nature of the patient's illness or diagnostic and treatment plan occurs with this type of consent. The scope of general consent is broad and allows the physician or nurse to perform a wide variety of actions on the patient's behalf. General consent is inadequate for procedures or tests that may be associated with a substantial risk of harm or injury to the patient.

Specific consent is obtained when a specific, often invasive, diagnostic test or therapeutic procedure is planned that may carry some risk to the patient. Examples include lumbar punctures, insertion of central lines, and surgery. When obtaining a specific consent to perform a test or other invasive intervention, the clinician should observe the usual formalities associated with seeking a patient's fully informed consent, discussed below. The scope of a patient's specific consent is narrowly tailored to a specific procedure and this type of consent may not be extended to other interventions not covered by the consent.

Informed consent is a patient's competent, voluntary, and understanding permission to proceed with the physician's proposed treatment. Obtaining a patient's informed consent is a dynamic process in which the physician provides the patient with information that will assist the patient in making an informed decision about the recommended treatment. The physician should disclose to the patient: (a) the indications for, and the nature of, the recommended treatment, (b) the risks associated with the recommended treatment, (c) the risks associated with not having the treatment, (d) any available alternative treatments (including no treatment) and (e) the risks associated with the alternative treatments. During the process of obtaining informed consent, the patient is given an opportunity to ask questions that are answered to his or her satisfaction. The act of merely asking a patient to sign a standardized form without the above discussion is not consistent with a properly executed informed consent and it wise to remember that obtaining a patient's informed consent is a process and not a paper.

Implied consent is a consent in which a patient's conduct would lead the physician or nurse to believe that he or she has the patient's permission to proceed with treatment. The time-honored example is of the patient who waits in line at the immunization clinic and when it is her turn to receive an immunization rolls up her sleeve and raises her arm to accept the immunization. In the emergency department, implied consent may occur when a patient with a laceration gets onto a gurney and presents the injured area to the physician for suturing without signing the usual consent forms for general or specific consent. Implied consent follows none of the usual formalities associated with the above consent types and it may create ambiguities regarding what the patient's actual intentions are. Implied consent is not informed.

Emergency implied consent allows emergency physicians to treat patients who are unable to provide consent for treatment of life-threatening illnesses. Many patients who are seen in emergency departments are unable to provide any of the above types of consent as a result of their conditions. Examples are patients who are suffering from intracranial injuries, diabetic ketoacidosis, septic shock, cardiac arrest, intoxication, and myriad other conditions, and who require emergent treatment for their illness or injury. Such patients are obviously in no condition to provide consent for emergency treatment, without which they may suffer serious adverse consequences. To avoid such tragic consequences, the law has created a legal fiction known as the emergency exception to the general consent rule that allows emergency medical personnel, including paramedics and emergency medical technicians in the field, to provide necessary stabilizing treatment on the patient's behalf. Three requirements must be met in order for the so-called "emergency privilege" to apply:

> (a) the patient must be unconscious or without capacity to make a decision, although no one legally authorized to act as an agent for the patient is available;
>
> (b) time must be of the essence, in the sense that it must reasonably appear that delay until such time as an effective consent could be obtained would subject the patient to a risk of a serious bodily injury or death which prompt action would avoid; and
>
> (c) under the circumstances, a reasonable person would consent, and the probabilities are that the patient would consent (17).

If there is any doubt regarding whether the emergency consent doctrine applies, it is best to err on the side of treatment and obtain the patient's (or the appropriate surrogate's) consent later but at the earliest opportune moment.

Refusals of Treatment

Patients who are brought to the emergency department and who refuse treatment are virtually guaranteed that their diagnosis will be missed and the danger of an adverse event in this setting cannot be overstated. It is incumbent on the emergency physician to ensure that the patient's treatment refusal is an informed refusal and based on a clear understanding of the associated risks. It is important to be aware that many patients who refuse treatment in the emergency department are suffering from an organic condition that impairs their sensorium and a delay in making the diagnosis can end in catastrophe.

The corollary to the informed consent theory is the doctrine of informed refusal. Just as a patient's informed consent must be based on knowledge of the material elements vital to an understanding and informed decision, so too must a patient's refusal of medical treatment be fully informed and based on a full understanding of the risks associated with that refusal (18).

In order for patients to provide a valid refusal they must be legally *competent* to do so and they must possess adequate decision-making *capacity*.

Competency

Competency is a legal concept and under the law all adult persons are presumed to be legally competent. A person may be declared incompetent only in the setting of a formal judicial proceeding in which a judge hears testimony from expert witnesses, usually psychiatrists or neurologists. If the judge determines by clear and convincing evidence that a person is mentally incompetent, a conservator or guardian is appointed by the court to manage the person's affairs. Once a person has been declared incompetent, he or she may not consent to or refuse treatment and only the court-appointed conservator or guardian ad litem may legally consent on the person's behalf. Minors, with some exceptions noted below, are legally incompetent and may neither consent to nor refuse treatment.

Capacity

Capacity is a medical concept and is the basis by which physicians determine whether patients are capable of understanding the nature of their disease and the ramifications of accepting or refusing treatment (19). The physician should ascertain the decision-making capacity of every patient who refuses treatment by performing a mental status examination and by inquiring regarding whether the patient has a full understanding of the nature of the illness and the risks associated with forgoing treatment (20). Patients who have adequate decision-making capacity and who understand the treatment recommendations of their physicians may refuse treatment, even if their refusal may result in death (21). If the physician determines that the patient does not have adequate decision-making capacity on the basis of the mental status examination and other information, the patient's refusal should be rejected and treatment should be initiated under the emergency consent doctrine.

Patients Who Leave Against Medical Advice

Physicians must carefully document in the medical record the basis for accepting a patient's treatment refusal and clearly indicate that the patient possessed adequate decision-making capacity based on a mental status examination (which is also carefully documented) and that all of the pertinent risks were fully explained to and understood by the patient. The patient should sign the hospital's "Leaving Against Medical Advice" (LAMA) form according to hospital policy. Signing the LAMA form memorializes the fact that the patient is refusing to accept the physician's recommendation that additional testing or treatment is indicated. The LAMA form also adds formality and solemnity to the patient's act of refusing treatment, which can prompt the patient to rethink the wisdom of his or her refusal. The LAMA form does not replace a physician's carefully drafted progress note documenting that the patient who has refused treatment possessed adequate decision-making capacity and was able to articulate understanding of the associated risks, which were fully explained. All patients who refuse emergency treatment must be given appropriate discharge instructions informing them to return to the emergency department immediately if they change their minds about treatment and when and where to go for follow-up. On the other hand, patients may not refuse emergency medical treatment if they do not possess decision-making capacity. Once the emergency physician has clinically determined that a patient does not have adequate decision-making capacity the physician must reject the patient's refusal, carefully document the basis for making that determination, and proceed with treatment on the basis of the emergency consent doctrine.

Finally, the emergency physician should not substitute his or her value system for the patient's value system. Physicians may not agree with their patients' decisions regarding emergency treatment but they must accept their patients' decisions if their patients have demonstrated adequate decision-making capacity and are able to articulate understanding of the associated risks.

Special Consent Issues

Issues of consent pertaining to surrogate decision makers and consent issues related to minors, psychiatric patients, prisoners, and intoxicated patients are other aspects with which the emergency physician should be familiar.

Advance Directives and Surrogate Decision Makers

An *advance directive* is a legal document that allows patients to notify their physicians of those therapeutic interventions they are willing to accept and those interventions they wish to forgo should they no longer possess adequate decision-making capacity to provide an informed consent to or refusal of treatment. The advance directive must be created while the individual executing the document is mentally competent. Advance directives permit patients to specify their wishes pertaining to a reasonably broad variety of treatment options. However, there is the possibility that a patient will later suffer from a medical condition that he or she did not contemplate or address at the time of executing the advance directive. In such cases, the patient's physicians may lack the guidance the patient had hoped the

advance directive would provide, giving rise to ambiguities regarding the patient's wishes. To address this deficiency, patients may appoint a "Durable Power of Attorney for Health Care" whereby the patient designates a *surrogate decision maker* who is legally authorized to consent to or refuse treatment on behalf of the patient. The durable power of attorney provision is triggered when a patient lacks decision-making capacity and when medical issues arise that are not adequately addressed in the patient's advance directive.

Unfortunately, few patients present to emergency departments with an advance directive in hand or with their designated durable power of attorney for health care in tow. If there is any question about whether to initiate or withhold emergency medical care pending delivery of a patient's advance directive, it is always wise to err on the side of providing treatment on the basis of the emergency consent doctrine until the issues related to the patient's advance directive or surrogate can be clarified.

Minors

The definition of "minor" is a person under the age of 18 years of age in all but a few states, and 19 years of age in the remaining states. With some exceptions, minors are not legally competent to provide consent for medical care and physicians ordinarily rely on the minor's surrogate, usually a parent, to obtain consent for treatment. Emergency medical care of a minor should never be withheld or delayed for lack of consent as unattended minor patients who suffer from emergency medical conditions meet the criteria for the emergency consent doctrine. Therefore, if a minor's surrogate is not immediately available, emergency physicians should initiate emergency treatment on the basis of the emergency consent doctrine and attempt to contact the surrogate as soon as practical. It should also be noted that the Emergency Medical Treatment and Active Labor Act (EMTALA) mandates that an emergency medical examination ("medical screening requirement") be performed on all patients who present to a hospital's emergency department and seek examination or treatment for a medical condition. Requesting the assistance of your hospital's social worker can be very helpful in contacting parents and documenting such efforts. If aggressive attempts to reach the minor's parents (or other appropriate surrogate) remain unsuccessful, the minor should be admitted to the hospital for protective custody irrespective of whether the medical condition warrants admission. In these cases, the social worker or physician should notify the state child protective services, who stand in the position of *parens patriae* regarding the child.

Certain classes of minors are legally competent to provide consent for treatment. Minors who live on their own, who are in the United States military, or who are pregnant or already a parent are *emancipated minors* and may legally consent to treatment. Minors who present for treatment for drug rehabilitation, for sexually transmitted diseases, or for pregnancy may also legally consent to treatment. You should be aware that state laws may differ and so it is wise to learn the specific laws governing the consent requirements pertaining to minors in your state.

A frequent issue that arises in the care of adolescents in the emergency department pertains to confidentiality of information elicited from the young patient or information generated during a diagnostic evaluation. It is widely accepted among emergency physicians and adolescent medicine specialists that candor vital to the adolescent's care is more forthcoming when the patient is assured of the confidentiality of the doctor-patient relationship. However, the provisions of the Health Insurance Portability and Accountability Act (HIPAA) allow access of medical records to parents of minor children, and physicians must be aware that only limited assurances of confidentiality are possible. The Act, however, does permit a licensed health care professional to deny parental access to medical records if he or she believes that the access requested is "reasonably likely to endanger the life or physical safety of the individual or another person" (22).

Psychiatric Patients

Patients with psychiatric disorders who possess adequate decision-making capacity may consent to or refuse treatment just as any other patient. There are two caveats to this general rule of which emergency physicians should be aware.

First, suicidal or homicidal patients who meet criteria for civil psychiatric commitment may not refuse treatment and they may not sign out of the hospital against medical advice. This rule includes patients who have actually proceeded with a suicide attempt or gesture and who are admitted to a medical service for stabilizing treatment prior to transfer to a psychiatric facility, irrespective of whether any formal civil commitment forms have been completed. Emergency treatment of a suicidal patient may proceed against the patient's wishes for as long as it takes to stabilize the patient medically. Also, state laws providing for the civil psychiatric commitment of suicidal patients expressly state that the legal basis of the commitment (the time frame of which varies by state but is usually 72–96 hours) is solely for the purpose of psychiatric evaluation, and not for the purpose of providing stabilizing medical treatment. Time devoted to the medical stabilization of postsuicide attempts or gestures is not included in the civil commitment time frame nor is the completion of a civil commitment form a condition necessary for the provision of emergency stabilizing treatment in such cases.

Second, some psychiatric patients have been declared mentally incompetent by a court order and placed under a conservatorship (in some states a guardianship). Any patient who has been declared mentally incompetent by a court may not legally consent to or refuse treatment and his or her court designated conservator or guardian ad litem should be contacted regarding medical treatment. Obviously, emergency medical treatment should not be delayed for lack of a consent and treatment should proceed on the basis of the emergency consent doctrine while efforts are made to contact the patient's conservator.

Prisoners

The right of prisoners and other patients in police custody to consent to or refuse emergency medical treatment does not differ from the nonprison patient population. When dealing with a prisoner who has refused emergency medical treatment, the physician should follow the usual guidelines pertaining to the management of treatment refusals that apply to the nonprison patient who has refused treatment. The prisoner's decision-making capacity must be carefully evaluated in the case of every treatment refusal and physicians should proceed to treat those who lack such capacity under the emergency consent doctrine. Although prisoners and those in police custody have the right to refuse medical treatment, they have no legal right to choose where they are incarcerated. A prisoner who has refused emergency medical treatment but who is suffering from a potentially significant medical condition may be admitted to the hospital's jail ward against his or her wishes at the request of law enforcement authorities responsible for the care of the prisoner.

Emergency physicians and nurses must also recognize that prisoners and others in police custody have an affirmative legal right to medical care under federal law and the failure to provide such care may be regarded by the courts as a violation of the prisoner's civil rights entitling the patient to monetary damages.

The Intoxicated Patient

Patients who are intoxicated present two primary challenges to emergency physicians. First, there is an increased risk that occult injuries, such as intracranial or spinal cord, will go undetected in a patient with an altered sensorium. Serial neurologic examinations may be nearly impossible to perform in the intoxicated patient and any deterioration in neurologic status, for example caused by a closed head injury, may be difficult to distinguish from alcohol-induced somnolence. Alcohol also impairs the ability to sense pain and an intoxicated patient with a spinal cord injury, for example, may deny having any neck pain by history or on examination. As a general principle, changes in an intoxicated patient's neurological status should be regarded as originating in the central nervous system until proved otherwise. Second, intoxicated patients are at increased risk of injury after discharge from the emergency department, and, if they attempt to drive, pose a hazard to the safety of others.

Although a blood alcohol level is useful under certain circumstances, it is not required to make a clinical determination that a patient is intoxicated and that treatment should be initiated against a patient's wishes. The emergency physician may determine that a patient is clinically sober or intoxicated based on the patient's conduct, mental status examination, speech, gait, and other elements of the physical examination. The physical examination findings that support a conclusion that the patient is either clinically sober or intoxicated should be documented in the record. Alcohol intoxication does not render a patient's treatment refusal invalid nor does it categorically indicate that the patient lacks decision-making capacity. Intoxication does, however, substantially lower the threshold for rejecting the patient's refusal and initiating treatment on the basis of the emergency consent doctrine. Intoxicated patients who are uncooperative or who verbally or physically refuse care are very difficult to evaluate and stabilize. An intoxicated patient cannot refuse emergency medical treatment or sign out against medical advice without exhibiting the ability to fully comprehend the risks associated with refusing treatment (23). The emergency physician is frequently confronted with the dilemma of accepting an intoxicated patient's treatment refusal and risking a delay in making the catastrophic diagnosis versus initiating treatment against the patient's wishes. In this situation the physician must assess the patient's ability to understand the risks and err on the side of treatment, if the patient's decision-making capacity is in doubt. Intoxicated patients represent the largest subgroup of restrained patients who require involuntary treatment orders (24).

Restraints

There are occasions when an emergency department patient who is suffering from a medical or psychiatric condition poses a risk to his own safety or to the safety of emergency department personnel and it is necessary to restrain him (25). The Center for Medicare and Medicaid Services (CMS) has adopted regulations pertaining to the use of restraint and seclusion as part of its conditions of participation, and hospitals must comply or risk losing their Medicare status. The CMS regulations state that any restraint of a patient cannot be punitive; that it respect the dignity of the patient; that less restrictive methods such as verbally calming the patient are attempted first, if possible; that frequent monitoring of the patient is performed; that the restraint of a patient is not extended beyond the time that restraint is no longer necessary; and that all orders for restraint and seclusion are signed by a physician (26).

Chemical restraint consists of using medication to control behavior or to restrict the patient's freedom of movement and is not a standard treatment for the patient's medical or psychiatric condition. A popular regimen is haloperidol 5 to 10 mg (intramuscularly [i.m.] or intravenously [i.v.]) or droperidol 2.5 mg to 5 mg (i.m. or i.v.) alone or in combination with lorazepam 2 to 4 mg i.m./i.v. This regimen has an excellent safety profile, although rarely some patients do experience dystonic reactions or orthostatic hypotension. See Chapter 123, "The Agitated or Violent Patient," for more information.

Some emergency physicians are reluctant to use droperidol in view of the black box warning issued by the Food and Drug Administration (FDA) in December 2001. Droperidol has long been known to cause cardiac dysrhythmias in high doses but little clinical significance was attached to this knowledge prior to the black box warning. When anecdotal reports of QT interval prolongation surfaced in the literature (27), the FDA issued a black box warning claiming that droperidol could cause serious cardiac events, including torsades des pointes and death. Clearly, adverse drug events remain a problem in emergency medicine and it is vital that emergency physicians and pharmacists remain vigilant in minimizing the risk to patients (28,29). The actual risks associated with droperidol use, however, are extremely remote and most clinicians familiar with the drug at the doses used in clinical practice have questioned the rationale of the FDA black box warning (30–32). A causal relationship between droperidol administration and sudden death is tenuous at best and based on uncontrolled anecdotal reports of twelve patient deaths. Droperidol remains a safe and effective drug in the emergency physician's pharmacopoeia.

Physical restraint ordinarily consists of using a mechanical device such as locking leather straps to restrict the patient's freedom of movement. This is most effective when applied by a team leader, who directs the team, and five team members, each of whom is responsible for restraining one extremity each and the torso, respectively. Great care must be employed to reduce the incidence of injury to the patient or to a staff member. Additionally, close patient monitoring and periodic assessment is required when physical restraint is employed. Patient deaths caused by asphyxiation have occurred when the prone position was used. Consequently, patients should always be restrained in the supine position.

The American College of Emergency Physicians' clinical policy pertaining to the use of patient restraints recommends the use of protocols to address observation and treatment during the period of restraint (33).

PATIENT TRANSFERS

A patient's transfer from one hospital to another represents the most vulnerable point along a continuum whereby any clinical deterioration en route will occur in the milieu of a lower level of clinical care. The Emergency Treatment and Active Labor Act (EMTALA) is the federal law that governs the transfer of patients from the emergency department (34). Under EMTALA, the transfer of an unstable patient to another facility is permitted if the following conditions are met: (a) the physician must certify that the expected benefits outweigh the risks; (b) the patient must consent to the transfer; (c) the receiving hospital agrees to accept the patient; (d) all of the patient's records are provided to the receiving hospital; and (e) the transfer employs qualified personnel and transportation equipment. EMTALA regulations pertaining to a patient transfer do not apply once the patient has been stabilized, nor does EMTALA apply to patients once they have been admitted even if they are later transferred (35). See Chapter 366, "Regulatory Issues," for more information.

COMMON PITFALLS

✔ Failure to educate patients about potential adverse outcomes and expected outcomes

✔ Failure to understand the concept of the right to refuse care and surrogate decision making

✔ Failure to carefully document in the medical record the basis for accepting a patient's treatment refusal

✔ Failure to document that all of the pertinent risks were fully explained to and understood by the patient who is leaving against medical advice

✔ Failure to document orders for and monitoring of physical restraints

Acknowledgment

We thank previous edition chapter author Abigail R. Williams, on whose chapters some of this was based.

References

1. Leape LL, Brennan TA, Laird N, et al. The nature of adverse events in hospitalized patients: results of the Harvard Medical Practice Study II. *N Engl J Med* 1991;324:377–384.
2. Cosby KS. A framework for classifying factors that contribute to error in the emergency department. *Ann Emerg Med* 2003;42:815–823.
3. Leape LL. Error in medicine. *JAMA* 1994;272:1851–1857.
4. Wears RL, Perry SJ. Human factors and ergonomics in the emergency department. *Ann Emerg Med* 2002;40:206–212.
5. Cook RI, Woods DD, Miller C. A tale of two stories: contrasting views on patient safety. National Patient Safety Foundation Conference, April 1998, Chicago. Available at www.npsf.org.
6. Keeton WP, Dobbs DB, Keeton RE, et al. *Prosser and Keeton on the law of torts,* 5th ed. St. Paul, Minnesota: West Publishing Co., 1984:164–165.
7. *Amoco Chemical Corp v Hill,* 318 A2d 614 (Del Super Ct 1974).
8. *Gillette v Tucker,* 65 NE 865 (1972).
9. Peth HA. Professional liability in emergency medicine. In: Sanbar S, ed. *Legal medicine,* 6th ed. St. Louis: Elsevier, 2004:468–473.
10. Henry GL, George JE. Specific high-risk clinical presentations. In: Henry GL, Sullivan DJ, eds. Emergency medicine risk management: a comprehensive review. Dallas: American College of Emergency Physicians, 1997:475–494.
11. Health Insurance Portability and Accountability Act (HIPAA) 45 CFR 164.524(a)(3)(i) (2000).
12. Peth HA, ed. High-Risk Presentations in Emergency Medicine. *Emerg Med Clin North Am* 2003.
13. Horowitz BZ, Bizovi K, Moreno R. Droperidol—behind the black box warning. *Acad Emerg Med* 2002;9:615–618.
14. Reason J. *Human error.* Cambridge, UK: Cambridge University Press, 1990.
15. *Cobbs v Grant,* 8 Cal. 3d 229 (Cal Sup Ct, 1972).
16. *Schloendorff v Society of New York Hospital,* 211 NY 125 (NY Ct App, 1914).
17. Keeton WP, Dobbs DB, Keeton RE, et al. *Prosser and Keeton on the law of torts,* 5th ed. St. Paul, MN: West Publishing, 1984:117.
18. *Truman v Thomas,* 27 Cal 3d 285 (1980).
19. Miller SS, Marin DB. Assessing capacity. *Emerg Med Clin North Am* 2000;233–242.
20. Etchells E, Darzins P, Silberfield M, et al. Assessment of patient capacity to consent to treatment. *J Gen Intern Med* 1999;14:27–34.
21. *Shine v Vega,* 429 Mass 456 (1999).
22. Karcz A, Korn R, Burke MC, et al. Malpractice claims against emergency physicians in Massachusetts: 1975–1993. *Am J Emerg Med* 1006;14:341–345.
23. *Miller v Rhode Island Hospital,* 625 A2d 778 (Sup Ct of Rhode Island, 1993).
24. Lavoie FW. Consent, involuntary treatment, and the use of force in an urban emergency department. *Ann Emerg Med* 1992;21:25–32.
25. Annas GJ. The last resort—the use of physical restraints in medical emergencies. *N Engl J Med* 1999;341:1408–1412.
26. Hospital Conditions of Participation. Patients' Rights 42 CFR 482 (1999).
27. Reilly JG, Ayis SA, Ferrier IN, et al. QTc-interval abnormalities and psychotropic drug therapy in psychiatric patients. *Lancet* 2000;355:1048–1052.
28. Peth HA. Medication errors in the emergency department: a systems approach to minimizing risk. In: Peth HA, (ed). High Risk Presentations in Emergency Medicine. *Emerg Med Clin North Am* 2003:141–158.
29. Roden DM. Drug-induced prolongation of the QT-interval. *N Engl J Med* 2004;350:1013–1022.
30. Chase PB, Biros MH. A retrospective review of the use and safety of droperidol in a large, high-risk, inner city emergency department patient population. *Acad Emerg Med* 2002;9:1402–1410.
31. Fischoff B. Hindsight does not equal foresight: the effect of outcome knowledge on judgment under uncertainty. *J Exper Psychol: Hum Perform Percept* 1975;1:288–299.

32. Shale JH, Shale CM, Mastin WD. A review of the safety and efficacy of droperidol for the rapid sedation of severely agitated and violent patients. *J Clin Psychiatry* 2003;64:500–505.

33. Policy Statements. Use of Patient Restraints. *Ann Emerg Med* 2001;38:199–200.

34. Emergency Medical Treatment and Active Labor Act (EMTALA) 42 USC 1395dd (1986).

35. Peth HA. The Emergency Medical Treatment and Active Labor Act (EMTALA): guidelines for compliance. In: Rice M, (ed). Emergency Department Administration and Management. *Emerg Med Clin North Am* 2004:225–240.

TABLE 366.1. JCAHO Functional Chapters
Chapter 1: Patient Rights and Organization Ethics
Chapter 2: Assessment of Patients
Chapter 3: Care of Patients
Chapter 4: Education of Patients and Family
Chapter 5: Continuum of care
Chapter 6: Improving Organization Performance
Chapter 7: Leadership
Chapter 8: Management of Environment of Care
Chapter 9: Management of Human Resources
Chapter 10: Management of Information
Chapter 11: Surveillance, Prevention, and Control of Infection

CHAPTER 366

Regulatory Issues

Jorge A. Martinez and Larry D. Weiss

The practice of medicine in the United States has become increasingly governed by state and federal regulations. Since 1965 the federal government has acted as a payer of health services through Medicaid and Medicare, through which it has issued numerous regulations governing the clinical and administrative practice of medicine. This chapter reviews the impact of the Joint Commission for the Accreditation of Healthcare Organizations, Emergency Medical Treatment and Active Labor Act, Health Insurance Portability and Accountability Act, and fraud and abuse legislation on the practice of emergency medicine.

JOINT COMMISSION FOR THE ACCREDITATION OF HEALTHCARE ORGANIZATIONS

In 1917 the American College of Surgeons (ACS) developed *Minimum Standards for Hospitals* establishing national standards for hospitals. In 1918 the ACS began on-site inspections of hospitals. In 1952 the ACS transferred its Hospital Standardization Program to the Joint Commission on Accreditation of Hospitals (JCAH), an independent nonprofit organization formed in 1951. In 1965 Congress established Medicare and provided that JCAH accreditation would certify that a hospital met conditions to participate in Medicare programs (10). In 1987, because its scope expanded to accrediting various types of health care organizations, it changed its name to the Joint Commission on Accreditation of Healthcare Organizations (JCAHO). In 1988 JCAHO began accrediting home care and managed care organizations. In 1994 it initiated health care networks certification, and in 1996 certification of ambulatory surgical centers began. The Health Care Financing Administration (HCFA) announced that JCAHO accreditation of these organizations would satisfy Medicare certification requirements.

JCAHO's *Accreditation Manual for Hospitals* includes eleven chapters containing standards necessary to maintain accreditation (Table 366.1). The intent of the standards is to promote appropriate medical care, protect patient safety, and enhance performance improvement within health care organizations. Over the last decade, JCAHO has established standards addressing such issues as pain management, restraint use, sentinel events, patient confidentiality, medication management, and adequate staffing. Approximately 50% of JCAHO standards relate to safety issues, including infection control, blood transfusion, restraint and seclusion, fire safety, and medical equipment.

Organizations must undergo JCAHO on-site accreditation every 3 years. Laboratories must be certified every 2 years. The 2004 JCAHO's *Shared Visions: New Pathways* initiative modifies its accreditation process placing more emphasis on safe and quality medical care, and less emphasis on rote compliance with standards. The accreditation process includes a periodic performance evaluation at eighteen months to assess compliance with JCAHO standards. The on-site survey reviews critical performance areas and track patients' treatment pathways within the organization. Unannounced random surveys will take place for all organizations by 2006.

Most JCAHO standards directly impact the emergency department (ED). For example, JCAHO requires an organization-wide, multidisciplinary policy regarding conscious sedation. Additionally, JCAHO requires a written restraint policy, including a restraint order form, which must be completed whenever a patient is restrained. JACHO also requires an organization-wide approach to pain management. The Sentinel Event Policy mandates organizations to identify adverse events and take corrective action to prevent their reoccurrence. Other standards involving the ED include patient safety, emergency and bioterrorism preparedness, best-practice identification, staff effectiveness and education, and emergency unit overcrowding. National Patient Safety Goals, effective January 1, 2004, were designed to enhance patient safety and prevent adverse outcomes. They include: (a) improving accuracy of patient identification; (b) improving communication among care givers; (c) improving safe use of high-alert medications, such as potassium chloride and 3% normal saline; (d) eliminating wrong site, wrong patient, wrong procedure surgery; (e) improving safety of infusion pumps; (f) improving effectiveness of clinical alarm systems; and (g) reducing the risk of health care-acquired infections.

THE EMERGENCY MEDICAL TREATMENT AND ACTIVE LABOR ACT

Until the 1960s, physicians and hospitals had no duty to provide medical care to patients requesting medical care. In situations in which an individual presented to a hospital ED for medical care without health insurance, no obligation existed requiring the hospital or its staff to provide medical care, even in emergencies. In 1946, Congress passed the Hill-Burton Act, which required hospitals to render emergency care if the hospital received federal funds (37). The majority of hospitals did not comply with the law. Nonetheless, litigation established that the failure to provide medical care, especially in emergency situations, could result in an action for negligence (15). In 1982, the Mississippi Supreme

Court ruled that if a patient presented to the ED for emergency care, and their condition deteriorated because therapy was delayed or denied as a result of a lack of ability to pay, the patient could bring a negligence action against the hospital (8). Courts also concluded that if a hospital held itself out as providing emergency care, a patient could reasonably rely on that representation (4). Courts also found that JCAHO standards established a duty to provide medical care (13). Eventually, the courts determined that hospitals had a duty to provide emergency care regardless of the ability to pay for it (7).

Despite the Hill-Burton Act and court decisions, hospitals continued to refuse to provide emergency care to those who could not pay for it. Hospitals simply refused to register, examine, or treat patients seeking emergency care without health insurance. Often, they refused to accept uninsured patients transported by local emergency medical services. Moreover, if after the patient arrived in the ED, it was determined that the patient did not have the means to pay for the medical care, services were suspended and the patient was transferred to another hospital with little or no medical care prior to the transfer. In many cases, the transferring ED did not contact the receiving ED to request a transfer, or to notify the ED that the patient was being transferred. It was not uncommon for a patient to arrive at a receiving ED without the staff knowing that the patient was being transferred; the reason for the transfer; the medical or surgical condition affecting the patient; or what treatment had been rendered prior to the transfer. The transfer of uninsured emergency patients to another facility because of the inability to pay for medical care became known as "patient dumping"(2).

In 1986, Congress enacted federal antidumping legislation, the Emergency Medical Treatment and Active Labor Act (EMTALA) (30). EMTALA was expanded in 1994 to require ED's to keep logs regarding individuals who came to the ED; to post signs in the ED informing individuals of their rights under EMTALA; to maintain physician on-call lists, and information on physicians who refused to provide timely treatment; to document an individual's refusal of treatment; and to inform HCFA if they were aware that a transferring facility had violated EMTALA (17). In 2000, HCFA declared that off-campus urgent care centers and on-campus clinics fell within EMTALA's purview (18). The 2003 Final Regulations, effective November 10, 2003, clarified definitions and provided guidance regarding EMTALA mandates (19).

EMTALA requires that any individual who presents to an ED seeking medical care must undergo a medical screening examination (MSE) designed to determine if the individual is suffering from an emergency medical condition (EMC). If the MSE reveals an EMC, the individual must be stabilized before being transferred. The evaluation and stabilization must be provided regardless of the individual's economic status or ability to pay for medical services. Furthermore, medical care may not be delayed to ascertain if the individual has health insurance (35).

The 2003 Final Regulations define a dedicated ED as any department or facility of a hospital, regardless of where it is located, if it is licensed as an emergency department; if it is held out to the public as a place that provides emergency care on an urgent basis without a scheduled appointment; or if one-third of its outpatient visits for emergency care occurred on an urgent basis without a scheduled appointment (22). The 2003 Final Rules also explain that an individual has come to the ED if (a) an individual presents to a dedicated ED or hospital property and requests an examination or treatment of a medical condition, a request is made on his behalf, or if a prudent layperson would believe that the individual needs an examination for or treatment of a medical condition, (b) an individual is transported by ground or air ambulance owned by the hospital, unless the ambulance is operating under community-wide protocols which directs the

transport of the individual to another hospital, or (c) an individual is transported by a nonhospital owned ambulance to the hospital's dedicated ED (22).

Medical Screening Examination

EMTALA's first mandate is that all individuals who present to the ED requesting emergency care must receive an MSE to determine whether an EMC exists. EMTALA does not define an MSE but does state that the MSE is based on the ED's capability, including ancillary services, such as diagnostic tests and specialty consultations typically available in the ED. An MSE is not triage, because it must include ancillary services (27). The MSE may not discriminate; it must be performed to the same extent for the same complaint for individuals who have insurance and those who do not (11). It may not be delayed in order to determine whether the individual has insurance coverage (24). A physician should perform the MSE, unless the hospital bylaws specifically authorize another level of provider (26). Finally, if the individual is admitted for treatment, the MSE requirement ends (20). In cases in which an individual is not seeking emergency care, a brief questioning by qualified personnel regarding the reason the individual presented to the ED will fulfill the MSE requirement (23).

Emergency Medical Condition

EMTALA defines an EMC as a medical condition manifesting as acute symptoms of sufficient severity (including severe pain, psychiatric disturbances, or substance abuse) such that the absence of immediate medical attention could result in placing the health of an individual or a pregnant woman or her unborn child in serious jeopardy; serious impairment to bodily functions; or serious dysfunction of any bodily organ or part (32). A pregnant woman having contractions is considered an EMC. The 2003 Final Regulations define labor as the process of childbirth beginning with the latent or early phase of labor and continuing through delivery of the placenta. A woman experiencing contractions is in true labor unless a physician clarifies, that, after a reasonable time of observation, the woman is in false labor (22).

Patient Stabilization

EMTALA's second mandate is that if an EMC exists, the individual must be stabilized before they can be transferred. Stabilization is defined as medical treatment necessary to assure, within reasonable medical probability, that no material deterioration will occur during the transfer of the individual from a facility, or that a pregnant woman having contractions delivers the child and placenta (22). Stabilization requires the provision of all necessary examination and treatment within the hospital's capabilities to stabilize the EMC and prevent any material deterioration (25). It does not require that the EMC be cured (3). Transfer is defined as the movement, including discharge, of a person outside the hospital's facilities. It does not include the movement of a person declared dead or who leaves the facility without permission (22).

EMTALA provides two exceptions to the rule that an EMC must be stabilized before transfer (28). First, a patient may request transfer to another institution before their EMC is stabilized. This request must be documented in writing on a transfer consent form. The signed transfer consent form verifies that the patient requested transfer and was informed of the risks of transfer. The patient may not be coerced into requesting a transfer because of the inability to pay for medical care. A copy of the signed transfer form must be sent with the patient. Second, a patient may also be transferred before being stabilized if the benefits of transfer outweigh the risks. For example, a patient with an open femur fracture presents to an ED that has no orthopaedic surgeon. The benefits of transferring the patient to a hospital with an orthopaedic surgeon would outweigh the risks of treating the injury without orthopaedic intervention. The physician must inform the patient of the reasons for the transfer, along with the benefits and risk of transfer. The patient must sign a transfer consent form confirming that they were given the information and agreed to the transfer. Importantly, the transferring ED must provide stabilization within its capabilities prior to transfer. A transfer to another ED for the convenience of an on-call physician does not fulfill the benefits versus risks analysis.

If a physician must transfer a patient before providing stabilizing treatment, specific steps must be taken (31). First, the physician must contact the receiving hospital and obtain approval for the transfer. Second, the patient's pertinent medical records and the signed transfer consent form must be sent. Third, an appropriate mode of transportation and personnel must be utilized to insure the patient's health and safety during transfer. Tertiary hospitals with specialized capabilities or facilities may not refuse to accept appropriate transfers if they have the capacity to treat the patient (29).

The 2003 Final Rules require hospitals to maintain an on-call list of physicians consistent with the needs of its patients and services available at the hospital. Hospitals must have policies addressing situations in which a particular specialty is not available or the on-call physician cannot respond. Hospitals must also assure that emergency services are available if its on-call physicians perform elective surgery while on-call, or if they schedule simultaneous on-call responsibilities at other hospitals (21).

EMTALA does not give rise to a federal medical malpractice action; its purpose is not to guarantee that all patients are properly diagnosed, or ensure that they receive adequate care (1). EMTALA simply protects patients from dumping, from improper screening for discriminatory reasons, and from failure to screen at all. Claims for faulty screening or negligence in screening or diagnosis are not actionable under EMTALA (12).

THE HEALTH INSURANCE PORTABILITY AND ACCOUNTABILITY ACT

Patient privacy and confidentiality is an essential part of the physician-patient relationship. Confidentiality is based on the right to privacy and autonomy in dealing with health care matters. Privacy has been defined as "the claim of individuals, groups, or institutions to determine for themselves when, how, and to what extent information about them is communicated to others" (14). Assurance of confidentiality and privacy encourages patients to seek medical care; fosters trust between patients and physicians; and prevents discrimination based on illness (6). Privacy and confidentiality of health information is a long-held moral and ethical obligation. The Hippocratic Oath states that whatever a physician learns from or about a patient is to be kept secret. The AMA's Code of Ethics maintains confidentiality as a patient right. Patient privacy and confidentiality has been upheld by the courts (5). Many states have enacted laws and patient bill of rights guaranteeing privacy and confidentiality of health information.

Assuring confidentiality of health information is often difficult as medicine becomes more technical, incorporates more specialties and paramedical providers, and involves regional or national institutions. Access to a patient's health information is essential to provide appropriate and comprehensive medical care. During treatment, a patient's health information is exposed to numerous health care providers, and support personnel and payers. It is not uncommon for persons not involved in the patient's medical care to obtain unauthorized access or exposure to health information. In 1993, Congress began to develop national standards for electronic health care transactions. In 1996, Congress enacted the Health Insurance Portability and Accountability Act (9).

The Health Insurance Portability and Accountability Act (HIPAA) consists of five titles: Health Insurance Access, Portability, and Renewal; Fraud and Abuse; Medical Savings Accounts; Group Health Plan Provisions; and Revenue Offset Provisions. The component of the HIPAA that most directly affects emergency physicians is *Administrative Simplification*, which deals with privacy and confidentiality of health information, and is contained in the Fraud and Abuse title. *Administrative Simplification* has four sections. The first section delineates codes and formats which must be used for all electronic health care transactions. The second section establishes unique identifiers for providers and payers. The third section mandates privacy and confidentiality of health care information, and security standards to prevent unauthorized access, alteration, destruction, or release of health information. The fourth section provides sanctions for HIPAA violations.

HIPAA governs any health care entity (HCE), public or private, that creates, stores, or transmits health information. Specifically, it regulates health care providers, health care plans, health care clearinghouses, and business associates. Health care providers include individual physicians, faculty practice groups, and hospitals. A health care clearinghouse is a public or private entity that processes or facilitates the exchange of health care data between health care providers and payers (38). Business associates include accountants, billing companies, collection agents or companies, practice managers, legal counsel, auditing firms, record copying services, and recycling services.

HIPAA provides rigid national standards for electronic health care transactions, including nine electronic data and transaction formats, and specific code sets for diagnosis, procedures, medications, and services. Providers and payers are required to use unique identifiers in all electronic transactions. HIPAA gives individuals more control over their health information by establishing standards to protect individuals' health information from unauthorized use, disclosure, or access. Privacy regulations went into effect on April 14, 2003. They apply to all information whether communicated, stored, or transmitted in oral, written, or electronic form. HIPAA also establishes security safeguards to protect health information. The privacy and security rules may be considered as a privacy triangle. The first angle of the privacy triangle explains how HCE's may use and disclose an individuals' health information. The second angle details privacy and security standards designed to safeguard the integrity, confidentiality, and availability of health information. The third angle grants specific rights to patients concerning their health information (Fig. 366.1).

Under HIPAA individual health information may only be utilized in specific manners and for specific reasons. HIPAA describes what health information is protected, the difference between use and disclosure, how information may be used or disclosed, the type of consent necessary for disclosure, and exceptions for disclosing information without authorization. Only the minimum information necessary to complete the action may be utilized. The rules do not restrict the use of information among doctors, nurses, or other health care providers evaluating or treating a patient.

Individually *Identifiable Health Information* is *protected health information* (PHI) under HIPAA. It includes all health information maintained or transmitted in any form, involving health information relating to an individual's health or mental condition, to

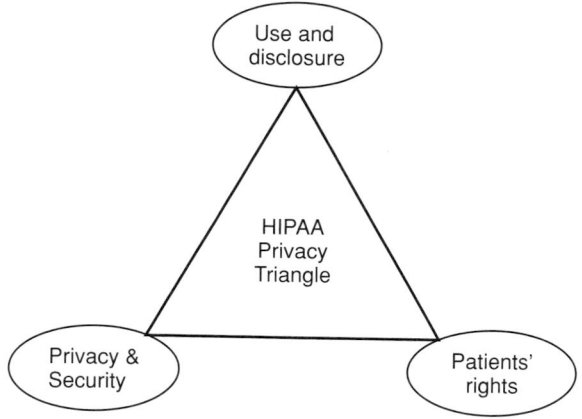

Figure 366.1. HIPAA Privacy Triangle.

TABLE 366.3. Examples of Disclosures Allowed Under HIPAA Without Authorization

- Judicial and administrative proceedings
- Reporting communicable diseases
- Required public health reporting, such as gunshot wounds, burns, dog bites
- Reporting victims of abuse, neglect, or domestic violence
- Identifying the body of a deceased person or cause of death
- Health care system oversight activities
- Law enforcement purposes
- Assisting in identifying or locating a suspect, fugitive, witness, or missing person
- Workers' compensation claims
- National defense and security

treatment, or to payment for treatment (Table 366.2). HIPAA defines the difference between use and disclosure of PHI. Use is defined as the sharing, employment, application, utilization, examination, or analysis of PHI within the HCE that maintains the PHI (39). Disclosure is the release of PHI to a person or agency outside of the HCE, such as the public, the press, or marketers (39).

In general, an HCE may use PHI for treatment, payment, and health care operations (TPO) without the individual's consent (41). Health care operations include such activities as quality assurance and quality improvement activities; credentialing; accreditation; certification; licensing; medical record review; legal services; auditing; fraud and abuse compliance; and business planning (39). HIPAA allows disclosure of PHI only if the individual gives authorization (42). However, certain exceptions do exist in which PHI may be released without authorization (44) (Table 366.3). The HCE may not decline to treat a patient who refuses to sign an authorization (43).

Incidental disclosure of PHI is a major concern in the ED. Examples of incidental disclosures include patients or family members overhearing a physician discussing patient orders with the nursing staff or patients overhearing the names of patients being called to examination rooms. HIPAA was not intended to impede normal communications or alter daily operations inherent in providing health care. Thus, incidental disclosures of PHI are permitted, but only if the HCE has implemented reasonable safeguards to limit them (40). Examples of safeguards in the ED include establishing visiting hours; rounding after visiting hours; speaking quietly in waiting rooms; moving x-ray view boxes and computer screens out of view of visitors; and posting signs to remind staff to protect patient confidentiality.

Each HCE must establish written policies describing how the HCE will comply with HIPAA privacy rules (48). Policies must list members of the HCE's workforce and detail each members access and limitations to PHI. The HCE must inform patients of their rights; how to obtain an accounting of disclosures of PHI; and how to file a complaint. When applicable, policies must address disclosure of PHI for research, marketing, and fund raising activities. The HCE must have a privacy officer or committee to oversee compliance and education regarding HIPAA privacy regulations.

The HCE must implement policies to address security issues. For example, computers should be turned off at the end of the work day and automatically log-off when left unattended. Areas with computers should be secured. Computer discs should be kept in secure compartments. File cabinets should be locked. The sharing of user names or passwords should be prohibited. Technical security mechanisms should control access to PHI, prevent unauthorized internal and external access, and monitor access.

HIPAA grants patients the right to receive notice of the HCE's privacy practices; to obtain access, inspect, and copy health information; to request corrections of health information; to request restrictions on the use and disclosure of health information; and to obtain an accounting of disclosures. Each patient must receive a Notice of Privacy Practices on their first visit to the physician's office or hospital, or on enrollment into a health plan (45). It must describe who has access to PHI and for what reasons. It must inform patients of their rights and the HCE's obligations under HIPAA. Patients are required to acknowledge that they received and reviewed the notice. A copy of the policy must be posted in the office or facility and on its website, and a written copy must be available to the patient. Patients have the right to access their medical records and obtain copies (46). They may be charged for copying and mailing costs. Patients may also request modifications or corrections of their medical record for inaccurate or incomplete information (47). The HCE may deny the request in writing, however it should have a policy in place through which patients may appeal the denial.

Patients may file HIPAA complaints with the HCE or the federal government. The Office of Civil Rights is charged with enforcing the HIPAA privacy standards. Sanctions for violation of privacy or security standards include civil monetary fines and incarceration of the offender (34). Routine fines are $100.00 per violation, not to exceed $25,000.00 in one year. For violations as a result of known unauthorized use or disclosure of PHI, fines of up to $50,000 per year can be levied, along with 1 year in prison. For violations resulting from acts under false pretenses, fines can be up to $100,000 with 5 years in prison. If the intent was to sell,

TABLE 366.2. Individually Identifiable Health Information

- Individual's name
- Geographic subdivisions smaller than the state
- Dates (except year) directly related to an individual, including birth date, admission date, discharge date, date of death
- Telephone numbers and facsimile numbers
- Electronic mail addresses
- Social security number
- Medical record numbers
- Health plan beneficiary numbers
- Account numbers
- Certificate, business, or license numbers
- Vehicle identifiers (including license plate numbers)
- Device identifiers and serial numbers
- Internet or extranet sites and URLs
- Internet protocol addresses
- Full face photograph images and other comparable images
- Biometric identifiers (including finger print or voice recognition)
- Any other unique identifier characteristic or code

use, or transfer PHI for commercial advantage, personal gain, or malicious harm, fines of up to $250,000 are allowed, along with imprisonment of 10 years.

FRAUD AND ABUSE

Fraud describes intentional behavior designed to induce another party to surrender something of value. Ordinarily, a prosecutor must show intent to act fraudulently. However, health care fraud means an unreasonable, improper, or excessive use of a process or procedure. Thus, health care fraud encompasses false claims, kickbacks, and self-referrals. The mere filing of an improper or inaccurate claim may constitute a false claim; payment of the claim is not necessary for liability to attach. The law only requires a false application for payment. Thus, courts may find culpability even if the health care provider did not intend to violate the law. Sanctions for fraudulent billing include fines of $25,000 and 5 years imprisonment. All criminal violations require exclusion from Medicare and Medicaid.

The False Claims Act (FCA) also addresses fraudulent behavior (16). The FCA prohibits a person or entity from knowingly submitting false claims to the federal government. Although fraud and abuse statutes involve Medicare and Medicaid, the FCA covers all federal spending programs. The FCA allows civil monetary penalties of up to $10,000 for each item or service, plus three times the amount claimed. Under the FCA, physicians have liability for all acts committed by their billing personnel whether intentional or not.

The criminal section of the Medicare Fraud and Abuse statutes contains the Anti-Kickback Statute enacted in 1972 (33). The statute prohibits the knowing and willful payment or solicitation of payment to induce patient referral. The Anti-Kickback statutes cover all federal health care programs. Parties offering and receiving payment have liability. Penalties include fines up to $50,000, five years imprisonment, and permanent exclusion from federal heath care programs.

Congress passed the Ethics in Patient Referrals Act known as Stark I, in 1989, known as Stark I, in response to its belief that physician self-referrals resulted in huge Medicare costs. Stark I prohibits physicians from referring Medicare or Medicaid patients to a provider in which the provider, or an immediate family member, has a financial interest in the entity receiving the referral (36). The Stark laws provide civil penalties against physicians only. Liability applies regardless of intent. Fines of $15,000 for each item or service, or up to $100,000 for schemes designed to circumvent the Stark prohibitions are possible.

COMMON PITFALLS

✔ Failure to provide a medical screening examination to determine if an EMC exists

✔ Failure to provide stabilizing treatment before transferring individuals with EMCs
✔ Failure to obtain authorization for disclosure of individually identifiable health information
✔ Failure to establish administrative, physical, and technical safeguards to protect the privacy and integrity of health information
✔ Failure to realize that laws governing fraud and abuse in health care apply when a relevant statute is violated even without specific intent to violate it

References

1. *Baber v Hospital Corp of America*, 977 F2d 872,880 (4th Cir 1992).
2. *Gatewood v Washington Healthcare Corp*, 933 F2d 1037 (DC Cir 1997).
3. *Green v Touro Infirmary*, 992 F2d 537 (5th Cir 1993).
4. *Guerro v Copper Queen Hospital*, 537 P2d 1329(Ariz 1975); *Stanturf v Sipes*, 447 SW 2d 558 (Mo1969).
5. *Horn v Patton*, 287 So2d 824 (Alabama 1974).
6. Lo B. Resolving ethical dilemmas: a guide for clinicians. Baltimore: Lippincott Williams & Wilkins, 1995.
7. *Mercy Medical Center of Oskosh v Winnebago City*, 206 NW 2d 198 (Wis 1975).
8. *New Biloxi Hospital v Frazier*, 146 So2d 882 (Miss 1982).
9. Public Law No 104–191, 110 Stat 1936 (1996).
10. Roberts JS, Coale JG, Redman RR. A history of the Joint Commission on the Accreditation of Hospitals. *JAMA* 1987;258(7):936–940.
11. Roberts v Galen of Virginia Inc., 525 US 249, 119 S ct 684, 142 L E 2d 648(1999).
12. *Summers v Baptist Medical Center, Arkadelphia*, 69 F3d 902 (8th Cir 1995), rev on reh 91 F3d 1132(1996).
13. *Thompson v Sun City Community Hospital*, 688 F2d 605 (Ariz 1984).
14. Westin A. *Privacy and Freedom*. New York: Antheneum Publishers, 1967.
15. *Wilmington General Hospital vs Manlove*, 174 A2d 135 (Del 1961).
16. 31 USC §3730(h) (1986).
17. 42 CFR §405 and 489.24 (1994).
18. 42 CFR §416.35 (2000).
19. 42 CFR §489.24 (2003).
20. 42 CFR §489.24(a)(1)(i) (2003).
21. 42 CFR §489.24(1) and (2) (2003).
22. 42 CFR §489.24(b) (2003).
23. 42 CFR §489.24(c) (2003).
24. 42 CFR §489.24(c)(4)(i) and (ii) (2003).
25. 42 CFR §489.24(d) (2003).
26. 42 CFR 489.24(e)(1)(ii)(c) (2003).
27. 42 CFR Parts 413, 482, and 489 (VII) (2003).
28. 42 USC §1395 dd(c)(1)(A)(i) & (ii) (1986).
29. 42 USC §1395 dd(g) (1986).
30. 42 USC §1395dd (1986).
31. 42 USC §1395dd(c)(2) (1986).
32. 42 USC §1395dd(e)(1) (1986).
33. 42 USC §1320a-7b (1999).
34. 42 USC §1320d-5.
35. 42 USC §1395dd(h) (1986).
36. 42 USC §1395nn (1999).
37. 42 USC §291–2910 (1988) and Supp II (1990).
38. 45 CFR §160.103.
39. 45 CFR §164.501.
40. 45 CFR §164.502(a)(1)(iii).
41. 45 CFR §164.506(c).
42. 45 CFR §164.508.
43. 45 CFR §164.508(c).
44. 45 CFR §164.512.
45. 45 CFR §164.520(a) and (b).
46. 45 CFR §164.524.
47. 45 CFR §164.526.
48. 45 FR §164.530.

Special Clinical Considerations

CHAPTER 367
Acute Pain Management

Steven Rosenzweig, Bernard Lopez, and Daniel Mines

Acute pain is the most common reason that patients seek emergency care. Patient survey studies consistently document that pain is often inadequately treated by physicians and that this problem is not limited to the emergency department (ED) (1). Providing expert and compassionate pain relief remains one of the greatest challenges in the practice of emergency medicine.

Drugs used to treat pain act by reversing the underlying cause of pain (e.g., nitrates for angina and sumatriptan for migraine) or by suppressing the symptom (i.e., the perception of pain). This chapter focuses on drugs used to treat the symptom of acute pain. Other medications that reverse the underlying cause of pain are discussed elsewhere in this book, such as the use of nitrates for angina. Related discussions elsewhere in this text include the chapters on conscious sedation (Chapter 369, "Procedural Sedation and Analgesia"), and chronic pain syndromes (Chapter 368, "Chronic Pain Syndromes").

PAIN ASSESSMENT

Current practice standards include pain assessment as the fifth vital sign. However, many challenges exist to the accurate assessment of pain in the ED.

Subjective Nature of Pain

Pain is an experience that has both physical and nonphysical dimensions. Physiologically, pain is mediated by a set of neurochemical events. At the level of consciousness, it is an event of personal anguish or suffering. The severity and quality of this suffering are highly individual; each person experiences and responds to pain in his or her own way.

Language of Pain

The subjective nature of pain presents a challenge to today's medical practice. It can be very difficult for anyone to find words to convey either the quality of pain or its severity. Descriptions lack the preferred exactness of clinical language. People resort to imagination and simile: "My back feels as if it is caught in a vise"; "my hand feels like it is on fire." Another problem is that patients and physicians use words differently. For example, a patient may use the word *sharp* to mean *severe,* whereas the physician may assume it to mean *knifelike.*

Meaning of Pain

One of the most important aspects of the pain experience is the *meaning* it holds for the sufferer. Pain is often greater when its cause is perceived to be life-threatening or when it is associated with emotional trauma. Conversely, pain that is perceived to offer some secondary gain can be easier to bear.

Objective Signs of Pain are Unreliable

The emergency physician cannot rely on objective findings in estimating pain severity. It is imperative for all emergency care providers to understand that the patient need not *appear* in pain to actually *be* in pain (7). There exist no objective signs for accurately gauging the magnitude of a patient's pain. Indicators such as heart rate, blood pressure, respiratory pattern, facial expression, and body posture are not reliable. The presentation of pain may be obscured by the effects of medication, a cultural bias toward stoicism, or complex coping mechanisms such as joking or maintaining a facade of being calm (1). Language and cultural barriers further confound pain assessment.

Equally unreliable is an estimate of pain severity based on its etiology. Can a toothache be more painful than salpingitis? Should an ankle sprain hurt less than pleurisy? These questions cannot be answered, because suffering depends on each individual's pain threshold and sensitivity to a particular condition.

Utilizing the Patient's Self-Report

Taking an accurate pain history, therefore, requires careful listening and clarification. Ultimately, the most reliable and valid means of assessing pain severity is the patient's self-report. Clinical judgment must always be guided by the patient's own assessment.

Patients can also be assisted in conveying pain intensity through descriptive scales. Using the visual analog scale (VAS), a patient would place a mark on a 10-cm line to indicate severity of pain. The numeric rating scale is a related tool by which a patient would report pain intensity as a representative number (usually from 0–10). Both VAS and numeric scales have been validated for use in the ED (4,5). The patient can also be asked to verbally rate pain severity (none-little-medium-severe-worst possible; or bearable-unbearable).

Pain in Children

Assessing pain in children, especially infants, is even more difficult than in adults (20). The experience and expression of pain are affected by the developmental age of the child, the child's previous pain experiences, the response of the child to the medical environment, and the quality of the relationship with parents or other care providers. Older children are able to describe their pain or point to pictures on a pain analogue scale. In infants and younger children, the quality of cry, facial expression, changes in vital signs, and impressions of the caretaker should all be taken into account.

Correcting Physician Attitudes and Beliefs

Appropriate evaluation of a patient's pain may be impaired by certain attitudes and beliefs held by the physician. One impediment is resistance to accepting the authority of the patient or the insight of a family member. The physician cannot be "in charge" of the assessment of pain. This situation in which the patient knows more than the doctor creates a reversal of roles that may be uncomfortable and even unacceptable for the treating physician.

Another impediment to accepting a patient's self-report of pain is the fear of being manipulated into giving narcotics to someone who is feigning illness. Bear in mind that *pain* is the most common reason for drug-seeking behavior. Even a legitimate patient may feel the need to dramatize distress in order to convince the doctor of his or her need. It may indeed be impossible to know for certain whether the patient's complaint is a sham. The physician must always weigh the gain of thwarting the possible abuser against the risk of withholding relief from the person who is truly suffering.

The diagnosis of drug abuse is based on a pattern of behavior that is unlikely to be established during a single ED encounter. Nevertheless, a few precautions can be taken:

1. Perform a detailed history and physical, being alert to inconsistencies.
2. Attempt to confirm the patient's history by contacting the personal physician or checking medical records.
3. Communicate with colleagues about problem patients in order to corroborate impressions and develop specific treatment strategies.
4. Substitute nonnarcotic agents when indicated.
5. Write prescriptions for only small amounts of medication, or dispense one or two doses rather than actually writing a prescription (9).

Children are much less likely than adults to be given adequate analgesia for the same painful condition (24). This observation has been attributed not only to the difficulties inherent to pain assessment, but also to the persistent myth that children do not experience or remember pain. As in any adult, pain in a child should be anticipated and aggressively treated.

Emotional desensitization and compassion fatigue also lead to suboptimal pain assessment. Emergency physicians habituate to crises and may become less attuned to the urgency of others' pain. Recurrent encounters with hostile patients, and physical and emotional fatigue, wear down the ability to respond compassionately. Facing our own vulnerability in the suffering of others may also lead physicians to withdraw from patients unintentionally. Compassion requires the physician to maintain an awareness of his or her own inner state in order to rise above these desensitizing factors. The capacity to remain compassionate in the midst of suffering and personal stressors can be strengthened through continuing medical education, accredited programs in physician self-care and stress reduction, and professional organizations such as the Institute for the Study of Health and Illness.

Even when pain assessment is accurate, physician attitudes may interfere with appropriate pain management. Withholding opioids for fear of creating an addiction in a patient is generally unwarranted. Studies have shown that the short-term prescription of narcotic analgesics for acute pain syndromes is not associated with future dependence (19). Personal prejudices also interfere with empathy; negative stereotyping and moral judgment lead to blaming the patient and under-treatment of pain. The extreme case of withholding analgesia as a punitive measure can only be considered inhumane.

EMERGENCY DEPARTMENT MANAGEMENT

Expediting Relief

Pain relief should be timely. Unnecessary delays can often be averted.

Patients should be treated before a definitive diagnosis is established. Pain can and should be treated before its underlying cause is known. Initial interventions can be nonpharmacologic (discussion follows). When the diagnosis depends solely on a laboratory or radiographic finding, there is no excuse for not offering pain medication while the evaluation is proceeding.

The belief that analgesics, particularly opioids, will obscure the underlying diagnosis is unfounded. Although it is common to withhold such medication from a patient with abdominal pain who may need surgical evaluation, this practice is not supported by clinical studies (2,17). On the contrary, the judicious use of short-acting agents can serve the needs of both the patient and the consulting surgeon. Providing pain relief may actually enhance the patient's cooperation and improve the accuracy of the examination. Factors to consider in the administration of analgesics include severity of abdominal pain and speed of the surgical consultation (16). The emergency physician should consider administering analgesics with the intent of reducing patient suffering but not completely eliminating the pain in order to allow a useful physical examination by the surgeon. Ironically, analgesics are often withheld in the ED, even after a decision has been made to take a patient to surgery. As the patient's most important advocate, the emergency physician must coordinate a rational and humane approach that takes into account the distress of the patient and the availability of the consultant.

Pain should be treated even if informed consent may subsequently be required. The practice of withholding opioids from a patient who might later need to sign a consent for surgery or other procedure should be reconsidered. Concern that these medications will compromise the competency of the patient are generally unfounded. First, pain can certainly be as mind-altering as medications. Second, it is possible to provide analgesia without clouding consciousness. Third, the implicit message that pain medication will be administered only after the consent is signed is itself coercive. And, finally, an opioid antagonist can be administered, if necessary.

The physician should anticipate and treat pain before it develops. Good pain management involves anticipating pain prior to its onset or recurrence. Medications should be given before painful procedures (see Chapter 369, "Procedural Sedation and Analgesia"). Similarly, patients should be given instructions and medication to help them cope with pain that may continue or recur following discharge.

Nonpharmacologic Therapy

A variety of simple and effective interventions can reduce pain.

Provide physical comfort measures. Attending to the overall physical comfort of the patient can alleviate factors that aggravate pain. This includes such actions as helping the patient find a more comfortable position, adjusting the lighting in the room, warming a patient who feels chilled, immobilizing injured extremities, and applying ice to closed bone and soft-tissue injuries.

Provide psychological support. Physical suffering is amplified by fear, anxiety and powerlessness. Fear often relates to the possibility that the cause of pain is life-threatening or permanently disabling. New pain in a cancer patient raises the specter of disease progression. Patients with chest pain often present with a fear of myocardial infarction. A laborer may associate an acute shoulder injury with the alarming possibility of permanent loss of income.

Information and reassurance, given whenever possible, reduce the need for analgesics. Family members of adult and pediatric patients should be included in this reassurance and support system. For unaccompanied patients, facilitating phone contact with a friend or family member may provide significant comfort.

Anxiety arises in response not only to sudden illness, but also to the ED experience itself. Unable to control their own pain, patients find themselves in a harsh and unfamiliar milieu, feeling exposed, vulnerable, and dependent on strangers. Building rapport, dignifying interactions, and restoring some sense of control to our patients are all essential in emergency pain management.

Muscular and mental tension arise out of pain, increasing distress even more. Both may respond to verbal and imagery techniques that relax the body and distract the mind. Music, videos, storytelling, and imagining favorite places or activities are techniques that are frequently used for pediatric patients.

It is also important to address the patient's expectations regarding pain medications. Let the patient know from the outset how much time it will take for the medication to work, and whether to anticipate partial or complete relief. This can allay a premature concern that the drug "isn't working."

Pharmacologic Therapy

Dozens of drugs are available to treat pain. To select the best regimen for an individual patient, several issues need to be explored. How intense is the pain? How quickly is pain relief required? Can the patient take oral medications? Are there contraindications to particular agents? The answers to these questions help direct the choice of drug, dose, and route of administration.

Aspirin and Acetaminophen

Aspirin and acetaminophen are equally effective for the relief of mild-to-moderate pain. Aspirin, the prototype NSAID, is believed to work by blocking cyclooxygenase (COX) enzymes, thereby inhibiting the synthesis of prostaglandins, which mediate both pain and inflammation. Unlike aspirin, acetaminophen lacks antiinflammatory properties, and its mechanism of action is poorly understood.

Aspirin also inhibits platelet function and commonly leads to gastrointestinal (GI) distress. It very rarely causes a hypersensitivity reaction (more common among asthmatics with nasal polyps), characterized by bronchospasm, urticaria, rhinitis, and even shock. Because acetaminophen is free of these side effects and hypersensitivity risk, it is often the preferable drug. Table 367.1 lists dosing recommendations for these drugs.

Nonsteroidal Antiinflammatory Drugs

At usual doses, NSAIDs are not as safe as acetaminophen but are generally better tolerated than aspirin. In addition to blocking COX enzymes, they may directly modulate neutrophil responses. More than a dozen are approved by the Food and Drug Administration (FDA) for analgesia, and still others are commonly used for pain relief (see Chapter 280, "Acetaminophen" and Chapter 282, "Nonsteroidal Antiinflammatory Drugs"). When given as a single full dose in the acute setting, most NSAIDs are more effective than aspirin or acetaminophen. In some settings, they provide analgesia equal or superior to certain oral opioids. Although no oral NSAID has emerged as a consistently superior analgesic, it is widely acknowledged that an individual patient may respond to one agent and not another (6).

The onset of analgesia is within 1 hour for the majority of NSAIDs. For drugs with a relatively long half-life, such as diflunisal and naproxen, onset of analgesia is considerably longer but can be hastened by administration of a loading dose. Note that doses in the higher range are generally required to achieve antiinflammatory effects, which may not be seen for a few days.

For patients who cannot swallow pills, several agents are available in a liquid form (see Table 367.1). For patients who are vomiting or for whom oral medications are contraindicated, rectal suppositories of aspirin, acetaminophen, naproxen, and indomethacin are available.

Costs of the NSAIDs vary considerably, ranging from pennies per dose of aspirin to more than a dollar per dose of newer, brand-name NSAIDs.

Selective COX-2 Inhibitors (COXIBs)

These drugs selectively block COX-2, the form of cyclooxygenase that mediates inflammation, without affecting COX-1, the inhibition of which can produce gastric injury. In comparison, older "nonspecific" NSAIDs block both COX isoenzymes (13).

Rofecoxib (Vioxx) and celecoxib (Celebrex) are FDA-approved for the treatment of acute pain. Both drugs appear to have an improved gastric safety profile compared with the older NSAIDs, but are not without any GI toxicity. It is also not yet clear how quickly they produce analgesia compared with older agents. These agents are not likely to be any more effective than the older, less costly NSAIDs (21). Because their major advantage is their safety profile, they should be reserved for patients at high risk of NSAID side effects (discussion follows). A disadvantage of these agents is their higher cost, and many insurance companies require precertification of need. Patients with sulfonamide allergy may not take celecoxib. Valdecoxib (Bextra) is a newer COXIB currently approved for the symptomatic treatment of osteoarthritis, rheumatoid arthritis, and primary dysmenorrhea.

Parenteral NSAID Agents

Ketorolac tromethamine (Toradol) is the only NSAID also available for parenteral administration in the ED, either i.m. or i.v.. It carries all the advantages and disadvantages of older NSAIDs. A single dose of i.v. ketorolac has been shown to be at least as effective as titrated i.v. meperidine in relieving pain in patients with renal colic, but its use was associated with fewer adverse effects and less functional impairment (25). Its efficacy is likely related to prostaglandin mechanisms in renal colic. However, it has not been compared to indomethacin, another NSAID also shown to be effective in renal colic.

Because of the drug's popularity in emergency medicine, practitioners need to be aware of its limitations. When studied in the ED setting, parenteral ketorolac does not provide superior

TABLE 367.1. Dosing Information for Nonopioids

Drug	Dosage	Comments	Generic Formula Available
Acetaminophen (Tylenol)	650 mg q4h 1,000 mg q6h	No antiinflammatory activity	yes
Aspirin	650–975 mg q4h		yes
Choline magnesium trisalicylate (Trilisate)	1,000–1,500 mg b.i.d.	Oral liquid available (brand name only)	yes
Celecoxib (Celebrex)	400 mg initially 200 mg BID	Selective COX-2 action Contraindicated in sulfonamide allergy	no
Diflunisal (Dolobid)	1,000-mg load; then 500 mg b.i.d.		yes
Etodolac (Lodine)	200–400 mg q6–8h		no
Fenoprofen (Nalfon)	200–600 mg q6–8h		yes
Ibuprofen (Motrin and others)	400 mg q4–6h, or 600 mg q6–8h or 800 mg q8h	Oral liquid available	yes
Indomethacin (Indocin)	25–50 mg t.i.d.	FDA approved only as an antiinflammatory Frequency of adverse effects higher than other NSAIDs. Available as a suppository	yes
Ketoprofen (Orudis)	25–75 mg q6–8h		yes
Ketorolac, oral (Toradol)	10 mg q6–8h	Not recommended for more than 5 d use	yes
Ketorolac, parenteral	30–60 mg i.m. or i.v. initially then 30 mg q6h i.m. or i.v.	Use lower dose in patients <50 kg or older than 65, or with renal impairment	yes
Naproxen (Naprosyn, Aleve), Naproxen sodium (Anaprox)	375–550 mg initially, then 250–375 mg b.i.d. to t.i.d.	Oral liquid available	yes
Rofecoxib (Vioxx)	12.5–50 mg qd or divided b.i.d	Selective COX-2 action Oral liquid available	no

analgesia to oral ibuprofen (15,23). Given parenterally, ketorolac does not act any faster than many oral NSAIDs, because the drug effect is limited by time to prostaglandin inhibition, not absorption. Ketorolac is relatively expensive—a parenteral dose costs more than about ten times as much as morphine 10 mg, and 45 times as much as a full dose of ibuprofen. Repetitive dosing of ketorolac carries a higher risk of upper GI bleeding when compared with other NSAIDs. Acute renal failure has also been described. It seems reasonable to reserve parenteral ketorolac only for patients in whom the oral administration of NSAIDs should be avoided.

Parecoxib is a parenteral COX-2 inhibitor that has been approved for dental and postoperative pain. Its analgesic effects seem similar to ketorolac, but the drug has not yet been studied in the ED setting. The potential advantage of parecoxib would be a higher safety profile as a COXIB.

The NSAIDs hold several advantages over the opioids. They do not cause respiratory depression and rarely cause mental clouding. Given their antiinflammatory properties, they treat the cause and the symptom of pain in conditions such as tendinitis, arthritis, or radiculitis. NSAIDs do not have abuse potential.

All NSAIDs can cause dyspepsia, the most common side effect. All NSAIDs can cause dyspepsia, the most common side effect. This can be minimized by administering the drug with food or an antacid. Less commonly, NSAIDs lead to ulcers and upper GI bleeding and perforation, complications that are seen more with chronic rather than short-term use and that may occur without warning (6). NSAIDs are thus strongly contraindi-

cated in patients with active ulcer disease, and should be given with caution to those with a history of upper GI bleeding. The incidence of GI bleeding may be dose-dependent; daily doses of ibuprofen above 1500 mg are associated with increased risk. Other risk factors for GI complications include patient age greater than 60 years and concurrent steroid or anticoagulant use (12). In such high-risk patients, the chance of GI bleeding can be reduced by coadministration of a proton pump inhibitor or misoprostol, at least with long-term NSAID use. The benefit these agents offer with short courses of NSAID is less well established. Other agents that were often used for prophylaxis of NSAID-related GI complications are either ineffective (antacids, sucralfate) or marginally effective (H₂ blockers) (12). COX-2 inhibitors—without gastroprotective drugs—represent another therapeutic option in patients with risk factors for GI bleeding.

All NSAIDs, including COXIBs, may affect the kidneys, causing fluid retention and renal insufficiency, which is usually reversible. Patients at greater risk for renal complications include those with chronic renal insufficiency, congestive heart failure, and cirrhosis, and patients taking diuretics or angiotensin converting enzyme inhibitors. NSAIDs should generally be prescribed for no more than a few days in this patient population.

Because they interfere with platelet function, the nonselective NSAIDs predispose toward bleeding and should not be given to patients with thrombocytopenia or intrinsic clotting abnormalities. They should generally not be used in patients receiving anticoagulant therapy and in those suspected of internal bleeding, as in the case of severe headache with possible subarachnoid hemorrhage. In contrast, because the COX-2 selective NSAIDs do not inhibit platelet function, they may be used in patients with low platelet counts or in those on warfarin.

Very rarely, NSAIDs cause hypersensitivity reactions; patients who are sensitive to aspirin are at greater risk. NSAIDs are generally contraindicated during pregnancy, particularly in the third trimester because of known effects on the fetal cardiovascular system (closure of the ductus arteriosus).

Opioid Analgesics

Opioids are usually the first-choice drugs for the prompt relief of severe, acute pain. Unlike the NSAIDs, they have no ceiling on analgesic effect. Given i.v., they work within minutes, and their effect can be titrated and reversed. Many patients treated with these agents, however, do not receive adequate pain relief because of physicians' misconceptions about correct dosing, route of administration, and adverse effects (18).

Dosing Considerations

In real life, the effective analgesic dose varies considerably among patients; the *correct* dose of narcotic is the dose that works. The "optimal initial dose" published in various references is only a general guideline; the "standard" 10-mg dose of parenteral morphine is inadequate analgesia for one-third of patients in severe pain (11). Therefore, in the initial treatment of severe pain it makes sense to titrate small frequent doses to effect (Tables 367.2 and 367.3).

Once satisfactory analgesia is achieved, another common pitfall is to withhold a subsequent dose until a "standard" dosing interval has elapsed. Statements about "average duration of action" provide only a rough estimate (1).

Route of Administration

Intravenous administration of opioids is preferable to the more commonly used intramuscular route for several reasons. Absorption is more reliable, and repeated dosing is painless. It also leads to more rapid onset of analgesia; intravenous morphine begins to work within 5 minutes (peaks in 10 to 20 minutes), whereas intramuscular morphine requires 10 to 30 minutes until an effect is seen (peaks in 30–60 minutes) (14,18). It is obviously easier to titrate the opioid dose using the i.v. route. It is also important to keep in mind that the frequency and severity of several side effects, such as respiratory depression, hypotension, histamine release, and nausea and vomiting, are related to the speed of intravenous injection. They can be minimized if drugs are injected over several minutes, rather than by rapid push. See Table 367.4 for a summary of safety guidelines for intravenous administration of opioids.

It is not clear which is the second best parenteral route for opioid administration. Although one authority (18) recommends subcutaneous (s.c.) injection as less painful than intramuscular, this benefit may be offset by an even more delayed onset of action (14).

Opioid analgesics can be given through a number of other routes as well. The oral route is most convenient and least expensive. When both i.v. and oral routes are unavailable, alternatives include rectal suppository (morphine, hydromorphone, and oxymorphone), sublingual tablet (buprenorphine), and even a nasal spray (butorphanol).

Adverse Effects

All opioid analgesics share certain side effects, although some occur more with one drug than another. A patient who has had a problem with one agent may be able to tolerate a second opioid without difficulty.

Of all the potential adverse effects, respiratory depression is the most dangerous. Using sophisticated testing, it is possible to show that therapeutic doses of most opiates cause some degree of respiratory depression in nearly all patients. Most of the time, this is not clinically important. However, patients with diminished respiratory reserve, such as those with severe chronic obstructive pulmonary disease or massive obesity, are liable to stop breathing after receiving these drugs. Even in those with normal reserve, removal of a painful stimulus, as occurs with the reduction of a dislocated joint, can precipitate respiratory depression; patients should be monitored closely after painful procedures. Except in the case of massive overdose, respiratory arrest does not occur suddenly but is heralded by a decreased respiratory rate and level of arousal.

Hypotension is the second major hazard of opioid use. Through a variety of mechanisms, opioids, particularly those given parenterally, may cause peripheral vasodilation. This seldom affects blood pressure in the supine patient, but the ambulatory patient may experience significant orthostatic hypotension. Volume-depleted individuals are at increased risk for hypotension regardless of body position. Hypotension from opioids generally resolves spontaneously within a few minutes; if necessary, i.v. fluids and possibly naloxone are effective.

Opiates occasionally trigger the release of histamine from mast cells. Because this occurs through a nonimmunologic mechanism, it is technically not an allergy. Clinical consequences include itching, urticaria, bronchospasm, and hypotension, which are not responsive to naloxone. The agents most frequently implicated in these reactions are morphine, followed by codeine and meperidine. Fentanyl has practically no potential for this complication.

Rapid administration of high-dose fentanyl has been associated with muscle rigidity, including chest wall spasm, which may require treatment with intravenous naloxone. This is usually seen in the context of fentanyl anesthesia and may be treated with a neuromuscular blocking agent.

Opiates commonly cause sedation and occasionally produce confusion. Therefore, ED patients should be warned not to drive vehicles or operate power tools when they take narcotics. Opioids present a special set of problems for head-injured patients. They may interfere with evaluation of central nervous system (CNS) function. The respiratory depressant effect of opioids is exaggerated in this group of patients, and the resultant hypoventilation may actually increase intracranial pressure, mediated by cerebral vasodilation in response to an elevated pCO_2 (14).

Opiates may cause spasm at the sphincter of Oddi and, in turn, precipitate biliary colic. Whether meperidine is less likely than morphine to do this remains unresolved. Among all opioids,

---

TABLE 367.2. Pediatric Dosing Guidelines for Drugs for Pain Management[a]

Drug	Route	Dosage (mg/kg/dose)
Morphine	i.v.	0.1–0.2
Meperidine	i.v./i.m.	1.0–1.5
Fentanyl	i.v.	0.001–0.003
	Oral/transmucosal	0.005–0.015
Codeine	Oral	0.5–1.0 q4–6h
Acetaminophen	Oral/rectal	10–15 q4–6 h
Ibuprofen	Oral	10 q6–8 h

[a]For further pediatric dosing guidelines, see Chapter 269, "Pediatric Sedation and Pain Management."

TABLE 367.3.   Dosing Guidelines for Parenteral Opioids

Drug	Route[a,b]	Dosage	Comments
Morphine	i.v.	Titrate 2–5-mg increments q5–10 min Peak analgesia in 10–20 min Average = 10 mg q3–4h	Preferred first-line agent in most situations
	i.m./s.c.	Average = 10 mg q3–4h	
Fentanyl	i.v.	Titrate 25–50-μg increments q2–3 min Peak analgesia in 3–5 min Duration 30–60 min	Ideal for short procedures No histamine release
	i.m./s.c.		Not suitable for the ED
Meperidine (Demerol)	i.v.	Titrate 12.5–50.0-mg increments Peak analgesia in 5–10 min Average = 100 mg q2–3h	Risk of unique CNS toxicity with repeated dosing
	i.m./s.c.	Average = 100 mg q3h	i.m./s.c. injection is very irritating to tissue
Hydromorphone (Dilaudid)	i.v.	Titrate 0.5–1.0 mg increments Peak analgesia in 5–15 min Average = 1.5 mg q3–4h	High solubility benefits s.c. injection
	i.m./s.c.	Average = 1.5 mg q3–4h	
Butorphanol (Stadol)	i.v.	Titrate 0.5–2.0-mg increments Peak analgesia in 4–5 min Average = 2 mg q3–4h	Mixed agonist-antagonist May be preferred in biliary colic
	i.m./s.c.	Average = 2 mg q3–4h	

Note: Intervals are approximate. Individual patients may require dosing either more or less frequently.
Caution: Dosing may need to be adjusted in the elderly, patients weighing less than 50 kg, and those with renal or hepatic insufficiency.
[a] Intravenous route is preferred for faster onset and ability to titrate to effect.
[b] Rapid i.v. administration increases incidence of respiratory depression, hypotension, nausea, and itching; i.v. administration should be slow (over 4–5 minutes), with the patient recumbent.

the agonists–antagonists appear to have the least potential for this complication (18). Paradoxically, even though it sometimes raises biliary tract pressures, morphine is usually successful in treating pain of biliary origin (18). Nitroglycerin and glucagon, drugs that relax smooth muscle, and naloxone, have been used to treat opioid-induced biliary colic (11,18).

Opioids have other effects on the genitourinary and GI systems. They may cause urinary retention, particularly in older men with underlying prostatism. They are constipating and can sometimes cause abdominal pain or dyspepsia. Nausea and vomiting can be minimized by administering the drug to the patient in the supine position and, if necessary, with an antiemetic (11). GI side effects, if severe, can be reversed with naloxone.

Opioids have the potential to mask the diagnosis of serious abdominal disease. Although they can be given safely to patients with abdominal pain who are under close observation, prescribing them for patients who are sent home with undiagnosed abdominal pain is potentially dangerous.

TABLE 367.4.   How to Give Intravenous Opioids Safely

1. Initiate infusion of normal saline before administering opioids.
2. Keep the patient in a recumbent position.
3. Have naloxone and airway management equipment at the bedside.
4. Avoid or adjust dose downward in patients with hypotension, COPD, or potential for airway compromise.
5. Give SLOWLY, over 3–5 minutes.
6. Titrate to pain relief.
7. Supplement careful observation with pulse oximetry and/or apnea monitoring.

Major Risks:
 • CNS depression leading to hypoventilation or aspiration
 • Hypotension

Choosing an Injectable Agent

A typical error in the use of opioids is to switch agents before the first one has been pushed to its limit, which is determined by unwanted side effects rather than an arbitrary "maximal" dose. Correct dosing is more important than the actual choice of agent.

Morphine is the traditional first-line parenteral narcotic. No other opioid is superior in relieving pain. It is also relatively inexpensive and has a relatively long duration of action.

Despite its widespread use, meperidine (Demerol) offers few, if any, advantages over morphine. Although it is less constipating, meperidine in equianalgesic doses produces the same degree of sedation, respiratory depression, and euphoria as does morphine (11). With repeated dosing, meperidine has its own peculiar CNS toxicity, caused by normeperidine, an active metabolite. Findings include irritable mood, agitation, myoclonus, and seizures. CNS toxicity is more common in patients with renal insufficiency. Meperidine should not be given to patients receiving monoamine oxidase (MAO) inhibitors because of the potential for a poorly understood interaction, characterized by delirium and hyperthermia, which may be fatal.

Meperidine is recommended as a second-line analgesic for brief courses in otherwise healthy patients who have had a problem with morphine. Intramuscular or s.c. injection causes local irritation. A common mistake in the use of meperidine is to use too small a dose and too long a dosing interval (1). Tables 367.2 and 367.3 list dosing guidelines.

Fentanyl is an ideal agent for performing short, painful procedures because of its very rapid onset and limited duration of action.

Partial agonist and agonist–antagonist opioids were developed to provide analgesia with less sedation, respiratory depression, nausea, and addiction potential (10). Practical benefits, however, have been limited (12). Pentazocine, the only drug of this class available in an oral form, produces psychotomimetic symptoms, including disorientation, paranoia, and hallucinations, in as many as 7% of treated patients. All drugs in this class can precipitate withdrawal when they are given to patients addicted to pure opioid agonist. These drugs really offer no advantages over the strong opioid agonists, except perhaps in the management of biliary pain.

Adjuvant Agents

A number of drugs have been administered along with parenteral opioids to minimize adverse effects by reducing the amount of opioid needed to treat pain. Phenothiazines can reduce GI side effects. When they are given along with an opioid, sedative effects are increased, but analgesia is not (11).

The antihistamine hydroxyzine (50–100 mg i.m. or 1 mg/kg i.m.) is often combined with opioids to potentiate analgesia and to provide limited antiemetic effects. Although hydroxyzine does have additive analgesic properties, this practice poses two problems. First, it requires an intramuscular injection. Second, it may not, in fact, decrease adverse effects because hydroxyzine itself is a mild respiratory depressant (8). No study has examined whether the combination of an opioid plus hydroxyzine produces respiratory depression less frequently than an equianalgesic dose of opioid alone.

Choosing an Oral Agent

Table 367.5 lists dosing guidelines for a number of commonly used oral opioids. Because opioids experience a significant first-pass hepatic metabolism, a higher oral than parenteral dose is necessary to achieve the same level of analgesia.

Codeine, which has gained widespread use, perhaps because of its low abuse potential, is a relatively weak analgesic with a relatively high incidence of GI side effects. The standard 60-mg dose alone is no more effective than 650 mg of aspirin or acetaminophen (3). At higher doses, the analgesic effect does not increase significantly, but the rate of side effects is higher.

Oxycodone and hydrocodone are excellent oral analgesics. They can produce euphoria, and, in certain patients, this is a liability.

Meperidine and propoxyphene (Darvon) are less satisfactory oral agents. Meperidine has a short analgesic duration, produces significant euphoria, and has a unique CNS toxicity. Its metabolite, normeperidine, is excitatory and may cause tremors, myoclonus, and seizures. Normeperidine has a longer half-life than its parent compound, accumulating with repeated dose administration of meperidine, thus increasing the risk of CNS toxicity. Propoxyphene's efficacy is arguable. In some studies, it has been no more effective than placebo, but combined with aspirin or acetaminophen, it produces additional analgesia (14). Overdose can result in seizures that are difficult to treat.

The main applications for oral morphine and hydromorphone (Dilaudid) are in cancer and sickle cell pain. Oral morphine is available as an immediate- and a sustained-release preparation.

Tramadol (Ultram) is an unscheduled, weak opioid agonist that also inhibits reuptake of serotonin and norepinephrine. It is a centrally acting synthetic analgesic compound with effects comparable to opioid analgesics, approved for the short-term treatment of acute pain in adults. The most common side effects are nausea, vomiting, dizziness, somnolence, and constipation. It does not appear to produce respiratory depression or hypotension, probably because of selective opioid receptor binding. It is as effective, or less effective, than codeine or hydrocodone in combination with acetaminophen (22). Tramadol is contraindicated in patients taking an MAO inhibitor as it inhibits monoamine uptake.

Combination Therapy

Rational pain management often involves combining analgesics of different classes (1). Adding acetaminophen (or an NSAID) to an opioid often produces better analgesia than a double dose of either agent alone (3). One possible explanation for this is that

---

TABLE 367.5.   Oral Opioid Dosing Information

Drug	Analgesic Equivalence[a]	Usual Starting Dose[b]	Usual Interval
Morphine (MSIR, Roxanol, others)	30 mg	15–30 mg[c]	3–4 h
Morphine: sustained release (MS Contin, Oramorph-SR)	30 mg	30 mg[c]	8–12 h
Meperidine (Demerol)[d]	300 mg	50–100 mg	2–3 h
Codeine (in Tylenol #3, others)[e]	200 mg	30–60 mg	3–4 h
Oxycodone (Roxicodone, also in Percocet, Percodan, Tylox, others)	20–30 mg	5–10 mg	3–6 h
Hydrocodone (in Lorcet, Lortab, Vicodin, others)	30 mg[f]	5–10 mg	3–6 h
Hydromorphone (Dilaudid)	7.5 mg	4–8 mg[c]	2–3 h
Tramadol (Ultram)	N/A	25–50 mg	4–6 h

Note: Addition of a nonopioid may allow lower dosing of an opioid. In using combination products, be careful not to exceed the allowable dose of the nonopioid constituent.

Note: Intervals are approximate. Individual patients may require dosing either more or less frequently.

Caution: Dosing may need to be adjusted in the elderly, patients weighing less than 50 kg, and those with renal or hepatic insufficiency.

[a] Doses equianalgesic to intravenous morphine 10 mg and intravenous meperidine 100 mg.

[b] Doses in this column are not equianalgesic.

[c] Usually reserved for chronic, severe pain.

[d] Meperidine has a unique CNS toxicity with repeated dosing and is not recommended as a first-line agent. See text.

[e] Doses greater than 60 mg are not recommended. See text.

[f] Limited data available.

the drugs work by different mechanisms. Combination therapy may permit a reduction in the opioid dose and a corresponding reduction in opioid-associated side effects.

Many formulations are commercially available that combine aspirin or acetaminophen with codeine, hydrocodone, or oxycodone. Although combination products containing codeine and hydrocodone are controlled substances, they are classified as schedule III (rather than II) and do not require duplicate or triplicate prescription paper. Therapy does not need to be restricted to these fixed-ratio products; prescribing the constituents separately may permit greater therapeutic flexibility. For very severe pain, the opioid dose can be increased without risking toxic doses of acetaminophen or aspirin. Conversely, as the pain improves, the patient can easily taper off the opioid but continue the nonnarcotic. For the outpatient treatment of severe pain, one common regimen is ibuprofen 2,400 mg/d in divided doses along with oxycodone 5 to 10 mg every 4 to 6 hours. An acetaminophen (120 mg) and codeine (12 mg/5 mL) elixir is available for use in children.

COMMON PITFALLS

✔ Relying too much on "objective" signs of pain severity and not enough on the patient's self-report
✔ Confusing pain avoidance behavior with drug-seeking behavior
✔ Withholding analgesia until a definitive diagnosis is made
✔ Withholding analgesia because consent for surgery or other procedure may later be necessary
✔ Failing to use an opioid for fear of creating addiction
✔ Administering opioids i.m. or s.c. when the intravenous route is superior
✔ Choosing a dose based on standard guidelines instead of individual patient response

References

1. Acute Pain Management Guideline Panel. *Acute pain management: Operative or medical procedures and trauma. Clinical practice guideline.* AHCPR Pub. No 92-0032. Rockville MD: Agency for Health Care Policy and Research, Public Health Service, U.S. Dept. of Health and Human Services, 1992.
2. Attard AR, Corlett MJ, Kidner NJ, et al. Safety of early pain relief for acute abdominal pain. *BMJ* 1992;305:554.
3. Beaver WT. Combination analgesics. *Am J Med* 1984;77[Suppl A]:38.
4. Bijur PR, Silver W, Gallagher EJ. Reliability of the visual analog scale for measurement of acute pain. *Acad Emerg Med* 2001;8:1153–1157.
5. Bijur PE, Latimer CT, Gallagher, JE. Validation of a verbally administered numerical rating scale of acute pain for use in the emergency department. *Acad Emerg Med* 2003;10:390–392.
6. Brooks PM, Day RO. Nonsteroidal antiinflammatory drugs—differences and similarities. *N Engl J Med* 1991;324:1716.
7. Cleeland CS. Measurement of pain by subjective report. In: Chapman CR, Loeser JD, eds. *Issues in pain management: Advances in pain research and therapy, vol 12.* New York: Raven Press 1989:399.
8. Glazier HS. Potentiation of pain relief with hydroxyzine: a therapeutic myth? *Ann Pharmacother* 1990;24:484.
9. Goldman B. Desperately seeking drugs: a clinical and risk management approach. *Emerg Physician Leg Bull* 1993;4:1.
10. Hoskin PJ, Hanks GW. Opioid agonist-antagonist drugs in acute and chronic pain states. *Drugs* 1991;41:326.
11. Jaffee JH, Martin WR.Opioid analgesics and antagonists. In: Goodman-Gilman A, Ball TW, Nies AS, et al, eds. *Goodman and Gilman's the pharmacologic basis of therapeutics* 8th ed. New York: Pergamon 1990:485.
12. Lanza FL. A guideline for the treatment and prevention of NSAID-induced ulcers. *J Gastroenterol* 1998;93:2037–2046.
13. Mandell BF. COX-2 selective NSAIDs. Biology, promises and concerns. *Cleve Clin J Med* 1999;66:285–291.
14. McEvoy GK, ed. *American hospital formulary service drug information.* Bethesda, MD: American Society of Hospital Pharmacists, 1993.
15. Neighbor ML, Puntillo KA. Intramuscular ketorolac vs. oral ibuprofen in emergency department patients with acute pain. *Acad Emerg Med* 1998;5:118–122.
16. Nissman SA, Kaplan LJ, Mann BD. Critical reappraising the literature-driven practice of analgesia administration for acute abdominal pain in the emergency room prior to surgical evaluation. *Am J Surg* 2003;185(4):291–296.
17. Pace S, Burke TF. Intravenous morphine for early pain relief in patients with acute abdominal pain. *Acad Emerg Med* 1996;3:1086–1092.
18. Paris PM, Weiss LD.Narcotic analgesics: The pure agonists. In: Paris PM, Stewart RD, eds. *Pain management in emergency medicine.* Norwalk, CT: Appleton & Lange 1988:125.
19. Porter J, Jick H. Addiction rare in patients treated with narcotics [Letter]. *N Engl J Med* 1980;302:123.
20. Sacchetti A, Schafermeyer R, Gerardi M, et al. Pediatric analgesia and sedation. *Ann Emerg Med* 1994;23:237.
21. Salo DF, Lavery R, Varma V, et al. A randomized, clinical trial comparing oral celecoxib 200 mg, celecoxib 400 mg, and ibuprofen 600 mg for acute pain. *Acad Emerg Med* 2003;10:22–30.
22. Turturro MA, Paris PM, Larkin GL. Tramadol versus hydrocodone-acetaminophen in acute musculoskeletal pain: a randomized, double-blind clinical trial. *Ann Emerg Med* 1998;32:139–143.
23. Turturro MA, Paris PM, Seaberg DC. Intramuscular ketorolac versus oral ibuprofen in acute musculoskeletal pain. *Ann Emerg Med* 1995;26:117–120.
24. Weisman SJ, Schechter NL. The management of pain in children. *Pediatr Rev* 1991;12:237.
25. Wood VM, et al. The NARC (nonsteroidal antiinflammatory in renal colic) trial: single-dose intravenous ketorolac versus titrated intravenous meperidine in acute renal colic. *Can J Emerg Med* 2000;2(2):83.

CHAPTER 368

Chronic Pain Syndromes

Michael A. Turturro and Paul M. Paris

Pain is typically defined as an unpleasant sensory and emotional phenomenon associated with actual or potential tissue damage. Chronic pain is defined as a sustained painful experience that persists beyond the time in which tissue damage occurs. Although acute pain typically has a rapid onset, coinciding with tissue damage, it typically resolves as tissue heals. It serves as a biologic warning of potential illness or injury, prompting the individual to protect the painful area and/or seek medical attention. Although distressing and anxiety provoking, it usually can be treated effectively with proper selection and use of analgesic drugs.

Chronic pain differs from acute pain in many respects (Table 368.1). In chronic pain, the symptom of pain itself often becomes more of a problem than its underlying cause, altering the patient's life and frequently causing both disability and depression. It has been estimated that the loss of productive time as a result of chronic pain costs over $60 billion a year in the United States (20); massive additional expenditures are also incurred from health care and litigation related to chronic pain syndromes. The treatment of chronic pain is complex and difficult. Success in treating chronic pain typically requires a multidisciplinary team approach, using various regimens of pharmacotherapy, physical therapy, and behavioral therapy to both reduce pain and restore function.

TABLE 368.1. Differences between Acute and Chronic Pain

Acute Pain	Chronic Pain
Usually as a result of tissue damage	Often no identifiable pathology
Is related to underlying illness	Is the problem itself
Has a biologic purpose	No biologic purpose
Responds to typical analgesics	May not respond to typical analgesics
Straightforward treatment	Complex treatment
Causes anxiety	Causes depression

CLINICAL PRESENTATION

Patients with chronic pain syndromes are often a management challenge for the emergency physician. Some present with vague signs and symptoms and often are not definitively diagnosed on the first encounter. Treatment is typically complex, requiring several regimens of varying effectiveness. Many patients have other psychological disturbances and a protracted course of exacerbations and remissions, with failures of assorted therapies. They may be demanding and frustrating, because their conditions are not easily managed. Patients may feel uncomfortable with a physician who has not been their regular caretaker. As a result, malingering or drug-seeking behavior may inappropriately be suspected. Establishing a rapport with the patient is essential, and the physician must not feel threatened by patient demands.

Each patient with chronic pain must also be evaluated for the development of progressive or new pathology. The physician should not assume that a patient's chronic pain exacerbation is nothing more than a worsening of an already existing disease process. For example, in a patient with increasing chronic low back pain one must consider new spinal cord pathology. Simply providing analgesics without an appropriate evaluation may result in missing serious disease.

Chronic pain syndromes typically fall into one of four categories:

1. Pain as a result of prolonged tissue destruction as a result of malignancy or other terminal illness (e.g., AIDS).
2. Pain as a result of dysfunction of the central or peripheral nervous system (e.g., trigeminal neuralgia).
3. Pain as a result of well known painful syndromes (e.g., fibromyalgia).
4. Pain with no objectively confirmed cause.

Although patients with pain as a result of prolonged tissue destruction are typically treated successfully with analgesics in the emergency department, patients in the remaining categories should also be referred to a chronic pain management center in which the manifestations of the chronic pain syndrome can be managed in a multidisciplinary manner. Communication between the emergency and pain service physicians fosters a team approach to the management of chronic pain exacerbations. For example, a contract may be developed between the patient, the pain service, and the emergency department regarding when the patient will be expected to present to the emergency department for a pain exacerbation, the analgesic that will be used after appropriate evaluation, and the quantity of analgesics prescribed on discharge.

Although chronic pain as a result of any cause may be exacerbated by psychological factors, the pathophysiology of chronic pain without obvious tissue pathology is unclear. Prolonged noxious sensory input from the periphery may result in self-sustaining central neural activity, possibly by reducing in-hibitory input into the central nervous system (CNS). This may produce a "memory" effect for pain perception in the CNS (13). These effects persist despite the lack of ongoing tissue injury. As a result, patients become increasingly more sensitive to painful stimuli.

Chronic pain patients should be considered valuable resources, because they often know the most effective therapies to treat their pain. Chronic pain commonly causes the patient to lose a sense of control over his or her environment. Allowing patients to become passively dependent on health care practitioners and medical therapy only feeds this vicious cycle of illness and the helpless victim.

Drug Abuse and Addiction

Drug abuse and addiction are unfortunate problems in our society, and drug abusers (whether or not they suffer from chronic pain) tend to patronize emergency departments on a frequent basis to obtain opioid analgesics. Because of this, emergency department staff members may develop a bias against many chronic pain patients. Because it may be difficult to differentiate patients with exacerbations of chronic pain from patients who are seeking drugs for abuse, many patients with real exacerbations of chronic pain are consequently labeled as drug abusers.

It is important to distinguish between opioid dependence, tolerance, and addiction. *Dependence* refers to the physical phenomenon in which sudden withdrawal of the drug results in a drug-specific withdrawal syndrome. This occurs in patients chronically using opioid analgesics, whether for legitimate or illicit purposes. *Tolerance* refers to the physical phenomenon of a decrease in drug effect at a specific dose over time, requiring increasing doses to produce the desired effect, whether that be analgesia or euphoria. Tolerance often occurs as a result of down-regulation or desensitization of opioid receptors, resulting in a physiologic resistance to opioid therapy (3). Additional physiologic changes may occur at the cellular level with chronic opioid therapy, which may result in abnormally increased sensitivity to painful stimuli.

Dependence and tolerance must be distinguished from *addiction*, which is the psychological state of compulsive use despite signs of toxicity, and inability to function as a result of this compulsive use. With legitimate prolonged use of opioid analgesics for chronic pain, dependence, and tolerance do occur, however addiction is rare. Conversely, when pain medication is withheld from patients with chronic pain, such patients may learn pain avoidance or maladaptive behaviors to obtain opioids. These drug-seeking behaviors do not imply addiction, but inappropriate techniques to satisfy a physiological need state, often referred to as *pseudoaddiction*. Giving pain medication on an as-needed basis for chronic pain, rather than around-the-clock dosing, contributes to this phenomenon, as the patient learns to express both symptoms and maladaptive behavior to obtain the reward of receiving pain medication.

Drug abusers often have a history of medical noncompliance, polysubstance abuse, multiple visits for treatment of various nonspecific painful conditions, an unusual reluctance to try new therapies, or a report that their primary physician is unreachable. They may have a history of selling prescription drugs, forging prescriptions, or using aliases. Because it is inappropriate and unethical to withhold analgesics from patients experiencing pain, unless the emergency physician is convinced that the patient is a drug abuser, the patient should be given the benefit of the doubt and a short course of analgesics should be prescribed. Sometimes, a known substance abuser may present with a truly painful condition. In these cases, pain should be adequately relieved in the emergency department, and judicious amounts of analgesics to be taken at regular intervals should be given on discharge. The use of opioid agonist–antagonists may be useful in these patients, as they are less likely to cause euphoria. However, they should not be given to a patient physically dependent on opioids, as they may precipitate withdrawal.

EMERGENCY DEPARTMENT MANAGEMENT

Although many of the concepts that apply to acute pain management (see Chapter 367, "Acute Pain Management") also apply to patients with chronic pain, the endpoint of total relief may not be attainable. Exacerbations of chronic pain are often as a result of a combination of both physical and psychological factors, and the primary goal in the emergency department is to reduce pain to the point in which the patient is functional, with pain service referral when appropriate. Additionally, certain pain syndromes (e.g., neuropathic pain) may not be effectively treated by the usual doses of typical analgesic agents. Therefore, an understanding of both the physical and psychological pathophysiology associated with these disorders will ensure optimal treatment.

The treatment of chronic pain includes the use of many modalities (Tables 367.2 and 367.3). Nonsteroidal antiinflammatory drugs and selective COX-2 inhibitors are often employed early in the patients course, however many patients are unable to be adequately controlled with these agents alone.

Opioid analgesics are the most useful drugs in treating exacerbations of chronic pain. The agents used are discussed in the chapter on acute pain (see Chapter 367, "Acute Pain Management"), but longer acting preparations such as sustained-release morphine (MS-Contin®), sustained-release oxycodone (OxyContin®), hydromorphone (Dilaudid®), and methadone are more appropriate for the treatment of chronic pain than acute pain. These agents also avoid the risk of aspirin or acetaminophen toxicity from the nonnarcotic component of combination products, which may occur when doses sufficient to provide adequate amounts of the opioid component are taken. Sustained-release oxycodone has gained considerable attention as a result of its potential for abuse. Its use should typically be reserved for patients with pain as a result of an advanced termi-

TABLE 368.2. Therapies for Chronic Pain

Therapy	Indications
Opioid analgesics	Most causes of chronic pain; limited effectiveness in neuropathic pain
Tricyclic antidepressants	Most causes of chronic pain
Anticonvulsants	Neuropathic pain
Transelectrical nerve stimulation (TENS)	Low back pain, neuropathic pain
Topical anesthetics	Neuropathic pain
Capsaicin	Neuropathic pain, arthritic pain
NMDA receptor antagonists	Neuropathic pain
Salmon calcitonin	Complex regional pain syndrome, phantom limb pain
Botulinum toxin	Myofascial pain, neuropathic pain
Behavioral therapy	Most causes of chronic pain
Physical therapy	Complex regional pain syndrome Temporomandibular disorders, tension myalgia
Surgery	Refractory trigeminal neuralgia, Complex regional pain syndrome, phantom limb pain

TABLE 368.3. Nonopioid Pharmacotherapy for Chronic Pain

Drug Class/Agent	Dosing
ANTIDEPRESSANTS	
Amitriptyline	50 mg PO q.h.s up to 150 mg/d
Imipramine	50 mg PO q.h.s.
Nortriptyline	25–50 mg p.o. q.h.s.
Doxepin	25–50 mg p.o. q.h.s.
Bupropion	150 mg p.o. b.i.d.
ANTICONVULSANTS	
Carbamazepine	100 mg p.o. q.h.s.;[a] increase to 100 mg p.o. b.i.d.; max. 1,200 mg/d
Clonazepam	1 mg p.o. q.h.s.; up to 1 mg p.o. t.i.d.
Gabapentin	300 mg p.o. t.i.d.; increase as necessary to maximum of 3,600 mg/d
Lamotrigine	25 mg q day; may double dose every 2 weeks to maximum of 200 mg q day
SKELETAL MUSCLE RELAXANTS	
Cyclobenzaprine	10 mg p.o. t.i.d.
Orphenadrine	100 mg p.o. b.i.d.
Carisoprodol	200–400 mg q.i.d.
Chlorzoxazone	250–750 mg p.o. t.i.d. or q.i.d.
Methocarbamol	1.5 g q.i.d.
Baclofen	5 mg p.o. t.i.d.; increase to 20 mg p.o. t.i.d.
TOPICAL ANESTHETICS	
Lidocaine patch	1–3 patches for 12 hours q day
Prilocaine/Lidocaine	2.5 g cream or 1 g disc
SUBSTANCE P INHIBITOR	
Capsaicin	Apply to affected area q.i.d.
NMDA RECEPTOR ANTAGONISTS	
Ketamine	0.4–0.5 mg/kg p.o. or i.v.
Dextromethorphan	60mg-240mg p.o. b.i.d., titrated to effect
OTHER AGENTS	
Salmon Calcitonin	200 I.U. Intranasal daily
Botulinum Toxin A	50–150 I.U. injection

[a] Obtain baseline complete blood count.

nal illness such as malignancy, as alternatives can be successfully used in other patients.

Pain as a result of malignancy, although chronic in nature, may be considered sustained acute pain because it is typically associated with progressive tissue damage. Although nonnarcotic analgesics and physical therapy are often used to treat malignant pain, progressively increasing doses of opioid analgesics remain the mainstay of therapy. Despite the risk of opioid dependence, opioid analgesics should never be withheld from patients with terminal malignant pain, as pain control is the most important factor contributing to overall quality of life. Acute exacerbations of malignant pain must be treated as an emergency, with aggressive opioid analgesia. Higher doses of opioids titrated more rapidly than in opioid-naive patients are typically needed, and this approach has been demonstrated to be safe and effective (10).

Tramadol is a centrally-acting oral analgesic that both activates opioid receptors in the CNS and also inhibits monoamine neurotransmitter reuptake (similar to tricyclic antidepressants). Tolerance and withdrawal symptoms appear to be absent with tramadol. However, it has been demonstrated to be less effective in the management of acute pain than other opioids (21) and is associated with a high incidence of side effects, including seizures. It appears to be most appropriate for adjunctive treatment in mild-to-moderate chronic pain.

Tricyclic antidepressants (TCAs) are useful in treating chronic pain, both by controlling depression and by altering nociceptive responses to painful stimuli, thereby altering the cerebral process in pain perception. They are effective in pain control even if no evidence of depression exists. TCAs are effective in various chronic pain syndromes, particularly neuropathic pain, face pain syndromes, fibromyalgia, and arthritis. TCAs act synergistically with opioids in controlling chronic pain. It is likely that all TCAs are effective in treating chronic pain, but amitriptyline has been the most extensively studied. The recommended starting dose for all TCAs in managing chronic pain is half the antidepressant dose, which may be titrated up if necessary. Analgesic effects may not be evident for several days. Referral for follow-up is essential in patients started on TCAs in the emergency department. Available evidence suggests that selective serotonin reuptake inhibitors (SSRIs) are less effective than TCAs in the management of chronic pain. Bupropion, an antidepressant unrelated to the TCAs or SSRIs, has shown promise in the treatment of neuropathic pain (17). The association between depression and chronic pain is clear, but in some patients the painful process produces depression, and in others chronic pain is a manifestation of a depressive disorder. In patients with chronic pain in whom no etiologic basis can be established, management is also focused on treating the underlying depression. Additionally, depression is also known to increase opioid analgesic requirements.

Transcutaneous electrical nerve stimulation (TENS) may be effective in certain acute and chronic pain syndromes. It is used most often in chronic low back pain and complex regional pain syndrome. Unfortunately, most patients note a decrease in the analgesic effect over time. The "gate control" theory of pain postulates that in the periphery small unmyelinated C fibers transmit nociceptive information, and large myelinated A fibers transmit light touch and pressure sensations. Both of these fibers synapse at the substantia gelatinosa in the dorsal horn of the spinal cord. Stimulation of the A fibers inhibits the transmission of nociceptive C fiber stimuli into the CNS, thereby "closing the gate." By using electricity to stimulate the A fibers preferentially, the pain stimulus entering the CNS can be controlled.

In neuropathic pain syndromes, pain originates from peripheral nerve dysfunction. Therefore, anticonvulsants play a primary role in treating most of these disorders. Additionally, because substance P may be the principal mediator of neuropathic pain, an effort to inhibit substance P may be beneficial. When applied topically, capsaicin, a substance derived from red chili peppers, releases substance P from primary afferent nerve fibers; with repeated application, capsaicin depletes substance P from these nerve fibers. Consequently, capsaicin may be useful in treating the neuropathic pain of postherpetic neuralgia, complex regional pain syndrome, and metabolic neuropathy, and other chronic pain syndromes such as psoriatic and rheumatoid arthritis. Capsaicin causes skin redness and burning. This may also contribute to its analgesic effect, as peripheral counter-irritation causes pain relief by a "gate-closing" effect, as described for TENS. However, this skin irritation also limits the concentration that may be used, thus reducing its potential efficacy (12). Botulinum toxin type A is a newer therapy currently being used in a variety of chronic pain syndromes, including neuropathic

pain and chronic myofascial pain. Its precise mechanism of action in treating acute pain is unclear, but it seems to involve both chemical denervation and inhibition of substance P (8).

It has recently been postulated that in chronic pain N-methyl-D-aspartate (NMDA) may play a central role in sensitizing the CNS to a prolonged painful stimulus, possibly by recruitment of C fibers. Consequently, substances that antagonize the NMDA receptor are gaining attention as possible agents in the management of chronic pain. Ketamine, dextromethorphan, methadone, and amantadine all antagonize the NMDA receptor and have been studied as agents for chronic pain management (particularly in neuropathic pain), however adverse effects may limit their utility (6).

Behavioral and physical therapy helps patients cope with chronic pain and regain a sense of self-control, thus improving overall day-to-day function. The focus with these therapies is rehabilitation, not total pain relief. However, patients must be motivated to be successful.

The most effective ways to treat these chronic pain syndromes are the multidisciplinary approaches used by pain clinics, in which combinations of the various therapies are coordinated. Thus, the emergency physician should confer with the patient's primary care or referring physician and make arrangements for follow-up before initiating or changing therapy.

Myofascial Pain and Fibromyalgia

Myofascial pain syndrome and fibromyalgia are conditions in which acute or chronic muscle pain, stiffness, and tenderness occur at specific anatomic sites ("trigger points"). A trigger point is an area within a taut band of skeletal muscle that, when palpated, produces referred pain in the area in which the patient complains of pain (a "reference zone"). It may be activated by physical trauma, other trigger points, or psychological stress.

Fibromyalgia and myofascial pain syndrome may be considered opposites in the spectrum of a single disorder (Table 368.4). Myofascial pain tends to be localized, and the involved muscle group may twitch involuntarily. Fibromyalgia pain tends to be diffuse and is associated with systemic symptoms such as chronic fatigue, sleep disturbance, headaches, vertigo, visual disturbances, and irritable bowel syndrome. Symptoms may begin after an acute viral illness, trauma, or psychological stress. Physical findings may be nonspecific, and the patient may be told that the symptoms are unexplained or psychogenic.

Although it has been postulated that psychological causes may underlie the pathophysiology of fibromyalgia (e.g., patients may not respond in a normal fashion to physical or psychological stress or may have a heightened perception of bodily discomfort), elevated levels of plasma substance P and decreased levels of serotonin have been demonstrated (14,15). Consequently, fibromyalgia patients may experience pain from stimuli that are below the painful threshold in normal patients as a result of

TABLE 368.4.   Myofascial Pain Syndrome versus Fibromyalgia

	Myofascial Pain	Fibromyalgia
Location	Regional	Generalized
Muscular twitch	Yes	No
Systemic symptoms	No	Possible
Sleep disturbances	No	Yes
Trigger-point injection useful	Yes	Sometimes
Physical therapy useful	Yes	No
Skeletal muscle relaxants useful	No	Yes

neurochemical alteration of pain pathways. Complicating matters is that depression is a frequent result of fibromyalgia, and somatization disorders are more frequent in fibromyalgia patients than the general population. Many patients seen in the emergency department for exacerbations of fibromyalgia pain may have failed traditional therapies, and may be using alternative treatments such as guaifenesin, magnetic therapy, diet therapy, acupuncture, herbal therapy, and zone therapy.

Other painful systemic illnesses such as systemic lupus erythematosus, polymyalgia rheumatica, polymyositis, metabolic myopathy, hypothyroidism, chronic fatigue syndrome, and irritable bowel syndrome should be considered. Because symptoms often overlap, the diagnosis is frequently one of exclusion.

The treatments of myofascial pain and fibromyalgia have certain similarities. Trigger-point injection of local anesthetics is a technique easily performed for both fibromyalgia and myofascial pain, often with rewarding results. Relief of local and referred pain and a decrease in muscle tension may be seen after injection. Topical vapor coolant sprays using fluoromethane or ethyl alcohol followed by stretch of the affected muscle may provide relief, however this mode of therapy is difficult to provide in the emergency department setting. Botulinum toxin therapy is a promising new treatment in the management of myofascial pain syndrome, but there is limited evidence of its effectiveness in treating fibromyalgia (19).

Although aerobic exercise may have some benefit in fibromyalgia, other physical techniques such as muscle stretching, biofeedback, and exercise, are useful in myofascial pain syndrome but are of limited value in fibromyalgia (18). In fibromyalgia patients, analgesics usually provide only partial relief, and additional therapy with antidepressants or muscle relaxants is often needed. Cyclobenzaprine, a skeletal muscle relaxant related to the TCAs, may be particularly useful in treating fibromyalgia (5). After initiating this therapy in the emergency department, follow-up care should be ensured.

Temporomandibular Disorders

Temporomandibular disorders affect the temporomandibular joint (TMJ) and surrounding facial structures, resulting in orofacial pain and dysfunction. Patients typically report facial pain and nonspecific headache, in addition to joint noise and difficulty in joint motion. Muscular and joint tenderness and limited TMJ range of motion may be found. The disorder is similar in many respects to both myofascial pain syndrome and fibromyalgia, and is often referred to as a form of myofascial pain. Many patients with TMJ dysfunction also are diagnosed with fibromyalgia or other myofascial pain syndromes.

The etiology is unclear. Some patients may exhibit signs of TMJ dysfunction but may not have troubling symptoms. Many patients have coexistent psychiatric diagnoses, which often leads to the assumption that emotional stress plays a role in this syndrome. Many patients show a greater sensitivity to certain noxious stimuli than do pain-free controls (16). Patients who clench or grind their teeth secondary to stress may develop masticatory muscle hyperactivity and fatigue, which can lead to pain and altered joint mechanics. Patients may present before definitive diagnosis with a complaint of nonspecific facial pain, or may present during a symptom exacerbation.

Facial neuralgias, myofascial pain syndrome, tension headache, and somatization disorder should be considered in the differential diagnosis.

As in other chronic pain syndromes, treatment frequently requires analgesics, antidepressants, and nonpharmacologic therapy. Physical therapy, biofeedback, and intraoral splinting help relax the afflicted muscles and reduce discomfort. Some patients improve with trigger point or TMJ joint injections, however pain control with analgesics is usually necessary. Patients should be discharged on TCAs if the diagnosis is certain and should be referred to a maxillofacial specialist so that an intraoral splint can be fitted and physical therapy started.

Neuropathic Pain Syndromes

Patients with neuropathic pain syndromes (Table 368.5) commonly present when symptoms first develop. The pain in these syndromes develops from nerve malfunction, sometimes as a result of physical damage to the involved nerve. In certain neuropathic pain syndromes, the pain is exacerbated by other stimuli that also stimulate the same nerve, such as light touch, temperature changes, or emotional stress. This phenomenon is known as allodynia. The pain is typically described as burning in nature, and treatment is often frustrating, because the usual doses of opioid and nonopioid analgesics are typically ineffective in relieving it.

Facial Neuralgias

Trigeminal neuralgia is a relatively common, often debilitating disorder. Typically older patients (over age 50) are affected, and the development of this disorder in patients under age 40 suggests a secondary cause, typically multiple sclerosis (9). Women develop this disorder more often than men do. The right side is more frequently involved, and bilaterality is rare. The second division of the fifth cranial nerve (V2) is most frequently affected. Attacks at the third division (V3) may also occur, but attacks at the first division (V1) are rare. The initial attacks are brief but severe and lancinating, often described as an "electric shock" sensation. Allodynia is prominent, and attacks may be triggered by touching the face, cold air blowing against the face, eating, shaving, or talking. Unlike other neuralgias, an objective sensory deficit is atypical and if found should alert the clinician to the possibility of nerve compression as a result of malignancy. As the condition progresses, the attacks become more frequent and a background ache may develop.

Glossopharyngeal neuralgia is less common and usually less severe than trigeminal neuralgia. It affects equal numbers of men and women. About 25% of cases are bilateral. Typically, a single episode of lancinating pain along the ninth cranial nerve sensory distribution (neck, throat, and ear) occurs. Atypical facial pain may occur, which is poorly localized but frequently involves the mandible. Unlike other facial pain syndromes, it is not clearly neuropathic and consequently does not respond and trigeminal neuralgia to anticonvulsants.

Cluster headache, maxillary sinusitis, postherpetic neuralgia (especially with V1 distribution), dental pain, and

---

TABLE 368.5. Neuropathic Pain Syndromes

Facial neuralgias
  Trigeminal
  Glossopharyngeal
Metabolic neuropathy
  Diabetic
  B_{12}
Nerve compression pain
  Radiculopathy
  Entrapment neuropathy
Postherpetic neuralgia
Complex regional pain syndrome
Phantom limb pain

temporomandibular disorders should be considered. Swallowing and chewing may trigger the pain from both facial neuralgias and TMJ dysfunction. Allodynia and the absence of TMJ tenderness suggest the former diagnosis.

The mainstay of treatment for the facial neuralgias is the administration of anticonvulsants, particularly carbamazepine. Unfortunately, patients typically present in extreme pain, and anticonvulsants usually require several days before a demonstrable effect is noticed. The recommended starting dose for carbamazepine is 100 mg q.h.s. for 3 days, then an increase to 100 mg twice a day. The dose may need to be titrated up to 1,200 mg per day. Other drugs, such as baclofen and clonazepam, may then need to be added. Because carbamazepine may cause neutropenia, a baseline complete blood count should be obtained. Carbamazepine may cause nausea, dizziness, or somnolence, which may limit patient compliance. Gabapentin and lamotrigine are newer anticonvulsants that have recently gained attention in the management of facial neuralgias, and are typically used in patients intolerant or refractory to carbamazepine (2). Follow-up with the patient's primary care physician or a neurologist should be arranged. Patients who fail medical therapy for trigeminal neuralgia often need surgical destruction of the sensory distribution of the trigeminal nerve, either by percutaneous thermocoagulation, cryosurgery, microvascular decompression, or glycerol injection.

Postherpetic Neuralgia

Postherpetic neuralgia is the most common neuropathic pain. It occurs in 10% of cases of herpes zoster, and it is more common in the elderly. It may begin during or after an attack of zoster; it typically persists for several weeks after the rash resolves, and it has no relation to the severity of the zoster attack. Burning pain occurs in the involved dermatome, which is most commonly thoracic (about 50%), ophthalmic (about 20%), and cervical (about 20%).

Diabetic neuropathy, demyelinating polyneuropathy, radiculopathy, and alcoholic neuropathy should be considered in the differential diagnosis.

Many treatments used in other neuropathic pain syndromes (e.g., diabetic neuropathy) have been recommended for the treatment of postherpetic neuralgia. However, it is difficult to determine what is truly effective because few well-designed, controlled clinical trials exist, and some cases may resolve with no treatment (1). The longer the condition is allowed to persist, the less likely that any one treatment will be effective.

Opioid analgesics may provide modest temporary improvement in pain, but they are typically are not useful alone in the treatment of postherpetic neuralgia. Tricyclic antidepressants are often used early in the course of therapy, and there is some evidence to suggest that preemptive treatment with antidepressants during an attack of herpes zoster may reduce the prevalence of postherpetic neuralgia (4).

Local anesthetics have been used in i.v. forms, in topical preparations such as lidocaine patch (Lidoderm®) and EMLA® (prilocaine/lidocaine) cream, and in nerve blocks. All of these methods appear to provide additional short-term relief of pain as a result of this condition. Capsaicin appears to provide temporary but effective relief if used four times a day for 3 to 4 weeks. Anticonvulsants reported to be useful in treating postherpetic neuralgia are primarily carbamazepine and gabapentin, however phenytoin, valproic acid, and the antispastic drug baclofen are occasionally used. Botulinum toxin, the NMDA antagonists dextromethorphan and ketamine have also been reported to treat postherpetic neuralgia, but the data on their effectiveness is limited.

Acyclovir, valacyclovir, and famciclovir are useful in the treatment of an acute attack of herpes zoster, particularly in the immunosuppressed host. These agents decrease viral shedding and the duration of lesions. Most evidence suggests that they also appear to have a modest effect on decreasing the incidence of postherpetic neuralgia, but are not effective treatments for postherpetic neuralgia (7). Although occasionally prescribed, there is no definite evidence that steroids are useful in preventing or treating postherpetic neuralgia (23).

Complex Regional Pain Syndrome

Complex regional pain syndrome (formerly referred to as reflex sympathetic dystrophy and causalgia), is a neuropathic pain syndrome characterized by a vicious cycle of pain, disuse atrophy, and peripheral autonomic dysfunction. Patients are usually 40 to 60 years old, although children are occasionally affected. It typically occurs after major extremity trauma, but it has also been related to minor trauma, cerebrovascular accident, myocardial infarction, arthritis, infection, and local tumor infiltration. Drugs such as isoniazid, ethanol, and phenobarbital have also been implicated as causative factors. It often occurs after prolonged extremity immobilization, presumably as a result of irritation of the sympathetic ganglia.

The term *causalgia* is reserved for complex regional pain syndrome related to a major peripheral nerve injury. After nerve damage as a result of an extremity injury, a positive feedback loop develops in which sympathetic efferent neurons stimulate afferent pain fibers and vice versa. Stimuli that cause sympathetic efferent outflow, such as temperature changes, often trigger this vicious cycle. Peripheral nociceptors are sensitized, and when stimulated they then stimulate sympathetic fibers. Thus, the cycle of pain and sympathetic overflow occurs.

The median, ulnar, and femoral nerves are most commonly affected. In patients with minor trauma, the degree of initial pain is often much greater than suggested by objective findings. The first (acute) stage occurs during the first several weeks of the disease process. Symptoms include pain, swelling, sympathetic underactivity, joint stiffness, warm skin, hypertrichosis, and edema. As the disease progresses, joint stiffness, hair loss, allodynia, sympathetic overreactivity, and muscular dystrophy occur, along with paroxysms of pain. After several months, decreased joint motion and muscle and skin atrophy occur. At this stage, the extremity appears cool, pale, shiny, and hairless. Radiographs are usually normal early in the disease and later show patchy osteopenia and erosions.

The differential diagnosis for complex regional pain syndrome includes collagen vascular disease, phlebitis, degenerative arthritis, and conversion hysteria.

Treatment is difficult, and most therapies provide only temporary relief. Medications that may be helpful include salmon calcitonin, tricyclic antidepressants, anticonvulsants, botulinum toxin, corticosteroids, β blockers, α blockers, calcium channel blockers, serotonin antagonists, capsaicin, N-methyl-D-aspartate (NMDA) receptor antagonists and type Ib antiarrhythmics (22). As with other forms of neuropathic pain, opioids and nonsteroidal antiinflammatory agents are often ineffective. Regional blocks using guanethidine may be effective but can exacerbate the pain before it improves. Physical therapy is essential, and other nonpharmacologic therapies, such as TENS, may be used. Sympathetic blocks may provide only temporary analgesia, but may allow aggressive physical therapy.

This disorder can be prevented by avoiding prolonged immobilization in patients with extremity trauma. Recognizing the early stages and intervening before the disease progresses is important. Patients should be referred for early physical therapy.

Phantom Limb Pain

Phantom limb pain is a poorly understood syndrome that occurs after extremity amputation. It too is difficult to treat. After amputation, phantom sensation is nearly universal, and usually resolves in less than a year. Persistent pain is thought to be related to neural damage in the postamputation period, and mechanisms in the peripheral nerve, spinal cord, and brain all contribute to the development of phantom limb pain. It has been postulated that the last impulses received by the limb before amputation may be stored in "memory," and if these impulses are painful, the sensation may persist (11). Consequently, the incidence of phantom limb pain is decreased in patients given preoperative regional anesthesia. As with other chronic pain syndromes, psychological stress exacerbates the degree of pain experienced.

The differential diagnosis includes complex regional pain syndrome, metabolic neuropathy, and neurosarcoma.

There are few well-designed studies that evaluate the various treatment regimens for phantom limb pain. Antidepressants, anticonvulsants, analgesics, capsaicin, and β-blocking agents all seem to provide temporary relief. Surgical techniques such as cordotomy, stump revision, and neuroma removal have been reported, with variable degrees of success. A combination of long-term behavioral therapy and antidepressants appears to be the most useful mode of therapy.

CRITICAL INTERVENTIONS

- Use nonanalgesic interventions that are specific for certain chronic pain syndromes
- Consult with the primary care physician or pain clinic before initiating or changing long-term therapy in patients with chronic pain syndromes. Arrange follow-up for these patients

COMMON PITFALLS

✔ Missing acute disease by assuming an exacerbation of chronic pain is due to preexisting disease

✔ Labeling chronic pain patients who have true pain as drug seekers

✔ Overreliance on analgesic drugs to treat neuropathic pain

✔ Failure to appreciate the risk of aspirin or acetaminophen toxicity when using escalating doses of combination opioid products to treat chronic pain

✔ Assuming the pain from fibromyalgia or temporomandibular disorders is psychogenic

References

1. Alper BS, Lewis PR. Treatment of postherpetic neuralgia: a systematic review of the literature. *J Fam Pract* 2002;51:121–128.
2. Backonja M. Use of anticonvulsants for treatment of neuropathic pain. *Neurology* 2002;59(Suppl 2):S14–S17.
3. Ballantyne JC, Jianren M. Opioid therapy for chronic pain *N Engl J Med* 2003;349:1943–1953.
4. Bowsher D. The effects or pre-emptive treatment of postherpetic neuralgia with amitriptyline: a randomized, double-blind placebo-controlled trial. *J Pain Symptom Manage* 1997;13:327–331.
5. Carette S, Bell MJ, Reynolds WJ, et al. Comparison of amitriptyline, cyclobenzaprine, and placebo in the treatment of fibromyalgia: a randomized, double-blind clinical trial. *Arthritis Rheum* 1994;37:32–40.
6. Hewitt DJ. The use of NMDA receptor antagonists in the treatment of chronic pain. *Clin J Pain* 2000;16(Suppl 2):S73–79.
7. Jackson JL, Gibbons R, Meyer G, et al. The effect of treating herpes zoster with oral acyclovir in preventing postherpetic neuralgia: a meta-analysis. *Arch Intern Med* 1997;157:909–912.
8. Lang AML. Botulinum toxin type A in chronic pain disorders. *Arch Phys Med Rehabil* 2003;84(Suppl 1):S69–73.
9. Marbach JJ. Medically unexplained chronic orofacial pain. *Med Clin North Am* 1999;83:691–710.
10. Moynihan TJ. Use of Opioids in the treatment of severe pain in terminally ill patients—dying should not be painful. *Mayo Clin Proc* 2003;78:1397–1401.
11. Nikolajsen L, Jensen TS. Phantom limb pain. *Br J Anaesth* 2001;87:107–116.
12. Robbins WR, Staats PS, Levine J, et al. Treatment of intractable pain with topical large-dose capsaicin: Preliminary report. *Anesth Analg* 1999;86:579–583.
13. Rosenow JM, Henderson JM. Anatomy and physiology of chronic pain. *Neurosurg Clin N Am* 2003;14:445–462.
14. Russell IJ, Orr MD, Littman B, et al. Elevated cerebrospinal fluid levels of substance P in patients with fibromyalgia syndrome. *Arthritis Rheum* 1994;37:1593–1601.
15. Russell IJ. Neurochemical pathogenesis of fibromyalgia syndrome. *J Musculoskel Pain* 1996;4:61–92.
16. Sarlani E, Greenspan JD. Evidence for generalized hyperalgesia in temporomandibular disorders patients. *Pain* 2003;102:221–226.
17. Semenchuk MR, Sherman S, Davis B. Double-blind, randomized trial of bupropion SR for the treatment of neuropathic pain. *Neurology* 2001;57:1583–1588.
18. Sim J, Adams N. Systematic review of randomized controlled trials of nonpharmacological interventions for fibromyalgia. *Clin J Pain* 2002;18:324–326.
19. Smith HS, Audette J, Royal MA. Botulinum toxin in pain management of soft tissue syndromes. *Clin J Pain* 2002;18(Suppl 6):S147–154.
20. Stewart WF, Ricci JA, Chee E, et al. Lost productive time and cost due to common pain conditions in the US workforce. *JAMA* 2003;290:2443–2454.
21. Stubhaug A, Grimstad J, Breivik H. Lack of analgesic effect of 50 and 100 mg oral tramadol after orthopaedic surgery: a randomized, double-blind, placebo and active standard drug comparison. *Pain* 1995;62:111–118.
22. Wasner G, Schattschneider J, Binder A, et al. Complex regional pain syndrome—diagnostic, mechanisms, CNS involvement and therapy. *Spinal Cord* 2003;41:61–75.
23. Whitley RJ, Weiss H, Gnann JW, et al. Acyclovir with and without prednisone for the treatment of herpes zoster: a randomized, placebo-controlled trial. *Ann Intern Med* 1996;125:376–383.

CHAPTER 369

Procedural Sedation and Analgesia

Robert J. Vissers

The care of patients with painful conditions and the performance of painful diagnostic and therapeutic procedures are routine aspects of emergency medicine care. Approximately half of emergency department visits are for pain-related chief complaints (14). Many of these conditions are also associated with anxiety. Accordingly, procedural sedation and analgesia (PSA) has become a fundamental skill of emergency physicians and an important part of emergency medicine resident training (1).

Despite the emphasis on PSA, oligoanalgesia has been well described in emergency care. Inadequate pain control has been ascribed to underestimation of patient pain, concern for patient safety, fear of delays associated with over-sedation and the alteration of physical findings (1,8,10). PSA can improve quality of care and patient satisfaction through the relief of pain and anxiety, and the facilitation of therapeutic or diagnostic procedures such as cardioversion, incision and drainage of abscesses, tube thoracostomy, lumbar punctures, fracture reduction, complex suturing, and imaging studies (1,15,20). Many drugs used for sedation and analgesia have the potential to cause respiratory, cardiovascular, and central nervous system (CNS) depression. The advent of shorter-acting, more effective drugs, the development of noninvasive monitoring devices, and published clinical policies for PSA have made it an extremely safe, practical procedure. The airway and critical care expertise of emergency physicians make them ideal providers of safe PSA.

The wide variety of procedures and patient types requires the ability to individualize PSA. This can only be achieved through a comprehensive understanding of the drugs used, and proper patient assessment. Protocols delineating staffing responsibilities, monitoring guidelines, approved medications, observation periods, and discharge criteria and instructions are recommended before implementing PSA in the emergency department.

Definitions

The term *conscious sedation* has previously been used to describe the process of providing analgesia, sedation, and amnesia for patients undergoing painful procedures. However, this term may be misleading (29). A more precise and preferred term is PSA. In a recent clinical policy published by the American College of Emergency Physicians, PSA was defined as "a technique of administering sedatives or dissociative agents with or without analgesics to induce a state that allows the patient to tolerate unpleasant procedures without undue pain and/or anxiety while maintaining cardiorespiratory function. Procedural sedation and analgesia is intended to result in a depressed level of consciousness that allows the patient to maintain oxygenation and airway control independently and continuously"(1).

The Joint Commission on Accreditation of Healthcare Organizations (JCAHO), in its 2003 Comprehensive Accreditation Manual for Hospitals, states that "the standards for sedation and anesthesia care apply when patients receive, in any setting, for any purpose, by any route, moderate or deep sedation and general, spinal, or other major regional anesthesia" (20). JCAHO has adopted the American Society of Anesthesiologists (ASA) definitions of sedation and analgesia created in 1999 to better describe the continuum of sedation and analgesia. *Moderate sedation* most closely approximates the replaced term *conscious sedation*.

Minimal sedation is primarily anxiolysis, during which patients respond normally to verbal commands. Ventilatory and cardiovascular function remain unaffected.

Moderate sedation/analgesia is a drug-induced depression of consciousness during which the patients respond purposefully to verbal commands, alone or accompanied by tactile stimulation. No interventions are required to maintain a patent airway. Spontaneous ventilation is adequate and cardiovascular function is maintained.

Deep sedation/analgesia is a drug-induced depression of consciousness during which patients cannot be easily aroused but respond purposefully following repeated or painful stimulation. Assistance may be needed to maintain a patent airway and independent ventilation may be inadequate. Cardiovascular function is usually maintained.

General anesthesia is a drug-induced loss of consciousness during which patients are not arousable, even by painful stimulation. Independent ventilatory function is often impaired and ventilatory and airway support is often required. Cardiovascular function may be impaired.

The response to medications can vary greatly between individuals and may be unpredictable. Therefore it is recommended that clinicians be competent in the skills required to manage patients at least one level greater than the intended sedation (3).

EMERGENCY DEPARTMENT EVALUATION

Careful patient selection is necessary to providing safe and effective PSA. The comorbid illness or injury, any underlying medical problems, patient age, the procedure, and the ability to manage the airway are important considerations in determining the indication and the method for PSA. Not all patients, or procedures, are appropriate candidates for PSA and may be best served in the operating room. A patient's physical status can be conveniently described using the American Society of Anesthesiologist's classification (Table 369.1) (3). This is frequently incorporated into the documentation of the preprocedure assessment and it has been suggested that anesthesiology be consulted for class III, IV, or V patients.

A history of prior problems with anesthesia or PSA should be elicited. Particular attention should be paid to underlying cardiorespiratory diseases, neurologic diseases, medications, and intoxicants. Physical examination should focus on the cardiovascular, respiratory, and neurological systems and performing an assessment of airway difficulty. There is no evidence to support the need for specific diagnostic testing before PSA. A discussion including the risks, benefits and potential side effects of PSA should take place before the procedure. Written consent is recommended when possible, however, patient condition may preclude this (1).

There is insufficient literature to recommend a necessary period of fasting prior to PSA. The combination of vomiting and loss of protective reflexes during PSA causing aspiration is considered to be a rare event (18). There is no evidence that gastric emptying or antacids reduces the incidence of PSA-associated complications. Recent food ingestion is not a contraindication but rather a consideration when choosing the targeted level of sedation.

EMERGENCY DEPARTMENT MANAGEMENT

Preparation

The necessary equipment and supplies should be gathered in an appropriate setting prior to the initiation of PSA. There does not have to be a specific dedicated area for PSA. However, the capability to provide cardiovascular and respiratory support, and availability of personnel, may dictate the location. Oxygen, suction, advanced life support equipment, a bag-valve-mask, and intubation equipment must be readily available. An i.v. should be placed in most circumstances. The most common exception would be the use of ketamine given intramuscularly, which has a wide safety margin with preservation of protective airway reflexes (19). Advanced life support medications should be accessible, and the antagonists naloxone and flumazenil, when opioids and benzodiazepines are being used (11,36).

JCAHO and compliant institutions insist that the PSA provider have adequate training to administer the agents effectively and safely and have the skills to manage all potential complications (20). Fortunately, these are all within the scope of the emergency physician's expertise. There is no clear guideline in the literature or organizational policies regarding the required

---

TABLE 369.1. ASA Physical Status Classification

I. Normal, healthy patient
II. Mild systemic disease
III. Severe systemic disease
IV. Severe systemic disease that is a constant threat to life
V. Moribund patient, not expected to survive the procedure

number of support personnel. It is essential that an individual is present who is monitoring and capable of recognizing the respiratory and hemodynamic responses to the medications. The performance of a procedure often precludes the continual clinical assessment of the patient. Therefore one individual not performing the procedure is usually recommended to monitor and document patient status (1).

The use of supplemental oxygen during PSA is somewhat controversial. Although its routine use may prevent hypoxemia in some patients, there is concern that it will delay the recognition of respiratory compromise and hypercarbia (27). There is little evidence to guide the use of oxygen in patients undergoing PSA, therefore institutional guidelines and physician discretion should be used.

Monitoring

The most important aspect of monitoring during PSA is the visual observation and assessment of physiologic changes and the level of consciousness. The patient's ability to follow commands, and the response to varied levels of stimulation are useful in quantifying the level of consciousness (20). Other components of monitoring may include respiratory rate, heart rate, blood pressure, oxygen saturation, capnometry, and cardiac rhythm.

The use of pulse oximetry is widely recommended in national and institutional PSA guidelines (1,3,20). Many studies have demonstrated its utility in identifying hypoxia, usually defined as a saturation less than 90%, however there is no clear demonstration that its use during PSA impacts patient outcome (2). This may be as a result of the extremely low risk of morbidity and mortality during PSA when the patient's respiratory efforts and level of consciousness are clinically monitored (5,12,19,26). Studies also demonstrate that decreases in oxygen saturation frequently occur without any clinical significance (1,9). Pulse oximetry should still be utilized as a reliable monitoring adjunct. However, it should not be a substitute for continuous clinical assessment.

Most medications used in PSA have the potential to cause hypoventilation and a subsequent rise in the patient's end-tidal CO_2. Capnometry measures end-tidal CO_2 and therefore may detect early cases of inadequate ventilation prior to the onset of hypoxia (23,25). Studies have demonstrated excellent correlation between rising end-tidal CO2 and dropping oxygen saturations, and earlier identification of possible hypoventilation through capnometry than oximetry (25,34). No study thus far has addressed whether earlier detection of hypoventilation has any impact on outcomes. The benefit of adding capnometry to oximetry and visual monitoring remains unclear, and may be considered useful in cases in which direct patient observation is not possible.

The Bispectral Index (BIS) is a noninvasive monitor attached to the forehead, which derives a sedation level from measures of frontal lobe electroencephalographic measures. It has been validated in the operating room as an objective measure of sedation, and it has been suggested that it may reduce time to discharge through the prevention of oversedation. At the present time its practical application in the emergency department requires more investigation before its role is defined (17).

Vital signs should be assessed frequently with patient observation. Patients are at the highest risk for complications within 5 to 20 minutes of receiving i.v. medications, and when noxious stimuli are removed (4,26). Continuous electrocardiographic monitoring is not routinely recommended. However, it should be used in older patients or those with a history of cardiovascular or pulmonary disease. Documentation of the

TABLE 369.2. Assessment of Sedation
Fully awake
Arouses easily
Arouses with tactile stimuli
Arouses to vigorous stimuli
Responsive to painful stimuli
Unresponsive

level of sedation can be quantified using a predefined sedation score, such as the Aldrete score or a simplified version suggested in Table 369.2.

Drug Selection and Administration

The ideal agent for PSA would provide analgesia, anxiolysis, amnesia, and somnolence rapidly and predictably with no adverse effects. Unfortunately this drug does not exist. As a result multiple sedative–hypnotics, opioids, and various anesthetic agents have been employed, singly and in combination, in an attempt to achieve the desired level of PSA (Table 369.3) (8). For example, many agents provide sedation without analgesia, therefore painful procedures require the addition of an opioid to a sedative–hypnotic. The therapeutic effects of these drugs in combination are often synergistic. However, the primary side effects of respiratory and cardiovascular depression are also exaggerated (26). Agent selection, dosing, and route of administration should be determined by the procedure and the specific patient. Drug availability and physician experience are also important determinants.

Regardless of the agent used, an important principle in PSA is the slow titration of drugs to the desired effect. Drugs given i.v. have a rapid onset with a more predictable response than agents given orally, transmucosally, or i.m (8). Drugs should be pushed slowly, because rapid administration is more likely to cause hypotension or respiratory depression. It is important to allow adequate time to achieve and assess peak effect before a second dose is given. A possible exception to the preferred i.v. route may exist in children, in whom i.v. access is often difficult and the i.m. response of ketamine is very predictable (19).

Analgesics

Fentanyl, a synthetic opioid, is about 1,000 times as potent as meperidine. It is short-acting, with a duration of action of 30 to 45 minutes (8,13). It does not cause histamine release and has minimal cardiovascular effects. It is highly lipophilic and rapidly crosses the blood–brain barrier. Redistribution then occurs into the peripheral tissues, in which it is metabolized by the liver. Like all opioids, fentanyl is reversed by naloxone. Respiratory depression is more likely at higher doses, when given rapidly i.v. push, or when combined with other CNS depressants, such as benzodiazepines or alcohol.

Fentanyl is best given in titrated intravenous doses until the desired level of sedation and analgesia is obtained. Dosing should begin at 0.5 to 1.0 μg/kg and is slowly titrated upward every 1 to 2 minutes until the desired effect is obtained. Adequate sedation and analgesia are usually obtained with doses of 2 to 3 μg/kg when fentanyl is used alone and 1 to 2 μg/kg when other medications, such as midazolam or etomidate, are used in combination (8). Lower doses should be used in elderly patients and when other CNS depressants may have been previously ingested (8,13). When mild sedation is needed and venous access may be difficult, such as in small children, i.m. injections of 2 to

TABLE 369.3. Agents Commonly Used in Procedural Sedation and Analgesia

Drug	Class	Effect	Side Effects	Dose	Peak	Clinical Duration
Morphine	Opioid	Analgesia Sedation	↓ Respirations N&V ↓ BP, HR ↑ Histamine	Children: i.v.: 0.05–0.1 mg/kg Adults: i.v.: 3–5 mg	i.v.: 20 m Oral: 60 m i.m.: 30–60 min	3–5 h
Fentanyl	Opioid	Analgesia Sedation	↓ Respirations N&V Chest wall rigidity	Children: i.v.: 1–2 mcg/kg Adults: i.v.: 1 mcg/kg	i.v.: 0.5–2 m	30–60 m
Midazolam	Benzodiazepine	Sedation Amnesia	↓ Respirations ↓ BP ↓ Pulse	Children i.v.: 0.05 mg/kg p.o.: 0.5 mg/kg Adults: i.v.: 0.5–5 mg	i.v.: 1–5 m p.o.: 30 m	1–2 h
Diazepam	Benzodiazepine	Sedation Amnesia	↓ Respirations ↓ BP ↓ Pulse	Children i.v.: 0.05 mg/kg p.o.: 0.2 mg/kg Adults: i.v.: 2.5–5 mg p.o.: 10 mg	i.v.: 5–15 m PO: 45–60 min	2–6 h
Methohexital	Barbiturate	Sedation Amnesia	↓ Respirations N&V ↓ BP ↑ Histamine	Adults: i.v.: 1–3 mg/kg Children: PR: 25mg/kg (max 500mg)	i.v.: 1 m PR: 8 m	i.v.: 8–10 m PR: 80 m
Pentobarbital	Barbiturate	Sedation Amnesia	↓ Respirations N&V ↓ BP ↑ Histamine	Children i.v.: 2 mg/kg p.o.: PR: 2–6 mg/kg i.m.: 2–6 mg/kg Adults: i.v.: 100 mg p.o.: 100 mg	i.v.: 1 m	6–10 m
Propofol	Imidazole derivative	Sedation Amnesia Antiemetic	↓ Respirations ↓ BP	1–2 mg/kg bolus 50–100 mcg/kg/ m i.v. continuous infusion	0.5 m	4–8 m
Etomidate	Isopropylphenol compound	Sedation Amnesia	↓ Respirations	0.1 mg/kg	1 m	5–8 m
Ketamine	Phencyclidine derivative	Dissociation Analgesia Sedation Amnesia	↑ BP, HR Laryngospasm Increased secretions	Adults: i.v.: 1–2 mg/kg Children: i.v.: 1 mg/kg i.m.: 2–5 mg/kg	i.v.: 1 m i.m.: 5 min	i.v.: 15–20 m i.m.: 30 m
Nitrous Oxide	Anesthetic gas	Analgesia Sedation		Self administered 50:50 mix NO$_2$ -O$_2$	1–2 m	5 m

3 μg/kg may suffice (21). As a result of its lack of amnesic effects, fentanyl is often combined with midazolam. Midazolam potentiates the effects of fentanyl and the potential for hypoxemia. It may also increase the incidence of hypotension. However, when the two drugs are carefully titrated, the incidence of significant cardiovascular side effects is very low.

Side effects of fentanyl include hypoxemia, apnea, vomiting, and pruritus. Hypotension is rare. Bradycardia may occur with high doses. Truncal rigidity and glottic spasm, which make ventilation difficult, are unique complications seen with doses above 10 μg/kg, or at lower doses if the drug is given rapidly.

Sedatives

Methohexital is an ultrashort-acting barbiturate with sedative and hypnotic effects. It produces deep sedation but provides no analgesia (37). Methohexital produces a state of deep sedation, which may be preferred for such procedures as cardioversion, chest tube insertion, or complicated orthopaedic reductions. It has a rapid onset of action of 30 to 60 seconds, a duration of action of 7 to 10 minutes, and a short recovery phase. Deep sedation is achieved with bolus doses of 1 to 2 mg/kg (37). Intramuscular

doses of 10 mg/kg produce effects that begin in 2 to 3 minutes and last almost 1 hour. Rectal methohexital is especially efficacious in children when a motionless state is needed. A dose of 20 to 30 mg/kg induces sleep within 10 minutes and lasts for about 45 to 80 minutes. Cardiorespiratory complications rarely occur with rectal administration (6). Adverse reactions associated with the use of methohexital include dose-dependent respiratory depression and apnea. Oxygen desaturation is especially common when concomitant respiratory depressants are used. Hypotension is uncommon but can occur, especially in patients with hypovolemia and sepsis. It is easily corrected by giving i.v. fluids (8,37). Hiccups can occur, and protective reflexes may be impaired. Methohexital induces epileptiform activity by electroencephalogram in seizure patients and should be avoided in patients with epilepsy (22).

Midazolam is a benzodiazepine with amnesic and anxiolytic properties. At physiologic pH, the drug's open-ring structure closes, making it lipophilic and able to cross the blood–brain barrier rapidly in which it interacts with the γ-aminobutyric acid receptors. Midazolam has a more rapid onset and shorter duration of action than diazepam and rarely causes phlebitis. Its amnesic properties also appear to be superior to those of diazepam (35). It is eliminated by hepatic metabolism. Like all benzodiazepines, midazolam has no analgesic properties and must be combined with analgesics such as fentanyl or morphine, or with regional or local anesthetics, when painful procedures are performed (8).

The i.v. dose is 0.03 to 0.1 mg/kg, with a starting dose of 1 mg. Onset of sedation is within 3 to 5 minutes, and the duration of action is about 30 to 60 minutes. With i.m. administration, the same dose is typically used, but the onset of sedation is delayed.

In children, oral, rectal, and intranasal routes are effective alternatives to i.v. sedation. Oral doses are 0.2 to 0.75 mg/kg, and sedation is achieved within 1 hour. Rectal administration is effective at doses of 0.3 to 0.5 mg/kg. The response by this route is variable as a result of the unpredictable effect of first-pass hepatic metabolism (28). It is not well tolerated or accepted by older children. Intranasal administration can be used when an intravenous line is not needed or when sedation is necessary to establish one (32). Doses of 0.2 to 0.4 mg/kg result in sedation in about 10 to 15 minutes.

Lower doses should be used when analgesic agents are given concomitantly, and in elderly patients. Prolonged effects may occur in elderly patients as a result of decreased metabolic clearance and decreased first-pass metabolism.

Side effects include dose-dependent hypoventilation and hypoxemia. At high doses, midazolam blunts the central respiratory center's sensitivity to hypercapnia (8). Apnea is rare, except when other CNS depressants, such as narcotics, are used. Hypotension can also occur with high doses.

Anesthetics

Etomidate is an ultrashort-acting, nonbarbiturate sedative–hypnotic with no analgesic properties. Like methohexital, it causes deep sedation, has a very rapid onset of less than 1 minute, and has a duration of action of 3 to 5 minutes. Etomidate has minimal cardiac effects. Although respiratory depression can occur, it is usually transient and associated with the use of other respiratory depressants (7).

The drug is given i.v. (0.1 mg/kg) and is currently not approved for children under age 10. Lower doses should be used when the drug is combined with analgesics.

Side effects are uncommon. Transient respiratory depression can occur. Myoclonic jerking can occur and has been mistaken for seizures. Using another agent, such as fentanyl, in conjunction with etomidate may prevent or minimize the jerking. Adrenal suppression only occurs after long term use and is not an issue in PSA. Published experience with the use and safety of etomidate in the emergency department is limited but suggests a relatively high rate of transient apnea (33).

Ketamine is an anesthetic that causes a dissociation between the thalamic and limbic systems. This, in turn, hinders the perception of visual, auditory, and painful stimuli, leaving the patient in a trancelike state (19). After absorption, ketamine is rapidly distributed and taken up by cerebral tissue. Effects are maintained until the drug redistributes into the peripheral tissues and is metabolized by the liver (8).

Ketamine can be given by multiple routes. An i.v. dose of 1 to 2 mg/kg, an i.m. dose of 2 to 6 mg/kg, a rectal dose of 5 to 15 mg/kg, an oral dose of 6 to 10 mg/kg, or an intranasal dose of 6 mg/kg provides adequate sedation and analgesia (8,18). Sedation is achieved within 1 minute when the drug is given intravenously, 5 minutes when given intramuscularly, and 5 to 20 minutes by other routes.

Ketamine's most common side effect is the emergence phenomenon, in which the patient wakes up hallucinating. This is more common in patients over age 10, females, and those with an underlying psychiatric disorder. It is less common with i.m. injection and can be attenuated with benzodiazepines.

Laryngospasm and emesis are infrequent complications. Patients given ketamine may develop nystagmus, and muscular hypertonicity. The pharyngeal–laryngeal reflexes remain intact, although laryngospasm sometimes occurs (18,19). Ketamine has minimal effects on oxygen delivery. Respiratory depression may occur with high doses or rapid i.v. infusion. The drug stimulates tracheobronchial and salivary secretions, however this effect can be minimized by the concomitant use of an anticholinergic such as atropine. Mild-to-moderate elevations in pulse rate and blood pressure may result from ketamine's ability to block the reuptake of catecholamines, especially with i.v. infusion. Twitching, hypertonus, and myoclonic jerking can occur and have been mistaken for seizures. Electroencephalographic studies, however, have shown that ketamine does not cause convulsions.

Ketamine is contraindicated in patients with cardiovascular disease, chronic obstructive pulmonary disease, intracranial and intraocular injuries, and increased intracranial or intraocular pressures. It is not recommended for use in patients with a history of psychiatric illness and children under 3 months of age.

Propofol is a very short acting sedative–hypnotic agent, with a rapid onset of action. It is currently approved for use in adults only, but its use in children is well described in the medical literature. Propofol is given intravenously as an initial bolus, followed by a continuous infusion or by intermittent bolus injections. It is metabolized by the liver and excreted by the kidneys. It is thought to have a secondary form of metabolism, because it can be used safely in patients with liver cirrhosis and renal failure. When propofol is used as the sole agent, patients fully recover from sedation 10 to 20 minutes after the infusion is discontinued.

Propofol is often used in combination with analgesics such as fentanyl. Studies comparing propofol with midazolam found them to have equivalent amnesic properties. However, patients receiving propofol did not demonstrate the residual grogginess associated with midazolam and were discharged sooner. Transient hypoxia appears to be common but without clinical sequelae (30,31). In an emergency department study, propofol had the lowest incidence of respiratory depression when compared to methohexital, fentanyl and midazolam, and etomidate (24).

Sedation is usually achieved with a bolus of 1 to 2 mg/kg. This should be titrated with a slow push at a rate of 10 to 40 mg every 10 seconds until the sedative effects are achieved. A continuous infusion of 3 to 6 mg/kg/h (50–100 μg/kg per minute) is then titrated to the desired level of sedation (31). Alternatively, intermittent boluses of 25 to 50 mg can be used to maintain sedation in adults. Lower doses should be used when sedating elderly patients or when administered with i.v. analgesics.

The major side effect noted with propofol is transient apnea, which occurs when the bolus is infused rapidly, or when propofol is given in conjunction with opioids. Hypotension and bradycardia may also occur but are easily reversed with fluids or by terminating the infusion. Propofol may cause transient pain on injection, but this can be prevented by giving lidocaine (1 mL of a 1% solution i.v.) first.

Nitrous oxide is a colorless gas that, when used in combination with oxygen, provides analgesia and sedation. The gas diffuses rapidly across membranes, providing a rapid onset and elimination (16). The level of sedation is often disproportional to the analgesia provided. The use of analgesics in combination with nitrous oxide appears to synergistically enhance the level of sedation and pain control, however potential side effects, such as hypoventilation also are compounded.

Nitrous oxide is given as a 50%/50% mixture with oxygen by a demand valve-mask or a mouthpiece, held by the patient.

Scavenger devices and adequate room ventilation are used to minimize the escape of the gas into the air, preventing potential acute and chronic adverse effects on the staff.

Because the gas rapidly diffuses into gas-filled pockets, it potentially can worsen conditions such as pneumothoraces, small-bowel obstructions, decompression sickness, chronic obstructive pulmonary disease, and ear effusions (16). Nitrous oxide has the potential for abuse, and every effort should be made to safeguard against this.

Reversal Agents

Naloxone is a competitive antagonist of opioids at the μ receptors, and is used primarily for the reversal of opioid-induced respiratory depression. The initial dose is 1 to 2 mg i.v. However if the patient is opioid-dependent, a titrated dosing of 0.1 to 0.2 mg i.v. every 1 to 2 minutes may prevent unpleasant withdrawal symptoms. Naloxone may have a shorter duration of action than the opioid used, therefore continued observation for delayed respiratory depression is required. It may not reverse the chest wall rigidity occasionally associated with high-dose fentanyl.

Flumazenil is a competitive antagonist of benzodiazepines and is given in titrated doses of 0.1 to 0.2 mg i.v., every 1 to 2 minutes to desired effect. It has a half-life of 45 to 100 minutes; therefore a similar caution must be exercised when used with benzodiazepines having a longer duration of effect. Flumazenil may not be effective at reversing respiratory depression. It should be used with caution in patients with benzodiazepine dependence or a history of seizures.

Elective reversal of PSA remains controversial. It has been proposed that reversal may reduce the time required for post-procedure observation. Several factors caution against this practice. Naloxone has a clinical effect of 30 minutes, which may be shorter than the continued duration of effect for the opioid (8), Its use may also preclude further opioid efficacy. Furthermore, flumazenil has not been shown to be effective at reversing the respiratory depression associated with benzodiazepines (11). No effect on discharge time has been demonstrated when reversal is used in the emergency department setting. Therefore, elective reversal is not recommended.

CRITICAL INTERVENTIONS

- Assess the patient's underlying medical conditions and potential airway difficulty prior to the initiation of PSA
- Continue to monitor the patient after the completion of the procedure until recovery to baseline. Patients may become more sedated after the removal of a painful stimulus

DISPOSITION

Patients must be observed after PSA to allow the sedative and analgesic effects to resolve sufficiently for safe discharge. Monitoring and documentation should continue in some form until the patient has returned to baseline. Elective reversal is not recommended for the reasons discussed above. Discharge criteria should be standardized and suggested formats are available on specialty Web sites, under clinical policies. At a minimum they should include documentation that the patient is conscious and responds appropriately, the vital signs are normal, pain and nausea have been minimized and no new problems exist. Patients should not drive or participate in dangerous activities for 24 hours until they are free of any residual sedative effects.

Standard discharge instructions for care pertaining to the presenting complaint should also be included.

COMMON PITFALLS

✔ Forgetting that the most important aspect of patient monitoring is visual inspection of sedation level and respiratory effort

✔ Using the "one-drug-fits-all" strategy. The selection and dosing of agents should be individualized to the patient and the procedure

✔ Failure to add an analgesic to drugs with only sedative properties when the condition or procedure is painful

Acknowledgment

We thank previous edition chapter author Daniel A. Muse.

References

1. American College of Emergency Physicians. Clinical policy for procedural sedation and analgesia in the emergency department. *Ann Emerg Med* 2004;publication pending.
2. American Medical Association, Council on Scientific Affairs. The use of pulse oximetry during procedural sedation and analgesia. *JAMA* 1993;270:1463–1468.
3. American Society of Anesthesiologists Task Force on Sedation and Analgesia by Non-Anesthesiologists. Practice guidelines for sedation and analgesia by non-anesthesiologists. *Anesthesiology* 2002;96:1004–1017.
4. Bailey P, Pace N, Ashburn M, et al. Frequent hypoxia and apnea after sedation with midazolam and fentanyl. *Anesthesiology* 1990;73:826–830.
5. Barsan WG, Tomassoni AJ, Seger D, et al. Safety assessment of high dose narcotic analgesia for emergency department procedures. *Ann Emerg Med* 1993;23:1444–1449.
6. Bauman LA, Kish I, Baumann RC, et al. Pediatric sedation with analgesia. *Am J Emerg Med* 1999;17(1):1.
7. Bergen JM, Smith DC. A review of etomidate for rapid sequence intubation in the emergency department. *J Emerg Med* 1997;15(2):221–227.
8. Blackburn P, Vissers RJ. Phamacologic advances of emergency department pain management and conscious sedation. *Emerg Med Clin North Am* 2000:18:803–826.
9. Block AJ, Boysen PG, Wynne JW, et al. Sleep apnea hypopnea and oxygen desaturation in normal subjects: a strong male predominance. *N Engl J Med* 1979;300:513–517.
10. Brown J, Klein E, Lewis C, et al. Emergency department analgesia for fracture pain. *Ann Emerg Med* 2003;42:197–205.
11. Chudnofsky CR. Safety and efficacy of flumazenil in reversing conscious sedation in the emergency department. Emergency Medicine Conscious Sedation Study Group. *Acad Emerg Med* 1997;4:944–950.
12. Chudnofsky CR, Weber JE, Stoyanoff PA, et al. A combination of midazolam and ketamine for procedural sedation and analgesia in adult emergency department patients. *Acad Emerg Med* 2000;7:228–235.
13. Chudnofsky CR, Wright SW, Dronen SC, et al. The safety of fentanyl use in the emergency department. *Ann Emerg Med* 1989;18:635.
14. Cordell WH, Keene KK, Giles BK, et al. The high prevalence of pain in emergency medical care. *Am J Emerg Med* 2002;20:165.
15. Cote CJ. Sedation for the pediatric patient. *Pediatr Clin North Am* 1994;41:31.
16. Gamis A, Knapp J, Glenski J, et al. Nitrous oxide analgesia in a pediatric emergency department. *Ann Emerg Med* 1989;18:177.
17. Gill M, Green S, Krauss B. A study of the bispectral index monitor during procedural sedation and analgesia in the emergency department. *Ann Emerg Med* 2003;41:234–241.
18. Green SM, Nakamura R, Johnson NE. Ketamine sedation for pediatric procedures: Part 2, review and implications. *Ann Emerg Med* 1990;19:1033.
19. Green SM, Rothrock SG, Lynch EL, et al. Intramuscular ketamine for pediatric sedation in the emergency department: Safety profile in 1022 cases. *Ann Emerg Med* 1998;31:688–697.
20. JCAHO. *Comprehensive Accreditation Manual for Hospitals, The Official Handbook.* Chicago, IL: JCAHO Publications, 2003.
21. Krauss B, Shannon M, Damian F, et al.*Guidelines for pediatric sedation.* Dallas: American College of Emergency Physicians, 1995.
22. Lerman B, et al. A prospective evaluation of the safety and efficacy of methohexital in the emergency department. *Am J Emerg Med* 1996;14(4):351.
23. McQuillen KK, Steel DW. Capnometry during sedation/analgesia in the pediatric emergency department. *Pediatr Emerg Care* 2000;16:401–404.
24. Miner JR, Biros M, Krieg S, et al. Randomized clinical trial of propofol versus methohexital for procedural sedation during fracture and dislocation reduction in the emergency department. *Acad Emerg Med* 2003;10:931–937.
25. Miner JR, Heegaard W, Plummer D. End tidal carbon dioxide monitoring during procedural sedation. *Acad Emerg Med* 2002;9:275–280.

26. Pohlgeers A, Friedland L, Keegan-Jones L. Combination fentanyl and diazepam for pediatric sedation and analgesia. *Acad Emerg Med* 1995;2:879–883.
27. Rubin D, Eiksig S, Freemen K, Kraut R. Effect of supplemental gases on end-tidal CO2 and oxygen saturation in patients undergoing fentanyl and midazolam outpatient sedation. *Anesth Prog* 1997;44:1–4.
28. Shane Sa, Fuchs SM, Khine H. Efficacy of rectal midazolam for the sedation of preschool undergoing laceration repair. *Ann Emerg Med* 1994;24:1065–1073.
29. Sklar DP. Joint Commission on the Accreditation of Healthcare Organizations requirements for sedation. *Ann Emerg Med* 1996;27:412–423.
30. Skokan EG, Pribble C, Bassett KE, et al. Use of propofol sedation in a pediatric emergency department: A prospective study. *Clin Pediatr (Phila)* 2001;40:663–671.
31. Swanson ER, Seaberg DC, Mathias S. The use of propofol for sedation in the emergency department. *Acad Emerg Med* 1996;3(3):234.
32. Theroux MC, West DW, Corddry DH, et al. Efficacy of intranasal midazolam in facilitating suturing of lacerations in preschool children in the emergency department. *Pediatrics* 1993;91:624.
33. Vinson DR, Bradbury DR. Etomidate for procedural sedation in emergency medicine. *Ann Emerg Med* 2002;39:592.
34. Wright SW. Conscious sedation in the emergency department: the value of capnography and pulse oximetry. *Ann Emerg Med* 1992;21:551–555.
35. Wright SW, Chudnofsky CR, Dronen SC, et al. Comparison of midazolam and diazepam for conscious sedation in the emergency department. *Ann Emerg Med* 1993;22:201.
36. Yaster M, Nichols D, Deshpande J, et al. Midazolam fentanyl intravenous sedation in children: Case report of respiratory arrest. *Pediatrics* 1990;86:463–467.
37. Zink B, Darfler K, Salluzzo R, et al. The efficacy and safety of methohexital in the emergency department. *Ann Emerg Med* 1991;20:1293.

CHAPTER 370
Interpersonal Violence

Debra Houry

The term *interpersonal violence* implies violence between two people with some relationship (partner, family, acquaintance, gang-related, patient, etc.). This chapter will focus specifically on partner violence and provider exposure to violence in the emergency department setting. Specific information on sexual assault (Chapter 93, "Sexual Assault"), trauma in the elderly (Chapter 203, "Trauma in the Elderly"), sexual abuse (Chapter 234, "Abuse: Sexual"), and physical abuse and neglect (Chapter 235, "Abuse and Neglect: Physical") can be found elsewhere in this textbook.

Also known as "domestic violence," "spousal abuse," or "battering," intimate partner violence (IPV) has been defined as "a pattern of coercive control, consisting of physical, sexual, or psychological assault against a former or current intimate partner" (7). A recent population-based study reported that 29% of women have experienced physical, sexual, or psychological IPV in their lifetime (3). In the United States, almost 2,000 women are murdered by their partner each year (18). Because of the scope of this problem, the surgeon general declared a decade ago that IPV is a national epidemic.

Many victims of IPV seek medical care for their injuries in emergency departments (EDs) (1,5). Others present to EDs for treatment of complaints related to IPV, such as depression or suicidal ideations; substance abuse; a range of somatic complaints; or complications of pregnancy secondary to abuse (1). In many cases, the ED is the primary access to health care for these patients (5). The incidence of acute physical or nonphysical abuse within the past 12 months among female ED patients has been reported to range from 12% to 20% (1,5). The lifetime prevalence of IPV exposure in ED patients has been estimated to be as high as 54% (1). With regards to special populations, current estimates are that over 2.5 million older adults, or 3% to 10% of the elderly, are mistreated annually in the United States. (15). Adult children are the most frequent perpetrators, although self-neglect is the most common form of abuse (42%) (16).

Currently, the Joint Commission on Accreditation of Healthcare Organizations (JCAHO) requires hospitals to have policies and procedures in place for identification and referral of victims of violence. However, compliance with these recommendations is poor. For example, only 54% of California EDs had written policies for screening and treating IPV victims, despite this requirement (17).

Violence within the ED is a problem that is likely underreported. Ninety-six percent of emergency physicians in one study reported verbal threats and 32% reported attempted assaults by their patients (19). Additionally, 62% of emergency medicine residents are concerned about their personal safety while working in the ED (2). The ED lends itself to promotion of a violent environment as a result of the volume of sick patients, waiting times, availability of drugs, 24-hour accessibility, and potentially violent psychiatric patients awaiting medical clearance. In one study, 77% of the perpetrators were patients, and almost one-third of the incidents occurred during the night shift (14).

The American College of Emergency Physicians (ACEP) recently reaffirmed their policy statement on protection from physical violence in the emergency department. ACEP stated that hospitals must ensure the provision of adequate security personnel, coordination of hospital security with local law enforcement agencies, the development of written protocols for violent situations in the ED, and education of staff on violent situations.

CLINICAL PRESENTATION

Intimate Partner Violence

Intimate partner violence crosses all sociodemographic levels. However, women who exhibit suicidal behavior or depressive symptoms, abuse alcohol (1), have a family history of IPV (5), or have recently become separated or divorced from their partner (8) are at an increased risk for partner violence. Women who are between 18 and 39 years of age, have a monthly income less than $1,000, and have children living at home also may be at increased risk for violence (4). Other specific populations at risk include children, disabled adults, and the elderly. Their reliance on a caregiver and their forced dependency on others heighten their risk of abuse. Elderly patients with low income, social isolation, low education, substance abuse (either caregiver or patient), previous history of family violence, and psychiatric disorders are at a particularly increased risk for abuse (16).

Intimate partner violence victims may present to the ED for treatment of an injury from IPV, evaluation of a chief complaint exacerbated by their situation (headache, anxiety, chronic pain), or with a history of IPV that is elucidated during universal screening. In addition to physical trauma, battered women may present with a variety of other medical problems, including chronic pain syndromes, posttraumatic stress disorder, suicidality, and substance abuse problems. Common presentations of battered women are listed in Table 370.1.

TABLE 370.1. Common Presentations of Women Experiencing IPV

Trauma to the face, neck, or throat
Trauma to the chest, breast, abdomen, or genitals
Bilateral or "pattern" injuries
Sexual assault
Chronic pain
Multiple injuries in various stages of healing
Extent or type of injury inconsistent with patient's explanation
Repeated use of the emergency department
Psychological or emotional complaints
Evidence of alcohol or drug abuse
Suicidal ideation or behavior

Violence in the Emergency Department

Patients may be physically violent, verbally abusive, exhibit psychiatric symptoms, or act in a bizarre manner. They may boast of prior acts of violence, a desire to commit violence, and feelings of inability to control impulse around others. Many patients will manifest changes in mental attitude, posture, speech, and motor activity before displaying violent behavior. They may pace the room or hallways, clench their fists, stand against the wall, grip bed rails, or appear anxious. The tone, volume, and character of the patients' voices may indicate the potential for violence. Health care providers may precipitate violent responses by argumentative, abrupt, or condescending attitudes, or failure to provide requested services.

DIFFERENTIAL DIAGNOSIS

Intimate partner violence should be considered in the differential diagnosis of every female ED patient, particularly in patients with substance abuse or psychiatric symptoms. Patients with recurrent visits to the ED for vague, somatic complaints should also be asked about IPV as this may be the underlying etiology. Patients with traumatic injuries should be questioned specifically about how the injury occurred, especially if the injury seems inconsistent with the stated mechanism. Without asking specifically about IPV, the diagnosis of abuse may not be made in these cases (13). This is especially true in the elderly patient who may feel embarrassed or fearful of their situation and the consequences if they discuss abuse (16).

Other causes for violent behavior in the emergency department should be considered. Metabolic abnormalities, infection, and trauma are among the life-threatening causes of altered mental status and agitation that must be ruled out. Table 370.2 lists several of these differential diagnoses.

TABLE 370.2. Organic Causes of Violent Behavior

Drug intoxication: PCP, LSD, cocaine, barbiturates, amphetamines, and alcohol
Trauma: closed head injury, subdural, tension pneumothorax
Infection: AIDS, encephalitis, meningitis
Metabolic: Hypoglycemia, thyroid storm, renal or liver failure, adrenal crisis, ketoacidosis, hypoxia, hypothermia, hyperthermia, and vitamin deficiency
Neurologic: tumors, epilepsy, cerebrovascular accidents, infections
Iatrogenic: medication induced delirium

EMERGENCY DEPARTMENT EVALUATION

Intimate Partner Violence

Studies have reported that patients will not disclose IPV unless prompted by a health provider (13). Thus, ED patients should be routinely screened for IPV. This can be done as part of the nurse's triage intake or during the physician's history and physical. Questioning should always be carried out in private and with a nonjudgmental manner.

Physicians have several specific areas of responsibility in the evaluation and management of patients who are experiencing IPV: to screen for IPV and to identify these patients; to provide medical treatment; to document findings and utterances; to facilitate appropriate referrals and follow-up; and to ensure the patient's safety.

Abused women or patients who are suspected to be victims of IPV should be interviewed in a secure area of the ED without their partner or children present. Patients should be asked in private if they want their companion to accompany them into the treatment area, to minimize the chances that they will feel coerced into silence by an abusive companion. If there is a concern for the patient's safety or a companion refuses to leave the patient in private, hospital security or police should be involved. A history of previous trauma, chronic complaints, psychological symptoms, or other red flags for IPV (inconsistent story, injury not consistent with chief complaint, multiple injuries in various stages of healing, partner who will not leave the patient's side) should be sought from direct history or from the medical record. If there is a language barrier, an interpreter should be provided. For IPV victims, a woman who is trained in medical interpretation and who will honor confidentiality is preferable to a family member. It is inappropriate to use a child as an interpreter when IPV is suspected.

Some hospitals have attempted to add a screening question on triage intake forms (12). Unfortunately, compliance with these policies is low (IPV screening rate of 29.5%) despite education and in-service training (11). Only with disciplinary actions did screening improve to 73% (12). Factors associated with screening included a lower severity of injury, nonpsychiatric complaint, and triage during the day shift. However, at least having a screening question on a triage intake form may prompt providers to ask about IPV.

Asking directly about IPV is more effective than an intake form, but it is only effective if providers inquire about IPV. The Partner Violence Screen has been previously validated in the ED setting. It is a simple, three-question screen for IPV that is easy and quick to administer. The screen is: "1. Have you been hit, kicked, punched, or otherwise hurt by someone in the past year? If so, by whom? 2. Do you feel safe in your current relationship? 3. Is there a partner from a previous relationship who is making you feel unsafe now?" It has a sensitivity of 65% to 71% and a specificity of 80% to 84% when compared to the Index of Spouse Abuse and Conflict Tactics Scale (6). Many other screens have been developed for the ED setting, although most have not been validated. What is most important, is simply to ask about violence in the patient's life.

If a patient discloses IPV, the physician needs to assess the patient's safety. It is important to determine if the patient has a safe place to stay and has a safety plan if she chooses to return home. Regardless of the severity of the presenting complaint or injury, the best indicator of danger is the patient's own assessment. The frequency and severity of previous attacks are also good guides to current danger. However, threats can be as important as the actual injury. Presence of a weapon in the home, prior battering episodes, and partner substance use may increase her risk of harm. Also, battered women are most likely to be killed when they are in the act of leaving or after they have left their abuser. Social work or an advocate can help with the safety plan and assess the patient's level of danger. Enlisting the services of a social worker can help bring victims into contact with resources such as shelters, social services, legal assistance, support groups, and other referrals that may benefit the patient.

Providers should also document the ED visit thoroughly. A review of IPV patient ED charts found that site of assault was not documented in 88% of charts, force/object use was not documented in 13% of charts, and police involvement was documented in only 54% of cases in a state that mandates reporting of IPV (9). It is also important to document the patient's exact words, as these utterances are admissible in court and are not considered hearsay. Additionally, photographs or body maps can be used to document injuries. An accurate and thoroughly documented medical record can be an asset to an IPV victim's case.

Violence in the Emergency Department

Many violent encounters in the ED can be prevented if a situation is recognized and controlled before an incident occurs. It is important to take steps to avoid confrontation as patients often act out of a sense of fear or danger. Health care providers should never respond to patients' threats with threats of their own. However, assaults against medical personnel should be reported to law enforcement agencies. Not doing so allows patients to think such behavior is acceptable and makes the staff feel they are not adequately protected.

The patient should be approached from the side, and should be watched for possible missiles or weapons. A nonoffensive posture, with hands out front but not raised, should be employed. The care provider should be cognizant of the patient's personal space and stay approximately two arm lengths away. It is important to acknowledge the patient's needs and ask him or her to discuss the problem. The patient should be informed in a low voice that help is available and that support will be provided but that the patient must take control of his or her own behavior. Expectations should be defined, and the consequences of aggressive behavior need to be clear. Frequently, talking to the patient and making offers of food and drinks may be calming and defuse the situation.

When possible, the patient should be interviewed alone and in private, but the provider should keep the door ajar and maintain space between the patient and the door should an escape be necessary. Some patients may not respond to these measures, and here a "show of force" may be needed. Prior to interviewing the patient, assemble a group of security personnel who will remain within calling distance. Frequently, this show of force may be sufficient to help disorganized patients gain control of their thoughts and behavior and back down.

The history may be difficult to obtain, and other sources, such as family members, friends, and medical records, should be used. A physical examination should be performed to exclude an organic cause of the patient's behavior (Table 370.2). Blood tests, including toxicology screen and a blood sugar, should be obtained. Vital signs and pulse oxygenation should be checked every 15 minutes while the patient is in restraints.

EMERGENCY DEPARTMENT MANAGEMENT

Interpersonal Violence

If the police are not already involved, the physician can offer to call them or help the victim to do so. The patient should be told

that battering is a crime and that he or she does not deserve to be treated in this manner. If a sexual assault occurred, state law requires providers to report all rapes and sexual assaults. Cases involving the abuse or neglect of elders (16), minors, and certain persons with disabilities must also be reported to the appropriate government agencies. Often a home visit (or assessment of nursing home care) can be arranged by social services or Adult Protective Services to assess abuse and the patient's safety. Some states may also require reporting of injuries from IPV. It is important to be familiar with the state laws that apply to reporting IPV, because these laws vary considerably. Currently, 45 states have laws that require providers to report violence-inflicted injuries; 42 states require reporting for injuries resulting from firearms, knives, or other weapons; 23 states require reporting for injuries from "crimes"; and 7 states specifically mandate reporting for injuries from IPV (10).

If the patient chooses not to talk with police or social work, it is important for the provider to be empathic and not to criticize the patient. Offer the patient information and contact numbers, which she may use later. Ensure that the patient is safe to go home and that she has a safety plan such as preparing an escape route should the situation at home escalate.

Violence in the Emergency Department

If a patient is or becomes combative or poses a danger to self or others, physical restraints may be needed. Explain clearly to the patient what is about to happen and why. Assemble a team, preferably with five members, four to restrain the limbs and one to act as team leader. Soft restraints (e.g., leather) are used to secure each limb to the stretcher. For the particularly violent patient, the team may employ mattresses, which are used to sandwich the patient. After the patient is restrained, he or she should be searched for weapons or objects that could inflict harm, and then moved to a quiet area. Zun reported that the most common complications of physical restraints were vomiting, injuring self, and increasing the patient's agitation (20).

Pharmacologic intervention may be required when the patient remains disorganized and uncooperative. Twenty-eight percent of patients in one study who were already physically restrained required chemical restraints (20). Frequently used agents include haloperidol (2–10 mg intramuscularly or intravenously in the young and 0.5–2.0 mg in the elderly) and benzodiazepines (e.g., diazepam 5–10 mg, or lorazepam 2–4 mg, intravenously or orally). Geodon (10 mg intramuscularly every 2 hours or 20 mg intramuscularly every 4 hours) was approved by the FDA for active psychosis. This medication became available in i.m. form in 2002 and recent studies have shown that it is effective in treating symptoms (hallucination, delusions, thought disorders) in schizophrenic patients. Droperidol is used less frequently, since the FDA recently issued a "blackbox" warning regarding QT prolongation and reports of sudden death with droperidol use. (See Chapter 123, "The Agitated or Violent Patient"). The reason for physical or chemical restraint and measures taken to ensure the patient's comfort while in restraints should be clearly documented in the medical record (20).

CRITICAL INTERVENTIONS

- Identify victims of violence
- Develop a safety plan and involve authorities and local agencies with victims
- Intervene early with potentially violent patients prior to escalation

DISPOSITION

A victim of intimate partner violence should be asked where they will go if they leave the ED, and who is waiting for them outside. If necessary, he/she can leave through a less visible exit. They should be given a list of emergency numbers and community resources. The option of overnight hospitalization should be discussed with the victim if he/she does not have an alternative safe place to go until placement can be arranged.

The discharge plan should include arrangements for a safe place to stay and other resources for daily living, such as money, personal papers, car keys, and a change of clothing for herself and her children. Victims should be informed that local programs for battered women provide free, confidential services, and that trained advocates from these programs can provide information regarding legal rights, police and court procedures for protective orders, shelter availability, support groups, and other essential resources. There are similar services for disabled and elderly victims of IPV. Physicians should discuss protection against sexually transmitted diseases and pregnancy, especially for those patients who have been raped or who have experienced coercive sexual activity as part of the violence. The physician should avoid prescribing tranquilizers or other sedating psychoactive medications, which could impair the victim's ability to respond appropriately should she need to leave quickly.

For patients with violent behavior in the ED, some may be discharged after a period of observation in the ED (e.g., those with alcohol- or drug-induced violent behavior). Some may require admission because of an underlying medical condition. Other patients may require further evaluation by mental health services and admission to psychiatric facilities. Patients without medical or psychiatric conditions requiring admission and who are under arrest may be discharged to the custody of law enforcement authorities after a medical evaluation.

COMMON PITFALLS

✔ Failure to make the diagnosis of IPV (especially in elderly patients who may not disclose abuse)

✔ Asking about IPV in the presence of a partner or family members

✔ Failure to provide appropriate referrals and follow-up for victims of IPV

✔ Failure to recognize the patient who is starting to escalate and who could have been calmed before the situation gets out of control

✔ Attributing violent behavior to drug or alcohol intoxication without looking for an organic cause

Acknowledgment

We thank previous edition author Taryn Kennedy.

References

1. Abbott J, Johnson R, Koziaol-Melain J, et al. Domestic violence against women: incidence and prevalence in an emergency department population. *JAMA* 1995;273:1763–1767.
2. Anglin D, Kyriacon DN, Hutson HR, et al. Residents' perspectives on violence and personal safety in the emergency department. *Ann Emerg Med* 1994;23:1082–1084.
3. Coker AL, Davis KE, Arias I, et al. Physical and mental health effects of intimate partner violence for men and women. *AM J Prev Med* 2002;23:260–268.
4. Dearwater SR, Cober JH, Campbell JC, et al. Prevalence of intimate partner violence in women treated at community hospital EDs. *JAMA* 1998;280:433–438.
5. Ernst AA, Nick TG, Weiss SJ, et al. Domestic violence among men and women in an inner city ED. *Ann Emerg Med* 1997;30:190–197.
6. Feldhaus KM, Koziol-Melain J, Ansburg HC, et al. Accuracy of 3 brief screening questions for detecting partner violence in the emergency department. *JAMA* 1997;277:1357–1361.
7. Flitcraft AH, Hadley SM, Hendricks MK, et al. Diagnosis and treatment guidelines for domestic violence. Chicago: American Medical Association, 1992.
8. Grisso JA, Schwartz DF, Hirschinger N, et al. Violent injuries among women in an urban area. *N Engl J Med* 1999;341:1899–1905.
9. Houry D, Feldhaus KM, Nyquist SR, et al. Emergency department documentation in cases of intentional assault. *Ann Emerg Med* 1999;34:715–719.
10. Houry D, Sachs CJ, Feldhaus KM, et al. Injury reporting laws in the fifty states. *Ann Emerg Med* 2002;39:56–60.
11. Larkin GL, Rolniak S, Hyman KB, et al. Effect of an administrative intervention on rates of screening for DV in an urban ED. *Am J Public Health* 2000;90:1444–1448.
12. Larkin GL, Hyman KB, Mathias SR, et al. Universal screening for intimate partner violence in the emergency department. *Ann Emerg Med* 1999;33:669–675.
13. McCauley J, Yurk RA, Jenckes MW, et al. Inside "Pandora's Box." *J Gen Intern Med* 1998;13:549–555.
14. Pane GA, Winiarski AM, Salness KA. Aggression directed toward emergency department staff at a university teaching hospital. *Ann Emerg Med* 1991;20:283–286.
15. Pavlik VN, Hyman DJ, Festa NA, et al. Quantifying the problem of abuse and neglect in adults: Analysis of a statewide database. *J Am Geriatr Soc* 2001;49:45–48.
16. Swagerty D. Elder mistreatment identification and assessment. *Clinics in Family Practice* 2003;5:195.
17. Emergency department response to domestic violence—California 1992. *MMWR Morb Mortal Wkly Rep* 1993;42:617–620.
18. U.S. Department of Justice. *Violence by Intimates.* Washington DC, March 1998. NCJ–167237.
19. Wyatt JP, Watt M, et al. Violence towards junior doctors in accident and emergency departments. *J Accid Emerg Med* 1995;12:40–42.
20. Zun LS. A prospective study of the complication rate of use of patient restraint in the emergency department. *J Emerg Med* 2003;24:119–124.

Christopher H. Linden

Appendices

APPENDIX A
Dermatomes

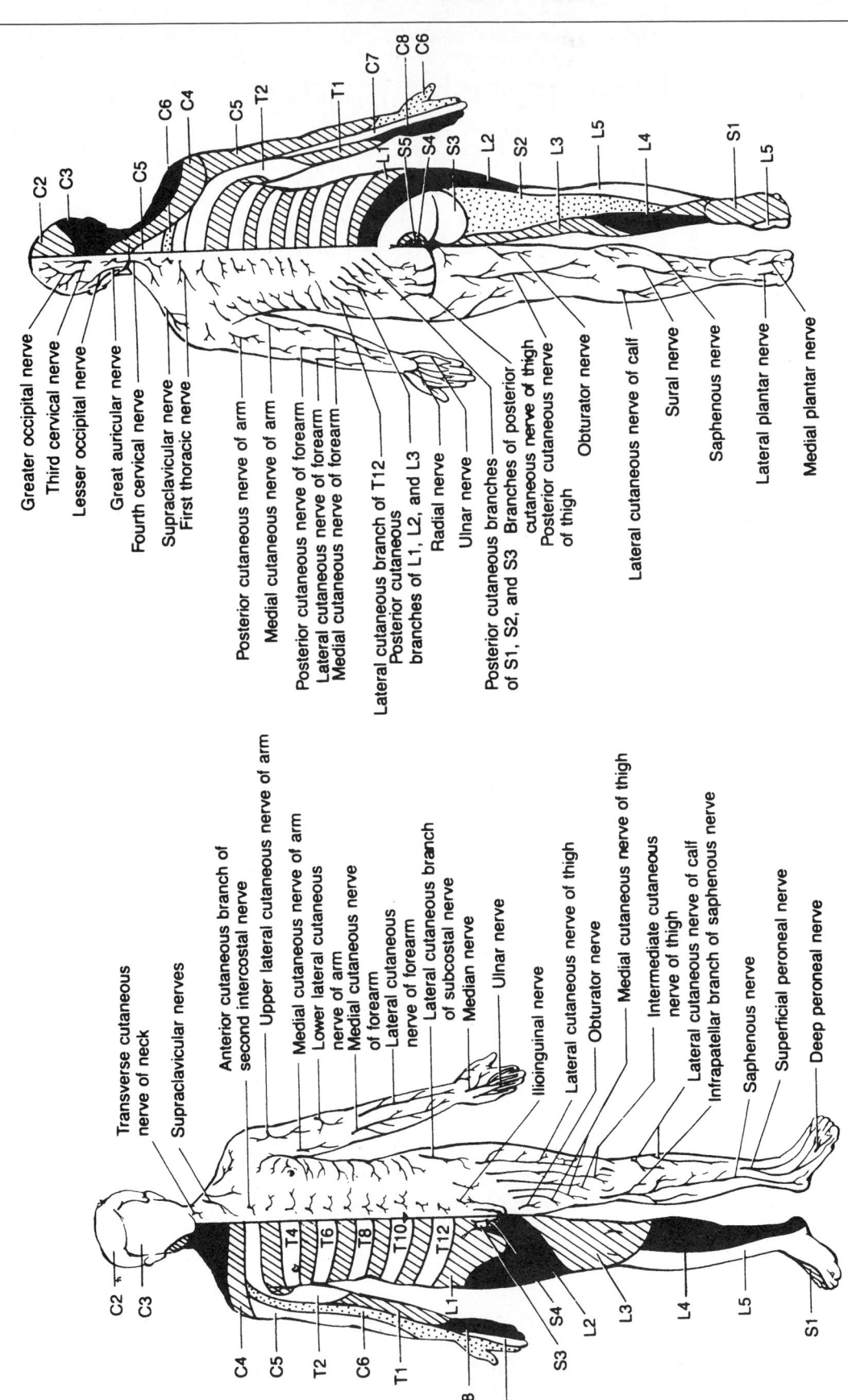

Sensory dermatomal segments.

APPENDIX B
Length-Based Equipment Chart

Item	Length (cm)						
	54–70 (4–7 kg)	70–85 (8–11 kg)	85–95 (12–14 kg)	95–107 (14–17 kg)	107–124 (18–23 kg)	124–138 (24–30 kg)	138–155 (>30 kg)
ET tube size (mm)	3.5	4.0	4.5	5.0	5.5	6.0	6.5
Lip–tip length (mm)	10.5	12.0	13.5	15.0	16.5	18.0	19.5
Laryngoscope	1 straight	1 straight	2 straight	2 straight or curved	2 straight or curved	2–3 straight or curved	3 straight or curved
Suction catheter	8F	8F–10F	10F	10F	10F	10F	12F
Stylet	6F	6F	6F	6F	14F	14F	14F
Oral airway	Infant/small child	Small child	Child	Child	Child/small adult	Child/adult	Medium adult
Bag-valve-mask	Infant	Child	Child	Child	Child	Child/adult	Adult
Oxygen mask	Newborn	Pediatric	Pediatric	Pediatric	Pediatric	Adult	Adult
Vascular access catheter/butterfly	22–24/23–25, intraosseous	20–22/23–25, intraosseous	18–22/21–23, intraosseous	18–22/21–23, intraosseous	18–20/21–23	18–22/21–22	16–20/18–21
Nasogastric tube	5F–8F	8F–10F	10F	10F–12F	12F–14F	14F–18F	18F
Urinary catheter	5F–8F	8F–10F	10F	10F–12F	10F–12F	12F	12F
Chest tube	12F–12F	16F–20F	20F–24F	20F–24F	24F–32F	28F–32F	32F–40F
Blood pressure cuff	Newborn/infant	Infant/child	Child	Child	Child	Child/adult	Adult

Directions
1. Measure patient length with centimeter tape.
2. Using measured length in centimeters, access appropriate equipment column.
Alternatively, this same information can be accessed from a single measurement directly from a Broselow tape.
Modified from Luten RC, Wears RL, Broselwo J, et al. Length-based endotracheal tube sizing for pediatric resuscitation. *Ann Emerg Med* 1995;21:900–904.

Subject Index

Note: *t* after page number denotes tabular material. Italic page numbers denotes figures. *Boldface* page numbers equal major chapter discussion.